HEART DISEASE

A Textbook of Cardiovascular Medicine

5TH EDITION

HEART DISEASE

A Textbook of Cardiovascular Medicine

Edited by

EUGENE BRAUNWALD A.B., M.D., M.A. (hon.), M.D. (hon.), Sc.D. (hon.), F.R.C.P.

Vice President for Academic Programs, Partners HealthCare System; Distinguished Hersey Professor of Medicine, Faculty Dean for Academic Programs at Brigham and Women's Hospital and Massachusetts General Hospital, Harvard Medical School, Boston, Massachusetts

W.B. SAUNDERS COMPANY

A Division of Harcourt Brace & Company

PHILADELPHIA / LONDON / TORONTO / MONTREAL / SYDNEY / TOKYO

W.B. SAUNDERS COMPANY
A Division of Harcourt Brace & Company

The Curtis Center
Independence Square West
Philadelphia, Pennsylvania 19106

Library of Congress Cataloging-in-Publication Data

Heart disease: a textbook of cardiovascular medicine /
[edited by] Eugene Braunwald.—5th ed.

p.   cm.

Includes bibliographical references and index.

ISBN 0–7216–5666–8 (single v.).—ISBN 0–7216–5663–3 (set).
ISBN 0–7216–5664–1 (v. 1).—ISBN 0–7216–5665–X (v. 2)

1. Heart—Diseases.   2. Cardiovascular system—Diseases.
   I. Braunwald, Eugene
       [DNLM: 1. Heart Diseases.   WG 200 H4364 1997]

RC681.H362   1997   616.1′2—dc20

DNLM/DLC   95-24767

ISBN 0–7216–5666–8 (single vol.)
ISBN 0–7216–5663–3 (2-vol. set)
ISBN 0–7216–5664–1 (vol. 1)
ISBN 0–7216–5665–X (vol. 2)

HEART DISEASE: A Textbook of
Cardiovascular Medicine, Fifth Edition

Printed in the United States of America

Last digit is the print number: 9   8   7   6   5   4   3

Dedicated to

ELAINE

KAREN, ALLISON, JILL

DANA, ALEX, MARA, ELISE, CARI, *and* BENJAMIN

CONTRIBUTORS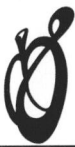

ELLIOTT M. ANTMAN, M.D.
Associate Professor of Medicine, Harvard Medical School. Director, Coronary Care Unit, Brigham and Women's Hospital, Boston, Massachusetts
Acute Myocardial Infarction; Medical Management of the Patient Undergoing Cardiac Surgery

S. SERGE BAROLD, M.D.
Professor of Medicine, University of Rochester School of Medicine and Dentistry. Chief, Cardiology Division, Department of Medicine, The Genesee Hospital, Rochester, New York
Cardiac Pacemakers and Antiarrhythmic Devices

JOHN A. BITTL, M.D.
Associate Professor of Medicine, Harvard Medical School. Director of Interventional Cardiology, Brigham and Women's Hospital, Boston, Massachusetts
Coronary Arteriography

ROBERT O. BONOW, M.D.
Goldberg Professor of Medicine and Chief, Division of Cardiology, Northwestern University Medical School. Chief, Division of Cardiology, Northwestern Memorial Hospital, Chicago, Illinois
Cardiac Catheterization

HARISIOS BOUDOULAS, M.D.
Professor of Medicine and Pharmacy, Ohio State University College of Medicine. Director, Overstreet Teaching and Research Laboratory (Division of Cardiology), Ohio State University Medical Center, Columbus, Ohio
Renal Disorders and Heart Disease

EUGENE BRAUNWALD, M.D.
Vice President for Academic Programs, Partners HealthCare System; Distinguished Hersey Professor of Medicine, Faculty Dean for Academic Programs at Brigham and Women's Hospital and Massachusetts General Hospital, Harvard Medical School, Boston, Massachusetts
The History; Physical Examination of the Heart and Circulation; Pathophysiology of Heart Failure; Assessment of Cardiac Function; Clinical Aspects of Heart Failure: High-Output Heart Failure; Pulmonary Edema; Management of Heart Failure; Pulmonary Hypertension; Valvular Heart Disease; Coronary Blood Flow and Myocardial Ischemia; Acute Myocardial Infarction; Chronic Coronary Artery Disease; The Cardiomyopathies and Myocarditides; Primary Tumors of the Heart; Traumatic Heart Disease; Hematological-Oncological Disorders and Heart Disease

BRUCE H. BRUNDAGE, M.D.
Professor of Medicine and Radiological Sciences, University of California, Los Angeles, School of Medicine, Los Angeles, California. Chief of Cardiology and Scientific Director, St. John's Cardiovascular Research Center, Harbor-UCLA Medical Center, Torrance, California
Relative Merits of Imaging Techniques

AGUSTIN CASTELLANOS, M.D.

Professor of Medicine, University of Miami School of Medicine. Director of Clinical Electrophysiology, Jackson Memorial Hospital, Miami, Florida
Cardiac Arrest and Sudden Cardiac Death

BERNARD R. CHAITMAN, M.D.

Professor of Medicine, St. Louis University School of Medicine. Chief of Cardiology, St. Louis University Health Sciences Center, St. Louis, Missouri
Exercise Stress Testing

KENNETH R. CHIEN, M.D., Ph.D.

Professor of Medicine and Member, Center for Molecular Genetics, University of California, San Diego, La Jolla, California. Attending Physician, University of California, San Diego, University Hospital, San Diego, California
Principles of Cardiovascular Molecular and Cellular Biology

JONATHAN S. COBLYN, M.D.

Assistant Professor of Medicine, Harvard Medical School. Associate Director, Robert B. Brigham Arthritis Center, Brigham and Women's Hospital, Boston, Massachusetts
Rheumatic Diseases and the Heart

PETER F. COHN, M.D.

Professor of Medicine and Chief, Cardiology Division, State University of New York Health Sciences Center, Stony Brook, New York
Traumatic Heart Disease

WILSON S. COLUCCI, M.D.

Professor of Medicine, Biochemistry and Physiology, Boston University School of Medicine. Associate Chief, Cardiovascular Division, and Director, Cardiomyopathy Program, Boston University Medical Center. Chief, Cardiology Section, Boston Veterans Affairs Medical Center, Boston, Massachusetts
Pathophysiology of Heart Failure; Clinical Aspects of Heart Failure: High-Output Heart Failure; Pulmonary Edema; Primary Tumors of the Heart

ADNAN S. DAJANI, M.D.

Professor of Pediatrics, Wayne State University School of Medicine. Director, Division of Infectious Diseases, Children's Hospital of Michigan, Detroit, Michigan
Rheumatic Fever

CHARLES J. DAVIDSON, M.D.

Associate Professor of Medicine, Northwestern University Medical School. Chief, Cardiac Catheterization Laboratories, Northwestern Memorial Hospital, Chicago, Illinois
Cardiac Catheterization

CHARLES DENNIS, M.D.

Chairman, Department of Cardiology, Deborah Heart and Lung Center, Browns Mills, New Jersey
Rehabilitation of Patients with Coronary Artery Disease

ROMAN W. DeSANCTIS, M.D.

Professor of Medicine, Harvard Medical School. Director of Clinical Cardiology and Physician, Massachusetts General Hospital, Boston, Massachusetts
Diseases of the Aorta

PAMELA S. DOUGLAS, M.D.
Associate Professor of Medicine, Harvard Medical School. Director, Noninvasive Cardiology, Beth Israel Hospital, Boston, Massachusetts
Coronary Artery Disease in Women

KIM A. EAGLE, M.D.
Associate Professor of Internal Medicine, University of Michigan School of Medicine. Director of Clinical Cardiology, University of Michigan Medical Center, Ann Arbor, Michigan
Diseases of the Aorta

URI ELKAYAM, M.D.
Professor of Medicine, Division of Cardiology, University of Southern California School of Medicine. Director, Heart Failure Program, and Director, High Risk Cardiology Perinatal Clinic, Los Angeles, California
Pregnancy and Cardiovascular Disease

JOHN A. FARMER, M.D.
Associate Professor of Medicine, Sections of Atherosclerosis and Cardiology, Baylor College of Medicine. Chief of Cardiology, Ben Taub General Hospital, Houston, Texas
Dyslipidemia and Other Risk Factors for Coronary Artery Disease

HARVEY FEIGENBAUM, M.D.
Distinguished Professor of Medicine, Indiana University School of Medicine. Senior Research Associate, Krannert Institute of Cardiology, Indianapolis, Indiana
Echocardiography

CHARLES FISCH, M.D.
Distinguished Professor Emeritus of Medicine, Indiana University School of Medicine, Indianapolis, Indiana
Electrocardiography

ROBERT F. FISHMAN, M.D.
Assistant Professor of Medicine, Northwestern University Medical School. Attending Physician, Northwestern Memorial Hospital, Chicago, Illinois
Cardiac Catheterization

WILLIAM F. FRIEDMAN, M.D.
J. H. Nicholson Professor of Pediatrics (Cardiology), Department of Pediatrics, and Senior Advisor, Clinical Affairs, to the Provost and Dean, University of California, Los Angeles, School of Medicine, Los Angeles, California
Congenital Heart Disease in Infancy and Childhood; Acquired Heart Disease in Infancy and Childhood

VALENTIN FUSTER, M.D., Ph.D.
Arthur M. and Hilda A. Master Professor of Medicine, Mount Sinai School of Medicine. Director, Cardiovascular Institute. Dean for Academic Affairs and Vice Chairman, Department of Medicine, Mount Sinai Medical Center, New York, New York
Hemostasis, Thrombosis, Fibrinolysis, and Cardiovascular Disease

PETER GANZ, M.D.
Associate Professor of Medicine, Harvard Medical School. Director of Research, Cardiac Catheterization Laboratory, Brigham and Women's Hospital, Boston, Massachusetts
Coronary Blood Flow and Myocardial Ischemia

BERNARD J. GERSH, M.B., D.Phil.

Professor of Medicine and Chief, Division of Cardiology, Georgetown University Medical Center, Washington, D.C.

Chronic Coronary Artery Disease

GARY GERSTENBLITH, M.D.

Professor of Medicine, Johns Hopkins University School of Medicine, Baltimore, Maryland

The Aging Heart: Structure, Function, and Disease

SAMUEL Z. GOLDHABER, M.D.

Associate Professor of Medicine, Harvard Medical School. Physician, Brigham and Women's Hospital, Boston, Massachusetts

Pulmonary Embolism

LEE GOLDMAN, M.D.

Julius Krevans Distinguished Professor and Chairman, Department of Medicine, and Associate Dean for Clinical Affairs, University of California, San Francisco, School of Medicine, San Francisco, California

Cost-Effective Strategies in Cardiology; General Anesthesia and Noncardiac Surgery in Patients with Heart Disease

ANTONIO M. GOTTO, Jr., M.D., D.Phil.

Distinguished Service Professor and Chairman, Department of Medicine, Baylor College of Medicine. Chief, Internal Medicine Service, Methodist Hospital, Houston, Texas

Dyslipidemia and Other Risk Factors for Coronary Artery Disease

ANDREW A. GRACE, Ph.D., M.R.C.P.

Senior Research Fellow, Departments of Medicine and Biochemistry, University of Cambridge, and Director, Cardiac Electrophysiology Service, Papworth Hospital, Cambridge, England. Visiting Scientist, Department of Medicine, University of California, San Diego, La Jolla, California.

Principles of Cardiovascular Molecular and Cellular Biology

WILLIAM GROSSMAN, M.D.

Adjunct Professor of Medicine, University of Pennsylvania School of Medicine, Philadelphia, Pennsylvania. Vice President, Clinical Research, Merck and Co., West Point, Pennsylvania

Clinical Aspects of Heart Failure: High-Output Heart Failure; Pulmonary Edema; Pulmonary Hypertension

CHARLES B. HIGGINS, M.D.

Professor and Vice-Chairman, Department of Radiology, University of California, San Francisco, San Francisco, California

Newer Cardiac Imaging Techniques: Magnetic Resonance Imaging and Computed Tomography

ERIC M. ISSELBACHER, M.D.

Instructor in Medicine, Harvard Medical School. Assistant in Medicine, Massachusetts General Hospital, Boston, Massachusetts

Diseases of the Aorta

NORMAN M. KAPLAN, M.D.

Professor of Internal Medicine and Head, Hypertension Division, University of Texas Southwestern Medical Center, Dallas, Texas

Systemic Hypertension: Mechanisms and Diagnosis; Systemic Hypertension: Therapy

WISHWA N. KAPOOR, M.D.

Falk Professor of Medicine, University of Pittsburgh. Chief, Division of Internal Medicine, Presbyterian-University Hospital, Pittsburgh, Pennsylvania
Syncope and Hypotension

ADOLF W. KARCHMER, M.D.

Professor of Medicine, Harvard Medical School. Chief, Division of Infectious Diseases, New England Deaconess Hospital, Boston, Massachusetts
Infective Endocarditis

RALPH A. KELLY, M.D.

Assistant Professor of Medicine, Harvard Medical School. Associate Physician, Division of Cardiology, Department of Medicine, Brigham and Women's Hospital, Boston, Massachusetts
Drugs Used in the Treatment of Heart Failure; Management of Heart Failure

EDWARD G. LAKATTA, M.D.

Professor of Medicine, Johns Hopkins School of Medicine. Professor of Physiology, University of Maryland School of Medicine. Chief, Laboratory of Cardiovascular Science, NIH/NIA/Gerontology Research Center, Baltimore, Maryland
The Aging Heart: Structure, Function, and Disease

THOMAS H. LEE, M.D., M.Sc.

Associate Professor of Medicine, Harvard Medical School and Brigham and Women's Hospital. Medical Director, Partners Community Health Care, Inc., Boston, Massachusetts
Practice Guidelines in Cardiovascular Medicine

CARL V. LEIER, M.D.

James W. Overstreet Professor of Medicine and Pharmacology, Ohio State University College of Medicine. Director, Division of Cardiology, and Director, Cardiac Transplantation Service, Ohio State University Medical Center, Columbus, Ohio
Renal Disorders and Heart Disease

DAVID C. LEVIN, M.D.

Professor of Radiology, Jefferson Medical College. Chairman, Department of Radiology, Thomas Jefferson University Hospital, Philadelphia, Pennsylvania
Radiology of the Heart; Coronary Arteriography

LEONARD S. LILLY, M.D.

Associate Professor of Medicine, Harvard Medical School. Associate Physician, Brigham and Women's Hospital, Boston, Massachusetts
The Heart in Endocrine and Nutritional Disorders

A. MICHAEL LINCOFF, M.D.

Assistant Professor of Medicine, Ohio State University. Director, Experimental Interventional Laboratory, Department of Cardiology, Center for Thrombosis and Vascular Biology, The Cleveland Clinic Foundation, Cleveland, Ohio
Interventional Catheterization Techniques

WILLIAM C. LITTLE, M.D.

Professor of Internal Medicine and Chief of Cardiology, Bowman-Gray School of Medicine of Wake Forest University. Chief of Cardiology and Associate Chief of Professional Services, North Carolina Baptist Hospital, Winston-Salem, North Carolina
Assessment of Cardiac Function

BEVERLY H. LORELL, M.D.
Associate Professor of Medicine, Harvard Medical School. Director, Hemodynamic Research Laboratory, and Associate Director, Cardiac Catheterization Laboratory, Beth Israel Hospital, Boston, Massachusetts
Pericardial Diseases

RICHARD A. MATTHAY, M.D.
Boehringer Ingelheim Professor of Medicine and Associate Director, Pulmonary and Critical Care Section, Department of Internal Medicine, Yale University School of Medicine, New Haven, Connecticut
Cor Pulmonale

ROBERT J. MYERBURG, M.D.
Professor of Medicine and Physiology and Director, Division of Cardiology, University of Miami School of Medicine. Chief of Cardiology, Jackson Memorial Medical Center, Miami, Florida
Cardiac Arrest and Sudden Cardiac Death

LIONEL H. OPIE, M.D., D.Phil., F.R.C.P.
Professor, Department of Medicine, University of Capetown. Director, Hypertension Clinic, Groote Schuur Hospital, Capetown, South Africa
Mechanisms of Cardiac Contraction and Relaxation

JOSEPH K. PERLOFF, M.D.
Streisand/American Heart Association Professor of Medicine and Pediatrics, University of California, Los Angeles, School of Medicine, Division of Cardiology, Departments of Medicine and Pediatrics, UCLA Center for the Health Sciences, Los Angeles, California
Physical Examination of the Heart and Circulation; Congenital Heart Disease in Adults; Neurological Disorders and Heart Disease

MARK G. PERLROTH, M.D.
Professor of Medicine, Division of Cardiovascular Medicine, Stanford University School of Medicine, Falk Cardiovascular Research Center. Professor of Medicine, Stanford University Medical Center and The Lucile Salter Packard Children's Hospital, Stanford, California. Consultant Cardiologist, Palo Alto Veterans Administration Medical Center, Palo Alto, California
Heart and Heart-Lung Transplantation

WILLIAM S. PIERCE, M.D.
Evan Pugh Professor of Surgery, Jane A. Fetter Professor of Surgery, and Chief, Division of Cardiothoracic Surgery, Department of Surgery, Pennsylvania State University College of Medicine, Hershey, Pennsylvania
Assisted Circulation and the Mechanical Heart

REED E. PYERITZ, M.D., Ph.D.
Chair, Department of Human Genetics, and Professor of Human Genetics, Medicine and Pediatrics, and Director, Institute for Medical Genetics, Medical College of Pennsylvania and Hahnemann University, Philadelphia and Pittsburgh, Pennsylvania. Director, Center for Medical Genetics, Allegheny General Hospital, Pittsburgh, Pennsylvania
Genetics and Cardiovascular Disease

BRUCE A. REITZ, M.D.
The Norman E. Shumway Professor and Chairman, Department of Cardiothoracic Surgery, Stanford University School of Medicine. Chief of the Cardiac Surgical Service, Stanford Health Services, Stanford, California. Chief of the Pediatric Cardiac Surgical Service, The Lucile Salter Packard Children's Hospital at Stanford, Palo Alto, California
Heart and Heart-Lung Transplantation

STUART RICH, M.D.
Professor of Medicine, University of Illinois, Chicago. Chief of Cardiology, University of Illinois, Chicago Medical Center, Chicago, Illinois
Pulmonary Hypertension

WAYNE E. RICHENBACHER, M.D.
Associate Professor, Division of Cardiothoracic Surgery, Department of Surgery, University of Iowa, Iowa City, Iowa
Assisted Circulation and the Mechanical Heart

DAVID S. ROSENTHAL, M.D.
Professor of Medicine, Harvard Medical School. Henry K. Oliver Professor of Hygiene, Harvard University. Physician, Brigham and Women's Hospital. Director and Physician, University Health Services, Harvard University, Cambridge, Massachusetts
Hematological-Oncological Disorders and Heart Disease

RUSSELL ROSS, Ph.D.
Professor, Department of Pathology, and Adjunct Professor, Department of Biochemistry, University of Washington School of Medicine, Seattle, Washington
The Pathogenesis of Atherosclerosis

JOHN D. RUTHERFORD, M.B., Ch.B., F.R.A.C.P.
Professor of Medicine, University of Texas, Gail Griffiths Hill Chair of Cardiology. Associate Director, Division of Cardiology, Southwestern Medical Center, Dallas, Texas
Chronic Coronary Artery Disease

HEINRICH R. SCHELBERT, M.D., Ph.D.
Professor of Pharmacology and Radiological Sciences and Vice Chairman, Department of Pharmacology, University of California, Los Angeles, School of Medicine, Los Angeles, California
Relative Merits of Imaging Techniques

FREDERICK J. SCHOEN, M.D., Ph.D.
Professor of Pathology, Harvard Medical School. Director, Cardiac Pathology, and Vice-Chairman, Department of Pathology, Brigham and Women's Hospital, Boston, Massachusetts
Primary Tumors of the Heart

ELLEN W. SEELY, M.D.
Assistant Professor of Medicine, Harvard Medical School. Director of Clinical Research, Endocrine-Hypertension Division, and Director, Ambulatory Clinical Research Center, Brigham and Women's Hospital, Boston, Massachusetts
The Heart in Endocrine and Nutritional Disorders

LAWRENCE N. SHULMAN, M.D.
Assistant Professor of Medicine, Harvard Medical School. Clinical Director, Hematology-Oncology Division, Brigham and Women's Hospital, Boston, Massachusetts
Hematological-Oncological Disorders and Heart Disease

DAVID J. SKORTON, M.D.

Professor of Medicine, College of Medicine, and Professor of Electrical and Computer Engineering, College of Engineering, University of Iowa. Co-Director, Adolescent and Adult Congenital Heart Disease Clinic. Staff Physician, University of Iowa Hospitals and Clinics. Consulting Physician, Department of Veterans Affairs Medical Center. Vice-President for Research, University of Iowa, Iowa City, Iowa

Relative Merits of Imaging Techniques

THOMAS W. SMITH, M.D.

Professor of Medicine, Harvard Medical School. Chief, Cardiovascular Division, and Senior Physician, Brigham and Women's Hospital, Boston, Massachusetts

Drugs Used in the Treatment of Heart Failure; Management of Heart Failure

ROBERT SOUFER, M.D.

Associate Professor of Diagnostic Radiology and Medicine (Cardiovascular Medicine), Yale University School of Medicine. Attending Physician, Internal Medicine, Yale-New Haven Hospital. Director, Positron Emission Tomography Center, Yale University-Veterans Administration PET Center, West Haven, Connecticut

Nuclear Cardiology

ROBERT M. STEINER, M.D.

Professor of Radiology and Medicine, Jefferson Medical College, Thomas Jefferson University Hospital, Philadelphia, Pennsylvania

Radiology of the Heart

LYNNE WARNER STEVENSON, M.D.

Associate Professor of Medicine, Harvard Medical School. Medical Director, Cardiomyopathy and Transplant Center, Brigham and Women's Hospital, Boston, Massachusetts

Management of Heart Failure

ERIC J. TOPOL, M.D.

Professor of Medicine, Cleveland Clinic Health Sciences Center, Ohio State University. Chairman, Department of Cardiology, and Director, Joseph J. Jacobs Center for Thrombosis and Vascular Biology, Cleveland Clinic Foundation, Cleveland, Ohio

Interventional Catheterization Techniques

MARC VERSTRAETE, M.D., Ph.D.

Professor of Medicine and Former Director, Center for Molecular and Vascular Biology, University of Leuven, Leuven, Belgium

Hemostasis, Thrombosis, Fibrinolysis and Cardiovascular Disease

FRANS J. TH. WACKERS, M.D.

Professor of Diagnostic Radiology and Medicine (Cardiology), Yale University School of Medicine. Director, Cardiovascular Nuclear Imaging and Exercise Laboratories, Yale-New Haven Hospital, New Haven, Connecticut

Nuclear Cardiology

HERBERT P. WEIDEMANN, M.D.

Chief, Pulmonary Department, The Cleveland Clinic Foundation, Cleveland, Ohio

Cor Pulmonale

MICHAEL E. WEINBLATT, M.D.
Associate Professor of Medicine, Harvard Medical School. Director of Clinical Rheumatology, Brigham and Women's Hospital, Boston, Massachusetts
Rheumatic Diseases and the Heart

MYRON L. WEISFELDT, M.D.
Samuel Bard Professor of Medicine and Chair, Department of Medicine, Columbia University College of Physicians and Surgeons. Director of the Medical Service and Attending Physician, Presbyterian Hospital, New York, New York
The Aging Heart: Structure, Function, and Disease

GORDON H. WILLIAMS, M.D.
Professor of Medicine, Harvard Medical School. Chief, Endocrine-Hypertension Division, and Director, Clinical Research Center, Brigham and Women's Hospital, Boston, Massachusetts
The Heart in Endocrine and Nutritional Disorders

GERALD L. WOLF, Ph.D., M.D.
Professor of Radiology, Harvard Medical School. Director, Center for Imaging and Pharmaceutical Research, Massachusetts General Hospital, Boston, Massachusetts
Relative Merits of Imaging Techniques

JOSHUA WYNNE, M.D.
Professor of Medicine and Chief, Division of Cardiology, Wayne State University. Chief, Section of Cardiology, Harper Hospital, Detroit Medical Center, Detroit, Michigan
The Cardiomyopathies and Myocarditides

BARRY L. ZARET, M.D.
Robert W. Berliner Professor of Medicine, Professor of Diagnostic Radiology, Chief, Section of Cardiovascular Medicine, and Associate Chair for Clinical Affairs, Department of Internal Medicine, Yale University School of Medicine. Chief of Cardiology, Yale-New Haven Hospital, New Haven, Connecticut
Nuclear Cardiology

DOUGLAS P. ZIPES, M.D.
Distinguished Professor of Medicine, Pharmacology, and Toxicology and Director, Division of Cardiology and Krannert Institute of Cardiology, Indiana University School of Medicine. Attending Physician, University Hospital, Wishard Memorial Hospital, and Roudebush Veterans Administration Hospital, Indianapolis, Indiana
Genesis of Cardiac Arrhythmias: Electrophysiological Considerations; Management of Cardiac Arrhythmias: Pharmacological, Electrical, and Surgical Techniques; Specific Arrhythmias: Diagnosis and Treatment; Cardiac Pacemakers and Antiarrhythmic Devices

PREFACE

As I complete the preparations of this new edition of *Heart Disease,* I am awed by the continued growth and progress in cardiovascular medicine. During my professional lifetime I have been privileged to observe the field's advance to a point at which the safe and accurate diagnosis and the effective treatment of most forms of heart disease is now feasible. While the overall population is aging and the total prevalence of heart disease rising, the age-adjusted mortality rate for cardiovascular disease in the United States has declined by approximately 1 per cent per year for the last 40 years, and this decline appears to be continuing.

The enormous advances in the field in the five years since the publication of the fourth edition have required the most extensive changes yet made in any revision of this text. Despite the need to include an enormous amount of new information, it was possible to retain the basic format of the previous edition of *Heart Disease.* The book is divided into five parts: Part I deals with the examination of the patient in the broadest sense, including clinical findings and the theory and application of modern noninvasive and invasive techniques to elicit information about the heart and circulation. Part II is concerned with the pathophysiology, diagnosis, and treatment of the principal abnormalities of circulatory function, including heart failure, arrhythmias, and abnormalities of arterial pressure. Part III, the longest in the book, consists of descriptions of the principal congenital and acquired diseases affecting the heart, pericardium, aorta, and pulmonary vascular bed in adults and children. Part IV deals with the interfaces between cardiology and broad fields such as genetics, aging, management of the postoperative cardiac patient, and the economics of cardiac care. Part V details the relationship between diseases of other organ systems and the circulation and vice versa.

Twenty-one new chapters—the most for any revision to date—have been added or substituted. Many other important new areas are covered in radically revised chapters.

A number of important areas are covered in this edition: The chapter on Physical Examination prepared with Perloff has been expanded and revised because the intelligent contemporary practice of cardiology requires careful integration of findings obtained from the clinical examination with those from the growing number of diagnostic modalities now available. The chapter on the Relative Merits of Imaging Techniques by Skorton and colleagues provides a rational approach to the intelligent selection among the several techniques now available to image the heart.

A new, and I believe unique, aspect of the fifth edition of *Heart Disease* is Lee's comprehensive chapter on Practice Guidelines in Cardiovascular Medicine. Increasingly, practice guidelines are influencing diagnosis and therapy and are rapidly becoming the basis for reimbursement of health care services. This new chapter provides a summary of the most important guidelines put together by authoritative groups—mostly key committees of the American Heart Association and the American College of Cardiology. In addition to a summary of the guidelines, Lee places them into the perspective of modern patient care. The chapter on Cost-Effective Strategies in Cardiology by Goldman explains how cost-conscious practice need not impair the quality of care.

Also of note is a new chapter on a subject that is attracting a great deal of interest—Coronary Artery Disease in Women—by Douglas, which complements the chapter on Aging in Cardiac Disease. This pair of chapters deals with two large groups of patients with special needs, problems, and issues, who together constitute an enormous percentage of the total population. Advances in interventional cardiology represent one of the most dramatic developments in the field and they are covered in an excellent new chapter by Lincoff and Topol. Cardiologists increasingly need an understanding of hemostasis, thrombosis, and fibrinolysis in their daily practice. Fuster and Verstraete have teamed up to provide a superb new chapter on this subject.

Because it is now clear that abnormalities of molecular processes may be the basis of many cardiovascular diseases and that genetic influences play critical roles in the development of these abnormalities, three new chapters have been included. Opie describes the basic mechanisms of cardiac contraction and relaxation. Chien and Grace present the impact of cell and molecular biology, while Pyeritz summarizes the genetics of cardiovascular disease. The important role played by genetics in cardiovascular disease is underscored by Figure 49–1, on pages 1652 and 1653, specially prepared for this book by Pyeritz, which shows the chromosomal location of 137 human genes whose mutations have been shown to produce deleterious effects on the cardiovascular system. This field is moving very swiftly indeed; undoubtedly many other genes will be identified and their chromosomal locations determined by the time the sixth edition of *Heart Disease* is published.

An important responsibility of an editor is to establish the boundaries of a book. In approaching this task, I have deliberately taken a broad approach—in the line with this book's subtitle "A Textbook of Cardiovascular Medicine." I believe that modern cardiologists will best serve their patients by being first broadly based physicians and second accomplished technical specialists. Cardiologists must remain the masters—not become the slaves—of the powerful new diagnostic and therapeutic tools now available. They must also understand the enormous influence that heart disease can exert on the function of other organ systems, as well as the equally important effect that disordered function of other organ systems can have on the circulation. Cardiologists must also be able to function effectively as a consultants to generalists, surgeons, and other specialists. The chapter on Pulmonary Embolism, and all of Part V (Heart Disease and Disorders of Other Organ Systems) explore the important interfaces between cardiology and other branches of medicine. The chapter by Antman on the medical management of the patient undergoing cardiac surgery should be helpful to the cardiologist and internist in what is a growing responsibility. Its companion chapter on noncardiac surgery in the patient with heart disease by Goldman provides an approach to an increasing challenge posed to the modern cardiologist and internist.

Considerable revisions have been made in both galley proofs and page proofs to include information about the most recent advances in the field. Particular emphasis has been placed on ensuring a comprehensive and up-to-date bibliography of more than 18,000 pertinent references, including hundreds to publications that appeared in 1996. Many of the 1,436 figures and 444 tables are new to this edition. The fifth edition of *Heart Disease* is approximately 15 per cent longer than the fourth. This has been accomplished with only a modest increase in the number of pages and bulk in the book through a more efficient page layout, the use of somewhat smaller illustrations, and the more liberal use of a special type face.

In order to allow the reader to keep pace with the enormous expansion of cardiovascular knowledge, the fifth edition is supplemented by a number of companion volumes. First, W.B. Saunders has just published the second edition of *Marcus Cardiac Imaging: A Companion to Braunwald's Heart Disease*, edited by Skorton, Schelbert, Wolf and Brundage, which provides an elegant analysis of the most important cardiovascular diagnostic imaging techniques now available. This companion book is especially useful given the profound advances in cardiovascular diagnosis made possible by modern imaging techniques. No area of cardiology has advanced more rapidly than therapeutics, and therefore it seems logical for the second companion to *Heart Disease* to be *Cardiovascular Therapeutics*. The editorial effort was ably led by my colleague at the Brigham, Thomas W. Smith, who enlisted the cooperation of a team of outstanding associate editors and authors.

Two other companions to *Heart Disease* are now in advanced stages of preparation—*Molecular Basis of Heart Disease*, edited by Chien, and *Clinical Trials in Cardiovascular Disease*, edited by Hennekens. In addition, a *Review and Assessment* book, prepared by Mendelsohn, will again accompany this edition of *Heart Disease*. It consists of 600 questions based on material discussed in the textbook and provides the answers as well as detailed explanations. This multipronged educational effort—*Heart Disease*, the growing number of companion volumes, as well as the *Review and Assessment* book, all appearing in print and electronic (CD-ROM) form—is designed to assist the reader with the awesome task of learning and remaining current in this dynamic field.

It is hoped that this textbook will prove useful to those who wish to broaden their knowledge of cardiovascular medicine. To the extent that it achieves this goal and thereby aids in the care of patients afflicted with heart disease, credit must be given to the many talented and dedicated persons involved in its preparation. My deepest appreciation goes to my fellow contributors for their professional expertise, knowledge and devoted scholarship, which are at the very "heart" of this book. At the W.B. Saunders Company, my editor, Richard Zorab, and the production team—Frank Polizzano, Edna Dick, Lorraine Kilmer, and Hazel Hacker—were enormously helpful. My editorial associate, Ms. Kathryn Saxon, rendered invaluable and devoted assistance.

This edition could not have become a reality were it not for the skillful and dedicated efforts of several other individuals. My responsibilities to the Harvard Medical School and the Brigham and Women's Hospital during the leave of absence that I required for much of my own writing were shouldered most effectively by my colleagues Drs. Dennis Kasper and Marshall Wolf, who provided the Department of Medicine with exemplary leadership. My administrative assistant, Ms. Diane Rioux, was enormously helpful in maintaining the orderly flow of activity essential to a busy Department of Medicine. I am especially indebted to Dr. Daniel C. Tosteson, Dean of the Harvard Medical School, and to Dr. H. Richard Nesson, President of the Partners HealthCare System and of the Brigham and Women's Hospital, for graciously allowing me the freedom to devote myself to this task. On a personal note, my wife, Elaine, provided the personal support, encouragement and understanding so essential for one who adds a task of this magnitude to an already full professional life.

EUGENE BRAUNWALD, 1996

Adapted from the PREFACE to the First Edition

Cardiovascular disease is the greatest scourge afflicting the population of the industrialized nations. As with previous scourges—bubonic plague, yellow fever, and smallpox—cardiovascular disease not only strikes down a significant fraction of the population without warning but causes prolonged suffering and disability in an even larger number. In the United States alone, despite recent encouraging declines, cardiovascular disease is still responsible for almost one million fatalities each year and more than one half of all deaths; almost 5 million persons afflicted with cardiovascular disease are hospitalized each year. The cost of this disease in terms of human suffering and of material resources is almost incalculable.

Fortunately, research focusing on the causes, diagnosis, treatment, and prevention of heart disease is moving ahead rapidly. In the last 25 years in particular we have witnessed an explosive expansion of our understanding of the structure and function of the cardiovascular system—both normal and abnormal—and of our ability to evaluate it in the living patient, sometimes by means of techniques that require penetration of the skin but also, with increasing accuracy, by noninvasive methods. Simultaneously, remarkable progress has been made in preventing and treating cardiovascular disease by medical and surgical means. Indeed, in the United States, the aforementioned steady reduction in mortality from cardiovascular disease during the past decade suggests that the effective application of this increased knowledge is beginning to prolong the human life span—the most valued resource on earth.

An attempt to summarize our present understanding of heart disease in a comprehensive textbook for the serious student of this subject is a formidable undertaking. Following the untimely death of Dr. Charles K. Friedberg, whose masterful text served as a bible to me and to a whole generation of cardiologists during the 1950's and 1960's, the W.B. Saunders Company invited me to accept this responsibility. Younger colleagues, particularly cardiology fellows and medical residents at the Brigham, convinced me of the need for such a book.

In order to provide a comprehensive, authoritative text in a field that has become as broad and deep as cardiovascular medicine, I chose to enlist the aid of a number of able colleagues. However, I hoped that my personal involvement in the writing of about half of the book would make it possible to minimize the fragmentation, gaps, inconsistencies, organizational difficulties, and impersonal tone that sometimes plague multiauthored texts. I also sought a compromise between a book that is too long as a result of excessive repetition and one in which all duplication is eliminated, resulting in fragmented coverage of certain subjects. To help achieve this objective, extensive cross references have been provided within the text.

Since the early part of this century, clinical cardiology has had a particularly strong foundation in the basic sciences of physiology and pharmacology. More recently, the disciplines of molecular biology, genetics, developmental biology, biophysics, biochemistry, experimental pathology, and bioengineering have also begun to provide critically important information about cardiac function and malfunction. Although *Heart Disease: A Textbook of Cardiovascular Medicine* is primarily a clinical treatise and not a textbook of fundamental cardiovascular science, an effort has been made to explain, in some detail, the scientific basis of cardiovascular diseases.

EUGENE BRAUNWALD, 1980

COLOR PLATES

CONTENTS

PART III DISEASES OF THE HEART, PERICARDIUM, AORTA, AND PULMONARY VASCULAR BED

PART IV BROADER PERSPECTIVES ON HEART DISEASE AND CARDIOLOGIC PRACTICE

PART V   HEART DISEASE AND DISORDERS OF OTHER ORGAN SYSTEMS

Part I
Examination of the Patient

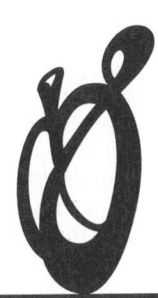

Chapter 1

The History

EUGENE BRAUNWALD

IMPORTANCE OF THE HISTORY

Specialized examinations of the cardiovascular system, presented in Chapters 3 to 11, provide a large portion of the data base required to establish a specific anatomical diagnosis of cardiac disease and to determine the extent of functional impairment of the heart. The development and application of these methods represent one of the triumphs of modern medicine. However, their appropriate use is to supplement but not to supplant a careful clinical examination. The latter remains the cornerstone of the assessment of the patient with known or suspected cardiovascular disease. There is a temptation in cardiology, as in many other areas of medicine, to carry out expensive, uncomfortable, and occasionally hazardous procedures to establish a diagnosis when a detailed and thoughtful history and physical examination are sufficient. Obviously, it is undesirable to subject patients to the unnecessary risks and expenses inherent in many specialized tests when a diagnosis can be made on the basis of an adequate clinical examination or when management will not be altered significantly as a result of these tests.[1] Intelligent selection of investigative procedures from the ever-increasing array of tests now available requires far more sophisticated decision-making than was necessary when the choices were limited to electrocardiography and chest roentgenography; some of the principles in such decision-making are dealt with in Chapters 11 and 53. The history and physical examination provide the critical information necessary for most of these decisions.

THE ROLE OF THE HISTORY. The overreliance on laboratory tests has increased as physicians attempt to utilize their time more efficiently by delegating responsibility for taking the history to a physician's assistant or nurse or even by limiting the history to a questionnaire—an approach that I consider to be an undesirable trend insofar as the patient with known or suspected heart disease is concerned.[2] First, it must be appreciated that the history remains the richest source of information concerning the patient's illness,[3,4] and any practice that might diminish the quality or quantity of information provided by the history is likely ultimately to impair the quality of care. Second, the physician's attentive and thoughtful taking of a history establishes a bond with the patient that may be valuable later in securing the patient's compliance in following a complex treatment plan, undergoing hospitalization for an intensive diagnostic work-up or a hazardous operation, and, in some instances, accepting that heart disease is not present at all.

Taking a history also permits the physician to evaluate the results of diagnostic tests that have strong subjective components, such as the determination of exercise capacity (Chap. 5). Perhaps most importantly, a careful history allows the physician to evaluate the impact of the disease, or the fear of the disease, on the various aspects of the patient's life and to assess the patient's personality, affect, and stability; often it provides a glimpse of the patient's responsibilities, fears, aspirations, and threshold for discomfort as well as the likelihood of compliance with one or another therapeutic regimen. Whenever possible, the physician should question not only the patient but also relatives or close friends to obtain a clearer understanding of the extent of the patient's disability and a broader perspective concerning the impact of the disease on both the patient and the family. (For example, the patient's spouse is much more likely than the patient to provide a history of Cheyne-Stokes [periodic] respiration.)

The combination of the widespread fear of cardiovascular disorders and the deep-seated emotional, symbolic, and sometimes even religious connotations surrounding the heart may, on the one hand, provoke symptoms that mimic those of organic heart disease in persons with normal cardiovascular systems. On the other, they cause so much fear that serious symptoms are repressed or denied by patients with established heart disease.

TECHNIQUE. Several approaches can be employed successfully in obtaining a medical history. I believe that patients should first be given the opportunity to relate their experiences and complaints in their own way. Although time-consuming and likely to include much seemingly irrelevant information, this technique has the advantage of providing considerable information concerning the patient's intelligence, emotional make-up, and attitude toward his or her complaints, as well as providing the patient with the satisfaction that he has been "heard" by the physician, rather than merely having had a few questions thrown at him and then been exposed to a battery of laboratory examinations. After the patient has given an account of the illness, the physician should direct the discussion and obtain information concerning the onset and chronology of symptoms; their location, quality, and intensity; the precipitating, aggravating, and alleviating factors, the setting in which the symptoms occur, and any associated symptoms; and the response to therapy.

Of course, a detailed general medical history including the personal past history, occupational history, nutritional history, and review of systems must be obtained. Of particular interest is a history of thyroid disease, recent dental extractions or manipulations, catheterization of the bladder, and earlier examinations that showed abnormalities of the cardiovascular system as reflected in restriction from physical activity at school and in rejection for life insurance, employment, or military service. Personal habits such as exercise, cigarette smoking, alcohol intake, and parenteral use of drugs—illicit and otherwise—should be ascertained. The exact nature of the patient's work, including the physical and emotional stresses, should be assessed. The increasing appreciation of the importance of genetic influences in many forms of heart disease (Chap. 49) underscores the importance of the family history.

A wide variety of disorders including, but not limited to, neurological (Chap. 60), endocrine (Chap. 61), and rheumatic (Chap. 56) may have important effects on the cardiovascular system; it is vital to ascertain the presence of these and other conditions that are not primarily cardiovascular. A history of the risk factors for ischemic heart disease—the history of cigarette smoking, hypertension, hypercholesterolemia, diabetes mellitus, artificial or early menopause, and long-term contraceptive pill ingestion, as well as the family history of ischemic heart disease (Chap. 35)—should always be sought.

Myocardial or coronary function that may be adequate at rest is often inadequate during exertion; therefore, specific attention should be directed to the influence of activity on the patient's symptoms. Thus, a history of chest discomfort and/or undue shortness of breath that appears only during activity is characteristic of heart disease, whereas the opposite pattern, i.e., the appearance of symptoms at rest and their remission during exertion, is almost never observed in patients with heart disease but is more characteristic of functional disorders. In attempting to assess the severity of functional impairment, both the *extent* of activity and the *rate* at which it is performed before symptoms develop should be determined and related to a detailed consideration of the therapeutic regimen. For example, the development of dyspnea after walking slowly up a flight of stairs in a patient receiving intensive treatment of heart failure denotes far more severe functional disability than does a similar symptom occurring in an untreated patient who has run up a flight of stairs.

As the patient relates the history, important nonverbal clues are often provided. The physician should observe the patient's attitude, reactions, and gestures while being questioned, as well as his or her choice of words or emphasis. Tumulty has aptly likened obtaining a meaningful clinical history to playing a game of chess:[5] "The patient makes a statement and based upon its content, and mode of expression, the physician asks a counter-question. One answer stimulates yet another question until the clinician is convinced that he understands precisely all of the circumstances of the patient's illness."

CARDINAL SYMPTOMS OF HEART DISEASE

The cardinal symptoms of heart disease include dyspnea, chest pain or discomfort, syncope, collapse, palpitation, edema, cough, hemoptysis, and excess fatigue. Cyanosis is more often a sign rather than a symptom, but it may be a key feature of the history, particularly in patients with congenital heart disease. Without doubt, history-taking is the most valuable technique available for determining whether or not these symptoms are caused by heart disease. Examples of the manner in which these symptoms may serve as a guide to diagnosis are given in the following pages, and reference is made to other portions of the book that contain more detailed information.

Dyspnea
(See also pp. 450 and 464)

Dyspnea is defined as an abnormally uncomfortable awareness of breathing; it is one of the principal symptoms of cardiac and pulmonary disease.[6] Since dyspnea is regularly caused by strenuous exertion in healthy, well-conditioned subjects and by only moderate exertion in those who are normal but unaccustomed to exercise, it should be regarded as abnormal only when it occurs at rest or at a level of physical activity not expected to cause this symptom. Dyspnea is associated with a wide variety of diseases of the heart and lungs, chest wall, and respiratory muscles as well as with anxiety[7-10]; the history is the most valuable means of establishing the etiology.[11,12] Table 1-1 provides a list of the various syndromes that may cause dyspnea and the primary pathophysiological mechanisms that are responsible.[13] Borg and Noble have developed a scale that is useful in quantitating the severity of dyspnea.[14]

The *sudden* development of dyspnea suggests pulmonary embolism, pneumothorax, acute pulmonary edema, pneumonia, or airway obstruction.[10] In contrast, in most forms of *chronic* heart failure, dyspnea progresses slowly over weeks or months. Such a protracted course may also occur in a variety of unrelated conditions, including obesity, pregnancy, and bilateral pleural effusion. *Inspiratory dyspnea* suggests obstruction of the upper airways, whereas *expiratory dyspnea* characterizes obstruction of the lower airways. Exertional dyspnea suggests the presence of organic diseases, such as left ventricular failure (Chap. 15) or chronic obstructive lung disease (Chap. 47), whereas dyspnea developing at rest may occur in pneumothorax, pulmonary embolism (Chap. 46), or pulmonary edema (Chap. 15), or it may be functional. Dyspnea that occurs only at rest and is absent on exertion is almost always functional. A *functional origin* is also suggested when dyspnea, or simply a heightened awareness of breathing, is accompanied by brief stabbing pain in the region of the cardiac apex or by prolonged (more than 2 hours) dull chest pain. It is often associated with difficulty in getting enough air into the lungs, claustrophobia, and sighing respirations that are relieved by exertion, by taking a few deep breaths, or by sedation. Dyspnea in patients with panic attacks is usually accompanied by hyperventilation. A history of relief of dyspnea by bronchodilators and corticosteroids suggests asthma as the etiology, whereas relief of dyspnea by rest, diuretics, and digitalis suggests left heart failure. Dyspnea accompanied by wheezing may be secondary to left ventricular failure (*cardiac* asthma) or primary bronchial constriction (*bronchial* asthma).

In patients with *chronic heart failure,* dyspnea is a clinical expression of pulmonary venous and capillary hyper-

TABLE 1–1 DISORDERS CAUSING DYSPNEA AND LIMITING EXERCISE PERFORMANCE; PATHOPHYSIOLOGY; AND DISCRIMINATING MEASUREMENTS

3

Ch 1

DISORDERS	PATHOPHYSIOLOGY	MEASUREMENTS THAT DEVIATE FROM NORMAL
Pulmonary		
Airflow limitation	Mechanical limitation to ventilation, mismatching of $\dot{V}_A/\dot{Q}$, hypoxic stimulation to breathing	$\dot{V}_E$ max/MVV, expiratory flow pattern, V_D, V_T; $\dot{V}_{O_2}$ max, $\dot{V}_E/\dot{V}_{O_2}$, $\dot{V}_E$ response to hyperoxia, $(A - a)P_{O_2}$
Restrictive	Mismatching $\dot{V}_A/\dot{Q}$, hypoxic stimulation to breathing	
Chest wall	Mechanical limitation to ventilation	$\dot{V}_E$ max/MVV, P_{ACO_2}, $\dot{V}_{O_2}$ max
Pulmonary circulation	Rise in physiological dead space as fraction of V_T, exercise hypoxemia	V_D/V_T, work-rate–related hypoxemia, V_{O_2} max, $\dot{V}_E/\dot{V}_{O_2}$, $(a - ET)P_{CO_2}$, O_2-pulse
Cardiac		
Coronary	Coronary insufficiency	ECG, $\dot{V}_{O_2}$ max, anaerobic threshold $\dot{V}_{O_2}$, $\dot{V}_E/\dot{V}_{O_2}$, O_2-pulse, BP (systolic, diastolic, pulse)
Valvular	Cardiac output limitation (decreased effective stroke volume)	
Myocardial	Cardiac output limitation (decreased ejection fraction and stroke volume)	
Anemia	Reduced O_2-carrying capacity	O_2-pulse, anaerobic threshold $\dot{V}_{O_2}$, $\dot{V}_{O_2}$ max, $\dot{V}_E/\dot{V}_{O_2}$
Peripheral circulation	Inadequate O_2 flow to metabolically active muscle	Anaerobic threshold $\dot{V}_{O_2}$, $\dot{V}_{O_2}$ max
Obesity	Increased work to move body; if severe, respiratory restriction and pulmonary insufficiency	$\dot{V}_{O_2}$-work-rate relationship, P_{AO_2}, P_{ACO_2}, $\dot{V}_{O_2}$ max
Psychogenic	Hyperventilation with precisely regular respiratory rate	Breathing pattern, P_{CO_2}
Malingering	Hyperventilation and hypoventilation with irregular respiratory rate	Breathing pattern, P_{CO_2}
Deconditioning	Inactivity or prolonged bed rest; loss of capability for effective redistribution of systemic blood flow	O_2-pulse, anaerobic threshold $\dot{V}_{O_2}$, $\dot{V}_{O_2}$ max

$\dot{V}_A$ = alveolar ventilation; $\dot{Q}$ = pulmonary blood flow; $\dot{V}_E$ = minute ventilation; MVV = maximum voluntary ventilation; V_D/V_T = physiological dead space/tidal volume ratio; O_2 = oxygen; V_{O_2} = O_2 consumption; $(A - a)P_{O_2}$ = alveolar-arterial P_{O_2} difference; $(a - ET)P_{CO_2}$ = arterial-end tidal P_{CO_2} difference.
Modified from Wasserman, D.: Dyspnea on exertion: Is it the heart or the lungs? JAMA *248*:2042, 1982. Copyright 1982 the American Medical Association.

tension (see p. 453). It occurs either during exertion or, in resting patients, in the recumbent position, and it is relieved promptly by sitting upright or standing (*orthopnea*). Patients with left ventricular failure soon learn to sleep on two or more pillows to avoid this symptom. In patients with heart failure, dyspnea is often accompanied by edema, upper abdominal pain (due to congestive hepatomegaly), and nocturia. The *sudden* occurrence of dyspnea in a patient with a history of mitral valve disease suggests the development of atrial fibrillation, rupture of chordae tendineae, or pulmonary embolism.

Paroxysmal nocturnal dyspnea is due to interstitial pulmonary edema and sometimes intraalveolar edema and is most commonly secondary to left ventricular failure (see p. 450). This condition, beginning usually 2 to 4 hours after the onset of sleep and often accompanied by cough, wheezing, and sweating, is quite frightening to the patient. Paroxysmal nocturnal dyspnea is often ameliorated by the patient's sitting on the side of the bed or getting out of bed; relief is not instantaneous but usually requires 15 to 30 minutes. Although paroxysmal nocturnal dyspnea secondary to left ventricular failure is usually accompanied by coughing, a careful history often discloses that the dyspnea *precedes* the cough, not vice versa. In contrast, patients with *chronic pulmonary disease* may also awaken at night, but cough and expectoration usually precede the dyspnea. These patients also often have a long history of smoking and a chronic cough with sputum production and wheezing and may be able to breathe more easily while leaning forward. Nocturnal dyspnea associated with pulmonary disease is usually relieved after the patient rids himself or herself of secretions rather than specifically by sitting up. Details of the value and limitations of the history of dysp-

nea in differentiating between primary diseases of the heart and lungs[15,16] are presented on page 451.

Patients with *pulmonary embolism* usually experience sudden dyspnea that may be associated with apprehension, palpitation, hemoptysis, or pleuritic chest pain (Chap. 46). The development or intensification of dyspnea, sometimes associated with a feeling of faintness, may be the only complaint of the patient with pulmonary emboli. *Pneumothorax* and *mediastinal emphysema* also cause dyspnea acutely, accompanied by sharp chest pain. Dyspnea accompanying thoracic pain occurs in *acute myocardial infarction.* Dyspnea is a common "anginal equivalent" (see p. 1290), i.e., a symptom secondary to myocardial ischemia that occurs in place of typical anginal discomfort.[16] This form of dyspnea may or may not be associated with a sensation of tightness in the chest, is present on exertion or emotional stress, is relieved by rest (more often in the sitting than in the recumbent position), is similar to angina in duration (i.e., 2 to 10 minutes), and is usually responsive to or prevented by nitroglycerin. The sudden development of severe dyspnea while sitting rather than lying, or whenever a particular position is assumed, suggests the possibility of a myxoma (see p. 1467) or ball-valve thrombus in the left atrium. When dyspnea is relieved by squatting, it is caused most commonly by tetralogy of Fallot or a variant thereof (see p. 929).

Chest Pain or Discomfort
(See also p. 1290)

Elucidation of the cause of chest pain is one of the key tasks of physicians, and this symptom is responsible for many cardiac consultations. The history remains the most important technique for distinguishing among the many causes of chest discomfort. Although chest pain or discomfort is one of the cardinal manifestations of cardiac disease, it is crucial to recognize that the pain may originate not only in the heart but also in (1) a variety of noncardiac intrathoracic structures, such as the aorta, pulmonary artery, bronchopulmonary tree, pleura, mediastinum, esophagus, and diaphragm; (2) the tissues of the neck or thoracic wall, including the skin, thoracic muscles, cervicodorsal spine, costochondral junctions, breasts, sensory nerves, and spinal cord; and (3) subdiaphragmatic organs such as the stomach, duodenum, pancreas, and gallbladder (Table 1–2). Pain of functional origin or factitious pain may also occur in the chest. Although a wide variety of laboratory tests is available to aid in the differential diagnosis of chest pain, without question the history remains the most valuable mode of examination. In obtaining the history of a patient with chest pain it is helpful to have a mental checklist and to ask the patient to describe the location, radiation, and character of the discomfort; what causes and relieves it; time relationships, including the duration, frequency, and pattern of recurrence of the discomfort; the setting in which it occurs; and associated symptoms. It is also particularly useful to observe the patient's gestures. Clenching the fist in front of the sternum while describing the sensation (Levine's sign) is a strong indication of an ischemic origin of the pain.

QUALITY. *Angina pectoris* may be defined as a discomfort in the chest and/or adjacent area associated with myocardial ischemia but without myocardial necrosis.[17–20] It is important to recognize that angina means *choking,* not pain. Thus, the discomfort of angina often is described not as pain at all but rather as an unpleasant sensation; "pressing," "squeezing," "strangling," "constricting," "bursting," and "burning" are some of the adjectives commonly used to describe this sensation (Table 1–3). "A band across the chest" and "a weight in the center of the chest" are other frequent descriptors. It is characteristic of angina that the intensity of effort required to incite it may vary from day to day and throughout the day in the same patient, but often a careful history will uncover explanations for this, such as

meals ingested, weather, emotions, and the like. The anginal threshold is lower in the morning than at any other time of day; thus patients note frequently that activities that may cause angina in the morning or when first undertaken do not do so later in the day. When the threshold for angina is quite variable, defies any pattern, and is prominent at rest, the possibility that myocardial ischemia is caused by coronary spasm should be considered (see p. 1189). Thus, a careful history not only may indicate the cause of the pain (i.e., myocardial ischemia) but can also provide a clue to the mechanism of the ischemia (spasm vs. organic obstruction).

A history of prolonged, severe anginal chest discomfort accompanied by profound fatigue often signifies acute myocardial infarction.[21] There is some relationship between location of the chest pain and the site of coronary artery occlusion[22]; patients with ischemic heart disease who complain of substernal or left chest pain with radiation to the left arm often have heart disease involving the left coronary artery, while those with epigastric pain radiating to the neck or jaw may *not* have disease of the left anterior descending coronary artery.

When dyspnea is an "anginal equivalent," the patient may describe the midchest as the site of the shortness of breath, whereas true dyspnea is usually not well localized. Other anginal equivalents are discomfort limited to areas that are ordinarily sites of secondary radiation, such as the ulnar aspect of the left arm and forearm, lower jaw, teeth, neck, or shoulders, and the development of gas and belching, nausea, "indigestion," dizziness, and diaphoresis. Anginal equivalents above the mandible or below the umbilicus are quite uncommon. It is useful to determine whether the patient has symptoms or complications caused by atherosclerosis of other vascular beds, e.g., intermittent claudication, transient ischemic attacks, or stroke. In patients with suspected angina, a history of one of these manifestations of extracardiac atherosclerosis lends weight to the diagnosis of myocardial ischemia.

The chest discomfort of *pulmonary hypertension* (see p. 788) may be identical to that of typical angina[23,24]; it is caused by right ventricular ischemia or dilation of the pul-

TABLE 1–2 DIFFERENTIAL DIAGNOSIS OF EPISODIC CHEST PAIN RESEMBLING ANGINA PECTORIS

	DURATION	QUALITY	PROVOCATION	RELIEF	LOCATION	COMMENT
Effort angina	5–15 minutes	Visceral (pressure)	During effort or emotion	Rest, nitroglycerin	Substernal, radiates	First episode vivid
Rest angina	5–15 minutes	Visceral (pressure)	Spontaneous (? with exercise)	Nitroglycerin	Substernal, radiates	Often nocturnal
Mitral prolapse	Minutes to hours	Superficial (rarely visceral)	Spontaneous (no pattern)	Time	Left anterior	No pattern, variable character
Esophageal reflux	10 minutes to 1 hour	Visceral	Recumbency, lack of food	Food, antacid	Substernal, epigastric	Rarely radiates
Esophageal spasm	5–60 minutes	Visceral	Spontaneous, cold liquids, exercise	Nitroglycerin	Substernal, radiates	Mimics angina
Peptic ulcer	Hours	Visceral, burning	Lack of food, "acid" foods	Foods, antacids	Epigastric, substernal	
Biliary disease	Hours	Visceral (waxes and wanes)	Spontaneous, food	Time, analgesia	Epigastric, ? radiates	Colic
Cervical disc	Variable (gradually subsides)	Superficial	Head and neck movement, palpation	Time, analgesia	Arm, neck	Not relieved by rest
Hyperventilation	2–3 minutes	Visceral	Emotion, tachypnea	Stimulus removal	Substernal	Facial paresthesia
Musculoskeletal	Variable	Superficial	Movement, palpation	Time, analgesia	Multiple	Tenderness
Pulmonary	30 minutes +	Visceral (pressure)	Often spontaneous	Rest, time, bronchodilator	Substernal	Dyspneic

Reproduced with permission from Christie, L.G., Jr., and Conti, C.R.: Systematic approach to the evaluation of angina-like chest pain. Am. Heart J. *102*:897, 1981.

TABLE 1–3 SOME FEATURES DIFFERENTIATING CARDIAC FROM NONCARDIAC CHEST PAIN

FAVORING ISCHEMIC ORIGIN	AGAINST ISCHEMIC ORIGIN
Character of Pain	
Constricting	Dull ache
Squeezing	"Knife-like," sharp, stabbing
Burning	"Jabs" aggravated by respiration
"Heaviness," "heavy feeling"	
Location of Pain	
Substernal	In the left submammary area
Across mid-thorax, anteriorly	In the left hemithorax
In both arms, shoulders	
In the neck, cheeks, teeth	
In the forearms, fingers	
In the interscapular region	
Factors Provoking Pain	
Exercise	Pain *after* completion of exercise
Excitement	Provoked by a specific body motion
Other forms of stress	
Cold weather	
After meals	

From Selzer, A.: Principles and Practice of Clinical Cardiology. 2nd ed. Philadelphia, W.B. Saunders Company, 1983, p. 17.

monary arteries. The chest discomfort of *unstable angina* and *acute myocardial infarction* (see p. 1198) is similar in quality to that of angina pectoris in location and character; however, it usually radiates more widely than does angina, is more severe, and therefore is generally referred to by the patient as true *pain* rather than *discomfort.* This pain generally develops unrelated to unusual effort or emotional stress, often with the patient at rest or even sleeping. Usually nitroglycerin does not provide complete or lasting relief.

Acute pericarditis (see p. 1481) is frequently preceded by a history of a viral upper respiratory infection. The inflammation causes pain that is sharper than is anginal discomfort, is more left-sided than central, and is often referred to the neck. The pain of pericarditis lasts for hours and is little affected by effort but is often aggravated by breathing, turning in bed, swallowing, or twisting the body; unlike angina, the pain of acute pericarditis may lessen when the patient sits up and leans forward.

Aortic dissection (see p. 1554) is suggested by the sudden development of persistent, severe pain with radiation to the back and into the lumbar region in a patient with a history of hypertension. An expanding *thoracic aortic aneurysm* may erode the vertebral bodies and cause localized, severe, boring pain that may be worse at night. An aneurysmally enlarged left atrium in patients with mitral valve disease rarely causes chest pain; instead, patients commonly complain of discomfort in the back or right side of the chest that intensifies on exertion.

Chest-wall pain due to *costochondritis* or *myositis* is common in patients who present with fear of heart disease.[25] It is associated with both local costochondral and muscle tenderness, which may be aggravated by moving or coughing. Chest-wall pain[26] may also accompany chest injury, or *Tietze syndrome* (i.e., discomfort localized in swelling of the costochondral and costosternal joints, which are painful on palpation). When *herpes zoster* affects the left chest it may mimic myocardial infarction. However, its persistence, its localization to a dermatome, the extreme sensitivity of the skin to touch, and the appearance of the characteristic vesicles allow recognition of this condition. Pain in the chest wall is quite common following cardiac or thoracic surgery and may be confused with myocardial ischemia. Postsurgical pain is usually localized to the incision or the site of insertion of a chest tube.

The pain of *pulmonary embolism* (Ch. 46) usually commences suddenly, and, when it occurs at rest, is seen in patients at high risk for this condition (heart failure, venous disease, the postoperative state), and is accompanied by shortness of breath. It is typically described as tightness in the chest and is accompanied or followed by *pleuritic* chest pain, i.e., sharp pain in the side of the chest that is intensified by respiration or cough. Chest pain associated with *spontaneous pneumothorax* develops suddenly, is associated with acute dyspnea, and is located in the lateral area of the chest. The chest pain associated with *mediastinal emphysema* also commences suddenly and is accompanied by dyspnea, sometimes severe; it is located in the center of the chest.

Functional or *psychogenic chest* pain may be one feature of an anxiety state called Da Costa syndrome or neurocirculatory asthenia.[27–29] It is localized typically to the cardiac apex and consists of a dull, persistent ache that lasts for hours and is often accentuated by or alternates with attacks of sharp, lancinating stabs of inframammary pain of 1 or 2 seconds' duration. The condition may occur with emotional strain and fatigue, bears little relation to exertion, and may be accompanied by precordial tenderness. Attacks may be associated with palpitation, hyperventilation, numbness and tingling in the extremities, sighing, dizziness, dyspnea, generalized weakness, and a history of panic attacks and other signs of emotional instability or depression. The pain may not be completely relieved by any medication other than analgesics, but it is often attenuated by many types of interventions, including rest, exertion, tranquilizers, and placebos. Therefore, in contrast to ischemic discomfort, functional pain is more likely to show variable responses to interventions on different occasions. Since functional chest pain is often preceded by hyperventilation, which in turn may cause increased muscle tension and be responsible for diffuse chest tightness, some instances of so-called functional chest pain may, in fact, have an organic basis. Chest pain is common in patients with prolapse of the mitral valve (see p. 1029). The nature of the pain varies considerably among patients with this condition; it may be similar to that of classic angina pectoris or may resemble the chest pain of neurocirculatory asthenia described above.

LOCATION. Embryologically the heart is a midline viscus; thus, cardiac ischemia produces anginal symptoms that are characteristically felt substernally or across both sides of the chest (Figs. 1–1 and 1–2). Some patients complain of discomfort only to the left or less commonly only to the right of the midline. If the pain or discomfort can be localized to the skin or superficial structures and can be reproduced by localized pressure, it generally arises from the chest wall. If the patient can point directly to the site of discomfort, and if that site is quite small (< 3 cm in diameter), it is usually not angina pectoris. Like other symptoms arising in deeper structures, angina tends to be diffuse and

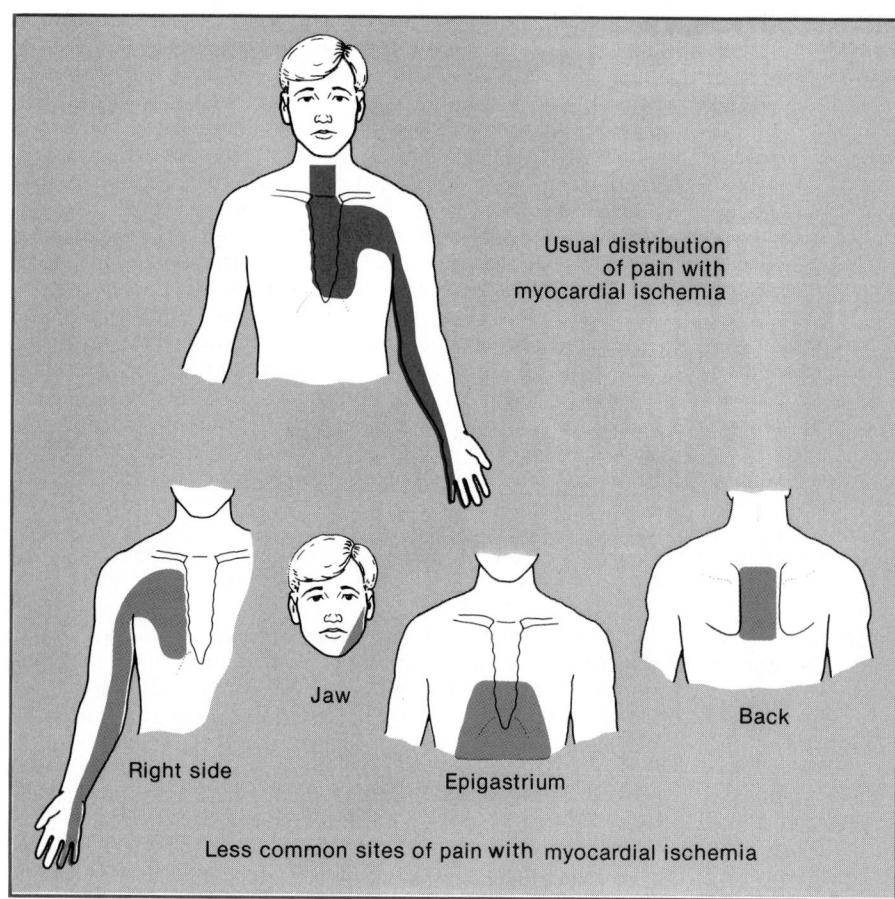

Usual distribution
of pain with
myocardial ischemia

Jaw

Back

Right side

Epigastrium

Less common sites of pain with myocardial ischemia

FIGURE 1–1. Pain patterns with myocardial ischemia. The usual distribution is referral to all or part of the sternal region, the left side of the chest, and the neck and down the ulnar side of the left forearm and hand. With severe ischemic pain, the right chest and right arm are often involved as well, although isolated involvement of these areas is rare. Other sites sometimes involved, either alone or together with other sites, are the jaw, epigastrium, and back. (From Horwitz, L. D.: Chest pain. *In* Horwitz, L. D., and Groves, B. M. [eds.]: Signs and Symptoms in Cardiology. Philadelphia, J. B. Lippincott, 1985, p. 9.)

eludes precise localization. Pain that is localized to the region of or under the left nipple or that radiates to the right lower chest[30] is usually noncardiac in origin and may be functional or due to osteoarthritis, gaseous distention of the stomach, or the splenic flexure syndrome. Although pain due to myocardial ischemia often radiates to the arm, especially the ulnar aspect of the left arm, wrist, epigastrium, or left shoulder, such radiation may also occur in pericarditis and disorders of the cervical spine. Radiation of pain from the chest to the neck and jaws is typical of myocardial infarction. Chest pain that radiates to the neck and jaw occurs in pericarditis as well as in myocardial ischemia. Dissection of the aorta or enlargement of an aortic aneurysm usually produces pain in the back in addition to the front of the chest.

DURATION. The duration of the pain is important in de-

FIGURE 1–2. Differential diagnosis of chest pain according to location where pain starts. Serious intrathoracic or subdiaphragmatic diseases are usually associated with pains that begin in the left anterior chest, left shoulder, or upper arm, the interscapular region, or the epigastrium. The scheme is not all-inclusive; e.g., intercostal neuralgia occurs in locations other than the left, lower anterior chest area. (From Miller, A. J.: Diagnosis of Chest Pain. New York, Raven Press, 1988, p. 175.)

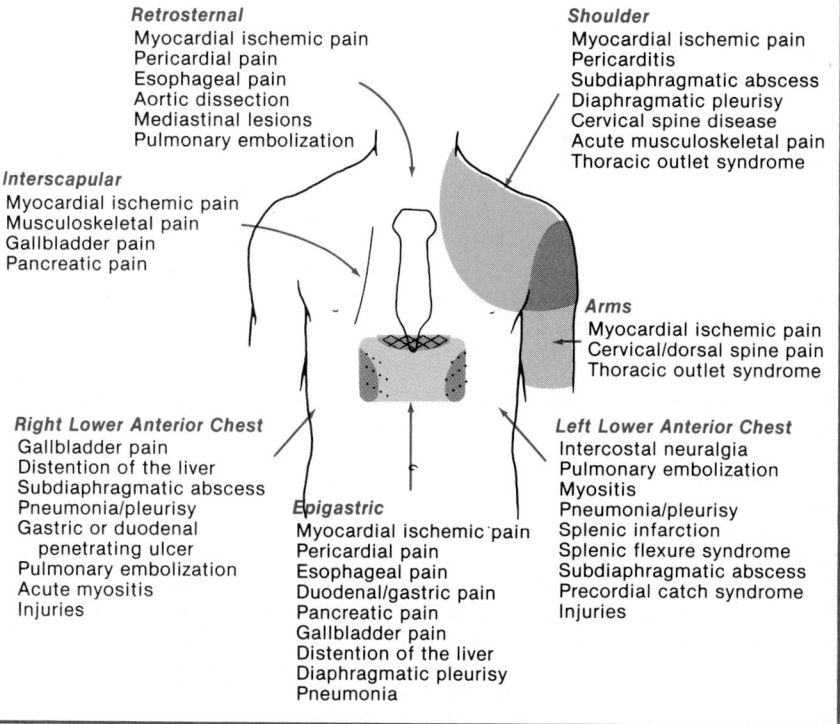

Retrosternal
Myocardial ischemic pain
Pericardial pain
Esophageal pain
Aortic dissection
Mediastinal lesions
Pulmonary embolization

Shoulder
Myocardial ischemic pain
Pericarditis
Subdiaphragmatic abscess
Diaphragmatic pleurisy
Cervical spine disease
Acute musculoskeletal pain
Thoracic outlet syndrome

Interscapular
Myocardial ischemic pain
Musculoskeletal pain
Gallbladder pain
Pancreatic pain

Arms
Myocardial ischemic pain
Cervical/dorsal spine pain
Thoracic outlet syndrome

Right Lower Anterior Chest
Gallbladder pain
Distention of the liver
Subdiaphragmatic abscess
Pneumonia/pleurisy
Gastric or duodenal
  penetrating ulcer
Pulmonary embolization
Acute myositis
Injuries

Left Lower Anterior Chest
Intercostal neuralgia
Pulmonary embolization
Myositis
Pneumonia/pleurisy
Splenic infarction
Splenic flexure syndrome
Subdiaphragmatic abscess
Precordial catch syndrome
Injuries

Epigastric
Myocardial ischemic pain
Pericardial pain
Esophageal pain
Duodenal/gastric pain
Pancreatic pain
Gallbladder pain
Distention of the liver
Diaphragmatic pleurisy
Pneumonia

termining its etiology. Angina pectoris is relatively short, usually lasting from 2 to 10 minutes. However, if the pain is very brief, i.e., a momentary, lancinating, sharp pain, "stitch," or other discomfort that lasts less than 15 seconds, angina can usually be excluded; such a short duration points instead to musculoskeletal pain, pain due to hiatal hernia, or functional pain. Chest pain that is otherwise typical of angina but that lasts for more than 10 minutes or occurs at rest is typical of unstable angina. Chest pain lasting for hours may be seen with acute myocardial infarction, pericarditis, aortic dissection, musculoskeletal disease, herpes zoster, and anxiety.

PRECIPITATING AND AGGRAVATING FACTORS. Angina pectoris occurs characteristically on exertion, particularly when the patient is hurrying or walking up an incline. Thus, the development of chest discomfort or pain during walking, typically in the cold and against a wind, and after a heavy meal, is characteristic of angina pectoris. Angina may be precipitated by strong emotion or fright, by a nightmare, by working with the arms over the head, by cold exposure, or smoking a cigarette. Prinzmetal's (variant) angina characteristically occurs at rest (see p. 1340), and may or may not be affected by exertion; however, it must be remembered that (nonvariant) angina, although most often precipitated by effort, not uncommonly may be experienced at rest, as in unstable angina (see p. 1331); in these patients exertion intensifies the discomfort.

DIFFERENTIAL DIAGNOSIS. Chest pain that occurs after protracted vomiting may be due to the Mallory-Weiss syndrome, i.e., a tear in the lower portion of the esophagus. Pain that occurs while the patient is bending over is often radicular and may be associated with osteoarthritis of the cervical or upper thoracic spine. Chest pain occurring on moving the neck may be due to a herniated intervertebral disc.

Esophageal Pain. Substernal and epigastric discomfort during swallowing may be due to esophageal spasm or esophagitis, often with acid reflux, with or without a hiatal hernia. These conditions may also be associated with substernal or epigastric burning pain that is brought on by eating or lying down after meals and that may be relieved by antacids. Pain due to esophageal spasm has many of the features of and may be difficult to differentiate from angina pectoris.[30] Indeed, it is a common cause of chest pain considered atypical of angina pectoris.[31-34] A history of acid reflux into the mouth (water brash) and/or dysphagia[35] may be a useful diagnostic clue pointing to esophageal disease.[36] The chest discomfort secondary to esophageal reflux is most common after meals and occurs in the supine position or on bending. The difficulty in distinguishing angina from esophageal disease is compounded by the frequent coexistence of these two common conditions, by the observation that esophageal reflux lowers the threshold for the development of angina,[37] and by the observation that esophageal spasm may be precipitated by ergonovine and relieved by nitroglycerin. Esophageal pain radiates to the back more frequently than does angina pectoris.[32]

The discomfort produced by *peptic ulcer disease* is characteristically located in the midepigastrium. It may also resemble angina pectoris, but its characteristic relationship to food ingestion and its relief by antacids are important differentiating features. While the pain of *acute pancreatitis* may mimic acute myocardial infarction, with the former there is usually a history of alcoholism or biliary tract disease. The pain of pancreatitis, like that of myocardial infarction, may be predominant in the epigastrium. However, unlike the pain of myocardial infarction, it is usually transmitted to the back, is position-sensitive, and may be relieved in part by leaning forward.[30] Chest pain aggravated by coughing may be due to pericarditis, bronchitis, or pleurisy or may be of radicular origin. *Congenital absence of the pericardium* (see p. 1522) produces chest pain that is relieved by changing position in bed, is brought on by

lying on the left side, and lasts a few seconds. Pain due to the *scalenus anticus (thoracic outlet) syndrome* may be confused with angina because it is often associated with paresthesias along the ulnar distribution of the arm and forearm. However, in contrast to angina, not only is it typically precipitated by abduction of the arm or lifting a weight, but it is not brought on by walking.

RELIEF OF PAIN. Rest and nitroglycerin characteristically relieve the discomfort of angina in approximately 1 to 5 minutes. If more than 10 minutes transpire before relief, the diagnosis of chronic stable angina becomes questionable and instead may be unstable angina, acute myocardial infarction, or pain not caused by myocardial ischemia at all. Although nitroglycerin commonly relieves the pain of angina pectoris, the discomfort of esophageal spasm and esophagitis may also be relieved by this drug. Angina pectoris is alleviated by quiet standing or sitting; sometimes resting in the recumbent position does not relieve angina. Chest pain secondary to *acute pericarditis* is characteristically relieved by leaning forward, whereas pain that is relieved by food or antacids may be due to *peptic ulcer disease* or esophagitis. Pain that is alleviated by holding the breath in deep expiration is commonly due to pleurisy. Some patients with upper gastrointestinal disease or anxiety report relief of symptoms after belching.

ACCOMPANYING SYMPTOMS. The physician should always be concerned about the patient who reports the presence of chest pain and profuse sweating. This combination of symptoms frequently signals a serious disorder, most often acute myocardial infarction, but also acute pulmonary embolism or aortic dissection. Severe chest pain accompanied by nausea and vomiting is also often due to myocardial infarction. The latter diagnosis, as well as pneumothorax, pulmonary embolism, or mediastinal emphysema, is suggested by pain associated with shortness of breath. Chest pain accompanied by palpitation may be due to the acute myocardial ischemia that results from a tachyarrhythmia-induced increase in myocardial oxygen consumption in the presence of coronary artery disease. Chest pain accompanied by hemoptysis suggests pulmonary embolism with infarction or lung tumor, whereas pain accompanied by fever occurs in pneumonia, pleurisy, and pericarditis. Functional pain is commonly accompanied by frequent sighing, anxiety, or depression.

Cyanosis

Cyanosis, both a symptom and a physical sign, is a bluish discoloration of the skin and mucous membranes resulting from an increased quantity of reduced hemoglobin or of abnormal hemoglobin pigments in the blood perfusing these areas[38,39] (see also pp. 885 and 891). There are two principal forms of cyanosis: (1) central cyanosis, characterized by decreased arterial oxygen saturation due to right-to-left shunting of blood or impaired pulmonary function, and (2) peripheral cyanosis, most commonly secondary to cutaneous vasoconstriction due to low cardiac output or exposure to cold air or water; if peripheral cyanosis is confined to an extremity, localized arterial or venous obstruction should be suspected. A history of cyanosis localized to the hands suggests Raynaud's phenomenon. Patients with central cyanosis due to congenital heart disease or pulmonary disease characteristically report that it worsens during exertion, whereas the resting peripheral cyanosis of congestive heart failure may be accentuated only slightly, if at all, during exertion.

Central cyanosis usually becomes apparent at a mean capillary concentration of 4 gm/dl reduced hemoglobin (or 0.5 gm/dl methemoglobin). In general, a history of cyanosis in light-skinned people is rarely elicited unless arterial saturation is 85 per cent or less; in pigmented races arterial saturation has to drop far lower before cyanosis is perceptible.

Although a history of cyanosis beginning in infancy suggests a congenital cardiac malformation with a right-to-left shunt, hereditary methemoglobinemia is another, albeit rare, cause of congenital cyanosis; the diagnosis of this condition is supported by a family history of cyanosis in the absence of heart disease.

A history of cyanosis limited to the neonatal period suggests the diagnosis of atrial septal defect with transient right-to-left shunting or, more commonly, pulmonary parenchymal disease or central nervous system depression. Cyanosis beginning at age 1 to 3 months may be reported when spontaneous closure of a patent ductus arteriosus causes a reduction of pulmonary blood flow in the presence of right-sided obstructive cardiac anomalies, most commonly tetralogy of Fallot. If cyanosis appears at age 6 months or later in childhood, it may be due to the development or progression of obstruction to right ventricular outflow in patients with ventricular septal defect. A history of the development of cyanosis in a patient with congenital heart disease between 5 and 20 years of age suggests an Eisenmenger reaction with right-to-left shunting as a consequence of a progressive increase in pulmonary vascular resistance (see p. 903). Cyanosis secondary to a pulmonary arteriovenous fistula also usually appears first in childhood.

Syncope

Syncope, which may be defined as a loss of consciousness (see also Chap. 28), results most commonly from reduced perfusion of the brain. The history is extremely valuable in the differential diagnosis of syncope (Table 1–4). Several daily attacks of loss of consciousness suggest (1) Stokes-Adams attacks, i.e., transient asystole or ventricular fibrillation in the presence of atrioventricular block; (2) other cardiac arrhythmias; or (3) a seizure disorder, i.e., petit mal epilepsy. These diagnoses are suggested when the loss of consciousness is abrupt and occurs over 1 or 2 seconds; a more gradual onset suggests vasodepressor syncope (i.e., the common faint) or syncope due to hyperventilation or, much less commonly, hypoglycemia.

CARDIAC SYNCOPE. This condition is usually of rapid onset without aura and is usually not associated with convulsive movements, urinary incontinence, and a postictal confusional state. Syncope in aortic stenosis[40,41] is usually precipitated by effort. Patients with epilepsy often have a prodromal aura preceding the seizure. Injury from falling is common, as are urinary incontinence and a postictal confusional state, associated with headache and drowsiness. Unconsciousness developing gradually and lasting for a few seconds suggests

vasodepressor syncope or syncope secondary to postural hypotension, whereas a longer period suggests aortic stenosis or hyperventilation. Hysterical fainting is usually not accompanied by any untoward display of anxiety or change in pulse, blood pressure, or skin color, and there may be a question whether any true loss of consciousness occurred. It is often associated with paresthesias of the hands or face, hyperventilation, dyspnea, chest pain, and feelings of acute anxiety.

A history of syncope independent of body position suggests Stokes-Adams attacks, hyperventilation, or a convulsive disorder, whereas syncope of other etiology usually occurs in the upright position. Syncope occurring upon bending, leaning, or assuming a particular body position should raise the possibility of a left atrial myxoma (see p. 1467) or a ball-valve thrombus. Since syncope is an unusual feature of mitral stenosis, when it does occur in a patient thought to have this condition, the possibility of left atrial myxoma or ball-valve thrombus should be considered. A history of syncope occurring during or immediately following exertion suggests aortic stenosis, hypertrophic obstructive cardiomyopathy, or primary pulmonary hypertension. Syncope is rare in patients with angina pectoris unless the latter is secondary to one of the aforementioned conditions. Syncope following insulin administration suggests a hypoglycemic etiology; a history of syncope occurring several hours after eating is characteristic of reactive hypoglycemia. Loss of consciousness following an emotional stress suggests that it is vasodepressor syncope or secondary to hyperventilation.

Patients with vasodepressor syncope often have a history of recurrent fainting, commonly associated with emotional or painful stimuli. This, the most common form of syncope, may be precipitated by the sight or loss of blood or by physical or emotional stress; it can be averted by promptly lying down, and it is characteristically preceded by symptoms of autonomic hyperactivity such as dim vision, giddiness, yawning, sweating, and nausea. A history of syncope in the erect position may also be elicited in patients who have become hypovolemic as a consequence of overly vigorous diuresis. Syncope secondary to *cerebrovascular disturbance* is often preceded by aphasia, unilateral weakness, or confusion. A history of fainting following sudden movements of the head, shaving the neck, or wearing a tight collar suggests carotid sinus syncope. Syncope associated with chest pain may be secondary to massive acute myocardial infarction or infarction associated with arrhythmias; occasionally, following recovery of consciousness, the associated chest pain may be forgotten, and the infarction may be recognized only by the characteristic changes in serum enzymes and on the electrocardiogram. A history of syncope following chest pain may also occur in patients with *acute pulmonary embolism*.

REGAINING CONSCIOUSNESS. Consciousness is usually regained quite promptly in syncope of cardiovascular origin, but more slowly in patients with convulsive disorders. When consciousness is regained after vasodepressor syncope, the patient is often pale and diaphoretic with a slow heart rate, whereas after a Stokes-Adams attack, the face is often flushed and there may be cardiac acceleration. Patients who report an injury when falling during a fainting spell usually have epilepsy or occasionally syncope of cardiac origin, but patients who have unconsciousness related to emotional disturbance rarely sustain physical trauma.

DIFFERENTIAL DIAGNOSIS. A family history of syncope or near-syncope can often be elicited in patients with hypertrophic cardiomyopathy (see p. 1414) or ventricular tachyarrhythmias associated with Q-T

TABLE 1–4 CLUES FROM THE HISTORY IN ELUCIDATING THE CAUSE OF SYNCOPE

PRECEDING EVENTS

Drugs:	Orthostatic hypotension (antihypertensives), hypoglycemia (insulin)
Severe pain, emotional stress:	Vasovagal syncope, hyperventilation
Movement of head and neck:	Carotid sinus hypersensitivity
Exertion:	Any form of obstruction to left ventricular outflow, Takayasu's arteritis
Upper extremity exertion:	Subclavian "steal"

TYPE OF ONSET

Sudden:	Neurological (seizure disorder); arrhythmia (ventricular tachycardia or fibrillation, Stokes-Adams)
Rapid with premonition:	Vasovagal, neurological (aura)
Gradual:	Hyperventilation, hypoglycemia

POSITION AT ONSET

Arising:	Orthostatic hypotension
Prolonged standing:	Vasovagal
Any position:	Arrhythmias, neurological, hypoglycemia, hyperventilation

POST-SYNCOPAL CLEARING OF SENSORIUM

Slow:	Neurological
Rapid:	All others

ASSOCIATED EVENTS

Incontinence, tongue biting, injury:	Neurological

Modified from Lindenfeld, J. A.: Syncope. *In* Horwitz, L. D., and Groves, B. M. (eds.): Signs and Symptoms in Cardiology. Philadelphia, J. B. Lippincott, 1985, 506 pp.

prolongation (see p. 685). A family history of epilepsy is positive in approximately 4 per cent of patients with convulsive disorders. A history of syncope associated with progressive intensification of cyanosis in an infant or child with cyanotic congenital heart disease is likely to be due to cerebral anoxia as a consequence of an increase in the right-to-left shunt, secondary to an increase in the obstruction to right ventricular outflow or a reduction in systemic vascular resistance (see p. 884). A history of syncope during childhood suggests the possibility of a cardiovascular anomaly obstructing left ventricular outflow—valvular, supravalvular, or subvalvular aortic stenosis. In patients with hypertrophic cardiomyopathy, syncope may be post-tussive and occurs characteristically in the erect position, when arising suddenly, after standing erect for long periods, and during or immediately after cessation of exertion.

Patients with syncope secondary to orthostatic hypotension may have a history of drug therapy for hypertension or of abnormalities of autonomic function, such as impotence, disturbances of sphincter function, peripheral neuropathy, and anhidrosis (see p. 865). When syncope is secondary to hypovolemia, there is often a history of melena, anemia, menorrhagia, or treatment with anticoagulants. Syncope due to cerebrovascular insufficiency is frequently associated with a history of unilateral blindness, weakness, paresthesias, or memory defects.

PALPITATION

This common symptom is defined as an unpleasant awareness of the forceful or rapid beating of the heart. It may be brought about by a variety of disorders involving changes in cardiac rhythm or rate, including all forms of tachycardia, ectopic beats, compensatory pauses, augmented stroke volume due to valvular regurgitation, hyperkinetic (high cardiac output) states, and the sudden onset of bradycardia. In the case of premature contractions the patient is more commonly aware of the postextrasystolic beat than of the premature beat itself, and it appears that it is the increased motion of the heart within the chest that is perceived. This explains why palpitation is not a characteristic feature of aortic or pulmonic stenosis or of severe systemic or pulmonary hypertension, conditions characterized by an increased force of cardiac contraction.

When episodes of palpitation last for an instant, they are described as "skipped beats" or a "flopping sensation" in the chest and most commonly are due to extrasystoles. On the other hand, the sensation that the heart has "stopped beating" often correlates with the compensatory pause following a premature contraction.

DIFFERENTIAL DIAGNOSIS. Palpitation characterized by a slow heart rate may be due to atrioventricular block or sinus node disease. When palpitation begins and ends abruptly, it is often due to a paroxysmal tachycardia such as paroxysmal atrial or junctional tachycardia, atrial flutter, or atrial fibrillation, whereas a gradual onset and cessation of the attack suggest sinus tachycardia and/or an anxiety state. A history of chaotic, rapid heart action suggests the diagnosis of atrial fibrillation; fleeting and repetitive palpitation suggests multiple ectopic beats. A history of multiple paroxysms of tachycardia followed by palpitation that occurs only with effort or excitement suggests paroxysmal atrial fibrillation that has become permanent—the palpitation being experienced only when the ventricular rate rises.

Some patients have taken their pulse during palpitation or have asked a companion to do so. A regular rate between 100 and 140 beats/min suggests sinus tachycardia, a regular rate of approximately 150 beats/min suggests atrial flutter, and a regular rate exceeding 160 beats/min suggests paroxysmal supraventricular tachycardia. As an adjunct to the history, it may be possible to ascertain the rhythm responsible for the palpitation by tapping the finger on the patient's chest in a variety of rhythms and asking the patient to identify the pattern that most closely resembles the abnormal feeling. Alternatively, patients can be asked to reproduce the arrhythmia by tapping

their fingers on a tabletop at the rate and rhythm they perceived during palpitation. As described on p. 640, these maneuvers may provide important clues to the etiology of the responsible arrhythmia.

A history of palpitation during strenuous physical activity is normal, whereas palpitation during mild exertion suggests the presence of heart failure, atrial fibrillation, anemia, or thyrotoxicosis, or that the individual is severely "out of condition." A feeling of forceful heart action accompanied by throbbing in the neck suggests aortic regurgitation. When palpitation can be relieved suddenly by stooping, breath-holding, or induced gagging or vomiting, i.e., by vagal maneuvers, the diagnosis of paroxysmal supraventricular tachycardia is suggested. A history of syncope *following* an episode of palpitation suggests either asystole or severe bradycardia following the termination of a tachyarrhythmia or a Stokes-Adams attack. A history of palpitation associated with anxiety, a lump in the throat, dizziness, and tingling in the hands and face suggests sinus tachycardia accompanying an anxiety state with hyperventilation. Palpitation followed by angina suggests that myocardial ischemia has been precipitated by increased oxygen demands induced by the rapid heart rate.

A directed history is also useful (Table 1–5). Is there a history of cocaine or amphetamine abuse? Thyrotoxicosis? Anemia? Do the palpitations occur after heavy cigarette smoking or caffeine ingestion? Is there a family history of syncope, arrhythmia, or sudden death?

In many individuals no obvious cause for palpitation emerges despite careful work-up, including a correlation between episodes of palpitation with a simultaneously recorded ambulatory electrocardiogram (see p. 578) or an electrocardiogram recorded by transtelephonic transmission. Anxiety is responsible for the symptom in many such patients, some of whom are known to have heart disease and may be receiving a vasodilator for the treatment of hypertension or nifedipine for the treatment of myocardial ischemia. In these patients palpitation may be due to postural hypotension resulting in reflex cardiac acceleration.

Edema

LOCALIZATION. This is helpful in elucidating the etiology of edema.[42,43] Thus a history of edema of the legs that is most pronounced in the evening is characteristic of heart failure or bilateral chronic venous insufficiency. Inability to fit the feet into shoes is a common early complaint. In most patients any visible edema of both lower extremities is preceded by a weight gain of at least 7 to 10 lb. Cardiac edema is generally symmetrical. As it progresses, it usually ascends to involve the legs, thighs, genitalia, and abdominal wall. In patients with heart failure who are confined largely to bed, the edematous fluid localizes particularly in the sacral area. Edema affecting both the abdomen and the legs is observed in heart failure and hepatic cirrhosis. Edema may be generalized (anasarca) in the nephrotic syndrome, severe heart failure, and hepatic cirrhosis. A history of edema around the eyes and face is characteristic of the nephrotic syndrome, acute glomerulonephritis, angioneurotic edema, hypoproteinemia, and myxedema. A history of edema limited to the face, neck, and upper arms may be associated with obstruction of the superior vena cava, most commonly by carcinoma of the lung, lymphoma, or aneurysm of the aortic arch. A history of edema restricted to one extremity is usually due to venous thrombosis or lymphatic blockage of that extremity.

ACCOMPANYING SYMPTOMS. A history of dyspnea asso-

TABLE 1–5   ITEMS TO BE COVERED IN HISTORY OF PATIENT WITH PALPITATION

DOES THE PALPITATION OCCUR:	IF SO, SUSPECT:
As isolated "jumps" or "skips"?	Extrasystoles
In attacks, known to be of abrupt beginning, with a heart rate of 120 beats per minute or over, with regular or irregular rhythm?	Paroxysmal rapid heart action
Independent of exercise or excitement adequate to account for the symptom?	Atrial fibrillation, atrial flutter, thyrotoxicosis, anemia, febrile states, hypoglycemia, anxiety state
In attacks developing rapidly though not absolutely abruptly, unrelated to exertion or excitement?	Hemorrhage, hypoglycemia, tumor of the adrenal medulla
In conjunction with the taking of drugs?	Tobacco, coffee, tea, alcohol, epinephrine, ephedrine, aminophylline, atropine, thyroid extract, monoamine oxidase inhibitors
On standing?	Postural hypotension
In middle-aged women, in conjunction with flushes and sweats?	Menopausal syndrome
When the rate is known to be normal and the rhythm regular?	Anxiety state

From Goldman, L., and Braunwald, E.: Chest discomfort and palpitation. *In* Isselbacher, K. J., Braunwald, E., et al. (eds.): Harrison's Principles of Internal Medicine. 13th ed. New York, McGraw-Hill, 1994.

ciated with edema is most frequently due to heart failure, but may also be observed in patients with large bilateral pleural effusions, elevation of the diaphragm due to ascites, angioneurotic edema with laryngeal involvement, and pulmonary embolism. When dyspnea precedes edema, the underlying disorder is usually left ventricular dysfunction, mitral stenosis, or chronic lung disease with cor pulmonale. A history of jaundice suggests that edema may be of hepatic origin, whereas edema associated with a history of ulceration and pigmentation of the skin of the legs is most commonly due to chronic venous insufficiency or postphlebitic syndrome. When cardiac edema is not associated with orthopnea, it may be due to tricuspid stenosis or regurgitation or constrictive pericarditis; in these conditions edema is not always most prominent in the lower extremities but may be generalized and may even involve the face. A history of leg edema after prolonged sitting (particularly in the elderly in wheelchairs) may be due to stasis and not be associated with disease at all.

A history of ascites preceding edema suggests cirrhosis, whereas a history of ascites following edema suggests cardiac or renal disease. Angioneurotic edema occurs intermittently, particularly after emotional stress or eating certain foods. Idiopathic cyclic edema is associated with menstruation. A history of edema on prolonged standing is observed in patients with chronic venous insufficiency.

Cough

Cough, one of the most frequent of all cardiorespiratory symptoms, may be defined as an explosive expiration that provides a means of clearing the tracheobronchial tree of secretions and foreign bodies.[44–46] It can be caused by a variety of infectious, neoplastic, or allergic disorders of the lungs and tracheobronchial tree. Cardiovascular disorders most frequently responsible for cough include those that lead to pulmonary venous hypertension, interstitial and alveolar pulmonary edema, pulmonary infarction, and compression of the tracheobronchial tree (aortic aneurysm). Cough due to pulmonary venous hypertension secondary to left ventricular failure or mitral stenosis tends to be dry, irritating, spasmodic, and nocturnal. When cough accompanies exertional dyspnea, it suggests either chronic obstructive lung disease or heart failure, whereas in a patient with a history of allergy and/or wheezing, cough is often a concomitant of bronchial asthma. A history of cough associated with expectoration for months or years occurs in chronic obstructive lung disease and/or chronic bronchitis.

The character of the sputum may be helpful in the differential diagnosis. Thus, a cough producing frothy, pink-tinged sputum occurs in pulmonary edema; clear, white, mucoid sputum suggests viral infection or longstanding bronchial irritation; thick, yellowish sputum suggests an infectious cause; rusty sputum suggests pneumococcal pneumonia; blood-streaked sputum suggests tuberculosis, bronchiectasis, carcinoma of the lung, or pulmonary infarction.

A history of a combination of cough with hoarseness without upper respiratory disease may be due to pressure of a greatly enlarged left atrium on an enlarged pulmonary artery compressing the recurrent laryngeal nerve.

HEMOPTYSIS

The expectoration of blood or of sputum, either streaked or grossly contaminated with blood, may be due to (1) escape of red cells into the alveoli from congested vessels in the lungs (acute pulmonary edema); (2) rupture of dilated endobronchial vessels that form collateral channels between the pulmonary and bronchial venous systems (mitral stenosis); (3) necrosis and hemorrhage into the alveoli (pulmonary infarction); (4) ulceration of the bronchial mucosa or the slough of a caseous lesion (tuberculosis); minor damage to the tracheobronchial mucosa, produced by excessive coughing of any cause, can result in mild hemoptysis; (5) vascular invasion (carcinoma of the lung);

or (6) necrosis of the mucosa with rupture of pulmonary-bronchial venous connections (bronchiectasis).

The history is often decisive in pinpointing the etiology of hemoptysis.[46] Recurrent episodes of minor bleeding are observed in patients with chronic bronchitis, bronchiectasis, tuberculosis, and mitral stenosis. Rarely, these conditions result in the expectoration of large quantities of blood, i.e., more than one-half cup. Massive hemoptysis may also be due to rupture of a pulmonary arteriovenous fistula; exsanguinating hemoptysis may occur with rupture of an aortic aneurysm into the bronchopulmonary tree.[47,48]

Hemoptysis associated with a history of expectoration of clear, gray sputum suggests chronic obstructive lung disease and of yellowish-green sputum, pulmonary infection. Hemoptysis associated with shortness of breath suggests mitral stenosis; in this condition the hemoptysis is often precipitated by sudden elevations in left atrial pressure during effort or pregnancy and is attributable to rupture of small pulmonary or bronchopulmonary anastomosing veins. Blood-tinged sputum in patients with mitral stenosis may also be due to transient pulmonary edema; in these circumstances it is usually associated with severe dyspnea.

A history of hemoptysis associated with acute pleuritic chest pain suggests pulmonary embolism with infarction. Recurrent hemoptysis in a young, otherwise asymptomatic woman favors the diagnosis of bronchial adenoma. Hemoptysis associated with congenital heart disease and cyanosis suggests Eisenmenger syndrome (see p. 799). A history of recurrent hemoptysis with chronic excessive sputum production suggests the diagnosis of bronchiectasis. Hemoptysis associated with the production of putrid sputum occurs in lung abscess, whereas hemoptysis associated with weight loss and anorexia in a male smoker suggests carcinoma of the lung. When blunt trauma to the chest is followed by hemoptysis, lung contusion is the probable cause.

A history of drug ingestion may be helpful in elucidating the etiology of hemoptysis; e.g., anticoagulants and immunosuppressive drugs can cause bleeding. A history of ingestion of contraceptive pills may be a risk factor for the development of deep vein thrombosis and subsequent pulmonary embolism and infarction.

FATIGUE AND OTHER SYMPTOMS

Cardiovascular disorders can cause symptoms emanating from every organ system. Several of these are mentioned here primarily to point out how detailed the history should be in providing a comprehensive evaluation of a patient suspected of having cardiovascular disease; fuller discussions are found elsewhere in this text.

FATIGUE. This is among the most common symptoms in patients with impaired cardiovascular function. However, it is also one of the most nonspecific of all symptoms in clinical medicine; in patients with impaired systemic circulation as a consequence of a depressed cardiac output, it may be associated with muscular weakness. In other patients with heart disease, fatigue may be caused by drugs, such as beta-adrenoceptor blocking agents. It may be the result of excessive blood pressure reduction in patients treated too vigorously for hypertension or heart failure. In patients with heart failure, fatigue may also be caused by excessive diuresis and by diuretic-induced hypokalemia. Extreme fatigue sometimes precedes or accompanies acute myocardial infarction.[20]

OTHER SYMPTOMS. *Nocturia* is a common early complaint in patients with congestive heart failure. *Anorexia*, abdominal fullness, right upper quadrant discomfort, weight loss, and cachexia are symptoms of advanced heart failure (see p. 452). Anorexia, *nausea, vomiting,* and *visual changes* are important signs of digitalis intoxication (see p. 484). Nausea and vomiting occur frequently in patients with acute myocardial infarction. Hoarseness may be caused by compression of the recurrent laryngeal nerve by an aortic aneurysm, a dilated pulmonary artery, or a greatly enlarged left atrium. A history of *fever* and *chills* is common in patients with infective endocarditis (see p. 1084).

The aforementioned symptoms are examples of the wide variety of symptoms that are not obviously associated with abnormalities of the cardiovascular system but that can be of critical importance in differential diagnosis when they are elicited in patients known to have or suspected of having heart disease. They serve to reemphasize that the physician whose responsibility is to care for patients with heart disease must be first and foremost a broadly based clinician.

THE HISTORY IN SPECIFIC FORMS OF HEART DISEASE

Just as the history is of central importance in determining whether or not a specific symptom is caused by heart disease, it is equally valuable in elucidating the etiology of recognized heart disease. A few examples are given below; considerably greater detail is provided in later chapters that deal with each specific disease entity.

Heart Disease in Infancy and Childhood

The history is particularly helpful in establishing a diagnosis of congenital heart disease. In view of the familial incidence of certain congenital malformations (Chaps. 29 and 49), a history of congenital heart disease, cyanosis, or heart murmur in the family should be ascertained. Rubella in the first 2 months of pregnancy is associated with a number of congenital cardiac malformations (patent ductus arteriosus, atrial and ventricular septal defect, tetralogy of Fallot, and supravalvular aortic stenosis [see p. 919]). A maternal viral illness in the last trimester of pregnancy may be responsible for neonatal myocarditis. Syncope on exertion in a child with congenital heart disease suggests a lesion in which the cardiac output is fixed, such as aortic or pulmonic stenosis. Exertional angina in a child suggests severe aortic stenosis, pulmonary stenosis, primary pulmonary hypertension, or anomalous origin of the left coronary artery. A history of syncope or faintness with straining and associated with cyanosis suggests tetralogy of Fallot (see p. 929).

In infants or children with cardiac murmurs, it is important to ascertain as precisely as possible when the murmur was first detected. Murmurs due to either aortic or pulmonic stenosis are usually audible within the first 48 hours of life, whereas those produced by a ventricular septal defect are usually apparent a few days or weeks later. On the other hand, the murmur produced by an atrial septal defect often is not heard until age 2 to 3 months.

Frequent episodes of pneumonia early in infancy suggest a large left-to-right shunt, and a history of excessive diaphoresis occurs in left ventricular failure, most commonly due to ventricular septal defect in this age group. A history of squatting is most frequently associated with tetralogy of Fallot or tricuspid atresia (see p. 932). Dysphagia in early infancy suggests the presence of an aortic arch anomaly such as double aortic arch or an anomalous origin of the right subclavian artery passing behind the esophagus. A history of headaches, weakness of the legs, and intermittent claudication is compatible with the diagnosis of coarctation of the aorta (see p. 965). Weakness or lack of coordination in a child with heart disease suggests cardiomyopathy associated with Friedreich's ataxia or muscular dystrophy (Chap. 60). Recurrent bleeding from the nose, lips, or mouth, associated with dizziness and visual disturbances, and a family history of bleeding in a cyanotic child suggest hereditary hemorrhagic telangiectasia (Osler-Weber-Rendu disease) with pulmonary arteriovenous fistula(s) (see p. 461). A cerebrovascular accident in a cyanotic patient may be due to cerebral thrombosis or abscess or paradoxical embolization (see p. 885).

MYOCARDITIS AND CARDIOMYOPATHY

Rheumatic fever (Chap. 55) is suggested by a history of sore throat followed by symptoms including rash and chorea (St. Vitus dance). This is manifested as a period of twitching or clumsiness for a few months in childhood, as well as by frequent episodes of epistaxis and growing pains, i.e., nocturnal pains in the legs. In patients suspected of having myocarditis or cardiomyopathy, a history of Raynaud's phenomenon, dysphagia, or tight skin suggests scleroderma (see p. 1781). A history of dyspnea following an influenza-like illness with myalgia suggests acute myocarditis. Pain in the hip or lower back that awakens the patient in the morning and is followed by morning back stiffness suggests rheumatoid spondylitis, which is often associated with aortic valve disease (see p. 1780). *Carcinoid heart disease* is associated with a history of diarrhea, bronchospasm, and flushing of the upper chest and head (see p. 1434). A history of diabetes, particularly if resistant to insulin and associated with bronzing of the skin, suggests *hemochromatosis* (see p. 1790), which may be associated with heart failure due to cardiac infiltration. *Amyloid heart disease* (see p. 1427) is often associated with a history of postural hypotension and peripheral neuropathy. *Hypertrophic cardiomyopathy* (see p. 1414) is often associated with a family history of this condition and sometimes with a family history of sudden death. The characteristic symptoms are angina, dyspnea, and syncope, which are often intensified paradoxically by digitalis and which occur during or immediately after exercise.

Patients with symptoms of heart failure (breathlessness and excess fluid accumulation) with warm extremities often have *high-output heart failure* (see p. 460). They should be questioned about a history of anemia and of its common causes and accompaniments, such as menorrhagia, melena, peptic ulcer, hemorrhoids, sickle cell disease, and the neurological manifestations of vitamin B_{12} deficiency. Also, in such patients an attempt should be made to elicit a history of thyrotoxicosis (see pp. 461 and 1894) (weight loss, polyphagia, diarrhea, diaphoresis, heat intolerance, nervousness, breathlessness, muscle weakness, and goiter). Patients with beriberi heart disease responsible for high-output heart failure often have a history characteristic of peripheral neuritis, alcoholism, poor eating habits, fad diets, or upper gastrointestinal surgery.

Patients with chronic cor pulmonale (see Chap. 47) frequently have a history of smoking, chronic cough and sputum production, dyspnea, and wheezing relieved by bronchodilators. Alternatively, they may have a history of pulmonary emboli, phlebitis, and the sudden development of dyspnea at rest with palpitations, pleuritic chest pain, and, in the case of massive infarction, syncope.

PERICARDITIS AND ENDOCARDITIS

In patients in whom *pericarditis* or *cardiac tamponade* is suspected (Chap. 43), an attempt should be made to elicit a history of chest trauma, a recent viral infection, recent cardiac surgery, neoplastic disease of the chest with or without extensive radiation therapy, myxedema, scleroderma, tuberculosis, or contact with tuberculous patients. The *sequence of development* of abdominal swelling, ankle edema, and dyspnea should be determined, since in patients with chronic constrictive pericarditis, ascites often precedes edema, which in turn usually precedes exertional dyspnea. A history of joint symptoms with a face rash suggests the possibility of systemic lupus erythematosus (SLE), an important cause of pericarditis, and it should be recalled that procainamide, hydralazine, and isoniazid can produce an SLE-like syndrome (see p. 604).

The diagnosis of infective endocarditis is suggested by a history of fever, severe night sweats, anorexia, and weight loss and embolic phenomena expressed as hematuria, back pain, petechiae, tender finger pads, and a cerebrovascular accident (see p. 1084).

Drug-Induced Heart Disease

Since a wide variety of cardiac abnormalities can be induced by drugs,[49] a meticulous history of drug intake is of great importance. Table 1–6 summarizes the major drugs responsible for various cardiovascular manifestations.

Catecholamines, whether administered exogenously or secreted by a pheochromocytoma (see p. 1897), may produce myocarditis and arrhythmias. *Digitalis glycosides* can be responsible for a variety of tachyarrhythmias and bradyarrhythmias as well as gastrointestinal, visual, and central nervous system disturbances (see p. 499). *Quinidine* may cause Q-T prolongation, ventricular tachycardia of the torsades de pointes variety, syncope, and sudden death, presumably due to ventricular fibrillation (see p. 602). Paradoxically, the administration of antiarrhythmic drugs is one of the major causes of serious cardiac arrhythmias (see p. 600).

Disopyramide (see p. 604), *beta-adrenoceptor blockers* (see p. 610), and the calcium channel antagonists *diltiazem* and *verapamil* (see p. 616) may depress ventricular performance, and in patients with ventricular dysfunction these drugs may intensify heart failure. *Alcohol* is also a potent myocardial depressant and may be responsible for the development of cardiomyopathy (see p. 1412), arrhythmias, and sudden death. *Tricyclic antidepressants* may cause orthostatic hypotension and arrhythmias. *Lithium,* also used in the treatment of psychiatric disorders, can aggravate preexisting cardiac arrhythmias, particularly in patients with heart failure in whom the renal clearance of this ion is impaired. *Cocaine* can cause coronary spasm with resultant myocardial ischemia, myocardial infarction, and sudden death.[50,51]

The *anthracycline compounds* doxorubicin (Adriamycin) and daunorubicin, which are widely used because of their broad spectrum of activity against various tumors, may cause or intensify left ventricular failure, arrhythmias, myocarditis, and pericarditis (see p. 1800). *Cyclophosphamide,* an antineoplastic alkylating agent, may also cause

TABLE 1-6 CARDIOVASCULAR MANIFESTATIONS OF ADVERSE REACTIONS TO DRUGS

Acute Chest Pain (nonischemic)	Arrhythmias	Fluid Retention/Congestive Heart Failure/Edema	Hypertension
Bleomycin	Adriamycin	Beta blockers	Clonidine withdrawal
Angina Exacerbation	Antiarrhythmic drugs	Calcium blockers	Corticotropin
Alpha blockers	Astemizole	Carbenoxolone	Cyclosporine
Beta-blocker withdrawal	Atropine	Diazoxide	Glucocorticoids
Ergotamine	Anticholinesterases	Estrogens	Monoamine oxidase inhibitors with sympathomimetics
Excessive thyroxine	Beta blockers	Indomethacin	NSAIDs (some)
Hydralazine	Daunorubicin	Mannitol	Oral contraceptives
Methysergide	Digitalis	Minoxidil	Sympathomimetics
Minoxidil	Emetine	Phenylbutazone	Tricyclic antidepressants with sympathomimetics
Nifedipine	Erythromycin	Steroids	**Pericarditis**
Oxytocin	Guanethidine	Verapamil	Emetine
Vasopressin	Lithium	**Hypotension** (see also Arrhythmias)	Hydralazine
	Papaverine	Amiodarone (perioperative)	Methysergide
	Phenothiazines, particularly thioridazine	Calcium channel blockers, e.g., nifedipine	Procainamide
	Sympathomimetics	Citrated blood	**Pericardial Effusion**
	Terfenadine	Diuretics	Minoxidil
	Theophylline	Interleukin-2	**Thromboembolism**
	Thyroid hormone	Levodopa	Oral contraceptives
	Tricyclic antidepressants	Morphine	
	Verapamil	Nitroglycerin	
	AV Block	Phenothiazines	
	Clonidine	Protamine	
	Methyldopa	Quinidine	
	Verapamil		
	Cardiomyopathy		
	Adriamycin		
	Daunorubicin		
	Emetine		
	Lithium		
	Phenothiazines		
	Sulfonamides		
	Sympathomimetics		

From Wood, A. J.: Adverse reactions to drugs. *In* Isselbacher, K. J., Braunwald, E., et al. (eds.): Harrison's Principles of Internal Medicine. 13th ed. New York, McGraw-Hill, 1994.

TABLE 1-7 A COMPARISON OF THREE METHODS OF ASSESSING CARDIOVASCULAR DISABILITY

CLASS	NEW YORK HEART ASSOCIATION FUNCTIONAL CLASSIFICATION	CANADIAN CARDIOVASCULAR SOCIETY FUNCTIONAL CLASSIFICATION	SPECIFIC ACTIVITY SCALE
I	Patients with cardiac disease but without resulting limitations of physical activity. Ordinary physical activity does not cause undue fatigue, palpitation, dyspnea, or anginal pain.	Ordinary physical activity, such as walking and climbing stairs, does not cause angina. Angina with strenuous or rapid or prolonged exertion at work or recreation.	Patients can perform to completion any activity requiring ≤7 metabolic equivalents, e.g., can carry 24 lb up eight steps; carry objects that weigh 80 lb; do outdoor work (shovel snow, spade soil); do recreational activities (skiing, basketball, squash, handball, jog/walk 5 mph).
II	Patients with cardiac disease resulting in slight limitation of physical activity. They are comfortable at rest. Ordinary physical activity results in fatigue, palpitation, dyspnea, or anginal pain.	Slight limitation of ordinary activity. Walking or climbing stairs rapidly, walking uphill, walking or stair climbing after meals, in cold, in wind, or when under emotional stress, or only during the few hours after awakening. Walking more than two blocks on the level and climbing more than one flight of ordinary stairs at a normal pace and in normal conditions.	Patients can perform to completion any activity requiring ≤5 metabolic equivalents, e.g., have sexual intercourse without stopping, garden, rake, weed, roller skate, dance fox trot, walk at 4 mph on level ground, but cannot and do not perform to completion activities requiring ≥7 metabolic equivalents.
III	Patients with cardiac disease resulting in marked limitation of physical activity. They are comfortable at rest. Less than ordinary physical activity causes fatigue, palpitation, dyspnea, or anginal pain.	Marked limitation of ordinary physical activity. Walking one to two blocks on the level and climbing more than one flight in normal conditions.	Patients can perform to completion any activity requiring ≤2 metabolic equivalents, e.g., shower without stopping, strip and make bed, clean windows, walk 2.5 mph, bowl, play golf, dress without stopping, but cannot and do not perform to completion any activities requiring ≥5 metabolic equivalents.
IV	Patient with cardiac disease resulting in inability to carry on any physical activity without discomfort. Symptoms of cardiac insufficiency or of the anginal syndrome may be present even at rest. If any physical activity is undertaken, discomfort is increased.	Inability to carry on any physical activity without discomfort—anginal syndrome *may be* present at rest.	Patients cannot or do not perform to completion activities requiring ≥2 metabolic equivalents. *Cannot* carry out activities listed above (Specific Activity Scale, Class III).

left ventricular dysfunction, while 5-fluorouracil and its derivatives (see p. 1803) may be responsible for angina secondary to coronary spasm (see p. 1189). Radiation therapy to the chest may cause acute and chronic pericarditis (see p. 1799), pancarditis, or coronary artery disease; further, it may enhance the aforementioned cardiotoxic effects of the anthracyclines.

Assessing Cardiovascular Disability
(Table 1–7)

One of the greatest values of the history is in categorizing the degree of cardiovascular disability, so that a patient's status can be followed over time, the effects of a therapeutic intervention assessed, and patients compared with one another. The Criteria Committee of the New York Heart Association has provided a widely used classification that relates functional activity to the ability to carry out "ordinary" activity.[52] The term "ordinary," of course, is subject to widely varying interpretation, as are terms such as "undue fatigue" that are used in this classification, and this has limited its accuracy and reproducibility. More recently, this Heart Association changed its evaluation from functional activity to a broader one, called Cardiac Status, which takes account of symptoms and other data gathered from the patient.[52] Cardiac status is classified as: (1) uncompromised, (2) slightly compromised, (3) moderately compromised, and (4) severely compromised.

Somewhat more detailed and specific criteria were provided by the Canadian Cardiovascular Society,[53] but this classification is limited to patients with angina pectoris. Goldman et al.[54] developed a specific activity scale in which classification is based on the estimated metabolic cost of various activities. This scale appears to be more reproducible and to be a better predictor of exercise tolerance than either the New York Heart Association Classification or the Canadian Cardiovascular Society Criteria.

A key element of the history is to determine whether the patient's disability is stable or progressive. A useful way to accomplish this is to inquire whether a specific task which now causes symptoms, e.g., dyspnea after climbing two flights of stairs, did so 3, 6, and 12 months previously. Precise questioning on this point is important since a gradual reduction of ordinary activity as heart disease progresses may lead to an underestimation of the apparent degree of disability.[55]

REFERENCES

IMPORTANCE OF THE HISTORY

1. Sandler, G.: The importance of the history in the medical clinic and the cost of unnecessary tests. Am. Heart J. 100:928, 1980.
2. Hickman, D. H., Soc, H. C., Jr., and Soc, C. H.: Systematic bias in recording the history in patients with chest pain. J. Chronic Dis. 38:91, 1985.
3. Sapira, J. D.: The history. In The Art and Science of Bedside Diagnosis. Baltimore, Urban Schwartzenberg, 1990, pp. 9–45.
4. Hampton, J. R., Harrison, M. J. G., Mitchell, J. R. A., et al.: Relative contributions of history-taking, physical examination, and laboratory investigation to diagnosis and management of medical outpatients. Br. Med. J. 2:486, 1975.
5. Tumulty, P. A.: Obtaining the history. In The Effective Clinician. Philadelphia, W. B. Saunders Company, 1973, pp. 17–28.

CARDINAL SYMPTOMS OF HEART DISEASE

6. Szidon, J. P., and Fishman, A. P.: The first approach to the patient with respiratory signs and symptoms. In Fishman, A. P. (ed.): Pulmonary Diseases and Disorders. 2nd ed. New York, McGraw-Hill, 1988, pp. 313–367.
7. Weber, K. T., and Szidon, J. P.: Exertional dyspnea. In Weber, K. T., and Janick, J. S. (eds.): Cardiopulmonary Exercise Testing. Philadelphia, W. B. Saunders Company, 1986, pp. 290–301.
8. Cherniack, N. S.: Dyspnea. In Murray, J. F., and Nadel, J. A. (eds.): Textbook of Respiratory Medicine. 2nd ed. Philadelphia, W. B. Saunders Company, 1995, pp. 430–465.
9. Simon, P. M., Schwartzstein, R. M., Weiss, J. W., et al.: Distinguishable types of dyspnea in patients with shortness of breath. Am. Rev. Respir. Dis. 142:1009, 1990.
10. Mahler, D. A.: Dyspnea: Diagnosis and management. Clin. Chest Med. 8:215, 1987.
11. Elliott, M. W., Adams, I., Cockcroft, A., et al.: The language of breathlessness: Use of verbal descriptors by patients with cardiopulmonary diseases. Am. Rev. Respir. Dis. 144:826, 1991.
12. Schwartzstein, R. M., et al.: Dyspnea: A sensory experience. Lung 169:543, 1991.
13. Wasserman, K.: Dyspnea on exertion. Is it the heart or the lungs? JAMA 248:2039, 1982.
14. Borg, G., and Noble, B.: Perceived exertion. In Wilmore, J. H. (ed.): Exercise and Sports. Science Reviews. New York, Academic Press, 1974, pp. 131–153.
15. Loke, J.: Distinguishing cardiac versus pulmonary limitation in exercise performance. Chest 83:441, 1983.
16. Schmitt, B. P., Kushner, M. S., and Weiner, S. L.: The diagnostic usefulness of the history of the patient with dyspnea. J. Gen. Intern. Med. 1:386, 1986.
17. Christie, L. G., and Conti, C. R.: Systematic approach to the evaluation of angina-like chest pain. Am. Heart J. 102:897, 1981.
18. Constant, J.: The clinical diagnosis of nonanginal chest pain: The differentiation of angina from nonanginal chest pain by history. Clin. Cardiol. 6:11, 1983.
19. Levine, H. J.: Difficult problems in the diagnosis of chest pain. Am. Heart J. 100:108, 1980.
20. Matthews, M. B., and Julian, D. G.: Angina pectoris: Definition and description. In Julian, D. G. (ed.): Angina Pectoris. New York, Churchill Livingstone, 1985, p. 2.
21. Appels, A., and Mulder, P.: Excess fatigue as a precursor of myocardial infarction. Eur. Heart J. 9:758, 1988.
22. Lichstein, E., Breitbart, S., Shani, J., et al.: Relationship between location of chest pain and site of coronary artery occlusion. Am. Heart J. 115:564, 1988.
23. Ross, R. S., and Babe, B. M.: Right ventricular hypertension as a cause of angina. Circulation 22:801, 1960.
24. Zimmerman, D., and Parker, B. M.: The pain of pulmonary hypertension: Fact or fancy? JAMA 246:2345, 1981.
25. Cook, D. G., and Shaper, A. G.: Breathlessness, angina pectoris and coronary artery disease. Am. J. Cardiol. 63:921, 1989.
26. Epstein, S. E., Gerber, L. N., and Boren, J. S.: Chest wall syndrome. A common cause of unexpected pain. JAMA 241:279, 1979.
27. Bass, C., Chambers, J. B., Kiff, P., et al.: Panic anxiety and hyperventilation in patients with chest pain: A controlled study. Q. J. Med. 69:260:949–959, 1988.
28. Beitman, B. D., Basha, I., Flaker, G. et al.: Atypical or nonanginal chest pain: Panic disorder or coronary artery disease? Arch. Intern. Med. 147:1548, 1987.
29. Kane, F. J., Jr., Harper, R. G., and Wittels, E.: Angina as a symptom of a psychiatric illness. South. Med. J. 81:1412, 1988.
30. Horwitz, L. D., and Groves, B. M. (eds.): Signs and Symptoms in Cardiology. Philadelphia, J. B. Lippincott, 1985, 506 pp.
31. Conte, M. R., Orzan, F., Magnacca, M., et al.: Atypical chest pain: Coronary or esophageal disease? Int. J. Cardiol. 13:135, 1986.
32. Schofield, P. M., Whorwell, P. J., Jones, P. E., et al.: Differentiation of "esophageal" and "cardiac" chest pain. Am. J. Cardiol. 62:315, 1988.
33. Hersh, T.: Gastrointestinal causes of chest discomfort. In Hurst, J. W. (ed.): The Heart, 7th ed. New York, McGraw-Hill, 1990, pp. 987–991.
34. Mellow, M. H.: A gastroenterologist's view of chest pain. Curr. Probl. Cardiol. 7:36, 1983.
35. Patterson, D. R.: Diffuse esophageal spasm in patients with undiagnosed chest pain. J. Clin. Gastroenterol. 4:415, 1982.
36. DeMeester, T. R., O'Sullivan, G. C., Bermudez, G. et al.: Esophageal function in patients with angina-type chest pain and normal coronary angiograms. Ann. Surg. 196:488, 1982.
37. Davies, H. A., Rush, E. M., Lewis, M. J., et al.: Oesophageal stimulation lowers exertional angina threshold. Lancet 1:1011, 1985.
38. Braunwald, E.: Cyanosis. In Isselbacher, K. J., Braunwald, E., et al. (eds.): Harrison's Principles of Internal Medicine. 13th ed. New York, McGraw-Hill, 1994, pp. 178–182.
39. Szidon, J. P., and Fishman, A. P.: Cyanosis and clubbing. In Fishman, A. (ed.): Pulmonary Diseases and Disorders. 2nd ed. Philadelphia, W. B. Saunders Company, 1988, p. 351.
40. Richards, A. M., et al.: Syncope in aortic valvular stenosis. Lancet 1:1113, 1984.
41. Brooks, R., et al.: Evaluation of the patient with unexplained syncope. In Zipes, D. P., and Jalife, J. (eds.): Cardiac Electrophysiology. Philadelphia, W. B. Saunders Company, 1990.
42. Braunwald, E.: Edema. In Isselbacher, K. J., Braunwald, E., et al. (eds.): Harrison's Principles of Internal Medicine. 13th ed. New York, McGraw-Hill, 1994, pp. 183–187.
43. Rose, B. D.: Edematous states. In Clinical Physiology of Acid-Base and Electrolyte Disorders. New York, McGraw-Hill, 1989, pp. 416–463.
44. Irwin, R. S., et al.: Chronic cough: The spectrum and frequency of causes, key components of the diagnostic evaluation, and outcome of specific therapy. Am. Rev. Respir. Dis. 141:640, 1990.
45. Poe, R. H., Harder, R. V., Israel, R. H., and Kallay, M. C.: Chronic persistent cough: Experience in diagnosis and outcome using an anatomic diagnostic protocol. Chest 95:723, 1989.
46. Braunwald, E.: Cough and hemoptysis. In Isselbacher, K. J., Braunwald, E., et al. (eds.): Harrison's Principles of Internal Medicine. 13th ed. New York, McGraw-Hill, 1994, pp. 171–174.

47. Thompson, A. B., et al.: Pathogenesis, evaluation, and therapy for massive hemoptysis. Clin. Chest Med. *13*:69, 1992.

48. Jones, D. K., and Davies, R.: Massive hemoptysis. Br. Med. J. *300*:299, 1990.

THE HISTORY IN SPECIFIC FORMS OF HEART DISEASE

49. Bristow, M. R. (ed.): Drug-Induced Heart Disease. Amsterdam, Elsevier, 1980, 476 pp.

50. Virmani, R., Robinowitz, M., Smialek, J. E., and Smyth, D. F.: Cardiovascular effect of cocaine: An autopsy study of 40 patients. Am. Heart J. *115*:1068, 1988.

51. Isner, J. M., and Chokshi, S. K.: Cocaine and vasospasm. N. Engl. J. Med. *321*:1604, 1989.

52. The Criteria Committee of the New York Heart Association: Nomenclature and Criteria for Diagnosis. 9th ed. Boston, Little, Brown, 1994.

53. Campeau, L.: Grading of angina pectoris. Circulation *54*:522, 1975.

54. Goldman, L., Hashimoto, B., Cook, E. F., and Loscalzo, A.: Comparative reproducibility and validity of systems for assessing cardiovascular functional class: Advantages of a new specific activity scale. Circulation *64*:1227, 1981.

55. Goldman, L., Cook, E. F., Mitchell, N., et al.: Pitfalls in the serial assessment of cardiac functional status. How a reduction in "ordinary" activity may reduce the apparent degree of cardiac compromise and give a misleading impression of improvement. J. Chronic Dis. *35*:763, 1982.

GENERAL REFERENCES

Constant, J.: The evolving check list in history-taking. *In* Bedside Cardiology. 4th ed. Boston, Little, Brown, 1993, pp. 1–22.

Dressler, W.: Clinical Aids in Cardiac Diagnosis. New York, Grune and Stratton, 1970.

Fowler, N. O.: The history in cardiac diagnosis. *In* Fowler, N. O. (ed.): Cardiac Diagnosis and Treatment. 3rd ed. Hagerstown, Md., Harper and Row, 1980, pp. 23–29.

Hurst, J. W.: Cardiovascular Diagnosis: The Initial Examination. St. Louis, C. V. Mosby, 1993, 556 pp.

Kraytman, J.: Cardiorespiratory system. *In* The Complete Patient History. New York, McGraw-Hill, 1979, pp. 11–112.

Chapter 2
Physical Examination of the Heart and Circulation

JOSEPH K. PERLOFF, EUGENE BRAUNWALD

Two of the most common pitfalls in cardiovascular medicine are the failure by the cardiologist to recognize the effects of systemic illnesses on the cardiovascular system and the failure by the noncardiologist to recognize the cardiac manifestations of systemic illnesses that have major effects on other organ systems. In order to avoid these pitfalls, patients known to have or suspected of having heart disease require not only a detailed examination of the cardiovascular system but a meticulous general physical examination as well.

For example, the presence of coronary artery disease should prompt a careful search for frequent noncardiac concomitants such as atherosclerosis of the carotid arteries and of the arteries of the lower extremities and aorta. Conversely, the very high incidence (approximately 50 per cent) of coronary artery disease in patients with cerebrovascular disorders must be considered in dealing with patients with these conditions.

THE GENERAL PHYSICAL EXAMINATION

GENERAL APPEARANCE

An assessment of the patient's general appearance is usually begun with a detailed inspection at the time when the history is being obtained.[1-4] The general build and appearance of the patient, the skin color, and the presence of pallor or cyanosis should then be noted, as well as the presence of shortness of breath, orthopnea, periodic (Cheyne-Stokes) respiration (see p. 455), and distention of the neck veins. If the patient is in pain, is he or she sitting quietly (typical of angina pectoris); moving about, trying to find a more comfortable position (characteristic of acute myocardial infarction); or most comfortable sitting upright (heart failure) or leaning forward (pericarditis)? Simple inspection also reveals whether the patient's whole body shakes with each heartbeat and whether Corrigan's pulses (bounding arterial pulsations, as occur with the large stroke volume of severe aortic regurgitation, arteriovenous fistula, or complete atrioventricular [AV] block) are present in the head, neck, and upper extremities. Marked weight loss, malnutrition, and cachexia, which occur in severe chronic heart failure (see p. 455), may also be readily evident on inspection. The cold, sweaty palms and frequent sighing respirations typical of *neurocirculatory asthenia* may be detected, as well as the marked obesity, somnolence, and cyanosis reflecting the *Pickwickian syndrome* (see p. 801). Abdominally localized obesity (diameter of waist/diameter of hips > 0.85; normal = 0.7) is associated with adult onset diabetes and coronary artery disease and should also be looked for.

The distinctive general appearance of the *Marfan syndrome* (see p. 1837) is often apparent, i.e., long extremities with an arm span that exceeds the height; a longer lower segment (pubis to foot) than upper segment (head to pubis);

and arachnodactyly (spider fingers). In *Cushing's syndrome,* a cause of secondary hypertension (see p. 1837), there is truncal obesity and rounding of the face, with disproportionately thin extremities.

HEAD AND FACE

Examination of the face often aids in the recognition of many disorders that can affect the cardiovascular system. For example, *myxedema* (see p. 1894) is characterized by a dull, expressionless face; periorbital puffiness; loss of the lateral eyebrows; a large tongue; and dry, sparse hair. An *earlobe crease* occurs more frequently in patients with coronary artery disease than in those without this condition.[5,6]

Bobbing of the head coincident with each heartbeat (de Musset's sign) is characteristic of severe aortic regurgitation. Facial edema may be present in patients with *tricuspid valve disease* or *constrictive pericarditis.*

The *muscular dystrophies,* the cardiac manifestations of which are described in Chapter 60, may also affect facial appearance profoundly. Patients with *myotonic dystrophy* exhibit a dull, expressionless face, with ptosis due to weakness of the levator muscles.

EYES

External ophthalmoplegia and ptosis due to muscular dystrophy of the extraocular muscles occur in the *Kearns-Sayre syndrome,* which may be associated with complete heart block (Fig. 60–16, p. 1876).

Exophthalmos and stare occur not only in hyperthyroidism, which can cause high-output cardiac failure (see p. 460), but also in advanced congestive heart failure, in which there is severe pulmonary venous hypertension and weight loss (see p. 455).[8] The stare is probably due to lid retraction caused by the increased adrenergic tone that accompanies heart failure. Severe tricuspid regurgitation can also cause pulsation of the eyeballs[9,10] (pulsatile exophthalmos), as well as of the earlobes.

Blue sclerae may be seen in patients with osteogenesis imperfecta[11] —a disorder that may be associated with aortic dilatation, regurgitation, and dissection and with prolapse of the mitral valve (Chap. 49).

FUNDI. Examination of the *fundi* allows classification of arteriolar disease in patients with hypertension (Fig. 2–1A), and may also be helpful in the recognition of arteriosclerosis. Beading of the retinal artery may be present in patients with hypercholesterolemia (Fig.

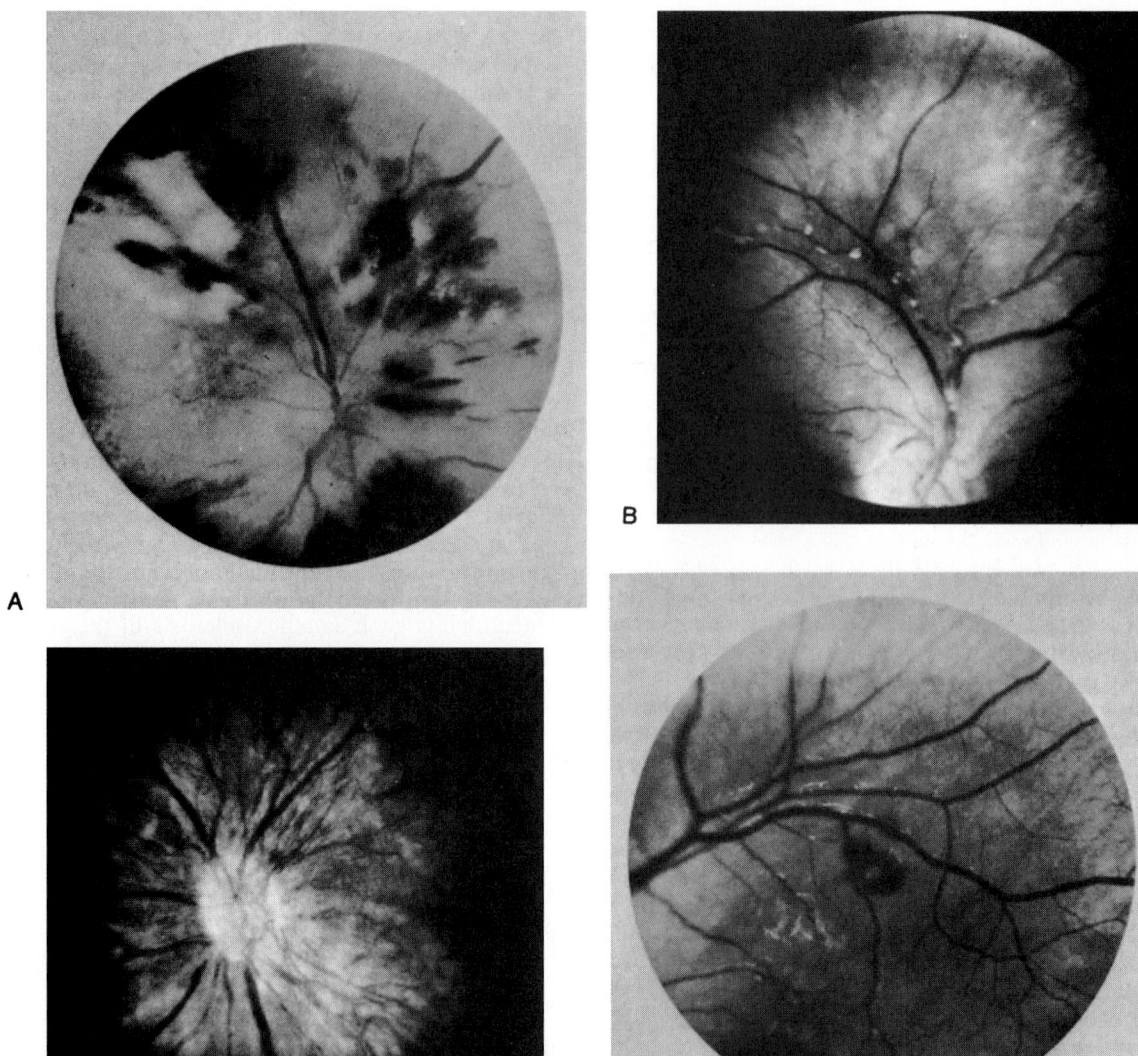

FIGURE 2–1. *A,* Severe hypertensive retinopathy. The patient was a 43-year-old man with the symptoms of malignant hypertension. He subsequently died of massive cerebral hemorrhage. *B,* Beading of the retinal artery in a patient with hypercholesterolemia. The patient was a 37-year-old man with a serum cholesterol level of 400 mg/100 ml. *C,* Proliferative retinopathy of Takayasu-Ohnishi disease. The patient was a 27-year-old Asian woman with postural amaurosis and hemiplegia. Brachial pulses were unobtainable. *D,* Roth spots (hemorrhage with white center) in a patient with subacute bacterial endocarditis. (From Cogan, D. G.: Ophthalmic Manifestations of Systemic Vascular Disease. Philadelphia, W. B. Saunders Company, 1974, p. 52.)

2–1*B*). Hemorrhages near the discs with white spots in the center (Roth's spots) occur in infective endocarditis (Fig. 33–7, p. 1085). Embolic retinal occlusions may occur in patients with rheumatic heart disease, left atrial myxoma, and atherosclerosis of the aorta or arch vessels. Papilledema may be present not only in patients with malignant hypertension (Chap. 26) but also in cor pulmonale with severe hypoxia.

SKIN AND MUCOUS MEMBRANES

Central cyanosis (due to intracardiac or intrapulmonary right-to-left shunting) involves the entire body, including warm, well-perfused sites such as the conjunctivae and the mucous membranes of the oral cavity, whereas peripheral cyanosis (due to reduction of peripheral blood flow, such as occurs in heart failure and peripheral vascular disease) is characteristically most prominent in cool, exposed areas that may not be well-perfused, such as the extremities, particularly the nailbeds and nose. Polycythemia can often be suspected from inspection of the conjunctivae, lips, and tongue, which in anemia are pale while in polycythemia are darkly congested.

Bronze pigmentation of the skin and loss of axillary and pubic hair occur in *hemochromatosis* (which may result in cardiomyopathy owing to iron deposits in the heart [see p. 1430]). Jaundice may be observed in patients following pulmonary infarction as well as in patients with congestive hepatomegaly or cardiac cirrhosis. *Lentigines,* i.e., small brown macular lesions on the neck and trunk that begin at about age 6 and do not increase in number with sunlight, are observed in patients with pulmonic stenosis and hypertrophic cardiomyopathy.[12]

Several types of *xanthomas,* i.e., cholesterol-filled nodules, are found either subcutaneously or over tendons in patients with hyperlipoproteinemia (Chap. 35). Premature atherosclerosis frequently develops in these individuals. *Tuberoeruptive xanthomas,* present subcutaneously or on the extensor surfaces of the extremities, and *xanthoma striatum palmare,* which produces yellowish, orange, or pink discoloration of the palmar and digital creases, occur most commonly in patients with Type III hyperlipoproteinemia. Patients with *xanthoma tendinosum* (Fig. 2–2), i.e., nodular swellings of the tendons, especially of the elbows, extensor surfaces of the hands, and Achilles' tendons, usually have Type II hyperlipoproteinemia (see p. 1143). *Eruptive xanthomas* are tiny yellowish nodules, 1 to 2 mm in diameter on an erythematous base, which may occur anywhere on the body and are associated with hyperchylomicronemia and are therefore often found in patients with Type I and Type V hyperlipoproteinemia.

Hereditary telangiectasias are multiple capillary hemangiomas occurring in the skin, lips (Fig. 2–3), nasal mucosa, and upper respiratory and gastrointestinal tracts and resemble the spider nevi seen in patients with liver disease. When present in the lung, they are associated with pulmonary arteriovenous fistulas and cause central cyanosis.

EXTREMITIES

A variety of congenital and acquired cardiac malformations are associated with characteristic changes in the extremities. Among the congenital lesions, short stature, cubitus valgus, and medial deviation of the extended forearm are characteristic of *Turner syndrome* (see p.

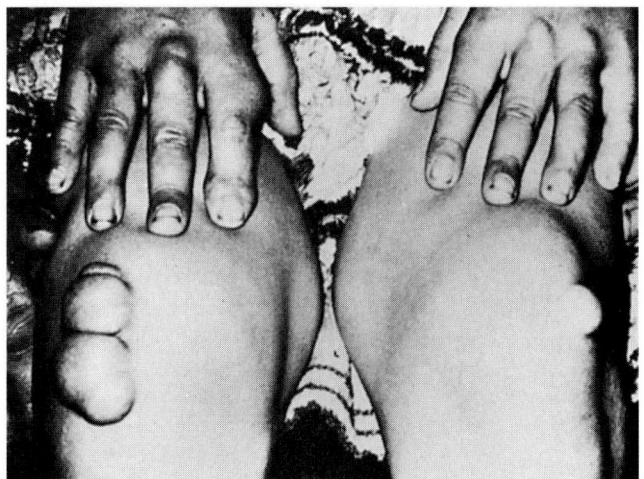

FIGURE 2–2. Tendinous xanthomas of the knees in a patient with familial hypercholesterolemia. The patient was a 10-year-old girl with a serum cholesterol level of 665 mg/100 ml. Several other members of the family had a similar syndrome. (From Cogan, D. G.: Ophthalmic Manifestations of Systemic Vascular Disease. Philadelphia, W. B. Saunders Company, 1974, pp. 14 and 15.)

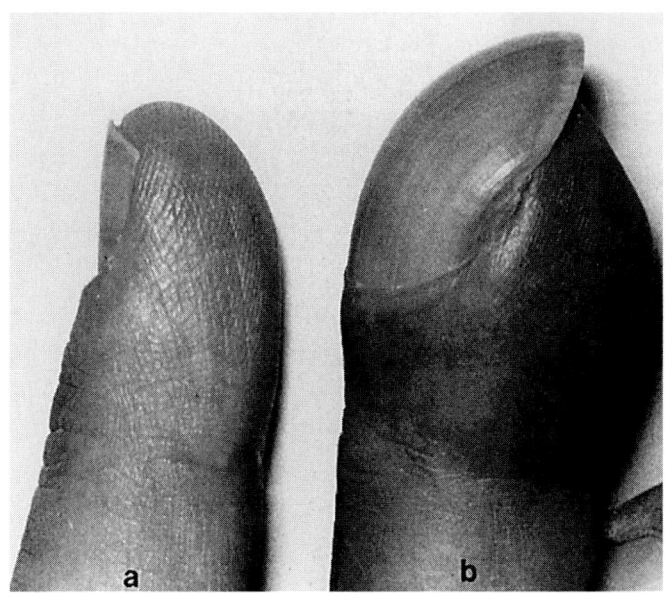

FIGURE 2–4. *A*, Normal finger. *B*, Advanced clubbing in a young cyanotic adult. (From Perloff, J. K.: The Clinical Recognition of Congenital Heart Disease. 4th ed. Philadelphia, W. B. Saunders Company, 1994, p. 7.)

1657). Patients with the *Holt-Oram syndrome*[13] (see p. 1661), i.e., atrial septal defect with skeletal deformities, often have a thumb with an extra phalanx, a so-called fingerized thumb, which lies in the same plane as the fingers, making it difficult to appose the thumb and fingers. In addition, they may exhibit deformities of the radius and ulna, causing difficulty in supination and pronation.

Arachnodactyly is characteristic of *Marfan syndrome* (p. 1669). Normally, when a fist is made over a clenched thumb, the latter does not extend beyond the ulnar side of the hand, but it usually does so in Marfan syndrome.

Systolic flushing of the nailbeds, which can be readily detected by pressing a flashlight against the terminal digits (Quincke's sign), is a sign of aortic regurgitation and of other conditions characterized by a greatly widened pulse pressure. *Differential cyanosis*, in which the hands and fingers (especially on the right side) are pink and the feet and toes are cyanotic, is indicative of patent ductus arteriosus with reversed shunt due to pulmonary hypertension (see p. 905); this finding can often be brought out by exercise. On the other hand, *reversed differential cyanosis*, in which cyanosis of the fingers exceeds that of the toes, suggests transposition of the great arteries, pulmonary hypertension, preductal narrowing of the aorta, and reversed flow through a patent ductus arteriosus.[14]

CLUBBING OF THE FINGERS AND TOES[15] (Fig. 2–4). Clubbing of the digits is characteristic of central cyanosis (cyanotic congenital heart disease or pulmonary disease with hypoxia). It may also appear within a few weeks of the development of infective endocarditis but usually develops after 2 or 3 years of central cyanosis. The earliest forms of clubbing are characterized by increased glossiness and cyanosis of the skin at the root of the nail.[16] Following obliteration of the normal angle between the base of the nail and the skin, the soft tissue of the pulp becomes hypertrophied, the nail root floats freely, and its loose proximal end can be palpated. In the more severe forms of clubbing, bony changes occur, i.e., *hypertrophic pulmonary osteoar-*

thropathy; these changes involve the terminal digits and in rare instances even the wrists, ankles, elbows, and knees. *Unilateral clubbing* of the fingers is rare but can occur when an aortic aneurysm interferes with the arterial supply to one arm.

Osler's nodes are small, tender, purplish erythematous skin lesions due to infected microemboli and occurring most frequently in the pads of the fingers or toes and in the palms of the hands or soles of the feet[17] (see p. 1085), whereas *Janeway lesions* are slightly raised, nontender hemorrhagic lesions in the palms of hands and soles of the feet; both these lesions as well as petechiae occur in infective endocarditis. When the latter occur under the nailbeds, they are termed *splinter hemorrhages*.

Edema of the lower extremities is a common finding in congestive heart failure; however, if it is present in only one leg, it is more likely due to obstructive venous or lymphatic disease than to heart failure. Firm pressure on the pretibial region for 10 to 20 seconds may be necessary for the detection of edema in ambulatory patients. In patients confined to bed, edema appears first in the sacral region. Edema may involve the face in children with heart failure of any etiology and in adults with heart failure associated with marked elevation of systemic venous pressure (e.g., constrictive pericarditis and tricuspid valve disease).

CHEST AND ABDOMEN

Examination of the thorax should begin with observations of the rate, effort, and regularity of respiration. The shape of the chest is important as well; thus, a barrel-shaped chest with low diaphragm suggests emphysema, bronchitis, and possibly cor pulmonale.

Inspection of the chest may reveal a bulging to the right of the upper sternum caused by an aortic aneurysm. This can also produce a venous collateral pattern caused by obstruction of the superior vena cava. *Kyphoscoliosis* of any etiology can cause cor pulmonale; this skeletal abnormality as well as pectus excavatum (funnel chest) and pectus carinatum (pigeon breast) is often present in Marfan syndrome.

Left ventricular failure and other causes of elevation of pulmonary venous pressure may cause pulmonary rales; wheezing is sometimes audible in pulmonary edema (cardiac asthma).

Painful enlargement of the *liver* may be due to venous congestion; the tenderness disappears in longstanding heart failure. Hepatic systolic expansile pulsations occur in patients with severe tricuspid regurgitation, and presystolic pulsations can be felt in patients with pure tricuspid stenosis and sinus rhythm. Patients with constrictive pericarditis

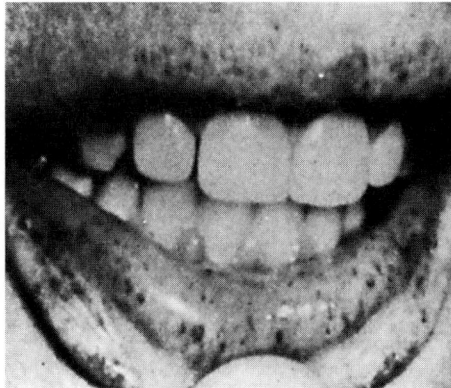

FIGURE 2–3. Hemorrhagic telangiectasia on the lips of a 25-year-old woman with pulmonary arteriovenous fistulas. (From Perloff, J. K.: The Clinical Recognition of Congenital Heart Disease. 4th ed. Philadelphia, W. B. Saunders Company, 1994, p. 719.)

also often have pulsatile hepatomegaly, the contour of the pulsations resembling those of the jugular venous pulse in this condition.[18,19] When firm pressure over the abdomen causes cervical venous distention, i.e., when there is *abdominojugular reflux*, right heart failure is usually present.[20] *Ascites* is also characteristic of heart failure, but is especially characteristic of tricuspid valve disease and chronic constrictive pericarditis.

Splenomegaly may occur in the presence of severe congestive hepatomegaly, most frequently in patients with constrictive pericarditis or tricuspid valve disease. The spleen may be enlarged and painful in infective endocarditis as well as following splenic embolization. Splenic infarction is frequently accompanied by an audible friction rub.

Both *kidneys* may be palpably enlarged in patients with hypertension secondary to polycystic disease. Auscultation of the abdomen should be carried out in all patients with hypertension; a systolic bruit secondary to renal artery stenosis may be audible near the umbilicus or in the flank.

Atherosclerotic aneurysms of the abdominal aorta are usually readily detected on palpation (see p. 1547), except in markedly obese patients. In patients with *coarctation of the aorta*, no abdominal pulsations are palpable despite the presence of prominent arterial pulses in the neck and upper extremities; arterial pulses in the lower extremities are reduced or absent.

JUGULAR VENOUS PULSE

Important information concerning the dynamics of the right side of the heart can be obtained by observation of the jugular venous pulse.[4,21,22,23] The *internal* jugular vein is ordinarily employed in the examination; the venous pulse can usually be analyzed more readily on the right than on the left side of the neck, because the right innominate and jugular veins extend in an almost straight line cephalad to the superior vena cava, thus favoring transmission of hemodynamic changes from the right atrium, while the left innominate vein is not in a straight line and may be kinked or compressed by a variety of normal structures, by a dilated aorta, or by an aneurysm.

The patient should be lying comfortably during the examination; clothing should be removed; although the head should rest on a pillow, it must not be at a sharp angle from the trunk. The jugular venous pulse may be examined effectively by shining a light tangentially across the neck. Most patients with heart disease are examined most effectively in the 45-degree position, but in patients in whom venous pressure is high, a greater inclination (60 or even 90 degrees) is required to obtain visible pulsations, while in those in whom jugular venous pressure is low, a lesser inclination (30 degrees) is desirable. In order to amplify the pulsations of the jugular veins, it may be helpful to place the patient in the supine position and try to increase venous return by elevating the patient's legs.

The internal jugular vein is located deep within the neck, where it is covered by the sternocleidomastoid muscle and is therefore not usually visible as a discrete structure, except in the presence of severe venous hypertension. However, its pulsations are transmitted to the skin of the neck, where they are usually easily visible. Sometimes difficulty may be experienced in differentiating between the carotid and jugular venous pulses in the neck, particularly when the latter exhibits prominent *v* waves, as occurs in patients with tricuspid regurgitation, in whom the valves in the internal jugular veins may be incompetent. However, there are several helpful clues[24]: (1) The arterial pulse is a sharply localized rapid movement that may not be readily visible but that strikes the palpating fingers with considerable force; in contrast, the venous pulse, while more readily visible, often disappears when the palpating finger is placed lightly on or below the pulsating area. (2) The arterial pulse usually exhibits a single upstroke while the venous pulse has two peaks and two troughs per cardiac cycle in sinus rhythm. (3) The arterial pulsations do not change when the patient is in the upright position or during respiration, whereas venous pulsations usually disappear or diminish greatly in the upright position and during inspiration, unless the venous pressure is greatly elevated. (4) Compression of the root of the neck does not affect the arterial pulse but usually abolishes venous pulsations, except in the presence of extreme venous hypertension.

Two principal observations can usually be made from examination of the neck veins: the level of venous pressure

and the type of venous wave pattern. In order to estimate jugular venous pressure, the height of the oscillating top of the distended proximal portion of the internal jugular vein, which reflects right atrial pressure, should be determined. The upper limit of normal is 4 cm above the sternal angle, which corresponds to a central venous pressure of approximately 9 cm H_2O, since the right atrium is approximately 5 cm below the sternal angle. When the veins in the neck collapse in a subject breathing normally in the horizontal

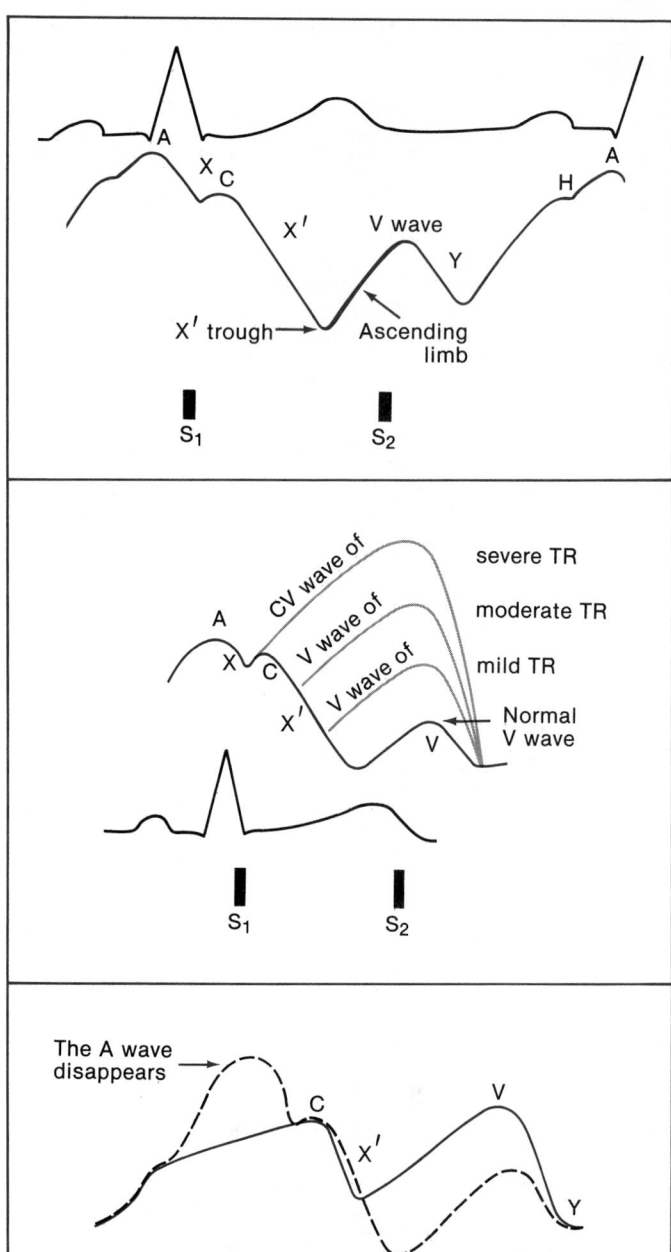

FIGURE 2–5. *Top,* Normal jugular venous pulse: the jugular *v* wave is built up during systole, and its height reflects the rate of filling and the elasticity of the right atrium. Between the bottom of the *y* descent (*y* trough) and beginning of the *a* wave is the period of relatively slow filling of the "atrioventricle" or diastasis period. The wave built up during diastasis is the *H* wave. The *H* wave height also reflects the stiffness of the right atrium. S_1 and S_2 refer to the first and second heart sounds, respectively. *Center,* As the degree of tricuspid regurgitation (TR) increases, the *x'* descent is increasingly encroached upon. With severe TR, no *x'* descent is seen, and the jugular pulse wave is said to be "ventricularized." *Bottom,* Black broken line = normal jugular venous pulse and sinus rhythm; red continuous line = following development of atrial fibrillation. The dominant descent in atrial fibrillation is almost always the *y* descent; i.e., it has the superficial appearance of the pulse wave of TR. (From Constant, J.: Bedside Cardiology. 4th ed. Boston, Little, Brown & Co., 1994, pp. 81 and 89.)

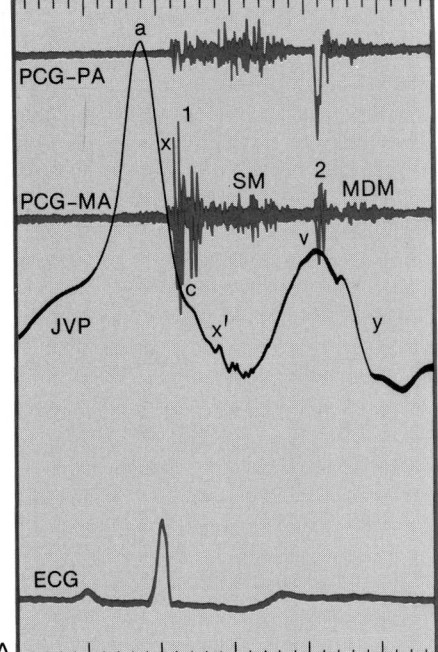
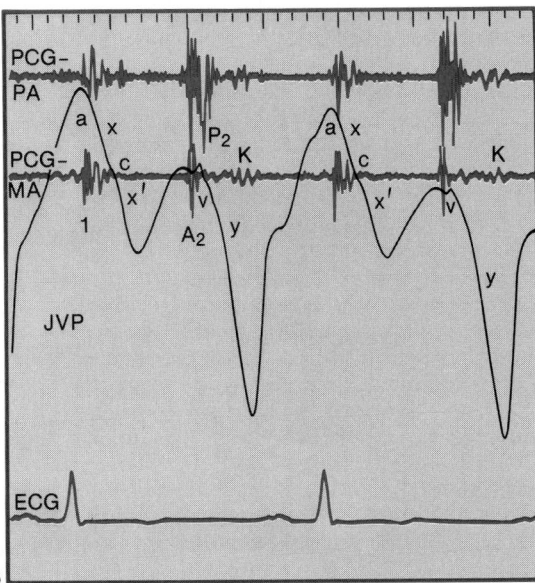

FIGURE 2–6. *A,* Jugular venous pressure (JVP) in mitral stenosis with pulmonary hypertension. The JVP is dominated by a very large *a* wave resulting from diminished compliance of the right ventricle associated with pulmonary hypertension. The peaked *a* wave represents a brief period of retrograde flow from right atrium to great veins. *B,* JVP in constrictive pericarditis. In this severe and longstanding case, the *x'* descent has become very shallow and the *y* descent is the principal feature, indicating that antegrade flow from the venous system to the right heart is now limited to early diastole. A pericardial knock (K) is seen at approximately the nadir of the *y* descent. (From Craige, E., and Smith, P.: Heart sounds. *In* Braunwald, E. [ed.]: Heart Disease: A Textbook of Cardiovascular Medicine. 3rd ed. Philadelphia, W. B. Saunders Company, 1988, pp. 61 and 62.)

position, it is likely that the central venous pressure is subnormal. When obstruction of veins in the lower extremities is responsible for edema, pressure in the neck veins is not elevated and the abdominal-jugular reflux is negative.

ABDOMINAL-JUGULAR REFLUX.[20,25] This can be tested by applying firm pressure to the periumbilical region for 10 to 30 seconds with the patient breathing quietly while the jugular veins are observed; increased respiratory excursions or straining should be avoided. In normal subjects, jugular venous pressure rises less than 3 cm H_2O and only transiently, while abdominal pressure is continued, whereas in right or left ventricular failure and/or tricuspid regurgitation the jugular venous pressure remains elevated. In the absence of these conditions a positive abdominal-jugular reflux suggests an elevated pulmonary artery wedge[21] or central venous pressure.[24]

PATTERN OF THE VENOUS PULSE. The events of the cardiac cycle, shown in Figure 12–22, p. 377, provide an explanation for the details of the jugular venous waveform (Fig. 2–5). The *a* wave in the venous pulse results from venous distention due to right atrial systole, while the *x* descent is due to atrial relaxation and descent of the floor of the right atrium during right ventricular systole; the latter, sometimes called the *x'* descent, interrupts the descent. The *c* wave, which occurs simultaneously with the carotid arterial pulse, is an inconstant wave in the jugular venous pulse and/or interruption of the descent following the peak of the *a* wave. (Many investigators refer to this wave as the *x* descent.) The *v* wave results from the rise in right atrial pressure when blood flows into the right atrium during ventricular systole when the tricuspid valve is shut, and the *y* descent, i.e., the downslope of the *v* wave, is related to the decline in right atrial pressure when the tricuspid valve reopens. Following the bottom of the *y* descent (the *y* trough) and beginning of the *a* wave is a period of relatively slow filling of the atrium or ventricle, the diastasis period, a wave termed the *H* wave.

While all or most of these events can usually be recorded, they may not be readily distinguishable on inspection. The descents or downward collapsing movements of the jugular veins are more rapid, produce larger excursions, and are therefore more prominent to the eye than are the ascents (Fig. 2–5). The normal dominant jugular venous descent, the *x'* descent, occurs just prior to the second heart sound, while the *y* descent ends after the second heart sound. With an increase in central venous pressure, the *v* wave becomes higher and the *y* collapse becomes more prominent. The *a* wave occurs just before the first sound or carotid pulse and has a sharp rise and fall. The *v* wave occurs just after the arterial pulse and has a slower, undulating pattern.

ALTERATIONS IN DISEASE. Elevation of jugular venous pressure reflects an increase in right atrial pressure and occurs in heart failure, reduced compliance of the right ventricle, pericardial disease, hypervolemia, obstruction of the tricuspid orifice, and obstruction of the superior vena cava. During inspiration, the jugular venous pressure normally declines but the *amplitude* of the pulsations increases. *Kussmaul's sign* is a paradoxical rise in the height of the jugular venous pressure during inspiration, which typically occurs in patients with chronic constrictive pericarditis and sometimes in congestive heart failure and tricuspid stenosis.

The *a* wave is particularly prominent in conditions in which the resistance to right atrial contraction is increased, such as right ventricular hypertrophy, pulmonary hypertension, and tricuspid stenosis (Fig. 2–6*A*). The *a* wave may also be tall in left ventricular hypertrophy when the thickened ventricular septum interferes with right ventricular filling. Tall *a* waves are present in patients with sinus rhythm and tricuspid stenosis or atresia, right atrial myxoma, or reduced compliance and/or marked hypertrophy of the right ventricle. Cannon (amplified) *a* waves are noted in patients with atrioventricular dissociation when the right atrium contracts against a closed tricuspid valve. In atrial fibrillation, the *a* wave and *x* descent disappear, and the x' descent becomes more prominent. In right ventricular failure and sinus rhythm, there may be increases in prominence of both the a and v waves. A steeply rising H wave is observed (or recorded) in restrictive cardiomyopathy, constrictive pericarditis, and right ventricular infarction. The a wave is absent in atrial fibrillation, accompanied by a diminished x' descent and a prominent v wave (Fig. 2–5, *Bottom*). The x descent may be prominent in patients with large a waves, as well as in patients with right ventricular volume overload (atrial septal defect).

Constrictive pericarditis (Fig. 2–6B) is characterized by a rapid and deep y descent followed by a rapid rise to a diastolic plateau (H wave) without a prominent a wave; occasionally, the x' descent is prominent in this condition as well, causing a "W"-shaped jugular venous pulse. However, it is in cardiac tamponade that the x descent is most prominent (Fig. 43–10, p. 1492). A prominent v wave or c-v wave, i.e., fusion of the c and v waves in the absence or attenuation of an x' descent, occurs in tricuspid regurgitation, sometimes causing a systolic movement of the ear lobe[29] (Figs. 2–5, *Center* and Fig. 32–46, p. 1058) and a right-to-left head movement with each ventricular systole. A prominent v wave and y descent are also seen in atrial septal defect; the y descent is gradual when right atrial emptying is impeded, as in tricuspid stenosis, and rapid when it is unimpeded, as in tricuspid regurgitation. A steep y descent is seen in any condition in which there is myocardial dysfunction, ventricular dilatation, and an elevated central venous pressure.

INDIRECT MEASUREMENT OF ARTERIAL PRESSURE

Systolic arterial pressure can be *estimated* without a sphygmomanometer cuff by gradually compressing the brachial artery while palpating the radial artery; the force required to obliterate the radial pulse represents the systolic blood pressure, and with practice, one can often estimate this level within 20 mm Hg. Ordinarily, however, a sphygmomanometer is used to obtain an indirect measurement of blood pressure.[26-28] The cuff should fit snugly around the arm, with its lower edge at least 1 inch above the antecubital space, and the diaphragm of the stethoscope should be placed close to or under the edge of the sphygmomanometer cuff. The width of the cuff selected should be at least 40 per cent of the circumference of the limb to be used.

The standard size, with a 5-inch-wide cuff, is designed for adults with an arm of average size. When this cuff is applied to a large upper arm or a normal adult thigh, arterial pressure is overestimated, leading to spurious hypertension in the obese (arm circumference >35 cm)[30,31]; when it is applied to a small arm, the pressure is underestimated. The cuff width should be approximately 1½ inches in infants and small children, 3 inches in young children (2 to 5 years), and 8 inches in obese adults. The rubber bag should be long enough to extend at least halfway around the limb (10 inches in adults). In patients with rigid, sclerotic arteries the systolic pressure may also be overestimated, by as much as 30 mm Hg. Mercury manometers are, in general, more accurate and reliable than the aneroid type; the latter should be calibrated at least once yearly.

BLOOD PRESSURE IN THE UPPER EXTREMITIES. In order to measure arterial pressure in an upper extremity,[32] the patient should be seated or lying comfortably and relaxed, the arm should be slightly flexed and at heart level, and the arm muscles should be relaxed. The cuff should be inflated rapidly to approximately 30 mm Hg above the anticipated systolic pressure.[33] These maneuvers, which diminish the volume of blood in the venous bed, decrease the tissue pressure distal to the cuff and thereby increase the flow into the occluded brachial artery. The cuff is then deflated slowly, no faster than 3 mm Hg/sec; the pressure at which the brachial pulse can be palpated is close to the systolic pressure.

The cuff should be deflated rapidly after the diastolic pressure is noted and a full minute allowed to elapse before pressure is remeasured in the same limb. Although excessive pressure on the stethoscope head does not affect systolic pressure, it does erroneously lower diastolic readings.[34] In one study, the anxiety associated with blood pressure measurement was shown to elevate arterial pressure by an average of 27/17 mm Hg[35]: ("white coat hypertension"). It is desirable for the patient to reduce anxiety and bladder distention and to avoid exercise, caffeine, eating, and smoking for a half hour preceding the screening. If doubt persists, a home blood pressure record should be obtained.

BLOOD PRESSURE IN THE LOWER EXTREMITIES. To measure pressure in the legs, the patient should lie on his or her abdomen, an 8-inch-wide cuff should be applied with the compression bag over the posterior aspect of the midthigh and should be rolled diagonally around the thigh to keep the edges snug against the skin, and auscultation should be carried out in the popliteal fossa. In order to measure pressure in the lower leg, an arm cuff is placed over the calf, and auscultation is carried out over the posterior tibial artery. Regardless of where the cuff is applied, care must be taken to avoid letting the rubber part of the balloon of the cuff extend beyond its covering and to avoid placing the cuff on so loosely that central ballooning occurs.

KOROTKOFF SOUNDS. There are five phases of Korotkoff sounds, i.e., sounds produced by the flow of blood as the constricting blood pressure cuff is gradually released. The first appearance of clear, tapping sound (phase I) represents the systolic pressure. These sounds are replaced by soft murmurs during phase II and by louder murmurs during phase III, as the volume of blood flowing through the constricted artery increases. The sounds suddenly become muffled in phase IV, when constriction of the brachial artery diminishes as arterial diastolic pressure is approached. Korotkoff sounds disappear in phase V, which is usually within 10 mm Hg of phase IV.

Diastolic pressure measured directly through an intraarterial needle and external manometer corresponds closely to phase V.[4] In severe aortic regurgitation, however, when the disappearance point is extremely low, sometimes 0 mm Hg, the sound of muffling (phase IV) is much closer to the intraarterial diastolic pressure than is the disappearance point (phase V). When there is a sizable difference between phases IV and V of the Korotkoff sounds (>10 mm Hg), both pressures should be recorded (e.g., 142/54/10 mm Hg).

Korotkoff sounds may be difficult to hear and arterial pressure difficult to measure when arterial pressure rises at a slow rate (as in severe aortic stenosis), when the arteries are markedly constricted (as in shock), and when the stroke volume is reduced (as in severe heart failure). Very soft or inaudible Korotkoff sounds can often be accentuated by dilating the blood vessels of the upper extremities simply by opening and closing the fist repeatedly. Sometimes in states of shock, the indirect method of measuring blood pressure is unreliable, and arterial pressure should be measured through an intraarterial needle.

The Auscultatory Gap. This is a silence that sometimes separates the first appearance of the Korotkoff sounds from their second appearance at a lower pressure. The phenomenon tends to occur when there is venous distention or reduced velocity of arterial flow into the arm. If the first muffling of sounds is considered to be the diastolic pressure, it will be overestimated. If the second appearance is taken as the systolic pressure, it will be underestimated. On the other hand, sounds transmitted through the arterial tree from prosthetic aortic valves may be responsible for falsely high readings.

BLOOD PRESSURE IN THE BASAL CONDITION. In order to determine arterial pressure in the basal condition, the patient should have rested in a quiet room for 15 minutes. It is desirable to record the arterial pressure in both arms at the time of the initial examination; differences in systolic pressure exceeding 10 mm Hg between the two arms when measurements are made simultaneously or in rapid sequence[36] suggest obstructive lesions involving the aorta or the origin of the innominate and subclavian arteries, or supravalvular aortic stenosis (in which pressure in the right arm exceeds that in the left). In patients with vertebral-basal artery insufficiency, a difference in pressure between the arms may signify that a subclavian "steal" is responsible for the cerebrovascular symptoms. In order to determine whether orthostatic hypotension is present, arterial pressure should be determined with the patient in both the supine and the erect positions. However, regardless of the patient's posture, the brachial artery should be at the level of the heart to avoid superimposition of the effects of gravity on the recorded pressure.

Normally, the systolic pressure in the legs is up to 20 mm Hg higher than in the arms, but the diastolic pressures are usually virtually identical. The recording of a higher diastolic pressure in the legs than in the arms suggests that the thigh cuff is too small. When systolic pressure in the popliteal artery exceeds that in the brachial artery by more than 20 mm Hg (Hill's sign), aortic regurgitation is usually present.[37] Blood pressure should be measured in the lower extremities in patients with hypertension to detect coarctation of the aorta or when obstructive disease of the aorta or its immediate branches is suspected.

To be *certain* from physical examination that the systolic pressure is different in the two arms or in the upper and lower extremities, two examiners should measure the pressures simultaneously, then switch extremities.[3]

ARTERIAL PULSE

The volume and contour of the arterial pulse are determined by a combination of factors, including the left ventricular stroke volume, the ejection velocity, the relative compliance and capacity of the arterial system, and the pressure waves that result from the antegrade flow of blood and reflections of the arterial pressure pulse returning from the peripheral circulation.[35] Bilateral palpation of the carotid, radial, brachial, femoral, popliteal, dorsalis pedis, and posterior tibial pulses should be part of the examina-

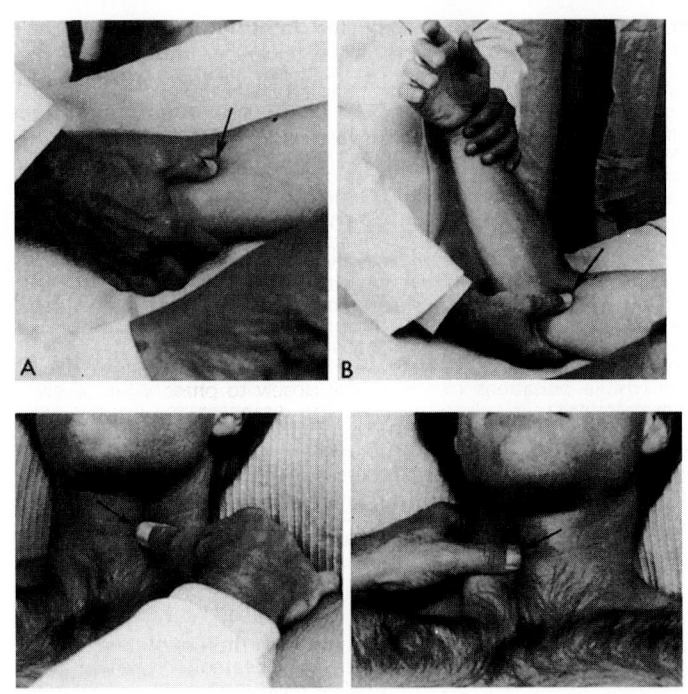

For palpation of the left carotid artery, the observer applies the right thumb to the patient's left carotid artery in the lower third of the neck[2] (Fig. 2–7*C*). The left femoral artery should be palpated with the right thumb. The patient should be supine with the head and chest at a 45-degree angle. The brachial artery is the vessel ordinarily most suitable for appreciating the rate of rise of the pulse and the contour, volume, and consistency of the peripheral vessels. This artery is located at the medial aspect of the elbow, and it may be helpful to flex the arm in order to improve palpation; palpation of the artery should be carried out with the thumb exerting pressure on the artery until its maximal movement is detected (Fig. 2–7*A* and *B*). A normal rate of rise of the arterial pulse suggests that there is no obstruction to left ventricular outflow, whereas a pulse wave of small amplitude with normal configuration suggests a reduced stroke volume.

THE NORMAL PULSE (Fig. 2–8). The pulse in the ascending aorta normally rises rapidly to a rounded dome; this initial rise reflects the peak velocity of blood ejected from the left ventricle. A slight anacrotic notch or pause is frequently recorded, but only occasionally felt, on the ascending limb of the pulse. The descending limb of the central aortic pulse is less steep than is the ascending limb, and it is interrupted by the incisura, a sharp downward deflection related to closure of the aortic valve. Immediately thereafter, the pulse wave rises slightly and then declines gradually throughout diastole. As the pulse wave is transmitted to the periphery, its upstroke becomes steeper, the systolic peak becomes higher, the anacrotic shoulder disappears, and the sharp incisura is replaced by a smoother, later dicrotic notch followed by a dicrotic wave.[41] Normally, the height of this dicrotic wave diminishes with age, hypertension, and arteriosclerosis. In the central arterial pulse (central aorta and innominate and carotid arteries), the rapidly transmitted impact of left ventricular ejection results in a peak in early systole, referred to as the *percussion wave;* a second, smaller peak, the *tidal wave,* presumed to represent a reflected wave from the periphery, can often be recorded but is not normally palpable. However, in older subjects, particularly those with increased peripheral resistance, as

FIGURE 2–7. *A,* Palpation of the right brachial pulse with the thumb while the patient's arm lies at the side with the palm up. *B,* Palpation of the right brachial pulse with the patient's elbow resting in the palm of the examiner's hand. The thumb explores the antecubital fossa (arrow), while the patient's forearm is passively raised and lowered to achieve maximum relaxation of muscles around the elbow. *C* and *D,* Palpation of the carotid pulse. The examiner places the right thumb (arrow) on the patient's left carotid artery *(C)*. The left thumb (arrow) is then applied separately to the right carotid *(D)*. (From Perloff, J. K.: Physical Examination of the Heart and Circulation. Philadelphia, W. B. Saunders Company, 1990.)

tion of all cardiac patients, although caution should be exercised in bilateral carotid palpation, especially in the aged. The frequency, regularity, and shape of the pulse wave and the character of the arterial wall should be deter-

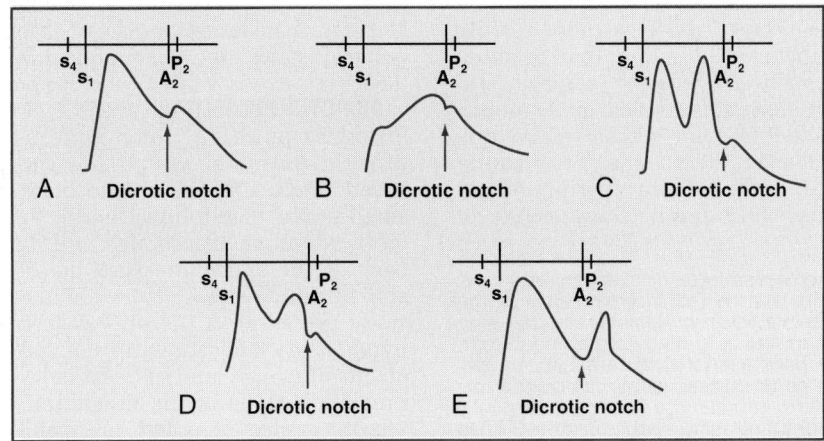

FIGURE 2–8. Schematic diagrams of the configurational changes in the carotid pulse and their differential diagnosis. Heart sounds are also illustrated. *A,* Normal. *B,* Anacrotic pulse with slow initial upstroke. The peak is close to the second heart sound. These features suggest fixed left ventricular outflow obstruction. *C,* Pulsus bisferiens with both percussion and tidal waves occurring during systole. This type of carotid pulse contour is most frequently observed in patients with hemodynamically significant aortic regurgitation or combined aortic stenosis and regurgitation with dominant regurgitation. It is rarely observed in mitral valve prolapse or in normal individuals. *D,* Pulsus bisferiens in hypertrophic obstructive cardiomyopathy. It is rarely appreciated at the bedside by palpation. *E,* Dicrotic pulse results from an accentuated dicrotic wave and tends to occur in sepsis, severe heart failure, hypovolemic shock, cardiac tamponade, and after aortic valve replacement. (S_4 = atrial sounds; S_1 = first heart sounds; A_2 = aortic component of the second heart sounds; P_2 = pulmonary component of the second heart sound). (From Chatterjee, K.: Bedside evaluation of the heart: The physical examination. *In* Chatterjee, K., et al. [eds.]: Cardiology: An Illustrated Text/Reference. Philadelphia, J. B. Lippincott, 1991, pp. 3.11–3.51.)

well as in patients with arteriosclerosis and diabetes, the tidal wave may be somewhat higher than the percussion wave; i.e., the pulse reaches a peak in late systole. In peripheral arteries, the pulse wave normally has a single sharp peak.

ABNORMAL PULSES. When peripheral vascular resistance and arterial stiffness are increased, as in hypertension or with the increased arterial stiffness that accompanies normal aging, there is an elevation in pulse wave velocity, and the pulse contour has a more rapid upstroke and greater amplitude. Reduced or unequal carotid arterial pulsations occur in patients with carotid atherosclerosis and with diseases of the aortic arch, including aortic dissection, aneurysm, and Takayasu's disease (see p. 1572). In *supravalvular aortic stenosis* there is a selective streaming of the jet toward the innominate artery, and the carotid and brachial arterial pulses are stronger and rise more rapidly on the right than on the left side, and pressures are higher in the right than in the left arm (see p. 919). The pulses of the upper extremities may be reduced or unequal in a variety of other conditions, including arterial embolus or thrombosis, anomalous origin or aberrant path of the major vessels, and cervical rib or scalenus anticus syndrome. Asymmetry of right and left popliteal pulses is characteristic of iliofemoral obstruction. Weakness or absence of radial, posterior tibial, or dorsalis pedis pulses on one side suggests arterial insufficiency. In *coarctation of the aorta* the carotid and brachial pulses are bounding, rise rapidly, and have large volumes, whereas in the lower extremities, the systolic and pulse pressures are reduced, their rate of rise is slow, and there is a late peak. This delay in the femoral arterial pulses can usually be readily detected by simultaneous palpation of the femoral and brachial arterial pulses.

In patients with fixed obstruction to left ventricular outflow (valvular aortic stenosis, and congenital fibrous subaortic stenosis), the carotid pulse rises slowly *(pulsus tardus)* (Fig. 2–8*B*); the upstroke is frequently characterized by a thrill (the *carotid shudder);* and the peak is reduced, occurs late in systole, and is sustained. There is a notch on the upstroke of the carotid pulse (anacrotic notch) that is so distinct that two separate waves can be palpated in what is termed an *anacrotic pulse. Pulsus parvus* is a pulse of small amplitude, usually because of a reduction of stroke volume. *Pulsus parvus et tardus* refers to a small pulse with a delayed systolic peak, which is characteristic of severe aortic stenosis. This type of pulse is more readily appreciated by palpating the carotid rather than a more peripheral artery. Patients with severe aortic stenosis and heart failure usually exhibit simply a reduced pulse amplitude, i.e., *pulsus parvus,* and the delay in the upstroke is not readily apparent. However, this delay is readily recorded. In elderly patients with inelastic peripheral arteries, the pulse may rise normally despite the presence of aortic stenosis.

The carotid arterial pulse may be prominent or exaggerated in any condition in which pulse pressure is increased, including anxiety, the hyperkinetic heart syndrome, anemia, fever, pregnancy, or other high cardiac output states (Chap. 15), as well as in bradycardia, and peripheral arteriosclerosis with reduction in arterial distensibility. In patients with *mitral regurgitation* or *ventricular septal defect,* the forward stroke volume (from the left ventricle into the aorta) is usually normal, but the fraction ejected during early systole is greater than normal; hence, the arterial pulse is of normal volume (the pulse pressure is normal), but the pulse may rise abnormally rapidly.[42] Exaggerated or bounding arterial pulses may be observed in patients with an elevated stroke volume, with sympathetic hyperactivity, and in patients with a rigid, sclerotic aorta. In *aortic regurgitation,* there is a very brisk rate of rise with an increased pulse pressure.

The *Corrigan* or *water-hammer pulse* of aortic regurgitation consists of an abrupt upstroke (percussion wave) followed by rapid collapse later in systole, but no dicrotic notch. Corrigan's pulse reflects a low resistance in the reservoir into which the left ventricle rapidly discharges an abnormally elevated stroke volume, and it can be exaggerated by raising the patient's arm. In *acute* aortic regurgitation, the left ventricle may not be significantly dilated, and premature closure of the mitral valve may occur and limit the volume of aortic reflux; therefore, the aortic diastolic pressure may *not* be very low, the

arterial pulse *not* bounding, and the pulse pressure *not* widened despite a serious abnormality of valve function (see p. 1048).

Signs characteristic of severe chronic aortic regurgitation include "pistol-shot" sounds heard over the femoral artery when the stethoscope is placed on it *(Traube's sign);* a systolic murmur heard over the femoral artery when the artery is gradually compressed proximally; a diastolic murmur when the artery is compressed distally *(Duroziez's sign[37,43])* and Quincke's sign (phasic blanching of the nail bed). Of these, Duroziez's sign is the most predictive. Bounding arterial pulses are also present in patients with patent ductus arteriosus or large arteriovenous fistulas; in hyperkinetic states such as thyrotoxicosis, pregnancy, fever, and anemia; in severe bradycardia; and in arteries proximal to coarctation of the aorta. In *Hill's sign* of aortic regurgitation (or any condition leading to an increased stroke volume, or the hyperkinetic circulatory state) the indirectly recorded systolic pressure in the lower extremities exceeds that in the arms by more than 20 mm Hg. Other signs of increased pulse pressure include *Becker's sign* (visible pulsations of the retinal arterioles) and *Mueller's sign* (pulsating uvula).

In the presence of AV dissociation, when atrial activity is irregularly transmitted to the ventricles, the strength of the peripheral arterial pulse depends on the time interval between atrial and ventricular contractions. In a patient with rapid heart action, the presence of such variations suggests ventricular tachycardia; with an equally rapid rate, an absence of variation of pulse strength suggests a supraventricular mechanism.

BISFERIENS PULSE (Fig. 2–8*C*). A bisferiens pulse is characterized by *two systolic peaks,* the percussion and tidal waves, separated by a distinct midsystolic dip; the peaks may be equal or either may be larger. This type of pulse is detected most readily by palpation of the carotid and less commonly of the brachial arteries. It occurs in conditions in which a large stroke volume is ejected rapidly from the left ventricle[44,45] and is observed most commonly in patients with pure aortic regurgitation or with a combination of aortic regurgitation and stenosis; it may disappear as heart failure supervenes.

A bisferiens pulse also occurs in patients with *hypertrophic obstructive cardiomyopathy,[46,47]* but the bifid nature may only be recorded, not palpated; on palpation there may merely be a rapid upstroke. In these patients the initial prominent percussion wave is associated with rapid ejection of blood into the aorta during early systole, followed by a rapid decline as obstruction becomes manifest in midsystole and by a tidal (reflected) wave. In some patients with hypertrophic cardiomyopathy with no or little obstruction to left ventricular outflow, the arterial pulse is normal or simply hyperkinetic in the basal state, but obstruction and a bisferiens pulse can be elicited by means of the Valsalva maneuver or inhalation of amyl nitrite. Occasionally, a bisferiens pulse is observed in hyperkinetic circulatory states, and very rarely it occurs in normal individuals.

DICROTIC PULSE (Fig. 2–8*E*). Not to be confused with a bisferiens pulse, in which both peaks occur in systole, is a dicrotic pulse, in which the second peak is in diastole immediately after the second heart sound.[39,40] The normally small wave that follows aortic valve closure (i.e., the dicrotic notch) is exaggerated and measures more than 50 per cent of the pulse pressure on direct pressure recordings and in which the dicrotic notch is low (i.e., near the diastolic pressure). A dicrotic wave may be present in normal hypotensive subjects with reduced peripheral resistance, as occurs in fever, and it may be elicited or exaggerated by inhalation alone or the inhalation of amyl nitrite. Rarely, a dicrotic pulse is noted in healthy adolescents or young adults, but it usually occurs in conditions such as cardiac tamponade, severe heart failure, and hypovolemic shock, in which a low stroke volume is ejected into a soft elastic aorta. In these conditions the dicrotic pulse is due to a reduction of the systolic wave with preservation of the incisura. A dicrotic pulse is rarely present when systolic pressure exceeds 130 mm Hg.

PULSUS ALTERNANS (alternating strong and weak pulses) (Fig. 2–9). Mechanical alternans is a sign of severe depression of myocardial function (see p. 455).[48] Although more readily recognized on sphygmomanometry, when the systolic pressure alternates by more than 20 mm Hg the

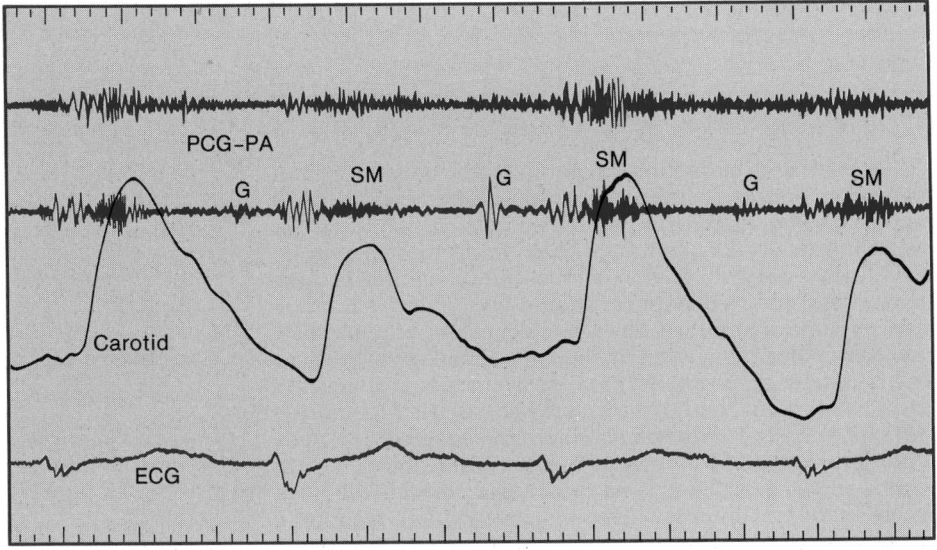

FIGURE 2–9. Pulsus alternans in a man with aortic stenosis and left ventricular failure. The first and third beats are of greater amplitude than the second and fourth beats. The stronger beats are also marked by a louder murmur (SM). The diastolic sound (G) is louder after the second (weak) beat. It is a summation sound caused by merging of S_3 and S_4, resulting from the combined effect of a rapid heart rate and a prolonged P-R interval. (From Craige, E., and Smith, D.: Heart sounds. *In* Braunwald, E. [ed.]: Heart Disease: A Textbook of Cardiovascular Medicine. 3rd ed. Philadelphia, W. B. Saunders Company, 1988, p. 57.)

alternans can be detected by palpation of a peripheral (femoral or brachial) pulse more frequently than by a more central pulse. Palpation should be carried out with light pressure and with the patient's breath held in midexpiration to avoid the superimposition of respiratory variation on the amplitude of the pulse. Pulsus alternans is generally accompanied by alternation in the intensity of the Korotkoff sounds and occasionally by alternation in intensity of the heart sounds. Rarely, pulsus alternans is so marked that the weak beat is not perceived at all. Aortic regurgitation, systemic hypertension, and reducing venous return by administration of nitroglycerin or by tilting the patient into the upright position all exaggerate pulsus alternans and assist in its detection. Pulsus alternans, which is frequently precipitated by a premature ventricular contraction, is characterized by a regular rhythm and must be distinguished from pulsus bigeminus (see below), which is usually irregular.

PULSUS BIGEMINUS. A bigeminal rhythm is caused by the occurrence of premature contractions, usually ventricular, after every other beat and results in alternation of the strength of the pulse, which can be confused with pulsus alternans. However, in contrast to the latter, in which the rhythm is regular, in pulsus bigeminus the weak beat always follows the shorter interval. In normal persons or in patients with fixed obstruction to left ventricular outflow, the compensatory pause following a premature beat is followed by a stronger-than-normal pulse. However, in patients with hypertrophic obstructive cardiomyopathy, the postpremature ventricular contraction beat is weaker than normal because of increased obstruction to left ventricular outflow[49] (see p. 1414).

PULSUS PARADOXUS (see p. 1489). This is an exaggerated reduction in the strength of the arterial pulse during normal inspiration or an exaggerated inspiratory fall in systolic pressure (more than 10 mm Hg during quiet breathing). When marked, i.e., an inspiratory reduction of pressure greater than 20 mm Hg, the paradoxical pulse can be detected by palpation of the brachial arterial pulse; in some instances there is inspiratory disappearance of the pulse. Milder degrees of a paradoxical pulse can be readily detected on sphygmomanometry: the cuff is inflated to suprasystolic levels and is deflated slowly at a rate of about 2 mm Hg per heartbeat; the peak systolic pressure during exhalation is noted. The cuff is then deflated even more slowly, and the pressure is again noted when Korotkoff sounds become audible throughout the respiratory cycle. Normally, the difference between the two pressures should not exceed 10 mm Hg during quiet respiration. (Pulsus alternans can also be detected by this maneuver by noting whether peak systolic pressure or the intensity of the Korotkoff sounds alternates when the breath is held.)

Pulsus paradoxus represents an exaggeration of the normal decline in systolic arterial pressure with inspiration. It results from the reduced left ventricular stroke volume and the transmission of negative intrathoracic pressure to the aorta. It is a frequent, indeed characteristic, finding in patients with cardiac tamponade (see p. 1486), occurs less frequently (in about half) in patients with chronic constrictive pericarditis (see p. 1496), and is also observed in patients with emphysema and bronchial asthma (who have wide respiratory swings of intrapleural pressure),[50] as well as in hypovolemic shock, pulmonary embolus, pregnancy, and extreme obesity. Aortic regurgitation tends to prevent the development of pulsus paradoxus despite the presence of cardiac tamponade. *Reversed* pulsus paradoxus (an inspiratory rise in arterial pressure) may occur in hypertrophic obstructive cardiomyopathy.[51]

THE ARTERIAL PULSE IN VASCULAR DISEASE. Examination of the arterial pulses is of critical importance in the diagnosis of extracardiac obstructive arterial disease. Systematic bilateral palpation of the common carotid, brachial, radial, femoral, popliteal, dorsalis pedis, and posterior tibial vessels, as well as palpation of the abdominal aorta (both above and below the umbilicus), should be part of every examination in patients suspected of having ischemic heart disease.[52] To diminish cold-induced vasoconstriction, peripheral pulses should be palpated after the patient has been in a warm room for at least 20 minutes.[53] Absent or weak peripheral pulses usually signify obstruction. However, the dorsalis pedis and posterior tibial arteries may be absent in approximately 2 per cent of normal persons because they pursue an abnormal course. Arterial bruits should be sought at specific anatomical sites. When the lumen diameter is reduced by approximately 50 per cent, a soft short systolic bruit is heard; as the obstruction becomes more severe, the bruit becomes high-pitched, louder, and longer. With approximately 80 per cent diameter reduction the murmur spills into early diastole, but disappears with very severe stenosis or complete occlusion. Arterial bruits are augmented by elevations of cardiac output (e.g., as occurs in anemia), by poor development of collaterals, and augmented arterial outflow (as occurs in regional exercise).

Auscultation over the spine in the interscapular region in patients with coarctation of the aorta may reveal a systolic or continuous murmur, and a systolic murmur may be heard over the lower abdomen in patients with aortic or iliofemoral obstructions.

INSPECTION

The cardiac examination proper should commence with inspection of the chest, which can best be accomplished with the examiner standing at the side or foot of the bed or examining table. Respirations—their frequency, regularity, and depth—as well as the relative effort required during inspiration and exhalation, should be noted. Simultaneously, one should search for cutaneous abnormalities, such as spider nevi (seen in hepatic cirrhosis and Osler-Weber-Rendu disease). Dilation of veins on the anterior chest wall with caudal flow suggests obstruction of the superior vena cava, whereas cranial flow occurs in patients with obstruction of the inferior vena cava. Precordial prominence is most striking if cardiac enlargement developed before puberty, but may also be present, although to a lesser extent, in patients in whom cardiomegaly developed in adult life, after the period of thoracic growth.[54,55]

A heavy muscular thorax, contrasting with less developed lower extremities, may occur in coarctation of the aorta, in which collateral arteries may be visible in the axillae and along the lateral chest wall. The upper portion of the thorax exhibits symmetrical bulging in children with stiff lungs in whom the inspiratory effort is increased. A "shield chest" is a broad chest in which the angle between the manubrium and the body of the sternum is greater than normal and is associated with widely separated nipples; shield chest is frequently observed in the Turner and Noonan syndromes. Careful note should be made of other deformities of the thoracic cage, such as *kyphoscoliosis*, which may be responsible for cor pulmonale (Chap. 47); *ankylosing spondylitis*, sometimes associated with aortic regurgitation (Chap. 56); and *pectus carinatum* (pigeon chest), which may be associated with Marfan syndrome but does not directly affect cardiovascular function.

Pectus excavatum, a condition in which the sternum is displaced posteriorly, is commonly observed in Marfan syndrome, homocystinuria, Ehlers-Danlos syndrome, Hunter-Hurler syndrome, and a small fraction of patients with mitral valve prolapse. This thoracic deformity rarely compresses the heart or elevates the systemic and pulmonary venous pressures, and the signs of heart disease are more often apparent rather than real. Displacement of the heart into the left thorax, prominence of the pulmonary artery, and a parasternal midsystolic murmur all may falsely suggest the presence of organic heart disease. Pectus excavatum may be associated with palpitations, tachycardia, fatigue, mild dyspnea, and some impairment of cardiac function.[56] Lack of normal thoracic kyphosis, i.e., the *straight back* syndrome,[1] is often associated with expiratory splitting of the second heart sound, a parasternal midsystolic murmur, and prominence of the pulmonary artery on radiography; less severe thoracic kyphosis is frequently associated with mitral valve prolapse.

CARDIOVASCULAR PULSATIONS. These should be looked for on the entire chest but specifically in the regions of the cardiac apex, the left parasternal region, and the third left and second right intercostal spaces. Prominent pulsations in these areas suggest enlargement of the left ventricle, right ventricle, pulmonary artery, and aorta, respectively. A thrusting apex exceeding 2 cm in diameter suggests left ventricular enlargement; systolic retraction of the apex may be visible in constrictive pericarditis. Normally, cardiac pulsations are not visible lateral to the midclavicular line; when present there, they signify cardiac enlargement unless there is thoracic deformity or congenital absence of the pericardium. Shaking of the entire precordium with each heartbeat may occur in patients with severe valvular regurgitation, large left-to-right shunts, especially patent ductus arteriosus, complete AV block, hypertrophic obstructive cardiomyopathy, and various hyperkinetic states (Chap. 15). Aortic aneurysms may produce visible pulsations of one of the sternoclavicular joints of the right anterior thoracic wall.

PALPATION

(Table 2–1)

Pulsations of the heart and great arteries that are transmitted to the chest wall are best appreciated when the examiner is positioned on the right side of a supine patient. In order to palpate the movements of the heart and great arteries, the examiner should use the fingertips or the area just proximal thereto. Precordial movements should be timed by using the simultaneously palpated carotid pulse or auscultated heart sounds.[58-60] The examination should be carried out with the chest completely exposed and ele-

TABLE 2–1 CHARACTERISTICS OF PRECORDIAL MOTION IN VARIOUS CARDIAC ABNORMALITIES

AORTIC REGURGITATION	ATRIAL SEPTAL DEFECT	CONGESTIVE CARDIOMYOPATHY	CORONARY ARTERY DISEASE
Apex impulse hyperdynamic in mild to moderate AR Severe AR: LV dilatation results in sustained impulse which is displaced laterally and downward (especially chronic AR) Systolic retraction medial to PMI Palpable *a* wave may be present	Hyperdynamic parasternal impulse PA impulse may be present RV impulse may be sustained if pulmonary hypertension is present and occasionally with large L to R shunt without elevated PA pressure	Sustained and displaced LV impulse, usually felt over 2 interspaces Palpable *a* wave (S₄) and S₃ common Parasternal lift, midsystolic bulge common	Usually normal at rest unless prior MI Palpable S₄ in left decubitus position Ectopic LV thrust if dyssynergy or LV aneurysm. May have transient abnormalities (e.g., bulge, heave) during acute infarction or attack of angina

HYPERTROPHIC CARDIOMYOPATHY	MITRAL REGURGITATION	MITRAL STENOSIS	VALVULAR AORTIC STENOSIS
Systolic thrill superior, medial to apex impulse Vigorous LV apical impulse, often sustained Large palpable *a* wave, especially in left decubitus position Occasional mid- or late systolic bulge—"triple ripple"	Apical systolic thrill in severe MR Apex impulse hyperdynamic Severe and/or chronic MR: apex is displaced laterally, sustained with amplitude Can have late parasternal impulse with severe MR without pulmonary hypertension Parasternal (RV) heave if significant pulmonary hypertension S₃ visible and palpable if severe MR S₄ palpable with acute onset MR	Small or impalpable apex impulse but S₁ typically palpable Opening snap palpable medial to apex Apical diastolic thrill in left decubitus position Parasternal lift is common; suggests pulmonary hypertension at rest or with effort	Systolic thrill—aortic area, 2 LICS. Or occasionally at apex Sustained and forceful LV apical impulse Little lateral (leftward) displacement of apex unless LV dilatation has occurred Palpable *a* wave (S₄) is common and indicates severe aortic obstruction

AR = aortic regurgitation; LV = left ventricular; PA = pulmonary artery; RV = right ventricular; MI = myocardial infarction; MR = mitral regurgitation; LICS = left intercostal space; L to R = left to right. Reproduced with permission from Abrams, J.: Examination of the precordium. Primary Cardiol. 8:156–158, 1982.

vated to 30 degrees, both with the patient supine and in the partial left lateral decubitus positions; the latter increases the detection and evaluation of the left ventricular impulse.[2] Rotating the patient into the left lateral decubitus position with the left arm elevated over the head causes the heart to move laterally and increases the palpability of both normal and pathological thrusts of the left ventricle. Obese, muscular, emphysematous, and elderly persons may have weak or undetectable cardiac pulsations in the absence of cardiac abnormality, and thoracic deformities (e.g., kyphoscoliosis, pectus excavatum) can alter the pulsations transmitted to the chest wall. In the course of cardiac palpation, precordial tenderness may be detected; this important finding (see p. 1291) may result from costochondritis (Tzietse's syndrome) and may be an important indication that chest pain is not due to myocardial ischemia.

THE LEFT VENTRICLE. The *apex beat*, also referred to as the cardiac impulse and the apical thrust, is normally produced by left ventricular contraction and is the lowest and most lateral point on the chest at which the cardiac impulse can be appreciated and is normally above the anatomic apex (Fig. 2–10*B*). Although the apex beat may also be the point of maximal impulse (PMI), this is not necessarily the case, because the pulsations produced by other structures, e.g., an enlarged right ventricle, a dilated pulmonary artery, or an aneurysm of the aorta, may be more powerful than the apex beat. Normally the left ventricular impulse is medial and superior to the intersection of the left midclavicular line and the fifth intercostal space and is palpable as a single, brief outward motion. Although it may not be palpable in the supine position in as many as half of all normal subjects more than 50 years of age, the left ventricular impulse can usually be felt in the left lateral decubitus position. Displacement of the apex beat lateral to the midclavicular line or more than 10 cm lateral to the midsternal line is a sensitive but not specific indicator of left ventricular enlargement. However, when the patient is in the left lateral decubitus position a palpable apical impulse that has a diameter of more than 3 cm is an accurate sign of left ventricular enlargement.[61] Thoracic deformities —particularly scoliosis, straight back, and pectus excavatum—can result in the lateral displacement of a normal-sized heart.

The patient should be examined both supine and then in the left lateral decubitus position. The examination should be carried out with both the fingertips and the distal metacarpals. The subxiphoid region, which allows palpation of the right ventricle, should be examined with the tip of the index finger during held inspiration.

The apex cardiogram, which reflects the movement of the chest wall, represents the pulsation of the entire left ventricle. Its contour differs from what is perceived on palpation of the apex or what is recorded by the kinetocardiogram, a device in which the motion of specific points on the chest wall is recorded relative to a fixed point in space[62] and which therefore presents a more faithful graphic registration of the movements of the palpating finger on the chest wall.

SYSTOLIC MOTION. During isovolumetric contraction, the heart normally rotates counterclockwise (as one faces the patient), and the lower anterior portion of the left ventricle strikes the anterior chest wall, causing a brief outward motion followed by medial retraction of the adjacent chest wall during ejection (Fig. 2-11). The segment of the left ventricle responsible for the apex beat is usually medial to the actual cardiac apex identified on radiological or angiographic examination. For timing purposes it is useful to correlate pulsations while simultaneously listening to heart sounds; a convenient way to do this is to correlate the observed motion of the stethoscope, placed lightly at the apex, with the auscultatory events.

The peak outward motion of the left ventricular impulse is brief and occurs simultaneously with, or just after, aortic valve opening; then the left ventricular apex moves inward. In asthenic persons, in patients with mild left ventricular enlargement, and in subjects with a normal left ventricle but an augmented stroke volume, as occurs in anxiety and other hyperkinetic states, and in mitral or aortic regurgitation, the cardiac impulse may be overactive but with a normal con-

tour; i.e., the outward thrust during systole is exaggerated in amplitude, but it is not sustained during ejection.

HYPERTROPHY AND DILATATION. With moderate or severe left ventricular concentric hypertrophy, the outward systolic thrust persists throughout ejection, often lasting up to the second heart sound (Fig. 2–11), and this motion is accompanied by retraction of the left parasternal region. This rocking motion can often be appreciated by placing the index finger of one hand on the apex beat and that of the other hand in the parasternal region and by observing the simultaneous outward motion of the former with retraction of the latter. The left ventricular heave or lift, which is more prominent in concentric hypertrophy than in left ventricular dilatation without volume overload, is characterized by a sustained outward movement of an area that is larger than the normal apex; i.e., it is more than 2 to 3 cm in diameter. In patients with left ventricular enlargement the systolic impulse is displaced laterally and downward into the sixth or seventh interspaces. In patients with ischemic heart disease a sustained apex beat is usually associated with a reduced ejection fraction.[63]

In patients with volume overload and/or sympathetic stimulation, the left ventricular impulse is *hyperkinetic*, i.e., it is brisker and larger than normal. It is hypokinetic in patients with reduced stroke volume, especially in acute myocardial infarction or dilated cardiomyopathy.

LEFT VENTRICULAR ANEURYSM. This produces a larger-than-normal area of pulsation of the left ventricular apex. Alternatively, it may produce a sustained systolic bulge several centimeters superior to the left ventricular impulse. In left ventricular pressure overload with normal ventricular function, the left ventricular impulse is prolonged and forceful. In patients with *left ventricular dyskinesia*, as occurs in acute myocardial ischemia following myocardial infarction, or left ventricular aneurysm, there may be two distinct impulses separated from each other by several centimeters; alternatively, a mid- or late systolic bulge may be palpated. In *mitral stenosis* there may be a brief prominent apical tap owing to an accentuated first sound, which must be distinguished from the apical thrust of the left ventricle.

OTHER CONDITIONS. A double systolic outward thrust of the left ventricle is characteristic of patients with hypertrophic obstructive cardiomyopathy (Fig. 2-12) who also often exhibit a typical presystolic cardiac expansion, thus resulting in three separate outward movements of the chest wall during each cardiac cycle.[46] In *aortic regurgitation* the apex exhibits a prominent outward thrust that may be followed by medial systolic retraction of the anterior chest wall as a consequence of the large stroke volume that evacuates the thorax during systole.

Constrictive pericarditis (as well as nonconstricting adherent pericarditis) is characterized by systolic retraction of the chest, particularly of the ribs in the left axilla (Broadbent's sign). This inward movement results from interference with the descent of the base of the heart and the compensatory exaggerated motion of the free wall of the left ventricle during ventricular ejection.[64] When left ventricular filling is very rapid during early diastole, outward movement of the chest wall may be particularly prominent and mistaken for systole, but it is usually accompanied by a third heart sound (see p. 35). A hypokinetic apical impulse is associated with a variety of low cardiac output states, including those secondary to hypovolemia, constrictive pericarditis, and pericardial effusion.

Diastolic Motion. The outward motion of the apex characteristic of rapid left ventricular diastolic filling is most readily palpated with the patient in the left lateral decubitus position and in full exhalation. The outward motion is accentuated when the inflow of blood into the left ventricle is accelerated, as occurs, for example, in mitral regurgitation, when the volume of the left ventricle is increased or its function is impaired.[55] This motion is the mechanical equivalent of and occurs simultaneously with a third heart sound. Prominent early diastolic left ventricular filling in constrictive pericarditis may be palpable.

When the atrial contribution to ventricular filling is augmented, as occurs in patients with reduced left ventricular compliance associated with concentric left ventricular hypertrophy, myocardial ischemia, and myocardial fibrosis, a presystolic pulsation (usually accompanying a fourth heart sound) is palpable, resulting in a double outward movement of the left ventricular impulse. This presystolic expansion is most readily discernible during exhalation, when the patient is in the left lateral decubitus position, and it can be confirmed by detecting the motion of the stethoscope placed over the left ventricular impulse or by observing the motion of an X mark over the left ventricular impulse. Presystolic expansion of the left ventricle can be enhanced by sustained handgrip, and is usually associated with marked elevation of left ventricular end-diastolic (rather than early diastolic) pressure. In contrast to prominence of early diastolic filling, in patients without ischemic

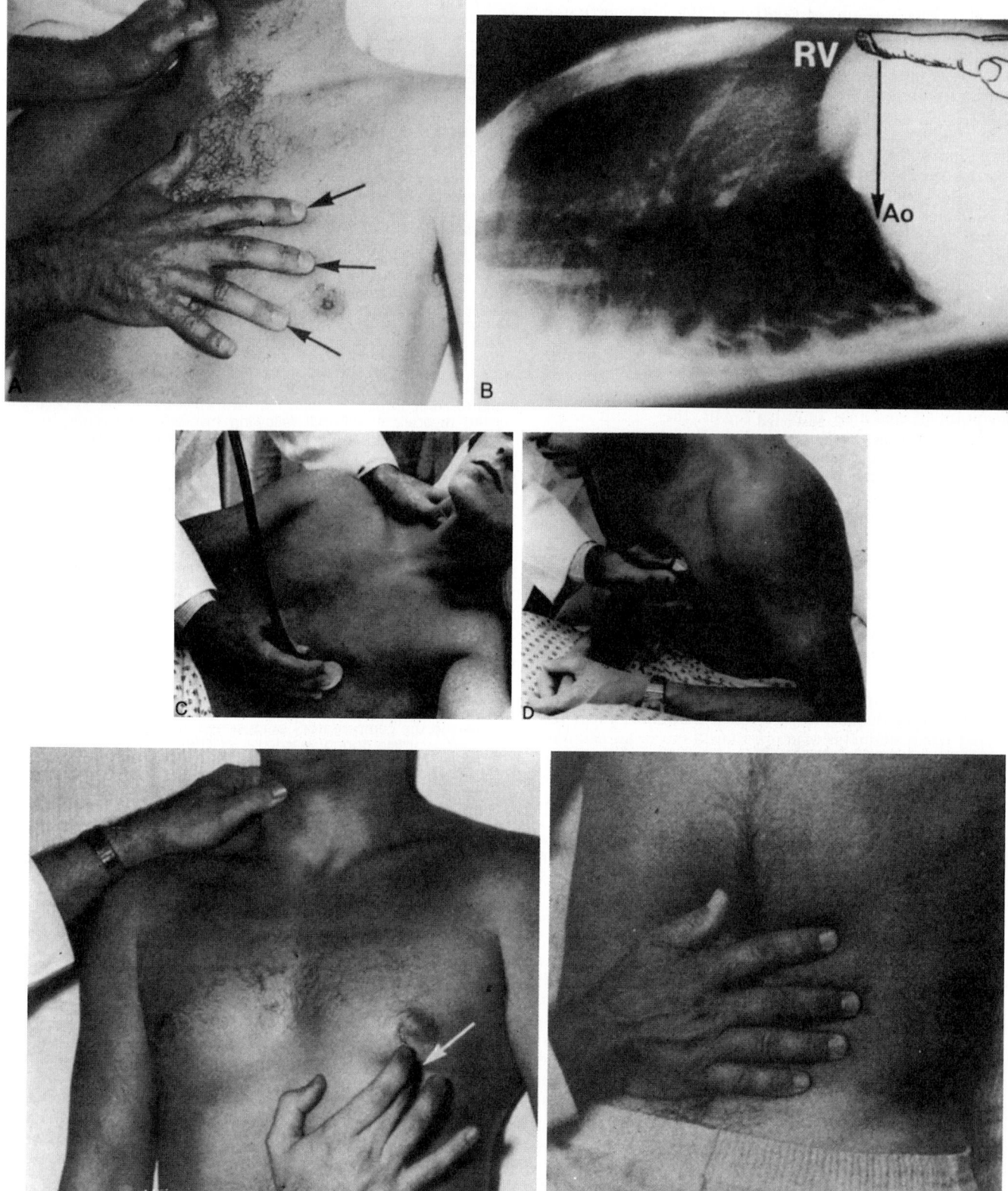

FIGURE 2–10.   *A,* Palpation of the anterior wall of the right ventricle by applying the tips of three fingers in the third, fourth, and fifth interspaces, left sternal edge (arrows), during full held exhalation. Patient is supine with the trunk elevated 30 degrees. *B,* Subxiphoid palpation of the inferior wall of the right ventricle (RV) with the relative position of the abdominal aorta (Ao) shown by the arrow. *C,* The bell of the stethoscope is applied to the cardiac apex while the patient lies in a partial left lateral decubitus position. The thumb of the examiner's free left hand is used to palpate the carotid artery for timing purposes. *D,* The soft, high-frequency early diastolic murmur of aortic regurgitation or pulmonary hypertensive regurgitation is best elicited by applying the stethoscopic diaphragm very firmly to the mid-left sternal edge. The patient leans forward with breath held in full exhalation. *E,* Palpation of the left ventricular impulse with a fingertip (arrow). The patient's trunk is 30 degrees above the horizontal. The examiner's right thumb palpates the carotid pulse for timing purposes. *F,* Palpation of the liver. The patient is supine with knees flexed to relax the abdomen. The flat of the examiner's right hand is placed on the right upper quadrant just below the expected inferior margin of the liver; the left hand is applied diametrically opposite. (From Perloff, J. K.: Physical Examination of the Heart and Circulation. 2nd ed. Philadelphia, W. B. Saunders Company, 1990.)

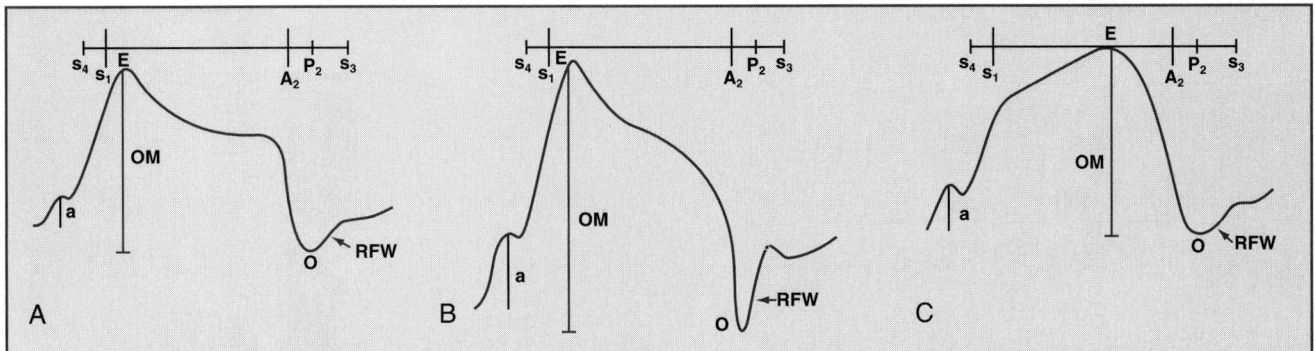

FIGURE 2–11. Schematic diagrams of normal hyperdynamic and sustained left ventricular impulse. Heart sounds are also illustrated. *A*, Normal apex cardiogram. The *a* wave, related to ventricular filling during atrial systole, usually does not exceed 15 per cent of the total height. E point usually coincides with the beginning of left ventricular ejection. Following E point, there is a gradual inward movement, explaining the brief duration of the normal left ventricular impulse. The O point approximately coincides with the mitral valve opening. *B*, Hyperdynamic left ventricular impulse is usually seen in left ventricular volume overloaded conditions such as primary mitral regurgitation and aortic regurgitation. Left ventricular ejection fraction is usually normal. Increased amplitude of *a* wave may be associated with palpable *a* waves, which are usually associated with increased left ventricular end-diastolic pressure. Accentuated rapid filling wave is frequently associated with audible S_3. *C*, Sustained left ventricular impulse (outward movement continued during ejection phase) is usually seen in the presence of decreased ejection fraction or when the left ventricle is markedly hypertrophied (S_4 = atrial sound; S_1 = first heart sound; A_2, = aortic component of the second heart sound; *a* = *a* wave; *E* = E point beginning of ejection; *OM* = outward movement; *O* = O point; *RFW* = rapid filling wave.) (From Chatterjee, K.: Bedside evaluation of the heart: The physical examination. *In* Chatterjee, K., et al. [eds.]: Cardiology: An Illustrated Text/Reference. Philadelphia, J. B. Lippincott, 1991, pp. 3.11–3.51.)

heart disease presystolic expansion is usually associated with normal or almost normal left ventricular function.[58] In patients with ischemic heart disease presystolic pulsation is usually associated with left ventricular dysfunction.[63] Presystolic expansion of the right ventricle occurs in right

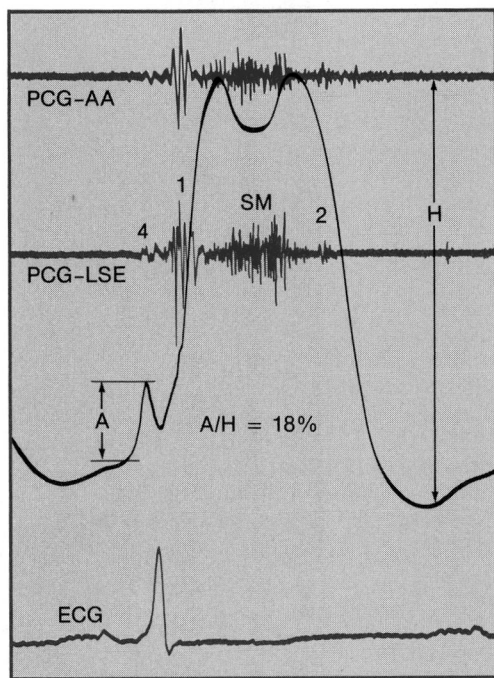

FIGURE 2–12. Apex cardiogram in hypertrophic obstructive cardiomyopathy. The *a* wave (A) is exaggerated in height, being 18 per cent of the entire amplitude of the apexcardiogram (H), and has an unusually rapid upstroke that culminates in a sharp peak, coinciding with the fourth heart sound (4). The systolic phase of the apexcardiogram has a bifid appearance with a prominent late systolic hump. The saddle-shaped decline in midsystole coincides in time with the systolic murmur and carotid pulse deformity, which, in turn, are related to the obstruction occasioned by the systolic anterior motion of the mitral valve. (From Craige, E., and Smith, D.: Heart sounds. *In* Braunwald, E. [ed.]: Heart Disease: A Textbook of Cardiovascular Medicine. 3rd ed. Philadelphia, W. B. Saunders Company, 1988, p. 59.)

ventricular hypertrophy and pulmonary hypertension and may be appreciated by subxiphoid palpation of the right ventricle during inspiration.

RIGHT VENTRICLE. Normally, neither this chamber, nor its motion, is palpable. A palpable anterior systolic movement (replacing systolic retraction) in the left parasternal region (Fig. 2–10*A*), best felt by the proximal palm or fingertips, and with the patient supine, usually represents *right ventricular enlargement* or hypertrophy.[65] In the absence of associated left ventricular enlargement, the right ventricular impulse is accompanied by reciprocal systolic retraction of the apex. In patients with pulmonary emphysema, even an enlarged right ventricle is not readily palpable at the left sternal edge but is better appreciated in the subxiphoid region. Exaggerated motion of the entire parasternal area, i.e., a hyperdynamic impulse with normal contour, usually reflects increased right ventricular contractility due to augmented stroke volume, as occurs in patients with atrial septal defect or tricuspid regurgitation, whereas a sustained left parasternal outward thrust reflects right ventricular hypertrophy due to pressure overload, as occurs in pulmonary hypertension or pulmonic stenosis. With marked right ventricular enlargement, this chamber occupies the apex because the left ventricle is displaced posteriorly.

When both ventricles are enlarged, both the left parasternal and the apical areas may rise with systole, but an area of systolic retraction between them can usually be appreciated. In patients with emphysema or obesity, an enlarged right ventricle is detected most readily in the subxiphoid region by palpating the epigastrium and pointing the fingers upward. With marked isolated right ventricular enlargement, the right ventricle may form the cardiac apex, and should not be confused with those of left or biventricular enlargement. When acute myocardial ischemia or myocardial infarction causes dyskinetic movement of the ventricular septum, there may be a transient left parasternal impulse not caused by right ventricular enlargement.

PULMONARY ARTERY. *Pulmonary hypertension* and/or increased pulmonary blood flow frequently produce a prominent systolic pulsation of the pulmonary trunk in the second intercostal space just to the left of the sternum. This pulsation is often associated with a prominent left parasternal impulse, reflecting right ventricular enlargement, or hypertrophy and a palpable shock synchronous with the second heart sound, reflecting forceful closure of the pulmonic valve.

LEFT ATRIUM. An enlarged left atrium or a large posterior left ventricular aneurysm can make right ventricular pulsations more prominent by displacing the right ventricle anteriorly against the left parasternal area, and in severe mitral regurgitation an expanding left atrium may be responsible for marked left parasternal movement, even in the absence of right ventricular hypertrophy. The systolic bulging of the left atrium, which is transmitted through the right ventricle, commences and terminates *after* the left ventricular thrust. Movement imparted by the systolic expansion of the left atrium can be appreciated by placing the index finger of one hand at the left ventricular apex and the index finger of the other in the left parasternal region in the third intercostal space; the movement of the latter finger begins and ends slightly later than that of the former. Although this difference in timing may be difficult to appreciate on palpation, particularly when the heart rate is rapid, recordings of chest wall motion in severe chronic mitral regurgitation demonstrate a delayed fall in the left lower precordium compared with the cardiac apex. Outward movement of the chest wall that is more marked to the right than to the left of the sternum is usually due to aneurysm of the aorta or to marked enlargement of the right atrium in the presence of tricuspid regurgitation. Occasionally, a giant left atrium is palpable in the right hemithorax. The left atrial appendage is sometimes visible and palpable in the third left intercostal space.

AORTA. Enlargement or aneurysm of the ascending aorta or aortic arch may cause visible or palpable systolic pulsations of the right or left sternoclavicular joint; and may also cause a systolic impulse in the suprasternal notch or the first or second right intercostal space.[1]

PALPABLE SOUNDS. Valve closure, if abnormally forceful or if normal in a patient with a thin chest wall, can be appreciated as a tapping sensation. A palpable sound occurs most prominently in the second left intercostal space in patients with pulmonary hypertension (pulmonic valve closure), in the second right intercostal space in patients with systemic hypertension (aortic valve closure), and at the cardiac apex in patients with mitral stenosis (mitral valve closure). Occasionally, in congenital aortic stenosis, aortic ejection sounds can be palpated at the cardiac apex; ejection sounds originating in a dilated aorta or pulmonary artery can sometimes be felt at the base of the heart.[61] Prominent third and fourth heart sounds are often palpable as diastolic movements at the cardiac apex. In patients with mitral stenosis an opening snap may be palpated at the apex.

THRILLS. The flat of the hand or the fingertips usually best appreciate thrills, vibratory sensations which are palpable manifestations of loud, harsh murmurs *having low-frequency to medium components.*[66] Because the vibrations must be quite intense before they are felt, far more information can be obtained from the auscultatory than from the palpatory features of heart murmurs. High-pitched murmurs such as those produced by valvular regurgitation, even when loud, are not usually associated with thrills.

PERCUSSION. Palpation is far more helpful than is percussion in determining cardiac size. However, in the absence of an apical beat, as in patients with pericardial effusion, or in some patients with dilated cardiomyopathy, heart failure, and marked displacement of a hypokinetic apical beat, the left border of the heart can be outlined by means of percussion. Also, percussion of dullness in the right lower parasternal area may, in some instances, aid in the detection of a greatly enlarged right atrium. Percussion aids materially in determining visceral situs, i.e., in ascertaining the side on which the heart, stomach, and liver are located. When the heart is in the right chest but the abdominal viscera are located normally, congenital heart disease is usually present. When both the heart and abdominal viscera are in the opposite side of the chest (situs inversus), congenital heart disease is uncommon.

CARDIAC AUSCULTATION

Principles and Technique

The modern binaural stethoscope is a well-crafted, airtight instrument with earpieces selected for comfort, with metal tubing joined to single flexible 12-inch-long, thick-walled rubber tubing (internal diameter of ⅛ inch) and with dual chest pieces—diaphragm for high frequencies, bell for low or lower frequencies—designed so that the examiner can readily switch from one chest piece to the other.[67,68] When the bell is applied with just enough pressure to form a skin seal, low frequencies are accentuated; when the bell is pressed firmly, the stretched skin becomes a diaphragm, damping low frequencies. Variable pressure with the bell provides a range of frequencies from low to medium.

Cardiac auscultation is best accomplished in a quiet room with the patient comfortable and the chest fully ex-

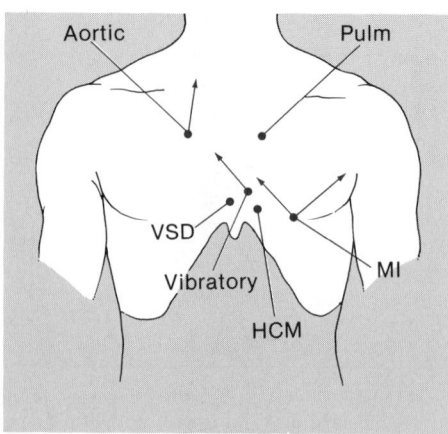

FIGURE 2–13. Maximal intensity and radiation of six isolated systolic murmurs. HCM = hypertrophic cardiomyopathy; MI = mitral incompetence; Pulm = pulmonary; VSD = ventricular septal defect. (From Barlow, J. B.: Perspectives on the Mitral Valve. Philadelphia, F. A. Davis, 1987, p. 140.)

posed. Percussion should precede auscultation in order to establish visceral and cardiac situs, so that auscultation can be carried out with confidence in the topographic anatomy of the heart. Terms such as "mitral area," "tricuspid area," "pulmonary area," and "aortic area" should be avoided because they assume situs solitus without ventricular inversion and with normally related great arteries. The topographic areas for auscultation (Fig. 2–13), irrespective of cardiac situs, are best designated by descriptive terms— cardiac apex, left and right sternal borders interspace by interspace, and subxiphoid. For patients in situs solitus with a left thoracic heart, auscultation should begin at the cardiac apex (best identified in the left lateral decubitus) and contiguous lower left sternal edge (inflow), proceeding interspace by interspace up the left sternal border to the left base and then to the right base (outflow). This topographic sequence permits the examiner to think physiologically by using a pattern that conforms to the direction of blood flow—inflow/outflow. In addition to the routine sites described above, the stethoscope should be applied regularly to certain nonprecordial thoracic areas, especially the axillae, the back, the anterior chest on the opposite side, and above the clavicles. In patients with increased anteroposterior chest dimensions (emphysema), auscultation is often best achieved by applying the stethoscope in the epigastrium (subxiphoid).

Information derived from auscultation benefits not only from knowledge of the cardiac situs, but also from identification of palpable and visible movements of the ventricles. During auscultation, the examiner is generally on the patient's right; three positions are routinely employed: left lateral decubitus (assuming left thoracic heart), supine, and sitting. Auscultation should begin by applying the stethoscope to the cardiac apex with the patient in the left lateral decubitus position (Fig. 2–14). If tachycardia makes identification of the first heart sound difficult, timing can be established, with few exceptions, by simultaneous palpation of the carotid artery with the thumb of the free left hand (Fig. 2–14). Once the first heart sound is identified, analysis then proceeds by systematic, methodical, sequential attention to early, mid, and late systole, the second heart sound, then early, mid, and late diastole (presystole), returning to the first heart sound. When auscultation at the apex has been completed, the patient is turned into the supine position. Each topographic area—lower to upper left sternal edge interspace by interspace and then the right base—is interrogated using the same systematic sequence of analysis.

Assessment of pitch or frequency ranging from low to moderately high can be achieved by variable pressure of

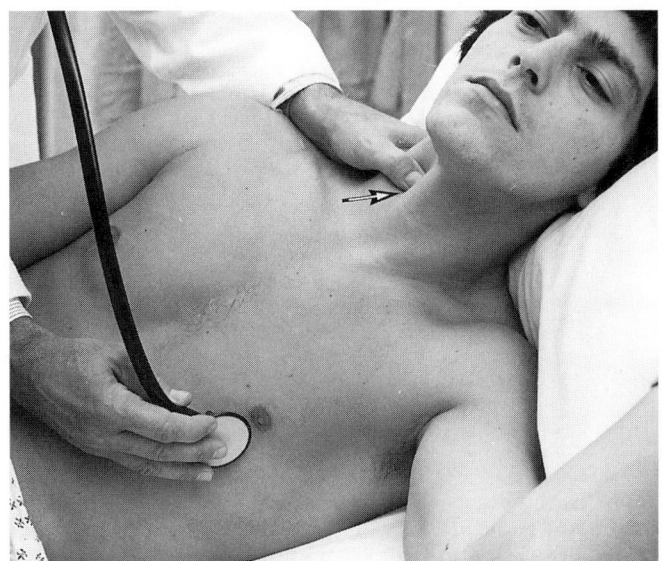

FIGURE 2–14. The bell of the stethoscope is applied to the cardiac apex while the patient lies in a left lateral decubitus position. The thumb of the examiner's free left hand palpates the carotid artery *(arrow)* for timing purposes.

the stethoscopic bell, whereas for high frequencies, the diaphragm should be employed. It is practical to begin by using the stethoscopic bell with varying pressure at the apex and lower left sternal edge, changing to the diaphragm when the base is reached. Low frequencies are best heard by applying the bell just lightly enough to achieve a skin seal. High frequency events are best elicited with firm pressure of the diaphragm, often with the patient sitting, leaning forward in full held exhalation.

The Heart Sounds

Heart sounds are relatively brief, discrete auditory vibrations of varying intensity (loudness), frequency (pitch), and quality (timbre). The first heart sound identifies the onset of ventricular systole, and the second heart sound identifies the onset of diastole. These two auscultatory events establish a framework within which other heart sounds and murmurs can be placed and timed.[1]

The basic heart sounds are the first, second, third, and fourth sounds (Fig. 2–15A). Each of these events can be normal or abnormal. Other heart sounds are, with few exceptions, abnormal, either intrinsically so or iatrogenic (e.g., prosthetic valve sounds, pacemaker sounds). A heart sound should first be characterized by a simple descriptive term that identifies where in the cardiac cycle the sound occurs. Accordingly, heart sounds within the framework established by the first and second sounds are designated as "early systolic, mid-systolic, late systolic," and "early diastolic, mid-diastolic, late diastolic (presystolic)" (Fig. 2–15B).[2] The next step is to draw conclusions based upon what a sound so identified represents. An *early systolic* sound might be an ejection sound (aortic or pulmonary) or an aortic prosthetic sound. Mid- and late systolic sounds are typified by the click(s) of mitral valve prolapse but occasionally are "remnants" of pericardial rubs. *Early diastolic* sounds are represented by opening snaps (usually mitral), early third heart sounds (constrictive pericarditis, less commonly mitral regurgitation), the opening of a mechanical inflow prosthesis, or the abrupt seating of a pedunculated mobile atrial myxoma ("tumor plop"). *Mid-diastolic* sounds are generally third heart sounds or summation sounds (synchronous occurrence of third and fourth heart sounds). *Late diastolic* or *presystolic* sounds are almost always fourth heart sounds, rarely pacemaker sounds.

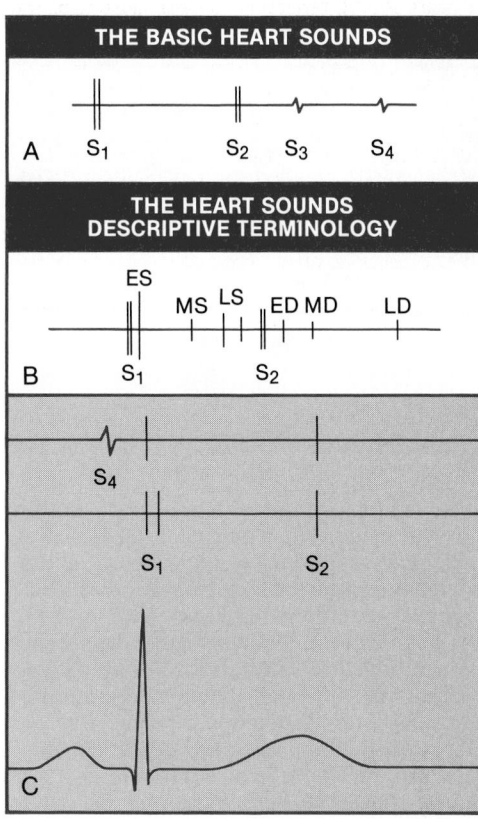

FIGURE 2–15. *A,* The basic heart sounds consist of the first heart sound (S$_1$), the second heart sound (S$_2$), the third heart sound (S$_3$), and the fourth heart sound (S$_4$). *B,* Heart sounds within the auscultatory framework established by the first heart sound (S$_1$) and the second heart sound (S$_2$). The additional heart sounds are designated descriptively as early systolic (ES), midsystolic (MS), late systolic (LS), early diastolic (ED), mid-diastolic (MD), and late diastolic (LD) or presystolic. *C,* Upper tracing illustrates a low-frequency fourth heart sound (S$_4$), and the lower tracing illustrates a split first heart sound (S$_1$), the two components of which are of the same quality.

The First Heart Sound

The first heart sound consists of two major components (Fig. 2–15C). The initial component is most prominent at the cardiac apex when the apex is occupied by the left ventricle.[69] The second component, if present, is normally confined to the lower left sternal edge, is less commonly heard at the apex, and is seldom heard at the base. The first major component is associated with closure of the mitral valve and coincides with abrupt arrest of leaflet motion when the cusps—especially the larger and more mobile anterior mitral cusp—reach their fully closed positions (maximal cephalad systolic excursion into the left atrium). The origin of the second major component of the first heart sound has been debated but is generally assigned to closure of the tricuspid valve based upon an analogous line of reasoning.[70] Opening of the semilunar valves with ejection of blood into the aortic root or pulmonary trunk usually produces no audible sound in the normal heart, although phonocardiograms sometimes record a low-amplitude sound following the mitral and tricuspid components and coinciding with the maximal opening excursion of the aortic cusps.[1] In complete right bundle branch block the first heart sound is widely split as a result of delay of the tricuspid component.[71] In complete left bundle branch block, the first heart sound is single as a result of delay of the mitral component.[72]

Because the two major audible components of the first heart sound are believed to originate in the closing movements of the atrioventricular valves, the quality of the two components (pitch) is similar (Fig. 2–15C). When the first heart sound is split, its first component is normally the

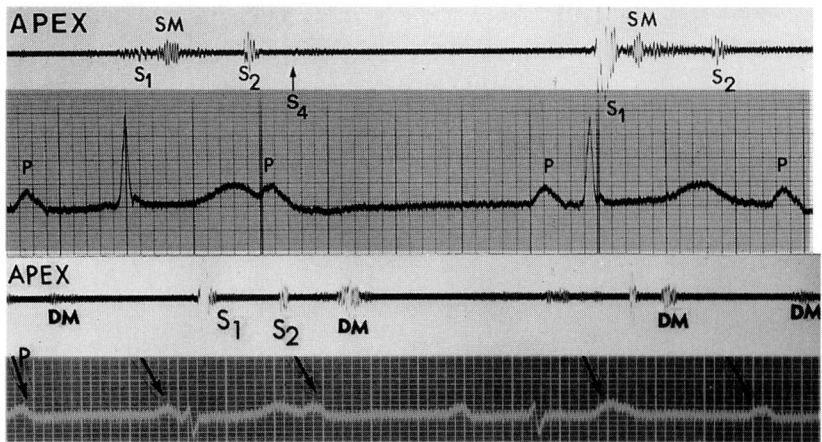

FIGURE 2–16. *Upper tracing,* Phonocardiogram and electrocardiogram (lead 2) from a 12-year-old girl with congenital complete heart block. The first heart sound (S₁) varies from soft (long P-R interval) to loud (short P-R interval). There is a grade 2/6 vibratory midsystolic murmur (SM). A soft fourth heart sound (arrow) follows the second P wave. *Lower tracing,* Phonocardiogram and electrocardiogram from a 15-year-old boy with congenital complete heart block. Arrows point to independent P waves. The first heart sound (S₁) varies from loud to soft depending upon the P-R interval. The short diastolic murmurs (DM) are especially prominent when atrial contraction (P wave) coincides with and reinforces the rapid filling phase (shortly after the T wave).

louder. The softer second component is confined to the lower left sternal edge but may also be heard at the apex. Only the louder first component is heard at the base. The intensity of the first heard sound, particularly its first major audible component, depends chiefly upon the position of the bellies of the mitral leaflets, especially the anterior leaflet, at the time the left ventricle begins to contract and less upon the rate of left ventricular contraction.[73] The first heart sound is therefore loudest when the onset of left ventricular systole finds the mitral leaflets maximally recessed into the left ventricular cavity, as in the presence of a rapid heart rate, a short P-R interval[74] (Fig. 2–16), short cycle lengths in atrial fibrillation, or mitral stenosis with a mobile anterior leaflet. In Ebstein's anomaly of the tricuspid valve, the first heart sound is widely split (delayed right ventricular activation), and the second component is loud provided the anterior tricuspid leaflet is large and mobile.[75]

Early Systolic Sounds

Aortic or pulmonary ejection sounds are the most common early systolic sounds.[76] "Ejection sound" is preferred to the term ejection "click," with the latter designation best reserved for the mid- to late systolic clicks of mitral valve prolapse (see p. 1032). Ejection sounds coincide with the fully opened position of the relevant semilunar valve, as in congenital aortic valve stenosis (Fig. 2–17A) or bicuspid aortic valve in the left side of the heart, or pulmonary valve stenosis (Fig. 2–18) in the right side of the heart.[75,77] Ejection sounds are relatively high frequency events, and depending upon intensity, have a pitch similar to that of the two major components of the first heart sound. An ejection sound originating in the aortic valve (congenital aortic stenosis or bicuspid aortic valve) or in the pulmonary valve (congenital pulmonary valve stenosis) indicates that the

valve is mobile because the ejection sound is caused by abrupt cephalad doming (Fig. 2–17B).[77] Less certain is the origin of an ejection sound within a dilated arterial trunk that is guarded by a normal semilunar valve. Origin of the sound is assigned either to opening movement of the leaflets that resonate in the arterial trunk or to the wall of the dilated great artery. Aortic ejection sounds do not vary with respiration except those that originate in the large biventricular aorta of Fallot's tetralogy with pulmonary atresia or truncus arteriosus (Fig. 2–18).[75] The mechanism responsible for the respiratory variation in this setting is unclear.

Pulmonary ejection sounds often selectively and distinctively decrease in intensity during normal inspiration (Fig. 2–19A). The mechanism responsible for respiratory variation of a pulmonary ejection sound is most convincing in the setting of typical pulmonary valve stenosis.[78] An inspiratory increase in right atrial contractile force is transmitted into the right ventricle and onto the ventricular surface of the mobile stenotic valve, moving its cusps upward *before* the onset of ventricular contraction. Cephalad excursion of the valve during ventricular systole is therefore diminished, accounting for the inspiratory decrease in intensity of the ejection sound. This mechanism cannot apply to the respiratory variation of a pulmonary ejection sound asso-

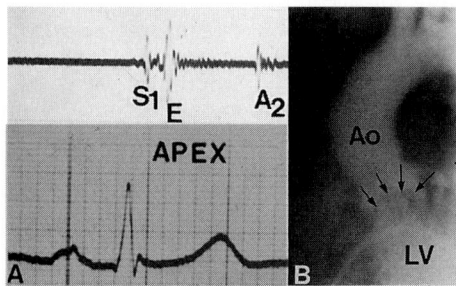

FIGURE 2–17. *A,* Phonocardiogram over the left ventricular impulse in a patient with mild congenital bicuspid aortic valve stenosis. The aortic ejection sound (E) is louder than the first heart sound (S₁). A₂ = Aortic component of the second heart sound. *B,* Left ventriculogram (LV) in another patient with congenital aortic valve stenosis. The cephalad systolic doming of the stenotic valve (arrows) produces the ejection sound.

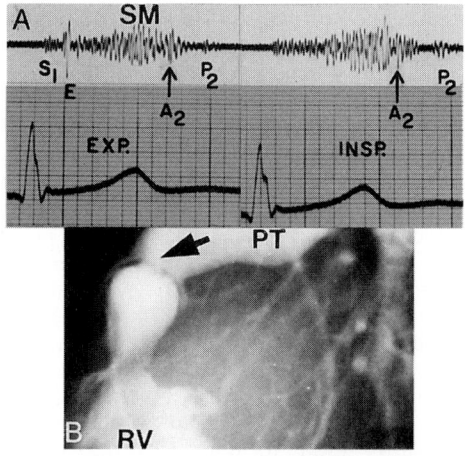

FIGURE 2–18. *A,* Phonocardiogram in the second left intercostal space of a patient with congenital pulmonary valve stenosis. The ejection sound (E) is obvious during exhalation (EXP) but disappears entirely during casual inhalation (INSP). The pulmonary component of the second heart sound (P₂) is delayed and soft. SM = Systolic murmur; S₁ = first heart sound. *B,* Right ventriculogram (RV) in another patient with pulmonary valve stenosis. The cephalad systolic doming of the mobile stenotic valve (arrow) produces the pulmonary ejection sound. There is post-stenotic dilatation of the pulmonary trunk (PT).

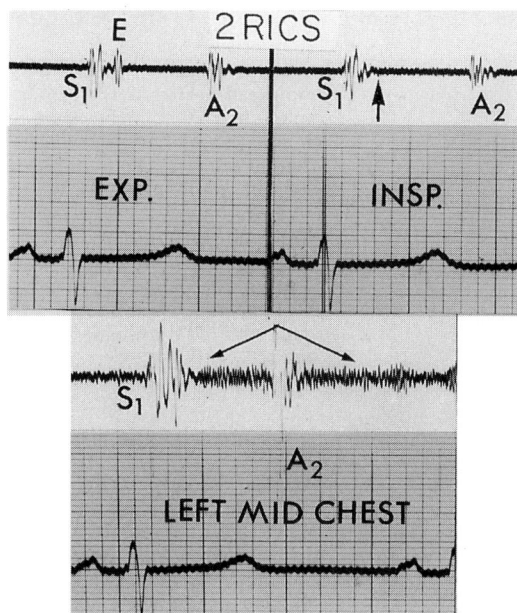

FIGURE 2–19. Phonocardiograms from an 11-year-girl with Fallot's tetralogy and pulmonary atresia. The upper tracing from the second right intercostal space (2RICS) shows an aortic ejection sound (E) that is prominent during exhalation (EXP) but absent during inspiration (INSP). The lower tracing from the left midchest shows a continuous murmur of aortopulmonary collaterals. The second heart sound is necessarily single and is represented by the aortic component (A₂). S₁ = First heart sound.

ciated with a dilated hypertensive pulmonary trunk (Fig. 2–20).[2,75]

Early systolic sounds accompany mechanical prostheses in the aortic location, especially the Starr-Edwards ball-in-cage valve, less so with a tilting disc valve such as the Björk-Shiley. Early systolic sounds do not occur with bioprosthetic valves (tissue valves) in either the aortic or pulmonary location.

Mid- to Late Systolic Sounds

Far and away the most common mid- to late systolic sound(s) are associated with mitral valve prolapse[2,79,80] (see p. 1029). The term "click" is appropriate because these mid- to late systolic sounds are of relatively high frequency and often, but not invariably, "clicking." Mid- to late systolic clicks of mitral valve prolapse coincide with maximal systolic excursion of a prolapsed leaflet (or scallop(s) of the posterior leaflet) into the left atrium and are ascribed to sudden tensing of the redundant leaflet(s) and elongated chordae tendinae. Variability epitomizes mitral systolic clicks, which from time-to-time may be replaced by a cluster of discrete late systolic "crackles." Physical or pharmacological interventions that *reduce* left ventricular volume, such as the Valsalva maneuver, or a change in position from squatting to standing (Fig. 2–21) causes the click(s) to occur earlier in systole.[79–82] Conversely, physical or pharmacological interventions that *increase* left ventricular volume, such as squatting (Fig. 2–21) or sustained hand grip, serve to delay the timing of the click(s). Multiple clicks are thought to arise from asynchronous tensing of different

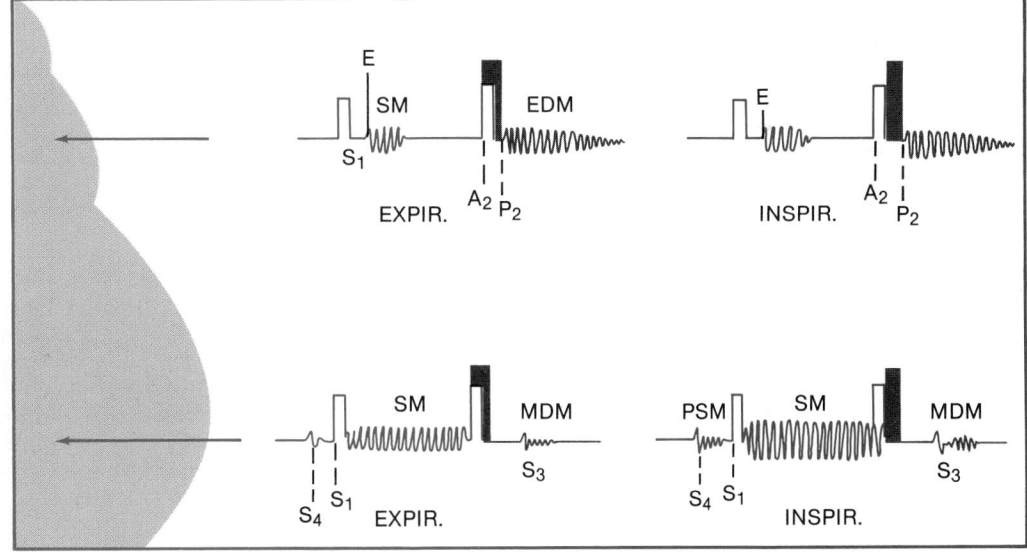

FIGURE 2–20. Composite of the principal auscultatory and phonocardiographic manifestations of pulmonary hypertension. (From Perloff, J. K.: Auscultatory and phonocardiographic manifestations of pulmonary hypertension. Prog. Cardiovasc. Dis. *9:*303, 1967.)

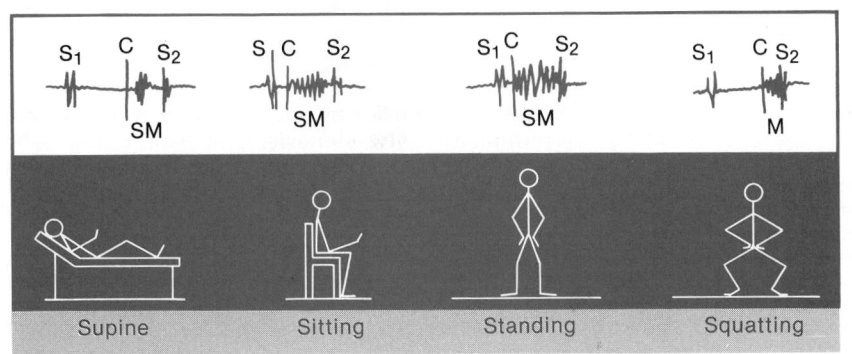

FIGURE 2–21. Postural maneuvers that affect the click(s) and late systolic murmur (SM) of mitral valve prolapse. A change from supine to sitting or standing causes the click to become earlier and the murmur longer although softer. Conversely, squatting delays the timing of the click, and the murmur becomes shorter but louder. (From Devereux, R., Perloff, J. K., Reichek, N., and Josephson, M.: Mitral valve prolapse. Circulation *54:*3, 1976, by permission of the American Heart Association.)

portions of redundant mitral leaflets, especially the triscalloped posterior leaflet.

On rare occasions, a pericardial friction rub leaves in its wake mid- to late systolic sounds—remnants of rubs—that persist after disappearance of the systolic phase of the rub. Carl Potain, in 1894, commented upon "small, short clicking sounds, well localized and such that one can scarcely attribute them to anything except the tensing of a pericardial adhesion." [83]

The Second Heart Sound

Respiratory splitting of the second heart sound was described by Potain in 1866,[84] and Leatham called the second heart sound the "key to auscultation of the heart." [85] The first component of the second heart sound is designated "aortic" and the second "pulmonary." [86,87] Each component coincides with the dicrotic incisura of its great arterial pressure pulse (Fig. 2–22).[69] Inspiratory splitting of the second heart sound is due chiefly to a delay in the pulmonary component, less to earlier timing of the aortic component.[88] During inspiration, the pulmonary arterial dicrotic incisura moves away from the descending limb of the right ventricular pressure pulse because of an inspiratory increase in capacitance of the pulmonary vascular bed, delaying the pulmonary component of the second heart sound.[89] Exhalation has the opposite effect. The earlier inspiratory timing of the aortic component of the second heart sound is attributed to a transient reduction in left ventricular volume coupled with unchanged impedance (capacitance) in the systemic vascular bed. Normal respiratory variations in the timing of the second heart sound are therefore ascribed principally to the variations in impedance characteristics (capacitance) of the pulmonary vascular bed, not to an inspiratory increase in right ventricular volume as originally proposed.[69,85] When an increase in capacitance of the pulmonary bed is lost because of a rise in pulmonary vascular resistance, inspiratory splitting of the second heart sound narrows and, if present at all, reflects an increase in right ventricular ejection time and/or earlier timing of the aortic component.[2]

The frequency compositions of the aortic and pulmonary components of the second heart sound are similar, but their normal amplitudes differ appreciably, reflecting the differences in systemic (aortic) and pulmonary arterial closing

TABLE 2–2   CAUSES OF SPLITTING OF THE SECOND HEART SOUND

NORMAL SPLITTING
DELAYED PULMONIC CLOSURE
Delayed electrical activation of the right ventricle
Complete RBBB (proximal type)
Left ventricular paced beats
Left ventricular ectopic beats
Prolonged right ventricular mechanical systole
Acute massive pulmonary embolus
Pulmonary hypertension with right heart failure
Pulmonic stenosis with intact septum (moderate to severe)
Decreased impedance of the pulmonary vascular bed (increased hang-out)
Normotensive atrial septal defect
Idiopathic dilatation of the pulmonary artery
Pulmonic stenosis (mild)
Atrial septal defect, postoperative (70%)
EARLY AORTIC CLOSURE
Shortened left ventricular mechanical systole (LVET)
Mitral regurgitation
Ventricular septal defect
REVERSED SPLITTING
DELAYED AORTIC CLOSURE
Delayed electrical activation of the left ventricle
Complete LBBB (proximal type)
Right ventricular paced beats
Right ventricular ectopic beats
Prolonged left ventricular mechanical systole
Complete LBBB (peripheral type)
Left ventricular outflow tract obstruction
Hypertensive cardiovascular disease
Arteriosclerotic heart disease
Chronic ischemic heart disease
Angina pectoris
Decreased impedance of the systemic vascular bed (increased hang-out)
Poststenotic dilatation of the aorta secondary to aortic stenosis or insufficiency
Patent ductus arteriosus
EARLY PULMONIC CLOSURE
Early electrical activation of the right ventricle
Wolff-Parkinson-White syndrome, type B

RBBB = right bundle-branch block; LVET = left ventricular ejection time; LBBB = left bundle-branch block.

Modified from Shaver, J. A., and O'Toole, J. D.: The second heart sound: Newer concepts. Parts 1 and 2. Mod. Concepts Cardiovasc. Dis. *46:*7 and 13, 1977.

pressures. Splitting of the second heart sound is most readily identified in the second left intercostal space, because the softer pulmonary component is normally confined to that site, whereas the louder aortic component is heard at the base, sternal edge, and apex.[2,86]

ABNORMAL SPLITTING OF THE SECOND HEART SOUND. Three general categories of abnormal splitting are recognized: (1) persistently single, (2) persistently split (fixed or nonfixed), and (3) paradoxically split (reversed). When the second heart sound remains single throughout the respiratory cycle, one component is absent or the two components are persistently synchronous. The most common cause of a single second heart sound is inaudibility of the *pulmonary* component in older adults with increased anteroposterior chest dimensions. In the setting of congenital heart disease, a single second heart sound due to absence of the pulmonary component is a feature of pulmonary atresia (Fig. 2–18), severe pulmonary valve stenosis, dysplastic pulmonary valve or complete transposition of the great arteries (pulmonary component inaudible because of the posterior position of the pulmonary trunk).[75] Conversely, a single second heart sound due to inaudibility of the *aortic* component occurs when the aortic valve is immobile (severe calcific aortic stenosis) or atretic (aortic atresia). A single second sound due to persistent synchrony of its two components is a feature of Eisenmenger's complex, in which the aortic

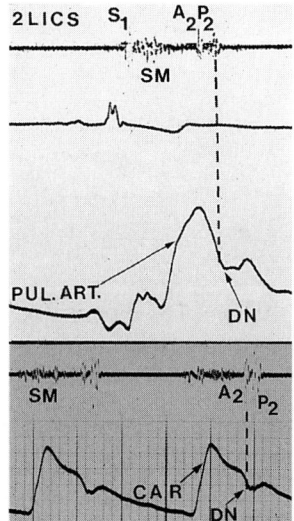

FIGURE 2–22. Tracings from a 28-year-old woman with an uncomplicated ostium secundum atrial septal defect. In the second left interspace (2LICS), the pulmonary component (P_2) of a widely split second heart sound is synchronous with the dicrotic notch (DN) of the pulmonary arterial pressure pulse. (S_1 = First heart sound; SM = midsystolic murmur). In the lower tracing, the aortic component (A_2) of the widely split second heart sound is synchronous with the dicrotic notch of the carotid arterial pulse (CAR).

and pulmonary arterial dicrotic incisurae are virtually identical in timing.[75]

Both components of the second heart sound are sometimes inaudible at *all* precordial sites. This is likely to be so in older adults in whom fibrocalcific changes limit mobility of the aortic valve, whereas the pulmonary component is inaudible because of a large anteroposterior chest dimension (see above).

A single semilunar valve, as in truncus arteriosus, does not necessarily generate what is judged on auscultation to be a single second heart sound. Instead, the second sound may be perceived as "split" because of asynchronous closure of the unequal cusps of a quadricuspid valve.[75] In systemic or pulmonary hypertension, the duration of a single loud second heart sound may be sufficiently prolonged and slurred (reduplicated) to encourage the mistaken impression of splitting.

Persistent Splitting of the Second Heart Sound. This term applies when the two components remain audible (or recordable) during both inspiration and exhalation. Persistent splitting may be due to a delay in the pulmonary component, as in simple complete right bundle branch block[69] or to early timing of the aortic component, as occasionally occurs in mitral regurgitation.[90] Normal directional changes in the interval of the split (greater with inspiration, lesser with exhalation) in the presence of persistent audibility of both components defines the split as *persistent* but not *fixed.*

Fixed Splitting of the Second Heart Sound. This term applies when the interval between the aortic and pulmonary components is not only wide and persistent, but remains unchanged during the respiratory cycle.[69] Fixed splitting is an auscultatory hallmark of uncomplicated ostium secundum atrial septal defect. The aortic and pulmonary components are widely separated during exhalation and exhibit little or no change in the degree of splitting during inspiration or with the Valsalva maneuver. The *wide* splitting is caused by a delay in the pulmonary component because a marked increase in pulmonary vascular capacitance prolongs the interval between the descending limbs of the pulmonary arterial and right ventricular pressure pulses ("hangout"), and therefore delays the pulmonary incisura and the pulmonary component of the second heart sound (Fig. 2–22). The capacitance (impedance) of the pulmonary bed is appreciably increased, so there is little or no additional increase during inspiration and little or no inspiratory delay in the pulmonary component of the second sound. Phasic changes in systemic venous return during respiration in atrial septal defect are associated with reciprocal changes in the volume of the left-to-right shunt, minimizing respiratory variations in right ventricular filling. The net effect is the characteristic wide fixed splitting of the two components of the second heart sound.[75]

Paradoxical Splitting of the Second Heart Sound. This term refers to a reversed sequence of semilunar valve closure, the pulmonary component (P_2) preceding the aortic component (A_2).[69] Common causes of paradoxical splitting are complete left bundle branch block[91] or a right ventricular pacemaker, both of which are associated with initial activation of the right side of the ventricular septum, and delayed activation of the left ventricle owing to transseptal (right-to-left) depolarization.[92] When the second heart sound splits paradoxically, its two components separate during *exhalation* and become single (synchronous) during *inspiration*. Inspiratory synchrony is achieved as the two components fuse because of a delay in the pulmonary component, less to earlier timing of the aortic component.

Abnormal Loudness (Intensity) of the Two Components of the Second Heart Sound. Assessment of intensity requires that both components be compared when heard simultaneously at the same site. The relative softness of the normal pulmonary component is responsible for its localization in the second left intercostal space, whereas the relative loudness of the normal aortic component accounts for its audibility at all precordial sites (see earlier).[2] An increase in intensity of the *aortic* component of the second sound occurs with systemic hypertension. The intensity of the aortic component also increases when the aorta is closer to the anterior chest wall owing to root dilatation or transposition of the great arteries, or when an anterior pulmonary trunk is small or absent, as in pulmonary atresia (Fig. 2–18).[75]

A loud *pulmonary* component of the second heart sound (Figs. 2–20 and 2–23A) is a feature of pulmonary hypertension, and the loudness is enhanced by dilatation of a hypertensive pulmonary trunk. Graham Steell, in describing the auscultatory signs of pulmonary hypertension, remarked that ". . . extreme accentuation of the pulmonary second sound is always present, the closure of the pulmonary semilunar valve being generally perceptible to the hand placed over the pulmonary area, as a sharp thud."[93] An accentuated pulmonary component can be transmitted to the mid or lower left sternal edge, and when very loud, throughout the precordium to the apex and right base. A loud pulmonary component in the second left interspace may obscure a closely preceding aortic component. In this eventuality, auscultation at other precordial sites often identifies the transmitted but attenuated pulmonary component and allows detection of splitting. A moderate increase in loudness of the pulmonary component of the second heart sound sometimes occurs in the absence of pulmonary hypertension when the pulmonary trunk is dilated, as with idiopathic dilatation or ostium secundum atrial septal defect, or when there is a decrease in anteroposterior chest dimensions (loss of thoracic kyphosis) that places the pulmonary trunk closer to the chest wall.[94]

Early Diastolic Sounds

The opening snap of rheumatic mitral stenosis is the best known early diastolic sound (Fig. 2–23B). The term "snap" was introduced in 1908 by W. S. Thayer as the English equivalent to the "claquement d'ouverture" of Rouchès.[95] The diagnostic value derived from the pitch, loudness, and

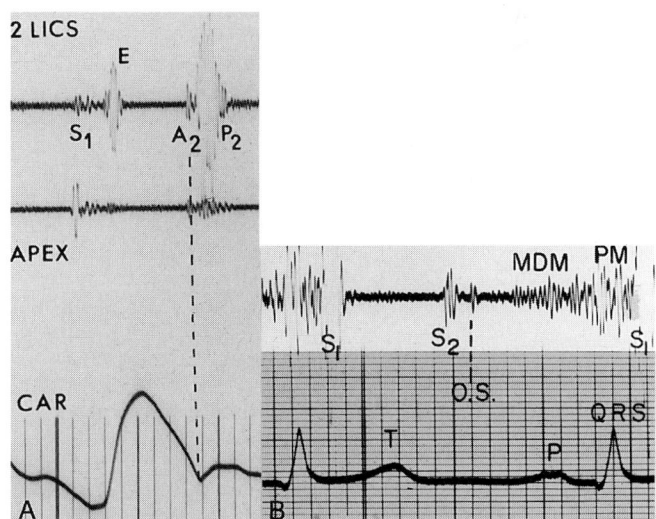

FIGURE 2–23. *A,* Tracings from a 32-year-old woman with an ostium secundum atrial septal defect, pulmonary hypertension, and a small right-to-left shunt. In the second left intercostal space (2LICS), the first heart sound is followed by a prominent pulmonary ejection sound (E). The second sound remains split. The pulmonary component (P_2) is very loud and is transmitted to the apex. (CAR = Carotid pulse). *B,* Phonocardiogram recorded in the left lateral decubitus position over the left ventricular impulse in a patient with pure rheumatic mitral stenosis. The first heart sound (S_1) is loud. The second heart sound (S_2) is followed by an opening snap (OS). There is a mid-diastolic murmur (MDM). The prominent presystolic murmur (PM) goes up to the subsequent loud first heart sound.

timing of the opening snap in the assessment of rheumatic mitral stenosis was established by Wood in his classic monograph, *An Appreciation of Mitral Stenosis*.[96] An audible opening snap indicates that the mitral valve is mobile, at least its longer anterior leaflet.[97] The snap is generated when superior systolic bowing of the anterior mitral leaflet is rapidly reversed toward the left ventricle in early diastole in response to high left atrial pressure. The mechanism of the opening snap is therefore a corollary to the loud first heart sound (Fig. 2–23*B*), which is generated by abrupt superior systolic displacement of a mobile anterior mitral leaflet that was recessed into the left ventricle during diastole by high left atrial pressure until the onset of left ventricular isovolumetric contraction (see earlier). The designation "snap" is appropriate because of the relatively high frequency of the sound.

The timing of the opening snap (OS) relative to the aortic component of the second heart sound (A$_2$) has important physiological meaning.[2] A short A$_2$-OS interval generally reflects the high left atrial pressure of *severe* mitral stenosis. However, in older subjects with systolic hypertension, mitral stenosis of appreciable severity can occur without a short A$_2$-OS interval because the elevated left ventricular systolic pressure takes longer to fall below the left atrial pressure. In the presence of atrial fibrillation, the A$_2$-OS interval varies inversely with cycle length, because (all else being equal) the higher the left atrial pressure (short cycle length), the earlier the stenotic valve opens and vice versa.

Early diastolic sounds are not confined to the opening snap of rheumatic mitral stenosis. In 1842, Dominic Corrigan, in a presentation to the Pathological Society of Dublin, described a "very loud bruit de frappement" in a patient with chronic constrictive pericarditis.[98] In French, "frapper" means "to knock," implying that Corrigan's "bruit de frappement" was what has come to be known as the pericardial "knock" of chronic constrictive pericarditis.[99] The term "knock" has also been applied to an early diastolic sound in pure severe mitral regurgitation with reduced left ventricular compliance. Both Corrigan's "pericardial knock" and the "knock" of mitral regurgitation are rapid filling sounds that are early and loud because a high-pressure atrium rapidly decompresses across an unobstructed AV valve into a recipient ventricle whose compliance is impaired.

Early diastolic sounds are sometimes caused by atrial myxomas.[100] The generation of such a sound, called a tumor "plop," requires a mobile myxoma attached to the atrial septum by a long stalk. The "plop" is believed to result from abrupt diastolic seating of the tumor within the right or left AV orifice.[100]

An early diastolic sound is generated by the opening movement of a mechanical prosthesis in the mitral location. This opening sound is especially prominent with a ball-in-cage prosthesis (Starr-Edwards) and less prominent with a tilting disc prosthesis (Björk-Shiley).

Mid-Diastolic and Late Diastolic (Presystolic) Sounds

Mid-diastolic sounds are, for all practical purposes, either normal or abnormal third heart sounds, and most if not all late diastolic or presystolic sounds are fourth heart sounds (Fig. 2–24). Each sound coincides with its relevant diastolic filling phase.[101] In sinus rhythm, the ventricles receive blood during two filling phases (Fig. 2–24). The first phase occurs when ventricular pressure drops sufficiently to allow the AV valve to open; blood then flows from atrium into ventricle. This flow coincides with the y descent of the atrial pressure pulse (Fig. 2–24) and is designated the "rapid filling phase," accounting for about 80 per cent of normal ventricular filling. The rapid filling phase is not a passive event in which the recipient ventricle merely expands in response to augmented inflow volume. Rather, ventricular relaxation is an active, complex, energy-dependent process.

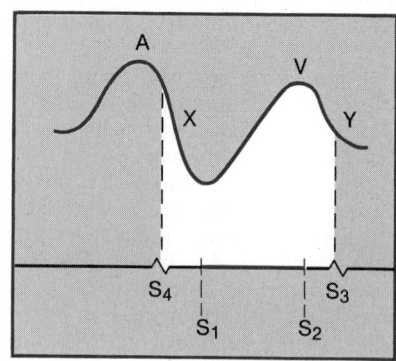

FIGURE 2–24. Atrial pressure pulse showing the *a* wave and *x* descent, and the *v* wave and *y* descent. The fourth heart sound (S$_4$) coincides with the phase of ventricular filling following atrial contraction. The third heart sound (S$_3$) coincides with the y descent (the phase of rapid ventricular filling). S$_1$ = First heart sound; S$_2$ = second heart sound.

The sound generated during the rapid filling phase is called the third heart sound (Fig. 2–24).[102] The second filling phase—diastasis—is variable in duration, usually accounting for less than 5 per cent of ventricular filling. The third phase of diastolic filling is in response to atrial contraction, which accounts for about 15 per cent of normal ventricular filling. The sound generated during the atrial filling phase is called the fourth heart sound (Fig. 2–24). Third and fourth heart sounds occur *within* the recipient ventricle as that chamber receives blood. Potain in 1876 attributed the third heart sound to sudden cessation of distention of the ventricle in early diastole, and he attributed the fourth heart sound to ". . . the abruptness with which the dilatation of the ventricle takes place during the presystolic period, a period which corresponds to the contraction of the auricle."[103] On both counts, he was not far from the mark.

The addition of either a third or a fourth heart sound to the cardiac cycle produces a *triple* rhythm. If both third *and* fourth heart sounds are present, a *quadruple* rhythm is produced. When diastole is short or the PR interval long, third and fourth heart sounds occur synchronously to form a summation sound.[2]

Children and young adults often have normal (physiological) *third* heart sounds but do not have normal fourth heart sounds.[104] Normal third heart sounds sometimes persist beyond age 40 years, especially in women.[105] After that age, however, especially in men, the third heart sound is likely to be abnormal.[106] Fourth heart sounds are sometimes heard in healthy older adults without clinical evidence of heart disease, particularly after exercise.[107] Such observations have led to the conclusion, still debated, that these fourth heart sounds are normal for age.

Because a fourth heart sound requires active atrial contribution to ventricular filling, the sound disappears when coordinated atrial contraction ceases, as in atrial fibrillation. When the atria and ventricles contract independently as in complete heart block (Fig. 2–16), fourth heart sounds or summation sounds occur randomly in diastole because the relationship between the P wave and the QRS of the electrocardiogram is random. Third and fourth heart sounds are events of ventricular filling, so obstruction of an AV valve, by impeding ventricular inflow, removes one of the prime preconditions for the generation of these filling sounds. Accordingly, the presence of a third or fourth heart sound implies an unobstructed (or relatively unobstructed) AV orifice on the side of the heart in which the sound originates. *Right ventricular* third or fourth heart sounds often respond selectively and distinctively to respiration, becoming more prominent during inspiration.[2] The inspiratory increase in right atrial flow is converted into an inspiratory augmentation of both mid-diastolic and presystolic filling.

Third and fourth heart sounds, either normal or abnormal, are relatively low-frequency events that vary considerably in intensity (loudness), that originate in either the left or right ventricle, and that are best elicited when the bell of the stethoscope is applied with just enough pressure to provide a skin seal. Left ventricular third and fourth heart sounds should be sought over the left ventricular impulse so identified with the patient in the left lateral decubitus position. Right ventricular third and fourth heart sounds should be sought over the right ventricular impulse (lower left sternal edge, occasionally subxiphoid) with the patient supine. An understanding of these simple principles sets the stage for bedside detection. The same principles can be used with advantage to distinguish a fourth heart sound preceding a single first heart sound from splitting of the two components of the first heart sound (Fig. 2–15C). The two components of the first heart sound are similar in frequency (pitch) although not in intensity (loudness), but differ in pitch from a preceding fourth heart sound. Selective pressure with the bell of the stethoscope enhances these distinctions.

Audibility of third heart sounds is improved by isotonic exercise that augments venous return and mid-diastolic AV flow. A few sit-ups usually suffice to produce the desired increase in venous return and acceleration in heart rate that increase the rate and volume of AV flow. Venous return can be increased by simple passive raising of both legs with the patient supine. The heart rate is also transiently increased by vigorous coughing. Left ventricular fourth heart sounds, especially in patients with ischemic heart disease, can be induced or augmented when resistance to left ventricular discharge is increased by sustained handgrip (isometric exercise, see later).

In the presence of sinus tachycardia, atrial contraction may coincide with the rapid filling phase, making it im-

possible to determine whether a given filling sound is a third heart sound, a fourth heart sound, or a summation sound. Carotid sinus massage transiently slows the heart rate, so the diastolic sound or sounds can be assigned their proper timing in the cardiac cycle.[2]

CAUSES OF THIRD AND FOURTH SOUNDS. The normal *third* heart sound is believed to be caused by sudden limitation of longitudinal expansion of the left ventricular wall during early diastolic filling.[108–111] The majority of *abnormal* third heart sounds are generated by altered physical properties of the recipient ventricle and/or an increase in the rate and volume of AV flow during the rapid filling phase of the cardiac cycle.[112] Abnormal *fourth* heart sounds occur when augmented atrial contraction generates presystolic ventricular distention (an increase in end-diastolic segment length) so that the recipient chamber can contract with greater force.[113,114] Typical substrates are the left ventricular hypertrophy of aortic stenosis or systemic hypertension in the left side of the heart,[115] or the right ventricular hypertrophy of pulmonary stenosis or pulmonary hypertension in the right side of the heart (Fig. 2–25).[113] Fourth heart sounds are also common in ischemic heart disease and are almost universal during angina pectoris or acute myocardial infarction because the atrial "booster pump" is needed to assist the relatively stiff ischemic ventricle.

A variation on the theme is the presystolic pacemaker sound.[116] A pacemaker electrode in the apex of the right ventricle may produce a presystolic sound that is relatively high-pitched and clicking and therefore different in pitch from a fourth heart sound. The presystolic pacemaker sound is believed to be extracardiac, resulting from contraction of chest wall muscle following spread of the electrical impulse from the pacemaker site.[116,117]

HEART MURMURS

According to O. H. Perry Pepper, *murmur* is a Latin word with probable onomatopoetic origins.[118] A cardiovascular murmur is a series of auditory vibrations that are more prolonged than a sound and are characterized according to intensity (loudness), frequency (pitch), configuration (shape), quality, duration, direction of radiation, and timing in the cardiac cycle. When these features are established, the stage is set for diagnostic conclusions that can be drawn from a murmur of a given description.

Intensity or loudness is graded from one to six, based upon the original recommendations of Samuel A. Levine in 1933.[119] A grade 1 murmur is so faint that it is heard only with special effort. A grade 2 is soft but readily detected; a grade 3 murmur is prominent but not loud; a grade 4 murmur is loud (and usually palpable); a grade 5 murmur is very loud. A grade 6 murmur is loud enough to be heard with the stethoscope just removed from contact with the chest wall. Frequency or pitch varies from high to low. The configuration or shape of a systolic murmur is best characterized as crescendo, decrescendo, crescendo-decrescendo (diamond-shaped), plateau (even), or variable (uneven). The duration of a murmur varies from short to long, with all gradations in between. A loud murmur radiates from its site of maximal intensity, and the direction of radiation is sometimes diagnostically useful. The timing of murmurs within the cardiac cycle is the basis for the following classification.

There are three categories of murmurs—systolic, diastolic, and continuous. A *systolic* murmur begins with or after the first heart sound and ends at or before the subsequent second heart sound on its side of origin. A *diastolic* murmur begins with or after the second heart sound and ends before the subsequent first heart sound. A *continuous* murmur begins in systole and continues without interruption through the timing of the second heart sound into all or part of diastole. The following classification of murmurs

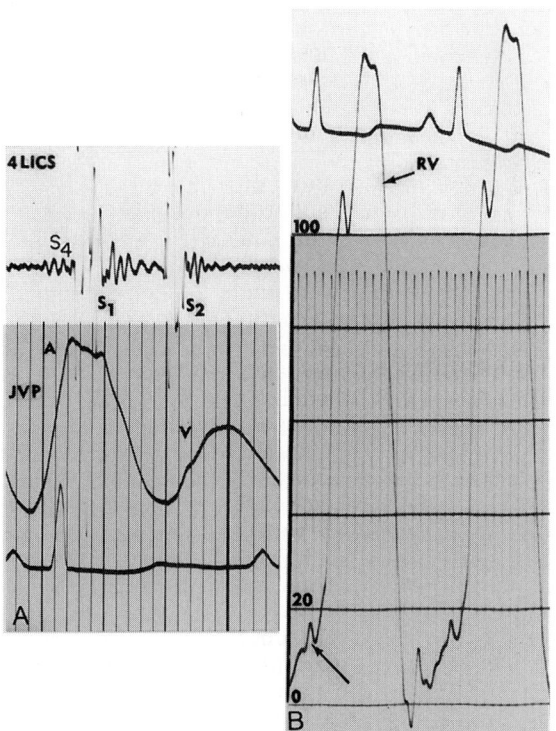

FIGURE 2–25. Tracings from an 18-year-old man with primary pulmonary hypertension. A, The phonocardiogram from the fourth left intercostal space (4LICS) shows a fourth heart sound (S_4). The jugular venous pulse (JVP) exhibits a prominent *a* wave. (S_1 = First heart sound; S_2 = second heart sound). B, The increased force of right atrial contraction, reflected in the large jugular venous *a* wave, results in presystolic distention (arrow) of the right ventricle (RV).

is based upon their timing relative to the first and second heart sounds.

Systolic Murmurs

Systolic murmurs are classified according to their time of onset and termination as midsystolic, holosystolic, early systolic, or late systolic (Fig. 2–26). A midsystolic murmur begins after the first heart sound and ends perceptibly before the second sound. The termination of a systolic murmur must be related to the relevant component of the second heart sound (Fig. 2–26). Accordingly, midsystolic murmurs originating in the *left* side of the heart end before the *aortic* component of the second heart sound; midsystolic murmurs originating in the *right* side of the heart end before the *pulmonary* component of the second sound. A *holosystolic* murmur begins with the first heart sound, occupies all of systole, and ends with the second heart sound on its side of origin. Holosystolic murmurs originating in the *left* side of the heart end with the *aortic* component of the second heart sound, and holosystolic murmurs originating in the *right* side of the heart end with the *pulmonary* component of the second sound.

The term "regurgitant systolic murmur," originally applied to murmurs that occupied all of systole,[69] has fallen out of use because "regurgitation" can be accompanied by holosystolic, midsystolic, early systolic, or late systolic murmurs.[2] Similarly, the term "ejection systolic murmur," originally applied to midsystolic murmurs, should be discarded, because midsystolic murmurs are not necessarily due to "ejection."[2]

MIDSYSTOLIC MURMURS. Midsystolic murmurs occur in five settings: (1) obstruction to ventricular outflow, (2) dilatation of the aortic root or pulmonary trunk, (3) accelerated

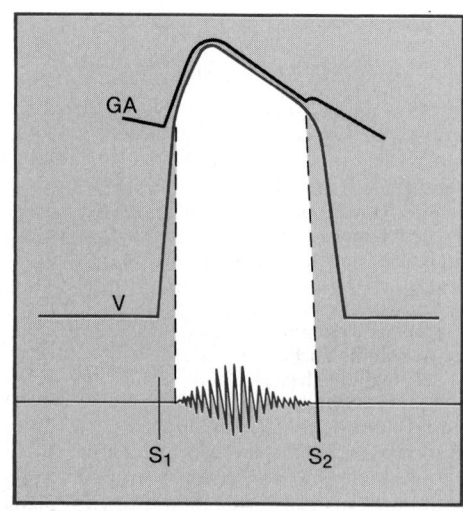

FIGURE 2–27. Illustration of the physiological mechanism of a midsystolic murmur generated by phasic flow into aortic root or pulmonary trunk. Ventricular (V) and great arterial (GA) pressure pulses are shown with phonocardiogram. The midsystolic murmur begins after the first heart sound (S₁), rises in crescendo to a peak as flow proceeds, then declines in decrescendo as flow diminishes, ending just before the second heart sound (S₂) as ventricular pressure falls below the pressure in the great artery.

systolic flow into the aorta or pulmonary trunk, (4) innocent (normal) midsystolic murmurs, and (5) some forms of mitral regurgitation. The physiological mechanism of *outflow* midsystolic murmurs reflects the pattern of phasic flow across the left or right ventricular outflow tract as originally described by Leatham (Fig. 2–27).[69] Isovolumetric contraction generates the first heart sound. Ventricular pressure rises, the semilunar valve opens, flow commences, and the murmur begins. As flow proceeds, the murmur increases in crescendo; as flow decreases, the murmur decreases in decrescendo. The murmur ends before ventricular pressure drops below the pressure in the central great artery, at which time the aortic and pulmonary valves close, generating the aortic and pulmonary components of the second heart sound.

Aortic valve stenosis is associated with a prototypical midsystolic murmur, which may have an early systolic peak and a short duration, a relatively late peak and a prolonged duration, or all gradations in between. Whether long or short, however, the murmur remains a symmetrical diamond beginning after the first heart sound (or with an aortic ejection sound), rising in crescendo to a systolic peak, and declining in decrescendo to end before the aortic component of the second heart sound. The high-velocity jet within the aortic root results in radiation of the murmur upward, to the right (second right intercostal space), and into the neck. An important variation occurs in older adults with previously normal trileaflet aortic valves rendered sclerotic or stenotic by fibrocalcific changes.[120] The accompanying murmur in the second right intercostal space is harsh, noisy, and impure, whereas the murmur over the left ventricular impulse is pure and often musical (Fig. 2–28). These two distinctive midsystolic murmurs—the noisy right basal and the musical apical—were described in 1925 by Gallavardin,[121] and the designation "Gallavardin dissociation" is still used. The impure right basal component of the murmur originates within the aortic root because of turbulence caused by the high-velocity jet. The pure musical component of the murmur heard over the left ventricular impulse originates from periodic high-frequency vibrations of the fibrocalcific aortic cusps (Fig. 2–29). The musical apical midsystolic murmur is sometimes dramatically loud. William Stokes (1855) reported that such a murmur was heard at a distance of 3 feet from the

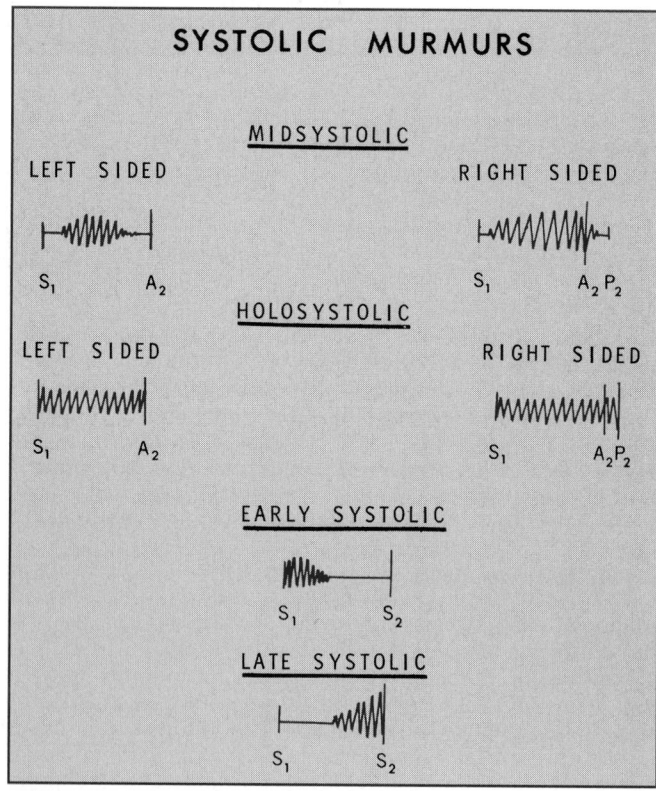

FIGURE 2–26. Systolic murmurs as illustrated here are descriptively classified according to their time of onset and termination as midsystolic, holosystolic, early systolic, and late systolic. The termination of the murmur must be related to the component of the second heart sound on its side of origin, that is, the aortic component (A₂) for systolic murmurs originating in the left side of the heart and the pulmonary component (P₂) for systolic murmurs originating in the right side of the heart.

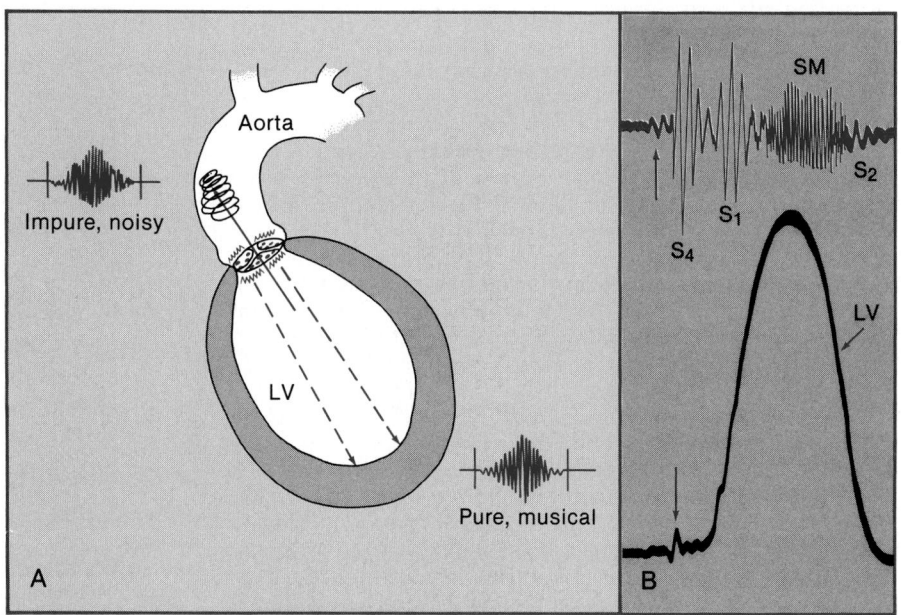

FIGURE 2–28. *A*, Illustration of "Gallavardin dissociation" of the basal and apical murmurs associated with a fibrocalcific trileaflet aortic valve in older adults. The impure, noisy midsystolic murmur at the right base originates within the aortic root because of turbulence caused by the high-velocity jet. The pure, musical midsystolic murmur at the apex results from high-frequency vibrations originating in the fibrocalcific but mobile aortic cusps and radiates selectively into the left ventricular cavity (LV). *B*, Left ventricular intracardiac phonocardiogram of an older adult with calcific aortic stenosis on a previously normal trileaflet valve. The pure, musical midsystolic murmur (SM) is recorded over the apex of the left ventricle (LV). A prominent fourth heart sound (S$_4$) coincides with presystolic distention of the left ventricle (lower vertical arrow). Upper vertical arrow identifies inaudible low-frequency vibrations preceding the fourth heart sound. S$_1$ = First heart sound; S$_2$ = second heart sound.

chest, and "this gentleman once observed to me that his entire body was one humming top."[122]

The high-frequency apical midsystolic murmur of aortic sclerosis or stenosis should be distinguished from the high-frequency apical murmur of mitral regurgitation, a distinction that may be difficult or impossible, especially if the aortic component of the second heart sound is soft or absent. However, when premature ventricular contractions are followed by pauses longer than the dominant cycle length, the apical midsystolic murmur of aortic stenosis or sclerosis increases in intensity in the beat following the premature contraction, whereas the intensity of the murmur of mitral regurgitation (whether midsystolic or holosystolic) remains relatively unchanged.[115] The same patterns hold following longer cycle lengths in atrial fibrillation. The validity of these observations assumes that aortic and mitral murmurs do not coexist at the apex.

The murmur of *pulmonary valve stenosis* is prototypical of a midsystolic murmur originating in the *right* side of the heart.[75] The murmur begins after the first heart sound or with a pulmonary ejection sound, rises in crescendo to a peak, then decreases in a slower decrescendo to end before a delayed or soft pulmonary component of the second heart sound (Fig. 2–19*A*). The length and configuration of the murmur are useful signs of the degree of obstruction.[75] The relative durations of right and left ventricular systole can be compared by relating the end of the pulmonary stenotic murmur (right-sided event) to the timing of the *aortic* component of the second heart sound (left-sided event) (Fig. 2–19*A*).

Short, soft midsystolic murmurs originate within a dilated aortic root or dilated pulmonary trunk. Midsystolic murmurs are also generated by rapid ejection into a *normal* aortic root or pulmonary trunk, as during pregnancy, fever, thyrotoxicosis, or anemia. The pulmonary midsystolic murmur of ostium secundum atrial septal defect results from *rapid* ejection into a *dilated* pulmonary trunk (Fig. 2–22). *Normal* (innocent) systolic murmurs are, except for the systolic mammary souffle, all midsystolic.[75]

The normal vibratory midsystolic murmur described by George Still in 1909[123] is short, buzzing, pure, and medium-frequency (Fig. 2–30) and is believed to be generated by low-frequency periodic vibrations of normal pulmonary leaflets at their attachments or periodic vibrations of a left ventricular false tendon. A second type of innocent midsystolic murmur occurs in children, adolescents, and young adults and represents an exaggeration of normal ejection vibrations within the pulmonary trunk. This normal pulmonary midsystolic murmur is relatively impure and is best heard in the second left intercostal space, in contrast to the vibratory midsystolic murmur of Still, which is typi-

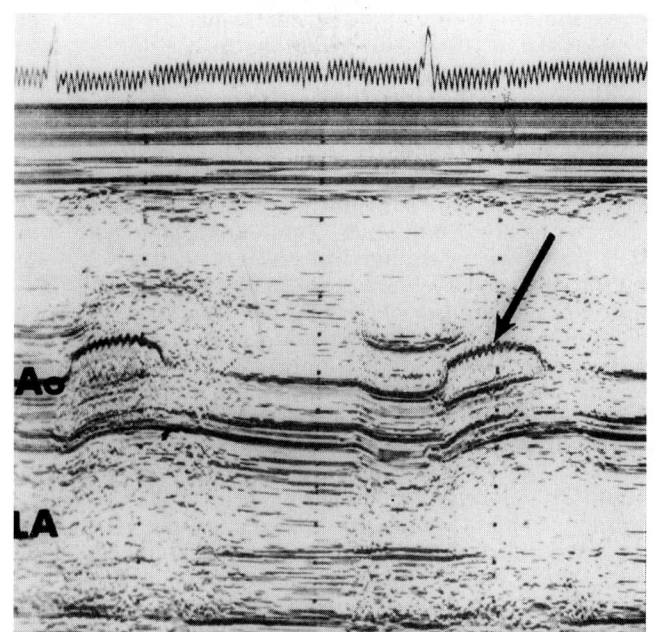

FIGURE 2–29. M-mode echocardiogram illustrating pure frequency vibrations of an open fibrocalcific mildly stenotic aortic valve (Ao) in a 64-year-old male with an apical musical midsystolic murmur of "Gallavardin dissociation" (see Fig. 2–28). LA = Left atrium.

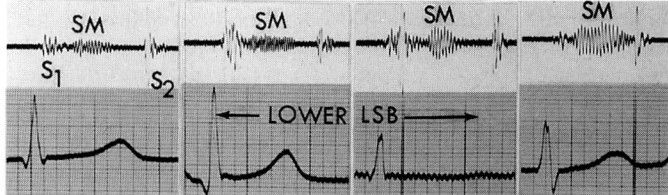

FIGURE 2–30. Four vibratory midsystolic murmurs (SM) from healthy children. These murmurs, designated "Still's murmur," are pure, medium frequency, relatively brief in duration, and maximal along the lower left sternal border (LSB). The last of the four murmurs was from a 5-year-old girl who was febrile. Following defervescence, the murmur decreased in loudness and duration.

cally heard between the lower left sternal edge and apex.[65] Normal pulmonary midsystolic murmurs are also heard in patients with diminished anteroposterior chest dimensions (loss of thoracic kyphosis, for example).[94]

The most common form of "innocent" midsystolic murmur in older adults has been designated the *"aortic sclerotic"* murmur (see above). The cause of this functionally benign murmur is fibrous or fibrocalcific thickening of the bases of otherwise normal aortic cusps as they insert into the sinuses of Valsalva.[75] As long as the fibrous or fibrocalcific thickening is confined to the *base* of the leaflets, the free edges remain mobile. No commissural fusion and no obstruction occurs. The Gallavardin dissociation phenomenon associated with such an aortic valve was described earlier.

It is not uncommon for *mitral regurgitation* to generate a midsystolic murmur.[90,124] The clinical setting is usually ischemic heart disease associated with left ventricular regional wall motion abnormalities. The physiological mechanism responsible for the midsystolic murmur of mitral regurgitation in this setting reflects impaired integrity of the muscular component of the mitral apparatus, with early systolic competence of the valve, midsystolic incompetence, followed by a late systolic decline in regurgitant flow. In any event, these midsystolic murmurs are unrelated to "ejection."

HOLOSYSTOLIC MURMURS.   Just as the term "midsystolic" is preferable to "ejection" systolic, the term "holosystolic" is preferable to "regurgitant" because holosystolic murmurs are not necessarily due to regurgitant flow. A holosystolic murmur begins with the first heart sound and occupies all of systole (Gr. *holos* = entire) up to the second sound on its side of origin (Fig. 2–26).[69] Such murmurs are generated by flow from a vascular bed whose pressure or resistance throughout systole is higher than the pressure or resistance in the vascular bed receiving the flow. Holosystolic murmurs occur in the left side of the heart with mitral regurgitation, in the right side of the heart with high-pressure tricuspid regurgitation, between the ventricles through a restrictive ventricular septal defect, and between the great arteries through aortopulmonary connections.

The timing of holosystolic murmurs within the framework established by the first and second heart sounds reflects the physiological and anatomical mechanisms responsible for their genesis. Figure 2–31 illustrates the mechanism of the holosystolic murmur of mitral regurgitation or high-pressure tricuspid regurgitation. Ventricular pressure exceeds atrial pressure at the very onset of systole (isovolumetric contraction), so regurgitant flow begins with the first heart sound. The murmur persists up to or slightly beyond the relevant component of the second heart sound, provided that ventricular pressure at end-systole exceeds atrial pressure and provided that the AV valve remains incompetent.

Direction of radiation of the intraatrial jet of mitral regurgitation determines the chest wall distribution of the murmur.[90,125] When the direction of the intraatrial jet is forward and medial against the atrial septum near the origin of the aorta, the murmur radiates to the left sternal edge, to the base, and even into the neck (Fig. 2–32). When the flow generating the murmur of mitral regurgitation is directed posterolaterally within the left atrial cavity, the murmur radiates to the axilla, to the angle of the left scapula, and occasionally to the vertebral column, with bone conduction from the cervical to the lumbar spine (Fig. 2–32).

The *murmur of tricuspid regurgitation* is holosystolic when there is a substantial elevation of right ventricular systolic pressure, as schematically illustrated in Figure 2–31. A distinctive and diagnostically important feature of the tricuspid murmur is its selective inspiratory increase in loudness—Carvallo's sign (Fig. 2–20).[126] The tricuspid murmur is occasionally audible only during inspiration. The increase in intensity occurs because the inspiratory

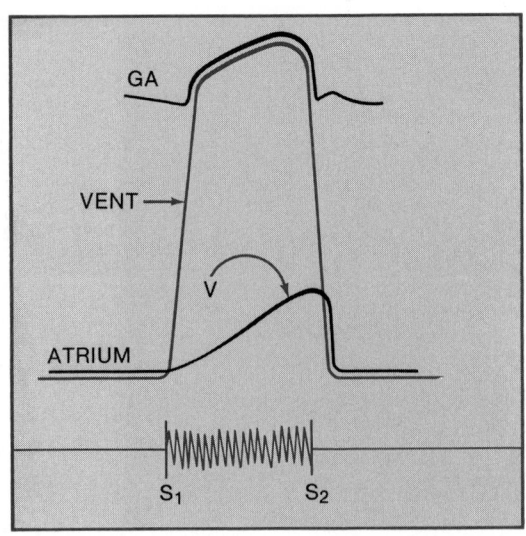

FIGURE 2–31.   Illustration of great arterial (GA), ventricular (VENT), and atrial pressure pulses with phonocardiogram showing the physiological mechanism of a holosystolic murmur in some forms of mitral regurgitation and in high-pressure tricuspid regurgitation. Ventricular pressure exceeds atrial pressure at the very onset of systole, so regurgitant flow and murmur commence with the first heart sound (S_1). The murmur persists up to or slightly beyond the second heart sound (S_2) because regurgitation persists to the end of systole (ventricular pressure still exceeds atrial pressure). V = Atrial v wave.

augmentation in right ventricular volume is converted into an increase in stroke volume and in the velocity of regurgitant flow.[127] When the right ventricle fails, this capacity is lost, so Carvallo's sign vanishes.

The murmur of an uncomplicated restrictive ventricular septal defect is holosystolic because left ventricular systolic pressure and systemic resistance exceed right ventricular systolic pressure and pulmonary resistance from the onset to the end of systole. Holosystolic murmurs are perceived as such in patients with large aortopulmonary connections (aortopulmonary window, patent ductus arteriosus) when a rise in pulmonary vascular resistance abolishes the diastolic portion of the continuous murmur, leaving a murmur that is holosystolic or nearly so.[75]

EARLY SYSTOLIC MURMURS.   Murmurs confined to early systole begin with the first heart sound, diminish in decrescendo, and end well before the second heart sound, generally at or before midsystole (Fig. 2–26). Certain types of mitral regurgitation, tricuspid regurgitation, or ventricular septal defects are the substrates.

Acute severe mitral regurgitation is accompanied by an early systolic murmur or a holosystolic murmur that is decrescendo, diminishing if not ending before the second heart sound (Fig. 2–33*A*).[128-130] The physiological mechanism responsible for this early systolic decrescendo murmur is acute severe regurgitation into a relatively normal-sized left atrium with limited distensibility. A steep rise in left atrial v wave approaches the left ventricular pressure at end-systole; a late systolic decline in left ventricular pressure favors this tendency (Fig. 2–33*B*). The stage is set for regurgitant flow that is maximal in early systole and minimal in late systole. The systolic murmur parallels this pattern, declining or vanishing before the second heart sound.

An early systolic murmur is a feature of tricuspid regurgitation with *normal* right ventricular systolic pressure.[131] An example is tricuspid regurgitation caused by infective endocarditis in drug abusers. The mechanisms responsible for the timing and configuration of the early systolic murmur of low-pressure tricuspid regurgitation are analogous to those just described for mitral regurgitation. The crest of the right atrial v wave reaches the level of normal right ventricular pressure in latter systole; the regurgitation and murmur are therefore chiefly, if not exclusively, *early* systolic. These murmurs are of medium frequency because

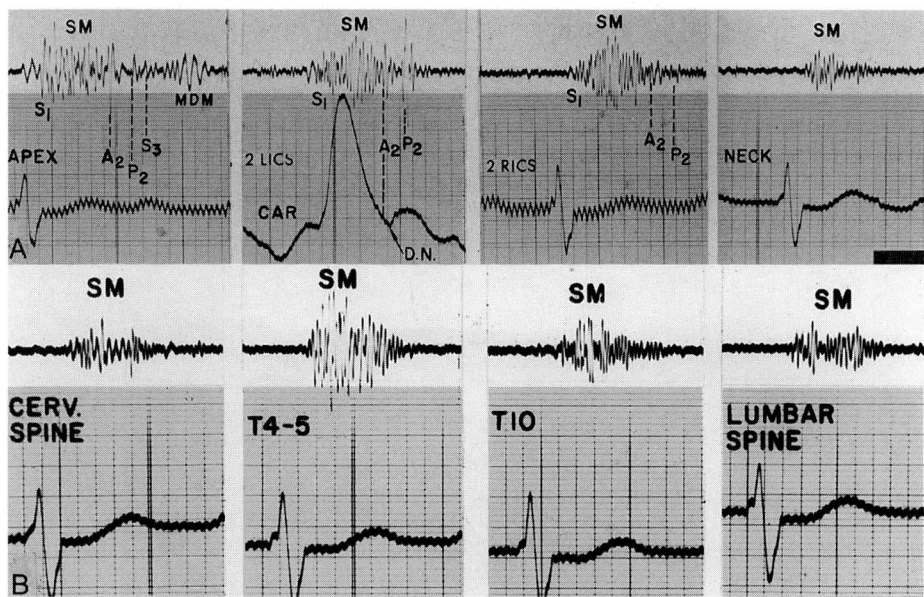

FIGURE 2–32. Phonocardiograms illustrating wide radiation of the murmur of mitral regurgitation. *A,* The holosystolic murmur (SM) radiates from the apex to the second left intercostal space (2LICS) to the second right intercostal space (2RICS) and into the neck. S_1 = First heart sound; A_2 = aortic component of the second sound; P_2 = pulmonary component of the second sound; S_3 = third heart sound; MDM = mid-diastolic murmur; CAR = carotid pulse; DN = dicrotic notch. *B,* The murmur of mitral regurgitation radiates to the cervical spine, down the thoracic spine (T4-5, T10) to the lumbar spine.

normal right ventricular systolic pressure generates comparatively low-velocity regurgitant flow in contrast to elevated right ventricular systolic pressure that generates a high-frequency holosystolic murmur (see earlier).

Early systolic murmurs also occur through ventricular septal defects, but under two widely divergent anatomical and physiological circumstances. A soft, pure, high-frequency, early systolic murmur localized to the mid- or lower left sternal edge is typical of a very small ventricular septal defect in which the shunt is confined to early systole.[75] A murmur of similar timing and configuration occurs through a nonrestrictive ventricular septal defect when an elevation in pulmonary vascular resistance decreases or abolishes late systolic shunting.[75]

LATE SYSTOLIC MURMURS. The term "late systolic" applies when a murmur begins in mid- to late systole and proceeds up to the second heart sound (Fig. 2–26). The late systolic murmur of *mitral valve prolapse* is prototypical (Fig. 2–33).[79,132] One or more mid- to late systolic clicks often introduce the murmur. The responses of the late systolic murmur and clicks to postural maneuvers (see earlier discussion) are illustrated in Figure 2–21. In response to a *diminution* in left ventricular volume, best achieved by prompt standing after squatting but also achieved by the Valsalva maneuver, the late systolic murmur becomes longer although softer.[79,82] In response to an *increase* in left ventricular volume associated with squatting or with sustained handgrip, the late systolic murmur becomes shorter but louder.[79,82] Pharmacological interventions that variably alter left ventricular volume, especially amyl nitrite (Fig. 2–34), produce analogous effects but are less practical at the bedside.

The late systolic murmur of mitral valve prolapse is occasionally replaced by an intermittent, striking, and sometimes disconcerting systolic whoop or honk, either spontaneously or in response to physical maneuvers.[79] The whoop is high-frequency, musical, widely transmitted, and

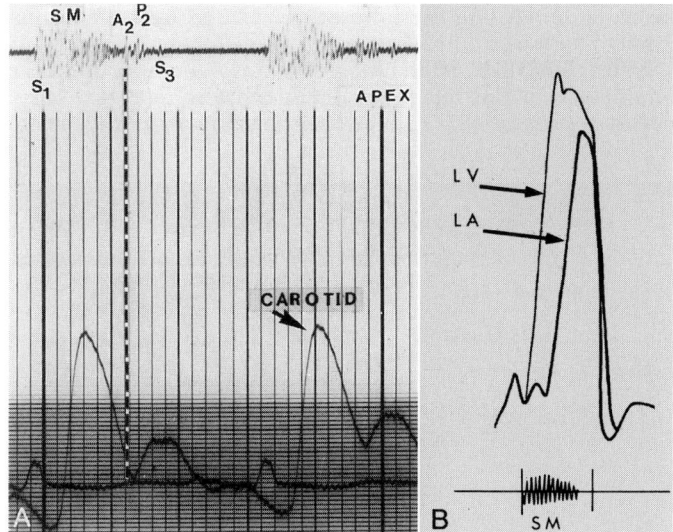

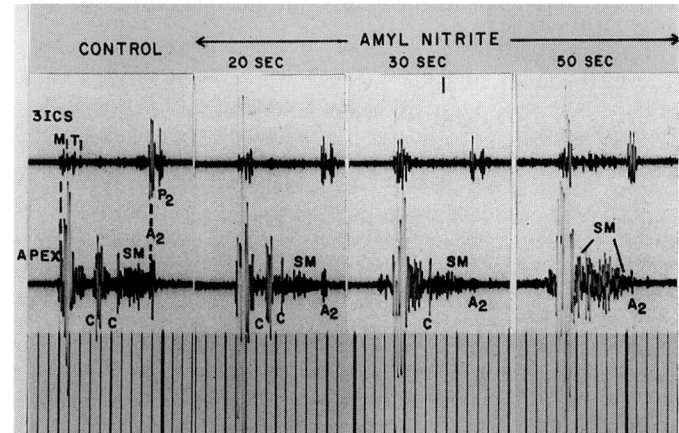

FIGURE 2–33. *A,* Phonocardiogram recorded from the cardiac apex of a patient with acute severe mitral regurgitation due to ruptured chordae tendineae. There is an early systolic decrescendo murmur (SM) diminishing if not ending before the aortic component (A_2) of the second heart sound. P_2 = Pulmonary component of the second heart sound; S_1 = first heart sound; S_3 = third heart sound. *B,* Left ventricular (LV) and left atrial (LA) pressure pulses with schematic illustration of the phonocardiogram showing the relationship between the decrescendo configuration of the early systolic murmur and late systolic approximation of the tall left atrial *v* wave and left ventricular end-systolic pressure. Regurgitant flow diminishes or ceases. The murmur therefore is early systolic and decrescendo, paralleling the hemodynamic pattern of regurgitation.

FIGURE 2–34. Phonocardiograms illustrating the response of the systolic clicks (C) and late systolic murmur (SM) of mitral valve prolapse to amyl nitrite inhalation. At 20 to 30 seconds, the clicks become earlier and the systolic murmur becomes longer but softer. At 50 seconds, the murmur is holosystolic and louder. M_1 = Mitral component of the first heart sound; T_1 = tricuspid component of the first heart sound; A_2 = aortic component of the second heart sound; P_2 = pulmonary component of the second sound.

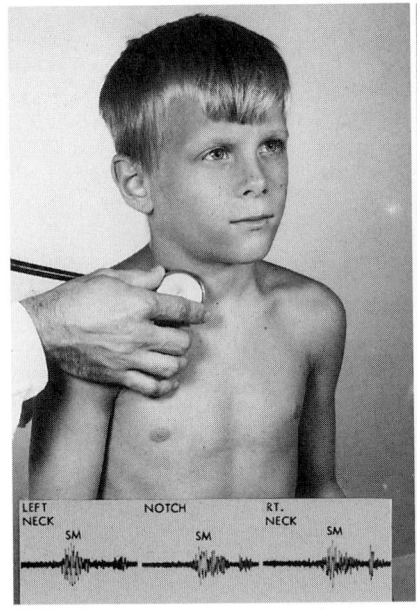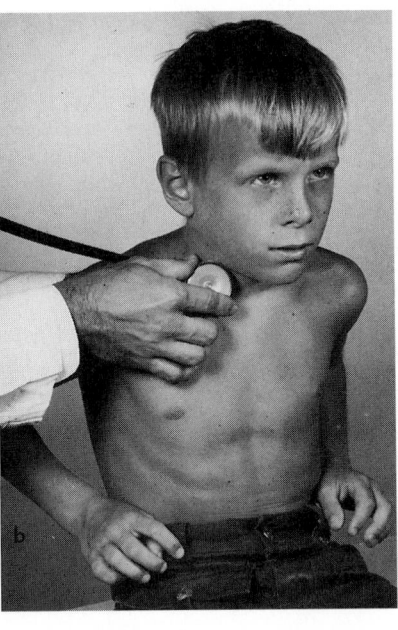

LEFT NECK   NOTCH   RT. NECK
SM   SM   SM

FIGURE 2–35. *Left*, Phonocardiogram showing a normal supraclavicular systolic arterial murmur maximal above the clavicles (left neck, right neck) and in the suprasternal notch. Auscultation is initially carried out while the patient sits with shoulders relaxed and arms resting in the lap. *Right*, When the elbows are brought well behind the back (hyperextension of the shoulders), the murmur markedly diminishes or disappears.

occasionally loud enough to be disturbing to the patient and sometimes to the physician.[133] The musical whoop is thought to arise from mitral leaflets and chordae tendineae set into high-frequency periodic vibration.

SYSTOLIC ARTERIAL MURMURS. Systolic murmurs can originate in anatomically normal arteries in the presence of normal or increased flow, or in abnormal arteries because of tortuosity or luminal narrowing. Detection of systolic arterial murmurs requires auscultation at nonprecordial sites. Timing with the first and second heart sounds is imprecise because the murmurs begin at variable distances from the heart. Nevertheless, the arterial murmurs dealt with here are essentially systolic and tend to have a crescendo-decrescendo configuration that reflects the rise and fall of pulsatile arterial flow.[2]

The "supraclavicular systolic murmur" (Fig. 2–35), often heard in children and adolescents, is believed to originate at the aortic origins of normal major brachiocephalic arteries.[75,134] The configuration of these murmurs is crescendo-decrescendo, the onset is abrupt, the duration is brief, and the intensity at times is surprisingly loud with radiation below the clavicles. Normal supraclavicular systolic murmurs decrease or vanish in response to hyperextension of the shoulders, which is achieved by bringing the elbows back until the shoulder girdle muscles are drawn taut (Fig. 2–35).[134]

In older adults, the most common cause of a systolic arterial murmur is atherosclerotic narrowing of a carotid, subclavian, or iliofemoral artery. A variation on this theme is the "compression artifact" that can be induced in the femoral artery in the presence of free aortic regurgitation. When the femoral artery is moderately compressed by the examiner's stethoscopic bell, a systolic arterial murmur is generated. Further compression causes the systolic murmur to continue into diastole, a sign described in 1861 by Duroziez.[75] The eponym is still in use.

A systolic "mammary souffle" is sometimes heard over the breasts because of increased flow through normal arteries during late pregnancy or more especially in the postpartum period in lactating women.[75,135] The murmur begins well after the first heart sound because of the interval between left ventricular ejection and arrival of flow at the artery of origin.

A systolic arterial murmur is present in the back between the scapulae over the site of coarctation of the aortic isthmus.[75] Transient systolic arterial murmurs originating in the pulmonary artery and its branches are occasionally heard in normal neonates because the angulation and disparity in size between the pulmonary trunk and its branches set the stage for turbulent systolic flow. These normal or innocent pulmonary arterial systolic murmurs disappear with maturation of the pulmonary bed, generally within the first few weeks or months of life.[75,136] Similar if not identical pulmonary arterial systolic murmurs are generated at sites of congenital stenosis of the pulmonary artery and its branches. Rarely, a pulmonary arterial systolic murmur is caused by luminal narrowing following a pulmonary embolus.[113]

Diastolic Murmurs

Diastolic murmurs are classified according to their time of *onset* as early diastolic, mid-diastolic, or late diastolic (presystolic) (Fig. 2–36). An *early* diastolic murmur begins with the aortic or pulmonary component of the second heart sound, depending upon its side of origin. A mid-diastolic murmur begins at a clear interval *after* the second heart sound. A late diastolic or presystolic murmur begins immediately before the first heart sound.

EARLY DIASTOLIC MURMURS. An early diastolic murmur originating in the left side of the heart is represented by *aortic regurgitation*. The murmur begins with the aortic

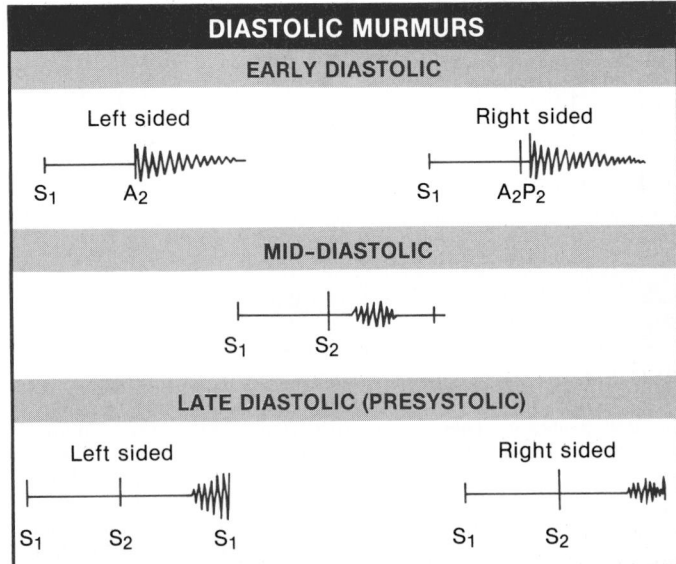

DIASTOLIC MURMURS

EARLY DIASTOLIC

Left sided   Right sided

S_1 A_2 S_1 A_2P_2

MID-DIASTOLIC

S_1 S_2

LATE DIASTOLIC (PRESYSTOLIC)

Left sided   Right sided

S_1 S_2 S_1 S_1 S_2

FIGURE 2–36. Diastolic murmurs are descriptively classified according to their time of *onset* as early diastolic, mid-diastolic, or late diastolic (presystolic). Diastolic murmurs originate in either the left or the right side of the heart.

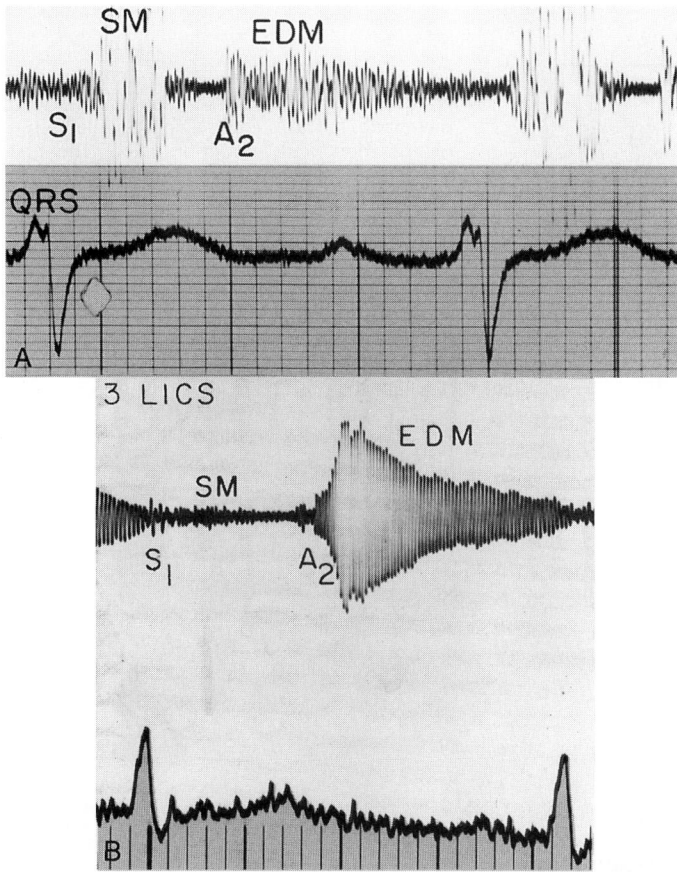

FIGURE 2–37. *A,* Phonocardiogram recorded from the mid-left sternal edge of a patient with chronic pure severe aortic regurgitation. An early diastolic murmur (EDM) proceeds immediately from the aortic component (A$_2$) of the second heart sound. The murmur has an early crescendo followed by a late long decrescendo. There is a prominent midsystolic flow murmur (SM) across an unobstructed aortic valve. S$_1$ = First heart sound. *B,* Phonocardiogram in the third left intercostal space (3LICS) records a high-frequency, musical, early diastolic decrescendo murmur (EDM) caused by eversion of an aortic cusp. S$_1$ = First heart sound; SM = midsystolic murmur; A$_2$ = aortic component of the second sound.

component of the second heart sound (Fig. 2–37*A*), i.e., as soon as left ventricular pressure falls below the aortic incisura. The configuration of the murmur tends to reflect the volume and rate of regurgitant flow. In chronic aortic regurgitation of moderate severity, the aortic diastolic pressure consistently and appreciably exceeds left ventricular diastolic pressure, so the decrescendo is subtle and the murmur is well heard throughout diastole. In chronic *severe* aortic regurgitation, the decrescendo is more obvious, paralleling the dramatic decline in aortic root diastolic pressure. Selective radiation of the murmur of aortic regurgitation to the *right* sternal edge implies aortic root dilatation, as in the Marfan syndrome. When an inverted cusp is set into high-frequency periodic vibration by aortic regurgitation, the accompanying murmur is musical, early diastolic, and decrescendo (Fig. 2–37*B*).

The diastolic murmur of *acute severe* aortic regurgitation differs importantly from the murmur of chronic severe aortic regurgitation as just described.[137] When regurgitant flow is both sudden *and* severe (bicuspid aortic valve infective endocarditis, aortic dissection), the diastolic murmur is relatively short because the aortic diastolic pressure rapidly equilibrates with the steeply rising diastolic pressure in the unprepared, nondilated left ventricle. The pitch of the murmur is likely to be medium rather than high because the velocity of regurgitant flow is less rapid than in chronic severe aortic regurgitation. This short, medium-frequency diastolic murmur of sudden severe aortic regurgitation may be disarmingly soft. These auscultatory features are in con-

trast to the long, pure, high-frequency, blowing early diastolic murmur of chronic severe aortic regurgitation (Fig. 2–37).

Early diastolic murmurs in the *right* side of the heart are represented by the Graham Steell murmur of pulmonary hypertensive pulmonary regurgitation described in 1888.[93] "I wish to plead for the admission among the recognized auscultatory signs of disease of a murmur due to . . . long-continuing excess blood pressure in the pulmonary artery. . . . When the second sound is reduplicated, the murmur proceeds from its latter part. That such a murmur as I have described does exist, there can, I think, be no doubt."[93]

The Graham Steell murmur begins with a loud *pulmonary* component of the second heart sound as Steell originally described (Fig. 2–20) because the elevated pressure exerted upon the incompetent pulmonary valve begins at the moment that right ventricular pressure drops below the pulmonary arterial incisura.[113] The high diastolic pressure generates high-velocity regurgitant flow and results in a high-frequency blowing murmur that may last throughout diastole. Because of the persistent and appreciable difference between pulmonary arterial and right ventricular diastolic pressures, the amplitude of the murmur is usually relatively uniform throughout most if not all of diastole.

MID-DIASTOLIC MURMURS. A mid-diastolic murmur begins at a clear interval after the second heart sound (Figs. 2–36 and 2–38). The majority of mid-diastolic murmurs originate across mitral or tricuspid valves during the rapid filling phase of the cardiac cycle (AV valve obstruction or abnormal patterns of AV flow) or across an incompetent pulmonary valve, provided that the pulmonary arterial pressure is not elevated.

The mid-diastolic murmur of rheumatic mitral stenosis is a prime example.[138,139] The murmur characteristically follows the mitral opening snap (Fig. 2–23*B*). Because the murmur originates within the left ventricular cavity, transmission to the chest wall is maximal over the left ventricular impulse. Care must be taken to place the bell of the stethoscope lightly against the skin precisely over the left ventricular impulse with the patient turned into the left lateral decubitus position (Fig. 2–14). Soft mid-diastolic murmurs are reinforced when the heart rate and mitral valve flow are transiently increased by vigorous voluntary coughs. In atrial fibrillation, the *duration* of the mid-diastolic murmur is a useful sign of the degree of obstruction at the mitral orifice (Fig. 2–38). A murmur that lasts up to the first heart sound even after long cycle lengths indicates that the stenosis is severe enough to generate a persistent gradient even at the end of long diastoles.

The mid-diastolic murmur of *tricuspid* stenosis occurs in the presence of atrial fibrillation. The tricuspid mid-diastolic murmur differs from the *mitral* mid-diastolic murmur in two important respects: (1) the loudness of the tricuspid murmur selectively and distinctively increases with inspiration; and (2) the tricuspid murmur is confined to a relatively localized area along the left lower sternal edge. The inspiratory increase in loudness occurs because inspiration is accompanied by an augmentation in right ventricular volume, by a fall in right ventricular diastolic pressure, and by an increase in gradient and flow rate across the stenotic tricuspid valve.[140] The murmur is localized to the lower left sternal edge because it originates within the inflow portion of the right ventricle and is transmitted to the overlying chest wall.

Mid-diastolic murmurs across *unobstructed* AV valves occur in the presence of augmented volume and velocity of flow. Examples in the left side of the heart are the mid-diastolic flow murmur of pure mitral regurgitation (Fig. 2–39) and the mid-diastolic mitral flow murmur that accompanies a large left-to-right shunt through a ventricular septal defect (Fig. 2–40*A*). Mid-diastolic murmurs due to augmented flow across unobstructed *tricuspid* valves are gen-

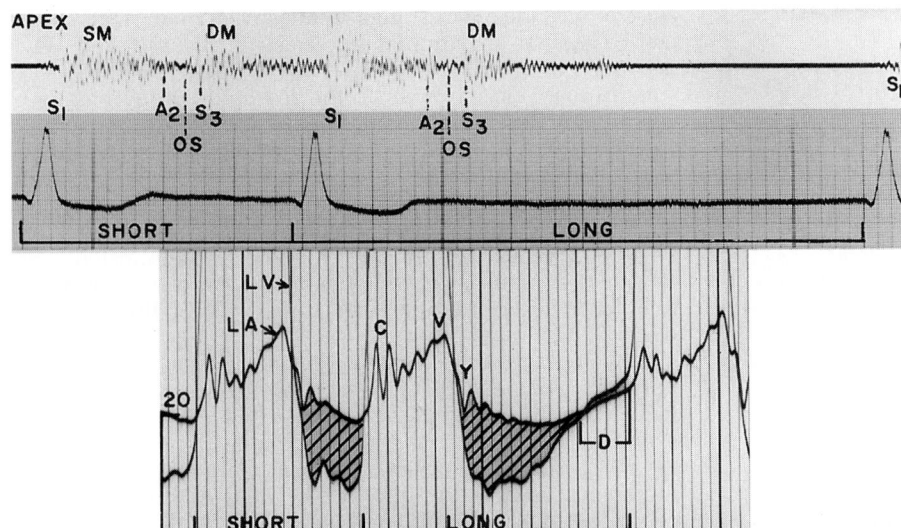

FIGURE 2-38. Tracings from a patient with rheumatic mitral stenosis, appreciable mitral regurgitation, and atrial fibrillation. The first heart sound (S_1) varies in intensity with cycle length. The aortic component of the second heart sound (A_2) is followed by a soft opening snap (OS), and a prominent third heart sound introduces a mid-diastolic murmur (DM). With a short cycle length, the murmur proceeds throughout diastole because there is an end-diastolic gradient between left atrium (LA) and left ventricle (LV). In the longer second cycle, the diastolic murmur ends, and the remainder of diastole is murmur-free, paralleling the equilibration of left atrial and left ventricular diastolic pressures (diastasis, D). C = c wave; V = v wave; Y = y descent.

FIGURE 2-39. Phonocardiogram recorded over the left ventricular impulse of a patient with pure mitral regurgitation. When regurgitant flow is augmented in response to a pressor amine, the holosystolic crescendo murmur (SM) becomes more prominent, and a mid-diastolic flow murmur (MDM) appears.

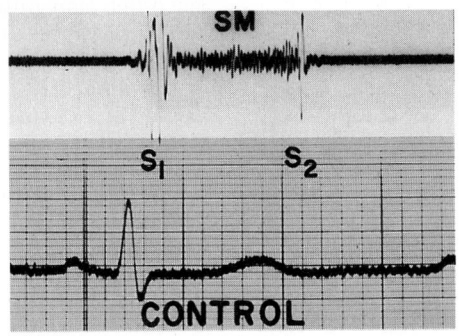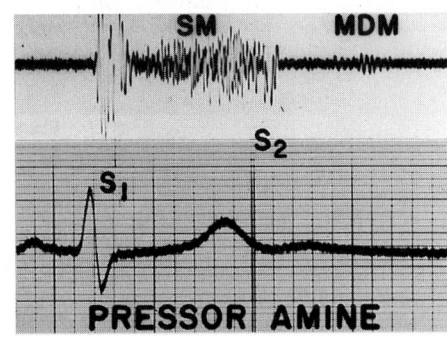

erated by severe tricuspid regurgitation or by a large left-to-right shunt through an atrial septal defect (Fig. 2–40B). These mid-diastolic murmurs indicate appreciable AV valve incompetence or large left-to-right shunts and are often preceded by third heart sounds, especially in the presence of mitral or tricuspid regurgitation.

Short, mid-diastolic AV flow murmurs occur intermittently in complete heart block when atrial contraction coincides with the phase of rapid diastolic filling (Fig. 2–16). These murmurs are believed to result from antegrade flow across AV valves that are closing rapidly during filling of the recipient ventricle.[138] A similar mechanism is believed

to be responsible for the Austin Flint murmur (Fig. 2–41), as Flint originally proposed (see below).[141-143]

A mid-diastolic murmur is a feature of pulmonary valve regurgitation, provided that the pulmonary arterial pressure is not elevated (Fig. 2–42A). The diastolic murmur typi-

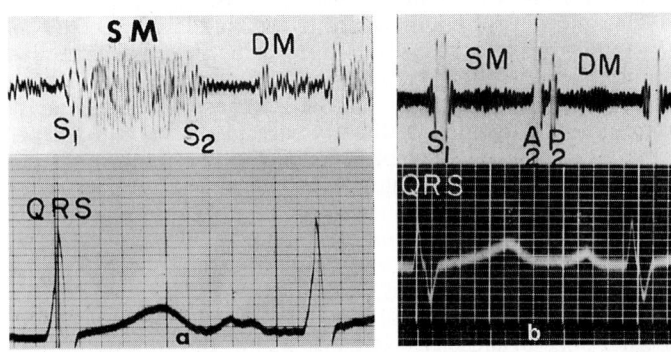

FIGURE 2-40. *a*, Phonocardiogram recorded at the apex of a patient with a moderately restrictive ventricular septal defect and increased pulmonary arterial blood flow. The mid-diastolic murmur (DM) results from augmented flow across the mitral valve. SM = Holosystolic murmur; S_1 = first heart sound; S_2 = second heart sound. *b*, Phonocardiogram at the lower left sternal edge of a patient with an ostium secundum atrial septal defect and increased pulmonary arterial blood flow. A mid-diastolic murmur (DM) resulted from augmented flow across the tricuspid valve. SM = Mid-systolic murmur; A_2 and P_2 = aortic and pulmonary components of a conspicuously split second heart sound.

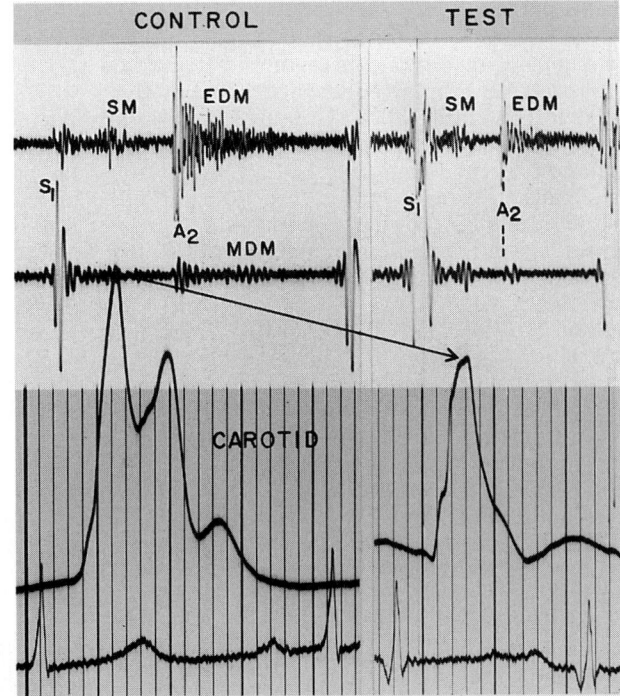

FIGURE 2-41. Phonocardiograms and simultaneous carotid pulse from a patient with chronic pure severe aortic regurgitation. Following amyl nitrite inhalation (test), the prominent early diastolic murmur (EDM) decreases, a mid-diastolic (MDM) Austin Flint murmur disappears, and the bisferiens carotid pulse becomes single-peaked.

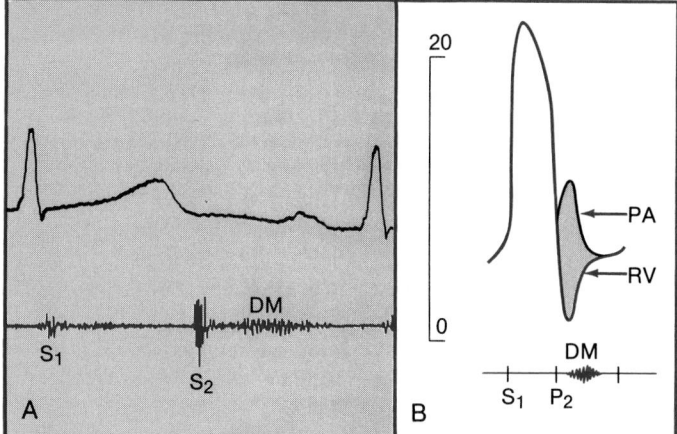

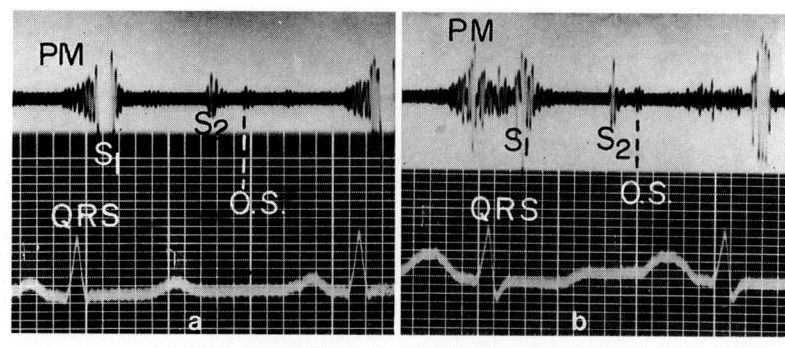

FIGURE 2–42. *A,* Phonocardiogram illustrating the mid-diastolic murmur (DM) of low-pressure pulmonary regurgitation in a heroin addict who had pulmonary valve infective endocarditis. The murmur begins well after the second heart sound (S_2), is medium-frequency and mid-diastolic, ending well before the subsequent first heart sound (S_1). *B,* Pressure pulses and phonocardiogram illustrate the physiological mechanism of the mid-diastolic murmur of low-pressure pulmonary regurgitation. Because the pressure exerted against the incompetent pulmonary valve is low, the murmur does not begin until well after the right ventricular (RV) and pulmonary arterial (PA) pressure pulses diverge. The murmur is maximal when the diastolic gradient *(cross-hatched area)* is greatest. Following an early diastolic dip in the RV pressure pulse, there is equilibration of the pulmonary arterial and right ventricular pressures in later diastole, so the regurgitant gradient is abolished and the murmur disappears.

cally begins at a perceptible interval after the pulmonary component of the second heart sound, is crescendo-decrescendo, ending well before the subsequent first heart sound.[75] The physiological mechanism responsible for the timing of this murmur is shown in Figure 2–42*B*. The diastolic pressure exerted upon the incompetent pulmonary valve is negligible at the inception of the pulmonary component of the second sound, so regurgitant flow is minimal. Regurgitation accelerates as right ventricular pressure dips below the diastolic pressure in the pulmonary trunk; at that point the murmur reaches its maximum (Fig. 2–42*B*). Late diastolic equilibration of pulmonary arterial and right ventricular pressures eliminates regurgitant flow and abolishes the murmur prior to the next first heart sound.

LATE DIASTOLIC OR PRESYSTOLIC MURMURS. A late diastolic murmur occurs immediately before the first heart sound, that is, in *presystole* (Fig. 2–26). With few exceptions, the late diastolic timing of the murmur coincides with the phase of ventricular filling that follows atrial systole and implies coordinated atrial contraction, generally sinus rhythm. Late diastolic or presystolic murmurs usually originate at the mitral or tricuspid orifice because of obstruction, but occasionally because of abnormal patterns of presystolic AV flow.

The best known presystolic murmur accompanies rheumatic mitral stenosis in sinus rhythm as AV flow is aug-

mented in response to an increase in the force of left atrial contraction (Figs. 2–23*B* and 2–43*A*).[96] "Presystolic" accentuation of a mid-diastolic murmur is occasionally heard in mitral stenosis with atrial fibrillation, especially during short cycle lengths,[144,145] but the timing is actually early systolic, and the mechanism differs from the true presystolic murmur as described above and as shown in Figure 2–43*A*.

In *tricuspid* stenosis with sinus rhythm, a late diastolic or presystolic murmur typically occurs in the absence of a perceptible mid-diastolic murmur (Fig. 2–43*B*). This is so because the timing of tricuspid diastolic murmurs reflects the maximal acceleration of flow and gradient, which is usually negligible until powerful right atrial contraction.[140] The presystolic murmur of tricuspid stenosis is crescendo-decrescendo and relatively discrete, fading before the first heart sound (Fig. 2–43*B*). This is in contrast to the presystolic murmur of mitral stenosis, which tends to rise in crescendo that is interrupted by the first heart sound (Fig. 2–43*A*). The most valuable auscultatory sign of tricuspid stenosis in sinus rhythm is the effect of respiration on the intensity of the presystolic murmur (Figs. 2–43 and 2–44). Inspiration increases right atrial volume, provoking an increase in right atrial contractile force that coincides with a fall in right ventricular end-diastolic pressure. The result is an increase in the tricuspid gradient, in the velocity of tricuspid flow, and in the intensity of the tricuspid stenotic presystolic murmur (Fig. 2–44).[140]

Short, crescendo-decrescendo presystolic murmurs are occasionally heard in *complete heart block* when atrial contraction falls in late diastole. However, the murmur is usually mid-diastolic, as already described, occurring when atrial contraction coincides with and reinforces the rapid filling phase of the cardiac cycle (Fig. 2–16).

In 1862, Austin Flint described a presystolic murmur in patients with aortic regurgitation and proposed a mechanism that was astonishingly perceptive.[141–143,146,147] "Now in cases of considerable aortic insufficiency, the left ventricle is rapidly filled with blood flowing back from the aorta as well as from the auricle, before the auricular contraction takes place. The distention of the ventricle is such that the mitral curtains are brought into coaptation, and when the auricular contraction takes place, the mitral direct current passing between the curtains throws them into vibration and gives rise to the characteristic blubbering murmur."[141]

Continuous Murmurs

The term "continuous" appropriately applies to murmurs that begin in systole and *continue* without interruption through the second heart sound into all or part of diastole (Fig. 2–45). The presence of murmurs throughout both phases of the cardiac cycle (holosystolic followed by holodiastolic) (Fig. 2–45) is not the criterion for the designation "continuous." Conversely, a murmur that fades completely before the subsequent first heart sound *is* continuous, provided that the systolic portion of the murmur proceeds without interruption through the second heart sound (Fig. 2–45).

FIGURE 2–43. *a,* Phonocardiogram from the cardiac apex of a patient with pure rheumatic mitral stenosis. A presystolic murmur (PM) rises in a crescendo that is interrupted by a loud first heart sound (S_1). S_2 = Second heart sound; OS = mitral opening snap. *b,* Phonocardiogram from the lower left sternal edge of a patient with rheumatic tricuspid stenosis. The first cycle is during inspiration and is accompanied by a prominent presystolic murmur (PM) that is crescendo-decrescendo, decreasing before the first heart sound (S_1). During exhalation (second cycle), the presystolic murmur all but vanishes.

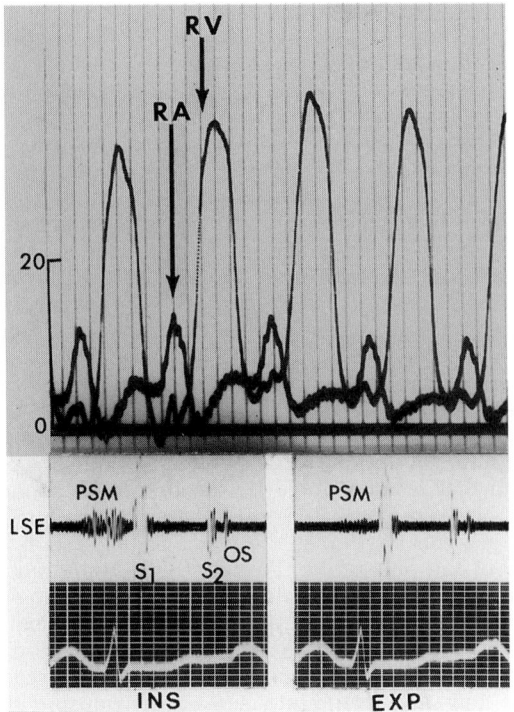

FIGURE 2–44. Pressure pulses and phonocardiogram illustrating the physiological mechanism of the respiratory variation in the presystolic murmur of tricuspid stenosis. During inhalation, a fall in intrathoracic pressure and an increase in systemic venous return result in an increase in the right atrial (RA) A wave and a decline in right ventricular (RV) end-diastolic pressure, so the presystolic murmur (PSM) increases in loudness. During exhalation, the right atrial A wave declines, the right ventricular diastolic pressure increases, the tricuspid gradient is at its minimum, and the presystolic murmur all but vanishes.

TABLE 2–3   DIFFERENTIAL DIAGNOSIS OF CONTINUOUS THORACIC MURMURS (IN ORDER OF FREQUENCY)

DIAGNOSIS	KEY FINDINGS
Cervical venous hum	Disappears on compression of the jugular vein
Hepatic venous hum	Often disappears with epigastric pressure
Mammary souffle	Disappears upon pressing hard with stethoscope
Patent ductus arteriosus	Loudest at 2nd left intercostal space
Coronary arteriovenous fistula	Loudest at lower sternal borders
Ruptured aneurysm of sinus of Valsalva	Loudest at upper right sternal border, sudden onset
Bronchial collaterals	Associated signs of congenital heart disease
High-grade coarctation	Brachial-pedal arterial pressure gradient
Anomalous left coronary artery arising from pulmonary artery	Electrocardiographic changes of myocardial infarction
Truncus arteriosus	
Pulmonary artery branch stenosis	Heard outside the area of cardiac dullness
Pulmonary AV fistula	Same as above
Atrial septal defect with mitral stenosis or atresia	Altered by the Valsalva maneuver
Aortic-atrial fistulas	

Adapted from Sapira, J. D.: The Art and Science of Bedside Diagnosis. Baltimore, Urban & Schwartzenberg, 1990.

Continuous murmurs are generated by uninterrupted flow from a vascular bed of higher pressure or resistance into a vascular bed of lower pressure or resistance without phasic interruption between systole and diastole. Such murmurs are due chiefly to (1) aortopulmonary connections, (2) arteriovenous connections, (3) disturbances of flow patterns in arteries, and (4) disturbances of flow patterns in veins.

The most celebrated continuous murmur is associated with the aortopulmonary connection of *patent ductus arteriosus* (Fig. 2–46). The murmur characteristically peaks just before and after the second heart sound which it envelops, decreases in late diastole—often appreciably, and may be soft or even absent before the subsequent first heart sound.[75] In 1847, the *London Medical Gazette* published the description of "a murmur accompanying the first heart sound . . . prolonged into the second sound so that there is no cessation of the murmur before the second sound had already commenced."[148] The author correctly assigned the cause of the murmur to patent ductus arteriosus and established the proper meaning of "continuous" as "no cessation of the murmur before the second sound had already commenced." George Gibson's description in 1900 was even more precise.[149] "It persists through the second sound

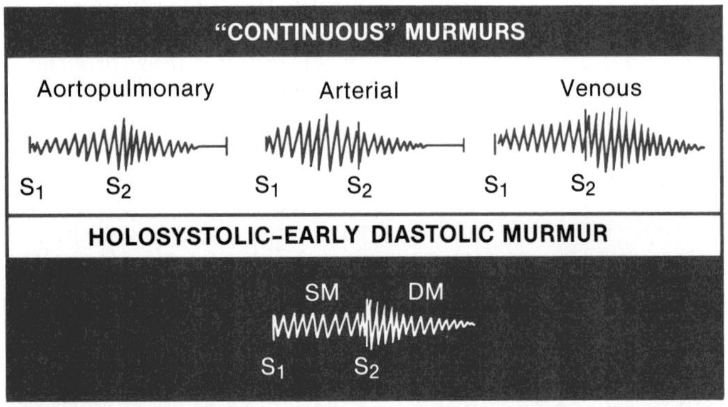

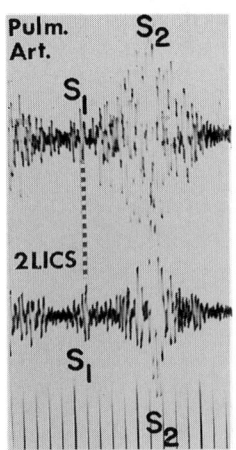

FIGURE 2–46. The classic continuous murmur of patent ductus arteriosus recorded from within the main pulmonary artery *(upper tracing)* and simultaneously on the chest wall at the second left intercostal space (2LICS). The murmur "begins softly and increases in intensity so as to reach its acme just about, or immediately after the incidence of the second sound, and from that point gradually wanes until its termination," as originally described by Gibson in 1900.[149]

FIGURE 2–45. Continuous murmurs begin in systole and *continue* without interruption through the timing of second heart sound (S₂) into all or part of diastole. The continuous murmurs shown here are aortopulmonary, systemic arterial, and systemic venous. A holosystolic murmur (SM) followed by a holodiastolic murmur (DM) represents two separate murmurs, not one continuous murmur.

and dies away gradually during the long pause. The murmur is rough and thrilling. It begins softly and increases in intensity so as to reach its acme just about, or immediately after, the incidence of the second sound, and from that point gradually wanes until its termination" (Fig. 2–46).

Arteriovenous continuous murmurs can be congenital or acquired and are represented in part by arteriovenous fistulas, coronary arterial fistulas, anomalous origin of the left coronary artery from the pulmonary trunk, and sinus of Valsalva–to–right heart communications.[75] The configuration, location, and intensity of arteriovenous continuous murmurs vary considerably among these different lesions. *Acquired* systemic arteriovenous fistulas are created surgically by forearm shunts for hemodialysis. *Congenital* arteriovenous continuous murmurs occur when a coronary arterial fistula enters the pulmonary trunk, right atrium, or right ventricle. At the latter site, the continuous murmur can be either softer or louder in systole, depending upon the degree of compression exerted on the fistulous coronary artery by right ventricular contraction.[75] Rupture of a congenital aortic sinus aneurysm into the right heart results in a continuous murmur that tends to be louder in either systole or diastole, sometimes creating a to-and-fro impression.[75]

Arterial continuous murmurs originate in either *constricted* or *nonconstricted* arteries. A common example of a continuous murmur arising in a constricted artery is carotid or femoral arterial atherosclerotic obstruction. Not surprisingly, these arterial continuous murmurs are characteristically louder in systole (Fig. 2–45) and more often than not are purely systolic.

Disturbances of flow patterns in *normal, nonconstricted* arteries sometimes produce continuous murmurs. The "mammary souffle" described earlier,[135] an innocent murmur heard during late pregnancy and the puerperium, is an arterial murmur which, when continuous, is typically louder in systole and maximal over either lactating breast. A distinct gap separates the first heart sound from the onset of the mammary souffle because of the relatively long interval that elapses before blood ejected from the left ventricle arrives at the artery of origin.[75] Light pressure with the stethoscope tends to augment the murmur and bring out its continuous features, whereas firm pressure with the stethoscope or by digital compression adjacent to the site of auscultation often abolishes the murmur.

Continuous murmurs in nonconstricted arteries originate in the large systemic-to-pulmonary arterial collaterals in certain types of cyanotic congenital heart disease, typically Fallot's tetralogy with pulmonary atresia (Fig. 2–19). These continuous murmurs are randomly located throughout the thorax because of the random location of the aortopulmonary collaterals.[75]

Continuous venous murmurs are well-represented by the innocent cervical venous hum (Fig. 2–47) described by Potain in 1867.[150] The hum is far and away the most common type of normal continuous murmur, universal in healthy children, and frequently present in healthy young adults, especially during pregnancy. Thyrotoxicosis and anemia, by augmenting cervical venous flow, initiate or reinforce the venous hum. The term "hum" does not necessarily characterize the quality of these cervical venous murmurs, which may be rough and noisy and are occasionally accompanied by a high-pitched whine.[75] The hum is truly continuous, although typically louder in diastole, as is generally the case with venous continuous murmurs (Fig. 2–47). The mechanism of the venous hum is unsettled. Silent laminar flow in the internal jugular vein may be disturbed by deformation of the vessel at the level of the transverse process of the atlas during head rotation designed to elicit the hum.[151]

Pericardial Rubs

In sinus rhythm, the typical pericardial rub is triple-phased, that is, midsystolic, mid-diastolic, and presystolic.[152] Recognition is simplest when all three phases are present, and when the characteristic superficial scratchy, leathery quality is evident. The term "rub" is appropriate because the auscultatory sign is generated by abnormal visceral and parietal pericardial surfaces "rubbing" against each other. In the supine position, firm pressure with the stethoscopic diaphragm during full held exhalation reinforces visceral and parietal pericardial contact and accentuates the rub. Apposition of visceral and parietal pericardium can be even better achieved by examination while the patient rests on elbows and knees.

Of the three phases of the pericardial rub, the systolic phase is the most consistent, followed by the presystolic phase. In atrial fibrillation, the presystolic component necessarily disappears. The diagnosis of a pericardial rub is least secure, and often impossible, when only one phase remains, typically the midsystolic. The most common clinical setting in which pericardial rubs are heard is immediately after open heart surgery. However, auscultation often detects instead a "crunch" synchronous with the heart beat, especially in the left lateral decubitus position. This is not a pericardial rub, but is Hamman's sign caused by air in the mediastinum.[153]

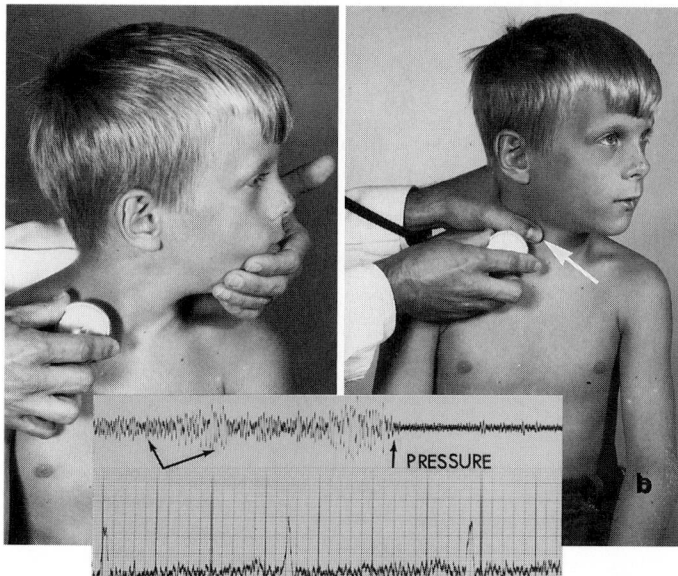

FIGURE 2–47. The phonocardiogram shows the continuous murmur of a normal venous hum. The *diastolic* component is louder (paired arrows). Digital pressure over the right internal jugular vein (vertical arrows) abolishes the murmur. The photographs show maneuvers used to elicit or abolish the venous hum. *Left,* The bell of the stethoscope is applied to the medial aspect of the *right* supraclavicular fossa as the examiner's left hand grasps the patient's chin from behind and pulls it tautly to the left and upward, stretching the neck. *Right,* The patient's head has returned to a more neutral position, and digital compression of the right internal jugular vein (arrow) abolishes the hum.

THE CARDIORESPIRATORY MURMUR

Thoracic auscultation occasionally detects what has been called a "cardiorespiratory murmur." Richard Cabot was aware that "Cardiorespiratory murmurs may be produced without any adhesion of the lung to the pericardium under conditions not at present understood."[154] Cabot went on to say that: "Such murmurs may be heard under the left clavicle or below the angle of the left scapula, as well as near the apex of the heart—less than in other parts of the chest. . . . Cardiorespiratory murmurs may be either systolic or diastolic, but the vast majority of cases are systolic. The area over which they are audible is usually a very limited one. They are greatly affected by position and by respiration, and are heard most distinctly if not exclusively during inspiration, especially at the end of that act." The mechanism responsible for the cardiorespiratory murmur remains unclear, but the location, timing, and relation to respiration remain as Cabot described.[154]

DYNAMIC AUSCULTATION

This term refers to the technique of altering circulatory dynamics by means of respiration and a variety of physiological and pharmacological maneuvers and determining the effects of these maneuvers on heart sounds and murmurs.[155-158] The interventions most commonly employed in dynamic auscultation include respiration, postural changes, the Valsalva maneuver, premature ventricular contractions, isometric exercise, and one of the vasoactive agents—amyl nitrite, methoxamine, or phenylephrine. The clinical applications of dynamic auscultation are summarized in Table 2–4.

TABLE 2–4   RESPONSE OF MURMURS AND HEART SOUNDS TO PHYSIOLOGICAL AND PHARMACOLOGICAL INTERVENTIONS

CLINICAL DISORDER	INTERVENTION AND RESPONSE
SYSTOLIC MURMURS	
Aortic outflow obstruction	
Valvular aortic stenosis	Louder with passive leg-raising, with sudden squatting, with Valsalva release (after five to six beats), following a pause induced by a premature beat, or after amyl nitrite; fades during Valsalva strain and with isometric handgrip
Hypertrophic obstructive cardiomyopathy	Louder with standing, during Valsalva strain, or with amyl nitrite; fades with sudden squatting, recumbency, or isometric handgrip
Pulmonic stenosis	Midsystolic murmur increases with amyl nitrite except with marked right ventricular hypertrophy; also increases during first few beats after Valsalva release
Mitral regurgitation	
Rheumatic	Murmur louder with sudden squatting, isometric handgrip, or phenylephrine; softens with amyl nitrite
Mitral valve prolapse	Midsystolic click moves toward S_1 and late systolic murmur starts earlier with standing, Valsalva strain, and amyl nitrite; click may occur earlier on inspiration; murmur starts later and click moves toward S_2 during squatting, with recumbency, and often after pause induced by a premature beat
Papillary muscle dysfunction	Late systolic murmur generally softer after a pause induced by a premature beat; response to amyl nitrite variable, depending on acute or chronic nature of this disorder
Tricuspid regurgitation	Murmur increases during inspiration, with passive leg-raising, and with amyl nitrite
Ventricular septal defect	
Small defect with pulmonary hypertension	Fades with amyl nitrite; increases with isometric handgrip or phenylephrine
Large defect with hyperkinetic pulmonary hypertension	Louder with amyl nitrite; fades with phenylephrine
Large defect with severe pulmonary vascular disease	Little change with any of above interventions
Tetralogy of Fallot	Murmur softens with amyl nitrite
Supraclavicular bruit	Altered by compression of subclavian artery; may be eliminated by extension of ipsilateral shoulder
DIASTOLIC MURMURS	
Aortic regurgitation	
Blowing diastolic murmur	Increases with sudden squatting, isometric handgrip, or phenylephrine
Austin Flint murmur	Fades with amyl nitrite
Pulmonary regurgitation	
Congenital	Early or mid-diastolic rumble increases on inspiration and with amyl nitrite
Pulmonary hypertension	High-frequency blowing murmur not altered by above interventions
Mitral stenosis	Mid-diastolic and presystolic murmurs louder with exercise, left lateral position, coughing, isometric handgrip, or amyl nitrite; phenylephrine widens A_2-OS interval; inspiration produces sequence of A_2-P_2-OS
Tricuspid stenosis	Mid-diastolic and presystolic murmurs increase during inspiration, with passive leg-raising, and with amyl nitrite
CONTINUOUS MURMURS	
Patent ductus arteriosus	Diastolic phase amplified with isometric handgrip or phenylephrine; diastolic phase fades with amyl nitrite
Cervical venous hum	Obliterated by direct compression of jugular veins or by Valsalva strain
ADDED HEART SOUNDS	
Gallop rhythm	
Ventricular gallop (S_3) and atrial gallop (S_4)	Accentuated by lying flat with passive leg-raising; decreased by standing or during Valsalva; right-sided gallop sounds usually increase during inspiration; left-sided during expiration
Summation gallop	Separates into ventricular gallop (S_3) and atrial gallop (S_4) sounds when heart rate slowed by carotid sinus massage
Ejection sounds	Ejection sound in pulmonary stenosis fades and occurs closer to the first sound during inspiration

OS = opening snap of mitral valve

From Criscitiello, M. G.: Physiologic and pharmacologic aids in cardiac auscultation. *In* Fowler, N. O. (ed.): Cardiac Diagnosis and Treatment. Hagerstown, MD, Harper and Row, 1980.

RESPIRATION

SECOND HEART SOUND. The splitting of S_2 is best audible along the left sternal border and can usually be appreciated when A_2 and P_2 are separated by more than 0.02 sec. The effects of respiration on the splitting of the second heart sound are discussed on p. 32.

THIRD AND FOURTH SOUNDS AND EJECTION SOUNDS. When third and fourth sounds originate from the right ventricle, they are characteristically diminished during exhalation and augmented during inspiration, whereas they exhibit the opposite response when they originate from the left side of the heart. Like other left-sided events, the opening snap of the mitral valve may become softer during inspiration and louder during exhalation owing to respiratory alterations in venous return, whereas the opening snap of the tricuspid valve behaves in the opposite fashion. Inspiration also diminishes the intensity of ejection sounds in pulmonary valve stenosis because the elevation of right ventricular diastolic pressure causes partial presystolic opening of the pulmonary valve and therefore less upward motion of the valve during systole. On the other hand, respiration does not affect the intensity of aortic ejection sounds, except in Fallot's tetralogy with pulmonary atresias.

Murmurs

Respiration exerts more pronounced and consistent alterations on murmurs originating from the right than from the left side of the heart. During inspiration, the diastolic murmurs of tricuspid stenosis (Fig. 2–44) and low pressure pulmonary regurgitation, the systolic murmurs of tricuspid regurgitation[159] (Carvallo's sign) and the presystolic murmur of Ebstein's anomaly may all be accentuated. The inspiratory reduction in left ventricular size in patients with mitral valve prolapse increases the redundancy of the mitral valve and therefore the degree of valvular prolapse; consequently, the midsystolic click and the systolic murmurs occur earlier during systole and may become accentuated.[160]

THE VALSALVA MANEUVER. This maneuver was described in 1704 as a method for expelling pus from the middle ear by straining with the mouth and nose closed.[75] The Valsalva maneuver is readily performed at the bedside and consists of a relatively deep inspiration followed by forced exhalation against a closed glottis for 10 to 12 seconds. The patient should be instructed on how to perform the maneuver. Simulation by the examiner is a simple means of doing so. The examiner then places the flat of the hand upon the abdomen to provide the patient with a force against which to strain and to permit assessment of the degree and duration of the straining effort.[161–163] The normal response to the Valsalva maneuver consists of four phases. *Phase I* is associated with a transient rise in systemic blood pressure as straining commences. This phase cannot, as a rule, be identified at the bedside. *Phase II* is accompanied by a perceptible decrease in systemic venous return, blood pressure, and pulse pressure (small pulse) and is readily detectable by reflex tachycardia. *Phase III* begins promptly with cessation of straining, is associated with an abrupt, transient decrease in blood pressure and in systemic venous return, and is generally not perceived at the bedside. *Phase IV* is characterized by an overshoot of systemic arterial pressure and relatively obvious reflex bradycardia. During phase II, third and fourth heart sounds are attenuated and the A_2-P_2 interval narrows or is abolished (Fig. 2–48). As stroke volume and systemic arterial pressure fall, the systolic murmurs of aortic and pulmonary stenosis and of mitral and tricuspid regurgitation diminish, and the diastolic murmurs of aortic and pulmonary regurgitation and of tricuspid and mitral stenosis soften. As left ventricular volume is reduced, the systolic murmur of hypertrophic

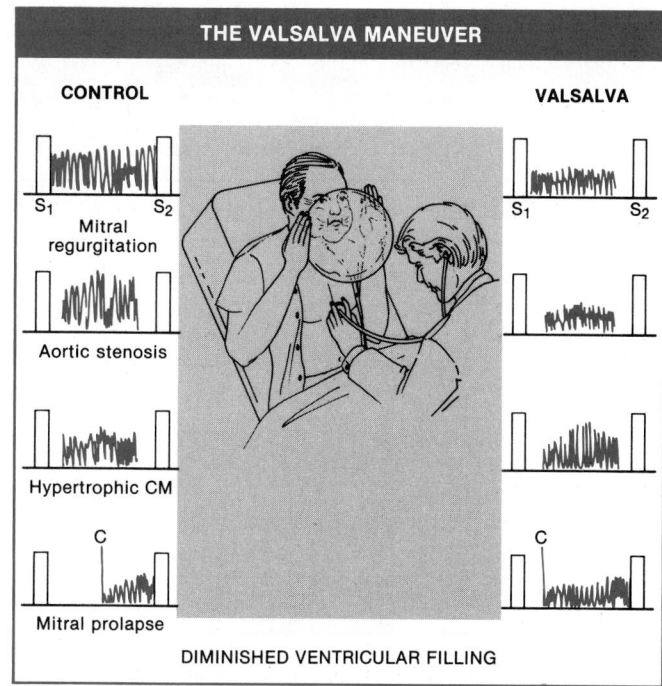

FIGURE 2–48. Changes in four left-sided systolic murmurs during the strain phase of the Valsalva maneuver. (From Grewe, K., Crawford, M. H., and O'Rourke, R. A.: Differentiation of cardiac murmurs by auscultation. Curr. Probl. Cardiol. *13*(10):669, 1988.)

obstructive cardiomyopathy amplifies, and the click and late systolic murmur of mitral valve prolapse begin earlier. In phase III, the sudden increase in systemic venous return is accompanied by wide splitting of the second heart sound and by augmentation of murmurs and filling sounds in the right side of the heart. Murmurs and filling sounds in the left side of the heart return to control levels and may transiently increase during the overshoot of phase IV.

In patients with atrial septal defect, mitral stenosis, or heart failure, the Valsalva maneuver provokes a "square wave" response, negating the four phases and their auscultatory equivalents. The Valsalva maneuver should not be performed in patients with ischemic heart disease because of the accompanying fall in coronary blood flow.

THE MÜLLER MANEUVER. This maneuver is the converse of the Valsalva maneuver but is less frequently employed because it is not as useful.[81] The maneuver is continued for about 10 seconds as the patient forcibly *inspires* while the nose is held closed and the mouth firmly sealed. The Müller maneuver exaggerates the inspiratory effort, widens the split second sound, and augments murmurs and filling sounds originating in the right side of the heart.

POSTURAL CHANGES AND EXERCISE

(Fig. 2–49)

Sudden assumption of the *lying* from the standing or sitting position or sudden passive elevation of both legs results in an increase in venous return, which augments first right ventricular and, several cardiac cycles later, left ventricular stroke volume. The principal auscultatory changes include widening of the splitting of S_2 in all phases of respiration and augmentations of right-sided S_3 and S_4 and, several cardiac cycles later, left-sided S_3 and S_4. The systolic murmurs of pulmonic valve stenosis and aortic stenosis, the systolic murmurs of mitral and tricuspid regurgitation and ventricular septal defect, and most functional systolic murmurs are augmented. On the other hand, because left ventricular end-diastolic volume is increased, the systolic murmur of hypertrophic obstructive

FIGURE 2–49. Diagrammatic representation of the character of the systolic murmur and of the second heart sound in five conditions. The effects of posture, amyl nitrite inhalation, and phenylephrine injection on the intensity of the murmur are shown. (Modified from Barlow, J. B.: Perspectives on the Mitral Valve. Philadelphia, F. A. Davis, 1987, p. 138.)

DIAGNOSIS	SYSTOLIC MURMUR	SECOND SOUND	EFFECT OF POSTURE		AMYL NITRATE	PHENYL-EPHRINE
			Erect	Squatting		
			Changes in intensity of systolic murmur			
1. Hypertrophic obstructive cardiomyopathy	◇	Variable ie - reversed partially reversed narrow or normal	↑	↓	↑	↓
2. Mitral incompetence a. Pure severe	◇	widely split	↓	↑	↓	↑
b. Papillary muscle dysfunction	◇	normal or partially reversed	↑↓	↑	↓	↑
c. Billowing posterior leaflet	◇	normal	↑↓	↑	↓	↑
d. Rheumatic of moderate degree	◇	slightly wide	↓	↑	↓	↑
3. Valvular aortic stenosis { mild to mod	◇	narrow or partially reversed	↓	↑	↑	−
marked	◇	reversed	↓	↑	↑	−
4. Ventricular septal defect	◇	slightly wide	−↓	↑	↓	↑
5. Innocent vibratory systolic murmur	◇	normal	↓	−	↑	↓

− No change from control

↓↑ Degree of increase

↓↓ Degree of decrease

cardiomyopathy is diminished, and the midsystolic click and late systolic murmur associated with mitral valve prolapse are delayed and sometimes attenuated (see p. 31) (Fig. 2–21).

Rapid standing or sitting up from a lying position or rapid standing from a squatting posture has the opposite effect; in patients in whom there is relatively wide splitting of S_2 during exhalation—a finding that may be confused with fixed splitting—the width of the splitting is reduced, so that a normal pattern emerges during the respiratory cycle. No change in splitting occurs in patients with true fixed splitting. The decrease in venous return reduces stroke volume and innocent pulmonary flow murmurs as well as the murmurs of semilunar valve stenosis and of AV valve regurgitation. The auscultatory changes in hypertrophic cardiomyopathy and mitral valve prolapse are opposite to those on assumption of the lying posture described above.

SQUATTING. A sudden change from standing to squatting increases venous return and systemic resistance simultaneously. Stroke volume and arterial pressure rise, and the latter may induce a transient reflex bradycardia. The auscultatory features include augmentation of S_3 and S_4 (from both ventricles) and as a consequence of an increase in stroke volume, the systolic murmurs of pulmonary and aortic stenosis and the diastolic murmurs of tricuspid and mitral stenosis become louder, with right-sided events preceding left-sided events. Squatting may make audible a previously inaudible murmur of aortic regurgitation.

The elevation of arterial pressure increases blood flow through the right ventricular outflow tract of patients with tetralogy of Fallot and increases the volume of mitral regurgitation and of the left-to-right shunt through a ventricular septal defect, thereby increasing the intensity of the systolic murmur in these conditions. Also, the diastolic murmur of aortic regurgitation is augmented consequent to an increase in aortic reflux. The combination of elevated arterial pressure and increased venous return increases left ventricular size, which reduces the obstruction to outflow and thus the intensity of the systolic murmur of hypertrophic obstructive cardiomyopathy[2]; the midsystolic click and the late systolic murmur of mitral valve prolapse are delayed.

OTHER POSITIONAL CHANGES. *Assumption of the left lateral recumbent position* accentuates the intensity of S_1, S_3, and S_4 originating from the left side of the heart; the opening snap and the murmurs associated with mitral stenosis and regurgitation; the midsystolic click and late systolic murmur of mitral valve prolapse; and the Austin Flint murmur associated with aortic regurgitation. *Sitting up and leaning forward* make the diastolic murmurs of aortic and pulmonary regurgitation more readily audible.

Hyperextension of the shoulders is an important positional maneuver that assists in assessing supraclavicular systolic murmurs.[134] The mechanism responsible for diminution in the intensity of normal supraclavicular systolic murmurs with hyperextension of the shoulders is apparently related to the effect of the maneuver on the site of origin of the murmurs in the proximal brachiocephalic arteries as they leave the aortic arch. *Stretching the neck* to elicit a venous hum is illustrated in Figure 2–50.

Passive elevation of the legs with the patient supine transiently increases venous return and augments third heart sounds. Pericardial rubs may be more readily detected when the patient is on elbows and knees (Fig. 2–51), a physical maneuver designed to increase the contact of visceral and parietal pericardium (see above).

ISOMETRIC EXERCISE. This can be carried out simply and reproducibly using a calibrated handgrip device or hand ball. (It is useful to carry out isometric exercise bilaterally simultaneously.) Isometric exercise should be avoided in patients with ventricular arrhythmias and myocardial ischemia, both of which can be intensified by this activity. Handgrip should be sustained for 20 to 30 seconds, but a Valsalva maneuver during the handgrip must be avoided. Isometric exercise results in transient but significant increases in systemic vascular resistance, arterial pressure, heart rate, cardiac output, left ventricular filling pressure, and heart size. As a consequence, (1) S_3 and S_4 originating from the left side of the heart become accentuated, (2) the

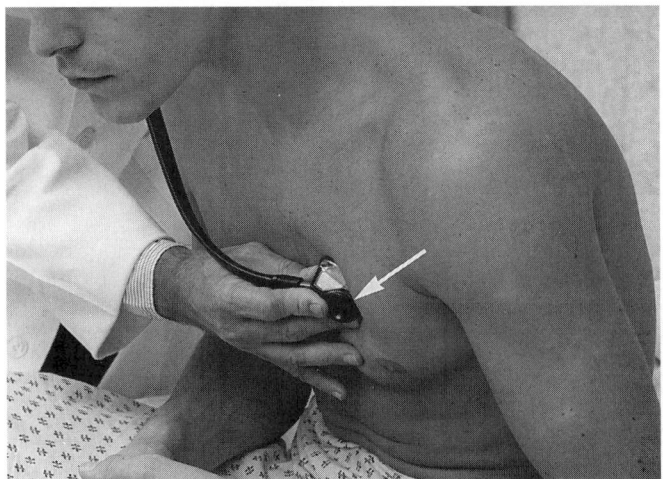

FIGURE 2–50. The soft, high-frequency early diastolic murmur of aortic regurgitation or pulmonary hypertensive regurgitation is best elicited by applying the diaphragm of the stethoscope very firmly to the mid-left sternal edge (arrow) as the patient sits and leans forward with breath held in full exhalation.

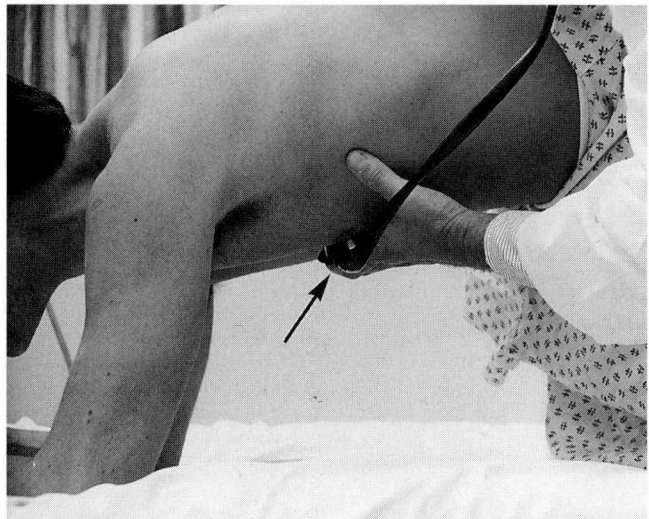

FIGURE 2–51. A technique for eliciting a pericardial rub. The diaphragm of the stethoscope is firmly applied to the precordium *(arrow)* while the patient rests on elbows and knees.

systolic murmur of aortic stenosis is diminished as a result of reduction of the pressure gradient across the aortic valve,[164,165] (3) the diastolic murmur of aortic regurgitation and the systolic murmurs of rheumatic mitral regurgitation and ventricular septal defect increase, (4) the diastolic murmur of mitral stenosis becomes louder consequent to the increase in cardiac output, and (5) the systolic murmur of hypertrophic obstructive cardiomyopathy diminishes and the systolic click and late systolic murmur of mitral valve prolapse are delayed because of the increased left ventricular volume.

PHARMACOLOGICAL AGENTS

(Fig. 2–49)

Inhalation of *amyl nitrite* is carried out by placing an ampule in gauze near the supine patient's nose and then crushing the ampule. The patient is asked to take three or four deep breaths over 10 to 15 seconds, after which the amyl nitrite is removed. The drug produces marked vasodilatation, resulting in the first 30 seconds in a reduction of systemic arterial pressure, and 30 to 60 seconds later in a reflex tachycardia, followed in turn by a reflex *increase* in cardiac output, velocity of blood flow, and heart rate.[2,155–158,166] The major auscultatory changes occur in the first 30 seconds following inhalation. S_1 is augmented and A_2 is diminished. The opening snaps of the mitral and tricuspid valves become louder, and as arterial pressure falls, the A_2-opening snap interval shortens. An S_3 originating in either ventricle is augmented, owing to greater rapidity of ventricular filling, but because mitral regurgitation is reduced, the S_3 associated with this lesion is diminished. The systolic murmurs of aortic valve stenosis, pulmonary stenosis, hypertrophic obstructive cardiomyopathy, tricuspid regurgitation, and functional systolic murmurs are all accentuated.

The reduction of arterial pressure increases the right-to-left shunt and decreases the blood flow from the right ventricle to the pulmonary artery and diminishes the midsystolic murmur in patients with tetralogy of Fallot. The increase in cardiac output augments the diastolic murmurs of mitral and tricuspid stenosis and of pulmonary regurgitation and the systolic murmur of tricuspid regurgitation. However, as a result of the fall in systemic arterial pressure, the systolic murmurs of mitral regurgitation and ventricular septal defect, the diastolic murmurs of aortic regurgitation (Fig. 2–41), and the Austin Flint murmur as well as the continuous murmurs of patent ductus arteriosus and of systemic arteriovenous fistula are all diminished.[164] The reduction of cardiac size results in an earlier appearance of

the midsystolic click and late systolic murmur of mitral valve prolapse; the intensity of the systolic murmur exhibits a variable response.

The response to amyl nitrite is useful in distinguishing (1) the systolic murmur of aortic stenosis (which is augmented) from that of mitral regurgitation (which is diminished),[166] (2) the systolic murmur of tricuspid regurgitation (augmented) from that of mitral regurgitation (diminished), (3) the systolic murmur of isolated pulmonary stenosis (augmented) from that of tetralogy of Fallot (diminished), (4) the diastolic rumbling murmur of mitral stenosis (augmented) from the Austin Flint murmur of aortic regurgitation (diminished), and (5) the early blowing diastolic murmur of pulmonary regurgitation (augmented) from that of aortic regurgitation (diminished).

Methoxamine and *phenylephrine* increase systemic arterial pressure and exert an effect opposite to that of amyl nitrite. In general, methoxamine, 3 to 5 mg intravenously, elevates arterial pressure by 20 to 40 mm Hg for 10 to 20 minutes, but phenylephrine is preferred because of its shorter duration of action; 0.3 to 0.5 mg of phenylephrine administered intravenously elevates systolic pressure by approximately 30 mm Hg for only 3 to 5 minutes. Both drugs cause reflex bradycardia and decreased contractility and cardiac output. They should not be used in the presence of congestive heart failure and systemic hypertension.

After administration, the intensity of S_1 is usually reduced, and the A_2-mitral opening snap interval becomes prolonged. The responses of S_3 and S_4 are variable. As a result of the increased arterial pressure, the diastolic murmur of aortic regurgitation; the systolic murmurs of mitral regurgitation (Fig. 2–39), ventricular septal defect, and tetralogy of Fallot; and the continuous murmurs of patent ductus arteriosus and systemic arteriovenous fistula all become louder.[164] On the other hand, as a consequence of the increase in left ventricular size, the systolic murmur of hypertrophic obstructive cardiomyopathy becomes softer, and the click and late systolic murmur of mitral valve prolapse are delayed. The reduction in cardiac output diminishes the systolic murmur of aortic valve stenosis, functional systolic murmurs, and the diastolic murmur of mitral stenosis. The rumbling diastolic murmurs of mitral regurgitation and the Austin Flint murmur also diminish.

REFERENCES

THE GENERAL PHYSICAL EXAMINATION

1. Marriott, H. J. L.: Bedside Cardiac Diagnosis. Philadelphia, J. B. Lippincott Co., 1993.
2. Perloff, J. K.: Physical Examination of the Heart and Circulation. 2nd ed. Philadelphia, W. B. Saunders Company, 1990.
3. Sapira, J. D.: The Art and Science of Bedside Diagnosis. Baltimore, Urban & Schwartzenberg, 1990.
4. Constant, J.: Bedside Cardiology, 4th ed. Boston, Little, Brown & Co., 1993.
5. Brady, P. M., Zive, M. A., Goldberg, R. J., et al.: A new wrinkle to the earlobe crease. Arch. Intern. Med. 147:65, 1987.
6. Kirkham, N., Murrels, T., Melcher, S. H., and Morrison, E. A.: Diagonal ear lobe creases and fatal cardiovascular disease: A necropsy study. Br. Heart J. 61:361, 1989.
7. Roberts, N. K., Perloff, J. K., and Kark, R. A. P.: Cardiac conduction in the Kearns-Sayre syndrome (a neuromuscular disorder associated with progressive external ophthalmoplegia and pigmentary retinopathy). Am. J. Cardiol. 44:1396, 1979.
8. Cogan, D. G.: Ophthalmic Manifestations of Systemic Vascular Disease. Philadelphia, W. B. Saunders Company, 1974.
9. Allen, S. J., and Naylor, D.: Pulsation of the eyeballs in tricuspid regurgitation. Can. Med. Assoc. J. 133:119, 1985.
10. Byrd, M. D.: Lateral systolic pulsation of the earlobe: A sign of tricuspid regurgitation. Am. J. Cardiol. 54:244, 1984.
11. Criscitiello, M. G., Ronan, J. A., Besterman, E. M., and Schoenwetter, W.: Cardiovascular abnormalities in osteogenesis imperfecta. Circulation 31:255, 1965.
12. St. John Sutton, M. G., Tajik, A. J., Giuliani, E. R., et al.: Hypertrophic obstructive cardiomyopathy and lentiginosis: A little known neural ectodermal syndrome. Am. J. Cardiol. 47:214, 1981.

13. Basson, C. T., Cowley, G. S., Solomon, S. D., et al.: The clinical and genetic spectrum of the Holt-Oram syndrome (heart-hand syndrome) N. Engl. J. Med. *330*:885, 1994; erratum, N. Engl. J. Med. *330*:1627, 1994.

14. Buckley, M. J., Mason, D. T., Ross, J., Jr., and Braunwald, E.: Reversed differential cyanosis with equal desaturation of the upper limbs. Syndrome of complete transposition of the great vessels with complete interruption of the aortic arch. Am. J. Cardiol. *15*:111, 1965.

15. Finger clubbing. Lancet *1*:1285, 1975.

16. Lanken, P. N., and Fishman, A. P.: Clubbing and hypertrophic osteoarthropathy. *In* Fishman, A. P. (ed.): Pulmonary Diseases and Disorders. New York, McGraw-Hill Book Co., 1980, pp. 84–91.

17. Yee, J., McAllister, C. K.: The utility of Osler's nodes in the diagnosis of infective endocarditis. Chest *92*:751, 1987.

18. Manga, P., Vythilingum, S., and Mitha, A. S.: Pulsatile hepatomegaly in constrictive pericarditis. Br. Heart J. *52*:465, 1984.

19. Coralli, R. J., and Crawley, I. S.: Hepatic pulsations in constrictive pericarditis. Am. J. Cardiol. *58*:370, 1986.

20. Ewy, G. A.: The abdominojugular test: Technique and hemodynamic correlates. Ann. Intern. Med. *109*:456, 1988.

21. Swartz, M. H.: Jugular venous pressure pulse: Its value in cardiac diagnosis. Primary Cardiol. *8*:197, 1982.

22. Stojnic, B. B., Brecker, S. J., Xiao, H. B., and Gibson, D. G.: Jugular venous "a" wave in pulmonary hypertension: New insights from a Doppler echocardiographic study. Br. Heart J. *68*:187, 1992.

23. Butman, S. M., Ewy, G. A., Standen, J. R., et al.: Bedside cardiovascular examination in patients with severe chronic heart failure: Importance of rest or inducible jugular venous distension. J. Am. Coll. Cardiol. *22*:968, 1993.

24. Ducas, J., Magder, S., and McGregor, M.: Validity of the hepatojugular reflux as a clinical test for congestive heart failure. Am. J. Cardiol. *52*:1299, 1983.

25. Sochowski, R. A., Dubbin, J. D., and Naqvi, S. Z.: Clinical and hemodynamic assessment of the hepatojugular reflux. Am. J. Cardiol. *66*:1002, 1990.

26. Petrie, J. C., et al.: Recommendations on blood pressure measurement. Br. Med. J. *293*:611, 1986.

27. Frohlich, E. D., et al.: Recommendations for human blood pressure determination by sphygmomanometers. Report of a special task force appointed by the steering committee, American Heart Association. Circulation *77*:501a, 1988.

28. O'Brien, E., et al.: Blood pressure measurement: Current practice and future trends. Br. Med. J. *290*:729, 1985.

29. Maisel, A. S., Atwood, J. E., Goldberger, A. L.: Hepatojugular reflux: Useful in the bedside diagnosis of tricuspid regurgitation. Ann. Intern. Med. *101*:781, 1984.

30. Linfors, E. W., Feussner, J. R., Blessing, C. L., et al.: Spurious hypertension in the obese patient. Effect of sphygmomanometer cuff size on prevalence of hypertension. Arch. Intern. Med. *144*:1482, 1984.

31. Manning, D. M., Kuchirka, C., and Kaminski, J.: Miscuffing: Inappropriate blood pressure cuff application. Circulation *68*:763, 1983.

32. Nelson, W. P., and Egbert, A. M.: How to measure blood pressure—accurately. Prim. Cardiol. *10*:14, 1984.

33. Kirkendall, W. M., Burton, A. C., Epstein, F. H., and Freis, E. D.: Recommendations for human blood pressure determination by sphygmomanometers. Circulation *36*:980, 1967.

34. Londe, S., and Klitzner, T. S.: Auscultatory blood pressure measurement—Effect of pressure on the head of the stethoscope. West. J. Med. *141*:193, 1984.

35. Mancia, G., Grassi, G., Pomidossi, G., et al.: Effects of blood-pressure measurement by the doctor on patient's blood pressure and heart rate. Lancet *2*:695, 1983.

36. Gould, B. A., Hornung, R. S., Kieso, H. A., et al.: Is the blood pressure the same in both arms? Clin. Cardiol. *8*:423, 1985.

37. Sapira, J. D.: Quincke, de Musset, Duroziez, and Hill: Some aortic regurgitations. South. Med. J. *74*:459, 1981.

38. Abrams, J.: The arterial pulse. Prim. Cardiol. *8*:138, 1982.

39. Schlant, R. C., and Feiner, J. M.: The arterial pulse—clinical manifestations. Curr. Probl. Cardiol. Vol. 1, No. 5, 1976, 50 pp.

40. Perloff, J. K.: The physiologic mechanisms of cardiac and vascular physical signs. J. Am. Coll. Cardiol. *1*:184, 1983.

41. Smith, D., and Craige, E.: Mechanism of the dicrotic pulse. Br. Heart J. *56*:531, 1986.

42. Elkins, R. C., Morrow, A. G., Vasko, J. S., and Braunwald, E.: The effects of mitral regurgitation on the pattern of instantaneous aortic blood flow. Clinical and experimental observations. Circulation *36*:45, 1967.

43. Rowe, G. G., Afonso, S., Castillo, C. A., and McKenna, D. H.: The mechanism of the production of Duroziez's murmur. N. Engl. J. Med. *272*:1207, 1965.

44. Fleming, P. R.: The mechanism of the pulsus bisferiens. Br. Heart J. *19*:519, 1957.

45. Talley, J. D.: Recognition, etiology, and clinical implications of pulsus bisferiens. Heart Dis. Stroke *3*:309, 1994.

46. Braunwald, E., Lambrew, C. T., Rockoff, S. D., et al.: Idiopathic hypertrophic subaortic stenosis. I. A description of the disease based upon an analysis of 64 patients. Circulation *30*(Suppl. 4):3, 1964.

47. Bartall, M., Auber, S., Desser, K. B., and Benchimol, A.: Normalization of the external carotid pulse tracing of hypertrophic subaortic stenosis during Müller's maneuver. Chest *74*:77, 1978.

48. Lab, M. J., and Seed, W. A.: Pulses alternans. Cardiovasc. Res. *27*:1407, 1993.

49. Brockenbrough, E. C., Braunwald, E., and Morrow, A. G.: A hemodynamic technic for the detection of hypertrophic subaortic stenosis. Circulation *23*:189, 1961.

50. Rebuck, A. S., and Pengelly, L. D.: Development of pulsus paradoxus in the presence of airways obstruction. N. Engl. J. Med. *288*:66, 1973.

51. Massumi, R. A., Mason, D. T., Zakauddin, V., et al.: Reversed pulsus paradoxus. N. Engl. J. Med. *289*:1272, 1973.

52. Kurtz, K. J.: Dynamic vascular auscultation. Am. J. Med. *76*:1066, 1984.

53. Linhart, J.: Bedside examination of peripheral vascular disease. Eur. Heart J. *4*:137, 1983.

THE CARDIAC EXAMINATION

54. Davies, H.: Chest deformities in congenital heart disease. Br. J. Dis. Chest *53*:151, 1959.

55. Perloff, J. K.: Diagnostic inferences drawn from observation and palpation of the precordium with special reference to congenital heart disease. Adv. Cardiopulm. Dis. *4*:13, 1969.

56. Beiser, G. D., Epstein, S. E., Stampfer, M., et al.: Impairment of cardiac function in patients with pectus excavatum. N. Engl. J. Med. *287*:267, 1972.

57. Ansari, A.: The "straight back" syndrome. Clin. Cardiol. *8*:290, 1985.

58. Abrams, J.: Precordial palpation. *In* Horwitz, L. D., and Groves, B. M. (eds.): Signs and Symptoms in Cardiology. Philadelphia, J. B. Lippincott, 1985, pp. 156–177.

59. O'Neill, T. W., Smith, M., Barry, M., and Graham, I. M.: Diagnostic value of the apex beat. Lancet *1*(8635):410, 1989.

60. Basta, I. L., and Bettinger, J. J.: The cardiac impulse: A new look at an old art. Am. Heart J. *97*:96, 1979.

61. Eilen, S. D., Crawford, M. H., and O'Rourke, R. A.: Accuracy of precordial palpation for detecting increased left ventricular volume. Ann. Intern. Med. *99*:628, 1983.

62. Bancroft, W. H., Jr., Eddleman, E. E., Jr., and Larkin, L. N.: Methods and physical characteristics of the kineto-cardiographic and apex cardiographic systems for recording low-frequency precordial motion. Am. Heart J. *73*:756, 1967.

63. Ranganathan, Juma, Z., and Sivaciyan, V.: The apical impulse in coronary heart disease. Clin. Cardiol. *8*:20, 1985.

64. Dressler, W.: Clinical Aids in Cardiac Diagnosis. New York, Grune and Stratton, 1970, 246 pp.

65. Gillam, P. M. S., et al.: The left parasternal impulse. Br. Heart J. *26*:726, 1964.

66. Counihan, T. B., Rappaport, M. B., and Sprague, H. B.: Physiologic and physical factors that govern the clinical appreciation of cardiac thrills. Circulation *4*:716, 1951.

67. Littmann, D.: An approach to the ideal stethoscope. JAMA *178*:504, 1961.

68. Kindig, J. R., Beeson, T. P., Campbell, R. W., et al.: Acoustical performance of the stethoscope: A comparative analysis. Am. Heart J. *104*:269, 1982.

HEART SOUNDS

69. Leatham, A.: Auscultation of the heart. Lancet *II*:703, 1958.

70. O'Toole, J. D., Reddy, P. S., Curtiss, E. L., et al.: The contribution of tricuspid valve closure to the first heart sound. An intracardiac micromanometer study. Circulation *53*:752, 1976.

71. Brooks, N., Leech, G., and Leatham, A.: Complete right bundle branch block: Echophonocardiographic study of the first heart sound and right ventricular contraction times. Br. Heart J. *41*:637, 1979.

72. Burggraf, G. W.: The first heart sound in left bundle branch block: An echophonocardiographic study. Circulation *63*:429, 1981.

73. Burggraf, G. W., and Craige E.: The first heart sound in complete heart block. Circulation *50*:17, 1974.

74. Leech, G., Brooks, N., Green-Wilkinson, A., and Leatham, A.: Mechanism of influence of PR interval on loudness of first heart sound. Br. Heart J. *43*:138, 1980.

75. Perloff, J. K.: The Clinical Recognition of Congenital Heart Disease, 4th ed. Philadelphia, W. B. Saunders Company, 1994.

76. Waider, W., and Craige, E.: The first heart sound and ejection sounds: Echophonocardiographic correlation with valvular events. Am. J. Cardiol. *35*:346, 1975.

77. Mills, P. G., Brodie, B., McLaurin, L., et al.: Echocardiographic and hemodynamic relationships of ejection sounds. Circulation *56*:430, 1977.

78. Hultgren, H. N., Reeve, R., Cohn, K., and McLeod, R.: The ejection click of valvular pulmonic stenosis. Circulation *40*:631, 1969.

79. Devereux, R., Perloff, J. K., Derchek, N., and Josephson, M.: Mitral valve prolapse. Circulation *54*:3, 1976.

80. Bank, A. J., Sharkey, S. W., Goldsmith, S. R., et al.: Atypical systolic clicks produced by prolapsing mitral valve masses. Am. J. Cardiol. *69*:1491, 1992.

81. Rothman, A., and Goldberger, A. L.: Aids to cardiac auscultation. Ann. Intern. Med. *99*:346, 1983.

82. Lembo, N. J., Dell'Italia, J. L., Crawford, M. H., and O'Rourke, R. A.: Bedside diagnosis of systolic murmurs. N. Engl. J. Med. *318*:1572, 1988.

83. Potain, P. C.: Clinique médicale de la Charité. Paris, Masson, 1894. *In* McKusick, V. A.: Cardiovascular Sound in Health and Disease. Baltimore, Williams and Wilkins Co., 1958.

84. Potain, P. C.: Note sur les dédoublements normaux des bruits du coeur. Bull. Mem. Soc. Med. Hop. Paris. *3*:138, 1866.

85. Leatham, A.: The second heart sound. Key to auscultation of the heart. Acta Cardiol. *19*:395, 1964.

86. Leatham, A.: Splitting of the first and second heart sounds. Lancet *II*:607, 1954.

87. Kupari, M.: Aortic valve closure and cardiac vibrations in the genesis of the second heart sound. Am. J. Cardiol. *52*:152, 1983.

88. Curtiss, E. I., Matthews, D. G., and Shaver, J. A.: Mechanism of normal splitting of the second heart sound. Circulation *51*:157, 1975.

89. Shaver, J. A., Nadolny, R. A., O'Toole, J. D., et al.: Sound-pressure correlates of the second heart sound. Circulation *49*:316, 1974.

90. Perloff, J. K., and Harvey, W. P.: Auscultatory and phonocardiographic manifestations of pure mitral regurgitation. Prog. Cardiovasc. Dis. *5*:172, 1962.

91. Xiao, H. B., Faiek, A. H., and Gibson, D. G.: Re-evaluation of normal splitting of the second heart sound in patients with classical left bundle branch block. Int. J. Cardiol. *45*:163, 1994.

92. Hultgren, H. N., Craige, E., Nakamura, T., and Bilisoly, J.: Left bundle branch block and mechanical events of the cardiac cycle. Am. J. Cardiol. *52*:755, 1985.

93. Steell, G.: The murmur of high pressure in the pulmonary artery. Med. Chron. (Manchester) *9*:182, 1888–1889.

94. de Leon, A. C., Perloff, J. K., Twigg, H., and Moyd, M.: The straight back syndrome. Circulation *32*:193, 1965.

95. Thayer, W. S.: On the early diastolic sound (the so-called third heart sound). Boston Med. Surg. J. *158*:713, 1908.

96. Wood, P.: An appreciation of mitral stenosis. I. Clinical features. Br. Med. J. *1*:1051, 1954; II. Investigations and results. *1*:1113, 1954.

97. Joyner, C. R., Jr., and Dear, W. E.: The motion of the normal and abnormal mitral valve. A study of the opening snap. J. Clin. Invest. *45*:1029, 1966.

98. Connolly, D. C., and Mann, R. J.: Dominic J. Corrigan (1802–1880) and his description of the pericardial knock. Mayo Clin. Proc. *55*:771, 1980.

99. Tyberg, T. I., Goodyer, A. V. N., and Langou, R. A.: Genesis of the pericardial knock in constrictive pericarditis. Am. J. Cardiol. *46*:570, 1980.

100. Bass, N. M., and Sharatt, G. J. P.: Left atrial myxoma diagnosed by echocardiography with observations on tumor movement. Br. Heart J. *35*:1332, 1973.

101. Van de Werf, F., Minten, J., Carmeliet, P., et al.: Genesis of the third and fourth heart sounds. J. Clin. Invest. *73*:1400, 1984.

102. Van de Werf, F., Boel, A., Geboers, J., et al.: Diastolic properties of the left ventricle in normal adults and in patients with third heart sounds. Circulation *69*:1070, 1984.

103. Potain, P. C.: Concerning the cardiac rhythm called gallop rhythm. Bull. Men. Soc. Med. Hop. (Paris) *12*:137, 1876.

104. Kupari, M., Koskinen, P., Virolainen, J., et al.: Prevalence and predictors of audible physiological third heart sound in a population sampled aged 36 to 37 years. Circulation *89*:1189, 1994.

105. Van de Werf, F., Geboers, J., Math, L., et al.: The mechanism of disappearance of the physiologic third heart sound with age. Circulation *73*:877, 1986.

106. Folland, E. D., Kriegel, B. J., Henderson, W. G., et al.: Implications of third heart sounds in patients with valvular heart disease. The Veterans Affairs Cooperative Study on Valvular Heart Disease. N. Engl. J. Med. *327*:458, 1992.

107. Aronow, W. S., Papageorge's, N. P., Uyeyama, R. R., and Cassidy, J.: Maximal treadmill stress test correlated with postexercise phonocardiogram in normal subjects. Circulation *43*:884, 1971.

108. Ozawa, Y., Smith D., and Craige, E.: Origin of the third heart sound. I. Studies in dogs. Circulation *67*:393, 1983.

109. Ozawa, Y., Smith, D., and Craige, E.: Origin of the third heart sound. II. Studies in human subjects. Circulation *67*:399, 1983.

110. Drzewiecki, G. M., Wasicko, M. J., and Li, J. K.: Diastolic mechanics and the origin of the third heart sound. Ann. Biomed. Engin. *19*:651, 1991.

111. Downes, T. R., Dunson, W., Stewart, K., et al.: Mechanism of physiologic and pathologic S_3 gallop sounds. Am. Soc. Echocardiol. *5*:211, 1992.

112. Ishimitsu, T., Smith, D., Berko, B., and Craige, E.: Origin of the third heart sound: Comparison of ventricular wall dynamics in hyperdynamic and hypodynamic types. J. Am. Coll. Cardiol. *5*:268, 1985.

113. Perloff, J. K.: Auscultatory and phonocardiographic manifestations of pulmonary hypertension. Prog. Cardiovasc. Dis. *9*:303, 1967.

114. Gibson, T. C., Madry, R., Grossman, W., et al.: The A wave of the apex cardiogram and left ventricular diastolic stiffness. Circulation *49*:441, 1974.

115. Perloff, J. K.: Clinical recognition of aortic stenosis. Progr. Cardiovasc. Dis. *10*:323, 1964.

116. Cheng, T. O., Ertem, G., and Vera, Z.: Heart sounds in patients with cardiac pacemakers. Chest *62*:66, 1972.

117. Harris, A.: Pacemaker "heart sound." Br. Heart J. *29*:608, 1967.

MURMURS

118. Pepper, O. H. P.: Medical Etymology. Philadelphia, W. B. Saunders Company, 1949.

119. Freeman, A. R., and Levine, S. A.: The clinical significance of the systolic murmur. A study of 1000 consecutive "non-cardiac" cases. Ann. Intern. Med. *6*:1371, 1933.

120. Roberts, W. C., Perloff, J. K., and Costantino, T.: Severe valvular aortic stenosis in patients over 65 years of age. Am. J. Cardiol. *27*:497, 1971.

121. Gallavardin, L., and Pauper-Ravault: Le souffle du rétré cissement aortique peut changer de timbre et devenir musical dans se propagation apexienne. Lyon Med. 1925, p. 523.

122. Stokes, W.: Diseases of the Heart in Aorta. Philadelphia, Lindsay and Blakiston, 1855.

123. Still, G. F.: Common Disorders and Diseases of Childhood. London, Henry Frowde, 1909.

124. Burch, G. E., DePasquale, N. P., and Phillips, J. H.: The syndrome of papillary muscle dysfunction. Am. Heart J. *75*:399, 1968.

125. Perloff, J. K., and Roberts, W. C.: The mitral apparatus: Functional anatomy of mitral regurgitation. Circulation *46*:227, 1972.

126. Rivero-Carvallo, J. M.: Sitno para el diagnostico de las insuficiencias tricuspideas. Arch. Inst. Cardiol. Mexico *16*:531, 1946.

127. Leon, D. F., Leonard, J. J., Lancaster, J. F., et al.: Effect of respiration on pansystolic regurgitant murmurs as studied by biatrial intracardiac phonocardiography. Am. J. Med. *39*:429, 1965.

128. Sanders, C. A., Scannell, J. G., Harthorne, J. W., and Austen, W. G.: Severe mitral regurgitation secondary to ruptured chordae tendineae. Circulation *31*:506, 1965.

129. Sutton, G. C., and Craige, E.: Clinical signs of acute severe mitral regurgitation. Am. J. Cardiol. *20*:141, 1967.

130. Ronan, J. A., Steelman, R. B., DeLeon, A. C., et al.: The clinical diagnosis of acute severe mitral insufficiency. Am. J. Cardiol. *27*:284, 1971.

131. Rios, J. C., Massumi, R. A., Breesman, W. T., and Sarin, R. K.: Auscultatory features of acute tricuspid regurgitation. Am. J. Cardiol. *23*:4, 1969.

132. Ronan, J. A., Perloff, J. K., and Harvey, W. P.: Systolic clicks and the late systolic murmur—intracardiac phonocardiographic evidence of their mitral valve origin. Am. Heart J. *70*:319, 1965.

133. Osler, W.: On a remarkable heart murmur, heard at a distance from the chest wall. Med. Times Gaz. Lond. *2*:432, 1980.

134. Nelson, W. P., and Hall, R. J.: The innocent supraclavicular arterial bruit—utility of shoulder maneuvers in its recognition. N. Engl. J. Med. *278*:778, 1968.

135. Grant, R. P.: A precordial systolic murmur of extracardiac origin during pregnancy. Am. Heart J. *52*:944, 1965.

136. Danilowicz, D. A., Rudolph, A. M., Hoffman, J. I. E., and Heyman, M.: Physiologic pressure differences between the main and branch pulmonary arteries in infants. Circulation *45*:410, 1972.

137. Morganroth, J., Perloff, J. K., Zeldis, S. M., and Dunkman, W. B.: Acute severe aortic regurgitation: Pathophysiology, clinical recognition and management. Ann. Intern. Med. *87*:223, 1977.

138. Fortuin, N. J., and Craige, E.: Echocardiographic studies of genesis of mitral diastolic murmurs. Br. Heart J. *35*:75, 1973.

139. Ross, R. S., and Criley, J. M.: Cineangiocardiographic studies of the origin of cardiovascular physical signs. Circulation *30*:255, 1964.

140. Perloff, J. K., and Harvey, W. P.: Clinical recognition of tricuspid stenosis. Circulation *22*:346, 1960.

141. Flint, A.: On cardiac murmurs. Am. J. Med. Sci. *44*:23, 1862.

142. Fortuin, N. J., and Craige, E.: On the mechanisms of the Austin Flint murmur. Circulation *45*:558, 1972.

143. Landzberg, J. S., Tflugfelder, P. W., Cassidy, M. M., et al.: Etiology of the Austin Flint murmur. J. Am. Coll. Cardiol. *20*:408, 1992.

144. Criley, J. M., and Hermer, H. A.: Crescendo pre-systolic murmur of mitral stenosis with atrial fibrillation. N. Engl. J. Med. *285*:1284, 1971.

145. Criley, J. M., Feldman, J. M., and Meredith, T.: Mitral valve closure and the crescendo presystolic murmur. Am. J. Med. *51*:456, 1971.

146. Reddy, P. S., Curtiss, E. L., and Salerni, R.: Sound-pressure correlates of the Austin Flint murmur: An intracardiac sound study. Circulation *53*:210, 1976.

147. Berman, P.: Austin Flint—America's Laënnec revisited. Arch. Intern. Med. *148*:2053, 1988.

148. Williams, X.: Comment in discussion of case of patent ductus arteriosus with aortic valve disease, coarctation of aorta and infective endocarditis reported by Babington. London Med. Gazette *4*:822, 1847.

149. Gibson, G. A.: Persistence of the arterial duct and its diagnosis. Edinb. Med. J. *8*:1, 1900.

150. Potain, P. C.: Des movements et de bruits qui se passent dans les veines jugulaires. Bull. Mem. Soc. Med. Hop. Paris *4*:3, 1867.

151. Cutforth, R., Wideman, J., and Sutherland, R. D.: The genesis of the cervical venous hum. Am. Heart J. *80*:488, 1970.

152. McGuire, J., Kotte, J. H., and Helm, R. A.: Acute pericarditis. Circulation *9*:425, 1954.

153. Hamman, L.: Mediastinal emphysema. JAMA *128*:1, 1945.

154. Cabot, R. C.: Physical Diagnosis. New York, William Wood and Co., 1915.

DYNAMIC AUSCULTATION

155. Grewe, K., Crawford, M. H., and O'Rourke, R. A.: Differentiation of cardiac murmurs by dynamic auscultation. Curr. Probl. Cardiol. *13*:671, 1988.

156. Lembro, N. J., Dell'Italia, L. J., Crawford, M. H., and O'Rourke, R. A.: Bedside diagnosis of systolic murmurs. N. Engl. J. Med. *318*:1572, 1988.

157. Baragan, J., Fernandez, F., and Thiron, J. M.: Dynamic Auscultation and Phonocardiography. Tavel, M. E., and Tavel, M. E. (eds.). Maryland, Charles Press, 1979.

158. Rothman, A., and Goldberger, A. L.: Aids to cardiac auscultation. Ann. Intern. Med. *99:*346, 1983.

159. Cha, S. D., and Gooch, A. S.: Diagnosis of tricuspid regurgitation. Arch. Intern. Med. *143:*1763, 1983.

160. Barlow, J. B.: Perspectives on the Mitral Valve, Philadelphia, F. A. Davis, 1987.

161. Vrewe, K., Crawford, M. H., and O'Rourke, R. A.: Differentiation of cardiac murmurs by dynamic auscultation. Curr. Probl. Cardiol. *13:*671, 1988.

162. Nishimura, R. A., and Tajik, A. J.: The Valsalva maneuver and response revisited. Mayo Clin. Proc. *61:*211, 1986.

163. Lembro, N. J., Dell'Italia, L. J., Crawford, M. H., and O'Rourke, R. A.: Bedside diagnosis of systolic murmurs. N. Engl. J. Med. *318:*1572, 1988.

164. Criscitiello, M.: Physiologic and pharmacologic aids in cardiac auscultation. *In* Fowler, N. O. (ed.): Cardiac Diagnosis and Treatment. 3rd ed. Hagerstown, Harper and Row, 1980, pp. 77–90.

165. McCraw, D. B., Siegel, W., Stonecipher, H. K., et al.: Response of the heart murmur intensity to isometric (handgrip) exercise. Br. Heart J. *34:*605, 1972.

166. Barlow, J., and Shillingford, J.: The use of amyl nitrite in differentiating mitral and aortic systolic murmurs. Br. Heart J. *20:*162, 1958.

167. Tavel, M. E.: Clinical Phonocardiography and External Pulse Recording. Chicago, Year Book Medical Publishers, 1985.

Chapter 3
Echocardiography

HARVEY FEIGENBAUM

PRINCIPLES OF ECHOCARDIOGRAPHY

CREATION OF IMAGES USING PULSED REFLECTED ULTRASOUND

The term *echocardiography* refers to a group of tests that utilize ultrasound to examine the heart and record information in the form of echoes, i.e., reflected sonic waves.[1-3] The upper limit for audible sound is 20,000 cycles/second, or 20 kiloHertz (kHz = 1000 cycles/second).[1] The sonic frequency used for echocardiography ranges from 1 to 10 million cycles/second, or 1 to 10 megaHertz (MHz).[2] In adults the frequencies commonly employed are 2.0 to 5.0 MHz, while in children they are usually higher, ranging from 3.5 to 10.0 MHz. The resolution of the recording, which is the ability to distinguish two objects that are spatially close together, varies directly with the frequency and inversely with the wavelength. High-frequency (short wavelength) ultrasound can identify separate objects that are less than 1 mm apart. Beams having lower frequencies and longer wavelengths have poorer resolution. However, the degree of penetration, which is the ability to transmit sufficient ultrasonic energy into the chest to provide a satisfactory recording, is inversely proportional to the frequency of the signal. Since a high-frequency ultrasonic beam (i.e., 5 or 10 MHz) is unable to penetrate a thick chest wall, lower frequency ultrasonic beams are used in adults. While this permits penetration through the chest wall, it partially sacrifices resolution; however, even with a transducer producing a beam of 2.50 MHz, which is commonly used in adult echocardiography, it is possible to resolve objects that are 1 to 2 mm apart.

Principles of Ultrasonic Imaging

The principles by which ultrasound creates an image are depicted in Figure 3–1. The transducer at the side of the beaker of water has a piezoelectric element that vibrates very rapidly and produces ultrasound when activated by an electrical field.[3] If a burst of electrical energy is imparted to the transducer, it will emit a burst of ultrasound, which travels through the beaker. As long as the medium through which the sound travels is homogeneous, the ultrasonic waves will travel in a straight line. When the ultrasound strikes an interface between two media that have different acoustical properties, the sound behaves according to the laws of reflection and refraction,[1,2] analogous to light. Whether or not ultrasound is reflected by an interface depends upon the difference in the acoustical impedances of the two media. Although acoustical impedance is the product of the density of the object and the velocity of sound through that object, for all practical purposes one can consider the acoustical impedance to be a function of density. Thus, if the interface is between a liquid and a solid, the ultrasonic wave will generally be reflected. If the interface is between two solids of different densities, the quantity of reflected ultrasound is usually less. Thus the quantity of energy reflected is directly proportional to the difference in the acoustical impedances (or densities) of the object and its surrounding media.

The left panel of Figure 3–1 shows diagrammatically an ultrasonic beam, which consists of individual bursts of ultrasound that leave the transducer, travel through the fluid, strike the far side of the beaker, are reflected by this interface, retrace their original path, and again strike the transducer. The piezoelectric element in the transducer not only converts electrical energy into ultrasonic impulses but also converts ultrasound back to electrical energy. Thus, when the reflected ultrasound (echo) strikes the piezoelectric element in the transducer, an electrical signal is produced. If the time it takes for (1) the ultrasound to leave the transducer and return and (2) the velocity of sound through the medium are both known, the distance between the transducer and the reflected interface can be calculated.

By calibration of the echograph for a velocity of sound in the medium under examination the time that it takes for the ultrasound to leave and return as an echo can be automatically converted to distance. Thus, the far wall of the beaker is depicted on the oscilloscope as being 6 cm from the transducer.

If a rod is placed in the water so that it transects the ultrasonic beam, part of the energy will strike it and be reflected by the rod before the beam strikes the far side of the beaker. Thus, the returning ultrasonic energy or echo from the rod will strike the transducer sooner than that returning from the far side of the beaker, and the corresponding electrical signal produced by the echo from the rod will be closer to the transducer than will that from the beaker. Also, since some of the ultrasonic energy is reflected by the rod, less energy will remain to strike the far wall of the beaker, and the magnitude of the echo (Fig. 3–1, center panel) will be reduced. If the interface is a very strong reflector of sound, no energy may transverse the object and no images are obtained behind the object, i.e., acoustic shadowing. There are adjustments in ultrasonic instrumentation that provide depth compensation and thereby correct for the usually gradual loss of ultrasonic energy from distant or far objects. From examination of the A-mode echo ("A" refers to amplitude) in

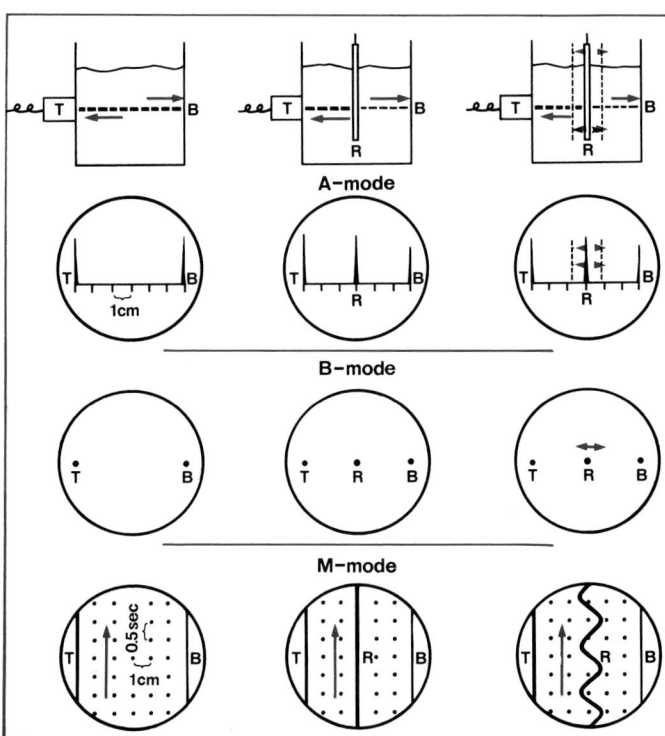

FIGURE 3–1. The principles of acoustic imaging using pulsed reflected ultrasound (see text for details). T = transducer; B = beaker; R = rod. (Modified from Feigenbaum, H., and Zaky, A.: Use of diagnostic ultrasound in clinical cardiology. J. Indiana State Med. Assoc. *59*:140, 1966.)

Figure 3–1 (center panel), one could deduce that the far wall of the beaker is 6 cm from the transducer and that an echo-reflecting object is present in the center of the beaker, 3 cm from the transducer.

Imaging a Moving Object

If the rod were moving back and forth as in the right panel of Figure 3–1, the ultrasonic examination would differ. The transducer functions as a transmitter of ultrasound for a very short time, just over 1 μsec in commercial echocardiographs. During the remaining time the transducer functions as a receiver, waiting for echoes to be converted into electrical signals. The rapidity of the repetition rate with which the transducer fires the 1 μsec impulses varies depending upon the design of the instrument. In most situations the transducer functions as a receiver for over 90 per cent of the time.

A-Mode, B-Mode, and M-Mode Presentations

In the left and center panels of Figure 3–1, the wall of the beaker and the rod are not moving. All the ultrasonic impulses firing at a rate of 1000/sec take the same time to leave the transducer and return as echoes. Therefore the signals or echoes seen on the oscilloscope are static. In the right panel, the object moves constantly, the time required for the ultrasound to leave the transducer and return as an echo varies correspondingly, and the echo signal on the oscilloscope moves. In the A-mode presentation the echo from the rod moves back and forth within the center of the beaker. To record the motion of the rod, one converts the amplitude of the echo to brightness, which changes the display from the A-mode to the B-mode ("B" refers to brightness), in which the returning echoes are displayed on the oscilloscope as dots rather than as spikes. Stronger signals are therefore taller on the A-mode and brighter on the B-mode presentation. On the M-mode presentation ("M" refers to motion), displayed in Figure 3–1, the oscilloscope sweeps from bottom to top. In the left and center panels the structures are fixed, and therefore the M-mode presentation shows simply a series of parallel lines. In the right panel the rod moves back and forth regularly, its echo inscribing a sinusoidal curve on the M-mode oscilloscope.

Thus, the M-mode presentation permits recording of amplitude and of the rate of motion of moving objects with great accuracy; the sampling rate is essentially 1000 pulses/sec, the repetition rate of the transducer. Because electrocardiograms and other cardiac parameters are conventionally displayed on the oscilloscope together with the echocardiographs, the oscilloscope usually sweeps from left to right rather than from bottom to top; therefore the transducer is generally displayed at the top of the oscilloscopic image rather than on the left side, as depicted in Figure 3–1.

M-Mode Echocardiography

TECHNIQUE. The ultrasonic transducer is ordinarily placed on the surface of the chest, usually along the left sternal border, and the ultrasonic beam is directed toward the part of the heart lobe examined. In Figure 3–2 the ultrasound is depicted as passing through a small portion of the right ventricle, the interventricular septum, and the cavity and posterior wall of the left ventricle. Structures such as the chest wall that do not move with cardiac activity are depicted as horizontal lines. Cardiac walls and valves that move with cardiac action inscribe wavy signals, while the blood-filled cavities are relatively echo free.

THE M-MODE TRACING. An M-mode recording is sometimes called a one-dimensional or an "ice pick" view of the heart. However, since time is the second dimension on M-mode tracings, this display is not truly one-dimensional. The information provided by an isolated M-mode view of the heart, as in Figure 3–2, can be augmented by changing the direction of the ultrasonic beam, as in an arc or sector. With the transducer placed along the left sternal border in approximately the third or fourth intercostal space, the ultrasonic beam can be swept in a sector between the apex and the base of the heart. When the transducer is pointed toward the apex of the heart, the ultrasonic beam traverses the left ventricular cavity at the level of the papillary muscles and passes through a small portion of the right ventricular cavity (Fig. 3–3, position 1). Tilting the transducer superiorly and medially causes the ultrasonic beam to traverse the left ventricular cavity at the level of the edges of the mitral valve leaflets or the chordae (position 2). The beam again passes through a small portion of the right

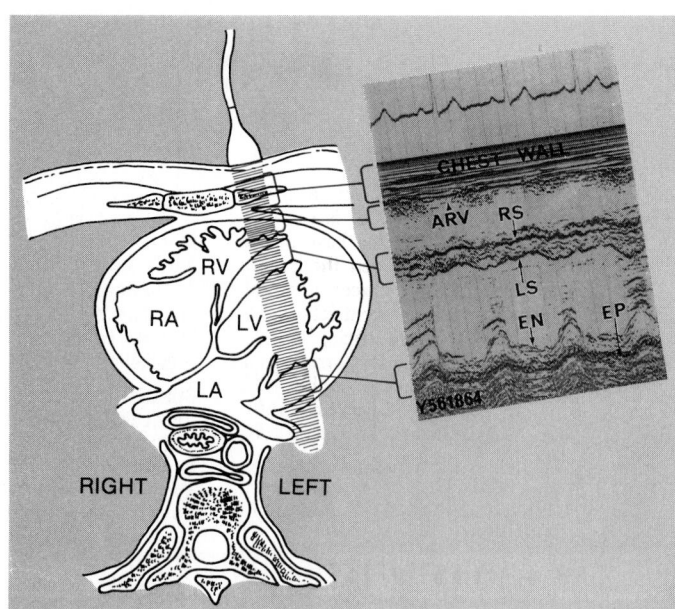

FIGURE 3–2. Cross-section of the heart and corresponding echocardiogram showing the cardiac structures transected by an ultrasonic beam directed toward the left ventricle. The ultrasound passes through the chest wall, the anterior right ventricular wall (ARV), a small portion of the right ventricular cavity, the interventricular septum, the cavity of the left ventricle, and the posterior left ventricular wall. RS = right side of the interventricular septum; LS = left side of interventricular septum; EN = posterior left ventricular endocardium; EP = posterior left ventricular epicardium. (Modified from Popp, R. L., et al.: Estimation of right and left ventricular size by ultrasound. A study of the echoes from the interventricular septum. Am. J. Cardiol. *24*:523, 1969.)

ventricle. By directing the transducer more superiorly and medially (position 3), more of the anterior leaflet of the mitral valve can be recorded and the beam may traverse part of the left atrial cavity. Further tilting of the transducer superiorly and medially (position 4) directs the beam through the root of the aorta, the leaflets of the aortic valve, and the body of the left atrium.

Figure 3–4 shows echoes from the aorta and aortic valve; by tilting the transducer medially from the aortic valve, it is possible to record the anterior leaflet of the tricuspid valve, which is similar in appearance to the recording from the anterior leaflet of the mitral valve. When the transducer is directed superiorly and laterally from the aortic valve, a posterior leaflet of the pulmonary valve can be recorded (Fig. 3–4).

Two-Dimensional Echocardiography

The principle of two-dimensional (2-D) echocardiography is depicted in Figure 3–5. The ultrasonic beam now moves in a sector so that a pie-shaped slice of the heart is interrogated. Most commercial 2-D echocardiographs move the ultrasonic beam so that approximately 30 slices/sec are obtained. The ultrasonic beam can be moved mechanically by oscillating a single transducer or by rotating a series of transducers. The ultrasound can also be steered electronically using the so-called phased array principles,[4] in which multiple ultrasonic elements are utilized to make up the beam and in which the firing sequence of the elements is controlled. A computer or microprocessor is necessary to control the firing of the elements and the direction of the beam. Figure 3–6 illustrates two individual frames representing stop-action sequences from a videotape recording of a normal heart in which the mitral and aortic valves and parts of the left ventricle, left atrium, and right ventricle are imaged.

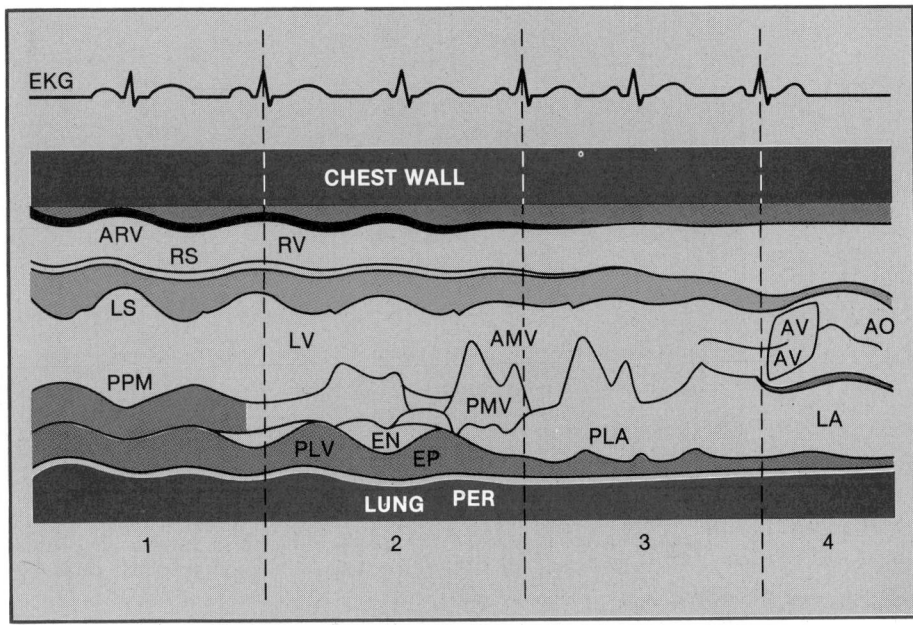

FIGURE 3–3. Presentation of an M-mode echocardiogram as the transducer is directed from the apex (position 1) to the base of the heart (position 4). Areas between the dotted lines correspond to the transducer position. EN = endocardium of the left ventricle; EP = epicardium of the left ventricle; PER = pericardium; PLA = posterior left atrial wall. (From Feigenbaum, H.: Clinical applications of echocardiography. Progr. Cardiovasc. Dis. 14:531, 1972, by permission of Grune and Stratton.)

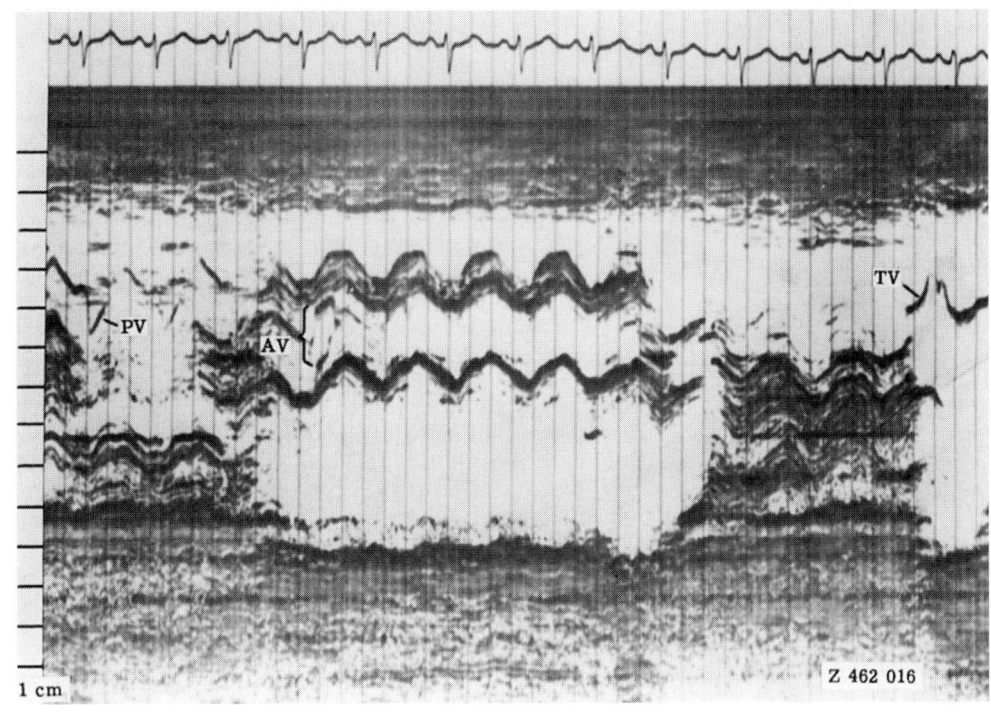

FIGURE 3–4. M-mode scan recording echoes from a pulmonic valve (PV), aortic valve (AV), and tricuspid valve (TV). (From Feigenbaum, H.: Echocardiography. 2nd ed. Philadelphia, Lea and Febiger, 1976.)

FIGURE 3–5. How to obtain a cross-sectional or 2-D image of the heart parallel to the long axis of the left ventricle. CW = chest wall.

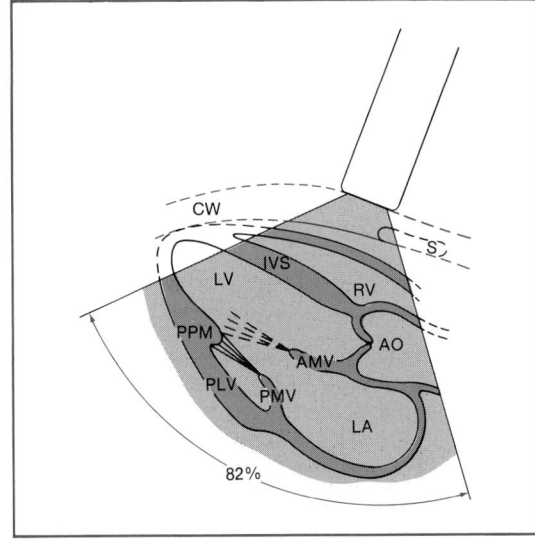

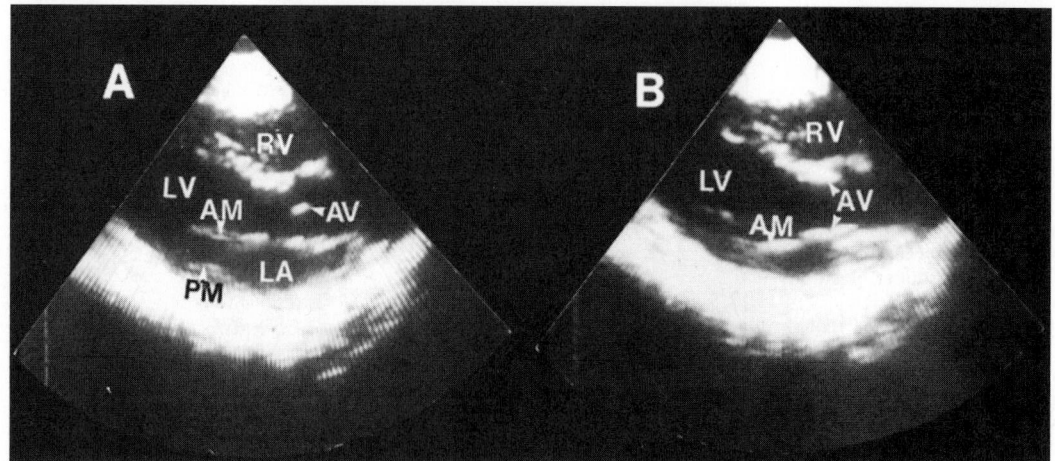

FIGURE 3–6. Long-axis 2-D echocardiographic images of the left ventricle (LV), right ventricle (RV), mitral valve, aortic valve, and left atrium (LA) during diastole *(A)* and systole *(B)*. During diastole the anterior (AM) and posterior (PM) mitral leaflets are apart and the aortic valve leaflets (AV) come together as a single echo in the midportion of the aorta *(A)*. With systole *(B)*, the mitral leaflets come together and the aortic valve leaflets separate.

Doppler Echocardiography

M-mode and 2-D echocardiography essentially create ultrasonic images of the heart. Doppler echocardiography utilizes ultrasound to record blood flow within the cardiovascular system. The principle of the Doppler effect is illustrated in Figure 3–7.[5,6] If the ultrasonic beam is reflected by a stationary object (Fig. 3–7), the transmitted frequency (f_t) and the reflected frequency (f_r) are equal. However, if the target reflecting the ultrasonic energy is moving toward the transducer (Fig. 3–7*B*), the reflected frequency is greater than the transmitted frequency. When

the target is moving away from the transducer (Fig. 3–7*C*), the reflected frequency is less than the transmitted frequency. The difference between the reflected and transmitted frequencies represents the Doppler shift or Doppler frequency. By knowing the Doppler frequency it is possible to calculate the velocity of the moving target. Figure 3–8 shows the Doppler equations that relate Doppler frequency (f_d) and the velocity of the moving target (v). To determine the velocity of blood flow it is necessary to know the Doppler frequency, the angle (Θ) between the paths of the ultrasonic beam and moving target, and the velocity of sound in the medium being examined; in Doppler echocardiography the targets are the red blood cells.

Figure 3–7 illustrates the principles of continuous-wave Doppler. There are two transducers, one of which continuously transmits ultrasonic energy, and the other, which continuously records the reflected ultrasonic signals. One can also use pulsed ultrasound to obtain the Doppler information (Fig. 3–9). With pulsed Doppler only one transducer is needed. In addition, pulsed Doppler permits creation of a simultaneous M-mode or 2-D image.[7] To derive the Doppler frequency, the frequencies of the reflected and transmitted bursts of ultrasound are subtracted.

Significant differences exist between continuous wave and pulsed Doppler. The velocity that can be recorded using pulsed Doppler is limited by the pulse repetition

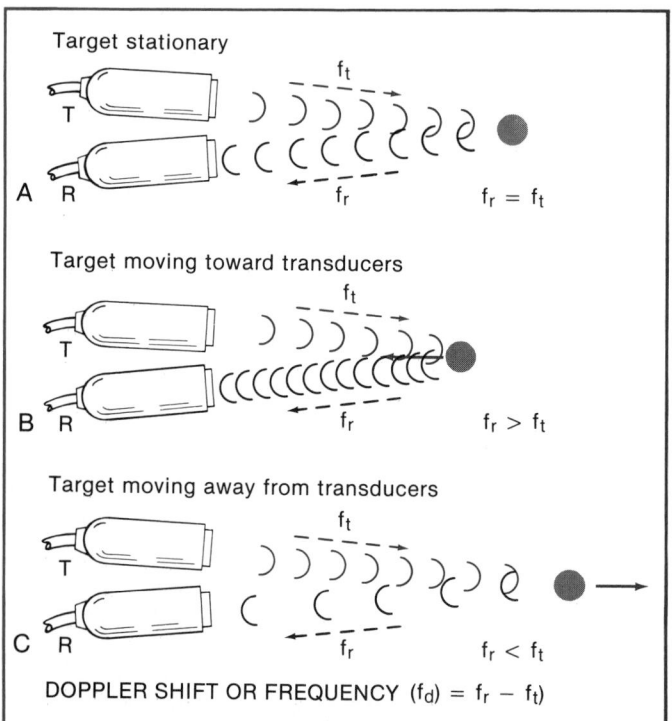

FIGURE 3–7. Demonstration of the Doppler effect using reflected sound from a target *(A)*. The reflected frequency (f_r) is greater than the transmitted frequency (f_t) when the target is moving toward the transducer *(B)*. The reflected frequency is smaller than the transmitted frequency when the target moves away from the transducer *(C)*. The Doppler shift or frequency (f_d) is the difference between the transmitted and reflected frequencies. (From Feigenbaum, H.: Echocardiography. 4th ed. Philadelphia, Lea and Febiger, 1986.)

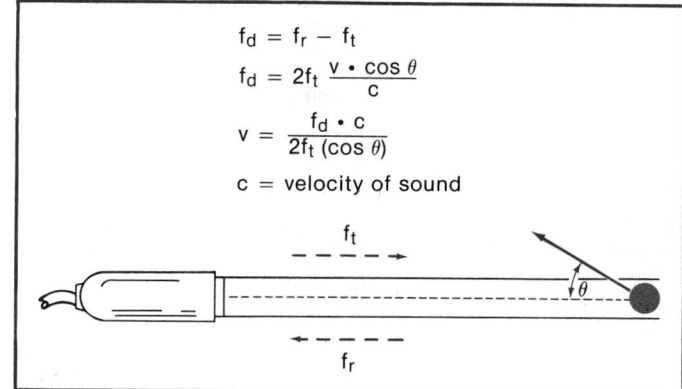

FIGURE 3–8. Doppler equations relating Doppler frequencies (f_d), received frequency (f_r), transmitted frequency (f_t), and the angle (θ) between the direction of the moving target and the path of the ultrasonic beam. (From Feigenbaum, H.: Echocardiography. 4th ed. Philadelphia, Lea and Febiger, 1986.)

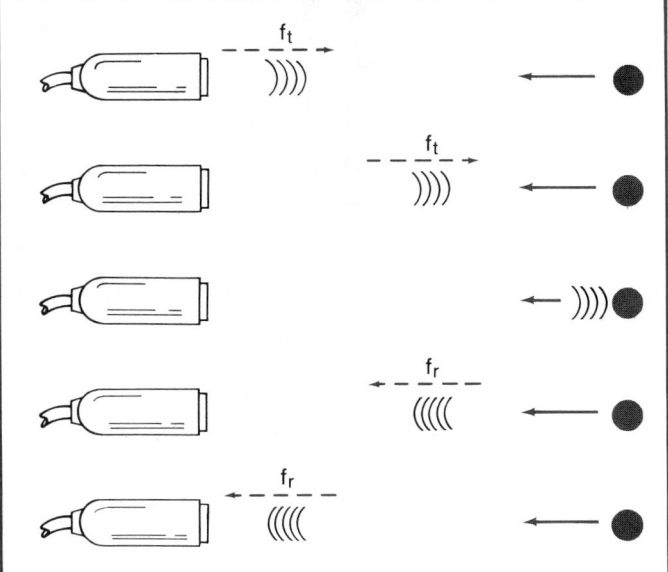

FIGURE 3–9. Demonstration of the principle of pulsed Doppler echocardiography. If the object reflecting the pulses with ultrasound is moving toward the transducer, the frequency of the received pulse (f_r) is greater than the transmitted frequency (f_t). (From Feigenbaum, H.: Echocardiography. 4th ed. Philadelphia, Lea and Febiger, 1986.)

frequency of the system. Thus, if the blood is moving very rapidly, as might occur when it is passing through a stenotic valve, then pulsed Doppler cannot sample rapidly enough to identify the Doppler frequency. This technical problem is known as *aliasing*.[8] As a result, continuous-wave Doppler is necessary for recording very high velocities within the cardiovascular system. An alternative way is to use a multiple pulsed or high pulse repetition frequency (high PRF) Doppler system. High PRF allows simultaneous imaging and recording of high flow rates; however, it is technically more difficult. The continuous wave approach is the more commonly used technique for recording high-frequency flows.[9]

The Doppler recording is a spectral display using fast Fourier analysis of the audible Doppler signal. The recording is usually on strip chart paper or videotape and is commonly referred to as *spectral Doppler*. The audio signal is helpful in interpreting the various types of flow and represents an important aspect of the Doppler examination.

COLOR DOPPLER. Doppler information from the cardiovascular system can also be recorded in a spatially correct format superimposed on an M-mode or 2-D echocardiogram. Doppler flow imaging is created by multiple Doppler gates that are spatially correct and display the moving blood within the 2-D or M-mode recording.[10] The direction of the blood is displayed in color as in Figure 3–10. With this particular instrument blood moving toward the transducer is depicted in shades of yellow and red, whereas blood moving away from the transducer is in shades of blue. Figure 3–11 shows an M-mode color Doppler or M/Q study of a patient with valvular disease. The tracing shows how turbulent flow can be displayed as green or as a mosaic of colors.[11]

Transesophageal Echocardiography

Although echocardiography is one of the most common noninvasive examinations, this ultrasonic examination need not be limited to merely placing the transducer on the surface of the chest. Transesophageal echocardiography has been available for many years. With the technical advances in placing a 2-D transducer at the end of a flexible endoscope, it is now possible to obtain high-quality 2-D images via the esophagus in multiple planes[12–14] (Figs. 3–12, 3–13). It is also possible to obtain Doppler information with this approach. Figure 3–14 demonstrates a transesophageal echocardiogram in a patient with mitral regurgitation. The regurgitant jet is multicolored instead of green.

FIGURE 3–10.   See color plate 1.

FIGURE 3–11.   See color plate 1.

FIGURE 3–12. Demonstration of the position of transesophageal probe and the horizontal images that can be obtained from the transgastric (2A, 2B), the midesophageal (3A, 3B), the upper esophageal (1A, 1B) positions. The echocardiographic images can be displayed with the apex of the sector up (1A, 2A, 3A) or with the apex of the sector down (1B, 2B, 3B). RPA = right pulmonary artery; SVC = superior vena cava; AO = aorta; LPA = left pulmonary artery; IVC = inferior vena cava; S = stomach; FO = fossa ovalis. (From Feigenbaum, H.: Echocardiography. 5th ed. Malvern, PA, Lea and Febiger, 1994.)

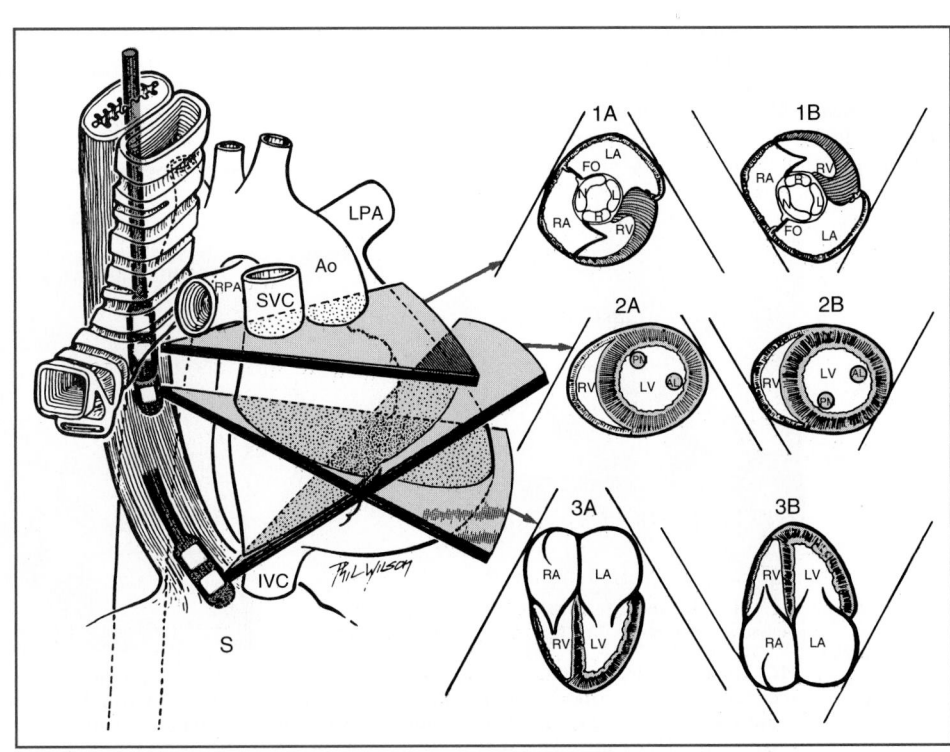

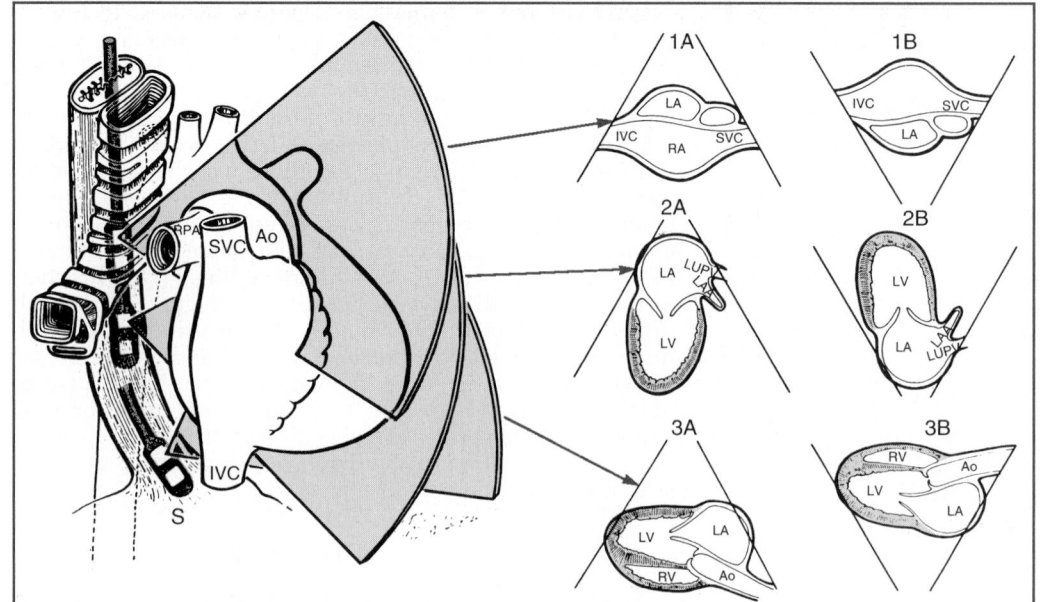

FIGURE 3–13. Views that can be obtained with the longitudinal transducer in the gastric (3A, 3B), midesophageal (2A, 2B), and upper esophageal (1A, 1B) positions. RPA =right pulmonary artery; SVC = superior vena cava; Ao = aorta; IVC = inferior vena cava; LA = left atrium; RA = right atrium; LUPV = left upper pulmonary vein; LAA = left atrial appendage; LV = left ventricle; RV = right ventricle. (From Feigenbaum, H.: Echocardiography. 5th ed. Malvern, PA, Lea and Febiger, 1994.)

Transesophageal echocardiography is useful in patients in whom the examination from the usual transthoracic approach is technically difficult or impossible.[15] This approach is particularly helpful in assessing prosthetic valves, vegetations, aortic disease, and intracardiac masses. Another major application for esophageal echocardiography is in the patient undergoing surgery. The esophageal ultrasonic probe can be used to monitor cardiac left ventricular function throughout the surgical procedure and into the postoperative state. Transesophageal echocardiography is being used in the operating room during open-heart surgery and to monitor myocardial ischemia during noncardiac surgery.[16] Cardiac surgeons are finding echocardiography helpful in assessing cardiac morphology and function before, during, and after surgical repair of valvular or congenital conditions.[17,18]

Echocardiography can also be used in conjunction with other invasive procedures such as pericardiocentesis[19] or diagnostic catheterization.[20] A similar type of monitoring has been useful to aid with endomyocardial biopsy.[21] Echocardiography may guide electrophysiological testing[22] and therapy.[23] Other therapeutic catheter techniques are also monitored effectively using echocardiography.[24–26]

INTRAVASCULAR ULTRASOUND. The ultrasonic transducer can be placed in a small catheter so that a vessel can be imaged via the lumen to provide an intravascular echocardiogram, a technique known as intravascular ultrasound. Several intravascular ultrasonic devices are currently being used.[27,28] The techniques utilize a rotating transducer, rotating ultrasonic mirror, or phased array multielement systems. These devices are generating considerable interest, especially for the ability to evaluate atherosclerosis from within the arteries (Fig. 3–15 and Figs. 39–12, p. 1381, and 39–13, p. 1383). Slightly larger intravascular ultrasonic devices are being used to visualize the heart from within cardiac chambers.[29,30]

CONTRAST ECHOCARDIOGRAPHY. Ultrasound is an extremely sensitive detector of intravascular bubbles. The injection of almost any liquid into the intravascular spaces will introduce many microbubbles that appear as a cloud of echoes on the echocardiogram. Figure 3–16 demonstrates a transesophageal echocardiogram of a patient with an atrial septal aneurysm (arrows) (Fig. 3–16A). With the intravenous injection of saline agitated with a small amount of air, one sees the right atrium (RA) filled with echo-producing bubbles. Some of these bubbles (arrowheads) pass through the atrial septal aneurysm into the left atrium (Fig. 3–16B).

FIGURE 3–14. See color plate 1.

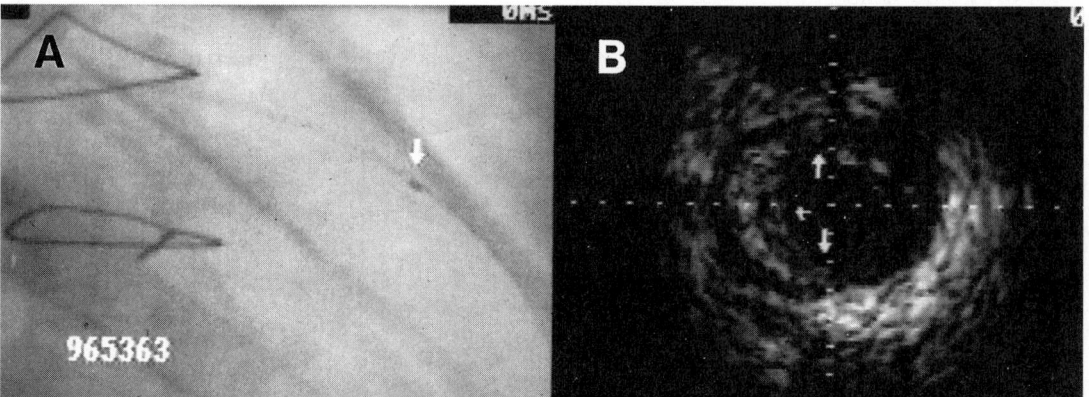

FIGURE 3–15. Intracoronary ultrasonic examination with the ultrasonic device within the left anterior descending coronary artery. The location of the transducer (arrow) can be seen in the angiogram (A). The ultrasonic image (B) shows extensive atherosclerotic plaque (arrows) on the left side of the arterial wall. (From Feigenbaum, H.: Echocardiography. 5th ed. Malvern, PA, Lea & Febiger, 1994.)

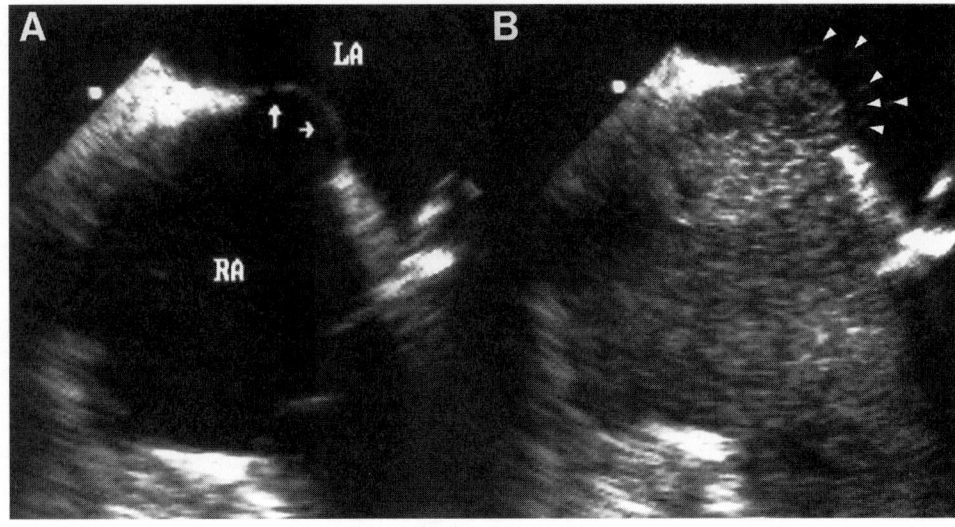

FIGURE 3–16. Transesophageal echo-cardiographic examination of an atrial septal aneurysm (arrows, *A*) with a small number of contrast bubbles (arrowheads, *B*) appearing in the left atrium (LA) following a right-sided contrast injection. RA = right atrium. (From Feigenbaum, H.: Echocardiography. 5th ed. Malvern, PA, Lea and Febiger, 1994.)

Contrast echocardiography is a very sensitive technique for detecting right-to-left shunts. The contrast agents that have been used include the patient's blood, saline, indocyanine green dye, agitated or sonicated angiographic contrast agents, and sonicated albumen. In all cases the contrast effect originates from suspended microbubbles in the fluid. Commercially manufactured microbubbles that traverse the pulmonary capillaries are now available.[31–33] The potential clinical uses for contrast echocardiography are numerous.[34–37]

FETAL ECHOCARDIOGRAPHY. Examination of the fetal heart in utero has become an important subspecialty of echocardiography. The examination is extremely demanding and requires great technical skill as well as an excellent understanding of fetal anatomy, physiology, and potential pathology.[38,39] The field is primarily in the hands of a few pediatric echocardiographers. Because of the highly specialized nature of this work it is beyond the scope of this particular discussion of echocardiography.

THREE-DIMENSIONAL ECHOCARDIOGRAPHY. A variety of approaches to recording echocardiograms that are oriented in three-dimensional (3-D) space have been proposed. One technique orients a 2-D transducer in 3-D space using spark gap sensors.[40–42] Most investigators are creating 3-D images of the heart using gated, reconstructed 2-D examinations.[43–45]

ADVANTAGES AND LIMITATIONS OF ECHOCARDIOGRAPHY. The advantages of echocardiography are numerous. The examination is painless, as best as can be determined it is virtually harmless,[46] and it is less costly than other sophisticated imaging techniques. However, some technical difficulties exist that require expertise on the part of the examiner and interpreter of the echocardiographic recordings. The principal problem is posed by the poor transmission of ultrasound through bony structures or air-containing lungs. The examiner must thus try to avoid these structures. A variety of techniques have been developed to circumvent this problem. The patient is commonly placed in the left recumbent position to move the heart from beneath the sternum. The subxiphoid or subcostal transducer position is frequently used in patients with hyperinflated lungs and a low diaphragm. Transesophageal echocardiography is available for the patient in whom the examination is extremely difficult. Thus, many examining techniques have been developed to minimize the technical difficulties in performing an echocardiographic examination.

EXAMINATION OF THE NORMAL HEART

TWO-DIMENSIONAL ECHOCARDIOGRAPHY. An infinite number of slices of the heart can theoretically be obtained using 2-D echocardiography. The American Society of Echocardiography has attempted to standardize and simplify the many 2-D examinations.[47] The Society thought that all views could be categorized into three orthogonal planes, as illustrated in Figure 3–17. These planes are the long-axis, short-axis, and four-chamber. The long-axis plane is the imaging plane that transects the heart perpendicular to the dorsal and ventral surfaces of the body and parallel to the long axis of the heart. The plane transecting the heart perpendicular to the dorsal and ventral surfaces of the body, but perpendicular to the long axis of the heart, is defined as the short-axis plane. The plane that transects the heart approximately parallel to the dorsal and ventral surfaces of the body is referred to as the four-chamber plan. It should be emphasized that these views or planes are with reference to the heart and not the thorax or body.

Transducer Locations. These ultrasonic planes or views can be obtained from more than one transducer location. Figure 3–18*A* demonstrates that the long-axis view can be obtained with the transducer in the apical position, in the parasternal position (left sternal border), or in the supra-

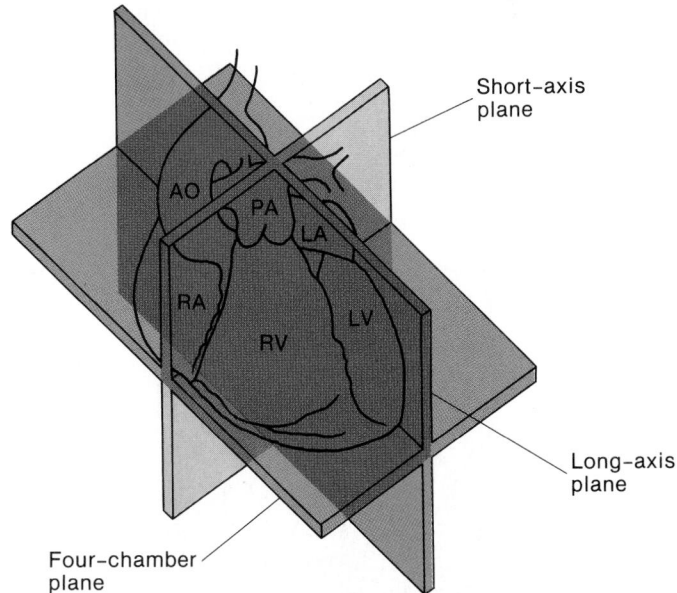

FIGURE 3–17. The three orthogonal planes for 2-D echocardiographic imaging. AO = aorta; PA = pulmonary artery; LA = left atrium; RA = right atrium; RV = right ventricle; LV = left ventricle. (Reproduced with permission from Henry, W. L., et al.: Report of the American Society of Echocardiography Nomenclature and Standards in Two-Dimensional Echocardiography. Circulation *62*:212, 1980. Copyright 1980 American Heart Association.)

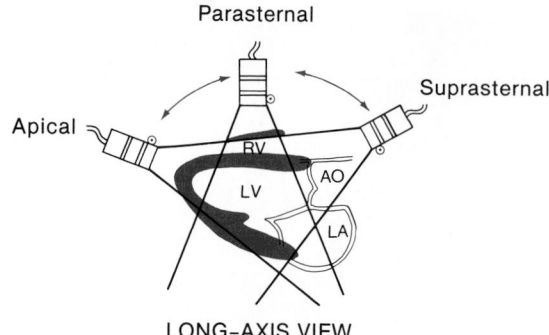

A **LONG-AXIS VIEW**

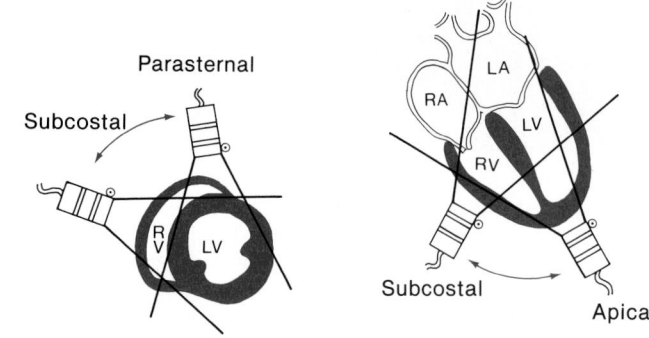

B **SHORT-AXIS VIEW** C **FOUR-CHAMBER VIEW**

FIGURE 3–18. How the various orthogonal planes can be obtained from different transducer positions. (Reproduced with permission from Henry, W. L., et al.: Report of the American Society of Echocardiography Nomenclature and Standards in Two-Dimensional Echocardiography. Circulation 62:212, 1980. Copyright 1980 American Heart Association.)

sternal notch. A short-axis view (Fig. 3–18B) cuts across the heart so that the left ventricle resembles a circle. The right ventricle can be seen curving around the left ventricle. Such an examination can be obtained with the transducer in the parasternal position or in the subcostal (subxiphoid) position. The four-chamber view is depicted in Figure 3–18C. Such a view permits the examination of all four cardiac chambers simultaneously. This type of examination can be obtained with the transducer over the cardiac apex or with the transducer in the subcostal position. Table 3–1 lists the various 2-D echocardiographic examinations cate-

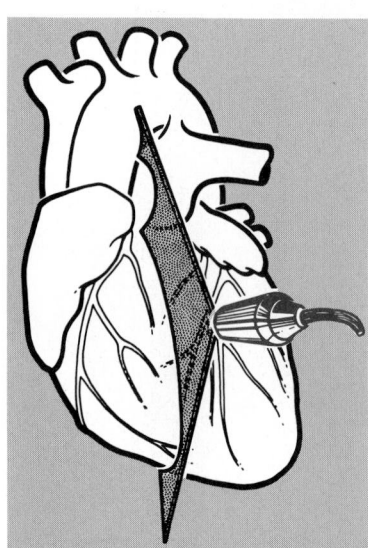

FIGURE 3–19. Transducer position for long-axis parasternal examination of the tricuspid valve, right atrium, and right ventricular inflow tract. (From Feigenbaum, H.: Echocardiography. 4th ed. Philadelphia, Lea and Febiger, 1986.)

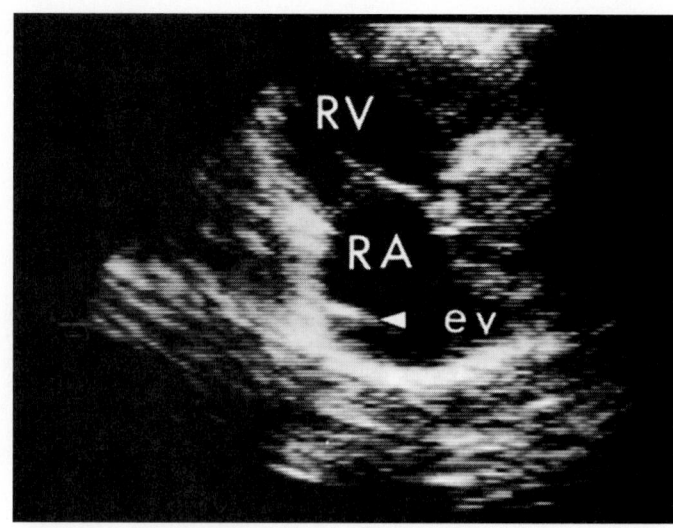

FIGURE 3–20. Two-dimensional echocardiogram of the right atrium (RA) and right ventricular inflow tract (RV). ev = eustachian valve. (From Feigenbaum, H.: Echocardiography. 4th ed. Philadelphia, Lea and Febiger, 1986.)

gorized according to the location of the transducer, the plane of the examination, and the cardiac structure being examined.

The right ventricle, right atrium, and tricuspid valve can be recorded with the transducer in the parasternal position (Fig. 3–19). The plane of the transducer does not exactly fit either the long axis or the short axis. However, the plane is closer to that of the long axis than that of the short axis and thus is categorized as a long-axis study. Figure 3–20 shows the right ventricular inflow tract and right atrium by way of such a parasternal examination.

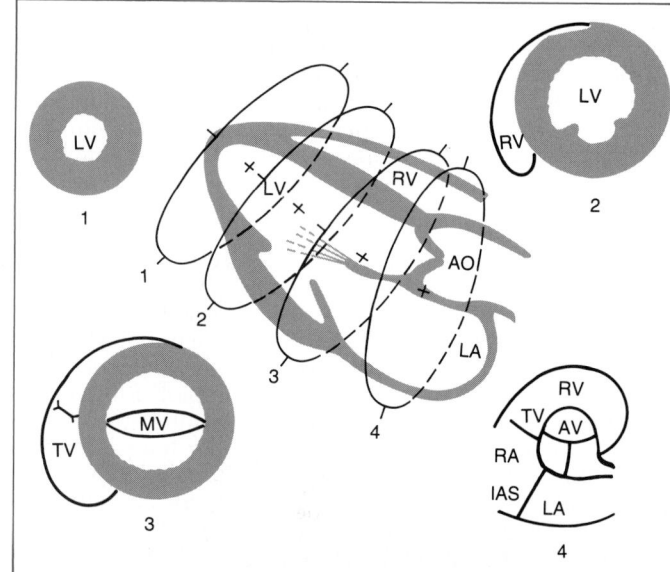

FIGURE 3–21. How short-axis echocardiographic cross-sectional images of the heart, which are perpendicular to the long axis of the left ventricle, are obtained. Diagram 1 shows a short-axis left ventricular echocardiogram near the cardiac apex. Diagram 2 demonstrates part of the right ventricle (RV) and the circular left ventricular cavity (LV) at the level of the papillary muscles, which can be seen to bulge into the LV cavity. Diagram 3 is closer to the base of the heart and shows the left ventricle at the level of the mitral valve (MV). Diagram 4 shows a short-axis cross-section of the base of the heart with the aorta, aortic valve (AV), left atrium (LA), interatrial septum (IAS), right atrium (RA), tricuspid valve (TV), and right ventricular outflow tract (RV). (From Feigenbaum, H.: Echocardiography. 4th ed. Philadelphia, Lea and Febiger, 1986.)

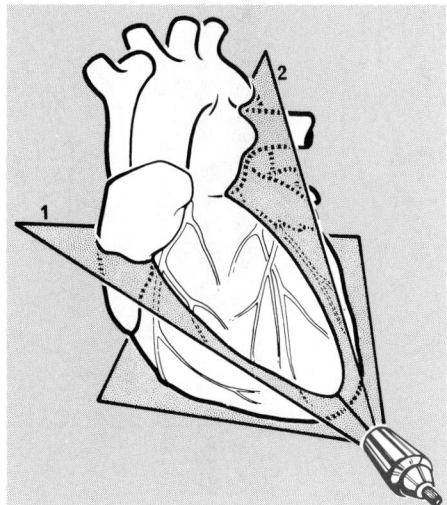

FIGURE 3–22. Transducer position and examining planes for apical 2-D echocardiograms. Plane 1 passes through the four-chamber plane of the heart. Plane 2 represents the path of the ultrasonic beam for the two-chamber apical examination. (From Feigenbaum, H.: Echocardiography. 4th ed. Philadelphia, Lea and Febiger, 1986.)

TABLE 3–1 TWO-DIMENSIONAL ECHOCARDIOGRAPHIC EXAMINATION

61

Ch 3

PARASTERNAL APPROACH
  Long-axis plane
    Root of aorta–aortic valve, left atrium, left ventricular outflow tract
    Body of left ventricle–mitral valve
    Left ventricular apex
    Right ventricular inflow tract–tricuspid valve
  Short-axis plane
    Root of the aorta–aortic valve, pulmonary valve, tricuspid valve, right ventricular outflow tract, left atrium, pulmonary artery, coronary arteries
    Left ventricle–mitral valve
    Left ventricle–papillary muscles
    Left ventricle–apex
APICAL APPROACH
  Four-chamber plane
    Four chamber
    Four chamber with aorta
  Long-axis plane
    Two chamber–left ventricle, left atrium
    Two chamber with aorta
SUBCOSTAL APPROACH
  Four-chamber plane–all four chambers and both septa
  Short-axis plane
    Left ventricle
    Right ventricle
    Inferior vena cava
SUPRASTERNAL APPROACH
  Four-chamber plane
    Arch of aorta–descending aorta
  Long-axis plane
    Arch of aorta–pulmonary artery, left atrium

Various short-axis examinations are diagrammatically illustrated in Figure 3–21. The short-axis views are commonly obtained at the level of the apex, the papillary muscles, the mitral valve, and the base of the heart. With slight variation in angulation the short-axis examination of the base of the heart can also record the pulmonary valve and the pulmonary artery with its bifurcation. It is also possible to use this examination to record the origins of the coronary arteries and the left atrial appendage.

Figure 3–22 diagrammatically illustrates two commonly used 2-D echocardiographic views with the transducer placed at the cardiac apex. Plane 1 demonstrates an apical four-chamber view of the heart and plane 2 is a longitudinal slice through the left ventricle and atrium, the so-called two-chamber view. The two-chamber view does not exactly fit the three-plane scheme, since it is between the four-chamber and long-axis planes. Figure 3–23 shows four common 2-D echocardiographic views. The long-axis (LX)

and short-axis (SX) echograms are with the transducer in the left parasternal position. The four chamber (4C) and two chamber (2C) views are obtained with the transducer at the apex.

The subcostal transducer location produces examinations roughly in the four-chamber and short-axis planes. The ultrasonic plane indicated in Figure 3–24A is similar to examining plane 1 in Figure 3–21. The resulting subcostal four-chamber echocardiogram appears in Figure 3–25A. Figures 3–24B and 3–25B show how the transducer can be rotated 90 degrees to provide a subcostal short-axis exami-

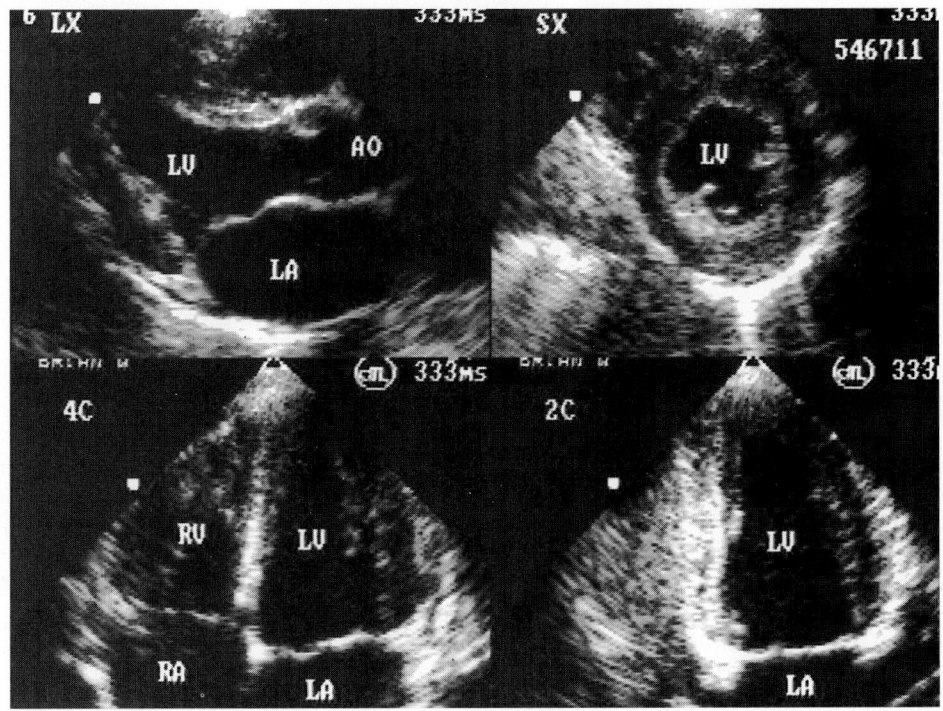

FIGURE 3–23. A quad screen display of four common 2-D echocardiographic views. LX = long axis; SX = short axis; 4C = four chamber; 2C = two chamber; LV = left ventricle; AO = aorta; LA = left atrium; RV = right ventricle; RA = right atrium. (From Feigenbaum, H.: Echocardiography. 5th ed. Malvern, PA, Lea and Febiger, 1994.)

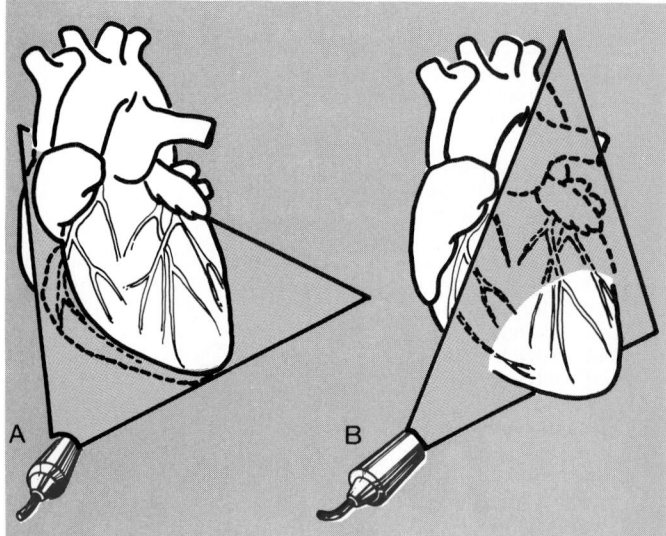

FIGURE 3–24. Transducer position and examining planes for a subcostal four-chamber examination (A) and a subcostal short-axis examination (B). (From Feigenbaum, H.: Echocardiography. 4th ed. Philadelphia, Lea and Febiger, 1986.)

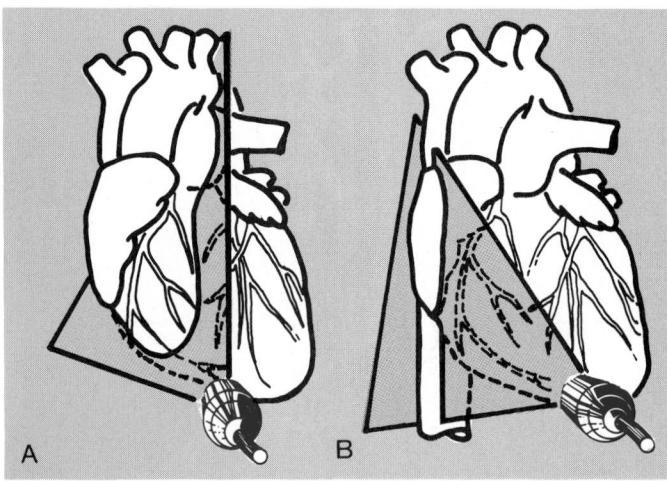

FIGURE 3–26. Examining planes and transducer positions for the subcostal examination of the right side of the heart (A) and the inferior vena cava (B). (From Feigenbaum, H.: Echocardiography. 4th ed. Philadelphia, Lea and Febiger, 1986.)

nation of the heart. The subcostal four-chamber view is particularly helpful in examining the interatrial and interventricular septa. By directing the transducer in a slightly modified short-axis examination, one can obtain an excellent view of the right side of the heart. The subcostal location also permits an opportunity to direct the ultrasonic beam through the inferior vena cava and hepatic veins (Figs. 3–26B and 3–27).

The two examining planes with the transducer in the suprasternal notch are depicted in Figure 3–28. The ultra-

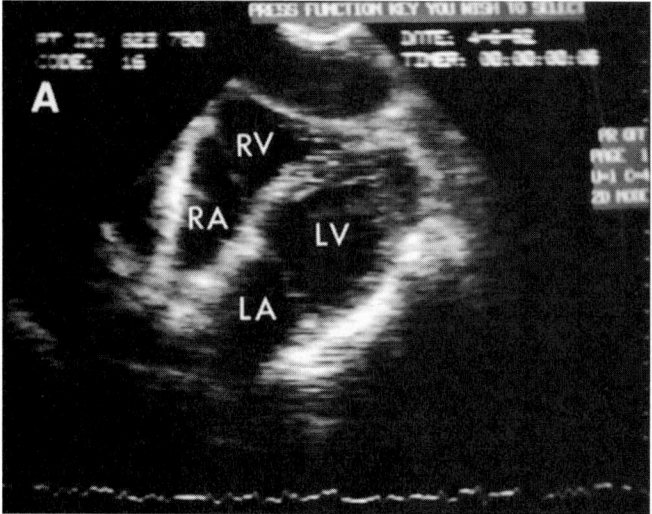

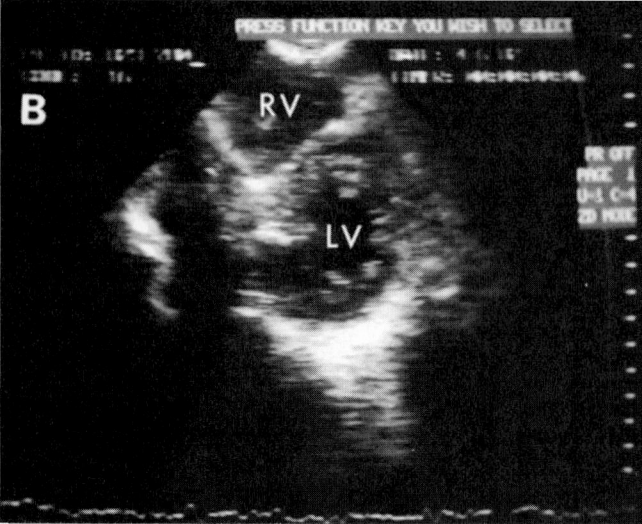

FIGURE 3–25. Two-dimensional echocardiograms obtained with the transducer in the subcostal position. Echocardiogram A represents a four-chamber view, and B is a short-axis examination. RV = right ventricle; RA = right atrium; LA = left atrium; LV = left ventricle.

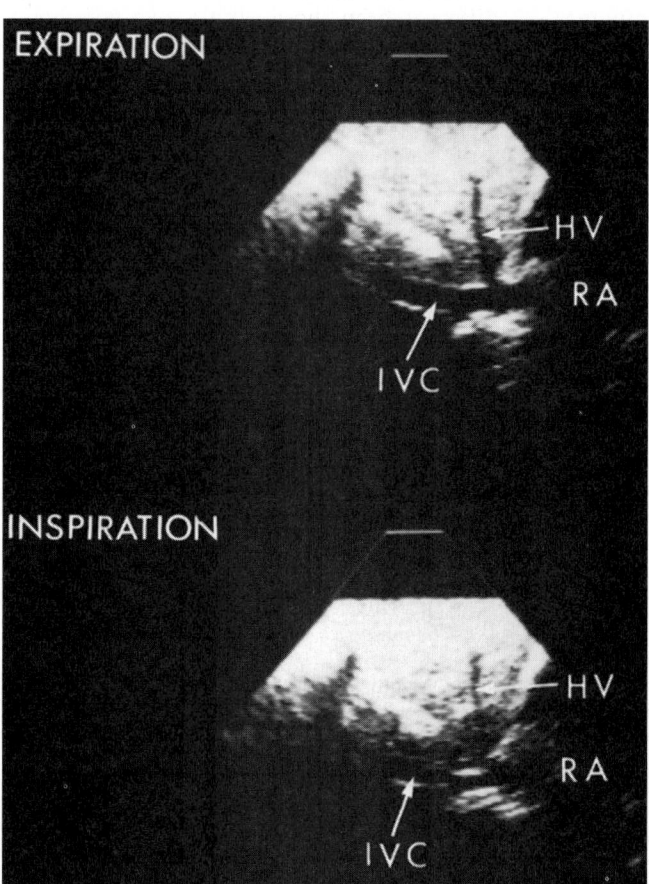

FIGURE 3–27. Subcostal 2-D echocardiograms of the inferior vena cava (IVC) and hepatic veins (HV). The inferior vena cava decreases in size with inspiration. RA = right atrium. (From Feigenbaum, H.: Echocardiography. 4th ed. Philadelphia, Lea and Febiger, 1986.)

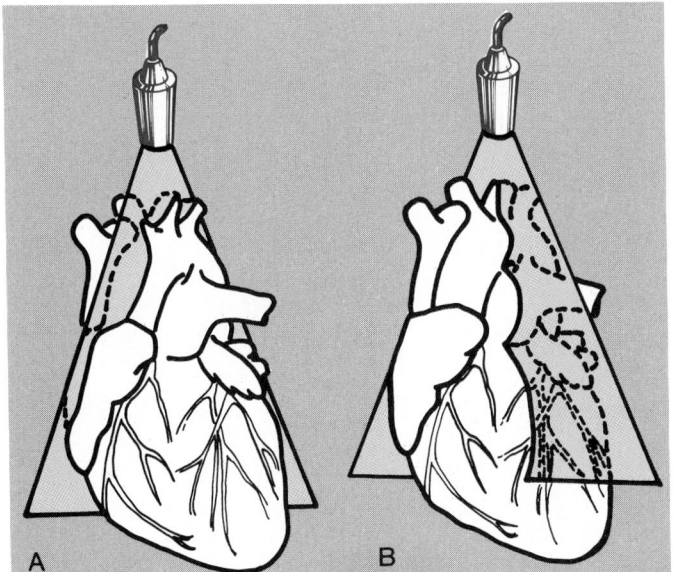

FIGURE 3–28. Transducer position in examining planes for the suprasternal examination parallel to the arch of the aorta *(A)* and perpendicular to the arch of the aorta *(B)*. (From Feigenbaum, H.: Echocardiography. 4th ed. Philadelphia, Lea and Febiger, 1986.)

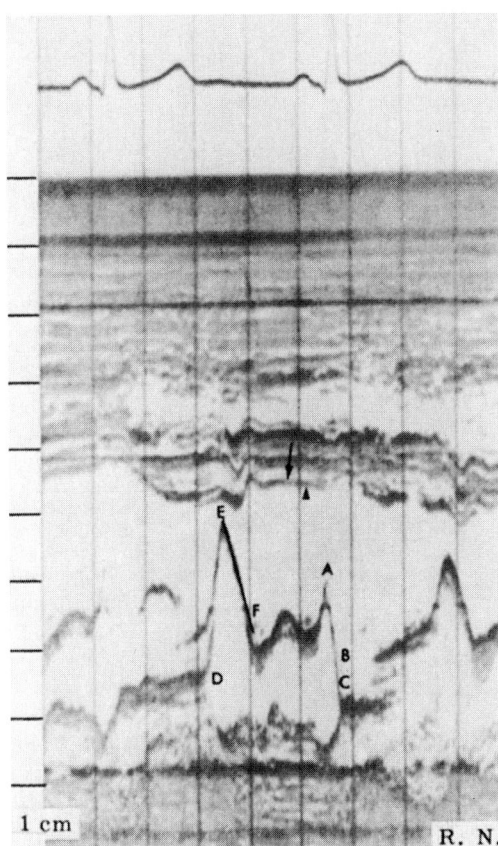

FIGURE 3–30. M-mode echocardiogram of a normal mitral valve. The letters A through F denote various portions of the anterior leaflet motion. The arrow indicates the leading edge of the echo from the left side of the interventricular septum; the arrowhead denotes the trailing edge of that echo. (From Feigenbaum, H.: Echocardiography. 2nd ed. Philadelphia, Lea and Febiger, 1976.)

sonic view in Figure 3–28*A* is roughly equivalent to that of a four-chamber plane, and the view in Figure 3–28*B* is somewhat comparable to that of the long-axis plane. However, it is probably best to orient the ultrasonic beam with regard to the arch of the aorta rather than to the heart, since one does not record much of the heart with the transducer in this position, especially in the adult. In addition, the planes are different from those with the transducer at the apex or subcostal region. Thus, better terminology with regard to the examining plane from the suprasternal location would be parallel or perpendicular to the arch of the aorta. Figure 3–29 shows a suprasternal examination parallel to the arch of the aorta.

M-MODE ECHOCARDIOGRAPHY. With the advent of 2-D echocardiography, and to some extent Doppler echocardiography, the M-mode examination now plays a lesser role in the ultrasonic examination of the heart.[48] The principal advantage of this examination is the high temporal resolution inherent in sampling cardiac motion at roughly 1000 times/second. One can utilize this examination to demonstrate subtle motion of cardiac structures. Figure 3–30 is an M-mode study of a normal mitral valve. One can appreciate the motion of the anterior and posterior leaflets with far greater detail than can be seen with a 2-D study that usu-

ally samples at 30 frames/sec. For example, the mid-diastolic reopening of the valve, which commonly is seen in normal persons, is rarely appreciated on a real-time 2-D examination. Figure 3–30 shows the usual labeling given to an M-mode mitral valve echogram.

One of the common uses of M-mode echocardiography is obtaining cardiac measurements. Figure 3–31 illustrates some of the M-mode measurements that are being used. The diastolic and systolic dimensions of the left ventricle can be used to calculate fractional shortening. One can also use an empirical formula to calculate volumes and provide ejection fraction. One can use M-mode dimensions for measuring septal and posterior wall thickness. These measurements can be combined to calculate left ventricular mass. Left atrial and aortic measurements are also commonly made with the M-mode examination. Table 3–2 shows some of the M-mode measurements and normal values for these determinations.[49]

DOPPLER ECHOCARDIOGRAPHY. Spectral Doppler echocardiographic recordings are basically of three types. There is the venous ventricular inflow and ventricular outflow pattern of Doppler flow (Fig. 3–32). Venous flow has both systolic and diastolic components. There will be some slight variation whether the recording is from systemic or pulmonary veins.[50] There is frequently reverse flow that moves downward or away from the transducer following atrial contraction.[51] Ventricular inflow is totally diastolic. There is an early component that peaks at the E wave and a late component following atrial contraction that peaks with an A wave. Ventricular outflow is entirely systolic in nature. Figure 3–33 shows the ventricular inflow or mitral flow pattern with the sample volume at the level of the mitral valve. One sees the early flow that peaks with the E

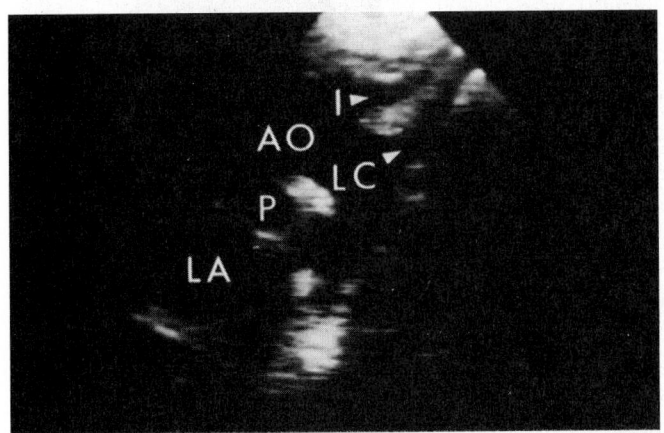

FIGURE 3–29. Suprasternal echocardiographic examination of the arch of the aorta (AO), pulmonary artery (P), and left atrium (LA). I = innominate artery; LC = left common carotid artery.

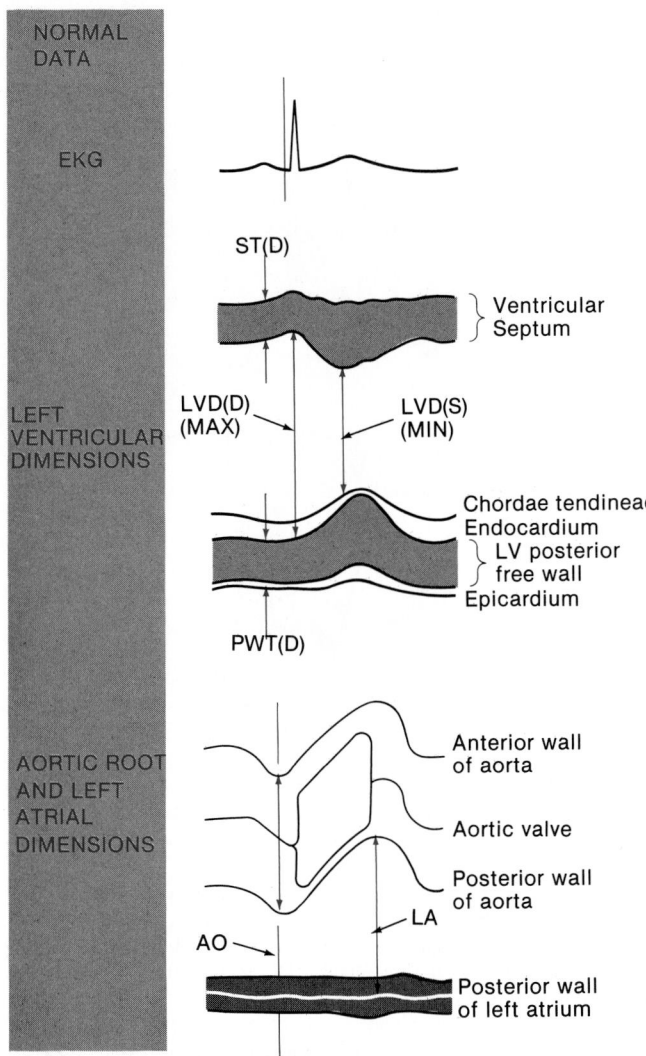

NORMAL DATA

EKG

LEFT VENTRICULAR DIMENSIONS

AORTIC ROOT AND LEFT ATRIAL DIMENSIONS

FIGURE 3–31. Methods for obtaining M-mode echocardiographic measurements. ST(D) = diastolic septal thickness; LVD (D) and LVD(S) = diastolic and systolic left ventricular diameters; PWT(D) = diastolic posterior wall thickness; AO = aorta; LA = left atrium. (Reproduced with permission from Henry, W. L., Gardin, J. M., and Ware, J. H.: Echocardiographic measurements in normal subjects from infancy to old age. Circulation 62:1054, 1980. Copyright 1980 American Heart Association.)

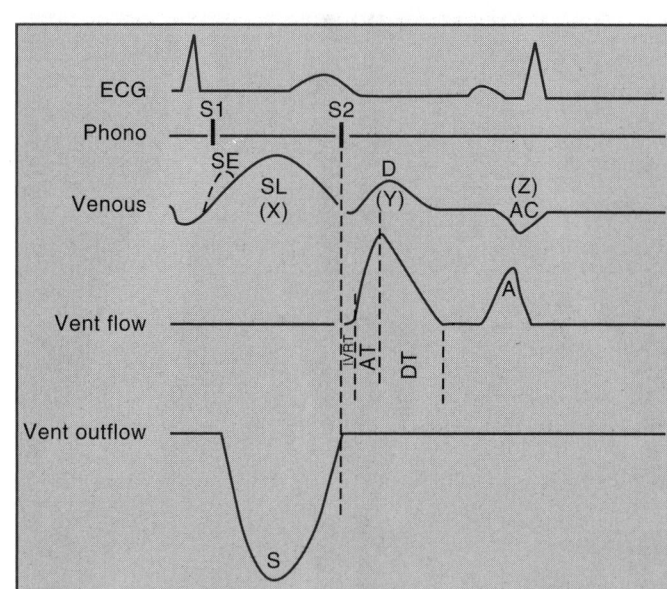

FIGURE 3–32. Relationship between the electrocardiogram (ECG), phonocardiogram (PHONO), venous, ventricular inflow, and ventricular outflow Doppler velocities. SE = early systole; SL = late systole; D = diastole; AC = atrial contraction; IVRT = isovolumic relaxation time; AT = acceleration time; DT = deceleration time. (From Feigenbaum, H.: Echocardiography. 5th ed. Malvern, PA, Lea and Febiger, 1994.)

wave and the late flow that peaks with the A wave. Figure 3–34 shows a pulsed Doppler recording of aortic flow taken with the transducer at the apex. With this "five-chamber" view one sees the systolic flow moving away from the transducer during systole. Doppler flow patterns on the right side of the heart are essentially the same except the velocities are lower. The peak mitral velocity in Figure 3–33 is about 100 cm/sec, and the aortic velocity in Figure 3–34 is about 120 cm/sec.

EVALUATION OF CARDIAC PERFORMANCE

M-MODE ECHOCARDIOGRAPHY. The ability to evaluate the function of the left ventricle by means of echocardiography has been one of the principal factors in the increasing ap-

TABLE 3–2 NORMAL VALUES OF M-MODE ECHOCARDIOGRAPHIC MEASUREMENTS IN ADULTS

	RANGE (CM)	MEAN (CM)	NUMBER OF SUBJECTS
Age (years)	13 to 54	26	134
Body surface area (M²)	1.45 to 2.22	1.8	130
RVD—flat	0.7 to 2.3	1.5	84
RVD—left lateral	0.9 to 2.6	1.7	83
LVID—flat	3.7 to 5.6	4.7	82
LVID—left lateral	3.5 to 5.7	4.7	81
Posterior LV wall thickness	0.6 to 1.1	0.9	137
Posterior LV wall amplitude	0.9 to 1.4	1.2	48
IVS wall thickness	0.6 to 1.1	0.9	137
Mid IVS amplitude	0.3 to 0.8	0.5	10
Apical IVS amplitude	0.5 to 1.2	0.7	38
Left atrial dimension	1.9 to 4.0	2.9	133
Aortic root dimension	2.0 to 3.7	2.7	121
Aortic cusps' separation	1.5 to 2.6	2.9	93
Percentage of fractional shortening*	34% to 44%	36%	20%
Mean rate of circumferential shortening (Vcf)† or mean normalized shortening velocity	1.02 to 1.94 circ/sec	1.3 circ/sec	38

* $\dfrac{\text{LVIDd} - \text{LVIDs}}{\text{LVIDd}}$

† $\dfrac{\text{LVIDd} - \text{LVIDs}}{\text{LVIDd} \times \text{Ejection time}}$

RVD = Right ventricular dimension
LVID = Left ventricular internal dimension; d = end diastole; s = end systole
LV = Left ventricle
IVS = Interventricular septum

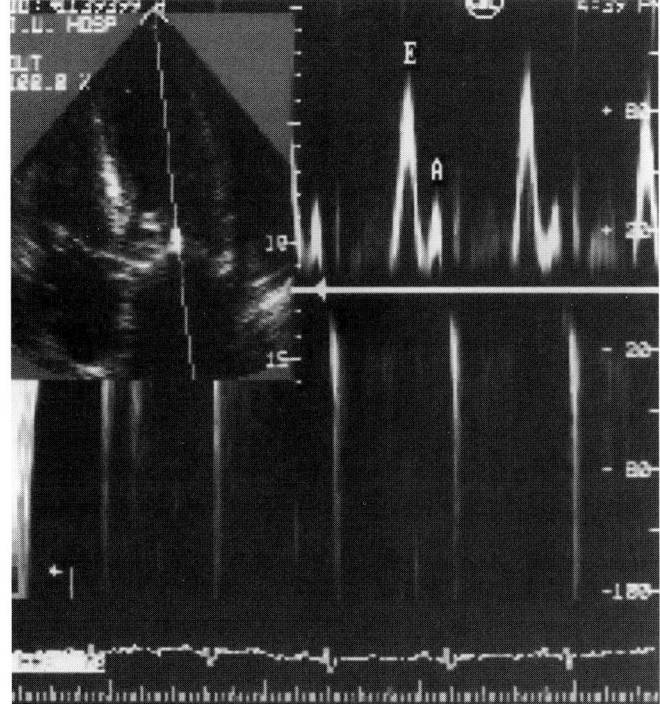

FIGURE 3–33. **Pulsed Doppler recording of mitral velocities showing the early diastolic flow (E) and late diastolic flow or velocity (A) following atrial systole.**

plication of this technique. The standard M-mode technique may be used to record a dimension of the left ventricle between the left side of the interventricular septum and the endocardial surface of the posterior left ventricular wall (Fig. 3–31).[52] This dimension may be measured in end diastole and end systole. Although these dimensions can be used to estimate ventricular volume, many errors can occur in such calculations,[53] since many assumptions that are not always valid are required to obtain the volume of a three-dimensional object from measurement of a single dimension. Irrespective of whether or not M-mode echocardiography can calculate true left ventricular volumes, simple dimensions of the left ventricle can provide an estimate of the overall size and performance of the left ventricle in many patients. Fractional shortening, i.e., the difference between the end-diastolic dimension, provides information

about left ventricular systolic function. The quotient of fractional shortening and ejection time provides the mean fractional or circumferential shortening.[54] While these measurements are useful in judging left ventricular performance (Table 3–1), it must be appreciated that the ventricle must be contracting uniformly for them to reflect global function. These echocardiographic measurements assess the status of only the basal portion of the chamber and must be interpreted with caution in patients with segmentally diseased left ventricles,[55] with left bundle branch block, with a dilated right ventricle, or with a low echocardiographic window so that the M-mode measurement is closer to the major axis than the minor axis.

Another useful M-mode echocardiographic technique for assessing ventricular size is to measure the distance between the E point of mitral valve and the left side of the interventricular septum.[56] Normally the mitral E point and the left side of the septum are within a few millimeters of each other. The upper limits of normal of the mitral E point septal separation (EPSS) is approximately 8 mm. As the left ventricular ejection fraction decreases, the EPSS increases. As the left ventricle dilates, the septum moves anteriorly. The opening of the mitral valve is largely dependent upon the volume of blood passing through that orifice. As the mitral valve flow or left ventricular stroke volume decreases, the amplitude of the E point is decreased. Thus, with a decreased stroke volume and/or left ventricular dilatation, the septum and anterior mitral leaflet would move in opposite directions. Naturally, if there is valvular disease, such as mitral stenosis, then the excursion of the mitral valve is not a reliable indicator of flow through that orifice. In patients with aortic regurgitation, mitral valve flow is not an indicator of total left ventricular stroke volume, and one would not be able to provide an assessment of ejection fraction.

TWO-DIMENSIONAL ECHOCARDIOGRAPHY. The limited number of sampling sites for the M-mode dimensions and the lack of spatial orientation limit the clinical usefulness of these measurements. Thus, it is not surprising that 2-D echocardiography is being used to assess cardiac chambers. Hesitancy to use the 2-D approach and continued reliance on M-mode measurements are partially due to convenience and familiarity with M-mode measurements and the difficulty of making measurements from videotape recordings. However, with the widespread use of computer analysis of the 2-D images both on-line and off-line, this inconvenience is no longer a problem.

FIGURE 3–34. **Pulsed Doppler recording of aortic flow with the transducer at the apex. The Doppler sample *(arrow)* is in the aorta in this apical five-chamber view. RV = right ventricle; RA = right atrium; LV = left ventricle; AV = aortic valve; LA = left atrium.**

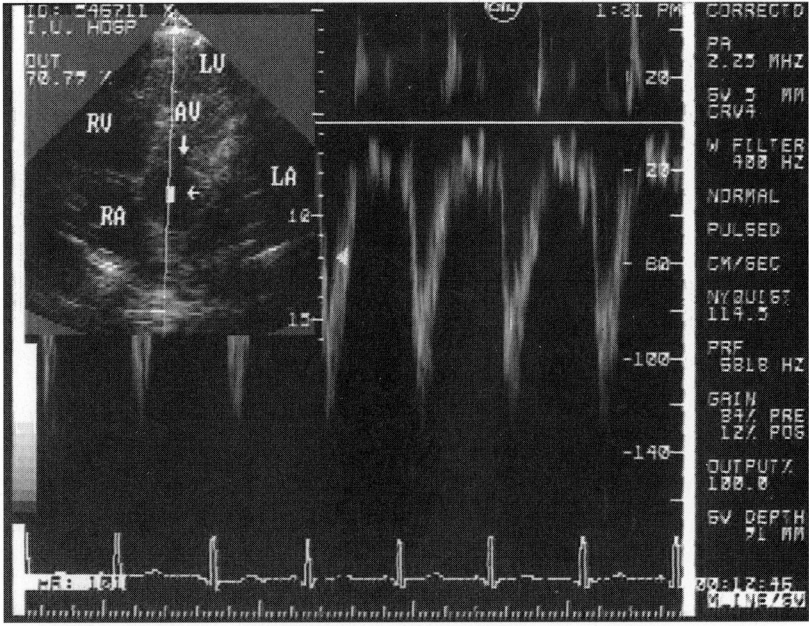

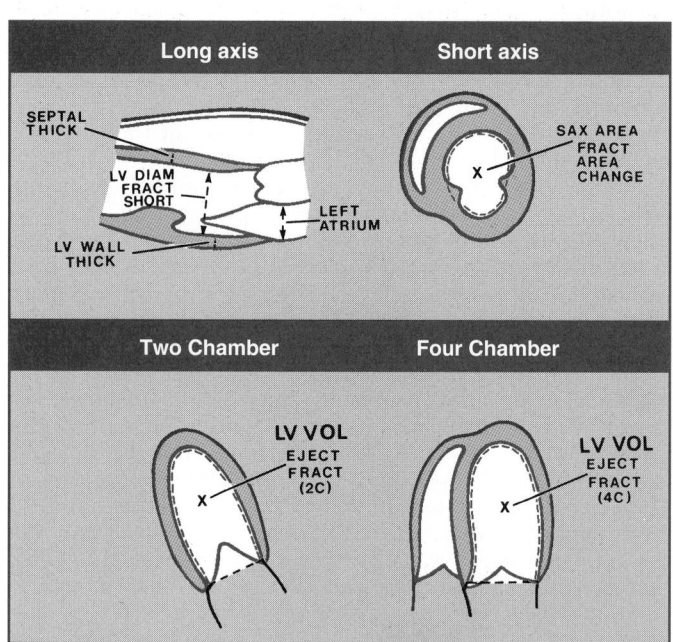

FIGURE 3–35. Some of the measurements that can be obtained from 2-D echocardiograms. The left ventricular diameter and fractional shortening provide an assessment of the size and systolic function of the base of the left ventricle. The short-axis (SAX) areas and fractional area change at the papillary muscle level give similar information for the midportion of the left ventricle. Left ventricular volumes (LV VOL) and ejection fraction can be determined from two-chamber and four-chamber echocardiograms using prolate ellipse or Simpson's rule formulas for calculating volumes. (From Feigenbaum, H.: Echocardiography. 5th ed. Malvern, PA, Lea and Febiger, 1994.)

Figure 3–35 shows some of the left ventricular measurements that are possible with 2-D echocardiography.[57] One can utilize the parasternal long-axis and short-axis views to obtain modified M-mode measurements. The long-axis examination permits measurements very similar to the M-mode measurements. The dimension between the interventricular septum and the posterior left ventricular wall provides an opportunity for calculating left ventricular dimensions and fractional shortening. It should be emphasized, however, that this dimension is not the same as the M-mode measurement. The M-mode dimension is usually not through the true minor dimension. The relationship of the M-mode measurement to the minor axis depends upon the available acoustic window. This window tends to be lower in older individuals. Thus the M-mode dimension changes with age. The dimensions from the long-axis view of the 2-D examination is truly through the minor dimension and is closer to the base of the heart. The 2-D fractional shortening essentially evaluates systolic function at the base of the left ventricle.[58] Septal thickness, posterior wall thickness, left atrial dimensions, and aortic dimensions are again possible using the long-axis 2-D examination as has been done with M-mode measurements. The short-axis view provides left ventricular area measurements and a systolic ejection index calculated as fractional area change.

To measure volumes the apical views are necessary. A variety of ways to calculate volumes have been proposed.[57] Probably the most accurate is to use a modified version of Simpson's rule because it minimizes the effect of geometric shape for calculating volumes. However, any of the angiographic techniques, such as the prolate ellipse or area-length methods, have also been used to calculate volumes using the apical 2-D echograms. A somewhat simplified formula for calculating volumes is the "bullet" formula, which takes five-sixths of the area in the short-axis view times the length of the left ventricle ($V = 5/6$ AL). This formula is attractive because of its simplicity and because the area of the left ventricle and the length of the left ventricle can be easily obtained with 2-D echocardiography. It is also common practice for the physician interpreting echocardiograms to merely estimate the ejection fraction on the basis of visual inspection.[59] This approach is attractive because it avoids the necessity to make any measurements. However, the measurement is obviously qualitative and is highly subjective.

There are attempts to automate the quantitation of left ventricular function using 2-D echocardiography. Figure 3–36 shows a technique whereby the endocardial border is automatically detected. The instrument provides an instantaneous measure of the cross-sectional area of the left ventricle.[60] This technique has also been extrapolated to attempt to give volumes as well as area changes.[61] As with all quantitative measurements, this technique is very dependent upon the quality of the image and clear identification of endocardial borders.[62] As a general rule, apical

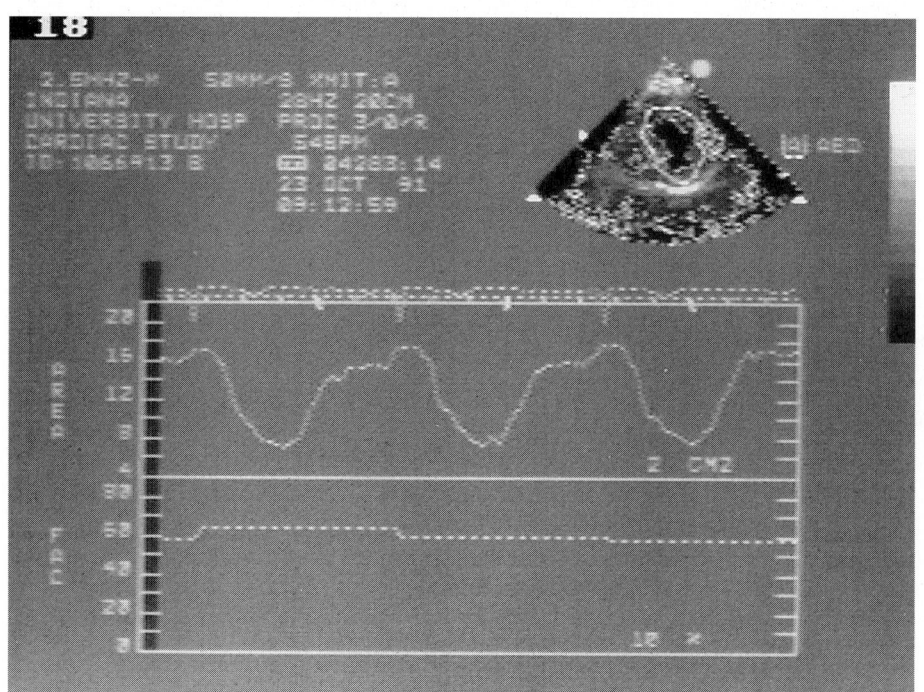

FIGURE 3–36. How a real-time edge detection device can produce a display of the cyclic variation in the area of the left ventricle. An area of interest is drawn around the left ventricular cavity, and an instrument automatically determines the area on a frame-to-frame basis. The graphic display shows change in area and fractional area change (FAC). (From Feigenbaum, H.: Echocardiography. 5th ed. Malvern, PA, Lea and Febiger, 1994.)

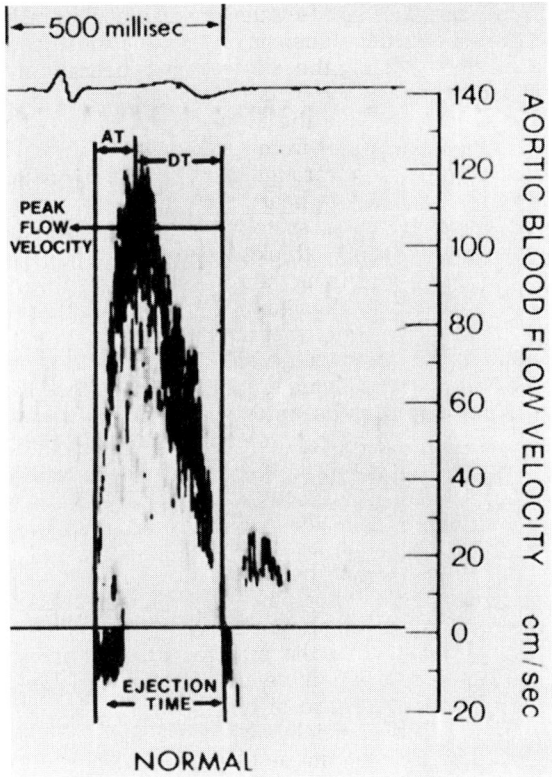

FIGURE 3–37. Pulsed Doppler recording of aortic blood flow velocity demonstrating how ejection time, peak flow velocity, acceleration time (AT), and deceleration time (DT) are measured. (From Gardin, J. M., et al.: Evaluation of blood flow velocity in the ascending aorta and main pulmonary artery of normal subjects by Doppler echocardiography. Am. Heart J. *107*:310, 1984.)

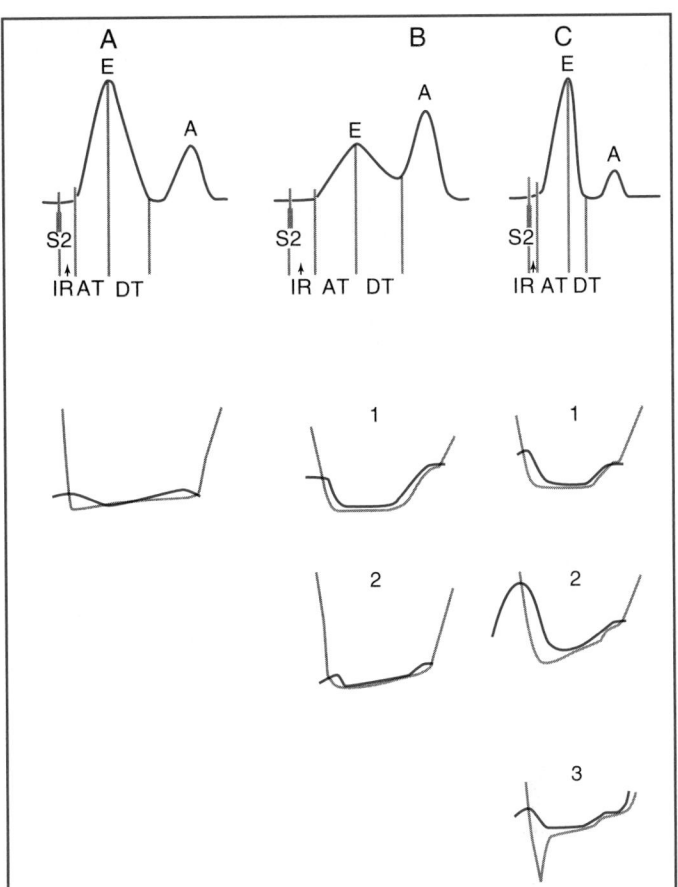

FIGURE 3–38. Relationship of mitral valve or left ventricular inflow Doppler velocities and left ventricular and left atrial pressures (see text for details). (From Feigenbaum, H.: Echocardiography. 5th ed. Malvern, PA, Lea and Febiger, 1994.)

views suffer more from loss of endocardial definition because the walls are parallel to the ultrasonic beam.

DOPPLER ECHOCARDIOGRAPHY. This technique can be used to evaluate left ventricular systolic function with a recording of flow in the ascending aorta. Acceleration time, from the onset of flow to the time of peak acceleration (Fig. 3–37), and peak acceleration have been shown to be related to global left ventricular systolic function.[63] The acceleration of the mitral regurgitant Doppler velocity may be an indicator of contractility.[64]

DIASTOLIC FUNCTION. Echocardiography has been used to evaluate left ventricular diastolic function. M-mode techniques have been used to record the rate of relaxation of the left ventricular cavity. This technique utilizes digitization of the borders of the left ventricular cavity, with the rapidity with which the left ventricular dimension increases in early diastole being noted.[66]

Doppler echocardiography currently is the primary technique used for evaluating left ventricular diastolic function.[67] Figure 3–38 shows the relationship between mitral flow and left ventricular and left atrial pressures.[68] With normal left-sided pressures the early diastolic mitral velocity (E) exceeds that following atrial systole (A). Under several conditions, one of which is normal aging,[69] the velocity in early diastole decreases and the late velocity increases (Fig. 3–38B). Among the pathologic states that produce this change are left ventricular hypertrophy and myocardial ischemia.[70] Both conditions produce abnormal relaxation and decreased early velocity into the left ventricle. This situation will commonly produce elevated left ventricular diastolic pressures (Fig. 3–38B-1). Unusually low filling pressures within the left atrium may also produce a similar pattern of flow (Fig. 3–38B-2).

If the left ventricular filling pressure is markedly elevated, as may occur with severe heart failure (Fig. 3–38C-1), then the left ventricular inflow velocity pattern changes

dramatically.[71] Now there is a marked increase in the early diastolic velocity with an increase in the E velocity (Fig. 3–38C). The atrial velocity is now reduced. A similar pattern may also occur if one has severe mitral regurgitation with an elevated V wave in the left atrial pressure (Fig. 3–38C-2). This type of mitral flow may also occur if there is a restrictive pattern of filling of the left ventricle, as may occur with constrictive pericarditis or restrictive cardiomyopathy (Fig. 3–38C-3). It is apparent that with an abnormal left ventricle the flow pattern may change from normal (A) to abnormal relaxation (B) early in the disease. As the problem progresses and heart failure and/or mitral regurgitation develops, then the pattern may change to C.[72] Between *B* and *C* one can have "pseudonormalization" whereby an apparent normal pattern *(A)* is really a transition between *B* and *C*. Investigators are also measuring various time intervals such as isovolumetric relaxation time from Doppler recordings to assess left ventricular diastolic function.[73]

STRESS ECHOCARDIOGRAPHY. Although echocardiography has been used primarily for evaluating the cardiac chambers at rest, there is increasing interest in performing the ultrasonic examination during or immediately after some form of stress. These studies have utilized supine[74] or upright bicycle exercise,[75] immediate post-treadmill exercise,[76] pharmacological stress, and atrial pacing.[77] Many of the technical difficulties involved in recording an echocardiogram while the patient is hyperventilating following exercise have been overcome by using digital techniques that record a single cardiac cycle or continuous loop display.[78] This digital approach eliminates respiratory artifacts and permits the resting and exercise studies to be presented side by side for ease of interpretation. This type of examination is being done primarily for detecting exercise-induced regional wall motion abnormalities in patients with coronary artery disease. Exercise studies using Doppler measurements during exercise have also been used to assess global changes in left ventricular function and hemodynamics in patients with valvular heart disease[79,80] or congenital heart disease.[81]

WALL THICKNESS. Echocardiography may also be employed to measure the thickness of the walls of the ventricle[82] (Figs. 3–32 and 3–35). The absolute thickness of the ventricle is important in determining the presence of left ventricular hypertrophy, in estimating left ventricular mass,[83,84] and in calculating left ventricular end-systolic stress.[85,86] Echocardiography also permits measurement of changes in left ventricular thickness during the cardiac cycle.[87] Normally the left ventricular wall thickens during systole, but in pathological conditions this thickening decreases and actual systolic thinning has been noted in acute ischemia or myocardial infarction.[88]

OTHER CHAMBERS

Left Atrium. Echocardiography offers the opportunity to evaluate all four cardiac chambers and not just the left ventricle. Left atrial dilatation is readily recognized on the M-mode[89] (Fig. 3–31) or 2-D echocardiogram (Fig. 3–35).[90] A variety of quantitative measurements have been introduced. A simple anteroposterior dimension of the chamber is usually sufficient for identifying patients with dilated left atria. Such measurements can be done with either the M-mode or parasternal long-axis 2-D view. In patients in whom the left atrium does not uniformly expand or if there is distortion by a dilated aorta,[91] other views, including the apical 2-D views, can be used to assess the size of the left atrium.[92,93] Transesophageal echocardiography provides an excellent view of the left atrium, especially the atrial appendage. Since this site is a common location for clot formation, it has been studied extensively for function[94] as well as for clots.[95]

Right Ventricle and Atrium. The right ventricle is more difficult to evaluate quantitatively because of its unusual shape.[96] However, gross dilatation is easily assessed with M-mode[97] or 2-D examinations. Probably the most common technique is to use the relative size of the right and left ventricles in the apical four-chamber view. The thickness of the right ventricle walls can also be detected using either M-mode or 2-D echocardiography.[98] With right ventricular dilatation there is frequently distortion of the shape of the interventricular septum.[99] Whether this distortion occurs primarily during diastole or systole will indicate whether or not there is primarily a pressure or volume overload of the right ventricle.[100] With a diastolic overload the septum is flat in diastole and assumes a more normal curvature in systole. With a pressure overload the flattened interventricular septum is seen with systole.[101]

The right atrium can also be evaluated with 2-D echocardiography using the apical four-chamber or parasternal right ventricular inflow view. Transesophageal echocardiography provides excellent examination of the right atrium.

Hemodynamic Information

DOPPLER ECHOCARDIOGRAPHY. This is now the principal ultrasonic technique for obtaining hemodynamic information. By recording the velocity of intracardiac blood flow, one can obtain quantitative data concerning both blood flow and intracardiac pressures. The principle is illustrated in Figure 3–39. To calculate flow the mean velocity passing through an orifice or vessel and the cross-sectional area of the orifice or vessel must be known. The mean velocity is acquired by measuring the velocity time integral of the Doppler signal, which is the area under the recording. The cross-sectional area of the orifice through which the blood is flowing can be obtained directly with 2-D echocardiography; alternatively the diameter can be measured with either 2-D[102] or M-mode[103] echocardiography, and then the area can be calculated. Such flow determinations are feasible through any orifice or vessel.[104]

Blood flow in the ascending aorta is commonly used for cardiac output calculations.[105] The integrated velocity from the ascending aorta is combined with the calculated cross-sectional area determined at any of three locations: the aortic annulus, the separation of the aortic valve leaflets, or just past the sinus of Valsalva. All three approaches have been used with reasonable success. In a similar manner, pulmonary blood flow can be measured by taking Doppler pulmonary artery velocity and multiplying it by the cross-sectional area of the pulmonary artery. Flow through the mitral[106,107] and tricuspid valves[108] has also been calculated. Atrioventricular valve flow is somewhat more complicated because the flow is phasic, and early and late diastolic flow must be allowed for.[109] Although the measurements are more complex, they have been reasonably accurate.[110]

The effectiveness of Doppler echocardiography for measuring flow has been validated; however, there are many technical details in making such calculations. The biggest limitation is the calculation of the orifice or vessel area.[111] It is difficult to obtain an accurate cross-sectional area of the various orifices. Because the measured diameter must be squared in the calculation of blood flow, any error would also be squared. For example, in many adult patients it is difficult to obtain an accurate orifice measurement of the main pulmonary artery.

Although the Doppler technique for measuring blood flow is not routinely done in many laboratories, the potential clinical utility is readily apparent. It can be used to measure cardiac output or stroke volume.[12] The technique is particularly useful for following directional changes in these variables in a given patient.[113,114] By calculating flow through different orifices, regurgitant fraction[115] and shunt ratios can be quantified.[116,117] For example, pulmonary to systemic flow ratios can be obtained by measuring aortic and pulmonary artery flows. Mitral regurgitant fraction can be calculated by measuring aortic flow and mitral valve flow. With the increasing availability of computer analysis, the difficulties of making these determinations have been resolved. However, some limitations still exist.[118]

DOPPLER MEASUREMENT OF PRESSURE GRADIENTS. Possibly the most important development in Doppler echocardiography has been the utilization of a modified version of the Bernoulli equation to calculate the pressure drop or

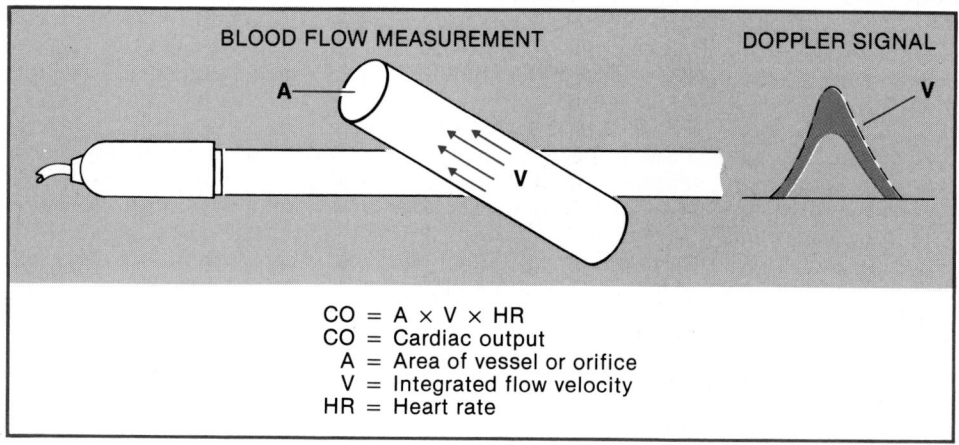

BLOOD FLOW MEASUREMENT   **DOPPLER SIGNAL**

A

V

V

CO = A × V × HR
CO = Cardiac output
 A = Area of vessel or orifice
 V = Integrated flow velocity
HR = Heart rate

FIGURE 3–39. Principles of using Doppler echocardiography to measure blood flow. (From Feigenbaum, H.: Echocardiography. 4th ed. Philadelphia, Lea and Febiger, 1986.)

PLATE 1

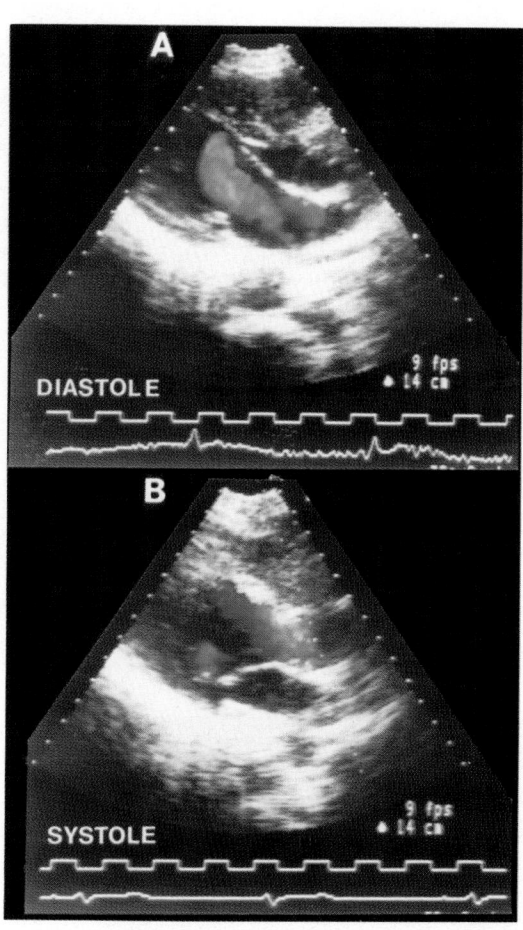

FIGURE 3–10. Two-dimensional color flow Doppler image of the left ventricular inflow (A) and outflow (B) in the parasternal long-axis view. The blood passing through the mitral valve during diastole (A) is moving toward the transducer and is encoded in red. During systole (B) the blood passes through the left ventricular outflow tract and is encoded in blue. As the velocity increases toward the aortic root, the intensity or brightness of the color increases.

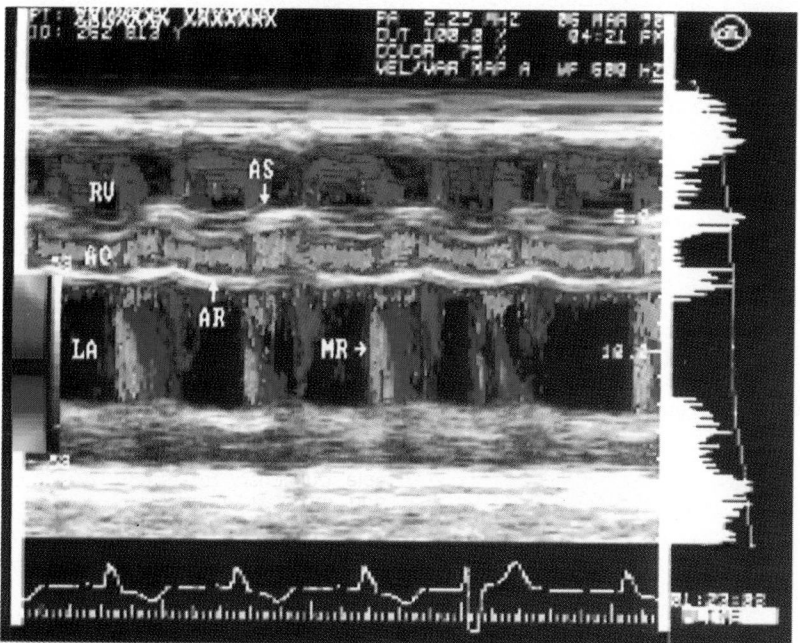

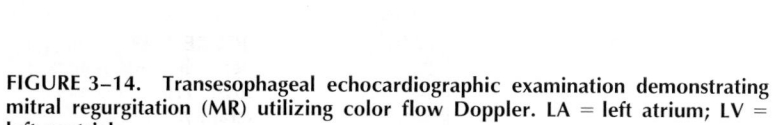

FIGURE 3–11. Color-encoded Doppler flow superimposed on an M-mode tracing in a patient with valvular heart disease. The high-velocity turbulent blood is encoded in green. Both the systolic aortic stenosis flow (AS) and the diastolic aortic regurgitation flow (AR) can be seen within the aorta (AO). The high-velocity mitral regurgitation jet (MR) is detected within the left atrium (LA) in systole. RV = right ventricle.

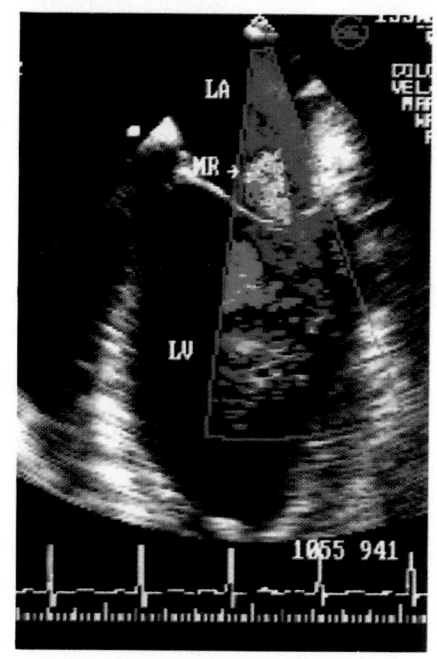

FIGURE 3–14. Transesophageal echocardiographic examination demonstrating mitral regurgitation (MR) utilizing color flow Doppler. LA = left atrium; LV = left ventricle.

PLATE 2

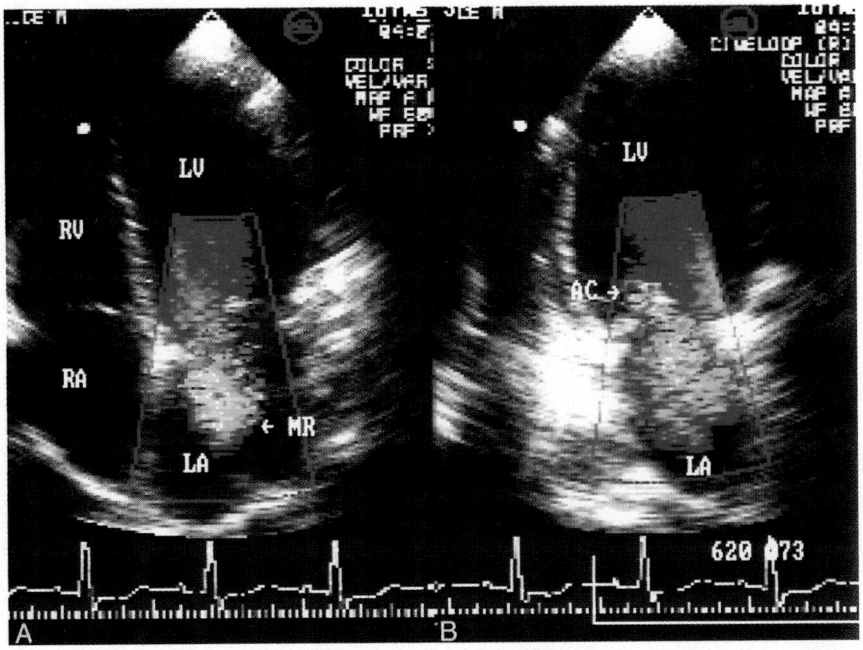

FIGURE 3–49. Color flow Doppler study of a patient with mitral regurgitation (MR) as viewed from the four-chamber *(A)* and two-chamber *(B)* views. There is acceleration of flow on the left ventricular side of the regurgitant mitral orifice (AC). LV = left ventricle; LA = left atrium; RV = right ventricle; RA = right atrium.

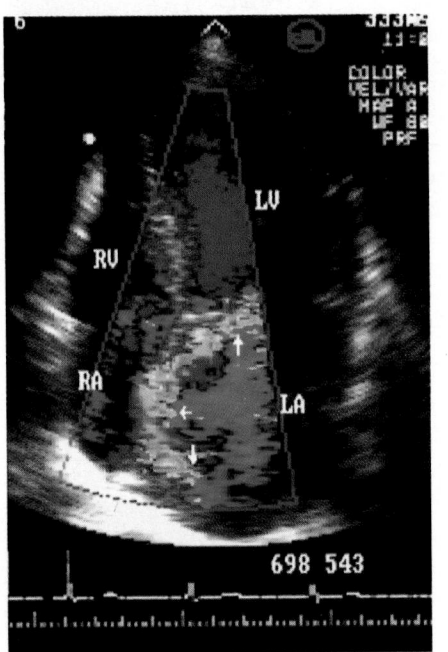

FIGURE 3–50. Color flow Doppler study of a patient with mitral regurgitation in whom the regurgitant jet (arrows) is eccentric and directed toward the interatrial septum. RV = right ventricle; LV = left ventricle; RA = right atrium; LA = left atrium.

FIGURE 3–58. Color flow mapping in a patient with aortic regurgitation. The brightly colored, high-velocity jet can be seen passing from the aorta (AO) to the left ventricle (LV). The center of the jet is white, and the edges are shades of blue. Even though the velocity is extremely high, most of the jet is blue because the flow is almost perpendicular to the ultrasonic beam, and the velocities are registered as being lower than they actually are.

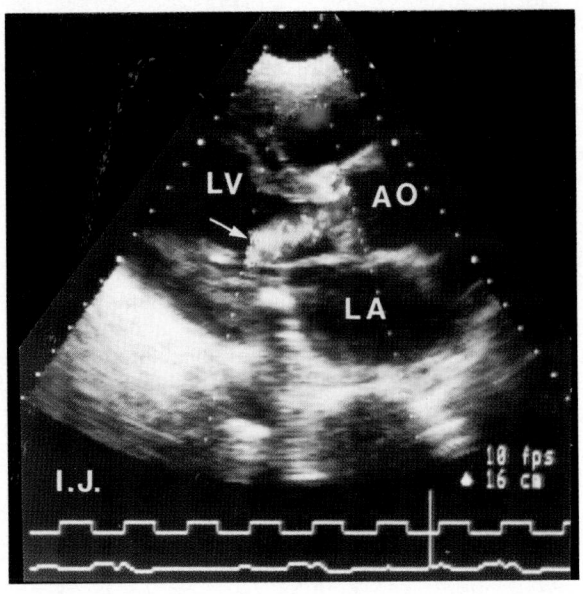

PLATE 3

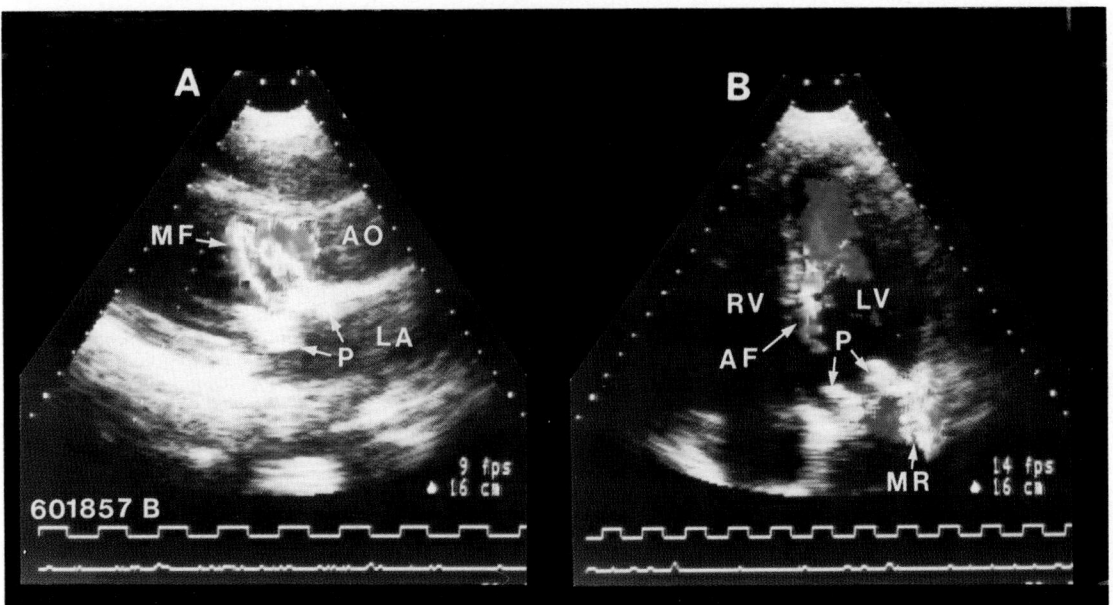

FIGURE 3–65. Color Doppler images in diastole *(A)* and systole *(B)* in a patient with a prosthetic mitral valve (P). During diastole *(A)*, turbulent multidirectional antegrade mitral flow (MF) is present. During systole *(B)*, a regurgitant jet (MR) is present within the left atrium along the lateral border of the prosthetic valve (P). Aortic flow (AF) exhibits aliasing in this patient who also had left ventricular outflow obstruction. The apical half of the left ventricular outflow tract is blue and the portion near the aorta is red. AO = aorta; LA = left atrium; RV = right ventricle; LV = left ventricle.

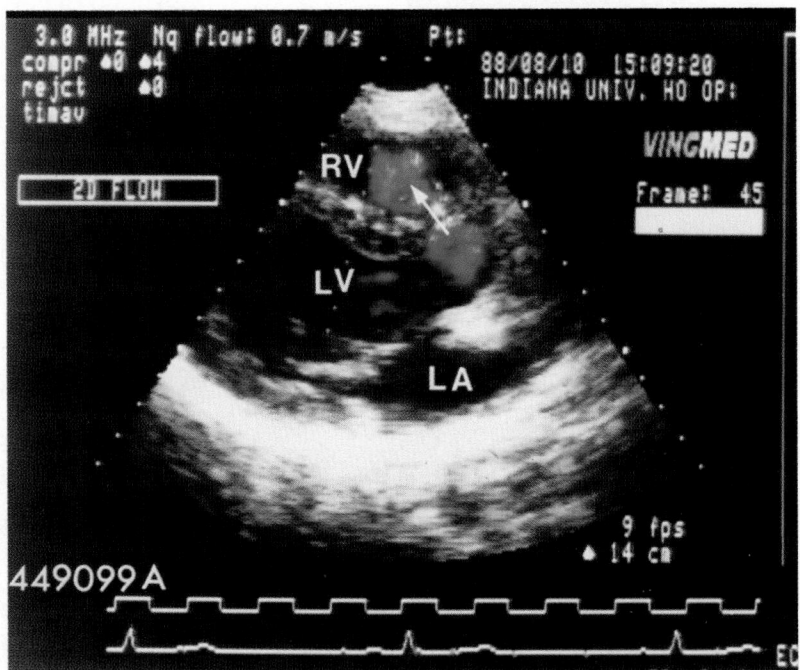

FIGURE 3–74. Color flow Doppler study of a patient with a membranous ventricular septal defect. The blood can be seen flowing toward the transducer and the right ventricle (RV) and is encoded in red (arrow). At the site of the defect the width of the jet is narrowed and the velocity is increased as noted by the multicolor nature of the flow map. LV = left ventricle; LA = left atrium.

PLATE 4

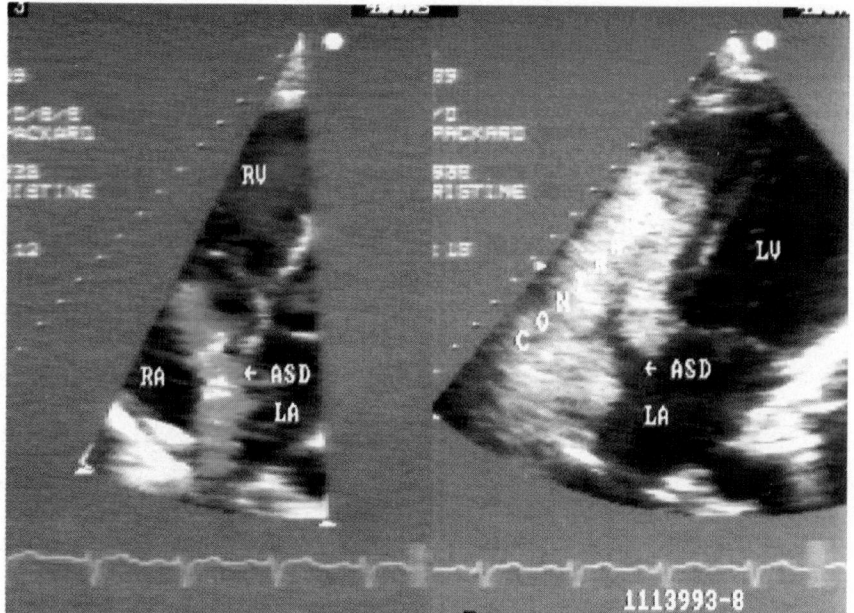

FIGURE 3–81. Color flow Doppler *(left)* and contrast echocardiogram *(right)* of a patient with a secundum atrial septal defect. The defect (ASD) is noted by red-encoded blood passing through the atrial septum on the color study and as a negative contrast with the contrast echocardiogram. RV = right ventricle; RA = right atrium; LA = left atrium; LV = left ventricle.

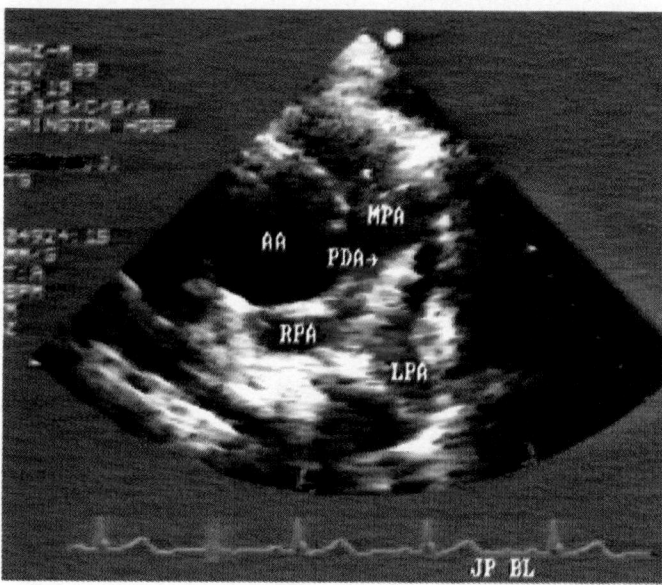

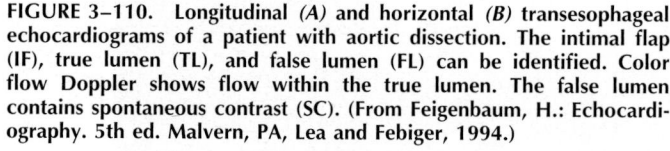

FIGURE 3–83. Color Doppler images in a patient with patent ductus arteriosus. The shunt flow passing from the aorta into the pulmonary artery can be seen as a blue jet (PDA) within the main pulmonary artery (MPA). RPA = right pulmonary artery; LPA = left pulmonary artery; AA = aorta.

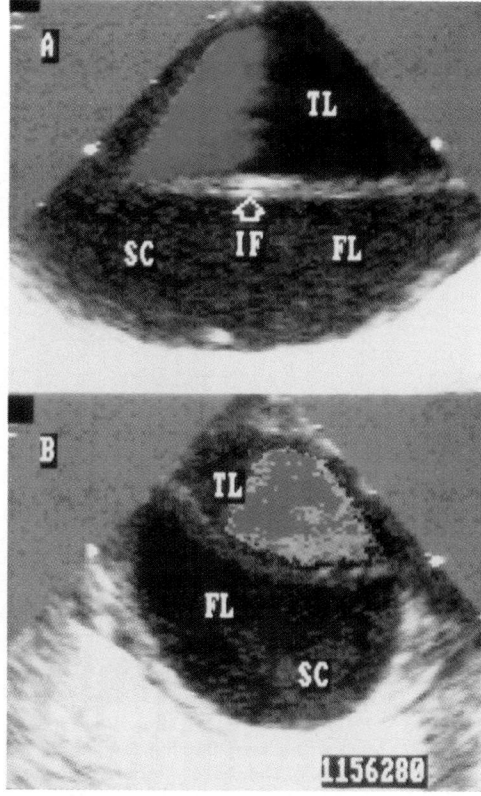

FIGURE 3–110. Longitudinal *(A)* and horizontal *(B)* transesophageal echocardiograms of a patient with aortic dissection. The intimal flap (IF), true lumen (TL), and false lumen (FL) can be identified. Color flow Doppler shows flow within the true lumen. The false lumen contains spontaneous contrast (SC). (From Feigenbaum, H.: Echocardiography. 5th ed. Malvern, PA, Lea and Febiger, 1994.)

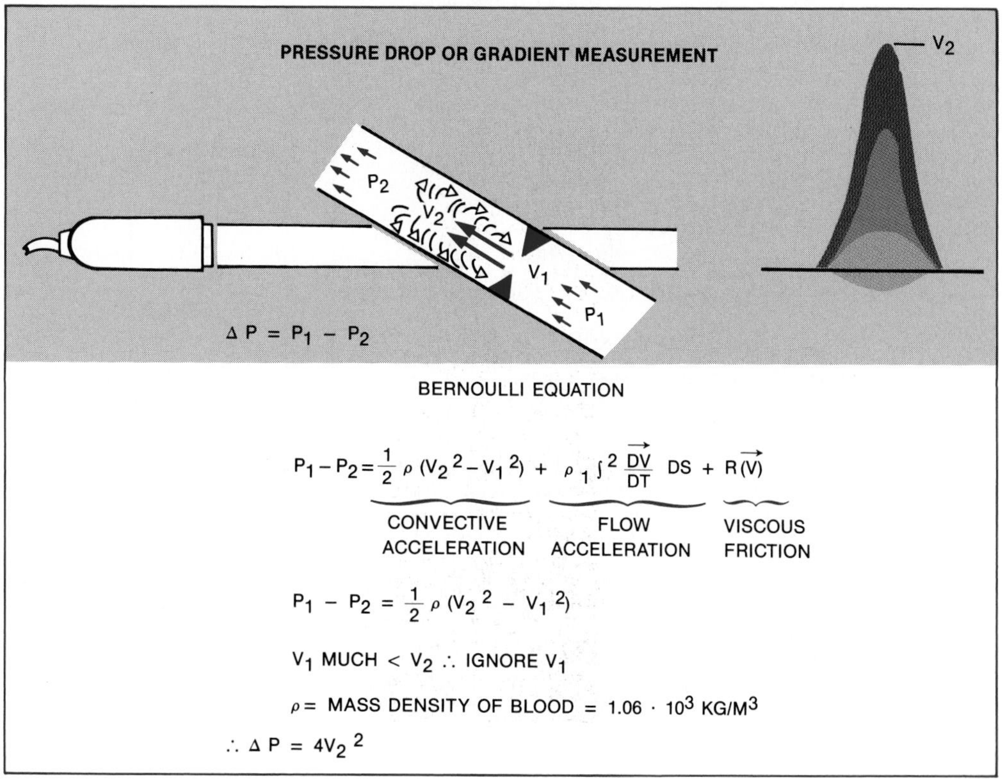

PRESSURE DROP OR GRADIENT MEASUREMENT

$\Delta P = P_1 - P_2$

BERNOULLI EQUATION

$$P_1 - P_2 = \frac{1}{2}\rho\,(V_2{}^2 - V_1{}^2) + \rho_1 \int 2\,\frac{\overrightarrow{DV}}{DT}\,DS + R(\overrightarrow{V})$$

CONVECTIVE   FLOW   VISCOUS
ACCELERATION   ACCELERATION   FRICTION

$$P_1 - P_2 = \frac{1}{2}\rho\,(V_2{}^2 - V_1{}^2)$$

V_1 MUCH $< V_2$ ∴ IGNORE V_1

$\rho =$ MASS DENSITY OF BLOOD $= 1.06 \cdot 10^3$ KG/M^3

$$\therefore \Delta P = 4V_2{}^2$$

FIGURE 3–40. Principles of using Doppler echocardiography to measure a pressure drop or gradient across an obstruction. P_2 = pressure distal to an obstruction; V_2 = blood velocity distal to an obstruction; V_1 = velocity proximal to an obstruction; P_1 = pressure proximal to an obstruction. (From Feigenbaum, H.: Echocardiography. 4th ed. Philadelphia, Lea and Febiger, 1986.)

gradient across a narrowed part of the cardiovascular system[5]; the principle is shown in Figure 3–40. Although the Bernoulli equation is fairly complex and involves convective acceleration, flow acceleration, and viscous friction, the equation can be limited to convective acceleration alone because flow acceleration and viscous friction are probably not relevant in the clinical setting. Essentially the equation relates the difference in pressure across a stenosis with the differences in velocities. As blood flows through a narrowed orifice, the velocity increases proportionally. With a few assumptions that seem to be clinically appropriate, a fairly complicated equation can be condensed to the difference in pressure (ΔP) equals 4 times the square of the velocity distal to the obstruction. The accuracy and validity of this approach have been confirmed in numerous laboratories.[119] This observation is now the basis for many clinical applications of Doppler echocardiography.

CLINICAL APPLICATIONS: THE ESTIMATION OF INTRACARDIAC PRESSURES. An early application of Doppler echocardiography was calculating a pressure gradient across a stenotic

mitral valve.[120] The approach was then used with stenotic semilunar valves.[119] This same technique can be used to assess the difference in pressure across a regurgitant valve as well as a stenotic valve. For example, in the presence of tricuspid regurgitation the difference in pressure between the right ventricle and the right atrium in systole can be assessed by noting the peak velocity of the regurgitant jet (Fig. 3–41).[121] By knowing the pressure differential between the right ventricle and right atrium and adding an estimate of the right atrial pressure, one can calculate right ventricular systolic pressure. If there is no obstruction to right ventricular outflow, the pulmonary artery systolic pressure is also known. If the velocity of blood flow across a ventricular septal defect is measured, the difference in pressure between the left and right ventricles can also be calculated. By knowing the left ventricular systolic pressure and the gradient between this chamber and the right ventricle, one can calculate right ventricular systolic pressure.[122] A similar approach is possible with aortic-pulmonary shunts.[123] With the help of the modified Bernoulli equation, Doppler

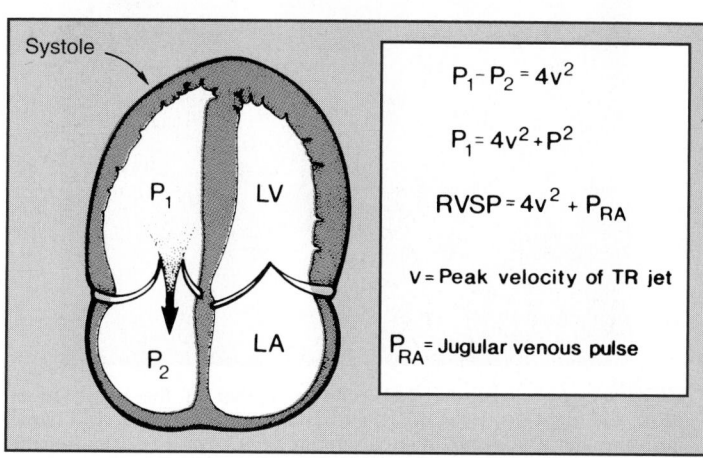

$$P_1 - P_2 = 4v^2$$

$$P_1 = 4v^2 + P^2$$

$$RVSP = 4v^2 + P_{RA}$$

$v =$ Peak velocity of TR jet

$P_{RA} =$ Jugular venous pulse

FIGURE 3–41. Measurement of right ventricular systolic pressure using Doppler recording of tricuspid regurgitation. Using the modified Bernoulli equation, one can calculate the pressure gradient across the regurgitant tricuspid valve ($P_1 - P_2$). The right ventricular systolic pressure of P_1 is equal to 4 times the square of the peak velocity of the tricuspid jet (v), plus the right atrial pressure (P_{RA}). (From Feigenbaum, H.: Echocardiography. 5th ed. Malvern, PA, Lea and Febiger, 1994.)

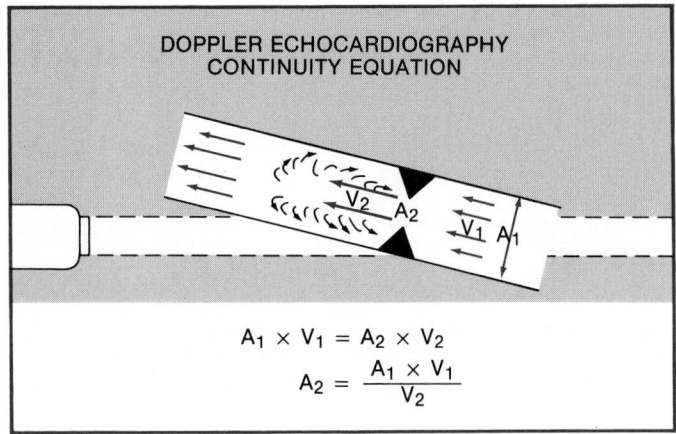

FIGURE 3–42. Principles of using Doppler echocardiography and the continuity equation for calculating the area of a stenotic orifice. A_1 = area proximal to the stenosis; A_2 = area of the stenosis; V_1 = velocity proximal to the stenosis; V_2 = velocity through the stenosis.

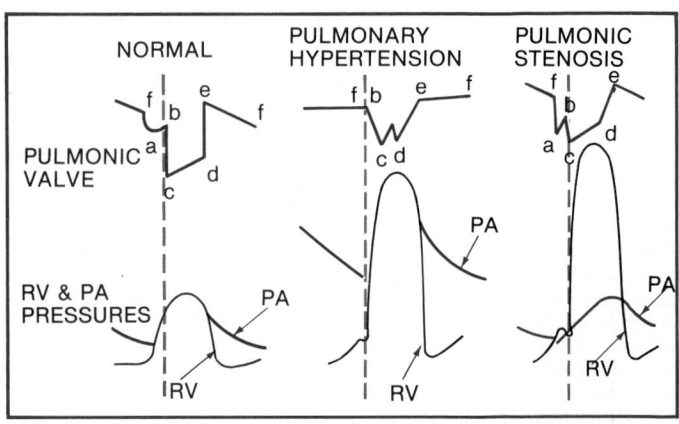

FIGURE 3–43. Relationship of the pulmonic valve echocardiogram and right-heart pressure in the normal state, with pulmonary hypertension and with pulmonic stenosis. PA = pulmonary artery pressure; RV = right ventricular pressure. (See text for details.) (From Feigenbaum, H.: Echocardiography. 2nd ed. Philadelphia, Lea and Febiger, 1976.)

echocardiography is playing an increasing role in estimating intracardiac pressures.

The pattern of the Doppler flow velocities can also provide hemodynamic information. Figure 3–38 shows the relationship between mitral flow and left-sided diastolic pressures. The flow pattern within the pulmonary artery can give clues to the presence of pulmonary hypertension.[124] However, this technique has been replaced by measurement of right ventricular systolic pressure.

DOPPLER MEASUREMENT OF VALVE AREA. Combining the Doppler principles for measuring blood flow and pressure gradient permits one to calculate a valve area utilizing the "continuity equation." Figure 3–42 shows the principle of how the area of a stenotic orifice can be calculated using a combination of Doppler and imaging ultrasound. From blood flow calculations (Fig. 3–39) stroke volume is a function of the product of the integrated velocity with the area. The continuity equation states that the blood flow proximal to the area of obstruction must equal the blood flow passing through the area of obstruction.[125] Thus, if the volume of blood proximal to an obstruction and the velocity of blood through the obstruction are known, the area of the stenotic orifice can be calculated (Fig. 3–42). In the case of aortic stenosis the velocity and the area of the left ventricular outflow tract must be measured to calculate blood flow proximal to a stenotic valve. Then by measuring the velocity of flow across the valve the aortic valve area can be calculated.

M-MODE VALVE RECORDINGS. M-mode recordings of the cardiac valves can also provide hemodynamic information. Abnormal closure of the mitral valve following atrial systole gives a qualitative assessment of elevated left atrial pressure. Normal valve motion between the A and C points (Fig. 3–30) is smooth and uninterrupted. If there is elevated left ventricular diastolic pressure secondary to a large increase with atrial systole, there will be interruption of this closure with a "B bump."[126,127] Premature closure of the mitral valve occurs with severe aortic regurgitation.[128] Analysis of the M-mode aortic valve recording is useful in patients with subaortic stenosis. With either dynamic or fixed obstruction one sees midsystolic closure of the aortic valve.[129] In patients with poor forward left ventricular stroke volume or severe mitral regurgitation there may be gradual closure of the aortic valve throughout systole. With severe aortic regurgitation and markedly elevated left ventricular diastolic pressure, the aortic valve may open before ventricular systole.[130]

Figure 3–43 diagrammatically shows the relationship of the M-mode pulmonary valve motion and right-sided pressures. Normally, atrial systole produces a slight downward motion of the pulmonary valve. With pulmonic stenosis,

the right ventricular systolic and diastolic pressures rise without any similar elevation in pulmonary artery pressure. As a result, atrial contribution to right ventricular pressure is exaggerated and is usually sufficient to open the pulmonary valve prior to ventricular systole (Fig. 3–43).[131] In patients with elevated right ventricular diastolic pressures due to right ventricular failure, tricuspid regurgitation, constrictive pericarditis, or communication between the aorta and right ventricle, the elevated pressure in the right ventricle in early diastole may cause opening of the pulmonary valve even before the onset of atrial systole.[132] An increase in pulmonary artery pressure may change pulmonary valve motion in several ways (Fig. 3–43). One of the most consistent changes is the elimination of atrial systolic motion and the absence of the pulmonary valve A wave.[133] This A wave may reappear if right ventricular failure occurs with pulmonary hypertension. Another sign of pulmonary hypertension is midsystolic closure of the pulmonary valve.[134] These M-mode findings are now secondary to the Doppler measurement of right ventricular systolic pressure.[135]

EXAMINATION OF THE INFERIOR VENA CAVA. A 2-D echocardiographic examination of the inferior vena cava and hepatic vein gives information concerning right-sided hemodynamics (Fig. 3–44).[136] This examination can be helpful in assessing the central venous pressure. An increase in

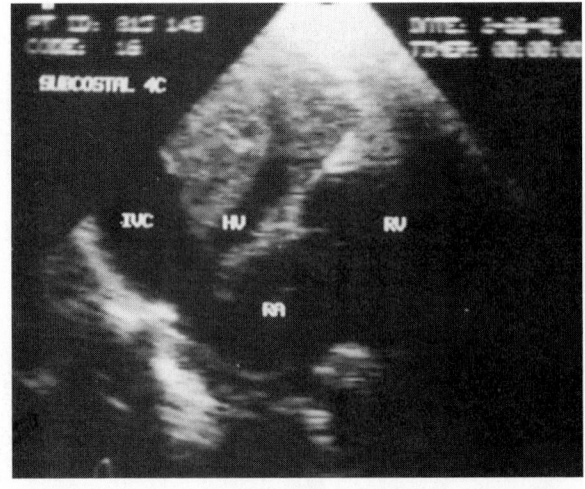

FIGURE 3–44. Subcostal 2-D echocardiogram of the right atrium (RA) and right ventricle (RV) in a patient with elevated right atrial pressure and a markedly dilated inferior vena cava (IVC) and hepatic vein (HV).

pressure dilates the veins[137] and eliminates the normal respiratory variation in the size of the inferior vena cava (Fig. 3–27).

ACQUIRED VALVULAR HEART DISEASE

(See also Chap. 32)

Mitral Stenosis

The detection of mitral stenosis (MS) was the first clinical application of echocardiography.[138] It remains an important technique in the evaluation of suspected mitral valve disease because echocardiography can allow visualization of the mitral valve in a manner not possible with any other procedure. The M-mode examination provides a sensitive assessment of the motion and thickness of the valve leaflets, while the 2-D technique provides a spatial image of the valve and allows direct measurement of the valve orifice.[139] Doppler echocardiography provides hemodynamic assessment of the stenotic orifice.

Figure 3–45 shows an M-mode echocardiogram of a patient with calcific MS. The motion of the mitral valve is considerably altered from the normal pattern seen in Figures 3–3 and 3–30; the normal M-shaped configuration during diastole is no longer present, since the presence of a holodiastolic atrioventricular pressure gradient (diastasis) prevents rapid closure of the valve in mid-diastole. Although sinus rhythm was present, there was no reopening of the valve with atrial contraction and no A wave. Thus, the M-mode echocardiographic hallmark of MS is the absence of valve closure in mid-diastole and of reopening in late diastole. Although this decreased (flat) diastolic (E-F) slope is characteristic of MS,[138] it is not specific. Other conditions such as decreased left ventricular compliance or low cardiac output may also reduce the diastolic slope of mitral valve motion.[140]

In addition to the change in motion of the valve, the number of echoes originating from the valve is increased when it is fibrotic or calcified, and another echocardiographic sign of MS is increased thickness of the valve leaflets. (Note that the quantity of echoes originating from the mitral valve in Figure 3–45 is considerably greater than in Figure 3–30.) Inadequate separation of the anterior and posterior leaflets of the valve occurs during diastole.[140] Normally the two leaflets move in opposite directions during diastole, but when fused, as in MS, they do not separate widely and may actually appear to move in the same direction (Fig. 3–45). The echocardiographic findings of reduced diastolic slope, increased thickness, and decreased separation of the valve leaflets provide a sensitive and accurate method for detection of MS.

The diagnosis of MS by 2-D echocardiography is made by noting thickening, doming, and restricted motion of the leaflets (Fig. 3–46). Doming of any valve on 2-D echocardiography is a characteristic sign of stenosis. This distortion in shape with opening of the valve indicates that the tips of the leaflets are restricted in their ability to open, whereas the bodies of the leaflets still wish to accommodate more blood flow; thus the leaflets are curved, or domed. The presence of doming distinguishes a valve that is truly stenotic from one that opens poorly because of low flow. Two-dimensional echocardiography provides an opportunity to visualize and measure the flow-restricting orifice of the stenotic mitral valve directly (Fig. 3–46B).[141]

Doppler echocardiography provides another means of quantitating the degree of MS.[142] Figure 3–47 shows a pulsed Doppler recording of a patient with MS and atrial fibrillation; there is no atrial contraction. The peak velocities are increased, and the fall in velocity in early diastole is decreased. The technique for quantitating the degree of MS depends on the rate of velocity decrease in early diastole. The time interval required for the peak velocity to reach half of its initial level is related directly to the severity of the obstruction of the mitral orifice.[143] This pressure half-time correlates reasonably well with the mitral valve area; however, there are some limitations to this technique.[144-146] The modified Bernoulli equation can also be used to calculate the mean gradient transmitral valve pressure gradient.[147] Mitral valve area can then be calculated using the Gorlin formula and a Doppler measurement for mitral blood flow.[148]

Echocardiography can help determine whether or not a stenotic valve is suitable for valvotomy by estimating its pliability and degree of calcification.[149] This ability is particularly valuable in evaluating patients for balloon valvuloplasty.[150,151] Two-dimensional echocardiography is the procedure of choice for assessing the fibrosis and pliability of the mitral valve apparatus, especially when subvalvular adhesions are present.[152] Secondary effects of mitral stenosis, such as left atrial dilatation and pulmonary hypertension, can be detected with various echocardiographic examinations.

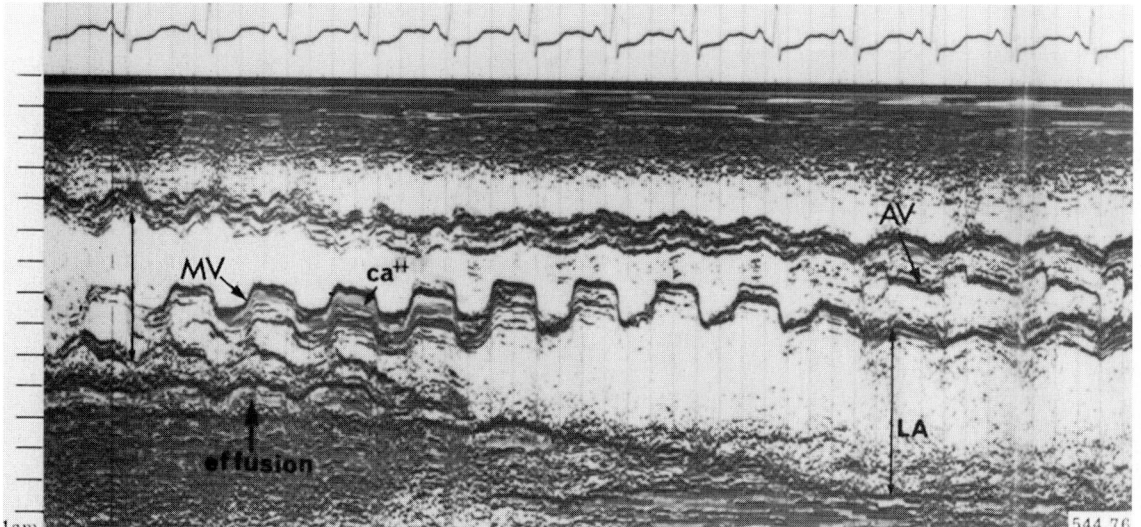

FIGURE 3–45. M-mode scan from a patient with mitral stenosis. The valve is calcified (Ca⁺⁺) and immobile. The left atrium (LA) is dilated, and there is moderate posterior pericardial effusion. AV = aortic valve. (From Chang, S.: M-Mode Echocardiographic Techniques and Pattern Recognition. Philadelphia, Lea and Febiger, 1976.)

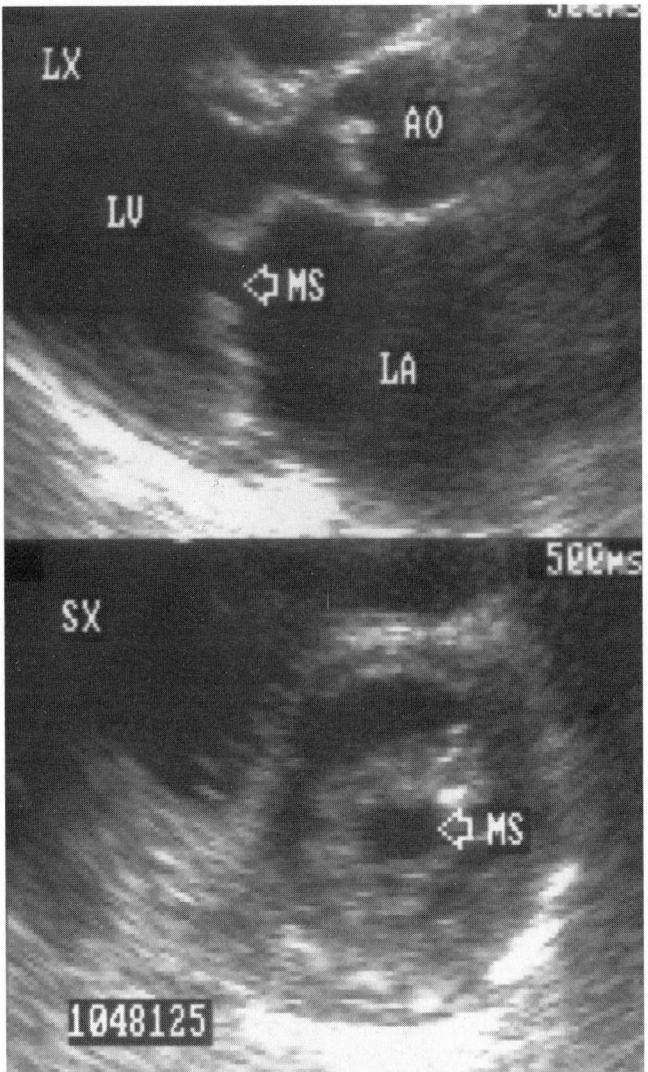

FIGURE 3–46. Long-axis (LX) and short-axis (SX) 2-D echocardiograms of a patient with mitral stenosis. The long-axis view shows typical doming of both leaflets with diminished separation (MS) between the anterior and posterior edges. The short-axis view shows the echo-free orifice in the center of the stenotic valve (MS). (From Feigenbaum, H.: Echocardiography. 5th ed. Malvern, PA, Lea and Febiger, 1994.)

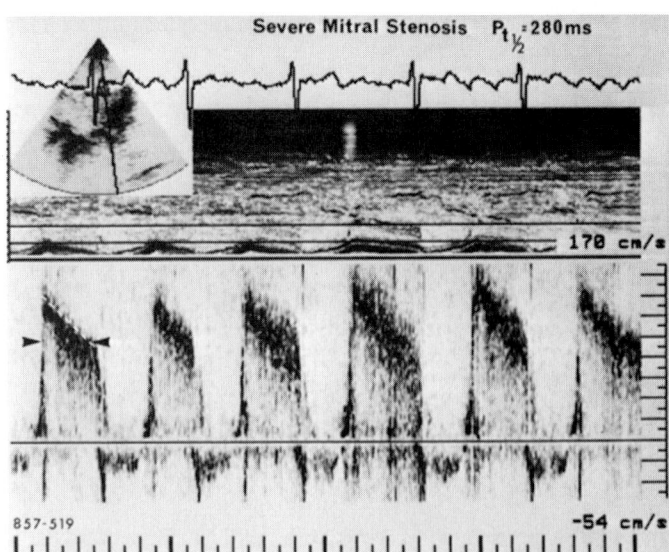

FIGURE 3–47. Pulsed Doppler echocardiogram of mitral flow in a patient with mitral stenosis, demonstrating how the pressure half-time ($P_{t_{1/2}}$) (arrowheads) is measured. (From Feigenbaum, H.: Echocardiography. 4th ed. Philadelphia, Lea and Febiger, 1986.)

Mitral Regurgitation

DOPPLER ECHOCARDIOGRAPHY. This is the ultrasonic procedure of choice for the detection of any valvular regurgitation.[153] Figure 3–48 shows a pulsed Doppler recording with the Doppler sample in the left atrium. With this type of examination, high-velocity flow which aliases is recorded during ventricular systole in the left atrium.

Color flow Doppler is the principal echocardiographic technique for assessing the presence and severity of mitral regurgitation (MR) (Fig. 3–49).[154] Transesophageal echocardiography is more sensitive in detecting MR than is the transthoracic approach.[155] The regurgitant blood flows into the left atrium during ventricular systole. The velocity is very high, and a mosaic, multicolored pattern is recorded because of aliasing. The location, direction, and size of the MR flow are readily depicted by the color flow system. There is a rough relationship between the size of the regurgitant jet and the extent of regurgitation,[156] but this relationship is influenced by many factors, such as the direction of the regurgant jet (Fig. 3–50). In Figure 3–49 the jet enters the center of the left atrium and fills much of the left

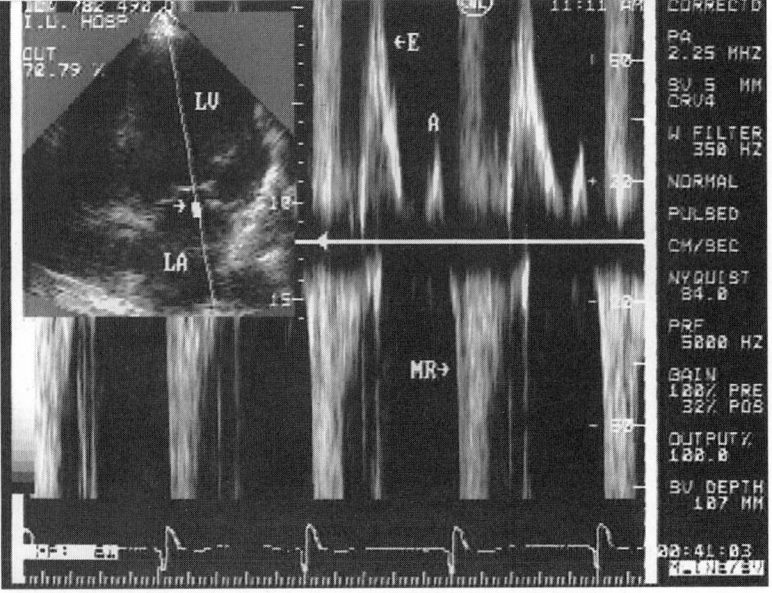

FIGURE 3–48. Pulsed Doppler examination of a patient with mitral regurgitation. The sample volume is within the left atrium (LA) and shows the high-velocity, aliasing mitral regurgitant jet (MR). LV = left ventricle. (From Feigenbaum, H.: Echocardiography. 5th ed. Malvern, PA, Lea and Febiger, 1994.)

FIGURE 3–49. See color plate 2.

FIGURE 3–50. See color plate 2.

atrium; it is known as a central jet. However, in Figure 3–50 the jet is directed toward the interatrial septum, and the flow curves around the atrial septum (arrows). Such Doppler flow is a wall jet.[157] The area of such a pattern underestimates the degree of regurgitation.

A useful sign when using color flow Doppler for valvular regurgitation is to look at the acceleration of flow proximal to the regurgitant orifice (AC) (Fig. 3–49). This acceleration is due to blood velocity increasing as it approaches the small regurgitant orifice.[158] This finding is usually indicative of significant blood flow or regurgitant flow. Techniques have been developed to use this proximal acceleration to calculate a proximal isovelocity area or PISA.[159] This area measurement has been used to quantitate the severity of MR.[160,161] Another technique is to record pulmonary venous Doppler velocities and noting systolic reverse flow.[162]

Unfortunately, all flow-mapping techniques with either color mapping or standard pulsed Doppler have only a limited relationship to the degree of MR.[163,164] Thus the quantitation of valvular regurgitation using Doppler flow mapping is at best semiquantitative. An alternative Doppler technique for quantifying MR is to calculate stroke volumes through two different orifices, one that reflects flow ejected from the left ventricle to the aorta and one measuring flow passing from the left atrium to the left ventricle.[165,166] The difference is the regurgitant volume, and regurgitant fraction can be calculated. This approach requires accurate stroke volume measurements and may not be possible in all patients.

Echocardiography is also helpful in assessing the hemodynamic consequences of the MR. The left atrium is invariably dilated, and left ventricular stroke volume increases with frequent left ventricular dilatation.[167] All of these findings are detectable on the echocardiogram. Possibly one of the most important uses of echocardiography is in identifying the etiology of the MR. Rheumatic MR almost always produces some thickening of the mitral valve and at least minimal echocardiographic evidence of MS. There are numerous other causes for MR, and echocardiography plays an important role in identifying these.

NONRHEUMATIC MITRAL REGURGITATION

Mitral Valve Prolapse (see p. 1029). Echocardiography is particularly useful in the diagnosis of this condition.[168] Figure 3–51 demonstrates the principal M-mode finding, a fairly abrupt posterior (downward) motion of the mitral valve apparatus in mid or late systole.[169] This motion often commences simultaneously with the mid or late systolic click (Fig. 3–51), a typical auscultatory and phonocardiographic finding in this condition (see p. 31). Although this mid or late systolic posterior motion of the mitral valve is a reasonably specific sign of mitral valve prolapse, it is not a very sensitive sign. Many patients with this lesion fail to show it, while in others the prolapse is a holosystolic event, i.e., there is posterior displacement of the valve throughout systole (Fig. 32–25, p. 1034).[170] Minor degrees of posterior displacement of the mitral valve can occur normally, and there is a troublesome "gray zone" in which it is difficult to determine whether the prolapse is normal or not.[171] Late or holosystolic prolapse, as in Figure 3–51, in which the leaflets move posteriorly by at least 5 mm, is generally accepted as abnormal. However, when

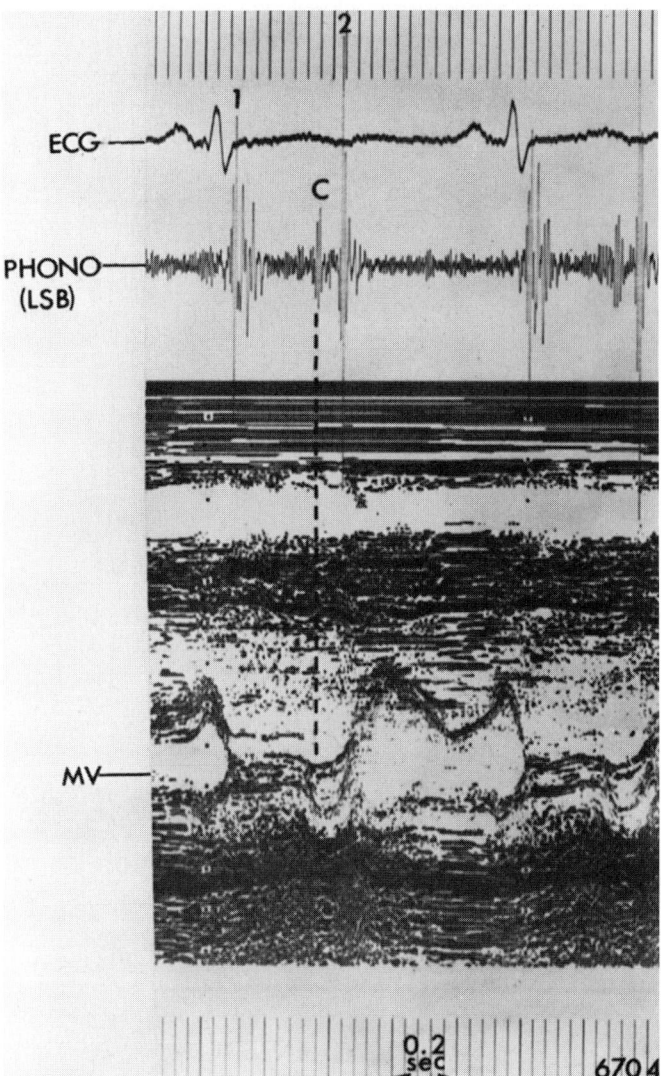

FIGURE 3–51. Phonocardiogram and M-mode echocardiogram from a patient with mitral valve prolapse. The late systolic click (C) on the phonocardiogram corresponds to late systolic posterior displacement of the mitral valve (MV). (From Tavel, M. E.: Clinical Phonocardiography and External Pulse Recordings. 3rd ed. Chicago, Year Book Medical Publishers, 1978.)

the holosystolic "hammocking" is less than 5 mm,[172] the diagnosis is not clear-cut.

Several findings on 2-D echocardiography have been suggested for the diagnosis of mitral valve prolapse,[173,174] including the recording of buckling of one or both mitral leaflets into the left atrium during systole. Figure 3–52 demonstrates a parasternal long-axis and a four-chamber examination of a patient with mitral valve prolapse. The posterior or mitral leaflet can be seen buckline or herniating into the left atrium in late systole. Unfortunately the amount of systolic prolapse noted on the 2-D echocardiograms also exhibits a continuum from normal to abnormal, and there may still be a problem in differentiating between prolapse and a normal variant with this technique.[175] The parasternal long-axis view is more specific for the diagnosis of prolapse[176] than is the four-chamber view.

Other echocardiographic findings in patients with mitral valve prolapse include excessive amplitude of motion of the valve during diastole that can be appreciated in both M-mode and 2-D examinations. Thickening of the leaflets is common and is presumably due to myxomatous degeneration.[177] The leaflets may also be redundant and seem to fold on themselves in diastole. When there is redundancy and thickening of the leaflets, the diagnosis of mitral valve

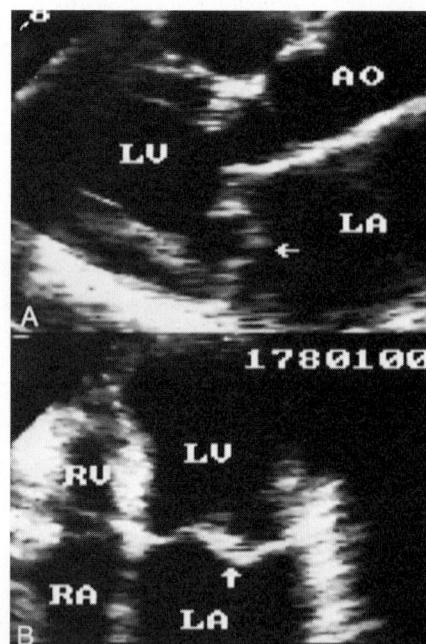

FIGURE 3–52. Two-dimensional echocardiogram in the parasternal long-axis *(A)* and apical four-chamber *(B)* views of a patient with mitral valve prolapse (arrows). LV = left ventricle; AO = aorta; LA = left atrium; RV = right ventricle; RA = right atrium.

prolapse is more secure than when the leaflets are seen to move into the left atrium only in systole.[178] It must be emphasized that although echocardiography can frequently be used to make a positive diagnosis of mitral valve prolapse, it is also difficult to distinguish minor degrees of prolapse from a normal variant.

Two-dimensional echocardiography is the examination of choice for establishing the presence of a flail mitral leaflet.[179] With this abnormality the leaflets are seen to protrude into the left atrium (Fig. 3–53).[180] The differentiation

between a flail mitral leaflet and mitral valve prolapse depends on whether the tips of the leaflet point toward the left atrium (flail valve) or curve back and point toward the left ventricle (prolapse).[181] Color Doppler almost always reveals an eccentric jet with a flail mitral valve.[182] As would be expected, transesophageal echocardiography is excellent in detecting and evaluating a flail mitral valve.[183]

PAPILLARY MUSCLE DYSFUNCTION. Two-dimensional echocardiography provides an opportunity to detect incomplete closure of the mitral valve because of left ventricular dilatation or scarring of the papillary muscles. In this condition the leaflets in the four-chamber view fail to reach the level of the mitral annulus.[184]

Aortic Stenosis

Doppler echocardiography has revolutionized the role of echocardiography and indeed the management of patients with aortic stenosis (AS). M-mode and 2-D echocardiography have always provided an excellent qualitative diagnosis of AS. Doppler echocardiography now provides an opportunity for the quantitative diagnosis. The 2-D echocardiographic diagnosis of valvular aortic stenosis is doming, thickening, and restricted motion of the leaflets (Fig. 3–54).[185] The valve may be heavily calcified and immobile, in which case only distorted, echo-producing, immobile valve leaflets are apparent.[186] It is possible to make a semiquantitative assessment of AS with 2-D echocardiography by judging the mobility of the leaflets, especially in the short-axis view (Fig. 3–54). Although transthoracic 2-D echocardiography is rarely used to quantitate AS, there is renewed interest in using transesophageal echocardiography to measure the cross-sectional area of the aortic valve and thus quantitating AS.[187,188]

The best ultrasonic technique for quantifying AS utilizes continuous-wave Doppler.[119,189] Using the modified Bernoulli equation (Fig. 3–40), it is possible to measure the pressure gradient across the aortic valve. Figure 3–55 shows a composite of simultaneous Doppler recordings and intracardiac pressure measurements in four patients with AS; an increase in the Doppler velocity occurs as the gradient increases. There is an excellent relationship between the instantaneous gradient across the stenotic valve as measured by both catheterization and Doppler techniques.[189]

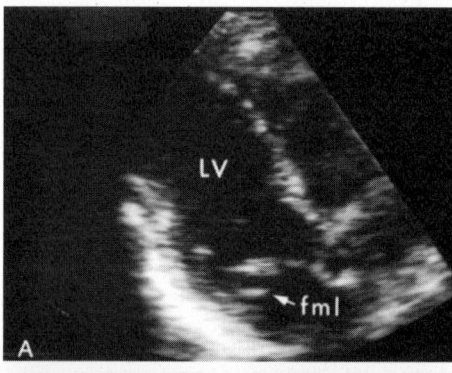

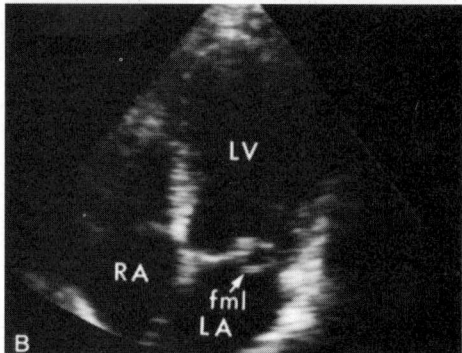

FIGURE 3–53. *A,* Apical two-chamber and *B,* four-chamber views of a patient with a flail mitral leaflet. The flail leaflet (fml) can be seen protruding into the left atrium (LA) during ventricular systole. LV = left ventricle; RA = right atrium. (From Feigenbaum, H.: Echocardiography. 4th ed. Philadelphia, Lea and Febiger, 1986.)

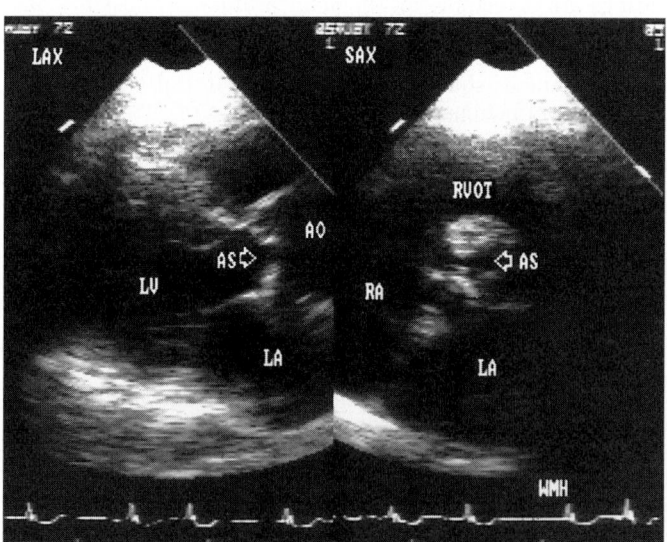

FIGURE 3–54. Long-axis (LAX) and short-axis (SAX) views from a patient with aortic stenosis (AS). The long-axis examination shows classic doming, restricted motion, and reduced separation of the leaflets. The elliptical orifice occasionally can be identified in the short-axis examination. LV = left ventricle; AO = aorta; LA = left atrium; RVOT = right ventricular outflow tract; RA = right atrium. (From Feigenbaum, H.: Echocardiography. 5th ed. Malvern, PA, Lea and Febiger, 1994).

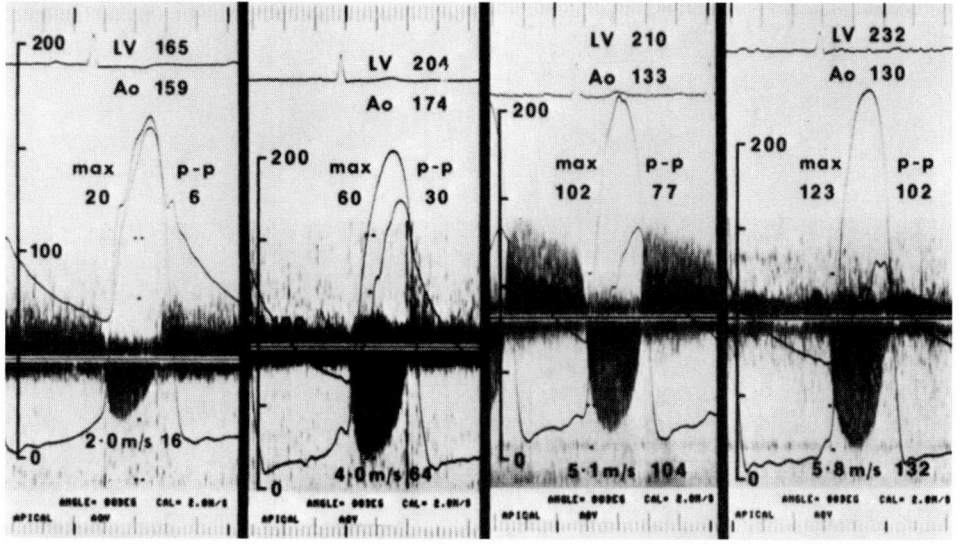

FIGURE 3–55. Simultaneous continuous wave Doppler and hemodynamic measurements in four different patients with valvular aortic stenosis. The peak velocity increases as the gradient between the left ventricular and aortic pressures increases. (Reproduced with permission from Currie, P. J., et al.: Continuous wave Doppler echocardiographic assessment of severity of calcific aortic stenosis: A simultaneous Doppler-catheter correlative study in 100 adult patients. Circulation 71:1162, 1985. Copyright 1985 American Heart Association.)

In the cardiac catheterization laboratory it is customary to measure the aortic valve gradient as the difference between the peak left ventricular pressure and the peak aortic pressure (the "peak-to-peak" gradient) (Fig. 3–56). This gradient actually does not exist at any instant in time because the peak aortic pressure occurs later than the peak left ventricular pressure. The peak instantaneous pressure gradient measured by the Doppler technique is invariably larger. If one measures the more accurate mean gradients both in the catheterization laboratory and with the Doppler examination, then the measurements are quite similar.

The Doppler technique thus gives a good estimate of the gradient across the aortic valve. Obviously the gradient is dependent on both the aortic valve area and the flow across the valve. With reduced cardiac output one can have a small gradient in a patient with severe AS. Cardiac output could be measured with a right-heart catheter and thermodilution techniques[190] or by use of one of the Doppler stroke volume measurements through an orifice that does not have a diseased valve. Another Doppler approach for calculating aortic valve area uses the "continuity equation"[191] (Fig. 3–42). This technique has been used with reasonable accuracy to calculate the aortic valve orifice in patients with valvular AS. A modification of the continuity

equation uses blood flow through the mitral orifice rather than the left ventricular outflow tract.[192]

The theoretical basis for using Doppler echocardiography for calculating the valve gradient is well established. However, there are technical details that must be recognized.[193,194] It is crucial that the maximal velocity be recorded and that the ultrasonic beam be parallel to the aortic stenotic jet. This requirement can make the examination fairly lengthy. Various ultrasonic windows must be tried to make certain that the optimal jet is identified.

From a practical point of view, if a high-velocity jet (in excess of 4 m/sec) is identified, the probability of critical AS is extremely high and the patient's condition can be managed accordingly. On the other hand, if the velocity is within normal limits or mildly elevated, the possibility of significant AS can be excluded. When the velocity is in an intermediate zone, which would indicate a pressure gradient between 23 and 50 mm Hg, additional hemodynamic information may be necessary for proper management.[195]

There are secondary signs of AS that can be noted on the echocardiogram. Both M-mode and 2-D echocardiography can detect left ventricular hypertrophy with increased thickness of the left ventricular walls. Although the degree of left ventricular hypertrophy has been used to assess the severity of AS,[196] this technique is not nearly as reliable as the use of Doppler for valve gradients and valve area.

Aortic Regurgitation

As with all valvular regurgitation, Doppler echocardiography is the examination of choice for detecting the presence of aortic regurgitation (AR).[197,198] Figure 3–57 shows a Doppler sample in the left ventricular outflow tract and the recording of high-velocity flow during diastole. This type of examination is both sensitive and specific for the presence of AR. Color flow Doppler provides a 2-D display of the AR jet (Fig. 3–58). The accuracy of Doppler flow mapping for quantitating AR is at best semiquantitative.[199,200] The same limitations pertain to AR as were discussed with MR (see p. 72). The width of the aortic jet at the valve orifice as judged by color flow Doppler is used to judge the severity of AR,[13,200] and is clinically useful. The rate of decrease in velocity of the regurgitant blood as recorded in the left ventricular outflow tract using continuous-wave Doppler has been used as a reflection of severity of the AR (Fig. 3–59). Severe AR produces a faster fall in velocity as the pressure difference between the aorta and left ventricle falls rapidly.[201] AR can also be judged by the difference between aortic flow and pulmonary artery flow or mitral flow.[202] One can calculate a regurgitant orifice size using Doppler continuity equation.[203]

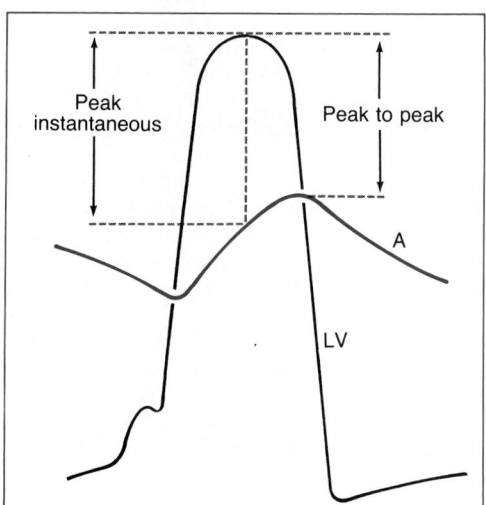

FIGURE 3–56. Left ventricular (LV) and aortic (A) pressures in aortic stenosis. The peak instantaneous pressure difference or gradient is greater than the peak-to-peak gradient because the peak aortic pressure occurs later than the peak left ventricular pressure. (From Feigenbaum, H.: Echocardiography. 4th ed. Philadelphia, Lea and Febiger, 1986.)

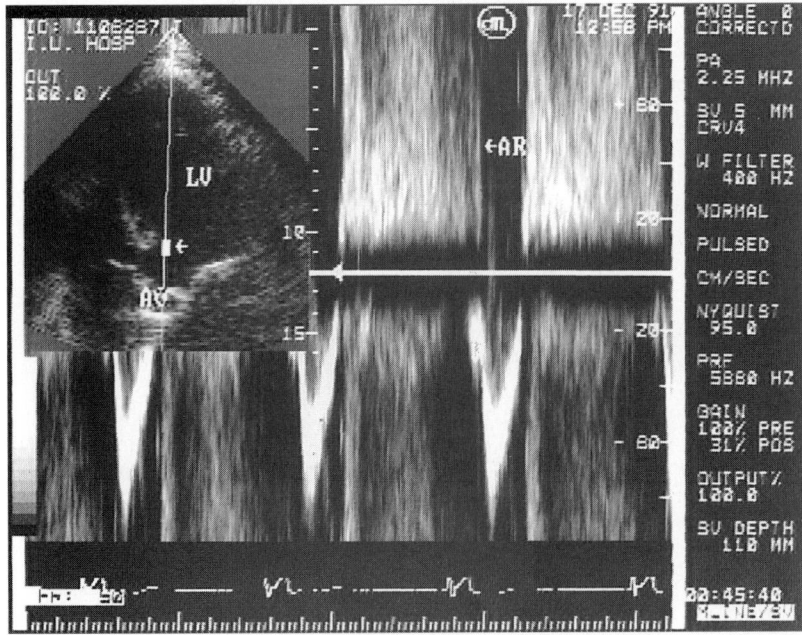

FIGURE 3–57. Pulsed Doppler echogram of a patient with aortic regurgitation. The Doppler sample *(arrow)* is within the left ventricular outflow tract, and the recording displays a high velocity, aliasing diastolic Doppler signal (AR). LV = left ventricle; AO = aorta. (From Feigenbaum, H.: Echocardiography. 5th ed. Malvern, PA, Lea and Febiger, 1994.)

FIGURE 3–58. See color plate 2.

One M-mode sign of AR that remains useful is premature closure of the mitral valve in the presence of severe, usually acute, AR[128] (see p. 1050). This premature mitral closure can also be noted on the Doppler recording.[204] With an elevated left ventricular diastolic pressure there may even be early opening of the aortic valve on the M-mode recording.[130] Both of these signs represent severe AR and markedly elevated left ventricular diastolic pressures. The secondary effects of AR on the left ventricle can be detected

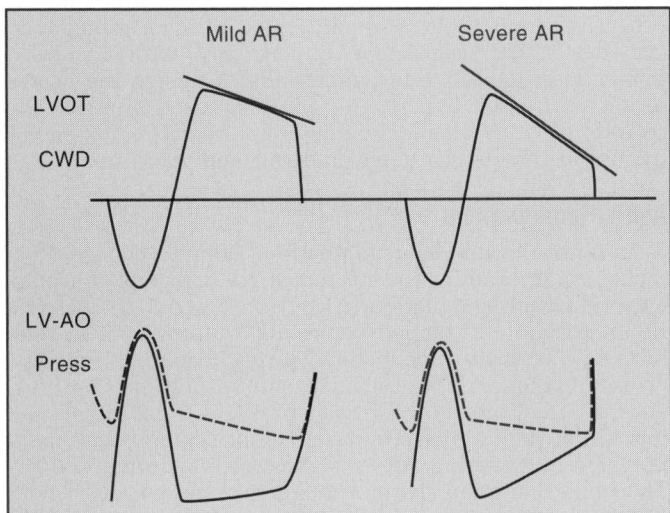

FIGURE 3–59. The principle of how the diastolic slope of the regurgitant jet can relate to the severity of aortic regurgitation (AR). The continuous-wave Doppler (CWD) signal is a function of the pressure difference between the left ventricle and the aorta (LV-AO). With relatively mild aortic regurgitation, the pressure difference gradually decreases as regurgitant blood is flowing into the left ventricle; however, with severe aortic regurgitation, the aortic pressure drops rapidly and the left ventricular pressure rises steeply as the large regurgitant volume increases the pressure. Thus the pressure differential decreases and the slope of the diastolic regurgitant jet increases. LVOT = left ventricular outflow tract. (From Feigenbaum, H.: Echocardiography. 5th ed. Malvern, PA, Lea and Febiger, 1994.)

with both M-mode and 2-D echocardiographic examinations. Serial measurements of left ventricular size and systolic function are important in observing patients with chronic AR or judging the efficacy of surgery.[205] Deterioration in left ventricular systolic function is one criterion for valve replacement[206] (see p. 1052).

Tricuspid Valve Disease

TRICUSPID STENOSIS. The echocardiographic findings of tricuspid stenosis and regurgitation are very similar to those for MS and MR. Two-dimensional and Doppler echocardiography are the procedures of choice for detecting tricuspid stenosis. Doming of the tricuspid valve on 2-D echocardiography is the hallmark of TS.[207] The Doppler findings of tricuspid stenosis are similar to those with MS.[208] The velocities passing through the orifice are increased, and the rate of diastolic decline in velocity is reduced. The pressure half-time can also be used to calculate the severity of the valvular obstruction.

TRICUSPID REGURGITATION. This abnormality is also best determined by pulsed, continuous wave, or color flow Doppler echocardiography.[209,210] As noted previously, the Doppler recording of tricuspid regurgitation can be used to estimate the pressure gradient across the tricuspid valve. This measurement provides an opportunity for estimating right ventricular systolic pressure by adding an estimate of right atrial pressure.

Two-dimensional echocardiography can help determine the etiology of tricuspid regurgitation. Rheumatic tricuspid regurgitation usually has an element of tricuspid stenosis and invariably exhibits MS. Pulmonary hypertension can be detected by estimating the right ventricular systolic pressure. Tricuspid valve prolapse gives an appearance similar to that of mitral valve prolapse (Fig. 3–60).[211] A flail tricuspid valve is indicated by the finding of parts of the tricuspid valve protruding into the right atrium in ventricular systole.[212] Carcinoid valve disease (see p. 1056) produces stiff immobile tricuspid leaflets that are continuously open.[213] Valve vegetations and Ebstein's anomaly are discussed on pp. 1083 and 934 respectively. As with all valvular disease, transesophageal echocardiography can provide higher quality images of tricuspid valve pathology.[214]

Secondary effects of tricuspid regurgitation can be noted on 2-D studies. Right ventricular and right atrial dilatation are invariably present. Abnormal diastolic motion of the interventricular septum indicates that right ventricular volume overload may be present.

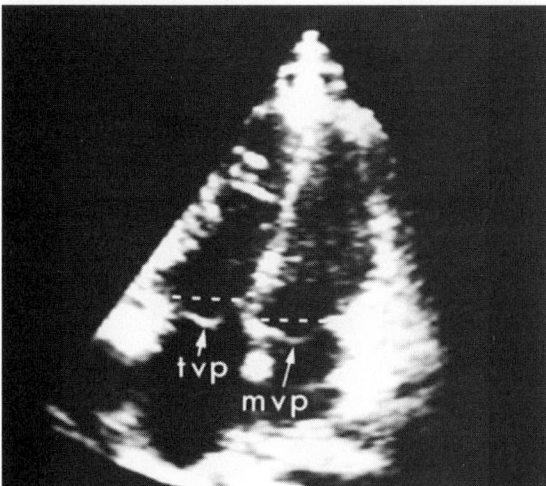

FIGURE 3-60. Apical four-chamber 2-D echocardiogram of a patient with tricuspid valve prolapse (tvp) and mitral valve prolapse (mvp). (From Feigenbaum, H.: Echocardiography. 4th ed. Philadelphia, Lea and Febiger, 1986.)

Infective Endocarditis
(See Chap. 33)

Echocardiography provides a means for visualizing the vegetations of infective valvular endocarditis, which appear as echo-producing masses attached to the infected valve (Fig. 3-61) (Fig. 33-4, p. 1084).[215] They are usually asymmetrical, commonly involving one leaflet more than another, but may be present on more than one valve. If the vegetation is associated with destruction of the valve or if it is on a long "stalk," it can be readily imaged; its excessive motion can be appreciated on both M-mode[216,217] and 2-D echocardiography.[218] Transesophageal echocardiography is proving to be much more sensitive than transthoracic echocardiography in detecting valvular vegetations.[219] Figure 3-62 shows a small vegetation on the aortic valve. This lesion was not seen on the routine transthoracic echocardiogram. (The greater sensitivity of transesophageal echocardiography for the detection of valvular vegetations may change our understanding as to why echocardio-

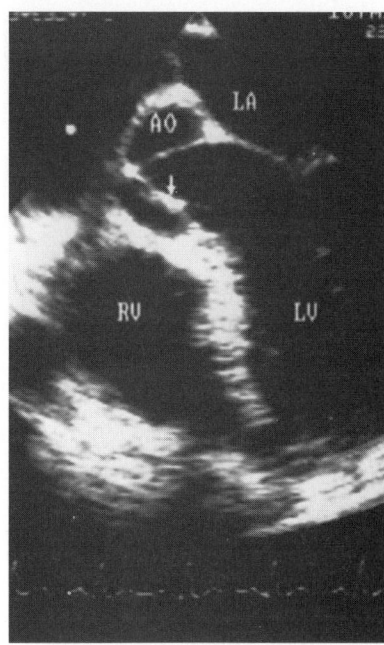

FIGURE 3-62. Transesophageal echocardiogram of a patient with a small vegetation (arrows) on the aortic valve. AO = aorta; LA = left atrium; RV = right ventricle; LV = left ventricle.

graphic vegetations are frequently seen in patients with endocarditis and whether or not this ultrasonic technique can exclude the diagnosis.[220])

Vegetations visualized echocardiographically need not be bacterial[221,222] or even infected. Infected vegetations may be difficult to distinguish from myxomatous degeneration of the valve,[218] although this differentiation is usually readily accomplished clinically.

One of the major applications of echocardiography in patients with endocarditis is in the identification of complications. When the valve is damaged to the point that it is grossly incompetent, echocardiography can both detect and assess the hemodynamic importance of the valvular regurgitation. When the aortic valve is involved, premature closure of the mitral valve because of the very high left ventricular diastolic pressure may be evident. Another serious complication of aortic valve endocarditis is the development of an aortic root abscess (Fig. 3-63).[223] This prob-

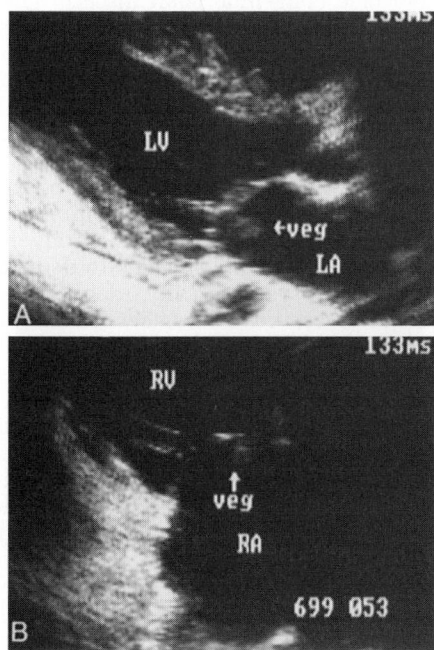

FIGURE 3-61. Two-dimensional echocardiograms of a patient with vegetation (veg) on the mitral (A) and tricuspid valves (B). LV = left ventricle; LA = left atrium; RV = right ventricle; RA = right atrium.

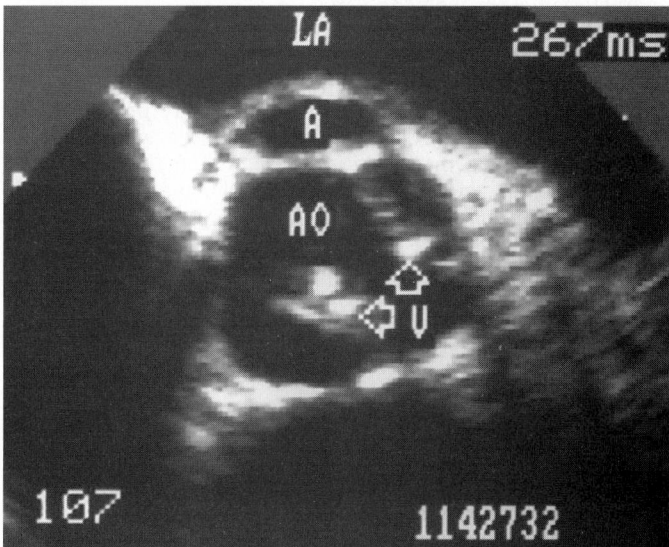

FIGURE 3-63. Transesophageal echocardiogram of a patient with vegetations (V) on the aortic valve and a periaortic abscess (A). LA = left atrium; AO = aorta. (From Feigenbaum, H.: Echocardiography. 5th ed. Malvern, PA, Lea and Febiger, 1994.)

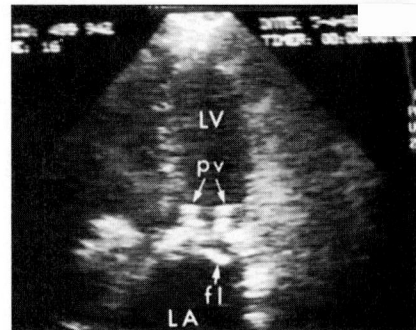

FIGURE 3–64. Apical four-chamber view in a patient with a degenerated flail porcine mitral prosthesis (pv). The flail leaflet (fl) can be seen protruding into the left atrium (LA) in systole. LV = left ventricle. (From Feigenbaum, H.: Echocardiography. 4th ed. Philadelphia, Lea and Febiger, 1986.)

lem is seen as a relatively echo-free space adjacent to the aortic root and is seen best with transesophageal echocardiography.[224] Mitral valve diverticulum can also be detected by means of esophageal echocardiography.[225]

Prosthetic Valves

There is a variety of echocardiographic signs of prosthetic valve malfunction. Most published reports of prosthetic valve malfunction represent isolated case studies.[226] Abnormal motion of a ball or disc usually results from a thrombus[227] or from ball variance.[228] A useful sign of a malfunctioning Björk-Shiley valve in the mitral position is a rounding of the E point on the M-mode echocardiogram.[229] An abnormal rocking motion of a prosthetic valve resulting from the sutures pulling loose from the annulus has been reported.[230] Thickening of the porcine valve leaflets is useful in judging deterioration of this valve.[231] A flail porcine valve, especially in the mitral position, can be easily identified with 2-D echocardiography (Fig. 3–64).[232]

DOPPLER ECHOCARDIOGRAPHY. This technique is very helpful in evaluating prosthetic valves.[233–235] Valvular regurgitation is detected readily with the Doppler technique. Color Doppler has the advantage of locating some of these unusually located valvular regurgitations (Fig. 3–65).[236] Doppler echocardiography can also assist in judging stenotic prosthetic valves. The technique is most effective with valves that have a central orifice, such as a tissue valve[237] or St. Jude mechanical valve.[238] Ball valves or tilting disc valves present more difficulties in judging the flow characteristics through the valve.

TRANSESOPHAGEAL ECHOCARDIOGRAPHY. This technique has made a major contribution to the detection of malfunctioning prosthetic valves, particularly in the mitral position.[239–241] Acoustic shadowing frequently prohibits the detection of MR involving a prosthetic valve when the examination is done through the chest. When the ultrasonic examination is performed via the esophagus, the view of the left atrium is unobstructed and the regurgitant jet is easily detected (Fig. 3–15).[242] In addition, the superior resolution inherent in the higher frequency transducer provides better visualization of the prosthetic valve, especially for the detection of minor abnormalities such as small thrombi or vegetations (Fig. 3–66).[243]

Calcified Mitral Annulus
(See p. 1017)

Calcification of a mitral annulus can be readily demonstrated by echocardiography.[244] The principal finding is a

FIGURE 3–65. See color plate 3.

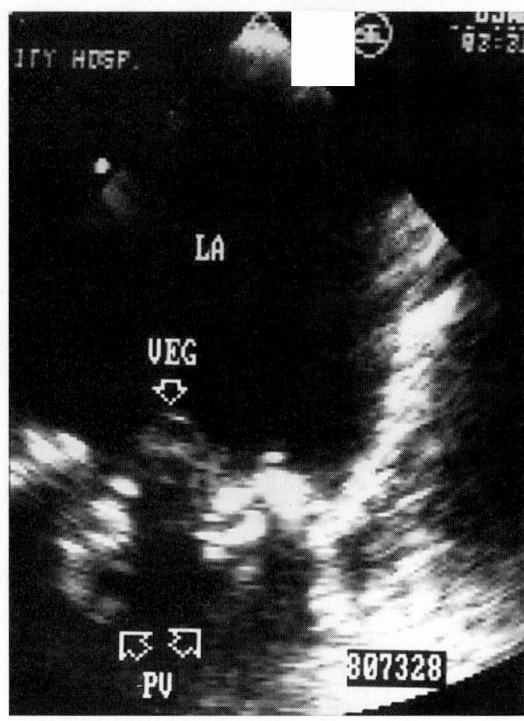

FIGURE 3–66. Transesophageal echocardiogram of a patient with a vegetation (VEG) on a porcine mitral valve (PV). LA = left atrium. (From Feigenbaum, H.: Echocardiography. 5th ed. Malvern, PA, Lea and Febiger, 1994.)

band of dense echoes between the mitral valve and the posterior left ventricular wall. Calcification can be extensive and involve the posterior mitral leaflet and much of the base of the heart.

CONGENITAL HEART DISEASE
(See also Chaps. 29 and 30)

Deductive Echocardiography

Echocardiography is an indispensable and frequently definitive examination for the evaluation of patients with known or suspected congenital heart disease. The availability of 2-D M-mode spectral Doppler, color Doppler, contrast and transesophageal echocardiography gives the clinician ample tools to decipher even the most complex congenital anomaly.[245] Echocardiography now can frequently obviate the need for more costly and dangerous invasive procedures.[246–248]

There are many ways in which echocardiography can be used to decipher the riddle of the congenitally malformed heart. The term *deductive echocardiography* refers to a technique by which an attempt is made to deduce the anatomy of the heart by systematically identifying the atria, atrioventricular valves, ventricles, semilunar valves, and great vessels. Several approaches can be used to identify the atria.[249,250] The right atrium contains the eustachian valve, has a different appearing appendage, and is not as round as the left atrium. Another technique is to identify the abdominal viscera and the venous drainage. Atrial and visceral situs are almost always concordant. The normal atrial relationship or atrial situs solitus can be determined by identifying a right-sided liver and left-sided stomach with an abdominal ultrasound examination from the subcostal position. The same examination can be used to identify the inferior vena cava, which almost invariably drains into the right atrium. One can also identify the pulmonary veins draining into the left atrium; however, this examination is technically more difficult, especially with the transthoracic examination.

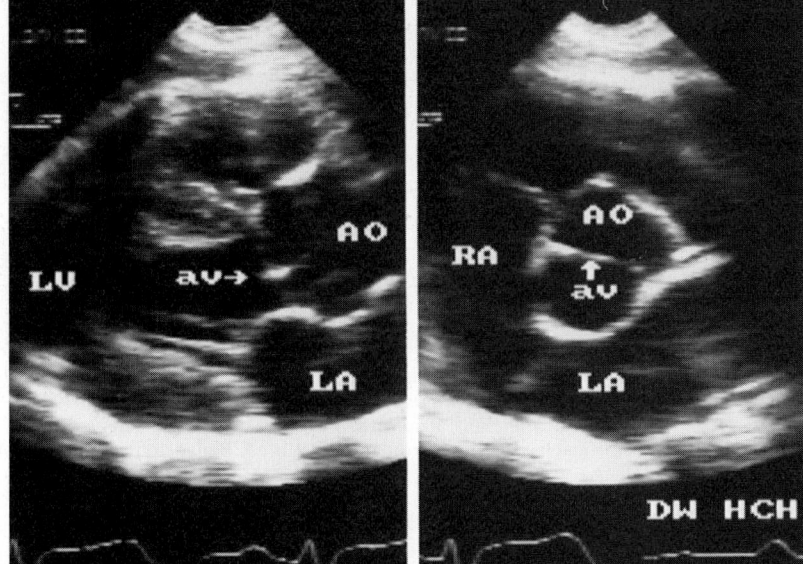

FIGURE 3–67. Long-axis *(A)* and short-axis *(B)* 2-D echocardiograms of a patient with a bicuspid aortic valve (av). LV = left ventricle; AO = aorta; LA = left atrium; RA = right atrium.

The ventricles are identified by the corresponding atrioventricular valve. The tricuspid valve is recognized by the fact that it inserts into the interventricular septum closer to the apex than does the mitral valve.[251] The right ventricle can also be identified by its trabeculations and the moderator band. The course of the great arteries and the bifurcation of the pulmonary artery help to distinguish the aorta from the pulmonary artery. The semilunar valves are always a part of the corresponding great vessel. This deductive approach can frequently unravel the mystery of even the most complex malformation.

Ventricular Inlet and Outlet Anomalies

VALVULAR STENOSIS. A bicuspid aortic valve (see p. 964) is probably the most common congenital cardiac anomaly. The best echocardiography criterion for making this diagnosis utilizes 2-D echocardiography. With this technique two cusps rather than the normal three cusps can be identified (Fig. 3–67). The diagnosis can be confusing, since occasionally a fused commissure may resemble a third leaflet echocardiographically. In addition, if the commissure is in an anterior-posterior direction, it is sometimes difficult to record echocardiographically.[252] The M-mode technique of identifying eccentric closure of the aortic valve within the aorta[253] is less reliable.

In aortic stenosis (see p. 1035), most echocardiographic findings are similar whether the valve is deformed on a congenital (see p. 914) or acquired basis. In the adult the valve is frequently heavily calcified, and the etiology is difficult to determine. The qualitative diagnosis is made by finding doming and/or restricted motion of the valve during systole. The quantitative diagnosis is now best obtained using continuous-wave Doppler (see p. 56).

A host of types of congenitally deformed mitral valves can be detected echocardiographically.[254] Congenital mitral stenosis is rare, but has been recognized by echocardiography. A parachute mitral valve has also a fairly characteristic echocardiographic appearance. Two-dimensional echocardiography can identify a double-orifice mitral valve.[255] The domed stenotic pulmonary valve resembles the congenitally stenotic aortic valve on 2-D echocardiography (Fig. 3–68A).[256] The M-mode recording of the pulmonary valve has an accentuated A wave (Fig. 3–43). The severity of congenital pulmonic stenosis may also be assessed by Doppler echocardiography.[257,258] If continuous-wave Doppler echocardiography and criteria similar to those for AS (see p. 74) are utilized, the gradient across the stenotic pulmonary valve can be estimated (Fig. 3–68B). A common abnormality associated with congenital pulmonic stenosis is pulmonic regurgitation. This abnormality is noted using Doppler recordings that reveal diastolic flow into the right ventricle.

EBSTEIN'S ANOMALY (see p. 934). The echocardiographic diagnosis of Ebstein's anomaly is based on the displacement of the tricuspid valve leaflets within the body of the right ventricle on the 2-D echocardiogram (Fig. 3–69).[259,260] Normally the tricuspid valve inserts on the interventricular septum slightly above the insertion of the mitral valve. However, with Ebstein's anomaly this displacement is marked, and much of the tricuspid valve lies within the body of the right ventricle. On M-mode echocardiography the diagnosis of Ebstein's anomaly is based on delayed closure of the tricuspid valve.[261] The 2-D echocardiogram is more specific and reliable for this diagnosis.

VALVULAR ATRESIA. Atresia of cardiac valves is generally associated with hypoplasia of the ipsilateral ventricle (Chap. 29). Thus, aortic or mitral atresia is associated with hypoplasia of the left ventricle.[262] Diminutive ventricles and the atretic valves have been imaged with both M-mode[263] and 2-D techniques (Fig. 3–70).[264,265]

SUBVALVULAR OBSTRUCTIONS. A variety of congenital subvalvular obstructions have been detected echocardiographically. Early systolic closure of the aortic valve has

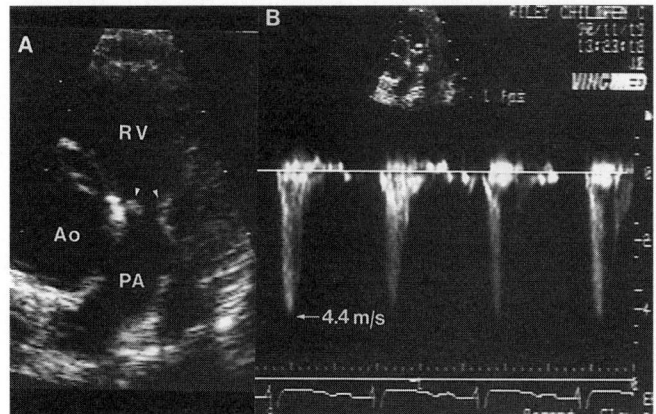

FIGURE 3–68. Two-dimensional *(A)* and continuous-wave Doppler *(B)* studies of a patient with valvular pulmonic stenosis. The 2-D study shows a thickened, domed pulmonary valve. The continuous-wave Doppler shows increased velocity that peaks at 4.4 M/sec, which is consistent with a systolic gradient of approximately 78 mm Hg. RV = right ventricle; Ao = aorta; PA = pulmonary artery. (From Feigenbaum, H.: Echocardiography. 5th ed. Malvern, PA, Lea and Febiger, 1994.)

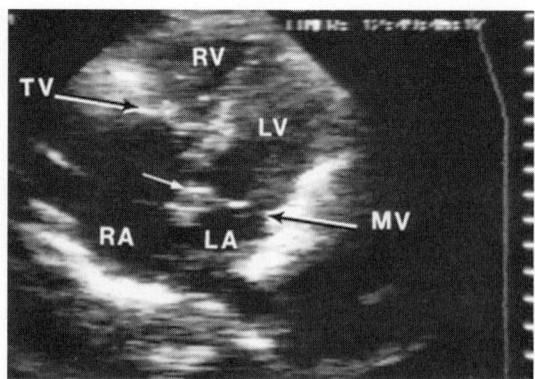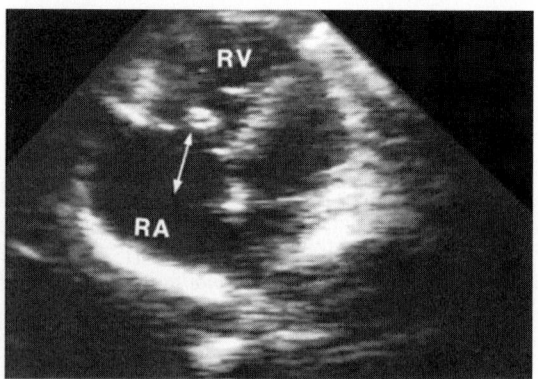

FIGURE 3–69. Apical four-chamber view in a patient with Ebstein's anomaly. The tricuspid valve (TV) is displaced from the tricuspid annulus (arrow). The effective right ventricular volume (RV) is decreased and the volume of the right atrium (RA) is increased. LV = left ventricle; LA = left atrium; MV = mitral valve. (From Feigenbaum, H.: Echocardiography. 4th ed. Philadelphia, Lea and Febiger, 1986.)

been observed in patients with both discrete (Fig. 3–71)[266] and hypertrophic obstructive cardiomyopathy (Fig. 41–17, p. 1418).[129] In addition, systolic fluttering of the aortic valve is often exaggerated, although some degree of aortic valve fluttering may be seen normally. Although midsystolic closure and fluttering of the aortic valve are not specific findings for subaortic stenosis, they can be very helpful in differentiating valvular from subvalvular obstruction, since they do not occur in the former condition.

Examination of the outflow tract is accomplished with transthoracic or transesophageal 2-D echocardiography, and the subvalvular obstruction can be identified directly by this technique (Fig. 3–72).[267,268] The 2-D technique also permits the classification of discrete obstruction into the discrete membranous and the diffuse types.[269] Distinguishing between them may be of considerable clinical importance, since their management may differ. The membranous form is frequently situated just below the aortic valve and may therefore be difficult to recognize at catheterization, since the short subvalvular chamber can be missed on a

pull-out pressure recording. Indeed, the thin membrane can even be missed on the angiogram, so that its recognition by 2-D echocardiography can be very helpful. Doppler echocardiography can be used to assess the severity of subvalvular as well as valvular stenosis.[270]

In subpulmonic obstruction the M-mode tracing exhibits coarse fluttering of the pulmonary valve.[271] The actual subpulmonic obstruction can be detected, and its severity quantified in patients with tetralogy of Fallot by means of

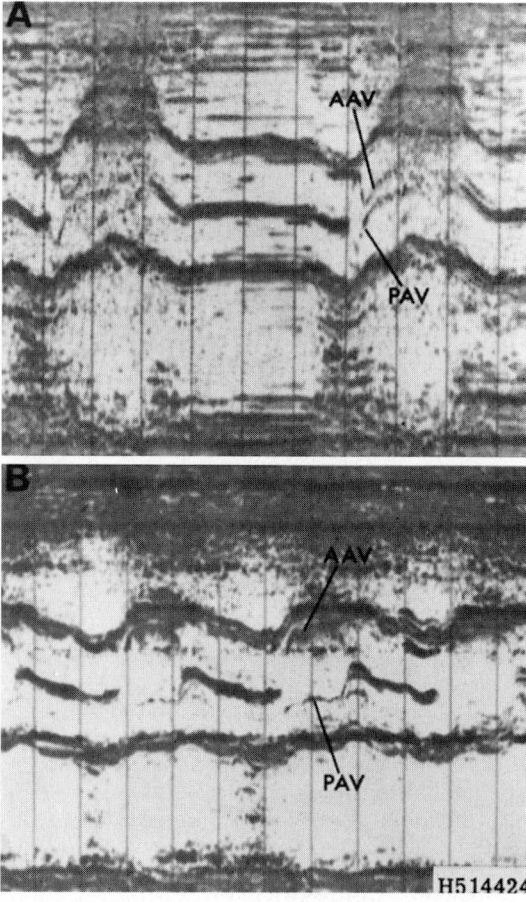

FIGURE 3–71. Aortic valve echocardiograms from a patient with discrete subaortic stenosis before *(A)* and *(B)* after surgery for the subaortic obstruction. Prior to surgery the aortic valve anterior (AAV) and posterior (PAV) leaflets come together shortly after the onset of ventricular ejection and remain essentially closed throughout systole. This systolic closure of the valve leaflets is no longer present after surgery. (From Davis, R. H., et al: Echocardiographic manifestation of discrete subaortic stenosis. Am. J. Cardiol. *33:277,* 1974.)

FIGURE 3–70. Apical four-chamber view in a patient with tricuspid atresia. The atretic tricuspid annulus is indicated by arrowheads. A large atrial septal defect is present. The hypoplastic right ventricle (RV) is seen. RA = right atrium; LA = left atrium; LV = left ventricle. (From Feigenbaum, H.: Echocardiography. 5th ed. Malvern, PA, Lea & Febiger, 1994.)

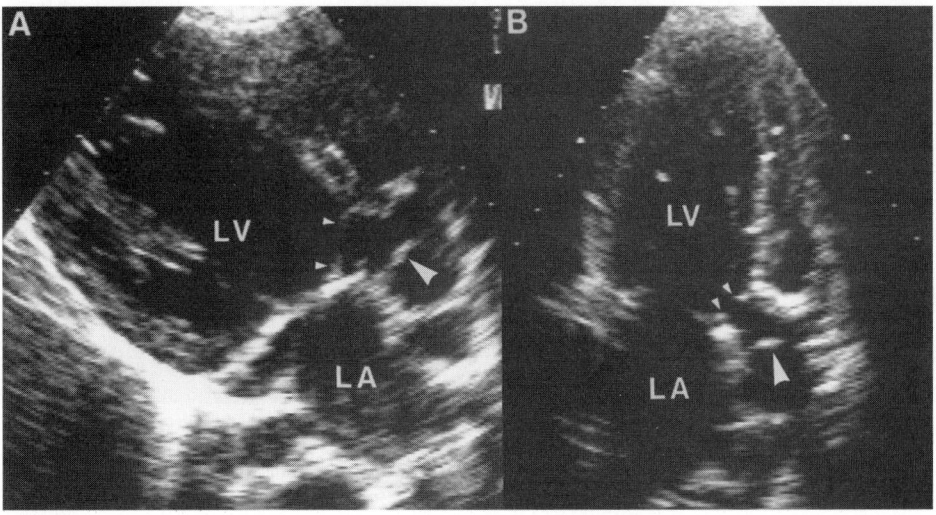

FIGURE 3–72. Parasternal *(A)* and apical *(B)* long-axis view from a patient with discrete, membranous subaortic stenosis. The aortic valve (large arrowhead) is thickened, but not stenotic. Immediately below the valve in the left ventricular outflow tract is a discrete membrane (small arrowheads). LA = left atrium; LV = left ventricle. (From Feigenbaum, H.: Echocardiography. 5th ed. Malvern, PA, Lea and Febiger, 1994.)

2-D examination of the right ventricular outflow tract and subpulmonic area.[272]

Subvalvular mitral obstruction can also occur. A fibrous membrane may be situated within the left atrial cavity (Fig. 3–73). Such a membrane obstructs flow and divides the left atrium into two chambers.[273] This anomaly is commonly known as *cor triatriatum* (see p. 923).[274] If the fibrous band is next to the mitral annulus, then the entity is known as a *supravalvular stenosing ring.*[275] Congenital stenoses of the pulmonary veins can also occur.

Cardiac Shunts

Echocardiography can be helpful in the diagnosis of cardiac shunts by detecting the actual defect between the two sides of the heart, by evaluating the hemodynamic consequences of the shunt, and by recording the shunted blood using color flow Doppler or contrast methods.

VENTRICULAR SEPTAL DEFECT (see also pp. 901 and 967). Pulsed Doppler is useful for detecting ventricular septal defects,[276] but color flow Doppler has become the technique of choice for visualizing these abnormalities[277,278] (Fig. 3–74). The examination is particularly helpful when multiple defects exist.[279] The defects can also be seen with 2-D echocardiography.[280] Figure 3–75 demonstrates a small membranous ventricular septal defect using 2-D echocardiography and contrast. Figure 3–76 demonstrates an apical four-chamber view in a patient with total absence of a ventricular septum or a single ventricle.[281] The continuous-wave Doppler velocity across the ventricular septal defect can reflect the pressure difference between the left and right ventricles during systole.[282] Subtracting the pressure gradient from the left ventricular systolic pressure provides an estimate of the right ventricular systolic pressure.

ATRIAL SEPTAL DEFECT (see also pp. 896 and 970). The 2-D echocardiographic examination, especially from the subcostal position, provides an opportunity for direct examination of the interarterial septum (Fig. 3–25A, p. 62).[283,284] Figure 3–77 demonstrates findings in a patient with an ostium secundum atrial septal defect. A remnant of the interatrial septum can be seen attached to the ventricular septum. In contrast, Figure 3–78 demonstrates an atrial septal defect in a patient with an ostium primum

---

FIGURE 3–74. See color plate 3.

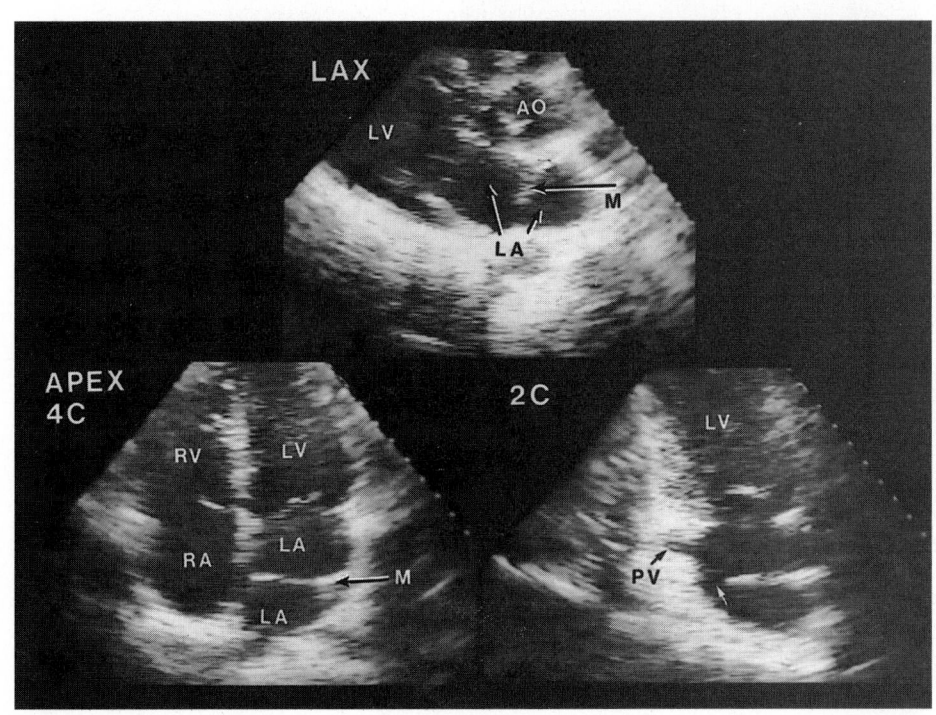

FIGURE 3–73. Parasternal long-axis and apical views from an asymptomatic patient with cor triatriatum. A linear echo courses posterior laterally within the left atrium, dividing it into two components. LA = left atrium; RA = right atrium; RV = right ventricle; LV = left ventricle; AO = aorta; M = left atrial membrane; PV = pulmonary vein. (From Feigenbaum, H.: Echocardiography. 5th ed. Malvern, PA, Lea and Febiger, 1994.)

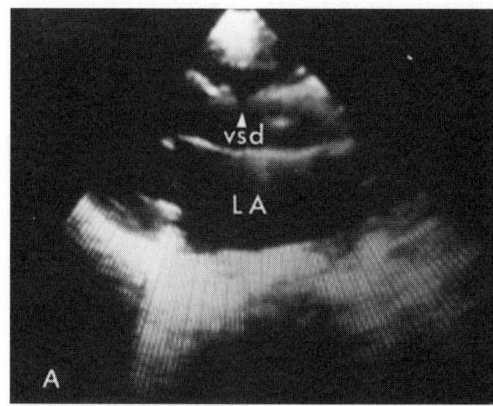
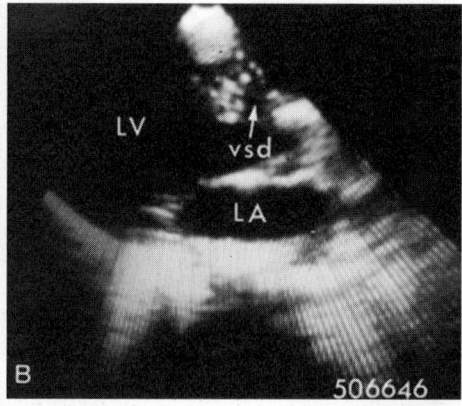

FIGURE 3–75. Two-dimensional long-axis echocardiograms of a patient with a membranous ventricular septal defect. A, The discontinuity of echoes from the ventricular septal defect (vsd) can be seen. B, A peripheral contrast injection fills the right ventricle, but an echo-free jet, i.e., negative contrast, can be seen anterior to the ventricular septal defect. LV = left ventricle; LA = left atrium. (From Feigenbaum, H.: Echocardiography. 4th ed. Philadelphia, Lea and Febiger, 1986.)

FIGURE 3–76. Cross-sectional echocardiogram of a patient with a single ventricle (SV). The ultrasonic probe is placed at the apex of the heart, and the plane of the scan transects the interatrial septum so that all chambers can be seen simultaneously. This view is particularly helpful in demonstrating the absence of the interventricular septum. RA = right atrium; LA = left atrium.

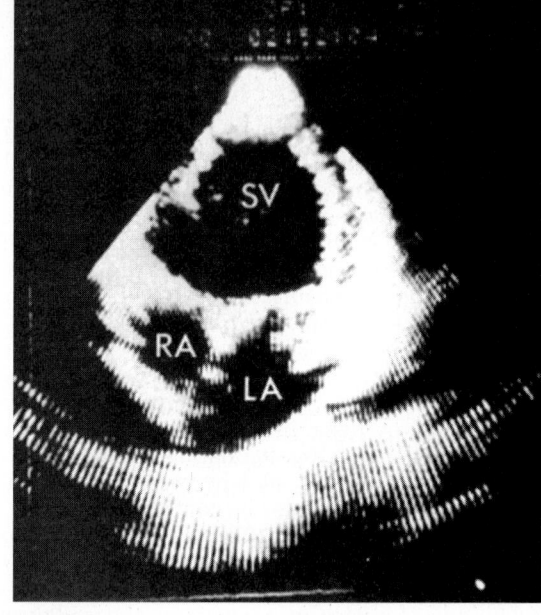

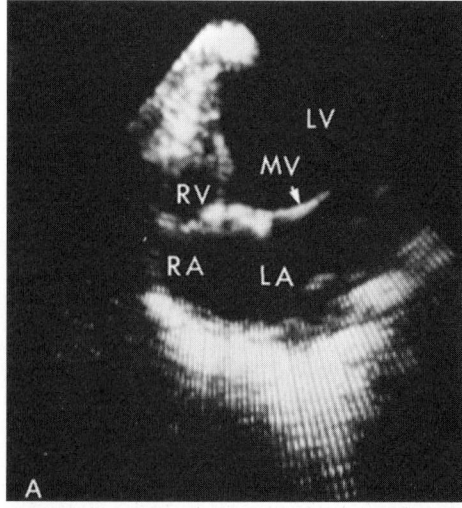
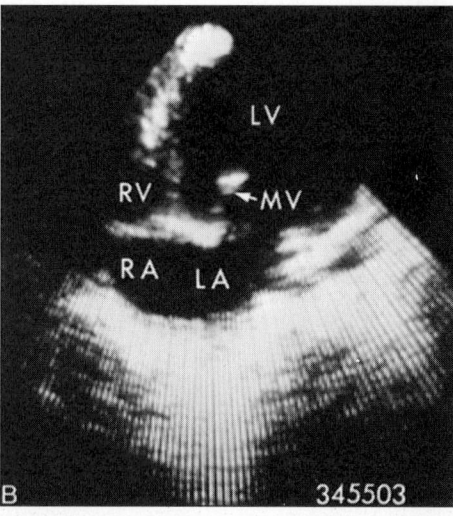

FIGURE 3–77. Subcostal 2-D echocardiogram of a patient with an ostium secundum atrial septal defect. Remnants of the interatrial septum are visible on both sides of the defect (ASD). RA = right atrium; LA = left atrium; LV = left ventricle. (From Feigenbaum, H.: Echocardiography. 3rd ed. Philadelphia, Lea and Febiger, 1981.)

defect. There is no residual septum attached to the ventricular septum. Thus, the 2-D technique not only helps to identify the presence of an atrial septal defect, but it is also an excellent means of differentiating a secundum from a primum type of abnormality. One can also identify more severe forms of an endocardial cushion defect with a coexistent ventricular septal defect (Fig. 3–79). A sinus venosus type of atrial septal defect is the most difficult type of atrial septal defect to detect with 2-D echocardiography[285] and is best seen with transesophageal echocardiography.[286] Actu-

ally, all atrial septal defects are better seen with the transesophageal approach[287] but such an examination is not always necessary.

Three-dimensional (3-D) echocardiography is an evolving technology that has great promise, especially in congenital heart disease.[288,289] Figure 3–80 shows a 3-D reconstructed echogram of a patient with both secundum and primum atrial septal defects. Figure 3–80A is equivalent to a 2-D four-chamber view cutting across the atrial septum. This 3-D examination permits one to appreciate the back walls

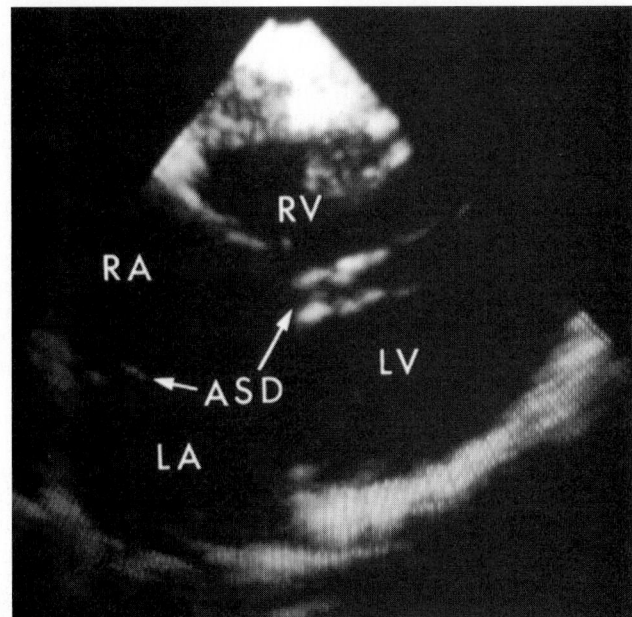

FIGURE 3–78. Subcostal 2-D echocardiogram of a patient with an ostium primum atrial septal defect. No residual septal tissue is apparent between the defect (ASD) and the interventricular septum. RA = right atrium; LA = left atrium; RV = right ventricle; LV = left ventricle. (From Feigenbaum, H.: Echocardiography. 3rd ed. Philadephia, Lea and Febiger, 1981.)

of the chambers as well as the cross-sectional appearance of the septa. By viewing the examination parallel to the septa (Fig. 3–80B), one now gains a new perspective of the atrial septum. Now as one examines the surface of the septum, what one sees is similar to what a surgeon might see in the operating room. With this approach one can appreciate the shape and size of the defects.

Color flow Doppler and contrast echocardiogram can both be used to demonstrate *atrial septal defects*. Figure 3–81 shows a color Doppler and a contrast echocardiogram in a patient with a secundum-type atrial septal defect.[290] With the Doppler study one can see the red-encoded blood passing from the left atrium to the right atrium through the defect. With the contrast examination one sees an echo-filled right atrium and right ventricle. The left atrium and left ventricle are echo free. As the non-contrast-containing left atrial blood passes through the atrial septal defect, a negative contrast effect within the right atrium (ASD) is

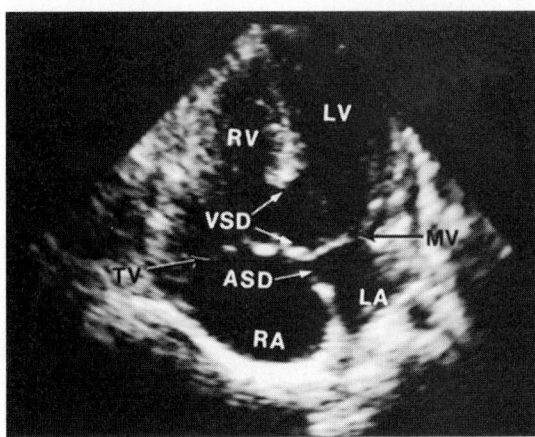

FIGURE 3–79. Apical four-chamber view in a patient with an endocardial cushion defect showing the perimembranous ventricular septal defect (VSD) and primum atrial septal defect (ASD). RA = right atrium; LA = left atrium; RV = right ventricle; LV = left ventricle; MV = mitral valve; TV = tricuspid valve. (From Feigenbaum, H.: Echocardiography. 4th ed. Philadelphia, Lea and Febiger, 1986.)

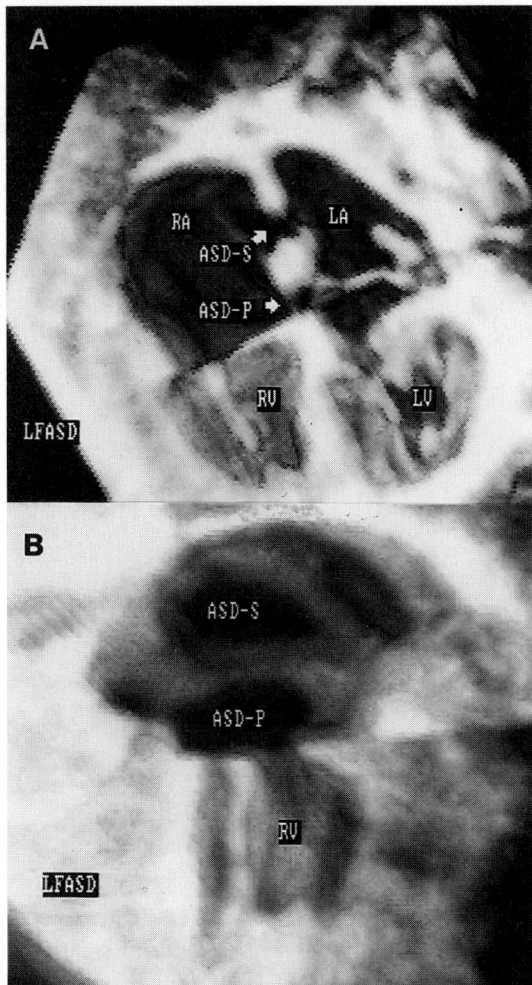

FIGURE 3–80. Three-dimensional reconstruction in an infant with a secundum (ASD-S) and primum (ASD-P) atrial septal defect. Figure A is comparable to a four-chamber view cutting through the atrial septal defects. The walls of the cardiac chambers are seen in the background. The 3-D view in B shows the surface of the atrial septa. Now one can better appreciate the size and shape of the two defects. RA = right atrium; LA = left atrium; RV = right ventricle; LV = left ventricle.

apparent.[291–293] If there were a right-to-left shunt, then contrast would be seen within the left atrium and left ventricle with such an injection.

In *total anomalous pulmonary venous return* all four pulmonary veins empty into a common pulmonary venous chamber behind the left atrium, which produces additional echoes posterior to the left atrium (Fig. 29–66, p. 944).[294,295]

Besides septal defects one can also record *septal aneurysms* frequently associated with septal defects. The aneurysm involving the membranous portion of the interventricular septum can be imaged on the right side of the septum.[296] Atrial septal aneurysms can also be detected by 2-D echocardiography and especially transesophageal echocardiography (Fig. 3–16).[297,298] These aneurysms are usually quite mobile and may be seen moving between the two atria throughout the cardiac cycle. These aneurysms frequently are fenestrated[299] and have been implicated in systemic emboli. Transesophageal echocardiography with contrast is proving to be a very sensitive way to identify a probe-patent foramen ovale.[300–302] (Fig. 3–16).

FIGURE 3–81. See color plate 4.

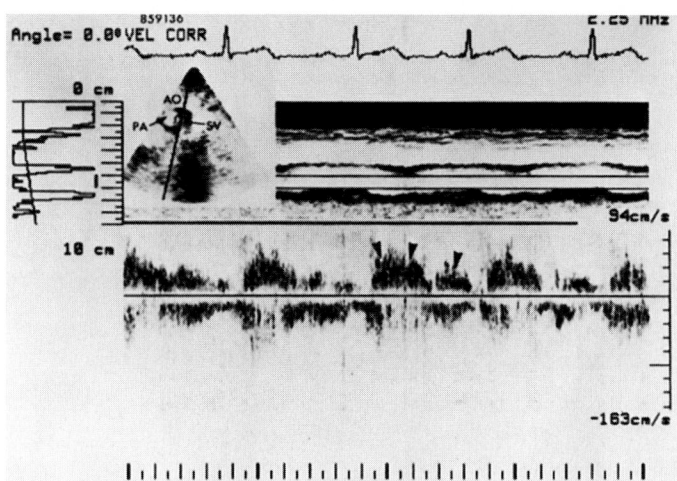

FIGURE 3–82. Pulsed Doppler examination with the sample volume (SV) placed in the wall of the pulmonary artery (PA) in the region of the presumed patent ductus. Note the presence of continuous flow in the region of the ductus *(arrowheads).* AO = aorta. (From Feigenbaum, H.: Echocardiography. 4th ed. Philadelphia, Lea and Febiger, 1986.)

FIGURE 3–83.   See color plate 4.

ASSOCIATED LESIONS. Intracardiac shunts are frequently associated with other anomalies of the heart that can be recognized echocardiographically. For example, in patients with defects of the atrioventricular canal, anomalies of the mitral and/or tricuspid valves can be appreciated on the echocardiogram.[303] The mitral valve appears to be closer than normal to the interventricular septum, a finding consistent with abnormal insertion of the mitral leaflet in this anomaly. The cleft in the mitral valve commonly present with ostium primum atrial septal may be detected using 2-D echocardiography.[304]

Another valvular anomaly that may be associated with an intracardiac shunt is a tricuspid valve that overrides the ventricular septum, which can pose major problems in the repair of a ventricular septal defect and which is therefore important to recognize preoperatively. The echocardiographic findings in this condition resemble those in atrioventricular canal defects in that the tricuspid valve is recorded to the left of the interventricular septum.[305]

PATENT DUCTUS ARTERIOSUS (see also p. 905). Although 2-D echocardiography can occasionally visualize the patent ductus between the aorta and pulmonary artery, Doppler is more sensitive and reliable in detecting the abnormal communication.[306] Although continuous flow within the ductus itself has been detected, since the ductus is frequently perpendicular to the sample volume the Doppler signal can be somewhat difficult to record. It is actually easier to make the diagnosis by obtaining Doppler recording from the aorta and pulmonary artery. By placing the sampling volume in the pulmonary artery, flow into this vessel can be noted in both systole and diastole as the shunted blood comes from the aorta (Fig. 3–82). Figure 3–83 shows a color Doppler study of a patient with a patent ductus arteriosus. The abnormal flow within the pulmonary artery can be readily detected.[307]

Abnormalities of the Great Arteries

Supravalvular aortic stenosis (see p. 919) can be detected using 2-D echocardiography.[264,308] The method of examination is similar to that used for the detection of valvular aortic stenosis, except that the scanning is carried out superior to the aortic valve. *Coarctation of the aorta*

(see p. 965) is detected with 2-D echocardiography by placing the probe in the suprasternal notch,[309] which allows imaging of both the narrowed segment of the aorta and the poststenotic dilation and detection of the excessive pulsation of the aorta proximal to the coarctation. Doppler echocardiography can be used to assess the hemodynamic obstruction across the coarctation.[310] Color flow Doppler is improving the ability to assess the severity of a coarctation.[311]

Tetralogy of Fallot (see p. 929) is detected echocardiographically by noting a membranous ventricular septal defect and a dilated aorta that overrides the interventricular septum (Fig. 3–84 and Fig. 29–48, p. 929). The short-axis view also demonstrates a narrowing of the right ventricular outflow tract, usually at the subpulmonic level.[272] *Double-outlet right ventricle* (see p. 941) is clinically similar to tetralogy of Fallot but can be differentiated echocardiographically from the more common anomaly when a mass of tissue can be noted betweeen the anterior mitral leaflet and the aorta.[312] This tissue indicates that the aorta is communicating directly with the right ventricle and cannot be repaired surgically as is possible in tetralogy of Fallot.

Two-dimensional echocardiography has greatly improved the ultrasonic detection of anomalies of the great arteries.[313] In the diagnosis of truncus arteriosus, 2-D echocardiography helps to establish the number of great arteries leaving the heart.[314] Normally, with a short-axis view of the great vessels, a circular aorta surrounded by a curved, tubular right ventricular outflow tract and pulmonary artery is recorded (Fig. 3–21, diagram 4); in truncus arteriosus only a single large circular vessel can be visualized. Actual recording of the branch of the truncus that supplies the lungs is more definitive in establishing the diagnosis of truncus arteriosus.

The 2-D technique for the detection of transposition of the great arteries (see p. 935) is based on determining the relationship between the two great arteries.[272,315] Normally the pulmonary artery twists around the aorta as the latter passes posteriorly. With transposition of the great arteries, on the other hand, the two arteries run parallel to each other, and with a 2-D view parallel to the arteries it is possible to appreciate how the transposed arteries do not twist around each other.[316] A perpendicular or short-axis view of the great vessels demonstrates two circular structures (Fig. 3–85) rather than the pulmonary artery normally wrapping around the circular aorta. Doppler examination

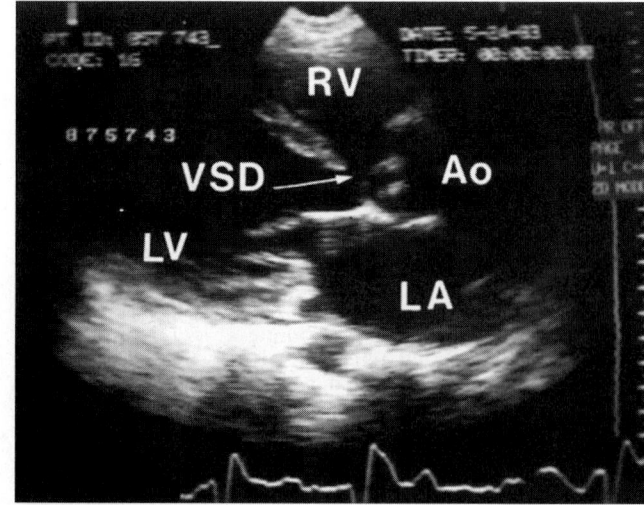

FIGURE 3–84. Parasternal long-axis examination in an adult with uncorrected tetralogy of Fallot. The ventricular septal defect (VSD) in the area of a membranous septum and overriding of the aorta (Ao) are apparent. LA = left atrium; LV = left ventricle; RV = right ventricle. (From Feigenbaum, H.: Echocardiography. 4th ed. Philadelphia, Lea and Febiger, 1986.)

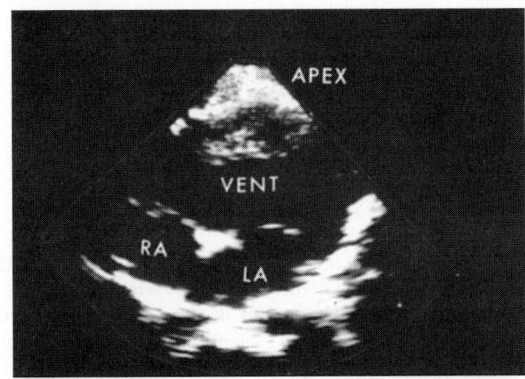

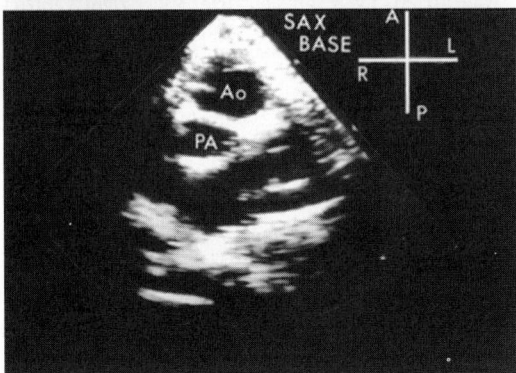

FIGURE 3–85. Apical four-chamber view *(top)* and short-axis (SAX) view *(bottom)* of the great vessels in a patient with a single ventricle and transposition of the great arteries. A single ventricular chamber (VENT) can be seen that received blood from both the right and left atria (RA, LA). In the short-axis view two great vessels oriented in a parallel direction can be seen. The aorta (Ao) is anterior and to the left of the pulmonary artery (PA). (From Feigenbaum, H.: Echocardiography. 4th ed. Philadelphia, Lea and Febiger, 1986.)

together with 2-D echocardiography helps in the recognition of corrected transposition.[317]

SURGICALLY CORRECTED CONGENITAL HEART DISEASE (see also p. 980). The adult cardiologist is increasingly being confronted with evaluating congenital anomalies that have been surgically repaired. In many ways these are far more difficult to evaluate than native congenital defects. It is frequently the role of echocardiography to try to evaluate the effectiveness and possible complications of the surgery.[318–320] The variety of procedures that are performed on these patients are too numerous to discuss in any detail at this time. Figure 3–86 gives one example of the type of challenge presented to the echocardiographer in examining surgically corrected congenital heart disease. In this illustration the patient had a Mustard procedure for *correction of transposition of the great arteries* (see p. 935). With this operation there are intra-atrial baffles diverting systemic venous flow into the left ventricle and pulmonary venous flow into the right ventricle. The echocardiogram in Figure

deliver blood into the appropriate ventricles. The evaluation of such iatrogenic anomalies requires a great deal of experience in identifying the surgically produced structures and recognizing malfunction when it occurs. As these patients live longer and well into adult life, this type of evaluation is becoming the responsibility of adult and pediatric cardiologists working together in adult congenital heart clinics.

ISCHEMIC HEART DISEASE

DETECTION OF MYOCARDIAL ISCHEMIA. Two-dimensional echocardiography can detect ischemic myocardium by evaluating the motion, thickening, and thickness of various segments of the heart.[321,322] Figure 3–87 shows diastolic and systolic frames in the long-axis and four-chamber views of a patient with ischemic heart disease. With systole the left ventricular cavity in both views becomes smaller. However, the smaller cavity is a function of hyperkinesis of the posterior wall in the long-axis view and the lateral wall in the four-chamber view. The anterior and medial septum and apex (arrows) fail to move from diastole to systole. This akinesis is a result of inadequate blood flow within the left anterior descending artery. One of the advantages of the 2-D examination in patients with coronary artery disease is that the various myocardial segments correlate fairly predictably to coronary artery perfusion. Figure 3–88 shows the relationship between four common 2-D echocardiographic views and the corresponding coronary artery perfusion. This diagram also shows the relationship between the short-axis view and the three longitudinal views (long-axis, two-chamber, and four-chamber). The recording of these four 2-D views can provide an excellent assessment of regional function in the setting of coronary artery disease.

Another advantage of 2-D echocardiography is that with chronic ischemia and scar formation there is frequently loss of myocardial tissue as well as increased intensity of the echoes from that segment. Figure 3–89 shows a patient with a scarred distal septum and apex. The chronically ischemic segments not only fail to move but also exhibit loss of diastolic wall thickness. Not all regional wall-motion abnormalities are due to coronary artery disease. Left bundle branch block,[323] right ventricular pacing, and open-heart surgery[325] can produce abnormal interventricular septal motion. It should also be emphasized that with acute ischemia the nonischemic myocardium is usually hyperkinetic.[326] This fact limits the usefulness of a global measurement such as ejection fraction.

Patients with coronary artery disease frequently have normal left ventricular function at rest. However, with stress there is inadequate blood flow, ischemia is produced,

FIGURE 3–86. A series of three modified, four-chamber views from a patient following an intraatrial baffle procedure for transposition of the great arteries. By tilting the transducer at different angles, various limbs of the baffle can be visualized. In *panel 1*, the systemic venous atrium (SVA) is seen in continuity with the mitral valve and left ventricle (LV). In *panel 2*, both the systemic pulmonary venous atria (PVA) are seen. In *panel 3*, by tilting the transducer to a more anterior plane, continuity between the pulmonary venous atrium and the tricuspid valve and right ventricle is demonstrated. (From Feigenbaum, H.: Echocardiography. 5th ed. Malvern, PA, Lea and Febiger, 1994.)

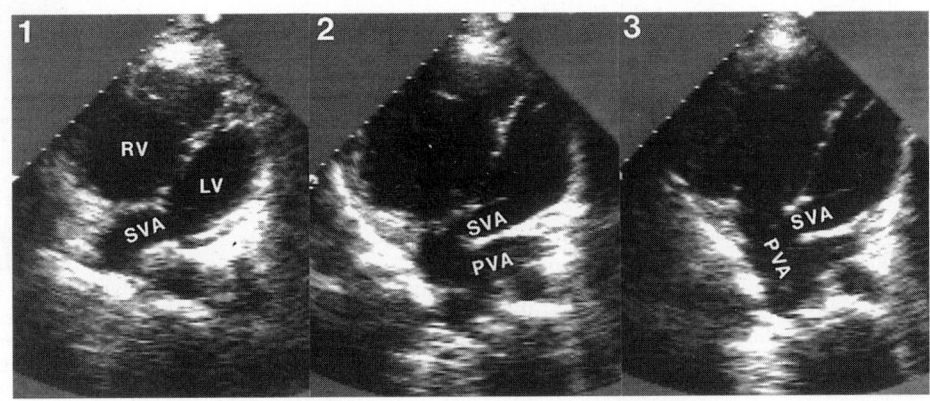

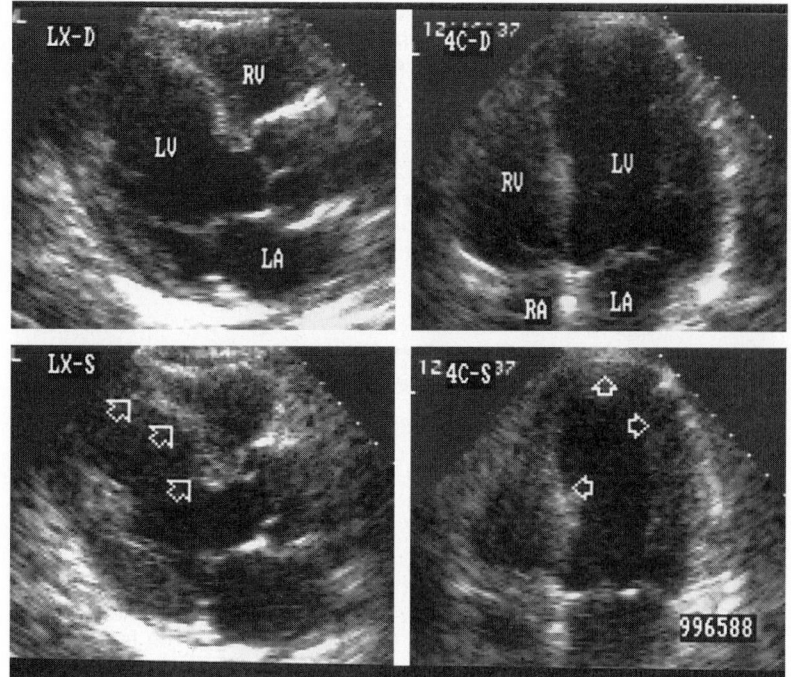

FIGURE 3–87. Long-axis (LX) and four-chamber 2-D echocardiogram of a patient with an anterior myocardial infarction secondary to occlusion of the left anterior descending artery. In systole there is akinesis (arrows) of the anterior system (LX-S) and distal septum, apex, and apical lateral wall (4C-S). LV = left ventricle; RV = right ventricle; LA = left atrium; RA = right atrium. (From Feigenbaum, H.: Echocardiography. 5th ed. Malvern, PA, Lea and Febiger, 1994.)

and the myocardium involved will stop moving. Figure 3–90 shows a patient before and immediately after exercise. At rest the long-axis and short-axis echocardiograms are normal at end-systole. Following exercise the septum stops moving (arrows) as noted in this end-systolic frame. A variety of stresses can be used with echocardiographic monitoring to identify stress-induced myocardial ischemia and regional dysfunction.[327–329] One can use immediate post-treadmill exercise,[330,331] supine[332] and upright[333] bicycle exercise, atrial pacing,[334] or a variety of pharmacological stresses.[335–338] The stress echocardiograms are frequently recorded digitally so that the resting and stress images are evaluated side by side on a computer screen.[339,340]

Not only is stress echocardiography being used for the detection and evaluation of coronary artery disease,[341,342] the examination is also valuable in establishing the prognosis following myocardial infarction,[343,344] for risk stratification of noncardiac surgery,[345,346] in establishing the prognosis in patients with high likelihood of coronary artery disease,[347–349] and in evaluating reperfusion procedures.[350,351]

ASSESSMENT OF LEFT VENTRICULAR PERFORMANCE. There are many echocardiographic techniques available for assessing left ventricular performance in patients with ischemic heart disease. Although the M-mode left ventricular dimensions are of limited value in patients with regional

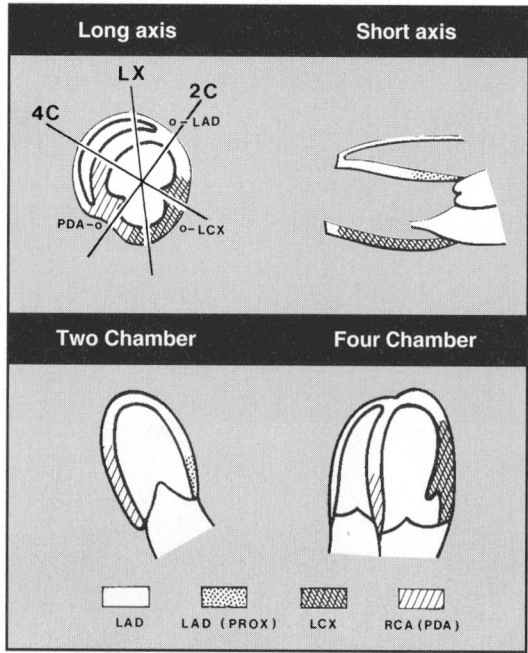

FIGURE 3–88. Relationship of 2-D echocardiographic views and coronary artery perfusion. 4C = four-chamber; LX = long-axis; 2C = two-chamber; LAD = left anterior descending; LCX = left circumflex artery; RCA = right coronary artery; PDA = posterior descending artery. (From Feigenbaum, H.: Echocardiography. 5th ed. Malvern, PA, Lea and Febiger, 1994).

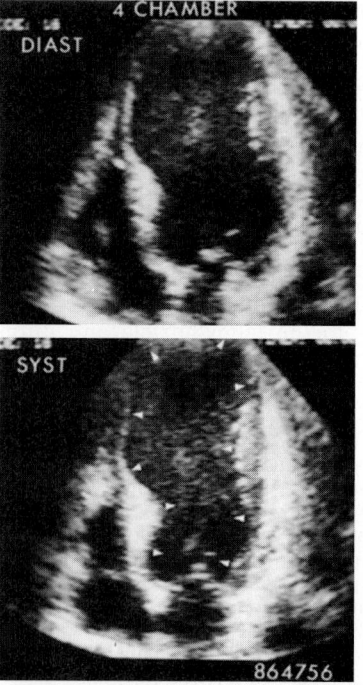

FIGURE 3–89. Apical four-chamber view in a patient with a scarred, dilated, aneurysmal apex and distal interventricular septum. The proximal half of the septum has normal thickness and contracts normally with systole. (From Feigenbaum, H.: Echocardiography. 4th ed. Philadelphia, Lea and Febiger, 1986.)

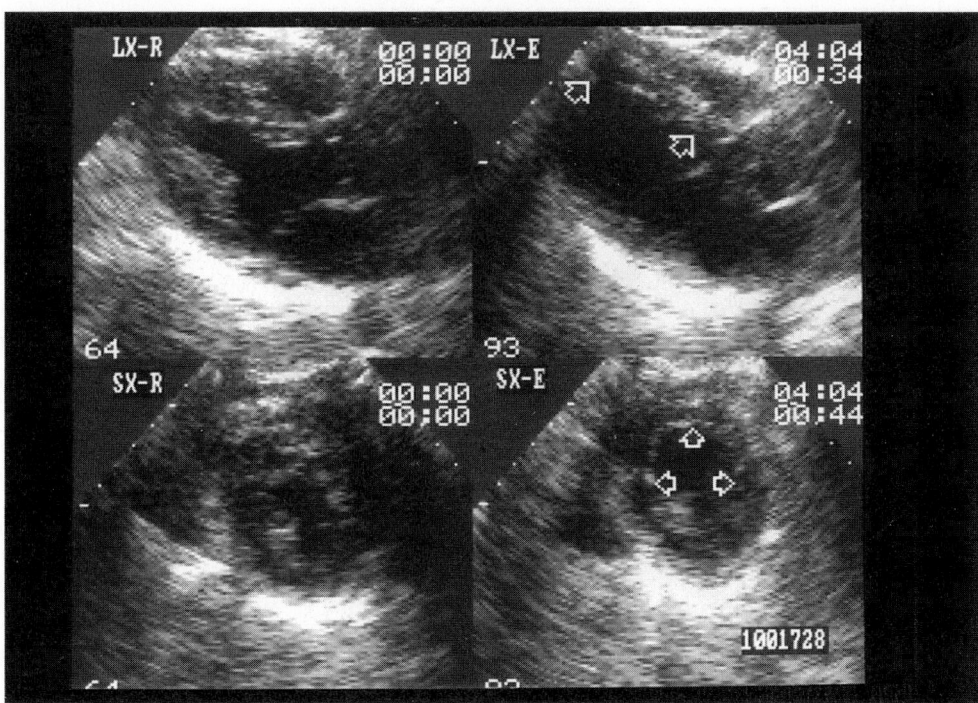

FIGURE 3–90. Exercise echocardiogram of a patient with an obstruction in the proximal left anterior descending coronary artery. The long-axis (LX-R) and short-axis (SX-R) resting images are normal. With exercise, however, the long-axis (LX-E) and short-axis (SX-E) examinations reveal that the septum and anterior wall (arrows) become akinetic. The heart rate is indicated in the left lower corner of each image; the numbers in the right upper corner indicate the exercise duration *(top)* and the postexercise duration *(bottom)*. In this example, the long-axis examination was obtained at 34 seconds after exercise; the short-axis study was recorded 45 seconds after exercise. (From Feigenbaum, H.: Echocardiography. 5th ed. Malvern, PA, Lea and Febiger, 1994).

heart disease, measurements such as mitral valve E point–septal separation and abnormal closure of the mitral valve can give reasonable assessment of altered left ventricular function in patients with ischemic heart disease. The E point–septal separation increases when left ventricular ejection fraction decreases and abnormal closure of the mitral valve occurs in patients with elevated atrial components of left ventricular diastolic pressure. Doppler echocardiography can also be used to evaluate global left ventricular function. Acceleration and peak velocity are reduced as global left ventricular function deteriorates. Instantaneous mitral valve flow can reflect altered left ventricular filling.[352] With ischemia the early diastolic flow or E point is reduced and the velocity of flow with atrial systole (A point) is increased. As a result the E/A ratio changes from a normal positive value to a negative one[353] (Fig. 3–38B).

The best echocardiographic technique for evaluating regional left ventricular performance utilizes 2-D echocardiography and the assessment of regional wall motion.[354,355] The left ventricle is divided into a number of segments. Determining the motion of each segment provides a wall motion score for the entire chamber.[57,356] A number of schemes have been suggested in the literature. Any or all of these techniques provide reasonable assessment of both regional and global left ventricular function. Standard ejection fractions can also be calculated from the apical two-chamber or four-chamber views in patients with ischemic heart disease.[357,358] Because of the frequently distorted shape of the ventricle in these patients, Simpson's rule technique is preferred.[57] Minor axis measurements using parasternal long-axis or short-axis views can also be very helpful in patients with coronary artery disease by providing regional systolic function. Frequently the status of the base of the left ventricle is a better predictor of prognosis than is global ejection fraction, especially in patients with apical aneurysms.[359,360]

Myocardial Infarction
(See also Chap. 37)

COMPLICATIONS. All of the common complications of acute myocardial infarction (AMI) may be detected with echocardiographic techniques.[361] A common problem is the development of a left ventricular aneurysm.[360,362] Figure

3–89 shows the echocardiographic findings characteristic of aneurysm. There is a loss of myocardial thickness, scar formation, localized dilatation, and frequently dyskinesis. A pseudoaneurysm (see p. 1242) is a serious complication of MI, which represents rupture of the free wall. The blood leaving the cavity of the left ventricle is trapped in the pericardium, clot forms within the pericardial sac, and an aneurysmal wall consisting of clot and pericardium prevents exsanguination. The echocardiographic appearance of this complication is fairly characteristic, with the neck of the aneurysm being smaller than the body (Fig. 3–91).[363] Doppler flow patterns, especially color flow Doppler, within the aneurysm can help differentiate between a true and a false aneurysm.[364,365] Transesophageal echocardiography can assist with the diagnosis at times.[366] Indications for surgery are more urgent with a pseudoaneurysm; therefore the diagnosis is crucial. On rare occasion the initial rupture of the free wall can be detected echocardiographically.[367]

Aneurysmal dilatation and subsequent perforation of the ventricular septum (see p. 1243) are another complication of MI.[368] The septal aneurysm may be seen on the 2-D echocardiogram.[369] On rare occasions the actual perforation can be visualized.[370] The echocardiographic diagnosis, however, is best made with Doppler.[371] When the sample volume is put on the right ventricular side of the interventricular septum, the high-velocity systolic flow from the left

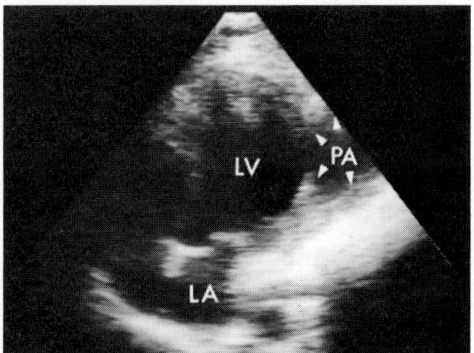

FIGURE 3–91. Four-chamber 2-D echocardiogram of a patient with a pseudoaneurysm (PA) adjacent to the posterior lateral free wall of the left ventricle (LV). LA = left atrium. (From Feigenbaum, H.: Echocardiography. 4th ed. Philadelphia, Lea and Febiger, 1986.)

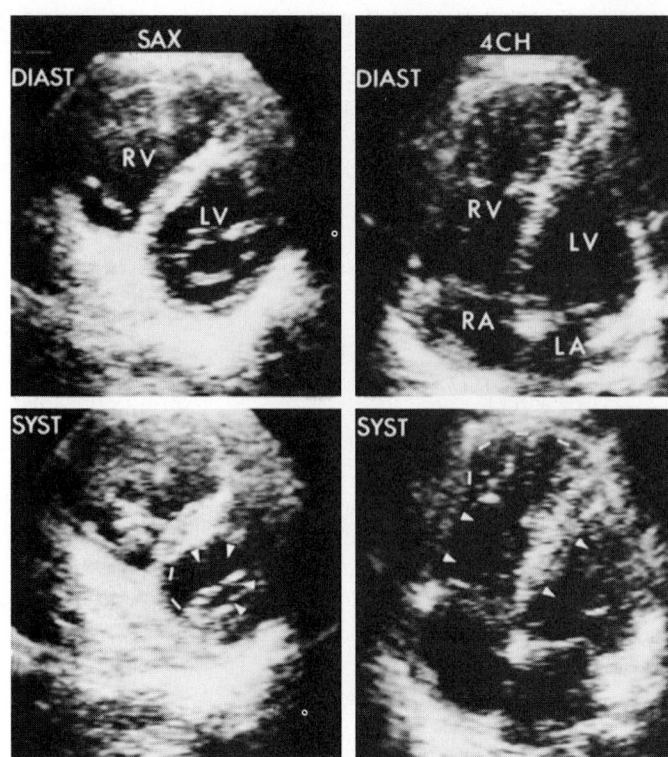

FIGURE 3-92. Short-axis (SAX) and four-chamber (4CH) 2-D echo-cardiograms of a patient with an inferior myocardial infarction complicated by right ventricular infarction. The posterior-inferior wall is akinetic (dashed line, SAX, SYST). In addition, the apical half of the right ventricular free wall is akinetic (dashed line, 4CH, SYST). The right ventricle (RV) is also dilated. RA = right atrium; LV = left ventricle; LA = left atrium. (From Feigenbaum, H.: Echocardiography. 4th ed. Philadelphia, Lea and Febiger, 1986.)

ventricle to the right ventricle through the ruptured septum can be recorded. Color flow Doppler recording of such a defect is the procedure of choice.[372,373] Transesophageal echocardiography may be useful in some patients.[374]

Right ventricular infarction (see p. 1192) is an increasingly recognized complication of MI and can have important clinical implications for management. Figure 3-92

shows the common echocardiographic findings with right ventricular infarction.[375,376] These patients usually have evidence of an inferior infarction. The inferior-posterior wall of the left ventricle is akinetic in systole (dashes) as noted in the short-axis view. The evidence for right ventricular infarction is right ventricular dilatation and right ventricular free wall motion akinesis (dashes) (Fig. 3-92). Premature pulmonary valve opening may occur with right ventricular infarction.[377] There may also be distortion of the interatrial septum so that it bulges toward the left atrium.[378]

Mural thrombus (see p. 1256) represents another common complication of AMI that can be detected with echocardiography.[379,380] These clots occur most often with aneurysms, especially those involving the anterior wall and apex. Figure 3-93 shows a variety of left ventricular clots. The thrombi may have various configurations. Those that protrude into the cavity and may be mobile, as in Figure 3-93*B* and *D*, are easier to detect echocardiographically and may have a greater likelihood of producing systemic emboli.[381-383] Other thrombi are layered along the wall and may not be as likely to break loose (Fig. 3-93*A*). Certain left ventricular echocardiographic flow patterns or spontaneous contrast may be precursors of thrombi.[384]

Other complications of AMI, such as mitral regurgitation[385-387] and pericardial effusion,[388] are easily detected echocardiographically.

NATURAL HISTORY AND PROGNOSIS. Echocardiography is ideal for serial studies in patients with MI.[389] Two-dimensional echocardiography carried out early in the course of an infarction is helpful in establishing the diagnosis.[390,391] and provides prognostic information as well.[392,393] This examination is useful in the assessment of the status of the myocardium not involved in the current infarction[394] because an unsuspected previous MI may be discovered. An early echocardiographic study also can serve as a baseline for detecting future ischemic events such as MI expansion[395,396] or other complications. The initial examination may even help identify the patients who are at high risk of experiencing complications.[397,398] A resting[399] or stress[400] 2-D echocardiogram before discharge can also provide long-term prognostic information.

Possibly one of the most important uses of echocardiography in patients with acute MI is to evaluate the efficacy of reperfusion therapy.[401,402] Figure 3-94 shows serial stud-

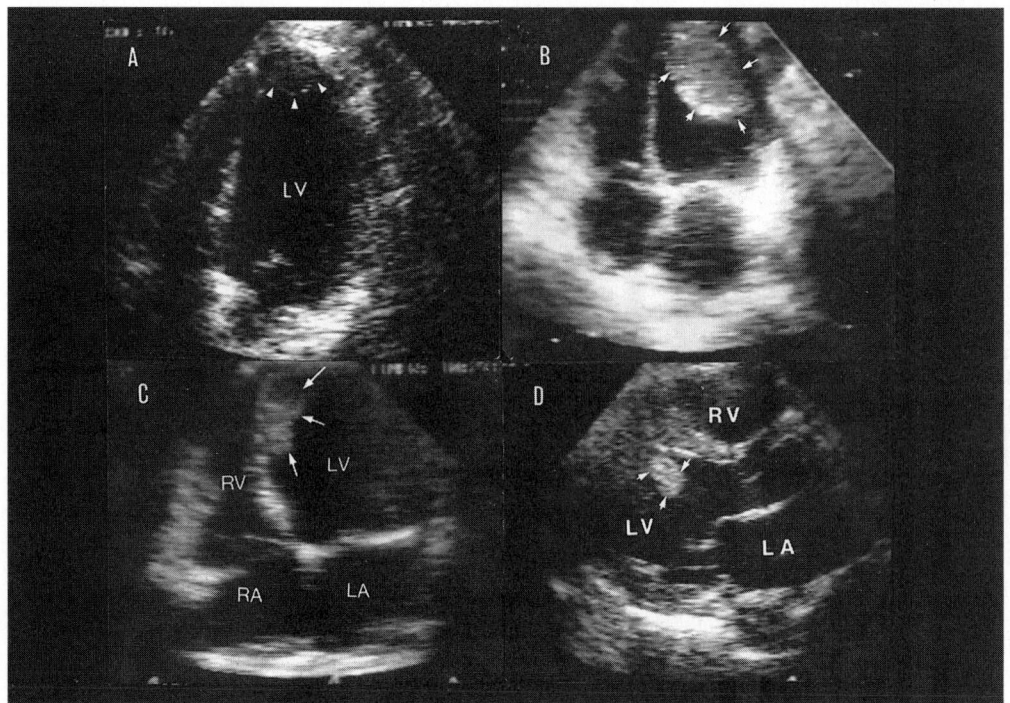

FIGURE 3-93. Echocardiograms demonstrating a variety of different left ventricular thrombi (arrows) that can be identified echocardiographically. The thrombi in *A* and *C* are relatively flat and adherent to the walls. The thrombus in *B* is large and protrudes into the cavity of the left ventricle. *D* demonstrates a relatively small (more mobile) thrombus attached to the interventricular septum. LV = left ventricle; RV = right ventricle; RA = right atrium; LA = left atrium. (From Feigenbaum, H.: Echocardiography. 5th ed. Malvern, PA, Lea and Febiger, 1994).

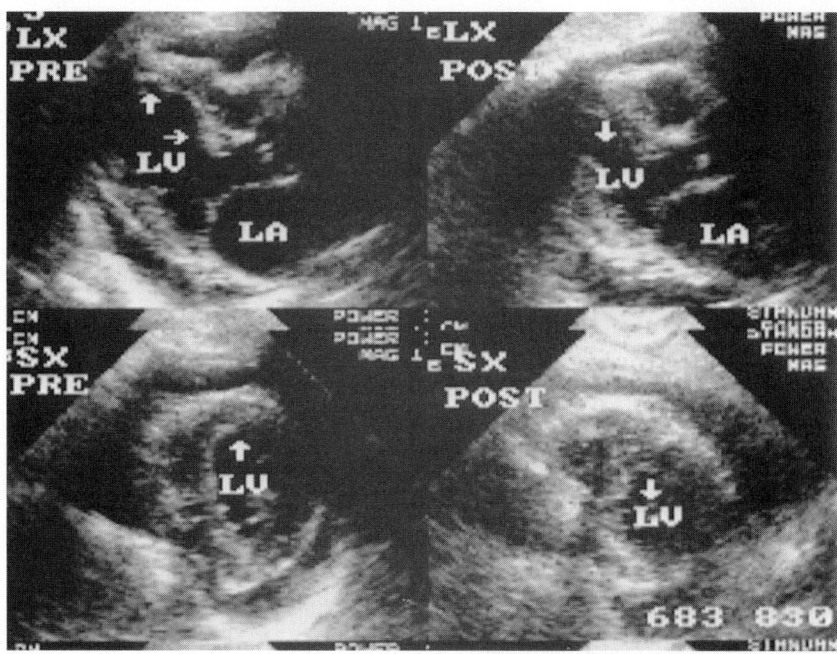

FIGURE 3–94. Long-axis (LX) and short-axis (SX) echocardiograms of a patient with an acute anterior myocardial infarction before (PRE) and after (POST) PTCA of the left anterior descending coronary artery. Before PTCA the anterior septum is dyskinetic (upward arrows). After successful PTCA the motion of the septum is normal (downward arrows).

ies of a patient who underwent angioplasty for an occluded left anterior descending coronary artery. During the acute infarction and before angioplasty the anterior septum was dyskinetic (reverse arrows). After successful reopening of the artery and recovery of the stunned myocardium, the septal motion returned to normal (arrows LX post, SX post).

STUNNED OR HIBERNATING MYOCARDIUM (see also p. 1176). Stunned or hibernating myocardium denotes viable but dysfunctional myocardial segments. It has been demonstrated that stressing the heart with dobutamine or dipyridamole can identify those segments that are viable and potentially functional by inducing them to contract, usually with low-dose pharmacologic agents.[403–405] With stunned myocardium the functional recovery will occur with time since the artery is already reopened. Reperfusion procedures are necessary to restore ventricular function with hibernating muscle.[406,407]

EXAMINATION OF THE CORONARY ARTERIES. Echocardiography is playing an increasing role in direct visualization of the coronary arteries. Ultrasonic transducers can be placed at the tip of an intracoronary catheter. These transducers are small enough to be inserted within the proximal coronary arteries (Fig. 3–15). The transducer then provides a cross-sectional picture of the artery.[408] This examination gives an excellent view of the arterial wall. The normal wall is very thin while atherosclerotic plaque has a thick crescent-shaped appearance (Fig. 3–15, arrows). Figure 3–95 illustrates the variety of coronary atherosclerotic lesions that can be detected with intravascular ultrasound. The ultrasonic technique has already changed our understanding of coronary artery disease.[409–413] The diffuse nature of this pathologic process is better appreciated with intracoronary ultrasound than is commonly noted with angiography.[414] This examination is being utilized with invasive angioplasty techniques.[415–417] Figure 3–96A illustrates two intracoronary echograms and accompanying diagrams of a patient with coronary atherosclerosis who underwent atherectomy for removal of the atherosclerotic plaque (A). Following atherectomy much of the atherosclerotic material has been removed (arrowheads). In Figure 3–96B an intravascular echogram and diagram show the deployment of a

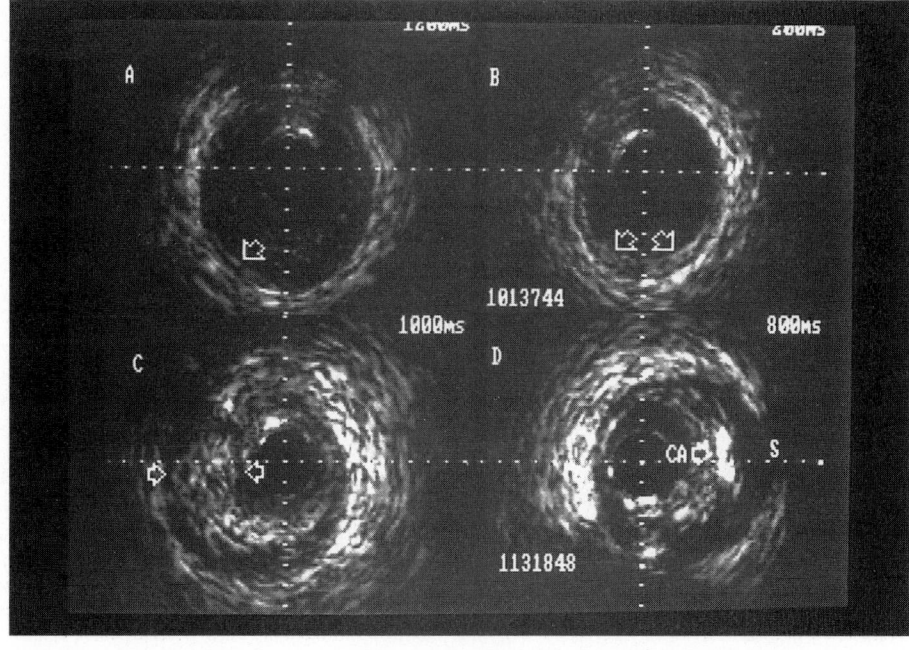

FIGURE 3–95. Intracoronary ultrasonic images demonstrating the different severity of coronary atherosclerosis: *A,* Small rim of thickened endothelium (arrow). *B,* Larger amount of eccentric endothelial thickening (arrows). *C,* Massive atherosclerotic plaque that is wider (arrows) than the residual lumen. *D,* Calcification in the plaque (CA) produces shadowing (S). (From Feigenbaum, H.: Echocardiography. 5th ed. Malvern, PA, Lea and Febiger, 1994).

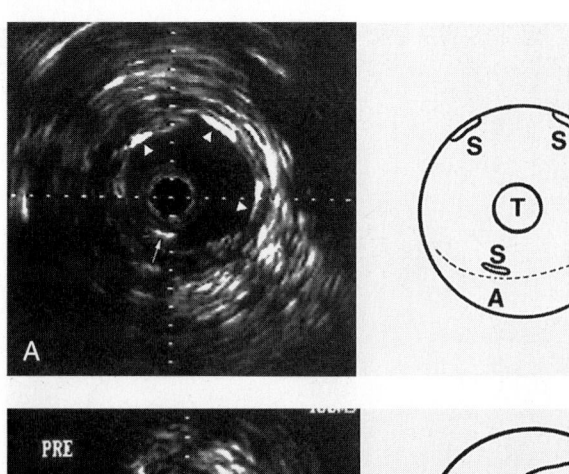

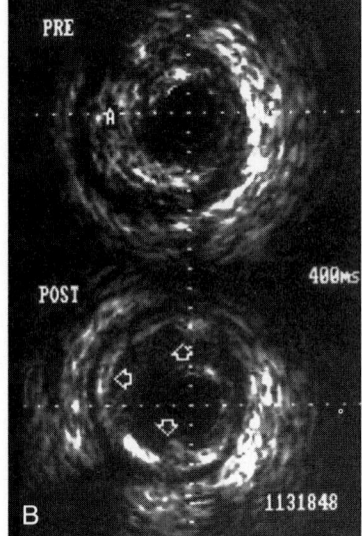

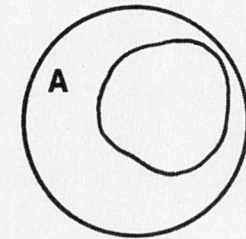

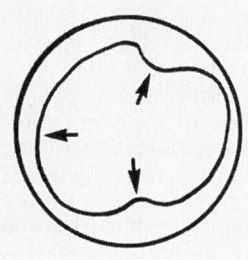

FIGURE 3–96. Intracoronary ultrasonic images and diagrams before (PRE) and after (POST) atherectomy and removal (arrows) of much of the preatherectomy atherosclerosis *(A).* (From Feigenbaum, H.: Echocardiography. 5th ed. Malvern, PA, Lea and Febiger, 1994.) *B,* Intracoronary echogram and diagram of a patient following elective placement of a Palmaz-Schatz stent. **Although the proper angiographic deployment was observed, a single strut (arrow) did not demonstrate full apposition to the wall, whereas the other struts (arrowheads) are fully deployed.** (Courtesy of R. L. Wilensky, M.D.)

Palmaz-Schatz stent (see p. 1380) in the vicinity of an atherosclerotic plaque. Three of the struts of the stent are in direct proximity to the arterial wall. However, one strut (arrow) abuts the atherosclerotic plaque but is not fully deployed against the arterial wall and may be prone to thrombose.

It is also possible to put a tiny Doppler transducer at the tip of an intracoronary catheter. In so doing one can record the blood velocities within the coronary arteries.[418,419] Using such a technique with a potent vasodilator provides an opportunity to record coronary flow reserve.[420,421] Normally there is a dramatic increase in the blood velocity with a vasodilator. In patients with reduced reserve this augmentation of flow is blunted.

Transesophageal and transthoracic echocardiography can also be used to examine the coronary arteries directly.[422,423] With the transesophageal approach one can record spatial Doppler velocities[424,425] and color flow imaging.[426] Both transthoracic and transesophageal imaging techniques can visualize the arterial walls. Figure 3–97 shows a transthoracic examination of a normal proximal left coronary artery. Atherosclerotic plaques within the proximal left coronary system can be identified as bright, segmental echoes that give an irregular appearance to the artery lumen.[427,428] Kawasaki's disease occurs in children and produces aneurysms of the coronary arteries.[429,430] These aneurysmal dila-

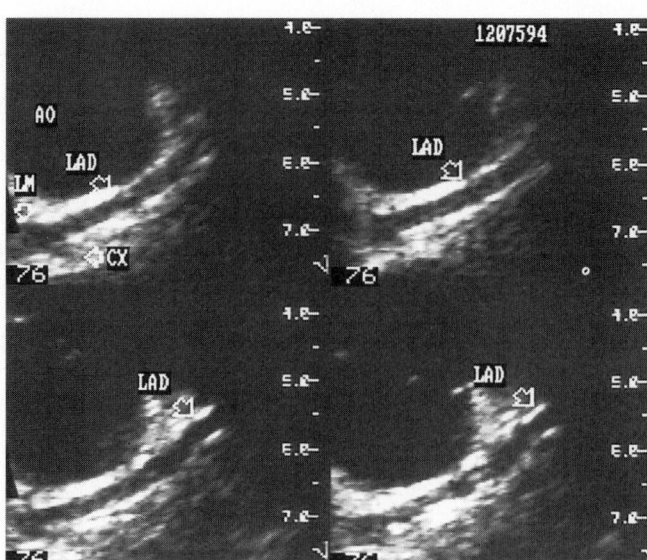

FIGURE 3–97. Left coronary artery examined with transthoracic echocardiography using a modified short-axis plane. LM = left main; AO = aorta; LAD = left anterior descending; CX = circumflex.

tations are identifiable with transthoracic echocardiography (Fig. 31–7, p. 996).[431] Congenital anomalies of the coronary arteries (pp. 909 and 966) can also be detected with both transthoracic and transesophageal 2-D, Doppler, and color Doppler echocardiography.[432–434] Coronary artery fistulas are also detected echocardiographically.[435]

MYOCARDIAL PERFUSION USING CONTRAST ECHOCARDIOG-RAPHY. Contrast echocardiography may also be employed to study myocardial perfusion.[436–438] If a fluid containing microbubbles is injected into the root of the aorta or directly into the coronary artery, the echogenicity of the myocardium will be increased (Fig. 3–98), provided that the blood supply is intact. When blood flow is impeded, the increase in echogenicity in that segment is reduced or absent. This examination has been done in a limited fashion in the catheterization laboratory or in the operating room. With the introduction of contrast agents that are visualized on the left side of the heart with intravenous injections, there is optimism for a less invasive recording of myocardial perfusion using this technique.[439,440]

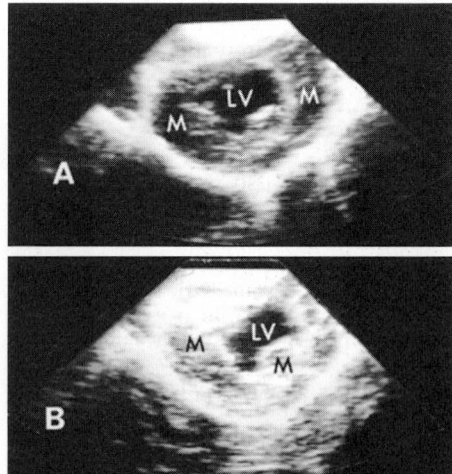

FIGURE 3–98. Short-axis 2-D echocardiogram of a dog before and after injection of contrast in the root of the aorta. **Before contrast injection *(A)* the myocardium (M) is relatively echo free. Following the injection of fluid containing tiny microbubbles *(B)* the myocardium becomes uniformly echogenic.**

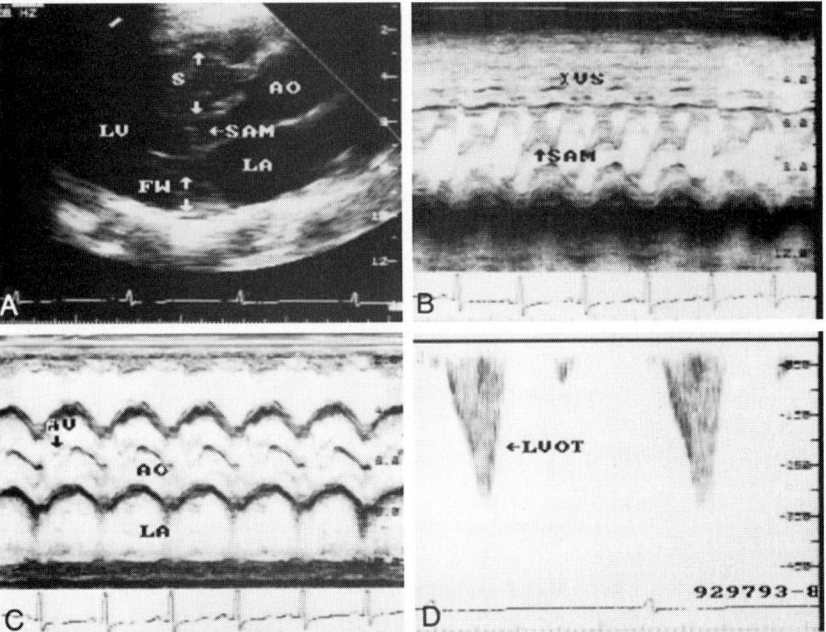

FIGURE 3–99. Two-dimensional, M-mode, and Doppler studies in a patient with hypertrophic obstructive cardiomyopathy. The 2-D long-axis study shows the thickened interventricular septum (S) and the systolic anterior motion of the mitral valve (SAM). The abnormal mitral motion and the thickened septum are also seen on the M-mode recording (B). The M-mode recording of the aortic valve shows midsystolic closure (AV). The Doppler recording of the left ventricular outflow tract shows how the velocity within the outflow tract increases in the latter half of systole. LV = left ventricle; AO = aorta; FW = left ventricular free wall; LA = left atrium; IVS = interventricular septum; LVOT = left ventricular outflow tract.

CARDIOMYOPATHIES

(See also Chap. 41)

HYPERTROPHIC CARDIOMYOPATHY (HCM) (see also p. 1414). Echocardiography is an important diagnostic tool in patients with HCM and has enriched our understanding of this abnormality. An early echocardiographic abnormality to be noted was systolic anterior motion of the mitral valve (termed *SAM*) (Fig. 3–99B),[441] which appeared to be related to and was correlated with the presence of obstruction to left ventricular outflow.[442,443] The shorter the distance between the septum and the leaflet and the longer the duration of apposition between these two structures, the more severe the obstruction.[444] This echocardiographic finding also demonstrated the critical importance of involvement of the mitral valve apparatus in the obstruction in this condition.[445] More recently SAM has been noted in a variety of other patients, some of whom had no evidence of left ventricular hypertrophy.[446,447] It has been observed in patients with anemia and hypovolemia as well as in patients with a hyperdynamic left ventricle.[446] It is possible that SAM is a nonspecific sign that occurs whenever the left ventricular systolic volume is reduced, either because of hypertrophy, as in HCM, or in the presence of a hyperdynamic state.[448]

A second echocardiographic finding in patients with obstructive HCM is midsystolic closure of the aortic valve (Fig. 3–99C). However, as noted earlier, this sign is not specific for HCM and is also present in patients with discrete subaortic stenosis. While this finding is not sensitive, when present it usually indicates a significant amount of obstruction.

Hypertrophy of the septum with abnormal organization of myocardial cells may be one of the basic abnormalities of HCM[449] (p. 1416), and a key echocardiographic finding is disproportionate hypertrophy of the septum in relation to the posterior wall of the left ventricle, so that the ratio of thickness of the septum to the free wall exceeds 1.3 : 1.0 (Fig. 3–98)[450] and the motion of the hypertrophied septum is reduced.[451] It has also been shown that asymmetrical septal hypertrophy (ASH) is frequently transmitted as an autosomal dominant trait and that there are patients with asymmetrical septal hypertrophy who do not show SAM and therefore do not have obstruction to left ventricular outflow.[452] These patients may be considered to have HCM without obstruction. While the concept of recognizing ASH

with or without obstruction to left ventricular outflow by echocardiography is an important one, there are limitations to echocardiographic diagnosis. First, the thickness of the septum may be difficult to measure precisely echocardiographically. (In Figure 3–99 the left side of the septum is clearly identified, but the right side is not as distinct.) Second, it must be appreciated that ASH is not pathognomonic for HCM and related myopathies and can occur in a variety of other disease states, including right ventricular hypertrophy. In addition, some patients with HCM may have concentric rather than asymmetrical hypertrophy, in which the septal and posterior left ventricular walls are equal in thickness (see p. 1415).

Two-dimensional echocardiography provides additional information by indicating the shape and location of the hypertrophied myocardium in patients with known or suspected HCM.[453,454] A variety of hypertrophied segments has been recorded by this technique. Figure 3–100 shows a hypertrophied septum limited to the basal two-thirds of the septum, while the apex is virtually free of muscular hyper-

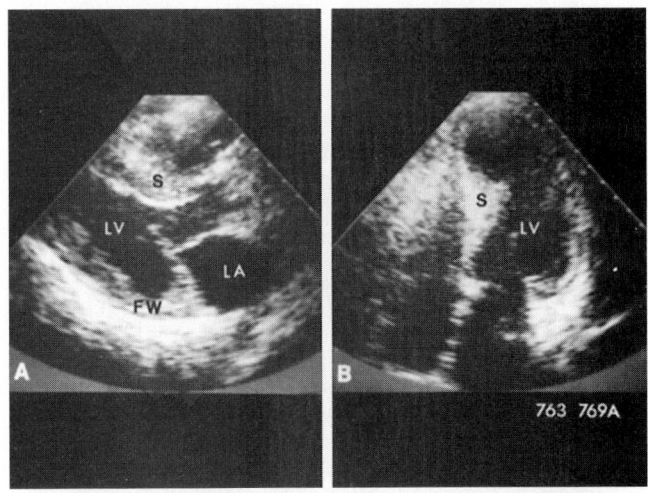

FIGURE 3–100. Long-axis (A) and apical four-chamber (B) echocardiograms of a patient with hypertrophic cardiomyopathy whose hypertrophy primarily involves the proximal two-thirds of the interventricular septum (S). The apex is spared from the hypertrophic process. LV = left ventricle; FW = left ventricular free wall; LA = left atrium. (From Feigenbaum, H.: Echocardiography. 4th ed. Philadelphia, Lea and Febiger, 1986.)

trophy. Other patients exhibit an apical form of hypertrophy with the proximal septum being relatively thin.[455,456] Concentric hypertrophy is also a fairly common form of hypertrophic myopathy (Fig. 3–101). Cavity obliteration with ventricular systole is almost always present with this type of disease. Two-dimensional echocardiography is useful in assessing the effectiveness of myotomy and myectomy. An intriguing observation is that the echoes from the diseased septum in HCM are more reflective or "speckled" than those from the free posterior wall.[457]

Doppler echocardiography may also be helpful in evaluating hypertrophic cardiomyopathy.[458,459] The Doppler recording of the left ventricular outflow may show an abnormal pattern with the abnormally high velocity occurring in late systole (Fig. 3–99D).[460] The systolic gradient can be estimated using the Doppler technique.[461] The left ventricular hypertrophy and reduced left ventricular compliance alter the Doppler recording of mitral valve flow. The early diastolic velocity or E point is reduced, and the late velocity with atrial systole is increased.[462] Color Doppler provides spatial visualization of the altered blood flow in patients with obstructive HCM.[463,464]

CONGESTIVE (DILATED) CARDIOMYOPATHY (see also p. 1407). The echocardiogram characteristically reveals a dilated poorly contracting left ventricle in patients with congestive cardiomyopathy.[465,466] Signs of reduced cardiac output include a poorly moving aorta, reduced opening of the mitral valve, and slow closure of the aortic valve. The left atrium is dilated, and the abnormal closure of the mitral valve indicative of elevated left diastolic pressure is frequently noted. Incomplete closure of the mitral valve or papillary muscle dysfunction and subsequent mitral regurgitation are common. Left ventricular filling on Doppler echograms changes as the disease progresses.[467,468] It must be appreciated that these findings are nonspecific and may also occur in patients with ischemic heart disease. However, at least one portion of the left ventricle continues to exhibit normal motion in most, although not all, patients with severe coronary artery disease.[465] In patients with cardiomyopathy the impairment of left ventricular wall motion is diffuse. If mitral regurgitation develops in patients with cardiomyopathy, septal motion may increase slightly in keeping with the left ventricular volume overload, although this increase in septal motion is certainly not as striking as that which occurs in primary mitral valve disease with secondary myocardial failure.

RESTRICTIVE (INFILTRATIVE) CARDIOMYOPATHY (see also p. 1426). The principal echocardiographic findings in patients with infiltrative cardiomyopathy are reduced wall motion and thickening of the left ventricular wall without dilatation.[469,470] These changes are usually uniform throughout the ventricle. There is also a characteristic left ventricular filling pattern with a tall E wave and short A wave on the mitral Doppler recording (Fig. 3–38C).[471] Obviously these findings are not specific for infiltrative cardiomyopathy, and like those obtained by means of electrocardiography, chest roentgenography, hemodynamics, and angiography, they must be interpreted in terms of the total clinical setting. In patients with amyloid heart disease (Fig. 3–102)[472] the echocardiographic findings are usually again nonspecific and show left ventricular hypertrophy. There are also frequently more specific findings in that the valves may be uniformly thickened in addition to the hypertrophy of the ventricular walls. The interatrial septum may also be unusually thick, and a peculiar speckled appearance of the myocardium may be noted, reflecting localized variations in echo density.[473] In the beginning course of amyloid heart disease early left ventricular filling is reduced. The Doppler mitral E wave is decreased and the A wave is

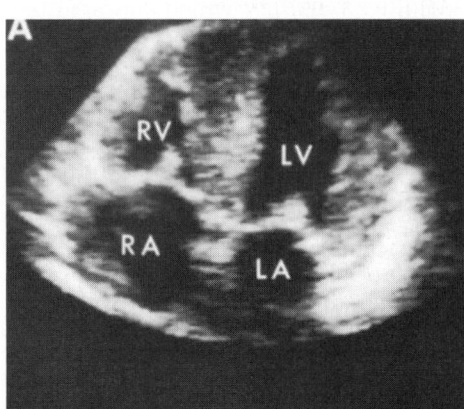

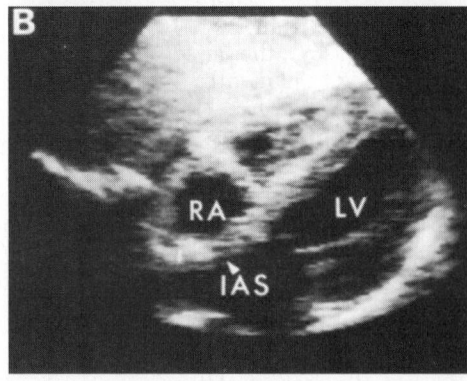

FIGURE 3–102. Four-chamber *(A)* and subcostal *(B)* 2-D echocardiograms of a patient with hereditary amyloidosis. The four-chamber view demonstrates markedly hypertrophied cardiac walls, especially the interventricular septum and free wall of the right ventricle. The tricuspid and mitral valve leaflets are also thickened. The left ventricle (LV) and right ventricle (RV) cavities are small. The subcostal examination demonstrates a thickened interatrial septum (IAS). RA = right atrium; LA = left atrium. (From Feigenbaum, H.: Echocardiography. 4th ed. Philadelphia, Lea and Febiger, 1986.)

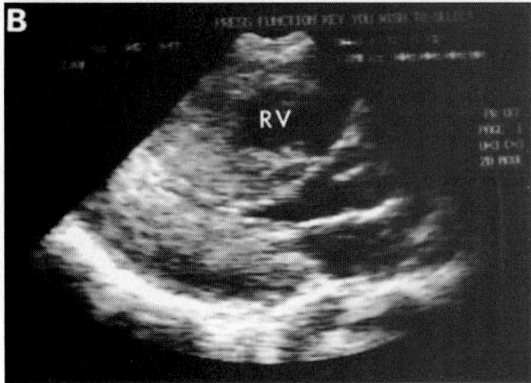

FIGURE 3–101. Long-axis 2-D echocardiogram of a patient with hypertrophic cardiomyopathy who exhibits uniform hypertrophy of the entire left ventricle (LV). RV = right ventricle; *A* = diastole; *B* = systole. (From Feigenbaum, H.: Echocardiography. 4th ed. Philadelphia, Lea and Febiger, 1986.)

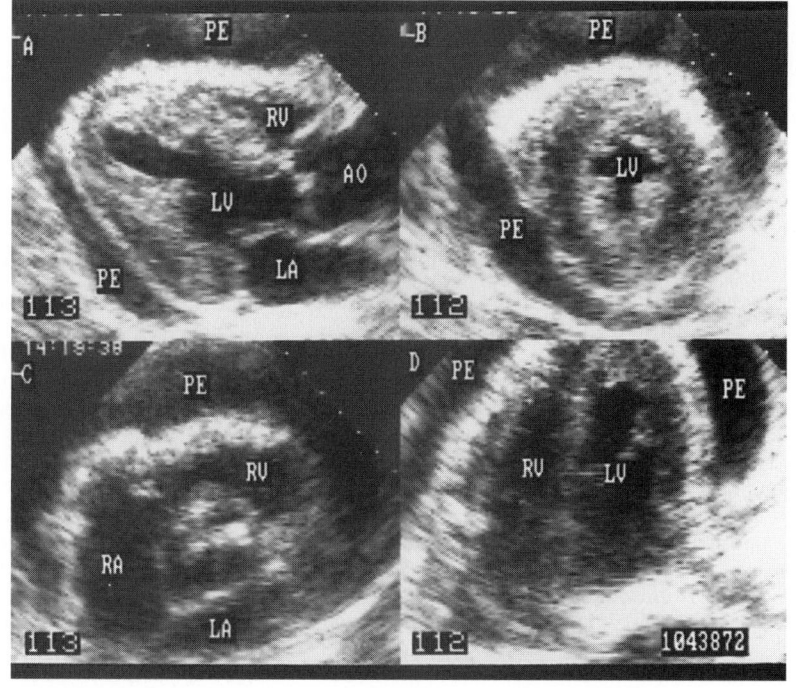

FIGURE 3–103. Long-axis (A), short-axis at the papillary muscle (B), short-axis at the base of the heart (C), and apical four-chamber (D) 2-D echocardiograms of a patient with a large pericardial effusion (PE). the relatively echo-free fluid can be seen surrounding the heart in all views. The visceral pericardium is echogenic and probably thickened. RV = right ventricle; LV = left ventricle; AO = aorta; LA = left atrium; RA = right atrium. (From Feigenbaum, H.: Echocardiography. 5th ed. Malvern, PA, Lea and Febiger, 1994.)

increased (Fig. 3–38B). Later, filling becomes more restrictive and the E and A waves are reversed (Fig. 3–38C), and in between there may be a pattern of "pseudonormalization."[474]

tion one finds an exaggerated increase in tricuspid flow and a decrease in mitral flow. The reverse occurs with expiration.

With very large effusions one can detect excessive motion of the heart within the pericardial sac. This excessive

PERICARDIAL DISEASE

(See also Chap. 43)

PERICARDIAL EFFUSION (see also p. 1485). The theory underlying the use of ultrasound in the recognition of pericardial effusion is relatively simple; since the acoustic properties of fluid differ significantly from those of cardiac muscle, the effusion surrounding the heart is less echogenic than is the myocardium. Accordingly, the detection of effusion was one of the first and has remained one of the most useful applications of echocardiography.[475]

Figure 3–103 shows a 2-D echocardiographic examination of a patient with a large pericardial effusion (PE). One can see the echo-free space both anteriorly and posteriorly in the long-axis (A) and short-axis (B) views. The four-chamber view (D) shows the fluid on both the medial and lateral aspects of the heart. There is very little if any fluid posterior to the left atrium (A and C). The size of the effusion is estimated by the amount of echo-free space surrounding the heart. Frequently with small effusions one sees only a posterior echo-free space and very little fluid anteriorly. As the fluid increases it distributes both anteriorly and posteriorly. With large effusions, as in Figure 3–103, one usually sees more anterior fluid than posterior fluid as the heart tends to sink posteriorly.

There are several echocardiographic signs for cardiac tamponade.[476] One of the most frequent findings is collapse of the anterior right ventricular free wall.[477,478] Figure 3–104 shows the collapse of the right ventricular wall (arrow) in the long-axis view (LX). In the four-chamber view one notes collapse of the right atrial free wall (arrow). Right atrial collapse is slightly more sensitive but less specific than right ventricular collapse.[478a,479] Occasionally one may see collapse of the left atrium[480,481] and even on rare occasion the left ventricle.[482,483] Right ventricular collapse occurs in early diastole and may be better appreciated on an M-mode recording. Doppler echocardiography can also be used to identify cardiac tamponade.[484,485] Under this hemodynamic setting one can see a respiratory cyclical variation of both tricuspid and mitral flow.[486,487] With inspira-

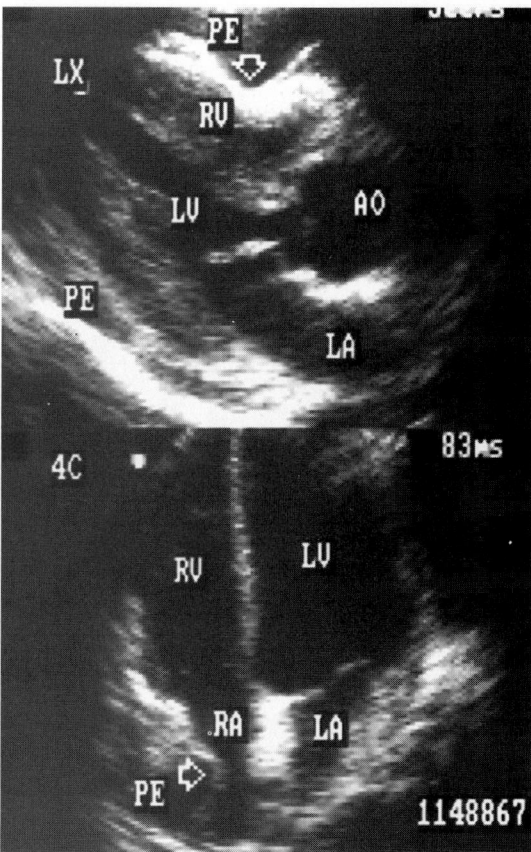

FIGURE 3–104. Long-axis (LX) and four-chamber (4C) 2-D echocardiographic views in a patient with pericardial effusion (PE) and cardiac tamponade. The long-axis view shows diastolic collapse of the right ventricular wall (arrow); the four-chamber view shows collapse of the right atrial free wall (arrow). RV = right ventricle; LV = left ventricle; AO = aorta; LA = left atrium; RA = right atrium. (From Feigenbaum, H.: Echocardiography. 5th ed. Malvern, PA, Lea and Febiger, 1994.)

motion has been noted as a "swinging heart."[488,489] If the motion is such that the heart does not resume its original position before the next electric depolarization occurs, then the axis of the QRS is altered and one notes electrical alternans on the electrocardiogram.

CONSTRICTIVE PERICARDITIS (see also p. 1496). Echocardiography is of some (albeit limited) value in the diagnosis of a thickened pericardium with constrictive pericarditis.[490,491] Although a thickened pericardium can be detected in many patients, particularly those who already have pericardial fluid (Fig. 3–103), this finding by itself does not imply the presence of constriction. The echocardiographic signs of constriction include lack of diastolic motion, i.e., a flat diastolic slope of the posterior left ventricular wall,[2,492,493] abnormal motion of the interventricular septum,[492] very short E to F slope of the mitral valve,[2] and a dilated inferior vena cava that does not get smaller with inspiration. Doppler studies of the tricuspid, mitral, pulmonary venous flow are probably the most useful current recordings for constriction.[494,495] One notes a typical restrictive filling pattern of the mitral valve flow with a tall E wave and very small A wave (Fig. 3–38C). In addition there is a respiratory variation that will distinguish this type of recording from restrictive cardiomyopathy.[496,497]

CONGENITAL ABSENCE OF THE PERICARDIUM (see p. 1522). On the M-mode echocardiogram, the right ventricle is usually dilated and there is paradoxical septal motion similar to a right ventricular volume overload. Two-dimensional echocardiography reveals bulging or displacement of part of the left ventricle or left atrium in a distorted manner that suggests absence of the pericardium.[498,499]

CARDIAC TUMORS AND THROMBI

(See also Chap. 42)

LEFT ATRIAL TUMORS. Left atrial myxoma (see p. 1467) is by far the most common cardiac tumor, and echocardiography has proved to be an extremely important diagnostic technique for its recognition.[500] Figure 3–105 demonstrates a 2-D echocardiogram of a patient with left atrial myxoma. The spatial orientation inherent in this examination provides additional useful information, and the size and shape of the mass are apparent. In addition, the site of attachment of the mass to the cardiac structure can frequently be detected. Transesophageal echocardiography provides an outstanding view of the left atrium[501,502] and has vastly improved our ability to detect all intracardiac masses.[503,504] Excellent definition of left atrial masses can be seen with this unobstructive view. Figure 3–106 shows four images of a small left atrial mass that is attached to the interatrial septum (IAS). Although this tumor was seen on a transthoracic 2-D echocardiogram, the clarity and detail were greater with the transesophageal examination[505] (Fig. 3–107).

LEFT ATRIAL THROMBI. Other space-occupying structures[506,507]—atrial thrombi—have been identified in the left atrium by means of echocardiography.[508] Since most are located near the left atrial appendage, transesophageal echocardiography is superior to conventional echocardiography in visualizing left atrial thrombi (Fig. 3–107). The transesophageal technique may detect spontaneous contrast in the left atrium, which is frequently associated with and may be a precursor of thrombus formation.[509,510]

RIGHT ATRIAL MASSES (see p. 1466). Right atrial myoma is not as common as the left atrial variety. Such tumors can also be detected echocardiographically.[511,512] They appear as a mass of echoes that are in the right atrium during systole and traverse the tricuspid valve during diastole. As on the left side of the heart, a large vegetation involving the tricuspid valve can simulate a right atrial myxoma. Bilateral atrial myxomas have been detected echocardiographically.[513] Right atrial thrombi that have the potential of producing massive pulmonary emboli have been detected with 2-D echocardiography.[514,515]

VENTRICULAR TUMORS. Myomas can occur in the ventricles as well as in the atria[516,517] (see p. 1466) and have been imaged in both ventricles. When the tumors are mobile, they can produce very dramatic echograms on both M-mode and 2-D examinations; they may move above the mitral valve into the left ventricular outflow tract during systole.[518] Pedunculated right ventricular masses can prolapse into the pulmonary artery[519] or simulate pulmonic stenosis.[520] Rhabdomyomas[521] and fibromas[522] can also in-

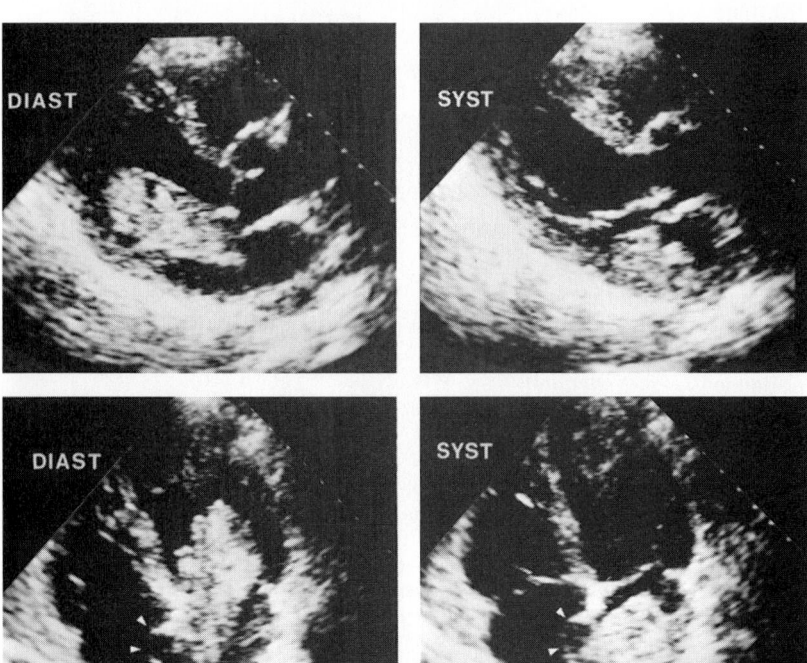

FIGURE 3–105. Long-axis *(top)* and apical four-chamber *(bottom)* 2-D echocardiograms in diastole and systole in a patient with a left atrial myxoma and an atrial septal aneurysm. The septal aneurysm (arrowheads) can be seen bulging toward the right atrium in both diastole and systole in the four-chamber view. (From Feigenbaum, H.: Echocardiography. 4th ed. Philadelphia, Lea and Febiger, 1986.)

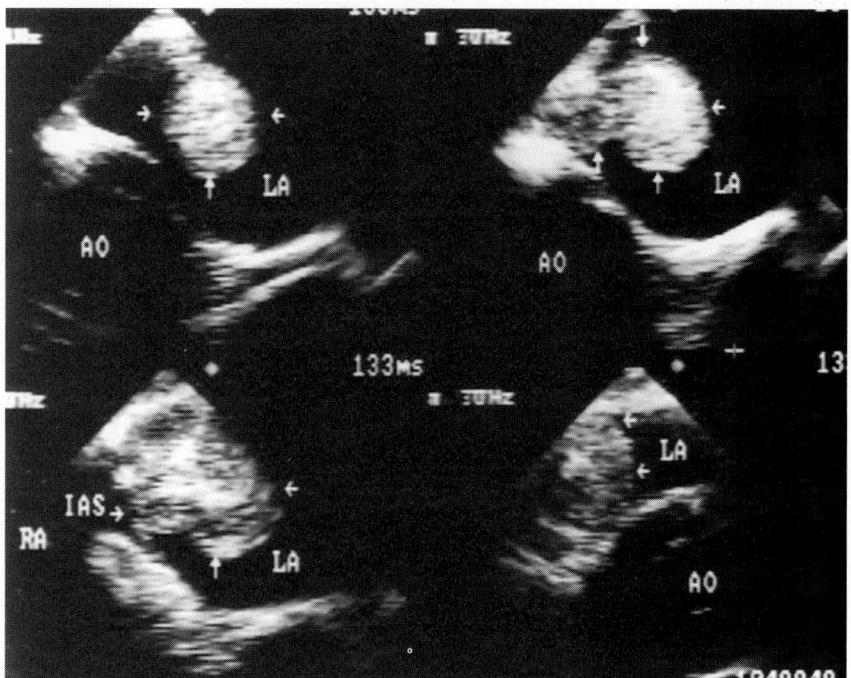

FIGURE 3–106. Transesophageal echocardiogram of a patient with a left atrial tumor (arrows). The tumor is attached to the interatrial septum (IAS). RA = right atrium; LA = left atrium; AO = aorta.

volve the ventricles; these two types of lesions have been imaged successfully.[523]

VALVULAR TUMORS. Neoplasms may involve the cardiac valves. Cardiac papillary fibroelastomas represent small

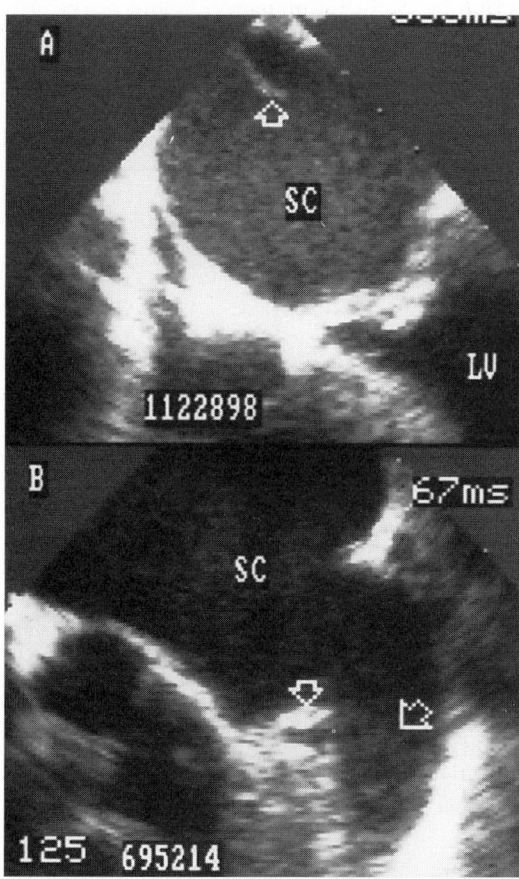

FIGURE 3–107. Transesophageal echocardiograms of two patients with spontaneous contrast (SC) and formed thrombi (arrows) in the left atrium. In *A* the thrombus is linear and immobile. In *B* a clot (small arrow) is attached to the junction of the left atrial appendage and the body of the left atrium. A less-dense echogenic mass (large arrow) is faintly seen within the left atrial appendage. LV = left ventricle. (From Feigenbaum, H.: Echocardiography. 5th ed. Malvern, PA, Lea and Febiger, 1994.)

tumors on the edges of the valve leaflets, primarily the mitral valve[524] and rarely the tricuspid valve.[525] Systemic emboli and stroke occur in patients with these neoplasms.[526] Other neoplasms, such as rhabdomyosarcoma, may also involve the mitral valve and can be detected echocardiographically.[527] Primary myxoma can also be attached to the mitral valve.[528]

OTHER INTRACARDIAC ECHOGENIC STRUCTURES. It should be kept in mind that not all echogenic structures in the heart are pathologic.[529] It is possible to detect various structures in the right atrium that are possibly normal variants. The so-called Chiari network may produce mobile echoes within the right atrium that may not be pathologic.[530,531] In addition, the eustachian valve may be prominent and simulate a pathologic mass.[532] Lipomatous hypertrophy of the interatrial septum may be striking but is benign.[533,534]

There are nonpathologic echo-producing structures on the left side of the heart as well.[535] Left ventricular bands or false tendons straddling the left ventricular chamber frequently can be imaged.[536] Moderator bands are routinely seen in the right ventricle. Iatrogenic masses, such as various catheters, are also easily detected on the 2-D echocardiogram. Occasionally this examination can help detect an incorrectly placed catheter or pacemaker catheter that may have perforated one of the cardiac walls.[537] Right atrial thrombi that have the potential of producing massive pulmonary emboli have been detected with 2-D echocardiography.[538,539]

INVASION AND METASTASIS TO THE HEART (see Ch. 57). Invasion of the wall of the heart[540,541] and compression of the heart[542] by neoplasms arising elsewhere have been imaged echocardiographically. Seeding of the pericardium with metastases and the production of pericardial effusion (see p. 1485) probably represent the most common types of cardiac involvement with malignant disease. Occasionally a massively thickened pericardium is produced. On echocardiography the position and configuration of the heart may be distorted by a large tumor mass in the mediastinum. Echocardiography has also been shown to be helpful in distinguishing between cystic and solid tumors involving the heart.[543] Transesophageal echocardiography can be very helpful in detecting paracardiac masses.[544]

PULMONARY ARTERY CLOTS. Transesophageal echocardiography now permits visualization of clots in the pulmonary arteries and is helpful in the diagnosis of pulmonary emboli.[545,546]

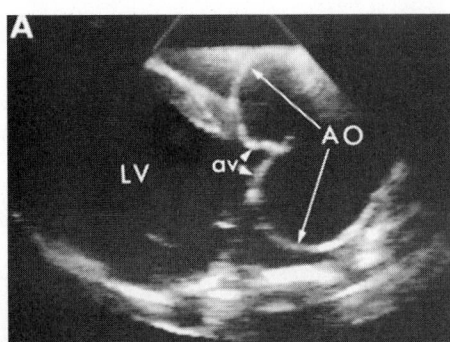

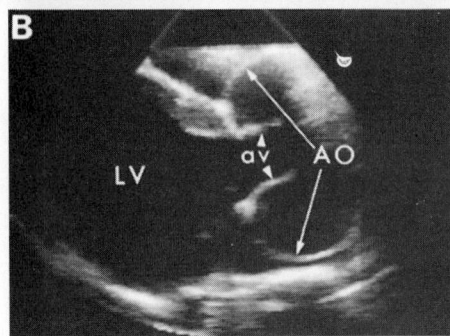

FIGURE 3–108. Diastolic *(A)* and systolic *(B)* long-axis, parasternal 2-D echocardiograms of a patient with Marfan syndrome. The aorta (AO) is markedly dilated. Note the marked discrepancy between the aortic valve (av) opening and the size of the aorta. LV = left ventricle. (From Feigenbaum, H.: Echocardiography. 3rd ed. Philadelphia, Lea and Febiger, 1981.)

DISEASES OF THE AORTA

(See also Chap. 45)

DILATATION AND ANEURYSM (see p. 1547). It is possible to examine almost the entire aorta using echocardiography.[547] The root of the aorta and proximal portion of the ascending aorta may be recorded with both M-mode and 2-D echocardiography. The 2-D technique utilizing the parasternal

long-axis examination permits recording of the descending aorta posterior to the left atrium and left ventricle.[548] The suprasternal approach provides visualization of the arch of the aorta and the proximal portion of the descending aorta. The abdominal aorta can then be imaged with the transducer in the subcostal position or over the abdomen itself. Transesophageal echocardiography provides the most spectacular images of the aorta. Aside from a small section of the arch of the aorta, all of the aorta can be imaged very accurately with the transesophageal approach.

As might be expected, dilatation of the aorta, as occurs in the Marfan syndrome and cystic medial necrosis, is imaged relatively easily (Fig. 3–108).[549] The echocardiographic detection of coarctation of the aorta has already been discussed (see p. 84). Aneurysms of the abdominal aorta are routinely examined quite successfully by 2-D echocardiography.

AORTIC DISSECTION (see p. 1554). Two-dimensional echocardiography has been used extensively for the detection of aortic dissection (Fig. 3–109, p. 96).[550,551] In addition to the usual transducer position, the right parasternal position may be useful in detecting dissection with its true and false lumina and in indicating systolic fluttering of the intimal flap.[552] Transesophageal echocardiography is becoming the procedure of choice in the diagnosis of aortic dissection (Fig. 3–110, p. 96).[553–555] Doppler echocardiography has also been useful in the diagnosis of aortic dissection.[556] The flow characteristics in the false channel are distinctly different from those in the true channel. Color flow Doppler helps in establishing the correct diagnosis by indicating the difference between the false and true lumina (Fig. 3–111, p. 97) and helps to identify the entry point of the dissection.[557,558]

ANEURYSM OF THE SINUS OF VALSALVA. Because examination of the root of the aorta is possible, 2-D and transesophageal echocardiography have been used to image the sinus of Valsalva, allowing detection of aneurysms of these sinuses.[559,560] Bulging of the sinus, usually the anterior or

FIGURE 3–110. See color plate 4.

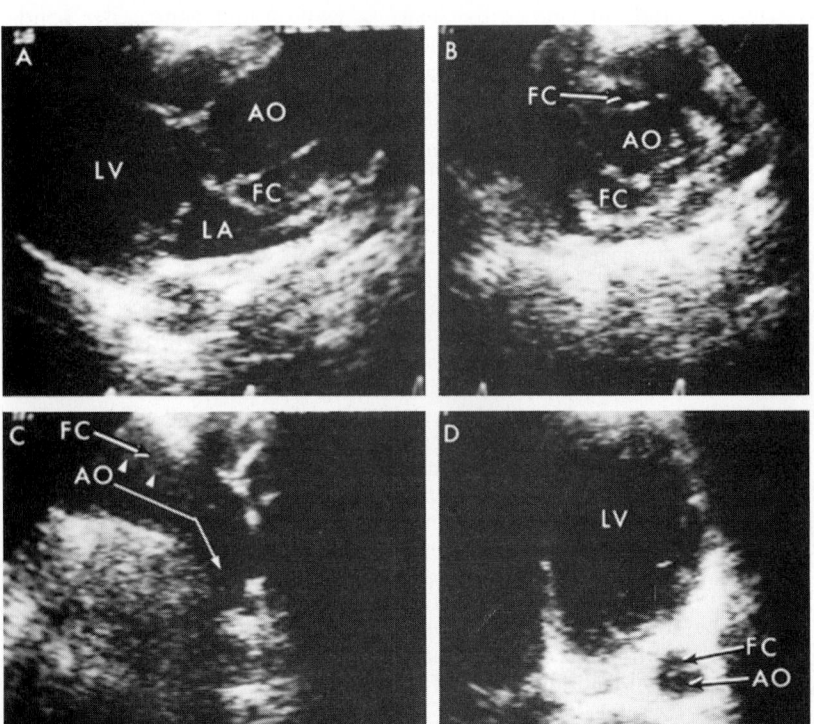

FIGURE 3–109. Parasternal long-axis *(A)*, short-axis *(B)*, suprasternal *(C)*, and apical *(D)* views in a patient with aortic dissection. The false channel (FC) can be seen in every view. The intimal flap (arrowheads) is only faintly seen in the suprasternal examination *(C)*. AO = true aortic lumen; LV = left ventricle; LA = left atrium. (From Feigenbaum, H.: Echocardiography. 4th ed. Philadelphia, Lea and Febiger, 1986.)

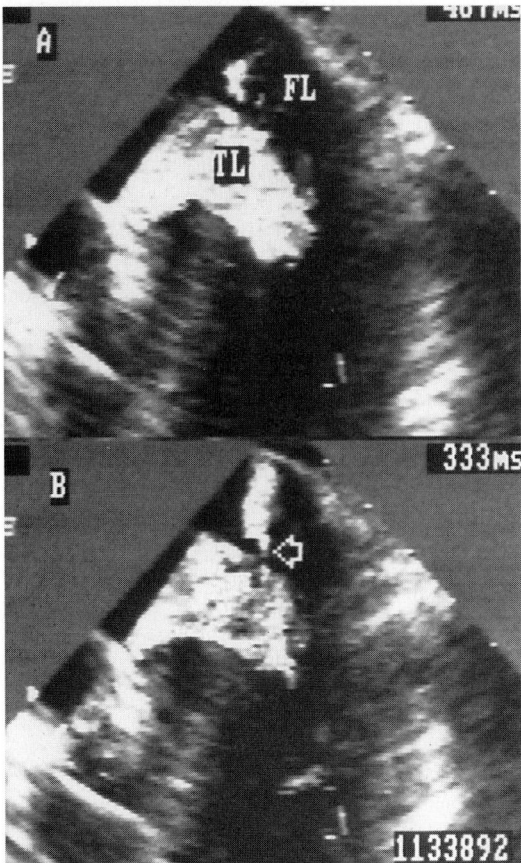

FIGURE 3-111. Doppler flow imaging in black and white showing an entry jet (arrow) passing from the true lumen (TL) into the false lumen (FL) of a patient with aortic dissection. (From Feigenbaum, H.: Echocardiography. 5th ed. Malvern, PA, Lea and Febiger, 1994.)

right coronary sinus, into the right ventricular outflow tract[561] or interventricular septum[562] has been recorded. With rupture there is discontinuity of the anterior wall of the sinus and mid-systolic closure and coarse fluttering of the right coronary cusp of the aortic valve.[563] With rupture of the sinus of Valsalva into the right side of the heart, fluttering of the tricuspid valve as well as premature opening of the pulmonary valve has been reported.[132] Doppler echocardiography, especially color flow, is the principal echocardiographic examination in the diagnosis of ruptured sinus of Valsalva aneurysms.[564] The abnormal jets of blood can be readily identified.

AORTIC ATHEROSCLEROSIS. Transesophageal echocardiography offers the opportunity to see atherosclerotic plaque within the thoracic aorta.[565,566] The masses vary in size and mobility[567] and may be responsible for systemic emboli.[568,569]

REFERENCES

PRINCIPLES OF ECHOCARDIOGRAPHY

1. Carlsen, E. N.: Ultrasound physics for the physician: A brief review. J. Clin. Ultrasound 3:69, 1975.
2. Feigenbaum, H.: Echocardiography. 5th ed. Malvern, PA, Lea and Febiger, 1994.
3. Wells, P. N. T.: Ultrasonics in Clinical Diagnosis. 2nd ed. New York, Churchill Livingstone, 1977.
4. Von Ramm, O.T., and Thurstone, F. L.: Cardiac imaging using a phased array ultrasound system. Circulation 53:258, 1976.
5. Hatle, L., and Angelsen, B.: Doppler ultrasound in cardiology: Physical principles and clinical applications. 2nd ed. Philadelphia, Lea and Febiger, 1984.
6. Goldberg, S. J., Allen, H. D., Marx, G. R., and Flinn, C. J.: Doppler Echocardiography. Philadelphia, Lea and Febiger, 1985.
7. Burns, P. N.: The physical principles of Doppler and spectral analysis. J. Clin. Ultrasound 15:567, 1987.
8. Bom, K., deBoo, J., and Rijsterborgh, H.: On the aliasing problem in pulsed Doppler cardiac studies. J. Clin. Ultrasound. 12:559, 1984.

97

Ch 3

9. Stewart, W. J., Galvin, K. A., Gillam, L. D., et al.: Comparison of high pulse repetition frequency and continuous wave Doppler echocardiography in the assessment of high flow velocity in patients with valvular stenosis and regurgitation. J. Am. Coll. Cardiol. 6:565, 1985.
10. Stevenson, J. G.: Appearance and recognition of basic concepts in color flow imaging. Echocardiography 6:451, 1989.
11. Ritter, S. B.: Red, green and blue: The flag of color flow mapping. Echocardiography 6:369, 1989.
12. Seward, J. B., Khandheria, B. K., Oh, J. K., et al.: Transesophageal echocardiography: Technique, anatomic correlations, implementation, and clinical applications. Mayo Clin. Proc. 63:649, 1988.
13. Tardif, J.-C., Schwartz, S. L., Vannan, M. A., et al.: Clinical usefulness of multiplane transesophageal echocardiography: Comparison to biplanar imaging. Am. Heart J. 128:156, 1994.
14. Seward, J. B., Khandheria, B. K., Edwards, W. D., et al.: Biplanar transesophageal echocardiography: Anatomic correlations, image orientation, and clinical applications. Mayo Clin Proc. 65:1193, 1990.
15. Schiller, N. B., Maurer, G., Ritter, S. B., et al.: Transesophageal echocardiography. J. Am. Soc. Echocardiogr. 2:354, 1989.
16. Eisenberg, M. J., London, M. J., Leung, J. M., et al.: Monitoring for myocardial ischemia during noncardiac surgery. A technology assessment of transesophageal echocardiography and 12-lead electrocardiography. The study of perioperative ischemia research group. JAMA 268:210, 1992.
17. Tee, S. D. C., Shiota, T., Weintraub, R., et al.: Evaluation of ventricular septal defect by transesophageal echocardiography: Intraoperative assessment. Am. Heart J. 127:585, 1994.
18. Cohen, G. I., Casale, P. N., Lytle, B. W., et al.: Transesophageal echocardiography guidance of closed mitral commissurotomy. J. Am. Soc. Echocardiogr. 6:332, 1993.
19. Callahan, J. A., Seward, J. B., Nishimura, R. A., et al.: Two-dimensional echocardiographically guided pericardiocentesis: Experience in 117 consecutive patients. Am. J. Cardiol. 55:476, 1985.
20. Koenig, P. R., Rossi, A., and Ritter, S. B.: Bedside cardiac catheterization using transesophageal echocardiographic guidance. Echocardiography 9:637, 1992.
21. Pytlewski, G., Georgeson, S., Burke, J., et al.: Endomyocardial biopsy under transesophageal echocardiographic guidance can be safely performed in the critically ill cardiac transplant recipient. Am. J. Cardiol. 73:1019, 1994.
22. Lee, M. S., Evans, S. J. L., Blumberg, S., et al.: Echocardiographically guided electrophysiologic testing in pregnancy. J. Am. Soc. Echocardiogr. 7:182, 1994.
23. Chu, E., Fitzpatrick, A. P., Chin, M. C., et al.: Radiofrequency catheter ablation guided by intracardiac echocardiography. Circulation 89:1301, 1994.
24. Thomas, M. R., Monaghan, M. J., Smyth, D. W., et al.: Comparative value of transthoracic and transesophageal echocardiography before balloon dilatation of the mitral valve. Br. Heart J. 68:493, 1992.
25. Boutin, C., Dyck, J., Benson, L., et al.: Balloon atrial septostomy under transesophageal echocardiographic guidance. Pediatr. Cardiol. 13:175, 1992.
26. VanDerVelde, M. E., Sanders, S. P., Keane, J. F., et al.: Transesophageal echocardiographic guidance of transcatheter ventricular septal defect closure. J. Am. Coll. Cardiol. 23:1660, 1994.
27. Nissen, S. E., Grines, C. L., Gurley, J. C., et al.: Application of a new phased-array ultrasound imaging catheter in the assessment of vascular dimensions. Circulation 81:660, 1990.
28. Pandian, N. G.: Intravascular and intracardiac ultrasound imaging. Circulation 80:1091, 1989.
29. Chen, C., Guerrero, J. L., dePrada, J. A. V., et al.: Intracardiac ultrasound measurement of volumes and ejection fraction in normal, infarcted, and aneurysmal left ventricles using a 10-MHz ultrasound catheter. Circulation 90:1481, 1994.
30. Chu, E., Kalman, J. M., Kwasman, M. A., et al.: Intracardiac echocardiography during radiofrequency catheter ablation of cardiac arrhythmias in humans. J. Am. Coll. Cardiol. 24:1268, 1994.
31. Smith, M. D., Elion, J. L., McClure, R. R., et al.: Left heart opacification with peripheral venous injection of a new saccharide echo contrast agent in dogs. J. Am. Coll. Cardiol. 13:1622, 1989.
32. Klein, A. L., Bailey, A. S., Moura, A., et al.: Reliability of echocardiographic measurements of myocardial perfusion using commercially produced sonicated serum albumin (Albunex). J. Am. Coll. Cardiol. 22:1983, 1993.
33. Goldberg, B. B., Liu, J.-B., and Forsberg, F.: Ultrasound contrast agents: A review. Ultrasound Med. Biol. 20:319, 1994.
34. Porter, T. R., Xie, F., Kricsfeld, A., et al.: Improved endocardial border resolution during dobutamine stress echocardiography with intravenous sonicated dextrose albumin. J. Am. Coll. Cardiol. 23:1440, 1994.
35. Terasawa, A., Miyatake, K., Nakatani, S., et al.: Enhancement of Doppler flow signals in the left heart chambers by intravenous injection of sonicated albumin. J. Am. Coll. Cardiol. 21:737, 1993.
36. Crouse, L. J., Cheirif, J., Hanly, D. E., et al.: Opacification and border delineation improvement in patients with suboptimal endocardial border definition in routine echocardiography. J. Am. Coll. Cardiol. 22:1494, 1993.
37. Von Bibra, H., Becher, H., Firschke, C., et al.: Enhancement of mitral regurgitation and normal left atrial color Doppler flow signals with peripheral venous injection of a saccharide-based contrast agent. J. Am. Coll. Cardiol. 22:521, 1993.

38. Martin, G. R., and Ruckman, R. N.: Fetal echocardiography: A large clinical experience and follow-up. J. Am. Soc. Echocardiogr 3:4, 1990.

39. Roberson, D. A., and Silverman, N. H.: Ebstein's anomaly: Echocardiographic and clinical features in the fetus and neonate. J. Am. Coll. Cardiol. 14:1300, 1989.

40. Sapin, P. M., Schroder, K. M., Gopal, A. S., et al.: Comparison of two- and three-dimensional echocardiography with cineventriculography for measurement of left ventricular volume in patients. J. Am. Coll. Cardiol. 24:1054, 1994.

41. Jiang, L., Vazquez de Prada, A., Handschumacher, M. D., et al.: Quantitative three-dimensional reconstruction of aneurysmal left ventricle. In vitro and in vivo validation. Circulation 91:222, 1995.

42. Handschumacher, M. D., Lethord, J.-P., Siu, S. C., et al.: A new integrated system for three-dimensional echocardiographic reconstruction: Development and validation for ventricular volume with application in human subjects. J. Am. Coll. Cardiol. 21:743, 1993.

43. Kupferwasser, I., Mohr-Kahaly, S., Erbel, R., et al.: Three-dimensional imaging of cardiac mass lesions by transesophageal echocardiographic computed tomography. J. Am. Soc. Endocardiogr. 7:561, 1994.

44. Roelandt, J. R. T. C., tenCate, F. J., Fletter, W. B., et al.: Ultrasonic dynamic three-dimensional visualization of the heart with a multiplane transesophageal imaging transducer. J. Am. Soc. Echocardiogr. 7:217, 1994.

45. Wang, X.-F., Li, Z.-A., Cheng, T. O., et al.: Clinical application of three-dimensional transesophageal echocardiography. Am. Heart J. 128:380, 1994.

46. Stewart, H. D., Stewart, H. F., Moore, R. M., and Garry, J.: Compilation of reported biological effects data and ultrasound exposure levels. J. Clin. Ultrasound 13:167, 1985.

EXAMINATION OF THE NORMAL HEART

47. Henry, W. L., DeMaria, A., Gramiak, R., et al.: Report of the American Society of Echocardiography Nomenclature and Standards in Two-Dimensional Echocardiography. Circulation 62:212, 1980.

48. Feigenbaum, H.: Current status of M-mode echocardiography. A.C.C. Current J. Review 3:58, 1994.

49. Huwez, F. U., Houston, A. B., Watson, J., et al.: Age and body surface area related normal upper and lower limits of M-mode echocardiographic measurements and left ventricular volume and mass from infancy to early adulthood. Br. Heart J. 72:276, 1994.

50. Kuecherer, H. F., Kusumoto, F., Muhiudeen, I. A., et al.: Pulmonary venous flow patterns by transesophageal pulsed Doppler echocardiography: Relation to parameters of left ventricular systolic and diastolic function. Am. Heart J. 122:1683, 1991.

51. Rossvoll, O., and Hatle, L. K.: Pulmonary venous flow velocities recorded by transthoracic Doppler ultrasound: Relation to left ventricular diastolic pressures. J. Am. Coll. Cardiol. 21:1687, 1993.

EVALUATION OF CARDIAC PERFORMANCE

52. Feigenbaum, H., Popp, R. L., Wolfe, S. B., et al.: Ultrasound measurements of the left ventricle: A correlative study with angiography. Arch. Intern. Med. 129:461, 1972.

53. Teichholz, L. E., Kreulen, T., Herman, M. V., et al.: Problems in echocardiographic volume determinations: Echocardiographic-angiographic correlations in the presence or absence of asynergy. Am. J. Cardiol. 37:7, 1976.

54. Quinones, M. A., Gaasch, W. H., and Alexander, J. K.: Echocardiographic assessment of left ventricular function: With special reference to normalized velocities. Circulation 50:42, 1974.

55. Feigenbaum, H.: Echocardiographic examination of the left ventricle. Circulation 51:1, 1975.

56. Ahmadpour, H., Shah, A. H., Allen, J. W., et al.: Mitral E point septal separation: A reliable index of left ventricular performance in coronary artery disease. Am. Heart J. 106:21, 1983.

57. Schiller, N. B., Shah, P. M., Crawford, M., et al.: Recommendations for qualitation of the left ventricle by two-dimensional echocardiography. J. Am. Soc. Echocardiogr. 5:362, 1989.

58. Ryan, T., Petrovic, O., Armstrong, W. F., et al.: Quantitative two-dimensional echocardiography assessment of patients undergoing left ventricular aneurysmectomy. Am. Heart J. 111:714, 1986.

59. Wong, M., Bruce, S., Joseph, D., et al.: Estimating left ventricular ejection fraction from two-dimensional echocardiograms: Visual and computer-processed interpretations. Echocardiography 8:1, 1991.

60. Waggoner, A. D., Miller, J. G., and Perez, J. E.: Two-dimensional echocardiographic automatic boundary detection for evaluation of left ventricular function in unselected adult patients. J. Am. Soc. Echocardiogr. 7:459, 1994.

61. Yvorchuk, K. J., Davies, R. A., and Chang, K.-L.: Measurement of left ventricular ejection fraction by acoustic quantification and comparison with radionuclide angiography. Am. J. Cardiol. 74:1052, 1994.

62. Katz, W. E., Gasior, T. A., and Reddy, S. C. B.: Utility and limitations of biplane transesophageal echocardiographic automated border detection for estimation of left ventricular stroke volume and cardiac output. Am. Heart J. 128:389, 1994.

63. Gardin, J. M.: Doppler measurements of aortic blood flow velocity and acceleration: Load-independent indexes of left ventricular performance? Am. J. Cardiol. 64:935, 1989.

64. Chen, C., Rodriguez, L., Lethord, J.-P., et al.: Continuous wave Doppler echocardiography for non-invasive assessment of left ventricular dP/dt

65. Kawai, H., Yokota, Y., and Yokoyama, M.: Noninvasive evaluation of contractile state by left ventricular dP/dtmax divided by end-diastolic volume using continuous-wave Doppler and M-mode echocardiography. Clin. Cardiol. 17:662, 1994.

66. Pandian, N. G., Nanda, N. C., Schwartz, S. L., et al.: Three-dimensional and four-dimensional transesophageal echocardiographic imaging of the heart and aorta in humans using a computed tomographic imaging probe. Echocardiography 9:677, 1992.

67. Taylor, R., and Waggoner, A. D.: Doppler assessment of left ventricular diastolic function. A review. J. Am. Soc. Echocardiogr. 5:603, 1992.

68. Thomas, J. D., and Weyman, A. E.: Echocardiographic Doppler evaluation of left ventricular diastolic function. Physics and physiology. Circulation 84:977, 1992.

69. Iwase, M., Nagata, K., Izawa, H., et al.: Age-related changes in left and right ventricular filling velocity profiles and their relationship in normal subjects. Am. Heart J. 126:419, 1993.

70. Pipilis, A., Meyer, T. E., Ormerdo, O., et al.: Early and late changes in left ventricular filling after acute myocardial infarction and the effect of infarct size. Am. J. Cardiol. 70:1397, 1992.

71. Ohno, M., Cheng, C.-P., and Little, W. C.: Mechanism of altered patterns of left ventricular filling during the development of congestive heart failure. Circulation 89:2241, 1994.

72. Oh, J. K., Ding, Z. P., Gersh, B. J., et al.: Restrictive left ventricular diastolic filling identifies patients with heart failure after acute myocardial infarction. J. Am. Soc. Echocardiogr. 5:497, 1992.

73. Thomas, J. D., Flachskampf, F. A., Chen, C., et al.: Isovolumic relaxation time varies predictably with its time constant and aortic and left atrial pressures: Implications for the noninvasive evaluation of ventricular relaxation. Am. Heart J. 124:1305, 1992.

74. Hecht, H. S., DeBord, L., Sotomayor, N., et al.: Truly silent ischemia and the relationship of chest pain and ST segment changes to the amount of ischemic myocardium: Evaluation of supine bicycle stress echocardiography. J. Am. Coll. Cardiol. 23:369, 1994.

75. Presti, C. F., Armstrong, W. F., and Feigenbaum, H.: Comparison of echocardiography at peak exercise and after bicycle exercise in evaluation of patients with known or suspected coronary artery disease. J. Am. Soc. Echocardiogr. 1:119, 1988.

76. Williams, M. J., Marwick, T. H., O'Gorman, D., et al.: Comparison of exercise echocardiography with an exercise score to diagnose coronary artery disease in women. Am. J. Cardiol. 74:435, 1994.

77. Iliceto, S., Sorino, M., D'Ambrosio, G., et al.: Detection of coronary artery disease by two-dimensional echocardiography and transesophageal atrial pacing. J. Am. Coll. Cardiol. 5:1188, 1985.

78. Feigenbaum, H.: Digital recording, display, and storage of echocardiograms. J. Am. Soc. Echocardiogr. 1:378, 1988.

79. Tischler, M. D., Battle, R. W., Saha, M., et al.: Observations suggesting a high incidence of exercise-induced severe mitral regurgitation in patients with mild rheumatic mitral valve disease at rest. J. Am. Coll. Cardiol. 25:128, 1995.

80. Otto, C. M., Pearlman, A. S., Kraft, C. D., et al.: Physiologic changes with maximal exercise in asymptomatic valvular aortic stenosis assessed by Doppler echocardiography. J. Am. Coll. Cardiol. 20:1160, 1992.

81. Kaplan, J. D., Foster, E., Redberg, R. F., et al.: Exercise Doppler echocardiography identifies abnormal hemodynamics in adults with congenital heart disease. Am. Heart J. 127:1572, 1994.

82. Feigenbaum, H., Popp, R. L., Chip, J. N., et al.: Left ventricular wall thickness measured by ultrasound. Arch. Intern. Med. 121:391, 1969.

83. Devereux, R. B., Alonso, D. R., Lutas, E. M., et al.: Echocardiographic assessment of left ventricular hypertrophy: Comparison to necropsy findings. Am. J. Cardiol. 57:450, 1986.

84. Byrd, B. F., Finkbeiner, W., Bouchard, A., et al.: Accuracy and reproducibility of clinically acquired two-dimensional echocardiographic mass measurements. Am. Heart J. 118:133, 1989.

85. Roman, M. J., Devereux, R. B., and Cody, R. J.: Ability of left ventricular stress-shortening relations, end-systolic stress/volume ratio and indirect indexes to detect severe contractile failure in ischemic or idiopathic dilated cardiomyopathy. Am. J. Cardiol. 64:1338, 1989.

86. Segar, D. S., Moran, M., Ryan, T., et al.: End-systolic regional wall stress-length and stress-shortening relations in an experimental model of normal, ischemic and reperfused myocardium. J. Am. Coll. Cardiol. 17:1651, 1991.

87. Goldberg, S. J.: Analysis and interpretation of thickening and thinning phases of left ventricular wall dynamics. Ultrasound Med. Biol. 10:797, 1984.

88. Corya, B. C., Rasmussen, S., Feigenbaum, H., et al.: Systolic thickening and thinning of the septum and posterior wall in patients with coronary artery disease, congestive cardiomyopathy, and atrial septal defect. Circulation 55:109, 1977.

89. Feigenbaum, H.: Estimation of left atrial size using ultrasound. Am. Heart J. 78:43, 1969.

90. Kircher, B., Abbott, J. A., Pau, S., et al.: Left atrial volume determination by biplane two-dimensional echocardiography: Validation by cine computed tomography. Am. Heart J. 121:864, 1991.

91. Lemire, F., Tajik, A. J., and Hagler, D. J.: Asymmetric left atrial enlargement: An echocardiographic observation. Chest 59:779, 1976.

92. Gehl, L. G., Mintz, G. S., Kotler, M. N., and Segal, B. L.: Left atrial volume overload in mitral regurgitation: A two-dimensional echocardiographic study. Am. J. Cardiol. 49:33, 1982.

93. Hiraishi, S., DiSessa, T. G., Jarmakani, J. M., et al.: Two-dimensional echocardiographic assessment of left atrial size in children. Am. J. Cardiol. 52:1249, 1983.

94. Mugge, A., Kuhn, H., Nikutta, P., et al.: Assessment of left atrial appendage function by biplane transesophageal echocardiography in patients with nonrheumatic atrial fibrillation: Identification of a subgroup of patients at increased embolic risk. J. Am. Coll. Cardiol. 23:599, 1994.

95. Salka, S., Saeian, K., and Sagar, K. B.: Cerebral thromboembolization after cardioversion of atrial fibrillation in patients without transesophageal echocardiographic findings of left atrial thrombus. Am. Heart J. 126:722, 1993.

96. Gibson, T. C., Miller, S. W., Aretz, T., et al.: Method for estimating right ventricular volume by planes applicable to cross-sectional echocardiography. Correlation with angiographic formulas. Am. J. Cardiol. 55:1584, 1985.

97. Popp, R. L., Wolfe, S. B., Hirata, T., et al.: Estimation of right and left ventricular size by ultrasound. A study of the echoes from the interventricular septum. Am. J. Cardiol. 24:523, 1969.

98. Baker, B. J., Scovil, J. A., Kane, J. J., et al.: Echocardiographic detection of right ventricular hypertrophy. Am. Heart J. 105:611, 1983.

99. King, M. E., Braun, H., Goldblatt, A., et al.: Interventricular septal configuration as a predictor of right ventricular systolic hypertension in children: A cross-sectional echocardiographic study. Circulation 68:68, 1983.

100. Ryan, T., Petrovic, O., Dillon, J. C., et al.: An echocardiographic index for separation of right ventricular volume and pressure overload. J. Am. Coll. Cardiol. 5:918, 1985.

101. Cheriex, E. C., Steeram, N., Eussen, Y. F. J. M., et al.: Cross-sectional Doppler echocardiography as the initial technique for the diagnosis of acute pulmonary embolism. Br. Heart J. 72:52, 1994.

102. Robson, S. C., Murray, A., Peart, I., et al.: Reproducibility of cardiac output measurement by cross-sectional and Doppler echocardiography. Br. Heart J. 59:680, 1988.

103. Bouchard, A., Blumlein, S., Schiller, N. B., et al.: Measurement of left ventricular stroke volume using continuous wave Doppler echocardiography of the ascending aorta and M-mode echocardiography of the aortic valve. J. Am. Coll. Cardiol. 9:75, 1987.

104. Sahn, D. J.: Determination of cardiac output by echocardiographic Doppler methods: Relative accuracy of various sites for measurement. J. Am. Coll. Cardiol. 6:663, 1985.

105. Moulinier, L., Venet, T., Schiller, N. B., et al.: Measurement of aortic blood flow by Doppler echocardiography: Day to day variability in normal subjects and applicability in clinical research. J. Am. Coll. Cardiol. 17:1326, 1991.

106. Ascah, K. J., Stewart, W. J., Gillam, L. D., et al.: Calculation of transmitral flow by Doppler echocardiography: A comparison of methods in a canine model. Am. Heart J. 117:402, 1989.

107. Shimamoto, H., Koto, H., Kawazoe, K., et al.: Transesophageal Doppler echocardiographic measurement of cardiac output by the mitral annulus method. Br. Heart J. 68:510, 1992.

108. Meijboom, E. J., Horowitz, S., Valdes-Cruz, L. M., et al.: A Doppler echocardiographic method for calculating volume flow across the tricuspid valve: Correlative laboratory and clinical studies. Circulation 71:551, 1985.

109. Valdes-Cruz, L. M., Horowitz, S., Goldberg, S. J., et al.: The mitral valve orifice method for noninvasive two-dimensional echo Doppler determinations of cardiac output. Circulation 67:872, 1983.

110. Miller, W. E., Richards, K. L., and Crawford, M. H.: Accuracy of mitral Doppler echocardiographic output determinations in adults. Am. Heart J., 119:620, 1990.

111. Lloyd, T. R., and Shirazi, F.: Nongeometric Doppler stroke volume determination is limited by aortic size. Am. J. Cardiol. 66:883, 1990.

112. Nishimuta, R. A., Callahan, M. J., Schaff, H. V., et al.: Non-invasive measurement of cardiac output by continuous-wave Doppler echocardiography: Initial experience and review of the literature. Mayo Clin. Proc. 59:484, 1984.

113. Ihlen, H., Myhre, E., Amlie, J. P., et al.: Changes in left ventricular stroke volume measured by Doppler echocardiography. Br. Heart J. 54:378, 1985.

114. Gorcsan, J., III, Ball, D. P., and Hattler, B. G.: Intraoperative determination of cardiac output by transesophageal continuous wave Doppler. Am. Heart J. 123:171, 1992.

115. Goldberg, S. J., and Allen, H. D.: Quantitative assessment by Doppler echocardiography of pulmonary or aortic regurgitation. Am. J. Cardiol. 56:131, 1985.

116. Jenni, R., Ritter, M., Vieli, A., et al.: Determination of the ratio of pulmonary blood flow to systemic blood flow by derivation of amplitude weighted mean velocity from continuous wave Doppler spectra. Br. Heart J. 61:167, 1989.

117. Jenni, R., Ritter, M., Vieli, A., et al.: Determination of the ratio of pulmonary blood flow to systemic blood flow by derivation of amplitude weighted mean velocity from continuous wave Doppler spectra. Br. Heart J. 61:167, 1989.

118. Meijboom, E. J., Rijsterborgh, H., Bot, H., et al.: Limits of reproducibility of blood flow measurements by Doppler echocardiography. Am. J. Cardiol. 59:133, 1987.

119. Stamm, R. B., and Martin, R. P.: Quantification of pressure gradients across stenotic valves by Doppler ultrasound. J. Am. Coll. Cardiol. 2:707, 1983.

120. Hatle, L., Brubakk, A., Tromsdal, A., et al.: Noninvasive assessment of pressure drop in mitral stenosis by Doppler ultrasound. Br. Heart J. 40:131, 1978.

121. Yock, P. G., and Popp, R. L.: Non-invasive estimation of right ventricular systolic pressure by Doppler ultrasound in patients with tricuspid regurgitation. Circulation 70:657, 1984.

122. Silbert, D. R., Brunson, S. C., Schiff, R., and Diamant, S.: Determination of right ventricular pressure in the presence of a ventricular septal defect using continuous wave Doppler ultrasound. J. Am. Coll. Cardiol. 8:379, 1986.

123. Marx, G. R., Allen, H. D., and Goldberg, S. J.: Doppler echocardiographic estimation of systolic pulmonary artery pressure in patients with aortic-pulmonary shunts. J. Am. Coll. Cardiol. 7:880, 1986.

124. Isobe, M., Yazaki, Y., Takaku, F., et al.: Prediction of pulmonary arterial pressure in adults by pulsed Doppler echocardiography. Am. J. Cardiol. 57:316, 1986.

125. Taylor, R.: Evaluation of the continuity equation in the Doppler echocardiographic assessment of the severity of valvular aortic stenosis. J. Am. Soc. Echocardiogr. 3:326, 1990.

126. Konecke, L. L., Feigenbaum, H., Chang, S.: Abnormal mitral valve motion in patients with elevated left ventricular diastolic pressures. Circulation 47:989, 1973.

127. Otsuji, Y., Toda, H., Ishigami, T., et al.: Mitral regurgitation during B bump of the mitral valve studied Doppler echocardiography. Am. J. Cardiol. 67:778, 1991.

128. Botvinick, E. H., Schiller, N. B., Wickramasekaran, R., et al.: Echocardiographic demonstration of early mitral valve closure in severe aortic insufficiency. Its clinical implications. Circulation 51:836, 1975.

129. Sabbah, H. N., and Stein, P. D.: Mechanism of early systolic closure of the aortic valve in discrete membranous subaortic stenosis. Circulation 65:399, 1982.

130. Nathan, M. P. R., Arora, R., and Rubenstein, H.: Mid-diastolic aortic valve opening in bacterial endocarditis of aortic valve. Clin. Cardiol. 5:294, 1982.

131. Weyman, A. E., Dillon, J. C., Feigenbaum, H., et al.: Echocardiographic patterns of pulmonic valve motion in pulmonic stenosis. Am. J. Cardiol. 34:644, 1974.

132. Wann, L. S., Weyman, A. E., Dillon, J. C., et al.: Premature pulmonary valve opening. Circulation 55:128, 1977.

133. Weyman, A. E., Dillon, J. C., Feigenbaum, H., et al.: Echocardiographic patterns of pulmonary valve motion with pulmonary hypertension. Circulation 50:905, 1974.

134. Turkevich, D., Groves, B.M., Micco, A., et al.: Early partial systolic closure of the pulmonic valve relates to severity of pulmonary hypertension. Am. Heart J. 115:409, 1988.

135. Stevenson, J. G.: Comparison of several noninvasive methods for estimation of pulmonary artery pressure. J. Am. Soc. Echocardiogr. 2:157, 1989.

136. Moreno, F. L. L., Hagan, A. D., Holman, J. R., et al.: Evaluation of size and dynamics of the inferior vena cava as an index of right-sided cardiac function. Am. J. Cardiol. 53:579, 1984.

137. Kircher, B. J., Himelman, R. B., Schiller, N. B.: Non-invasive estimation of right atrial pressure from the inspiratory collapse of the inferior vena cava. Am. J. Cardiol. 66:493, 1990.

ACQUIRED VALVULAR HEART DISEASE

138. Edler, I.: Ultrasound cardiogram in mitral valve disease. Acta Chir. Scand. 111:230, 1956.

139. Wann, L. S., Weyman, A. E., Dillon, J. C., et al.: Determination of mitral valve area by cross-sectional echocardiography. Ann. Intern. Med. 88:337, 1978.

140. Duchak, J. M., Jr., Chang, S., and Feigenbaum, H.: The posterior mitral valve echo and the echocardiographic diagnosis of mitral stenosis. Am. J. Cardiol. 29:628, 1972.

141. Riggs, T. W., Lapin, G. D., Paul, M. H., et al.: Measurement of mitral valve orifice area in infants and children by two-dimensional echocardiography. J. Am. Coll Cardiol. 1:873, 1983.

142. Hatle, L., Brubakk, A., Tromsdal, A., et al.: Noninvasive assessment of pressure drop in mitral stenosis by Doppler ultrasound. Br. Heart J. 40:131, 1978.

143. Smith, M. D., Handshoe, R., Handshoe, S., et al.: Comparative accuracy of two-dimensional echocardiography and Doppler pressure half-time methods in assessing severity of mitral stenosis in patients with and without prior commissurotomy. Circulation 73:100, 1986.

144. Loyd, D., Ask, P., and Wranne, B.: Pressure half-time does not always predict mitral valve area correctly. J. Am. Soc. Echocardiogr. 1:313, 1988.

145. Thomas, J. D., Wilkins, G. T., Choong, C. Y. P., et al.: Inaccuracy of mitral pressure half-time immediately after percutaneous mitral valvotomy. Circulation 78:980, 1988.

146. Yoneda, Y., Suwa, M., Hanada, H., et al.: Noninvasive detection of left ventricular diastolic dysfunction using M-mode echocardiography to assess left ventricular posterior wall kinetics in hypertrophic cardiomyopathy. Am. J. Cardiol. 70:1583, 1992.

147. Nishimura, R. A., Rihal, C. S., Tajik, A. J., et al.: Accurate measurement of the transmitral gradient in patient with mitral stenosis: A simultaneous catheterization and Doppler echocardiographic study. J. Am. Coll. Cardiol. 24:152, 1994.

148. Fredman, C. S., Pearson, A. C., Labovitz, A. J., et al.: Comparison of hemodynamic pressure half-time method and Gorlin formula with Doppler and echocardiographic determination of mitral valve area in

patients with combined mitral stenosis and regurgitation. Am. Heart J. *119*:121, 1990.

149. Abascal, V. M., Wilkins, G. T., O'Shea, J. P., et al.: Prediction of successful outcome in 130 patients undergoing percutaneous balloon mitral valvotomy. Circulation *82*:448, 1990.

150. Chen, C., Wang, X., Wang, Y., et al.: Value of two-dimensional echocardiography in selecting patients and balloon sizes for percutaneous balloon mitral valvuloplasty. J. Am. Coll. Cardiol. *14*:1651, 1989.

151. Reid, C. L., Otto, C. M., Davis, K. B., et al.: Influence of mitral valve morphology on mitral balloon commissurotomy: Immediate and six-month results from the NHLBI balloon valvuloplasty register. Am. Heart J. *123*:657, 1992.

152. Zaretskii, V. V., Kuznetsoa, L. M., Bobkov, V. V., et al.: Diagnosis of subvalvular adhesions in mitral stenosis by 2-dimensional echocardiography. Kardiologiia *25*:68, 1985.

153. Patel, A. K., Rowe, G. G., Thomsen, J. H., et al.: Detection and estimation of rheumatic mitral regurgitation in the presence of mitral stenosis by pulsed Doppler echocardiography. Am. J. Cardiol. *51*:986, 1983.

154. Rivera, J. M., Vandervoort, P. M., Morris, E., et al.: Visual assessment of valvular regurgitation: Comparison with quantitative Doppler measurements. J. Am. Soc. Echocardiogr. *7*:480, 1994.

155. Castello, R., Fagan, L., Lenzen, P., et al.: Comparison of transthoracic and transesophageal echocardiography for assessment of left-sided valvular regurgitation. Am. J. Cardiol. *68*:1677, 1991.

156. Spain, M. B., Smith, M. D., Grayburn, P. A., et al.: Quantitative assessment of mitral regurgitation by Doppler color flow imaging: Angiographic and hemodynamic correlations. J. Am. Coll. Cardiol. *13*:585, 1989.

157. Enriquez-Sarano, M., Tajik, A. J., Bailey, K. R., et al.: Color flow imaging compared with quantitative Doppler assessment of severity of mitral regurgitation: Influence of eccentricity of jet and mechanism of regurgitation. J. Am. Coll. Cardiol. *21*:1211, 1993.

158. Appleton, C. P., Hatle, L. K., Nellesen, U., et al.: Flow velocity acceleration in the left ventricle: A useful Doppler echocardiographic sign of hemodynamically significant mitral regurgitation. J. Am. Soc. Echocardiogr. *3*:35, 1990.

159. Utsunomiya, T., Ogawa, T., Doshi, R., et al.: Doppler color flow: "Proximal isovelocity surface area" method for estimating volume flow rate: Effects of orifice shape and machine factors. J. Am. Coll. Cardiol. *17*:1103, 1991.

160. Shiota, T., Jones, M., Teien, D. E., et al.: Evaluation of mitral regurgitation using a digitally determined color Doppler flow convergence "centerline" acceleration method. Circulation *89*:2879, 1994.

161. Grayburn, P. A., Fehske, W., Omran, H., et al.: Multiplane transesophageal echocardiographic assessment of mitral regurgitation by Doppler color flow mapping of the vena contracta. Am. J. Cardiol. *74*:912, 1994.

162. Kamp, O., Huitink, H., vanEenige, M. J., et al.: Value of pulmonary venous flow characteristics in the assessment of severity of native mitral valve regurgitation: An angiographic correlated study. J. Am. Soc. Echocardiogr. *5*:239, 1992.

163. McCully, R. B., Enriquez-Sarano, M., Tajik, A. J., et al.: Overestimation of severity of ischemic/functional mitral regurgitation by color Doppler jet area. Am. J. Cardiol. *74*:790, 1994.

164. Rivera, J. M., Mele, D., Vendervoort, P. M., et al.: Physical factors determining mitral regurgitation jet area. Am. J. Cardiol. *74*:515, 1994.

165. Ascah, K. J., Stewart, W. J., Jiang, L., et al.: A Doppler two-dimensional echocardiographic method for quantitation of mitral regurgitation. Circulation *72*:377, 1985.

166. Tribouilloy, C., Shen, W. F., Slama, M. A., et al.: Non-invasive measurement of the regurgitant fraction by pulsed Doppler echocardiography in isolated pure mitral regurgitation. Br. Heart J. *66*:290, 1991.

167. Burwash, I. G., Blackmore, G. L., and Koilpillai, C. J.: Usefulness of left atrial and left ventricular chamber sizes as predictors of the severity of mitral regurgitation. Am. J. Cardiol. *70*:774, 1992.

168. Shah, P. M.: Echocardiographic diagnosis of mitral valve prolapse. J. Am. Soc. Echocardiogr. *7*:286, 1994.

169. Dillon, J. C., Haine, C. L., Chang, S., et al.: Use of echocardiography in patients with prolapsed mitral valve. Am. J. Cardiol. *43*:503, 1971.

170. DeMaria, A. N., King, J. F., Bogren, H. G., et al.: The variable spectrum of echocardiographic manifestations of the mitral valve prolapse syndrome. Circulation *50*:33, 1974.

171. Sahn, D. J., Wood, J., Allen, H. D., et al.: Echocardiographic spectrum of mitral valve motion in children with and without mitral valve prolapse. The nature of false positive diagnosis. Am. J. Cardiol. *39*:422, 1977.

172. Markiewicz, W., Stoner, J., London, E., et al.: Mitral valve prolapse in one hunderd presumably healthy young females. Circulation *53*:464, 1976.

173. Sahn, D. J., Allen, H. D., Goldberg, S. J., et al.: Mitral valve prolapse in children. A problem defined by real-time cross-sectional echocardiography. Circulation *53*:651, 1976.

174. Morganroth, J., Jones, R. H., Chen, C. C., et al.: Two dimensional echocardiography in mitral, aortic and tricuspid valve prolapse. The clinical problem, cardiac nuclear imaging considerations and a proposed standard for diagnosis. Am. J. Cardiol. *46*:1164, 1980.

175. Krivokapich, J., Child, J. S., Dadourian, B. J., et al.: Reassessment of echocardiographic criteria for diagnosis of mitral valve prolapse. Am. J. Cardiol. *61*:131, 1988.

176. Levine, R. A., Stathogiannis, E., Newell, J. B., et al.: Reconsideration of echocardiographic standards for mitral valve prolapse: Lack of association between leaflet displacement isolated to the apical four chamber

177. Chun, P. K. C., and Sheehan, M. W.: Myxomatous degeneration of mitral valve M-mode and two-dimensional echocardiographic findings. Br. Heart J. *47*:404, 1982.

178. Ballester, M., Presbitero, P., Foale, R., et al.: Prolapse of the mitral valve in secundum atrial septal defect: A functional mechanism. Eur. Heart J. *4*:472, 1983.

179. Avgeropoulou, C. C., Rahko, P. S., and Patel, A. K.: Reliability of M-mode, two-dimensional, and Doppler echocardiography in diagnosing a flail mitral valve leaflet. J. Am. Soc. Echocardiogr. *2*:433, 1988.

180. Ballester, M., Foale, R., Presbitero, P., et al.: Cross-sectional echocardiographic features of ruptured chordae tendineae. Eur. Heart J. *4*:795, 1983.

181. Mintz, G. S., Kotler, M. N., Segal, B. L., et al.: Two-dimensional echocardiographic recognition of ruptured chordae tendineae. Circulation *57*:244, 1978.

182. Pearson, A. C., St. Vrain, J., Mrosek, A., et al.: Color Doppler echocardiographic evaluation of patients with a flail mitral leaflet. J. Am. Coll. Cardiol. *16*:232, 1990.

183. Shyu, K.-G., Lei, M.-H., Hwang, J.-J., et al.: Morphologic characterization and quantitative assessment of mitral regurgitation with ruptured chordae tendineae by transesophageal echocardiography. Am. J. Cardiol. *70*:1152, 1992.

184. Godley, R. W., Wann, L. S., Rogers, E. W., et al.: Incomplete mitral leaflet closure in patients with papillary muscle dysfunction. Circulation *63*:565, 1981.

185. Weyman, A. E., Feigenbaum, H., Dillon, J. C., et al.: Cross-sectional echocardiography in assessing the severity of valvular aortic stenosis. Circulation *52*:828, 1975.

186. Godley, R. W., Green, D., Dillon, J. C., et al.: Reliability of two-dimensional echocardiography in assessing the severity of valvular aortic stenosis. Chest *79*:657, 1981.

187. Tribouilloy, C., Shen, W. F., Peltier, M., et al.: Quantitation of aortic valve area in aortic stenosis with multiplane transesophageal echocardiography: Comparison with monoplane transesophageal approach. Am. Heart J. *128*:526, 1994.

188. Hoffmann, R., Flachskampf, F. A., and Hanrath, P.: Planimetry of orifice area in aortic stenosis using multiplane transesophageal echocardiography. J. Am. Coll. Cardiol. *22*:529, 1993.

189. Currie, P. J., Seward, J. B., Reeder, G. S., et al.: Continuous-wave Doppler echocardiographic assessment of severity of calcific aortic stenosis: A simultaneous Doppler-catheter correlative study in 100 adult patients. Circulation *71*:1162, 1985.

190. Warth, D. C., Stewart, W. J., Block, P. C., et al.: A new method to calculate aortic valve area without left heart catheterization. Circulation *70*:978, 1984.

191. Taylor, R.: Evolution of the continuity equation in the Doppler echocardiographic assessment of the severity of valvular aortic stenosis. J. Am. Soc. Echocardiogr. *3*:326, 1990.

192. Richards, K. L., Cannon, S. R., Miller, J. F., et al.: Calculation of aortic valve area by Doppler echocardiography: A direct application of the continuity equation. Circulation *73*:964, 1986.

193. Danielsen, R., Nordrehaug, J. E., and Vik-Mo, H.: Factors affecting Doppler echocardiographic valve area assessment in aortic stenosis. Am. J. Cardiol. *63*:1107, 1989.

194. Danielsen, R., Nordrehaug, J. E., Strangeland, L., et al.: Limitations in assessing the severity of aortic stenosis by Doppler gradients. Br. Heart J. *59*:551, 1988.

195. Yeager, M., Yock, P. G., and Popp, R. L.: Comparison of Doppler-derived pressure gradient to that determined at cardiac catheterization in adults with aortic valve stenosis: Implications of management. Am. J. Cardiol. *57*:644, 1986.

196. Reichek, N., and Devereux, R. B.: Reliable estimation of peak left ventricular systolic pressure by M-mode echographic-determined end-diastolic relative wall thickness: Identification of severe valvular aortic stenosis in adult patients. Am. Heart J. *103*:202, 1982.

197. Ciobanu, M., Abbasi, A. S., Allen, M., et al.: Pulsed Doppler echocardiography in the diagnosis and estimation of severity of aortic insufficiency. Am. J. Cardiol. *49*:339, 1982.

198. Grayburn, P. A., Smith, M. D., Handshoe, R., et al.: Detection of aortic insufficiency by standard echocardiography, pulsed Doppler echocardiography, and auscultation. Ann. Intern. Med. *104*:599, 1986.

199. Bouchard, A., Yock, P., Schiller, N. B., et al.: Value of color Doppler estimation of regurgitant volume in patients with chronic aortic insufficiency. Am. Heart J. *117*:1099, 1989.

200. Perry, G. J., Helmcke, F., Nanda, N. C., et al.: Evaluation of aortic insufficiency by Doppler color flow mapping. J. Am. Coll. Cardiol. *9*:952, 1987.

201. Samstad, S. O., Hegrenaes, L., Skjaerpe, T., et al.: Half time of the diastolic aortoventricular pressure difference by continuous wave Doppler ultrasound: A measure of the severity of aortic regurgitation? Br. Heart J. *61*:336, 1989.

202. Nishimura, R. A., Vonk, G. D., Rumberger, J. A., et al.: Semiquantitation of aortic regurgitation by different Doppler echocardiographic techniques and comparison with ultrafast computed tomography. Am. Heart J. *124*:995, 1992.

203. Yeung, A. C., Plappert, T., and St. John Sutton, M. G.: Calculation of aortic regurgitation orifice area by Doppler echocardiography: An application of the continuity equation. Br. Heart J. *68*:236, 1992.

204. Marcus, R. H., Neumann, A., Borow, M. K., et al.: Transmitral flow

velocity in symptomatic severe aortic regurgitation: Utility of Doppler for determination of preclosure of the mitral valve. Am. Heart J. 120:449, 1990.

205. Fioretti, P., Roelandt, J., Sclavo, M., et al.: Postoperative regression of left ventricular dimensions in aortic insufficiency: A long-term echocardiographic study. J. Am. Coll. Cardiol. 5:856, 1985.

206. Bonow, R. O., Rosing, D. R., Kent, K. M., et al.: Timing of operation for chronic aortic regurgitation. Am. J. Cardiol. 50:325, 1982.

207. Guyer, D. E., Gillam, L. D., Foale, R. A., et al.: Comparison of the echocardiographic and hemodynamic diagnosis of rheumatic tricuspid stenosis. J. Am. Coll. Cardiol. 3:1135, 1984.

208. Parris, T. M., Panidis, I. P., Ross, J., et al.: Doppler echocardiographic findings in rheumatic tricuspid stenosis. Am. J. Cardiol. 60:1414, 1987.

209. Blanchard, D., Diebold, B., Guermonprez, J. L., et al.: Doppler echocardiographic diagnosis and evaluation of tricuspid regurgitation. Arch. Mal. Coeur. 75:1357, 1982.

210. Mugge, A., Danile, W. G., Herrmann, G., et al.: Quantification of tricuspid regurgitant by Doppler color flow mapping after cardiac transplantation. Am. J. Cardiol. 66:884, 1990.

211. Ogawa, S., Hayashi, J., Sasaki, H., et al.: Evaluation of combined valvular prolapse syndrome by two-dimensional echocardiography. Circulation 65:174, 1982.

212. Eckfeldt, J. H., Weir, E. K., and Chesler, E.: Echocardiographic findings in ruptured chordae tendineae of the tricuspid valve. Am. Heart J. 105:1033, 1983.

213. Forman, M. B., Byrd, B. F., Oates, J. A., et al.: Two-dimensional echocardiography in the diagnosis of carcinoid heart disease. Am. Heart J. 107:492, 1984.

214. Winslow, T., Redberg, R., and Schiller, N. B.: Transesophageal echocardiography in the diagnosis of flail tricuspid valve. Am. Heart J. 123:1682, 1992.

215. Yvorchuk, K. J., and Chan, K.-L.: Application of transthoracic and transesophageal echocardiography in the diagnosis and management of infective endocarditis. J. Am. Soc. Echocardiogr. 7:294, 1994.

216. Dillon, J. C., Feigenbaum, H., Konecke, L. L., et al.: Echocardiographic manifestations of valvular vegetations. Am. Heart J. 86:698, 1973.

217. Roy, P., Tajik, A. J., Giuliani, E. R., et al.: Spectrum of echocardiographic findings in bacterial endocarditis. Circulation 53:474, 1976.

218. Gallis, H. A., Johnson, M. L., and Kisslo, J. A.: Two-dimensional echocardiographic assessment of vegetative endocarditis. Circulation 55:346, 1977.

219. Lowry, R. W., Zoghbi, W. A., Baker, W. B., et al.: Clinical impact of transesophageal echocardiography in the diagnosis and management of infective endocarditis. Am. J. Cardiol. 73:1089, 1994.

220. Sochowski, R. A., and Chan, K.-L.: Implication of negative results on a monoplane transesophageal echocardiographic study in patients with suspected infective endocarditis. J. Am. Coll. Cardiol. 21:216, 1993.

221. Blanchard, D. G., Ross, R. S., and Dittrich, H. C.: Non-bacterial thrombotic endocarditis. Assessment by transesophageal echocardiography. Chest 102:954, 1992.

222. Appelbe, A. F., Olson, D., Mixon, R., et al.: Libman-Sacks endocarditis mimicking intracardiac tumor. Am. J. Cardiol. 68:817, 1991.

223. Pollak, S. J., and Felner, J. M.: Echocardiographic identification of an aortic valve ring abscess. J. Am. Coll. Cardiol. 7:1167, 1986.

224. Leung, D. Y. C., Cranney, G. B., Hopkins, A. P., et al.: Role of transesophageal echocardiography in the diagnosis and management of aortic root abscess. Br. Heart J. 72:175, 1994.

225. Teskey, R. J., Chan, K.-L., and Beanlands, D. S.: Diverticulum of the mitral valve complicating bacterial endocarditis: Diagnosis by transesophageal echocardiography. Am. Heart J. 118:1063, 1989.

226. Wann, L. S., Pyhel, H. J., Judson, W. E., et al.: Ball variance in a Harken mitral prosthesis. Echocardiographic and phonocardiographic features. Chest 72:785, 1977.

227. Pfeifer, J., Goldschlager, N., Sweatman, T., et al.: Malfunction of mitral ball valve prosthesis due to thrombus. Am. J. Cardiol. 29:95, 1972.

229. Clements, S. D., and Perkins, J. V.: Malfunction of a Bjork-Shiley prosthetic heart valve in the mitral position producing an abnormal echocardiographic pattern. J. Clin. Ultrasound 6:334, 1978.

230. Mehta, A., Kessler, K. M., Tamer, D., et al.: Two-dimensional echographic observations in major detachment of a prosthetic aortic valve. Am. Heart J. 101:231, 1981.

231. Alam, M., Goldstein, S., and Lakier, J. B.: Echocardiographic changes in the thickness of porcine valves with time. Chest 79:663, 1981.

232. Bansal, R. C., Morrison, D. L., and Jacobsen, J. G.: Echocardiography of porcine aortic prostheses with flail leaflets due to degeneration and calcification. Am. Heart J. 107:591, 1984.

233. Burstow, D. J., Nishimura, R. A., Bailey, K. R., et al.: Continuous wave Doppler echocardiographic measurement of prosthetic valve gradients. Circulation 80:504, 1989.

234. Ryan, T., Armstrong, W. F., Dillon, J. C., et al.: Doppler echocardiographic evaluation of patients with porcine mitral valves. Am. Heart J. 111:237, 1986.

235. Ferrara, R. P., Labovitz, A. J., Wiens, R. D., et al.: Prosthetic mitral regurgitation detected by Doppler echocardiography. Am. J. Cardiol. 55:229, 1985.

236. Chambers, J., Monaghan, M., and Jackson, G.: Colour Doppler mapping in the assessment of prosthetic valve regurgitation. Br. Heart J. 62:1, 1989.

237. Rothbart, R. M., Castriz, J. L., Harding, L. V., et al.: Determination of aortic valve area by two-dimensional and Doppler echocardiography in patients with normal and stenotic bioprosthetic valves. J. Am. Coll. Cardiol. 15:817, 1990.

238. Weinstein, I. R., Marbarger, J. P., and Perez, J. E.: Ultrasonic assessment of the St. Jude prosthetic valve: M-mode, two-dimensional and Doppler echocardiography. Circulation 68:897, 1983.

239. Khandheria, B. K., Seward, J. B., Oh, J. K., et al.: Value and limitations of transesophageal echocardiography in assessment of mitral valve prostheses. Circulation 83:1956, 1991.

240. Daniel, W. G., Mugge, A., Grote, J., et al.: Comparison of transthoracic and transesophageal echocardiography for detection of abnormalities of prosthetic and bioprosthetic valves in the mitral and aortic positions. Am. J. Cardiol. 71:210, 1993.

241. Gueret, P., Vignon, P., Fournier, P., et al.: Transesophageal echocardiography for the diagnosis and management of nonobstructive thrombosis of mechanical mitral valve prosthesis. Circulation 91:103, 1995.

242. Taams, M. A., Gussenhoven, E. J., Cahalan, M. K., et al.: Transesophageal Doppler color flow imaging in the detection of native and Bjork-Shiley mitral valve regurgitation. J. Am. Coll. Cardiol. 13:95, 1989.

243. Alam, M., Rosman, H. S., and Sun, I.: Transesophageal echocardiographic evaluation of St. Jude Medical and bioprosthetic valve endocarditis. Am. Heart J. 123:236, 1992.

244. Nair, C. K., Thomson, W., Ryschon, K., et al.: Long-term follow-up of patients with echocardiographically detected mitral annular calcium and comparison with age- and sex-matched control subjects. Am. J. Cardiol. 63:465, 1989.

CONGENITAL HEART DISEASE

245. VanPraagh, R.: Diagnosis of complex congenital heart disease: Morphologic-anatomic method and terminology. Cardiovasc. Intervent. Radiol. 7:115, 1984.

246. Lipshultz, S. E., Sanders, S. P., Mayer, J. E., et al.: Are routine preoperative cardiac catheterization and angiography necessary before repair of ostium primum atrial septal defect? J. Am. Coll. Cardiol. 11:373, 1988.

247. Huhta, J. C., Glasow, P., Murphy, D. J., et al.: Surgery without catheterization for congenital heart defects: Management of 100 patients. J. Am. Coll. Cardiol. 9:823, 1987.

248. Santoro, G., Marino, B., DiCarlo, D., et al.: Echocardiographically guided repair of tetralogy of Fallot. Am. J. Cardiol. 73:808, 1994.

249. Foale, R., Stefanini, L., Rickards, A., et al.: Left and right ventricular morphology in complex congenital heart disease defined by two dimensional echocardiography. Am. J. Cardiol. 49:93, 1982.

250. Silverman, N. H.: An ultrasonic approach to the diagnosis of cardiac situs, connections, and malpositions. Cardiol. Clin. 1:473, 1983.

251. Hagler, D. J., Tajik, A. J., Seward, J. B., et al.: Atrioventricular and ventriculoarterial discordance (corrected transposition of the great arteries). Wide-angle two-dimensional echocardiographic assessment of ventricular morphology. Mayo Clin. Proc. 56:591, 1981.

252. Lesbre, J. P., Scheuble, C., Kalisa, A., et al.: Echocardiography in the diagnosis of severe aortic valve stenosis in adults. Arch. Mal. Coeur. 76:1, 1983.

253. Brandenburg, R. O., Jr., Tajik, A. J., Edwards, W. D., et al.: Accuracy of 2-dimensional echocardiographic diagnosis of congenitally bicuspid aortic valve: Echocardiographic-anatomic correlation in 115 patients. Am. J. Cardiol. 51:1469, 1983.

254. Smallhorn, J., Tommasini, G., Deanfield, J., et al.: Congenital mitral stenosis. Anatomical and functional assessment by echocardiography. Br. Heart J. 45:527, 1981.

255. Trowitzsch, E., Bano-Rodrigo, A., Burger, B. M., et al.: Two-dimensional echocardiographic findings in double orifice mitral valve. J. Am. Coll. Cardiol. 6:383, 1985.

256. Weyman, A. E., Hurwitz, R. A., Girod, D. A., et al.: Cross-sectional echocardiographic visualization of the stenotic pulmonary valve. Circulation 56:769, 1977.

257. Johnson, G. L., Kwan, O. L., Handshoe, S., et al.: Accuracy of combined two-dimensional echocardiography and continuous wave Doppler recordings in the estimation of pressure gradient in right ventricular outlet obstruction. J. Am. Coll. Cardiol. 3:1013, 1984.

258. Hagler, D. J., Tajik, A. J., Seward, J. B., et al.: Noninvasive assessment of pulmonary valve stenosis, aortic valve stenosis, and coarctation of the aorta in critically ill neonates. Am. J. Cardiol. 57:369, 1986.

259. Shiina, A., Seward, J. B., Edwards, W. D., et al.: Two-dimensional echocardiographic spectrum of Ebstein's anomaly: Detailed anatomic assessment. J. Am. Coll. Cardiol. 3:356, 1984.

260. Radford, D. J., Graff, R. F., and Neilson, G. H.: Diagnosis and natural history of Ebstein's anomaly. Br. Heart J. 54:517, 1985.

261. Milner, S., Meyer, R. A., Venables, A. W., et al.: Mitral and tricuspid valve closure in congenital heart disease. Circulation 53:513, 1976.

262. Meyer, R. A., and Kaplan, S.: Echocardiography in the diagnosis of hypoplasia of the left or right ventricle in the neonate. Circulation 46:55, 1972.

263. Lundstrom, N. R.: Ultrasound cardiographic studies of the mitral valve region in young infants with mitral atresia, mitral stenosis, hypoplasia of the left ventricle and cor triatriatum. Circulation 45:324, 1972.

264. Weyman, A. E., Caldwell, R. L., Hurwitz, R. A., et al.: Cross-sectional echocardiographic characterization of aortic obstruction: I. Supravalvular aortic stenosis and aortic hypoplasia. Circulation 57:491, 1978.

265. Cabrera, A., Pastor, E., and Lekuona, I.: Congenital aortic atresia with intact ventricular septum and normal left ventricle. Diagnosis by cross-sectional echocardiography. Int. J. Cardiol. 8:339, 1985.

266. Davis, R. A., Feigenbaum, H., Chang, S., et al.: Echocardiographic manifestations of discrete subaortic stenosis. Am. J. Cardiol. *33*:277, 1974.

267. DiSessa, T. G., Hagan, A. D., Isabel-Jones, J. B., et al.: Two-dimensional echocardiographic evaluation of discrete subaortic stenosis from the apical long axis view. Am. Heart J. *101*:774, 1981.

268. Gnanapragasam, J. P., Houston, A. B., Doig, W. B., et al.: Transesophageal echocardiographic assessment of fixed subaortic obstruction in children. Br. Heart J. *66*:281, 1991.

269. Sreeram, N., Franks, R., and Walsh, K.: Aortic-ventricular tunnel in a neonate: Diagnosis and management based on cross sectional and colour Doppler ultrasonography. Br. Heart J. *65*:161, 1991.

270. Valdes-Cruz, L. M., Jones, M., Scagnelli, S., et al.: Prediction of gradients in fibrous subaortic stenosis by continous wave two-dimensional Doppler echocardiography: Animal studies. J. Am. Coll. Cardiol. *5*:1363, 1985.

271. Weyman, A. E., Dillon, J. C., Feigenbaum, H., et al.: Echocardiographic differentiation of infundibular from valvular pulmonary stenosis. Am. J. Cardiol. *36*:21, 1975.

272. Caldwell, R. L., Weyman, A. G., Hurwitz, R. A., et al.: Right ventricular outflow tract assessment by cross-sectional echocardiography in tetralogy of Fallot. Circulation *59*:395, 1979.

273. Horowitz, M. D., Zager, W., Bilsker, M., et al.: Cor triatriatum in adults. Am. Heart J. *126*:472, 1993.

274. Lengyel, M., Arvay, A., and Biro, V.: Two-dimensional echocardiographic diagnosis of cor triatriatum. *59*:484, 1987.

275. Sullivan, I. D., Robinson, P. J., DeLeval, M., et al.: Membranous supravalvular mitral stenosis: A treatable form of congenital heart disease. J. Am. Coll. Cardiol. *8*:159, 1986.

276. Magherini, A., Azzolina, G., Weichmann, V., et al.: Pulsed Doppler echocardiography for diagnosis of ventricular septal defects. Br. Heart J. *43*:143, 1980.

277. Helmcke, F., deSouza, A., Nanda, N. C., et al.: Two-dimensional and color Doppler assessment of ventricular septal defect of congenital origin. Am. J. Cardiol. *63*:1112, 1989.

278. Sommer, R. J., Golinko, R. J., and Ritter, S. B.: Intracardiac shunting in children with ventricular septal defect: Evaluation with Doppler color flow mapping. J. Am. Coll. Cardiol. *16*:1437, 1990.

279. Sutherland, G. S., Smyllie, J. H., Ogilvie, B. C., et al.: Colour flow imaging in the diagnosis of multiple ventricular septal defects. Br. Heart J. *62*:43, 1989.

280. Sharif, D. S., Huhta, J. C., Maranttz, P., et al.: Two-dimensional echocardiographic determination of ventricular septal defect size: Correlation with autopsy. Am. Heart J. *117*:1333, 1989.

281. Rigby, M. L., Anderson, R. H., Gibson, D., et al.: Two dimensional echocardiographic categorisation of the univentricular heart. Br. Heart J. *46*:603, 1981.

282. Houston, A. B., Lim, M. K., Doig, W. B., et al.: Doppler assessment of the interventricular pressure drop in patients with ventricular septal defects. Br. Heart J. *60*:50, 1988.

283. Shub, C., Dimopoulos, I. N., Seward, J. B., et al.: Sensitivity of two-dimensional echocardiography in the direct visualization of atrial septal defect utilizing the subcostal approach: Experience with 154 patients. J. Am. Coll. Cardiol. *2*:127, 1983.

284. Mehta, R. H., Helmcke, F., Nanda, N. C., et al.: Uses and limitations of transthoracic echocardiography in the assessment of atrial septal defect in the adult. Am. J. Cardiol. *67*:288, 1991.

285. Nasser, F. N., Tajik, A. J., Stewart, J. B., et al.: Diagnosis of sinus venosus atrial septal defect by two-dimensional echocardiography. Mayo Clin. Proc. *56*:568, 1981.

286. Sonoda, M., Wang, Y., Sakamoto, T., et al.: Visualization of sinus venosus-type atrial septal defect by biplane transesophageal echocardiography. J. Am. Soc. Echocardiogr. *7*:179, 1994.

287. Hausmann, D., Daniel, W. G., Mugge, A., et al.: Value of transesophageal color Doppler echocardiography for detection of different types of atrial septal defects in adults. J. Am. Soc. Echocardiogr. *5*:481, 1992.

288. Bartel, T., Muller, S., and Geibel, A.: Preoperative assessment of cor triatriatum in an adult by dynamic three dimensional echocardiography was more informative than transesophageal echocardiography or magnetic resonance imaging. Br. Heart J. *72*:4989, 1994.

289. Vogel, M., and Losch, S.: Dynamic three-dimensional echocardiography with a computed tomography imaging probe: Initial clinical experience with transthoracic application in infants and children with congenital heart defects. Br. Heart J. *71*:462, 1994.

290. Pollick, C., Sullivan, H., Cujec, B., et al.: Doppler color-flow imaging assessment of shunt size in atrial septal defect. Circulation *78*:522, 1988.

291. Weyman, A. E., Wann, L. S., Caldwell, R. L., et al.: Negative contrast echocardiography: A new method for detecting left-to-right shunts. Circulation *59*:498, 1979.

292. VanHare, G. G., and Silverman, N. H.: Contrast two-dimensional echocardiography in congenital heart disease: Techniques, indications and clinical utility. J. Am. Coll. Cardiol. *13*:673, 1989.

293. Konstantinides, S., Kasper, W., Geibel, A., et al.: Detection of left-to-right shunt in atrial septal defect by negative contrast echocardiography: A comparison of transthoracic and transesophageal approach. Am. Heart J. *126*:909, 1993.

294. Goswami, K. C., Shrivastava, S., Saxena, A., et al.: Echocardiographic diagnosis of total anomalous pulmonary venous connection. Am. Heart J. *126*:433, 1993.

295. Romero-Cardenas, A., Vargas-Barron, J., Rylaarsdam, M., et al.: Total anomalous pulmonary venous return: Diagnosis by transesophageal echocardiography. Am. Heart J. *121*:1831, 1991.

296. Barron, J. V., Sahn, D. J., Valdes-Cruz, L. M., et al.: Two-dimensional echocardiographic features of ventricular septal aneurysm paradoxically bulging into the left ventricular outflow tract. Am. Heart J. *104*:156, 1982.

297. Schneider, B., Hofmann, T., Meinertz, T., et al.: Diagnostic value of transesophageal echocardiography in atrial septal aneurysm. Int. J. Cardiac Imaging *8*:143, 1992.

298. Wolf, W. J., Casta, A., and Sapire, D. W.: Atrial septal aneurysms in infants and children. Am. Heart J. *113*:1149, 1987.

299. Belkin, R. N., Waugh, R. A., and Kisslo, J.: Interatrial shunting in atrial septal aneurysm. Am. J. Cardiol. *57*:310, 1986.

300. Belkin, R. N., Pollack, B. D., Ruggiero, M. L., et al.: Comparison of transesophageal and transthoracic echocardiography with contrast and color flow Doppler in the detection of patent foramen ovale. Am. Heart J. *128*:520, 1994.

301. Stoddard, M. D., Keedy, D. L., Dawkins, P. R., et al.: The cough test is superior to the Valsalva maneuver, the delineation of right-to-left shunting through a patent foramen ovale during contrast transesophageal echocardiography. Am. Heart J. *125*:185, 1993.

302. Stollberger, C., Schneider, B., Abzieher, F., et al.: Diagnosis of patent foramen ovale by transesophageal contrast echocardiography. Am. J. Cardiol. *71*:604, 1993.

303. Beppu, S., Nimura, Y., Nagata, S., et al.: Diagnosis of endocardial cushion defect with cross-sectional and M-mode scanning of echocardiography. Differentiation from secundum atrial septal defect. Br. Heart J. *38*:911, 1976.

304. Beppu, S., Nimura, Y., Saka, H., et al.: Mitral cleft in ostium primum atrial septal defect assessed by cross-sectional echocardiography. Circulation *62*:1099, 1980.

305. Rice, M. J., Seward, J. B., Edwards, W. D., et al.: Straddling atrioventricular valve: Two-dimensional echocardiographic diagnosis, classification and surgical implications. Am. J. Cardiol. *55*:505, 1985.

306. Milne, M. J., Sung, R. Y. T., Fok, T. F., et al.: Doppler echocardiographic assessment of shunting via the ductus arteriosus in newborn infants. Am. J. Cardiol. *64*:102, 1989.

307. Liao, P.-K., Su, W.-J., and Hung, J.-S.: Doppler echocardiographic flow characteristics of isolated patent ductus arteriosus: Better delineation by Doppler color flow mapping. J. Am. Coll. Cardiol. *12*:1285, 1988.

308. Vogt, J., Rupprath, G., Grimm, T., et al.: Qualitative and quantitative evaluation of supravalvular aortic stenosis by cross-sectional echocardiography. Pediatr. Cardiol. *3*:13, 1982.

309. Snider, A. R., and Silverman, N. H.: Suprasternal notch echocardiography: A two-dimensional technique for evaluating congenital heart disease. Circulation *63*:165, 1981.

310. Rao, P. S., and Carey, P.: Doppler ultrasound in the prediction of pressure gradients across aortic coarctation. Am. Heart. J. *118*:299, 1989.

311. Simpson, I. A., Sahn, D. J., Valdes-Cruz, L. M., et al.: Color Doppler flow mapping in patients with coarctation of the aorta: New observations and improved evaluation with color flow diameter and proximal acceleration as predictors of severity. Circulation *77*:736, 1988.

312. Hagler, D. J., Tajik, A. J., Seward, J. B., et al.: Double-outlet right ventricle: Wide-angle two dimensional echocardiographic observations. Circulation *63*:419, 1981.

313. Daskalopoulos, D. A., Edwards, W. D., Driscoll, D. J., et al.: Correlation of two-dimensional echocardiographic and autopsy findings in complete transposition of the great arteries. J. Am. Coll. Cardiol. *2*:1151, 1983.

314. Marin-Garcia, J., and Tonkin, I. L. D.: Two-dimensional echocardiographic evaluation of persistent truncus arteriosus. Am. J. Cardiol. *50*:1376, 1982.

315. Marino, B., DeSimone, G., Pasquini, L., et al.: Complete transposition of the great arteries: Visualization of left and right outflow tract obstruction by oblique subcostal two-dimensional echocardiography. Am. J. Cardiol. *55*:1140, 1985.

316. Sahn, D. J., Terry, R., O'Rourke, R., et al.: Multiple crystal cross-sectional echocardiography in the diagnosis of cyanotic congenital heart disease. Circulation *50*:230, 1974.

317. Meissner, M. D., Panidis, I. P., Eshaghpour, E., et al.: Corrected transposition of the great arteries: Evaluation by two-dimensional and Doppler echocardiography. Am. Heart J. *111*:599, 1986.

318. Chin, A. J., Larsen, R. L., Seliem, M. A., et al.: Noninvasive imaging of intraatrial baffles in infants and children. J. Am. Soc. Echocardiogr. *6*:45, 1993.

319. Arisawa, J., Morimoto, S., Ikezoe, J., et al.: Pulsed Doppler echocardiographic assessment of portal venous flow patterns in patients after the Fontan operation. Br. Heart J. *69*:41, 1993.

320. Nascimento, R., Cunha, D. L., Bastos, P., et al.: Echo-Doppler study of right ventricular filling in asymptomatic patients with Senning operation for transposition of the great arteries. Am. J. Cardiol. *68*:693, 1991.

ISCHEMIC HEART DISEASE

321. Buda, A. J., Zotz, R. J., Pace, D. P., et al.: Comparison of two-dimensional echocardiographic wall motion and wall thickening abnormalities in relation to the myocardium at risk. Am. Heart J. *111*:587, 1986.

322. Heger, J. J., Weyman, A. E., Wann, L. S., et al.: Cross-sectional echocardiographic analysis of the extent of left ventricular asynergy in acute myocardial infarction. Circulation *61*:1113, 1980.

323. Xiao, H. B., Lee, C. H., and Gibson, D. G.: Effect of left bundle branch block on diastolic function in dilated cardiomyopathy. Br. Heart J. 66:443, 1991.

325. Lehmann, K. G., Lee, F. A., McKenzie, W. B., et al.: Onset of altered interventricular septal motion during cardiac surgery. Circulation 82: 1325, 1990.

326. Buda, A. J., Lefkowitz, C. A., and Gallagher, K. P.: Augmentation of regional function in nonischemic myocardium during coronary occlusion measured with two-dimensional echocardiography. J. Am. Coll. Cardiol. 16:175, 1990.

327. Previtali, M., Lanzarini, L., Fetiveau, R., et al.: Comparison of dobutamine stress echocardiography, dipyridamole stress echocardiography and exercise stress testing for diagnosis of coronary artery disease. Am. J. Cardiol. 72:865, 1993.

328. Beleslin, B. D., Ostojic, M., Stepanovic, J., et al.: Stress echocardiography in the detection of myocardial ischemia. Head-to-head comparison of exercise, dobutamine, and dipyridamole tests. Circulation 90:1168, 1994.

329. Roger, V. L., Pellikka, P. A., Oh, J. K., et al.: Stress echocardiography: I. Exercise echocardiography: Techniques, implementation, clinical applications, and correlations. Mayo Clin. Proc. 70:5, 1995.

330. Quinones, M. A., Verani, M. S., Haichin, R. M., et al.: Exercise echocardiography versus 201 T1 single photon emission computed tomography in evaluation of coronary artery disease. Circulation 85:1026, 1992.

331. Rober, V. L., Pellikka, P. A., Oh, J. K., et al.: Identification of multivessel coronary artery disease by exercise echocardiography. J. Am. Coll. Cardiol. 24:109, 1994.

332. Hecht, H. S., et al.: Digital supine bicycle stress echocardiography: A new technique for evaluating coronary artery disease. J. Am. Coll. Cardiol. 21:950, 1993.

333. Ryan, T., Segar, D. S., Sawada, S. G., et al.: Detection of coronary artery disease with upright bicycle exercise echocardiography. J. Am. Soc. Echocardiogr. 6:186, 1993.

334. Anselmi, M., Golia, G., Marino, P., et al.: Usefulness of transesophageal atrial pacing combined with two-dimensional echocardiography (echopacing) in predicting the presence and site of residual jeopardized myocardium after uncomplicated acute myocardial infarction. Am. J. Cardiol. 73:534, 1994.

335. Pellikka, P. A., Roger, V. L., Oh, J. K., et al.: Stress echocardiography: II. Dobutamine stress echocardiography: Techniques, implementation, clinical applications, and correlations. Mayo Clin. Proc. 70:16, 1995.

336. Takeishi, Y., Chiba, J., Abe, S., et al.: Adenosine-echocardiography for the detection of coronary artery disease. J. Cardiol. 24:1, 1994.

337. Picano, E., Parodi, O., Lattanzi, F., et al.: Assessment of anatomic and physiological severity of single-vessel coronary artery lesions by dipyridamole echocardiography. Circulation 89:753, 1994.

338. Segar, D. S., Brown, S. E., Sawada, S. G., et al.: Dobutamine stress echocardiography: Correlation with coronary lesion severity as determined by quantitative angiography. J. Am. Coll. Cardiol. 19:1197, 1992.

339. Madu, E. C., Ahmar, W., Arthur, J., et al.: Clinical utility of digital dobutamine stress echocardiography in the noninvasive evaluation of coronary artery disease. Arch. Intern. Med. 154:1065, 1994.

340. Marangelli, V., Iliceto, S., Piccinni, G., et al.: Detection of coronary artery disease by digital stress echocardiography: Comparison of exercise, transesophageal atrial pacing and dipyridamole echocardiography. J. Am. Coll. Cardiol. 24:117, 1994.

341. Marcovitz, P. A., and Armstrong, W. F.: Accuracy of dobutamine stress echocardiography in detecting coronary artery disease. Am. J. Cardiol. 69:1269, 1992.

342. Sawada, S. G., Segar, D. S., Ryan, T., et al.: Echocardiographic detection of coronary artery disease during dobutamine infusion. Circulation 83:1605, 1991.

343. Camerieri, A., Picano, E., Landi, P., et al.: Prognostic value of dipyridamole echocardiography early after myocardial infarction in elderly patients. J. Am. Coll. Cardiol. 22:1809, 1993.

344. Takeuchi, M., Araki, M., Nakashima, Y., et al.: The detection of residual ischemia and stenosis in patients with acute myocardial infarction with dobutamine stress echocardiography. J. Am. Soc. Echocardiogr. 7:242, 1994.

345. Lalka, S. G., Sawada, S. G., Dalsing, M. C., et al.: Dobutamine stress echocardiography as a predictor of cardiac events associated with aortic surgery. J. Vasc. Surg. 15:831, 1992.

346. Dávila-Román, V. G., Waggoner, A. D., Sicard, G. A., et al.: Dobutamine stress echocardiography predicts surgical outcome in patients with an aortic aneurysm and peripheral vascular disease. J. Am. Coll. Cardiol. 21:957, 1993.

347. Sawada, S. G., Ryan, T., Conley, M. J., et al.: Prognostic value of a normal exercise echocardiogram. Am. Heart J. 120:49, 1990.

348. Maseika, P. K., Nadazdin, A., and Oakley, C. M.: Prognostic value of dobutamine echocardiography in patients with high pretest likelihood of coronary artery disease. Am. J. Cardiol. 71:33, 1993.

349. Krivokapich, J., Child, J. S., Gerber, R. S., et al.: Prognostic usefulness of positive or negative exercise stress echocardiography for predicting coronary events in ensuing twelve months. Am. J. Cardiol. 71:646, 1993.

350. Akosah, K. O., Porter, T. R., Simon, R., et al.: Ischemia-induced regional wall motion abnormality is improved after coronary angioplasty: Demonstration by dobutamine stress echocardiography. J. Am. Coll. Cardiol. 21:584, 1993.

351. Hecht, H. S., DeBord, L., Shaw, R., et al.: Usefulness of supine bicycle stress echocardiography for detection of restenosis after percutaneous transluminal coronary angioplasty. Am. J. Cardiol. 71:293, 1993.

352. Stoddard, M. F., Pearson, A. C., Kern, M. J., et al.: Left ventricular diastolic function: Comparison of pulsed Doppler echocardiographic and hemodynamic indexes in subjects with and without coronary artery disease. J. Am. Coll. Cardiol. 13:327, 1989.

353. Fujii, J., Yazaki, Y., Sawada, H., et al.: Noninvasive assessment of left and right ventricular filling in myocardial infarction with a two-dimensional Doppler echocardiographic method. J. Am. Coll. Cardiol. 5:1155, 1985.

354. Erbel, R., Schweizer, P., Meyer, J., et al.: Sensitivity of cross-sectional echocardiography in detection of impaired global and regional left ventricular function: Prospective study. Int. J. Cardiol. 7:375, 1985.

355. Ren, J-F., Kotler, M. N., Hakki, A-H., et al.: Quantitation of regional left ventricular function by two-dimensional echocardiography in normals and patients with coronary artery disease. Am. Heart J. 110:552, 1985.

356. Shiina, A., Tajik, A. J., Smith, H. C., et al.: Prognostic significance of regional wall motion abnormality in patients with prior myocardial infarction: A prospective correlative study of two-dimensional echocardiography and angiography. Mayo Clin. Proc. 61:254, 1986.

357. Van Reet, R. E., Quinones, M. A., Poliner, L. R., et al.: Comparison of two-dimensional echocardiography with gated radionuclide ventriculography in the evaluation of global and regional left ventricular function in acute myocardial infarction. J. Am. Coll. Cardiol. 3:243, 1984.

358. Iliceto, S., Ricci, A., Sorino, M., et al.: Evaluation of the ejection fraction using two simplified echocardiographic methods in patients with ischemic heart disease and left ventricular asynergy. G. Ital. Cardiol. 15:142, 1985.

359. Ryan, T., Petrovic, O., Armstrong, W. F., et al.: Quantitative two-dimensional echocardiographic assessment of patients undergoing left ventricular aneurysmectomy. Am. Heart J. 111:714, 1986.

360. Visser, C. A., Kan, G., Meltzer, R. S., et al.: Assessment of left ventricular aneurysm resectability by two-dimensional echocardiography. Am. J. Cardiol. 56:857, 1985.

361. Katz, A. S., Harrigan, P., and Parisi, A. F.: The value and promise of echocardiography in acute myocardial infarction and coronary artery disease. Clin. Cardiol. 15:401, 1992.

362. Matsumoto, M., Watanabe, F., Goto, A., et al.: Left ventricular aneurysm and the prediction of left ventricular enlargement studied by two-dimensional echocardiography: Quantitative assessment of aneurysm size in relation to clinical course. Circulation 72:280, 1985.

363. Hamilton, K., Ellenbogen, K., Lowe, J. E., et al.: Ultrasound diagnosis of pseudoaneurysm and contiguous ventricular septal defect complicating inferior myocardial infarction. J. Am. Coll. Cardiol. 6:1160, 1985.

364. Sutherland, G. R., Smyllie, J. H., and Croelandt, J. R. T.: Advantages of colour flow imaging in the diagnosis of left ventricular pseudoaneurysm. Br. Heart J. 61:59, 1989.

365. Bansal, R. C., Pai, R. G., Hauck, A. J., et al.: Biventricular apical rupture and formation of pseudoaneurysm: Unique flow patterns by Doppler and color flow imaging. Am. Heart J. 124:497, 1992.

366. Burns, C. A., Paulsen, W., Arrowood, J. A., et al.: Improved identification of posterior left ventricular pseudoaneurysms by transesophageal echocardiography. Am. Heart J. 124:796, 1992.

367. Deshmukh, H. G., Khosla, S., and Jefferson, K. K.: Direct visualization of left ventricular free wall rupture by transesophageal echocardiography in acute myocardial infarction. Am. Heart J. 126:475, 1993.

368. Mascarenhas, D. A. N., Benotti, J. R., Daggett, W. M., et al.: Postinfarction septal aneurysm with delayed formation of left-to-right shunt. Am. Heart J. 122:226, 1991.

369. Stephens, J. D., Giles, M. R., and Banim, S. O.: Ruptured postinfarction ventricular septal aneurysm causing chronic congestive cardiac failure. Detection by two-dimensional echocardiography. Br. Heart J. 46:216, 1981.

370. Smith, G., Endresen, K., Sivertssen, E., and Semb, G.: Ventricular septal rupture diagnosed by simultaneous cross-sectional echocardiography and Doppler ultrasound. Eur. Heart J. 6:631, 1985.

371. Panidis, I. P., Mintz, G. S., Goel, I., et al.: Acquired ventricular septal defect after myocardial infarction: Detection by combined two-dimensional and Doppler echocardiography. Am. Heart J. 111:427, 1986.

372. Maurer, G., Czer, L. S. C., Shah, P. K., et al.: Assessment by Doppler color flow mapping of ventricular septal defect after acute myocardial infarction. Am. J. Cardiol. 64:668, 1989.

373. Smyllie, J. H., Sutherland, G. R., Geuskins, R., et al.: Doppler color flow mapping in the diagnosis of ventricular septal rupture and acute mitral regurgitation after myocardial infarction. J. Am. Coll. Cardiol. 15:1449, 1990.

374. Ballal, R. S., Sanyal, R. S., Nanda, N. C., et al.: Usefulness of transesophageal echocardiography in the diagnosis of ventricular septal rupture secondary to acute myocardial infarction. Am. J. Cardiol. 71:367, 1993.

375. Jugdutt, B. I., Sussex, B. A., Sivaram, C. A., et al.: Right ventricular infarction: Two-dimensional echocardiographic evaluation. Am. Heart J. 107:505, 1984.

376. Goldberger, J. J., Himelman, R. B., Wolfe, C. L., et al.: Right ventricular infarction: Recognition and assessment of its hemodynamic significance by two-dimensional echocardiography. J. Am. Soc. Echocardiogr. 4:140, 1991.

377. Doyle, T., Troup, P. J., and Wann, L. S.: Mid-diastolic opening of the

pulmonary valve after right ventricular infarction. J. Am. Coll. Cardiol. 5:366, 1985.

378. Lopez-Sendon, J., DeSa, E. L., Roldan, I., et al.: Inversion of the normal interatrial septum convexity in acute myocardial infarction: Incidence, clinical relevance and prognostic significance. J. Am. Coll. Cardiol. 15:801, 1990.

379. Asinger, R. W., Mikell, F. L., Elsperger, J., et al.: Incidence of left-ventricular thrombosis after acute transmural myocardial infarction. Serial evaluation by two-dimensional echocardiography. N. Engl. J. Med. 305:297, 1981.

380. Sharma, B., Carvalho, A., Wyeth, R., et al.: Left ventricular thrombi diagnosed by echocardiography in patients with acute myocardial infarction treated with intracoronary streptokinase followed by intravenous heparin. Am. J. Cardiol. 56:422, 1985.

381. Keren, A., Goldberg, S., Gottlieb, S., et al.: Natural history of left ventricular thrombi: Their appearance and resolution in the posthospitalization period of acute myocardial infarction. J. Am. Coll. Cardiol. 15:790, 1990.

382. Weintraub, W. S., and Ba'albaki, H. A.: Decision analysis concerning the application of echocardiography to the diagnosis and treatment of mural thrombi after anterior wall acute myocardial infarction. Am. J. Cardiol. 64:708, 1989.

383. Jugdutt, B. I., Sivaram, C. A., Wortman, C., et al.: Prospective two-dimensional echocardiographic evaluation of left ventricular thrombus and embolism after acute myocardial infarction. J. Am. Coll. Cardiol. 13:554, 1989.

384. Delemarre, B. J., Visser, C. A., Bot, H., et al.: Prediction of apical thrombus formation in acute myocardial infarction based on left ventricular spatial flow pattern. J. Am. Coll. Cardiol. 15:355, 1990.

385. Barzilai, B., Gessler, C., Perez, J. E., et al.: Significance of Doppler-detected mitral regurgitation in acute myocardial infarction. Am. J. Cardiol. 61:220, 1988.

386. Kono, T., Sabbah, H. N., Rosman, H., et al.: Mechanism of functional mitral regurgitation during acute myocardial ischemia. J. Am. Coll. Cardiol. 19:1101, 1992.

387. Hanlon, J. T., et al.: Echocardiography recognition of partial papillary muscle rupture. J. Am. Soc. Echocardiogr. 6:101, 1993.

388. Pierard, L. A., Albert, A., Henrard, L., et al.: Incidence and significance of pericardial effusion in acute myocardial infarction as determined by two-dimensional echocardiography. J. Am. Coll. Cardiol. 8:517, 1986.

389. Berning, J., Launbjerg, J., and Appleyard, M.: Echocardiographic algorithms for admission and predischarge prediction of mortality in acute myocardial infarction. Am. J. Cardiol. 69:1538, 1992.

390. Horowitz, R. S., Morganroth, J., Parrotto, C., et al.: Immediate diagnosis of acute myocardial infarction by two dimensional echocardiography. Circulation 65:323, 1982.

391. Sabia, P., Abbott, R. D., Afrookiteh, A., et al.: Importance of two-dimensional echocardiographic assessment of left ventricular systolic function in patients presenting to the emergency room with cardiac-related symptoms. Circulation 84:1615, 1991.

392. Kan, G., Visser, C. A., Koolen, J. J., et al.: Short and long term predictive value of admission wall motion score in acute myocardial infarction. Br. Heart J. 56:422, 1986.

393. Abernethy, M., Sharpe, N., Smith, H., et al.: Echocardiographic prediction of left ventricular volume after myocardial infarction. J. Am. Coll. Cardiol. 17:1527, 1991.

394. Ginzton, L. E., Conant, R., Rodrigues, D. M., et al.: Functional significance of hypertrophy of the noninfarcted myocardium after myocardial infarction in humans. Circulation 80:816, 1989.

395. Weiss, J. L., Marino, P. N., and Shapiro, E. P.: Myocardial infarction expansion: Recognition, significance and pathology. Am. J. Cardiol. 68:35D, 1991.

396. Jugdutt, B. I.: Identification of patients prone to infarct expansion by the degree of regional shape distortion on an early two-dimensional echocardiogram after myocardial infarction. Clin. Cardiol. 13:28, 1990.

397. Nishimura, R. A., Tajik, A. J., Shib, C., et al.: Role of two-dimensional echocardiography in the prediction of in-hospital complications after acute myocardial infarction. J. Am. Coll. Cardiol. 4:1080, 1984.

398. Abrams, D. S., Starling, M. R., Crawford, M. H., et al.: Value of noninvasive techniques for predicting early complications in patients with clinical class II acute myocardial infarction. J. Am. Coll. Cardiol. 2:818, 1983.

399. Bhatnagar, S. K., and Al-Yusuf, A. R.: The role of prehospital discharge two-dimensional echocardiography in determining the prognosis of survivors of first myocardial infarction. Am. Heart J. 109:472, 1985.

400. Ryan, T., Armstrong, W. F., O'Donnell, J. A., et al.: Risk stratification after acute myocardial infarction by means of exercise two-dimensional echocardiography. Am. Heart J. 114:1305, 1987.

401. Bourdillon, P. D. V., Broderick, T. M., Williams, E. S., et al.: Early recovery of regional left ventricular function after reperfusion in acute myocardial infarction assessed by serial two-dimensional echocardiography. Am. J. Cardiol. 63:641, 1989.

402. Otto, C. M., Stratton, J. R., Maynard, C., et al.: Echocardiographic evaluation of segmental wall motion early and late after thrombolytic therapy in acute myocardial infarction: The Western Washington tissue plasminogen activator emergency room trial. Am. J. Cardiol. 65:132, 1990.

403. Smart, S. C., Sawada, S., Ryan, T., et al.: Low-dose dobutamine echocardiography detects reversible dysfunction after thrombolytic therapy of acute myocardial infarction. Circulation 88:405, 1993.

404. Barilla, F., Gheorghiade, M., Alam, M., et al.: Low-dose dobutamine in

patients with acute myocardial infarction identifies viable but not contractile myocardium and predicts the magnitude of improvement in wall motion abnormalities in response to coronary revascularization. Am. Heart J. 122:1522, 1991.

405. Pierard, L. A., DeLandsheere, C. M., Berthe, C., et al.: Identification of viable myocardium by echocardiography during dobutamine infusion in patients with myocardial infarction after thrombolytic therapy: Comparison with positron emission tomography. J. Am. Coll. Cardiol. 15:1021, 1990.

406. Charney, R., Schwinger, M. E., Chun, J., et al.: Dobutamine echocardiography and resting-redistribution thallium-201 scintigraphy predicts recovery of hibernating myocardium after coronary revascularization. Am. Heart J. 128:864, 1994.

407. Cigarroa, C. G., deFilippi, C. R., Brickner, E., et al.: Dobutamine stress echocardiography identifies hibernating myocardium and predicts recovery of left ventricular function after coronary revascularization. Circulation 88:430, 1993.

408. Hausmann, D., Lundkvist, A.-J.S., Friedrich, G. J., et al.: Intracoronary ultrasound imaging: Intraobserver and interobserver variability of morphometric measurements. Am. Heart J. 128:674, 1994.

409. Hausmann, D., Lundkvist, A.-J. S., Friedrich, G., et al.: Lumen and plaque shape in atherosclerotic coronary arteries assessed by in vivo intracoronary ultrasound. Am. J. Cardiol. 74:573, 1994.

410. Rasheed, Q., Nair, R., Sheehan, H., et al.: Correlation of intracoronary ultrasound plaque characteristics in atherosclerotic coronary artery disease in patients with clinical variables. Am. J. Cardiol. 73:753, 1994.

411. Gerber, T. C., Erbel, R., Gorge, G., et al.: Extent of atherosclerosis and remodeling of the left main coronary artery determined by intravascular ultrasound. Am. J. Cardiol. 73:666, 1994.

412. Pinto, F. J., Chenzbraum, A., Botas, J., et al.: Feasibility of serial intracoronary ultrasound imaging for assessment of progression of intimal proliferation in cardiac transplant recipients. Circulation 90:348, 1994.

413. Yamagishi, M., Nissen, S. E., Booth, D. C., et al.: Coronary reactivity to nitroglycerin: Intravascular ultrasound evidence for the importance of plaque distribution. J. Am. Coll. Cardiol. 25:224, 1995.

414. Ge, J., Erbel, R., Gerber, T., et al.: Intravascular ultrasound imaging of angiographically normal coronary arteries: A prospective study in vivo. Br. Heart J. 71:572, 1994.

415. Nakamura, S., Colombo, A., Galione, A., et al.: Intracoronary ultrasound observations during stent implantation. Circulation 89:2026, 1994.

416. Mintz, G. S., Potkin, B. N., Keren, G., et al.: Intravascular ultrasound evaluation of the effect of rotational atherectomy in obstructive atherosclerotic coronary artery disease. Circulation 86:1383, 1992.

417. Hodgson, J. M., et al.: Intracoronary ultrasound imaging: Correlation of plaque morphology with angiography, clinical syndrome and procedural results in patients undergoing coronary angioplasty. J. Am. Coll. Cardiol. 21:35, 1993.

418. Kern, M. J., Aguirre, F. V., Donohue, T. J., et al.: Continuous coronary flow velocity monitoring during coronary interventions: Velocity trend patterns associated with adverse events. Am. Heart J. 128:426, 1994.

419. DiMario, C., Krams, R., Gil, R., et al.: Slope of the instantaneous hyperemic diastolic coronary flow velocity-pressure relation. A new index for assessment of the physiological significance of coronary stenosis in humans. Circulation 94:1315, 1994.

420. Deychak, Y. A., Segal, J., Reiner, J. S., et al.: Doppler guide wire–derived coronary flow reserve distal to intermediate stenoses used in clinical decision making regarding interventional therapy. Am. Heart J. 128:178, 1994.

421. Rossen, J. D., and Winniford, M. D.: Effect of increases in heart rate and arterial pressure on coronary flow reserve in humans. J. Am. Coll. Cardiol. 21:343, 1993.

422. Tardif, J.-C., Vannan, M. A., Taylor, K., et al.: Delineation of extended lengths of coronary arteries by multiplane transesophageal echocardiography. J. Am. Coll. Cardiol. 24:909, 1994.

423. Memmola, C., Iliceto, S., and Rizzon, P.: Detection of proximal stenosis of left coronary artery by digital transesophageal echocardiography: Feasibility, sensitivity, and specificity. J. Am. Soc. Echocardiogr. 6:149, 1993.

424. Isaaz, K., Bruntz, J. F., Ethevenot, G., et al.: Abnormal coronary flow velocity pattern in patients with left ventricular hypertrophy, angina pectoris, and normal coronary arteries: A transesophageal Doppler echocardiographic study. Am. Heart J. 128:500, 1994.

425. Isaaz, K., Bruntz, J. F., Ethevenot, G., et al.: Noninvasive assessment of coronary flow dynamics before and after coronary angioplasty using transesophageal Doppler. Am. J. Cardiol. 72:1238, 1993.

426. Yamagishi, M., Yasu, T., Ohara, K., et al.: Detection of coronary blood flow associated with left main coronary artery stenosis by transesophageal Doppler color flow echocardiography. J. Am. Coll. Cardiol. 17:87, 1991.

427. Faletra, F., Cipriani, M., Corno, R., et al.: Transthoracic high-frequency echocardiographic detection of atherosclerotic lesions in the descending portion of the left coronary artery. J. Am. Soc. Echocardiogr. 6:290, 1993.

428. Sawada, S. G., Ryan, T., Segar, D., et al.: Distinguishing ischemic cardiomyopathy from nonischemic dilated cardiomyopathy with coronary echocardiography. Am. Heart J. 19:1223, 1992.

429. Ching, K. J., Fulton, D. R., and Lapp, R.: One-year follow-up of cardiac and coronary artery disease in infants and children with Kawasaki disease. Am. Heart J. 115:1263, 1988.

430. Eteedgui, J. A., Neches, W. H., and Pahl, E.: The role of cross-sectional echocardiography in Kawasaki disease. Cardiol. Young. 1:221, 1991.

431. Capannari, T. E., Daniels, S. R., Meyer, R. A., et al.: Sensitivity, specificity, and predictive value of two-dimensional echocardiography in detecting coronary artery aneurysms in patients with Kawasaki disease. J. Am. Coll. Cardiol. 7:355, 1986.

432. Sanders, S. P., Parness, I. A., and Colan, S. D.: Recognition of abnormal connections of coronary arteries with the use of Doppler color flow mapping. J. Am. Coll. Cardiol. 13:922, 1989.

433. Oda, H., Kawada, Y., Toeda, T., et al.: Assessment of a coronary artery fistula to the pulmonary artery by transesophageal echocardiography. Am. Heart J. 125:1460, 1993.

434. Maire, R., Gallino, A., and Jenni, R.: Initial detection in a teenager of anomalous left coronary artery from the pulmonary artery by color Doppler echocardiography. Am. Heart J. 125:1803, 1993.

435. Thomas, M. R., Monaghan, M. J., Michalis, L. K., et al.: Aortoatrial fistulae diagnosed by transthoracic and transesophageal echocardiography: Advantages of the transesophageal approach. J. Am. Soc. Echocardiogr. 6:21, 1993.

436. Agati L., Voci P., Bilotta F., et al.: Influence of residual perfusion within the infarct zone on the natural history of left ventricular dysfunction after acute myocardial infarction: A myocardial contrast echocardiographic study. J. Am. Coll. Cardiol. 24:336, 1994.

437. Porter, T. R., D'Sa, A., Turner, C., et al.: Myocardial contrast echocardiography for the assessment of coronary blood flow reserve: Validation in humans. J. Am. Coll. Cardiol. 21:349, 1993.

438. Ito, H., Tomooka, T., Sakai, N., et al.: Lack of myocardial perfusion immediately after successful thrombolysis. Circulation 85:1699, 1992.

439. Voci, P., Bilotta, F., Merialdo, P., et al.: Myocardial contrast enhancement after intravenous injection of sonicated albumin microbubbles: A transesophageal echocardiography dipyridamole study. J. Am. Soc. Echocardiogr. 7:337, 1994.

440. Skyba, D. M., Jayaweera, A. R., Goodman, N. C., et al.: Quantification of myocardial perfusion with myocardial contrast echocardiography during left atrial injection of contrast. Implications for venous injection. Circulation 90:1513, 1994.

CARDIOMYOPATHIES

441. Shah, P. M., Taylor, R. D., and Wong, M.: Abnormal mitral valve coaptation in hypertrophic obstructive cardiomyopathy: Proposed role in systolic anterior motion of mitral valve. Am. J. Cardiol. 48:258, 1981.

442. Henry, W. L., Clark, C. E., Glancy, D. L., et al.: Echocardiographic measurement of the left ventricular outflow gradient in idiopathic hypertrophic subaortic stenosis. N. Engl. J. Med 288:989, 1973.

443. Panza, J. A., Maris, T. J., and Maron, B. J.: Development and determinants of dynamic obstruction to left ventricular outflow in young patients with hypertrophic cardiomyopathy. Circulation 85:1398, 1992.

444. Pollick, C., Rakowski, H., and Wigle, E. D.: Muscular subaortic stenosis: The quantitative relationship between systolic anterior motion and the pressure gradient. Circulation 69:43, 1984.

445. Henry, W. L., Clark, C. E., Griffith, J. M., et al.: Mechanism of left ventricular outflow obstruction in patients with obstructive aysmmetric septal hypertrophy (idiopathic hypertrophic subaortic stenosis). Am. J. Cardiol. 35:337, 1975.

446. Mintz, G. S., Kotler, M. N., Segal, B. L., et al.: Systolic anterior motion of the mitral valve in the absence of asymmetric septal hypertrophy. Circulation 57:256, 1978.

447. Maron, B. J., Epstein, S. E., Bonow, R. O., Wyngaarden, M. K., and Wesley, Y. E.: Obstructive hypertrophic cardiomyopathy associated with minimal left ventricular hypertrophy. Am. J. Cardiol. 53:377, 1984.

448. Jiang, L., Levine, R. A., King, M. E., et al.: An integrated mechanism for systolic anterior motion of the mitral valve in hypertrophic cardiomyopathy based on echocardiographic observations. Am. Heart J. 113:633, 1987.

449. Henry, W. L., Clark, C. E., Roberts, W. C., et al.: Difference in distributions of myocardial abnormalities in patients with obstructive and nonobstructive asymmetric septal hypertrophy (ASH): Echocardiographic and gross anatomic findings. Circulation 50:447, 1974.

450. Henry, W. L., Clark, C. E., and Epstein, S. E.: Asymmetric septal hypertrophy (ASH). Echocardiographic identification of the pathognomonic anatomic abnormality of IHSS. Circulation 47:225, 1973.

451. TenCate, F. J., Hugenholtz, P. G., and Roelandt, J.: Ultrasound study of dynamic behaviour of left ventricle in genetic asymmetric septal hypertrophy. Br. Heart J. 39:627, 1977.

452. Clark, C. E., Henry, W. L., and Epstein, S. E.: Familial prevalence and genetic transmission of idiopathic hypertrophic subaortic stenosis. N. Engl. J. Med. 289:709, 1973.

453. Lewis, J. F., and Maron, B. J.: Hypertrophic cardiomyopathy characterized by marked hypertrophy of the posterior left ventricular free wall: Significance and clinical implications. J. Am. Coll. Cardiol. 18:421, 1991.

454. Maron, B. J., Gottdiener, J. S., and Epstein S. E.: Patterns and significance of distribution of left ventricular hypertrophy in hypertrophic cardiomyopathy. A wide angle, two-dimensional echocardiographic study of 125 patients. Am. J. Cardiol. 48:418, 1981.

455. Webb, J. G., Sasson, Z., Rakowski, H., et al.: Apical hypertrophic cardiomyopathy: Clinical follow-up and diagnostic correlates. J. Am. Coll. Cardiol. 15:83, 1990.

456. Ko, Y.-L., Lei, M.-H., Chiang, F.-T., et al.: Apical hypertrophic cardiomyopathy of the Japanese type: Occurrence with familial hypertrophic cardiomyopathy in a family. Am. Heart J. 124:1626, 1992.

457. Lattanzi, F., Spirito, P., Picano, E., et al.: Quantitative assessment of ultrasonic myocardial reflectivity in hypertrophic cardiomyopathy. J. Am. Coll. Cardiol. 17:1085, 1991.

458. Maron, B. J., Gottdiener, J. S., Arce, J., et al.: Dynamic subaortic obstruction in hypertrophic cardiomyopathy: Pulsed Doppler echocardiography. J. Am. Coll. Cardiol. 6:1, 1985.

459. Zoghbi, W. A., Haichin, R. N., and Quinones, M. A.: Mid-cavity obstruction in apical hypertrophy: Doppler evidence of diastolic intraventricular gradient with higher apical pressure. Am. Heart J. 116:1469, 1988.

460. Panza, J. A., Petrone, R. K., Fananapazir, L., et al.: Utility of continuous wave Doppler echocardiography in the noninvasive assessment of left ventricular outflow tract pressure gradient in patients with hypertrophic cardiomyopathy. J. Am. Coll. Cardiol. 19:91, 1992.

461. Sasson, Z., Yock, P. G., Hatle, L. K., et al.: Doppler echocardiographic determination of the pressure gradient in hypertrophic cardiomyopathy. J. Am. Coll. Cardiol. 11:752, 1988.

462. Spirito, P., and Maron, B. J.: Relation between extent of left ventricular hypertrophy and diastolic filling abnormalities in hypertrophic cardiomyopathy. J. Am. Coll. Cardiol. 15:808, 1990.

463. Hoit, B. D., Penonen, E., Dalton, N., et al.: Doppler color flow mapping studies of jet formation and spatial orientation in obstructive hypertrophic cardiomyopathy. Am. Heart J. 117:1119, 1989.

464. Schwammental, E., Block, M., Schwartzkopff, B., et al.: Prediction of the site and severity of obstruction in hypertrophic cardiomyopathy by flow mapping and continuous wave Doppler echocardiography. J. Am. Coll. Cardiol. 20:964, 1992.

465. Douglas, P. S., Morrow, R., Ioli, A., et al.: Left ventricular shape, afterload and survival in idiopathic dilated cardiomyopathy. J. Am. Coll. Cardiol. 13:311, 1989.

466. Goldberg, S. J., Valdes-Cruz, L. M., Sahn, D. J., et al.: Two dimensional echocardiographic evaluation of dilated cardiomyopathy in children. Am. J. Cardiol. 52:1244, 1983.

467. Pinamonti, B., DiLenarda, A., Sinagra, G., et al.: Restrictive left ventricular filling pattern in dilated cardiomyopathy assessed by Doppler echocardiography: Clinical, echocardiographic and hemodynamic correlations and prognostic implications. J. Am. Coll. Cardiol. 22:808, 1993.

468. Werner, G. S., Schaefer, C., Dirks, R., et al.: Doppler echocardiographic assessment of left ventricular filling in idiopathic dilated cardiomyopathy during one-year follow-up: Relation to the clinical course of disease. Am. Heart J. 126:1408, 1993.

469. Siegel, R. J., Shah, P. K., and Fishbein, M. C.: Idiopathic restrictive cardiomyopathy. Circulation 70:165, 1984.

470. Gross, D. M., Williams, J. C., Caprilio, C., et al.: Echocardiographic abnormalities in the mucopolysaccharide storage diseases. Am. J. Cardiol. 61:170, 1988.

471. Spirito, P., Lupi, G., Melevendi, C., et al.: Restrictive diastolic abnormalities identified by Doppler echocardiography in patients with thalassemia major. Circulation 82:88, 1990.

472. Simons, M., and Isner, J. M.: Assessment of relative sensitivities of noninvasive tests for cardiac amyloidosis in documented cardiac amyloidosis. Am. J. Cardiol. 69:425, 1992.

473. Chandrasekaran, K., Aylward, P. E., Fleagle, S. R., et al.: Feasibility of identifying amyloid and hypertrophic cardiomyopathy with the use of computerized quantitative texture analysis of clinical echocardiographic data. J. Am. Coll. Cardiol. 13:832, 1989.

474. Klein, A. L., Hatle, L. K., Taliercio, C. P., et al.: Prognostic significance of Doppler measures of diastolic function in cardiac amyloidosis. Circulation 83:808, 1991.

PERICARDIAL DISEASE

475. Feigenbaum, H., Waldhausen, J. A., and Hyde, L. P.: Ultrasound diagnosis of pericardial effusion. JAMA 191:107, 1965.

476. Levine, M. J., Lorell, B. H., Diver, D. J., et al.: Implications of echocardiographically assisted diagnosis of pericardial tamponade in contemporary medical patients: Detection before hemodynamic embarrassment. J. Am. Coll. Cardiol. 17:59, 1991.

477. Armstrong, W. F., Schilt, B. F., Helper, D. J., et al.: Diastolic collapse of the right ventricle with cardiac tamponade: An echocardiographic study. Circulation 65:1491, 1982.

478. Singh, S., Wann, L. S., Klopfenstein, H. S., et al.: Usefulness of right ventricular diastolic collapse in diagnosing cardiac tamponade and comparison to pulsus paradoxus. Am. J. Cardiol. 57:652, 1986.

478a. Gillam, L. D., Guyer, D. E., Gibson, T. C., et al.: Hydrodynamic compression of the right atrium: A new echocardiographic sign of cardiac tamponade. Circulation 68:294, 1983.

479. Kochar, G. S., Jacobs, L. E., and Kotler, M. N.: Right atrial compression in postoperative cardiac patients: Detection by transesophageal echocardiography. J. Am. Coll. Cardiol. 16:511, 1990.

480. Torelli, J., Marwick, T. H., and Salcedo, E. E.: Left atrial tamponade: Diagnosis by transesophageal echocardiography. J. Am. Soc. Echocardiogr. 4:413, 1991.

481. Brodyn, N. E., Rose, M. R., Prior, F. P., et al.: Left atrial diastolic compression in a patient with a large pericardial effusion and pulmonary hypertension. Am. J. Med. 88:1, 1990.

482. Fusman, B., Schwinger, M. E., Charney, R., et al.: Isolated collapse of

left-sided heart chambers in cardiac tamponade: Demonstration by two-dimensional echocardiography. Am. Heart J. *121*:613, 1991.

483. Chuttani, K., Pandian, N. G., Mohanty, P. K., et al.: Left ventricular diastolic collapse. An echocardiographic sign of regional cardiac tamponade. Circulation *83*:1999, 1991.

484. Burstow, D. J., Oh, J. K., Bailey, K. R., et al.: Cardiac tamponade: Characteristic Doppler observations. Mayo Clin. Proc. *64*:312, 1989.

485. Schutzman, J. J., Obarski, T. P., Pearce, G. L., et al.: Comparison of Doppler and two-dimensional echocardiography for assessment of pericardial effusion. Am. J. Cardiol. *70*:1353, 1992.

486. Leeman, D. E., Levine, M. J., and Come, P. C.: Doppler echocardiography in cardiac tamponade: Exaggerated respiratory variation in transvalvular blood flow velocity integrals. J. Am. Coll. Cardiol. *11*:572, 1988.

487. Appleton, C. P., Hatle, L. K., and Popp, R. L.: Cardiac tamponade and pericardial effusion: Respiratory variation in transvalvular flow velocities studied by Doppler echocardiography. J. Am. Coll. Cardiol. *11*: 1020, 1988.

488. Feigenbaum, H., Zaky, A., and Grabhorn, L.: Cardiac motion in patients with pericardial effusion: A study using ultrasound cardiography. Circulation *34*:611, 1966.

489. Kreuger, S. K., Zucker, R. P., Dzindzio, B. S., et al.: Swinging heart syndrome with predominant anterior pericardial effusion. J. Clin. Ultrasound *4*:113, 1976.

490. Lewis, B. S.: Real time two dimensional echocardiography in constrictive pericarditis. Am. J. Cardiol. *49*:1789, 1982.

491. Engel, P. J., Fowler, N. O., Tei, C., et al.: M-mode echocardiography in constrictive pericarditis. J. Am. Coll. Cardiol. *6*:471, 1985.

492. Morgan, J. M., Raposo, L., Clague, J. C., et al.: Restrictive cardiomyopathy and constrictive pericarditis: Non-invasive distinction by digitised M mode echocardiography. Br. Heart J. *61*:29, 1989.

493. Voelkel, A. G., Pietro, D. A., Folland, E. D., et al.: Echocardiographic features of constrictive pericarditis. Circulation *58*:871, 1978.

494. Oh, J. K., Hatle, L. K., Seward, J. B., et al.: Diagnostic role of Doppler echocardiography in constrictive pericarditis. J. Am. Coll. Cardiol. *23*:154, 1994.

495. Hatle, L. K., Appleton, C. P., and Popp, R.L.: Differentiation of constrictive pericarditis and restrictive cardiomyopathy by Doppler echocardiography. Circulation *80*:357, 1989.

496. Klein, A. L., Cohen, G. I., Pietrolungo, J. F., et al.: Differentiation of constrictive pericarditis from restrictive cardiomyopathy by Doppler transesophageal echocardiographic measurements of respiratory variations in pulmonary venous flow. J. Am. Coll. Cardiol. *22*:1935, 1993.

497. Vaitkus, P. T., and Kussmaul, W. G.: Constrictive pericarditis versus restrictive cardiomyopathy: A reappraisal and update of diagnostic criteria. Am. Heart J. *122*:1431, 1991.

498. Ruys, F., Paulus, W., Stevens, C., et al.: Expansion of the left atrial appendage is a distinctive cross-sectional echocardiographic feature of congenital defect of the pericardium. Eur. Heart J. *4*:738, 1983.

499. Kansal, S., Roitman, D., and Sheffield, L. T.: Two-dimensional echocardiography of congenital absence of pericardium. Am. Heart J., *109*:912, 1985.

500. Obeid, A. I., Marvasti, M., Parker, F., et al.: Comparison of transthoracic and transesophageal echocardiography in diagnosis of left atrial myxoma. Am. J. Cardiol. *63*:1006, 1989.

501. Tway, K. P., Shah, A. A., and Rahimtoola, S. H.: Multiple bilateral myxomas demonstrated by two-dimensional echocardiography. Am. J. Med. *71*:896, 1981.

502. Alam, M., and Sun, I.: Transesophageal echocardiographic evaluation of left atrial mass lesions. J. Am. Soc. Echocardiogr. *4*:323, 1991.

503. Reeder, G. S., Khandheria, B. K., Seward, J. B., et al.: Transesophageal echocardiography and cardiac masses. Mayo Clin. Proc. *66*:1101, 1991.

504. Pearson, A. C., Labovitz, A. J., Tatineni, S., et al.: Superiority of transesophageal echocardiography in detecting cardiac sources of embolism in patients with cerebral ischemia of uncertain etiology. J. Am. Coll. Cardiol. *17*:66, 1991.

505. Shyu, K.-G., Chen, J.-J., Cheng, J.-J., et al.: Comparison of transthoracic and transesophageal echocardiography in the diagnosis of intracardiac tumors in adults. J. Clin. Ultrasound *22*:381, 1994.

506. Saxon, L. A., Stevenson, W. G., Fonarow, G. C., et al.: Transesophageal echocardiography during radiofrequency catheter ablation of ventricular tachycardia. Am. J. Cardiol. *72*:658, 1993.

507. Brickner, M. E., Friedman, D. B., Cigarroa, C. G., et al.: Relation of thrombus in the left atrial appendage by transesophageal echocardiography to clinical risk factors for thrombus formation. Am. J. Cardiol. *74*:391, 1994.

508. Bansal, R. C., Heywood, J. T., Applegate, P. M., et al.: Detection of left atrial thrombi by two-dimensional echocardiography and surgical correlation in 148 patients with mitral valve disease. Am. J. Cardiol. *64*:243, 1989.

509. Hwang, J.-J., Kuan, P., Chen, J.-J., et al.: Significance of left atrial spontaneous echo contrast in rheumatic mitral valve disease as a predictor of systemic arterial embolization: A transesophageal echocardiographic study. Am. Heart J. *127*:880, 1994.

510. Fatkin, D., Kelly, R. P., and Feneley, M. P.: Relations between left atrial appendage blood flow velocity, spontaneous echocardiographic contrast and thromboembolic risk in vivo. J. Am. Coll. Cardiol. *23*:961, 1994.

511. Riggs, T., Paul, M. H., DeLeon, S., et al.: Two dimensional echocardiography in evaluation of right atrial masses: Five cases in pediatric patients. Am. J. Cardiol. *48*:961, 1981.

512. Sommariva, L., Auricchio, A., Polisca, P., et al.: Right atrial myxoma with atypical features of syndrome myxoma. Am. Heart J. *126*:256, 1993.

513. Dittmann, H., Voelker, W., Karsch, K. R., et al.: Bilateral atrial myxomas detected by transesophageal two-dimensional echocardiography. Am. Heart J. *118*:172, 1989.

514. Cameron, J., Pohlner, P. G., Stafford, E. G., et al.: Right heart thrombus: Recognition and management. J. Am. Coll. Cardiol. *5*:1239, 1985.

515. Sans, P., Provansal, D., Balansard, P., et al.: Large right intracardiac thrombus cause of recurrent pulmonary embolism. Arch. Mal. Coeur. *78*:650, 1985.

516. Meller, J., Teichholz, L. E., Pichard, A. O., et al.: Left ventricular myxoma. Echocardiographic diagnosis and review of the literature. Am. J. Med. *63*:816, 1977.

517. Roelandt, J., Bletter, W. B., Leuftink, E. W., et al.: Ultrasonic demonstration of right ventricular myxoma. J. Clin. Ultrasound *5*:191, 1977.

518. Levisman, J. A., MacAlpin, R. N., Abbasi, A. S., et al.: Echocardiographic diagnosis of a mobile, pedunculated tumor in the left ventricular cavity. Am. J. Cardiol. *36*:957, 1975.

519. Nanda, N. C., Barold, S. S., Gramiak, R., et al.: Echocardiographic features of right ventricular outflow tumor prolapsing into the pulmonary artery. Am. J. Cardiol. *40*:272, 1977.

520. Grantham, N.: Echocardiographic, angiocardiographic, and surgical correlations in right ventricular myxoma simulating valvular pulmonic stenosis. Circulation *55*:619, 1977.

521. Bass, J. L., Breningstall, G. N., and Swaiman, K. F.: Echocardiographic incidence of cardiac rhabdomyoma in tuberous sclerosis. Am. J. Cardiol. *55*:1379, 1985.

522. Yabek, S. M., Isabel-Jones, J., Gyepes, M. T., et al.: Cardiac fibroma in a neonate presenting with severe congestive heart failure. J. Pediatr. *91*:310, 1977.

523. Ports, T. A., Schiller, N. B., and Strunk, B. L.: Echocardiography of right ventricular tumors. Circulation *56*:439, 1977.

524. Topol, E. J., Biern, R. O., and Reitz, B. A.: Cardiac papillary fibroelastoma and stroke. Am. J. Med. *80*:129, 1986.

525. Schwinger, M. E., Katz, E. Rotterda, H., et al.: Right atrial papillary fibroelastoma: Diagnosis by transthoracic and transesophageal echocardiography and percutaneous transvenous biopsy. Am. Heart J. *118*:1047, 1989.

526. Fowles, R. E., Miller, D. C., Egbert, B. M., et al.: Systemic embolization from mitral valve papillary endocardial fibroma detected by two dimensional echocardiography. Am. Heart J. *102*:128, 1981.

527. Hajar, R., Roberts, W. C., and Folger, G. M.: Embryonal botryoid rhabdomyosarcoma of the mitral valve. Am. J. Cardiol. *57*:376, 1986.

528. Grosse, P., Herpin, D., Roudaut, R., et al.: Myxoma of the mitral valve diagnosed by echocardiography. Am. Heart J *111*:803, 1986.

529. Stoddard, M. F., Liddell, N. E., Longacker, R. A., et al.: Transesophageal echocardiography: Normal variants and mimickers. Am. Heart J. *124*:1587, 1992.

530. Cujec, B., Mycyk, T., and Khouri, M.: Identification of Chiari's network with transesophageal echocardiography. J. Am. Soc. Echocardiogr. *5*:96, 1992.

531. Cloez, J. L., Neimann, J. L., Chivoret, G., et al.: Echocardiographic rediscovery of an anatomical structure: The Chiari network. Apropos of 16 cases. Arch. Mal. Coeur *76*:1284, 1983.

532. Limacher, M. C., Gutgesell, H. P., Vick, G. W., et al.: Echocardiographic anatomy of the eustachian valve. Am. J. Cardiol. *57*:363, 1986.

533. Pochis, W. T., Saeian, K., and Sagar, K. B.: Usefulness of transesophageal echocardiography in diagnosing lipomatous hypertrophy of the atrial septum with comparison to transthoracic echocardiography. Am. J. Cardiol. *70*:396, 1992.

534. Cohen, I. S., and Raiker, K.: Atrial lipomatous hypertrophy: Lipomatous atrial hypertrophy with significant involvement of the right atrial wall. J. Am. Soc. Echocardiogr. *6*:30, 1993.

535. Keren, A., Billingham, M. E., and Popp, R. L.: Echocardiographic recognition and implications of ventricular hypertrophic trabeculations and aberrant bands. Circulation *70*:836, 1984.

536. Casta, A., and Wolf, W. J.: Left ventricular bands (false tendons): Echocardiographic and angiocardiographic delineation in children. Am. Heart J. *111*:321, 1986.

537. Chazal, R. A., and Feigenbaum, H.: Two-dimensional echocardiographic identification of epicardial pacemaker wire perforation. Am. Heart J. *107*:165, 1984.

538. Cameron, J., Pohlner, P. G., Stafford, E. G., et al.: Right heart thrombus: Recognition and management. J. Am. Coll. Cardiol. *51*:1239, 1985.

539. Sans, P., Provansal, D., Balansard, P., et al.: Large right intracardiac thrombus cause of recurrent pulmonary embolism. Arch. Mal. Coeur *78*:650, 1985.

540. Weg, I. L., Mehra, S., Azueta, V., et al.: Cardiac metastasis from adenocarcinoma of the lung. Am. J. Med. *80*:108, 1986.

541. Sobue, T., Iwase, M., Iwase, M., et al.: Solitary left ventricular metastasis of renal cell carcinoma. Am. Heart J. *125*:1801, 1993.

542. Cueto-Garcia, L., Shub, C., Sheps, S. G., et al.: Two-dimensional echocardiographic detection and mediastinal pheochromocytoma. Chest *87*:834, 1985.

543. Kruger, S. R., Michaud, J., and Cannom, D. S.: Spontaneous resolution of a pericardial cyst. Am. Heart J. *109*:1390, 1985.

544. Lestuzzi, C., Nicolosi, G. L., Mimo, R., et al.: Usefulness of transesophageal echocardiography in evaluation of paracardiac neoplastic masses. Am. J. Cardiol. *70*:247, 1992.

545. Torbicki, A., Tramarain, R., and Morpurgo, M.: Role of echo/Doppler in the diagnosis of pulmonary embolism. Clin. Cardiol. *15*:805, 1992.

546. Rittoo, D., Sutherland, G. R., Samuel, L., et al.: Role of transesophageal echocardiography in diagnosis and management of central pulmonary artery thromboembolism. Am. J. Cardiol. 71:1115, 1993.

547. Goldstein, S. A., Mintz, G. S., and Lindsay, J., Jr.: Aorta: Comprehensive evaluation by echocardiography and transesophageal echocardiography. J. Am. Soc. Echocardiogr. 6:634, 1993.

548. Come, P. C., Sacks, B., Vine, H., et al.: Ultrasonic visualization of the posterior thoracic aorta in long axis: Diagnosis of a saccular mycotic aneurysm. Chest 79:470, 1981.

549. Simpson, I. A., deBelder, M. A., Treasure, T., et al.: Cardiovascular manifestations of Marfan's syndrome: Improved evaluation by transesophageal echocardiography. Br. Heart J. 69:104, 1992.

550. Cigarroa, J. E., Isselbacher, E. M., DeSanctis, R. W., and Eagle, K. A.: Diagnostic imaging in the evaluation of suspected aortic dissection. Old standards and new directions. N. Engl. J. Med. 328:35, 1993.

551. Granato, J. E., Dee, P., and Gibson, R. S.: Utility of two-dimensional echocardiography in suspected ascending aortic dissection. Am. J. Cardiol. 56:123, 1985.

552. D'Cruz, I. A., Jain, M., Campbell, C., et al.: Ultrasound visualization of aortic dissection by right parasternal scanning, including systolic flutter of the intimal flap. Chest 80:239, 1981.

553. Banning, A. P., Masani, N. D., Ikram, S., et al.: Transesophageal echocardiography as the sole diagnostic investigation in patients with suspected thoracic aortic dissection. Br. Heart J. 72:461, 1994.

554. Chirillo, F., Cavallini, C., Longhini, C., et al.: Comparative diagnostic value of transesophageal echocardiography and retrograde aortography in the evaluation of thoracic aortic dissection. Am. J. Cardiol. 74:590, 1994.

555. Duch, P. M., Chandrasekaran, K., Karalis, D. G., et al.: Improved diagnosis of coexisting types II and III aortic dissection with multiplane transesophageal echocardigraphy. Am. Heart J. 127:699, 1994.

556. Hashimoto, S., Kumada, T., Osakada, G., et al.: Assessment of transesophageal Doppler echography in dissecting aortic aneurysm. J. Am. Coll. Cardiol. 14:1252, 1989.

557. Iliceto, S., Nanda, N. C., Rizzon, P., et al.: Color Doppler evaluation of aortic dissection. Circulation 75:748, 1987.

558. Chia, B. L., Yan, P. C., Ee, B. K., et al.: Two-dimensional echocardiography and Doppler color flow abnormalities in aortic root dissection. Am. Heart J. 116:192, 1988.

559. Cabanes, L., Garcia, E., VanDamme, C., et al.: Aneurysm of the noncoronary sinus of Valsalva ruptured into the left atrium. Am. Heart J. 124:1659, 1992.

560. Dev, V., Goswami, K. C., Shrivastava, S., et al.: Echocardiographic diagnosis of aneurysm of the sinus of Valsalva. Am. Heart J. 126:930, 1993.

561. Kiefaber, R. W., Tabakin, B. S., Coffin, L. H., et al.: Unruptured sinus of Valsalva aneurysm with right ventricular outflow obstruction diagnosed by two-dimensional and Doppler echocardiography. J. Am. Coll. Cardiol. 7:438, 1986.

562. Hands, M. E., Lloyd, B. L., and Hung, J.: Cross-sectional echocardiographic diagnosis of unruptured right sinus of Valsalva aneurysm dissecting into the interventricular septum. Int. J. Cardiol. 9:380, 1985.

563. Terdjman, N., Bourdarias, J. P., Farcot, J. C., et al.: Aneurysms of sinus of Valsalva: Two-dimensional echocardiographic diagnosis and recognition of rupture into the right heart cavities. J. Am. Coll. Cardiol. 3:1227, 1984.

564. Chia, B. L., Ee, B. K., Choo, M. H., et al.: Ruptured aneurysm of sinus of Valsalva: Recognition of Doppler color flow mapping. Am. Heart J. 115:686, 1988.

565. Nihoyannopoulos, P., Jayshree, J., Athanasopoulos, G., et al.: Detection of atherosclerotic lesions in the aorta by transesophageal echocardiography. Am. J. Cardiol. 71:1208, 1993.

566. Nishino, M., Masugata, H., Yamada, Y., et al.: Evaluation of thoracic aortic atherosclerosis by transesophageal echocardiography. Am. Heart J. 127:336, 1994.

567. Dee, W., Geibel, A., Kasper, W., et al.: Mobile thrombi in atherosclerotic lesions of the thoracic aorta: The diagnostic impact of transesophageal echocardiography. Am. Heart J. 126:707, 1993.

568. Horowitz, D. R., Tuhrim, S., Budd, J., et al.: Aortic plaque in patient with brain ischemia: Diagnosis by transesophageal echocardiography. Neurology 42:1602, 1992.

569. Tunick, P. A., Rosenzweig, B. P., Katz, E. S., et al.: High risk for vascular events in patients with protruding aortic atheromas: A prospective study. J. Am. Coll. Cardiol. 23:1085, 1994.

Chapter 4
Electrocardiography

CHARLES FISCH

The clinical electrocardiogram (ECG) records the changing potentials of the electrical field imparted by the heart. The ECG *does not record directly the electrical activity of the source itself.* Such activity is registered only when an electrode is in immediate contact with the tissue generating the current and at the moment when the electrode senses the edge of the wave of activation or recovery. In all other circumstances only potential differences in an electrical field are registered. It is important to appreciate that the ECG, while recording the changes of an electrical field, often provides only an *approximation of the actual* voltage generated by the heart. Efforts to predict surface potentials from the knowledge of behavior of the cardiac generator—the so-called electrocardiographic *forward problem*—or to predict the electrical behavior of the cardiac generator from the body surface potentials—the so-called electrocardiographic *inverse problem*—have to date been unsuccessful.[1]

Despite this basic limitation, the ECG has evolved into an extremely useful clinical laboratory tool and is the only practical means of recording the electrical behavior of the heart.[2] Its usefulness as a diagnostic method is the result of careful, often purely deductive analysis of innumerable patient records and of studies correlating the ECG with basic electrophysiological properties of the heart; with clinical and laboratory findings; and with anatomical, pathological, and experimental observations.[3] As a result, electrocardiography can be used, within limits, to identify anatomical, metabolic, ionic, and hemodynamic changes. It is often an independent marker of cardiac disease, occasionally the only indicator of a pathological process, and not infrequently a guide to therapy.[4–11]

Electrocardiography serves as a gold standard for the diagnosis of arrhythmias, which are discussed in detail in Chapters 20 to 24. Although arrhythmias have been studied by a variety of methods for centuries, none has approached the levels of sensitivity and specificity offered by the ECG.[12] Free of the assumptions required for interpreting the electrocardiographic waveforms, arrhythmias recorded from the surface of the body, with rare exceptions, accurately reflect intracardiac events. However, while most arrhythmias are due to disordered impulse formation or conduction (or both) of the specialized tissue, the ECG reflects the electrical behavior of the myocardium and not of the specialized tissue. This limitation, once appreciated as inherent in the ECG, rarely interferes with proper analysis of even the most complex arrhythmias.[11]

As with any other laboratory procedure, the sensitivity and specificity of the ECG and of its individual components are critical determinants of its clinical usefulness. This is far more complex for the ECG than for other laboratory techniques developed for any single purpose, since its multiple waveforms may be identically or differentially influenced by a wide spectrum of physiological, pathophysiological, or anatomical changes. Thus, it may be difficult—if not impossible—to identify a single cause for any given ECG abnormality.

THE NORMAL ELECTROCARDIOGRAM

Theoretical Considerations

Essential to an understanding of the derivation and interpretation of the clinical ECG is information about (1) the physical and electrophysiological events responsible for the electrical potential recorded as the transmembrane action potential and the spread of excitation, (2) the role of the volume conductor, and (3) the theoretical basis of the lead systems.

ELECTRICAL BASES AND THEORY

At any instant, the cardiac generator can be viewed as a dipole consisting of a positive and a negative charge separated by a small distance. Since the dipole generates a force that has magnitude and direction, it can be expressed as a vector. By convention, the arrowhead of the vector indicates the positive pole. When such a dipole is immersed in a volume conductor, an electrical field is generated.[13,14] In a homogeneous volume conductor, the field is symmetrically distributed. The lines of the electrical field are symmetrical in relation to a line that is perpendicular to and transects the dipole at its midpoint.

At any instant, the magnitude of the potential at a given point (P) in the volume conductor can be estimated using the solid-angle concept, or the concept relating the potential to an angle formed by a line drawn from P to the midpoint of the dipole axis and the dipole axis itself (Fig. 4–1).

The electrical surface with its boundary projected to P results in a cone and defines the solid angle subtended by the area in question. The segment of a sphere inscribed by a radius of unity drawn about point P, with P as the center of the sphere and its border delineated by the cone, is proportional to the area of electrical activity. With variables such as tissue resistance and geometry being constant, the voltage at P can be expressed as $Ep = \phi \cdot \Omega$, where ϕ is voltage per unit of the solid angle and Ω is the solid angle. An alternative and perhaps clinically more applicable approach to estimating Ep considers the distance (r) of P from the source, the strength of the source (m), and the cosine of the angle formed by a line drawn from P to the midpoint of the dipole axis and the dipole axis (Θ), with the magnitude of the angle estimated in reference to the positive pole of the dipole. This relationship can be expressed as

$$Ep = \frac{m \cos \Theta}{r^2}$$

According to this formula, when the angle is 90 degrees, the line drawn from P is perpendicular to the dipole axis, and the Ep is zero. In the ECG the inscription would be isoelectric or equiphasic. On the other hand, with the angle becoming smaller, the point P is closer to the positive pole of the dipole, and the voltage becomes greater.

Assuming that the volume conductor is homogeneous and infinite and has a uniform boundary and that the generator is located in the center of the volume conductor, both approaches for estimation of Ep at P are correct. Such assumptions, however, are not entirely valid in humans (see below).

The influence of polarity of the dipole, the distance of the electrode from the dipole, and the strength of the electrical field on waveform are important in analysis of the ECG. These relationships can be studied using a hypothetical dipole or tissue immersed in a homogeneous volume conductor. An electrode, located outside the electrical field, when moved into the negative field records a gradually increasing negativity. Halfway between the two poles, a sharp reversal of polarity is registered (intrinsic deflection), and the electrode enters the positive field. As the electrode is moved, positive voltage declines gradually until a potential difference is no longer registered. A similar sequence of events is registered with the electrode stationary and the electrical field moving relative to the electrode. When the positive field moves toward the electrode, a positive

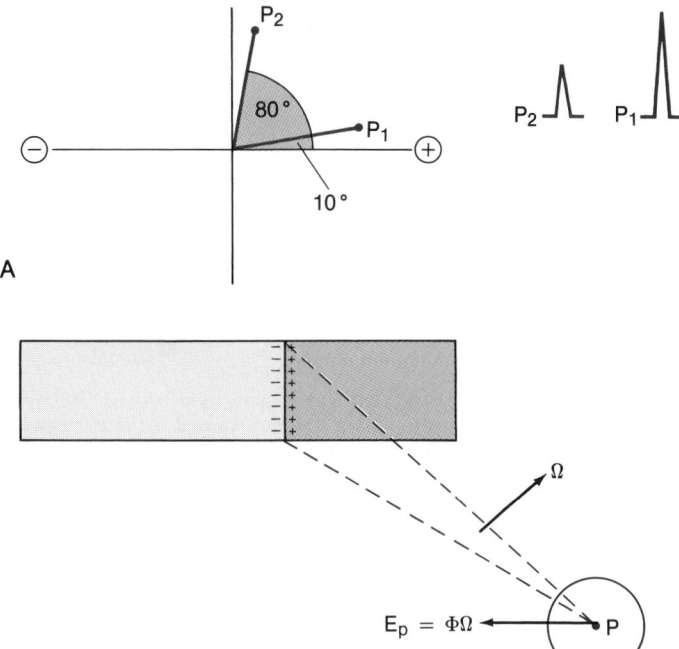

A

B

FIGURE 4–1. *A,* The potentials at points P_1 and P_2 are inversely proportional to the square of the distance from the source and proportional to the cosine of angle formed by a line drawn from point P to the midpoint of the dipole axis and the axis itself. *B,* The potential E is proportional to the solid angle Ω and the strength of the charged surface. (Modified from Wolff, L: Electrocardiography: Fundamentals and Clinical Application. 3rd ed. Philadelphia, W. B. Saunders Company, 1962, p. 15.)

potential is recorded; when the electrode finds itself in the negative field, a negative potential is recorded.

Transmembrane ionic fluxes are responsible for voltage differences between activated and resting tissue. These ionic fluxes are reflected as the transmembrane action potential, the cellular counterpart of the clinical ECG. The ECG counterparts of the phases 0, 1, 2, 3, and 4 of the transmembrane action potential are the QRS complex, the ST segment, the T wave, and the isoelectric baseline, respectively (see Chap. 20).

DEPOLARIZATION AND REPOLARIZATION. To progress logically toward an understanding of the ECG, we will review the effect of a muscle strip immersed in a homogenous volume conductor on the electrical field generated by the muscle strip and on the electrode immersed in the field.

A muscle strip, when uniformly positive on the outside, is in a resting or polarized state. Because it exhibits no difference of potential and fails to impart an electrical field, an electrode immersed in the volume conductor registers an isoelectric line. Stimulation of the muscle strip at any given point increases membrane permeability, and positive ions, largely sodium, enter the cell. The result is depolarized muscle whose external field is relatively negative in apposition to polarized muscle whose external field is relatively positive, with a potential difference across a boundary. In the surrounding medium the current flows from the positively (source) to the negatively (sink) charged muscle. The moving boundary between the polarized (positive) and the depolarized (negative) muscle can be represented by a dipole or vector. This dipole or vector moves along the muscle fiber from the point of excitation, leaving in its wake tissue that is electrically negative (depolarized) in relation to the still polarized (resting) muscle. When the wave of depolarization reaches the end of the muscle strip, the surface becomes uniformly negative, and the strip is now completely depolarized. Since a difference of potential no longer exists, an isoelectric baseline is inscribed. The most intense difference of potential exists at the boundary

between depolarized and resting tissue, and the recorded voltage changes reflect the events taking place at this boundary.[13,14]

Restitution of membrane polarity, *repolarization,* can be viewed as a "wave" of positivity sweeping across the cells or tissue. As a result, the outside of the cell is again uniformly positive. Since the boundary moves in the direction of the depolarized, negative muscle, an electrode located at the point of origin of repolarization records a positive potential, while an electrode placed at the opposite end records a negative potential. In a preparation of *isolated myocardial tissue* (not the intact heart), the direction of repolarization is the same as that of depolarization but is preceded by the negative pole of the dipole. The repolarization inscribes an area equal to that inscribed by depolarization but of opposite polarity.

EFFECT OF THE BOUNDARY OF DEPOLARIZATION ON POLARITY OF THE RECORDED POTENTIAL. Three electrodes placed on a muscle strip will illustrate the effect of a boundary potential, which can be represented as a dipole or vector, on the recording electrode (Fig. 4–2). Electrode A is located at the point of excitation, electrode B at the midpoint of the muscle strip, and electrode C at the opposite end of the muscle strip. Immediately after excitation, electrode A is in the most intensively negative field. As the dipole moves away, the potential becomes less negative, and at the end of depolarization the inscription returns to the baseline. Thus, the electrode at point A inscribes a negative deflection. At the moment of excitation, electrode B is located in the positive field of the dipole, and as the dipole moves toward the recording electrode, the latter registers a gradually increasing positivity and records an upright deflection. When the dipole passes the electrode, there is a sudden reversal of polarity, termed the *intrinsic deflection,* and the electrode finds itself in a strongly negative field. A downward, negative deflection is recorded. With the dipole moving away, the electrode at point B registers a less negative potential, and finally, when the strip is completely depolar-

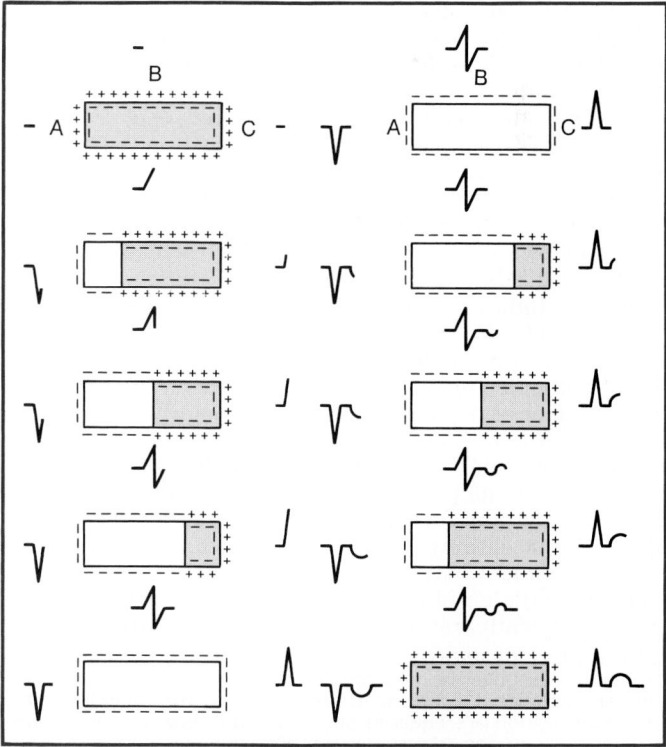

FIGURE 4–2. Potential generated during depolarization (left vertical sequence of panels) and repolarization (right vertical sequence of panels) recorded with an exploring electrode located at the endocardium (A), epicardium (C), and midway between the two (B). (Modified from Barker, J. M.: The Unipolar Electrocardiogram: A Clinical Interpretation. New York, Appleton-Century-Crofts, Inc., 1952.)

ized, an isoelectric baseline is recorded. Thus, the electrode at point B registers a positive-negative deflection. Electrode C is located in the positive field throughout the entire process of depolarization. As the dipole approaches the electrode, the field becomes more intensively positive, with the most intense positivity occurring at the moment immediately before completion of depolarization. Thus, the electrode at point C records an upright deflection.

SEQUENCE OF CARDIAC ACTIVATION. The sequence of cardiac activation has been studied in animals, primarily in the dog, and in the isolated perfused human heart.[15] The normal impulse originates in the sinoatrial (SA) node and traverses the atria in a wavelike front with a velocity of approximately 1000 mm/sec. The wave of atrial activation resembles a wavefront seen when a pebble is thrown into water. The sinoatrial node is located in the right atrium and initially activates the right atrium in a right and anterior direction, followed by excitation of the left atrium in a left and posterior direction. It has been suggested that preferential internodal pathways connect the SA node and the atrioventricular (AV) junctional tissue and that these specialized internodal pathways are capable of conducting an impulse in the presence of a quiescent atrium.

The impulse arrives at the AV node, where it is delayed, most probably because of decremental conduction (see p. 569). Study of the sequence of ventricular activation in the dog reveals an early (0 to 5 msec) and almost simultaneous activation of the central left side of the septum and the high anterior and apical posterior paraseptal areas of the left ventricle. At 5 to 10 msec after the onset of ventricular activation, the wave of activation envelops left and right ventricular walls and the remainder of the septum; the latter is completely activated at 12 msec. The earliest epicardial breakthrough occurs at the anterior right epicardial surface near the apex, followed by anterior and posterior paraseptal areas of the left ventricle. At 18 msec, activation of the central portion of the two ventricles is complete. Excitation continues along the lateral and basal aspects of the left ventricle, with the basal portion of the septum the last to become depolarized.

Studies of perfused human heart indicate that its path of activation closely follows that of the canine heart (Fig. 4–3).[15] The results obtained from the resuscitated human heart were validated by comparing the process of activation with that of a perfused and in situ dog heart. The only difference was that the activation proceeded more rapidly in the perfused dog preparation. Intracardiac mapping during surgery indicates that initial epicardial breakthrough occurs in the right ventricle followed by activation of the anterior and inferior left ventricle.

Human studies indicate that atrial repolarization follows approximately the same path as atrial depolarization, with the polarity of repolarization opposite to that of depolarization. Ventricular repolarization proceeds in a direction *opposite* to that of depolarization, and its polarity is therefore the *same* as that of depolarization. The process of repolarization in the intact ventricle begins at the epicardium—a sequence opposite to that observed in isolated muscle strip. The reason for the reversal in vivo of the order of repolarization is not entirely clear. The presence of a transmural pressure gradient may be an important factor, since it prolongs the duration of the excited state of the endocardium, and consequently, recovery begins at the epicardium.

VENTRICULAR GRADIENT. The ventricular gradient (G), introduced by Wilson, describes the relationships between depolarization (QRS) and repolarization (T).[16] In an isolated muscle strip, depolarization and repolarization are equal in duration and follow the same path. The net areas of the QRS complex (AQRS) and the T wave (AT) are equal but of opposite polarity so that their sum is zero and there is no gradient. In the intact heart, on the other hand, repolarization proceeds from the epicardium to endocardium, in a direction *opposite* to that of depolarization; the algebraic sum of their respective areas is no longer zero; and a gradient is said to exist. AQRS, AT, and G can be expressed as a vectorial quantity from any two of the three bipolar limb leads of the ECG. AQRS and AT are expressed in the form

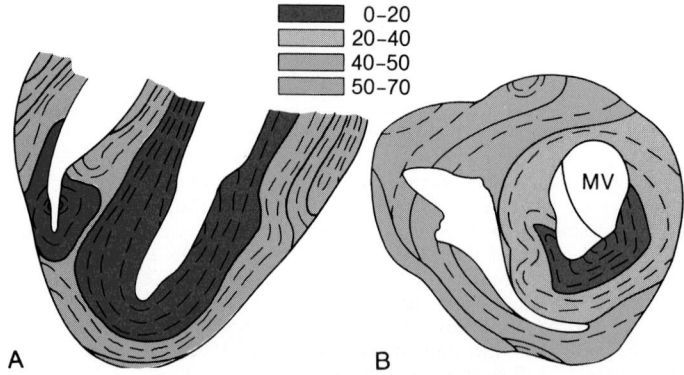

FIGURE 4–3. Sequence of ventricular activation of an isolated human heart. *A* and *B* represent sagittal and coronal sections, respectively. The dotted lines denote 5-msec sequences, while changes in pattern represent 20-msec intervals. (Reproduced with permission from Durrer, D., et al.: Total excitation of the isolated human heart. *Circulation 41:*899, 1970. Copyright 1970 American Heart Association, Inc.)

of vectors and are plotted using the Einthoven triangle or Bayley triaxial reference system. A parallelogram of the AQRS and the AT is constructed, with the resultant diagonal vector being the manifest AQRST vector or gradient (G). The G vector and the mean QRS vector are located in about the same plane. The G forms an angle of approximately 30 degrees with the mean spatial QRS vector.

THEORETICAL BASES OF SURFACE LEADS. At any instant the surface leads reflect projection of the electrical field of the equivalent or "net" dipole expressed as the mean instantaneous spatial vector. Orientation of a lead axis is defined as one that records a maximal voltage when its axis is parallel to that of the axis or vector of the equivalent dipole. The voltage registered in any lead, having magnitude and direction, can be expressed as a vector (lead vector), with the amplitude of deflection in any lead paralleling the magnitude of the vector. Since more than one dipole may exist at any instant, the net potential and consequently the resultant lead vector reflect the contribution of all such dipoles. Furthermore, because dipole vectors may vary in magnitude and direction, the equivalent or "net" dipole is an approximation of these forces, and consequently, its expression on a lead axis is also an approximation.

LEADS. *Bipolar limb leads,* introduced by Einthoven, register the direction, magnitude, and duration of voltage changes in the frontal plane. The three bipolar leads—I, II, and III—record the differences in potential between left arm (LA) and right arm (RA), left leg (LF) and RA, and LF and LA, respectively.

Unipolar limb leads are constructed by connecting all three extremities to a "central terminal" (Fig. 4–4A). Although in reality the central terminal registers a small voltage, for practical purposes it is considered to have a zero potential and serves as the *indifferent* or *reference electrode.* The potential differences recorded by the positive terminal, the *exploring electrode,* are dominated by local electrical events. When placed on the right arm, left arm, or left foot, the exploring electrode registers the potential from the respective limb. The letter *V* identifies a unipolar lead and the letters *r, l,* and *f* the respective extremities. If one disconnects the central terminal from the extremity from which the potential is being recorded, the amplitude registered by the respective unipolar limb lead is augmented, and the leads are designated as aV$_r$, aV$_l$, and aV$_f$.

Locations of the exploring electrode for the *precordial leads* are as follows: V$_1$—fourth interspace to the right of the sternum; V$_2$—fourth interspace to the left of the sternum; V$_3$—midway between leads V$_2$ and V$_4$; V$_4$—fifth interspace at the midclavicular line; V$_5$—anterior axillary line at the level of lead V$_4$; and V$_6$—midaxillary line at the level of lead V$_4$ (Fig. 4–4A).[17]

In the absence of major thoracic deformity or cardiac malposition, three pairs of precordial leads, i.e., leads V$_1$ and V$_2$, V$_3$ and V$_4$, and V$_5$ and V$_6$, face the right side of the septum, the septum itself, and the left side of the septum, respectively, and are referred to as *right ventricular, septal* or *transitional,* and *left ventricular leads,* respectively.

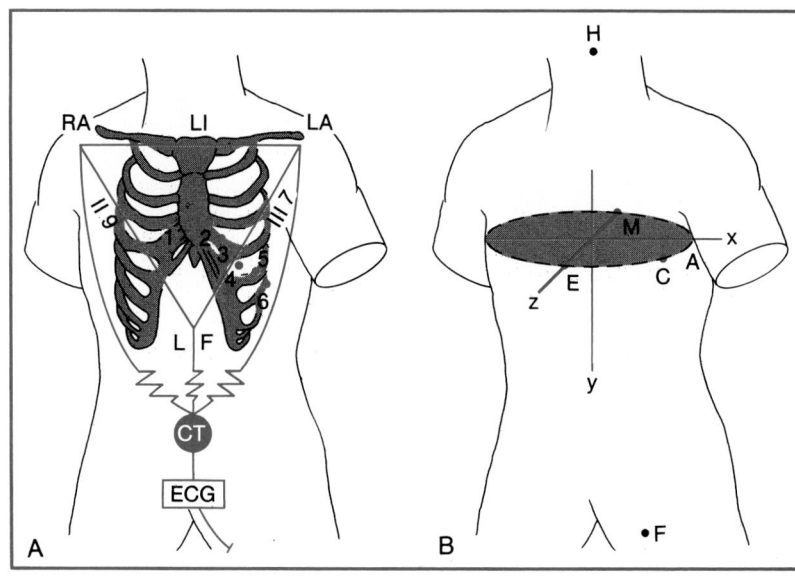

FIGURE 4–4. *A,* ECG lead system. Leads I, II, and III are formed by connecting RA-LA, RA-LF, and LA-LF, respectively. The indifferent electrode of the unipolar system is obtained by connecting RA, LA, and LF through 50,000-ohm resistance into a central terminal (CT). (For details about positioning of the exploring unipolar electrode, see discussion under Leads.) *B,* Frank electrode system. Five horizontal electrodes are placed at the level where the fifth intercostal space intersects the sternal line. Specific locations include fifth intercostal space and sternum (E), the midaxillary line (A,I) and the vertebral column (M). Electrode C is located halfway between points E and A, while electrodes H and F are on the back of the neck and left lower extremity, respectively.

Right precordial leads are of increasing interest because of their importance in the diagnosis of right ventricular infarction. The leads are recorded from the following positions on the right chest: V_3R—between V_1 and V_4R; V_4R—right midclavicular line in the fifth intercostal space; V_5R—right anterior axillary line in the same horizontal plane as V_4R; V_6R—right midaxillary line in the same horizontal plane as V_4R. Normally, an rS configuration is present in 98 per cent of V_3R leads. Secondary R wave (R') increases in frequency and amplitude in the right lateral leads (for details see ref. 18).

The Standard 12-Lead Electrocardiogram

The P Wave

The cardiac impulse originating in the SA node activates the right and left atria in the general direction from right to left, inferiorly and posteriorly. Initial activation of the right atrium, an anterior chamber, is directed anteriorly and inferiorly and is followed by activation of the left or posterior atrium, directed to the left, posteriorly, and inferiorly.

The P wave is rounded with a notch corresponding to the separation between right and left atrial activation. Amplitude of the P wave is normally less than 0.20 mV (2.0 mm) with a duration less than 0.12 sec (Table 4–1). The P wave and the *Ta segment,* or atrial repolarization, define atrial electrical systole. The P vector varies from −50 to +60 degrees. In the precordial leads the P wave is positive except in lead V_1, where the P wave may be upright, biphasic, or negative.

The Ta segment may be inscribed during the P-R segment, the QRS complex, and the early part of the ST segment (Fig. 4–5). It is best seen in the presence of AV block. Duration of the Ta segment varies from 0.15 to 0.45 sec,

TABLE 4–1   P WAVE: AMPLITUDE AND DURATION IN NORMAL ADULTS

	LEAD I	LEAD II	LEAD III	LEAD V_1*
P Amplitude (mV)				
Mean	0.049	0.103	0.069	0.040
Range	0.02 to 0.10	0.03 to 0.20	0 to 0.20	0.005 to 0.080
P Duration (sec)				
Mean	0.08	0.09	0.16	0.05
Range	0.05 to 0.12	0.05 to 0.12	0.12 to 0.20	0 to 0.08
P-R Interval (sec)				
Mean	0.16	0.16		
Range	0.12 to 0.20	0.12 to 0.20		

AMPLITUDE OF Q, R, S, AND T WAVES IN SCALAR ELECTROCARDIOGRAM OF 100 NORMAL ADULTS†

	I	II	III	aV$_r$	aV$_l$	aV$_f$	V$_1$	V$_5$	V$_6$
Patients with Q Wave	38%	41%	50%	—	38%	40%	0%	60%	75%
Q Amplitude									
Mean	0.4	0.6	0.09	—	0.04	0.07	0	0.03	0.03
Range	0 to 0.1	0 to 0.16	0 to 0.23		0 to 0.11	0 to 0.17	0	0 to 0.18	0 to 0.18
R Amplitude									
Mean	0.56	0.89	0.45	0.13	0.34	0.6	0.19	1.2	1.0
Range	0.1 to 1.0	0.2 to 1.6	0.1 to 1.2	0 to 0.29	0 to 0.82	0 to 1.38	0.1 to 0.6	0.7 to 2.1	0.5 to 1.8
S Amplitude									
Mean	0.2	0.2	0.24	0.7	0.26	—	0.8	0.25	0.13
Range	0 to 0.5	0 to 0.37	0 to 0.64	0.22 to 1.18	0 to 0.58	—	0.3 to 1.3	0 to 0.5	0 to 0.2
T Amplitude									
Mean	0.19	0.23	0.1	—	0.03	0.17	0.1	0.33	0.1
Range	0.1 to 0.3	0.1 to 0.2	−0.2 to 0.2	—	−0.1 to 0.2	0 to 0.4	−0.2 to 0.2	0.2 to 0.7	0.1 to 0.4

* Twenty-five per cent of the series had a small terminal negative deflection of the P wave in lead V_1.
† Amplitude values are in millivolts (0.1 mV = 1 mm).
From Cooksey, J. D., et al.: Clinical Vectorcardiography and Electrocardiography. 2nd ed. Chicago, Year Book Medical Publishers, 1977.

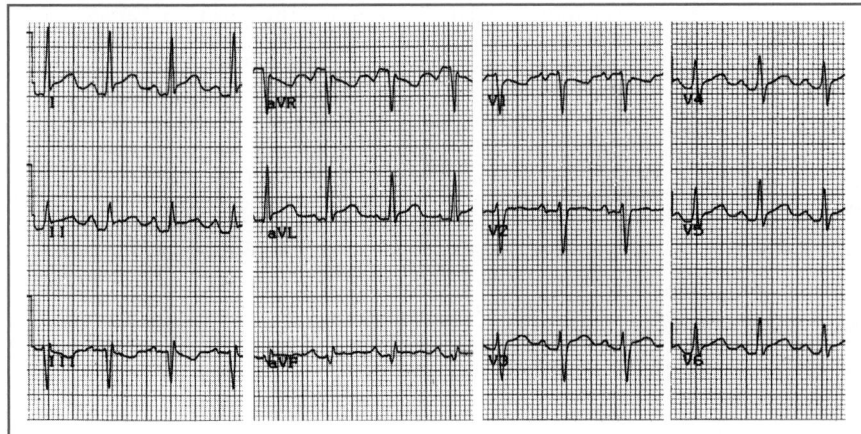

FIGURE 4–5. Acute pericarditis indicated by the diffuse ST-segment elevation without QRS or T-wave abnormality and with the highly diagnostic Ta segment depression in leads I, II, V_4, V_5, and V_6 and elevation in lead aV_r.

and its amplitude is low, reaching 0.08 mV. The magnitude of the Ta is directionally related to the area of the P wave. The orientation of the Ta segment is opposite to that of the P wave. The P wave and Ta areas are equal and opposite in direction, and the resultant gradient is zero. In the presence of atrial enlargement, the Ta segment may result in displacement of the ST segment.

P-R INTERVAL. The P-R interval includes the time for intraatrial, AV nodal, and His-Purkinje conduction, and its duration varies from 0.12 to 0.20 or 0.22 sec (Table 4–1; Chap. 20).

The QRS Complex

Ventricular activation proceeds chiefly symmetrically about the septum and from the endocardium to the epicardium. Consequently, much of its voltage is canceled; in fact, only 10 to 15 per cent of the potential generated by the heart is ultimately recorded on the surface ECG.

The normal QRS complex can be described by four vectors (Fig. 4–6): (1) initial septal activation from left to right, anteriorly, inferiorly, or superiorly, followed by further septal activation from left to right (0.01 sec); (2) an overlapping wave of excitation involving both ventricles, with the vector directed inferiorly and slightly to the left (0.02 sec); (3) unopposed activation of the apical and central portions of the left ventricle, the thin right ventricular wall having been depolarized, with a resultant vector directed posteriorly, inferiorly, and to the left (0.04 sec); and finally, (4) activation of the posterior basal portion of the left ventricle

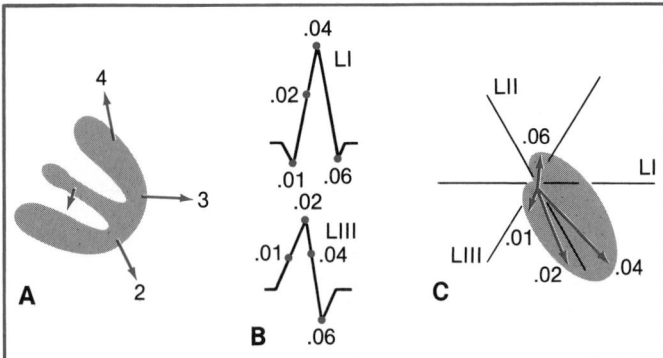

FIGURE 4–6. Correlation between the order of ventricular activation (A), scalar ECG (B), and vectorcardiogram (C). A, The sequence of ventricular activation is represented by four instantaneous frontal plane vectors. B, The four vectors plotted on leads I and III at the appropriate time during inscription of the QRS. C, Using the method of construction of vectors described in Figure 4-7, one can derive each of the four vectors in the frontal plane. A line joining the ends of the vectors results in a frontal plane QRS loop. The same method can be used to derive the orthogonal X, Y, and Z leads from the frontal, transverse, or sagittal planes. (Times given are in seconds.)

and septum, with a vector directed superiorly and posteriorly (0.06 sec).

Septal activation from left to right and anteriorly results, normally, in an initial Q wave in leads I, II, III, aV_1, V_5, and V_6 and an R wave in the right precordial and septal leads V_1 to V_4. Lead aV_f registers an R or Q wave depending on whether the septal vector is directed superiorly or inferiorly. The ventricular vector directed inferiorly and to the left is reflected by an R wave in leads II and III and in the transitional or septal leads V_3 and V_4. The third vector, that of the unopposed force directed to the left, posteriorly, and somewhat inferiorly, gives rise to an R wave in leads I, II, III, aV_1, aV_f, V_5, V_6, and occasionally V_4, with an S wave in leads aV_r, V_1, V_2, V_3, and at times V_4. The terminal force directed superiorly and posteriorly and perhaps to the right may result in a terminal S wave in leads I, V_5, and V_6. A lead positioned in the right fourth interspace in the midclavicular line (V_{4r}) may record a terminal R wave (R'), which also may occasionally be recorded in lead V_1.[17] The magnitudes of the Q, R, and S waves are given in Table 4–1.

One hundred msec is considered the upper limit of normal QRS duration. In a recent study of 1254 normal white males, however, a QRS complex of 100 to 120 msec in duration, some with R' in leads V_1 and V_2, was present in 21 per cent of the group. This indicates that a QRS duration of 100 to 120 msec may be normal and does not necessarily indicate pathological intraventricular conduction defect.[19]

THE QRS AXIS, POSITION, AND ROTATION. The electrical position of the heart can be described by the QRS axis and the rotation of the heart on the anteroposterior and longitudinal (apex-to-base) axes. Because the *order* of activation can be viewed as a sequence of instantaneous dipoles or vectors, *total* cardiac activation can be presented as a mean QRS vector. When such a vector is placed within the triangle formed by leads I, II, and III, which define the frontal plane, and assuming that this triangle is equilateral, that the heart is located in its center, and that the thorax is a homogeneous volume conductor with a uniform boundary, projection of the vector on the respective leads permits an estimate of the magnitude of voltage recorded in each lead. Similarly, if the voltage in each of the leads is known, the mean QRS vector can be reconstructed and the axis of the QRS complex can be estimated (Fig. 4–7).

The preceding assumptions—the Einthoven postulates—are applicable in the experimental setting. In the human, however, the heart is a large organ; it is not a point generator nor is it centrally located, and the thorax is not a homogeneous conductor within a uniform boundary. Burger, using a model of a human torso, with nonhomogeneous conduction to reflect the nature of human organs and an eccentrically located generator, found that the triangle formed by the axes of leads I, II, and III is not equilateral

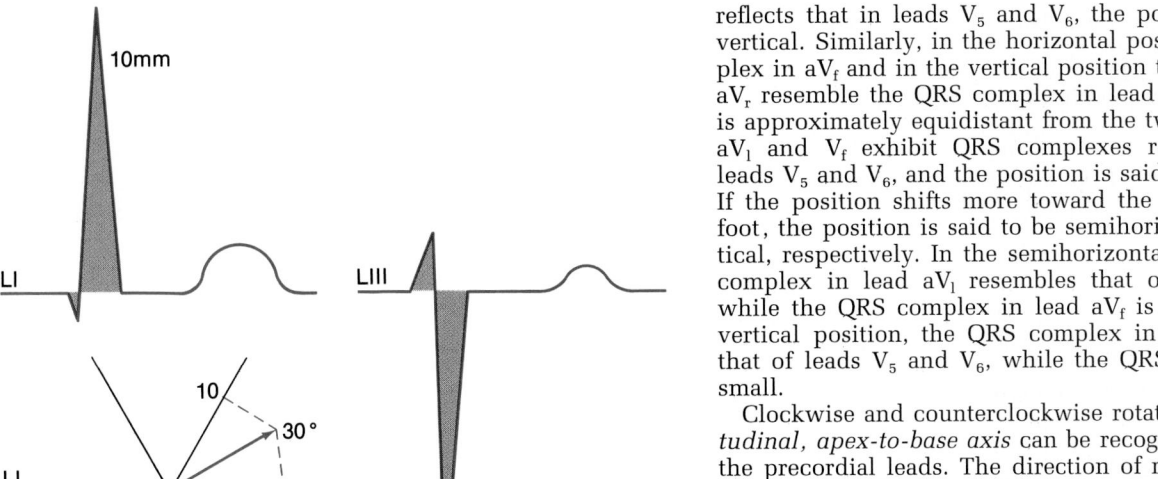

FIGURE 4-7. Electrical axis plotted in leads I and II of the Einthoven triangle. Peak amplitudes of the R wave in lead I and of the S wave in lead III—in this instance each measuring 10 mm—are plotted on their respective leads. Perpendicular lines are dropped and the point at which these cross is identified. A line drawn from the point where leads I, II, and III cross to the point where the two "perpendicular" lines intersect identifies the electrical axis of the QRS (30 degrees). The same approach is used for plotting the P and T axes. When the P, QRS, or T wave area is plotted on the respective lead, the mean P, QRS, or T vector is identified. The latter represents the mean magnitude, direction, and polarity of the entire period of depolarization. This is a more accurate but impractical method of estimating the electrical axis. Although the direction of the QRS axis and of the mean QRS vector differ, as a rule both lie in the same quadrant.

but is scalene, with lead I being shortest and lead III longest.[20] The scalene triangle configuration is more consistent with clinical electrocardiography.

The most accurate method for determining the QRS axis is based on estimation of the QRS area in each of the limb leads and a plot of these as vectors on the respective lead axis of a triaxial reference system. From the positive end of the vector, lines perpendicular to the lead axis are dropped. A vector is drawn from the center of the triaxial reference system to the point where the perpendicular lines cross. This vector defines the direction and magnitude of the mean QRS vector. The same method is used to estimate the T vector. Normally, the angle between the QRS and T vectors does not exceed 30 degrees. For practical purposes, however, the assumption that the magnitude of the force projected on a given lead axis is directionally related to the cosine of the angle subtended by the lead vector and lead axis allows a rapid and reasonably accurate estimate of the QRS axis. Thus, if the mean QRS vector is perpendicular to a given lead axis, the angle between the two is 90 degrees, the cosine of the angle is zero, and the QRS will be iso-electric, very small, or equiphasic. On the other hand, when the mean QRS vector is parallel to a lead axis, the angle between the two is zero, the cosine of the angle is one, and the amplitude of the QRS will be greatest in that lead.

Plotted on a hexaxial reference system, axes of −30 to +90 degrees, −30 to −90 degrees, +90 to 180 degrees, and −90 to 180 degrees are normal, left, right, and inde-terminate, respectively (Fig. 4–8).[21]

An *anteroposterior axis* allows the apex to face either the left arm or the left foot or to assume a position between the two. Thus, when a QRS complex in aV_1 resembles that in leads V_5 and V_6, the electrical position is said to be hori-zontal. On the other hand, when the QRS complex in aV_f

reflects that in leads V_5 and V_6, the position is said to be vertical. Similarly, in the horizontal position the QRS com-plex in aV_f and in the vertical position the QRS complex in aV_r resemble the QRS complex in lead V_1. When the apex is approximately equidistant from the two extremities, both aV_1 and V_f exhibit QRS complexes resembling those in leads V_5 and V_6, and the position is said to be intermediate. If the position shifts more toward the left arm or the left foot, the position is said to be semihorizontal and semiver-tical, respectively. In the semihorizontal position, the QRS complex in lead aV_1 resembles that of leads V_5 and V_6, while the QRS complex in lead aV_f is small. In the semi-vertical position, the QRS complex in lead aV_f resembles that of leads V_5 and V_6, while the QRS complex in aV_1 is small.

Clockwise and counterclockwise rotation along the *longi-tudinal, apex-to-base axis* can be recognized by analysis of the precordial leads. The direction of rotation is described by viewing the heart from the diaphragmatic surface. *Clockwise rotation* shifts the transitional zone (the position at which the rS complex changes to a qR complex) to the left, and consequently, the right ventricular QRS complex (rS) is displaced to the left and occasionally may be regis-tered in all the precordial positions. *Counterclockwise rota-tion* results in a more anterior shift of the left ventricle and a more posterior displacement of the right ventricle. Conse-quently, the transitional zone is shifted to the right, and the left precordial QRS (qR) pattern may be registered, for example, in the V_3 position.

THE ST SEGMENT. The ST segment reflects phase 2 of the transmembrane action potential (see p. 109). Because there is little change in the potential during this phase, the ST segment is usually isoelectric in normal sub-jects.

THE T WAVE. The mechanism and sequence of ventricu-lar repolarization were described on page 109. The right and left precordial T waves are upright in 75 and 50 per cent of newborns, respectively. Often, after about 8 hours, and invariably after 60 to 90 hours, the left precordial T waves become upright. The right precordial T waves usu-ally become upright after the age of 16, but occasionally the negative T waves persist into early adulthood—a normal variant—termed the *juvenile* T wave.

In the adult, all the unipolar leads inscribe an upright T

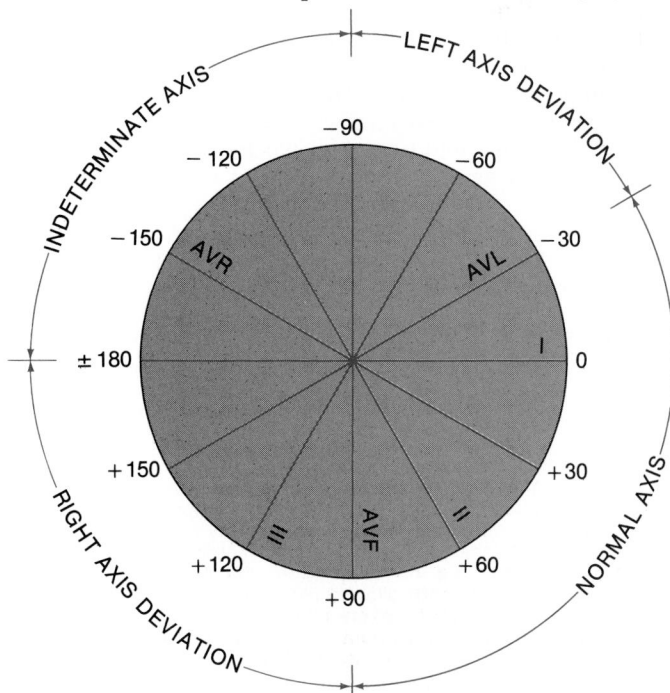

FIGURE 4-8. The frontal plane hexaxial reference system and the respective ranges of axis deviation.

wave except for aV_r and occasionally V_1. The amplitude of T waves is given in Table 4–1.

THE U WAVE. The genesis of the U wave, which follows the T wave, is not clear. It has been suggested that it represents a surface reflection of a negative afterpotential. The two prevailing concepts of the mechanism of the U wave include repolarization of the Purkinje fibers and a mechanical event, presumably ventricular relaxation.

The U wave is upright, and its amplitude is 5 to 50 per cent that of the T wave. The tallest U wave is recorded in leads V_2 and V_3, where its amplitude may reach 0.2 mV. Ordinarily the U and T waves are clearly separated. However, under conditions in which the U wave appears early, such as with abbreviated ventricular filling and ejection or when the Q-T interval is prolonged (as with hypocalcemia or after administration of drugs such as quinidine), the U wave may be difficult to separate from the T wave; on the other hand, when the Q-T interval is abbreviated, as with digitalis or hypercalcemia, the U wave is easily identifiable.

The Q-T Interval

The Q-T interval, measured from the beginning of the QRS complex to the end of the T wave, reflects, within limits, the duration of depolarization and repolarization. Importantly, the Q-T interval may not always accurately reflect the recovery time of the ventricles. In some portions of the ventricles repolarization is complete before the end of the Q-T interval, while in other areas repolarization may continue after the end of the Q-T interval, but because of the small magnitude of the potential or because of cancellation, it cannot be identified in the surface tracing. In addition, because the onset of the QRS complex or the end of the T wave or both may be difficult to define, one cannot always obtain an accurate measurement of the Q-T interval.[21a] The point at which the line of maximal downslope of the T wave crosses the baseline helps to identify the end of the T wave.

Duration of the Q-T interval varies with cycle length, and numerous formulas have been suggested to correct for heart rate. Bazett proposed a formula for estimating the Q-T interval corrected for heart rate,[22] or the *Q-T$_c$ interval:* Q-T/√R-R. The upper limit of the Q-T$_c$ interval is 0.39 sec for men and 0.44 sec for women. The earlier correction equations give conflicting results at low and high heart rates. This is especially true for the Bazett formula. An improved method for adjusting the Q-T interval for heart rate has been proposed using a linear regression model.[23] Similarly, a nomogram giving the number of milliseconds by which the Q-T interval should be corrected for the different heart rates results in an excellent adjustment of the Q-T for the heart rate.[24]

Because of the variability of measurements and potential influences other than heart rate, different ranges of normal are accepted by different investigators.[25] For practical purposes, therefore, minor deviations from the expected Q-T$_c$ interval should be disregarded as being of questionable clinical significance.

The Normal Vectorcardiogram

The concept of vectorcardiography, introduced in 1920 by Mann,[26] can be defined as registration of the time course of mean instantaneous spatial cardiac vectors. By plotting on a triaxial reference system a number of vectors derived simultaneously from leads I and III, and by connecting the ends of the derived vectors, Mann recorded a loop, which he termed a *monocardiogram* (Fig. 4–6C). The advent of the cathode-ray oscilloscope allowed for direct recording of the loop.

Vectorcardiogram (VCG) loops are recorded in three planes: frontal, transverse, and sagittal. Both right and left sagittal views are in use (Fig. 4–9). Any two of the three leads of the orthogonal system will define a plane and will inscribe a loop in a given plane. The combination of *X* and *Y*, *X* and *Z*, *Y* and *Z* will register the VCG loop in the frontal, transverse, or sagittal planes, respectively. To correct for nonuniformity of the conducting medium, eccentricity of the heart as a source, presence of a number of dipoles, and variation in vector-

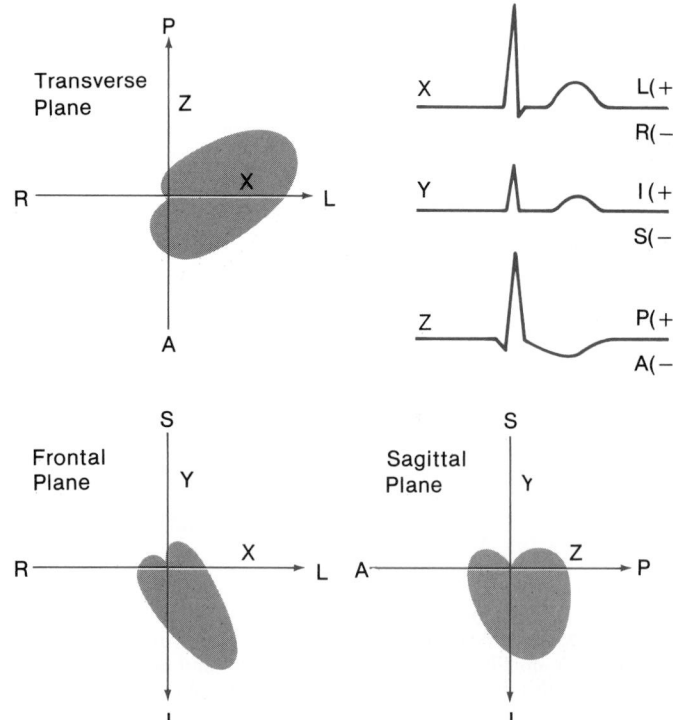

FIGURE 4–9. The transverse, frontal, and sagittal planes and the respective orthogonal leads XZ, XY, and YZ that define the planes. The arrow indicates the positive pole. Normal transverse, frontal, and right sagittal loops are diagrammed. The right upper panel diagrams the orthogonal X, Y, and Z leads. When the vector points to the left (L), inferiorly (I), or posteriorly (P), a positive or upright deflection is recorded. Similarly, if the current flows to the right (R), superiorly (S), or anteriorly (A), a negative or downward deflection is recorded. In this instance the mean vector is oriented to the left, inferiorly, and posteriorly.

ial expression of the magnitude of an electrical signal and to ensure that the three leads are perpendicular, a number of corrected orthogonal leads have been devised. Although none is ideal, the Frank system, because of its relative simplicity, is most widely used[27] (Fig. 4–4B).

The VCG differs from the ECG only in the method of display of the electrical field generated by the heart. *While the ECG reflects best the changes in time and amplitude, the VCG adds the important dimension of direction.* Despite the corrected nature of the orthogonal leads, the assumptions and limitations implicit in the ECG are also applicable to the VCG.

Whether because of the relative complexity of recording the VCG compared with the ECG or because of its failure to add significant information to that gained from the ECG, routine use of the VCG is no longer favored. The spatial VCG, however, is an excellent teaching tool, especially for the analysis of the QRS complex. It is for this reason that the QRS loop is discussed briefly in this chapter.

In a three-dimensional projection, the major portion of the normal QRS loop is located in the left, inferior, and posterior octant[27] (Fig. 4–9). In the frontal plane, the loop is narrow and elongated, and in about one-third of subjects the inscription is clockwise; in the remaining two-thirds the inscription is counterclockwise or a figure-of-eight. The loop is most frequently located in the left inferior quadrant. In the transverse plane, the loop is inscribed counterclockwise and is oval in appearance, and the major portion is located in the left posterior quadrant. In the right sagittal plane, the loop is inscribed clockwise and is located in the anterior and posterior quadrants.

Although the QRS loop is routinely inscribed in the three orthogonal planes, with few exceptions, the characteristic patterns can be recognized in the transverse plane. Patterns with a superior or inferior orientation require frontal projection for analysis. Of these, the most commonly encountered abnormalities include block of the divisions of the left bundle and inferior myocardial infarction. Normal values for the QRS loop are given in Table 4–2.

BODY SURFACE POTENTIAL MAPPING

Body surface potential mapping may contribute information not available from the 12-lead ECG or the VCG; i.e., it provides regional electrophysiological information that cannot be extracted using these methods. Analysis of surface potentials has been applied to the diagnosis of old inferior myocardial infarction, localization of the by-

TABLE 4–2   SOME CHARACTERISTICS OF THE NORMAL QRSsÊ LOOP

115

Ch 4

CHARACTERISTIC	TRANSVERSE PLANE		RIGHT SAGITTAL PLANE		FRONTAL PLANE	
	Mean	95% Range	Mean	95% Range	Mean	95% Range
Max QRS vector						
Direction (degrees)	− 10	− 80 to 20.0	100	50 to 165	35	10 to 65
Magnitude (mV)	1.30	0.85 to 1.95	1.00	0.3 to 1.9	1.50	0.9 to 2.2
0.02-sec vector						
Direction	55	0 to 120.0	15	− 30 to 75	20	Widely scattered
Magnitude	0.40	0.15 to 0.75	0.30	0.10 to 0.55	0.25	0.05 to 0.7
0.04-sec vector						
Direction	− 20	− 90 to 25.0	110	60 to 170	35	− 10 to 70
Magnitude	1.15	0.55 to 1.90	0.90	0.25 to 1.80	1.25	0.4 to 2.2
0.06-sec vector						
Direction	− 90	− 125 to − 35	160	115 to 220	85	Widely scattered
Magnitude	0.45	0 to 0.9	0.55	0.1 to 1.0	0.25	0 to 0.6
Time of occurrence of max						
QRS vector (msec)	38	30 to 48	Same as transverse		Same as transverse	
Direction of inscription		Counterclockwise	Clockwise		Clockwise 65%	
					Figure-of-eight 25%	
					Counterclockwise 10%	

From Chou, T. C., et al.: Clinical Vectorcardiography. 2nd ed. New York, Grune and Stratton, 1974, p. 60.

pass pathway in the Wolff-Parkinson-White syndrome, recognition of ventricular hypertrophy, estimation of the size of a myocardial infarction, and the effects of different interventions designed to reduce infarct size. The limiting factor at present is the complexity of the recording and analysis, which requires 100 or more electrodes, sophisticated instrumentation, and dedicated personnel. Initial efforts toward reducing the number of electrodes without loss of pertinent information are promising. Once the technical obstacles are overcome, large numbers of patients can be studied, and the ultimate utility of this procedure can be evaluated.

THE ABNORMAL ELECTROCARDIOGRAM

Abnormal P Wave and the Ta Segment

Although an atrial abnormality often implies atrial enlargement or hypertrophy, P-wave changes may reflect altered intraatrial pressure, volume, or conduction. Furthermore, shift of the site of origin of the P wave with an intraatrial conduction disturbance may simulate a pathological state. *Right atrial enlargement* or preponderance is manifested by an atrial vector that is increased in magnitude and shifted to the right. The P wave is normal in duration, low or isoelectric in lead I, and tall—but more importantly, peaked or pointed—in leads II, III, and aV$_f$ (Fig. 4–10B). P waves in leads V$_{4r}$, V$_1$, and V$_2$ may be upright and increased in amplitude. A P-wave axis of + 90 degrees or greater, with an isoelectric P wave in lead I, is rarely, if ever, a normal finding. Using two-dimensional echocardiography as a reference, it appears that the most powerful predictor of right atrial enlargement is a P wave in lead V$_2$ greater than 1.5 mm, especially when associated with a QRS axis of + 90 degrees and an R/S ratio greater than 1 in lead V$_1$. While P pulmonale alone detected only 6 per cent of patients with right atrial enlargement, the combined sensitivity of the three criteria was 49 per cent and the specificity was 100 per cent.[28]

In the adult the most common cause of right atrial abnormality is chronic obstructive lung disease (see p. 135). The predictive value of P wave amplitude for detecting right atrial enlargement diagnosed with two-dimensional echocardiography is low. P pulmonale pattern in the absence of right atrial enlargement, termed *pseudo–P pulmonale*, has been found in association with a variety of disorders of the left heart, including coronary artery disease with angina pectoris, and less often in the absence of heart disease. It has been suggested that in the presence of left heart disease, pseudo–P pulmonale reflects an increase of the left atrial component of the P waves.[29] This suggestion is supported by a recent observation that damage to the left atrium increases the right atrial vector and damage to the right atrium simulates left atrial enlargement.[30]

Left atrial enlargement is manifested by prolongation of the P wave, shortening or absence of the P-R segment, and a shift of the P vector to the left and posteriorly (Fig. 4–10A). The duration of the P wave is 0.12 sec or longer, the prolongation is at the expense of the P-R segment, the P wave is notched, and its axis is shifted to the left. Because the vector is increased in magnitude and oriented posteriorly, lead V$_1$ registers a prominent negative P wave. A negative P wave in lead V$_1$, 0.04 sec in duration and 0.1 mV in depth, is consistent with left atrial preponderance, the so-called *P mitrale*. In a study of 57 patients with

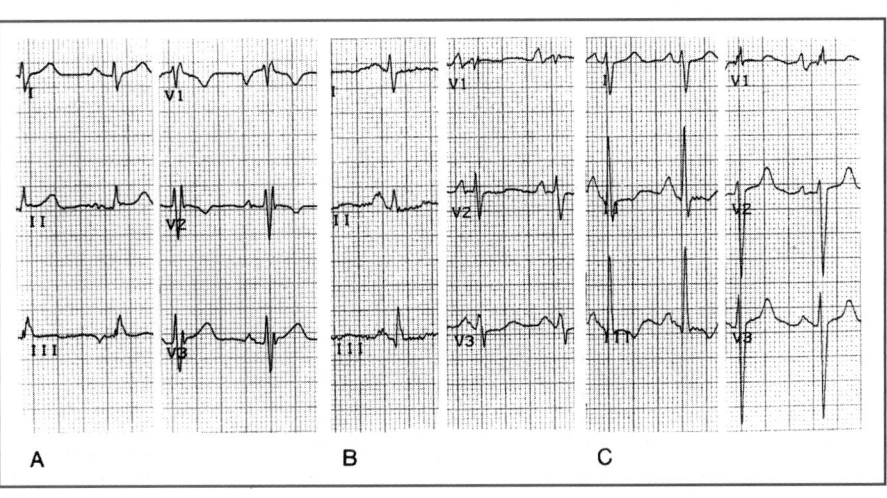

FIGURE 4–10. *A*, Left atrial enlargement manifest by prolonged notched P wave with left axis and the highly specific negative P wave in lead V$_1$. A common feature, not evident in this figure, is foreshortening or absence of the P-R segment. *B*, Right atrial enlargement with the diagnostic prominent positive P waves in leads V$_1$ and V$_2$. The other characteristic features of the P wave in the frontal plane, namely, right-axis deviation and prominent, pointed P waves in leads II and III, are shown in Figure 4–14. *C*, Biatrial enlargement manifest by a tall, broad P wave in lead II, a notched P wave in lead III, and a large biphasic P in lead V$_1$.

echocardiographically confirmed left atrial enlargement, the sensitivity of the various ECG criteria for left atrial enlargements varied from as low as 15 per cent for notched P wave with interpeak duration more than 0.04 sec to as high as 83 per cent for negative P wave of more than 0.04 sec in lead V_1. The specificity varied from 64 per cent for a foreshortened P-R segment to nearly 100 per cent for notched P wave with interpeak more than 0.04 sec.[31] Although P mitrale is common in mitral valve disease, the most frequent cause is left ventricular disease, with the increased left ventricular end-diastolic pressure reflected in the atrium.

In *biatrial* enlargement, both anterior and posterior forces are increased. The abnormality includes a prominent initial part of the P wave coupled with the left axis of the terminal portion of the P wave and a biphasic P wave in leads V_1 and occasionally in V_2 (Fig. 4–10C).

In the presence of atrial fibrillation, atrial disease can occasionally be suspected from an analysis of the QRS complex. With severe tricuspid regurgitation, right atrial enlargement displaces the tricuspid valve down and to the left. As a result, lead V_1 (and sometimes V_2), normally subtended by the right ventricle, now reflects the intracavitary (qR) right atrial potential as indicated by QR, qR, or qrs complexes in leads V_1 or V_1 and V_2 followed by a normal progression of R-wave amplitude from leads V_2 or V_3 to V_6 (Fig. 4–AE1, p. 146). Atrial enlargement also can be suspected when coarse, relatively large fibrillatory waves are present, especially in lead V_1. This is in contrast to atrial fibrillation complicating arteriosclerotic and hypertensive heart disease, in which the fibrillatory waves are fine and frequently unidentifiable.

Alteration of atrial repolarization (Ta), recognized by deviation from the T-P segment, can be either secondary or primary. Secondary changes appear in response to and are obligatory to atrial depolarization, while primary Ta changes are independent of atrial depolarization and indicate nonuniformity of atrial repolarization (Fig. 4–5). The usual pathological causes of secondary Ta-segment depression, which may exceed 1 mm (0.1 mV), include atrial dilation, hypertrophy, and intraatrial block. In chronic obstructive lung disease, for example, depression of the Ta segment may be exaggerated and mistaken for ST-segment displacement.

The usual causes of *primary* Ta-segment changes are pericarditis (Fig. 4–5), atrial infarction, and atrial injury due to penetrating wounds. *Pericarditis* exaggerates the normally negative Ta segment, and Ta-segment depression is recorded in all leads except aV_r, in which it is elevated. Occasionally, a Ta-segment abnormality may be the only convincing evidence of acute pericarditis.

The incidence of *atrial infarction* in myocardial infarction (see p. 1192) is difficult to estimate, and the reported numbers vary widely. In a study of 304 consecutive patients with Q-wave myocardial infarction, displacement of the Ta segment was noted in 10 per cent. However, in 12 patients the Ta depression was associated with a pericardial friction rub, making a differentiation of Ta abnormality due to infarction from that due to pericarditis difficult. A Ta depression suggested a larger infarct size and an increased in-hospital mortality.[32] Isolated atrial infarction in the absence of ventricular infarction is a most unlikely event. The manifestations of infarction may include elevation of the Ta segment in leads I, II, III, V_5, or V_6 or a depression that may exceed 0.15 mV in precordial leads and 0.1 mV in leads I, II, and III. Displacement of Ta segment in an opposite direction, a reciprocal change, may be recorded in "distal" leads, i.e., those facing noninfarcted areas of the atrium. Attempts to localize the site of atrial infarction by ECG have been unsuccessful. Supraventricular arrhythmias frequently accompany atrial infarction.

Penetrating injury of the atria due to gunshot wounds (see p. 1539) or perforation in the course of cardiac catheterization may be associated with diagnostic Ta-segment depression. Ta-segment displacement is also frequently observed following open heart surgery, and whether or not the displacement reflects mechanical injury, associated pericarditis, hemopericardium, or a combination of these factors is still unclear.

Ventricular Hypertrophy

Left Ventricular Hypertrophy (LVH)

ECG manifestations of LVH include an increase in voltage; shift of the mean QRS axis posteriorly, superiorly, and to the left; prolongation of depolarization (delayed intrinsicoid deflection); and gradual shift of the ST segment and T wave in a direction opposite to that of the QRS complex. The exact mechanism of the voltage increase is not clear.[33] In addition to the muscle mass, other factors may play a role, such as intracavitary blood volume, proximity to the chest wall, conducting properties of intrathoracic organs, location of the heart within the thorax, intraventricular and transmural pressures, and perhaps unopposed inscription of a portion of the QRS complex due to delayed activation.

The left superior and posterior orientation of the mean QRS vector in LVH is most likely related to hypertrophy of the basal portion of the left ventricle with delayed, and at times unopposed, activation. Variables that may be responsible for delayed depolarization include increased muscle mass, decreased Purkinje activation, and localized intraventricular conduction delays. Marked superior orientation is noted in association with left anterior divisional block.

Prolongation of the excited state through the myocardium and prolongation of activation result in a change in the order of repolarization, which proceeds from endocardium to epicardium, resulting in a reversal of T-wave polarity. Of the mechanisms responsible for this reversal of repolarization, increased muscle mass without a concomitant increase in the capillary bed, the so-called relative coronary insufficiency, may be an important factor. It is also possible that as the muscle mass outgrows the Purkinje fiber mass, more of the activation proceeds through the myocardium, and this can contribute to a change in the T-wave vector. ST-segment depression may be due to the onset of repolarization before the completion of depolarization.

The mean QRS vector, increased in magnitude and oriented toward the left, posteriorly and superiorly, results in a positive deflection in leads I, II, aV_1, V_5, and V_6 and a positive or negative deflection in leads III and aV_f. The precordial transitional zone is shifted to the left. Leads V_1 and V_2 record an rS pattern, but in some instances the initial R wave may be absent, most likely due to posterior rotation of the QRS loop (Fig. 4–11). Lack of the initial R wave may be erroneously interpreted as an anteroseptal myocardial infarction.

QRS voltage criteria for LVH include $R_I + S_{III} \geq 2.5$ mV, R in $aV_1 > 1.2$ mV, R in $aV_f > 2.0$ mV, S in $V_1 \geq 2.4$ mV, R in V_5 or $V_6 > 2.6$ mV, and R in V_5 or V_6 + S in $V_1 > 3.5$ mV.[34] The following point system for diagnosing LVH has been suggested. Amplitude of R or S wave in limb leads ≥ 2.0 mV *or* S wave in V_1 or $V_2 \geq 3.0$ mV *or* R wave

Transverse

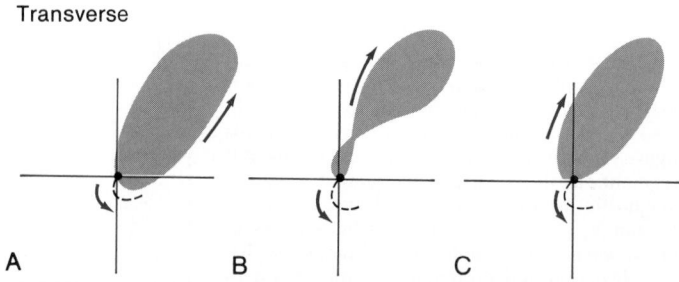

FIGURE 4–11. VCG loops in the transverse plane in left ventricular hypertrophy. The loops illustrate the occasional loss of the initial rightward force (*A*) and rightward and anterior forces (*B, C*) as a result of LVH. Such changes are reflected in the precordial ECG by diminution or loss of the initial R wave in right precordial leads, which could mistakenly suggest myocardial infarction. The dashed lines represent the initial normal forces.

in V_5 or $V_6 \geq 3.0$ mV = 3 points. ST segment changes with or without digitalis = 1 or 2 points, respectively. Left atrial enlargement = 3 points. Left-axis deviation of -30 degrees or more = 2 points. QRS duration ≥ 0.09 sec and intrinsicoid deflection in V_5 and $V_6 \geq 0.05$ sec = 1 point each. Left ventricular hypertrophy is considered to be likely if the points total 4 and to be present if the total is 5 or more. It also has been suggested that the strongest independent variables for LVH, when compared with the echocardiogram, include the S wave in lead V_3 and the R wave in aV_l. In men, the sum of R wave in aV_l and S wave in V_3 (the Cornell index) exceeding 35 mm indicates LVH.[35]

The diagnosis of LVH is strengthened by a delayed intrinsicoid deflection in lead V_5 or V_6, measuring more than 0.05 sec in the adult. The *intrinsicoid deflection,* based on the concept of intrinsic deflection (see p. 109) and applied to the indirect surface leads, is theoretically related to muscle mass. In the clinical ECG the time from the onset of the QRS to the peak of the R wave is an estimate of the intrinsicoid deflection. In the right (namely, V_1, V_2) and left (namely, V_5, V_6) precordial leads, the time from onset of the QRS to appearance of the intrinsicoid deflection is 0.035 and 0.055 sec or less, respectively. For practical purposes in the study of conduction delays, the term *R peak time* is preferred.[21]

The direction of the ST segment and T wave is opposite to that of the QRS complex in LVH. Characteristically, the T wave is negative and asymmetrical, its ascending limb being steeper with an occasional terminal positive inscription. The J point and the ST segment are depressed in leads I, aV_l, V_5, and V_6. The T-wave inversion is greater in lead V_6 than in V_4. In the presence of a vertical position, these changes are recorded in leads II, III, and aV_f. It has been suggested that depression of the J point, asymmetry of the T wave with a more rapid return to the baseline, terminal positivity of the T wave ("overshoot"), T-wave inversion in lead V_6 greater than 3 mm, and T-wave change greater in lead V_6 than V_4 support the diagnosis of LVH and help to distinguish LVH from coronary artery disease in the absence of voltage criteria for LVH.[36] Left atrial dilatation is common with LVH.

The limitations of the sensitivity of the ECG criteria for LVH are recognized. This is true for both the voltage criteria and the point system.[37] Anatomical and echocardiographic studies suggest a sensitivity of about 25 per cent for Sokolow-Lyons voltage criteria and approximately 50 per cent for Romhilt-Estes point score. The specificity is approximately 95 per cent for both. Sensitivity of the criteria for LVH varies depending on the etiology of the underlying heart disease, with the sensitivity lowest in the presence of coronary artery disease.

In a population with a true prevalence of LVH of less than 10 per cent, there are more false-positive than true-positive diagnoses. Similarly, autopsy data indicate that voltage changes consistent with LVH can be present in the absence of LVH.

The concept of *diastolic overload* may be useful clinically.[38] It may point to such lesions as patent ductus arteriosus, ventricular septal defect, or aortic or mitral valve regurgitation, in which there is volume overload. The ECG pattern is one of LVH but with a prominent Q wave in the leads facing the left side of the septum, namely, I, aV_l, V_5, and V_6, and a reciprocal, prominent R wave in the leads facing the right side of the septum, namely, V_1 and V_2. As a rule, the Q wave is narrow, measuring 0.025 sec or less, and its depth is 0.2 mV or greater (Figs. 4–AE2 and 4–AE3, p. 146). Systolic or "pressure" overload is characterized by high-amplitude R waves and ST-segment and T-wave changes in the left ventricular leads and may be present in disorders with an increased resistance to left ventricular outflow. However, the accuracy of the LVH pattern in predicting the hemodynamic abnormality is limited.

VECTORCARDIOGRAM. The VCG changes in LVH are due to an increase in and rotation of the forces farther to the left and posteriorly. These events are best reflected in the transverse plane. The VCG loop is increased in magnitude, elongated, inscribed counterclockwise as a rule, and shifted posteriorly. The occasional posterior orientation of the initial part of the loop simulates anteroseptal myocardial infarction (Fig. 4–11).

Right Ventricular Hypertrophy (RVH)

In contrast to LVH, RVH is not simply an exaggeration of the normal. For RVH to become manifested, the right ventricular mass must be sufficiently large to overcome the left ventricular forces (Fig. 4–12). For this reason, the specificity of the ECG pattern of RVH is much greater, but the sensitivity is relatively low, varying from 25 to 40 per cent depending on the criteria used.[33] While the ECG changes of RVH result largely from the chamber's anatomical dominance, the cause of the heart disease and associated hemodynamic alterations often contribute to the abnormal ECG pattern. At times, the etiology of the cardiac disorder and the severity of right ventricular pressure can be estimated from an analysis of the ECG.

In RVH the axis shifts to the right, the degree of axis deviation varying with the clinical disorder, and this is accompanied by vertical position and clockwise rotation. Based on the QRS pattern in lead V_1, RVH can generally be separated into three groups, namely, a dominant R wave (qR, rR, rsR') (Figs. 4–12 and 4–AE4, p. 146), RS complex (Rs, Rsr'), and rS or rsr' complex. The different QRS patterns may provide a clue to the degree of elevation in right ventricular pressure. In general, a qR complex, a prominent R wave with a slur on the upstroke, or an rsR' complex (incomplete right bundle branch block) suggests that right ventricular pressure exceeds (qR), is equal to (R or rR), or is lower than (rsR') left ventricular pressure, respectively. Ex-

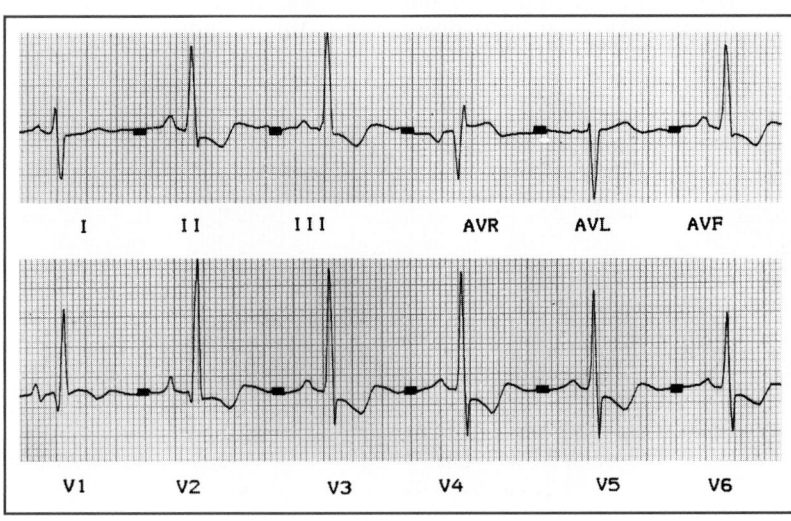

FIGURE 4–12. Right ventricular hypertrophy with marked right-axis deviation and vertical position of the QRS complex, a qR pattern in leads V_1 and V_2, and tall R wave in lead V_1. The qR pattern in leads V_1 and V_2 suggests that the right ventricular pressure exceeds the left ventricular pressure. Absence of the typical P wave changes in leads I, II, and III is compatible with pulmonary hypertension due to pulmonary fibrosis (see text). The ST-T changes are secondary to the right ventricular hypertrophy.

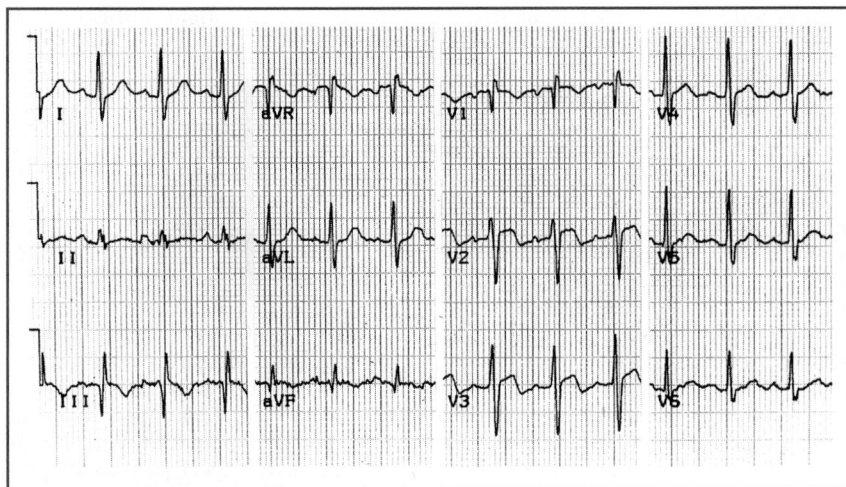

FIGURE 4–13. Acute massive pulmonary embolus with the characteristic S_1Q_3 pattern and the more common but nonspecific changes including incomplete right bundle branch block and ST segment elevation in leads V_1 to V_3 with terminal T wave inversion.

amples include severe pulmonary stenosis or primary pulmonary hypertension (qR), tetralogy of Fallot or Eisenmenger complex (R or rR), and atrial septal defect (rsR'), respectively. In the latter, hypertrophy of the outflow tract of the right ventricle is responsible for the R' wave.

In the presence of RVH the delay of ventricular activation results in earlier recovery of the endocardium, and as in LVH, repolarization proceeds from endocardium to epicardium. The ST segment is thereby depressed and the T wave inverted in lead V_1 and occasionally in V_2. Significant ST-segment depression and T-wave inversion are, as a rule, indicative of moderate or severe right ventricular hypertension.

In the adult with acquired RVH the most commonly encountered ECG changes include right-axis deviation and an R/S ratio equal to or greater than 1 in V_1, with an R wave 0.5 mV or greater. Isolated right-axis deviation of +100 to −90 degrees is considered by some to be indicative of RVH, but this criterion alone is less sensitive (Fig. 4–AE5, p. 146). An R/S ratio greater than 1 in lead V_1 alone is not diagnostic of RVH, since it may be recorded in patients with a posterior infarction or occasionally in the absence of heart disease.

ACUTE PULMONARY EMBOLISM (ACUTE COR PULMONALE) (see Chap. 46). The most characteristic ECG feature of this disorder is probably the transient nature of the changes, and for this reason serial tracings are most helpful.[39] In 49 proven cases of acute pulmonary embolism, the ECG diagnosis was considered probable in 37 patients (76 per cent). This was based on the presence of three or more of the following ECG changes: (1) incomplete or complete RBBB ($n = 33$); associated with ST elevation ($n = 17$) and positive T wave in lead V_1 ($n = 3$); (2) S wave in leads I and aV_1 of >1.5 mm ($n = 36$); (3) clockwise rotation ($n = 25$); (4) Q waves in leads III and aV_f but not in lead II ($n = 24$); (5) right-axis deviation >90 degrees ($n = 16$) or indeterminate axis ($n = 15$); (6) low-voltage QRS complex of <5 mm in limb leads ($n = 10$); and (7) T wave inversion in leads III and aV_f ($n = 16$) or leads V_1 to V_4 ($n = 13$) (Fig. 4–13). Of the 12 patients with normal ECG on admission, only 3 became positive on serial tracings.[40] The ECG changes are most likely related to acute pulmonary hypertension with right atrial and ventricular dilation, hypoxia, and perhaps myocardial ischemia. Acute atrial dilation coupled with myocardial ischemia is probably responsible for the frequent atrial arrhythmias. Despite the high incidence of abnormal tracings, the diagnosis is difficult because of the nonspecific nature of the ECG changes. While a single ECG is rarely helpful, a comparison with a tracing obtained before the acute episode and serial tracings after the episode increase significantly the sensitivity of the ECG.

CHRONIC OBSTRUCTIVE LUNG DISEASE (COLD) AND COR PULMONALE (see Chap. 47). The ECG pattern of COLD and COLD with pulmonary hypertension (cor pulmonale) can be ascribed to a combination of positional changes, increased lung volume, and RVH. ECG changes include right-axis deviation of the P wave, increased amplitude and "peaked" appearance of the P wave in the limb leads, and "peaked" and biphasic morphology wave in leads V_1 and V_2 (Figs. 4–10B and 4–14). A P-wave axis of +90 degrees is highly suggestive of COLD. The shift of the P-wave axis is most likely due to overinflation of the lungs. While right-axis deviation of the P wave is present in about 80 per cent of patients with obstructive lung disease, only 7 per cent of the patients with restrictive lung disease manifest right-axis deviation of the P wave. Similarly, 53 per cent of patients with restrictive lung disease manifest a horizontal P-wave axis as contrasted with only 8 per cent of the patients with obstructive lung disease.[41] Because of the large P-wave area, the Ta segment is exaggerated and occasionally interpreted as ST-segment depression. Right-

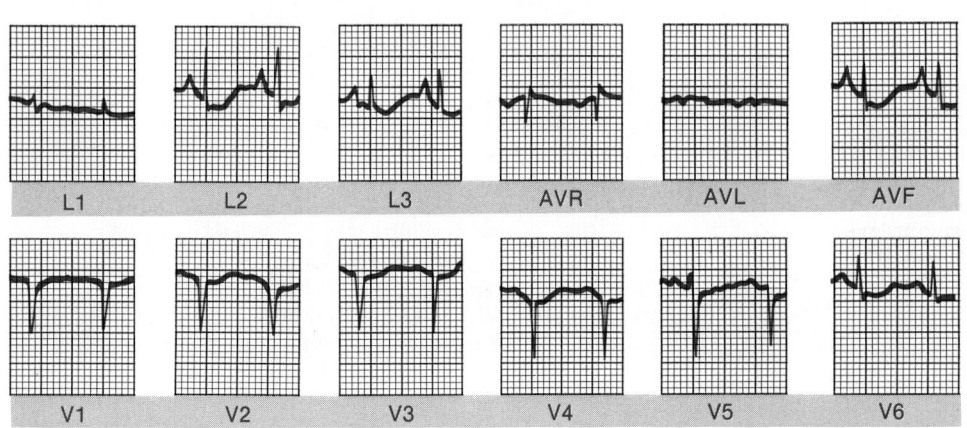

FIGURE 4–14. A case of chronic obstructive lung disease (COLD) simulating an anteroseptal myocardial infarction. The characteristic features of COLD include "pointed" tall P waves in leads 2, 3, AV_f with right-axis deviation (+90 degrees), tendency to right axis of the QRS, clockwise rotation, and "pseudo–ST segment" depression. The latter reflects atrial repolarization. The clockwise rotation simulates anteroseptal myocardial infarction.

axis deviation and clockwise rotation are characteristic findings. Occasionally, an $S_1S_2S_3$ pattern may be present.[42] Amplitude of the precordial R wave is reduced in leads V_5 and V_6, often measuring less than 0.7 mV. When the clockwise rotation is marked, absence of the R wave in precordial leads simulates an anterior myocardial infarction. With progression to pulmonary hypertension and RVH, prominent R waves may appear in leads V_1 and V_2. These changes are probably due to unopposed late activation of the crista terminalis and right ventricular free wall. Right atrial dilatation is probably responsible for the QR pattern in V_1, with the Q wave reflecting right atrial intracavitary potential (as occurs also in tricuspid regurgitation) (Fig. 4–AE1). As indicated, the sensitivity of the ECG for cor pulmonale is relatively low, the test being diagnostic in about 25 to 40 per cent of patients with confirmed RVH.

In *biventricular hypertrophy*, the LV forces are dominant and often obscure the RVH.

VECTORCARDIOGRAM. In RVH, the characteristic VCG changes of the QRS loop are recorded in the transverse plane, and these fall into three general types (Fig. 4–15). In type A, the configuration varies considerably. It may be oval, narrow, or figure-of-eight. The major segment of the loops is located anteriorly and to the right. The loop is inscribed clockwise or, as in the case of the figure-of-eight loop,

initially counterclockwise with the latter component recorded clockwise. An oval loop is illustrated in Figure 4–15. In type B, the loop is inscribed clockwise or counterclockwise, is often figure-of-eight, and is located primarily in the left anterior and to a lesser extent in the left and right posterior quadrants. In type C, the loop is inscribed counterclockwise, with 50 per cent of the loop located in posterior left and right quadrants. Of the three, type A usually reflects severe RVH, while type B is most often encountered in patients with atrial septal defect and mitral stenosis. Type C can be recorded with chronic obstructive lung disease.

VENTRICULAR HYPERTROPHY IN THE PRESENCE OF CONDUCTION DEFECTS

The diagnosis of ventricular hypertrophy in the presence of intraventricular conduction defect is difficult, if not impossible, owing in part to the fact that a portion of cardiac activation may be unopposed for a period of time, resulting in misleading voltage changes[43] (Fig. 4–AE6, p. 146). It has been suggested that in the presence of right bundle branch block (RBBB), an R' greater than 1.0 to 1.5 mV indicates associated RVH. However, it is not unusual to record preoperatively a normal QRS complex in lead V_1, only to register postoperatively an RBBB with an R' wave greater than 1.0 or 1.5 mV, indicating that this criterion of RVH may not be valid in the presence of RBBB (Fig. 4–AE7, p. 147). Left bundle branch block (LBBB) makes a diagnosis of RVH and LVH essentially impossible. In the presence of RBBB, LVH may be suspected when the S wave in lead V_1 and the R wave in lead V_6 satisfy voltage criteria for LVH. However, such an interpretation is subject to the limitations imposed by the relatively low sensitivity and specificity of the voltage criteria. It also has been suggested that the QRS is significantly longer in LBBB with LVH than with isolated LBBB.

In a study of 50 patients with left anterior fascicular block, the sum of S in lead III and the maximal R + S in any precordial lead equal to or exceeding 3 mV (30 mm) showed a specificity of 87 per cent, a sensitivity of 96 per cent, a positive predictive value of 89 per cent, and a negative predictive value of 95 per cent for LVH.[44]

Intraventricular Conduction Defects

The bundle of His bifurcates into right and left bundles (see Fig. 20–5, p. 551). The ribbon-like right bundle descends subendocardially on the right side of the septum. At the base of the right ventricular anterior papillary muscle, it divides and supplies fibers to the free right ventricular wall and the right side of the septum. The left bundle divides into an anterior division (LAD) and posterior division (LPD), which supply the left ventricular wall and left side of the septum. Discrete anatomical lesions, asynchrony of conduction in the bundles or its branches, nonuniformity of refractoriness, changes in membrane responsiveness, and a decrease in the magnitude of phase 4 of the transmembrane action potential (see p. 109) may, singly or in combination, cause block of conduction in the bundle branches (BBB) and the divisions of the left bundle. However, most commonly BBB is due to an anatomical lesion. In transient BBB, the specific underlying electrophysiological mechanism may be difficult to define.

Left Bundle Branch Block (LBBB)

Interruption of the left bundle branch results in early activation of the right side of the septum and of the right ventricular myocardium. Transseptal activation from right to left is transmyocardial and thus slow, and probably a major cause of the prolonged ventricular activation. Initial activation of the ventricles proceeds from right to left, inferiorly, and more often anteriorly than posteriorly. This is followed by continued activation of the septum and of the adjacent free left ventricular wall, with the activation proceeding to the left, posteriorly, and inferiorly. This phase of activation is rapid, presumably because the impulse enters the Purkinje system below the site of the BBB. Last to be activated are the lateral wall and basal aspect of the left ventricle, with a vector oriented posteriorly, superiorly, and, less frequently, inferiorly.

In complete LBBB, the QRS complex is prolonged, measuring 0.12 to 0.18 sec (Fig. 4–16).[45] An upright notched or slurred R wave reflecting the right-to-left myocardial activation is recorded in leads I, aV_l, and V_6. A small R wave followed by an S wave is present in aV_f; the R wave and

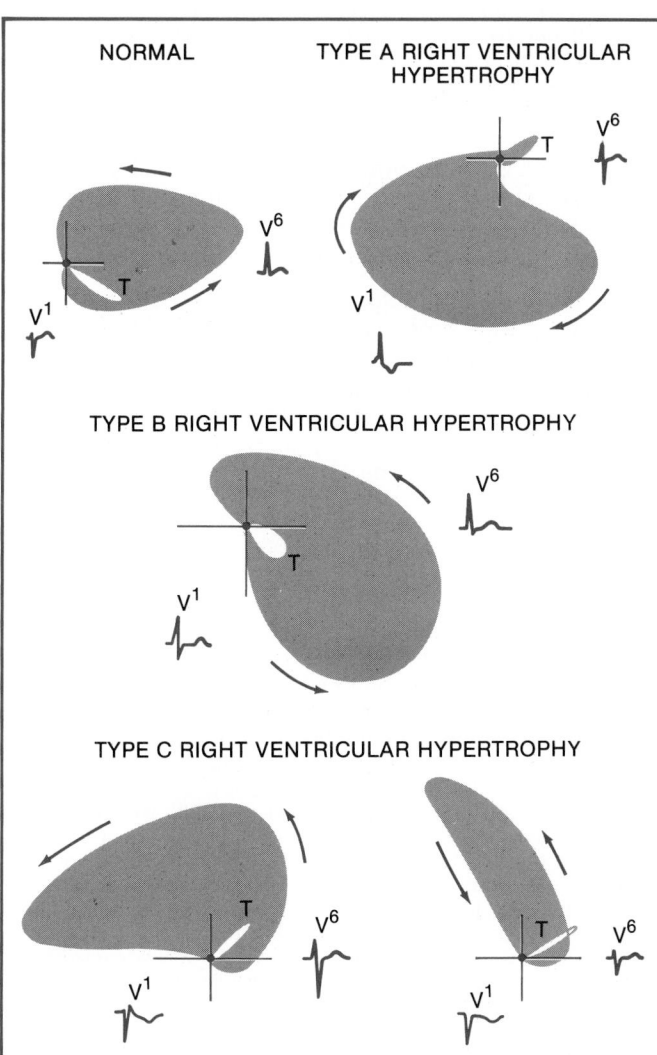

FIGURE 4–15. Diagrammatic representation of the three common, but not exclusive, VCG patterns of right ventricular hypertrophy recorded in the horizontal plane. When compared with the normal, the QRS loops are located in the right and left anterior quadrants in type A and in the left anterior and to a lesser extent left and right posterior quadrants in type B; a major portion of the loop is located in the left and right posterior quadrants in type C. (Modified from Chou, T. C., Helm, R. A., and Kaplan, S.: Clinical Vectorcardiography. 2nd ed. New York, Grune and Stratton, 1974, pp. 87, 99, 102.)

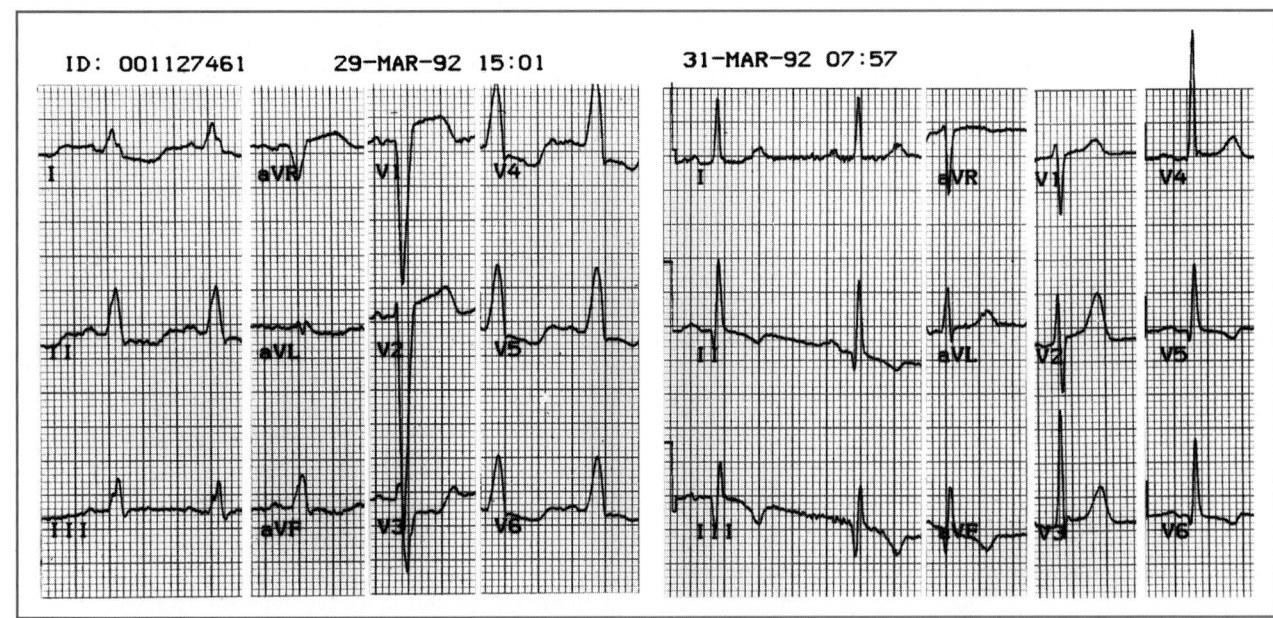

FIGURE 4–16. Left bundle branch block (LBBB) obscuring an inferior myocardial infarction. LBBB is present in the left panel at a heart rate of 100 beats/min. With slowing of the heart rate to 75 beats/min in the right panel, the intraventricular conduction normalizes with appearance of an inferior myocardial infarction and most likely ischemic T waves in leads V_5 and V_6. With LBBB, the septum depolarizes from right to left, and the left ventricular intracavitary potential is initially positive, thus in keeping with the "window" concept of ECG changes of myocardial infarction, precluding recording of a Q wave.

the S wave reflect, respectively, the initial septal activation directed inferiorly and the superior orientation of the final vector. An rS or a QS complex, depending on whether the initial activation is oriented anteriorly or posteriorly, is recorded in lead V_1, with the S wave reflecting activation of the left ventricle from right to left. An initial R wave in lead V_1 is present in about 45 per cent of cases of LBBB. The precordial leads V_1 to V_4 may exhibit a small R wave, with the R waves in the midprecordial leads occasionally lower in amplitude than those in the right precordial leads. One clinically important feature of LBBB is an absence of a

septal Q, owing to the initial right-to-left septal activation. Similarly, a Q wave fails to register when either myocardial infarction complicates preexisting LBBB or when LBBB complicates an acute myocardial infarction (see p. 127) (Fig. 4–16). The frontal axis in LBBB may be either normal or directed to the left (− 30 to − 90 degrees), the prevalence of the two being about equal. Although it has been accepted that an abnormal left axis in excess of − 45 degrees is nearly always due to a left anterior divisional block, LBBB per se also may result in pronounced left-axis deviation.

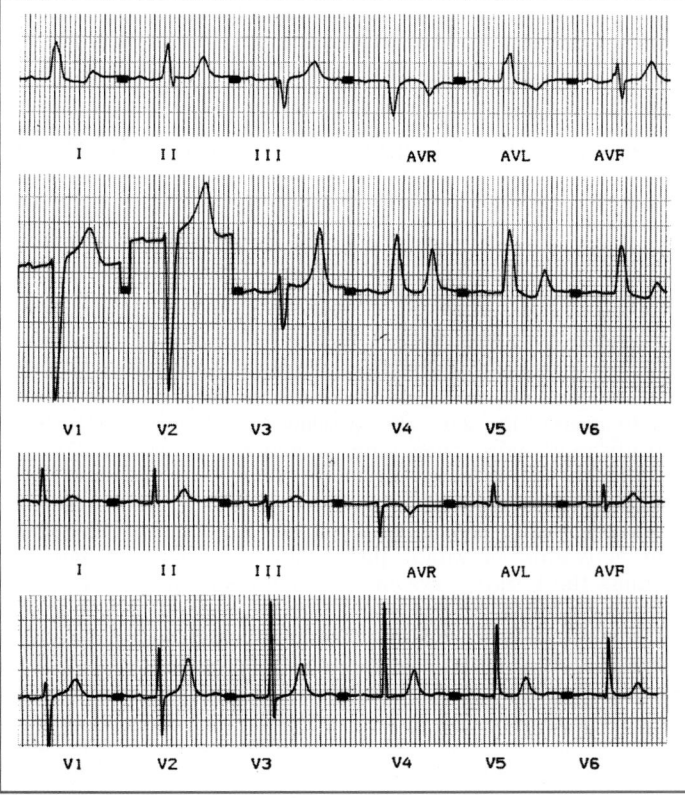

FIGURE 4–17. Left bundle branch block (LBBB) with primary T wave changes; i.e., the T waves are upright rather than being inverted and opposite to the QRS area. Such primary T waves suggest a primary myocardial disorder that is not secondary to the bundle branch block. In approximately 15 per cent, however, with normalization of the intraventricular conduction the electrocardiogram is normal *(lower panel)*. In this instance the LBBB was rate-related.

In LBBB, the direction of the ST-segment and T-wave vectors is opposite to that of the QRS vector. In the presence of an upright QRS complex in leads I, aV_l, and V_6, the ST segment is depressed and the T waves are inverted. The opposite is true in leads V_1, V_2, and V_3, in which a predominantly negative QRS complex is recorded. The ST-segment and T-wave changes are secondary to the conduction disturbance, and the magnitude of the change parallels the magnitude of the QRS aberration. Occasionally LBBB is associated with an isoelectric ST segment and a T-wave vector concordant with the QRS vector. Such primary T-wave changes suggest a myocardial abnormality independent of the LBBB, which may be due, for example, to accompanying myocardial ischemia. However, this is not always a reliable sign of a primary myocardial disorder (Fig. 4–17).

Incomplete LBBB implies a greater delay of conduction in the left than in the right bundle, with initial right-to-left septal activation and loss of the septal Q wave. In contrast to complete LBBB, the left bundle ultimately contributes to activation of the septum and left ventricular wall. ECG criteria for incomplete LBBB include a QRS complex of 0.10 to 0.12 sec, loss of the initial septal Q wave, slurring or notching, and often high voltage of the QRS complex.

In the transverse plane of the VCG, the QRS loop of LBBB is oriented to the left and posteriorly. The initial portion of the loop reflects septal activation and is inscribed slowly from right to left and anteriorly. The remainder of the loop is inscribed clockwise with slow inscription of the midportion, most likely reflecting slow intramyocardial conduction through the left ventricular wall. The T loop points in a direction opposite to that of the QRS.

Right Bundle Branch Block (RBBB)

In RBBB the septum is activated normally, from left to right. While the left ventricle is activated normally, right ventricular depolarization is delayed, the right ventricle being last to be activated, and this terminal activation is unopposed. Prolongation of the QRS complex is largely due to delayed activation of the right ventricular wall. The initial dominant septal force is directed from left to right, anteriorly and superiorly, followed by a vector dominated by the left ventricle, oriented to the left, inferiorly, and either somewhat anteriorly or posteriorly. The final vector representing activation of the right ventricle is directed to the right, anteriorly, and either superiorly, inferiorly, or horizontally.

The characteristic ECG changes of RBBB are recorded in lead V_1. The initial normal septal activation inscribes an R wave, followed by an S wave reflecting left ventricular activation and a final R' wave due to depolarization of the right ventricle from left to right and anteriorly. The depth of the S wave in lead V_1 varies depending on whether the left ventricular activation generates a more posteriorly or anteriorly oriented vector. In the former, a prominent S wave separates the R wave from the R' wave, while in the latter, the S wave may be shallow or a slur or, indeed, may be absent. Leads facing the left side of the septum, namely, I, aV_l, V_5, and V_6, record an initial Q wave followed by an R wave of normal duration and a prolonged, relatively shallow S wave. The latter reflects delayed activation of the right ventricle (Figs. 4–18 to 4–20). Because the initial septal activation is normal, namely, left to right, RBBB, in contrast to LBBB, does not obscure myocardial infarction.

The T wave is usually inverted in lead V_1 and occasionally in V_2, while it is upright in the remaining precordial and limb leads, a direction opposite to the *terminal* portion of the QRS complex.

Preliminary evidence suggests that patients with RBBB with a normal QT interval but persistent ST-segment elevation in leads V_1 to V_3 not explainable by electrolyte disturbances, ischemia, or structural heart disease are prone to rapid polymorphic ventricular tachycardia and sudden death.[46] Others propose that the terminal "delay" in the right precordial leads represents a J wave rather than delay due to RBBB. The mechanism of the J wave is unclear and may vary depending on the underlying clinical condition.[47]

The characteristic VCG feature is evident in the transverse plane and consists of a slowly inscribed terminal appendage directed to the right and anteriorly. The initial septal and left ventricular portion of the loop is normal.

Divisional (Fascicular) Blocks

The ventricular conduction system, including the right bundle branch and the two divisions of the left bundle, can be considered for purposes of clinical electrocardiography to consist of three divisions (fascicles) (Fig. 4–21). Divisional blocks are, with rare exception, acquired. Although the evidence for the existence of anatomically discrete divisions of the left bundle branch is not convincing, experimental data support a functional divisional conduction system.[48]

Furthermore, nearly simultaneous early endocardial activation at two sites—the middle anterior and posterior paraseptal areas—is consistent with the concept of functional divisions of the left bundle. This concept is also supported by distinctive and predictable ECG patterns. Thus, from the ECG standpoint, the concept of divisions of the left bundle is a useful one.[49]

BLOCK OF ANTERIOR DIVISION OF THE LEFT BUNDLE BRANCH (ANTERIOR FASCICULAR BLOCK). In the presence of left anterior divisional block, the initial septal activation proceeds inferiorly, anteriorly, to the right, and occasionally to the left. This is followed by activation of inferior and apical

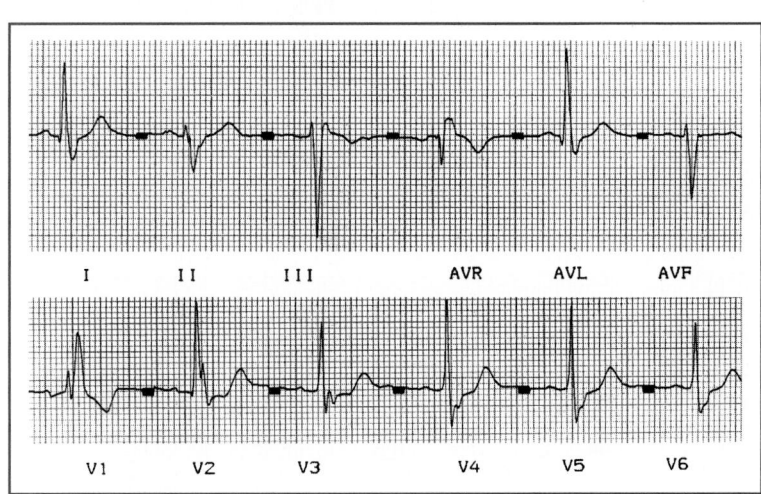

FIGURE 4–18. Right bundle branch block manifest by prominent S wave in leads I, aV_l, and the left ventricular precordial leads and an rsR pattern in lead V_1. The left anterior fascicular block is indicated by the marked left-axis deviation in the frontal leads.

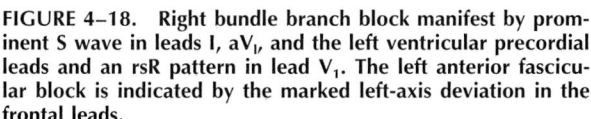

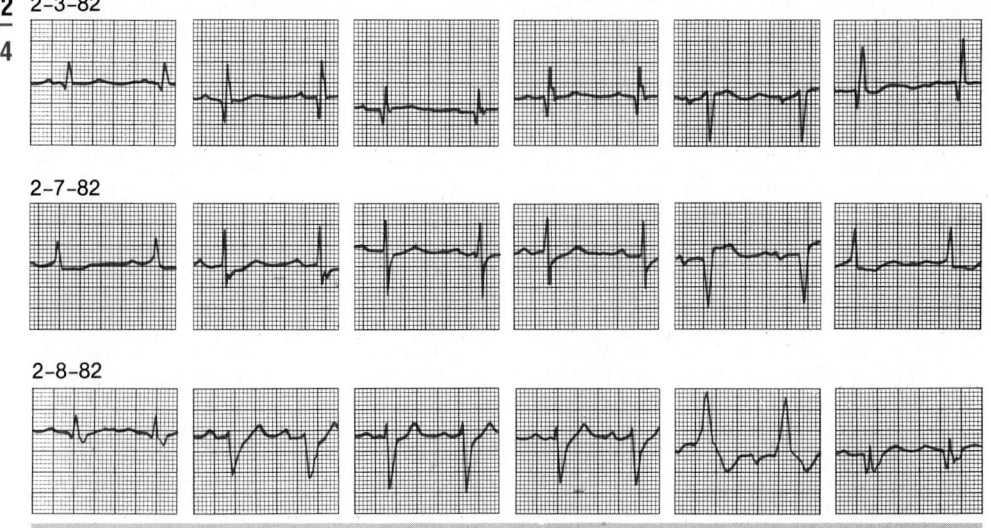

2-3-82

2-7-82

2-8-82

| L1 | L2 | L3 | AVF | V1 | V6 |

FIGURE 4–19. Masking of myocardial infarction Q waves by intraventricular conduction defects. Top trace (2-3-82) illustrates an inferolateral infarction manifested by Q waves in leads II, III, aV$_f$, and V$_6$. Incomplete LBBB and LAFB (left anterior fascicular block) in the middle trace (2-7-82) mask the inferior and lateral infarction. In the bottom trace (2-8-82), the LAFB masks the inferior infarction. The RBBB, in contrast to the incomplete LBBB in the middle trace, does not obscure the lateral infarction. (From Fisch, C.: Evolution of the clinical electrocardiogram. Reprinted with permission of the American College of Cardiology. J. Am. Coll. Cardiol. *14*:1127, 1989.)

areas with the vector oriented inferiorly, to the left, and anteriorly. Final activation is that of the anterolateral and posterobasal left ventricular wall, the vector oriented superiorly, posteriorly, and to the left (Fig. 4–AE8, p. 147).

The resultant ECG pattern is characteristic (Figs. 4–18 through 4–21). Lead I records a dominant R wave, with or without an initial Q wave. The criterion of a small Q wave in leads I and aV$_1$ is the subject of continued controversy.[21] The presence or absence of a Q wave depends on whether the initial septal activation is directed to the right or to the left. Since the initial activation is directed inferiorly, leads II, III, and aV$_f$ inscribe an R wave followed by a deep S wave reflecting activation of the anterolateral and posterobasal segments of the left ventricle. The QRS axis varies from −45 to −90 degrees. The duration of the QRS is less than 0.12 sec[21] (Figs. 4–18 and 4–20).

The precordial transitional zone is frequently displaced to the left. The amplitude of the R wave is diminished, with a prominent S wave in V$_5$ and V$_6$ reflecting the superior orientation of the mean left ventricular vector. The S wave is exaggerated when the final order of activation is directed to the right. Because of the inferior orientation of the initial vector, the right and midprecordial leads may register an initial Q wave. Such patterns could be mistaken

for anteroseptal myocardial infarction were it not for the fact that an R wave is recorded when the leads are placed an interspace lower (Fig. 4–AE9, p. 147). The T waves are normally upright except in lead aV$_r$ and occasionally in leads aV$_1$ and V$_1$.

BLOCK OF POSTERIOR DIVISION OF THE LEFT BUNDLE BRANCH (POSTERIOR FASCICULAR BLOCK). Left posterior divisional block is a rare finding, and its pattern is nonspecific. It can be recorded in asthenic individuals and patients with emphysema, RVH, and extensive lateral infarction.[49] Diagnosis is secure only if a normal or a different ECG pattern is recorded before appearance of the block (Fig. 4–AE82, p. 147).

In the presence of left posterior divisional block, activation begins in the midseptal and paraseptal areas, with the vector directed to the left, anteriorly, and superiorly. This is followed by activation of the left ventricular anterior and anterolateral walls, with the vector directed to the left and anteriorly. Final activation is of the inferior and posterior walls with the vector directed inferiorly, posteriorly, and to the right. The QRS duration is less than 0.12 sec.[21] In the limb leads, the initial superior and left orientation of septal vectors is reflected as R waves in leads I and aV$_1$ and a narrow, 0.025-msec Q wave in leads II, III, I, and aV$_f$. The

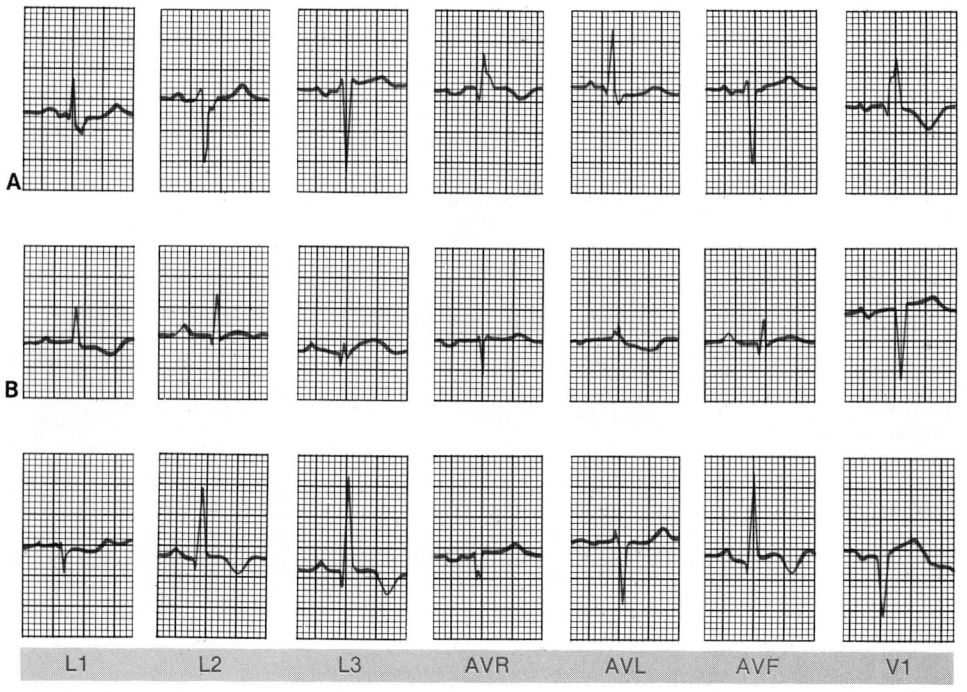

| L1 | L2 | L3 | AVR | AVL | AVF | V1 |

FIGURE 4–20. *A,* Right bundle branch block with left anterior divisional block. *B,* Upper trace, the control trace, illustrates an inferior myocardial infarction with a normal QRS axis. The bottom trace demonstrates left posterior divisional block (LPDB). Because the latter may be due to causes other than LPDB a diagnosis of LPDB requires evidence of normal conduction prior to appearance of LPDB such as illustrated in upper trace of panel B.

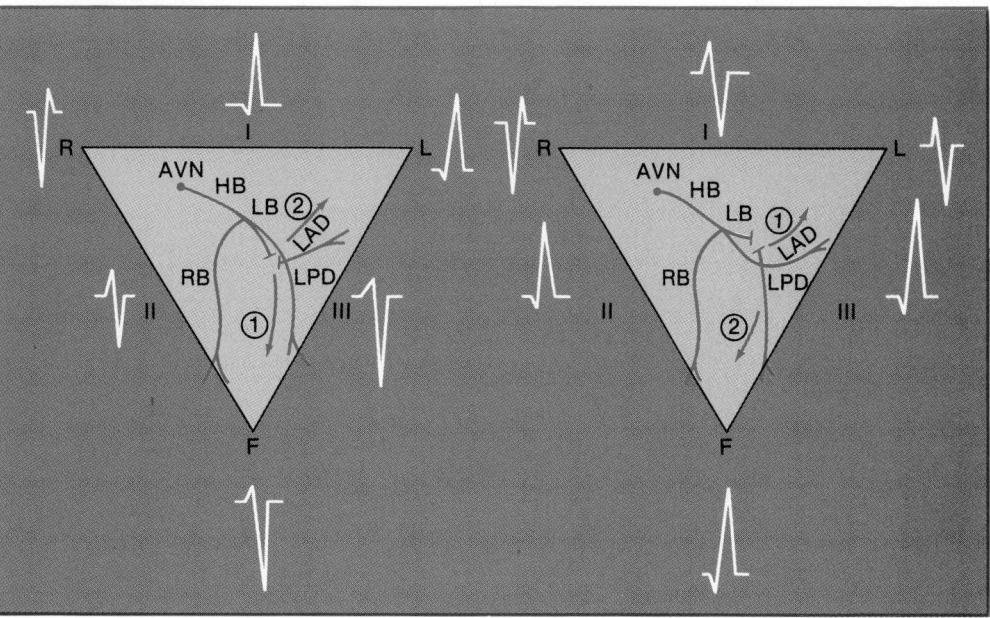

FIGURE 4–21. Diagrammatic representation of the conduction system. Interruption of the LAD (left) results in an initial inferior (1) followed by a dominant superior (2) direction of activation; interruption of the LPD (right) results in an initial superior (1) followed by a dominant inferior (2) direction of activation. AVN = atrioventricular node; HB = His bundle; LB = left bundle; RB = right bundle; LAD = left anterior division; LPD = left posterior division.

R waves in leads I and aV_l are small and followed by deep S waves reflecting the inferior, posterior, and right orientation of the wave of activation (Figs. 4–20 and 4–21). The initial superior force and final inferior force result in a QR complex in leads II, III, and aV_f. The amplitude of the R wave in lead III exceeds the R wave in lead II. The frontal axis varies from about +90 to +120 degrees, or perhaps +80 to +140 degrees. The T wave is usually normal.

RIGHT BUNDLE BRANCH BLOCK AND DIVISIONAL BLOCKS. RBBB with left anterior divisional block is the most common combination (Fig. 4–18). The activation during the first 0.08 sec determines the axis and identifies the left anterior divisional block. The delay of depolarization due to RBBB results in a final activation of the right ventricle to the right and anteriorly (Figs. 4–20 and 4–AE8, p. 147).

RBBB with left posterior divisional block is a rare combination. The initial 0.08 sec defines the axis and divisional block, while the final delayed activation, oriented to the right and anteriorly, reflects RBBB (Fig. 4–AE8).

Block of the right bundle and both divisions of the left bundle (trifascicular block) can occur in the presence of RBBB with alternating left anterior and posterior divisional blocks. Such patterns are usually associated with Mobitz (type II) AV block. It has been suggested that RBBB with either hemiblock and a prolonged P-R interval may be a manifestation of trifascicular block. Although the prolonged P-R interval may be due to delayed conduction in the remaining division, the delay also may reflect AV nodal delay.

NONSPECIFIC INTRAVENTRICULAR CONDUCTION DEFECT (IVCD). The QRS complex may be abnormally prolonged but without the characteristic pattern of either RBBB or LBBB. Such conduction delays are referred to as *nonspecific* IVCD. These often resemble LBBB or LBBB with an abnormal left-axis deviation, a combination suggesting left anterior hemiblock with peripheral conduction delay. Presence of a normal Q wave supports peripheral delay as the cause of QRS prolongation. Although such a nonspecific prolongation may be due to drugs or electrolyte abnormalities, it is most often due to organic heart disease. An interesting form of right ventricular conduction delay has been described in patients with arrhythmogenic ventricular dysplasia. The delayed activation is inscribed in the form of a sharp deflection after termination of the QRS, during the ST segment or upstroke of the T wave.[50]

MASQUERADING BUNDLE BRANCH BLOCK. This form of BBB is rare. It is manifest by RBBB, marked left-axis deviation, and absence of a significant S wave in leads I, aV_l, and V_6. In essence, it can be described as LBBB in the limb leads and RBBB in the chest leads. In contrast to the ordinary RBBB with left anterior fascicular block, or bifascicular block, the masquerading BBB is usually associated with significant heart disease and a relatively poor long-term prognosis. (Fig. 4–22).[51]

BILATERAL BUNDLE BRANCH BLOCK. This diagnosis can be considered when alternating RBBB and LBBB are present. Any other combination of conduction delays cannot be differentiated from block in the AV junction. For example, simultaneous block in both bundles results in complete AV block. Similarly, intermittent delay or block in one bundle and complete block of conduction in the contralateral bundle will manifest either as BBB with a prolonged P-R interval or intermittent AV block. In the presence of BBB, a superimposed AV block due to failure of conduction in the contralateral bundle branch cannot be differentiated from block in the AV junction (Fig. 4–23).

BUNDLE BRANCH BLOCK ALTERNANS. Bundle branch block (BBB) alternans is a rare finding and may be manifested as alternans of (1) RBBB or LBBB with a normal QRS, (2) RBBB and LBBB (see Bilateral BBB), or (3) complete and incomplete RBBB or LBBB.[52]

FIGURE 4–22. Anterolateral myocardial infarction with a "masquerading" bundle branch block. The latter is indicated by the right bundle branch block (RBBB)–like pattern in leads V_1 and V_2 but without the characteristic, diagnostic S wave in leads I and aV_l. The exact mechanism of this type of intraventricular conduction is unclear. It is possible that the changes in right precordial leads are not due to RBBB.

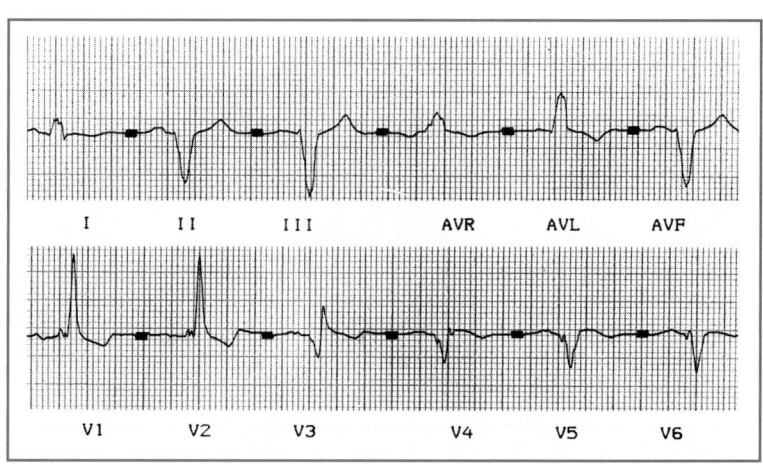

I   II   III   AVR   AVL   AVF

V1   V2   V3   V4   V5   V6

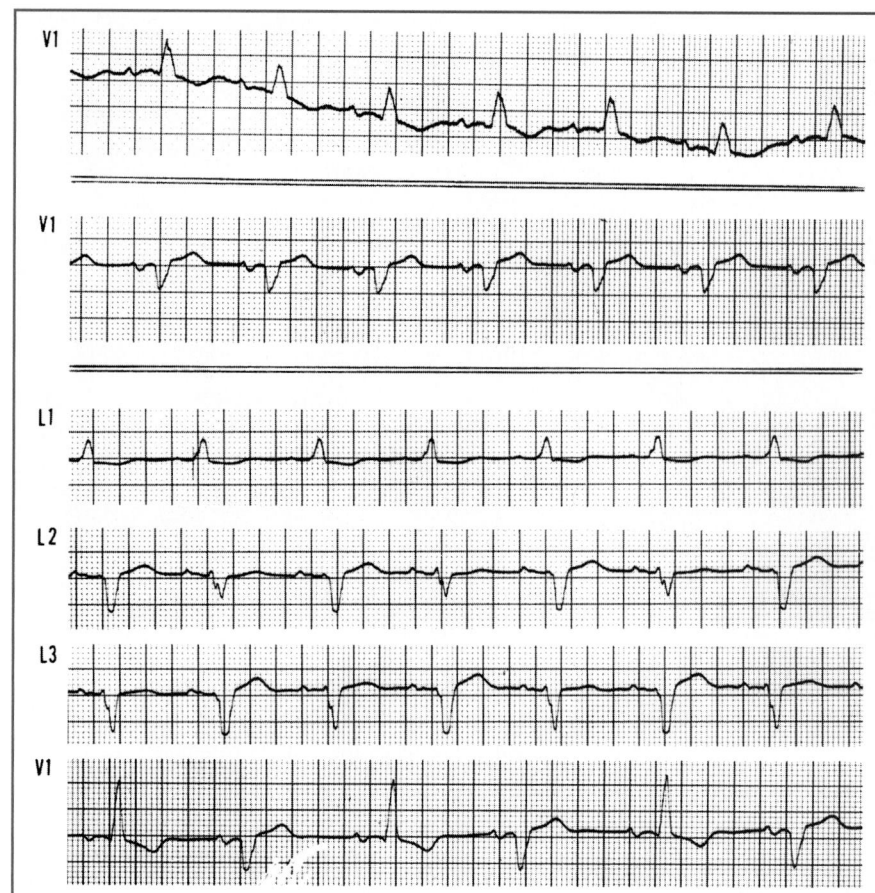

FIGURE 4-23. Alternating P-R interval and bundle branch block (BBB). *Top tracing,* V1 Right bundle branch block (RBBB) with a P-R interval of 280 msec. *Middle panel,* V1 Left bundle branch block (LBBB) with a P-R interval of 180 msec. *Lower panel,* RBBB alternating with LBBB with alternation of the P-R interval. Leads 1, 2, and 3 exhibit left anterior fascicular block. (From Fisch, C.: Electrocardiography of Arrhythmias. Philadelphia, Lea and Febiger, 1990, p. 433, with permission.)

Aberration

Intraventricular aberration describes a supraventricular impulse with abnormal, bizarre intraventricular conduction (Fig. 4-24).[53] It refers to intraventricular conduction abnormalities related to changing heart rate or other functional alterations in electrophysiological properties, anomalous AV conduction, metabolic and electrolyte abnormalities, and toxic effects of drugs. The term *aberration,* as used currently, does not include fixed organic conduction defects.

The mechanisms responsible for, or contributory to, aberration with changing cycle length include (1) excitation prior to completion of repolarization (i.e., in the presence of a reduced transmembrane potential), (2) unequal refractoriness of conducting tissue resulting in local delay or block of conduction, (3) prolongation of the action potential due to prolongation of the preceding cycle length, (4) failure of restitution of transmembrane electrolyte concentration during diastole, (5) failure of the refractory period to

shorten in response to acceleration of the heart rate, (6) a reduced take-off potential secondary to diastole depolarization, (7) concealed transseptal conduction with delay or block of bundle branch conduction, and (8) diffuse depression of intraventricular conduction including that of specialized as well as myocardial tissue.

Aberration may result when any of these mechanisms alter conduction in the bundle branches or the divisions of the left bundle branch (or a combination of the two), the Purkinje fibers, or the myocardium. RBBB is the most common form of aberrancy and is frequently associated with left anterior divisional block. Aberrancy due to LBBB is much less common and in our experience often due to heart disease, although the heart disease may not be clinically evident. An abnormality of intraventricular conduction due to diffuse depression of conduction in the Purkinje system and in the myocardium should be suspected when both the initial and terminal portions of the QRS complex are abnormal.

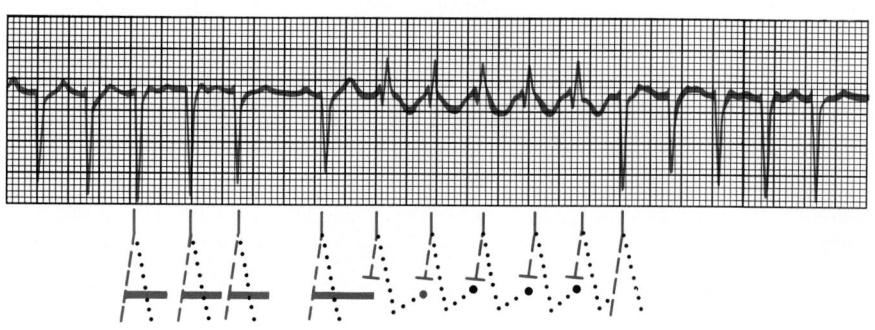

FIGURE 4-24. Atrial tachycardia with Wenckebach (type I) AV block, ventricular aberration due to the Ashman phenomenon, and probably concealed transseptal conduction. The long pause of the atrial tachycardia is followed by five QRS complexes with RBBB morphology. The RBBB of the first QRS reflects the Ashman phenomenon. The aberration is perpetuated by concealed transseptal activation from the left bundle into the right bundle with block of the anterograde conduction of the subsequent sinus impulse in the right bundle. Foreshortening of the R-R cycle, a manifestation of the Wenckebach structure, disturbs the relationship between transseptal and anterograde sinus conduction, and RBB conduction

is normalized. In the ladder diagram below the tracing, the solid lines represent the His bundle, the dashes the RBB and the dots the LBB, while the solid horizontal bars denote the refractory period. Neither the P waves nor the AV node is identified in the diagram.

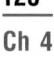

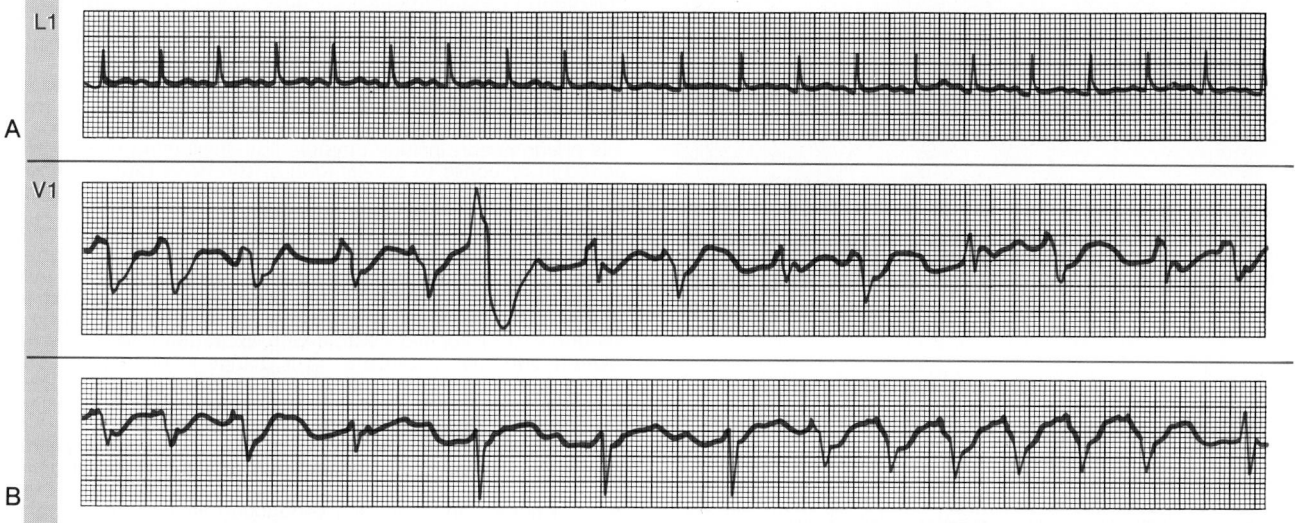

FIGURE 4–25. Intraventricular aberration due to quinidine and acceleration of the heart rate. In panel *A,* control tracing, the ECG is normal with a sinus rate of 130 beats/min. After administration of quinidine (panel *B),* the heart rate is 120 beats/min and the QRS widened to 0.20 sec with a 3:2 Wenckebach (type I) AV block interrrupted by one VPC. P wave duration is prolonged and the P-R interval is increased to 0.28 sec. The QRS complex which follows the longer pauses are narrower, probably owing to a longer period of recovery. In the bottom trace 1:1 AV conduction is interrupted by 2:1 AV conduction. P waves measure 0.20 sec in duration, the P-R interval is 0.40 sec, and the QRS complexes at onset of 2:1 AV block are foreshortened to 0.16 sec. The QRS prolongation to 0.16 sec is due to quinidine, while further widening of the QRS complexes to 0.20 sec in presence of 1:1 AV conduction reflects both the effect of quinidine and the accelerated heart rate.

Of the mechanisms and manifestations of aberration, seven will be considered in further detail: (1) premature excitation, (2) the Ashman phenomenon, (3) acceleration-dependent aberrancy, (4) deceleration-dependent aberrancy, (5) concealed conduction, (6) diffuse myocardial depression of conduction, and (7) postextrasystolic aberrancy.

PREMATURE EXCITATION. Conduction will fail or be delayed if the stimulus falls during the effective or the relative refractory period of recovery. When the impulse falls during the relative refractory period of a single bundle branch, the unilateral delay results in a bundle branch block. The duration of the refractory period may equal that of the transmembrane action potential, so-called voltage-dependent refractoriness, or it may exceed it, so-called time-dependent refractoriness. Duration of the refractory period depends to a great extent on the basic heart rate and on the duration of the immediately preceding cycle(s). Normally, the refractory period shortens with acceleration of the heart rate and lengthens with slowing of the heart rate. With all variables affecting conduction being constant, the degree of aberration is usually a function of prematurity of excitation.

The site of conduction depression and thus the morphology of the aberrant QRS complex is determined by the length of the refractory period of the AV node, the bundle of His, and the bundle system itself. Normally, at slow heart rates, the right bundle branch has the longest refractory period, with the left bundle and the AV node somewhat shorter and the bundle of His the shortest. Only at very rapid rates may the duration of the refractory period of the left bundle exceed that of the right bundle.

EFFECT OF CHANGING CYCLE LENGTH ON REFRACTORINESS (ASHMAN PHENOMENON). This form of aberrancy, also a function of premature excitation, differs from that due to early excitation just described in that the abnormal conduction is a function of an altered duration of the refractory period rather than of changing prematurity of stimulation. Since the duration of the refractory period is a function of the immediately preceding cycle length, the longer the preceding cycle, the longer the refractory period that follows. Consequently, with a relatively constant heart rate, sudden prolongation of the immediately preceding cycle length may result in aberration. This relationship of aberrancy to changes in the preceding cycle length is known as the *Ashman phenomenon.*[54] Aberrancy so initiated may persist for a number of cycles (Fig. 4–24), usually exhibits RBBB morphology, and may be associated with left anterior or rarely with left posterior divisional block.

In the presence of irregular supraventricular rhythms, such as atrial fibrillation, repetitive atrial tachycardia, or atrial tachycardia with Wenckebach (type 1) AV block (Fig. 4–24), aberration due to the Ashman phenomenon is suggested by the following: (1) a relatively long cycle immediately preceding the cycle terminated by the aberrant QRS complex, (2) RBBB aberrancy with normal orientation of the initial QRS vector, (3) irregular coupling of the aberrant QRS complex, and (4) lack of a compensatory pause following the aberrant QRS complex.

ACCELERATION-DEPENDENT ABERRATION (TACHYCARDIA-DEPENDENT ABERRANCY, PHASE 3 ABERRANCY). This form of aberration has been recognized since 1913.[55] At certain critical heart rates, impaired intraventricular conduction results in aberrancy (Figs. 4–25 and 4–26). This phenomenon has been described as tachycardia-dependent aberrancy or phase 3 aberrancy; however, the term *acceleration-dependent aberrancy* appears most appropriate. Aberration often appears at relatively slow rates, frequently below 75 beats/min; similarly, because of the slow rate at which the conduction fails, one would have to postulate an extremely long transmembrane action potential in order to accept excitation during phase 3 as the cause of the impaired conduction. Finally, conduction also will fail with excitation during phase 2 of the action potential.

The appearance and disappearance of aberration often depends on very small changes in cycle length, a change frequently difficult if not impossible to detect in the ECG. Assuming that a reasonably long recording is available, a comparison of the earliest available cycle length terminated by a normal QRS complex with the cycle length terminated by the first aberrant QRS complex will aid in the diagnosis

1527 L

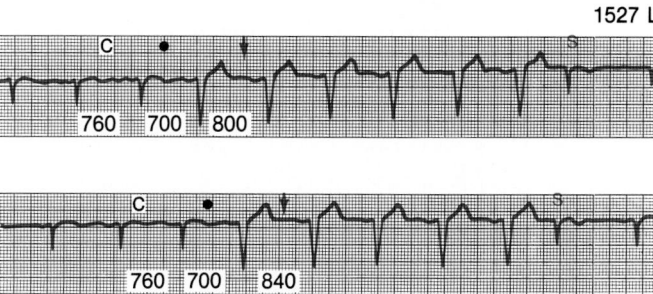

FIGURE 4–26. Acceleration-dependent QRS aberration with the paradox of persistence at a longer cycle and normalization at a shorter cycle than that which initiated the aberration. The duration of the basic cycle (C) is 760 msec. LBBB appears at a cycle length of 700 msec (·) and is perpetuated at cycle lengths of 800 (↓) and 840 (↓) msec; conduction normalizes after a cycle length of 600 msec. Perpetuation of LBBB at a cycle length of 800 and 840 (↓) msec is probably due to transseptal concealment, similar to that described in Figure 4–24. Unexpected normalization of the QRS (S) following the atrial premature contraction is probably due to equalization of conduction in the two bundles; however, supernormal conduction in the left bundle cannot be excluded. (Reproduced with permission from Fisch, C., et al.: Rate dependent aberrancy. *Circulation 48:*714, 1973. Copyright 1973 American Heart Association.)

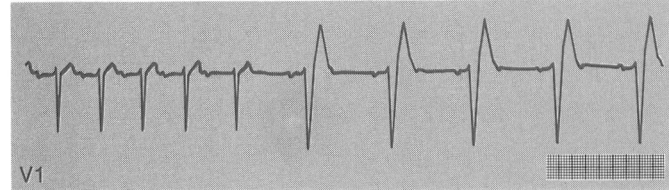

V1

FIGURE 4–27. Deceleration-dependent aberration. The basic rhythm is sinus with Wenckebach (type I) AV block. With 1:1 AV conduction, the QRS complexes are normal in duration; with 2:1 AV block or after the longer pause of a Wenckebach sequence, LBBB appears. Slow diastolic depolarization (phase 4) of the transmembrane action potential during the prolonged cycle is implicated as the cause of the LBBB.

of acceleration-dependent aberrancy. The difference in the duration of two such cycles is often less than 0.04 sec.

Acceleration-dependent aberration differs from the physiological aberrancy observed in a normal heart. Differences include (1) appearance of aberrancy at relatively slow heart rates, (2) predominance of LBBB morphology, (3) independence from the immediately preceding cycle length, (4) occasional appearance without or with only a slight change in cycle length, and (5) association with heart disease.

QRS aberrancy may persist at an R-R interval considerably longer than the interval that initiated the aberrancy (Fig. 4–26). Three mechanisms have been suggested to explain this paradox: (1) concealed transseptal activation blocking conduction in the contralateral bundles, (2) "fatigue" of the bundle, and (3) concealed transseptal conduction coupled with suppression of conduction due to the increased heart rate, somewhat analogous to suppression of pacemakers by an ectopic tachycardia. A discrepancy of as much as 210 msec between the cycles initiating and terminating the aberration suggests that concealed transseptal conduction may not be the sole factor responsible for the unexpected persistence of aberrancy at the longer cycle lengths. The difference cannot be explained solely on the basis of time consumed by conduction along the contralateral bundle and across the septum. Normal transseptal activation in the human heart is about 40 to 45 msec; in the diseased heart, it may be prolonged to 115 msec.[56–59] It is likely, therefore, that a combination of mechanisms is operative.

One mechanism that would explain the unexpected delay in normalization of intraventricular conduction is *fatigue,* a descriptive term that may reflect failure of restitution of transmembrane ionic gradients and lowering of the transmembrane resting potential and/or a shift of the membrane responsiveness to the right. The latter denotes a decrease in upstroke velocity of phase 0 for any given magnitude of transmembrane resting potential. A different mechanism, namely, concealed conduction, may explain the delayed nor-

malization of bundle branch conduction in patients with atrial fibrillation. Concealed conduction of atrial fibrillatory impulses into the blocked bundle may result in a true bundle-to-bundle interval that is consistently shorter than the manifest QRS interval.

Occasionally, paradoxical normalization of the QRS complex without a change in heart rate—or, in fact, with acceleration of the heart rate—has been documented (Fig. 4–26). Mechanisms that may explain this phenomenon include physiological shortening of the refractory period in response to acceleration of the heart rate, equalization of conduction in the two bundles and conduction during the supernormal period, and the gap phenomenon.

DECELERATION-DEPENDENT ABERRANCY (BRADYCARDIA-DEPENDENT ABERRANCY, PHASE 4 ABERRANCY). A prolonged cycle may be terminated by an aberrant QRS and foreshortening of the cycle may normalize the QRS (Fig. 4–27).[60] It has been suggested that this form of aberrancy is due to a gradual loss of transmembrane resting potential during a prolonged diastole with excitation from a less negative take-off potential. Because a small change in resting potential may have a pronounced effect on the rate of rise of phase 0 of the action potential, deceleration aberrancy may be seen with a relatively small prolongation of the cycle length.

CONCEALED CONDUCTION. Conduction in the bundle branches may be impaired by concealed penetration of a supraventricular impulse or by transseptal activation from the contralateral bundle (Fig. 4–24). In atrial fibrillation, concealed conduction into a bundle branch can be considered when acceleration-dependent aberrancy persists at a QRS cycle that is longer than a cycle terminated by a normal QRS. Transseptal concealed conduction into a bundle branch from the contralateral bundle should be suspected if aberrancy, once initiated, persists at rates slower than the rate that initiated the aberrancy (Fig. 4–26).

MYOCARDIAL DEPRESSION. Drugs and metabolic and electrolyte disorders are frequent causes of QRS aberrancy (Fig. 4–25). The severity of depression of conduction varies, and the QRS may exhibit RBBB or LBBB, divisional block, or any combination. As indicated previously, aberrancy can be differentiated from ordinary BBB by the presence of distortion in the initial and terminal components of the QRS complex. The appearance of aberration is often rate related (Fig. 4–25).

POSTEXTRASYSTOLIC ABERRATION. Aberrant intraventricular conduction of a sinus impulse terminating a compensatory pause is rare and must be differentiated from an aberrant escape complex. The exact mechanism of the postpausal aberrancy is not clear. It may be due to slow diastolic depolarization, unequal recovery of conducting or myocardial tissue, or increased diastolic volume.

Wolff-Parkinson-White (WPW) Syndrome
(See pp. 574 and 667)

WPW, or preexcitation,[61] syndrome is an electrocardiographic syndrome characterized by a short P-R (≤ 0.12 sec) interval, prolonged QRS (≥ 0.12 sec) complex, a slur on the

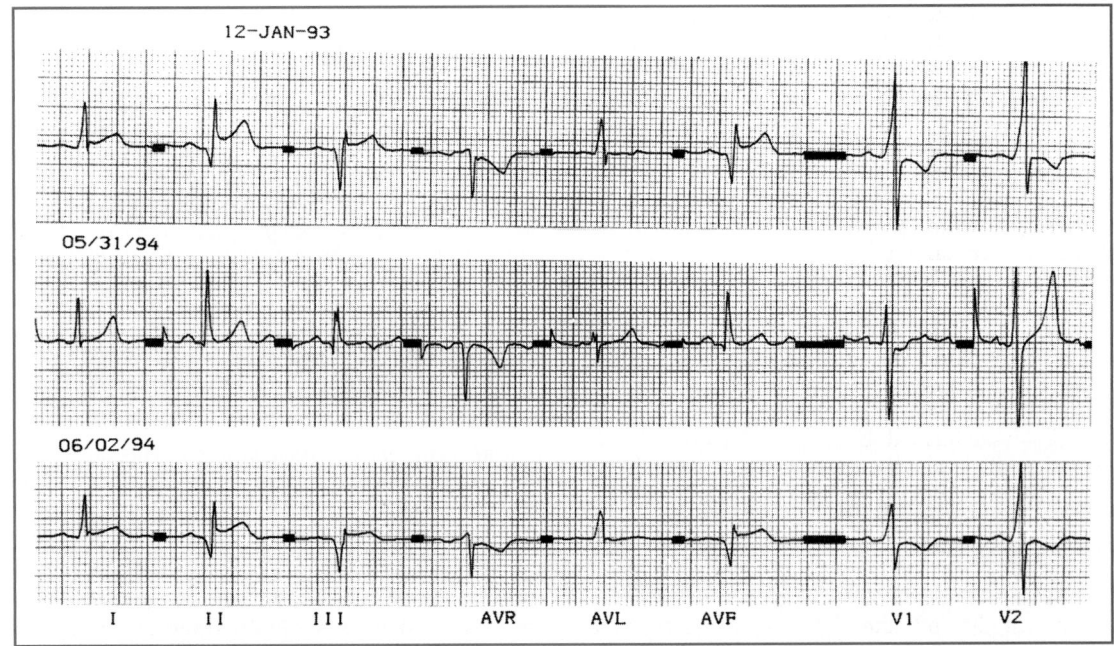

FIGURE 4–28. WPW syndrome simulating an inferior myocardial infarction. 1/12/93, WPW syndrome with negative delta wave suggestive of inferior infarction. 5/31/94, Normal AV conduction with normal QRS complexes. 6/2/94, Recurrence of WPW syndrome with negative delta wave, again simulating an inferior infarction. The normalization of the QRS in the recurrence of the pseudoinfarction Q wave on 6/2/94 rules out a myocardial infarction.

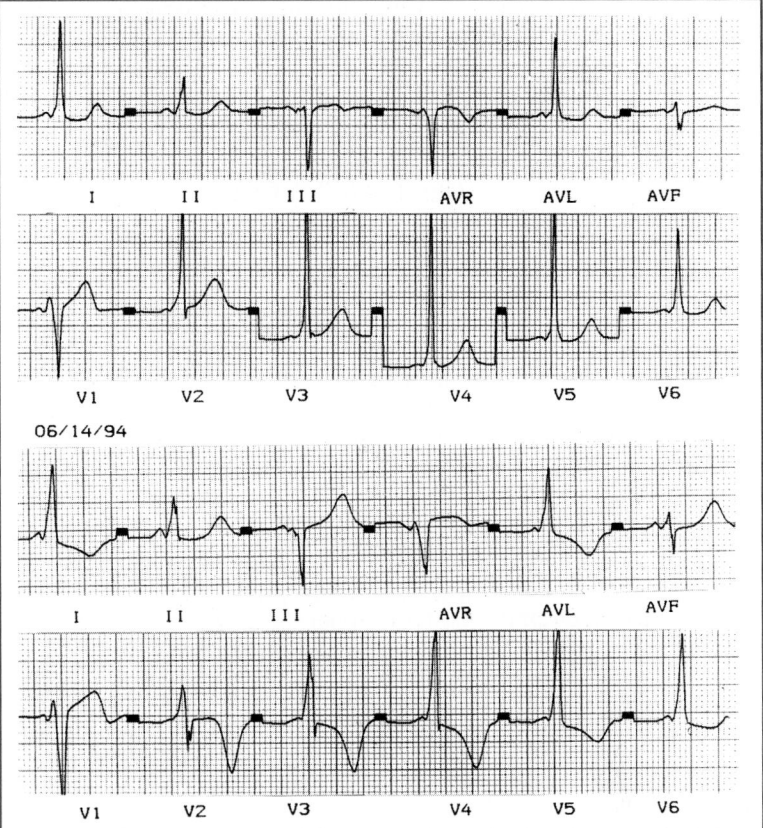

FIGURE 4–29. WPW syndrome and acute myocardial infarction. 1/12/93, WPW syndrome with a short P-R interval and a delta wave. The tracing of 6/14/94 was recorded during an acute myocardial infarction. The latter manifest by the negative T waves. Because of the conduction via the bypass toward the left ventricle, the left ventricular cavity is initially positive, thus precluding registration of the diagnostic Q wave (see Fig. 4–16).

upstroke of the QRS (delta wave), and (as a rule) a normal P-J interval (Figs. 4–28, 4–29, and 4–AE6). Secondary ST-segment and T-wave changes are nearly always present. Paroxysmal supraventricular tachycardia is recorded in about 50 per cent of patients with WPW. The characteristic pattern of WPW can be altered by abnormalities of AV and intraventricular conduction. The prevalence of WPW in the general population is approximately 3 per 1000.

Although Wilson is credited with the initial report of WPW[62] it was Cohn who brought the electrocardiograph to America and first described an ECG pattern to become known as WPW. His patient, described in 1913, exhibited the WPW pattern and supraventricular tachycardia.[63] In 1930, this pattern was recognized as a discrete ECG syndrome. Shortly thereafter the bypass concept of WPW was proposed, and this concept has stood the test of time.[64]

In WPW the QRS complex is a fusion between the impulse traversing the bypass and the normal AV junction. The bypass component of the QRS complex, or *delta wave,* varies depending on the size of the ventricular muscle mass activated through the bypass. In some instances, especially in the presence of AV conduction delay, the entire ventricular mass may be activated by the impulse propagated through the bypass, and the entire QRS complex becomes essentially a delta wave.

Traditionally, WPW has been classified into type A and type B. *Type A* is characterized by a prominent positive initial QRS deflection in leads V_1 and V_2 and *type B* by a predominantly negative deflection in leads V_1 and V_2.[65] In type A, the initial inscription of the QRS complex, the delta wave, reflects early activation of the posterior left ventricle and, in type B, early activation of the anterior superior right ventricle. *Type C WPW,* characterized by a negative delta wave in the left lateral leads, also has been described. Studies using surface potential mapping, epicardial mapping during surgery, and electrophysiological studies have identified a number of preexcitation sites.[66] Presence of more than one QRS pattern in an individual patient suggests the possibility of multiple bypass tracts. A short

P-R interval with a normal QRS complex accompanied by paroxysmal supraventricular tachycardia has been suggested as a variant of WPW (see p. 667).

First-, second-, and third-degree AV block have been reported with WPW, as have right and left BBB. In the presence of a BBB, an ipsilateral bypass, by preexciting the ventricle normally activated by the blocked bundle branch, will obscure the BBB. Both supernormal and concealed conduction have been invoked to explain unexpected patterns of behavior of bypass conduction.

WPW often complicates ECG interpretation because it may obscure or simulate a variety of patterns. It may mask (Fig. 4–29) or simulate myocardial infarction (Fig. 4–28). When the QRS vector is directed toward the left ventricular cavity, the cavity becomes initially positive, and a Q wave will not be recorded. A diagnosis of ventricular hypertrophy in the presence of WPW (as in BBB) may be difficult if not impossible (Fig. 4–AE6). WPW has been mistaken for RBBB, LBBB, and RVH. Supraventricular arrhythmias with aberration, resulting from conduction through the bypass, have been mistaken for ventricular tachycardia. Aberration due to WPW should be suspected when the ventricular rate is rapid, often approaching 300 beats/min, or when the QRS morphology of the bizarre complexes is upright in leads V_1 and V_2 as well as in V_5 and V_6.

Myocardial Infarction
(See Chap. 37)

The ECG changes of myocardial infarction, first described in humans in 1920,[67] are those of ischemia, injury, and cellular death and are, within limits, reflected by T-wave changes, ST-segment displacement, and the appearance of Q waves, respectively. Such a clear-cut differentiation, although clinically useful, may be overly simplistic and artificial. For example, T-wave changes may be due to ischemia, injury, or death of muscle. Similarly, a Q wave may be due to impairment of transmembrane ionic fluxes and not necessarily cellular death. However, for the purpose of this discussion, T-wave changes, ST-segment displacement, and appearance of a Q wave are assumed to reflect ischemia, injury, and cell death, respectively.

ISCHEMIA. In the dog, the earliest change following ligation of a coronary artery is the almost immediate appearance of a primary, as a rule negative, T wave. After 60 or 90 seconds, there is a maximal shift of the ST segment. The T wave becomes positive and peaked, and the change is as a rule a primary change. The amplitude of the R wave decreases during the first 30 seconds after experimental occlusion. This is followed by an increase in the amplitude, which peaks 20 to 30 seconds after the maximal increase of the left ventricular volume. In humans, unless an ECG is recorded at the moment of occlusion, the initial T wave change is usually missed (Figs. 4–AE10 and 4–AE11, p. 147). Occasionally, a giant R wave is recorded early during the ischemic episode (Fig. 4–AE12, p. 147). Such changes in the QRS could contribute to the T-wave abnormality, and the abnormal T wave would reflect both primary and secondary changes of repolarization.

Normally the process of repolarization proceeds from the epicardium to the endocardium, and an upright T wave is recorded. Ischemia prolongs the regional duration of recovery, with the ischemic area being last to repolarize. If the ischemia is subendocardial, the direction of repolarization remains unchanged and the polarity of the T wave remains upright. In the presence of subepicardial ischemia, the duration of the excited state is longer in the epicardium; the normal order of repolarization is reversed, proceeding from endocardium to epicardium, and an inverted T wave is inscribed. Because of local prolongation of recovery, the late phase of repolarization may be unopposed, and a large and prolonged T wave may be registered.

INJURY. Two concepts based on systolic and diastolic phenomena have been suggested to explain the ST-segment displacement. One postulates local reduction or loss of resting potential, resulting in a *diastolic current of injury*. The second concept assumes an unopposed current flowing from the injured area during the isoelectric ST segment, resulting in a *systolic current of injury*. These systolic and diastolic phenomena cannot be differentiated with the ordinary clinical alternating-current (AC) electrocardiograph but can be recorded experimentally with direct-current (DC) equipment (Fig. 4–30).

The concept of the *diastolic current* of injury proposes that localized injury is associated with a flow of current from the uninjured to the injured area. As a result, the T-Q segment is displaced downward but is automatically shifted to control level by the capacitor-coupled amplifier of the ECG. When the entire heart (including the injured area) is depolarized, the ST segment is elevated with respect to the depressed but rectified (isoelectric) diastolic T-Q segment (Fig. 4–31).

The concept of the *systolic current* of injury proposes that during the ST segment, the normal heart is depolarized, but the injured area undergoes early repolarization. The result is a current flow from the more positive, injured area to a more negative, uninjured area. The result is true elevation of the ST segment. Similarly, if, rather than repolarizing early, the injured area fails to depolarize with the normal myocardium, a current of injury would exist and an elevated ST segment would be recorded (Fig. 4–31).

Earlier experimental studies indicate that during injury both systolic and diastolic currents are present,[68] and at times the systolic precedes the diastolic current of injury. Subsequent studies, however, indicate that the diastolic current predominates while the systolic current plays a lesser role and that the magnitude of the current is modified by the heart rate[69] (Fig. 4–30). As indicated, the clinical ECG does not differentiate between systolic and diastolic currents of injury. Furthermore, unless the onset of the injury is recorded, even a DC-coupled ECG would not identify the mechanism of the ST-segment shift.

An electrode facing subendocardial injury registers an elevated ST segment, while an epicardial electrode subtended by the normal myocardium registers ST-segment depression. Similarly, an electrode facing epicardial injury registers elevation of the ST segment, while the endocardial electrode inscribes ST-segment depression.

INFARCTION. The diagnostic feature of infarction (myocardial necrosis) is the *Q wave*. Two concepts have been invoked to explain the appearance of the Q wave. The theory of proximity, the "window" theory, suggests that the

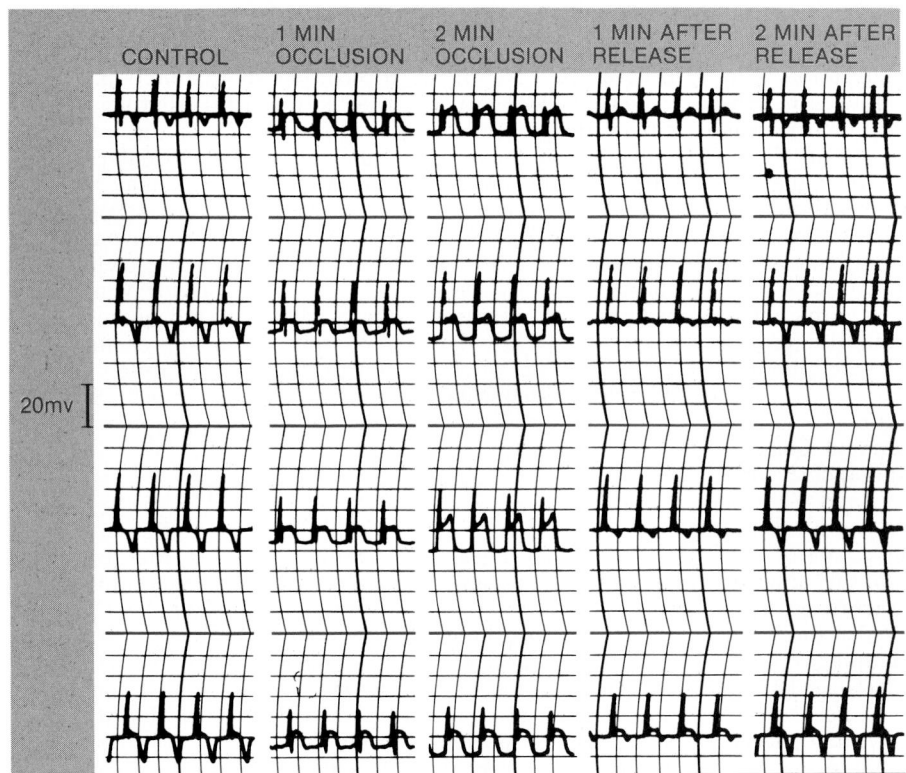

|CONTROL | 1 MIN OCCLUSION | 2 MIN OCCLUSION | 1 MIN AFTER RELEASE | 2 MIN AFTER RELEASE|

20mv

FIGURE 4–30. A series of simultaneous epicardial electrograms recorded from four sites. The electrodes were distributed randomly in the ischemic area, with some closer to the center of the ischemic area than others. After 1 minute of occlusion, TQ segment depression is apparent in all recordings. After 2 minutes of occlusion, TQ segment depression has increased. The ST segment take-off is slightly elevated or isoelectric in all recordings. The polarity of the T wave is changed from negative during the control period to positive. These recordings emphasize that major changes in action potential downstroke, shape, and timing can occur without significant alteration of phase 2 and of the action potential. Similarly, T wave changes can occur without a significant shift of the true ST segment. True TQ segment depression appears to be the major cause of ST segment displacement and the true ST segment shift of lesser magnitude and variable. T waveform is markedly altered with occlusion. (From Vincent, G. M., et al.: Mechanisms of ischemic ST-segment displacement. Circulation *56*:559, 1977, by permission of the American Heart Association, Inc.)

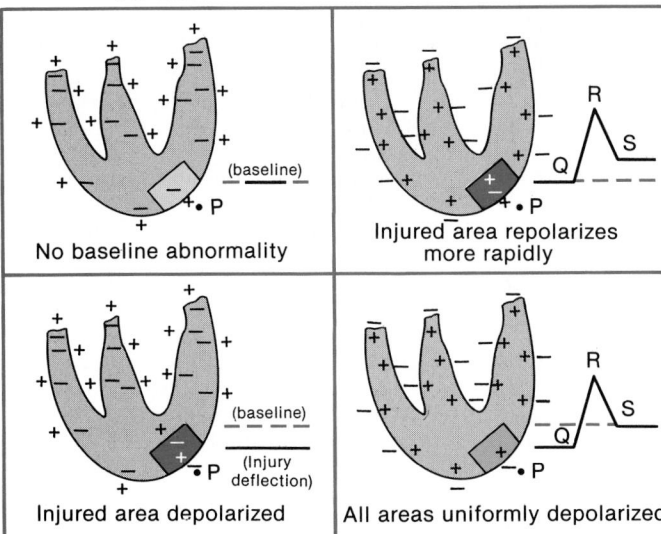

AT REST	AFTER DEPOLARIZATION
No baseline abnormality	Injured area repolarizes more rapidly
Injured area depolarized	All areas uniformly depolarized

FIGURE 4–31. Systolic *(upper row)* and diastolic *(lower row)* currents of injury. *Upper row,* The ischemic area (pink) is electrically identical to the nonischemic heart at rest, and there is no shift of the baseline potential. During repolarization, however, the ischemic area (red) has repolarized early and is positive relative to the depolarized heart, the baseline is shifted upward (positive), and the ECG records an elevated ST segment. Similarly, if the ischemic area fails to depolarize with the remainder of the heart, it would be positive relative to the remainder of the heart and a positive ST segment would be recorded. This latter mechanism also may be operative. *Lower row,* The ischemic area (red) is depolarized at rest, thus negative relative to the remainder of the heart, and the baseline is shifted down (negative). This shift is not recognizable on ECG. However, with completion of depolarization the injured area is also depolarized; its potential becomes identical to that of the rest of the heart; and the ST segment, although isoelectric, is elevated relative to the depressed baseline; so that an elevated ST segment is registered. These two mechanisms cannot be differentiated with the ECG, and although both contribute to the current of injury, the systolic is thought to dominate (Fig. 4–30). (From Scher, A. M.: Electrocardiogram. *In* Ruch, I. C., and Patton, H. D. (eds.): Physiology and Biophysics. Philadelphia, W. B. Saunders Company, 1974, p. 94.)

electrically inert myocardium allows an electrode to record the intracavitary negativity. There is ample evidence, however, to suggest that a Q wave can be recorded in the absence of a transmural infarction. Heterogeneity of electrophysiological changes associated with the dynamic events of ischemic and subsequent healing, with intermingling of fibrous and viable tissue, has been suggested as an explanation.

According to the vectorial concept, the electrically inert myocardium fails to contribute to the normal electrical forces, and the result is a vector that points away from the area of infarction, reflected by a Q wave. Theoretically, the infarction vector represents the force that alters the normal vector. It is equal to but opposite in direction from the vector generated by the infarcted myocardium before infarction. If the net vector is directed normally but is reduced in magnitude, a Q wave will not be recorded, but the amplitude of the QRS complex will be reduced, indicating loss of myocardium. However, the specificity of such a change for infarction is low (Table 4–3).

Diagnosis

One of the most valuable contributions of the ECG is in the diagnosis of myocardial infarction. Usually it is the first laboratory test performed; the technique is reliable and reproducible, can be applied serially, and when properly interpreted is the cornerstone of the laboratory diagnosis of myocardial infarction and often dictates the initial therapy.[70]

THE INITIAL ECG. The initial ECG is "diagnostic" of acute infarction in approximately 50 per cent of patients, abnormal but not diagnostic in approximately 40 per cent, and normal in about 10 per cent. Serial tracings increase the sensitivity to near 95 per cent. A single ECG may never be "diagnostic." However, a pattern of ST-segment displacement, especially with associated Q-wave and T-wave changes, and a clinical history suggestive of ischemic heart disease is highly suggestive—if not diagnostic—of acute myocardial infarction.

CLASSIC PATTERN AND EVOLUTION OF INFARCTION. As in the experimental animal, if the ECG is inscribed at the

TABLE 4–3 SUMMARY OF VECTORCARDIOGRAPHIC CRITERIA FOR DIAGNOSIS OF MYOCARDIAL INFARCTION (MI)

Anteroseptal MI (1 and 2)*
1. Initial anterior QRS forces absent
2. 0.02-sec QRS vector directed posteriorly

Localized Anterior MI (1, 2, and 3)
1. Initial anterior septal forces present
2. 0.02-sec QRS vector directed posteriorly
3. Voltage criteria for left ventricular hypertrophy absent

Anterolateral MI (1, 2, and 3)
1. Initial anterior septal forces normal
2. Initial rightward QRS forces > 0.022 sec
3. Efferent limb of transverse plane QRS loop inscribed clockwise
4. Initial rightward QRS forces > 0.16 mV
5. Maximum frontal plane QRS vector > 40°, QRS loop inscribed counterclockwise

Extensive Anterior MI (1 and 2)
1. Initial anterior QRS forces absent
2. Transverse plane QRS loop inscribed clockwise

Inferior MI (1 or more)
1. Initial superior QRS forces > 0.025 sec
2. Initial superior QRS forces ≥ 0.020 sec, maximum left superior force ≥ 0.25 mV
3. Maximum frontal plane QRS vector < 10°, efferent limb of frontal QRS loop inscribed clockwise
4. Bites in afferent limb of frontal QRS loop

Inferolateral MI (1 and 2)
1. Initial rightward QRS forces > 0.022 sec
2. Initial superior QRS forces > 0.025 sec

* Numbers in parentheses after each type of infarction indicate the minimum requirements for the diagnosis.
From Chou, T. C., et al.: Clinical Vectorcardiography. 2nd ed. New York, Grune and Stratton, 1974, p. 229.

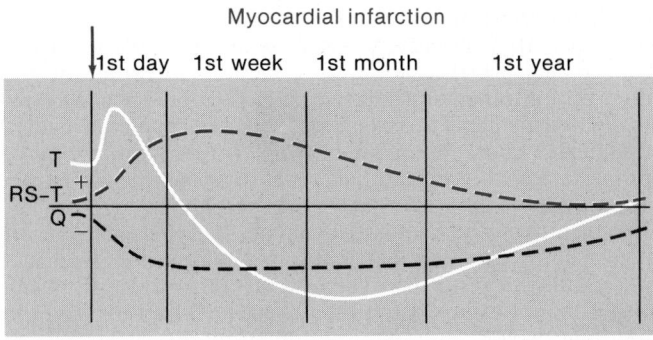

1st day   1st week   1st month   1st year

FIGURE 4–32. Evolution of the T wave, ST segment, and Q wave after myocardial infarction. (From Lepeschkin, E.: Modern Electrocardiography. Baltimore, Williams and Wilkins Co., 1951.)

onset of myocardial infarction, the characteristic early change—namely, an abnormal T wave—is often recorded (Figs. 4–AE10 and 4–AE11, p. 147). The T wave may be prolonged, increased in magnitude, and either upright or inverted. This is followed by ST segment elevation in leads facing the area of injury, with reciprocal depression in the "remote" opposite leads. The upright T wave may exhibit terminal inversion at a time when the ST segment is still elevated. A Q wave may be present in the first ECG or may not appear for hours or sometimes days.[70a] The amplitude of the QRS complex may diminish and may be replaced by a QS pattern. As the ST segment returns to the baseline, symmetrically inverted T waves evolve.[67] The time of appearance and the magnitude of the changes vary among patients (Fig. 4–32).

Occasionally, early in the course of evolution of acute infarction, a very tall R wave merging with an elevated ST segment with reduction or loss of the S wave may be

present. The pattern resembles a monophasic action potential (Fig. 4–AE12, p. 147).[71]

The classic evolution of acute myocardial infarction is documented in approximately one-half to two-thirds of the patients (Fig. 4–33), while in those remaining the infarct is manifested by ST-segment, T-wave, and non-Q QRS changes (Fig. 4–34).

SUBTLE, ATYPICAL, NONSPECIFIC PATTERNS OF INFARCTION. Atypical features and characteristics of early infarction seen in about 40 to 50 per cent of the first ECG's include a normal ECG, subtle ST-segment and T-wave changes, isolated T-wave abnormality, transient normalization of the ST-segment, T-wave, or QRS complex, involvement of electrically "silent" areas (see Fig. 4–35 and 4–AE18), or the masking effect of conduction defects (Figs. 4–16, 4–19, and 4–29). Awareness and recognition of the early, nondiagnostic, "atypical" or subtle abnormalities will improve the diagnostic sensitivity of the ECG.

Although ECG changes can be documented within seconds after experimental coronary occlusion and in humans during angioplasty, such changes may be delayed. A normal initial ECG in a patient with evolving clinical acute myocardial infarction may be due to absence of ischemia at the time of the initial tracing, a delay in evolution of the characteristic pattern, an initially small infarct that produces diagnostic ECG changes only after extension, transient normalization of the ECG in the course of evolution of acute myocardial infarction, or infarction of an electrocardiographically "silent" area of the myocardium (Fig. 4–35).

Early changes of myocardial infarction may alter the terminal part of the QRS (Fig. 4–34). With an inferior infarction these may be manifested by an increase of the R wave amplitude in lead III and appearance of an S wave in aV$_l$. There also may be an associated increase in S wave amplitude in leads V$_2$ and V$_3$.[72] These changes are most likely due to conduction delays in the ischemic and injured

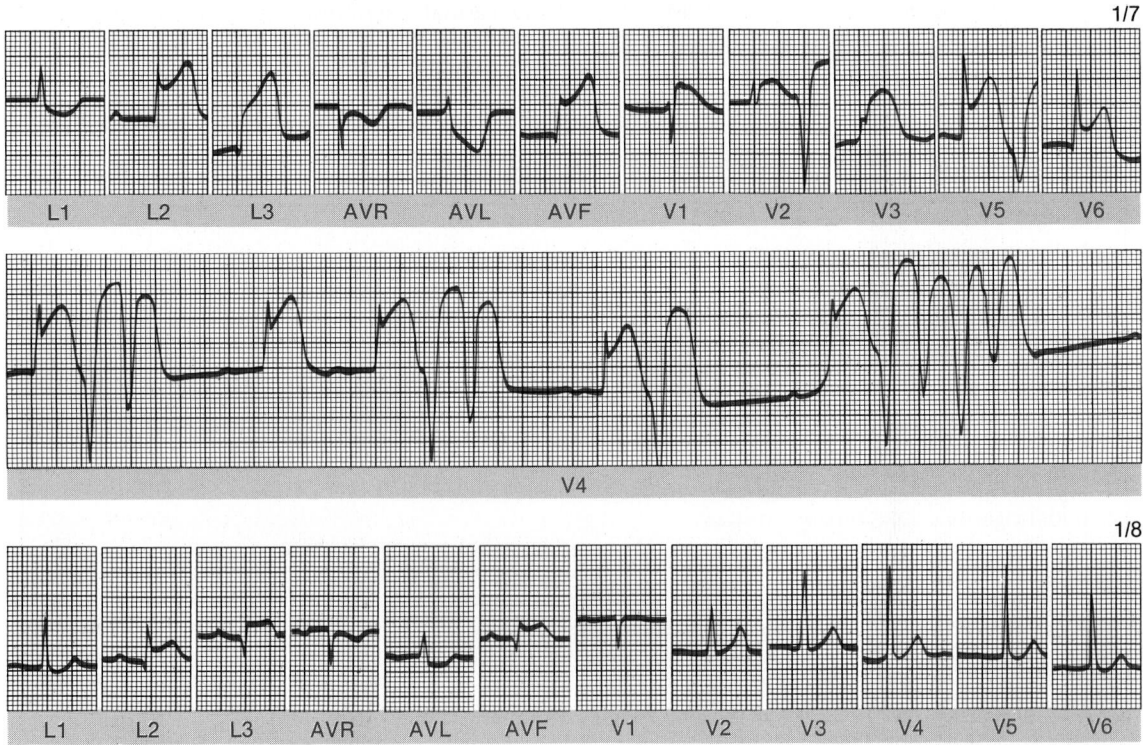

1/7

| L1 | L2 | L3 | AVR | AVL | AVF | V1 | V2 | V3 | V5 | V6 |

V4

1/8

| L1 | L2 | L3 | AVR | AVL | AVF | V1 | V2 | V3 | V4 | V5 | V6 |

FIGURE 4–33. Acute inferior myocardial infarction and transient extensive anterior injury. Tracing made on 1/7 shows elevation of the ST segment in leads II, III, and aV$_f$, V$_1$ through V$_6$ with reciprocal depression of the ST segment in leads I and aV$_l$. In the second row the acute injury is accompanied by ventricular premature complexes (isolated and couplets) and a short run of ventricular tachycardia. In the tracing of 1/8, the anterior current of injury is no longer present, and the residual pattern is that of an acute inferior myocardial infarction manifest by a Q wave and ST segment elevation in leads II, III, and aV$_f$. The tall R in lead V$_2$ and upright right precordial R waves suggest an associated posterior infarction.

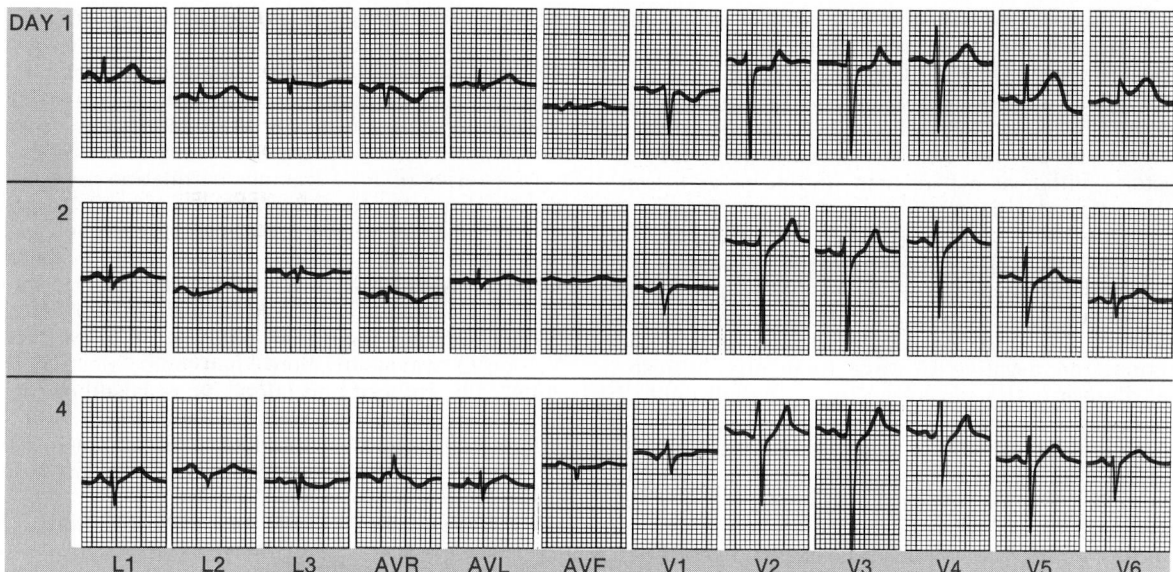

FIGURE 4–34. Acute myocardial infarction manifested by an altered sequence of ventricular activation. Tracing recorded on day 1 suggests a lateral infarction with reciprocal ST segment depression in leads V_1 to V_3. A shift of axis to right with prominent S waves in leads V_5 and V_6 is noted in the middle trace (Day 2). The Q waves in leads II, III, and aV_f with R waves of higher amplitude in leads V_1 and V_2 suggest that the infarct is inferior and probably posterior (Day 4). The marked right-axis duration and the prominent S waves in leads V_5 and V_6 indicate an inferior and posterior periinfarction block with the terminal ventricular excitation directed toward the infarction.

areas, in some way similar to periinfarction block (see p. 1251).

Evolution of the characteristic ST-segment and T-wave changes coupled with appearance of Q waves is highly specific for acute myocardial infarction. In the first ECG, the sensitivity and specificity of the ST-segment change alone, especially when marked, is high. With the passage of 4 to 12 hours, however, *evolving* changes in the ST segment need to be demonstrated, since conditions such as pericarditis, early repolarization, and ventricular aneurysm (Fig. 4–AE19) also may manifest ST-segment elevation, but it is usually persistent. Transient hyperkalemia (Fig. 4–45) and Prinzmetal's angina (see below) (Fig. 4–44), like acute myocardial infarction, also can cause transient ST-segment elevations. Although subtle, minor ST-segment elevation can be easily overlooked, it is a relatively common, isolated early finding.

ST-segment depression may reflect subendocardial ischemia, infarction, or reciprocal changes secondary to infarction at a "remote" (opposite) site.[73–75] It also has been suggested that depression of the ST segment in leads V_1 to V_4 in the presence of an inferior infarction may indicate ischemia secondary to significant obstruction of the left anterior descending coronary artery. However, evidence indicates that the ST-segment depression is reciprocal to the inferior or posterolateral infarction and that the severity of the anterior wall ST-segment depression may be related to the severity and extent of the inferior ischemia rather than to anterior wall ischemia. There is evidence that inferior ST-segment depression noted with anterior ischemia is also a reciprocal phenomenon and does not reflect inferior ischemia.[76–80]

Minor, subtle ST-segment depression is a common early finding of acute myocardial infarction, especially non-Q wave infarction. However, since ST-segment depression is often a nonspecific change, it should be evaluated in light of other clinical and laboratory findings.

Tall, peaked T waves seen in experimental coronary occlusion are occasionally recorded in humans and are thought to reflect subendocardial ischemia (Fig. 4–AE10). More often, initially the T waves are isoelectric, negative (Fig. 4–AE11, p. 147), or biphasic. While subtle T-wave changes are often the earliest recorded signs of infarction, their value is limited because of nonspecificity. In about 20 to 30 percent of patients with myocardial infarction, a T-wave abnormality is the only sign of acute infarction.

In patients with ischemic heart disease, ST alternans is usually noted in limb leads and anterior precordial leads. It is characteristically associated with vasospastic angina

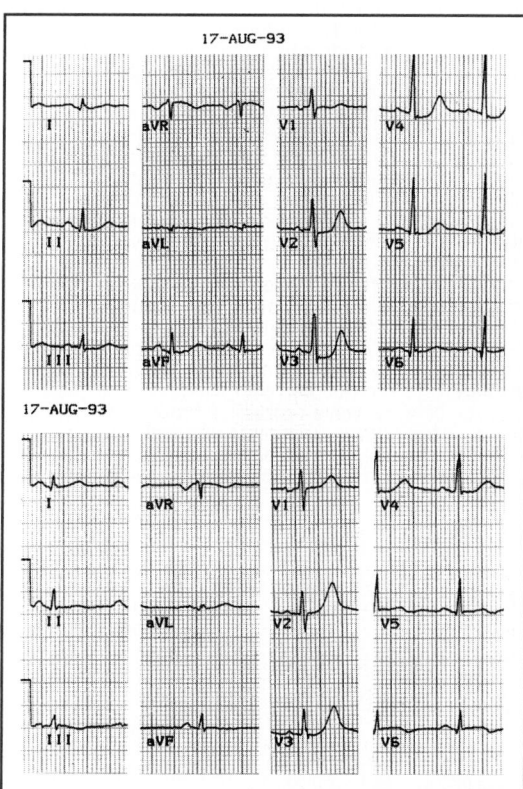

FIGURE 4–35. The top tracing illustrates what appears to be a "pure" posterior myocardial infarction manifest by tall R waves in leads V_1 and V_2 with ST segment depression in leads V_2 to V_4. The bottom tracing, however, discloses inferoapical changes. Pure posterior infarction without a concomitant inferior or lateral infarction or both is extremely rare (see Fig. 4–AE16, p. 149).

(Printzmetal's angina, p. 1340) but has been reported during acute infarction, during exercise tests, after subarachnoid hemorrhage, and rarely with other conditions.[52]

An *abnormal U wave* is a frequent marker of ischemic heart disease.[80a] Negative or biphasic U waves have been reported in up to 30 per cent of patients with chronic angina pectoris, either as a persistent finding or as a transient manifestation during an episode of angina. It is most often recorded in leads I, II, and V_4 to V_6. Appearance of a negative U wave during exercise-induced ischemia has been appreciated for some time and is highly specific for disease of the left anterior descending coronary artery.[81] When accompanying unstable angina or anterior myocardial infarction, the negative U wave frequently indicates multivessel disease with a severe lesion in the left anterior descending artery.[82] A negative U wave is seen in 10 to 60 per cent of patients with anterior infarction and in up to 30 per cent of patients with inferior infarction. When present in a setting of a previous myocardial infarction, the negative U waves are a sign of extensive infarction involving the apex and a marker of significant impairment of left ventricular function.[83] Appearance of a negative U wave may precede other ECG changes of infarction by several hours (Fig. 4–36), an observation supported by changes noted during PTCA.

An abnormal QRS complex, ST segment, and T wave may normalize transiently in the course of evolution of acute myocardial infarction. This may be due to reversible ischemia or injury or conduction defects, but it is also frequently observed in the normal evolution of acute myocardial infarction. Presence of an upright T wave longer than 48 hours after infarction or an early reversal of an inverted T wave to a positive deflection is indicative of postinfarction pericarditis with or without pericardial effusion and suggests the presence of transmural infarction.[84]

A premature ventricular complex with a qR or QR morphology even in the absence of ECG findings of infarction suggests the presence of myocardial infarction. This finding may prove particularly useful when the myocardial infarction is masked, for example, by LBBB or WPW. A recent study, however, questions the value of this finding in the absence of other ECG findings of myocardial infarction.

OLD INFARCTION. ECG diagnosis of old myocardial infarction is often difficult and frequently impossible without the availability of tracings documenting the acute episode. A definitive diagnosis of old infarction depends on the presence of a pathological Q wave. Only rarely can it be based on T-wave changes alone. While abnormal Q waves may be absent in transmural infarction and present in nontransmural infarction, the sensitivity and specificity of the ECG for diagnosis of an old myocardial infarction still depend on Q waves. The specificity of abnormal Q waves for myocardial infarction is relatively high; however, the sensitivity is quite low. Within 6 to 12 months after an acute myocardial infarction, about 30 per cent of the tracings,

although abnormal, are no longer diagnostic of infarction, because the Q wave(s) are absent. Similarly, by the end of 10 years, or sooner, some 6 to 10 per cent of the cardiograms revert to normal. There is evidence to suggest that regression of Q waves following anterior myocardial infarction is associated with smaller areas of infarction.[85]

In a series of 1184 tracings correlating myocardial infarction with postmortem findings, the specificity and sensitivity of the Q wave were 89 and 61 per cent, respectively, and varied with location of the infarction. Anteriorly located Q waves (leads V_1 to V_4) and inferiorly located Q waves (leads II, III, and aV_f) were falsely positive in 46 per cent. Q waves longer than 0.03 sec in lateral leads (V_5 and V_6) or Q waves in more than one "electrocardiographic zone," i.e., inferior and lateral, were false positive in only 4 per cent. The sensitivity of the Q wave was lowest for infarction located in the lateral basal portion of the left ventricle.[86] This anatomical area is usually reflected in leads I and aV_1.[86a]

MYOCARDIAL INFARCTION AND CONDUCTION DELAYS. Conduction defects may not interfere with, may mask, or may falsely suggest the diagnosis of myocardial infarction. In RBBB, the initial order of activation is normal, and thus the pattern of infarction is unaltered. Rarely, the development of RBBB will unmask an anteroseptal infarction.[87] In LBBB the sequence of early activation is altered, with the initial septal vector directed from right to left. As a result, the earliest left ventricular intracavitary potential is positive. In keeping with the "window" concept of infarction, a Q wave cannot be registered except when there is extensive septal infarction. Restated in terms of the dipole or vector concept, since the free wall infarct is inscribed during the latter part of the QRS complex after the septal activation is complete, the direction of initial activation expressed as a dipole or vector is unaltered by the infarction, and the infarct is masked (Figs. 4–16 and 4–19).

LEFT BUNDLE BRANCH BLOCK. Numerous attempts at defining diagnostic criteria for myocardial infarction in the presence of LBBB have proven unsuccessful. The proposed criteria rarely correlate with autopsy findings. In a study of 52 patients with LBBB and autopsy findings of myocardial infarction, the following ECG findings were thought to correlate with myocardial infarction: (1) a Q wave 0.04 sec or greater in leads I, aV_1, V_5, or V_6; (2) rapid serial ST-segment and T-wave changes; (3) acute ST-segment elevation disproportionate to the area of the QRS complex; and (4) a Q wave of any size in lead V_6. Others suggest that a deep S wave in leads V_5 and V_6, a qRs complex with a slurred S wave in leads V_5 and V_6, loss of the R wave in the precordial leads, or a Q wave in leads II, III, and aV_f is consistent with myocardial infarction complicating LBBB. However, in another study of patients with LBBB, the significance of Q waves, broad R waves, notched middle and left precordial S waves, rsR' complexes, ST-segment elevation, and T-wave changes was found to lack significant correlation with myocardial infarction.

In patients with LBBB, ischemia, and infarction, the following criteria were found highly specific and predictive for myocardial infarction in a range of 90 to 100 per cent: Q wave in at least two leads, leads I, aV_1, V_5, or V_6; R-wave regression from V_1 to V_4; notching on the upstroke of the S wave in at least two leads (leads V_3, V_4, or V_5), and primary ST-T changes in two or more adjacent leads (Fig. 4–17).[88] A somewhat better correlation was noted between an ECG sugges-

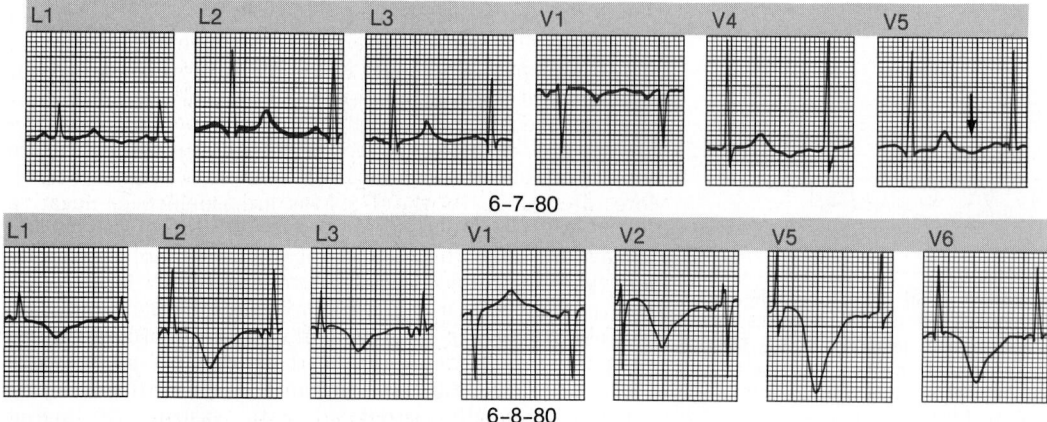

6-7-80

6-8-80

FIGURE 4–36. Negative U wave as the only marker of an acute ischemic episode. On 6/7/80 a negative U wave ($\downarrow$) was recorded in leads I, V_4 and V_5, and an upright reciprocal U wave was present in lead V_1. In the tracing of 6/8/80 a prolonged Q-T interval and deeply inverted T waves are present in all the leads—evolutionary changes consistent with an acute myocardial infarction. At necropsy a subendocardial infarction was found.

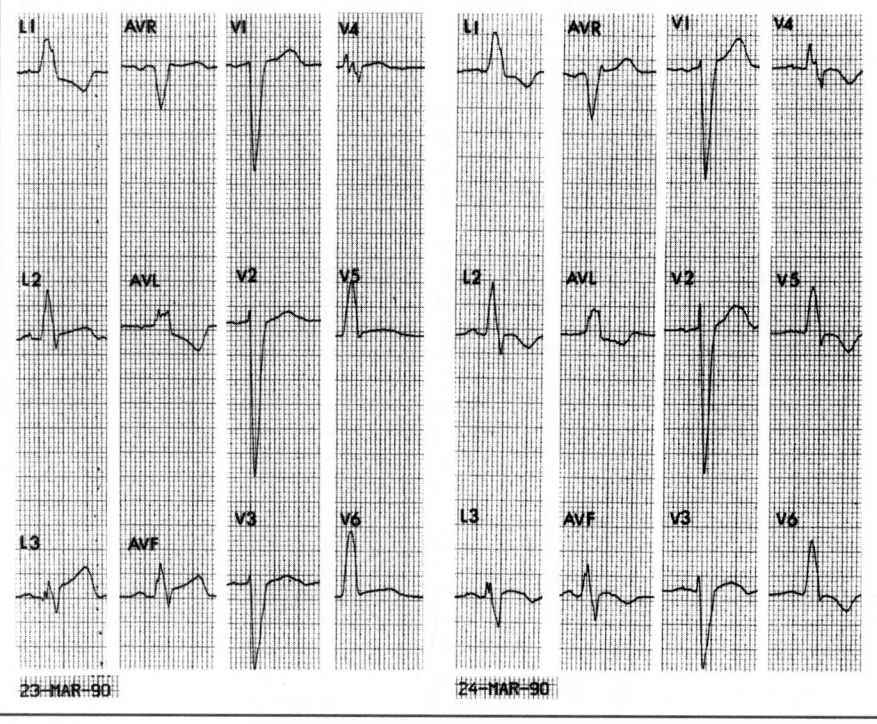

FIGURE 4–37. Acute myocardial infarction and LBBB. 3/23/90, The LBBB is accompanied by elevated ST segments in leads II, III, aV$_f$, and V$_6$ and depressed in leads I and aV$_l$. 3/24/90, Symmetrically inverted T waves are present in leads II, III, aV$_f$, V$_4$, V$_5$, and V$_6$. Although Q waves are not recorded, the evolution of the ST-T changes is consistent with the clinical history of acute myocardial infarction.

tive of acute inferior myocardial infarction and postmortem findings (Fig. 4–37). Observations made during angioplasty indicate that in the presence of LBBB with acute transmural ischemia, the ST segment becomes elevated over the area of the acute ischemia; this is a change similar to that observed with normal intraventricular conduction[89] (Fig. 4–AE13).

Studies of patients with intermittent LBBB and myocardial infarction provide additonal evidence that LBBB masks myocardial infarction (Fig. 4–16). It should be noted, however, that occasionally when acute infarction is evident during normal intraventricular conduction, acute changes are also recognizable in the presence of LBBB (Figs. 4–AE13, p. 148, and 4–37).

Block of the divisions of the LBBB may simulate or obscure myocardial infarction. Left anterior fascicular block (LAFB) may simulate an anterior infarction and obscure an inferior infarction (Fig. 4–19). In LAFB the R wave in lead aV$_f$ is taller than in lead III and the R wave in lead II is taller than in lead aV$_f$ (II > aV$_f$ > III). A reversal of this progression, namely III > aV$_f$ > II, is highly suggestive of a previous myocardial infarction.[90]

In WPW syndrome as in LBBB, the initial vector may be directed toward the left ventricular cavity, precluding the appearance of a Q wave (Fig. 4–29). The ECG pattern of infarction masked by WPW is recognizable in the presence of normal intraventricular conduction by ST-segment and T-wave changes.

PERIINFARCTION BLOCK. As originally defined, periinfarction block is a specific conduction abnormality due to myocardial infarction.[91–94] The ECG changes include a Q wave of 0.04 sec and a QRS complex in the limb leads of 0.10 sec, with a slurred prolonged terminal component facing the site of infarction. Peri-infarction block is not synonymous with left anterior divisional block. Peri-infarction block may be of help in the diagnosis of old inferior infarction when the characteristic changes are no longer evident. Presence of terminal, somewhat

delayed activation facing leads II, III, or aV$_f$ and a terminal negative wave in leads I, V$_5$, and V$_6$ (signs of peri-infarction block) strengthen the diagnosis of inferior myocardial infarction (Fig. 4–38).

In acute anterior infarction, slowing of conduction in the ischemic area is manifest by a decrease of the S wave in leads V$_2$ and V$_3$. In inferior infarction, the slowing of conduction is manifested by an increase in R wave in leads III and aV$_f$ and S wave in lead aV$_l$.[95]

An RSR' complex not related to RBBB but due to terminal conduction delay has been shown to be associated with severe segmental motion abnormality consistent with myocardial infarction scar tissue.[96]

THE ECG AND SITE OF CORONARY ARTERY OBSTRUCTION. The correlation of ECG pattern and site of obstruction early in the course of myocardial infarction was investigated arteriographically in 152 patients. The sensitivity, specificity, and predictive value for (1) ECG indicative of anterior infarction and occlusion of the left anterior descending coronary was 90, 95, and 96 per cent, respectively; (2) ECG indicative of inferior infarction and occlusion of the right coronary artery was 56, 97, and 80 per cent, respectively; (3) ECG indicative of posterior or lateral infarction and obstruction of the left circumflex coronary was 24, 98, and 75 per cent, respectively; (4) ECG indicative of inferior infarction and obstruction of the right or left circumflex coronary was 53, 98, and 94 per cent, respectively; and (5) ECG indicative of posterior or lateral infarction and obstruction of the right or left circumflex coronary was 53, 98, and 94 per cent, respectively.[97]

FIGURE 4–38. Inferior myocardial infarction and peri-infarction block. The inferior infarction is manifest by the Q waves in leads II, III, and aV$_f$. There is a terminal delay of depolarization toward the inferior infarction, as indicated by an S wave in leads I and aV$_l$ and a terminal positive deflection of the QRS in leads III and aV$_f$. This terminal vector is due to an unopposed depolarization in the direction of the infarction. The delayed, slow depolarization is due to loss of the Purkinje fibers.

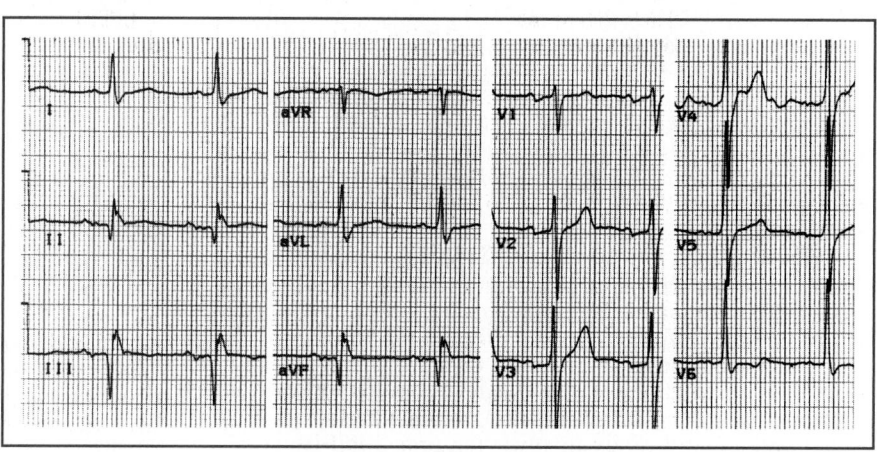

In acute inferior myocardial infarction, changes in the lateral leads (aV_L, V_5, and V_6) with an isoelectric or elevated ST in lead I identified obstruction of the circumflex coronary artery with a sensitivity, specificity, and predictive value of 83, 96, and 93, respectively. Changes in the lateral leads are rare, with inferior infarction resulting from obstruction of the right coronary artery.[98] There is evidence that lateral ECG abnormalities with an abnormal R wave in lead V_1 indicate a proximal left circumflex lesion.[99]

Two hundred and four consecutive patients with unstable angina manifesting abnormal ST-segment and terminal T-wave inversion in leads V_2 and V_3 without abnormal Q waves were found to have more than 50 per cent narrowing of proximal left anterior descending artery. Of this group, 33 had complete obstruction and 75 had collateral circulation to the affected vessel.[100] Others have made similar observations.

Presence of ST-segment elevation equal to or greater than 1 mm in lead V_4R has a sensitivity of 100 per cent and specificity of 87 per cent and a predictive accuracy of 92 per cent for occlusion of right coronary above the first right ventricular branch. The absence of ST-segment elevation of 1 mm excludes such lesions. Similarly, presence of ST-segment elevation in V_4R excluded isolated obstruction of left circumflex artery.[101]

THE ECG AND LOCATION OF INFARCTION. A precise anatomical location of anterior myocardial infarction based on ECG is not always possible.[101a] Accuracy of such localization is influenced, for example, by distance of the electrode from the heart, which varies considerably among individuals. The area subtending a given precordial electrode varies with the anteroposterior (AP) diameter of the chest and is greater in individuals with an increased diameter. Consequently, the same size anterior infarct would be recorded in more leads than in an individual with a normal AP diameter.

The diagnosis of transmural and nontransmural infarction when based on presence or absence of a Q wave shows a poor correlation with autopsy findings. Experimental and autopsy findings indicate that while nontransmural lesions may be accompanied by a Q wave, the Q wave may be absent in transmural infarction. It has been suggested that as many as 50 per cent of nontransmural myocardial infarctions manifest Q waves, making differentiation of nontransmural and transmural infarction based on the Q wave highly tenuous. It appears, therefore, that the terms Q and non-Q wave infarction (Fig. 4–36) may be preferable to transmural and nontransmural, unless necropsy findings are available.[102,103] Early elevation of the ST segment is a poor predictor of subsequent Q wave evolution.[104]

Septal Infarction. On the basis of the presence of Q waves, an infarct is considered septal when a Q wave is present in leads V_1 and V_2 (Fig. 4–AE14, p. 148); anterior when they are present in leads V_3 and V_4; anteroseptal if present in V_1 to V_4; lateral when present in leads I, aV_L, and V_6; anterolateral when present in leads I, aV_L, and V_3 to V_6; extensive anterior when present in leads I, aV_L, and V_1 to V_6, high lateral when present in leads I and aV_L (Fig. 4–AE15), and inferior when present in leads II, III, and aV_f (see Figs. 4–16, 4–33, and 4–34); and anteroinferior, or apical, when present in leads II, III, aV_L, and in one or more of the V_1 to V_4 leads. A posterior infarct is recognized by prominent R waves in lead V_1 or V_2 (Figs. 4–35 and 4–AE16 and 4–AE17, p. 149).

Loss of R waves in leads V_1 and V_2 indicates infarction of the septum and left anterior ventricular wall. Studies in isolated human hearts[18] suggest that the loss of the R wave is due to loss of the early excitation of the middle of the left side of the septum (Fig. 4–AE14).[105]

Isolated obstruction of the diagonal branch of the left anterior descending artery results in changes localized to leads I and aV_l and rarely involves the precordial leads.[106]

Right Ventricular Infarction. This is likely when an elevated ST segment in lead V_1 or V_2 complicates a Q-wave inferior left ventricular septal infarction (Fig. 4–39).[107] It has been suggested that simultaneous ST-segment elevation in lead V_1 and depression in lead V_2 is an important and specific sign for right ventricular infarction.[108] Although Q waves and ST elevation may appear in leads V_1 through V_3, their specificity is too low to be useful in the diagnosis of right ventricular infarction. Right ventricular infarction is more likely when the changes are recorded in right precordial leads, especially V_4R (Fig. 4–AE18, p. 149). The sensitivity and specificity of ST segment elevation in lead V_4R alone has been estimated between 82 to 100 and 68 to 77 per cent, respectively. ST-segment elevation equal to or greater than 1 mm in one or more leads V_4R to V_6R has been shown to have a sensitivity and specificity for infarction of the right ventricle of 90 and 91 per cent, respectively. It has been suggested that ST-segment elevation when greater in lead V_4R than in V_1, V_2, and V_3 reaches a specificity of 100 per cent, but its sensitivity is somewhat lower (78 per cent) than that of an elevated ST segment in V_4R alone.[109,110] During the acute phase of inferior infarction, ST segment elevation in right precordial leads V_4R to V_6R is a most reliable sign of right ventricular infarction. Q waves are superior to ST-segment elevation in patients admitted 12 hours or longer after onset of symptoms. Right ventricular infarction was recorded in 57 per cent of the 187 patients with inferior myocardial infarction.[111] Right ventricular conduction delay is a frequent finding in patients with right ventricular ischemia with an elevated ST segment.[112]

Posterior Left Ventricular Infarction. This is rarely detected. This area of the left ventricle, the last to be depolarized, is inscribed during the terminal 0.04 to 0.06 sec of the QRS complex. Theoretically, therefore, it cannot be expressed as an initial positive wave in leads V_1 and V_2. In keeping with the dipole concept, however, the S wave may become smaller, a sign that lacks any degree of specificity. In a small number of patients, posterior myocardial infarction may be suspected when there is ST-segment depression in lead V_1 or V_2 or both, an R wave in lead V_1 of 0.04 sec, and an R/S ratio greater than 1. The exact mechanism of the change in the initial QRS forces in leads V_1 and V_2 is not clear. Some have suggested that posterior myocardial infarction is not manifested in the ECG but that the find-

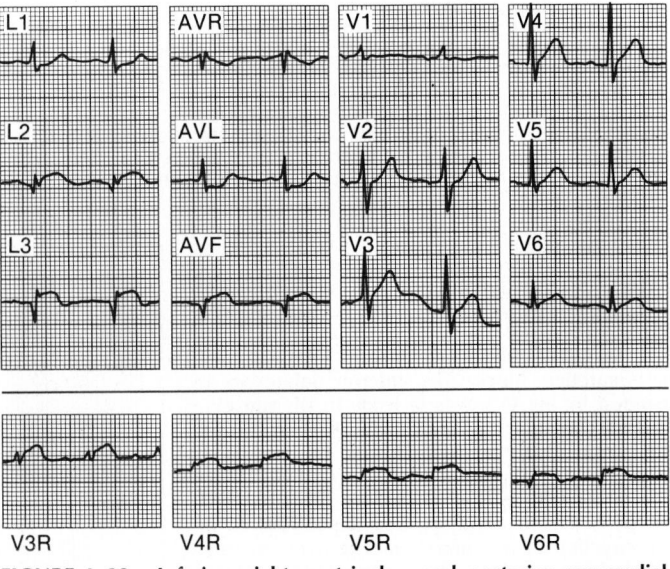

FIGURE 4–39. Inferior, right ventricular, and posterior myocardial infarction. The inferior infarct is manifested by Q waves and elevated ST segments in leads II, III, and aV_f, the posterior by the prominent R waves in leads V_1 and V_2, and the right ventricular by ST segment elevation in leads V_3R to V_6R.

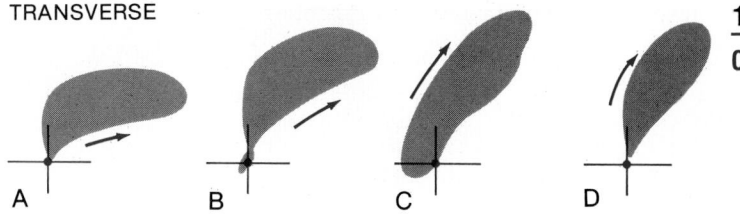

FIGURE 4–40. Vectorcardiogram (diagram) of anterior myocardial infarction. *A,* Anteroseptal; *B,* localized anterior; *C,* anterolateral; *D,* extensive anterior. (Modified from Chou, T. C., et al.: Clinical Vectorcardiography. 2nd ed. New York, Grune and Stratton, 1974, pp. 191, 196, 199.)

ings in lead V_1 or V_2 or both reflect an associated lateral infarction. In patients with an inferior or lateral myocardial infarction, an R wave of increased amplitude 0.04 sec in duration in leads V_1 and V_2 and an upright T wave in lead V_1 suggest concomitant posterior wall involvement (Figs. 4–35, 4–36, 4–AE16, and 4–AE17, p. 149). On occasion, ST-segment depression in leads V_2 and V_3 may be the early evidence of an evolving posterolateral myocardial infarction.[113]

In an effort to estimate the size of infarction, a QRS scoring system based on duration of the Q and R waves and loss of R-wave amplitude expressed in amplitude ratio of R/Q or R/S has been proposed.[114]

THE VCG IN MYOCARDIAL INFARCTION

The appearance of the vector loop in myocardial infarction depends on the site and size of the infarction. Deviation from normal reflects loss of forces normally generated by the infarcted area and resultant dominance of the noninfarcted myocardium. Anterior myocardial infarction is best visualized in the transverse plane, while inferior infarction is best displayed in the frontal or sagittal planes (Fig. 4–40 and 4–41).

Anteroseptal myocardial infarction is recognized in the transverse plane by loss of the first 10- to 20-msec forces, with the initial position of the loop oriented posteriorly and to the left. The entire loop is displaced posteriorly with loss of the anterior convexity. In the vast majority of cases, the loop is inscribed in a counterclockwise direction. The initial posterior and leftward orientation of the loop is reflected in the ECG as a QS complex in leads V_1 to V_4 (Fig. 4–40).

In *localized anterior infarction,* the transverse loop is similar in appearance to that present in anteroseptal myocardial infarction except for a normally inscribed initial force in a left and anterior direction. This initial inscription is displayed in the ECG as an R wave in lead V_1 and at times in V_2 (Fig. 4–40). In *extensive anterior infarction,* the transverse loop reflects loss of both the septal and free left ventricular walls. The initial normal anteriorly inscribed portion of the loop is lost, and the loop is shifted posteriorly and inscribed clockwise. The ECG shows a loss of R wave, at times, in all precordial leads.

Anterolateral infarction is inscribed clockwise or as a figure-of-eight in the transverse plane. The initial normal part of the loop is followed by posterior and somewhat rightward displacement, reflecting the more extensive loss of left ventricular wall. Loss of the lateral wall may result in an increase in magnitude of the initial left-to-right portion of the loop, reflected in the ECG as a tall R wave inscribed in the right precordial leads (Fig. 4–40).

Inferior myocardial infarction is best displayed in the frontal and sagittal planes (Fig. 4–41). In the frontal plane, the loop is most often inscribed in a clockwise direction. The initial portion is directed superiorly, the superior displacement exceeding 25 to 30 msec. The loop

crosses the X axis to the left of the point of origin. It has been suggested that when the above diagnostic findings are absent, a shift to the left of the QRS loop combined with clockwise rotation is strongly indicative of an inferior infarction. Occasionally, when the inferior septum is spared, the initial loop may have a normal orientation, that is, to the right and inferiorly. This is followed by clockwise inscription and superior displacement of the remainder of the loop. In such instances the ECG will record small initial R waves in leads II, III, and aV_f.

In *posterior myocardial infarction* the initial forces are normal in the transverse plane, but more than half the loop is ultimately displaced anteriorly. In the majority of cases, inscription of the loop is counterclockwise. The anterior displacement of the loop is reflected in the ECG by a prominent R wave in lead V_1 or V_2 that may exceed 0.04 sec in duration (Fig. 4–41).

A summary of VCG criteria for myocardial infarction is presented in Table 4–3 and Figures 4–40 and 4–41.

Noninfarction Q Waves

While the vast majority of abnormal Q waves are due to myocardial infarction, a significant number are due to other causes.

Noninfarction Q waves may be transient or permanent. Transient Q waves have been produced experimentally in animals and observed in patients during ischemic episodes.[115] Such Q waves have been explained by a transient loss of electrophysiological function, but without irreversible cellular damage, a phenomenon referred to by some as "myocardial concussion."[116,117] Q waves have been recorded with severe metabolic disturbances accompanying shock or pancreatitis. Similarly, transient Q waves have been noted during cardiac surgery and ascribed variously to transient ischemia and hypoxia, coronary spasm, localized metabolic and electrolyte disturbances, and possible hypothermia. Rarely a transient Q wave may result from tachycardia.

The largest group of noninfarction Q waves is due to myocardial disease, including myocarditis, AIDS (Fig. 4–AE19, p. 149), cardiac amyloidosis,[118] neuromuscular disorders such as progressive muscular dystrophy,[119] myotonia atrophica, Friedreich's ataxia, scleroderma, postpartum myopathy, myocardial replacement by tumor (Fig. 4–42), sarcoidosis, idiopathic cardiomyopathy, anomalous coronary artery, and coronary embolism.

Noninfarction Q waves are common in hypertrophic cardiomyopathy[120,121] and may simulate anterior or inferior myocardial infarction (Figs. 4–43 and 4–AE20, p. 149). Although the exact mechanism of the abnormal Q waves in this condition is unclear, increased septal mass or abnormal depolarization because of anomalous architecture of the septal myocardium, or both, have been proposed as the cause.

Abnormal Q waves can be associated with chronic obstructive lung disease (COLD) with or without cor pulmonale, pulmonary embolism, and pneumothorax. In COLD, findings in the precordial leads frequently simulate anterior myocardial infarction (Fig. 4–14). The mechanism responsible for the QS complex is clockwise rotation and downward displacement of the diaphragm and of the heart. As a result, the electrodes are located superior to the initial vector; when this vector is directed inferiorly, a QS pattern results. By placing the electrode one interspace lower, it is often possible to record an R wave and thus provide strong evidence against myocardial infarction. Occasionally in COLD the Q wave may simulate inferior myocardial infarction. The positional origin of the anterior or inferior Q

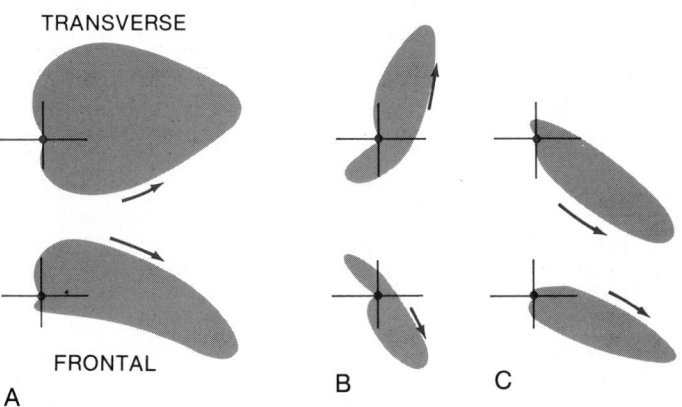

TRANSVERSE

FRONTAL

A   B   C

FIGURE 4–41. Vectorcardiogram of inferior and posterior myocardial infarction. *A,* Inferior; *B,* inferolateral; *C,* true posterior. (Modified from Chou, T. C., et al.: Clinical Vectorcardiography. 2nd ed. New York, Grune and Stratton, 1974, pp. 208, 220, 226.)

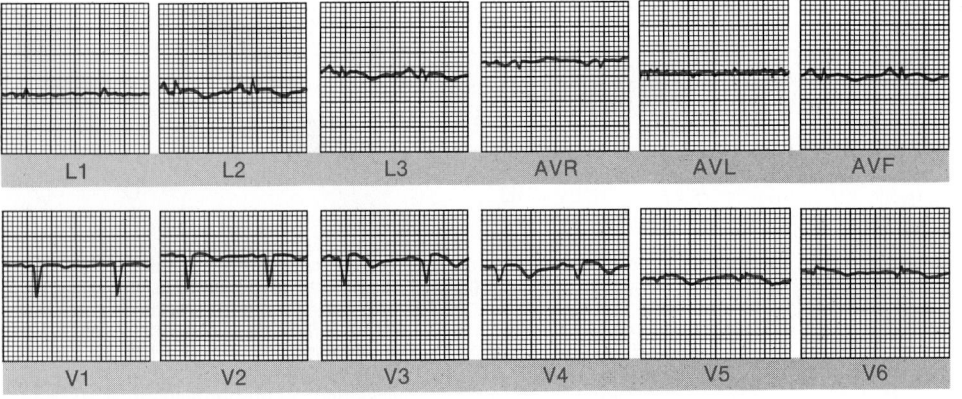

FIGURE 4–42. Extensive anterior and inferior myocardial infarction simulated by extensive myocardial metastasis of carcinoma of the breast.

waves may be suspected when the Q wave is accompanied by other ECG findings of COLD (see p. 115). However, since both COLD and myocardial infarction frequently coexist, differential diagnosis may at times be difficult or impossible.

Abnormal Q waves, especially in lead III and rarely in lead aV$_f$, with an S wave in lead I, can be recorded in acute cor pulmonale due to *pulmonary embolism* (Fig. 4–13). Clockwise rotation with superior orientation of the initial vector is most likely responsible for the Q waves in lead III. A Q wave in lead II is rarely recorded. Occasionally acute pulmonary embolus may simulate anterior myocardial infarction.

Spontaneous pneumothorax, particularly on the left, may result in a pattern simulating anterior myocardial infarction with occasional absence of the R wave in all the precordial leads.

In LBBB the initial forces are directed from right to left and either superiorly or inferiorly. When the inferiorly directed forces dominate, a QS complex may be recorded in the precordial leads, simulating an anterior myocardial infarction. If the initial vector is oriented to the left and superiorly, a QS complex may be registered in the inferior leads, suggesting inferior myocardial infarction.

With left anterior divisional block, the transitional zone is shifted to the left, and an initial Q wave may appear in the right precordial leads. Loss of the forces normally contributed by the left anterior division results in a vector directed inferiorly, posteriorly, and to the right. Consequently, right precordial leads may register a qrS complex suggestive of an anteroseptal infarction. By placement of the electrodes one interspace lower, an rS complex can be recorded attesting to the positional nature of the Q wave.

Noninfarction Q waves are frequent in WPW (see p. 667). WPW type B, with the initial forces directed from right to left, registers a QS complex in the right precordial leads and may be mistaken for anteroseptal or anterior myocardial infarction. Rarely, preexcitation of the left lateral wall, with the vector oriented anteriorly and to the right, simulates lateral infarction. Most often, however, WPW simulates inferior infarction (Fig. 4–28). The Q waves recorded in leads II, III, and aV$_f$ are due to superior orientation of the initial vector and may be seen with either type A or type B WPW.

In LVH, failure to record an R wave in leads V$_1$ to V$_4$ may suggest an anteroseptal myocardial infarction (Fig. 4–11). Similarly, reciprocal elevation of the ST segments in these leads may contribute to an erroneous diagnosis of myocardial infarction. The exact mechanism of the initial negative deflection of the QRS is not clear, but it may be related to posterior rotation or inferior orientation of the initial vector (Fig. 4–11).

ST-Segment and T-Wave Changes

ST-SEGMENT ELEVATION. In addition to the three most common organic causes of ST-segment elevations—acute myocardial infarction, pericarditis, and Prinzmetal's angina (Fig. 4–44)—ST-segment elevation is occasionally observed in acute cor pulmonale, hyperkalemia (Fig. 4–45), cerebrovascular accidents, LVH, LBBB, hypertrophic cardiomyopathy, invasion of the heart by neoplastic tissue, hypothermia, and cocaine abuse.[122] Elevation of the ST segment also may be an artifact caused by excessive inertia of the stylus of the electrocardiograph. In the normal heart the most common cause of ST-segment elevation is so-called *early repolarization*, a normal variant (Fig. 4–46).

T-WAVE ABNORMALITIES. A *primary T wave change* indicates a regional alteration in the duration of the depolarized state. Some common clinical conditions associated with primary T-wave changes include myocardial ischemia, ventricular aneurysm (Fig. 4–AE21), electrolyte abnormalities (Fig. 4–45), drugs, and a variety of primary myocardial and extracardiac disorders such as myocarditis and subarachnoid hemorrhage. A clinically important sequence of T-wave changes is one of abnormal baseline with normalization of the T wave during ischemia and return to the abnormal baseline after ischemia subsides. Lack of a control tracing could lead to an erroneous conclusion of non-Q wave infarction (Fig. 4–47).

Global, diffuse symmetrical T-wave inversion is a nonspecific finding[123] most often seen with patients with myocardial ischemia (Fig. 4–36), or infarction, following

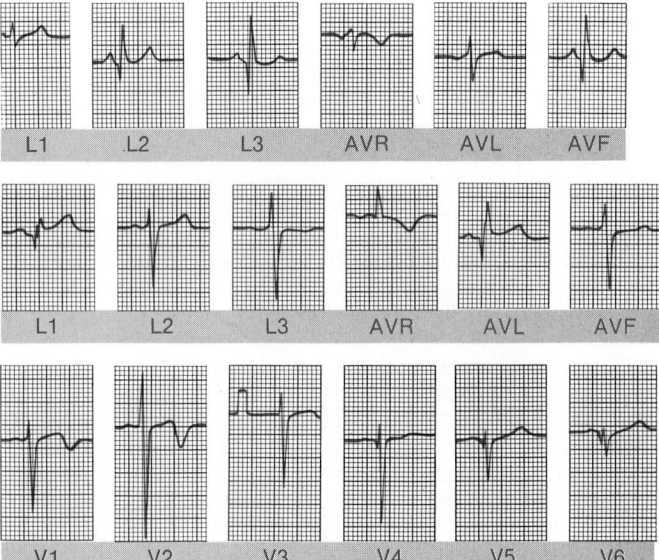

FIGURE 4–43. Hypertrophic cardiomyopathy simulating an inferior, high lateral (precordial leads, not shown, are normal) and anterolateral myocardial infarction in the upper, middle, and lower trace, respectively. (From Fisch, C.: Evolution of the clinical electrocardiogram. J. Am. Coll. Cardiol. *14*:1127, 1989. Reprinted by permission of the American College of Cardiology.)

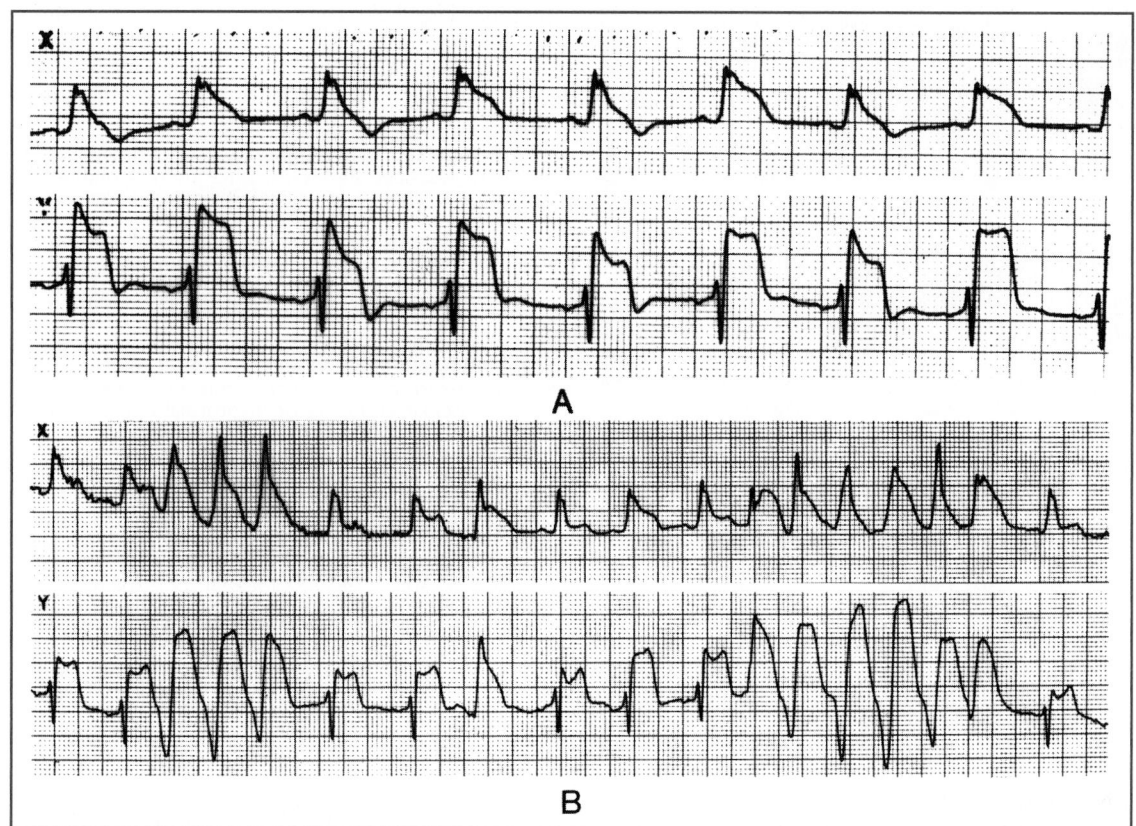

FIGURE 4–44. Printzmetal's angina with ST segment and T wave alternans in panel *A* and ST segment and T wave alternans and nonsustained VT in panel *B.*

cardiac resuscitation, cerebrovascular accidents, apical hypertrophic nonobstructive cardiomyopathy (Fig. 4–AE22, p. 150),[124,125] acute pulmonary embolism,[126] and rarely pheochromocytoma.[127] In a series of 29 patients, it was present in 6 individuals without evidence of organic heart disease. There is an unexplained female preponderance. This striking diffuse T-wave inversion does not in itself imply a poor prognosis. The prognosis is that of the disease.[123]

There is an interesting form of T-wave inversion ascribed to cardiac "memory." It was first noted following cardiac pacing, with the T-wave inversion persisting long after resumption of normal sinus rhythm.[128] Similar T-wave inversion has been recorded following radiofrequency ablation of the accessory pathway in WPW (Fig. 4–AE23, p. 150).[129,130]

Secondary T-wave changes result from alterations of the

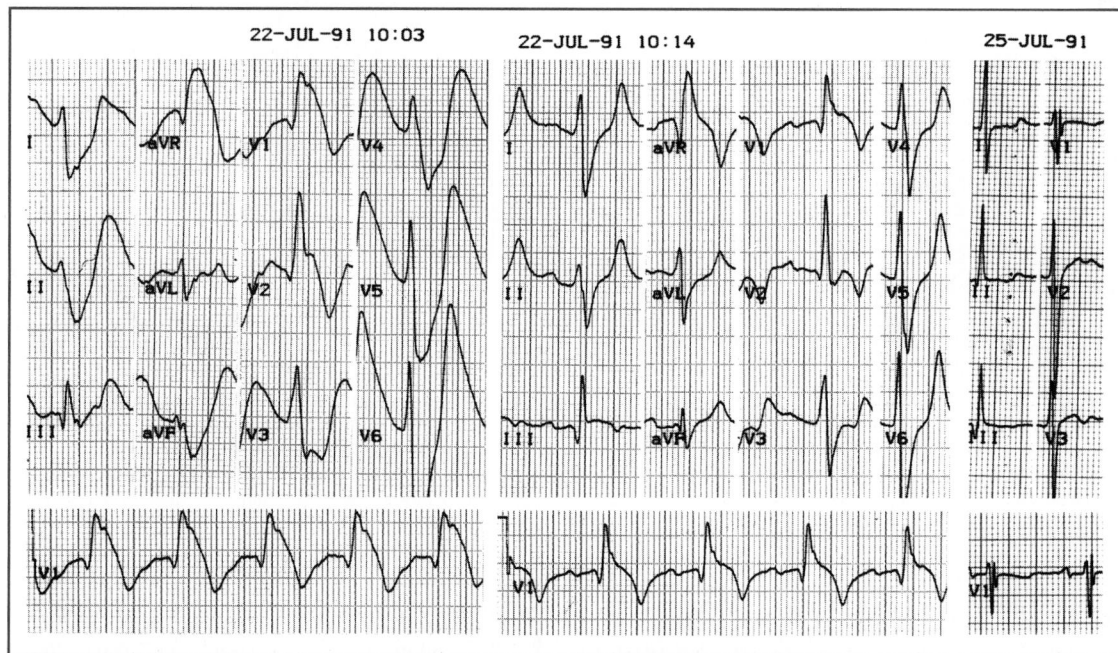

FIGURE 4–45. Severe hyperkalemia. 7/22/91, 10:03, P waves are absent, and there is a marked and diffused prolongation of the QRS with a "dialyzable" current of injury in leads V_1 and V_2. 7/22/91, 10:14, P waves are now present with a P-R interval of 0.24 sec. The QRS pattern is that of right bundle branch block with Q waves in leads V_1 and V_2 simulating a septal infarction. Elevation of the ST segment in lead V_1 is less pronounced. 7/25/91, The tracing is normal except for nonspecific ST-T changes in leads I, II, and III.

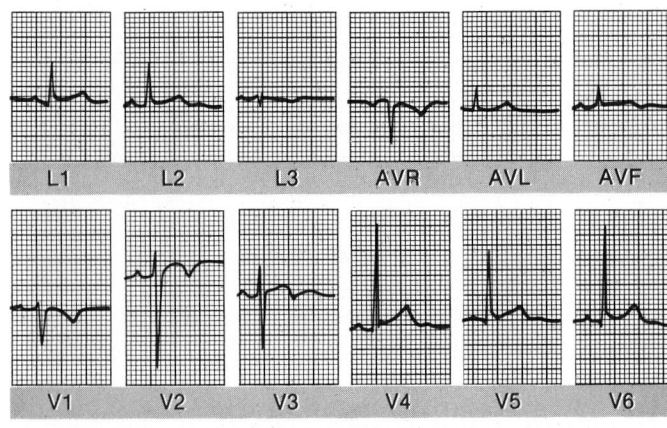

FIGURE 4–46. Normal tracing with juvenile T wave inversion in leads V₁, V₂, and V₃ and early repolarization manifested by ST-segment elevation in leads I, II, aV_f, V₄, V₅, and V₆.

timing or sequencing of depolarization or both, with an obligatory change of the order of repolarization. For example, in LBBB, left ventricular epicardial activation is delayed because of slow conduction through the ventricualr myocardium. As a result, repolarization begins in the subendocardium and an inverted T wave is recorded in precordial leads. The change in the area of the QRS complex and T waves is identical but opposite in direction. Oc-

casionally LBBB is associated with an upright T wave in the left ventricular leads, suggesting that in addition to altered activation due to LBBB, regional abnormalities of repolarization contribute to the T-wave morphology (Fig. 4–17).

RATE-RELATED T-WAVE CHANGES. Postextrasystolic T-wave change was first described in 1915.[131] Since then, a number of mechanisms have been proposed to explain this observation, including an abnormal pathway of repolarization, prolonged diastolic filling time, and an abrupt change in the cycle length. Minor T-wave changes following an abrupt cycle change or after an interpolated ventricular premature complex may be recorded in normal tissue, while more pronounced T-wave alterations suggest an underlying myocardial disorder.

T-wave inversion is occasionally noted following supraventricular or ventricular tachycardia. The magnitude of the T-wave inversion varies, and when extreme, it may resemble the T-wave changes seen with cerebrovascular accidents or myocardial ischemia. The exact mechanism of the posttachycardia T wave is obscure.

T-WAVE ALTERNANS. Isolated T-wave alternans, i.e., without a change in either the QRS complex or the P wave, was first noted in the cat papillary muscle.[132] It is relatively rare and its mechanism not clear. Alternans of phases 2 and 3 of the action potential of the T wave has been recorded without any demonstrable change in phase 0, supporting the concept that isolated alternation of repolarization reflected in the T wave is possible. T-wave alternans of the type already mentioned is most often present during tachycardia or during a sudden change in cycle length. Isolated T-wave alternans, independent of tachycardia or premature systole, is nearly always associated with advanced heart disease or severe electrolyte disturbance (Fig. 4–48) following cardiac resuscitation, rarely with administration of amiodarone, acute pulmonary embolism, and idiopathic long Q-T syndrome. When T-wave alternans is associated with idiopathic pro-

B08

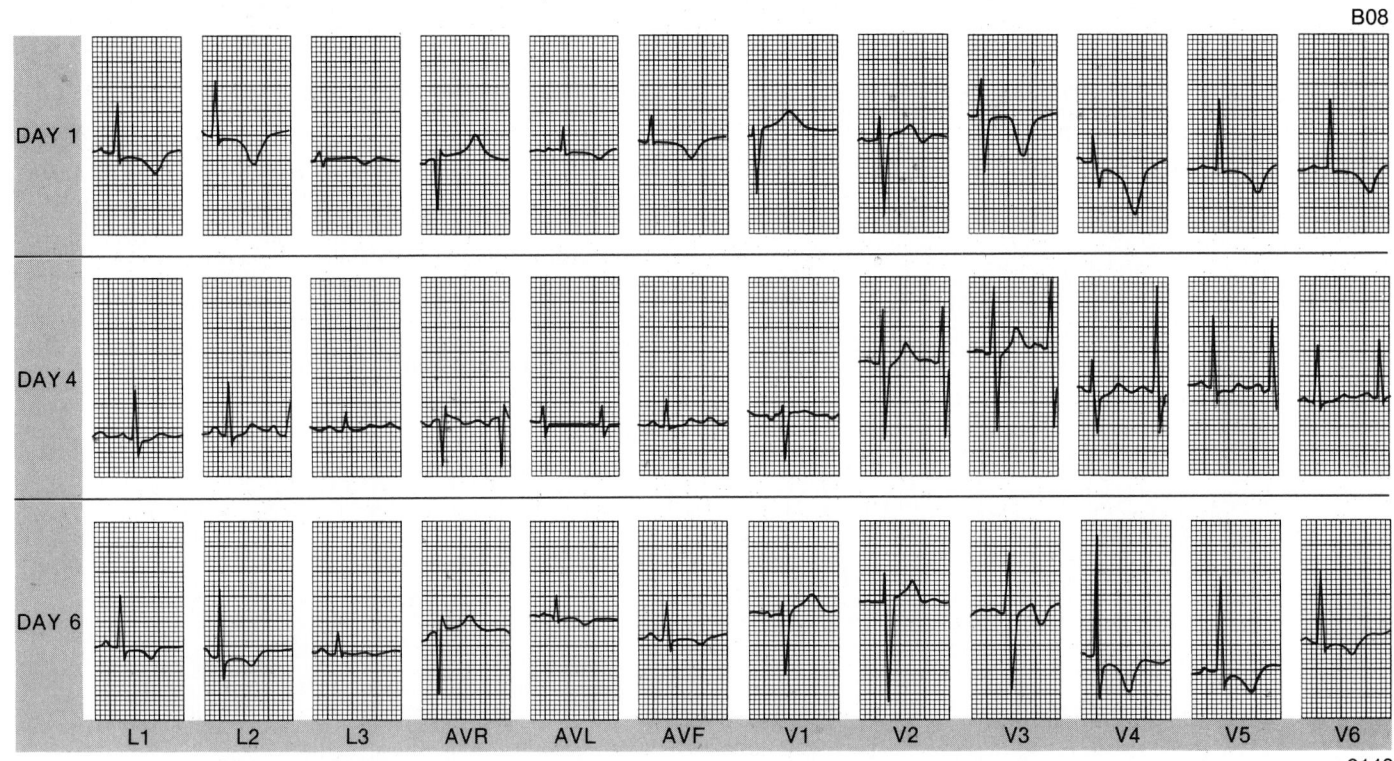

2146

FIGURE 4–47. The top, control, trace recorded when the patient was asymptomatic illustrates symmetrical T wave inversion consistent with ischemic heart disease. During pain, on day 4, the T waves normalized, only to return to control after the pain subsided. If the top trace had been unavailable, the sequence of changes noted in the middle and lower traces coupled with the history could have been mistaken for a new non-Q-wave infarction.

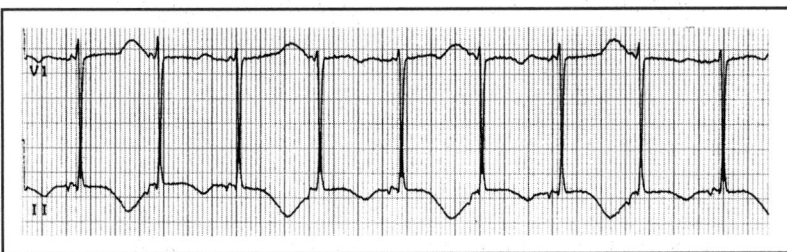

FIGURE 4–48. The QT interval is prolonged, measuring approximately 600 msec with T-wave alternans. The tracing was recorded in a patient with chronic renal disease shortly following dialysis.

longation of the Q-T interval, the risk is related to the prolonged Q-T interval rather than the T-wave alternans.[133-137]

NOTCHED, BIFID T WAVES. Notched, bifid T waves are relatively common in the absence of heart disease, especially in children. These waves also may be present in congenital organic heart disease, the prolonged Q-T syndrome, central nervous system disorders, alcoholic cardiomyopathy, and following the administration of drugs, especially the phenothiazines. The mechanism of bifid or notched T waves is unclear. It has been suggested that in some instances they are caused by nonuniform repolarization secondary to differential innervation of the anterior and posterior ventricular walls. it also has been proposed that in patients with left ventricular disease they may reflect regional delay of repolarization of the left ventricle. Notched or bifid T waves are much more common in association with a long Q-T interval and identify patients at higher risk for syncope or cardiac arrest.[138]

NONSPECIFIC ST-SEGMENT AND T-WAVE CHANGES.

Although the ST segment and T wave represent different electrophysiological events and their respective changes may have different clinical connotations, the widespread practice among electrocardiographers is to refer to either one or both as *ST-T changes*. While it is more appropriate to discuss the two separately, it should be recognized that abnormalities of the ST segment and T wave frequently coexist.

Nondiagnostic ST-segment and T-wave changes are the most common ECG abnormality and account for about 50 per cent of the abnormal tracings recorded in a general hospital population and in 2.4 per cent of all cardiograms.[139] An abnormal T wave is extremely common because the wave is highly sensitive to physiological, pharmacological, and organic changes and therefore is least likely to suggest a specific diagnosis. This fact has been recognized since 1923, when Wilson first recorded inversion of the T wave following the ingestion of cold water.[140]

Although an abnormal T wave suggests the presence of an abnormal or, more appropriately, an altered state, it is recorded with relative frequency in the absence of any disorder (Fig. 4–45), as a reflection of physiological influences, e.g., in highly trained athletes,[141] or during paroxysmal supraventricular tachycardia.[142] For these reasons, an isolated T-wave change must be interpreted with caution and must *always* be correlated with all available clinical and laboratory information. Misinterpretation of the significance of a T-wave abnormality is the most common cause of "iatrogenic ECG heart disease." Attempts to identify the etiology of an abnormal ST segment, T wave, or ST-T segment in isolation from clinical and other laboratory findings often fail.

CLASSIC ST-T CHANGES. The specificity of the purported "classic" ST-T changes, such as those seen with LVH, digitalis administration, and ischemic heart disease, is relatively low. For example, a negative T wave reflecting persistence of a juvenile pattern cannot be differentiated from the symmetrically inverted T wave due to myocardial ischemia. The "classic" ST-T change of LVH also may be due to ischemic heart disease or digitalis, while the marked ST-segment depression due to ischemia or subendocardial infarction may be simulated by the administration of digitalis in the presence of moderate or severe disease. However, when correlated with clinical and other laboratory data, ST-T changes assume a greater predictive value. In a series of 410 abnormal tracings analyzed without regard to clinical data, 70 per cent could be interpreted only as "nonspecific ST-T change." This number was reduced to 10 per cent when such changes were correlated with available clinical information.[139]

The nonspecific and labile nature of the ST segment and the T wave, especially the latter, is expected. Repolarization is a much more diverse process than depolarization. Depolarization is rapid, with a reasonably uniform potential difference across the boundary of activation, and is reflected in the rate of rise of phase 0 and the amplitude of the action potential (see p. 555). Repolarization, displayed as the ST segment and T wave, reflects phases 2 and 3 of the action potential, is considerably longer, and is nonuniform, with many simultaneous boundaries and with differing potentials across various boundaries. It has been shown that shortening of the monophasic action potential by as little as 12 to 18 msec will alter the morphology of the T wave, and importantly, the change can be seen with involvement of 10 per cent or less of the myocardial mass.[143] The magnitude of the T-wave changes, unlike that of the QRS complex, is not related to the mass of the myocardium. The difference has been ascribed to cancellation of repolarization voltages and to uneven contributions from the different regions of repolarization to the genesis of the T wave. Such experimental findings explain, at least partially, the nonspecific character of ST-segment and T-wave changes.

A number of the clinical conditions that may alter the ST segment and T waves are listed in Table 4–4.

U WAVE ABNORMALITIES. An abnormal U wave may be increased in amplitude, inverted, or prolonged. A negative U wave is documented in about 1 per cent of cardiograms recorded in a general hospital. An exaggerated upright U wave may be due to hypokalemia, a variety of drugs (particularly digitalis), and some of the antiarrhythmic agents (e.g., amiodarone).

The most common causes of a *negative U wave* are hypertension (Fig. 4–AE24, p. 150), aortic and mitral valve disease, RVH, and myocardial ischemia (Fig. 4–36).[81,144] A negative U wave can occasionally be found in other metabolic or organic diseases. In hypertension, a negative U wave may be the earliest sign of myocardial involvement, appearing long before any change in the T wave, and has been reported in about 16 per cent of ECGs with an upright T wave and 45 per cent with negative T waves. It may revert to normal with control of the hypertension.[145] The majority of patients with aortic regurgitation and about 10 per cent of patients with aortic stenosis manifest negative U waves. Approximately 5 and 80 per cent of patients with systolic and diastolic overload of the right ventricle, respectively, manifest negative U waves in leads II, III, V_1, and V_2. While high-amplitude positive U waves are the usual finding in hypokalemia, on rare occasions profound hypokalemia may result in large negative U waves obscuring the hypokalemia.[146] In essence, a negative U wave, even as an isolated finding in an otherwise normal ECG, is strongly suggestive of a pathophysiological state.

Q-T INTERVAL ABNORMALITY (see also p. 114). *Shortening of the Q-T interval* may be recorded with hyperkalemia, digitalis, hypercalcemia, and acidosis. *Prolongation of the Q-T interval* may be primary and independent of the QRS, or it may reflect secondary changes of repolarization due to abnormal depolarization, or a combination of the two. Prolongation of the Q-T interval, independent of QRS duration, can be congenital (Figs. 4–49 and 4–AE25, p. 150) or acquired. Acquired disorders include ischemic heart disease, hypothermia, cardiomyopathy, mitral valve prolapse, complete heart block, the condition following cardiac resuscitation, electrolyte changes, and administration of drugs.[147-152] Q-T interval prolongation is a relatively frequent complication of acquired cerebral lesions, especially subarachnoid

TABLE 4–4   CAUSES OF ST-SEGMENT AND T WAVE
CHANGES (SELECTED)

Physiological Position, temperature, hyperventilation, anxiety, food (glucose), tachycardia, neurogenic influences, physical training
Pharmacological Digitalis, antiarrhythmic and psychotrophic drugs (phenothiazines, tricyclics, lithium)
Extracardiac Disorders Electrolyte abnormalities, cerebrovascular accidents, shock, anemia, allergic reactions, infections, endocrine disorders, acute abdominal disorders, pulmonary embolism
Primary Myocardial Disease Congestive, hypertrophic, postpartum cardiomyopathy, myocarditis
Secondary Myocardial Disease Amyloidosis, hemochromatosis, neoplasm, sarcoidosis, connective tissue, neuromuscular disorders
Ischemic Heart Disease Myocardial infarction

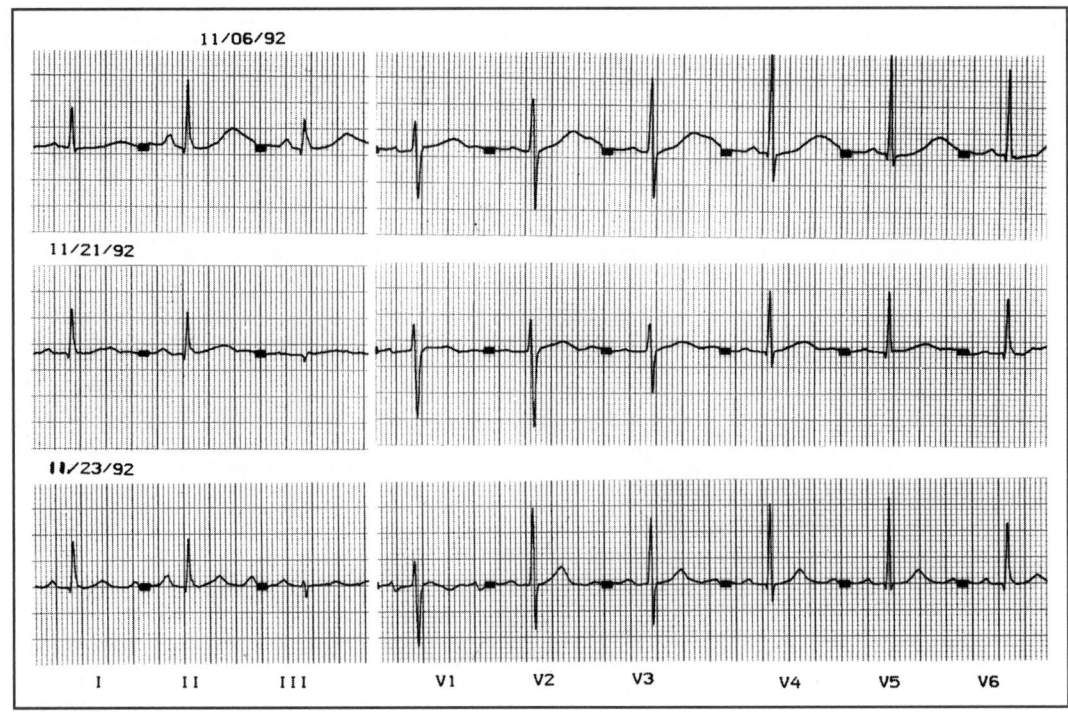

FIGURE 4–49. CVA with marked prolongation of the Q-T interval on 11/6/92. The Q-T interval is shorter but still prolonged on 11/21/92. On 11/23/92 the Q-T interval is normal.

hemorrhage, and also can be present during and following neurosurgical procedures.

ELECTRICAL ALTERNANS. Alternation of amplitude and direction of the QRS complex was noted in the experimental animal and humans as early as 1909 and 1910, respectively,[153] followed by documentation of alternation of the P wave, ST segment, and T wave[52] (Fig. 4–48). Isolated *alternation of the P wave* is seen frequently in the experimental setting but is rare in humans. Most often it accompanies alternation of the QRS complex and occasionally the QRS complex and the T wave. The latter is referred to as *total alternans* and suggests pericardial effusion, usually due to malignancy and frequently associated with tamponade or impending tamponade.

Although pericardial effusion is the most common cause of alternation of the QRS complex (see p. 112), *QRS alternans* is also seen with myocardial ischemia and myocardial disease due to other causes. Two mechanisms of QRS alternans have been proposed: positional oscillation and aberrancy of intraventricular conduction. The

early suggestion that oscillation or alternation of position is the mechanism of alternans of the QRS complex was proved by means of echocardiography. The concept of oscillation also explains the fact that P-wave alternans is seen predominantly with massive pericardial effusion.

ST-segment alternans has been described in dogs after ligation of the coronary artery, in severely ill infants with congenital heart disease, and in patients with Prinzmetal's angina. *T-wave alternans* is discussed on page 137. *U-wave alternans* is least common and very difficult to recognize.

The mechanism of alternans in severe myocardial disorders but in the absence of pericardial effusion is obscure. It has been ascribed to uneven duration of the excited state or to two alternating foci of impulse formation. However, the fact that alternation of depolarization, activation, and repo-

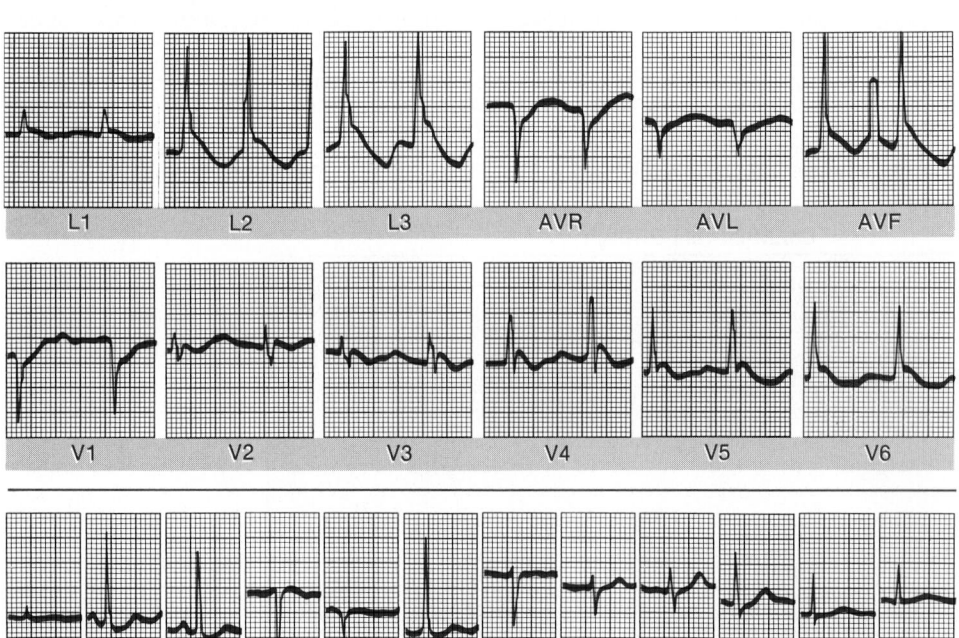

FIGURE 4–50. Osborne wave. Upper panel was recorded during hypothermia. The P-R interval is 0.28 sec; the QRS complex measures 0.10 sec and is followed by a wave (the Osborne wave) that merges with the ST segment: The T wave is inverted in leads I, II, III, aV$_f$, V$_5$, and V$_6$. It is difficult to separate the Osborne wave from the initial part of the ST segment. Bottom panel was recorded after the temperature returned to normal. The tracing is normal. The prolongation and increase in QRS amplitude noted during hypothermia, although within normal limits, are evident when compared with the normal ECG.

larization can be recorded in a single cell suggests that the mechanism is probably related to transmembrane ionic fluxes. Alternans of a human atrial monophasic action potential adds further credence to the primary role of transmembrane ionic events.[52]

THE OSBORNE WAVE. An Osborne wave, seen in hypothermia, is a deflection inscribed between the QRS complex and the beginning of the ST segment (Fig. 4–50).[154] It has been variously suggested that this wave reflects delay of depolarization, a current of injury, or early repolarization. In the left ventricular leads the polarity of the wave is positive and its amplitude is inversely related to body temperature. The electrophysiological mechanism of the Osborne wave remains unclear.

Abnormal ECG in Absence of Clinical Heart Disease

Abnormal ECGs may be recorded in patients with clinically normal hearts.[155,156] The abnormalities may be those of the QRS, ST segment, or T wave. Common abnormalities of the QRS include QS complexes in lead aV_l or QS or QR complexes in leads III and aV_f, a QS complex in leads V_1 and V_2, a tall R wave in leads V_1 and V_2, and high voltage of the R wave over the left ventricle. A frequent "normal" alteration of the ST segment is an elevation, the so-called early repolarization, which may be recorded in the inferior, left precordial, and rarely right precordial leads. Abnormal T waves include persistence of juvenile T-wave inversion over the right precordium (Fig. 4–45), isolated midprecordial T-wave inversion, and terminal T-wave inversion associated with ST-segment elevation due to early repolarization and right precordial T-wave inversion in middle-aged women. A variety of physiological influences alter the T wave of a normal heart (Table 4–4).

An abnormal ECG in the absence of clinical evidence of heart disease in the young should be evaluated carefully, because the prevalence of true heart disease in this setting is low and the chances are high that the tracing is false positive for disease.

Limb lead reversal is a relatively common error of technique and may result in an erroneous diagnosis of arrhythmias, myocardial ischemia or infarction, fascicular blocks, and ventricular hypertrophy. Lead reversal should be suspected when the limb leads exhibit significant changes while the precordial leads are normal and unchanged. The most common form of lead reversal is that of the right and left arms with a resultant "mirror image" of lead I. Right arm and right leg and left arm and right leg reversal should be suspected when lead II and III are isoelectric.[157] Not infrequently the sequence of leads V_1, V_2, and V_3 is reversed, and the computer will inevitably interpret the tracing as an anterior myocardial infarction (Fig. 4–AE25, p. 150). Such lead reversal is easily detected by analysis of the P wave. The inverted or biphasic P wave will identify lead V_1. However, when there is doubt, the cardiogram should be repeated.

The ECG and Electrolyte Abnormalities

HYPERKALEMIA. There is a good correlation between plasma K and the surface ECG in experimental hyperkalemia. The earliest ECG change, at a plasma level of about 5.7 mEq/liter, is a tall, peaked, most often symmetrical T wave with a narrow base and a normal or decreased $Q-T_c$ interval. The QRS complex widens uniformly at a level of 9 to 11 mEq/liter and an occasional acute current of injury resembling myocardial infarction may be present. Reduction in P-wave amplitude, intraatrial conduction delay, and P-R interval prolongation are recorded at a plasma level of about 7.0 mEq/liter. At plasma K levels of about 8.4 mEq/liter or higher, the P wave is no longer recognizable. When the plasma concentration exceeds 12 mEq/liter, either ventricular fibrillation or arrest follows. SA node fibers, being more resistant to the depressive action of K than is atrial

myocardium, continue to generate impulses that are now delayed in their exit or may fail to propagate because of depressed intraatrial conduction. The result may be Wenckebach (type I) or Mobitz (type II) sinoatrial (SA) block (see p. 687). Junctional escape and junctional rhythm are relatively common in experimental hyperkalemia.

In clinical hyperkalemia, abnormalities of impulse information and conduction appear at K levels lower than those observed in the experimental animal, and the correlation between plasma K and the ECG is less reliable. A tall, peaked, symmetrical T wave with a narrow base, the so-called "tented" T wave, is the earliest ECG abnormality, usually best seen in leads II, III, V_2, V_3, and V_4. The pointed, symmetrical appearance and narrow base of the T wave help to differentiate the effect of hyperkalemia from other causes of tall T waves, including normal variants. The tented appearance and the narrow base are probably more characteristic of hyperkalemia than is the amplitude of the T wave. A decrease in amplitude of the R wave, appearance of a prominent S wave, widening of the QRS complex, depression of the ST segment, and an occasional elevation of the ST segment evolve as plasma K continues to rise and approaches 8 to 9 mEq/liter (Fig. 4–51). A decrease in amplitude and prolongation of the P wave and lengthening of the P-R interval followed by disappearance of the P wave often make recognition of arrhythmias in hyperkalemia difficult, if not impossible. At times hyperkalemia induces a current of injury called *dialyzable current of injury,* which may be mistaken for acute ischemia (Fig. 4–45).

With hyperkalemia, depression of intraventricular conduction is characteristically diffuse and fairly uniform and results in prolongation of both the initial and terminal parts of the QRS complex. The resulting pattern may resemble RBBB, LBBB, left anterior or posterior divisional block, or a combination of the four. When the ECG resembles RBBB, the initial phase of the QRS complex is prolonged, in contrast to the conventional RBBB, in which only the terminal portion of the QRS complex is delayed

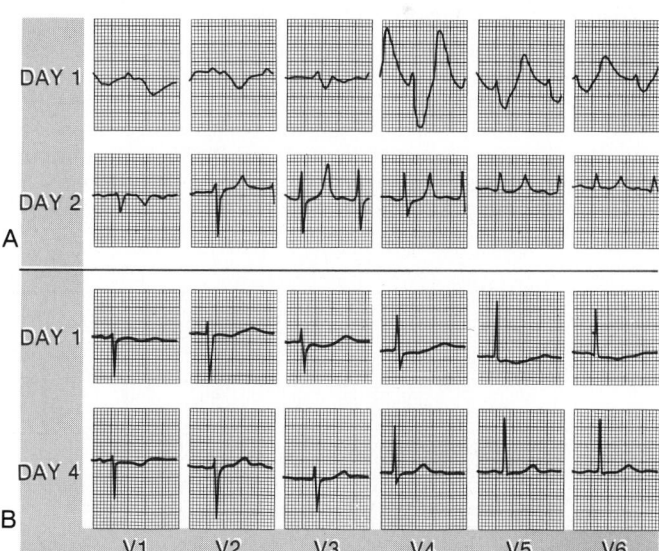

FIGURE 4–51. ECG changes in hyperkalemia *(A)* and hypokalemia *(B)*. Panel *A*, On day 1, at a K⁺ level of 8.6 mEq/liter, the P wave is no longer recognizable and the QRS complex is diffusely prolonged. Initial and terminal QRS delay is characteristic of K⁺-induced intraventricular conduction and is best illustrated in leads V_2 and V_6. On day 2, at a K⁺ level of 5.8 mEq/liter, the P wave is recognizable with a P-R interval of 0.24 sec, the duration of the QRS complex is approximately 0.10 sec, and the T waves are characteristically "tented." Panel *B*, On day 1, at a K⁺ level of 1.5 mEq/liter, the T and U waves are merged. The U wave is prominent and the Q-U interval prolonged. On day 4, at a K⁺ level of 3.7 mEq/liter, the tracing is normal.

(Fig. 4–AE26, p. 150). Similarly, when the ECG simulates LBBB, an S wave indicates slowing of the terminal portion of the QRS (Fig. 4–51). In conventional LBBB, on the other hand, prolongation involves only the initial component of the QRS complex.

In humans, as in animals, SA block (see p. 687), either Wenckebach (type I) or Mobitz (type II), passive or accelerated junctional or ventricular escape rhythms may be present. Potassium may normalize physiologically or functionally inverted T waves, but as a rule it has no effect on T-wave inversion due to organic disorders or drugs.

HYPOKALEMIA. The ECG in *hypokalemia* is characterized by gradual depression of the ST segment, decrease of T-wave amplitude, occasionally inversion of the T wave, and a prominent U wave but without a significant change in the Q-T interval (Figs. 4–51 and 4–AE27, p. 151). In advanced hypokalemia the ST segment gradually fuses with the U wave, the latter greater in amplitude than the T wave. An increase in amplitude of the QRS complex may be present. There is reasonable correlation between ECG changes and K concentrations below 2.3 or 3.0 mEq/liter. Prominent U waves with ST-segment and T-wave changes are not specific for hypokalemia, however. Such abnormalities can be the result of administration of digitalis and other drugs, ventricular hypertrophy, and bradycardia.

CALCIUM. The effects of Ca on the ECG were recognized in 1922.[158] In general, the ECG changes due to alteration in Ca concentrations correlate with the effect of Ca ions on the transmembrane action potential. Changes in duration of phase 2 parallel the altered duration of the ST segment and the Q-T interval.

Hypocalcemia prolongs phase 2, reflected by prolongation of the ST segment and Q-T interval (Figs. 4–52 and 4–AE29). The Q-aT (Q to the apex of the T wave) and the Q-T intervals are prolonged, but the Q-T$_c$ interval rarely exceeds 140 per cent of the normal. If longer, the U wave is likely to be included in the measurement. Hypocalcemia does not affect phase 3 of the action potential or the T wave. Hypocalcemia with hyperkalemia, most often seen in patients with chronic renal disease, results in a prolonged ST segment and a "tented" T wave. Hypocalcemia and hypokalemia exhibit a prolonged ST segment and a prominent terminal wave that includes both T and U waves.

Hypercalcemia shortens phase 2 of the action potential and the ST segment. The Q-T interval is shortened (Fig. 4–AE28, p. 151), the ST segment occasionally depressed, and the T wave inverted (Fig. 4–52).[159,160] A prominent J wave similar to that of hypothermia has been observed.

The correlation between the Q-T interval and serum Ca

concentration is unpredictable, largely because the Q-T duration is affected by factors other than calcium levels, such as age, sex, heart rate, myocardial disease, drugs, and other electrolytes. It has been suggested that when factors known to alter the Q-T interval are eliminated, a reasonably good correlation is found between the ECG and calcium levels. This assumption is supported by the fact that Ca levels in pure hypocalcemia induced by EDTA show a reasonably good correlation with the Q-T interval. Of the three intervals—Q-T, Q-oT (Q to the onset of the T wave), and Q-aT (Q to the apex of the T wave)—the Q-aT interval can be measured with greatest accuracy and correlates best with the Ca level.

MAGNESIUM. Administration of magnesium may result in shortening of the Q-T interval and prolongation of the P-R interval, QRS complex, and intraatrial conduction. As a rule, however, abnormalities of the ST segment due to hypermagnesemia cannot be identified on the ECG because the changes are dominated by calcium.[161] Hypomagnesemia cannot be recognized on the ECG.

Effects of Drugs on the ECG

The effect of antiarrhythmic drugs on the ECG is considered in Chapter 21.

Digitalis
(See p. 664)

Alterations of the ST segment and the T wave are the earliest recognizable changes due to the digitalis glycosides. The T wave amplitude is lowered, and the ST segment is depressed and shortened, with occasional appearance of a prominent U wave.[162] While the "characteristic" digitalis-induced ST segment is described as sagging, it is often difficult if not impossible to differentiate it from ST-segment depresseion of other causes. When the ST segment is also shortened, digitalis is the likely cause of the depression. ST-segment displacement due to digitalis may be greatly exaggerated by myocardial disease, tachycardia, and high-amplitude QRS complexes. Rarely, digitalis causes symmetrical inversion of the T wave similar to that in pericarditis and ischemia, but there is usually associated shortening of the Q-T interval. A peaked, "tented" T wave, probably due to concomitant hyperkalemia, also can be present. Digitalis has no significant effect on depolarization of the atrium or ventricle. Consequently, prolongation of intraatrial and intraventricular conduction is rare.

DIGITALIS-INDUCED ARRHYTHMIAS. Digitalis has been known to induce nearly every known arrhythmia.[163,164]

1. Ectopic rhythms due to enhanced automaticity, reentry, or delayed diastolic afterdepolarizations: atrial tachycardia with block (Fig. 22-17, p. 657), atrial fibrillation and flutter, nonparoxysmal junctional tachycardia, ventricular premature contractions, ventricular tachycardia, ventricular flutter and fibrillation, multiple ectopic rhythms (Figs. 4–AE29 and AE30, p. 151), bidirectional ventricular tachycardia, or accelerated escape.
2. Depression of pacemaker: SA node arrest.
3. Depression of conduction: SA block, AV block, exit block, or reciprocation.
4. AV dissociation: Suppression of the dominant pacemaker with passive escape of the lower junctional focus or inappropriate acceleration of a subsidiary pacemaker, or, rarely, dissociation within the AV function (double junctional tachycardia).

Arrhythmias identical to those due to digitalis toxicity also can be caused by heart disease, drugs other than digitalis, and a variety of extracardiac factors.

THERAPEUTIC AND TOXIC EFFECTS (See p. 484). Appearance of ectopic rhythms in the course of digitalis administration is nearly always a sign of toxicity. On the other hand, depression of AV conduction may at times be a desirable therapeutic endpoint. Acknowledging that some degree of overlap is unavoidable and that the clinical significance of an arrhythmia may differ depending on the setting, the effects of digitalis on the ECG can be divided into three general groups—therapeutic, excessive and/or toxic, and unequivocally toxic.

The wide spectrum of arrhythmias induced by digitalis and the coexistence of a number of different arrhythmias in the same tracing can be explained by the interplay between digitalis and myocardial and extracardiac factors on the electrophysiological properties of cardiac tissues. The drug may have different effects on the same specialized tissue; i.e., it may depress conduction or enhance automaticity, or both. Also, digitalis may act directly on the specialized tissue or its action may be mediated through the sympathetic or parasympathetic system or both. In addition, the sensitivity of the tissues to digitalis may be altered by factors such as a changing

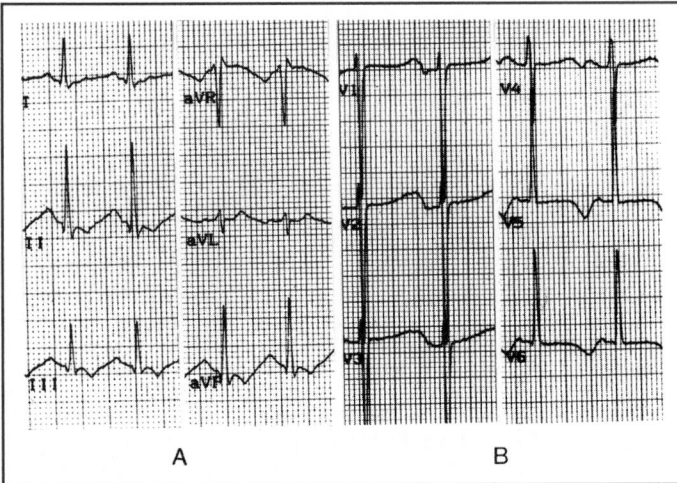

FIGURE 4–52. *A,* Hypercalcemia with a short Q-T interval (0.22 sec) and inverted T waves, the latter a rare manifestation of hypercalcemia. *B,* Hypocalcemia with a prolonged Q-T interval.

acid-balance, plasma and intracellular electrolyte levels, oxygen tension, and mechanical stretch.

The arrhythmias most commonly caused by digitalis include atrial tachycardia with block, nonparoxysmal junctional tachycardia, ventricular tachyarrhythmias, AV dissociation, and AV conduction delay (see Ch.22).

ACCELERATED JUNCTIONAL ESCAPE. This arrhythmia is seen in the same clinical conditions as is nonparoxysmal junctional tachycardia, and its clinical significance is probably the same. Accelerated junctional escape follows the rules set for cardiac arrhythmias induced by delayed afterdepolarization and may be the clinical counterpart of the arrhythmias induced in the Purkinje fiber and the intact animal.

REFERENCES

1. Macfarlane, P. W., and Lawrie, V. T. D.: Comprehensive Electrocardiology. Vol. 1. New York, Pergamon Press, 1989.
2. Fye, W. B.: A history of the origin, evolution, and impact of electrocardiography. Am. J. Cardiol. 73:937, 1994.
3. Horan, I. G.: Manifest orientation: The theoretical link between the anatomy of the heart and the clinical electrocardiogram. J. Am. Coll. Cardiol. 9:1049, 1987.
4. Burch, G. E., and DePasquale, N. P.: A History of Electrocardiography. Chicago, Year Book Medical Publishers, 1964.
5. Fisch, C.: Evolution of the clinical electrocardiogram. J. Am. Coll. Cardiol. 14:1127, 1989.
6. Waller, A. D.: A demonstration on man of electromotive changes accompanying the heart's beat. J. Physiol. 8:229, 1887.
7. Einthoven, W.: Selected Papers on Electrocardiography. Snellen, A. (ed.). Leiden, University Press. 1977.
8. Lewis, T.: The Mechanism and Graphic Registration of the Heart Beat. London, Shaw and Sons, Ltd., 1920, p. 228.
9. Wilson, F. N.: Selected Papers of FD Johnston. Lepeschkin, F. D. E. (ed.). Ann Arbor, Edward Brothers, Inc., 1954.
10. Durrer, D.: Selected Papers. Meijler, F. L., and Burchell, H. B. (eds.). Amsterdam, North Holland Publishing Co., 1986.
11. Fisch, C.: Electrocardiography of Arrhythmias. Philadelphia, Lea and Febiger, 1989.
12. Fye, W. B.: Disorders of the Heartbeat: A historical overview from antiquity to mid-20th century. Am. J. Cardiol. 72:1055, 1993.

THE NORMAL ELECTROCARDIOGRAM

13. Craib, W. H.: A study of the electrical field surrounding active heart muscle. Heart 14:71, 1927.
14. Wilson, F. N., MacLeod, A. G., and Barker, P. S.: The distribution of the action currents produced by the heart muscle and other excitable tissues immersed in extensive conducting media. J. Gen. Physiol. 16:423, 1933.
15. Durrer, D., VanDam, R. T., Freud, G. E., et al.: Total excitation of the isolated human heart. Circulation 41:899, 1970.
16. Wilson, F. N., MacLeod, A. G., Barker, P. S., and Johnston, F. D.: The determination and the significance of the areas of the ventricular deflections of the electrocardiogram. Am. Heart J. 10:46, 1934.
17. Wilson, F. N., Johnston, F. D., Rosenbaum, F. F., et al.: The precordial electrocardiogram. Am. Heart J. 27:19, 1944.
18. Andersen, H. R., Nielsen, D., and Hansen, I. G.: The normal right chest electrocardiogram. J. Electrocardiol. 20:27, 1987.
19. Selvester, R. H., Velasquez, D. W., Elko, P. P., and Cady, L. D.: Intraventricular conduction defect (IVCD), real or fancied, QRS duration in 1,254 normal adult white males by a multi-lead automated algorithm. J. Electrocardiol. 23:118, 1990.
20. Burger, H. C., and Van Millaan, J. B.: Heart—Vector and leads. Br. Heart J. 9:154, 1947.
21. Willems, J. L., Robles de Medina, E., Bernard, R., et al.: WHO task force on criteria for intraventricular conduction disturbances and pre-excitation. J. Am. Coll. Cardiol. 5:1261, 1985.
21a. McLaughlin, N. B., Campbell, R. W. F., Murray, D.: Comparison of automatic QT measurement techniques in the normal 12 lead electrocardiogram. Br. Heart J. 74:85, 1995.
22. Bazett, H. C.: An analysis of the time-relations of electrocardiograms. Heart 7:353, 1920.
23. Sagie, A., Larson, M. G., Goldberg, R. J., et al.: An improved method for adjusting the QT interval for heart rate (the Framingham Heart Study). Am. J. Cardiol. 70:797, 1992.
24. Karjalainen, J., Viitasalo, M., Manttari, M., and Manninen, V.: Relation between QT intervals and heart rates from 40 to 120 beats/min in rest electrocardiograms of men and a simple method to adjust QT interval values. J. Am. Coll. Cardiol. 23:1547, 1994.
25. Schweitzer, P.: The values and limitations of the QT interval in clinical practice. Am. Heart J. 124:1121, 1992.
26. Mann, H.: A method of analyzing the electrocardiogram. Arch. Intern. Med. 25:283, 1920.
27. Frank, E.: An accurate, clinically practical system for spatial vectorcardiography. Circulation 13:737, 1956.

28. Kaplan, J. D., Evans, G. T., Foster, E., et al.: Evaluation of electrocardiographic criteria for right atrial enlargement by quantitative two-dimensional echocardiography. J. Am. Coll. Cardiol. 23:747, 1994.
29. Chou, T. C., and Helm, R. A.: The pseudo P pulmonale. Circulation 32:96, 1965.
30. Medrano, G. A., De Micheli, A., and Osornio, S.: Interatrial conduction and STa in experimental atrial damage. J. Electrocardiol. 20:357, 1987.
31. Munuswamy, K., Alpert, M. A., Martin, R. H., et al.: Sensitivity and specificity of commonly used electrocardiographic criteria for left atrial enlargement determined by M-mode echocardiography. Am. J. Cardiol. 53:829, 1984.
32. Nagahama, Y., Sugiura, T., Takehana, K., et al.: Clinical significance of PQ segment depression in acute Q wave anterior wall myocardial infarction. J. Am. Coll. Cardiol. 23:885, 1994.
33. Surawicz, B.: Electrocardiographic diagnosis of chamber enlargement. J. Am. Coll. Cardiol. 8:714, 1986.
34. Sokolow, M., and Lyon, T. P.: The ventricular complex in left ventricular hypertrophy as obtained by unipolar precordial and limb leads. Am. Heart J. 37:161, 1949.
35. Schillaci, G., Verdecchia, P., Borgioni, C., et al.: Improved electrocardiographic diagnosis of left ventricular hypertrophy. Am. J. Cardiol. 74:714, 1994.
36. Huwez, F. U., Pringle, S. D., and Macfarlane, P. W.: Variable patterns of ST-T abnormalities in patients with left ventricular hypertrophy and normal coronary arteries. Br. Heart J. 67:304, 1992.
37. Levy, D., Labib, S. B., Anderson, K. M., et al.: Determinants of sensitivity and specificity of electrocardiographic criteria for left ventricular hypertrophy. Circulation 81:815, 1990.
38. Cabrera, E., and Gaxiola, A.: A critical reevaluation of systolic and diastolic overloading patterns. Prog. Cardiovasc. Dis. 2:219, 1959.
39. Goldberger, A. L.: Myocardial Infarction. 3rd ed. St. Louis, C. V. Mosby Co., 1984.
40. Sreeram, N., Cheriex, E., Smeets, J. L. R. M., et al.: Value of the 12-lead electrocardiogram at hospital admission in the diagnosis of pulmonary embolism. Am. J. Cardiol. 73:298, 1994.
41. Shah, N. S., Velury, S., Mascarenhas, D., and Spodick, D. H.: Electrocardiographic features of restrictive pulmonary disease, and comparison with those of obstructive pulmonary disease. Am. J. Cardiol. 70:394, 1992.
42. Delise, P., Piccolo, E., O'Este, D., et al.: Electrogenesis of the S1S2S3 electrocardiographic pattern. J. Electrocardiol. 23:23, 1990.
43. Xiao, H. B., Brecker, S. J. D., and Gibson, D. G.: Relative effects of left ventricular mass and conduction disturbance on activation in patients with pathological left ventricular hypertrophy. Br. Heart J. 71:548, 1994.
44. Gertsch, M., Theier, A., and Foglia, E.: Electrocardiographic detection of left ventricular hypertrophy in the presence of left anterior fascicular block. Am. J. Cardiol. 61:1098, 1988.
45. Flowers, N. C.: Left bundle branch block: A continuously evolving concept. J. Am. Coll. Cardiol. 9:684, 1987.
46. Brugada, P., and Brugada, J.: Right bundle branch block, persistent ST segment elevation and sudden cardiac death: A distinct clinical and electrocardiographic syndrome. Am. Coll. Cardiol. 20:1391, 1992.
47. Bjerregaard, P., Gussak, I., Kotar, S. L., et al.: Recurrent syncope in a patient with prominent J wave. Am. Heart J. 127:1426, 1994.
48. Watt, T. B., Jr., Freud, G. E., Durrer, D., and Pruitt, R. D.: Left anterior arborization block combined with right bundle branch block in canine and primate hearts. An electrocardiographic study. Circ. Res. 22:57, 1968.
49. Rosenbaum, M. B., Elizari, M. V., and Lazzari, J. O.: The Hemiblocks: New Concepts of Intraventricular Conduction Based on Human Anatomical Physiological, and Clinical Studies. Oldsmar, FL, Tampa Tracings, 1970.
50. Angelini, P., Springer, A., Sulbaran, T., and Livesay, W. R.: Right ventricular myopathy with an unusual intraventricular conduction defect (Epsilon potential). Am. Heart J. 101:680, 1981.
51. Garcia-Moll, X. G., Guindo, J., Vinolas, X., et al.: Intermittent masked bifascicular block. Am. Heart J. 127:214, 1994.
52. Surawicz, B., and Fisch, C.: Cardiac alternans: Diverse mechanisms and clinical manifestations. J. Am. Coll. Cardiol. 120:483, 1992.
53. Lewis, T.: Observations upon disorders of the heart's action. Heart 3:279, 1912.
54. Gouaux, J. L., and Ashman, R.: Auricular fibrillation with aberration simulating ventricular paroxysmal tachycardia. Am. Heart J. 34:366, 1947.
55. Lewis, T.: Certain physical signs of myocardial involvement. Br. Med. J. 1:484, 1913.
56. Katz, A., and Pick, A.: The transseptal conduction time in the human heart. Circulation 27:1061, 1963.
57. Fisch, C., and Knoebel, S. B.: Vagaries of acceleration dependent aberration. Br. Heart J. 67:16, 1992.
58. Moore, E. N., Spear, J. F., and Fisch, C.: "Supernormal" conduction and excitability. J. Cardiovasc. Electrophysiol. 4:320, 1993.
59. Oreto, G., Smeets, J. L. R. M., Rodriguez, L. M., et al.: Supernormal conduction in the left bundle branch. J. Cardiovasc. Electrophysiol. 5:345, 1994.
60. Dressler, W.: Transient bundle branch block occurring during slowing of the heart beat and following gagging. Am. Heart J. 58:750, 1959.
61. Wolff, L., Parkinson, J., and White, P. D.: Bundle branch block with

short P-R interval in healthy young people prone to paroxysmal tachycardia. Am. Heart J. *5*:685, 1930.

62. Wilson, F. N.: A case in which the vagus influenced the form of the ventricular complex of the electrocardiogram. Arch. Intern. Med. *16*:1008, 1915.

63. Cohn, A. E., and Fraser, F. R.: Paroxysmal tachycardia and the effect of stimulation of the vagus nerves by pressure. Heart *5*:93, 1913.

64. Holzmann, N., and Scherf, D.: Ueber Elekrokardiogramme mit ver kuerzter Vornot-Kammer-Distanz und positiven P. Zacken Z Klin Med *121*:404, 1932.

65. Rosenbaum, F. F., Hecht, H. H., Wilson, F. N., and Johnston, F. D.: The potential variations of the thorax and the esophagus in anomalous atrioventricular excitation (Wolff-Parkinson-White syndrome). Am. Heart J. *29*:281, 1945.

66. Yuan, S., Iwa, T., Bando, T., and Bando, H.: Comparative study of eight sets of ECG criteria for the localization of the accessory pathway in Wolff-Parkinson-White syndrome. J. Electrocardiol. *25*:203, 1992.

67. Pardee, H. E. B.: An electrocardiographic sign of coronary artery obstruction. Arch. Intern. Med. *26*:244, 1920.

68. Samson, W. E., and Scher, A. N.: Mechanism of ST segment alteration during myocardial injury. Circ. Res. *8*:780, 1960.

69. Vincent, G. M., Abildskov, J. A., and Burgess, M. J.: Mechanisms of ischemic ST-segment displacement. Evaluation by direct current recordings. Circulation *56*:559, 1977.

70. Sharkey, S. W., Berger, C. R., Brunette, D. D., and Henry, T. D.: Impact of the electrocardiogram on the delivery of thrombolytic therapy for acute myocardial infarction. Am. J. Cardiol. *73*:550, 1994.

70a. Raitt, M. H., Maynard, C., Wagner, G. S., et al.: Appearance of abnormal Q waves early in the course of acute myocardial infarction: Implications for efficacy of thrombolytic therapy. J. Am. Coll. Cardiol. *25*:1084, 1995.

71. Madias, J. E.: The "Giant R Waves" ECG pattern of hyperacute phase of myocardial infarction. J. Electrocardiol. *26*:77, 1993.

72. Barnhill, J. E., III, Tendera, M., Cade, H., et al.: Depolarization changes early in the course of myocardial infarction: Significance of changes in the terminal portion of the QRS complex. J. Am. Coll. Cardiol. *14*:143, 1989.

73. Strasberg, B., Pinchas, A., Barbash, G. L., et al.: Importance of reciprocal ST segment depression in leads V5 and V6 as an indicator of disease of the left anterior descending coronary artery in acute inferior wall myocardial infarction. Br. Heart J. *63*:339, 1990.

74. Kracoff, O. S., Adelman, A. G., Marquis, J. F., et al.: Twelve-lead electrocardiogram recording during percutaneous transluminal coronary angioplasty. J. Electrocardiol. *23*:191, 1990.

75. Stevenson, R. N., Ranjadayalan, K., Umachandran, V., and Timmis, A. D.: Significance of reciprocal ST depression in acute myocardial infarction: A study of 258 patients treated by thrombolysis. Br. Heart J. *69*:211, 1993.

76. Sato, H., Kodama, K., Masuvama, T., et al.: Right coronary artery occlusion: Its role in the mechanism of precordial ST segment depression. J. Am. Coll. Cardiol. *14*:297, 1989.

77. Norell, M. S., Lyons, J. P., Gardener, J. E., et al.: Significance of "reciprocal" ST segment depression: Left ventriculographic observations during left anterior descending coronary angioplasty. J. Am. Coll. Cardiol. *13*:1270, 1989.

78. Edmunds, J. J., Gibbons, R. J., Bresnahan, J. F., and Clements, I. P.: Significance of anterior ST depression in inferior wall acute myocardial infarction. Am. J. Cardiol. *73*:143, 1994.

79. Kracoff, O. H., Adelman, A. G., Oettinger, M., et al.: Reciprocal changes as the presenting electrocardiographic manifestation of acute myocardial ischemia. Am. J. Cardiol. *71*:1359, 1993.

80. Birnbaum, Y., Solodky, A., Herz, I., et al.: Implications of inferior ST-segment depression in anterior acute myocardial infarction: Electrocardiographic and angiographic correlation. Am. Heart J. *127*:1467, 1994.

80a. Chikamori, T., Takata, J., Furuno, T., et al.: Usefulness of U wave analysis in detecting significant narrowing limited to a single coronary artery. Am. J. Cardiol. *75*:508, 1995.

81. Jain, A., Jenkins, M. G., and Gettes, L. S.: Lack of specificity of new negative U waves for anterior myocardial ischemia as evidenced by intracoronary electrogram during balloon angioplasty. J. Am. Coll. Cardiol. *15*:1007, 1990.

82. Gurick, A., Oral, D., Pamir, G., and Akyol, T.: Significance of resting U wave polarity in patients with atherosclerotic heart disease. J. Electrocardiol. *27*:157, 1994.

83. Kanemoto, N., Imaoka, C., and Suzuki, Y.: Significance of U wave polarities in previous anterior myocardial infarction. J. Electrocardiol. *24*:169, 1991.

84. Oliva, P. B., Hammill, S. C., and Talano, J. V.: T wave changes consistent with epicardial involvement in acute myocardial infarction. J. Am. Cardiol. *24*:1073, 1994.

85. Bergovec, M., Prpic, H., Zigman, M., et al.: Regression of ECG signs of myocardial infarction related to infarct size and left ventricular function. J. Electrocardiol. *26*:1, 1993.

86. Horan, L. G., Flowers, N. C., and Johnson, J. C.: Significance of the diagnostic Q wave of myocardial infarction. Circulation *43*:428, 1971.

86a. Parker, A. B. III, Waller, B. F., and Gering, L. E.: Usefulness of the 12-lead electrocardiogram in detection of myocardial infarction: Electrocardiographic-anatomic correlations—Part I. Clin. Cardiol. *19*:55, 1996.

87. Rosenbaum, M. B., Girotti, L. A., Lazzari, J. O., et al.: Abnormal Q

waves in right sided chest leads provoked by onset of right bundle branch block in patients with anteroseptal infarction. Br. Heart J. *47*:227, 1982.

88. Hands, M. E., Cook, E. F., Stone, P. H., et al.: Electrocardiographic diagnosis of myocardial infarction in the presence of complete bundle branch block. Am. Heart J. *116*:23, 1988.

89. Cannon, A., Freedman, S. B., Bailey, B. P., and Bernstein, L.: ST-segment changes during transmural myocardial ischemia in chronic left bundle branch block. Am. J. Cardiol. *64*:1216, 1989.

90. Oreto, G., Saporito, F., Donato, G., et al.: The "Inverse" R wave progression in inferior leads in the presence of left anterior hemiblock: A clinical study. J. Electrocardiol. *24*:277, 1991.

91. First, S. R., Bayley, R. H., and Bedford, D. R.: Peri-infarction block electrocardiographic abnormality occasionally resembling bundle branch block and local ventricular block of other types. Circulation *2*:31, 1950.

92. Grant, R. P.: Peri-infarction block. Prog. Cardiovasc. Dis. *2*:237, 1959.

93. Babbitt, D. G., Binkley, P. F., and Schaal, S. F.: Clinical significance of terminal QRS abnormalities in the setting of inferior myocardial infarction. J. Electrocardiol. *24*:85, 1991.

94. Flowers, N. C., Horan, L. G., Wyids, A. C., et al.: Relation of peri-infarction block to ventricular late potentials in patients with inferior wall myocardial infarction. Am. J. Cardiol. *66*:568, 1990.

95. Barnhill, J. E., Tendera, M., Cade, H., et al.: Depolarization changes early in the course of myocardial infarction: Significance of changes in the terminal portion of the QRS complex. J. Am. Coll. Cardiol. *14*:143, 1989.

96. Varriale, P., and Chryssos, B. E.: The RSR' complex not related to right bundle branch block: Diagnostic value as a sign of myocardial infarction scar. Am. Heart J. *123*:369, 1992.

97. Blanke, H., Cohen, M., Schlueter, G. V., et al.: Electrocardiographic and coronary arteriographic correlations during acute myocardial infarction. Am. J. Cardiol. *54*:249, 1984.

98. Hiasa, Y., Morimoto, S., Wada, T., et al.: Differentiation between left circumflex and right coronary artery occlusions: Studies on ST-segment deviation during percutaneous transluminal coronary angioplasty. Clin. Cardiol. *13*:783, 1990.

99. Shen, W. F., Tribouilloy, C., and Lesbre, J. P.: Relationship between electrocardiographic patterns and angiographic features in isolated left circumflex coronary artery disease. Clin. Cardiol. *14*:720, 1991.

100. de Zwaan, C., Bar, F. W., Janssen, J. J. A., et al.: Angiographic and clinical characteristics of patients with unstable angina showing an ECG pattern indicating critical narrowing of the proximal LAD coronary artery. Am. Heart J. *117*:557, 1989.

101. Braat, S. H., Brugada, P., Dulk, K., et al.: Value of lead V4R for recognition of the infarct coronary artery in acute inferior myocardial infarction. Am. J. Cardiol. *53*:1538, 1984.

101a. Shalev, Y., Fogelman, R., Oettinger, M., et al.: Does the electrocardiographic pattern of "anteroseptal" myocardial infarction correlate with anatomic location of myocardial surgery? Am. J. Cardiol. *75*:763, 1995.

102. Baer, M. F., Theissen, P., and Voth, E.: Morphologic correlate of pathologic Q waves as assessed by gradient-echo magnetic resonance imaging. Am. J. Cardiol. *74*:430, 1994.

103. Antaloczy, Z., Barcsak, J., and Magyar, E.: Correlation of electrocardiologic and pathologic findings in 100 cases of Q wave and non-Q wave myocardial infarction. J. Electrocardiol. *21*:331, 1988.

104. Boden, W. E., Gibson, R. S., Schechtman, K. B., et al.: ST segment shifts are poor predictors of subsequent Q wave evolution in acute myocardial infarction. Circulation *79*:537, 1989.

105. Tamura, A., Katooka, H., and Mikuriya, Y.: Electrocardiographic findings in a patient with pure septal infarction. Br. Heart J. *65*:166, 1991.

106. Iwasaki, K., Kusachi, S., Kita, T., and Taniguchi, G.: Prediction of isolated first diagonal branch occlusion by 12-lead electrocardiography: ST segment shift in leads I and aVL. J. Am. Coll. Cardiol. *23*:1557, 1994.

107. Kataoka, H., Kanzaki, K., and Mikuriva, Y.: Massive ST-segment elevation in precordial and inferior leads in right ventricular myocardial infarction. J. Electrocardiol. *21*:115, 1988.

108. Mak, K. H., Chia, B. L., Tan, A. T. H., and Johan, A.: Simultaneous ST segment elevation in lead V1 and depression in lead V2. A discordant ECG pattern indicating right ventricular infarction. J. Electrocardiol. *27*:203, 1994.

109. Andersen, H. R., Falk, E., and Nielsen, D.: Right ventricular infarction: Diagnostic accuracy of electrocardiographic right chest leads V3R to V7R investigated prospectively in 43 consecutive fatal cases from a coronary care unit. Br. Heart J. *62*:328, 1989.

110. Lopez-Sendon, J., Coma-Cannella, J., Alcasena, S., et al.: Electrocardiographic findings in acute right ventricular infarction: Sensitivity and specificity of electrocardiographic alterations in right precordial leads V_4R, V_3R, V_1, V_2 and V_3. J. Am. Coll. Cardiol. *8*:1273, 1985.

111. Zehender, M., Kasper, W., Kauder, E., et al.: Comparison of diagnostic accuracy, time dependency, and prognostic impact of abnormal Q waves, combined electrocardiographic criteria, and ST abnormalities in right ventricular infarction. Br. Heart J. *72*:119, 1994.

112. Kataoka, H., Tamura, A., Yano, S., and Kazaki, K.: Intraventricular conduction delay in acute right ventricular ischemia. Am. J. Cardiol. *64*:94, 1989.

113. Sclarovsky, S., Topaz, O., Rechavia, E., et al.: Ischemic ST segment depression in leads V_2–V_3 as the presenting electrocardiographic fea-

ture of posterolateral wall myocardial infarction. Am. Heart J. *113:*1085, 1987.

114. Bounous, E. P., Jr., Califf, R. M., Harrell, F. E., Jr., et al.: Prognostic value of the simplified Selvester QRS score in patients with coronary artery disease. J. Am. Coll. Cardiol. *11:*35, 1988.

115. Ascher, E. K., Stauffer, J. E., and Gaasch, W. H.: Coronary artery spasm, cardiac arrest, transient electrocardiographic Q waves and stunned myocardium in cocaine-associated acute myocardial infarction. Am. J. Cardiol. *61:*941, 939, 1988.

116. DePasquale, N. P., Burch, G. E., and Phillips, J. H.: Electrocardiograph alterations associated with electrically "silent" areas of myocardium. Am. Heart J. *68:*697, 1964.

117. Braunwald, E., and Kloner, R. A.: The stunned myocardium: Prolonged postischemic ventricular dysfunction. Circulation *66:*1146, 1982.

118. Hesse, A., Altland, K., Linke, R. P., et al.: Cardiac amyloidosis: A review and report of a new transthyretin (prealbumin) variant. Br. Heart J. *70:*111, 1993.

119. Yotsukura, M., Miyagawa, M., Tsuya, T., et al.: A 10-year follow-up study by orthogonal Frank lead ECG on patients with progressive muscular dystrophy of the Duchenne type. J. Electrocardiol. *25:*(4)345, 1992.

120. Lemery, R., Kleinebenne, A., Nihoyannopoulos, P., et al.: Q waves in hypertrophic cardiomyopathy in relation to the distribution and severity of right and left ventricular hypertrophy. J. Am. Coll. Cardiol. *16:*388, 1990.

121. Pelliccia, F., Clantrocca, C., Cristotani, R., et al.: Electrocardiographic findings in patients with hypertrophic cardiomyopathy. J. Electrocardiol. *23:*213, 1990.

122. Chakko, S., Sepulveda, S., Kessler, K. M., et al.: Frequency and type of electrocardiographic abnormalities in cocaine abusers. Am. J. Cardiol. *74:*710, 1994.

123. Walder, L. A., and Spodick, D. H.: Global T wave inversion: Long-term follow-up. J. Am. Coll. Cardiol. *21:*1652, 1993.

124. Usui, M., Inoue, H., Suzuki, J., et al.: Relationship between distribution of hypertrophy and electrocardiographic changes in hypertrophic cardiomyopathy. Am. Heart J. *126:*177, 1993.

125. Suzuki, J., Watanabe, F., Takenaka, K., et al.: New subtype of apical hypertrophic cardiomyopathy identified with nuclear magnetic resonance imaging as an underlying cause of markedly inverted T waves. J. Am. Coll. Cardiol. *22:*1175, 1993.

126. Lui, C. Y.: Acute pulmonary embolism as the cause of global T wave inversion and QT prolongation. J. Electrocardiol. *26:*91, 1993.

127. Trevethan, S., Castilla, R., Medrano, G., and Michelli, A.: Giant T waves simulating apical hypertrophic myocardiopathy that disappear with sodium nitroprusside administration. J. Electrocardiol. *24:*267, 1991.

128. Balzo, U., and Rosen, M. R.: T wave changes persisting after ventricular pacing in canine hearts are altered by 4-aminopyridine but not by lidocaine. Implications with respect to phenomenon of cardiac "memory." Circulation *85:*1464, 1992.

129. Wood, M. A., DiMarco, J. P., and Haines, D. E.: Electrocardiographic abnormalities after radiofrequency catheter ablation of accessory bypass tracts in the Wolff-Parkinson-White syndrome. Am. J. Cardiol. *70:*200, 1992.

130. Helguera, M. E., Pinski, S. L., Sterba, R., and Throman, R. G.: Memory T wave after radiofrequency catheter ablation of accessory atrioventricular connections in W-P-W syndrome. J. Electrocardiol. *27:*243, 1994.

131. White, P. D.: Alternation of the pulse: A common clinical condition. Am. J. Med. Sci. *150:*82, 1915.

132. Taussig, H. B.: Electrograms taken from isolated strips of mammalian ventricular cardiac muscle. Bull. Johns Hopkins Hosp. *43:*81, 1928.

133. Verrier, R. L., and Nearing, B. D.: Electrophysiologic basis for T wave alternans as an index of vulnerability to ventricular fibrillation. J. Cardiovasc. Electrophysiol. *5:*445, 1994.

134. Bardaji, A., Vidal, F., and Richart, C.: T wave alternans associated with amiodarone. J. Electrocardiol. *26:*155, 1993.

135. Tighe, D. A., Chung, E. K., and Park, C. H.: Electric alternans associated with acute pulmonary embolism. Am. Heart J. *128:*188, 1994.

136. Zareba, W., Moss, A. J., le Cessie, S., and Hall, W. J.: T wave alternans in idiopathic long QT syndrome. J. Am. Coll. Cardiol. *23:*1541, 1994.

137. Rosenbaum, D. S., Jackson, L. E., Smith, J. M., et al.: Electrical alternans

and vulnerability to ventricular arrhythmias. N. Engl. J. Med. *330:*235, 1994.

138. Malfatto, G., Beria, G., Sala, S., et al.: Quantitative analysis of T wave abnormalities and their prognostic implications in the idiopathic long QT syndrome. Am. J. Cardiol. *23:*296, 1994.

139. Friedberg, C. K., and Zager, A.: "Nonspecific" ST and T-wave changes. Circulation *23:*655, 1961.

140. Wilson, F. N., and Finch, R.: The effect of drinking iced-water upon the form of the T deflection of the electrocardiogram. Heart *10:*275, 1923.

141. Balady, G. J., Cadigan, J. B., and Ryan, T. J.: Electrocardiogram of the athlete: An analysis of 289 professional football players. Am. J. Cardiol. *53:*1339, 1984.

142. Nelson, S. D., Kou, W. H., Annesiey, T., et al.: Significance of ST segment depression during paroxysmal supraventricular tachycardia. J. Am. Coll. Cardiol. *12:*383, 1988.

143. Autenrieth, G., Surawicz, B., Kuo, C. S., and Arita, M.: Primary T wave abnormalities caused by uniform and regional shortening of ventricular monophasic action potential in the dog. Circulation *51:*568, 1975.

144. Miwa, K., Miyagi, Y., Fujita, M., et al.: Transient terminal U wave inversion as a more specific marker for myocardial ischemia. Am. Heart J. *125:*981, 1993.

145. Twidale, N., Gallagher, A. W., and Tonkin, A. M.: Echocardiographic study of U wave inversion in the electrocardiograms of hypertensive patients. J. Electrocardiol. *22:*365, 1989.

146. Kanemoto, N., Nakayama, K., Ide, M., and Goto, Y.: Giant negative U waves in a patient with uncontrolled hypertension and severe hypokalemia. J. Electrocardiol. *25:*163, 1992.

147. Garson, A., Jr., Dick, M., 2d, Fournier, A., et al.: The long QT syndrome in children. An international study of 287 patients. Circulation *87*(6):1866, 1993.

148. Ward, O. C.: New familial cardiac syndrome in children. JAMA *54:*103, 1964.

149. Vincent, G. M., Timothy, K. W., Leppert, M., and Keating, M.: The spectrum of symptoms and QT intervals in carriers of the gene for the long QT syndrome. N. Engl. J. Med. *327:*846, 1992.

150. Martin, A. B., Garson, A., Jr., and Perry, J. C.: Prolonged QT interval in hypertrophic and dilated cardiomyopathy in children. Am. Heart J. *127:*64, 1994.

151. Schwartz, P. J., Moss, A. J., Vincent, G. M., et al.: Diagnostic criteria for the long QT syndrome. An update. Circulation *88:*782, 1993.

152. Surawicz, B., and Knoebel, S. B.: Long QT, good, bad or indifferent? J. Am. Coll. Cardiol. *4:*138, 1983.

153. Lewis, T.: Notes upon alternation of the heart. Q. J. Med. *4:*141, 1910.

154. Osborn, J. J.: Experimental hypothermia. Respiratory and blood pH changes in relation to cardiac function. Am. J. Physiol. *175:*389, 1953.

155. Fisch, C.: Abnormal ECG in clinically normal individuals. JAMA *250:*1321, 1983.

156. Zehender, M., Meinertz, T., Kaui, J., et al.: ECG variants and cardiac arrhythmias in athletes: Clinical relevance and prognostic importance. Am. Heart J. *119:*1378, 1990.

157. Haisty, W. K., Pahlm, O., Edenbrandt, L., and Newman, K.: Recognition of electrocardiographic electrode misplacements involving the ground (right leg) electrode. Am. J. Cardiol. *71:*1490, 1993.

158. Carter, E. P., and Andrus, E. C.: Q-T interval in human electrocardiogram in absence of cardiac disease. JAMA *78:*1922, 1922.

159. Ahmed, R., Yano, K., Mitsuoka, T., et al.: Changes in T wave morphology during hypercalcemia and its relations to the severity of hypercalcemia. J. Electrocardiol. *22:*125, 1989.

160. Lind, L., and Ljunghall, S.: Serum calcium and the ECG in patients with primary hyperparathyroidism. J. Electrocardiol. *27:*99, 1994.

161. Mosseri, M., Porath, A., Ovsyshcher, I., and Stone, D.: Electrocardiographic manifestations of combined hypercalcemia in hypermagnesemia. J. Electrocardiol. *23:*235, 1990.

162. Cohn, A. E., Fraser, F. R., and Jamieson, A.: The influence of digitalis on the T wave of the human electrocardiogram. J. Exp. Med. *21:*593, 1915.

163. Fisch, C., Knoebel, S. B.: Digitalis cardiotoxicity. J. Am. Coll. Cardiol. *5:*91A, 1985.

164. Smith, T. W., Antman, E. M., Friedman, P. L., et al.: Digitalis glycosides: Mechanisms and manifestations of toxicity. Prog. Cardiovasc. Dis. *26:*413, 1984.

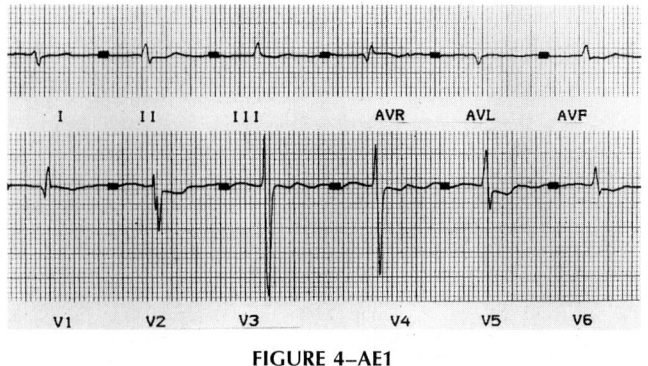

FIGURE 4–AE1

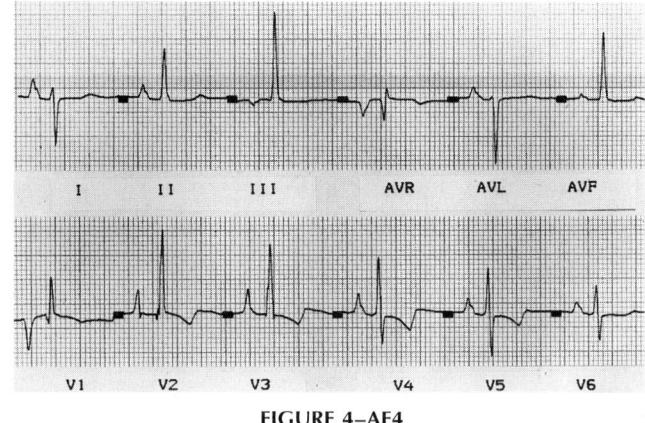

FIGURE 4–AE4

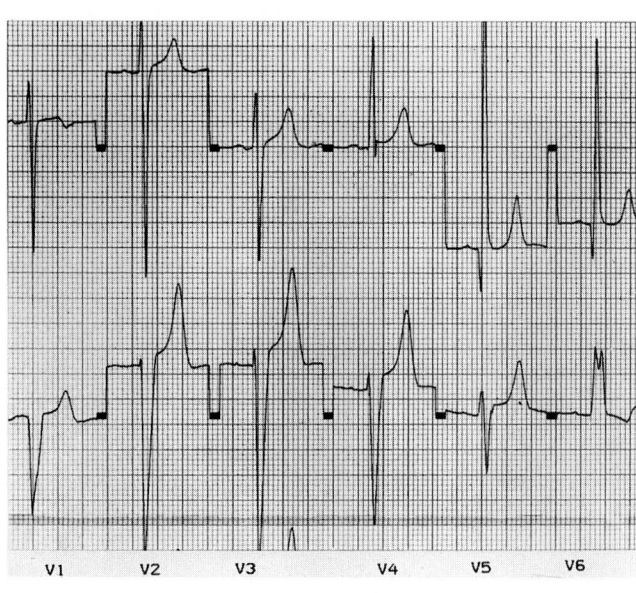

FIGURE 4–AE2

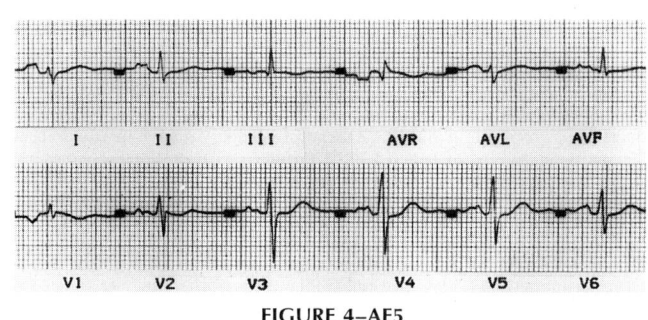

FIGURE 4–AE5

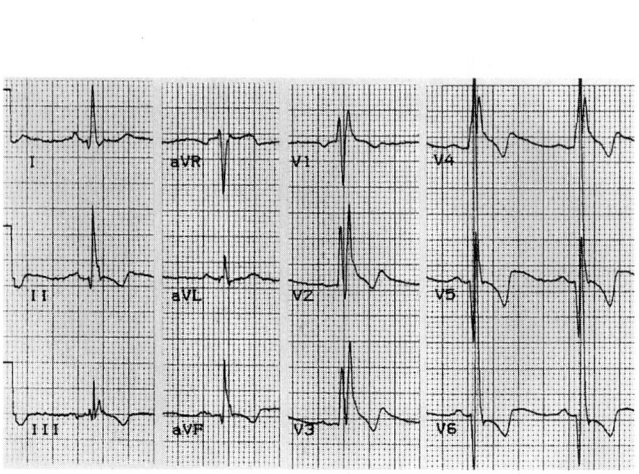

FIGURE 4–AE3

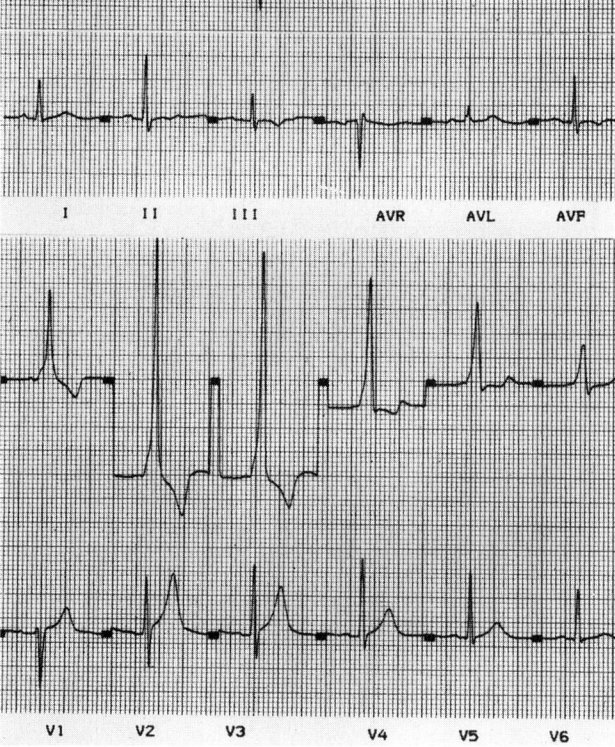

FIGURE 4–AE6

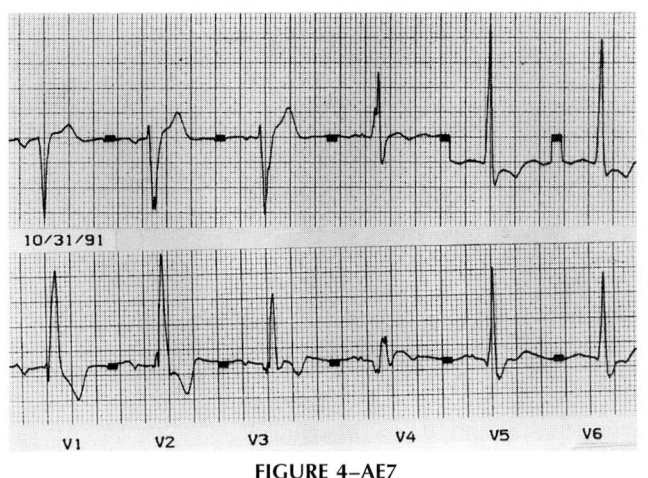

10/31/91

V1 V2 V3 V4 V5 V6

FIGURE 4–AE7

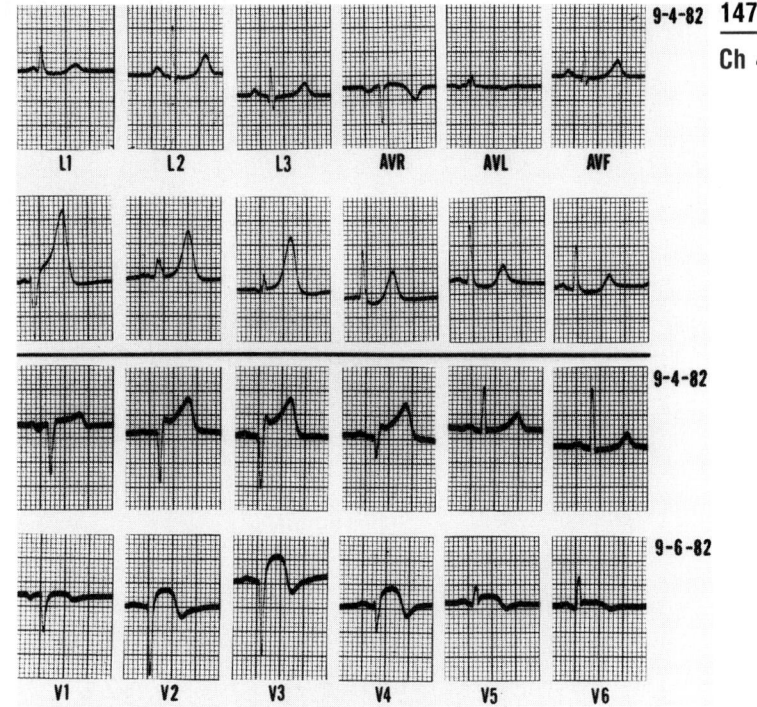

9-4-82

L1 L2 L3 AVR AVL AVF

9-4-82

9-6-82

V1 V2 V3 V4 V5 V6

FIGURE 4–AE10

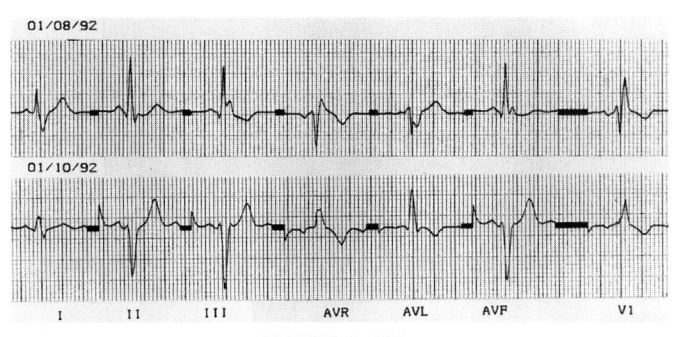

01/08/92

01/10/92

I II III AVR AVL AVF V1

FIGURE 4–AE8

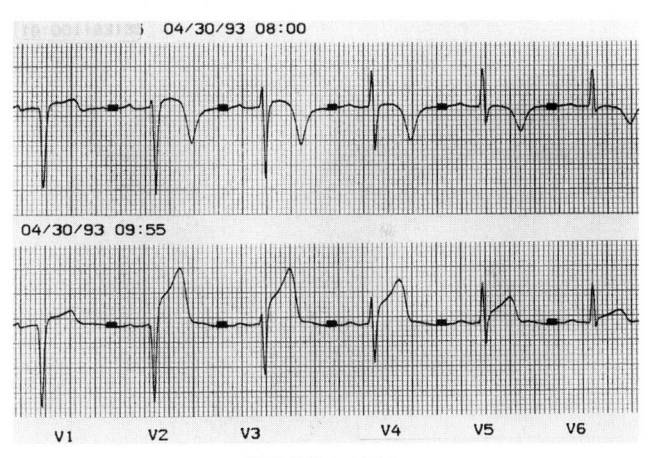

04/30/93 08:00

04/30/93 09:55

V1 V2 V3 V4 V5 V6

FIGURE 4–AE11

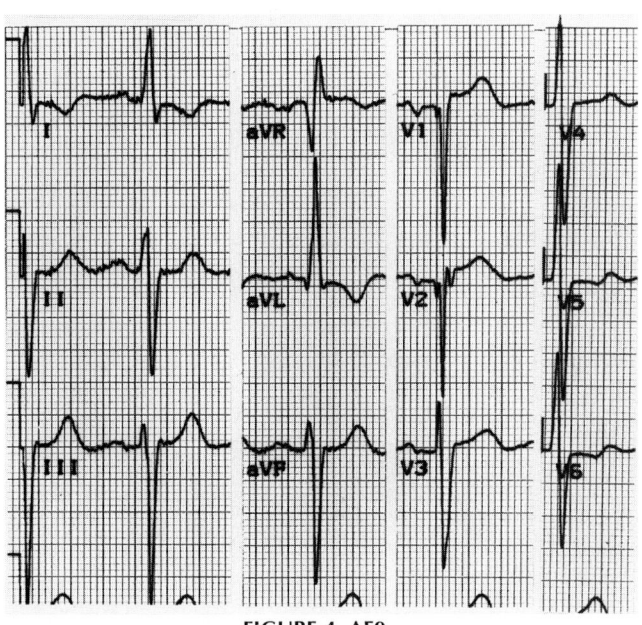

I aVR V1 V4

II aVL V2 V5

III aVF V3 V6

FIGURE 4–AE9

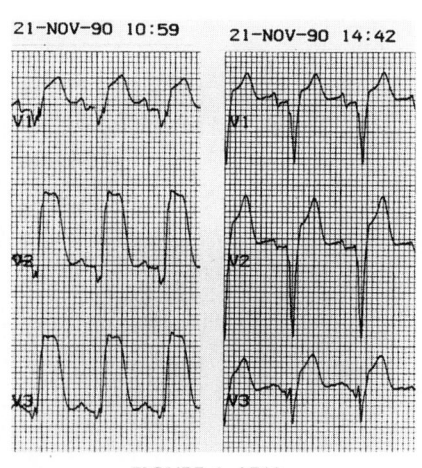

21-NOV-90 10:59   21-NOV-90 14:42

V1 V1

V2 V2

V3 V3

FIGURE 4–AE12

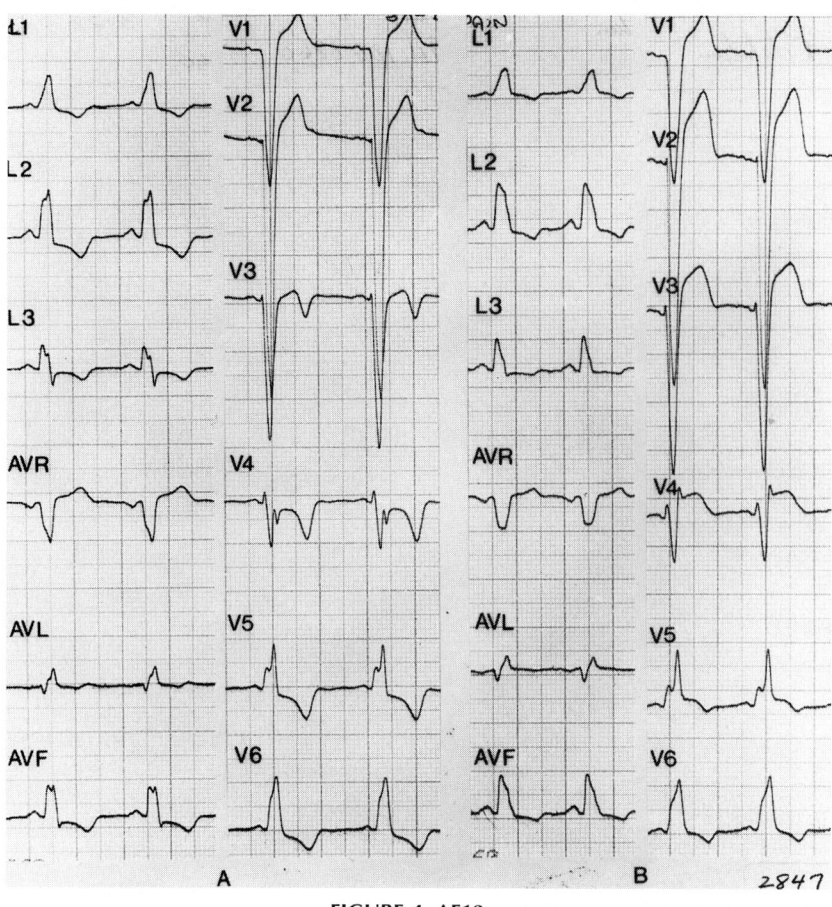

FIGURE 4–AE13

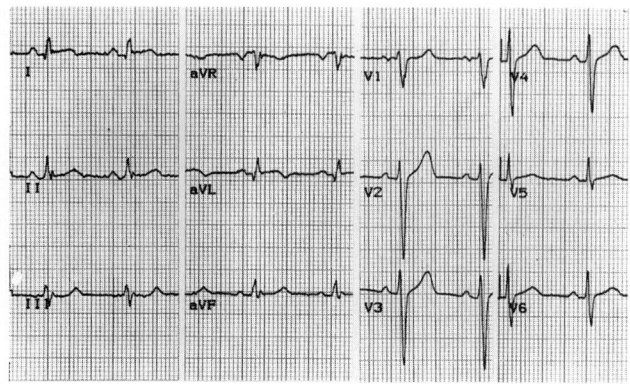

FIGURE 4–AE14

FIGURE 4–AE15

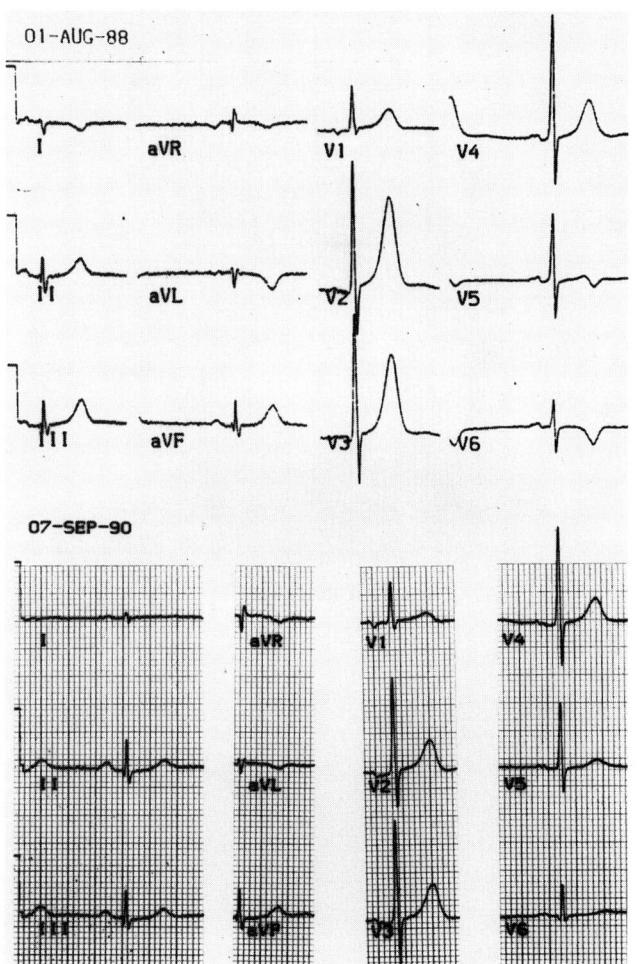

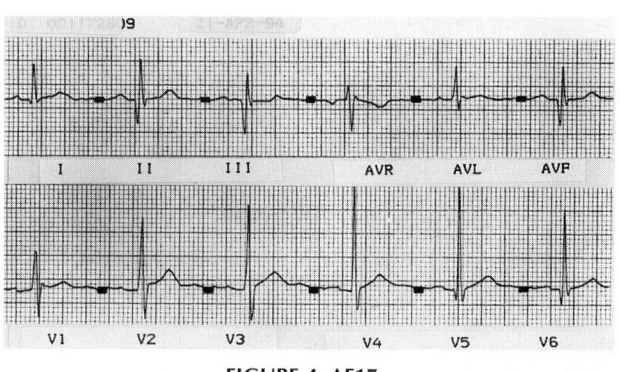

FIGURE 4–AE16

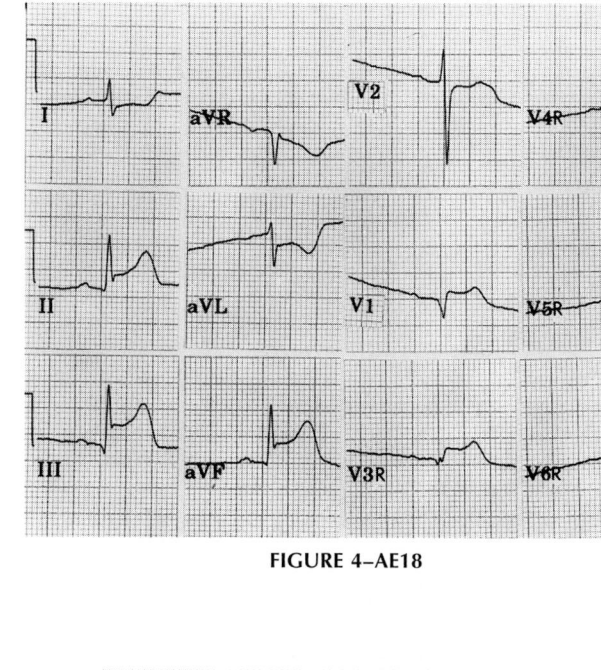

FIGURE 4–AE18

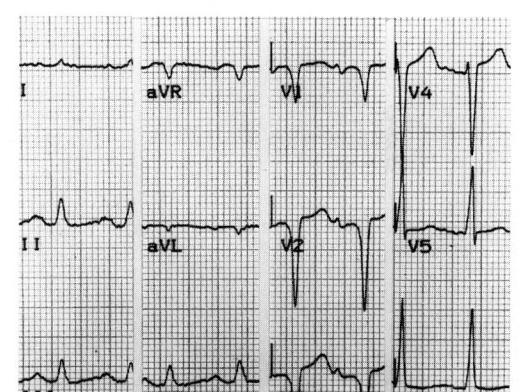
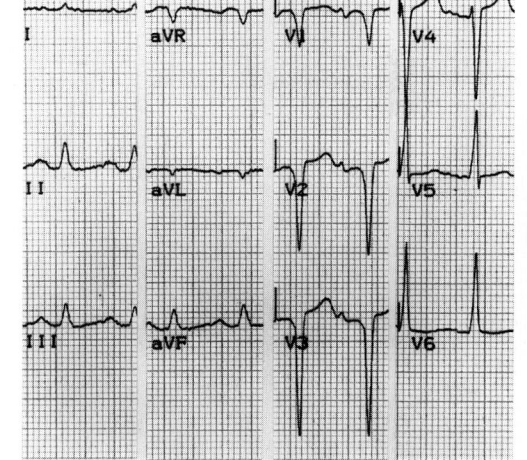
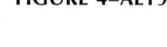

FIGURE 4–AE19

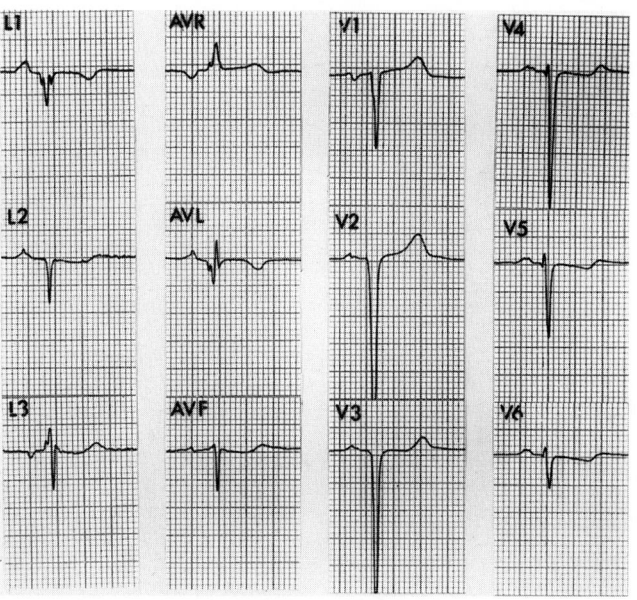

FIGURE 4–AE17

FIGURE 4–AE20

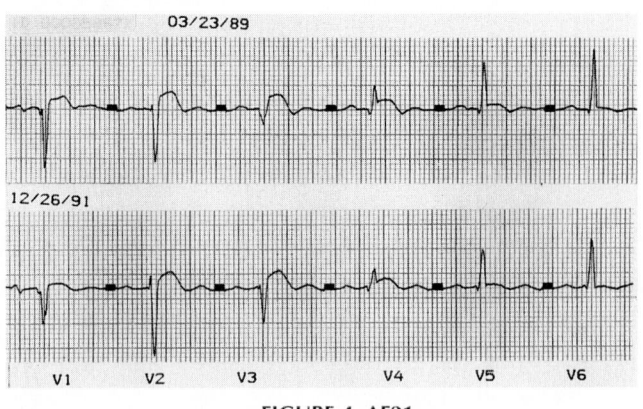

FIGURE 4–AE21

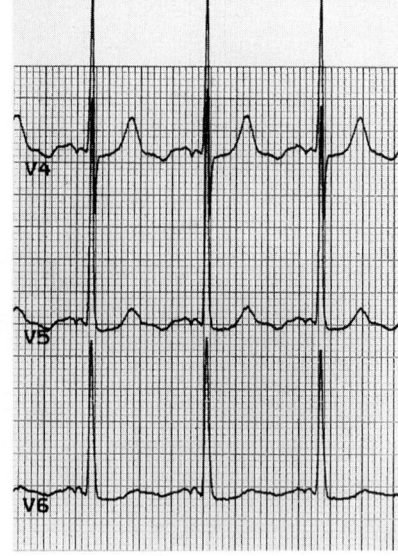

FIGURE 4–AE24

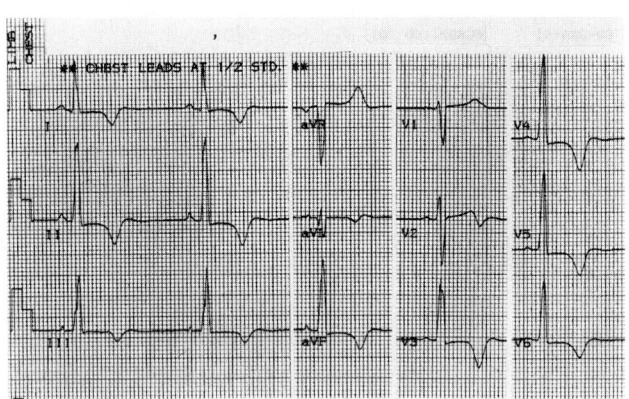

FIGURE 4–AE22

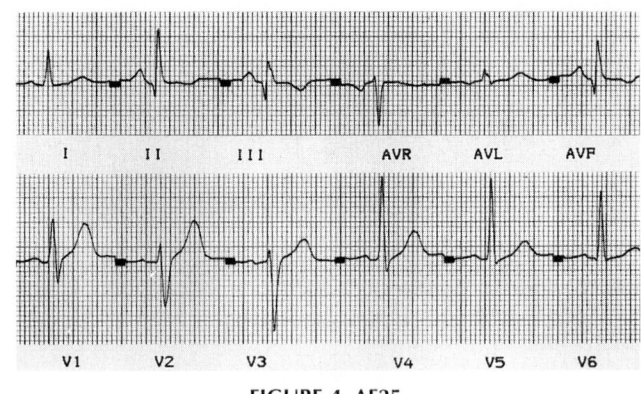

FIGURE 4–AE25

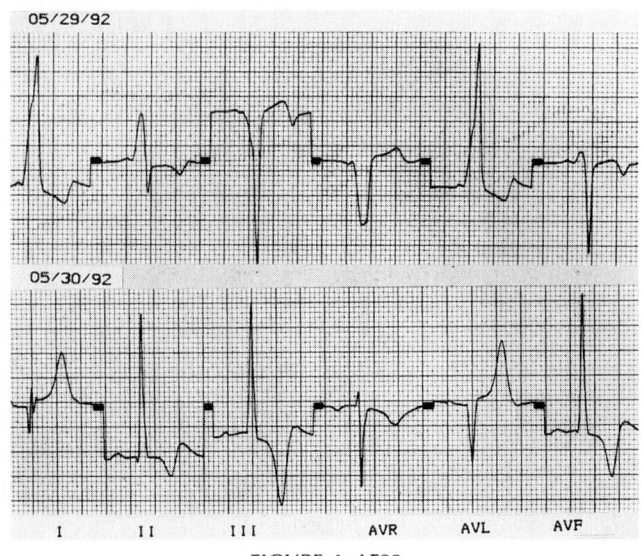

FIGURE 4–AE23

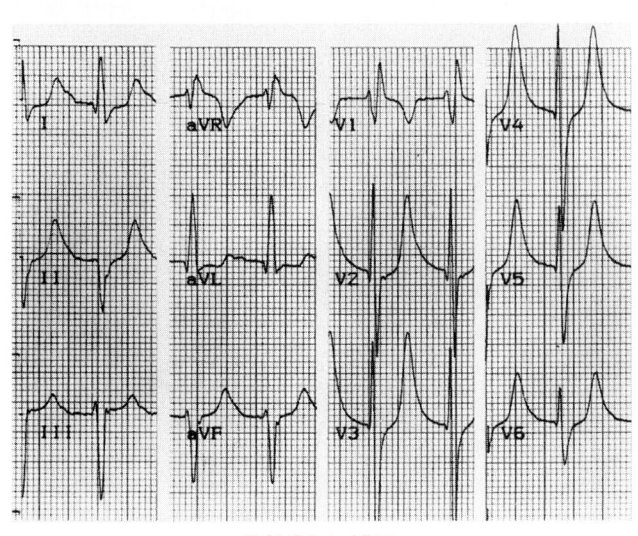

FIGURE 4–AE26

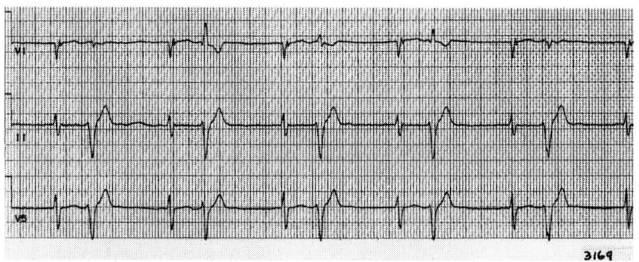

FIGURE 4–AE29

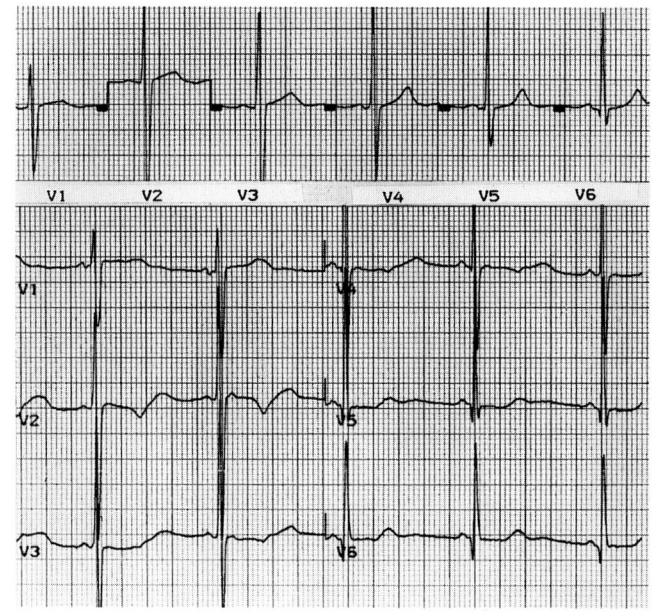

FIGURE 4–AE27

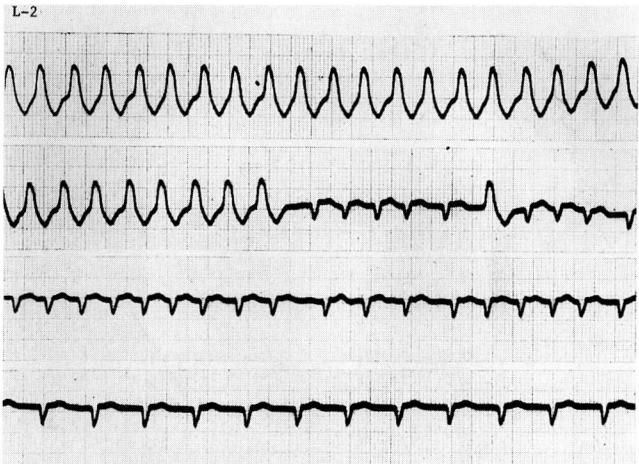

FIGURE 4–AE30

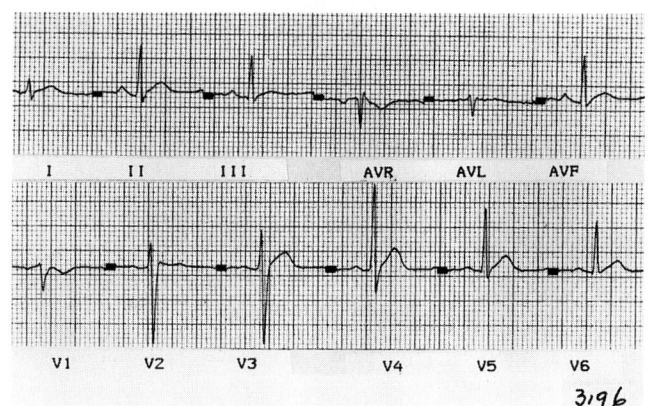

FIGURE 4–AE28

AF–Atrial fibrillation
LVH–Left ventricular hypertrophy
RVH–Right ventricular hypertrophy
LBBB–Left bundle branch block
RBBB–Right bundle branch block

IVCD–Intraventricular conduction delay
LAFB–Left anterior fascicular block
LPFB–Left posterior fascicular block
MI–Myocardial infarction

Figure 4–AE1

AF. The qR in lead V_1, in essence, a right atrial electrogram, is followed by a normal right-to-left R wave progression. The qR with a normal R wave progression beginning with lead V_2 is diagnostic of severe tricuspid insufficiency with a large right atrium subtending the V_1 electrode.

Figure 4–AE2

In the top tracing the large-amplitude QRS complexes with prominent Q waves in leads V_5 and V_6 indicates LVH due to a diastolic overload consistent with aortic regurgitation. In the lower tracing the LBBB obscures the Q waves and diminishes the R wave amplitude in leads V_4 to V_6. An IVCD, in this instance LBBB, makes a diagnosis of ventricular hypertrophy difficult if not impossible.

Figure 4–AE3

RBBB and LVH with a diastolic overload manifest by the high amplitude R waves, deep Q waves, and secondary ST-T changes recorded in a patient with a large patent ductus arteriosus.

Figure 4–AE4

Severe RVH. The q wave in V_1 suggests that the right ventricular pressure exceeds the left ventricular pressure. The left axis of the P wave and the prominent negative P wave in lead V_1 are unusual and most likely are due to a markedly enlarged right atrium projecting to the left and posteriorly. The prominent P waves in leads V_2 and V_3 are diagnostic of right atrial enlargement.

Figure 4–AE5

Mitral stenosis with pulmonary hypertension manifest by P mitrale, right-axis deviation, "squatty" QRS with a prominent R wave in V_1, and clockwise rotation.

Figure 4–AE6

Top row of each panel illustrates WPW with large-amplitude R waves in leads V_1 to V_4. In the lower row the AV conduction is normal with normal amplitude of the R waves. This tracing emphasizes the lack of specificity of QRS amplitude for ventricular hypertrophy in the presence of IVCD.

Figure 4–AE7

Top, IVCD with normal R wave amplitude in leads V_1, V_2, and V_3. 10/31/91 *(bottom).* Postoperative RBBB with large-amplitude R waves in leads V_1, V_2, and V_3 stresses a lack of specificity of the tall R waves for RVH in presence of IVCD, in this instance RBBB. Q waves in leads V_3 and V_4 are consistent with an anterior MI.

Figure 4–AE8

1/8/92, RBBB with LPFB. 1/10/92, RBBB with LAFB. Both recorded from the same patient.

Figure 4–AE9

IVCD with LAFB simulating septal MI.

Figure 4–AE10

Prominent, tall, upright T waves in leads V_1 to V_4 recorded early during acute MI are illustrated in the top panel. Evolution of an acute anteroseptal MI is recorded in the lower panel.

Figure 4–AE11

The earliest tracing (8:00) recorded in the course of evolution of an acute MI illustrates T wave inversion due to ischemia. This is followed (9:55) by ST elevation and Q waves in leads V_1 and V_2 indicative of a current of injury and "death" of muscle respectively.

Figure 4–AE12

Acute MI with early high-amplitude R waves recorded at 10:59 and loss of R waves at 14:42.

Figure 4–AE13

A, LBBB with primary T waves in leads V_3 and V_4. *B,* LBBB with acute MI manifest by ST segment elevation in leads V_1 to V_5. While LBBB precludes recording of a Q wave, acute MI may occasionally be recognized by ST segment elevation.

Figure 4–AE14

Septal MI with the highly specific qrS pattern in lead V_2. The qrS pattern indicates reversal of septal activation, namely, from right to left, followed by right and left ventricular activation, respectively. Changes in leads III and aV_f are consistent with an inferior MI.

Figure 4–AE15

Isolated high lateral MI with changes confined to leads I and aV_l. The S waves in leads V_5 and V_6 are most likely due to peri-infarction block with the terminal activation directed toward the area of the MI.

Figure 4–AE16

Upper panel, Posterior and anterolateral MI manifest by the tall R waves in leads V_1 and V_2 and T wave changes in leads I, aV_l, V_5, and V_6. *Lower panel,* Suggests a pure posterior infarction were it not for the earlier evidence of the lateral infarction. Isolated posterior infarction is extremely rare.

Figure 4–AE17

Posterior MI manifest by delayed and large-amplitude R in leads V_1 and V_2 with an inferior MI, the latter manifest by Q waves in leads II, III, and aV_f.

Figure 4–AE18

Acute inferior and right ventricular MI. The latter is manifested by Q waves and elevated ST segments in leads V_1 to V_6R.

Figure 4–AE19

AIDS myocarditis simulating an anteroseptal MI.

Figure 4–AE20

Hypertrophic cardiomyopathy simulating an anteroseptal MI.

Figure 4–AE21

Anteroseptal myocardial infarction with persistence of ST segment elevation over a period of more than $2\frac{1}{2}$ years is characteristic of a ventricular aneurysm.

Figure 4–AE22

This tracing was recorded at $\frac{1}{2}$ standard and illustrates giant negative T waves occasionally present in patients with localized hypertrophic cardiomyopathy.

Figure 4–AE23

WPW recorded on 5/29/92. The tracing recorded on 5/30/92, after ablation of an accessory pathway illustrates inverted T waves in leads II, III, and aV_f. The latter is thought by some to reflect T wave "memory."

Figure 4–AE24

LVH with negative U waves. The latter are rarely, if ever, recorded in a normal heart.

Figure 4–AE25

Faulty technique with reversal of the order of recording of leads V_1, V_2, and V_3, invariably interpreted by the computer as an anterior MI. Analysis of the P wave leads to a correct diagnosis. Q waves in leads II, III, and aV_f indicate an inferior MI.

Figure 4–AE26

Hyperkalemia with a prolonged P-R interval best seen in lead I, depression of intraventricular conduction with the pattern of a RBBB with LAFB, and tall "tented" T waves.

Figure 4–AE27

Long Q-U interval due to hypokalemia. The prominent U waves are best seen in leads II, III, aV_f, V_2, and V_3. Although the T waves in hypokalemia are as a rule upright, on rare occasion the T wave may be inverted.

Figure 4–AE28

Hypercalcemia manifested by a short QT interval.

Figure 4–AE29

AF with a junctional rhythm and multiform VPC with fixed coupling. The presence of more than one ectopic rhythm and multiform VPC with fixed coupling is highly specific for digitalis intoxication.

Figure 4–AE30

AF treated with large doses of digitoxin which not only fails to slow the ventricular rate *(middle row)* but also induces a ventricular *(top row)* and junctional *(bottom row)* tachycardia. Recorded in a patient with pneumococcic pneumonia.

Chapter 5
Exercise Stress Testing

BERNARD R. CHAITMAN

Exercise testing is an important diagnostic and prognostic procedure in the assessment of patients with ischemic heart disease. The diagnostic utility of the electrocardiogram was recognized by Feil and Siegel as early as 1928, when ST- and T-wave changes following exercise were reported in three of four patients with chronic stable angina.[1] Master and Oppenheimer developed a standardized exercise protocol to assess functional capacity and hemodynamic response in 1929.[2] Continued research into causal mechanisms of ST-segment displacement, effect of lead position, refinement of exercise protocols, and determination of diagnostic and prognostic exercise variables in clinical patient subsets characterized the subsequent 30 years. Shortly after the advent of coronary angiography, the limitation of exercise-induced ST-segment depression as a diagnostic marker for obstructive coronary disease in patient populations with a low disease prevalence became apparent. The test is now most frequently used to estimate prognosis and to determine functional capacity, likelihood and extent of coronary disease, and effects of therapy.[3–10] Ancillary techniques such as metabolic gas analysis, radionuclide imaging, and echocardiography enhance the information content of exercise testing in selected patients.

EXERCISE PHYSIOLOGY

Anticipation of dynamic exercise results in an acceleration of ventricular rate due to vagal withdrawal, increase in alveolar ventilation, and increased venous return as a result of sympathetic vasoconstriction. In normal subjects, the net effect is to increase resting cardiac output before the start of exercise. The magnitude of hemodynamic response during exercise depends on the severity and amount of muscle mass involved. In the early phases of exercise in the upright position, cardiac output is increased by an augmentation in stroke volume mediated through the use of the Frank-Starling mechanism and heart rate; the increase in cardiac output in the latter phases of exercise is primarily due to an increase in ventricular rate (see p. 381). During strenuous exertion, sympathetic discharge is maximal and parasympathetic stimulation is withdrawn, resulting in vasoconstriction of most circulatory body systems, except for that in exercising muscle and in the cerebral and coronary circulations. Venous and arterial norepinephrine release from sympathetic postganglionic nerve endings is increased, and epinephrine levels are increased at peak exertion; this enhances ventricular contractility. As exercise progresses, skeletal muscle blood flow is increased, oxygen extraction increases by as much as threefold, total calculated peripheral resistance decreases, and systolic blood pressure, mean arterial pressure, and pulse pressure usually increase. Diastolic blood pressure is unchanged or may increase or decrease by approximately 10 mm Hg. The pulmonary vascular bed can accommodate as much as a sixfold increase in cardiac output with only modest increases in pulmonary artery pressure, pulmonary capillary wedge pressure, and right atrial pressure; in normal subjects, this is not a limiting determinant of peak exercise capacity.

Cardiac output increases by four- to sixfold above basal levels during strenuous exertion in the upright position, depending on genetic endowment and level of training.[3]

The maximum heart rate and cardiac output are decreased in older individuals related in part to decreased beta-adrenergic responsivity[11] (see p. 1692). Maximum heart rate can be calculated from the formula 220 − age (years) with a standard deviation of 10 to 12 beats per minute.[6] The age-predicted maximum heart rate is a useful measurement for safety reasons. However, the wide standard deviation seen in the various regression equations used and the impact of drug therapy limit the usefulness of this parameter in arbitrary selection of limits of age-predicted maximum heart rate to define the adequacy of cardiac reserve in individual patients.

In the postexercise phase, hemodynamics return to baseline within minutes of termination. Vagal reactivation is an important cardiac deceleration mechanism after exercise and is accelerated in well-trained athletes but blunted in patients with chronic heart failure.[12] Intense physical work or important cardiorespiratory impairment may interfere with achievement of a steady state, and an oxygen deficit occurs during exercise. The total oxygen uptake in excess of the resting oxygen uptake during the recovery period is the oxygen debt.

PATIENT POSITION. At rest, the cardiac output and stroke volume are higher in the supine than in the upright position. With exercise in normal supine subjects, the elevation of cardiac output results almost entirely from an increase in heart rate with little augmentation of stroke volume. In the upright posture, the increase in cardiac output in normal subjects results from a combination of elevations in stroke volume and heart rate. A change from supine to upright posture causes decrease in venous return, left ventricular end-diastolic volume and pressure, stroke volume, and cardiac index. Renin and norepinephrine levels are increased. End-systolic volume and ejection fraction are not significantly changed. In normal individuals, end-systolic volume decreases and ejection fraction increases to a similar extent from rest to exercise in the supine and upright positions. The magnitude and direction of change in end-diastolic volume from rest to maximum exercise in both positions are small and may vary according to the patient population studied. The net effect on exercise performance is an approximate 10 per cent increase in exercise time, cardiac index, heart rate, and rate pressure product at peak exercise in the upright as compared with the supine position.

Cardiopulmonary Exercise Testing

Cardiopulmonary exercise testing involves measurements of respiratory oxygen uptake ($\dot{V}_{O_2}$), carbon dioxide production ($\dot{V}_{CO_2}$), and ventilatory parameters during a symptom-limited exercise test. During testing, the patient usually wears a nose clip and breathes through a nonrebreathing valve that separates expired air from room air. Important measurements of expired gas are O_2 tension, CO_2 tension, and airflow. A flowmeter is used to determine airflow. Ventilatory measurements include respiratory rate, tidal volume, and minute ventilation (VE). O_2 and CO_2 tension are sampled breath by breath or by use of a mixing chamber. The $\dot{V}_{O_2}$ and $\dot{V}_{CO_2}$ can be computed on-line from ventilatory volumes and differences between inspired and expired gases.[13] Under steady-state (equilibrium) conditions, $\dot{V}_{O_2}$ and $\dot{V}_{CO_2}$ measured at the mouth are equivalent to total-body oxygen consumption and CO_2 production. The relationship between work output, oxygen consumption, heart rate, and cardiac output during exercise is linear (Fig. 5–1). $\dot{V}_{O_2max}$ is the product of maximal arterial venous oxygen difference and cardiac output. In untrained persons, the arterial–mixed venous O_2 difference at peak exercise is relatively constant (14 to 17 vol per cent), and $\dot{V}_{O_2max}$ is an approximation of maximum cardiac output. $\dot{V}_{O_2max}$ does not reliably predict degree of systolic left ventricular dysfunction measured by ejection fraction.[14] Measured $\dot{V}_{O_2max}$ can be compared with predicted values from empirically derived formulas based on age, sex, weight, and height.[13,15,16] Peak exercise capacity is decreased when the ratio of measured to predicted $\dot{V}_{O_2max}$ is <85 to 90 per cent. Oximetry, determined noninvasively, can be used to monitor arterial oxygen saturation and normally does not decrease by more than 5 per cent during exercise. Estimates of oxygen saturation during strenuous exercise using pulse oximetry may be unreliable in some patients.[17]

ANAEROBIC THRESHOLD. *Anaerobic threshold* is a theoretical point during dynamic exercise when muscle tissue switches over to anaerobic metabolism as an additional energy source. All tissues do not shift simultaneously, and there is a brief interval during which exercising muscle tissue shifts from predominantly aerobic to anaerobic metabolism.[3,13,15,16,18] (Fig. 5–1). Lactic acid begins to accumulate when a healthy untrained subject reaches about 50 to 60 per cent of the maximal capacity for aerobic metabolism. The increase in lactic acid becomes greater as exercise becomes more intense, resulting in metabolic acidosis.

As lactate is formed, it is buffered in the serum by the bicarbonate system, resulting in increased CO_2 excretion, which causes reflex hyperventilation. The gas exchange anaerobic threshold (AT_{ge}) is the point at which VE increases disproportionately relative to $\dot{V}_{O_2}$ and work; it occurs at 40 to 60 per cent of $\dot{V}_{O_2max}$ in normal, untrained individuals.[13] Below the anaerobic threshold, CO_2 production is proportional to oxygen consumption. Above the anaerobic threshold, CO_2 is produced in excess of oxygen consumption. There are several methods to determine AT_{ge}, which include (1) the V-slope method, the point at which the rate of increase in $\dot{V}_{CO_2}$ relative to $\dot{V}_{O_2}$ increases (Fig. 5–1), (2) the point at which the $\dot{V}_{O_2}$ and $\dot{V}_{CO_2}$ slopes intersect, and (3) the point at which the ratio of VE/$\dot{V}_{O_2}$ and end-tidal O_2 tension begins to increase systematically without an immediate increase in the VE/$\dot{V}_{O_2}$. The AT_{ge} is a useful parameter because work below AT_{ge} encompasses most activities of daily living. Anaerobic threshold is often reduced in patients with important cardiovascular disease. An increase in anaerobic threshold with training can greatly enhance an individual's capacity to perform sustained submaximal activities with consequent improvement in quality of life and daily living. Changes in anaerobic threshold with repeat testing can be used to assess disease progression, response to medical therapy, and improvement in cardiovascular fitness with training.

METABOLIC EQUIVALENT. The current usage of the term *MET* refers to the resting $\dot{V}_{O_2}$ for a 70-kg, 40-year-old male, and 1 MET is equivalent to 3.5 ml/min/kg of body weight. Work activities can be calculated in multiples of METs;

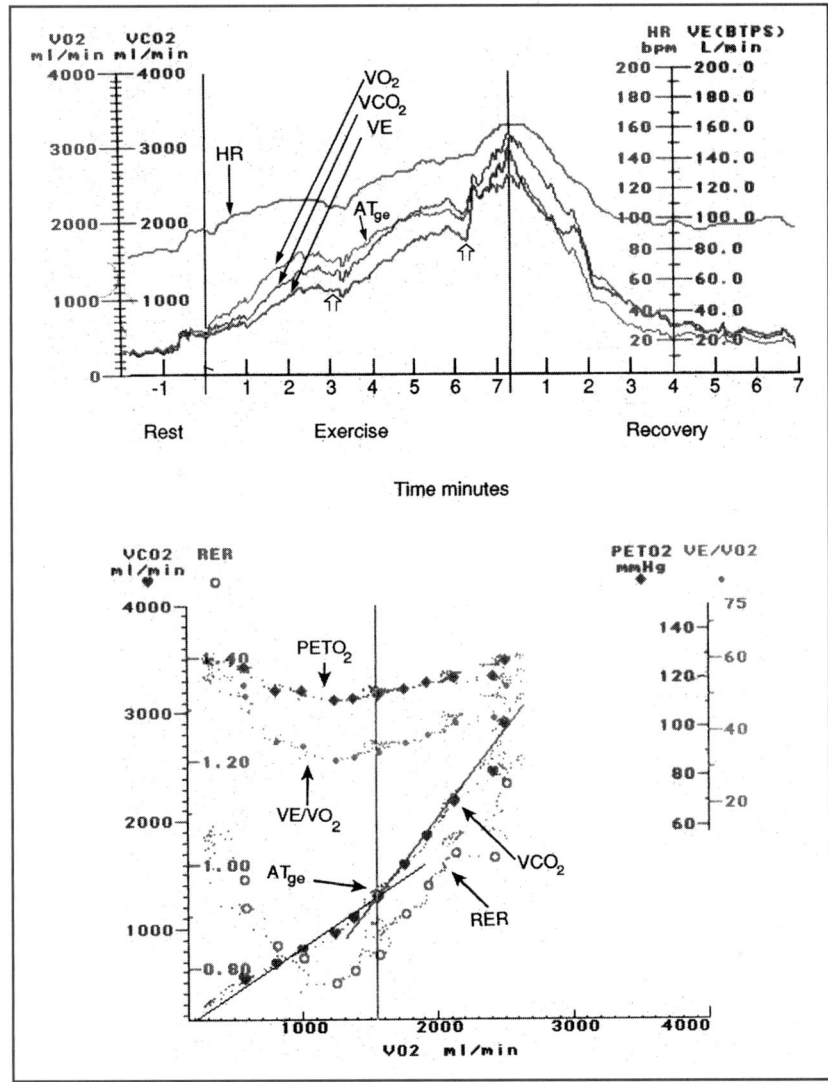

FIGURE 5–1. Cardiopulmonary exercise test in a 53-year-old, healthy man using the Bruce protocol. The progressive linear increase in work output, heart rate, and oxygen consumption ($\dot{V}_{O_2}$) is noted with steady-state conditions reached after 2 minutes in each of the first two stages *(top panel)*. Open arrows indicate the beginning of each new 3-minute stage. The subject completed 7 minutes and 10 seconds of exercise, and peak $\dot{V}_{O_2}$ was 3.08 liters/min. The anaerobic threshold (AT_{ge}), determined by the $\dot{V}$-slope method is the point at which the slope of the relative rate of increase in $\dot{V}_{CO_2}$ relative to $\dot{V}_{O_2}$, changes, and occurred at a $\dot{V}_{O_2}$ of 1.3 liters/min, or 42 per cent of peak $\dot{V}_{O_2}$, within predicted values for a normal sedentary population *(bottom panel)*. The AT_{ge} determined by the point at which the $\dot{V}_{O_2}$ and $\dot{V}_{CO_2}$ slopes intersect (1.8 liters/min) *(top panel)* is slightly greater than the AT_{ge} determined by the $\dot{V}$-slope method *(bottom panel)*. The $\dot{V}$-slope method usually provides a more reproducible estimate of AT_{ge}. PET_{O_2} = end-tidal pressure of oxygen; RER = respiratory exchange ratio; VE/$\dot{V}_{O_2}$ = ratio ventilation to oxygen uptake.

this measurement is useful to determine exercise prescriptions, assess disability, and standardize the reporting of submaximal and peak exercise workloads when different protocols are employed. An exercise workload of 3 to 5 METs is consistent with activities such as raking leaves, light carpentry, golf, and walking at 3 to 4 miles per hour. Workloads of 5 to 7 METs are consistent with exterior carpentry, singles tennis, and light backpacking. Workloads in excess of 9 METs are compatible with heavy labor, handball, squash, and running at 6 miles per hour (see p. 3004). Estimating $\dot{V}_{O_2}$ from work rate or treadmill time in individual patients may lead to misinterpretation of data if exercise equipment is not correctly calibrated or if the patient fails to achieve steady state, is obese, or has peripheral vascular disease, pulmonary vascular disease, or cardiac impairment. $\dot{V}_{O_2}$ does not increase linearly in some patients with cardiovascular or pulmonary disease as work rate is increased and may lead to overestimation of $\dot{V}_{O_2}$.[13] The measurements obtained with cardiopulmonary exercise testing are useful in understanding an individual patient's response to exercise and can be quite useful in the diagnostic evaluation of a patient with dyspnea.[19]

PATHOPHYSIOLOGY OF THE MYOCARDIAL ISCHEMIC RESPONSE

Myocardial oxygen consumption (M_{O_2}) is determined by heart rate, systolic blood pressure, left ventricular end-diastolic volume, wall thickness, and contractility.[6,10] The rate-pressure or double product (heart rate × systolic blood pressure) increases progressively with increasing work and can be used to estimate the myocardial perfusion requirement in normal subjects and in many patients with coronary artery disease. The heart is an aerobic organ with little capacity to generate energy through anaerobic metabolism. O_2 extraction in the coronary circulation is nearly maximal at rest. The only significant mechanism available to the heart to increase oxygen consumption is to increase perfusion, and there is a direct linear relationship between M_{O_2} consumption and coronary blood flow in normal individuals. The principal mechanism for increasing coronary blood flow during exercise is to decrease resistance at the coronary arteriolar level.[20] In patients with progressive atherosclerotic narrowing of the epicardial vessels, an ischemic threshold occurs beyond which exercise can produce abnormalities in diastolic and systolic ventricular function, electrocardiographic changes, and chest pain. The subendocardium is more susceptible to myocardial ischemia than the subepicardium because of increased wall tension, causing a relative increase in myocardial O_2 demand.

Dynamic changes in coronary artery tone at the site of an atherosclerotic plaque may result in diminished coronary flow during static or dynamic exercise; i.e., perfusion pressure distal to the stenotic plaque actually falls during exercise, resulting in reduced subendocardial blood flow[21] (see p. 404). Thus regional left ventricular myocardial ischemia may result not only from an increase in myocardial O_2 demand during exercise but also from a limitation of coronary flow as a result of coronary vasoconstriction and inability to vasodilate near the site of an atherosclerotic plaque.

EXERCISE PROTOCOLS

The main types of exercise are dynamic or isotonic exercise and static or isometric exercise. In daily living, a person frequently performs both types simultaneously. Dynamic protocols most frequently are used to assess cardiovascular reserve, and those suitable for clinical testing should include a low-intensity "warmup" phase. In general, 6 to 10 minutes of continuous progressive exercise during which the myocardial O_2 demand is elevated to the patient's maximal level is optimal for diagnostic and prognostic purposes. The protocol should include a suitable recovery or "cool-down" period. If the protocol is too strenuous for an individual patient, early test termination will result and will not allow an opportunity to observe clinically important responses. If the exercise protocol is too easy for an individual patient, the prolonged procedure will test endurance and not aerobic capacity. Thus exercise protocols should be individualized to accommodate the patient's limitations. Protocols may be set up at a fixed duration of exercise for a certain intensity to meet minimal qualifications for certain industrial tasks or sports programs.

STATIC EXERCISE. This form of isometric exercise generates force with little muscle shortening and produces a greater pressor response than with dynamic exercise. In a common form, the patient's maximal force on a hand dynamometer is recorded. The patient then sustains 25 to 33 per cent of maximal force for 3 to 5 minutes while ECG and blood pressures are recorded. The increase in myocardial $\dot{V}_{O_2}$ is often insufficient to initiate an ischemic response.

ARM ERGOMETRY. Arm crank ergometry protocols involve arm cranking at incremental workloads of 10 to 20 watts for 2 or 3 minute stages.[22] The heart rate and blood pressure responses to a given workload of arm exercise usually are greater than those for leg exercise. A bicycle ergometer with the axle placed at the level of the shoulders is used, and the subject sits or stands and cycles the peddles so that the arms are alternately fully extended. The most common frequency is 50 rpm's. In normal subjects, maximum $\dot{V}_{O_2}$ and VE for arm cycling approximates 50 to 70 per cent of leg cycling. Peak heart rate is approximately 70 per cent of that during leg testing.

BICYCLE ERGOMETRY. Bicycle protocols involve incremental workloads calibrated in watts or kilopond (KPD) meters/min. One watt is equivalent to 6 KPD meters/min in mechanically braked bicycles, work is determined by force and distance and requires a constant pedaling rate of 60 to 80 rpm, according to subject preference. Electronically braked bicycles provide a constant workload in spite of changes in pedaling rate and are less dependent on patient cooperation; although they are more costly than a mechanically braked bicycle, they are preferred for diagnostic and prognostic assessment. Most protocols begin at a workload of 25 watts and increase in 25-watt increments every 2 minutes. Younger subjects may start at 50 watts, with 50-watt increments every 2 minutes. A ramp protocol differs from the staged protocols in that the patient starts at 3 minutes of unloaded pedaling at a cycle speed of 60 rpm. Work rate is increased by a uniform amount each minute ranging from 5- to 30-watt increments depending on expected patient performance.[6,13] Exercise is terminated if the patient is unable to maintain a cycling frequency above 40 rpm. In the cardiac catheterization laboratory, hemodynamic measurements may be made during supine bicycle ergometry at rest and at one or two submaximal workloads.

In subjects unfamiliar with bicycle exercise, the muscles required for optimal performance are not as well developed as for treadmill exercise, and early fatigue may be a limiting factor. The bicycle ergometer is associated with a lower maximal $\dot{V}_{O_2}$ and anaerobic threshold than the treadmill, although maximal heart rate, maximal VE, and maximal lactate values are often similar. The metabolic requirements of ergometric workloads are inversely related to body mass, whereas the requirements of treadmill exercise are relatively independent of body mass. The bicycle ergometer has the advantage of requiring less space than a treadmill, is quieter, and permits sensitive precordial measurements without much motion artifact. However, in North America, treadmill protocols are more widely used in the assessment of patients with coronary disease.

TREADMILL PROTOCOL. The treadmill protocol should be consistent with the patient's physical capacity and the purpose of the test. In healthy individuals, the standard Bruce protocol is popular, and a large diagnostic and prognostic data base has been published.[6,10,23] In older individuals, or those whose exercise capacity is limited by cardiac disease, the Bruce protocol can be modified by two 3-minute warmup stages at 1.7 mph and 0 per cent grade and 1.7 mph and 5 per cent grade. The Bruce multistage maximal treadmill protocol has 3-minute periods to allow achievement of a steady state before workload is increased (Fig. 5–1). A limitation of the Bruce protocol is the relatively large increase in $\dot{V}_{O_2}$ between stages and the additional energy cost of running as compared with walking at stages in excess of Bruce stage III. The *Naughton* and *Weber* protocols use 1- to 2-minute stages with 1-MET increments between stages; these protocols may be more suitable for patients with limited exercise tolerance such as patients with congestive heart failure. The ACIP and modified ACIP (mACIP) protocols use 2-minute stages with 1.5-MET increments between stages after two 1-minute warmup stages with 1.0-MET increments. The ACIP protocols test patients with established coronary disease and result in a linear increase in heart rate and $\dot{V}_{O_2}$, permitting the time to occurrence of ST-segment depression over a wider range of heart rate and exercise time than protocols with more abrupt

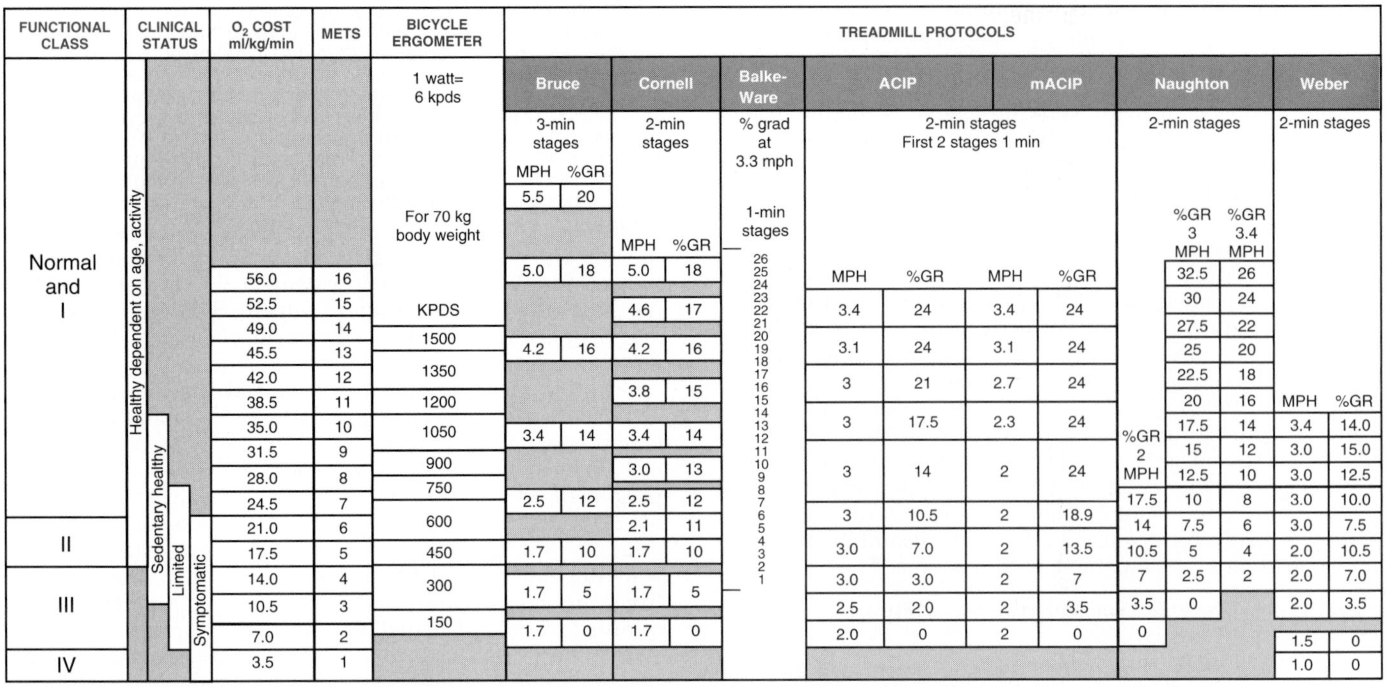

FUNCTIONAL CLASS	CLINICAL STATUS	O₂ COST ml/kg/min	METS	BICYCLE ERGOMETER (1 watt = 6 kpds; For 70 kg body weight)	Bruce (3-min stages) MPH	Bruce %GR	Cornell (2-min stages) MPH	Cornell %GR	Balke-Ware (% grad at 3.3 mph, 1-min stages)	ACIP (2-min stages; first 2 stages 1 min) MPH	ACIP %GR	mACIP MPH	mACIP %GR	Naughton (2-min stages) %GR 3 MPH	Naughton %GR 3.4 MPH	Weber (2-min stages) MPH	Weber %GR
Normal and I	Healthy (dependent on age, activity)				5.5	20			26								
		56.0	16		5.0	18	5.0	18	25					32.5	26		
		52.5	15	KPDS 1500			4.6	17	24 / 23 / 22	3.4	24	3.4	24	30	24		
		49.0	14						21 / 20	3.1	24	3.1	24	27.5	22		
		45.5	13	1350	4.2	16	4.2	16	19 / 18	3	21	2.7	24	25	20		
		42.0	12				3.8	15	17 / 16	3	17.5	2.3	24	22.5	18		
		38.5	11	1200					15 / 14					20	16		
	Sedentary healthy	35.0	10	1050	3.4	14	3.4	14	13 / 12	3	14	2	24	17.5	14		
		31.5	9	900					11 / 10					15	12		
		28.0	8	750			3.0	13	9	3	10.5	2	18.9	12.5	10		
II		24.5	7		2.5	12	2.5	12	8 / 7					%GR 2 MPH 17.5 / 14		3.4	14.0
	Limited	21.0	6	600			2.1	11	6 / 5					15 / 12		3.0	15.0
		17.5	5	450	1.7	10	1.7	10	4	3.0	7.0	2	13.5	12.5 / 10		3.0	12.5
III	Symptomatic	14.0	4	300					3	3.0	3.0	2	7	17.5 / 8		3.0	10.0
		10.5	3		1.7	5	1.7	5	2	2.5	2.0	2	3.5	14 / 6		3.0	7.5
		7.0	2	150	1.7	0	1.7	0	1	2.0	0	2	0	10.5 / 4		2.0	10.5
IV		3.5	1											7 / 2		2.0	7.0
														3.5 / 0		2.0	3.5
														0		1.5	0
																1.0	0

FIGURE 5–2. Estimated oxygen cost of bicycle ergometer and selected treadmill protocols. The standard Bruce protocol starts at 1.7 mph and 10 per cent grade (5 METs) with a larger increment between stages than protocols such as the Naughton, ACIP, and Weber protocols, which start at less than 2 METs at 2 mph and increase by 1- to 1.5-MET increments between stages. The Bruce protocol can be modified by two 3-minute warmup stages at 1.7 mph and 0 per cent grade and 1.7 mph and 5 per cent grade. (Adapted with permission from Fletcher, G. F., Balady, G., Froelicher, V. F., et al: Exercise standards. A statement for healthcare professionals from the American Heart Association. Circulation 91:580, 1995. Copyright 1995 American Heart Association.)

increments in workload between stages. The mACIP protocol produces a similar aerobic demand as the standard ACIP protocol for each minute of exercise and is well suited for short or elderly individuals who cannot keep up with a walking speed of 3 mph (Fig. 5–2).[24,25]

Ramp protocols start the patient at relatively slow treadmill speed, which is gradually increased until the patient has a good stride. The ramp angle of incline is progressively increased at fixed intervals (e.g., 10 to 60 seconds) starting at zero grade with the increase in grade calculated on the patient's estimated functional capacity such that the protocol will be complete at between 6 and 10 minutes.[6,10] In this type of protocol, the rate of work increase is continuous, and steady-state conditions are not reached. A limitation of ramp protocols is the requirement to estimate functional capacity from an activity scale; occasionally, under- or overestimation of functional capacity will result in an endurance test or premature cessation. One formula for estimating $\dot{V}_{O_2}$ from treadmill speed and grade is $\dot{V}_{O_2}$ (mlO₂/kg/min) = (mph × 2.68) + (1.8 × 26.82 × mph × grade ÷ 100) + 3.5.[26] $\dot{V}_{O_2}$ max is usually the same regardless of treadmill protocol used; the difference is the rate of time at which $\dot{V}_{O_2}$ is achieved.

It is important to encourage the patient not to grasp the handrails of the treadmill during exercise. Functional capacity can be overestimated by as much as 20 per cent in tests in which handrail support is permitted, and $\dot{V}_{O_2}$ is decreased. Since the degree of handrail support is difficult to quantify from one test to another, more consistent results can be obtained during serial testing when handrail support is not permitted.

The *6-minute walk test* can be used in patients with marked left ventricular dysfunction who cannot perform bicycle or treadmill exercise.[27] Patients are instructed to walk down a 100-foot corridor at their own pace, attempting to cover as much ground as possible in 6 minutes. At the end of the 6-minute interval, the total distance walked is determined and the symptoms experienced by the patient are recorded.

ELECTROCARDIOGRAPHIC MEASUREMENTS

LEAD SYSTEMS. The Mason-Likar modification of the standard 12-lead electrocardiogram requires that the extremity electrodes be moved to the torso to reduce motion artifact. The arm electrodes should be located in the lateral-most aspects of the infraclavicular fossae and the leg electrodes in a stable position above the anterior iliac crest and below the rib cage (Fig. 5–3). The Mason-Likar modification results in a right-axis shift and increased voltage in the inferior leads and may produce a loss of inferior Q waves and the development of new Q waves in lead aVl. Thus, the body torso limb lead positions cannot be used to interpret a diagnostic rest 12-lead ECG. The more cephalad the leg electrodes are placed, the greater is the degree of change and the greater is the augmentation of R-wave amplitude, potentiating exercise-induced ST-segment changes.

Bipolar lead groups place the negative or reference electrode over the manubrium (CM₅), right scapula (CB₅), RV₅ (CC₅), or on the forehead (CH₅), and the active electrode at V₅ or proximate location to optimize R-wave amplitude. In bipolar lead ML, which reflects inferior wall changes, the negative reference is at the manubrium and the active electrode in the left leg position. Bipolar lead groups may provide additional diagnostic information, and in some medical centers lead CM₅ is substituted for lead aV_r in the Mason-Likar modified lead system (Fig. 5–3). Bipolar leads are frequently used when only a limited ECG set is required (e.g., in cardiac rehabilitation programs). The use of more elaborate lead set systems is usually reserved for research purposes.

Types of ST Segment Displacement

In normal subjects, the P-R, QRS, and Q-T intervals shorten as heart rate increases. P amplitude increases and the P-R segment becomes progressively more downsloping in the inferior leads. J point, or junctional, depression is a normal finding during exercise (Fig. 5–4). However, in patients with myocardial ischemia, the ST segment usually becomes more horizontal (flattens) as the severity of the ischemic response worsens. With progressive exercise, the depth of ST-segment depression may increase, involving more ECG leads, and the patient may develop angina. In the immediate postrecovery phase, the ST-segment displacement may persist, with downsloping ST segments and T wave inversion, gradually returning to baseline after 5 to 10 minutes (Figs. 5–5 and 5–6). However, ischemic ST-segment displacement may be seen only during exercise, emphasizing the importance of adequate skin preparation and electrode placement to capture high-quality recordings during maximum exertion (Fig. 5–7). In about 10 per cent of patients, the ischemic response may appear only in the recovery phase.[27] The patient should not leave the exercise laboratory area until the postexercise ECG has returned to baseline. Figure 5–8 illustrates different ECG patterns seen during exercise testing.

MEASUREMENT OF ST-SEGMENT DISPLACEMENT. For purposes of interpretation, the PQ junction is usually chosen as the isoelectric point. The TP segment represents a true isoelectric point but is an impractical choice for most routine clinical measurements. The development of ≥ 0.10 mV (1 mm) of J point depression measured from the PQ junction, with a relatively flat ST-segment slope (< 1 mV/sec), depressed ≥ 0.10 mV 60 to 80 msec after the J point in the three consecutive beats with a stable baseline is considered to be an abnormal response (Fig. 5–9). Occasionally, the ST segment at rest may be depressed. When this occurs, the J point and ST60 to ST80 measurements should be de-

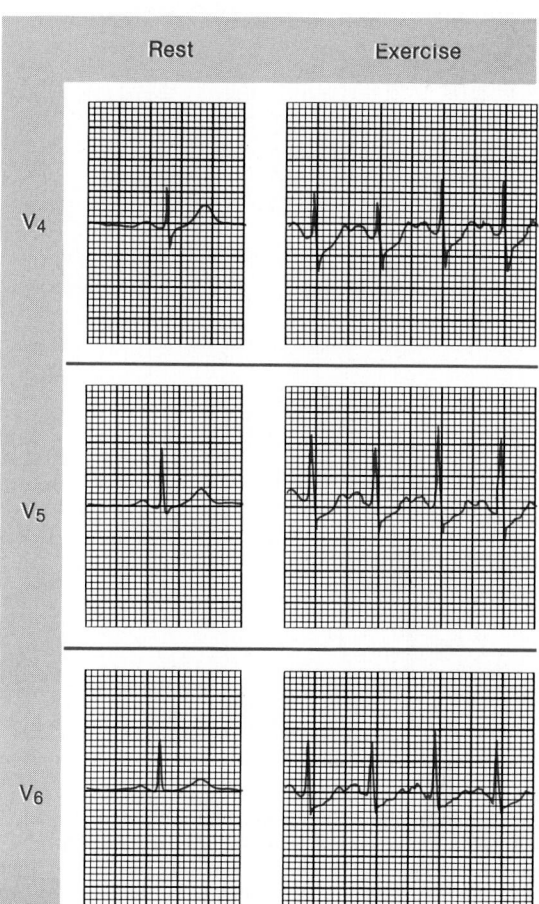

FIGURE 5–4. J point depression of 2 to 3 mm in leads V_4 to V_6 with rapid upsloping ST segments depressed approximately 1 mm 80 msec after the J point. The ST segment slope in leads V_4 and V_5 is ≥ 3.0 mV/sec. This response should not be considered abnormal.

pressed an additional ≥ 0.10 mV to be considered abnormal. In patients with early repolarization and resting ST-segment elevation, return to the PQ junction is normal. Abnormal ST-segment depression in a patient with early repolarization should be measured from the PQ junction. A slow, upsloping ST segment is defined as J point depression with an upsloping ST segment (> 1 mV/sec), depressed ≥ 0.15 mV at 60 to 80 msec after the J point, in three consecutive beats (Fig. 5–6).

Exercise-induced ST segment elevation may occur in Q wave or non-Q wave leads. The development of ≥ 0.10 mV (1 mm) of J point elevation, persistently elevated ≥ 0.10 mV at 60 to 80 msec after the J point in three consecutive beats, is considered an abnormal response (Figs. 5–8 and 5–10).

Exercise-induced ST segment depression does *not* localize the site of myocardial ischemia, *nor* does it provide a clue as to which coronary artery is involved.[29] For example, it is not unusual for patients with isolated right coronary disease to exhibit exercise-induced ST-segment depression only in leads V_4 to V_6, nor is it unusual for patients with disease of the left anterior descending coronary artery to exhibit exercise-induced ST-segment displacements in leads II, III, and aV_f. Exercise-induced ST-segment elevation is relatively specific for the territory of myocardial ischemia and the coronary artery involved.

T-WAVE CHANGES. The morphology of the T wave is influenced by body position, respiration, and hyperventilation. Occasionally, a patient may be referred for exercise testing who has T-wave inversion on the resting 12-lead ECG. Pseudonormalization of T waves (inverted at rest and becoming upright with exercise) is a nondiagnostic finding.[6] Although in rare instances this finding may be a marker for myocardial ischemia in a patient with docu-

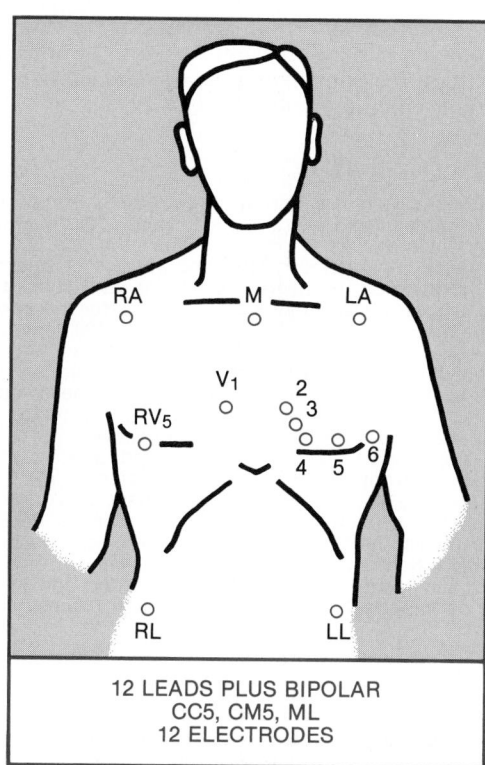

FIGURE 5–3. This lead group set reflects the Mason-Likar leads with the precordial electrodes in standard position and the arm and leg electrodes moved proximally to the subclavicular fossa and just above the anterior iliac crest. The position of the negative reference manubrial electrode and RV_5 electrode illustrates the position required for lead CM_5 and lead CC_5. In lead ML, the active electrode is in the left leg position.

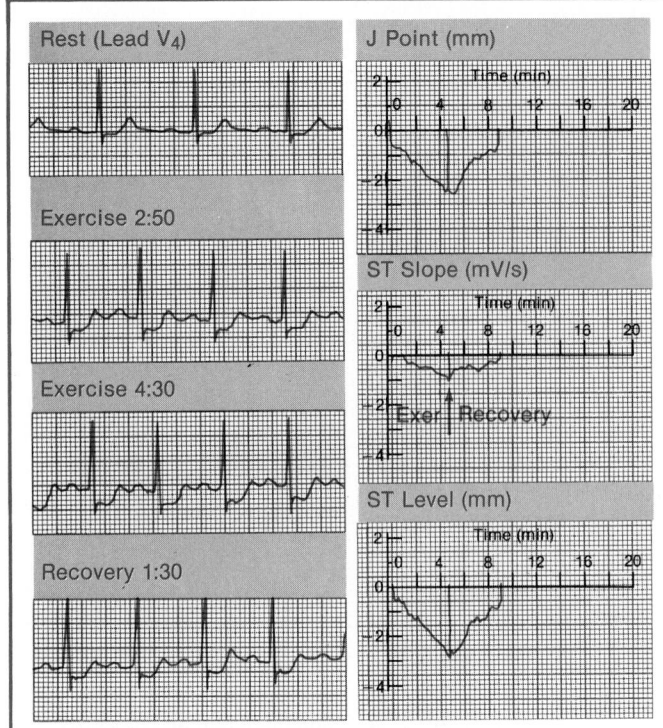

FIGURE 5–5. Bruce protocol. In lead V$_4$, the exercise ECG is abnormal early in the test, reaching 3 mm (0.3 mV) of horizontal ST-segment depression at the end of exercise. The ischemic changes persist for at least 1 min and 30 sec into the recovery phase. The right panel provides a continuous plot of the J point, ST slope, and ST-segment displacement at 80 msec after the J point (ST level) during exercise and in the recovery phase. Exercise ends at the vertical line at 4.5 min. The computer trends permit a more precise identification of initial onset and offset of ischemic ST-segment depression. This type of ECG pattern, with early onset of ischemic ST-segment depression, reaching more than 3 mm of horizontal ST-segment displacement, and persisting several minutes into the recovery phase, is consistent with a severe ischemic response.

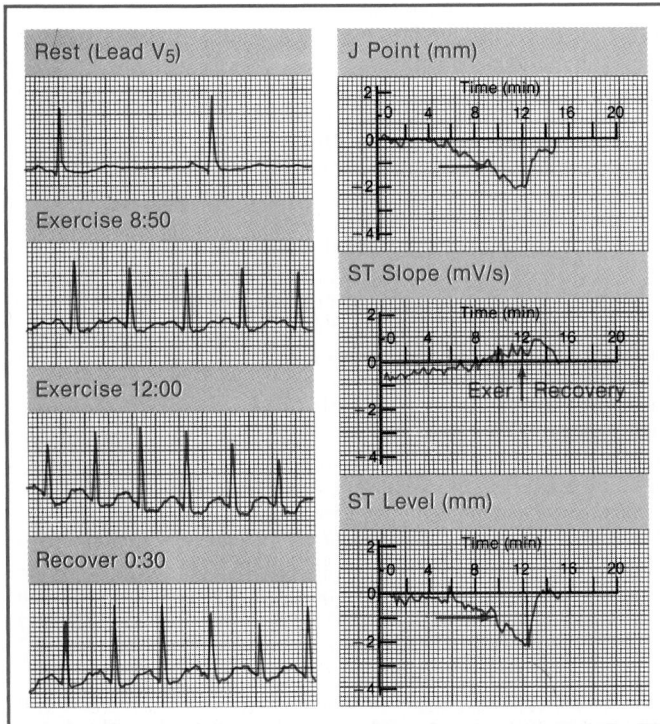

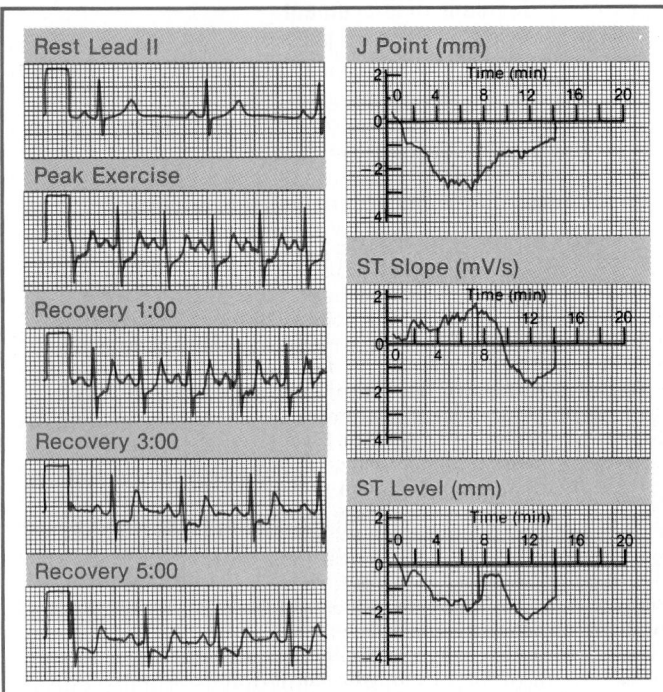

FIGURE 5–6. Bruce protocol. In this type of ischemic pattern, the J point at peak exertion is depressed 2.5 mm, the ST-segment slope is 1.5 mV/second, and the ST-segment level at 80 msec after the J point is depressed 1.6 mm. This "slow upsloping" ST segment at peak exercise indicates an ischemic pattern in patients with a high coronary disease prevalence pretest. A typical ischemic pattern is seen at 3 minutes of the recovery phase when the ST segment is horizontal and 5 minutes postexertion when the ST segment is downsloping. Exercise is discontinued at the vertical line in the right panels at 7.5 min.

mented coronary disease, it would need to be substantiated by an ancillary technique, such as the concomitant finding of a reversible thallium defect.

COMPUTER-ASSISTED ANALYSIS

The use of computers has facilitated the routine analysis and measurements required from exercise electrocardiography and can be performed on-line as well as off-line.[30] When the raw ECG data are high quality, the computer can filter and average or select median complexes from which the degree of J point displacement, ST-segment slope, and ST displacement 60 to 80 msec after the J point (ST60 to 80) can be measured. The selection of ST60 or ST80 depends on the heart rate response. At ventricular rates ≥130 beats/min, the ST80 measurement may fall on the upslope of the T wave, and the ST60 measurement should be employed instead. In some computerized systems, the PQ junction or isoelectric interval is detected by scanning before the R wave for the 10-msec interval with the least slope. J point, ST slope, and ST levels are determined, and the ST integral can be calculated from the area below the isoelectric line from the J point to ST60 to ST80. Computerized treatment of ECG complexes permits reduction of motion and myographic artifacts. However, the averaged or median beats occasionally may be erroneous because of ECG signal distortion caused by noise, baseline wander, or changes in conduction, and identification of the PQ junction and ST-segment onset may be imperfect. Therefore, it is crucial to ensure that the

FIGURE 5–7. Bruce protocol. The exercise ECG becomes abnormal at 9:30 min of a 12 min exercise (horizontal panel, arrow *right*) and resolves in the immediate recovery phase. This ECG pattern in which the ST segment becomes abnormal only at high exercise workloads and returns to baseline in the immediate recovery phase may indicate a false-positive test in an asymptomatic subject without atherosclerotic risk factors. Exercise thallium scintigraphy would provide more diagnostic and prognostic information if this were an older person with several atherosclerotic risk factors.

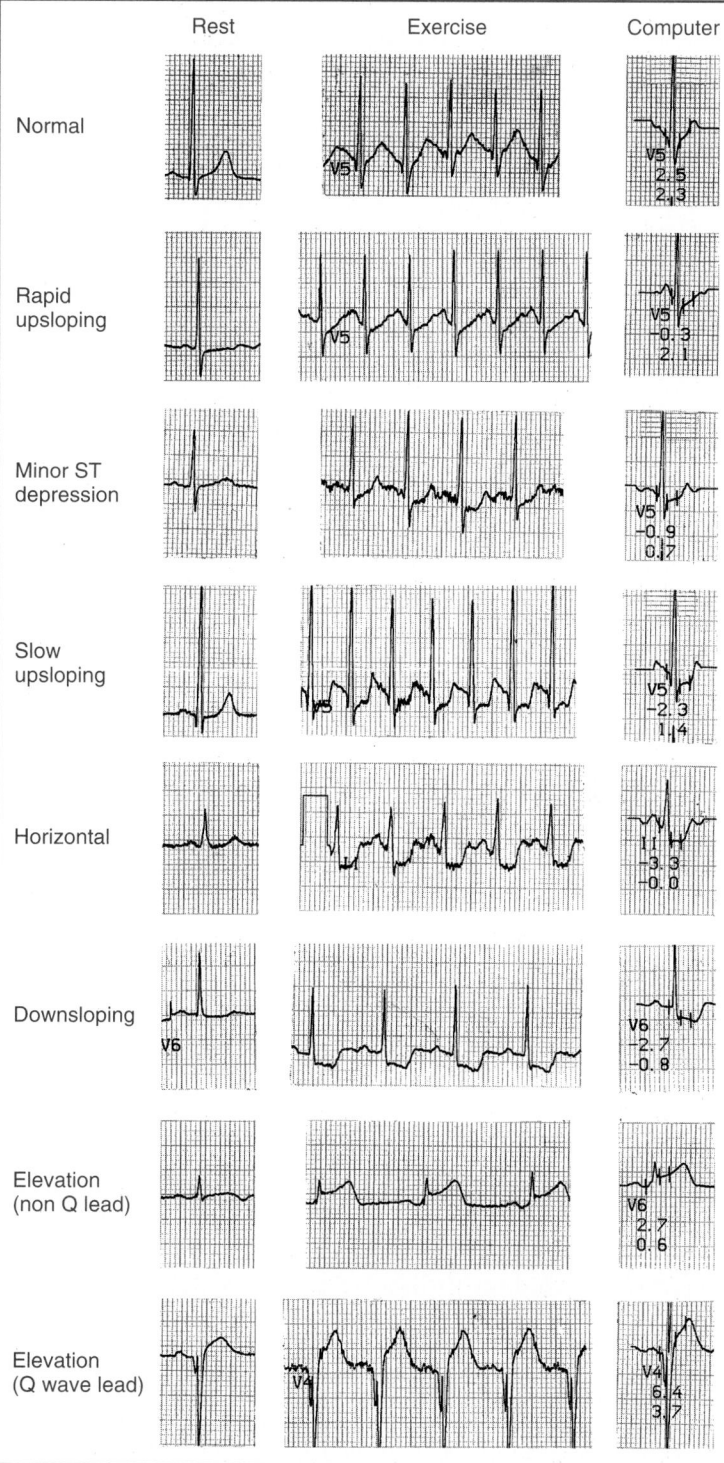

FIGURE 5-8. Illustration of typical exercise electrocardiographic patterns at rest and at peak exertion. The computer processed incrementally averaged beat corresponds with the raw data taken at the same time point during exercise and is illustrated in the last column. The patterns represent worsening ECG responses during exercise. In the column of computer-averaged beats, ST80 displacement (top number) indicates the magnitude of ST segment displacement 80 msec after the J point relative to the PQ junction or E point. ST segment slope measurement (bottom number) indicates the ST segment slope at a fixed time point after the J point to the ST80 measurement. At least three noncomputer average complexes with a stable baseline should meet criteria for abnormality before the exercise ECG can be considered abnormal (see Fig. 5-9). The normal and rapid upsloping ST segment responses are normal responses to exercise. J-point depression with rapid upsloping ST segments is a common response in an older, apparently healthy population. Minor ST depression can occur occasionally at submaximal workloads in patients with coronary disease; in this illustration, the ST segment is depressed 0.9 mm (0.09 mV) 80 ms after the J point. The slow upsloping ST segment pattern often demonstrates an ischemic response in patients with known coronary disease or those with a high pretest clinical risk of coronary disease. Criteria for slow upsloping ST segment depression include J-point and ST80 depression of 0.15 mV or more and ST segment slope of more than 1.0 mV/sec. Classic criteria for myocardial ischemia include horizontal ST-segment depression observed when both the J point and ST80 depression are 0.1 mV or more and ST segment slope is within the range of ± 1.0 mV/sec. Downsloping ST segment depression occurs when the J-point and ST80 depression are > 0.1 mV and ST segment slope is > − 1.0 mV/sec. ST segment elevation in a non–Q-wave, noninfarct lead occurs when the J point and ST60 are 1.0 mV or greater and represents a severe ischemic response. ST segment elevation in an infarct territory (Q-wave lead) indicates a severe wall motion abnormality and in most cases is not considered an ischemic response. (From Chaitman, B. R.: Exercise electrocardiographic stress testing. *In* Beller, G. A. (ed.): Chronic Ischemic Heart Disease. *In* Braunwald, E. (series ed.): Atlas of Heart Diseases. Vol. 5. Chronic Ischemic Heart Disease. Philadelphia, Current Medicine, 1995, pp 2.1–2.30.)

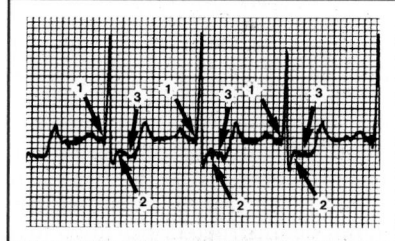

FIGURE 5-9. Magnified ischemic exercise-induced ECG pattern. Three consecutive complexes with a relatively stable baseline are selected. The PQ junction (1) and J point (2) are determined; the ST80 (3) is determined at 80 msec after the J point. In this example, average J point displacement is 2 mm (0.2 mV) and ST80 is 2.4 mm (0.24 mV). The average slope measurement from the J point to ST80 is − 1.1 mV/sec.

computer-determined averages or median complexes reflect the raw ECG data, and physicians should program the computer to print out raw data during exercise and inspect the raw data to be certain that the QRS template is accurately reproduced before accepting the automatic measurements.

MECHANISM OF ST-SEGMENT DISPLACEMENT

The mechanism of exercise-induced ST-segment displacement is not completely understood (see also Fig. 4–30, p. 128). In normal persons, the action potential duration of the endocardial region is longer than that of the epicardial region, and ventricular repolarization is from epicardium to endocardium. The action potential duration is shortened in the presence of myocardial ischemia, and electrical gradients are created, resulting in ST-segment depression or elevation, depending on the surface ECG leads.[31] Increased myocardial oxygen demand associated with a failure to increase or an actual decrease in regional coronary blood flow will usually cause ST-segment depression; occasionally, ST-segment elevation may occur, depending on the severity of coronary flow reduction. ST-segment ele-

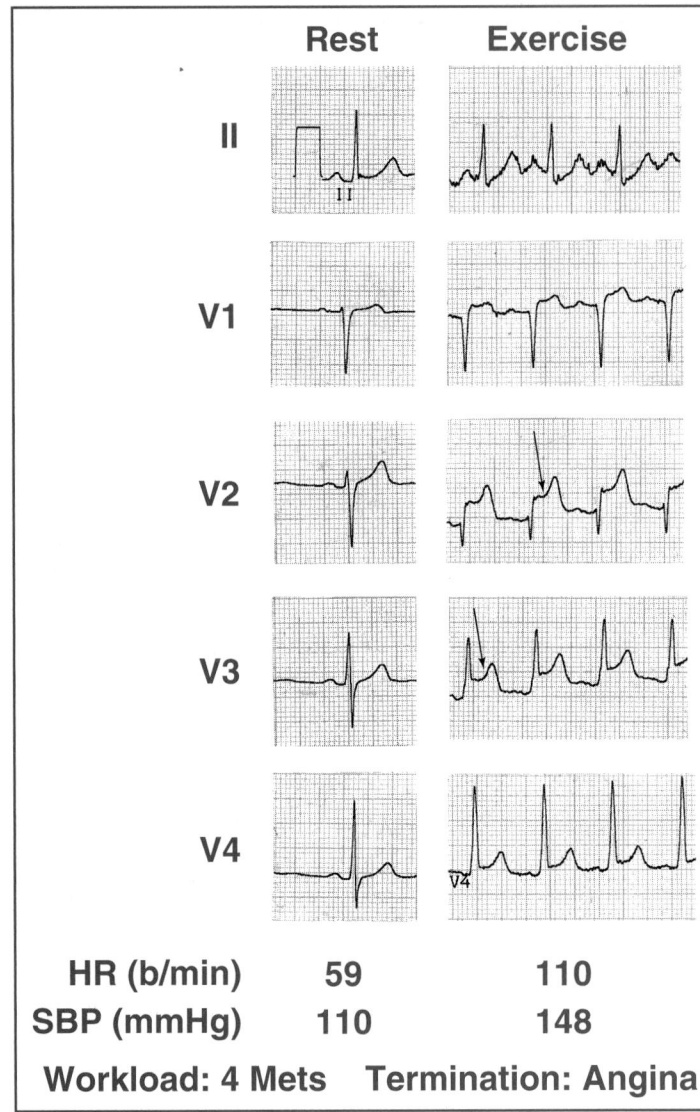

FIGURE 5–10. A 48-year-old man with several atherosclerotic risk factors and a normal rest ECG developed marked ST segment elevation (4 mm, [arrows]) in leads V_2 and V_3 with lesser degrees of ST-segment elevation in leads V_1 and V_4 and J point depression with upsloping ST segments in lead II, associated with angina. This type of ECG pattern is usually associated with a full-thickness, reversible myocardial perfusion defect in the corresponding left ventricular myocardial segments and high-grade intraluminal narrowing at coronary angiography. Rarely, coronary vasospasm will produce this result in the absence of significant intraluminal atherosclerotic narrowing. (From Chaitman, B. R.: Exercise electrocardiographic stress testing. *In* Beller, G. A., (ed.): Chronic Ischemic Heart Disease. *In* Braunwald, E. (series ed.): Atlas of Heart Diseases. Vol. 5. Chronic Ischemic Heart Disease. Philadelphia, Current Medicine, 1995, pp 2.1–2.30.)

vation in a non-Q wave lead is associated with a more severe degree of myocardial ischemia than is ST-segment depression.

EXERCISE TESTING

INDICATIONS. The most frequent indications for exercise testing are to aid in establishing the diagnosis of coronary artery disease in determining functional capacity and in estimating prognosis. The indications continue to evolve, with some that are uniformly accepted and others that are more controversial. The AHA and ACC Exercise Task Force determined several categories of test indications drawn from a large body of published literature on exercise testing[32] (Table 5–1). A class I indication indicates general agreement that exercise testing is justified; a class II indication indicates a condition for which exercise testing is frequently used but in which there is a divergence of opinion with respect to value and appropriateness; class III indicates general agreement that exercise testing is of little or no value or inappropriate. Exercise testing should not be used to screen very low-risk, asymptomatic individuals because the test has limited diagnostic and prognostic value in this situation, and the resultant undesirable consequences of a false-positive exercise test result in unnecessary follow-up, additional procedures, anxiety, and exercise restrictions.[7,8,32] Most asymptomatic subjects in an exercise screening program for coronary disease who die suddenly of cardiac causes have had a previous normal exercise test.

TECHNIQUES. The patient should be instructed not to eat, drink caffeinated beverages, or smoke for 3 hours prior to testing and to wear comfortable shoes and loose-fitting clothes. Unusual physical exertion should be avoided prior to testing. A brief history and physical examination should be performed, and the patient should be advised about the risks and benefits of the procedure. A written informed consent form is usually required. The indication for the test should be known. In many laboratories, the presence or absence of atherosclerotic risk factors is noted and cardioactive medication recorded. A 12-lead ECG should be obtained with the electrodes at the distal extremities.

Following recording of the standard 12-lead ECG, a torso ECG should be obtained in the supine position and in the sitting or standing position. Postural changes can bring out labile ST-T wave abnormalities. Hyperventilation is not recommended before exercise. If a false-positive test is suspected, hyperventilation should be performed after the test, and the hyperventilation tracing compared with the maximum ST segment abnormalities observed. The ECG and blood pressure should be recorded in both positions, and the patient should be instructed on how to perform the test.

Adequate skin preparation is essential for high-quality recordings, and the superficial layer of skin needs to be removed to augment signal-to-noise ratio. The areas of electrode application are rubbed with an alcohol-saturated pad to remove oil and rubbed with fine sandpaper or a rough material to reduce skin resistance to 5000 ohms or

TABLE 5-1 INDICATIONS FOR EXERCISE TESTING

161

Ch 5

CLASS 1 (CLEAR INDICATION)
Patients with suspected or proven coronary artery disease:
1. Diagnosis: patients with exercise related complaints of palpitations, dizziness, or syncope
2. Diagnosis: men with atypical symptoms
3. Prognostic assessment and functional capacity evaluation in patients with chronic stable angina or post-myocardial infarction
4. Symptomatic recurrent exercise-induced arrhythmias
5. Evaluation after revascularization procedure

CLASS 2 (TEST MAY BE INDICATED)
1. Diagnosis: women with typical or atypical angina pectoris
2. Functional capacity evaluation to monitor cardiovascular therapy in patients with CAD* or heart failure
3. Evaluation of patients with variant angina
4. Follow-up of patients with known CAD
5. Evaluation of asymptomatic men over 40 who are in special occupations (pilots, firefighters, police officers, bus or truck drivers, and railroad engineers), or who have two or more atherosclerotic risk factors or who plan to enter a vigorous exercise program

CLASS 3 (TEST PROBABLY NOT INDICATED)
1. Evaluation of patients with isolated premature ventricular beats and no evidence of CAD
2. Multiple serial testing during the course of cardiac rehab program
3. Diagnosis of CAD in patients, who have preexcitation syndrome or complete left bundle branch block or are on digitalis therapy
4. Evaluation of young or middle-aged asymptomatic men or women, who have no atherosclerotic risk factors or who have noncardiac chest discomfort

INDICATIONS FOR EXERCISE TESTING IN PATIENTS WITH VALVULAR HEART DISEASE OR HYPERTENSION
Test in common usage:
1. Evaluation of functional capacity in selected patients with valvular heart disease
2. Evaluation of blood pressure of hypertensive patients who wish to engage in vigorous dynamic or static exercise

* CAD = coronary artery disease
Data from ACC and AHA Subcommittee Report on Exercise Testing. Circulation 74:653A, 1986.

less. Silver chloride electrodes with a fluid column to avoid direct metal-to-skin contact produce high-quality tracings; these electrodes have the lowest offset voltage.

Cables connecting the electrodes and recorders should be light, flexible, and properly shielded. In a small minority of patients, a fishnet jersey may be required over the electrodes and cables to reduce motion artifact. The electrode-skin interface can be verified by tapping on the electrode and examining the cathode-ray screen or by measuring skin impedance. Excessive noise indicates that the electrode needs to be replaced; replacement before the test rather than during exercise can save time. The ECG signal can be digitized systematically at the patient end of the cable by some systems, reducing powerline artifact. Exercise equipment should be calibrated regularly. Room temperature should be between 64 and 72°F (18 and 22°C) and humidity <60 per cent.

Treadmill walking should be demonstrated. The heart rate, blood pressure, and ECG should be recorded at the end of each stage of exercise, immediately before and immediately after stopping exercise, at the onset of an ischemic response, and for each minute for at least 5 to 10 minutes in the recovery phase. A minimum of three leads should be displayed continuously on the cathode-ray screen during the test. There is some controversy regarding optimal patient position in the recovery phase. In the sitting position, less space is required for a stretcher, and patients are more comfortable immediately after exertion. The supine position increases end-diastolic volume and has the potential to augment ST-segment changes.[33]

DIAGNOSTIC USE OF EXERCISE TESTING

Appreciation of the exercise test literature requires an understanding of standard terminology such as sensitivity, specificity, and test accuracy (Table 5-2). The literature on the use of diagnostic exercise testing is extensive. The sensitivity of exercise ECG for single-vessel disease ranges from 25 to 71 per cent, with exercise-induced ST segment displacement most frequent in patients with left anterior descending coronary artery disease, followed by those with right coronary artery disease and those with isolated left circumflex coronary disease. An obstruction in an isolated

TABLE 5-2 TERMS USEFUL IN EVALUATION OF TEST RESULTS

True-positive (TP) = abnormal test result in individual with disease

False-positive (FP) = abnormal test result in individual without disease

True-negative (TN) = normal test result in individual without disease

False-negative (FN) = normal test result in individual with disease

Sensitivity: percentage of patients with CAD who have an abnormal test = TP/(TP + FN)

Specificity: percentage of patients without CAD who have a normal test = TN/(TN + FP)

Predictive value (+ test): percentage of patients with abnormal test who have CAD = TP/(TP + FP)

Predictive value (− test): percentage of patients with normal test and of normal test without CAD = TN/(TN + FN)

Test accuracy: percentage of true test results = (TP + TN)/total number tests performed

Likelihood ratio: odds of a test result being true: of an abnormal test: sensitivity/(1 − specificity); of a normal test: specificity/(1 − sensitivity)

Relative risk: $\dfrac{\text{disease rate in persons with a positive test result}}{\text{disease rate in persons with a negative test result}}$

left circumflex coronary artery has the tendency to exaggerate the depth of ST-segment depression when the ECG is abnormal, most likely related to the fact that the ischemic territory underlies the lateral precordial leads. Approximately 75 to 80 per cent of the diagnostic information on exercise-induced ST-segment depression is contained in leads V_4 to V_6. The ability to detect ECG changes in patients with right coronary disease can be augmented by recording lead V_5R.[34]

Gianrossi et al. performed an overview or meta-analysis of 147 consecutive published reports involving 24,074 patients who underwent both coronary angiography and exercise testing.[35] The mean sensitivity was 68 (range 23 to 100) per cent and mean specificity was 77 (range 17 to 100)

TABLE 5-3 NONCORONARY CAUSES OF ST-SEGMENT DEPRESSION

Severe aortic stenosis	Glucose load
Severe hypertension	Left ventricular hypertrophy
Cardiomyopathy	Hyperventilation
Anemia	Mitral valve prolapse
Hypokalemia	Intraventricular conduction disturbance
Severe hypoxia	Preexcitation syndrome
Digitalis	Severe volume overload (aortic, mitral regurgitation)
Sudden excessive exercise	Supraventricular tachyarrhythmias

per cent. In patients with multivessel coronary disease, the mean sensitivity was 81 (range 40 to 100) per cent and mean specificity was 66 (range 17 to 100) per cent.[36] The weighted mean sensitivity was 86 ± 11 per cent and mean specificity was 53 ± 24 per cent for left main or three-vessel coronary disease. The exercise ECG tends to be less sensitive in patients with extensive Q wave anterior wall myocardial infarction and when a limited-exercise ECG lead set is used.[37]

Selective referral of patients with a positive test for further study both decreases the rate of detection of true negative tests and increases the rate of detection of false-positive results, thus increasing sensitivity and decreasing specificity.[38] A positive exercise test cannot be considered false-positive for myocardial ischemia simply because angiography fails to reveal epicardial coronary disease. In patients with normal-appearing coronary arteries but abnormal coronary vasodilator reserve, ischemic ST-segment changes during exercise testing and abnormalities of left ventricular systolic and diastolic function during exercise have been reported (Table 5-3).[39]

SEVERITY OF ELECTROCARDIOGRAPHIC ISCHEMIC RESPONSE. The exercise ECG is more likely to be abnormal in patients with more severe coronary arterial obstruction, more extensive coronary disease, and after more strenuous levels of exercise. Early onset of angina, ischemic ST-segment depression, and fall in blood pressure at low exercise workloads are the most important exercise parameters associated with an adverse prognosis and multivessel coronary artery disease. Additional adverse markers include profound ST-segment displacement, ischemic changes in five or more ECG leads, and persistence of the changes late in the recovery phase of exercise (Table 5-4).

CORRELATION OF EXERCISE TEST RESULTS WITH CORONARY ANGIOGRAPHY. The traditional reference standard against which the exercise ECG has been measured is a qualitative assessment of the coronary angiogram using 50 to 70 per cent obstruction of the luminal diameter as the angiographic cutpoint. There are limitations of the angiographic

TABLE 5-4 EXERCISE PARAMETERS ASSOCIATED WITH AN ADVERSE PROGNOSIS AND MULTIVESSEL CORONARY ARTERY DISEASE

Duration of symptom-limiting exercise (< 6 METs)
Failure to increase systolic blood pressure ≥ 120 mm Hg, or a sustained decrease ≥ 10 mm Hg, or below rest levels, during progressive exercise
ST segment depression ≥ 2 mm, downsloping ST segment, starting at < 6 METs, involving ≥ 5 leads, persisting ≥ 5 minutes into recovery
Exercise-induced ST segment elevation (aV$_r$ excluded)
Angina pectoris during exercise
Reproducible sustained (> 30 sec) or symptomatic ventricular tachycardia

classification of patients into one-, two-, and three-vessel coronary disease, and the length of the coronary artery narrowing and the impact of serial lesions are not accounted for in correlative studies comparing diagnostic exercise testing with coronary angiographic findings. Other approaches, including intracoronary Doppler flow studies and quantitative coronary angiography, have been proposed to assess coronary vascular reserve which may be more accurate than qualitative assessment of the angiogram.[40,41]

BAYESIAN THEORY (see also p. 1744). The depth of exercise-induced ST-segment depression and the extent of the myocardial ischemic response can be thought of as continuous variables. Cutpoints such as 1 mm of horizontal or downsloping ST-segment depression as compared with baseline cannot completely discriminate patients with disease from those without disease, and the requirement of more severe degrees of ST-segment depression to improve specificity will decrease sensitivity. Sensitivity and specificity are inversely related, and false-negative and false-positive results are to be expected when ECG or angiographic cutpoints are selected to optimize the diagnostic accuracy of the test.[38]

The use of Bayesian theory incorporates the pretest risk of disease and the sensitivity and specificity of the test (likelihood ratio) to calculate the posttest probability of coronary disease (Fig. 5-11). The results of the patient's clinical information and exercise test results are used to make a final estimate of the probability of coronary disease. The diagnostic power of the exercise test is maximal when the pretest probability of coronary artery disease is inter-

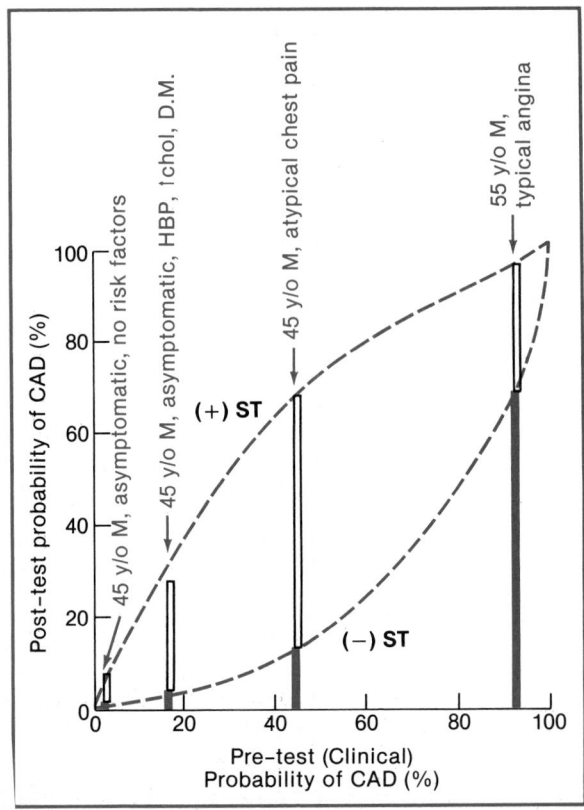

FIGURE 5-11. Use of Bayes theorem to calculate the probability of coronary artery disease (CAD). Four specific patient examples are shown by vertical bars where the height of the solid dark bar illustrates results for a negative exercise electrocardiogram (ECG) (−) ST, and a clear bar shows the results for a positive exercise ECG (+) ST. The posttest probability of coronary disease is optimal in patients with an intermediate coronary disease prevalence. (From Patterson, R. E., and Horowitz, S. F.: Importance of epidemiology and biostatistics in deciding clinical strategies for using diagnostic tests: A simplified approach using examples from coronary artery disease. Reprinted by permission of the American College of Cardiology. J. Am. Coll. Cardiol. *13*:1653, 1989.)

mediate (30 to 70 per cent). Exercise testing to diagnose coronary artery disease in young or middle-aged asymptomatic subjects without atherosclerotic risk factors is not useful, since the pretest risk is very low and a normal or abnormal exercise ECG result does not alter significantly the posttest risk of coronary artery disease[42] (Fig. 5–11).

MULTIVARIATE ANALYSIS. Multivariate analysis of exercise test variables to estimate posttest risk also can provide important diagnostic information. There is some controversy concerning whether to use Bayesian theory or multivariate analysis to estimate final posttest risk. Multivariate analysis offers the potential advantage that it does not require that the tests be independent of each other or that sensitivity and specificity remain constant over a wide range of disease prevalence rates. However, the multivariate technique depends critically on how patients are selected to establish the reference data base. Both Bayesian and multivariate techniques are acceptable.[43]

UPSLOPING SEGMENTS. Junctional or J point depression is a normal finding during maximum exercise, and a rapid upsloping ST segment (>1 mV/sec) depressed <1.5 mm (0.15 mV) after the J point should be considered to be normal. Occasionally, however, the ST segment will be depressed ≥ 1.5 mm (0.15 mV) at 80 msec after the J point. This type of "slow upsloping" ST segment may be the only ECG finding in patients with well-defined obstructive coronary disease and may depend on the lead set employed (Fig. 5–6). In patient subsets with a high disease prevalence, a slow upsloping ST segment depressed ≥ 1.5 mm at 80 msec after the J point should be considered to be abnormal. The importance of this finding in asymptomatic subjects or those with a low coronary disease prevalence is less certain. Increasing the degree of ST-segment depression at 80 msec after the J point to ≥ 2.0 mm (0.20 mV) in patients with a slow upsloping ST segment increases specificity but decreases sensitivity.[44]

ST-SEGMENT ELEVATION. Exercise-induced ST segment elevation in an infarct territory with abnormal Q waves is a marker for more severe left ventricular wall motion abnormalities and an adverse prognosis.[45] This finding occurs in approximately 30 per cent of patients with anterior myocardial infarctions and 15 per cent of those with inferior ones tested early (within 2 weeks) after the index event (Fig. 5–8) and decreases in frequency by 6 weeks. As a group, patients with exercise-induced ST-segment elevation have a lower ejection fraction than those without and greater severity of resting wall motion abnormalities. Exercise-induced ST-segment elevation in leads with abnormal Q waves is *not* a marker of more extensive coronary artery disease and rarely indicates myocardial ischemia. Occasionally, exercise-induced ST-segment elevation may occur in a patient who has regenerated R waves after an acute myocardial infarction; the clinical significance of this finding is similar to that observed when Q waves are present.

When ST-segment elevation develops during exercise in a non-Q wave lead in a patient without a previous myocardial infarction, the finding should be considered as likely evidence of transmural myocardial ischemia caused by coronary vasospasm or a high-grade coronary narrowing (Fig. 5–10). This finding is relatively uncommon, occurring in approximately 1 per cent of patients with obstructive coronary disease. The ECG site of ST-segment elevation is relatively specific for the coronary artery involved, and thallium scintigraphy will usually reveal a defect in the territory involved.

OTHER ELECTROCARDIOGRAPHIC MARKERS. Changes in R wave amplitude during exercise are relatively nonspecific and are related to the level of exercise performed. When the R wave amplitude meets voltage criteria for left ventricular hypertrophy, the ST-segment response *cannot* be used reliably to diagnose coronary disease, even in the absence of a left ventricular strain pattern. Loss of R wave amplitude, commonly seen after myocardial infarction, reduces the sensitivity of the ST-segment response in that lead to diagnose obstructive coronary artery disease. Occasionally, U wave inversion may be

seen in the precordial leads at heart rates <120 beats/min. While this finding is relatively specific for coronary artery disease, it is relatively insensitive.[46]

ST/HEART RATE SLOPE MEASUREMENTS. Heart rate adjustment of ST-segment depression appears to improve the sensitivity of the exercise test, particularly the prediction of multivessel coronary disease.[47,48] The ST/heart rate slope depends on the type of exercise performed, number and location of monitoring electrodes, method of measuring ST-segment depression, and clinical characteristics of the study population. Calculation of maximal ST/heart rate slope in mV/beats/min is performed by linear regression analysis relating the measured amount of ST-segment depression in individual leads to the heart rate at the end of each stage of exercise, starting at end exercise. An ST/heart rate slope ≥ 2.4 mV/beats/min is considered abnormal, and values ≥ 6 mV/beats/min[47] are suggestive evidence of three-vessel coronary disease.[47] The use of this measurement requires modification of the exercise protocol such that increments in heart rate are gradual, as in the Cornell protocol, as opposed to more abrupt increases in heart rate between stages, as in the Bruce or Ellestad protocols, which limit the ability to calculate statistically valid ST-segment heart rate slopes. The measurement is not accurate in the early postinfarction phase. A modification of the ST-segment/heart rate slope method is the ΔST-segment/heart rate index calculation, which represents the average change of ST-segment depression with heart rate throughout the course of the exercise test. The ΔST/heart rate index measurements are less than the ST/heart rate slope measurements, and a ΔST/heart rate index ≥ 1.6 is defined as abnormal. The incremental additional prognostic content of ST-segment/heart rate slope measurements as compared with standard criteria is required before these measurements can be widely adopted for prognostic purposes.[49]

NONELECTROCARDIOGRAPHIC OBSERVATIONS

The ECG is only one part of the exercise response, and abnormal hemodynamics or functional capacity is just as important if not more so than ST-segment displacement.

BLOOD PRESSURE. The normal exercise response is to increase systolic blood pressure progressively with increasing workloads to a peak response ranging from 160 to 200 mm Hg, with the higher range of the scale seen in older patients with less compliant vascular systems.[6,10] As a group, black patients tend to have a higher systolic blood pressure response than do whites.[50] At high exercise workloads, it is sometimes difficult to obtain an accurate determination of systolic blood pressure.[51] In normal subjects the diastolic blood pressure does not change significantly, fluctuating ± 10 mm Hg as compared with that at rest. Failure to increase systolic blood pressure ≥ 120 mm Hg, or a sustained decrease ≥ 10 mm Hg repeatable within 15 seconds, or a fall in systolic blood pressure below standing rest values is abnormal and reflects either inadequate elevation of cardiac output because of left ventricular systolic pump dysfunction or an excessive reduction in systemic vascular resistance.[52] The prevalence of exertional hypotension ranges from 2.7 to 9.3 per cent and is higher in patients with three-vessel or left main coronary disease. The finding of an abnormal systolic blood pressure response in patients with a high prevalence of coronary artery disease is associated with more extensive coronary disease and more extensive thallium defects. Conditions other than myocardial ischemia that have been associated with the failure to increase or an actual decrease in systolic blood pressure during progressive exercise are cardiomyopathy, cardiac arrhythmias, vasovagal reactions, left ventricular outflow tract obstruction, ingestion of antihypertensive drugs, hypovolemia, and prolonged vigorous exercise.[53]

It is important to make the distinction between a decline in blood pressure in the *postexercise* phase and a decrease or failure to increase systolic blood pressure *during* progressive exercise. The incidence of postexertional hypotension in asymptomatic subjects was 1.9 per cent in 781 asymptomatic volunteers in the Baltimore Longitudinal Study on Aging, with a 3.1 per cent incidence noted in subjects younger than age 55 and 0.3 per cent incidence in patients older than age 55.[54] In this series, most hypotensive episodes were symptomatic, and only two patients had hypotension associated with bradycardia and vagal symptoms. Although ST-segment abnormalities suggestive of ischemia occurred in one-third of the patients with hypotension, none of the patients had a cardiac event during 4 years of follow-up. Rarely, in young patients, vasovagal syncope can occur in the immediate postexercise phase, progressing through sinus bradycardia to several seconds of asystole and hypotension before reverting to sinus rhythm.

POSTEXERCISE SYSTOLIC BLOOD PRESSURE RATIOS. In the postexercise phase, there is a progressive decline in systolic and diastolic blood pressure. An abnormal postexercise systolic blood pressure response has been defined as a paradoxical increase in systolic blood pressure within minutes of stopping exercise. Some authors have reported a greater extent of exercise-induced myocardial ischemia, left ventricular dysfunction, and more extensive coronary disease with this finding.[55] Other investigators have not found this response to enhance diagnostic accuracy as compared with exercise-induced ST-segment depression alone.

MAXIMAL WORK CAPACITY. This variable is one of the most important prognostic measurements obtained from an exercise test.[56-60] Maximal work capacity in normal individuals is influenced by familiarization with the exercise test equipment, level of training, and environmental conditions at the time of testing. In patients with known or suspected coronary artery disease, a limited exercise capacity is associated with an increased risk of cardiac events, and in general, the more severe the limitation, the worse the coronary disease extent and prognosis. In estimating functional capacity, the amount of work performed (or exercise stage achieved) should be the parameter measured and not the number of minutes of exercise. Estimates of peak functional capacity for age and gender have been well established for most of the exercise protocols in common usage, subject to the limitations described in the section on cardiopulmonary testing.[61,62] Comparison of an individual's performance against normal standards provides an estimate of the degree of exercise impairment. There is a rough correlation between observed peak functional capacity during exercise treadmill testing and estimates derived from clinical data and specific activity questionnaires.[61]

Serial comparison of functional capacity in individual patients to assess significant interval change requires a careful examination of the exercise protocol used during both tests, of drug therapy and time of ingestion, of systemic blood pressure, and of other conditions that might influence test performance. All these variables need to be considered before attributing changes in functional capacity to progression of coronary artery disease or worsening of left ventricular function. Major reductions in exercise capacity usually indicate significant worsening of cardiovascular status; modest changes may not.

SUBMAXIMAL EXERCISE. The interpretation of an exercise test for diagnostic and prognostic purposes requires consideration of maximum work capacity. When a patient is unable to complete moderate levels of exercise or reach at least 85 to 90 per cent of age-predicted maximum, the level of exercise performed may be inadequate to test cardiac reserve. Thus, ischemic ECG, scintigraphic, or ventriculographic abnormalities may not be evoked and the test may be nondiagnostic.[63] Nondiagnostic tests are more common in patients with peripheral vascular disease, orthopedic limitation, or neurological impairment and in patients with poor motivation.

HEART RATE RESPONSE. The sinus rate increases progressively with exercise, mediated in part through sympathetic and parasympathetic innervation of the sinoatrial node and circulating catecholamines. In some patients who may be anxious about the exercise test, there may be an initial overreaction of heart rate and systolic blood pressure at the beginning of exercise with stabilization after approximately 30 to 60 seconds. Maximum heart rate during exercise is

highest in childhood, decreases with age, and is slightly reduced in a trained athlete.

There are two types of abnormal heart rate responses to exercise. In patients with chronotropic incompetence, the heart rate increment per stage of exercise is less than normal and the heart rate may plateau at submaximal workloads.[12] This finding may indicate sinus node disease, may be present with drug therapy such as beta blockers, or may indicate a myocardial ischemic response. The second type of abnormal heart rate response is an inappropriate increase in heart rate of low exercise workloads. This response may occur in patients who are physically deconditioned, hypovolemic, or anemic or who have marginal left ventricular function and may persist for several minutes in the recovery phase.

RATE-PRESSURE PRODUCT. The heart rate–systolic blood pressure product, an indirect measure of myocardial oxygen demand (see p. 1162), increases progressively with exercise, and the peak rate pressure product can be used to characterize cardiovascular performance. Most normal subjects develop a peak rate pressure product of 20 to 35 mm $Hg \times beats/min \times 10^{-3}$. In many patients with significant ischemic heart disease, rate-pressure products exceeding 25 mm $Hg \times beats/min \times 10^{-3}$ are unusual. However, the cutpoint of 25 mm $Hg \times beats/min \times 10^{-3}$ is not a useful diagnostic parameter; significant overlap exists between patients with disease and those without disease. Furthermore, cardioactive drug therapy will significantly influence this measurement.

CHEST DISCOMFORT. Characterization of chest discomfort during exercise can be a useful diagnostic finding, particularly when the symptom complex is compatible with typical angina pectoris. In some patients, the exercise level during the test may exceed that which the patient exhibits in day-to-day activities. Exercise-induced chest discomfort usually occurs after the onset of ischemic ST-segment abnormalities and may be associated with diastolic hypertension.[55,64] However, in some patients, chest discomfort may be the only marker that obstructive coronary artery disease is present. In patients with chronic stable angina, exercise-induced chest discomfort occurs less frequently than ischemic ST-segment depression. The severity of myocardial ischemia in a patient with exercise-induced angina and a normal ECG can often be assessed using thallium scintigraphy. The new development of an S_3 holosystolic apical murmur or basilar rates in the early recovery phase of exercise will enhance the diagnostic accuracy of the test.

EXERCISE TESTING IN DETERMINING PROGNOSIS

ASYMPTOMATIC POPULATION. The prevalence of an abnormal exercise electrocardiogram in middle-aged asymptomatic men ranges from 5 to 12 per cent.[64-69] The risk of developing a cardiac event such as angina, myocardial infarction, or death in men is 9 times greater when the test is abnormal as when it is normal; however, over 5 years of follow-up, only one in four such men will suffer a cardiac event, and this will most commonly be the development of angina. The risk is slightly greater when the test is strongly positive. In the LRC Prevention Trial, a strongly positive test was defined as one in which the ST response was ≥ 2 mm (0.2 mV) or occurred during the first 6 minutes of exercise or at heart rate at or below $163 - 0.66 \times$ age. Of 3806 middle-aged asymptomatic men who had a total cholesterol ≥ 265 mg/dl at entry, 3 per cent had a strongly positive test; the event rate was 2 per cent per year over an average of 4 years of follow-up.[66] A positive test was *not* significantly associated with nonfatal myocardial infarction; this indicates the difficulty in identifying patients destined to develop abrupt changes in plaque morphology.

In the Seattle Heart Watch, Bruce noted that an abnormal ST response to exercise in asymptomatic men did *not* increase the likelihood of developing cardiac events within 6 years in the absence of conventional risk factors. However, the likelihood of developing a cardiac event was increased when the patient had any conventional atherosclerotic risk factor (see Chap. 35) and two or more abnormal responses to exercise, with an abnormal exercise response defined as chest discomfort during the test, exercise duration <6 minutes or two stages, failure to achieve 90 per cent of age-predicted maximum heart rate, or ≥1 mm (0.1 mV) of horizontal or downsloping ST depression with exercise in early recovery. Only 1.1 per cent of the asymptomatic healthy men in this study were in a high-risk category.[68] The lead set and criteria for an abnormal ECG response were different in both studies. In the Baltimore Longitudinal Study on Aging, Fleg et al. performed maximal treadmill exercise electrocardiography and thallium scintigraphy in 407 asymptomatic volunteers whose mean age was 60 years. The only combination of test results predictive of subsequent cardiac events occurred in the 6 per cent of patients who had *both* an abnormal exercise ECG and thallium scan; 48 per cent had a cardiac event over an average 4-year follow-up.[69]

In asymptomatic middle-aged or older men with several atherosclerotic risk factors, a markedly abnormal exercise response is associated with a significant increased risk of subsequent cardiac events, particularly when there is additional supporting evidence for underlying coronary artery disease (e.g., coronary calcification, abnormal thallium scan, and the like).[69,70] Serial change of a negative exercise ECG to a positive one in an asymptomatic subject carries the same prognostic importance as an initially abnormal test.[71] However, when an asymptomatic subject with an initially abnormal test has significant worsening of the ECG abnormalities at lower exercise workloads, this finding may indicate significant coronary artery disease progression and warrants a more aggressive diagnostic workup.

The prevalence of an abnormal exercise ECG in middle-aged asymptomatic women ranges from 20 to 30 per cent.[6,23] In general, the prognostic value of an ST segment shift in women is less than in men. However, there are few prognostic data on large series of asymptomatic women stratified by age and atherosclerotic risk factors.

SYMPTOMATIC PATIENTS. Exercise testing should be routinely performed (unless this is not feasible or unless there are contraindications) before coronary angiography in patients with chronic ischemic heart disease. Patients who have excellent exercise tolerance (e.g., >10 METs) usually have an excellent prognosis regardless of the anatomical extent of coronary artery disease. The test provides an estimate of the functional significance of angiographically documented coronary artery stenoses. The impact of exercise testing in patients with proven or suspected coronary artery disease was studied by Weiner et al. in 4083 medically treated patients in the CASS study.[72] A high-risk patient subset was identified (12 per cent of the population) with an annual mortality ≥5 per cent a year when exercise workload was <Bruce stage I and the exercise ECG exhibited ≥1 mm (0.1 mV) ST-segment depression. A low-risk patient subset (34 per cent of the population) able to exercise into ≥ Bruce stage III who had a normal exercise ECG had an annual mortality <1 per cent per year over 4 years of follow-up. Similar ECG and workload parameters were useful in risk stratifying patients with three-vessel coronary artery disease likely to benefit from coronary bypass grafting.[73]

Mark et al. developed a treadmill score based on 2842 consecutive patients in the Duke data bank with chest pain who had treadmill testing using the Bruce protocol and cardiac catheterization.[74] Patients with left bundle branch block or those with exercise-induced ST elevation in a Q wave lead were excluded. The treadmill score is calculated

as follows: exercise time – (5 × ST deviation) – (4 × treadmill angina index). Angina index was assigned a value of 0 if angina was absent, 1 if typical angina occurred during exercise, and 2 if angina was the reason the patient stopped exercising. Exercise-induced ST deviation was defined as the largest net ST displacement in any lead. The 13 per cent of patients with a treadmill score ≤ – 11 had a 5-year survival of 72 per cent compared with 97 per cent in the 34 per cent of patients at low risk with a treadmill score ≥ + 5. The score added independent prognostic information to that provided by clinical data, coronary anatomy, and left ventricular ejection fraction. The stratified annual mortality rates predicted from the treadmill score were less in 613 outpatients referred for exercise testing from the same institution[75] (Fig. 5–12).

Morrow et al. developed a treadmill score based on 2546 male veterans who underwent exercise testing for prognostic purposes and were followed for 2.75 years. The scoring system uses a history of congestive heart failure or digoxin use and three exercise test variables (exercise-induced ST-segment depression, peak exercise capacity, and change in systolic blood pressure). The scoring system identified 77 per cent of patients at low risk (annual cardiac mortality rate <2 per cent), 18 per cent at moderate risk (annual cardiac mortality rate 7 per cent), and 6 per cent at high risk (annual cardiac mortality rate 15 per cent)[76,77] (Fig. 5–13).

Exercise scoring systems can be used to identify prognostic, intermediate–high-risk patients in whom coronary angiography would be indicated to define coronary anatomy. In patients with less extensive coronary disease (e.g., one to two vessels narrowed) and well-preserved left ventricular function, a similar degree of exercise-induced myocardial ischemia does not carry the same significant increased risk of cardiac events as in patients with more extensive disease (e.g., three vessels narrowed) or those with impaired left ventricular function.[60,78–80]

SILENT MYOCARDIAL ISCHEMIA (see p. 1344). In patients with documented coronary artery disease, the presence of exercise-induced ischemic ST-segment depression confers increased risk of subsequent cardiac events regardless of whether angina occurs during the test.[25,81–85] Exercise-induced chest pain tends to lose its apparent value as a clinical predictor when its analysis is restricted to coronary artery disease populations with a greater a priori likelihood of manifesting inducible ischemia.[83] The magnitude of the prognostic gradient in patients with an abnormal exercise ECG with or without angina varies considerably in the published literature, most likely a feature of patient selection.[84,85] In the CASS data bank, 7-year survival in patients with silent or symptomatic exercise-induced myocardial ischemia was similar in patients stratified by coronary anatomy and left ventricular function.[84] In the Asymptomatic Cardiac Ischemia Pilot (ACIP) trial, coronary revascularization was a more effective treatment strategy to reduce exercise-induced myocardial ischemia than medical therapy.[25]

UNSTABLE ANGINA (see p. 1331). The incidence of exercise-induced angina or ischemic ST-segment abnormalities in patients with unstable angina who undergo a predischarge low-level protocol ranges from 30 to 40 per cent. The finding of ischemic ST-segment changes or limiting chest pain is associated with a significantly increased risk of subsequent cardiac events. The *absence* of these findings identifies a low-risk patient subset.[86–88] Exercise testing should be considered in the outpatient evaluation of low-risk patients with unstable angina and should be performed in hospitalized low-to-intermediate-risk ambulatory patients who are free of angina or heart failure symptoms for at least 48 hours.[88]

MYOCARDIAL INFARCTION (see also Ch. 37). A low-level exercise test (achievement of 5 to 6 METs or 70 to 80 per cent of age-predicted maximum) is frequently performed before hospital discharge to establish the hemodynamic re-

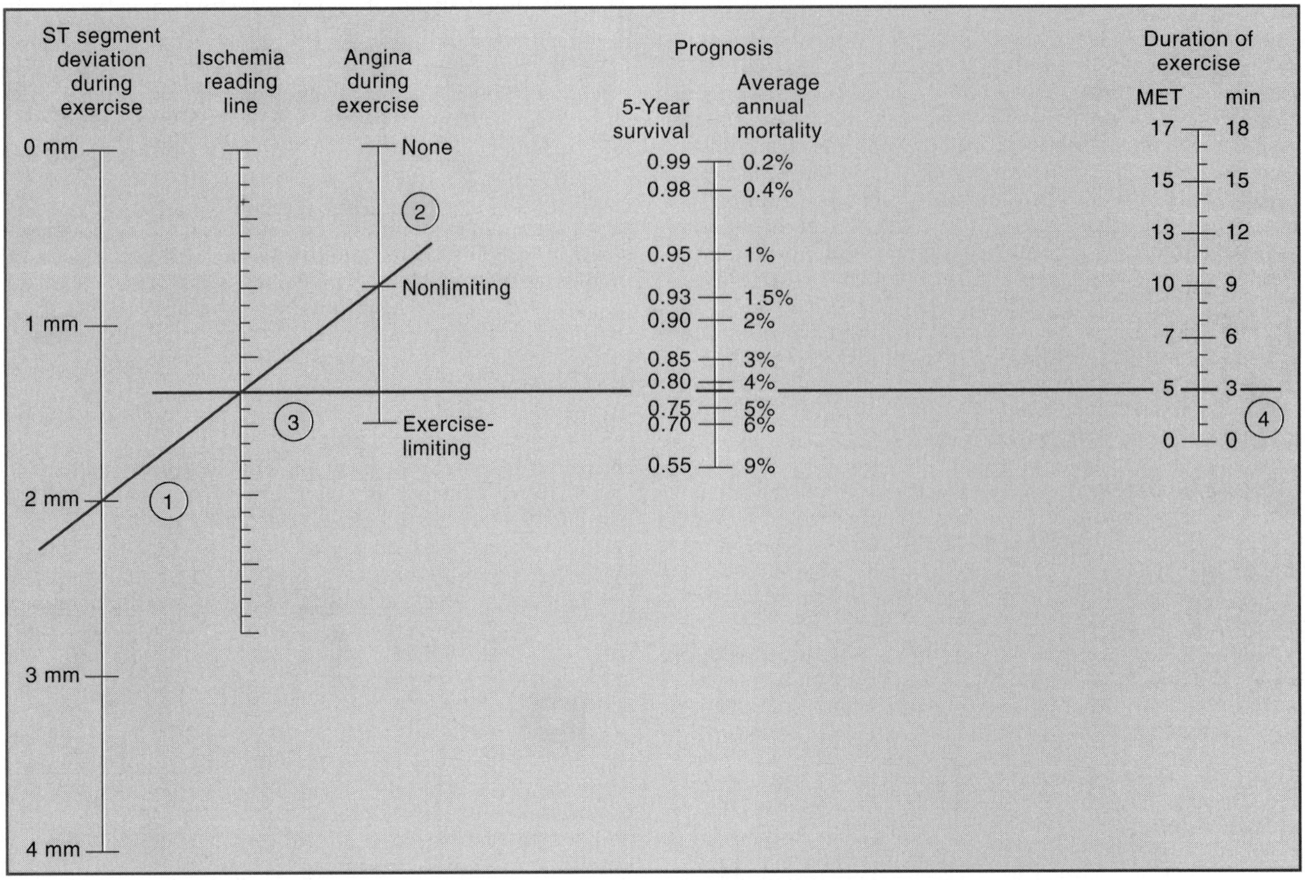

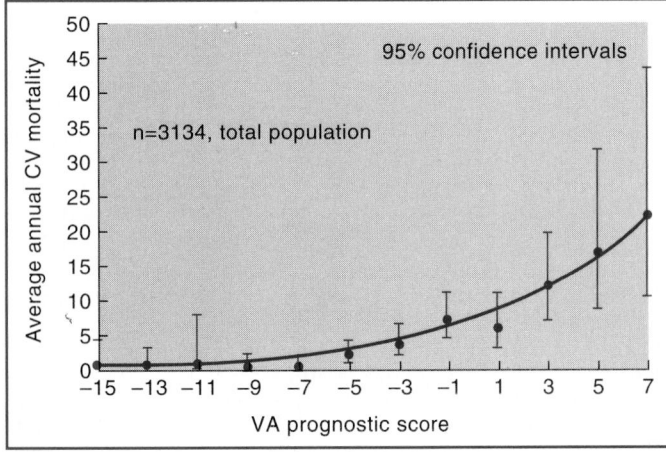

ST segment deviation during exercise	Ischemia reading line	Angina during exercise	Prognosis		Duration of exercise

FIGURE 5–12. Nomogram of prognostic relations using the Duke treadmill score, which incorporates duration of exercise (in minutes) − (5 × maximal ST segment deviation during or after exercise) (in mm) − (4 × treadmill angina index). Treadmill angina index is 0 for no angina, 1 for nonlimiting angina, and 2 for exercise limiting angina. The nomogram can be used to assess the prognosis of ambulatory outpatients referred for exercise testing. In this example, the observed amount of exercise-induced ST-segment deviation (minus resting changes) is marked on the line for ST-segment deviation during exercise (1). The degree of angina during exercise is plotted (2), and the points are connected. The point of intersect on the ischemia reading line is noted (3). The number of METs (or minutes of exercise if the Bruce protocol is used) is marked on the exercise duration line (4). The marks on the ischemia reading line and duration of exercise line are connected, and the intersect on the prognosis line determines 5-year survival rate and average annual mortality for patients with these selected specific variables. In this example the 5-year prognosis is estimated at 78 per cent in this patient with exercise-induced 2-mm ST-depression, nonlimiting exercise angina, and peak exercise workload of 5 METs. (Adapted from Mark, D. B., et al.: Prognostic value of a treadmill exercise score in outpatients with suspected coronary artery disease. N. Engl. J. Med. *325*:849, 1991. Copyright Massachusetts Medical Society.)

FIGURE 5–13. Plot of average cardiovascular mortality against the Veterans Affairs Prognostic Score including 95 per cent confidence intervals. A score of less than − 2 is associated with an annual cardiac mortality rate of less than 2 per cent per year. (Reproduced with permission from Froelicher, V., et al.: Prediction of atherosclerotic cardiovascular death in men using a prognostic score. Am. J. Cardiol. *73*:133, 1994.)

sponse and functional capacity for exercise prescriptions, to identify serious ventricular arrhythmia, and to identify patients at increased risk of cardiac events.[37,89–95] The ability to complete 5 to 6 METs of exercise or 70 to 80 per cent of age-predicted maximum in the absence of abnormal ECG or blood pressure abnormalities is associated with a 1-year mortality of 1 to 2 per cent[6,37,60] (Fig. 5–14). Parameters associated with increased risk include inability to perform the low-level predischarge exercise test, poor exercise capacity, inability to increase or a decrease in exercise systolic blood pressure, and angina or exercise-induced ST-segment depression at low workloads.[37,60,90] The prognostic importance of painless ST-segment depression in postinfarct patients able to complete a low-level predischarge exercise test is less than in patients unable to complete the protocol.[91,93,95] The prognostic importance of exercise-induced ST-segment changes is influenced by the fact that many patients who have an abnormal test undergo coronary angiography and revascularization, which may alter the natural history of the disease process.[56] The performance of a predischarge maximum, symptom-limited test as opposed to a submaximal low-level test is gaining in popularity and is associated with an increased incidence of ischemic ST-segment depression and angina.[89] However, the

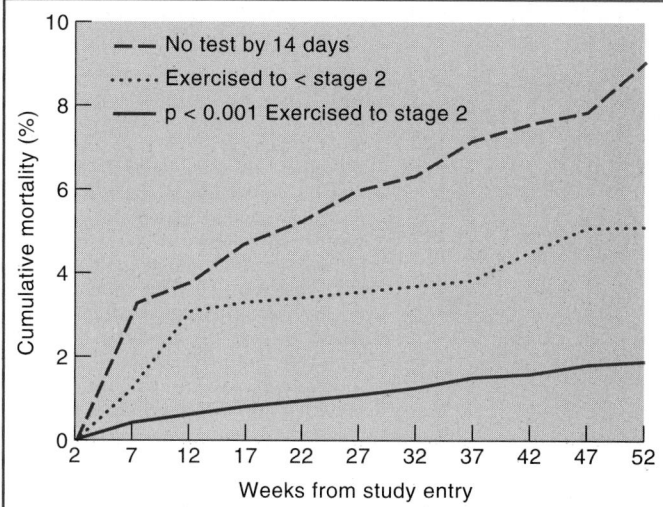

The additional value of exercise testing in patients with a left ventricular ejection fraction < 35 per cent by gated radionuclide scans 1 month after acute myocardial infarction was examined by Pilote et al.[97] Patients with an exercise capacity < 4 METs have a 3.5-fold greater risk of dying than patients with an exercise capacity ≥ 7 METs.

FIGURE 5–14. One-year mortality of patients assigned to the conservative strategy enrolled in the Thrombolysis in Myocardial Infarction (TIMI) II trial. All patients were treated with thrombolytic therapy within 4 hours of symptom onset. Patients unable to perform the exercise test were compared with individuals able to complete 200 kpm (< stage II) or 200 to 400 kpm (stage II) on a supine bicycle ergometry study performed within 2 weeks of the index event. Although the absolute mortality rates are less than patient series studied in the prethrombolytic era, a similar gradient of worsening prognosis is noted in patients unable to perform the low-level exercise test within 2 weeks of the index event, patients able to perform the test but unable to complete the protocol, and patients able to complete the low-level exercise test. (Reproduced with permission from Chaitman, B. R.: Impact of treatment strategy on predischarge exercise test in the Thrombolysis in Myocardial Infarction (TIMI) II trial. Am. J. Cardiol. 71:131, 1993.)

safety and incremental increase in prognostic information in this approach require further study.

The relative prognostic value of a 6-week postdischarge exercise test is minimal once clinical variables and the results of the low-level predischarge test are adjusted for. For this reason, the timing of the exercise test after the infarct event favors predischarge exercise testing to allow implementation of a definitive treatment plan in patients in whom coronary anatomy is known as well as risk stratification of patients in whom coronary anatomy has not yet been determined.[37,92] A 6-week test is useful in clearing patients to return to work in occupations involving physical labor and to provide a better estimate of cardiovascular reserve at peak exercise performance.

The goals and basic principles of the predischarge evaluation have not been changed by the advent of reperfusion or direct PTCA therapy for acute infarction. The patient's clinical presentation and course during hospitalization are required to determine the indications for testing and to determine prognostic estimates.[37,95–98] After receiving intravenous thrombolytic therapy, uncomplicated myocardial infarct patients tend to exhibit exercise-induced angina and ST-segment depression less frequently than in consecutive postinfarct patients before thrombolysis was widely applied.[37] The indication to perform exercise testing in patients who have undergone coronary angiography or revascularization during hospital admission is to define the patient's functional status as part of the rehabilitation process and detect residual ischemia from incomplete revascularization or reocclusion of the infarct vessel. In the Primary Angioplasty Myocardial Infarct (PAMI) trial, a predischarge modified Bruce test was positive in 9 per cent of patients who received thrombolytic therapy versus 3 per cent of patients who received direct coronary angioplasty.[96] Left ventricular ejection fraction is one of the most important prognostic determinants of mortality following acute myocardial infarction (see also pp. 1238 and 1260).

CARDIAC ARRHYTHMIAS AND CONDUCTION DISTURBANCES

The genesis of cardiac arrhythmias includes reentry, delayed afterpotentials, and enhanced automaticity of ectopic foci (Chap. 20). Increased catecholamines during exercise accelerate impulse conduction velocity, shorten the myocardial refractory period, increase the amplitude of delayed afterpotentials, and increase the slope of phase 4 spontaneous depolarization of the action potential. Other potentiators of cardiac rhythm disturbance include metabolic acidosis and exercise-induced myocardial ischemia.[99] Ventricular premature beats occur frequently during exercise testing and increase with age.[100] Repetitive forms occur in 0 to 5 per cent of asymptomatic subjects without suspected cardiac disease and are not associated with an increased risk of cardiac death. Exercise-induced ventricular ectopic activity is not a useful diagnostic marker of ischemic heart disease in the absence of ischemic ST-segment depression. Suppression of ventricular ectopic activity during exercise is a nonspecific finding and may occur in patients with coronary artery disease as well as in normal subjects. The prognostic importance of ventricular arrhythmias in patients with chronic ischemic heart disease after adjustment for baseline, clinical, and left ventricular function characteristics is small.[101] Approximately 20 per cent of patients with known heart disease and 50 to 75 per cent of sudden cardiac death survivors have repetitive ventricular beats induced by exercise. In patients with a recent myocardial infarction, the presence of exercise-induced repetitive forms is associated with an increased risk of subsequent cardiac events.

Exercise-induced ventricular arrhythmias tend to be more frequent in the recovery phase of exercise because peripheral plasma norepinephrine levels continue to increase for several minutes after cessation of exercise and vagal tone is high in the immediate recovery phase. Beta-adrenergic blocking drugs may suppress exercise-induced ventricular arrhythmias. Continuous recording of the exercise test will enhance documentation of the cardiac arrhythmia.

EVALUATION OF VENTRICULAR ARRHYTHMIAS (see also Chap. 22). Exercise testing is useful in the assessment of patients with ventricular arrhythmias and has an important adjunctive role along with ambulatory monitoring and electrophysiological studies. Exercise testing provokes repetitive ventricular premature beats in most patients with a history of sustained ventricular tachyarrhythmia, and in approximately 10 to 15 per cent of such patients, spontaneously occurring arrhythmias are observed only during exercise testing (Fig. 5–15). The test is useful in the evaluation of the effects of antiarrhythmic drugs, the detection of supraventricular arrhythmias, the management of patients with chronic atrial fibrillation, and exposing possible drug toxicity in patients placed on antiarrhythmic drugs. Paradoxical prolongation of the QT_C interval ≥ 10 msec with exercise identifies patients likely to develop a proarrhythmic effect on type 1A antiarrhythmic drugs.[101] Exercise-induced widening of the QRS complex in patients using type 1C drugs may favor reentry induction of ventricular tachycardia.

SUPRAVENTRICULAR ARRHYTHMIAS. Supraventricular premature beats induced by exercise are observed in 4 to 10 per cent of normal subjects and up to 40 per cent of patients with underlying heart disease. Sustained supraven-

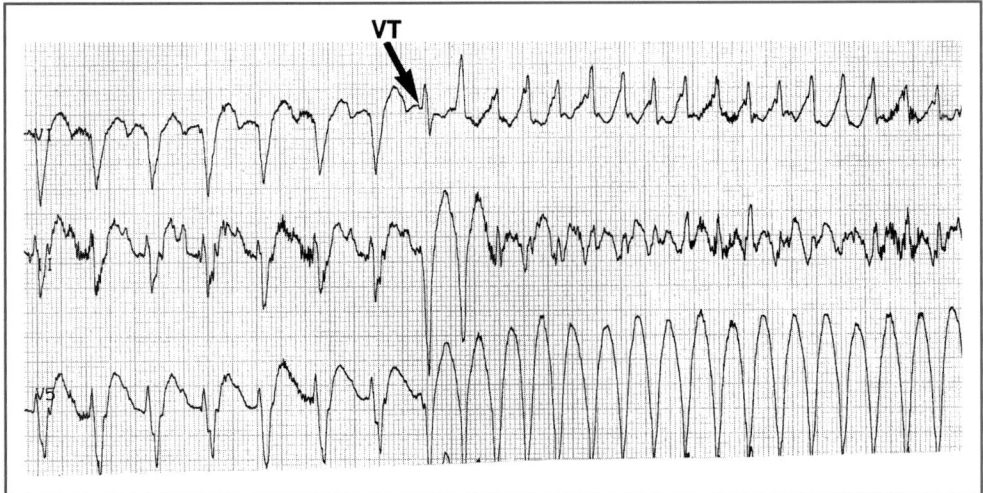

FIGURE 5–15. A 67-year-old man with ischemic cardiomyopathy referred for exercise testing had a left bundle branch block and first-degree AV block on the resting ECG. There was no worsening of the AV conduction disturbance immediately prior to ventricular tachycardia (VT) onset (arrow). At 4:55 minutes into the test, a 27-beat run of VT was noted, reproducing the patient's symptoms of dizziness and chest pounding. The exercise test proved useful in directing subsequent patient management to treatment of the ventricular arrhythmia.

tricular tachyarrhythmias occur in only 1 to 2 per cent of patients, although the frequency may approach as much as 10 to 15 per cent in patients referred for management of episodic supraventricular arrhythmias. The presence of supraventricular arrhythmias is not diagnostic for ischemic heart disease.

ATRIAL FIBRILLATION (see p. 654). Patients with chronic atrial fibrillation tend to have a rapid ventricular response in the initial stages of exercise and 60 to 70 per cent of the total change in heart rate usually occurs within the first few minutes of exercise (Fig. 5–16). The effect of digitalis preparations and beta-adrenergic and calcium antagonists on attenuating this rapid increase in heart rate for individual patients can be measured using exercise testing. Pharmacological control of the ventricular rate does not necessarily result in a significant increase in exercise capacity, which in many patients is related to the underlying cardiac disease process and not adequacy of control of the ventricular rate.

SICK SINUS SYNDROME (see p. 648). In general, patients with sick sinus syndrome have a lower heart rate at submaximal and maximal workloads compared with control subjects. However, as many as 40 to 50 per cent of patients will have a normal exercise heart rate response.

AV BLOCK. Exercise testing may help determine the need for AV sequential pacing in selected patients. In patients with congenital AV block, exercise-induced heart rates are

low and some patients develop symptomatic rapid junctional rhythms which can be suppressed with DDD devices. In patients with acquired conduction disease, exercise can occasionally bring out advanced AV block.

LEFT BUNDLE BRANCH BLOCK (LBBB) (see also p. 119). Exercise-induced ST-segment depression is seen in most patients with LBBB and cannot be used as a diagnostic or prognostic indicator regardless of the degree of ST-segment abnormality. In patients referred to a tertiary center in whom exercise testing is carried out, the new development of exercise-induced transient left hemiblock is 0.3 per cent and left bundle branch block is 0.4 per cent, with a slightly greater incidence in older patients.[102] The development of ischemic ST-segment depression before the LBBB pattern appears or in the recovery phase after the LBBB has resolved does not attenuate the diagnostic yield of the ST-segment shift. The ventricular rate at which the LBBB appears and disappears can be significantly different (Fig. 5–17). In one series, permanent LBBB was reported in approximately half the patients who developed transient LBBB during exercise and who were followed for an average 6.6 years. High-grade AV block did not develop in any of the patients in this 15-patient series.[103]

RIGHT BUNDLE BRANCH BLOCK (RBBB). The resting ECG in RBBB is frequently associated with T wave and ST segment changes in the early anterior precordial leads (V_1 to V_3). Exercise-induced ST depression in leads V_1 to V_4 is a com-

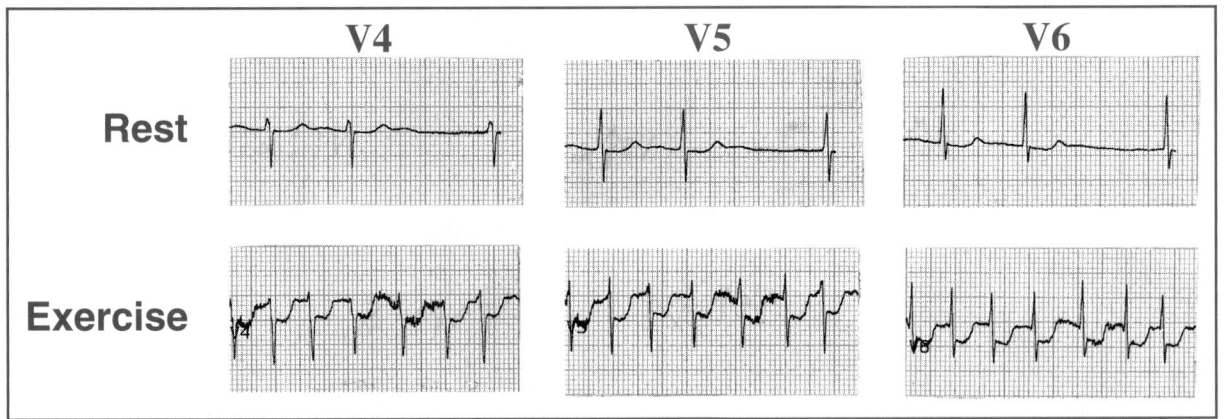

FIGURE 5–16. A 75-year-old woman with chronic atrial fibrillation and a 6-month history of atypical chest pain underwent mitral valve repair 1 year before testing, at which time nonobstructive coronary disease was noted. The patient exercised for 6 minutes, achieving a peak heart rate of 176 beats/min and peak blood pressure of 170/90 mm Hg. The resting ECG shows atrial fibrillation with a controlled ventricular response and minor ST-segment depression. At peak exertion, marked ST-segment depression is seen in the anterior leads, consistent with either digitalis effect or myocardial ischemia. In this type of patient, initial exercise testing with myocardial perfusion tracers or echocardiography would provide more useful diagnostic information than exercise testing alone.

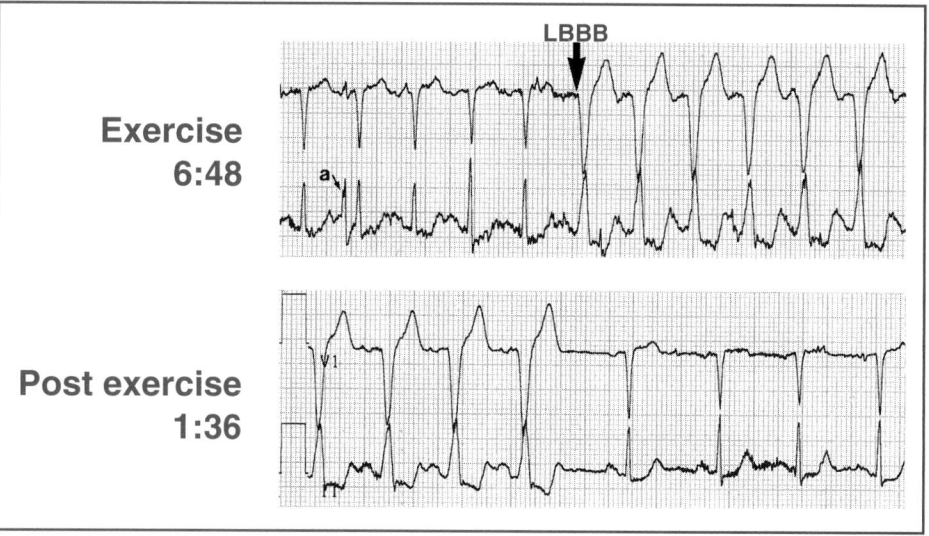

FIGURE 5–17. A 58-year-old hypertensive diabetic man with prior history of cigarette smoking was referred for evaluation of dyspnea and early fatigability during exercise. At 6:48 min into the test the patient developed a rate-related left bundle branch block (LBBB) at a heart rate of 133 beats/min which persisted during exercise and resolved at 1:36 min into the postexercise phase. The test was stopped because of dyspnea at a peak heart rate of 138 beats/min (85 per cent of predicted) and estimated workload of 6 METs. Peak blood pressure at end exercise was 174/94 mm Hg. Time to onset and offset of LBBB occurred at different ventricular rates related to fatigue in the left bundle, a common finding.

mon finding in patients with RBBB and is nondiagnostic. The new development of exercise-induced ST-segment depression in leads V_5 and V_6, reduced exercise capacity, and inability to adequately increase systolic blood pressure are useful in detecting patients with coronary artery disease who have a high clinical pretest risk of disease. The presence of RBBB decreases the sensitivity of the test.[104] The new development of exercise-induced RBBB is relatively uncommon, occurring in approximately 0.1 per cent of tests.

PREEXCITATION SYNDROME (see p. 693). The presence of WPW syndrome invalidates the use of ST-segment analysis as a diagnostic method for detecting coronary artery disease in preexcited as well as normally conducted beats; false-positive ischemic changes are frequently registered (Fig. 5–18). In patients with persistent preexcitation, exercise may normalize the QRS complex with disappearance of the delta wave in 20 to 50 per cent of cases dependent on the series studied.[105] Abrupt disappearance of the delta wave is presumptive evidence of a longer anterograde effective refractory period of the accessory pathway. Progressive disappearance of the delta wave is less reassuring and occurs when the improvement in AV node conduction is greater than in the accessory pathway; this finding does not exclude a possible significant or even critical shortening of the anterograde effective refractory period in the accessory pathway under the influence of sympathetic stimulation. Exercise-induced disappearance of the delta wave is more frequent with type A than type B WPW patterns. Although tachyarrhythmias appearing during an exercise test in pa-

tients with WPW are rare, when they do occur, they provide an opportunity to evaluate AV conduction velocity. The presence of WPW does not cause a limitation of physical work capacity.

SPECIFIC CLINICAL APPLICATIONS

WOMEN (see also Chap. 51). The specificity of exercise-induced ST-segment depression for obstructive coronary artery disease is less in women than in men. The decreased diagnostic accuracy results in part from a lower prevalence and extent of coronary artery disease in young and middle-aged women.[106] Women tend to have a greater release of catecholamines during exercise, which could potentiate coronary vasoconstriction and augment the incidence of abnormal exercise ECGs, and false-positive tests have been reported to be more common during menses or preovulation.[107]

The increased false-positive rate in women may potentiate gender differences in the use of follow-up diagnostic testing in women who have an initially abnormal noninvasive stress test result. In an 840-patient series evaluated for clinically suspect coronary disease using noninvasive tests, 62 per cent of women compared with only 38 per cent of men with an initial abnormal test result did not go on for additional diagnostic testing, even though the rates of initial abnormal test results were similar in both[108] (Fig. 5–19). Additional research to determine optimal diagnostic and prognostic algorithms for women is needed.[109]

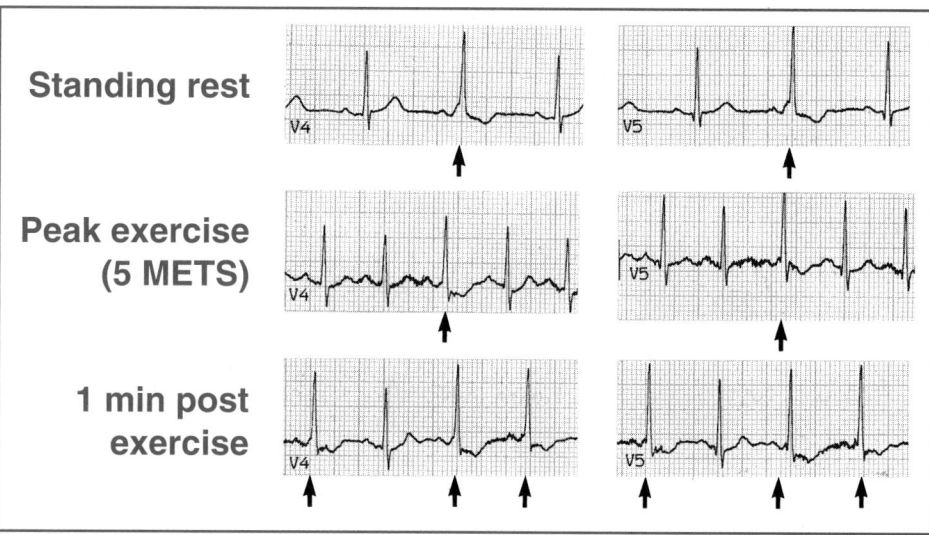

FIGURE 5–18. A 61-year-old man with atypical angina and a hiatal hernia was referred for diagnostic exercise testing. The test was stopped because of dyspnea. The standing rest ECG shows an intermittent WPW pattern (arrows). In the non-preexcited beats, ST-segment depression does not occur either at peak exercise or in the postexercise phase. However, in the preexcited beats (arrows) an additional 1.3 mm of downsloping ST-segment depression is noted as compared with baseline during and after exertion.

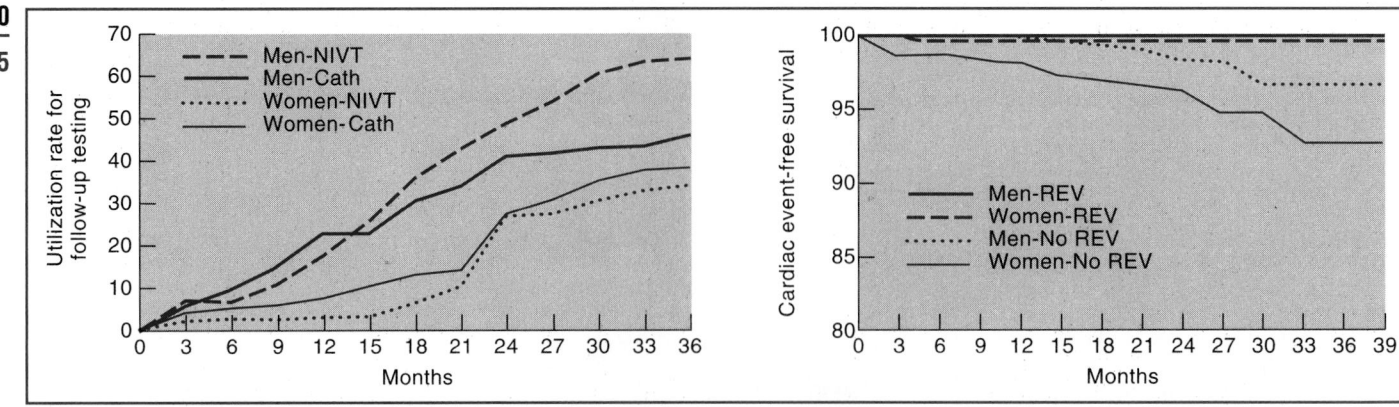

FIGURE 5–19. *Left panel,* A gender-based comparison of noninvasive test use rates over time. A greater percentage of men with initially abnormal test results received follow-up noninvasive testing (NIVT) compared with women (*p* < 0.001). Similarly, a comparison of use of coronary arteriography during the 2-year follow-up period showed that a greater percentage of men than women subsequently had catheterization (cath) (*p* < 0.001). *Right panel,* Cardiac events by gender. Patients who were revascularized (REV) had better cardiac event–free survival (*p* < 0.001). In patients with REV, cardiac events were more frequent in women. (From Shaw, L. J., et al.: Gender differences in the noninvasive evaluation and management of patients with suspected coronary artery disease. Ann. Intern. Med. *120:*559, 1994.)

HYPERTENSION. Exercise testing has been used in an attempt to identify patients with abnormal blood pressure response destined to subsequently develop hypertension. The optimal exercise protocol, and consensus on what constitutes an abnormal exercise response, requires additional study.[9] Different criteria may be required for blacks and whites, men and women, and younger versus older patients.[50] Severe systemic hypertension may interfere with subendocardial perfusion and cause exercise-induced ST-segment depression in the absence of atherosclerosis, even when the rest ECG does not show significant ST- or T-wave changes.[110] Beta and calcium channel blocking drugs decrease submaximal and peak systolic blood pressure in many hypertensive patients.

CONGESTIVE HEART FAILURE. Cardiac and peripheral compensatory mechanisms are activated in patients with chronic congestive heart failure to partly or fully restore impaired left ventricular performance.[108–112] There is a wide range of exercise capacity in patients who have a markedly reduced ejection fraction, with some patients having near-normal peak exercise capacity.[14] Symptoms in patients with congestive heart failure are related to an excessive increase in blood lactate during low exercise levels, reduction in quantity of oxygen consumed at peak exertion, and disproportionate increase in ventilation at submaximal and peak workloads. The increased ventilatory requirement assessed by the hyperventilatory response to exercise and increase in pulmonary dead space leads to rapid and shallow breathing during exercise. Fatigue may be related to altered skeletal muscle metabolism secondary to chronic physical deconditioning as well as impaired perfusion.[116] Dyspnea and fatigue are the usual reasons for exercise termination. Peak $\dot{V}_{O_2}$ measurements in patients with compensated congestive heart failure are useful in risk stratifying patients with congestive heart failure to determine subsequent incidence of cardiac events (Fig. 5–20). The ability to achieve a peak $\dot{V}_{O_2}$ of > 20 ml/min/kg and AT_{ge} > 14 ml/min/kg is associated with a relatively good long-term prognosis and a maximum cardiac output > 8 liters/min/m². Patients who are unable to achieve a peak $\dot{V}_{O_2}$ of 10 ml/min/kg and AT_{ge} of 8 ml/min/kg have a poor prognosis, and their maximum exercise cardiac output is usually < 4 liters/min/m². Failure of $\dot{V}_{O_2}$ to decrease within 30 sec after peak exertion is associated with more severe reductions in left ventricular ejection fraction and moderate to severe impairment of pulmonary gas exchange. Inability to increase oxygen pulse is related to lack or minimal increase of stroke volume. A blunted heart rate response is not uncommon in patients

with congestive heart failure caused by postsynaptic desensitization of beta-adrenergic receptors[12,111] (see p. 411).

Exercise protocols that limit exercise duration to 5 to 7 minutes are associated with the most reproducible peak $\dot{V}_{O_2}$ measurements in patients with heart failure. The interpretation of cardiopulmonary exercise tests in patients with heart failure can occasionally be difficult, because some patients hyperventilate during exercise, producing falsely low peak oxygen consumption, and it can be difficult to distinguish patients who are deconditioned from those who have impaired exercise performance and low peak $\dot{V}_{O_2}$ due to cardiac pathology. A 6-minute walk test also can be used to evaluate functional capacity in patients unable to exercise on a bicycle ergometer or treadmill.[27]

DRUGS. Digitalis glycosides can produce exertional ST segment depression even if the effect is not evident on the resting ECG and can accentuate ischemic exercise-induced ST segment changes (see p. 500). Absence of ST-segment deviation during an exercise test in a patient receiving a cardiac glycoside is considered a valid negative response. Hypokalemia in patients on long-term diuretic therapy may be associated with exercise-induced ST-segment depression. Antiischemic drug therapy with nitrates, beta-blocking drugs, or calcium channel blocking drugs will prolong the time to onset of ischemic ST-segment depression, increase exercise tolerance, and, in a small minority of patients (10 to 15 per cent), may normalize the exercise ECG response in patients with documented coronary artery disease.[6,23,25,117] The time and dose of drug ingestion may affect exercise performance. In some laboratories, cardioactive drug therapy is withheld for 3 to 5 half-lives and digitalis for 1 to 2 weeks before diagnostic testing. However, this is impractical in many cases. Heparin therapy may increase total exercise duration and ability to achieve a higher rate pressure product before the onset of angina, and at peak exertion.[118] The onset of ischemic ST-segment depression in patients with chronic ischemic heart disease occurs earlier in patients who are cold sensitive and who are exposed to low levels of carbon monoxide.[119,120] Amiodarone therapy increases the QRS duration during exercise by approximately 6 per cent in patients with a QRS duration < 110 msec compared with 15 per cent in patients with a QRS duration > 110 msec.[121]

CORONARY REVASCULARIZATION PROCEDURES. The degree of improvement in exercise-induced myocardial ischemia and aerobic capacity after coronary bypass grafting depends in part on the degree of revascularization achieved and left ventricular function.[25,59] Exercise-induced ischemic ST-seg-

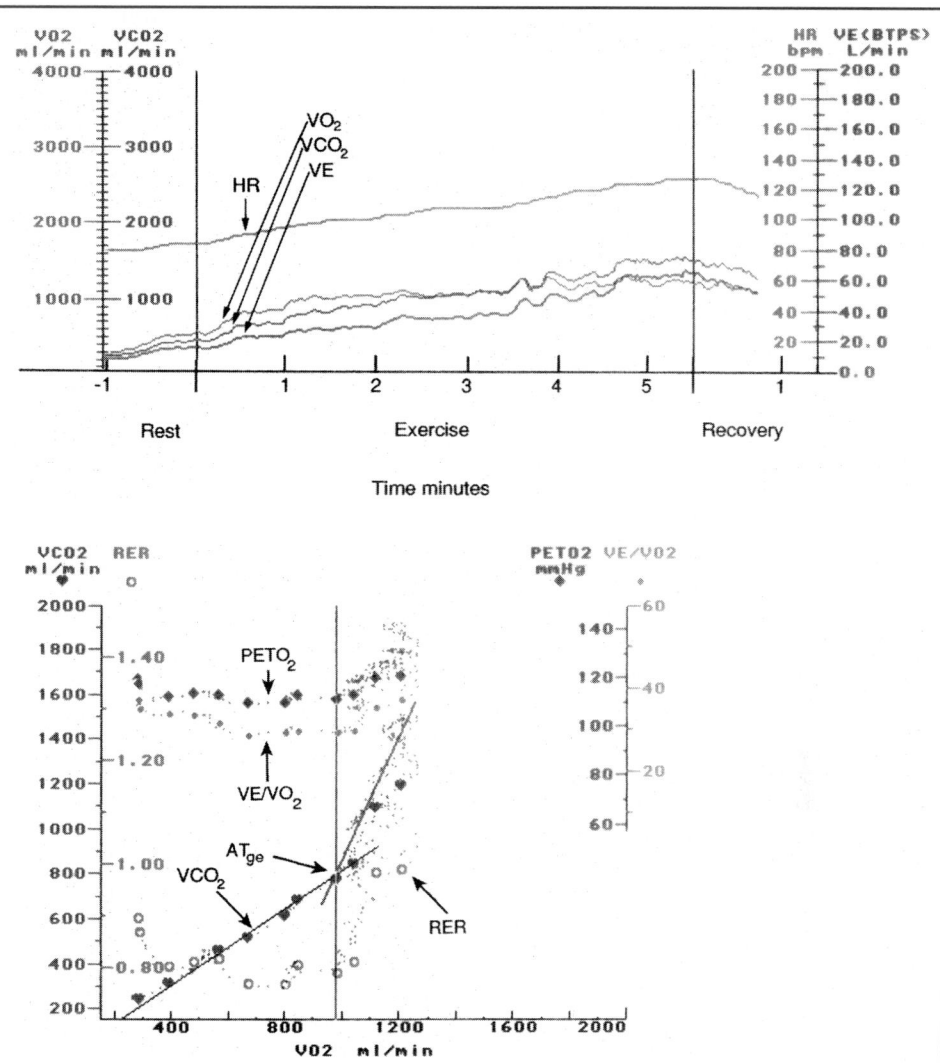

FIGURE 5–20. Cardiopulmonary exercise test in a 51-year-old man with cardiomyopathy in NYHA class III. A modified Bruce protocol was used. The patient reached a peak $\dot{V}_{O_2}$ of 14 ml/min/kg (4 METs), 44 per cent of predicted for age, size, and weight *(top panel)*. Anaerobic threshold (AT_{ge}) occurred at a $\dot{V}_{O_2}$ of 977 ml/min *(bottom panel)*. The blunted cardiopulmonary response is typical for a patient with severe cardiomyopathy and marked impairment of cardiac reserve. This patient was listed for cardiac transplantation.

ment depression may persist when incomplete revascularization is achieved, albeit at higher exercise workloads, and in approximately 5 per cent of patients in whom complete revascularization has been achieved.[122–124] It usually takes at least 6 weeks of convalescence before maximum exercise can be performed. The natural history of saphenous vein grafts and internal mammary artery conduits is different, and serial conversion from an initially normal to abnormal exercise ECG over time will depend in part on the type of conduit used and coronary disease progression in nongrafted vessels. The diagnostic and prognostic utility of exercise testing late after coronary revascularization (e.g., 5 to 10 years) is much greater than early (< 1 year) testing, since a late abnormal exercise response is more likely to indicate graft occlusion, stenosis, or progression of coronary artery disease.

After coronary angioplasty (PTCA), restenosis occurs in approximately 20 to 40 per cent of patients, usually within the first 6 months, and is more common in patients with proximal LAD disease, long coronary artery narrowings, diabetic patients, patients with multivessel or multilesion dilation, and those in whom post PTCA luminal obstruction is > 50 per cent. In the early post-PTCA phase (< 1 month) an abnormal exercise ECG may be secondary to a suboptimal PTCA result, impaired coronary vascular reserve in a successfully dilated vessel, or incomplete revascularization.[125] The optimal time to perform an exercise test following PTCA depends in part on the success of the procedure and the degree of revascularization obtained. Exercise testing early after PTCA (within days) often can be used to help determine the need for a staged procedure and to

provide a reference baseline for subsequent follow-up. In an otherwise asymptomatic patient, a 6-month postprocedure test allows a sufficient amount of time to document restenosis should it occur and allows the dilated vessel an opportunity to heal. In the absence of significant epicardial stenosis after PTCA, exercise-induced ST-segment depression may be associated with the presence of preprocedure regional left ventricular dysfunction that has recovered during follow-up.[126] Serial conversion of an initially normal exercise test post PTCA to an abnormal test in the initial 6 months after the procedure, particularly when it occurs at a lower exercise workload, is usually associated with restenosis. The use of thallium scintigraphy in selected patients enhances greatly the diagnostic content of the test and can help localize the territory of myocardial ischemia and guide indications for repeat coronary angiography in patients who have undergone multivessel/multilesion PTCA.

CARDIAC TRANSPLANTATION (see also Chap. 18). Cardiopulmonary exercise testing is useful in selecting patients with end-stage heart failure for cardiac transplantation. A peak oxygen uptake of less than 12 to 14 ml/kg/min or 40 to 50 per cent of predicted $\dot{V}_{O_2}$ is associated with 2-year survival rates of approximately 32 per cent. In patients awaiting heart transplantation, with initial poor exercise capacity, ability to increase peak oxygen uptake with increased peak oxygen pulse identifies a relatively lower-risk group in whom cardiac transplantation may be able to be deferred if the patient's clinical status is stable (Fig. 5–21).[129] Exercise performance in post-transplant recipients is influenced by the fact that the donor heart is surgically denervated without efferent parasympathetic or sympa-

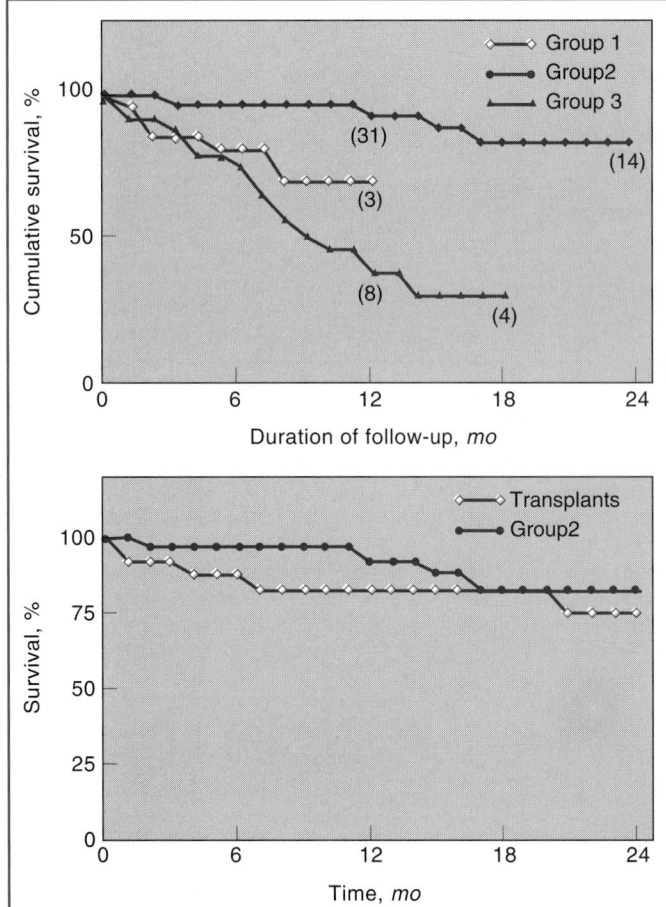

FIGURE 5–21. Cardiopulmonary exercise testing enhances the selection process for congestive heart failure patients considered for cardiac transplantation. The 2-year survival of 122 patients with an average ejection fraction of 19 per cent considered for heart transplantation was analyzed according to peak oxygen uptake ($\dot{V}_{O_2}$) and ability to reach anaerobic threshold *(top panel).* The survival of 35 patients accepted for cardiac transplantation with a peak $\dot{V}_{O_2}$ of 14 ml/kg/min or less (group 1) is compared with that of 52 patients for whom transplantation was considered unnecessary because of a peak $\dot{V}_{O_2} > 14$ ml/kg/min (group 2) and 27 patients with a peak $\dot{V}_{O_2}$ of 14 ml/kg/min or less rejected for transplantation because of noncardiac problems (group 3). *Bottom panel:* Group 2 patients had cumulative 1- to 2-year survival rates of 94 and 84 per cent, respectively, similar to survival levels after transplantation. Group 3 patients (not shown) had survival rates of only 47 and 32 per cent at 1 and 2 years, respectively. The data indicate that cardiac transplantation can be deferred safely in ambulatory patients with moderate-to-severe left ventricular dysfunction and a peak $\dot{V}_{O_2}$ of > 14 ml/kg/min. (Adapted with permission from Mancini, D. M.: Value of peak exercise oxygen consumption for optimal timing of cardiac transplantation in ambulatory patients with heart failure. Circulation 83:778, 1991. Copyright 1991 American Heart Association.)

thetic innervation and by the occurrence of rejection and scar formation, donor-recipient size mismatch, systemic and pulmonary vascular resistance, and development of coronary atherosclerosis in the graft.[127,128] Maximum oxygen uptake and work capacity are reduced after cardiac transplantation compared with age-matched controls but are usually markedly improved compared with preoperative findings. Abnormalities of the ventricular rate response include a resting tachycardia due to parasympathetic denervation, a slow heart rate response during mild-to-moderate exercise, a more rapid response during more strenuous exercise, and a more prolonged time for the ventricular rate to return to baseline during recovery. The transplanted heart relies heavily on the Frank-Starling mechanism to increase cardiac output during mild-to-moderate exercise. Systemic vascular resistance may be increased because of

cyclosporine therapy. The exercise electrocardiogram is relatively insensitive to detect coronary artery vasculopathy after cardiac transplantation.[130,131] However, the new development of an abnormal exercise ECG several years following cardiac transplantation may indicate focal intraluminal narrowing.

VALVULAR HEART DISEASE (see also Chap. 32). The hemodynamics of exercise provide an excellent opportunity to measure gradients across stenotic valves, to assess ventricular function in patients with primary valvular regurgitation or mixed lesions, and to assess pulmonary and systemic vascular resistance. The use of echocardiographic Doppler techniques is particularly valuable in evaluating patients whose symptoms are out of proportion to the degree of valvular disease observed and in assessing the results of valvulotomy or valve replacement.[132] Clinical and exercise noninvasive assessment of patients with valvular heart disease can provide very useful information on the timing of operative intervention and help achieve a more precise estimate of a patient's degree of incapacitation than can assessment of symptoms alone.[133]

CARDIAC PACEMAKERS (see also Chap. 23). The exercise protocol used to assess chronotropic responsiveness in patients before and after cardiac pacemaker insertion should adjust for the fact that many such patients are older individuals and may not tolerate high exercise workloads or abrupt and relatively large increments in work between stages of exercise. An optimal physiological cardiac pacemaker should normalize the heart rate response to exercise in proportion to oxygen uptake and increase heart rate 2 to 4 beats/min for an increase in $\dot{V}_{O_2}$ of 1 ml/min/kg, with a slightly steeper slope for patients with severe left ventricular function impairment.[134,135]

ELDERLY PATIENTS (see also Chap. 50). The exercise protocol in elderly patients should be selected according to estimated aerobic capacity. In patients with limited exercise tolerance, the test should be started at the slowest speed with a 0 per cent grade and adjusted according to the patient's ability. Older patients may need to grasp the handrails for support. Limited exercise tolerance is to be expected in many persons ≥ 80 years old. The frequency of abnormal exercise ECG patterns is greater in older than younger individuals, and the risk of cardiac events is significantly increased because of a concomitant increase in prevalence of more extensive coronary disease.[136,137]

Termination of Exercise

The use of standard test indications to terminate an exercise test will reduce risk (Table 5–5). Termination of exercise should be determined in part by the patient's recent activity level. The rate of perceived patient exertion can be estimated by the Borg scale (Table 40–2, p. 1396).[138] The

TABLE 5–5 INDICATIONS FOR TERMINATING EXERCISE TEST

Severe fatigue or dyspnea
Ataxia
Grade III/IV chest pain
Ischemic ST-segment depression ≥ 3.0 mm
Ischemic ST-segment elevation ≥ 1 mm in a non-Q wave lead
Unsuspected appearance of ventricular tachycardia
Ectopic supraventricular tachycardia
Progressive reproducible decrease in systolic blood pressure
Abnormal elevation of systolic blood pressure
Decreasing heart rate
Technical problems interfering with ECG or blood pressure interpretation

scale is linear with values of 7, very, very light; 9, very light; 11, fairly light; 13, somewhat hard; 15, hard; 17, very hard; and 19, very, very hard. Borg readings of 14 to 16 approximate anaerobic threshold, and readings ≥ 18 approximate a patient's maximum exercise capacity. Ataxia may indicate cerebral hypoxia. It is helpful to grade exercise-induced chest discomfort on a 1 to 4 scale, with 1 indicating the initial onset of chest discomfort and 4 the most severe chest pain the patient has ever experienced. The exercise technician should note the onset of grade 1 chest discomfort on the worksheet, and the test should be stopped when the patient reports grade 3 chest pain. In the absence of symptoms, it is prudent to stop exercise when a patient demonstrates ≥ 3 mm (0.3 mV) of ischemic ST-segment depression or ≥ 1 mm (0.1 mv) of ST-segment elevation in a lead without an abnormal Q wave. Significant worsening of ambient ventricular ectopy during exercise or the unsuspected appearance of ventricular tachycardia is an indication to terminate exercise. A progressive, reproducible decrease in systolic blood pressure of 10 mm Hg or more may indicate transient left ventricular dysfunction or an inappropriate decrease in systemic vascular resistance and is an indication to terminate exercise. The test should be stopped if the arterial blood pressure is ≥ 250 to 270/ 120–130 mm Hg.

A resuscitory cart and defibrillator should be available in the room where the test procedure is carried out and appropriate cardioactive medication available to treat cardiac arrhythmias, atrioventricular block, hypotension, and persistent chest pain. An intravenous line should be started in high-risk patients such as those being tested for adequacy of control of life-threatening ventricular arrhythmias. The equipment and supplies in the cart should be checked on a regular basis. A previously specified routine for cardiac emergencies needs to be determined which includes patient transfer and admission to a coronary care unit if necessary.

Clinical judgment is required to determine which patients can be tested safely in an office as opposed to a hospital-based setting. High-risk patients, such as those with evident left ventricular dysfunction, severe angina pectoris, history of cardiac syncope, and significant ambient ventricular ectopy on the pretest examination, should be tested in the hospital. Low-risk patients, such as asymptomatic subjects and those with a low pretest risk of disease, may be tested by specially trained nurses or physician assistants who have received ACLS certification, *with a physician in close proximity.*[139]

The exercise test report should contain basic demographic data, the indication for testing, a brief description of the patient profile, and exercise test results (Table 5–6).

TABLE 5–6 EXERCISE TEST REPORT INFORMATION

1. **Demographic data: name, patient identifier, date of birth/ age, gender, weight, height, test date**
2. **Indication(s) for test**
3. **Patient descriptors: atherosclerotic risk profile, drug usage, resting ECG findings**
4. **Exercise test results**
   a. **Protocol used**
   b. **Reason(s) for stopping exercise**
   c. **Hemodynamic data: rest and peak heart rate, rest and peak blood pressure, per cent maximum achieved heart rate, maximum rate of perceived exertion (Borg scale), peak workload, peak METs, total exercise duration in minutes**
   d. **Evidence for myocardial ischemia: time to onset and offset of ischemic ST-segment deviation or angina, maximum depth of ST-segment deviation, number of abnormal exercise ECG leads, abnormal systemic blood pressure response**
5. **General comments**

TABLE 5–7 CONTRAINDICATIONS TO EXERCISE TESTING

173

Ch 5

Unstable angina with recent rest pain
Untreated life-threatening cardiac arrhythmias
Uncompensated congestive heart failure
Advanced atrioventricular block
Acute myocarditis or pericarditis
Critical aortic stenosis
Severe hypertrophic obstructive cardiomyopathy
Uncontrolled hypertension
Acute systemic illness

Safety and Risks of Exercise Testing

Exercise testing has an excellent safety record. The risk is determined by the clinical characteristics of the patient referred for the procedure. In nonselected patient populations, the mortality is < 0.01 per cent and morbidity < 0.05 per cent.[140] The risk is greater when the test is performed soon after an acute ischemic event. In a survey of 151,941 tests conducted within 4 weeks of an acute myocardial infarction, mortality was 0.03 per cent, and 0.09 per cent of patients had either a nonfatal reinfarction or were resuscitated from cardiac arrest.[141] The relative risk of a major complication is about twice as great when a symptom-limited protocol is used as compared with a low-level protocol. Nevertheless, in the early postinfarction phase, the risk of a fatal complication during symptom-limited testing is only 0.03 per cent. The use of exercise testing as a screening procedure for low-risk patients who present to the emergency room with atypical angina or typical angina who have a normal ECG or minimal ST- and T-segment abnormalities at rest needs to be evaluated further in larger patient series. In a study of 93 patients who had a negative initial total CK and were considered clinically low risk, no complications of exercise testing were observed as a result of early exercise testing.[142] Exercise testing can be performed safely in patients with compensated congestive heart failure, with no major complications reported in 1286 tests in which a bicycle ergometer was used.[143] The risk of exercise testing in patients referred for life-threatening ventricular arrhythmias was examined by Young et al.[144] in a series of 263 patients who underwent 1377 tests; 2.2 per cent developed sustained ventricular tachyarrhythmias that required cardioversion, cardiopulmonary resuscitation, or antiarrhythmic drugs to restore sinus rhythm. The ventricular arrhythmias were more frequent in tests performed on antiarrhythmic drug therapy as compared with the baseline drug-free state.[144] In contrast to the high risk in the aforementioned patient subsets, the risk of complications in asymptomatic subjects is extremely low, with no fatalities reported in several series.[66,139]

The risk of incurring a major complication during exercise testing can be reduced by performing a careful history and physical examination before the test and observing the patient closely during exercise with monitoring of the electrocardiogram, arterial pressure, and symptoms. The standard 12-lead ECG should be verified before the test for any acute or recent change. There are well-defined contraindications to exercise testing (Table 5–7). After an episode of unstable angina, patients should be free of rest pain, of other evidence of ischemia, or of heart failure for at least 48 to 72 hours before testing. After an uncomplicated acute myocardial infarction, it is wise to wait at least 4 to 6 days before testing. Patients with critical obstruction to left ventricular outflow are at increased risk of cardiac events during exercise. In selected patients, low-level exercise can be quite useful in determining the severity of the left ventricular outflow tract gradient. The "cool-down" period should be prolonged to at least 2 minutes in patients with stenotic valves or those who have exertional hypotension, to avoid sudden pressure-volume shifts that occur in the immediate postexercise phase.

Uncontrolled systemic hypertension is a contraindication to exercise testing. Patients who present with systemic arterial pressure readings of $\geq 220/120$ mm Hg should rest for 15 to 20 minutes and the blood pressure should be remeasured. If blood pressure remains at these levels, the test should be postponed until the hypertension is better controlled.

REFERENCES

EXERCISE TESTING FOR CARDIAC DISEASE

1. Feil, H., and Siegel, M. L.: Electrocardiographic changes during attacks of angina pectoris. Am. J. Med. Sci. 175:255, 1928.
2. Master, A. M., and Oppenheimer, E. T.: A simple exercise tolerance test for circulatory efficiency with standard tables for normal individuals. Am. J. Med. Sci. 177:223, 1929.
3. Guyton, A. C.: Textbook of Medical Physiology. 9th ed. Philadelphia, W. B. Saunders Company, 1995.
4. Pina, I. L., Balady, G. J., Hanson, P., et al: Guidelines for clinical exercise testing laboratories. A statement for healthcare professionals from the Committee on Exercise Cardiac Rehabilitation, American Heart Association. Circulation 91:912, 1995.
5. Froelicher, V. F.: Manual of Exercise Testing. 2nd ed. St. Louis, Mosby–Year Book, 1994.
6. Froelicher, V. F., Myers, J., Follansbee, W. P., and Labovitz, A. J.: Exercise and the Heart. 3rd ed. St. Louis, Mosby–Year Book, 1993.
7. ESC Working Group on Exercise Physiology, Physiopathology and Electrocardiography: Guidelines for cardiac exercise testing. Eur. Heart J. 14:969, 1993.
8. Gordon, N. F., Kohl, H. W., Scott, C. B., et al.: Reassessment of the guidelines for exercise testing. What alterations to current recommendations are required? Sports Med. 13:293, 1992.
9. Washington, R. L., Bricker, J. T., Alpert, B. S., et al.: Guidelines for exercise testing in the pediatric age group. From the Committee on Atherosclerosis and Hypertension in Children, Council on Cardiovascular Disease in Young, the American Heart Association. Circulation 90:2166, 1994.
10. Fletcher, G. F., Balady, G., Froelicher, V. F., et al.: Exercise standards. A statement for healthcare professionals from the American Heart Association. Circulation 91:580, 1995.

EXERCISE PHYSIOLOGY

11. Fleg, J. L., Schulman, S., O'Connor, F., et al.: Effects of acute β-adrenergic receptor blockade on age-associated changes in cardiovascular performance during dynamic exercise. Circulation 90:2333, 1994.
12. Imai, K., Sato, H., Hori, M., et al.: Vagally mediated heart rate recovery after exercise is accelerated in athletes but blunted in patients with chronic heart failure. J. Am. Coll. Cardiol. 24:1529, 1994.
13. Wasserman, K., Hansen, J. E., Sue, D. Y., et al.: Principles of Exercise Testing and Interpretation. 2nd ed. Philadelphia, Lea and Febiger, 1994.
14. Smith, R. F., Johnson, G., Ziesche, S., et al.: Functional capacity in heart failure: Comparison of methods for assessment and their relation to other indexes of heart failure. The V-HeFT VA Cooperative Studies Group. Circulation 87:VI88, 1993.
15. Weber, K. T., Janicki, J. S., McElroy, P. A., and Reddy, H. K.: Concepts and applications of cardiopulmonary exercise testing. Chest 93:843, 1988.
16. Wasserman, K., Beaver, W. L., and Whipp, B. J.: Gas exchange theory and the lactic acidosis (anaerobic) threshold. Circulation 81:II-14, 1990.
17. Norton, L. H., Squires, B., Craig, N. P., et al.: Accuracy of pulse oximetry during exercise stress testing. Int. J. Sports Med. 13:523, 1992.
18. Cohen-Solal, A., Aupetit, J. F., Gueret, P., et al.: Can anaerobic threshold be used as an end-point for therapeutic trials in heart failure? Lessons from a multicentre randomized placebo-controlled trial. The $\dot{V}_{O_2}$ French Study Group. Eur. Heart J. 15:236, 1994.
19. Eliasson, A. H., Phillips, Y. Y., Rajagopal, K. R., and Howard, R. S.: Sensitivity and specificity of bronchial provocation testing: An evaluation of four techniques in exercise-induced bronchospasm. Chest 102:347, 1992.
20. Berdeaux, A., Ghaleh, B., Dubois-Rande, J. L., et al.: Role of vascular endothelium in exercise-induced dilation of large epicardial coronary arteries in conscious dogs. Circulation 89:2799, 1994.
21. Kaufmann, P., Vassalli, G., Utzinger, U., and Hess, O. M.: Coronary vasomotion during dynamic exercise: Influence of intravenous and intracoronary nicardipine. J. Am. Coll. Cardiol. 26:624, 1995.
22. Balady, G. J., Weiner, D. A., Rose, L., and Ryan, T. J.: Physiology responses to arm ergometry exercise relative to age and gender. J. Am. Coll. Cardiol. 16:130, 1990.
23. Ellestad, M. H.: Stress Testing: Principles and Practice. 4th ed. Philadelphia, F. A. Davis Co., 1995.
24. Tamesis, B., Stelken, A., Byers, S., et al.: Comparison of the Asymptomatic Cardiac Ischemia Pilot and modified Asymptomatic Cardiac Ischemia Pilot versus Bruce and Cornell exercise protocols. Am. J. Cardiol. 72:715, 1993.
25. Chaitman, B. R., Stone, P. H., Knatterud, G. L., et al.: Asymptomatic Cardiac Ischemia Pilot (ACIP) study: Impact of anti-ischemia therapy on 12-week rest ECG and exercise test outcomes. J. Am. Coll. Cardiol. 26:585, 1995.
26. Blair, S. N., Gibbons, L. W., Painter, P., Pate, R. R., Taylor, C. B., and Will, J.: Guidelines for Exercise Testing and Prescriptions. 3rd ed. Philadelphia, Lea and Febiger, 1986.
27. Bittner, V., Weiner, D. H., Yusuf, S., et al.: Prediction of mortality and morbidity with a 6-minute walk test in patients with left ventricular dysfunction. JAMA 270:1702, 1993.
28. Lachterman, B., Lehmann, K. G., Abrahamson, D., and Froelicher, V. F.: "Recovery only" ST-segment depression and the predictive accuracy of the exercise test. Ann. Intern. Med. 112:11, 1990.

DIAGNOSTIC TESTING

29. Mark, D. B., Hlatky, M. A., Lee, K. L., Harrell, F. E., Califf, R. M., and Pryor, D. B.: Localizing coronary artery obstructions with the exercise treadmill test. Ann. Intern. Med. 106:53, 1987.
30. Caralis, D. G., Shaw, L., Bilgere, B., et al.: Application of computerized exercise ECG digitization: Interpretation in large clinical trials. J. Electrocardiogr. 25:101, 1992.
31. Kubota, I., Yamaki, M., Shibata, T., et al.: Role of ATP-sensitive K^+ channel on ECG ST segment elevation during a bout of myocardial ischemia: A study on epicardial mapping in dogs. Circulation 88:1845, 1993.
32. Schlant, R. C., Blonqvist, C. G., Brandenburg, R. O., et al.: Guidelines for exercise testing: A report of the Joint American College of Cardiology–American Heart Association Task Force on Assessment of Cardiovascular Procedures (Subcommittee on Exercise Testing). Circulation 74 (Suppl. III): 653a, 1986.
33. Shaw, L. J., Younis, L. T., Stocke, K. S., et al.: Effects of posture on metabolic and hemodynamic predischarge exercise response after acute myocardial infarction. Am J. Cardiol. 66:134, 1990.
34. Couhan, L., Krone, R. J., Keller, A., and Eisenkramer, G.: Utility of lead V_4R in exercise testing for detection of coronary artery disease. Am. J. Cardiol. 64:938, 1989.
35. Gianrossi, R., Detrano, R., Mulvihill, D., et al.: Exercise-induced ST depression in the diagnosis of coronary artery disease: A meta-analysis. Circulation 80:87, 1989.
36. Detrano, R., Gianrossi, R., Mulvihill, D., et al.: Exercise-induced ST segment depression in the diagnosis of multivessel coronary disease: A metaanalysis. J. Am. Coll. Cardiol. 14:1501, 1989.
37. Mark, D. B., and Froelicher, V. F.: Exercise treadmill testing and ambulatory monitoring. In Califf, R. M., Mark, D. B., and Wagner, G. S. (eds.): Acute Coronary Care. St. Louis, Mosby–Year Book, 1995, p. 767.
38. Patterson, R. E., and Horowitz, S. F.: Importance of epidemiology and biostatistics in deciding clinical strategies for using diagnostic tests: A simplified approach using examples from coronary artery disease: J. Am. Coll. Cardiol. 13:1653, 1989.
39. Chauhan, A., Mullins, P. A., Petch, M. C., and Schofield, P. M.: Is coronary flow reserve in response to papaverine really normal in syndrome X? Circulation 89:1998, 1994.
40. Folland, E. D., Vogel, R. A., Hartigan, P., et al.: Relation between coronary artery stenosis assessed by visual, caliper, and computer methods and exercise capacity in patients with single-vessel coronary artery disease. Circulation 89:2005, 1994.
41. Kern, M. J., Donohue, T. J., Aguirre, F. V., et al.: Clinical outcome of deferring angioplasty in patients with normal translesional pressure-flow velocity measurements. J. Am. Coll. Cardiol. 25:178, 1995.
42. Pryor, D. B., Shaw, L., McCants, C. B., et al.: Value of the history and physical in identifying patients at increased risk for coronary artery disease. Ann. Intern. Med. 118:81, 1993.
43. Detrano, R., Leatherman, J., Salcedo, E. E., et al.: Bayesian analysis versus discriminant function analysis: Their relative utility in the diagnosis of coronary disease. Circulation 73:970, 1986.
44. Chaitman, B. R.: The changing role of the exercise electrocardiogram as a diagnostic and prognostic test for chronic ischemic heart disease. J. Am. Coll. Cardiol. 8:1195, 1986.
45. Bruce, R. A., Fisher, L. D., Pettinger, M., et al.: ST segment elevation with exercise: A marker for poor ventricular function and poor prognosis. Coronary Artery Surgery Study (CASS) confirmation of Seattle Heart Watch results. Circulation 77:897, 1988.
46. Chikamori, T., Yamada, M., Takata, J., et al.: Exercise-induced prominent U waves as a marker of significant narrowing of the left circumflex or right coronary artery. Am. J. Cardiol. 74:495, 1994.
47. Kligfield, P., Ameisen, O., and Okin, P. M.: Heart rate adjustment of ST segment depression for improved detection of coronary artery disease. Circulation 79:245, 1989.
48. Kligfield, P., Okin, P. M., and Goldberg, H. L.: Value and limitations of heart rate–adjusted ST segment depression criteria for the identification of anatomically severe coronary obstruction: Test performance in relation to method of ST correction, definition of extent of disease, and β-blockade. Am. Heart J. 125:1262, 1993.
49. Lachterman, B., Lehmann, K. G., Detrano, R., et al.: Comparison of ST segment/heart rate index to standard ST criteria for analysis of exercise electrocardiogram. Circulation 82:44, 1990.
50. Ekelund, L. G., Suchindran, C. M., Karon, J. M., et al.: Black-white differences in exercise blood pressure. Circulation 31:1568, 1990.
51. White, W. B., Lund-Johansen, P., and Omvik, P.: Assessment of four

ambulatory blood pressure monitors and measurements by clinicians versus intraarterial blood pressure at rest and during exercise. Am. J. Cardiol. 65:60, 1990.

52. Lele, S. S., Scalia, G., Thomson, H., et al.: Mechanism of exercise hypotension in patients with ischemic heart disease: Role of neurocardiogenically mediated vasodilation. Circulation 90:2701, 1994.

53. Derman, W. E., Sims, R., and Noakes, T. D.: The effects of antihypertensive medications on the physiological response to maximal exercise testing. J. Cardiovasc. Pharmacol. 19:S122, 1992.

54. Fleg, J. L., and Lakatta, E. G.: Prevalence and significance of postexercise hypotension in apparently healthy subjects. Am. J. Cardiol. 57:1380, 1986.

55. Hashimoto, M., Okamoto, M., Yamagata, T., et al.: Abnormal systolic blood pressure response during exercise recovery in patients with angina pectoris. J. Am. Coll. Cardiol. 22:659, 1993.

EXERCISE TESTING DETERMINING PROGNOSIS

56. Chaitman, B. R., McMahon, R. P., Terrin, M., et al.: Impact of treatment strategy on predischarge exercise test in the Thrombolysis in Myocardial Infarction (TIMI) II trial. Am. J. Cardiol. 71:131, 1993.

57. Morris, C. K., Ueshima, K., Kawaguchi, T., et al.: The prognostic value of exercise capacity: A review of the literature. Am. Heart J. 122:1423, 1991.

58. Stevenson, L. W., Steimle, A. E., Fonarow, G., et al.: Improvement in exercise capacity of candidates awaiting heart transplantation. J. Am. Coll. Cardiol. 25:163, 1995.

59. Vanhees, L., Fagard, R., Thijs, L., et al.: Prognostic significance of peak exercise capacity in patients with coronary artery disease. J. Am. Coll. Cardiol. 23:358, 1994.

60. Younis, L. T., and Chaitman, B.R.: The prognostic value of exercise testing. Cardiol. Clin. 11:229, 1993.

61. Myers, J., Do, D., Herbert, W., et al.: A nomogram to predict exercise capacity from a specific activity questionnaire and clinical data. Am. J. Cardiol. 73:591, 1994.

62. Morris, C. K., Myers, J., Froelicher, V. F., et al.: Nomogram based on metabolic equivalents and age for assessing aerobic exercise capacity in men. J. Am. Coll. Cardiol. 22:175, 1993.

63. Iskandrian, A. S., Heo, J., Kong, B., and Lyons, E.: Effect of exercise level on the ability of thallium-201 tomographic imaging in detecting coronary artery disease: analysis of 461 patients. J. Am. Coll. Cardiol. 14:1477, 1989.

64. McCance, A. J., and Forfar, J. C.: Selective enhancement of the cardiac sympathetic response to exercise by anginal chest pain in humans. Circulation 80:1642, 1989.

66. Ekelund, L. G., Suchindran, C. M., McMahon, R. P., et al.: Coronary heart disease morbidity and mortality in hypercholesterolemic men predicted from an exercise test: The Lipid Research Clinics Coronary Primary Prevention Trial. J. Am. Coll. Cardiol. 14:556, 1989.

67. Rautaharju, P. M., Prineas, R. J., Eifler, W. J., et al.: Prognostic value of exercise electrocardiogram in men at high risk of future coronary heart disease: Multiple Risk Factor Intervention Trial experience. J. Am. Coll. Cardiol. 8:1, 1986.

68. Bruce, R. A., and Fisher, L. D.: Exercise-enhanced assessment of risk factors for coronary heart disease in healthy men. J. Electrocardiol. (Suppl. October) 20:162, 1987.

69. Fleg, J. L., Gerstenblith, G., Zonerman, A. B., et al.: Prevalence and prognostic significance of exercise-induced silent myocardial ischemia detected by thallium scintigraphy and electrocardiography in asymptomatic volunteers. Circulation 81:428, 1990.

70. Fagan, L. F., Shaw, L., Kong, B. A., et al.: Prognostic value of exercise thallium scintigraphy in patients with good exercise tolerance and a normal or abnormal exercise electrocardiogram and suspected or confirmed coronary artery disease. Am. J. Cardiol. 69:607, 1992.

71. Josephson, R. A., Shefrin, E., Lakatta, E. G., et al.: Can serial exercise testing improve the prediction of coronary events in asymptomatic individuals? Circulation 81:20, 1990.

72. Weiner, D. A., Ryan, T. J., McCabe, C. H., et al.: Prognostic importance of a clinical profile and exercise test in medically treated patients with coronary artery disease. J. Am. Coll. Cardiol. 3:772, 1984.

73. Weiner, D. A., Ryan, T. J., McCabe, C. H., et al.: Value of exercise testing in determining the risk classification and the response to coronary artery bypass grafting in three-vessel coronary artery disease: A report from the Coronary Artery Surgery Study (CASS) registry. Am. J. Cardiol. 60:262, 1987.

74. Mark, D. B., Hlatky, M. A., Harrell, F. E., et al.: Exercise treadmill score for predicting prognosis in coronary artery disease. Ann. Intern. Med. 106:793, 1987.

75. Mark, D. B., Shaw, L., Harrell, F. E. Jr., et al.: Prognostic value of a treadmill exercise score in outpatients with suspected coronary artery disease. N. Engl. J. Med. 325:849, 1991.

76. Morrow, K., Morris, C. K., Froelicher, V. F., et al.: Prediction of cardiovascular death in men undergoing noninvasive evaluation for coronary artery disease. Ann. Intern. Med. 118:689, 1993.

77. Froelicher, V., Morrow, K., Brown, M., et al.: Prediction of atherscolerotic cardiovascular death in men using a prognostic score. Am. J. Cardiol. 73:133, 1994.

78. Chang, J., Atwood, J. E., and Froelicher, V.: Prognostic impact of myocardial ischemia. J. Am. Coll. Cardiol. 23:225, 1994.

79. Miller, T. D., Christian, T. F., Taliercio, C. P., et al.: Severe exercise-induced ischemia does not identify high risk patients with normal left

ventricular function and one- or two-vessel coronary artery disease. J. Am. Coll. Cardiol. 23:219, 1994.

80. Quyyumi, A. A., Panza, J. A., Diodati, J. G., et al.: Prognostic implications of myocardial ischemia during daily life in low risk patients with coronary artery disease. J. Am. Coll. Cardiol. 21:700, 1993.

81. Hecht, H. S., DeBord, L., Sotomayor, N., et al.: Truly silent ischemia and the relationship of chest pain and ST segment changes to the amount of ischemic myocardium: Evaluation by supine bicycle stress echocardiography. J. Am. Coll. Cardiol. 21:369, 1994.

82. Benhorin, J., Pinsker, G., Moriel, M., et al.: Ischemic threshold during two exercise testing protocols and during ambulatory electrocardiographic monitoring. J. Am. Coll. Cardiol. 22:671, 1993.

83. Klein, J., Chao, S. Y., Berman, D. S., and Rozanski, A.: Is "silent" myocardial ischemia really as severe as symptomatic ischemia? The analytical effect of patient selection biases. Circulation 89:1958, 1994.

84. Weiner, D. A., Ryan, T. J., McCabe, C. H., et al.: Significance of silent myocardial ischemia during exercise testing in patients with coronary artery disease. Am. J. Cardiol. 59:725, 1987.

85. Mark, D. B., Hlatky, M. A., Califf, R. M., et al.: Painless exercise ST deviation on the treadmill: Long-term prognosis. J. Am. Coll. Cardiol. 14:885, 1989.

86. Nyman, I., Larsson, H., Areskog, J., et al. and the RISC Study Group: The predictive value of silent ischemia at an exercise test before discharge after an episode of unstable coronary artery disease. Am. Heart J. 123:324, 1992.

87. Fruergaard, P., Launbjerg, J., Jacobsen, H. L., and Madsen, J. K.: Seven-year prognostic value of the electrocardiogram at rest and an exercise test in patients admitted for, but without, confirmed myocardial infarction. Eur. Heart J. 14:499, 1993.

88. U.S. Department of Health and Human Services, Public Health Service Agency for Health Care Policy and Research, National Heart, Lung and Blood Institute: Clinical Practice Guideline. Unstable Angina: Diagnosis and Management. AHCPR Publication No. 94-0602, Number 10, March 1994.

89. Juneau, M., Colles, P., Theroux, P., et al.: Symptom-limited versus low level exercise testing before hospital discharge after myocardial infarction. J. Am. Coll. Cardiol. 20:927, 1992.

90. Froelicher, E. S.: Usefulness of exercise testing shortly after acute myocardial infarction for predicting 10-year mortality. Am. J. Cardiol. 74:318, 1994.

91. Khoury, Z., Keren, A., and Stern, S.: Correlation of exercise-induced ST depression in precordial electrocardiographic leads after inferior wall acute myocardial infarction with thallium-201 stress scintigraphy, coronary angiography and two-dimensional echocardiography. Am. J. Cardiol. 73:868, 1994.

92. Morgan, C. D., Gent, M., Daly, P. A., et al.: Graded exercise testing following thrombolytic therapy for acute myocardial infarction: The importance of timing and infarct location. Can. J. Cardiol. 10:897, 1994.

93. Moss, A. J., Goldstein, R. E., Hall, J., et al.: Detection and significance of myocardial ischemia in stable patients after recovery from an acute coronary event. J.A.M.A. 269:2379, 1993.

94. Stevenson, R., Umachandran, V., Ranjadayalan, K., et al.: Reassessment of treadmill stress testing for risk stratification in patients with acute myocardial infarction treated by thrombolysis. Br. Heart J. 70:415, 1993.

95. Arnold, A. E. R., Simoons, M. L., Detry, J. M. R., et al.: Prediction of mortality following hospital discharge after thrombolysis for acute myocardial infarction: Is there a need for coronary angiography? Eur. Heart J. 14:306, 1993.

96. Grines, C. L., Browne, K. F., Marco, J., et al.: A comparison of immediate angioplasty with thrombolytic therapy for acute myocardial infarction: The Primary Angioplasty in Myocardial Infarction Study Group. N. Engl. J. Med. 328:673, 1993.

97. Pilote, L., Silberberg, J., Lisbona, R., and Sniderman, A.: Prognosis in patients with low left ventricular ejection fraction after myocardial infarction. Circulation 80:1636, 1989.

98. Aguirre, F. V., McMahon, R. P., Mueller, H., et al.: Impact of age on clinical outcome and postlytic management strategies in patients treated with intravenous thrombolytic therapy: Results from the TIMI II study. Circulation 90:78, 1994.

99. Buckingham, T. A., and Chaitman, B. R.: Stress testing. In Zipes, D. P., and Rowlands, D. J. (eds.): Progress in Cardiology. Philadelphia, Lea and Febiger, 1988, p. 289.

100. Busby, M. J., Shefrin, E. A., and Fleg, J. L.: Prevalence and long-term significance of exercise-induced frequent or repetitive ventricular ectopic beats in apparently healthy volunteers. J. Am. Coll. Cardiol. 14:1659, 1989.

101. Kadish, A. H., Weisman, H. F., Veltri, E. P., et al.: Paradoxical effects of exercise on the QT interval in patients with polymorphic ventricular tachycardia receiving type 1a antiarrhythmic agents. Circulation 81:14, 1990.

CLINICAL APPLICATIONS

102. Williams, M. A., Esterbrooks, D. J., Nair, C. K., et al.: Clinical significance of exercise-induced bundle branch block. Am. J. Cardiol. 61:346, 1988.

103. Heinsimer, J. A., Irwin, J. M., and Basnight, L. L.: Influence of underlying coronary artery disease on the natural history and prognosis of exercise-induced left bundle branch block. Am. J. Cardiol. 60:1065, 1987.

104. Yen, R. S., Miranda, C., and Froelicher, V. F.: Diagnostic and prognostic accuracy of the exercise electrocardiogram in patients with preexisting right bundle branch block. Am. Heart J. *127*:1521, 1994.

105. Yamabe, H., Okumura, K., and Yasue, H.: Comparison of the effects of exercise and isoproterenol on the antegrade refractory period of the accessory pathway in patients with Wolff-Parkinson-White syndrome. Jpn. Circ. J. *58*:22, 1994.

106. Chaitman, B. R., Bourassa, M. G., Davis, K., et al.: Angiographic prevalence of high-risk coronary artery disease in patient subsets (CASS). Circulation *64*:360, 1981.

107. Clark, P. I., Glasser, S. P., Lyman, G. H., et al.: Relation of results of exercise tests in young women to phases of the menstrual cycle. Am. J. Cardiol. *61*:197, 1988.

108. Shaw, L. J., Miller, D. D., Romeis, J. C., et al.: Gender differences in the noninvasive evaluation and management of patients with suspected coronary artery disease. Ann. Intern. Med. *120*:559, 1994.

109. Mark, D. B., Shaw, L. K., DeLong, E. R., et al.: Absence of sex bias in the referral of patients for cardiac catheterization. N. Engl. J. Med. *330*:1101, 1994.

110. Otterstad, J. E., Davies, M., Ball, S. G., et al.: Left ventricular hypertrophy and myocardial ischaemia in hypertension: The THAMES study. Eur. Heart J. *14*:1622, 1993.

111. Colucci, W. S., Ribeiro, J. P., Rocco, M. B., et al.: Impaired chronotropic response to exercise in patients with congestive heart failure: Role of postsynaptic β-adrenergic desensitization. Circulation *80*:314, 1989.

112. Coats, A. J. S., Adamopoulos, S., Radaelli, A., et al.: Controlled trial of physical training in chronic heart failure: Exercise performance, hemodynamics, ventilation, and autonomic function. Circulation *85*:2119, 1992.

113. LeJemtel, T. H., Liang, C., Stewart, D. K., et al.: Reduced peak aerobic capacity in asymptomatic left ventricular systolic dysfunction: A substudy of the Studies of Left Ventricular Dysfunction (SOLVD). Circulation *90*:2757, 1994.

114. Myers, J., and Froelicher, V. F.: Hemodynamic determinants of exercise capacity in chronic heart failure. Ann. Intern. Med. *115*:377, 1991.

115. Waagstein, F., Bristow, M. R., Swedberg, K., et al.: Beneficial effects of metoprolol in idiopathic dilated cardiomyopathy: Metoprolol in Dilated Cardiomyopathy (MDC) Trial Study Group. Lancet *342*:1441, 1993.

116. Mancini, D. M., Walter, G., Reichek, N., et al.: Contribution of skeletal muscle atrophy to exercise intolerance and altered muscle metabolism in heart failure. Circulation *85*:1364, 1992.

117. Mahmarian, J. J., Fenimore, N. L., and Marks, G. F.: Transdermal nitroglycerin patch therapy reduces the extent of exercise-induced myocardial ischemia: Results of a double-blind, placebo-controlled trial using quantitative thallium-201 tomography. J. Am. Coll. Cardiol. *24*:25, 1994.

118. Melandri, G., Semprini, F., Cervi, V., et al.: Benefit of adding low molecular weight heparin to the conventional treatment of stable angina pectoris: A double-blind, randomized, placebo-controlled trial. Circulation *88*:2517, 1993.

119. Juneau, M., Johnstone, M., Dempsey, E., and Waters, D. D.: Exercise-induced myocardial ischemia in a cold environment: Effect of antianginal medications. Circulation *79*:1015, 1989.

120. Allred, E. N., Bleecker, E. R., Chaitman, B. R., et al.: Acute effects of carbon monoxide exposure on exercise performance in subjects with coronary artery disease. N. Engl. J. Med. *321*:1426, 1989.

121. Cascio, W. E., Woefel, A., Knisley, S. B., et al.: Use dependence of amiodarone during the sinus tachycardia of exercise in coronary artery disease. Am. J. Cardiol. *61*:1042, 1988.

122. Yli-Mayry, S., Huikuri, H. V., Airaksinen, K. E., et al.: Usefulness of a postoperative exercise test for predicting cardiac events after coronary artery bypass grafting. Am. J. Cardiol. *70*:56, 1992.

123. Parisi, A. F., Folland, E. D., and Hartigan, P.: A comparison of angioplasty with medical therapy in the treatment of single-vessel coronary artery disease: Veterans Affairs ACME Investigators. N. Engl. J. Med. *326*:10, 1992.

124. Weiner, D. A., Ryan, T. J., Parsons, L., et al.: Prevalence and prognostic significance of silent and symptomatic ischemia after coronary bypass surgery: A report from the Coronary Artery Surgery Study (CASS) randomization population. J. Am. Coll. Cardiol. *18*:343, 1991.

125. Uren, N. G., Crake, T., Lefroy, D. C., et al.: Delayed recovery of coronary resistive vessel function after coronary angioplasty. J. Am. Coll. Cardiol. *21*:612, 1993.

126. Beregi, J. P., Bauters, C., McFadden, E. P., et al.: Exercise-induced ST-segment depression in patients without restenosis after coronary angioplasty: Relation to preprocedural impaired left ventricular function. Circulation *90*:148, 1994.

127. Ehrman, J., Keteyian, S., Fedel, F., et al.: Cardiovascular responses of heart transplant recipients to graded exercise testing. J. Appl. Physiol. *73*:260, 1992.

128. Kao, A. C., Trigt, P. V., Shaeffer-McCall, G. S., et al.: Central and peripheral limitations to upright exercise in untrained cardiac transplant recipients. Circulation *89*:2605, 1994.

129. Mancini, D. M., Eisen, H., Kussmaul, W., et al.: Value of peak exercise oxygen consumption for optimal timing of cardiac transplantation in ambulatory patients with heart failure. Circulation *83*:778, 1991.

130. Smart, F. W., Ballantyne, C. M., Cocanougher, B., et al.: Insensitivity of noninvasive tests to detect coronary artery vasculopathy after heart transplant. Am. J. Cardiol. *67*:243, 1991.

131. Smart, F. W., Grinstead, W. C., Cocanougher, B., et al.: Detection of transplant arteriopathy: Does exercise thallium scintigraphy improve noninvasive diagnostic capabilities? Transplant. Proc. *23*:1189, 1991.

132. Burwash, I. G., Pearlman, A. S., Kraft, C. D., et al.: Flow dependence of measures of aortic stenosis severity during exercise. J. Am. Coll. Cardiol. *24*:1342, 1994.

133. Siemienczuk, D., Greenberg, B., Morris, C., et al.: Chronic aortic insufficiency: Factors associated with progression to aortic valve replacement. Ann. Intern. Med. *110*:587, 1989.

134. Hayes, D. L., Von Feldt, L., and Higano, S. T.: Standardized informal exercise testing for programming rate adaptive pacemakers. PACE *14*;1772, 1991.

135. McElroy, P. A., Janicki, J. S., and Weber, K. T.: Physiologic correlates of the heart rate response to upright isotonic exercise: relevance to rate-responsive pacemakers. J. Am. Coll. Cardiol. *11*:94, 1988.

136. Hilton, T. C., Shaw, L. J., Chaitman, B. R., et al.: Prognostic significance of exercise thallium-201 testing in patients aged greater than or equal to 70 years with known or suspected coronary artery disease. Am. J. Cardiol. *69*:45, 1992.

137. Ciaroni, S., Delonca, J., and Righetti, A.: Early exercise testing after acute myocardial infarction in the elderly: Clinical evaluation and prognostic significance. Am. Heart J. *126*:304, 1993.

138. Borg, G.: Perceived exertion as an indicator of somatic stress. Scand. J. Rehabil. Med. *2–3*:92, 1970.

139. Cahalin, L. P., Blessey, R. L., Kummer, D., and Simard, M.: The safety of exercise testing performed independently by physical therapists. J. Cardiopulmonary Rehabil. *7*:269, 1987.

140. Stuart, R. J., and Ellestad, M. H.: National survey of exercise stress testing facilities. Chest *77*:94, 1980.

141. Hamm, L. F., Crow, R. S., Stull, G. A., and Hannan, P.: Safety and characteristics of exercise testing early after acute myocardial infarction. Am. J. Cardiol. *63*:1193, 1989.

142. Lewis, W. R., and Amsterdam, E. A.: Utility and safety of immediate exercise testing of low-risk patients admitted to the hospital for suspected acute myocardial infarction. Am. J. Cardiol. *74*:987, 1994.

143. Tristani, F. E., Hughes, C. V., Archibald, D. G., et al.: Safety of graded symptom-limited exercise testing in patients with congestive heart failure. Circulation *76*:VI-54, 1987.

144. Young, D.Z., Lampert, S., Graboys, T. B., and Lown, B.: Safety of maximal exercise testing in patients at high risk for ventricular arrhythmia. Circulation *70*:184, 1984.

Chapter 6
Cardiac Catheterization

CHARLES J. DAVIDSON, ROBERT F. FISHMAN, ROBERT O. BONOW

HISTORICAL PERSPECTIVE

Procedures in the cardiac catheterization laboratory have evolved from purely diagnostic and research techniques to potentially life-saving interventional procedures. In 1733, Stephen Hales described the mechanics of blood circulation and went on to directly measure blood pressure and its response to various physiological conditions in animals and humans. Almost 200 years later, in 1929, Werner Forss-mann performed the first human cardiac catheterization. During his training as a surgeon in Eberswalde, Germany, he used fluoroscopic guidance to advance a urethral catheter through his own left ante-cubital vein into the right atrium. In an attempt to develop a technique for direct delivery of drugs into the heart, he performed right heart catheterizations on himself on at least six occasions. He tried to opacify the heart with contrast medium injection into the right atrium, but because of poor fluoroscopic imaging, he was unable to visualize the heart structures. Although intense criticism eventually caused him to abandon this pursuit and to undertake a career as a urologist, he was awarded the Nobel prize in medicine in 1956 for his pioneering work. It was not until 1941 that right heart catheterization was routinely undertaken in humans to study cardiac physiology. Right heart catheterization was facilitated in 1970 when balloon-tipped flow-directed catheters that could be inserted without fluoroscopy were introduced by Swan and Ganz.[1]

Zimmerman and coworkers[2] undertook the first retrograde left heart catheterization in 1950 using a No. 6 French catheter inserted through the ulnar artery. The technique was facilitated greatly when Seldinger in 1953 described the method of percutaneous needle puncture and catheter exchange over a guidewire. In 1945, Radner visualized coronary arteries by nonselective injection of radiopaque contrast medium into the ascending aorta, but it was not until 1958 that the first selective injection of contrast medium into the coronary arteries was performed by Sones.[3] The following year, transseptal heart catheterization with interatrial puncture of the septum was described by Ross and by Cope.[4,5] Various retrograde percutaneous femoral artery coronary angiographic techniques were developed by Ricketts and Abrams,[6] Amplatz and colleagues,[7] and Judkins.[8] The catheter created by Judkins permits relatively easy and safe selective coronary arteriography. One of Judkins' favorite phrases was that the left coronary catheter will seek the lumen of the coronary artery unless thwarted by the operator.[9] The percutaneous femoral technique introduced by Judkins and the brachial arteriotomy technique pioneered by Sones are the most widely used today. Each method has its own set of advantages and disadvantages, which will be discussed later in greater detail.

Dotter and Judkins developed the technique of transluminal angio-plasty in 1964. In 1977, Andreas Gruentzig performed the first percu-taneous balloon coronary angioplasty in humans. Percutaneous re-vascularization strategies have evolved to include the use of intracoronary stents, various atherectomy methods, and laser technology. Technology is advancing to the point that genetic manipulation may be feasible in the catheterization laboratory.

INDICATIONS FOR DIAGNOSTIC CARDIAC CATHETERIZATION

As with any procedure, the decision to recommend cardiac catheterization is based on an appropriate risk-benefit ratio. In general, diagnostic cardiac catheterization is recommended whenever it is clinically important to define the presence or severity of a suspected cardiac lesion that cannot be adequately evaluated by noninvasive techniques. In-tracardiac pressure measurements and coronary arteriography are procedures that can be performed only by catheterization as of this writing, although some intracardiac pressures and rudimentary coronary artery anatomy can be evaluated with echocardiography and magnetic resonance imaging, respectively. Since the mortality from cardiac catheterization is approximately 0.1 per cent in most laboratories, there are few patients who cannot be studied safely in an active laboratory.

The guidelines for diagnostic coronary angiography have been reported by a joint task force of the American College of Cardiology and the American Heart Association[10] (see p. 3012). These guidelines describe a three-tiered priority classification for specific disease states. Class I applications exist for those conditions in which there is general agreement that coronary angiography is justified, although this may not be the only appropriate diagnostic procedure. Class II indications apply to those conditions in which coronary angiography is frequently performed, but there is divergence of opinion with respect to justification of the value and appropriateness of the procedure. Class III conditions are those in which there is general agreement that cardiac catheterization is not ordinarily justified. Diseases are grouped under several categories: known or suspected coronary heart disease, atypical chest pain, acute myocardial infarction, valvular heart disease, congenital heart disease, and other conditions. Table 6–1 summarizes the recommendations of the task force.

The indications for cardiac catheterization are changing and are likely to continue to evolve. The trend during the last 10 years in the United States has been in two divergent directions. At the one extreme, many critically ill and hemodynamically unstable patients are being studied during acute myocardial ischemia. At the other end of the spectrum, an increasing number of studies are being performed in an outpatient setting. The result has been the expansion of traditional indications for cardiac catheterization to include both seriously ill patients and ambulatory patients.

Cardiac catheterization should be considered to be a diagnostic test for use in combination with other complementary noninvasive tests in cardiology. For example, cardiac catheterization in valvular or congenital heart disease is best done with full knowledge of the echocardiographic and any other functional information. Then, catheterization can be directed and simplified without obtaining redundant anatomical information.

Identification of coronary artery disease and assessment of its extent and severity are the most common indications for cardiac catheterization in adults. The information obtained by catheterization is crucial to optimize the care of patients with various chest pain syndromes. In addition, the presence of dynamic coronary vascular lesions, such as spasm or thrombosis, may be identified. The consequences of coronary heart disease, such as ischemic mitral regurgi- **177**

TABLE 6–1 INDICATIONS FOR CORONARY ANGIOGRAPHY

KNOWN OR SUSPECTED CORONARY DISEASE (Known: previous myocardial infarction, or coronary bypass surgery or PTCA. Suspected: rest- or exercise-induced ECG abnormalities suggesting silent ischemia.)

ASYMPTOMATIC PATIENTS
Class I indications
1. Evidence for high risk on noninvasive testing
2. Individuals in high-risk occupations (airline pilots, bus drivers)
3. Following successful resuscitation from cardiac arrest
Class II indications
1. Positive noninvasive test in non–high-risk patient
2. Multiple risk factors for coronary artery disease
3. Prior MI with positive noninvasive testing
4. Following cardiac transplantation
5. After CABG or PTCA with positive ischemia
6. Before noncardiac surgery with positive noninvasive test

SYMPTOMATIC PATIENTS
Class I indications
1. Inadequate response to medical treatment
2. Unstable angina
3. Printzmetal's or variant angina
4. Canadian Cardiovascular Society functional Class I or II angina associated with the following:
   a. Positive exercise test
   b. History of MI or hypertension with ECG changes
   c. Side effects of medical therapy
   d. Occupational or lifestyle "need to know"
   e. Episodic pulmonary edema
5. Before major vascular surgery if angina present or noninvasive positive test results
6. After resuscitation from cardiac arrest
Class II indications
1. Any angina in the following groups:
   a. Female patients < 40 yr of age with positive noninvasive testing
   b. Male patients < 40
   c. Patients < 40 with prior MI
   d. Patients requiring major nonvascular surgery
2. Class 3 or 4 angina that improves on medical therapy
3. Patients who cannot be risk-stratified by other techniques

ATYPICAL CHEST PAIN OF UNCERTAIN ORIGIN
Class I indications
1. When noninvasive stress test reveals high risk for coronary disease
2. Suspected coronary artery
3. Associated symptoms or signs of abnormal LV function or failure
Class II indications
1. Patients in whom coronary disease cannot be excluded by noninvasive studies
2. Severe symptoms despite negative noninvasive tests

ACUTE MYOCARDIAL INFARCTION
Acute, Evolving MI
Class I indications
1. None*
Class II indications
1. Within the first 6 hr in candidates for revascularization therapy
2. After IV thrombolytic therapy when PTCA contemplated (see text)

Completed Myocardial Infarction (after 6 hr and before discharge evaluation)
Class I indications
1. Recurrent episodes of ischemic chest pain
2. Suspected ruptured septum or acute mitral regurgitation with CHF
3. Suspected left ventricular pseudoaneurysm
Class II indications
1. Thrombolytic therapy during evolving MI period
2. CHF and/or hypotension during intensive medical therapy
3. Recurrent VT and/or VF
4. Cardiogenic shock
5. MI due to coronary embolism

Convalescent Myocardial Infarction (predischarge to 8 wks)
Class I indications
1. Angina at rest or with minimal activity
2. CHF, recurrent ischemia, or ventricular arrhythmias
3. Positive noninvasive study
4. Non-Q-wave infarction
Class II indications
1. Mild angina
2. Asymptomatic and younger than 50
3. Need to return to unusually active or vigorous activity
4. Previous history of MI or angina for > 6 mo before the current MI
5. Thrombolytic therapy given during evolving phase

VALVULAR HEART DISEASE
Class I indications
1. Before valve surgery in an adult with chest discomfort and/or ECG changes
2. Before valve surgery in a male patient ≥ 35
3. Before valve surgery in postmenopausal women
Class II indications
1. During left heart catheterization in men < 35 or women > 40 when aortic or mitral valve surgery is being considered
2. Multiple risk factors for coronary disease
3. Reoperation for valve surgery when angiography > 1 year
4. In infective endocarditis when coronary embolization occurs

CONGENITAL HEART DISEASE
Class I indications
1. Signs or symptoms of angina
2. Suspected congestive coronary anomaly
3. Male patient > 40 or postmenopausal woman
Class II indications
1. Presence of a congenital lesion with high frequency of coronary anomalies

MISCELLANEOUS
Class I indications
1. Disease of the aorta in which the presence or extent of coronary disease will affect management
2. LV failure without obvious cause
3. Angina associated with hypertrophic cardiomyopathy in patients ≥ 35 or postmenopausal women with angina
Class II indications
1. Dilated cardiomyopathy
2. Recent blunt chest trauma
3. Male patients > 35 or postmenopausal women to undergo other cardiac surgery
4. Prospective transplant donors
5. Kawasaki's disease (coronary aneurysms)

Data from Ross J, Brandenburg RO, Dinsmore RE, and members of the subcommittee task force on coronary angiography of the AHA/ACC. J Am Coll Cardiol 10:935, 1987.

* Revised ACC/AHA task force guidelines indicate a clinical role (Class I) for PTCA during acute myocardial infarction (Circulation 88:2987, 1993). See text for details.

tation or left ventricular dysfunction and aneurysm, can be defined. In the current era of acute catheter intervention for coronary artery disease, patients may be studied during myocardial infarction or in the early period after acute myocardial injury. The aggressiveness of individual centers in approaching such patients depends on local facilities and treatment philosophies as well as the availability of appropriate therapy and surgical support.

According to the ACC/AHA task force recommendations, coronary angiography has no indications during the acute phase of myocardial infarction. However, several recent prospective randomized trials have demonstrated that immediate cardiac catheterization with direct percutaneous transluminal coronary angiography (PTCA) of the infarct-related artery produces clinical outcomes that are equivalent to and possibly superior to thrombolytic therapy[11] (see p. 1313). In certain patient subgroups, particularly those not at low risk, PTCA appears to be safer and more effective than thrombolytic therapy. The task force guidelines also suggest that coronary angiography is desirable during the evolving phase of acute myocardial infarction after thrombolytic therapy has been administered. Data from several large randomized prospective trials indicate that emergent catheterization should not be routinely performed after successful thrombolytic therapy.[12,13] Thus, the recommendations of the 1987 task force for cardiac catheterization during acute evolving myocardial infarction may be outdated based on the current literature.

The 1993 ACC/AHA task force recommendations regarding the use of PTCA in the setting of acute myocardial infarction and acute ischemic syndromes more accurately reflect current practice guidelines[14] (see p. 1221). These recommendations acknowledge that acute cardiac catheterization and PTCA are appropriately indicated (i.e., Class I) for evolving acute myocardial infarction and after acute myocardial infarction during initial hospitalization.

In patients with myocardial disease, cardiac catheterization may provide crucial information. It can exclude coronary artery disease as the cause of symptoms and evaluate left ventricular dysfunction in patients with cardiomyopathy. Cardiac catheterization also permits quantification of the severity of both diastolic and systolic dysfunction, differentiation of myocardial restriction from pericardial constriction, assessment of the extent of valvular regurgitation, detection of active myocarditis by endomyocardial biopsy, and observation of the cardiovascular response to acute pharmacological intervention.

In patients with valvular heart disease, cardiac catheterization provides both confirmatory and complementary data to noninvasive echocardiography and nuclear studies. Roberts[15] and Rahimtoola[16] have emphasized that the risk-benefit ratio of preoperative cardiac catheterization is weighted heavily in favor of the cardiac catheterization. Catheterization may be unnecessary in some preoperative situations, such as in patients with an atrial myxoma or young patients with endocarditis or acute mitral or acute aortic regurgitation. Nevertheless, additional confirmation of the severity of the valvular lesion, identification of associated coronary disease, quantification of the hemodynamic consequences of the valvular lesions (such as pulmonary hypertension), and occasionally the acute hemodynamic response to pharmacological therapy all provide useful preoperative information that fully defines the operative risk and permits a more directed surgical approach.

The current role of cardiac catheterization in certain congenital disease states is less well defined, as echocardiography, Doppler techniques, and cardiac magnetic resonance imaging have improved in accuracy and image quality. Because gross cardiac anatomy can generally be well defined by these methods, catheterization is required only if certain hemodynamic information (e.g., shunt size or pulmonary vascular resistance) is important in determining the indications for surgical procedures, if catheter interventional methods are contemplated, or if coronary anomalies are suspected.

COMPLICATIONS ASSOCIATED WITH CARDIAC CATHETERIZATION

(Table 6–2)

Cardiac catheterization is a relatively safe procedure but has a well-defined risk of morbidity and mortality.[17–22] The potential risk of major complications during cardiac catheterization may be difficult to ascertain due to the confounding aspects of comorbid disease and disparities in methodology used to collect complication data. Recent advances including the use of nonionic contrast media, lower profile diagnostic catheters, and extensive operator experience all serve to reduce further the incidence of complica-

TABLE 6–2 RISK GROUPS FOR CARDIAC CATHETERIZATION

179

Ch 6

	MORTALITY RATE (%)
Overall mortality	**0.14**
Age-related mortality	
Less than 1 year	1.75
More than 60 years	0.25
Coronary artery disease	
One-vessel disease	0.03
Three-vessel disease	0.16
Left main disease	0.86
Coronary heart failure	
NYHA functional Class I or II	0.02
NYHA functional Class III	0.12
NYHA functional Class IV	0.67
Valvular heart disease	**0.28**

PATIENTS AT HIGHEST RISK FOR COMPLICATIONS AND UNSUITABLE FOR CATHETERIZATION IN AN AMBULATORY SETTING
Coronary artery disease
   Unstable or progressive angina
   Recent myocardial infarction (< 7 days)
   Pulmonary edema thought due to ischemia
   High risk for left main disease by noninvasive testing
Congestive heart failure
   NYHA functional Class III or IV
   Severe right heart failure
Valvular heart disease
   Suspected severe AS
   Suspected severe AI (pulse pressure ≥ 80 mm Hg)
Congenital heart disease
   Suspected severe pulmonary hypertension
   Severe right heart failure

PATIENTS WHO REQUIRE PROLONGED MONITORING AFTER CARDIAC CATHETERIZATION AND MAY BE UNSUITABLE FOR AMBULATORY CARDIAC CATHETERIZATION
Severe peripheral vascular disease
General debility, mental confusion, or cachexia
Need for continuous anticoagulation or a bleeding diathesis
Uncontrolled systemic hypertension
Poorly controlled diabetes mellitus
Recent stroke (< 1 month)
Renal insufficiency (creatinine ≥ 2 mg/dl)

Modified from Bashore, TM: Traditional and nontraditional cardiac catheterization laboratory settings. *In* Pepine, C. J., Hill, J. A., and Lambert, C. R.: Diagnostic and Therapeutic Cardiac Catheterization. 2nd ed. Baltimore, Williams and Wilkins, 1994, pp. 18, 19.
* Adapted from ACC/AHA Ad Hoc Task Force on Cardiac Catheterization. Guidelines for cardiac catheterization and cardiac catheterization laboratories. J Am Coll Cardiol 1991; 84:2213–2247.

tions. Several large trials including the American Heart Association's Cooperative Study on cardiac catheterization,[17] the Society for Cardiac Angiography's Registry,[18] and others[19,21,22] permit insight into the incidence of major events and delineate patient cohorts that are at increased risk. Two studies evaluating the specific risk of coronary angiography are also available—a survey of 46,904 patients[23] and the report from the Collaborative Study of Coronary Artery Surgery that included 7553 patients who were studied prospectively.[20]

Death from diagnostic cardiac catheterization occurs in 0.14 to 0.75 per cent of patients, depending on the population studied. Data from the Society for Cardiac Angiography identified subsets of patients with an increased mortality rate.[19] These include patients with >50 per cent stenosis of the left coronary artery (0.94 per cent), left ventricular ejection fraction < 30 per cent (0.54 per cent), New York Heart Association (NYHA) functional class III or IV heart failure (0.24 per cent), age greater than 60 years (0.23 per cent), aortic valvular disease (0.23 per cent), and three-vessel coronary artery disease (0.13 per cent).[18] In an analysis of 58,332 patients studied in 1990, multivariate predictors of significant complications were moribund status, advanced NYHA functional class, hypertension, shock, aortic valve disease, renal insufficiency, unstable angina, mitral valve disease, acute myocardial infarction within 24 hours, congestive heart failure, and cardiomyopathy.[21] The risk of cardiac catheterization appears to be further increased in octogenarians,[24] in whom overall mortality is approximately 0.8 per cent and the risk of nonfatal major complications, which are primarily peripheral vascular, is about 5 per cent.

The risk of myocardial infarction varies from 0.07 to 0.6 per cent, cerebrovascular accidents from 0.03 to 0.2 per cent, and significant brady- or tachyarrhythmias from 0.56 to 1.3 per cent. Reports of the incidence of major vascular complications have varied widely, with most series suggesting a slightly higher frequency when the brachial approach is used. Recent data suggest the incidence of major vascular complications to be approximately 0.40 per cent.[21] Major vascular complications include occlusion requiring arterial repair or thrombectomy, retroperitoneal bleeding, hematoma formation, pseudoaneurysm, arteriovenous fistula formation, and infection. The risk of requiring surgical repair for vascular injury is related to advanced age, congestive heart failure, and larger body surface area.[25]

Systemic complications can vary from mild vasovagal responses to severe vagal reactions that lead to cardiac arrest. Prolonged hypotension during the procedure may also occur as a result of various mechanisms that include the vasodepressor vagal response, contrast medium–induced vasodilation or osmotic diuresis, cardiac tamponade due to myocardial perforation or coronary laceration, myocardial infarction, and an acute anaphylactoid reaction to the contrast media. Minor complications occur in approximately 4 per cent of patients undergoing routine cardiac catheterization.[26] The most common untoward effects are transient hypotension and brief episodes of angina lasting less than 10 minutes. However, with the use of low osmolar contrast media, bradycardia is infrequent and usually responds to cough. Rarely, administration of intravenous atropine is necessary.

After the procedure, diuresis from the radiographic contrast load and subsequent hypotension can be common. Intravenous hydration given before and after the procedure can usually restore the intravascular volume to compensate for the anticipated diuresis. A recent prospective trial evaluated the effects of saline, mannitol, and furosemide in preventing acute decreases in renal function due to contrast media–induced nephrotoxicity.[27] The authors concluded that saline alone was most effective in reducing the acute increase in serum creatinine. The incidence of acute renal dysfunction in patients with baseline renal insufficiency was 28 and 40 per cent with mannitol and furosemide, respectively, compared with 11 per cent with saline hydration alone.

Controversy exists regarding the use of low osmolar nonionic or hemionic versus high osmolar ionic contrast media for routine cardiac catheterization and angiography. Consensus is growing regarding the types of patients in whom use of low osmolar contrast agents should be considered (Table 6–3). Several reviews have suggested that contrast media–related toxicity occurs in 1.4 to 2.3 per cent of patients receiving ionic contrast media.[28,29] High osmolar ionic contrast media produce various adverse hemodynamic and electrophysiologic effects during coronary angiography. Most of these adverse events are clearly related to the osmolality, sodium content, and calcium binding characteristics of the ionic contrast solutions. In addition, myocardial depression, peripheral vasodilation, and increased coronary blood flow occur.[30] Nonionic low osmolar contrast agents clearly reduce acute adverse hemodynamic and electrophysiological reactions[31,32] and may reduce nephrotoxicity in patients at highest risk. They appear to release less histamine from mast cells and potentially reduce allergic reactions.[33] Clinical studies suggest no advantage of low osmolar contrast over ionic contrast media in the prevention of nephrotoxicity in patients with normal renal function.[26,34] However, other data indicate that the risk of contrast media–induced nephropathy may be reduced in patients with baseline renal insufficiency if nonionic contrast medium is utilized.[35]

Baseline renal insufficiency has been consistently shown to be an independent predictor of subsequent contrast nephrotoxicity.[26] Contrast media–induced renal dysfunction can be minimized if the dosage of contrast medium is kept below 30 ml for the entire study.[36] The question of some inherent thrombogenicity of nonionic agents has also been raised,[37] and this possibility may relate to the formation of "thin" fibrin in the thrombus.[38] Because a substantial difference in costs exists between ionic and nonionic media, the controversy regarding the exclusive use of nonionic contrast media for routine cardiac catheterization is unresolved.

TABLE 6–3   INDICATIONS FOR USE OF LOW OSMOLAR CONTRAST AGENTS

Unstable ischemic syndromes
Congestive heart failure
Diabetes mellitus
Renal insufficiency
Hypotension
Severe bradycardia
History of contrast allergy
Severe valvular heart disease
Internal mammary artery injection

From Hill JA, Lambert CR, Pepine CJ: Radiographic contrast agents. In Pepine CJ, Hill JA, and Lambert CR: Diagnostic and Therapeutic Cardiac Catheterization. 2nd ed. Baltimore, Williams and Wilkins, 1994, p. 192.

TECHNICAL ASPECTS OF CARDIAC CATHETERIZATION

CATHETERIZATION LABORATORY FACILITIES

Cardiac catheterization facilities have evolved to include traditional hospital-based laboratories with in-house cardiothoracic surgical programs, hospital-based laboratories without on-site surgical programs, free-standing laboratories, and mobile laboratories. The relative merits of each type of facility have been discussed in detail by a task force of the American Heart Association and the American College of Cardiology,[39] and guidelines for development of a mobile facility have been outlined by the Society for Cardiac Angiography and Interventions.[40] The goals of the free-standing and mobile cardiac catheterization facilities are to reduce cost while offering services in a convenient location for low-risk patients. In one study evaluating the safety of mobile catheterization involving 1001 low-risk patients, no patient died, 0.9 per cent required urgent referral for clinical instability, 0.6 per cent had major complications, and 27 per cent required further referral to a tertiary site for additional diagnostic or therapeutic procedures.[41] The issue of cost-saving potential of mobile and free-standing laboratories, as well as quality of patient care and ethical issues, remains unresolved. Because the majority of patients in the United States live within 30 to 60 minutes of a hospital-based facility,[39] it is generally recommended that catheterization be performed in traditional settings.

Because of cost containment considerations and the documented safety of diagnostic cardiac catheterization, there has been increasing pressure to perform catheterization on an ambulatory outpatient basis.[42,43] Criteria for ambulatory catheterization have been reported.[39,44] In general, patients who are not appropriate candidates for ambulatory catheterization include those with severe peripheral vascular disease, mechanical prosthetic valves, severe congestive heart failure, bleeding disorders, severe ischemia during stress testing, ischemia at rest, known or highly suspected severe left main or proximal three-vessel disease, critical aortic stenosis, and severe comorbid disease. Despite careful screening for low-risk patients, 12 per cent of patients may require hospitalization.[45]

PERSONNEL

Personnel in the catheterization laboratory include the director, physicians, nurses, and radiologic technologists. All members should be trained in cardiopulmonary resuscitation and preferably in advanced cardiac life support. It is desirable for facilities to be associated with a cardiothoracic surgical program. In general, high-risk diagnostic studies and all elective percutaneous interventions should be performed in laboratories with on-site surgical facilities. The re-

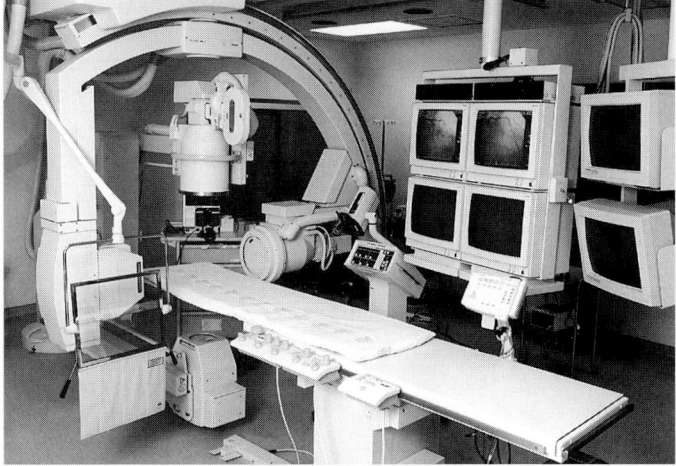

FIGURE 6–1. Cardiac catheterization laboratory at Northwestern University, Northwestern Memorial Hospital. Biplane radiographic equipment including x-ray tube and image intensifier assembly, hemodynamic physiological monitors, power injector, and emergency cart are shown.

cent American Heart Association/American College of Cardiology task force assessment of diagnostic and therapeutic cardiovascular procedures suggests that PTCA of high-risk patients with acute myocardial infarction may be performed by trained physicians without on-site surgical backup if the patient cannot be transferred to a more traditional setting without additional risk.[14]

In order to maintain proficiency, laboratories for adult studies should perform a minimum of 300 procedures per year, and physicians performing diagnostic catheterization should perform a minimum of 150 procedures per year.[39,46] Regular evaluation of laboratory and physician performance is also mandatory.[47]

EQUIPMENT

The physical requirements for the catheterization facility have been described in detail elsewhere.[39] Necessary equipment includes the radiographic system, physiological data monitoring and acquisition instrumentation, sterile supplies, and an emergency cart. Also included are support equipment consisting of a power injector, cineangiographic film or digital archiving, film processors, and viewing equipment (Fig. 6–1).

RADIOGRAPHIC EQUIPMENT. High-resolution x-ray imaging is required for optimal performance of catheterization procedures. The necessary equipment includes a generator, x-ray tube, image intensifier, video system, and usually a cinecamera.[48] While most facilities continue to use traditional film-based cineangiography, many laboratories have made the transition to using digital technology, thus becoming "cinefilm-less" laboratories.[49,50] The advantages of digital acquisition and archiving include the ability to have on-line review, quantitative computer analysis of high-quality images, image manipulation capabilities, and flicker-free images at very low frame rates thereby minimizing radiation exposure. Using these technologies, transfer of images between cardiac catheterization laboratories, hospitals, and physician offices could be accomplished using a common network. In order for this goal to be achieved, however, the digital archiving systems must be compatible.[51]

PHYSIOLOGICAL MONITORS. Continuous monitoring of blood pressure and the electrocardiogram (ECG) is required during cardiac catheterization. Systemic, pulmonary, and intracardiac pressures are generally recorded using fluid-filled catheters connected to strain-gauge pressure transducers and then transmitted to a monitor. Equipment for determination of cardiac output and blood gas determination, as well as a standard 12-lead ECG machine, are necessary.

RADIATION SAFETY

The patient and catheterization laboratory personnel must be protected from the harmful effects of radiation. Installing and maintaining optimal x-ray imaging equipment will reduce unnecessary radiation exposure. The amount of radiation exposure to the patient can be reduced by limiting fluoroscopic and image acquisition time, collimation of the beam to the anatomical region of interest, using low-intensity fluoroscopy, acquiring images at lower frame rates (i.e., 15 frames/sec), maintaining a minimum distance between the image intensifier and the x-ray tube, and using lead shielding when appropriate. Personnel in the laboratory can limit radiation exposure by minimizing acquisition and fluoroscopy times and by using low-dose fluoroscopy and 15 frames/sec acquisition rates. The most important factors are maximizing distance from the source of x-rays and using appropriate shielding (lead aprons, lead thyroid collars, lead eyeglasses, and moveable leaded glass barriers). A method for measuring radiation exposure for personnel is required. The maximum allowable

radiation dose per year for those working with radiation is 5 roentgen-equivalents–man (rem). A full discussion of radiation safety has been presented by the Society for Cardiac Angiography and Interventions and others.[39,52,53]

181

Ch 6

Catheterization Laboratory Protocol

PREPARATION OF THE PATIENT FOR CARDIAC CATHETERIZATION. Before arrival in the catheterization laboratory, the cardiologist responsible for the procedure should fully explain the procedure including its risk and benefits to the patient and answer questions that the patient and/or family may have. Precatheterization evaluation includes a patient history, physical examination, laboratory evaluation (complete blood count, platelet count, blood urea nitrogen, serum creatinine, serum electrolytes, blood glucose, prothrombin time, and partial thromboplastin time), chest x-ray, and ECG. Important components of the history that need to be addressed include possible insulin-dependent diabetes mellitus, renal insufficiency, chronic anticoagulation, and peripheral vascular disease as well as previous contrast media reactions. A full knowledge of any prior procedures, including prior cardiac catheterizations, percutaneous interventions, and cardiac surgery, are necessary before the procedure. The patient should be fasting and an intravenous line should be established. Usually, oral or intravenous sedation should be administered (e.g., benzodizepine). Many laboratories routinely premedicate patients with antihistamines such as diphenhydramine (25 mg intravenous push) to decrease allergic reactions and prolong mild sedation.

CATHETERIZATION PROTOCOL. Each physician should develop an individual routine for performing diagnostic catheterization to ensure efficient acquisition of all pertinent data. The particular technical approach and necessary procedures should be individualized for each patient so that the specific clinical questions can be addressed (Table 6–4). In general, hemodynamic measurements and cardiac output determination should be made before angiography to most accurately reflect basal conditions and to guide angiography. When angiography is performed, the vessel or chamber with most clinical importance should be visualized first, in case an untoward reaction to the contrast media or another complication of the procedure should occur.

Controversy exists regarding whether right heart catheterization should be performed in *all* patients undergoing routine coronary angiography. Some physicians believe that right heart catheterization including screening oximetric analysis, measurement of right heart pressures, and determination of cardiac output should be performed in every patient because the risks are limited and potential benefits exist (uncovering an unsuspected problem). A prospective study evaluated 200 patients undergoing left heart catheterization for suspected coronary artery disease in whom data from right heart catheterization were not considered necessary for clinical management before the procedure.[54] The right heart catheterization took approximately 6 additional minutes of procedure time and 86 seconds of fluoroscopy time. Management was altered in only 1.5 per cent of patients as a result of the data obtained by right heart catheterization. While routine right heart catheterization does not appear necessary for patients undergoing routine coronary angiography, it is clearly indicated when the clinical question cannot be answered by isolated left heart catheterization or when there is left ventricular dysfunction, congestive heart failure, complicated acute myocardial infarction, valvular disease, suspected pulmonary hypertension, congenital anomaly, or pericardial disease.[39]

While the use of a temporary pacemaker is not indicated for routine cardiac catheterization, operators should understand the techniques for proper insertion and setting of the pacemaker if needed (Chap. 24). Even in patients with isolated left bundle branch block, right heart catheterization

CLINICAL ISSUE	LHC	RHC	CORO	LV	AO	RV	PA	BX	PROVO	IABP	PTCA
Known or suspected coronary artery disease											
stable angina	✔		✔	✔							
positive stress test	✔		✔	✔							
preoperative evaluation	✔		✔	✔							
atypical chest pain	✔		✔	✔					±		
unstable or new-onset angina	✔		✔	✔							±
acute myocardial infarction	✔	✔	✔	±						±	±
failed thrombolysis	✔	✔	✔	±						±	±
post-infarction angina	✔		✔	±						±	±
cardiogenic shock	✔	✔	✔	±						±	±
mechanical complications	✔	✔	✔	✔						±	±
sudden cardiac death	✔	✔	✔	✔							
Valvular heart disease	✔	✔	✔	✔	✔						
Myocardial disease	✔	✔	✔	✔	✔			±			
Pericardial disease	✔	✔	✔	✔							
Congenital heart disease	✔	✔	✔	✔	±	±	±				
Aortic dissection	✔	±	✔	±	✔						
Pulmonary disease	✔	✔	✔	✔		±	±				

AO, aortogram; BX, biopsy; CORO, coronary angiography; IABP, intra-aortic balloon pump; LHC, left heart catheterization, including measurement of left ventricular end-diastolic pressure and aortic valve gradient; LV, left ventriculography; PA, pulmonary angiography or wedge pulmonary angiography; PROVO, provocative challenge (i.e., ergot alkaloids, acetylcholine); PTCA, percutaneous transluminal coronary angioplasty; RHC, right heart catheterization including pressure measurement, determination of cardiac output, oximetric analysis; RV, right ventriculography; ✔, appropriate; ±, may be appropriate in certain clinical circumstances.

can generally be performed safely with balloon flotation catheters without causing additional conduction disturbance.

CATHETERS AND ASSOCIATED EQUIPMENT. Physicians performing cardiac catheterization should be familiar with technical aspects of the equipment used during the procedure.[55] Catheters used for cardiac catheterization come in various lengths, sizes, and shapes. Typical catheter lengths vary between 50 and 125 centimeters, with 100 centimeters being the most commonly used length for adult left heart catheterization via the femoral approach. The outer diameter of the catheter is specified using French units where one French unit (F) = 0.33 mm. The inner diameter of the catheter is smaller than the outside diameter due to the thickness of the catheter material. Guidewires used during the procedure must be small enough to pass through the inner diameter of both the introducer needle and the catheter. Guidewires are described by their length in centimeters, diameter in inches, and tip conformation. A commonly used wire is a 150-cm, 0.035-inch J-tipped wire. The introducer sheaths are specified by the French number of the largest catheter that will pass freely through the inner diameter of the sheath, rather than its outer diameter. Therefore, a No. 7F introducer sheath will accept a 7F catheter but will have an outer diameter of more than 7F or 2.31 mm.

The choice of the size of the catheters to be used is made by balancing the need to opacify the coronary arteries and cardiac chambers adequately, to have adequate catheter manipulation, to limit vascular complications, and to permit early ambulation. While the larger catheters (7F and 8F) allow greater catheter manipulation and excellent visualization, the smaller catheters (5F and 6F) permit earlier ambulation after catheterization. Catheter technology has advanced such that 5 French systems may be used for routine angiography without significant compromise of angiographic quality.[56] Use of the smaller-sized catheters requires greater technical skill of manipulation in order to achieve adequate angiography and thus may be less appropriate for the training of students of catheterization. The 6F diagnostic catheter is most widely used for routine angiography as this size catheter appears to most appropriately balance the needs outlined above. The relationship between sheath size and vascular complications is not clear.

Rather, anticoagulation status and operator experience are more important factors related to vascular complications.[57]

Techniques

Right Heart Catheterization

Right heart catheterization allows for measurement and analysis of right heart, pulmonary artery, and pulmonary capillary wedge pressures, measurement of cardiac output by thermodilution, screening for intracardiac shunts, temporary ventricular pacing, assessment of arrhythmias, and pulmonary wedge angiography.[58] Right heart catheterization is performed antegrade through either the inferior or superior vena cava. Percutaneous entry is achieved via the femoral, subclavian, jugular, or antecubital vein. The anatomy of the major arteries and veins used for cardiac catheterization are shown in Figures 6–2 and 6–3. In the cardiac catheterization laboratory, the femoral venous access is used most often because the Judkins technique of left heart catheterization is performed concurrently. Balloon flotation catheters are the simplest and most widely employed. If thermodilution cardiac outputs are necessary, catheters that contain thermistors, such as Swan-Ganz catheters, should be used. These catheters have balloon tips, proximal and distal ports, and thermistors. Therefore, intracardiac pressures and oxygen saturation to evaluate intracardiac shunts can be obtained. Screening blood samples for oximetric analysis should be obtained from the superior vena cava and the pulmonary artery to evaluate for intracardiac shunts. Cardiac output can also be determined by thermodilution techniques. These catheters are both flexible and flow-directed, but when the femoral approach is employed, fluoroscopic guidance is almost always necessary to cannulate the pulmonary artery and to obtain pulmonary capillary wedge position. While most right heart catheters have a J-shaped curvature distally to facilitate passage from the superior vena cava to the pulmonary artery, a catheter with an S-shaped distal end has been designed for femoral insertion. Although manipulation is limited, the balloon flotation catheters are the safest and most rapid method to obtain right heart pressures and blood samples. Other balloon flotation end hole catheters that are stiffer and therefore allow better manipulation are available for right heart

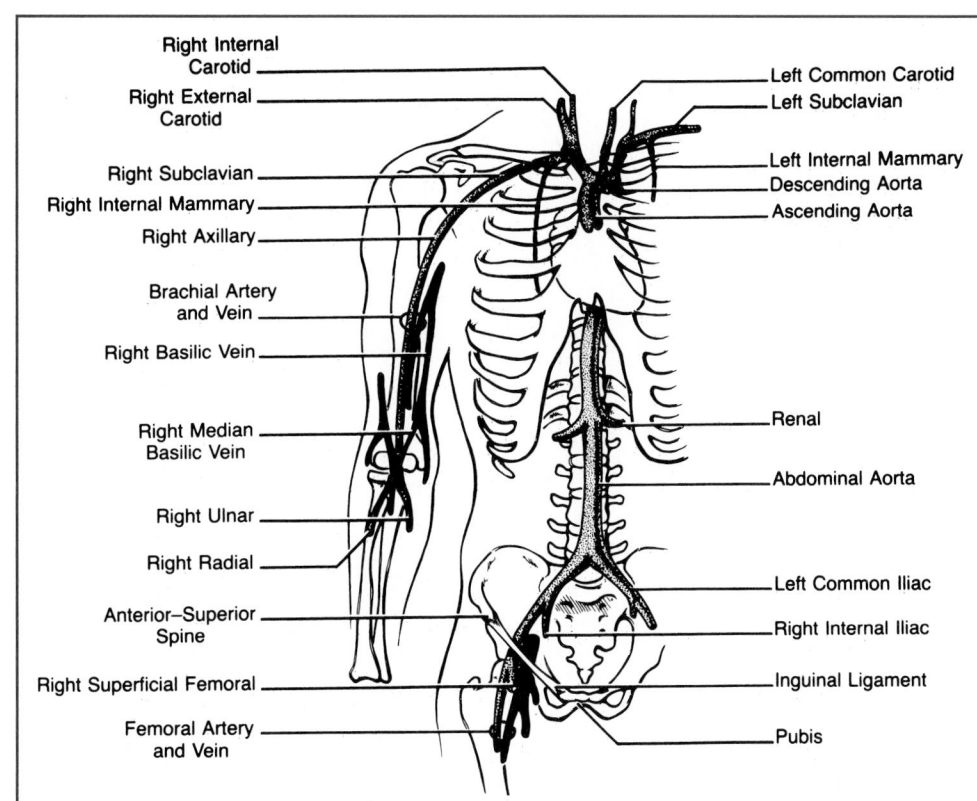

FIGURE 6-2. Principal arteries used for access during cardiac catheterization. Only the superficial veins are shown on the forearm. (Modified from Anthony, C. P.: Textbook of Anatomy and Physiology. 11th ed. St. Louis, C. V. Mosby, 1983. *In* Kern M. J.: The Cardiac Catheterization Handbook. 2nd ed. St. Louis, C. V. Mosby, 1995.)

catheterization. These lack the ability to obtain thermodilution cardiac outputs but yield better pressure fidelity, due to less catheter whip artifact and a larger end hole.

There are two methods to advance a balloon flotation

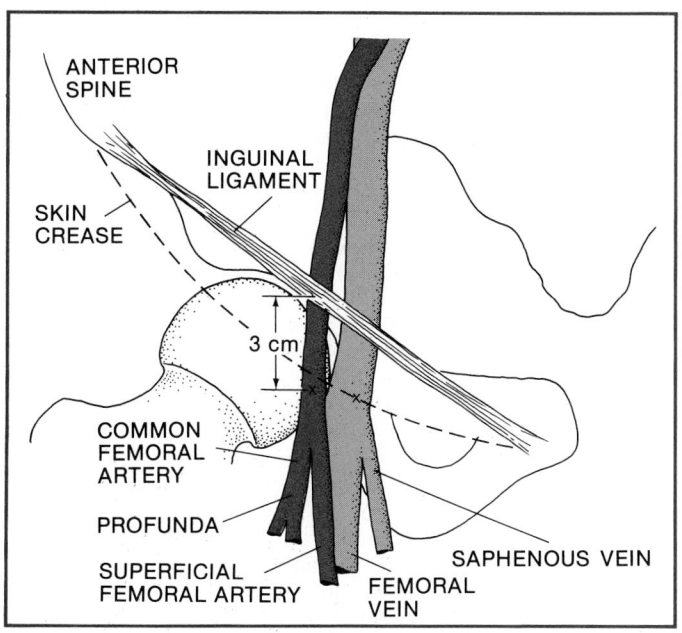

FIGURE 6-3. Anatomy relevant to percutaneous catheterization of femoral artery and vein: the right femoral artery and vein run underneath the inguinal ligament, which connects the anterior-superior iliac spine and pubic tubercle. The arterial skin nick (indicated by X) should be placed approximately 1½ to 2 fingerbreadths (3 cm) below the inguinal ligament and directly over the femoral artery pulsation. The venous skin nick should be placed at the same level, but approximately 1 fingerbreadth medial. (From Baim, D. S., and Grossman, W.: Percutaneous approach. *In* Grossman, W., and Baim, D. S. [eds.]: Cardiac Catheterization, Angiography, and Intervention. 4th ed. Philadelphia, Lea and Febiger, 1991.)

catheter from the femoral vein. On many occasions, the catheter can be advanced directly through the right atrium and across the tricuspid valve. Once in the right ventricle, the catheter is manipulated to point superiorly and directly into the right ventricular outflow tract. This can usually be achieved while the catheter is advanced with slight clockwise rotation. Once in the outflow tract, the balloon tip should allow flotation into the pulmonary artery and wedge positions. When necessary, deep inspiration or cough can facilitate this maneuver and assist in crossing the pulmonic valve. If the catheter continues to point inferiorly toward the right ventricular apex, another technique should be employed, because further advancement can risk perforation of the right ventricular apex.

One such additional technique for performing right heart catheterization with a balloon flotation catheter is shown in Figure 6-4. A loop is formed in the right atrium with the catheter tip directed laterally. The loop can be created by hooking the catheter tip on the hepatic vein or by advancing the catheter while it is directed laterally in the right atrium. Once the loop is formed, the catheter should be advanced further; this will direct the tip inferiorly and then medially across the tricuspid valve. Antegrade blood flow should then direct the catheter into the pulmonary artery. After the catheter is placed into the wedge position, the redundant loop should be removed by slow withdrawal.

When an end hole catheter that does not have a balloon tip is used, the technique for cannulating the pulmonary artery is markedly different. Manipulation and torquing of the nonflotation catheter are necessary to advance into the pulmonary artery. The catheter should be directed inferiorly across the tricuspid valve and then superiorly into the right ventricular outflow tract. It is generally recommended to attempt to form a loop in the right atrium before advancement into the right ventricle in order to lessen the risk of perforation. These stiffer catheters can often prolapse into the left atrium with mild pressure against the interatrial septum in patients with a probe-patent foramen ovale. Left atrial position can be verified by the pressure

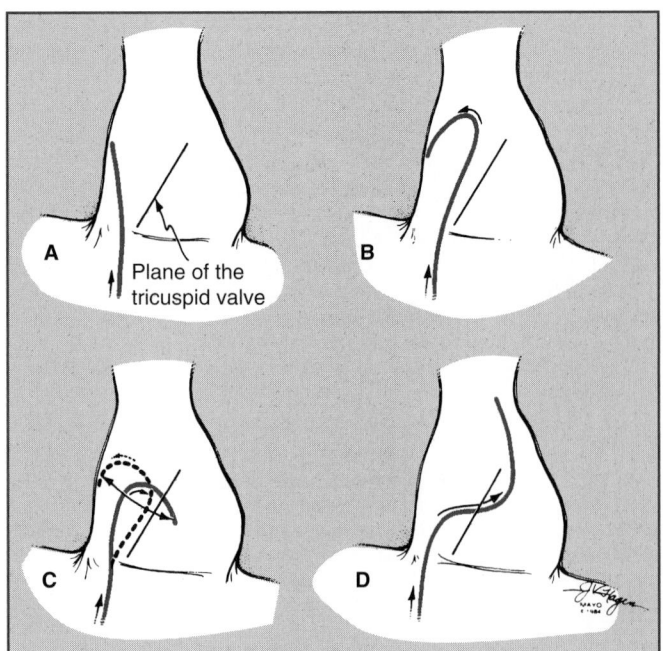

FIGURE 6-4. Technique of right heart catheterization from the femoral approach. *A,* The catheter is advanced through the inferior vena cava. *B,* A loop is created in the catheter by hooking on the hepatic vein or lateral right arterial wall. *C,* Clockwise rotation and advancement of catheter cross the tricuspid valve. *D,* Additional rotation and withdrawal straightens the catheter and directs it superiorly so that it may be advanced through the right ventricular outflow tract. (From Schwartz, R. S., et al.: Cardiac catheterization and angiography. *In* Giuliani, E. R., Fuster, V., Gersh, B. J., McGoon, M. D., and McGoon, D. C. [eds.]: Cardiology Fundamentals and Practice. 2nd ed. St. Louis, C. V. Mosby, 1991. By permission of Mayo Foundation.)

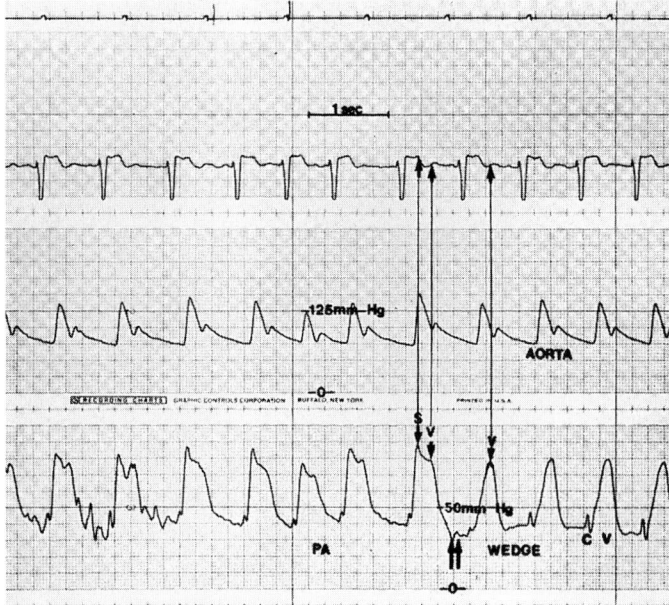

FIGURE 6-5. Arterial, pulmonary artery (PA) and pulmonary capillary wedge waveforms in a patient with acute mitral regurgitation. A prominent *v* wave is present in both the pulmonary artery and wedge tracings. The *v* wave occurs after the ECG T wave. Inflation of the balloon of the right heart catheter (double arrows) obliterates the pulmonary artery systolic (*s*) wave when the catheter wedges. The large *v* wave can cause the wedge to be mistaken for the PA tracing if the difference in timing between the *s* and *v* waves is not noticed. (From Sharkey, S. W.: Beyond the wedge: Clinical physiology and the Swan-Ganz catheter. Am. J. Med. *83:*115, 1987.)

waveform, by blood samples demonstrating arterial saturation, or by hand contrast injection.

The most common complications of right heart catheterization are nonsustained atrial and ventricular arrhythmias. Major complications associated with right heart catheterization are infrequent. These include pulmonary infarction, pulmonary artery or right ventricular perforation, and infection. Pulmonary artery rupture can be avoided by the combined use of fluoroscopic guidance and constant evaluation of the pressure waveform. Confusion as to the location of the distal end of the catheter may arise in the setting of large *v* waves in the pulmonary capillary wedge pressure tracing, which the operator may mistake for a pulmonary artery waveform. Careful attention to the timing of the peak pulmonary artery systolic pressure and the *v* wave with respect to the ECG along with the use of fluoroscopy will prevent inadvertent inflation of the balloon in the wedged position, which can cause pulmonary artery rupture (Fig. 6-5).

Left Heart Catheterization and Coronary Arteriography

THE JUDKINS TECHNIQUE. Because of its relative ease, speed, reliability, and low complication rate,[20] the Judkins technique[8] has become the most widely used method of left heart catheterization and coronary arteriography in the United States. After local anesthesia with 1 per cent lidocaine (Xylocaine), percutaneous entry of the femoral artery is achieved by puncturing the vessel 1 to 3 cm (or 1 to 2 fingerbreadths) below the inguinal ligament. The ligament can be palpated as it courses from the anterior superior iliac spine to the superior pubic ramus. It should be used as the landmark and not the inguinal crease; use of this crease is misleading. A transverse skin incision is made over the femoral artery with a scapel. Using a modified Seldinger technique (Fig. 6-6), an 18-gauge thin-walled needle (Fig. 6-7) is inserted at a 30- to 45-degree angle into the femoral artery, and a 0.035- or 0.038-inch J-tip Teflon-coated guidewire is advanced through the needle into the artery. The wire should pass freely up the aorta. After obtaining arterial access, a sheath at least equal in size to the coronary catheter is usually inserted into the femoral artery. It is generally recommended that the patient receive 3000 to 5000 units of heparin after access is obtained. The technique of coronary arteriography using this approach is described on p. 249.

Left ventricular systolic and end-diastolic pressures can be obtained by advancing a pigtail catheter into the left ventricle (Fig. 6-8). In assessing valvular aortic stenosis, left ventricular and aortic pressures should be recorded simultaneously. In suspected mitral stenosis, left ventricular and wedge or left atrial pressures should be obtained simultaneously. Left ventriculography is performed in the 30-degree RAO and 45- to 50-degree LAO views. A pigtail catheter is most commonly used for this purpose. Power injection of 30 to 50 ml of contrast medium into the ventricle is used to assess left ventricular function and the severity of mitral regurgitation. After ventriculography, pressure measurements may be repeated and the systolic pressure should be recorded as the catheter is withdrawn from the left ventricle into the aorta. If an aortic transvalvular gradient is present, recording these pressures will detect it. For measurement of suspected intraventricular gradients, a multipurpose catheter with an end hole is desirable to localize the gradient in the left ventricle. Pigtail catheters contain side holes, which will obscure the capacity to define whether the gradient is intraventricular or transvalvular.

After coronary arteriography and left heart catheterization have been completed, the catheters are removed and firm pressure is applied to the femoral area for 15 to 20 minutes, either by hand or by a mechanical clamp. The patient should be instructed to lie in bed for several hours, with the leg remaining straight to prevent hematoma formation.

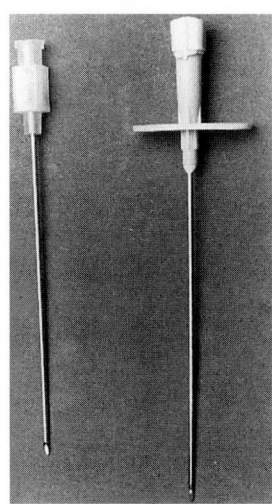

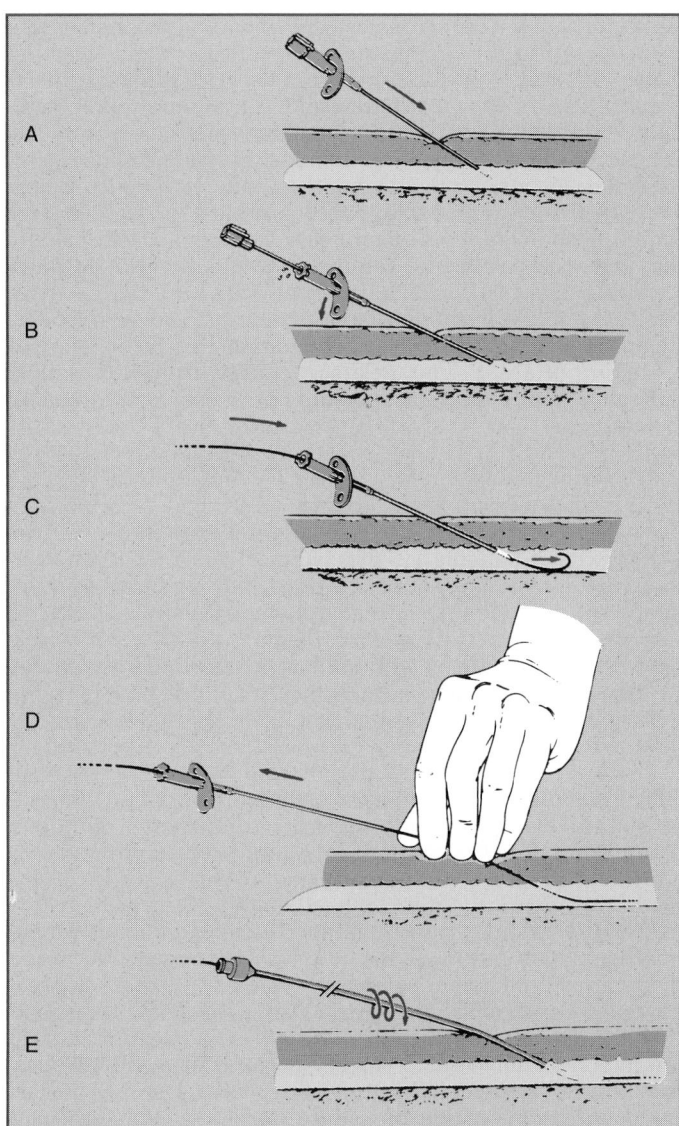

FIGURE 6–7. Two most commonly used needle types for vascular access. On the left, a single-piece, thin-walled "frontwall needle"; on the right, a two-component, thin-walled Seldinger needle. (From Mac-Donald, R. G.: Catheters, sheaths, guidewires, needles and related equipment. *In* Pepine, C. J., Hill, J. A., and Lambert, C. R. [eds.]: Diagnostic and Therapeutic Cardiac Catheterization. 2nd ed. Baltimore, Williams and Wilkins, 1994, p. 112.)

entry. A No. 5F or 6F sheath is placed into the brachial artery, and 5000 units of heparin are infused into the side port. A guidewire is then advanced to the ascending aorta under fluoroscopic control. A No. 5F or 6F left, right, and pigtail catheters are passed over the guidewire for routine arteriography and ventriculography. Occasionally the guidewire may be necessary to direct the left coronary catheter into the left sinus of Valsalva and the ostium of the left main coronary artery.

The main advantage of the percutaneous brachial technique is that it avoids a brachial artery cutdown and repair. The main disadvantage is that manipulation of catheters can be difficult. When this tech-

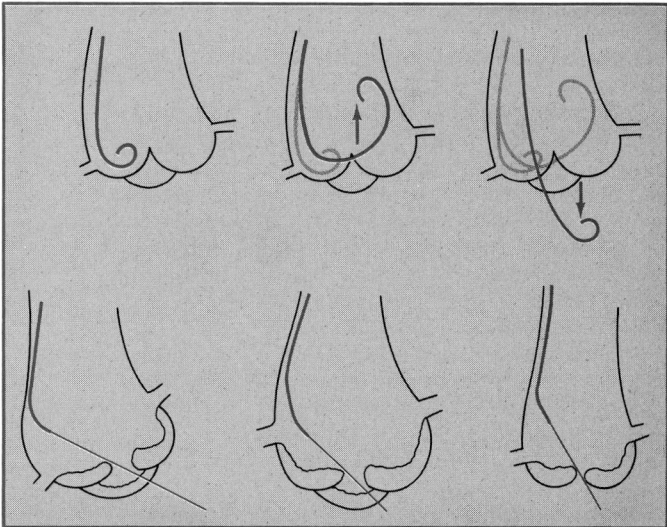

FIGURE 6–6. Basic procedure for the Seldinger technique. *A,* The vessel is punctured with the needle at a 30- to 40-degree angle. *B,* The stylet is removed and free blood flow is observed; the angle of the needle is then reduced. *C,* The flexible tip of the guidewire is passed through the needle into the vessel. *D,* The needle is removed over the wire while firm pressure is applied at the site. *E,* The tip of the catheter is passed over the wire and advanced into the vessel with a rotating motion. (From Tilkian, A. G., and Dailey, E. K.: Cardiovascular Procedures: Diagnostic Techniques and Therapeutic Procedures. St. Louis, C. V. Mosby, 1986.)

With No. 5F catheters, 2 hours of bed rest is usually sufficient, whereas use of 6F catheters usually involves at least 3 to 4 hours.

The main advantage of the Judkins technique is the speed and ease of selective catheterization. However, these attributes do not preclude the importance of extensive operator experience to ensure quality studies with acceptable safety. The main disadvantage of this technique is its use in patients with ileofemoral atherosclerotic disease in whom retrograde passage of catheters through areas of extreme narrowing or tortuosity may be difficult or impossible.

BRACHIAL ARTERY TECHNIQUE—SONES TECHNIQUE. Sones and colleagues[3] introduced the first technique for coronary artery catheterization by means of a brachial artery cutdown. The Sones technique is still popular in many centers and is described on p. 244.

PERCUTANEOUS BRACHIAL ARTERY TECHNIQUE

A modification of Sones technique is the percutaneous brachial artery technique utilizing pre-formed Judkins catheters. This technique uses the Seldinger method of percutaneous brachial artery

FIGURE 6–8. Technique for retrograde crossing of an aortic valve using a pigtail catheter. The upper row shows the technique for crossing a normal aortic valve. In the bottom row, the use of a straight guidewire and pigtail catheter in combination is shown. Increasing the length of protruding guidewire straightens the catheter curve and causes the wire to point more toward the right coronary ostium; reducing the length of protruding wire restores the pigtail contour and deflects the guidewire tip toward the left coronary artery. Once the correct length of wire and the correct rotational orientation of the catheter have been found, repeated advancement and withdrawal of catheter and guidewire together will allow retrograde passage across the valve. In a dilated aortic root, the angled pigtail catheter is preferable. In a small aortic root (bottom row, right) a right coronary Judkins catheter may have advantages. (From Baim, D. S., and Grossman, W.: Percutaneous approach. *In* Grossman, W., and Baim, D. S. [eds.]: Cardiac Catheterization, Angiography, and Intervention. 4th ed. Philadelphia, Lea and Febiger, 1991.)

nique was compared with the femoral technique, patient comfort, hemostasis time, and time to ambulation favor the brachial technique, while procedural efficiency, time of radiation exposure, and diagnostic film quality were more favorable with the femoral approach.[59] Complication rates appear similar.

PERCUTANEOUS RADIAL ARTERY TECHNIQUE

Left heart catheterization via the radial artery approach was developed as an alternative to the percutaneous transbrachial approach in an attempt to limit vascular complications.[60] The inherent advantages of the transradial approach are that the hand has a dual arterial supply connected via the palmar arches and that there are no nerves or veins at the site of puncture. In addition, prolonged bedrest is unnecessary after the procedure, thus allowing for more efficient outpatient angiography.

The procedure requires a normal Allen test: Following manual compression of both the radial and ulnar arteries during fist clenching, normal color returns to the opened hand within 10 seconds after releasing pressure over the ulnar artery, and significant reactive hyperemia is absent upon releasing pressure over the radial artery.[61] The arm is abducted and the wrist hyperextended over a gauze roll. Routine skin anesthesia is used, a small incision is made just proximal to the styloid process of the radius, and the subcutaneous tissue is tunneled using a forceps. An 18-gauge needle is introduced at a 45-degree angle and an exchange-length 0.035- or 0.038-inch J-tip guidewire is inserted. A 23-cm long 5F sheath is then introduced. Heparin, 5000 units, is administered through the side arm of the sheath. No. 5F coronary catheters are then advanced over the exchange wire into the ascending aorta. The left coronary artery is intubated using a left 4-cm tip Judkins (JL 4.0), a left Amplatz, or a brachial Castillo type II catheter. The right coronary artery is intubated using a 4-cm right Judkins (JR 4.0), a left Amplatz, or a multipurpose catheter. Left ventriculography can be performed using a multipurpose catheter with side holes or a pigtail catheter. Exchanges are best performed over the guidewire. Hemostasis is obtained at the end of the procedure after sheath removal using digital pressure. It is recommended that the arterial puncture site be allowed to bleed for several beats before maintaining digital pressure. The radial pulse should be monitored regularly for several hours after the procedure.

The potential limitations of this procedure include the inability to cannulate the radial artery owing to its smaller size and propensity to develop spasm, poor visualization of the coronary arteries resulting from the small-caliber catheters with limited manipulation potential, and risk of arterial occlusion caused by dissection or thrombus formation. In addition, when right heart catheterization is required, other approaches are necessary. While there is little debate that the femoral approach is the simplest and probably the safest technique for left heart catheterization, the transradial approach for left heart catheterization could gain in popularity with refinements in technique and equipment.

Transseptal Catheterization

Transseptal left-sided heart catheterization has received renewed interest recently with the growth of percutaneous balloon mitral commissurotomy as a viable option to surgical commissurotomy and with increasing utilization of disc valves in the aortic position. These mechanical prosthetic valves cannot be crossed safely and prohibit retrograde left heart catheterization.

The original technique of transseptal heart catheterization has been well described[4,5,62] and various techniques currently exist. The transseptal catheter is a short, curved catheter with a tapered tip and side holes. One approach is to place a 0.032-inch guidewire via the femoral vein through the right atrium and into the superior vena cava. A Mullins transseptal sheath and dilator are then advanced over the wire into the superior vena cava. The guidewire is removed and replaced with a Brokenbrough needle, and the distal port is connected to a pressure manifold. With the needle tip just proximal to the Mullins sheath tip, the entire catheter system is withdrawn. The catheter is simultaneously rotated from a 12 o'clock to 5 o'clock position. The operator experiences two abrupt rightward movements. The first occurs as the catheter descends from the superior vena cava to the right atrium. The second occurs as the Mullins dilator tip passes over the limbic edge into the fossa ovalis. The curve of the sheath and needle should be oriented slightly anteriorly. The dilator and needle can then be advanced as a unit. Steady pressure often is adequate to advance the system into the left atrium. If not, the needle should be advanced sharply across the interatrial septum, while holding the Mullins sheath.

Left atrial position can be confirmed by the increase in pressure with left atrial a and v waveforms, hand injection of contrast medium, or measurement of arterial oxygen saturation. Once position is confirmed, the dilator and sheath can be safely advanced 2 to 3 cm into the left atrium. The sheath is held firmly and the dilator and needle are removed. Left atrial pressure measurements may then be repeated. If measurement of left ventricular pressure and/or left ventriculography is necessary, the catheter can usually be advanced easily into the left ventricle after slight counterclockwise rotation. The risk of major morbidity with skilled operators should be less than 2 per cent.[63] The major risk of transseptal catheterization lies in inadvertent puncture of atrial structures, such as the atrial free wall or coronary sinus, or entry into the aortic root or pulmonary artery.

Direct Transthoracic Left Ventricular Puncture

The sole indication for direct left ventricular puncture is to measure left ventricular pressure and to perform ventriculography in patients with mechanical prosthetic valves in both the mitral and aortic positions, thus preventing retrograde arterial and transseptal catheterization. Crossing tilting disc valves with catheters should be avoided as this may result in catheter entrapment, occlusion of the valve, or possible dislodgment of the disc with embolization. The procedure is performed after localizing the left ventricular apex via palpation or preferably using echocardiography.[64] After local anesthesia is administered, a 3½-inch-long 18-gauge needle is inserted at the upper rib margin and directed slightly posteriorly and toward the right shoulder. An 0.035-inch J-tip guidewire is introduced into the ventricle under fluoroscopic guidance, followed by a No. 4F dilator and then a 4F pigtail catheter.[65] The risks of this procedure include cardiac tamponade, hemothorax, pneumothorax, laceration of the left anterior descending coronary artery, embolism of left ventricular thrombus, vagal reactions, and ventricular arrhythmias. The risk of pericardial tamponade, however, is limited in patients who have undergone prior cardiac surgery because mediastinal fibrosis will be present. With the advent of transesophageal echocardiography, this procedure is now infrequently performed.

Endomyocardial Biopsy

Endomyocardial biopsy can be performed using a variety of bioptomes (Fig. 6-9). The most common devices in use as of this writing include the stiff-shaft Caves-Schulz Stanford bioptome[66,67] and the floppy-shaft King's bioptome.[68,69] Right ventricular biopsy may be performed using the internal jugular vein,[67,70] the subclavian vein,[71] or the femoral vein.[72] Left ventricular biopsy may be performed using the femoral arterial approach.[69]

For performing right ventricular biopsy via the right internal jugular vein, a No. 7-9F sheath is introduced using the usual Seldinger technique. A No. 7-9F bioptome is advanced under fluoroscopic guidance to the lateral wall of the right atrium. Using counterclockwise rotation, the device is advanced across the tricuspid valve and toward the interventricular septum. Position of the bioptome against the interventricular septum is confirmed using 30-degree right anterior oblique and 60-degree left anterior oblique fluoroscopic projections. Alternatively, two-dimensional echocardiography has been used to guide the position of the bioptome with good results.[73] Contact with the myocardium is confirmed by the presence of premature ventricular contractions, lack of further advancement, and transmission of ventricular impulse to the operator. The bioptome is then withdrawn from the septum slightly, the forceps jaws are opened, the bioptome is readvanced to contact the myocardium, and the forceps is closed. A slight tug is felt upon removal of the device. Approximately four to six samples of myocardium are required

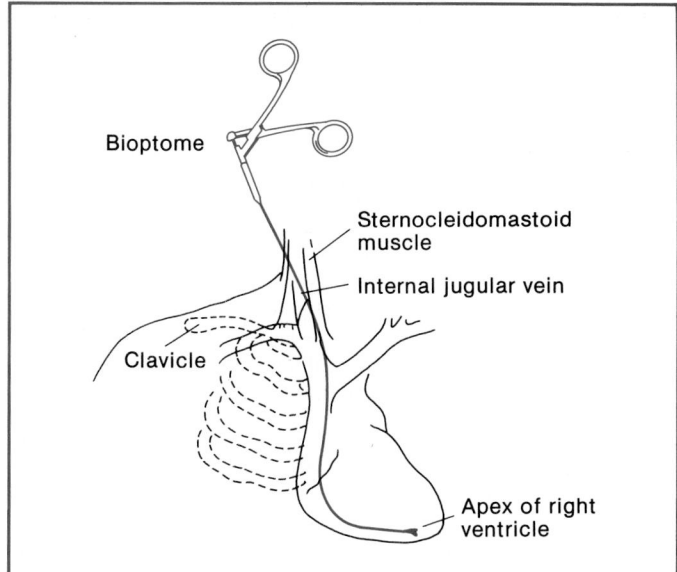

FIGURE 6–9. Endomyocardial biopsy. The bioptome is introduced by way of the right internal jugular vein and is passed across the tricuspid valve into the right ventricle. With the bioptome, a small segment of right ventricular endocardium is removed from the interventricular septum for microscopic examination. (From Mason, J. W., et al.: Myocardial biopsy. *In* Willerson, J. T., and Sanders, C. A. [eds.]: Clinical Cardiology. New York, Grune and Stratton, 1977.)

for adequate pathological analysis. Consultation with a pathologist should be obtained to ensure appropriate specimen collection and processing.

Right or left ventricular biopsy from the femoral vein or artery requires insertion of a long No. 6F or 7F sheath directed toward the portion of the ventricle to be sampled. The sheath used for right ventricular biopsy has a 45-degree angle on its distal end to allow for easier access to the right ventricle. An angled pigtail catheter and long guidewire system are used to enter the right ventricle. The sheath is then advanced over the pigtail catheter into the right ventricle, the catheter is withdrawn, the sheath is flushed, and pressure is measured. The bioptome is advanced through the sheath as flush solution is being continuously infused through the sheath. Samples of myocardium are taken in a manner similar to that described above. If left ventricular biopsy is to be performed, the biopsy sheath is generally positioned over a multipurpose or pigtail catheter which has been positioned in the ventricle. The sheath is advanced below the mitral apparatus and away from the posterobasal wall. The catheter is then withdrawn and either a long King's bioptome or the Stanford left ventricular bioptome is inserted. Care must be taken when left ventricular biopsy is performed to prevent air embolism while introducing the bioptome into the sheath. A constant infusion of flush solution through the sheath minimizes the risk of air or thrombus embolism.

Complications of endomyocardial biopsy include cardiac perforation with cardiac tamponade, emboli (air, tissue, or thromboembolus), arrhythmias, electrical conduction disturbances, injury to heart valves, vasovagal reactions, and pneumothorax.[74] The overall complication rate is between 1 and 2 per cent, with the risk of cardiac perforation with tamponade generally reported in less than 0.05 per cent.[75] Systemic embolization and ventricular arrhythmias are more common with left ventricular biopsy. Left ventricular biopsy should generally be avoided in patients with right bundle branch block because of the potential for developing complete atrioventricular block, and in patients with known left ventricular thrombus.

The indications for endomyocardial biopsy remain controversial.[76–78] Generally, there is agreement that endomyocardial biopsy is indicated to monitor cardiac allograft rejection and may also be useful to monitor for anthracycline cardiotoxicity.[76] However, considerable controversy persists regarding endomyocardial biopsy to evaluate the cause of dilated cardiomopathy.[78,79] Other possible indications for endomyocardial biopsy include differentiation between restrictive and constrictive myopathies,[80,81] determination of whether myocarditis is the cause of ventricular arrhythmias,[76,78] and assessment of patients with left ventricular dysfunction associated with human immunodeficiency virus infection.[82–84]

Percutaneous Intraaortic Balloon Pump Insertion

The intraaortic balloon counterpulsation devices available for adult usage are positioned in the descending thoracic aorta. They have a balloon volume of 30 to 50 ml, use helium as the inflation gas, and are timed to inflate during diastole and deflate during systole. Details of the technique of balloon insertion have been well described.[85] Briefly, the device is inserted via the femoral artery using the standard Seldinger technique. The device is placed such that the tip is just below the level of the left subclavian artery. Optimal positioning requires fluoroscopic guidance. Timing of the balloon is adjusted during 1:2 pumping such that inflation of the balloon will occur at the aortic dicrotic notch and deflation will occur immediately before systole to ensure maximal augmentation of diastolic flow and maximal systolic unloading.

Favorable hemodynamic effects include reduction in left ventricular afterload and improvement in myocardial oxygenation.[86,87] Therefore, intraaortic balloon pump (IABP) insertion is indicated for patients with angina refractory to medical therapy, cardiogenic shock, mechanical complications of myocardial infarction (including severe mitral regurgitation, ventricular septal defect), or those with severe left main coronary artery stenosis who will be undergoing cardiac surgery. IABP may also be valuable in patients undergoing high-risk angioplasty and after primary angioplasty in the setting of acute myocardial infarction.[88–90] IABP insertion is contraindicated in patients with moderate or severe aortic insufficiency, aortic dissection, aortic aneurysm, patent ductus arteriosus, severe peripheral vascular disease, bleeding disorders, or sepsis.

Complications of IABP insertion include limb ischemia requiring early balloon removal or vascular surgery, balloon rupture, balloon entrapment, hematomas, and sepsis.[91–93] The incidence of vascular complications ranges from 12 per cent[92] to over 40 per cent.[91] Most patients who develop limb ischemia after insertion of a balloon pump device have resolution of the ischemia upon balloon removal and do not require surgical intervention (thrombectomy, vascular repair, fasciotomy, or amputation). The risk of limb ischemia is heightened in patients with diabetes or peripheral vascular disease, in women, and in patients with a postinsertion ankle-brachial index of less than 0.8.[91] With the development of smaller size catheters (No. 8.5F to 9.5F) and the advent of the sheathless insertion techniques, vascular complications have been reduced.[93,94]

HEMODYNAMIC DATA

The hemodynamic component of the cardiac catheterization procedure focuses on pressure measurements, the measurement of flow (cardiac output, shunt flows, flow across a stenotic orifice, regurgitant flows, coronary blood flow, and so on), and the determination of vascular resistances. Simply stated, flow through a blood vessel is determined by the pressure difference within the vessel and the vascular resistance as described by Ohm's law: $Q = \Delta P/R$.

Pressure Measurements

The accurate recording of pressure waveforms and the correct interpretation of physiological data derived from these waveforms is a major goal of cardiac catheterization. A pressure wave is the cyclical force generated by cardiac muscle contraction, and its amplitude and duration are influenced by various mechanical and physiological parameters. The pressure waveform from a particular cardiac chamber is influenced by the force of the contracting chamber and its surrounding structures including the contiguous chambers of the heart, the pericardium, the lungs, and the vasculature. Physiological variables of heart rate and the respiratory cycle also influence the pressure waveform. An understanding of the various components of the cardiac cycle is essential to the correct interpretation of hemodynamic data obtained in the catheterization laboratory (Fig. 12–22).

PRESSURE MEASUREMENT SYSTEMS. Intravascular pressures are typically measured using a fluid-filled catheter that is attached to a pressure transducer. The pressure wave is transmitted from the catheter tip to the transducer by the fluid column within the catheter. The majority of pressure transducers used currently are disposable electrical strain-gauges. The pressure wave distorts the diaphragm or wire within the transducer. This energy is then converted to an electric signal proportional to the pressure being applied using the principle of the Wheatstone bridge. This signal is then amplified and recorded as an analog signal.[95]

There are a number of sources of error when pressures are measured using a fluid-filled catheter/transducer system.[96] Distortion of the output signal occurs as a result of the frequency response characteristics and damping characteristics of the system. The frequency response of the system is the ratio of the output amplitude to input amplitude over a range of frequencies of the input pressure wave. The natural frequency is the frequency that the system oscillates when it is shock-excited in the absence of friction. If the energy of the system is dissipated, such as by friction, this is called *damping*. In order to ensure a high-frequency response range, the pressure measurement system should have the highest possible natural frequency and optimal damping. Optimal damping dissipates the energy gradually, thus maintaining the frequency response curve as close to an output/input ratio of 1 as it approaches the system's natural frequency. This is achieved by using a short wide-bore, noncompliant catheter/tubing system that is directly connected to the transducer using a low-density liquid from which all air bubbles have been removed.[95]

The pressure transducer must be calibrated against a known pressure, and the establishment of a zero reference must be undertaken at the start of the catheterization procedure. In order to "zero" the transducer, the tranducer is placed at the level of the heart, which is approximately midchest. If the transducer is attached to the manifold and is therefore at variable positions during the procedure, a second fluid-filled catheter system should be attached to the transducer and positioned at the level of the heart. All transducers being used during the procedure should be zeroed and calibrated simultaneously.

Other sources of error include catheter whip artifact (motion of the tip of the catheter within the measured chamber), end pressure artifact (an end hole catheter measures an artificially elevated pressure on account of streaming or high velocity of the pressure wave), catheter impact artifact (when the catheter is impacted by the walls or valves of the cardiac chambers), and catheter tip obstruction within small vessels or valvular orifices occurring because of the size of the catheter itself. The operator must be aware of the many sources of potential error, and when there is a discrepancy between the observed data and the clinical scenario, the system should be examined for errors or artifacts.

Use of micromanometer catheters, which have the pressure transducer mounted at their catheter tip, greatly reduces many of these errors in measurement. However, their utility is limited by the additional cost and time to properly calibrate and utilize the system. These catheters have higher natural frequencies and more optimal damping characteristics because the interposing fluid column is eliminated. In addition, there is a decrease in catheter whip artifact. The pressure waveform is less distorted and is without the 30- to 40-millisecond delay seen in the fluid-filled catheter/transducer system. Commercially available high-fidelity micromanometer systems (Millar Instruments, Houston, TX) have both an end hole and side holes to allow for an over-the-wire insertion into the circulation while also permitting angiography. Catheters that have two transducers separated by a short distance are useful for accurate measurement of gradients across valvular structures and within ventricular chambers. The micromanometer system has been used for research purposes to measure the rate of ventricular pressure rise (dP/dt), wall stress, the rate of ventricular pressure decay (− dP/dt), and the time constant of relaxation, and to determine ventricular pressure-volume relationships.[97]

There are several disadvantages of the micromanometer catheter systems including their expense and fragility and the need for sterilization between usage. In addition, the zero level of these systems may drift after the pressure is zeroed to the fluid-filled lumen within the catheter.

Normal Pressure Waveforms

An understanding of the normal pressure waveform morphologies is necessary to comprehend the abnormalities that characterize certain pathological conditions. Normal pressures in the cardiac chambers and great vessels are given in Table 6–5. Simply stated, whenever fluid is added

TABLE 6–5 NORMAL PRESSURES AND VASCULAR RESISTANCES

PRESSURES	AVERAGE (mm Hg)	RANGE (mm Hg)
Right atrium		
a wave	6	2–7
v wave	5	2–7
mean	3	1–5
Right ventricle		
peak systolic	25	15–30
end-diastolic	4	1–7
Pulmonary artery		
peak systolic	25	15–30
end-diastolic	9	4–12
mean	15	9–19
Pulmonary capillary wedge		
mean	9	4–12
Left atrium		
a wave	10	4–16
v wave	12	6–21
mean	8	2–12
Left ventricle		
peak systolic	130	90–140
end-diastolic	8	5–12
Central aorta		
peak systolic	130	90–140
end-diastolic	70	60–90
mean	85	70–105

VASCULAR RESISTANCES	MEAN (dyne-sec-cm^{-5})	RANGE (dyne-sec-cm^{-5})
Systemic vascular resistance	1100	700–1600
Total pulmonary resistance	200	100–300
Pulmonary vascular resistance	70	20–130

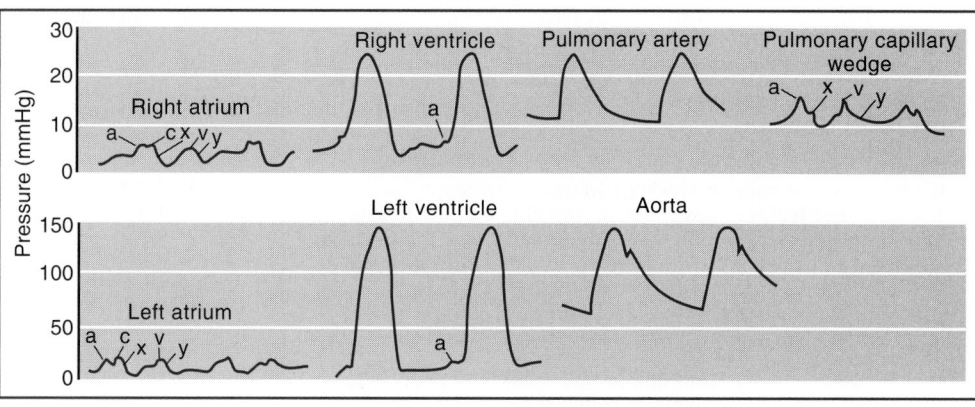

FIGURE 6–10. Normal right and left heart pressures recorded from fluid-filled catheter systems in a human. (From Pepine, C.: Diagnostic and Therapeutic Cardiac Catheterization. Baltimore, Williams and Wilkins, 1989.)

to a chamber or compressed within a chamber, the pressure usually rises; conversely, whenever fluid exits from a chamber or the chamber relaxes, the pressure usually falls. One exception to this rule is the early phase of ventricular diastolic filling when ventricular volume increases after mitral valve opening but ventricular pressure continues to decrease because of active relaxation.[98] Examples of normal pressure waveforms are given in Figure 6–10.

ATRIAL PRESSURE. The *right atrial pressure waveform* has three positive deflections, the *a*, *c*, and *v* waves. The *a* wave is due to atrial systole and follows the P wave of the ECG. The height of the *a* wave depends on atrial contractility and the resistance to right ventricle filling. The *x* descent follows the *a* wave and represents relaxation of the atrium and the downward pulling of the tricuspid annulus by right ventricular contraction. The *x* descent is interrupted by the *c* wave, which is a small positive deflection due to protrusion of the closed tricuspid valve into the right atrium. Pressure in the atrium rises after the *x* descent owing to passive atrial filling. The atrial pressure then peaks as the *v* wave, which represents right ventricular systole. The height of the *v* wave is related to atrial compliance and the amount of blood returning to the atrium from the periphery. The right atrial *v* wave is generally smaller than the *a* wave. The *y* descent occurs after the *v* wave and reflects tricuspid valve opening and right atrial emptying into the right ventricle. During spontaneous respiration, there is a decline in right atrial pressure during inhalation as intrathoracic pressure falls. Right atrial pressure rises during exhalation as intrathoracic pressures increase. The opposite effect is seen when patients are mechanically ventilated.

The *left atrial pressure waveform* is similar to that of the right atrium, although normal left atrial pressure is higher, reflecting the high pressure system of the left side of the heart. In the left atrium, as opposed to the right atrium, the *v* wave is generally higher than the *a* wave. This occurs because the left atrium is constrained posteriorly by the pulmonary veins, while the right atrium can easily decompress throughout the inferior and superior venae cavae. The height of the left atrial *v* wave most accurately reflects left atrial compliance.

PULMONARY CAPILLARY WEDGE PRESSURE. The pulmonary capillary wedge pressure waveform is similar to the left atrial pressure waveform but is slightly damped and delayed as a result of transmission through the lungs. The *a* and *v* waves with both *x* and *y* descents are visible, but *c* waves may not be seen. In the normal state, the pulmonary artery diastolic pressure is similar to the mean pulmonary capillary wedge pressure because the pulmonary circulation has low resistance. In certain disease states that are associated with an elevated pulmonary vascular resistance (hypoxemia, pulmonary embolism, and chronic pulmonary hypertension), and occasionally after mitral valve surgery, the pulmonary capillary wedge pressure may not accurately reflect left atrial pressure. Pulmonary capillary wedge may overestimate true left atrial pressure in this circumstance.

Thus, accurate measurement of mitral valve gradient may require obtaining direct left atrial pressure.

VENTRICULAR PRESSURE. Right and left ventricular waveforms are similar in morphology. They differ mainly with respect to their magnitudes, with left ventricular systolic and diastolic pressures being higher. The duration of systole and isovolumic contraction and relaxation are longer, and the ejection period shorter in the left than in the right ventricle. There may be a small (≤5 mm Hg) systolic gradient between the right ventricle and the pulmonary artery. Ventricular diastolic pressure is characterized by an early rapid filling wave during which most of the ventricle fills, a slow-filling phase and the *a* wave denoting atrial systolic activity. End-diastolic pressure is generally measured at the *c* point, which is the rise in ventricular pressure at the onset of isovolumic contraction (Fig. 12–22). When the *c* point is not well seen, a line is drawn from the R wave on the simultaneous ECG to the ventricular pressure waveform, and this is used as the end-diastolic pressure.

GREAT VESSEL PRESSURES. The contour of the *central aortic pressure* and the *pulmonary artery pressure* tracing consists of a systolic wave, the incisura (indicating closure of the semilunar valves), and a gradual decline in pressure until the following systole. The pulse pressure reflects the stroke volume and compliance of the arterial system. The mean aortic pressure more accurately reflects peripheral resistance. As the systemic pressure wave is transmitted through the length of the aorta, the systolic wave increases in amplitude and becomes more triangular in shape, while the diastolic wave decreases until it reaches the midthoracic aorta and then increases. The mean aortic pressures, however, are usually similar, with the mean *peripheral arterial pressure* typically ≤5 mm Hg lower than the mean central aortic pressure. The difference in systolic pressures between the central aorta and the periphery (femoral, brachial, or radial arteries) is greatest in younger patients due to their increased vascular compliance. These potential differences between proximal aorta and peripheral artery must be considered in order to measure and interpret the peak systolic pressure gradient between the left ventricle and systemic arterial system in patients with suspected aortic stenosis.

ABNORMAL PRESSURE CHARACTERISTICS. Abnormal pressure waveforms may be diagnostic of specific pathological conditions. Although these conditions are discussed in greater detail elsewhere in this book, Table 6–6 summarizes the more commonly encountered waveforms.

Cardiac Output Measurements

There is no totally accurate method to measure cardiac output, but it can be estimated on the basis of various assumptions. The two most commonly used methods are the Fick method and thermodilution method. For comparison among patients, cardiac output is often corrected for the patient's size based on the body surface area and expressed as cardiac index.

TABLE 6–6 PATHOLOGICAL WAVEFORMS

I. RIGHT ATRIAL PRESSURE WAVEFORMS

A. Low mean atrial pressure
   1. Hypovolemia
   2. Improper zeroing of the transducer
B. Elevated mean atrial pressure
   1. Intravascular volume overload states
   2. Right ventricular failure due to valvular disease (tricuspid or pulmonic stenosis or regurgitation)
   3. Right ventricular failure due to myocardial disease (right ventricular ischemia, cardiomyopathy)
   4. Right ventricular failure due to left heart failure (mitral stenosis/regurgitation, aortic stenosis/regurgitation, cardiomyopathy, ischemia)
   5. Right ventricular failure due to increased pulmonary vascular resistance (pulmonary embolism, chronic obstructive pulmonary disease, primary pulmonary hypertension)
   6. Pericardial effusion with tamponade physiology
   7. Obstructive atrial myxoma
C. Elevated a wave (any increase to ventricular filling)
   1. Tricuspid stenosis
   2. Decreased ventricular compliance due to ventricular failure, pulmonic valve stenosis, or pulmonary hypertension
D. Cannon a wave
   1. Atrial-ventricular asynchrony (atria contract against a closed tricuspid valve, as during complete heart block, following premature ventricular contraction, during ventricular tachycardia, with ventricular pacemaker)
E. Absent a wave
   1. Atrial fibrillation or atrial standstill
   2. Atrial flutter
F. Elevated v wave
   1. Tricuspid regurgitation
   2. Right ventricular heart failure
   3. Reduced atrial compliance (restrictive myopathy)
G. a wave equal to v wave
   1. Tamponade
   2. Constrictive pericardial disease
   3. Hypervolemia
H. Prominent x descent
   1. Tamponade
   2. Subacute constriction and possibly chronic constriction
   3. Right ventricular ischemia with preservation of atrial contractility
I. Prominent y descent
   1. Constrictive pericarditis
   2. Restrictive myopathies
   3. Tricuspid regurgitation
J. Blunted x descent
   1. Atrial fibrillation
   2. Right atrial ischemia
K. Blunted y descent
   1. Tamponade
   2. Right ventricular ischemia
   3. Tricuspid stenosis
L. Miscellaneous abnormalities
   1. Kussmaul's sign (inspiratory rise or lack of decline in right atrial pressure): constrictive pericarditis, right ventricular ischemia
   2. Equalization (≤ 5 mm Hg) of mean right atrial, right ventricular diastolic, pulmonary artery diastolic, pulmonary capillary wedge, and pericardial pressures in tamponade
   3. M or W patterns: right ventricular ischemia, pericardial constriction, congestive heart failure
   4 Ventricularization of the right atrial pressure: severe tricuspid regurgitation
   5. Saw tooth pattern: atrial flutter
   6. Dissociation between pressure recording and intracardiac ECG: Ebstein's anomaly

II. LEFT ATRIAL PRESSURE/PULMONARY CAPILLARY WEDGE PRESSURE WAVEFORMS

A. Low mean pressure
   1. Hypovolemia
   2. Improper zeroing of the transducer
B. Elevated mean pressure
   1. Intravascular volume overload states
   2. Left ventricular failure due to valvular disease (mitral or aortic stenosis or regurgitation)
   3. Left ventricular failure due to myocardial disease (ischemia or cardiomyopathy)
   4. Left ventricular failure due to systemic hypertension
   5. Pericardial effusion with tamponade physiology
   6. Obstructive atrial myxoma
C. Elevated a wave (any increase to ventricular filling)
   1. Mitral stenosis
   2. Decreased ventricular compliance due to ventricular failure, aortic valve stenosis, or systemic hypertension
D. Cannon a wave
   1. Atrial-ventricular asynchrony (atria contract against a closed mitral valve, as during complete heart block, following premature ventricular contraction, during ventricular tachycardia, with ventricular pacemaker)
E. Absent a wave
   1. Atrial fibrillation or atrial standstill
   2. Atrial flutter
F. Elevated v wave
   1. Mitral regurgitation
   2. Left ventricular heart failure
   3. Ventricular septal defect
G. a wave equal to v wave
   1. Tamponade
   2. Constrictive pericardial disease
   3. Hypervolemia
H. Prominent x descent
   1. Tamponade
   2. Subacute constriction and possibly chronic constriction
I. Prominent y descent
   1. Constrictive pericarditis
   2. Restrictive myopathies
   3. Mitral regurgitation
J. Blunted x descent
   1. Atrial fibrillation
   2. Atrial ischemia
K. Blunted y descent
   1. Tamponade
   2. Ventricular ischemia
   3. Mitral stenosis
L. Pulmonary capillary wedge pressure not equal to left ventricular end-diastolic pressure
   1. Mitral stenosis
   2. Left atrial myxoma
   3. Cor triatriatum
   4. Pulmonary venous obstruction
   5. Decreased ventricular compliance
   6. Increased pleural pressure
   7. Placement of catheter in a nondependent zone of lung

III. PULMONARY ARTERY PRESSURE WAVEFORMS

A. Elevated systolic pressure
   1. Primary pulmonary hypertension
   2. Mitral stenosis or regurgitation
   3. Congestive heart failure
   4. Restrictive myopathies
   5. Significant left to right shunt
   6. Pulmonary disease (pulmonary embolism, hypoxemia, chronic obstructive pulmonary disease)
B. Reduced systolic pressure
   1. Hypovolemia
   2. Pulmonary artery stenosis
   3. Sub- or supravalvular stenosis
   4. Ebstein's anomaly
   5. Tricuspid stenosis
   6. Tricuspid atresia
C. Reduced pulse pressure
   1. Right heart ischemia
   2. Right ventricular infarction
   3. Pulmonary embolism
   4. Tamponade
D. Bifid pulmonary artery waveform
   1. Large left atrial v wave transmitted backward (i.e., MR)
E. Pulmonary artery diastolic pressure greater than pulmonary capillary wedge pressure
   1. Pulmonary disease
   2. Pulmonary embolus
   3. Tachycardia

TABLE 6–6 PATHOLOGICAL WAVEFORMS—Continued

IV. VENTRICULAR PRESSURE WAVEFORMS

A. Systolic pressure elevated
   1. Pulmonary or systemic hypertension
   2. Pulmonary valve or aortic valve stenosis
   3. Ventricular outflow tract obstruction
   4. Supravalvular obstruction
   5. Right ventricular pressure elevation with significant:
     a. Atrial septal defect
     b. Ventricular septal defect
   6. Right ventricular pressure elevation due to factors that increase pulmonary vascular resistance (see factors that increase right atrial pressure)
B. Systolic pressure reduced
   1. Hypovolemia
   2. Cardiogenic shock
   3. Tamponade
C. End-diastolic pressure elevated
   1. Hypervolemia
   2. Congestive heart failure
   3. Diminished compliance
   4. Hypertrophy
   5. Tamponade
   6. Regurgitant valvular disease
   7. Pericardial constriction
D. End-diastolic pressure reduced
   1. Hypovolemia
   2. Tricuspid or mitral stenosis
E. Diminished or absent *a* wave
   1. Atrial fibrillation or flutter
   2. Tricuspid or mitral stenosis
   3. Tricuspid or mitral regurgitation when ventricular compliance is increased
F. Dip and plateau in diastolic pressure wave
   1. Constrictive pericarditis
   2. Restrictive myopathies
   3. Right ventricular ischemia
   4. Acute dilatation associated with:
     a. Tricuspid regurgitation
     b. Mitral regurgitation
G. Left ventricular end-diastolic pressure > right ventricular end-diastolic pressure
   1. Restrictive myopathies

V. AORTIC PRESSURE WAVEFORMS

A. Systolic pressure elevated
   1. Systemic hypertension
   2. Arteriosclerosis
   3. Aortic insufficiency
B. Systolic pressure reduced
   1. Aortic stenosis
   2. Heart failure
   3. Hypovolemia
C. Widened pulse pressure
   1. Systemic hypertension
   2. Aortic insufficiency
   3. Significant patent ductus arteriosus
   4. Significant ruptures sinus of Valsalva aneurysm
D. Reduced pulse pressure
   1. Tamponade
   2. Congestive heart failure
   3. Cardiogenic shock
   4. Aortic stenosis
E. Pulsus bisferiens
   1. Aortic insufficiency
   2. Obstructive hypertrophic cardiomyopathy
F. Pulsus paradoxus
   1. Tamponade
   2. Chronic obstructive airway disease
   3. Pulmonary embolism
G. Pulsus alternans
   1. Congestive heart failure
   2. Cardiomyopathy
H. Pulsus parvus et tardus
   1. Aortic stenosis
I. Spike and dome configuration
   1. Obstructive hypertrophic cardiomyopathy

INDICATOR-DILUTION TECHNIQUES. The indicator-dilution method has been used to measure cardiac output since its introduction by Stewart in 1897 and subsequent modification by Hamilton and associates in 1932. The basic equation, commonly referred to as the Stewart-Hamilton equation, is shown below:

$$\text{Cardiac output (1/min)} = \frac{\text{amount of indicator injected (mg)} \times 60 \text{ sec/min}}{\text{mean indicator concentration (mg/ml)} \times \text{curve duration}}$$

The assumption is made that after the injection of a certain quantity of an indicator into the circulation, the indicator appears and disappears from any downstream point in a manner commensurate with the cardiac output. For example, if the indicator rapidly appears at a specific location downstream and then washes out quickly, the assumption is that the cardiac output is high. Although variation can occur, the site of injection is usually a systemic vein or the right side of the heart, and the sampling site is generally a systemic artery. The normal curve itself has an initial rapid upstroke followed by a slower downstroke and eventual appearance of recirculation of the tracer. In practice, this recirculation creates some uncertainty on the tail of the curve, and assumptions are required to correct for this distortion. Because the indicator concentration declines exponentially in the absence of recirculation, the initial data points from the descending limb are used to extrapolate the remainder of the descending limb. The area under both the ascending and descending limbs is then determined along with the total curve duration. The area of the curve is assumed to be a function of the mean indicator concentration. Both variables can be substituted in the Stewart-Hamilton equation to calculate the cardiac output.

There are several sources of error in this determination. Because the dye is unstable over time and can be affected by light, fresh preparations of indocyanine green dye are necessary. The exact amount of dye must be accurately measured, as it is crucial to the performance of the study. It is generally administered through a tuberculin syringe and injected rapidly as a single bolus. After injection, the indicator must mix well before reaching the sampling site, and the dilution curve must have an exponential decay over time so that extrapolation can be performed. If, for example, there is severe valvular regurgitation or a low cardiac output state in which the washout of the indicator is prolonged and recirculation begins well before an adequate decline in the indicator curve occurs, determinations will be erroneous. Intracardiac shunts may also greatly affect the shape of the curve.

THERMODILUTION TECHNIQUES. Because of the rather tedious and time-consuming nature of the indicator-dilution method, it has been replaced by thermodilution techniques in many laboratories. The development of balloon flotation (e.g., Swan-Ganz) catheters with a proximal port and distal thermistor has greatly expanded the ability to obtain thermodilution cardiac outputs in many clinical settings.

The thermodilution procedure requires the injection of a bolus of liquid (saline or dextrose) into the proximal port of the catheter. The resultant change in temperature in the liquid is measured by a thermistor mounted in the distal end of the catheter. The change in temperature versus time can be plotted in a manner similar to the dye-dilution method described above (in which the indicator is now the cooler liquid). The cardiac output is then calculated using an equation that considers the temperature and specific gravity of the injectate and the temperature and specific gravity of the blood, along with the injectate volume. A calibration factor is also used. The cardiac output is inversely related to the area under a thermodilution curve, plotted as a function of temperature versus time, with a smaller area indicative of a higher cardiac output.

The thermodilution method has several advantages. It obviates the need for withdrawal of blood from an arterial site and is less affected by recirculation. Perhaps its greatest advantage is the rapid display of results using computerized methods. Computers use the washout rate represented by the downslope of the curve to obtain a decay constant to correct the descending limb and compute the cardiac output.

Thermodilution cardiac outputs are susceptible to pitfalls similar to those encountered with indicator-dilution methods using indocyanine green. Because the data represent right-sided heart output, tricuspid regurgitation can be a particular problem as the bolus of saline is subsequently broken up. The thermodilution method tends to overestimate cardiac output in low-output states, because the dissipation of the cooler temperature to the surrounding cardiac structures results in reduction in the total area under the curve, causing a falsely elevated cardiac output value. Other difficulties include fluctuations in blood temperature during respiratory or cardiac cycles and the warming of the temperature of the injectate before its injection into the catheter. Because of these possible limitations, the general practice is to calculate the average of several (usually 3 to 5) cardiac output determinations.

From a practical viewpoint, thermodilution cardiac outputs have become standard practice. Their variability can be relatively large; thus small changes should not be over-interpreted. Practically, cardiac output data can be defined only to within a 15 per cent range.[99]

FICK TECHNIQUE. The Fick principle was first described by Adolph Fick in 1870. It assumes that the rate in which oxygen is consumed is a function of the rate of blood flow times the rate of oxygen pickup by the red blood cells. The basic assumption is that the flow of blood in a given period of time is equal to the amount of substance entering the stream of flow in the same period of time divided by the difference between the concentrations of the substance in the blood upstream and downstream from its point of entry into the circulation[100] (Fig. 6–11). The same number of red blood cells that enter the lung must leave the lung, if no intracardiac shunt is present. Thus, if certain parameters were known (the number of oxygen molecules that were attached to the red blood cells entering the lung, the number of oxygen molecules that were attached to the red blood cells leaving the lung, and the number of oxygen molecules consumed during travel through the lung), then the rate of flow of these red blood cells as they pass through the lung could be determined. This can be expressed in the following terms:

$$\text{Cardiac output (L/min)} = \frac{O_2 \text{ consumption (ml/min)}}{A - VO_2 \text{ difference (vol \%)} \times 10}$$

Measurements must be done in steady state. Automated methods can accurately determine the oxygen content within the blood samples. Thus, the greatest source of measurement variability is that of the oxygen consumption. Traditional Fick determinations used Van Slyke's method, in which expiratory gas samples were collected in a large bag over a specified period of time. By measuring the oxygen consumption within the bag and by knowing the concentration of oxygen in room air, the quantity of oxygen consumed over time could be determined. Newer techniques now allow for the measurement of oxygen consumption by a polargraphic method in which expired oxygen can be quantified by calculating the change in electrical current between a gold cathode and silver anode embedded in a potassium chloride gel. These devices can be connected to the patient by use of a plastic hood or by a mouthpiece and tubing.

The Fick method suffers primarily from the difficulty in obtaining accurate oxygen consumption measurements and the inability to obtain a steady state under certain conditions. Since the method assumes mean flow over a period of time, it is not suitable during rapid change in flow. It requires considerable time and effort on the part of the catheterization laboratory to obtain the appropriate data. Many laboratories use an "assumed" Fick method in which oxygen consumption index is assumed on the basis of the patient's age, gender, and body surface area or an estimate made (125 ml/m²) on the basis of body surface area. The advantage of the Fick method is that it is the most accurate method in patients with low cardiac output and thus is preferred over the thermodilution method in these circumstances. It is also independent of the factors that affect curve shape and cause errors in thermodilution cardiac output. The inaccuracy of oxygen consumption measurements results in up to 10 per cent variability in the calculated cardiac output, which may be even greater when assumed oxygen consumption, rather than measured oxygen consumption, is used.

ANGIOGRAPHIC CARDIAC OUTPUT. Angiographic stroke volume can be calculated from tracing the end-diastolic and end-systolic images. Stroke volume is the amount of blood ejected with each beat. End-diastolic volume is the maximum left ventricular volume and occurs immediately before the onset of systole. This occurs immediately after atrial contraction in patients in sinus rhythm. End-systolic volume is the minimum volume during the cardiac cycle. Calibration of the images with calibrated grids or ventricular phantoms is necessary to obtain accurate ventricular volumes. Angiographic cardiac output and stroke volume are derived from the equation:

$$\text{Stroke volume} = EDV - ESV$$

$$\text{Cardiac output} = (EDV - ESV) \times \text{heart rate}$$

where EDV = end-diastolic volume and ESV = end-systolic volume. The inherent inaccuracies of calibrating angiographic volumes often make this method of measurement unreliable. In cases of valvular regurgitation or atrial fibrillation, angiographic cardiac output will not accurately measure true systemic outputs. However, the angiographic cardiac output is preferred over the Fick or thermodilution outputs for calculation of stenotic valve areas in patients with significant aortic or mitral regurgitation.

DETERMINATION OF VASCULAR RESISTANCE. Vascular resistance calculations are based on hydraulic principles of

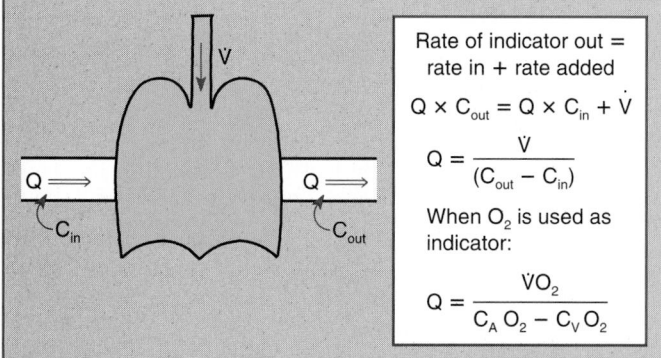

FIGURE 6–11. Schematic illustration of flow measurement using the Fick principle. Fluid containing a known concentration of an indicator (C_{in}) enters a system at flow rate, Q. As the fluid passes through the system, indicator is continuously added at rate $\dot{V}$, raising the concentration in the outflow to C_{out}. In a steady state, the rate of indicator leaving the system (QC_{out}) must equal the rate at which it enters (QC_{in}) plus the rate at which it is added ($\dot{V}$). When oxygen is used as the indicator, cardiac output can be determined by measuring oxygen consumption ($\dot{V}O_2$), arterial oxygen content (C_AO_2), and mixed venous oxygen content (C_VO_2). (From Winniford, M. D., and Lambert, C. R. [eds.]: Blood flow measurement. In Pepine, C. J., Hill, J. A., and Lambert, C. R. [eds.]: Diagnostic and Therapeutic Cardiac Catheterization. 2nd ed. Baltimore, Williams and Wilkins, 1994, p. 322.)

Within the figure:

Rate of indicator out = rate in + rate added

$$Q \times C_{out} = Q \times C_{in} + \dot{V}$$

$$Q = \frac{\dot{V}}{(C_{out} - C_{in})}$$

When O_2 is used as indicator:

$$Q = \frac{\dot{V}O_2}{C_A O_2 - C_V O_2}$$

fluid flow, in which resistance is defined as the ratio of the decrease in pressure between two points in a vascular segment and the blood flow through the segment. Although this straightforward analogy to Ohm's law represents an oversimplification of the complex behavior of pulsatile flow in dynamic and diverse vascular beds, the calculation of vascular resistance based on these principles has proven to be of value in a number of clinical settings.

The determination of the resistance in a vascular bed requires measurement of the mean pressure of the proximal and distal ends of the vascular bed and accurate measurement of cardiac output. For this purpose, measurement of cardiac output by the Fick, the indicator-dilution, or the thermodilution method is preferred. Vascular resistance (R) is usually defined in absolute units (dynes-sec-cm^{-5}) and is defined as R = [mean pressure gradient (dyne/cm^2)]/[mean flow (cm^3/sec)]. Hybrid units (Wood units) are less often used.[101]

Systemic vascular resistance in absolute units is calculated using the equation:

$$SVR = \frac{80(Ao_m - RA_m)}{Q_s}$$

where Ao_m and RA_m are the mean pressures (in mm Hg) in the aorta and right atrium, respectively, and Q_s is the systemic cardiac output (in liters/min). The constant 80 is used to convert units from mm Hg/liters/min (Wood units) to the absolute resistance units dynes-sec-cm^{-5}. If the right atrial pressure is not known, the term RA_m can be dropped, and the resulting value is called the *total peripheral resistance* (TPR).

$$TPR = \frac{80(Ao_m)}{Q_s}$$

Similarly, the pulmonary vascular resistance is derived from the equation:

$$PVR = \frac{80(PA_m - LA_m)}{Q_p}$$

where PA_m and LA_m are the pulmonary artery and left atrial pressures, respectively, and Q_p is the pulmonary blood flow. Mean pulmonary capillary wedge pressure is commonly substituted for mean left atrial pressure if the latter has not been measured directly.[102-104] In the absence of an intracardiac shunt, Q_p is equal to the systemic cardiac output.

Elevated resistances in the systemic and pulmonary circuits may represent reversible abnormalities or may be fixed owing to irreversible anatomical changes. In several clinical situations, such as congestive heart failure, valvular heart disease, primary pulmonary hypertension, and congenital heart disease with intracardiac shunting, determination of whether elevated systemic or pulmonary vascular resistance can be lowered transiently in the catheterization laboratory may provide important insights into potential management strategies. Interventions that may be used in the laboratory for this purpose include the administration of vasodilating drugs (e.g., nifedipine, sodium nitroprusside), exercise, and (in patients with pulmonary hypertension) oxygen inhalation.

Vascular impedance measurements account for blood viscosity, pulsatile flow, reflected waves, and arterial compliance. Hence, vascular impedance has the potential to describe the dynamic relation between pressure and flow more comprehensively than is possible using the simpler calculations of vascular resistance. However, because the simultaneous pressure and flow data required for the calculation of impedance are complex and difficult to obtain, the concept of impedance has failed to gain widespread acceptance, and vascular impedance has not been adopted as a routine clinical index in most laboratories.

(See also Chap. 32)

Determining the severity of valvular stenosis based on the pressure gradient and flow across the valve is one of the most important aspects of evaluation in the catheterization laboratory of patients with valvular heart disease. In most patients, the magnitude of the pressure gradient alone is sufficient to distinguish clinically significant from insignificant valvular stenosis.

DETERMINATION OF PRESSURE GRADIENTS. In patients with *aortic stenosis* (see p. 1035), the transvalvular pressure gradient should be measured, whenever possible, with a catheter in the left ventricle and another in the proximal aorta. Although it is convenient to measure the gradient between the left ventricle and the femoral artery, downstream augmentation of the pressure signal and delay in pressure transmission between the proximal aorta and femoral artery may alter the pressure waveform substantially and introduce errors into the measured gradient.[105]

Left ventricular–femoral artery pressure gradients may suffice in many patients as an estimate of the severity of aortic stenosis to confirm the presence of a severely stenotic valve. If the side port of the arterial introducing sheath is used to monitor femoral pressure, the inner diameter of the sheath should be 1F size larger than the outer diameter of the catheter being used. The left ventricular–femoral artery gradient should not be relied on in the calculation of valve orifice area in patients with equivocal valve gradients. Thus, measurements obtained with two catheters, one positioned in the body of the left ventricle and the other in the proximal aorta, or in a careful single catheter pullback from left ventricle to aorta, are preferable to simultaneous measurement of left ventricular and femoral artery pressures. Alternatively, a single catheter with distal and proximal lumens, or a micromanometer catheter with distal and proximal transducers, may be used for simultaneous measurement of left ventricular pressure and central aortic pressure.

In patients with very severe aortic stenosis, the left ventricular catheter itself may reduce the effective orifice area, resulting in an artifactual increase in the measured pressure gradient.[106] This overestimation of the severity of aortic stenosis is rarely an important issue, as the diagnosis of severe aortic stenosis is usually already apparent in such patients.

The mean pressure gradient across the aortic valve is determined by planimetry of the area separating the left ventricular and aortic pressures using multiple beats (Fig. 6–12), and it is this gradient that is applied to calculation of the valve orifice area. The peak-to-peak gradient, measured as the difference between peak left ventricular pressure and peak aortic pressure, is commonly used to quantify the valve gradient, because this measurement is rapidly obtained and can be estimated visually. However, there is no physiological basis for the peak-to-peak gradient, since the maximum left ventricular and aortic pressures rarely occur simultaneously. The peak-to-peak gradient measured in the catheterization laboratory is generally lower than the peak instantaneous gradient measured in the echocardiography laboratory. This is because the peak instantaneous gradient represents the maximum pressure difference between the left ventricle and aorta when measured simultaneously. This occurs on the upslope of the aortic pressure tracing (Fig. 6–12). Therefore, apparent disparities between cardiac catheterization and echocardiographic measures of peak gradient occur because cardiac catheterization uses peak-to-peak gradient determinations, whereas Doppler echocardiography reports peak instantaneous gradient. Mean aortic transvalvular gradient and aortic valve area are well correlated with both techniques (r = 0.86 − 0.90 and r = 0.88 − 0.95, respectively).[107]

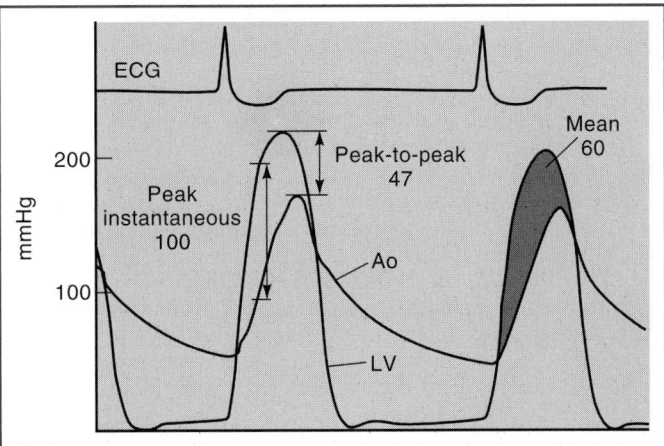

FIGURE 6–12. Various methods of describing an aortic transvalvular gradient. The peak-to-peak gradient (47 mm Hg) is the difference between the maximal pressure in the aorta (Ao) and the maximal left ventricle (LV) pressure. The peak instantaneous gradient (100 mm Hg) is the maximal pressure difference between the Ao and LV when the pressures are measured in the same moment (usually during early systole). The mean gradient *(shaded area)* is the integral of the pressure difference between the LV and Ao during systole (60 mm Hg). (From Bashore, T. M.: Invasive Cardiology: Principles and Techniques. Philadelphia, B. C. Decker Inc., 1990.)

In patients with *mitral stenosis* (see p. 1007), the most accurate means of determining mitral valve gradient is the measurement of left atrial pressure using the transseptal technique with simultaneous measurement of left ventricular pressure and with planimetry of the area bounded by the left ventricular and left atrial pressures in diastole using multiple cardiac cycles (Fig. 6–13). In most laboratories, the pulmonary capillary wedge pressure is substituted

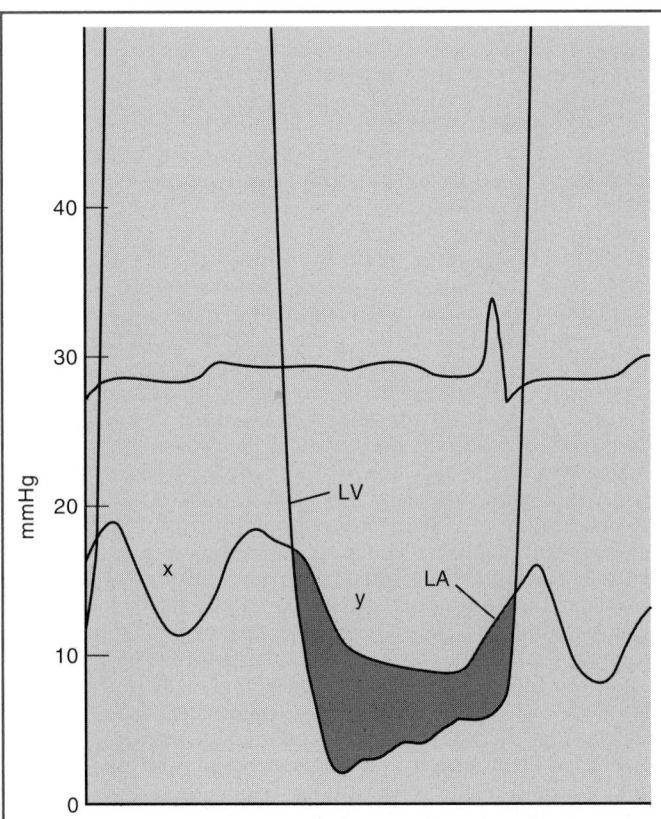

FIGURE 6–13. Pressure gradient in a patient with mitral stenosis. The pressure in the left atrium (LA) exceeds the pressure in the left ventricle (LV) during diastole, producing a diastolic pressure gradient *(shaded area)*. (From Bashore, T. M.: Invasive Cardiology: Principles and Techniques. Philadelphia, B. C. Decker Inc., 1990.)

for the left atrial pressure, as the pulmonary wedge pressure is more readily obtained. The pulmonary wedge pressure tracing must be realigned with the left ventricular tracing for accurate mean gradient determination. Although it has been generally accepted that pulmonary capillary wedge pressure is a satisfactory estimate of left atrial pressure,[102–104] other studies indicate that the pulmonary wedge pressure may systematically overestimate the left atrial pressure by 2 to 3 mm Hg (up to 53 per cent), thereby increasing the measured mitral valve gradient.[108,109] In addition, accurate wedge tracings may be difficult to obtain in patients with mitral stenosis because of pulmonary hypertension or dilated right-sided heart chambers. Improperly wedged catheters, resulting in damped pulmonary artery pressure recordings, will further overestimate the severity of mitral stenosis. If there is doubt about the accurate position of the catheter in the wedge position, the position can be confirmed by slow withdrawal of blood for oximetric analysis. An oxygen saturation equal to that of the systemic circulation confirms the wedge position.

In *pulmonic stenosis*, the valve gradient is usually obtained by a catheter pullback from the pulmonary artery to the right ventricle, although multilumen catheters are available for simultaneous pressure recordings. Tricuspid valve gradients should be assessed with simultaneous recording of right atrial and right ventricular pressures.

CALCULATION OF STENOTIC VALVE ORIFICE AREAS. The stenotic orifice area is determined from the pressure gradient and cardiac output using the formula developed by Gorlin and Gorlin from the fundamental hydraulic relationships linking the area of an orifice to the flow and pressure drop across the orifice.[110] Flow (F) and orifice area (A) are related by the fundamental formula $F = cAV$, where V is velocity of flow and c is a constant accounting for central streaming of fluid through an orifice which tends to reduce the effective orifice size. Hence,

$$A = F/cV$$

Velocity is related to the pressure gradient through the relation $V = k\sqrt{2g\Delta P}$, where k is a constant accounting for frictional energy loss, g is the acceleration due to gravity (980 cm/s²), and ΔP is the mean pressure gradient (mm Hg). Substituting for V in the orifice area equation and combining c and k into one constant C:

$$A = \frac{F}{C\sqrt{1960\Delta P}} = \frac{F}{44.3C\sqrt{\Delta P}}$$

Gorlin and Gorlin determined the value of the constant C by comparing the calculated valve area to actual valve area measured at autopsy or at surgery in 11 mitral valves. The maximal discrepancy between the actual mitral valve area and calculated values was only 0.2 cm² when the constant 0.85 was used. No data were obtained for aortic valves, a limitation noted by the Gorlins, and a constant of 1.0 was assumed. Because flow across the aortic valve occurs only in systole, the flow value for calculating aortic valve area (cm²) is the cardiac output in ml/minute divided by the systolic ejection period (SEP) in seconds/beat times the heart rate (HR) in beats/min. The systolic ejection period is defined from aortic valve opening to closure. Hence, the aortic valve area is calculated from the Gorlin formula using the equation:

$$\text{Aortic valve area} = \frac{\text{cardiac output}}{44.3(\text{SEP})(\text{HR})\sqrt{\text{mean gradient}}}$$

Similarly, as mitral flow occurs only in diastole, the cardiac output is corrected for the diastolic filling period (DFP) in seconds/beat in the equation for mitral valve area, where the diastolic filling period is defined from mitral valve opening to mitral valve closure:

$$\text{Mitral valve area} = \frac{\text{cardiac output}}{37.7(\text{DFP})(\text{HR})\sqrt{\text{mean gradient}}}$$

The normal aortic valve area is 2.6 to 3.5 cm² in adults. Valve areas of 0.8 cm² or less represent severe aortic stenosis. The normal mitral valve area is 4 to 6 cm², and severe mitral stenosis is present with valve areas less than 1.0 to 1.5 cm².

The calculated valve area often is crucial in management decisions in patients with aortic stenosis or mitral stenosis. Hence, it is essential that accurate and simultaneous pressure gradient and cardiac output determinations be made, especially in patients with borderline or low pressure gradients. As the square root of the mean gradient is used in the Gorlin formula, the valve area calculation is more strongly influenced by errors in the cardiac output measurement than by errors in the pressure gradient. Thus, errors in measuring cardiac output may have profound effects on the calculated valve area, particularly in patients with low cardiac outputs in whom the calculated valve area is often of greatest importance.

The Fick method of determining cardiac output is the most accurate for assessing cardiac output, especially in low-output states. As noted previously, both the dye-dilution technique and the thermodilution technique may provide inaccurate cardiac output data when cardiac output is reduced or when concomitant aortic, mitral, or tricuspid regurgitation is present. In patients with mixed valvular disease (stenosis and regurgitation) of the same valve, the use of forward flow as determined by the Fick method or thermodilution technique will overestimate the severity of the valvular stenosis. This is because the Gorlin formula depends on total forward flow across the stenotic valve, not net forward flow. If valvular regurgitation is present, the angiographic cardiac output is the most appropriate measure of flow. If both aortic and mitral regurgitation are present, flow across a single valve cannot be determined and neither aortic valve area nor mitral valve area can be assessed accurately.

There are other potential errors and limitations in the use of the Gorlin formula,[111,112] related both to inaccuracies in measurement of valve gradients and to more fundamental issues regarding the validity of the assumptions underlying the formula. In low-output states the Gorlin formula may systematically predict smaller valve areas than are actually present. Several lines of evidence indicate that the aortic valve area by the Gorlin formula increases with increases in cardiac output.[113–116] Although this may represent an actual greater opening of stenotic valves by the higher proximal opening pressures that result from increases in transvalvular flow, the flow dependence of the calculated valve area may also reflect inherent errors in the assumptions underlying the Gorlin formula, particularly with respect to the aortic valve.[111,117]

Cannon et al.[115] demonstrated in valves of fixed orifice size that the constant in the Gorlin formula is actually not constant but varies with the square root of the mean pressure gradient ($C = k\sqrt{mean\ gradient}$). This concept would transform the Gorlin formula such that the square root disappears and the valve area varies inversely with the mean gradient:

$$Valve\ area = \frac{Flow}{44.3C\sqrt{\Delta P}} = \frac{Flow}{44.3(k\sqrt{\Delta P})\sqrt{\Delta P}} = \frac{Flow}{K\Delta P} + h$$

This concept has particular implications in aortic stenosis, in which the higher valve gradients have a greater effect on the Gorlin constant than the considerably smaller gradients encountered in mitral stenosis. The constant h was added to correct for a small offset between predicted and measured valve areas. The values of the new constants K and h have not been fully determined or validated, and the complete independence of these constants from transvalvular flow has not been fully investigated.

Other alternative formulas for determining valve areas have been proposed. Hakki[118] observed empirically that the effects of the systolic ejection period and the diastolic filling period were relatively constant at normal heart rates and proposed eliminating this term from the equation. This assumes that $(HR \times SEP \times 44.3) \approx 1000$ in most circumstances. In this modified and simplified approach, the aortic valve area would be determined by the formula:

$$Aortic\ valve\ area = \frac{cardiac\ output\ (L/min)}{\sqrt{mean\ gradient\ (mm\ Hg)}}$$

Angel et al.[119] tested this approach at various heart rates and proposed adding an empiric constant for heart rates less than 75 beats/min for mitral stenosis and more than 90 beats/min for aortic stenosis. As is the case with the Cannon modification of the Gorlin formula, this alternate approach to determining valve area has not been fully validated.

To surmount the limitations of the Gorlin formula in low-flow states, a number of investigators have advocated maneuvers in the cardiac catheterization laboratory to increase cardiac output and calculate valve area at the higher output and valve gradient. However, definitive data are lacking to indicate that this is a valid approach that actually yields more accurate valve area calculations. A second approach to the patient with a low aortic transvalvular gradient and low cardiac output is to calculate the aortic valve resistance using the formula:

$$Aortic\ valve\ resistance = \frac{mean\ gradient}{flow}$$
$$= \frac{1.33\ (mean\ gradient)(HR)(SEP)}{cardiac\ output}$$

where HR is heart rate, SEP is systolic ejection period, and valve resistance is expressed in dynes-sec-cm^{-5}.[116,120] The limited data available using aortic valve resistance suggest that this measure may be a helpful adjunct in distinguishing those patients with borderline aortic valve areas (0.6 to 0.8 cm²) who have severe from those with mild aortic stenosis.

Measurement of Intraventricular Pressure Gradients

The demonstration of an intracavitary pressure gradient is among the most interesting and challenging aspects of diagnostic catheterization. Simultaneous pressure measurements are usually obtained in the central aorta and from within the ventricular cavity. Pullback of the catheter from the ventricular apex to a posterior position just beneath the aortic valve will demonstrate an intracavitary gradient. An erroneous intracavitary gradient may be seen if the catheter becomes entrapped by the myocardium.

The intracavitary gradient is distinguished from aortic valvular stenosis due to the loss of the aortic–left ventricular gradient when the catheter is still within the left ventricle yet proximal to the myocardial obstruction. In addition, careful analysis of the upstroke of the aortic pressure waveform will distinguish a valvular from a subvalvular stenosis, as the aortic pressure waveform demonstrates a slow upstroke in aortic stenosis. Other methods to localize intracavitary gradients include the use of a dual-lumen catheter or a double-sensor micromanometer catheter, or placement of an end hole catheter in the left ventricular outflow tract while a transseptal catheter is advanced into the left ventricle, with pressure measured simultaneously. An intracavitary gradient may be increased by various provocative maneuvers including the Valsalva maneuver, inhalation of amyl nitrate, introduction of a premature ventricular beat, or isoproterenol infusion (see section on physiological maneuvers).

Assessment of Valvular Regurgitation

The severity of valvular regurgitation is generally graded by visual assessment, although calculation of the regurgitant fraction is used occasionally. A full description of the techniques of left ventriculography and aortography can be found elsewhere in this textbook (see Chap. 7).

VISUAL ASSESSMENT OF REGURGITATION. Valvular regurgitation may be assessed visually by determining the relative amount of radiographic contrast medium that opacifies the chamber proximal to its injection. The estimation of regurgitation depends on the regurgitant volume as well as the size and contractility of the proximal chamber. The original classification scheme devised by Sellers remains the standard in most catheterization laboratories:[121]

+   Minimal regurgitant jet seen. Clears rapidly from proximal chamber with each beat.

++   Moderate opacification of proximal chamber, clearing with subsequent beats.

+++   Intense opacification of proximal chamber, becoming equal to that of the distal chamber.

++++ Intense opacification of proximal chamber, becoming more dense than that of the distal chamber. Opacification often persists over the entire series of images obtained.

REGURGITANT FRACTION. A gross estimate of the degree of valvular regurgitation may be obtained by determining the regurgitant fraction. The difference between the angiographic stroke volume and the forward stroke volume can be defined as the regurgitant stroke volume. The regurgitant fraction (RF) is that portion of the angiographic stroke volume that does not contribute to the net cardiac output.

$$\text{Regurgitant stroke volume} = \text{angiographic stroke volume} - \text{forward stroke volume}$$

$$RF = \frac{\text{angiographic stroke volume} - \text{forward stroke volume}}{\text{angiographic stroke volume}}$$

Forward stroke volume is the cardiac output determined by the Fick or thermodilution method divided by the heart rate. Thermodilution cardiac output cannot be used if there is significant concomitant tricuspid regurgitation.

An RF of ≤ 20 per cent is roughly equivalent to $1+$ regurgitation as detected visually; an RF of 21 to 40 per cent is equivalent to $2+$ regurgitation; an RF of 41 to 60 per cent is equivalent to $3+$ regurgitation; and an RF of 60 per cent or more is equivalent to $4+$ regurgitation. The assumption underlying regurgitation fraction determination is that the angiographic and forward cardiac outputs are accurate and comparable, a state requiring similar heart rates, stable hemodynamic states between measurements, and only a single regurgitant valve. Given these conditions, the equation yields only a gross approximation of regurgitant flow.

Shunt Determinations

Normally, pulmonary blood flow and systemic blood flow are equal. When there is an abnormal communication between intracardiac chambers or great vessels, blood flow is shunted either from the systemic circulation to the pulmonary circulation (left-to-right shunt), from the pulmonary circulation to the systemic circulation (right-to-left shunt), or in both directions (bidirectional shunt). While many shunts are suspected before cardiac catheterization, physicians performing the procedure should be vigilant in determining the cause of unexpected findings. For example, an unexplained pulmonary artery oxygen saturation exceeding 80 per cent should raise the operator's suspicion of a left-to-right shunt, whereas unexplained arterial desaturation (< 95 per cent) may indicate a right-to-left shunt.[122] Arterial desaturation commonly results from alveolar hypoventilation and associated "physiological

shunting," the causes of which include oversedation from premedication, pulmonary disease, pulmonary venous congestion, pulmonary edema, and cardiogenic shock. If arterial desaturation persists after the patient takes several deep breaths or coughs, or following administration of 100 per cent oxygen, a right-to-left shunt must be highly suspected.

Several noninvasive and invasive methods are available for detection of intracardiac shunts. Noninvasive methods include echocardiographic, radionuclide, and magnetic resonance imaging techniques. The most commonly used method in the cardiac catheterization laboratory is the oximetric method.

OXIMETRIC METHOD. The oximetric method is based on blood sampling from various cardiac chambers for oxygen saturation determination. A left-to-right shunt is detected when there is a significant increase in blood oxygen saturation between two right-sided vessels or chambers.[123,124]

A screening oxygen saturation measurement for any left-to-right shunt should be performed with every right heart catheterization by sampling blood in the superior vena cava (SVC) and the pulmonary artery. If the difference in oxygen saturation between these samples is 8 per cent or more, a left-to-right shunt may be present, and a full oximetry "run" should be performed.[122] This includes obtaining blood samples from all right-sided locations including the superior vena cava (SVC), inferior vena cava (IVC), right atrium, right ventricle, and pulmonary artery. In cases of interatrial or interventricular shunts, it may be helpful to obtain multiple samples from the high, middle, and low right atrium or the right ventricular inflow tract, apex, and outflow tract in order to localize the level of the shunt. One may miss a small left-to-right shunt using the right atrium for screening purposes rather than the SVC because of incomplete mixing of blood in the right atrium, which receives blood from the IVC, SVC, and coronary sinus. Oxygen saturation in the IVC is higher than in the SVC because the kidneys use less oxygen relative to their blood flow than do other organs, while coronary sinus blood has very low oxygen saturation. Mixed venous saturation is most accurately measured in the pulmonary artery after complete mixing has occurred.

A full saturation run involves obtaining samples from the high and low IVC; high and low SVC; high, mid, and low right atrium; right ventricular inflow, outflow tracts, and mid-cavity; main pulmonary artery; left or right pulmonary artery; pulmonary vein and left atrium if possible; left ventricle; and distal aorta. When a right-to-left shunt must be localized, oxygen saturation samples must be taken from the pulmonary veins, left atrium, left ventricle, and aorta. While the major weakness of the oxygen step-up method is its lack of sensitivity, clinically significant shunts are generally detected by this technique. Another method of oximetric determination of intracardiac shunts uses a balloon-tipped fiberoptic catheter that allows for continuous registration of oxygen saturation as it is withdrawn from the pulmonary artery through the right heart chambers into the SVC and IVC.

SHUNT QUANTIFICATION. The principles used to determine Fick cardiac output are used to quantify intracardiac shunts. To determine the size of a left-to-right shunt, pulmonary blood flow and systemic blood flow determinations are required. Pulmonary blood flow (PBF) is simply oxygen consumption divided by the difference in oxygen content across the pulmonary bed, while systemic blood flow (SBF) is oxygen consumption divided by the difference in oxygen content across the systemic bed. The effective blood flow (EBF) is the fraction of mixed venous return received by the lungs without contamination by the shunt flow. In the *absence* of a shunt, PBF, SBF, and EBF are all equal. These equations are shown below:

$$PBF = \frac{O_2 \text{ consumption (ml/min)}}{(PV\ O_2 - PA\ O_2)}$$

$$SBF = \frac{O_2 \text{ consumption (ml/min)}}{(SA\ O_2 - MV\ O_2)}$$

$$EBF = \frac{O_2 \text{ consumption (ml/min)}}{(PV\ O_2 - MV\ O_2}$$

where $PV\ O_2$, $PA\ O_2$, $SA\ O_2$, and $MV\ O_2$ are the oxygen contents (in milliliters of oxygen per liter of blood) of pulmonary venous, pulmonary arterial, systemic arterial, and mixed venous bloods, respectively. The oxygen content is determined as outlined in the section on Fick cardiac output.

If a pulmonary vein is not sampled, systemic arterial oxygen content may be substituted, assuming systemic arterial saturation is 95 per cent or more. As discussed above, if systemic arterial saturation is less than 95 per cent, a right-to-left shunt may be present. If arterial desaturation is present but not secondary to a right-to-left shunt, systemic arterial oxygen content is used. If a right-to-left shunt is present, pulmonary venous oxygen content is calculated as 98 per cent of the oxygen capacity.

The mixed venous oxygen content is the average oxygen content of the blood in the chamber proximal to the shunt. When assessing a left-to-right shunt at the level of the right atrium, one must calculate mixed venous oxygen content on the basis of the contributing blood flow from the IVC, SVC, and coronary sinus. The most common formula used is the Flamm formula:[125]

Mixed venous oxygen content
$$= \frac{3(SVC\ O_2 \text{ content}) + 1(IVC\ O_2 \text{ content})}{4}$$

Assuming conservation of mass, the size of a left-to-right shunt, when there is no associated right-to-left shunt, is simply:

$$L \to R \text{ shunt} = PBF - SBF$$

When there is evidence of a right-to-left shunt in addition to a left-to-right shunt, the approximate left to right shunt size is:

$$L \to R \text{ shunt} = PBF - EBF$$

while the approximate right-to-left shunt size is:

$$R \to L \text{ shunt} = SBF - EBF$$

The flow ratio PBF/SBF (or QP/QS) is used clinically to determine the significance of the shunt. A ratio of less than 1.5 indicates a small left-to-right shunt. A ratio of 2.0 or more indicates a large left-to-right shunt and generally requires repair in order to prevent future pulmonary and/or right ventricular complications. A flow ratio of less than 1.0 indicates a net right-to-left shunt. If oxygen consumption is not measured, the flow ratio may be calculated as follows:

$$\frac{PBF}{SBF} = \frac{(SA\ O_2 - MV\ O_2)}{(PV\ O_2 - PA\ O_2)}$$

where $SA\ O_2$, $MV\ O_2$, $PV\ O_2$, and $PA\ O_2$ are systemic arterial, mixed venous, pulmonary venous, and pulmonary arterial blood oxygen saturations, respectively.

Indicator-Dilution Method

While the indicator-dilution method is more sensitive than the oximetric method in detection of small shunts, it cannot be used to localize the level of a left-to-right shunt (Fig. 6–14). An indicator such as indocyanine green dye is injected into a proximal chamber while a sample is taken from a distal chamber using a densitometer and the density of dye is displayed over time. In order to detect a left-to-right shunt, dye is injected into the pulmonary artery and sampling is performed in a systemic artery. Presence of a shunt is indicated by early recirculation of the dye on the *downslope* of the curve.[126] The presence of aortic or mitral regurgitation may distort the downslope of the curve, thereby yielding a false positive result. In adults, the indocyanine green method provides estimates of shunt magnitude that are somewhat smaller than those of the oximetric method, although they are in general agreement with one another concerning the QP/QS.[127,128] In order to detect a right-to-left shunt, dye is injected into the right heart proximal to the presumed shunt and sampling is performed in a systemic artery. If there is a right-to-left shunt, a distinctive early peak is seen on the *upslope* of the curve.[129] The level of the right-to-left shunt may be localized by injecting more distally until the early peak disappears. Shunts may also be quantified using this technique.

Miscellaneous Techniques

A sensitive method for detection and localization of a left-to-right shunt is to check systematically within the various right heart chambers for the early appearance of an indicator that is injected distal to the presumed shunt. Indicators that have been used for this

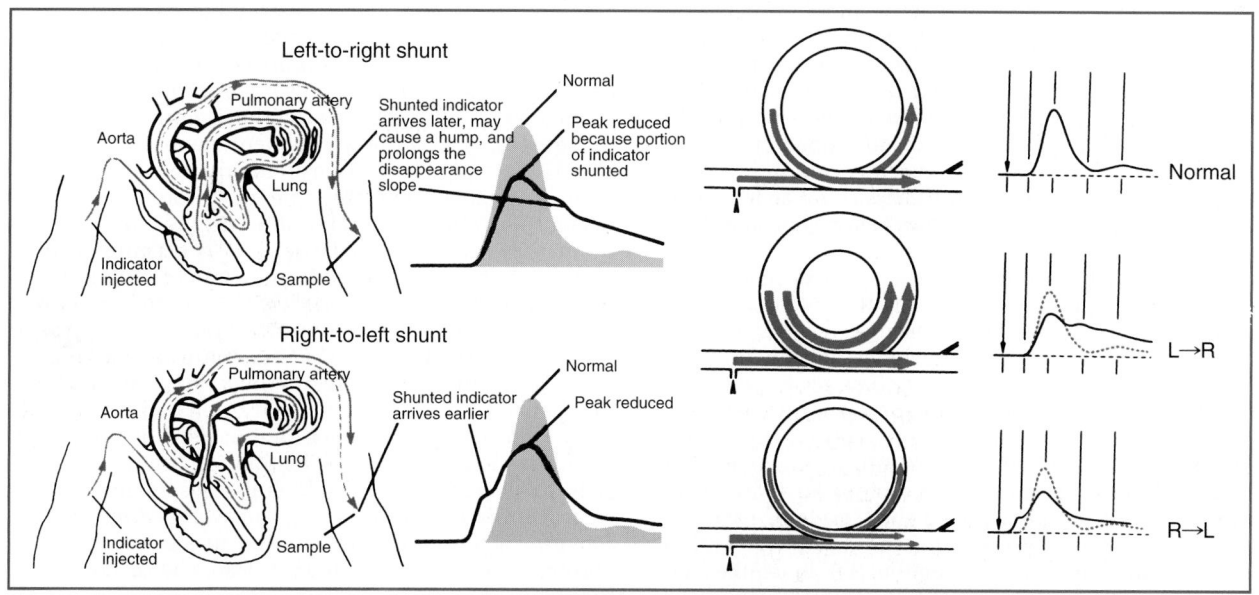

FIGURE 6–14. Left-to-right shunt (increased pulmonic flow). Indicator is not cleared rapidly but recirculates through central circulation via defect. Based on magnitude of shunt, a constant fraction leaves the central pool with each circulation. Maximal deflection is reduced and the disappearance is prolonged as a result of slow clearance. Right-to-left shunt (decreased pulmonic flow). A portion of the indicator passes directly to the arterial circulation via the defect without passing through the lungs and arrives at the arterial sampling site before the portion that did traverse the pulmonary circulation. (From Kern, M. J., Deligonul, U., Donohue, T., et al.: Hemodynamic data. *In* Kern, M. J.: The Cardiac Catheterization Handbook. 2nd ed. St. Louis, Mosby–Year Book, 1995, p. 142.)

purpose include indocyanine green dye, inhaled hydrogen, hydrogen dissolved in saline, and ascorbic acid. Platinum-tipped electrodes are used for detection when hydrogen and ascorbic acid are used. These techniques may also be used to detect small right-to-left shunts by altering of the sites of injection and sampling.

Selective injection of radiographic contrast (angiocardiography) can detect both left-to-right and right-to-left shunts, although these cannot be quantified. Angiocardiography is a useful adjunct to transesophageal echocardiography as part of a preoperative evaluation. It is also very useful in detecting pulmonary arteriovenous fistulas that may not be detected by other methods.

Physiological and Pharmacological Maneuvers

Potentially significant cardiac abnormalities may be silent in the resting condition. Abnormal hemodynamics may not be shown without physiological stresses in valvular, myocardial, and coronary disease states. Therefore, if the physician performing a cardiac catheterization procedure cannot elucidate the cause of the patient's symptoms at rest, various physiological and pharmacological maneuvers can be considered.

DYNAMIC EXERCISE. Dynamic exercise in the catheterization laboratory is most commonly performed using supine bicycle ergometry, although straight leg raises or arm or upright bicycle exercise may be used. Upright treadmill exercise may also be performed outside the catheterization laboratory, using a balloon flotation catheter inserted through an antecubital vein to measure pulmonary artery and wedge pressure and cardiac output. The associated changes in the heart rate, cardiac output, oxygen consumption, and intracardiac pressures are monitored at steady state during progressive stages of exercise. Normally, the increased oxygen requirements of exercise are met by an increase in cardiac output and an increase in oxygen extraction from arterial blood.[130] Patients with cardiac dysfunction are unable to increase their cardiac output appropriately in response to exercise and must meet the demands of the exercising muscle groups by increasing the extraction of oxygen from arterial blood, thereby increasing the arteriovenous oxygen difference. Dexter and colleagues found that the relationship between cardiac output and oxygen consumption was linear and that a regression formula may be used to calculate the predicted cardiac index at a given level of oxygen consumption.[131] The actual cardiac index divided by the predicted cardiac index is defined as the *exercise index*. A value of 0.8 or more indicates a normal cardiac output response to exercise.[130] The *exercise factor* is another method of describing the same relationship between the cardiac output and oxygen consumption. The exercise factor is the increase in cardiac output divided by the increase in oxygen consumption. Normally, for every 100 ml/min increase in oxygen consumption with exercise, the cardiac output should increase by at least 600 ml/min. Therefore, a normal exercise factor should be 0.6 or more.[130]

Supine exercise will normally cause a rise in mean arterial and pulmonary pressures. There will be a proportionally greater decrease in systemic vascular resistance compared with pulmonary vascular resistance and an increase in heart rate. Myocardial contractility increases owing to both the increase in heart rate and increased sympathetic tone. Left ventricular ejection fraction rises. During early levels of exercise, increased venous return augments left ventricular end-diastolic volume, leading to an increase in stroke volume.[132] At progressively higher levels of exercise, both left ventricular end-systolic and end-diastolic volumes decrease such that there is a negligible rise in stroke volume. Thus, the augmentation in cardiac output during peak supine exercise in the catheterization laboratory is generally caused by an increase in heart rate. For this reason, all agents that may impair the chronotropic response should be discontinued before catheterization if exercise is contemplated during the procedure.

Exercise may provoke symptoms in a patient who had been diagnosed as having valvular disease of borderline significance in the resting state. Exercise increases the gradient across the mitral valve in mitral stenosis and may provoke symptoms not experienced at rest. The hemodynamic response to exercise is also useful in evaluating regurgitant valvular lesions. Clinically significant valvular regurgitation exists if an increase occurs in left ventricular end-diastolic pressure, pulmonary capillary wedge pressure, and systemic vascular resistance, in conjunction with a reduced exercise index and abnormal exercise factor. Simultaneous echocardiographic data may also be useful in equivocal cases. Patients with myocardial disease, ischemic or otherwise, may have pronounced increases in left ventricular end-diastolic pressure with exercise.[133]

ISOMETRIC EXERCISE. Isometric handgrip exercise causes an increase in heart rate, mean arterial pressure, and cardiac output. Since the systemic vascular resistance does not rise, the elevation in arterial pressure is due to the rise in cardiac output rather than a vasoconstrictor response. Patients with left ventricular dysfunction respond abnormally to isometric exercise (i.e., significant increase in left ventricular end-diastolic pressure, a failure to increase stroke work appropriately, and a blunted rise in left ventricular peak dP/dT).[130]

PACING TACHYCARDIA. Rapid atrial or ventricular pacing increases myocardial oxygen consumption and myocardial blood flow.[134] In distinction from dynamic or isometric exercise, left ventricular end-diastolic volume decreases with pacing and there is little change in cardiac output.[135] This method may be used to determine the significance of coronary artery disease or valvular abnormalities. For example, the gradient across the mitral valve increases with rapid atrial pacing owing to the increase in heart rate. Pacing has the advantage of allowing for greater control and rapid termination of the induced stress.

PHYSIOLOGICAL STRESS. The *Valsalva maneuver* (forcible expiration against a closed glottis) should increase the systolic subaortic pressure gradient in patients with obstructive hypertrophic cardiomyopathy in the strain phase, during which there is a decrease in venous return and decreased left ventricular volume (see p. 1420). This maneuver is often abnormal in patients with heart failure.[136] The *Mueller maneuver* (forced inspiration against a closed glottis) causes the opposite effect on the systolic pressure gradient in patients with obstructive hypertrophic cardiomyopathy. Another useful maneuver in patients with hypertrophic obstructive cardiomyopathy is the introduction of a *premature ventricular beat* (Brockenbrough maneuver). Premature ventricular contractions normally increase the pulse pressure of the subsequent ventricular beat. In obstructive hypertrophic cardiomyopathy, the outflow gradient is increased during the postpremature beat with a decrease in the pulse pressure of the aortic contour. A premature ventricular beat may also accentuate the spike-and-dome configuration of the aortic pressure waveform. *Rapid volume loading* may reveal occult pericardial constriction, when atrial and ventricular filling pressures are relatively normal under baseline conditions owing to hypovolemia,[137] and may help distinguish pericardial constriction from myocardial restriction. *Kussmaul's sign* occurs in pericardial constriction (see p. 1497). This is demonstrated when, with inspiration, right atrial pressure fails to decrease or actually increases related to impaired right ventricular filling. *Cold pressor testing,* whereby the forearm of the patient is exposed to ice water, may induce coronary vasoconstriction in patients with coronary artery disease.[138]

PHARMACOLOGICAL MANEUVERS. *Isoproterenol infusion* may be used to simulate supine dynamic exercise, although untoward side effects may limit its applicability. This drug's positive inotropic and chronotropic effects may increase the gradients in obstructive hypertrophic cardiomyopathy and mitral stenosis. *Nitroglycerin* and *amyl nitrate* decrease preload and accentuate the systolic gradient in patients with obstructive hypertrophic cardiomyopathy. Amyl nitrate is generally inhaled and its onset of action is very rapid. Agents that increase systemic vascular resistance, such as *phenylephrine*, reduce the gradient in obstructive hypertrophic cardiomyopathy. Infusion of *sodium nitroprusside* may improve the cardiac output and filling pressures in patients with dilated cardiomyopathies and in patients with mitral regurgitation by lowering systemic and pulmonary vascular resistances. A favorable response to sodium nitroprusside infusion may predict a good clinical outcome. The use of *ergonovine* for provocation of coronary spasm as a diagnostic tool is limited by its lack of specificity.[139] In addition, production of this drug has recently been halted because of limited use.

Coronary Blood Flow Determinations

Four methods are generally used to measure human coronary blood flow in the cardiac catheterization laboratory: thermodilution, digital subtraction angiography, and the use of electromagnetic flow meters, and of Doppler velocity probes. Although most current methods measure relative changes in coronary blood flow, useful information regarding the physiological significance of stenosis,[140] cardiac hypertrophy,[141] and pharmacological interventions[142] can be obtained from these measurements.

Ganz and colleagues[143] introduced thermodilution methods for measuring coronary sinus flow in humans (Fig. 6–15). This inexpensive, widely available technique is the most frequently applied method for measuring global coronary blood flow in humans.[144] By injecting iced saline in the distal end of the catheter placed in the coronary sinus and measuring the temperature change from a proximal thermistor, the rate of change in temperature can be used to define coronary flow. The frequency response of this system is sufficient to measure flow changes that occur in 2 to

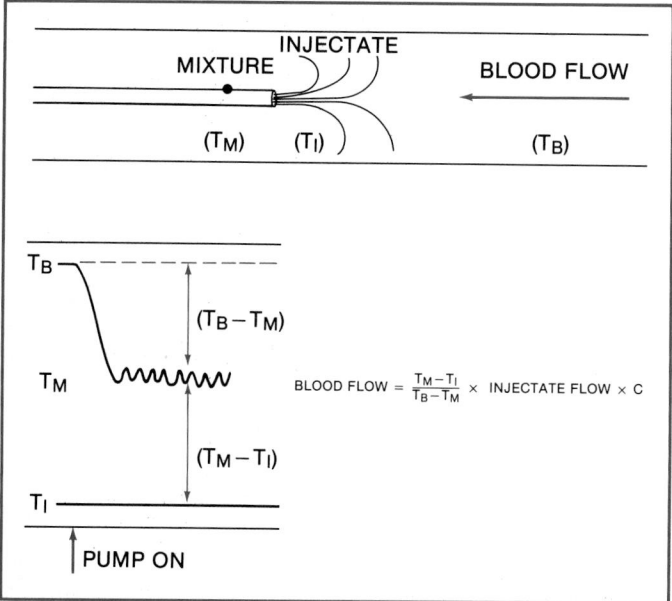

FIGURE 6–15. Schematic illustration of venous thermodilution method for measurement of coronary blood flow. The thermal indicator (injectate) at temperature T_I is infused at a constant rate (e.g., 15 ml/min). Turbulence causes mixing of the injectate with coronary venous blood at temperature T_B, resulting in a blood-injectate mixture at temperature T_M. The catheter tip thermistor monitors T_B and T_M, while an internal thermistor monitors T_I, and these are recorded continuously on a uniform temperature scale *(lower left).* Because heat loss by blood is gained by injectate, coronary venous flow is calculated using the measured temperatures, the rate of indicator injection, and the constant derived from the specific heats of blood and injectate. (From Bradley, A. B., and Baim, D. S.: Measurement of coronary blood flow in man. Methods and implications for clinical practice. Cardiovasc. Clin. *14:*67, 1984.)

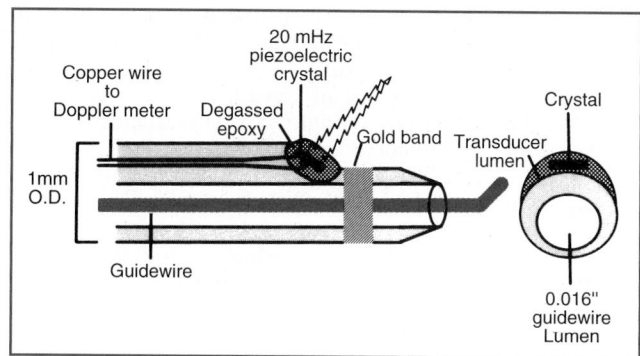

FIGURE 6–16. Schematic diagram of the distal portion of a 3F intracoronary Doppler catheter with side-mounted piezoelectric crystal. The copper wires attached to the crystal exit from the proximal end of the catheter and are connected to a 20 mHz pulsed Doppler velocimeter. The catheter is advanced into the coronary artery over an 0.014-inch angioplasty guidewire. O.D., outer diameter. (Modified from Wilson, R. F., Laughlin, D. E., and Ackell, P. H., et al.: Transluminal, subselective measurement of coronary artery blood flow velocity and vasodilator reserve in man. Circulation *72:*82, 1985. Copyright 1985 American Heart Association.)

3 seconds and are greater than 30 per cent.[143] This technique has several serious limitations, however.[144] Although the method has been validated in vitro with the thermodilution catheter attached to the coronary sinus,[143] weaker correlations have been shown when the thermodilution catheter is allowed to move within the coronary sinus.[145] Meanwhile, no studies have clearly demonstrated the accuracy of this method in patients with severe coronary artery disease or myocardial infarction. Other fundamental limitations include the fact that (1) rapid changes in flow cannot be assessed because of the slow time constant of the technique, (2) right atrial and ventricular perfusion cannot be evaluated because the venous drainage does not occur by means of the coronary sinus, and (3) regional function and specifically transmural coronary flow cannot be assessed.

To measure coronary flow with digital subtraction angiography, contrast medium is power injected into a coronary artery at a rate sufficient to replace blood within the artery completely. It is assumed that the contrast bolus is undiluted until the peak concentration has been imaged distally in the arterial segment. Regional flow reserve can be calculated in a number of ways, including the use of downstream appearance time and maximal contrast concentration before and during reactive hyperemia.[146] The assumption is that transit time within a region is inversely proportional to coronary blood flow in that region. This is true if the volume of distribution is constant. The technique is limited by a slow time constant and the inability to measure absolute flow. Evaluation of coronary flow reserve has been validated for this method in dogs by comparing digital flow ratio estimates with electromagnetic flow ratio measurements.[147,148] In humans, flow reserve has been shown to be abnormal in stenosed coronary arteries and bypass grafts and after coronary angioplasty.[149] Further human validation is necessary.

The electromagnetic flow meter is based on Faraday's induction law, which states that a conductor moving in an electric field produces current. A major advantage of electromagnetic flow meters is the high-frequency response.[141] Although these flow meters have been used to measure aortic blood flow velocity in humans,[150] they have not been developed to the point at which they are useful for measuring coronary blood flow at catheterization, in part because most methods require placement directly around the coronary artery. Electromagnetic flow meters are still in occasional use intraoperatively to evaluate flow in aortocoronary bypass grafts.

The Doppler flow meter is based on the principle of the Doppler effect (Fig. 6–16). It is the most widely applied technique for measurement of coronary flow in humans. High-frequency sound waves are reflected from moving red blood cells and undergo a shift in sound frequency that is proportional to the velocity of the blood flow. In pulsed-wave Doppler methods, a single piezoelectric crystal can both transmit and receive high-frequency sound waves. These methods have been applied successfully in humans by using miniaturized crystals fixed to the tip of catheters. Recent developments in technology have further miniaturized steerable 12-mHz Doppler guidewires to 0.014 inch in diameter. Therefore, flow can be assessed distal and proximal to a stenosis. The Doppler guidewire measures phasic flow velocity patterns and tracks linearly with flow rates in small, straight coronary arteries.[151] It has been advocated for use in determining the severity of intermediate stenosis (40 to 60 per cent) and in evaluating whether normal blood flow has been restored after PTCA. Validation studies have been performed that compare Doppler flow probes with labeled microspheres[152] and electromagnetic flow probes.[153] The use of this technique in 200 patients in the cardiac catheterization laboratory has been reported.[154] It has the advantage of permitting repeated sampling and at high frequency, thus allowing measurements after physiological or pharmacological interventions. The use of smaller Doppler catheters allows selective coronary artery flow velocity to be measured. By noting the increase in flow velocity following a strong coronary vasodilator, such as papaverine, the coronary flow reserve can be defined. Coronary flow reserve (CFR) provides an index of the functional significance of coronary lesions that obviates some of the ambiguity of anatomical description.[154]

Animal data indicate that stenosis exceeding 50 per cent is associated with a reduction in absolute flow reserve. It has been suggested that stenosis flow reserve (SFR) is a more reliable method of functional severity.[155] For a fixed arterial dimension and stenosis geometry, directly measured arterial CFR can be zero if no aortic perfusion is present or may change with other physiological conditions. Thus, CFR can be broken into its component parts of SFR, i.e., the flow reserve of the proximal arterial stenosis, and myocardial perfusion reserve (MPR), the flow reserve of the distal vascular bed. SFR is defined by geometric quantitative coronary dimensions using standard physiological conditions. MPR is directly or indirectly measured and is affected by geometric as well as physiological variables. The equation relating pressure change across a lesion and flow is:

$$\Delta P = Pa - Pc = A(Q/Qrest) + B(Q/Qrest)^2$$

where ΔP is the translesional gradient, Pc is distal coronary pressure, Pa is aortic pressure, Q and Qrest are flow and rest flow, and A and B are related to lesion geometry. A and B are defined by lesion length, minimal cross-sectional area of the lesion and reference segment, and blood viscosity.

The limitation of the current Doppler probe method is that only changes in flow velocity, rather than absolute velocity or volumetric flow, are measurable. The change in flow velocity is directly proportional to changes in volumetric flow only when vessel dimensions are constant at the site of the sample volume. Furthermore, there is concern that changes in luminal diameter and arterial cross-sectional area during interventions are not reflected in measurements of flow velocity, thus potentially causing underestimation of the true volume flow.[146]

REFERENCES

HISTORICAL PERSPECTIVE

1. Swan, H. J. C., Ganz, W., Forrester, J. S., et al.: Catheterization of the heart in man with use of a flow-directed balloon-tipped catheter. N. Engl. J. Med. 283:447, 1970.
2. Zimmerman, H. A., Scott, R. W., and Becker, N. O.: Catheterization of the left side of the heart in man. Circulation 1:357, 1950.
3. Sones, F. M., Jr., Shivey, E. K., Proudfit, W. L., and Westcott, R. N.: Cinecoronary arteriography (Abstract). Circulation 20:773, 1959.
4. Ross, J., Jr.: Transseptal left heart catheterization: A new method of left atrial puncture. Ann. Surg. 1949:395, 1959.
5. Cope, C.: Technique for transseptal catheterization of the left atrium: Preliminary report. J. Thorac. Surg. 37:482, 1959.
6. Ricketts, H. J., and Abrams, H. L.: Percutaneous selective coronary cine arteriography. JAMA 181:140, 1962.
7. Amplatz, K., Formonek G., Stranger, P., and Wilson, W.: Mechanics of selective coronary artery catheterization via the femoral approach. Radiology 89:1040, 1967.
8. Judkins, M. P.: Selective coronary arteriography. I: A percutaneous transfemoral technique. Radiology 89:815, 1967.
9. Acierno, L. J.: The History of Cardiology. 1st ed. Pearl River, NY, The Parthenon Publishing Group Inc., 1994.

INDICATIONS FOR DIAGNOSTIC CARDIAC CATHETERIZATION

10. Ross, J., Jr., Pepine, C. J., Brandenburg, R. O., et al.: Guidelines for coronary angiography. A report of the American College of Cardiology/American Heart Association Task Force on Assessment of Diagnostic and Therapeutic Cardiovascular Procedures (Subcommittee on Coronary Angiography). J. Am. Coll. Cardiol. 10:935, 1987.
11. Grines, C. L., Browne, K. F., Marco, J., et al.: A comparison of immediate angioplasty with thrombolytic therapy for acute myocardial infarction. N. Engl. J. Med. 328:673, 1993.
12. Topol, E. J., Califf, R. M., George, B. S., et al.: A randomized prospective trial of immediate versus delayed elective angioplasty after intravenous tissue plasminogen activator in acute myocardial infarction. N. Engl. J. Med. 317:581, 1987.
13. The TIMI Study Group: Comparison of invasive and conservative strategies after treatment with intravenous tissue plasminogen activatorin acute myocardial infarction: Results of the Thrombolysis in Acute Myocardial Infarction (TIMI) Phase II Trial. N. Engl. J. Med. 320:618, 1989.
14. Ryan, T. J., Bauman, W. B., Kennedy, J. W., et al.: Guidelines and indications for percutaneous transluminal coronary angioplasty. A report of the American College of Cardiology/American Heart Association Task Force on Assessment of Diagnostic and Therapeutic Cardiovascular Procedures (Subcommittee on Percutaneous Transluminal Coronary Angioplasty). Circulation 88:2987, 1993.
15. Roberts, W. C.: Reasons for cardiac catheterization before cardiac valve replacement. N. Engl. J. Med. 306:1291, 1982.
16. Rahimtoola, S. H.: The need for cardiac catheterization and angiography in valvular heart disease is not disproven. Ann. Intern. Med. 97:433, 1982.

COMPLICATIONS ASSOCIATED WITH CARDIAC CATHETERIZATION

17. Braunwald, E., and Swan, H. J. C.: Cooperative study on cardiac catheterization. Circulation 37(Suppl.III):1, 1968.
18. Kennedy, J. W.: Complication associated with cardiac catheterization and angiography. Cathet. Cardiovasc. Diagn. 8:13, 1982.
19. Johnson, L. W., Lozner, E. C., Johnson, S., et al.: Coronary arteriography 1984–1987: A report of the Registry of the Society for Cardiac Angiography and Interventions. Results and complications. Cathet. Cardiovasc. Diagn. 17:5, 1989.
20. Davis, K., Kennedy, J. W., Kemp, H. G., et al.: Complications of coronary arteriography from the collaborative study of coronary artery surgery (CASS). Circulation 59:1105, 1979.
21. Laskey, W., Boyle, J., Johnson, L. W., and the Registry Committee of the Society for Cardiac Angiography and Interventions: Multivariable model for prediction of risk of significant complication during diagnostic cardiac catheterization. Cathet. Cardiovasc. Diagn. 30:185, 1993.
22. Davidson, C. J., Mark, D. B., Pieper, K. S., et al.: Thrombotic and cardiovascular complications related to nonionic contrast media during cardiac catheterization. Analysis of 8517 patients. Am. J. Cardiol. 65:1481, 1990.
23. Adams, D. F., Fraser, D. B., and Abrams, H. L.: The complications of coronary arteriography. Circulation 48:609, 1973.
24. Clark, V. L., and Khaja, F.: Risk of cardiac catheterization in patients aged >80 years without previous cardiac surgery. Am. J. Cardiol. 74:1076, 1994.
25. McCann, R. L., Schwartz, L. B., Pieper, K. S.: Vascular complications of cardiac catheterization. J. Vasc. Surg. 14:375, 1991.
26. Davidson, C. J., Hlatky, M., Morris, G. G., et al.: Cardiovascular and renal toxicity of a nonionic radiographic contrast agent after cardiac catheterization. Ann. Intern. Med. 110:119, 1989.
27. Solomon, R., Werner, C., Mann, D., D'Elia, J., and Silva, P.: Effects of saline, mannitol, and furosemide on acute decreases in renal function induced by radiocontrast agents. N. Engl. J. Med. 331:1416, 1994.
28. Fareed, J., Moncada, R., Messmore, H. L., et al.: Molecular markers of contrast media–induced adverse reactors. Semin. Thromb. Hemost. 10:306, 1984.
29. Shehadi, W. H.: Contrast media adverse reactions: Occurrence, recurrence and distribution patterns. Radiology 143:11, 1982.
30. Fischer, H. W., and Thomson, K. R.: Contrast media in coronary arteriography: A review. Invest. Radiol. 13:450, 1978.
31. Bashore, T. M., Davidson, C. J., Mark, D. B., et al.: Iopamidol use in the cardiac catheterization laboratory: A retrospective analysis of 3,313 patients. Cardiology 5(Suppl.):6, 1988.
32. Higgins, C. B., Sovak, M., Schmidt, W. S., et al.: Direct myocardial effects of intracoronary administration of new contrast agents with low osmolality. Invest. Radiol. 15:39, 1980.

33. Salem, D. N., Findlay, S. R., Isner, J. M., et al.: Comparison of histamine release effects of ionic and nonionic radiographic contrast media. Am. J. Med. *80:*382, 1986.

34. Schwab, S., Hlatky, M. A., Pieper, K. S., et al.: Contrast nephrotoxicity: A randomized study of the nephrotoxicity of ionic versus nonionic contrast following cardiac catheterization. N. Engl. J. Med. *320:*149, 1989.

35. Hill, J. A., Winniford, M., Van Fossen, D. B., et al.: Nephrotoxicity following cardiac angiography: A randomized double blind multicenter trial of ionic and nonionic contrast media in 1194 patients. Circulation *84:*II-333, 1991.

36. Manske, C. L., Sprafka, J. M., Strony, J. T., Wang, Y.: Contrast nephrotoxicity in an azotemic diabetic patient undergoing coronary angiography. Am. J. Med. *89:*615, 1990.

37. Grollman, J. H., Liu, C. K., Astone, R. A., and Lurie, M. D.: Thromboembolic complications in coronary angiography associated with the use of nonionic contrast medium. Cathet. Cardiovasc. Diagn. *14:*159, 1988.

38. Granger, C. B., Gabriel, D. A., Reece, N. S., et al.: Fibrin modification by ionic and non-ionic contrast media during cardiac catheterization. Am. J. Cardiol. *69:*8217, 1992.

TECHNICAL ASPECTS OF CARDIAC CATHETERIZATION

39. Pepine, C. J., Allen, H. D., Bashore, T. M., et al.: ACC/AHA guidelines for cardiac catheterization and cardiac catheterization laboratories. J. Am. Coll. Cardiol. *18:*1149, 1991.

40. Goss, J. E., and Cameron, A., for the Society for Cardiac Angiography and Interventions Laboratory Performance Standards Committee: Mobile cardiac catheterization laboratories. Cathet. Cardiovasc. Diagn. *26:*71, 1992.

41. Bersin, R. M., Elliott, C. M., Fedor, J. M., et al.: Mobile cardiac catheterization registry: Report of the first 1,001 patients. Cathet. Cardiovasc. Diagn. *31:*1, 1994.

42. Lee, J. C., Bengtson, J. R., Lipscomb, J., et al.: Feasibility and cost-saving potential of outpatient cardiac catheterization. J. Am. Coll. Cardiol. *15:*378, 1990.

43. Clements, S. D., Jr., and Gatlin, S.: Outpatient cardiac catheterization: A report of 3,000 cases. Clin. Cardiol. *14:*477, 1991.

44. Clark, D. A., Moscovich, M. D., Vetrovec, G. W., and Wexler, L.: Guidelines for the performance of outpatient catheterization and angiographic procedures. Cathet. Cardiovasc. Diagn. *27:*5, 1992.

45. Block, P., Ockene, I., Goldberg, R. J., et al.: A prospective randomized trial of outpatient versus inpatient cardiac catheterization. N. Engl. J. Med. *319:*1252, 1988.

46. Cameron, A., for the Society for Cardiac Angiography and Interventions Laboratory Performance Standards Committee: Guidelines for professional staff privileges in the cardiac catheterization laboratory. Cathet. Cardiovasc. Diagn. *21:*203, 1990.

47. Heupler, F. A., Al-Hani, A. J., Dear, W. E., and Members of the Laboratory and Performance Standards Committee of the Society for Cardiac Angiography and Interventions: Guidelines for continuous quality improvement in the cardiac catheterization laboratory. Cathet. Cardiovasc. Diagn. *30:*191, 1993.

48. Holmes, D. R., Jr., Wondrow, M. S., and Tulsrud, P. R.: Radiographic techniques used in cardiac catheterization. *In* Pepine, C. J., Hill, J. A., and Lambert, C. R. (eds.): Diagnostic and Therapeutic Cardiac Catheterization. 2nd ed. Baltimore, Williams and Wilkins, 1994, p. 141.

49. Tobis, J. M.: The future of digital angiography. Cathet. Cardiovasc. Diagn. *27:*14, 1992.

50. Nissen, S. E.: Principles and applications of digital imaging in cardiac and coronary angiography. *In* Pepine, C. J., Hill, J. A., and Lambert, C. R. (eds.): Diagnostic and Therapeutic Cardiac Catheterization. 2nd ed. Baltimore, Williams and Wilkins, 1994, p. 162.

51. Nissen, S. E., Pepine, C. J., Bashore, T. M., et al.: Cardiac angiography without cine film: Erecting a "Tower of Babel" in the cardiac catheterization laboratory. J. Am. Coll. Cardiol. *24:*834, 1994.

52. Balter, S., and Members of the Laboratory and Performance Standards Committee of the Society for Cardiac Angiography and Interventions: Guidelines for personnel radiation monitoring in the cardiac catheterization laboratory. Cathet. Cardiovasc. Diagn. *30:*277, 1993.

53. Johnson, L. W., Moore, R. J., and Balter, S.: Review of radiation safety in the cardiac catheterization laboratory. Cathet. Cardiovasc. Diagn. *25:*186, 1992.

54. Hill, J. A., Miranda, A. A., Keim, S. G., et al.: Value of right-sided cardiac catheterization in patients undergoing left-sided cardiac catheterization for evaluation of coronary artery disease. Am. J. Cardiol. *65:*590, 1990.

55. MacDonald, R. G.: Catheters, sheaths, guidewires, needles and related equipment. *In* Pepine, C. J., Hill, J. A., and Lambert, C. R. (eds.): Diagnostic and Therapeutic Cardiac Catheterization. 2nd ed. Baltimore, Williams and Wilkins, 1994, p. 111.

56. Kern, M. J., Cohen, M., Talley, J. D., et al.: Early ambulation after 5 French diagnostic cardiac catheterization: Results of a multicenter trial. J. Am. Coll. Cardiol. *15:*1475, 1990.

57. Popma, J. J., Satler, L. F., Pichard, A. D., et al.: Vascular complications after balloon and new device angioplasty. Circulation *88*(part I):1569, 1993.

58. Sharkey, S. W.: Beyond the wedge: Clinical physiology and the Swan-Ganz catheter. Am. J. Med. *83:*111, 1987.

59. Bush, C. A., Van Fossen, D. B., Kolibash, A. J., et al.: Cardiac catheterization and coronary angiography using 5F preformed (Judkins) cath-

eters from the percutaneous right brachial approach. Cathet. Cardiovasc. Diagn. *29:*267, 1993.

60. Campeau, L.: Percutaneous radial artery approach for coronary angiography. Cathet. Cardiovasc. Diagn. *16:*3, 1989.

61. Kieffer, R. W., and Dean, R. H.: Complications of intra-arterial monitoring. Problems Gen. Surg. *2:*116, 1985.

62. Braunwald, E.: A new technique for left ventricular angiography and transseptal left heart catheterization. Am. J. Cardiol. *6:*1062, 1960.

63. Clugston, R., Lau, F. Y. K., and Ruiz, C.: Transseptal catheterization update 1992. Cathet. Cardiovasc. Diagn. *26:*266, 1992.

64. Vignola, P. A., Swaye, P. S., and Gosselin, A. J.: Safe transthoracic left ventricular puncture performed with echocardiographic guidance. Cathet. Cardiovasc. Diagn. *6:*317, 1980.

65. Baim, D. S., and Grossman, W.: Percutaneous approach, including transseptal catheterization and apical left ventricular puncture. *In* Grossman, W. and Baim, D. S. (eds.): Cardiac Catheterization, Angiography, and Intervention. 4th ed. Philadelphia, Lea and Febiger, 1991, p. 62.

66. Caves, P. K., Schulz, W. P., and Dong, E., Jr.: New instrument for transvenous cardiac biopsy. Am. J. Cardiol. *33:*264, 1974.

67. Mason, J. W.: Techniques for right and left ventricular endomyocardial biopsy. Am. J. Cardiol. *41:*887, 1978.

68. Richardson, P. J.: King's endomyocardial bioptome. Lancet *1:*660, 1974.

69. Brooksby, I. A. B., Jenkins, B. S., Coltast, D. J., et al.: Left ventricular endomyocardial biopsy. Lancet *2:*1222, 1974.

70. Hauptman, P. J., Selwyn, A. P., and Cooper, C. J.: Use of the left internal jugular vein approach in endomyocardial biopsy. Cathet. Cardiovasc. Diagn. *32:*42, 1994.

71. Corley, D. D., and Strickman, N.: Alternative approaches to right ventricular endomyocardial biopsy. Cathet. Cardiovasc. Diagn. *31:*236, 1994.

72. Anderson, J. L. and Marshall, H. W.: The femoral venous approach to endomyocardial biopsy: Comparison with internal jugular and transarterial approaches. Am. J. Cardiol. *53:*833, 1984.

73. Miller, L. W., Labovitz, A. J., McBride, L. A., et al.: Echocardiography-guided endomyocardial biopsy: A 5-year experience. Circulation *78*(suppl III):III-99, 1988.

74. Sekiguchi, M., and Take, M.: World survey of catheter biopsy of the heart. *In* Sekiguchi, M., and Olsen, E. G. J. (eds.): Cardiomyopathy. Clinical, Pathological, and Theoretical Aspects. Baltimore, University Park Press, 1980, p. 217.

75. Fowler, R. E., and Mason, J. W.: Role of cardiac biopsy in the diagnosis and management of cardiac disease. Prog. Cardiovasc. Dis. *27:*153, 1984.

76. Mason, J. W., and O'Connell, J. B.: Clinical merit of endomyocardial biopsy. Circulation *79:*971, 1989.

77. Abelmann, W. H., Baim, D. S., and Schnitt, S. J.: Endomyocardial biopsy: Is it of clinical value? Postgrad. Med. J. *68*(suppl. 1):S44, 1992.

78. Mason, J. W.: Endomyocardial biopsy and the causes of dilated cardiomyopathy. J. Am. Coll. Cardiol. *23:*591, 1994.

79. Kasper, E. K., Agema, W. R. P., Hutchins, G. M., et al.: The causes of dilated cardiomyopathy: A clinicopathologic review of 673 consecutive patients. J. Am. Coll. Cardiol. *23:*586, 1994.

80. Schoenfeld, M. H., Supple, E. W., Dec, G. W., et al.: Restrictive cardiomyopathy versus constrictive pericarditis: Role of endomyocardial biopsy in avoiding unnecessary thoracotomy. Circulation *75:*1012, 1987.

81. Vaitkus, P. T., and Kussmaul, W. G.: Constrictive pericarditis versus restrictive cardiomyopathy: A reappraisal and update of diagnostic criteria. Am. Heart J. *122:*1431, 1991.

82. Hershkowitz, A., Vlahov, D., Willoughby, S. B., et al.: Prevalence and incidence of left ventricular dysfunction in patients with human immunodeficiency syndrome. Am. J. Cardiol. *71:*955, 1993.

83. Cohen, I. S., Anderson, D. W., Virmani, R., et al.: Congestive cardiomyopathy in association with the acquired immunodeficiency syndrome. N. Engl. J. Med. *315:*628, 1986.

84. Beschorner, W. E., Baughman, K., Turnicky, R. P., et al.: HIV-associated myocarditis, pathology and immunopathology. Am. J. Pathol. *137:*1365, 1990.

85. Nanas, J. N., and Moulopoulos, S. D.: Counterpulsation: Historical background, technical improvements, hemodynamic and metabolic effects. Cardiology *84:*156, 1994.

86. Weber, K. T., and Janick, J. S.: Intraaortic balloon counterpulsation: a review of physiologic principles, clinical results, and device safety. Ann. Thorac. Surg. *17:*602, 1974.

87. Kern, M. J., Aguirre, F. V., Jatineni, S., et al.: Enhanced coronary blood flow velocity during intraaortic balloon counterpulsation in critically ill patients. J. Am. Coll. Cardiol. *21:*359, 1993.

88. Aguire, F. V., Kern, M. J., Bach, R., et al.: Intraaortic balloon pump support during high-risk coronary angioplasty. Cardiology *84:*175, 1994.

89. Mueller, H. S.: Role of intra-aortic counterpulsation in cardiogenic shock and acute myocardial infarction. Cardiology *84:*186, 1994.

90. Ohman, E. M., George, B. S., White, C. J., et al.: Use of aortic counterpulsation to improve sustained coronary artery patency during acute myocardial infarction: Results of a randomized trial. Circulation *90:*792, 1994.

91. Alderman, J. D., Gabliani, G. I., McCabe, C. H., et al.: Incidence and management of limb ischemia with percutaneous wire guided intraaortic balloon catheters. J. Am. Coll. Cardiol. *9:*524, 1987.

92. Barnett, M. G., Swartz, M. T., Peterson, G. J., et al.: Vascular complications from intraaortic balloons: Risk analysis. J. Vasc. Surg. *19:*81, 1994.

93. Eitchaninoff, H., Dimas, A. P., and Whitlow, P. L.: Complications associated with percutaneous placement and use of intraaortic balloon counterpulsation. Am. J. Cardiol. 71:328, 1993.

94. Nash, I. S., Lorell, B. H., Fishman, R. F., et al.: A new technique for sheathless percutaneous intraaortic balloon catheter insertion. Cathet. Cardiovasc. Diagn. 23:57, 1991.

HEMODYNAMIC DATA

95. Grossman, W.: Pressure measurement. In Grossman, W., and Baim, D. S. (eds.): Cardiac Catheterization, Angiography, and Intervention. 4th ed. Philadelphia, Lea and Febiger, 1991, p. 123.

96. Milnor, W. R.: Hemodynamics. Baltimore, Williams and Wilkins, 1982.

97. Gersh, B. J., Hahn, C. E. W., and Prys-Roberts, C.: Physical criteria for measurement of left ventricular pressure and its first derivative. Cardiovasc. Res. 5:32, 1971.

98. Bonow, R. O., and Udelson, J. E.: Left ventricular diastolic dysfunction as a cause of congestive heart failure: Mechanisms and management. Ann. Intern. Med. 117:502, 1992.

99. Grondelle, A. van, Ditchey, R. V., Groves, B. M., et al.: Thermodilution method overestimates low cardiac low output in humans. Am. J. Physiol. 245:H690, 1983.

100. Fargard, R., and Conway, J.: Measurement of cardiac output: Fick principle using catheterization. Eur. Heart J. 11:1, 1990.

101. Nichols, W. W., and O'Rourke, M. F. (eds.): McDonald's Blood Flow in Arteries. 3rd ed. Philadelphia, Lea and Febiger, 1990.

102. Werko, L., Varnauskas, E., Eliasch, H., et al.: Further evidence that the pulmonary capillary wedge pressure pulse in man reflects cyclic pressure changes in the left atrium. Circ. Res. 1:337, 1953.

103. Luchsinger, P. C., Seipp, H. W., and Patel, D. J.: Relationship of pulmonary artery-wedge pressure to left atrial pressure in man. Circ. Res. 11:315, 1962.

104. Lange, R. A., Moore, D. M., Jr., Cigarroa, R. G., and Hillis, L. D.: Use of pulmonary capillary wedge pressure to assess severity of mitral stenosis. Is true left atrial pressure needed in this condition? J. Am. Coll. Cardiol. 13:825, 1989.

105. McDonald, D. A., and Taylor, M. G.: The hydrodynamics of the arterial circulation. Prog. Biophys. Chem. 9:107, 1959.

106. Carabello, B. A., Barry, W. H., and Grossman, W.: Changes in arterial pressure during left heart pullback in patients with aortic stenosis: A sign of severe aortic stenosis. Am. J. Cardiol. 44:424, 1979.

107. Otto, C. M.: Echo-Doppler evaluation of aortic stenosis and the effect of percutaneous balloon aortic valvuloplasty. In Bashore, T. M. and Davidson, C. J. (eds.): Percutaneous Balloon Valvuloplasty and Related Techniques. Baltimore, Williams and Wilkins, 1991, p. 67.

108. Schoenfield, M. H., Palacios, I. F., Hutter, A. M., Jr., et al.: Underestimation of prosthetic mitral valve areas: Role of transseptal catheterization in avoiding unnecessary repeat mitral valve surgery. J. Am. Coll. Cardiol. 5:1387, 1985.

109. Nishimura, R. A., Rihal, C. S., Tajik, A. J., and Holmes, D. R.: Accurate measurement of the transmitral gradient in patients with mitral stenosis: A simultaneous catheterization and Doppler echocardiographic study. J. Am. Coll. Cardiol. 24:152, 1994.

110. Gorlin, R., and Gorlin, S. G.: Hydraulic formula for calculation of the area of the stenotic mitral valve, other cardiac valves, and central circulatory shunts. Am. Heart J. 41:1, 1951.

111. Gorlin, R.: Calculations of cardiac valve stenosis: Restoring an old concept for advanced applications. J. Am. Coll. Cardiol. 19:920, 1987.

112. Kass, D.: Hemodynamic assessment of valvular stenosis. In Bashore, T. M. and Davidson, C. J. (eds.): Percutaneous Balloon Valvuloplasty and Related Techniques. Baltimore, Williams and Wilkins, 1991, p. 37.

113. Bache, R. J., Wang, Y., and Jorgensen, C. R.: Hemodynamic effects of exercise in isolated valvular aortic stenosis. Circulation 44:1003, 1971.

114. Ubago, J. L., Figueroa, A., Colman, T., et al.: Hemodynamic factors that affect calculated orifice areas in the mitral Hancock xenograft valve. Circulation 61:388, 1980.

115. Cannon, S. R., Richards, K. L., and Crawford, M.: Hydraulic estimation of stenotic orifice area: A correction of the Gorlin formula. Circulation 71:1170, 1985.

116. Cannon, J. D., Zile, M. R., Crawford, F. A., and Carabello, B. A.: Aortic valve resistance as an adjunct to the Gorlin formula in assessing the severity of aortic stenosis in symptomatic patients. J. Am. Coll. Cardiol. 20:1517, 1992.

117. Carabello, B. A.: Advances in the hemodynamic assessment of stenotic cardiac valves. J. Am. Coll. Cardiol. 10:912, 1987.

118. Hakki, A. H.: A simplified valve formula for the calculation of stenotic cardiac valve areas. Circulation 63:1050, 1981.

119. Angel, J., Soler-Soler, J., Anivarro, I., and Domingo, E.: Hemodynamic evaluation of stenotic cardiac valves. II: Modification of the simplified formula for mitral and aortic valve calculation. Cathet. Cardiovasc. Diagn. 11:127, 1985.

120. Ford, L. E., Feldman, T., Chiu, Y. C., and Carroll, J. D.: Hemodynamic resistance as a measure of functional impairment in aortic valvular stenosis. Circ. Res. 66:1, 1990.

121. Sellers, R. D., Levy, M. J., Amplatz, K., and Lillehei, C. W.: Left retrograde cardioangiography in acquired cardiac disease: Technique, indications and interpretations in 700 cases. Am. J. Cardiol. 14:437, 1964.

122. Grossman, W.: Shunt detection and measurement. In Grossman, W. and Baim, D. S. (eds.): Cardiac Catheterization, Angiography, and Intervention. 4th ed. Philadelphia, Lea and Febiger, 1991, p. 166.

123. Dexter, L., Haynes, F. W., Burwell, C. S., et al.: Studies of congenital heart disease. II. The pressure and oxygen content of blood in the right auricle, right ventricle, and pulmonary artery in control patients, with observations on the oxygen saturation and source of pulmonary capillary blood. J. Clin. Invest. 26:554, 1947.

124. Antman, E. M., Marsh, J. D., Green, L. H., and Grossman, W.: Blood oxygen measurements in the assessment of intracardiac left to right shunts: A critical appraisal of methodology. Am. J. Cardiol. 46:265, 1980.

125. Flamm, M. D., Cohn, K. E., and Hancock, E. W.: Measurement of systemic cardiac output at rest and exercise in patients with atrial septal defect. Am. J. Cardiol. 23:258, 1969.

126. Swan, H. J. C., and Wood, E. H.: Localization of cardiac defects by dye-dilution curves recorded after injection of T-1824 at multiple sites in the heart and great vessels during cardiac catheterization. Proc. Staff Meet. Mayo Clin. 28:95, 1953.

127. Daniel, W. C., Lange, R. A., Willard, J. E., et al.: Oximetric versus indicator dilution techniques for quantitating intracardiac left-to-right shunting in adults. Am. J. Cardiol. 75:199, 1995.

128. Dehmer, G. J., and Rutala, W. A.: Current use of green dye curves. Am. J. Cardiol. 75:170, 1995.

129. Castillo, C. A., Kyle, J. C., Gilson, W. E., and Rowe, G. G.: Simulated shunt curves. Am. J. Cardiol. 17:691, 1966.

130. Lorell, B. H., and Grossman, W.: Dynamic and isometric exercise during cardiac catheterization. In Grossman, W. and Baim, D. S. (eds.): Cardiac Catheterization, Angiography, and Intervention. 4th ed. Philadelphia, Lea and Febiger, 1991, p. 267.

131. Dexter, L., Whittenberger, F. W., Haynes, W. T., et al.: Effects of exercise on circulatory dynamics of normal individuals. J. Appl. Physiol. 3:439, 1951.

132. Bonow, R. O.: Left ventricular response to exercise. In Fletcher, G. F. (ed.): Cardiovascular Response to Exercise. American Heart Association Monograph Series. Mount Kisco, NY, Futura Publishing Co., 1993, p. 31.

133. Carroll, J. D., Hess, O. M., and Krayenbuehl, H. P.: Diastolic function during exercise-induced ischemia in man. In Grossman, W., and Lorell, B. H. (eds.): Diastolic Relaxation of the Heart. Boston, Martinus Nijhoff, 1986, p. 217.

134. Forrester, J. S., Helfart, R. H., Pasternac, A., et al.: Atrial pacing in coronary heart disease. Effects on hemodynamics, metabolism, and coronary circulation. Am. J. Cardiol. 27:237, 1971.

135. Udelson, J. E., Bacharach, S. L., Cannon, R. O., and Bonow, R. O.: Minimum left ventricular pressure during beta-adrenergic stimulation in human subjects: Evidence for elastic recoil and diastolic "suction" in the normal heart. Circulation 82:1174, 1990.

136. Gorlin, R., Knowles, J. H., and Storey, C. F.: The Valsalva maneuver as a test of cardiac function. Pathologic physiology and clinical significance. Am. J. Med. 22:197, 1957.

137. Buch, C. A., Stang, J. M., Wooley C. F., and Kilman, J. W.: Occult constrictive pericardial disease: Diagnosis by rapid volume expansion and correction by pericardiectomy. Circulation 56:924, 1977.

138. Mudge, G. H., Grossman, W., Mills, R. M., Jr., et al.: Reflex increase in coronary vascular resistance in patients with ischemic heart disease. N. Engl. J. Med. 295:1333, 1976.

139. Harding, M. B., Leithe, M. E., Mark, D. B., et al.: Ergonovine maleate testing during cardiac catheterization: A 10-year perspective in 3447 patients without significant coronary artery disease or Prinzmetal's variant angina. J. Am. Coll. Cardiol. 20:107, 1992.

140. Wilson, R. F., Marcus, M. L., and White, C. W.: Prediction of the physiologic significance of coronary artery lesions by quantitative lesion geometry in patients with limited coronary artery disease. Circulation 75:723, 1987.

141. Marcus, M. L.: Effects of cardiac hypertrophy on the coronary circulation. In Marcus, M. L. (ed.): The Coronary Circulation in Health and Disease. New York, McGraw-Hill Book Company, 1983, p. 285.

142. Klocke, F. J., Ellisa, K., and Canty, J. M., Jr.: Interpretation of changes in coronary flow that accompany pharmacologic interventions. Circulation 75(suppl. V):34, 1987.

143. Ganz, W., Tamura, K., Marcus, H. S., et al.: Measurement of coronary sinus blood flow by continuous thermodilution in man. Circulation 44:181, 1971.

144. Marcus, M. L., Wilson, R. F., and White, C. W.: Methods of measurement of myocardial blood flow in patients: A critical review. Circulation 76:245, 1987.

145. Mathey, D. G., Chatterjee, K., Tyberg, J. V., et al.: Coronary sinus reflux: A source of error in the measurement of thermodilution coronary sinus flow. Circulation 57:778, 1978.

146. Klocke, F. J.: Measurement of coronary flow reserve: Defining pathophysiology versus making decisions about patient care. Circulation 76:1183, 1987.

147. Cusma, J. T., Toggart, E. J., Folts, J. D., et al.: Digital subtraction angiographic imaging of coronary flow reserve. Circulation 75:461, 1987.

148. Hodgson, J. M., LeGrand, V., Bates, E. R., et al.: Validation in dogs of a rapid digital angiographic technique to measure relative coronary blood flow during routine cardiac catheterization. Am. J. Cardiol. 55:188, 1985.

149. Vogel, R. A.: Digital radiographic assessment of coronary flow reserve. In Buda, A. J., and Delp, E. J. (eds.): Digital Cardiac Imaging. Boston, Martinus Nijhoff, 1985, p. 106.

150. Klinke, W. P., Christie, L. G., Nichols, W. W., et al.: Use of catheter-tip

velocity-pressure transducer to evaluate left ventricular function in man: Effects of intravenous propranolol. Circulation *61*:946, 1980.

151. Doucette, J. W., Cori, P. D., Payne, H. M., et al.: Validation of a Doppler guidewire for intravascular measurement of coronary artery flow velocity. Circulation *85*:1899, 1992.

152. Wangler, R. D., Peters, K. G., Laughlin, D. E., et al.: A method for continuously assessing coronary velocity in the rat. Am. J. Physiol. *10*:H816, 1981.

153. Marcus, M., Wright, C., Doty, D., et al.: Measurement of coronary velocity and reactive hyperemia in the coronary circulation in humans. Circ. Res. *49*:877, 1981.

154. Wilson, R. F., and White, C. W.: Measurement of maximal coronary flow reserve: A technique for assessing the physiologic significance of coronary arterial lesions in humans. Herz *12*:163, 1987.

155. Dehmer, L., Gould, K. L., and Kirkeeide, R.: Assessing stenosis severity, coronary flow reserve, collateral function, quantitative coronary arteriography, position imaging, and digital subtraction angiography. A review and analysis. Prog. Cardiovasc. Dis. *30*:307, 1988.

Chapter 7
Radiology of the Heart

ROBERT M. STEINER, DAVID C. LEVIN

HISTORICAL PERSPECTIVE

The history of cardiac imaging is almost as old as radiology itself. Within one year of Roentgen's discovery, Francis H. Williams of Boston published two articles on cardiac imaging.[1] He reported, "I found that the outline of the heart as seen . . . through the fluoroscope corresponded to the outline drawn on the skin with percussion as a guide." Williams was a true pioneer. Using fluoroscopy, he was the first to describe the difference in pulsations between pericardial effusion and an enlarged heart.[2] By 1899 Williams concluded that radiography was the best method of determining heart size based on a comparison of radiographic findings, digital percussion, and autopsy specimens in 546 patients.[2]

During the decades that followed, dramatic developments in imaging technology occurred, highlighted by the Coolidge hot cathode ray tube in 1913, kymography in the 1920's, angiocardiography in the early 1930's, and the image intensifier in 1952.[3] Since the 1950's, a number of new modalities including radioisotope scanning, ultrasound, computed tomography (CT) and magnetic resonance imaging (MRI) have revolutionized cardiac imaging, allowing real-time anatomically detailed examination of the heart not possible with plain film techniques. In spite of these advances, the plain chest radiograph continues to yield unique and valuable information about the structure and function of the heart and the great vessels. As a screening examination patients undergo on entering the hospital or at an outpatient office for a wide variety of cardiopulmonary as well as other disorders, the chest radiograph presents an opportunity to identify subtle or overlooked cardiac pathology, including significant vascular calcification, chamber enlargement, and evidence of pulmonary arterial or venous hypertension. Adult-onset congenital heart disease, which may be overlooked clinically, is often identified by plain film chest radiography. The chest film frequently helps to confirm a clinical impression of valvular heart disease, acute or chronic pericarditis, ischemic heart disease, left ventricular failure, or pulmonary edema.

The former mainstay of cardiac diagnosis, the four-view heart series with a barium esophagram and cardiac fluoroscopy, has been supplanted by more sensitive and specific imaging modalities such as angiography,[4,5] CT (Chap. 10),[4,6–10] nuclear cardiology (Chap. 9),[11–12] MRI (Chap. 10),[6,11,13–18a] and echocardiography (Chap. 3).[19–21]

In recent years, the bedside portable chest roentgenogram has gained special importance in the evaluation and monitoring of patients with cardiac disease in the intensive care unit, including the postoperative cardiac patient.[5,22,23]

In this chapter we discuss the role of plain film chest radiology, emphasizing cardiovascular anatomy and alterations of that anatomy in a variety of pathological disorders. Correlation with cross-sectional imaging is used to clarify important anatomical questions.

NORMAL CARDIAC ANATOMY

Plain Chest Radiography

There is excellent contrast between the air-filled lung and the adjacent soft tissue structures in the normal chest radiograph. As a result, the pulmonary arteries and veins and the interlobar fissures are visualized in great detail. For this reason, the chest film remains the study of first choice for the evaluation of pulmonary parenchymal and vascular disease. On the other hand, the heart and other mediastinal structures appear as a featureless, opaque silhouette. Blood, myocardium, pericardium, coronary arteries and great vessels, valves, and mediastinal fat cannot be separated because they have similar radiographic attenuation characteristics, so that there is little or no contrast available to differentiate these structures. However, the cardiac borders are clearly outlined, and deviation from the normal configuration does suggest disease. Thus, knowledge of the appearance of the normal and pathological cardiac silhouettes is essential for the initial evaluation of the cardiac patient.

FRONTAL VIEW. In a well-positioned posteroanterior (PA) or frontal chest roentgenogram, the normal cardiac and other vascular structures are predictably outlined against the lung as a series of indentations and bulges along the right and left mediastinal borders (Fig. 7–1).

Left Subclavian Artery. The left subclavian artery is the border-forming structure along the upper left mediastinum above the aortic arch. Although the left innominate vein is actually lateral in position to the left subclavian artery, it is adjacent to the anterior chest wall so that there is no available contrast in the frontal view to single out the left innominate vein as a distinct structure. The left subclavian artery usually forms a concave border with the lung, extending from the clavicle to the aortic arch. The left subclavian artery may bulge laterally when there is increased blood flow through the vessel, as in postductal coarctation of the aorta or when the vessel is tortuous due to atherosclerosis or hypertension. A straight or a convex left supraaortic border is found in patients with persistent left superior vena cava (Fig. 7–2).

Aortic Arch. The aortic arch or "knob" forms a sharply marginated convex border immediately below the left subclavian artery. It is usually small in the young patient, with a diameter of 2.0 ± 1.0 cm, and represents the left posterior-lateral portion of the aortic arch. The trachea is displaced slightly to the right at the level of the aortic arch. When a right aortic arch is present, the trachea is displaced slightly to the left, a clear indication of that anomaly. A small bump or "nipple" measuring about 2 to 3 mm in diameter, representing the left superior intercostal vein, can be seen along the aortic arch in a minority of individuals (4 to 10 per cent) (Fig. 7–3).[23,24] When enlarged, the left superior intercostal vein has the same significance as a dilated azygos vein; i.e., it is due to increased central venous pressure or increased blood flow resulting from diversion from other major venous structures, as may occur in superior vena cava syndrome, inferior vena caval obstruction, or deep mediastinal venous obstruction.

The aortic arch is prominent on the frontal view in older individuals with pronounced aortic regurgitation, systemic hypertension, or atherosclerosis (Fig. 7–4). It is wider and higher than in the normal aorta and may even reach the level of the clavicle. The ascending aorta protrudes farther to the right side. The descending aorta assumes a tortuous or serpentine configuration (Fig. 7–4A). Aortic dissection (Fig. 7–4B) and aneurysm of the aortic arch (Fig. 7–4C) are evident on the frontal view. The brachiocephalic vessels also dilate and become tortuous. At times, a dilated right brachiocephalic artery may mimic the appearance of a substernal thyroid or other superior mediastinal mass and may require CT or MRI for diagnosis. In one of 1500 patients there is a right-sided aortic arch related to either an

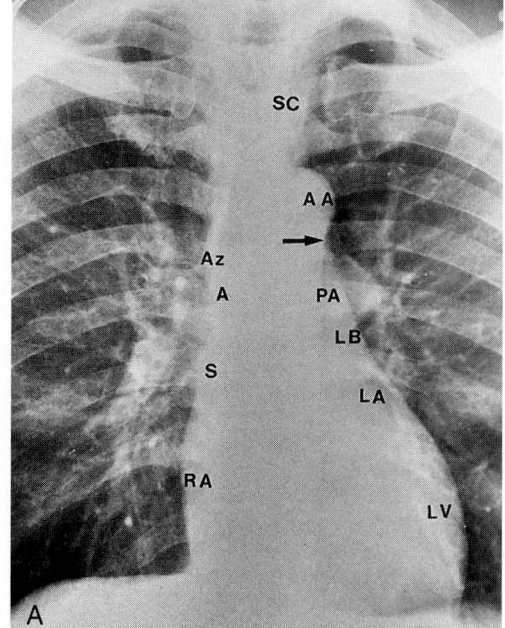 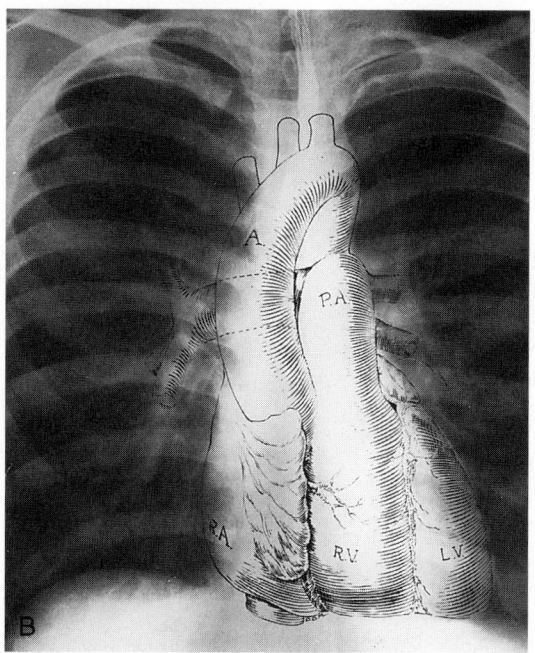

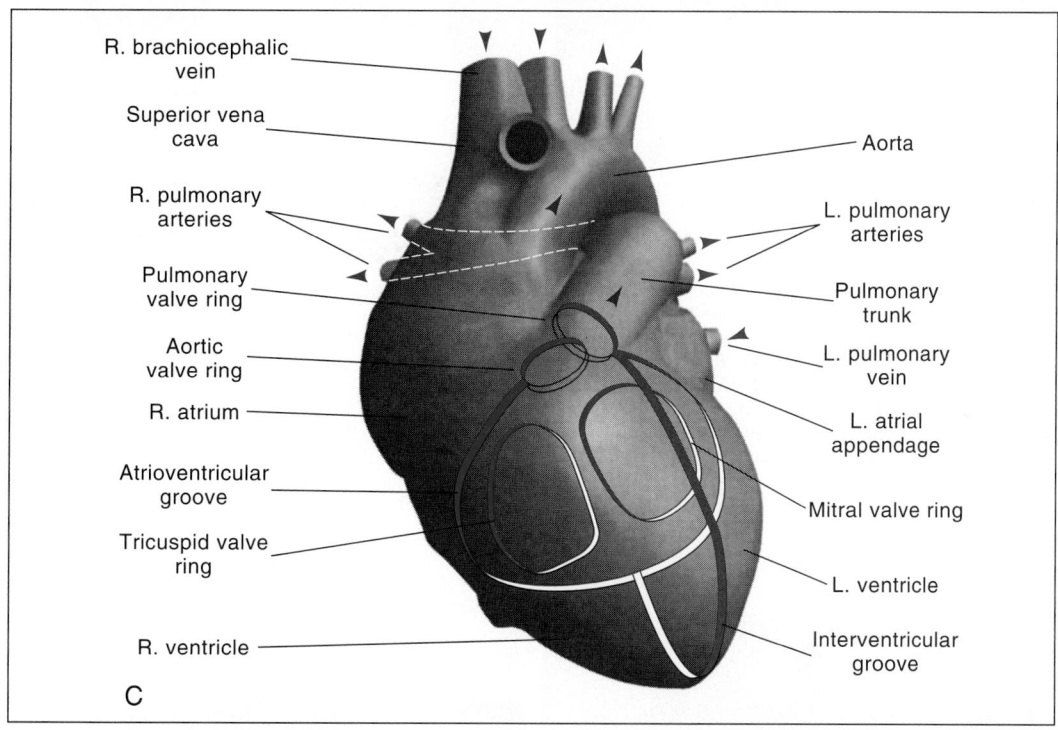

FIGURE 7–1. Frontal projection of the heart and great vessels. *A,* Left and right heart borders in the frontal projection. SC = left subclavian artery; A = ascending aorta; LV = left ventricle; B = left bronchus; LA = left atrial appendage; PA = main pulmonary artery; RA = right atrium; S = superior vena cava; AA = aortic arch; Az = azygos vein; arrow = aorticopulmonary window. *B,* Superimposed line drawing demonstrates the position of the heart and great vessels. PA = pulmonary artery; RV = right ventricle; A = aorta; LV = left ventricle; RA = right atrium. (*A* and *B* from Van Houten, F. X., et al.: Radiology of valvular heart disease. *In* Sonnenblick, E., and Lesch, M. [eds.]: Valvular Heart Disease. New York, Grune and Stratton, 1974.) *C,* Line drawing in the frontal projection demonstrates the relationship of the cardiac valves, rings, and sulci to the cardiac silhouette.

aberrent left subclavian artery or a mirror image arch. When no aortic knob is visible on the left side, displacement of the trachea to the left and an aortic arch on the right should lead to the diagnosis of right aortic arch[25,26] (Fig. 7–5).

The left mediastinal border immediately below the aortic arch is characterized by a variable-sized indentation of the lung into the mediastinum. This indentation is the aorticopulmonary window (Fig. 7–6). It is bordered superiorly by the inferior margin of the aortic arch and inferiorly by the upper margin of the left pulmonary artery. This small space contains, in addition to fat and soft tissue, several important anatomical structures. These include the left recurrent laryngeal nerve, the ligamentum or ductus arteriosus, and the ductus node. Lymphadenopathy or a ductus diverticulum may cause a convex bulge in the normally concave mediastinal reflection of the aorticopulmonary window.[27,28] Encroachment on the recurrent laryngeal nerve within the aorticopulmonary window by a neoplasm, a ductus diverticulum, or an enlarged lymph node or extrinsic pressure on the nerve from an aortic aneurysm or large left atrium can cause paralysis of the left vocal cord.

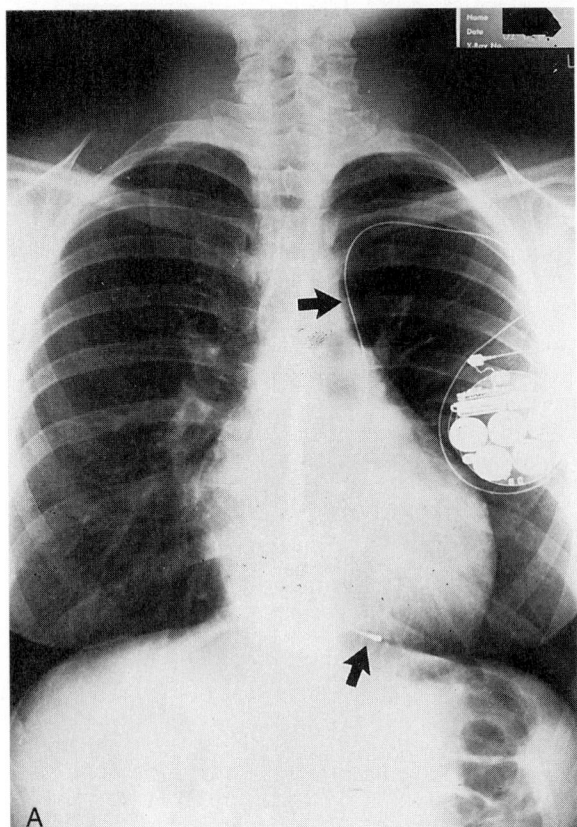

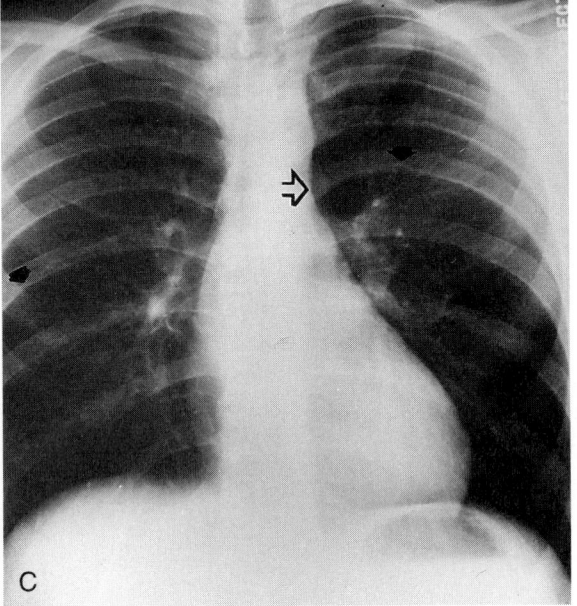

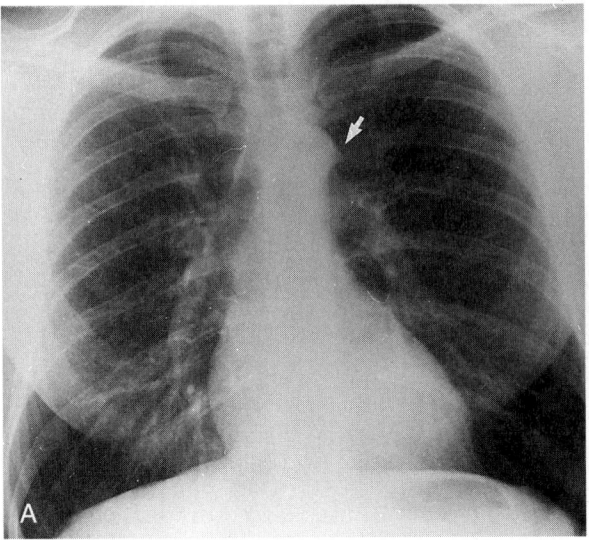

FIGURE 7–2. Persistent left superior vena cava (LSVC). *A,* PA chest film in a man with a normally functioning intravenous cardiac pacemaker. The course of the lead is as follows: LSVC (upper arrow) to coronary sinus, to right atrium and right ventricular apex (lower arrow). *B,* Left subclavian venogram illustrates the course of the LSVC: the subclavian vein (one arrow), the LSVC (two arrows), and the coronary sinus (three arrows). *C,* The left subclavian artery is prominent (open arrow) in this patient with coarction of the aorta. Rib notching is present (arrows).

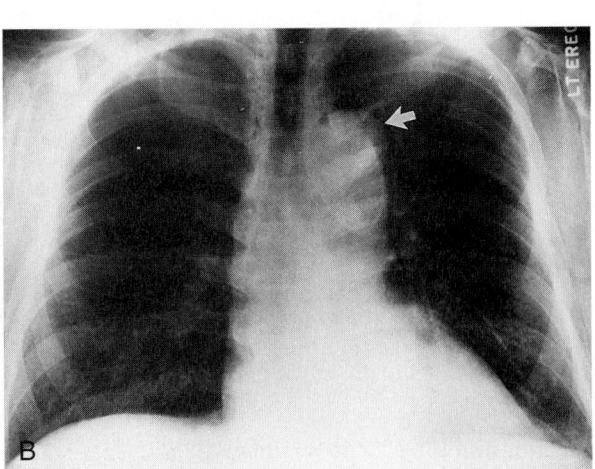

FIGURE 7–3. Left superior intercostal vein (LSIV). A small nipple or bulge is visible on the aortic knob. The LSIV normally measures 2 to 3 mm in diameter. Enlargement may be due to deep venous obstruction or altered hemodynamics. *A,* PA projection in a young woman. LSIV is a beak-like bulge that extends to the left at the aortic knob (arrow). *B,* A larger convex "mass" than that shown in *A* overlying the aortic knob (arrow).

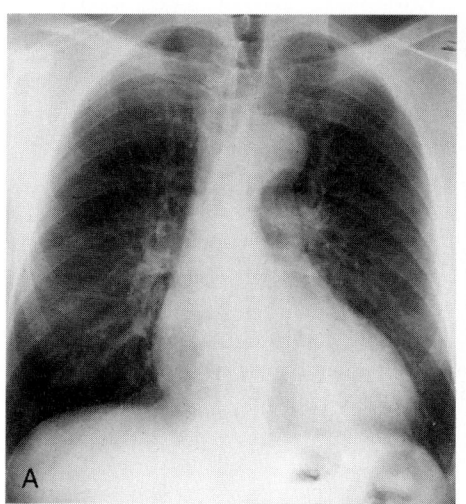
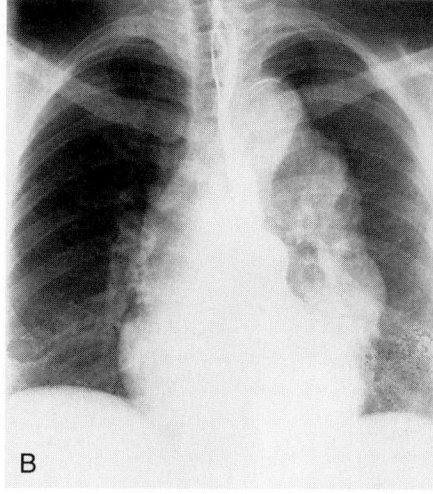
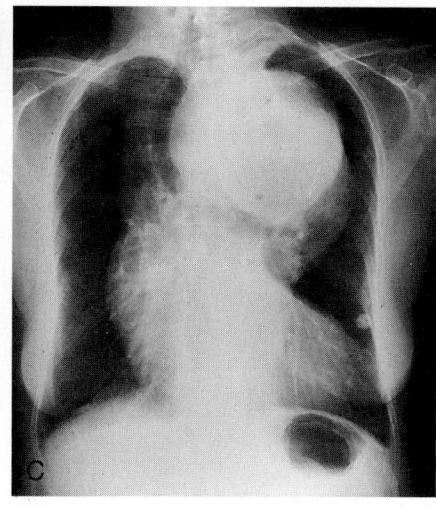

FIGURE 7–4. *A,* Aortic enlargement. A 63-year-old man with longstanding systemic hypertension and aortic regurgitation. There is marked dilatation and uncoiling of the aortic arch and descending aorta. *B,* Chronic aortic dissection. Marked dilation and elongation of the arch and descending aorta. The barium-filled esophagus follows the aorta and cannot be used to evaluate left atrial size. *C,* Giant aneurysm of the aortic arch with marked displacement of the trachea to the right.

Main Pulmonary Artery. The origin of the left main pulmonary artery is located immediately below the aortico-pulmonary window and is border-forming with the left lung (Fig. 7–1*A, B*). It is identified as a small to moderate-sized, smoothly marginated arc at the level where the left pulmonary artery branches. Another indication of the location of the main pulmonary artery is the position of the left main stem bronchus. The left pulmonary artery arches over the left main stem bronchus, unlike the right pulmonary artery, which is located between the right upper lobe and right middle lobe bronchus. When enlarged, the normally slightly convex main pulmonary artery will form a prominent convex bulge. Enlargement of the main pulmonary artery is caused by increased flow, as in patients with anemia or a left-to-right shunt. A large main pulmonary artery may also be related to turbulent blood flow, as in pulmonary valvular stenosis, or to increased pressure related to Eisenmenger physiology, pulmonary hypertension associated with scleroderma, or primary pulmonary hyperten-

sion. Finally, a large main pulmonary artery may be found in disorders of vascular wall collagen such as Marfan syndrome or "idiopathic pulmonary artery dilatation." On the other hand, the main pulmonary artery border may be flat or not seen at all in patients with transposition of the great vessels, truncus arteriosus, tetralogy of Fallot, or pulmonary atresia (Fig. 7–7).

Left Atrium. The left atrial appendage or auricle lies immediately below the left main stem bronchus in the frontal projection. The left atrial appendage normally forms a smooth and slightly concave segment of the left heart border. When the left atrial border is straightened or bulges laterally, atrial enlargement should be suspected. Nonvascular pathology may simulate enlargement of the left atrial appendage. For example, a pericardial fibroma or cyst, lymphoma, or other mediastinal or pleural neoplasms may present as a convexity of the upper left mediastinal border. Congenital absence of the pericardium also causes bulging of the left atrial appendage. An important sign of left atrial

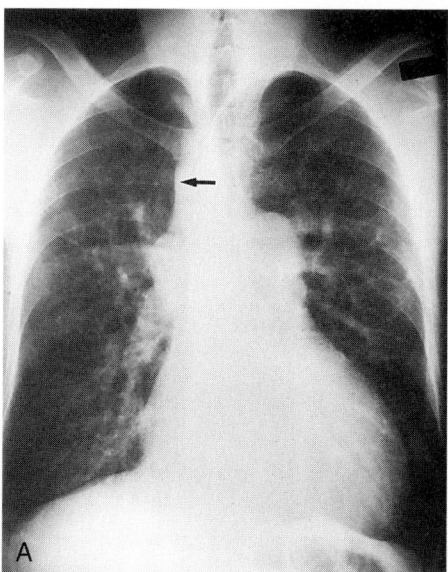
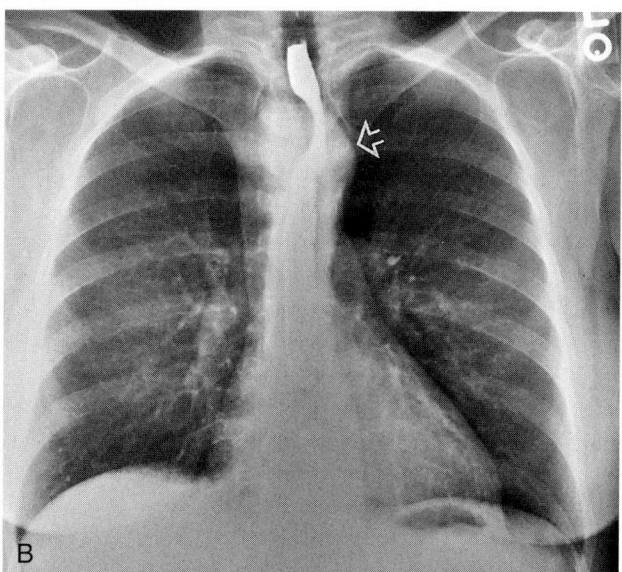

FIGURE 7–5. Right aortic arch. *A,* There is no evidence of a left-sided aortic knob in this patient with a right-sided arch (arrow). The pulmonary arteries are enlarged in this cyanotic 25-year-old man with truncus arteriosus type I. *B,* Frontal view of the chest in an adult female. The barium column is displaced to the left by the right aortic arch. The bulge on the left is due to the wide origin of the aberrant left subclavian artery (the diverticulum of Kommerall) (arrow).

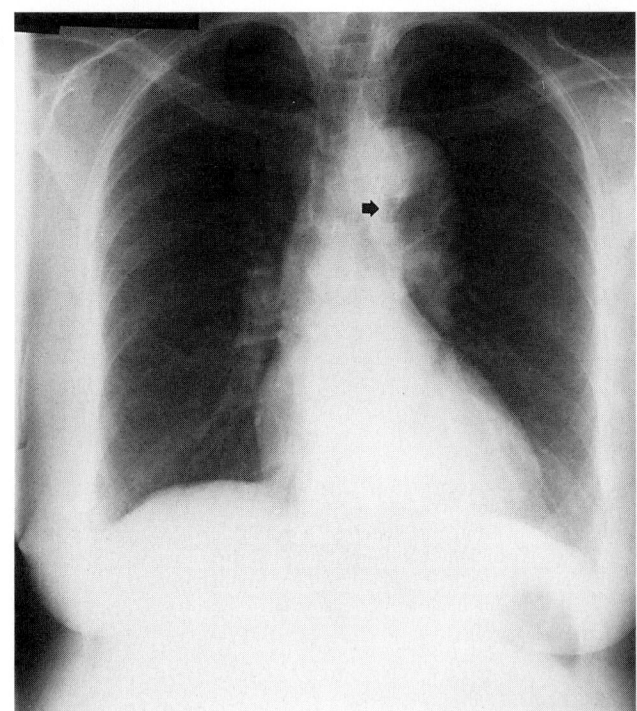

FIGURE 7–6. The deep recess between the inferior margin of the aortic arch and the superior edge of the left pulmonary artery represents the aorticopulmonary window (arrow).

enlargement in the frontal projection is elevation of the main stem bronchus so that the carinal angle is greater than the normal value of up to 75 degrees[29,30] (Figs. 7–8, 7–9).

Left Ventricle. The left ventricular border seamlessly blends with the left atrial border (Fig. 7–1A) without a specific landmark to differentiate between the two chambers. The left ventricular border is mildly convex extending to the diaphragm. It may be rounded and the apex elevated with hypertrophy due to aortic stenosis or hypertrophic cardiomyopathy. When the left ventricle is enlarged because of dilatation, as may occur with aortic regurgitation or aneurysm, the apex is displaced downward and laterally. Much of the downward displaced apex may be obscured by the overlying left diaphragmatic dome (Fig. 7–10).

With dilatation of the left ventricle due to volume overload as occurs, for example, in mitral regurgitation, the dimensions of the chamber increase markedly and the heart assumes a globular appearance. The left ventricular border extends to the left and may even reach the rib convexities. As the left ventricle enlarges, it obscures the left atrial border. The left anterior oblique projection helps to separate the two chambers so that their relative sizes can be discerned. The ability to separate the left heart chambers assumes importance when the differential diagnosis lies between ischemic cardiomyopathy (in which case the left ventricle is larger than the left atrium) and mitral regurgitation (in which case the left atrium may be larger than the left ventricle).

Right Atrium. The right atrial border forms a gentle convex interface with the adjacent right middle lobe. In the frontal projection, the inferior vena caval border below the right atrium is usually straight, and in a good inspiratory film it can be separated from the convex right atrial border.[30] The outline of the normal left atrium is seen deep to the right atrial border as an additional convex density.

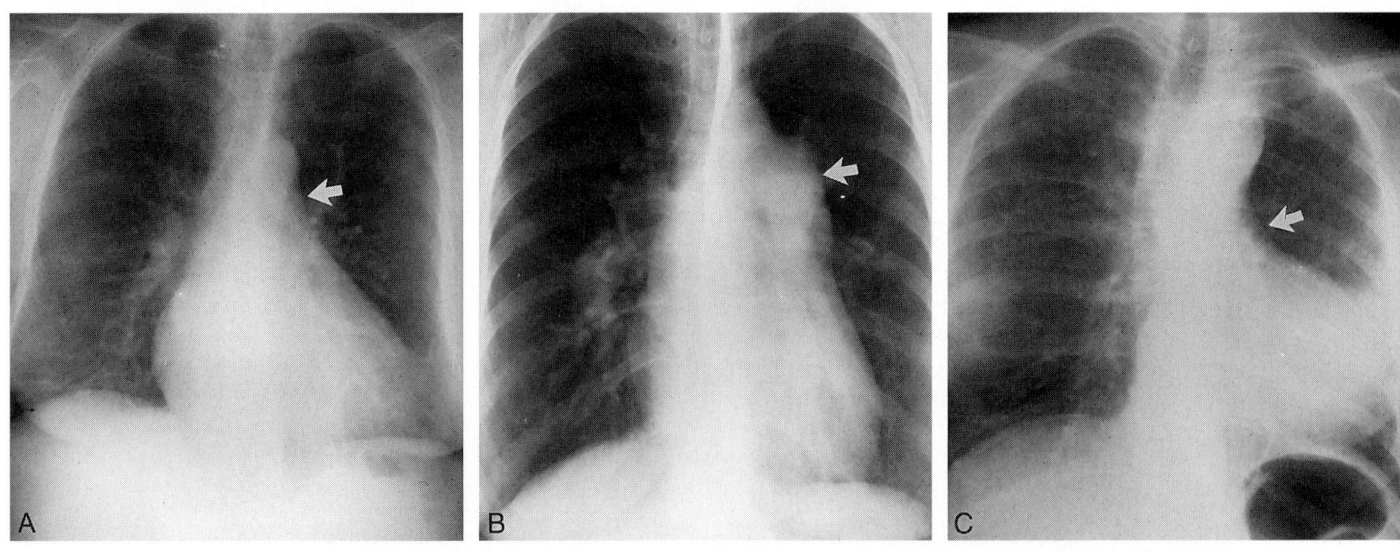

FIGURE 7–7. The pulmonary artery contour. A, Normal pulmonary artery segment in a 36-year-old woman with sickle cell anemia and moderate cardiomegaly (arrow). B, The main pulmonary artery is grossly enlarged in this patient with primary pulmonary hypertension (arrow). C, The pulmonary artery contour is small in this 16-year-old with tetralogy of Fallot and moderate pulmonary infundibular stenosis (arrow).

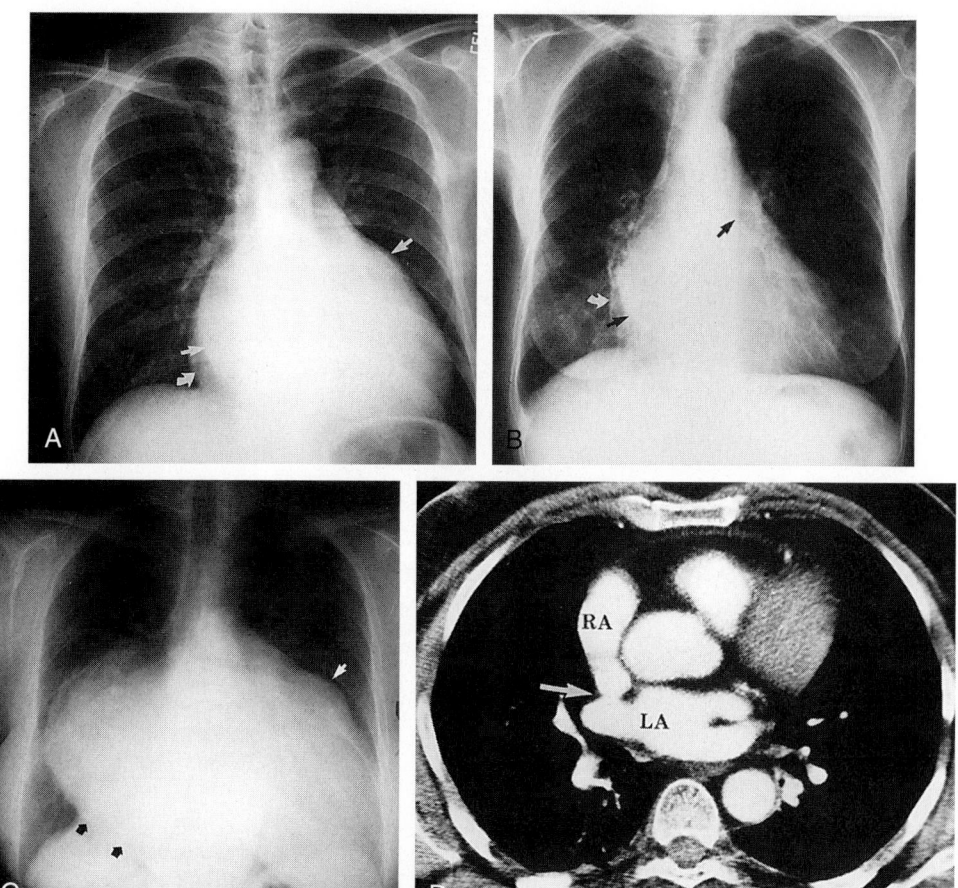

FIGURE 7–8. Prominent left atrial (LA) contour. *A,* The left atrial appendage bulges laterally to the left in this patient with multivalvular rheumatic heart disease (arrow). The double convex contour of enlarged right (curved arrow) and left (arrow) atria is present along the right atrial border (arrow). *B,* A 40-year-old woman with mitral stenosis. There is left atrial enlargement with a double right-sided heart border (white arrow = right atrium; black arrow = left atrial border). The left main stem bronchus is elevated (black arrow). *C,* Left atrial (LA) enlargement. A large convex bulge is seen in the area of the LA appendage (white arrow). The LA is grossly enlarged and is border-forming on the right side after traversing the smaller right atrium. The inferior border of the left atrium is visualized (black arrows) as it extends back toward the midline. If this were the right atrial border instead, it would have blended imperceptibly with the right hemidiaphragm and inferior vena cava. *D,* Enhanced CT demonstrates the anatomical relationship between the anterior RA and the posterior LA. The indentation of lung and fat between the atria (arrow) permits separation of the right-sided borders of both atria as seen in the PA chest radiograph.

The confluence of the right pulmonary veins is directed toward the epicenter of this bulge. The left atrium is clearly visualized within the right atrial shadow because of an interface of lung between the posteriorly positioned left atrium and the more anteriorly positioned right atrium. If the left atrium is markedly enlarged, the left atrial border may actually be lateral to the right atrium (Fig. 7–8). The borders of the right and left atria can be differentiated because the inferior border of the right atrium blends with the inferior vena cava while the left atrial shadow crosses the midline toward the left side of the heart. The upper right atrial border blends superiorly with the superior vena cava, which forms a straight interface with the adjacent lung as it continues toward the neck (Fig. 7–1). The right

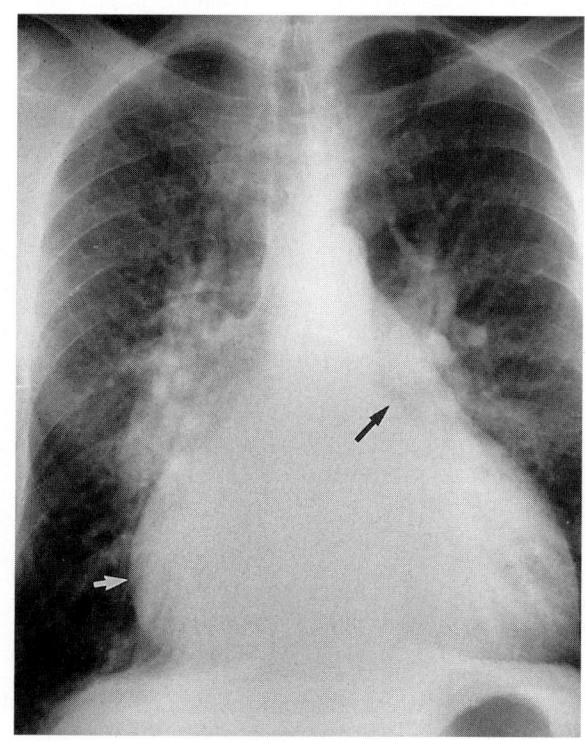

FIGURE 7–9. Prominent right atrial contour (white arrow). The RA border is prominent and convex (white arrow). There is cephalization of the pulmonary vasculature. The left atrium is deep to the enlarged right atrium. The left main stem bronchus is elevated (black arrow) in this patient with a dilated cardiomyopathy with mitral and tricuspid regurgitation.

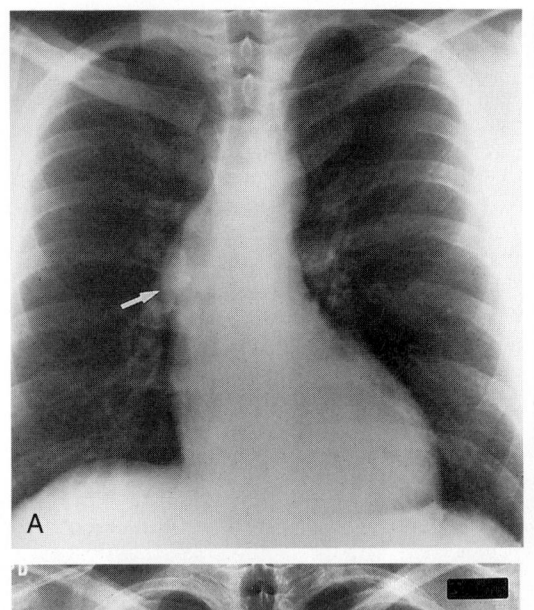
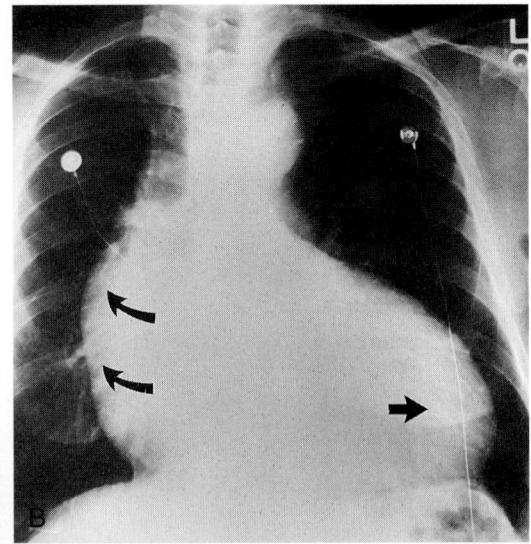
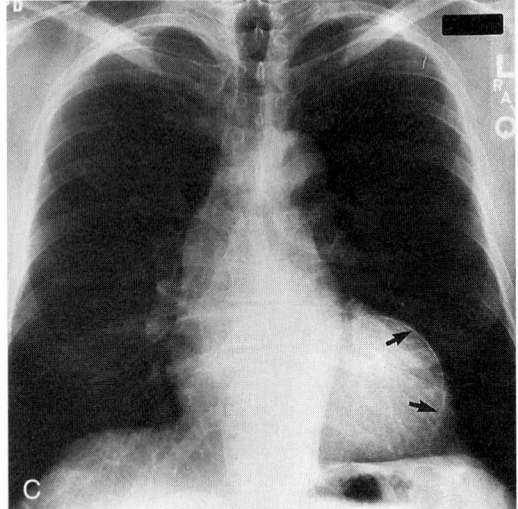

FIGURE 7-10. *A,* Aortic stenosis. The left ventricular border is rounded and prominent due to left ventricular hypertrophy. The proximal ascending aorta is prominent due to poststenotic dilatation (arrow). *B,* Aortic regurgitation in a patient with Marfan syndrome. Prominent left ventricular border (arrow). The LV chamber is dilated due to aortic regurgitation and the ascending aorta is convex (curved arrows). The descending aorta is dilated. *C,* The ascending aorta is enlarged, and there is a thin mural calcification within the left ventricle due to a large aneurysm (arrows).

atrial border is considered enlarged when it bulges more than 5.5 cm to the right of the midline[8] (Fig. 7-9).

Right Ventricle. The right ventricle is not border-forming in the frontal projection and cannot be directly viewed (Fig. 7-11; see also Fig. 7-1). As the right ventricle dilates, the left ventricle is displaced posteriorly and to the left, causing widening of the cardiac shadow. In selected cases such as tetralogy of Fallot, the enlarged right ventricle displaces the left ventricle laterally and superiorly, creating a high round left ventricular border.

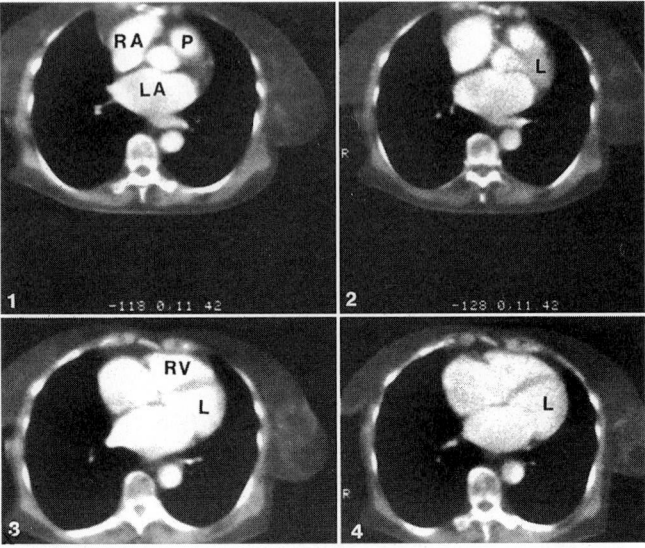

FIGURE 7-11. Enhanced ultrafast CT shows the anatomic relationships of the right ventricle. *Frame 1,* The main pulmonary artery is border-forming on the left and the right atrium is border-forming on the right. *Frame 2,* The left ventricle borders the left side of the heart. *Frames 3 and 4,* The right ventricle is border-forming anteriorly but not border-forming laterally or posteriorly. (RA = right atrium; LA = left atrium; P = pulmonary artery; L = left ventricle; RV = right ventricle.)

Ascending Aorta. This structure is superimposed on the superior vena cava and forms a convex border above the right atrium (Fig. 7–1). The aortic valve and annulus, the proximal ascending aorta, and the coronary arteries are not visible on plain films unless they are calcified, since their attenuation characteristics are similar to those of the rest of the heart. Enlargement of the aorta is shown in Figure 7–4.

Azygos Vein. The azygos vein is an elliptical structure at the right tracheobronchial angle. The azygos vein ascends in the right paravertebral sulcus and arches forward over the right main stem bronchus to enter the back of the superior vena cava (Fig. 7–12). The azygos vein and its left-sided equivalent, the hemiazygos vein, receive intercostal veins and act as an important collateral pathway when the deep mediastinal veins are obstructed.[30] Normally measuring 0.7 to 1 cm in the erect and 1 to 1.3 cm in the supine anteroposterior position, the azygos vein is a good indicator of changing cardiovascular dynamics. It is enlarged in superior vena caval and inferior vena caval obstruction, in the absence of the intrahepatic portion of the inferior vena cava, in portal vein obstruction, and in both left- and right-sided cardiac failure.[31] A change in diameter of the azygos vein will parallel changes in pulmonary venous pressure, making it a useful guide to the development of congestive heart failure on plain film x-rays. There is an azygos fissure in 3 per cent of the population. When this occurs the azygos vein is displaced laterally and superiorly and will dilate for the same reasons as a normally positioned azygos vein.[30]

LATERAL VIEW (Fig. 7–13). Proper positioning of the patient in the lateral projection is critical for accurate identification of cardiac structures.[32] The need for accurate positioning is exemplified by the right atrium. The normal right atrium is not border-forming in this projection, but if the patient is rotated backward the right atrium will form part of the lower posterior cardiac border, simulating enlargement.[30] The right ventricle is border-forming in the subxyphoid area and usually extends superiorly to a point about one-third of the distance between the diaphragm and the thoracic apex. As the right ventricle dilates, it encroaches further upon the retrosternal space.[33] The relationship between the size of the right ventricle and the extent of retro-

sternal encroachment is affected by body habitus and lung volume. For example, in the patient with emphysema, right ventricular enlargement may coexist with an expanded retrosternal space (Fig. 7–14A). In a patient with a small anterior-posterior (AP) diameter and/or a pectus excavatum deformity, the retrosternal space may be obliterated despite the absence of right ventricular enlargement (Fig. 7–14B). CT and MRI as well as echocardiography, unlike the chest film, portray relationships of the right ventricle to nearby structures with great accuracy and permit a clear analysis of right ventricular volume and function.[8,33,34]

The anterior margin of the pulmonary artery and the ascending aorta lie above the right ventricle; however, because of abundant mediastinal fat, neither structure is visualized clearly in the normal patient. In patients with severe emphysema, however, the increased lung volume permits the main pulmonary artery and the ascending aorta to be well outlined. The arch of the aorta is usually clearly seen except at the level where the superior vena cava crosses the aorta and where the brachiocephalic arteries enter the aorta. The inferior margin of the posterior aortic arch is often visible because of the indentation of the lung into the aorticopulmonary window. The semilunar lucency of the aorticopulmonary window also outlines the superior margin of the left pulmonary artery. The descending aorta is usually not clearly discernible in the normal individual because it lies adjacent to the spine and the posterior mediastinal fat. However, in patients with hyperaeration or those with a tortuous or calcified aorta, the descending aorta is better seen.

The normal *left atrium* forms a shallow convex bulge at the upper aspect of the posterior border of the heart on the lateral view. It may be easily identified because the posterior border of the left atrium lies immediately anterior to the pulmonary venous confluence.

The normal *left ventricle* forms a long convexity at the posterior inferior heart border just above the diaphragm. Enlargement of the left ventricle is suggested by the use of the Hoffman-Rigler sign—a measurement determined by drawing a 2-cm line upward along the inferior vena cava from the point where the left ventricle and inferior vena cava cross in the lateral projection. At this point a second line is drawn parallel to the vertebral bodies. The distance between the left ventricle and the inferior vena cava should not exceed 1.8 cm. If it does, left ventricular enlargement is suggested. Although this sign is helpful, it is far from accurate because a poor positioning for a lateral chest film or backward displacement of the left ventricle due to right ventricular enlargement may influence this measurement.[32,35]

The *esophagus* lies immediately behind the left atrium and, when filled with contrast medium, can be used to locate the posterior border of the left atrial chamber. Normally the left atrium does not displace the esophagus, but when the left atrium is enlarged, posterior displacement of the esophagus from the area of the left main stem bronchus to the level of the left ventricle will occur (Fig. 7–14C). The normal left ventricle usually does not displace the esophagus but extends posterior and lateral to the esophagus. When both the left atrium and left ventricle are enlarged, the barium-filled esophagus may be pushed backward in one long curve.[36] Sometimes the left atrium enlarges without displacing the barium-filled esophagus because the esophagus may slide off the back of the left atrium to the left or right. When the aorta is tortuous and dilated (Fig. 7–4B) or when there is a scoliosis, the esophagus parallels the spinal curvature and cannot be used to evaluate left atrial size.

RIGHT ANTERIOR OBLIQUE (RAO) PROJECTION (Fig. 7–15). Chest radiography in this projection is performed with the patient in a 45-degree right anterior oblique relationship to the film cassette (right shoulder toward the cassette). In this view there is elongation of the ventricles; the long axes

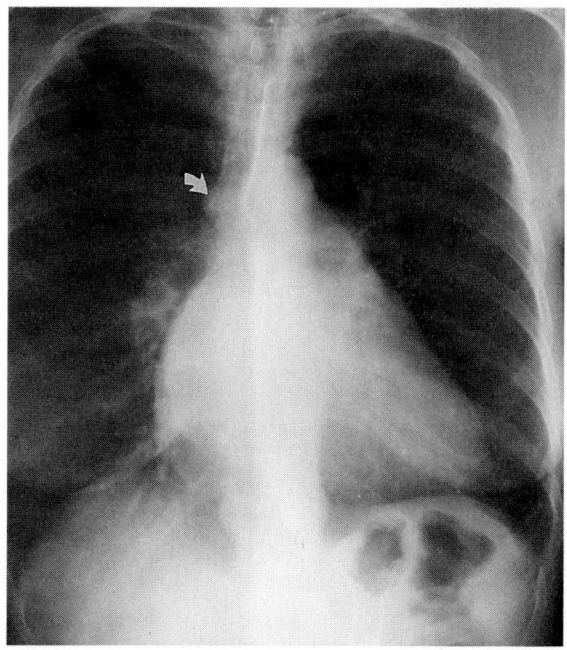

FIGURE 7–12. The azygos vein forms an elliptical opacity at the junction of the trachea and right main stem bronchus. It is enlarged in this patient with mitral and tricuspid regurgitation (arrow).

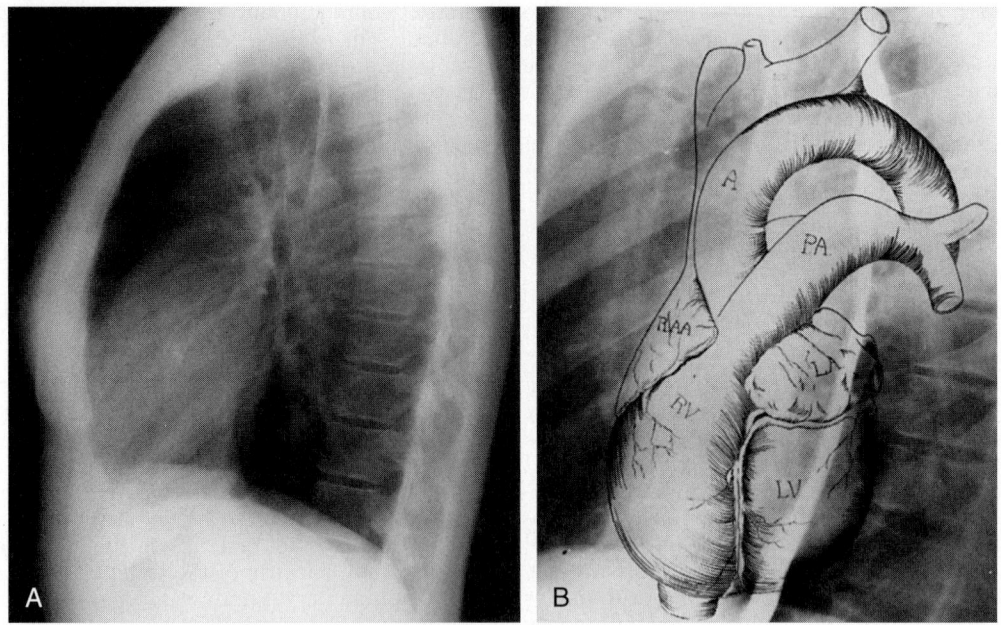

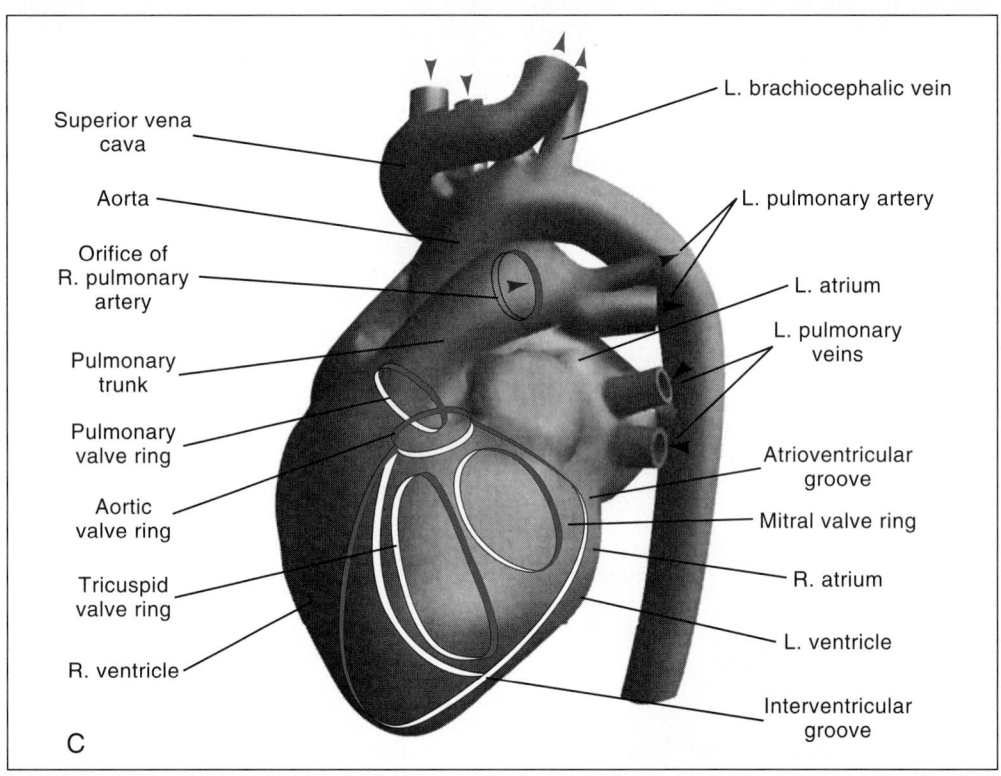

FIGURE 7–13. *A,* Lateral chest film. *B,* Superimposed anatomical drawing of the cardiac chambers and great vessels. (*A, B* from Van Houten, F. X., et al: Radiology of valvular heart disease. *In* Sonnenblick, E., and Lesch, M. [eds.]: Valvular Heart Disease. New York, Grune and Stratton, 1974.) *C,* Lateral projection of the heart showing position of valve rings.

of the ventricles are in view and the atrioventricular groove is in profile. This position permits optimal visualization of a calcified mitral or tricuspid valve. The right anterior oblique view is used by angiographers to determine the presence of left atrial enlargement, a common feature in mitral stenosis (Fig. 7–16). It is also helpful to the fluoroscopist when studying the function of a mechanical mitral valve prosthesis. The aortic arch is foreshortened in this view, so that the arch and proximal descending aorta are often superimposed and obscured. The anterior border of the heart consists of the sinus portion of the right ventricle inferiorly and the right ventricular outflow tract and the main pulmonary artery superiorly. The right-sided or posterior heart border consists of the right atrium superiorly and the left atrium inferiorly.[36,37]

LEFT ANTERIOR OBLIQUE (LAO) PROJECTION (Fig. 7–17). The left anterior oblique projection is performed with the patient in a 60-degree oblique relationhip to the cassette. This is a useful angiographic view to diagnose the presence of left ventricular enlargement. Since the ventricular septum is in profile in the LAO projection, septal defects, dyskinesia, and displacement, due to right heart enlargement, can be identified. In this projection the aortic and pulmonary valves are in profile, so that aortic valve calcifi-

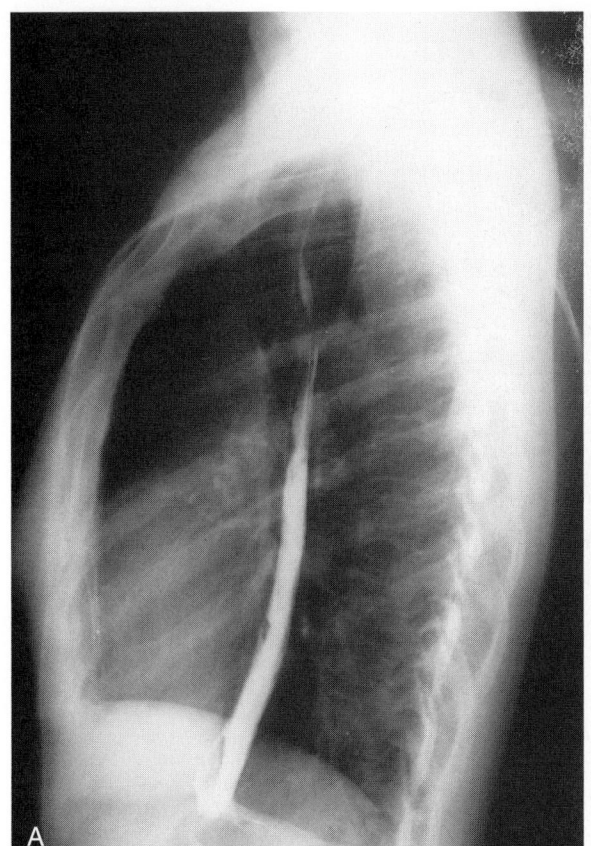

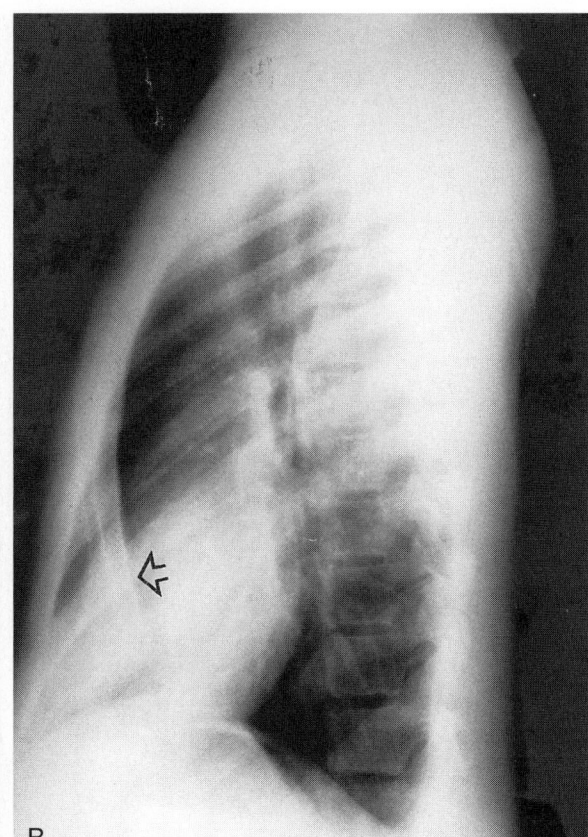

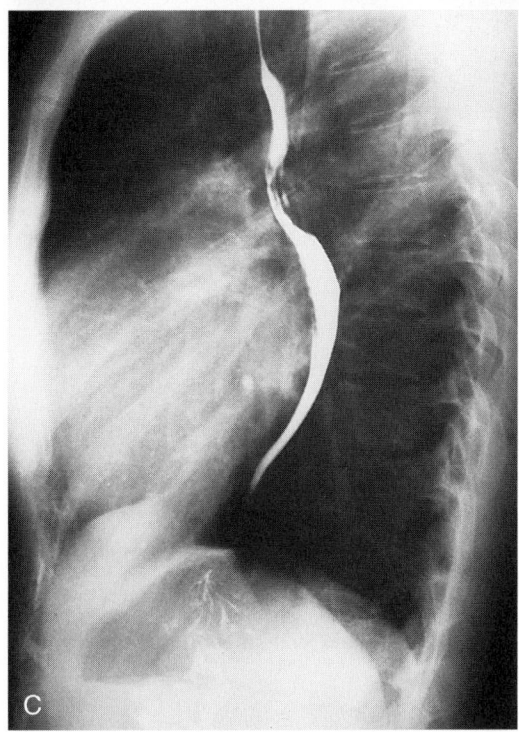

FIGURE 7–14. *A,* The extent of right ventricular encroachment on the retrosternal space is reduced by the hyperinflated lung due to emphysema. *B,* Severe pectus excavatum in patient with prolapsed mitral valve (arrow). The deformity exaggerates the extent of retrosternal encroachment. *C,* There is discrete posterior displacement of the barium column due to left atrial enlargement in a patient with mitral stenosis.

cations can be clearly visualized and aortic or pulmonary stenosis and regurgitation can be assessed.[32,37,38] The aortic arch is also in profile in the LAO projection so that abnormalities of the arch including dissection, contained rupture, aortitis, aneurysm, and coarctation can be detected with aortography or cross-sectional imaging.[30,39,40] The anterior (right) heart border consists of the right atrium above and right ventricle below. Along the left posterior heart border, the left atrium is border-forming superiorly and the left ventricle inferiorly.[41] The LAO projection is superior to other projections for detecting right ventricular enlargement, characterized by an increase in the convexity of the anterior border of the cardiac silhouette. An enlarged right atrium may cause bulging of the upper anterior border of the cardiac shadow, producing a shelf-like configuration.[30]

Fluoroscopy of the Heart

Fluoroscopy is performed to study cardiac motion and to identify cardiac and other mediastinal calcifications.[42]

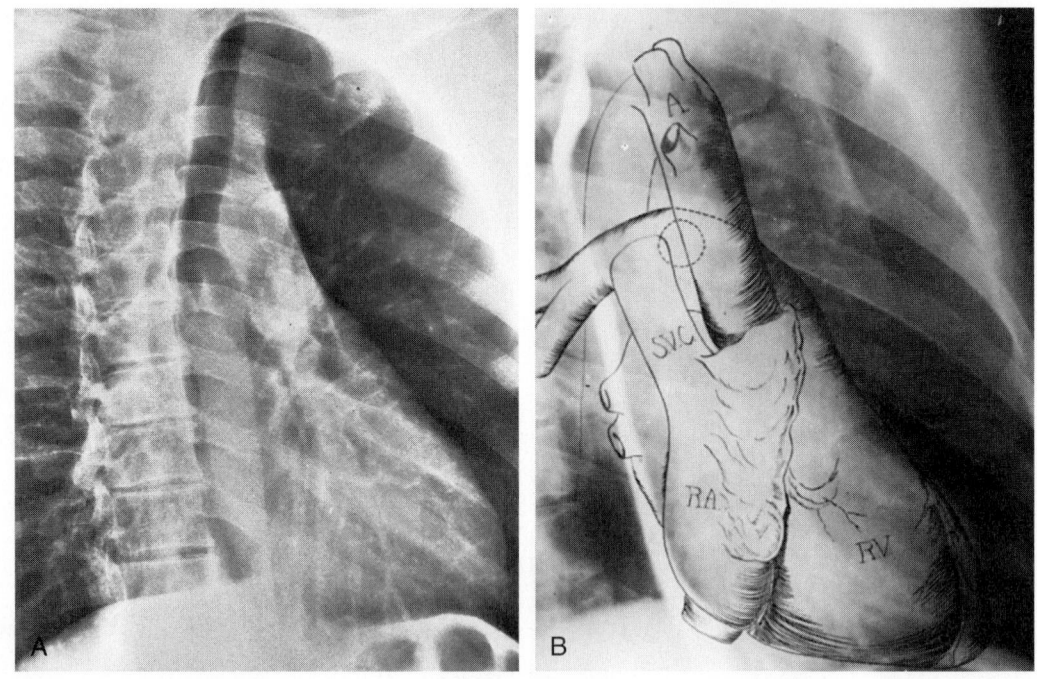

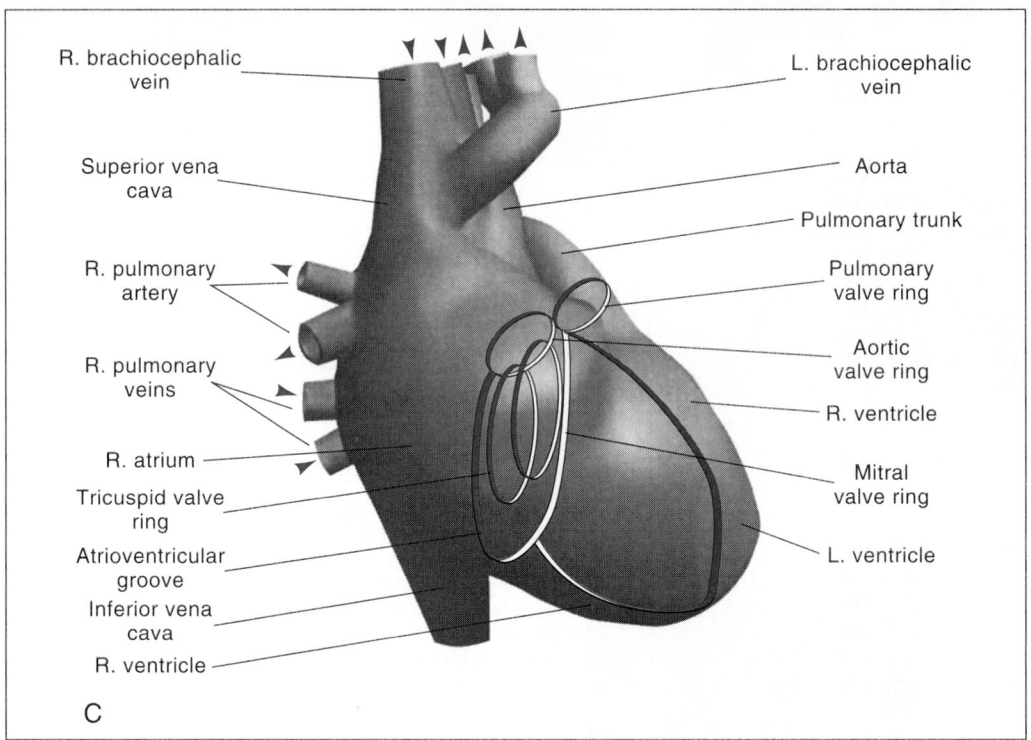

FIGURE 7–15. **Right anterior oblique (45-degree) projection.** *A,* Chest radiograph. *B,* Line drawing shows position of cardiac chambers. (*A, B* from Van Houten, F. X., et al.: Radiology of valvular heart disease. *In* Sonnenblick, E., and Lesch, M. [eds.]: Valvular Heart Disease. New York, Grune and Stratton, 1974.) *C,* Drawing shows position of valve rings.

Today, cardiac fluoroscopy is no longer performed routinely but is used largely to solve specific clinical questions. Because fluoroscopy potentially causes significant radiation risk to the patient, it should be used selectively, with careful beam collimation. Exposure time should be kept to a minimum, preferably not more than 5 minutes.[43] Perhaps the most important applications of fluoroscopy today are to evaluate prosthetic valve function and to detect coronary artery, valvular, and pericardial calcifications.[44–53]

Cardiac fluoroscopy is usually performed with the patient in the upright position at 68 to 75 kVp to enhance contrast and reduce mottle. The patient's position is deter-

mined by the structure to be studied. For example, if the presence or absence of aortic valve calcification is to be determined, positioning for a LAO projection is optimal. If the function of a mitral valve prosthesis is in question, or if the presence of mitral calcification is suspected, the RAO projection is most suitable. Coronary calcifications are best studied in the left and right oblique projections. In the 60-degree LAO projection, the right coronary artery, left circumflex, and left main coronary artery are seen to advantage. In the lateral and RAO projections, calcification of the left anterior descending artery is easily discernible.[49]

Although large calcifications may be seen on the chest film, small calcifications are often obscured because of mo-

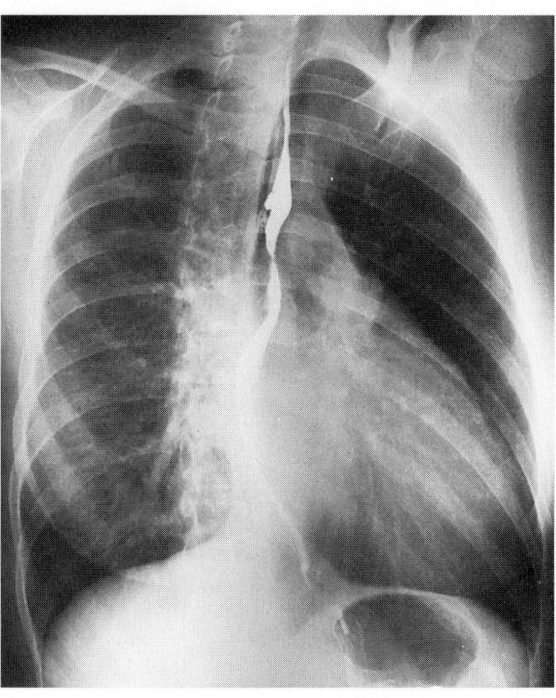

FIGURE 7–16. Right anterior oblique view. There is posterior displacement of the barium column by an enlarged LA in this patient with mitral stenosis.

tion. On the other hand, motion is an advantage with fluoroscopy and even small coronary artery calcifications are seen clearly as opaque tracks of calcification moving perpendicular to their long axes in a "to and fro" motion. The right main and circumflex coronary arteries move more vigorously than the anterior and posterior descending arteries. Subepicardial fat represents an important landmark for the identification of vascular and valvular anatomy and is best seen with fluoroscopy. Fat surrounding the coronary arteries and within the atrioventricular groove is well visualized so that the location of the mitral and tricuspid valves, the coronary sinus, and circumflex and right coronary arteries can be determined.

Fluoroscopy with videotape recording is useful in analyzing the integrity of the radiopaque components of prosthetic valves.[45,46] Excursion of the sewing ring exceeding 9 to 12 degrees between systole and diastole is associated with significant dehiscence (Fig. 7–18). Limitation of poppet or disc occluder motion suggests the presence of thrombus or vegetation. The results of fluoroscopic analysis of mechanical components compare favorably with echocardiography and phonocardiography but do not yield useful information about the degree of valvular regurgitation as will Doppler echocardiography, MRI, and angiography.[45,54,55]

Measuring Cardiac Size

Measurement of the size of the heart with plain film radiography has been de-emphasized in recent years because more accurate analyses of cardiac chamber dimensions and volume are available with echocardiography, radioisotope scanning, CT, and MRI. However, since an enlarged heart is abnormal, estimation of the cardiothoracic ratio remains a valuable yardstick to gain an impression of cardiac size and particularly serial changes in heart size coinciding with cardiac events. This may be done subjectively by estimating whether a heart is normal in size, enlarged, or grossly enlarged on the basis of an average cardiothoracic ratio of ≤0.50 with a range of 0.39 to 0.55.[37,56] Using more objective criteria, the cardiothoracic ratio may be expressed as the ratio between the maximum transverse diameter of the heart divided by the maximum width of the thorax. To obtain these diameters, a vertical line is drawn on the radiograph through the midpoint of the spine from

the sternum to the diaphragm. The maximum transverse diameter of the heart is obtained by adding the widest distance of the heart border from the midline on the right and the left side (Fig. 7–19A). This value is then divided by the maximum transverse diameter of the thorax.[57,58] The normal range of the transverse diameter of the heart is 10 cm in a small, thin individual to 16.5 cm in a tall, heavy person. A measurement 10 per cent beyond these values represents the upper limits of normal.[59] Normal differences of transverse cardiac diameter in systole and diastole of 0.3 to 0.9 cm must be taken into account when analyzing cardiac size.[58] While the cardiothoracic ratio is helpful, it serves only as a guide. The normal heart may appear large in the frontal projection because of a small AP diameter of the thorax caused by pectus excavatum deformity or straight back. A large heart may appear smaller than it really is because of a downwardly displaced cardiac apex in patients with aortic regurgitation. The heart will be truly small in patients with Addison's disease, or anorexia nervosa due to the absence of brown fat (Fig. 7–19B).

Because of cardiac magnification on AP films (including portable radiographs), a visual correction must be made in order to avoid overdiagnosis of heart enlargement.[60] A correction of 10 to 12.5 per cent, depending on the anode-to-tube distance, will amend this discrepancy. High-kilovoltage PA airgap films also magnify the mediastinum approximately 6.6 per cent when compared with low-kV films in which an airgap is not used.[61] For the most part, calculated cardiothoracic ratios are of historical or research interest. In practice, these calculations are seldom performed because they are time consuming, and more accurate estimations of cardiac volume and size may be obtained with other imaging techniques.[13,14,62]

THE PULMONARY VASCULATURE

Normal Radiographic Anatomy

The pulmonary blood flow mirrors the hemodynamics of the heart itself. Because the pulmonary blood vessels are clearly visualized on the chest film, both normal and abnormal patterns of pulmonary blood flow can be identified. Increased, decreased, redistributed, or asymmetrical flow can be identified and correlated with other indications of

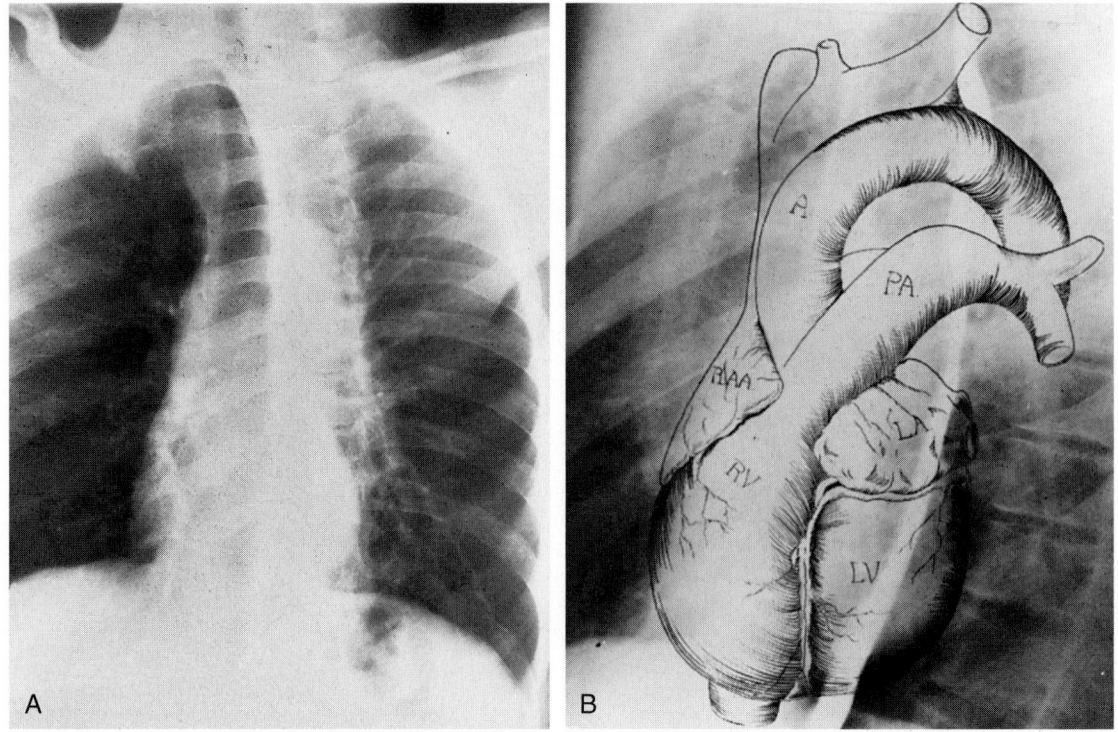

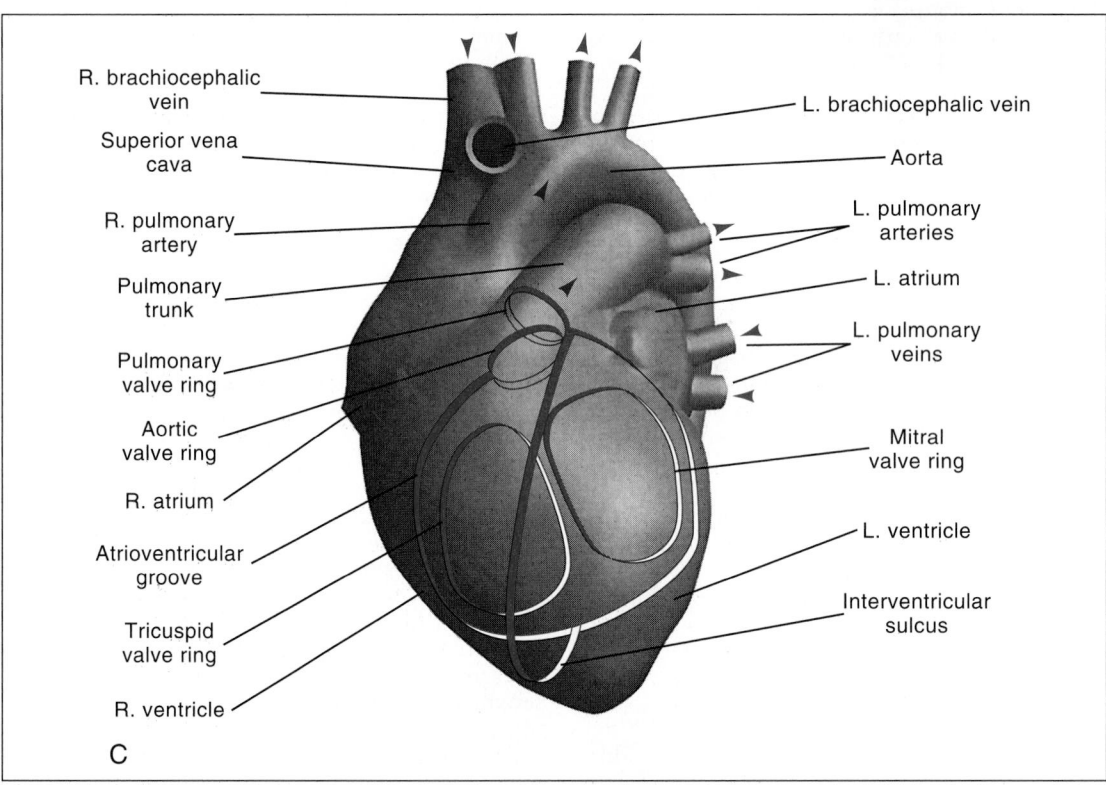

FIGURE 7–17. Sixty-degree left anterior oblique projection. *A,* Chest film. *B,* Superimposed line drawing in the same patient. (*A* and *B* from Van Houten, F. X., et al: Radiology of valvular heart disease. *In* Sonnenblick, E., and Lesch, M. [eds.]: Valvular Heart Disease. New York, Grune and Stratton, 1974.) *C,* Diagram in the left anterior oblique projection showing valves, rings, and sulci.

disease. The main pulmonary artery bifurcates within the mediastinum. The left pulmonary artery then courses to the left and backward, and its borders are visible just above the center of the left hilum (Fig. 7–1). In the lateral view, the left pulmonary artery passes over the left main stem bronchus paralleling the aortic arch (Fig. 7–13). The right pulmonary artery follows a horizontal course within the mediastinum, forming a round or elliptical opacity anterior to the right main stem bronchus on the lateral view. The right pulmonary artery divides within the mediastinum proximal to the right hilum. The intrapulmonary branches parallel the bronchi, divide in an orderly manner, and gradually taper toward the periphery of the lung. The arteries and bronchi subtending the same segment are of ap-

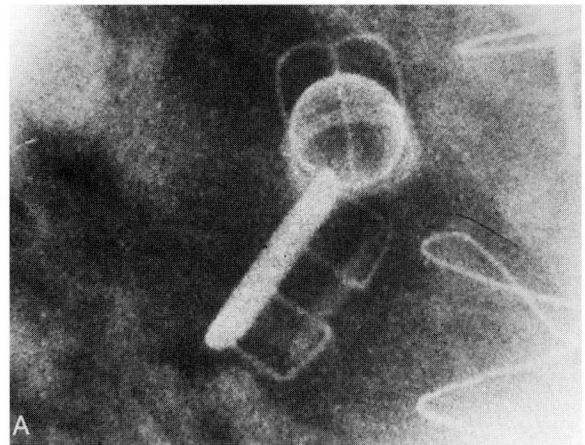

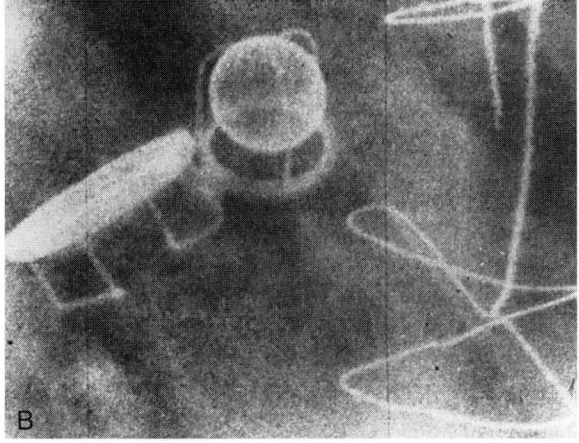

FIGURE 7–18. Abnormal excursion of a Beall mitral valve prosthesis due to partial dehiscence at the sewing ring. *A,* Diastole; *B,* systole.

proximately the same diameter at any particular level, with a ratio of 1.2 : 1.0. This relationship assumes importance when objective criteria are needed to support the impression of increased or redistributed blood flow (Fig. 7–20).

In the erect position, blood flow is greater to the lower lobes than to the upper lobes, partly because of the effects of gravity.[63,64] Another contributing factor affecting the normal distribution of pulmonary blood flow is differential intraalveolar pressures, as described by West.[63] In the supine and prone chest films, blood flow appears equal in both the upper and lower lung zones. Actually, flow is greatest in the dependent position or posterior third of each lung in the recumbent position, best appreciated with axial CT images.

In normal individuals, the pulmonary arteries and veins in the outer third of the lung are too small to be seen clearly on chest roentgenograms. The central pulmonary veins usually can be distinguished from pulmonary arteries because they follow different pathways. Pulmonary veins course centrally in the interlobular septa, converging in the left atrium 2 to 3 cm below the hila. The pulmonary arteries radiate from the hila several centimeters above the pulmonary venous confluences. The veins of the upper lobes are usually lateral to or superimposed on their companion pulmonary arteries, and for the most part, the veins are larger and branch less frequently than arteries. In practice, because the venous drainage and arterial supply to the upper lobes are so variable, it is often difficult to distinguish vein from artery.

Abnormal Pulmonary Blood Flow

INCREASED PULMONARY FLOW. The size of the pulmonary arteries is proportional to the volume of pulmonary blood flow so that if there is an increase in right-sided cardiac output the vessels will enlarge as long as the reserve of the

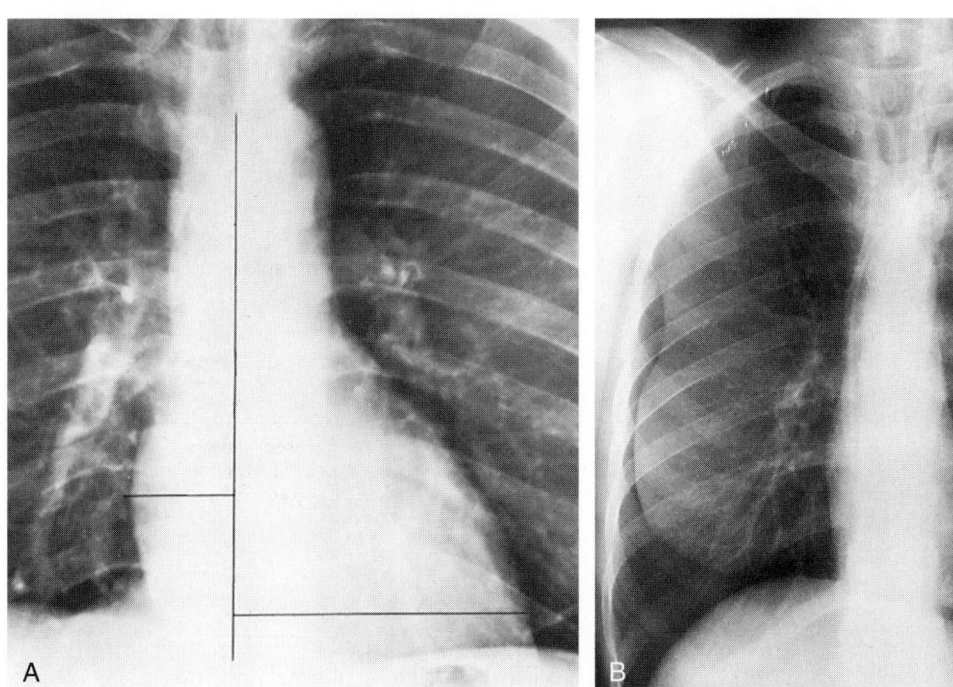

FIGURE 7–19. *A,* Measurement of the transverse cardiac diameter. A vertical reference line is drawn through the spinous processes of the vertebrae. The greatest distance from this line to the right and left margins of the cardiac shadow are then measured. The sum is the transverse cardiac diameter. *B,* The heart is unusually small in this young woman with anorexia nervosa.

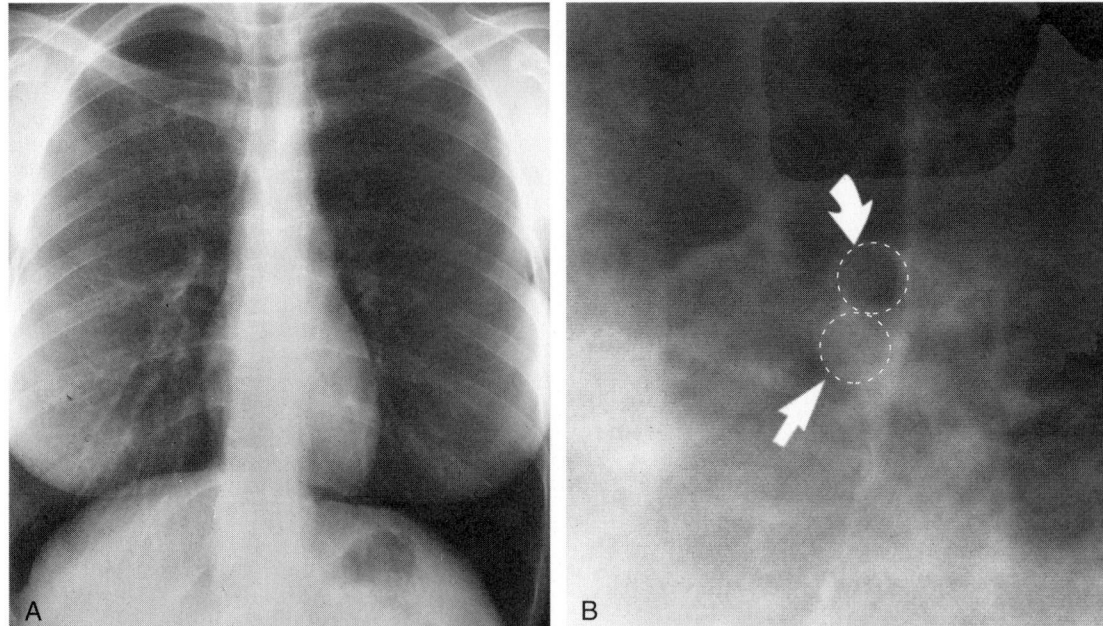

FIGURE 7–20. *A,* Normal pulmonary blood flow. The lower lobe vessels are two to three times greater in diameter than upper lobe vessels due to gravity and relative lung volumes. *B,* Magnification of paired anterior segment right upper lobe bronchus and pulmonary artery in a normal erect patient. The bronchus *(top)* and vessel *(bottom)* are of approximately the same size. This arterial-bronchial ratio is helpful in analyzing alterations in pulmonary vasculature.

pulmonary vascular bed (8 times normal flow) is not exceeded. When the reserve volume is overwhelmed or reduced because of vascular disease, the size of the vessels will be related to both blood flow and blood pressure or to pressure alone[37] (Fig. 7–21). The pulmonary veins also enlarge as pulmonary arterial blood flow rises. Enlarged pulmonary branches are found in a variety of conditions including left-to-right shunt, admixture lesions such as transposition of the great arteries, and conditions that produce an increase in cardiac output, such as chronic anemia, hyperthyroidism, arteriovenous fistula, and pregnancy. As pulmonary artery flow increases, radiographs demonstrate enlarged pulmonary arteries clearly seen to the edge of the lung. In a small left-to-right shunt, the increase may appear

confined to the lower lobes, but in larger shunts there is recruitment of the upper lobe vessels as well, so that the differential flow between the upper and lower lobe vessels is lost. In left-to-right shunts smaller than 1.8/1, pulmonary vascular abnormalities may not be detected at all.

The size of the pulmonary vessels can be measured objectively by determining the transverse diameter of the right descending pulmonary artery immediately above the origin of the right middle lobe branch. The normal transverse diameter of this vessel is 10 to 15 mm in males and 9 to 14 mm in females. A variation of ±1.0 mm beyond these limits is abnormal.[65]

PULMONARY ARTERIAL HYPERTENSION. As the pulmonary vascular reserve is fully recruited by increased blood flow

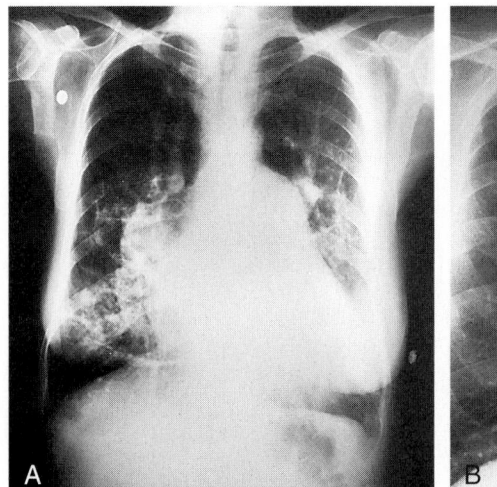
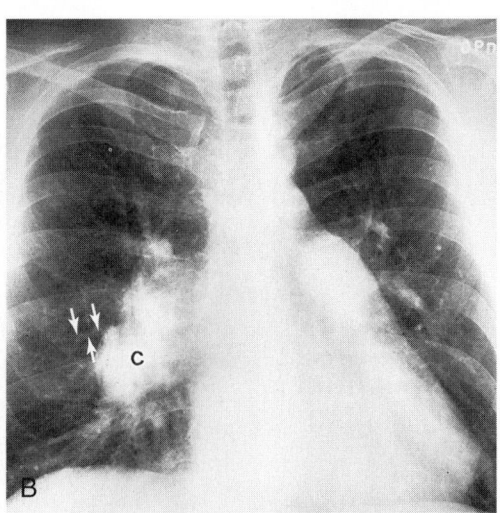
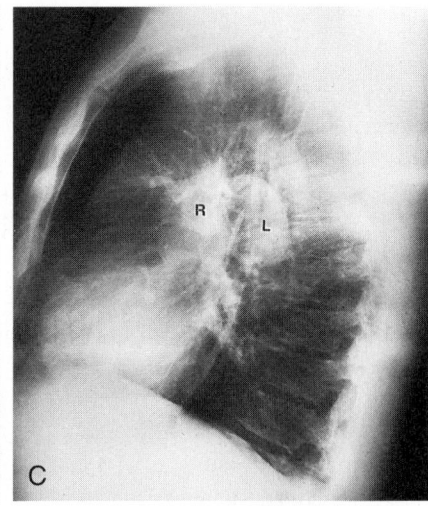

FIGURE 7–21. *A,* Increased pulmonary blood flow. This 41-year-old woman has an atrial septal defect, ostium primum type, with a pulmonary to systemic flow ratio of 5:1. There is secondary mitral regurgitation due to a cleft aortic leaflet of the mitral valve. There is moderate pulmonary hypertension with disparity between central and peripheral arterial branches. The right atrial border, the main pulmonary artery, and the upper and lower lobe vessels are enlarged and their branches are visible in the outer third of both lungs. *B,* There is a disparity between large central and smaller peripheral vessels in this patient with ventricular septal defect and pulmonary arterial hypertension (Eisenmenger physiology). C = central pulmonary arteries. Arrows indicate peripheral pulmonary artery. *C,* In the same patient as in *B,* the large pulmonary arteries are clearly seen on the lateral view. (L = left pulmonary artery; R = right pulmonary artery.)

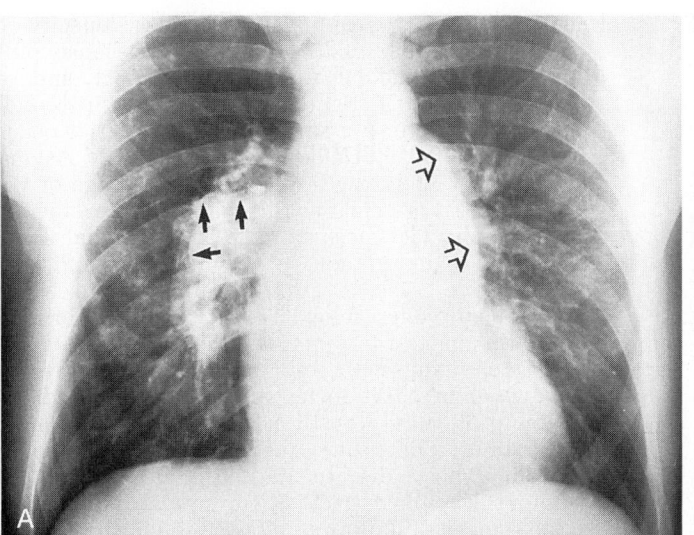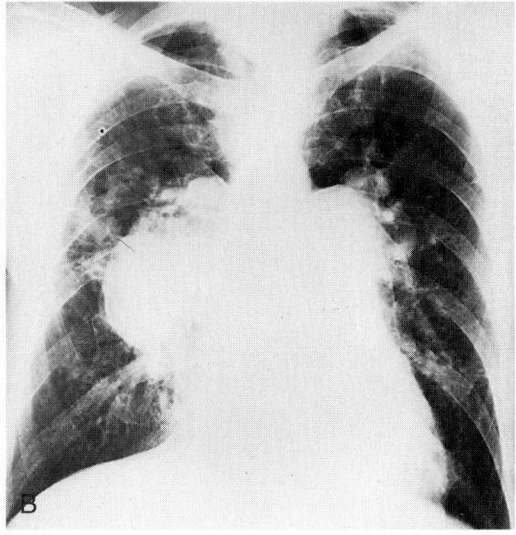

FIGURE 7–22. Pulmonary arterial hypertension. *A,* PA projection of chest of a 50-year-old male with a known membranous ventricular septal defect and cyanosis. There is calcification of the large right central pulmonary artery (arrows). The main pulmonary artery is enlarged in this patient with pulmonary hypertension and Eisenmenger physiology (open arrows). *B,* Severe longstanding pulmonary hypertension in a 64-year-old patient with an atrial septal defect and Eisenmenger physiology. The pulmonary arteries are calcified and aneurysmal.

or reduced by pulmonary arteritis or emphysema, pulmonary arterial pressure rises. The vascular engorgement that characterizes increased pressure is accompanied by vasospasm, peripheral vasoconstriction, and vessel wall thickening. Eventually, there is a decrease in peripheral blood flow, and the outer one-third of the lungs appears more lucent radiographically. The central elastic vessels enlarge, including the main pulmonary artery, the right and left pulmonary arteries, and second-order branching vessels. Calcification of the main pulmonary artery and the proximal branches may develop in longstanding and severe pulmonary arterial hypertension[66] (Fig. 7–22). Pulmonary arterial hypertension may be primary, particularly in women in the childbearing age group. It may also be secondary to chronic recurrent pulmonary thromboembolic disease, a longstanding left-to-right shunt, or pulmonary venous hypertension.[25,67,68]

PULMONARY VENOUS HYPERTENSION. Left ventricular failure, mitral stenosis, and other causes of vascular obstruction distal to the pulmonary arterial bed cause an increase in pulmonary venous pressure above the normal range of 8 to 12 mm Hg. As pressure rises to between 12 mm Hg and 18 mm Hg, pulmonary blood flow is directed into the upper lobes in the erect position and anteriorly in the supine position so that there is reversal of the normal difference in size between the small upper lobe and larger lower lobe vessels. With further elevation of pulmonary venous pressure above 18 mm Hg, pulmonary interstitial edema occurs. With pressure above 25 mm Hg, alveolar edema is seen (Fig. 7–23).

Radiographically, "cephalization" or redistribution of pulmonary venous and arterial flow to the upper lobes is the earliest sign of pulmonary venous hypertension (Fig. 7–24). A clue to the recognition of pulmonary venous hypertension is the diameter of vessels in the first anterior interspace. Normally, they do not measure more than 3 mm in diameter. If they are larger, increased or redirected flow should be considered.

Although the exact mechanism of vascular redistribution remains unresolved, one explanation has been proposed by several authors.[36,37,69–71] With an increase in pulmonary venous pressure, there is leakage of fluid from the pulmonary veins into the interlobular spaces, occurring first in the lower lobes because of gravitational effects. Fluid accumulation in the interlobular spaces decreases pulmonary compliance and increases interstitial pressure. These two

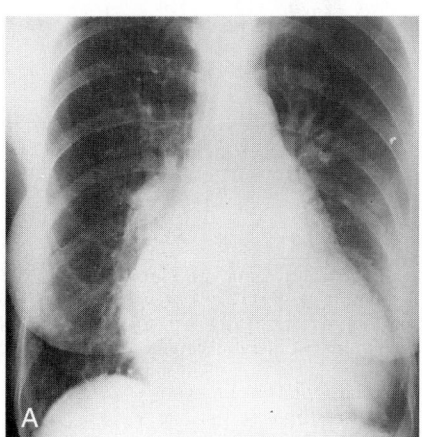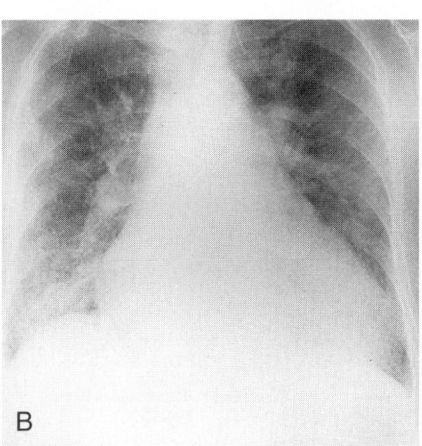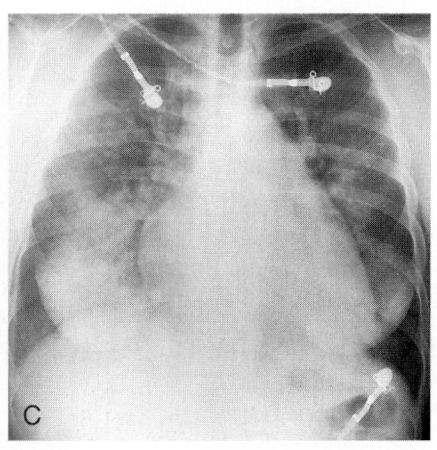

FIGURE 7–23. *A,* Pulmonary blood flow redistribution. Enlargement of the upper lobe vessels in this patient with ischemic cardiomyopathy and elevated pulmonary venous pressure. *B,* Pulmonary interstitial edema. The vessels are indistinct and enlarged. There is peribronchial cuffing. *C,* Pulmonary alveolar edema in a patient with congestive cardiomyopathy. The central parahilar distribution of edema, termed "bat wing" edema, is typical of cardiovascular or fluid overload (uremic) pulmonary alveolar edema.

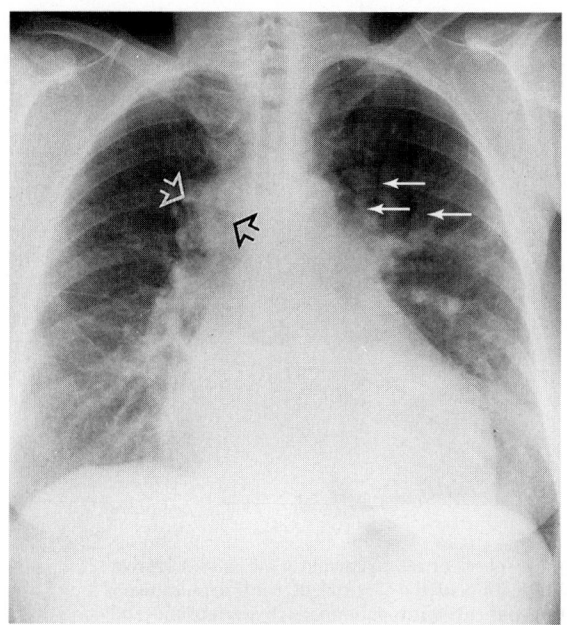

FIGURE 7–24. Congestive heart failure. There is vascular redistribution to the upper lung zones. The vessels in the lung at the first anterior interspaces are enlarged (small arrows) due to "cephalization." The prominent bulge at the right tracheobronchial angle is a dilated azygous vein (open arrows).

phenomena restrict flow to the lower lobes. Arterial spasm may also be a factor. Since these processes first develop in the lower lobes, redistribution of blood flow to the upper lobes follows.

DECREASED PULMONARY BLOOD FLOW. When blood flow is reduced, usually because of pulmonary outflow tract obstruction or an intracardiac right-to-left shunt, the pulmonary arteries and veins are reduced in size. The central vessels narrow and the peripheral vessels are not visible. Reduced pulmonary blood flow may be generalized, as in tetralogy of Fallot, or may be regional as a result of pulmonary embolus, emphysema, and narrowing of vessels due to tumor invasion or to the reduced perfusion of arteritis. When pulmonary perfusion is reduced, as in pulmonary atresia with ventricular septal defect or chronic pulmonary thromboembolism, there is an increase in bronchial and other collateral arterial circulation. Radiographically, bronchial vessels are tortuous, small, and nontapered, and because they emanate from the aorta they do not radiate from the hilum. Otherwise normal but small pulmonary arteries

and veins also contribute to pulmonary opacity in lungs with significant bronchial circulation because pulmonary arteries and bronchial arteries interconnect, and preferential flow from the higher pressure systemic bronchial arteries to the lower pressure pulmonary arteries occurs.[66,72]

ASYMMETRICAL PULMONARY BLOOD FLOW. Asymmetrical pulmonary blood flow is due to the presence of vessels in one lung that are smaller than those in the other lung. As already indicated, these patterns of differential flow may be localized, as in pulmonary embolism, chronic obstructive pulmonary disease, or arteritis. Unilateral decrease or absence of pulmonary blood flow may also occur in patients with pulmonary artery branch atresia, hemitruncus, and tetralogy of Fallot with unilateral pulmonary artery branch narrowing. In addition, asymmetrical increased flow may be found after creation of a Blalock-Taussig, Waterston, or Potts shunt. Sometimes, the differences in blood flow in congenital heart disease are caused by orientation of the pulmonary outflow tract. For example, in pulmonary valvular stenosis, the flow of blood through the stenotic valve may be directed toward the left pulmonary artery[73] (Fig. 7–25). In patent ductus arteriosus, the preferential flow is often toward the left because the ductus is oriented toward the left pulmonary artery.

PULMONARY EDEMA (Fig. 7–23C). In the normal individual, there is continuous passage of fluid from the pulmonary veins into adjacent interlobular lymphatics that return the fluid to the central mediastinal veins. If the lymphatic reserve is overcome by increased transudate as a result of elevated pulmonary venous pressure, the interlobular septa are thickened and become visible radiographically. Redistribution of blood flow to the upper lung zone, or "cephalization," will occur following reduction in compliance or vasoconstriction in the lower lobes roughly paralleling the increase in pulmonary venous pressure.[67,69,74,75] Interlobular septal lines, or Kerley B lines, are visible as thin horizontal lines present at both lung bases perpendicular to the lateral pleural surface on the frontal chest film.[74,75] Prominent interstitial linear opacities throughout the lung reflect additional thickened septal lines. If the origin of the pulmonary interstitial edema is related to the cardiovascular system, the heart may be normal or enlarged, depending upon the chronicity of cardiac failure. In addition to cardiac failure, prominent interstitial lines may occur in a wide variety of noncardiac diseases including sarcoidosis, lymphatic spread of tumor, interstitial pneumonia, and asbestosis. When pulmonary interstitial edema is present, the lungs may be clear to auscultation—a clue that the extravascular fluid is confined to the interstitium. With further increases in pulmonary venous pressure above 25 mm Hg, there is

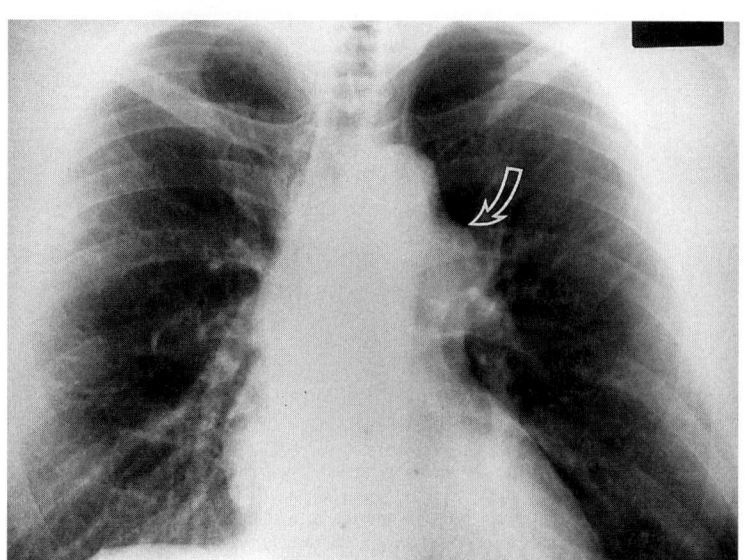

FIGURE 7–25. Asymmetrical pulmonary blood flow in a 51-year-old male with pulmonary valvular stenosis. The left pulmonary artery is larger than the right because the jet of blood is directed to the left pulmonary artery (arrow).

leakage of fluid into the pulmonary air spaces leading to alveolar edema.

Radiographically, pulmonary alveolar edema typically involves the inner two-thirds of the lung, producing a "butterfly" or "bat wing" appearance (Fig. 7–23C). An explanation for this pattern is that the outer third of the lung or cortex has better aeration, better compliance, and more efficient lymphatic drainage than the inner two-thirds, and for this reason fluid concentrates in the central portion of the lung.[69,73] Distinguishing pulmonary edema caused by congestive heart failure from that caused by increased "capillary permeability" or "overhydration" pulmonary edema is often difficult. Recent studies have attempted to separate cardiovascular pulmonary edema from the other forms by definable characteristics such as change in heart size, width of the pulmonary vascular pedicle, blood flow distribution, interstitial thickening, and regional distribution of pulmonary edema. In these studies, cardiovascular pulmonary edema is characteristically associated with a large heart, vascular redistribution, diffuse distribution of pulmonary edema fluid, a widened vascular pedicle, and increased pulmonary blood volumes, septal lines, and pleural effusions. Overhydration pulmonary edema is characterized by a balanced blood flow and perihilar pulmonary edema. In capillary permeability pulmonary edema, there is no cardiac enlargement, the vascular pedicle is normal or reduced in size, no septal lines are found, and the pulmonary edema has a peripheral rather than central pattern.[76,77]

CARDIAC CALCIFICATION

MYOCARDIAL CALCIFICATION. Dystrophic calcification of the heart is usually caused by a large myocardial infarction and is reported to occur in 8 per cent of infarcts more than 6 years old.[37,44] It has also been described following cardiac trauma, particularly in the anterior wall of the right ventricle.[78] The deposition of calcium is related to the slow production of carbon dioxide in slowly metabolizing tissue. Consequently, there is development of relative alkalinity and reduced solubility of calcium.[79] Myocardial calcification occurs most frequently in a left ventricular aneurysm and in the apical and anterior lateral aspects of the left ventricular wall. The calcium deposits are usually curvilinear in shape within the periphery of the infarct or aneurysm and occasionally may be homogeneous when an entire infarcted area calcifies.

Calcification may also occur within the left atrium and left atrial appendage, particularly in patients with rheumatic heart disease associated with mitral stenosis or regurgitation. Left atrial calcification is most often found in the endo- or subendocardial layers and is seen less often within an organized thrombus adherent to the chamber wall. Left atrial calcification is usually thin-walled and curvilinear, forming a shell around the circumference of the left atrial chamber or confined to the left atrial appendage[37,44,80,81] (Fig. 7–26).

VALVULAR CALCIFICATION. The radiographic presence of calcification within a cardiac valve suggests the presence of hemodynamically significant stenosis.[45,82] In the mitral valve, calcification appears clump-like or linear, usually measuring about 2 to 4 cm in diameter, and is most often caused by rheumatic heart disease.[44,83,84] Isolated aortic valve calcification in patients under age 40 generally signifies marked aortic stenosis related to a bicuspid valve (Fig. 7–27). In patients over 65 years of age, aortic valve calcification can be due to sclerosis with degeneration of normal valve leaflets or may be a manifestation of hemodynamically significant aortic stenosis.[54,82,82a]

The radiographic appearance of the calcification may help to determine the origin of the valvular deformity. For example, a thick, irregular semilunar ring pattern with a

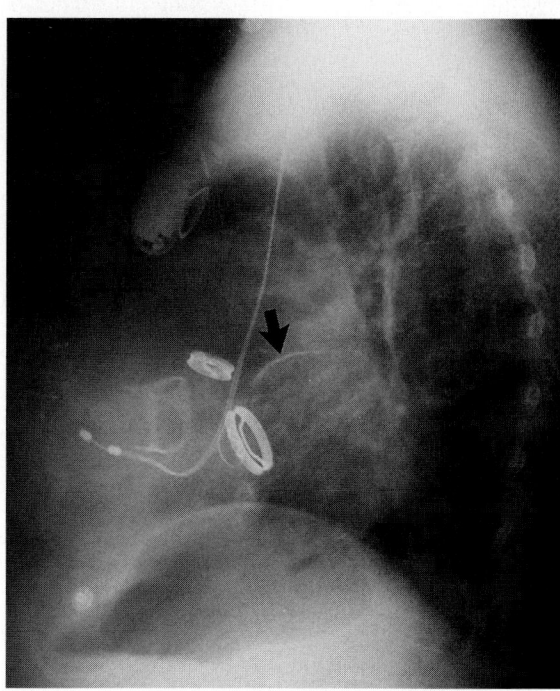

FIGURE 7–26. Left atrial calcification. A thin curvilinear calcification (arrow) is present in the superior and anterior wall of the left atrium in this patient with multivalvular rheumatic heart disease and atrial fibrillation. Prosthetic valves are seen in the tricuspid, mitral, and aortic areas.

central bar or knob is typical of stenotic bicuspid valve and is found in 65 per cent of patients with congenital aortic stenosis[25,48,85] (Fig. 7–27). This pattern is due to calcification of the valve ring and the dividing ridge or raphe of one of the two cusps or the conjoint leaflet. The abundance of calcification in this entity is thought to be due to constant wear and tear from the abnormal tension-producing motion of the bicuspid valve leaflets. Occasionally three-leaflet aortic valves will mimic bicuspid valves because of fusion of two of the three leaflets. In these patients, three sinuses of Valsalva are present.[36] Calcification of the pulmonary valve occurs occasionally in pulmonary valvular stenosis with gradients in excess of 80 mm Hg or in long-standing severe pulmonary hypertension. Calcification of the tricuspid valve is unusual and is caused most frequently by rheumatic disease.[86]

ANNULAR CALCIFICATION. Annular calcification is found in the valve rings or fibroskeleton of the heart. It is a degenerative process occurring with aging and is found most often in individuals above the age of 40 years and especially in women.[83,86,87] Mitral annular calcification (see p. 1017) presents radiographically as a wavy O-, J-, or C-shaped opacity[87] (Fig. 7–28). When calcification is limited to the posterior-medial portion of the annulus at the base of the posterior leaflet there are usually no complications.[83] When the calcification is more extensive it may involve the valve leaflets and cause limitation of motion leading to regurgitation or, occasionally, an obstructive gradient during diastole.[84,87,88] Aortic annular calcification may also extend into the ascending aorta and down into the interventricular septum (Fig. 7–28B, C). Atrial fibrillation, conduction abnormalities, endocarditis, and mitral valve incompetence are associated findings.[83] Tricuspid annular calcification is rare, usually occurring in patients with longstanding pulmonary valvular stenosis, atrial septal defect, and/or right ventricular hypertension.[86]

Several methods have been suggested to identify the location of valvular calcification on plain films. A line drawn on the lateral chest film from the junction of the anterior chest wall and the diaphragm through the hilum to the lung apex will separate anterior superior aortic calcifica-

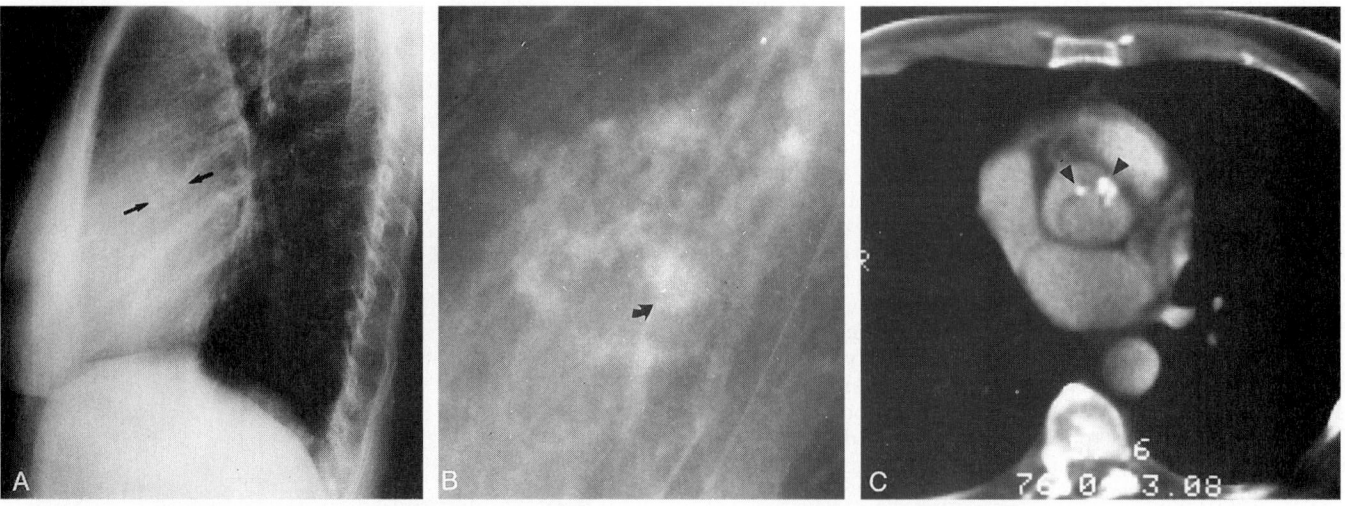

FIGURE 7–27. Aortic valve calcification. *A,* Lateral projection shows the typical pattern of calcification of congenital bicuspid aortic valve in a 60-year-old woman with secondary aortic regurgitation (arrows). *B,* A fluoroscopic spot film shows the calcified valve to better advantage (curved arrow indicates calcified raphe). *C,* Cine CT demonstrates calcification of the aortic valve leaflets in a different patient with congenital bicuspid aortic valve (arrowheads). (Courtesy of Stephanie Flicker, M.D.)

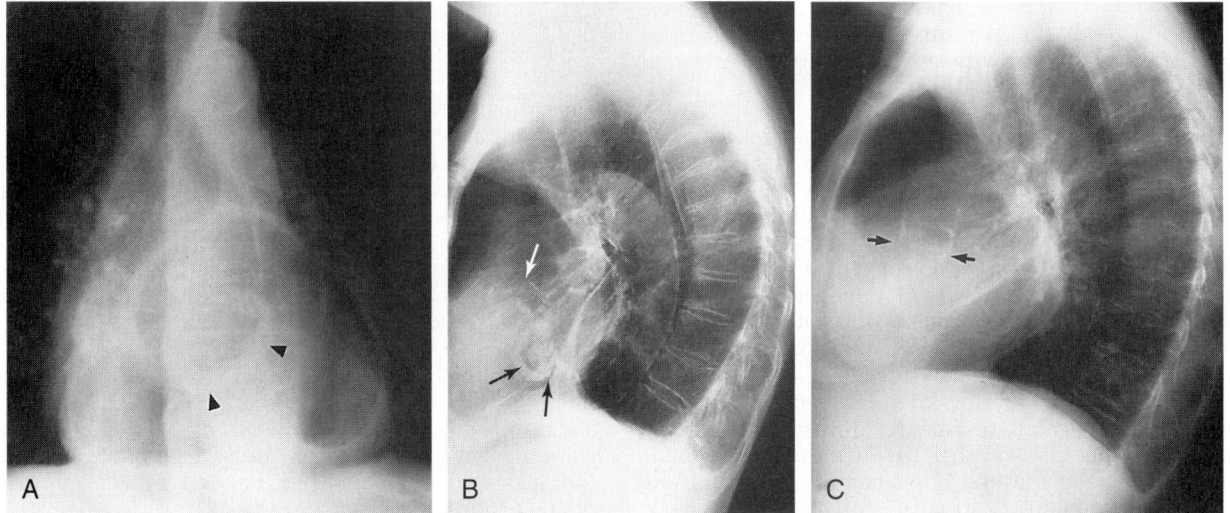

FIGURE 7–28. *A,* Calcified aortic and mitral annulus in an elderly woman. The air in a large hiatal hernia permits excellent visualization of the mitral annulus (arrowheads) in the PA projection. *B,* In the lateral projection, calcification can be seen in both the aortic (white arrow) and mitral (black arrows) annuli. *C,* Aortic annular calcification (arrows) in an elderly patient without signs or symptoms of aortic stenosis.

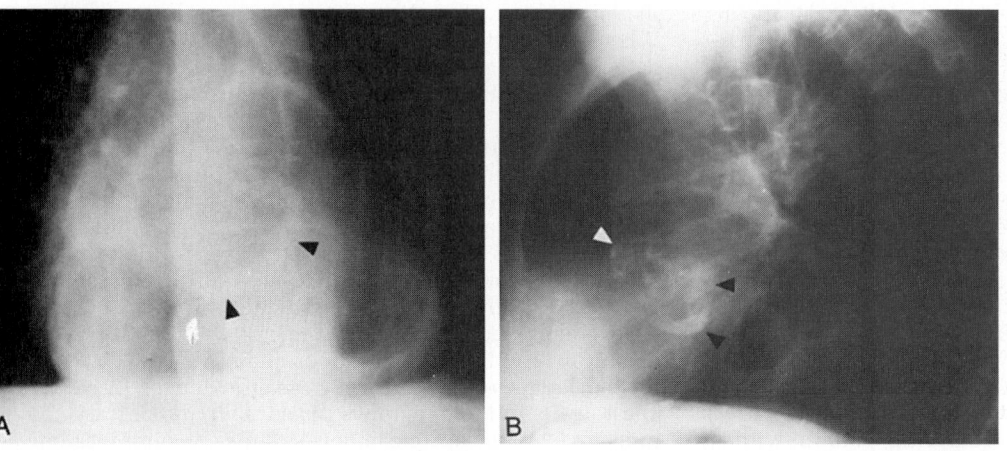

FIGURE 7–29. Mitral valve calcification. In the lateral projection, *(B),* the valve calcification (black arrows) lies below the line drawn from the left main bronchus to the anterior costophrenic sulcus, localizing it to the mitral valve. The aortic valve in this projection lies more anteriorly and above the line (open arrows).

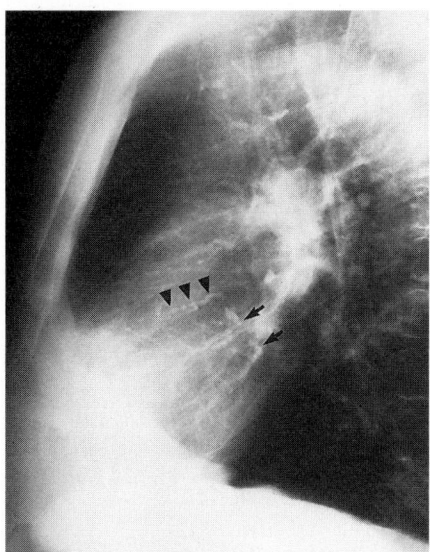

FIGURE 7-30. Lateral projection demonstrates the "tram track" pattern of coronary artery calcifications involving the left anterior descending (arrowheads) and circumflex coronary arteries (arrows).

tions from posterior inferior mitral calcifications (Fig. 7–29). Another approach is to divide the heart on the lateral view into six sections; this will permit identification of the aortic valve in the upper row middle section and mitral calcification in the lower row posterior section.

CORONARY ARTERY CALCIFICATION. Calcium is deposited early in the formation of an atherosclerotic plaque in the coronary arteries, and calcification can be used to monitor the evolution of the atherosclerotic process. Coronary artery calcification can be detected by a number of imaging modalities including plain radiography, fluoroscopy, ultrafast CT, and ultrasonography[89-93] (Fig. 7–30). Of these modalities, fluoroscopy has been studied most intensively.[89]

A number of studies have compared the efficacy of fluoroscopy with arteriography and exercise testing for the identification of significant coronary artery disease.[4,49,53,89] As a result of these studies, a direct relationship between fluoroscopically identified coronary calci-

fication and the frequency and severity of stenotic lesions has been established. In one study of 360 patients undergoing arteriography for coronary artery disease who also underwent cardiac fluoroscopy, 97 per cent of those with calcified coronary arteries on fluoroscopy had significant (≥70 per cent occlusion) coronary artery stenosis of at least one major vessel on arteriography. Of those with significant coronary disease on arteriography, 56 per cent had calcification at fluoroscopy.[53] Another study was performed in asymptomatic patients with type II hyperlipidemia who were under the age of 55 years. Of those with both positive exercise tests and coronary calcification on fluoroscopy, 92 per cent had angiographically determined coronary artery disease. Fluoroscopy had an 82 per cent accuracy in the detection of significant (≥50 per cent occlusion) coronary artery disease.[89] In yet a third study in a randomly selected group of 108 asymptomatic men who underwent cardiac fluoroscopy and exercise testing, 81 per cent of those with a positive exercise test had coronary calcifications, and 35 per cent of these had a positive exercise test. Only 4 per cent of those without calcified coronary arteries had a positive exercise test. Finally, in this same series 92 per cent had at least one stenosed (≥50 per cent occlusion) coronary artery diagnosed by angiography.[51] Bartel et al. showed that approximately 90 per cent of patients with fluoroscopically detectable coronary calcifications had significant coronary disease.[53]

Since exercise tests alone yield 10 to 20 per cent positive results in an asymptomatic middle-aged male population without coronary artery disease (false-positives), fluoroscopy has been suggested as an effective additional screening test for identification of patients with critical coronary artery disease. Fluoroscopy is most valuable when there is atypical chest pain or cardiomyopathy or for screening asymptomatic patients. Those at particular risk are cigarette smokers, have hyperlipidemia, or have other positive prognostic indicators.

Coronary calcifications in the proximal left coronary artery may be identified with plain chest radiography or fluoroscopy in the frontal projection medial to the left atrial appendage. In the lateral view, calcification of the left anterior descending artery is often seen vividly as a double line of calcification extending along the anterior border of the cardiac silhouette (Fig. 7–30). Circumflex and right coronary artery calcification may also be identified by means of chest radiography, particularly oblique views.

CT is superior to fluoroscopy for the detection of coronary calcification.[4,52,90] In fact, approximately twice as many patients will be found to have calcified coronary arteries with CT than with fluoroscopy.[91-93] There is a similar detection yield of critical coronary artery disease when compared with those obtained by fluoroscopy. Although CT has been considered impractical as a screening test because of cost and limited availability, recent studies with cine CT have emphasized its value as a highly sensitive screening procedure in three selected populations.[90,93] Since CT is performed routinely for other disease indications, it is important to make note of coronary calcifications and their distribution on CT to alert the clinician to their significance.

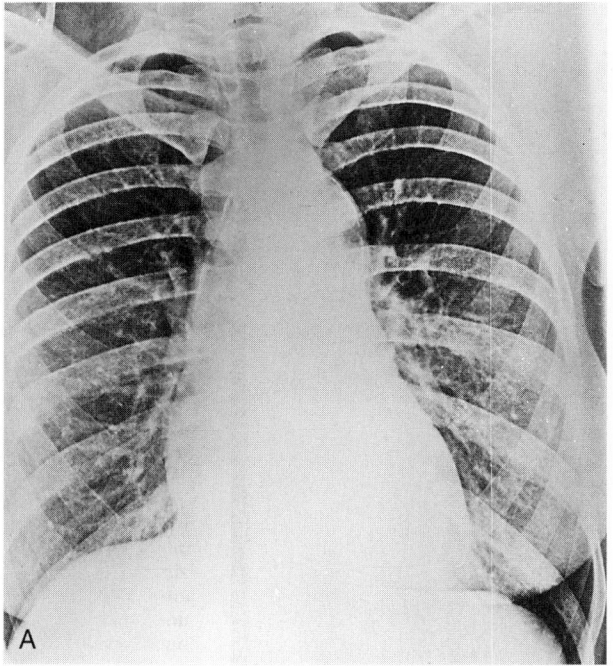

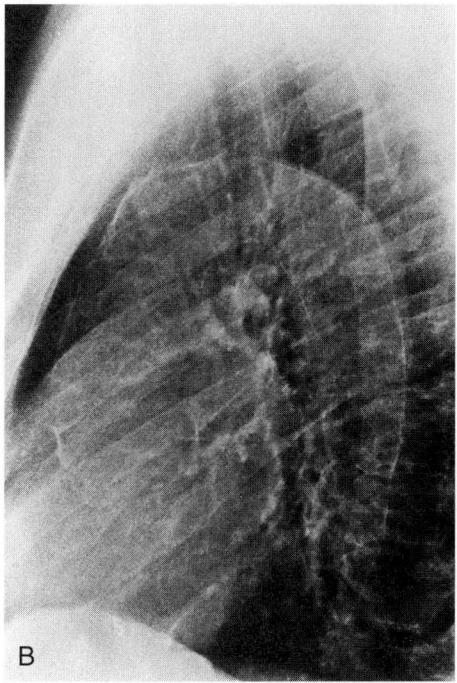

FIGURE 7–31. *A,* PA projection. *B,* Lateral projection. Abundant thin line calcification extending from the aortic root to the distal descending thoracic aorta in a 30-year-old woman. Biopsy demonstrated Takayasu's arteritis.

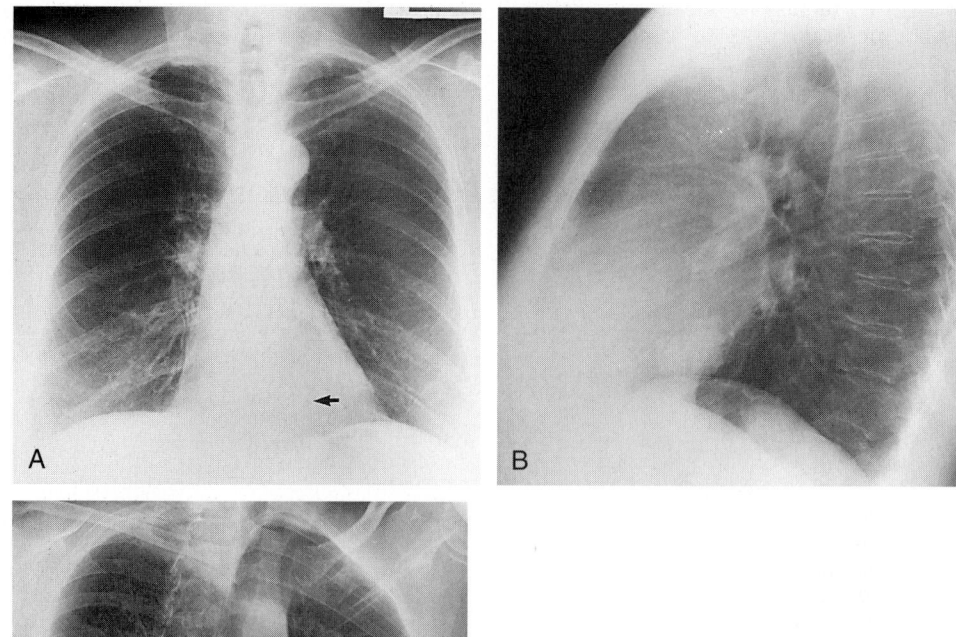

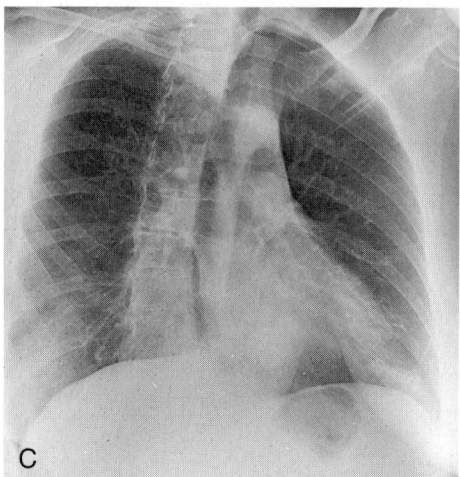

FIGURE 7–32. Tumor calcification. *A,* A large clump of calcification is present in the left atrium, faintly seen on the PA projection (arrow) and well demonstrated on the *(B)* lateral and *(C)* RAO projections of the chest. A myxoma was found at surgery.

CALCIFICATION OF THE GREAT VESSELS. Aortic calcification, particularly in the region of the arch, is almost ubiquitous in individuals over the age of 50. It is usually noted on chest radiographs as a thin curvilinear opacity near the lateral border of the arch. When the calcification is located deep to the aortic border, dissection may be present. Other causes of aortic calcification are syphilis (usually involving the ascending aorta), sinus of Valsalva aneurysm, and Takayasu's arteritis[86,94] (Fig. 7–31). The main pulmonary artery occasionally calcifies following right ventricular out-

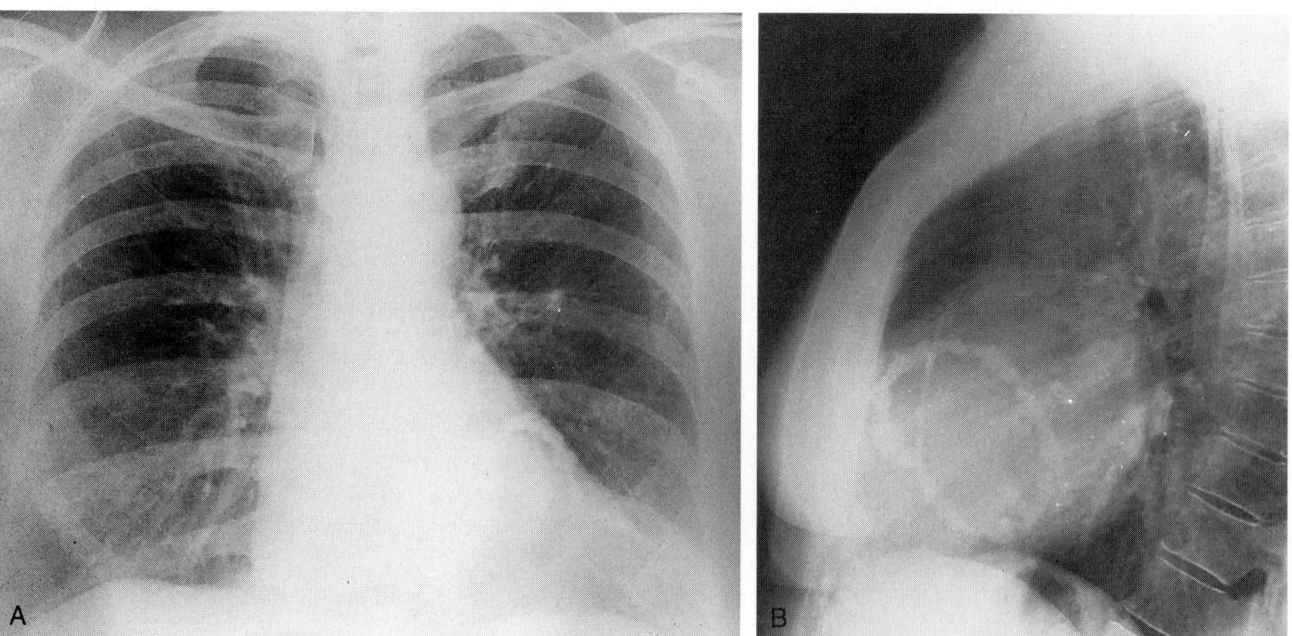

FIGURE 7–33. Pericardial calcification. *A,* PA projection. *B,* Lateral projection. Both show extensive calcification of the pericardium in the atrioventricular groove in a patient with a history of rheumatic heart disease. (From Moncada, R., et al.: Multimodality approach to pericardial imaging. *In* Kotler, M. N., and Steiner, R. M. (eds.): Cardiac Imaging: New Technologies and Clinical Applications. Philadelphia, F. A. Davis, 1986.)

flow tract surgery for total correction of tetralogy of Fallot. Calcification of the main pulmonary artery also occurs in severe longstanding pulmonary hypertension.

TUMOR CALCIFICATION. The most common primary tumor of the heart is myxoma (see p. 1467), a polypoid mass occurring most frequently in the left atrium (Fig. 7–32). About 10 per cent of myxomas calcify sufficiently to be seen radiographically.[95,96] Calcifications in cardiac tumors vary from a speckled pattern to a round clump of calcium mimicking mitral annular or valve calcification. Calcification may be visible on plain film or may be seen only with fluoroscopy or CT. With fluoroscopy or cine CT, a calcified atrial tumor may be seen to prolapse through the atrioventricular valve during diastole and cause obstructive symptoms. Echocardiography and cine MRI will demonstrate prolapse of a noncalcified myxoma.[96,96a]

PERICARDIAL CALCIFICATION (see also Chap. 43). Pericardial calcification occurs most often in association with previous acute pericarditis or trauma.[78,97] The most common causes are viral illness, especially Coxsackie or influenza A and B virus infection, granulomatous disease including tuberculosis and histoplasmosis, hemopericardium following trauma, and autoimmune disease—particularly systemic lupus erythematosus and rheumatic heart disease[98] (Fig. 7–33).

Occasionally, pericardial tumors (among them intrapericardial teratomas and cysts) calcify.[98] Calcification is present in up to 50 per cent of patients with constrictive pericarditis. On the other hand, extensive calcification may be present without the signs and symptoms of pericardial constriction.[99,100] Pericardial and myocardial calcifications are frequently confused with each other.[79] However, pericardial calcifications can be distinguished from myocardial calcification by differences in their distribution. Pericardial calcifications are most abundant along the right atrial and ventricular borders and in the area of the atrioventricular groove. The pericardium adjacent to the left ventricle is usually free of calcification, probably because of its vigorous pulsations, and calcification rarely occurs in the left atrial pericardium because of the absence of pericardium behind the left atrium.[80] On the other hand, myocardial calcification is usually localized to the left ventricle and is rare in the right atrium or ventricle.[79] Pericardial calcification is often obscured on a frontal chest film because of underexposure of the mediastinum. Overpenetrated films or fluoroscopy studies are helpful for localizing mediastinal calcifications, and CT may demonstrate calcium not seen on plain chest films.

ACQUIRED HEART DISEASE

The diagnosis and assessment of the severity of acquired heart disease is assisted by a combination of imaging studies including plain chest radiography.[54] The chest film is particularly useful to assess cardiac size and pulmonary vascularity. At the same time it offers important clues to the enlargement of individual cardiac chambers, although cineangiography, echocardiography, and other cross-sectional imaging techniques are more reliable.[101–104] Nevertheless, the plain film remains a useful first examination in the work-up of the cardiac patient.[51]

Valvular Heart Disease

AORTIC STENOSIS (see also p. 1035). In critical aortic stenosis the size of the aortic valve orifice is reduced from a normal cross-sectional area of 2.5 to 3.5 cm^2 to a cross-sectional area of less than 0.7 cm.^{2}[2,25] With mild to moderate constriction of the aortic valve orifice, there is compensatory concentric hypertrophy of the left ventricle (Fig. 7–10). With further increases in the severity of the stenosis, cardiac output and left ventricular contractility decrease,

resulting in left ventricular dilatation, elevated left ventricular end-diastolic pressure, and pulmonary venous hypertension together with the signs and symptoms of congestive heart failure.

The typical radiographic changes of mild to moderate aortic stenosis include a normal-sized heart with rounding of the left ventricular border or an elongated cardiac silhouette with downward displacement of the cardiac apex due to concentric left ventricular hypertrophy[38,82] (Fig. 7–10). There is a characteristic discrete bulge on the right side of the ascending aorta just above the sinus of Valsalva due to poststenotic dilatation best visualized in the LAO or PA projection.[37] In pure aortic stenosis, the aortic arch and descending aorta remain normal in size and aortic valve calcification is frequent. It increases with the severity of stenosis and the age of the patient so that by the age of 40 years, more than 90 per cent of patients with aortic stenosis have visible aortic calcification (Fig. 7–27). Aortic valvular calcification has also been associated with a peak systolic gradient at the aortic valve of greater than 30 mm Hg in 97 per cent of patients.[37]

With severe aortic stenosis, the left atrium and ventricle will decompensate and enlarge.[79] The degree of enlargement of both chambers is correlated with the severity of aortic stenosis and with mitral regurgitation due to left ventricular dilatation or to associated intrinsic mitral valve disease. Isolated aortic stenosis is usually nonrheumatic in origin and is most often due to degeneration, scarring, and fusion of a congenital bicuspid valve (see p. 1036). Additional causes of left ventricular outflow tract narrowing, causing left ventricular enlargement without valvular calcification, are hypertrophic cardiomyopathy and supravalvular and subvalvular aortic stenosis.

Congenital aortic stenosis may take two principal forms. The more common is a bicuspid valve with congenital commissural fusion and a central or eccentric orifice. The second form is a bicuspid valve that is initially nonobstructive but undergoes commissural fusion with time. Turbulent blood flow traumatizes the valve and causes irregular nodular scarring of both leaflets, which subsequently undergo gradual fusion and calcification[48,82a] (Fig. 7–27). With time, these valves may also become insufficient due either to incomplete closure of the deformed valve leaflets or to infective endocarditis.

Degenerative and rheumatic aortic valvular stenosis may be found in normally tricuspid valves. On the chest film, linear or clumped calcifications may be found in the area of the aortic valve leaflets or annulus. In patients with rheumatic aortic stenosis, mitral calcifications also are frequently present.[37,105]

Both the obstructive and nonobstructive forms of hypertrophic cardiomyopathy and membranous subaortic stenosis are characterized radiographically by left ventricular enlargement alone.[19,101] Although the plain film findings are suggestive, a specific diagnosis of hypertrophic cardiomyopathy can be established with MRI, echocardiography, and/or radionuclide studies[19] (see p. 1421). Since the aortic leaflets are uninvolved, blood flow is normal during ventricular systole, and as a result, the ascending aorta does not dilate and the aortic valve does not calcify. Left atrial enlargement, when present, is usually associated with mitral regurgitation.[101,105]

AORTIC REGURGITATION (see also p. 1045). Aortic regurgitation may result from a stenotic bicuspid valve that developed insufficiency due to endocarditis or degeneration (Fig. 7–10B). *Rheuma*tic valvulitis and infective endocarditis are other important primary causes. A secondary cause of aortic regurgitation is dilatation of the aortic annulus in diseases preferentially affecting the ascending aorta, such as ankylosing spondylitis, annuloaortic ectasia, Marfan syndrome, Reiter syndrome, psoriatic arthritis, and others (Chap. 45).[106] The aortic regurgitation due to rheumatic heart disease is commonly associated with mitral disease

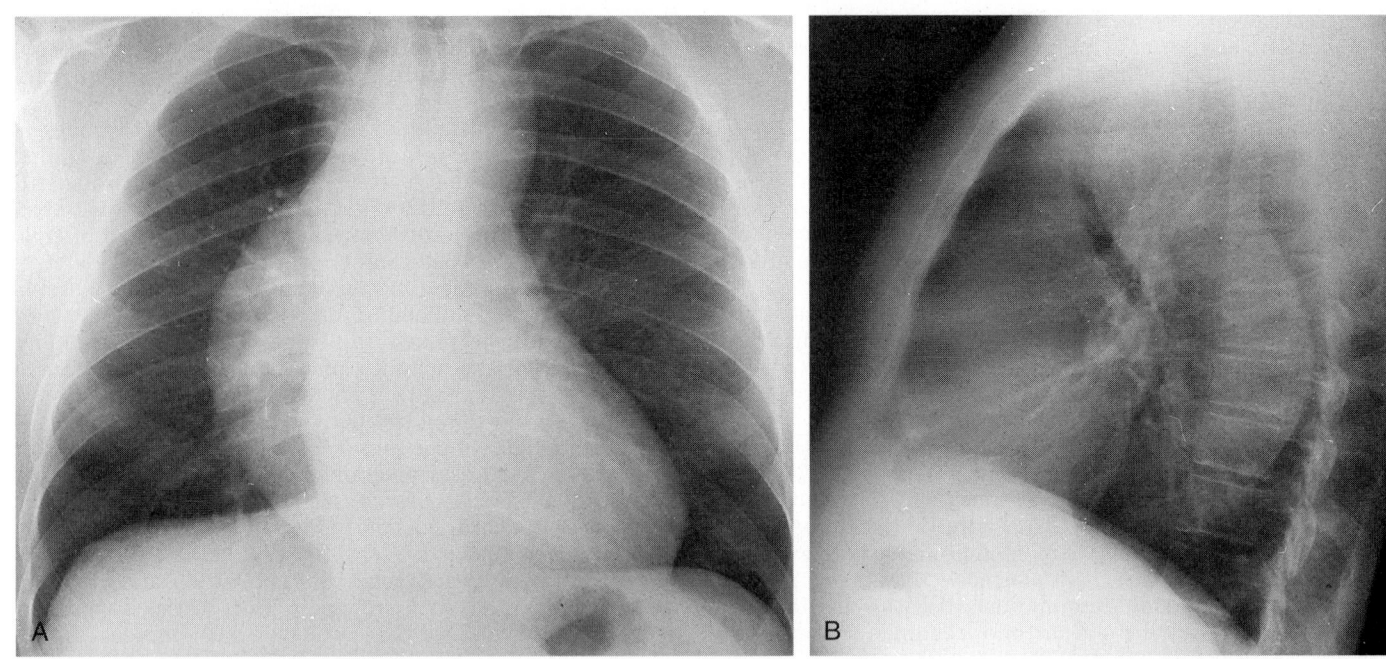

FIGURE 7–34. Aortic regurgitation. There is massive aortic dilatation in this man with severe aortic regurgitation related to annuloaortic ectasia. *A,* PA projection. *B,* Lateral projection.

alone or may involve all four cardiac valves (see p. 1045). Aortic regurgitation may also be due to trauma or may accompany dissection of the ascending aorta.[106]

In mild aortic regurgitation, the aorta is radiographically normal or mildly enlarged and the left ventricle remains normal in size. With moderate or severe regurgitation, there is increased dilatation of the left ventricle, and the cardiothoracic ratio usually exceeds 0.55. The aorta is diffusely and often massively dilated, unlike in aortic stenosis, in which only the ascending aorta is involved (Fig. 7–34). If the sinus portion of the ascending aorta is the only portion selectively dilated, Marfan syndrome (annuloaortic ectasia) is the most likely diagnosis. If the ascending aorta is also calcified, syphilis or, occasionally, Takayusu's aortitis is the likely diagnostic possibility. If the valve itself is calcified, aortic regurgitation secondary to a congenital bicuspid aortic valve or rheumatic disease should be considered.[105] If the mitral valve is also regurgitant, the left atrium may

be markedly enlarged visually, obscuring the enlarged left ventricle. When aortic regurgitation occurs acutely due to infective endocarditis, trauma, or dissection, the left ventricle remains normal in size, but because end-diastolic pressure is dramatically increased, the pulmonary venous pressure rises and pulmonary interstitial and/or alveolar edema may be observed. In chronic compensated aortic regurgitation, progressive volume overload occurs with left ventricular dilatation and increase in overall cardiac size but with normal-appearing lungs.[106]

As is true of aortic stenosis, aortic regurgitation is best diagnosed by Doppler echocardiography (see p. 1051) or cine MRI (see p. 1051). In selected cases, however, analysis of the plain chest radiograph will often establish the diagnosis or reveal specific findings that support the diagnosis of this abnormality.

MITRAL STENOSIS (see also p. 1007). Rheumatic carditis is the most common cause of mitral stenosis. Left atrial

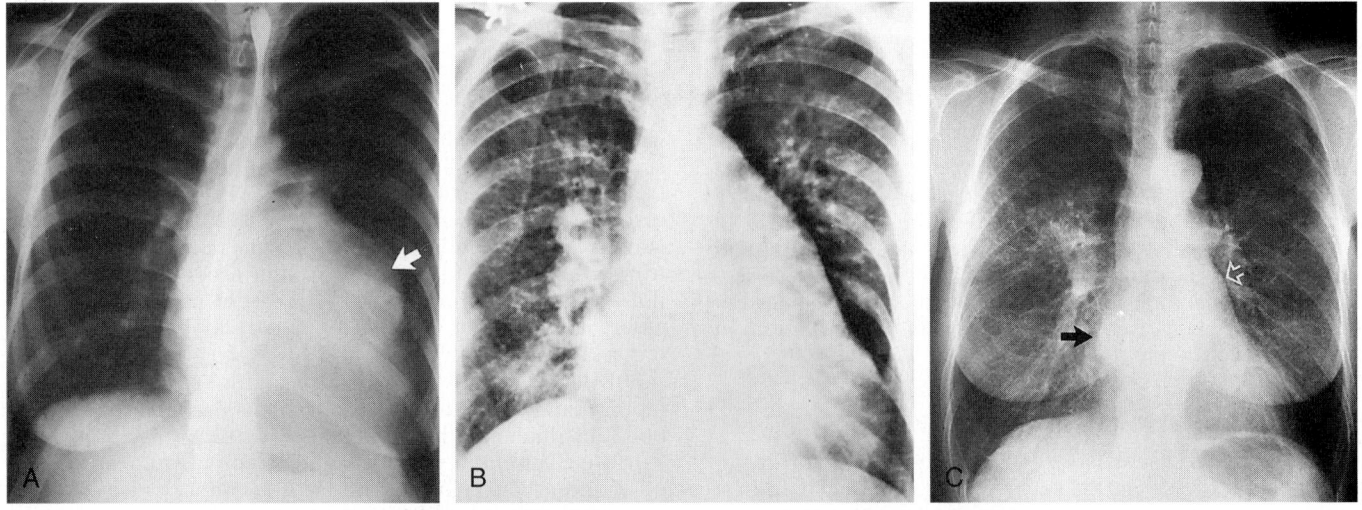

FIGURE 7–35. Mitral stenosis. *A,* The left atrial border is prominently convex. The aorta is small in this 19-year-old patient with mitral stenosis (arrow). *B,* In another patient, the lungs are studded with small nodules of moderate radiodensity due to hemosiderosis. The left atrium and left ventricle are enlarged. Kerley B lines are present in the lateral basal portions of the lungs. *C,* There is a subtle convex bulge at the level of the left atrial appendage (open arrow). A double atrial shadow is present on the right atrial border (black arrow). The heart is not enlarged in this 54-year-old woman with mitral stenosis.

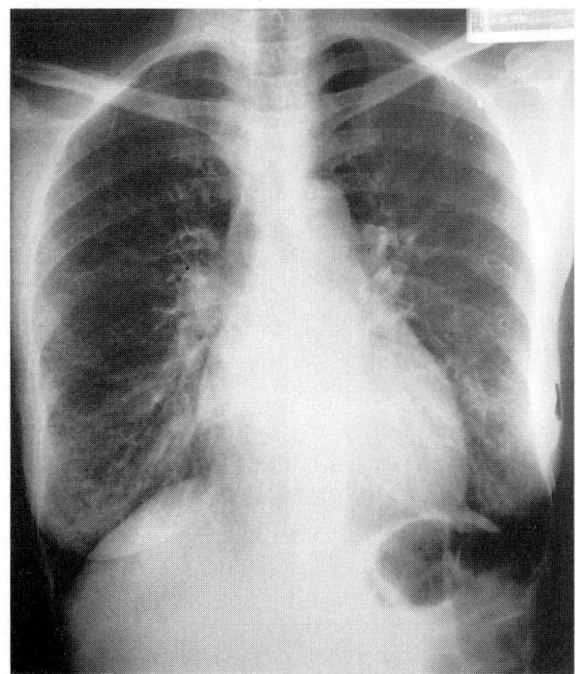

FIGURE 7–36. Mitral stenosis. There is chronic interstitial pulmonary edema with small punctate opacities representing small islands of ossification within the alveoli.

myxoma and, rarely, congenital mitral stenosis are also causes of mitral valve obstruction. The early roentgenographic signs of mitral stenosis are often subtle and include mild left atrial enlargement and posterior or posterior-lateral displacement of the barium-filled esophagus on the lateral chest. In most patients with mitral stenosis, the left ventricle and the pulmonary vessels are normal in appearance.

With more severe mitral stenosis, the left atrium usually increases further in size; however, in any given patient there is poor correlation between the severity of mitral stenosis and the size of the left atrial chamber[69,107] (Fig. 7–35). The left atrial appendage can be disproportionately enlarged, but the shape of the appendage appears to bear no relationship to the presence or absence of thrombosis.[81,108,109] The left main stem bronchus may be displaced upward by the enlarged left atrium. The right atrium is displaced to the right, and there is evidence of vascular redistribution of pulmonary blood flow to the upper lobes.

The main pulmonary artery is enlarged, the left ventricle and aorta are usually normal or small, and the mitral valve is often calcified. In addition, calcification of the left atrial wall (often associated with atrial fibrillation) may be seen. The enlarged left atrium displaces the barium-filled esophagus posteriorly (Fig. 7–16). Left atrial wall calcification is most common in the posterior portion of the left atrial chamber as well as the appendage in patients with rheumatic heart disease (Fig. 7–26). There is evidence of pulmonary interstitial edema, characterized by "hilar haze" or central vascular indistinctness, Kerley B lines at the lung bases, and cephalization as pulmonary venous pressure rises to the range of 25 mm Hg.[70,107]

Interlobular effusions are also seen and are described as Kerley C lines or a reticular pattern representing superimposed Kerley B lines. Kerley A lines are best observed in the lateral projection as long, opaque lines merging into the hila, representing thickened perivascular connective tissue planes.[74,75] Hemosiderosis, due to recurrent small hemorrhages related to chronically elevated capillary pressure, is often associated with chronic mitral stenosis (Fig. 7–35B). The radiographic appearance in hemosiderosis is that of interstitial or miliary lung disease most prominent in the mid and lower lung zones.[36] With chronic pulmonary interstitial edema, small punctate pulmonary opacities may be found which represent small islands of bone within the alveoli and are visible as dense nodules on the chest radiograph (Fig. 7–36).

MITRAL REGURGITATION (see also p. 1017). Acute mitral regurgitation may be related to ruptured chordae tendineae, rupture of the papillary muscles, ischemic dysfunction, or infective endocarditis. While the heart may not be enlarged in acute mitral regurgitation, severe pulmonary edema is frequently present as a result of left-sided cardiac failure (Fig. 7–37). Although pulmonary edema secondary to mitral regurgitation[110,111] is usually symmetrical, selective right upper lobe pulmonary edema has been described in as many as 9 per cent of patients with acute or chronic mitral regurgitation. It is probably due to selective retrograde flow from the mitral valve to the right upper lobe pulmonary veins[110,112] (Fig. 7–38). Chronic mitral regurgitation may be secondary to rheumatic heart disease, mitral prolapse due to myxomatous degeneration, infective endocarditis, ischemic cardiomyopathy, hypertrophic cardiomyopathy, extensive mitral annulus calcification, Marfan syndrome, and other causes (see p. 1669).

Radiographically, in chronic mitral regurgitation, the left atrium as well as the left ventricle is enlarged and may be massive in size because of volume overload and increased

FIGURE 7–37. A, Acute post–myocardial infarction papillary muscle dysfunction. Acute pulmonary interstitial edema is present but there is no cardiac enlargement. B, Dilated cardiomyopathy. There is diffuse dilatation of the heart in this woman with systemic lupus erythematosus.

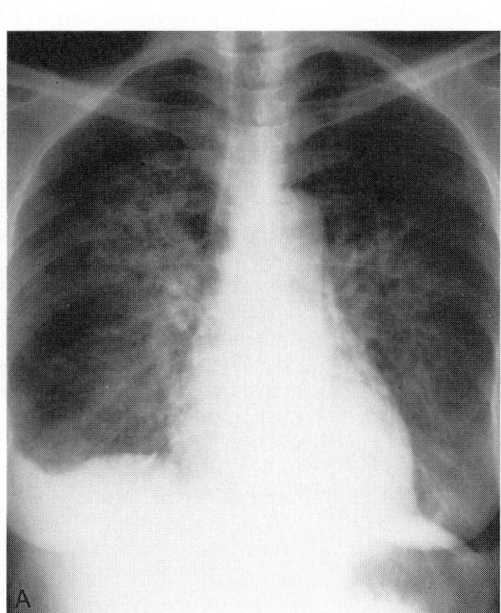

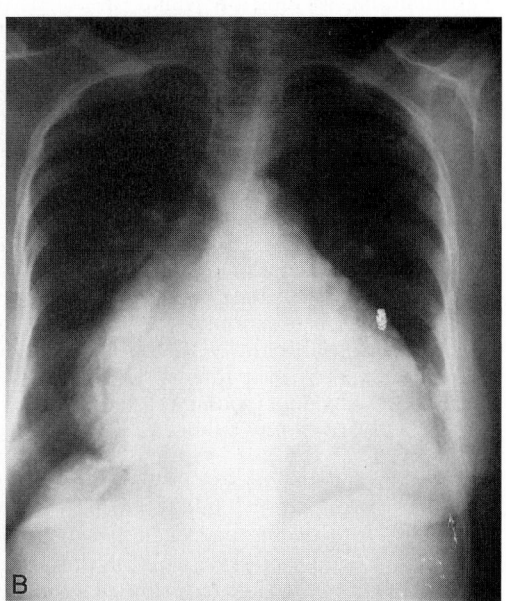

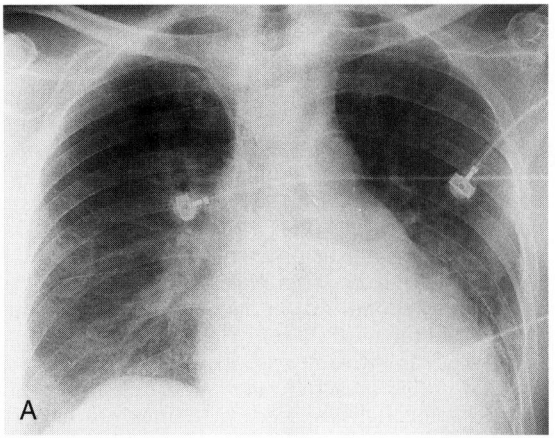 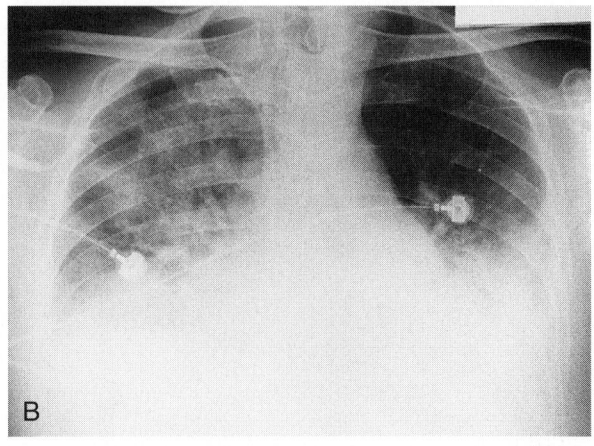

FIGURE 7–38. Mitral regurgitation. This 53-year-old patient developed mitral regurgitation secondary to dilated cardiomyopathy. He was admitted in congestive failure. There is localized development of alveolar edema in the right upper lobe. This phenomenon is due to preferential regurgitant flow toward the right upper lobe pulmonary vein. *A*, Portable AP chest film on admission. *B*, Three days later, patient is clinically in congestive heart failure.

pressure.[113] When the left atrium is enlarged, it may extend toward the right side and may be observed as a double shadow along the right atrial border. In the LAO projection, the large atrium causes upward displacement of the left main stem bronchus. Coexistent pulmonary arterial hypertension or tricuspid regurgitation may cause dilatation of the right atrium and ventricle and enlargement of the pulmonary arteries.[8,114,115] MRI and echocardiography can demonstrate the abnormality of the valve apparatus and evaluate the amount of regurgitant flow.

Ischemic Heart Disease

Many imaging modalities contribute to the diagnosis of ischemic heart disease, including coronary arteriography, radionuclide scintigraphy, echocardiography, CT, and MRI.[115,116] In ischemic cardiomyopathy, the chest roentgenogram can be entirely normal, even in patients with advanced disease; however, left ventricular enlargement and/ or aneurysm are often present. Following infarction of 25 per cent or more of left ventricular muscle mass, pulmonary edema may occur, even in patients with a normal-sized heart.[116] When congestive heart failure persists in spite of treatment, complications of myocardial infarction, such as aneurysm, pseudoaneurysm, ventricular wall or papillary muscle rupture, and interventricular septal defect must be excluded.[10,115–120]

MYOCARDIAL INFARCTION (Chap. 37). An interventricular septal defect occurs in 0.5 to 1.0 per cent of patients with recent septal infarction and is characterized by cardiomegaly, pulmonary edema, and poor myocardial contractility (see p. 1243). On the plain film radiograph, the typical shunt pattern may not be appreciated because of pulmonary edema but can emerge months later if the patient survives. Such defects usually involve the muscular septum and occur within 7 to 12 days after myocardial infarction. The radiographic picture of post–myocardial infarction syndrome (Dressler syndrome) is that of an enlarged heart due to pericardial effusion. Unilateral or, less often, bilateral pleural effusions are common, and lower lobe consolidation, particularly on the left side, occurs in fewer than 20 per cent of patients. It generally occurs 2 to 6 weeks following myocardial infarction and is analogous to the postpericardiotomy syndrome.[116]

Aneurysm of the left ventricle is an abnormal bulge or outpouching of the myocardial wall that develops in 12 to 15 per cent of patients following myocardial infarction[115] (see p. 1256). It occurs most commonly at the cardiac apex or along the anterior free wall of the left ventricle. The chest film shows a localized bulge along the ventricular

wall near the apex, with or without a thin rim of calcification. Angiography, CT, MRI, and echocardiography will also demonstrate the filling defect of a mural thrombus (if one is present) in the aneurysm. The differential diagnosis of left ventricular aneurysm includes pericardial cyst, mediastinal or pleural tumor, thymoma, and other mediastinal masses.

Cardiac rupture usually occurs in patients who have had an acute transmural infarction[119–121] (see p. 1241). Most die immediately, but in a minority of patients the rupture is contained or enclosed by the surrounding extracardiac soft tissues and a pseudoaneurysm is formed. Radiographically, a paracardiac mass is present, with sharply marginated edges free of calcification. The mass is usually posterior on the lateral projection, unlike the more anterior position of a true aneurysm.[121] A firm diagnosis is made by echocardiography, MRI, or contrast ventriculography. Coronary arteriography will show a complete absence of vessels in the wall of the pseudoaneurysm, unlike a true aneurysm, which may have a rim of mural vessels.[120]

Papillary muscle rupture following myocardial infarction occurs in approximately 1 per cent of patients (Fig. 7–37A) (see p. 1243). Plain film radiographic findings vary from a normal chest to gross cardiomegaly with left atrial and ventricular enlargement and pulmonary edema. Left ventriculography, MRI, or Doppler echocardiography will demonstrate the flail mitral valve leaflets and estimate the degree of mitral regurgitation.[45]

THE CARDIOMYOPATHIES (Chap. 41). The term cardiomyopathy describes a spectrum of myocardial disorders of varying etiology and pathophysiology. They are classified as dilated or congestive, infiltrative, restrictive, hypertrophic, and ischemic cardiomyopathies.[36,122]

In congestive, dilated, and ischemic cardiomyopathy, the left ventricular ejection fraction is reduced, often severely. Chest radiographs exhibit a wide spectrum of findings from a normal heart to diffuse nonspecific enlargement, which may resemble a large pericardial effusion (Fig. 7–37B). Echocardiography will demonstrate decreased ventricular contraction and enlargement of the left atrium and ventricle. With time, the right atrium and ventricle also enlarge. Doppler echocardiography or MRI may reveal mitral or tricuspid regurgitation caused by dilatation of the valve annulus.[123] Left-sided and later biventricular failure occur in most patients, an important predictive indicator of shortened survival time.

The radiographic appearance of *hypertrophic cardiomyopathy* (see p. 1414) is variable. Chest roentgenograms may demonstrate a normal heart or enlargement of the left ventricle, which can be focal or diffuse. If mitral regurgitation is present, the left atrium is also enlarged. Unlike in aortic valvular stenosis, no ascending aortic dilatation is present unless the patient has coincidental systemic hypertension or atherosclerotic uncoiling of the aorta.[82] The diagnosis is usually established by echocardiography, and cardiac catheterization with angiography is reserved for those cases in which noninvasive techniques are technically inadequate, coronary disease is suspected, or surgery is contemplated.[19] Angiography demonstrates, during systole, a narrow slit-like left ventricular chamber, marked wall thickening, and hyperdynamic contractions. CT and MRI are less invasive alternatives to angiography (Chap. 10).[19,123–126]

Restrictive cardiomyopathy (see p. 1426) is characterized by marked myocardial rigidity with poor left ventricular diastolic relaxation.[127] Radiographically, there are no consistent features of restrictive cardiomyopathy. The heart is normal in size or may be moderately or, more rarely, even markedly enlarged. The left atrium may also be enlarged when mitral regurgitation is present. Pulmonary congestion occurs in most patients, and calcification of the right or left ventricular wall may be seen. Contrast ventriculography (and radionuclide angiography) demonstrates rapid relaxation during early diastole followed by "plateauing" and absence of an "atrial kick".

POSTOPERATIVE CARDIAC RADIOLOGY

(See also Chap. 52)

With the unrelenting growth of coronary bypass graft surgery and the increased frequency of other cardiac surgical procedures during the last three decades, the postoperative supine portable chest roentgenogram has become one of the most frequently ordered examinations. In the Department of Radiology at Thomas Jefferson University Hospital, over 50 per cent of inpatient chest roentgenograms are performed at the bedside, usually in the intensive care unit. About one-third of these studies are of postsurgical cardiac patients. In order to interpret properly the postoperative chest film, special attention must be given to optimization of technique.[128–130] Adequate complementary film-screen combinations as well as careful patient positioning are needed to overcome the effects of low-capacity portable equipment and motion artifacts. Knowledge of the appearance of the preoperative film often aids in clarifying abnor-

malities seen on the postoperative portable roentgenogram. When the pre- and postoperative films are compared, the differences in vascularity, cardiac size, and degree of inspiration between the preoperative erect PA and the postoperative supine AP films must be taken into account.[131] For example, an 11 per cent increase in cardiac diameter, a 9 per cent increase in cardiothoracic ratio, and a 15 per cent increase in mediastinal width when an inspiratory PA film is compared with an inspiratory AP chest film have been described. For this reason, many surgeons and radiologists recommend that a preoperative supine AP film be taken prior to operation to guarantee the availability of a comparative film.[132]

Most cardiac surgery is performed through an extrapleural median sternotomy with the use of cardiopulmonary bypass. Except for specific problems related to the patient's preexisting cardiac disorder or to the specific surgical procedure, alterations found in the postoperative chest film are common to all cardiac surgical procedures.[133–136]

Immediately after operation, the lungs appear normal or there are varying degrees of subsegmental left lower lobe atelectasis related to incomplete reexpansion of the lungs after cardiopulmonary bypass. There may be mediastinal widening due to intraoperative edema or hemorrhage, and a small pneumomediastinum may also be present.

A number of tubes, wires, and catheters are present in or overlie the postoperative chest[23,133–137] (Fig. 7-39). These include an endotracheal tube, which should be positioned 5 to 7 cm above the carina to allow excursion in both flexion and extension of the neck. If the endotracheal tube is too close to the carina, flexion of the head or neck may force the distal end of the tube into the right or, less often, the left main stem bronchus, causing varying degrees of atelectasis of the opposite lung and barotrauma if assisted ventilation is used.[128] If the tube is too high, the patient may run the risk of aspiration, and dead space is increased.

The central venous pressure catheter is ideally placed in the superior vena cava. However, its distal tip is often found in the right atrium, in which case pressure measurements remain accurate, but there is an increased risk of cardiac perforation when the catheter is placed in the thin-walled right atrium.[23] In addition to malposition, compression or "pinch-off" of the catheter by the clavicle and first rib may produce narrowing or kinking of the catheter. Pinch-off occurs in 1 per cent of catheter placements.[138] When pinch-off occurs, the catheter should be removed and replaced with a more rigid catheter, one that is oval rather than round in cross section.

A Swan-Ganz catheter is usually placed in either major pulmonary artery (ideally with the tip lying within a dependent branch) to monitor pulmonary artery or pulmonary capillary wedge pressure and to obtain mixed venous blood samples. If the catheter is too peripheral in position, the inflated balloon near the tip of the catheter may

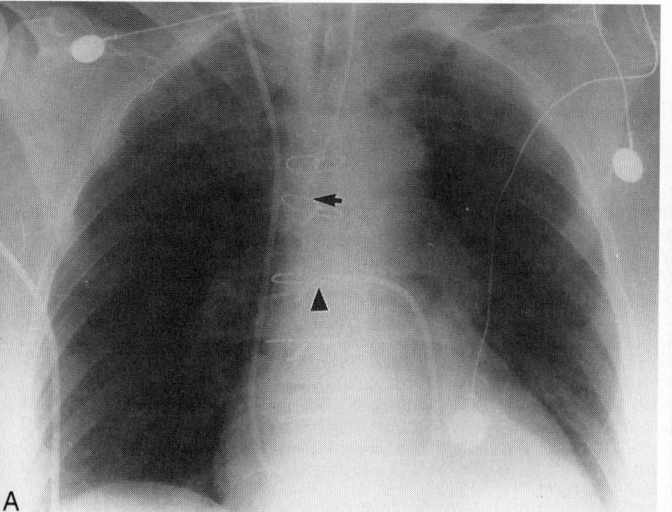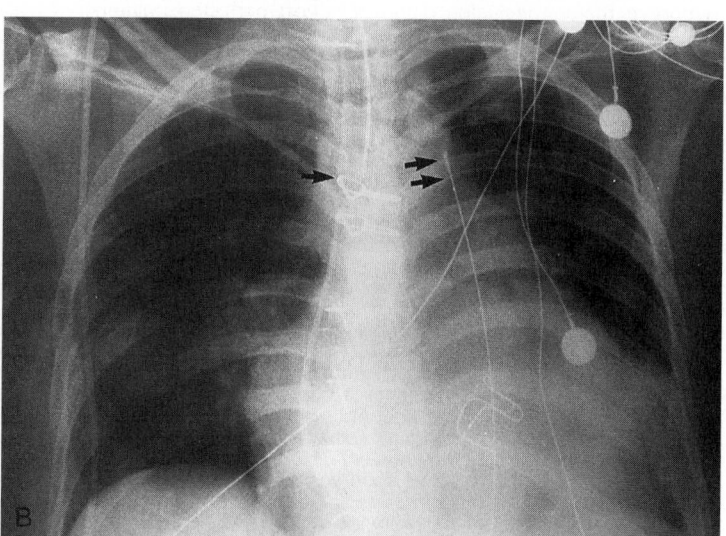

FIGURE 7–39. *A,* An early postoperative chest radiograph. There is a Swan-Ganz catheter in the right pulmonary artery (arrowhead). The endotracheal tube lies 2 cm above the carina (arrow). It should be repositioned proximally to prevent selective bronchial placement. *B,* This 60-year-old man developed a massive myocardial infarction. The endotracheal tube lies just above the carina (left arrow). The intraaortic balloon catheter is located at the top of the arch near the orifice of the left subclavian artery (double arrows on right) and required at least 2 cm of retraction.

damage the pulmonary artery wall and cause a perforation leading to a pseudoaneurysm.[137] The tip should lie in a large central branch from which it can float distally to a wedged position, whereupon the balloon is inflated.

Anterior mediastinal drainage catheters are located in the parasternal area, and posterior mediastinal drainage catheters usually lie on the left side behind the heart. Epicardial pacing wires or pacemaker wires project over the heart and lungs.[135,136] When circulatory assistance is needed, an intraaortic counterpulsation balloon catheter may be positioned with its tip just below the level of the left subclavian artery within the proximal descending aorta[136] (Fig. 7–39B). Pacemaker leads,[23,133] prosthetic valves,[46] and implantable cardioverter-defibrillators[139] require careful observation for lead or component malposition, pouch infection, or fracture.[133] A nasogastric tube is also usually present. It may be inadvertently placed in a bronchus and pass into the lung or even the pleura. If malposition of a nasogastric tube is unrecognized, aspiration of fluid may occur, causing a chemical pulmonary edema or pneumonia. Early recognition of the normal and abnormal positions of the large number of catheters, wires, and tubes found on the postoperative chest radiograph requires rapid interpretation by a physician thoroughly familiar with both the appearance of the postoperative chest and the possible complications that may frequently occur.

EARLY POSTOPERATIVE FILM. The first postoperative chest film usually demonstrates varying degrees of lower lobe atelectasis, mediastinal widening, pulmonary edema, and pleural effusion.[130,140] Unilateral or bilateral lower lobe atelectasis, usually accompanied by small pleural effusions, is the source of lower lung zone opacities found in almost all cardiac surgery patients.[135] Elevation of the involved hemidiaphragm is also present.[141] The lower lobe opacities usually appear within 8 hours after surgery and clear within 5 to 7 days. Although pneumonia can occur as a complication, it is unusual. These changes occur most commonly on the left side. The mechanisms for preferential left lower lobe atelectasis include paralysis of the phrenic nerve caused by cardioplegic solutions or crushed ice administered for myocardial preservation or retained secretions.[141] Decreased diaphragmatic motion may persist for many weeks after operation but will eventually resolve in most patients.

Pleural Effusion. Radiographically, pleural effusions manifested by blunting of the costophrenic angle, loss of sharpness of the diaphragmatic contour, and increased opacity behind the diaphragmatic dome are seen. Postoperative effusions are probably related to pericardial fluid that leaks into the pleural space through the surgically created pericardial window or to irritation of the pleura during operation. Postpericardiotomy syndrome and congestive heart failure are the sources of pleural effusion in some patients.[142] Increasingly larger or persistent pleural effusions may be due to hemomediastinum, with blood escaping into the pleural space through a pleural tear. Large pleural effusions are more common after left internal mammary bypass surgery because the pleural space is entered in that procedure.

Pulmonary Consolidation. Patchy or occasionally diffuse consolidation in both lungs following cardiac surgery is usually caused by pulmonary edema. Pulmonary edema due to increased capillary permeability or adult respiratory distress syndrome is common after cardiac surgery because of vasoactive substances released during cardiopulmonary bypass, which affect capillary permeability. Pulmonary edema usually occurs within 2 days of surgery and is reversible with supportive therapy including diuretics.[135] Post-perfusion pulmonary edema occurs after cardiopulmonary bypass, which causes a marked increase in fluid in the extravascular space. The mechanism for post-perfusion pulmonary edema is thought to be related to the contact of circulating blood with foreign surfaces during bypass.[131] Congestive heart failure following cardiac bypass surgery occurs in patients with poor cardiac output. Typically, vascular redistribution to the upper lobes, Kerley B lines, small bilateral pleural effusions, and patchy opacities due to pulmonary edema are present.

Other early complications of cardiac surgery identified by plain film chest radiography include sternal dehiscence, pneumothorax, pneumomediastinum, mediastinal hematoma, pneumopericardium, subcutaneous emphysema, and the findings of pulmonary embolism[143–145] (Fig. 7–40). Rib fractures occur in 2 to 4 per cent of patients and are usually identified by plain films. Their importance lies in the possible misdiagnosis of chest pain of another cause, including angina or aortic dissection.

Pneumothorax is often difficult to identify in the supine patient.[129] It is characterized radiographically as a poorly defined radiolucency overlying the lower lung zones. Decubitus views are helpful in clearly defining the presence of a pleural air collection. Pneumomediastinum may occur when the mediastinum is entered during surgery. In most cases the mediastinal air resolves spontaneously within several days. A radiolucency overlying the center of the sternum following median sternotomy is due to a small gap in the sternum and soft tissues at the surgical site; this occurs in approximately one-third of patients. There is no proven correlation between this thin radiolucency and sternal dehiscence.[143]

Mediastinal Hemorrhage. This complication is common after cardiac surgery but is seldom serious enough to require reoperation. In the typical postoperative patient the mediastinum is widened by up to 35 per cent compared with preoperative PA chest films. Katzberg et al. found that if the mediastinum is widened more than 70 per

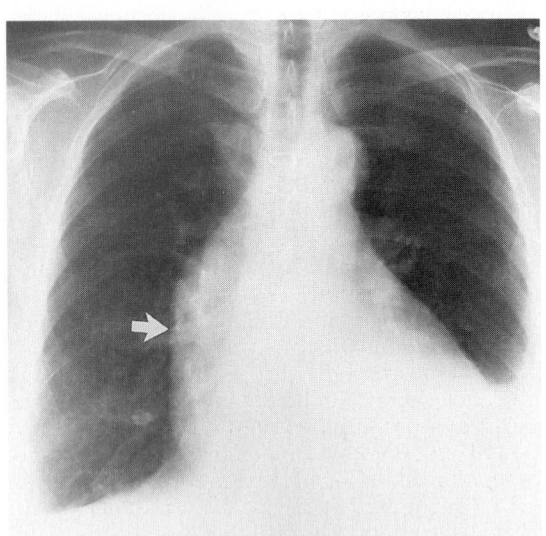

FIGURE 7–40. Mediastinal hemorrhage. There is marked widening of the right side of the mediastinum in the area of the ascending aorta (arrow). A large left pleural effusion is also present. Three days after CABG surgery.

cent compared with the baseline radiograph, surgery is usually required to remove the hematoma.[130] However, considerable bleeding may be present without visible mediastinal widening, especially if the patient is receiving positive end-expiratory pressure support, which may compress the mediastinum. Moreover, some patients may have a wide mediastinum but are hemodynamically stable, have no significant bloody drainage, and do not require reoperation.

Both CT and echocardiography can be helpful in establishing the diagnosis of intrapericardial hematoma. With echocardiography the hematoma has an echo-free center and a refractile margin. CT, with and without contrast enhancement, is also useful to differentiate hematoma from other masses. On nonenhanced CT the hematoma is denser than other soft tissues and the pericardium is visualized alongside the collection.[131,146]

Enlargement of the cardiac silhouette occurring during the early postoperative period may be due to cardiac failure with or without myocardial infarction or to a mediastinal or pericardial fluid collection. In some patients, pericardial tamponade occurs from bleeding of small arteries in the area of the sternal incision. Equalization of diastolic pressures and elevation of the pulmonary capillary wedge pressure without pulmonary redistribution or edema, together with diffuse enlargement of the cardiac silhouette, suggest pericardial tamponade. Although the chest roentgenogram is suggestive, both CT and echocardiography will clearly reveal the presence of pericardial fluid, while CT is the procedure of choice to detect a mediastinal fluid collection.[145]

LATE COMPLICATIONS OF CARDIAC SURGERY. **Postpericardiotomy Syndrome** (see p. 1520). This common late complication of cardiac surgery is characterized by pleuritis, pericarditis, and fever. It is believed to be the result of an immune response to the necrotic epicardium. It generally occurs several weeks after operation and is self-limited.[142] Occasionally, cardiac tamponade or constrictive pericarditis occurs as a complication of the postpericardiotomy syndrome. Radiographically, unilateral or bilateral pleural effusions, diffuse enlargement of the cardiac silhouette caused by pericardial effusion, and small basilar pulmonary opacities are found. Echocardiography or CT will identify the pleural or pericardial fluid collections.[142,145] Other late postoperative complications of cardiac surgery include sternal osteomyelitis, especially after internal mammary artery surgery,[147] dehiscence,[143] mediastinitis, and cardiac rupture.[119]

Pseudoaneurysm of the Thoracic Aorta (Fig. 7–41). This complication is associated with sternal and mediastinal inflammation following median sternotomy.[148–150] Pseudoaneurysm is a rare but serious complication of cardiac surgery and may occur at the site of an aortic cannulation or vent, the aortic clamp line, or the saphenous graft-aortic anastomosis.[150] Cardiac pseudoaneurysms can also occur at sites where full-thickness cardiac incisions were made. Although plain film radiographs will demonstrate a mass in the cardiac or aortic region, enhanced CT or MRI is diagnostic and should be performed before reoperation.[148,150]

Aortic Dissection. Although aortic dissection rarely occurs in patients who have undergone surgery of the aorta and aortic valve replacement, it should be considered in the differential diagnosis of mediastinal widening or anterior mediastinal mass. A dissection may appear immediately after operation but is more likely to occur weeks to months later. Although aortography is diagnostic, contrast-enhanced CT is helpful to distinguish between dissection on the one hand, and hematoma, abscess, tumor, or prominent mediastinal fat on the other.[148]

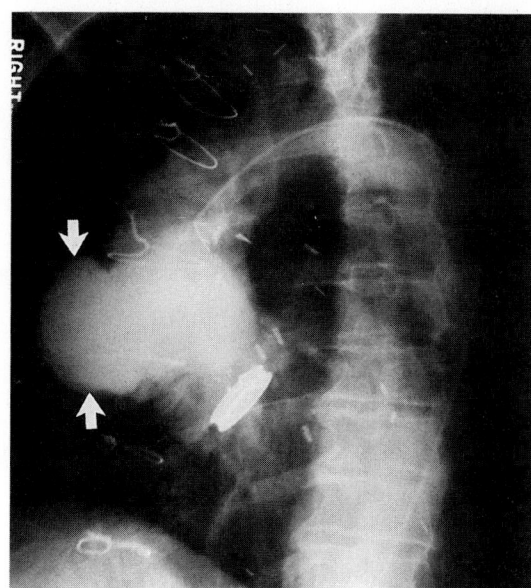

FIGURE 7–41. Pseudoaneurysm of the ascending aorta. This saccular pseudoaneurysm (arrows) developed 5 months after valve replacement at the aortotomy site in a 78-year-old man. (From Sullivan, K. L., et al.: Pseudoaneurysm of the ascending aorta following cardiac surgery. Chest 93:138, 1988.)

PROSTHETIC VALVE SURGERY (see also p. 1065). The chest roentgenogram is helpful in following patients for the potential complications of valve implantation. Identification of the site of the prosthetic valve is not as simple as that of calcified native cardiac valves because only an AP film may be available during the early postoperative period and the prosthetic valves vary in position and often overlap each other.[151] If the patient fails to improve clinically after valve replacement or if there is pulmonary edema after a brief period of improvement, malfunction of the prosthetic valve may be the cause. Major malfunctions result from sewing ring dehiscence, strut fracture, tissue encroachment into the ring orifice, disc- or poppet-induced thrombosis, and infective endocarditis.[45,46] Plain chest film may show enlargement of the adjacent cardiac chambers or pulmonary edema. Calcification of a heterograft or homograft valve may be seen and is usually caused by tissue degeneration. Fracture and separation of radiopaque components and their distal migration may be identified by fluoroscopy or on radiographs of the chest and abdomen.[47,55]

Fluoroscopy documents prosthetic valve motion, the integrity of the mechanical components, and the presence of calcification. If there is more than 12 degrees of rocking of the mitral or aortic sewing ring in systole and diastole, prosthesis dehiscence at the ring should be considered.[54] Reduced or absent excursion of the valve occluder suggests thrombus, tissue intrusion, or vegetation. Doppler echocardiography will document regurgitant blood flow proximal to the valve. Enhanced cine CT and cine MRI are complementary studies to diagnose valvular regurgitation.

CORONARY ARTERY SURGERY (Chap. 30). The early plain film radiographic findings after coronary bypass surgery are nonspecific and are similar to those of other cardiac surgical procedures.[62,130,152] Radiographic evaluation of coronary bypass grafts utilizing ultrafast CT or MRI sometimes aids in distinguishing graft occlusion from other causes of postoperative chest pain.[132,153,154] MRI has an accuracy of 91 per cent for determination of patency and is 72 per cent accurate for determination of occlusion[154] (Fig. 10–10, p. 323). In comparison, CT exhibits 85 to 95 per cent accuracy in demonstrating occlusions and up to 100 per cent accuracy in demonstrating patency (Fig. 10–36, p. 338).[152] A drawback to these noninvasive techniques is that they neither exclude nonocclusive stenosis of the grafts nor document progression of disease in native vessels. Moreover, they do not eliminate the need to perform cardiac catheterization in patients in whom reoperation is contemplated.

CARDIAC TRANSPLANTATION (Chap. 18). Most transplant candidates have a history of end-stage cardiac failure caused by ischemic heart disease or cardiomyopathy. The heart is invariably enlarged, and pulmonary vascular redistribution or edema is generally present. In orthotopic cardiac transplantation, the recipient heart is removed and the donor heart, with intact aorta and pulmonary arteries, is attached to a cuff of native left atrium containing the pulmonary veins. Following transplant surgery, typical radiographic changes associated with median sternotomy are found, including a widened mediastinum, pleural effusion, left lower lobe consolidation, and atelectasis. Within 2 months after transplantation, the heart becomes smaller and reaches stability 6 months after surgery. Persistent cardiomegaly most likely is caused by pericardial effusion, which may result from cyclosporine therapy or placement of a small donor heart in a large pericardial sac. Following transplantation the radiograph often has a double density in the vicinity of the right atrial border because of the overlapping donor and recipient atria. MRI or CT can clearly depict postoperative transplantation anatomy as well as the presence of pericardial effusion and lymphadenopathy.[155]

If graft rejection occurs, the heart enlarges, but pulmonary edema does not usually develop. The diagnosis of rejection, made by endomyocardial biopsy, demonstrates lymphocytic infiltration and myocytic necrosis.[156] MRI can demonstrate alterations in signal intensity in moderate and severe rejection.[157] Accelerated coronary atherosclerosis can lead to myocardial infarction and left ventricular enlargement. Pulmonary infection due to immunosuppressive therapy is common and may be bacterial, viral, or protozoan in origin.

Heart-lung transplantation is usually performed in patients with a history of primary pulmonary hypertension, end-stage chronic pulmonary disease with right ventricular decompensation, or Eisenmenger physiology. Early complications in this group of patients include cytomegalovirus and bacterial pneumonia. Long-term sequelae include accelerated coronary atherosclerosis and bronchiolitis obliterans with or without organizing pneumonia. Radiographically, the parenchymal pattern of bronchiolitis obliterans is characterized by coarse, asymmetrical nodular or reticular-nodular densities throughout the lungs with relative sparing of the upper lobes.[158–160]

CONGENITAL HEART DISEASE IN THE ADULT

Adults with congenital cardiac disorders (see Chap. 30) fall into three different clinical groups: those whose cardiac disorder was recognized in childhood and surgically treated, those whose cardiac abnormalities were recognized but did not undergo surgery and were followed medically, and those patients who survived into adulthood with unrecognized or misdiagnosed congenital cardiac disease.

The radiographic findings in adult congenital heart disease can be classified in a number of ways, based on the frequency of the disorder or a combination of the hallmarks of disease including the state of the pulmonary vasculature, the position of the aortic arch, cardiac size, and abdominal situs. Combining the radiographic findings with a history of the presence or absence of cyanosis, the time of onset of the cardiac murmur, and the clinical state of the patient should narrow the diagnostic choices. Several of the more common congenital cardiovascular disorders found with some frequency in adults are discussed below.

Coarctation of the Aorta

Coarctation of the aorta (see p. 965) is a common anomaly, accounting for 8 per cent of congenital heart defects in children and about 6 per cent of adult congenital heart disease.[25] In the adult patient, localized postductal narrowing of the aorta is most common. It represents a deformity in the aortic media that narrows the lumen by a curtain-like unfolding of the vessel wall.[161,162] The clinical presentation is highly variable and ranges from left ventricular failure in infancy to hypertension in otherwise asymptomatic adult patients, depending on the site and severity of the coarctation and the presence of associated abnormalities.[163,164] The most common associated anomaly is bicuspid aortic valve, which occurs in as many as 85 per

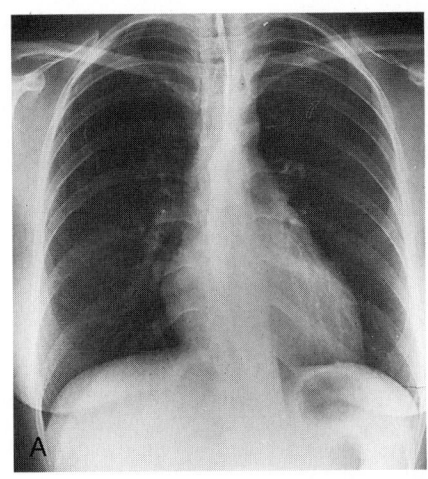
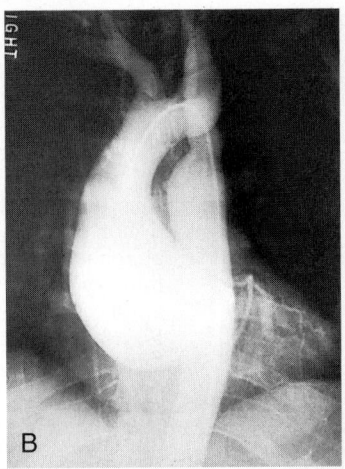
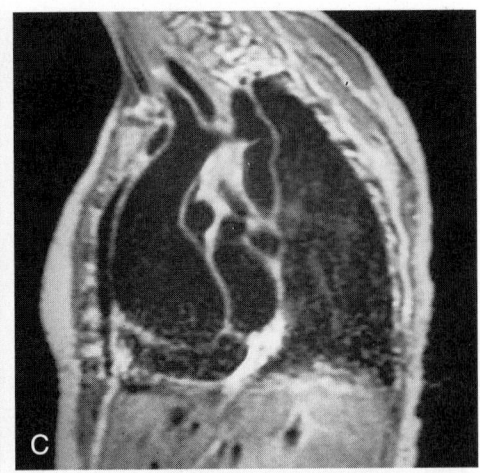

FIGURE 7–42. Coarctation of the aorta. *A,* There is displacement of the barium column to the right above and below the coarctation. *B,* Thoracic aortography. The luminal narrowing at the isthmus and enlargement of the LSCA are characteristic of coarctation. It may be described as a "3" sign or "E" sign becaue of the precoarctation bulge of the LSCA, the coarctation itself, and postcoarctation aortic dilatation. The dilatation of the ascending aorta is due to a regurgitant bicuspid aortic valve. *C,* Sagittal T1-weighted MRI in the same patient shows the same findings as the aortogram but without contrast media, radiation, or catheterization.

cent of patients with coarctation of the aorta.[25] Other associated congenital anomalies include ventricular septal defect, stenosis or atresia of the left subclavian artery, patent ductus arteriosus, Turner syndrome, or mitral valve prolapse.[165]

ROENTGENOGRAPHIC FINDINGS. The diagnosis of coarctation of the aorta can be established from the PA chest film alone in up to 92 per cent of patients.[161] The most useful radiographic sign is an abnormal contour of the aortic arch, which may appear as a double bulge above and below the usual site of the aortic knob.[166] This pattern has been described as a "figure 3" sign. The upper arc of the "3" is the dilated arch proximal to the coarctation and/or a dilated left subclavian artery (Fig. 7–42). The lower arc or bulge is the poststenotic dilatation of the aorta immediately below the coarctation. The indentation between the two bulges is the coarctation itself. When the esophagus is filled with barium, a reverse "3" or "E" sign is often seen, representing a mirror image of the areas of pre- and poststenotic dilatation. The "3" sign is variable in that the upper arc may be small and the lower arc large or vice versa (Fig. 7–42). Superior mediastinal widening due to large internal mammary collateral arteries is visible in some patients.[167] The aortic arch may also be obscured in the frontal view due to overlapping of the aorta by an enlarged left subclavian artery.[166] Left ventricular enlargement usually occurs with coarctation, particularly when there is an associated bicuspid aortic valve and aortic stenosis.

Bilateral symmetrical rib notching, readily appreciated on the chest film, is diagnostic of aortic coarctation. It is due to obstruction to blood flow at the narrowed aortic segment with collateral blood flow through the intercostal vessels. Rib notching is unusual in infancy, but it becomes more prominent with increased age and is present in 75 per cent of adults with coarctation. Rib notching occurs along the inferior margin of the third to the eighth ribs due to the pulsations of the dilated intercostal arteries. The major pathways of collateral flow include (1) subclavian artery to internal mammary artery to intercostal arteries, (2) subclavian artery to the costovertebral trunk to the intercostal arteries, and (3) transverse cervical and suprascapular arteries to the intercostal arteries. Dilatation of the internal mammary arteries acting as a collateral pathway may cause scallop-edged retrosternal notching.[167]

Cardiac catheterization and angiography are diagnostic, demonstrating both the site of the coarctation and associated anomalies, including aortic valvular disease (Fig. 7–42B). Cross-sectional imaging modalities yield important diagnostic information. Echocardiography, for example, demonstrates the presence or absence of bicuspid aortic and mitral valve deformities. MRI is useful in demonstrating both the coarctation itself and restenosis of the aorta following surgery or angioplasty[164,165,168,169] (Fig. 7–42C).

Left-to-Right Shunts

OSTIUM SECUNDUM ATRIAL SEPTAL DEFECT (ASD) (see also p. 966). This is the most common left-to-right shunt diagnosed in adult life, accounting for over 40 per cent of adult congenital heart defects.[170–171a] Although the chest radiograph may be normal in a patient with a small shunt, typically the main pulmonary artery, the peripheral pulmonary branches, the right atrium, and right ventricu-

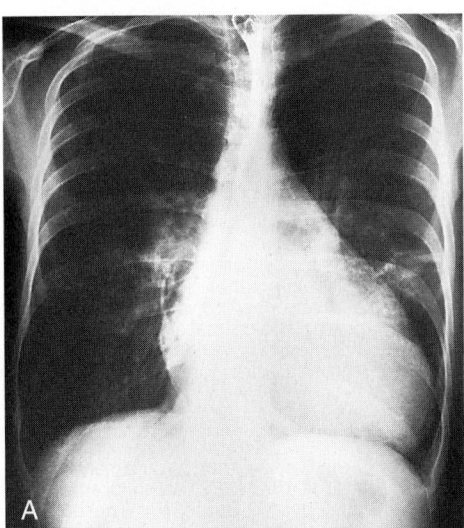
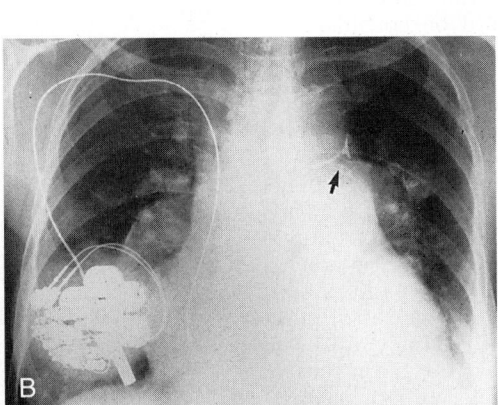
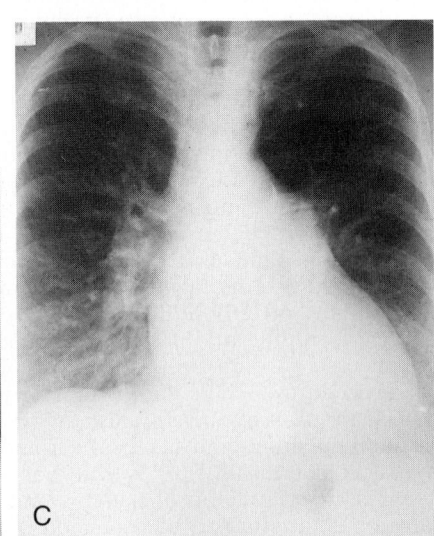

FIGURE 7–43. *A,* Atrial septal defect. A 45-year-old woman with an ostium secundum defect. The pulmonary artery is enlarged and there is prominence of the right atrial border. The enlargement of the right ventricle causes rounding of the left heart border. *B,* Patent ductus arteriosus in a patient with a cardiac pacemaker. An inverted "Y" calcification is present above an enlarged pulmonary artery (arrow). *C,* Ventricular septal defect. There is an increase in the size of the central pulmonary arteries in this patient with VSD and Eisenmenger physiology.

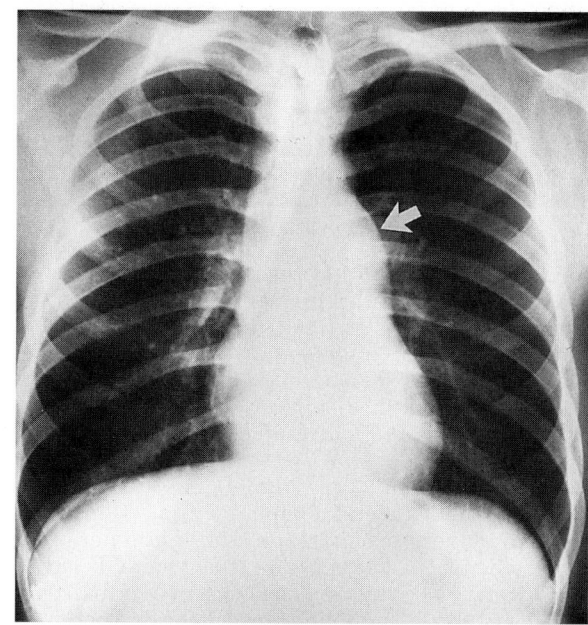

FIGURE 7-44. Pulmonary valvular stenosis. Pulmonary blood flow and cardiac size are normal, but the main pulmonary artery is enlarged (arrow) in this young woman with pulmonary valvular stenosis.

is small or normal in size, whereas the aorta is enlarged in PDA. Cine CT, MRI, and echocardiography will demonstrate the site of the defect.[162,164,173]

PULMONARY VALVULAR STENOSIS (see also p. 968). Pulmonary valvular stenosis in adults is usually an isolated anomaly.[174] Most patients are asymptomatic even with severe obstruction. There is mild to moderate enlargement of the main pulmonary artery due to post-stenotic dilatation resulting from the jet effect of blood flow through the narrowed pulmonary valve orifice (Fig. 7-44). Since the jet is directed toward the left, the left pulmonary artery is often preferentially enlarged. Calcification of the pulmonary valve is rare in this condition. The differential diagnosis of pulmonary valvular stenosis includes primary and secondary pulmonary hypertension and idiopathic pulmonary artery dilatation.

CONGENITAL CORRECTED TRANSPOSITION OF THE GREAT ARTERIES (see also p. 966). In this condition ventricular inversion and transposition of the pulmonary artery and aorta result from formation of a left (levo or l) rather than a right (dextro or d) bulboventricular loop. The systemic venous flow is transmitted to the lungs by way of a right-sided anatomical left ventricle and the transposed pulmonary artery. Pulmonary venous flow traverses the left atrium and a left-sided anatomical right ventricle en route to the aorta.

Radiographically, the ascending aorta is positioned to the left, forming a long continuous shadow along the left cardiac border from the ventricular apex to the aortic arch[175] (Fig. 7-45A,B). The main pulmonary artery lies behind and to the right of the aorta and is not border-forming with the lung in the PA view. A left-to-right shunt may or may not be present, and left atrioventricular valve regurgitation and conduction abnormalities leading to heart block are fairly common. The heart is normal to enlarged in size, depending on the degree of atrioventricular valve regurgitation. Cross-sectional imaging supports the plain film diagnosis, showing an anterior left-sided aorta and a pulmonary artery lying behind and medial to the aorta.[176,177]

Cyanotic Congenital Heart Disease in the Adult

TETRALOGY OF FALLOT (see also p. 968). This is the most common cyanotic congenital cardiac lesion in adults as well as in children. Most adults with tetralogy of Fallot demonstrate mild to moderate pulmonary hypovascularity. Those with mild infundibular pulmonary stenosis have normal pulmonary blood flow (Fig. 7-7C). Small tortuous bronchial arteries are found in both lungs when severe pulmonary outflow tract stenosis or atresia is present. There is a right aortic arch in 25 per cent of patients.[178] The combination of right aortic arch and cyanosis should always suggest the diagnosis of tetralogy of Fallot, although the same combination can also be seen in the rare examples of truncus arteriosus or double-outlet right ventricle in the adult patient. Echocardiography often demonstrates a high and large ventricular septal defect, overriding of the ventricular septum by the aorta, and right ventricular hypertrophy. Cine CT and MRI can demonstrate the septal defect and the large ascending aorta, as well a right aortic arch.[164,169] Plain films show a boot-shaped heart in some adult patients, but this is less common than in children because those who survive into adulthood are less likely to have severe right ventricular outflow tract stenosis.

EBSTEIN'S ANOMALY (see also p. 969). In this condition the tricuspid valve is malformed and partially fused to the walls of the right ventricle. This results in downward displacement of the tricuspid orifice, and regurgitation ensues. There is a right-to-left shunt at the atrial

lar borders are enlarged (Fig. 7-21A). Differentiation from other left-to-right shunts is often possible. There is usually less pulmonary artery dilatation in patent ductus arteriosus (PDA) than in ASD, and both PDA and ventricular septal defect (VSD) are associated with enlarged left-sided cardiac chambers. In the adult over the age of 50 years, the radiographic findings of ASD are often atypical and may include left atrial enlargement, evidence of pulmonary venous hypertension, and pulmonary edema (Fig. 7-43A). These changes are associated with smaller shunts and a higher prevalence of left ventricular dysfunction and pulmonary arterial hypertension.[172] Echocardiography is diagnostic in ASD (Fig. 3-77, p. 82); right ventricular chamber dilation and paradoxical anterior systolic motion of the interventricular septum are seen. The size and the location of the ASD can often be visualized, as well as associated abnormalities including mitral valve prolapse. Cine CT and MRI also demonstrate the defect of the atrial septum.[169]

VENTRICULAR SEPTAL DEFECT (see also p. 967). VSD accounts for 30 per cent of cardiac malformations in the newborn but comprises only 10 per cent of adult-onset congenital heart defects. The relatively small incidence in adults is due to spontaneous closure of the defect in childhood or surgical repair.[173] If the VSD is small, the chest film is normal. However, if there is a large left-to-right shunt or secondary pulmonary hypertension, the pulmonary arteries are enlarged, as are both ventricles and the left atrium (Fig. 7-43C). The ascending aorta

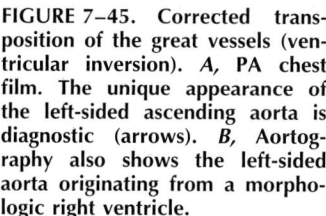

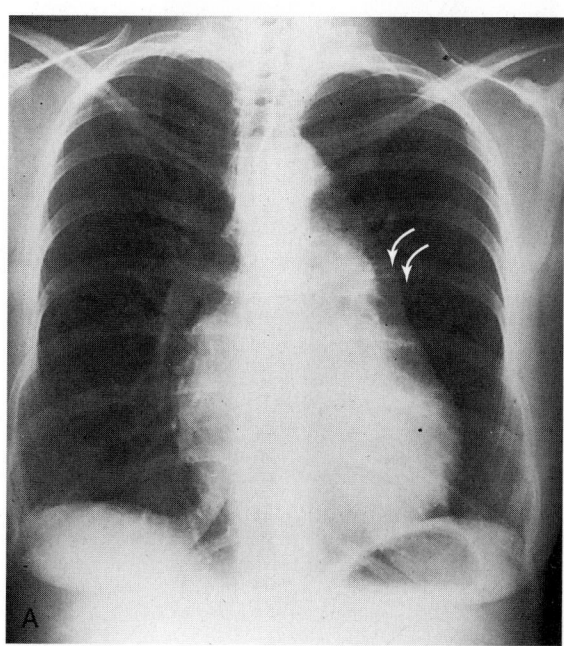

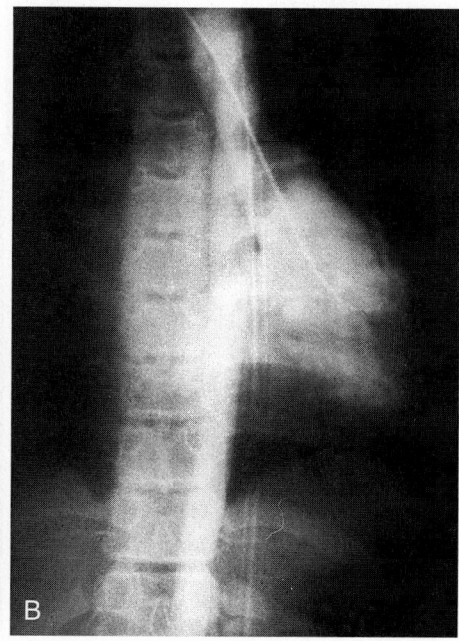

FIGURE 7-45. Corrected transposition of the great vessels (ventricular inversion). *A,* PA chest film. The unique appearance of the left-sided ascending aorta is diagnostic (arrows). *B,* Aortography also shows the left-sided aorta originating from a morphologic right ventricle.

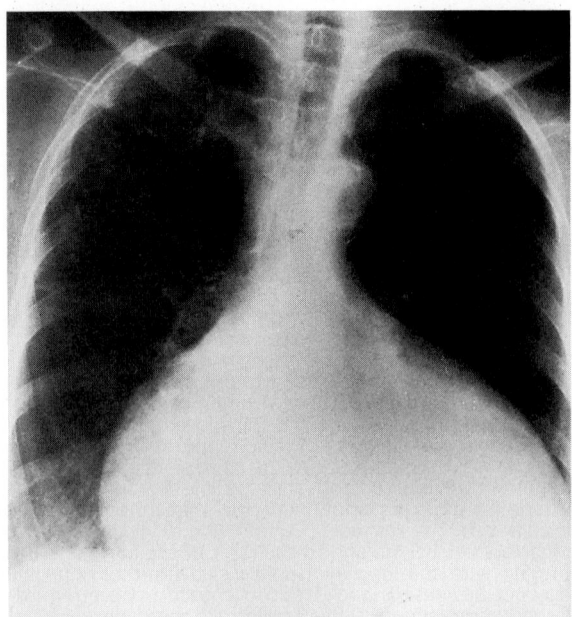

FIGURE 7–46. Ebstein's anomaly. There is globular cardiac enlargement due to severe tricuspid regurgitation and right heart enlargement. The pulmonary blood flow is reduced.

level, causing cyanosis. The right heart chambers are enlarged, often markedly, as a manifestation of the tricuspid regurgitation. The typical roentgenographical findings are those of a large rounded or triangular heart with a narrow vascular pedicle.[179,180] The pulmonary vasculature is reduced, depending on the degree of right-to-left shunting. The greater the shunt, the more diminished the vascularity. Echocardiography shows the abnormal placement of the tricuspid

valve with downward displacement of the septal and posterior leaflets. Tricuspid regurgitation can be evaluated by two-dimensional and Doppler echocardiography. MRI and CT also demonstrate the downward displacement of the valve and enlargement of the right atrium[169,179,180] (Fig. 7–46).

THE PERICARDIUM

(See also Chap. 43)

The incidence of pericardial disease in the patient with cardiac disease parallels the frequency of cardiac surgery, multisystem inflammatory disease, thoracic irradiation, and the use of an array of therapeutic agents that affect the pericardium. There is also increasing recognition of the presence of pericardial disease because of modalities, such as echocardiography, which portray pericardial disease with great accuracy.

NORMAL PERICARDIUM. The normal pericardium is frequently identified on lateral plain film projections of the chest as a thin linear opacity separating the anterior subxiphoid mediastinal fat from the subepicardial fat[181–183] (Fig. 7–47B). The pericardium may also be visualized in the frontal projection paralleling the left heart border. The extent of the normal and abnormal pericardium is best appreciated with CT and MRI in most patients because of the superior contrast resolution of both techniques.[183,184] With both CT and MRI, the anterior, lateral, and posterior pericardium are clearly separated from mediastinal fat, and subtle discontinuous areas of mild pericardial thickening and loculated effusions may be clearly seen.[185–187] One disadvantage of MRI and CT is that while the pericardial recesses are clearly defined, they may on occasion mimic an aortic dissection or mediastinal lymphadenopathy.[186]

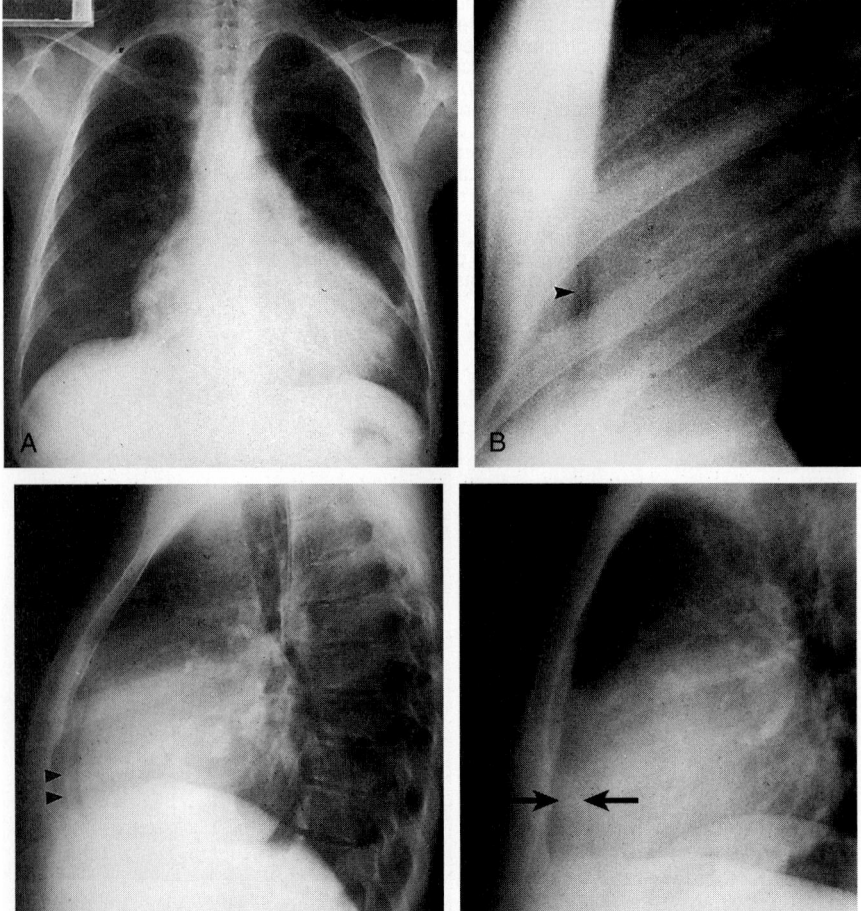

FIGURE 7–47. Pericardial effusion. *A,* The heart assumes a globular rounded shape following development of a pericardial effusion. The normal indentations along the heart borders are effaced so that the cardiac silhouette is smooth and featureless. *B,* The subepicardial radiolucent fat stripe is separated from the subxiphoid fat by the thin, higher density stripe of pericardial fluid (arrowhead). *C,* The pericardial stripe (arrowheads) is wider than in *B* because of a small pericardial effusion. *D,* A large pericardial effusion is present (arrows).

Echocardiography is probably the most sensitive technique for the diagnosis of small pericardial effusions. It is most often the imaging study of choice when pericardial effusion is clinically suspected or is considered as a possibility by plain film radiograph.[186]

PERICARDIAL EFFUSION (see also p. 1485). The effusion may be a transudate or exudate, hemorrhagic, gaseous, or chylous and may be due to a wide variety of causes.[37,186,187] When fluid accumulates in the pericardial space, the cardiac silhouette develops a "flask-like," triangular, or "globular" silhouette (Fig. 7–47). The normal indentations and prominences along both the left and right heart borders are effaced so that the shape of the cardiac silhouette becomes smooth and featureless. Since the pericardium extends up to the pulmonary bifurcation, when a large pericardial effusion is present, the hilar structures are draped and obscured by the distended pericardial cavity. This radiographic appearance should help to distinguish a large pericardial effusion from massive cardiomegaly, which will not obscure the hilar vessels.

In the lateral chest radiograph in the patient with pericardial effusion, the retrosternal space is typically narrowed or obliterated by the expanding cardiac silhouette. Normally the low-density subepicardial fat merges imperceptibly with the mediastinal fat since the two fat planes are separated only by the 2-mm-thick stripe of the pericardium.[182] When pericardial effusion is present the subepicardial fat is displaced posteriorly by the higher-density fluid, which may be visible as a wide opaque vertical band between the anterior border of the heart and the mediastinum (Fig. 7–47). This "epicardial fat pad sign" is visualized best on the lateral projection and is highly specific for pericardial effusion.[182,183,185]

Echocardiography is the most efficient method for the detection of simple pericardial effusion and/or thickening[188] (Fig. 3–104, p. 93). A major advantage of echocardiography is that the ultrasound apparatus can be transported to the bedside to examine critically ill patients. The technique is noninvasive and is diagnostically sensitive to fluid-filled structures. When the pericardial fluid volume is small, it appears as an elliptical hypoechoic region behind the left ventricle. When the effusion is large, the pericardial hypoechoic zone expands to surround the right ventricular apex. In some cases echocardiography may fail to identify pericardial thickening when constrictive pericarditis, neoplasm, or hemorrhage is present.

If echocardiography is inconclusive, CT can be helpful in detecting pericardial thickening, diffuse or loculated effusion, calcification, and adjacent mediastinal and pulmonary disease, as well as neoplasm[145,185,189] (Fig. 10–40, p. 340). The nature of the fluid may be identified by an analysis of CT density numbers. For example, there are higher CT density values in hemopericardium than in serous effusions. Chylous pericardial effusions may have a lower attenuation value than normal pericardial fluid.[185]

MRI and CT can clearly detect pericardial effusion.[190] On T1-weighted images, MRI will show the pericardial cavity as a dark signal void because of the motion of the fluid in the pericardial sac. On the other hand, the pericardial effusion is bright on a gradient echo sequence.[185] Pericardial fibrosis will present with a medium-intensity signal on T1-weighted or dark signal on T2-weighted images. Intrapericardial masses, cysts, and diffuse thickening are well demonstrated with MRI.[189] Furthermore, MRI can clearly define pericardial recesses, mediastinal fat, and other anatomical landmarks that may present pitfalls for the echocardiographer.[189–191a]

PERICARDIAL CONSTRICTION (see also p. 1496). Pericardial constriction may complicate viral or tuberculous pericarditis, hemopericardium, pericarditis associated with radiation, and postpericardiotomy syndrome.[186,187] In patients with chronic pericardial constriction, the overall heart size is large when the pericardium is thickened to 2 cm or

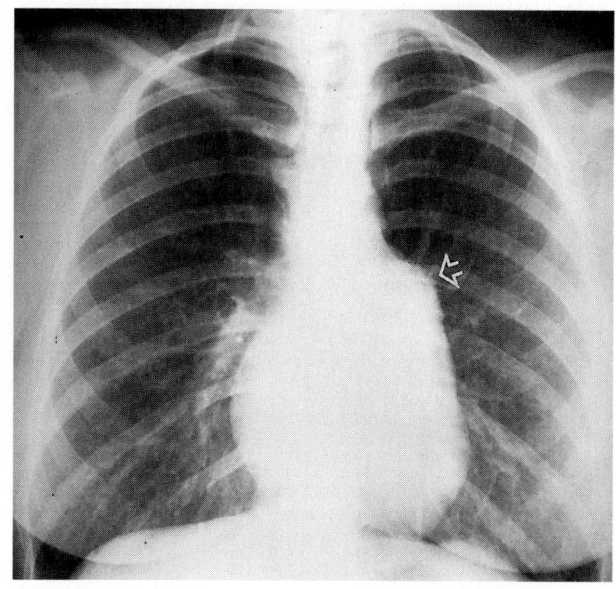

FIGURE 7–48. Partial absence of the pericardium: There is a convex bulge (open arrow) along the left atrial border due to herniation of the left atrial appendage through the pericardial defect.

more; otherwise the cardiac silhouette remains normal or small. The right atrial border is flattened, and there may be pulmonary vascular redistribution.[182,191]

Small to large pleural effusions are found in 60 per cent of patients with pericardial constriction, and enlargement of the azygos vein and left atrium occurs in 20 per cent of patients. In the past, tuberculous pericarditis was a frequent cause of pericardial calcification and constriction. But today tuberculosis is relatively uncommon. As a result, pericardial calcification occurs in fewer than 20 per cent of patients with chronic pericardial constriction[145] (Fig. 7–33). Pericardial calcification is best appreciated along the anterior and inferior cardiac borders or in the atrioventricular groove. While it is important to appreciate that the presence of pericardial calcification indicates chronic pericarditis, it does not in itself establish a diagnosis of pericardial constriction.

Pericardial constriction is often confused with restrictive cardiomyopathy, and MRI and CT are particularly helpful in differentiating between these entities (see p. 1501). The pericardium in patients with restrictive cardiomyopathy is normal in thickness and no calcification is present. In addition, there is diffuse limitation of global cardiac excursion in systole and diastole together with myocardial thickening in hearts with restrictive cardiomyopathy.[187]

CONGENITAL ANOMALIES (see also p. 1522). Congenital absence of the pericardium may be partial or complete. Complete absence is less common than partial absence and is usually left-sided.[192,193] Partial absence most frequently occurs along the upper border of the pericardium on either side.[183] If the left-sided defect is small, herniation of the left atrial appendage and/or the pulmonary trunk may occur. On the frontal chest film, herniation through a pericardial defect may resemble the appearance of pulmonary stenosis, mitral stenosis, or a mediastinal tumor (Fig. 7–48). When there is complete absence of the left pericardium, the aortic knob remains in its usual position, but the remainder of the cardiac silhouette shifts to the left and rotates toward the right, so that the right ventricle may become border-forming and the pulmonary artery and left atrial appendage become prominent.[192,193]

In patients with absence of the left pericardium, the plain film shows the lung interposed between the medial border of the pulmonary artery and the thoracic aorta outlining the pulmonary artery on both its medial and lateral sides, so that the lung may be visible between the heart and the diaphragm.[192] CT and MRI demonstrate to best

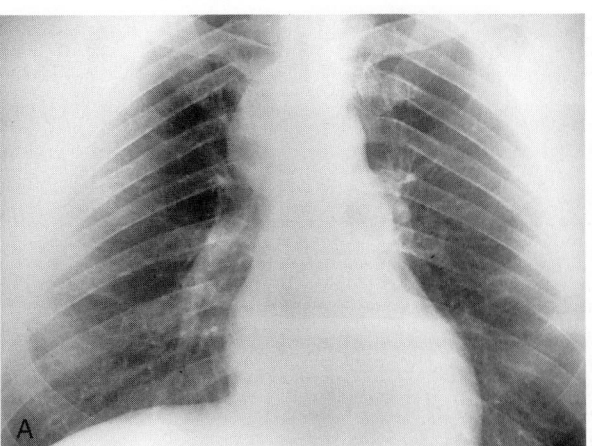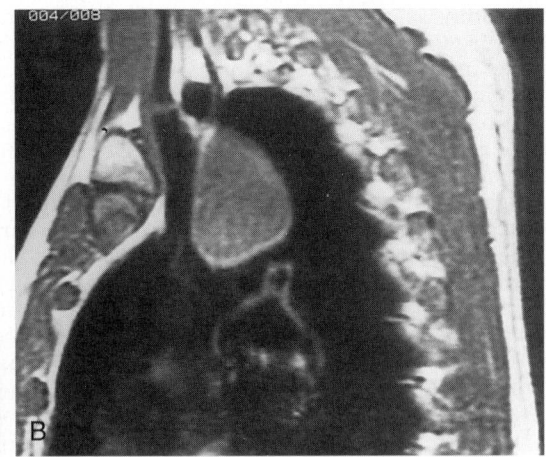

FIGURE 7–49. Pericardial recess cyst. *A,* PA chest film shows a mediastinal bulge along the right paratracheal line. *B,* MRI in sagittal plane shows the cyst as a homogeneous-intensity structure.

advantage the absence of the left anterior pericardium between ascending aorta and the main pulmonary artery. Displacement of the main pulmonary artery laterally and anteriorly is often a clue to the diagnosis.

PERICARDIAL CYST. A pericardial cyst generally appears as a smooth convex bulge along the middle or lower right heart border near the cardiophrenic sulcus. However, 20 per cent of pericardial cysts lie along the left heart border, sometimes mimicking a prominent left atrial appendage or left ventricular aneurysm.[194] Occasionally, pericardial recess cysts present as a soft tissue mass along the right superior mediastinal border in the area of the superior vena cava[194] (Fig. 7–49). While pericardial cysts are usually asymptomatic, chest pain has been described due to torsion or rapid increase in pericardial cyst volume due to intracystic bleeding.[195] Pericardial cysts rarely calcify and do not communicate with the pericardial space. Their clinical importance lies in the need to differentiate pericardial cysts from other masses with a similar appearance, such as fibroma, lymphoma, postoperative hematoma,[146,196] bronchogenic cyst, and cardiac neoplasm. Pericardial cysts are best diagnosed by echocardiography, CT, or MRI as smoothly marginated, fluid-filled structures adjacent to the right heart border.[194,195]

PERICARDIAL NEOPLASM. Pericardial tumors are demonstrated best by CT, MRI, or echocardiography[183] (Fig. 43–23, p. 1514). They generally do not cause a discrete bulge on the plain chest radiograph, but rather infiltrate the heart. When there is associated pericardial effusion, the cardiac silhouette will globally enlarge. CT can clearly identify associated pleural and parenchymal disease including metastatic lesions in the pleural space.

Metastatic neoplasm of the pericardium is far more common than primary tumor. The most common sources of pericardial metastases are the lung, breast, lymphoma, leukemia, and melanoma. Benign masses are unusual and include teratomas, bronchogenic cysts, lipomas, and fibromas.[98,189,195] The principal primary pericardial malignancy is mesothelioma, a rare pericardial tumor without a clear relationship to asbestos exposure (p. 1514). The tumor may be a single mass, multicentric, or diffuse with extensive encasement. Typically, pericardial mesothelioma is manifested by a clinical picture of pericardial constriction.[185]

REFERENCES

HISTORICAL PERSPECTIVE

1. Williams, F. H.: Notes on x-rays in medicine. Trans. Assoc. Am. Physicians *11:*375, 1896.
2. Williams, F. H.: A method for more fully determining the outline of the heart by means of a fluoroscope together with other uses of this instrument in medicine. Boston Med. Surg. J. *135:*335, 1896.

3. Eisenberg, R. L.: Radiology: An Illustrated History. St. Louis, Mosby-Year Book, 1992.
4. Schultz, K. W., Thorsen, M. K., Gurney, J. W., et al.: Comparison of fluoroscopy, angiography and CT in coronary artery calcification. Appl. Radiol. *6:*38, 1989.
5. Henry, D. A., Jolles, H., Berberich, J. J., and Schmelzer, V.: The postcardiac surgery chest radiograph: A clinically integrated approach. J. Thorac. Imaging *4:*20, 1989.
6. Bank, E. R., and Hernandez, R. J.: CT and MR of congenital heart disease. Radiol. Clin. North Am. *26:*241, 1988.
7. Thompson, B. H., and Stanford, W.: Evaluation of cardiac function with ultrafast computed tomography. Radiol. Clin. North Am. *32:*537, 1994.
8. Stanford, W., and Galvin, J. R.: The radiology of right heart dysfunction: Chest roentgenogram and computed tomography. J. Thorac. Imaging *4:*7, 1989.
9. Holt, W. W., Wong, E., and Lipton, M. J.: Conventional and ultra-fast cine-computed tomography in cardiac imaging. Curr. Opin. Radiol. *1:*159, 1989.
10. Budoff, M. J., Georgiou, D., Brody, A., et al.: Number of calcified coronary vessels by ultrafast computed tomography as a mediator of angiographic coronary artery disease in a symptomatic population. Am. J. Card. Imaging *8*(51):6, 1994.
11. Ahmad, M., Johnson, R. F., Jr., Fawcett, H. D., et al.: Left ventricular aneurysm in short axis: A comparison of magnetic resonance, ultrasound and thallium-201 SPECT images. Magn. Reson. Imaging *5:*293, 1987.
12. Brown, K. A., Altland, E., and Rowen, M.: Prognostic value of normal technetium 99m-sestamibi cardiac imaging. J. Nucl. Med. *35:*554, 1994.
13. Utz, J. A., Herfkens, R. J., Heinsimer, J. A., et al.: Cine MR determination of left ventricular ejection fraction. A.J.R. *148:*839, 1987.
14. Sechtem, U., Pflugfelder, P. W., Gould, R. G., et al.: Measurement of right and left ventricular volumes in healthy individuals with cine MR imaging. Radiology *163:*697, 1987.
15. Kersting-Sommerhoff, B. A., Diethelm, L., Stanger, P., et al.: Evaluation of complex congenital ventricular anomalies with magnetic resonance imaging. Am. Heart J. *120:*133, 1990.
16. Mitchell, L., Jenklins, J. P. R., Watson, Y., et al.: Diagnosis and assessment of mitral and aortic valve disease by cine-flow magnetic resonance imaging. Magn. Reson. Med. *12:*181, 1989.
17. Higgins, C. B., and Caputo, G. R.: Role of MR imaging in acquired and congenital cardiovascular disease. A.J.R. *161:*13, 1993.
18. Davis, C. P., McKinnow, G. C., Debatin, J. F., et al.: Normal heart: Evaluation with echo-planar MR imaging. Radiology *191:*691, 1994.
18a. Wetter, D. R., McKinnow, G. C., Debatin, J. F., and Von Schulthess, G. K.: Cardiac echo-planar MR imaging: Comparison of single and multiple shot techniques. Radiology *194:*765, 1995.
19. Needleman, L., Gardiner, G. A., Jr., and Levin, D. C.: Hypertrophic cardiomyopathy: Changing concepts over the last two decades. A.J.R. *150:*1219, 1988.
20. Gordon, S., and Butler, M.: Echocardiography in cardiac tamponade. J. Clin. Ultrasound *17:*428, 1989.
21. Hartnell, G. G.: Developments in echocardiography. Radiol. Clin. North Am. *32:*461, 1994.
22. Wandtke, J. C.: Bedside chest radiography. Radiology *190:*1, 1994.
23. Wechsler, R. J., Steiner, R. M., and Kinori, I.: Monitoring the monitors: The radiology of thoracic catheters, wires and tubes. Semin. Roentgenol. *23:*61, 1988.

NORMAL CARDIAC ANATOMY

24. Ball, J. B., and Proto, A. V.: The variable appearance of the left superior intercostal vein. Radiology *144:*445, 1982.
25. Steiner, R. M., Gross, G., Flicker, S., et al.: Congenital heart disease in the adult patient. J. Thorac. Imaging *10:*1, 1995.

26. Benedikt, R. A., Jellnec, J. S., Schaefer, P. S., et al.: Right-side aortic arch with aneurysm of aberrant left subclavicular artery: MR imaging appearance. J. Magn. Reson. Imaging *1*:485, 1991.

27. Danza, F. M., Fusco, C. A., Breda, M., et al.: Ductus arteriosus aneurysm in an adult. A.J.R. *143*:131, 1984.

28. Salomonowitz, E., Edwards, J. E., Hunter, D. W., et al.: The three types of aortic diverticula. A.J.R. *142*:673, 1984.

29. Carlsson, E., Gross, R., and Hold, R. G.: The radiological diagnosis of cardiac valvar insufficiencies. Circulation *55*:921, 1977.

30. Jefferson, K., and Rees, S.: Clinical Cardiac Radiology. 2nd ed. London, Butterworths, 1980.

31. Berdon, W. E., and Baker, D. H.: Plain film findings in azygos continuation of the inferior vena cava. A.J.R. *104*:452, 1968.

32. Bachman, D. M., Ellis, K., and Austin, J. H. M.: The effect of minor degrees of obliquity on the lateral chest radiograph. Radiol. Clin. North Am. *16*:465, 1978.

33. Murphy, M. L., Blue, L. R., Ferris, E. J., et al.: Sensitivity and specificity of chest roentgenogram criteria for right ventricular hypertrophy. Invest. Radiol. *23*:853, 1988.

34. Marzullo, P., L'Abbate, A. L., and Marcus, M.: Patterns of global and regional systolic and diastolic function in the normal right ventricle assessed by ultrafast computed tomography. J. Am. Coll. Cardiol. *17*:1318, 1991.

35. Hoffman, R. B., and Rigler, L. G.: Evaluation of left ventricular enlargement in the lateral projection of the chest. Radiology *85*:93, 1965.

36. Baron, M. G.: Radiological and angiographic examination of the heart. *In* Braunwald, E. (ed.): Heart Disease: A Textbook of Cardiovascular Medicine. 3rd ed. Philadelphia, W. B. Saunders Co., 1988, p. 140.

37. Chen, J. T. T.: Essentials of Cardiac Roentgenology. Boston, Little Brown, 1987.

38. Van Houten, F. X., Adams, D. F., and Abrams, H. L.: Radiology of valvular heart disease. *In* Sonnenblick, E., and Lesch, M. (eds.): Valvular Heart Disease. New York, Grune and Stratton, 1974.

39. Mandalam, K. R., Subramanyan, R., Joseph, S., et al.: Natural history of aortoarteritis: Angiographic study in 26 survivors. Clin. Radiol. *49*:38, 1994.

40. Morgan, P. W., Goodman, L. R., Aprahamian, C., et al.: Evaluation of traumatic aortic injury: Does dynamic contrast enhanced CT play a role? Radiology *182*:661, 1992.

41. Baron, M.: Left anterior oblique view for evaluation of left atrial size. Circulation *44*:926, 1971.

42. Sos, T. A., Levin, D. C., Sniderman, K. W., et al.: Cinefluoroscopy in evaluating left ventricular contractility and aneurysms. Circulation *56* (Suppl. III):18, 1977.

43. Benson, J. S.: Patient and physician radiation during fluoroscopy. Radiology *182*:286, 1992.

44. Freundlich, L. M., and Lind, T. A.: Calcification of the heart and great vessels. C.R.C. Crit. Rev. Clin. Radiol. Nucl. Med. *6*:171, 1975.

45. Kotler, M. N., Mintz, G. S., Panidis, I., et al.: Noninvasive evaluation of normal and abnormal prosthetic valve function. J. Am. Coll. Cardiol. *2*:151, 1983.

46. Steiner, R. M., Mintz, G., Morse, D., et al.: Radiology of cardiac valve prosthesis. Radiographics *8*:277, 1988.

47. Guit, G. L., Van Voorthuisen, A. E., and Steiner, R. M.: Outlet strut fracture of the Björk-Shiley mitral prosthesis. Radiology *154*:298, 1985.

48. Spindola-Franco, H., Fish, B. G., Dachman, A., et al.: Recognition of bicuspid aortic valve by plain film calcification. A.J.R. *139*:867, 1982.

49. Green, C. E., and Kelley, M. J.: A renewed role for fluoroscopy in the evaluation of cardiac disease. Radiol. Clin. North Am. *18*:345, 1980.

50. Schultz, K. W., Thorsen, M. K., Gurney, J. W., et al.: Comparison of fluoroscopy, angiography and CT in coronary artery calcification. Appl. Radiol. *19*:38, 1989.

51. Kelley, M. J., Huang, E. K., and Langou, R. A.: Correlations of fluoroscopically detected coronary artery calcification with exercise stress testing in asymptomatic men. Radiology *729*:1, 1978.

52. Stanford, W., Thompson, B. H., Weiss, R. M., and Galvin, J. R.: Coronary artery visualization using ultrafast computed tomography. Am. J. Card. Imaging *7*:243, 1993.

53. Bartel, A. G., Chen, J. T. T., Peter, R. H., et al.: The significance of coronary calcification detected by fluoroscopy: A report of 360 patients. Circulation *49*:1247, 1974.

54. Duerinckx, A. J., and Higgins, C. B.: Valvular heart disease. Radiol. Clin. North Am. *32*:613, 1994.

55. Bordeleau, R. P.: Cardiac valve reconstruction and replacement: A brief review. Radiographics *12*:659, 1992.

56. Van der Jagt, E. J., and Smits, H. J.: Cardiac size in the supine chest film. Eur. J. Radiol. *14*:173, 1992.

57. Kabala, J. E., and Wilde, P.: Measurement of heart size in the anteroposterior chest radiograph. Br. J. Radiol. *60*:981, 1987.

58. Gammill, S. L., Krebs, C., Meyers, P., et al.: Cardiac measurements in systole and diastole. Radiology *94*:115, 1970.

59. Glover, L., Baxley, W. A., and Dodge, H. T.: A quantitative evaluation of heart size measurements from chest roentgenograms. Circulation *47*:1289, 1973.

60. Milne, E. N. C., Burnett, K., Aufrichtig, D., et al.: Assessment of cardiac size on portable chest films. J. Thorac. Imaging *3*:64, 1988.

61. Peerry, M. M., Irfan, A. Y., Simmons, S. P., et al.: Heart size in high-kilovoltage chest radiography. Clin. Radiol. *36*:335, 1985.

62. Righetti, A., Crawford, M. H., O'Rourke, R. A., et al.: Echocardiographic and roentgenographic determination of left ventricular size after coronary arterial bypass graft surgery. Chest *72*:455, 1977.

63. West, J. B.: Regional differences in gas exchange in the lung in erect man. J. Appl. Physiol. *17*:893, 1963.

64. Milne, E. N. C.: A physiological approach to reading critical care unit films. J. Thorac. Imaging *1*:60, 1986.

65. Chang, C. H.: The normal roentgenographic measurement of the right descending artery in 1085 cases. A.J.R. *87*:929, 1962.

66. Gutierrez, F. R., Moran, C. J., Ludbrook, P. A., et al.: Pulmonary arterial calcification with reversible pulmonary hypertension. A.J.R. *135*:177, 1980.

67. Harrison, M. O., Conte, P. J., and Heitzman, E. R.: Radiological detection of clinically occult cardiac failure following myocardial infarction. Br. J. Radiol. *44*:265, 1971.

68. Auger, W. R., Fedullo, P. F., Moser, K. M., et al.: Chronic major vessel thromboembolic pulmonary artery obstruction appearance at angiography. Radiology *182*:393, 1992.

69. Milne, E. N. C., Pistolesi, M., Miniati, M., et al.: The radiologic distinction of cardiogenic and noncardiogenic edema. A.J.R. *144*:879, 1985.

70. Chen, J. T. T., Behar, V. S., Morris, J. J., Jr., et al.: Correlation of roentgen findings with hemodynamic data in pure mitral stenosis. A.J.R. *102*:280, 1968.

71. Herman, P. C., Khan, A., Kallman, C. E., et al.: Limited correlation of left ventricular end-diastolic pressure with radiographic assessment of pulmonary hemodynamics. Radiology *174*:721, 1990.

72. Tanaka, F., Hayakawa, K., Satol, Y., et al.: Evaluating bronchial drainage in patients with lung disease using digital subtraction and angiography. Invest. Radiol. *28*:434, 1993.

73. Chen, J. T. T., Robinson, A. E., Goodrich, F. K., et al.: Uneven distribution of pulmonary blood flow between left and right lungs in isolated valvular pulmonary stenosis. A.J.R. *107*:343, 1969.

74. Grainger, R. G.: Interstitial pulmonary oedema and its radiological diagnosis. A sign of pulmonary venous and capillary hypertension. Br. J. Radiol. *31*:201, 1958.

75. Kerley, P. J.: Radiology in heart disease. Br. Med. J. *2*:594, 1933.

76. Milne, E. N. C., Pistolesi, M., Miniati, M., et al.: The vascular pedicle of the heart and the vena azygos. I: The normal subject. Radiology *152*:1, 1984.

77. Pistoles, M., Milne, E. N. C., Miniati, M., et al.: The vascular pedicle and the vena azygos. II: Acquired heart disease. Radiology *152*:9, 1984.

CARDIAC CALCIFICATION

78. Soulen, R. L., and Freeman, E.: Radiologic evaluation of traumatic heart disease. Radiol. Clin. North Am. *9*:285, 1971.

79. Lasser, A.: Calcification of the myocardium. Hum. Pathol. *14*:824, 1983.

80. Leonard, J. J., Katz, S., and Nelson, D.: Calcification of the left atrium: Its anatomic location, diagnostic significance, and roentgenologic demonstration. N. Engl. J. Med. *256*:629, 1957.

81. Matsuyama, S., Watabe, T., Kuribayashi, S., et al.: Plain film diagnosis of thrombosis of left atrial appendage in mitral valve disease. Radiology *146*:15, 1983.

82. Rodan, B. A., Chen, J. T. T., Halber, M. D., et al.: Chest roentgenographic evaluation of the severity of aortic stenosis. Invest. Radiol. *17*:453, 1982.

82a. Lippert, J. A., White, C. S., Mason, A. C., and Plotnick, G. D.: Calcification of aortic valve detected incidentally on CT scans: prevalence and clinical significance. A.J.R. *164*:73, 1995.

83. Pounder, D. J.: Calcification of the mitral annulus and its complications. Am. J. Forensic Med. Pathol. *3*:109, 1982.

84. Osterberger, L. E., Goldstein, S., Khaja, F., and Lakier, J. B.: Functional mitral stenosis in patients with massive annular calcification. Circulation *64*:472, 1981.

85. Spindola-Franco, H., and Fish, B. G.: Radiology of the Heart. New York, Springer-Verlag, 1985, p. 259.

86. Rogers, J. V., Chandler, N. W., and Franch, R. H.: Calcification of the tricuspid annulus. A.J.R. *106*:550, 1969.

87. Roberts, W. C., and Waller, B. F.: Mitral valve "anular" calcium forming a complete circle or "O" configuration. Clinical and necropsy observations. Am. Heart J. *101*:619, 1981.

88. Fulkerson, P. K., Beaver, B. M., Auseon, J. C., et al.: Calcification of the mitral annulus: Etiology, clinical associations, complications, and therapy. Am. J. Med. *66*:967, 1979.

89. Aldrich, R. F., Brensike, J. F., Battaglini, J. W., et al.: Coronary calcification in the detection of coronary artery disease and comparison with electrocardiographic exercise testing. Circulation *59*:113, 1979.

90. Stanford, W., Rooholamini, M., Rumberger, J., et al.: Evaluation of coronary bypass graft patency by ultrafast computed tomography. J. Thorac. Imaging *3*(2):52, 1988.

91. Stanford, W., Thompson, B. H., and Weiss, R. M.: Coronary artery calcification: Clinical significance and current methods of detection. A.J.R. *161*:1139, 1993.

92. Shemesh, J., Tenenbaum, A., Fisman, E. Z., et al.: Coronary calcium as a reliable tool for differentiating ischemic from nonischemic cardiomyopathy. Am. J. Cardiol. *77*:191, 1996.

93. Moore, E. H., Greenberg, R. W., Merrick, S. H., et al.: Coronary artery calcifications: Significance of incidental detection on CT scans. Radiology *172*:711, 1989.

94. Sharma, S., Rajani, M., and Talwar, K. K.: Angiographic morphology in

nonspecific aortoarteritis (Takayasu's arteritis). Cardiovasc. Intervent. Radiol. *15*:160, 1992.

95. Nomeir, A. M., Watts, L. E., Seagle, R., et al.: Intracardiac myxomas: Twenty-year echocardiographic experience with review of the literature. J. Am. Soc. Echocardiogr. *2*:139, 1989.

96. Pucillo, A. L., Schechter, A. G., Kay, R. H., et al.: Identification of calcified intracardiac lesions using gradient echo MR imaging. J. Comput. Assist. Tomogr. *14*:743, 1990.

96a. Masui, T., Takahashi, M., Miura, K., et al. Cardiac myxoma: Identification of intratumoral hemorrhage and calcification on MR images. A.J.R. *164*:850, 1995.

97. McComb, B. L., and Steiner, R. M.: Pericardial disease. *In* Goodman, L., and Putman, C. (eds.): Critical Care Imaging. 3rd. ed. Philadelphia, W.B. Saunders Co., 1992.

98. Moncada, R., Baker, M., Salinas, M., et al.: Diagnostic role of computed tomography in pericardial heart disease: Congenital defects, thickening, neoplasms and effusions. Am. Heart J. *103*:263, 1982.

99. Crawley, I. S.: Noninvasive diagnosis of pericardial disease. *In* Miller, D. D., Burns, R. J., Gill, J. B., Ruddy, T. D. (eds.): Clinical Cardiac Imaging. New York, McGraw-Hill, 1988, p. 521.

100. Doppman, J. L., Rienmuller, R., Lissner, J., et al.: Computed tomography in constrictive pericardial disease. J. Comput. Assist. Tomogr. *5*:1, 1981.

ACQUIRED HEART DISEASE

101. Braunwald, E., Morrow, A. G., Cornell, W. P., et al.: Idiopathic hypertrophic subaortic stenosis: Clinical, hemodynamic and angiographic manifestations. Am. J. Med. *29*:924, 1960.

102. Lipton, M. J.: Quantitation of cardiac function by cine CT. Radiol. Clin. North Am. *23*:613, 1985.

103. de Roos, A., Reichek, N., Axel, L., et al.: Cine MR imaging in aortic stenosis. J. Comput. Assist. Tomogr. *13*:421, 1989.

104. Utz, J. A., Herfkens, R. J., Heinsimer, J. A., et al.: Valvular regurgitation: Dynamic MR imaging. Radiology *168*:91, 1988.

105. Raphael, M. J.: Acquired valvular heart disease. *In* Grainger, R. G., and Allison, J. (eds.): Diagnostic Radiology. 2nd ed. London, Churchill Livingstone, 1992.

106. Follman, D. F.: Aortic regurgitation. Postgrad. Med. *93*:1, 1993.

107. Probst, P., Goldschlager, N., and Selzer, A.: Left atrial size and atrial fibrillation in mitral stenosis: Factors influencing their relationship. Circulation *48*:1282, 1973.

108. Green, C. E., Kelley, M. J., and Higgins, C. B.: Etiologic significance of enlargement of the left atrial appendage in adults. Radiology *142*:21, 1982.

109. Sharma, S., Kumar, M. V., Aggarwal, S., et al.: Chest radiographs are unreliable in predicting thrombi in the left atrium or its appendage in rheumatic mitral stenosis. Clin. Radiol. *43*:337, 1991.

110. Gurney, J. W., and Goodman, L. R.: Pulmonary edema localized to the right upper lobe accompanying mitral regurgitation. Radiology *171*:397, 1989.

111. Raphael, M. J., Steiner, R. E., and Raftery, E. B.: Acute mitral incompetence. Clin. Radiol. *18*:126, 1967.

112. Schnyder, P., Sarraj, A. M., Duvoisin, B. E., et al.: Pulmonary edema associated with mitral regurgitation. A.J.R. *161*:33, 1993.

113. Rubin, S. A., Hightower, C. W., and Flicker, S.: Giant right atrium after mitral valve replacement: Plain film findings in 15 patients. A.J.R. *149*:257, 1987.

114. Gal, R. A., Shalev, Y., and Schmidt, D. H.: Mitral regurgitation: Parameters that affect the correlation between Doppler echocardiography and contrast ventriculography. Int. J. Cardiol. *28*:87, 1990.

115. Higgins, C. B., and Lipton, M. J.: Radiography of acute myocardial infarction. Radiol. Clin. North Am. *18*:359, 1980.

116. Watanabe, A. M.: Ischemic heart disease. *In* Kelly, N. W. (ed.): Essentials of Internal Medicine. Philadelphia, J. B. Lippincott, 1994.

117. Revel, D., and Higgins, C. B.: Magnetic resonance imaging of ischemic heart disease. Radiol. Clin. North Am. *23*:719, 1985.

118. Björk, L.: Radiology in diagnosis of mitral valve prolapse. Ann. Radiol. *245*:327, 1981.

119. Oliva, P. B., Hammill, S. C., and Edwards, W. D.: Cardiac rupture, a clinically predictable complication of acute myocardial infarction: Report of 70 cases with clinicopathologic correlations. J. Am. Coll. Cardiol. *22*:720, 1993.

120. Topaz, O., DiSciascio, G., and Vetrovec, G. W.: Acute ventricular septal rupture: Perspectives on the current role of ventriculography and coronary arteriography and their implication for surgical repair. Am. Heart J. *120*:412, 1990.

121. Higgins, C. B., Lipton, M. J., Johnson, A. D., et al.: False aneurysms of the left ventricle. Radiology *127*:21, 1978.

122. Johnson, R. A., and Palacios, I.: Dilated cardiomyopathies of the adult. N. Engl. J. Med. *307*:1051, 1119, 1982.

123. Sardenelli, F., Molinari, G., Petillo, A., et al.: MRI in hypertrophic cardiomyopathy: Morphofunctional study. J. Comput. Assist. Tomogr. *17*:862, 1993.

124. Higgins, C. B., Byrd, B. F., III, and Stark, D.: Magnetic resonance imaging in hypertrophic cardiomyopathy. Am. J. Cardiol. *55*:1121, 1985.

125. Wojtowicz, J., Pawlak, B., Lehman, Z., et al.: Cardiac chambers and their walls in cardiomyopathies as evaluated with CT. Eur. J. Radiol. *4*:93, 1984.

126. Bisset, G. S., III, and Meyer, R. A.: Obstructive left heart lesions. Semin. Roentgenol. *20*:244, 1985.

127. Chiles, C., Adams, G. W., and Ravin, C. E.: Radiographic manifestations of cardiac sarcoid. A.J.R. *145*:711, 1985.

POSTOPERATIVE CARDIAC RADIOLOGY

128. Goodman, L. R.: Postoperative chest radiograph: II. Alterations after major intrathoracic surgery. A.J.R. *134*:803, 1980.

129. Tocino, I. M., Miller, M. H., and Fairfax, W. R.: Distribution of pneumothorax in the supine and semi-recumbent critically ill adult. A.J.R. *144*:901, 1985.

130. Katzberg, R. W., Whitehouse, G. H., and deWeese, J. A.: The early radiologic findings in the adult chest after cardiopulmonary bypass surgery. Cardiovasc. Radiol. *1*:205, 1978.

131. Henry, D. A., Jolles, H., Berberich, J. J., and Schmelzer, V.: The post-cardiac surgery chest radiograph: A clinically integrated approach. J. Thorac. Imaging *4*:20, 1989.

132. Harris, R. S.: The preoperative chest film in relation to postoperative management—some effects of different projection, posture and lung inflation. Br. J. Radiol. *53*:96, 1950.

133. Steiner, R. M., Tegtmeyer, C. J., Morse, D., et al.: Radiology of cardiac pacemakers. Radiographics *6*:373, 1986.

134. Goodman, L. R., Conrardy, P. A., Laing, F., et al.: Radiologic evaluation of endotracheal tube position. A.J.R. *127*:433, 1976.

135. Thorsen, M. K., and Goodman, L. R.: Extracardiac complications of cardiac surgery. Semin. Roentgenol. *23*:32, 1988.

136. Landay, M. J., Mootz, A. R., and Estrera, A. S.: Apparatus seen on chest radiographs after cardiac surgery in adults. Radiology *174*:477, 1990.

137. Dieden, J. D., Friloux, L. A., and Renner, J. W.: Pulmonary artery false aneurysms secondary to Swan-Ganz pulmonary artery catheters. A.J.R. *149*:901, 1987.

138. Ramsen, W. H., Coehn, A. T., and Blanshard, K. S.: Case report: Central venous catheter fracture due to compression between the clavicle and first rib. Clin. Radiol. *50*:59, 1995.

139. Anderson, M. H., Ward, D. E., Camm, A. J., and Wilson, A.: Radiological appearance of implantable defibrillator systems. Clin. Radiol. *50*:29, 1995.

140. Peng, M-J., Vargas, F. S., Cukier, A., et al.: Postoperative pleural changes after coronary revascularization. Chest *10*:32, 1992.

141. Wheeler, W. E., Rubis, L. J., and Jones, C. W.: Etiology and prevention of topical cardiac hypothermia-induced phrenic nerve injury and left lower lobe atelectasis during cardiac surgery. Chest *88*:680, 1985.

142. Kaminsky, M. E., Rodan, B. A., Osborne, D. R., et al.: Postpericardiotomy syndrome. A.J.R. *138*:503, 1982.

143. Ziter, F. M.: Major thoracic dehiscence: Radiographic considerations. Radiology *122*:587, 1977.

144. Josa, M., Siouffi, S. Y., Silverman, A. B., et al.: Pulmonary embolism after cardiac surgery. J. Am. Coll. Cardiol. *21*:990, 1993.

145. Moncada, R., Kotler, M. N., Churchill, R. J., et al.: Multimodality approach to pericardial imaging. *In* Kotler, M. N., and Steiner, R. M. (eds.): Cardiac Imaging: New Technologies and Clinical Applications. Philadelphia, F. A. Davis, 1986, p. 409.

146. Fyke, F. E., Tancredi, R. G., Shub, C., et al.: Detection of intrapericardial hematoma after open heart surgery: The role of echocardiography. J. Am Coll. Cardiol. *5*:1496, 1985.

147. Grossi, E. A., Esposito, R., Harris, L. J., et al.: Sternal wound infections and the use of internal mammary artery grafts. J. Thorac. Cardiovasc. Surg. *102*(3):342, 1991.

148. Goodwin, J. D.: Conventional CT of the aorta. J. Thorac. Imaging *5*:18, 1990.

149. Thorsen, M. K., Goodman, L. R., Sagel, S. S., et al.: Ascending aorta complications of cardiac surgery: CT evaluation. J. Comput. Assist. Tomogr. *10*:219, 1986.

150. Sullivan, K. L., Steiner, R. M., Smullens, S. N., et al.: Pseudoaneurysm of the ascending aorta following cardiac surgery. Chest *93*:138, 1988.

151. Gross, B. H., Shirazi, K. K., and Slater, A. D.: Differentiation of aortic and mitral valve prosthesis based on postoperative frontal chest radiographs. Radiology *149*:389, 1983.

152. Goodwin, J. D., Califf, R. M., Korobkin, M., et al.: Clinical value of coronary bypass graft evaluation with CT. A.J.R. *140*:649, 1983.

153. Sherry, C. S., and Harms, S. E.: MR imaging of pseudoaneurysms in aorticocoronary bypass graft. J. Comput. Assist. Tomogr. *13*(3):426, 1989.

154. White, R., Caputo, G., Mark, A., et al.: Coronary bypass graft patency: Noninvasive evaluation with MR imaging. Radiology *164*:681, 1987.

155. Henry, D. A., Corcoran, H. L., Lewis, T. D., et al.: Orthotopic cardiac transplantation: Evaluation with CT. Radiology *170*:343, 1988.

156. Florence, S. H., Hutton, L. C., McKenzie, F. N., et al.: Cardiac transplantation: Postoperative chest radiographs. J. Can. Assoc. Radiol. *39*:115, 1989.

157. Aherne, T., Tscholakoff, D., Finkbeiner, W., et al.: Magnetic resonance imaging of cardiac transplants: The evaluation of rejection of cardiac allografts with and without immunosuppression. Circulation *74*(1):145, 1986.

158. Griffith, J. P., Hardesty, R. L., Trento, A., et al.: Heart-lung transplantation: Lessons learned and future hopes. Ann. Thorac. Surg. *43*:6, 1987.

159. Bonser, R. S., Fragomeni, L. S. U., and Jamieson, S. W.: Heart-lung transplantation. Invest. Radiol. *24*:310, 1989.

160. Holland, S. A., Hutton, L. C., and McKenzie, F. N.: Radiologic findings in heart-lung transplantation: A preliminary experience. J. Can. Assoc. Radiol. *40*:94, 1989.

161. Martin, E. C., Stratford, M. A., and Gersony, W. M.: Initial detection of

coarctation of the aorta: An opportunity for the radiologist. A.J.R. *127*:1015, 1981.

162. Gross, G. W., and Steiner, R. M.: Radiologic manifestations of congenital heart disease in the adult patient. Radiol. Clin. North Am. *29*:293, 1991.

163. Perloff, J. K., and Child, J. S.: Congenital Heart Disease in Adults. Philadelphia, W. B. Saunders Co., 1991.

164. Perloff, J. K.: Congenital heart disease in the adult: Clinical approach. J. Thorac. Imaging *9*:260, 1994.

165. Greenberg, B., Balsara, R. K., and Faerber, E. N.: Coarctation of the aorta: Diagnostic imaging after corrective surgery. J. Thorac. Imaging *10*:36, 1995.

166. Chen, J. T. T., Khoury, M., and Kirks, D. R.: Obscured aortic arch on the lateral view as a sign of coarctation. Radiology *153*:595, 1984.

167. Woodring, J. H., and Rhodes, R. A.: Posterior superior mediastinal widening in aortic coarctation. A.J.R. *144*:23, 1985.

168. Gomes, A. S.: MR imaging of congenital anomalies of the thoracic aorta and pulmonary arteries. Radiol. Clin. North Am. *27*:1171, 1989.

169. Wexler, L., Higgins, C. B., and Herfkens, R. J.: Magnetic resonance imaging in adult congenital heart disease. J. Thorac. Imaging *9*:219, 1994.

170. Whittemore, R., Wells, J. A., and Castellsague, X.: A second-generation study of 427 probands with congenital heart disease and their 837 children. J. Am. Coll. Cardiol. *23*:1459, 1994.

171. Green, C. E., Gottdiener, J. S., and Goldstein, H. A.: Atrial septal defect. Semin. Roentgenol. *20*:214, 1985.

171a. Eichhorn, P., Vogt, P., Ritter, M., et al.: Malformations of the interatrial septum: Recognition, prevalence and clinical relevance in adults. Schweiz. Med. Wochenschr. *125*:1336, 1995.

172. Sanders, C., Bittner, V., Nath, P. H., et al.: Atrial septal defects in older adults: Atypical radiographic appearances. Radiology *167*:123, 1988.

173. Soto, B., Bergeron, L. M., Jr., and Dethlein, E.: Ventricular septal defect. Semin. Roentgenol. *20*:200, 1985.

174. Hoeffel, J. C., Dally, P., Legras, B., et al.: Roentgen aspects of isolated pulmonary valvular stenosis. Radiology *26*:248, 1986.

175. Guit, G. L., Kroon, H. M., Van Voorthuisen, A., et al.: Congenitally corrected transposition in adults with left atrioventricular valve incompetence. Radiology *155*:567, 1985.

176. Takasugi, J. E., Godwin, J. D., and Chen, J. T. T.: CT in congenitally corrected transposition of the great vessels. Comput. Radiol. *11*:215, 1987.

177. Soulen, R. L., Donner, R. M., and Capitanio, M.: Postoperative evaluation of complex congenital heart disease by magnetic resonance imaging. Radiographics *7*:975, 1987.

178. Greenberg, B., Faerber, E. N., and Balsara, R. K.: Tetralogy of Fallot: Diagnostic imaging after palliative and corrective surgery. J. Thorac. Imaging *10*:26, 1995.

179. Deutsch, V., Wexler, L., Blieden, L. C., et al.: Ebstein's anomaly of tricuspid valve: Critical review of roentgenological features and additional angiographic signs. A.J.R. *125*:395, 1985.

180. Mu-sheng, T., Partridge, J., and Radford, D.: The plain film chest radiograph in uncomplicated Ebstein's disease. Clin. Radiol. *37*:551, 1986.

THE PERICARDIUM

181. Levy-Ravetch, M., Auh, Y. H., Rubenstein, W. A., et al.: CT of the pericardial recesses. A.J.R. *144*:707, 1985.

182. Carsky, E. W., Mauceri, R. A., and Azimi, R.: The epicardial fat pad sign. Radiology *137*:303, 1980.

183. Steiner, R. M., and Rao, V. M.: Radiology of the pericardium. *In* Grainger, R. G., and Allison, J. (eds.): Diagnostic Radiology. London, Churchill Livingstone, 1991.

184. Olson, M. C., Posniak, H. V., McDonald, V., et al.: Computed tomography and magnetic resonance imaging of the pericardium. Radiographics *9*:633, 1989.

185. Miller, S. W.: Imaging pericardial disease. Radiol. Clin. North Am. *27*:1113, 1989.

186. Boxt, L. M., and Katz, J.: Effect of drugs on the radiographic appearance of the heart. J. Thorac. Imaging *6*(1):76, 1991.

187. Vaitkus, P. T., and Kussmaul, W. G.: Constrictive pericarditis versus restrictive cardomyopathy: A reappraisal and update of diagnostic criteria. Am. Heart J. *122*:1431, 1991.

188. Engel, P. J.: Echocardiography in pericardial disease. Cardiovasc. Clin. *13*(2):181, 1993.

189. Brown, J. J., Barakos, J. A., and Higgins, C. B.: Magnetic resonance imaging of cardiac and paracardiac masses. J. Thorac. Imaging *4*(2):58, 1989.

190. Sechtem, U., Tscholakoff, D., and Higgins, C. B.: MRI of the abnormal pericardium. A.J.R. *147*:245, 1986.

191. Sutton, F. J., Whitley, N. O., and Applefield, M. M.: The role of echocardiography and computed tomography in the evaluation of constrictive pericarditis. Am. Heart J. *109*:350, 1985.

191a. Protopapas, Z., and Westcott, J. L.: Left pulmonic recess of the pericardium: Findings at CT and MR imaging. Radiology *196*:85, 1995.

192. Gutierrez, F. R., Shackelford, G. D., McKnight, R. C., et al.: Diagnosis of congenital absence of left pericardium by MR imaging. J. Comput. Assist. Tomogr. *9*:551, 1985.

193. Decanay, S., Hsieh, A. M., Fitzgerald, S. W., et al.: Diagnosis of congenital absence of the left pericardium. Am. J. Card. Imaging *6*:267, 1992.

194. Vinee, P., Stover, B., Sigmund, G., et al.: MR imaging of the pericardial cyst. J. Magn. Reson. Imaging *2*:593, 1992.

195. Feigin, D. S., Fenoglio, J. J., McAllister, H. A., et al.: Pericardial cysts. A radiologic-pathologic correlation and review. Radiology *125*:15, 1977.

196. Ellis, K., Malm, J. R., Bowman, F. O., Jr., and King, D. L.: Roentgenographic findings after pericardial surgery. *9*:327, 1971.

Chapter 8
Coronary Arteriography

JOHN A. BITTL, DAVID C. LEVIN

Coronary arteriography is the imaging method of choice for establishing the presence or absence of coronary artery disease and for providing the most reliable information for making critical decisions about the need for medical therapy, angioplasty, or bypass surgery. First performed by Sones in 1959,[1] coronary arteriography has become one of the most widely performed and accurate tests in cardiovascular medicine. Almost one million coronary arteriograms are performed every year in the United States[2] in 1537 of the 6044 acute care hospitals (25 per cent).[3] The growing use of coronary arteriography over the past 35 years has increased the need for universal standards to ensure optimal utilization and performance of this procedure.[4] Although the original purpose of coronary arteriography was limited to defining the presence or absence of significant narrowings in the epicardial coronary arteries, newer interventional cardiovascular therapies have increased the importance of precise anatomical assessment of lesion characteristics before and after interventional cardiovascular procedures, thus placing greater demands on the angiographer for ensuring high-quality imaging with optimal spatial and contrast resolution. The physician performing coronary arteriography should thus be an expert in angiography and in cardiovascular medicine and must consult carefully with the referring physician before carrying out the procedure. The aims of this chapter are to provide the serious angiographer with a discussion of the indications and techniques of coronary arteriography with emphasis on interventional arteriography, to present a detailed review of normal and pathological coronary anatomy, and to highlight the relations between coronary arteriographic anatomy and clinical outcome.

INDICATIONS FOR CORONARY ARTERIOGRAPHY

The primary indications for coronary arteriography are to establish the presence or absence of coronary artery disease, define therapeutic options, and determine prognosis (see Table 63–6, p. 3012). Coronary arteriography is thus recommended for patients with a history of stable angina refractory to medical management. Patients with a history of angina and an exercise treadmill test showing high-risk features such as hypotension, more than 2 mm of ST-segment depression associated with decreased exercise capac-

ity,[5] or myocardial perfusion scanning showing increased lung uptake or multiple perfusion defects ordinarily should undergo coronary arteriography.[6] Coronary arteriography is also recommended for middle-aged and older patients scheduled to undergo surgery for valvular heart disease or congenital heart disease. Patients with a history of angina or provocable ischemia who are scheduled for vascular surgery should undergo coronary arteriography.

Coronary arteriography is important in certain patients who present with chest pain of unclear etiology. In patients with cardiac risk factors and chest pain atypical for angina, the finding of angiographically normal coronary arteries provides important information about therapy and prognosis. The diagnosis of coronary artery spasm relies on the clinical presentation, but coronary arteriography remains useful in patients with clinical evidence of coronary spasm to exclude the presence of fixed atherosclerotic lesions (see p. 264). Provocative testing for coronary artery spasm with ergonovine has recently been reintroduced in the United States. Provocative testing with other agents such as acetylcholine is too sensitive, because coronary artery spasm can be provoked in almost all patients with coronary atherosclerosis.[7]

Patients with unstable angina often require urgent coronary arteriography (see p. 288). Recurrent symptoms after initial medical management are an indication of refractory unstable angina and should initiate the referral for urgent coronary arteriography. Coronary arteriography should be carried out in most patients judged to be at high risk for complications of unstable angina, including those with prolonged chest pain lasting more than 20 minutes, pulmonary edema, new mitral regurgitation, dynamic ST-segment changes, S_3 or rales, hypotension, impaired left ventricular function with an ejection fraction of less than 50 per cent, or significant ventricular arrhythmias or atrioventricular block.[8] The rationale for using coronary arteriography in patients with unstable angina is supported by the Thrombolysis in Myocardial Ischemia (TIMI) IIIB study.[9] Although major complications of death or myocardial infarction, or positive exercise tests occurred with similar frequencies in patients randomized to early coronary arteriography and in patients managed conservatively, fewer postdischarge procedures and hospitalizations were required in the patients who underwent early coronary arteriography (7.8 versus 14.1 per cent; P < 0.001).[9] Thus patients managed with early diagnostic coronary arteriography and revascularization techniques had greater relief of angina without increasing the risk of major complications. Coronary arteriography also should be carried out in most patients with unstable angina if they have had prior angioplasty or bypass surgery.

Coronary arteriography is performed increasingly in the setting of acute myocardial infarction without antecedent thrombolytic therapy as a prelude to direct angioplasty because of reports that direct angioplasty results in a greater reduction in the incidence of death or nonfatal reinfarction at 6 weeks as compared with thrombolytic therapy[10] (see p. 1221). Coronary arteriography is also performed increasingly as a prelude to "rescue" angioplasty in patients who have received thrombolytic therapy but show no evidence of reperfusion[11] (see p. 1221). Coronary arteriography should be performed in many patients with non-Q-wave myocardial infarction or when myocardial infarction is complicated by congestive heart failure, cardiac arrest, mitral regurgitation, or ventricular septal rupture. Patients with angina or provocable ischemia after myocardial infarction also benefit from coronary arteriography, because revascularization may reduce the high risk of reinfarction in this group of patients.[5]

Coronary arteriography is commonly performed annually in patients after cardiac transplantation in the absence of clinical symptoms because of the diffuse nature of graft atherosclerosis[12] (see p. 525). Coronary arteriography is useful in potential donors for cardiac transplantation whose age or cardiac risk profile increases the likelihood of coronary artery disease. Coronary arteriography often provides important diagnostic information about the presence of coronary artery disease in patients with intractable arrhythmias who are scheduled to undergo electrophysiological testing. Coronary arteriography is also useful for establishing the presence of coronary artery disease associated with ischemic cardiomyopathy in patients with dilated cardiomyopathy of unknown etiology. Patients with severe coronary artery disease and impaired left ventricular function may benefit from revascularization.

Contraindications to coronary arteriography include unexplained fever, untreated infection, severe anemia with hemoglobin less than 8 gm/dl, severe electrolyte imbalance, severe active bleeding, uncontrolled systemic hypertension, digitalis toxicity, previous contrast material allergy but no pretreatment with glucocorticoids, and active stroke. Risk factors for significant complications after catheterization include advanced age, as well as several general medical, vascular, and cardiac characteristics (Table 8–1). Patients with these characteristics should be monitored closely after coronary arteriography for a minimum of 18 to 24 hours.

PREPARATION OF THE PATIENT

The optimal timing of coronary arteriography is one of the most important features of the diagnostic management of patients with coronary artery disease. The study should be performed at a time when problems such as congestive heart failure, renal failure, or mental status changes are stable or improving. Otherwise, the risk of complications increases. Under many circumstances, however, coronary arteriography must be performed under emergency conditions with increased risk of complications. The study should be performed after careful consultation between the referring physician and the angiographer so that all important information can be obtained from the procedure. Under all circumstances, the physician performing the study must review the history, physical examination, and laboratory data and then obtain informed consent from the patient after describing the procedure and explaining its benefits and potential complications.

A baseline electrocardiogram, measurement of serum electrolytes and creatinine, complete blood count, and coagulation parameters must be obtained and reviewed, ideally within 24 hours before the procedure. All cardiac medications, including aspirin, should be continued before the procedure. Warfarin sodium should be discontinued 2 days before elective coronary arteriography is performed. Elective studies can be undertaken safely when the international normalized ratio (INR) is less than 2.0. For patients at increased risk for systemic thromboembolism upon withdrawal of warfarin sodium, such as those with atrial fibrillation and mitral stenosis or those with a prior history of systemic thromboembolism, admission to the hospital 1 day before the procedure for full heparinization is necessary.

Coronary arteriography is often performed along with other invasive procedures such as right-heart catheterization or left ventriculography at the time of cardiac catheterization. The sequence of procedures depends on priority. For patients in whom the diagnosis or treatment of coronary artery disease is the primary indication for cardiac catheterization, coronary arteriography should be performed before left ventriculography. For patients with valvular or congenital heart disease, on the other hand, hemodynamic measurements, oximetric determinations, and left ventriculography or aortography should be performed before coronary arteriography.

TECHNIQUE OF CORONARY ARTERIOGRAPHY

Equipment for Coronary Arteriography

JUDKINS CATHETERS. The Judkins catheters are shaped specifically to aid entry into the coronary ostia (Fig. 8–1). The catheters are constructed of polyethylene or polyurethane with a fine wire braid within the wall to allow advancement and directional control (torque ability) and yet prevent kinking. The size of the catheters ranges from No. 4 French (4F) to 8F (each French number = 0.33 mm in diameter), but 6F catheters are used most commonly. Diagnostic catheter dimensions are given by the outer diameter. Most diagnostic catheters have a 0.45-inch inner lumen diameter.

The shape or configuration of the catheters varies (Fig. 8–2). Selection of catheter shape is based on the body habitus of the patient and size of the aortic root. Whereas the left coronary artery is easily intubated with the Judkins left

TABLE 8–1 PATIENTS AT INCREASED RISK FOR COMPLICATIONS AFTER CORONARY ARTERIOGRAPHY

INCREASED GENERAL MEDICAL RISK
Age >70 years
Complex congenital heart disease
Morbid obesity
General debility or cachexia
Uncontrolled glucose intolerance
Arterial oxygen desaturation
Severe chronic obstructive lung disease
Renal insufficiency with creatinine greater than 1.5 mg/dl

INCREASED CARDIAC RISK
Three-vessel coronary artery disease
Left main coronary artery disease
Functional class IV
Significant mitral or aortic valve disease or mechanical prosthesis
Low ejection fraction less than 35 per cent
High-risk exercise treadmill test results (hypotension or severe ischemia)
Pulmonary hypertension
Pulmonary artery wedge pressure greater than 25 mm Hg

INCREASED VASCULAR RISK
Anticoagulation or bleeding diathesis
Uncontrolled systemic hypertension
Severe peripheral vascular disease
Recent stroke
Severe aortic insufficiency

242

Ch 8

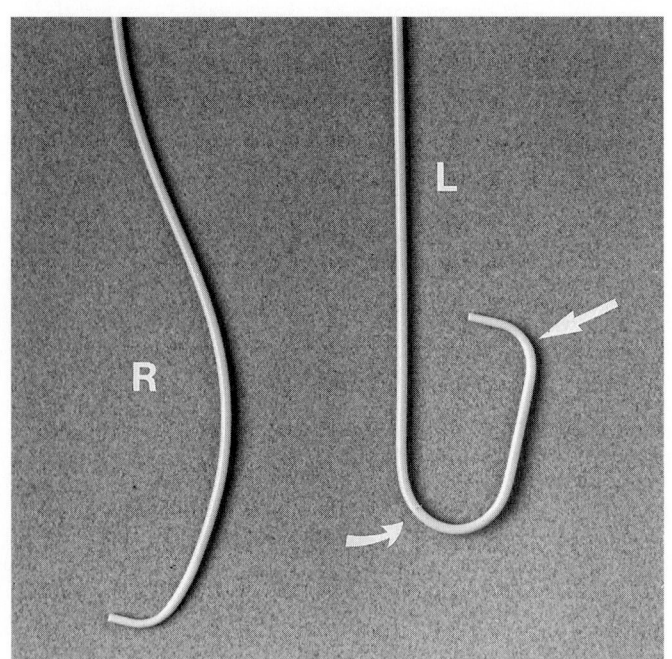

FIGURE 8–1. Judkins catheters. The right (R) and left (L) Judkins are shown. The primary (straight arrow) and secondary (curved arrow) curves of the left Judkins catheter are shown. (Photograph courtesy of Cordis Corporation.)

to folding or re-forming of the catheter. The best technique for removing a re-formed Judkins left catheter from the body involves withdrawing the reshaped catheter into the descending aorta and advancing a guidewire anterograde in the contralateral common iliac artery. Upon withdrawal of the catheter and guidewire together, the catheter will straighten and can be removed safely from the body without disrupting the arterial access site.

AMPLATZ CATHETERS. Amplatz catheters[13] can be used for the femoral or brachial approach to coronary arteriography (Fig. 8–3). Although the Amplatz catheters are used less commonly than the Judkins catheters, they are an excellent alternative in cases in which the Judkins catheter is not appropriately shaped to enter the coronary arteries.

MULTIPURPOSE CATHETERS. A single catheter that can be used for selective left and right coronary arteriography, as well as for left ventriculography, via the femoral approach was originally described by Schoonmaker and King.[14] The catheter shape is similar to that of the Sones catheter, but the tip is shorter (Fig. 8–4). The maneuvers required are also similar to those for the Sones catheter via the brachial approach.

MANIFOLD. The coronary catheter is attached to a three-way manifold, which enables the angiographer to switch among pressure measurement, saline flushing, and contrast injection all in a closed system that allows for speed and maintenance of sterility. In addition to the three side ports, the manifold has a rotating adapter for attachment to the catheter itself, while the other end has a locking fitting to which a fingertip-control syringe is attached for contrast or saline injection.

FEMORAL SHEATH. The Judkins catheters are usually inserted into the femoral artery through a side arm sheath (Fig. 8–5). The sheath is inserted into the femoral artery over a polyethylene dilator, which has been advanced over a guidewire previously inserted in the femoral artery through the entry needle. The sheath is constructed of Teflon and contains a hemostatic valve at its external end. It

4.0 catheter in most patients, patients with a dilated ascending aorta (e.g., in the setting of congenital aortic stenosis and poststenotic dilatation) may require the use of a Judkins left 5.0 or 6.0 catheter, and the patient with an ascending aortic aneurysm may require catheterization with shapes modified by use of a sterile metal guide and steam to achieve a Judkins left 7.0 to 10.0 shape. Use of a Judkins shape that is too small for the ascending aorta often leads

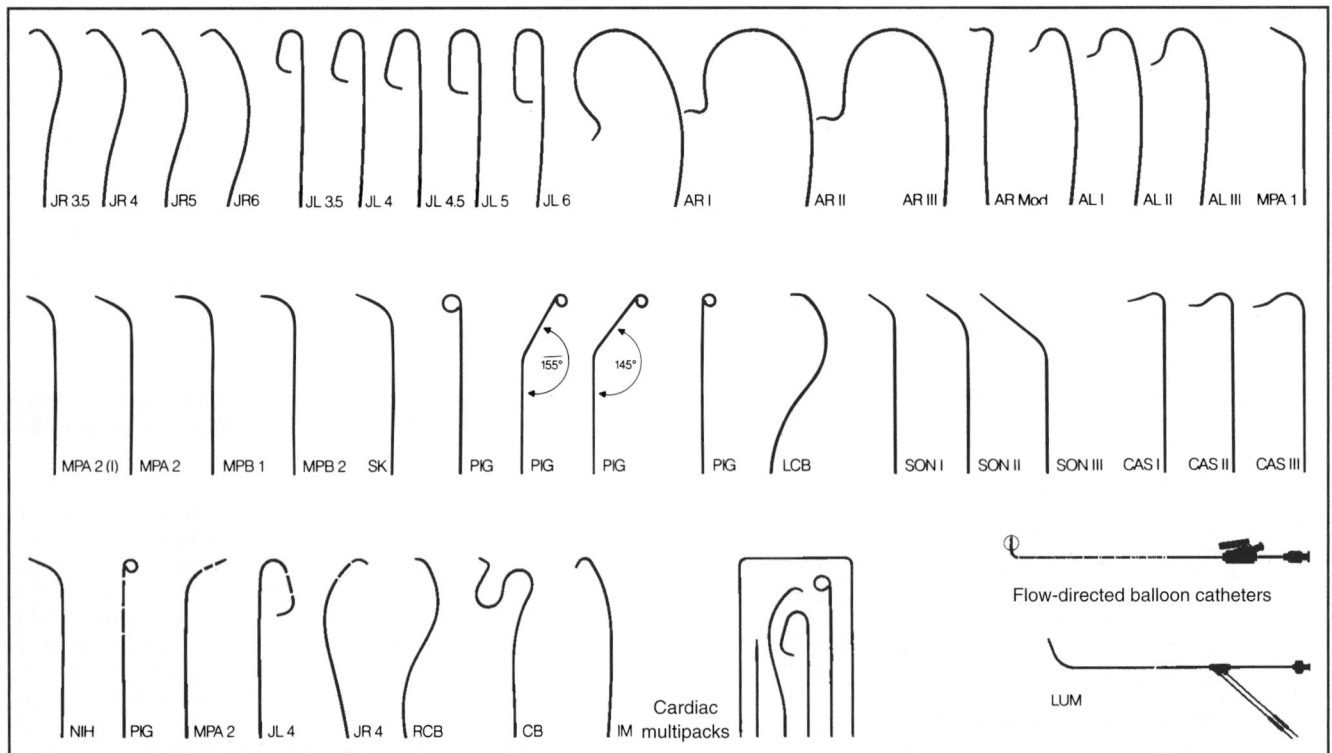

FIGURE 8–2. Coronary catheters. The tip configurations for several catheters useful in coronary arteriography are shown. JR = Judkins right; JL = Judkins left; AR = Amplatz right; Mod = modified; AL = Amplatz left; MP = multipurpose; PIG = pigtail; LCB = left coronary bypass graft; SON = Sones; CAS = Castillo; NIH = National Institutes of Health; RCB = right coronary bypass graft; CB = coronary bypass catheter; IM = internal mammary; LUM = lumen. (Photograph courtesy of Cordis Corporation.)

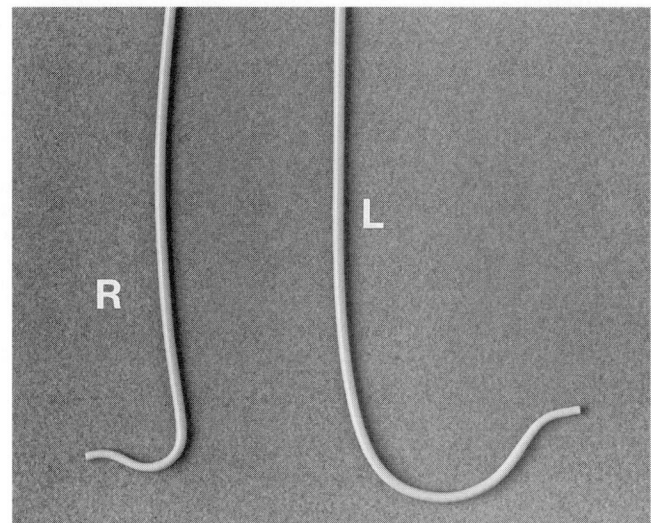

FIGURE 8–3. Amplatz catheters. The right (R) and left (L) Amplatz catheters are shown. (Photograph courtesy of Cordis Corporation.)

also has a side arm through which femoral artery pressure can be measured. The advantage of the sheath is that it permits multiple catheter exchanges without femoral site compression. The inner diameter of the sheath must permit easy passage of the diagnostic catheter, so the outer diameter of the sheath is approximately 1.5F larger than the sheath itself (i.e., a 6F sheath has an outer diameter of approximately 7.5F). Although the sheath requires a larger arteriotomy, the protection provided by the sheath minimizes arterial injury from multiple catheter exchanges and manipulations and reduces patient discomfort from manual compression during catheter exchange.

After the procedure, the sheath can be removed if the patient has not been treated with heparin. Compression of the femoral puncture site manually or with a compression device usually results in stable hemostasis after 20 minutes. Patients can sit up approximately 6 to 8 hours after coronary arteriography if no hematoma or bleeding has developed at the puncture site.

GUIDEWIRES. The standard guidewire for coronary arteriography is the 180-cm, 0.035-inch diameter, Teflon-coated

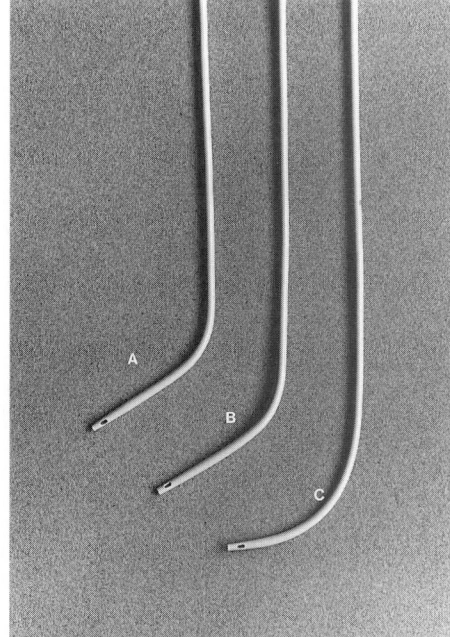

FIGURE 8–4. Multipurpose catheters. The multipurpose A, B, and C type catheters are shown. (Photograph courtesy of Cordis Corporation.)

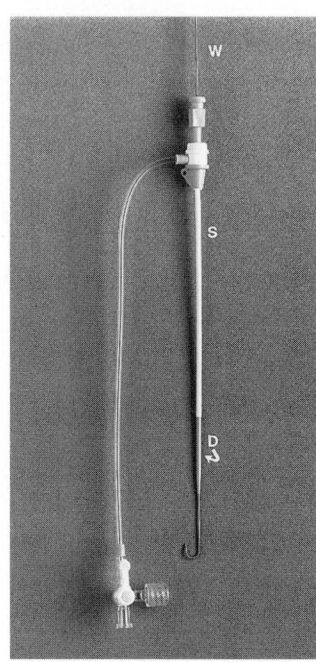

FIGURE 8–5. Side arm sheath. The side arm sheath (S) consists of a dilator (D) for entry into the artery over a guidewire (W). (Photograph courtesy of Cordis Corporation.)

guidewire with a 3-mm J-tip. The J configuration allows the guidewire to be advanced atraumatically through most iliac and brachial arteries. Occasionally, a 0.15-mm J-tip is required for advancement through small brachial arteries. In the presence of atherosclerotic disease in the iliac or subclavian arteries, other wire configurations such as those containing either a 15-mm J-tip, a long floppy distal segment, or a hydrophilic coating are required for successful passage.

Catheterization of the Coronary Arteries

FEMORAL APPROACH. A combination of physical and radiographic landmarks is used to identify the common femoral artery for arterial puncture. The common femoral artery should be punctured several centimeters below the inguinal ligament at the point of maximal impulse by palpation (Fig. 6–3, p. 183). This is usually located approximately 1 to 2 cm below the inguinal crease, which has a variable relation with the inguinal ligament. To confirm the location of the common femoral artery, the radiographic landmark of the femoral head is very useful. With 1 to 2 seconds of fluoroscopy, the course of the common femoral artery across the junction between the middle and medial thirds of the femoral head can be ascertained. If the puncture site is proximal to the inguinal ligament, hemostasis after the procedure may be impossible to achieve with manual compression, and retroperitoneal hemorrhage may ensue. If the puncture site is at the bifurcation of the common femoral artery, a pseudoaneurysm may appear.

After infiltration of the skin, subcutaneous tissue, and perivascular space surrounding and deep to the common femoral artery with 1 per cent lidocaine, the common femoral artery is entered either upon withdrawal of the Seldinger needle (Fig. 6–6, p. 185) or advancement of an 18-gauge thin-walled needle puncturing only the anterior wall of the artery. The guidewire is then passed through the needle into the aorta. The needle is removed over the guidewire, and the sheath and its dilator are advanced into the vessel with slight rotating motion and firm axial support to prevent buckling. Once the sheath is positioned correctly in the artery, the guidewire and dilator are quickly removed, and the side arm is connected to a two-

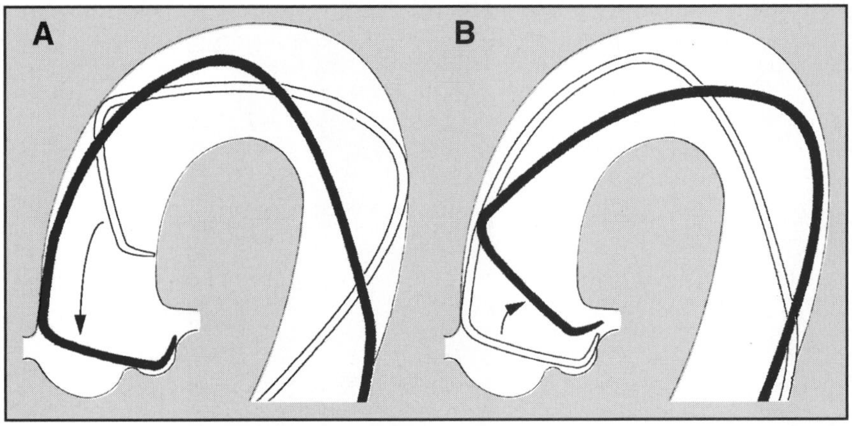

FIGURE 8–6. The push-pull technique for catheterizing the left coronary artery with the Judkins left catheter. In the left anterior oblique view, the coronary catheter is positioned in the ascending aorta over a guidewire, and the guidewire is removed. The catheter is advanced so that the tip enters the left sinus of Valsalva. If the catheter does not selectively enter the ostium of the left coronary artery, further slow advancement forces the tip deep into the left sinus of Valsalva and imparts a temporary acute angle at the catheter tip (A). Prompt withdrawal of the catheter over a short distance allows easy entry into the ostium of the left coronary artery (B).

way manifold for pressure monitoring and flushing of the system with saline.

The guidewire is then loaded into the Judkins coronary catheter so that the flexible tip of the wire protrudes beyond the tip of the catheter. The guidewire is barely retracted into the catheter, and both are inserted together through the femoral sheath. The guidewire is then advanced from the femoral sheath into the aorta under fluoroscopic guidance, and both the guidewire and catheter are advanced together to the ascending aorta. After the guidewire has been advanced to the aortic valve, its position is fixed while the catheter tip is advanced to a position approximately 10 cm above the aortic valve in the ascending aorta. The guidewire is removed, blood is aspirated from the catheter and discarded, and the catheter is connected to the three-way manifold and flushed with saline to remove all traces of blood or air bubbles.

To catheterize either coronary artery, the angiographer should position the image intensifier so that the patient's heart is viewed in the left anterior oblique (LAO) view. Viewed in this position, the left main coronary artery (LMCA) originates from the left sinus of Valsalva, while the right coronary artery (RCA) originates from the right side of the aorta (Fig. 8–6). From a true anatomical point of view, the LMCA originates from the left posterolateral aspect of the aorta, while the RCA originates from its anterior part inferior to the origin of the LMCA (for abbreviations, see Table 8–2).

Other Approaches to Coronary Arteriography

BRACHIAL TECHNIQUE

The brachial artery can be approached by cutdown with blunt dissection or by percutaneous entry. If cutdown is used, the brachial pulsation is identified 1 cm proximal to the antecubital crease, and the skin, subcutaneous tissue, and perivascular tissue are infiltrated carefully with 1 per cent lidocaine to avoid injection of the median nerve or brachial artery itself. The artery is identified, isolated with Silastic tubing, and entered after a small transverse nick is made with a No. 11 blade. A sheath can be inserted into the artery to prevent injury to the vessel during catheter manipulation or exchanges, or the procedure can be carried out without a sheath.

The technique most commonly used from the right brachial artery involves use of the Sones catheter, the multipurpose catheter, or preformed Amplatz catheters. From the left brachial artery, preformed Judkins catheters can be used. The Sones and the multipurpose catheters have an end hole and two to four small side holes near the catheter tip (Fig. 8–4). The multipurpose catheter forms an open loop on the right aortic cusp so that the shaft of the catheter and its tip form a 45-degree angle directed toward the left aortic cusp. Rapid advancement and withdrawal of the catheter will permit entry into the left sinus of Valsalva, and slow advancement with gentle catheter rotation will permit selective engagement of the left coronary ostium.

In some cases, slight withdrawal of the catheter results in deep engagement of the left main coronary artery, which can be detected by observing catheter advancement and the presence of an abnormal pressure recording at the tip of the catheter, and by practicing deep intubation during test injections with small amounts of contrast medium. If deep engagement is detected, the catheter should be withdrawn, and selective arteriography of the left coronary artery may be performed. After left coronary arteriography, the catheter tip is withdrawn into the left sinus of Valsalva. A slightly smaller open loop is formed, and the catheter is rotated clockwise to enter the right sinus of Valsalva anteriorly. Advancement and further rotation will allow the catheter to enter the right coronary artery.

Catheterization of bypass grafts via the brachial artery is straightforward and involves the same catheters used for the femoral approach. Catheterization of the internal mammary artery, however, is most easily performed from the ipsilateral brachial artery. Contralateral catheterization of the left internal mammary artery from the right brachial artery is technically more challenging and may require the use of an H1H or "headhunter" catheter for selective entry into the left subclavian artery.

RADIAL TECHNIQUE. Coronary arteriography can be performed via the radial artery with 5F and 6F catheters in adults. Before the procedure is performed, the Allen test should be carried out to ensure that the ulnar artery is patent.

Drugs Used During Coronary Arteriography

Adequate *premedication* of the patient is important for safe and comfortable coronary arteriography. The goal of premedication is to achieve a state of *conscious sedation*, defined as a "minimally depressed level of consciousness that allows a patient to respond appropriately to verbal commands and to maintain a patent airway."[15] The minimum number of personnel required to evaluate the patient during conscious sedation is two: the cardiologist performing the procedure and a clinical monitor trained to evaluate appropriate physiological variables and to provide support if resuscitation is required. Several different sedation regimens are recommended, but most involve the use of diazepam in doses of 2.5 to 10 mg orally and diphenhydramine in doses of 25 to 50 mg orally 1 hour before the procedure. For the elderly or frail patient, one or both premedications may be used in lower doses or skipped altogether. During the procedure, midazolam in doses of 1 to 2 mg can be given intravenously, but respiratory failure and arrest have been reported, especially when this agent is administered concurrently with a narcotic.[16] If midazolam is not used, conscious sedation may be achieved safely with the combi-

TABLE 8–2 ABBREVIATIONS

ABBREVIATION	DEFINITION
Vessels	
LCA	Left coronary artery
LMCA	Left main coronary artery
LAD	Left anterior descending artery
LCx	Left circumflex coronary artery
RCA	Right coronary artery
IMA	Internal mammary artery
SVG	Saphenous vein bypass graft
Angiographic projections	
LAO	Left anterior oblique
AP	Anteroposterior
RAO	Right anterior oblique

nation of fentanyl 25 μg and promethazine 12.5 mg, both given intravenously and repeated if necessary.

HEPARIN. The need for *heparin* for coronary arteriography performed via the femoral artery is controversial. Data from the Coronary Artery Surgery Study (CASS) Registry suggested that this was not beneficial.[17] For patients at increased risk for thromboembolic complications, however, 5000 units of heparin should be administered after the catheters have entered the central circulation. Patients at increased risk for thromboembolic complications include those who have severe, progressive peripheral arterial disease, arterial atheroembolic disease, or a need for prolonged use of guidewires in the central circulation for catheterization of the internal mammary arteries, bypass grafts, or the stenotic aortic valve. For catheter manipulation in the central circulation not requiring guidewires, frequent flushing of the catheter with contrast medium or heparinized saline approximately every 30 to 60 seconds avoids the formation of microthrombi within the catheter tip and reduces the risk of thromboembolism. It should be emphasized that prolonged use of guidewires in the central circulation (greater than 1 minute of uninterrupted guidewire use) should be accompanied by systemic anticoagulation with approximately 5000 units of heparin administered intravenously to reduce the risk of systemic thromboembolism. After heparin has been administered, guidewires should not remain in the central circulation for more than 2 minutes without removal and catheter flushing. For patients undergoing cardiac catheterization and coronary arteriography via the brachial or radial artery, 5000 units of heparin is administered before the arteriotomy is performed.

After the procedure, the anticoagulant effect of heparin can be reversed with *protamine*, in a dose of approximately 1 mg for every 100 units of heparin. It should be noted, however, that the use of protamine is associated with a risk of anaphylaxis or serious hypotensive episodes in approximately 2 per cent of patients. The risk of protamine reactions is increased in patients with prior exposure to neutral protamine H (NPH) insulin. Thus, protamine should not be administered to patients with prior exposure to NPH insulin. Protamine should not be used in patients with a history of unstable angina, those with high-risk coronary anatomy such as left main coronary artery disease, or those who have undergone coronary arteriography via the brachial or radial artery. If heparin is not reversed with protamine, femoral sheaths can be removed after the anticoagulant effect of heparin has dissipated, as evidenced by an activated clotting time of less than 180 seconds.

Although *atropine* frequently was recommended in the past to prevent vagal reactions and heart rate slowing during radiographic contrast injection, skillful technique and selective use of radiographic contrast agents have decreased the consequences of heart rate slowing during coronary arteriography. Atropine is used now only for circumstances of persistent bradycardia and hypotension and is not recommended as a prophylactic agent because of the risk of exacerbating unstable angina in patients with severe coronary disease.

Nitroglycerin diminishes the tone of the epicardial coronary arteries. For patients with adequate blood pressure greater than 100 mm Hg, this drug can be administered at a dose of 0.4 mg sublingually, 50 to 200 μg intracoronary, or 25 μg/min in a constant intravenous infusion.

Beta blockers frequently are required during coronary arteriography in patients with unstable angina and severe coronary artery disease. For patients with heart rates greater than 80 beats per minute and no contraindication to beta blockers such as bronchospastic disease or left ventricular dysfunction, an agent such as metoprolol can be administered in a dose of 5 mg intravenously over 1 minute.

Prednisone in a dose of 60 mg should be administered

approximately 12 hours before coronary arteriography in any patient with a history of contrast allergy.[18]

Mechanical ventilation before coronary arteriography is required for all patients with respiratory failure, refractory pulmonary edema, or inability to protect the airway.

Intraaortic balloon counterpulsation is a useful adjunct for performing coronary arteriography in patients with cardiogenic shock or refractory pulmonary edema. The capability for this treatment must exist in any laboratory performing coronary arteriography.

Support equipment for coronary arteriography includes hemodynamic and electrocardiographic monitoring, oxygen and suction ports, general anesthesia cart, intraaortic balloon console, resuscitation cart, activated clotting time analyzer, blood gas analyzer or hemoglobin-oxygen saturation analyzer, and close proximity of Doppler echocardiography capability and expertise.

Continuous electrocardiographic, pressure, and oximetric monitoring is required for the safe performance of coronary arteriography.[4] Electrocardiographic monitoring involves the continuous display of standard limb lead I or II. Physiological measurements of blood pressure must be calibrated against a mercury manometer in every case. Transcutaneous monitoring of arterial hemoglobin-oxygen saturation with pulse oximetry should be used to ensure adequate oxygenation.

RADIOGRAPHIC CONTRAST AGENTS. These agents may produce a number of adverse hemodynamic, electrophysiological, and renal effects consequent to coronary arteriography. The monomeric ionic contrast agents that have been used in coronary arteriography for many years are high-osmolar methylglucamine and sodium salts of diatrizoic acid. These substances dissociate into cations and iodine-containing anions,[19] resulting in aqueous solutions of 1940 mOsmol/kg, as compared with the osmolality of human plasma of 300 mOsmol/kg. The hypertonicity of these compounds produces sinus bradycardia, heart block, Q-T interval and QRS prolongation, ST-segment depression, giant T-wave inversion, decreased left ventricular contractility, decreased systolic pressure, and increased left ventricular end-diastolic pressure. One cause of these hemodynamic and electrocardiographic effects is the presence of calcium-chelating properties of some of these agents. If the contrast agents are injected into a damped coronary catheter with ventricular pressure tracing or given too rapidly in too great a volume (e.g., more than approximately 5 ml for opacification of the right coronary artery), ventricular tachycardia or fibrillation may ensue.

Non-ionic agents such as iohexol and iopamidol also are available. Because they go into solution as single neutral molecules, their osmolality is substantially reduced (<850 mOsmol/kg). They also do not contain calcium-chelating agents. The standard ionic contrast agents have an inhibitory effect on clot formation when mixed with blood, whereas non-ionic agents exhibit less of this inhibitory effect. Because contrast agents and blood are in direct contact in syringes and tubing for varying time intervals during arteriography, clots are more likely to form when non-ionic agents are used. Serious thromboembolic complications have been reported anecdotally. The risk of such complications may be reduced, however, with careful attention to catheter technique.

The low-osmolality ionic dimer methylglucamine–sodium ioxaglate is another alternative to the high-osmolar agents. Ioxaglate retains most of the anticoagulant properties of diatrizoate sodium[20-22] and may have advantages in the unstable patient with hemodynamic compromise.

Radiographic contrast agents can lead to worsening azotemia. Patients with preexisting renal impairment or diabetes mellitus are at increased risk for developing radiocontrast-induced renal failure.[23] Other risk factors for radiocontrast-induced renal failure include advanced age, intravascular volume depletion, congestive heart failure, and the volume of contrast media administered.[24] In patients with renal insufficiency who undergo coronary arteriography, hydration with intravenous saline provides better protection against radiocontrast-induced renal failure than does mannitol or furosemide.[25]

Contrast agents produce several syndromes characterized as allergic. The incidence of anaphylaxis (bronchospasm, angioedema, urticaria, and hypotension) is approximately 0.15 per cent in individuals given intraarterial contrast agents.[24] In patients with a prior allergic reaction, pretreatment with steroids 12 and 2 hours before repeat challenge reduced the likelihood of allergic reaction.[18]

STANDARD VERSUS LOW-OSMOLAR AGENTS. The major drawback of the low-osmolar, low-ionic and non-ionic contrast agents is their 20-fold increase in cost relative to ionic agents. Although some laboratories routinely use low-osmolar agents, it appears that most have avoided doing so because of the associated high costs and lack of clear benefit. A rational and cost-effective policy is to use the standard ionic agents for most elective procedures. The use of low-osmolar, low-ionic, or non-ionic agents should be reserved for patients with resting heart rates of less than 55 to 60 beats per minute, unstable angina, acute myocardial infarction, renal failure, age older than 65 to 70, congestive heart failure, or a previous reaction to contrast agents. When ionic agents are selected, additional precautions are needed to avoid complications. Patients should be "coached" about coughing before the first selective coronary arteriogram is performed, and use of the minimal amount of contrast agent to fill the entire coronary artery for two cardiac cycles and allow brief reflux of contrast into the aortic root is needed. Often, only 4 to 5 ml of contrast agent for the left coronary artery and 1 to 2 ml for the right coronary artery is needed for optimal yet safe selective coronary arteriography.

Cineangiographic Equipment

ANGIOGRAPHIC EQUIPMENT. Cineangiographic equipment is composed of several components (Fig. 8–7): (1) An x-ray generator with an output of 80 to 100 kW with the potential applied preferably by a technique known as "secondary switching" is used in order to reduce preexposure and postexposure radiation release from stored radiation in the capacitance of high-voltage cables. A cine pulse system with exposure settings in the range of 5 to 8 msec is needed to optimize image quality. Longer exposures are associated with motion artifact, whereas shorter exposures may require increased voltage, which results in decreased image resolution. Automatic exposure control sets the brightness level of the image intensifier by varying voltage, current, and exposure duration. (2) An x-ray tube for the conversion of electrical energy to x-radiation is usually mounted in a **C**-arm configuration for multiaxial projection. Radiographic carbon fiber grids are commonly used to improve contrast by decreasing the scatter of radiation. (3) A dual- or triple-mode cesium iodide image intensifier with a resolution capability of approximately 5 line pairs per millimeter, a contrast ratio of greater than 15:1, and a conversion factor of greater than 50 for the small mode is recommended for coronary arteriography. The intensifier should have at least two modes, the large mode approximating 9 inches to be able to image large ventricles and a small mode (magnified mode) of 6 inches or less. (4) An optical system consisting of an objective lens, an image-distributing mirror, and a cine camera lens should be engineered to maximize image quality. The focal length of the camera lens should allow the proper degree of overframing. A diaphragm should be interposed in front of the cine camera lens, and ideally, the entire system should be set up so that the lens can operate at two f-stops above maximum aperture. (5) A cine camera capable of operating at either 30 or

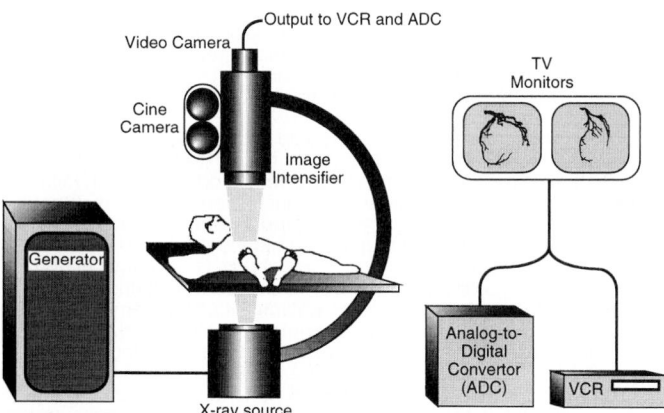

FIGURE 8–7. Cineangiographic equipment. The major components include a generator, x-ray tube, image intensifier attached to a positioner such as a C-arm, optical system, cine camera, video camera, videocassette recorder (VCR), analog-to-digital convertor, and television monitors. The x-ray tube is the source of the x-ray beam, which passes superiorly through the patient.

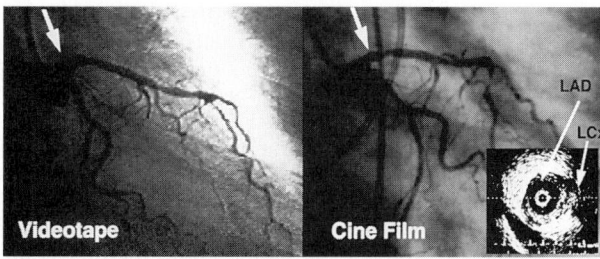

FIGURE 8–8. Comparison of analog videotape with 35-mm cinefilm. Nearly simultaneous recordings of the left coronary artery of an 82-year-old patient were made with both analog videotape and 35-mm cinefilm. Although both images were transferred using identical image-processing parameters such as line resolution, gray-scale range, and gamma curves, the videotape image has significant degradation in image quality as compared with cinefilm. An artifact representing a possible stenosis at the origin of the left anterior descending artery (*A*, arrow) was found to be a minor stenosis on cinefilm (*B*, arrow) and confirmed by intravascular ultrasound (*inset*).

60 frames per second with low vibration levels is required to record coronary arteriography with the optimal recording medium. (6) Cinefilm with a speed and average gradient appropriate for the system should be chosen carefully. (7) A cinefilm processor should be selected that can maintain highly stable developer temperature and immersion time; it also must provide adequate replenishment of chemical solutions, proper agitation, and recirculation. (8) A television system must be used that has excellent image clarity and minimal lag. A high-quality television camera and 525- or 1023-line monitor with a signal/noise ratio of at least 45 dB are suggested.[4] The 1023-line television system results in reduced raster line artifact.

IMAGE RECORDING AND STORAGE

The medium of choice for recording and storage of coronary arteriograms is 35-mm cinefilm. Despite its relative expense, 35-mm cinefilm currently meets the desirable criteria of exchangeability, adherence to a standard format, high quality of resolution, a permanent record format, and suitability for quantitative analysis. So long as quality control in film development is adequate, no other recording medium can compete with the spatial resolution or the dynamic contrast range of 35-mm cinefilm. Optimal radiographic imaging is crucial to the success of coronary arteriography. Under ideal circumstances, modern radiographic imaging techniques provide spatial resolution of 5 line pairs per millimeter, a level of resolution that must be considered of borderline adequacy for imaging coronary vessels as small as 1 mm.

Despite being the industry standard, use of 35-mm cinefilm has certain drawbacks, including high cost, delay in access, and inability for processing of data directly on film. Therefore, several other modalities, including analog videotape, digital tape, and optical discs, are currently being developed as possible replacements for cinefilm.[26] A few laboratories have already replaced cinefilm storage with analog videotape using super-VHS videotapes as the storage medium. Unfortunately, much of the spatial resolution is lost in the transfer of digital images to analog tape, which is caused by the poor signal/noise ratio and limited bandwidth of videotape.[27] The corresponding deterioration in image quality strongly interferes with decision-making regarding the need for revascularization (Fig. 8–8). Thus, analog videotape cannot be recommended as a replacement for cinefilm at the current time.[28]

Another alternative to cinefilm is digital tape or optical disc recording. Although these media may overcome most of the limitations of image degradation seen with analog videotape, requirements for storage (1 to 2.5 gigabytes per study)[29] and difficulties with later retrieval are shortcomings.[29] In addition, no set of uniform standards exists for digital formats, so a digital arteriogram recorded in one laboratory may not be interpretable in another. Despite the current limitations of digital formats, further development of uniform standards can be expected eventually to identify a recording medium that may ultimately supplant 35-mm cinefilm.

Quantitative Coronary Arteriography

The role of quantitative coronary arteriography in judging the severity of coronary artery stenoses is one of the most controversial subjects in the field of invasive cardiology. It

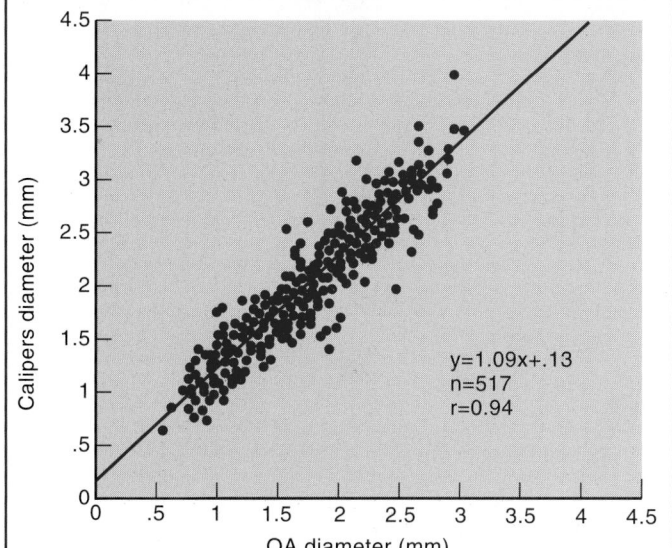

FIGURE 8–9. Coronary artery lumen diameter. The relationship between coronary artery lumen diameter measured with electronic digital calipers as compared with that measured with computerized quantitative coronary angiography (QA) shows excellent correlation and agreement. (Reproduced with permission from Uehata, A., Matsugushi, T., Bittl, J. A., et al.: The accuracy of electronic digital calipers compared with quantitative angiography in measuring arterial diameters. Circulation **88**:1724, 1993. Copyright 1993 American Heart Association.)

has been suggested that no technique in invasive cardiology is discussed more but utilized less than quantitative coronary arteriography.[30] Despite the development of several computer-assisted approaches to quantitative coronary arteriography, the standard method for interpreting the presence and severity of stenoses in the epicardial coronary arteries continues to be visual assessment. Several studies have suggested, however, that visual assessment of lesion severity suffers from a suboptimal degree of interobserver variability and accuracy.[31–34] Therefore, several computer-assisted systems have been promoted, but lack of uniform standards and unclear relation between quantitative measures of stenosis severity and clinical outcome have made recommendations difficult.

Quantitative angiography defines the edge of the vessel at the points of maximal rate of change of density of contrast, whereas visual assessment defines the minimal lumen diameter at the point where any gradient is detected. An approach that benefits from excellent interobserver variability and yet maintains the ability of the angiographer to integrate the visual information from several frames relies on the use of hand-held electronic digital calipers, which have been found to have acceptable agreement with computer-assisted methods (Fig. 8–9).[36]

CORONARY ARTERY ANATOMY

Coronary arteriography visualizes only a small portion of the coronary circulation: the major epicardial branches and their second-, third-, and perhaps fourth-order branches. The myriad small intramyocardial branches are not visualized because of their small size, cardiac motion, and limitations in resolution of cine imaging systems. Although these small "resistance" vessels play a major role in regulation of coronary blood flow, they are thought to play a small role in human coronary artery disease, limiting blood flow and contributing to ischemia in patients with left ventricular hypertrophy or systemic hypertension in the absence of epicardial coronary artery stenosis.

Because the heart is oriented obliquely in the thoracic cavity, the direct frontal and lateral views are not commonly used during coronary arteriography. Instead, the coronary circulation is imaged in the right anterior oblique (RAO) and left anterior oblique (LAO) views (Figs. 8–10 and 8–11). The major coronary arteries traverse the atrioventricular and interventicular grooves, which in turn are aligned with the long and short axes of the heart. Thus, the best angiographic projections to visualize these vessels in profile are the oblique views. Because the straight RAO and LAO views of the heart have serious shortcomings caused by foreshortening and superimposition of branches,[37,38] the rotation of the x-ray beam about the patient in the transverse plane for RAO and LAO projections is almost always accompanied by rotation of the x-ray beam about the patient in the sagittal plane for cranial and caudal angulation.

General recommendations about routine views, however, can be made for most patients, and tailored views are required to accommodate possible variations. During coronary arteriography, the anteroposterior (AP) view with shallow caudal angulation is often performed first to evaluate the possibility of left main coronary artery disease. Other important views include the LAO view with cranial angulation to evaluate the left anterior descending artery. This view should have sufficient leftward positioning of the image intensifier to prevent overlap between the left anterior descending artery (LAD) and the spine. This is followed by the LAO caudal view to evaluate the proximal segment of the left circumflex coronary artery (LCx), RAO view with caudal angulation to assess the LCx and marginal branches in full profile, and shallow RAO or AP cranial view to evaluate the midportion of the LAD. Although the foregoing sequence of views is recommended for the minimal assessment of the left coronary artery (LCA), a rigid sequence of views is not mandated. Instead, the views must be selected based on the rotation of the heart and the presence of lesions that may be targeted for revascularization techniques.

TERMINOLOGY OF VIEWS. The terminology originally proposed to describe these views was somewhat confusing, because several different terms were introduced by different authors. A simple nomenclature has evolved that defines the cineangiographic projection as the relation between the image intensifier and the patient. In most cardiac catheterization laboratories, the x-ray tube is under the patient table, and the image intensifier, with its coupled video and cinecameras, is over the patient table (Fig. 8–7). If the over-table image intensifier is tilted up toward the head of the patient, the resulting projection is referred to as the "cranial" view. The images recorded in this view appear as if the angiographer were looking down at the heart from the patient's head. Conversely, if the image intensifier is tilted down toward the feet of the patient, this is referred to as the "caudal" view and provides images as if the angiographer were looking up at the heart from the patient's feet. Cranial and caudal angulations have become a standard part of coronary arteriography and are used routinely in most laboratories that have the necessary U- or C-arm mounting units for their cine systems.

It is difficult to predict which angulated views will be most useful in any given patient. The usefulness of the angiographic projections depends largely on body habitus, variations in the coronary anatomy, and location of lesions. For this reason, it is recommended that coronary angiographers routinely use both cranial and caudal angulation views in both the LAO and RAO projections of the left coronary system. These views also can be helpful on occasion during examination of the right coronary system, especially in visualizing the origin of the posterior descending artery in the LAO cranial projection.

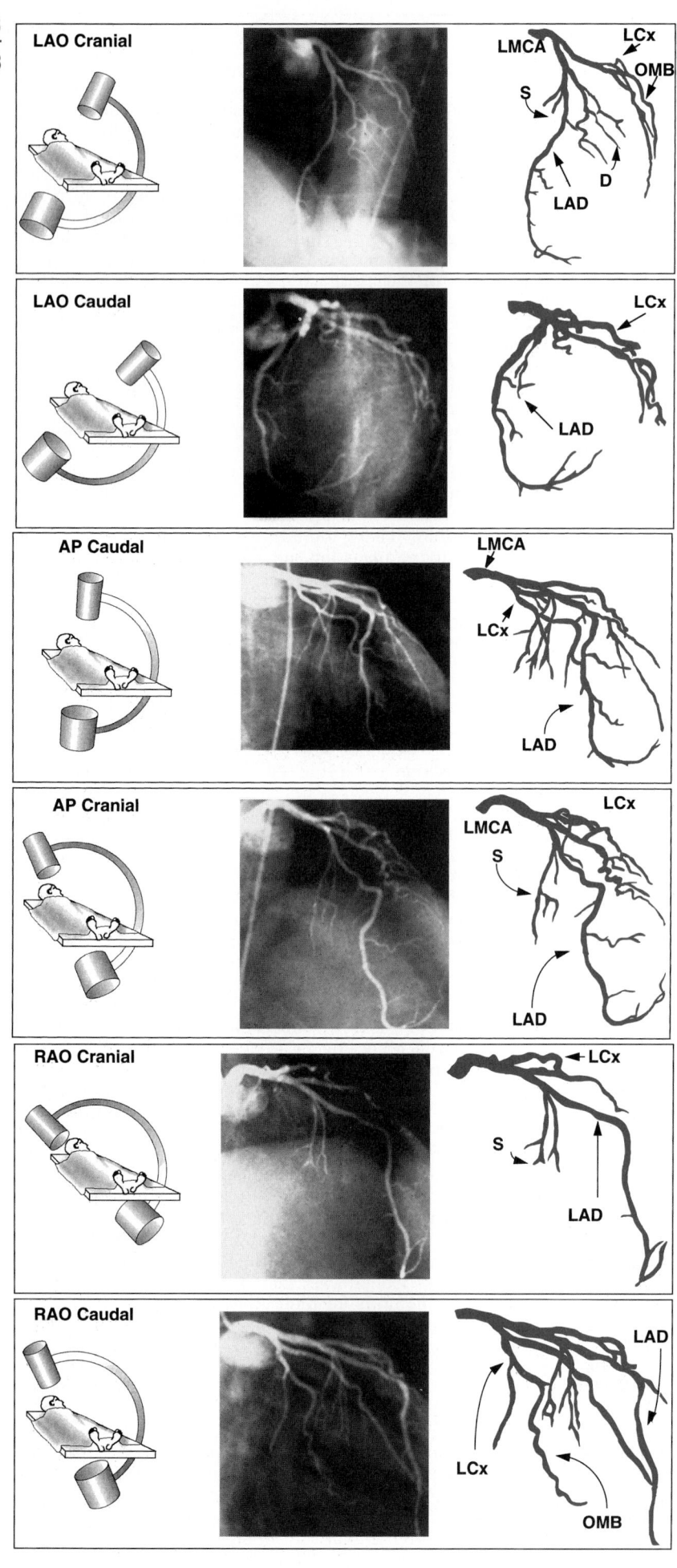

FIGURE 8–10. Angiographic views of the left coronary artery. The approximate positions of the x-ray tube and image intensifier are shown for each of the commonly used angiographic views. The 60-degree left anterior oblique view with 20 degrees of cranial angulation (LAO cranial) shows the ostium and occasionally the distal portion of the LMCA, the middle and distal portions of the LAD, septal perforators (S), diagonal branches (D), the proximal LCx and superimposed obtuse marginal branch (OMB). The 60-degree left anterior oblique view with 25 degrees of caudal angulation (LAO caudal) shows the proximal LMCA and the proximal segments of the LAD and LCx. The anteroposterior projection with 20 degrees of caudal angulation (AP caudal) shows the distal LMCA and proximal segment of the LAD and LCx. The proximal segment of the LCx is characterized by a 75- to 90-degree angle, but the midportion of the LCx and septal branches are superimposed. The anteroposterior projection with 20 degrees of cranial angulation (AP cranial) displays the midportion of the LAD and its septal (S) and diagonal branches. The 30-degree right anterior oblique projection with 20 degrees of cranial angulation (RAO cranial) shows the course of the LAD and its diagonal branches. The 30-degree right anterior oblique projection with 25 degrees of caudal angulation (RAO caudal) shows the LCx and marginal branches.

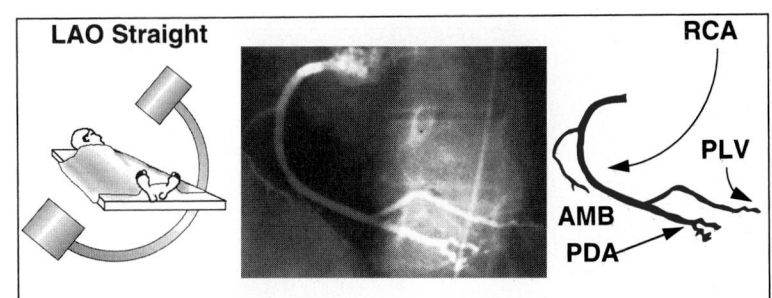

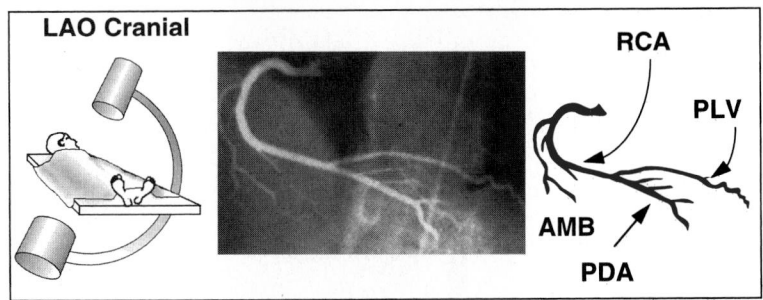

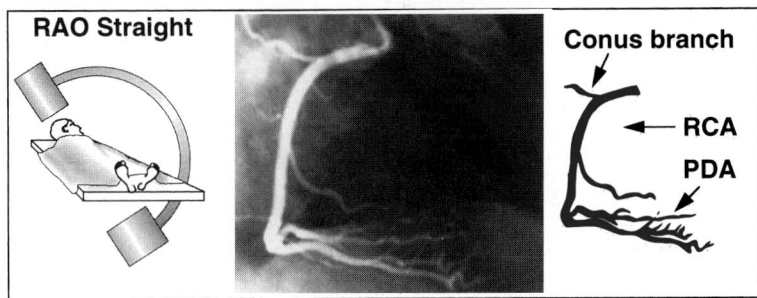

FIGURE 8–11. Angiographic views of the right coronary artery. The approximate positions of the x-ray tube and image intensifier are shown for each of the commonly used angiographic views. The 60-degree left anterior oblique view (LAO straight) shows the proximal and midportions of the right coronary artery (RCA), as well as the acute marginal branch (AMB). The 60-degree left anterior oblique view with 25-degree cranial angulation (LAO cranial) shows the midportion of the RCA and the origin and course of the PDA. The 30-degree right anterior oblique view (RAO straight) shows the conus branch, the midportion of the RCA, and the course of the PDA.

Dominance

The term "dominance" often is used to describe coronary artery anatomy. With this nomenclature, the dominant vessel is the one that supplies the posterior diaphragmatic portion of the interventricular septum and the diaphragmatic surface of the left ventricle (Figs. 8–12, 8–13, and 8–14). The right coronary artery (RCA) is dominant in about 85 per cent of humans. Use of the term dominance is somewhat misleading because it implies that the RCA is the more important vessel in 85 per cent of patients. Because human coronary artery disease (CAD) is primarily the result of interruption of blood supply to the left ventricular myocardium, a nondominant left coronary artery (LCA) is almost always more important than the dominant RCA. With this understanding, the term dominance nevertheless is used because it is a commonly accepted anatomical concept. Dominance is most easily assessed in the LAO cranial view.

Left Coronary Artery Catheterization Technique

The technique for catheterizing the left main coronary artery involves advancing the Judkins left coronary catheter toward the left coronary ostium (Fig. 8–6). If the catheter begins to turn out of profile (so that one or both curves of the catheter are no longer visualized en face), it can be rotated very slightly and advanced slowly to enter the left sinus of Valsalva. Overrotation of the left Judkins catheter "will only thwart attempts" to enter the left coronary ostium.[39] Further slow advancement will permit the catheter tip to engage the ostium of the left coronary artery. In conditions of a large ascending aorta, advancement of the Judkins left coronary catheter is associated with formation of an acute secondary angle. Further advancement should be avoided, because this would re-form the catheter shape and prevent catheterization of the left coronary artery. In the

presence of a mildly dilated ascending aorta, the guidewire can be temporarily reinserted into the catheter to straighten the secondary bend and permit the catheter to be advanced to the left sinus of Valsalva.

If the ascending aorta is significantly dilated, however, the catheter should be exchanged for a larger size (e.g., Judkins left 5.0 or 6.0). If the tip of the Judkins left catheter advances beyond the ostium of the left coronary artery without engagement, the primary bend of the catheter can be reshaped within the patient's body by further careful advancement and prompt withdrawal of the catheter, allowing the tip to "pop" into the ostium of the left coronary artery. This maneuver, along with gentle clockwise or counterclockwise rotation, frequently permits selective engagement of the left coronary artery when the initial attempt has failed. It is imperative, however, to ensure that the catheter tip has not entered the left main coronary artery before further advancement is made.

To catheterize the left main coronary artery with the Amplatz catheter, the broad secondary curve of the appropriately sized left Amplatz catheter is positioned so that it rests on the right aortic cusp with its tip pointing toward the left aortic cusp. Alternating advancement and retraction of the catheter with slight clockwise or counterclockwise rotation allows the catheter tip to enter the left coronary ostium. Once the tip enters the ostium, the position of the catheter usually can be stabilized with slight retraction.

After the left coronary ostium is entered, the pressure at the tip of the catheter should be checked immediately to ensure that it matches femoral artery pressure. If this is the case, the catheter tip is most likely aligned coaxially with the origin of the coronary artery and free within its lumen. This can be verified by the gentle injection of a small amount of contrast medium. If a damped or ventricularized pressure tracing is obtained, the catheter should be removed immediately from the left coronary artery, and an attempt at repositioning should be made. If abnormal pressure recordings persist, it is reasonable to withdraw the catheter slightly from the coronary artery and perform a nonselective injection of contrast medium into the left coronary artery in the anteroposterior view to evaluate the possibility of left main coronary artery disease. If the pressure measured at the catheter tip is normal and a small test injection of contrast medium suggests the absence of left main coronary artery disease, left coronary arteriography is then performed using multiple projections.

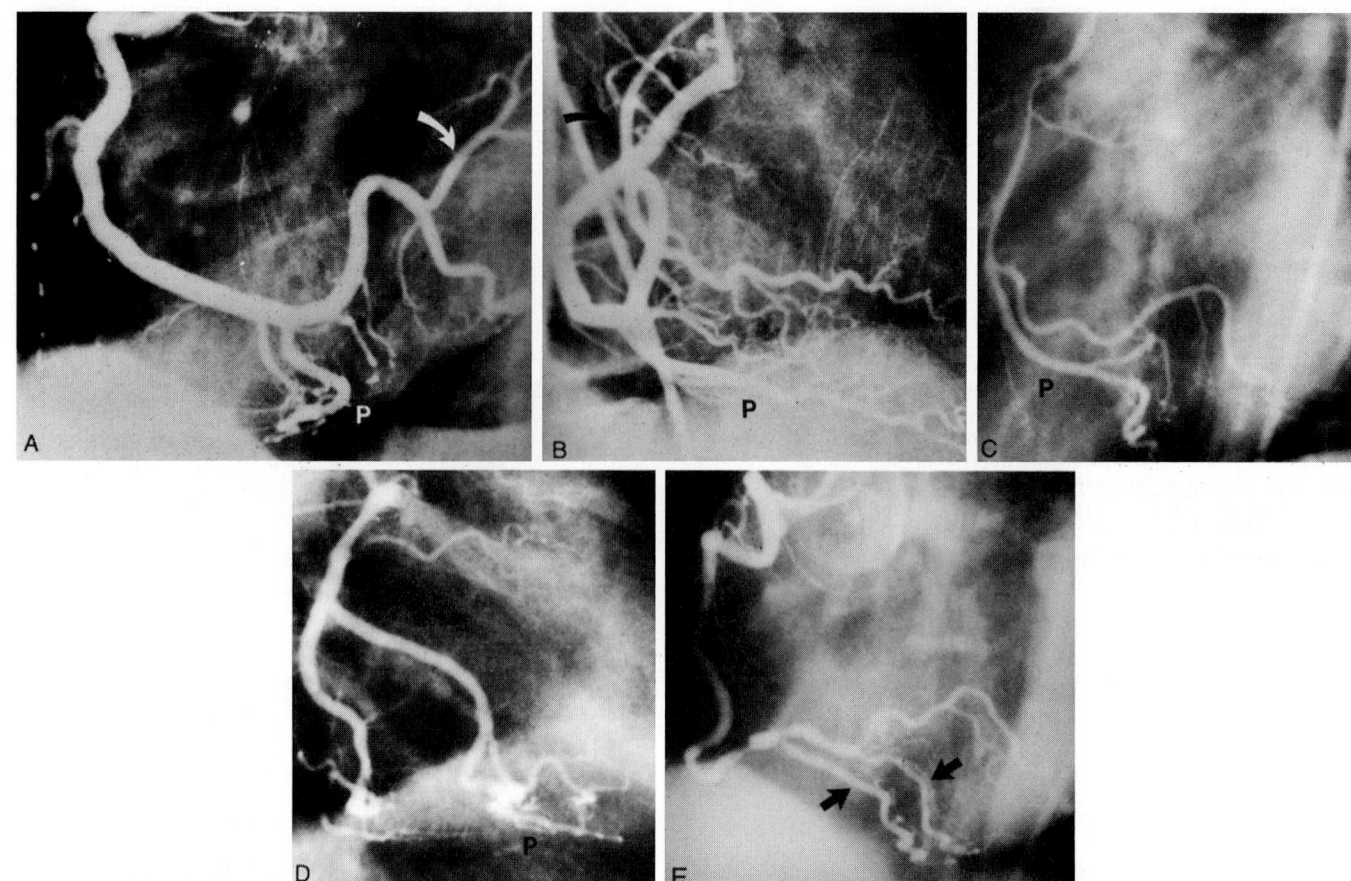

FIGURE 8–12. Strongly dominant right coronary artery. *A* and *B*, LAO and RAO views of the RCA show that the distal segment (arrows) extends to the left atrioventricular groove. After giving rise to the posterior descending artery, the RCA gives rise to multiple posterior left ventricular and obtuse marginal branches. *C*, A variation in the origin of the posterior descending artery, which originates early from the RCA, runs parallel to it, and enters the posterior interventricular groove. (From Levin, D. C., and Baltaxe, H. A.: Angiographic demonstration of important anatomic variations of the posterior descending artery. A. J. R. *116:*41, 1972, with permission). *D,* RAO right coronary arteriogram showing the posterior descending artery arising from a right ventricular branch of the RCA. *E,* LAO right coronary arteriogram showing duplicated posterior descending arteries (arrows). (From Levin, D. C., and Baltaxe, H. A.: Angiographic demonstration of important anatomic variations of the posterior descending artery. A. J. R. *116:*41, 1972, copyright 1972, American Roentgen Ray Society.)

Left Coronary Artery Anatomy

Left Main Coronary Artery (LMCA)

The LMCA arises from the upper portion of the left aortic sinus, just below the sinotubular ridge of the aorta, which defines the border separating the left sinus of Valsalva from the smooth (tubular) portion of the aorta. The diameter of the LMCA ranges from 3 to 6 mm. Quantitative analysis has shown that the diameter of the LMCA is greater for patients with entirely normal coronary arteries (4.5 ± 0.5 mm [$\pm$ S.D.]) than in those with disease in the distal LCA (4.0 ± 0.3 mm) or disease in the adjacent segment of the LCA (3.8 ± 0.3 mm).[40] The LMCA passes behind the right ventricular outflow tract and may extend for 0 to 10 mm. It usually then bifurcates into the LAD and LCx branches.

Left Anterior Descending Artery (LAD)

The LAD passes down the anterior interventicular groove toward the cardiac apex. In the RAO projection, it extends toward the anterior aspect of the heart. In the LAO projection, it passes down the cardiac midline, between the right and left ventricles (Fig. 8–10). Its major branches are the septal and diagonal branches.

The septal branches emanate from the LAD at approximately 90-degree angles and pass into the interventricular

septum. They vary in size, number, and distribution. In some cases there is a large first septal branch, which is vertically oriented and divides into a number of secondary branches that ramify throughout the septum. In other cases a more horizontally oriented, large first septal branch is present, which passes parallel to and below the LAD itself. In still other cases a number of septal arteries are roughly comparable in size. These septal branches interconnect with similar septal branches passing upward from the posterior descending branch of the RCA to produce a network of potential collateral channels. The interventicular septum is the most densely vascularized area of the heart, and the first septal branch is its most important potential collateral channel.

The diagonal branches of the LAD pass over the anterolateral aspect of the heart. Although virtually all patients have a single LAD in the anterior interventicular groove, there is wide variability in the number and size of diagonal branches. More than 90 per cent have one to three such branches.[41] Because less than 1 per cent of patients have no diagonal branches, the angiographer should suspect the presence of acquired atherosclerotic occlusion of the diagonal branch(es) if none are seen. This is particularly true in cases in which there are unexplained contraction abnormalities of the anterolateral left ventricle. Visualization of the origin of the diagonal branches often requires very

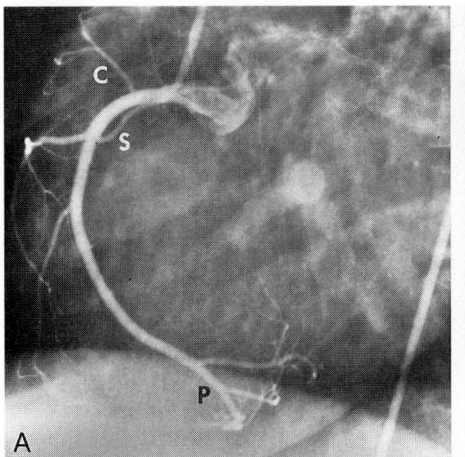
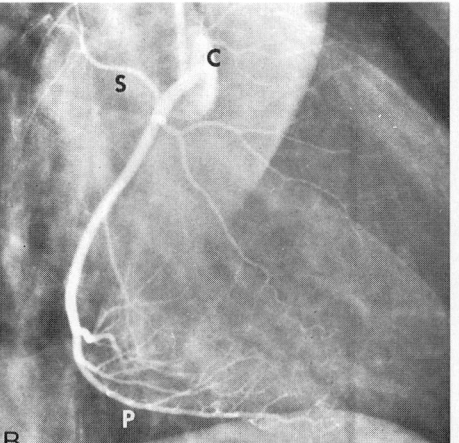
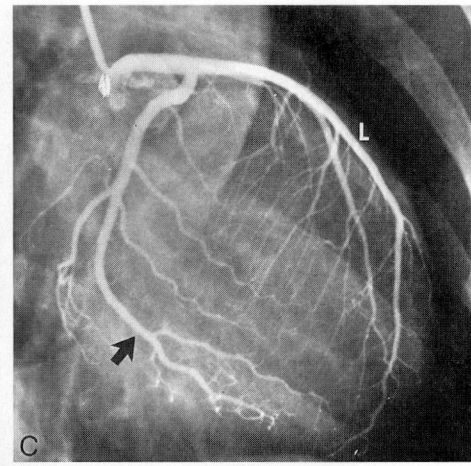

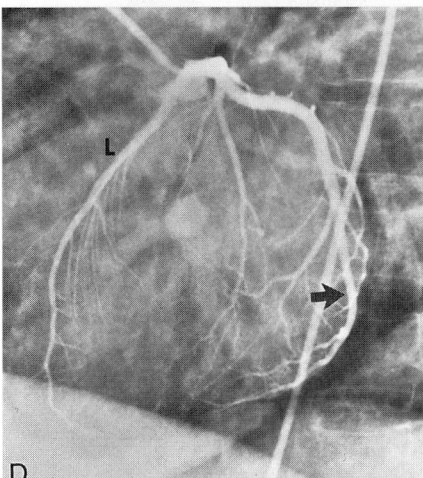
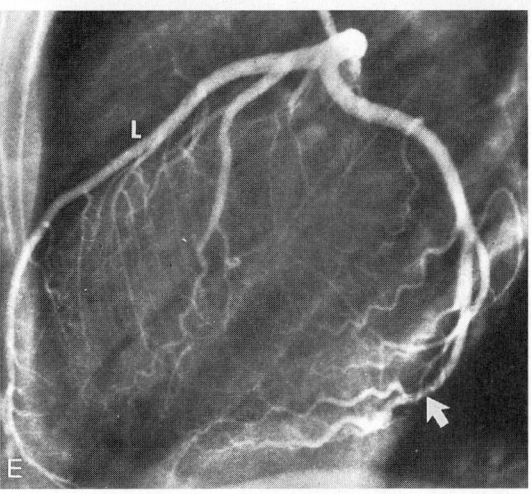

FIGURE 8–13. Weakly dominant right coronary artery. A and B, LAO and RAO views of the RCA. Both the conus and sinoatrial node artery arise from the RCA. The distal portion of the RCA beyond the origin of the posterior descending artery is short and gives rise to a single small posterior left ventricular branch. C, D, and E, LCA in the RAO, LAO, and left lateral projections, respectively. Note that the circumflex artery gives rise to four obtuse marginal branches, the most distal of which (arrow) supplies some of the diaphragmatic surface of the left ventricle. The LAD gives rise to two small and one medium-sized diagonal branches. C = conus branch; L = left anterior descending artery; P = posterior descending artery; S = sinoatrial nodal artery.

steep LAO cranial views involving as much as 80 degrees of leftward angulation and 20 to 40 degrees of cranial skew for optimal projection. The origin of the diagonal branches often can be brought into relief with less severely angulated RAO cranial or caudal projections.

In 37 per cent of patients, the LMCA trifurcates into the LAD, LCx, and *ramus medianus*.[41] In these cases, the ramus arises between the LAD and LCx arteries. This vessel is analogous to a diagonal branch and usually supplies the free wall along the lateral aspect of the left ventricle.

In 78 per cent of patients, the LAD courses beyond the left ventricular apex and terminates along the diaphragmatic aspect of the left ventricle. In 22 per cent of patients, however, the LAD fails to reach the diaphragmatic surface, terminating instead either at or before the cardiac apex.[42] In these latter cases, the posterior descending branch of the RCA is larger and longer than usual, supplies the apex, and may be informally termed "superdominant." In these patients, the LAD does not supply the cardiac apex, and its distal segment is smaller and shorter than usual. Early attenuation and a distal narrow segment in these cases do not necessarily signify LAD disease if some or all of the cardiac apex is supplied by the posterior descending artery.

The LAD requires carefully constructed projections to assess the ostium of the vessel and to separate it from its multiple septal and diagonal side branches. The best angiographic projections for viewing the course of the LAD are the cranially angulated views. The LAO caudal view (Fig. 8–10), however, will display the origin of the LAD in a horizontally oriented heart, and the AP caudal or shallow RAO caudal view also will project the proximal LAD well. The LAO cranial view displays the midportion of the LAD and origins of the diagonal branches but superimposes the LAD and the septal branches. The RAO cranial view displays the proximal, middle, and distal segments of the LAD but often superimposes the midportion of the LAD and the diagonal branches. The left lateral view often shows the midportion of the LAD only. Views designed to assess the origin of the diagonal branches and define ostial lesions of these branches are often tailored LAO cranial or RAO cranial views. Lastly, variations of the AP view requiring 20 to 40 degrees of cranial skew often will project the midportion of the LAD in best relief, separating the vessel from its diagonal branches.

In some patients, no LMCA is present. In these cases, separate ostia for the LAD and LCx are present, which can be separately engaged for selective arteriography. In general, the LAD has a more anterior origin than the LCx. The LAD can be engaged with the left Judkins catheter in this setting with paradoxical counterclockwise rotation, which rotates the secondary bend of the catheter to a posterior position in the aorta and turns the primary bend and tip of the catheter to an anterior position. The opposite maneuver may be used to engage the LCx selectively in the setting of separate LAD and LCx ostia. On the other hand, a Judkins catheter such as the Judkins left 5.0 with a larger curve will selectively engage the downward-coursing left circumflex, and a catheter with a shorter curve such as the Judkins left 3.5 will tend to engage selectively the more anterior and superior left anterior descending coronary artery.

Left Circumflex Artery (LCx)

The left circumflex artery originates at the bifurcation (or trifurcation) of the LMCA and passes down the left atrioventricular groove (Fig. 8–10). In about 85 per cent of human hearts, the LCx artery is the nondominant vessel and varies in size and length, depending on the actual degree of right coronary dominance. The LCx usually gives

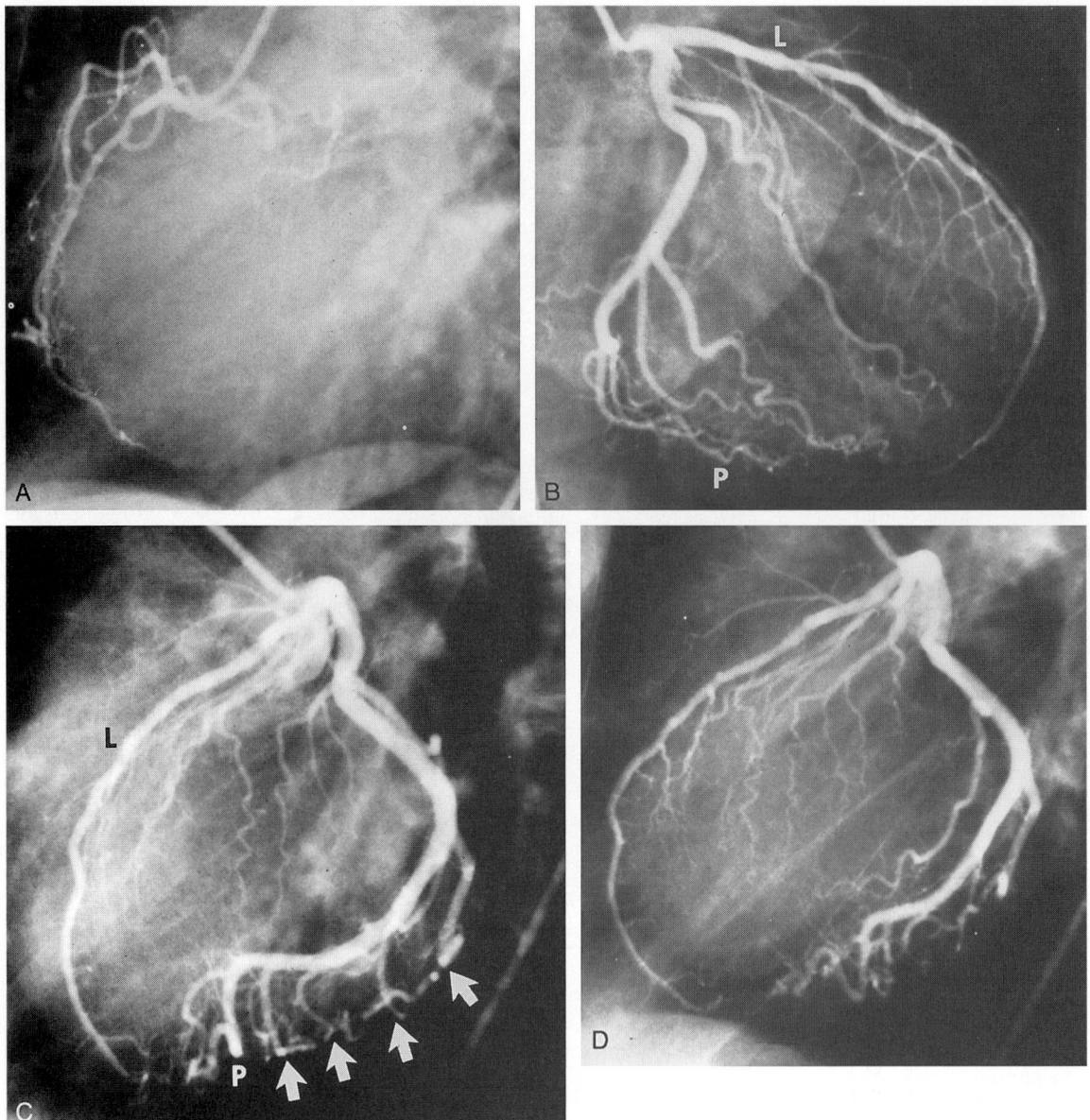

FIGURE 8–14. Dominant left coronary system. *A,* The LAO projection shows that the RCA is small and terminates before reaching the crux. *B, C,* and *D.* The RAO, LAO, and left lateral projections show that the LCx is large and gives rise to the posterior descending artery at the crux of the heart, and to several posterior descending arteries.

off one to three large *obtuse marginal branches* (OMBs) as it passes down the atrioventricular groove. These are the principal branches of the LCx, since they supply the free wall of the left ventricle along its lateral aspect. Beyond the origins of the obtuse marginal branches, the distal LCx tends to be small. The actual position of the LCx can be determined on the late phase of a left coronary injection, when the coronary sinus becomes opacified with diluted contrast material. The position of the coronary sinus identifies the position of the left atrioventricular groove and the proper LCx artery, which runs along the left ventricular side of the coronary sinus. The optimal projections for viewing the LCx and obtuse marginal branches usually involve caudal angulation to project the posteriorly and inferiorly coursing LCx into the plane of the angiographic film. The ostium of the LCx often requires the LAO caudal or RAO caudal view. The midportion of the LCx and the origins of the obtuse marginal branches are often best viewed in the AP caudal views or RAO caudal view with only 5 to 15 degrees of rightward angulation. More severe rightward angulation often superimposes the origins of the obtuse marginal branches on the LCx. If the LCA is dominant, the

optimal projection for the posterior descending artery is the LAO cranial view.

The LCx also gives rise to one or two left atrial circumflex branches. These branches supply the lateral and posterior aspects of the left atrium.

Right Coronary Artery Catheterization Technique

Catheterization of the RCA is also performed in the LAO position, but this requires different maneuvers than catheterization of the LMCA. Whereas the left Judkins catheter naturally seeks the ostium of the LMCA, the right coronary catheter must be rotated by the angiographer to engage the vessel. This usually is accomplished by first passing the catheter to a point just above the aortic valve in the left sinus of Valsalva and then rotating the catheter clockwise, which forces the tip to move anteriorly from the left sinus of Valsalva to the right sinus of Valsalva. Entry into the right coronary ostium is signified by a sudden rightward and downward movement of the catheter tip. If the ostium of the RCA is not easily located, the most common reason is that the ostium has a higher and more anterior origin than anticipated. Repeat attempts to engage the RCA should be made at a level slightly more distal to the aortic valve. Nonselective contrast medium injections in the right sinus of Valsalva may reveal the site of origin of the RCA. Positioning an Amplatz catheter in the ostium of the RCA requires a catheterization technique similar to that used with the right Judkins catheter. If a gentle attempt to withdraw the Amplatz catheter results in paradoxical deep entry into the coronary artery, removal of the catheter can be achieved by clockwise or counterclockwise rotation and advancement to prolapse the catheter into the aortic sinus.

The catheter-tip pressure should be checked to ensure that damping or ventricularization has not occurred. An abnormal pressure tracing may suggest the presence of an ostial stenosis or spasm, selective engagement of the conus branch, or deep intubation of the RCA. If an abnormal pressure tracing has been encountered, the catheter tip should be rotated gently counterclockwise and withdrawn slightly in an effort to free the tip of the catheter. If persistent damping occurs, a very small amount of contrast medium (<1 ml) can be injected carefully and the catheter immediately withdrawn in a "shoot-and-run" maneuver, which may allow the cause of damping to be identified.

If the pressure tracing is normal on entry into the RCA, the vessel should be imaged in at least two projections. The initial injection should be gentle, because of the possibility that forceful injection through a catheter whose tip is immediately adjacent to the vessel wall may lead to dissection. The standard LAO and RAO projections usually will suffice, but on occasion cranial angulation should be added to view the origin and course of the posterior descending artery.

The ideal angiographic projections for evaluating the right coronary artery are the standard LAO and RAO views. The ostium of the RCA is best evaluated in the LAO view, with or without cranial angulation. If the standard Judkins catheter encounters a lesion at the ostium, this catheter should be replaced by a right Amplatz catheter or a short-tipped Judkins catheter to decrease the likelihood of vessel dissection. The origin of the posterior descending artery (PDA) is evaluated in the LAO cranial view, whereas the midportion of the RCA occasionally requires the left lateral view.

Right Coronary Artery Anatomy

The RCA originates from the right aortic sinus at a point somewhat lower than the origin of the LCA from the left aortic sinus (Fig. 8–11). It passes down the right atrioventricular groove toward the crux (a point on the diaphragmatic surface of the heart where the right atrioventricular groove, the left atrioventricular groove, and the posterior interventricular groove come together).

The first branch of the RCA is considered to be the *conus artery*. In about 50 per cent of hearts, this vessel arises at the right coronary ostium or within the first few millimeters of the RCA. It passes anteriorly and upward over the right ventricular outflow tract toward the LAD. The Judkins right coronary catheter frequently engages the conus artery subselectively, and this almost always produces a damped or ventricularized pressure tracing. Gentle withdrawal and further clockwise rotation may allow the catheter to enter the proper RCA. The primary importance of the conus artery is to serve as a source of collateral circulation in patients with LAD occlusion. In the other 50 per cent of hearts, the conus artery is not actually a branch of the RCA but arises from a separate ostium in the right aortic sinus just above the right coronary ostium.[43] In this group of patients, subselective conus branch arteriography may fail to opacify the RCA proper unless sufficient reflux of contrast medium occurs to fill the separate ostium.

The second branch of the RCA usually is the *sinoatrial node artery*. It has been found that this vessel arises from the RCA in 59 per cent, from the LCx in 38 per cent, and from both arteries with a dual blood supply in 3 per cent.[44] When it originates from the RCA, it passes obliquely backward through the upper portion of the atrial septum and the anteromedial wall of the right atrium. It sends branches to the sinus node and usually also to the right atrium or both atria. When the sinoatrial node artery originates from the LCx, it may pass backward in the atrial septum or around the posterolateral wall of the left atrium to reach the area of the sinus node.

The midportion of the RCA usually gives rise to one or more medium-sized acute marginal branches. These branches supply the anterior wall of the right ventricle and are relatively unimportant, except insofar as they also may serve as sources of collateral circulation in patients with LAD occlusion.

The next important branch of the RCA is the *posterior descending artery* (PDA) (Fig. 8–11). When the RCA is dominant, as it is in about 85 per cent of patients, the PDA originates at or shortly before the crux and passes forward in the posterior interventricular groove. During its course along this groove, it gives rise to a number of small inferior septal branches which pass upward to supply the lower portion of the interventricular septum and interdigitate with superior septal branches passing down from the LAD. After giving rise to the PDA, a dominant RCA continues beyond the crux and begins to pass upward along the distal portion of the left atrioventricular groove. Here it usually terminates by giving rise to one or several posterior left ventricular (PLV) branches, which supply the diaphragmatic surface of the left ventricle.

About 15 per cent of patients do not have RCA dominance; about half these patients have LCA dominance. With this anatomical pattern, the LCx artery is large and continues down to the diaphragmatic surface of the left ventricle, where it gives rise to the PLV branches and then reaches the crux and turns forward to become the PDA. In these cases, the RCA is very small, terminating before reaching the crux, and therefore does not supply any blood to the left ventricular myocardium. The other half of patients without RCA dominance have a mixed or "balanced" circulation, wherein the RCA gives rise to the PDA, while the LCx gives rise to the PLV branches.

At or near the crux, the dominant artery gives rise to a small atrioventricular node artery, which passes upward to supply the node.

In about 25 per cent of patients with RCA dominance, there are significant anatomical variations in the origin of the PDA. These variations include partial supply of the PDA territory by acute marginal branches, double PDA, and early origin of the PDA proximal to the crux.

Coronary Bypass Angiography

Angiography after coronary bypass is commonly performed to evaluate the cause of recurrent angina in surgically treated patients. It is estimated that more than 300,000 bypass operations are performed each year in the United States.[2] Although bypass surgery may achieve 99 per cent revascularization of target segments initially,[45] only 87 per cent of saphenous vein grafts (SVGs) remain open at 6 months,[46] and only 75 per cent of target segments remain revascularized 3 years after surgery.[45] The short- and long-term patency rates for SVGs have been reported in several large clinical studies (see p. 1319). In the CASS trial, patency of SVGs was 90 per cent within 60 days of surgery, 82 per cent at 18 months, and about 80 per cent at 3 years.[47] Similar results were seen in the European Coronary Surgery Study, in which SVGs were found to have a 77 per cent patency rate 9 to 18 months after surgery.[48] In patients at the Montreal Heart Institute, SVG patency at 1 year was about 80 per cent, and there was no further reduction in patency between 1 and 6 years after operation.[47] By the time 10 to 12 years had elapsed after surgery, the patency rate of SVGs had dropped to 63 per cent. Moreover, almost half the grafts still patent showed significant atherosclerotic changes. In 161 patients undergoing bypass surgery in the German Angioplasty Bypass Surgery Investigation (GABI),[46] 92 per cent were discharged from the hospital angina-free, but this proportion decreased to 84 per cent at 3 months and to 74 per cent at 6 months.

The patency of SVGs and internal mammary artery (IMA) grafts has been compared (see p. 1318). After a mean follow-up period of 36 months, the patency rate for IMA grafts was 96 per cent, whereas the patency rate for SVGs at a mean follow-up period of 39 months was 77 per cent.[49] At 6 months after bypass surgery, 93 per cent of IMA grafts were functioning.[46] At 7 to 10 years after surgery, IMA graft patency was in the range of 85 to 95 per cent.

The right gastroepiploic artery (GEA) has been used increasingly as a conduit for coronary artery bypass surgery. The right GEA has a slightly greater tendency to develop atherosclerosis than the IMA, with moderate to severe atherosclerosis seen in 12 per cent of right GEAs versus 0 per cent of IMAs at pathological examination.[50] Late GEA graft patency has been documented in 94 per cent of patients 2 to 5 years after surgery.[51]

Several mechanisms lead to failure of bypass grafts. The development of symptoms in the immediate postoperative period after bypass surgery may be due to incomplete revascularization, spasm of the internal mammary artery, or early thrombotic graft occlusion of saphenous vein grafts. The development of symptoms within 1 year of bypass surgery may be due to fibrointimal hyperplasia of saphenous vein grafts.[52] Symptoms in patients more than 1 year after bypass surgery may be due to development of atherosclerosis[52] in the bypass grafts[53] or progression of native vessel disease.[53]

Coronary Bypass Graft Catheterization Technique

Selective catheterization of coronary bypass grafts may be more difficult than catheterization of the native coronary arteries because the locations of graft ostia are more variable, even when surgical clips or ostia markers are used. The experienced angiographer, however, can easily locate graft ostia because the sites of origin for grafts leading to each coronary artery are very predictable. It is therefore crucial for the angiographer to review the operative note describing the number, course, and types of bypass grafts before performing graft arteriography.

Saphenous vein grafts (SVGs) from the aorta to the distal right coronary artery or posterior descending artery originate from the right anterolateral aspect of the aorta approximately 2 cm above the origin of the sinotubular ridge, whereas SVGs to the LAD originate from the anterior portion of the aorta about 4 cm above the sinotubular ridge, and SVGs to the obtuse marginal branches arise from the left anterolateral aspect of the aorta about 5 to 6 cm above the sinotubular ridge (Fig. 8–15). In most patients, all SVGs can be engaged with a single catheter. Use of the Amplatz right 2.0 catheter results in a very high rate of successful SVG catheterizations. Other catheters useful for engaging bypass grafts include the right and left bypass graft catheters (Fig. 8–2).

The eye-hand coordination of the angiographer contributes to the success of graft angiography. Viewed in the LAO projection, the Amplatz catheter will rotate anteriorly from the leftward position as the angiographer turns the catheter in a clockwise direction at the femoral artery. The relation between movement of the catheter shaft at the femoral artery, and the response of the catheter tip on fluoroscopy immediately informs the angiographer whether the catheter tip is positioned anteriorly in the aorta and thus likely to enter a graft ostium or positioned posteriorly and thus unlikely to engage an SVG. Steady advancement and withdrawal of the catheter tip proximal and distal in the ascending aorta, approximately 2 to 6 cm above the sinotubular ridge, with varying degrees of rotation usually results in entry into the graft.

Entry into the graft is associated with abrupt outward motion of the tip of the catheter. When this occurs, a small test injection of contrast material verifies that the catheter is in the SVG. Even if the graft is occluded, a well-circumscribed "stump" is almost always present. Each graft or stump must be viewed in nearly orthogonal views. The relation between the origin of the grafts and surgical clips confirms whether all targeted SVGs have been visualized. If neither a patent graft nor a stump can be located, it may be necessary to

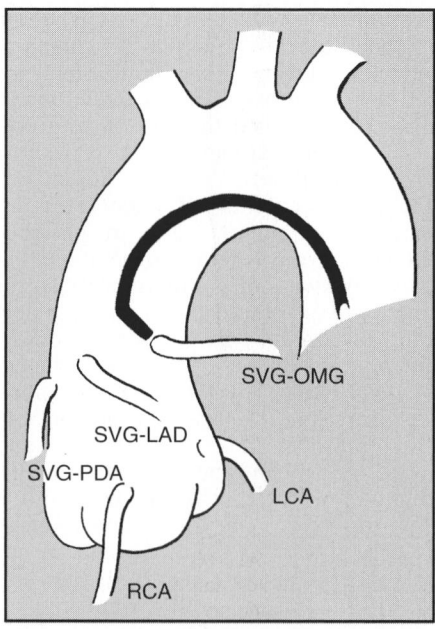

FIGURE 8–15. Catheterization of saphenous vein bypass grafts. In the LAO projection, saphenous vein bypass grafts to the native coronary arteries are positioned and oriented in a predictable manner. Bypass grafts anastomosing to the obtuse marginal branches (SVG-OMB) are characteristically the most leftward and superior of the grafts, those anastomosing primarily with posterior descending artery (SVG-PDA) are the most rightward and inferior, and those to the left anterior descending artery (SVG-LAD) are intermediate in position and orientation. (From Judkins, M. W.: Coronary arteriography. In Douglas, J. S., Jr., King, S. B., III [eds.]: Coronary Arteriography and Intervention. New York, McGraw-Hill, 1985, p. 229, with permission.)

perform an ascending aortogram (preferably in biplane) in an attempt to visualize all SVGs.

GOAL OF BYPASS GRAFT ANGIOGRAPHY. This is to provide an assessment of the ostium of the graft, its entire course, and the distal insertion site at the anastomosis between the bypass graft and the native coronary vessel. The ostium of a bypass graft must be evaluated by achieving a parallel relation between the tip of the catheter and the origin of the graft. The midportion (body) of the graft must be evaluated in the absence of contrast streaming, because inadequate opacification produces an angiographic artifact suggestive of friable filling defects. It is critical to assess the graft insertion site in full profile without any overlap of the distal graft or the native vessel. Angiographic assessment of the native vessels beyond graft anastomotic sites requires views that are conventionally used for the native segments themselves but modified to avoid overlap with the graft itself.

INTERNAL MAMMARY ARTERY CATHETERIZATION

The left IMA arises inferiorly from the left subclavian artery approximately 10 cm from its origin. Catheterization of the left IMA is easily performed (Fig. 8–16) with a specially designed J-tip catheter, referred to as the "IM catheter" (Fig. 8–2). Advancement of the catheter into the aortic arch distal to the origin of the left subclavian artery in the LAO projection, counterclockwise rotation of the catheter, and gentle withdrawal of the catheter with the tip pointing in a cranial direction will easily allow entry into the left subclavian artery, which is usually located immediately under the head of the clavicle. If a small injection of contrast material or guidewire position confirms catheter position in the left subclavian artery, the guidewire is advanced to the left subclavian artery under the distal third of the clavicle. The artery is then viewed "down the barrel" in the RAO projection as the catheter is withdrawn and rotated slightly anteriorly and inferiorly (counterclockwise), tip down, to selectively engage the left IMA.

CATHETERIZATION OF THE RIGHT IMA. This also involves use of the IM catheter. The innominate artery is entered in the LAO projection. The guidewire must be advanced cautiously because of easy entry into the right common carotid artery. Once the guidewire is advanced to the distal right subclavian artery, the catheter is advanced to a point distal to the expected origin of the right IMA. The catheter is withdrawn in the LAO view, while the angiographer looks "down the barrel" of the right IMA.

Often, selective catheterization of the IMAs is compromised by tortuosity of the subclavian arteries. Another catheter that may be use-

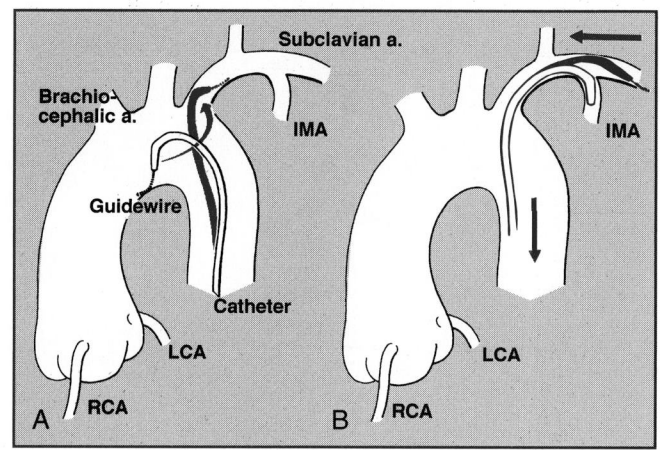

FIGURE 8–16. Catheterization of the left internal mammary artery. The internal mammary catheter is positioned in the aortic arch and visualized in the LAO position. The catheter tip is rotated so that it engages the origin of the left subclavian artery immediately subjacent to the head of the left clavicle (A). This is followed by gentle advancement of the guidewire into subclavian artery to a point distal to the origin of the left internal mammary artery. After the guidewire is removed, the left subclavian is visualized in the RAO projection, the catheter is gently withdrawn, and the catheter tip engages the ostium of the left internal mammary artery selectively (B). (From Judkins, M. W.: Coronary arteriography. In Douglas, J. S., Jr., King, S. B., III [eds.]: Coronary Arteriography and Intervention. New York, McGraw-Hill, 1985, p. 231, with permission.)

ful to enter the left subclavian or the innominate artery is the Headhunter catheter. The ability to advance the guidewire and catheter through the subclavian system also may be compromised by tortuosity and require the use of floppy-tip or hydrophilic-coated guidewire.

As the IMA has been used increasingly because of its superiority as a bypass conduit, the need for selective IMA arteriography also has increased. The IMA itself is rarely affected by atherosclerosis, which may be attributable to superior endothelial properties of anticoagulation, vasodilatation, and growth inhibition as compared with SVGs and native coronary arteries.[54] The distal insertion site, however, is subject to focal stenosis. Thus angiographic studies of the IMAs must assess not only the patency of the graft itself but also the distal anastomosis, where most of IMA graft compromise occurs.[47]

The LAO cranial view is often disappointing in projecting the anas-

tomosis of the IMA with the LAD because of overlap, but the straight LAO and LAO caudal views are often helpful. The risk of catheter-induced dissection of the origin of the IMA can be reduced by careful manipulation of the catheter tip and avoidance of forceful advancement without the protection of the guidewire. If the IMA cannot be selectively engaged because of tortuosity of the subclavian artery, nonselective arteriography can be enhanced by placing a blood pressure cuff on the ipsilateral arm and inflating it to a pressure above systolic arterial pressure. The occurrence of IMA spasm can be treated with 50 to 200 μg of intraarterial nitroglycerin or 50 to 100 μg of intraarterial verapamil.

GASTROEPIPLOIC ARTERY CATHETERIZATION

The right gastroepiploic artery (GEA) is the largest terminal artery of the gastroduodenal artery. The other terminal branch of the gastroduodenal artery is the superior pancreaticoduodenal artery. The gastroepiploic artery arises from the common hepatic artery in 75 per cent of cases, but it also may arise from the right or left hepatic artery or the celiac trunk. Catheterization of the right GEA is carried out by first entering the common hepatic artery with a cobra catheter (Fig. 8–17). The angiographer then gently advances a torquable, hydrophilic-coated guidewire to the gastroduodenal artery and then to the right GEA. Exchange of the cobra for a multipurpose or Judkins right coronary catheter will then permit selective arteriography of the right GEA.

Pitfalls of Coronary Arteriography

GENERAL PRINCIPLES OF ARTERIOGRAPHIC INTERPRETATION. A systematic approach based on a few common sense principles is needed to avoid pitfalls in the performance and interpretation of coronary arteriography. It should be recalled that the normal coronary artery tapers gradually from proximal to distal and has smooth walls completely free of irregularities. Although it is tempting in some cases to invoke the diagnosis of an anatomical variant to account for a particular arteriographic finding, it must be emphasized that the prevalence of acquired coronary artery disease is several orders of magnitude greater than the rare occurrence of congenital variants. Thus, attention to the following three rules of congenital variations[55] is needed: (1) acquired atherosclerotic coronary artery disease is far more frequent than are the unusual anatomical variations; (2) there are thousands of collaterals for any one anomalous vessel; and (3) before an unusual vessel is accepted as a variant, an occlusion or large collateral channel should be suspected.

LEFT MAIN CORONARY ARTERY STENOSIS. The left main coronary artery should be viewed in several projections with the vessel off the spine. Catheter pressure damping and the absence of reflux suggest the presence of LMCA disease (Figs. 8–18 and 8–19). Unrecognized LMCA stenosis often results in inappropriate referral of patients for coronary intervention.[56]

INADEQUATE OPACIFICATION. Inadequate filling of the coronary artery with contrast medium may result in streaming of contrast medium and give the impression of ostial stenoses, missing side branches, or thrombus. Similarly, superselective injection of contrast medium into the left circumflex artery through a short left main coronary artery may give the impression of total occlusion of the left anterior descending coronary artery. Adequate filling of the coronary arteries and bypass grafts is required to overcome the native flow of unopacified blood and produce high-quality coronary arteriograms. Stenoses may be under- or overassessed if incomplete filling is achieved. The causes of incomplete filling include competition from increased native coronary blood flow in the setting of left ventricular hypertrophy associated with aortic insufficiency or anemia and inadequate placement of the diagnostic catheter with subselective injection. The problem of underfilling can be overcome by more forceful contrast material injection as long as the catheter-tip position and pressure recording confirm the safety of such a maneuver. Under some conditions, switching to an angioplasty guiding catheter with a soft, short tip and a larger lumen than a diagnostic catheter

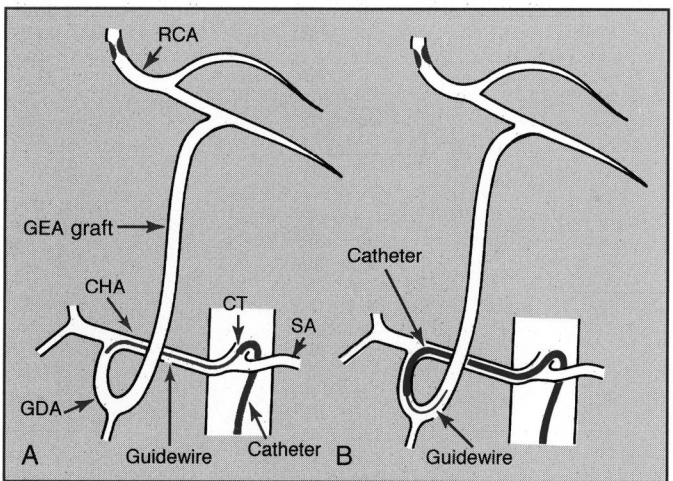

FIGURE 8–17. Catheterization of the right gastroepiploic artery graft. The celiac trunk (CT) is selectively engaged with a cobra catheter, and a torquable, hydrophilic-coated guidewire is gently advanced to the gastroduodenal artery (GDA) and the GEA (gastroepiploic) artery (A). The catheter is advanced over the guidewire for selective arteriography of the GEA graft (B). CHA = common hepatic artery; RCA = right coronary artery; SA = splenic artery. (From Isshiki, T., Yamaguchi, T., Tamura, T., et al.: Percutaneous angiography of stenosed gastroepiploic artery grafts. J. Am. Coll. Cardiol. 21:727, 1993. Reprinted with permission from the American College of Cardiology.)

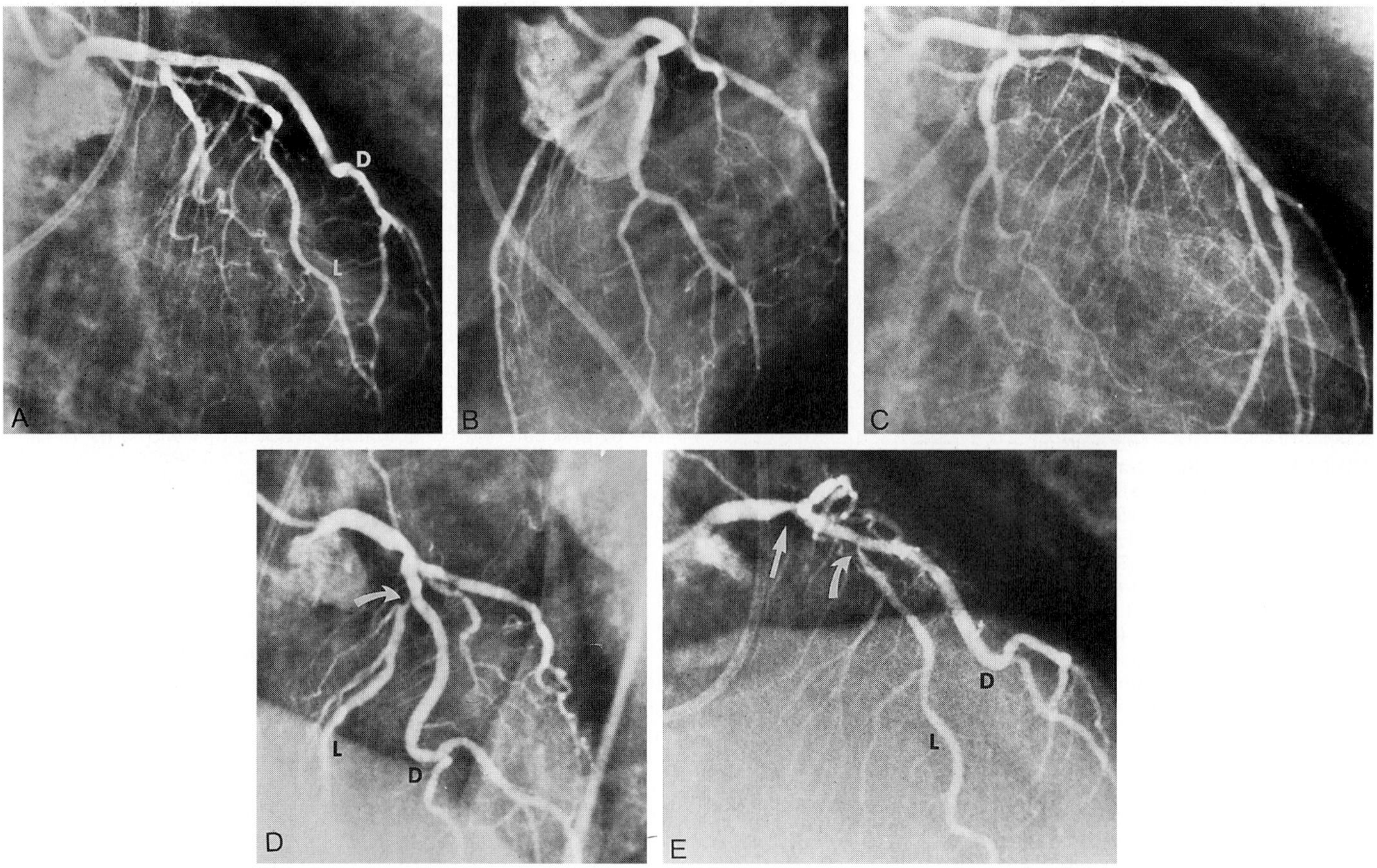

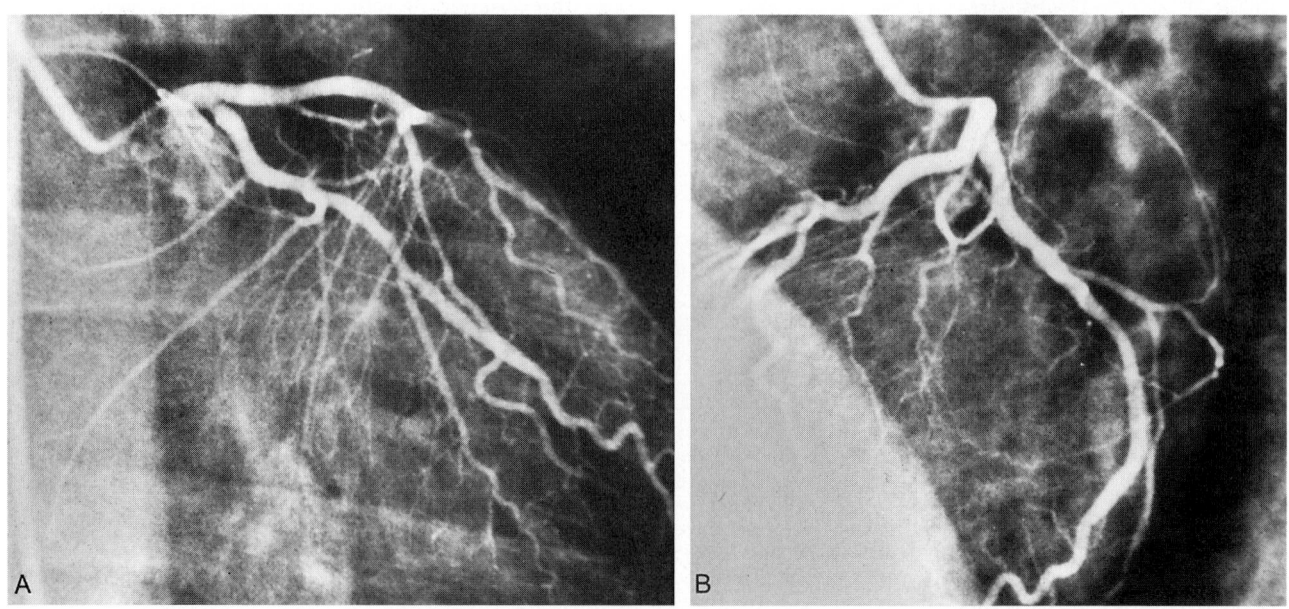

FIGURE 8–18. Missed left main coronary artery stenosis. *A–C,* left coronary arteriography in the standard RAO, LAO, and RAO caudal views fails to demonstrate significant stenoses of the LMCA or LAD. *D,* LAO cranial view shows severe stenosis (curved arrow) of the LAD (L) immediately beyond the origin of the diagonal branch (D). *E,* RAO cranial view shows the LAD stenosis (curved arrow) but also shows a severe stenosis of the LMCA (straight arrow) at its bifurcation.

may allow for more complete opacification of the target coronary artery or bypass graft.

ECCENTRIC STENOSES. Coronary atherosclerosis more often leads to eccentric or slit-like atherosclerotic narrowings than to concentric narrowings. If, in such cases, the long axis of the eccentric lumen is projected, the vessel may appear to have a normal or near-normal caliber. Only if the short axis of the stenotic lumen is projected will the narrowing be visible (Fig. 8–20). For this reason, coronary arteries must be viewed in at least two projections approximately 90 degrees apart.

A related problem is that of the band-like or membranous

FIGURE 8–19. Difficulty in detecting ostial left main coronary artery stenosis. *A,* Shallow RAO views of the LAD with the catheter not well seated in the vessel result in poor visualization of the ostial stenosis of the LMCA. *B,* LAO cranial view shows the catheter tip selectively positioned in the LMCA without reflux of contrast around the tip.

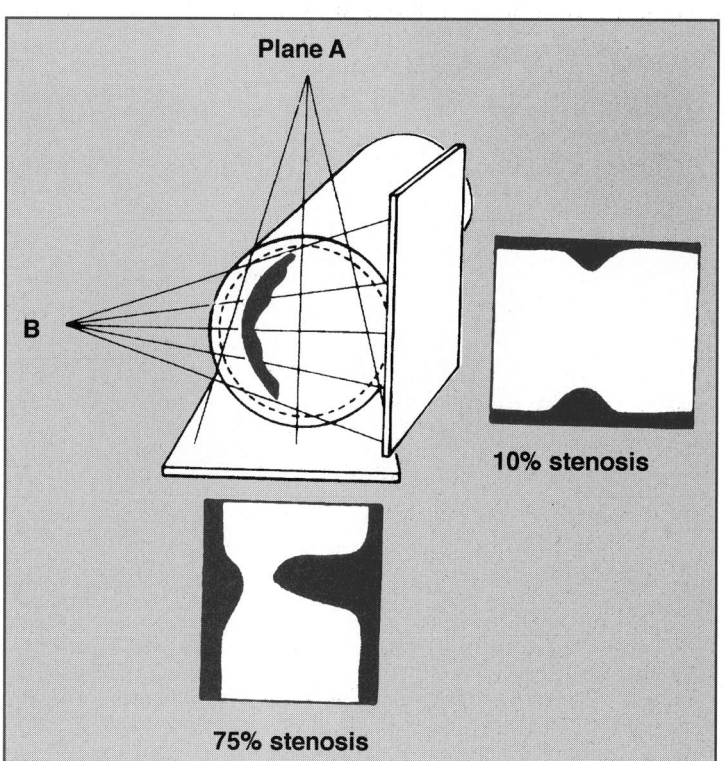

FIGURE 8–20. Importance of orthogonal projections. Each vascular segment of the coronary artery must be recorded in two orthogonal or nearly orthogonal views to avoid missing important diagnostic information about eccentric stenoses. In plane A the image is associated with a 75 per cent stenosis, but in plane B the image results in 10 per cent stenosis. (From Miller, S. W.: Coronary artery disease. *In* Miller, S. W. [ed.]: Cardiac Angiography. Boston, Little, Brown, 1984, p. 87, with permission.)

stenosis. Lesions such as this may be exceedingly difficult to detect. It is not clear whether these peculiar lesions represent pure atherosclerotic stenosis or are caused in some instances by congenital membranous bands.[57] Aside from the difficulty in detecting these lesions, it is difficult to ascertain their hemodynamic significance. Measurement of the pressure gradient across the lesion through a small inner catheter inserted through the angiographic catheter may be useful in this regard. The use of intravascular ultrasound also may be very helpful.

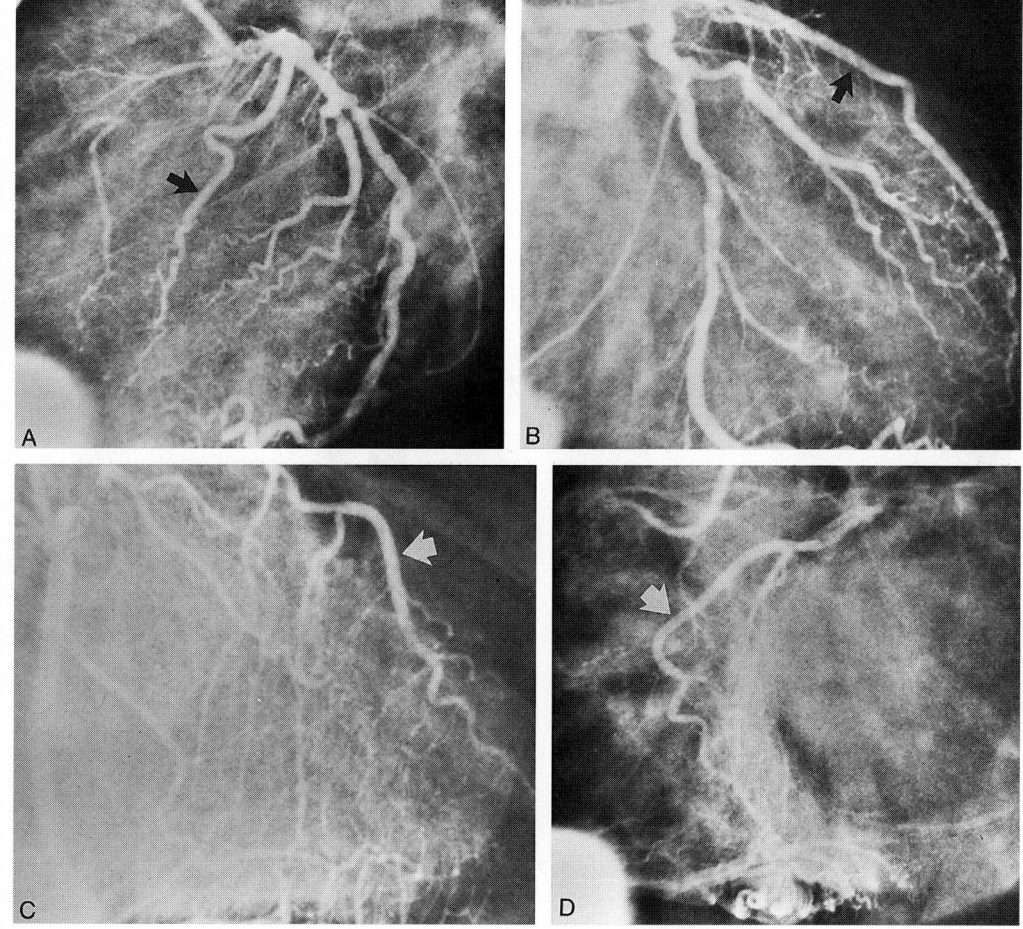

FIGURE 8–21. Superimposition of branches. *A, B,* LAO and RAO views of the left coronary arteriogram show that the LAD is totally occluded, although the point of occlusion is not visualized. There is a large diagonal branch (black arrows) that closely parallels the LAD in both projections and could be mistaken for the LAD. Late-phase frames from an RAO *(C)* and LAD *(D)* right coronary arteriogram show filling of the LAD (white arrows) via septal collaterals.

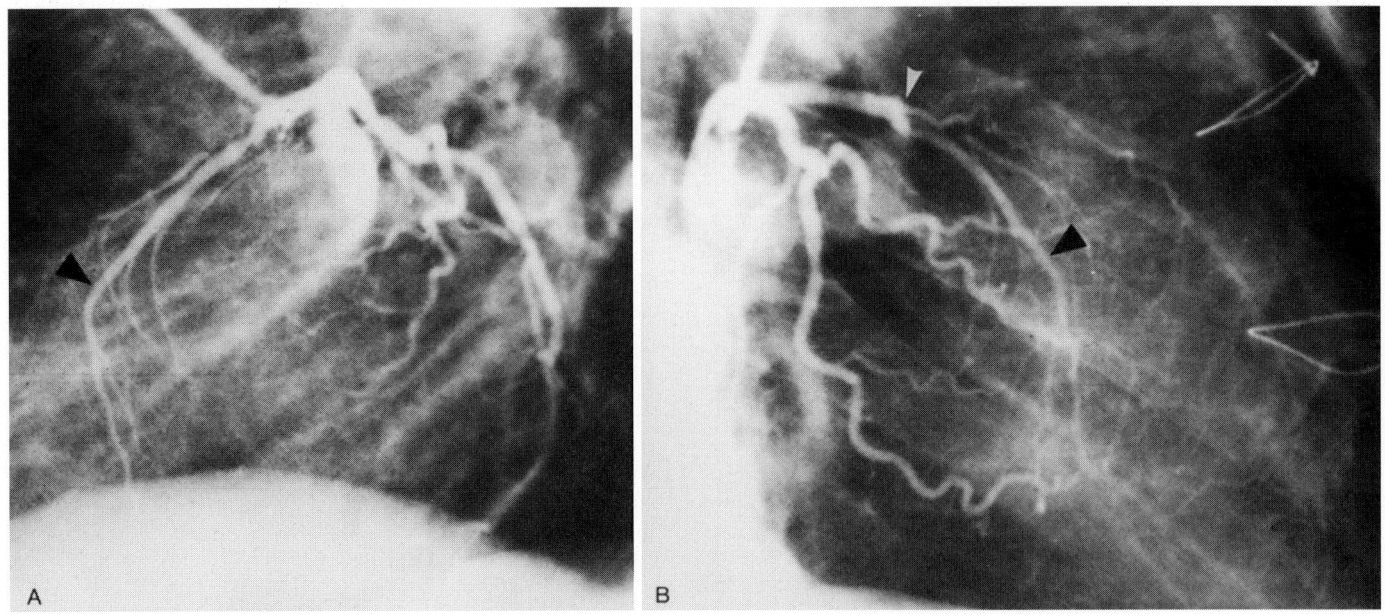

FIGURE 8–22. Septal branch mimicking the LAD. *A,* LAO left coronary arteriogram shows an enlarged septal branch (arrowhead) occupying the expected course of the LAD. *B,* The RAO view shows that the LAD is totally occluded (white arrowhead). The septal branch (black arrowhead) runs in a course approximately parallel to the LAD but below it and within the interventricular septum. (From Levin, D. C., Baltaxe, H. A., and Sos, T. A.: Potential sources of error in coronary arteriography. II. Interpretation of the study. *A.J.R. 124:*386, 1975, copyright 1975 American Roentgen Ray Society.)

UNRECOGNIZED OCCLUSIONS. Flow disturbances associated with branch points predispose to the development of atherosclerosis and total occlusions of major arteries at these locations.[58,59] Because of this fact and the variability in the number and distribution of side branches in the normal coronary circulation, it is possible for occlusions at branch origins to escape detection. In some cases, occlusion of a branch can be recognized only by late filling of the distal segment of this branch by means of collateral circulation (Fig. 8–21).

SUPERIMPOSITION OF BRANCHES. Superimposition of major branches of the left coronary tree in the LAO and RAO projections can result in failure to detect stenoses or total occlusions of these branches. Although this problem most commonly affects the LAD and parallel diagonal branches (Fig. 8–19), it is alleviated by the use of cranial and caudal angulation. It should be noted that septal branches may mimic the LAD in the LAO cranial projection (Fig. 8–22). When the LAD is occluded beyond the

origin of the first septal branch, this branch often enlarges in an attempt to provide collateral circulation to the vascular bed of the distal LAD.

MYOCARDIAL BRIDGING. The major coronary arteries pass over the epicardial surface of the heart. In some cases, however, short segments descend into the myocardium for a variable distance. This occurs in 5 to 12 per cent of humans and is almost always confined to the LAD.[60] Because a "bridge" of myocardial fibers passes over the involved segment of the LAD, each systolic contraction of these fibers can cause narrowing of the artery. Myocardial bridging has a characteristic appearance on cineangiography (Fig. 8–23). The bridged segment is of normal caliber during diastole but abruptly narrows with each systole. Systolic narrowing caused by myocardial bridging should not be confused with an atherosclerotic plaque. Although bridging is not thought to have any hemodynamic significance in most cases, some have suggested that when it produces severe systolic narrowing, ischemia or infarction

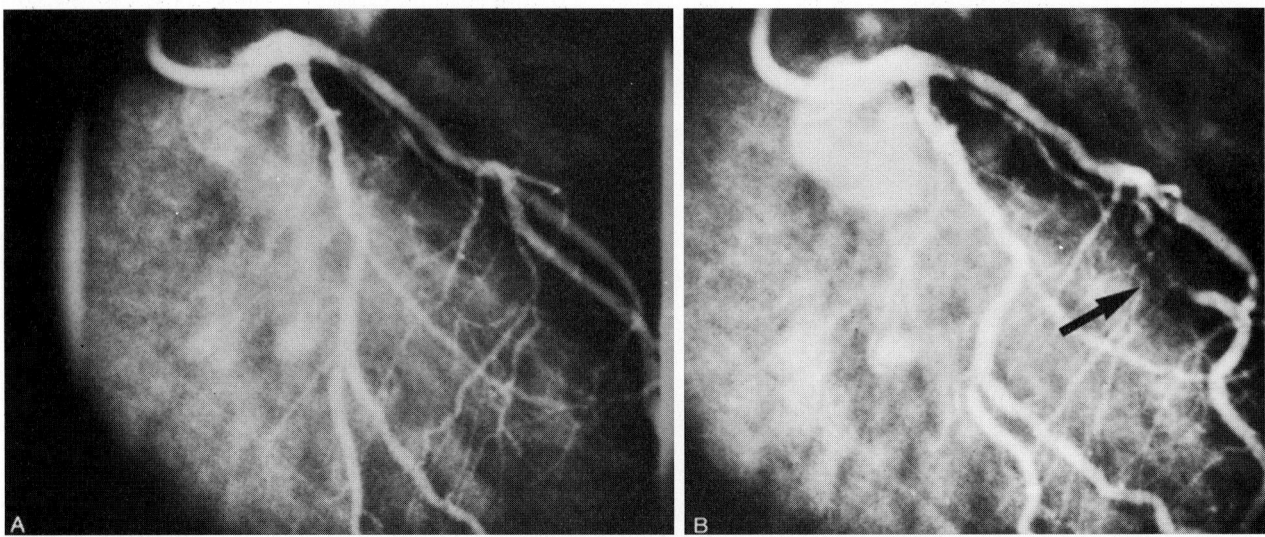

FIGURE 8–23. Myocardial bridging. *A,* RAO left coronary arteriogram shows a normal LAD during diastole. *B,* During systole, there is pronounced narrowing of the LAD (arrow).

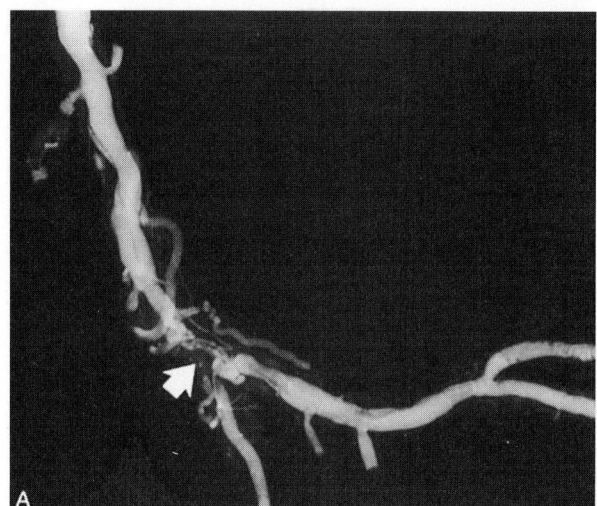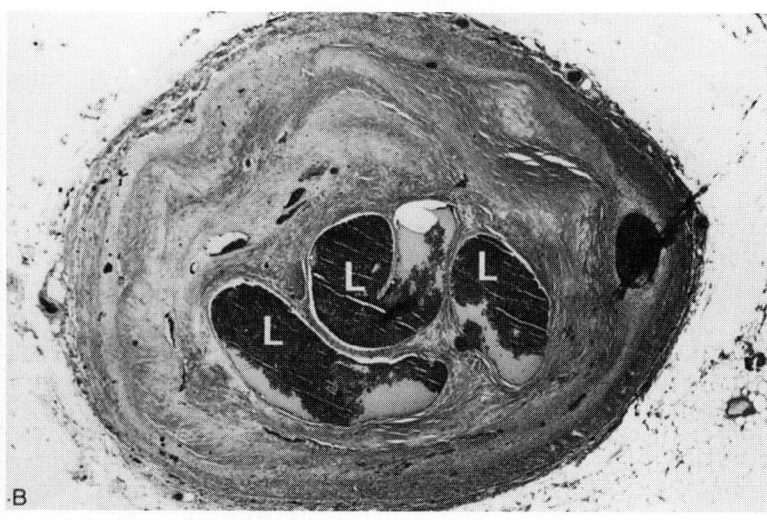

FIGURE 8-24. Recanalization of a total occlusion. *A,* Postmortem injection specimen. The RCA was injected with barium-gelatin mixture and then dissected from the epicardial surface of the heart. The recanalized segment (arrow) demonstrates several irregular channels. It is likely that angiography of such a segment in a living patient would not have sufficient resolution to demonstrate these channels. The angiographic appearance would likely be a total occlusion. *B,* Histologic section of the recanalized segment. L = recanalized lumina filled with the barium-gelatin mixture.

may result. The presence of myocardial bridging has important implications for interventional cardiovascular therapy because bridges do not respond to angioplasty.

RECANALIZATION. Although a narrowed segment of a coronary artery seen on arteriography usually is considered a "stenosis," such lesions may actually be segments which were once totally occluded but have recanalized. Pathological studies suggest that approximately one-third of totally occluded coronary arteries ultimately recanalize.[61] The arteriographic appearances of stenosis and recanalization may be indistinguishable. Recanalization usually results in the development of multiple tortuous channels, which are quite small and close to one another, creating an impression on cineangiography of a single, slightly irregular channel (Fig. 8-24). The spatial resolution of cineangiography is insufficient to demonstrate this degree of detail in most patients with recanalized total occlusions, but this has important implications for interventional cardiovascular treatments, because they are unlikely to be successful in the setting of multiple small channels.

COMPLICATIONS

The incidence of complications of coronary arteriography has been given in several large, multicenter reports. Data on complications for coronary arteriography for the 13 institutions participating in the CASS Registry involved a total of 7553 consecutive procedures.[17] The complications in 1087 patients undergoing coronary arteriography via the brachial approach were compared with those in 6328 patients undergoing the femoral approach. Death occurred in 0.51 per cent of the brachial patients and in 0.14 per cent of the femoral patients. Cerebral ischemia occurred in 0.17 per cent of the brachial patients and in 0.08 per cent of the femoral patients. Local vascular complications such as thrombosis occurred in 1.85 per cent of the brachial patients and in 0.24 per cent of the femoral patients.

The complications of outpatient coronary arteriography via the femoral approach have been reported.[62] In 3071 consecutive patients, death occurred in 0.13 per cent, nonfatal myocardial infarction in 0.07 per cent, neurological complications in 0.14 per cent, and local vascular complications in 0.35 per cent. The most extensive analysis of complications of coronary arteriography is the report of the Registry of the Society for Cardiac Angiography and Inter-

ventions.[63] Among 222,553 patients entered into this registry between 1984 and 1987, death occurred in 0.10 per cent, myocardial infarction in 0.06 per cent, stroke in 0.07 per cent, vascular complications in 0.46 per cent, and contrast reactions in 0.23 per cent. Major complications (death, myocardial infarction, and stroke) occurred with similar frequencies using the femoral and brachial approaches, but vascular complications were increased fourfold with the brachial approach. The incidence of death was increased in the presence of left main coronary artery disease (0.55 per cent), with ejection fraction less than 30 per cent (0.30 per cent), and in NYHA functional class IV (0.29 per cent). More recent registries have identified equivalent complication rates despite increasing age and acuity of illness in the patients undergoing coronary arteriography.[64]

The risk of clinically significant coronary air embolus during diagnostic coronary arteriography is low, probably occurring in less than 0.1 per cent of cases. If the syndrome of coronary air embolus and air lock does occur, 100 per cent O_2 should be administered to encourage rapid resorption of N_2, morphine sulfate is given for pain relief, and ventricular arrhythmias are anticipated and treated with lidocaine and direct-current (DC) cardioversion. Small amounts of air are usually resorbed within 2 to 4 minutes on 100 per cent oxygen.

ABNORMALITIES OF THE CORONARY CIRCULATION

Congenital Anomalies That Cause Myocardial Ischemia
(See also Chap. 29)

CORONARY ARTERY FISTULAS (see p. 908). A review of a large series of patients with congenital anomalies of the coronary arteries revealed that coronary artery fistula is by far the most common.[65] Although about half the patients with large fistulas remain asymptomatic, the other half develop congestive heart failure, infective endocarditis, myocardial ischemia, or rupture of an aneurysmal fistula. About half these fistulas arise from the RCA or its branches, slightly fewer than half arise from the LAD or LCx artery or their branches, and in the remaining cases there are multiple origins (Fig. 8-25). Drainage occurs into the right ventricle in 41 per cent, into the right atrium in 26 per cent, into the pulmonary artery in 17 per cent, into the left ven-

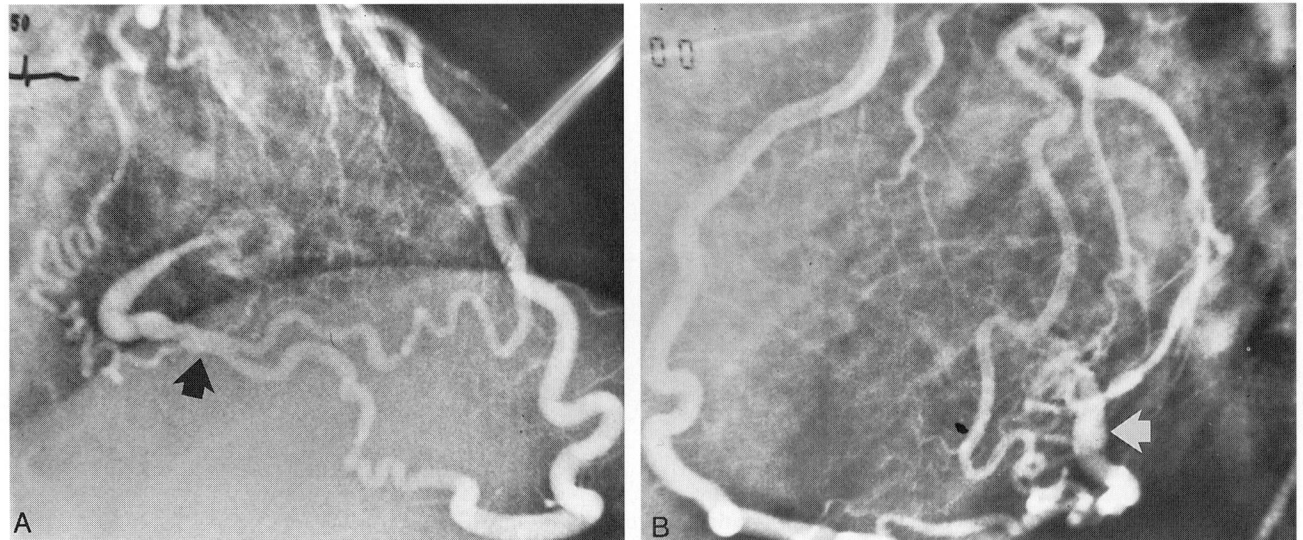

FIGURE 8–25. Congenital fistula. *A,* RAO cranial view of the left coronary arteriogram shows a congenital fistula (arrow) arising from branches of both the LAD and LCx and draining into the left ventricle. *B,* LAO view of the left coronary arteriogram shows the fistula (arrow).

tricle in 3 per cent, and into the superior vena cava in 1 per cent.[65] Thus a left-to-right shunt exists in more than 90 per cent of cases. Selective coronary arteriography is the only way to demonstrate the origin of these fistulas.

ORIGIN OF THE LEFT CORONARY ARTERY FROM THE PULMONARY ARTERY. Most patients with origin of the LCA from the main pulmonary artery develop myocardial ischemia early in life. About 25 per cent survive to adolescence or adulthood but frequently experience mitral regurgitation, angina, or congestive heart failure.[66] Aortography typically shows a large RCA with absence of a left coronary ostium in the left aortic sinus. During the late phase of the aortogram, patulous LAD and LCx branches fill by means of collateral circulation from RCA branches. Still later in the filming sequence, retrograde flow from the LAD and LCx opacifies the main LCA and its origin from the main pulmonary artery (Fig. 8–26). The clinical course of the patient tends to be more favorable if extensive collateral circulation exists. In rare instances, the RCA rather than the LCA may arise from the pulmonary artery.

CONGENITAL CORONARY STENOSIS OR ATRESIA. Congenital stenosis or atresia of a coronary artery can occur as an isolated lesion or in association with other congenital diseases such as calcific coronary sclerosis, supravalvular aortic stenosis, homocystinuria, Friedreich's ataxia, Hurler's syndrome, progeria, and rubella syndrome.[65] In these latter cases, the atretic vessel usually fills by means of collateral circulation from the contralateral side.

ANOMALOUS ORIGIN OF EITHER CORONARY ARTERY FROM THE CONTRALATERAL SINUS. Origin of the LCA from the proximal RCA or the right aortic sinus with subsequent passage between the aorta and the right ventricular outflow tract has been associated with sudden death during or shortly after exercise in young persons.[67-71] After its aberrant origin, the LCA takes an abrupt leftward turn and tunnels between the aorta and the right ventricular outflow tract. Sudden death is thought to result from transient occlusion of the anomalous LCA caused by an increase in blood flow through the aorta and pulmonary artery that occurs during exercise and creates either a kink at the sharp leftward bend or a pinchcock mechanism in the tunnel. Origin of the RCA from the LCA or left aortic sinus with passage between the aorta and the right ventricular outflow tract is somewhat less dangerous. This anomaly, however, also has been associated with myocardial ischemia or sudden death, presumably through the same mechanism.[69,71,72] In rare cases of anomalous origin of the LCA from the right aortic sinus, myocardial ischemia may occur even if the LCA passes anterior to the right ventricular outflow tract

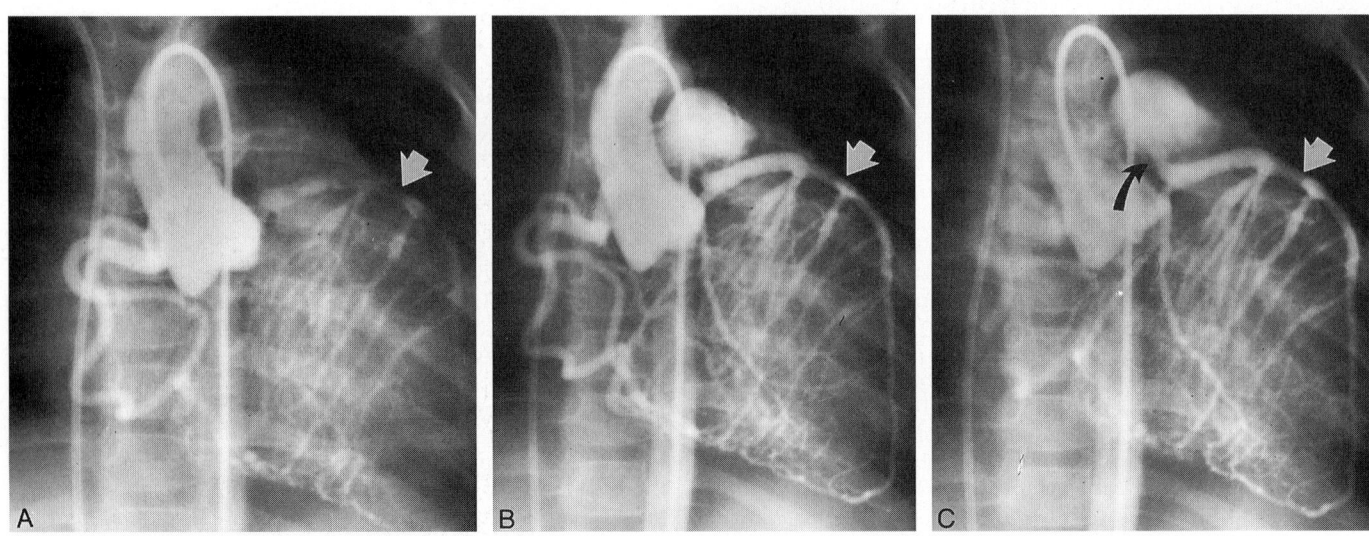

FIGURE 8–26. Anomalous origin of the LCA from the pulmonary artery. *A, B,* and *C,* The thoracic aortogram shows a large RCA and no antegrade filling of the LCA. The LCA fills primarily through extensive collaterals from the RCA to the LAD (white arrows). The anomalous origin of the LCA from the pulmonary artery is demonstrated in late phases of the aortogram (*C,* curved arrow).

or posterior to the aorta (i.e., not through a tunnel between the two great vessels),[73] but the cause of the defect is not clear.

The course of the anomalous coronary arteries is easily assessed by angiography in the RAO view (Fig. 8–27). There are four common courses for the anomalously arising LCA from the right sinus of Valsalva, one common course for the anomalous RCA arising from the left sinus of Valsalva, and one common course for the anomalous LCx arising from the right sinus of Valsalva. The anomalous LCA arising from the right sinus of Valsalva may take either a septal, anterior, interarterial, or posterior course (Fig. 8–27).[74] The posterior course of the anomalous LCA arising from the left sinus of Valsalva is similar to the almost unvarying course of the anomalous LCx arising from the right sinus of Valsalva, whereas the common interarterial course of the anomalous RCA from the left sinus of Valsalva (Fig. 8–28) is by symmetry similar to the interarterial course of the anomalous LCA arising from the right sinus of Valsalva.

When either the LCA or the LAD arises anomalously from the right aortic sinus, an alternative angiographic method to identify the course of the anomalous vessel is first to pass a catheter into the main pulmonary artery and then to perform an arteriogram of the aberrant coronary artery in the steep AP caudal projection. This places the aberrant coronary artery, the rightward and anterior pulmonary valve, and the leftward and posterior aortic valve all in one plane (see Fig. 8–27). From this "laid-back arteriogram," which can be used even in mapping the course of anomalous coronary arteries in transposition of the great vessels, it is usually possible to confirm whether the course of the aberrant coronary artery is between the great vessels.

Although angiography is useful for establishing the presence of anomalous coronary arteries, transesophageal echocardiography may be an important adjunctive diagnostic tool for defining the course of the vessels.[75]

CONGENITAL CORONARY ANOMALIES NOT CAUSING MYOCARDIAL ISCHEMIA

In this category of anomalies, the coronary arteries originate from the aorta, but their origins are in unusual locations. Although myocardial perfusion is normal, the angiographer may have trouble locating the arteries. These anomalies occur in about 0.5 to 1.0 per cent of adult patients undergoing coronary arteriography.[76]

ORIGIN OF THE LEFT CIRCUMFLEX ARTERY FROM THE RIGHT AORTIC SINUS. Anomalous origin of the LCx from the right aortic sinus is the most common of these anomalies (Fig. 8–29). In a series of almost

FIGURE 8–27. Anomalous origin of the left coronary artery from the right sinus of Valsalva. Each panel includes a caudo-cranial cross-sectional schematic representation at the level of the semilunar valves, showing the course of the anomalous coronary. The RAO angiograms and bitmaps show examples of each of four most common courses of the anomalous left coronary artery aberrantly arising from the right sinus of Valsalva: posterior (retroaortic), interarterial, anterior, and septal (subpulmonic) courses.

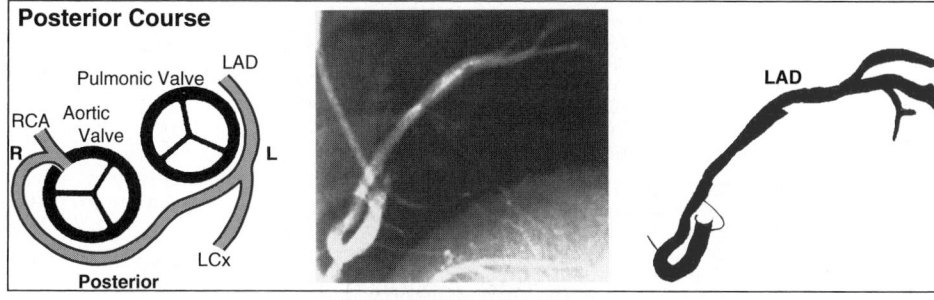

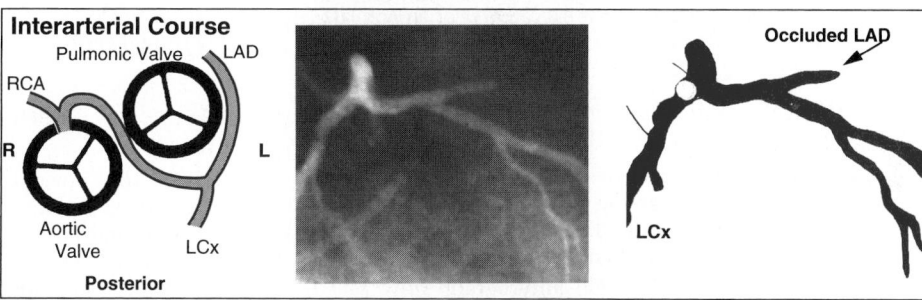

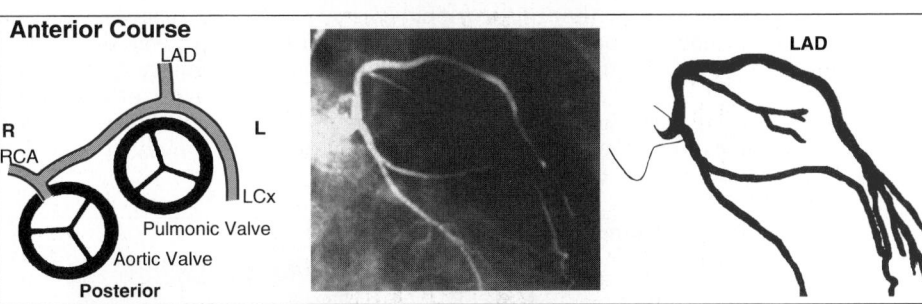

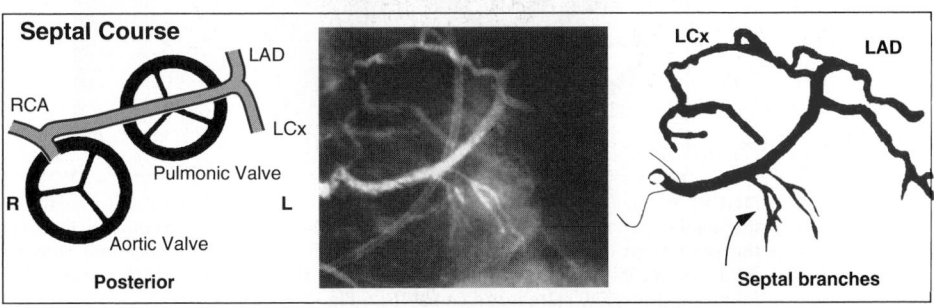

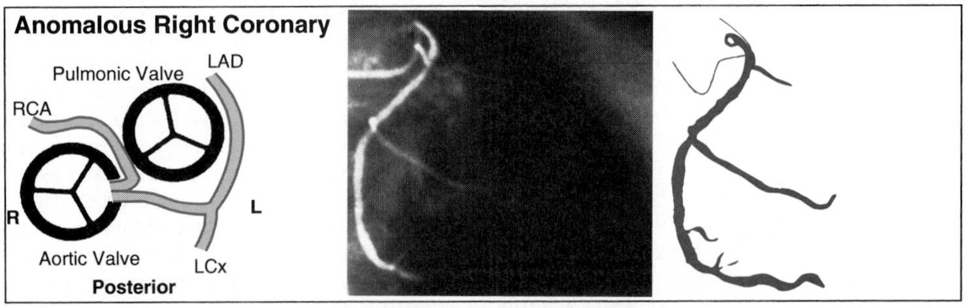

Anomalous Right Coronary

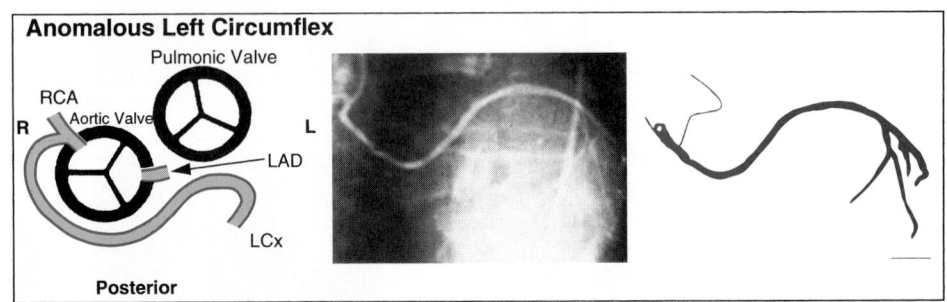

FIGURE 8–28. Anomalous origin of the right coronary artery. RAO coronary arteriogram shows an anomalous RCA arising from left sinus of Valsalva. The origin of the aberrantly arising artery, which is engaged with a left Judkins catheter, arises immediately anterior to the origin of the left coronary artery (not shown in the arteriogram). The anomalous right coronary follows an interarterial course opposite but analogous to that for the anomalous LCA arising from the right sinus of Valsalva (see Fig. 8–27).

3000 patients, this anomaly was found in 0.67 per cent.[77] In virtually every case, the anomalous LCx arises posterior to the right coronary artery and courses inferiorly and posteriorly to the aorta to enter the left atrioventricular groove. An interarterial course for an anomalously arising LCx from the right sinus of Valsalva would be almost unprecedented.

SINGLE CORONARY ARTERY. Although there are numerous variations of this anomaly,[78] it assumes hemodynamic significance when a major branch passes between the aorta and the right ventricular outflow tract, as described earlier.

ORIGIN OF ALL THREE CORONARY ARTERIES FROM EITHER THE RIGHT OR LEFT AORTIC SINUS VIA MULTIPLE SEPARATE OSTIA. This rare anomaly is similar to single coronary artery. There is absence of a coronary ostium in either the left or right aortic sinus. The missing vessels arise in the contralateral aortic sinus, but instead of arising as a single coronary artery, they arise through two or even three separate ostia.

HIGH ANTERIOR ORIGIN OF THE RIGHT CORONARY ARTERY. This anomaly is commonly encountered but of no hemodynamic significance. The inability to engage the ostium of the RCA selectively from conventional catheter manipulation raises the question of superior origin of the RCA above the sinotubular ridge. Forceful, nonselective injection of contrast medium into the right sinus of Valsalva may reveal the anomalous takeoff of the RCA, which can then be selectively engaged with a Judkins right 5.0 catheter or an Amplatz left 1.0 or 1.5 catheter.

Angiographic Assessment of Myocardial Blood Flow

Angiographic evidence of coronary artery perfusion can be based on the flow grades first proposed by the Thrombolysis in Myocardial Infarction (TIMI) study group.[79] With this scheme, coronary perfusion is classified as follows:

Grade 0: No perfusion. No anterograde flow of contrast medium is detected beyond the point of occlusion.

Grade 1: Penetration without perfusion. Contrast medium passes through the point of obstruction, but anterograde flow fails to opacify the distal portion of the vessel at any time.

Grade 2: Partial perfusion. Contrast material penetrates through the point of obstruction but enters the distal vessel at a rate slower than that for nonobstructed arteries in the same patient.

Grade 3: Complete perfusion. Anterograde flow into the distal coronary bed is rapid and complete.

The rate of coronary flow as assessed by the TIMI flow grade is determined by two major factors: the severity of the stenosis in the vessel and the status of the microvasculature. The clinical outcome after thrombolysis for acute myocardial infarction is related to TIMI flow grade. After receiving thrombolytic therapy for acute myocardial infarction, patients with TIMI grade 3 flow at 90 minutes had lower mortality rates than those with TIMI grade 2 flow.[80] A method for quantifying the angiographic rates of coronary artery perfusion has been proposed using the TIMI frame count. With this method, the number of cinefilm frames required for opacification of the involved vessel is counted by means of an automated frame counter, which is present on most cineprojectors. The quantitative frame count method offers the advantages of being more objective, more reproducible, and more strongly correlated with clinical outcomes than conventional methods.[81]

Coronary Collateral Circulation
(See also p. 1174)

In the normal human heart, myriad tiny anastomotic branches interconnect the major coronary arteries.[82] Most of these anatomical vessels are less than 200 μm in diameter, and they are the precursors of the collateral circulation. In coronary arteriograms of patients with normal or mildly diseased coronary arteries, they cannot be visualized because they carry only minimal flow and their small caliber is well beyond the spatial resolution capabilities of cine imaging systems. If, however, obstruction of a major coronary artery occurs, a pressure gradient is created in the anastomotic vessels connecting the distal segment of the involved artery with either its proximal segment or the

Anomalous Left Circumflex

FIGURE 8–29. Anomalous origin of the left circumflex. The caudo-cranial cross-sectional view at the level of the semilunar valves shows the common course of the left circumflex coronary artery aberrantly arising from the right sinus of Valsalva. The LCx passes behind the aortic root and runs to the left atrioventricular groove following an initial course identical to that for the anomalous LCA arising from the right sinus of Valsalva that follows a posterior, retroaortic course (see Fig. 8–27).

nearby segments of other vessels. With the creation of this gradient, an increased volume of blood is propelled through the anastomotic vessels, which progressively dilate and eventually become visible angiographically as collateral channels. The reason this process seems to occur effectively in some patients and ineffectively in others is not entirely clear, but it may involve the rate at which obstruction develops. The most favorable clinical circumstance is gradual development of the obstruction, thereby allowing collateral channels to enlarge and become functional before the native vessel becomes totally occluded.

Other factors that affect collateral development are patency of the feeding arteries and the size and vascular resistance of the postobstructive segment.[83] Some interesting observations on the temporal sequence of collateral development resulted from an angiographic study of patients who showed persistent occlusion of the infarct artery after acute myocardial infarction.[84] Among patients studied within 6 hours of infarction, about half demonstrated angiographically visible collaterals. Among those studied more than 24 hours after infarction, virtually all had visible collaterals. This suggests that collateral flow may develop more quickly than previously thought, perhaps within hours after total occlusion. In any event, collateral circulation does not represent the formation of new vessels but rather the utilization of vessels that already exist but carry little blood flow until the need arises. Collaterals usually cannot be demonstrated at coronary arteriography unless the recipient vessel has developed at least 90 per cent diameter stenosis by visual estimates.[82,85]

A large number of collateral pathways exist in patients with severe coronary artery disease (Figs. 8–30 to 8–32). The functional role of coronary collateral circulation has been debated for many years. In patients with total occlusions, regional left ventricular contraction was significantly better in segments supplied by adequate collateral circulation than in those segments supplied by inadequate or no collateral circulation.[82] In another study, patients with acute myocardial infarction undergoing emergency coronary arteriography without antecedent thrombolytic therapy were divided into those with adequate collateral circulation to the infarct-related vessel and those with inadequate or no collateral circulation to the infarct vessel.[86] The group with adequate collaterals had significantly lower left ventricular end-diastolic pressures, higher cardiac index, higher ejection fraction, and lower percentage of area dyssynergy. None of the patients with adequate collaterals died, whereas the majority with inadequate or no collaterals died. Patients with severe coronary obstruction without collateral circulation were found to have a significantly higher incidence of thallium-201 myocardial perfusion defects than those with collateral circulation.[87] This suggests that collaterals may improve myocardial perfusion in the ischemic zone.

The advent of percutaneous transluminal coronary angioplasty (PTCA, see Chap. 39) has provided opportunities to study hemodynamic aspects and angiographic patterns of the coronary collateral circulation, since balloon inflation during PTCA simulates abrupt occlusion of a previously stenotic vessel. Using bilateral coronary angiography, Rentrop and Cohen[88] developed a grading system of 0 to 3 for collateral filling classified as follows:

Grade 0: No collaterals present
Grade 1: Barely detectable collateral flow. Contrast medium passes through collateral channels but fails to opacify the epicardial vessel at any time.
Grade 2: Partial collateral flow. Contrast material enters but fails to opacify the target epicardial vessel completely.
Grade 3: Complete perfusion. Contrast material enters and completely opacifies the target epicardial vessel.

With balloon inflation during PTCA, patients with well-developed collaterals experienced less pain, less left ventricular dyssynergy, and less summed ST-segment elevation than those with poorly developed collaterals.[88] Distal coronary perfusion pressure during balloon inflation is higher in patients with well-developed collaterals than in those with poorly developed collateral circulation.[89–91]

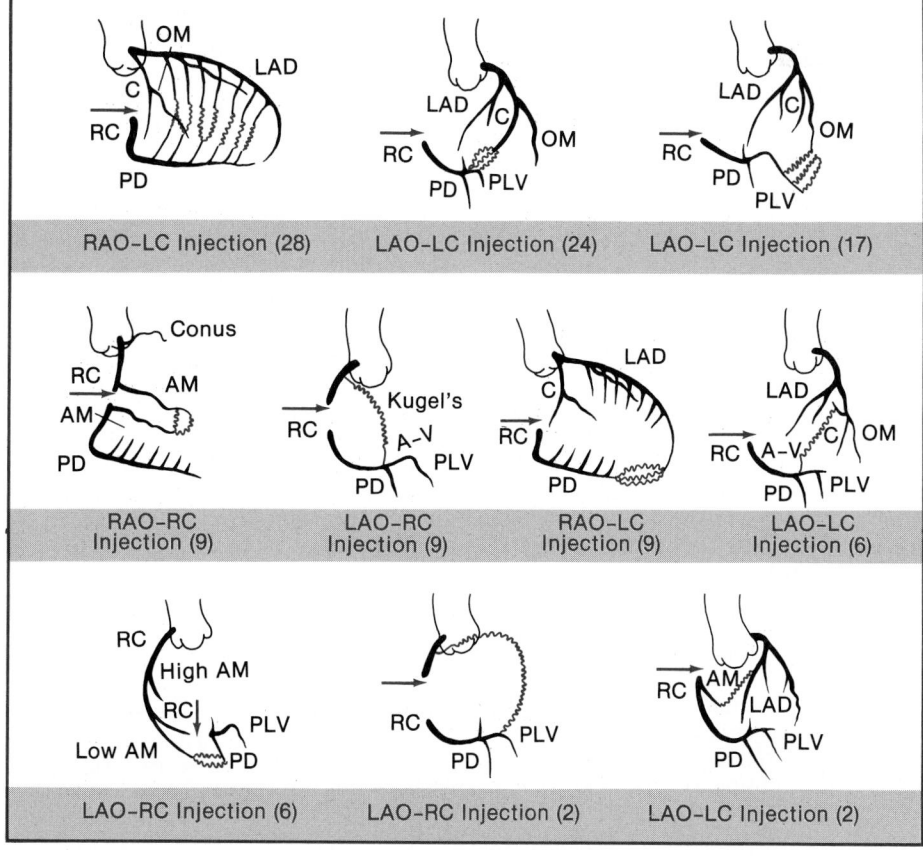

FIGURE 8–30. Coronary collaterals seen with RCA occlusion. Common collateral pathways seen with RCA occlusion. The arrows point to the site of obstruction. The small tortuous channels represent the collateral connections. Numbers in parentheses refer to the frequency with which each pathway was visualized in a series of 200 patients with significant coronary disease. RC = right coronary artery, C = circumflex artery, OM = obtuse marginal branch of the circumflex artery, PD = posterior descending branch of the right coronary artery, PLV = posterior left ventricular branch of the right coronary artery, AM = acute marginal branch of the right coronary artery, A-V = artery to the atrioventricular node. (Reproduced with permission from Levin, D. C.: Pathways and functional significance of the coronary collateral circulation. Circulation 50:831, 1974, Copyright 1974 American Heart Association.)

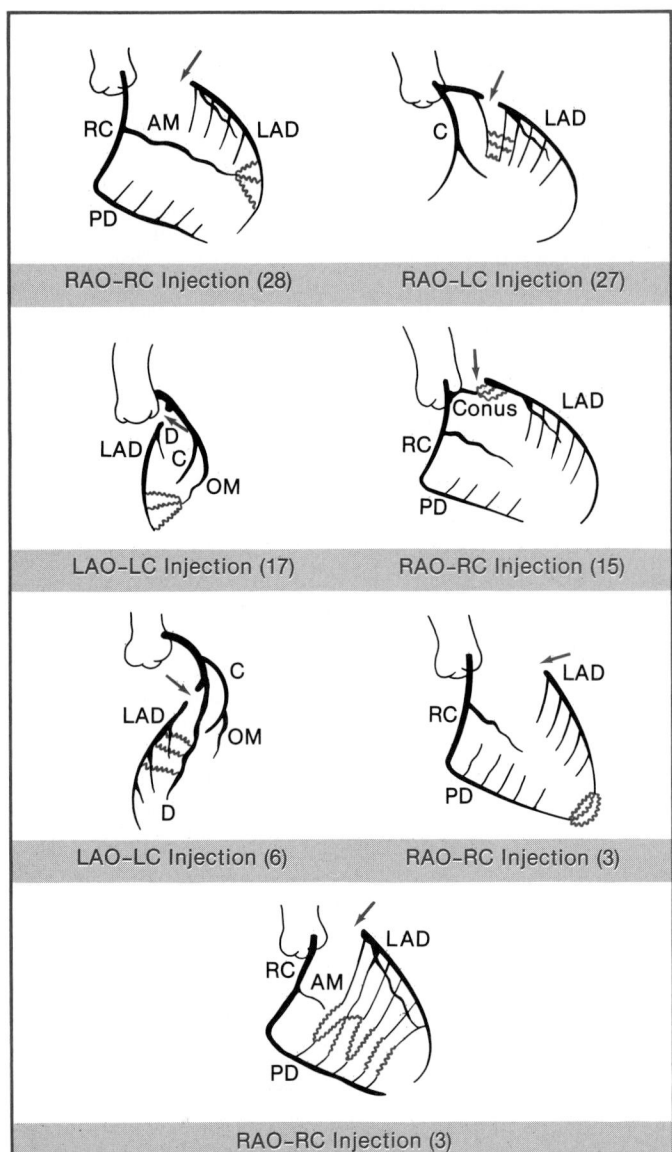

FIGURE 8–31. Common collateral pathways seen with LAD occlusion. (See Fig. 8–30 legend for abbreviations.) (From Levin, D. C.: Pathways and functional significance of the coronary collateral circulation. Circulation *50:*831, 1974. Copyright 1974 American Heart Association.)

Coronary Artery Spasm

(See also p. 1340)

Almost four decades have elapsed since Prinzmetal and coworkers[92] described an unusual or variant form of angina in which the onset of chest pain was not provoked by the usual factors, such as exercise, emotional upset, cold, or ingestion of a meal. According to currently accepted theories, patients considered to have variant angina are those in whom chest pain commences at rest or occurs both at rest and during exertion.[93] The pain often occurs in a cyclical pattern at the same time every day, generally in the morning, and usually is accompanied by ST-segment elevation if an electrocardiogram is recorded. Symptoms may occur many times daily, cease for weeks or months, and then recur. Although the ST-segment elevation often is striking, it rapidly reverts to normal when the pain disappears spontaneously or is terminated by the administration of nitroglycerin. Ischemic episodes may be accompanies by atrioventricular block, ventricular ectopic activity, ventricular tachycardia, or ventricular fibrillation. Although the original description of this syndrome emphasized its transient nature and its onset at rest, it has become apparent through further studies that coronary spasm also can play a

role in exercise-induced angina, unstable angina, acute myocardial infarction, and sudden death.[92]

The mechanisms of coronary vasospasm are varied. Current evidence suggests that the presence of coronary atherosclerosis interferes with the normal ability of the endothelium to reduce resting tone of the coronary artery. The normal endothelium releases nitric oxide and prostacyclin (PGI_2), which relax the underlying smooth muscle cells and produce vasodilatation. Aggregating platelets release vasoconstrictor substances such as thromboxane A_2 and serotonin (5-hydroxytryptamine). Atherosclerosis interferes with the synthesis and action of the vasoactive substances produced by the endothelium. Thrombin has antithrombotic properties in intact endothelium. It is able to release enough nitric oxide and prostacyclin to overcome platelet-induced contraction resulting from the direct activation of platelets by thrombin.[54]

Coronary arteriography has played an important role in understanding the pathophysiology and clinical consequences of coronary artery spasm. In the early 1970's, several angiographic studies demonstrated spasm in patients with clinical variant angina.[94] These studies showed that although spasm usually was superimposed on areas of fixed stenosis, in some cases it occurred in segments of coronary arteries that appeared angiographically normal. Postmortem studies, however, have essentially confirmed the relation between spasm and coronary atherosclerosis, with only one case serving as an exception to the general rule that coronary artery spasm is associated with coronary atherosclerosis. In the late 1970's, intravenous ergonovine maleate was used to provoke spasm in patients with suspected variant angina who were undergoing coronary arteriography.[95] A comprehensive angiographic study of the frequency of coronary spasm was carried out by Bertrand

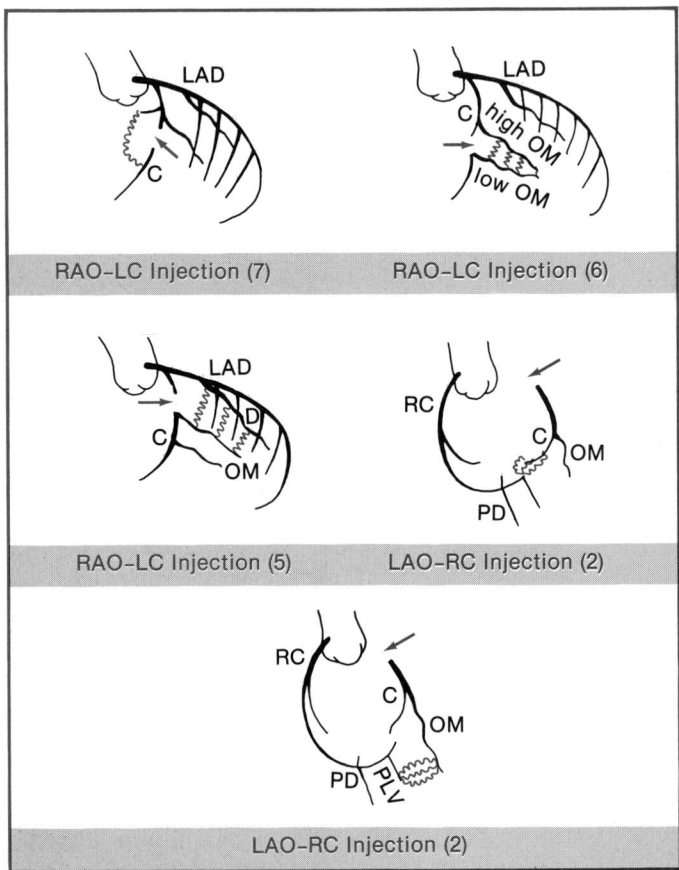

FIGURE 8–32. Common collateral pathways seen with LCx occlusion. (See Fig. 8–30 legend for abbreviations.) (From Levin, D. C.: Pathways and functional significance of the coronary collateral circulation. Circulation *50:*831, 1974. Copyright 1974 American Heart Association.)

and coworkers[96] in 1089 consecutive patients undergoing coronary arteriography for chest pain. Patients with left main coronary artery disease, severe three-vessel disease, NYHA functional class III or IV symptoms, or spontaneously occurring spasm were excluded. Of the 1089 patients, 134 exhibited spasm after ergonovine; in 59 per cent of these patients spasm was associated with angiographic evidence of a coronary stenosis, whereas in 41 per cent it occurred in an angiographically normal segment. Although ergonovine-induced spasm occurred rarely (less than 5 per cent) in patients with atypical chest pain or exertional angina, it occurred in 14 per cent of patients with symptoms of both exertional and resting angina. Ergonovine-induced coronary spasm was seen in 85 per cent of patients with primarily rest angina who were observed to have episodes of ST-segment elevation. In patients with recent myocardial infarction (less than 6 weeks), ergonovine-induced spasm was noted in 20 per cent.

Serious complications, including irreversible occlusion,[97] occur on rare occasions during ergonovine testing. The use of acetylcholine for diagnosing spasm is limited by the increased sensitivity and lack of specificity of the test; almost all patients with coronary atherosclerosis show evidence of at least mild constriction upon treatment with acetylcholine.[7] The diagnosis of coronary artery spasm must be supported by clinical features and response to treatment with nitrate compounds and calcium channel blockers.

INTERVENTIONAL CORONARY ARTERIOGRAPHY

(See also Chap. 39)

The introduction of balloon angioplasty by Grüntzig and coworkers[98] in 1977 and the subsequent development of atherectomy, coronary stenting, and laser angioplasty for specific lesion types have placed new demands on coronary arteriography for accurate characterization of lesion morphology. The angiographer must identify projections that show each target lesion clearly without foreshortening. In addition, the approach to the target lesion must be clearly delineated. For most cardiologists, this is probably a natural goal of the arteriographic procedure because approximately two-thirds of angiographers also perform angioplasty.[99] Several recommendations for interventional coronary arteriography can thus be made:

1. Before an intervention is planned, disease in the unprotected LMCA must be excluded. If pressure damping with a diagnostic catheter is detected, this probably reflects significant narrowing of the LMCA and predicts the likelihood of significant pressure damping when larger coronary guide catheters are used.

2. The course to the target lesion must be displayed conspicuously.

3. The target lesion itself should be projected in at least two views before interventional therapy.

4. The morphology of the lesion should be plainly defined by the angiographic procedure.

5. The lesion after angioplasty must be viewed in multiple projections after all intracoronary guidewires are retracted to assess adequacy of treatment, residual thrombus, and vessel dissection.

Lesion Morphology

In the American College of Cardiology/American Heart Association classification for coronary angioplasty,[100] lesion types are defined as simple (Type A), moderately complex (Type B), and complex (Type C) (Table 39–3, p. 1370). In a recent series of patients undergoing conventional balloon angioplasty,[101] most lesions were found to be moderately complex (Table 8–3).

TABLE 8–3 LESION CHARACTERISTICS OF PATIENTS UNDERGOING ANGIOPLASTY

N	733 (%)
Lesion complexity (ACC-AHA score)*	
A	227 (31)
B	314 (43)
C	192 (26)
Specific lesion types	
Saphenous vein graft lesion	517 (70)
Eccentric stenosis	169 (23)
Tubular lesion (10–20 mm)	121 (17)
Diffuse disease (>20 mm)	56 (7.6)
Total occlusion	60 (8.2)
Ostial stenosis	10 (1.4)
Bifurcation lesion	31 (4.2)
Ulcerated lesion	56 (7.6)
Thrombus present	21 (2.9)
Lesion in bend >45 degrees	16 (2.2)
Lesion in bend >90 degrees	4 (0.5)
Severely calcified stenosis	9 (1.2)

*ACC-AHA = American College of Cardiology/American Heart Association Task Force on PTCA.[100]

Wolfe, M. W., Roubin, G. S., Schweiger, M., et al.: Length of hospital stay and complications after percutaneous transluminal coronary angioplasty: Clinical and procedural predictors. Circulation 92:311, 1995. Copyright 1995 American Heart Association.

Lesion eccentricity is assessed in a nonforeshortened projection and is evident by asymmetry. Although a quantitative assessment of the eccentricity index as the percentage deviation of the stenosis centerline from the vessel centerline has been used in some studies,[102] it is more common to use qualitative assessment.

Lesion angulation also must be assessed in a nonforeshortened end-diastolic projection. Visual assessment is frequently used but is less accurate than the semiquantitative method, in which the angle between 20-mm arterial centerlines originating at the stenosis is calculated to define the angle between the proximal and distal segments.[103] Although a hand-held protractor may be useful to measure the angle,[104] some angiographers measure the angle of the noninflated balloon catheter positioned across the stenosis.[104] Lesions associated with bends of 45 degrees or more are simply classified as "angulated," and lesions with bends of 90 degrees or more are commonly classified as "severely angulated."

CORONARY THROMBUS. Because coronary angiography provides a silhouette of lesion edges, it has limited ability to identify intracoronary thrombus as compared with other imaging modalities such as angioscopy.[105] Despite its limitations, the angiographic detection of complex lesions or thrombus in unstable angina has important prognostic and therapeutic implications. Angiographic-pathological correlations have suggested that an eccentric stenosis with a narrow neck, overhanging edge, or scalloped border corresponds to plaque rupture or hemorrhage, with superimposed partially occlusive or recanalized thrombus.[106] The most specific angiographic hallmark of intracoronary thrombus, however, is the presence of a globular filling defect, completely surrounded by contrast material and usually located distal to the point of most severe stenosis (Figs. 8–33 and 8–34). When an eccentric lesion is associated with contrast retention, thrombolytic intervention is often unsuccessful, suggesting that these lesions may actually represent areas of microvascular channels and not thrombus.[107]

The angiographic detection of thrombus varies from 6 to 17 per cent in angioplasty series and from 16 to 57 per cent in angiographic series.[107–116] The variation in the reporting of coronary thrombus in angiography is attributed to the type of study performed, the patient population studied, and definitions used. Patients in angioplasty series have a lower incidence of intracoronary thrombus than those in

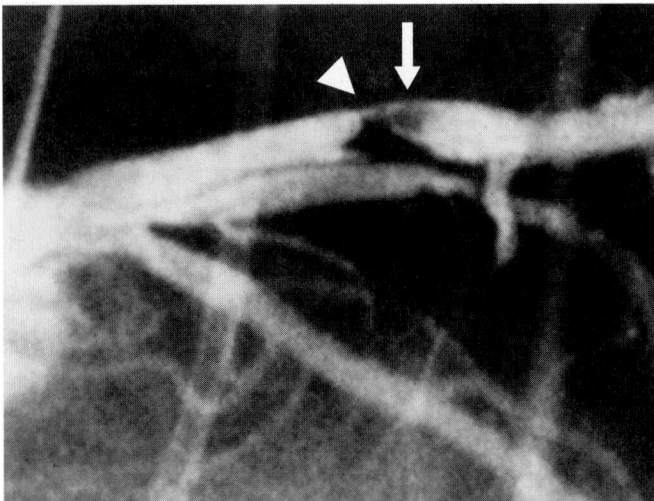

FIGURE 8–33. Intracoronary thrombus in acute myocardial infarction. In the setting of acute myocardial infarction, this RAO caudal left coronary arteriogram shows an eccentric lesion (arrowhead) in the proximal left anterior descending artery, immediately followed by a globular filling defect (arrow) surrounded by contrast medium on all sides.

angiographic series because angioplasty is often postponed when thrombus is detected.[104,110,113–118] Patients with rest angina or postinfarction angina have been found to have a higher likelihood of intracoronary thrombus than those with crescendo angina.[108,110] Angiographic detection of complex or ulcerated lesions in unstable angina is associated with an increased likelihood of thrombosis and an increased risk of adverse cardiac events.[119]

CORONARY DISSECTION. Interventional cardiovascular treatments occasionally are associated with the formation of vessel dissection, and rarely the performance of diagnostic coronary arteriography may be associated with vessel dissection. Thus, the angiographer must be familiar with the angiographic patterns of vessel dissection. Patients with severe dissections associated with contrast retention or propagation are more likely to experience complications

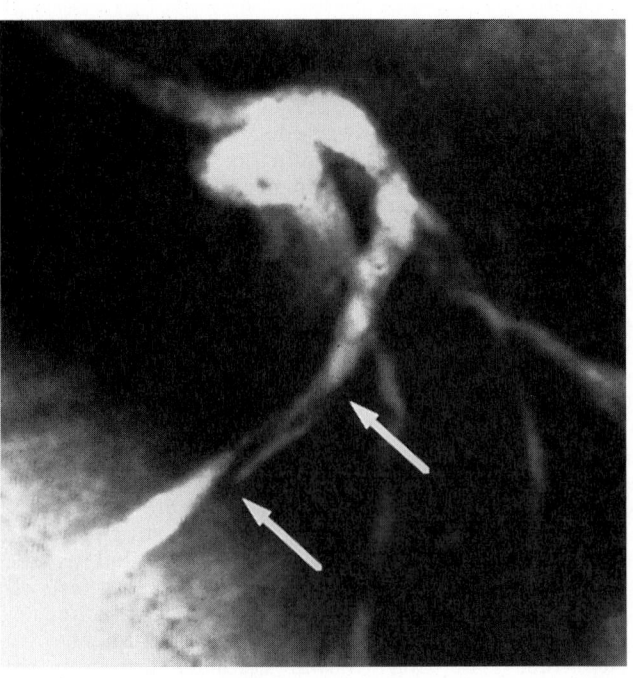

FIGURE 8–35. Moderately severe coronary dissection. This LAO cranial left coronary arteriogram shows a large intramural collection of contrast medium (arrows) at the site of angioplasty in the proximal LAD. Although contrast medium cleared rapidly from LAD itself, contrast medium persisted within the dissection itself, thus meeting criteria for a Grade C dissection (see text discussion).[120,121]

outside the cardiac catheterization laboratory than those with mild dissections[120] (Fig. 8–35). The National Heart, Lung, and Blood Institute (NHLBI) Registry scoring system for vessel dissection has been modified to provide a uniform scale for rating dissections[120,121]:

Grade A: A radiolucent area, often linear, within the coronary lumen during contrast injection with minimal or no persistence of contrast after the dye has cleared.

Grade B: Parallel tracts or double lumen separated by a

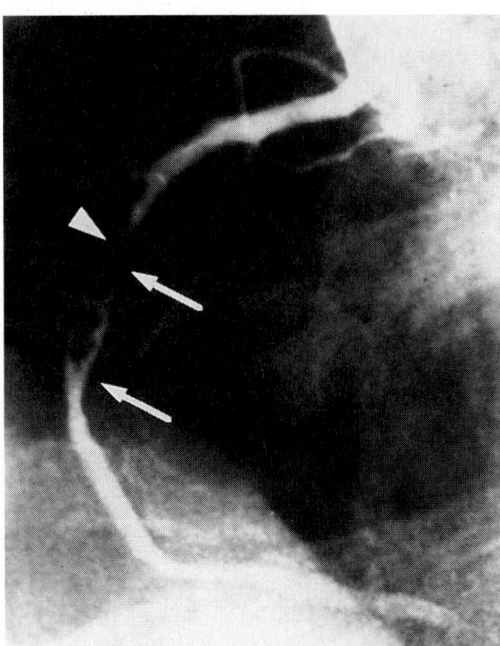

FIGURE 8–34. Intracoronary thrombus in unstable angina. This LAO right coronary arteriogram shows a severe stenosis in the mid-portion of the RCA (arrowhead), followed by a large filling defect surrounded by contrast medium on all sides (arrows).

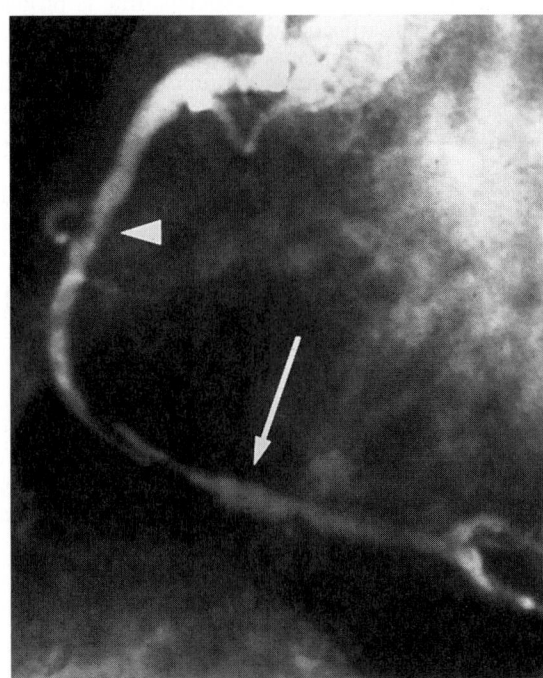

FIGURE 8–36. Spiral dissection. This LAO right coronary arteriogram shows evidence of a vessel dissection emanating from the site of angioplasty in the midportion of the RCA (arrowhead) and extending to the distal RCA (arrow), thus meeting criteria for a severe Grade D dissection.[120,121]

radiolucent area during contrast injection with minimal or no persistence after dye clearance.

Grade C: Contrast material immediately outside the coronary lumen but within the vessel wall with persistence of contrast material in the area after clearance of dye from the coronary lumen.

Grade D: Spiral luminal filling defects, frequently with extensive contrast material staining of the vessel (Fig. 8–36).

Dissection is more commonly detected than thrombus by angiography and by angioscopy in patients experiencing abrupt vessel closure. In 109 patients with abrupt vessel closure, 39 (34 per cent) had angiographic evidence of dissection, but 30 had evidence of thrombus (27 per cent).[122] In 65 patients with abrupt vessel closure, 31 (48 per cent) had dissection, but 27 (42 per cent) had evidence of thrombus.[101] In an angioscopic evaluation of abrupt vessel closure, 14 of 17 patients had evidence of dissection or extruded atheromatous plaque, but only 3 of 17 patients had evidence of thrombus.[123]

TOTAL OCCLUSIONS. Angiography of total occlusions requires detailed assessment of the anatomy at the site of the occlusion, the extent of collateral development, and the length of the totally occluded segment. The morphology at the point of total occlusion influences the likelihood of success with interventional cardiovascular procedures. Total occlusions associated with a blunt occlusion (Fig. 8–37) are less likely to result in successful angioplasty than those with a tapering funnel[124] (Fig. 8–38). The vascular segment distal to the obstruction occasionally requires visualization via contralateral collaterals.

PSEUDOLESIONS. When a tortuous coronary artery is straightened with an angioplasty wire, the redundant intimal tissue may compress via a "concertina effect" to produce coronary "pseudonarrowings"[125] or intimal intussusception (Fig. 8–39). These narrowings are not responsive to nitroglycerin and usually are resistant to balloon angioplasty. The characteristic appearance of sharply angulated protrusions of tissue into the lumen in a staircase pattern is a clue to the presence of coronary pseudonarrowings. Removal of the guidewire abolishes this angiographic finding.

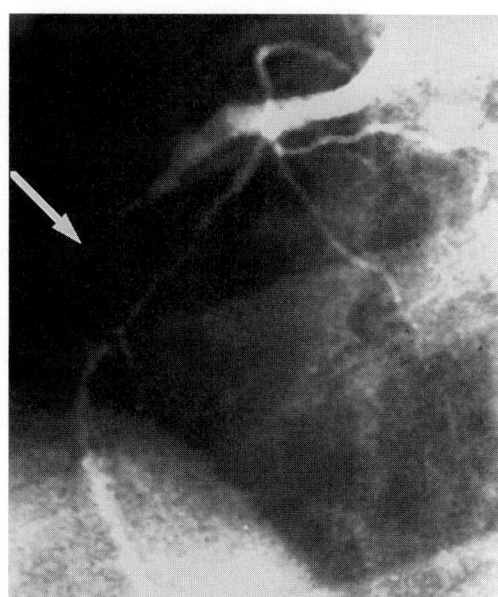

FIGURE 8–38. Total occlusion with taper. The LAO right coronary arteriogram shows a total occlusion (arrow) of the midportion of the RCA, but the smoothly tapering appearance of the site of total occlusion suggests that attempts with angioplasty may be successful.

RELATION BETWEEN ARTERIOGRAPHIC FINDINGS AND CLINICAL OUTCOME

Numerous studies have determined that the strongest predictors of survival in patients with coronary artery disease are (1) extent of coronary artery disease, (2) left ventricular function, and (3) exercise tolerance measured as time on the treadmill test (Chap. 38).

In the CASS Registry, the 7-year survival rate was 96 per cent among patients with completely smooth coronary arteries and 92 per cent among patients with luminal irregularities associated with less than 50 per cent stenosis of one or more coronary segments.[126] Among 1977 patients followed in the Duke University Cardiovascular Disease Databank, those with completely normal vessels had an infarct-free 10-year survival rate of 98 per cent, whereas those with less than a 75 per cent stenosis of any coronary artery

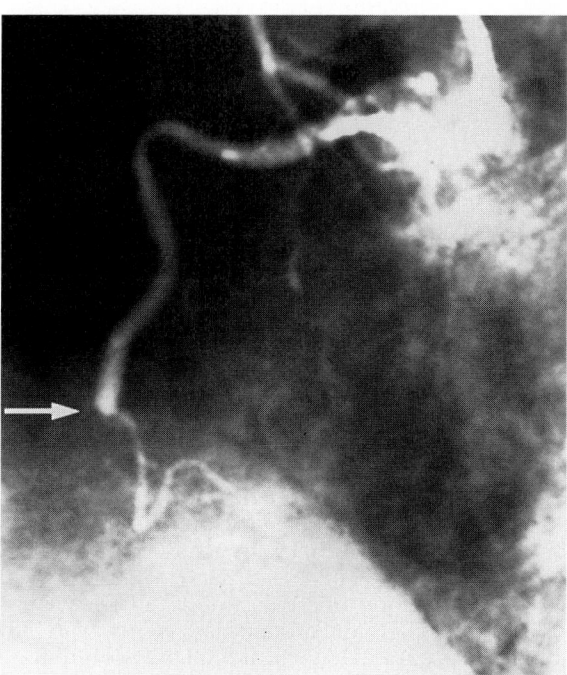

FIGURE 8–37. Total occlusion with blunt appearance. The LAO right coronary arteriogram shows a blunt total occlusion (arrow) of the midportion of the right coronary artery associated with a side branch. The blunt appearance and the presence of the side branch are characteristics that suggest that angioplasty may be unsuccessful.

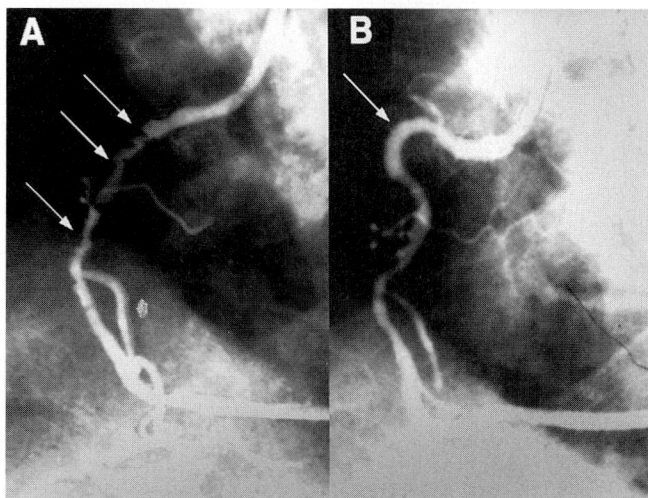

FIGURE 8–39. Coronary pseudolesions. The LAO coronary arteriogram shows evidence of multiple, sharply angulated narrowings (arrows) in the proximal RCA when an angioplasty guidewire is present with its tip in the distal RCA *(A).* These areas were unresponsive to intracoronary nitroglycerin but immediately resolved upon removal of the guidewire *(B),* revealing a very tortuous RCA with a prominent shepherd's crook (arrow) in the proximal segment.

TABLE 8–4   RELATION BETWEEN 4-YEAR SURVIVAL (%) AND EXTENT OF CORONARY ARTERY DISEASE AND LEFT VENTRICULAR DYSFUNCTION

EXTENT OF CAD	EF > 50%	EF 35 – 49%	EF < 35%
One-vessel CAD	95	91	74
Two-vessel CAD	93	83	57
Three-vessel CAD	82	71	50

Reproduced from Mock, M. B., Ringqvist, I., Fisher, L.D., et al.: Survival of medically treated patients in the Coronary Artery Surgery Study (CASS) registry. Circulation *66*:562, 1982. Copyright 1982 American Heart Association.

had an infarct-free 10-year survival rate of 90 per cent.[127] Patients with significant left main coronary artery disease are at increased risk. The cumulative survival among a group of medically treated patients with more than 70 per cent stenosis of the left main coronary artery was 72 per cent at 1 year and 41 per cent at 3 years.[128] For patients with left main coronary artery stenosis between 50 and 70 per cent, the prognosis was more favorable, with 91 per cent survival at 1 year and 66 per cent survival at 3 years. For patients with at least 75 per cent left main coronary artery stenosis on medical therapy, 42-month survival was 48 per cent for medically treated patients and 75 per cent for patients undergoing coronary artery bypass surgery.[129] Thus left main coronary artery disease is an indication for bypass surgery (see p. 1322).

The relations among survival, coronary artery disease, and left ventricular function have been assessed in the CASS Registry in 20,088 patients.[130] The 4-year survival rate for patients with more than 70 per cent diameter stenosis of one coronary artery was 92 per cent, for two coronary arteries 84 per cent, and for three coronary arteries 68 per cent. Left ventricular ejection fraction (EF), however, was found to be a more important predictor of survival (Table 8–4). Four-year survival was 95 per cent for patients with one-vessel disease and an EF greater than 50 per cent, 91 per cent for patients with an EF in the range of 35 to 49 per cent, and 74 per cent for patients with an EF of less than 35 per cent. Similar relations between survival and left ventricular dysfunction were seen for patients with two-vessel and three-vessel disease as well.

Relation Between Coronary Lesion Morphology and Clinical Presentation

It has been accepted from angiographic,[106,108,109,119,131] angioscopic,[105,132,133] and histological[134–139] observations that plaque inflammation, rupture, and nonocclusive thrombus formation precipitate unstable angina (see p. 1333). However, there is wide variability in the detection of these pathogenic events with angiographic and angioscopic methods. For example, only 10 to 26 per cent of patients with unstable angina have angiographic evidence of thrombus,[9,107–110,119,131] whereas the majority of such patients show angioscopic findings of intracoronary thrombus.[105,132,133] New information from the examination of atherectomy specimens[112,138] confirms the role of coronary thrombus formation in a significant proportion of patients with unstable angina but raises important questions about pathophysiology in the remaining patients. Although many episodes of unstable angina are undoubtedly caused by plaque rupture and thrombus formation, other mechanisms that alter the balance between myocardial oxygen supply and demand must be considered. For example, vasoconstriction may occur in the absence of deep arterial injury if endothelial function is abnormal.[140]

Several studies have suggested that angiographic plaque morphology is correlated with the clinical status and prognosis of the patient. In a study of 110 patients with stable or unstable angina, Ambrose and coworkers[131] classified lesions into four categories: concentric stenoses with smooth borders, eccentric stenoses with smooth borders, eccentric stenoses with complex borders (narrow base or neck caused by overhanging edges, or scalloped borders), and lesions with multiple irregularities. Among patients with stable angina, complex angiographic stenoses were present in 18 per cent of coronary arteries. Among the patients with unstable angina, complex lesions were seen in 56 per cent. These data show that in patients with unstable angina, lesions characterized by overhanging edges, scalloped or irregular borders, or multiple irregularities were more than three times as common than in patients with stable angina.

UNSTABLE ANGINA (see also p. 1331). Because a broad spectrum of patients with myocardial ischemia varying widely in cause, prognosis,

and responsiveness to therapy are lumped together under the single diagnosis of "unstable angina pectoris," a new clinical classification that depends on the timing of rest pain and its relation to previous myocardial infarction has been proposed.[141] The new classification is based on the acuity of presentation (presence and timing of rest pain) and the clinical presentation. In 246 consecutive patients with unstable angina and 50 patients with stable angina, the severity of angina was based on a score derived from the clinical circumstances (0 = stable angina, 1 = unstable angina secondary to a noncardiac condition such as anemia, 2 = unstable angina de novo, and 3 = postinfarction angina) and the acuity of presentation (0 = stable angina, 1 = no rest pain, 2 = rest pain occurring more than 48 hours before evaluation, and 3 = rest pain occurring 48 hours or less before evaluation).

Angiographic findings varied widely.[108] Depending on both the acuity and clinical circumstances of presentation, the probability of minimal obstruction (< 50 per cent stenosis) ranged from 2.1 to 20.0 per cent, and the incidence of intracoronary filling defects varied from 0.0 to 22.2 per cent. The unstable angina score was identified as the most important predictor of presence of intracoronary filling defects. Multiple regression analysis showed that the unstable angina score also predicted lesion complexity in the ischemia-related vessel ($P = 0.001$). The multiple regression model, which included unstable angina score and quantitative measurements of lesion severity such as minimal lumen diameter and flow, may account for about 55 per cent of the variability in lesion complexity ($r^2 = 0.55$, $P = 10^{-6}$). Thus, unstable angina pectoris is a heterogeneous syndrome with a wide range of clinical presentations and underlying coronary morphology. The classification of unstable angina[141] predicts underlying angiographic anatomy and may thus aid in the decision regarding diagnostic procedures as well as provide a sound basis for evaluating the response to therapy in patients with unstable angina.

Relation Between Stenosis Severity and Clinical Outcome

(See also Chap. 38)

It was long assumed that the risk posed to the patient with a given coronary artery stenosis is related to the severity of the obstruction: The greater the degree of narrowing, the greater is the degree of risk of myocardial infarction and death. Conversely, mild or moderate stenoses (less than 50 per cent) were assumed to cause less risk. Investigations using sequential coronary arteriograms with or without lipid-lowering interventions have disproved this notion.

Angiographic studies of cholesterol reduction have provided additional insights into the relation between lesion severity and clinical events. In the National Heart, Lung, and Blood Institute Type II Coronary Intervention Study,[142] a total of 116 men with elevated low-density lipoprotein (LDL) cholesterol levels were randomly assigned to treatment with dietary modification alone or dietary modification plus cholestyramine. Coronary arteriography was performed at baseline and at 5 years. Although cholestyramine resulted in a 17 per cent reduction in cholesterol levels, coronary artery disease progressed in 32 per cent of cholestyramine patients versus 49 per cent of control patients.[142]

In the Familial Atherosclerosis Treatment Study (FATS),[143] 120 men with coronary artery disease were given dietary counseling and randomly assigned to treatment with lovastatin plus colestipol, niacin plus colestipol, or placebo. After 2.5 years of treatment, total cholesterol levels were reduced by 34 per cent in the group receiving lovastatin plus colestipol, by 23 per cent in the group receiving niacin plus colestipol, and by 4 per cent in the control group. Progression of coronary artery disease was detected in 21 per cent in the group receiving lovastatin plus colestipol, 25 per cent in the group receiving niacin plus colestipol, and 46 per cent in the control group. Regression of disease was detected in 32 per cent in the group receiving lovastatin plus colestipol, 39 per cent in the group receiving niacin plus colestipol, and 11 per cent in the control group. Although stenosis severity was reduced by a modest 0.3 and 1.1 per cent in the two groups with active treatment, there was a striking difference in clinical events: fatal or nonfatal myocardial infarction occurred in 4 per cent in the group receiving lovastatin plus colestipol, 6 per cent in the group receiving niacin plus colestipol, but in 19 per cent in the control group.[143]

A similar relation between quantitative angiography and clinical events after cholesterol reduction has been observed in several other studies. In the St. Thomas' Atherosclerosis Regression Study (STARS),[144] cholestyramine and dietary modification reduced stenosis severity by 1.5 per cent. This was associated with a substantial reduction in death and cardiovascular events.[144] Thus, cholesterol-lowering therapy results in modest reductions in stenosis severity but striking reductions in the incidence of cardiovascular events. One possible explanation for this apparent discrepancy may relate to endothelial function and the propensity for plaque rupture.[145,146]

The relation between stenosis severity and the likelihood of myocardial infarction has been evaluated in several studies. Ambrose and colleagues[147] compared the degree of baseline coronary stenoses in 38 patients who underwent two separate coronary arteriograms and had experienced either myocardial infarction or new total occlusion without infarction during the interval. In the infarct group, only 22 per cent of the culprit lesions were initially greater than 70 per cent, whereas in the noninfarct group, 61 per cent of the lesions that subsequently progressed to total occlusion were initially greater than 70 per cent. The lesions responsible for Q-wave myocardial infarction were characterized by a mean stenosis of only 34 per cent.

In another similar study of the progression of coronary artery disease, it was found that only 15 per cent of lesions that produced myocardial infarctions were severe (greater than 75 per cent) and half were mild (less than 50 per cent) on the initial angiogram.[148] Most patients who developed new total occlusion did not experience infarcts; 48 per cent of these stenoses were greater than 75 per cent on the initial coronary arteriograms. Little and colleagues[149] in a separate report reviewed coronary arteriograms in 42 consecutive patients who had been studied both before and shortly after acute myocardial infarction. In 29 patients a new total occlusion was observed on the second arteriogram. Among these 29 patients, 66 per cent of the culprit stenoses had been less than 50 per cent on the initial arteriogram, and almost all of them had been less than 70 per cent.

These observations are inconsistent with the simplistic notion that the severity of obstruction is proportional to an increased risk of myocardial infarction and cardiac death. Rather, the angiographic evidence of the presence of coronary artery disease provides more clinical information than the severity of the obstruction itself. This lack of correlation may be related to the inability of angiography to identify unstable plaques that are at high risk of rupture and to distinguish them from critically obstructive stenoses that are stable.

REFERENCES

1. Sones, F. M., and Shirey, E. K.: Cine coronary arteriography. Med. Concepts Cardiovasc. Dis. 31:735, 1962.
2. Graves, E. J.: Vital and Health Statistics: National Hospital Discharge Survey: Annual Summary 1991. Hyattsville, Md., National Center for Health Statistics, 1993.
3. American Hospital Association guide to the health care field. Chicago, American Hospital Association, 1993.
4. Pepine, C. J., Allen, H. D., Bashore, T. M., et al.: ACC/AHA guidelines for cardiac catheterization and cardiac catheterization laboratories: American College of Cardiology/American Heart Association Ad Hoc Task Force on Cardiac Catheterization. Circulation 84:2213, 1991.

INDICATIONS FOR CORONARY ARTERIOGRAPHY

5. Fletcher, G. F., Baladay, G., Froelicher, V. F., et al.: Exercise standards: A statement for healthcare professionals from the American Heart Association. Circulation 91:580, 1995.
6. Travin, M. I., Boucher, C. A., Newell, J. B., et al.: Variables associated with a poor prognosis in patients with an ischemic thallium-201 exercise test. Am. Heart J. 125:335, 1993.
7. Ludmer, P. L., Selwyn, A. P., Shook, T. L., et al.: Paradoxical vasoconstriction induced by acetylcholine in atherosclerotic coronary arteries. N. Engl. J. Med. 315:1046, 1986.
8. Braunwald, E., Jones, R. H., Mark, D. B., et al.: Diagnosing and managing unstable angina. Circulation 90:613, 1994.
9. The TIMI IIIB Investigators: Effects of tissue plasminogen activator and a comparison of early invasive and conservative strategies in unstable angina and non–Q-wave myocardial infarction. Circulation 89:1545, 1994.
10. Michels, K. B., and Yusuf, S.: Does PTCA in acute myocardial infarction affect mortality and reinfarction rates? A quantitative overview (meta-analysis) of the randomized clinical trials. Circulation 91:476, 1995.
11. Ellis, S. G., Ribeiro da Silva, E., Heyndrickx, G., et al.: Randomized comparison of rescue angioplasty with conservative management of patients with early failure of thrombolysis for acute anterior myocardial infarction. Circulation 90:2280, 1994.
12. Fish, R. D., Nabel, E. G., Selwyn, A. P., et al.: Responses of coronary arteries of cardiac transplant patients to acetylcholine. J. Clin. Invest. 81:21, 1988.
13. Amplatz, K., Formanek, G., Stanger, P., and Wilson, W.: Mechanics of selective coronary artery catheterization via femoral approach. Radiology 89:1040, 1967.
14. Schoonmaker, F. W., and King, S. B., III: Coronary arteriography by the single catheter percutaneous femoral technique. Circulation 50:735, 1974.
15. Holzman, R. S., Cullen, D. J., Eichhorn, J. H., and Philip, J. H.: Guidelines for sedation by nonanesthesiologists during diagnostic and therapeutic procedures. J. Clin. Anesthesiol. 6:265, 1994.
16. Bailey, P. L., Pace, N. L., Ashburn, M. A., et al.: Frequent hypoxemia and apnea after sedation with midazolam and fentanyl. Anesthesiology 73:826, 1990.
17. Davis, K., Kennedy, J. W., Kemp, H. G., Jr., et al.: Complications of coronary arteriography. Circulation 59:1105, 1979.
18. Lasser, E. D., Berry, C. C., Talner, L. B., et al.: Pretreatment with corticosteroids to alleviate reactions to intravenous contrast material. N. Engl. J. Med. 317:845, 1987.
19. Bettmann, M. A.: Radiographic contrast agents—A perspective. N. Engl. J. Med. 317:891, 1987.
20. Levi, M., Pascucci, C., Agnelli, G., et al.: Effect on thrombus growth and thrombolysis of two types of osmolar contrast media in rabbits. Invest. Radiol. 25:533, 1990.
21. Ing, J. J., Smith, D. C., and Bull, B. S.: Differing mechanisms of clotting inhibition by ionic and nonionic contrast agents. Radiology 172:345, 1989.
22. Rasuli, P., McLeish, W. A., and Hammond, D. I.: Anticoagulant effects of contrast materials: In vitro study of iohexol, ioxaglate, and diatrizoate. A.J.R. 152:309, 1989.
23. Taliercio, C. P., McCallister, B. H., Holmes, D. R., Jr., et al.: Nephrotoxicity of nonionic contrast media after cardiac angiography. Am. J. Cardiol. 64:815, 1989.
24. Brogan, W. C., III, Hillis, L. D., and Lange, R. A.: Contrast agents for cardiac catheterization: Conceptions and misconceptions. Am. Heart J. 122:1129, 1991.
25. Solomon, R., Werner, C., Mann, D., et al.: Effects of saline, mannitol, and furosemide to prevent acute decreases in renal function induced by radiocontrast agents. N. Engl. J. Med. 331:1416, 1994.
26. Holmes, D. R., Jr., Wondrow, M. A., and Julsrud, P. R.: Radiographic techniques used in cardiac catheterization. In Pepine, C. J., Hill, J. A., Lambert, C. R. (eds.): Diagnostic and Therapeutic Cardiac Catheterization. Baltimore, Williams and Wilkins, 1994, p. 141.
27. Gurley, J. C., Nissen, S. E., Booth, D. C., et al.: Comparison of simultaneously performed digital and film-based angiography in the assessment of coronary artery disease. Circulation 78:1411, 1988.
28. Nissen, S. E.: Principles and applications of digital imaging in cardiac and coronary angiography. In Pepine, C. J., Hill, J.A., Lambert, C. R. (eds.): Diagnostic and Therapeutic Cardiac Catheterization. Baltimore, Williams and Wilkins, 1994, p. 162.
29. Nissen, S. E.: Principles of Radiographic Imaging. In Roubin, G. S., Califf, R. M., O'Neill, W. W., et al. (eds.): Interventional Cardiovascular Medicine. New York, Churchill Livingstone, 1994, p. 409.
30. King, S. B., III: Foreword. In Serruys, P. W., Foley, D. P., and De Feyter, P. J. (eds.): Quantitative Coronary Angiography in Clinical Practice. Boston, Kluwer Academic Publishers, 1994, p. xvii.
31. Folland, E. D., Vogel, R. A., Hartigan, P., et al.: Relation between coronary artery stenosis assessed by visual, caliper, and computer methods and exercise capacity in patients with single-vessel coronary artery disease. Circulation 89:2005, 1994.
32. Beauman, G. J., and Vogel, R. A.: Accuracy of individual and panel visual interpretations of coronary arteriograms: Implications for clinical decisions. J. Am. Coll. Cardiol. 16:108, 1990.
33. Kalbfleisch, S. J., McGillem, M. J., Pinto, I. M. F., et al.: Comparison of automated quantitative coronary angiography with caliper measurements of percent diameter stenosis. Am. J. Cardiol. 65:1181, 1990.
34. White, C. W., Wright, C. B., Doty, D. B., et al.: Does the visual interpretation of the coronary arteriogram predict the physiologic significance of a coronary stenosis? N. Engl. J. Med. 310:819, 1984.
35. Stadius, M. L., and Alderman, A. L.: Coronary artery revascularization: Critical need for, and consequences of, objective angiographic assessment of lesion severity. Circulation 82:2231, 1990.
36. Uehata, A., Matsugushi, T., Bittl, J. A., et al.: The accuracy of electronic digital calipers compared with quantitative angiography in measuring arterial diameters. Circulation 88:1724, 1993.

37. Bunnell, I. L., Greene, D. G., Tandon, R. N., and Arani, D. T.: The half axial projection: A new look at the proximal left coronary artery. Circulation 48:151, 1973.

38. Arani, D. T., Bunnell, I. L., and Greene, D. G.: Lordotic right posterior oblique projection of the left coronary artery: A special view for special anatomy. Circulation 52:504, 1975.

39. Judkins, M. W.: Coronary arteriography. In Douglas, J. S., Jr., and King, S. B., III (eds.): Coronary Arteriography and Intervention. New York, McGraw-Hill, 1985.

40. Leung, W.-H., Alderman, E. L., Lee, T. C., and Stadius, M. L.: Quantitative arteriography of apparently normal coronary segments with nearby or distant disease suggests the presence of occult, nonvisualized atherosclerosis. J. Am. Coll. Cardiol. 25:311, 1995.

41. Levin, D. C., Harrington, D. P., Bettmann, M. A., et al.: Anatomic variations of the left coronary arteries supplying the anterolateral aspect of the left ventricle: Possible explanation for the "unexplained" left ventricular aneurysm. Invest. Radiol. 17:458, 1982.

42. Perlmutt, L. M., Jay, M. E., and Levin, D. C.: Variations in the blood supply of the left ventricular apex. Invest. Radiol. 18:138, 1983.

43. Levin, D. C., Bechmann, C. F., Garnic, J. D., et al.: Frequency and clinical significance of failure to visualize the conus artery during coronary arteriography. Circulation 63:833, 1981.

44. Kyriakidis, M. K., Kouraouklis, C. B., Papaioannou, J. T., et al.: Sinus node coronary arteries studied with angiography. Am. J. Cardiol. 51:749, 1983.

45. King, S. B., III, Lembo, N. J., Weintraub, W. S., et al.: A randomized trial comparing coronary angioplasty with coronary bypass surgery. N. Engl. J. Med. 331:1044, 1994.

46. Hamm, C. W., Reimers, J., Ischinger, T., et al.: A randomized study of coronary angioplasty compared with bypass surgery in patients with symptomatic multivessel coronary disease. N. Engl. J. Med. 331:1037, 1994.

47. Bourassa, M. G., Fisher, L. D., Campeua, L., et al.: Long-term fate of bypass grafts: The Coronary Artery Surgery Study (CASS) and the Montreal Heart Institute experiences. Circulation 72 (Suppl. V):V-71, 1985.

48. European Coronary Surgery Study Group: Long-term results of prospective randomized study of coronary artery bypass surgery in stable angina pectoris. Lancet 2:1173, 1982.

49. Loop, F. D., Lytle, B. W., Cosgrove, D. M., et al.: Influence of the internal-mammary-artery graft on 10-year survival and other cardiac events. N. Engl. J. Med. 314:1, 1986.

50. Suma, H., and Takanashi, R.: Arteriosclerosis of the gastroepiploic and internal thoracic arteries. Ann. Thorac. Surg. 50:413, 1990.

51. Suma, H., Wanibuchi, Y., and Terada, Y.: The right gastroepiploic artery graft: Clinical and angiographic mid-term results in 200 patients. J. Thorac. Cardiovasc. Surg. 105:615, 1993.

52. de Feyter, P. J., van Suylen, R.-J., de Jaegere, P. P. T., et al.: Balloon angioplasty for the treatment of lesions in saphenous vein bypass grafts. J. Am. Coll. Cardiol. 21:1539, 1993.

53. Hwang, M. H., Meadows, W. R., Palac, R. T., et al.: Progression of native coronary artery disease at 10 years: Insight from a randomized study of medical versus surgical therapy for angina. J. Am. Coll. Cardiol. 16:1066, 1990.

54. Luscher, T. F., Diederich, D., Siebenmann, R., et al.: Difference between endothelium-dependent relaxation in arterial and in venous coronary bypass grafts. N. Engl. J. Med. 319:462, 1988.

55. Gensini, G. G.: Coronary arteriography. In Braunwald, E. (ed.): Heart Disease: A Textbook of Cardiovascular Medicine. Philadelphia, W. B. Saunders Company, 1984, p. 337.

56. Hermiller, J. B., Buller, C. E., Taneglia, A. N., et al.: Unrecognized left main coronary artery disease in patients undergoing interventional procedures. Am. J. Cardiol. 71:173, 1993.

57. Haraphongse, M., and Rossall, R. E.: Diaphragmatic coronary lesion mimics significant coronary stenosis: Report of 4 cases. Cathet. Cardiovasc. Diagn. 11:173, 1985.

58. Zarins, C. K., Giddens, D. P., Bharadvaj, B. K., et al.: Carotid bifurcation atherosclerosis: Quantitative correlation of plaque localization with flow velocity profiles and wall shear stress. Circ. Res. 53:502, 1983.

59. Fuster, V., Badimon, J. J., and Badimon, L.: Clinical-pathological correlations of coronary disease progression and regression. Circulation 86 (Suppl. III):III-1, 1992.

60. Kramer, J. R., Kitazume, H., Proudfit, W. L., and Sones, F. M., Jr.: Clinical significance of isolated coronary bridges: Benign and frequent condition involving the left anterior descending artery. Am. Heart J. 103:282, 1982.

61. Friedman, M.: The coronary canalized thrombus: Provenance, structure, function and relationship to death due to coronary artery disease. Br. J. Exp. Pathol. 48:556, 1967.

62. Klinke, W. P., Kubac, G., Talibi, T., and Lee, S. J. K.: Safety of outpatient catheterizations. Am. J. Cardiol. 56:639, 1985.

63. Johnson, L. W., Lozner, E. C., Johnson, S., et al.: Coronary arteriography 1984–1987: A report of the Registry of the Society for Cardiac Angiography and Interventions: I. Results and complications. Cathet. Cardiovasc. Diagn. 17:5, 1989.

64. Johnson, L. W., and Krone, R.: Cardiac catheterization 1991: A report of the Registry of the Society for Cardiac Angiography and Interventions. Cathet. Cardiovasc. Diagn. 28:219, 1993.

65. Levin, D. C., Fellows, K. E., and Abrams, H. L.: Hemodynamically significant primary anomalies of the coronary arteries: Angiographic aspects. Circulation 58:25, 1978.

66. Wilson, C. L., Dlabal, P. W., Holeyfield, R. W., et al.: Anomalous origin of left coronary artery from pulmonary artery: Case reports and review of literature concerning teenagers and adults. J. Thorac. Cardiovasc. Surg. 73:887, 1977.

67. Cheitlin, M. D., Decastro, D. M., and McAllister, H. A.: Sudden death as a complication of anomalous left coronary origin from the anterior sinus of Valsalva. Circulation 50:780, 1974.

68. Liberthson, R. R., Dinsmore, R. E., and Fallon, J. T.: Aberrant coronary artery origin from the aorta: Report of 18, review of literature and delineation of natural history and management. Circulation 59:748, 1979.

69. Roberts, W. C.: Major anomalies of coronary artery origin seen in adulthood. Am. Heart J. 111:941, 1986.

70. Roberts, W. C., Siegel, R. J., and Zipes, D. P.: Origin of the right coronary artery from the left sinus of Valsalva and its functional consequences: Analysis of 10 necropsy patients. Am. Heart J. 49:863, 1982.

71. Kragel, A. H., and Roberts, W. C.: Anomalous origin of either the right or left main coronary artery from the aorta with subsequent coursing between aorta and pulmonary trunk: Analysis of 32 necropsy cases. Am. J. Cardiol. 62:771, 1988.

72. Brandt, B., III, Martins, J. B., and Marcus, M. L.: Anomalous origin of the right coronary artery form the left sinus of Valsalva. N. Engl. J. Med. 309:596, 1983.

73. Kimbiris, D., Iskandrian, A. S., Segal, B. L., and Bemis, C. E.: Anomalous aortic origin of coronary arteries. Circulation 58:606, 1978.

74. Serota, H., Barth, C. W., III, Seuc, C. A., et al.: Rapid identification of the course of anomalous coronary arteries in adults: The "dot and eye" method. Am. J. Cardiol. 65:891, 1990.

75. Fernandes, F., Alam, M., Smith, S., and Khaja, F.: The role of transesophageal echocardiography identifying anomalous coronary arteries. Circulation 88:2532, 1993.

76. Click, R. L., Holmes, D. R., Jr., Vlietstra, R. E., et al.: Anomalous coronary arteries: Location, degree of atherosclerosis and effect on survival—A report from the Coronary Artery Surgery Study. J. Am. Coll. Cardiol. 12:531, 1988.

77. Page, H. L., Jr., Engel, H. J., Campbell, W. B., and Thomas, C. S., Jr.: Anomalous origin of the left circumflex coronary artery: Recognition, angiographic demonstration and clinical significance. Circulation 50:768, 1974.

78. Lipton, M. J., Barry, W. H., Obrez, I., et al.: Isolated single coronary artery: Diagnosis, angiographic classification, and clinical significance. Radiology 130:39, 1979.

79. TIMI Study Group: The Thrombolysis in Myocardial Infarction (TIMI) trial: Phase I findings. N. Engl. J. Med. 312:932, 1985.

80. The GUSTO Angiographic Investigators: The effects of tissue plasminogen activator, streptokinase, or both on coronary artery patency, ventricular function, and survival after acute myocardial infarction. N. Engl. J. Med. 329:1615, 1993.

81. Gibson C. M.: TIMI frame count: A new standardization of infarct-related artery flow grade, and its relationship to clinical outcomes in the TIMI-4 trial. Circulation 90 (Abs.):I-220, 1994.

82. Levin, D. C.: Pathways and functional significance of the coronary collateral circulation. Circulation 50:831, 1974.

83. Newman, P. E.: Coronary collateral circulation: Determinants and functional significance in ischemic heart disease. Am. Heart J. 102:431, 1981.

84. Schwartz, H., Leiboff, R. H., and Bren, G. B.: Temporal evolution of the human coronary collateral circulation following acute myocardial infarction. J. Am. Coll. Cardiol. 4:1088, 1984.

85. Freedman, S. B., Dunn, R. F., Bernstein, L., et al.: Influence of coronary collateral blood flow on the development of exertional ischemia and Q wave infarction in patients with severe single-vessel disease. Circulation 71:681, 1985.

86. Williams, D. O., Amsterdam, E. A., Miller, R. R., and Mason, D. T.: Functional significance of coronary collateral vessels in patients with acute myocardial infarction: Relation to pump performance, cardiogenic shock, and survival. Am. J. Cardiol. 37:345, 1976.

87. Tubau, J. F., Chaitman, B. R., Bourassa, M. G., et al.: Importance of coronary collateral circulation in interpreting exercise test results. Am. J. Cardiol. 47:27, 1981.

88. Cohen, M., and Rentrop, P.: Limitation of myocardial ischemia by collateral circulation during sudden controlled coronary artery occlusion in human subjects. Circulation 74:469, 1986.

89. Mizuno, K., Horiuchi, K., Matui, H., et al.: Role of coronary collateral vessels during transient coronary occlusion during angioplasty assessed by hemodynamic, electrocardiographic, and metabolic changes. J. Am. Coll. Cardiol. 12:624, 1988.

90. Meier, B., Luethy, P., Fincy, L., et al.: Coronary wedge pressure in relation to spontaneously visible and recruitable collaterals. Circulation 75:906, 1987.

91. Probst, P., Zangl, W., and Pachinger, O.: Relation of coronary arterial occlusion pressure during percutaneous transluminal coronary angioplasty to presence of collaterals. Am. J. Cardiol. 55:1264, 1985.

92. Prinzmetal, M., Kennamer, R., Merliss, R., et al.: Angina pectoris: I. Variant form of angina pectoris. Am. J. Med. 27:375, 1959.

93. Braunwald, E.: Coronary artery spasm: Mechanisms and clinical relevance. JAMA 256:1957, 1981.
94. Olivas, P. B., Potts, D. E., and Pluss, R. G.: Coronary arterial spasm in Prinzmetal angina: Documentation by coronary arteriography. N. Engl. J. Med. 288:745, 1973.
95. Curry, R. C., Jr., Pepine, C. J., Varnell, J. H., et al.: Clinical usefulness and safety of the ergonovine test in patients with chest pain. Am. J. Cardiol. 41:369, 1978.
96. Bertrand, M. E., LaBlanche, J. M., Tilmant, P. Y., et al.: Frequency of provoked coronary arterial spasm in 1089 consecutive patients undergoing coronary arteriography. Circulation 65:1299, 1982.
97. Crevey, B. J., Owen, S. F., and Pitt, B.: Irreversible coronary occlusion related to administration of ergonovine. Circulation 66:252, 1982.

INTERVENTIONAL CORONARY ARTERIOGRAPHY

98. Grüntzig, A. R., Senning, A., and Siegenthaler, W. E.: Nonoperative dilatation for coronary artery stenosis—Percutaneous transluminal coronary angioplasty. N. Engl. J. Med. 301:61, 1979.
99. Ritchie, J. L., Phillips, K. A., and Luft, H. S.: Coronary angiopasty: Statewide experience in California. Circulation 88:2735, 1993.
100. Ryan, T. J., Bauman, W. B., Kennedy, J. W., et al.: Guidelines for percutaneous transluminal coronary angioplasty: A report of the American Heart Association/American College of Cardiology Task Force on Assessment of Diagnostic and Therapeutic Cardiovascular Procedures (Subcommittee on Percutaneous Transluminal Coronary Angioplasty). Circulation 88:2987, 1993.
101. Wolfe, M. W., Roubin, G. S., Schweiger, M., et al.: Length of hospital stay and complications after percutaneous transluminal coronary angioplasty: Clinical and procedural predictors. Circulation 92:311, 1995.
102. Ghazzal, Z. M. B., Hearn, J., Litvack, F., et al.: Morphological predictors of acute complications after percutaneous excimer laser coronary angioplasty. Results of a comprehensive angiographic analysis: Importance of the eccentricity index. Circulation 86:820, 1992.
103. Ellis, S. G., and Topol, E. J.: Results of percutaneous transluminal coronary angioplasty of high-risk angulated stenoses. Am. J. Cardiol. 66:932, 1990.
104. Ellis, S. G., Roubin, G. S., King, S. B., III, et al.: Angiographic and clinical predictors of acute closure after native vessel coronary angioplasty. Circulation 77:372, 1988.
105. Sherman, C. T., Litvack, F., Grundfest, W., et al.: Coronary angioscopy in patients with unstable angina pectoris. N. Engl. J. Med. 315:913, 1986.
106. Holmes, D. R., Hartzler, G. O., Smith, H. C., and Fuster, V.: Coronary artery thrombosis in patients with unstable angina. Br. Heart J. 45:411, 1981.
107. The TIMI IIIA Investigators: Early effects of tissue-type plasminogen activator added to conventional therapy on the culprit coronary lesion in patients presenting with ischemia cardiac pain at rest: Results of the Thrombolysis in Myocardial Ischemia (TIMI IIIA) trial. Circulation 87:38, 1993.
108. Ahmed, W. H., Bittl, J. A., and Braunwald, E.: Relation between clinical presentation and angiographic findings in unstable angina pectoris, and comparison with that in stable angina. Am. J. Cardiol. 72:544, 1993.
109. Gotoh, K., Minamino, T., Katoh, O., et al.: The role of intracoronary thrombus in unstable angina: Angiographic assessment and thrombolytic therapy during ongoing anginal attacks. Circulation 77:526, 1988.
110. Bentivoglio, L. G., Detre, K., Yeh, W., et al.: Outcome of percutaneous transluminal coronary angioplasty in subsets of unstable angina pectoris: A report of the 1985–1986 National Heart, Lung, and Blood Institute Percutaneous Transluminal Coronary Angioplasty Registry. J. Am. Coll. Cardiol. 24:1195, 1994.
111. Ellis, S. G., Topol, E. J., Gallison, L., et al.: Predictors of success for coronary angioplasty performed for acute myocardial infarction. J. Am. Coll. Cardiol. 12:1407, 1988.
112. Sullivan, E., Kearney, M., Isner, J. M., et al.: Pathology of unstable angina: Analysis of biopsies obtained by directional coronary atherectomy. J. Thromb. Thrombol. 1:63, 1994.
113. Sutton, J. M., Ellis, S. G., Roubin, G. S., et al.: Major clinical events after coronary stenting: The multicenter registry of acute and elective Gianturco-Roubin stent placement. Circulation 89:1126, 1994.
114. Popma, J. J., Leon, M. B., Mintz, G. S., et al.: Results of coronary angioplasty using the transluminal extraction catheter. Am. J. Cardiol. 70:1526, 1992.
115. Safian, R. D., Grines, C. L., May, M. A., et al.: Clinical and angiographic results of transluminal extraction coronary atherectomy in saphenous vein bypass grafts. Circulation 89:302, 1994.
116. Mabin, T. A., Holmes, D. R., Jr., Smith, H. C., et al.: Intracoronary thrombus: Role in coronary occlusion complicating percutaneous transluminal coronary angioplasty. J. Am. Coll. Cardiol. 5:198, 1985.
117. Grassman, E. D., Leya, F., Johnson, S. A., et al.: Percutaneous transluminal coronary angioplasty for unstable angina: Predictors of outcome in a multicenter study. J. Thromb. Thrombol. 1:73, 1994.
118. Estella, P., Ryan, T. J., Jr., Landzberg, J. S., and Bittl, J. A.: Excimer laser-assisted angioplasty for lesions containing thrombus. J. Am. Coll. Cardiol. 21:1550, 1993.
119. Freeman, M. R., Williams, A. E., Chisholm, R. J., and Armstrong, P. W.: Intracoronary thrombus and complex morphology in unstable angina: Relation of timing of angiography and in-hospital cardiac events. Circulation 80:17, 1989.
120. Huber, M. S., Mooney, J. F., Madison, J., and Mooney, M. R.: Use of a morphologic classification to predict clinical outcome after dissection from coronary angioplasty. Am. J. Cardiol. 68:467, 1991.
121. Dorros, G., Cowley, M. J., Simpson, J., et al.: Percutaneous transluminal coronary angioplasty: Report of complications from the National Heart, Lung, and Blood Institute PTCA Registry. Circulation 67:723, 1983.
122. Lincoff, A. M., Popma, J. J., Ellis, S. G., et al.: Abrupt vessel closure complicating coronary angioplasty: Clinical, angiographic and therapeutic profile. J. Am. Coll. Cardiol. 19:926, 1992.
123. White, C. J., Ramee, S. R., Collins, T. J., et al.: Coronary angioscopy of abrupt occlusion after angioplasty. J. Am. Coll. Cardiol. 25:1681, 1995.
124. Stone, G. W., Rutherford, B. D., McConahay, D. R., et al.: Procedural outcome of angioplasty for total coronary artery occlusion: An analysis of 971 lesions in 905 patients. J. Am. Coll. Cardiol. 15:849, 1990.
125. Tenaglia, A. N., Tcheng, J. E., Phillips, H. R., III, and Stack, R. S.: Creation of a pseudonarrowing during coronary angioplasty. Am. J. Cardiol. 67:658, 1991.

RELATION BETWEEN ARTERIOGRAPHIC FINDINGS AND CLINICAL OUTCOME

126. Kemp, H. G., Kronmal, R. A., Vlietstra, R. E., et al.: Seven-year survival of patients with normal or near normal coronary arteriograms: A CASS Registry study. J. Am. Coll. Cardiol. 7:479, 1986.
127. Papanicolaou, M. N., Califf, R. M., Hlatky, M. A., et al.: Prognostic implications of angiographically normal and insignificantly narrowed coronary arteries. Am. J. Cardiol. 58:1181, 1986.
128. Conley, M. J., Ely, R. L., Kisslo, J., et al.: The prognostic spectrum of left main stenosis. Circulation 57:947, 1978.
129. Takaro, T., Peduzzi, P., Detre, K. M., et al.: Survival in subgroups of patients with left main coronary artery disease: Veterans Administration Cooperative Study of Surgery for Coronary Arterial Occlusive Disease. Circulation 66:14, 1982.
130. Mock, M. B., Ringqvist, I., Fisher, L. D., et al.: Survival of medically treated patients in the Coronary Artery Surgery Study (CASS) Registry. Circulation 66:562, 1982.
131. Ambrose, J. A., Winters, S. L., Stern, A., et al.: Angiographic morphology and the pathogenesis of unstable angina pectoris. J. Am. Coll. Cardiol. 5:609, 1985.
132. Mizuno, K., Satomura, K., Miyamoto, A., et al.: Angioscopic evaluation of coronary-artery thrombi in acute coronary syndromes. N. Engl. J. Med. 326:287, 1992.
133. Forrester, J. S., Litvack, F., Grundfest, W., and Hickey, A.: A perspective of coronary disease seen through the arteries of living man. Circulation 75:505, 1986.
134. Falk, E.: Unstable angina with fatal outcome: Dynamic coronary thrombosis leading to infarction and/or sudden death. Circulation 71:699, 1983.
135. Davies, M. J., and Thomas, A. C.: Plaque-fissuring: The cause of acute myocardial infarction, sudden ischaemic death, and crescendo angina. Br. Heart J. 53:363, 1985.
136. Davies, M. J., Thomas, A. C., Knapman, P. A., and Hangartner, J. R.: Intramyocardial platelet aggregation in patients with unstable angina suffering ischemic cardiac death. Circulation 73:418, 1986.
137. Lendon, C. L., Davies, M. J., Born, G. V., and Richardson, P. D.: Atherosclerotic plaque caps are locally weakened when macrophage density is increased. Atherosclerosis 87:87, 1991.
138. Flugelman, M. Y., Virmani, R., Correa, R., et al.: Smooth muscle cell abundance and fibroblast growth factors in coronary lesions of patients with nonfatal unstable angina. Circulation 88:2493, 1993.
139. van der Wal, A. C., Becker, A. E., van der Loos, C. M., and Das, P. K.: Site of intimal rupture or erosion of thrombosed coronary atherosclerotic plaques is characterized by an inflammatory process irrespective of the dominant plaque morphology. Circulation 89:36, 1994.
140. Fuster, V., Badimon, L., Badimon, J. J., and Chesebro, J. H.: The pathophysiology of coronary artery disease and the acute coronary syndromes. N. Engl. J. Med. 326:242, 1992.
141. Braunwald, E.: Unstable angina: A classification. Circulation 80:410, 1989.
142. Brensike, J. F., Levy, R. I., Kelsey, S. F., et al.: Effects of therapy with cholestyramine on progression of coronary arteriosclerosis: Results of the NHLBI Type II Coronary Intervention Study. Circulation 69:313, 1984.
143. Brown, G., Albers, J. J., Fisher, L. D., et al.: Regression of coronary artery disease as a result of intensive lipid-lowering therapy in men with high levels of apolipoprotein B. N. Engl. J. Med. 323:1289, 1990.
144. Watts, G. F., Lewis, B., Brunt, J. N. H., et al.: Effects on coronary artery disease of lipid-lowering diet, or diet plus cholestyramine, in the St. Thomas' Atherosclerosis Regression Study (STARS). Lancet 339:563, 1992.
145. Treasure, C. B., Klein, J. L., Weintraub, W. S., et al.: Beneficial effects of cholesterol-lowering therapy on the coronary endothelium in patients with coronary artery disease. N. Engl. J. Med. 332:481, 1995.
146. Anderson, T. J., Meredith, I. T., Yeung, A. C., et al.: The effect of cholesterol-lowering and antioxidant therapy on endothelium-dependent coronary vasomotion. N. Engl. J. Med. 332:488, 1995.
147. Ambrose, J. A., Tannenbaum, M. A., and Alexopoulos, D.: Angiographic

progression of coronary artery disease and the development of myocardial infarction. J. Am. Coll. Cardiol. *12*:56, 1988.

148. Webster, M. W., Chesebro, J. H., Smith, H. C., et al.: Myocardial infarction and coronary artery occlusion: A prospective 5-year angiographic study. J. Am. Coll. Cardiol. *15*(Abs.):218A, 1990.

149. Little, W. C., Constantinescu, M., Applegate, R. J., et al.: Can coronary angiography predict the site of a subsequent myocardial infarction in patients with mild-to-moderate coronary artery disease? Circulation *78*:1157, 1988.

150. Bär, F. W., Raynaud, P., Renkin, J. P., et al.: Coronary angiographic findings do not predict clinical outcome in patients with unstable angina. J. Am. Coll. Cardiol. *24*:1453, 1994.

151. Isshiki, T., Yamaguchi, T., Tamura, T., et al.: Percutaneous angioplasty of stenosed gastroepiploic artery grafts. J. Am. Coll. Cardiol. *21*:727, 1993.

152. Miller, S. W.: Coronary artery disease. *In* Miller, S. W. (ed.): Cardiac Angiography. Boston, Little, Brown, 1984, p. 87.

Chapter 9
Nuclear Cardiology

FRANS J. TH. WACKERS, ROBERT SOUFER, BARRY L. ZARET

Nuclear cardiology has been an active clinical discipline for more than two decades. Since the initial evolution from investigative studies to clinical studies, new techniques have evolved progressively. Major advances have occurred in both instrumentation and radiopharmaceutical development. In a parallel fashion, studies have actively pursued issues relating to clinical relevance, efficacy, and outcomes. The discipline has moved from the primary diagnostic sphere to an equally intense involvement in the functional categorization of patients with known disease. This has provided numerous insights into risk stratification and prognosis. In this chapter, following an introduction of some principles of instrumentation, the major techniques of nuclear cardiology are discussed. In each section, relevant technical issues necessary for adequate test performance are presented together with the clinical and investigative impact of the derived data.

INSTRUMENTATION

The acquisition and display of a nuclear image depend on the detection of radiation emitted from the patient following the administration of a radionuclide. In radionuclide cardiac imaging, the radionuclides are either extracted by the myocardium or remain in the cardiac blood pool. Several components are required to acquire gamma rays and to produce an image. These include a scintillation device such as the sodium iodide (NaI) crystal, which absorbs the gamma rays and generates photons that are converted to an electrical signal by photomultiplier tubes. The electrical signal then is amplified and accelerated such that the energy of the gamma ray initially absorbed by the crystal is directly proportional to the height of the generated electrical pulse. Different radionuclides emit at different energies. This allows discrimination between photons from the target and scatter.

THE SCINTILLATION (GAMMA) CAMERA

Nuclear cardiology studies are performed with a scintillation camera interfaced with a computer. Radionuclide images are the result of gamma rays passing through several principal camera components: a collimator, a large NaI crystal, and a hexagonal array of 37 to 91 photomultiplier tubes. The gamma camera provides an image of the location and intensity of a radiopharmaceutical in the body. The image is the result of the interaction between gamma rays and the camera crystal, which converts part of this energy into light (scintillation).

The photomultiplier tubes translate these scintillations into voltage pulses; these are measured as an electrical signal that defines the position at which gamma ray and crystal interact. This is accomplished by electronic circuits that compute x and y coordinates of crystal interaction and display this interaction in a two-dimensional matrix anatomically analogous to the site of occurrence within the patient. A multichannel analyzer defines the appropriate energy of the event; thus, low-energy (Compton) scatter events are not accepted.

COLLIMATION. Collimation is important for radionuclide imaging. It can be thought of as comparable to a focusing lens on a photographic camera. A collimator is composed of lead channels designed in either a parallel or diverging manner. Gamma rays must pass through the collimator before reaching the crystal. The purpose of the collimator is to approximate the origin of the photon emission within the patient to an analogous location within the crystal. Parallel-hole collimators are of either the high-resolution or the high-sensitivity variety. The high-resolution collimator permits better spatial resolution (the ability of the detector source to discriminate between neighboring sources of activity and visually resolve various components within the field of view), but with a loss of count sensitivity (the number of counts acquired per unit time).

Alternatively, a high-sensitivity collimator maximizes count sensitivity at the expense of spatial resolution. A compromise between the two types of collimators is the low-energy all-purpose or general all-purpose collimator, which is intermediate with respect to sensitivity and resolution. The thickness of the crystal and the type of collimation determine the sensitivity of a gamma camera. The type of collimation used for a particular study is based on these simple concepts. For instance, a parallel-hole high-sensitivity is appropriate for rapidly acquired studies such as first-pass blood pool studies.

Characteristics that influence the overall performance of the gamma camera are intrinsic and partial resolution, field uniformity, and count rate linearity. Most scintillation cameras have a spatial resolution of 10 to 12 mm, with a count rate linearity of approximately 75,000 counts per second and a flood of uniformity of ± 5 per cent.

COMPUTING. The computer is a principal component of all nuclear imaging systems. These data processing systems are interfaced with the gamma camera. The routine use of computers makes radionuclide imaging intrinsically quantitative. The computers have software containing algorithms for quantification of both static and dynamic digital images. The principal hardware components of the computer include analog digital convertor, central processing unit, image memory, mass storage, an array processor, and a display monitor. The scintigraphic matrix is generally 64×64 or 128×128 pixels (picture elements).

SINGLE-PHOTON EMISSION COMPUTED TOMOGRAPHY (SPECT)

Over the past several years SPECT acquisition has been used more commonly in cardiovascular nuclear medicine imaging. With SPECT, a series of planar images is obtained over a 180-degree arc around the patient's thorax. Transaxial images are recreated using a technique called filtered backprojection. These transaxial images are reconstructed into short axis and horizontal and vertical long axis orientations relative to the anatomical axis of the heart. The overall result is an improvement in anatomical resolution and contrast. Alternatively, SPECT imaging requires more attention to detail with regard to the parameters set for acquisition and more stringent quality control measures.

TECHNICAL ADVANCES. Conventional gamma cameras have one detector head. In planar imaging the detector head remains in position and acquires the projection of radioactivity in one plane. For SPECT imaging the detector head rotates around the patient while acquiring multiple projection images. From these planar projection images a three-dimensional image is constructed by backprojection. Recently, gamma cameras with multiple detector heads have been developed. These systems have improved electronics and count sensitivities, which improve image resolution and decrease SPECT imaging time. The optimal detector configuration is two camera crystal heads separated by 90 degrees. Because two camera heads are used simultaneously, the full 180-degree orbit may be required, with only a 90-degree motion resulting in half the acquisition time. Optimal 360-degree acquisition may be performed with triple head systems, in which each head is separated by 120-degrees. The increased count sensitivity of these detectors allows high-resolution collimation and improved image quality and quantification.

FUTURE DEVELOPMENTS. A significant limitation of traditional single-photon imaging is inhomogeneous attenuation of radiation by soft tissue. Attenuation artifacts are most commonly located in the anterior wall owing to breast or chest wall attenuation or in the inferior wall owing to diaphragmatic attenuation. Attenuation correction systems currently are under clinical investigation. Another problem with SPECT imaging is patient motion. Motion correction software has been developed but as yet is not widely used clinically. Finally, scatter photons are a major source of degraded image quality. Scatter correction signifies a major improvement of radionuclide image quality. A more detailed discussion of instrumentation used in cardiovascular nuclear medicine is beyond the scope of this chapter and may be found elsewhere.[1,2]

MYOCARDIAL PERFUSION IMAGING

The regional distribution of myocardial perfusion can be visualized using radiopharmaceuticals that accumulate proportional to regional myocardial blood flow. The first scintigraphic images of myocardial perfusion were acquired in 1964 by Carr et al.[3] using cesium-131. Exercise-induced myocardial ischemia was initially visualized with potassium-43 in 1973 by Zaret et al.[4] Thallium-201 (^{201}Tl), a potassium analog, became available in 1974 and has since been employed successfully.[5-8] Recently, new technetium-99m (^{99m}Tc)–labeled compounds with better imaging characteristics and novel biological properties have been introduced for visualization of myocardial perfusion.[10-16] Employing any of these imaging agents, the *relative* distribution of myocardial blood flow can be visualized. *Absolute* quantification of myocardial blood flow is not feasible using single-photon emitting radioisotopes but can be achieved with positron emission tomography.

The most important clinical application of myocardial perfusion imaging is in conjunction with stress testing for evaluation of ischemic heart disease. Numerous investigators have shown the diagnostic usefulness of exercise myocardial perfusion imaging[8,9] using either ^{201}Tl or the ^{99m}Tc-labeled imaging agents.[10-16] Generally good agreement is found between the results of stress myocardial perfusion imaging and findings on contrast coronary angiography. More importantly, it has been demonstrated that findings on stress myocardial perfusion images reflect the hemodynamic and functional significance of coronary artery stenoses and thus provide important prognostic information. Finally, the information derived from radionuclide myocardial perfusion imaging has independent and incremental value over that derived by other diagnostic methods.

RADIOPHARMACEUTICALS

THALLIUM-201. Thallium-201 is cyclotron-produced and emits mercury x-rays at 69 to 83 keV (88 per cent) and gamma rays at 135, 165, and 167 keV (12 per cent). Its physical half-life is 74 hours; however, its biological half-life is approximately 58 hours. The estimated absorbed radiation dose to the whole body is 0.21 rad/mCi, to the kidney 0.24 rad/mCi, and to the large intestine 0.54 rad/mCi. Because of the relatively long half-life of ^{201}Tl, only a relatively small amount of radioactivity can be administered. For planar imaging, usually 2 to 2.5 mCi is administered, whereas for tomographic imaging is 3.5 to 4.0 mCi is given. The first-pass myocardial extraction fraction of ^{201}Tl of 85 per cent is relatively high.[17] The initial myocardial accumulation of ^{201}Tl is proportional to myocardial blood flow. Once ^{201}Tl has entered the myocyte, a continuous exchange of ^{201}Tl takes place across the cell membrane. This process involves the Na$^+$, K$^+$-ATPase pump. The intrinsic half-life of ^{201}Tl within the myocardial cell is approximately 85 minutes. However, because of continued cellular reaccumulation of ^{201}Tl, the effective half-life of ^{201}Tl in the heart is 7.5 hours. A unique aspect of ^{201}Tl

studies is that images obtained *early* and *late* after injection provide different pathophysiologic information:

1. Images immediately after injection reflect the flow-dependent initial distribution and thus regional myocardial blood flow.

2. Images taken after a delay of 2 to 24 hours reflect the distribution of the potassium pool and hence myocardial viability.

TECHNETIUM-99m–LABELED COMPOUNDS. A number of ^{99m}Tc-labeled compounds have been introduced in recent years for myocardial imaging. The first to be approved by the Food and Drug Administration and the most widely used compound in this class is ^{99m}Tc-sestamibi,[10,11] a lipophilic monovalent cation. Technetium-99m–tetrofosmin[14,15] and ^{99m}Tc-furifosmin[16] have at the time of this writing been tested in phase-two and phase-three clinical trials but have not yet been approved for routine clinical use. The ^{99m}Tc label emits gamma rays at 140 keV and has a physical half-life of 6 hours. Because of the slow body clearance, the biological half-life of sestamibi, tetrofosmin, and furifosmin is approximately the same. The whole-body absorbed radiation dose for these agents is approximately 0.02 rad/mCi. The target organ is the gallbladder, which receives approximately 0.29 rad/mCi.

Because of favorable dosimetry of the ^{99m}Tc-labeled compounds compared with ^{201}Tl, up to 30 mCi of these agents can be administered per day (see imaging protocols). The initial myocardial distribution of ^{99m}Tc-labeled agents is similar to that of ^{201}Tl and is proportional to regional distribution of myocardial blood flow. However, in contrast to ^{201}Tl, simultaneous rapid accumulation in the liver and subsequent clearance into the biliary tract occur. Myocardial extraction of ^{99m}Tc-sestamibi with an extraction fraction of 65 per cent, is substantially less efficient than that of ^{201}Tl. Sestamibi enters the myocyte by passive diffusion and binds stably to intracellular membranes. Because of intracellular retention and additional subsequent myocardial uptake during recirculation, the *absolute net retention* of ^{99m}Tc agents at several minutes after administration is comparable to that of ^{201}Tl.[18] Because myocardial distribution of ^{99m}Tc agents remains relatively fixed over time and no significant redistribution occurs, the distribution of myocardial blood flow *at the time of injection* is "frozen" over time and can be imaged for several hours. In addition, two separate injections are required to evaluate myocardial uptake at rest and exercise.

Technetium-99m–Teboroxime. Another recently developed ^{99m}Tc-labeled myocardial perfusion imaging agent with markedly different physiological characteristics is teboroxime. Technetium-99m–teboroxime is a neutral cation and a boronic acid adduct of technetium oxime (BATO). In contrast to the other ^{99m}Tc-labeled compounds, this imaging agent has both the rapid and efficient myocardial extraction (80 to 90 per cent myocardial extraction fraction) and subsequent rapid washout from the heart.[12] In addition, intense early hepatic activity may hinder complete evaluation of myocardial uptake, particularly of the inferior wall.

	^{201}Tl	^{99m}Tc-SESTAMIBI ^{99m}Tc-TETROFOSMIN ^{99m}Tc-FURIFOSMIN	^{99m}Tc-TEBOROXIME
Energy emissions	69–83 keV (x-rays) 135, 165, 167 keV	140 keV	140 keV
Physical half-life	74 hr	6 hr	6 hr
Biological half-life	58 hr	6 hr	<6 hr
Heart half-life	3–4 hr	6–7 hr	<10 min
Dose	2–4.0 mCi	30 mCi	30 mCi
Radiation dose			
Whole body	0.21 rad/mCi	0.02 rad/mCi	0.02 rad/mCi
Intestines	0.54 rad/mCi	0.18 rad/mCi	0.11 rad/mCi
Myocardial EF	85%	65%	80–90%
% ID heart	4%	1.5%	?
Visualizes			
Blood flow	+	+	+
Viability	+ (delayed image)	+	–
Redistribution	+	Minimal	–
LVEF (first pass)	–	+	+
ECG gating	–	+	–
Imaging time/views			
Planar	10 min	5 min	1–2 min
Tomography	21 min	11 min	1 min

Abbreviations: EF = Extraction fraction; % ID = Per cent of injected dose; LVEF = Left ventricular ejection fraction

Myocardial washout of teboroxime is biexponential: At 5 minutes after injection only 25 per cent of the initial activity remains in the heart. The estimated whole-body absorbed radiation dose is 0.02 rad/mCi. The target organs are liver and large intestine, which receive 0.12 rad/mCi and 0.11 rad/mCi, respectively. This imaging agent requires rapid serial imaging during the 5 minutes immediately following injection.[13] The main characteristics of the various imaging agents are summarized in Table 9–1.

Technical Considerations

GAMMA CAMERA. For planar imaging, a camera with 10-inch diameter detector and a ¼-inch thick crystal is preferred. Low-energy photons of ^{201}Tl do not adequately penetrate thicker crystals, resulting in images of inadequate count density. Tomographic cameras with large field of view (20-inch diameter) generally have a ⅜-inch thick crystal and are thus not ideally suited for ^{201}Tl imaging but are ideally suited for imaging of ^{99m}Tc-labeled agents.

COLLIMATION. For both planar and SPECT imaging with ^{201}Tl, a general all-purpose parallel-hole collimator is preferred to ensure adequate count density. Owing to the higher photon flux with ^{99m}Tc-labeled imaging agents, good-quality images are obtained with a high-resolution parallel-hole collimator.

ENERGY WINDOW. For ^{201}Tl imaging, a dual window is preferred: 25 per cent window over the 80-keV mercury x-ray peak and 20 per cent window over the 167-keV gamma-ray peak. The latter window accounts for approximately 10 per cent additional counts. For ^{99m}Tc-labeled imaging agents, a 20 per cent window is placed over the 140-keV peak.

COMPUTER ACQUISITION. Radionuclide images are acquired on computer and stored on computer disk or magnetic tape for data processing. For planar myocardial perfusion imaging, acquisition in 128 × 128 matrix is preferred, whereas for SPECT imaging a 64 × 64 matrix is commonly used.

IMAGING PROTOCOLS

Because of the introduction of new imaging agents and new insights in ^{201}Tl biokinetics, imaging protocols have recently been modified considerably. Figure 9–1 provides a schematic representation of the most frequently used imaging protocols at the time of this writing. For a more detailed discussion of various imaging protocols, see a recent review by Wackers.[19]

For Tl-201 stress imaging (Fig. 9–1A), one single dose of ^{201}Tl is injected at peak exercise. Initial stress imaging should be started *within 5 minutes* of the injection. Delayed or redistribution imaging is performed *2 to 4 hours later* (timing of delayed imaging should be standardized in each laboratory). For complete assessment of viable myocardium, a second injection of ^{201}Tl is administered at rest in selected patients. The repeat rest injection can be given either following redistribution imaging or on a different day (see p. 294).

For imaging with ^{99m}Tc-labeled perfusion imaging agents (Fig. 9–1B, C) two separate injections are given: one during exercise and a second at rest. Employing ^{99m}Tc-sestamibi, imaging is started approxi-

mately *15 minutes after injection during exercise and 60 minutes after injection at rest.* Because ^{99m}Tc-tetrofosmin and ^{99m}Tc-furifosmin clear more rapidly from the liver after rest injection, rest imaging with these compounds can be started relatively early *(15 minutes after injection).* Thus, with these latter agents both rest and exercise imaging is started at 15 minutes after injection.

With ^{99m}Tc-teboroxime the patient should be imaged rapidly, starting at *1 minute after injection.* After 5 to 10 minutes not enough teboroxime remains in the heart to allow adequate quality imaging.

DUAL ISOTOPE IMAGING (Fig. 9–1D). This is a "hybrid" imaging protocol, designed to overcome the disadvantage of a relatively lengthy imaging protocol using two injections of sestamibi.[20] Using the dual-isotope protocol a rest injection of ^{201}Tl (3.5 mCi) is given first, followed by rest ^{201}Tl imaging. The patient is then stressed and injected

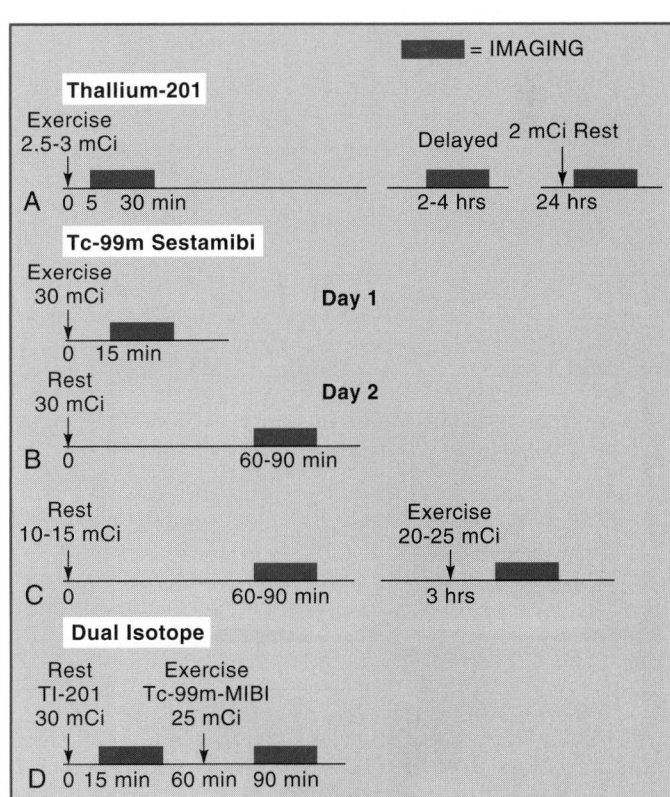

FIGURE 9–1. Schematic representation of preferred myocardial perfusion imaging protocols using either ^{201}Tl, ^{99m}Tc-sestamibi, or dual isotope imaging (see text).

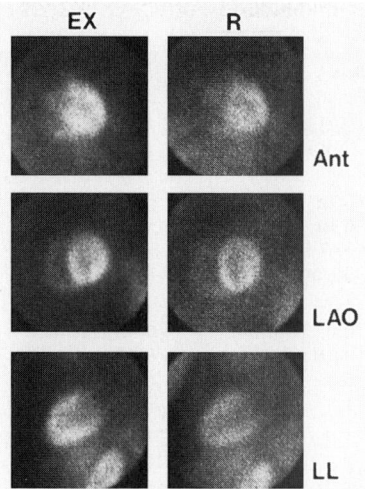

EX R

Ant

LAO

LL

FIGURE 9–2. Normal planar exercise (EX) and redistribution (R) planar ²⁰¹Tl images. Ant = Anterior view; LAO = left anterior oblique view; LL = left lateral view.

with 25 to 30 mCi of sestamibi at peak stress, followed after 15 minutes by sestamibi imaging. This imaging protocol can be completed in 1½ to 2 hours.

Imaging Techniques

PLANAR IMAGING. Although SPECT imaging at the present time is the predominant imaging technique used in clinical nuclear cardiology, the technical basis for good-quality SPECT imaging remains the ability to perform good-quality planar imaging. To acquire optimal planar myocardial perfusion images, some basic requirements should be met.[21,22] The most frequent reasons for suboptimal quality images are (1) insufficient count density within the heart, (2) inconsistent *patient positioning and repositioning*, (3) the use of *too large a zoom factor*, and (4) inadequate display of images.

ADEQUATE COUNT DENSITY. Images should have at least 600,000 counts in the field of view. However, when extracardiac activity is present, such as in lungs or subdiaphragmatic organs, the count density in the field of view does not reflect the count density in the heart. Longer imaging time is needed to obtain adequate counts from the heart. Therefore, it is recommended to acquire images for a certain *preset time*. For planar ²⁰¹Tl imaging, 8- to 10-minute acquisitions per view usually results in adequate count density imaging. Using ⁹⁹ᵐTc-labeled imaging agents, adequate count density is readily achieved because 20 to 30 mCi is administered. Employing the latter

agents, 1.5 to 2 million counts per field of view can be obtained with 5-minute acquisitions per view.

PATIENT POSITIONING. Planar imaging is routinely performed in three positions. The *left anterior oblique* (LAO) view usually is obtained with the patient lying supine. An optimal LAO is the projection that shows best separation of right and left ventricular cavities with the septum straight and vertical. This angulation should be used as a reference angle for the other views. The *anterior view* is obtained with the patient lying supine, 45 degrees to the right of the LAO view. For the *left lateral view* the patient should be turned on his *right side*, with the camera head in the same position as for the anterior view. The detector head should be angled in such a way that it is as close as possible to the patient's chest wall.

On all views the heart should be in the *center* of the field of view. *Repositioning* of the patient at delayed imaging should be performed with great care. The position of heart on the exercise images should be reproduced as close as possible.

ZOOM FACTOR. When a large field of view camera is used, the *zoom factor* (magnification) should not exceed 1.2 times. On an optimal image, the heart is approximately one-third to one-fourth of the diameter of the field of view.

PLANAR IMAGE DISPLAY. The *display* of myocardial perfusion images is important for reproducible and consistent interpretation. Color display of *planar* images should be discouraged. "White on black" display using a linear gray scale is preferred (Fig. 9–2). On these images the heart is white (radioactivity). When interpretation is performed from a computer screen, standardization of display is important. Arbitrarily changing contrast intensity and gray scales should be limited to a minimum. We recommend use of the test pattern designed by the Society for Motion Picture and Television Engineers (SMPTE) for quality control. The linear gray scale should be normalized to the "hottest pixel" within the heart (Fig. 9–3). In this manner the gray scale is fully utilized in the representation of the heart. This is particularly important for display of images acquired with ⁹⁹ᵐTc-labeled agents. Exercise and rest/delayed images should be displayed side by side for comparison.

TOMOGRAPHIC (SPECT) IMAGING. Careful attention to technical details is even more important for SPECT imaging than for planar imaging. Energy settings are the same as for planar imaging. Usually a general all-purpose collimator is used. For imaging with ⁹⁹ᵐTc-labeled myocardial perfusion agents, a high-resolution parallel-hole collimator is preferred because of higher count rate.[23] During cardiac SPECT imaging, the gamma camera rotates thorough a 180-degree arc with 32 stops. For imaging with ²⁰¹Tl, the duration of each stop is 40 seconds. Employing ⁹⁹ᵐTc-sestamibi, the time for each stop can be shortened to 25 seconds for a high-dose (22 to 25 mCi) study. For the low-dose (8 to 10 mCi) study, 40 seconds per stop is recommended.

The basic principle of tomographic reconstruction involves the acquisition of multiple planar projection images around an object and the reconstruction of the three-dimensional object by "filtered backprojection."[24] For cardiac SPECT, because the heart lies eccentrically in the chest, 180-degree image acquisition may be used. The pos-

NORMALIZATION Tc-99m SESTAMIBI IMAGE

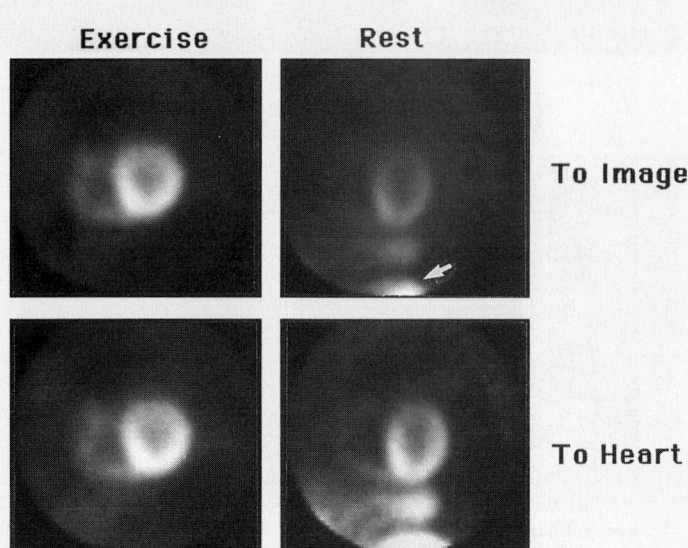

Exercise Rest

To Image

To Heart

FIGURE 9–3. Normalization of exercise/rest ⁹⁹ᵐTc-sestamibi images. Intense subdiaphragmatic activity (arrow) may cause problems with adequate display of the image of the heart. Radionuclide images are usually normalized to the "hottest" area in the field of view. On the exercise sestamibi images the heart is the hottest organ. However, on the rest image the gastrointestinal tract is the hottest area (arrow). Consequently, when the rest image is normalized to subdiaphragmatic activity, the heart is only faintly visualized *(top)*. Using ⁹⁹ᵐTc-labeled myocardial perfusion imaging agents, images should be normalized to the heart, as shown in the bottom panel, for adequate visualization of the heart. (From Wackers, F. J. Th.: Myocardial perfusion imaging. *In* Sandler, M. P., Coleman, R. E., Wackers, F. J. Th., et al.: Diagnostic Nuclear Medicine. 3rd ed. Baltimore, Williams and Wilkins, 1995.)

terior 180-degree arch is not used with ^{201}Tl because it contains low count data as a result of greater distance from the heart and substantial attenuation. Using ^{99m}Tc-labeled radiotracers that are better suited for gamma camera imaging and the new multihead gamma cameras, data acquired over a 360-degree orbit can be used for reconstruction. After backprojection, filtering techniques are used to correct for reconstruction artifacts and enhance the image quality. Tomographic slices are generated perpendicular to the anatomical axis of the heart, rather than those of the body.

PATIENT POSITIONING

Patient positioning and patient preparation are extremely important for optimal SPECT imaging. Patient motion is a common cause for artifacts on SPECT imaging.[30] *Motion* may involve movement of the patient's upper body but may also result from a change in position of the heart within the chest. Immediately after exercise, because of deeper breathing, the heart may be in a vertical position. While the patient recovers from exercise, the heart may move into a horizontal position. This phenomenon of "upward creep" can cause artifactual inferior wall defects on reconstructed slices.[25] This can be avoided by delaying the start of SPECT imaging after termination of exercise for approximately 10 minutes. This allows for acquisition of one *planar* image immediately after exercise, which is useful for evaluation of increased lung uptake. Because SPECT imaging with ^{99m}Tc-labeled agents is not started before 15 minutes after exercise, upward creep is not an issue using these radiotracers.

Adequate count density is a frequently ignored aspect of tomographic perfusion imaging. As mentioned above, gamma cameras used for SPECT imaging have a ¾-inch thick crystal, which is not optimal for ^{201}Tl imaging. Therefore, a relatively high dose of at least 3.5 mCi (129.5 MBq) of ^{201}Tl should be administered. Using ^{99m}Tc-labeled compounds, 10 to 30 mCi (370 to 1110 MBq) is administered. Consequently, count densities are usually adequate for good-quality SPECT images. Unfortunately, most commercially available computer software does not provide information on count density of unprocessed planar projection images. Poor count density on reconstructed and filtered SPECT images should be suspected when the distribution of radiopharmaceutical appears to occur in multiple "patches" of apparent higher and lower activity, a pattern that does not match the usual anatomy of coronary artery disease.

SPECT ORBIT. Many cameras provide a choice of various acquisition orbits. The camera may rotate around the patient in a perfect *circle*, or may follow the *body contour* of the patient. A body-contour orbit may cause artifacts because of varying gamma camera resolution with varying distance of the detector head from the target organ. These artifacts are characteristic and consist of small 180-degree diametrical defects on the short-axis slices.[26] High-resolution collimation reduces the effect of varying spatial resolution and resulting artifacts. Therefore, a circular orbit is preferred for cardiac SPECT imaging.

SPECT IMAGE DISPLAY. The display of reconstructed SPECT slices has been standardized (Fig. 9–4).[27] Images should be displayed "white on black" using a linear gray scale (Fig. 9–5). Three sets of slices are reconstructed: short-axis slices, horizontal long-axis slices, and vertical long-axis slices. The exercise and rest (or delayed) images are displayed side by side to facilitate comparison. Because of the multitude of images, it is useful to "condense" all information into one color-coded polar map, or "bull's-eye" image[28] (see Figs. 9–17B and 9–18B, p. 284).

Normal Planar Myocardial Perfusion Images

In planar imaging, perfusion is visualized as the projection of myocardial radioactivity on a plane parallel to the crystal surface of the gamma camera. The "left ventricular cavity" as it appears on planar images is in part an optical illusion.[21] The familiar horseshoe appearance of the left ventricle on ^{201}Tl images is a result of attenuation of radiation from the distant myocardial wall by ventricular blood pool and the relatively greater myocardial mass of the walls perpendicular to the plane of view. The "facing" myocardial wall contains relatively less radiopharmaceutical, which creates the illusion of visualization of the ventricular cavity.

Because of overprojection of myocardial regions in one plane, it is necessary to obtain multiple planar images from different angles to visualize all segments of left ventricular myocardium. The anatomy of the heart as projected on various planar views and the various coronary artery territories are shown in Figure 9–6.

NORMAL VARIATIONS OF PLANAR MYOCARDIAL PERFUSION IMAGES. The interpretation of myocardial perfusion images may be difficult at times because of normal variations in the pattern of radiotracer uptake.[21]

Apex. A well-recognized area of normally decreased tracer activity is at the apex of the left ventricle. In patients with a vertical position of the heart, this may be a prominent feature. An apical variant appears as a narrow slit or cleft-like area, aligned with the long axis of the left ventricle.

Aortic Valve Plane. On the LAO view the membranous septum and aortic valve plane are projected at the open end of the horseshoe, at times causing an apparent high septal defect. This may be seen prominently in patients with a horizontal position of the heart.

Mitral Valve Plane. The mitral valve plane is seen as the open end of the horseshoe in all three views.

ARTIFACTS ON PLANAR IMAGES

ANTERIOR VIEW. In most normal subjects the intensity of radiotracer uptake in the inferoseptal wall on the planar anterior view is approximately equal to that of the anterolateral wall. However, in a patient with enlargement of the right ventricle (e.g., in chronic obstructive pulmonary disease), the right ventricular blood pool may attenuate inferoseptal activity and produce an apparent defect. Such artifacts can be unmasked by imaging the patient in the upright position, thereby changing the position of the right ventricle in the chest.

LEFT ANTERIOR OBLIQUE VIEW. The appearance of the heart in the planar LAO view depends on both the position of the heart in the chest and the size of the heart. Patients with left ventricular dilatation may have clockwise rotation. In the latter situation a routine 45-degree LAO view may display an image similar to that usually seen in the anterior projection. The (normal) open end of the horseshoe could be misinterpreted as a septal defect. A steeper (60-degree)

FIGURE 9–4. *Standardized display of SPECT myocardial perfusion images. The short-axis slices are displayed with the right ventricle left and the left ventricle right. The short-axis slices are displayed as a horizontal row of images, starting with the apical slice on the left and the basal slices on the right. The vertical long-axis slices are cut from the septum toward the lateral wall, displaying the septal slices on the left and the lateral slices on the right. The horizontal long-axis slices are cut from the inferior wall toward the anterior wall, displaying the inferior wall slices on the left and the anterior wall slices on the right. (From the Cardiovascular Imaging Committee, American College of Cardiology; the Committee on Advanced Cardiac Imaging and Technology, Council of Clinical Cardiology, American Heart Association; and the Board of Directors, Cardiovascular Council Society of Nuclear Medicine: ACC/AHA/SNM Policy Statement: Standardization of cardiac tomographic imaging. J. Nucl. Cardiol. 1:117, 1994.)*

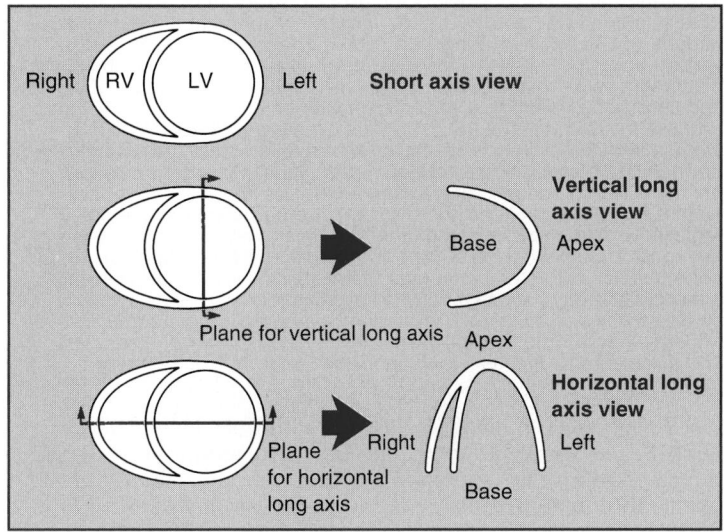

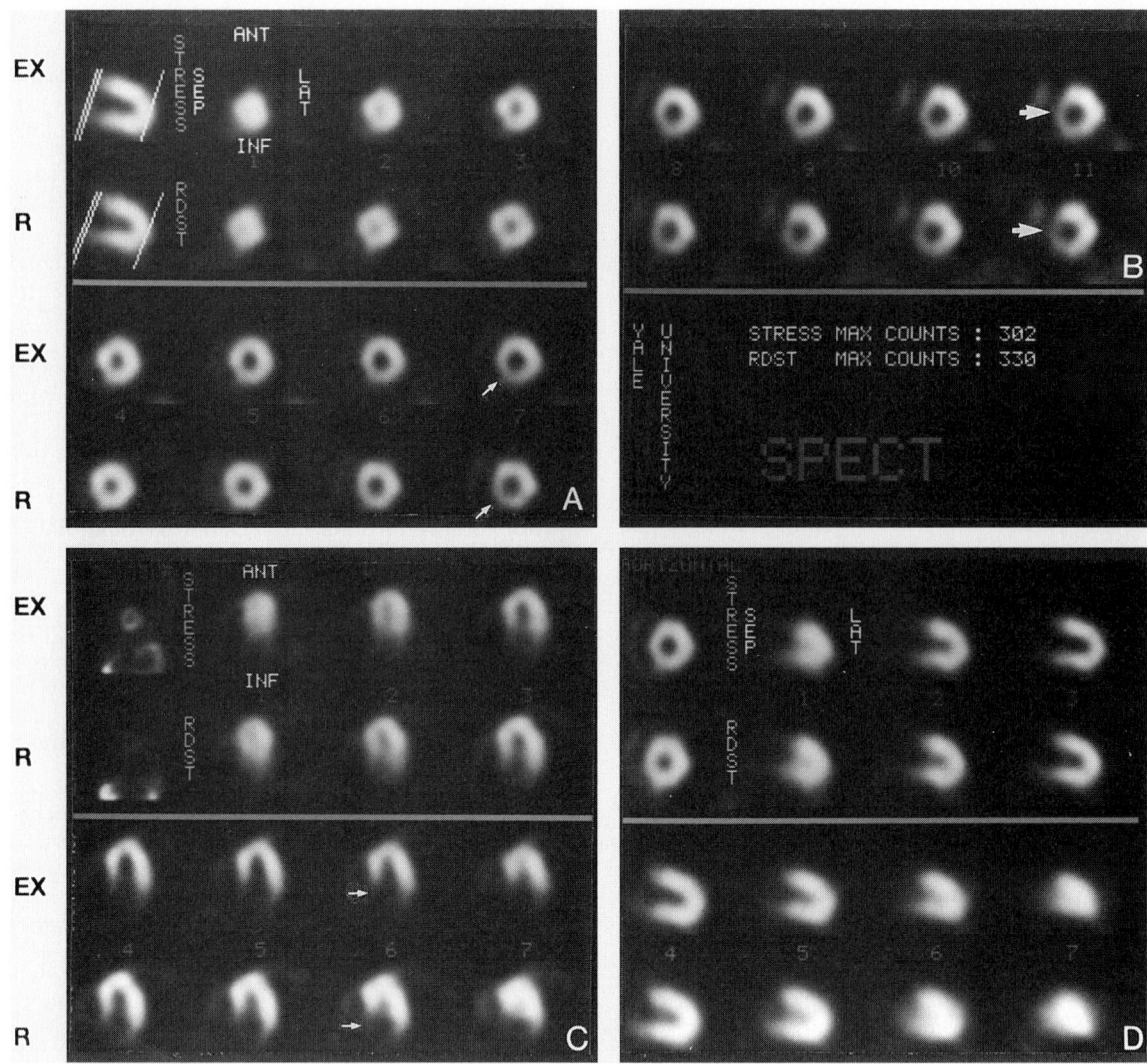

FIGURE 9–5. SPECT 99mTc-sestamibi myocardial images after exercise and at rest in a normal subject, showing normal variations of radiopharmaceutical distribution. On the midventricular short-axis slices (A) the inferior septal areas (small arrows) have slightly less activity than the lateral wall. This is a normal variation. The hottest area is in the lateral wall. On the basal slices (B) an apparent septal defect is present (large arrow). This is the membranous portion of the septum. This "septal defect" and normal variation are also seen in the horizontal long-axis slices (C), where the septum is shorter (arrows) than the lateral wall. Vertical long-axis slices are shown in D. (From Wackers, F. J. Th.: Artifacts in planar and SPECT myocardial perfusion imaging. Am. J. Cardiac Imaging 6:42, 1992.)

angulation may project the left ventricle correctly along the long axis, thereby restoring the "typical" doughnut-shaped configuration.

LEFT LATERAL VIEW. Acquisition of a steep LAO or left lateral image with the patient *supine* may cause artifactual inferior wall defects. This artifact is seen in approximately one-fourth of the patients imaged in the supine position.[29] This artifact is caused by attenuation of the inferior wall activity by the left hemidiaphragm. Turning the patient on his or her right side causes the heart to shift into a vertical position (Fig. 9–7). Moreover, in this position of the left hemidiaphragm makes larger excursions. This results in less attenuation and improved projection of the inferoposterior wall.

OBESE PATIENTS/LARGE BREASTS. In extremely obese patients or in women with large breasts, attenuation of radiation may cause apparent defects. These artifactual defects often appear as anterior defects on the anterior and left lateral views, whereas the location of artifacts is less predictable on the LAO view. We find it useful to employ radioactive string markers to outline the breasts and thus define the relationship between the breasts and cardiac defects (Fig. 9–8). Superimposition of breast tissue over the heart may also result in linear areas of relatively *increased* activity. This linear artifact is believed to be caused by a small-angle scatter from the breast tissue fold. Breast artifacts are the most frequent cause of false-positive 201Tl studies. The use of breast markers is an important aid in correctly interpreting 201Tl images.[21,22,30]

NORMAL PLANAR IMAGES WITH TECHNETIUM-99m–LABELED AGENTS.

Images with 99mTc-labeled myocardial perfusion imaging agents are generally of better quality than 201Tl images. Compared with 201Tl, these images have substantially less low-radiation background scatter and are there-

fore clearer than 201Tl images. The normal variants and artifacts described above can also be observed on images with 99mTc-labeled compounds. The most important difference from 201Tl is the amount of subdiaphragmatic uptake, such as in liver, gallbladder, and large intestine (Fig. 9–9). The liver clearance of sestamibi, tetrofosmin, and furifosmin after exercise is relatively rapid. Postexercise imaging can be started at 15 minutes after injection. However, there is a difference in liver clearance *after rest injection* between various 99mTc-labeled compounds. The clearance of sestamibi is slow and rest imaging often has to be postponed until 60 to 90 minutes after injection.[10] In contrast, tetrofosmin and furifosmin clear relatively rapidly after rest injection, and rest imaging can be started at 15 minutes after injection.

Because of significant extracardiac activity, images with 99mTc-labeled compounds should be displayed with the gray scale normalized to the "hottest" pixel within the heart (Fig. 9–3). Nevertheless, planar images with 99mTc-labeled compound may be difficult to interpret, particularly the inferior wall in the left lateral view, owing to intense subdiaphragmatic activity.

Technetium-99m-Teboroxime. Images with this radiopharmaceutical are characterized by rapid initial accumulation of the radiotracer within the heart and subsequent fast

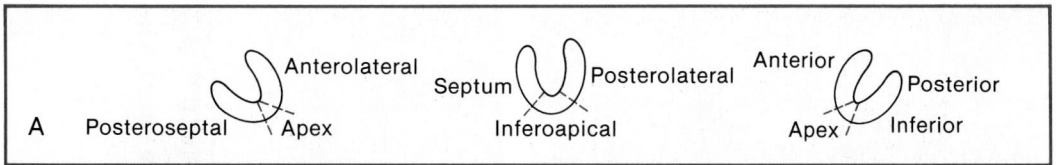

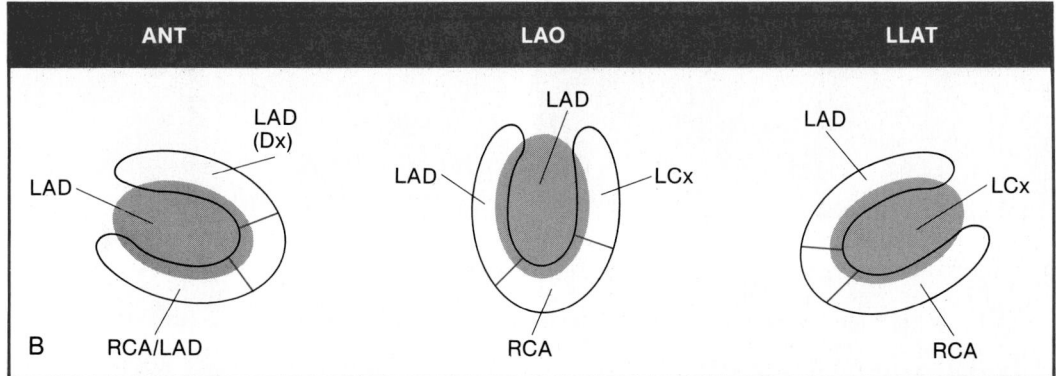

FIGURE 9–6. *A,* Anatomy of the heart as projected on planar views. *B,* Coronary artery territories on three planar views. The shaded area indicates the facing myocardium overlying the left ventricular cavity. LAD = Left anterior descending coronary artery; RCA = right coronary artery; Dx = diagonal artery; LCx = left circumflex artery; ANT = anteroposterior; LAO = left anterior oblique; LLAT = left lateral.

clearance (within 2 to 3 minutes) from the heart and intensive accumulation (within 2 to 3 minutes) in the liver.[12] Consequently, the heart can be imaged only for a few minutes after administration of the radiopharmaceutical (Fig. 9–10). The appearance of the heart is very similar in quality to that with ^{201}Tl. The intense subdiaphragmatic activity also may interfere with analysis of the inferior wall.

Characteristics of Normal SPECT Myocardial Perfusion Images

SPECT images are reconstructed as multiple slices oriented along the anatomical axis of the left ventricle. For interpretation of the short-axis slices it is convenient to divide the slices into three groups: apical slices, midventricular slices, and basal slices. To avoid apical artifacts by partial volume effect, only apical slices that clearly show the ventricular cavity should by analyzed. When interpreting basal slices, slices showing that membranous septum are excluded. SPECT anatomy and coronary territories are shown in Figure 9–11.

NORMAL VARIATIONS OF SPECT MYOCARDIAL PERFUSION IMAGES. A useful practical rule for interpreting a SPECT study is that a perfusion defect should be seen on at least three consecutive slices in order to be considered a true abnormality.

The *vertical long-axis slices* and the *horizontal long-axis* slices contain the same information shown on the short-axis slices. However, the apex and base of the heart can be analyzed in these views without partial volume artifacts. Only slices that clearly show the left ventricular cavity should be analyzed.

Slightly less inferoseptal uptake can be noted in male patients as a normal variant (Fig. 9–5). In females radiotracer distribution is usually more homogeneous. The basal short-axis slices usually show a septal defect. This is a normal finding and represents the membranous portion of the septum.

ARTIFACTS ON SPECT IMAGES

Motion artifacts and how to avoid them have been discussed above (Patient Positioning). Although computer software has been developed to correct for patient motion, this is not widely used in clinical practice.

Other common artifacts are caused by *attenuation.* The supine position of the patient may cause inferior wall defects by attenuation by the left hemidiaphragm (Figs. 9–7 and 9–12). To avoid such artifacts, alternative patient positioning has been proposed. For instance, the patient can be imaged prone (lying on the stomach),[31,32] turned on the right side,[33] or sitting in an upright position.[34]

Attenuation by breast tissue can cause artifacts on SPECT imaging as well. Breast artifacts are in general easier to recognize on planar images than on reconstructed SPECT images.[35] It is important to be alert to the potential presence of artifact *before* the interpretation of images. For SPECT imaging, images with breast markers cannot be obtained as is done for planar imaging. For SPECT imaging careful

FIGURE 9–7. Artifactual inferoposterior defect in the supine position. ^{201}Tl images following exercise in a patient with angiographically normal coronary arteries. A definite inferoposterior myocardial perfusion defect (arrow) is seen on the left lateral (LL) supine projection. A LL view obtained with the patient lying on his right side demonstrates a normal inferoposterior wall. The two left lateral images were acquired immediately after each other. (From Wackers, F. J. Th.: Artifacts in planar and SPECT myocardial perfusion imaging. Am. J. Cardiac Imaging 6:42, 1992.)

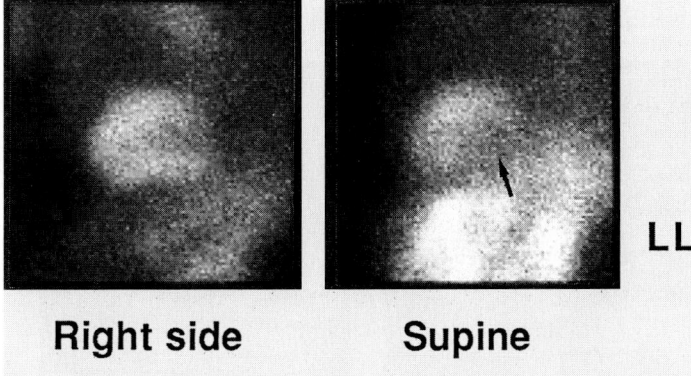

Right side   **Supine**   LL

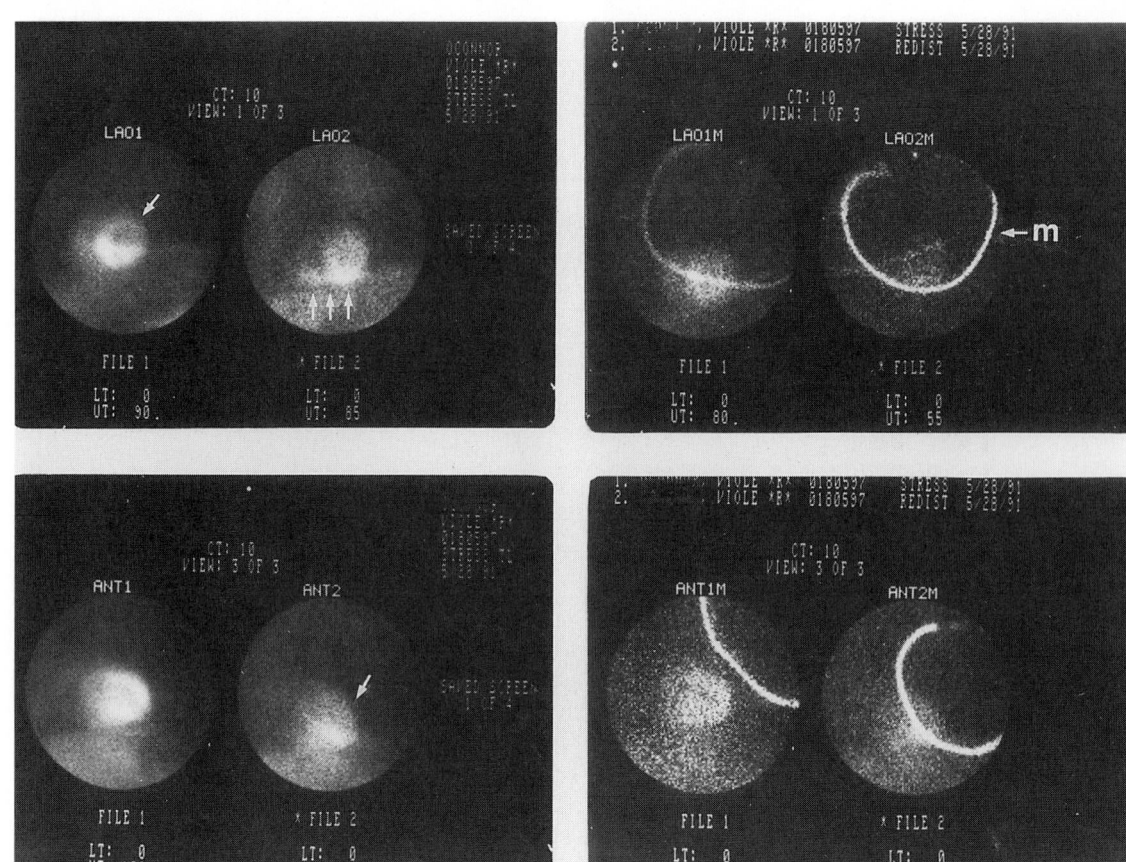

FIGURE 9–8. Planar ^{201}Tl left anterior oblique (LAO) and anterior (ANT) images in a woman with large breasts (LAO1, ANT1 = exercise images; LAO2, ANT2 = delayed images). The breasts are marked with radioactive line markers (m) in the images on the right. On the LAO exercise images *(top)*, a definite attenuation artifact is present (arrow). At delayed imaging, the breast contour is lower and is visualized as a linear area (arrow) with increased activity due to "small-angle scatter." The exercise anterior view *(bottom)* is normal because the breast did not cover the heart. However, at delayed imaging, the contour of the breast is across the heart, causing an attenuation artifact (arrow). This is an example of how breast attenuation artifacts can vary in the same view owing to different breast positions. Note that on the delayed LAO image, unequal attenuation mimics an image with increased lung uptake of ^{201}Tl. (From Wackers, F. J. Th.: Artifacts in planar and SPECT myocardial perfusion imaging. Am. J. Cardiac Imaging 6:42, 1992.)

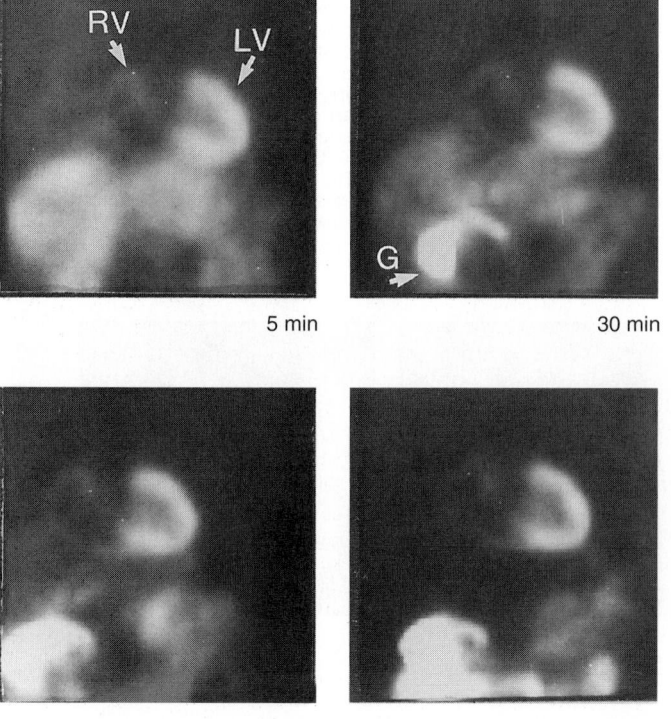

5 min

30 min

60 min

180 min

FIGURE 9–9. Planar myocardial perfusion images with ^{99m}Tc-sesta-mibi. Images of normal volunteer after exercise. The images are taken with a large field-of-view camera. Both the right *(RV)* and left *(LV)* ventricles are well visualized. The imaging agent initially accumulated in the liver and cleared into the gallbladder *(G)*. After 30 minutes there is no significant liver accumulation. Solid-colored line, 10 to 19 per cent; broken line, < 10 per cent; p = 0.0032; white line, > 20 per cent. (Reprinted by permission of the Society of Nuclear Medicine from Wackers, F. J. Th., Berman, D. S., Maddahi, J., et al.: Technetium-99m Hexakis 2-methoxyisobutyl isonitrile: Human biodistribution, dosimetry, safety and preliminary comparison to thallium-201 for myocardial perfusion imaging. J. Nucl. Med. 30:301, 1989.)

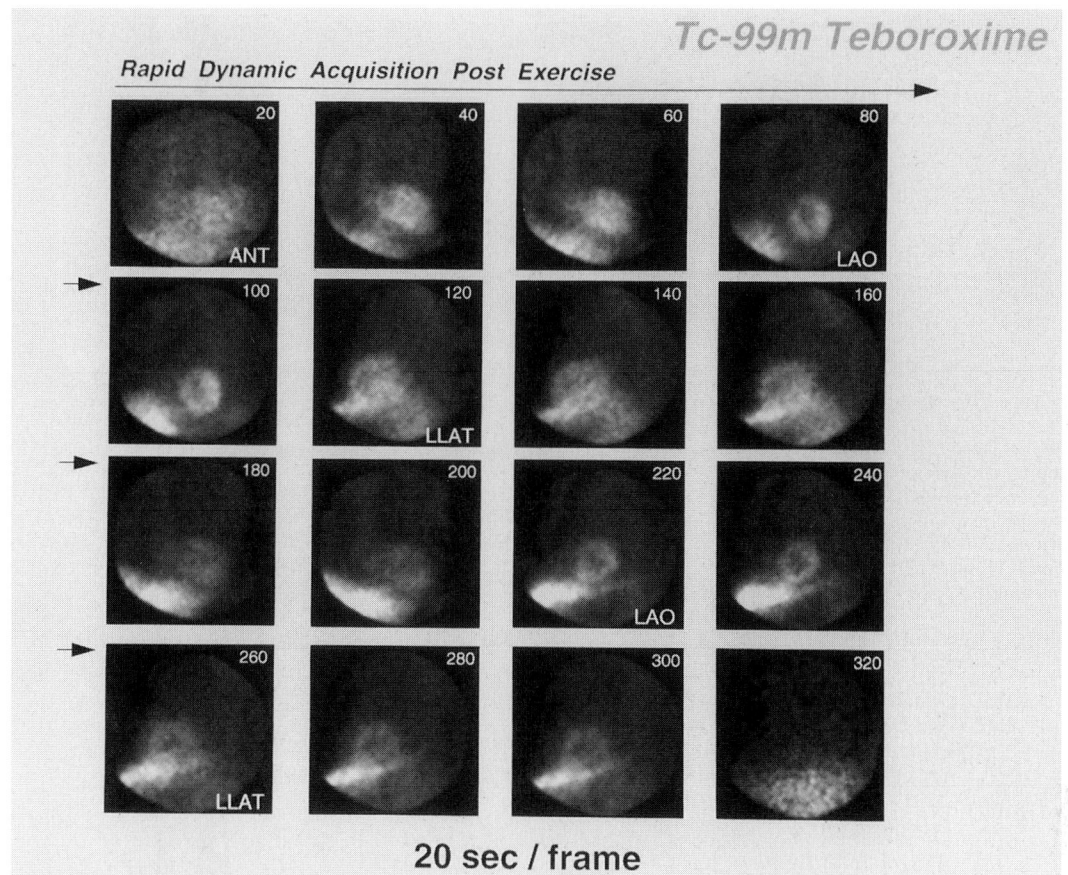

Rapid Dynamic Acquisition Post Exercise

20 sec / frame

FIGURE 9–10. Rapid serial planar imaging with ^{99m}Tc-teboroxime. Each planar image is taken for 20 seconds, starting in the anterior (ANT) position immediately after termination of exercise. The patient was seated upright on a swivel chair and rotated from the anterior to the left anterior oblique (LAO) and left lateral (LLAT) position and again ANT, LAO, and LLAT. Note the rapid disappearance of ^{99m}Tc-teboroxime from the heart in 260 seconds and intensive liver uptake. (From Wackers, F. J. Th.: Artifacts in planar and SPECT myocardial perfusion imaging. Am. J. Cardiac Imaging *6:*42, 1992.)

inspection of the *cine display of unprocessed projection images* may help to anticipate a potential attenuation problem. The breast can often be recognized as a shadow moving over the heart in certain projections and therefore may cause attentation artifacts. Attenuation artifacts are the most common source of error in SPECT imaging. Attenuation correction software is currently being developed but as yet has not been clinically validated.

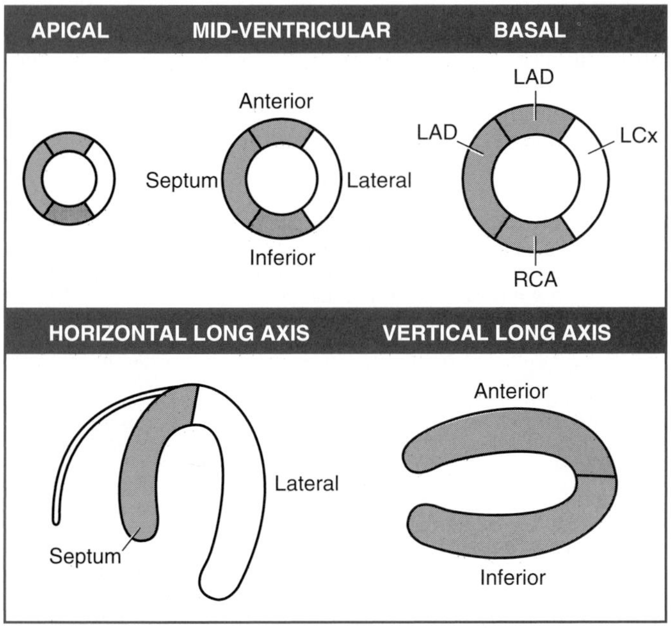

Quality control should be performed systematically as a part of the interpretation of a SPECT study and should involve the following:

1. Inspection of cine display of 32 planar projection images to assess motion of the patient or of the heart and identify the presence of a breast shadow. The cine display also allows one to evaluate whether the heart is in the center of rotation.

2. A check for adequate count density—*at least 100 counts* within the "hottest" pixel of the heart in one of the unprocessed anterior projection images.

3. Assessment of the presence of diaphragmatic attenuation of the inferoposterior wall. This can be done readily by comparing a planar left lateral supine view with a planar left lateral right side down view (Figs. 9–7 and 9–12).

Image Interpretation

Planar and SPECT images are interpreted qualitatively by visual analysis, often aided by computer quantification. Image interpretation can be described as follows (Fig. 9–13):

NORMAL. Homogeneous uptake of the radiopharmaceutical throughout the myocardium.

DEFECT. A localized myocardial area with a relative decrease in radiotracer uptake. Defects may vary in intensity, from slightly reduced activity to almost absent activity.

REVERSIBLE DEFECT. A defect present on the initial stress images is no longer present or is present to a lesser degree on the resting or delayed images. This pattern indicates myocardial ischemia. Improvement over time on ^{201}Tl imaging is referred to as *redistribution*. It is not appropriate to use this terminology for ^{99m}Tc-labeled agents.

Fixed Defect. A defect is unchanged and present on both exercise and rest (delayed) images. This pattern generally indicates infarction and scar tissue. However, in some patients with fixed ^{201}Tl defects on 2- to 4-hour delayed

FIGURE 9–11. Left ventricular anatomy and coronary artery territories on SPECT slices.

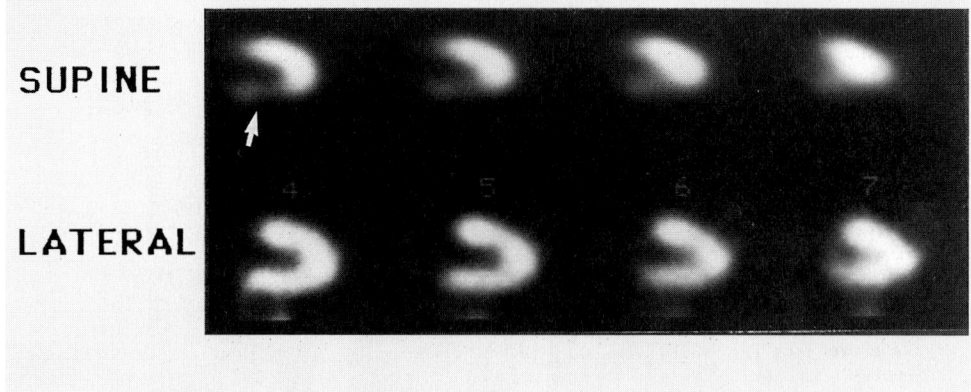

SUPINE

LATERAL

FIGURE 9–12. Vertical long-axis ²⁰¹Tl SPECT images of the patient shown in Figure 9–7. Images acquired with the patient lying on his back *(supine)* are shown in the top panel. An inferior wall myocardial perfusion defect is present (arrow). The patient was turned on the right side *(lateral)* and SPECT imaging was repeated. This time the vertical long-axis images are normal. The erroneous inferior wall defect on supine imaging is caused by attenuation by the left hemidiaphragm. Turning the patient on the right side diminishes diaphragmatic attenuation. (From Wackers, F. J. Th.: Artifacts in planar and SPECT myocardial perfusion imaging. Am. J. Cardiac Imaging 6:42, 1992.)

imaging, improved uptake can be noted on 24-hour redistribution imaging or after a new resting injection (see below).[36,37] It is controversial at the time of this writing whether a fixed defect with ⁹⁹mTc-labeled agents (which involves a rest injection) at times may underestimate myocardial viability.

REVERSE REDISTRIBUTION. This pattern occurs only with ²⁰¹Tl imaging. The initial stress images either are normal or show a defect, whereas the delayed images show a new or a more severe defect.[38] This pattern is frequently observed in patients with infarction who have undergone thrombolytic therapy or percutaneous coronary angioplasty. The phenomenon is thought to be caused by initial *excess* of tracer uptake in a reperfused area with a mixture of scar tissue and viable myocytes. Initial accumulation is followed by rapid clearance from scar tissue. Although the significance of this finding is controversial, it does *not* represent evidence of exercise-induced ischemia. With positron emission tomography with F18-deoxyglucose, the presence of residual viable myocardium has been demonstrated within areas with reverse redistribution.[39]

RADIOTRACER LUNG UPTAKE. Normally very little or no radiotracer is noted in the lung fields on postexercise images. Increased lung uptake can be quantitated as lung/heart ratio (normal < 0.5 for ²⁰¹Tl) or as lung washout (normal < 42 per cent for ²⁰¹Tl). This abnormal pattern has been well documented for ²⁰¹Tl and indicates exercise-induced left ventricular dysfunction.[40] Increased lung uptake has also been noted in occasional patients with ⁹⁹mTc-la-

beled agents,[41] but less frequently than with ²⁰¹Tl. At the time of this writing it is still unclear whether increased lung uptake of ⁹⁹mTc-labeled compounds has the same significance as noted for ²⁰¹Tl.

TRANSIENT LEFT VENTRICULAR DILATION. Occasionally the left ventricle is noted to be larger following exercise than on the rest or delayed image. This pattern indicates exercise-induced left ventricular dysfunction.[42]

Image Quantification

Myocardial perfusion images are relatively difficult to interpret. As with visual interpretation of any data set, considerable intraobserver and interobserver variability exists for subjective interpretation, even among experienced readers.[43] Reproducibility of interpretation is related to a number of factors: (1) overall quality of raw data, (2) quality of image display, (3) degree of abnormality, (4) degree of change between exercise and rest images, and (5) familiarity with normal variations.

Computer quantification of myocardial perfusion images provides an important means of improving consistency of image interpretation and decreasing reader variability.[43] Several approaches to image quantification have been described. Irrespective of planar or SPECT imaging, the output of computer quantification generally consists of the following: (1) graphic or polar map display of relative myocardial distribution of radiotracer, (2) quantitative comparison of relative radiotracer distribution with a normal reference data base, (3) quantitative comparison of stress defect size with rest (delayed) defect size and quantification of defect reversibility, and (4) quantification of myocardial kinetics (applicable only for ²⁰¹Tl).

MYOCARDIAL KINETICS OF THALLIUM-201. Quantitative analysis of ²⁰¹Tl kinetics has become of decreasing importance over the last few years with the increased use of SPECT imaging and the introduction of ⁹⁹mTc-labeled radiopharmaceuticals that show no significant redistribution. After injection at peak exercise, ²⁰¹Tl accumulates rapidly in myocardium supplied by normal coronary arteries and subsequently clears slowly from the myocardium (Fig. 9–14). In normal patients washout at 2 hours after injection is approximately 30 per cent, and at 4 hours 35 per cent. The rate of ²⁰¹Tl washout is related to peak exercise heart rate, exercise duration, and ²⁰¹Tl blood level. The kinetics of ²⁰¹Tl in *ischemic myocardium* is variable.[44]

When a significant coronary artery stenosis is present, the initial uptake of ²⁰¹Tl during exercise is lower than in normal myocardium. Subsequently, the washout of ²⁰¹Tl from ischemic tissue is lower than normal, and accumulation of ²⁰¹Tl may even occur over time. The initial uptake of ²⁰¹Tl in infarcted or scarred myocardium is considerably lower than in normal myocardium. On planar images ²⁰¹Tl clearance from an infarct parallels that of normal myocardium. This is very likely explained by overlap of normal myocardium on planar images.

MYOCARDIAL KINETICS OF TECHNETIUM-99m–LABELED AGENTS. During the first 3 hours after injection, approximately 30 per cent of a

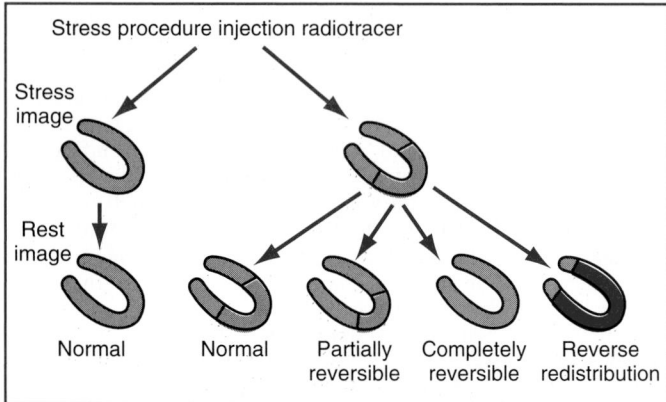

FIGURE 9–13. Schematic representation of interpretation of myocardial perfusion images. The shaded areas indicate myocardial perfusion defects.

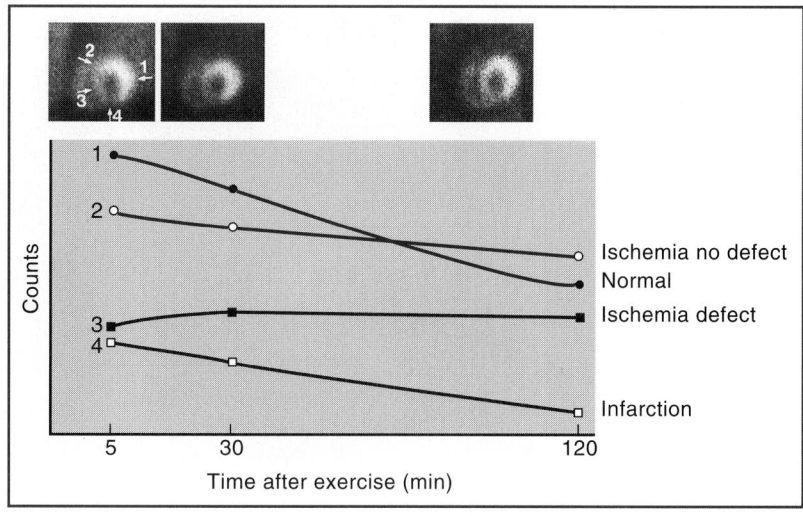

FIGURE 9–14. ^{201}Tl time activity curves after exercise in normal myocardium (1), transiently ischemic myocardium without visual defect (2), transiently ischemic myocardium with a visible defect (3), and old myocardial infarction (4). Normal myocardium (1) shows a gradual decrease of ^{201}Tl activity over time. After transient ischemia, ^{201}Tl clearance is slower than normal (2), or ^{201}Tl uptake may increase (3) in the myocardium over time. An old infarct area (4) without exercise-induced myocardial ischemia shows gradual decrease in ^{201}Tl activity over time similar to that in normal myocardium. The images show an example of a septal defect that gradually fills in over time, except at the apex where an old scar is present (4).

^{99m}Tc-labeled myocardial perfusion imaging agent clears from the heart (Fig. 9–15). Although redistribution of sestaMIBI in ischemic defects has been demonstrated in experimental animals[45] and in selected patients, the degree of redistribution in humans is minimal and does not have clinical significance. For practical clinical imaging, two separate injections are required to assess reversibility of stress-induced defects.

QUANTIFICATION OF PLANAR IMAGES

Planar exercises and rest images usually show marked differences in background radiotracer activity.[21] Accordingly, before quantification, interpolative background correction is performed.[46] After background correction, the relative distribution of radiopharmaceutical in the myocardium can be displayed in several ways: either as traverse count profiles or as circumferential count profiles.[47–49]

For the transverse count profile method, usually four profiles are generated across the left ventricle in each planar view. The count profiles are normalized to the pixel with maximal activity and compared with the lower limit of normal radiotracer distribution. In addition, myocardial clearance can be assessed by measuring the change in absolute myocardial count density over time.

With circumferential count profiles (Fig. 9–16), the mean regional distribution of radiopharmaceutical is displayed, sampling the entire left ventricle in 36 or more segments. Exercise and rest circumferential profiles are normalized to the segment with highest tracer activity, and the patient's profiles are compared with those of a normal data base. A normal data base is usually not derived from patients with normal angiographic coronary arteries but rather from subjects with a low (<3 per cent) likelihood of coronary artery disease.

In a normal image, all data points of either transverse or circumferential profiles are above the lower limit of normal. In a patient with a myocardial perfusion defect, the count profile is below the lower limit of normal in the anatomical location corresponding to the visually perceived defect. With circumferential profiles, a defect can be quantified as a *defect integral*, that is, the area below the lower limit of normal curve proportional to the total potentially visualized normal myocardium (Fig. 9–16). The reproducibility of these methods has been well established.[50]

QUANTIFICATION OF SPECT IMAGING

In SPECT imaging a multitude of reconstructed images are available for analysis. A typical SPECT study consists of approximately 32 paired (stress and rest) images in short-axis, vertical long-axis, and horizontal long-axis slices (Figs. 9–17A and 9–18A). Computer quantification is usually performed on reconstructed short-axis slices.

THE POLAR MAP (BULL'S EYE DISPLAY). The most widely used and commercially available approach is that of polar map or bull's-eye display (Figs. 9–17B and 9–18B). The purpose of a polar map is to generate one single image that encompasses the relative radiopharmaceutical distribution in the entire heart.[28] Relative radiopharmaceutical uptake on short-axis images is compressed to color-coded concentric rings, with the apical slice in the center and the basal slices on the periphery of the polar map.

It is important to understand that a polar map is not a true image but a simplified color-coded derivative of analog images. The bull's-eye image can be compared with a normal reference polar map. As mentioned above, a normal data base is usually derived from subjects with a low likelihood of coronary artery disease. Considerable variation exists with regard to the generation of a SPECT normal data base. In some software packages, the lower limit is a uniform mean minus two standard deviations. In other approaches, different criteria are applied for each coronary artery territory. Gender-specific data bases also have been recommended.[28]

Areas with a significant myocardial perfusion defect (i.e., relative count distribution below the lower limit of normal) can be highlighted on a polar map as a "black-out area" (Fig. 9–18C). By comparing stress and rest polar maps and image subtraction, the amount of defect reversibility can be visualized and quantified.[51] Although several commercially available software packages exist for generation of polar maps, manufacturers often do not supply a normal data base. Consequently, in many laboratories, SPECT polar maps are inter-

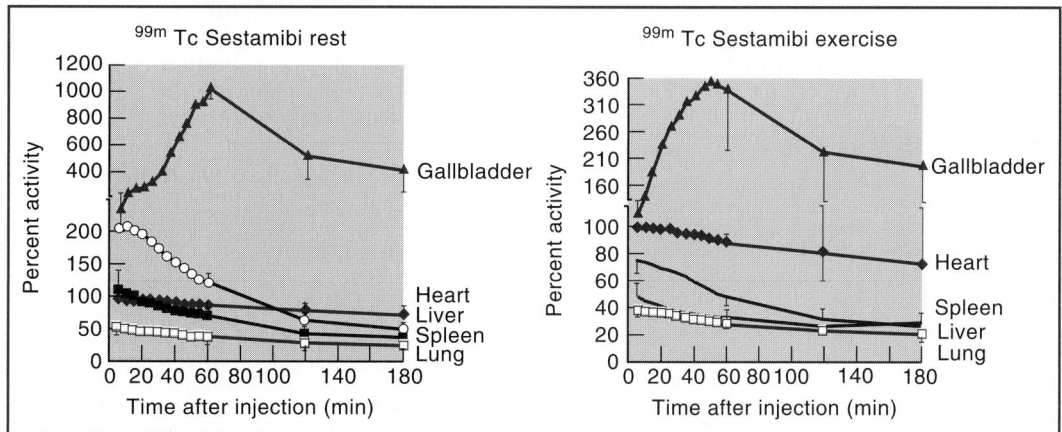

FIGURE 9–15. ^{99m}Tc-sestamibi organ time activity curves after injection at rest and after exercise in 5 normal volunteers (mean ± standard deviation). The data are normalized at cardiac activity at 5 minutes after injection. For clarity, standard deviations are shown only at 5, 60, 120, and 180 minutes. ^{99m}Tc-hexamibi is obsolete nomenclature for ^{99m}Tc-sestamibi. (Reprinted by permission of the Society of Nuclear Medicine from Wackers, F. J. Th., Berman, D. S., Maddahi, J., et al.: Technetium-99m Hexakis 2-methoxyisobutyl isonitrile: Human biodistribution, dosimetry, safety and preliminary comparison to Thallium-201 for myocardial perfusion imaging. J. Nucl. Med. *30*:301, 1989.)

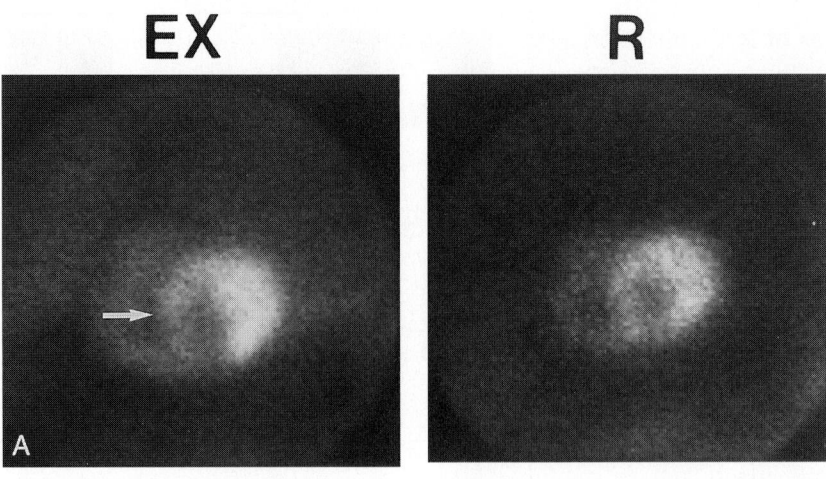

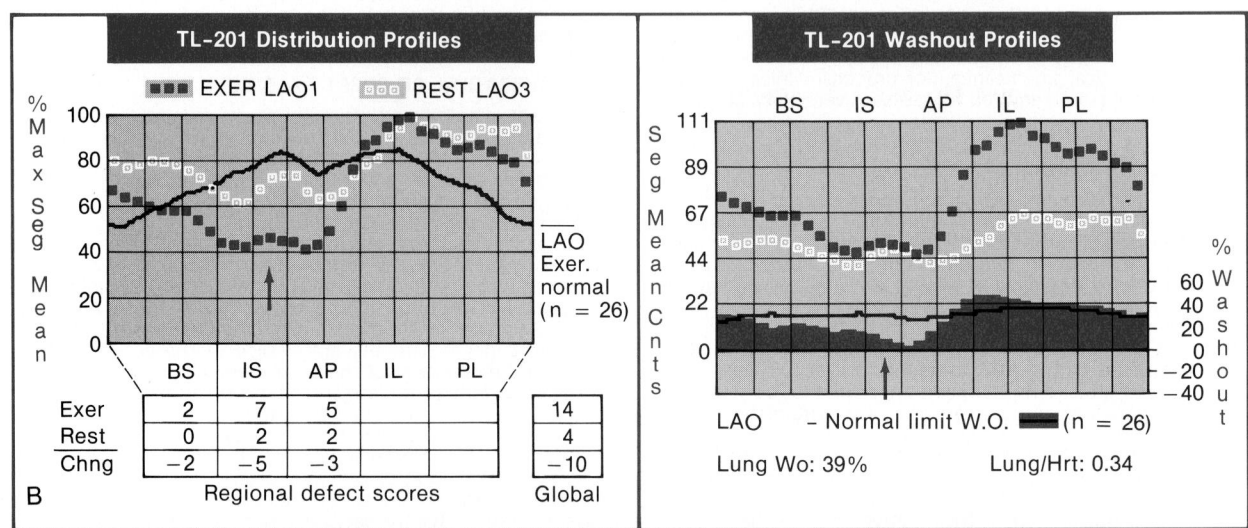

FIGURE 9–16. Left anterior oblique (LAO) images after exercise (EX) and at redistribution (R) imaging, and circumferential count distribution and washout profiles generated from these images. *A,* The analog images show a reversible exercise-induced inferoseptal defect (arrow). *B, Left,* Circumferential count distribution profiles display myocardial activity from basal septum (BS) to posterolateral (PL) wall. The continuous black line indicates the lower-limit-of-normal ^{201}Tl distribution (mean − 2 deviations). The exercise (colored dots) and delayed (white dots) profiles are normalized to the area with maximal counts (i.e., PL wall). The exercise profile is below the lower limit of normal in the basal septal (BS), inferoseptal (IS), and apical septal (AP) segments. This exercise defect (arrow) is quantified as an integral of 14. The delayed profile shows the graphic representation of a reversible defect (closer to the lower limit of normal). The defect on the delayed images is 4. The change in defect size (reversibility) is 10. *Right,* The washout (WO) profiles show thallium distribution as absolute counts. In the (normal) inferolateral and posterolateral area absolute counts decreased over time, with a measured washout of approximately 40 per cent. This is shown as the colored histogram on the bottom. The continuous black line indicates the lower limit of normal washout. In the ischemic BS, IS, and AP areas there is no change in absolute counts. In these areas the washout is below the lower-limit-of-normal curve (arrow). The patient's lung washout is normal at 39 per cent, and the lung/heart ratio is normal at 0.34.

FIGURE 9–17.   See color plate 5.

FIGURE 9–18.   See color plates 6 and 7.

---

preted visually without normal reference file and without quantification.

CIRCUMFERENTIAL PROFILES. An alternative approach to the polar map display for quantification of SPECT images is the use of circumferential profiles (Fig. 9–17C), similar to that described for planar images. Multiple circumferential profiles are generated over each of the short-axis slices and compared with those of a normal reference data base.[52] In a normal image, all data points of circumferential profiles are above the lower limit of normal. In a patient with a myocardial perfusion defect (Fig. 9–18C), the count profile is below the lower limit of normal in the areas corresponding to visually perceived defect. With circumferential profiles, a defect can be quantified as an integral, i.e., the area below the lower limit of a normal curve proportional to the total potentially visualized normal myocardium.

The total size of a myocardial perfusion defect can be expressed as a percentage of the entire left ventricle. The computed defect size is adjusted for slice thickness and varying diameter of each short-axis slice from base to apex. This approach provides quantification of total exercise defect size, rest defect size, and per cent defect reversibility.

Regardless of the quantitative approach used, the advantage of computer quantification is in providing a graphic display of the relative distribution of radiopharmaceutical uptake in the myocardium and the degree of perfusion abnormality compared with a normal reference data base.

Clinical Use of Quantification of Myocardial Perfusion Imaging

Computer quantification of myocardial perfusion imaging enhances the overall accuracy of the detection of coronary artery disease and also enhances reproducibility of interpretation. However, quantification should be used astutely. In general, from a standpoint of diagnostic interpretation, quantification should confirm the impression derived from visual analysis of analog images. If quantitative information appears to be discordant, one should inspect the analog images again. Frequently, one may recognize that quantification was correct. However, sometimes artifacts cause abnormal quantitative results. The process of integrating analog and quantitative information can be referred to as "quantitative analysis with visual overread." It is important to realize that artifacts, such as those caused by attenuation due to overlying soft tissue or diaphragm or resulting from patient motion, often have an unpredictable effect on the appearance of reconstructed slices. Although a normal data base, to a certain extent, incorporates normal variations, computer quantification per se should not be expected to distinguish between true perfusion defects and artifacts.

Electrocardiograph (ECG)-Gated Myocardial Perfusion Imaging

The high photon flux of ^{99m}Tc-sestamibi and of other ^{99m}Tc-labeled compounds makes it feasible to acquire myocardial perfusion images in ECG-gated mode.[53] ECG-gated myocardial perfusion images can be displayed as an endless-loop cine, similar to that commonly used for ECG-gated equilibrium radionuclide angiocardiography. The interpretation of ECG-gated *planar* images is not always unequivocal because of confluence of "endocardial edges" due to thickening of the facing myocardial wall.[53] However, interpretation of ECG-gated *SPECT* images is usually easier.[54] ECG-gated SPECT images allow assessment of regional wall motion and regional wall thickening. ECG gating is usually applied to the study in which the agent is injected during stress. However, because the acquisition is performed at rest, it is possible to evaluate *resting* wall motion and *resting* wall thickening in areas with exercise-induced myocardial perfusion defects (Figs. 9–17*D* and 9–18*D*). Combined interpretation of perfusion and function of ECG-gated images substantially increases confidence of interpretation. ECG-gated images are also useful for the recognition of artifactual defects due to attenuation (breast and diaphragm). Several investigators have demonstrated the feasibility of determining left ventricular ejection fraction ventricular volumes and regional wall thickening from ECG-gated SPECT slices.[55,56]

CLINICAL APPLICATIONS OF MYOCARDIAL PERFUSION IMAGING

Acute Myocardial Infarction
(See also Chap. 37)

DETECTION. Myocardial perfusion imaging with either ^{201}Tl or ^{99m}Tc-labeled compounds is an extremely sensitive and reliable means for early visualization of acute myocardial infarction (Figs. 9–19 and 9–20*A* and *B*). The timing of imaging after the onset of acute chest pain is relevant for the results of imaging. Images obtained during the first 6 hours after the onset of myocardial infarction show perfusion abnormalities at the anatomical location of infarction almost without exception.[57] However, as the time interval after onset of chest pain increases, some patients may have normal perfusion images. Serial imaging in patients with acute myocardial infarction revealed that in some patients the size of myocardial perfusion defect may decrease over time. These observations, initially made in 1974 with ^{201}Tl, are currently better understood. In approximately 20 per cent of patients with acute infarction, spontaneous throm-

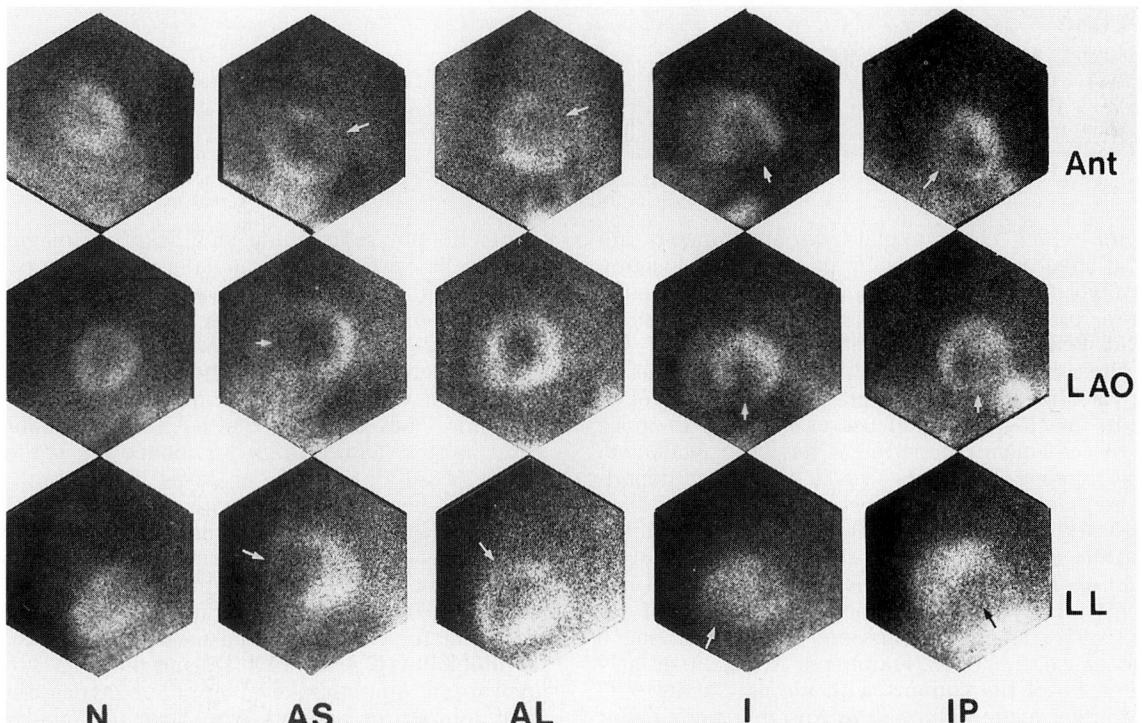

FIGURE 9–19. Planar ^{201}Tl images in acute myocardial infarction. Typical images of acute myocardial infarction in three projections. The first column shows normal ^{201}Tl images (N), the second to fourth columns show typical images of acute myocardial infarcts at anteroseptal (AS), anterolateral (AL), inferior (I), and inferoposterior (IP) locations. The defects are marked by arrows. (From Wackers, F. J. Th., Busemann Sokole, E., Samson, G., et al.: Value and limitations of thallium-201 scintigraphy in the acute phase of myocardial infarction. N. Engl. J. Med. *295*:1, 1976. Copyright Massachusetts Medical Society.)

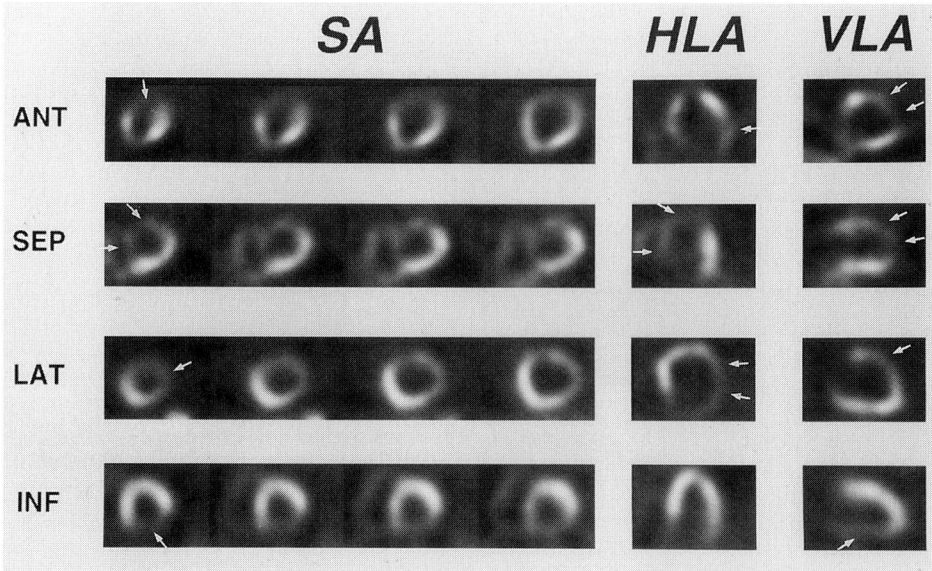

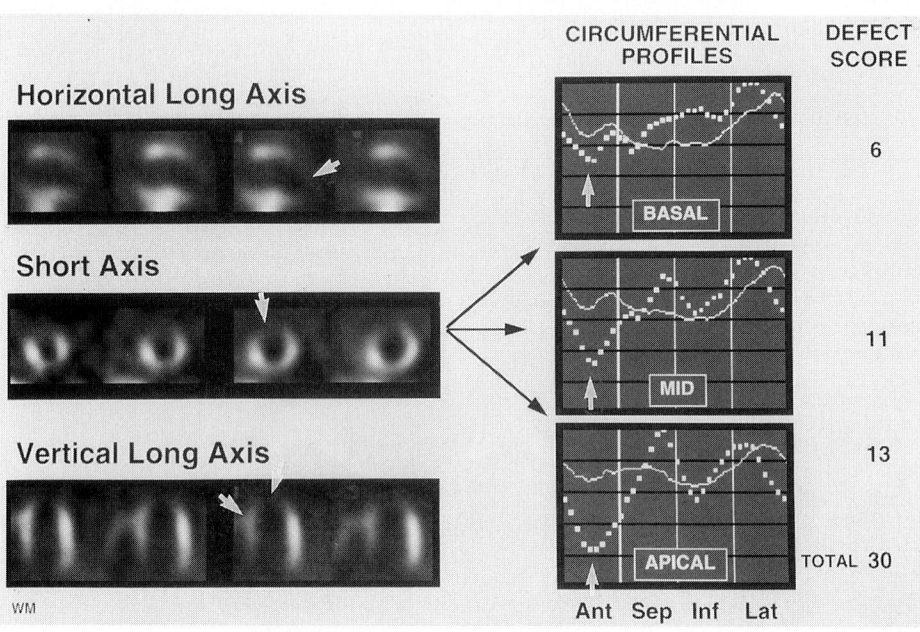

FIGURE 9–20. *Top*, SPECT ^{99m}Tc-sestamibi images of acute myocardial infarction. Typical ^{99m}Tc-sestamibi SPECT images of acute myocardial infarction in short-axis (SA), horizontal long-axis (HLA), and vertical long-axis (VLA) slices. From top to bottom: anterior (ANT), anteroseptal (SEP), lateral (LAT), and inferior (INF) infarctions. Defects are indicated by arrows. (From Wackers, F. J. Th.: Myocardial perfusion imaging. *In* Sandler, M. P., Coleman, R. E., Wackers, F. J. Th. (eds.): Diagnostic Nuclear Medicine. Baltimore, Williams & Wilkins, 1995.) *Bottom*, Quantification of infarct size on SPECT myocardial perfusion images. ^{99m}Tc-sestamibi images in a patient with anteroseptal myocardial infarction are shown. The images on the left show horizontal long-axis, short-axis, and vertical long-axis slices. An anterior apical myocardial perfusion defect (arrow) is present. On the right, circumferential profiles count distribution. The thin line represents the lower-limit-of-normal distribution of sestamibi. The white data points represent patient's circumferential profile. The circumferential profile is below the lower limit of normal in the anteroseptal and lateral areas. The defect is quantified as 30 per cent of the total left ventricle.

bolysis occurs, which could explain the spontaneous improvement of myocardial perfusion images. The location and size of myocardial perfusion defects in acute myocardial infarction correlate well with findings at postmortem.[58]

MYOCARDIAL PERFUSION IMAGING IN THE EMERGENCY DEPARTMENT. Because acute regional myocardial hypoperfusion can be visualized almost instantaneously with myocardial perfusion imaging, potential use as a means to triage patients in the emergency department has been evaluated. A substantial number of patients seen in emergency departments with complaints of acute chest pain have a nondiagnostic electrocardiogram. These patients are often admitted to rule out acute myocardial infarction. However, in only a small proportion of these patients (15 to 20 per cent) can acute coronary disease be confirmed. The majority of patients have costly hospital admissions without having a true cardiac cause for their symptoms. Wackers et al.[59] showed that none of the patients with normal "acute ^{201}Tl images" had either acute infarction or unstable angina after further clinical evaluation. In contrast, more than 80 per cent of patients who later were proven to have either acute infarction or unstable angina had abnormal ^{201}Tl perfusion images on admission in the emergency room.[59]

The new ^{99m}Tc-labeled myocardial perfusion imaging agents are better suited than ^{201}Tl for imaging patients with chest pain in the emergency department. Because these agents do not redistribute significantly, imaging does not have to be performed immediately, and myocardial perfusion during chest pain can be imaged at a convenient time. Moreover, SPECT imaging can be performed, which allows more detailed evaluation of various coronary vascular territories. Varetto et al.[60] and Hilton et al.[61] injected sestamibi in patients with chest pain and nondiagnostic electrocardiograms. They observed that patients with abnormal sestamibi images had a high incidence of coronary events (death, acute infarction, or revascularization) during follow-up, whereas patients with normal acute myocardial perfusion images in general had a favorable outcome. If these observations are confirmed in larger series of patients, myocardial perfusion imaging in the emergency department could become an important and cost-effective means for the triage of patients with acute chest pain.[62]

THROMBOLYTIC THERAPY. During the early hours of acute myocardial infarction, evaluation of myocardial perfusion is of interest in patients who have thrombolytic therapy. Serial myocardial perfusion imaging can demonstrate a decrease in myocardial perfusion defect size over time in patients who had successful reperfusion. Imaging with ^{201}Tl is not practical in this setting. Because of ^{201}Tl redistribution, myocardial imaging has to be performed *before* initiation of therapy. This would cause a clinically unacceptable delay in treatment. A more practical approach is the use of

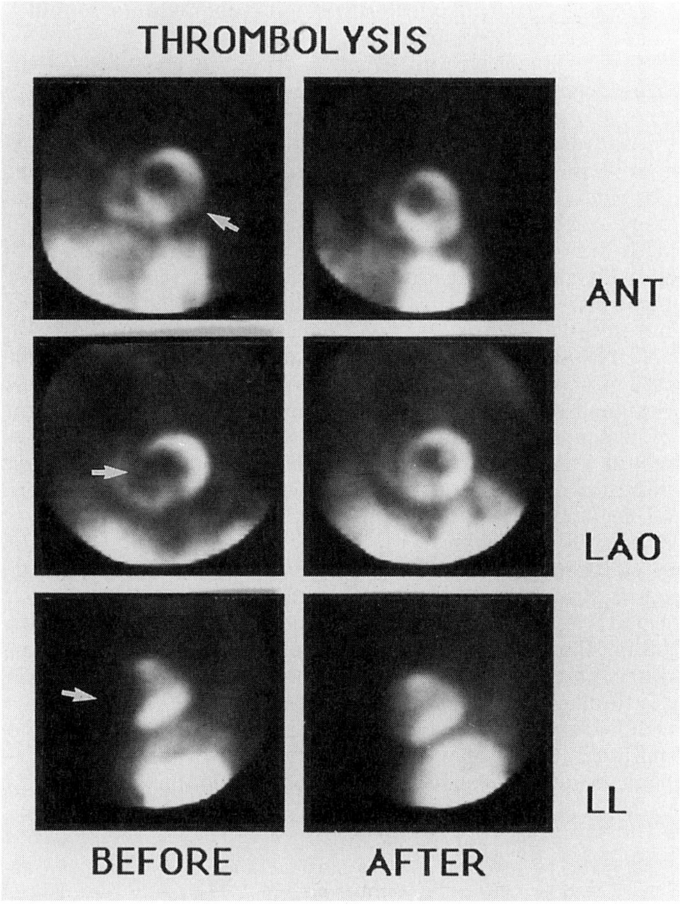

THROMBOLYSIS

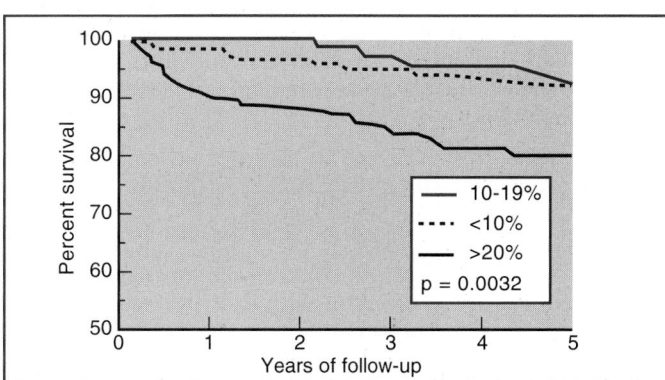

ANT

LAO

LL

BEFORE   AFTER

FIGURE 9-21. Planar myocardial perfusion imaging with ^{99m}Tc-sestamibi before and after thrombolytic therapy in a patient with an acute anteroseptal myocardial infarct. ^{99m}Tc-sestamibi was injected immediately before initiation of thrombolytic therapy and imaging was performed 2 hours later. Because of the lack of significant redistribution of ^{99m}Tc-sestamibi, the distribution of myocardial blood flow at the time of injection is "frozen" in time. The images before thrombolytic therapy show an anteroseptal myocardial perfusion defect (arrows) that was quantified as 53. The patient was reinjected with ^{99m}Tc-sestamibi when thrombolytic therapy was completed. These images show improved perfusion of the anteroseptal segments, indicating successful reperfusion of the infarcted artery. The perfusion defect size after thrombolytic therapy was 35. Therefore, 33 per cent of myocardium was salvaged by thrombolytic therapy in this patient. (From Wackers, F. J. Th., Gibbons, R. J., Verani, M. S., et al.: Serial quantitative planar technetium-99m-isonitrile imaging in acute myocardial infarction: Efficacy for noninvasive assessment of thrombolytic therapy. Reprinted with permission from the American College of Cardiology. J. Am. Coll. Cardiol. *14*:861, 1989.)

^{99m}Tc-sestamibi. Because of the lack of significant redistribution, this imaging agent can be injected *before* initiation of thrombolytic therapy, and imaging of myocardial perfusion can be performed later using either planar imaging at the bedside or SPECT imaging in the nuclear cardiology laboratory.[63-68] Gibbons et al.[63] and Wackers et al.[64] showed that successful thrombolysis of the infarct artery can be predicted by a decrease of the size of myocardial perfusion defects on serial ^{99m}Tc-sestamibi imaging (Fig. 9-21).

The noninvasive demonstration of successful myocardial reperfusion by thrombolysis could be useful in defining management of individual patients. For example, patients who apparently had failure of thrombolytic therapy (i.e., no change in myocardial perfusion defect) may be candidates for a more aggressive and invasive approach, whereas patients who had apparently successful reperfusion, as demonstrated by improvement of myocardial perfusion, may be more appropriate candidates for conservative management. With the use of a "split-dose" technique (i.e., a small dose initially followed by a larger dose later), it is feasible to obtain the same information on risk area and salvage within a few hours after the patient's arrival in the emergency room.

Serial myocardial perfusion imaging with sestamibi has provided new insights on the pathophysiology of acute human myocardial in-

farction. Gibbons et al. conducted a series of important clinical studies with sestamibi in patients with acute infarction. Their experience can be summarized as follows.

The myocardial area at risk varies greatly in individual patients.[63,64] Little correlation exists between extent of the risk area as demonstrated with sestamibi imaging and the anatomic site of occlusion of the infarct artery, i.e., distal or proximal.[69] The area at risk in acute anterior myocardial infarction is usually larger than that in acute inferior infarction.[71] Patients with collateral coronary circulation to the infarct artery have smaller ultimate infarct size than patients without collateral vessels.[71]

A decrease in myocardial perfusion defect size on serial imaging before and after thrombolytic therapy is a reliable predictor of reperfusion on the infarct artery and subsequent improvement of left ventricular regional wall motion.[72] Serial myocardial perfusion imaging has further shown that in many patients (approximately 40 per cent) myocardial perfusion defect size continues to decrease during the days after thrombolytic therapy was administered.[64] Others have confirmed this observation.[73,74]

Marcassa et al.[75] observed the same phenomenon of continued decreasing resting defect size in stable patients late (7 months) after anterior wall infarction. This may cause an apparent increase of stress-induced ischemia. The pathophysiological basis of this phenomenon remains unclear. Ito et al.[76] demonstrated delayed recovery from microvascular damage after acute infarction. This could be a potential explanation for late improvement in defect size.

Serial myocardial perfusion imaging with ^{99m}Tc-labeled myocardial perfusion imaging agents is now recognized as a potentially useful clinical research tool to assess the efficacy of various thrombolytic strategies in acute myocardial infarction.[77] The patient serves as his own control, and fewer patients needed to be recruited for a clinical trial. In a comparative trial of primary angioplasty versus thrombolysis for acute myocardial infarction, Gibbons et al.[78] demonstrated with acute sestamibi imaging that the area at risk in both patient groups was the same.

EARLY ASSESSMENT OF PROGNOSIS AFTER ACUTE INFARCTION. The size of myocardial perfusion defects in stable patients after acute myocardial infarction has been shown to be of prognostic significance. Silverman et al.[79] showed that patients with large resting myocardial perfusion defects had a significantly poorer prognosis and survival than patients with small myocardial perfusion defects. This outcome appeared to be independent of other clinical parameters. Similar prognostic information on the size of SPECT myocardial perfusion defect was reported by Cerqueira et al.[80] after thrombolytic therapy (Fig. 9-22).

Visualization of the right ventricle at rest[81] and increased ^{201}Tl uptake in the lung at rest in patients with recent infarction[82] have been reported as additional indicators of an unfavorable course after myocardial infarction.

Brown et al.[83] evaluated the potential of pharmacological vasodilation and myocardial perfusion imaging for early (first to fourth day) risk stratification in patients with recent acute myocardial infarction. Patients who had evi-

FIGURE 9-22. ^{201}Tl SPECT infarct size and per cent survival during follow-up after thrombolytic therapy for acute myocardial infarction. Patients with large (> 20 per cent of left ventricle) myocardium perfusion defects after thrombolytic therapy for myocardial infarction had significantly poorer prognosis than patients with a small (< 10 per cent) or moderate (10 to 19 per cent) sized myocardial perfusion defect. (From Cerqueira, M. D., Maynard, C., Ritchie, J. L., et al.: Long-term survival in 618 patients from the Western Washington streptokinase in myocardial infarction trials. Reprinted with permission from the American College of Cardiology. J. Am. Coll. Cardiol. *20*:1452, 1992.)

dence of residual jeopardized myocardium (i.e., partially reversible defects) had a significantly higher in-hospital complication rate than patients who had fixed myocardial perfusion defects.

UNSTABLE ANGINA (see p. 1331). In patients with unstable angina without prior myocardial infarction, rest myocardial perfusion defects have been demonstrated. These perfusion defects are demonstrable not only when the radiopharmaceutical is injected *during* chest pain but also for considerable time *after* the angina has subsided.[84-86] Resting ^{201}Tl defects in patients with unstable angina are invariably reversible, indicating transient hypoperfusion of viable myocardium.

Technetium-99m–labeled myocardial perfusion imaging agents that do not redistribute have a particular advantage in patients with unstable angina. The lack of redistribution makes it possible to inject the radiotracer during pain and acquire images at a later time when the patient is pain free and stable. Bilodeau et al.[86] reported similar observations in patients with unstable angina using sestamibi SPECT imaging as described above with [201]Tl. Patients with abnormal electrocardiographic findings during pain had larger myocardial perfusion defects than those who did not. The observations with myocardial perfusion imaging in patients with unstable angina indicate that impaired regional myocardial blood flow persists longer than can be judged from the clinical status or electrocardiogram. Patients with reversible resting myocardial perfusion defects usually have severe multivessel coronary artery disease. Resting myocardial perfusion imaging during pain was more sensitive and more specific for significant coronary artery disease than the resting electrocardiogram.

Resting imaging in patients with recurrent chest pain after infarction or with unstable angina is useful for objectively demonstrating the presence of transient myocardial hypoperfusion and viable myocardium. This information can be very helpful when myocardial revascularization is considered. In patients with unstable angina who have been stabilized, subsequent exercise myocardial perfusion defect size has been shown to be a reliable predictor of the extent of coronary artery disease.[87]

DETECTION OF OLD MYOCARDIAL INFARCTION. Myocardial perfusion imaging does not differentiate between acute myocardial infarction, acute ischemia, or old scar. A substantial number of patients with small or old myocardial infarction may have normal perfusion images. Frequently, prior myocardial infarction can be recognized only as "thinner" myocardial segments. In approximately one-half of patients with old infarction, planar myocardial perfusion images may become normal. This occurs particularly in patients with old inferior wall myocardial infarcts. SPECT imaging appears to be more sensitive in detecting such small myocardial scars.

Chronic Coronary Artery Disease
(See also Chap. 38)

In patients with chronic stable coronary artery disease who are capable of physical exercise, myocardial perfusion imaging is used in conjunction with exercise testing. Physical exercise can be performed either on a treadmill, which is most popular in the United States, or on an upright bicycle, which is frequently used in Europe and other countries. Physical exercise has the advantage of providing additional useful clinical and physiological parameters, such as duration of exercise, total workload, maximum heart rate, exercise-induced symptoms, electrocardiographic changes, and blood pressure response. However, a substantial number of patients referred for evaluation cannot physically exercise because of orthopedic, neurological, or peripheral vascular problems. In the latter group of patients pharmacological vasodilatation with dipyridamole or aden-

osine or pharmacological stress with dobutamine provides useful alternative approaches.

The basic principle of using various modes of stress in conjunction with radionuclide myocardial perfusion imaging is to create *heterogeneity of myocardial blood flow* between vascular territories supplied by normal coronary arteries and that supplied by an artery with significant obstructive coronary artery stenosis (Fig. 9–23). Heterogeneity of regional myocardial blood flow can be visualized with radionuclide myocardial perfusion agents. Heterogeneity of regional myocardial blood flow is a requirement for abnormal images. However, regional hypoperfusion does not necessarily imply myocardial ischemia.

PHYSICAL EXERCISE. Several standardized treadmill exercise protocols exist. The most widely used protocol was designed by Bruce. Nonimaging endpoints are reproduction of the patient's symptoms, exhaustion, hypotension or decrease in systolic blood pressure of 20 mm Hg or more, ventricular arrhythmias, and electrocardiographic severe ST-segment depression on electrocardiography. An intravenous line should be in place in a large antecubital vein for injection of the radiopharmaceutical agent. When the endpoint of exercise is reached, the radiopharmaceutical is injected rapidly in the intravenous line and flushed with saline. The patient is then encouraged to exercise for another 1 to 2 minutes at the same level of exercise. This continuation of exercise after injection of the radiotracer is crucial for diagnostic stress imaging. It is important to maintain heart rate, and thus myocardial blood flow, at peak exercise level to allow for accumulation of the radio-

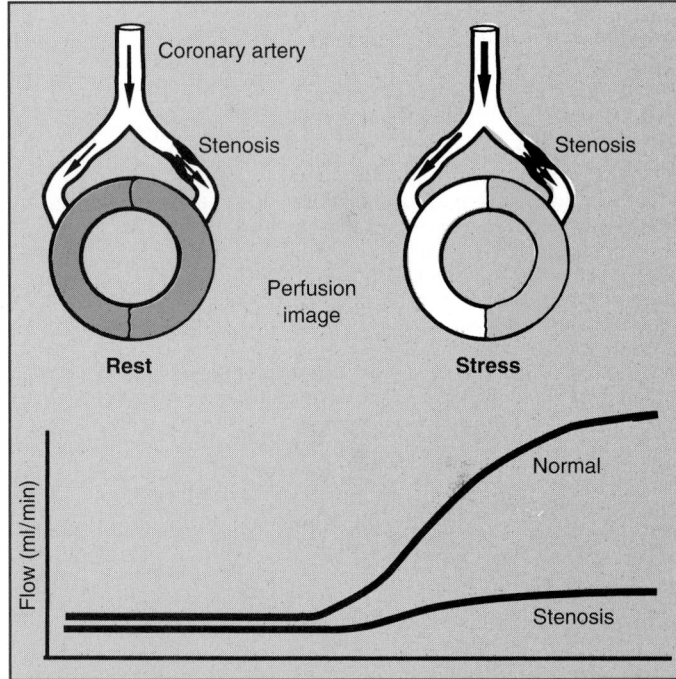

FIGURE 9–23. Schematic representation of the principle of rest/stress myocardial perfusion imaging. *Top,* Two branches of a coronary artery are schematically shown; the left branch is normal, and the right branch has a significant stenosis *(middle).* Myocardial perfusion images of the territories supplied by two branches. *Bottom,* Schematic representation of coronary blood flow in the branches at rest and during stress. At rest, myocardial blood flow is similar in both coronary artery branches. When a myocardial perfusion imaging agent is injected at rest, myocardial uptake is homogeneous (normal image). During stress, coronary blood flow increases 2.0 to 2.5 times in the normal branch, but not to the same extent in the stenosed branch, resulting in heterogeneous distribution of blood flow. This heterogeneity of blood flow can be visualized with ^{201}Tl or ^{99m}Tc-sestamibi as an area with relatively decreased radiotracer uptake (myocardial perfusion defect). (Reprinted by permission of the Society of Nuclear Medicine from Wackers, F. J. Th.: Exercise myocardial perfusion imaging. J. Nucl. Med. *35:*726, 1994.)

tracer during a "steady ischemic state." If the patient is unable to continue exercising at the same level, the speed and grade of the treadmill can be decreased to a lower level.

For bicycle exercise a similar graded exercise protocol is used. Usually the patient starts at 25 kpm, and the resistance is increased every 3 minutes until an exercise endpoint is reached.

The purpose of exercise is to increase cardiac metabolic demands and to test the ability of the coronary circulation to meet these demands with an appropriate increase of myocardial blood flow. Consequently, myocardial ischemia is frequently provoked with physical exercise.

PHARMACOLOGICAL VASODILATION. Patients with orthopedic, neurological, or peripheral vascular problems are incapable of exercising adequately on a treadmill or bicycle. These patients can be evaluated for the presence of significant coronary artery disease by use of pharmacological vasodilation in combination with radionuclide myocardial perfusion imaging. Furthermore patients on beta-blocking medication who are unable to increase their heart rate adequately by physical exercise have been studied successfully with pharmacological coronary vasodilation. In addition, patients with complete left bundle branch block are preferably studied with dipyridamole to avoid artifactual perfusion defects.

Intravenous infusion of *dipyridamole* blocks the cellular reabsorption of adenosine and thus increases the concentrations of adenosine, an endogenous vasodilator that activates specific receptors. Coronary blood flow is autoregulated by adenosine to meet myocardial metabolic demands.[88] In patients without coronary artery disease dipyridamole infusion creates vasodilatation and increases coronary blood flow three to five times above baseline levels. In patients with significant coronary artery disease the resistance vessels distal to a stenosis are already dilated, often maximally, in order to maintain normal resting flow. In these patients, infusion of dipyridamole does not cause further significant vasodilatation in the diseased vascular bed. However, in the adjacent myocardium supplied by normal coronary arteries, a substantial increase in myocardial blood flow occurs. In this manner, *heterogeneity of regional myocardial blood flow is created:* Territories supplied by diseased arteries are relatively hypoperfused compared with normal regions (Fig. 9–23). Pharmacological vasodilation by dipyridamole or adenosine infusion usually does not provoke myocardial ischemia.

DIPYRIDAMOLE INFUSION PROTOCOL. Dipyridamole is infused over a 4-minute period (0.142 mg/kg/min).[88] At approximately 4 minutes after completion of the infusion, maximal dilatory effect is achieved. At this time the radiotracer is injected intravenously. Maximal vasodilatory effect is usually associated with a modest increase in heart rate (10 beats per minute) and slight decrease (10 mm Hg) in systolic blood pressure. In some laboratories dipyridamole infusion is combined with low-level exercise. This appears to decrease the incidence of side effects, which occur in about 50 per cent of patients during infusion of dipyridamole.[89] Approximately 10 per cent may have electrocardiographic changes, and 20 per cent may experience angina, although most frequent complaints are headache, flushing, and nausea (Table 9–2).[90,91]

Ischemia may be caused by "coronary steal." In this situation, the marked increase in blood flow in the *normal* myocardial zones "steals" blood away via collaterals from the vascular bed supplied by significantly diseased coronary arteries. This and other undesirable side effects can usually be reversed quickly by blocking adenosine receptor sites with intravenous aminophylline.

ADENOSINE INFUSION. Clinical experience of direct intravenous infusion of adenosine (maximal 140 μg/kg/min) has been comparable to that reported for dipyridamole.[92,93] The coronary vasodilatory effect of adenosine appears to be more potent and more consistent than that of dipyridamole.[94] However, side effects are more common, occurring in about 75 per cent of patients (Table 9–2). Approximately 50 per cent of patients may have chest pain, and many have headache, nausea, and flushing. Atrioventricular conduction abnormalities have been reported occasionally in patients using adenosine infusion. This has been of some concern. However, because of the short half-life of adenosine, side effects can be reversed almost instantaneously by termination infusion of adenosine. Samuels et al.[95] observed that adenosine-SPECT imaging was well tolerated by patients with moderate to severe aortic valvular stenosis who were evaluated for coexisting coronary artery disease.

DOBUTAMINE STRESS. For patients who have contraindications to dipyridamole or adenosine infusion, such as those with bronchospastic pulmonary disease, or for patients who are on xanthine derivatives or who have consumed caffeine, dobutamine infusion offers an alternative diagnostic approach.[96,97] Dobutamine increases myocardial oxygen demand by increasing myocardial contractility, heart rate, and blood pressure. The increase in coronary blood flow is comparable to that during physical exercise (two- to three-fold) but less than that with adenosine or dipyridamole.

Nevertheless dobutamine infusion should not be considered equivalent to physical exercise. Useful clinical information such as duration of exercise, exercise capacity, and reproduction of symptoms is not obtained. The increase in heart rate is usually lower than with exercise. Thus, dobutamine pharmacological stress should be considered

TABLE 9–2   REPORTED SIDE EFFECTS (% OF PATIENTS) OF INTRAVENOUS DIPYRIDAMOLE, ADENOSINE, AND DOBUTAMINE MYOCARDIAL PERFUSION IMAGING

	DIPYRIDAMOLE (RANHOSKY AND RAWSON[90])	ADENOSINE (VERANI et al.[92])	DOBUTAMINE (HAYS et al.[97])
Cardiac			
Fatal myocardial infarction	0.05	0	0
Nonfatal myocardial infarction	0.05	0	0
Chest pain	19.7	57	31
ST-T changes on ECG	7.5	12	50
Ventricular ectopy	5.2	?	43
Tachycardia	3.2	?	1.4
Hypotension	4.6	?	0
Blood pressure lability	1.6	?	?
Hypertension	1.5	?	1.4
Atrioventricular block	0	10	0.6
Noncardiac			
Headache	12.2	35	14
Dizziness	11.8	?	4
Nausea	4.6	?	9
Flushing	3.4	29	14
Pain (nonspecific)	2.6	?	7
Dyspnea	2.6	15	14
Paresthesia	1.3	?	12
Fatigue	1.2	?	?
Dyspepsia	1.0	?	?
Acute bronchospasm	0.15	0*	?

*Patients with history of bronchospasm excluded
? = Not reported

TABLE 9–3   SENSITIVITY AND SPECIFICITY FOR DETECTION OF CORONARY ARTERY DISEASE BY QUANTITATIVE PLANAR ²⁰¹Tl SCINTIGRAPHY

AUTHOR	NUMBER OF PATIENTS	SENSITIVITY (%)	SPECIFICITY (%)
Berger et al. 1981[99]	140	91	90
Maddahi et al. 1981[100]	67	93	91
Wackers et al. 1985[49]	150	89	95
Kaul et al. 1986[102]	325	90	80
van Train et al. 1986[101]	157	84	88
TOTAL	839	89	89

a last resort in patients who cannot exercise, rather than a substitute for exercise.

Dobutamine Infusion Protocol. Infusion of dobutamine is started with a low dose of 5 μg/kg/min. The dose is increased each 3 minutes, if tolerated, to a maximal dose of 40 μg/kg/min. The radiopharmaceutical is injected during infusion of maximal dose, and infusion is continued for 2 to 3 minutes. Table 9–2 shows the incidence of side effects during dobutamine infusion.[97] A similar infusion protocol is used for dobutamine stress echocardiography. In a recent review of 2942 patients who had dobutamine-atropine stress echocardiography, nine patients (0.3 per cent) had serious cardiac side effects, including two nonfatal infarctions, two instances of ventricular fibrillation, two instances of sustained ventricular tachycardia, two cases of sustained severe hypotension, and one case of prolonged severe myocardial ischemia.[98]

Clinical Results of Exercise Testing and Myocardial Perfusion Imaging

Each year more than 2.5 million patients undergo stress myocardial perfusion imaging in the United States. Currently, approximately 70 per cent of all studies are performed with ²⁰¹Tl, and the remaining studies are obtained with ⁹⁹ᵐTc-sestamibi. About 60 to 70 per cent of studies are performed in conjunction with physical exercise and 30 per cent with pharmacological vasodilation. Eighty per cent of all studies in the United States use SPECT imaging.

Over the last 20 years the clinical usefulness of stress myocardial perfusion imaging has been well established. Although the majority of data in the literature are based on planar ²⁰¹Tl imaging, recent published reports indicate that similar results are obtained with SPECT imaging and ⁹⁹ᵐTc-labeled agents.

The introduction of computer processing and quantification of *planar* myocardial perfusion images improved overall detection of coronary artery disease substantially (Table 9–3). For instance, the detection of single-vessel disease with ²⁰¹Tl improved from 55 per cent by visual analysis to 84 per cent by quantitative analysis. Almost all patients with double- or triple-vessel coronary artery disease are detected by quantitative myocardial perfusion imaging.[49,99–102]

ASSESSMENT OF MYOCARDIAL PERFUSION. In 1994 the American Medical Association performed a Diagnostic And Therapeutic Technology Assessment (DATTA) of SPECT myocardial perfusion imaging.[103] This extensive review of the literature revealed sensitivities for planar imaging ranging from 67 to 96 per cent and sensitivities for SPECT imaging ranging from 83 to 98 per cent. The range of specificities for planar imaging varied from 40 to 100 per cent and from 53 to 100 per cent for SPECT imaging. The report did not address the potential contribution of image quantification on improvement of diagnostic accuracy. The DATTA panel of experts considered ²⁰¹Tl SPECT myocardial perfusion imaging a well-established and proven technology. Representative results of qualitative and quantitative SPECT imaging are shown in Table 9–4.[104–112]

The ability to accurately predict coronary disease in specific individual vessels has been consistently suboptimal by planar imaging and reflects an inherent limitation of planar technology. Using SPECT imaging, detection of coronary artery disease in individual vessels, in particular the left circumflex coronary artery, is significantly improved.[105] Consequently, SPECT stress myocardial perfusion imaging is particularly useful in following patients who had coronary angioplasty (see below).

VALUE OF TECHNETIUM-99m RADIOPHARMACEUTICALS. Since the introduction of ⁹⁹ᵐTc-sestamibi in 1989, thousands of patients have been evaluated with this new myocardial perfusion agent. Several comparative studies, both by planar and SPECT technique, have shown that the detection of coronary artery disease with ⁹⁹ᵐTc-sestamibi is comparable to that with ²⁰¹Tl.[10,11,113–116] Similar results have been reported recently for ⁹⁹ᵐTc-tetrofosmin[15,117,118] and ⁹⁹ᵐTc-furifosmin.[119,120]

The relatively high dose of ⁹⁹ᵐTc administered makes it feasible to acquire images in ECG-gated mode and to perform first-pass angiocardiography in combination with myocardial perfusion imaging.[54,114] The feasibility of acquiring simultaneous myocardial perfusion and myocardial contraction data (*"one-stop shop"*) using the same radiopharmaceutical injection is one of the major advantages of the ⁹⁹ᵐTc-labeled compounds over ²⁰¹Tl (Fig. 9–24). Combined analysis of "still" slices and perfusion wall motion images further improves accuracy and confidence of interpretation. The clinical importance of acquiring both resting and peak exercise left ventricular ejection fraction is discussed elsewhere in this chapter.

Technetium-99m–Teboroxime. The clinical experience with ⁹⁹ᵐTc-teboroxime is still limited to a relatively small number of patients (Fig. 9–10). The diagnostic yield of this agent to detect coronary artery disease appears to be comparable to that of ²⁰¹Tl.[12,13,121,122] This imaging agent is of

TABLE 9–4   SENSITIVITY AND SPECIFICITY FOR DETECTION OF CORONARY ARTERY DISEASE BY ²⁰¹Tl SINGLE-PHOTON EMISSION COMPUTERIZED TOMOGRAPHY

AUTHOR	NUMBER OF PATIENTS	SENSITIVITY (%)	SPECIFICITY (%)	NORMALCY RATE
Tamaki et al. 1984[109]	104	91	92	
De Pasquale et al. 1988[105]	210	95	71	
Borges-Neto et al. 1988[112]	100	92	69	
Maddahi et al. 1989[104]	110	96	56	86
Fintel et al. 1989[106]	112	91	90	
Iskandrian et al. 1989[110]	164	88	62	93
Go et al. 1990[108]	202	76	80	
Mahmarian et al. 1990[107]	360	93	87	
van Train et al. 1990[111]	242	95	56	
TOTAL	1901	91	73	90

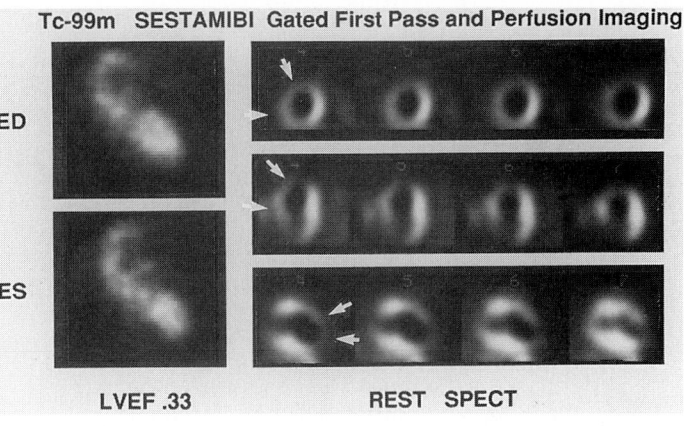

ED

ES

LVEF .33   REST SPECT

FIGURE 9-24. Simultaneous assessment of myocardial perfusion and function. ^{99m}Tc-sestamibi imaging in acute myocardial infarction allows assessment of both function and perfusion. In this patient with large anteroseptal infarction, the resting injection of sestamibi was used for first-pass radionuclide angiography (left). The end-diastolic and systolic frames are shown. Global left ventricular ejection fraction was severely depressed at 0.33. On the right are resting SPECT sestamibi images in short-axis and vertical and horizontal long-axis slices. A large anteroseptal myocardial perfusion defect is present (arrows).

particular interest because the relatively short residence time in the heart allows for multiple injections and repeat simultaneous assessment of left ventricular function by first-pass radionuclide angiocardiography and myocardial perfusion. Preliminary data suggest that it may be feasible to derive pathophysiological information with regard to the presence of significant coronary artery disease by analysis of regional differences in myocardial washout of ^{99m}Tc-teboroxime.[123,124] The sensitivities and specificities to detect coronary artery disease using pharmacological vasodilation with various myocardial perfusion imaging agents have been reported to be similar to those used for physical exercise.[125,131]

REFERRAL BIAS. As mentioned above, many investigators report a relatively low specificity of stress SPECT myocardial perfusion imaging. The reported specificities range from 53 to 100 per cent. This lack of specificity has been explained by "referral bias."[132] That is, since stress myocardial imaging has become accepted in the clinical practice of cardiology, patients with normal stress radionuclide images are no longer referred for cardiac catheterization. Thus, the occasional patient who has normal coronary arteries on angiography almost always is referred because of abnormal stress myocardial perfusion images. The true specificity of stress SPECT imaging therefore can no longer be assessed in patients undergoing coronary angiography because of this referral bias.

Specificity should, however, be tested in patients with low likelihood of coronary artery disease. In such patients the "normalcy rate" is determined. The normalcy rate of planar imaging using ^{201}Tl and ^{99m}Tc-labeled compounds is generally over 95 per cent. With SPECT imaging, normalcy rate ranges from 85 per cent for ^{201}Tl to 95 to 100 per cent for ^{99m}Tc-labeled agents.

DETECTION OF HIGH-RISK CORONARY ARTERY DISEASE. The greater the functional severity of coronary artery disease, the more abnormal exercise myocardial perfusion images are likely to be. Most patients (approximately 95 per cent) with left main coronary disease have abnormal stress myocardial perfusion images.[133] However, the expected typical left main pattern, i.e., defects in the anteroseptal and posterolateral walls, is found in only a minority (approximately 14 per cent) of patients with left main coronary artery disease.[133-135] The majority (approximately 75 per cent) of patients have multiple perfusion defects and frequently abnormally increased lung uptake of [201]Tl.[136]

Although most patients with triple-vessel disease have abnormal stress images, approximately 60 per cent have multiple defects in two or more vascular regions. Most frequently, disease in the left circumflex coronary artery is not detected on planar stress myocardial perfusion images.

High-risk myocardial perfusion images (Figs. 9-18 and 9-25) can be characterized by (1) multiple reversible defects in two or more coronary artery territories[137]; (2) quantitatively large myocardial perfusion defects[138-142]; (3) increased pulmonary radiotracer uptake after exercise[40,41];

and (4) transient dilatation of the left ventricle immediately after exercise.[42]

This high-risk pattern is highly specific (approximately 95 per cent) for multivessel coronary artery disease; however, the sensitivity is only about 70 per cent. Therefore, in the absence of the above-mentioned scintigraphic characteristics, the presence of multivessel disease cannot be ruled out.

SEVERITY OF MYOCARDIAL PERFUSION DEFECTS. Myocardial perfusion defects vary in intensity. A defect can be very dense (severe), i.e., almost without any radiotracer uptake. On the other hand, some residual activity may still be present within the defect. The severity of perfusion defects is often assessed using a semiquantitative visual scoring system: 0 = normal, 1 = mildly reduced or equivocal, 2 = moderately reduced, and 3 = severely reduced. Computer quantification of circumferential count distribution profiles provides a means of quantifying precisely the extent (the number of angles below the lower limit) and severity (area below the lower limit) of a perfusion defect. This measurement can be expressed as an integrated defect score.[50-52]

Stress Myocardial Perfusion Imaging and Prognosis

The detection of coronary artery disease is only one aspect of the clinical value of stress myocardial perfusion imaging. An important additional feature is the ability to

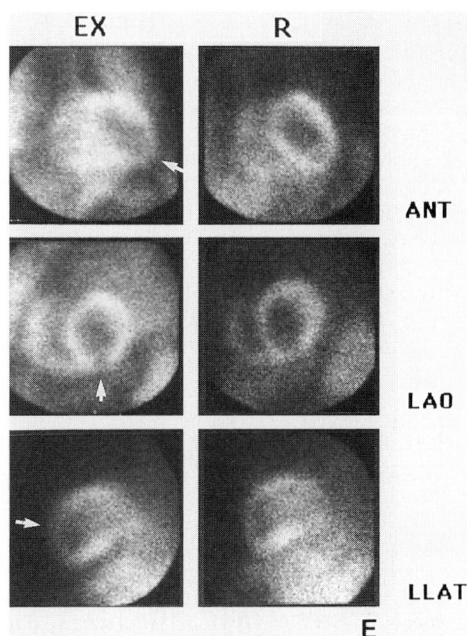

EX   R

ANT

LAO

LLAT

E

FIGURE 9-25. High risk ^{201}Tl images. After exercise the heart is enlarged and there is increased lung uptake of [201]Tl. Furthermore, there is a partially reversible anteroapical myocardial perfusion defect (arrows).

predict prognosis and to identify high- and low-risk patients. The first critical finding on myocardial perfusion images is the presence or absence of defect reversibility, i.e., ischemia.[141] Patients with evidence of transient ischemia on planar ^{201}Tl images have been shown to have a higher incidence of future cardiac events than patients with fixed defects. In patients with suspected or known chronic coronary artery disease, semiquantitative and quantitative assessment of the number or extent of myocardial perfusion defects and the magnitude of defect reversibility are predictive of cardiac events during follow-up (Figs. 9–26 and 9–27).[138,143]

Gibson et al.[137] evaluated patients who had uncomplicated myocardial infarction at the time of hospital discharge by planar quantitative ^{201}Tl stress imaging. Patients with a fixed single ^{201}Tl stress defect and without washout abnormalities (i.e., normal clearance of ^{201}Tl from the heart) at hospital discharge had only a 6 per cent cardiac event rate (death, recurrent infarction, or unstable angina), whereas patients who had high-risk findings on predischarge ^{201}Tl stress images (multiple defects in more than one vascular region, abnormal washout, or increased lung uptake) had a 51 per cent cardiac event rate. Numerous other investigators have since reported similar prognostic value of stress myocardial perfusion imaging after myocardial infarction using either physical or pharmacological stress.[144–147] Brown et al.[145] reported that patients with recurrent chest pain *after myocardial infarction* frequently had ischemia *within* the infarct region (75 per cent of patients), whereas only 25 per cent of patients had ischemia at distance. Patients with evidence of reversibility had a substantially poorer prognosis and higher incidence of revascularization procedures than patients who did not have demonstrable defect reversibility. Evidence of transient left ventricular dysfunction during stress (i.e., transient postexercise dilatation and/or increased radiotracer lung uptake) constitutes an important additional scintigraphic marker of adverse outcome.[148]

Bateman et al.[149] showed that categorization of results of SPECT imaging in high- and low-risk subsets is an effective strategy to select appropriate patients for coronary angiography, as well as to avoid unnecessary cardiac catheterization. Recently Nallamother et al.[149a] reported similar results, suggesting a future role for SPECT imaging as a "gatekeeper" for coronary angiography.

Alternatively, the presence of *quantitatively normal planar or SPECT stress myocardial perfusion images,* even

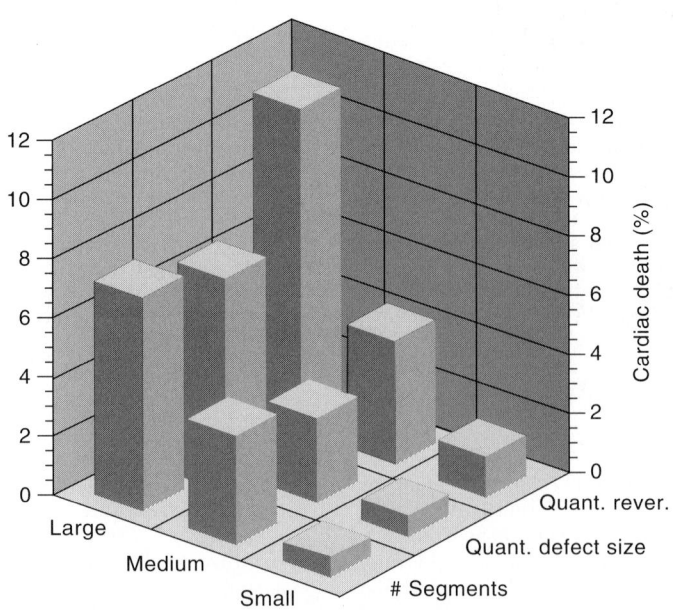

FIGURE 9–27. **Prognostic importance of size and type of myocardial perfusion abnormality. Data are from 816 patients with stable coronary artery disease enrolled in the Multicenter Study on Silent Myocardial Ischemia (MSSMI). The patients had 26 months follow-up. All patients had quantitative planar** [201]**Tl stress imaging. The graph relates the size of exercise defects, defect reversibility, and number of abnormal segments to cardiac death rate during follow-up. The highest cardiac death rate occurred in patients with most abnormal images. In particular, patients with greatest defect reversibility had highest cardiac death rate. (Modified from Bodenheimer, M. M., Wackers, F. J. Th., Schwartz, R. G., et al.: Prognostic significance of a fixed thallium defect one to six months after onset of acute myocardial infarction or unstable angina. Am. J. Cardiol. 74:1196, 1994.)**

when coronary artery stenosis is angiographically documented, indicates favorable prognosis with low subsequent cardiac event rate.[150–156] Patients with quantitatively normal myocardial perfusion images have a yearly nonfatal myocardial infarction rate of 0.6 per cent and a mortality rate of 0.5 per cent per year.

These data on abnormal and normal stress myocardial perfusion images indicate that the extent of myocardial perfusion defects, or the lack thereof, provide significant physiological and prognostic information that surpasses the anatomical information obtained from coronary angiograms. Recent data in the literature suggest that the prognostic predictive value of stress myocardial perfusion imaging is independent of the imaging technique applied (planar or SPECT) or the radiopharmaceutical used (^{201}Tl or ^{99m}Tc-sestamibi).[157,158]

INDEPENDENT INCREMENTAL VALUE OF STRESS MYOCARDIAL PERFUSION IMAGING. In clinical practice diagnostic tests are usually used in conjunction with each other. The clinician usually has other clinical and diagnostic information available. The pathophysiological prognostic value of stress myocardial perfusion imaging as outlined above is important. However, if similar information can be derived from other less costly and readily available tests, it may not be cost-effective to perform radionuclide myocardial perfusion imaging. The incremental prognostic value of various diagnostic data obtained in succession (clinical data, exercise ECG, planar ^{201}Tl stress imaging, and coronary angiography) was assessed by Pollock et al.[159] and Melin et al.[160] The combination of clinical and exercise ^{201}Tl variables provide greater prognostic information than the combination of clinical and angiographic data. Iskandrian et al.[161] observed similar independent and incremental prognostic information using SPECT ^{201}Tl stress imaging, even when cardiac catheterization data are available (Fig. 9–28).

Bodenheimer et al.[140] reported that the extent of myocardial perfusion abnormality on quantitative SPECT was the

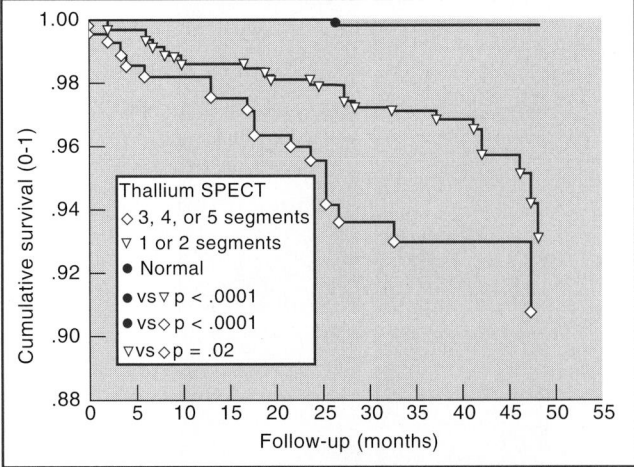

FIGURE 9–26. **Cardiovascular cumulative survival and number of abnormal segments on SPECT** [201]**Tl stress scintigraphy. (From Machecourt, J., Longere, P., Fagret, D., et al.: Prognostic value of thallium-201 single-photon emission computed tomographic myocardial perfusion imaging according to extent of myocardial defect. Reprinted with permission from the American College of Cardiology. J. Am. Coll. Cardiol. 23:1096, 1994.)**

PLATE 5

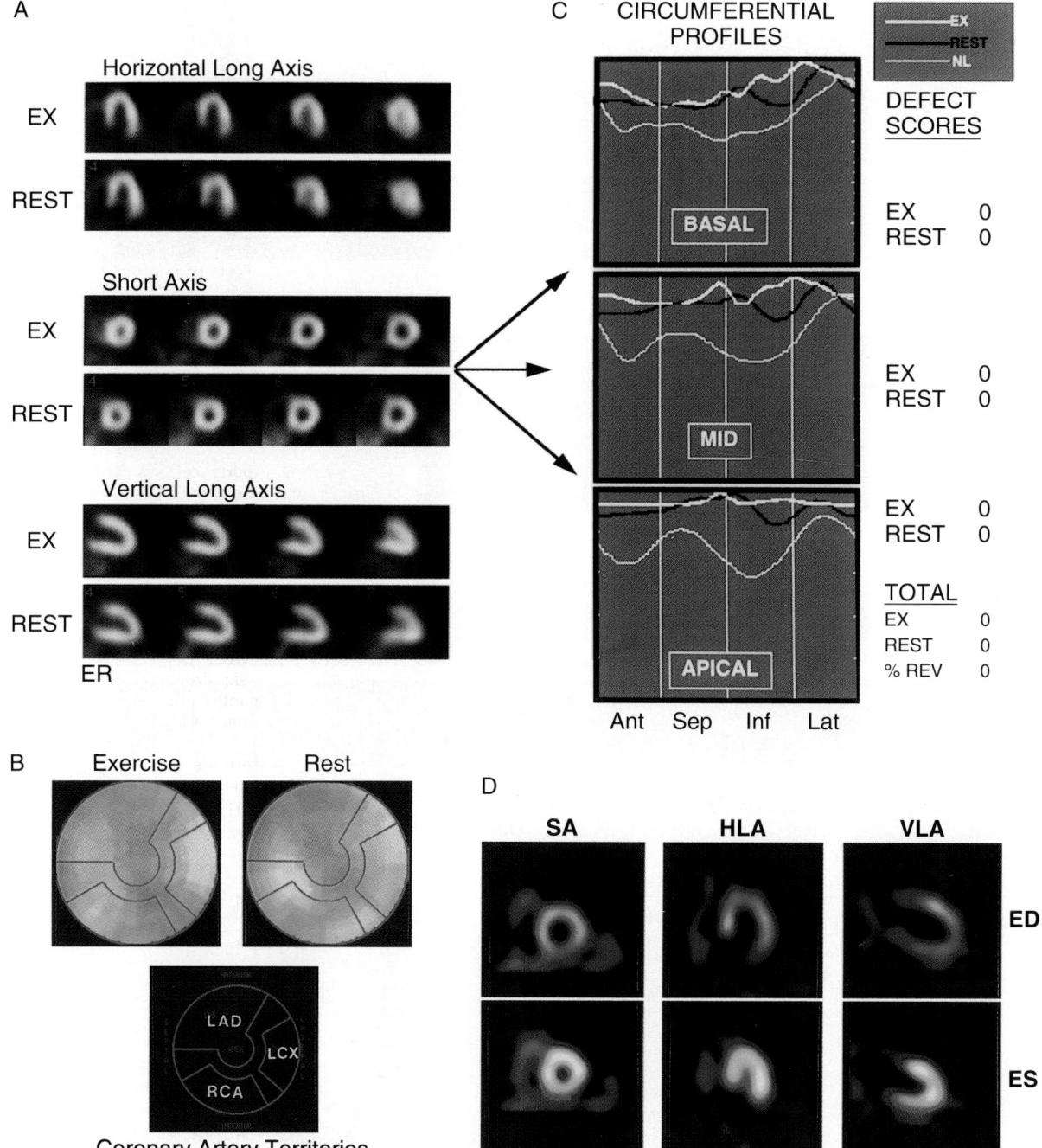

FIGURE 9–17. Exercise and rest SPECT myocardial perfusion imaging with ^{99m}Tc-sestamibi in a normal subject.

A, Horizontal long-axis, short-axis, and vertical long-axis slices. Normal distribution of ^{99m}Tc-sestamibi is noted.

B, Exercise and rest polar maps (bull's-eye display) of tomographic slices in *A.* On both the exercise and rest polar map, distribution of radiopharmaceutical is approximately homogeneous. Color scale: White represents the area with highest activity; yellow, orange, red, violet blue, and black indicate gradually decreasing count activity. The coronary artery territories of the LAD (left anterior coronary artery), LCX (left circumflex coronary artery), and RCA (right coronary artery) are indicated. The yellow, white, and orange colors represent normal perfusion.

C, Circumferential count profiles. Relative activity of sestamibi on the exercise images is displayed as a white line. The relative activity of sestamibi of the rest images is displayed as a black line. The lower-limit-of-normal sestamibi distribution is indicated as the thin white line. The relative radiotracer activity in the anterior (ANT), septum (SEP), interior (INF), and lateral (LAT) walls is shown in representative basal, midventricular, and apical short-axis slices. In this normal subject the relative distribution of sestamibi is above the lower-limit-of-normal distribution, indicating absence of perfusion defects and thus normal images.

D, ECG-gated exercise myocardial perfusion images of the same patient. End-diastolic and end-systolic frames of the short-axis slices (SA), horizontal long-axis slices (HLA), and vertical long-axis slices (VLA) are shown. The color coding is the same as in *B.* Comparison of the end-diastolic and end-systolic frames allow assessment of regional wall motion and regional wall thickening. In this normal subject wall motion and thickening are homogeneous: The color in the anterior wall, septum, and lateral wall changes from yellow to white; in the inferior wall color changes from orange to yellow. The relatively lesser activity in the inferior wall is due to diaphragmatic attenuation.

PLATE 6

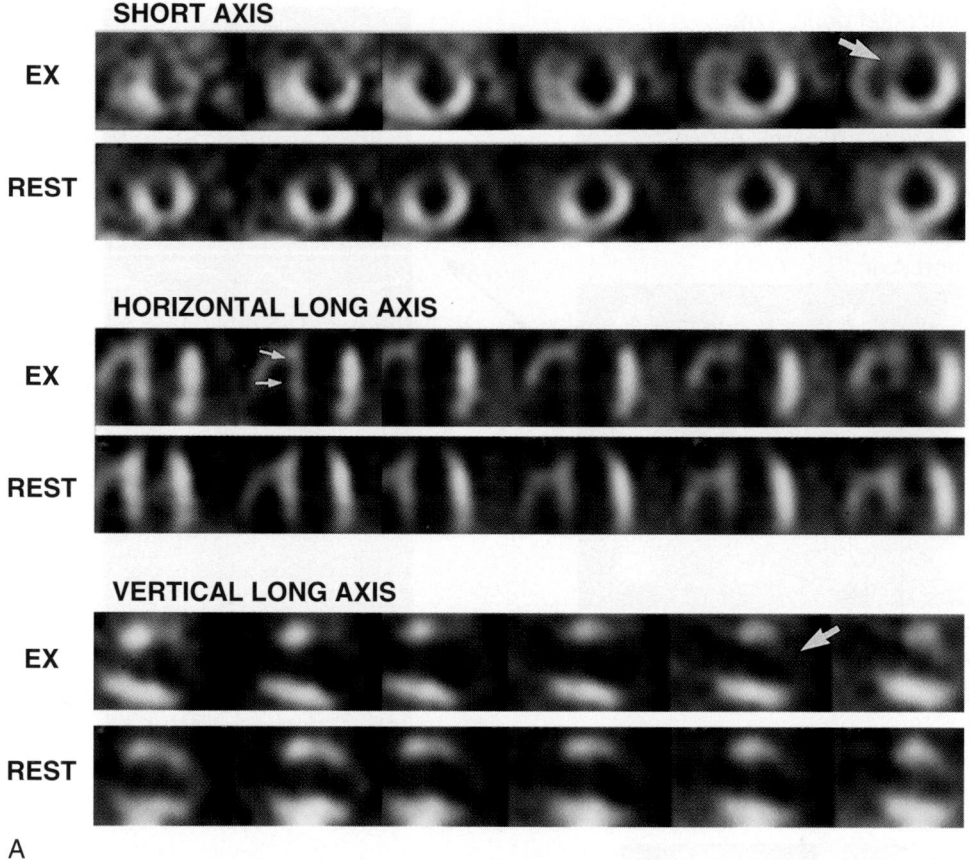

SHORT AXIS

EX

REST

HORIZONTAL LONG AXIS

EX

REST

VERTICAL LONG AXIS

EX

REST

A

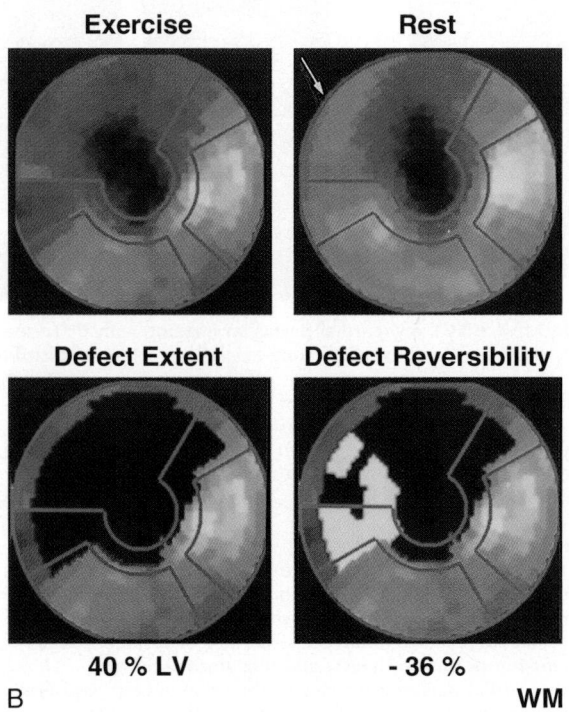

Exercise   Rest

Defect Extent   Defect Reversibility

40 % LV   - 36 %

B   WM

Legend on opposite page

PLATE 7

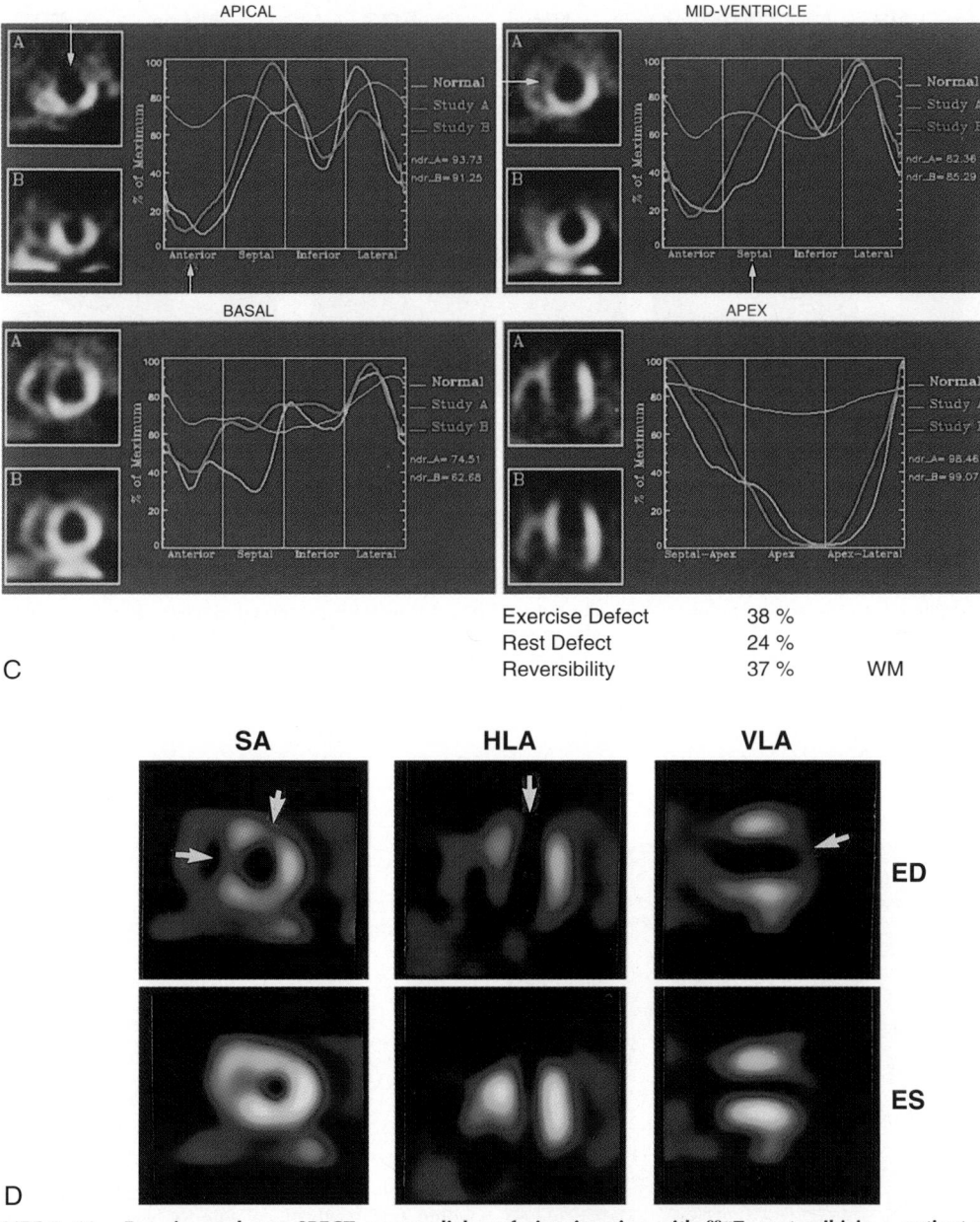

FIGURE 9–18. Exercise and rest SPECT myocardial perfusion imaging with ^{99m}Tc-sestamibi in a patient with anterior infarction and extensive triple-vessel coronary artery disease.

A, Reconstructed short-axis, horizontal long-axis, and vertical long-axis slices. On the exercise (EX) short-axis images an extensive anteroseptal myocardial perfusion defect (arrow) is present, which is partially reversible on the basal rest images. On the horizontal long-axis slices, a fixed apical defect is present with some reversibility in the septal area (arrows). On the vertical long-axis slices an extensive anteroapical myocardial perfusion defect is present which shows only minimal reversibility at rest.

B, Polar map display of short-axis slices in *A*. The color coding is the same as in Figure 9–17. On the exercise polar map an extensive anteroseptal myocardial perfusion defect is present. On the rest polar map, improvement in the septum (arrow) can be appreciated. On the bottom polar map, defect extent is compared with a normal data base. The abnormal area is black. The extent of the defect is calculated as 40 per cent of the left ventricle. On the reversibility polar map defect (white), reversibility is quantified as 36 per cent of the exercise defect.

C, Circumferential profiles analysis. The relative distribution of radiopharmaceutical is displayed for representative apical, midventricular, and basal short-axis slices. The yellow line represents the exercise study, the orange line the rest study, and the thin white line the lower-limit-of-normal distribution. The apical slice *(top left)* shows no significant improvement on the resting study. In contrast, the septal defect reversibility is demonstrated in the midventricular slice *(top right)* and the basal slice *(bottom left)*. The apical defect *(bottom right)* is fixed. Total exercise myocardial perfusion defect size is quantified as 38 per cent of total left ventricle. The rest defect is 24 per cent. Defect reversibility is 34 per cent.

D, ECG-gated exercise SPECT images. End-diastolic and end-systolic frames are shown for the short-axis slices (SA), horizontal long-axis slices (HLA), and vertical long-axis slices (VLA). On the end-diastolic frames an extensive anteroapical and septal myocardial perfusion defect (arrow) is present. Analysis of wall motion shows absence of thickening in the anteroapical segment on the vertical long-axis and horizontal long-axis slices. On the short-axis slice and horizontal long-axis slice, in spite of the presence of an exercise-induced anteroseptal myocardial perfusion defect, thickening (change from orange and blue to yellow) of the anteroseptal segment can be appreciated.

PLATE 8

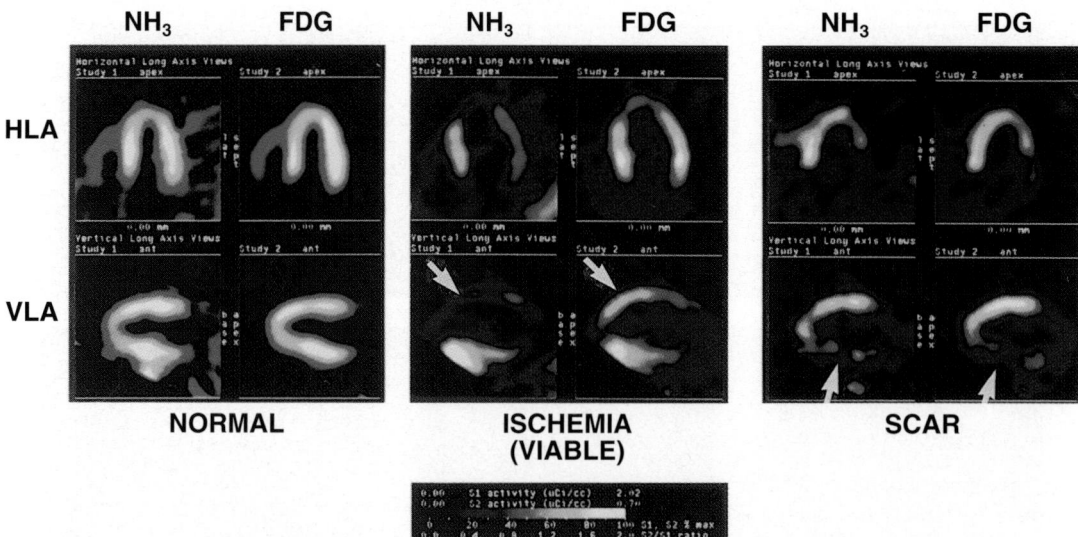

| NH₃ | FDG | NH₃ | FDG | NH₃ | FDG |

HLA

VLA

NORMAL **ISCHEMIA (VIABLE)** **SCAR**

FIGURE 9–40.   Three PET scintigraphic presentations are shown. On each panel, perfusion is represented by NH₃ and glucose metabolism by FDG. The left panel shows normal homogeneous uptake of NH₃ and FDG. In the middle panel, the arrows point to markedly reduced blood flow with preserved glucose uptake in a patient with myocardial viability in an area of an old anterior wall myocardial infarction. On the right, the arrows point to concordant reduction of blood flow and FDG in a patient with remote inferior wall myocardial infarction. (From Zaret, B. L., and Wackers, F. T.: Nuclear Cardiology (I). N. Engl. J. Med. *329*:775, 1993. Copyright 1993 Massachusetts Medical Society.)

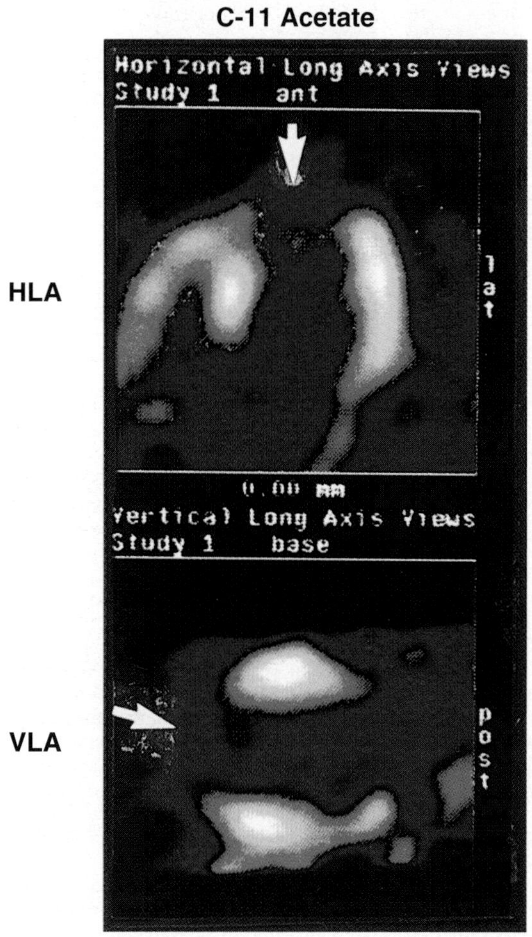

C-11 Acetate

HLA

VLA

FIGURE 9–41.   Static ¹¹C acetate images in a patient within one week of an anterior wall myocardial infarction are shown. The white arrows point to marked decrease of ¹¹C acetate in the anteroapical region. Serial data acquisition over time revealed marked decrease of ¹¹C acetate washout in these regions.

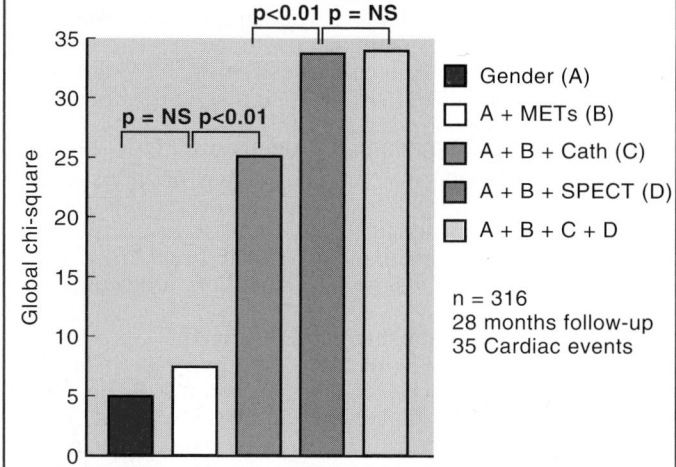

FIGURE 9–28. Independent and incremental prognostic power of clinical, exercise, catheterization, and quantitative ^{201}Tl SPECT variables. Data shown represent the global chi-square statistics of various clinical and diagnostic variables. SPECT imaging provides independent and incremental information to identify high-risk patients. Note that angiography (Cath) has less incremental value over clinical variables than ^{201}Tl-SPECT imaging. (From Iskandrian, A. S., Chae, S. C., Heo, J., et al.: Independent and incremental prognostic value of exercise single-photon emission computed tomographic (SPECT) thallium imaging in coronary artery disease. Reprinted with permission from the American College of Cardiology. J. Am. Coll. Cardiol. 22:665, 1993.)

single most important prognostic predictor. Petretta et al.[162] and Fagan et al.[163] noted that the exercise ECG should be taken into consideration when the exercise ECG is normal and the additive prognostic value of stress myocardial perfusion imaging is less than when the exercise ECG is abnormal or nondiagnostic.

STRESS MYOCARDIAL PERFUSION IMAGING AFTER THROMBOLYIS. Several investigators[164,165] reported apparent diminished sensitivity of stress myocardial perfusion imaging for predicting multivessel coronary artery disease and cardiac events after treatment with thrombolysis for acute myocardial infarction. There may be several potential explanations for this observation. It is well recognized that patients eligible for thrombolytic therapy constitute a patient cohort at relatively low risk. These patients are generally younger and have fewer prior myocardial infarctions, fewer non-Q-wave infarctions, and less multivessel coronary artery disease than patients with acute infarction in the prethrombolytic era.

Because of the favorable outcome and low mortality in these patients, one would predict, based on Bayesian principles, diminished predictive value for stress myocardial perfusion imaging. Another confounding factor is that patients with abnormal stress perfusion images after acute myocardial infarction are generally referred for coronary angiography and revascularization if coronary anatomy is suitable. Accordingly, Gimple and Beller[166] have suggested that "the excellent outcome in patients treated with thrombolytic therapy and risk stratified with exercise testing provides strong empiric support for the continued use of noninvasive testing of patients without complication after thrombolytic therapy." Dakik et al.[167] reported that quantitative predischarge SPECT ^{201}Tl imaging in patients who had thrombolytic therapy for acute infarction provided a reliable means of identifying patients at high, intermediate, and low risk for future adverse events.

DETECTION OF CORONARY ARTERY DISEASE IN WOMEN (see also p. 1705). Exercise electrocardiography has been reported to be less accurate in women than in men to detect coronary artery disease. This can be explained in part by differences in disease prevalence in men and women.[168] Moreover, women more often have an abnormal baseline electrocardiogram, which affects accuracy of interpretation of the exercise electrocardiograms. Although breast attenuation artifacts may make the interpretation of stress myocardial perfusion images in women more difficult, Desmarais et al.[169] demonstrated that experienced interpreters usually recognize artifacts and can avoid false-positive interpretations.

Several investigators have examined the performance of stress myocardial perfusion imaging in women. Although women in general achieve lower exercise workload, the detection of significant coronary artery disease using radionuclide stress perfusion imaging[170–172] is similar to that in men. Moreover, Chae et al. and others showed that low- and high-risk patients are identified without gender differences.[155,171,173] Hendel et al.[174] reported that long-term outcome for vascular surgery patients also can be predicted by dipyridamole ^{201}Tl imaging irrespective of gender.

Syndrome X (typical exertional angina pectoris, positive ECG response to exercise, and angiographically normal coronary arteries (see p. 1343), occurs predominantly in postmenopausal women.[175] These patients, who have a good prognosis, generally have normal myocardial perfusion images, although myocardial perfusion abnormalities have been noted in an occasional patient.

PATIENTS WITH LEFT BUNDLE BRANCH BLOCK. In patients with complete left bundle branch block, the conduction abnormality precludes the use of conventional electrocardiographic criteria for the diagnosis of infarction or exercise-induced ischemia. It was expected that myocardial distribution of myocardial perfusion imaging agents would be unaffected by the electrocardiographic abnormality.[176] Indeed, in patients with left bundle branch block without prior myocardial infarction, *resting* myocardial perfusion images are generally normal. However, the septum is frequently thin and in older patients the left ventricle is often dilated.

A number of investigators have reported exercise-induced myocardial perfusion defects in anteroapical and anteroseptal areas in patients with complete left bundle branch block and angiographic normal coronary arteries.[177,178] In some patients partial or complete reversibility of these defects have been observed. Hirzel et al.[179] proposed, based upon experimental animal data with right ventricular pacing, that diminished septal myocardial blood flow during abnormal sequence of electrical ventricular depolarization caused septal defects. Shefcyk et al.[180] compared regional myocardial uptake of ^{201}Tl during rapid atrial pacing (normal conduction) with that during rapid right ventricular pacing (left bundle branch block). These investigators found no significant quantitative difference in regional ^{201}Tl uptake. Thus, it appears that the altered sequence of ventricular depolarization *itself* is not a principal cause of myocardial perfusion defects in left bundle branch block.

We noted a relationship between the presence of exercise-induced myocardial perfusion defects in left bundle branch block and degree of *left ventricular dilatation* at rest. Patients with left bundle branch block often have clinically unexpected cardiomyopathy with ventricular dilation and depressed left ventricular ejection fraction. Thus, altered geometry and partial volume effect may be other plausible explanations for observed defects. The use of pharmacological vasodilation with dipyridamole has been shown to reduce the incidence of artifactual perfusion defects in left bundle branch block.[181] We recommend that patients with electrocardiographic left bundle branch block be studied with pharmacologic vasodilation with dipyridamole or adenosine rather than with physical exercise to avoid false-positive results.

THALLIUM-201 STRESS IMAGING IN NONCORONARY ARTERY DISEASE. Thallium-201 imaging has been used in a number of clinical conditions that may be present with symptoms of chest pain but angiographically normal epicardial arteries.[182,183] In a number of these patients abnormal and "false-positive" [201]Tl images have been observed. LeGrand et al.[184] demonstrated that in patients with syndrome X, abnormal coronary reserve also could be demonstrated. Cannon et al.[185] found that these patients also had abnormal global and regional systolic and diastolic function. At least some of the so-called false-positive ^{201}Tl images in patients with angiographic normal coronary arteries may in fact reveal true abnormalities in myocardial microcirculation.[185a] In patients with mitral valve prolapse and atypical chest pain, several investigators have demonstrated normal ^{201}Tl stress images.

MYOCARDIAL PERFUSION IMAGING FOR PREOPERATIVE SCREENING (see also p. 1759). An important clinical application of myocardial perfusion imaging is the preoperative evaluation of patients undergoing noncardiac surgery. This has had its most meaningful application in the study of patients prior to revascularization surgery involving the descending aorta and the lower extremities. This group of patients has a strong likelihood coexisting coronary artery disease. Boucher et al.[186] were the first to show that dipyridamole thallium imaging is predictive of subsequent perioperative cardiac events in this patient's subgroup. The findings of reversibility on the dipyridamole thallium study were the single most important prognostic indicator.

Subsequent studies have indicated that the total cohort of patients can be stratified prior to perfusion scintigraphy based upon clinical variables. Eagle et al.[187] demonstrated that, based upon simple clinical assessment of specified risk factors, those with high risk of coronary disease and those with very low risk of coronary disease did not require perfusion studies for appropriate risk stratification. However, the majority of patients fell into an intermediate clinical group who were categorized quite effectively by perfusion studies. Further studies in this area have also demonstrated that the simple qualitative characterization of a perfusion study as either positive or negative for ischemia may be insufficient. However, appropriate categorization can be obtained using quantitative techniques that allow definition of a large potential ischemic burden as well as the identification of specific "high-risk" findings.[188,191] It has also recently been shown that dipyridamole thallium scintigraphy is of value in predicting long-range outcomes, beyond the perioperative period, in this group of patients.[191]

The predictive value of dipyridamole thallium imaging in preoperative assessment has been questioned in two recent studies.[192,193] However, it should be noted that both studies had potential for significant selection bias in the populations studied. It should also be noted that at the present time further prospective analysis of efficacy may be somewhat difficult because clinicians use the results of perfusion studies in routine preoperative management.[191] Consequently, those with substantial abnormalities are often evaluated further with preoperative coronary angiography which, if found to be abnormal, often lead to additional procedures such as coronary angioplasty or bypass surgery prior to vascular surgery.

MYOCARDIAL PERFUSION IMAGING BEFORE AND AFTER REVASCULARIZATION. A main purpose for performing stress myocardial perfusion imaging is not only to detect significant coronary artery disease, but also to aid in patient management decisions. Patients with markedly abnormal and high-risk stress myocardial perfusion images are usually considered candidates for coronary revascularization, either by coronary bypass surgery or percutaneous transluminal coronary angioplasty. Myocardial perfusion imaging is not routinely performed after coronary bypass surgery and is indicated only when symptoms recur. Because many patients have nonspecific ST-T segment changes on the baseline electrocardiogram after surgery, myocardial perfusion imaging is preferred over the exercise electrocardiography in the evaluation of these patients.

Coronary Angioplasty. Stress myocardial perfusion imaging is particularly useful after coronary angioplasty because often only one vessel is dilated and its vascular territory can be evaluated readily with SPECT imaging. The optimal timing of imaging after angioplasty is controversial. Some investigators[194] reported a high incidence of false-positive myocardial perfusion abnormalities early after angioplasty, presumably because of delayed return of coronary reserve. This is not a general experience. Most patients have normal myocardial perfusion images within the first week of successful angioplasty. At approximately 4 weeks after coronary angioplasty, a good correlation has been demonstrated between stress-induced myocardial perfusion abnormalities and the presence or absence of restenosis, independent of clinical symptoms.[195–197] In our own laboratory we perform electrocardiographic treadmill stress testing shortly after angioplasty to assess functional status and exercise-induced symptoms. Stress myocardial perfusion imaging is performed in patients who develop symptoms supportive of restenosis, or at 6 months in those who are asymptomatic.[190]

SPECT imaging is particularly useful in patients with known coronary artery disease. Tomographic localization of perfusion abnormalities allows us to determine whether clinical ischemia is likely to be caused by coronary graft closure, restenosis at the site of angioplasty, or progression of disease in other coronary arteries.

ASSESSMENT OF MYOCARDIAL VIABILITY (see also p. 1296). In patients with recurrent angina, known previous infarction(s), and left ventricular dysfunction, a reliable method for assessing the presence, extent, and location of viable myocardium is of considerable clinical importance when therapeutic decisions on revascularization procedures are made.

It is now well established that, using the conventional 201Tl imaging protocol with 2- to 4-hour delayed imaging, myocardial viability occasionally may be underestimated in patients who appear to have "scintigraphic scar," i.e., a fixed perfusion defect.[36,37] Apparently fixed defects may improve after coronary bypass surgery or coronary angioplasty. Depending on patient selection, approximately 30 to 50 per cent of patients with a fixed 201Tl stress defect on 2- to 4-hour delayed imaging may show "late filling-in" on either 24-hour redistribution imaging or after reinjection at rest (Fig. 9–29).[199–201] Because 24-hour redistribution images are generally of suboptimal quality, reinjection of 201Tl at rest is preferred. Reinjection of 201Tl can be done either *on the same day* of the stress test by administration of a new dose (1 mCi) of 201Tl immediately after completion of the 2- to 4-hour delayed images or *on a different day* by injection of a new dose (2 mCi) of 201Tl at rest (Fig. 9–1). In some laboratories, delayed 201Tl imaging has been abolished and 1 mCi of 201Tl is reinjected at rest as soon as stress imaging is completed. Rest imaging is then performed 3 hours later.

The phenomenon of "rest filling-in" with 201Tl cannot be predicted readily by clinical parameters such as the presence of prior infarction, the presence of angina, or electrocardiographic signs of ischemia. Rest filling-in correlates in selected patients with improvement of wall motion after revascularization and shows substantial concordance with the demonstration of metabolically viable myocardium on positron F18-deoxyglucose imaging.[202] Although in most laboratories rest 201Tl imaging is performed at approximately 15 to 45 minutes after injection, the highest yield for detection of myocardial viability is probably obtained by 3- to 4-hour rest-delayed imaging.[203]

Comparison with PET imaging showed further that 201Tl defect intensity was predictive of the presence of viable myocardium.[204] Mild to moderate fixed defects (on 2- to 4-hour delayed imaging) with greater than 50 per cent of normal 201Tl uptake showed evidence of viability on PET imaging in more than 95 per cent of cases. In contrast, only one-half of defects with less than 50 per cent of normal uptake had evidence of viable myocardium. However, on rest reinjection of 201Tl in patients with fixed defects with

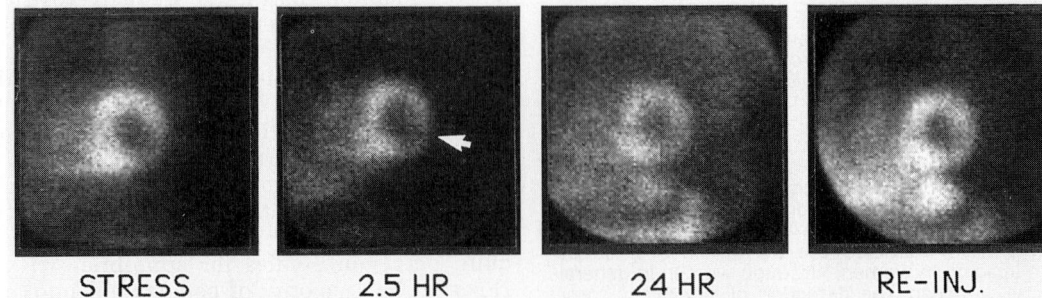

| STRESS | 2.5 HR | 24 HR | RE-INJ. |

FIGURE 9–29. 201Tl images after exercise (stress), 2.5-hr delayed imaging, 24-hr delayed imaging, and a reinjection of 201Tl at rest. This patient has an apparently fixed defect (arrow) at 2.5-hr delayed imaging. However, on 24-hr redistribution imaging, filling-in of the defect can be appreciated. After reinjection of 201Tl at rest, further normalization of the image can be appreciated.

less than 50 per cent of normal uptake, concordance of "filling-in" and "no filling-in" with PET evidence of metabolic activity was 88 per cent. Zimmerman et al.[205] demonstrated that the level of residual ^{201}Tl activity in defects after reinjection is significantly related to the mass of preserved viable myocytes in myocardial biopsies.

Thus, for assessment of myocardial viability on myocardial perfusion images one should consider two aspects: (1) the quantitative reduction in radiotracer uptake relative to normal myocardium and (2) the presence of defect reversibility. Thallium-201 uptake greater than 50 per cent of normal and/or defect reversibility (complete or partial) suggests viable myocardium. When clinical decisions on revascularization are to be made, the extent of viable myocardium that can be revascularized should be taken into account[206] (see p. 1313). Revascularization of only small quantities of viable myocardium cannot be expected to result in substantial improvement of global ventricular function, although ischemia may be abolished. At the time of this writing, no well-defined quantitative imaging criteria have been developed to guide such clinical decisions on revascularization.

There is considerable (and, at the time of this writing, inconclusive) debate in the literature whether *resting ^{99m}Tc-sestamibi imaging* is comparable to resting ^{201}Tl imaging for detecting myocardial viability. Experimental studies have shown that only viable myocardial cells with preserved membrane integrity accumulate and retain sestamibi.[207] However, the delivery of sestamibi is primarily flow dependent and only minimal redistribution occurs.[45] Other confounding factors are the physical and imaging differences between the two radiotracers.[208] Thus far, comparative studies involve only a relatively small number of patients. Although differences in uptake between ^{201}Tl and sestamibi are noted, the predictive accuracy of sestamibi uptake for improved wall motion after revascularization is similar to that of [201]Tl.[199–201] Udelson et al.[212] reported similar quantitative uptake of the two radiotracers in patients with unstable angina and left ventricular dysfunction. Dilsizian et al.[213] stressed the potential importance of 4-hour rest-redistribution sestamibi images. Because of known differences in tracer kinetics, one should probably use different tracer uptake threshold values when evaluating myocardial viability. Several investigators[214,215] have suggested resting sestamibi imaging in conjunction with nitrate administration as an improved means to predict accurately myocardial viability. In summary, the role of sestamibi and other ^{99m}Tc-labeled radiotracers for evaluating myocardial viability has not been as yet fully elucidated. More properly designed studies using an appropriate adequate gold standard for myocardial viability are needed.[216]

Selection of Patients for Myocardial Perfusion Stress Imaging

Although the sensitivity and specificity of myocardial perfusion imaging for detection of coronary artery disease is better than that of electrocardiographic stress testing, false-negative and false-positive results occur. According to Bayes' theorem, the significance of test results relates not only to the sensitivity and specificity of a test but also to the prevalence of disease in the population under study.[217,218] Quantitative planar ^{201}Tl and ^{99m}Tc-sestamibi stress imaging has a reported sensitivity of approximately 90 per cent and a specificity of approximately 95 per cent.

A positive result obtained in a population with a very low prevalence of coronary disease (e.g., less than 3 per cent) has a predictive value of only 36 per cent because, compared with expected true-positive results, a relatively large absolute number of false positives can be anticipated. However, in a patient population with a high prevalence of coronary disease, e.g., 90 per cent, a positive result has a predictive value of 99 per cent. In this setting, relative to the true-positive results, only a few false-positive results are obtained. On the other hand, in a population with a high prevalence of disease, a relatively large number of false-negative results are also obtained, and the predictive value of the negative test for absence of coronary disease is only 51 per cent.

Thus, in a population with a low prevalence of coronary disease (such as young asymptomatic subjects) a positive test is of little predictive value, whereas in a population with a high prevalence of coronary artery disease (50- to 60-year-old males with typical angina pectoris), a negative test is of little practical diagnostic value. The difference between pretest probability of disease (determined by the patient's age, symptoms, and stress ECG) and post-test probability (determined by the results of myocardial perfusion stress imaging) indicates the practical value of the test. Stress myocardial perfusion imaging has optimal discriminative value in a patient population with a pretest probability of coronary artery disease ranging from about 40 to 70 per cent. This population includes patients with atypical chest pain, asymptomatic patients with major risk factors, or asymptomatic patients with a positive stress electrocardiogram.[219]

When ordering a stress test for diagnostic purposes, the baseline electrocardiogram should be considered. In patients with normal baseline electrocardiograms, the ST-T segment response to maximal exercise is of diagnostic value. We and others[220,221] observed that patients with a normal ST-segment response to maximal exercise almost without exception also had normal exercise myocardial perfusion images. Thus, *myocardial perfusion imaging did not provide additional new information.* However, of patients with positive or equivocal exercise electrocardiograms, a substantial number had normal exercise myocardial perfusion images. Thus, in certain patient populations it may be cost-effective to perform exercise electrocardiography as a first test in patients with normal baseline electrocardiograms and repeat the exercise test with added myocardial perfusion imaging only in patients with abnormal exercise electrocardiograms. However, Nallamothu et al.[222] showed that in patients with an intermediate to high likelihood of coronary artery disease and normal baseline ECG, SPECT is superior to the electrocardiographic response in detecting coronary artery disease.

UNIQUE VALUE OF RADIONUCLIDE IMAGING COMPARED WITH OTHER DIAGNOSTIC MODALITIES. Compared with other diagnostic modalities, radionuclide imaging has certain unique characteristics: (1) Radionuclide imaging provides information regarding the physiological significance of disease that surpasses anatomical information. (2) Radionuclide imaging provides information that has independent and incremental prognostic value over other clinical and diagnostic information, including the contrast coronary angiogram. (3) Radionuclide images are digital count-based images that can be quantified readily. (4) Quantitative radionuclide imaging has been shown to be highly reproducible. (5) Diagnostic quality radionuclide images can be acquired in almost all patients, regardless of body habitus or patient cooperation. The above attributes are uniquely related to the use of radiotracers for imaging.

From the early days of nuclear cardiology, myocardial infarction was visualized either as a "cold spot" (perfusion defect) or as a "hot spot." Cold-spot imaging has been extensively discussed above. When a radiopharmaceutical localizes specifically in an area of recent infarction, the infarct is visualized as a "hot spot." The advantage of hot-spot imaging is that it is generally easier to image the presence of a tracer than its absence. The clinical usefulness of infarct imaging still requires clear definition. The diagnosis of acute myocardial infarction in the majority of patients can readily be made on the basis of simple and inexpensive tests, such as electrocardiography and cardiac enzyme analysis.

TECHNETIUM-99m-Sn—PYROPHOSPHATE

The first clinically useful hot spot imaging of acute infarction was performed using ^{99m}Tc-Sn-pyrophosphate (Fig. 9–30). This imaging agent was very sensitive for detecting acute myocardial infarction from 24 hours to 5 days after the onset of chest pain.[223] However, small and nontransmural infarcts were often not detected. Although as a rule scintigraphy was negative very early after infarction, some infarcts were positive within a few hours after onset of chest pain. Based upon present knowledge, it seems likely that spontaneous reperfusion occurred in these patients.[224] On the other hand, some very large acute infarcts remained scintigraphically negative, apparently because of absence of residual flow to the infarct region. The intensity and pattern of ^{99m}Tc-Sn-pyrophosphate uptake were found to be of prognostic significance. At the present time ^{99m}Tc-pyrophosphate infarct imaging is mainly of historic interest and is performed infrequently in most laboratories. In occasional patients who are suspected of having sustained an acute infarction 2 to 3 days prior to the hospital admission ^{99m}Tc-pyrophosphate imaging may be useful to establish the diagnosis at a time when plasma enzyme levels have returned to normal. SPECT imaging appears to be more sensitive than planar imaging.

Technetium-99m–pyrophosphate is also a specific but not very sensitive imaging agent to detect cardiac amyloidosis.[225]

INDIUM-111 LEUKOCYTES. Another approach to hot-spot infarct imaging, which has never come to routine clinical application, involves the use of ^{111}In-labeled leukocytes.[226] The patient's own white blood cells are labeled in vitro with ^{111}In and then reinjected. On the second or third day after acute infarction, migration of white cells occurs into the infarct area and can be visualized by imaging with ^{111}In.

INDIUM-111–ANTIMYOSIN. More recently, imaging with a monoclonal antibody specific for intracellular myosin has shown promising clinical results. Indium-111 murine monoclonal antimyosin binds selectively to irreversibly damaged myocytes.[227] Imaging is performed after administration of approximately 2 mCi of ^{111}In-antimyosin. Planar or SPECT imaging is performed 24 hours after antibody injection. The gamma camera is peaked on both photopeaks (171 and 245 keV) of ^{111}In. A medium-energy collimator is used. Either the conventional three planar views—anterior, LAO, and left lateral—or 360-degree SPECT is obtained.

Typical ^{111}In-antimyosin images of an acute infarct demonstrate discrete uptake in the myocardium. In addition, substantial liver and spleen uptake may be seen. Initial clinical duties have been encouraging. Indium-111–labeled antimyosin appears highly specific (100 per cent) and sensitive (92 per cent) for the detection of acute myocardial necrosis.[228] In addition to positive images in patients with acute myocardial infarction, uptake of ^{111}In-antimyosin has been noted in patients with unstable angina. The intensity and extent of ^{111}In-antimyosin accumulation appears to be of prognostic significance, both in patients with acute infarction and in those with unstable angina. Patients with extensive antimyosin uptake, i.e., greater than 50 per cent of the myocardium, had a four- to nine-fold increased risk for future cardiac events (cardiac death and nonfatal myocardial infarction) than patients with less or no uptake. The positive uptake seen in patients with unstable angina probably should be interpreted as the noninvasive demonstration of small, clinically undetectable focal areas of necrosis.

The potential prognostic significance of the extent of antimyosin uptake is important and has to be investigated in a larger number of patients. It has been proposed that simultaneous dual tracer imaging (^{201}Tl and ^{111}In-antimyosin) may have a role in the assessment of myocardial salvage after thrombolytic therapy (Fig. 9–31).

In addition to imaging of acute myocardial infarction, ^{111}In-antimyosin may have a role in cardiac transplant patients for detection of cardiac rejection.[229] Furthermore, in patients with active myocarditis, diffuse ^{111}In-antimyosin uptake has been observed.[230] More patients (55 per cent) had abnormal ^{111}In-antimyosin images than abnormal endomyocardial biopsies (22 per cent). Nearly all patients with abnormal myocardial biopsies had abnormal ^{111}In-antimyosin images. More than half of the patients with positive antimyosin images

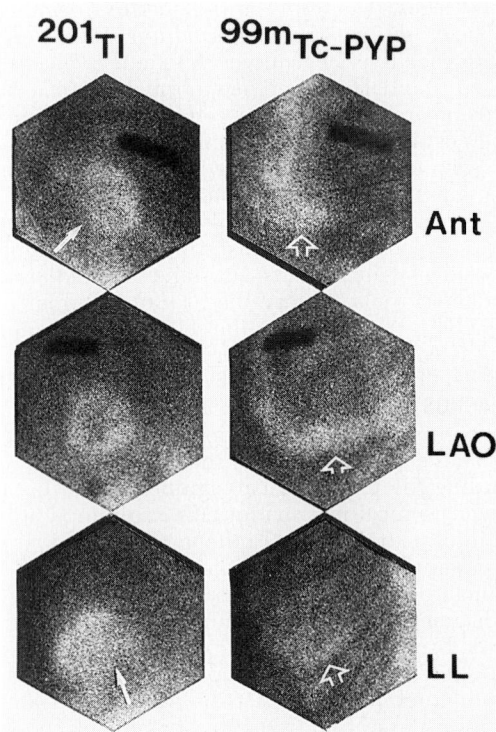

FIGURE 9–30. *Left,* ^{201}Tl images in a patient with acute inferior wall myocardial infarction. An inferior ^{201}Tl myocardial perfusion defect can be seen (arrow). Right, ^{99m}Tc-Sn-pyrophosphate (PYP) imaging in the same patient. Uptake of ^{99m}Tc-pyrophosphate occurred in matching area (open arrow). On the LAO view, intense uptake of ^{99m}Tc-pyrophosphate is present in the inferior wall and extends into the right ventricle. This patient had, in addition to left ventricular infarction, right ventricular involvement.

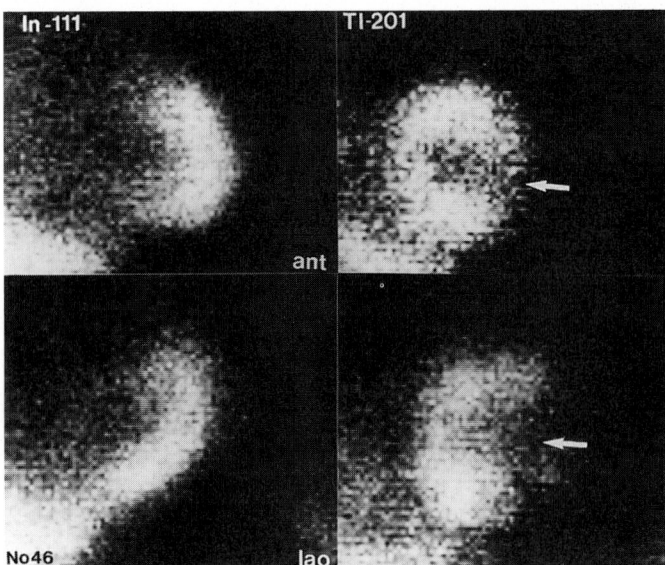

FIGURE 9–31. ^{111}In-antimyosin *(left)* and ^{201}Tl imaging in a patient with acute anterolateral infarction. The ^{201}Tl defects (arrow) correspond with areas of ^{111}In-antimyosin accumulation. (From Lahiri, A., and Jain, D.: New radionuclide imaging in cardiovascular disease. Curr. Opin. Cardiol. 2:1070, 1986.)

showed improvement of left ventricular function over time, whereas only 18 per cent of patients with normal scans improved. This clinical course was independent of biopsy results. These observations suggest that imaging with ¹¹¹In-antimyosin provides independent impor-

tant clinical information in myocarditis. Further studies are needed to define the usefulness of ¹¹¹In-antimyosin imaging in acute ischemic syndromes and other cardiac diseases associated with cellular necrosis.[231]

ASSESSMENT OF CARDIAC PERFORMANCE

Cardiac performance can be assessed with radionuclide techniques by either of two generic approaches. The first involves analysis of the first transit of a radionuclide bolus through the central circulation (first-pass radionuclide angiocardiogram). The second, more widely applied method involves analysis following equilibrium intravascular labeling, which allows repeat imaging over several hours (equilibrium radionuclide angiocardiogram).

Variations of each technique involve assessment of the right and left ventricles, diastolic as well as systolic function, regional or global performance, ventricular volumes, and adaptations for longer term or ambulatory monitoring. Although the radionuclide approach for the evaluation of ventricular function has been challenged recently by echocardiography, these techniques continue to play an important role in the quantitative assessment of cardiac performance. These specific approaches, their clinical implications, and applications are discussed below.

EQUILIBRIUM RADIONUCLIDE ANGIOCARDIOGRAPHY

The concept of utilizing a physiological signal such as the electrocardiogram to "gate," or physiologically control, the otherwise static imaging of the cardiac blood pool was initially proposed in 1971.[232,233] The ERNA utilizes electrocardiographic events to define the temporal relationship between the acquisition of nuclear data and the volumetric components of the cardiac cycle. Sampling is performed repetitively over several hundred heartbeats with physiological segregation of nuclear data according to occurrence within the cardiac cycle (Fig. 9–32). Data are accumulated until radioactivity count density is sufficient for statistically meaningful analysis. The electrocardiogram provides a reasonably sensitive and easily defined physiological signal with which to link the static imaging technique. Data are quantified and displayed in an endless loop cine format for additional qualitative visual interpretation and analysis.

TECHNICAL CONSIDERATIONS. Because analysis involves the summation of several hundred cardiac cycles, a number of factors must be considered for the study to be deemed adequate. First, the patient must be able to remain relatively still beneath the detector during the period of data acquisition. In general, studies should be obtained in multiple views for interpretation to be complete. These include the standard anterior and LAO views, as well as the left lateral and/or left posterior oblique views (Figs. 9–33 and 9–34).

The need for multiple views is inherent in this form of imaging because overlying radioactivity in multiple cardiac and noncardiac structures can obscure a given ventricular region in any one view. In addition, specific abnormalities in regional left ventricular performance, such as ventricular aneurysms or akinesis of the posterobasal segment, may be appreciated only in lateral or posterior oblique views.[234] It is also assumed that cardiac performance remains relatively stable during the entire period of acquisition. This obviously is not the case in the presence of substantial arrhythmia such as atrial fibrillation or frequent premature beats.

The presence of major arrhythmia must be accounted for in interpretation; otherwise, the potential exists for substantially underestimating ventricular performance. Some currently available programs routinely exclude premature beats. Finally, the radionuclide label also must remain stable during the period of analysis, and the interval of data acquisition (framing interval) must be sufficiently short to allow adequate temporal resolution for definition of both systolic and diastolic performance parameters.

PERFORMANCE. Equilibrium blood pool labeling is achieved using ⁹⁹ᵐTc. The intravascular label is established with the patient's own red blood cells, using an in vitro or modified in vitro technique. Unlabeled stannous pyrophosphate is used to facilitate this reaction. The labeling techniques are now well standardized and quality control can be assured.[235] Following a single labeling procedure, serial studies can be readily obtained for periods ranging from 4 to 6 hours. If necessary, additional labeling can be achieved and the duration of observation extended.

Conventional Anger scintillation cameras are employed for these studies. Equipment is sufficiently portable to be brought to the bed-

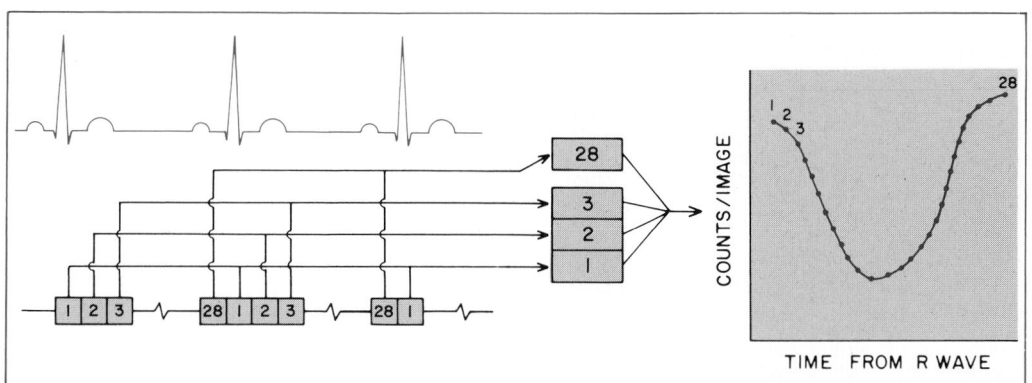

FIGURE 9–32. Diagrammatic representation of the technique for equilibrium radionuclide angiocardiography. Each cardiac cycle is divided into 28 equal segments. For each heartbeat, data are accumulated and then stored in a separate file. To the right, these data for the 28 portions of the cycle are displayed as a single summed ventricular volume curve. The numbers 1 to 28 refer to the temporal sequence within the cardiac cycle. (From Zaret, B. L., and Berger, H. J.: Nuclear cardiology. In Hurst, J. W. (ed.): The Heart, Arteries and Veins. 7th ed. New York, McGraw-Hill Book Co., 1990, p. 1899.)

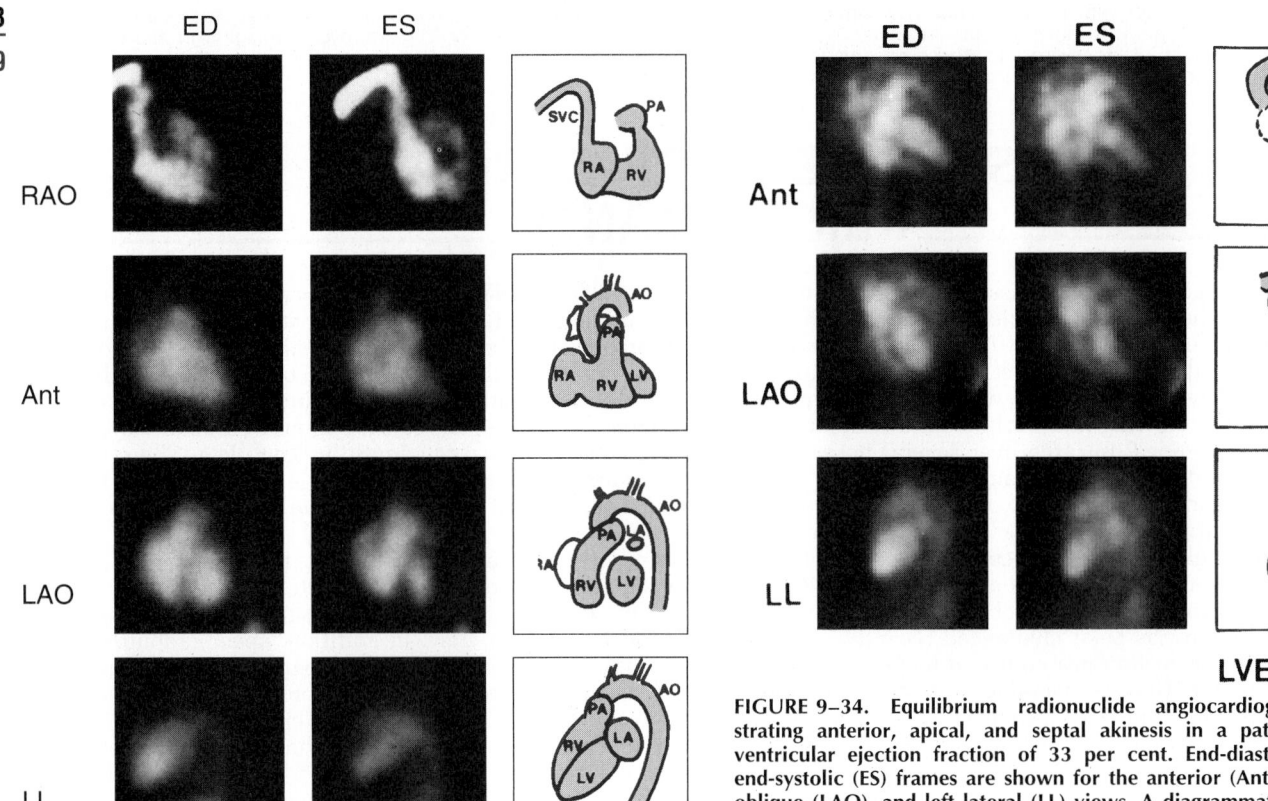

ED   ES

RAO

Ant

LAO

LL

RL

FIGURE 9–33. End-diastolic (ED) and end-systolic (ES) images obtained from a gated first-pass and equilibrium radionuclide angiocardiogram study. The anatomical configuration is shown diagrammatically to the right. In the upper panel, a gated first-pass study for evaluating the right ventricle is shown in the right anterior oblique (RAO) view. In the lower three panels (the equilibrium radionuclide angiocardiogram), images are shown for the anterior (Ant), left anterior oblique (LAO), and left lateral (LL) views. Note a normal contraction pattern in each view. (AO = aorta, LA = left atrium, LV = left ventricle, PA = pulmonary artery, RA = right atrium, RV = right ventricle, SVC = superior vena cava.)

side of acutely ill patients. Data are analyzed by computer, generally with some operator interaction. Analysis may be obtained in either the "frame" or "list" mode.[235] Radionuclide data are collected and segregated temporally. In the frame mode, which is employed most frequently, the R-R interval of electrocardiogram is divided into 20- to 50-msec portions, depending upon the patient's intrinsic heart rate and the conditions of the study, i.e., rest or exercise. If one is interested in defining diastolic filling events, a relatively short framing interval is required. The process generally requires 3 to 10 minutes for completion of each view. Following data acquisition, the data from the several hundred individual beats are summed, processed, and displayed as a single "representative cardiac cycle."

Data from the LAO view also are utilized for qualitative analysis of global left ventricular function. In this view, there is minimal overlap of the two ventricles. Using a count-based approach, left ventricular ejection fraction as well as other indices of filling and ejection are calculated from the left ventricular radioactivity present at various points throughout the cardiac cycle (Fig. 9–35). Measurements obtained in this manner correlate well with other defined standards, such as contrast left ventricular angiography.

BACKGROUND ACTIVITY. Because radioactivity is present within the entire intravascular space, it is necessary to correct for contribution of activity in adjacent intravascular structures to the overall measured left ventricular radioactivity. Major contributions to this "background" come from lungs and left atrium. Because the left atrium is posterior to the left ventricle in the LAO view, its background contribution is attenuated substantially by the more anterior left ventricular blood pool. Semiautomated methods are now routine for determining regions of interest as well as background zones. With the equilibrium technique, a variable region of interest is used for determining the left ventricular blood pool for each frame of the cardiac cycle. This is necessary because using a so-called fixed or single region of interest throughout the cardiac cycle introduces error and results in an underestimation of ejection fraction.

INTERPRETATION. Interpretation of ERNA requires both visual and

ED   ES

Ant

LAO

LL

LVEF: 33%

FIGURE 9–34. Equilibrium radionuclide angiocardiogram demonstrating anterior, apical, and septal akinesis in a patient with left ventricular ejection fraction of 33 per cent. End-diastolic (ED) and end-systolic (ES) frames are shown for the anterior (Ant), left anterior oblique (LAO), and left lateral (LL) views. A diagrammatic representation of superimposed end-diastolic and end-systolic contours are shown to the right of each image pair.

quantitative analysis. The approximate 45-degree LAO view provides data for the quantitative count-based assessment of left ventricular function. In the equilibrium study, quantitative analysis of right ventricular function is difficult because of contamination from overlying anterior right atrial activity. For this reason, right ventricular function is best evaluated by first-pass techniques. The degree of left anterior obliquity must be individualized based upon specific patient anatomy and cardiac orientation within the thorax. The degree of obliquity is determined in a manner providing optimal separation of right and left ventricles ("best septal view"). This is a relatively straightforward approach that can be used by the technologist without physician interaction. The LAO view also provides qualitative information concerning contraction of the septal, inferoapical, and lateral walls. The anterior view provides data concerning regional motion of the anterior and apical segments. The left lateral or left posterior oblique views provide optimal qualitative information concerning contraction of the inferior wall and posterobasal segment.

Ventricular aneurysm can be assessed best in the lateral views as

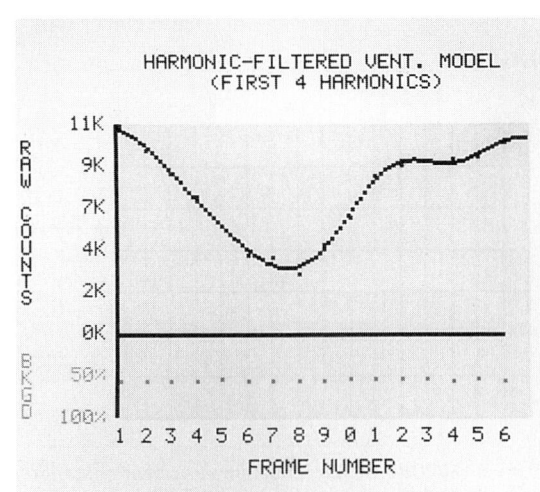

HARMONIC-FILTERED VENT. MODEL
(FIRST 4 HARMONICS)

FRAME NUMBER

FIGURE 9–35. Ventricular volume curve derived from an equilibrium radionuclide angiocardiographic study. The raw data have been smoothed using a Fourier filter technique to four harmonics. Note the discrimination of the period of rapid diastolic filling as well as the atrial contribution to diastolic filling.

well. Analysis of only the anterior and LAO views may give the false impression of an enlarged, diffusely hypokinetic ventricle, when in fact there are additional obscured zones of normally contracting myocardium. In addition to a purely visual assessment, a point scoring system can be utilized for assessing regional function. This is generally done with a 5-point score for each segment, with specific numerical grades assigned for dyskinesis, akinesis, mild and severe hypokinesis, and normal function.[236]

An advantage of labeling the entire intravascular blood pool involves visualization of all cardiac and vascular structures. Such a visual assessment can provide information concerning relative cardiac chamber sizes and the relative adequacy of contraction of each chamber. In addition, the size, orientation, and pathology of the great vessels can be defined. The relative thickness of the interventricular septum can be appreciated, as can the presence of filling defects representing intracardiac masses such as left atrial myxoma or intraventricular thrombus.

The ERNA can easily be combined with additional physiological stress testing or provocation. This may be in the form of either physiological stress such as exercise, pharmacological stress with positive ionotropic agents such as dobutamine or isoproterenol, or psychological stress.[237] Because equilibrium labeling is stable for the short term, studies can be repeated, allowing for multiple stress and control measurements.

VENTRICULAR VOLUMES. Ventricular volume also can be determined by count-based methods.[238,239] Because radioactivity at equilibrium is directly proportional to volume, it is straightforward to establish a relationship between volume of a chamber and counts emanating from a region of interest representing that chamber in the two-dimensional display. The study also requires a blood sample to serve as a calibration standard. In addition, radiation attenuation must be accounted for.[238] Attenuation measurement represents the major source of error of the technique. However, volumes measured in this manner correlate well with other analyses. Because analysis is count-based, data are independent of the constraints and errors associated with fitting a deformed left ventricle to a geometrically ideal shape. There are now available new count-based approaches to measuring volume that do not involve attenuation correction.[239] This innovative new approach simplifies substantially current volumetric analyses.

The ability to measure ventricular volumes is quite important, because volumetric changes may be critical for analysis of patients with heart failure and severely depressed systolic function. In such individuals, therapeutic benefit may be documented by a reduction in ventricular size while ejection fraction does not change. Measurement of volume is also key to understanding the process of ventricular remodeling. Furthermore, linking volumetric analysis to concomitantly obtained pressure measurements can provide important insights into ventricular pressure–volume relations during both systole and diastole. This particular approach has been employed using both nonimaging nuclear probes and gamma camera equilibrium studies in the cardiac catheterization laboratory in which direct intracavitary pressure measurements are available.[240]

Marmor et al. have utilized equilibrium blood pool studies in conjunction with a noninvasive Doppler technique for accurately measuring central aortic systolic pressure from peripheral signals. With this procedure, an assessment of systolic pressure-volume relationships as well as a measure of ventricular power can be obtained noninvasively. Ventricular power is a measurement that is relatively independent of afterload and appears suitable for following patients with depressed ventricular function receiving a variety of interventions.[242]

QUANTIFICATION OF REGIONAL FUNCTION. The equilibrium technique has been adapted for quantitative measurement of regional left ventricular function. In the LAO view, this is best done using a regional ejection fraction technique.[242,243] This technique is based upon the same principles utilized for measuring global ejection fraction. However, when regional function is assessed, the left ventricular blood pool is divided into several discrete regions with well-established anatomical correlates. The best

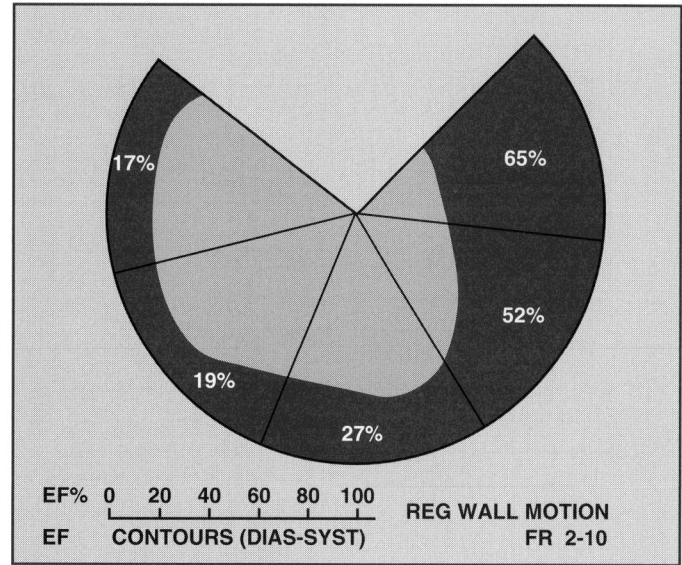

FIGURE 9–36. A typical regional ejection fraction display obtained from a left anterior oblique equilibrium study. The left ventricle is divided into five sectors. An upper sector involving the valve planes is excluded. These sectors, from upper left to upper right counterclockwise, involve upper septum, lower septum, apex, and inferolateral and posterolateral segments. In this particular study, there is a decrease of regional ejection fraction in the upper and lower septum as well as the apex, with maintained contraction of the two lateral segments.

approach involves division of the left ventricular blood pool into five regions of equal size (Fig. 9–36). These are upper and lower septal regions and inferoapical, inferolateral, and posterolateral regions. An upper zone involving the valve planes is excluded. This particular technique has been utilized in the TIMI multicenter trial and has provided meaningful insights into regional left ventricular function at rest and exercise following thrombolytic therapy.[243]

PHASE ANALYSIS OF CONTRACTION. Regional function can also be assessed from phase analysis based upon the onset, timing, and extent of contraction.[244] The phase and amplitude images also can be used for specific localization of bypass tracts in Wolff-Parkinson-White syndrome, as well as for definition of the site of sustained ventricular ectopy or tachycardia.[245]

OTHER CIRCULATORY BEDS. With the same study in which an ERNA is obtained, it is also possible to gather quantitative data concerning circulatory beds other than the heart. Since counts are proportional to volume, relative change in counts provides information concerning alterations in volume of various capacitance beds. This approach has been utilized to assess the effects of exercise and of drugs.[246,247]

Nonimaging Probe Studies

A variation of the equilibrium technique involves application of nonimaging probes for longer term (several hours) ventricular function monitoring.[248] The probes employed initially were high-sensitivity devices that provided beat-by-beat analysis as well as equilibrium analysis. High temporal resolution also allowed relatively easy assessment of diastolic filling.[249] The nonimaging probe has been utilized in a number of clinical studies; one example involved evaluation of graded infusions of intravenous nitroglycerin in patients with unstable angina.[250] The principle of monitoring ventricular function in unstable intensive care unit patients is appealing. The initial nonimaging probe called the "nuclear stethoscope" is no longer commercially available. However, new miniaturized devices have been developed.[251] This device can be affixed easily to the patient's chest and allows for serial monitoring in the intensive care unit environment. Preliminary data indicate that ejection fraction measured in this manner correlates well with that measured with conventional gamma cameras.

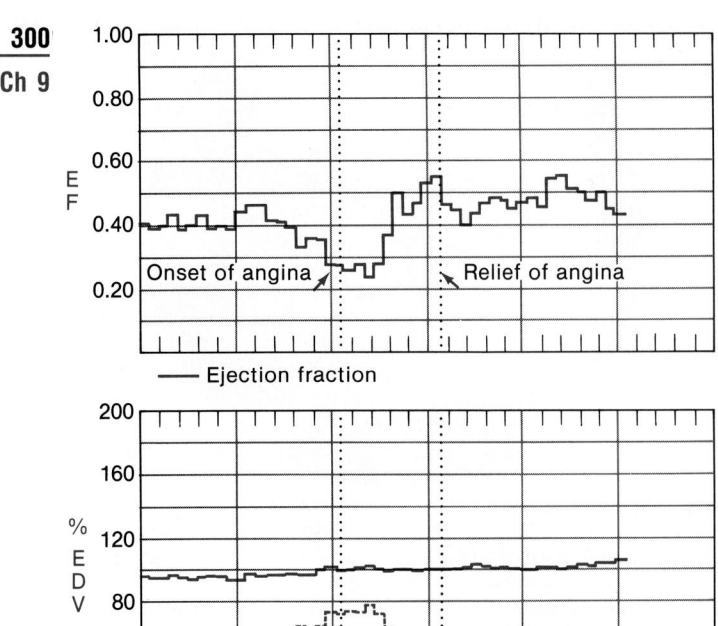

—— Ejection fraction

—— End diastolic volume   ---- End systolic volume

FIGURE 9–37.   Trended data obtained with the VEST in a patient developing postmyocardial infarction ischemia. Data for ejection fraction are shown in the upper panel and data for relative end-diastolic volume and end-systolic volume are shown in the lower panel. Continuous data are shown for a 25-minute period. The times of onset and relief of angina are indicated. The fall in ejection fraction precedes the clinical occurrence of angina. This fall is associated predominantly with a rise in end-systolic volume, with minimal change in end-diastolic volume. (From Kayden, D. S., Wackers, F. J., and Zaret, B. L.: Silent left ventricular dysfunction during routine activity after thrombolytic therapy for acute myocardial infarction. Reprinted by permission of the American College of Cardiology. J. Am. Coll. Cardiol. 15:1500, 1990.)

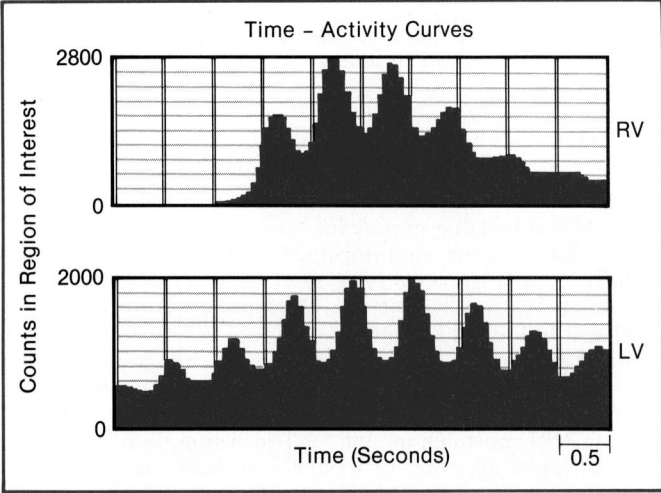

FIGURE 9–38.   Radionuclide time activity curves obtained from a right ventricular (RV) and left ventricular (LV) region of interest during a first-pass radionuclide angiocardiogram. Each peak and valley represents a single cardiac cycle. Data from this study are summed to provide right and left ventricular ejection fractions. (From Zaret, B. L., and Berger, H. J.: Nuclear Cardiology. In Hurst, J. W. (ed.): The Heart, Arteries and Veins. 7th ed. New York, McGraw-Hill Book Co., 1990, p. 1899.)

Ambulatory Monitoring

Further application of the technique of equilibrium angiocardiography relates to utilization of miniaturized equipment suitable for monitoring patients during routine activities. A newly developed instrument, called the VEST, allows for monitoring over several hours following blood pool labeling.[252] It again employs the basic principles of ERNA. The device is worn by patients so that they are fully ambulatory (Fig. 9–37). Radionuclide and electrocardiographic data are stored on tape in a manner comparable to that of the Holter monitor employed for arrhythmia detection. Offline analysis provides trended data concerning ventricular function (Fig. 9–38). This instrumentation has been validated and standardized in several laboratories and is ready for broader clinical application. Initial studies suggest a potential major role for this device in the assessment of silent myocardial ischemia and mental stress.[253–255]

SPECT Studies

The equilibrium radionuclide technique may also be suitable for application to SPECT studies. At this time, work in this area is still relatively early and experimental.[256] However, tomographic studies may provide optimal radionuclide three-dimensional assessment of global and regional function.[257]

FIRST-PASS RADIONUCLIDE ANGIOCARDIOGRAPHY

First-pass radionuclide angiocardiography was the first radionuclide technique applied to the study of cardiac physiology. The initial reports of Blumgart and Weiss occurred in 1927.[258] However, it was not until the early 1970's that the clinical and investigative impact of the measurement was appreciated.[259] The first-pass approach remains a viable alternative to equilibrium studies. At present, it is performed much less frequently than ERNA. However, with the recent availability and use of technetium-labeled myocardial perfusion agents (see p. 274), the first-pass technique may take on new significance because ventricular function can be assessed by first-pass methods at the time of injection of the perfusion agent before subsequent static perfusion imaging.

TECHNICAL CONSIDERATIONS

The FPRNA technique involves sampling for only seconds during the initial transit of the bolus through the central circulation. The high-frequency components of this radioactive passage are recorded and analyzed quantitatively.[234] It is assumed that there is sufficient mixing of the indicator with blood such that changes in count rates are proportional to volumetric changes. During the initial passage, there should be temporal and anatomical separation of radioactivity within each ventricle. Because of this, it is possible to analyze right and left ventricular function independently during this brief transit. Regional function also can be assessed from generated outlines of ventricular silhouettes.

THE SCINTILLATION CAMERA. In contrast to the equilibrium study, the choice of scintillation camera for the first-pass study is critical. Instrumentation must be utilized that provides high sensitivity with respect to count rate acquisition. If system linearity is lacking and there are major dead time losses, then data are inaccurate. For this reason the multicrystal scintillation camera was initially developed. This instrument has since been replaced by second- and third-generation digital cameras that are suitable for rapid acquisition of the high count rate data necessary for first-pass studies.

Several technical issues are relevant to performance of first-pass studies. First, the injection technique must be impeccable; it is necessary to have a compact radionuclide bolus without streaming. Injections can be made from either the jugular or the antecubital venous systems. Injections at more peripheral sites are not suitable. The presence of major arrhythmia during the evaluation invalidates the data. Because analysis is based upon at most 8 to 10 cardiac cycles, the presence of rhythmic irregularity or premature beats negates the validity of the study.

RADIOPHARMACEUTICALS. ^{99m}Tc radiopharmaceuticals are used for first-pass studies; for the most part, in the past technetium pertechnetate or technetium complexed to either DTPA or sulfur colloid was used. Thus, based on the clearance of individual tracers, multiple injections can be made during a single study. Again, with the advent of technetium-labeled perfusion agents, it is now possible also to utilize these perfusion agents for several purposes including first-pass functional evaluation. In the past, attempts were made to develop additional radiopharmaceuticals suitable for first-pass techniques. However, these short-lived generator systems have been purely investigational and have been employed for the most part only in individual laboratories with a specific research interest in their use.

PROCESSING OF FIRST-PASS STUDIES. The first-pass study is computer-processed in frame mode. Regions of interest are selected over either the right or left ventricle; generally, a fixed region of interest is used. Activity is analyzed only when the initial bolus passes through the specific chamber of interest. This temporal segregation of radioactivity compensates for the potential problem of overlapping regions of interest. Background corrections are necessary for which a variety of approaches have been described. The same approach utilized for the equilibrium study can be applied to the first-pass technique. In such a manner, global and regional left ventricular performance can be assessed. The first-pass technique is the radionuclide modality of choice for assessing *right* ventricular function.[260] This can be carried out in concert with left ventricular analysis as part of a total first-pass evaluation.

GATED FIRST-PASS TECHNIQUE. Alternatively, a gated first-pass technique can be employed at the time of tracer injection for a subsequent equilibrium study. With this latter technique, first-pass data are acquired synchronously with the electrocardiogram. They are stored temporally and several beats are subsequently summed, forming a representative cardiac cycle obtained during the right heart phase. This particular approach provides higher count rate data than could be obtained with simple bolus injection and conventional Anger camera acquisition. The data from this study also can be viewed in endless loop cine format. Unlike the case for the left ventricle, poor contrast angiographic standards exist with which right ventricular radionuclide data can be compared. For this reason, normal values for right ventricular ejection fraction have been established independently and the technique standardized.[260] Right ventricular ejection fraction is a highly afterload-dependent measure. The finding of abnormal right ventricular ejection in the absence of intrinsic right ventricular disease is excellent evidence of acquired pulmonary hypertension.[260]

Shunt Studies

The first-pass study also can be used to detect and quantify intracardiac shunts.[261] With this particular approach, a region of interest is selected over the lung field. A pulmonary time-activity curve from the region is analyzed. Normally, there is a sharp rise and subsequent fall-off of radioactivity as it enters and leaves the pulmonary vasculature. A second, lower amplitude peak occurs as a result of normal recirculation of the bolus. In the presence of a significant left-to-right shunt, persistent activity remains in the lungs and there is relatively slow washout. Techniques have been developed for applying this approach to quantification of the degree of shunting. By deconvolution of the pulmonary time-activity curve using a gamma-variate fit, the magnitude of shunting can be determined. This correlates extremely well with oximetry measures of left-to-right shunting. From right-to-left shunting, qualitative assessment demonstrating early appearance of activity in the aorta is often sufficient. Quantitative approaches also exist for defining the degree of right-to-left shunts.

Comparison of First-Pass and Equilibrium Techniques

Both the ERNA and FPRNA techniques have advantages and limitations. In addition, any one laboratory should perform that study with which it is most familiar and for which its equipment is optimal. The ERNA has several distinct advantages: (1) multiple studies can be performed following a single radionuclide injection; (2) regional assessment can be done in as many views as are relevant for analysis; (3) sequential and serial data can be obtained during a variety of control, physiological, and/or pharmacolog-

ical states; (4) the statistical reliability of high count rate equilibrium studies is superior to that of the first-pass technique; (5) the entire cardiovascular blood pool may be viewed at equilibrium; and (6) the equilibrium study is less prone to invalidation because of transient arrhythmia than is the first-pass study. On the other hand, additional activity from adjacent or overlying tissues can hinder optimal visualization of a specific ventricular segment in the ERNA. Evaluation of right ventricular performance, as well as shunt detection, is better achieved with the first-pass than the equilibrium technique. While equipment necessary for performing first-pass studies is more complex, as already stated, first-pass techniques will likely achieve resurgent popularity when combined with perfusion studies involving technetium-labeled agents.

CLINICAL ASSESSMENT OF CARDIAC PERFORMANCE

Diastolic Function

Diastolic function of the ventricles (see pp. 385 and 448) can be evaluated from either the equilibrium or first-pass study, although the former has been more frequently used. A number of indices have been described for assessing diastolic function. The most widely employed are the peak filling rate and the time-to-peak filling rate.[262] Filling fraction also has been recently studied.[263] High temporal resolution is necessary for performing these studies. Equilibrium studies have often been obtained in list mode so that ectopic or irregular beats can be eliminated from analysis. It is crucial that there be high temporal resolution and reliability of the diastolic filling phase if accurate data are to be obtained. Fourier filtering techniques, in conjunction with polynomial mathematical algorithms, have been applied to volume curves obtained by frame mode equilibrium studies of lower temporal resolution in a manner that provides accurate data. High temporal resolution nuclear probe studies also provide excellent analyses of diastole.[249]

Assessment of diastolic function has achieved increasing importance with clinical recognition of the entity of congestive heart failure associated with normal systolic and abnormal diastolic function (see p. 448). This has been most commonly observed in left ventricular hypertrophy and coronary artery disease,[262,264] as well as in restrictive cardiomyopathies. Abnormal peak filling rates have been noted in a majority of patients with coronary disease, even in the presence of normal systolic function.[262] Improvement in filling parameters has been noted following successful coronary angioplasty or after the institution of antianginal therapy. Abnormal diastolic function has been estimated to occur in as many as 30 to 40 per cent of patients hospitalized with congestive heart failure.[265]

A group of 54 such patients was described. The majority of patients with unequivocal heart failure and intact systolic performance had hypertensive or coronary disease, alone or in combination.[249] Follow-up of these patients over a 5-year period has indicated substantial cardiovascular morbidity and mortality that is not dissimilar to that of individuals manifesting systolic dysfunction alone.[266] Treatment with verapamil has been shown to improve objective and clinical parameters of heart failure as well as left ventricular filling in such patients.[267] Measurement of diastolic function is an important dimension in the assessment of ventricular performance in patients with heart failure. However, it must be noted that parameters of diastolic filling are age-dependent. Abnormal filling is noted, proportional to age, in the absence of disease.[268]

RESTING VENTRICULAR PERFORMANCE. Measurement of right and left ventricular performance at rest is clearly of value in the evaluation of patients with congestive heart failure. In the simplest assessment, this particular study can be utilized to distinguish cardiac from pulmonary or other noncardiac causes of the symptom complex. Resting function is valuable in assessing preoperative surgical risk.[269] The cause of heart failure may be inferred from the involvement of the right and/or the left ventricle as well as the presence of diffuse left ventricular dysfunction as opposed to regional dysfunction.[235] Systolic versus diastolic heart failure may be differentiated by this study. Relative chamber size may also provide important insights concerning the occurrence of concomitant or primary valvular disease.

Coronary Artery Disease

Perhaps the widest clinical and investigative application of resting radionuclide ventricular function studies has been in the assessment of patients with myocardial infarction. Several reports have documented the importance of prognostic stratification on the basis of global ventricular function as measured by ejection fraction. Ejection fraction, certainly in the prethrombolytic era, was a key factor in defining prognosis (see also p. 425).[270-274] In the thrombolytic era, ejection fraction at rest still remains an important prognostic index; however, for any level of ejection fraction, mortality is substantially lower than noted in the prethrombolytic period (Fig. 9–39).[270a] The CASS trial has also shown the importance of prognostic stratification based upon ejection fraction in patients with multivessel disease when survival was compared in patients assigned to surgical as opposed to medical therapy.[275] In patients who have survived out-of-hospital cardiac arrest, the single best prognostic factor also has been the degree of impairment in global function as measured by ejection fraction.[276]

In addition, the finding of a postinfarction functional left ventricular aneurysm carries further prognostic significance. In one study involving patients with an anterior wall infarction, the finding of aneurysm formation, as defined by nuclear data, provided relevant prognostic information not available from the ejection fraction alone.[277] In the setting of acute infarction, radionuclide studies at rest also are of major value in distinguishing true aneurysm from pseudoaneurysm and in distinguishing right from left ventricular infarction.

EXERCISE STUDIES. Ventricular performance during exercise can be assessed with either equilibrium or first-pass techniques. In general, exercise may be performed in the supine, semisupine, or nearly upright position. A normal exercise response is generally defined by an increment of at least 5 per cent (in absolute terms) in global ejection fraction of both right and left ventricles. In patients with coronary artery disease, abnormal ventricular reserve is manifested by failure of such augmentation. The finding of a major fall (>5 per cent) in ejection fraction from rest to exercise carries with it a poor prognosis.[278] Lee and colleagues have defined the prognostic impact of exercise ejection fraction data.[279] They have noted that the exercise ejection fraction itself as an absolute number provides the most relevant prognostic information. The ventricular response to exercise in patients with abnormal resting function may have greater prognostic significance than the extent of coronary disease.[280] The exercise response may also be used effectively to monitor the prognostic effects of medical therapy.[281]

SILENT MYOCARDIAL ISCHEMIA (see also p. 1344). The prognosis associated with ischemia appears not to be affected by the presence or absence of a concomitant pain syndrome.[282] Because it is recognized that radionuclide exercise studies generally add to the sensitivity and specificity of the exercise ECG, it is not surprising that the study of left ventricular function during rest and exercise provides additional information concerning prognosis in silent ischemia.[283] The ability to detect silent myocardial ischemia during routine activities (as opposed to exercise in the laboratory) is of additional importance. It is within this context that ambulatory ventricular function monitoring has achieved prominence (Fig. 9–38). Transient abnormalities in global left ventricular function during routine activity frequently occur silently.[254] Abnormal VEST responses have also been noted in the absence of symptoms during balloon occlusion at the time of coronary angioplasty, a situation producing transient transmural ischemia.[284]

Silent ventricular dysfunction also is relatively common under conditions of mental stress. This phenomenon has been demonstrated in studies using the gamma camera or nuclear probe during several forms of induced mental stress.[237,255] Regional wall motion abnormalities were readily demonstrated during mental stress in patients with coronary artery disease, with or without an associated abnormal global ejection fraction response. These responses occurred in the absence of major increments in heart rate; this suggests that altered myocardial oxygen supply is the major mechanism. Jain et al. recently demonstrated the independent prognostic significance of mental stress–induced ventricular dysfunction.[285]

Congestive Heart Failure

Analysis of left ventricular function is cardinal for the assessment of patients with known or presumed congestive heart failure. Radionuclide studies provide systolic and diastolic data of relevance. The finding of diastolic dysfunction as the primary pathophysiological abnormality may necessitate use of a different therapeutic regimen (see p. 507) from that used when systolic dysfunction alone is noted. The radionuclide study also can provide insight into the presence of valvular problems complicating or mimicking heart failure. Serial radionuclide studies provide a basis for monitoring the effects of therapy. In the presence of unexplained congestive heart failure, the demonstration of intact right ventricular function with abnormal left ventricular function speaks against primary cardiomyopathy as a cause. Generally, the most likely culprits in such a circumstance are coronary artery disease (ischemic cardiomyopathy), hypertensive heart disease, or aortic valvular disease. However, it should be noted that the converse is not necessarily true; patients with advanced left ventricular dysfunction may develop secondary pulmonary hypertension and, with this, secondary right ventricular dysfunction.

DOXORUBICIN CARDIOTOXICITY (see also p. 1800). A major role for serial radionuclide left ventricular function studies involves the moni-

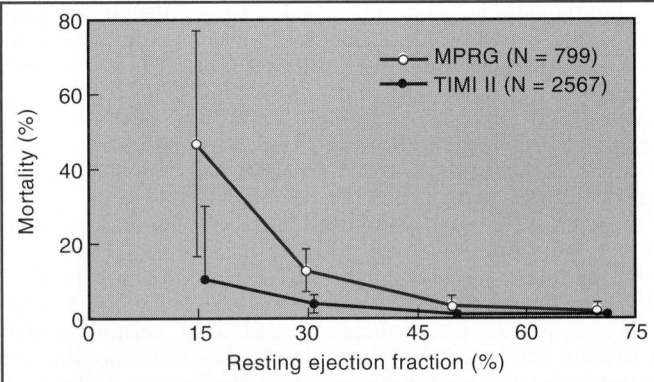

FIGURE 9–39. Relationship of rest ejection fraction to cardiac mortality in the TIMI II study *(black circles)* and MPRG (Multicenter Post Infarction Research Group Study *(open circles)*. Note the comparable shape of both mortality curves and the significantly lower mortality noted in the TIMI II study of the lower ejection fraction levels. (From Zaret, B. L., Wackers, F. J., Terrin, M. L., et al.: Value of radionuclide rest and exercise left ventricular ejection fraction to assess survival of patients following thrombolytic therapy for acute myocardial infarction: Results of the Thrombolysis in Myocardial Infarction (TIMI) Phase II study. Reprinted with permission of the American College of Cardiology. J. Am. Coll. Cardiol. *26:*73, 1995.

TABLE 9-5 GUIDELINES FOR MONITORING PATIENTS RECEIVING DOXORUBICIN

Perform baseline radionuclide angiocardiography at rest for LVEF prior to administration of 100 mg/m² doxorubicin. Subsequent studies at least 3 weeks after the indicated total cumulative doses have been given, but before next dose.

A. PATIENTS WITH NORMAL BASELINE LVEF (≥50%)
Perform the second study after 250 to 300 mg/m²
Repeat study after 400 mg/m² in patients with known heart disease, radiation exposure, abnormal electrocardiogram, or cyclophosphamide therapy; or after 450 mg/m² in the absence of any of these risk factors
Perform sequential studies thereafter before each dose
Discontinue doxorubicin if absolute decrease in LVEF ≥10% (EF units) with a decline to a level ≤50% (EF units)

B. PATIENTS WITH ABNORMAL BASELINE LVEF (<50%)
Doxorubicin therapy should not be initiated with baseline LVEF ≤30%
In patients with LVEF >30% and <50%, sequential studies should be obtained before each dose
Discontinue doxorubicin if absolute decrease in LVEF ≥10% (EF units) and/or final LVEF ≤30%

Modified from Schwartz, R. G., McKenzie, W. B., Alexander, J., et al.: Congestive heart failure and left ventricular dysfunction complicating doxorubicin therapy: Seven-year experience using serial radionuclide myocardiography. Am. J. Med. 82:1109, 1987.

toring of patients with neoplastic disease for drug-induced cardiotoxicity. Doxorubicin, a commonly employed antineoplastic agent, may be associated with development of a severe cardiomyopathy that is often both irreversible and ultimately fatal. Radionuclide ventriculography has become established as a means of detecting presymptomatic cardiotoxicity.[286-288]

Guidelines for patient management with doxorubicin based upon resting ejection fraction data have been developed and are now currently employed (Table 9-5). Retrospective analysis noted marked differences in outcome between individuals who were managed

with adherence to the radionuclide guidelines and those who were not.

It appears that resting ejection fraction provides an optimal means of assessing patients receiving cardiotoxic medication. The addition of exercise stress does not appear to add significantly to this prognostic assessment.

VALVULAR HEART DISEASE (see also Chap. 32). Rest and exercise ventricular performance studies have been employed in the study of valvular heart disease. It has been suggested that exercise left ventricular responses are of value in patients with aortic regurgitation with respect to defining the indications for aortic valve replacement, even in the asymptomatic state.[289] At the present time, this general approach is not popular. Resting studies of ventricular performance clearly play a role in the assessment of patients with suspected or known valvular disease in whom surgery is being contemplated. In the context of the mitral regurgitation, such an evaluation may be particularly relevant clinically with respect to the definition of operability.

CHRONIC OBSTRUCTIVE PULMONARY DISEASE (see also Chap. 47). Patients with chronic obstructive pulmonary disease were studied intensively when radionuclide techniques for assessing the right ventricle were developed initially.[260] It is recognized that the right ventricle is an extremely afterload-dependent structure. The presence of abnormal right ventricular ejection fraction in such patients strongly suggests the presence of significant pulmonary hypertension. Abnormalities in right ventricular performance also can be related to the degree of ventilatory and physiological impairment.[260] Right ventricular performance, as measured by ejection fraction, is responsive to agents that both augment inotropic performance as well as serve as pulmonary vasodilators.

The impact of positive end-expiratory pressure (PEEP) upon right ventricular function has also been evaluated.[290] Therapy involving PEEP is now routine in patients with severe respiratory insufficiency. Patients with normal baseline right ventricular function have no change in right ventricular volumetric status or contractile performance with PEEP. In contrast, those with depressed baseline right ventricular function manifest abnormal right ventricular hemodynamic responses to PEEP. On the basis of such data, a baseline evaluation of right ventricular performance before the institution of PEEP therapy seems reasonable. In addition, the impact of right coronary flow upon right ventricular responses to PEEP has been studied. Abnormal right ventricular performance during PEEP frequently occurs under conditions of coronary stenosis or obstruction.[290] This also has been confirmed in experimental animal preparations.[291]

SPECIAL IMAGING TECHNIQUES

ASSESSMENT OF MYOCARDIAL FATTY ACID METABOLISM BY SPECT

Long-chain fatty acids are important substrates for myocardial oxidative metabolism. Approximately 60 to 80 per cent of ATP produced derives from fatty acid oxidation.[292] In the presence of myocardial ischemia, oxidation of fatty acids is generally suppressed, with a more active role played by glucose metabolism. The study of fatty acid metabolism involves radioactive iodine labeling of free fatty acids and has been an area of active research since the early 1970's. Initially research in this area was limited by problems with loss of the radioiodine label and the subsequent introduction of substantial artifact. Recently a number of [123I]-labeled fatty acids have been introduced for imaging.[293]

There are two general groups of iodinated fatty acid compounds utilized: straight-chain fatty acids and branched-chain fatty acids. The straight-chain fatty acids are metabolized via beta-oxidation and released from the myocardium. Therefore fatty acid utilization can be assessed directly by evaluation of the washout kinetics of the radioactive tracer. This requires rapid dynamic acquisition. In the presence of ischemia, washout is slowed substantially. Consequently, by evaluating the initial degree of uptake and the subsequent washout, one can assess metabolism. The prototype straight-chain fatty acid used for imaging is [123I] phenyl pentadecanoic acid (IPPA).[293]

In order to measure absolute regional uptake of the fatty acid and quantify the initial distribution in the most precise manner, the regional uptake of the tracer must be maintained for a substantial period of time. In order to do this, the fatty acid compound can be modified with the introduction of a branched chain. This leads to metabolic trapping and allows for the acquisition of metabolic images of high quality without change in distribution during the imaging period. The methyl branching of the fatty acid chain protects the compounds from metabolism via beta-oxidation while retaining some of the physiological properties such as uptake and turnover rate in the triglyceride pool.

Currently, there are two iodinated branched chain fatty acids with which one can effectively image uptake distribution patterns: [123I]-methyl-pentadecanoic acid (BMIPP) and [123I]-dimethyl-pentadecanoic acid (DMIBP).[294]

Initial studies using both types of fatty acids have demonstrated potential for assessing myocardial viability in the presence of left

ventricular dysfunction as well as myocardial ischemia in association with stress. Combined imaging with a perfusion agent allows for appropriate assessment of regional metabolism and regional perfusion in a manner comparable to that performed with PET.[294]

IODINE-123-LABELED METAIODOBENZYLGUANIDINE IMAGING

Metaiodobenzylguanidine (MIBG) may be labeled with [125I], [131I], or [123I]. The analog participates in the same uptake and storage mechanisms as norepinephrine.[295] It is not metabolized by catechol-O-methyltransferase or monoamine oxidase. MIBG uptake for imaging involves mainly the specific uptake-1 path by which norepinephrine is stored in presynaptic vesicles. Imaging of this uptake consequently provides evidence of the intactness of sympathetic cardiac innervation as assessed by the uptake-1 pathway.[296] Doses of 4 to 10 mCi of [123I] MIBG are used for either planar or SPECT modes. Cardiac uptake can be quantified on both a global and regional basis.[296] Decreased MIBG uptake has been noted in congestive heart failure. This is consistent with the pathophysiological observations involving depletion of cardiac stores of norepinephrine in association with this condition (see p. 409).

Scintigraphic measurements of cardiac MIBG uptake have been used to evaluate patients with idiopathic cardiomyopathy. Scintigraphically determined [123I] MIBG activity correlates with that measured from endomyocardial biopsy samples.[297] Diminished MIBG uptake has been repeatedly related to various indices of left ventricular dysfunction, including left ventricular ejection fraction, cardiac index, and intraventricular pressures. In a study of 90 patients with heart failure, MIBG uptake was related inversely to prognosis. Uptake, measured as a heart/mediastinum activity ratio, had a high predictive value for survival. Multivariate analysis showed that MIBG cardiac uptake was an independent predictor.[298]

Abnormalities of regional MIBG uptake have been noted in the presence of acute ischemia, both in experimental animals and in humans.[296] Iodine-123 MIBG has been used to delineate the denervated area after myocardial infarction. Studies have demonstrated the zone of denervation to be larger than the comparable perfusion defect associated with the infarct. Altered MIBG uptake may also play a significant role in the assessment of arrhythmogenic potential in patients with heart disease as well as cardiomyopathy.

Currently, the most commonly used radiotracers reflect physiological or biochemical processes that respond to changes in cellular viability and integrity. Because oxygen supply to the heart is fundamental for cardiac function, an assessment of tissue oxygen content by tracers extracted readily by and retained significantly in the myocardium in direct response to tissue oxygen levels may provide a means of imaging hypoxic myocardium.

A class of compounds with high electron affinity, the radiolabeled nitroimidazoles, is under active evaluation for this purpose. These lipophilic compounds diffuse across the cell membrane and undergo reduction in the cytoplasm to form a radical.[299-301] When oxygen is abundant in the cell, nitroimidazol reacts with the radical anion formed to yield superoxide and noncharged nitroimidazole that then diffuses out of the cell. When intracellular hypoxia is present, the nitroimidazole radical anion is reduced further to form nitrous com-pounds that combine covalently with cytosolic macromolecules and are trapped intracellularly.

Enhanced retention of nitroimidazoles in hypoxic cells has been demonstrated in intact dogs[302,303] and perfused hearts[304] using [18F]fluoromisonidazole and in isolated adult rat myocytes[305] and dogs[306] using [3H]fluoromisonidazole. In order to have wider clinical applications, 99mTc-nitroimidazole (BMS-181321) has been developed recently to be used as a potential hypoxic marker in SPECT. Preliminary studies in dogs,[307,308] perfused hearts,[309] and isolated myocytes[309] indicate that 99mTc-nitroimidazole (BMS-181321) may serve as a sensitive marker for hypoxic myocardium. Ng et al. evaluated myocardial kinetics of 99mTc-nitroimidazole. They confirmed that tissue retention of nitroimidazol was inversely proportional to perfusate oxygen level. This report found the threshold for myocellular binding to be 60 per cent or less of the perfusate oxygen level.[310] In the future, hypoxic compounds that are more lipophilic and thus have greater myocardial retention will be developed.

POSITRON EMISSION TOMOGRAPHY

Positron emission tomography (PET), long viewed as primarily a research imaging modality, is currently becoming a clinically important technique.[311] The uniqueness of PET imaging lies in its ability to image and quantify metabolic processes, receptor occupancy, and blood flow. The main advantages of positron imaging are the ability to label and thus image biologically active compounds and drugs. A major result of these advantages is the ability to derive absolute quantitative measurements with the appropriate kinetic model.

TECHNICAL CONSIDERATIONS

Conventional single-photon emitters such as 99mTc, 123I, 201Tl, and 111In have several limitations. These isotopes decay with the emission of a single photon traveling in a random direction. The percentage of photons reaching the detector depends upon scatter attenuation and the distance between photon source and detector. These factors result in loss of relevant physiological information, which precludes accurate quantification of volumes, blood flow, and metabolism. Positron-emitting isotopes overcome these limitations. Positron-emitting radionuclides are characterized by excess protons. This unstable structure results in the conversion of an excess proton to a neutron; in the process, a positron (antielectron) is emitted. The positron travels a few millimeters in tissue; when it encounters an electron, an annihilation ensues. This results in the release of a photon pair with characteristic energy of 511 keV. These photon gamma rays travel at 180 degrees from each other. Using detectors that are paired and aligned, the photon pairs emitted from the positron annihilation can be detected by coincidence counting.

Images are obtained in a tomographic manner similar to SPECT imaging. However, in SPECT studies a single or several camera head(s) (each containing NaI crystal) are used, which rotate on a gantry. In contrast, PET imaging utilizes 1200 to 1500 small stationary crystal/detectors arranged in a circle, allowing photons to be detected in coincidence. This principle provides for correction for body attenuation and for the ability of this technology to electronically, not structurally, collimate data. These factors result in better count statistics and the ability to quantify various metabolic processes. With present technology, up to 21 simultaneous tomographic slices may be obtained, with reconstruction along cardiac planes similar to those displayed in cardiac SPECT imaging.

PROCEDURES. Current PET imaging protocols depend on both the positron emitter and detector source. Briefly, the heart must be localized by either fluoroscopy or various transmission scan programs. The patient is positioned with arms above the head or at the sides so that the heart is within the 12-cm detector range. After the patient is made comfortable, a 10- to 30-minute attenuation scan (depending on the ring source) is acquired. This allows subtraction of activity in noncardiac structures from the overall field of view, thereby providing an isolated image of only cardiac activity. The positron-emitting radionuclide then is injected. Allowance must be made for individual variation in the time needed for accumulation and subsequent acquisition of each radiopharmaceutical. For example, metabolic imaging with 18FDG (fluorodeoxyglucose) requires injection of 5 to 10 mCi. Then 30 to 40 minutes must elapse before FDG image acquisition is initiated for an additional 20 to 30 minutes.

RADIOPHARMACEUTICALS. Many positron emitters are unique because their naturally occurring counterparts (hydrogen, carbon, nitrogen, and oxygen) are predominant constituents of natural compounds. Positron-emitting isotopes of carbon, nitrogen, and oxygen may replace stable counterparts in the synthesis of metabolic substrate, receptor ligands, drugs, and other biologically active compounds without disrupting biochemical properties or activity. Fluorine-18 is also a suitable substitute for naturally occurring hydrogen because of its strong carbon-fluorine bond and stearic effect similar to that of hydrogen. Positron-emitting tracers generally have shorter physical half-lives than most single-photon emitters. This property allows for repeat injections as a means of observing rapidly changing events over time. Table 9-6 summarizes the PET radioisotopes, half-lives, and synthesized radiopharmaceuticals suitable for use in cardiovascular medicine.

Clinical Indications

PET studies are recommended for the identification of myocardial viability in patients with established coronary

TABLE 9-6 POSITRON EMITTERS IN CARDIOVASCULAR IMAGING

ISOTOPE	HALF-LIFE	LABELED COMPOUND	APPLICATION
18F	109 min	18F Fluoro-2-deoxyglucose (18FDG)	Carbohydrate metabolism
		18F Fluorodopamine	Adrenergic neuronal imaging
		18F-6 Fluorometaraminol	Adrenergic neuronal imaging
		18F Misonidazole	Tissue hypoxia
13N	10 min	13N Ammonia	Perfusion
		13N Amino acids (glutamate, alanine, leucine, aspartate)	Amino acid metabolism
11C	20 min	11C Amino acids (alanine, leucine, tryptophan)	Amino acid metabolism
		11C Palmitate	Fatty acid metabolism
		11C Acetate	Myocardial oxygen consumption
		11C Butanol	Perfusion
		11C Hydroxyephedrine	Adrenergic neuronal imaging
		11C CGP 12177	Muscarinic receptor density
		11C Carazolol	Beta-receptor imaging
15O	2 min	15O Oxygen	Oxygen utilization
		15O Water	Blood flow quantification
82Rb	75 sec	82Rb Chloride	Perfusion
68Ga	68 min	68Ga Platelets	Thrombus formation

artery disease and regional or global left ventricular dysfunction[311,312] and for the noninvasive diagnosis of coronary artery disease. Other readily available imaging alternatives have limited PET application for these indications. These include conventional perfusion imaging, reinjection thallium imaging, and the development of new classes of [99mTc]-perfusion agents.[313] Although [201Tl] and PET both have high accuracies for predicting recovery of regional and global left ventricular dysfunction after revascularization, PET has a higher positive and negative predictive accuracy for improvement in left ventricular function and is considered the gold standard for detection of viability.[314] Specific comparisons between various modalities are discussed below.

Assessment of Myocardial Viability

An accurate assessment of the presence and extent of viable yet poorly contractile myocardium and its discrimination from purely infarcted tissue are of clinical importance.[315] Myocardial viability is particularly relevant to current cardiology practice because revascularization and reperfusion can be established by surgery or by a variety of catheter-based techniques (see p. 286). An assessment of viability is important with respect to establishing the appropriateness of these procedures as well as their ultimate efficacy. Available imaging techniques must be able to differentiate "stunned" or "hibernating" myocardium from true infarcted tissue.

For institutions without PET facilities, myocardial viability is generally assessed with [201Tl] scintigraphy (see p. 294). The assessment of myocardial viability with [99mTc]-sestaMIBI still is under active investigation, and results are variable with regard to the positive and negative predictive accuracies for reversal of wall motion abnormalities after revascularization or to direct comparison with thallium scintigraphy.[209,316–318] Although modified single-photon imaging protocols for detecting viable myocardium have been performed, the results are still suboptimal. PET imaging generally is regarded as the gold standard and final arbiter in decisions regarding viability. Viable but dysfunctional myocardium can be assessed by metabolic PET imaging with [18F]-FDG as a marker of glucose utilization, [11C]-acetate as a marker of oxidative metabolism, and [15O]-H_2O (water-perfusable tissue index) to assess the rate of water exchange.

FLUORINE-18 DEOXYGLUCOSE. Assessment of myocardial viability by PET imaging involves comparison of regional myocardial perfusion with regional glucose utilization. Myocardial perfusion can be visualized and quantified with flow tracers such as [82Rb], [13N] ammonia, and [15O] water. Regional myocardial metabolism is visualized with [18F]-fluorodeoxyglucose (FDG). Experimental studies have demonstrated that glucose utilization is *augmented* in segments that are hypoperfused and ischemic but nevertheless viable. During ischemia energy production shifts from the oxidation of free fatty acids to that of glucose. Under normal conditions, glycolysis (glucose utilization) predominantly results in CO_2 production with minimal lactate generation. However, during ischemia, lactate production is increased relative to CO_2 production; glucose may contribute up to 70 per cent of the total energy production during ischemia.[319]

Metabolism as assessed with [18F]-FDG, traces exogenous glucose utilization. When FDG exchanges across the cellular membrane in proportion to glucose exchange, it competes for the enzyme hexokinase. The phosphorylated glucose analog, FDG-6-phosphate, unlike the native glucose-6-phosphate, is a poor substrate for glycolysis, glycogen synthesis, or the fructose-pentose shunt. It also is relatively impermeable to cell membranes, because the enzyme that catalyzes the reverse reaction, glucose-6-phosphatase, is absent or present in only negligible quantities. Therefore, the tracer becomes trapped in the myocardium

and its persistent activity reflects regional rates of exogenous glucose uptake and utilization.[320] In myocardial segments with irreversible injury, tissue glucose utilization declines linearly with blood flow. Thus, in patients with ischemic heart disease, PET imaging with [18F] deoxyglucose has been useful in discriminating hypoperfused but viable tissue from regions with irreversible injury.[321–325]

Cross-sectional left ventricular images are acquired 2 to 5 minutes following intravenous injection of a flow tracer. Then, 5 to 15 mCi of FDG are injected and metabolic images obtained 30 to 50 minutes after injection. These images can be analyzed by circumferential activity profile analysis similar to that employed in SPECT thallium image processing.[326]

Three basic patterns of comparative blood flow and metabolism activity distribution are demonstrable (Fig. 9–40). First, there may be a match between flow and metabolic activity with homogeneous myocardial distribution of each tracer (normal). Second, regional blood flow may be decreased while glucose utilization in the same area is normal or increased relative to normally perfused myocardium or to the regions with reduced blood flow. This pattern of blood flow–metabolism mismatch is the PET scintigraphic signature of myocardial viability in the presence of ventricular dysfunction. Third, regional myocardial blood flow and glucose utilization may be concordantly decreased. This pattern is the marker of myocardial scar and irreversible damage.

CLINICAL APPLICATIONS. There have been several clinical investigations demonstrating that blood flow–metabolism mismatch on PET images is representative of hypoperfused but viable myocardium. These studies are based on the demonstration of improvement in regional wall motion after revascularization in regions demonstrating flow-metabolism mismatch (diminished flow, increased glucose uptake).[202,325,327,328]

Tillisch and colleagues evaluated 17 patients with a total of 73 regions with abnormal resting wall motion.[202] Those myocardial segments that showed preserved glucose uptake in regions of abnormal wall motion predicted reversibility of wall motion abnormalities following bypass surgery. In contrast, abnormal motion in regions with depressed glucose uptake did not improve following revascularization. Abnormal contraction in 35 of 41 segments was correctly predicted to be reversible (85 per cent predictive accuracy). Abnormal contraction in 24 of 26 regions was correctly predicted to be irreversible (92 per cent predictive accuracy). In the 17 patients, left ventricular ejection fraction averaged 32 ± 14 per cent before and 41 ± 15 per cent after revascularization. This improvement was more marked in 11 patients with two or more regions that were either normal or revealed glucose activity in hypoperfused segments. Left ventricular ejection fraction increased in these patients from 30 ± 11 per cent to 45 ± 14 per cent ($P < 0.05$), compared with no improvement in the remaining 6 patients with only one or no mismatched FDG/blood flow regions.

In a comparable study, Tamaki et al. performed PET myocardial perfusion and FDG metabolic imaging before and 5 to 7 weeks after coronary artery bypass surgery in 22 patients.[325] Postoperative improvement in wall motion abnormalities was observed more often in the metabolically active segments (78 per cent) than in the metabolically inactive segments (22 per cent) ($P < 0.001$). Thus, the persistence of metabolic activity with FDG identifies viable, dysfunctional myocardium. An alternative approach using postexercise FDG PET imaging was used by Marwick et al. to determine the spectrum of metabolic responses of hibernating myocardium, as well as to predict improvement in exercise capacity after revascularization.[327,328]

These studies reinforce the concept that metabolic imaging with PET is a useful tool to predict the reversal of preoperative wall motion abnormalities after successful revascularization. These studies also point out that although a subgroup shows improvement in wall motion and perfusion after revascularization, myocardial metabolism may remain abnormal. The latter occurred in segments with extensive perfusion and metabolic changes preoperatively.[328] In a separate study by the same author, postexercise FDG uptake in patients with previous myocardial infarction predicted improvement in regional systolic function as well as in exercise tolerance after revascularization.[327] Studies addressing the ability of modified SPECT camera systems to accept 511-keV photons, specifically [18FDG], have been performed.[329,330] These preliminary studies suggest that [18FDG] SPECT

FIGURE 9–40. See color plate 8.

TABLE 9–7 POSITRON IMAGING PATTERNS AND MORTALITY IN CORONARY ARTERY DISEASE AND LEFT VENTRICULAR DYSFUNCTION

STUDY	NUMBER OF PATIENTS	VIABLE		NONVIABLE	
		Medical	Revascularization	Medical	Revascularization
Eitzman et al.[331]	83	6/18	1/26	2/24	0/14
DiCarli et al.[332]	93	7/17	3/26	3/33	1/17
Lee et al.[333]	137	10/21	4/49	2/40	2/19
TOTAL	313	23/56	8/101	7/97	3/50
% mortality		41%	8%	7%	6%

imaging may be a clinical and cost-effective means for the metabolic assessment of left ventricular myocardial viability.

PROGNOSIS AND PET IMAGING FOR MYOCARDIAL VIABILITY. Prognostic stratification of patients with coronary artery disease and left ventricular dysfunction recently has been addressed with metabolic PET imaging. There are three reports (one retrospective, two prospective) that address this issue using paired perfusion-FDG metabolic PET studies (Table 9–7).[331–333] In each of these studies patients were characterized as FDG viable or nonviable and then according to treatment with medical therapy or revascularization. Both studies then looked at mortality among four subgroups. The mortality rate was significantly lower in patients with a PET mismatch pattern who were revascularized. When these three studies are combined in a total of 313 patients, patients with a PET scintigraphic marker of viability had significantly lower mortality following revascularization compared with medical therapy (8 per cent versus 41 per cent). The patients were followed for approximately 1 year in two studies[331,332] and for a mean of 18 months in the remaining study.[333]

Another study also determined the prognostic value of PET in patients who underwent either revascularization or medical therapy.[334] This study was based on infarct size and viability measured by rubidium PET. The extent of scar and the presence of viable myocardium by PET in vascular areas at risk in patients with myocardial infarction were highly predictive of 3-year mortality. This study differed from the others discussed above because it included patients with a normal ejection fraction.[334] In a study by Tamaki et al., 158 patients with myocardial infarction were referred for FDG PET and stress thallium imaging.[335] Eighty-four patients were followed for a mean interval of 23 months. This study confirmed that an increase in FDG uptake was the best predictor of future cardiac events when compared with clinical, angiographic, and radionuclide variables. An increase in FDG uptake was also predictive even when a stress thallium-201 scan did not show redistribution.

COMPARISON OF PET FDG WITH THALLIUM-201-REDISTRIBUTION/REINJECTION SCINTIGRAPHY. Studies directly comparing ^{201}Tl redistribution scintigraphy and PET have been performed.[336–339] As detailed above, standard ^{201}Tl redistribution imaging underestimates the amount of viable myocardium compared with reinjection imaging. Thus, although these studies indicate that PET metabolic imaging is superior to standard thallium scintigraphy without reinjection in the delineation of viable myocardium, they currently are not particularly relevant.

Two reports have compared thallium reinjection and PET FDG imaging.[204,340] In the study by Bonow et al., PET FDG scintigraphic findings correlated a high percentage of the time with ^{201}Tl reinjection scintigraphy in severe irreversible defects that had less than 50 per cent of maximum counts on the initial post-stress image. However, moderate and mild irreversible thallium defects, when imaged with PET FDG and subsequent thallium reinjection, showed a greater discordance.[204] This was confirmed in a study by Tamaki et al., in which the thallium reinjection defect scores were not segregated according to the magnitude of the defect, and an overall discordance rate of 25 per cent was noted.[340]

COMPARISON OF PET FDG WITH SESTAMIBI SCINTIGRAPHY. Several studies have been performed comparing FDG and MIBI in the assessment of myocardial viability in patients with chronic coronary artery disease.[213,316–318, 341, 342] Some authors found FDG uptake in 23 per cent of the resting perfusion defects as assessed with sestamibi.[317] FDG is most helpful in distinguishing viability in those MIBI defects that were 31 to 50 per cent of peak normalized counts, clinically considered to be severe defects.

The potential for sestamibi to underestimate viability has been addressed by two additional studies.[318,342] In the study by Sawada et al., FDG evidence of viability was present in 50 per cent of segments with ^{99m}Tc-sestamibi activity less than 40 per cent. Moderate defects (50 to 59 per cent of peak activity) were viable as assessed by FDG.[342] These results were reinforced by another study, which revealed that a major portion of the discordance was contributed by the inferior wall myocardial segments.[318] The latter suggests that inferior wall attenuation artifact on sestamibi SPECT imaging may contribute significantly to the underestimation of viability by sestamibi.

A study by Dilsizian et al. showed that same-day rest/stress sestaMIBI imaging incorrectly identified 36 per cent of myocardial regions as irreversibly impaired and nonviable compared with both thallium redistribution/reinjection and PET FDG imaging.[213]

OTHER CONSIDERATIONS. Several aspects of FDG metabolic imaging require resolution. The dietary state of patients undergoing metabolic imaging is to be standardized. Some investigators studied patients with FDG in the fasting state and others after feeding and glucose loading. We recommend PET imaging using ^{13}N-ammonia and [18]FDG in the glucose-loaded state.[343] It also is not clear how accurate PET assessments of viability will be when tomography is performed early in the postinfarct period. Most studies to date have been performed late after the acute event. Other issues concern the accuracy of this technique in patients with diabetes and the lack of data concerning interobserver and intraobserver variability.

ADDITIONAL PET MARKERS OF MYOCARDIAL METABOLISM

The study of flow/FDG relationships is only one approach for the assessment of myocardial metabolism in ischemic conditions. Metabolic perturbation may occur on a cellular level as a result of acute or chronic ischemia and not be detected by flow/FDG relationships. Cardiac work depends on the availability of high-energy phosphate production, which is derived normally from the oxidation of long-chain fatty acids.[319] Only when fatty acid levels are low and glucose levels are high (as in the postprandial state) does the heart utilize glucose oxidation as a major source of energy. Therefore, it is relevant to evaluate other markers of myocardial metabolism in patients with coronary artery disease.[344–348]

[11]C-ACETATE. Dynamic PET studies of ^{11}C-acetate kinetics provide a noninvasive measurement of regional myocardial oxygen consumption.[349] Furthermore, myocardial blood flow may be quantified using the same tracer injection. Clearance of ^{11}C-acetate from the myocardium is bi-exponential.[350] The decay constant of the initial component of the clearance curve is linearly related to myocardial oxygen consumption. Analysis of ^{11}C kinetics is thought to accurately reflect myocardial oxygen consumption and thus mitochondrial oxidative flux in human subjects.[351]

Gropler et al. quantified myocardial oxidative metabolism by analysis of the rate of myocardial clearance of ^{11}C-acetate in 35 patients with ischemic myocardial dysfunction who were undergoing coronary revascularization. Glucose metabolism was assessed preoperatively and by analysis of FDG uptake. The predictive value for recovery of regional function based on measurements of oxidative and glucose metabolism was compared. In myocardial segments with initially severe dysfunction, ^{11}C-acetate clearance appeared to have better positive and negative predictive values than FDG, although the difference did not reach statistical significance.[352] The complementary role of ^{11}C-acetate in PET myocardial viability imaging may be its ability to distinguish viable from nonviable myocardium in acute infarction (Fig. 9–41). In this setting where myocardial stunning may be predominant, an index of overall oxidative metabolism may be more accurate than FDG.[320] Additionally, because ^{11}C-acetate is not influenced by substrate availability, it may be more useful than FDG imaging in diabetic patients with chronic coronary artery disease. Imaging with ^{11}C-acetate in this setting would make unnecessary the titration of serum insulin levels with an insulin clamp and/or serial serum glucose measurements titrated by insulin administration.[353]

RUBIDIUM-82. Myocardial viability also can be assessed by dynamic measurements of resting myocardial kinetics of [82]Rb. [82]Rb is extracted

FIGURE 9–41. See color plate 8.

and retained by viable and normal myocardium, whereas it clears rapidly from necrotic myocardium, resulting in a defect.[354] Further studies addressing the functional outcome after revascularization are needed to establish the clinical usefulness of [82]Rb as a marker of myocardial viability.

WATER-PERFUSABLE TISSUE INDEX. The water-perfusable tissue index assesses myocardial viability based on the principle that normal or viable myocardium, and not scar, exchanges water rapidly.[355] Preliminary data by DeSilva et al. in patients with chronic coronary artery disease and previous myocardial infarction who underwent revascularization show that the perfusable tissue index accurately predicted contractile recovery after revascularization, and that there was good agreement with FDG in this regard. This study should be considered preliminary until performed in a larger group of patients.[356]

ASSESSMENT OF MYOCARDIAL BLOOD FLOW

The assessment of myocardial blood flow with PET can be performed with either [82]Rb, ^{13}N ammonia, ^{15}O-labeled water, or copper pyruvaldehyde bis (N[4]-methylthiosemicarbazonate) (PTSM). [82]Rb and ^{13}N ammonia are transiently trapped in the myocardium proportional to regional distribution of blood flow.[357–359] [15]O water is an inert diffusible tracer that accumulates in and clears from the myocardium as a function of blood flow.[358] Rubidium is a potassium analog that in part requires the sodium-potassium transport pump for uptake and thus utilizes energy for its myocardial trapping.[360,361] Its first-pass extraction fraction is 65 per cent.[359] [82]Rb is a unique and convenient radiopharmaceutical to use because it is generator-produced and does not depend upon a cyclotron for production. Because its half-life is only 76 seconds, repeated measurements may be performed to assess the effects of rapid physiological interventions.[359]

Copper PTSM is another noncyclotron, generator-produced tracer with a high single pass extraction, and it may prove to be another alternative for measuring blood flow with PET.[362,363] [13]N ammonia has a first-pass extraction fraction of 80 per cent and requires energy for myocardial trapping.[357] [13]N ammonia is converted to ^{13}N glutamine by the glutamine synthetase reaction.[326] Myocardial uptake of ^{13}N is linear over a wide range of myocardial blood flow (44 and 200 ml/min/100 g). However, at flows higher than 200 ml/min/100 g, uptake is not linear and flow measurement is inaccurate in this range. Similar lack of linearity at high blood flow has been observed for [82]Rb.[360] This characteristic is true for all myocardial perfusion agents, including ^{201}Tl, sestaMIBI, and tetrofosmin.

It has not been firmly established that flow measurements with either of these positron emitters are totally independent of metabolic conditions. Accumulation of these tracers depends upon some level of tissue viability following the ischemic insult.[323,364,365] Therefore, absolute quantification of blood flow with these two tracers may be limited by the nonlinear uptake at high flow rates and the extent to which metabolic factors affect the myocardial retention of these tracers. In contrast, water labeled with [15]O (half-life = 2.1 minutes) is a diffusible tracer of myocardial blood flow. Its extraction fraction is independent of the metabolic state of the myocardium.[366] Accurate measurements of absolute myocardial blood flow may be performed across a wide spectrum of flow values[367]; however, measurements with this tracer may be more technically challenging.

CORONARY BLOOD FLOW. The noninvasive absolute quantification of myocardial blood flow in vivo is a major advantage of positron imaging. The relationship between myocardial blood flow and the severity of coronary artery stenosis has been measured by positron emission tomography with ^{15}O-labeled water at rest and during hyperemia induced with intravenous adenosine.[368] Absolute quantitative basal myocardial blood flow remained constant regardless of the severity of coronary artery stenosis. In contrast, during hyperemia there was a progressive decrease in flow reserve when the degree of stenosis was 40 per cent or more. This study supports the high degree of sensitivity for PET to detect the functional significance of subcritical stenosis during pharmacological intervention.

The augmentation of myocardial perfusion reserve after coronary angioplasty has been quantified by PET H$_2$ [15]O studies.[369] The high concentration of [15]O water in the intracavitary blood pool occurs concomitantly with myocardial activity. This necessitates subtraction of the blood pool activity in order to obtain an accurate assessment of myocardial perfusion.[370,371]

Diagnosis of Coronary Artery Narrowing

The anatomical delineation of coronary artery luminal narrowing by coronary angiography may not accurately reflect the functional significance of coronary artery disease.[372] PET imaging with [13]NH$_3$ and [82]Rb has identified abnormal flow reserve in patients with coronary artery disease. The term "flow reserve" is meaningful to the extent that absolute measurement before and after pharmacological intervention is measured. Absolute flow reserve reflects the cumulative effects of physiological factors such as vasomotor tone, workload, hypertrophy, and stenosis. Relative flow reserve measurement reflects more specifically

TABLE 9–8 DIAGNOSTIC ASSESSMENT OF CORONARY ARTERY DISEASE WITH POSITRON EMISSION TOMOGRAPHY

STUDY	NUMBER OF PATIENTS	SENSITIVITY (%)	SPECIFICITY (%)
Gupta[377]	48	94	95
Stewart et al.[381]	81	84	88
Williams[378]	208	98	93
Go et al.[108]	132	95	82
Stewart[379]	60	87	82
Demer et al.[376]	193	94	95
Tamaki et al.[375]	51	88	90
Yonekura et al.[382]	60	97	100
Gould et al.[374]	50	95	100
Schelbert et al.[373]	32	97	100
TOTAL	915	93%	93%

coronary stenosis independent of these other physiological variables and thus is comparable (with regard to mechanism) to reversible/nonreversible SPECT flow tracers for the assessment of CAD. PET myocardial perfusion imaging using either [82]Rb, ^{13}N ammonia, or ^{15}O-labeled water has identified abnormal perfusion reserve in patients with coronary artery disease with high sensitivity and specificity[108,373–382] (Table 9–8). Cardiac PET detects coronary artery disease with similar accuracy in asymptomatic as well as symptomatic subjects[375] and is equal to or better than arteriography for following changes in stenosis severity.[359]

In another study, 50 patients were studied with either [82]Rb or ^{13}N ammonia after intravenous dipyridamole and isometric handgrip stress. Quantitative coronary arteriography was obtained to determine coronary flow reserve. Those patients with a coronary flow reserve of less than 3 were identified accurately by PET imaging.[374]

Limited coronary artery perfusion reserve can also be delineated with ^{15}O-labeled water. Abnormalities in myocardial perfusion reserve have been reported in relative and absolute terms.[358,369,380] In one study, perfusion distal to a coronary stenosis after dipyridamole increased to only 64 per cent of that in normal anatomical areas. However, as quantified with PET, areas with successfully dilated arteries had postdipyridamole perfusion similar to areas supplied by nonstenotic vessels.[371]

COMPARISON WITH THALLIUM-201 SCINTIGRAPHY. The higher-energy photons released from positron-emitting tracers in conjunction with attenuation correction and higher resolution overcome to a major extent the photon attenuation problems commonly encountered with thallium studies. Three studies directly compared ^{201}Tl stress scintigraphy and PET perfusion studies in the same patient.[375,379,381]

Tamaki and colleagues studied 51 patients (48 with coronary artery disease) with exercise thallium SPECT and PET employing dipyridamole and ^{13}N ammonia. Both qualitative and semiquantitative image interpretation and qualitative analysis of the coronary arteriogram were employed. Of the 48 coronary artery disease patients, SPECT showed abnormal perfusion in 46 (96 per cent), and PET detected abnormalities in 47 (98 per cent). The sensitivity for detecting disease in individual coronary arteries (>50 per cent stenosis) was similar for SPECT (81 per cent) and PET (88 per cent). However, preliminary data in 60 patients who underwent [82]Rb PET and Tl-SPECT imaging within a 4-week interval recorded a higher specificity for PET.[381]

GATED PET PERFUSION STUDIES. Gated myocardial PET also has been performed, quantified, and compared with magnetic resonance imaging in controls and with left ventriculography in patients with coronary artery disease.[383] In controls, percentage of wall thickening showed a good correlation with percentage of count increase. In coronary artery disease patients, count increase decreased significantly as wall motion worsened. This investigational technique could eventually provide assessment of left ventricular regional function at the time of PET perfusion imaging.

NEUROCARDIOLOGIC POSITRON EMISSION TOMOGRAPHIC IMAGING

Several reports utilizing single-photon imaging with radioiodinated M-iodobenzylguanidine (MIBG) have underscored the usefulness of evaluating presynaptic adrenergic neuronal function.[384–386] However, this agent defines activity only in the presynaptic system and requires several hours for detection and resolution of MIBG-derived radioactivity in cardiac tissue compared with that in blood.[387] Thus, conventional MIBG imaging is not suited for kinetic analysis and quantification of sympathetic function.

PET neurocardiac studies may develop into a new approach focusing on sympathetic and parasympathetic interactions, neural regulation of the coronary circulation, adrenergic mechanisms in the genesis of arrhythmias, cardiac reflexes, and sympathetic innervation in the failing heart. Currently, PET imaging may assess preganglionic and postganglionic neurochemistry, providing the opportunity to gain insights in cardiovascular neurohormonal interactions. ^{18}F-fluorodopamine can be used to visualize sympathetic innervation and function in vivo.[388] ^{18}F-fluorodopamine is converted to ^{18}F-fluoronorepinephrine in synaptic adrenergic vesicles. Imaging with this agent allows depiction of tissue sites of uptake, retention, and excretion for 3 hours after injection. The homogeneous uptake of the tracer occurs within 2 to 5 minutes after injection and is independent of blood flow because displacement with reserpine and desipramine inhibit uptake and retention of the tracer.

Visualization of the cardiac sympathetic nervous system has also been performed with ^{11}C hydroxyephedrine (^{11}C HED), an analog of norepinephrine.[389] Comparative studies were performed in six normal volunteers and five cardiac transplant patients, the latter representing a model of global cardiac denervation. The normal volunteers showed homogeneous uptake of ^{11}C HED and of [82]Rb. However, the transplant patients, while demonstrating normal blood flow with [82]Rb, had a markedly reduced uptake of ^{11}C HED.

Other cardiac neuronal agents such as [^{18}F] 6-fluorometaraminol are under investigation.[390] Furthermore, true postganglionic receptor imaging may be possible with the ongoing development of muscarinic and beta-receptor ligands. In a recent study by Valette et al., PET was used serially in dogs to assess changes in ventricular muscarinic and beta-adrenergic densities following chemical and surgical denervation with the ligand CGP 12177. Their results showed an up-regulation of beta-adrenergic receptor densities following chemical or surgical denervation without any serial changes in muscarinic receptor density.[391] Adrenergic receptor imaging has direct clinical applicability in patients with left ventricular dysfunction, heart failure, and painful or silent myocardial ischemia. In patients with heart failure, quantification of specific beta-adrenergic receptor binding may provide a useful index for beta-blocker therapy in congestive heart failure.[392]

The reason for the lack of pain perception in silent myocardial ischemia is unclear. Although peripheral levels of circulating endorphins correlate with pain threshold, recent observations indirectly measuring central nervous system modulation of opiate receptor outflow challenge the contribution of opiate pathways in silent myocardial ischemia.[393,394] The quantification of regional opiate receptors with tracers such as ^{11}C diprenorphine may deliver important insights into silent myocardial ischemia and the central nervous system modulation of specific cardiovascular presentations.[395]

NONINVASIVE ASSESSMENT OF CHOLESTEROL LOWERING

Evidence supports the benefits of aggressive cholesterol lowering in secondary prevention studies, which results in a decrease in coronary events.[396–399] Longitudinal noninvasive management with dipyridamole PET has been shown to demonstrate a decrease in the size and severity of perfusion abnormalities in patients with successful vigorous cholesterol lowering during a 90-day intensive lowering treatment plan.[400] These same patients had a final control period off their lipid-lowering regimens, with repeat rest-dipyridamole PET which showed significant increases (worsening) in the size and severity of perfusion abnormalities. The pathophysiological mechanisms that may account for improved perfusion defects over such a short period of cholesterol lowering are not likely explained by anatomical regression of atherosclerosis but may be more consistent with restoration of endothelium-dependent vasodilatation by a reduction and/or pharmacological manipulation of serum lipids.[401] These provocative observations provide a basis for future studies with larger populations that would address absolute serial changes in perfusion.

Future of Clinical Cardiovascular PET Imaging

The initial capital costs and maintenance of PET technology have limited its availability. In those institutions where both PET and SPECT are available, established referral patterns suggest that PET is used in situations where conventional modalities render equivocal results (for example, attenuation artifacts on SPECT imaging or questions about the presence of viable myocardium). The higher spatial resolution and attenuation correction may justify direct PET referrals when the pretest likelihood of coronary artery disease is low.[402] Socioeconomic changes have influenced institutions with PET capability to offer PET imaging at competitive cost compared with SPECT and conventional nuclear cardiology studies. In institutions where SPECT and PET are both available, for reasons stated above PET

viability studies frequently are a final resort for making difficult clinical decisions in high-risk coronary artery disease patients after conventional myocardial perfusion imaging, echocardiography, and coronary angiography have been performed.[318,322,323,332]

In the future, the clinical indications for cardiac PET may be more widely used if the prices of PET studies decline, and regional distribution of PET radiopharmaceuticals or generator-produced radiopharmaceuticals becomes available. These trends already are in place in some locales and may play an important role in the wider future use of PET in clinical cardiology. Patterson et al. addressed economic aspects of a multimodality approach to the diagnosis of coronary artery disease with a comparison of stress PET, SPECT, coronary angiography, and stress ECG.[403] Their analysis suggested that stress PET is most economical with lowest cost per use in patients with a less than 70 per cent pretest likelihood of coronary artery disease. Two future diagnostic indications may provide an expanded role for PET in clinical cardiology. These include absolute quantification of regional myocardial blood flow and the assessment of adrenergic neuronal integrity.

To the extent that endothelial dysfunction represents the results of lipid deposition and is expressed clinically by altered vasomotor control, the absolute quantification of myocardial blood flow with interventions designed to detect early coronary artery disease with PET may emerge.[404,405] In addition, the interaction between flow and mechanical left ventricular function may be addressed in various clinical situations such as ventricular remodeling and in those instances in which mechanical dysfunction exceeds the extent of coronary artery disease.

Adrenergic receptor density in the myocardium may be of increasing importance in the future. Given the neurohormonal contribution to presentations such as congestive heart failure,[406] acute myocardial infarction,[407] long Q-T syndrome,[408] and sudden death,[409] PET may play an important role in identifying, stratifying, and monitoring therapy in these patients.

REFERENCES

INSTRUMENTATION

1. Garcia, E. V.: Quantitative myocardial perfusion single-photon emission computed tomographic imaging: Quo vadis? (Where do we go from here?) J. Nucl. Cardiol. 1:83, 1994.
2. Rullo, F., and Patton, J. A.: Instrumentation and information portrayal. In Freeman, L. M. (eds.): Freeman and Johnson's Clinical Radionuclide Imaging. Orlando, Grune & Stratton, 1988, p. 203.

MYOCARDIAL PERFUSION IMAGING

3. Carr, E. A., Gleason, G., Shaw, J., et al.: The direct diagnosis of myocardial infarction by photoscanning after administration of cesium-131. Am. Heart J. 68:627, 1964.
4. Zaret, B. L., Strauss, H. W., Martin, N. D., et al.: Noninvasive regional myocardial perfusion with radioactive potassium. N. Engl. J. Med. 288:809, 1973.
5. Bradley-Moore, P. R., Lebowitz, E., Greene, M. W., et al.: Thallium-201 for medical use. II: Biologic behavior. J. Nucl. Med. 16:156, 1975.
6. Strauss, H. W., Harrison, K., Langan, J. K., et al.: Thallium-201 for myocardial imaging. Relation of thallium-201 to regional myocardial perfusion. Circulation 51:641, 1975.
7. Wackers, F. J. Th., van der Schoot, J. B., Busemann Sokole, E., et al.: Noninvasive visualization of acute myocardial infarction in man with thallium-201. Br. Heart J. 37:741, 1975.
8. Kaul, S.: A look at 15 years of planar thallium-201 imaging. Am. Heart J. 118:581, 1989.
9. Brown, K. A.: Prognostic value of thallium-201 myocardial perfusion imaging: A diagnostic tool comes of age. Circulation 83:363, 1991.
10. Wackers, F. J. Th., Berman D. S., Maddahi, J., et al.: Technetium-99m Hexakis 2-methyoxyisobutyl isonitrile: Human biodistribution, dosimetry, safety and preliminary comparison to thallium-201 for myocardial perfusion imaging. J. Nucl. Med. 30:301, 1989.
11. Kiat, H., Maddahi, J., Roy, L. T., et al.: Comparison of technetium-99m-methyoxy isobutyl isonitrile and thallium-201 for evaluation of coronary artery disease by planar and tomographic methods. Am. Heart J. 117:1, 1989.
12. Seldin, D. W., Johnson, L. L., Blood, D. K., et al.: Myocardial perfusion imaging with technetium-99m SQ30217: Comparison with thallium-201 and coronary anatomy. J. Nucl. Med. 30:312, 1989.

13. Hendel, R. C., McSherry, B., Karimeddini, M., et al.: Diagnostic value of a new myocardial perfusion agent, teboroxime (SQ30,217), utilizing a rapid planar imaging protocol: Preliminary results. J. Am. Coll. Cardiol. 16:855, 1990.

14. Jain, D., Wackers, F. J. Th., Mattera, J., et al.: Biokinetics of 99mTc-tetrofosmin, a new myocardial perfusion imaging agent: Implications for a one day imaging protocol. J. Nucl. Med. 34:1254, 1993.

15. Zaret, B. L., Rigo, P., Wackers, F. J. Th., et al.: The Tetrofosmine International Trial Study Group: Myocardial perfusion imaging with 99mTc-tetrofosmin. Comparison to 201Tl imaging and coronary angiography in a phase III multicenter trial. Circulation 91:313, 1995.

16. Gerson, M. C., Millard, R. W., Roszell, N. J., et al.: Kinetic properties of 99mTc-Q12 in canine myocardium. Circulation 89:1291, 1994.

17. Weich, H. F., Strauss, H. W., and Pitt, B.: The extraction of thallium-201 by the myocardium. Circulation 56:188, 1977.

18. Marshall, R. C., Leidholdt, E. M., Zhang, D. Y., et al.: Technetium-99m hexakis 2-methoxy-2-isobutyl isonitrile and thallium-201 extraction, washout, and retention at varying coronary flow rates in rabbit heart. Circulation 82:998, 1990.

19. Wackers, F. J. Th.: The maze of myocardial perfusion imaging protocols anno 1994. J. Nucl. Cardiol. 1:180, 1994.

20. Berman, D. S., Kiat, H., Friedman, J. D., et al.: Separate acquisitions rest thallium–201/stress technetium–99m sestamibi dual-isotope myocardial perfusion single-photon emission computed tomography: A clinical validation study. J. Am. Coll. Cardiol. 22:1455, 1993.

21. Wackers, F. J. Th.: Myocardial perfusion imaging. In Sandler, M. P., Coleman, R. E., Wackers, F. J. Th., et al. (eds.): Diagnostic Nuclear Medicine. 3rd ed. Baltimore, Williams & Wilkins, 1995.

22. Wackers, F. J. Th., and Mattera, J. A.: Optimizing planar Tl-201 imaging: Computer quantification. Cardiology 7:103, 1990.

23. Berman, D. S., Kiat, H. S., Van Train, K. F., et al.: Myocardial perfusion imaging with technetium-99m sestamibi: Comparative analysis of available imaging protocols. J. Nucl. Med. 35:681, 1994.

24. DePuey, E. G., Berman, D. S., and Garcia, E. V.: Cardiac SPECT Imaging. New York, Raven Press, 1995.

25. Friedman, J., Van Train, K., Maddahi, J., et al.: "Upward creep" of the heart: A frequent source of false positive reversible defects during thallium-201 stress-distribution SPECT. J. Nucl. Med. 30:1718, 1989.

26. Maniawski, P. J., Morgan, H. T., Wackers, F. J. Th.: Orbit related variation in spatial resolution as a source of artifactual defects in Tl201 SPECT. J. Nucl. Med. 32:871, 1991.

27. The Cardiovascular Imaging Committee, American College of Cardiology; The Committee on Advanced Cardiac Imaging and Technology, Council of Clinical Cardiology, American Heart Association; and the Board of Directors, Cardiovascular Council, Society of Nuclear Medicine: ACC/AHA/SNM Policy Statement: Standardization of cardiac tomographic imaging. J. Am. Coll. Cardiol. 1:117, 1994.

28. Eisner, R. I., Tammas, M. J., Colinger, K., et al.: Normal SPECT thallium-201 bull's eye display: Gender differences. J. Nucl. Med. 29:1901, 1988.

29. Johnstone, D. E., Wackers, F. J. Th., Berger, H. J., et al.: Effect of patient positioning on left lateral thallium-201 myocardial images. J. Nucl. Med. 20:183, 1979.

30. Wackers, F. J. Th.: Artifacts in planar and SPECT myocardial perfusion imaging. Am. J. Cardiac Imaging 6:42, 1992.

31. Segal, G. M., and Davis, M. J.: Prone versus supine thallium myocardial SPECT: A method to decrease artifactual inferior wall defects. J. Nucl. Med. 30:548, 1989.

32. Esquerre, J. P., Coca, F. J., Martinez, S. J., et al.: Prone decubitus: A solution to inferior wall attenuation in thallium-201 myocardial tomography. J. Nucl. Med. 30:398, 1989.

33. Suzki, A., Muto, S., Oshima, M., et al.: A new scanning method for thallium-201 myocardial SPECT: Semi-decubital position method. Clin. Nucl. Med. 14:736, 1989.

34. Barr, S. A., Shen, M. Y. H., Sinusas, A. J., et al.: Reduced inferior attenuation on rest SPECT myocardial perfusion imaging in the upright position using a rotating chair: Comparison with standard supine SPECT imaging. J. Nucl. Med. 35:91P, 1994.

35. DePuey, E. G., and Garcia, E. V.: Optimal specificity of thallium-201 SPECT through recognition of imaging artifacts. J. Nucl. Med. 30:441, 1989.

36. Cloninger, K. G., DePuey, E. G., Garcia, E. V., et al.: Incomplete redistribution of delayed thallium-201 single photon emission computed tomographic (SPECT) images: An overestimation of myocardial scarring. J. Am. Coll. Cardiol. 12:955, 1988.

37. Kiat, H. K., Berman, D. S., Maddahi, J., et al.: Late reversibility of tomographic myocardial thallium-201 defects: An accurate marker of myocardial viability. J. Am. Coll. Cardiol. 12:1456, 1988.

38. Weiss, A. T., Maddahi, J., Lew, A. S., et al.: Reverse redistribution of thallium-201: A sign of nontransmural myocardial infarction with patency of the infarct-related coronary artery. J. Am. Coll. Cardiol. 7:61, 1986.

39. Soufer, R., Dey, H. M., Lawson, A. J., et al.: Relationship between reverse redistribution on planar thallium scintigraphy and regional myocardial viability: A correlative PET study. J. Nucl. Med. 36:180, 1995.

40. Gill, J. B., Ruddy, T. D., Newell, J. B., et al.: Prognostic importance of thallium uptake by the lungs during exercise in coronary artery disease. N. Engl. J. Med. 317:1485, 1987.

41. Giubbini, R., Campini, R., Milan, E., et al.: Evaluation of technetium-99m-sestamibi lung uptake: Correlation with left ventricular function. J. Nucl. Med. 36:58, 1995.

42. Weiss, A. T., Berman, D. S., Lew, A. S., et al.: Transient ischemic dilation of the left ventricle on stress thallium-201 scintigraphy: A marker of severe and extensive coronary artery disease. J. Am. Coll. Cardiol. 9:752, 1987.

43. Wackers, F. J. Th., Bodenheimer, M., Fleiss, J. L., et al.: Factors affecting uniformity in interpretation of planar Tl-201 imaging in a multicenter trial. J. Am. Coll. Cardiol. 21:1064, 1993.

44. Beller, G. A., Watson, D. D., and Pohost, G. M.: Kinetics of thallium distribution and redistribution: Clinical applications in sequential myocardial imaging. In Strauss, H. W., and Pitt, B. (eds.): Cardiovascular Nuclear Medicine, 2nd ed. St. Louis, C. V. Mosby Co., 1979.

45. Sinusas, A. J., Bergin, J. D., Edwards, N. C., et al.: Redistribution of 99mTc-Sestamibi and 201Tl in presence of a severe coronary artery stenosis. Circulation 89:2332, 1994.

46. Goris, M. L., Daspit, S. G., McLaughlin, P., et al.: Interpolative background subtraction. J. Nucl. Med. 17:744, 1976.

47. Watson, D. D., Campbell, N. P., Read, E. K., et al.: Spatial and temporal quantitation of plane thallium myocardial images. J. Nucl. Med. 22:577, 1981.

48. Garcia, E., Maddahi, J., Berman, D. S., et al.: Space/time quantitation of thallium-201 myocardial scintigraphy. J. Nucl. Med. 22:309, 1981.

49. Wackers, F. J. Th., Fetterman, R. C., Mattera, J. A., et al.: Quantitative planar thallium-201 stress scintigraphy: A critical evaluation of the method. Semin. Nucl. Med. 15:46, 1985.

50. Sigal, S. L., Soufer, R., Fetterman, R. C., et al.: Reproducibility of quantitative planar thallium-201 scintigraphy. Quantitative criteria for reversibility of myocardial perfusion defects. J. Nucl. Med. 32:759, 1991.

51. Klein, J. L., Garcia, E. V., DePuey, G., et al.: Reversibility bulls-eye: A new polar bulls-eye may quantify reversibility of stress-induced SPECT thallium-201 myocardial perfusion defects. J. Nucl. Med. 31:1240, 1990.

52. Wackers, F. J. Th.: Science, art and artifacts: How important is quantification for the practicing physician interpreting myocardial perfusion studies. J. Nucl. Cardiol. 1:S109, 1994.

53. Wackers, F. J. Th., Maniawski, P., and Sinusas, A. J.: Evaluation of left ventricular wall function by ECG-gated Tc-99m-Sestambi imaging. In Beller, G. A., and Zaret, B. L. (eds.): Nuclear Cardiology: State of the Art and Future Direction. St. Louis, C. V. Mosby Co., 1993, p. 85.

54. Chua, T., Kiat, H., Germano, G., et al.: Gated technetium-99m sestamibi for simultaneous assessment of stress myocardial perfusion, postexercise regional ventricular function and myocardial viability. J. Am. Coll. Cardiol. 23:1107, 1994.

55. Germano, G., Kavanaugh, P. B., Kiat, H., et al.: Automated analysis of gated myocardial SPECT: Development and initial validation of a method. J. Nucl. Med. 35:816, 1994.

56. DePuey, E. G., Nichols, K., and Dobrinsky, C.: Left ventricular ejection fraction assessed from gated technetium-99m-sestamibi SPECT. J. Nucl. Med. 34:1871, 1993.

CLINICAL APPLICATIONS OF MYOCARDIAL PERFUSION IMAGING

57. Wackers, F. J. Th., Busemann Sokole, E., Samson, G., et al.: Value and limitations of thallium-201 scintigraphy in the acute phase of myocardial infarction. N. Engl. J. Med. 295:1, 1976.

58. Wackers, F. J. Th., Becker, A. E., Samson, G., et al.: Location and size of acute transmural myocardial infarction estimated from thallium-201 scintiscans. Circulation 56:71, 1977.

59. Wackers, F. J. Th., Lie, K. I., Liem, K. I., et al.: Potential value of thallium-201 scintigraphy as a means of selecting patients for the coronary care unit. Br. Heart J. 41:111, 1979.

60. Varetto, T., Cantalupi, D., Altiero, A., et al.: Emergency room technetium-99m-sestamibi imaging to rule out acute myocardial ischemic events in patients with nondiagnostic electrocardiograms. J. Am. Coll. Cardiol. 22:1804, 1993.

61. Hilton, T. C., Thompson, R. C., Williams, H. J., et al.: Technetium-99-sestamibi myocardial perfusion imaging in the emergency room evaluation of chest pain. J. Am. Coll. Cardiol. 23:1016, 1994.

62. Radensky, P. W., Stowers, S. A., Hilton, T. C., et al.: Cost-effectiveness of acute myocardial perfusion imaging with Tc-99m-sestamibi for risk stratification of emergency room patients with acute chest pain. Circulation 90(Abs.):528, 1994.

63. Gibbons, R. J., Verani, M. S., Behrenbeck, T., et al.: Feasibility of tomographic 99mTc-hexakis-2-methoxy-2-methylpropyl-isonitrile imaging for the assessment of myocardial area at risk and the effect of treatment in acute myocardial infarction. Circulation 80:177, 1989.

64. Wackers, F. J. Th., Gibbons, R. J., Verani, M. S., et al.: Serial quantitative planar technetium-99m-isonitrile imaging in acute myocardial infarction: Efficacy for noninvasive assessment of thrombolytic therapy. J. Am. Coll. Cardiol. 14:861, 1989.

65. Santoro, G. M., Bisi, G., Sciagra, R., et al.: Single photon emission computed tomography with technetium-99m-hexakis 2-methoxy isobutyl isonitrile in acute myocardial infarction before and after thrombolytic treatment: Assessment of salvaged myocardium and prediction of late functional recovery. J. Am. Coll. Cardiol. 15:301, 1990.

66. Decoster, P. M., Wijns, W., Cauwe, F., et al.: Area-at-risk determination by technetium-99m-hexakis-2-methoxyisobutyl isonitrile in experimental reperfused myocardial infarction. Circulation 82:2152, 1990.

67. Bisi, G., Sciagra, R., Santoro, G. M., et al.: Comparison of tomography and planar imaging for the evaluation of thrombolytic therapy in acute myocardial infarction using pre- and post-treatment myocardial scintigraphy with technetium-99m sestamibi. Am. Heart J. 122:13, 1991.

68. Faraggi, M., Assayag, P., Messian, O., et al.: Early isonitrile SPECT in acute myocardial infarction: Feasibility and results before and after fibrinolysis. Nucl. Med. Communications 10:539, 1989.

69. Gibbons, R. J.: Perfusion imaging with 99mTc-sestamibi for the assessment of myocardial area at risk and the efficacy of acute treatment in myocardial infarction. Circulation 84(Suppl I.):1, 1991.

70. Christian, T. F., Gibbons, R. J., and Gersh, B. J.: Effect of infarct location on myocardial salvage assessed by technetium-99m isonitrile. J. Am. Coll. Cardiol. 17:1303, 1991.

71. Christian, T. F., Schwartz, R. S., and Gibbons, R. J.: Determinants of infarct size in reperfusion therapy for acute myocardial infarction. Circulation 86:81, 1992.

72. Christian, T. F., Behrenbeck, T., Pellikka, P. A., et al.: Mismatch of left ventricular function and infarct size demonstrated by technetium-99m isonitrile imaging after reperfusion therapy for acute myocardial infarction: Identification of myocardial stunning and hyperkinesia. J. Am. Coll. Cardiol. 16:1632, 1990.

73. Pellikka, P. A., Behrenbeck, T., Verani, M. S., et al.: Serial changes in myocardial perfusion using tomographic technetium-99m-hexakis-2-methoxy-2-methylpropyl-isonitrile imaging following reperfusion therapy of myocardial infarction. J. Nucl. Med. 31:1269, 1990.

74. Gibbons, R. J.: Technetium-99m sestamibi in the assessment of acute myocardial infarction. Semin. Nucl. Med. 21:213, 1991.

75. Marcassa, C., Galli, M., Luigi, P., et al.: Technetium-99m-sestamibi tomographic evaluation of residual ischemia after anterior myocardial infarction. J. Am. Coll. Cardiol. 25:590, 1995.

76. Ito, H., Iwakura, K., Oh, H., et al.: Temporal changes in myocardial perfusion patterns in patients with reperfused anterior wall myocardial infarction. Their relation to myocardial viability. Circulation 91:656, 1995.

77. Gibbons, R. J., Christian, T. F., Hopfenspringer, M., et al.: Myocardium at risk and infarct size after thrombolytic therapy for acute myocardial infarction: Implications for the design of randomized trials of acute intervention. J. Am. Coll. Cardiol. 24:616, 1994.

78. Gibbons, R. J., Holmes, D. R., Reeder, G. S., et al.: Immediate angioplasty compared with the administration of a thrombolytic agent followed by conservative treatment for myocardial infarction. N. Engl. J. Med. 328:685, 1993.

79. Silverman, K. J., Becker, L. C., Bulkley, B. H., et al.: Value of early thallium-201 scintigraphy for predicting mortality in patients with acute myocardial infarction. Circulation 61:996, 1980.

80. Cerqueira, M. D., Maynard, C., Ritchie, J. L., et al.: Long-term survival in 618 patients from the Western Washington streptokinase in myocardial infarction trials. J. Am. Coll. Cardiol. 20:1452, 1992.

81. Nestico, P. E., Hakki, A., Felsher, J., et al.: Implications of abnormal right ventricular thallium uptake in acute myocardial infarction. Am. J. Cardiol. 58:230, 1986.

82. Jain, D., Lahiri, A., Raftery, E. B., et al.: Clinical and prognostic significance of lung thallium uptake on rest imaging in acute myocardial infarction. Am. J. Cardiol. 65:154, 1990.

83. Brown, K. A., O'Meara, J., Chambers, C. E., et al.: Ability of dipyridamole-thallium-201 imaging one to four days after acute myocardial infarction to predict in-hospital and late recurrent myocardial ischemic events. Am. J. Cardiol. 65:160, 1990.

84. Wackers, F. J. Th., Lie, K. I., Liem, K. L., et al.: Thallium-201 scintigraphy in unstable angina pectoris. Circulation 57:738, 1978.

85. Berger, B. C., Watson, D. D., Burwell, L. R., et al.: Redistribution of thallium at rest in patients with stable and unstable angina and the effect of coronary artery bypass surgery. Circulation 60:1114, 1979.

86. Bilodeau, L., Theroux, P., Gregoire, J., et al.: Technetium-99m sestamibi tomography in patients with spontaneous chest pain: Correlations with clinical, electrocardiographic and angiographic findings. J. Am. Coll. Cardiol. 18:1684, 1991.

87. Freeman, M. R., Chisholm, R. J., and Armstrong, P. W.: Usefulness of exercise electrocardiography and thallium scintigraphy in unstable angina pectoris in predicting the extent and severity of coronary artery disease. Am. J. Cardiol. 62:1164, 1988.

88. Gould, K. L.: Noninvasive assessment of coronary stenoses by myocardial perfusion imaging during pharmacologic coronary vasodilatation. I. Physiologic basis and experimental validation. Am. J. Cardiol. 41:267, 1978.

89. Casale, P. N., Guiney, T. E., Strauss, H. W., et al.: Simultaneous low level treadmill exercise and intravenous dipyridamole stress thallium imaging. Am. J. Cardiol. 62:799, 1988.

90. Ranhosky, A., and Rawson, J.: The safety of intravenous dipyridamole thallium myocardial perfusion imaging. Circulation 81:1205, 1990.

91. Lette, J., Tatum, J. L., Fraser, S., et al.: Safety of dipyridamole testing in 73,806 patients: The multicenter dipyridamole safety study. J. Nucl. Cardiol. 2:3, 1995.

92. Verani, M. S., Mahmarian, J. J., Hixson, J. B., et al.: Diagnosis of coronary artery disease by controlled coronary vasodilation with adenosine and thallium-201 scintigraphy in patients unable to exercise. Circulation 82:80, 1990.

93. Nguyen, T., Heo, J., Ogilby, J. D., et al.: Single photon emission computed tomography with thallium-201 during adenosine-induced coronary hyperemia: Correlation with coronary arteriography, exercise thallium imaging and two-dimensional echocardiography. J. Am. Coll. Cardiol. 16:1375, 1990.

94. Wilson, R. F., Wyche, K., Christensen, B. V., et al.: Effects of adenosine on human coronary arterial circulation. Circulation 82:1595, 1990.

95. Samuels, B., Kiat, H., Friedman, J. D., et al.: Adenosine pharmacologic stress myocardial perfusion tomographic imaging in patients with significant aortic stenosis. Diagnostic efficacy and comparison of clinical, hemodynamic and electrocardiographic variables with 100 age-matched control subjects. J. Am. Coll. Cardiol. 25:99, 1995.

96. Pennell, D. J., Underwood, R., Swanton, R. H., et al.: Dobutamine thallium myocardial perfusion tomography. J. Am. Coll. Cardiol. 18:147, 1991.

97. Hays, J. T., Mahmarian, J. J., Cochran, A. J., et al.: Dobutamine thallium-201 tomography for evaluating patients with suspected coronary artery disease unable to undergo exercise or vasodilator pharmacologic stress testing. J. Am. Coll. Cardiol. 21:1583, 1993.

98. Picano, E., Mathias, W., Pingitore, A., et al.: Safety and tolerability of dobutamine-atropine stress echocardiography: A prospective, multi-centre study. Lancet 344:1190, 1994.

99. Berger, B. C., Watson, D. D., Taylor, G. J., et al.: Quantitative thallium-201 exercise scintigraphy for detection of coronary artery disease. J. Nucl. Med. 22:585, 1981.

100. Maddahi, J., Garcia, E. V., Berman, D. S., et al.: Improved noninvasive assessment of coronary artery disease by quantitative analysis of regional stress myocardial distribution and washout of thallium-201. Circulation 64:924, 1981.

101. van Train, K. F., Berman, D. S., Garcia, E. V., et al.: Quantitative analysis of stress thallium-201 myocardial scintigrams: A multicenter trial. J. Nucl. Med. 27:17, 1986.

102. Kaul, S., Boucher, C. A., Newell, J. B., et al.: Determination of the quantitative thallium imaging variables that optimize detection of coronary artery disease. J. Am. Coll. Cardiol. 7:527, 1986.

103. Henkin, R. E., Kalousdian, S., Kikkawa, R. M., et al.: Diagnostic and therapeutic technology assessment (DATTA) myocardial perfusion imaging utilizing single-photon emission-computed tomography (SPECT). Washington Manual of Therapeutic Technology, 1994, p. 2850.

104. Maddahi, J., van Train, K., Prigent, F., et al.: Quantitative single photon emission computed thallium-201 tomography for detection and localization of coronary artery disease: Optimization and prospective validation of a new technique. J. Am. Coll. Cardiol. 14:1689, 1989.

105. DePasquale, E. E., Nody, A. C., DePuey, E. G., et al.: Quantitative rotational thallium-201 tomography for identifying and localizing coronary artery disease. Circulation 77:316, 1988.

106. Fintel, D. J., Links, J. M., Brinker, J. A., et al.: Improved diagnostic performance of exercise thallium-201 single photon emission computed tomography over planar imaging in the diagnosis of coronary artery disease: A receiver operating characteristic analysis. J. Am. Coll. Cardiol. 13:600, 1989.

107. Mahmarian, J. J., Boyce, T. M., Goldberg, R. K., et al.: Quantitative exercise thallium-201 single photo emission computed tomography for the enhanced diagnosis of ischemic heart disease. J. Am. Coll. Cardiol. 15:318, 1990.

108. Go, R. T., Marwick, T. H., MacIntyre, W. J., et al.: A prospective comparison of rubidium-82 PET and thallium-201 SPECT myocardial perfusion imaging utilizing a single dipyridamole stress in the diagnosis of coronary artery disease. J. Nucl. Med. 31:1899, 1990.

109. Tamaki, N., Yonekura, Y., Mukai, T., et al.: Stress thallium-201 transaxial emission computed tomography: Quantitative versus qualitative analysis for evaluation of coronary artery disease. J. Am. Coll. Cardiol. 4:1213, 1984.

110. Iskandrian, A. S., Heo, J., Kong, B., et al.: Effect of exercise level on the ability of thallium-201 tomographic imaging in detecting coronary artery disease: Analysis of 461 patients. J. Am. Coll. Cardiol. 14:1477, 1989.

111. van Train, K. F., Maddahi, J., Berman, D. S., et al.: Quantitative analysis of tomographic stress thallium-201 myocardial scintigrams: A multicenter trial. J. Nucl. Med. 31:1168, 1990.

112. Borges-Neto, S., Mahmarian, J. J., Jain, A., et al.: Quantitative thallium-201 single photon emission computed tomography after oral dipyridamole for assessing the presence, anatomic location and severity of coronary artery disease. J. Am. Coll. Cardiol. 11:962, 1988.

113. Taillefer, R., Lambert, R., Dupras, G., et al.: Clinical comparison between thallium-201 and Tc-99m-methoxyisobutyl isonitrile (hexamibi) myocardial perfusion imaging for the detection of coronary artery disease. Eur. J. Nucl. Med. 15:280, 1989.

114. Iskandrian, A., Heo, J., Kong, B., et al.: Use of technetium-99m isonitrile (RP-30A) in assessing left ventricular perfusion and function at rest and during exercise in coronary artery disease, and comparison with coronary arteriography and exercise thallium-201 SPECT imaging. Am. J. Cardiol. 64:270, 1989.

115. Maddahi, J., Kiat, H., Friedman, J. D., et al.: Technetium-99m-sestamibi myocardial perfusion imaging for evaluation of coronary artery disease. In Zaret, B. L., and Beller, G. A. (eds.): Nuclear Cardiology. St. Louis, C. V. Mosby Co., 1993, p. 191.

116. van Train, K. F., Garcia, E. V., Maddahi, J., et al.: Multicenter trial validation of quantitative analysis of same-day rest stress technetium-99m-sestamibi myocardial tomograms. J. Nucl. Med. 35:609, 1994.

117. Rigo, P., Leclercq, B., Itti, R., et al.: Technetium-99m-tetrofosmin myocardial imaging: A comparison with thallium-201 and angiography. J. Nucl. Med. 35:587, 1994.

118. Heo, J., Cave, V., Wasserleben, V., et al.: Planar and tomographic imaging with technetium 99m-labeled tetrofosmin: Correlation with thallium 201 and coronary angiography. J. Nucl. Cardiol. 1:317, 1994.

119. Gerson, M. C., Lukes, J., Deutsh, E., et al.: Comparison of technetium 99m Q12 and thallium-201 for detection of angiographically docu-

mented coronary artery disease in humans. J. Nucl. Cardiol. 1:499, 1994.

120. Hendel, R. C., Gerson, M. C., Verani, M. S., et al.: Perfusion imaging with Tc-99m furisfosmin (Q12): Multicenter phase III trial to evaluate safety and comparative efficacy. Circulation 90(Abs.):449, 1994.

121. Iskandrian, A. S., Heo, J., Nguyen, T., et al.: Tomographic myocardial perfusion imaging with technetium-99m teboroxime during adenosine-induced coronary hyperemia: Correlation with thallium-201 imaging. J. Am. Coll. Cardiol. 19:307, 1992.

122. Serafini, A. N., Topchik, S., Jiminez, H., et al.: Clinical comparison of technetium-99m-teboroxime and thallium-201 utilizing a continuous SPECT imaging protocol. J. Nucl. Med. 33:1304, 1992.

123. Henzlova, M. J., and Machac, J.: Clinical utility of technetium-99m-teboroxime myocardial washout imaging. J. Nucl. Med. 35:575, 1994.

124. Stewart, R. E., Heyl, B., O'Rourke, R. A., et al.: Demonstration of differential post-stenotic myocardial technetium-99m-teboroxime clearance kinetics after experimental ischemia and hyperemic stress. J. Nucl. Med. 32:2000, 1991.

125. Albro, P. C., Gould, K. L., Westcott, R. J., et al.: Noninvasive assessment of coronary stenoses by myocardial imaging during pharmacologic coronary vasodilatation. III. Clinical trial. Am. J. Cardiol. 42:751, 1978.

126. Sochor, H., Pachinger, O., Ogris, E., et al.: Radionuclide imaging after coronary vasodilation: Myocardial scintigraphy with thallium-201 and radionuclide angiography after administration of dipyridamole. Eur. Heart J. 5:400, 1984.

127. Francisco, D. A., Collins, S. M., Go, R. T., et al.: Tomographic thallium-201 myocardial perfusion scintigrams after maximal coronary artery vasodilation with intravenous dipyridamole: Comparison of qualitative and quantitative approaches. Circulation 66:370, 1982.

128. Kong, B. A., Shaw, L., Miller, D. D., et al.: Comparison of accuracy for detecting coronary artery disease and side-effect profile of dipyridamole thallium-201 myocardial perfusion imaging in women versus men. Am. J. Cardiol. 70:168, 1992.

129. Verani, M. S., Mahmarian, J. J., Hixson, J. B., et al.: Diagnosis of coronary artery disease by controlled coronary vasodilation with adenosine and thallium-201 scintigraphy in patients unable to exercise. Circulation 82:80, 1990.

130. Iskandrian, A. S., Heo, J., Nguyen, T., et al: Assessment of coronary artery disease using single photon emission computed tomography with thallium-201 during adenosine induced coronary hyperemia. Am. J. Cardiol. 67:1190, 1991.

131. Santos-O'Campos, C. D., Herman, S. D., Travin, M. I., et al.: Comparison of exercise, dipyridamole, and adenosine by use of technetium 99m sestamibi tomographic imaging. J. Nucl. Cardiol. 1:57, 1994.

132. Rozanski, A., Diamond, G., Forrester, J. S., et al.: Declining specificity of exercise radionuclide ventriculography. N. Engl. J. Med. 309:518, 1983.

133. Maddahi, J., Abdulla, A., Garcia, E. V., et al.: Noninvasive identification of left main and triple vessel coronary artery disease: Improved accuracy using quantitative analysis of regional myocardial stress distribution and washout of thallium-201. J. Am. Coll. Cardiol. 7:53, 1986.

134. Dash, H., Massie, B. M., Botvinick, E. H., et al.: The noninvasive identification of left main and three-vessel coronary artery disease by myocardial stress perfusion scintigraphy and treadmill exercise electrocardiography. Circulation 60:276, 1979.

135. Nygaard, T. W., Gibson, R. S., Ryan, J. M., et al.: Prevalance of high-risk thallium-201 scintigraphic findings in left main coronary artery stenosis: Comparison with patients with multiple and single-vessel coronary artery disease. Am. J. Cardiol. 53:462, 1984.

136. Kushner, F. G., Okada, R. D., Kirshenbaum, H. D., et al.: Lung thallium-201 uptake after stress testing in patients with coronary artery disease. Circulation 63:341, 1981.

137. Gibson, R. S., Watson, D. D., Craddock, G. B., et al.: Prediction of cardiac events after uncomplicated myocardial infarction: A prospective study comparing predischarge exercise thallium-201 scintigraphy and coronary angiography. Circulation 68:321, 1983.

138. Brown, K. A., Boucher, C. A., Okada, R. D., et al.: Prognostic value of exercise thallium-201 imaging in patients presenting for evaluation of chest pain. J. Am. Coll. Cardiol. 1:994, 1983.

139. Abraham, R. D., Freedman, S. B., Dunn, R. F., et al.: Prediction of multivessel coronary artery disease and prognosis early after acute myocardial infarction by exercise electrocardiography and thallium-201 myocardial perfusion scanning. Am. J. Cardiol. 58:423, 1986.

140. Bodenheimer, M. M., Wackers, F. J. Th., Schwartz, R. G., et al.: Prognostic significance of a fixed thallium defect one to six months after onset of acute myocardial infarction or unstable angina. Am. J. Cardiol. 74:1196, 1994.

141. Kaul, S., Finkelstein, D. M., Homma, S., et al.: Superiority of quantitative exercise thallium-201 variables in determining long-term prognosis in ambulatory patients with chest pain: A comparison with cardiac catheterization. J. Am. Coll. Cardiol. 12:25, 1988.

142. Manchecourt, J., Longere, P., Fagret, D., et al.: Prognostic value of thallium-201 single-photon emission computed tomographic myocardial perfusion imaging according to extent of myocardial defect. J. Am. Coll. Cardiol. 23:1096, 1994.

143. Miller, D. D., Stratmann, H. G., Shaw, L., et al.: Dipyridamole technetium 99m sestamibi myocardial tomography as an independent predictor of cardiac event-free survival after acute ischemic events. J. Nucl. Cardiol. 1:172, 1994.

144. Leppo, J. A., O'Brien, J., Rothendler, J. A., et al.: Dipyridamole-thal-

lium-201 scintigraphy in the prediction of future cardiac events after acute myocardial infarction. N. Engl. J. Med. 310:1014, 1984.

145. Brown, K. A., Weiss, R. M., Clements, J. P., et al.: Usefulness of residual ischemic myocardium within prior infarct zone for identifying patients at high risk late after acute myocardial infarction. Am. J. Cardiol. 60:15, 1987.

146. Kamal, A., Fattah, A. A., Pancholy, S., et al.: Prognostic value of adenosine single-photon emission computed tomographic thallium imaging in medically treated patients with angiographic evidence of coronary artery disease. J. Nucl. Cardiol. 1:254, 1994.

147. Olona, M., Candell-Riera, J., Permanyer-Miralda, G., et al.: Strategies for prognostic assessment of uncomplicated first myocardial infarction: 5 year follow-up study. J. Am. Coll. Cardiol. 25:815, 1995.

148. Krawczynska, E. G., Weintraub, W. S., Garcia, E. V., et al.: Left ventricular dilation and multivessel coronary artery disease on thallium-201 SPECT are important prognostic indicators in patients with large defects in the left anterior descending distribution. Am. J. Cardiol. 74:1233, 1994.

149. Bateman, T. M., O'Keefe, J. H., Dong, V. M., et al.: Coronary angiography rates following stress SPECT scintigraphy. J. Nucl. Cardiol. 2:217, 1995.

149a. Nallamothu, N., Pancholy, S. B., Lee, K., et al.: Impact of exercise single-photon emission computed tomographic thallium imaging on patient management and outcome. J. Nucl. Cardiol. 2:334, 1995.

150. Wackers, F. J. Th., Russo, D. J., Russo, D., et al.: Prognostic significance of normal quantitative planar thallium-201 stress scintigraphy in patients with chest pain. J. Am. Coll. Cardiol. 6:27, 1985.

151. Pamelia, F. X., Gibson, R. S., Watson, D. D., et al.: Prognosis with chest pain and normal thallium-201 exercise scintigrams. Am. J. Cardiol. 55:920, 1985.

152. Wahl, J., Hakki, A. H., and Iskandrian, A. S.: Prognostic implications of normal exercise thallium-201 images. Arch. Intern. Med. 145:253, 1985.

153. Staniloff, H. M., Forrester, J. S., Berman, D. S., et al.: Prediction of death, myocardial infarction, and worsening chest pain using thallium scintigraphy and exercise electrocardiography. J. Nucl. Med. 27:1842, 1986.

154. Brown, K. A., Altland, E., and Rowen, M.: Prognostic value of normal Tc-99m sestamibi cardiac imaging. J. Nucl. Med. 35:554, 1994.

155. Raiker, K., Sinusas, A. J., Zaret, B. L., et al.: One year prognosis of patients with normal Tc-99m-sestamibi stress imaging. J. Nucl. Cardiol. 1:449, 1994.

156. Berman, D. S., Kiat, H., Cohen, J., et al.: Prognosis of 1044 patients with normal exercise Tc-99m sestamibi myocardial perfusion SPECT. J. Am. Coll. Cardiol. 1A:63A, 1994.

157. Miller, D. D., Stratmann, H. G., Shaw, L., et al.: Dipyridamole technetium-99m-sestamibi myocardial tomography as an independent predictor of cardiac event-free survival after acute ischemic events. J. Nucl. Cardiol. 1:172, 1994.

158. Stratmann, H. G., Williams, G. A., Wittry, M. D., et al.: Exercise technetium-99m sestamibi tomography for cardiac risk stratification of patients with stable chest pain. Circulation 89:615, 1994.

159. Pollock, S. G., Abbott, R. D., Boucher, C. A., et al.: Independent and incremental prognostic value of tests performed in hierarchical order to evaluate patients with suspected coronary artery disease. Circulation 85:237, 1992.

160. Melin, J. A., Robert, A., Luwaert, R., et al.: Additional prognostic value of exercise testing and thallium-201 scintigraphy in catheterized patients without previous myocardial infarction. Int. J. Cardiol. 27:235, 1990.

161. Iskandrian, A. S., Chae, S. C., Heo, J., et al.: Independent and incremental prognostic value of exercise single-photon emission computed tomographic (SPECT) thallium imaging in coronary artery disease. J. Am. Coll. Cardiol. 22:665, 1993.

162. Petretta, M., Cuocolo, A., Carpinelli, A., et al.: Prognostic value of myocardial hypoperfusion indexes in patients with suspected or known coronary artery disease. J. Nucl. Cardiol. 1:325, 1994.

163. Fagan, L. F., Shaw, L., Kong, B. A., et al.: Prognostic value of exercise thallium scintigraphy in patients with good exercise tolerance and a normal or abnormal exercise electrocardiogram and suspected or confirmed coronary artery disease. Am. J. Cardiol. 69:607, 1992.

164. Tilkemeier, P. L., Guiney, T. E., LaRaia, P. J., et al.: Prognostic value of predischarge low-level exercise thallium testing after thrombolytic treatment of acute myocardial infarction. Am. J. Cardiol. 66:1203, 1990.

165. Sutton, J. M., Topol, E. J.: Significance of a negative exercise thallium test in the presence of a critical residual stenosis after thrombolysis for acute myocardial infarction. Circulation 83:1278, 1991.

166. Gimple, L. W., and Beller, G. A.: Assessing prognosis after acute myocardial infarction in the thrombolytic era. J. Nucl. Cardiol. 1:198, 1994.

167. Dakik, H. A., Kimball, K. T., Koutelou, M., et al.: Prognostic value of exercise thallium-201 tomography after myocardial infarction in the thrombolytic era. Circulation 88(Abs.):487, 1993.

168. Weiner, D. A., Ryan, T. J., McCabe, C. H., et al.: Correlations among history of angina, ST-segment response and prevalence of coronary artery disease in the coronary artery surgery study (CASS). N. Engl. J. Med. 301:230, 1979.

169. Desmarais, R. L., Kaul, S., Watson, D. D., et al.: Do false positive thallium-201 scans lead to unnecessary catheterization? Outcome of patients with perfusion defects on quantitative planar thallium-201 scintigraphy. J. Am. Coll. Cardiol. 21:1058, 1993.

170. Kong, B. A., Shaw, L., Miller, D. D., et al.: Comparison of accuracy for detecting coronary artery disease and side-effect profile of dipyrida-

mole thallium-201 myocardial perfusion imaging in women versus men. Am. J. Cardiol. 70:168, 1992.

171. Chae, S. C., Heo, J., Iskandrian, A. S., et al.: Identification of extensive coronary artery disease in women by exercise single-photon emission computed tomographic (SPECT) thallium imaging. J. Am. Coll. Cardiol. 21:1305, 1993.

172. Shaw, L. J., Miller, D. D., Romeis, J. C., et al.: Gender differences in the noninvasive evaluation and management of patients with suspected coronary artery disease. Ann. Intern. Med. 120:559, 1994.

173. Travin, M. I., Rama, P. R., Arthur, A. L., et al.: The relationship of gender to the use and prognostic value of stress technetium-99m sestamibi myocardial SPECT scintigraphy. J. Nucl. Med. 35:60P, 1994.

174. Hendel, R. C., Chen, M. H., L'Italien, G. J., et al.: Sex differences in perioperative and long term cardiac event-free survival in vascular surgery patients. An analysis of clinical and scintrigraphic variables. Circulation 91:1044, 1995.

175. Kaski, J. C., Rosano, G. M. C., Collins, P., et al.: Cardiac syndrome X: Clinical characteristics and left ventricular function. J. Am. Coll. Cardiol. 25:807, 1995.

176. Wackers, F. J. Th.: Complete left bundle branch block: Is the diagnosis of myocardial infarction possible? Int. J. Cardiol. 2:521, 1983.

177. McGowan, R. L., Welch, T. G., Zaret, B. L., et al.: Noninvasive myocardial imaging with potassium-43 and rubidium-81 in patients with left bundle branch block. Am. J. Cardiol. 38:422, 1976.

178. DePuey, E. G., Guertler-Krawczynska, E., and Robbins, W. L.: Thallium-201 SPECT in coronary artery disease patients with left bundle branch block. J. Nucl. Med. 29:1479, 1988.

179. Hirzel, H. O., Senn, M., Neusch, K., et al.: Thallium-201 scintigraphy in complete left bundle branch block. Am. J. Cardiol. 53:764, 1984.

180. Shefcyk, D. I., Gingrich, S., Nino, A. F., et al.: Altered left ventricular depolarization sequences in left bundle branch block is not a cause for false-positive thallium-201. J. Am. Coll. Cardiol. 17:II-78A, 1991.

181. Burns, R. J., Galligan, L., Wright, L. M., et al.: Improved specificity of myocardial thallium-201 single-photon emission computed tomography in patients with left bundle branch block by dipyridamole. Am. J. Cardiol. 68:504, 1991.

182. Berger, H. J., Sands, M. J., Davies, R. A., et al.: Exercise left ventricular performance in patients with chest pain, ischemic-appearing exercise electrocardiograms, and angiographically normal coronary arteries. Ann. Intern. Med. 94:186, 1981.

183. Berger, B. C., Abramowitz, R., Park, C. H., et al.: Abnormal thallium-201 scans in patients with chest pain and angiographically normal coronary arteries. Am. J. Cardiol. 52:365, 1983.

184. Legrand, V., Hodgson, J. M., Bates, E. R., et al.: Abnormal coronary flow reserve and abnormal radionuclide exercise test results in patients with normal coronary angiograms. J. Am. Coll. Cardiol. 6:1245, 1985.

185. Cannon, R. O., Bonow, R. O., Bacharach, S. L., et al.: Left ventricular dysfunction in patients with angina pectoris, normal epicardial coronary arteries, and abnormal vasodilator reserve. Circulation 71:218, 1985.

185a. Zeiher, A. M., Krause, T., Schächinger, V., et al.: Impaired endothelium-dependent vasodilation of coronary resistance vessels is associated with exercise-induced myocardial ischemia. Circulation 91:2345, 1995.

186. Boucher, C. A., Brewster, D. C., Darling, R. C., et al.: Determination of cardiac risk by dipyridamole-thallium imaging before peripheral vascular surgery. N. Engl. J. Med. 312:389, 1985.

187. Eagle, K. A., Singer, D. E., Brewster, D. C., et al.: Dipyridamole thallium scanning in patients undergoing vascular surgery. Optimizing preoperative evaluation of cardiac risk. JAMA 257:2185, 1987.

188. Lane, S. E., Lewis, S. M., Pippin, J. J., et al.: Predictive value of quantitative dipyridamole thallium scintigraphy and assessing cardiovascular risk after vascular surgery in diabetes mellitus. Am. J. Cardiol. 64:1275, 1989.

189. Lette, J., Waters, D., Bernier, H., et al.: Preoperative and long term risk cardiac assessment. Predictive value of 23 clinical descriptors, 7 multivariates scoring systems and quantitative dipyridamole imaging in 360 patients. Ann. Surg. 216:192, 1992.

190. Levinson, J. R., Boucher, C. A., Coley, C. M., et al.: Usefulness of semiquantitative analysis of dipyridamole thallium-201 redistribution from proving risk stratification before vascular surgery. Am. J. Cardiol. 66:406, 1990.

191. Fleisher, L. A., Rosenbaum, S. H., Nelson, A. H., et al.: Preoperative dipyridamole thallium imaging and ambulatory electrocardiographic monitoring as a predictor of perioperative cardiac events and long term outcome. Anesthesiology 83:906, 1995.

192. Mangano, D. T., London, M. J., Tubau, J. F., et al.: Dipyridamole thallium-201 scintigraphy as a preoperative screening test. A re-examination of its predictive potential. Circulation 84:493, 1991.

193. Baron, J. F., Mundler, O., Bertran, D., et al.: Dipyridamole thallium scintigraphy and gated radionuclide angiography to assess cardiac risk before abdominal aortic surgery. N. Engl. J. Med. 330:663, 1994.

194. Manyari, D. E., Knudson, M., Kloiber, R., et al.: Sequential thallium-201 myocardial perfusion studies after successful percutaneous transluminal coronary artery angioplasty: Delayed resolution of exercise-induced scintigraphic abnormalities. Circulation 77:86, 1988.

195. Hecht, H. S., Shaw, R. E., Bruce, T. R., et al.: Usefulness of tomographic thallium-201 imaging for detection of restenosis after percutaneous transluminal coronary angioplasty. Am. J. Cardiol. 66:1314, 1990.

196. Jain, A., Mahmarian, J. J., Borges-Neto, S., et al.: Clinical significance of perfusion defects by thallium-201 single photon emission tomography following oral dipyridamole early after coronary angioplasty. J. Am. Coll. Cardiol. 11:970, 1988.

197. Miller, D. D., Liu, P., Strauss, H. W., et al.: Prognostic value of computer-quantitated exercise thallium imaging early after percutaneous transluminal coronary angioplasty. J. Am. Coll. Cardiol. 10:275, 1987.

198. Miller, D. D., and Verani, M. S.: Current status of myocardial perfusion imaging after percutaneous transluminal coronary angioplasty. J. Am. Coll. Cardiol. 24:260, 1994.

199. Dilsizian, V., Rocco, T. P., Freedman, N. M. T., et al.: Enhanced detection of ischemic but viable myocardium by the reinjection of thallium after stress-redistribution imaging. N. Engl. J. Med. 323:141, 1990.

200. Rocco, T. P., Dilsizian, V., McKusick, K. A., et al.: Comparison of thallium redistribution with rest "reinjection" imaging for the detection of viable myocardium. Am. J. Cardiol. 66:158, 1990.

201. Kayden, D. S., Zaret, B. L., Wackers, F. J. Th., et al.: 24 hour planar thallium-201 delayed imaging: Is reinjection necessary? Circulation 80(Abs.):376, 1991.

202. Tillisch, J., Brunken, R., Marshall, R., et al.: Reversibility of cardiac wall-motion abnormalities predicted by positron tomography. N. Engl. J. Med. 314:884, 1986.

203. Favaro, L., Masini, F., Serra, W., et al.: Thallium-201 for detection of viable myocardium: Comparison of different reinjection protocols. J. Nucl. Cardiol. 1:515, 1994.

204. Bonow, R. O., Dilsizian, V., Cuocolo, A., et al.: Identification of viable myocardium in patients with chronic coronary artery disease and left ventricular dysfunction and PET imaging with ^{18}F-fluorodeoxyglucose. Circulation 83:26, 1991.

205. Zimmerman, R., Mall, G., Rauch, B., et al.: Residual ^{201}Tl activity in irreversible defects as a marker of myocardial viability. Clinicopathological study. Circulation 91:1016, 1995.

206. Ragosta, M., Beller, G. A., Watson, D. D., et al.: Quantitative planar rest-redistribution ^{201}Tl imaging in detection of myocardial viability and prediction of improvement in left ventricular function after coronary bypass surgery in patients with severely depressed left ventricular function. Circulation 87:1630, 1993.

207. Piwnica-Worms, D., Chiu, M. L., and Kronauge, J. F.: Divergent kinetics of ^{201}Tl and ^{99m}Tc-sestamibi in cultured chick ventricular myocytes during ATP depletion. Circulation 85:1531, 1992.

208. Weinstein, H., King, M. A., Reinhardt, C. P., et al.: A method of simultaneous dual-radionuclide cardiac imaging with technetium-99m and thallium-201. I: Analysis of interradionuclide crossover and validation in phantoms. J. Nucl. Cardiol. 1:39, 1994.

209. Cuocolo, A., Pace, L., Ricciardell, B., et al.: Identification of viable myocardium in patients with chronic coronary artery disease: Comparison of thallium 201 scintigraphy with reinjection and technetium-99m-methoxyisobutyl isonitrile. J. Nucl. Med. 33:505, 1992.

210. Maurea, S., Cuocolo, A., Pace, L., et al.: Left ventricular dysfunction in coronary artery disease: Comparison between rest-redistribution thallium-201 and resting technetium 99m methoxyisobutyl isonitrile cardiac imaging. J. Nucl. Cardiol. 1:165, 1994.

211. Marzullo, P., Sambuceti, G., and Parodi, O.: The role of sestamibi scintigraphy in the radioisotopic assessment of myocardial viability. J. Nucl. Med. 33:1925, 1992.

212. Udelson, J. E., Coleman, P. S., Metherall, J., et al.: Predicting recovery of severe regional ventricular dysfunction: Comparison of resting scintigraphy with ^{201}Tl and ^{99m}Tc-sestamibi. Circulation 89:2552, 1994.

213. Dilsizian, V., Arrighi, J. A., Diodati, J. G., et al.: Myocardial viability in patients with chronic coronary artery disease. Comparison of ^{99m}Tc-sestamibi with thallium reinjection and [^{18}F]Fluorodeoxyglucose. Circulation 89:578, 1994.

214. Galli, M., Marcassa, C., Imparato, A., et al.: Effects of nitroglycerin by technetium-99m sestamibi tomoscintigraphy of resting regional myocardial hypoperfusion in stable patients with healed myocardial infarction. Am. J. Cardiol. 74:843, 1994.

215. Bisi, G., Sciagra, R., Santoro, G. M., et al.: Rest technetium-99m sestamibi tomography in combination with short-term administration of nitrates: Feasibility and reliability for prediction of postrevascularization outcome of asynergic territories. J. Am. Coll. Cardiol. 24:1282, 1994.

216. Udelson, J. E.: Can technetium-99m-labeled sestamibi track myocardial viability? J. Nucl. Cardiol. 1:571, 1994.

217. Diamond, G. A., and Forrester, J. S.: Analysis of probability as an aid in the clinical diagnosis of coronary artery disease. N. Engl. J. Med. 300:1350, 1979.

218. Epstein, S. E.: Implications of probability analysis on the strategy used for noninvasive detection of coronary artery disease. Role of single or combined use of exercise electrocardiographic testing, radionuclide cineangiography and myocardial perfusion imaging. Am. J. Cardiol. 46:491, 1980.

219. Hamilton, G. W., Trobaugh, G. B., Ritchie, J. C., et al.: Myocardial imaging with ^{201}Thallium: An analysis of clinical usefulness based on Bayes' theorem. Semin. Nucl. Med. 8:358, 1978.

220. Arain, S. A., Mattera, J. A., Sinusas, A. J., et al.: Is myocardial perfusion imaging necessary in patients with normal baseline ECG referred for stress testing? J. Nucl. Med. 36(Abs.):110P, 1995.

221. Christian, T. F., Miller, T. D., Bailey, K. R., et al.: Exercise tomographic thallium-201 imaging in patients with severe coronary artery disease and normal electrocardiograms. Ann. Intern. Med. 121:825, 1994.

222. Nallamothu, N., Ghods, M., Heo, J., et al.: Comparison of thallium-201 single photon emission computed tomography and electrocardiographic

response during exercise in patients with normal rest electrocardiographic results. J. Am. Coll. Cardiol. 25:830, 1995.

INFARCT IMAGING

223. Rude, R. E., Parkey, R. W., Bonte, F. J., et al.: Clinical implications of the technetium-99 stannous pyrophosphate myocardial scintigraphic "doughnut" pattern in patients with acute myocardial infarcts. Circulation 59:721, 1979.
224. Schofer, J., Spielmann, R. P., Bromel, T., et al.: Thallium-201/technetium-99m pyrophosphate overlap in patients with acute myocardial infarction after thrombolysis: Prediction of depressed wall motion despite thallium uptake. Am. Heart J. 112:291, 1986.
225. Gertz, M. A., Brown, M. L., Hauser, M. F., et al.: Utility of technetium-99m pyrophosphate bone scanning in cardiac amyloidosis. Arch. Intern. Med. 147:1039, 1987.
226. Davies, A. D., Thakur, M. L., Berger, H. J., et al.: Imaging the inflammatory response to acute myocardial infarction in man using Indium-111 labeled autologous leukocytes. Circulation 63:826, 1981.
227. Narula, J., Torchilin, V. P., Petrov, A. N., et al.: In vivo targeting of acute myocardial infarction with negative-charge, polymer-modified antimyosin antibody: Use of different cross-linkers. J. Nucl. Cardiol. 2:26, 1995.
228. Johnson, L. L., Seldin, D. W., Becker, L. C., et al.: Antimyosin imaging in acute transmural myocardial infarctions: Results of a multicenter clinical trial. J. Am. Coll. Cardiol. 13:27, 1989.
229. Carrio, I., Bernia, L., Ballester, M., et al.: Indium-111 antimyosin scintigraphy to assess myocardial damage in patients with suspected myocarditis and cardiac rejection. J. Nucl. Med. 29:1900, 1988.
230. Dec, G. W., Palacios, I., Yasuda, T., et al.: Antimyosin antibody cardiac imaging: Its role in the diagnosis of myocarditis. J. Am. Coll. Cardiol. 16:97, 1990.
231. Lahiri, A., Jain, D.: New radionuclide imaging in cardiovascular disease. Curr. Opin. Cardiol. 2:1070, 1987.

ASSESSMENT OF CARDIAC PERFORMANCE

232. Zaret, B. L., Strauss, H. W., Hurley, P. J., et al.: A noninvasive scintiphotographic method for detecting regional ventricular dysfunction in man. N. Engl. J. Med. 284:1165, 1971.
233. Strauss, H. W., Zaret, B. L., Hurley, P. J., et al.: A scintiphotographic method for measuring left ventricular ejection fraction in man without cardiac catheterization. Am. J. Cardiol. 28:575, 1971.
234. Berger, H. J., and Zaret, B. L.: Radionuclide assessment of cardiovascular performance. In Freeman, L. M. (ed.): Freeman and Johnson's Clinical Radionuclide Imaging. 3rd ed. New York, Grune and Stratton, 1984, p. 364.
235. Zaret, B. L., and Berger, H. J.: Nuclear cardiology. In Hurst, J. W. (ed.): The Heart, Arteries and Veins. 7th ed. New York, McGraw-Hill Book Co., 1990, p. 1899.
236. Kimchi, A., Rozanski, A., Fletcher, C., et al.: Reversal of rest myocardial asynergy during exercise: A radionuclide scintigraphic study. J. Am. Coll. Cardiol. 6:1004, 1985.
237. Rozanski, A., Bairey, C. N., Krantz, D. S., et al.: Mental stress and the induction of silent myocardial ischemia in patients with coronary artery disease. N. Engl. J. Med. 318:1005, 1988.
238. Links, J. M., Becker, L. C., Shindledecker, J. G., et al.: Measurement of absolute left ventricular volume from gated blood pool studies. Circulation 65:82, 1982.
239. Massardo, T., Gal, R. A., Grenier, R. P., et al.: Left ventricular volume calculation using a count-based ratio method applied to multigated radionuclide angiography. J. Nucl. Med. 31:450, 1990.
240. Gerson, M. C.: Radionuclide ventriculography: Left ventricular volumes and pressure-volume relations. In Gerson M. C. (ed.): Cardiac Nuclear Medicine. New York, McGraw-Hill Book Co., 1991, p. 81.
241. Marmor, A., Jain, D., Cohen, L. S., et al.: Left ventricular peak power during exercise: A noninvasive approach for assessment of contractile reserve. J. Nucl. Med. 34:1877, 1993.
242. Marmor, A., Jain, D., and Zaret, B. L.: Beyond ejection fraction. J. Nucl. Med. 1:477, 1994.
243. Zaret, B. L., Wackers, F. J., Terrin, M., et al.: Assessment of global and regional left ventricular performance at rest and during exercise after thrombolytic therapy for acute myocardial infarction: Results of the Thrombolysis in Myocardial Infarction (TIMI II) study. Am. J. Cardiol. 69:1, 1992.
244. Starling, M. R., Walsh, R. Z., Lasher, J. C., et al.: Quantification of left ventricular regional dyssynergy by radionuclide angiography. J. Nucl. Med. 28:1725, 1987.
245. Botvinick, E. H., Dae, M. W., O'Connell, J. W., et al.: First harmonic Fourier (phase) analysis of blood pool scintigrams for the evaluation of cardiac contraction and conduction. In Gerson, M. D. (ed.): Cardiac Nuclear Medicine. New York, McGraw-Hill Book Co., 1991, p. 81.
246. Robinson, V. J. B., Smiseth, O. A., Scott-Douglas, N. W., et al.: Assessment of splanchnic vascular capacity and capacitance using quantitative equilibrium blood pool scintigraphy. J. Nucl. Med. 31:154, 1990.
247. Flamm, S. D., Taki, J., Moore, R., et al.: Redistribution of regional and organ blood volume and effect on cardiac function in relation to upright exercise intensity in healthy human subjects. Circulation 81:1550, 1990.
248. Zaret, B. L., and Jain, D.: Continuous monitoring left ventricular function with miniaturized nonimaging detectors. In Zaret, B. L., and

Beller, G. A. (eds.): Nuclear Cardiology: State-of-the-Art and Future Directions. St. Louis, C. V. Mosby Co., 1993, p. 136.
249. Soufer, R., Wohlgelernter, D., Vita, N. A., et al.: Intact systolic left ventricular function in clinical congestive heart failure. Am. J. Cardiol. 55:1032, 1985.
250. Breisblatt, W. M., Vita, N. A., Armuchastegui, M., et al.: Usefulness of serial radionuclide monitoring during graded nitroglycerin infusion for unstable angina pectoris for determining left ventricular function and individualized therapeutic dose. Am. J. Cardiol. 61:685, 1988.
251. Broadhurst, P., Cashman, P., Crawley, J., et al.: Clinical validation of a miniature nuclear probe system for continuous on-line monitoring of cardiac function and ST-segment. J. Nucl. Med. 32:37, 1991.
252. Tamaki, N., Yasuda, T., Moore, R., et al.: Continuous monitoring of left ventricular function by an ambulatory radionuclide detector in patients with coronary artery disease. J. Am. Coll. Cardiol. 12:669, 1988.
253. Kayden, D. S., Wackers, F. J., and Zaret, B. L.: Silent left ventricular dysfunction during routine activity after thrombolytic therapy for acute myocardial infarction. J. Am. Coll. Cardiol. 15:1500, 1990.
254. Zaret, B. L., and Kayden, D. S.: Ambulatory monitoring of left ventricular function: A new modality for assessing silent myocardial ischemia. In Kellerman, J. J., and Braunwald, E. (eds.): Silent Myocardial Ischemia: A Critical Appraisal. Basel, Karger, 1990, p. 105.
255. Berg, M. M., Jain, D., Soufer, R., et al.: Role of behavioral and psychological factors in mental stress induced silent left ventricular dysfunction in coronary artery disease. J. Am. Coll. Cardiol. 22:440, 1993.
256. Corbett, J. R.: Tomographic radionuclide ventriculography: Opportunity ignored? J. Nucl. Cardiol. 1:567, 1994.
257. Lu, P., Liu, X, Shi, R., et al.: Comparison of tomographic and planar radionuclide ventriculography in the assessment of regional left ventricular function in patients with left ventricular aneurysm before and after surgery. J. Nucl. Cardiol. 1:537, 1994.

FIRST-PASS RADIONUCLIDE ANGIOCARDIOGRAPHY

258. Blumgart, H. L., and Weiss, S.: Studies on the velocity of blood flow. VII. The pulmonary circulation time in normal resting individuals. J. Clin. Invest. 4:399, 1927.
259. Van Dyke, D. C., Anger, H. O., Sullivan, R. W., et al.: Cardiac evaluation for radioisotope dynamics. J. Nucl. Med. 13:585, 1972.
260. Zaret, B. L., and Wackers, F. J.: Measurement of right ventricular function. In Gerson, M. C. (ed.): Cardiac Nuclear Medicine. New York, McGraw-Hill Book Co., 1991, p. 183.
261. Gelfand, M. J., and Hannon, D. W.: Pediatric Nuclear Cardiology. In Gerson, M. C. (ed.): Cardiac Nuclear Medicine. New York, McGraw-Hill Book Co., 1991, p. 551.
262. Bonow, R. O., Bacharach, S. L., Green, M. V., et al.: Impaired left ventricular diastolic filling in patients with coronary artery disease: Assessment with radionuclide angiography. Circulation 64:315, 1981.
263. Bashore, T. M., Leithe, M. E., and Shaffer, P.: Diastolic function. In Gerson, M. C. (ed.): Cardiac Nuclear Medicine. New York, McGraw-Hill Book Co., 1991, p. 195.
264. Fouad, F. M., Slominski, J. M., and Tarazi, R. C.: Left ventricular diastolic function in hypertension: Relation to left ventricular mass and function. J. Am. Coll. Cardiol. 3:1500, 1984.
265. Cohn, J. N., Johnson, G., and the Veterans Administration Cooperative Study Group: Heart failure with normal ejection fraction. Circulation 82(Suppl. III):4A, 1990.
266. Setaro, J., Soufer, R., Remetz, M. S., et al.: Long term outcome in patients with congestive heart failure and intact systolic left ventricular performance. Am. J. Cardiol. 69:1212, 1992.
267. Setaro, J. F., Zaret, B. L., Schulman, D. S., et al.: Usefulness of verapamil for congestive heart failure, abnormal diastolic filling and normal left ventricular systolic performance. Am. J. Cardiol. 66:981, 1990.
268. Iskandrian, A. S., and Hakki, A.: Age-related changes in left ventricular diastolic performance. Am. Heart J. 112:75, 1986.

CLINICAL APPLICATIONS OF CARDIAC PERFORMANCE STUDIES

269. Kazmers, A., Cerqueira, M. D., and Zierler, R. E.: The role of preoperative radionuclide ejection fraction in direct abdominal aortic aneurysm repair. J. Vasc. Surg. 8:128, 1988.
270. The Multicenter Postinfarction Research Group: Risk stratification and survival after myocardial infarction. N. Engl. J. Med. 309:331, 1983.
270a. Zaret, B. L., Wackers, F. J., Terrin, M. L., et al.: Value of radionuclide rest and exercise left ventricular ejection fraction to assess survival of patients following thrombolytic therapy for acute myocardial infarction: Results of the Thrombolysis in Myocardial Infarction (TIMI) Phase II study. J. Am. Coll. Cardiol. 26:73, 1995.
271. Abraham, R. D., Harris, P. G., Rubin, G. S., et al.: Usefulness of ejection fraction response to exercise one month after acute myocardial infarction in predicting coronary anatomy and prognosis. Am. J. Cardiol. 60:225, 1987.
272. Ahnve, S., Gilpin, E., Henning, H., et al.: Limitations and advantages of the ejection fraction for defining high risk after acute myocardial infarction. Am. J. Cardiol. 58:872, 1986.
273. Kuchard, L., Frund, J., Yates, M., et al.: Enhanced prediction of major cardiac events after myocardial infarction using exercise radionuclide ventriculography. Aust. N.Z. J. Med. 17:228, 1987.
274. Mazzotta, G., Camerini, A., Scopinaro, G., et al.: Predicting cardiac mortality after uncomplicated myocardial infarction by exercise radio-

nuclide ventriculography and exercise-induced ST-segment elevation. Eur. Heart J. 13:330, 1992.

275. CASS Principal Investigators: Coronary artery surgery study (CASS): A randomized trial of coronary bypass surgery. Survival data. Circulation 68:939, 1983.

276. Ritchie, J. L., Hallstrom, A. P., Troubaugh, C. B., et al.: Out-of-hospital sudden coronary death: Rest and exercise left ventricular function in survivors. Am. J. Cardiol. 55:645, 1985.

277. Meizlish, J., Berger, H. J., Plankey, R. T., et al.: Functional left ventricular aneurysm formation following acute anterior transmural myocardial infarction: Incidence, natural history and prognostic implications. N. Engl. J. Med. 311:101, 1984.

278. Bonow, R. O., Kent, K. M., Rosing, D. R., et al.: Exercise-induced ischemia in mildly symptomatic patients with coronary artery disease and preserved left ventricular function: Identification of subgroups at risk of death during medical therapy. N. Engl. J. Med. 311:1339, 1984.

279. Lee, K. L., Pryor, D. B., Pieper, K. S., et al.: Prognostic value of radionuclide angiography in medically treated patients with coronary artery disease: A comparison with clinical and catheterization variables. Circulation 82:1705, 1990.

280. Mazzotta, G., Pace, L., and Bonow, R. O.: Risk stratification of patients with coronary artery disease and left ventricular dysfunction by exercise radionuclide angiography and exercise electrocardiography. J. Nucl. Cardiol. 1:529, 1994.

281. Lim, R., Dyke, L., and Dymond, D. S.: Objective assessment of "cardioprotective" efficacy as a prognostic guide in the management of mildly symptomatic revascularisible coronary artery disease. J. Am. Coll. Cardiol. 1995 (in press).

282. Schlant, R. C.: The prognosis of individuals with silent myocardial ischemia. In Kellerman, N. J. J., and Braunwald, E. (eds.): Silent Myocardial Ischemia: A Critical Appraisal. Vol. 37. Basel, Karger, 1990, p. 187.

283. Breitenbucher, A., Pfisterer, M., Hoffman, A., et al.: Long-term follow-up of patients with silent ischemia during exercise radionuclide angiography. J. Am. Coll. Cardiol. 15:999, 1990.

284. Kayden, D. S., Remetz, M. S., Cabin, H. S., et al.: Validation of continuous radionuclide left ventricular function monitoring in detecting myocardial ischemia during balloon angioplasty of the left anterior descending artery. Am. J. Cardiol. 67:1339, 1991.

285. Jain, D., Burg, M., Soufer, R., et al.: Prognostic implications of mental stress induced silent left ventricular dysfunction of patients with stable angina pectoris. Am. J. Cardiol. 76:31, 1995.

286. Alexander, J., Dainiak, N., Berger, H. J., et al.: Serial assessment of doxorubicin cardiotoxicity with quantitative radionuclide angiocardiography. N. Engl. J. Med. 300:278, 1979.

287. Schwartz, R. G., McKenzie, W. B., Alexander, J., et al.: Congestive heart failure and left ventricular dysfunction complicating doxorubicin therapy: Seven-year-experience using serial radionuclide angiocardiography. Am. J. Med. 82:1109, 1987.

288. Schwartz, R. G., and Zaret, B. L.: The diagnosis and treatment of drug-induced myocardial disease. In: Muggia, F. M., Green, M. D., and Speyer, J. L. (eds.): Cancer Treatment and the Heart. Baltimore, John Hopkins University Press, 1992, p. 173.

289. Borer, J. S., Bacharach, S. L., Green, M. V., et al.: Exercise-induced left ventricular dysfunction in symptomatic and asymptomatic patients with aortic regurgitation: Assessment by radionuclide cineangiography. Am. J. Cardiol. 42:351, 1978.

290. Schulman, D. S., Biondi, J. W., Matthay, R. A., et al.: Differing responses in ventricular filling, loading, and volumes during positive and expiratory pressure in man. Am. J. Cardiol. 64:772, 1989.

291. Schulman, D. S., Biondi, J. W., Zohgbi, S., et al.: Coronary flow limits right ventricular performance during positive and exploratory pressure. Am. Rev. Respir. Dis. 141:1531, 1990.

OTHER SPECIAL IMAGING STUDIES

292. Tamaki, N., Fujibayas, H. I. Y., Magata, Y., et al.: Radionuclide assessment of myocardial fatty acid metabolism by PET and SPECT. J. Nucl. Cardiol. 2:256, 1995.

293. Iskandrian, A. S., Powers, J., Cave, E. V., et al.: Assessment of myocardial viability by dynamic tomographic I-123 iodophenyl pentadecanoic acid imaging: Comparison to rest-redistribution thallium-201 imaging. J. Nucl. Cardiol. 2:101, 1995.

294. Nishimura, T., Uehara, T., Shimonagata, T., et al.: Clinical results with beta-methyl iodolphenylpentadecanoic acid single photon emission computer tomography in cardiac disease. J. Nucl. Cardiol. 1:S65, 1994.

295. Dae, M. W., O'Connell, J. W., and Botvinick, E. H.: Scintigraphic assessment of regional cardiac adrenergic innervation. Circulation 79:634, 1989.

296. Merlet, P. T., Valette, H., DuBois-Rande, J. L., et al.: Iodine 123-labeled metaiodobenzylguanidine imaging in heart disease. J. Nucl. Cardiol. 1:S79, 1994.

297. Schofer, J., Spielmann, R., Schubert, A., et al.: Iodine-123 metaiodobenzylguanidine scintigraphy: A non-invasive method to demonstrate myocardial adrenergic system disintegrity in patients with idiopathic dilated cardiomyopathy. J. Am. Coll. Cardiol. 12:1252, 1988.

298. Merlet, P., Vailette, H., DuBois-Rande, J. L., et al.: Prognostic value of cardiac MIBG imaging in patients with congestive heart failure. J. Nucl. Med. 33:471, 1992.

HYPOXIA IMAGING

299. Chapman, J. D.: Hypoxic sensitizers: Implications for radiation therapy. N. Engl. J. Med. 301:1429, 1979.

300. Frank, A. J., Chapman, J. D., and Doch, C. J.: Binding of misonidazole to EMT6 and V79 spheroids. Int. J. Radiat. Oncol. Biol. Phys. 8:737, 1982.

301. Miller, G. G., Ngan-Lee, J., and Chapman, J. D.: Intracellular localization of radioactivity labeled misonidazole in EMT-6 tumor cells in vitro. Int. J. Radiat. Oncol. Biol. Phys. 8:741, 1982.

302. Martin, G. V., Caldwell, J. H., Graham, M. M., et al.: Noninvasive detection of hypoxic myocardium using fluorine-18-fluoromisonidazole and positron emission tomography. J. Nucl. Med. 33:2202, 1992.

303. Shelton, M. E., Dence, C. S., Hwang, D. R., et al.: In vivo delineation of myocardial hypoxia during coronary occlusion using fluorin-18-fluoromisonidazole and positron emission tomography: A potential approach for identification of jeopardized myocardium. J. Am. Coll. Cardiol. 16:477, 1990.

304. Shelton, M. E., Dence, C. S., Hwang, D. R., et al.: Myocardial kinetics of fluorine-18 misonidazole: A marker for hypoxic myocardium. J. Nucl. Med. 30:351, 1989.

305. Martin, G. V., Cerqueira, M. D., Caldwell, J. H., et al.: Fluoromisonidazole a metabolic marker for myocyte hypoxia. Circ. Res. 67:240, 1990.

306. Martin, G. V., Caldwell, J. H., Rasey, J. S., et al.: Enhanced binding of the hypoxic cell marker [3H]Fluoromisonidazole in ischemic myocardium. J. Nucl. Med. 30:194, 1989.

307. Rumsey, W. L., Patel, B., Kuczynski, B., et al.: Planar and SPECT imaging of ischemic canine myocardium using a novel ^{99m}Tc-nitroimidazole. J. Nucl. Med. 34(Abs.):(5):15P, 1993.

308. Shi, W., Dione, D. P., Singer, M. J., et al.: Technetium-99m nitroimidazole: A positive imaging agent for the detection of myocardial ischemia. Circulation 88(Abs.)(4):1, 1993.

309. Rumsey, W. L., Cyr, J. E., Raju, N., et al.: A novel [99m]technetium-labeled nitroheterocycle capable of identification of hypoxia in heart. Biochem. Biophys. Res. Comm. 193:1239, 1993.

310. Ng, C. K., Sinusas, A. J., Zaret, B. L., et al.: Kinetic analysis of technetium-99m labeled nitroimidazole (BMS-181321) as a tracer of myocardial hypoxia. Circulation 92:1261, 1995.

POSITRON EMISSION TOMOGRAPHY

311. Schelbert, H., Bonow, R. O., Geltman, E., et al.: Position statement: Clinical use of cardiac positron emission tomography. Position paper of the Cardiovascular Council of the Society of Nuclear Medicine. J. Nucl. Med. 34:1385, 1993.

312. ACC/AHA Task Force Report: Guidelines for clinical use of cardiac radionuclide imaging. Report of the ACC/AHA task force on assessment of diagnostic and therapeutic procedures (committee on radionuclide imaging), developed in collaboration with the American Society of Nuclear Cardiology. J. Am. Coll. Cardiol. 25:521, 1995.

313. Bonow, R. O., Berman, D. S., Gibbons, R. J., et al.: Cardiac positron emission tomography. A report for health professionals from the committee on advanced cardiac imaging and technology of the Council on Clinical Cardiology, American Heart Association. Circulation 84:447, 1991.

314. Maddahi, J., Schelbert, H., Brunken, R., et al.: Role of thallium-201 and PET imaging in evaluation of myocardial viability and management of patients with coronary artery disease and left ventricular dysfunction. J. Nucl. Med. 35:707, 1994.

315. Mody, F. V., Brunken, R. C., Stevenson, L. W., et al.: Differentiating cardiomyopathy of coronary artery disease from nonischemic dilated cardiomyopathy utilizing positron emission tomography. J. Am. Coll. Cardiol. 17:373, 1991.

316. vom Dahl, J., Altehoefer, C., Biedermann, M., et al.: Technetium-99m methoxy-isobutyl-isonitrile as a tracer of myocardial viability? A quantitative comparison with F-18 FDG in 100 patients with coronary artery disease. J. Am. Coll. Cardiol. 21(Suppl A):283A, 1993.

317. Altehoefer, C., Hans-Jurgen, K., Dorr, R., et al.: Fluorine-18 deoxyglucose PET for assessment of viable myocardium in perfusion defects in Tc-99m MIBI SPECT: A comparative study in patients with coronary artery disease. Eur. J. Nucl. Med. 19:334, 1992.

318. Soufer, R., Dey, H. M., Ng, C. K., et al.: Comparison of sestamibi single photon emission computed tomography to positron emission tomography for estimating left ventricular myocardial viability. Am. J. Cardiol. 75:1214, 1995.

319. Camici, P., Ferrannini, E., and Opie, L. H.: Myocardial metabolism in ischemic heart disease: Basic principles and application to imaging by positron emission tomography. Prog. Cardiovasc. Dis. 32:217, 1989.

320. Bergmann, S. R.: Use and limitations of metabolic tracers labeled with positron-emitting radionuclides in the identification of viable myocardium. J. Nucl. Med. 35(Suppl):15S, 1994.

321. Marshall, R. C., Tillisch, J. H., Phelps, M. E., et al.: Identification and differentiation of resting myocardial ischemia and infarction in man with positron computed tomography, 18F-labeled fluorodeoxyglucose and N-13 ammonia. Circulation 67:766, 1983.

322. Brunken, R., Tillisch, J., Schwaiger, M., et al.: Regional perfusion, glucose metabolism and wall motion in patients with chronic electrocardiographic Q wave infarctions: Evidence for persistence of viable tissue in some infarct regions by positron emission tomography. Circulation 73:951, 1986.

323. Schelbert, H. R., and Buxton, D.: Insights into coronary artery disease gained from metabolic imaging. Circulation *78*:496, 1988.

324. Fudo, T., Kambara, H, Hashimoto, T., et al.: F-18 deoxyglucose and stress N-13 ammonia positron emission tomography in anterior wall healed myocardial infarction. Am. J. Cardiol. *61*:1191, 1988.

325. Tamaki, N., Yonekura, Y., Yamashita, K., et al.: Positron emission tomography using F-18 deoxyglucose in evaluation of coronary artery bypass grafting. Am. J. Cardiol. *64*:860, 1989.

326. Brunken, R. C., and Schelbert, H. R.: Positron emission tomography in clinical cardiology. Cardiol. Clin. *7*:607, 1989.

327. Marwick, T. H., Nemec, J. J., Lafont, A., et al.: Prediction by post exercise fluoro-18-deoxyglucose positron emission tomography of improvement in exercise capacity after revascularization. Am. J. Cardiol. *69*:854, 1992.

328. Marwick, T. H., MacIntyre, W. J., Lafont, A., et al.: Metabolic responses of hibernating and infarcted myocardium to revascularization: A follow-up study of regional perfusion, function, and metabolism. Circulation *85*:1347, 1992.

329. Burt, R. W., Perkins, O. W., Oppenheim, B. E., et al.: Direct comparison of fluorine-18-FDG SPECT, fluorine-18-FDG PET and rest thallium-201 SPECT for detection of myocardial viability. J. Nucl. Med. *36*:176, 1995.

330. Bax, J. J., Visser, F. C., van Lingen, A., et al.: Feasibility of assessing regional myocardial uptake of 18F-fluorodeoxyglucose using single photon emission computed tomography. Eur. Heart J. *14*:1675, 1993.

331. Eitzman, D., Al-Aouar, Z., Kanter, H. L., et al.: Clinical outcome of patients with advanced coronary artery disease after viability studies with positron emission tomography. J. Am. Coll. Cardiol. *20*:559, 1992.

332. DiCarli, M. F., Davidson, M., Little, R., et al.: Value of metabolic imaging with positron emission tomography for evaluating prognosis in patients with coronary artery disease and left ventricular dysfunction. Am. J. Cardiol. *73*:527, 1994.

333. Lee, K. S., Marwick, T. H., Cook, S. A., et al.: Prognosis of patients with left ventricular dysfunction, with and without viable myocardium after myocardial infarction: Relative efficacy of medical therapy and revascularization. Circulation *90*:2687, 1994.

334. Yoshida, K., and Gould, K. L.: Quantitative relation of myocardial infarct size and myocardial viability by positron emission tomography to left ventricular ejection fraction and 3-year mortality with and without revascularization. J. Am. Coll. Cardiol. *22*:984, 1993.

335. Tamaki, N., Kawamoto, M., Takahashi, N., et al.: Prognostic value of an increase in fluorine-18-deoxyglucose uptake in patients with myocardial infarction: Comparison with stress thallium imaging. J. Am. Coll. Cardiol. *22*:1621, 1993.

336. Brunken, R., Schwaiger, M., Grover-McKay, M., et al.: Positron emission tomography detects tissue metabolic activity in myocardial segments with persistent thallium perfusion defects. J. Am. Coll. Cardiol. *10*:557, 1987.

337. Brunken, R. C., Kottou, S., Nienabar, C. A., et al.: PET detection of viable tissue in myocardial segments with persistent defects at Tl-201 SPECT. Radiology *172*:65, 1989.

338. Tamaki, N., Yonekura, Y., Yamashita, K., et al.: Relation of left ventricular perfusion and wall motion with metabolic activity in persistent defects on thallium-201 tomography in healed myocardial infarction. Am. J. Cardiol. *62*:202, 1988.

339. Tamaki, N., Yonekura, Y., Yamashita, K., et al.: SPECT thallium-201 tomography and positron tomography using N-13 ammonia and F-18 fluorodeoxyglucose in coronary artery disease. Am. J. Cardiac Imag. *3*:3, 1989.

340. Tamaki, N., Ohtani, H., Yamashita, K., et al.: Metabolic activity in the areas of new fill-in after thallium-201 reinjection: Comparison with positron emission tomography using fluorine-18-deoxyglucose. J. Nucl. Med. *32*:673, 1991.

341. Altehoefer, C., vom Dahl, J., Biedermann, M., et al.: Significance of defect severity in technetium-99m-MIBI SPECT at rest to assess myocardial viability: Comparison with fluorine-18-FDG PET. J. Nucl. Med. *35*:569, 1994.

342. Sawada, S. G., Allman, K. C., Muzik, O., et al.: Positron emission tomography detects evidence of viability in rest technetium-99m sestamibi defects. J. Am. Coll. Cardiol. *23*:92, 1994.

343. Berry, J. J., Baker, J. A., Pieper, K. S., et al.: The effect of metabolic milieu on cardiac PET imaging using fluorine-18-deoxyglucose and nitrogen-13-ammonia in normal volunteers. J. Nucl. Med. *32*:1518, 1991.

344. Schwaiger, M., Schelbert, H. R., Ellison, D., et al.: Sustained regional abnormalities in cardiac metabolism after transient ischemia in the chronic dog model. J. Am. Coll. Cardiol. *6*:336, 1985.

345. Sobel, B. E., Geltman, E. M., Tiefenbrunn, A. J., et al.: Improvement of regional myocardial metabolism after coronary thrombolysis induced with tissue-type plasminogen activator or streptokinase. Circulation *69*:983, 1984.

346. Schwaiger, M., Schelbert, H. R., Keen, R., et al.: Retention and clearance of C-11 palmitic acid in ischemic and reperfused canine myocardium. J. Am. Coll. Cardiol. *6*:310, 1985.

347. Grover-McKay, M., Schelbert, H. R., Schwaiger, M., et al.: Identification of impaired metabolic reserve in patients with significant coronary artery stenosis by atrial pacing. Circulation *74*:281, 1986.

348. Rosamond, T. L., Abendschein, D. R., Sobel, B. E., et al.: Metabolic fate of radiolabeled palmitate in ischemic canine myocardium: Implications for positron emission tomography. J. Nucl. Med. *28*:1322, 1987.

349. Armbrecht, J. J., Buxton, D. B., Brunken, R. C., et al.: Regional myocardial oxygen consumption determined noninvasively in humans with [1-^{11}C] acetate and dynamic positron tomography. Circulation *80*:863, 1989.

350. Buxton, D. B., Nienaber, C. A., Luxen, A., et al.: Noninvasive quantitation of regional myocardial oxygen consumption in vivo with [1-11C]acetate and dynamic positron emission tomography. Circulation *79*:134, 1989.

351. Ng, C. K., Huang, S. C., Schelbert, H. R., et al.: Validation of a model for [1-^{11}C]acetate as a tracer of cardiac oxidative metabolism. Am. J. Physiol. *255*:H1304, 1994.

352. Gropler, R. J., Geltman, E. M., Sampathkumaran, K., et al.: Comparison of carbon-11-acetate with fluorine-18-fluorodeoxyglucose for delineating viable myocardium by positron emission tomography. J. Am. Coll. Cardiol. *22*:1587, 1993.

353. Vom Dahl, J., Herman, W. H., Hicks, R. J., et al.: Myocardial glucose uptake in patients with insulin-dependent diabetes mellitus assessed quantitatively by dynamic positron emission tomography. Circulation *88*:395, 1993.

354. Gould, L., Yoshida, K., Hess, M., et al.: Myocardial metabolism of fluorodeoxyglucose compared to cell membrane integrity for the potassium analogue rubidium-82 for assessing infarct size in man by PET. J. Nucl. Med. *32*:1, 1991.

355. Yamamoto, Y., deSilva, R., Rhodes, C., et al.: A new strategy for the assessment of viable myocardium and regional myocardial blood flow using ^{15}O-water and dynamic positron emission tomography. Circulation *86*:167, 1992.

356. DeSilva, R., Yamamoto, Y., Rhodes, C., et al.: Detection of hibernating myocardium using H$_2$^{15}O and positron emission tomography (PET). Circulation *86*:1738, 1992.

357. Shah, A., Schelbert, H. R., Schwaiger, M., et al.: Measurement of regional myocardial blood flow with N-13 ammonia and positron emission tomography in intact dogs. J. Am. Coll. Cardiol. *5*:92, 1985.

358. Bergmann, S. R., Herrero, P., Markham, J., et al.: Noninvasive quantitation of myocardial blood flow in human subjects with oxygen-15-labeled water and positron emission tomography. J. Am. Coll. Cardiol. *14*:639, 1989.

359. Gould, K. L.: PET perfusion imaging and nuclear cardiology. J. Nucl. Med. *32*:579, 1991.

360. Goldstein, R. A., Mullani, N. A., Marani, S. K., et al.: Myocardial perfusion with rubidium-82. II. Effects and pharmacologic intervention. J. Nucl. Med. *24*:907, 1983.

361. Mullani, N. A., Goldstein, R. A., Gould, K. L., et al.: Myocardial perfusion with rubidium-82. I. Measurement of extraction fraction and flow with external detectors. J. Nucl. Med. *24*:898, 1983.

362. Shelton, M. E., Green, M. A., Mathias, C. J., et al.: Kinetics of copper-PTSM in isolated hearts: A novel tracer for measuring blood flow with positron emission tomography. J. Nucl. Med. *30*:1843, 1989.

363. Shelton, M. E., Green, M. A., Mathias, C. J., et al.: Assessment of regional myocardial and renal blood flow with copper-PTSM and positron emission tomography. Circulation *82*:990, 1990.

364. Goldstein, R. A.: Kinetics of rubidium-82 after coronary occlusion and reperfusion: Assessment of patency and viability in open-chested dogs. J. Clin. Invest. *75*:1131, 1985.

365. Goldstein, R. A.: Rubidium-82 kinetics after coronary occlusion: Temporal relation of net myocardial accumulation and viability in open-chested dogs. J. Nucl. Med. *27*:1456, 1986.

366. Bergmann, S. T., Hack, S., Tweson, T., et al.: Dependence of accumulation of ^{13}NH$_3$ by myocardium on metabolic factors and its implications for the quantitative assessment of perfusion. Circulation *61*:34, 1980.

367. Bergmann, S. R., Fox, K. A. A., Rand, A. L., et al.: Quantification of regional myocardial blood flow in vivo with H$_2$^{15}O. Circulation *70*:724, 1984.

368. Uren, N. G., Melin, J. A., DeBruyne, B., et al.: Relation between myocardial blood flow and the severity of coronary artery stenosis. N. Engl. J. Med. *330*:1782, 1994.

369. Walsh, M. N., Geltman, E. M., Steele, R. L., et al.: Augmented myocardial perfusion reserve after coronary angioplasty quantified by positron emission tomography with H$_2$^{15}O. J. Am. Coll. Cardiol. *15*:119, 1990.

370. Soufer, R., and Zaret, B. L.: Positron emission tomography and the quantitative assessment of regional myocardial blood flow (editorial). J. Am. Coll. Cardiol. *15*:128, 1990.

371. Huang, S. C., Schwaiger, M., Carson, R. E., et al.: Quantitative measurement of myocardial blood flow with oxygen-15 water and positron computed tomography: An assessment of potential and problems. J. Nucl. Med. *26*:616, 1985.

372. Gould, K. L.: Percent coronary stenosis: Battered gold standard, pernicious relic or clinical practicality. J. Am. Coll. Cardiol. *11*:886, 1988.

373. Schelbert, H. R., Wisenberg, C., Phelps, M. E., et al.: Noninvasive assessment of coronary stenosis by myocardial imaging during pharmacologic coronary vasodilation. VI. Detection of coronary artery disease in human beings with intravenous N-13 ammonia and positron computed tomography. Am. J. Cardiol. *49*:1197, 1982.

374. Gould, K. L., Goldstein, R. A., Mullani, N. A., et al.: Noninvasive assessment of coronary stenosis by myocardial perfusion imaging during pharmacologic coronary vasodilation. VIII. Clinical feasibility of positron cardiac imaging without a cyclotron using generator-produced rubidium-82. J. Am. Coll. Cardiol. *7*:775, 1986.

375. Tamaki, N., Yonekura, Y., Senda, M., et al.: Value and limitation of stress thallium-201 single photon emission computed tomography:

Comparison with nitrogen-13 positron tomography. J. Nucl. Med. *29*:1181, 1988.

376. Demer, L. L., Gould, K. L., Goldstein, R. A., et al.: Assessment of coronary artery disease severity by positron emission tomography. Comparison with quantitative arteriography in 193 patients. Circulation *79*:825, 1989.

377. Gupta, N. C.: Adenosine in myocardial perfusion imaging using positron emission tomography. Am. Heart J. *122*:293, 1991.

378. Williams, B. R.: Positron emission tomography for the assessment of ischemia and myocardial viability. J. Myocard. Ischemia *2*(4):38, 1990.

379. Stewart, R.: Comparison of rubidium-82 positron emission tomography and thallium-201 SPECT imaging for detection of coronary artery disease. Am. J. Cardiol. *67*:1303, 1991.

380. Walsh, M. N., Bergmann, S. R., Steele, R. L., et al.: Delineation of impaired regional myocardial perfusion by positron emission tomography with H$_2$^{15}O. Circulation *78*:620, 1988.

381. Stewart, R., Kalus, M., Molina, E., et al.: Rubidium-82 PET versus thallium-201 SPECT for the diagnosis of regional coronary artery disease. Circulation *80*:209, 1989.

382. Yonekura, Y., Tamaki, N., Senda, M., et al.: Detection of coronary artery disease with N-13 ammonia and high-resolution positron emission computed tomography. Am. Heart J. *113*:645, 1987.

383. Yamashita, K., Tamaki, N., Yonekura, Y., et al.: Quantitative analysis of regional wall motion by gated myocardial positron emission tomography: Validation and comparison with left ventriculography. J. Nucl. Med. *30*:1775, 1989.

384. Sisson, J. C., and Wieland, D. M.: Radiolabeled meta-iodobenzylguanidine: Pharmacology and clinical studies. Am. J. Physiol. Imaging *1*:96, 1986.

385. Glowniak, J. V., Turner, F. E., Gray, L. L., et al.: Iodine-123-metaiodobenzylguanidine imaging of the heart in idiopathic congestive cardiomyopathy and cardiac transplants. J. Nucl. Med. *30*:1182, 1989.

386. Fagret, D., Wolf, J. E., Vanzetto, G., et al.: Myocardial uptake of metaiodobenzylguanidine in patients with left ventricular hypertrophy secondary to valvular aortic stenosis. J. Nucl. Med. *34*:57, 1993.

387. Dae, M. W., O'Connell, J. W., Botvinick, E. H., et al.: Scintigraphic assessment of regional cardiac innervation. Circulation *79*:634, 1989.

388. Goldstein, D. S., Chang, P. C., Eisenhofer, G., et al.: Positron emission tomographic imaging of cardiac sympathetic innervation and function. Circulation *81*:1606, 1990.

389. Schwaiger, M., Kalff, V., Rosenspire, K., et al.: Noninvasive evaluation of sympathetic nervous system in human heart by positron emission tomography. Circulation *82*:457, 1990.

390. Rosenspire, K. C., Gildersleeve, D. L., Massin, C. C., et al.: Metabolic fate of the heart agent [18F]6-Fluorometaraminol. Nucl. Med. Biol. *16*:735, 1989.

391. Valette, H., Deleuze, P., Syrota, A., et al.: Canine myocardial beta-adrenergic, muscarinic receptor densities after denervation: A PET study. J. Nucl. Med. *36*:140, 1995.

392. Berridge, M. S., Nelson, A. D., Zhen, L., et al.: Specific beta-adrenergic receptor binding of carazolol measured with PET. J. Nucl. Med. *35*:1665, 1994.

393. Droste, C., and Roskamm, H.: Pain perception and endogenous pain modulation in angina pectoris. Adv. Cardiol. *37*:142, 1990.

394. Marchant, B., Umachandran, V., Wilkinson, P., et al.: Reexamination of the role of endogenous opiates in silent myocardial ischemia. J. Am. Coll. Cardiol. *23*:645, 1994.

395. Johes, A. K. P., Luthra, S. K., Maziere, B., et al.: Regional cerebral opioid receptor studies with [^{11}C]diprenorphine in normal volunteers. J. Neurosci. Methods *23*:121, 1988.

396. Haskell, W. L., Alderman, E. L., Fair, J. M., et al.: Effects of intensive multiple risk factor reduction on coronary atherosclerosis and clinical cardiac events in men and women with coronary artery disease: The Standard Coronary Risk Intervention Project (SCRIP). Circulation *89*:975, 1994.

397. National Cholesterol Education Program: Second report of the expert panel on detection, evaluation and treatment of high blood cholesterol in adults (adult treatment panel II). Circulation *89*:1329, 1994.

398. Buchwald, H., Matts, J. P., Fitch, L. L., et al.: Changes in sequential coronary arteriograms and subsequent coronary events: Program on the Surgical Control of the Hyperlipidemias (POSCH) Group. JAMA *268*:1429, 1992.

399. Superko, H. R., and Drauss, R. M.: Coronary artery disease regression: Convincing evidence for the benefit of aggressive lipoprotein management. Circulation *90*:1056, 1994.

400. Gould, K. L., Martucci, J. P., Goldberg, D. I., et al.: Short-term cholesterol lowering decreases size and severity of perfusion abnormalities by positron emission tomography after dipyridamole in patients with coronary artery disease: A potential noninvasive marker of healing coronary endothelium. Circulation *89*:1530, 1994.

401. Harrison, D. G., Armstrong, M. L., Frieman, P. C., et al.: Restoration of endothelium-dependent relaxation by dietary treatment of atherosclerosis. J. Clin. Invest. *80*:1801, 1987.

402. Schelbert, H. R., and Maddahi, J.: Clinical cardiac PET: Quo vadis? J. Nucl. Cardiol. *1*:429, 1994.

403. Patterson, R. E., Eisner, R. L., and Horowitz, S. F.: Comparison of cost-effectiveness and utility of exercise ECG, single photon emission computed tomography, positron emission tomography and coronary angiography for diagnosis of coronary artery disease. Circulation *91*:54, 1995.

404. Zeiher, A., Drexler, H., Wollschlager, H., et al.: Endothelial dysfunction of the coronary microvasculature is associated with impaired coronary blood flow regulation in patients with early atherosclerosis. Circulation *84*:1984, 1991.

405. Grambow, D., Dayanikli, F., Muzik, O., et al.: Assessment of endothelial function with PET cold pressure test in patients with various degrees of coronary atherosclerosis. J. Nucl. Med. *34*:P36, 1993.

406. Packer, M.: The neurohormonal hypothesis: A theory to explain the mechanism of disease progression in heart failure (editorial). J. Am. Coll. Cardiol. *20*:248, 1992.

407. Allman, K., Wieland, D., Muzik, O., et al.: Carbon-11 hydroxyephedrine with positron emission tomography for serial assessment of cardiac adrenergic neuronal function after acute myocardial infarction in humans. J. Am. Coll. Cardiol. *22*:368, 1993.

408. Calkins, H., Lehmann, M. H., Allman, K., et al.: Scintigraphic pattern of regional cardiac sympathetic innervation in patients with familial long QT syndrome using positron emission tomography. Circulation *87*:1616, 1993.

409. Calkins, H., Allman, K., Bolling, S., et al.: Correlation between scintigraphic evidence of regional sympathetic neuronal dysfunction and ventricular refractoriness in the human heart. Circulation *88*:172, 1993.

Chapter 10
Newer Cardiac Imaging Techniques: Magnetic Resonance Imaging and Computed Tomography

CHARLES B. HIGGINS

MAGNETIC RESONANCE IMAGING OF THE HEART

Magnetic resonance imaging (MRI) has several important attributes that make it intrinsically advantageous for cardiovascular diagnosis. First, a high natural contrast exists between the blood pool and the cardiovascular structures because of the lack of signal from flowing blood with the spin-echo MRI technique or the bright signal from blood with the gradient-echo (cine MRI) technique. When the spin-echo technique is used, blood appears black on images; therefore, internal structures of the heart can be visualized within the signal void of the cardiac chambers. Using the gradient-echo technique, the blood pool appears white and has substantially higher signal than the myocardium, again providing good edge definition of the endocardial margin. Consequently, contrast medium is not required for discrimination of the blood pool, as MRI is an entirely noninvasive imaging technique. Second, a wide range of soft tissue contrast provides the potential for the characterization of myocardial tissue. This contrast among tissues depends on proton (hydrogen nuclei) density, magnetic relaxation times of the protons, and magnetic susceptibility effects. Third, imaging can be done in any plane, including those parallel and perpendicular to the major axis of the ventricles.

MAGNETIC RESONANCE GLOSSARY

Brief descriptions of the MRI process, general imaging techniques, and specific imaging techniques for the heart are given below, along with some useful terminology for MRI. A more detailed description of the principles underlying MRI is available elsewhere.

ECHOPLANAR IMAGING. A method for obtaining MR images in 30 to 50 msecs. Data for all points in the image matrix are obtained with a single pulse repetition (single TR). In echoplanar imaging, a very rapid series of echoes is generated by rapidly switching a strong phase-encoding gradient in the presence of a weaker read gradient.
FREE INDUCTION DECAY. The signal produced by the release of energy absorbed by the nuclei from a previously applied radiofrequency (RF) pulse. The free induction decay is the signal analyzed in MRI and spectroscopy.
GRADIENT-ECHO IMAGING SEQUENCE. A method by which images are acquired more rapidly than with spin-echo imaging by substantially reducing the repetition time (TR). The technique uses a flip angle of 90 degrees or less and a short TR. This reduction is achieved by switching the read gradient to focus the signal rather than by a time-consuming refocusing RF pulse. Contrast on these images is very different from that for spin-echo images. A major difference is that flow blood produces strong signal and appears bright.
HYDROGEN DENSITY (SPIN DENSITY, PROTON DENSITY). Density of protons at a site in a sample which are resonating as part of the magnetic resonance process. From the point of view of quantum mechanics, these are the protons making transitions from high-energy states to lower ones and vice versa, when energy just equal to the difference between these two states is applied.
MAGNETIC MOMENT. Intensity and direction of the net magnetic field of spinning nuclei. In a magnetic field, nuclei align to produce a net magnetic moment parallel to the field.
MAGNETIC RESONANCE IMAGING (MRI). Spatial two- or three-dimensional map of nuclei resonating at a characteristic frequency when placed in a magnetic field and subjected to intermittently applied RF pulses.
PROTON MRI. Imaging dependent on the concentration and relaxation time of hydrogen nuclei.
MULTINUCLEAR MRI. Imaging using nuclei other than hydrogen, such as sodium-23 and phosphorus-31.
MAGNETIC RESONANCE SIGNAL. During relaxation after cessation of an RF pulse, energy absorbed from this pulse is released and provides an RF signal.
RELAXATION. Return of nuclei to the original state of alignment with a magnetic field after having been tilted by an RF pulse.
MAGNETIC RESONANCE SPECTROSCOPY. Spectrum of resonant frequencies of a specific nucleus contained within a sample. This spectrum results from the chemical shift of a nucleus caused by the influence of the local chemical environment. Consequently, the resonant frequency of phosphorus in the inorganic state is slightly different from its frequency in creatine phosphate. Magnetic resonance spectroscopy detects and maps these chemical shifts of a nucleus.
PROTON SPECTROSCOPY. Spectrum of resonant frequencies of hydrogen nuclei (protons) in relation to the chemical environment. Proton spectroscopy can define chemical peaks representative of substances such as fats, water, lactic acid, choline, and carnitine.
PARAMAGNETIC SUBSTANCES. Substances that alter the natural relaxation times of nuclei undergoing the magnetic resonance process. These are usually molecules with unpaired electrons which reduce the relaxation times of resonating nuclei. These substances are being used and developed as contrast media for magnetic resonance imaging.

RELAXATION TIMES. Relaxation of nuclei undergoing the magnetic resonance process has two components called T1 and T2 relaxation times. These relaxation times are time-constant, measured as the magnetization vector processes into alignment with the magnetic field after perturbation by an RF pulse.

RESONANT FREQUENCY. Each nucleus that is sensitive to the magnetic resonance process must be tilted in the magnetic field by a specific frequency (resonant frequency) in order to induce resonance. When this frequency is applied, the nucleus is rotated away from its equilibrium alignment with the magnetic field. When the RF pulse ceases, the nucleus realigns with the magnetic field through a process of magnetic relaxation.

SPIN-ECHO IMAGING SEQUENCE. Images are produced by sampling signal after an initial 90-degree RF pulse, followed by one or more 180-degree pulses. The 180-degree pulse refocuses spins and thereby enhances the signal from them. Signal is sampled some time after the 180-degree pulse.

SURFACE COILS. RF receiver coils placed upon the surface of the subject or upon an organ of interest in order to detect the magnetic resonance signal. These coils increase the efficiency and signal strength for both MRI and spectroscopy.

T1 RELAXATION TIME. Also called spin-lattice or longitudinal relaxation time. T1 relaxation is a measure of the exponential rate of growth of the magnetization vector along the direction of the external magnetic field after the nuclei have been tilted (flipped) by an RF pulse.

T1-WEIGHTED IMAGE. Image in which the intensity of image voxels depends greatly on the T1 relaxation time of tissues. For the spin-echo technique, this is done with a short TR and TE.

T2 RELAXATION TIME. Also called spin-spin or transverse relaxation time. Immediately after cessation of a 90-degree RF pulse, the nuclei process in phase, resulting in a magnetization vector in the transverse plane. There is gradual dephasing of nuclei, leading to cancellation of the magnetization vector in the transverse plane.

T2-WEIGHTED IMAGE. Image in which the intensity of image voxels depends heavily upon the T2 relaxation time of tissues. For the spin-echo technique, this is done with a long TR and TE.

TE. Echo delay time. Time between the initiation of a pulse sequence (90-degree pulse) and the sampling of the spin-echo signal. For the spin-echo sequence, this sampling is done after the 180-degree pulse. For example, the first spin-echo signal is sampled at a time that is twice the duration between the initial 90-degree pulse and the 180-degree refocusing pulse.

Technical Aspects

Atomic nuclei with a net charge have a magnetic moment. A net charge exists when a nucleus contains unpaired (an odd number) of protons, neutrons, or both. The hydrogen nucleus contains only a proton; it is positively charged and has a strong magnetic moment. The magnetic properties of nuclei are expressed when they are placed in an external magnetic field. When protons or other nuclei with magnetic moment lie within a magnetic field and are then exposed to electromagnetic radiation (RF waves), energy is absorbed and subsequently emitted. This absorption and release of energy causes resonance—nuclear magnetic resonance. The RF necessary to induce resonance has to be proportional to the local magnetic field (H_L) and a constant (magnetogyric ratio) related to the specific nucleus involved. The relationship between frequency (f) and magnetic field is expressed by the following equation:

$$f = \delta H_L / 2\pi$$

When nuclei at equilibrium in a magnetic field are irradiated at the resonant frequency, they attain a higher energy state. When they return to equilibrium, they emit energy at the same frequency if the magnetic field remains constant. If the magnetic field changes between the time of excitation and emission, then the emission occurs at a frequency corresponding to the new field strength as expressed by this equation.

Localization of Magnetic Resonance Signal

MRI depends on the reception of the emitted RF signal from resonating nuclei and on the capability of locating these nuclei in space. Location of the resonating nuclei can be achieved by spatially varying the field strength in a known manner. Because resonance frequency of a nucleus at a specific site is related to local field strength, the emitted frequency characterizes the spatial location of the nu-

cleus when a magnetic gradient exists in one or more planes.

Selection of a transverse section for imaging is done by applying a magnetic gradient along the Z axis (long axis of the body). In such a gradient, each transverse plane (XY plane) has a specific and different resonant frequency. If the body is irradiated with a 90-degree RF pulse consisting of a narrow range of frequencies corresponding to the resonance frequency of a single plane, only the nuclei in that plane resonate *selective irradiation*, and the image plane is delineated.

Once a plane is excited by selective irradiation, spatial localization is attained in that plane by another gradient oriented parallel to that plane. After the selective 90-degree RF pulse is applied, a magnetic field gradient is produced in the X or Y direction. Nuclei at the stronger end of the field gradient resonate at a higher frequency than those at the weaker end of the gradient. This provides spatial localization within the selected plane.

The magnetic signal from a sample undergoing MRI is detected by an RF receiver coil. The intensity of the signal at foci in the imaging plane depends on the concentration of resonating nuclei at the site and the magnetic relaxation times of the nuclei. The relaxation times are measures of the interaction of the resonating protons with the static magnetic field and the intermittently applied RF pulses.

The net magnetic moment of nuclei at any site can be expressed as a vector with length (intensity) and direction. At equilibrium, the vector points along the main static magnetic field. The vector can be tipped 90 degrees by the application of an RF pulse. The component of the net magnetic moment that points along the main magnetic field is called *longitudinal magnetization*. The component at 90 degrees to the main field is the *transverse magnetization*. The component at 90 degrees to the main field is fully aligned with the magnetic field (equilibrium); the vector varies continuously between longitudinal and transverse magnetization and gradually approaches full longitudinal magnetization.

MAGNETIC RELAXATION TIMES

After the application of a 90-degree RF pulse, net magnetization is rotated from the longitudinal direction (ZY plane) into the transverse direction (XY plane). At this instant, transverse magnetization is maximum and longitudinal magnetization is zero. Immediately after this, longitudinal magnetization gradually recovers toward its equilibrium value. This exponential growth has a time constant called *T1*. Likewise, after the 90-degree pulse, transverse magnetization exponentially decays; the time constant is called *T2*. In tissues, T2 is much shorter than T1. These relaxation times are related to several characteristics of tissues, including temperature. Tissues have different relaxation times, and these differences contribute to contrast among tissues during imaging. Contrast between two tissues can be accentuated by sampling signal at an instant when the difference between the relaxation times of the two tissues is maximal.

IMAGING, TR, AND TE. The MR image is produced by applying the sets of RF pulses many times over several minutes; generally, 128 to 512 pulse sequences are used. The time between application of sets of RF pulses is called the *repetition time* (TR). Depending on the technique employed for imaging, each set consists of one or more RF pulses. The time between the initial pulse in a sequence and the instant when signal is acquired from the sample is called the *echo delay time* (TE). It is possible to alter the pulse sequences in such a way that differences in T1 and T2 relaxation times among the tissues can be accentuated to produce contrast among these tissues. This is referred to as *T1* or *T2 weighting* of the images. T1-weighted images have short TR and TE intervals, while T2-weighted images have long TR and TE intervals when using the spin-echo technique. T1 and T2 weighting for new fast-imaging techniques is achieved to some extent by variations in the flip angles induced in the nuclei by the initial RF pulses.

EFFECTS OF MOVING BLOOD. During an imaging sequence, the motion of nuclei through the region that is being imaged greatly influences signal intensity. Although the influence of blood flow on MR images is complex, motion of the excited nuclei causes either a loss or increase of signal intensity, depending upon the RF pulse sequence employed. For the spin-echo sequence, moving blood in the lumina of vessels appears dark (no signal), providing considerable natural contrast for visualization of the internal surfaces of the blood vessels and walls of the cardiac chambers (Fig. 10–1). Because contrast medium is not required to mark the blood pool, MRI is a totally noninvasive technique for cardiovascular diagnosis. When blood veloc-

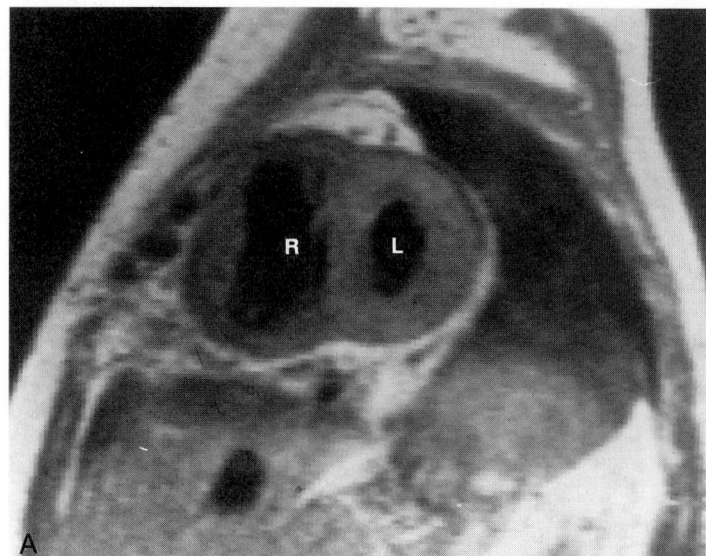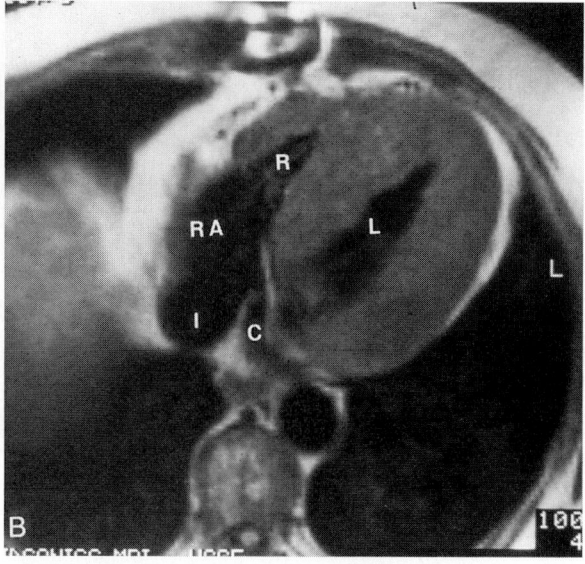

FIGURE 10–1. *A,* ECG-gated spin-echo MR image acquired in the short-axis plane through the middle of the ventricles. On this type of image the moving blood within the chambers of the heart produces little or no signal, resulting in high contrast between the blood pool and myocardial walls. The right ventricular wall is thickened in this patient. L = left ventricle; R = right ventricle. *B,* ECG-gated spin-echo image acquired in the transverse plane. The endocardial border is sharply demarcated owing to the contrast between the blood pool and the myocardium. There is severe left ventricular hypertrophy. I = inferior vena cava; L = left ventricle; RA = right atrium; R = right ventricle; C = coronary sinus. Note that the cardiac short-axis image transects the heart perpendicular to the long axis of the heart while the transverse plane sections the ventricles obliquely.

ity is such that protons move through the thickness of the tomogram (usually 5 to 10 mm) in the time between the 90-degree and 180-degree pulses of the spin-echo sequence, signal is lost from the blood. Using standard spin-echo sequences, this time (TE/2) is usually 7 to 15 msec for the first such image. For the gradient-echo pulse sequence, signal is received from blood flowing at normal velocities in the cardiac chambers and all blood vessels. The signal of flowing blood increases in proportion to the rate of flow (velocity) over a moderate range of velocities until a plateau of nearly constant signal is reached. In this circumstance, blood appears substantially brighter (white) than the cardiac walls (Fig. 10–2). With jet flow at very high velocities, signal is lost. This loss of signal from high-velocity disturbed flow in jets can be minimized by the use of short TE (<5 msec). High-velocity jets produced by flow across stenotic or regurgitant valves can be recognized as a signal void within the signal-filled cardiac chambers.

Techniques for MRI of the Heart

Cardiac imaging requires some form of physiological gating of the imaging sequence. Acquisition of MR signals of the thorax without gating results in poor cardiac images owing to loss of the signal from moving structures and to the variable position of the cardiac structure relative to imaging pixels when data are acquired indiscriminantly throughout the cardiac cycle.

GATING WITH MRI. This is associated with unique problems. Sensors, wire leads, and transducers are usually composed of ferromagnetic materials, which can generate noise or may grossly distort the images within the RF-shielded room containing the MRI device. Consequently, gating with MRI requires the use of a nonferromagnetic physiological signal-sensing circuit. An electronically isolated electrocardiogram (ECG) electrode-lead circuit containing very little metal has been used for repetitive synchronization, i.e., ECG gating, of pulse sequences to fixed segments of the cardiac cycle.

MULTISLICE TECHNIQUES. Several imaging strategies have been used, depending upon the information desired. For anatomical diagnosis, the *ECG-gated multislice technique* is used. This technique is economical in time, requiring less than 10 minutes for the acquisition of tomograms (0.3 to 1.0 cm in thickness) at multiple, usually 10 to 12, anatomical levels, which encompasses the entire heart and root of the great vessels. A difference of about 30 to 50 msec exists between each adjacent level, so the images are obtained at different phases of the cardiac cycle. Images can be obtained at multiple anatomical levels during a single imaging sequence because the time required to

complete a set of RF pulses and sample the emitted signal for each line on that image is usually 15 to 30 msec (TE interval) for T1-weighted images, while the time between the application of repetitive sets of pulses is approximately 500 to 1000 msec (TR interval). Consequently, the inactive time for each cycle is long, frequently greater than 90 per cent of the cycle. Efficiency is improved by applying the set of spin-echo pulses at other levels during the magnetization recovery period. For example, upon completion of a 50-msec duty cycle at one level, the full set of pulses is selectively applied at the next adjacent tomographic level and then the next, and so forth. With this multislice technique, the total number of tomographic levels that can be imaged is approximately TR/TE. As indicated earlier, TR equals the length of the cardiac cycle (R-R interval) when using ECG gating.

The *multiphasic multislice technique* can be used for the evaluation of cardiac dimensions and function. With this technique, each anatomical section is imaged at 5 to 10 phases of the cardiac cycle. From end-diastolic and end (late)-systolic images of each anatomical level, measurement can be made of diastolic and systolic volumes, stroke volume, ejection fraction, myocardial mass, and extent of left ventricular regional wall thickening. With this technique, wall thickening dynamics have been measured for various regions of the left ventricle in normal subjects and patients with global and regional myocardial dysfunction and in patients with focal and generalized hypertrophy.

CINE MRI. This can be accomplished by ECG referencing of gradient-echo sequences. This approach can produce a set of images corresponding to multiple evenly spaced phases of the cardiac cycle. The temporal window for each phasic image is usually 20 to 30 msec for acquisition at a single anatomical level, but double or triple the time if acquisitions are done simultaneously at two or three levels. Acquisitions are usually done at two levels simultaneously, and 16 phasic images are produced at each level. These images are laced together in a cinematic display so that wall motion of the ventricles, valve motion, and blood flow patterns in the heart and great vessels can be visualized.

FAST GRADIENT-ECHO MRI. These fast gradient-echo imaging techniques are important for MRI of the heart. For conventional spin-echo and gradient-echo techniques, one line of the imaging matrix (usually 128 to 256 lines compose an imaging matrix) is acquired for each TR interval (R-R interval for gated acquisitions). With fast gradient-echo imaging, multiple lines (usually eight) are acquired for each TR interval. This reduces the acquisition time by a factor of 8 (number of lines acquired), so that a cine acquisition can be done in a breath hold period of about 12 to 14 seconds (breath-hold cine MR imaging).[1] Because multiple lines or a segment of the image matrix (K space) is acquired rather than a single line, this technique is sometimes called segmented fast gradient-echo imaging. Because the respiration is suspended during the acquisition, cine MR images are produced which are free of motion artifacts associated with breathing.

Another fast imaging method uses very short TR and TE intervals for gradient-echo acquisition with a course matrix (64 to 128 lines) to produce low spatial resolution images in about 600 to 2000 msec. These are sometimes called fast gradient-echo or turbo gradient-

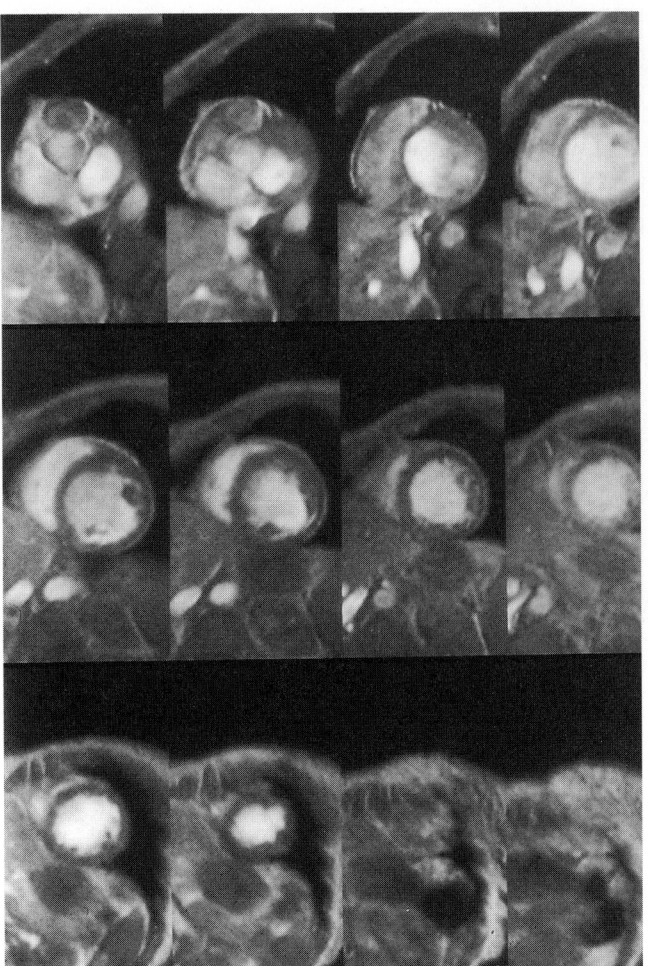

FIGURE 10–2. Series of cine MR images extending from base *(upper left)* to apex *(lower right)* of the heart. Images are acquired at the same phase of the cardiac cycle. From such a set of images acquired at end-diastole and end-systole, direct measurements of right and left ventricular volumes and mass can be done. With this type of imaging sequence (gradient-echo), the blood pool produces higher signal than the myocardium, resulting in substantial contrast between the two, and sharp delineation of the endocardial margin.

echo images. These can be weighted for T1 or T2 contrast by applying a preparation pulse before the imaging sequence, such as an inversion recovery (180-degree) pulse before the image sequence. These sequences have been initially applied to provide 1- to 2-second monitoring of the initial passage of injected contrast medium through the central circulation and myocardium in order to evaluate regional myocardial perfusion.[2,3]

Echo planar imaging (EPI) is the fastest MRI technique.[4] It can provide an image in an acquisition time of 40 to 50 msec. The acquisition can be done so that all lines in the image matrix or K space are acquired in a single TR interval (single-shot EPI) or in a few (usually two to four) sequential TR intervals (multishot or interleaved EPI).[5] Echoplanar imaging sequences can be either spin-echo EPI or gradient-echo EPI. In addition, preparatory pulses can be used to increase the T1 weighting of the imaging; inversion recovery EPI is very sensitive to T1 contrast effects such as those produced by low doses of MR contrast medium.[6]

EVALUATION OF SPECIFIC CARDIAC DISEASES

The clinical use of MRI has been primarily for the demonstration of pathological anatomy. However, in the past few years cine MRI has been used for the quantification of global and regional function of the right and left ventricles, for the quantification of valvular heart disease, for the measurement of blood flow in the heart and great arteries, and for the assessment of myocardial perfusion and even coronary blood flow. Precise demonstration of anatomical ab-

normalities has been useful for the evaluation of patients with ischemic heart disease, cardiomyopathies, pericardial disease, neoplastic disease, congenital heart disease, and thoracic aortic disease.

Ischemic Heart Disease

The role of MRI in ischemic heart disease has been quite minor up to the current time. However, recent advances in technology provide capabilities by which MRI could evolve as a comprehensive imaging technique for ischemic heart disease.[7] In this regard, morphology can be assessed with the ECG-gated spin-echo and cine MRI techniques, permitting determination of the extent of wall thinning caused by previous infarctions and depiction of complications of infarctions, such as true and false aneurysms. Segmental myocardial function can be quantified by measuring the extent of regional wall thickening or wall motion on standard or breath-hold cine MRI. Moreover, regional myocardial ischemia can be demonstrated by analysis of regional myocardial wall thickening in the basal state and during pharmacological stress induced by dipyridamole or dobutamine.[8,9] Using breath-hold cine MRI, images of the major coronary arteries can be produced.[10,11] Breath-hold velocity-encoded techniques can be applied for measuring coronary blood flow or velocity at rest and during interventions intended to test coronary flow reserve.[12,13] Finally, contrast-prepared fast gradient-echo imaging can be used to evaluate myocardial perfusion in the basal and vasodilated states to identify myocardium jeopardized by coronary arterial stenosis.[14,15]

MORPHOLOGY. MRI provides direct visualization of the myocardium with excellent delineation of the epicardial and endocardial interfaces. Consequently, it can define accurately segmental wall thinning that is indicative of previous myocardial infarction.[16–18] In some patients with a history of transmural infarction, residual myocardium can be demonstrated at the site of the infarction. In others, MRI shows virtually complete absence of remnant muscle. Direct visualization of the myocardium can be used to determine whether there is sufficient residual myocardium in the region jeopardized by a coronary arterial lesion to warrant a bypass graft (Fig. 10–3). Regional wall thickening can also be assessed.[19] It has been shown that a wall thickness of less than 6 mm at end-diastole and wall thickening of less than 1 mm are indicative of myocardial scar when

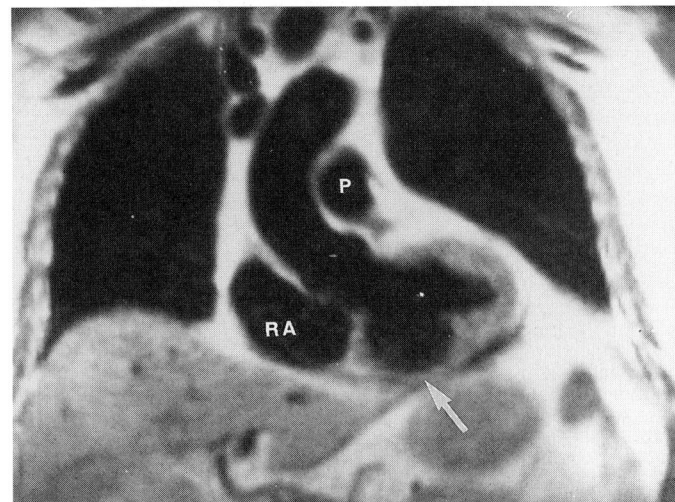

FIGURE 10–3. ECG-gated spin-echo image in the coronal plane displays a chronic transmural myocardial infarction (arrow) of the diaphragmatic wall of the left ventricle, which has caused severe wall thinning and aneurysmal bulging. P = pulmonary artery; RA = right atrium.

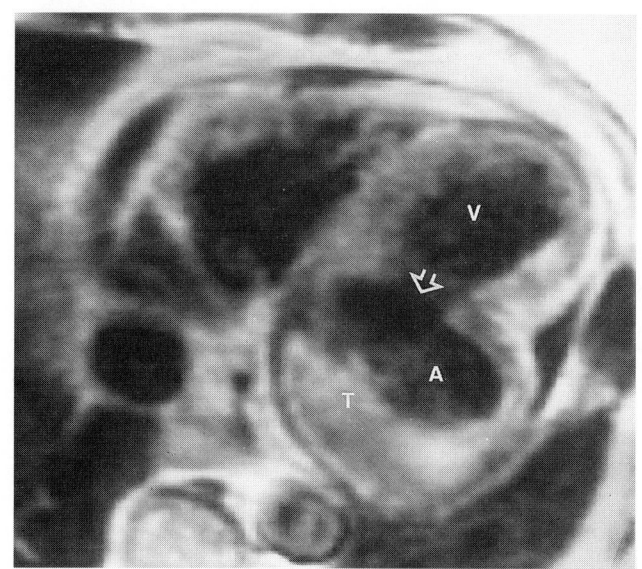

FIGURE 10–4. ECG-gated spin-echo image of a false aneurysm of the left ventricle. There is a narrow ostium (open arrow) connecting the large posterior aneurysm (A) to the ventricular (V) chamber. There is thrombus (T) in the aneurysm.

compared with uptake of ^{99m}Tc-sestamibi single-photon emission tomography.

The recognition of decreased signal intensity of the myocardial wall at the site of old myocardial infarction suggests that MRI can identify the replacement of myocardium by fibrous scar.[17] Gated MRI has also demonstrated complications of myocardial infarctions, such as left ventricular thrombus and aneurysms[16,17] (Fig. 10–4). Transverse or short-axis tomography facilitates the recognition of the small ostium connecting the left ventricular chamber and the false aneurysm (Fig. 10–4); this is a distinguishing feature of the false compared with the true left ventricular aneurysm.

Acute myocardial infarctions have been demonstrated by gated MRI. The region of ischemically damaged myocardium displays increased signal intensity compared with normal myocardium.[21-25] Contrast between infarcted and normal myocardium increases on images with greater T2 contribution to signal intensity. Because cardiac pulsations

and respiration can cause high-intensity artifacts projected over the myocardial region, caution must be used in the interpretation of this finding.[25] Comparison of changes in contrast among images with increasing TE value and estimation of T2 relaxation times can alleviate this problem.[22] Administration of MR contrast medium (gadolinium chelates) with T1-weighted spin-echo images causes greater enhancement of infarcted than of normal myocardium (Fig. 10–5).

Regional Contraction Abnormalities. The major role of noninvasive imaging techniques in ischemic heart disease is the detection of ischemic myocardium and other features indicative of the presence of obstructive coronary arterial disease. Ischemic myocardium can be demonstrated directly or indirectly by MRI. Indirectly, it is shown by demonstrating a regional contraction abnormality, usually by wall thickening measurement, at rest or during pharmacological stress. Cine MRI in the basal state and during pharmacological intervention with dobutamine or dipyridamole has correlated closely with nuclear perfusion imaging and/ or coronary arteriography for demonstrating potentially ischemic myocardial segments.[7-9] Directly, the monitoring of the first-pass distribution of MR contrast medium with T1-sensitive fast GRE imaging in basal and vasodilated states has shown regions of decreased myocardial perfusion in association with coronary arterial stenosis[14,15] (Fig. 10–6).

Visualization of Coronary Arteries. The unique information provided by MRI relevant to ischemic heart disease is visualization of the major coronary arteries using newly developed MR angiographic techniques[10,11] (Fig. 10–7). One report has shown approximately 90 per cent correlation between coronary MRA and coronary x-ray angiography for identifying hemodynamically significant coronary arterial stenoses or occlusions.[26] Equally intriguing is the possibility of measuring volume or velocity of flow in the major coronary arteries using breath-hold gradient-echo or echo planar velocity-encoded techniques[12,13] (Figs. 10–8 and 10–9). These techniques have already been used in human subjects to document an increase in volume flow or flow velocity in response to vasodilators; the exclusion or confirmation of coronary arterial disease by the noninvasive assessment of coronary flow may be an important future application of MRI in ischemic heart disease.

CORONARY ARTERY BYPASS GRAFTS. Gated MRI has been used to evaluate the patency of bypass grafts. Because blood usually flows rapidly through the grafts, they appear

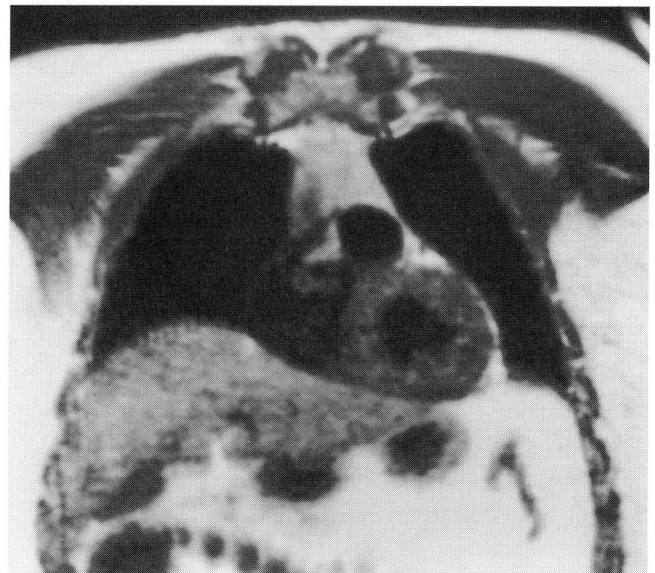

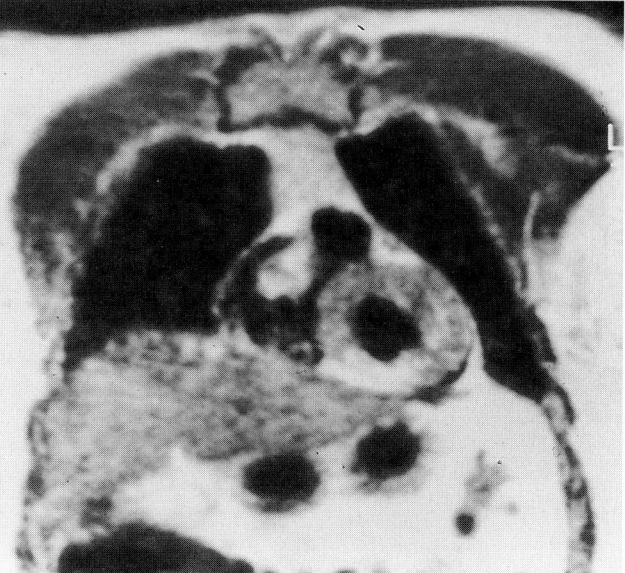

FIGURE 10–5. ECG-gated spin-echo image in the coronal plane before *(left)* and after *(right)* the administration of MR contrast medium (gadolinium chelate). The contrast medium causes greater enhancement of the infarcted area and demarcates it on the postcontrast image.

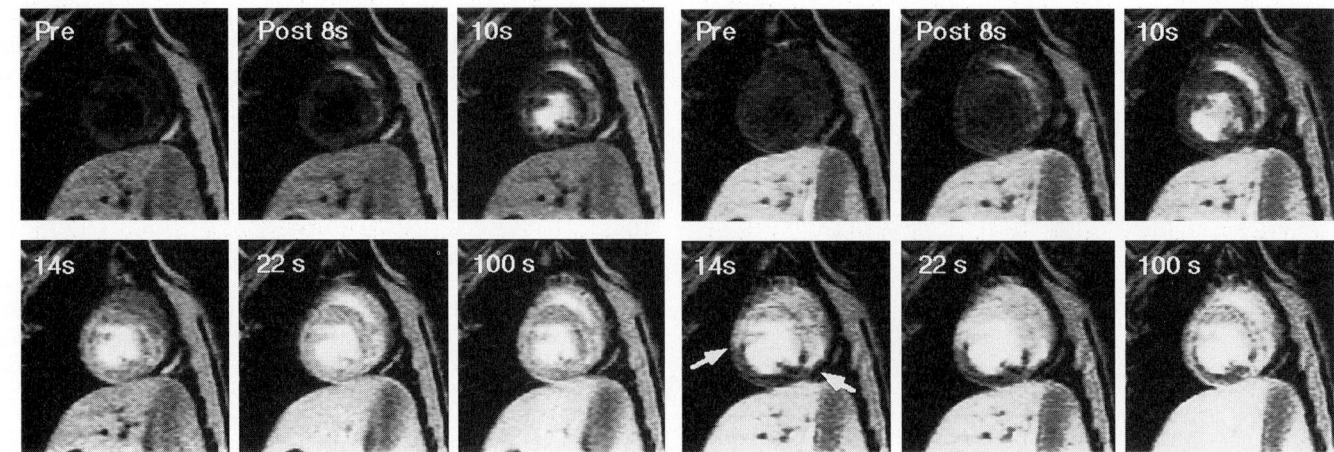

FIGURE 10–6. Sequential inversion recovery fast gradient-echo images acquired during the first passage of MR contrast medium (gadolinium chelate) through the heart. The series of images was performed in the basal (left) and vasodilated (right) states. In this animal model of a nonocclusive coronary arterial stenosis, the potentially ischemic region is not evident in the basal state. After dipyridamole the ischemic region is demarcated as a low-intensity zone (arrows) compared with normal myocardium.

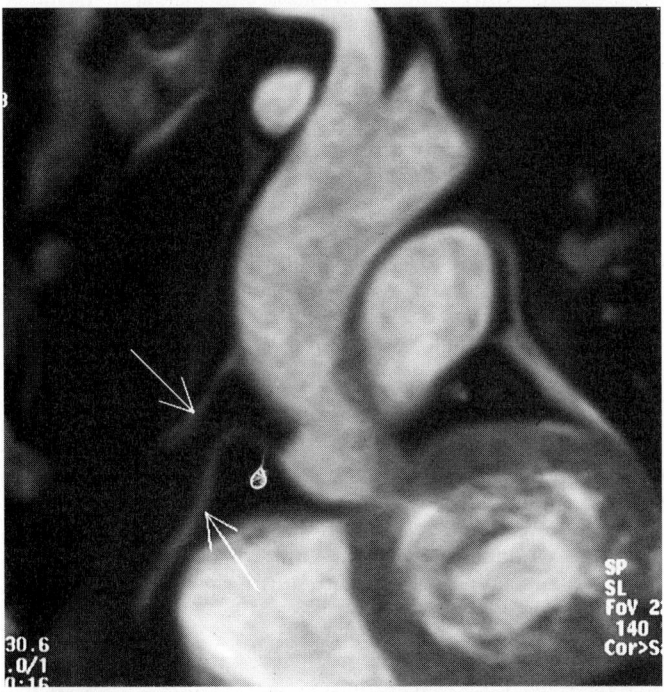

FIGURE 10–7. Breath-hold cine MR image demonstrates the proximal portion of the right coronary artery (arrow) and a bypass graft (arrow) to the right coronary artery. (Courtesy of Robert Edelman, M.D.)

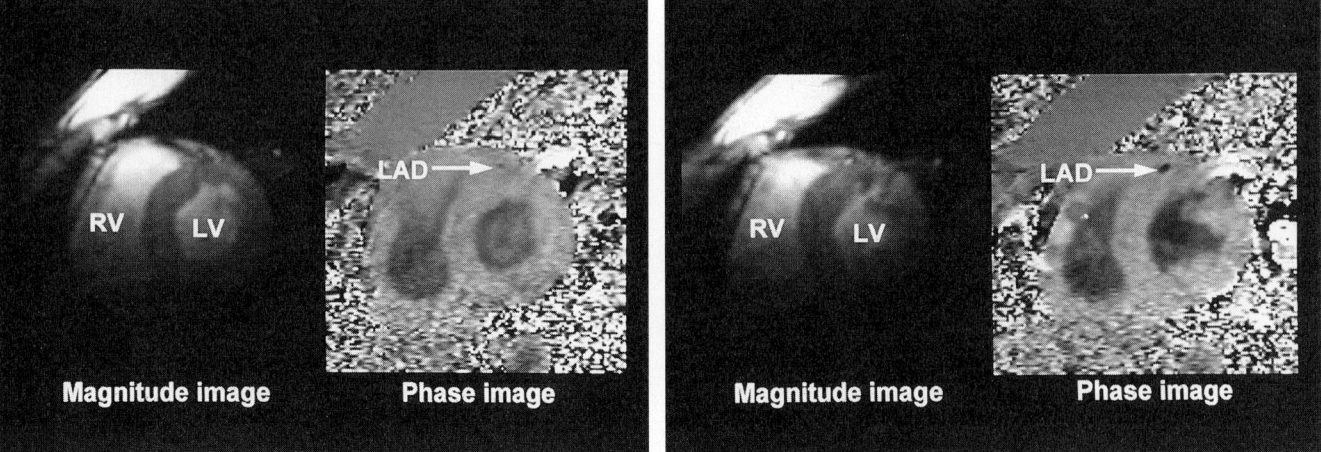

FIGURE 10–8. Magnitude and phase images in the short-axis planes display the left anterior descending coronary artery (LAD, arrow) in the basal (left) and vasodilated (right) states. Signal of the artery is increased in the vasodilated state due to increased flow induced by dipyridamole. These images were derived from breath-hold velocity-encoded MR sequences.

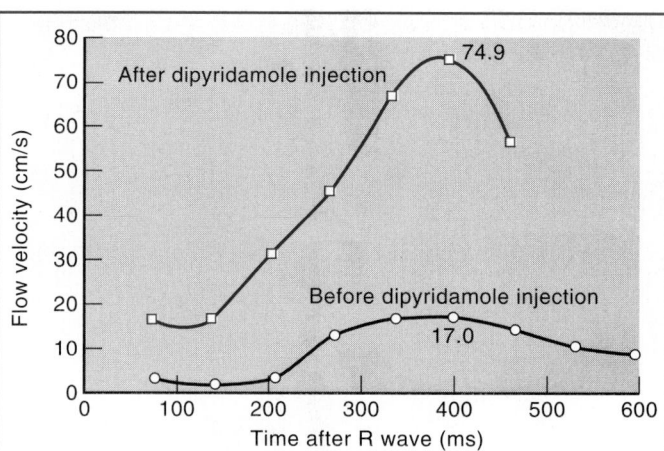

FIGURE 10–9. Graph showing left anterior descending coronary flow velocity in basal and vasodilated states.

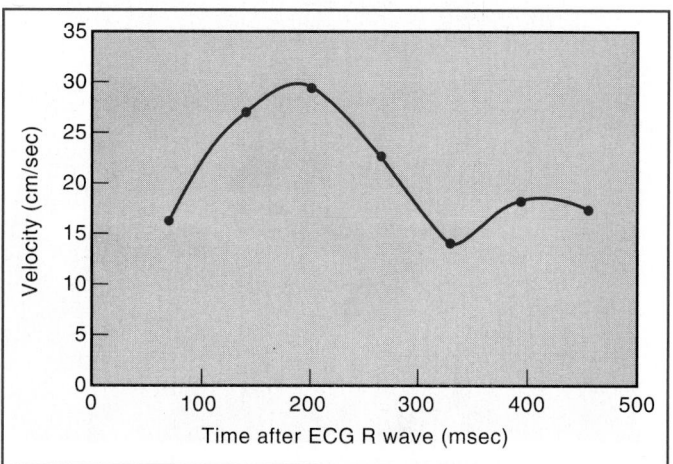

FIGURE 10–11. Plot of the flow velocity versus time curve from an internal mammary artery bypass conduit.

as small circular structures with absence of a luminal signal. For visualization of grafts, ECG-gated images are acquired in order to minimize the effect of motion of the grafts. Generally, images are acquired at each anatomical level during multiple phases of the cardiac cycle to ensure that an image is acquired at a phase when the rate of flow through the graft is rapid. High flow rate in the graft produces a flow void in the lumen of the graft using spin-echo MRI and thus indicates patency of the graft. With the cine (gradient-echo) MRI and MR angiographic techniques, flowing blood causes bright signal intensity; therefore, bright signal rather than flow void indicates graft patency with this technique (Fig. 10–10). MRI has an accuracy of 80 to 90 per cent for defining graft patency.[27–31] Phase-contrast gradient-echo techniques have been used to demonstrate flow and to estimate flow velocity in coronary bypass conduits[32,33] (Fig. 10–11).

Cardiomyopathies
(See also Chap. 41)

HYPERTROPHIC CARDIOMYOPATHIES (see also p. 1414). MRI has been used to define the presence, distribution, and severity of hypertrophic cardiomyopathies.[34,35] It has displayed the extent of septal involvement (Fig. 10–12) and has been particularly useful for identifying the unusual distribution of hypertrophy in the variant forms of hypertrophic cardiomyopathy. Left ventricular[36,37] and right ventricular[37,38] mass and wall thickness have been quantified using spin-echo and cine MRI. Substantial right ventricular hypertrophy has been shown by MRI measurements in pa-

tients with hypertrophic cardiomyopathy.[37,38] Cine MRI has also been used to assess ventricular diastolic parameters by constructing volume-time curves during the cardiac cycle; reduced filling rate and time to peak filling have been demonstrated in patients with hypertrophic cardiomyopathy.[38]

DILATED CARDIOMYOPATHY (see also p. 1407). MRI has depicted the morphologic[39] and functional[40] alterations in congestive (dilated) cardiomyopathy. It has been used to quantify left ventricular volume and systolic wall stress in patients with congestive cardiomyopathies.[41,42] Cine MRI has also been performed sequentially in order to monitor the effect of drug therapy in patients with congestive cardiomyopathy; it has demonstrated significant decreases in left ventricular volume, mass, and systolic wall stress during 3 months of treatment with an angiotensin-converting enzyme inhibitor.[42] Because MRI provides excellent discrimination of the edges of the myocardium, it can also be used to assess myocardial mass and wall thickness in patients with cardiomyopathies; several studies have indicated the accuracy of MRI for quantifying myocardial mass in both normally and abnormally shaped left ventricles.[43,44] Cine MRI has also been found to be highly reproducible in measuring left ventricular mass and volumes between two studies in the same subject.[43,44] The interstudy variability of mass measurements is less than 5 per cent. Cine MRI has demonstrated considerable increase in left ventricular mass and markedly elevated end-systolic wall stress in patients with dilated cardiomyopathy.[41,42,44] Cine MRI has demonstrated both a decrease in the extent of wall thickening and a change in the regional pattern of wall thickening

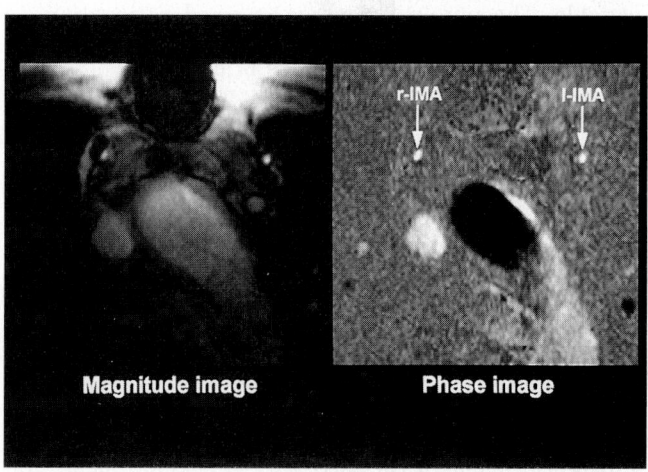

FIGURE 10–10. Magnitude and phase images of right (R-IMA) and left (L-IMA) internal mammary bypass grafts.

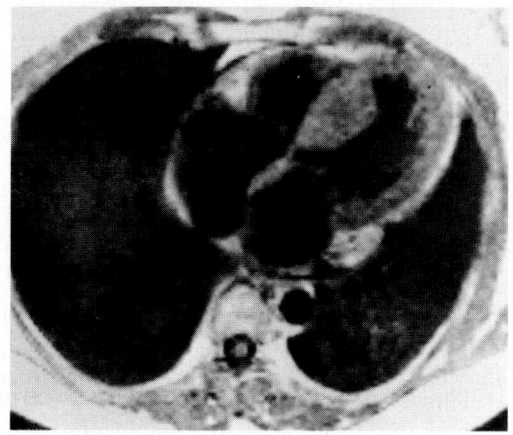

FIGURE 10–12. Hypertrophic cardiomyopathy. MRI displays severe hypertrophy of the entire septum and normal thickness of the lateral wall.

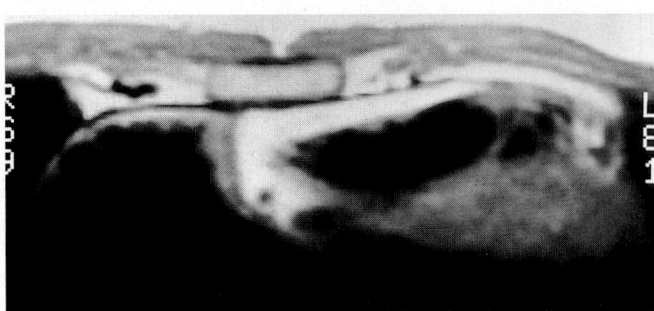
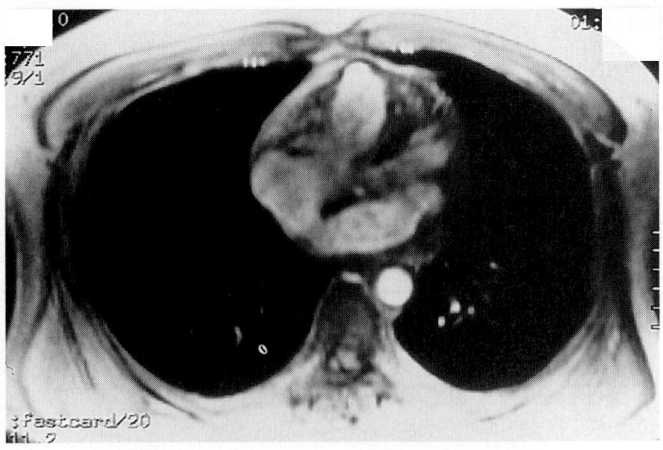

FIGURE 10–13. Spin-echo image *(left)* in a patient with right ventricular dysplasia shows transmural fat in the right ventricular free wall. Cine MR image *(right)* shows wall thinning and aneurysmal bulging of the right ventricular free wall in another patient with right ventricular dysplasia.

in patients with dilated cardiomyopathy compared with normal subjects.[40]

RESTRICTIVE CARDIOMYOPATHY (see also p. 1426). ECG-gated spin-echo MRI has displayed features considered to be characteristic for restrictive cardiomyopathy.[45] There is substantial enlargement of the atria and the inferior vena cava, with usually less prominent ventricular enlargement. Because of resistance caused by the noncompliant ventricles to atrial emptying during diastole, prominent signal is observed in the atrial blood. Such intra-atrial signal originates from slowly moving blood on spin-echo MR images. The major contribution of MRI to establishing the diagnosis of restrictive cardiomyopathy is the demonstration of normal pericardial thickness, which essentially excludes the alternate diagnosis of constrictive pericarditis. In *amyloid heart disease,* MRI has demonstrated thickened myocardial walls and diminished wall thickening during the cardiac cycle.[46,47] Cine MRI indicates apparent hypertrophy of the left ventricle with normal or decreased left ventricular contraction rather than hypercontractile left ventricle expected in left ventricular hypertrophy. MRI has also demonstrated infiltration of the myocardium by tumorous and inflammatory processes[48]; detection of such myocardial infiltrates can be useful for the diagnosis of specific forms of restrictive myocardial diseases.

The MRI findings in cardiomyopathies have thus far been limited to *anatomical* and *functional* abnormalities. No consistent changes in MRI relaxation times have been found for the myocardium in hypertrophic or congestive cardiomyopathies or in amyloid heart disease.

RIGHT VENTRICULAR DYSPLASIA (see also p. 749). Right ventricular dysplasia is represented pathologically by variable replacement or infiltration of right ventricular myocardium by fatty or fibrous tissue. Aside from suggestive clinical and electrophysiological features, the diagnosis has been definitively established by tissue examination after endomyocardial biopsy. The major differential diagnoses for ventricular arrhythmias of right ventricular origin in the presence of a grossly normal right ventricle are right ventricular dysplasia and right ventricular outflow tract tachycardia. ECG-gated spin-echo MRI has been used to identify transmural or focal fat in the right ventricular free wall in order to establish the diagnosis of right ventricular dysplasia[49] (Fig. 10–13). Focal or generalized wall thinning of the right ventricle also is consistent with this diagnosis[49] (Fig. 10–13). Focal wall thinning and focal bulging (aneurysm) of the right ventricular outflow tract has been shown also on MRI in right ventricular outflow tract tachycardia.[50] One report has shown that MRI actually demonstrates fat in the right ventricular free wall in less than half of patients with right ventricular dysplasia, but a regional contractile abnormality is demonstrated by cine MRI in a majority.[51]

Pericardial Disease

(See also Chap. 43)

Gated MRI provides direct visualization of the pericardium.[52] It has been effective for the assessment of patients with suspected pericardial disease. Normal pericardium is composed primarily of fibrous tissue and has low MRI signal intensity. The thickness of pericardial line measured in normal subjects was 1.5 ± 0.4 mm (S.D.) with a range from 0.8 to 2.6 mm.[52] A variation of thickness of the low-intensity line has been observed during the cardiac cycle in normal subjects. These latter observations, along with information from postmortem studies, indicate that the normal pericardium measures less than 3.0 mm and suggest that the low-intensity pericardial line consists of pericardium and some adherent pericardial fluid. A thickness of 4 mm or greater is abnormal (Fig. 10–14). This is probably responsible for the pericardial line observed on CT as well because normal CT measurements of pericardial thickness are similar to MRI measurements. On spin-echo MR images, pericardial effusion causes a low signal intensity space separating the heart and pericardium (Fig. 10–15). The distinction between the pericardium itself and pericardial fluid can also be achieved on cine MR images, on which the fluid has bright signal and the pericardium is a dark line (Fig. 10–15). MRI has been used to establish the diagnosis of congenital absence of the left pericardium.[53] Pericardial thickening and effusions are characteristic features of acute pericarditis.

Gated MRI has been useful for demonstrating pericardial thickness in patients with suspected constrictive pericarditis.[52,54,55] The signal intensity of the thickened pericardium is variable. The purely fibrous or calcified pericardium in chronic constrictive pericardial disease has low signal intensity. However, in subacute forms of constrictive pericarditis caused by irradiation, surgical trauma, or uremia, the thickened pericardium has moderate to high intensity on spin-echo images.[52] The effusive-constrictive form of pericardial disease has thickened pericardium and pericardial effusion. One study[55] has demonstrated a diagnostic accuracy of 93 per cent for MRI in distinguishing between constrictive pericarditis and restrictive cardiomyopathy by demonstrating thickened pericardium (≥4 mm) in the former disease.

MRI demonstrates even the small amount of pericardial fluid present in normal subjects. Fluid in the superior pericardial recesses is commonly seen even when fluid is not evident posterior to the left ventricle. The appearance of pericardial fluid is different on spin-echo and cine MRI (gradient-echo) images (Fig. 10–15). Nonhemorrhagic fluid shows low intensity on short-TR, short-TE sequences (T1-weighted) and has high intensity on long-TR, long-TE se-

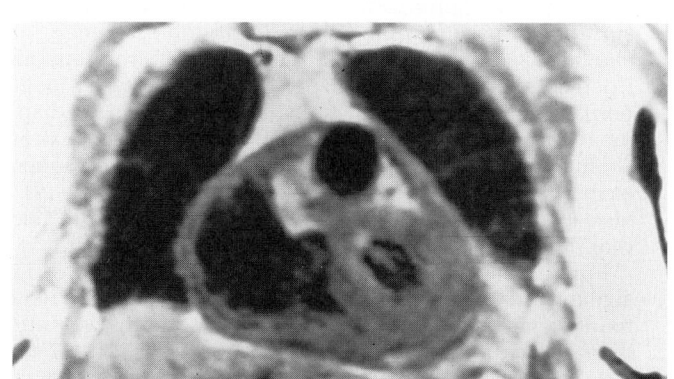
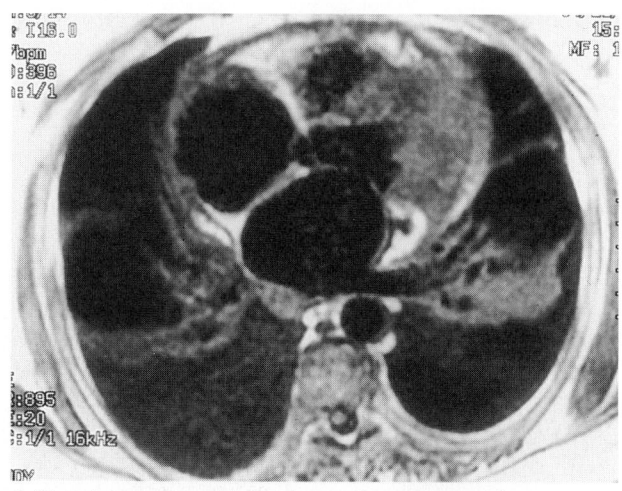

FIGURE 10–14. ECG-gated spin-echo images in coronal *(left)* and transverse *(right)* planes of a patient with constrictive pericarditis. The pericardium is substantially thickened. Thick pericardium can be visualized extending over the pulmonary artery on the coronal image.

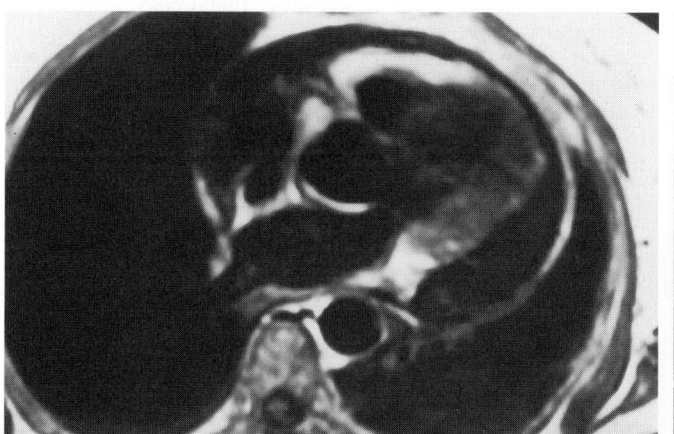
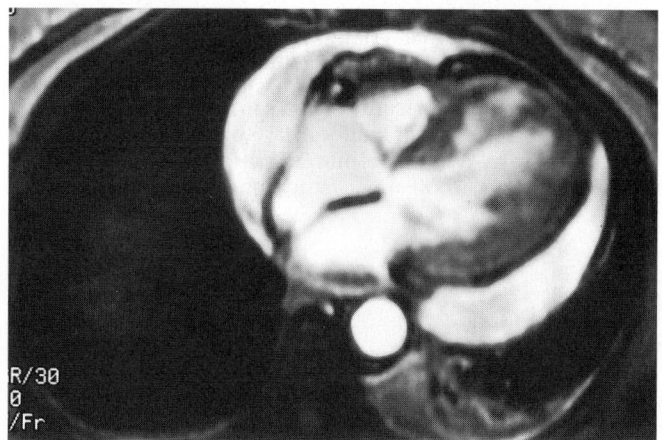

FIGURE 10–15. Spin-echo *(left)* and gradient-echo (cine MR) *(right)* images of a patient with a large pericardial effusion.

quences (T2-weighted). On the other hand, pericardial hematoma has high intensity on T1-weighted images (Fig. 10–16) and may have high intensity on T2-weighted images, depending on the age of the hematoma and the magnetic field strength of the imager. On cine MRI, the nonhemorrhagic effusion is bright and the hemorrhagic one may be low intensity.

In pericardial disease the role of MRI must be considered in the light of the established effectiveness of echocardiography. An advantage of MRI over echocardiography is the capability to differentiate pericardial hematoma from other types of effusions. Because of the wide field of view, MRI seems to be useful in locating loculated effusions. Determination of pericardial thickening seems to be a clear indication for the use of MRI.

Neoplastic Disease
(See also Chaps. 42 and 57)

Several reports have documented the clinical utility of gated MRI for the evaluation of intracardiac and paracardiac masses.[56–60] Because of the unequivocal delineation of the pericardium, myocardial walls, and chambers of the heart on MR images, the precise relationship of tumors to cardiovascular structures can be defined. Tumors within the myocardial wall may be identified by virtue of a difference in signal intensity (usually higher) compared with the myocardium. In this regard, MR contrast media can be used in an attempt to accentuate differences in signal intensity between tumor and myocardium.[61]

Secondary cardiac involvement by tumors (see p. 1794) is about 40 times more frequent than primary tumors (see p. 1464). Secondary involvement occurs by three routes: direct extension from the mediastinum and lungs (Fig. 10–

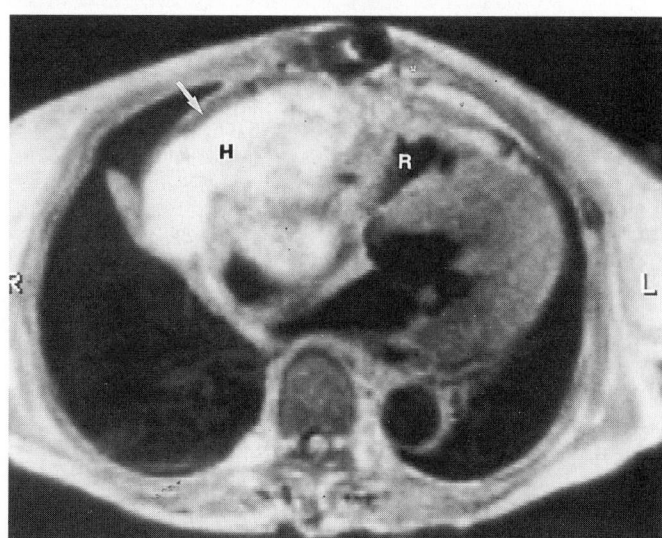

FIGURE 10–16. ECG-gated spin-echo images show a pericardial hematoma (H). The hemorrhagic pericardial effusion causes bright signal intensity on the T1-weighted (TE = 30 msec) image. The right atrium and right ventricle are compressed by the hematoma. Pericardium (arrow) is thickened. R = right ventricle.

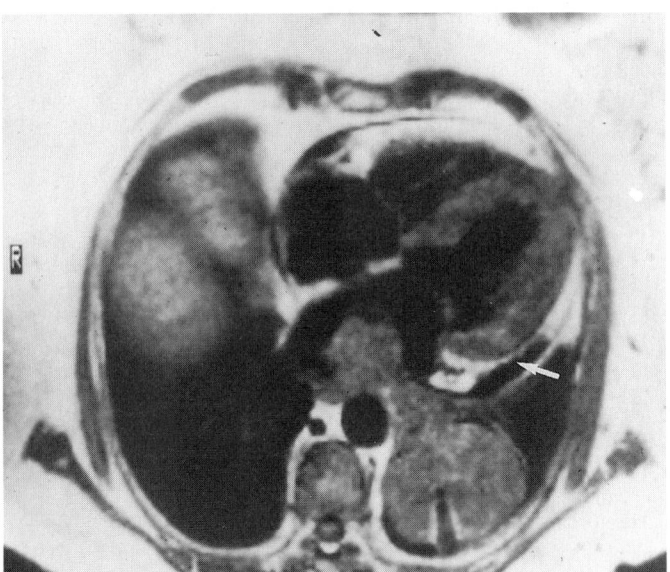

FIGURE 10–17. ECG-gated spin-echo image shows a lung tumor extending through the pericardium and into the left atrial chamber. The MR image clearly displays the extracardiac and intracardiac parts of the mass and a small pericardial effusion (arrow).

(CT) for assessing the extent and effect of mediastinal masses adjacent to cardiovascular structures.[60,62] Gated MRI is the imaging procedure of choice for identifying paracardiac masses, defining their nature, and determining invasion of the pericardium. The intensity on spin-echo images can be used to differentiate such masses from innocuous lipomas, the pericardial fat pad, pericardial cysts, loculated pericardial effusions, and unusual enlargement or displacement of cardiac chambers. Gated MRI has been extremely useful for demonstrating invasion of cardiac chambers by pulmonary and mediastinal malignancies (Fig. 10–17). Metastases to the pericardium and the accompanying pericardial effusion can be readily depicted by gated MRI.

Intracardiac tumors can be clearly identified within the signal void of the cardiac blood pool. Because of its wide field of view, MRI is ideal for defining both the intracardiac and extracardiac extent of masses (Figs. 10–17 to 10–19). For the evaluation of intracardiac masses, it is advisable to acquire spin-echo and gradient-echo MR images and to obtain images with at least two planes perpendicular to each other. A recent investigation has suggested that intracardiac or intravascular tumors can be distinguished from thrombus using cine MRI in most instances[63] (Fig. 10–19). Tumors are represented by medium signal (higher signal or similar signal compared with myocardium), whereas thrombus produces very low signal (less than myocardium). This low signal is due to elements in the thrombus (e.g., hemosiderin, deoxyhemoglobin) that induce a magnetic susceptibility effect and vitiate signal from the region. The cine MRI sequence is very sensitive to this effect.

17, metastases to the pericardium or cardiac chambers, and direct extension of upper abdominal tumors through the inferior vena cava or lung tumors through the pulmonary veins. MRI appears to be superior to computed tomography

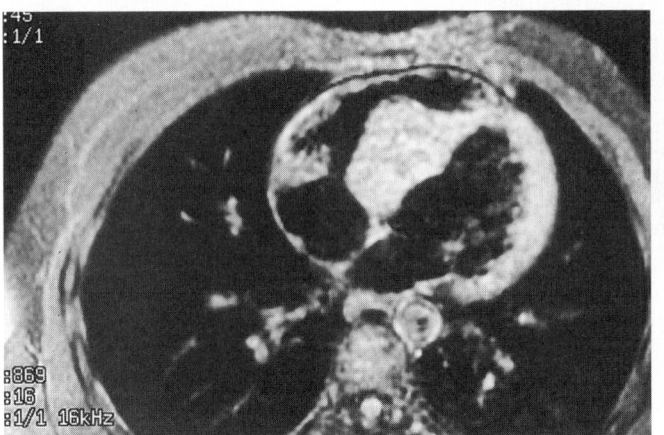
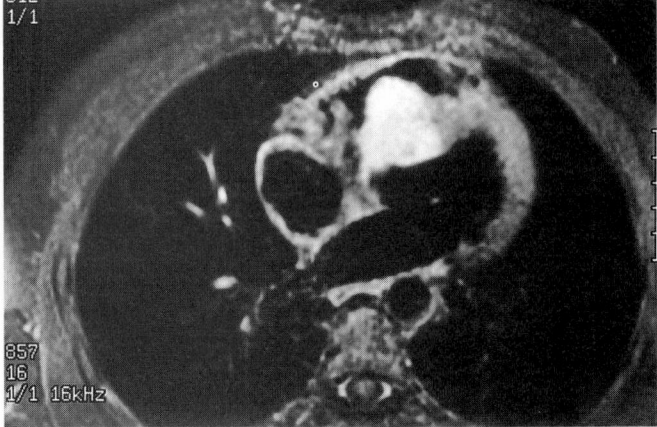

FIGURE 10–18. ECG-gated spin-echo images before *(left)* and after *(right)* injection of gadolinium chelate in a patient with a sarcoma of the ventricular septum. A fat saturation technique was used after contrast medium in order to accentuate the effect of the contrast medium. The tumor is contrast-enhanced to a greater degree than myocardium.

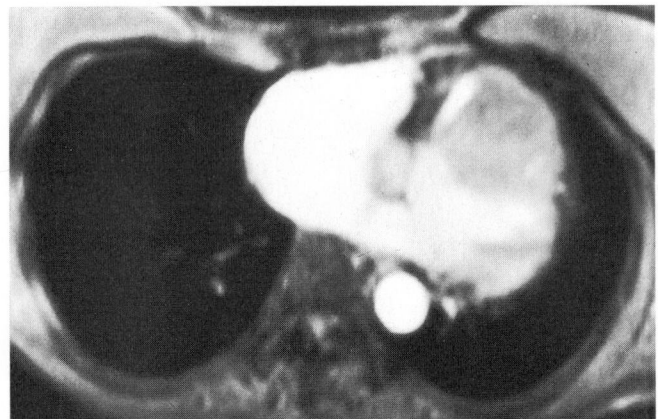
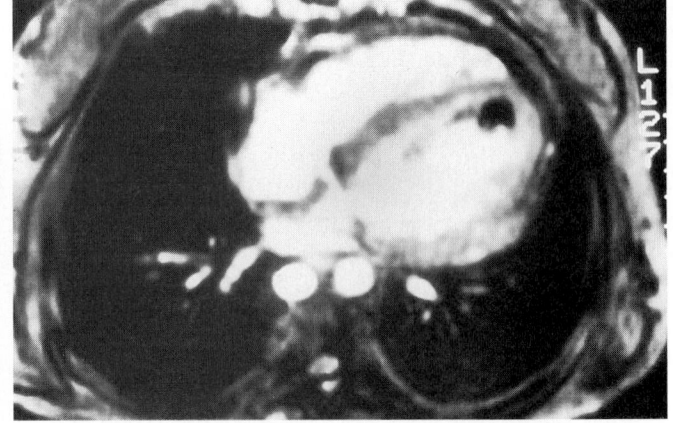

FIGURE 10–19. Gradient-echo (cine MR) images in two patients with intracardiac masses. *Left,* Metastatic tumor in the right ventricle has medium intensity. *Right,* Thrombus at the left ventricular apex has low intensity. (From Higgins, C. B., Hricak, H., and Helms, C. A.: MRI of the Body, 2nd ed. New York, Raven Press, 1992.)

Some myxomas contain a considerable amount of iron and can show the same effect, so confident distinction between myxoma and clot may not always be possible. Differentiation between tumor and thrombus has not been possible using the ECG-gated spin-echo sequence. Differentiation between tumor and blood clots can also be done using MR contrast media. The contrast media enhances the signal of tumor but not that of clots.[61]

Congenital Heart Disease
(See also Chaps. 29 and 30)

MRI has multiple capabilities for the evaluation of congenital heart disease. Morphological information is provided by ECG-gated spin-echo and cine MRI. Ventricular volumes, mass, and function can be obtained using cine MRI. The volumes of shunts, valvular function, and pressure gradients across valves and conduits can be estimated using velocity-encoded cine MRI (velocity-flow mapping). However, the clinical use of these capabilities is influenced by the widespread application of echocardiography and Doppler techniques for many of these same purposes. Consequently, the current clinical role of MRI is to supplement the information acquired by echocardiography.

Reports from several centers indicate encouraging results with MRI for the evaluation of patients with congenital heart disease.[64–82] In several studies in which the results of MRI were corroborated by angiography and/or two-dimensional echocardiography, accurate anatomical diagnosis of anomalies was achieved by MRI in more than 90 per cent of patients.[66,70,72]

Visceroatrial situs, the type of ventricular loop, and the relationship of the great vessels could be identified in all patients in whom studies encompassing the entire heart were done.[72] The diagnostic accuracy of MRI exceeded 90 per cent for abnormalities of arterioventricular connections; great vessel anomalies such as coarctation and vascular rings; ventricular and atrial septal defects, and abnormalities of venous connections.[72] Likewise, determination of visceroatrial situs and type of ventricular loop reached an accuracy of nearly 100 per cent with MRI.[72] The major limitation of spin-echo MRI was the determination of stenosis and regurgitation of the semilunar and atrioventricular valves; however, valvular atresia was accurately defined. The limitation of spin-echo MRI for valvular disease can be overcome with the use of cine MRI.

In another report,[70] blinded analysis of MR images has shown a sensitivity and specificity of over 90 per cent for the identification of atrial level abnormalities, including ostia secundum and primum atrial septal defects as well as anomalous pulmonary venous connection. However, it is recognized that a thin fossa ovalis can be confused with an atrial septal defect on static MR images. It may be possible to avoid this misinterpretation by using cine MRI techniques.

Much of the diagnostic information provided by MRI can also be shown by two-dimensional echocardiography (see p. 78). The role of MRI must therefore be considered in respect to the established role of echocardiography. The unique capabilities of MRI in congenital heart disease are visualization of the central pulmonary arteries in cases of pulmonary atresia[76] (Fig. 10–20) and assessment of anomalies of the thoracic aorta[65,68] (Fig. 10–21): complete definition of complex anomalies involving both the great vessels and ventricles[69,73] and the postoperative evaluation of patients who have undergone complicated supracardiac operations for cyanotic congenital heart disease.[74,75,77–80] MRI has been shown to be reliable for both preoperative and postoperative evaluation of coarctation of the aorta[65,68]; angiography can be obviated in most patients (Fig. 10–21). Several reports[74–80] have shown the effectiveness of MRI for the postoperative evaluation of the Fontan, Rastelli, Norwood, Damus, Glenn, and Jatene procedures. MRI has been used to quantitatively monitor the size of the pulmonary arteries after surgical procedures that either involve the pulmonary arteries or are intended to increase their size by altering pulmonary blood flow.[79,81] A comparative study between echocardiography and MRI for the evaluation of the pulmonary arteries after surgery showed that MRI was superior for the evaluation of right and left pulmonary stenoses and dimensions.[81] MRI has been used to monitor pulmonary arteries through multiple staged surgeries such as the Fontan[79] and Norwood[77] procedures. Velocity-encoded MRI has been effective for estimating and monitoring the gradient across Rastelli conduits.[80]

Therefore, the major indications for MRI in patients with congenital heart disease are evaluation of thoracic aortic anomalies such as coarctation and aortic arch anomalies, determination of pulmonary arterial size in patients with

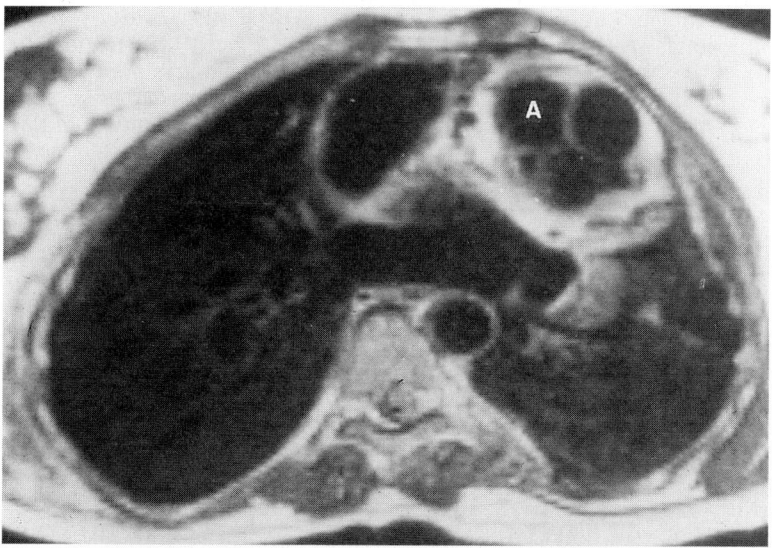
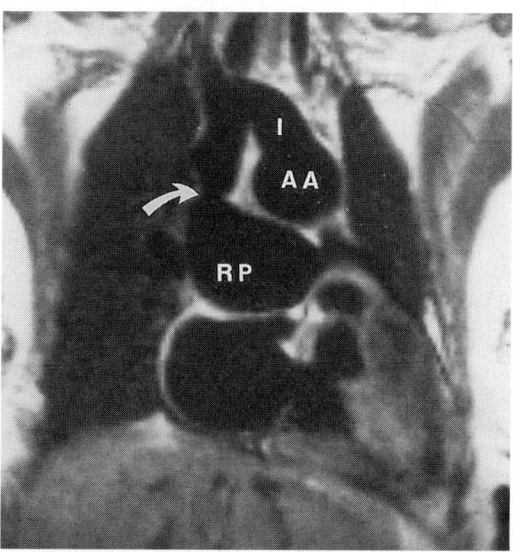

FIGURE 10–20. Transverse *(left)* and coronal *(right)* spin-echo images of a patient with transposition of the great arteries, pulmonary atresia, and ventricular septal defect. The transverse image acquired at the base of the heart shows only the aortic valve (A). Coronal image shows the right subclavian to pulmonary arterial anastomosis (curved arrow). The right pulmonary artery is aneurysmal while the left pulmonary artery is absent. The heart is shifted to the left owing to decreased size of the left lung. AA = aortic arch; I = innominate artery; RP = right pulmonary artery.

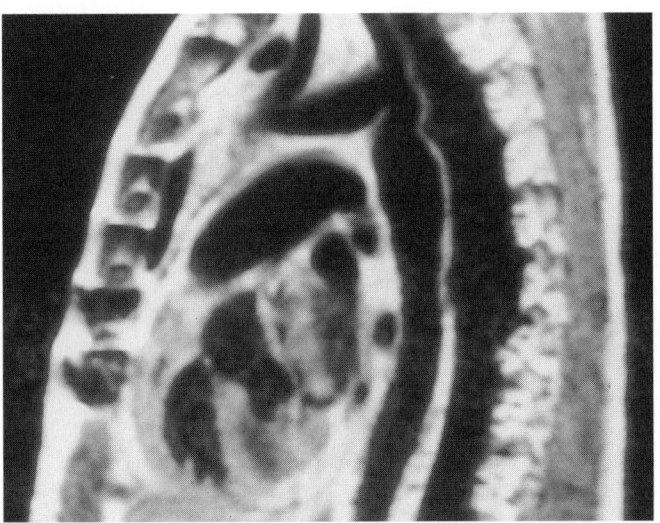

FIGURE 10–21. ECG-gated spin-echo image in oblique sagittal plane in a patient with re-coarctation of the aorta. Three-millimeter slice thickness was used for this image.

pulmonary atresia or severe obstruction, definition of complex cyanotic lesions in which precise definition of septal size and chamber size are needed, and assessment of the status of surgically created shunts, anastomoses, and conduits. MRI more completely depicts the segmental anatomy of the heart and great vessels in patients with complex cyanotic anomalies than is possible with angiography.[73] Likewise, a comparative study also showed that MRI was at least as effective as angiography for demonstrating the anatomy and complications associated with surgical procedures involving supracardiac structures.[74] Because echocardiography is limited for the demonstration of supracardiac anatomy, MRI may be the most effective technique for the monitoring of patients after various operations such as the Rastelli, Damus, Fontan, Jatene, and Norwood procedures.

The role of MRI in the evaluation of congenital heart disease is evolving rapidly. Experience at many institutions in large numbers of patients has not been achieved, so widespread familiarity with the technique and its attributes, limitations, and indications does not exist. As reliance upon angiography as the definitive diagnostic procedure for congenital heart disease wanes, it seems likely that echocardiography and MRI will be used increasingly for this purpose and will eventually obviate angiography, both for preoperative analysis and for postoperative monitoring of the morphology of congenital heart disease. Because the tomographic thickness can be reduced to 2 to 3 mm, MRI can be used to display morphology of the heart of infants.

However, limitations exist for its use in critically ill neonates because of lack of portability and difficulties in management of such patients in the MR environment.

The capability of MRI in congenital heart disease has been extended by cine MRI and velocity-encoded cine MRI. The former technique can provide multiple images per cardiac cycle so that ventricular function can be evaluated, whereas the latter technique permits measurement of blood flow and velocity in the aorta and pulmonary artery and across valves and conduits. High-velocity flow causes a signal void within the blood pool on cine MRI images; this enables the recognition of flow through sites of stenosis,[80] as well as depiction of valvular regurgitant flow. Functional evaluation of congenital heart disease using MR techniques is discussed below.

Diseases of the Thoracic Aorta
(See also Chap. 45)

A number of reports attest to the effectiveness of MRI for the evaluation of aortic dissection, true and false aneurysms, periaortic abscess and hematoma, aortic arch anomalies, and coarctation of the aorta.[83–93] In aortic dissection, MRI can depict the intimal flap and the proximal extent of the dissection, and it can distinguish true from false channels (Fig. 10–22). On spin-echo MR images, intraluminal signal is usually seen in the false channel as a result of thrombus, slow blood flow, or both. Differentiation between slow flow and thrombus is evident on cine MRI (gradient-echo) images because the former produces high or moderate intraluminal signal whereas thrombus causes low signal on this type of image (Fig. 10–22). Velocity-encoded cine MRI provides a measurement of the differential flow velocity in the true and false channels.[90] Using multiple images per cardiac cycle, a velocity-time curve can be generated to display the disparate flow pattern in the two channels.

The recent availability of *breath-hold cine MRI* (segmental fast gradient-echo imaging) can provide multiple evenly spaced images through the cardiac cycle at a single anatomical level in a period of about 14 seconds.[11] The patient usually suspends respiration during this rapid acquisition. Because the entire thoracic aorta can be imaged in less than 5 minutes with this technique, it is attractive for providing a rapid evaluation of the thoracic aorta in patients with suspected aortic dissection[91] (Fig. 10–23).

A recent report[93] has shown high sensitivity for transesophageal echocardiography, CT, and MRI for the diagnosis of *aortic dissection*. However, the specificity of CT and MRI was significantly better than that of transesophageal echocardiography. The wide field of view of CT and MRI is

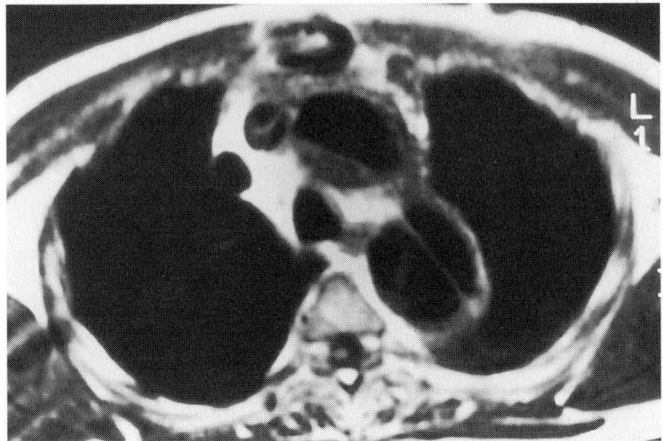
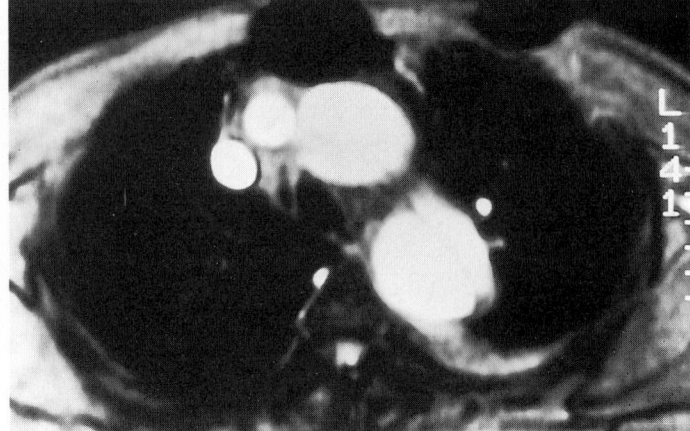

FIGURE 10–22. Spin-echo *(left)* and gradient-echo (cine MR) *(right)* images in a patient with type A aortic dissection.

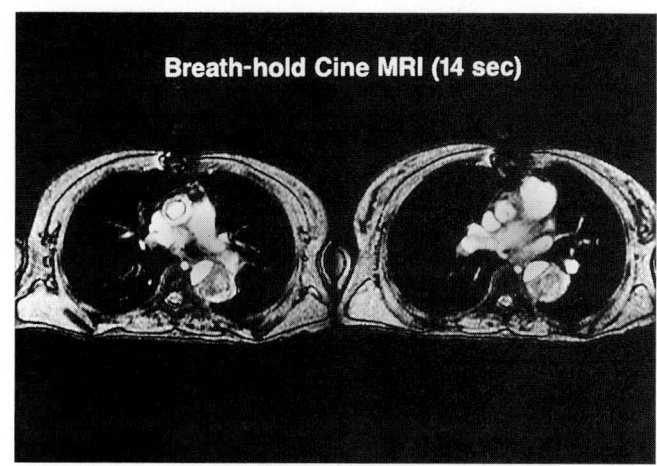

Breath-hold Cine MRI (14 sec)

FIGURE 10–23. Breath-hold cine MR images of a patient after repair of type A aortic dissection. Images are taken from a series of cine MR images acquired during a 14-second breath-hold period.

an additional advantage for showing the extent of the dissection. On the other hand, transesophageal echocardiography has the important advantage of portability.

MRI has been used to monitor the size of the thoracic aorta in patients with the *Marfan syndrome* and to exclude the presence of an occult dissection.[88] Dimensions at various segments of the thoracic aorta have been defined for normal subjects and patients with aneurysmal dilatation due to Marfan syndrome and other causes. Because MRI is a completely noninvasive technique, it is ideal for monitoring patients with aortic diseases and patients who have undergone surgical or medical treatment of aortic dissection.[89] MRI is also the most logical technique for the study of patients whose chest roentgenogram suggests a substantial increase in the size of the thoracic aorta.

MRI has been used to detect periaortic abscess complicating bacterial endocarditis.[92] The three-dimensional tomographic nature of the technique permits precise localization of these abscesses. MRI can also demonstrate the presence of intramural[93] or periaortic hematoma. Using T1-weighted spin-echo images, mediastinal intramural or pericardial blood has high intensity.

Evaluation of Cardiovascular Function
(See also Chap. 14)

A variety of MRI techniques has been employed for the evaluation of several aspects of cardiovascular function. These include standard cine MRI for the quantitation of global and regional contraction of the left and right ventricles.[94,95] The cine MRI technique usually produces gradient-echo images at 16 to 30 evenly spaced intervals through the cardiac cycle (Fig. 10–24). With standard cine MRI, the data acquisition period occupies 256 cardiac cycles. A fast version can be performed in only 16 cardiac cycles and has been called breath-hold cine MRI or segmental fast cine gradient-echo imaging.[1]

Blood flow volume and flow velocity can be quantified using velocity-encoded cine MRI (velocity flow mapping).[96–99] This technique provides a velocity image (velocity map, phase image) at evenly spaced intervals, usually 16, throughout the cardiac cycle. Analysis of the velocity image can be done to measure peak velocity or average velocity in any selected region of interest in the flow channel. Velocity-encoded sequences can be coupled with either standard cine MRI or breath-hold cine MRI. Using the multiple phase images collected over the cardiac cycle, flow or velocity versus time curve can be made.[98,99]

ECHOPLANAR IMAGING. The most attractive technique for evaluating cardiovascular function is *echoplanar imaging* (EPI), which essentially constitutes real-time MRI. It can be used in "single shot" or "multishot" modes.[5,100,101] The "single-shot" mode acquires the entire image in about a 40- to 80-msec interval of a single heart beat. The "multishot" mode acquires the image in 20- to 40-msec intervals of

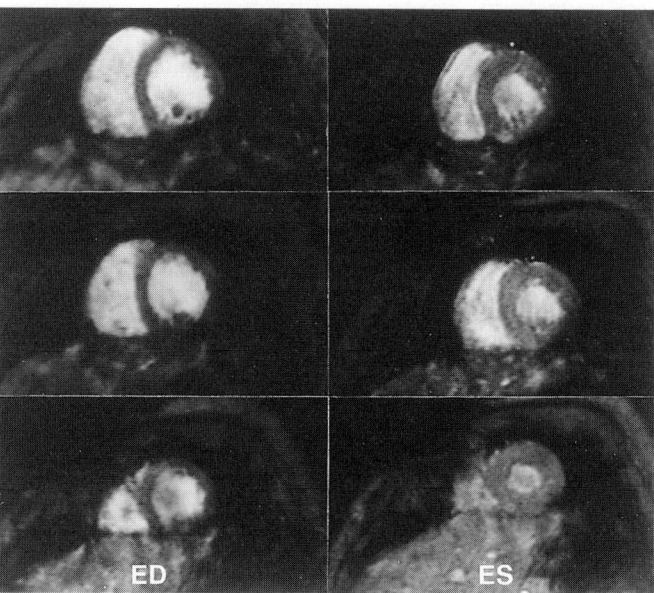

FIGURE 10–24. Cine MR images in the short-axis plane acquired at end-diastole (ED) and end-systole (ES) near the base *(upper panels)*, middle *(middle panels)*, and apex *(lower panels)* of the left ventricle. These images demonstrate symmetrical wall thickening of the left ventricle. From such images encompassing the length of both ventricles, measurement of ventricular volume and global function can be made.

two to four consecutive heart beats. Thus, a cine version of EPI can be done during a single cardiac cycle or acquired over two to four cardiac cycles. Velocity-encoded EPI can also be done. Thereby, analysis of contractile function of the ventricles and blood flow quantification are possible in essentially real time and on a nearly beat-to-beat basis using cine and velocity-encoded cine versions of EPI.

Because MRI is a three-dimensional imaging technique, it can provide direct measurements upon which the clinical evaluation of global left ventricular function has been based. Using sets of images encompassing the left ventricle, it is possible to calculate end-diastolic, end-systolic, and stroke volumes, and ejection fraction (Fig. 10–24). This can be done directly and does not depend upon the geometric assumptions used for such measurements from echocardiograms and x-ray angiograms. Moreover, MRI provides a three-dimensional direct visualization of the myocardium with excellent mural edge discrimination, thereby allowing quantitation of left ventricular mass.[1,43,44,102,103] MRI measurements have correlated closely with postmortem measurements of left ventricular mass.[102,103] Measurements of volumes and mass using a single MR image acquired in the long-axis plane of the left ventricle or in two perpendicular long- or short-axis planes, assuming various geometrical models, have been validated.[104–106]

RIGHT VENTRICULAR FUNCTION. Because MRI also defines the right ventricular myocardium, it may serve as the preferred technique for the accurate determination of right ventricular mass.[107] Reasonable accuracy has been shown for the measurement of right ventricular end-diastolic, end-systolic, and stroke volumes as well as ejection fraction.[107–109] Moreover, comparison of right and left ventricular stroke volumes has been used to estimate the regurgitant fraction in patients with aortic and mitral regurgitation.[109]

REGIONAL LEFT VENTRICULAR FUNCTION. Acquisition of MR images at various phases of the cardiac cycle provides a noninvasive method of assessing regional myocardial function.[46,110] Using various MR techniques, the extent of regional wall thickening in normal subjects has been defined.[46,110] Diminished regional wall thickening has been demonstrated in patients with acute myocardial infarction,[46,110] and generalized wall-thickening abnormalities have been demonstrated in patients with congestive cardiomyopathy and concentric left ventricular hypertrophy.[46]

Regional function is usually assessed with standard or breath-hold cine MRI because of the ability to segment the cardiac cycle into multiple frames (usually 16 to 30 per cycle) (Fig. 10–24). A study in normal individuals and patients with prior myocardial infarction demonstrated that cine MRI readily distinguished the site of previous injury by a diminution or absence of wall thickening during systole.[110] Systolic wall thickening of less than 2 mm was found in 31 of 40 abnormal segments (shown to be abnormal by angiography or echocardiography) and was found in only 3 of 78 segments of normal subjects. In addition, dyskinetic segments showed significantly thinned walls at end-diastole compared with normal values, whereas hypokinetic and akinetic segments did not show such severe wall thinning. Therefore, residual systolic wall thickening and nearly normal wall thickness at end diastole may indicate the presence of residual viable myocardium in a previously infarcted region. Infarcted segments as defined by ^{99m}Tc-sestamibi single-photon emission tomography have generally correlated with the cine MRI characteristics of wall thickness less than 6 mm and wall thickening of 1 mm or less.[20] Pharmacological stress has been successfully applied with cine MRI to provoke regional wall thickening abnormalities in patients with hemodynamically significant coronary arterial stenosis.[8,9]

Wall Thickening. For accurate measurements of wall thickness, imaging planes perpendicular to the long axis of the left ventricular wall (cardiac short-axis plane) are used (Fig. 10–24). These cardiac imaging planes (short- or long-axis) can minimize the problem of overestimation of wall thickness caused by oblique sectioning of the heart using the standard transverse planes. However, because of the ellipsoid shape of the left ventricle, some obliquity is unavoidable even when using planes oriented to the intrinsic axes of the left ventricle. This may be even more pronounced during systole because of shortening of the left ventricle along its long axis, resulting in possible overestimation of wall thickening at the apical level. A study with cine MRI acquired in short-axis planes showed a gradient of wall thickening increasing progressively from the base to the apex.[40] The influence of the imaging plane on this finding is not clear, but a similar gradient in the extent of regional myocardial shortening has been observed using sonomicrometer measurements in dogs.[111]

Although cine MRI provides an accurate means to quantify wall thickening, the major limiting factor to its widespread clinical implementation will be the time required to manually create the ventricular epicardial and endocardial contours. With the future development of a computerized automated contour-detection algorithm, time efficient, accurate, and reproducible analysis of ventricular volumes and wall thickening dynamics by cine MRI can be implemented clinically.

MYOCARDIAL TAGGING. Recently, myocardial tagging, a new method for quantitation of myocardial motion with MRI, has been developed.[112,113] Specified regions of the myocardium can be labeled by restricted localized RF pulses; these are placed perpendicular to the myocardial wall. These RF pulses are followed by a conventional imaging sequence after a short, specified delay. The labeled or "tagged" myocardial regions can be tracked precisely during systolic contraction. Myocardial motion occurring between RF excitation of the tag and image formation can be expressed as the displacement and distortion of the tagged regions, which appear as dark stripes (Fig. 10–25). The extent of the displacement of the tagged myocardium can be measured as the distance between a given tag and its original position at end-diastole. Heterogeneous myocardial motion among various segments of the left ventricle has been shown in normal subjects.[112] The longitudinal displacement of the tag during systole is significantly greater at the basal layer than at the mid or apical layers of the left ventricle. Short-axis images with tagging showed heterogeneous rotation of the wall with an increasing degree of counterclockwise rotation from the base to the apex. This technique has been used to characterize abnormal contraction and twist-

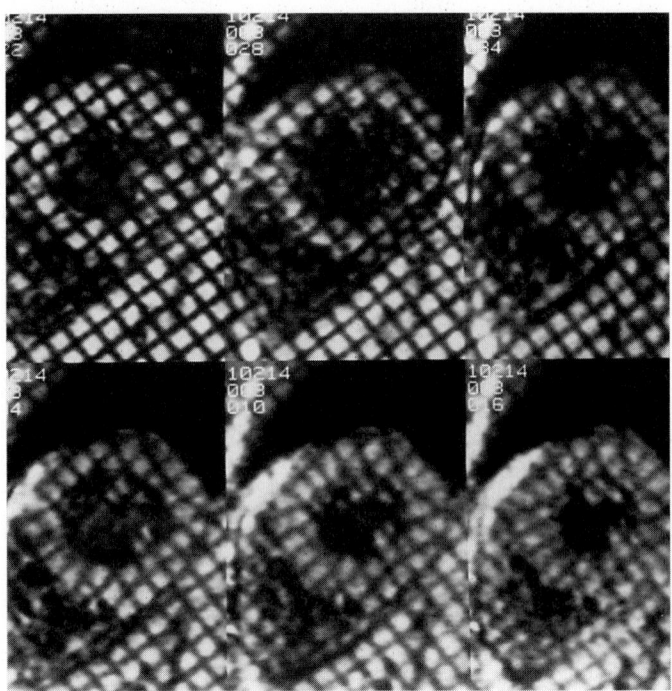

FIGURE 10–25. Composite of six short-axis views of the left ventricle (LV) from end-diastole *(upper left)* to end-systole *(lower right)* in a patient with left ventricular hypertrophy. The pattern of diagonal lines is a magnetic grid created in the tissue with spatial modulation of magnetization (SPAMM). Initially the grid moves with the underlying tissue, enabling analysis of regional wall motion within separate delineated elements of the wall. (Courtesy of Leon Axel, M.D., University of Pennsylvania Medical School.)

ing of various myocardial regions in hypertrophic cardiomyopathy.[114] It has also demonstrated tethering and compensatory regional contraction of normal myocardial segments after acute myocardial infarction.[115] This technique may provide the first noninvasive method for quantitating the complex multidirectional motion of myocardial segments.

Quantification of Valvular Regurgitation
(See also Chap. 32)

Accurate determination of the severity of valvular regurgitation is important for the evaluation of medical therapy and timing of surgical interventions. Among various methods, Doppler echocardiography has been used as the main diagnostic tool to detect valvular regurgitation because of its high sensitivity and specificity. However, quantification of severity has been less successful. Mapping of the spatial extent of the disturbed flow in the regurgitant chamber with pulse Doppler or color Doppler is useful for routine serial evaluation but provides only a semiquantitative estimate of the severity of valvular regurgitation. In this regard, cine MRI provides several methods for quantifying the extent of valvular regurgitation, including measurement of signal void on cine MRI and determination of the difference in stroke volumes of the two ventricles. In addition, velocity-encoded cine MRI can be used to measure the volume of retrograde flow in the ascending aorta or pulmonary artery in aortic and pulmonary regurgitation, respectively.

THE SIGNAL VOID IN REGURGITATION. The high-velocity jet caused by regurgitation can be readily identified on cine MR images because it produces a signal void in the recipient cardiac chamber[116–123] (Fig. 10–26). Mitral regurgitation causes a systolic signal void extending from the incompetent mitral valve into the left atrium, whereas aortic regurgitation causes a diastolic signal void extending from the

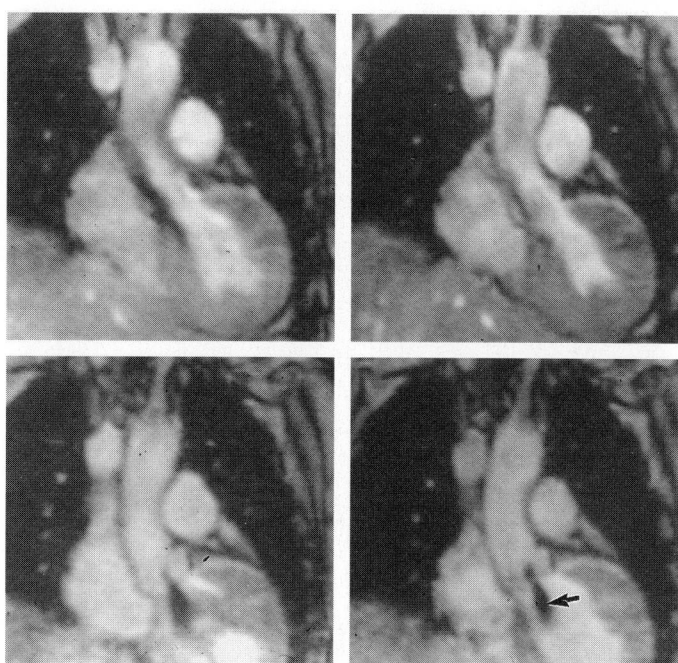

FIGURE 10–26. Series of cine MR images obtained in the coronal plane. Images in upper panels are from systole and those in the lower panels are from diastole. A signal void (arrow) originates from the closed aortic valve during diastole, indicating aortic regurgitation.

aortic valve *into* the left ventricle. Measurements of the signal void have been used to provide a semiquantitative estimation of the severity of mitral or aortic regurgitation.[117,119,121,123] The area of signal loss roughly corresponds to the extent of turbulent retrograde flow and has been correlated with the severity of regurgitation established by angiography, echocardiography,[117,119] or regurgitant volumes calculated as the difference between right and left ventricular stroke volumes using cine MRI.[119]

Some possible pitfalls should be considered in measuring signal void on cine MRI. The size of the flow void can be affected by the velocity of the jet flow and the relationship between the direction of regurgitant flow and orientation of the imaging plane. The signal void is influenced also by the size of the aperture in the closed valve and pressure differential between the two chambers or artery. In addition, the size of the void varies relative to the echo delay time (TE) used for imaging. With shortening of the TE, the size of the void is reduced. Therefore, serial quantification of valvular regurgitation or direct comparison of results among groups may be possible only if identical imaging parameters are used.

STROKE VOLUME RATIO AND REGURGITANT VOLUME. The difference between end-diastolic and end-systolic volume for a ventricle with a regurgitant valve includes both the forward stroke volume and the regurgitant volume. Because the forward or net stroke volume is equal to the volume ejected from normal ventricle, the difference in stroke volumes between a regurgitant ventricle (e.g., left ventricle with aortic and mitral regurgitation) and normal ventricle (e.g., right ventricle) is the regurgitant volume. The sum of the forward and regurgitant volume is called total stroke volume of the regurgitant ventricle.

Several reports have verified that ventricular volume can be accurately measured from cine MRI images.[40,108] In the absence of regurgitation, the stroke volumes of the right and left ventricle are nearly equal.[108] However, in patients with aortic and/or mitral regurgitation, the stroke volume of the left ventricle exceeds that of the right ventricle by a value equivalent to the regurgitant volume. The regurgitant fraction can be calculated as the regurgitant volume divided by the total stroke volume of the regurgitant ventri-

cle. The stroke volume ratio can also be calculated from the stroke volumes of the two ventricles. These measurements derived from cine MRI have distinguished patients with mild, moderate, and severe left-sided regurgitant lesions, as shown by independent imaging techniques.[109]

The major limitation of utilizing stroke volume difference for quantification of regurgitation is in the presence of multiple valve disease. If both aortic and mitral regurgitation are present, the calculation determines only the total volume of regurgitation. If regurgitation coexists on both sides of the heart, this calculation is not meaningful.

VELOCITY-ENCODED CINE MRI. The most effective MR technique for quantifying valvular function is velocity-encoded cine MRI or velocity-flow mapping. It has been used to quantify the volumes of aortic[124] and mitral[125] regurgitation and to estimate the pressure gradients in aortic[126,127] and mitral[127,128] stenosis. The methodology, validation, and applications of velocities accorded cine MRI are discussed below.

Quantification of *aortic regurgitation* by velocity-encoded cine MRI has been accomplished in two ways. Measurement of blood flow in the ascending aorta and main pulmonary artery provides stroke volume for the left and right ventricles, respectively. The difference between the two stroke volumes is the aortic regurgitant volume. Moreover, because retrograde as well as antegrade flow can be determined from the instantaneous flow changes throughout the cardiac cycle using velocity-encoded cine MRI, the volume of aortic regurgitation or pulmonary regurgitation can be measured directly by the time integration of diastolic regurgitant flow[124] (Fig. 10–27).

Mitral regurgitation has been quantified by measuring diastolic inflow to the left ventricle by a velocity-encoded cine MR acquisition in a short-axis plane positioned at the level of the mitral annulus, and systolic outflow by a velocity-encoded cine MR acquisition positioned at the level of the proximal ascending aorta. The difference between the two volumes is the volume of mitral regurgitation.[125]

Measurement of Blood Flow

Measurement of blood flow velocity with MRI has been achieved in several laboratories using a technique originally proposed by Moran[129] and introduced clinically by Underwood and associates.[130] The version used in the laboratory of the author is called "velocity-encoded cine MRI." This method is principally based on the phase shifts of moving spins in the magnetic field gradient.[131,132] The extent of phase shifts of moving spins is proportional to velocity along the velocity-encoding direction. Velocity encoding is performed by using bipolar gradient pulses. The direction of velocity encoding can be done in any orthogonal or oblique axis of the body.

Velocity encoding of blood flow in each pixel provides two-dimensional quantitative velocity mapping of the vascular system (Figs. 10–27 to 10–29). The instantaneous flow in the ascending aorta can be determined by the product of the cross-sectional area and mean velocity of the blood within the aorta. The integration of the instantaneous flow at the base of the aorta through the cardiac cycle provides a measure of left ventricular stroke volume and the same done at the proximal pulmonary artery is a measure of right ventricular stroke volume (Fig. 10–29). The stroke volumes measured in this manner have correlated well with ventricular stroke volumes measured by planimetry of the multiple adjacent cine MR images.[97]

VELOCITY-ENCODED CINE MRI. Measurement of flow by velocity-encoded cine MRI should be very accurate provided that the flowing blood generates enough signal to calculate phase; the velocity phase-encoding gradients are accurately calibrated; and the correct range of velocity in the vessels being interrogated has been selected. The calculation of blood flow in the main pulmonary artery by the velocity-encoded cine MRI technique has shown nearly equivalent values to the sum of the flow in the right and left pulmonary arteries.[133] A distinctly different flow pattern in the pulmonary artery has been observed in patients with pulmonary hypertension than in normal subjects using this technique.[134,135]

Velocity-encoded cine MRI has been tested for an array of applications, including measurement of stroke volume of both ventricles,[97] quantification of valvular regurgitation[124,125] (Figs. 10–27 and 10–28), estimation of the gradient across valvular and vascular stenoses,[126–128] and the measurement of the volume of left-to-right shunts[136] (Fig. 10–29). Velocity encoding can be used with the breath-hold cine MRI sequence[12,13] (Fig. 10–8) and with EPI. Some pitfalls accompany the

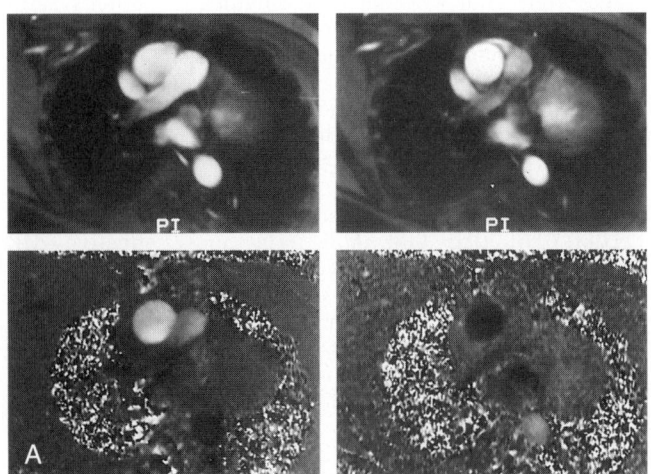

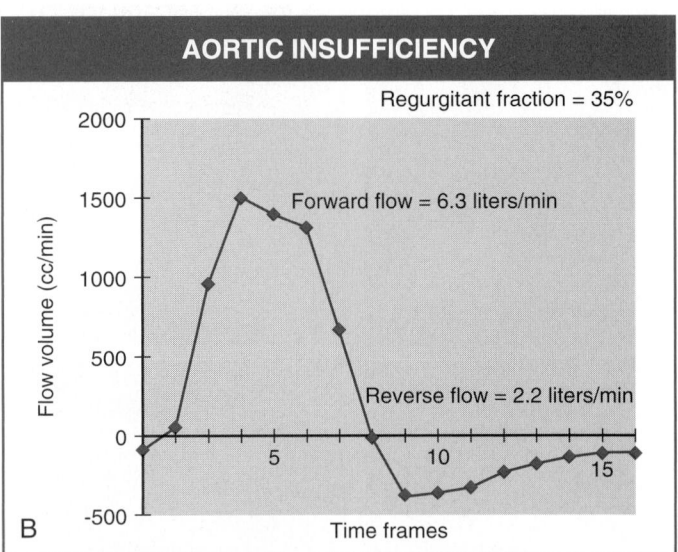

FIGURE 10–27. *A,* magnitude *(above)* and phase *(below)* images in systole *(left)* and diastole *(right)* of a patient with aortic regurgitation on phase images. Bright signal in the ascending aorta in systole represents antegrade flow. In diastole, dark signal in the ascending aorta represents retrograde flow due to aortic regurgitation. *B,* Flow versus time curve in a patient with aortic regurgitation. Reverse flow in diastole represents aortic insufficiency. The area under this curve provides a direct measurement of the volume of aortic regurgitation. (From Higgins, C. B., and Caputo, G. R.: MRI of valvular heart disease. *In* Pohost, G. M., (ed.): Cardiovascular Applications of Magnetic Resonance. Mt. Kisco, NY, Futura Publishing, 1993.)

use of the velocity-encoded cine MRI technique for measuring blood flow. These include aliasing due to setting of the maximum velocity range to less than the actual velocity. The finite slice thickness also results in volume averaging, causing underestimation of peak velocity. Furthermore, orientation may not provide optimal interrogation of the jet, so that velocity is underestimated.

ESTIMATION OF PRESSURE GRADIENTS AND SHUNTS. Doppler echocardiography has been found to be effective for measuring peak velocity across valvular stenoses and for estimating the pressure gradient with the modified Bernoulli equation (peak pressure gradient = $4 \times$ peak velocity^2; $\Delta P = 4V^2$) (see Fig. 3–41, p. 69). By the same principle, velocity-encoded cine MRI can provide estimates of the gradients of aortic and mitral stenoses. The velocity-encoded cine estimates have correlated with measurements obtained via catheterization and/or echocardiography.[126-128]

Velocity-encoded cine MRI can be used to measure flow in the ascending aorta and pulmonary artery simultaneously in order to quantify the volume of some left-to-right shunts and to calculate the pulmonary-to-systemic flow ratio (Qp/Qs) of cardiovascular shunts (Fig. 10–29). The MR measurement of Qp/Qs has correlated closely with that derived from oximetric data acquired during cardiac catheterization in patients with atrial septal defects.[136] Measurement of blood flow separately in the right and left pulmonary arteries can be used to quantify the distribution of pulmonary blood flow in lesions causing unequal flow. This technique can also be applied to estimate the gradient across pulmonary vascular stenosis, stenosis of branches of the pulmonary artery, coarctation of the aorta, and Rastelli conduits.[80]

Recently, velocity-encoded cine MRI has been used to provide an estimate of the collateral circulation in coarctation.[137] In healthy subjects the total flow in the distal part of the descending aorta is slightly decreased compared with the flow in the proximal part of the descending aorta because of runoff through the intercostal arteries. In patients with hemodynamically significant coarctation, the MR measurements have revealed a substantial increase in flow in the distal compared with the proximal part of the descending aorta. This increase in flow is presumably due to retrograde flow in the branches of the descending aorta.

CORONARY FLOW VELOCITY. Velocity-encoded cine MR images can also be acquired during a single breath hold and have been used to measure coronary flow velocity in humans[12,13] (Fig. 10–8). Volume flow and flow velocity in the coronary circulation can be augmented severalfold in response to increased oxygen demands caused by exercise or in response to vasodilators. Coronary vasodilator reserve is ablated or attenuated in the presence of a hemodynamically significant stenosis of the coronary arteries. Breath-hold velocity-encoded MRI has shown an increase in coronary flow velocity in response to the vasodilator adenosine[12] and dipyridamole.[13] Thus, MRI has the potential to provide noninvasive imaging of the major coronary arteries and, additionally, to test the physiological integrity of the coronary circulation by quantifying coronary vasodilator reserve. Breath-hold velocity-encoded MRI can also be used to determine the adequacy of flow in internal mammary arterial and saphenous venous bypass grafts. The normal flow pattern in grafts and in native coronary arteries has a characteristic biphasic pattern with substantial flow velocity in dias-

tole (Figs. 10–9 and 10–10). Loss of the phasic pattern and/or loss of vasodilator reserve may indicate failing coronary bypass conduits.

Characterization of Myocardial Tissue

Characterization of myocardial tissue depends on estimation of signal intensity on images with varying TR and TE values, hydrogen density, and T1 and T2 relaxation times. The measurements of relaxation times from gated images are approximations rendered inexact by cardiac and respiratory motion.[138] Despite these limitations, the T2 relaxation times have been found to discriminate between normal and pathological myocardium of the in situ beating heart.

Ex vivo measurements have revealed that several myocardial diseases, including ischemic myocardial injury[139,140] and cardiac transplant rejection[141] produce significant alteration of relaxation time. Increases in signal intensity and T2 relaxation times have been found in experimental animals[21,142,143] with acute myocardial infarction and in humans with acute and subacute infarction.[22,23] The utility of MR for myocardial tissue characterization is not clear, and little attention has been focused on this topic in recent years.

MRI CONTRAST MEDIA FOR MYOCARDIAL ENHANCEMENT. ECG-gated spin-echo MRI can demonstrate the presence of acute myocardial infarction without the use of contrast agents. However, this ability to detect acute infarction depends on the prolongation of T1 and T2 relaxation times, which is caused by increased tissue water content and does not reach a detectable level until several hours after coronary artery occlusion. Therefore, acute ischemia is not visible until the onset of myocardial edema. Consequently, contrast agents seem to be necessary for identifying acute ischemia. Moreover, contrast agents may be useful to enhance the contrast between myocardial infarction and normal myocardium by differently altering the relaxation times of the two regions. The current status of myocardial contrast media has been reviewed recently.[144]

Contrast agents currently used can be classified by the mechanisms of action.[144] The first class of MRI contrast agents are *relaxivity agents,* which affect signal by enhancing relaxation of neighboring protons. In this class, paramagnetic compounds mainly decrease T1 relaxation time

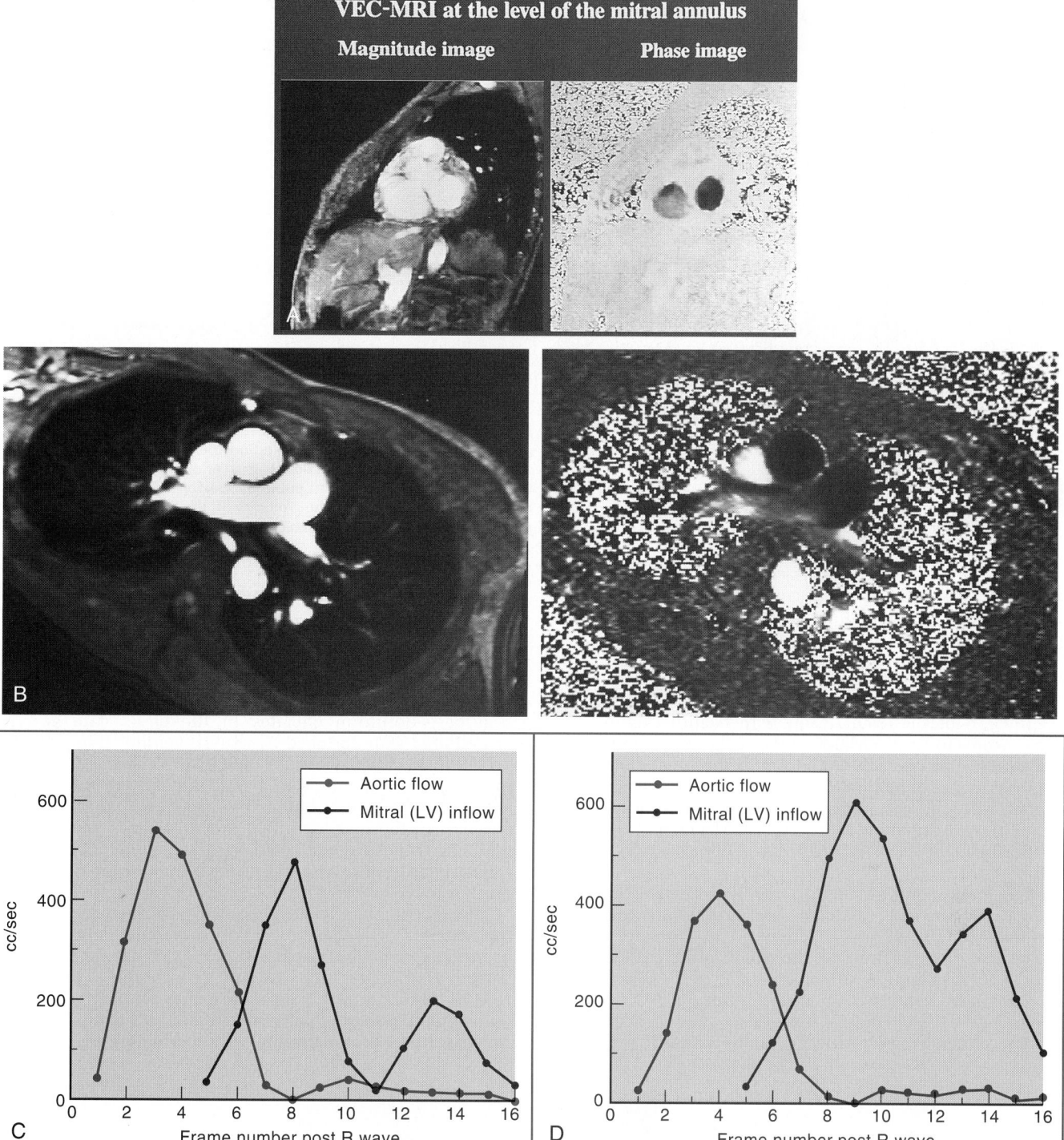

FIGURE 10–28. *A,* Magnitude and phase images at the level of the mitral annulus. The phase image is used to measure mitral inflow. *B,* Magnitude *(left)* and phase *(right)* images at the level of the proximal aorta. *C,* Flow versus time curve for mitral inflow and aortic outflow in a normal subject. *D,* Flow versus time curve in a patient with mitral regurgitation. Using phase images, flow is calculated as the spatial average velocity in the region of interest (i.e., aorta) and the cross-sectional area of the region of interest. The areas under the two curves in *C* are nearly equal. In *D,* the area under the mitral inflow curve is considerably greater than the area of the aortic outflow curve. The difference between the two areas is the volume of mitral regurgitation. (From Fujita, N., Chazouilleres, A. F., Hartiala, J. J., et al.: Quantification of mitral regurgitation by velocity-encoded cine magnetic resonance imaging. J. Am. Coll. Cardiol. *23:*951–958, 1994.)

and thereby enhance the regional intensity of tissues. The effect is maximal on T1-weighted images (Fig. 10–6). Examples of relaxivity agents are gadolinium chelates. The second class of MRI contrast media are *magnetic susceptibility agents;* these agents cause inhomogeneity in the local magnetic field within tissues and by this mechanism decrease signal intensity. The effect of this agent is maximal

on T2-weighted images. Examples of susceptibility agents are dysprosium chelates[145] and iron oxide particles.

PARAMAGNETIC AGENTS. Most MR contrast agents used to date for myocardial imaging have been predominantly paramagnetic agents. They are soluble, aqueous substances much like x-ray contrast media. The magnitude of relaxation enhancement is influenced by magnetic field strength

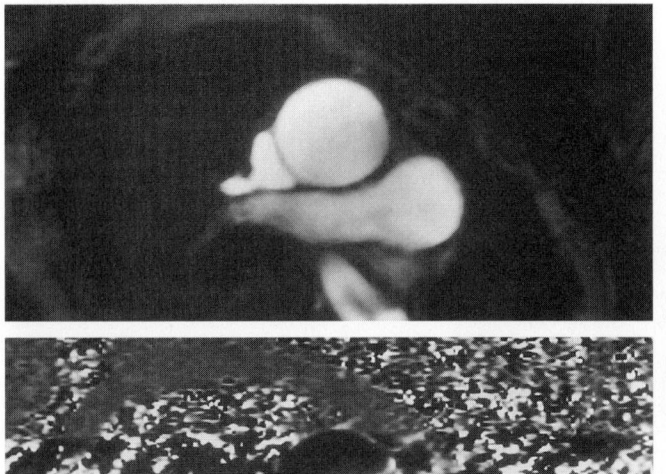

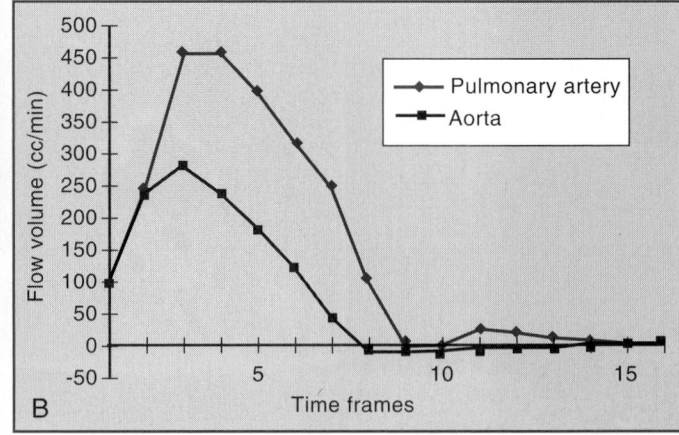

FIGURE 10–29.   *A,* Phase image at level of ascending aorta and main pulmonary artery. Flow is calculated on the spatial average velocity of the vessel and the cross-sectional area of the vessel. *B,* Flow versus time curves for the aorta and pulmonary artery. The difference in area under the two curves is the volume of the left-to-right shunt in a patient with an atrial septal defect.

and the concentration of the paramagnetic agents. Although they can cause shortening of both T1 and T2 relaxation times, T1 shortening predominates at lower doses and T2 effects are dominant at higher doses. Myocardial intensity after administration of a paramagnetic agent depends upon myocardial perfusion as well as other factors, including diffusion of the agent through the capillaries, affinity of the agent for myocardial cells, volume of the interstitial space, and rate of elimination of the agent from myocardial tissue and bloodstream. The currently used paramagnetic MR contrast media are ionic or nonionic chelates of gadolinium (Gd) such as Gd DTPA (Magnevist, Schering AG, Berlin), and Gd DTPA-BMA (Omniscan Nycomed, Oslo).

Paramagnetic contrast media have been used to improve demarcation between infarcted and normal myocardium; the infarcted myocardium is enhanced to a greater degree than normal myocardium on images acquired during the steady-state distribution of the media[144,146,147] (Fig. 10–5). This has been observed both in animals[144,146] and in humans.[147–149] These media have also shown a different intensity enhancement pattern for reperfused compared

with occlusive myocardial infarctions in experimental animals using spin-echo imaging[150] and a different early distribution pattern using EPI.[151]

Regional myocardial perfusion has been assessed using T1-sensitive fast gradient-echo imaging (images acquired at the rate of one every 1 or 2 seconds) after the bolus injection of gadolinium chelates in the basal state and in a vasodilated state induced by dipyridamole[15] (Fig. 10–6).

MAGNETIC SUSCEPTIBILITY AGENTS. These MR contrast media cause a decrease in signal intensity of the tissues to which they are distributed because they induce local differences in the magnetic field of the tissues. Acute myocardial ischemia is demarcated as a region of high signal in the myocardium owing to greater reduction of signal of the normal myocardium.[145]

The recent experience with MRI contrast media in animal models of ischemic heart disease indicates that these agents expand the capability of MRI for characterizing various tissue alterations caused by ischemia. The potential role of MRI contrast media in ischemic heart disease includes distinguishing between normal and acutely ischemic myocardium; demonstration of reperfusion of myocardial

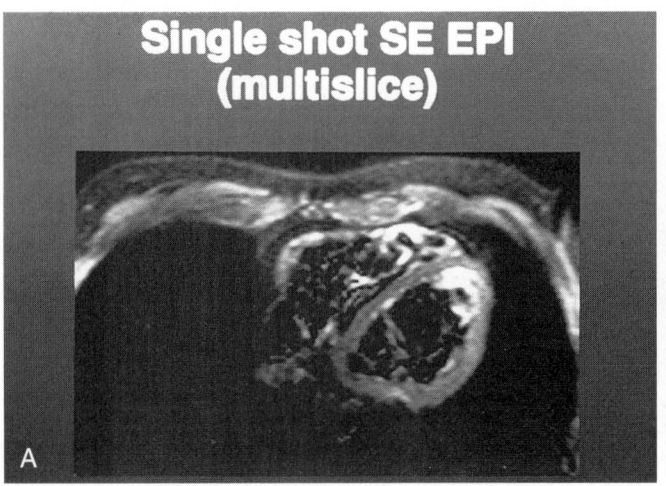

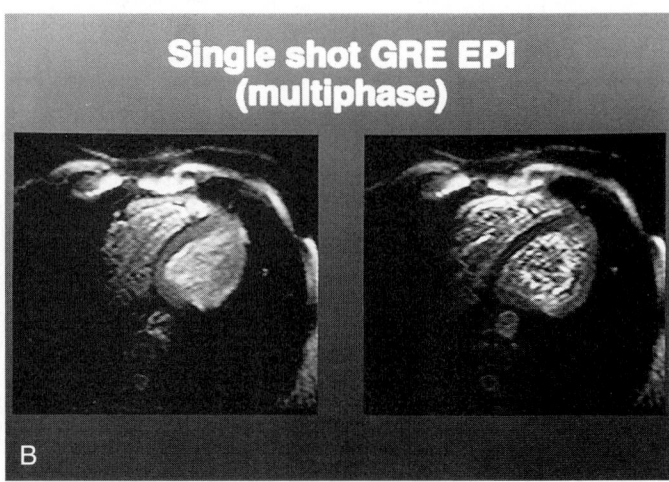

FIGURE 10–30.   Single-shot echoplanar images. Each image was acquired in approximately 50 msec. *A,* Spin-echo pulse sequence. *B,* Gradient-echo pulse sequence.

infarctions; and possibly differentiation between reperfused reversibly injured and irreversibly injured myocardium. It is reasonable to expect considerable progress in this area of research in the next few years.

ECHOPLANAR IMAGING. In the past 2 years MR imagers capable of producing MR images in approximately 50 msec (Fig. 10–30) have been put into operation at a few centers around the world. The EPI technique provides the possibil-ity of imaging the entire heart in a single heart beat. More-over, it can be used to assess myocardial perfusion of the entire left ventricle at a temporal resolution of 1 second during the first passage of MR contrast media. It can be applied to measure blood flow on a beat-to-beat basis. Consequently, this technique is expected to have an im-portant impact on the cardiovascular applications of MRI.

COMPUTED TOMOGRAPHY

Technical Aspects

Computed tomographic (CT) scanning of the heart usu-ally requires modification of the standard CT techniques used for investigating other parts of the body. For some purposes, such as evaluation of thoracic aortic disease, pericardial disease, paracardiac and intracardiac tumors, and patency of coronary arterial bypass grafts, newer stan-dard CT scanners with exposure times of less than 2 sec-onds are usually adequate.[152–155] Continuously rotating (spiral) CT scanners have an exposure time of 1 second for each image with no interscan delay between images at se-quential anatomical levels, producing images of the entire heart in approximately 12 to 20 seconds. Although ade-quate anatomical depiction of cardiovascular anatomy is attained with spiral CT, scans corresponding to precise phases of the cardiac cycle cannot be obtained. For the assessment of cardiac dimensions and function in addition to morphology, millisecond CT scanners are required.[156,157] The evolution of CT scanning of the heart in the early stages also involved ECG gating of CT data acquisition. However, such gating techniques proved to be cumbersome and never received clinical acceptance. This approach has been discarded.

SPIRAL CT SCANNER. CT scans at multiple adjacent ana-tomical levels are obtained during a breath-hold period. Each CT scan is acquired in approximately 1 second. This is accomplished by multiple rotations of the CT scanner gantry while the table is continuously incremented through the gantry. This permits multiple transaxial scans, 4 mm to 10 mm in thickness, of most or the entire thorax during a single breath-hold period at the time of peak contrast en-hancement of the cardiovascular structures. Approximately 80 to 100 ml of contrast medium at a rate of 2 to 3 ml/sec is injected intravenously, and CT acquisition is started at 20 to 30 seconds after the start of the injection (circulation time).

ULTRAFAST (CINE, ELECTRON BEAM) CT SCANNER. The ul-trafast CT scanner employs a scanning focused x-ray beam, which provides complete cardiac imaging in 50 msec with-out the need for ECG gating (Fig. 10–31). This CT scanner is not limited by the inertia associated with moving me-chanical parts. It uses a focused electron beam that is suc-cessively swept across four cadmium tungstate target arcs at the speed of light. Each of the four targets generates a fan beam of photons that pass from beneath the patient to a bank of photon detectors arranged in a semicircle above the patient.

The ultrafast CT scanner can be operated in three different modes: (1) the *cine mode* is used to assess global and regional myocardial function. The scans are obtained at an exposure time of 50 msec and at a rate of 17 scans per second[153] (Fig. 10–32). The *triggered mode*, used for flow analysis, employs a series of 20 to 40 successive scans in which each 50-msec exposure is triggered at a specific phase of the cardiac cycle of successive heart beats or every other heart beat. From such a series of scans, time-density curves can be constructed for specific regions of interest in the cardiac chamber or myocar-dium, providing an estimate of transit time, perfusion, or blood flow.[154] The *volume mode* provides eight scans by the use of all four target arcs in an imaging period of approximately 200 msec. These eight transverse scans can sometimes encompass the entire left ven-tricular chamber and thereby provide an estimate of left ventricular volume and mass. Usually 10 to 12 tomographic levels are needed to entirely encompass the heart.

Because multiple images can be acquired at multiple levels, ultra-fast CT permits the acquisition of images at end-diastole and end-systole because both are approximately 60 msec in duration. Real-time sequential imaging is accomplished within a single heart beat at multiple levels, and these images can then be displayed in a close-loop cine format (cine CT display).

CONTRAST ENHANCEMENT. For nearly all purposes, intravenous in-jection of iodinated contrast medium is used to delineate the blood pool on CT scans. The contrast medium can be given as an intrave-nous bolus injection or a rapid infusion. For evaluation of the heart and great vessels, contrast medium is usually delivered in a bolus over several seconds and in a volume of approximately 30 to 60 ml. Scans are exposed at the estimated time of peak enhancement of the structure of interest. In order to identify the time of arrival of con-trast medium in the left-sided cardiac chamber and aorta, a prelimi-nary bolus injection of indocyanine dye can be given in order to define circulation time. This time is then used to specify the time of acquisition of the series of ultrafast CT scans. Scans are sometimes obtained without contrast medium in order to identify calcification of cardiac structures.

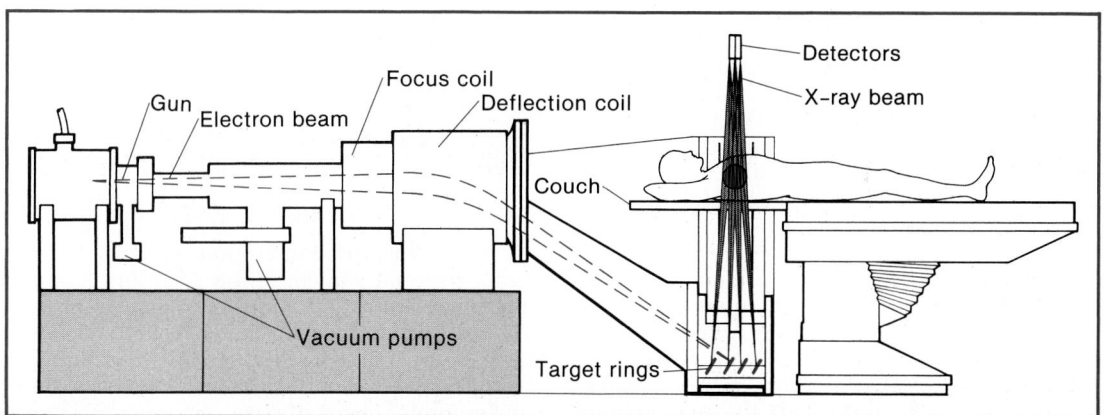

FIGURE 10–31. Diagram of cine CT scanner. Electron gun produces a stream of electrons that are magneti-cally focused and directed onto four tungsten target rings. Each target ring emits two fan beams of x-ray. Transmission of x-rays through the subject is registered by detectors arranged over a 180-degree arc.

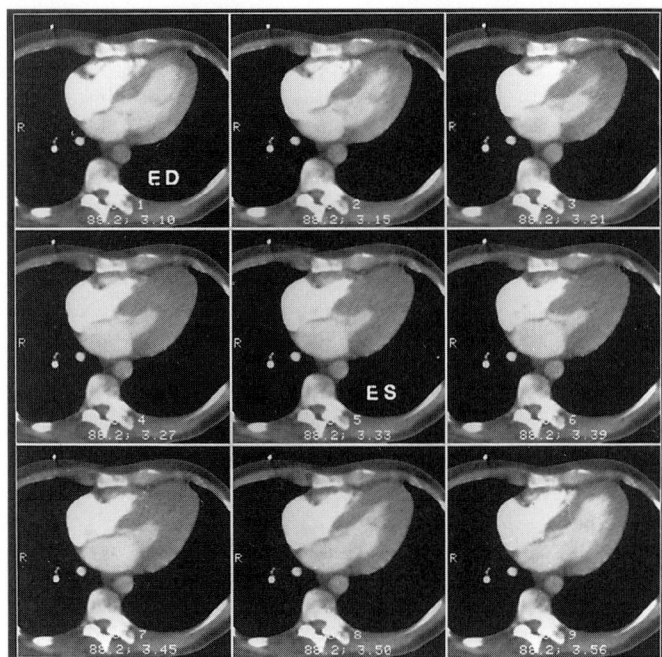

FIGURE 10–32. Series of CT scans of the same anatomical level acquired every 50 msec during a single cardiac cycle in a patient with hypertrophic cardiomyopathy. These are 9 of 17 scans acquired in approximately one cardiac cycle. Frame at upper left is near end-diastole (ED) and middle frame is near end-systole (ES). Note the change in ventricular volumes during the cardiac cycle and wall thickening during systole. (Courtesy of J. Rumberger, Ph.D., M.D., Mayo Clinic.)

Evaluation of Cardiac Dimensions and Function

CT scans have the capability of identifying not only the inner endocardial wall but also the epicardial surface. Wall thickness and myocardial mass have been estimated accurately with ultrafast CT[162] (Fig. 10–33). A close correlation has been found between CT measurements and postmortem anatomical measurements of wall thickness and mass[158,159] (Fig. 10–33). It has also been employed to estimate right ventricular mass by measuring the mass of the free wall.[160,161] Right ventricular mass was demonstrated to be substantially increased in patients with pulmonary arterial hypertension compared with measurements in normal subjects.[161]

CT scanning can be used in the assessment of the dynamics of *regional myocardial wall-thickening*.[162–164] A series of tomograms in a short-axis plane acquired during multiple phases of the cardiac cycle provides the capability to measure area ejection fraction and wall thickening at various levels of the left ventricle, extending from the base to the apex. In normal human subjects, a variation in both regional ejection fraction and extent of wall thickening has been defined; a gradient in both area ejection fraction and extent of wall thickening increases progressively from basal to apical layers.[164] Cine CT has demonstrated dysfunction of wall thickening and wall motion in global and regional myocardial abnormalities.[165–167]

Left ventricular volumes and *ejection fraction* can be estimated by contrast angiography, echocardiography, and gated blood pool nuclear images. While the quantitation of ventricular volumes and ejection fraction by cine CT is not a unique capability, the accuracy of CT can potentially exceed that of the other techniques. Other cardiac imaging techniques such as echocardiography and LV angiography estimate left ventricular volume, making geometric assumptions from measurements performed in one or two planes. These assumptions lead to inaccuracies of volume mea-

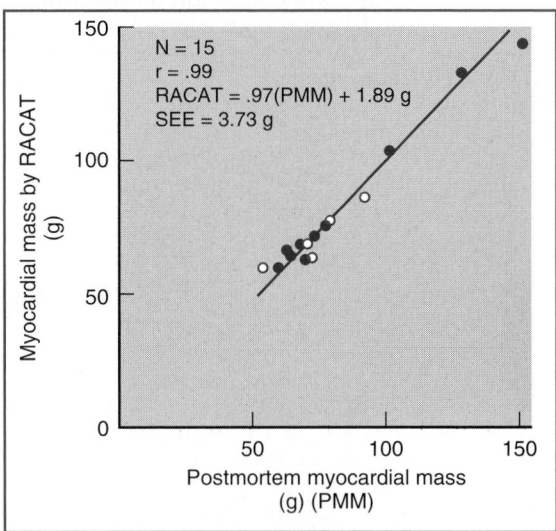

FIGURE 10–33. Graph plots mass determined by rapid-acquisition computer-assisted tomography (RACAT) versus postmortem measurement of left ventricular mass (PMM). RACAT is another denotation for cine CT. This study was done in anesthetized dogs. (Reproduced with permission from Feiring, A., et al.: Determination of left ventricular mass in dogs with rapid-acquisition cardiac CT scanning. *Circulation* 72:1355, 1985. Copyright 1985 American Heart Association.)

surement in the presence of left ventricular conformational abnormalities. Ultrafast CT directly measures chamber volumes by planimetry of the cardiac blood pool on each tomogram, allowing precise volume determination. It has been demonstrated that left ventricular volume, ejection fraction, and stroke volume can be acquired by ultrafast CT with high accuracy and close reproducibility among observers and among studies on different occasions in the same subject.[168,169] In normal subjects the stroke volumes of the right and left ventricle as measured by ultrafast CT were equal.[169]

Ultrafast CT provides a measurement of total ventricular *stroke volume*. If an independent technique is used for the measurement of forward (effective) stroke volume, then these measurements can be combined to estimate regurgitant volume; regurgitant volume is the difference between total stroke volume and forward stroke volume. Ultrafast CT can also be applied for the simultaneous quantification of the right and left ventricular stroke volumes.[169,170] The difference in the stroke volume between the ventricles is equal to the total regurgitant volume of valves on one side of the heart. This method has been shown to be highly accurate for measuring the regurgitant volume in an animal model of acute aortic regurgitation.[170] The method is not relevant for circumstances in which valvular regurgitation is present in both the right and left ventricles.

EVALUATION OF SPECIFIC CARDIAC DISEASES

Ischemic Heart Disease

After myocardial infarction, CT can be used to demonstrate regional wall thinning[171–174] and complications of infarction, such as left ventricular aneurysm (Figs. 10–34 and 10–35) and mural thrombus. Gated CT and ultrafast CT have demonstrated reduced wall thickening and wall motion as evidence of left ventricular segmental dysfunction in ischemic heart disease. In one large series in which ECG-gated CT was compared with left ventricular cineangiography, a sensitivity of 94 per cent and a specificity of 87 per cent were shown for the detection of a regional wall

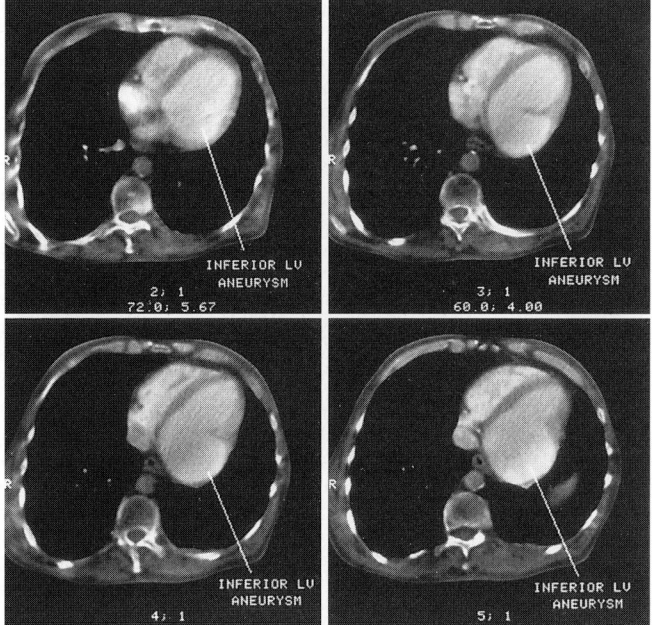

FIGURE 10–34. Cine (ultrafast) CT images at four adjacent anatomical levels *(upper left,* cranial to *lower right,* caudal) in a patient with inferior left ventricular aneurysm. The CT images demonstrate the location and extent of the aneurysm. (Courtesy of Imatron, Inc.)

abnormality.[171] The accuracy of detecting the anatomical and functional sequelae of infarction was substantially better for the anterior wall than for the posterior and diaphragmatic walls of the left ventricle because of the orientation of the heart in relation to the fixed transverse imaging. The ability of present-day methodology to acquire images in a plane approximating the cardiac short axis by elevating and tilting the table has considerably alleviated this limitation.

CT provides unequivocal spatial separation between various regions of the left ventricle, enabling better localization and estimation of the extent of wall thinning after

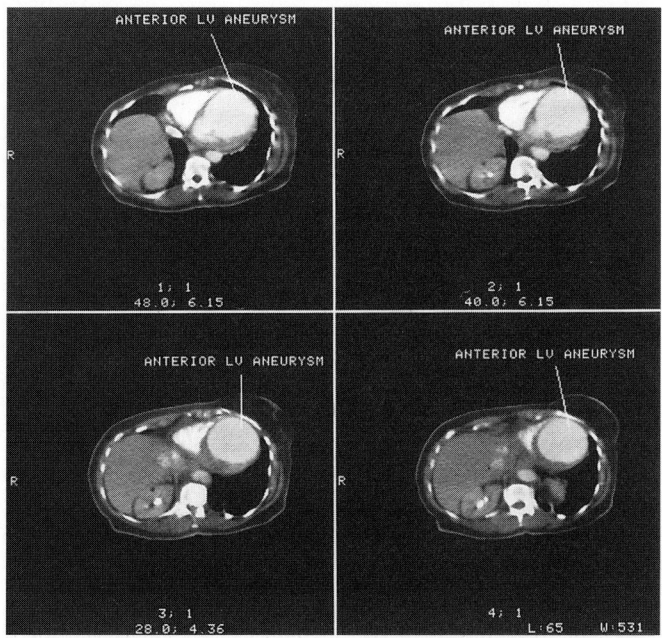

FIGURE 10–35. Cine (ultrafast) CT images at four adjacent anatomical levels *(upper left,* cranial to *lower right,* caudal) demonstrate an anterior left ventricular aneurysm. There is severe thinning of the anteroseptal and anterior walls and bulging of the left ventricle anteriorly. (Courtesy of Imatron, Inc.)

infarction compared with projectional techniques such as left ventriculography and most scintigraphic techniques. Likewise, the site and extent of anterior (Fig. 10–35) and posterior aneurysms of the left ventricle can be well demonstrated. The differentiation by CT between true aneurysm and pseudoaneurysm depends on the identification of the small ostium connecting the left ventricular cavity and the aneurysm. False aneurysms are usually substantially larger than true aneurysms and frequently arise from the posterior or inferior wall of the left ventricle.

CT has been found to be as accurate as two-dimensional echocardiography for identifying left ventricular *mural thrombus.*[175,176] Moreover, comparative studies have shown greater accuracy of CT compared with two-dimensional echocardiography in demonstration of thrombus in the left atrium.[177] The comparative accuracy of CT and transesophageal echocardiography has not been established.

REGIONAL WALL MOTION. For the evaluation of regional myocardial function, the cine mode of the ultrafast CT scanner is used to acquire images at 17 scans per second at the time of peak opacification of the left ventricle (Fig. 10–34). Quantitation of systolic myocardial wall thickening appears to be a particularly useful technique for evaluating regional myocardial contractile function in patients with ischemic heart disease. Ultrafast CT has been effective in identifying the region of ischemia by demonstrating loss of regional wall thickening during acute coronary occlusion in a canine experimental model.[165] Using ultrafast CT scanning with contrast enhancement for demonstrating regional contraction abnormalities in patients with prior infarctions, a 91 per cent correlation with left ventriculography for identifying abnormal myocardial segments has been reported.[173] Regional wall thickening and inward motion were used as the parameters of regional function on CT scans; they correlated well with wall motion abnormalities demonstrated on left ventriculography and critical coronary stenoses shown by coronary angiography.[174]

MYOCARDIAL PERFUSION. Ultrafast CT may also be able to provide an indication of *regional myocardial perfusion.*[178–181] Estimates of myocardial perfusion are obtained by drawing regions of interest over various sites of the myocardium displayed on the transverse CT scans. The density of the myocardial regions is measured on sequential 50-msec scans acquired during an appropriate duration of the myocardial contrast-enhancement phase. From these measurements, time-density curves are constructed; analyses of these curves in regard to contrast appearance and wash-out are used to estimate regional myocardial perfusion. Thus, fast CT has the potential of providing both regional function and perfusion in a single study. Experiments have shown that flow can be reliably estimated under variable physiological (vasodilatation) and pathological (stenosis) states in comparison to radiolabeled microspheres.[179,181] Measurements of regional flow in response to a vasodilator could be used to test coronary flow reserve in various regions and to identify a region served by an artery with a critical stenosis by failure of flow to rise in response to a vasodilator.

MYOCARDIAL INFARCTION. CT with contrast enhancement provides direct visualization of the infarction because of differences between normal and infarcted myocardium in the distribution kinetics of iodinated contrast media.[182] After intravenous administration of contrast material, temporally distinct phases of enhancement of normal and ischemically damaged myocardium have been depicted on CT. During the perfusion phase, normal myocardium is maximally enhanced (maximum increase in x-ray attenuation value), whereas the area of damage is nonenhanced or minimally enhanced. Several minutes after administration of contrast material, enhancement of normal myocardium has declined and the damaged myocardium is nearly maximally enhanced. In the perfusion phase, the ischemically damaged area appears as a low-density defect within the myocardium, whereas in the later phase it appears as a high-density region.

In animal studies quantitation of infarct volume or mass from a series of transverse CT scans encompassing the full extent of the left ventricle has been found to correlate closely with postmortem measurements.[182,183] In a canine model, sequential CT scans have been utilized to monitor the mass of the infarct and of the remaining normal myocardium during the initial month after coronary occlusion.[182] The noninfarcted myocardial mass in animals with infarcts was found to increase during the initial month after occlusion, presumably representing compensatory hypertrophy. CT scans have also been used to document the beneficial effects of reperfusion 2 hours after occlusion in the dog.[183]

CORONARY ARTERY BYPASS GRAFTS. The patency of coronary artery bypass grafts can be assessed by sequential CT scans during the transit of intravenously administered contrast medium through the arterial side of the circulation. An early study[152] showed 93 per cent sensitivity and 95 per cent specificity for defining graft patency using coronary angiography as the standard of reference. Subsequent reports in larger numbers of patients have shown somewhat lower diagnostic accuracy of standard CT in defining graft patency.[153,154] Although all reports show high diagnostic accuracy for evaluation of grafts to the left anterior descending coronary artery system, the accuracy for assessing grafts to the circumflex and right coronary arterial systems is poorer.[152-154] Another limitation of the technique is the inability to identify grafts with significant stenoses.[184] Several reports have indicated high accuracy of ultrafast CT for defining the patency of coronary artery bypass grafts.[185-187] The diagnostic accuracy of ultrafast CT for defining the patency of saphenous grafts and internal mammary bypasses has been shown to be greater than 90 per cent in a multicenter study.[185] High accuracy was shown for defining patency of grafts to the left anterior descending, circumflex branches, and right coronary arterial branches. CT scanning has been used to assess graft patency within the first several days after bypass surgery with a view to reoperation in the event of documented early occlusion.[188,189]

The site of the bypass graft on contrast-enhanced CT scans can be related to a clock. The grafts to the right coronary artery are situated between 9 and 11 o'clock; grafts to the left anterior descending artery system are situated at 12 to 2 o'clock, and the graft to the circumflex coronary system is located at 2 to 4 o'clock (Fig. 10–36). Diagnostic confidence is enhanced by visualizing the grafts at two adjacent anatomical levels and by showing contrast enhancement of the graft simultaneously with aortic opacification.

CORONARY ARTERIAL CALCIFICATION. Calcification in the coronary arteries usually indicates the presence of atherosclerosis (p. 1298). Although the early stages of atherosclerosis exist without calcification and calcification can exist in the coronary arteries in the absence of hemodynamically significant arterial obstruction, the detection of calcification increases the likelihood of significant coronary arterial obstructive disease in a specified population of patients. Older studies[190-192] have revealed that in patients being studied by coronary arteriography, the absence of fluoroscopically detectable coronary arterial calcification is usually associated with no significant arterial stenoses and the presence of calcification with significant stenoses (>50 per cent reduction in luminal diameter). Because the population of patients used in these studies contained a preponderance of patients with symptomatic disease, the role of detection of calcium as an indicator of occult disease was an unresolved question. Hamby et al.[190] demonstrated in a large group of patients that fluoroscopically detectable calcification increased the likelihood of significant coronary arterial disease by severalfold in patients less than 60 years of age. The positive predictive value was highest in younger subjects and in women. In comparison with exercise electrocardiography, fluoroscopic detection of calcification has been shown to be more sensitive for defining the presence of some degree of atherosclerotic disease but less specific than exercise electrocardiography for identifying patients with hemodynamically significant lesions.[192]

Ultrafast CT has been used in the past few years for the detection of calcification in the coronary arteries. It can be performed more rapidly than can fluoroscopy, without the presence of a physician, which potentially makes it feasible as a low-cost screening test. It is more sensitive than fluoroscopy in detecting calcification, with excellent intra- and interobserver and interstudy reproducibility.[193,194] Several studies using excised hearts or excised coronary arteries have shown a nearly one-to-one correlation between sites of coronary calcification depicted by ultrafast CT and postmortem histomorphometry.[195-198]

A close correlation has been found between the total mass of calcium in the coronary arteries as reflected in the calcium score (area of calcium on scan × density of calcium as expressed by the range of CT density numbers) and the total mass of atherosclerotic plaques, numbers of arterial segments with stenosis, and numbers of arteries and segments with greater than 75 per cent reduction in luminal diameter.[195-198] In one postmortem study, greater than 97 per cent of arterial segments without calcification were free of hemodynamically significant stenosis (<75 per cent area stenosis), and no hemodynamically significant stenosis was shown in any vessel without calcification in any segment.[195] Thus, ultrafast CT examination of postmortem specimens shows that the technique detects coronary calcification when it is present and can accurately quantify the mass of calcium in the coronary arteries. The mass of the calcium as mea-

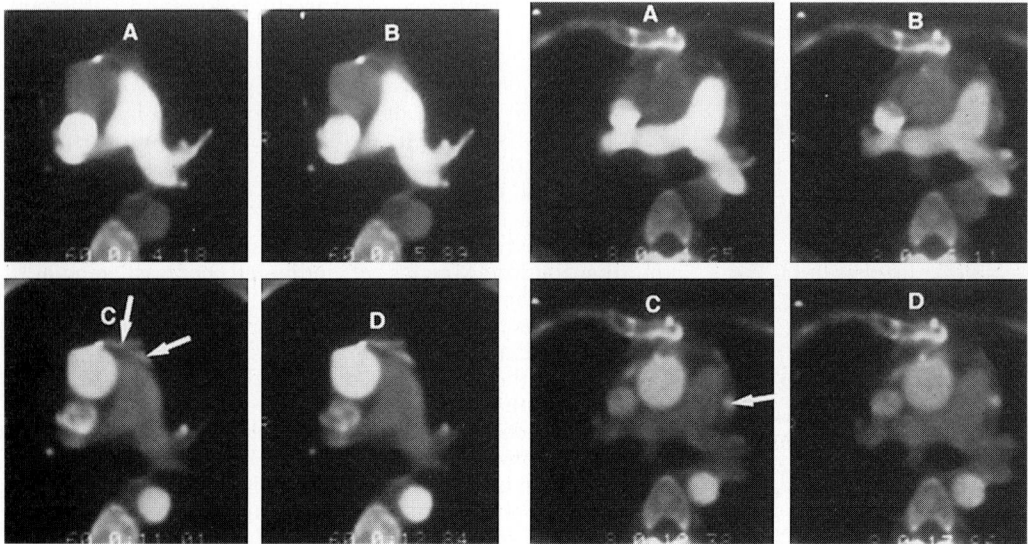

FIGURE 10–36. *Left,* Sequential cine CT scans show patent bypass grafts (arrows) to the left anterior descending artery and acute diagonal. *Right,* Graft to the obtuse marginal branch of the circumflex artery (arrow). Note that the grafts opacify simultaneously with the ascending aorta. Each set of four images was obtained at the same anatomical level. The images were done with the passage of contrast medium through the central circulation. Early images *(A,B)* show contrast in the pulmonary artery and later images *(C,D)* show contrast in the aorta and bypass grafts.

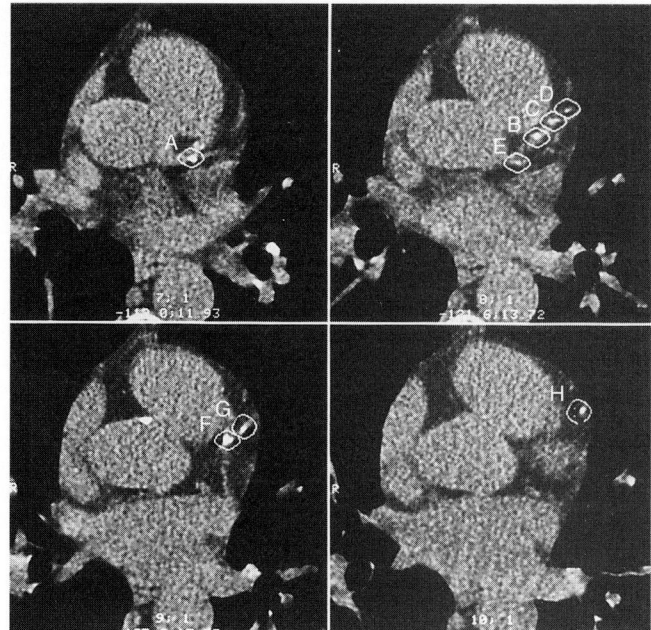

FIGURE 10–37. Cine CT scans obtained without contrast medium used to detect the presence, severity, and extent of coronary arterial calcification. Adjacent images extending from cranial (upper left) to caudal (lower right). Sites of calcification are labeled A to H. There are multiple sites of calcification in the proximal and mid left anterior descending artery.

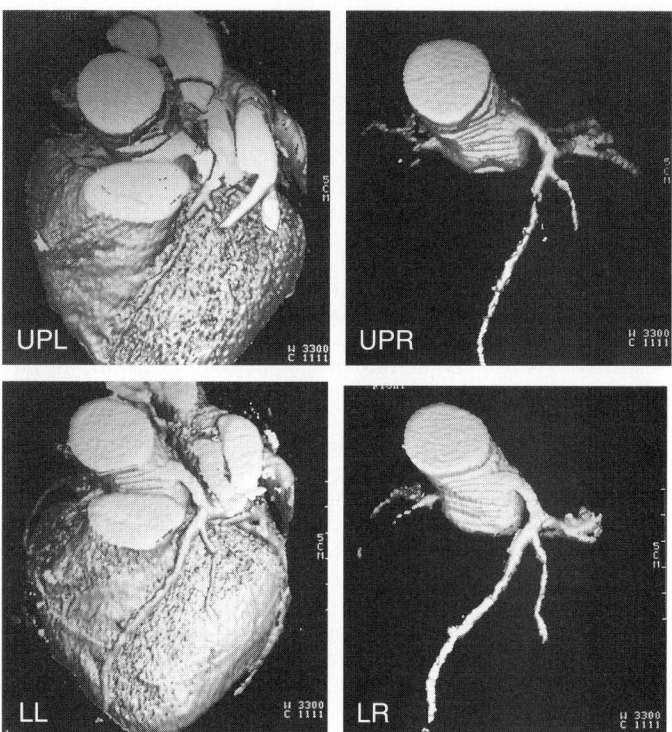

FIGURE 10–39. Reconstructed image of the left anterior ascending coronary artery produced from contiguous ultrafast CT scans acquired in diastole. Postprocessing of data shows three-dimensional reconstructions (left) of the images and isolated projectional images (right) of the artery before (above) and after angioplasty (below). (Courtesy of Imatron, Inc., and Werner Moshage, M.D., University of Erlangen.)

sured by ultrafast CT is closely related to the number of arterial segments and number of arteries containing nonobstructive and obstructive atherosclerotic plaques and the total atherosclerotic burden of the coronary arterial system.

PREDICTION OF PRESENCE OF CORONARY STENOSIS. The presence of coronary arterial calcification, the number of coronary arteries with calcification, and the total mass of coronary calcification in the coronary circulation have been used to predict the presence of any degree of coronary arterial stenosis and hemodynamically significant stenosis compared with coronary arteriography.[199–201] The sensitivity for predicting any degree of stenosis or hemodynamically significant stenosis has been high, usually exceeding 90 per cent, but the specificity is only fair. The mass of calcium is quantified by calculating the calcium score (total area of calcium × density weighting) (Fig. 10–37).[193]

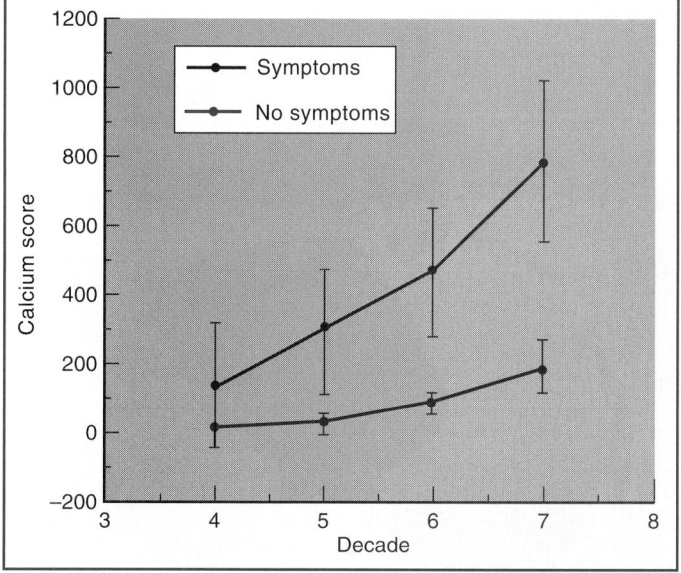

FIGURE 10–38. Plot of coronary arterial calcium score versus decade of age for groups of patients with and without known (symptomatic) coronary disease. (From Agatston, A. S., Janowitz, W. R., Hildner, E. J., et al.: Quantification of coronary artery calcium using ultrafast computed tomography. Reprinted with permission of the American College of Cardiology. J. Am. Coll. Cardiol. 15:827, 1990.)

The prevalence of coronary arterial calcification detected by ultrafast CT in women is half that of men until the age of 60; the distribution of calcium scores of men between the ages 40 and 69 years was nearly identical to that of women between ages 50 and 79.[201] Because the presence of coronary calcification and the calcium score increase with age,[193] the usefulness of ultrafast CT for identifying patients at a higher risk for significant coronary arterial disease decreases with increasing age (Fig. 10–38). Although the sensitivity remains high even in patients under 50 years, the specificity for predicting significant stenosis is still only fair.[202]

The role of ultrafast CT in identifying patients at higher risk for the development of symptomatic coronary arterial disease, cardiac morbidity, and death remains somewhat controversial. As a potential screening test, it does have high sensitivity and can be performed rapidly, inexpensively, and noninvasively. Perhaps its role at the current time is to indicate patients with some degree of atherosclerotic coronary arterial disease who should enter strict risk-reduction programs. The absence of coronary arterial calcification by ultrafast CT makes the presence of significant coronary arterial disease very unlikely. However, it does not totally exclude such disease.[202]

CORONARY ANGIOGRAPHY. Recently, ultrafast CT has been used to image the coronary arteries. This is done by acquiring contiguous or overlapping thin CT scans at the same phase of diastole during breath holding. From this three-dimensional data set, projectional images are produced which display the major coronary arterial branches (Fig. 10–39). Postprocessing of the data set can be done to subtract the heart from the image and thereby provide an isolated projectional image of the coronary arteries (Fig. 10–39).

Pericardial Disease
(See also Chap. 43)

Computed tomography provides distinct visualization of the pericardium in most patients. Discrimination of the pericardial line from the myocardium depends upon the presence of some epicardial and pericardial fat; it has been reported to be visible on CT scans of 95 per cent of normal subjects.[203] Although visible over the right atrium and ventricle in most subjects, it is frequently not detectable on the lateral and posterior walls of the left ventricle. The mean width of the line in normal subjects is 2.2 mm at its thinnest portion and is always less than 4 mm. Pericardial thickness is usually normal near its diaphragmatic attachments. CT also frequently demonstrates the superior recesses of the pericardium extending over the ascending aorta and lateral to the main pulmonary artery. These recesses may be distended in the presence of a pericardial effusion.

Two-dimensional echocardiography is an extremely effective technique for the diagnosis of pericardial abnormalities and is the primary modality for evaluation of suspected pericardial disease (p. 93). Although it is extremely sensitive for the detection of pericardial effusion, it has some limitations in defining loculated effusions, hemorrhagic effusions, and especially pericardial thickening. CT is especially effective in depicting these entities.[204,205] Consequently, it is complementary to echocardiography in the diagnosis and assessment of pericardial disease.

CONGENITAL ABNORMALITIES AND CYSTS OF THE PERICARDIUM (see also p. 1522). Congenital abnormalities, such as absence of the pericardium[206] and pericardial cyst[204,205,207,208] can be well demonstrated by CT. Pericardial defect (usually partial or complete absence of left-sided pericardium) is recognized on CT by the discontinuity of the pericardial line over the left aspect of the heart, with shift of the heart leftward or bulging of the left atrial appendage through the defect. CT demonstrates interposition of a tongue of lung tissue between the proximal ascending aorta and main pulmonary artery at the base of the heart in the absence of the left-sided pericardium.

A pericardial cyst appears as a paracardiac mass with a thin capsule that is occasionally partially or completely calcified and has a homogeneous internal density nearly equivalent to that of water. However, rarely the cyst contains mucoid material, causing the density to be higher than water; such a cyst usually cannot be reliably distinguished from a solid mass. *Thymic* and *bronchogenic cysts,* which may be adjacent to the pericardium, also may show homogeneous water density on CT densitometry and may be indistinguishable from pericardial cysts.

PERICARDIAL FLUID (see also p. 1485). Fluid in the pericardial space may be reliably detected by CT.[204,209] This technique can also provide an accurate estimate of the volume of this fluid.[209] Although two-dimensional echocardiography is sufficient and, for economic and logistic reasons, more clinically efficacious for the primary evaluation of most pericardial effusions, CT is indicated in some special situations. Loculated effusions (especially anterior loculations), which may pose difficulty for echocardiography,

are readily demonstrated on CT[205] because of the wide field of view provided and the potentially three-dimensional nature of the technique. CT can be effective not only for diagnosing loculated effusions but also for guiding pericardiocentesis.[210] CT density measurements provide some degree of characterization of pericardial fluid.[204,205,209] Density numbers (Hounsfield numbers) exceeding water density (water density = 0 to 12 units) are suggestive of hemopericardium, purulent exudate, or effusions associated with hypothyroidism. Low-density pericardial effusions have been reported in the presence of chylopericardium.[209]

CONSTRICTIVE PERICARDITIS (see also p. 1501). The establishment of the diagnosis of constrictive pericarditis can be substantially aided by CT. Because CT shows the pericardium, it can document pericardial thickening, defined as thickness greater than 4 mm. Focal plaques of thickening or the greater thickness of the pericardium near the diaphragm should not be confused with the more extensive pericardial thickening associated with constrictive pericarditis. However, the pericardial thickening may be limited to the right side of the heart, a form that appears to be more prevalent in patients who have undergone coronary arterial bypass surgery.

The documentation of pericardial thickening is the major discriminatory feature between constrictive pericarditis and restrictive cardiomyopathy (Fig. 10–40). However, thickened pericardium per se is not indicative of constrictive disease. Pericardial thickening without constriction is frequently observed in the early postoperative period and may persist for several months following operation in patients with the postpericardiotomy syndrome.[204] Thickened pericardium without constriction has also been observed in association with inflammation of the pericardium caused by a variety of conditions, including uremia, rheumatic heart disease, rheumatoid arthritis, sarcoidosis, and postmediastinal irradiation. Pericardial thickening may also be caused by metastatic carcinoma, thymoma,[211] and lymphoma[204] and mesothelioma. These conditions are usually associated with effusion. Likewise, primary sarcoma of the heart and mediastinal and lung malignant tumors extending to the pericardium produce local or diffuse pericardial thickening and loculated or generalized pericardial effusion. Moreover, thickened pericardium is to be expected in many patients for several weeks after cardiac surgery. It may be present for a prolonged period in patients afflicted by the postpericardiotomy syndrome (Dressler's syndrome).

EFFUSIVE-CONSTRICTIVE PERICARDITIS (see also p. 1505). This condition is demonstrated by an effusion in association with thickened pericardium; however, it may not

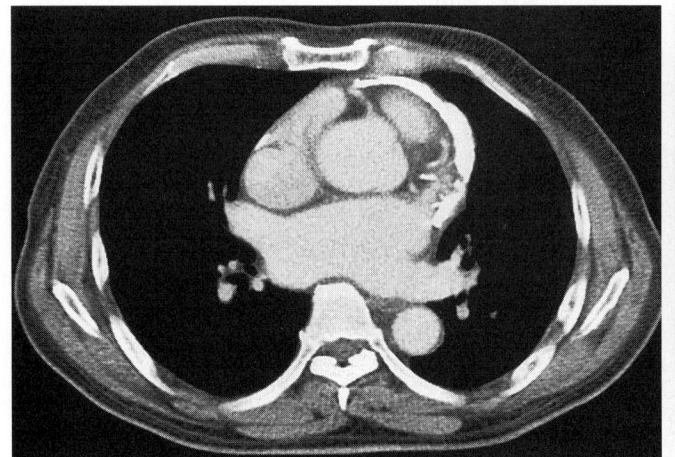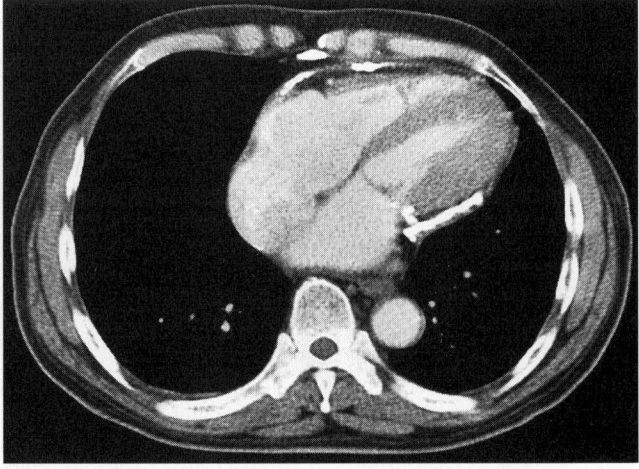

FIGURE 10–40. Calcific constrictive pericarditis. Cine CT scans at the base of the heart *(left)* and at mid ventricular level *(right)*. Note the heavy calcification at multiple sites of the pericardium and extending into the posterior atrioventricular grove. (Courtesy of Imatron, Inc.)

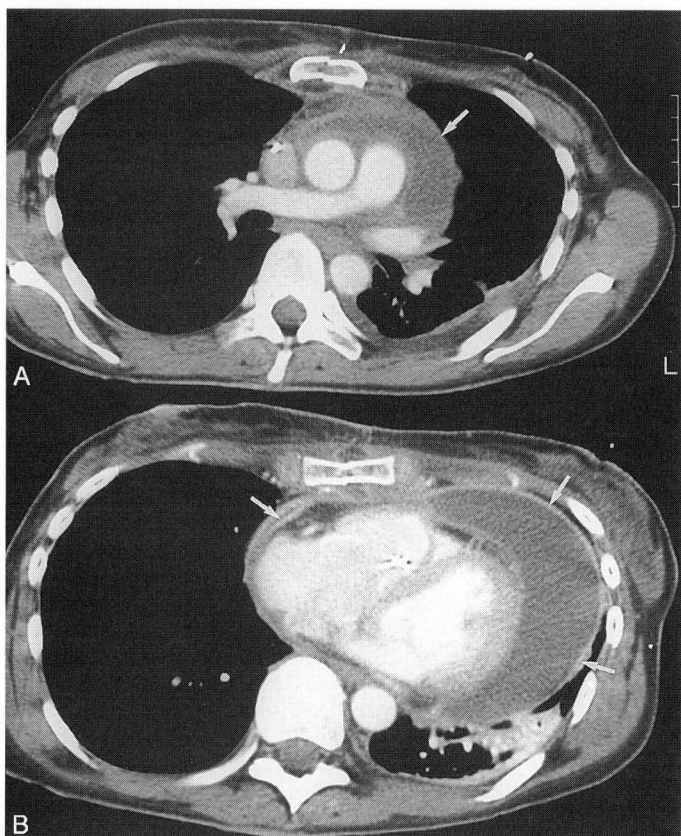

FIGURE 10–41. Cine CT scans at the levels of the right pulmonary artery *(A)* and at the ventricles *(B)* in a patient with a pericardial inflammation and large effusion (outlined by the arrows). The effusion extends over the pulmonary artery as well as the ventricles. There is contrast enhancement of the pericardium, suggesting pericardial inflammation. (Courtesy of Imatron, Inc.)

convexity of the septum has been observed. Unusual contours, such as straightening or focal indentation of the free wall of either the right or left ventricle, have been noted on CT scans.[213]

The density resolution of CT makes it the most sensitive technique for identifying pericardial calcification. Pericardial calcific deposits are usually residuals of pericardial inflammation and are most commonly found in the visceral layer along the atrioventricular and interventricular grooves. Extensive calcification of the pericardium suggests but does not prove the presence of cardiac constriction.

Paracardiac, Pericardial, and Cardiac Masses
(See also Chaps. 42 and 57)

CT is useful for the evaluation of pericardial and paracardiac masses. CT and more recently MRI have emerged as the preferential techniques for defining the site and extent of such masses and in some cases even indicate their nature.[204,205,207,208,215,216] CT may show the water density of pericardial cysts; this is an especially useful finding when the cyst is located in an unusual mediastinal location[209] or when it protrudes inwardly, displacing the atrial wall.[217] In one series CT detected eight of eight intrapericardial masses compared with echocardiography, which identified only one.[216] CT and MRI are currently the best techniques for defining the extension of mediastinal neoplasms (including lymphoma) and of carcinoma of the lung into the pericardium. Metastatic involvement of the pericardium is suggested by the CT findings of effusion with an irregularly thickened pericardium or the actual demonstration of a mass involving the pericardium.[204,205,216] An effusion with high CT density (hemopericardium) along with pericardial thickening also suggests metastatic pericardial involvement.[205]

CT sometimes provides insight into the nature of the mass by demonstrating the shape, defining the density measurements, or showing multiple masses. The CT demonstration of multiple pericardial nodules suggests metastatic tumor or, rarely, multicentric mesothelioma. Pericardial cysts have water density, whereas lipomas have a very low density value (−55 or fewer Hounsfield units). Demonstration of calcium or bone and fat in a paracardiac mass by CT suggests teratoma.

Intracardiac masses can be detected very well by echocardiography (Fig. 3–105, p. 94) and angiography. However, CT not only can detect masses within the cardiac chambers but also can define fully their extent (Fig. 10–42). CT can demonstrate components of the mass within the myocardial wall and extending outside of the heart. The contrast resolution of CT may provide some insight

always be possible to distinguish a small effusion from thickened pericardium.[204] Pericardial thickening alone usually measures between 5 and 20 mm, while greater thickening generally indicates associated effusion or effusion alone. Contrast enhancement of the thickened pericardium is indicative of pericardial inflammation[212] (Fig. 10–41). Additional CT findings in constrictive pericarditis often reflect the anatomical and physiological consequences of the thickened pericardium on the cardiac chambers.[213,214] CT shows substantial dilatation of the inferior vena cava and some enlargement of the atria, especially the right atrium (Fig. 10–40). The ventricles tend to have a small volume and a narrow tubular configuration.[213] In some cases, a sigmoid-shaped ventricular septum or prominent leftward

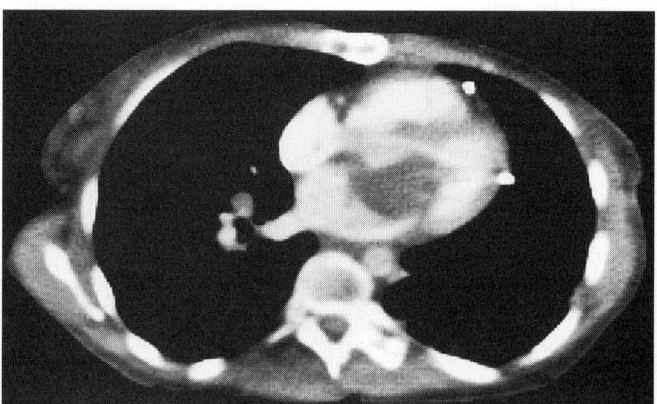
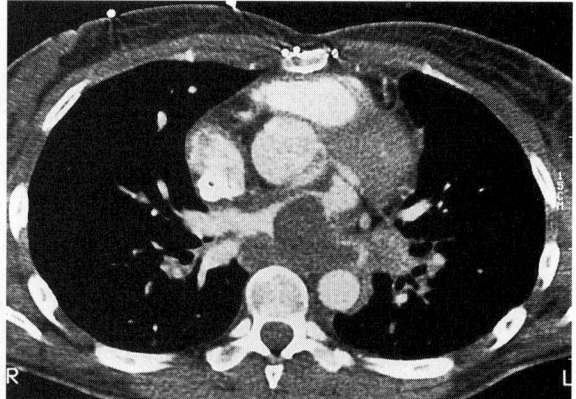

FIGURE 10–42. *Left,* Cine CT scans of left atrial myxoma. The attachment of the myxoma to the atrial septum and prolapsing across the mitral valve are shown. *Right,* Malignant tumor invading the left atrium.

into the composition of the mass, such as demonstrating the presence of fat or calcium. CT has detected simple intracardiac masses such as atrial myxoma[171,218,219] and complex masses involving the myocardial wall with extracardiac extension.[171] Finally, by defining clearly the myocardial wall, CT allows distinguishing of the extracardiac location of tumors which produce compression and invagination of cardiac walls, simulating an intracardiac origin.[217]

INTRACARDIAC THROMBUS. The most frequent intracardiac mass is a thrombus. Intracardiac thrombi are usually located in the left atrium in patients with mitral valve disease or patients with atrial fibrillation from any cause; and in the left ventricle in patients with recent myocardial infarction or patients with dilated (congestive) cardiomyopathy. Although transthoracic echocardiography is usually the initial study used to detect intracardiac thrombi or an intracardiac source of peripheral embolism, recent studies have revealed that CT is as sensitive but more specific for identifying ventricular thrombus[176] and more sensitive for defining left atrial thrombus.[177] Thrombi in the left atrial appendage and lateral wall of the atrium are more readily detected with MRI and CT than with transthoracic echocardiography. MRI and CT are very effective techniques for the detection of intracardiac thrombus; however, their accuracy compared with transesophageal echocardiography has yet to be systematically evaluated.

Congenital Heart Disease
(See also Chaps. 28 and 29)

Standard CT, ultrafast CT (cine CT), and MRI are useful noninvasive techniques for the visualization of cardiovascular anatomy in patients with congenital heart disease (CHD). Ultrafast CT and MRI can also provide assessment of cardiovascular function in these patients. MRI appears to be the most suitable of these techniques for assessing congenital heart disease. The x-ray exposure, contrast media requirement, and inability to image in multiple plane are limitations of CT for the evaluation of CHD.

STANDARD CT. This technique has been found to be useful for evaluation of suspected *anomalies of the aortic arch*.[220-222] Contrast-enhanced CT is usually required to show the vascular tissue surrounding the trachea in the presence of double aortic arch and the retroesophageal vascular structure indicating anomalous origin of the subclavian artery. Double arch is also suggested by the presence of four paratracheal vessels arranged symmetrically at the cervicothoracic junction.[220]

Although many cardiac anomalies such as septal defects, tetralogy of Fallot, Ebstein's anomaly, abnormal arterioventricular connections, and others have been demonstrated by CT,[221,223,224] the technique has not found widespread use owing to the ease and the usual diagnostic superiority of two-dimensional echocardiography and more recently MRI. An exception is the definitive demonstration of systemic veins, liver, and spleen possible with CT; this is important for complete evaluation of situs-splenic syndromes.[223]

ULTRAFAST CT. At a few centers ultrafast CT has also been tested for its potential for the evaluation of congenital heart disease.[223-225] Ultrafast CT has been found to be accurate in defining systemic and pulmonary venous connections. Likewise, it has demonstrated atrial and ventricular septal defects. Transverse tomograms provide clear spatial separation of the inflow and outflow portions of the ventricular septum. This permits localization of defects and facilitates the detection of multiple ventricular septal defects.[223,224] In addition, an assessment of the hemodynamic effects of septal defects (and of other lesions) can be made by evaluation of chamber dimension and wall thickness. Because of the absence of overlying structures defined on CT scans and the three-dimensional nature of ultrafast CT acquisition, the size of the ventricles can be measured.

Normal and abnormal atrioventricular valves can be demonstrated by ultrafast CT,[223,224] which can be used to diagnose both tricuspid and mitral atresia. It can also demonstrate the size of the atrium above the atretic valve.

Ultrafast CT has been effective for demonstrating abnormal arterioventricular connections, including transposition complexes and double-outlet right ventricle.[223,224] Abnormalities of the pulmonary arteries, such as congenital absence, peripheral coarctations, and hypoplasia, have been demonstrated by this technique.[224] However, cine CT is not recommended for this purpose because multiplanar MRI has been shown in recent years to be the most effective technique for assessing pulmonary arterial anomalies.

Congenital anomalies of the coronary arteries (see p. 967) have been demonstrated very well using ultrafast CT scans positioned at the base of the heart.[226] Ectopic origin of coronary arteries and coronary arteriovenous fistulae have been effectively demonstrated by this technique.[226] Contrast-enhanced ultrafast CT is probably the noninvasive procedure of choice for the diagnosis and exclusion of major or minor anomalies of origin and course of the coronary arteries.

EVALUATION OF CARDIAC FUNCTION IN CONGENITAL HEART DISEASE. This can be accomplished in patients with congenital heart disease by ultrafast CT which, along with cine MRI, may be the best technique for quantitating right ventricular volumes and ejection fraction. In addition, ultrafast CT can be used to estimate the volume of shunts; its accuracy has been documented in an experimental right-to-left shunt model in the dog.[225] This is accomplished by measuring density of contrast medium within a cardiac chamber receiving shunt flow on sequential CT scans obtained during passage of contrast medium through the central circulation. A density-versus-time curve can be generated for such a region of interest. The normal curve is unimodal as contrast medium enters and leaves a cardiac chamber. A bimodal time-density curve may be generated from the region-of-interest cursor placed over any chamber involved in a shunt. Using a gamma variate fit method, the areas under the primary and secondary portions of the curve can be measured in order to calculate pulmonary-to-systemic flow ratios. A close correlation has been found for the measurement of pulmonary-to-systemic flow ratio by cine CT and oximetry in experimental animals[225] and in patients.[224]

Another method for calculating the net shunt is to compare the difference in stroke volume between the two ventricles. For a left-to-right shunt at the ventricular level, the difference between the larger left ventricular stroke volume and right ventricular stroke volume indicates the net shunt value. Such an approach can be used also to calculate net volume and fraction of regurgitant lesions.

Cine CT appears to be an excellent technique for the evaluation of both right and left ventricular function in surgically corrected congenital heart disease. Because volumes[164,168,169] and mass[159,160] of both ventricles can be measured accurately by CT, this technique can be used to evaluate the expected regression of ventricular dilatation and hypertrophy after corrective procedures.

Disease of the Thoracic Aorta
(See also Chap. 45)

CT has been shown to be extremely accurate for the diagnosis of thoracic aortic aneurysm and dissection.[227-231] **AORTIC DISSECTION.** In one prospective study in 26 patients with suspected aortic dissection there were no false-negative or false-positive CT scans for this diagnosis.[229] In this study CT correctly indicated the true extent of dissection in some patients in whom it was underestimated by angiography. In general, CT has an accuracy of greater than 90 per cent and is equivalent to MRI and better than x-ray

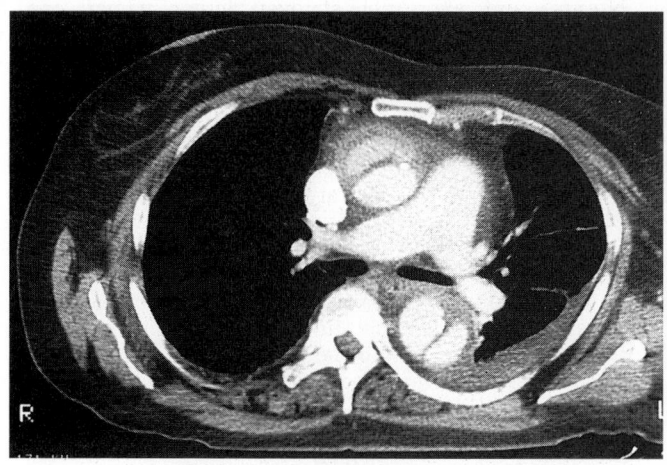 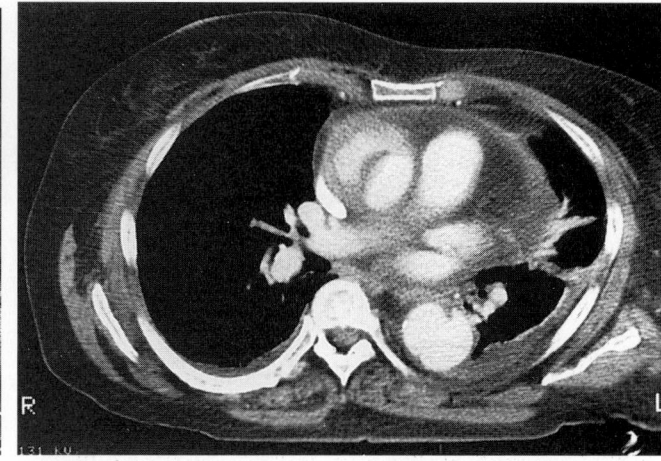

FIGURE 10–43. Type A aortic dissection, cine CT scans at level of right pulmonary artery *(left)* and 1 cm caudal *(right)* demonstrate intimal flap in ascending and descending aorta. Note also the pericardial effusion, indicating probable leakage from the false channel. (Courtesy of Imatron, Inc.)

angiography for the diagnosis of a variety of diseases of the thoracic aorta.[230,232] A recent study comparing CT, MRI, and transesophageal and transthoracic echocardiography has shown greater diagnostic accuracy of CT and MRI than of the echocardiographic techniques.[232] However, some instances of false-negative CT examination in aortic dissection have been reported.[227,230] Diagnosis of dissection requires the demonstration of the intimal flap, appearing as a lucency within the lumen of the contrast-enhanced aortic lumen on CT scans (Fig. 10–43). Intramural hematoma has been reported as a feature of aortic dissection without entry into the lumen of the aorta.[233] This has been reported in approximately 30 per cent of patients with dissection in a report from Japan.[232] It is likely that this is an early stage of some acute dissections, but not all intramural hematomas progress to the typical feature of acute dissection. Supportive findings for the diagnosis of aortic dissection are differential temporal enhancement of the true and false aortic channels or compression of the opacified true lumen by a thrombosed false channel. Inward displacement of calcium in the aortic wall is also a sign of aortic dissection. CT can distinguish between dissections that involve the ascending aorta and those that are limited to the descending aorta. In the former, the intimal flap can be demonstrated in the ascending aorta. It may be difficult to differentiate a dissection with thrombus of the false channel from an aortic

aneurysm with mural thrombus. A dissection is more likely when CT scans at multiple levels show the thrombus extending for more than 10 cm longitudinally. Also, dissection usually results in a compressed true aortic lumen whereas aneurysm has a normal or increased lumen.

CT also may be used for following the course of thoracic aortic dissections after initial treatment.[234–237] After surgical placement of an ascending aortic graft, the false channel beyond the distal anastomosis of the graft frequently remains patent. Sequential CT studies have also revealed persistent patency of the false channel after medical as well as surgical therapy: Eventual thrombosis of the false channel or even its disappearance is seen in some patients.[236,237] CT has also been used to follow the alterations in the false channel of untreated type B dissections; in a minority of patients the aorta reverts to a normal appearance after months to years.[235]

AORTIC ANEURYSM. This is characterized by an increase in aortic diameter and by outward displacement of calcium of the aortic wall (Fig. 10–44). CT is an effective method for defining the maximum diameter of the aneurysm and monitoring the diameter over time. A diameter exceeding 4 cm is considered aneurysmal and one exceeding 6 cm is usually an indication for surgery of thoracic aortic aneurysm.

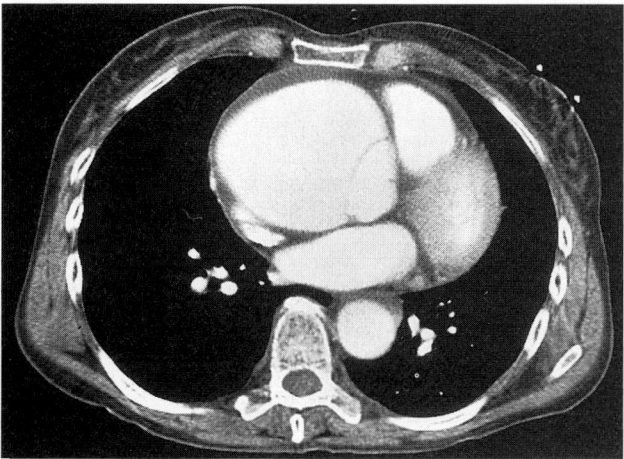 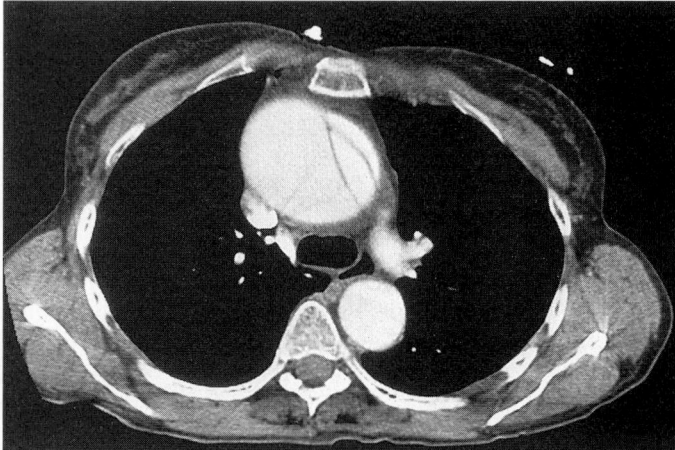

FIGURE 10–44. Thoracic aortic aneurysm and type A dissection, cine CT scans at the level of the sinus of Valsalva *(left)* and distal ascending aorta *(right)*. There is aneurysmal dilatation of the sinuses of Valsalva and ascending aorta. Note also the intimal flap in the ascending aorta. There is no dissection of the descending aorta. (Courtesy of Imatron, Inc.)

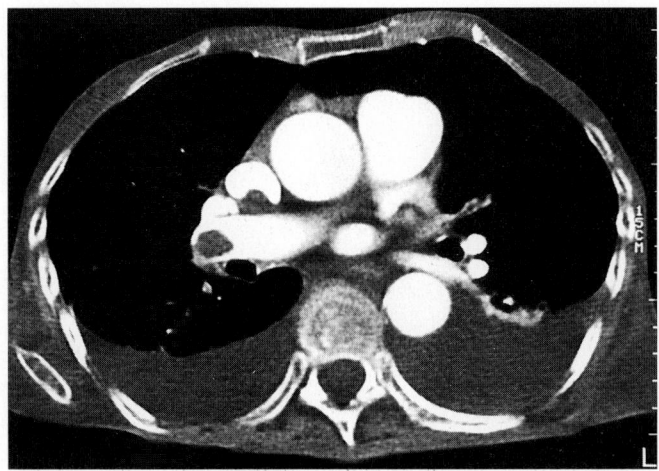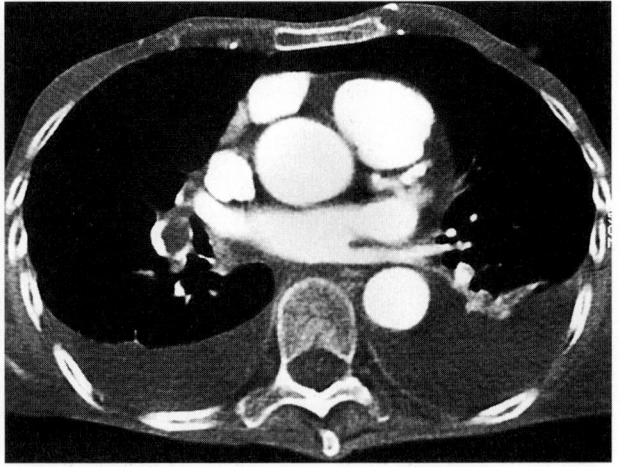

FIGURE 10–45. Ultrafast CT scans of pulmonary arteries demonstrate a thrombus in the central right pulmonary artery *(left)* and extending into the descending branch of the right pulmonary artery *(right)*. (Courtesy of Imatron, Inc.).

PULMONARY EMBOLISM. Ultrafast[238] and spiral[239] CT have been used in recent years for establishing or excluding the diagnosis of pulmonary embolism (Fig. 10–45). Both techniques have been shown to provide high diagnostic accuracy for this purpose. It has been proposed that CT scanning be used to confirm the diagnosis of pulmonary embolism in patients with intermediate likelihood of the diagnosis by nuclear pulmonary perfusion scans. At some centers, ultrafast or spiral CT has substantially replaced x-ray angiography for the definitive diagnosis of pulmonary embolism.

REFERENCES

MAGNETIC RESONANCE IMAGING

1. Sakuma, H., Fujita, N., Foo, T. K., et al.: Evaluation of LV volume and mass with breath hold cine MR imaging. Radiology *188:*377, 1993.
2. Atkinson, D. J., Burstein, D., and Edelman, R. R.: First pass cardiac perfusion: Evaluation with ultrafast MR imaging. Radiology *174:*757, 1990.
3. Saeed, M., Wendland, M. F., Lauerma, K., et al.: First pass contrast-enhanced inversion recovery and driven equilibrium fast GRE imaging studies: Detection of acute myocardial ischemia. J. Magn. Reson. Imag. *5:*515, 1995.
4. Mansfield, P.: Real time echo planar imaging by NMR. Br. Med. Bull. *40:*187, 1984.
5. McKinnon, G. C.: Ultrafast interleaved gradient echoplanar imaging on a standard scanner. Magn. Reson. Med. *30:*609, 1993.
6. Wendland, M. F., Saeed, M., Masui, T., et al.: Echoplanar MR imaging of normal and ischemic myocardium with gadodiamide injection. Radiology *186:*535, 1993.

EVALUATION OF SPECIFIC CARDIAC DISEASES

7. Steffens, J. C., Bourne, M. W., Sakuma, H., et al.: MR imaging of ischemic heart disease. Am Heart J. *(in press).*
8. Pennell, D. J., Underwood, S. R., and Langmore, D. B.: Detection of coronary artery disease using MR imaging with dipyridamole. J. Comput. Assist. Tomogr. *14:*167, 1990.
9. Baer, F. M., Smolarz, K., Jungebulsing, M., et al.: Feasibility of high dose dipyridamole-magnetic resonance imaging for the detection of coronary disease and comparison with coronary angiography. Am. J. Cardiol. *69:*51, 1992.
10. Edelman, R. R., Manning, W. J., Burstein, D., et al.: Coronary arteries: Breath hold MR angiography. Radiology *181:*641, 1991.
11. Sakuma, H., Caputo, G. R., Steffens, J. C., et al.: Breath-hold MR cine angiography of coronary arteries in healthy volunteers: Value of multiangle oblique imaging planes. A.J.R. *163:*533, 1994.
12. Edelman, R. R., Manning, W. L., Gervino, E., et al.: Flow velocity quantification in human coronary arteries with breath hold MR angiography. J. Magn. Reson. Imag. *3:*699, 1993.
13. Sakuma, H., Blake L. M., Amidon, T. M., et al.: Noninvasive measurement of coronary flow reserve in humans using breath-hold velocity encoded cine MR imaging. Radiology. *(submitted for publication).*
14. Wilke, N., Simm, C., Zhong, J., et al.: Contrast enhanced first pass myocardial perfusion imaging: Correlation between myocardial blood flow in dogs at rest and during hyperemia. Magn. Reson. Med. *29:*485, 1993.

15. Saeed, M., Wendland, M. F., Sakuma, H., et al.: Coronary artery stenosis: Detection with contrast-enhanced MR imaging in dogs. Radiology *196:*79, 1995.
16. Higgins, C. B., Lanzer, P., Stark, D., et al.: Imaging by nuclear magnetic resonance in patients with chronic ischemic heart disease. Circulation *69:*523, 1984.
17. McNamara, M. T., and Higgins, C. B.: Magnetic resonance imaging of chronic myocardial infarctions in man. A.J.R. *146:*315, 1986.
18. Akins, E. W., Hill, J. A., Sievers, K. W., et al.: Assessment of left ventricular wall thickness in healed myocardial infarction by magnetic resonance imaging. Am. J. Cardiol. *59:*24, 1987.
19. Sechtem, U., Sommerhoff, B. A., Markiewicz, W., et al.: Assessment of regional left ventricular wall thickening by magnetic resonance imaging: Evaluation in normal persons and patients with global and regional dysfunction. Am. J. Cardiol. *59:*145, 1987.
20. Sechtem, U., Voth, E., Schneider, C., et al.: Assessment of myocardial viability in patients with myocardial infarction using magnetic resonance imaging. Int. J. Card. Imaging. *9:*31, 1993.
21. Wesbey, G., Higgins, C. B., Lanzer, P., et al.: In vivo imaging and characterization of acute myocardial infarction using gated nuclear magnetic resonance. Circulation *69:*125, 1984.
22. McNamara, M. T., Higgins, C. B., Schechtmann, N., et al.: Detection and characterization of acute myocardial infarctions in man using gated magnetic resonance imaging. Circulation *71:*717, 1985.
23. Wisenberg, G., Finnie, K., Jablonsky, G., et al.: Nuclear magnetic resonance and radionuclide angiographic assessment of acute myocardial infarction in a randomized trial of intravenous streptokinase. Am. J. Cardiol. *62:*1011, 1988.
24. Wisenberg, G., Proto, F. S., Carrol, S. E., et al.: Serial NMR imaging of acute myocardial infarction with and without reperfusion. Am. Heart. J. *115:*510, 1988.
25. Filipchuk, N. G., Peshock, R. M., Malloy, C. R., et al.: Detection and localization of recent myocardial infarction by MRI. Am. J. Cardiol. *58:*214, 1986.
26. Manning, W. J., Lil, W., and Edelman, R. R.: A preliminary report comparing magnetic resonance coronary angiography with conventional angiography. N. Engl. J. Med. *328:*828, 1993.
27. White, R. D., Caputo, G. R., Mark, A. S., et al.: Noninvasive evaluation of coronary artery bypass graft patency using magnetic resonance imaging. Radiology *164:*681, 1987.
28. White, R. D., Pflugfelder, P. W., Lipton, M. J., et al.: Coronary artery bypass grafts: Evaluation of patency with cine MR imaging. A.J.R. *150:*1271, 1988.
29. Gomes, A. S., Lois, J. F., Drinkwater, D. C., et al.: Coronary artery bypass grafts: Visualization with MR imaging. Radiology *162:*175, 1987.
30. Frija, G., Schouman-Clays, E., Lacombe, P., et al.: A study of coronary artery bypass graft patency using MR imaging. J. Comput. Assist. Tomogr. *13:*226, 1989.
31. Aurigemma, G. R., Reichek, N., Axel, L., et al.: Noninvasive determination of coronary artery bypass graft patency by cine magnetic resonance imaging. Circulation *80:*1595, 1989.
32. Underwood, S. R., Firmin, D. W., Klipstein, R. H., et al.: The assessment of coronary artery bypass grafts using MRI with velocity mapping. Br. Heart. J. *57:*93, 1982.
33. Debatin, J. F., Strong, J. A., Sostman, H. D., et al.: MR characterization of blood flow in native and grafted internal mammary arteries. J. Magn. Resn. Imag. *3:*443, 1993.
34. Higgins, C. B., Byrd, B. F., McNamara, M. T., et al.: Magnetic resonance imaging of the heart: A review of the experience in 172 subjects. Radiology *155:*671, 1985.
35. Higgins, C. B., Byrd, B. F., and Stark, D.: Magnetic resonance imaging of hypertrophic cardiomyopathy. Am. J. Cardiol. *55:*1121, 1985.

36. Wagner, S., Chew, W. M., Semelka, R., et al.: Integrative analysis of cardiac function and metabolism in patients with idiopathic hypertrophic cardiomyopathy with cine MR imaging and P-31 spectroscopy. Radiology 173:238, 1989.

37. Suzuki, J-I., Chang, J-M., Caputo, G. R., et al.: Evaluation of right ventricular early diastolic filling by cine nuclear magnetic resonance imaging in patients with hypertrophic cardiomyopathy. J. Am. Coll. Cardiol. 18:809, 1991.

38. Suzuki, J. I., Sakamoto, T., Takenaka, K., et al.: Assessment of the thickness of the right ventricular free wall by MRI in patients with hypertrophic cardiomyopathy. Br. Heart J. 60:440, 1988.

39. Byrd, B. F., Schiller, N. B., Botvinick, E. H., et al.: Magnetic resonance imaging and 2D echocardiography in dilated cardiomyopathy. Circulation 72(Suppl III):III22, 1985.

40. Buser, P. T., Auffermann, W., Holt, W. W., et al.: Noninvasive evaluation of the global left ventricular function using cine MR imaging. J. Am. Coll. Cardiol. 13:1294, 1989.

41. Wagner, S., Auffermann, W., Buser, P., et al.: Functional description of the left ventricle in patients with volume overload, pressure overload and myocardial disease using cine nuclear magnetic resonance imaging (NMRI). Am. J. Cardiac. Imaging 5:87, 1991.

42. Doherty, N. E. III, Seelos, K. C., Suzuki, J-I., et al.: Application of cine NMR imaging for sequential evaluation of response to angiotensin converting enzyme inhibitor therapy in dilated cardiomyopathy. J. Am. Coll. Cardiol. 19:1294, 1992.

43. Semelka, R. C., Tomei, E., Wagner, S., et al.: Normal left ventricular dimensions and function: Interstudy reproducibility of measurements with cine MR imaging. Radiology 174:763, 1990.

44. Semelka, R. C., Tomei, E., Wagner, S., et al.: Interstudy reproducibility of dimensional and functional measurements between cine magnetic resonance studies in the morphologically abnormal left ventricle. Am. Heart J. 119:1367, 1990.

45. Sechtem, U., Higgins, C. B., Sommerhoff, B. A., et al.: Magnetic resonance imaging of restrictive cardiomyopathy: A report of 3 cases. Am. J. Cardiol. 59:480, 1987.

46. Sechtem, U., Sommerhoff, B. A., Markiewicz, W., et al.: Assessment of regional left ventricular wall thickening by MRI. Am. J. Cardiol. 59:149, 1987.

47. O'Donnell, J. K., Go, R. T., Bolt-Silverman, C., et al.: Cardiac amyloidosis: Comparison of MR imaging and echocardiography. Radiology 153(Abs.):261, 1984.

48. Riedy, K., Fisher, M., Belic, N., et al.: MR imaging of myocardial sarcoidosis. A.J.R. 151:915, 1988.

49. Blake, L. M., Scheinman, M. M., and Higgins, C. B.: MR features of arrhythmogenic right ventricular dysplasia. A.J.R. 162:809, 1994.

50. Carlson, M. D., White, R. D., Trohman, R. G., et al.: Right ventricular outflow tract tachycardia: Detection of previously unrecognized abnormalities using cine MRI. J. Am. Coll. Cardiol. 24:720, 1994.

51. Auffermann, W., Wichter, T., Bretthardt, G., et al.: Arrhythmogenic right ventricular disease: MR imaging vs angiography. A.J.R. 161:549, 1993.

52. Sechtem, U., Tscholakoff, D., and Higgins, C. B.: Pericardial disease: Diagnosis by MRI. A.J.R. 147:245, 1986.

53. Guttierrez, F. R., Shackleford, G. D., McKnight, R. L., et al.: Diagnosis of congenital absence of left pericardium by MR imaging. J. Comput. Assist. Tomogr. 9:551, 1985.

54. Soulen, R. L., Stark, D. D., and Higgins, C. B.: Magnetic resonance imaging of constrictive pericardial disease. Am. J. Cardiol. 55:480, 1985.

55. Masui, T., Finck, S., and Higgins, C. B.: Constrictive pericarditis and restrictive cardiomyopathy: Evaluation with MR imaging. Radiology 182:369, 1992.

56. Amparo, E. G., Higgins, C. B., Farmer, D., et al.: Gated MRI of cardiac and paracardiac masses: Initial experiment. A.J.R. 143:1151, 1984.

57. Go, R. T., O'Donnell, J. K., Underwood, D. A., et al.: Comparison of gated cardiac MRI and 2D echocardiography of intracardiac neoplasms. A.J.R. 145:21, 1985.

58. Conces, D. J., Vox, V. A., and Klatte, E. C.: Gated MR imaging of left atrial myxomas. Radiology 156:445, 1985.

59. Fujita, N., Caputo, G. R., and Higgins, C. B.: Diagnosis and characterization of intracardiac masses by magnetic resonance imaging. Am. J. Cardiac Imaging 8:69, 1994.

60. Barakos, J. A., Brown, J. J., and Higgins, C. B.: Magnetic resonance imaging of secondary cardiac and paracardiac masses. A.J.R. 153:48, 1989.

61. Funari, M., Fujita, N., Peck, W. W., et al.: Cardiac tumors: Assessment with Gd-DTPA enhanced MR imaging. J. Comput. Assist. Tomogr. 15:953, 1992.

62. von Schulthess, G. K., McMurdo, K., Tscholakoff, D., et al.: Mediastinal masses: MR imaging. Radiology 158:289, 1986.

63. Seelos, K., Caputo, G. R., Carrol, C. L., et al.: Cine gradient refocused (GRE) echo imaging of intravascular masses: Differentiation between tumor and nontumor thrombus. J. Comput. Assist. Tomogr. 16:169, 1992.

64. Higgins, C. B., Byrd, B. F. III, Farmer, D., et al.: Magnetic resonance imaging in patients with congenital heart disease. Circulation 70:851, 1984.

65. Rees, S., Sommerville, J., Ward, C., et al.: Coarctation of the aorta: MR imaging in late postoperative assessment. Radiology 173:499, 1989.

66. Didier, D., Higgins, C. B., Fisher, M. R., et al.: Congenital heart disease in 72 patients. Radiology 158:227, 1986.

67. Didier, D., and Higgins, C. B.: Identification and localization of ventricular septal defects by gated magnetic resonance imaging. Am. J. Coll. Cardiol. 57:1363, 1986.

68. von Schulthess, G. K., Higashino, S. M., Higgins, S. S., et al.: Coarctation of the aorta: MR imaging. Radiology 158:474, 1986.

69. Peshock, R. M., Parrish, M., Fixler, D., et al.: MR imaging in the evaluation of single ventricle. Radiology 158:474, 1986.

70. Diethelm, L., Dery, R., Lipton, M. J., et al.: Atrial level shunts: Sensitivity and specificity of MR diagnosis. Radiology 162:181, 1987.

71. Hirsch, R., Kilner, P. J., Connelly, M. S., et al.: Diagnosis in adolescents and adults with congenital heart disease: Prospective of individual and combined roles of MRI and TEE. Circulation 90:2937, 1994.

72. Kersting-Sommerhoff, B. A., Diethelm, L., Teitel, D. F., et al.: Magnetic resonance imaging of congenital heart disease: Sensitivity and specificity using receiver operating characteristic curve analysis. Am. Heart. J. 118:155, 1989.

73. Kersting-Sommerhoff, B. A., Diethelm, L., Stanger, P., et al.: Evaluation of complex congenital ventricular anomalies with magnetic resonance imaging. Am. Heart J. 120:133, 1990.

74. Kersting-Sommerhoff, B. A., Seelos, K. C., Hardy, C., et al.: Evaluation of surgical procedures for cyanotic congenital heart disease using MR imaging. A.J.R. 155:259, 1990.

75. Julsrud, P. P., Ehman, R. L., Hagler, D. J., et al.: Extracardiac vasculature in candidates for Fontan surgery: MR imaging. Radiology 173:503, 1989.

76. Sommerhoff, B. K., Sechtem, U. P., and Higgins, C. B.: Evaluation of pulmonary blood supply by nuclear magnetic resonance imaging in patients with pulmonary atresia. J. Am. Coll. Cardiol. 11:166, 1988.

77. Kondo, C., Hardy, C., Higgins, S. S., et al.: MR imaging of the palliative operation for hypoplastic left heart syndrome. J. Am. Coll. Cardiol. 18:809, 1991.

78. Blankenberg, F., Rhee, J., Hardy, C., et al.: MRI vs echocardiography in the evaluation of the Jatene procedure. J. Comput. Assist. Tomogr. 18:749, 1994.

79. Fogel, M. A., Donofrio, M. T., Romaciotti, C., et al.: Magnetic resonance and echocardiographic imaging of pulmonary artery size throughout stages of Fontan reconstruction. Circulation 90:2927, 1994.

80. Martinez, J. E., Mohiaddin, R. H., Kilner, P. J., et al.: Obstruction in extracardiac ventriculopulmonary conduits: Value of NMR imaging with velocity mapping and Doppler echocardiography. J. Am. Coll. Cardiol. 20:338, 1992.

81. Duerinckx, A. J., Wexler, L., Banerjee, A., et al.: Postoperative evaluation of pulmonary arteries in congenital heart surgery by MR imaging: Comparison with echocardiography. Am. Heart J. 128:1139, 1994.

82. Sechtem, U., Pflugfelder, P., Cassidy, M. C., et al.: Ventricular septal defect: Visualization of shunt flow and determination of shunt size by cine magnetic resonance imaging. A.J.R. 149:689, 1987.

83. Amparo, E. G., Higgins, C. B., Hricak, H., et al.: Aortic dissection: Magnetic resonance imaging. Radiology 155:399, 1985.

84. White, R. C., Dooms, G. C., and Higgins, C. B.: Advances in imaging thoracic aortic disease. Invest. Radiol. 21:761, 1986.

85. Dinsmore, R. E., Liberthson, R. R., Wismer, G. L., et al.: Magnetic resonance imaging of thoracic aortic aneurysms. A.J.R. 146:309, 1986.

86. Kersting-Sommerhoff, B. A., Higgins, C. B., White, R. D., et al.: Aortic dissection: Sensitivity and specificity of MR imaging. Radiology 3:651, 1988.

87. Laissy, J-P., Blanc, F., Soyer, P., et al.: Thoracic aortic dissection: Diagnosis with transesophageal echocardiography vs MR imaging. Radiology 194:331, 1995.

88. Sommerhoff, B. A., Sechtem, U. P., Schiller, N. B., et al.: MRI of thoracic aorta in Marfan patients. J. Comput. Assist. Tomogr. 11:633, 1987.

89. White, R. D., Ullyot, D. J., and Higgins, C. B.: MR imaging of the aorta after surgery for aortic dissection. A.J.R. 150:87, 1988.

90. Chang, J-M., Friese, K., Caputo, G. R., et al.: MR measurement of blood flow in the true and false channel in chronic aortic dissection. J. Comput. Assist. Tomogr. 15:418, 1991.

91. Sakuma, H., Globits, S., O'Sullivan, M., et al.: Flow velocity measurements in native internal mammary arteries and coronary artery bypass grafts with breath-held velocity encoded cine MR imaging. J. Magn. Reson. Imaging (in press).

92. Winkler, M. L., and Higgins, C. B.: Magnetic resonance imaging of perivalvular infectious pseudoaneurysms. A.J.R. 147:153, 1986.

93. Nienaber, C. A., Spielmann, R. P., Von Kodolitsch, Y., et al.: Diagnosis of thoracic aortic dissection: Magnetic resonance imaging vs transesophageal echocardiography. Circulation 85:434, 1992.

94. Higgins, C. B., and Caputo, G. R.: Role of MR imaging in acquired and congenital cardiovascular disease. A.J.R. 161:13, 1993.

95. Szolar, D., Sakuma, H., and Higgins, C. B.: Cardiovascular application of magnetic resonance flow and velocity measurements. J. Magn. Reson. Imaging (in press).

96. Firmin, D. N., Naigler, G. L., Klipstein, R. H., et al.: In vivo validation of MR velocity mapping. J. Comput. Assist. Tomogr. 11:751, 1987.

97. Kondo, C., Caputo, G. R., Semelka, R., et al.: Right and left ventricular stroke volume measurements with velocity encoded cine NMR imaging: In vitro and in vivo validation. A.J.R. 157:9, 1991.

98. Mostbeck, G. H., Caputo, G. R., and Higgins, C. B.: MR measurement of blood flow in the cardiovascular system. A.J.R. 159:453, 1992.

99. Mohiaddin, R. H., and Longmore, D. B.: Functional aspects of cardio-

vascular nuclear magnetic resonance imaging. Circulation 88:264, 1993.

100. Wetter, D. R., McKinnon, G. C., Debatin, J. F., and von Schulthess, G. K.: Cardiac echo-planar MR imaging: Comparison of single- and multiple-shot techniques. Radiology 194:765, 1995.

101. Untermerger, M., Debatin, J. F., Leung, D. A., et al.: Cardiac volumetry: Comparison of echoplanar and conventional cine MR data acquisition strategies. Invest. Radiol. 29:994, 1994.

102. Caputo, G. R., Tscholakoff, D., Sechtem, U., et al.: Measurement of canine left ventricular mass using gated magnetic resonance imaging. A.J.R. 148:33, 1987.

103. Maddahi, J., Crues, J., Berman, D. S., et al.: Noninvasive quantitation of left ventricular mass by gated proton NMR imaging. J. Am. Coll. Cardiol. 10:682, 1987.

104. Underwood, S. R., Firmin, D. N., Klipstein, H., et al.: Rapid measurement of left ventricular volume from single oblique MR images. Radiology 157:309, 1986.

105. Cranney, G. B., Lotan, C. S., Dean, L., et al.: Left ventricular volume measurement using cardiac axis NMR imaging. Circulation 82:154, 1990.

106. Dulce, M-C., Mostbeck, G. H., Friese, K. K., et al.: Quantification of the left ventricular volumes and function with cine MRI: Comparison of geometric models with three-dimensional data. Radiology 188:371, 1993.

107. Doherty, N. E., Fujita, N., Caputo, G. R., et al.: Measurement of right ventricular mass in normal and dilated cardiomyopathic ventricles using cine MRI. Am. J. Cardiol. 69:1225, 1992.

108. Sechtem, U., Pflugfelder, P., Gould, R., et al.: Measurement of right and left ventricular volumes in healthy individuals with cine MR imaging. Radiology 163:697, 1987.

109. Sechtem, U., Pflugfelder, P. W., Cassidy, M. M., et al.: Mitral or aortic regurgitation: Quantification of regurgitant volumes with cine MR imaging. Radiology 167:425, 1988.

110. Pflugfelder, P. W., Sechtem, U. P., White, R. D., et al.: Quantification of regional myocardial function by rapid (cine) magnetic resonance imaging. A.J.R. 150:523, 1988.

111. LeWinter, M. M., Kent, R. S., Kroener, J. M., et al.: Regional differences in myocardial performance in the left ventricle of the dog. Circ. Res. 37:191, 1975.

112. Zerhouni, E. A., Parish, D. M., Roger, W. J., et al.: Human heart: Tagging with MR imaging—a method for noninvasive assessment of myocardial motion. Radiology 169:59, 1988.

113. Axel, L., and Dougherty, L.: MR imaging of motion with spatial modulation of magnetization. Radiology 171:841, 1989.

114. Maier, S. E., Fischer, S. E., McKinnon, G. C., et al.: Evaluation of left ventricular segmental wall motion in hypertrophic cardiomyopathy with myocardial tagging. Circulation 86:1919, 1992.

115. Lima, J. A. C., Jeremy, R., Guier, W., et al.: Accurate systolic wall thickening by MRI with tissue tagging: Correlation with sonomicrometers in normal and ischemic myocardium. J. Am. Coll. Cardiol. 21:1741, 1993.

116. Sechtem, U., Pflugfelder, P. W., White, R. D., et al.: Cine MRI: Potential for the evaluation of cardiovascular function. A.J.R. 148:239, 1987.

117. Pflugfelder, P. W., Sechtem, U. P., White, R. D., et al.: Noninvasive evaluation of mitral regurgitation by analysis of left atrial signal loss in cine magnetic resonance. Am. Heart J. 117:1113, 1989.

118. Pflugfelder, P. W., Landzberg, J. S., Cassidy, M. M., et al.: Comparison of cine MR imaging with Doppler echocardiography for the evaluation of aortic regurgitation. A.J.R. 152:729, 1989.

119. Wagner, S., Auffermann, W., Buser, P., et al.: Diagnostic accuracy and estimation of the severity of valvular regurgitation from the signal void on cine magnetic resonance images. Am. Heart J. 118:760, 1989.

120. Underwood, S. R., Klipstein, P. H., Firmin, D. N., et al.: Magnetic resonance assessment of aortic and mitral regurgitation. Br. Heart J. 56:455, 1986.

121. Higgins, C. B., Wagner, S., Kondo, C., et al.: Evaluation of valvular heart disease using cine GRE magnetic resonance imaging. Circulation (Suppl.) 84(3):I-198, 1991.

122. Cranney, G. B., Lotan, C. S., and Pohost, G. M.: Nuclear magnetic resonance imaging for assessment and follow up of patients with valve disease. Circulation (Suppl.) 84:216, 1991.

123. Globits, S., and Higgins, C. B.: Assessment of valvular heart disease using magnetic resonance imaging. Am. Heart J. 129:369, 1995.

124. Dulce, M-C., Mostbeck, G., O'Sullivan, M. M., et al.: Severity of aortic regurgitation: Interstudy reproducibility of measurements with velocity-encoded cine MR imaging. Radiology 185:235, 1992.

125. Fujita, N., Chazouilleres, A. F., Hartiala, J. J., et al.: Quantification of mitral regurgitation by velocity-encoded cine magnetic resonance imaging. J. Am. Coll. Cardiol. 23:951, 1994.

126. Eichenberger, A. C., Jenni, R., and von Schulthess, G. K.: Aortic valve pressure gradients in patients with aortic valve stenosis: Quantification with velocity encoded cine MRI. A.J.R. 160:971, 1992.

127. Kilner, P. J., Firmin, D. N., Rees, R. S. O., et al.: Valve and great vessel stenosis: Assessment with MR jet velocity mapping. Radiology 178:229, 1991.

128. Hendenreich, P. A., Steffens, J. C., Fujita, N., et al.: The evaluation of mitral stenosis with velocity-encoded cine magnetic resonance imaging. Am. J. Cardiol. 75:365, 1995.

129. Moran, P. R.: A flow zeugmatographic interface for NMR imaging in humans. Magn. Reson. Imaging 1:197, 1982.

130. Underwood, S. R., Firmin, D. N., Klipstein, R. H., et al.: Magnetic resonance velocity mapping: Clinical application of a new technique. Br. Heart J. 57:404, 1987.

131. Meier, D., Meier, S., and Böseger, P.: Quantitative flow measurements on phantoms and on blood vessels with MR. Magn. Reson. Med. 8:25, 1988.

132. Moran, P. R., Moran, R. A., and Karstaedt, N. K.: Verification and evaluation of internal flow and motion. Radiology 154:433, 1985.

133. Caputo, G. R., Kondo, C., Masui, T., et al.: Right and left lung perfusion: In vitro and in vivo validation with oblique-angle, velocity-encoded cine MR imaging. Radiology 180:693, 1991.

134. Bogren, H. G., Klipstein, R. H., Mohiaddin, R. H., et al.: Pulmonary artery distensibility and blood flow patterns: A magnetic resonance study of normal subjects and of patients with pulmonary arterial hypertension. Am. Heart J. 118:990, 1989.

135. Kondo, C., Caputo, G. R., Masui, T., et al.: Pulmonary hypertension: Pulmonary flow quantification and flow profile analysis with velocity-encoded cine MR imaging. Radiology 183:751, 1992.

136. Brenner, L. D., Caputo, G. R., Mostbeck, G., et al.: Quantification of left to right atrial shunts with velocity encoded cine nuclear magnetic resonance imaging. J. Am. Coll. Cardiol. 20:1246, 1992.

137. Steffens, J. C., Bourne, M. W., Sakuma, H., et al.: Quantification of collateral blood flow in coarctation of the aorta by velocity encoded cine MRI. Circulation 90:937, 1994.

138. Ehman, R. L., McNamara, M. T., Brasch, R. C., et al.: Influence of physiologic motion on the appearance of tissue in MR images. Radiology 159:777, 1986.

139. Higgins, C. B., Herfkens, R., Lipton, M. J., et al.: Nuclear magnetic resonance imaging of acute myocardial infarction in dogs: Alterations in magnetic relaxation times. Am. J. Cardiol. 52:184, 1983.

140. Johnston, D. L., Brady, T. J., Ratner, A. V., et al.: Assessment of myocardial ischemia with proton magnetic resonance: Effects of a three hour coronary occlusion with and without perfusion. Circulation 71:595, 1985.

141. Tscholakoff, D., Aherne, T., Yee, E. S., et al.: Cardiac transplantation in dogs: Evaluation with MRI. Radiology 157:697, 1985.

142. Tscholakoff, D., Higgins, C. B., McNamara, M. T., et al.: Early phase myocardial infarction: Evaluation by magnetic resonance imaging. Radiology 159:667, 1986.

143. Pflugfelder, P. W., Wisenberg, G., Prato, F. S., et al.: Early detection of canine myocardial infarction by magnetic resonance imaging in vivo. Circulation 71:587, 1985.

144. Saeed, M., Wendland, M. F., and Higgins, C. B.: Contrast media for MR imaging of the heart. J. Magn. Reson. Imag. 4:269, 1994.

145. Saeed, M., Wendland, M. F., and Tomei, E.: Demarcation of myocardial ischemia: Magnetic susceptibility effect of contrast medium in MR imaging. Radiology 173:763, 1989.

146. Saeed, M., Wendland, M. F., Yu, K. K., et al.: Dual effects of gadodiamide injection in depiction of the region of myocardial ischemia. J. Magn. Reson. Imag. 3:21, 1993.

147. Dulce, M-C., Duerinckx, A. J., Hartiala, J., et al.: MR imaging of the myocardium using nonionic contrast medium: Signal intensity changes in patients with subacute myocardial infarction. A.J.R. 160:1, 1993.

148. Eichstaedt, H. W., Felix, R., Dougherty, F. C., et al.: Magnetic resonance imaging (MRI) in different stages of myocardial infarction using the contrast agent gadolinium-DTPA. Clin. Cardiol. 9:527, 1986.

149. de Roos, A., van Rossum, A. C., van der Wall, E., et al.: Reperfused and nonreperfused myocardial infarction: Diagnostic potential of Gd-DTPA-enhanced MR imaging. Radiology 172:717, 1989.

150. Saeed, M., Wendland, M. F., Takehara, Y., et al.: Reperfusion and irreversible myocardial injury: Identification with a nonionic MR imaging contrast medium. Radiology 182:675, 1991.

151. Wendland, M. F., Saeed, M., Masui, T., et al.: Echo-planar MR imaging of normal and ischemic myocardium with gadodiamide injection. Radiology 186:535, 1993.

COMPUTED TOMOGRAPHY

152. Brundage, B., Lipton, M. J., Herfkens, R. J., et al.: Detection of patent coronary artery bypass grafts by computed tomography: A preliminary report. Circulation 61:826, 1980.

153. Moncada, R., Salinas, M., Churchill, R., et al.: Patency of saphenous aortocoronary grafts demonstrated by computed tomography. N. Engl. J. Med. 303:503, 1980.

154. Kohl, F. C., Wolfman, N. T., and Watts, L. E.: Evaluation of aortocoronary bypass graft status by computed tomography. Am. J. Cardiol. 48:304, 1981.

155. Higgins, C. B., Carlsson, E., and Lipton, M. J. (eds.): CT of the Heart and Great Vessels. Mt. Kisco, N.Y., Futura Publishing Co., 1983, p. 167.

156. Lipton, M. J., Higgins, C. B., Farmer, D., et al.: Cardiac imaging with a high-speed cine-CT scanner: Preliminary results. Radiology 152:579, 1983.

157. Sinak, L. F., and Ritman, E. L.: Dynamic spatial reconstructor. In CT of the Heart and Great Vessels. Mt. Kisco, N.Y., Futura Publishing Co., 1983, p. 61.

158. Rumberger, J. A., Feiring, A. J., Reiter, S. J., et al.: Ultrafast computed tomography: Evaluation of global left ventricular anatomy and function. In Pohost, G. M., Higgins, C. B., Morganroth, J., et al. (eds.): New Con-

cepts in Cardiac Imaging. Chicago, Year Book Medical Publishers, 1988, p. 195.

159. Feiring, A., Rumberger, J. A., Reiter, S. J., et al.: Determination of left ventricular mass in dogs with rapid-acquisition cardiac CT scanning. Circulation 72:1355, 1985.

160. Hajkuczok, Z. D., Weiss, R. M., Stanford, W., et al.: Determination of right ventricular mass in humans and dogs with ultrafast cardiac computed tomography. Circulation 82:202, 1990.

161. Himelman, R. B., Abbott, J. A., Lipton, M. J., et al.: Cine CT compared with echocardiography in the evaluation of cardiac function in emphysema. Am. J. Cardiac Imaging 2:283, 1988.

162. Lanzer, P., Garrett, J., Lipton, M. J., et al.: Quantitation of regional myocardial function by cine computed tomography: Pharmacologic changes in wall thickness. J. Am. Coll. Cardiol. 8:682, 1986.

163. Caputo, G. R., and Lipton, M. J.: Evaluation of regional left ventricular function using ultrafast CT. In Pohost, G. L., Higgins, C. B., Morganroth, J., et al. (eds.): New Concepts in Cardiac Imaging. Chicago, Year Book Medical Publishers, 1988, p. 231.

164. Feiring, A. J., Rumberger, J. A., Reiter, S. J., et al.: Sectional and segmental variability of left ventricular function: Experimental and clinical studies using ultrafast computed tomography. J. Am. Coll. Cardiol. 12:415, 1988.

165. Farmer, D. W., Lipton, M. J., Higgins, C. B., et al.: In vivo assessment of left ventricular wall and chamber dynamics during transient myocardial ischemia using cine CT. Am. J. Cardiol. 55:560, 1985.

166. Marcus, M. L., and Weiss, R. M.: Evaluation of cardiac structures and function with ultrafast computed tomography. In Marcus, M. L., Schelbert, H. R., Skorton, D. J., et al. (eds.): Cardiac Imaging. Philadelphia, W.B. Saunders Company, 1991, p. 669.

167. Roig, E., Chomka, E. V., Costaner, A., et al.: Exercise ultrafast computed tomography for the detection of coronary artery disease. J. Am. Coll. Cardiol. 13:1073, 1989.

168. McMillan, R. M., and Rees, M. R.: Determinants of left ventricular ejection fraction by ultrafast CT. Angiology 39:203, 1988.

169. Reiter, S. J., Rumberger, J. A., Feiring, A. J., et al.: Precision of right and left ventricular stroke volume measurements by rapid acquisition cine CT. Circulation 74:890, 1986.

170. Reiter, S. J., Rumberger, J. A., Stanford, W., et al.: Quantitative determination of aortic regurgitant volumes in dogs by ultrafast computed tomography. Circulation 76:728, 1987.

EVALUATION OF SPECIFIC CARDIAC DISEASES

171. Lackner, K., and Thurn, P.: Computed tomography of the heart: ECG gated and continuous scans. Radiology 140:413, 1981.

172. Kramer, P., Goldstein, J., Herfkens, R., et al.: Imaging of acute myocardial infarction in man with contrast enhanced computed transmission tomography. Am. Heart J. 108:1514, 1984.

173. Lipton, M. J., Farmer, D. W., Killebrew, E. J., et al.: Regional myocardial dysfunction: Evaluation of patients with prior myocardial infarction with fast CT. Radiology 157:735, 1985.

174. Lackner, K.: Clinical application of CTT for evaluation of ischemic heart disease—comparison with other imaging methods. In Higgins, C. B. (ed.): CTT of the Heart and Great Vessels. Mt. Kisco, N.Y., Futura Publishing Co., 1982, p. 267.

175. Tomoda, H., Hoshiai, M., Furuya, H., et al.: Evaluation of intracardiac thrombus with computed tomography. Am. J. Cardiol. 51:843, 1983.

176. Tomoda, H., Hoshiai, M., Furuya, H., et al.: Evaluation of left ventricular thrombus with computed tomography. Am. J. Cardiol. 48:573, 1981.

177. Tomoda, H., Hoshiai, M., Tozawa, R., et al.: Evaluation of left atrial thrombus with computed tomography. Am. Heart J. 100:306, 1980.

178. Rumberger, J. A., Feiring, A. J., Lipton, M. J., et al.: Use of ultrafast computed tomography to quantitate regional myocardial perfusion: A preliminary report. J. Am. Coll. Cardiol. 9:59, 1987.

179. Gould, R. G., Lipton, M. J., McNamara, M. T., et al.: Measurement of regional myocardial flow in dogs using ultrafast CT. Invest. Radiol. 23:348, 1988.

180. Wolfkiel, C. J., Ferguson, J. L., Chomka, E. V., et al.: Measurement of myocardial blood flow by ultrafast computed tomography. Circulation 76:1262, 1987.

181. Rumberger, J. A., Bell, M. R., Feiring, A. J., et al.: Measurement of myocardial perfusion using fast computed tomography. In Marcus, M. L., Schelbert, H. R., Skorton, D. J., et al. (eds.): Cardiac Imaging. Philadelphia, W.B. Saunders Company, 1991, p. 688.

182. Peck, W. A., Mancini, G. B. J., Mattrey, R. F., et al.: In vivo assessment by CT of natural progression of infarct size, left ventricular mass, and function after myocardial infarction in the dog. Am. J. Cardiol. 53:929, 1984.

183. Mancini, G. B. J., Peck, W. W., Ross, J., Jr., et al.: Use of computerized tomography to assess myocardial infarct size and ventricular function in dogs during acute coronary occlusion and reperfusion. Am. J. Cardiol. 53:282, 1984.

184. Daniel, W. G., Doring, W., Stender, H. S., et al.: Value and limitations of computed tomography in assessing aortocoronary bypass graft patency. Circulation 67:983, 1983.

185. Stanford, W., Brundage, B. H., MacMillan, R., et al.: Sensitivity and specificity of assessing coronary bypass graft patency with ultrafast computed tomography: Results of a multicenter study. J. Am. Coll. Cardiol. 12:1, 1988.

186. Bateman, T. M., Gray, R. J., Whiting, J. S., et al.: Ultrafast computed tomographic evaluation of aortocoronary bypass graft patency. J. Am. Coll. Cardiol. 8:693, 1986.

187. Bateman, T. M., Gray, R. J., Whiting, J. S., et al.: Prospective evaluation of ultrafast CT for determination of coronary bypass graft patency. Circulation 75:1018, 1987.

188. Ullyot, D. J., Turley, K., McKay, C. R., et al.: Assessment of saphenous vein graft patency by contrast enhanced computed tomography. J. Thorac. Cardiovasc. Surg. 83:512, 1982.

189. McKay, C. R., Brundage, B. H., Ullyot, D. J., et al.: Evaluation of early postoperative coronary artery bypass graft patency by contrast enhanced computed tomography. J. Am. Coll. Cardiol. 2:312, 1963.

190. Hamby, R. I., Tabrah, F., Wisoff, B. G., et al.: Coronary artery calcification: Clinical implications and angiographic correlates. Am. Heart J. 87:565, 1974.

191. Bartel, A. G., Chen, J. T., Peter, R. H., et al.: The significance of coronary arterial calcification detected by fluoroscopy. Circulation 49:1247, 1974.

192. Aldrich, R. F., Brensike, J. F., Battaglini, J. W., et al.: Coronary calcification in the detection of coronary artery disease and comparison with electrocardiographic exercise testing. Circulation 59:113, 1979.

193. Agatston, A. S., Janowitz, W. R., Hildner, F. J., et al.: Quantification of coronary artery calcium using ultrafast computed tomography. J. Am. Coll. Cardiol. 15:827, 1990.

194. Kaufman, R. B., Sheedy, P. F., Breen, J. F., et al.: Detection of heart calcification with electron beam CT: Interobserver and intraobserver reliability for scoring quantification. Radiology 190:347, 1994.

195. Simon, D. B., Schwartz, R. S., Edwards, W. O., et al.: Noninvasive detection of anatomic coronary artery disease by ultrafast tomographic scanning: A quantitative pathologic comparison study. J. Am. Coll. Cardiol. 20:1118, 1992.

196. Mautner, S., Mautner, G., Frolich, J., et al.: Coronary artery disease: Prediction with in vitro electron beam CT. Radiology 192:625, 1994.

197. Mautner, G., Mautner, S. L., Frolich, J., et al.: Coronary artery calcification: Assessment with electron beam CT and histomorphometric correlation. Radiology 192:619, 1994.

198. Rumberger, J. A., Schwartz, R. S., Simons, D. B., et al.: Relation of coronary calcium determined by electron beam computed tomography and lumen narrowing by autopsy. Am. J. Cardiol. 74:1169, 1994.

199. Breen, J. F., Sheedy, P. F., Schwartz, R. S., et al.: Coronary artery calcification detected by ultrafast CT as an indication of coronary artery disease. Radiology 185:435, 1992.

200. Agatson, A. S., Janowitz, W. R., Kaplan, G., et al.: Ultrafast computed tomography detected coronary calcium reflects the angiographic extent of coronary arterial stenosis. Am. J. Cardiol. 74:1272, 1994.

201. Janowitz, W. R., Agathson, A. S., Kaplan, G., et al.: Differences in prevalence and extent of coronary artery calcium detected by ultrafast computed tomography in asymptomatic men and women. Am. J. Cardiol. 72:247, 1993.

202. Fallavolleta, J. A., Brody, A. S., Bannell, I., et al.: Fast detection of coronary calcification in the diagnosis of coronary artery disease. Circulation 72:247, 1993.

203. Silverman, P. M., and Harell, G. S.: Computed tomography of the normal pericardium. Invest. Radiol. 18:141, 1983.

204. Moncada, R., Baker, M., Salinas, M., et al.: Diagnostic role of computed tomography in pericardial heart disease: Congenital defects, thickening, neoplasms and effusions. Am. Heart J. 103:263, 1981.

205. Isner, J. M., Carter, B. L., Bankoff, M. S., et al.: Computed tomography in the diagnosis of pericardial heart disease. Ann. Intern. Med. 97:473, 1982.

206. Baim, R. S., MacDonald, I. L., Wise, D. J., et al.: Computed tomography of absent left pericardium. Radiology 135:127, 1980.

207. Roger, C. I., Seymour, Q., and Brock, G. I.: Atypical pericardial cysts location: The value of computed tomography. J. Comput. Assist. Tomogr. 4:583, 1980.

208. Pugatch, R. D., Braver, J. H., Robbins, A. H., et al.: CT diagnosis of pericardial cysts. A.J.R. 131:515, 1978.

209. Tomoda, H., Hoshiai, M., Furuya, H., et al.: Evaluation of pericardial effusion with computed tomography. Am. Heart J. 99:701, 1980.

210. Higgins, C. B., Mattrey, R. F., and Shea, P.: CT localization and aspiration of postoperative pericardial fluid collection. J. Comput. Assist. Tomogr. 7:734, 1983.

211. Zerhouni, E. A., Scott, W. W., Baker, R. R., et al.: Invasive thymomas: Diagnosis and evaluation by computed tomography. J. Comput. Assist. Tomogr. 6:92, 1982.

212. Hackney, D., Mattrey, R., Peck, W. W., et al.: Experimental pericardial inflammation evaluated by computed tomography. Radiology 151:145, 1984.

213. Doppman, J. C., Reinmuller, R., Lissner, J., et al.: Computed tomography in constrictive pericardial disease. J. Comput. Assist. Tomogr. 5:1, 1981.

214. Isner, J. M., Carter, B. L., Bankoff, M. S., et al.: Differentiation of constrictive pericarditis from restrictive cardiomyopathy by computed tomographic imaging. Am. Heart J. 105:1019, 1983.

215. Handler, J. B., Higgins, C. B., Warrent, S. E., et al.: Computerized tomographic diagnosis of paracardiac masses. West. J. Med. 135:271, 1981.

216. Glazer, G. M., Gross, B. H., Oringer, M. B., et al.: Computed tomography of pericardial masses. J. Comput. Assist. Tomogr. 8:895, 1984.

217. Patel, B. K., Markivee, C. R., and George, E. A.: Pericardial cyst simulating intracardiac mass. A.J.R. 141:292, 1983.

218. Norlindh, T., Lilja, B., Nyman, U., et al.: Left atrial myxoma demonstrated by CT. A.J.R. *137*:153, 1981.

219. Huggins, T. J., Huggins, M. J., Schnopf, D. J., et al.: Left atrial myxoma: Computed tomography as a diagnostic modality. Invest. Radiol. *12*:559, 1977.

220. Baron, R. L., Guitterez, F. R., and McKnight, R. C.: Computed tomographic evaluation of the great arteries and aortic arch anomalies. *In* Freedman, W. F., and Higgins, C. B. (eds.): Pediatric Cardiac Imaging. Philadelphia, W.B. Saunders Company, 1984, pp. 135–156.

221. Farmer, D. W., Lipton, M. J., Webb, W. R., et al.: Computed tomography in congenital heart disease. J. Comput. Assist. Tomogr. *8*:677, 1984.

222. Webb, W. R., Gamsu, G., Speckman, G., et al.: CT demonstration of mediastinal aortic arch anomalies. J. Comput. Assist. Tomogr. *6*:445, 1982.

223. Eldridge, W. J.: Comprehensive evaluation of congenital heart disease using ultrafast computed tomography. *In* Marcus, M. L., Schelbert, H. R., Skorton, D. J., et al. (eds.): Cardiac Imaging. Philadelphia, W.B. Saunders Company, 1991, p. 714.

224. Eldridge, W. J., Flicker, S., and Steiner, R. M.: Cine CT in the anatomical evaluation of congenital heart disease. *In* Pohost, G., Higgins, C. B., Morgenroth, J., et al. (eds.): New Concepts in Cardiac Imaging. Vol. 3. Chicago, Year Book Medical Publishers, 1987, p. 265.

225. Garrett, J. S., Jaschke, W., Aherne, T., et al.: Quantitation of intracardiac shunts by cine CT. J. Comput. Assist. Tomogr. *12*:82, 1988.

226. MacMillan, R. M., Shakriari, A., Sumithisena, F., et al.: Contrast enhanced cine computed tomography for the diagnosis of right coronary to coronary sinus arteriovenous fistulae. Am. J. Cardiol. *56*:997, 1985.

227. Helberg, E., Wolverson, M., Sundaram, M., et al.: CT finding in thoracic aortic dissection. A.J.R. *136*:13, 1981.

228. Thorsten, M. K., San Drelto, M. A., Lawson, T. L., et al.: Dissecting aortic aneurysms: Accuracy of computed tomographic diagnosis. Radiology *148*:773, 1983.

229. Dudkerk, M., Overbosch, E., and Dee, P.: CT recognition of acute aortic dissection. A.J.R. *141*:671, 1983.

230. White, R. C., Lipton, M. J., Higgins, C. B., et al.: Noninvasive evaluation of suspected thoracic aortic disease by contrast-enhanced computed tomography. Am. J. Cardiol. *57*:282, 1986.

231. Cizarros, J. E., Isselbacher, E. M., DeSanctis, R. W., et al.: Diagnostic imaging in the evaluation of suspected aortic dissection: Old standards and new directions. N. Engl. J. Med. *328*:35, 1993.

232. Nienaber, C. A., Von Kodolitsch, Y., Nichols, V., et al.: The diagnosis of thoracic aortic dissection by noninvasive imaging procedures. N. Engl. J. Med. *328*:1, 1993.

233. Yamada, T., Toda, S., and Harada, J.: Aortic dissection without intimal rupture: Diagnosis with MR imaging and CT. Radiology *168*:347, 1988.

234. Guthaner, D. F., Miller, D. C., Silverman, J. F., et al.: Fate of the false lumen following surgical repair of aortic dissection: An angiographic study. Radiology *133*:1, 1979.

235. Yamaguchi, T., Naito, H., Ohta, M., et al.: False lumens in type III aortic dissection: Progress in CT study. Radiology *156*:757, 1985.

236. Yamaguchi, T., Guthaner, D. F., and Wexler, L.: Natural history of the false channel of type A aortic dissection after surgical repair: CT study. Radiology *170*:743, 1989.

237. Mathieu, D., Keita, K., Loisance, D., et al.: Postoperative CT follow-up of aortic dissection. J. Comput. Assist. Tomogr. *10*:216, 1986.

238. Teigen, C. L., Maus, T. P., Sheedy, P. F., et al.: Pulmonary embolism: Diagnosis with contrast enhanced electron beam CT and comparison with pulmonary angiography. Radiology *194*:313, 1995.

239. Remy-Jardin, M., Remy, J., Wattinne, L., et al.: Central pulmonary thromboembolism: Diagnosis with spiral volumetric CT with single breath hold technique—comparison with pulmonary angiography. Radiology *185*:381, 1992.

Chapter 11
Relative Merits of Imaging Techniques

DAVID J. SKORTON, BRUCE H. BRUNDAGE,
HEINRICH R. SCHELBERT, GERALD L. WOLF

Evaluation of the patient with known or suspected cardiovascular disease is becoming both more accurate and more precise due to the availability of an already broad and still growing array of diagnostic methods (described in the first 10 chapters of this book). The process of diagnosis in the mid-1990's still begins with a careful and thorough history (Chap. 1) and physical examination (Chap. 2). Often, these are followed by a resting 12-lead electrocardiogram (Chap. 4) and chest roentgenogram (Chap. 7). At this point in the diagnostic process, the clinician usually forms presumptive diagnostic hypotheses. To confirm or refute these hypotheses, the clinician can turn to a range of laboratory examinations, including measurements made on blood and urine, exercise electrocardiographic testing (Chap. 5), electrophysiological monitoring or testing, and a large number of sophisticated imaging techniques. With the exception of evaluating arrhythmias and conduction disturbances, methods of imaging the heart are the predominant laboratory diagnostic methods in cardiology.[1,2] Thus, the clinician needs to be conversant with the several methods of imaging the heart and circulation. However, because of the wealth of sometimes redundant information offered by these methods, in the interest of efficient and cost-effective diagnosis, the clinician also needs to be aware of the relative strengths and weaknesses of these techniques under particular clinical circumstances. In Chapters 3 and 7 through 10, details regarding the use and interpretation of each of the individual imaging techniques are presented. It is the purpose of this chapter to offer some insights into the relative advantages and disadvantages of these several modalities.

SCOPE OF CARDIAC IMAGING

The several available and developing methods of cardiac imaging may be categorized in various ways; we choose to divide them, somewhat arbitrarily, into "standard" and "evolving" methods (Table 11–1). The basis of this distinction is the general availability of and clinical experience with the methods. Only a few investigative centers have all these methods available for routine clinical use. In general, those we classify as standard are widely available and thus are methods with which most clinicians have at least some experience. The modalities classified as evolving are relatively new or not widely employed, so most clinicians have relatively little direct experience with them.

Projection versus Tomographic Imaging

The distinction between *projection* and *tomographic* imaging is of theoretical and practical importance. The standard chest roentgenogram is a good example of a projection imaging method. The patient is placed between an x-ray source and an x-ray detector (a film-screen system). The x-rays are launched; they pass through the patient and are then received and detected on film. Thus, the imaging energy is *projected* through the patient so that attenuation of x-rays occurs not only due to the structure of interest (e.g., the heart) but also due to other structures interposed along the path taken by the x-rays (such as chest wall and lung). Because of this projection phenomenon, x-ray shadows in the resulting roentgenogram represent a superimposition of wanted and unwanted information. Plain-film

TABLE 11–1   STANDARD AND EVOLVING METHODS OF
CARDIAC IMAGING

STANDARD METHODS
Chest roentgenography
Echocardiography
Radionuclide methods
Planar and single-photon emission computed tomography
Myocardial perfusion scintigraphy (thallium-201 and technetium-99m agents)
Radionuclide ventriculography (technetium-99m-labeled red blood cells)
Infarct-avid imaging (technetium-99m pyrophosphate or indium-111 antimyosin antibody)
Selective angiography
Ventriculography/aortography
Pulmonary angiography
Coronary angiography
EVOLVING METHODS
Computer-assisted echocardiography
Perfusion (contrast) studies
Ultrasound tissue characterization
Three-dimensional reconstructions
Radionuclide methods
Newer imaging tracers
Positron emission tomography
Digital angiography
Fast computed tomography
Electron beam
Slip-ring
Magnetic resonance methods
Magnetic resonance imaging
Magnetic resonance spectroscopy

roentgenography, fluoroscopy, and angiography are all examples of projection imaging methods.

Projection radionuclide images are usually referred to as *planar.* In the case of planar radionuclide images (see p. 276), the basic data consist of photons emitted by the injected radionuclide; these photons are detected externally by a gamma camera. The resulting images may be degraded by interactions of the photons with other tissues interposed along the paths taken by the photons as they travel from the tissue of interest to the gamma camera.

The other basic approach to imaging is the selective depiction of a slice, or *tomogram,* through the patient. For example, in the case of x-ray computed tomography (CT) (Chap. 10), the production of a tomogram is accomplished by acquiring x-ray attenuation measurements from many different angles around the patient within a selected plane. At each angle, x-rays are sent from an x-ray source through the patient and are then received by a detector on the opposite side of the patient. This process is repeated for many angles around the patient, yielding a set of x-ray attenuation profiles. By computer reconstruction methods,[3] these many x-ray attenuation profiles are combined to produce an image depicting the two-dimensional distribution of x-ray attenuation data for a slice, or tomogram, through the patient. Since the resulting data selectively represent x-ray attenuation only in the "slice" under study, the problem of superimposition found in projection methods does not occur. Thus, the tomographic imaging techniques permit clearer delineation of physical characteristics and anatomical features of selected body regions than is possible with nontomographic, projection methods. Two-dimensional echocardiography, single-photon emission radionuclide CT, x-ray CT, and magnetic resonance imaging (MRI) are all examples of tomographic imaging methods. Tomographic imaging methods virtually all depend on digital computer image processing methods for image generation, display, and analysis.

Standard Imaging Methods

Standard widely available imaging methods include chest roentgenography, fluoroscopy, echocardiography, myocardial perfusion scintigraphy employing thallium-201 (^{201}TI) or agents labeled with technetium-99m (^{99m}Tc) (including both planar scintigraphy and single-photon emission computed tomography [SPECT]), radionuclide ventriculography, infarct scans, and selective angiocardiography. The information content of these several imaging methods varies widely, because the method of image formation is different in each type of technique. Each imaging method

represents the use of a particular energy source to produce an image containing anatomical and/or physiological information. As the energy sources vary, so do the types of information that may be extracted by application of the different methods. Table 11–2 lists the basic energy forms used to produce medical image data with an indication of some of the biophysical bases of image formation by each technique. Standard radiographic techniques (including chest roentgenography, fluoroscopy, and selective angiocardiography) are based on differential attenuation of x-rays by tissues of varying density. In angiography, attenuation of x-rays by blood is increased selectively by the infusion of iodinated contrast media. Ultrasonographic imaging is based on differential reflection and absorption of ultrasound (mechanical) energy by structures of varying density and elasticity. Radionuclide image data depend on both the radioisotope used as a label and the biologically relevant compound to which the label is attached. The regional image intensity reflects the regional distribution of that particular radiotracer in the body or the organ under study at the time of imaging.

Evolving Imaging Methods

Evolving and/or less commonly used imaging methods include newer, computer-assisted ultrasound applications (including contrast-based perfusion imaging,[4] tissue characterization,[5] and three-dimensional reconstruction[6]), positron emission tomography (PET)[7] (Chap. 9), digital angiography,[8], magnetic resonance methods[9] (both imaging [MRI][10] and spectroscopy[11] [Chap. 10]), and fast x-ray computed tomography (fast CT).[12] (We use the term "fast CT" to include at least two methods of rapid acquisition CT: slip-ring methods and electron beam CT [the latter previously referred to as "ultrafast CT"].) As discussed already for standard imaging methods, the information content of the evolving methods also varies widely and is based on the energy form used to produce the image. The newer computer-assisted ultrasound applications depend on standard ultrasound interactions with tissue and therefore share the determinants of image intensity noted for standard echocardiography, but they employ new image data acquisition and processing methods. Similarly, PET image data are related to unique radionuclides and biologically relevant ligands. CT and digital angiography remain x-ray–based techniques in which image intensity is related to tissue density, but signal detection and image formation allow new capabilities. Image intensity in MRI (for proton images, the only widely available type) is a complex function of several variables, including regional water content, flow, motion, so-called nuclear magnetic resonance (NMR) relaxation times (both spin-lattice, or T_1, and spin-spin, or T_2, relaxation times), chemical shift and possibly other factors not fully understood[13] (Chap. 10). To summarize, the evolving and standard imaging methods are based on production of pictures using a wide variety of energy forms and biophysical determinants. Thus, these methods should be considered potentially complementary in the information they may offer.

A final general point to be emphasized is that the evolving imaging methods depend to a greater degree than do the standard methods on digital computer image processing technology for data acquisition, image production, display, storage, and analysis.[14,15] For example, chest roentgenography and selective angiocardiography may be performed without the aid of computer storage or manipulation of image data, although digital applications are becoming more common in these two modalities. However, computed tomographic techniques (including x-ray CT, SPECT, and PET) depend completely on computer technology for acquisition of basic image data, reconstruction of these data into tomographic images, and display, enhancement, and storage of the resulting images. Similarly, modern echocardiographic and MRI systems depend on computer methods for

TABLE 11–2 SOME DETERMINANTS OF IMAGE INTENSITY

ENERGY FORM	IMAGE INTENSITY DETERMINANTS

X-ray based methods
  Plain-film radiography
  Angiography
  Computed tomography
	Density of tissue
	Local contrast (iodine) concentration

Ultrasound	Acoustic velocity Density of tissue Tissue elasticity Contrast agent
Radionuclides	Tracer concentration (depends on biological activity of ligand) Photon energy
Magnetic resonance methods	Proton (spin) density (i.e., water content) Nuclear magnetic resonance relaxation times Chemical shift Blood flow Contrast agent effect

TABLE 11–3 RELATIVE USEFULNESS OF CONVENTIONAL IMAGING TECHNIQUES IN ACHIEVING DIAGNOSTIC GOALS*

DIAGNOSTIC GOAL	CXR	ANGIO†	ECHO	RADIONUCLIDE VENTRICULOGRAPHY	MYOCARDIAL SCINTIGRAPHY
CARDIAC ANATOMY					
Chamber size	+	+++	+++	++	+
Myocardial mass	0	+	+++	0	+
Intracardiac masses	0	+++	++++	+	0
Valvular anatomy	0	++	++++	0	0
Pericardial disease	+	++	+++	0	0
Coronary anatomy	0	++++	+	0	0
Graft patency	0	++++	+	0	0
CARDIAC PHYSIOLOGY					
Ventricular systolic function	+	+++	+++	++	+
Ventricular diastolic function	0	++++	+++	++	0
Valvular stenosis/insufficiency	+	++++	+++	+	0
Intracardiac shunt	+	++++	+++	++	0
Myocardial blood flow	0	+	+	0	+++
Tissue characterization	0	0	+	0	0
Myocardial metabolism	0	0	0	0	+

* 0, no information; ++++, maximum information; angio, angiography; CXR, chest roentgenogram; echo, echocardiography.
† Angio includes both imaging and hemodynamic evaluation.
Modified and updated from Grover-McKay, M., and Skorton D. J.: Comparative aspects of modern imaging techniques. *In* Zipes, D. P., and Rowlands, D. J. (eds.): Progress in Cardiology. Philadelphia, Lea and Febiger, 1990, p. 3.

image generation and display. Once images are produced, digital computer technology is feasible for quantitative image analyses.

MEETING THE GOALS OF CARDIAC IMAGING

The complete assessment of a patient with known or suspected heart disease ideally should include information on cardiac anatomy (including the detailed anatomy of the coronary arteries), the function of the heart chambers and valves, myocardial perfusion and metabolism and their responses to exercise stress and/or pharmacologic agents, and tissue characteristics such as the replacement of normal myocardium by scar or infiltration by abnormal substances.

Standard imaging methods give very useful information on cardiovascular anatomy and on chamber and valvular function (Table 11–3). In addition, information on relative regional deficits in myocardial perfusion is offered by myocardial perfusion scintigraphy employing thallium-201 or agents labeled with technetium-99m. However, none of the standard imaging methods offers information on the *absolute* level of regional myocardial perfusion, the details of regional myocardial metabolism, or the definition of tissue characteristics. Thus, development of the evolving imaging methods has been based in part on the perceived need to realize all the goals of cardiac imaging in clinical practice (Table 11–4). No single standard or evolving imaging modality is likely to be capable of optimal achievement of all the goals of cardiac imaging. Conversely, several techniques permit assessment of cardiac anatomy and function; there-

TABLE 11–4 RELATIVE USEFULNESS OF EVOLVING IMAGING TECHNIQUES IN ACHIEVING DIAGNOSTIC GOALS*

DIAGNOSTIC GOAL	DIGITAL ANGIO†	COMPUTER-ASSISTED ECHO	MRI	MRS	FCT	PET
CARDIAC ANATOMY						
Chamber size	+++	+++	++++	0	++++	++
Myocardial mass	+	+++	++++	0	++++	++
Intracardiac masses	+++	++++	++++	0	++++	0
Valvular anatomy	++	++++	+++	0	+++	0
Pericardial disease	++	+++	++++	0	++++	0
Coronary anatomy	++++	++	++	0	++	0
Graft patency	++++	+	++	0	+++	++
CARDIAC PHYSIOLOGY						
Ventricular systolic function	+++	+++	++++	0	++++	++
Ventricular diastolic function	++++	+++	++	0	++	0
Valvular stenosis/insufficiency	++++	+++	+++	0	++	0
Intracardiac shunt	++++	+++	+++	0	+++	0
Myocardial blood flow	++	++	+	0	++	++++
Tissue characterization	0	++	++	+++	+	+++
Myocardial metabolism	0	0	0	++++	0	++++

* 0, no information; ++++, maximum information; angio, angiography; echo, echocardiography; MRI, magnetic resonance imaging; MRS, magnetic resonance spectroscopy; PET, positron emission tomography; FCT, fast computed tomography.
† Angio includes both imaging and hemodynamic evaluation.
Modified and updated from Grover-McKay, M., and Skorton D. J.: Comparative aspects of modern imaging techniques. *In* Zipes, D. P., and Rowlands, D. J. (eds.): Progress in Cardiology. Philadelphia, Lea and Febiger, 1990, p. 3.

fore, redundant information will be obtained if these techniques are used additively without consideration of their relative strengths in the attainment of all imaging goals.

Assessment of Anatomy

Cardiac chamber and great vessel anatomy can be evaluated accurately with the use of any of several imaging techniques, including echocardiography, selective angiocardiography, CT, and MRI. An estimate of chamber size and shape also can be obtained from radionuclide ventriculograms. However, because of relatively coarse spatial resolution (on the order of several millimeters to 1 cm), the radionuclide techniques are not the methods of choice for assessing the detailed aspects of cardiac morphology. Selective angiocardiography has been the traditional standard for chamber volume against which other techniques have been judged. Tomographic methods, however, are superior in assessment of cardiac size and shape because of their ability to delineate wall thickness clearly, because of their relative freedom from problems caused by superimposition, and because their use in assessing chamber volume or mass does not require simplified geometric assumptions. Thus, echocardiography, CT, and MRI are the best methods for determining chamber and great vessel morphology. Fast CT permits enormously accurate and precise determination of cardiac anatomy.[16] However, CT has the disadvantages of not being portable and of having the problems associated with the need for iodinated contrast medium and radiation exposure. In the patient who can lie relatively still for several minutes, MRI can produce exquisitely detailed images of cardiac anatomy.[17] More recent, rapid methods of MRI image acquisition are increasing the utility of MRI in assessment of cardiac anatomy.[18] However, like CT, MRI is not portable. Because of these considerations, echocardiography is often considered the initial procedure of choice for assessment of chamber and great vessel morphology in patients in whom studies of diagnostic quality can be achieved. Particularly with the advent of transesophageal echocardiography (see p. 57), it is possible to assess accurately cardiac chamber and great vessel anatomy in the vast majority of patients by using ultrasound methods.

Determination of the detailed anatomy of the coronary arteries in routine clinical practice continues to be the domain of selective coronary arteriography (Chap. 8). Whether recorded on 35-mm cine film or in digital format, selective coronary angiograms exhibit the high spatial and temporal resolution necessary to image the coronary arteries sufficiently accurately to plan and evaluate catheter and/or surgical interventions. This is true particularly for the distal portions of the coronary vasculature or severely diseased vessels in which arterial lumen diameters may be 1 mm or smaller. CT shows potential for visualization of selected portions of the coronary arteries.[19] Both transesophageal echocardiography[20] and MRI[21] also may be used to visualize portions of the coronary tree and to assess flow within the vessels. However, it is unlikely that any technique other than selective coronary angiography will be capable within the next few years of defining the details of coronary anatomy throughout the epicardial coronary tree in the great majority of patients. The one exception to this statement may be intravascular ultrasound imaging (see p. 58), which offers unique information on not only luminal but also vessel wall anatomy.

Delineation of the anatomy of coronary bypass grafts (whether of internal mammary or saphenous vein origin) is also best done using angiography with selective graft injections (Fig. 8–17, p. 255). However, CT[22] (Fig. 10–36, p. 338) and MRI[23] (Fig. 10–10, p. 323) have substantial utility in identification of bypass graft patency.

Evaluation of Chamber and Valvular Function

LEFT VENTRICULAR FUNCTION. Global systolic and diastolic function of the left ventricle can be assessed with echocardiography, radionuclide ventriculography, selective angiocardiography, CT, and MRI. Because of its portability, safety, and high patient acceptance, echocardiography (including both imaging and Doppler approaches) is commonly used as the initial tool to assess left ventricular global and regional function. Echocardiography permits accurate assessment of left ventricular function[24] when studies of adequate quality are obtained; with the widespread availability of transesophageal echocardiography, this includes most patients. However, clinicians may not wish to undertake transesophageal echocardiography strictly for the assessment of left ventricular function. Echocardiograms of sufficient quality for at least semiquantitative analysis of left ventricular function can be obtained by the transthoracic approach in most patients. However, echocardiography has some inherent problems that limit its ability to define precisely left ventricular volume, mass, and ejection fraction. Among these problems is the fact that echocardiographic images are not acquired in mutually parallel or perpendicular orientations but are obtained at somewhat arbitrary angles, dictated by the constraints of the intercostal spaces and other aspects of thoracic anatomy. As opposed to these problems of echocardiography, CT and MRI permit the acquisition of multiple parallel, high-resolution tomograms from the apex to the base of the left ventricle, yielding quite precise and accurate assessment of chamber volume,[25–27] mass,[16,25,28] and function[29,30] (Figs. 10–34 and 10–35, p. 337). Whether the additional precision and accuracy afforded by CT and MRI justify the additional expense of these techniques and the biological hazards of CT (contrast media and small radiation exposure) remains to be proved. Nonetheless, in terms of theoretical and practical experience, the newer tomographic methods should be considered the most precise and accurate in this application.

Radionuclide methods, while not extremely precise for the calculation of left ventricular mass or volume, nonetheless offer acceptable accuracy for the determination of left ventricular systolic and diastolic performance[31] (see p. 434). Radionuclide determinations of left ventricular function are achieved without the necessity of the geometrical assumptions common to echocardiography and without the requirements for detailed definition of endocardial and epicardial contours (by hand or computer tracing) that are characteristic of echocardiographic, CT, and MRI methods.

Echocardiographic or radionuclide techniques can be used at the bedside and thus are the techniques of choice in the assessment of left ventricular function in the critical care unit or the emergency department. Overall, radionuclide techniques appear to offer a good balance of accuracy, ease of use, portability, and cost-effectiveness for the quantitative determination of left ventricular function. In situations in which extremely precise determinations of left ventricular mass or volume are desired, the use of CT or MRI may be justified (Fig. 10–2, p. 320).

RIGHT VENTRICULAR FUNCTION. Assessment of the function of the right ventricle is more difficult than that of the left ventricle because of the complex shape of the right ventricle, which defies easy representation by simple geometrical models. Although echocardiographic methods of quantitatively assessing right ventricular function have been developed,[32] there has not been widespread use of these techniques. Fast CT is extremely precise and accurate in the derivation of right ventricular volumes[33] and stroke volumes,[34] and MRI methods also appear to have impressive accuracy for assessment of right ventricular function[27,35] and mass.[35,36] First-pass radionuclide ventriculography[37] (see p. 300) is a relatively inexpensive and simple method that can determine right ventricular ejection fraction accurately at the bedside or in the clinical imaging area.

VALVULAR FUNCTION. A complete assessment of valvular function requires determining the anatomical and physiological characteristics of the valve itself (such as the degree of stenosis or regurgitation) as well as defining the effect of the valvular abnormality on ventricular or atrial anatomy and performance. For the determination of valvular anatomy, transvalvular gradient, and the severity of valvular regurgitation, echocardiographic methods (including imaging and Doppler approaches) are the current procedures of choice.[38] Particularly with the wide availability of high-quality pulsed, continuous-wave, and color flow Doppler systems, coupled with transesophageal echocardiography in selected patients, the assessment of valvular heart disease in general falls within the domain of echocardiography (Figs. 3–55, p. 75, and 3–63, p. 77). With regard to determining the effect of the valvular abnormality on chamber size and function, the previous comments concerning the relative precision and accuracy of radionuclide, ultrasound, CT, and MRI methods apply.

Assessment of Myocardial Perfusion

At present, the only approach widely used clinically to identify regional deficits in perfusion is radionuclide imaging with thallium-201 or with the more recently developed technetium-99m–labeled perfusion agents, performed at rest and with exercise stress or pharmacological vasodilation (Figs. 9–19, p. 285, and 9–20, p. 286). Unfortunately, these techniques have shortcomings in terms of both the physics of the imaging agents and the inability of conventional radionuclide imaging to estimate absolute values of regional myocardial perfusion. Therefore, several additional methods of determining perfusion are being developed. As shown in Figure 11–1, the various methods of assessing perfusion or indices related to perfusion can be considered systematically on the basis of the anatomical level at which data are acquired, beginning at the level of the epicardial coronary arteries. Clinicians commonly interpret the sever-

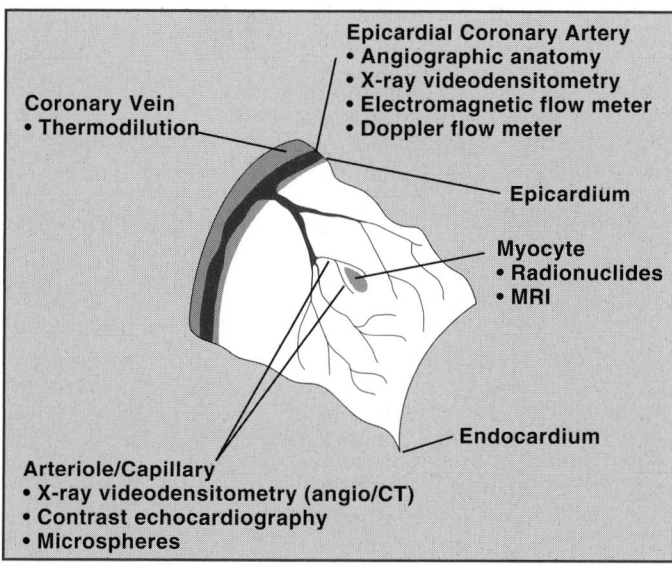

FIGURE 11–1. Current and evolving approaches to the assessment of coronary artery flow and myocardial perfusion. A schematic cross section of the left ventricular wall is shown, along with an indication of the anatomical levels at which various methods are used to evaluate perfusion. At the level of the epicardial coronary arteries, angiographic anatomy is commonly used to identify hydraulically significant stenoses, thereby inferring the potential for hypoperfusion with stress. X-ray videodensitometry and electromagnetic and Doppler flowmeters also may be used to assess perfusion at the level of the coronary arteries. (Some of these methods can be used only with an open chest.) Coronary venous thermodilution methods offer some insight into global or regional perfusion. At the arteriolar/capillary level, x-ray videodensitometry, contrast echocardiography, and microspheres may be employed. Finally, radionuclide and magnetic resonance imaging (MRI) methods attempt to assess perfusion at the level of the myocyte. Angio, angiography; CT, computed tomography.

In the figure:

Epicardial Coronary Artery
• Angiographic anatomy
• X-ray videodensitometry
• Electromagnetic flow meter
• Doppler flow meter

Coronary Vein
• Thermodilution

Epicardium

Myocyte
• Radionuclides
• MRI

Endocardium

Arteriole/Capillary
• X-ray videodensitometry (angio/CT)
• Contrast echocardiography
• Microspheres

ity of narrowing of a particular coronary artery on the cine-angiogram as an indicator of the likelihood of hypoperfusion distal to that stenosis. Thus arterial stenoses in excess of 50 to 75 per cent diameter narrowing are commonly assumed to represent hydraulically significant stenoses, capable of limiting flow at high rates.[39] Unfortunately, percentage diameter stenosis is an imperfect estimator of the functional significance of individual coronary lesions.[40] Further, this approach gives no information on *absolute* levels of regional perfusion. Videodensitometric techniques evaluate transit time or other measures of flow rate through an epicardial coronary artery based on angiograms and showed some potential in early studies.[41,42] However, due in part to the relative complexity of the measurements, quantitative assessment of coronary angiographic transit time has not gained widespread acceptance. Doppler ultrasound devices, either mounted on intracoronary catheters or placed directly on the epicardial coronary arteries in the operating room, have been used to measure velocity of coronary flow.[43] These devices may be used to estimate relative coronary flow at rest and after a hyperemic stimulus, giving a measure of coronary flow reserve. Once again, these methods do not yield absolute measures of myocardial perfusion or regional perfusion data and are not widely employed in routine clinical practice.

The next anatomical level to consider is that of the coronary microvasculature. Several densitometric methods use various indicators and the principles of indicator-dilution theory to assess myocardial perfusion. Thus the kinetics of indicator entry into and washout from the myocardium may be assessed utilizing angiography[44] or CT[45] (in which an iodinated contrast medium is the indicator) or echocardiography[4,46] (in which "microbubbles" or other echogenic material is used as the indicator) (Fig. 3–98, p. 90). Perhaps most relevant to the clinician and physiologist would be the determination of nutrient flow at the level of the myocyte, utilizing indicators that are taken up by normally perfused cells. Thus radionuclides such as thallium-201[47] or technetium-99m–labeled perfusion agents[48] are used for the qualitative assessment of regional perfusion because of their relatively avid uptake by myocardial cells.

The most promising radionuclide approach to quantitative myocardial perfusion imaging is PET (see p. 304). The combination of the high-energy photons released during positron annihilation (511 keV) and the method of coincidence detection for image formation permits high-resolution depiction of the distribution of a perfusion tracer. The high temporal resolution, together with a quantitative imaging capability, combined with the use of multicompartment tracer kinetic models permits accurate estimates of absolute levels of myocardial perfusion.[49–52]

MRI methods, coupled with paramagnetic contrast agents, also show promise for the delineation of myocardial perfusion (Fig. 10–6, p. 322). For example, regional myocardial concentration of manganese has been shown to correlate with microsphere-determined blood flow.[53] Recent studies using gadolinium-based MRI contrast agents or other substances also appear promising for the assessment of myocardial perfusion.[54–56]

As of this writing, PET and fast CT appear to be the methods most capable of accurate, absolute measurements of regional myocardial perfusion at rest and with stress.

Assessment of Myocardial Metabolism

Two general approaches to the assessment of myocardial metabolism appear to be possible through imaging techniques: PET and MR spectroscopy. These two methods should be viewed as complementary,[57] since they offer different insights into the biochemistry of the myocardium. PET offers a wide range of metabolic information. Chief among these are studies of the uptake of fuel substrates such as glucose[58] and fatty acids.[59] Further, oxidative metabolism may be assessed quantitatively using PET.[60] Measurements of receptor density and function[61] and of other aspects of intermediary metabolism also may be performed utilizing PET (Fig. 9–40, Color plate 7).

MR spectroscopy of the myocardium is still in its infancy compared with PET. Nonetheless, MR spectroscopy shows promise and potentially can be performed using a variety of nuclei including protons (hydrogen nuclei), phosphorus-31, carbon-13, fluorine-19, and sodium-23.[62–64] Currently, whole-body spectroscopy seems most feasible with phosphorus-31 or proton methods. Phosphorus-31 spectroscopy allows quantitation of the relative amounts of myocardial high-energy phosphates, including phosphocreatine, inorganic phosphate, and adenosine triphosphate.[62,63,65] In addition to a "snapshot" assessment of the relative amounts of various high-energy phosphate compounds at a given point in time, magnetization transfer techniques show promise for the assessment of enzyme kinetics in vivo.[66] Finally, phosphorus-31 spectroscopy offers the potential of assessing intracellular pH, and MR spectroscopy using carbon-13 or protons offers insights into aspects of intermediary metabolism.

Delineation of Tissue Characteristics

In selected patients, clinicians will wish to have information on the physical characteristics or composition of the myocardium. For example, identification of the amount of scar tissue versus viable myocardium present after myocardial infarction is of great clinical interest. Similarly, knowledge of the degree of myocardial fibrosis attendant to long-standing volume overload in aortic regurgitation likely would be of use in the timing of valve replacement. The two techniques that appear to be most promising in the assessment of tissue characteristics are ultrasonography and MRI.

Myocardial reflection or absorption of ultrasound depends in part on tissue composition. Thus, acoustic characteristics of injured tissue may differ from those of normal myocardium. For example, edema related to acute ischemia and infarction, necrosis attendant to acute infarction, collagen deposition in chronic infarction, and atherosclerosis in vessel walls have all been identified using acoustic ultrasonographic analyses.[67] Further, diffuse cardiomyopathies, such as amyloidosis (Fig. 41–21, p. 1428) and hypertrophic cardiomyopathy, have been identified and differentiated from each other and from hypertensive left ventricular hypertrophy utilizing ultrasonographic tissue characterization methods.[68] Although many technical problems related to the acquisition of ultrasound data remain to be solved before these methods will be widely useful clinically, the general approach appears promising.

MRI techniques also may identify alterations in tissue composition based on differing image brightness in appropriately weighted images or on measurement of tissue NMR relaxation times. For example, alterations in image intensity, in myocardial T_1 and T_2 relaxation times, or in proton spectra have been demonstrated in infarction,[69–71] scar,[72] and "stunned" myocardium.[73] Paramagnetic contrast agents such as gadolinium appear to accentuate the image intensity and relaxation time differences and thus improve identification of myocardial abnormalities with MRI.[74]

EVALUATING SPECIFIC CATEGORIES OF CARDIAC DISEASE WITH IMAGING METHODS

In Table 11–5 and the following paragraphs is a summary of our opinions on the relative current utility of the various imaging methods in specific patient groups.

Ischemic Heart Disease
(See also Chaps. 37 and 38)

CORONARY ATHEROSCLEROSIS. The presence and extent of coronary atherosclerosis can be characterized most definitively utilizing selective coronary angiography. Particularly in the present era of aggressive interventional techniques to reduce the severity of coronary atherosclerotic narrowing, a large percentage of patients with ischemic heart disease will continue to be candidates for selective coronary angiography. As sophisticated methods of analyzing coronary arteriograms are further developed and validated, some advantages may accrue to the acquisition of coronary arteriographic data in digital format so that the newer computer analysis algorithms may be easily applied.[75]

Two other imaging approaches also make contributions to the diagnosis of coronary atherosclerosis. Intravascular ultrasound (see p. 58) permits extremely high resolution imaging of coronary lumen and adjacent wall thickness and composition (e.g., the presence of calcified plaque).[76,77] Recent intravascular ultrasound studies have demonstrated atherosclerosis in regions of coronary arteries judged normal on angiography.[76] CT also can contribute to the diagnosis of coronary atherosclerosis by the identification of coronary calcification[78,79] (Fig. 10–37, p. 339).

ACUTE FLOW DISTURBANCE AND TRANSIENT ISCHEMIA. In many patients with ischemic heart disease, coronary angiography is not indicated, particularly upon initial presentation. Thus, methods of identifying reduced coronary flow reserve or transient ischemia, particularly with exercise stress or pharmacological coronary vasodilation, are of great interest to clinicians. Thallium-201 scintigraphy (employing exercise stress or pharmacological vasodilation[47]) remains a useful procedure for the identification of regional myocardial ischemia, including the approximate severity of ischemia (Fig. 9–29, p. 294) and, in some patients, the identification of multivessel disease. The newer ^{99m}Tc-based myocardial perfusion tracers (Fig. 9–1, p. 275) and PET will ensure a continued important role for radionuclide methods in the assessment of transient ischemia.

Exercise or pharmacological stress radionuclide ventriculography and echocardiography offer an indirect but especially useful marker for acute ischemia: the appearance of new regional wall motion disturbances resulting from acute hypoperfusion of the myocardium. Although it does not give direct information on myocardial perfusion, the delineation of new regional wall motion disturbances (particu-

**TABLE 11–5   RELATIVE USEFULNESS OF CARDIAC IMAGING METHODS
IN SPECIFIC PATIENT GROUPS***

DISORDER	CXR	ECHO/DOPPLER	ANGIO†	RADIONUCLIDES	FCT	MRI
Ischemic	+	++	++++	+++	++	++
Valvular	++	++++	++++	++	+++	+++
Congenital	++	++++	++++	++	++++	++++
Traumatic	++	+++	+++	++	++	++
Cardiomyopathy	+	++++	+++	++	+++	+++
Pericardial	+	+++	++	0	++++	++++
Endocarditis	+	++++	++	0	++	+++
Masses	0	++++	+++	+	++++	++++

* 0, no information; ++++, maximum information; CXR, chest x-ray; echo, echocardiography; angio, angiography; FCT, fast computed tomography; MRI, magnetic resonance imaging.
† Angio includes both imaging and hemodynamic evaluation.

larly systolic ventricular wall thinning) will likely make stress echocardiography a more widely used technique in the future[80] (Fig. 3–90, p. 87). CT methods are much less widely used in the identification of transient ischemia because of the relatively small number of installed systems capable of performing high-speed CT imaging with pharmacologic stress. MRI may prove useful in the diagnosis of ischemia if paramagnetic contrast agents are found to be efficacious in identifying regional deficits in perfusion[81] or if spectroscopy becomes widely available.[82] However, because of the widespread availability of radionuclide methods and echocardiography, MRI probably will *not* be a first-line method for assessing acute or transient ischemia in the near future.

INFARCTION/REPERFUSION (see Chap. 37).   The only clinically available imaging methods capable of directly identifying acutely necrotic myocardium are ⁹⁹ᵐTc pyrophosphate scintigraphy and labeled monoclonal antimyosin-specific antibody[83] scintigraphy (Fig. 9–19, p. 285). Although these methods permit the identification of acute necrosis, their clinical applicability is somewhat limited by their poor spatial resolution, which precludes detailed assessment of the size of myocardial infarction. Nonetheless, infarct-avid scintigraphy is, in selected patients, a useful method of infarct identification. Metabolic imaging with PET (see p. 306) shows great promise in the identification and quantitation of acute myocardial infarction.[84] MR spectroscopy using ³¹P also may prove to be useful in identifying infarction.[65]

Analysis of regional wall motion is also a useful method of indirectly identifying acute myocardial infarction. If a patient is known to have had normal wall motion in a particular region before an infarction, echocardiographic delineation of regional wall motion disturbances in that region permit some assessment of the size of infarction, as do similar wall motion analyses utilizing radionuclide, CT, or MRI techniques. However, the assessment of regional wall motion abnormalities is plagued by the inherent biological heterogeneity of contraction in normal subjects,[85] by the fact that regional wall motion patterns appear to be load-dependent,[86] and by the nonspecificity of regional wall motion abnormalities. Acute ischemia, infarction, and scar may all be associated with similar wall motion abnormalities. Thus, in the future, these indirect techniques may have a lesser place in the identification of infarction than more direct methods.

Discrimination among reperfused, nonreperfused but viable, and irreversibly injured tissue is important, particularly with the availability of potent thrombolytic agents and other interventional procedures. The reversal of a regional wall motion disturbance identified by echocardiography, radionuclide ventriculography, CT, or MRI is a good marker for reperfusion of viable myocardium. Wall motion may not immediately return to normal, however, because the myocardium may be "stunned" (see p. 388) or "hibernating" (see p. 388). Echocardiography performed before and after pharmacological stimulation of the myocardium (e.g., with dobutamine) (see p. 289) may reveal an increase in regional contraction after stimulation. This approach is showing promise as a method of determining myocardial viability.[87] The most direct method available to help the clinician negotiate the quandary of assessing myocardial viability is metabolic imaging with PET. For example, the combination of PET scans of fuel substrate uptake and perfusion offers a unique strategy to differentiate viable from irreversibly injured myocardium (Fig. 9–41, Color plate 8). Fatty acids are the preferred substrate for normal myocardium; nonetheless, normal myocardium does take up glucose. Ischemic but viable myocardium may take up increased amounts of glucose as it operates in an oxygen-limited environment. Thus, the combination of PET scans showing preserved or *increased* glucose uptake in a region of *decreased* perfusion (a "mismatch") suggests that

the region is, in fact, potentially viable. A concordant decrement in perfusion and fuel substrate uptake identifies irreversibly injured myocardium.[88]

The assessment of high-energy phosphate stores by MR spectroscopy also offers the potential for identification of the presence and extent of irreversibly injured myocardial tissue, although this approach remains investigative.

CHRONIC INFARCTION/SCAR FORMATION (see Chap. 38).   As already described, the combination of lack of perfusion and lack of fuel substrate uptake on PET identifies a region as infarcted, although scar tissue from earlier infarction may produce the same pattern (Fig. 9–40, Color plate 8). Fibrosis may be identified directly in the future by the use of echocardiographic[89] or MRI tissue characterization[90] techniques or by PET as the fraction of tissue unable to exchange water rapidly.[91] As of this writing, however, no widely available imaging method is capable of identifying directly the presence and extent of myocardial fibrosis in the clinical setting. Thus, clinicians must depend on persistent abnormalities of regional contraction and decreased wall thickness (as delineated by echocardiography, radionuclide ventriculography, CT, or MRI) to identify chronic infarction.

Valvular Heart Disease
(See also Chap. 32)

Echocardiography remains the procedure of choice for the initial assessment of patients with valvular heart disease. Frequently, decisions regarding medical and surgical management are based on echocardiography without the need for invasive evaluation. In selected patients, angiography and cardiac catheterization are still quite useful, particularly in the identification of concomitant coronary artery disease and when ultrasound examinations yield equivocal results. CT and MRI methods offer the ability to determine left ventricular mass more precisely than does echocardiography. Regurgitant volume also can be determined accurately with CT[34] (see p. 336). This may prove useful in selected patients with valvular heart disease.

Congenital Heart Disease
(See also Chaps. 29 and 30)

Clinicians caring for patients with congenital heart disease require accurate information on cardiac morphology, often in settings of extremely complex spatial relationships among atria, ventricles, and great vessels. Methods capable of high-resolution anatomical assessment are of paramount importance in congenital heart disease. Currently, echocardiography is the initial method of choice in evaluating the anatomy of the heart and great vessels, whether in fetus, newborn, child, adolescent, or adult with established or suspected congenital heart disease. In addition to echocardiography, first-pass radionuclide angiography also offers information of use in congenital heart disease by permitting accurate noninvasive quantitation of cardiac shunts.[92] CT[93] and MRI[94] also permit shunt identification and quantitation.

Echocardiographic methods (including Doppler techniques) frequently yield diagnostic information of sufficient reliability to obviate the need for cardiac catheterization in relatively simple abnormalities, such as atrial septal defects in patients younger than 40 years of age. Invasive angiographic, oximetric, and hemodynamic studies will be needed, however, in many complex anomalies before surgical intervention. For abnormalities of the great vessels, particularly disorders of the aorta and pulmonary arteries, CT (Fig. 10–41, p. 341) and MRI (Fig. 10–20, p. 327) offer extremely useful information in selected patients. Finally, assessment of patients who have undergone complex repairs, particularly those involving the placement of conduits or baffles, is greatly aided by CT and especially MRI studies. The three-dimensional imaging characteristics of

MRI and the ability to assess intracardiac, great vessel, and conduit flow may make MRI of increasing importance in these patients.[95-97]

Traumatic Heart Disease and Aortic Disease
(See also Chaps. 44 and 45)

Assessment of the trauma patient with suspected cardiovascular sequelae generally involves a search for myocardial contusion, deceleration injuries (e.g., chordal rupture, aortic dissection), and, in the case of penetrating wounds, a wide variety of problems (including hemopericardium, tricuspid valve damage, and coronary artery laceration). While echocardiography is of use in the identification of acute valvular disruption, it may be difficult to perform after major thoracic trauma. Transesophageal echocardiography,[98] CT,[99] and MRI[100] are useful in identifying acute aortic dissection or rupture; of these three methods, only echocardiography can be performed at the bedside (Fig. 45-15, p. 1562).

Echocardiography, CT, or MRI may be used to identify abnormalities of regional ventricular contraction that indirectly suggest myocardial contusion. Technetium-99m pyrophospate scintigraphy identifies myocardial contusion directly (Fig. 44-7, p. 1541) but has a temporal limitation: the need to wait at least 24 hours after injury for acceptable scan sensitivity.

Cardiac catheterization may be required to assess the condition of selected patients after trauma, particularly those with suspected coronary injuries. Most, however, will be evaluated adequately using echocardiography, CT, and/or MRI.

Cardiomyopathies
(See also Chap. 41)

Although echocardiography is capable of differentiating among dilated, hypertrophic, and restrictive cardiomyopathies in most patients, it offers limited insight into the specific causes of these disorders. Observations of unusual echocardiographic textural appearance of the myocardium in amyloidosis (Fig. 3-102, p. 92) and hypertrophic cardiomyopathy have led to investigative quantitative approaches to discrimination among these disorders with ultrasound tissue characterization methods.[68] Although as of this writing these are not clinically applicable, tissue characterization may become available in the future. Perhaps more promising in selected disorders will be metabolic studies with PET and MR spectroscopy. As of this writing, invasive studies, including hemodynamic evaluation and sometimes endomyocardial biopsy, also are required in selected cases for complete characterization of the type and severity of cardiomyopathy.

Pericardial Disease
(See also Chap. 43)

Echocardiographic methods can ascertain the presence of pericardial effusion as well as give some indication of the existence of tamponade; therefore, echocardiography is the initial procedure of choice in investigating the patient with suspected pericardial effusion (Fig. 3-104, p. 93). In selected cases, echocardiography may be supplemented by CT or MRI. Due to the wider field of view of these latter methods, in some patients a better appreciation of the quantity and anatomical distribution of the effusion may be gained (Figs. 10-15, p. 325, and 10-41, p. 341). However, echocardiography, CT, and MRI give limited information on the cause of the effusion. Positron emission tomography and MRI may eventually offer assistance in this regard.

Echocardiographic images are of only limited value in identifying pericardial thickening and delineating the physiology of constrictive pericarditis. CT[101] and MRI[102] offer excellent visualization of the pericardium (Fig. 10-14, p. 325, and 10-40, p. 340) and are probably more useful than echocardiography in precise measurement of the thickness

of the pericardium. Recent investigations with Doppler echocardiography,[103] CT,[104] and MRI[105] suggest that these noninvasive techniques may give information relevant to the diagnosis of constrictive pericarditis. Thus noninvasive assessment of diastolic filling may offer some help in the diagnosis of constrictive pericarditis, but these methods are still not as well established as hemodynamic data obtained at cardiac catheterization (see p. 187).

Infective Endocarditis
(See also Chap. 33)

The presence of vegetations may be established in the majority of patients using echocardiography (Fig. 3-61, p. 77). The advent of transesophageal echocardiography has substantially improved the sensitivity of ultrasonic identification of vegetations.[106] Thus, ultrasound is the initial imaging technique of choice in the patient suspected of having infective endocarditis. It should be emphasized, however, that failure to identify a vegetation by echocardiography should not be used to exclude definitively a diagnosis of endocarditis, since false-negative examination results do occur, even with transesophageal echocardiography.

The complications of endocarditis, including valve disruption and abscess formation, often can be identified with echocardiography (Fig. 3-63, p. 77), and likely with CT or MRI as well. Catheterization and angiocardiography are rarely necessary to identify either the presence of endocarditis or its attendant complications.

Intracardiac Masses
(See also Chaps. 42 and 57)

In addition to vegetations, clinicians will encounter other varieties of intracardiac mass lesions, including thrombi, myxomata, and metastatic tumors. Once again, echocardiography is quite useful in assessment of these patients (Fig. 3-105, p. 94). Transesophageal echocardiography has proved particularly helpful in identifying thrombi in areas that are difficult to image by other methods, such as the left atrial appendage in patients with a suspected cardiogenic source of cerebral emboli.[107] CT and MRI are also excellent methods of identifying intracardiac masses (Figs. 10-18, p. 326, and 10-42, p. 341) and should be considered when the results of echocardiography are equivocal. The determination of the nature of an intracardiac mass is best made currently by indirect evidence, such as the anatomical position and attachment of the mass, but such methods as characterization of the tissue by ultrasonography or MRI may prove helpful in this regard in the future.

COST CONSIDERATIONS IN CARDIAC IMAGING

A major, global change is occurring in the practice of medicine, wherein the intellectual challenge is framed less by what we *can* do and more by what we *should* do. Increasingly, the physician is faced with the dilemma that the best possible care for the patient is not necessarily aligned with the optimal use of resources for society. Even when imaging is likely to be beneficial, recommendations can be expected to differ between a managed care organization concerned with "covered lives" and a physician who has responsibility for an individual patient. The clinician strives to do the right thing for a patient even when outcomes data, cost-effectiveness information, and practice guidelines are of dubious relevance to the individual case. Only the personal physician can be aware of the diverse factors impacting the patient's care at any given time.

The several methods of imaging the heart and circulation vary widely in their costs. In considering these variations, several types of expenses should be considered (Table 11-6). These include the initial purchase price of the system

TABLE 11–6 SOME COSTS ASSOCIATED WITH CARDIAC IMAGING METHODS

Purchase price of system
Site preparation
Power, water, and environmental costs
Personnel
   Physicians
   Nurses
   Technicians
   Support personnel (physicists, engineers, pharmacists, others)

and any necessary expenditures for site preparation. Once the system is installed, consideration must be given to power and environmental costs. Personnel costs to be considered include the physicians, technicians, and nurses who deal with the day-to-day operation of the system, as well as support personnel for maintenance and quality control testing. Overall, in terms of establishing and operating a particular imaging system, excluding chest roentgenography, echocardiography falls at the least expensive end of the spectrum, although a complete modern echocardiographic system costs about $250,000. At the other end of the spectrum are CT, MRI, and PET, all of which cost in excess of $1 million. Conventional radionuclide imaging falls between these extremes of the cost spectrum.

Currently evolving changes in the health care reimbursement system, however, may render some of these cost comparisons less relevant. The total cost of a complete diagnostic evaluation for a particular disorder will likely become the factor of key interest. Thus a relatively more expensive technique that eliminates other tests may reduce the overall cost of an individual patient workup. An a priori expensive test may become, thereby, a rather cost-effective test. This approach, however, will necessitate discipline on the part of the responsible clinician to choose only those imaging tests which add unique information that will significantly impact patient management decisions.

SUMMARY AND CONCLUSION

A large, at times bewildering set of choices in diagnostic imaging methods confronts clinicians evaluating patients with known or suspected cardiovascular disease. The varying biophysical bases of the several available imaging approaches suggest their complementarity in patient evaluation. We have offered our consensus opinions on the relative merits of available and evolving imaging methods in general and for specific patient groups. In the individual practice setting, availability and local expertise are additional, critical factors to be considered.

REFERENCES

SCOPE OF CARDIAC IMAGING

1. Skorton, D. J., Schelbert, H. R., Wolf, G. L., and Brundage, B. H. (eds.): Marcus Cardiac Imaging. 2nd ed. (A companion to E. Braunwald, Heart Disease.) Philadelphia, W. B. Saunders Company, 1996.
2. Pohost, G. M., and O'Rourke, R. A.: Principles and Practice of Cardiovascular Imaging. Boston, Little, Brown, 1991.
3. Hounsfield, G. N.: Computed medical imaging (Nobel lecture, December 8, 1979). J. Comput. Assist. Tomogr. 4:665, 1980.
4. Jayaweera, A. R., and Kaul, S.: Quantifying myocardial blood flow with contrast echocardiography. Am. J. Cardiac Imaging 7:317, 1993.
5. Wickline, S. A., Verdonk, E. D., Wong, A. K., et al.: Structural remodeling of human myocardial tissue after infarction: Quantification with ultrasonic backscatter. Circulation 85:259, 1992.
6. Siu, S. C., Rivera, J. M., Guerrero, J. L., et al.: Three-dimensional echocardiography: In vivo validation for left ventricular volume and function. Circulation 88 (Part 1):1715, 1993.
7. Schelbert, H. R.: Blood flow and metabolism by PET. In Verani, M. S. (ed.): Cardiology Clinics, Nuclear Cardiology: State of the Art. Vol. 12. Philadelphia, W.B. Saunders Company, 1994, p. 303.
8. Koning, G., Brandvanden, M., Zorn, I., et al.: Usefulness of digital angiography in the assessment of left ventricular ejection fraction. Cathet. Cardiovasc. Diagn. 21:185, 1990.
9. Edelman, R. R., and Warach, S.: Magnetic resonance imaging. N. Engl. J. Med. 328:708, 1993.
10. Mohiaddin, R. H., and Longmore, D. B.: Functional aspects of cardiovascular nuclear magnetic resonance imaging: Techniques and application. Circulation 88:264, 1993.
11. Weiss, R. G., Bottomley, P. A., Hardy, C. J., and Gerstenblith, G.: Regional myocardial metabolism of high-energy phosphates during isometric exercise in patients with coronary artery disease. N. Engl. J. Med. 323:1593, 1990.
12. Brundage, B. H.: Myocardial imaging with ultrafast computed tomography. In Zoreb, B. L., Kaufman, L., Berson, A. S., and Dunn, R. A. (eds.): Frontiers in Cardiovascular Imaging. New York, Raven Press, 1993, p. 35.
13. Jones, J. P.: Physics of the MR image: From the basic principles to image intensity and contrast. In Partain, C. L., Price, R. R., Patton, J. A., et al. (eds.): Magnetic Resonance Imaging. 2nd ed. Vol. 2: Physical Principles and Instrumentation. Philadelphia, W.B. Saunders Company, 1988, p. 1003.
14. Collins, S. M., and Skorton, D. J. (eds.): Cardiac Imaging and Image Processing. New York, McGraw-Hill Book Co., 1986.
15. Buda, A. J., and Delp, E. J.: Digital Cardiac Imaging. Boston, Martinus Nijhoff, 1985.

MEETING THE GOALS OF CARDIAC IMAGING

16. Feiring, A. J., Rumberger, J. A., Reiter, S. J., et al.: Determination of left ventricular mass in dogs with rapid-acquisition cardiac computed tomographic scanning. Circulation 72:1355, 1985.
17. Pattynama, P. M. T., de Roos, A., van der Wall, E. E., and van der Voorthuisen, A. D. E.: Evaluation of cardiac function with magnetic resonance imaging. Am. Heart J. 128:595, 1994.
18. Pearlman, J. D., and Edelman, R. R.: Ultrafast magnetic resonance imaging: Segmented turboflash, echo-planar, and real-time nuclear magnetic resonance. Radiol. Clin. North Am. 32:593, 1994.
19. Napel, S., Rutt, B. K., and Pflugfelder, P.: Three-dimensional images of the coronary arteries from ultrafast computed tomography: Method and comparison with two-dimensional arteriography. Am. J. Cardiac Imaging 3:237, 1989.
20. Iliceto, S., Marangelli, V., Memmola, C., and Rizzon, P.: Transesophageal Doppler echocardiography evaluation of coronary blood flow velocity in baseline conditions and during dipyridamole-induced coronary vasodilation. Circulation 83:61, 1991.
21. Manning, W. J., Li, W., and Edelman, R. R.: A preliminary report comparing magnetic resonance coronary angiography with conventional angiography. N. Engl. J. Med. 328:828, 1993.
22. Stanford, W., Brundage, B. H., MacMillan, R., et al.: Sensitivity and specificity of assessing coronary bypass graft patency with ultrafast computed tomography: Results of a multicenter study. J. Am. Coll. Cardiol. 12:1, 1988.
23. Stanford, W., Galvin, J. R., Thompson, B. H., Grover-McKay, M., and Skorton, D. J.: Nonangiographic assessment of coronary artery bypass graft patency. Int. J. Cardiac Imaging 9:77, 1993.
24. Schiller, N. B., Shah, P. M., Crawford, M., DeMaria, A., et al.: American Society of Echocardiography Committee on Standards, Subcommittee on Quantitation of Two-Dimensional Echocardiograms: Recommendations for quantitation of the left ventricle by two-dimensional echocardiography. J. Am. Soc. Echocardiogr. 2:358, 1989.
25. Roig, E., Georgiou, D., Chomka, E. V., Wolfkiel, C., LoGalbo-Zak, C., Rich, S., and Brundage, B. H.: Reproducibility of left ventricular myocardial volume and mass measurement by ultrafast computed tomography. J. Am. Coll. Cardiol. 18:990, 1991.
26. Hunter, G. J., Hamberg, L. M., Weisskoff, R. M., Halpern, E. F., and Brady, T. J.: Measurement of stroke volume and cardiac output within a single breath hold with echo-planar MR imaging. J. Magn. Reson. Imaging 4:51, 1994.
27. Kondo, C., Caputo, G. R., Semelka, R., et al.: Right and left ventricular stroke volume measurements with velocity-encoded cine MR imaging: In vitro and in vivo validation. A.J.R. 157:9, 1991.
28. Florentine, M. S., Grosskreutz, C. L., Chang, W., et al.: Measurement of left ventricular mass in vivo using gated nuclear magnetic resonance imaging. J. Am. Coll. Cardiol. 8:107, 1986.
29. Rumberger, J. A., Weiss, R. M., Feiring, A. J., et al.: Patterns of regional diastolic function in the normal human left ventricle: An ultrafast computed tomography study. J. Am. Coll. Cardiol. 14:119, 1989.
30. Beache, G. M., Wedeen, V. J., and Dinsmore, R. E.: Magnetic resonance imaging evaluation of left ventricular dimensions and function and pericardial and myocardial disease. Coronary Artery Dis. 4:328, 1993.
31. Gibbons, R. J.: Equilibrium radionuclide angiography. In Skorton, D. J., Schelbert, H. R., Wolf, G. L., and Brundage, B. H. (eds.): Marcus Cardiac Imaging. 2nd ed. (A companion to E. Braunwald, Heart Disease.) Philadelphia, W.B. Saunders Company, 1996.
32. Aebischer, N. M., and Czegledy, F.: Determination of right ventricular volume by two-dimensional echocardiography with a crescentic model. J. Am. Soc. Echocardiogr. 2:110, 1989.
33. Mahoney, L. T., Smith, W., Noel, M. P., et al.: Measurement of right ventricular volume using cine computed tomography. Invest. Radiol. 22:451, 1987.
34. Reiter, S. J., Rumberger, J. A., Feiring, A. J., et al.: Precision of measurements of right and left ventricular volume by cine computed tomography. Circulation 74:890, 1986.
35. Pattynama, P. M. T., Lamb, H. J., Van der Geest, R., et al.: Reproducibil-

ity of MRI-derived measurements of right ventricular volumes and myocardial mass. J. Magn. Reson. Imaging 13:53, 1995.

36. Doherty, N. E., Fujita, N., Caputo, G. R., and Higgins, C. B.: Measurement of right ventricular mass in normal and dilated cardiomyopathic ventricles using cine magnetic resonance imaging. Am. J. Cardiol. 69:1223, 1992.

37. Rezai, K., Weiss, R., Stanford, W., et al.: Relative accuracy of three scintigraphic methods for determination of right ventricular ejection fraction: A correlative study with ultrafast CT. J. Nucl. Med. 32:429, 1991.

38. van den Brink, R. B., Verheul, H. A., Hoedemaker, G., et al.: The value of Doppler echocardiography in the management of patients with valvular heart disease: analysis of one year of clinical practice. J. Am. Soc. Echocardiogr. 4:109, 1991.

39. Gould, K. L., and Lipscomb, K.: Effects of coronary stenoses on coronary flow reserve and resistance. Am. J. Cardiol. 34:48, 1974.

40. White, C. W., Wright, C. B., Doty, D. B., et al.: Does the visual interpretation of the coronary arteriogram predict the physiological importance of a coronary stenosis? N. Engl. J. Med. 310:819, 1984.

41. Rutishauser, W., Noseda, G., Bussman, W. D., and Preter, B.: Blood flow measurements through single coronary arteries by roentgen densitometry: II. Right coronary artery flow in conscious man. A.J.R. 109:21, 1970.

42. Smith, H. C., Sturm, R. E., and Wood, E. H.: Videodensitometric system for measurement of vessel blood flow, particularly in the coronary arteries, in man. Am. J. Cardiol. 32:144, 1973.

43. Wilson, R. F., Laughlin, D. E., Ackell, P. H., et al.: Transluminal subselective measurement of coronary artery blood flow velocity and vasodilator reserve in man. Circulation 72:82, 1985.

44. Hodgson, J. M., LeGrand, V., Bates, E. R., et al.: Validation in dogs of a rapid digital angiographic technique to measure relative coronary blood flow during routine cardiac catheterization. Am. J. Cardiol. 5:188, 1985.

45. Wolfkiel, C. J., and Brundage, B. H.: Measurement of myocardial blood flow by UFCT: Towards clinical applicability. Int. J. Cardiac Imaging 7:89, 1991.

46. Feinstein, S. B., Lang, R. M., Dick, C., et al.: Contrast echocardiography during coronary arteriography in humans: Perfusion and anatomic studies. J. Am. Coll. Cardiol. 11:59, 1988.

47. Beller, G.: Myocardial perfusion imaging with thallium-201. J. Nucl. Med. 35:674, 1994.

48. van Train, K.: Multicenter trial validation for quantitative analysis of same-day rest-stress technetium-99m-sestamibi myocardial tomograms. J. Nucl. Med. 35:609, 1994.

49. Kuhle, W., Porenta, G., Huang, S. C., et al.: Quantification of regional myocardial blood flow using ^{13}N-ammonia and reoriented dynamic positron emission tomographic imaging. Circulation 86:1004, 1992.

50. Bergmann, S. R., Herrero, P., Markham, J., et al.: Noninvasive quantitation of myocardial blood flow in human subjects with oxygen-15–labeled water and positron emission tomography. J. Am. Coll. Cardiol. 14:639, 1989.

51. Krivokapich, J., Smith, G. T., Huang, S. C., et al.: N-13 ammonia myocardial imaging at rest and with exercise in normal volunteers: Quantification of absolute myocardial perfusion with dynamic positron emission tomography. Circulation 80:1328, 1989.

52. Czernin, J., Müller, P., Chan, S., et al.: Influence of age and hemodynamics on myocardial blood flow and flow reserve. Circulation 88:62, 1993.

53. Schaefer, S., Lange, R. A., Kulkarni, P. V., et al.: In vivo nuclear magnetic resonance imaging of myocardial perfusion using the paramagnetic contrast agent manganese gluconate. J. Am. Coll. Cardiol. 14:472, 1989.

54. Edelman, R. R., and Li, W.: Contrast-enhanced echo-planar MR imaging of myocardial perfusion: Preliminary study in humans. Radiology 190:771, 1994.

55. Wendland, M. F., Saeed, M., Masui, T., Derugin, N., and Higgins, C. B.: First pass of an MR susceptibility contrast agent through normal and ischemic heart: Gradient-recalled echo-planar imaging. J. Magn. Reson. Imaging 3:755, 1993.

56. Saeed, M., Wendland, M. F., Masui, T., et al.: Dual mechanisms for change in myocardial signal intensity by means of a single MR contrast medium: Dependence on concentration and pulse sequence. Radiology 186:175, 1993.

57. Syrota, A., and Jehenson, P.: Complementarity of magnetic resonance spectroscopy, positron emission tomography and single photon emission tomography for the in vivo investigation of human cardiac metabolism and neurotransmission. Eur. J. Nucl. Med. 18:897, 1991.

58. Choi, Y., Brunken, R., Hawkins, R., et al.: Factors affecting myocardial 2-[F-18]fluoro-2-deoxy-D-glucose uptake in positron emission tomography studies of normal humans. Eur. J. Nucl. Med. 20:308, 1993.

59. Schelbert, H. R., Henze, E., Sochor, H., et al.: Effects of substrate availability on myocardial C-11 palmitate kinetics by positron emission tomography in normal subjects and patients with ventricular dysfunction. Am. Heart J. 111:1055, 1986.

60. Armbrecht, J. J., Buxton, D. B., Brunken, R. C., et al.: Regional myocardial oxygen consumption determined noninvasively in humans with [1-^{11}C]acetate and dynamic positron tomography. Circulation 80:863, 1989.

61. Merlet, P., Delforge, J., Syrota, A., et al.: Positron emission tomography with ^{11}C CGP-12177 to assess β-adrenergic receptor concentration in idiopathic dilated cardiomyopathy. Circulation 87:1169, 1993.

62. Bottomley, P. A.: Noninvasive study of high-energy phosphate metabolism in human heart by depth-resolved P-31 NMR spectroscopy. Science 229:769, 1985.

63. Bottomley, P. A., Hardy, C. J., and Roemer, P. B.: Phosphate metabolite imaging and concentration measurements in human heart by nuclear magnetic resonance. Magn. Reson. Med. 14:425, 1990.

64. Jelicks, L. A., and Gupta, R. K.: Nuclear magnetic resonance measurement of intracellular sodium in the perfused normotensive and spontaneously hypertensive rat heart. Am. J. Hypertens. 7:429, 1994.

65. Scholz, T. D., Grover-McKay, M., Fleagle, S. R., and Skorton, D. J.: Quantitation of the extent of acute myocardial infarction by phosphorus-31 nuclear magnetic resonance spectroscopy. J. Am. Coll. Cardiol. 18:1380, 1991.

66. Zahler, R., and Ingwall, J. S.: Estimation of heart mitochondrial creatine kinase flux using magnetization transfer NMR spectroscopy. Am. J. Physiol. 262:H1022, 1992.

67. Pérez, J. E., and Miller, J. G.: Ultrasonic backscatter tissue characterization in cardiac diagnosis. Clin. Cardiol. 14 (Suppl V):V-4, 1991.

68. Chandrasekaran, K., Aylward, P. E., Fleagle, S. R., et al.: Feasibility of identifying amyloid and hypertrophic cardiomyopathy with the use of computerized quantitative texture analysis of clinical echocardiographic data. J. Am. Coll. Cardiol. 13:832, 1989.

69. Johnston, D. L.: Myocardial tissue characterization with magnetic resonance imaging techniques. Am. J. Cardiac Imaging 8:140, 1994.

70. de Roos, A., van der Wall, E. E., Bruschke, A. V. G., and van Voorthuisen, A. E.: Magnetic resonance imaging in the diagnosis and evaluation of myocardial infarction. Magn. Reson. Q. 7:191, 1991.

71. Saeed, M., Wendland, M. R., Yu, K. K., et al.: Identification of myocardial reperfusion with echo planar magnetic resonance imaging: Discrimination between occlusive and reperfused infarctions. Circulation 90:1492, 1994.

72. Wisenberg, G., Prato, F. S., Carroll, S. E., et al.: Serial nuclear magnetic resonance imaging of acute myocardial infarction with and without reperfusion. Am. Heart J. 115:510, 1988.

73. Reeves, R. C., Evanochko, W. T., Canby, R. C., et al.: Demonstration of increased myocardial lipid with postischemic dysfunction ("myocardial stunning") by proton nuclear magnetic resonance spectroscopy. J. Am. Coll. Cardiol. 13:739, 1989.

74. Saeed, M., Wendland, M. F., and Higgins, C. B.: Contrast media for MR imaging of the heart. J. Magn. Reson. Imaging 4:269, 1994.

EVALUATING SPECIFIC CATEGORIES OF CARDIAC DISEASE

75. Rensing, B. J., Hermans, W. R. M., Deckers, J. W., et al.: Lumen narrowing after percutaneous transluminal coronary balloon angioplasty follows a near gaussian distribution: A quantitative angiographic study in 1445 successfully dilated lesions. J. Am. Coll. Cardiol. 19:939, 1992.

76. St.Goar, F. G., Pinto, F. J., Alderman, E. L., et al.: Intracoronary ultrasound in cardiac transplant recipients: In vivo evidence of "angiographically silent" intimal thickening. Circulation 85:979, 1992.

77. Linker, D. T., Kleven, A., Grønningsaether, Å., et al.: Tissue characterization with intra-arterial ultrasound: Special promise and problems. Int. J. Cardiac Imaging 6:255, 1991.

78. Agatston, A. S., Janowitz, W. R., Hildner, F. J., Zusmer, N. R., Viamonte, M., and Detrano, R.: Quantification of coronary artery calcium using ultrafast computed tomography. J. Am. Coll. Cardiol. 15:827, 1990.

79. Mautner, S. L., Mautner, G. L., Froelich, J., Feurstein, I. M., Proschan, M. A., Roberts, W. C., and Doppman, J. L.: Predicting coronary artery disease by electron beam tomography. Radiology 192:625, 1994.

80. Ryan, T., Segar, D. S., Sawada, S. G., et al.: Detection of coronary artery disease using upright bicycle exercise echocardiography. J. Am. Soc. Echocardiogr. 6:186, 1993.

81. Wendland, M. F., Saeed, M., Masui, T., Derugin, N., Moseley, M. E., and Higgins, C. B.: Echo-planar MR imaging of normal and ischemic myocardium with gadodiamide injection. Radiology 186:535, 1993.

82. Yabe, T., Mitsunami, K., Okada, M., Morikawa, S., Inubushi, T., and Kinoshita, M.: Detection of myocardial ischemia by ^{31}P magnetic resonance spectroscopy during handgrip exercise. Circulation 89:1709, 1994.

83. Maddahi, J.: Clinical applications of antimyosin monoclonal antibody imaging. Am. J. Cardiac Imaging 8:249, 1994.

84. Hicks, R., Melon, P., Kalff, V., et al.: Metabolic imaging by positron emission tomography early after myocardial infarction as a predictor of recovery of myocardial function after reperfusion. J. Nucl. Cardiol. 1:124, 1994.

85. Pandian, N. G., Skorton, D. J., Collins, S. M., et al.: Heterogeneity of left ventricular segmental wall thickening and excursion in two-dimensional echocardiograms of normal human subjects. Am. J. Cardiol. 51:1667, 1983.

86. Weiss, R. M., Shonka, M. D., Kinzey, J. E., et al.: Effects of loading alterations on the pattern of heterogeneity of regional left ventricular function (Abs.). FASEB J 2:1494A, 1988.

87. LaCanna, G., Alfieri, O., Giubbini, R., et al.: Echocardiography during infusion of dobutamine for identification of reversible dysfunction in patients with chronic coronary artery disease. J. Am. Coll. Cardiol. 23:617, 1994.

88. Tillisch, J., Brunken, R., Marshall, R., et al.: Reversibility of cardiac wall-motion abnormalities predicted by positron tomography. N. Engl. J. Med. 314:884, 1986.

89. Hoyt, R. H., Collins, S. M., Skorton, D. J., et al.: Assessment of fibrosis

in infarcted human hearts by analysis of ultrasonic backscatter. Circulation 71:740, 1985.

90. Hsu, J. C. M., Johnson, G. A., and Smith, W. M.: Magnetic resonance imaging of chronic myocardial infarcts in formalin-fixed human autopsy hearts. Circulation 89:2133, 1994.

91. Yamamoto, Y., De Silva, R., Rhodes, C., et al.: A new strategy for the assessment of viable myocardium and regional myocardial blood flow using 15O-water and dynamic positron emission tomography. Circulation 86:167, 1992.

92. Alazraki, N.: Nuclear imaging of valvular disease, left atrial myxoma, and shunts. In Elliott, L. P. (ed.): Cardiac Imaging in Infants, Children and Adults. Philadelphia, J. B. Lippincott Co., 1991, p. 796.

93. Garrett, J., Jaschke, W., Aherue, T., et al.: Quantitation of intracardiac shunts by cine-CT. J. Comput. Asst. Tomogr. 12:82, 1988.

94. Sieverding, L., Jung, W. I., Klose, U., and Apitz, J.: Noninvasive blood flow measurement and quantification of shunt volume by cine magnetic resonance in congenital heart disease: Preliminary results. Pediatr. Radiol. 22:48, 1992.

95. Link, K. M., and Lesko, N. M.: Magnetic resonance imaging in the evaluation of congenital heart disease. Magn. Reson. Q. 7:173, 1991.

96. Fellows, K. E., Weinberg, P. M., Baffa, J. M., and Hoffman, E. A.: Evaluation of congenital heart disease with MR imaging: Current and coming attractions. A.J.R. 159:925, 1992.

97. White, R. D.: Magnetic resonance imaging of congenital heart disease. In Pohost, G. M. (ed.): Cardiovascular Applications of Magnetic Resonance. Mount Kisco, N.Y., Futura, 1993, p. 59.

98. Smith, M. D., Cassidy, J. M., Souther, S., et al.: Transesophageal echocardiography in the diagnosis of traumatic rupture of the aorta. N. Engl. J. Med. 332:356, 1995.

99. Stanford, W., Rooholamini, S. A., and Galvin, J. R.: Ultrafast computed tomography in the diagnosis of aortic aneurysms and dissections. J. Thoracic Imaging 5:32, 1990.

100. Link, K. M., and Lesko, N. M.: The role of MR imaging in the evaluation of acquired disease of the thoracic aorta. A.J.R. 158:1115, 1992.

101. Grover-McKay, M., Burke, S., Thompson, S. A., et al.: Measurement of pericardial thickness by cine computed tomography. Am. J. Cardiac Imaging 5:98, 1991.

102. Didier, D., Terrier, R., and Grossholz, M.: Imaging of the pericardium using magnetic resonance (German). Radiologe 33:87, 1993.

103. Oh, J. K., Hatle, L. K., Seward, J. B., et al.: Diagnostic role of Doppler echocardiography in constrictive pericarditis. J. Am. Coll. Cardiol. 23:154, 1994.

104. Oren, R. M., Grover-McKay, M., Stanford, W., and Weiss, R. M.: Accurate preoperative diagnosis of pericardial constriction using cine computed tomography. J. Am. Coll. Cardiol. 22:832, 1993.

105. Masui, T., Finck, S., and Higgins, C. B.: Constrictive pericarditis and restrictive cardiomyopathy: Evaluation with MR imaging. Radiology 182:369, 1992.

106. Erbel, R., Rohmann, S., Drexler, M., et al.: Improved diagnostic value of echocardiography in patients with infective endocarditis by transesophageal approach: A prospective study. Eur. Heart J. 9:43, 1988.

107. Pearson, A. C., Labovitz, A. J., Tatineni S., and Gomez, C. R.: Superiority of transesophageal echocardiography in detecting cardiac source of embolism in patients with cerebral ischemia of uncertain etiology. J. Am. Coll. Cardiol. 17:66, 1991.

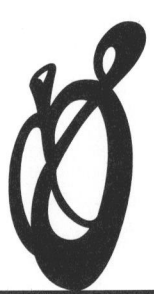

Part II
Normal and Abnormal Circulatory Function

Chapter 12

Mechanisms of Cardiac Contraction and Relaxation

LIONEL H. OPIE

MICROANATOMY OF CONTRACTILE CELLS AND PROTEINS

Ultrastructure of Contractile Cells

The contractile proteins of the heart lie within the muscle cells (cardiomyocytes), which constitute about 75 per cent of the total volume of the myocardium, although only about one-third in number of all the cells.[1] About half of each ventricular myocyte is occupied by myofibrils and about one-quarter to one-third by mitochondria (Table 12–1).[2] A myofiber is a group of myocytes (Fig. 12–1) held together by surrounding collagen connective tissue. Further strands of collagen connect myofibers to each other,[3] and excess collagen, as in left ventricular (LV) hypertrophy, may cause LV diastolic dysfunction.[1]

The individual cardiomyocytes that account for more than half of the heart's weight are roughly cylindrical in shape (Fig. 12–1). Those in the atrium are quite small, less than 10 microns in diameter and about 20 microns in length. Relative to atrial cells, human ventricular myocytes are large, measuring about 17 to 25 microns in diameter and 60 to 140 microns in length (Table 12–1).

When examined under the light microscope, the atrial and ventricular muscle cells have cross-striations and are branched.[2] Each cell is bounded by a complex cell membrane, the sarcolemma (sarco = flesh; lemma = thin husk), and is filled with rodlike bundles of myofibrils (Fig. 12–1). The latter are the contractile elements. The sarcolemma of the myocyte invaginates to form an extensive tubular network (T tubules) that extends the extracellular space into the interior of the cell (Figs. 12–1 and 12–2). The nucleus, which contains almost all of the cell's genetic information, is often centrally located. Some myocytes have several nuclei. Interspersed between the myofibrils and immediately beneath the sarcolemma are many mitochondria, the main function of which is to generate the energy in the form of adenosine triphosphate (ATP) needed to maintain the heart's contractile function and the associated ion gradients. Of the other organelles, the sarcoplasmic reticulum (SR), is most important (Fig. 12–3).

Anatomically, the SR is a fine network spreading throughout the myocytes, demarcated by its lipid bilayer which is rather similar to that of the sarcolemma. Parts of the SR lie in very close apposition to the T tubules.[2] Here the tubules of the SR expand into bulbous swellings, still hollow, which lie along the inner surface of the sarcolemma or are wrapped around the T tubules (Fig. 12–1). These expanded areas of the SR have several names: subsarcolemmal cisternae (baskets, Latin) or junctional SR. Sometimes the cisternae occur in pairs (dyads) lying astride the T tubule, the whole having the appearance of triads. Their function is to release calcium from the calcium release channel (also called the ryanodine receptor) to initiate the contractile cycle (Fig. 12–3 and Fig. 16–5, p. 481).

The second part of the SR, the longitudinal or network SR, consists of ramifying tubules (Fig. 12–1) and is concerned with the uptake of calcium that initiates relaxation. This uptake is achieved by the ATP-requiring calcium pump, also called SERCA (sarcoendoplasmic reticulum Ca^{++}-ATPase), that increases its activity in response to beta-adrenergic stimulation (see p. 405). Calcium taken up

TABLE 12–1   CHARACTERISTICS OF CARDIAC CELLS, ORGANELLES, AND CONTRACTILE PROTEINS

MICROANATOMY OF HEART CELLS			
	Ventricular Myocyte	Atrial Myocyte	Purkinje Cells
Shape	Long and narrow	Elliptical	Long and broad
Length (microns)	60–140	About 20	150–200
Diameter (microns)	About 20	5–6	35–40
Volume (microns³)	15–45,000	About 500	135,000–250,000
T tubules	Plentiful	Rare or none	Absent
Intercalated disc	Prominent end-to-end transmission	Side-to-side as well as end-to-end transmission	Very prominent; abundant gap junctions. Fast end-to-end transmission
General appearance	Mitochondria and sarcomeres very abundant Rectangular branching bundles with little interstitial collagen	Bundles of atrial tissue separated by wide areas of collagen	Fewer sarcomeres, paler

COMPOSITION AND FUNCTION OF VENTRICULAR CELL		
Organelle	Percentage of Cell Volume	Function
Myofibril	About 50–60	Interaction of thick and thin filaments during contraction cycle
Mitochondria	16 in neonate 33 in adult rat 23 in adult man	Provide ATP chiefly for contraction
T system	About 1	Transmission of electrical signal from sarcolemma to cell interior
Sarcoplasmic reticulum (SR)	33 in neonate 2 in adult	Takes up and releases Ca⁺⁺ during contraction cycle
Terminal cisternae of SR	0.33 in adult	Site of calcium storage and release
Rest of network of SR	Rest of volume	Site of calcium uptake en route to cisternae
Sarcolemma	Very low	Control of ionic gradients; channels for ions (action potential); maintenance of cell integrity; receptors for drugs and hormones
Nucleus	About 5	Protein synthesis
Lysosomes	Very low	Intracellular digestion and proteolysis
Sarcoplasm (= cytoplasm) (+ nuclei + other structures)	About 12 in adult rat, 18 in humans	Provides cytosol in which rise and fall of ionized calcium occurs; contains other ions and small molecules

is then stored at high concentration in a number of storage proteins, including *calsequestrin,* before being released again.

The *cytoplasm* is the intracellular fluid and proteins therein, contained within the sarcolemma but excluding the contents of organelles such as mitochondria and the SR. The fluid component of the cytoplasm, minus the proteins, is called the *cytosol.* It is in the cytosol that the concentrations of calcium ions rise and fall to cause cardiac contraction and relaxation. The proteins of the sarcoplasm include many specialized molecules, the *enzymes,* that act to accelerate the conversion of one chemical form to another, thereby eventually producing energy.

Contractile Proteins

The major function of myocardial myocytes lies in the contraction-relaxation cycle. The major molecules involved include the two chief contractile proteins, the thin *actin* filament and the thick *myosin* filament. The molecular structure of the myosin head is now well understood (Fig. 12–4). Of note is the concept that it is the elongated basal part of the head that changes configuration during the contractile cycle, and not flexion and extension at the head-tail junction, as previously thought. Calcium ions interact with troponin-C at binding sites now identified to relieve the inhibition otherwise exerted by troponin-I (Fig. 12–4). *Titin* is a newly discovered large elastic molecule that supports myosin. During contraction, the filaments slide over each other without the individual molecules of actin or myosin actually shortening. As they slide, they pull together the two ends of the fundamental contractile unit called the *sarcomere.* On electron microscopy, the sarcomere is limited on either side by the *Z line* (Z, abbreviation for German *Zückung,* contraction), to which the actin filaments are attached (Fig. 12–2). Conversely, the myosin filaments extend from the center of the sarcomere in either direction toward but not actually reaching the Z lines (Fig. 12–1).

The myosin heads interact with actin filaments when sufficient calcium is present (Fig. 12–5). The process is called *crossbridge cycling.* As the actin filaments move inward toward the center of the sarcomere, drawing the Z lines closer together, the sarcomere shortens. The energy for this shortening is provided by the breakdown of ATP, chiefly made in the mitochondria.

Titin (also called *connectin*), the largest protein molecule yet described, is an extraordinarily long, flexible, and slender myofibrillar protein.[4] It acts as a third filament and provides elasticity.[5] Between 0.6 and 1.2 μm in length, the titin molecule extends from the Z line, stopping just short of the M line (Fig. 12–1). It has two distinct segments: an inextensible segment that interacts with myosin and an extensible segment that stretches as sarcomere length increases.[6] Titin has two functions: It tethers the myosin molecule to the Z line, and as it stretches its elasticity explains the stress-strain elastic relation of striated muscle, without having to postulate a major role for nonmyofibrillar structures such as extracellular connective tissue.[6]

ACTIN AND TROPONIN-C.   To understand the indispensable role of calcium ions in providing a crucial switch-on signal to the crossbridge cycle requires a brief outline of the molecular structure of the actin filament. Thin filaments are composed of *two actin units,* which intertwine in a helical pattern, both being carried on a heavier tropomyosin molecule that functions as a "backbone" (Fig. 12–4). At regular intervals of 38.5 nm along this twisting structure is a closely bound group of three regulatory proteins called the *troponin complex.*[7] Of these three, it is troponin-C that

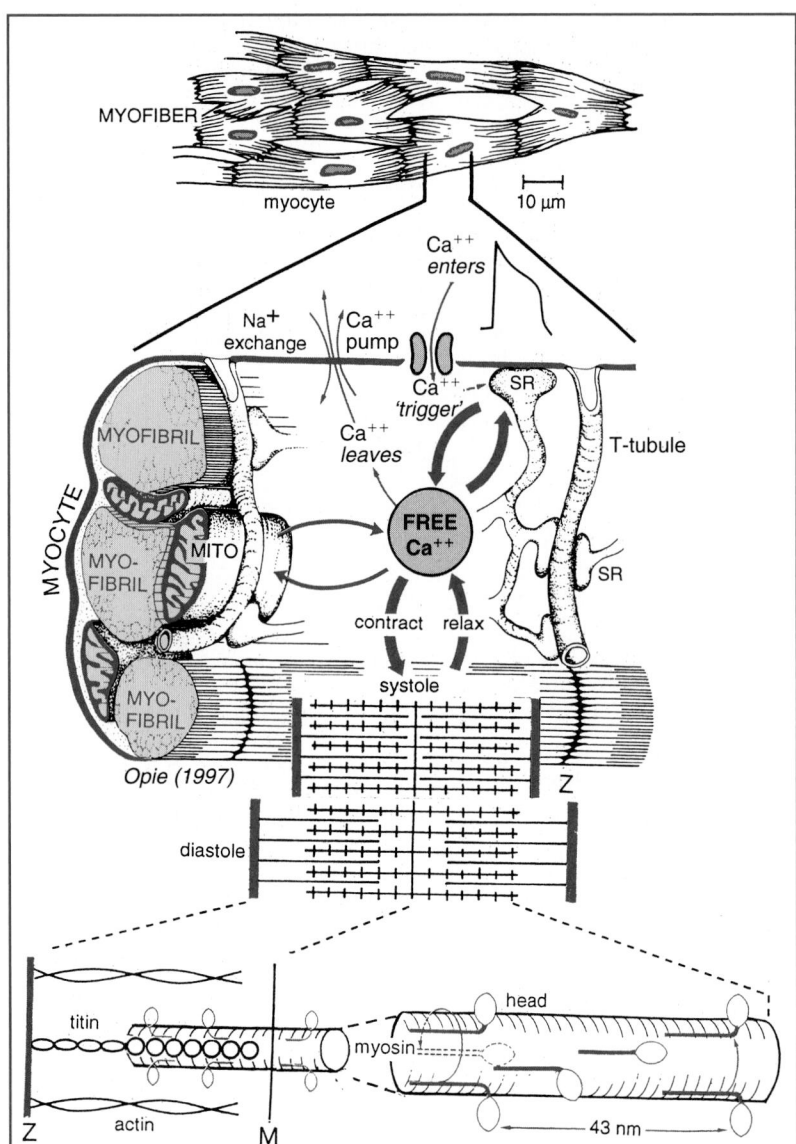

MYOFIBER

myocyte

10 μm

FIGURE 12–1. The crux of the contractile process lies in the changing concentrations of Ca⁺⁺ ions in the myocardial cytosol. Ca⁺⁺ ions are schematically shown as entering via the calcium channel, which opens in response to the wave of depolarization that travels along the sarcolemma. These Ca⁺⁺ ions "trigger" the release of more calcium from the sarcoplasmic reticulum (SR) and thereby initiate a contraction-relaxation cycle. Eventually the small amount of calcium that has entered the cell leaves, predominantly by a Na⁺/Ca⁺⁺ exchanger with a lesser role for the sarcolemmal calcium pump. The varying actin-myosin overlap is shown for systole and diastole. The myosin heads, attached to the thick filaments, interact with the thin actin filaments, as shown in Figure 12–6. For role of titin, see Figure 12–4. (Upper panel reproduced with permission from Braunwald E., et al.: Mechanisms of Contraction of the Normal and Failing Heart. 2nd ed. Boston, Little, Brown, & Co., 1976; middle and lower panels reprinted with permission. Copyright ©1997 L. H. Opie.)

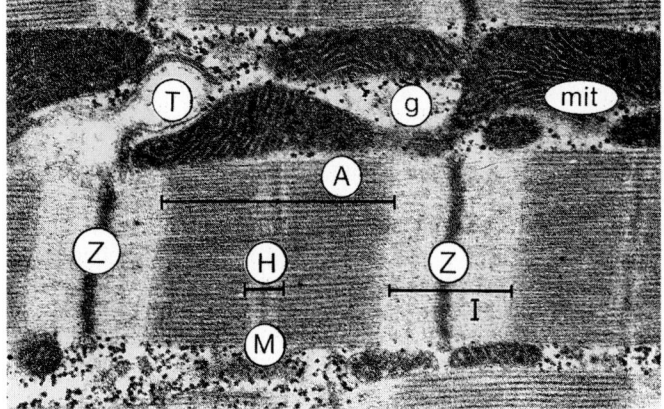

FIGURE 12–2. The sarcomere is the distance between the two Z lines. Note the presence of numerous mitochondria (mit) sandwiched between the myofibrils, and the presence of T tubules (T), which penetrate into the muscle at the level of the Z lines. This two-dimensional picture should not disguise the fact that the Z line is really a "Z disc," as is the M line (M). H = Central clear zone containing only myosin filament bodies and the M line; A = band of actin-myosin overlap; I = band of actin filaments, titin, and Z line; g = glycogen granules. ×32,000 rat papillary muscle. (Courtesy of Dr. J. Moravec, Dijon, France.)

responds to the calcium ions that are released in large amounts from the SR to start the crossbridge cycle.

Schematically, when the cytosolic calcium level is low, the *tropomyosin* molecule is twisted in such a way that the myosin heads cannot interact with actin (Fig. 12–5). When more calcium ions arrive at the start of the contractile cycle and interact with troponin-C, then the activated troponin-C binds tightly to the inhibitory molecule, *troponin-I*. This process repositions troponin-M (tropomyosin) on the thin filament,[8] which removes the inhibition exerted by tropomyosin on the actin-myosin interaction. Thus, the crossbridge cycle is initiated. When troponin-I is phosphorylated by beta-adrenergic stimulation, then the rate of relaxation is enhanced.[9]

STRONG AND WEAK BINDING STATES. Although at a molecular level the events underlying the crossbridge cycle are exceedingly complex, one simple current hypothesis is a revival of a two-state model first proposed by Huxley.[10] According to this proposal, the crossbridges exist in either a strong or a weak binding state (Fig. 12–5).[8] The arrival of calcium ions at the contractile proteins is a crucial link in the series of events known as *excitation-contraction coupling*. The ensuing interaction of calcium with troponin-C and the deinhibition of troponin-I puts the crossbridges in the strong binding state. As long as enough calcium ions are present, the strong binding state potentially dominates (Fig. 12–5). If, however, the strong binding state were con-

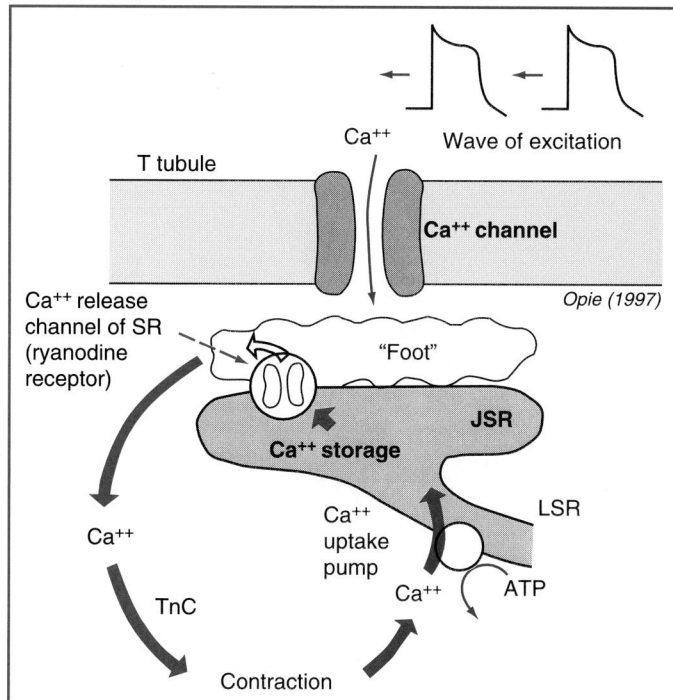

Opie (1997)

FIGURE 12–3. The sarcoplasmic reticulum (SR) plays an essential role in the contraction-relaxation cycle. When the wave of excitation opens the Ca^{++} channel of the T tubule, the Ca^{++} ions thus entering release much more Ca^{++} from the SR. The function of the "foot" is shown in Figure 12–10. This Ca^{++} is released from the ryanodine receptor located in the junctional SR (JSR), and is also called the Ca^{++} release channel of the SR. The Ca^{++} thus released into the cytosol interacts with troponin-C to trigger the contractile process (Figs. 12–4 to 12–7). Ca^{++} ions are then taken up from troponin-C into the longitudinal SR (L-SR) to be stored at high concentrations in the JSR in association with calsequestrin and other storage proteins. Then the Ca^{++} ions can once again be released when more Ca^{++} triggers the process during the next wave of excitation. (Reprinted with permission. Copyright ©1997 L. H. Opie.)

tinuously present, then the contractile proteins could never relax. Thus, the proposal is that the binding of ATP to the myosin head puts the crossbridges into a weak binding state even when the calcium concentration is high.[8] Conversely, when ATP is hydrolyzed to ADP and P$_i$, the strong binding state again predominates. Thus, the ATP-induced changes in the molecular configuration of the myosin head result in corresponding variations in the physical properties (a similar concept is common in metabolic regulation).

When cytosolic calcium levels fall at the start of diastole, a master switch is turned off as the calcium ions leave troponin-C and tropomyosin again assumes the inhibitory configuration. The weak binding state now predominates.

MODEL FOR MOLECULAR BASIS OF MUSCULAR CONTRACTION. Each myosin head is the terminal part of a heavy chain. The bodies of two of these chains intertwine, and each terminates in a short "neck" that carries the elongated myosin head (Fig. 12–4). It is the base of the head, also sometimes called the neck, that changes configuration in the contractile cycle. Together with the "bodies" of all the other heads, the myosin thick filament is formed. Each lobe of the bilobed head has an *ATP-binding pocket* (also called nucleotide-pocket) and a narrow cleft that extends from the base of this pocket to the actin-binding face.[11] ATP and its breakdown products ADP and P$_i$ bind to the nucleotide pocket, which has in close proximity the myosin ATPase activity that breaks down ATP to its products (Fig. 12–6). According to the revised Rayment model,[12] the narrow cleft that splits the central 50-kDA segment of the myosin head responds to the binding of ATP or its breakdown products to the nucleotide pocket in such a way that the confor-

mational changes necessary for movement of the head are produced. Starting with the rigor state (Fig. 12–6*A*), the binding of ATP to its pocket changes the molecular configuration of the myosin head so that the head detaches from actin to terminate the rigor state (Fig. 12–6*B*). Next, the ATPase activity of the myosin head splits ATP into ADP and P$_i$ and the head flexes (Fig. 12–6*C*). As ATP is hydrolyzed, the cleft extending from the nucleotide pocket to the actin-binding face starts to close, and, once it is closed, the myosin head transiently binds weakly to an actin unit. Then P$_i$ is released from the head, the cleft finally closes, and there is strong binding of the myosin head to actin (Fig. 12–6*D*). Next, the head extends, i.e., straightens. A power stroke takes place, the actin molecule moves by 5 to 10 nm,[11,13] and the myosin head is now in the rigor state. The pocket then releases ADP, ready for acceptance of ATP, and repetition of the cycle. A major point of emphasis is that it is straightening and not flexion of the light chain region of the head (i.e., the "neck") that produces the power stroke; however, the angle between the straightened head and the myosin body does decrease to give the appearance of flexion of head on the body.

Myosin ATPase activity normally responds to calcium in such a way that an increase of calcium ion concentration from 10^{-7} M to 5×10^{-5} M results in a fivefold increase in activity.[14] Similar calcium concentrations are associated with contraction in the whole heart (Fig. 12–7).

Myosin heavy chain isoforms help regulate myosin ATPase activity. Each myosin filament consists of two heavy chains, the bodies of which are intertwined and each ending in one head, and four light chains, two in apposition to each head. The heavy chains, containing the myosin ATPase activity on the heads, occur in two isoforms, alpha and beta of the same molecular weight, but with substantially different ATPase activities. The beta-heavy chain (β-MHC) isoform has lower ATPase activity and is the predominant form in the adult human. In small animals, the faster α-MHC form changes to a predominant β-MHC pattern in experimental heart failure. A mutant gene for β-MHC is thought to be responsible for some kindreds of patients with human hypertrophic cardiomyopathy (see p. 1664).[15] Less commonly, mutants for tropomyosin or troponin-T are responsible[15] (see p. 1664).

Two *myosin light chains* surround the elongated base of each myosin head (four per bilobed head). The *essential myosin light chain* (MLC-1), an integral part of the structure of the myosin head, appears to inhibit the contractile process by a newly described interaction with actin.[16] The other *regulatory myosin light chain* (MLC-2) is a potential site for phosphorylation, for example in response to beta-adrenergic stimulation. Such phosphorylation (i.e., the gaining of a phosphate grouping) promotes crossbridge cycling by increasing the affinity of myosin for actin.[8] In vascular smooth muscle, a similar phosphorylation occurs under the influence of the enzyme, myosin light chain kinase (MLCK), and is an obligatory step in the initiation of the contractile process.

Effects of Increased Cytosolic Calcium Levels on Crossbridge Cycle

Calcium ions stimulate the contractile process at multiple control sites.[8,17,18] Their interaction with troponin-C is essential for crossbridge cycling.[7] Two major models are proposed to account for increased force development at greater calcium ion concentrations (Figs. 12–7 and 12–8). First, it has been held that calcium acts as an on-off switch, and, therefore, the enhanced force development in the presence of calcium ions must be due to recruitment of additional crossbridge sites.[19] The alternate point of view is that the crossbridges react to calcium in a graded manner.[18,20]

The cellular mechanisms in the "graded model" may involve (1) a graded response of troponin-C to calcium ions,

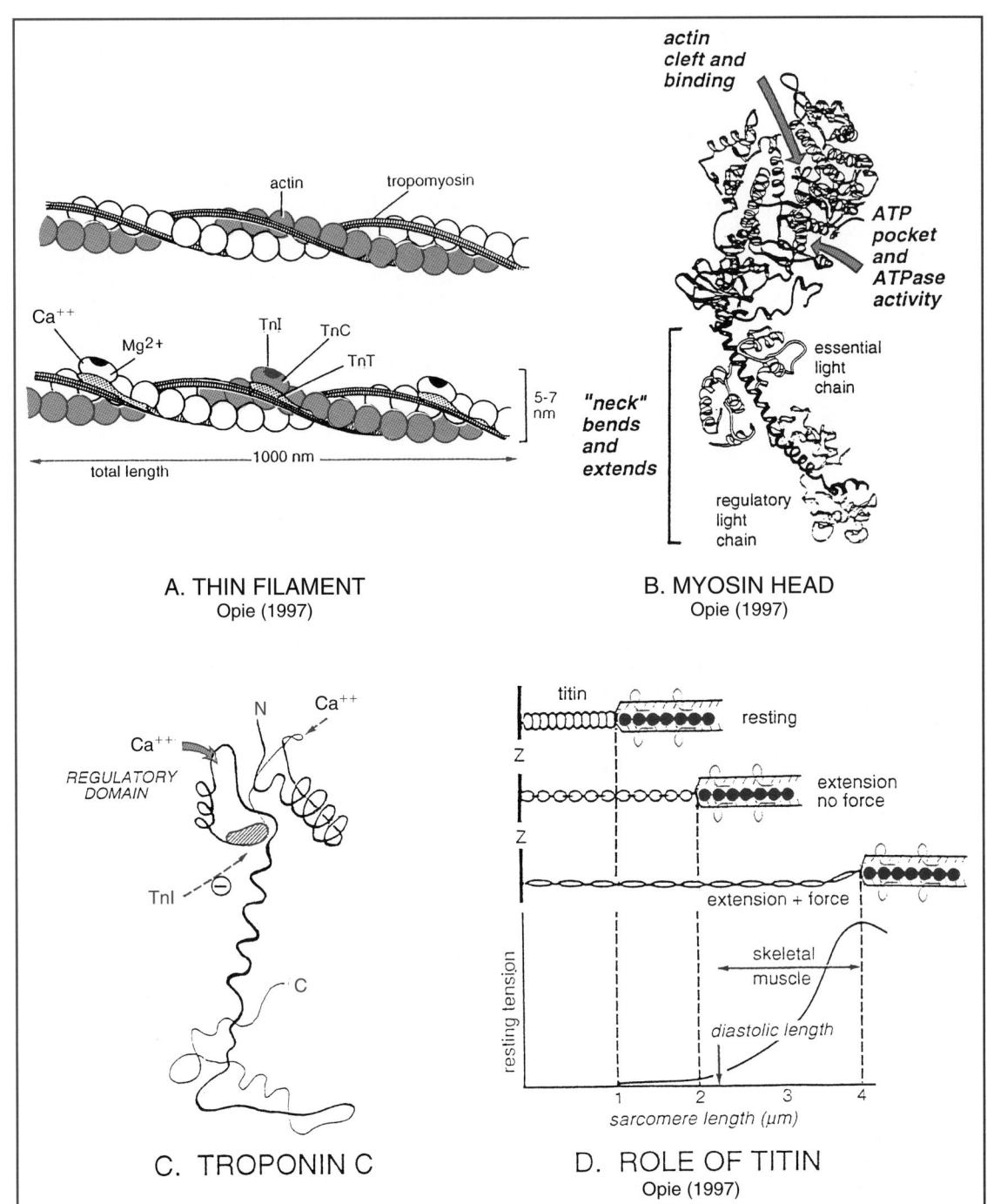

actin
cleft and
binding

ATP
pocket
and
ATPase
activity

essential
light
chain

"neck"
bends
and
extends

regulatory
light
chain

actin   tropomyosin

Ca++

Mg2+

TnI   TnC

TnT

5-7
nm

1000 nm

total length

A. THIN FILAMENT
Opie (1997)

B. MYOSIN HEAD
Opie (1997)

N   Ca++

Ca++

REGULATORY
DOMAIN

TnI ⊖

C

C. TROPONIN C

titin   resting

Z

extension
no force

Z

extension + force

skeletal
muscle

resting tension

diastolic length

1   2   3   4

sarcomere length (μm)

D. ROLE OF TITIN
Opie (1997)

FIGURE 12–4. The major molecules of the contractile system. The thin actin filament *(A)* interacts with the myosin head *(B)* when Ca++ ions arrive at troponin-C *(C)*. The giant molecule titin *(D)* provides structural support by linking myosin to the Z line. The molecular aspects are as follows: The thin actin filament *(A)* contains troponin-C (TnC) and its Ca++ binding sites. When TnC is not activated by Ca++, then troponin-I (TnI) inhibits the actin-myosin interaction. The role of troponin-T (TnT) is less well defined. *B,* Myosin head molecular structure, based on Rayment et al.,[11] is composed of heavy and light chains. The heavy head chain in turn has two major domains: one of 70 kDA (i.e., 70,000 molecular weight) that interacts with actin at the actin cleft and has an ATP-binding pocket. The other domain of 20 kDA is elongated, extends and bends, and has two light chains attached to it. The essential light chain (ELC) is part of the structure. The other regulatory light chain (RLC) influences the extent of the actin-myosin interaction. *C,* TnC with sites in the regulatory domain for activation by calcium and for interaction with TnI. *D,* Titin, the very large elongated protein with elasticity that binds myosin to the Z line. (Modified from Wang, K., McCarter, R., Wright, J., et al.: Regulation of skeletal muscle stiffness and elasticity by titin isoforms: A test of the segmental extension model of resting tension. Proc. Natl. Acad. Sci. *88:*7101–7105, 1991; with permission.) As the sarcomere is stretched to its maximum diastolic length of 2.2 microns (Fig. 12–24), titin is increasingly stretched and contributes to the elastic properties of the sarcomere. For differences between cardiac and skeletal titin, see reference 6. (Reprinted with permission. Copyright ©1997 L. H. Opie.)

which is unlikely in view of the very steep relationship between force development; (2) a graded response of myosin ATPase to calcium[14] (Fig. 12–7); and/or (3) increased myosin light chain phosphorylation—this is still specula-

tive. Additional possibilities are, first, that there could be "near neighbor" self-activation whereby actin-myosin interaction activates additional crossbridges even in the absence of binding of calcium to the troponin-C of those cross-

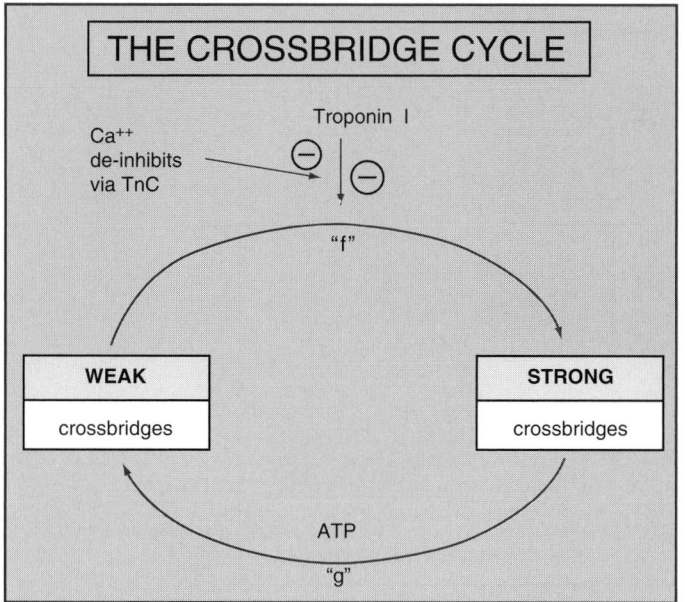

THE CROSSBRIDGE CYCLE

FIGURE 12–5. Hypothesis for crossbridge cycle based on concepts of Brenner.[20] Strong crossbridges are required for the power stroke (Fig. 12–6). The probability of such crossbridges forming is decreased by troponin-I. When Ca^{++} interacts with troponin-C (TnC), de-inhibition occurs and the strong crossbridges form more easily. ATP, when attached to the myosin head, causes the strong binding state to change to the weak state and, therefore, inhibits rigor formation (Fig. 12–6). During force generation, the molecular force-generators (myosin crossbridges) cycle between weak and strong states with apparent rate constants, f and g. According to Brenner,[20] calcium, by activating TnC, increases the probability of forming strong, force-generating crossbridges. The responsiveness to calcium depends on the relative values of f and g, as well as on the calcium affinity of TnC. For original concepts, see Rüegg.[24]

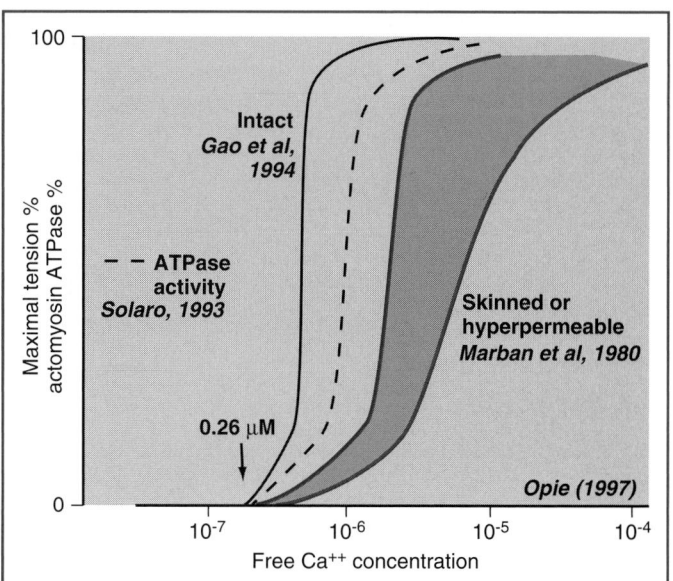

FIGURE 12–7. Relation of free ionized Ca^{++} to tension development in (1) intact rat trabeculae, at fixed diastolic fiber lengths of 2.2 μm, shown on left, and taken from Gao et al.[17] and (2) a variety of skinned and hyperpermeable preparations from Gao et al.[17] and Marban et al.,[25] shown in slashes. The dashed line indicates the effect of $[Ca^{++}]_i$ on actomyosin ATPase activity from Solaro et al.[14] Note the steep curve of activation of intact fibers and of actomyosin ATPase activity. Also note that the myofibrils of intact preparations are much more sensitive to calcium than those of skinned preparations. (Reprinted with permission. Copyright ©1997 L. H. Opie.)

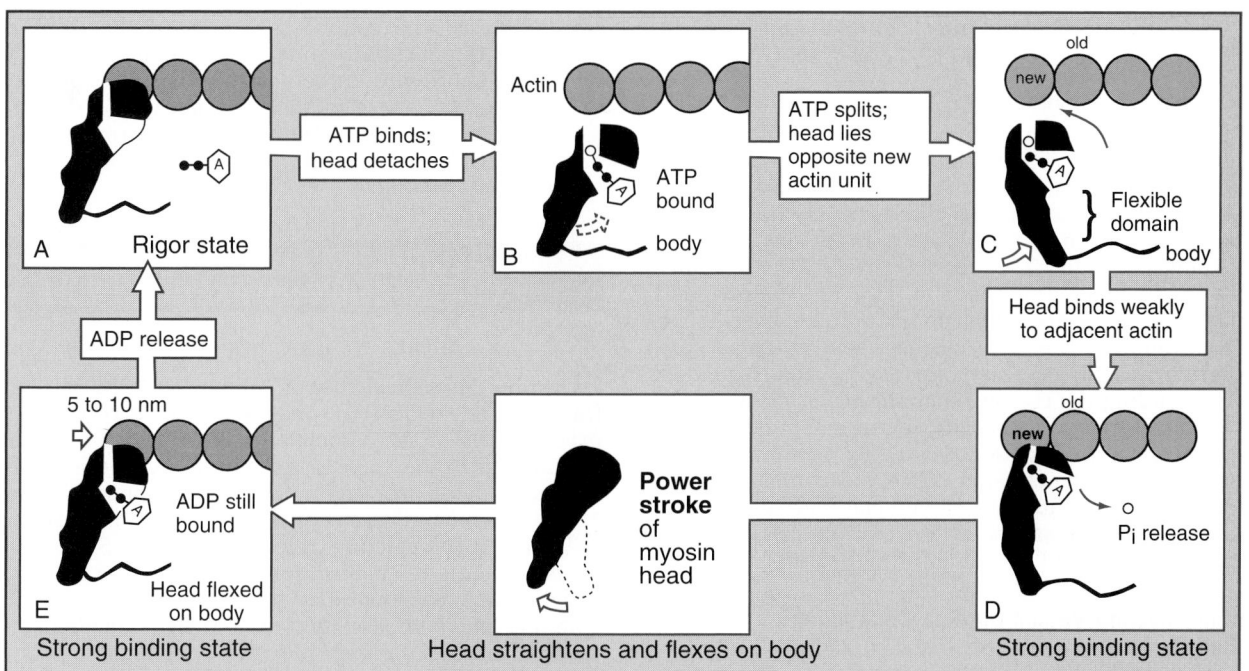

FIGURE 12–6. Schema modified from the Rayment[11] five-step model for interaction between the myosin head and the actin filament, taking into account revisions[12] and additional changes proposed by the present author. The cycle starts with the rigor state (A), in which the myosin head is still attached to actin at the end of the power stroke. ATP binds to the ATP-binding pocket to cause the head to assume the same molecular configuration as before the power stroke. Binding of the head to an adjacent actin monomer occurs first weakly and then strongly. Myosin ATPase activity splits the ATP into ADP (adenosine diphosphate) and P_i (inorganic phosphate). As P_i is released, the power stroke occurs, and the actin filament is moved by 5 to 10 nm. The actin monomer with which the myosin head is interacting is dotted. (Professor J. C. Rüegg of Heidelberg University, Germany, is thanked for comments.)

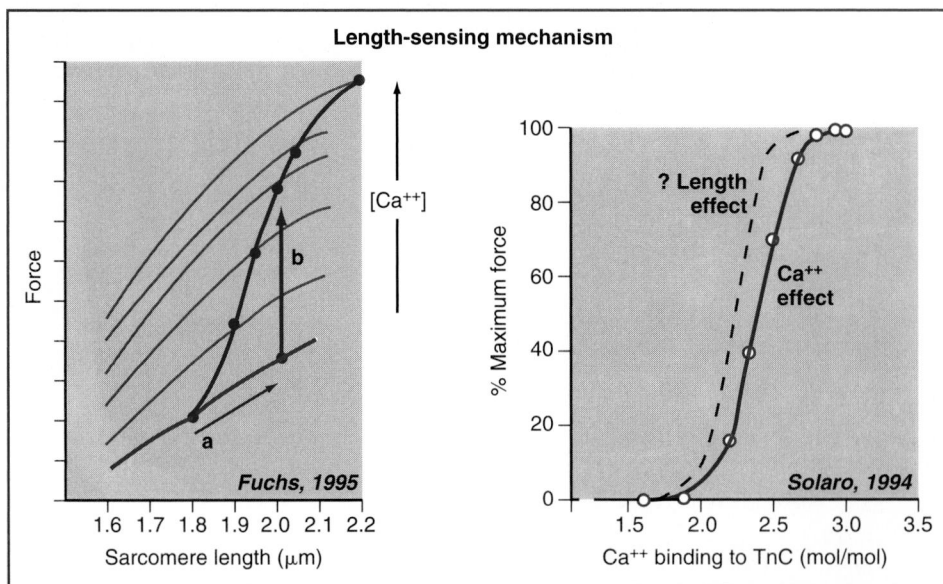

FIGURE 12–8. The proposed explanation for the Starling effect, whereby a greater end-diastolic fiber length develops a greater force. The left panel shows how the steep ascending limb of the cardiac force-length curve is explained by an interaction between sarcomere length and calcium ions. Light lines show a family of hypothetical force-length curves for increasing free Ca^{++} concentrations, each drawn on the assumption that the shape of the curve is determined solely by the degree of overlap of thin and thick filaments (Fig. 12–1). It is postulated that a change in end-diastolic fiber length (a) at any given free Ca^{++} concentration would increase force by the Starling effect and would, in addition, cause cooperative interactions within the thin filament, the latter leading to a greater binding of Ca^{++} to the thin filament. Hence there would be a greater force (b) than would be expected simply on the basis of the change in filament overlap (a). The right panel proposes that the effects of Ca^{++} and length can be explained by the properties of troponin-C (TnC) and the binding of calcium to TnC. As more Ca^{++} ions bind to TnC in a skinned fiber preparation, more force is developed. There is a steep relation, similar to that shown in the left panel. When the fiber is stretched and the sarcomere length increased, it is postulated that for any given number of Ca^{++} ions binding to TnC there is a greater force development, so that TnC has become sensitized to Ca^{++}. (Modified from Fuchs, F.: Mechanical modulation of the Ca^{2+} regulatory protein complex in cardiac muscle. NIPS *10*:6–12, 1995; and Solaro, R. J., Wolska, B. M., and Westfall, M.: Regulatory proteins and diastolic relaxation. *In* Lorell, B. H., and Grossman, W. (eds.): Diastolic Relaxation of the Heart. Norwell, MA, Kluwer Academic Publishers, 1994, pp. 43–53.)

bridges.[14] Second, once crossbridge attachment has occurred, the affinity of troponin-C for calcium may increase.[21,22]

Length-Dependent Activation

The other major factor influencing the strength of contraction is the length of the muscle fiber at the end of diastole, just before the onset of systole. Starling observed that the greater the volume of the heart in diastole, the more forceful the contraction (see p. 464). The increased volume translates into an increased muscle length, which acts by a length-sensing mechanism (Fig. 12–8). Previously this relation was ascribed to a more optimal overlap between actin and myosin. The current view is that a complex interplay occurs between anatomical and regulatory factors,[23] including the concept that an increased sarcomere length leads to greater sensitivity of the contractile apparatus to the prevailing cytosolic calcium,[8] thereby explaining length-dependent activation. The mechanism for this regulatory change, although not yet clarified, may hypothetically involve increased sensitivity of the calcium-binding domain of troponin-C to calcium (Fig. 12–8).[8]

Crossbridge Cycling Versus Cardiac Contraction-Relaxation Cycle

The crossbridge and the cardiac cycles must be distinguished. The former cycle is the repetitive interaction between myosin heads and actin, according to the five-step model (Fig. 12–6). So long as enough calcium ions are bound to troponin-C, many repetitive cycles of this nature occur. Thus, at any given moment, some myosin heads are flexing or have flexed, some are extending or have extended, some are attached to actin, and some are detached from actin. Numerous such crossbridge cycles, each lasting

only a few microseconds, actively move the thin actin filaments toward the central bare area of the thick myosin filaments, thereby shortening the sarcomere. The sum total of all the shortening sarcomeres leads to systole, which is the contraction phase of the cardiac cycle. When calcium ions depart from their binding sites on troponin-C, crossbridge cycling cannot occur, and the diastolic phase of the cardiac cycle sets in.

CALCIUM ION FLUXES IN CARDIAC CONTRACTION-RELAXATION CYCLE

Pattern of Calcium Movements

Despite the critical role of calcium in regulating the contraction and relaxation phases of the cardiac cycle, the exact details of the associated calcium ion fluxes that link contraction to the wave of excitation are not yet fully clarified, although a working model can be conceptualized (Fig. 12–9). A generally accepted hypothesis is based on the critical role of calcium release from the SR.[26] Relatively small amounts of calcium ions actually enter and leave the cell during each cardiac cycle, whereas much larger amounts move in and out of the SR. The theory of *calcium-induced calcium release*[27] explains most of the current available data.[26] The basic proposal is that the SR releases relatively large amounts of calcium ions into the cytosol in response to the much smaller amounts entering the cardiac myocyte with each wave of depolarization.[28] This process elevates by about tenfold the concentration of calcium ions in the cytosol.[27] The result is the increasing interaction of calcium ions with troponin-C to trigger the contractile process. This theory, also called the *chemical synapse theory*,[29] has recently received strong support from

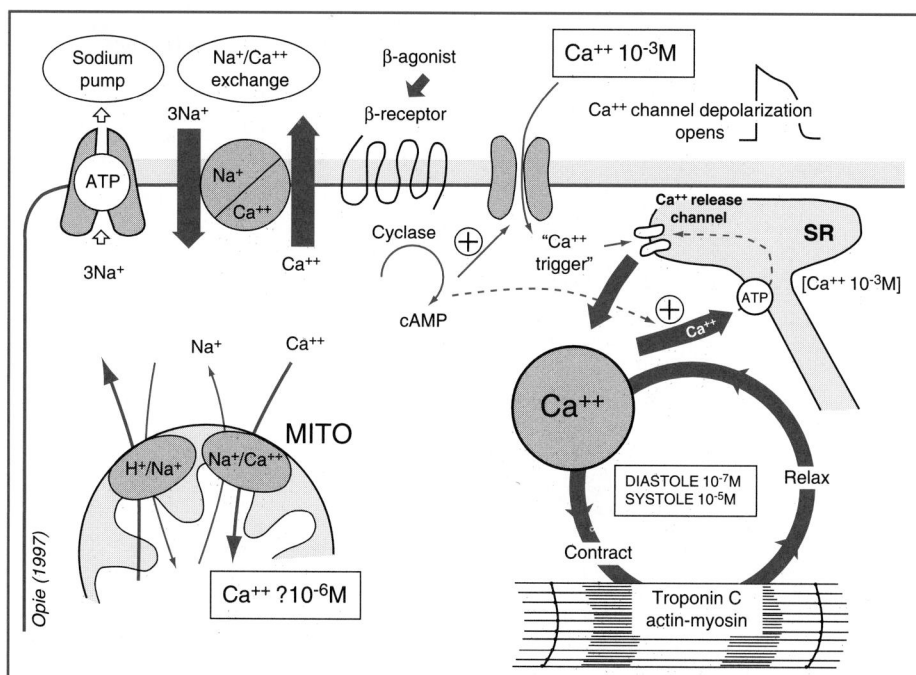

FIGURE 12–9. Calcium fluxes in the myocardium. Crucial features are (1) entry of Ca++ ions via the voltage-sensitive Ca++ channel, acting as a trigger to the release of Ca++ ions from the sarcoplasmic reticulum (SR) as shown in Figure 12–3; (2) the effect of beta-adrenergic stimulation with adenylate cyclase forming cyclic AMP, the latter both helping to open the Ca++ channel and to increase the rate of uptake of Ca++ into the SR; and (3) exit of Ca++ ions chiefly via the Na+/Ca++ exchange, with the sodium pump thereafter extruding the Na+ ions thus gained. The latter process requires ATP. Note the much higher extracellular (10^{-3} M) than intracellular values (Fig. 12–7) and a hypothetical mitochondrial value of about 10^{-6} M. The mitochondria can act as a buffer against excessive changes in the free cytosolic calcium concentration. MITO = Mitochondria. (Reprinted with permission. Copyright ©1997 L. H. Opie.)

the molecular characterization of the receptor on the SR that releases calcium[30] from the anatomical proximity of the junctional SR to the sarcolemma of the T tubule (Fig. 12–10), and from electrophysiological evidence closely

linking the duration of the action potential with the extent of Ca++ release.[28]

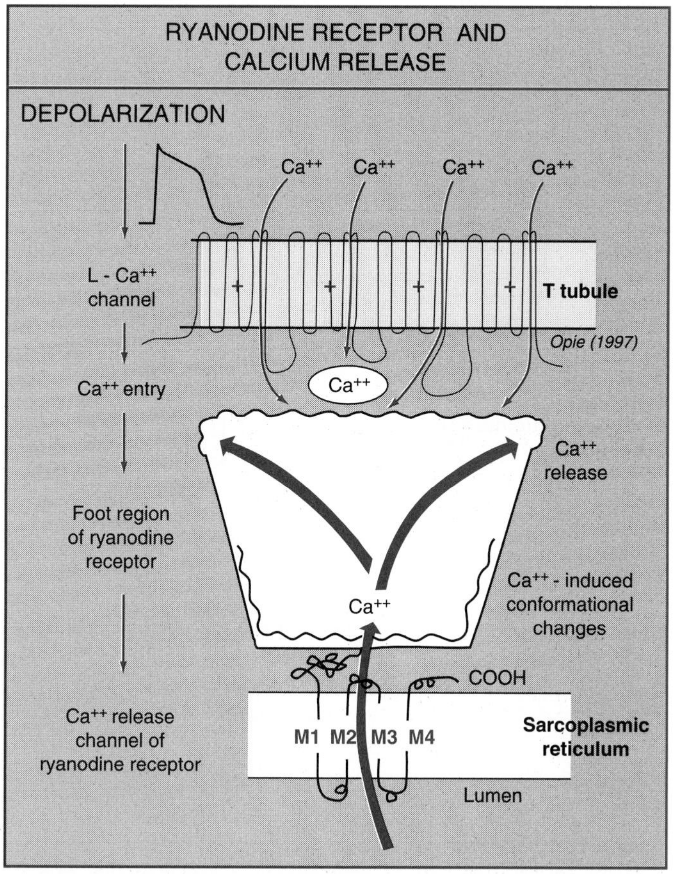

The rise of cytosolic calcium concentration comes to an end as the wave of excitation passes, no more calcium ions enter, and the release of calcium from the SR ceases. The latter event could be explained by one or more of several proposals, namely (1) that the cytosolic calcium ion concentration has risen high enough to inhibit the process of calcium-induced calcium release[27]; (2) the release of calcium from the SR is tightly linked to opening of the calcium channel, so that when the latter closes the release of calcium from the SR ceases[31]; (3) the rising cytosolic calcium ion concentration can activate the calcium uptake pump of the SR[32]; or (4) calcium release from the SR continues only for the duration of action potential duration.[28] The overall effect of these mechanisms is that the cytosolic calcium ion concentration starts to fall and relaxation is initiated. As the cytosolic calcium decreases, tropomyosin again starts to inhibit the interaction between actin and myosin, and relaxation proceeds.

To balance the small amount of calcium ions entering the heart cell with each depolarization, a similar quantity must leave the cell by one of two processes. First, calcium can be exchanged for sodium ions entering by the Na+/Ca++ exchange, and, second, an ATP-consuming sarcolemmal calcium pump can transfer calcium into the extracellular space against a concentration gradient.

Calcium Release Channel of the Sarcoplasmic Reticulum

Each sarcolemmal voltage-operated calcium channel is thought to control a cluster of SR release channels[31,33] by virtue of close anatomical proximity of the sarcolemmal calcium channels, situated on the T tubules, to the calcium release channels, situated on the SR. The calcium release channel is part of the complex structure known as the *ryanodine receptor,* so called because it coincidentally binds the potent insecticide ryanodine.[32] Part of this receptor extends from the membrane of the SR toward the T tubule to constitute the *foot structure* or *junctional channel complex* that bridges the gap between the SR and the T tubule.[34] After the wave of depolarization has reached the T tubule and induced the voltage-operated calcium channels to open, the calcium ions enter the cardiac myocyte to reach the foot regions of the ryanodine receptors (Fig. 12–10). The result is a change in the molecular configuration

RYANODINE RECEPTOR AND CALCIUM RELEASE

DEPOLARIZATION

L - Ca++ channel

Ca++ entry

Foot region of ryanodine receptor

Ca++ release channel of ryanodine receptor

T tubule

Opie (1997)

Ca++ release

Ca++ - induced conformational changes

COOH

M1 M2 M3 M4

Sarcoplasmic reticulum

Lumen

FIGURE 12–10. Proposed crucial role of T tubule, the feet and calcium release channel of the sarcoplasmic reticulum (SR) in excitation-contraction coupling. Depolarization stimulates the L-type calcium channel of the T tubule to allow calcium ion entry, which interacts with the "foot" region of the ryanodine receptor to cause molecular conformational changes that eventually result in calcium release from the calcium-release channel of the ryanodine receptor of the SR. For molecular structure of the foot, see Wagenknecht et al.[34] (Reprinted with permission. Copyright ©1997 L. H. Opie.)

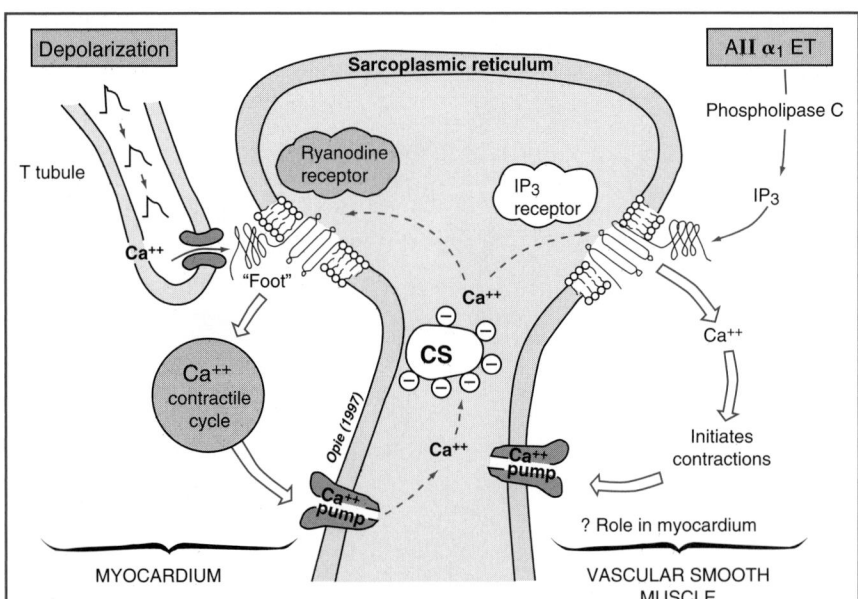

FIGURE 12–11. In the *myocardium* (left side of figure), calcium is released from the sarcoplasmic reticulum (SR) via the calcium release channel (part of the ryanodine receptor), chiefly in response to calcium that has entered during voltage depolarization. Calcium is taken up again by the calcium pump of the longitudinal SR, to interact with the storage protein calsequestrin (CS), thence to be released again. In contrast, in *vascular smooth muscle*, stimulation of vasoconstrictor receptors, such as angiotensin II (AII), alpha$_1$-adrenergic (α_1), and endothelin (ET), leads to release of inositol trisphosphate (IP$_3$) that acts on its receptor to release calcium from the SR. The role of IP$_3$ as a signal in the myocardium is still under evaluation. (Reprinted with permission. Copyright ©1997 L. H. Opie.)

of the ryanodine receptor that opens the calcium release channel of the SR to discharge calcium ions, probably into the subsarcolemmal space between the foot and the T tubule[34] and thence into the cytosol.

From the molecular point of view, the calcium release channel of the SR has been analyzed by cloning and sequencing the complementary DNA.[35] The predicted structure is that of a large protein comprising over 5000 amino acids, with two major components. The larger part is the foot, which links the T tubules and the SR, and the smaller structure is the C-terminal region, which constitutes the actual pore-containing channel of the SR.[34,35] The density of this channel, as measured by ryanodine binding, is very high with nearly 800 receptors per μm^2 of the junctional SR.[36]

IP$_3$-Induced Release of Calcium from Sarcoplasmic Reticulum

A totally different calcium release signal system may also be involved. In addition to the ryanodine receptor on the SR, there is a second receptor, that for inositol trisphosphate (IP$_3$) (Fig. 12–11). This IP$_3$ receptor has a high degree of molecular homology with the ryanodine receptor, although only about half its size. IP$_3$ is one of the messengers of the phosphatidylinositol pathway, responding to certain agonists with vasoconstriction as their major physiological role, namely alpha$_1$-adrenergic stimulation, angiotensin II, and endothelin.[30] Calcium released from the SR by IP$_3$ may stimulate Na$^+$/Ca^{++} exchange directly.[37] In vascular smooth muscle, this IP$_3$ messenger system is of fundamental importance in regulating the release of calcium from the SR. In cardiac muscle, the role of IP$_3$ is still sufficiently controversial to question its role in the inotropic response.[38] An attractive possibility is that in human heart failure, the IP$_3$ receptor becomes upregulated in relation to the ryanodine receptor, perhaps to help maintain release of calcium from the SR.[39]

Calcium Uptake by the Calcium ATPase of the Sarcoplasmic Reticulum

Calcium ions are taken up into the SR by the activity of the calcium pump, that is, the *calcium-pumping ATPase* of the SR (also called SERCA), that constitutes nearly 90 per cent of the protein component of the SR.[40,41] Its molecular weight is about 115 kDA, and it straddles the SR membrane in such a way that part of it actually protrudes into the cytosol.[42] It exists in several isoforms.[40] For each mole of ATP hydrolyzed by this enzyme, two calcium ions are taken up to accumulate within the SR (Fig. 12–12).

Phospholamban, which means "phosphate receiver," is the major regulator of this calcium pump.[32] Phospholamban is a pentamer protein, consisting of five subunits, each

with a molecular weight of 6 kDA, found in a 1:1 molar ratio to the ATPase of the calcium pump. The activity of phospholamban is governed by its state of phosphorylation, a process that alters the molecular configuration of the calcium pump in such a way that the normal inhibition exerted by unphosphorylated phospholamban on the calcium uptake pump is removed (Fig. 12–12). Each of the five

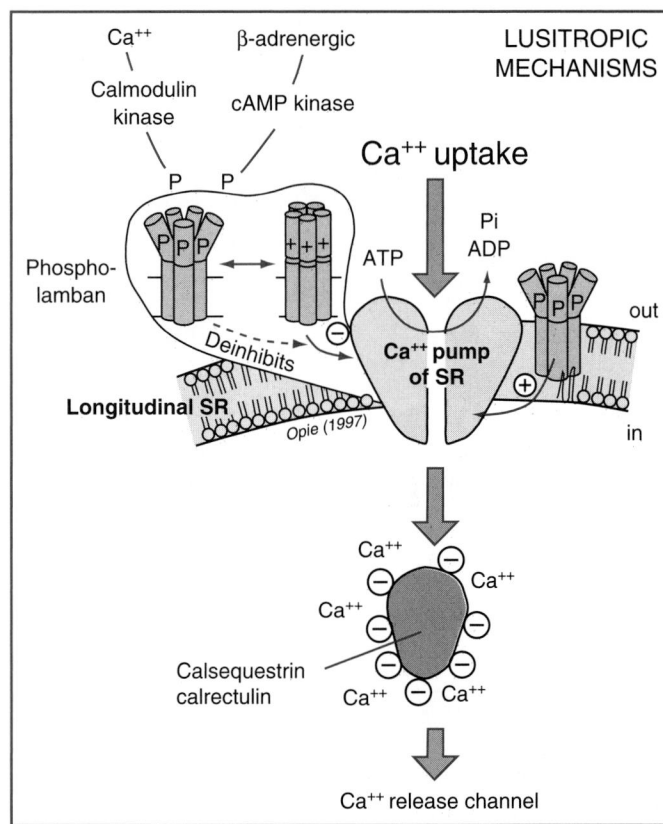

FIGURE 12–12. Calcium uptake by the energy-requiring calcium pump into the sarcoplasmic reticulum (SR). Phospholamban can be phosphorylated (P) to remove the inhibition exerted by its unphosphorylated form (positive charges) on the calcium pump. Calcium uptake is thereby increased either in response to an enhanced cytosolic calcium or in response to beta-adrenergic stimulation. Thus, two phosphorylations activate phospholamban at distinct sites and their effects are additive. An increased rate of uptake of calcium into the SR enhances the rate of relaxation (lusitropic effect). (Reprinted with permission. Copyright ©1997 L. H. Opie.)

subunits of phospholamban can be phosphorylated at two different sites[43] by at least two and possibly three protein kinases.[41] Of specific interest is that one of the two major protein kinases involved, the one activated by cyclic AMP, responds to beta-adrenergic stimulation of the cardiac myocyte by enhancing the uptake of calcium into the SR to increase the rate of relaxation.[41] The further proposal is that the increased store of calcium in the SR is then released by the subsequent waves of depolarization with an increased rate and force of contraction. This sequence is strongly supported by the transgenic mouse model, totally deficient in phospholamban, in which rates of contraction and relaxation are maximal and do not vary in response to beta-adrenergic stimulation by isoproterenol.[41]

The calcium taken up into the SR by the calcium pump is stored prior to further release. The highly charged storage protein, *calsequestrin,* is found in that part of the SR that lies near the T tubules.[44] Calcium stored with calsequestrin is thought to become available for the release process as calsequestrin discharges calcium ions into the inner mouth of the calcium release channel. This process replaces those calcium ions liberated from the outer mouth into the cytosol. *Calrectulin* is another Ca^{++}-storing protein, very similar in structure to calsequestrin, and probably similar in function.[32]

Role of Sarcoplasmic Reticulum in Heart Failure
(See also p. 405)

In heart failure, the force of cardiac contraction is reduced and there is an abnormal delayed pattern of cardiac relaxation. Because the SR is so intimately concerned in both of these phases of the cardiac contractile cycle, it is not surprising that abnormalities of the SR are thought to play a fundamental role in heart failure. The calcium release channel of the SR of the failing heart is diminished in activity and markedly less sensitive to caffeine.[45] Furthermore, the levels of the messenger RNAs of the proteins regulating calcium uptake and release are decreased in end-stage human heart failure. The mRNAs for the ryanodine receptor, the calcium uptake pump, and phospholamban are all abnormally deficient.[46] One hypothesis currently favored is that abnormal calcium handling by the SR of the failing myocardium is due to impaired expression of the genes encoding these specific SR proteins. These proposals tie in with the downgraded state of the ryanodine receptor in SR from patients in severe heart failure.[39]

SARCOLEMMAL CONTROL OF CALCIUM AND OTHER IONS

Ion Channels
(See also Chap. 20)

All current models of excitation-contraction coupling ascribe a crucial role to the voltage-induced opening of the sarcolemmal L-type calcium channels in the initiation of the contractile process.[28] Channels are pore-forming macromolecular proteins that span the sarcolemmal lipid bilayer to allow a highly selective pathway for ion transfer into the heart cell when the channel changes from a closed to an open state.[47,48] Ion channels have two major properties: gating and permeation. Guarding each channel are two or more hypothetical gates that control its opening. Ions can permeate through the channel only when both gates are open. In the case of the sodium and calcium channels, which are best understood, the activation gate is shut at the normal resting membrane potential and the inactivation gate is open, so that the channels are *voltage-gated.* Depolarization opens the activation gate.

MOLECULAR STRUCTURE OF L-TYPE CALCIUM CHANNELS. There is a striking molecular similarity between the sodium

and calcium channels.[48] "This finding shows a conservation of structure probably among all the voltage-gated ion channels and suggests a common gene family."[49] Both channels contain a major alpha-subunit with four transmembrane subunits or domains, very similar to each other in structure. In addition, both sodium and calcium channels include in their overall structure a number of other subunits whose function is less well understood, such as the beta-subunit. Each of the four transmembrane domains of the alpha-subunit is made up of six helices. In each domain, one specific helical segment, called S4, is rich in amino acids, is highly positively charged, and is the proposed site of the voltage sensor (Fig. 12–13).

Activation is now understood in molecular terms as the change in charge on the fourth transmembrane segment, S4, called the *voltage sensor,* of each of the four subunits of the sodium or calcium channel.[50] *Inactivation* is the process whereby the current initially elicited by depolarization decreases with time despite continuation of the original stimulus.[50] For the Na$^+$ channel and hypothetically also for the calcium channel, it is the intracellular linker region between subunits 3 and 4 that inactivates (Fig. 12–13). This linker chain is the proposed molecular explanation for the

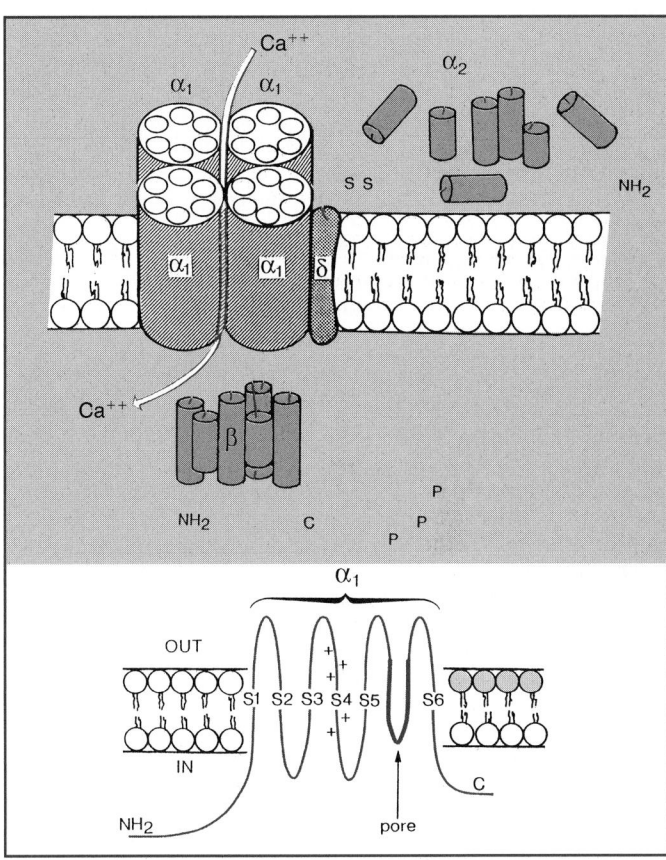

FIGURE 12–13. **Simplified model of Ca^{++} channel showing the alpha$_1$-subunit (α_1) forming the central pore, the regulatory beta-subunit (β), and α_2 and delta-subunits of unknown function. Beta-adrenergic stimulation, via cyclic AMP, promotes phosphorylation (P) and the opening probability of the Ca^{++} channel. The proposal is that four domains, each similar to that shown in the righthand panel and composed of six spanning segments, combine to form the α_1-subunit. Segment S$_4$ is thought to respond to voltage depolarization (+ = positive charges) by altering the molecular configuration of the loop between S$_5$ and S$_6$ (part of the pore), so that there is a greater probability of Ca^{++} ions entering (channel opens). For more details, see Heinemann and Stuhmer.[50] (Upper panel modified from Varadi, G., et al.: Molecular determinants of Ca^{2+} channel function and drug action. Trends Pharmacol. Sci. *16*:43–49, 1995, with permission of the authors and Elsevier Science Ltd. Lower panel modified from Tomaselli, G. F., et al.: Molecular basis of permeation in voltage-gated ion channels. Circ. Res. *72*:491–496, 1993. Copyright 1993 American Heart Association.)**

previous concept of the internal inactivation gate (f). The actual channel pore is probably contained in the alpha₁-subunit, lying between helices S5 and S6, where calcium ions are potentially admitted. Each of the four domains of the alpha₁-subunit appears to be folded in on itself, so that the four S5-S6 spans structurally combine to form the single functioning pore of each calcium channel. The beta-subunit acts to enhance the calcium current flow through the alpha-subunit pores.[51] The amino acid structure of the channel pores has critical properties. For example, the presence of the glutamate residue helps determine the presence of high-affinity calcium binding and therefore the calcium ion specificity of the pore.[52]

Channels are not simply open or closed. Rather, the open state is the last of a sequence of many molecular states, varying from a fully closed to a fully open configuration. Therefore, it is more correct to speak of the *probability of channel opening*.

CALCIUM CHANNEL PHOSPHORYLATION. The alpha₁-subunit (the organ-specific subunit) of the sarcolemmal calcium channel can be phosphorylated at several sites, especially in the C-terminal tail.[53] During beta-adrenergic stimulation, cyclic AMP increases within the cell and phosphate groups are transferred from ATP to the alpha₁-subunit. Thereby, the electrical charges near the inner mouth of the nearby pores are altered to induce changes in the molecular conformation of the pores, so that there is an increased probability of opening of the calcium channel.[48] Either the time that the channel remains in the open state is increased so that more calcium ions flow with the same degree of voltage activation, or phosphorylation activates calcium channels that were otherwise inactive.

T- AND L-TYPE CALCIUM CHANNELS. There are two major subpopulations of sarcolemmal calcium channels relevant to the cardiovascular system, namely the T channels and the L channels.[53,54] The T (transient) channels open at a more negative voltage, have short bursts of opening and do not interact with conventional calcium antagonist drugs.[53] The T channels presumably account for the earlier phase of the opening of the calcium channel, which may also give them a special role in the early electrical depolarization of the sinoatrial node, and hence of initiation of the heart beat. Although T channels are found in atrial cells,[54] their existence in normal ventricular cells is controversial.

The sarcolemmal L (longlasting) channels are the standard calcium channels found in the myocardium and are involved in calcium-induced calcium release. The L channels have two patterns in which their gates work (modes of gating). Mode 1 has short bursts of opening, and mode 2 has longer periods of opening. The sites to which the calcium channel antagonist drugs bind are located in those transmembrane-spanning helices that are close to the pores, mostly on segment S6.[53]

Ion Exchangers

Sodium-Calcium Exchanger

During relaxation, the sarcoplasmic calcium uptake pump and the Na⁺/Ca⁺⁺ exchanger compete for the removal of cytosolic calcium, with the SR pump normally being dominant.[55] Restitution of calcium balance takes place by the activity of a series of transsarcolemmal exchangers, the chief of which is the Na⁺/Ca⁺⁺ exchanger[56] (Fig. 12–14). The exchanger (molecular weight of 108 kDa) consists of 970 amino acids[57] and does not have substantial homology to any other known protein.[56] A specific inhibitory peptide (XIP = exchange inhibitor peptide) has been identified.[58] The direction of ion exchange is responsive to the membrane potential and to the concentrations of sodium and calcium ions on either side of the sarcolemma. Because sodium and calcium ions can exchange either inward or outward in response to the membrane potential, there must be a specific membrane potential, called the reversal or equilibrium potential, at which the ions are so distributed that they can move as easily one way as the other.[56] The reversal potential may lie about halfway between the resting membrane potential and the potential of the fully depolarized state.[59] Changing the membrane potential from the resting value of, say, −85 mV to +20 mV in the phase of rapid depolarization of the action potential may therefore briefly affect the direction of Na⁺/Ca⁺⁺ exchange.[56] During depolarization the charge on the inner side of the sarcolemma becomes positive, which tends to hinder the entrance of sodium ions with their positive charge. Thus, the sodium ions that have just entered during the opening of the sodium channel tend to leave, and calcium ions tend to enter. This process, still controversial, is termed "reverse mode Na⁺/Ca⁺⁺ exchange"[60] to distinguish it from the standard "forward mode" (Na⁺ in, Ca⁺⁺ out) (compare Figs. 12–14 and 12–15).

A major unsolved problem in relation to the activity of the Na⁺/Ca⁺⁺ exchanger is the true value of the internal sodium or calcium ion concentrations, which may differ in the subsarcolemmal "fuzzy space" from the bulk cytosol (Fig. 12–15). Using a sophisticated computer model, very different patterns for the operation of this exchanger during the action potential can be obtained.[61] In particular, if the subsarcolemmal sodium ion concentration is low enough, then the early "reversed mode" exchange with outward movement of sodium ions does not occur, and the exchanger does not contribute to the action potential plateau.

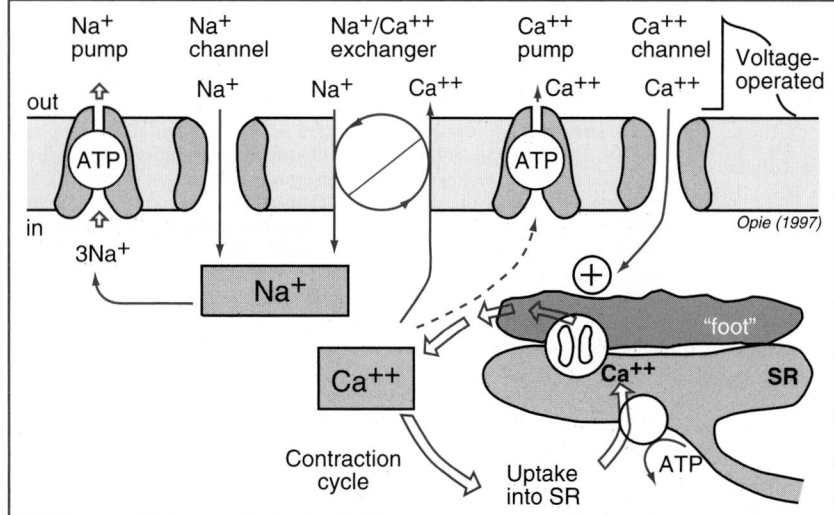

FIGURE 12–14. Regulation of Ca⁺⁺ balance within myocardial cell, showing role of sarcoplasmic reticulum (SR) in contraction-relaxation cycle, as in Figure 12–3. There is a balance between the Ca⁺⁺ ions entering upon depolarization (*right*) and those leaving the cell by the Na⁺/Ca⁺⁺ exchange mechanism. A smaller number of Ca⁺⁺ ions leave by an ATP-dependent sarcolemmal Ca⁺⁺ pump. Ion gradients for Na⁺ and K⁺ are maintained by the operation of the sodium pump (Na⁺/K⁺-ATPase). An increased internal Ca⁺⁺ following Ca⁺⁺ release from the SR is reduced by competition among one of three routes: uptake into the sarcoplasmic reticulum (SR), Na⁺/Ca⁺⁺ exchange, and outward pumping by the membrane Ca⁺⁺-ATPase. The dominant uptake mechanism is into the SR, followed by the exchanger, followed by the membrane pump. (Reprinted with permission. Copyright ©1997 L. H. Opie.)

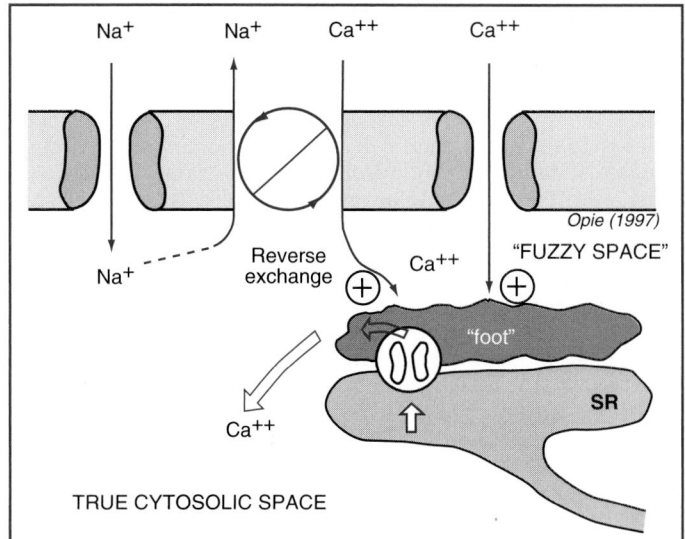

FIGURE 12–15. Proposal for "reverse mode" Na+/Ca++ exchange in the direction of calcium entry following accumulation of sodium ions in the "fuzzy space."[71] According to this proposal, the Na+/Ca++ exchange may play a role in the liberation of calcium involved in the cardiac contractile cycle. For criticism of proposal, see Johnson and Lemieux.[72] (Reprinted with permission. Copyright ©1997 L. H. Opie.)

PHYSIOLOGICAL SIGNIFICANCE OF SODIUM-CALCIUM EXCHANGER.

First, transsarcolemmal calcium entry during reversed mode exchange may participate in calcium-induced calcium release.[37,62,63] Second, the exchanger participates in the restitution of ionic balances.[56] Third, this exchanger may participate in the force-frequency relationship (Treppe or Bowditch phenomenon).[62] According to the "sodium pump lag" hypothesis, the rapid accumulation of calcium ions during rapid stimulation of the myocardium outstrips the ability of the Na+/Ca++ exchanger and the sodium pump to achieve return to ionic normality. The result is an accumulation of calcium ions within the SR and an increased force of contraction.[64]

Sodium-Proton Exchange and Acid-Base Homeostasis

The internal pH, pH_i, is more alkaline than can be expected if protons (H+) were passively distributed across the cardiac cell membrane. To achieve transport of protons out of the myocyte, the electroneutral 1-for-1 exchange of Na+ and H+ is driven by the gradient of Na+ ions, much higher outside than inside the myocyte (Fig. 12–16). The exchanger can be inhibited by the diuretic amiloride and its more specific derivatives, and also by the novel highly specific inhibitor HOE 694.

Physiologically, Na+/H+ exchange is thought to play a role in the regulation of protein synthesis, because cytoplasmic alkalinization, for example by insulin, may regulate certain crucial steps in protein synthesis. Alkalinization may also explain why angiotensin II opens Ca++ channels in rabbit myocardium.[65]

This exchanger also corrects an acid load during ischemia and acidosis, or during early *postischemic reperfusion,* by transporting protons (H+) out of the cell while transporting Na+ into the cell. The resultant increase of internal Na+ can be dealt with either by the operation of the Na+/Ca++ exchanger or by Na+/K+ pump or by sodium-bicarbonate cotransport or by Na+/K+ cotransport. Alternatively, the exchanger could operate in the reverse direction to extrude Na+ from the cells at the expense of a gain of protons that in turn could be dealt with by decreasing the activity of the bicarbonate-chloride exchanger.

The *sodium/bicarbonate cotransporter* helps the Na+/H+ exchanger to correct acidosis by the inward transport of bicarbonate, at the cost, however, of a simultaneous gain of Na+ ions.[66] Such Na+ gain must be offset by the activity of the Na+/K+ pump at the cost of ATP.

The *bicarbonate/chloride exchanger* acidifies by outward movement of the bicarbonate ion, leaving behind protons.[66] In contrast, the Na+/H+ exchanger acts chiefly as an alkalinizing mechanism. When acidification is required, the bicarbonate-chloride exchanger transports HCO_3^- outward, leaving H+ behind. The steady-state pH of cardiac cells is, therefore, controlled at about 7.0 to 7.2 by a balance between the alkalinizing and acidifying exchangers and the metabolic production of acids.[67] Recently, the bicarbonate-chloride exchanger has been cloned from the human heart.[67] Beta-adrenergic stimulation causes acidification by increasing the activity of this exchanger.[68]

Sodium Pump

The sarcolemma becomes highly permeable to Na+ only during the opening of the Na+ channel during early depolarization, and Na+ also enters during the exit of Ca++ by Na+/Ca++ exchange. Most of this influx of Na+ across the sarcolemma must be corrected by the activity of the Na+/K+ pump, also called the Na+/K+-ATPase or simply the Na+ pump.[69] The pump is activated by internal Na+ or external K+.[69] One ATP molecule is used per transport cycle. The ions are first secluded within the pump protein and then extruded to either side. Although there has been some dispute about the exact ratio of Na+ to K+ that are pumped, a generally accepted model is that for every three Na+ ex-

FIGURE 12–16. The difference between extracellular pH (7.40) and intracellular pH (7.15) is maintained by the activity of a series of exchanges and transporters. Intracellular pH is lower because of the generation of CO_2 and H_2O by metabolism, and hence formation of H+ and HCO_3^-. Note the crucial role of H+ extrusion by Na+/H+ exchange with subsequent activity of the Na+/Ca++ exchanger to transport outward the Na+ ions gained from Na+/H+ exchange. Further adjustments are possible by varying the rates of bicarbonate entry *(bottom left)* and exit *(bottom right).* During intracellular acidosis as in ischemia, the necessity to extrude H+ means that there is a gain of Na+ and hence indirectly of Ca++. (Reprinted with permission. Copyright ©1997 L. H. Opie.)

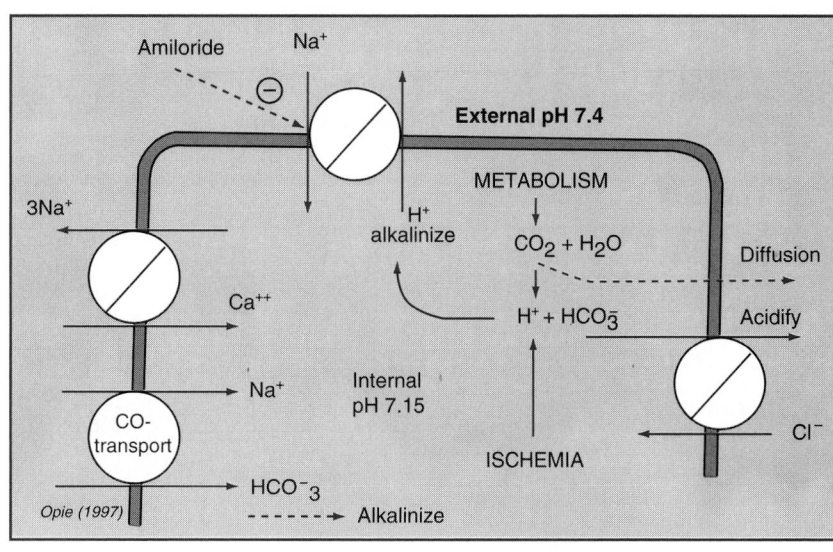

ported, two K$^+$ are imported.[70] During this process, one positive charge must leave the cell. Hence, the pump is electrogenic and is also called the electrogenic Na$^+$ pump.[69] The current induced by sustained activity of the pump may contribute about -10 mV to the resting membrane potential.[69] Because the pump must extrude Na$^+$ ions entering by either Na$^+$/Ca^{++} exchange or by the Na$^+$ channel, its sustained activity is essential for the maintenance of normal ion balance (Fig. 12–14).

RECEPTORS AND SIGNAL SYSTEMS

The autonomic nervous system can initiate signal systems that profoundly alter the fluxes of calcium and other ions. Thus, adrenergic or cholinergic stimulation of the sarcolemmal receptors inaugurates the activity of a complex system of sarcolemmal and cytosolic messengers.[73] Occupancy of the beta-adrenergic receptor is coupled by a G-protein complex (Fig. 12–17) to activation of a sarcolemmal enzyme, adenylate cyclase.[74,75] The G-protein complex involved, being stimulatory, is called G$_s$.[75] Situated in the

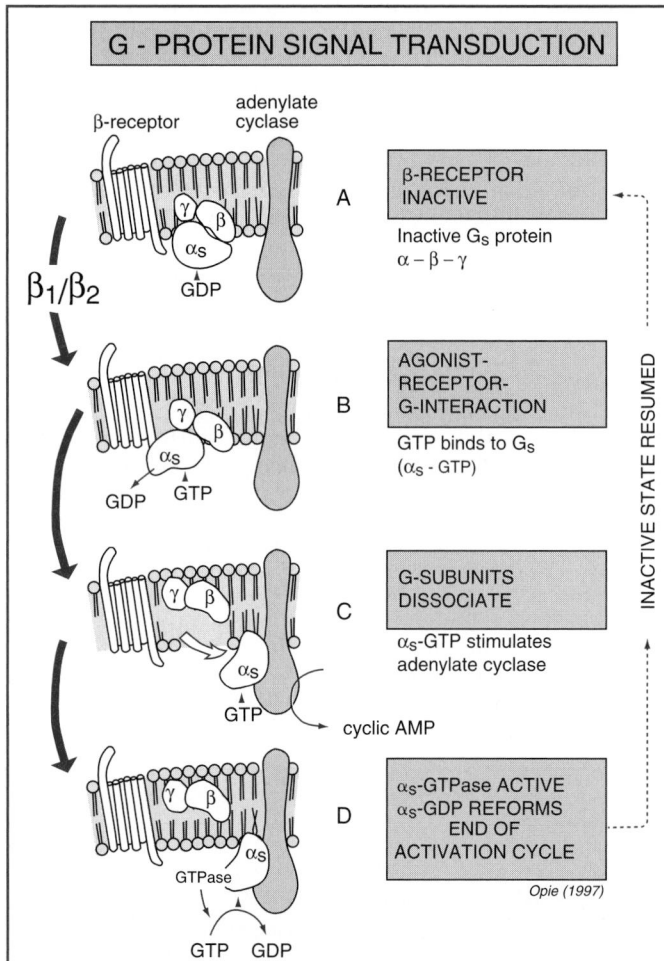

FIGURE 12–17. G proteins and their role in signal transduction in response to beta-adrenergic stimulation. Steps in G$_s$ protein cycle: *(A)* inactive beta-receptor, inactive G$_s$ protein $(\alpha + \beta + \gamma)$; *(B)* beta-receptor occupancy, GTP binds to alpha-subunit of G$_s$(α_s) to displace GDP; *(C)* the G-subunits dissociate. Affinity of receptor for agonist decreases. α_s-GTP stimulates activity of adenylate cyclase with formation of cyclic AMP; *(D)* GTPase becomes active; converts GTP to GDP, α_s-GDP reforms. End of activation cycle. Inactive state resumed. α_s = stimulatory alpha-subunit of G protein; β = beta-subunit of G protein; γ = gamma-subunit of G protein; GDP = guanine diphosphate; G$_s$ = stimulatory G-protein; GTP = guanine triphosphate. (Reprinted with permission. Copyright ©1997 L. H. Opie.)

sarcolemma, G$_s$ passes on the signal from the beta-receptor to adenylate cyclase.[74,76] In the sinus node, a similar messenger system increases the heart rate. Adenylate cyclase, stimulated by G$_s$, produces the second messenger, cyclic AMP, which then acts through a further series of intracellular signals and specifically the third messenger protein kinase A, to increase cytosolic calcium transients. In contrast, cholinergic stimulation exerts inhibitory influences, largely on the heart rate, but also on atrial contraction, acting at least in part by decreasing the rate of formation of cyclic AMP.[73]

Other cardiac receptors, such as the alpha-adrenergic receptor, have an alternate dual messenger system involving inositol trisphosphate (IP$_3$) and diacylglycerol, with the latter activating protein kinase C.[30,77] Such signals are of established importance in controlling calcium flux in vascular smooth muscle, thereby regulating vascular tone and indirectly the blood pressure. In the case of cardiac myocytes, it is now appreciated that receptors coupled to protein kinase C, such as angiotensin II, may play a major role in the regulation of cardiac myocyte growth[78] and sometimes have inotropic effects.

Yet other messenger systems exist to convey different signals. For example, in blood vessels, nitric oxide formed in the inner endothelial layer stimulates the formation of cyclic GMP in the smooth muscle layer, thereby causing relaxation (vasodilation).

The sum total of these processes converting an extracellular hormonal or neural stimulus to an intracellular physiological change is called *signal transduction,* which typically starts with the agonist binding to a receptor site.[30,75]

Beta-Adrenergic Receptors and G Proteins

Cardiac beta-adrenergic receptors are chiefly the beta$_1$-subtype, whereas most noncardiac receptors are beta$_2$. There are also beta$_2$-receptors in the human heart, about 20 per cent of the total beta-receptor population in the left ventricle and about twice as high a percentage in the atria.[79] These beta$_2$-receptors appear to have greater efficacy in their capacity to activate the G-protein–adenylate cyclase system than do the beta$_1$-receptors.[80]

The receptor site is highly stereospecific, the best fit among catecholamines being obtained with the synthetic agent isoproterenol (ISO) rather than with the naturally occurring catecholamines, norepinephrine (NE), and epinephrine (E). In the case of beta$_1$-receptors, the order of agonist activity is ISO > E = NE, whereas in the case of beta$_2$-receptors, the order is ISO > E > NE.[81] The structure of the beta$_2$-receptor has been particularly well studied. The transmembrane domains are held to be the site of agonist and antagonist binding, whereas the cytoplasmic domains interact with G proteins. One of the phosphorylation sites lies on the terminal COOH tail and may be involved in the process of desensitization (see next section).

THE STIMULATORY G PROTEIN. G proteins are a superfamily of proteins that bind guanine triphosphate (GTP) and other guanine nucleotides, a process that is crucial in linking the effect of the first messenger on the receptor to the activity of the membrane-bound enzyme system that produces the second messenger (Fig. 12–17).[74] The triple combination of the beta-receptor, the G-protein complex, and adenylate cyclase is termed the *beta-adrenergic system.*[82] The G protein itself is a heterotrimer composed of G$_\alpha$, G$_\beta$, and G$_\gamma$, which upon receptor stimulation splits into the alpha-subunit that is bound to GTP, and the beta-gamma-subunit.[83] Either of these subunits may regulate differing effectors such as adenylate cyclase, phospholipase C, and ion channels. The activity of adenylate cyclase is controlled by two different G-protein complexes, namely G$_s$ which stimulates and G$_i$ which inhibits.[84] The alpha-subunit of G_s (α_s) combines with GTP and then separates from the other two subunits to enhance activity of adenylate cyclase. The beta- and gamma-subunits appear to be linked structurally and in function.

THE INHIBITORY G PROTEIN. In contrast, a second trimeric GTP-binding protein, G_i, is responsible for inhibition of adenylate cyclase.[83] During cholinergic signaling, the muscarinic receptor is stimulated and GTP binds to the inhibitory alpha-subunit, α_i.[75] The latter then dissociates from the other two components of the G-protein complex, which are, as in the case of G_s, the combined beta-gamma-subunits. Whereas the role of α_i is not clear, the beta-gamma-subunits act as follows. By stimulating the enzyme GTPase,[85] they break down the active alpha$_s$-subunit (α_s-GTP), so that the activation of adenylate cyclase in response to beta-stimulation becomes less. Furthermore, the beta-gamma-subunit activates the K_{ACh} channel[86] that, in turn, can inhibit the sinoatrial node to contribute to the bradycardic effect of cholinergic stimulation. The alpha$_i$-subunit activates another potassium channel (K_{ATP})[86] whose physiological function is still under discussion.

A third G protein, G_q, is involved in linking myocardial alpha-adrenergic receptors to another membrane-associated enzyme, phospholipase C (see p. 375). G_q has at least four isoforms, of which two have been found in the heart. This G protein, unlike G_i, is not susceptible to inhibition by pertussis toxin.[75]

Adenylate cyclase is the only enzyme system producing cyclic AMP and specifically requires low concentrations of ATP (and magnesium) as substrate. Surprisingly, the proposed molecular structure resembles certain channel proteins, such as that of the calcium channel. Most of the protein is located on the cytoplasmic side,[87] the presumed site of interaction with the G protein.

Cyclic AMP acts as the second messenger of beta-adrenergic receptor activity (Fig. 12–18), while another cyclic nucleotide, cyclic GMP, acts as a second messenger for some aspects of vagal activity (Fig. 12–19). In vascular smooth muscle, cyclic GMP is the second messenger of the nitric oxide messenger system. These messenger chemicals are present in the heart cell in minute concentrations, that of cyclic AMP being roughly about 10^{-9} M and that of cyclic GMP about 10^{-11} M.[88] Cyclic AMP has a very rapid turnover as a result of a constant dynamic balance between its formation by adenylate cyclase and removal by another enzyme, phosphodiesterase. In general, directional changes in the tissue content of cyclic AMP can be related to directional changes in cardiac contractile activity (Table 7–3[89]). For example, beta-adrenergic stimulation increases both, whereas beta-blockade inhibits the increases induced by beta-agonists. *Forskolin*, a direct stimulator of adenylate cy-

FIGURE 12–18. Signal systems involved in positive inotropic and lusitropic (enhanced relaxation) effects of beta-adrenergic stimulation. When the beta-adrenergic agonist interacts with the beta-receptor, a series of G protein–mediated changes (Fig. 12–17) lead to activation of adenylate cyclase and formation of cyclic AMP (cAMP). The latter acts via protein kinase A to stimulate metabolism *(left)* and to phosphorylate the calcium channel protein (Fig. 12–13). The result is an enhanced opening probability of the calcium channel, thereby increasing the inward movement of Ca^{++} ions through the sarcolemma (SL) of the T tubule. These Ca^{++} ions release more calcium from the sarcoplasmic reticulum (SR) (Fig. 12–3) to increase cytosolic calcium and to activate troponin-C. Calcium ions also increase the rate of breakdown of ATP to ADP and inorganic phosphate (P$_i$). Enhanced myosin ATPase activity explains the increased rate of contraction, with increased activation of troponin-C explaining increased peak force development. An increased rate of relaxation is explained because cyclic AMP also activates the protein phospholamban, situated on the membrane of the SR, that controls the rate of uptake of calcium into the SR (Fig. 12–12). The latter effect explains enhanced relaxation (lusitropic effect). P = phosphorylation; PL = phospholamban; SL = sarcolemma; SR = sarcoplasmic reticulum. (Reprinted with permission. Copyright ©1997 L. H. Opie.)

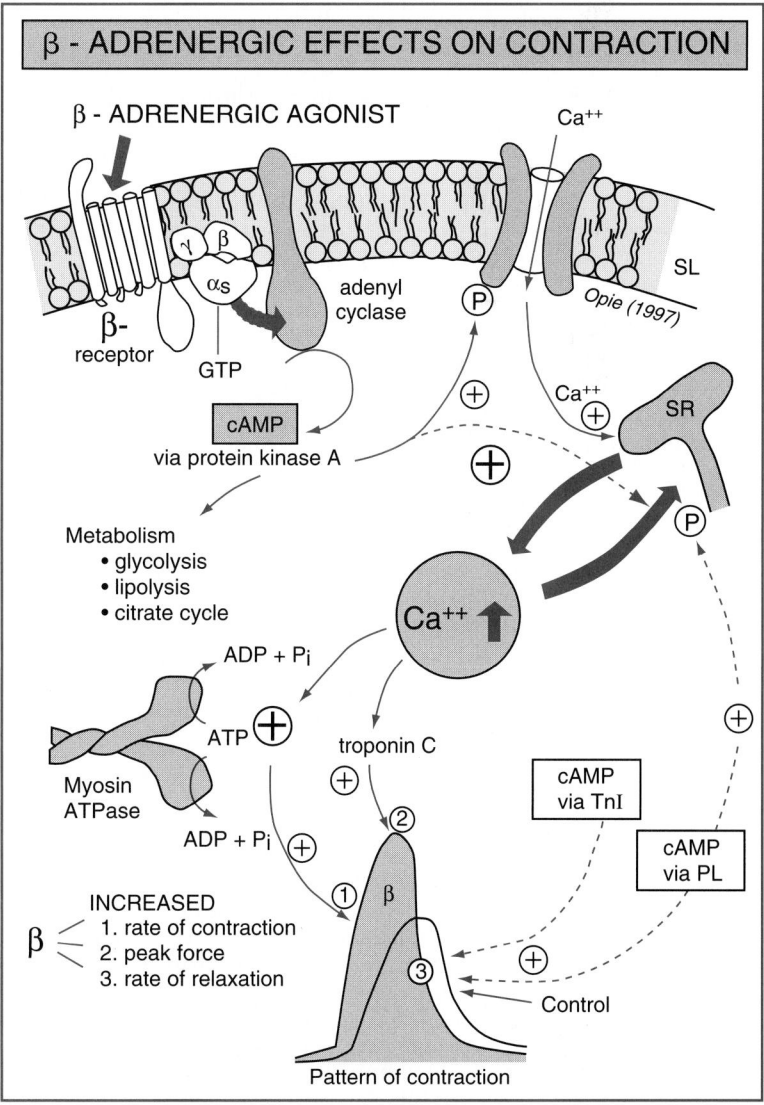

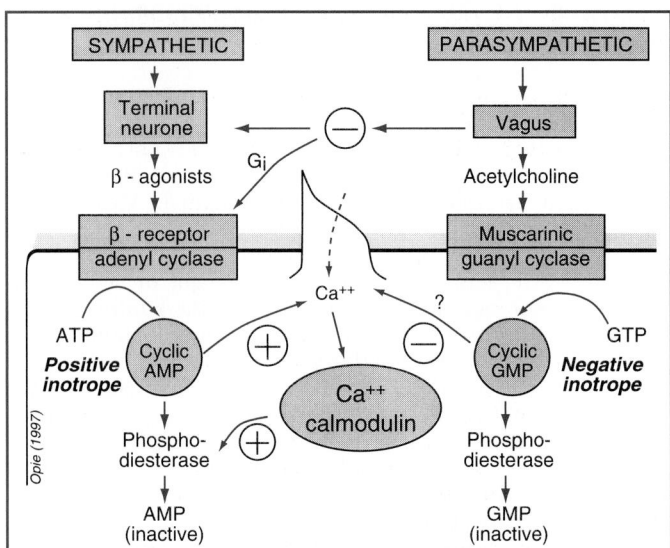

FIGURE 12–19. Interaction between parasympathetic and sympathetic systems at a cellular level may involve two opposing cyclic nucleotides, cyclic AMP and cyclic GMP. Many effects of vagal stimulation could best be explained by the inhibitory effect on the formation of cyclic AMP, including formation of inhibitory G protein, G_i, in response to M_2-receptor stimulation (Fig. 12–21). (Reprinted with permission. Copyright ©1997 L. H. Opie.)

clase, increases cyclic AMP and contractile activity. Adenosine, acting through A_1-receptors, inhibits adenylate cyclase, decreases cyclic AMP, and lessens contractile activity.

A number of hormones can couple to myocardial adenylate cyclase independently of the beta-adrenergic receptor. These are glucagon, thyroid hormone, prostacyclin (PGI_2), and the calcitonin gene-related peptide.

INHIBITION OF CYCLIC AMP FORMATION. The major physiological stimulus to G_s is thought to be vagal muscarinic receptor stimulation (Fig. 12–19). There are two additional inhibitory agonists. First, adenosine, interacting with A_1-receptors, couples to G_i to inhibit contraction and heart rate.[90] The adenosine A_2-receptor, also found in the heart, paradoxically increases cyclic AMP. The latter effect is thought to be of major importance in vascular smooth muscle but of only ancillary significance in the heart.[90] Second, endothelin may also inhibit cyclic AMP formation through a G_s-linked receptor[91] to have a potentially negative inotropic effect, in contrast to the possible positive effect generated by the coupling of the endothelin receptor to phospholipase C.

CYCLIC AMP–DEPENDENT PROTEIN KINASES. It is now clear that most if not all of the effects of cyclic AMP are ultimately mediated by the protein kinases that phosphorylate various important proteins and enzymes.[92,93] *Phosphorylation* is the donation of a phosphate group to the enzyme concerned, acting as a fundamental metabolic switch that can extensively amplify the signal.

Each protein kinase is composed of two subunits, regulatory (R) and catalytic (C). When cyclic AMP interacts with the inactive protein kinase, it binds to the R-subunit to liberate the active kinase, which is the C-subunit:

$$(R_2 + C_2) + 2\ cAMP \rightarrow 2\ RcAMP + 2\ C$$

At a molecular level, this active kinase catalyzes the transfer of the terminal phosphate of ATP to serine and threonine residues of the protein substrates, leading to phosphorylation and modification of the properties of the proteins concerned, thereby leading to further key reactions. Protein kinase A occurs in different cells in two isoforms: *protein kinase II* predominates in cardiac cells.[93] The proposed anchorage of this kinase to specific organelles could help explain the phenomenon of *cyclic AMP*

compartmentation.[94] In addition, the G-protein system may not be evenly spread throughout the sarcolemma but localized to certain focal areas.[83] Thus, it is very likely that there is a specific compartment of cyclic AMP available to increase contractile activity.[95,96]

Physiological Beta-Adrenergic Effects

The probable sequence of events describing the positive inotropic effects of catecholamines is shown in Figure 12–18 and is as follows[89]:

Catecholamine stimulation → beta-receptor → molecular changes → binding of GTP to alpha$_s$-subunit of G protein → GTP-alpha$_s$-subunit stimulates adenylate cyclase → formation of cyclic AMP from ATP → activation of cyclic AMP–dependent protein kinase (PKA) → phosphorylation of a sarcolemmal protein p27 → increased entry of calcium ion through increased opening of the voltage-dependent L-type calcium channels → greater calcium-induced calcium release via ryanodine receptor of sarcoplasmic reticulum → more rise of intracellular free calcium ion concentration → increased calcium–troponin-C interaction with deinhibition of tropomyosin effect on actin-myosin interaction → increased rate and number of crossbridges interacting with increased myosin ATPase activity → increased rate and peak force development.

The increased lusitropic (relaxant) effect is the consequence of increased protein kinase A–mediated phosphorylation of phospholamban (Fig. 12–18).

Cholinergic Receptors

In the case of the parasympathetic system, signaling is again an extracellular first messenger (acetylcholine), a receptor system (the muscarinic receptor), and a sarcolemmal signaling system (the G-protein system). The myocardial *muscarinic receptor (M_2)* is associated specifically with the activity of the vagal nerve endings. Receptor stimulation produces a negative chronotropic response that is inhibited by atropine.

Regarding the *negative inotropic effect of vagal stimulation* (Fig. 12–19), the mechanism is multiple, including (1) heart rate slowing (negative Treppe phenomenon); (2) an inhibition of the formation of cyclic AMP; and (3) a direct negative inotropic effect mediated by cyclic GMP.[97] It should be noted that ventricular tissue is much less responsive to muscarinic agonists than atrial tissue, although the receptor populations are similar in density.[73] Thus, there must be postreceptor differences between atrial and ventricular tissue, probably in the degree of G-protein coupling. In general, the negative inotropic effect has been best observed in the presence of beta-stimulation (Table 12–2) when vagal effects counteract those of prior beta-stimulation.[73,98] The proposal is that muscarinic stimulation inhibits the G_s activation that results from beta-receptor occupation.

Cyclic GMP may act as a second messenger to vagal stimulation just as cyclic AMP does to beta-adrenergic stimulation. Thus, the vagus may have a dual effect on second messengers, inhibiting the formation of cyclic AMP and increasing that of cyclic GMP.[97] Cyclic GMP may in turn inhibit the activity of the L-calcium channel by a cyclic GMP–dependent kinase (G kinase).[99,100] Favoring this view is the finding that cell-permeable analogs of cyclic GMP have antiadrenergic effects. The problem with this hypothesis is the inconstant increase in ventricular cyclic GMP in response to vagal stimulation. The explanation could lie in cell compartmentation of cyclic GMP, as postulated for cyclic AMP. Also the effects of cyclic GMP on contractility may be more subtle than changes in the pattern of peak force development. Rather, there may be decreased sensitivity of the myofilaments to Ca^{++} and earlier relaxation.[101]

Yet another mechanism for parasympathetic-sympathetic interaction lies at the level of the sympathetic terminal

TABLE 12–2 IONIC EFFECTS OF ADRENERGIC AND CHOLINERGIC STIMULATION: RELATION TO HEART RATE AND CONTRACTILE ACTIVITY

AGONIST	IONIC CURRENT	EFFECT
Beta-adrenergic stimulation[1,2]	I_{Ca} increased	+ inotropic
	I_k increased	− inotropic
	I_{to} increased	− inotropic
	I_f increased	Heart rate +
	I_{Na} increased	Contraction +
		Conduction +
ACh during beta-stimulation[1,3]	I_{Ca} decreased	− inotropic
	I_{Na} decreased	− dromotropic
	I_f decreased	− chronotropic
ACh direct effect on K^+ currents[4]	I_{kACh} and I_{kATP} increased	Heart rate decreased
Alpha₁-adrenergic stimulation[5]	I_{to} decreased	+ inotropic
	I_k decreased	+ inotropic
	I_{kACh} decreased	Atrial current, effects not clear

− = negative; + = positive
[1] Matsuda et al.[98]
[2] Matsuda et al.[130]
[3] Chang and Cohen[131]
[4] Kurachi[86]
[5] Fedida[108]

neuronse, where a *presynaptic muscarinic M₂ receptor* inhibits the release of norepinephrine.[73]

Additionally, both adrenergic and cholinergic stimuli exert complex and potentially important effects on ion channels that can be translated into opposing effects on cardiac function (Table 12–2). The presence of such multiple mechanisms for the inhibitory effects of vagal stimulation on the heart rate and inotropic state suggest that "braking" of beta-adrenergic stimulation is desirable. Otherwise, the risk may be that intense beta-adrenergic stimulation would excessively increase the heart rate or inotropic state.

Receptors Linked to Phospholipase C

There is an important group of receptors previously thought to act chiefly on the myocardium at the presynaptic level to enhance release of norepinephrine, and on postsynaptic vascular receptors to cause vasoconstriction. Such receptors include those for alpha₁-adrenergic catecholamines, angiotensin II, and endothelin. They are all linked to phospholipase C by a G protein, G_q (Fig. 12–20). Currently, two aspects of their action are under intense

focus. First, the signaling system involved is clearly different from that involved in beta-adrenergic effects.[30] Second, these receptors have been identified in ventricular myocytes, posing the question of their physiological role—a problem that is still not fully clarified.[77]

PHOSPHATIDYLINOSITOL SYSTEM. When any of these agonists occupies its receptor, then the link to phospholipase C is by one of the G-protein family, namely G_q. The exact steps involved are not as well understood as is the coupling of the beta-receptor to adenylate cyclase, but similar components of the G-protein complex appear to be involved.[102] First, G_q activates phospholipase C to split the compound phosphatidylinositol bisphosphate (PIP₂), part of the membrane phospholipid system, into two second messengers, *inositol trisphosphate* (IP₃) and 1,2-diacylglycerol (DAG). IP₃, in turn, stimulates the slow release of calcium from the SR and increases calcium oscillations.[103] This calcium acts on the next messenger in the system, protein kinase C, by promoting the translocation of this enzyme from cytosol to sarcolemma.[104] Once translocated, protein kinase C becomes activated by DAG, the other second messenger of phospholipase C activity. DAG, being highly lipophilic, stays in the cell membrane and, together with a resident serine component of the membrane lipids, stimulates protein kinase C into activity by reducing the calcium requirement of the protein kinase C to micromolar values.[93]

PROTEIN KINASE C. Protein kinase C has at least nine isoforms, the functions of which are poorly understood.[105] Some of the isoforms may hypothetically be associated with enhanced growth via proto-oncogenes.[106] Other isoforms may be concerned with inotropy.[107] The involvement of different isoforms may be concerned with inotropy.[107] The involvement of different isoforms may explain variable effects on contraction, mostly positive with some negatives.[73,108,109] Hypothetically, protein kinase C is an effector of preconditioning,[110] perhaps activating potassium channels (Fig. 12–20).[111]

Other Signals

Nitric Oxide as Messenger with Cyclic GMP as Target

In the myocardium, the proposal is that cyclic GMP can, by stimulation of the appropriate protein G kinases (PKG), result in a decreased heart rate and in a negative inotropic effect.[100] Formation of cyclic GMP, under the influence of guanylate cyclase, is thought to occur in response to (1) cholinergic stimulation, as already discussed, and (2) the nitric oxide signaling path.

In vascular smooth muscle, soluble guanylate cyclase responds to stimulation by nitric oxide, released by the vascular endothelium, by formation of cyclic GMP.[112] The latter vasodilates through a mechanism not fully understood but thought to involve G kinase and a decrease of cytosolic calcium. Until recently it was thought that nitric oxide played no role in the regulation of myocardial cell function. Yet, in ventricular myocytes, production of nitric oxide enhances the negative inotropic effect of acetylcholine and decreases the positive inotropic effects of beta-stimulation.[113] Therefore, the nitric oxide system, it is proposed, may have a negative modulatory role on the cardiac effects of autonomic stimulation in keeping with the proposed formation of cyclic GMP. Nonetheless, in cardiac muscle not undergoing beta-adrenergic stimulation, physiological concentrations of nitric oxide do not appear to alter cardiac contractile behavior.[114] Thus, the physiological role of the nitric oxide messenger system in the myocardium remains controversial.

Adenosine Signaling

Adenosine, like nitric oxide, is a physiological vasodilator. It is formed from the breakdown of ATP both physiologically (as during an increased heart load) and pathologi-

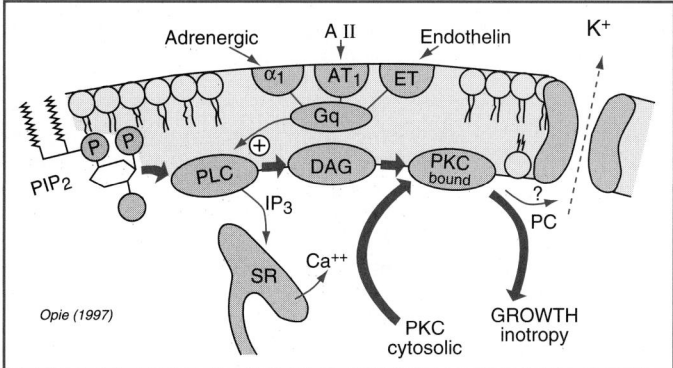

FIGURE 12–20. Phospholipase C (PLC) signaling system in myocardium, coupled to alpha₁-adrenergic, angiotensin AT₁, and endothelin (ET) receptors by G proteins G_q. PLC splits phosphatidylinositol bisphosphate (PIP₂) to inositol trisphosphate (IP₃) and diacylglycerol (DAG), the latter being membrane-bound. IP₃ (and IP₄) release Ca⁺⁺ from the sarcoplasmic reticulum (SR) to activate protein kinase C (PKC) by translocating it from a cytosolic to a membrane-bound situation. PKC plays a role in growth regulation and possibly in inotropy and ion channel control. Hypothetically, PKC is an effector of preconditioning (PC) and activates potassium channels. (Reprinted with permission. Copyright ©1997 L. H. Opie.)

cally (as in ischemia). Adenosine can diffuse from myocardial cells to act on coronary arterial smooth muscle to cause vasodilation (see p. 386). The mechanism of the latter effect is reasonably well understood and involves the stimulation of vascular adenylate cyclase and cyclic AMP formation. A_2-Receptors mediate such vasodilation. Although A_2-receptors have also been identified in cardiomyocytes, stimulation of such receptors does not appear to have functional consequences.[115] Therefore only the A_1-receptors coupled to adenylate cyclase by the inhibitory G protein (alpha$_i$-subunit) are functional in the myocardium.

Other signal systems are also involved.[116] First, A_1-receptors couple to the acetylcholine-sensitive potassium channel (current I_{kACh}) to stimulate channel opening and thereby to exert inhibitory effects on the sinus and AV nodes, the latter inhibition being the basis for the use of adenosine in the treatment of supraventricular nodal reentry arrhythmias (see p. 618). Second, A_1-receptors may in some circumstances couple to phospholipase C, which hypothetically explains their role in preconditioning.

Stretch Receptors

Both myocardial and vascular cells can respond to stretch by activation of a group of poorly understood mechanoreceptors, also called stretch receptors. Activation of these receptors is linked to a series of phosphorylations, including those of two crucial enzymes in the growth cascade, namely MAP (mitogen-activated protein) kinase and S6 kinase.[117] Stretch may initiate a series of conformational changes in ion channels or receptors to allow increased entry of a specific ion, such as sodium, which could then be converted to a calcium signal by Na^+/Ca^{++} exchange. Another example of a mechanoreceptor is the response of the ATP-sensitive potassium channel of atrial muscle.[118] Of considerable interest is the concept that an early event in the sequence leading from muscle stretch to hypertrophy is release of angiotensin II from the stretched muscle.[78] The mechanism of this stretch-induced release of angiotensin II is not known but may include stimulation of formation of the cardiac mRNA for renin.[119]

Signaling Systems in Heart Failure
(See also Chap. 13)

In congestive heart failure (Fig. 12–21), changes to the beta-adrenergic–cyclic AMP system include (1) major beta$_1$-receptor downregulation[79,120]; (2) beta$_2$-receptor uncoupling

from adenylate cyclase[120]; (3) decreased adenylate cyclase activity[120,121]; and (4) increased levels of inhibitory G_i proteins.[122] In combination, these changes may explain the poorly developed and low-amplitude calcium transients in human tissue from severe heart failure subjects.[123] There is a major (50 to 70 per cent) *downregulation* of the beta$_1$-receptor with decreased receptor density, especially when the heart failure is caused by idiopathic cardiomyopathy.[120] Of the beta-receptor subtypes in the human ventricle, the normal ratio of the beta$_1$ to beta$_2$ of about 80:20 is changed to a ratio of about 60:40,[79,124] so that beta$_2$-mediated inotropic effects may become relatively more important. The previous proposal that the beta$_1$-receptor downregulation occurs in response to the excess level of circulating catecholamines seems not valid.[120] Rather, a poorly understood local mechanism translates into a decrease of the mRNA for the beta$_1$-receptor.[120,125] In addition, both Beta$_1$- and beta$_2$-receptors become moderately uncoupled from their signaling systems, so that even beta$_2$-stimulation is less positively inotropic than expected.[79,120] In this context, although it might be anticipated that alpha$_1$-mediated positive inotropic effects would become more prominent as a compensatory mechanism, nonetheless the response to alpha$_1$-stimulation in heart failure is much diminished.[124]

Uncoupling of the beta-receptor from the signaling system may be explained as follows.[125,126] Sustained beta-agonist stimulation rapidly induces the activity of the beta-agonist receptor kinase (βARK) that is involved in the transfer of the phosphate group to the phosphorylation site on the terminal COOH tail of the receptor, which of itself does not markedly affect the signaling properties. Rather, βARK increases the affinity of the beta-receptor for another protein family, the *arrestins*,[125,127] that cause the uncoupling. Hypothetically, the molecular configuration of the receptor is changed in such a way that the G proteins cannot interact optimally with it. Resensitization of the receptor occurs if the phosphate group is split off by a phosphatase and the receptor may then more readily be linked to G_s.[81]

Physiologically, the βARK-arrestin mechanism causes a very rapid desensitization of beta-receptor within minutes to seconds, yet this mechanism also plays a role in long-term desensitization as in heart failure.[125,127]

Also causing physiological (but not pathological) desensitization is phosphorylation of the beta-receptor by protein kinase A,[127] occurring within minutes and acting as a feedback mechanism to prevent adverse effects of excess cyclic AMP elevation and protein kinase activation such as severe arrhythmias.[128] Long-term desensitization may be associated with receptor internalization, sequestration,[127] and even lysosomal degradation.[129]

CONTRACTILE PERFORMANCE OF THE INTACT HEART

There are three main determinants of myocardial mechanical performance, namely the Frank-Starling mechanism, the contractile state, and the heart rate. This section describes the cardiac cycle and then the determinants of left ventricular (LV) function.

The Cardiac Cycle

The cardiac cycle, fully assembled by Lewis[132] but first conceived by Wiggers,[133] yields important information on the temporal sequence of events in the cardiac cycle. The three basic events are (1) LV contraction, (2) LV relaxation, and (3) LV filling (Table 12–3). Although similar mechanical events occur in the right side of the heart, those on the left side are the focus.

LV CONTRACTION. LV pressure starts to build up when the arrival of calcium ions at the contractile proteins starts to trigger actin-myosin interaction. On the electrocardio-

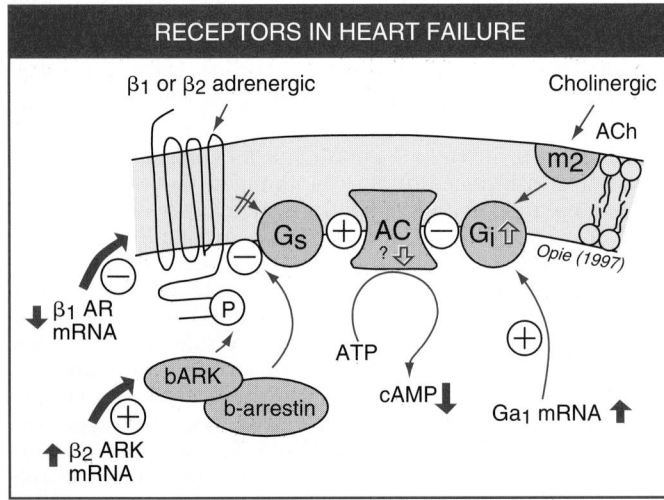

FIGURE 12–21. Proposed changes in beta-adrenergic receptor signal system in severe congestive heart failure (CHF). For concepts, see Lohse.[125] AC = Adenylate cyclase; β_1AR = beta$_1$-adrenergic receptor; β_2AR = beta$_2$-adrenergic receptor; βARK = beta-adrenergic receptor kinase; M$_2$ = muscarinic receptor; ACh = acetylcholine; G$_i$ = inhibitory G protein; G$_s$ = stimulatory G protein. (Reprinted with permission. Copyright ©1997 L. H. Opie.)

TABLE 12-3 THE CARDIAC CYCLE

LV CONTRACTION
Isovolumic contraction (b)
Maximal ejection (c)
LV RELAXATION
Start of relaxation and reduced ejection (d)
Isovolumic relaxation (e)
LV filling: rapid phase (f)
Slow LV filling (diastasis) (g)
Atrial systole or booster (a)

The letters a to g refer to the phases of the cardiac cycle shown in Wiggers' diagram (Fig. 12–22). These letters are arbitrarily allocated so that atrial systole (a) coincides with the A wave and (c) with the C wave of the jugular venous pressure.

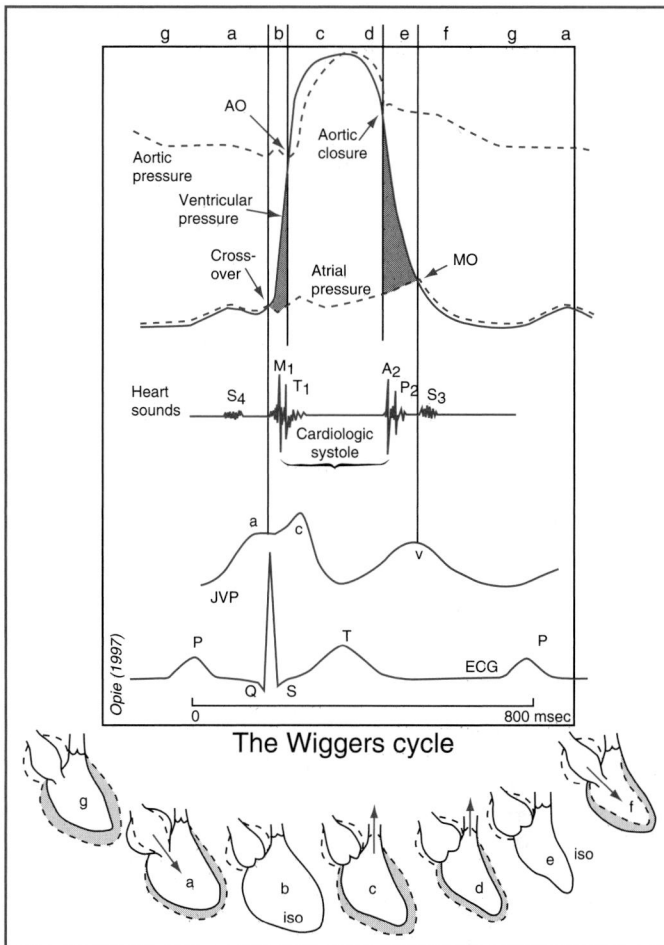

FIGURE 12-22. The mechanical events in the cardiac cycle, first assembled by Lewis in 1920 but first conceived by Wiggers in 1915.[133] Note that mitral valve closure occurs *after* the crossover point of atrial and ventricular pressures at the start of systole. (Visual phases of the ventricular cycle in bottom panel are modified from Shepherd J. T., and Vanhoutte P. M.: The Human Cardiovascular System. New York, Raven Press, 1979, p. 68.) For explanation of phases a to g, see Table 12–3. ECG = Electrocardiogram; JVP = jugular venous pressure; M_1 = mitral component of first sound at time of mitral valve closure; T_1 = tricuspid valve closure, second component of first heart sound; AO = aortic valve opening, normally inaudible; A_2 = aortic valve closure, aortic component of second sound; P_2 = pulmonary component of second sound, pulmonary valve closure; MO = mitral valve opening, may be audible in mitral stenosis as the opening snap; S_3 = third heart sound; S_4 = fourth heart sound; a = wave produced by right atrial contraction; c = carotid wave artifact during rapid LV ejection phase; v = venous return wave which causes pressure to rise while tricuspid valve is closed. Cycle length of 800 msec for 75 beats per minute. (Copyright ©1997 L. H. Opie.)

gram (ECG), the advance of the wave of depolarization is indicated by the peak of the R wave (Fig. 12–22). Soon after LV pressure in the early contraction phase builds up and exceeds that in the left atrium (normally 10 to 15 mm Hg), followed about 20 msec later by M_1, the mitral component of the first sound. The exact relation of M_1 to mitral valve closure is open to debate.[134,135] Although mitral valve closure is often thought to coincide with the crossover point at which the LV pressure starts to exceed the left atrial pressure,[132,133,136] in reality mitral valve closure is delayed because the valve is kept open by the inertia of the blood flow.[135,137] Shortly thereafter, pressure changes in the right ventricle, similar in pattern but lesser in magnitude to those in the left ventricle, cause the tricuspid valve to close, thereby creating T_1, which is the second component of the first heart sound.

During this phase of contraction between mitral valve and aortic valve opening, the LV volume is fixed *(isovolumic contraction)*, because both aortic and mitral valves are shut. As more and more myofibers enter the contracted state, pressure development in the left ventricle proceeds. The interaction of actin and myosin increases, and cross-bridge cycling augments. When the pressure in the left ventricle exceeds that in the aorta, the aortic valve opens. Opening of the aortic valve is followed by the phase of *rapid ejection,* determined not only by the pressure gradient across the aortic valve, but also by the elastic properties of the aorta and the arterial tree, which undergoes systolic expansion. LV pressure rises to a peak and then starts to fall.

LV RELAXATION. As the cytosolic calcium ion concentration starts to decline because of uptake of calcium into the SR under the influence of phospholamban, more and more myofibers enter the state of relaxation and the rate of ejection of blood from the left ventricle into the aorta falls (phase of *reduced ejection*). During this phase, blood flow from the LV to the aorta rapidly diminishes but is maintained by aortic distensibility—the Windkessel effect.[138] The pressure in the aorta exceeds the falling pressure in the LV. The aortic valve closes, creating the first component of the second sound, A_2 (the second component, P_2, results from closure of the pulmonary valve as the pulmonary artery pressure exceeds that in the right ventricle). Thereafter, the ventricle continues to relax. Because the mitral valve is closed during this phase, the LV volume does not change *(isovolumic relaxation).* When the LV pressure falls to below that in the left atrium, the mitral valve opens and the filling phase of the cardiac cycle starts (Fig. 12–22). Mitral valve opening is normally silent, but in mitral stenosis there may be an audible opening snap.

LV FILLING. As LV pressure drops below that in the left atrium, just after mitral valve opening, the *phase of rapid or early filling* occurs to account for most of ventricular filling.[139] Active diastolic relaxation of the ventricle may also contribute to early filling (see section on Ventricular Suction). Such rapid filling may cause the physiological third heart sound (S_3), particularly when there is a hyperkinetic circulation.[140] As pressures in the atrium and ven-

tricle equalize, LV filling partially stops (*diastasis,* separation). Renewed filling requires that the pressure gradient from the atrium to the ventricle should increase. This is achieved by *atrial systole* (or the *left atrial booster*), which is especially important when a high cardiac output is required as during exercise, or when the LV fails to relax normally as in LV hypertrophy.[139]

DEFINITIONS OF SYSTOLE AND DIASTOLE. *Systole* means contraction in Greek, and *diastole* is derived from two Greek words, *to send* and *apart*. For the physiologist, systole lasts from the start of isovolumic contraction (where LV pressure crosses over atrial pressure, Fig. 12–22) to the peak of the ejection phase, so that physiological diastole commences as the LV pressure starts to fall (Table 12–4). In contrast, *cardiological* systole is demarcated by the heart sounds and extends from the first heart sound (M_1) to the closure of the aortic valve (A_2), with the rest of the cardiac cycle being defined as cardiological diastole. Mitral valve

TABLE 12–4 PHYSIOLOGICAL VERSUS CARDIOLOGICAL SYSTOLE AND DIASTOLE

PHYSIOLOGICAL SYSTOLE	CARDIOLOGICAL SYSTOLE
Isovolumic contraction	From M_1 to A_2
Maximal ejection	Only part of isovolumic contraction*
	Maximal ejection
	Reduced ejection
PHYSIOLOGICAL DIASTOLE	**CARDIOLOGICAL DIASTOLE**
Reduced ejection	A_2-M_1 interval (Filling phases included)
Isovolumic relaxation	
Filling phases	

* Note that M_1 occurs with a definite delay after the start of LV contraction.

closure (M_1) actually occurs about 20 msec after the onset of physiological systole at the crossover point of pressure.[135] The term *protodiastolic* (early diastole) for the physiologist is the early part of the relaxation phase—from when aortic flow begins to fall until the aortic valve shuts. For the cardiologist, protodiastole is the early phase of rapid filling, the time when the third heart sound (S_3) can be heard. This sound probably reflects ventricular wall vibrations during rapid filling and becomes audible with an increase in LV diastolic pressure or wall stiffness or rate of filling.

Frank-Starling Relationship

PRELOAD. The preload, literally the load before contraction has started, is provided by the venous return that fills the left atrium, which in turn empties into the LV during diastole.[141] When the preload increases, the LV distends, the LV pressure development becomes more rapid and rises to a higher peak pressure,[142] and the stroke volume augments. Because the heart rate also increases (see later in this section), the cardiac output rises as the venous pressure rises, as originally described by Starling. An example of such increases in the venous return are the increased cardiac output of exercise or of volume expansion as during an infusion of excess intravenous fluids. The preload is physiologically determined by the *venous return,* which in turn is influenced by venous compliance. There is also a lesser effect of a hemodynamically inactive "venous storage" component, also called the "unstressed volume," which is increased in size by venodilators.[143]

AFTERLOAD. During systole, the LV contracts against the afterload (the load *after* the onset of contraction, against which the LV contracts during LV ejection). It is less well known that Starling also studied the effect of an acute increase in afterload on LV performance. He and his co-workers abruptly increased the blood pressure of the heart-lung preparation and found that LV performance increased to overcome the greater peripheral resistance. Both systolic and diastolic LV volumes rose, indicating that the left ventricle did not empty completely. The increased diastolic volume acted in a manner similar to an increased preload to prevent the stroke volume from falling as the afterload increased. Such an afterload-dependent myocardium was probably the result of experimental conditions in which the left ventricle was in a state of incipient failure. In experimental preparations and in normal humans, a sudden increase in blood pressure is compensated for by an increased force of contraction (see Anrep effect) and by a reflex decrease of the peripheral vascular resistance mediated by the baroreflexes.

FORCE-LENGTH RELATIONSHIPS IN CALCIUM TRANSIENTS. The temptation is to link "optimal sarcomere length" with Starling's law and the force-length relationship, by supposing that ventricular stretch gives rise to such optimal overlap of actin and myosin. Whereas the overlap theory explains the force-length relationship in skeletal muscle, in cardiac muscle the situation is different (Fig. 12–23). In the

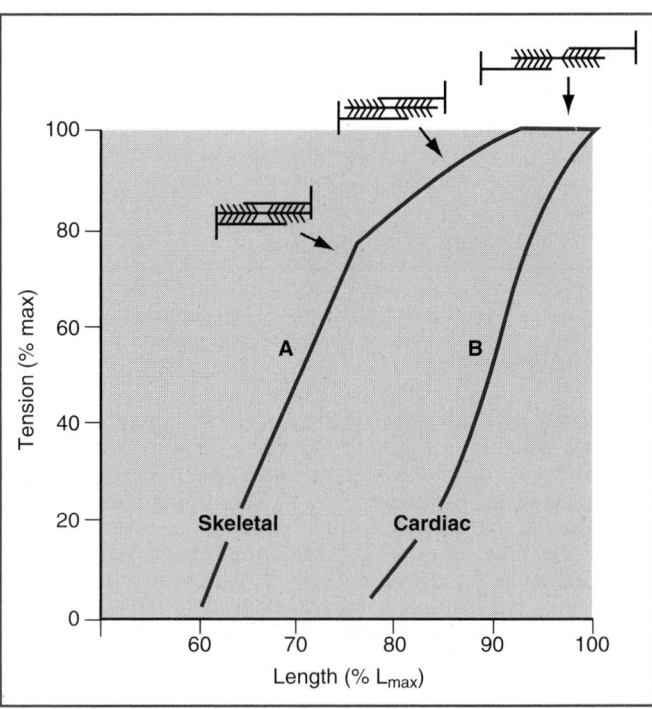

FIGURE 12–23. Schematic drawing illustrating general shape of ascending limb of *force-length relationship* in skeletal (A) and cardiac (B) muscle. Normalized force is plotted as a function of normalized length, i.e., length relative to length at which maximum force is generated (L_{max}). Also shown is approximate disposition of thick and thin filaments at different points along the physiologically relevant portion of the ascending limb. The maximum length (L_{max} 100 per cent) corresponds to the situation at maximum sarcomere lengths (2.2 microns, Fig. 12–24) or 2.15 microns (Fig. 12–25). (From Fuchs, F.: Mechanical modulation of the Ca^{2+} regulatory protein complex in cardiac muscle. NIPS *10*:6–12, 1995.)

case of skeletal muscle, the argument is as follows: "Because each actin filament projects about 1 micron from each side of the Z-disc, active force would decline when the sarcomere length was less than the sum of the lengths of the individual actin filaments, i.e., less than 2.0–2.2 microns."[23] In cardiac muscle, however, even at 80 per cent of the optimal length, only 10 per cent or less of the maximal force is developed (Fig. 12–23). Thus, it can be predicted that cardiac sarcomeres must function near the upper limit of their maximal length (L_{max}). Rodriguez et al.[144] have tested this prediction by relating sarcomere length changes to volume changes of the intact heart. By implanting small radiopaque beads in only about 1 cm^3 of the LV free wall and using biplane cineradiography, the motion of the markers can be tracked through various cardiac cycles with allowances made for local myocardial deformation. Thus, the change in sarcomere length from approximately 85 per cent of L_{max} to L_{max} itself is able to effect physiological LV volume changes (Fig. 12–24).

The favored explanation for the steep length-tension relation of cardiac muscles is *length-dependent activation,* whereby an increase in calcium sensitivity is the major factor explaining the steep increase of force development as the initial sarcomere length increases.[8,145] At a molecular level, it is supposed that an increased length sensitizes troponin-C to the prevailing cytosolic calcium transient.[23] Proof that there is no increase in the calcium transient as the sarcomere length increases is provided by direct measurements (Fig. 12–25).

It should be noted that Starling did not relate sarcomere length nor LV end-diastolic pressure nor the pulmonary capillary wedge pressure but rather the *LV volume* to cardiac output. The relation between LV end-diastolic volume and LV end-diastolic pressure is curvilinear depending on the LV compliance.

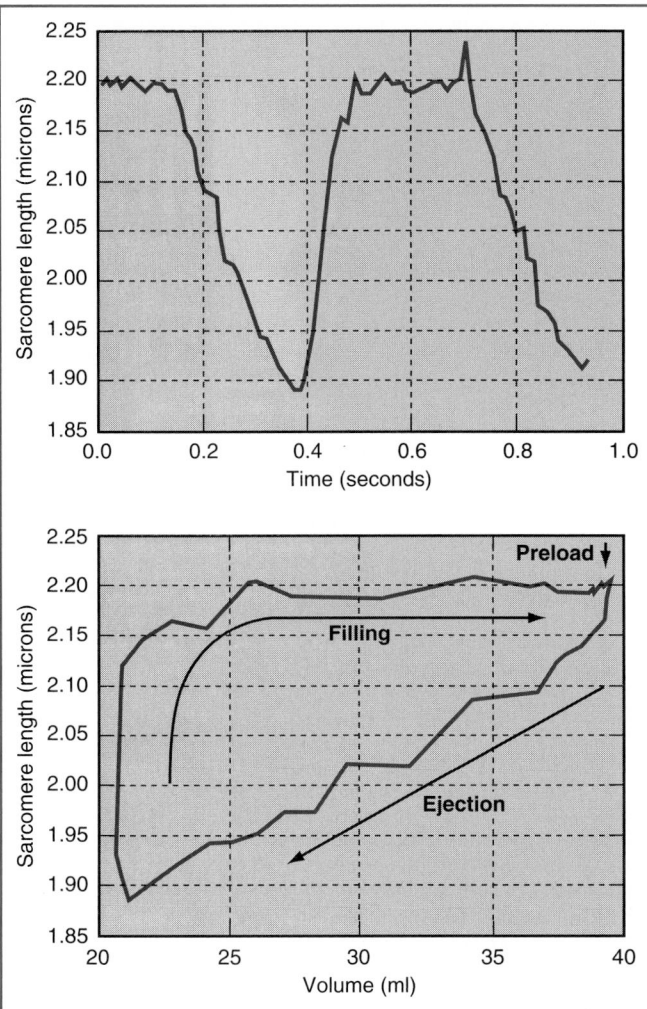

FIGURE 12–24. Changes in sarcomere length during a typical cardiac contraction-relaxation cycle in the intact dog heart. Top panel shows that during diastole the sarcomere length is 2.2 microns, reducing to 1.90 microns during systole. Bottom panel relates sarcomere length to LV volume. Starting at the top right, the preload is the maximum sarcomere length just before the onset of contraction. Then ejection decreases the LV volume, in this case by about half. Sarcomere length falls from 2.20 to 1.90 microns. Then, during the rapid phase of filling (Fig. 12–32), the sarcomere length increases from 1.90 to 2.15 microns, to be followed by the phase of constant sarcomere length (diastasis). (Modified from Rodriguez, E. K., Hunter, W. C., Royce, M. J., et al.: A method to reconstruct sarcomere lengths and orientations at transmural sites in beating canine hearts. Am J. Physiol. *263*:H293–H306, 1992.)

ANREP EFFECT: ABRUPT INCREASE IN AFTERLOAD. When the aortic pressure is elevated abruptly, a positive inotropic effect follows within 1 or 2 minutes. This was called *homeometric* autoregulation (*homeo* = the same; *metric* = length) because it was apparently independent of muscle length and by definition a true inotropic effect. A reasonable speculation would be that increased LV wall tension could act on myocardial stretch receptors to increase cytosolic sodium[146] and then, by Na^+/Ca^{++} exchange, cytosolic calcium. Thus, this effect would differ from that of an increase in preload (which acts by length-activation).

Wall Stress

Stress develops when tension is applied to a cross-sectional area, and the units are force per unit area (Fig. 14–6, p. 426). According to the *Laplace law* (Fig. 12–26):

$$\text{Wall stress} = \frac{\text{pressure} \times \text{radius}}{2 \times \text{wall thickness}}$$

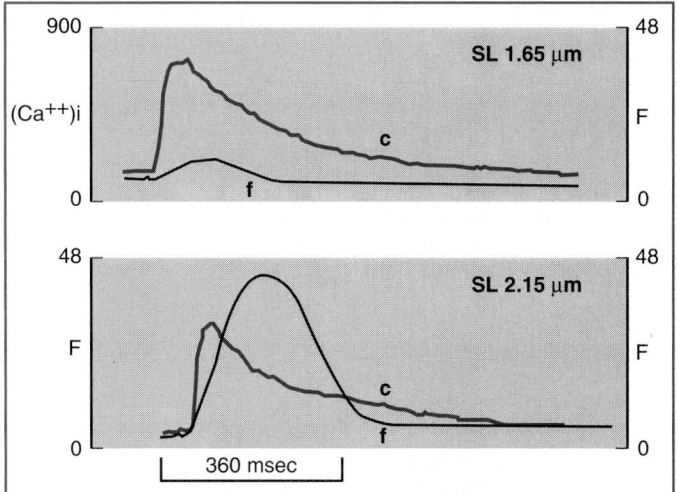

FIGURE 12–25. Length-sensitization of the sarcomere. *Top,* the sarcomere length (SL) is 1.65 microns, which gives very little force (f) development (Fig. 12–8). *Bottom,* at a near maximum sarcomere length (Figs. 12–8 and 12–24), the same $[Ca^{2+}]$ transient (c) with the same peak value and overall pattern causes a much greater force development. Therefore, there has been length-induced calcium sensitization. (Modified from Backx, P. H., and ter Keurs, H. E. D. J.: Fluorescent properties of rat cardiac trabeculae microinjected with fura-2 salt. Am. J. Physiol. *264*:H1098–H1110, 1993.)

This equation, although an oversimplification, emphasizes two points. First, the bigger the left ventricle and the greater its radius, the greater the wall stress. Second, at any given radius (LV size), the greater the pressure developed by the LV, the greater the wall stress. An increase in wall stress achieved by either of these two mechanisms (LV size or intraventricular pressure) increases myocardial oxygen uptake. This is because a greater rate of ATP use is required, as the myofibrils develop greater tension. (For more details and formulas for circumferential and meridional wall stress, see Chapter 14, pp. 426 and 427).

In cardiac hypertrophy, Laplace's law explains the effects of changes in wall thickness on wall stress (Fig. 12–26). The increased wall thickness due to hypertrophy balances

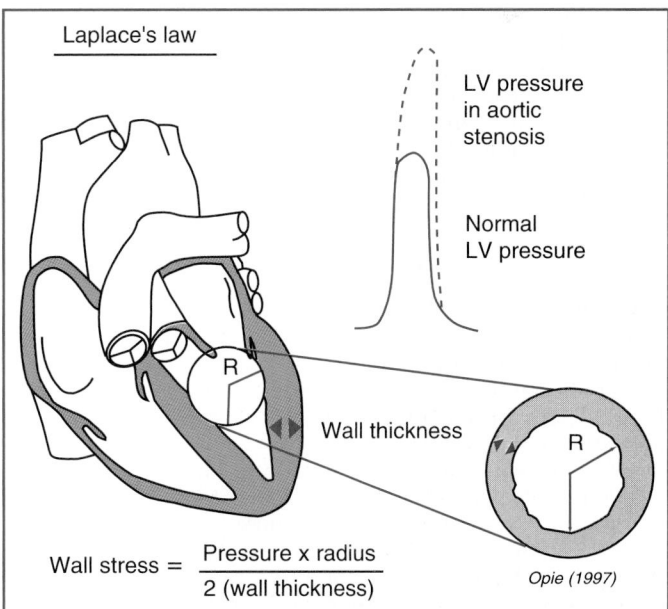

FIGURE 12–26. Wall stress increases as the afterload increases. The formula shown is derived from the Laplace law. The increased LV pressure in aortic stenosis is compensated for by LV wall hypertrophy, which decreases the denominator on the right side of the equation, thereby maintaining wall stress at control levels. (Reprinted with permission. Copyright ©1997 L. H. Opie.)

the increased pressure, and the wall stress remains unchanged during the phase of compensatory hypertrophy. In congestive heart failure, the heart dilates so that the increased radius elevates wall stress. Furthermore, because ejection of blood is inadequate, the radius stays too large throughout the contractile cycle, and both end-diastolic and end-systolic tensions are higher.

WALL STRESS, PRELOAD, AND AFTERLOAD. *Preload* can now be defined more exactly as the wall stress at the end of diastole and therefore at the maximal resting length of the sarcomere (Fig. 12–24). Measurement of wall stress in vivo is difficult because the radius of the left ventricle (see preceding sections) neglects the confounding influence of the complex anatomy of the left ventricle.[147] Surrogate measurements of the indices of preload include LV end-diastolic pressure or dimensions (the latter being the major and minor axes of the heart in a two-dimensional echocardiographic view). The *afterload,* being the load on the contracting myocardium, is also the wall stress during LV ejection. Increased afterload means that an increased intraventricular pressure has to be generated first to open the aortic valve and then during the ejection phase. These increases translate themselves into an increased myocardial wall stress, which can be measured either as an average value or at a given phase of systole, such as end-systole. Systolic wall stress reflects the two major components of the afterload, namely the arterial blood pressure and the arterial compliance. Decreased arterial compliance and increased afterload can be anticipated when there is aortic dilation as in severe systemic hypertension or in the elderly. Generally, in clinical practice, it is a sufficient approximation to take the arterial blood pressure as a measure of the afterload, provided that there is no significant aortic stenosis nor change in arterial compliance.

The *aortic impedance,* also termed the arterial input impedance, gives another accurate measure of the afterload. The aortic impedance is the aortic pressure divided by the aortic flow at that instance, so that this index of the afterload varies at each stage of the contraction cycle. Factors reducing aortic flow, such as high arterial blood pressure or aortic stenosis or loss of aortic compliance, increase impedance and hence the afterload. During systole, when the aortic valve is open, an increased afterload communicates itself to the ventricles by increasing wall stress. In LV failure, aortic impedance is augmented not only by peripheral vasoconstriction but by decreases in aortic compliance.[148] The problem with the clinical measurement of aortic impedance is that invasive instrumentation is required. An approximation can be found by using transesophageal echocardiography to determine aortic blood flow at, for example, the time of maximal increase of aortic flow just after aortic valve opening.

Heart Rate and Force-Frequency Relation

TREPPE OR BOWDITCH EFFECT. An increased heart rate progressively increases the force of ventricular contraction, even in an isolated papillary muscle preparation (Bowditch staircase phenomenon[149]). Alternative names are the *treppe* (steps, German) phenomenon or positive inotropic effect of activation or force-frequency relation (Figs. 12–27 and 12–28). Conversely, a decreased heart rate has a negative staircase effect. When stimulation becomes too rapid, force decreases.[150] The proposal is that during rapid stimulation, more sodium and calcium ions enter the myocardial cell than can be handled by the sodium pump and the mechanisms for calcium exit. Opposing the force-frequency effect is the negative contractile influence of the decreased duration of ventricular filling at high heart rates. The longer the filling interval, the better the ventricular filling and the stronger the subsequent contraction. This phenomenon can be shown in patients with mitral stenosis and atrial fibrillation with a variable filling interval.

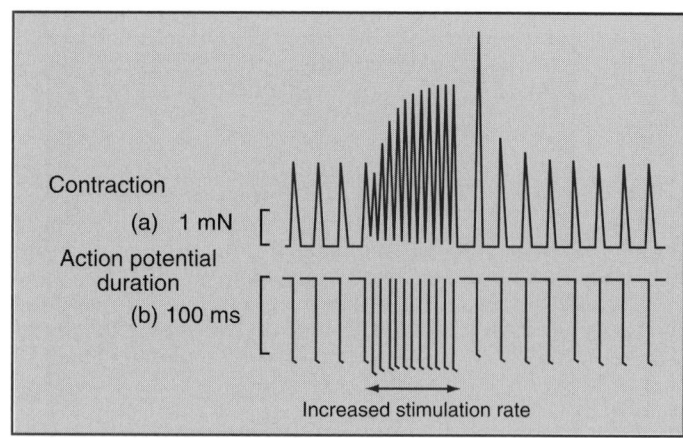

FIGURE 12–27. The Bowditch or *treppe* phenomenon, whereby a faster stimulation rate *(bottom panel)* increases the force of contraction *(top panel).* The stimulus rate is shown as the action potential duration on an analog analyzer (ms = milliseconds). The tension developed by papillary muscle contraction is shown in milliNewtons (mN) in the top panel. On cessation of rapid stimulation, the contraction force gradually declines. Hypothetically, the explanation for the increased contraction during the increased stimulation is repetitive Ca++ entry with each depolarization and, hence, an accumulation of cytosolic calcium. (From Noble, M. I. M.: Excitation-contraction coupling. *In* Drake-Holland, A. J., and Noble, M. I. M. (eds.): Cardiac Metabolism. Chichester, John Wiley, 1983, pp. 49–71.)

Post-extrasystolic potentiation and the inotropic effect of *paired pacing* can be explained by the same model,[151] again assuming an enhanced contractile state after the prolonged interval between beats. Nonetheless, the exact cellular mechanism remains to be clarified.[152]

FORCE-FREQUENCY RELATIONSHIP IN HUMANS. Muscle strips prepared from patients with mitral regurgitation behave very differently from normal muscle in response to an increased stimulation of frequency (Fig. 12–28). Normally, peak contractile force at a fixed muscle length (isometric contraction) is reached at about 150 to 180 stimuli per minute.[150] This is the human counterpart of the *treppe*

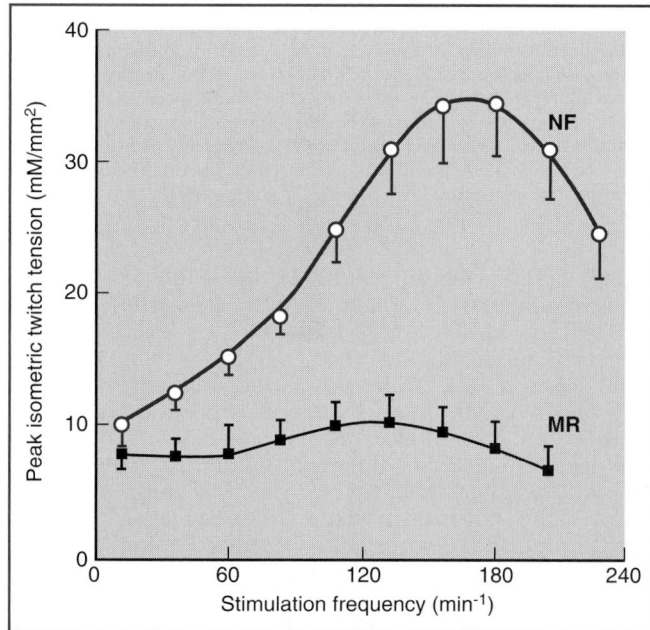

FIGURE 12–28. Plot of average steady-state isometric twitch tension versus stimulation frequency. Each point represents the mean ± SEM of eight nonfailing, control preparations (NF) and eight failing, mitral regurgitation preparations (MR). Temperature 37°C. (Data from Mulieri, L. A., et al.: Myocardial force-frequency defect in mitral regurgitation heart failure is reversed by forskolin. Circulation *88*:2700, 1993. Copyright 1993 American Heart Association.)

phenomenon. In severe mitral regurgitation there is hardly any response to an increased stimulation frequency. In another study on muscle strips from normal hearts, optimal force development was reached at rates of about 120 to 150 beats per minute,[153] whereas in patients with cardiomyopathy, an increased heart rate produced a decreased twitch tension.

HEART RATE IN SITU. In situ, the optimal heart rate is not only the rate that would give maximal mechanical performance of an isolated muscle strip, but is also determined by the need for adequate time for diastolic filling. In normal humans, it is not possible to attach exact values to the heart rate required to decrease rather than increase cardiac output or to keep it steady. Pacing rates of up to 150 per minute can be tolerated whereas higher rates cannot because of the development of AV block. In contrast, during exercise, indices of LV function still increase up to a maximum heart rate of about 170 beats per minute, presumably because of enhanced contractility and peripheral vasodilation.[154] It is presumed that the increased heart rate during exercise produces an increase in contractile force in keeping with the *treppe* phenomenon and in response to (1) adrenergic discharge and (2) activation of mechanoreceptors in the left atrium.

Myocardial Oxygen Uptake

The myocardial oxygen demand can be increased by heart rate, preload, or afterload (Fig. 12–29), factors that can all precipitate myocardial ischemia in those with coronary artery disease. A less commonly known but equally important concept is that the oxygen uptake can be augmented by increased contractility as during beta-adrenergic stimulation.[155]

Because myocardial oxygen uptake ultimately reflects the rate of mitochondrial metabolism and of ATP production, any increase of ATP requirement is reflected in an increased oxygen uptake. In general, factors increasing wall stress increase the oxygen uptake. An increased afterload causes an increased systolic wall stress, which needs a greater oxygen uptake. An increased diastolic wall stress, resulting from an increased preload, also requires more oxygen because the greater stroke volume must be ejected against the afterload. In states of enhanced contractility, the rate of change of wall stress is increased. Thus, thinking in terms of wall stress provides a comprehensive approach to the problem of myocardial oxygen uptake. Because the systolic blood pressure is an important determinant of the

afterload, a practical index of the oxygen uptake is systolic blood pressure × heart rate, the *double-product*.[156] In addition, there may be a metabolic component to the oxygen uptake which is usually small but may be prominent in certain special conditions, such as the "oxygen wastage" found during abnormally high circulating free fatty acid values.[157,158] The concept of wall stress in relation to oxygen uptake also explains why heart size is such an important determinant of the myocardial oxygen uptake (because the larger radius increases wall stress).

WORK OF THE HEART. External work is done when, for example, a mass is lifted a certain distance. In terms of the heart, the cardiac output is the mass moved, and the resistance against which it is moved is the blood pressure. Because volume work needs less oxygen than pressure work,[151,159] it might be supposed that external work is not an important determinant of the myocardial oxygen uptake. However, three determinants of the myocardial oxygen uptake are involved: preload (because this helps determine the stroke volume), afterload (in part determined by the blood pressure), and heart rate, as can be seen from the following formula:

$$\text{Minute work} = \text{SBP} \times \text{SV} \times \text{heart rate}$$

where SBP = systolic blood pressure and SV = stroke volume. Thus, it is not surprising that heart work is related to oxygen uptake.[156] The *pressure-work index* takes into account both the double-product (SBP × HR) and the HR × stroke volume, i.e., cardiac output.[156] The *pressure-volume area* is another index of myocardial oxygen uptake, requiring invasive monitoring for accurate measurements.[151] External cardiac work can account for up to 40 per cent of the total myocardial oxygen uptake.[156]

In strict terms, the work performed *(power production)* needs to take into account not only pressure but kinetic components.[160] It is the pressure work that has been discussed (product of cardiac output and peak systolic pressure). The kinetic work is the component required to move the blood against the afterload. Normally kinetic work is less than 1 per cent of the total. In aortic stenosis, kinetic work increases sharply as the cross-sectional area of the aorta narrows, whereas pressure work increases as the gradient across the aortic valve rises. Currently, noninvasive measures of peak power production are being assessed as indices of cardiac contractility.[161]

Efficiency of work is the relation between the work performed and the myocardial oxygen uptake.[151] Exercise increases the efficiency of external work, an improvement that offsets any metabolic cost of the increased contractility.[162] Certain pharmacological agents, such as dobutamine, also improve efficiency in the failing heart.[163] The subcellular basis for changes in efficiency of work are not fully understood. Because as little as 12 to 14 per cent of the oxygen uptake may be converted to external work,[162] it is probably the "internal work" that becomes less demanding. Internal ion fluxes ($Na^+/K^+/Ca^{++}$) account for about 20 to 30 per cent of the ATP requirement of the heart,[89] so that most ATP is spent on actin-myosin interaction, and much of that on generation of heat rather than on external work. An increased initial muscle length is known to sensitize the contractile apparatus to calcium, thereby theoretically increasing the efficiency of contraction by diminishing the amount of calcium flux required. In addition, muscle shortening in itself appears to increase efficiency, again by an unknown mechanism.[164]

Contractility or the Inotropic State

Although difficult to define with precision, increased contractility results in a greater velocity of contraction, which reaches a greater peak force or pressure when other factors influencing the myocardial oxygen uptake, such as the heart rate, the preload, and the afterload, are kept con-

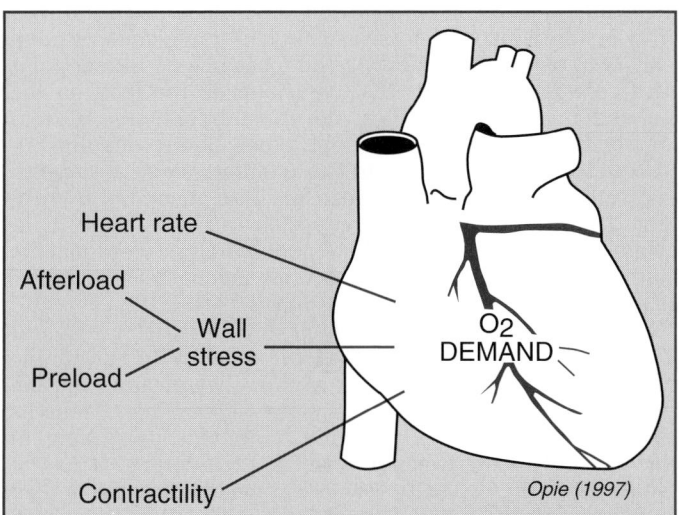

FIGURE 12–29. Major determinants of the oxygen demand of the normal heart are heart rate, wall stress, and contractility. For use of pressure-volume area as index of oxygen uptake, see Figure 12–33. (Reprinted with permission. Copyright ©1997 L. H. Opie.)

stant. An alternate name for contractility is the *inotropic state* (*ino* = fiber; *tropos* = to move). Contractility is one of the major determinants of the myocardial oxygen uptake (Fig. 12–29). Factors that increase contractility include adrenergic stimulation (exercise, emotion), digitalis, and other inotropic agents. *A useful hypothesis is that the factor common to all situations with an increased inotropic state is enhanced interaction between calcium ions and the contractile proteins.* Such interaction could result from either an increased systolic rate of rise and peak of the cytosolic calcium ion concentration or from sensitization of the contractile proteins to a given level of cytosolic calcium, as during the action of certain positively inotropic drugs acting through this mechanism.[165] Some experimental data suggest that sensitization may be a physiological mechanism for the increase in contractility in response, for example, to alpha-adrenergic stimulation.[108]

Conversely, contractility is decreased whenever calcium transients are depressed, as when beta-adrenergic blockade decreases calcium entry through the L-type calcium channel, when the ATP required for the activity of the calcium uptake pump of the SR is impaired as during anoxia or ischemia, or when there are abnormalities of the SR as in congestive heart failure.

The concept of contractility has at least two serious defects, including (1) the absence of any potential index that can be measured in situ and is free of significant criticism and, in particular, the absence of any acceptable noninvasive index; and (2) the impossibility of separating the cellular mechanisms of contractility changes from those of load or heart rate. Thus, an increased heart rate through the sodium pump lag mechanism gives rise to an increased cytosolic calcium, which is thought to explain the *treppe* phenomenon. An increased preload involves increased fiber stretch, which in turn causes length activation, explicable by sensitization of the contractile proteins to the prevailing cytosolic calcium concentration. An increased afterload may increase cytosolic calcium through stretch-sensitive channels. Thus, there is a clear overlap between contractility, which should be independent of load or heart rate, and the effects of load and heart rate on the cellular mechanisms. Hence, the traditional separation of inotropic state from load/heart rate effects as two independent regulators of cardiac muscle performance is no longer simple now that the underlying cellular mechanisms have been uncovered.[166] In clinical terms, it nonetheless remains important to separate the effects of a primary increase of load or heart rate from a primary increase in contractility (Fig. 14–2, p. 422). This distinction is especially relevant when attempting to dissect the multiple abnormalities found in congestive heart failure, where a decreased contractility could indirectly or directly result in increased afterload, preload, and heart rate, all of which factors then predispose to a further decrease in myocardial performance. Thus, decreased contractility is eventually self-augmenting.

FORCE-VELOCITY RELATIONSHIP AND MAXIMUM CONTRACTILITY IN MUSCLE MODELS. If the concept of contractility is truly independent of the load and the heart rate, then unloaded heart muscle stimulated at a fixed rate should have a maximum value of contractility for any given magnitude of the cytosolic calcium transient. This value, the V_{max} of muscle contraction, is defined as the *maximal velocity of contraction* when there is no load on the isolated muscle or no afterload to prevent maximal rates of cardiac ejection (Fig. 12–30). Beta-adrenergic stimulation increases V_{max}, and converse changes are found in the failing myocardium. V_{max} is also termed V_0 (the maximum velocity at zero load). The problem with this relatively simple concept is that V_{max} cannot be measured directly but is extrapolated from the peak rates of force development in unloaded muscle obtained from the intercept on the velocity axis.[167] In another extreme condition, there is no muscle shortening at all (zero shortening), and all the energy goes into develop-

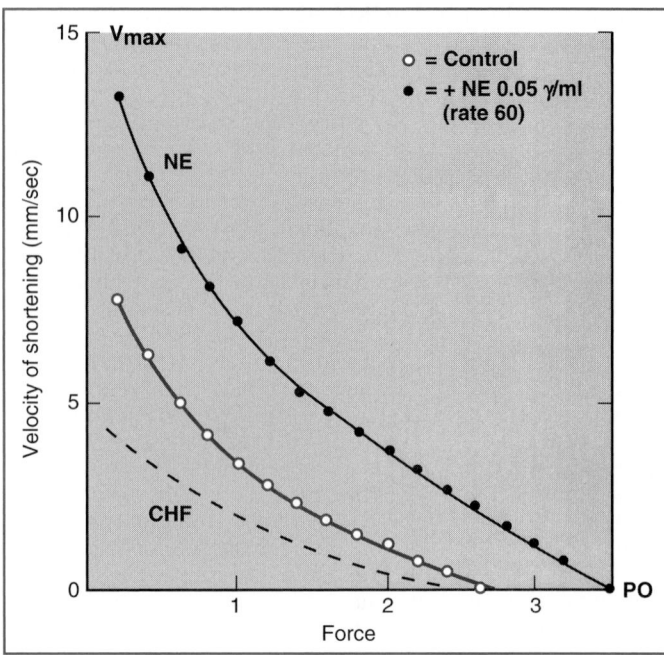

FIGURE 12–30. Effects of the addition of norepinephrine (NE) on the force-velocity relation of the cat papillary muscle. NE induces an increase in the velocity of shortening at any load, in the force of isometric contraction (P_0) and in the maximum velocity of zero-load shortening (V_{max}). The dashed line adds hypothetical data from congestive heart failure (CHF). (Modified from Braunwald, E., Sonnenblick, E. H., and Ross, J.: Normal and abnormal circulatory function. *In* Braunwald, E. (ed.): Heart Disease: A Textbook of Cardiovascular Medicine. 4th ed. Philadelphia, W. B. Saunders Company, 1992, pp. 351–392.)

ment of pressure (P_0) or force (F_0). This situation is an example of *isometric shortening* (*iso* = the same; *metric* = length). Because the peak velocity is obtained at zero load when there is no external force development, the relationship is usually termed the *force-velocity relationship*.

The concept of V_{max} has been subject to much debate over many years, chiefly because of the technical difficulties in obtaining truly unloaded conditions. Braunwald et al.[168] used cat papillary muscle to define a hyperbolic force-velocity curve, with V_{max} relatively independent of the initial muscle length, but increased by the addition of norepinephrine (Fig. 12–30).

Another preparation used to examine force-velocity relations uses single cardiac myocytes isolated by enzymatic digestion of the rat myocardium and then permeabilized with a staphylococcal toxin. Again, the force-velocity relation is hyperbolic, suggesting the existence of intracellular *passive elastic elements* that contribute to the load on the isolated myocyte.[169] In fact, the more hyperbolic and increased curvilinear nature of the force-velocity relationship in isolated myocytes than in the papillary muscle suggests that internal passive forces such as those generated by titin (Fig. 12–4) are greater than expected in the isolated myocytes. In the intact heart, the noncontractile components contribute relatively little to overall mechanical behavior, at least in physiological circumstances.[170]

Do similar relations hold at the level of the sarcomere? Ter Keurs[171] carefully measured the velocity of shortening of the central sarcomeres in a maximally unloaded muscle and found that V_{max} was the same at sarcomere lengths between 1.85 and 2.35 microns, although decreasing at shorter lengths to become zero at 1.6 microns. Thus, it seems as if V_{max} is truly length-independent at the longer and more physiological sarcomere lengths. Both the work on papillary muscle and that on sarcomeres suggest that in unloaded conditions the intrinsic contractility as assessed by V_{max} does not change with initial fiber or sarcomere length.

MECHANISM OF BETA-ADRENERGIC EFFECTS ON FORCE-VELOCITY RELATIONSHIP. The data on papillary muscles showing that norepinephrine can increase V_{max} could be explained by either an effect of beta-adrenergic stimulation on enhancing calcium ion entry or a direct effect on the contractile proteins, or both. Strang et al.[172] showed that either isoproterenol (beta-stimulant) or protein kinase A (intracellular messenger) increased V_{max} by about 40 per cent, concurrently with phosphorylation of troponin-I and C protein in an isolated ventricular myocyte preparation. Hypothetically, such phosphorylations increase the rate of crossbridge cycling, possibly by promoting release of ADP from myosin, or else by increasing myosin ATPase activity.[169] In contrast, de Tombe and ter Keurs[173] emphasize the dominant role of calcium ion entry, because they could find the expected increase V_{max} with beta-stimulation only when the external calcium ion concentration of their preparation was suboptimal.

The overall concept is that beta-adrenergic stimulation mediates the major component of its inotropic effect through increasing the cytosolic calcium transient and the factors controlling it, such as the rate of entry of calcium ions through the sarcolemmal L-type channels, the rate of calcium uptake under the influence of phospholamban into the SR, and the rate of calcium release from the ryanodine receptor in response to calcium entry in association with depolarization. Of all these factors, phosphorylation of phospholamban may be most important (see p. 368).

ISOMETRIC VERSUS ISOTONIC CONTRACTION. Despite the similarities in the force-velocity patterns between the data obtained on papillary muscle and isolated myocytes, it should be considered that a number of different types of muscular contraction may be involved. For example, data for P_0 are obtained under isometric conditions (length unchanged). When muscle is allowed to shorten against a steady load, the conditions are *isotonic* (*iso* = same; *tonic* = contractile force). Yet measurements of V_{max} have to be under totally unloaded conditions, both in the papillary muscles and in permeabilized myocytes.[167] Thus, the force-velocity curve may be a combination of initial isometric conditions followed by isotonic contraction and then may follow abrupt and total unloading to measure V_{max}. Although isometric conditions can be found in the whole heart as an approximation during isovolumic contraction, isotonic conditions cannot prevail because the load is constantly changing during the ejection period, and complete unloading is impossible. Therefore, the application of force-velocity relations to the heart in vivo is limited.

PRESSURE-VOLUME LOOPS. Accordingly, measurements of pressure-volume loops are among the best of the current approaches to the assessment of the contractile behavior of the intact heart (Figs. 14–1 and 14–2, p. 422). Major criticisms arise when it is assumed that the slope of the pressure-volume relationship (E_S) is necessarily linear (it may be curvilinear[174]) or when E_S is used as an index of "absolute" contractility (for E_S, see Fig. 12–31). Also in clinical practice, the need to change the loading conditions and the requirement for invasive monitoring lessen the usefulness of this index.[175] Invasive measurements of the LV pressure are required for the full loop, which is an indirect measure of the Starling relationship between the force (as measured by the pressure) and the muscle length (measured indirectly by volume). Measuring LV volume adequately and continuously throughout the cardiac cycle is not easy.

During a positive inotropic intervention, the pressure-volume loop reflects a smaller end-systolic volume and a higher end-systolic pressure, so that E_S has moved upward and to the left (Fig. 12–31). When the positive inotropic intervention is by beta-adrenergic stimulation, then enhanced relaxation (lusitropic effect) results in a lower pressure-volume curve during ventricular filling than in controls.

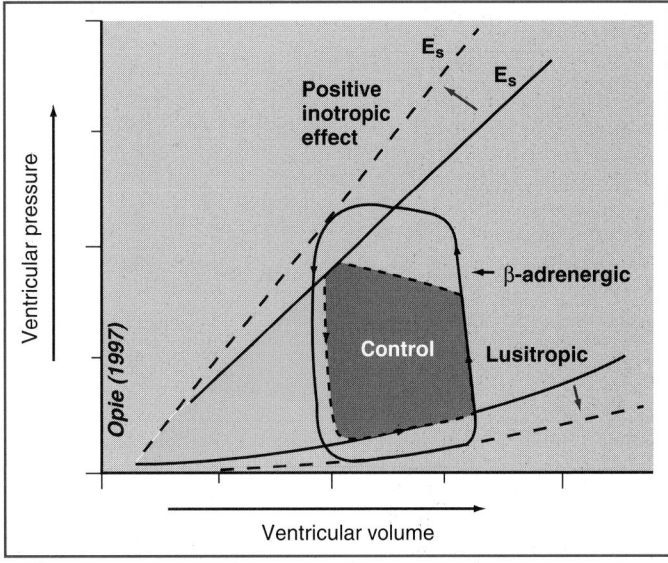

FIGURE 12–31. Note the effects of beta-adrenergic catecholamines with both positive inotropic (increased slope of line E_s) and increased lusitropic (relaxant) effects. E_s = Slope of pressure-volume relationship. The total pressure-volume area (sum of slashed and dotted areas for control) is closely related to the myocardial oxygen uptake.[151] (Reprinted with permission. Copyright ©1997 L. H. Opie.)

Ventricular Relaxation and Diastolic Dysfunction
(See also p. 402)

Among the many complex cellular factors influencing relaxation, four are of chief interest. First, the cytosolic calcium level must fall to cause the relaxation phase, a process requiring ATP and phosphorylation of phospholamban for uptake of calcium into the SR. Second, the inherent viscoelastic properties of the myocardium are important. In the hypertrophied heart, relaxation occurs more slowly. Third, increased phosphorylation of troponin-I enhances the rate of relaxation.[9] Fourth, relaxation is influenced by the systolic load. The history of contraction affects crossbridge relaxation.[176,177] Within limits, the greater the systolic load, the faster the rate of relaxation.

This complex relationship has been explored in detail by Brutsaert and Sys[178] and Brutsaert et al.[179] but could perhaps be simplified as follows. When the workload is high, peak cytosolic calcium is also thought to be high. A high end-systolic cytosolic calcium means that the rate of fall of calcium also can be greater, provided that the uptake mechanisms are functioning effectively. In this way a systolic pressure load and the rate of diastolic relaxation can be related. Furthermore, a greater muscle length (when the workload is high) at the end of systole should produce a more rapid rate of relaxation by the opposite of length-dependent sensitization, so that there is a more marked response to the rate of decline of calcium in early diastole. Yet, when the systolic load exceeds a certain limit, the rate of relaxation is delayed,[177] perhaps because of too great a mechanical stress on the individual crossbridges. Thus, in congestive heart failure caused by an excess systolic load, relaxation becomes increasingly afterload-dependent, so that therapeutic reduction of the systolic load should improve LV relaxation.[180]

IMPAIRED RELAXATION AND CYTOSOLIC CALCIUM. Hemodynamically, diastole can be divided into four phases (Fig. 12–32). For these purposes, this chapter has used the clinical definition of diastole according to which diastole extends from aortic valve closure to the start of the first heart sound. The first phase of diastole is the isovolumic phase, which, by definition, does not contribute to ventricular filling. The second phase of rapid filling provides most of

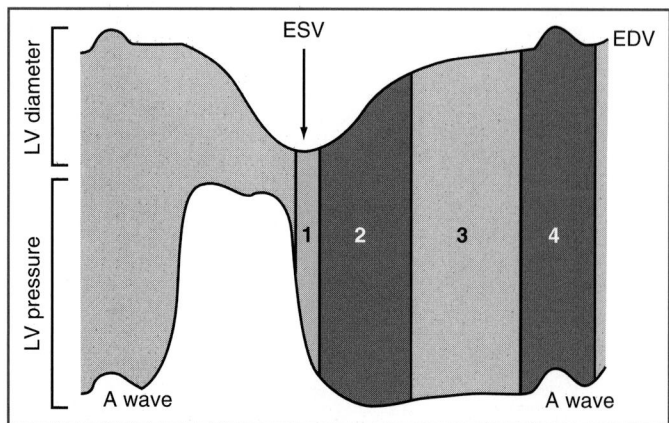

FIGURE 12–32. Phases of left ventricular (LV) diastole. 1, Isovolumic relaxation period, from aortic valve closure to mitral valve opening. 2, Rapid filling period, from mitral valve opening to onset of plateau (diastasis) of LV volume curve. 3, Diastasis, from onset of plateau on volume curve to atrial systole. 4, Atrial systole with end-diastolic volume. Arrow, end-systolic volume. (Modified from Harizi, R. C., Bianco, J. A., and Alpert, J. S.: Diastolic function of the heart in clinical cardiology. Arch. Intern. Med. *148:*99–109, 1988.) For A wave, see Figure 12–22. For further details, see Figure 14–22.

ventricular filling. The third phase of slow filling or diastasis accounts for only 5 per cent of the total filling. The final atrial booster phase accounts for the remaining 15 per cent. The first phase of isovolumic relaxation is energy-dependent.

ISOVOLUMIC RELAXATION. This phase of the cardiac cycle is energy-dependent, requiring ATP for the uptake of calcium ions by the SR (Fig. 12–33) which is an active, not a passive, process. Impaired relaxation is an early event in angina pectoris. A proposed metabolic explanation is that there is impaired generation of energy, which diminishes the supply of ATP required for the early diastolic uptake of calcium by the SR. The result is that the cytosolic calcium level, at a peak in systole, delays its return to normal in the early diastolic period. In other conditions, too, there is a

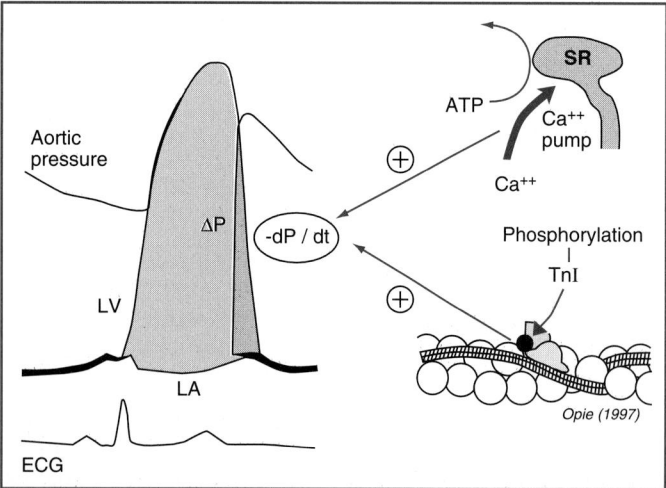

FIGURE 12–33. Factors governing the isovolumic relaxation phase of the cardiac cycle (see Fig. 12–32). This period of the cycle extends from the aortic second sound (A_2) (Fig. 12–22) to the crossover point between the left ventricular and left atrial pressures. The maximum negative rate of pressure development ($-dP/dt_{max}$), which gives the isovolumic relaxation rate, is measured either invasively or by a continuous wave Doppler velocity spectrum in aortic regurgitation.[183] Isovolumic relaxation is increased (+ sign) when the rate of calcium uptake into the sarcoplasmic reticulum (SR) is enhanced, for example during beta-adrenergic stimulation (Fig. 12–18). Isovolumic relaxation is also enhanced when phosphorylation of troponin I (TnI), as in response to beta-adrenergic stimulation, decreases the affinity of the contractile system for calcium. Copyright ©1997 L. H. Opie.)

relationship between the rate of diastolic decay of the calcium transient and diastolic relaxation, with a relation to impaired function of the SR.[181] When the rate of relaxation is prolonged by hypothyroidism, the rate of return of the systolic calcium elevation is likewised delayed, whereas opposite changes occur in hyperthyroidism.[182] In congestive heart failure, diastolic relaxation also is delayed and irregular, as is the rate of decay of the cytosolic calcium elevation.[182] Most patients with coronary artery disease have a variety of abnormalities of diastolic filling, probably related to those also found in angina pectoris. Theoretically, such abnormalities of relaxation are potentially reversible because they depend on changes in patterns of calcium ion movement. Indices of the isovolumic phase and other indices of diastolic function are shown in Table 12–5. Of interest is the echocardiographic determination in patients with regurgitant valve disease of $-dP/dt_{max}$[183] and of *tau*, the time constant of relaxation.[184]

DOES THE LEFT VENTRICLE "SUCK" DURING EARLY FILLING? Whether the LV suction by active relaxation could increase the pressure gradient from left atrium to LV during the early filling phase remains controversial, although well supported by the data. An LV suction effect can be found by carefully comparing LV and left atrial pressures, and it occurs especially in the early diastolic phase of rapid filling. The sucking effect may be of most importance in mitral stenosis, when the mitral valve does not open as it otherwise should in response to diastolic suction. During catecholamine stimulation, the rate of relaxation may increase to enhance the sucking effect[185] and to prolong the period of filling. The proposed mechanism of sucking is as follows.[186] When the end-systolic volume is less than the equilibrium volume, the shortened muscle fibers and collagen matrix may act as a compressed spring, to generate recoil forces in diastole.

ATRIAL FUNCTION. The left atrium, besides its well-known function as a blood-receiving chamber, also acts as follows: First, by presystolic contraction and its booster function, it helps to complete LV filling.[187] Second, it is the volume sensor of the heart, releasing atrial natriuretic peptide (ANP) in response to intermittent stretch and several other stimuli, including angiotensin II[188] and endothelin.[189] Third, the atrium contains receptors for the afferent arms of various reflexes, including mechanoreceptors that increase sinus discharge rate, thereby contributing to the tachycardia of exercise as the venous return increases (Bainbridge reflex).

The atria have a number of differences in structure and function from the ventricles, having smaller myocytes with a shorter action potential duration as well as a more fetal type of myosin (both in heavy and light chains). Furthermore, the atria are more reliant on the phosphatidylinositol signal transduction pathway,[190] which may explain the relatively greater positive inotropic effect in the atria than in

TABLE 12–5 SOME INDICES OF DIASTOLIC FUNCTION

ISOVOLUMIC RELAXATION
$(-)\ dP/dt_{max}$ (Fig. 12–33)
Aortic closing–mitral opening interval
Peak rate of LV wall thinning
Time constant of relaxation, *tau**
EARLY DIASTOLIC FILLING
Relaxation kinetics on ERNA (rate of volume increase)
Early filling phase (E phase) on Doppler transmitral velocity trace
DIASTASIS
Pressure-volume relation indicates compliance
ATRIAL CONTRACTION
Invasive measurement of atrial and ventricular pressures
Doppler transmitral pattern (E to A ratio)

* For noninvasive measurements by continuous-wave Doppler velocity profile in mitral regurgitation, see Chen et al.[184]

ERNA = Equilibrated radionuclide angiography

the ventricles in response to angiotensin II.[191] The more rapid atrial repolarization is thought to be due to increased outward potassium currents, such as I_{to} and I_{kACh}.[192,193] In addition, some atrial cells have the capacity for spontaneous depolarization.[194] In general, these histological and physiological changes can be related to the decreased need for the atria to generate high intrachamber pressures, rather than being sensitive to volume changes, while retaining enough contractile action to help with LV filling and to respond to inotropic stimuli.[187]

MEASUREMENT OF DIASTOLIC FUNCTION (see also p. 434). The rate of isovolumic relaxation can be measured by negative dP/dt_{max} at invasive catheterization. *Tau,* the time constant of relaxation, describes the rate of fall of LV pressure during isovolumic relaxation and also requires invasive techniques for precise determination.[184] *Tau* is increased as the systolic LV pressure rises.[177] Another index of relaxation can be obtained echocardiographically from the peak rate of wall thinning.[195] The isovolumic relaxation time lies between aortic valve closure and mitral valve opening measured by signals of valve movements taken by Doppler echocardiography.[196] In mitral regurgitation, the Doppler velocity profile can be used to calculate *tau.*[184] In each case, precise measurement is difficult, and the range of normality is large.

DIASTOLIC DYSFUNCTION IN HYPERTROPHIC MYOCARDIUM. In hypertrophic hearts, as in chronic hypertension or severe aortic stenosis,[197] abnormalities of diastole are common and may precede systolic failure. The mechanism is not clear, although it is thought to be related to the extent of ventricular hypertrophy or indirectly to a stiff left atrium.[198] Conceptually, impaired relaxation must be distinguished from prolonged systolic contraction with delayed onset of normal relaxation.[179] Experimentally, there are several defects in early hypertensive hypertrophy, including decreased rates of contraction and relaxation, and decreased peak force development.[181] Of specific interest is the concept that the loss of the load-sensitive component of relaxation is due to impaired activity of the SR. Impaired relaxation is associated with an increase of the late (atrial) filling phase, so that E/A ratio on the mitral Doppler pattern declines. In time, with both increased hypertrophy and the development of fibrosis, chamber compliance decreases (Fig. 14–20, p. 435). Such multiple abnormalities are difficult to detect in the transmitral flow pattern (Fig. 14–23, p. 437).

Vascular Compliance

Because vascular compliance is one of the two major factors influencing the afterload (the other being arterial blood pressure), increasing attention is being paid to its changes in disease states and during drug therapy. For example, severe hypertension decreases arterial compliance while nitrates increase large arterial diameter, thereby showing that compliance has increased.[199] Some workers distinguish between the distensibility of the arteries, taken as a measure of the elastic properties, and the compliance, a measure of the buffering capacity.[199]

Aortic-Ventricular Coupling

The interaction between physical properties of the arterial tree and the mechanical function of the left ventricle is influenced by numerous factors, including distensibility of the ascending aorta.[200] The latter can be measured noninvasively by the change in aortic diameter in relation to the pulse pressure using echocardiography[200] or magnetic resonance imaging.[201]

From the conceptual point of view, the aorta functions as a Windkessel, i.e., as a pressure chamber, which provides compliance to act as a buffer.[202] If aortic pressure oscillations can be measured, then aortic flow can be calculated and hence the cardiac output measured noninvasively. In practice, models and extrapolations from the radial pulse

pressure patterns can be used to estimate aortic pressure pulsations.[202]

Ventricular Interaction

Thus far, LV function has been discussed as if the left ventricle were working in isolation. In reality, its function is intimately linked to that of the right ventricle, both functionally and anatomically. The cardiac output of the left ventricle must equal that of the right ventricle unless there is a state of imbalance, as in conditions of acute LV failure when blood may accumulate in the lungs to cause pulmonary edema. In general, the right ventricle is working against a low resistance circuit, and afterload is not a major problem in physiological conditions. What the right ventricle receives by means of its filling pressure in the venous system, it empties in response to the Starling effect. The amount of pressure work generated by the right ventricle is relatively low, which explains the thinner right ventricular wall and the dominance of LV function in calculations of pressure work or of myocardial oxygen uptake.

Anatomically, the two ventricles are interlinked. They share a common septum. That septum constitutes part of the load against which each ventricle must work. In LV hypertrophy, which includes the septum, the right ventricle must, therefore, work harder and tends to become hypertrophied. This is *systolic ventricular interaction.* One type of diastolic ventricular interaction is the *Bernheim effect,* whereby a large left ventricle compresses the right ventricle, the volume on the left side being so great that the right side is unable to fill properly. A converse ventricular interaction can occur in severe heart failure, when the dilated right ventricle may impinge on the left. When the right ventricle is unloaded by the venodilator agent nitroglycerin, it can decrease in size and allow the LV function to improve. Similarly, following surgical thromboendarterectomy for chronic thromboembolic pulmonary hypertension, LV diastolic function improved as the interventricular septum changed position.[203]

When there is a physical impairment of the mechanical function of one ventricle on the other as a result of volume overloading with blood, the result is *diastolic ventricular interference.*[204]

Pericardium
(See also Chap. 43)

The normal pericardium has an important restraining effect on the diastolic properties of the ventricles, especially the right ventricle.[205] Without the pericardium, the right ventricle would dilate by about 40 per cent and the right atrium by about 70 per cent. Therefore, the physical properties of the pericardium help to determine ventricular pressure-volume relations and, indirectly, the compliance. Normally LV diastolic pressure is greater than that in the other chambers by the amount of its transmural pressure (5 to 10 mm Hg), the low pericardial pressure being equally applied to all chambers. During pericardial disease with cardiac tamponade, the pressure within the pericardial cavity rises as the volume increases, especially with a volume above 200 ml,[206] so that the intrapericardial pressure equals or exceeds the normal diastolic filling pressure. When this happens, diastole is interrupted and ventricular diastolic collapse can be seen on echocardiography.[207]

Endocardium

The vascular and endocardial endothelium constitute "one continuous sheet of tissue."[208] A current proposal is that there is intracavity autoregulation by endocardial endothelial cells. Release of an endothelin-like agent, endocardin, from the stretched endocardium could, it is proposed, increase the duration of contraction.[209] The dilated failing left ventricle could thereby generate an autoregulating inotropic stimulus. Yet there is thought to be a defect in the endocardial endothelium in heart failure causing, for example, a decreased response to alpha$_2$-adrenergic inotropic stimulation.[208] What is thus far not explained is how, if the properties of endocardin resemble those of endothelin, a preferential positive inotropic effect rather than vasoconstriction could be achieved unless endocardin preferentially stimulates adjacent endocardial papillary muscle cells.

EFFECTS OF ISCHEMIA AND REPERFUSION ON CONTRACTION AND RELAXATION

Contractile Impairment in Ischemia
(See p. 1162)

Despite experimental differences, there is now widespread agreement that early contractile failure (Fig. 12–34) can occur even when *calcium transients* are normal or near normal,[212–214] and, therefore, a metabolic cause must be sought. The latter could be either decreased sensitivity of the contractile proteins to calcium, as for example caused by acidosis, or inhibition of the crossbridge cycle, as for example from the early rise in inorganic phosphate. As creatine phosphate falls, the activity of the creatine phosphate shuttle decreases so that "local" ATP, required for calcium movements in the contractile cycle, falls.[215] In addition, the free energy of hydrolysis of ATP decreases during ischemia.[216,216a] The large increase in P$_i$, as a result of creatine phosphate breakdown, decreases free energy of hydrolysis, as do the smaller decreases in ATP and increases in ADP. Creatine phosphate fall can also indirectly inhibit contractility by accumulation of inorganic phosphate, which decreases the contractile effects of any given cytosolic calcium level.[217] Inorganic phosphate may act by promotion of formation of weak rather than strong crossbridges.

Accumulation of neutral lactate can promote mitochondrial damage, decrease the action potential duration, and inhibit glyceraldehyde-3-phosphate dehydrogenase.[218] The mechanism of these lactate effects is not clarified and may include extracellular acidosis with Na$^+$/H$^+$ exchange, a subsequent gain in cell Na$^+$, and then Na$^+$/Ca^{++} exchange with gain of harmful Ca^{++}.[219]

Potassium Efflux. The mechanism of early potassium efflux in ischemia is not well understood, and there are three major theories. First, the ATP-inhibited potassium channel (K$_{ATP}$) may open as a result of cytosolic ATP deficiency (Fig. 12–35).[220] Not all potassium loss can be blocked by sulfonylureas,[221] so that other potassium channels such as those activated by sodium or by fatty acids may play a role. Second, inhibition of the sodium-potassium pump has long been suspected, but the onset of such inhibition is probably too late to explain early potassium egress, although probably contributing to the later phase of potassium loss. Third, co-ionic loss of potassium with negatively charged lactate and phosphate ions has often been proposed, but the evidence is scanty.[222] For example, inhibition of lactate transport by alpha-cyanohydroxycinnamic acid does not change extracellular potassium accumulation in ischemia.[220] The importance of potassium loss is that because the action potential duration is shortened, calcium influx may be diminished.[28]

Adenosine. This substance is formed during ischemia from the breakdown of ATP. It is potentially recyclable as a building block of ATP during resynthesis. Besides being the probable origin of the ischemic anginal pain,[223] adenosine has complex cardioprotective qualities. In response to stimulation of the A$_1$-receptor,[115] adenosine increases the inhibitory G protein G$_i$, which, in turn, lessens the activity of adenylate cyclase and increases the opening probability of two types of potassium channels. The consequences include negative inotropic, chronotropic, and dromotropic effects, as well as coronary vasodilation. Adenosine may also play an important role in preconditioning.[224]

SUPPLY VERSUS DEMAND ISCHEMIA. Apstein and Grossman[225] proposed that ischemia has different effects on the systolic and diastolic properties of the left ventricle, depending on how ischemia is produced. In *supply ischemia,* with a decreased oxygen supply as the dominant metabolic change, there is an early increase in diastolic distensibility (compliance increases, ischemic area bulges). The proposed mechanism is lack of washout of ischemic metabolites that impair the interaction of the increased cytosolic calcium with the myofilaments. In contrast, when *demand ischemia* is precipitated, for example by rapid atrial pacing in the presence of experimental coronary stenosis, the diastolic distensibility acutely decreases, so that there is stiffening and the failure of the ischemic tissue to relax, with a rise in LV end-diastolic pressure. The proposed metabolic explanation is that intracellular calcium is thought to increase without a significant acidosis so that ischemia-induced loss of compliance takes place and the myocardium stiffens.

In reality, these distinctions between supply and demand ischemia are not absolute. The real differences may lie more in the severity of ischemia than in the mode of its

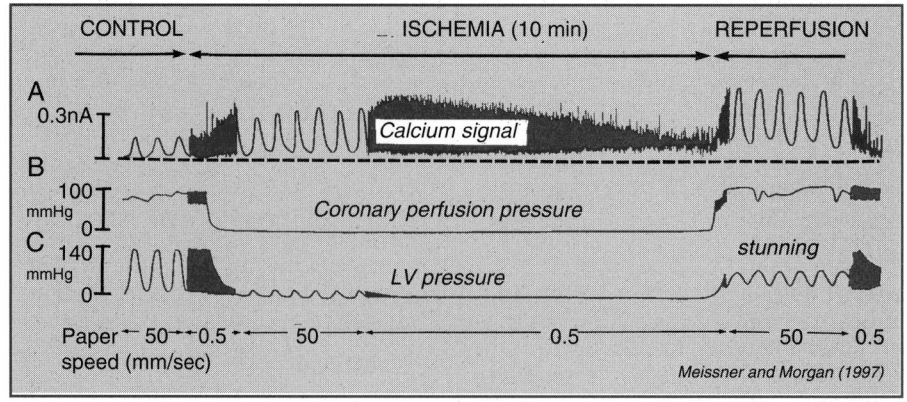

FIGURE 12–34. Can LV mechanical failure during severe ischemia be explained by changes in the cytosolic calcium? These data show that when there is abrupt ischemic LV failure (LV pressure falls to zero in *C*), the calcium signal *(A)* increases before it falls. Ischemia is designated by the abrupt fall of coronary perfusion pressure to zero in this isolated rat heart preparation. During reperfusion there is also a dissociation between the cytosolic calcium oscillations, which are augmented (righthand panel of A) in contrast to LV contraction which is decreased (righthand aspect of bottom panel), so that there is mechanical stunning. It is thought that excess calcium oscillations damage the contractile proteins (Fig. 12–38). (From Meissner, A., and Morgan, J. P.: Contractile dysfunction and abnormal Ca^{2+} modulation during postischemic reperfusion in rat heart. *Am. J. Physiol.* **268:**H100–H111, 1995.)

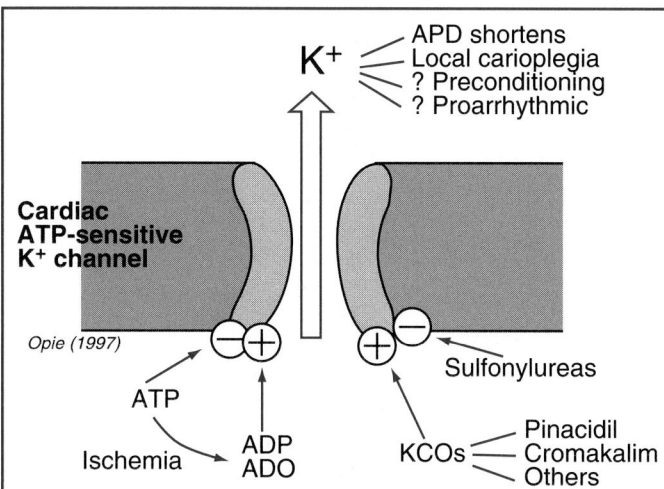

FIGURE 12–35. Proposed role of ATP-sensitive potassium channel in promotion of potassium loss in early ischemia. As ATP decreases and breaks down in ischemia to ADP and adenosine (ADO), the probability is greater that this potassium channel is open. The consequences include shortening of the action potential duration (APD), low cardioplegia, and possibly preconditioning and proarrhythmic effects. The potassium channel openers (KCOs) act on a site integral to the channel pore to promote the probability of channel opening, whereas the sulfonylureas act on a site not integral to the pore, to inhibit the potassium channel opening. For further details, see Edwards and Weston.[265] (Reprinted with permission. Copyright ©1997 L. H. Opie.)

production.[226] Thus, balloon occlusion in angioplasty is more likely to produce severe ischemia and increased distensibility than is pacing ischemia in the same patient.[227,228]

ISCHEMIC CONTRACTURE. After 5 to 20 minutes of severe ischemia, but depending on variable metabolic circumstances, including the cardiac glycogen reserve,[229] there is the gradual onset of ischemic contracture with a rise in diastolic pressure virtually without systolic activity. In general, even complete reperfusion never fully relieves ischemic contracture. The mechanisms for contracture include ATP depletion and a rise in cytosolic calcium (Fig. 12–36). Of interest is the proposal that continued glycolysis and production of glycolytic ATP have roles in the maintenance of intracellular calcium homeostasis, probably acting indirectly by maintaining activity of the sodium pump.[230] As glycolysis is inhibited, diastolic tension increases.[231]

INTERMITTENT ISCHEMIA AND PRECONDITIONING. Whereas many repetitive episodes of ischemia should produce cumulative damage, relatively few episodes or even one burst of short-lived severe ischemia followed by complete reperfusion causes preconditioning. The latter is a condition in which the myocardium is protected against a greater subsequent ischemic insult, with less threat of infarction.[232,233] The mechanism of the protective effect of preconditioning is still speculative. Of note is the important proposal that G_i is upregulated (Fig. 12–37) so that activation of receptors coupled to it, such as adenosine A_1- and muscarinic M_2-receptors, leads to greater inhibition of adenylate cyclase and hence to an indirect antiadrenergic effect.[234–236] In addition, G_i may mediate other potentially protective mechanisms, such as direct inhibition of L-calcium channels and activation of the ATP-sensitive potassium channels in the ventricles.[224] An alternate hypothesis is that adenosine formed during the preconditioning ischemic period activates protein kinase C, which mediates the subsequent protection by an unknown mechanism (Fig. 12–20).[110,237]

Preconditioning is an important phenomenon, probably with clinical implications, because repetitive anginal episodes in patients may develop into full-fledged infarction. Patients with preinfarction angina may suffer from a less

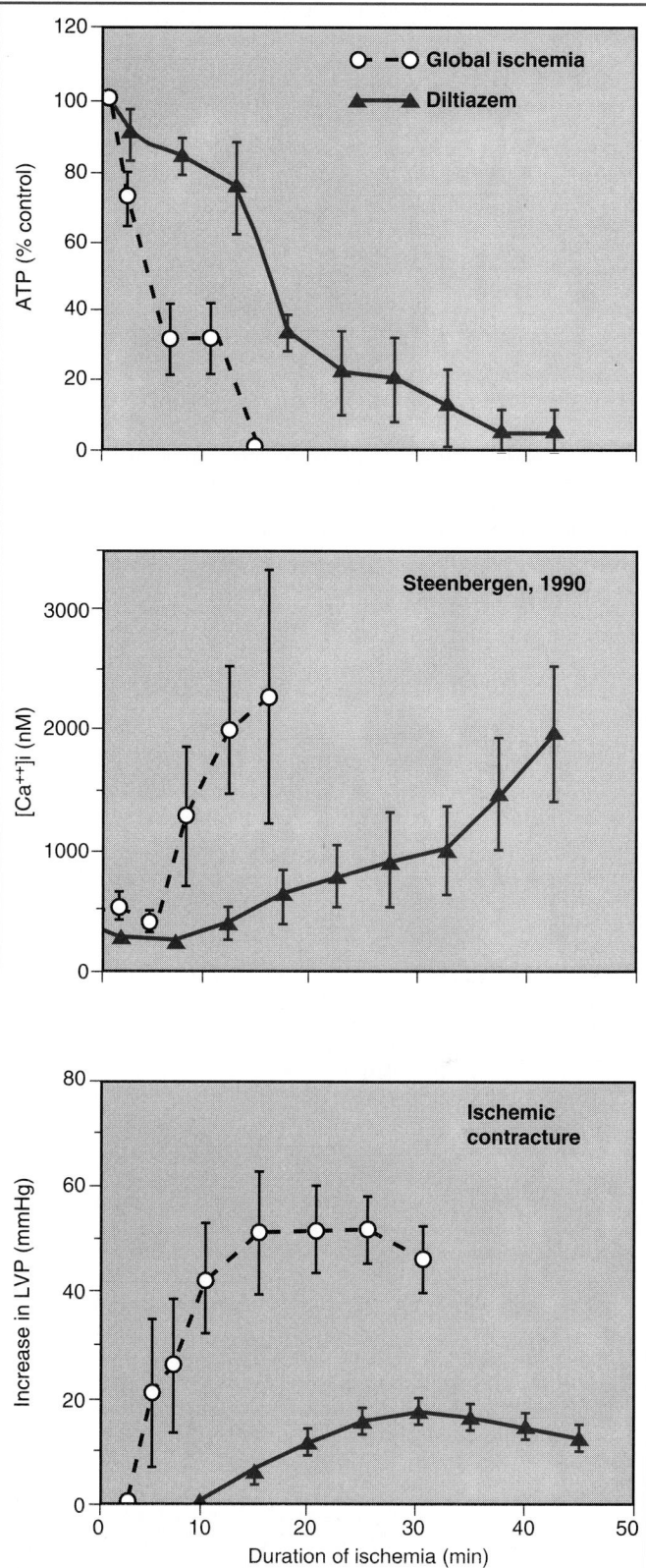

FIGURE 12–36. Ischemic contracture in isolated rat hearts under control conditions and in the presence of diltiazem (0.9 μm). In control hearts, note rapid fall of ATP followed by rise of internal Ca++ at time of onset of ischemic contracture. Diltiazem (and K+ cardioplegia, not shown) reduced the rate of fall of ATP and delayed the onset of rise in [Ca++]$_i$ and in ischemic contracture. Preservation of ATP and in particular glycolytically generated ATP delays ischemic contracture. (Data from Figures 2 and 7 of Steenbergen, C., et al.: Correlation between cytosolic free calcium, contracture, ATP, and irreversible ischemic injury in perfused rat heart. Circ. Res. *66*:135–146, 1990. Copyright 1990 American Heart Association.)

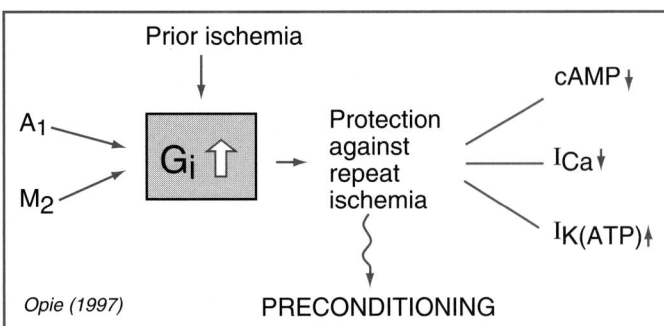

FIGURE 12–37. Proposed role of inhibitory G protein, G_i, in mediating effects of preconditioning.[234] The proposal is that prior ischemia (preconditioning episode) upregulates G_i according to Niroomand et al.[236] G_i, by inhibiting formation of cyclic AMP, lessens L-type calcium channel activity and promotes opening of the ATP-dependent K^+ channel. Thus, when ischemia is repeated, there is relative protection. A_1 = Subtype 1 of adenosine receptor; M_2 = subtype 2 of muscarinic receptor; I_{Ca} = L-type calcium current; $I_{k(ATP)}$ = ATP-dependent potassium current. (Reprinted with permission. Copyright ©1997 L. H. Opie.)

severe infarct than those thought to undergo sudden coronary occlusion without the opportunity for preconditioning.[238,239] In contrast, patients with multiple short-lived attacks of ischemia might become tolerant to the development of protective preconditioning, according to animal data.[240]

Hibernating Heart
(See also pp. 89 and 1176)

The hibernating myocardium, like the hibernating animal, is temporarily asleep and can wake up to function normally when the blood supply is fully restored (Table 12–6). The proposal is that the fall of myocardial function to a lower level copes with the reduced myocardial oxygen supply and leads to self-preservation, the so-called smart heart.[241] However, a greater flow reduction should lead to true ischemia. When the myocardium is blood-perfused, the exact limit to hibernation is not so clearly defined but could be only about 70 to 80 per cent of normal coronary flow, judging from human data.[242] Hibernation is a complex clinical situation without a good animal model. When ischemia in patients is delineated echocardiographically as depressed regional wall motion, the hypocontractile segments that still have a sustained glucose extraction, as shown by positron emission tomography (PET), have a high chance of recovery after coronary artery bypass surgery. In contrast, those segments with a decreased glucose extraction almost uniformly fail to recover.[243]

An alternative point of view, gaining ground, is that hibernation can occur even when the resting coronary flow is normal despite the presence of coronary disease. The proposed mechanism is that recurrent episodes of ischemia leave behind stunned myocardium, so that hibernation is the sum of repetitive and cumulative stunning.[244,245]

Stunning
(See also pp. 89 and 1176)

The first observation was that the recovery of mechanical function following transient coronary occlusion was not instant but delayed.[246] Thereafter, Braunwald and Kloner[247] defined the "stunned myocardium" as one characterized by prolonged postischemic myocardial dysfunction with eventual return of normal contractile activity. In addition, the "diagnosis of reversible impairment of contractility requires simultaneous measurements of regional myocardial function and flow."[248] Thus, either coronary angiography or some other measurement of flow, such as PET, would need to be performed. In practice, myocardial stunning is often inferred from circumstantial evidence. By such criteria, stunning is thought to occur in several clinical situations, including delayed recovery from effort angina, unstable angina, after thrombolytic reperfusion, and following ischemic cardioplegia. The two chief explanations for stunning are an increased cytosolic calcium[249–251] and formation of free radicals upon reperfusion.[248,252]

MECHANISM OF INCREASED CYTOSOLIC CALCIUM DURING EARLY REPERFUSION. In view of the excess cytosolic calcium found in prolonged severe ischemia,[214,253] the $[Ca^{++}]_i$ is high at the start of reperfusion. Thus, restoration of energy with reperfusion induces excess oscillations (Fig. 12–38). Second, opening of the voltage-sensitive calcium channels during early reperfusion may also be important.[254] The highly specific L-calcium channel antagonist, nisoldipine, when given only at the time of reperfusion, lessens stunning, as do the nonorganic ions, magnesium and manganese.[254] Third, release of calcium from the SR is also likely,[255,256] probably in response to free radicals.[257,258] Fourth, considerable evidence indicates that calcium may enter the reperfused cells via the process of Na^+/Ca^{++} exchange, consequent on Na^+/H^+ exchange.[254,259] Fifth, it may be predicted that all agents stimulating the phosphatidylinositol cycle and increasing inositol trisphosphate[103] at the time of reperfusion should worsen stunning. These would include angiotensin II, endothelin,[260] and alpha$_1$-adrenergic stimulation.[261] Increased calcium transients may also explain reperfusion arrhythmias.[103,251,262] Decreased systolic force generation may be linked to a calcium-induced abnormality in the thin filaments.[251]

CHRONIC STUNNING. Although experimental stunning typically lasts for hours, full mechanical recovery can sometimes take much longer. Full recovery from thrombolytic reperfusion in patients with acute myocardial infarction may be delayed over weeks. To explain this finding, a current proposal is that there is a condition of late or chronic stunning,[263] hypothetically the end-result changes

TABLE 12–6 CHARACTERISTICS OF STUNNING, HIBERNATION, AND ISCHEMIA

PARAMETER	STUNNING	HIBERNATION	TRUE ISCHEMIA
Myocardial function	Reduced	Reduced	Reduced
Coronary blood flow	Normal/high	Modestly reduced	Most severely reduced
Myocardial energy metabolism	Normal or excessive	Reduced; in steady state	Reduced; increasingly severe as ischemia proceeds
Duration	Hours to days	Days to hours to months	Minutes to hours
Outcome	Full recovery	Recovery if blood flow restored	Infarction if severe ischemia persists
Proposed change in metabolic regulation of calcium	Cytosolic overload of calcium in early reperfusion	Possibly just enough glycolytic ATP to prevent contracture	Insufficient glycolytic ATP to prevent ischemic contracture and irreversibility

Modified from Opie, L. H.: Stunning, Hibernation and Calcium in Myocardial Ischemia and Reperfusion. Norwell, MA, Kluwer Academic Publishers, 1992.

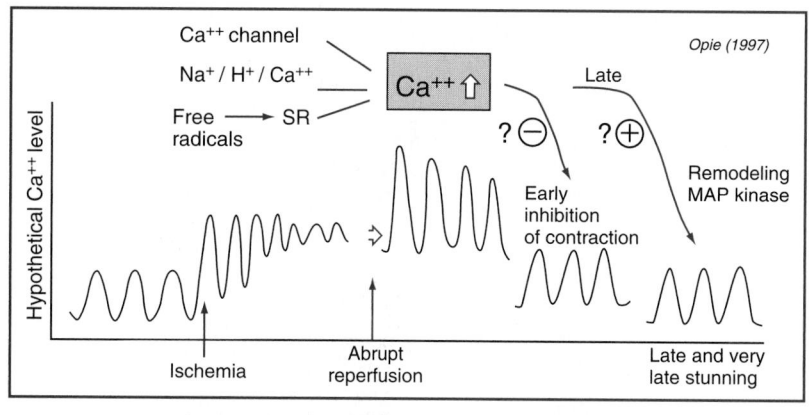

FIGURE 12–38. Proposed role of increased cytosolic calcium in causing early stunning after reperfusion and in hypothetically playing a role in late remodeling by stimulation of protein synthesis, possibly at the level of MAP kinase (mitogen-actived protein kinase). Na+/H+/Ca++ = Sodium/proton and sodium/calcium exchange mechanisms; SR = sarcoplasmic reticulum. (Reprinted with permission. Copyright ©1997 L. H. Opie.)

in cytosolic calcium, perhaps acting as a trigger to complex changes in protein synthesis and degradation.[264] Chronic stunning may be the explanation for some aspects of hibernation. For example, repetitive ischemia precipitated by excitement in pigs with severe coronary stenosis can cause depressed mechanical function even in the absence of any measurable reduction of coronary blood flow at rest.[245]

REFERENCES

MICROANATOMY OF CONTRACTILE PROTEINS

1. Brilla, C. G., Janicki, J. S., and Weber, K. T.: Impaired diastolic function and coronary reserve in genetic hypertension. Role of interstitial fibrosis and medial thickening of intramyocardial coronary arteries. Circ. Res. 69:107–115, 1991.
2. Forbes, M. S., and Sperelakis, N.: Ultrastructure of mammalian cardiac muscle. In Sperelakis, N. (ed.): Physiology and Pathophysiology of the Heart. 3rd ed. Boston, Kluwer Academic Publishers, 1995, pp. 1–35.
3. Weber, K. T., Sun, Y., Tyagi, S. C., and Cleutjens, J. P. M.: Collagen network of the myocardium: Function, structural remodeling and regulatory mechanisms. J. Mol. Cell. Cardiol. 26:279–292, 1994.
4. Wang, K., Ramirez-Mitchell, R., and Palter, D.: Titin is an extraordinarily long, flexible, and slender myofibrillar protein. Proc. Natl. Acad. Sci. 81:3685–3689, 1984.
5. Hein, S., Scholz, D., Fujitani, N., et al.: Altered expression of titin and contractile proteins in failing human myocardium. J. Mol. Cell Cardiol. 26:1291–1306, 1994.
6. Trombitas, K., Jin, J.-P., and Granzier, H.: The mechanically active domain of titin in cardiac muscle. Circ. Res. 77:856–861, 1995.
7. Perry, S. V.: The regulation of contractile activity in muscle. Biochem. Soc. Trans. 7:593–617, 1979.
8. Solaro, R. J., Wolska, B. M., and Westfall, M.: Regulatory proteins and diastolic relaxation. In Lorell, B. H., and Grossman, W. (eds.): Diastolic Relaxation of the Heart. Boston, Kluwer Academic Publishers, 1994, pp. 43–53.
9. Zhang, R., Zhao, J., Mandveno, A., and Potter, J. D.: Cardiac troponin-I phosphorylation increases the rate of cardiac muscle relaxation. Circ. Res. 76:1028–1035, 1995.
10. Huxley, A. F.: Muscle structure and theories of contraction. Prog. Biophys. Chem. 7:255–318, 1957.
11. Rayment, I., Holden, H. M., Whittaker, M., et al.: Structure of the actin-myosin complex and its implications for muscle contraction. Science 261:58–65, 1993.
12. Fisher, A. J., Smith, C. A., Thoden, J., et al.: Structural studies of myosin: Nucleotide complexes: A revised model for the molecular basis of muscle contraction. Biophys. J. 68:19s–28s, 1995.
13. Irving, M., Lombardi, V., Piazzesi, G., and Ferenczi, M. A.: Myosin head movements are synchronous with the elementary force-generating process in muscle. Nature 357:156–158, 1992.
14. Solaro, R. J., Powers, F. M., Gao, L., and Gwathmey, J. K.: Control of myofilament activation in heart failure. Circulation 87(Suppl VII):38–43, 1993.
15. Watkins, H., McKenna, W. J., Thierfelder, L., et al.: Mutations in the genes for cardiac troponin-T and alpha-tropomyosin in hypertrophic cardiomyopathy. N. Engl. J. Med. 332:1058–1064, 1995.
16. Morano, I., Ritter, O., Bonz, A., et al.: Myosin light chain–actin interaction regulates cardiac contractility. Circ. Res. 76:720–725, 1995.
17. Gao, W. D., Backx, P. H., Azan-Backx, M., and Marban, E.: Myofilament Ca2+ sensitivity in intact versus skinned rat ventricular muscle. Circ. Res. 74:408–415, 1994.
18. Wolff, M. R., McDonald, K. S., and Moss, R. L.: Rate of tension development in cardiac muscle varies with level of activator calcium. Circ. Res. 76:154–160, 1995.
19. Hancock, W. O., Martyn, D. A., and Huntsman, L. L.: Ca2+ and segment length dependence of isometric force kinetics in intact ferret cardiac muscle. Circ. Res. 73:603–611, 1993.

20. Brenner, B.: Effect of Ca2+ on crossbridge turnover kinetics in skinned rabbit psoas fibers. Proc. Natl. Acad. Sci. U.S.A. 85:3265–3269, 1988.
21. Hofmann, P. A., and Fuchs, F.: Evidence for a force-dependent component of calcium binding to cardiac troponin-C. Am. J. Physiol. 253:C541–C546, 1987.
22. Hannon, J. D., Martyn, D. A., and Gordon, A. M.: Effects of cycling and rigor crossbridges on the conformation of cardiac troponin-C. Circ. Res. 71:984–991, 1992.
23. Fuchs, F.: Mechanical modulation of the Ca2+ regulatory protein complex in cardiac muscle. News Physiol. Sci. 10:6–12, 1995.
24. Rüegg, J. C.: Towards a molecular understanding of contractility. Cardioscience 1:163–167, 1990.
25. Marban, E., Rink, T. J., Tsien, R. W., and Tsien, R. Y.: Free calcium in heart muscle at rest and during contraction measured with Ca2+-sensitive microelectrodes. Nature 286:845–850, 1980.

CALCIUM ION FLUXES IN CARDIAC CONTRACTION-RELAXATION CYCLE

26. Gibbons, W. R., and Zygmunt, A. C.: Excitation-contraction coupling in heart. In Fozzard, H. A., et al. (eds.): The Heart and Cardiovascular System. 2nd ed. New York, Raven Press, 1992, pp. 1249–1279.
27. Fabiato, A.: Calcium-induced release of calcium from the cardiac sarcoplasmic reticulum. Am. J. Physiol. 245:C1–C14, 1983.
28. Bouchard, R. A., Clark, R. B., and Giles, W. R.: Effects of action potential duration on excitation-contraction coupling in rat ventricular myocytes. Action potential voltage-clamp measurements. Circ. Res. 76:790–801, 1995.
29. Kohmoto, O., Levi, A. J., and Bridge, J. H. B.: Relation between reverse sodium-calcium exchange and sarcoplasmic reticulum calcium release in guinea pig ventricular cells. Circ. Res. 74:550–554, 1994.
30. Berridge, M. J.: Inositol trisphosphate and calcium signalling. Nature 361:315–325, 1993.
31. Wier, W. G., Egan, T. M., Lopez-Lopez, J. R., and Balke, C. W.: Local control of excitation-contraction coupling in rat heart cells. J. Physiol. 474:463–471, 1994.
32. Lytton, J., and MacLennan, D. H.: Sarcoplasmic reticulum. In Fozzard, H. A., et al. (eds.): The Heart and Cardiovascular System. 2nd ed. New York, Raven Press, 1992, pp. 1203–1222.
33. Sipido, K. R., Callewaert, G., and Carmeliet, E.: Inhibition and rapid recovery of Ca2+ current during Ca2+-release from sarcoplasmic reticulum in guinea pig ventricular myocytes. Circ. Res. 76:102–109, 1995.
34. Wagenknecht, T., Grassucci, R., Frank, J., et al.: Three-dimensional architecture of the calcium channel/foot structure of sarcoplasmic reticulum. Nature 338:167–170, 1989.
35. Takeshima, H., Nishimura, S., Matsumoto, T., et al.: Primary structure and expression from complementary DNA of skeletal muscle ryanodine receptor. Nature 339:439–445, 1989.
36. Wibo, M., Bravo, G., and Godraind, T.: Postnatal maturation of excitation-contraction coupling in rat ventricle in relation to the subcellular localization and surface density of 1,4-dihydropyridine and ryanodine receptors. Circ. Res. 68:662–673, 1991.
37. Gilbert, J. C., Shirayama, T., and Pappano, A. J.: Inositol trisphosphate promotes Na-Ca exchange current by releasing calcium from sarcoplasmic reticulum in cardiac myocytes. Circ. Res. 69:1632–1639, 1991.
38. Brown, J. H., and Martinson, E. A.: Phosphoinositide-generated second messengers in cardiac signal transduction. Trends Cardiovasc. Med. 2:209–214, 1992.
39. Go, L. O., Moschella, M. C., Handa, K. K., et al.: Differential regulation of two types of intracellular calcium-release channels during end-stage human heart failure. Circulation 90(Abs.):I-L, 1994.
40. Arai, M., Matsui, H., and Periasamy, M.: Sarcoplasmic reticulum gene expression in cardiac hypertrophy and heart failure. Circ. Res. 74:555–564, 1994.
41. Luo, W., Grupp, I. L., Harrer, J., et al.: Targeted ablation of the phospholamban gene is associated with markedly enhanced myocardial contractility and loss of beta-agonist stimulation. Circ. Res. 75:401–409, 1994.

42. Tada, M., and Katz, A. M.: Phosphorylation of the sarcoplasmic reticulum and sarcolemma. Ann. Rev. Physiol. 44:401–423, 1982.

43. Gasser, J., Paganetti, P., Carafoli, E., and Chiesi, M.: Heterogeneous distribution of calmodulin- and cAMP-dependent regulation of Ca²⁺ uptake in cardiac sarcoplasmic reticulum subfractions. Eur. J. Biochem. 176:535–541, 1988.

44. McLeod, A. G., Shen, A. C. Y., Campbell, K. P., et al.: Frog cardiac calsequestrin. Identification, characterization, and subcellular distribution in two structurally distinct regions of peripheral sarcoplasmic reticulum in frog ventricular myocardium. Circ. Res. 69:344–359, 1991.

45. D'Agnolo, A., Luciani, G. B., Mazzucco, A., et al.: Contractile properties and Ca²⁺ release activity of the sarcoplasmic reticulum in dilated cardiomyopathy. Circulation 85:518–525, 1992.

46. Arai, M., Alpert, N. R., MacLennan, D. H., et al.: Alterations in sarcoplasmic reticulum gene expression in human heart failure. A possible mechanism for alterations in systolic and diastolic properties of the failing myocardium. Circ. Res. 72:463–469, 1993.

SARCOLEMMAL CONTROL OF CALCIUM AND OTHER IONS

47. Katz, A. M.: Cardiac ion channels. N. Engl. J. Med. 328:1244–1251, 1993.

48. Tomaselli, G. F., Backx, P. H., and Marban, E.: Molecular basis of permeation in voltage-gated ion channels. Circ. Res. 72:491–496, 1993.

49. Schwartz, A.: Calcium antagonists: Review and perspective on mechanism of action. Am. J. Cardiol. 64(Suppl.):3I–9I, 1989.

50. Heinemann, S. H., Stuhmer, W.: Molecular structure of potassium and sodium channels and their structure-function correlation. In Sperelakis, N. (ed.): Physiology and Pathophysiology of the Heart. 3rd ed. Boston, Kluwer Academic Publishers, 1995, pp. 101–114.

51. Pragnell, M., De Waard, M., Mori, Y., et al.: Calcium channel beta-subunit binds to a conserved motif in the I-II cytoplasmic linker of the alpha₁-subunit. Nature 368:67–70, 1994.

52. Yatani, A., Bahinski, A., Mikala, G., et al.: Single amino acid substitutions within the ion permeation pathway alter single-channel conductance of the human L-type cardiac Ca²⁺ channel. Circ. Res. 75:315–323, 1994.

53. Flockerzi, V., and Hofmann, F.: Molecular structure of the cardiac calcium channel. In Sperelakis, E. (ed.): Physiology and Pathophysiology of the Heart. 3rd ed. Boston, Kluwer Academic Publishers, 1995, pp. 91–99.

54. Bean, B. P.: Two kinds of calcium channels in canine atrial cells. Differences in kinetics, selectivity and pharmacology. J. Gen. Physiol. 86:1–30, 1985.

55. Bers, D. M., Bassani, J. W. M., and Bassani, R. A.: Competition and redistribution among calcium transport systems in rabbit cardiac myocytes. Cardiovasc. Res. 27:1772–1777, 1993.

56. Reeves, J. P.: Cardiac sodium-calcium exchange sytstem. In Sperelakis, N. (ed.): Physiology and Pathophysiology of the Heart. 3rd ed. Boston, Kluwer Academic Publishers, 1995, pp. 309–318.

57. Nicoll, D. A., Longoni, S., and Philipson, K. D.: Molecular cloning and functional expression of the cardiac sarcolemmal Na⁺–Ca²⁺ exchanger. Science 250:562–565, 1990.

58. Chin, T. K., Spitzer, K. W., Philipson, K. D., and Bridge, J. H. B.: The effect of exchanger inhibitory peptide (XIP) on sodium-calcium exchange current in guinea-pig ventricular cells. Circ. Res. 72:497–503, 1993.

59. Bers, D. M.: Excitation-Contraction Coupling and Cardiac Contractile Force. Boston, Kluwer Academic Publishers, 1991.

60. Leblanc, N., and Hume, J. R.: Sodium current-induced release of calcium from cardiac sarcoplasmic reticulum. Science 248:372–376, 1990.

61. Noble, D., Noble, S. J., Bett, C. L., et al.: The role of sodium-calcium exchange during the cardiac action potential. Ann. N. Y. Acad. Sci. 639:334–353, 1991.

62. Sheu, S.-S., and Blaustein, M. P.: Sodium/calcium exchange and control of cell calcium and contractility in cardiac and vascular smooth muscles. In Fozzard, H. A., et al. (eds.): The Heart and Cardiovascular System. 2nd ed. New York, Raven Press, 1992, pp. 903–943.

63. Levi, A. J., Brooksby, P., and Hancox, J. C.: A role for depolarisation-induced calcium entry on the Na-Ca exchange in triggering intracellular calcium release and contraction in rat ventricular myocytes. Cardiovasc. Res. 27:1677–1690, 1993.

64. Han, S., Schiefer, A., and Isenberg, G.: Ca²⁺ load of guinea-pig ventricular myocytes determines efficacy of brief Ca²⁺ currents as trigger for Ca²⁺ release. J. Physiol. 480:411–421, 1994.

65. Kaibara, M., Mitarai, S., Yano, K., and Kameyama, M.: Involvement of Na⁺/H⁺ antiporter in regulation of L-type Ca²⁺ channel current by angiotensin-II in rabbit ventricular myocytes. Circ. Res. 75:1121–1125, 1994.

66. Vandenberg, J. I., Metcalfe, J. C., Grace, A. A.: Mechanisms of pHᵢ recovery after global ischemia in the perfused heart. Circ. Res. 72:993–1003, 1993.

67. Yanoukakos, D., Stuart-Tilley, A., Fernandez, H. A., et al.: Molecular cloning, expression, and chromosomal localization of two isoforms of the AE3 anion exchanger from human heart. Circ. Res. 75:603–614, 1994.

68. Desilets, M., Puceat, M., and Vassort, G.: Chloride dependence of pH modulation by beta-adrenergic agonist in rat cardiomyocytes. Circ. Res. 75:862–869, 1994.

69. Eisner, D. A., and Smith, T. W.: The Na-K pump and its effectors in

cardiac muscle. In Fozzard, H. A., et al. (eds.): The Heart and Cardiovascular System. 2nd ed. New York, Raven Press, 1992, pp. 863–902.

70. Lelievre, L., and Charlemagne, D.: The myocyte sarcolemma in cardiac hypertrophy: Na⁺/K⁺-ATPase, Ca²⁺-ATPase, Na⁺/Ca²⁺ exchange and phospholipids. In Swynghedauw, B. (ed.): Research in Cardiac Hypertrophy and Failure. INSERM/John Libbey Eurotext, London, 1990, pp. 171–184.

71. Carmeliet, E.: A fuzzy subsarcolemmal space for intracellular Na⁺ in cardiac cells? Cardiovasc. Res. 26:433–442, 1992.

72. Johnson, E. A., and Lemieux, R. D.: Sodium-calcium exchange. Science 251:1370, 1991.

RECEPTORS AND SIGNAL SYSTEMS

73. Lindemann, J. P., and Watanabe, A. M.: Mechanisms of adrenergic and cholinergic regulation of myocardial contractility. In Sperelakis, N. (ed.): Physiology and Pathophysiology of the Heart. 3rd ed. Boston, Kluwer Academic Publishers, 1995, pp. 467–494.

74. Fleming, J. W., Wisler, P. L., and Watanabe, A. M.: Signal transduction by G-proteins in cardiac tissues. Circulation 85:420–433, 1992.

75. Neer, E. J., and Clapham, D. E.: Signal transduction through G-proteins in the cardiac myocyte. Trends Cardiovasc. Med. 2:6–11, 1992.

76. Lefkowitz, R. J.: Clinical implications of basic research. N. Engl. J. Med. 332:186–187, 1995.

77. De Jonge, H. W., Van Heugten, H. A. A., and Lamers, J. M. J.: Signal transduction by the phosphatidylinositol cycle in myocardium. J. Mol. Cell Cardiol. 27:93–106, 1995.

78. Sadoshima, J., Xu, Y., Slayter, H. S., and Izumo, S.: Autocrine release of angiotensin-II mediates stretch-induced hypertrophy of cardiac myocytes in vitro. Cell 75:977–984, 1993.

79. Bristow, M. R., Hershberger, R. E., Port, J. D., and Rasmussen, R.: Beta₁ and beta₂ adrenergic receptor–mediated adenylate cyclase stimulation in nonfailing and failing human ventricular myocardium. Mol. Pharmacol. 35:295, 1989.

80. Levy, F. O., Zhu, X., Kaumann, A. J., and Birnbaumer, L.: Efficacy of β₁-adrenergic receptors is lower than that of β₂-adrenergic receptors. Proc. Natl. Acad. Sci. 90:10798–10802, 1993.

81. Raymond, J. R., Hantowich, M., Lefkowitz, R. J., and Caron, M. G.: Adrenergic receptors. Models for regulation of signal transduction processes. Hypertension 15:119–131, 1990.

82. Spinale, F. G., Tempel, G. E., Mukherjee, R., et al.: Cellular and molecular alterations in the β-adrenergic system with cardiomyopathy induced by tachycardia. Cardiovasc. Res. 28:1243–1250, 1994.

83. Neubig, R. R.: Membrane organization in G-protein mechanisms. FASEB J. 8:939–946, 1994.

84. Port, J. D., and Malbon, C. C.: Integration of transmembrane signaling. Cross-talk among G-protein–linked receptors and other signal transduction pathways. Trends Cardiovasc. Med. 3:85–92, 1993.

85. Coleman, D. E., Berghuis, A. M., Lee, E., et al.: Structures of active conformations of G_{iα1} and the mechanism of GTP hydrolysis. Science 265:1405–1412, 1994.

86. Kurachi, Y.: G-protein control of cardiac potassium channels. Trends Cardiovasc. Med. 4:64–69, 1994.

87. Schofield, P. R., and Abbott, A.: Molecular pharmacology and drug action: Structural information casts light on ligand binding. TIPS 10:207–212, 1989.

88. Kumar, R., Joyner, R. W., Hartzell, H. C., et al.: Postnatal changes in the G-proteins, cyclic nucleotides and adenylyl cyclase activity in rabbit heart cells. J. Mol. Cell Cardiol. 26:1537–1550, 1994.

89. Opie, L. H.: The Heart: Physiology and Metabolism. 2nd ed. New York, Raven Press, 1991, pp. 67–126, 147–175.

90. Liang, B. T., and Haltiwanger, B.: Adenosine A_{2a} and A_{2b} receptors in cultured fetal chick heart cells. High- and low-affinity coupling to stimulation of myocyte contractility and cAMP accumulation. Circ. Res. 76:242–251, 1995.

91. Ono, K., Eto, K., Sakamoto, A., et al.: Negative chronotropic effect of endothelin 1 mediated through ET_A receptors in guinea pig atria. Circ. Res. 76:284–292, 1995.

92. Shabb, J. B., and Corbin, J. D.: Protein phosphorylation in the heart. In Fozzard, H. A., et al.: The Heart and Cardiovascular System. 2nd ed. New York, Raven Press, 1992, pp. 1539–1562.

93. Walsh, D. A., and Van Patten, S. M.: Multiple pathway signal transduction by the cAMP-dependent protein kinase. FASEB J. 8:1227–1236, 1994.

94. Scott, J. D., and Carr, D. W.: Subcellular localization of the Type II cAMP-dependent protein kinase. NIPS 7:143–148, 1992.

95. Hohl, C. M., and Li, Q.: Compartmentation of cAMP in adult canine ventricular myocytes. Relation to single cell free Ca²⁺ transients. Circ. Res. 69:1369–1379, 1991.

96. Worthington, M., and Opie, L. H.: Contrasting effects of cyclic AMP increase caused by beta-adrenergic stimulation or by adenylate cyclase activation on ventricular fibrillation threshold of isolated rat heart. J. Cardiovasc. Pharmacol. 20:595–600, 1992.

97. Bartel, S., Karczewski, P., and Krause, E.-G.: Protein phosphorylation and cardiac function: Cholinergic-adrenergic interaction. Cardiovasc. Res. 27:1948–1953, 1993.

98. Matsuda, J. J., Lee, H. C., and Shibata, E. F.: Acetylcholine reversal of isoproterenol-stimulated sodium currents in rabbit ventricular myocytes. Circ. Res. 72:517–525, 1993.

99. Sumii, K., and Sperelakis, N.: cGMP-dependent protein kinase regula-

tion of the L-type Ca²⁺ current in rat ventricular myocytes. Circ. Res. 77:803–812, 1995.

100. Lohmann, S. M., Fischmeister, R., and Walter, U.: Signal transduction by cGMP in heart. Basic Res. Cardiol. 86:503–514, 1991.

101. Shah, A. M., Spurgeon, H. A., Sollott, S. J., et al.: 8-Bromo-cGMP reduces the myofilament response to Ca²⁺ in intact cardiac myocytes. Circ. Res. 74:970–978, 1994.

102. Deckmyn, H., Ven Geet, C., and Vermylen, J.: Dual regulation of phospholipase C activity by G-proteins. NIPS 8:61–63, 1993.

103. Du, X.-J., Anderson, K.E., Jacobsen, A., et al.: Suppression of ventricular arrhythmias during ischemia-reperfusion by agents inhibiting Ins(1, 4,5)P₃ release. Circulation 91:2712–2716, 1995.

104. Rogers, T. B., and Lokuta, A. J.: Angiotensin-II signal transduction pathways in the cardiovascular system. Trends Cardiovasc. Med. 4:110–116, 1994.

105. Hug, H., and Sarre, T. F.: Protein kinase C isoenzymes: Divergence in signal transduction? Biochem. J. 291:329–343, 1993.

106. Gu, X., and Bishop, S. P.: Increased protein kinase C and isozyme redistribution in pressure-overload cardiac hypertrophy in the rat. Circ. Res. 75:926–931, 1994.

107. Johnson, J. A., and Mochly-Rosen, D.: Inhibition of the spontaneous rate of contraction of neonatal cardiac myocytes by protein kinase C isozymes. Circ. Res. 76:654–663, 1995.

108. Fedida, D.: Modulation of cardiac contractility by α₁-adrenoceptors. Cardiovasc. Res. 27:1735–1742, 1993.

109. Steinberg, S. F., Goldberg, M., and Rybin, V. O.: Protein kinase C isoform diversity in the heart. J. Mol. Cell Cardiol. 27:141–153, 1995.

110. Mitchell, M. B., Meng, X., Brown, J. M., et al.: Preconditioning of isolated rat heart is mediated by protein kinase C. Circ. Res. 76:73–81, 1995.

111. Tomai, F., Crea, F., Gaspardone, A., et al.: Ischemic preconditioning during coronary angioplasty is prevented by glibenclamide, a selective ATP-sensitive K⁺ channel blocker. Circulation 90:700–705, 1994.

112. Forstermann, U., Pollock, J. S., and Nakane, M.: Nitric oxide synthases in the cardiovascular system. Trends Cardiovasc. Med. 3:104–110, 1993.

113. Balligand, J.-L., Kelly, R. A., Marsden, P. A., et al.: Control of cardiac muscle cell function by an endogenous nitric oxide signaling system. Proc. Natl. Acad. Sci. 90:347–351, 1993.

114. Weyrich, A. S., Ma, X., Buerke, M., et al.: Physiological concentrations of nitric oxide do not elicit an acute negative inotropic effect in unstimulated cardiac muscle. Circ. Res. 75:692–700, 1994.

115. Shryock, J., Song, Y., Wang, D., et al.: Selective A₂-adenosine receptor agonists do not alter action potential duration, twitch shortening, or cAMP accumulation in guinea pig, rat, or rabbit isolated ventricular myocytes. Circ. Res. 72:194–205, 1993.

116. Stiles, G. L.: Adenosine receptors. J. Biol. Chem. 267:6451–6454, 1992.

117. Komuro, I., and Yazaki, Y.: Intracellular signaling pathways in cardiac myocytes induced by mechanical stress. Trends Cardiovasc. Med. 4:117–121, 1994.

118. Van Wagoner, D. R.: Mechanosensitive gating of atrial ATP-sensitive potassium channels. Circ. Res. 72:973–983, 1993.

119. Boer, P. H. Ruzicka, M., Lear, W., et al.: Stretch-mediated activation of the cardiac renin gene. Am. J. Physiol. 267:H1630–H1636, 1994.

120. Bristow, M. R., Anderson, F. L., Port, D., et al.: Differences in beta-adrenergic neuroeffector mechanisms in ischemic versus idiopathic dilated cardiomyopathy. Circlation 84:1024–1039, 1991.

121. Böhm, M., Reiger, B., Schwinger, R. H. G., and Erdmann, E.: cAMP concentrations, cAMP dependent protein kinase activity, and phospholamban in non-failing and failing myocardium. Cardiovasc. Res. 28:1713–1719, 1994.

122. Böhm, M., Eschenhagen, T., Gierschik, P., et al.: Radioimmunochemical quantification of Giα in right and left ventricles from patients with ischaemic and dilated cardiomyopathy and predominant left ventricular failure. J. Mol. Cell Cardiol. 26:133–149, 1994.

123. Beuckelmann, D. J., Nabauer, M., and Erdmann, E.: Intracellular calcium handling in isolated ventricular myocytes from patients with terminal heart failure. Circulation 85:1046–1055, 1992.

124. Steinfath, M., Danielsen, W., von der Leyen, H., et al.: Reduced α₁- and β₂-adrenoceptor-mediated positive inotropic effects in human end-stage heart failure. Br. J. Pharmacol. 105:463–469, 1992.

125. Lohse, M. J.: G-protein-coupled receptor kinases and the heart. Trends Cardiovasc. Med. 5:63–68, 1995.

126. Hausdorff, W. P., Caron, M. G., and Lefkowitz, R. J.: Turning off the signal: Desensitization of beta-adrenergic receptor function. FASEB J. 4:2881–2889, 1990.

127. Ungerer, M., Böhm, M., Elce, J. S., et al.: Altered expression of β-adrenergic receptor kinase and β₁-adrenergic receptors in the failing human heart. Circulation 87:454–463, 1993.

128. Lubbe, W. F., Podzuweit, T., and Opie, L. H.: Potential arrhythmogenic role of cyclic AMP and cytosolic calcium overload: Implications for prophylactic effects of beta-blockers and proarrhythmic effects of phosphodiesterase inhibitors. J. Am. Coll. Cardiol. 19:1622–1633, 1992.

129. Muntz, K. H., Zhao, M., and Miller, J. C.: Downregulation of myocardial β-adrenergic receptors. Receptor subtype selectivity. Circ. Res. 74:369–375, 1994.

130. Matsuda, J. J., Lee, H., and Shibata, E. F.: Enhancement of rabbit cardiac sodium channels by β-adrenergic stimulation. Circ. Res. 70:199–207, 1992.

131. Chang, F., and Cohen, I. S.: Mechanism of acetylcholine action on pacemaker current (I_f) in canine Purkinje fibers. Pflugers Arch. 420:389–392, 1992.

CONTRACTILE PERFORMANCE OF THE INTACT HEART

132. Lewis, T.: The Mechanism and Graphic Registration of the Heart Beat. London, Shaw and Sons, 1920, p. 24.

133. Wiggers, C. J.: Modern Aspects of the Circulation in Health and Disease. Philadelphia, Lea and Febiger, 1915, p. 98.

134. Laniado, S., Yellin, E. L., Miller, H., and Frater, R. W. M.: Temporal relation of the first heart sound to closure of the mitral valve. Circulation 47:1006–1014, 1973.

135. Parisi, A. F., and Milton, B. G.: Relation of mitral valve closure to the first heart sound in man. Echocardiographic and phonocardiographic assessment. Am. J. Cardiol. 32:779–782, 1973.

136. Rhodes, J., Udelson, J. E., Marx, G. R., et al.: A new noninvasive method for the estimation of peak dP/dt. Circulation 88:2693–2699, 1993.

137. Hirschfeld, S., Meyer, R., Korfhagen, J., et al.: The isovolumic contraction time of the left ventricle. An echographic study. Circulation 54:751–756, 1976.

138. Belz, G. G.: Elastic properties and Windkessel function of the human aorta. Cardiovasc. Drugs Ther. 9:73–83, 1995.

139. Ohno, M., Cheng, C.-P., and Little, W. C.: Mechanism of altered patterns of left ventricular filling during the development of congestive heart failure. Circulation 89:2241–2250, 1994.

140. Glower, D. D., Murrah, R. L., Olsen, C. O., et al.: Mechanical correlates of the third heart sound. J. Am. Coll. Cardiol. 19:450–457, 1992.

141. Starling, E. H.: The Linacre Lecture on the Law of the Heart. London, Longmans, Green and Co., 1918.

142. Frank, O.: Zur Dynamik des Herzmuskels. Z. Biol. 32:370–447, 1895. Translated in Am. Heart J. 58:282–317, 467–478, 1958.

143. Greenway, C. V., and Wayne Lautt, W.: Blood volume, the venous system, preload and cardiac output. Can. J. Physiol. Pharmacol. 64:383–387, 1986.

144. Rodriguez, E. K., Hunter, W. C., Royce, M. J., et al.: A method to reconstruct myocardial sarcomere lengths and orientations at transmural sites in beating canine hearts. Am. J. Physiol. 263:H293–H306, 1992.

145. Backx, P. H., ter Keurs, H. E. D. J.: Fluorescent properties of rat cardiac trabeculae microinjected with fura-2 salt. Am J. Physiol. 264:H1098–H1110, 1993.

146. Kent, R. L., Hoober, K., and Cooper, G.: Load responsiveness of protein synthesis in adult mammalian myocardium: Role of cardiac deformation linked to sodium influx. Circ. Res. 64:74–85, 1989.

147. Borow, K. M.: Clinical assessment of contractility in the symmetrically contracting left ventricle: Part I. Mod. Concepts Cardiovasc. Dis. 57:29–34, 1988.

148. Eaton, G. M., Cody, R. J., and Binkley, P. F.: Increased aortic impedance precedes peripheral vasoconstriction at the early stage of ventricular failure in the paced canine model. Circulation 88:2714–2721, 1993.

149. Bowditch, H.: Uber die Eigenthumlickkeiten der Reizbarkeit, welche die Muskelfasern des Herzens Zeigen. Arb. Physiol. Inst. Lpz. 6:139, 1871.

150. Mulieri, L. A., Leavitt, B. J., Martin, B. J., et al.: Myocardial force-frequency defect in mitral regurgitation heart failure is reversed by forskolin. Circulation 88:2700–2704, 1993.

151. Suga, H.: Ventricular energetics. Physiol. Rev. 70:247–277, 1990.

152. Cooper, M. W.: Postextrasystolic potentiation. Do we really know what it means and how to use it? Circulation 88:2962–2971, 1993.

153. Hasenfuss, G., Reinecke, H., Studer, R., et al.: Relation between myocardial function and expression of sarcoplasmic reticulum Ca²⁺-ATPase in failing and nonfailing human myocardium. Circ. Res. 75:434–442, 1994.

154. Pierard, L. A., Serruys, P. W., Roelandt, J., and Meltzer, R. S.: Left ventricular function at similar heart rates during tachycardia induced by exercise and atrial pacing: An echocardiographic study. Br. Heart J. 57:154–160, 1987.

155. Braunwald, E., and Sobel, B. E.: Coronary blood flow and myocardial ischemia. In Braunwald, E. (ed.): Heart Disease. A Textbook of Cardiovascular Medicine. 4th ed. Philadelphia, W. B. Saunders Company, 1992, pp. 1161–1199.

156. Rooke, G. A., and Feigl, E. O.: Work as a correlate of canine left ventricular oxygen consumption, and the problem of catecholamine oxygen wasting. Circ. Res. 50:273–286, 1982.

157. Simonsen, S., and Kjekshus, J. K.: The effect of free fatty acids on myocardial oxygen consumption during atrial pacing and catecholamine infusion in man. Circulation 58:484–491, 1978.

158. Burkhoff, D., Weiss, R. G., Schulman, S. P., et al.: Influence of metabolic substrate on rat heart function and metabolism at different coronary flows. Am. J. Physiol. 261:H741–H750, 1991.

159. Braunwald, E.: Control of myocardial oxygen consumption. Physiologic and clinical considerations. Am. J. Cardiol. 27:416–432, 1971.

160. Kannengiesser, G. J., Opie, L. H., and van der Werff, T. J.: Impaired cardiac work and oxygen uptake after reperfusion of ischaemic myocardium. J. Mol. Cell Cardiol. 11:197–207, 1979.

161. Kass, D. A., and Beyar, R.: Evaluation of contractile state by maximal ventricular power divided by the square of end-diastolic volume. Circulation 84:1698–1708, 1991.

162. Nozawa, T., Cheng, C.-P., Noda, T., and Little, W. C.: Effect of exercise on left ventricular mechanical efficiency in conscious dogs. Circulation 90:3047–3054, 1994.

163. Beanlands, R. S. B., Bach, D. S., Raylman, R., et al.: Acute effects of dobutamine on myocardial oxygen consumption and cardiac efficiency measured using carbon-11 acetate kinetics in patients with dilated cardiomyopathy. J. Am. Coll. Cardiol. 22:1389–1398, 1993.

164. Burkhoff, D., de Tombe, P. P., Hunter, W. C., and Kass, D. A.: Contractile strength and mechanical efficiency of left ventricle are enhanced by physiological afterload. Am. J. Physiol. 260:H569–H578, 1991.

165. Opie, L. H.: Regulation of myocardial contractility. J. Cardiovasc. Pharmacol. 26(Suppl. 1):S1–S9, 1995.

166. Lakatta, E. G.: Starling's Law of the heart is explained by an intimate interaction of muscle length and myofilament calcium activation. J. Am. Coll. Cardiol. 10:1157–1164, 1987.

167. Schlant, R. C., and Sonnenblick, E. H.: Normal physiology of the cardiovascular system. In Schlant, R. C., and Alexander, R. W. (eds.): The Heart, Arteries and Veins. New York, McGill Inc., 1994, pp. 113–151.

168. Braunwald, E., Sonnenblick, E. H., and Ross, J.: Normal and abnormal circulatory function. In Braunwald, E. (ed.): Heart Disease. A textbook of Cardiovascular Medicine. 4th ed. Philadelphia, W. B. Saunders Company, 1992, pp. 351–392.

169. Sweitzer, N. K., and Moss, R. L.: Determinants of loaded shortening velocity in single cardiac myocytes permeabilized with alpha-hemolysin. Circ. Res. 73:1150–1162, 1993.

170. Campbell, K. B., Kirkpatrick, R. D., Tobias, A. H., et al.: Series coupled non-contractile elements are functionally unimportant in the isolated heart. Cardiovasc. Res. 28:242–251, 1994.

171. Ter Keurs, H. E. D. J.: Calcium and contractility. In Drake-Holland, A. J., and Noble, M. I. M. (eds.): Cardiac Metabolism. Chicester, John Wiley, 1983, pp. 73–99.

172. Strang, K. T., Sweitzer, N. K., Greaser, M. L., and Moss, R. L.: Beta-adrenergic receptor stimulation increases unloaded shortening velocity of skinned single ventricular myocytes from rats. Circ. Res. 74:542–549, 1994.

173. de Tombe, P. P., and ter Keurs, H. E. D. J.: Lack of effect of isoproterenol on unloaded velocity of sarcomere shortening in rat cardiac trabeculae. Circ. Res. 68:382–391, 1991.

174. Kass, D. A., Beyar, R., Lankford, E., et al.: Influence of contractile state on curvilinearity of in situ end-systolic pressure-volume relations. Circulation 79:167–178, 1989.

175. Carabello, B. A.: The role of end-systolic pressure-volume analysis in clinical assessment of ventricular function. Trends Cardiovasc. Med. 1:337–341, 1991.

176. Hori, M., Kitakaze, M., Ishida, Y., et al.: Delayed end ejection increases isovolumic ventricular relaxation rate in isolated perfused canine hearts. Circ. Res. 68:300–308, 1991.

177. Leite-Moreira, A. F., and Gillebert, T. C.: Nonuniform course of left ventricular pressure fall and its regulation by load and contractile state. Circulation 90:2481–2491, 1994.

178. Brutsaert, D. L., and Sys, S. U.: Relaxation and diastole of the heart. Physiol. Rev. 69:1228–1315, 1989.

179. Brutsaert, D. L., Sys, S. U., and Gillebert, T. C.: Diastolic failure: Pathophysiology and therapeutic implications. J. Am. Coll. Cardiol. 22:318–325, 1993.

180. Eichhorn, E. J., Willard, J. E., Alvarez, L., et al.: Are contraction and relaxation coupled in patients with and without congestive heart failure? Circulation 85:2132–2139, 1992.

181. Cory, C. R., Grange, R. W., and Houston, M. E.: Role of sarcoplasmic reticulum in loss of load-sensitive relaxation in pressure overload cardiac hypertrophy. Am. J. Physiol. 266:H68–H78, 1994.

182. Morgan, J. P., and Morgan, K. G.: Intracellular calcium and cardiovascular function in heart failure: Effects of pharmacologic agents. Cardiovasc. Drugs Ther. 3:959–970, 1989.

183. Yamamoto, K., Masuyama, T., Doi, Y., et al.: Noninvasive assessment of left ventricular relaxation using continuous wave Doppler aortic regurgitant velocity curve. Its comparative value to the mitral regurgitation method. Circulation 91:192–200, 1995.

184. Chen, C., Rodriguez, L., Levine, R. A., et al.: Noninvasive measurement of the time constant of left ventricular relaxation using the continuous-wave Doppler velocity profile of mitral regurgitation. Circulation 86:272–278, 1992.

185. Udelson, J. E., Bacharach, S. L., Cannon, R. O., and Bonow, R. O.: Minimum left ventricular pressure during beta-adrenergic stimulation in human subjects. Circulation 82:1174–1182, 1990.

186. Gilbert, J. C., and Glantz, S. A.: Determinants of left ventricular filling and of the diastolic pressure-volume relation. Circ. Res. 64:827–852, 1989.

187. Hoit, B. D., Shao, Y., Gabel, M., and Walsh, R. A.: In vivo assessment of left atrial contractile performance in normal and pathological conditions using a time-varying elastance model. Circulation 89:1829–1838, 1994.

188. Focaccio, A., Volpe, M., Ambrosio, G., et al.: Angiotensin-II directly stimulates release of atrial natriuretic factor in isolated rabbit hearts. Circulation 87:192–198, 1993.

189. Fyrhquist, F., Sirvio, M.-L., Helin, K., et al.: Endothelin antiserum decreases volume-stimulated and basal plasma concentration of atrial natriuretic peptide. Circulation 88:1172–1176, 1993.

190. Mouton, R., Lochner, J. De V., and Lochner, A.: New emphasis on atrial cardiology. S. Afr. Med. J. 82:222–223, 1992.

191. Holubarsch, C., Hasenfuss, G., Schmidt-Schweda, S., et al.: Angiotensin-I and II exert inotropic effects in atrial but not in ventricular human myocardium. An in vitro study under physiological experimental conditions. Circulation 88:1228–1237, 1993.

192. Wang, Z., Fermini, B., and Nattel, S.: Delayed rectifier outward current and repolarization in human atrial myocytes. Circ. Res. 73:276–285, 1993.

193. Koumi, S.-I., and Wasserstrom, J. A.: Acetylcholine-sensitive muscarinic K+ channels in mammalian ventricular myocytes. Am. J. Physiol. 266:H1812–H1821, 1994.

194. Rozanski, G. J., Lipsius, S. L., and Randall, W. C.: Functional characteristics of sinoatrial and subsidiary pacemaker activity in the canine right atrium. Circulation 67:1378–1387, 1983.

195. Douglas, P. S., Berko, B., Lesh, M., and Reichek, N.: Alterations in diastolic function in response to progressive left ventricular hypertrophy. J. Am. Coll. Cardiol. 13:461–467, 1989.

196. Myreng, Y., and Smiseth, O. A.: Assessment of ventricular relaxation by Doppler echocardiography. Comparison of isovolumic relaxation time and transmitral flow velocities with time constant of isovolumic relaxation. Circulation 81:260–266, 1990.

197. Villari, B., Vassalli, G., Monrad, E. S., et al.: Normalization of diastolic dysfunction in aortic stenosis late after valve replacement. Circulation 91:2353–2358, 1995.

198. Mehta, S., Charbonneau, F., Fitchett, D. H., et al.: The clinical consequences of a stiff left atrium. Am. Heart J. 122:1184–1191, 1991.

199. Kool, M. J., Spek, J. J., Struyker Boudier, H. A., et al.: Acute and subacute effects of nicorandil and isosorbide dinitrate on vessel wall properties of large arteries and hemodynamics in healthy volunteers. Cardiovasc. Drugs Ther. 9:331–337, 1995.

200. Stefanadis, C., Stratos, C., Boudoulas, H., et al.: Distensibility of the ascending aorta: Comparison of invasive and non-invasive techniques in healthy men and in men with coronary artery disease. Eur. Heart J. 11:990–996, 1990.

201. Adams, J. N., Brooks, M., Redpath, T. W., et al.: Aortic distensibility and stiffness index measure by magnetic resonance imaging in patients with Marfan's syndrome. Br. Heart J. 73:265–269, 1995.

202. Wesseling, K. H., Jansen, J. R. C., Settels, J. J., and Schreuder, J. J.: Computation of aortic flow from pressure in humans using a nonlinear, three-element model. J. Appl. Physiol. 74:2566–2573, 1993.

203. Dittrich, H. C., Chow, L. C., and Nicod, P. H.: Early improvement in left ventricular diastolic function after relief of chronic right ventricular pressure overload. Circulation 80:823–830, 1989.

204. Feneley, M. P., Olsen, C. O., Glower, D. D., and Rankin, J. S.: Effect of acutely increased right ventricular afterload on work output from the left ventricle in conscious dogs. Systolic ventricular interaction. Circ. Res. 65:135–145, 1989.

205. Hamilton, D. R., Dani, R. S., Semlacher, R. A., et al.: Right atrial and right ventricular transmural pressures in dogs and humans. Effects of the pericardium. Circulation 90:2492–2500, 1994.

206. Refsum, H., Junemann, M., Lipton, M. J., et al.: Ventricular diastolic pressure-volume relations and the pericardium. Effects of changes in blood volume and pericardial effusion in dogs. Circulation 64:997–1004, 1981.

207. Chuttani, K., Pandian, N. G., Mohanty, P. K., et al.: Left ventricular diastolic collapse. An echocardiographic sign of regional cardiac tamponade. Circulation 83:1999–2006, 1991.

208. Li, K., Rouleau, J. L., Calderone, A., et al.: Endocardial function in pacing-induced heart failure in the dog. J. Mol. Cell Cardiol. 25:529–540, 1993.

209. Brutsaert, D. L., and Andries, L. J.: The endocardial endothelium. Am. J. Physiol. 263:H985–H1002, 1992.

210. Noble, M. I. M.: Excitation-contraction coupling. In Drake-Holland, A. J., and Noble, M. I. M. (eds.): Cardiac Metabolism. New York, John Wiley, 1983, pp. 49–71.

211. Harizi, R. C., Bianco, J. A., and Alpert, J. S.: Diastolic function of the heart in clinical cardiology. Arch. Intern. Med. 148:99–109, 1988.

EFFECTS OF ISCHEMIA AND REPERFUSION ON CONTRACTION AND RELAXATION

212. Figueredo, V., Brandes, R., Weiner, M. W., et al.: Endocardial versus epicardial differences of intracellular free calcium under normal and ischemic conditions in perfused rat hearts. Circ. Res. 72:1082–1090, 1993.

213. Urthaler, F., Harris, K., Walker, A. A., et al.: Beat to beat $[Ca^{2+}]_i$ and left ventricular function during brief bouts of ischemia in rats. J. Am. Coll. Cardiol. 22(Abs.):317A, 1994.

214. Meissner, A., and Morgan, J. P.: Contractile dysfunction and abnormal Ca^{2+} modulation during postischemic reperfusion in rat heart. Am. J. Physiol. 268:H100–H111, 1995.

215. Korge, P., Byrd, S. K., and Campbell, K. B.: Functional coupling between sarcoplasmic reticulum-bound creatine kinase and Ca^{2+}-ATPase. Eur. J. Biochem. 213:973–980, 1993.

216. Cross, H. R., Clarke, K., Opie, L. H., and Radda, G. K.: Is lactate-induced myocardial ischaemic injury mediated by decreased pH or increased intracellular lactate? J. Mol. Cell Cardiol. 27:1369–1381, 1995.

216a. Sata, M., Sugiura, S., Yamashita, H., et al.: Coupling between myosin ATPase cycle and creatine kinase cycle facilitates cardiac actomyosin sliding in vitro. A clue to mechanical dysfunction during myocardial ischemia. Circulation 93:310, 1996.

217. Kentish, J. C.: The effects of inorganic phosphate and creatine phosphate on force production in skinned muscles from rat ventricle. J. Physiol. 370:585–604, 1986.

218. Opie, L. H.: Myocardial metabolism in ischemia. In Heusch, G. (ed.): Pathophysiology and Rational Therapy of Myocardial Ischemia. Darmstadt, Steinkopff Verlag, 1990, pp. 37–57.

219. Turvey, S. E., and Allen, D. G.: Changes in myoplasmic sodium concentration during exposure to lactate in perfused rat heart. Cardiovasc. Res. 28:987–993, 1994.

220. Gasser, R. N. A., and Klein, W.: Contractile failure in early myocardial ischemia: Models and mechanisms. Cardiovasc. Drugs Ther. 8:813–822, 1994.

221. Kantor, P., Coetzee, W. A., Carmeliet, E., et al.: Reduction of ischemic K+ loss and arrhythmias in rat hearts. Effects of glibenclamide, a sulfonylurea. Circ. Res. 66:478–485, 1990.

222. Weiss, J. N., and Shieh, R.-C.: Potassium loss during myocardial ischaemia and hypoxia: Does lactate efflux play a role? Cardiovasc. Res. 28:1125–1132, 1994.

223. Sylven, C.: Mechanisms of pain in angina pectoris—A critical review of the adenosine hypothesis. Cardiovasc. Drugs Ther. 7:745–759, 1993.

224. Yao, Z., and Gross, G. J.: A comparison of adenosine-induced cardioprotection and ischemic preconditioning in dogs. Efficacy, time course, and role of K_{ATP} channels. Circulation 89:1229–1236, 1994.

225. Apstein, C. S., and Grossman, W.: Opposite initial effects of supply and demand ischemia on left ventricular diastolic compliance: The ischemic-diastolic paradox. J. Mol. Cell Cardiol. 19:119–128, 1987.

226. Applegate, R. J., Walsh, R. A., and O'Rourke, R. A.: Comparative effects of pacing-induced and flow-limited ischemia on left ventricular function. Circulation 81:1380–1392, 1990.

227. De Bruyne, B., Bronzwaer, J. G. F., Heyndrickx, G. R., and Paulus, W. J.: Comparative effects of ischemia and hypoxemia on left ventricular systolic and diastolic function in humans. Circulation 88:461–471, 1993.

228. Takano, H., and Glantz, S. A.: Left ventricular contractility predicts how the end-diastolic pressure-volume relation shifts during pacing-induced ischemia in dogs. Circulation 91:2423–2434, 1995.

229. King, L. M., Boucher, F., and Opie, L. H.: Coronary flow rate and glucose delivery as determinants of contracture in the ischaemic myocardium. J. Mol. Cell Cardiol. 27:701–720, 1995.

230. Cross, H. R., Radda, G. K., and Clarke, K.: The role of Na+/K+ ATPase activity during low flow ischemia in preventing myocardial injury: A 31P, 23Na and 87Rb NMR spectroscopic study. Mag. Res. Med. in press.

231. Owen, P., Dennis, S., and Opie, L. H.: Glucose flux rate regulates onset of ischemic contracture in globally underperfused rat hearts. Circ. Res. 66:344–354, 1990.

232. Murry, C. E., Jennings, R. B., and Reimer, K. A.: Preconditioning with ischemia: A delay of lethal cell injury in ischemic myocardium. Circulation 74:1124–1136, 1986.

233. Schott, R. J., Rohmann, S., Braun, E. R., and Schaper, W.: Ischemic preconditioning reduces infarct size in swine myocardium. Circ. Res. 66:1133–1142, 1990.

234. Thornton, J. D., Liu, G. S., and Downey, J. M.: Pretreatment with pertussis toxin blocks the protective effects of preconditioning: Evidence for a G-protein mechanism. J. Mol. Cell Cardiol. 25:311–320, 1993.

235. Ashraf, M., Suleiman, J., and Ahmad, M.: Ca2+ preconditioning elicits a unique protection against the Ca2+ paradox injury in rat heart. Role of adenosine. Circ. Res. 74:360–367, 1994.

236. Niroomand, F., Weinbrenner, C., Weis, A., et al.: Impaired function of inhibitory G proteins during acute myocardial ischemia of canine hearts and its reversal during reperfusion and a second period of ischemia. Possible implications for the protective mechanism of ischemic preconditioning. Circ. Res. 76:861–870, 1995.

237. Ytrehus, K., Liu, Y., and Downey, J.: Preconditioning protects ischemic rabbit heart by protein kinase C activation. Am. J. Physiol. 266:H1145–H1152, 1994.

238. Ottani, F., Galvani, M., Ferrini, D., et al.: Prodromal angina limits infarct size. A role for ischemic preconditioning. Circulation 91:291–297, 1995.

239. Kloner, R. A., Shook, T., Przyklenk, K., and TIMI-4 Investigators: Previous angina alters in-hospital outcome in TIMI-4. A clinical correlate to preconditioning? Circulation 91:37–45, 1995.

240. Cohen, M. V., Yang, X.-M., and Downey, J. M.: Conscious rabbits become tolerant to multiple episodes of ischemic preconditioning. Circ. Res. 74:998–1004, 1994.

241. Rahimtoola, S. H.: The hibernating myocardium. Am. Heart J. 117:211–221, 1989.

242. Maes, A., Flameng, W., Nuyts, J., et al.: Histological alterations in chronically hypoperfused myocardium. Correlation with PET findings. Circulation 90:735–745, 1994.

243. vom Dahl, J., Eitzman, D. T., Al-Aouar, Z. R., et al.: Relation of regional function, perfusion, and metabolism in patients with advanced coronary artery disease undergoing surgical revascularization. Circulation 90:2356–2366, 1994.

244. Vanoverschelde, J.-L., Wijns, W., Depre, C., et al.: Mechanisms of chronic regional post-ischemic dysfunction in humans. New insights from the study of noninfarcted collateral-dependent myocardium. Circulation 87:1513–1523, 1993.

245. Shen, Y.-T., and Vatner, S. F.: Mechanism of impaired myocardial function during progressive coronary stenosis in conscious pigs. Hibernation versus stunning? Circ. Res. 76:479–488, 1995.

246. Heyndrickx, G. R., Baig, H., Nellens, P., et al.: Depression of regional blood flow and wall thickening after brief coronary occlusions. Am. J. Physiol. 234:H653–H659, 1978.

247. Braunwald, E., and Kloner, R. A.: The stunned myocardium: Prolonged, postischemic ventricular dysfunction. Circulation 66:1146–1149, 1982.

248. Bolli, R., Hartley, C. J., and Rabinovitz, R. S.: Clinical relevance of myocardial "stunning." In Opie, L. H. (ed.): Stunning, Hibernation, and Calcium in Myocardial Ischemia and Reperfusion. Boston, Kluwer Academic Publishers, 1992, pp. 56–82.

249. Opie, L. H.: Reperfusion injury and its pharmacological modification. Circulation 80:1049–1062, 1989.

250. Kusuoka, H., and Marban, E.: Cellular mechanism of myocardial stunning. Annu. Rev. Physiol. 54:243–256, 1992.

251. Gao, W. D., Atar, D., Backx, P. H., and Marban, E.: Relationship between intracellular calcium and contractile force in stunned myocardium. Direct evidence for decreased myofilament Ca2+ responsiveness and altered diastolic function in intact ventricular muscle. Circ. Res. 76:1036–1048, 1995.

252. Hearse, D. J.: Stunning: A radical re-view. Cardiovasc. Drugs Ther. 5:853–876, 1991.

253. Lee, J. A., and Allen, D. G.: Mechanisms of acute ischemic contractile failure of the heart. Role of the intracellular calcium. J. Clin. Invest. 88:361–367, 1991.

254. Du Toit, E. F., and Opie, L. H.: Modulation of severity of reperfusion stunning in the isolated rat heart by agents altering calcium flux at onset of reperfusion. Circ. Res. 70:960–967, 1992.

255. Du Toit, E. F., and Opie, L. H.: Role for the Na+/H+ exchanger in reperfusion stunning in isolated perfused rat heart. J. Cardiovasc. Pharmacol. 22:877–883, 1993.

256. Smart, S., Schultz, J., Sagar, K., and Warltier, D.: Intracoronary doxorubicin, but not intracoronary verapamil, improves recovery of postischemic function. J. Am. Coll. Cardiol. 21(Abs.):164A, 1993.

257. Matsuura, H., and Shattock, M. J.: Membrane potential fluctuations and transient inward currents induced by reactive oxygen intermediates in isolated rabbit ventricular cells. Circ. Res. 68:319–329, 1991.

258. Jabr, R. I., and Cole, W. C.: Alterations in electrical activity and membrane currents induced by intracellular oxygen-derived free radical stress in guinea pig ventricular myocytes. Circ. Res. 72:1229–1244, 1993.

259. Kusuoka, H., Camilion de Hurtado, M. C., and Marban, E.: Role of sodium-calcium exchange in the mechanism of myocardial stunning: Protective effect of reperfusion with high sodium solution. J. Am. Coll. Cardiol. 21:240–248, 1993.

260. Brunner, F., Du Toit, E. F., and Opie, L. H.: Endothelin release during ischaemia and reperfusion of isolated perfused rat hearts. J. Mol. Cell Cardiol. 24:1291–1305, 1993.

261. Mouton, R., Genade, S., Huisamen, B., et al.: The effect of ischaemia-reperfusion on [3H]inositol phosphates and Ins(1,4,5)P3 levels in cardiac atria and ventricles—a comparative study. Mol. Cell Biochem. 115:195–202, 1992.

262. Du Toit, E. F., and Opie, L. H.: Antiarrhythmic properties of specific inhibitors of sarcoplasmic reticulum calcium ATPase in the isolated perfused rat heart after coronary artery litigation. J. Am. Coll. Cardiol. 23:1505–1510, 1994.

263. Opie, L. H.: Chronic stunning: The new switch in thought. Invited Comment. Basic Res. Cardiol. 90:303–304, 1995.

264. Sadoshima, J., Qiu, Z., Morgan, J. P., and Izumo, S.: Angiotensin-II and other hypertrophic stimuli mediated by G protein–coupled receptors activate tyrosine kinase, mitogen-activated protein kinase, and 90-kD S6 kinase in cardiac myocytes. The critical role of Ca2+-dependent signaling. Circ. Res. 76:1–15, 1995.

265. Edwards, G., and Weston, A. H.: Pharmacology of the potassium channel openers. Cardiovasc. Drugs Ther. 9:185–193, 1995.

266. Opie, L. H.: Stunning, Hibernation, and Calcium in Myocardial Ischemia and Reperfusion. Boston, Kluwer Academic Publishers, 1992.

Chapter 13
Pathophysiology of Heart Failure

WILSON S. COLUCCI, EUGENE BRAUNWALD

Heart (or cardiac) failure is the pathophysiological state in which the heart is unable to pump blood at a rate commensurate with the requirements of the metabolizing tissues or can do so only from an elevated filling pressure. It is usually, but not always, caused by a defect in myocardial contraction, i.e., by *myocardial failure.* However, in some patients with heart failure, a similar clinical syndrome is present, but there is no detectable abnormality of *myocardial* function. In many such cases heart failure is caused by conditions in which the normal heart is suddenly presented with a load that exceeds its capacity or in which ventricular filling is impaired.[1] *Heart failure* should be distinguished from *circulatory failure,* in which an abnormality of some component of the circulation—the heart, the blood volume, the concentration of oxygenated hemoglobin in the arterial blood, or the vascular bed—is responsible for the inadequate cardiac output.

Thus, the terms myocardial failure, heart failure, and circulatory failure are not synonymous, but refer to progressively more inclusive entities. Myocardial failure, when sufficiently severe, always causes heart failure, but the converse is not necessarily the case, because a number of conditions in which the heart is suddenly overloaded (e.g., acute aortic regurgitation secondary to acute infective endocarditis) can cause heart failure in the presence of normal myocardial function, at least early in the course of the illness. Also, conditions such as tricuspid stenosis and constrictive pericarditis, which interfere with cardiac filling, can cause heart failure without myocardial failure. Heart failure, in turn, always causes circulatory failure, but again the converse is not necessarily the case, because a variety of noncardiac conditions, e.g., hypovolemic shock, can produce circulatory failure at a time when cardiac function is normal or only modestly impaired.

The hemodynamic, contractile, and wall motion disorders in heart failure are discussed in the chapters on echocardiography (Chap. 3), cardiac catheterization (Chap. 6), radionuclide imaging (Chap. 9), and assessment of cardiac function (Chap. 14). In this chapter, the focus is on the physiological, neurohumoral, biochemical, and cellular changes characteristic of heart failure.

ADAPTIVE MECHANISMS

In the presence of a primary disturbance in myocardial contractility or an excessive hemodynamic burden placed on the ventricle, or both, the heart depends on a number of adaptive mechanisms for maintenance of its pumping function[2,3] (Table 13–1). Most important among these are (1)

the Frank-Starling mechanism, in which an increased preload helps to sustain cardiac performance (see p. 378); (2) myocardial hypertrophy with or without cardiac chamber dilatation, in which the mass of contractile tissue is augmented (see p. 399); and (3) activation of neurohumoral systems, especially the release of the neurotransmitter norepinephrine (NE) by adrenergic cardiac nerves (see p. 408), which augments myocardial contractility and the activation of the renin-angiotensin-aldosterone system (see p. 446), and other neurohumoral adjustments (see p. 414) that act to maintain arterial pressure and perfusion of vital organs. In acute heart failure, these adaptive mechanisms may be adequate to maintain the overall pumping performance of the heart at relatively normal levels. However, the capacity of each of these mechanisms to sustain cardiac performance in the face of hemodynamic overload relative to myocardial contractility is finite and, when chronically maintained, becomes maladaptive (Fig. 13–1).

Cardiac output is often depressed and the arterial–mixed venous oxygen difference is widened in the basal state in patients with the common forms of heart failure secondary to ischemic heart disease, hypertension, primary myocardial disease, valvular disease, and pericardial disease (so-called low-output heart failure).[4,5] In cases of mild heart failure, the cardiac output may be normal at rest but fails to rise normally during exercise (see p. 451).[5] When the volume of blood delivered into the systemic arterial bed is chronically reduced, and/or when one or both ventricles has an elevated filling pressure, a complex sequence of adjustments occurs that ultimately results in the retention of sodium and water in the intravascular and interstitial compartments (see Chap. 62).[6] Many of the clinical manifestations of heart failure such as dyspnea and edema are secondary to this excessive retention of fluid (see Chap. 15).

Interactions Between Frank-Starling Mechanism and Adrenergic Nervous System in Heart Failure

It may be useful to consider the function of the normal and failing heart within the framework of the Frank-Starling mechanism, in which an increase in preload, reflected in an elevation of end-diastolic volume, augments ventricular performance. The normal relationship between ventricular end-diastolic volume and performance is shown in Figure 13–2, curve 1. During exercise and other stresses, the increases in adrenergic nerve impulses to the myocardium, the concentration of circulating catecholamines (see p. 374), and tachycardia all augment myocardial contractil-

TABLE 13-1 SHORT-TERM AND LONG-TERM RESPONSES TO IMPAIRED CARDIAC PERFORMANCE

RESPONSE	SHORT-TERM EFFECTS*	LONG-TERM EFFECTS†
Salt and water retention	Augments preload	Causes pulmonary congestion, anasarca
Vasoconstriction	Maintains blood pressure for perfusion of vital organs (brain, heart)	Exacerbates pump dysfunction (afterload mismatch); increases cardiac energy expenditure
Sympathetic stimulation	Increases heart rate and ejection	Increases energy expenditure
Sympathetic desensitization	—	Spares energy
Hypertrophy	Unloads individual muscle fibers	Leads to deterioration and death of cardiac cells; cardiomyopathy of overload
Capillary deficit	—	Leads to energy starvation
Mitochondrial density	Increase in density helps meet energy demands	Decrease in density leads to energy starvation
Appearance of slow myosin	—	Increases force, decreases shortening velocity and contractility; is energy-sparing
Prolonged action potential	—	Increases contractility and energy expenditure
Decreased density of sarcoplasmic reticulum calcium-pump sites	—	Slows relaxation; may be energy-sparing
Increased collagen	May reduce dilatation	Impairs relaxation

* Short-term effects are mainly adaptive and occur after hemorrhage and in acute heart failure.

† Long-term effects are mainly deleterious and occur in chronic heart failure.

Reprinted by permission from Katz, A. M.: Cardiomyopathy of overload: A major determinant of prognosis in congestive heart failure. N. Engl. J. Med. *322*:100, 1990. Copyright Massachuetts Medical Society.

ity with a shift from curve 1 to curve 2. Ventricular performance, as reflected in stroke work or cardiac output, increases with little change in end-diastolic pressure and volume. This is represented by a shift from point A to point B in Figure 13-2. Vasodilation occurs in the exercising muscles, reducing peripheral vascular resistance and aortic impedance. This ultimately allows achievement of a greatly elevated cardiac output during exercise, at an arterial pressure only slightly greater than in the resting state. During intense exercise, cardiac output can rise to a maximal level if use is made of the Frank-Starling mechanism, as reflected in modest increases in the left ventricular end-diastolic volume and pressure (point B to point C).

In moderately severe systolic heart failure, as represented by curve 3, cardiac output and external ventricular performance at rest are within normal limits but are maintained at these levels only because the end-diastolic fiber

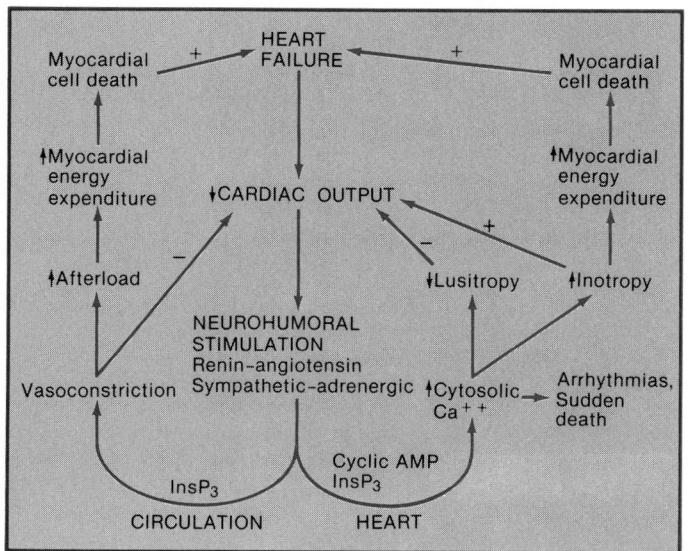

FIGURE 13-1. The low-output state can accelerate the rate of cell death in the failing heart by stimulating the renin-angiotensin and sympathetic-adrenergic systems, which act on both the circulation and the heart. Vasoconstriction increases afterload, which further decreases cardiac output; the increased afterload may also accelerate the rate of myocardial cell death by increasing the work of the heart. In the heart, increased concentrations of cyclic AMP and inositol-1,4,5-tris phosphate ($InsP_3$) promote calcium entry, augmenting contractility; along with a chronotropic response (not shown), this inotropic response increases cardiac output and is thus compensatory. However, the increased amount of calcium that enters the cytosol can overload the systems that pump this ion out of the cell during diastole, thus impairing relaxation. Calcium overload may also induce arrhythmias and lead to sudden death. Because the inotropic and chronotropic responses to sympathetic-adrenergic stimulation increase myocardial energy expenditure, they may also accelerate the rate of cell death in the failing heart. Thus, when the initial adaptive responses of both the circulation and the heart to a chronic low-output state become sustained, they can have deleterious long-term effects in patients with congestive heart failure. (Reprinted with permission from Katz, A. M.: Cardiomyopathy of overload: A major determinant of prognosis in congestive heart failure. N. Engl. J. Med. *322*:100, 1990. Copyright Massachuetts Medical Society.)

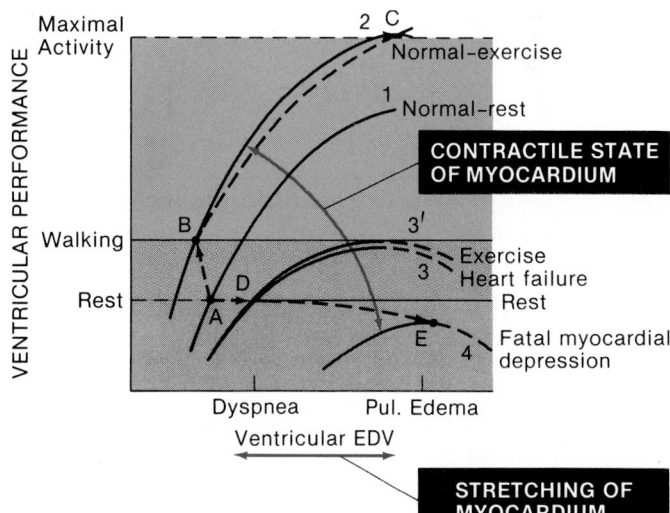

FIGURE 13-2. Diagram showing the interrelationship of influences on ventricular end-diastolic volume (EDV) through stretching of the myocardium and the contractile state of the myocardium. Levels of ventricular EDV associated with filling pressures that result in dyspnea and pulmonary edema are shown on the abscissa. Levels of ventricular performance required during rest, walking, and maximal activity are designated on the ordinate. The dotted lines are the descending limbs of the ventricular performance curves, which are rarely seen during life but which show what the level of ventricular performance would be if end-diastolic volume could be elevated to very high levels. (Modified from Braunwald, E., Ross, J., Jr., and Sonnenblick, E. H.: Mechanisms of Contraction of the Normal and Failing Heart. Boston, Little, Brown and Co., 1968.)

length and the ventricular end-diastolic volume (ventricular preload) are elevated, i.e., through the operation of the Frank-Starling mechanism. The elevations of left ventricular diastolic pressure are associated with abnormally high levels of pulmonary capillary pressure, contributing to the dyspnea experienced by patients with heart failure, sometimes even at rest (point D).

Heart failure is frequently accompanied by reductions in NE stores and myocardial beta-adrenoceptor density (see p. 410) and therefore in the inotropic response to impulses in the cardiac adrenergic nerves. As a consequence, ventricular function (performance) curves cannot be elevated to normal levels by the adrenergic nervous system, and the normal improvement of contractility that takes places during exercise is attenuated (curves 3 and 3'). The factors that tend to augment ventricular filling during exercise push the failing ventricle even farther along its flattened, depressed function curve, and there is an inordinate elevation of ventricular end-diastolic volume and pressure and therefore of pulmonary capillary pressure.[7] The elevation of the latter intensifies dyspnea and plays an important role in limit-

ing the intensity of exercise that the patient can perform. According to this formulation, left ventricular failure becomes fatal when the left ventricular function curve becomes depressed (curve 4) to the point at which either cardiac output is insufficient to satisfy the requirements of the peripheral tissue at rest or the left ventricular end-diastolic and pulmonary capillary pressures are elevated to levels that result in pulmonary edema, or both (point E).

REDISTRIBUTION OF LEFT VENTRICULAR OUTPUT. Heart failure is characterized by generalized adrenergic activation (see p. 412) and parasympathetic withdrawal[8] (see p. 413), as illustrated in Figure 13–3. This leads to tachycardia, sodium retention, renin release, and generalized systemic vasoconstriction. Maintenance of arterial pressure in the presence of a reduced cardiac output is a primitive but effective compensatory mechanism. In hypovolemia and heart failure, this important mechanism is brought into play in order to allow the limited cardiac output to be most useful for survival. Vasoconstriction, mediated in part by the adrenergic nervous system, plays an important role in

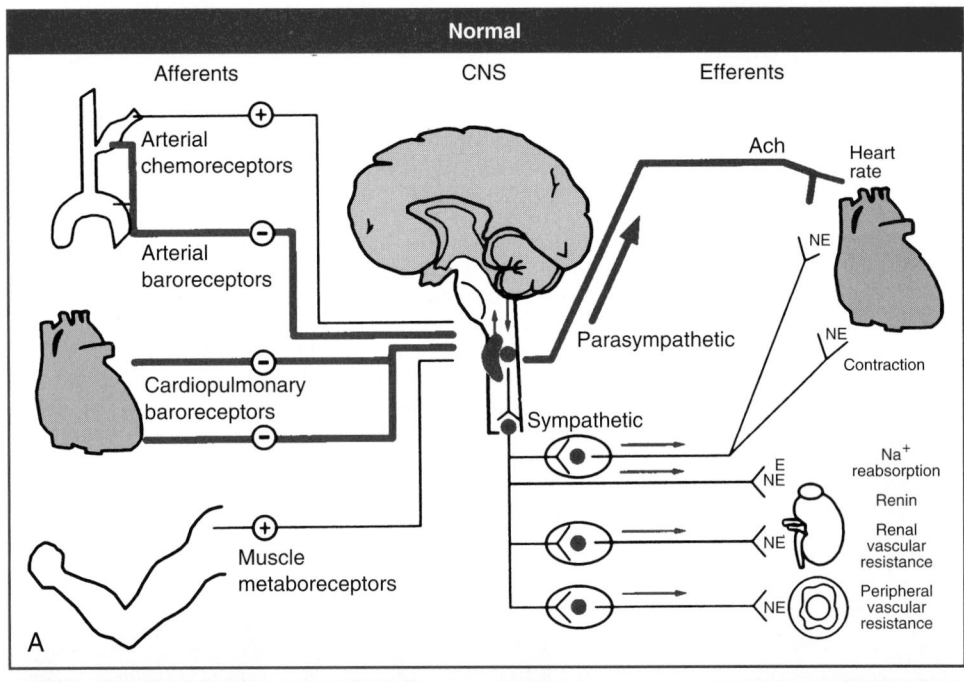

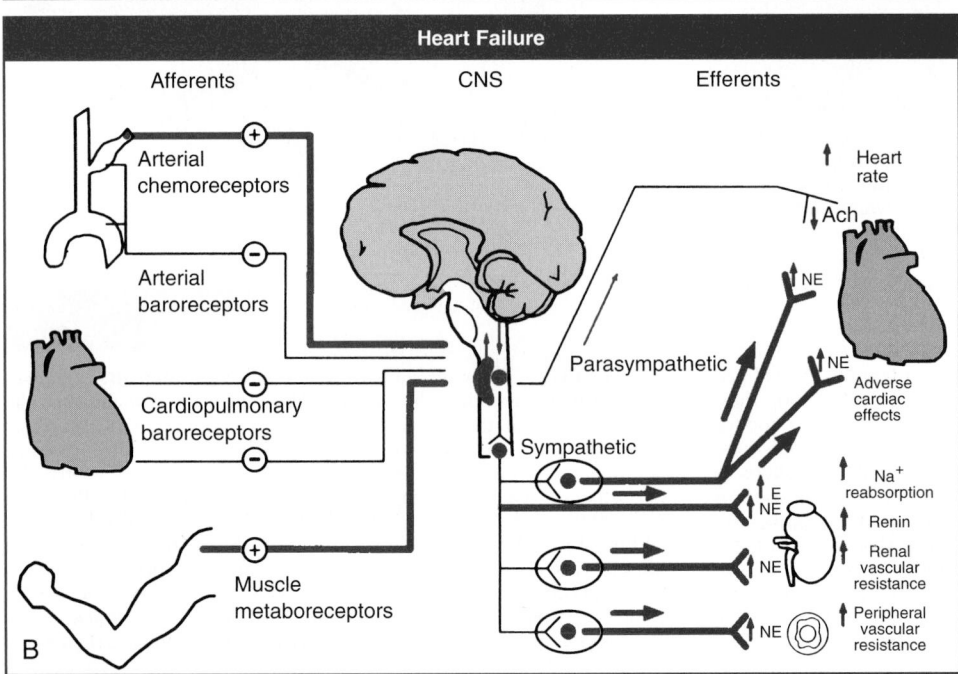

FIGURE 13–3. Mechanisms for generalized sympathetic activation and parasympathetic withdrawal in heart failure. *A,* Under normal conditions, inhibitory (−) inputs from arterial and cardiopulmonary baroreceptor afferent nerves are the principal influence on sympathetic outflow. Parasympathetic control of heart rate is also under potent arterial baroreflex control. Efferent sympathetic traffic and arterial catecholamines are low and heart rate variability high. *B,* As heart failure progresses, inhibitory input from arterial and cardiopulmonary receptors decreases and excitatory (+) input increases. The net response to this altered balance includes a generalized increase in sympathetic nerve traffic, blunted parasympathetic and sympathetic control of heart rate, and impairment of the reflex sympathetic regulation of vascular resistance. Anterior wall ischemia has additional excitatory effects on efferent sympathetic nerve traffic. See text for details. Ach = acetylcholine; CNS = central nervous system; E = epinephrine; Na$^+$ = sodium; NE = norepinephrine. (From Floras, J. S.: Clinical aspects of sympathetic activation and parasympathetic withdrawal in heart failure. Reprinted with permission from the American College of Cardiology. J. Am. Coll. Cardiol. *22:*72A, 1993.)

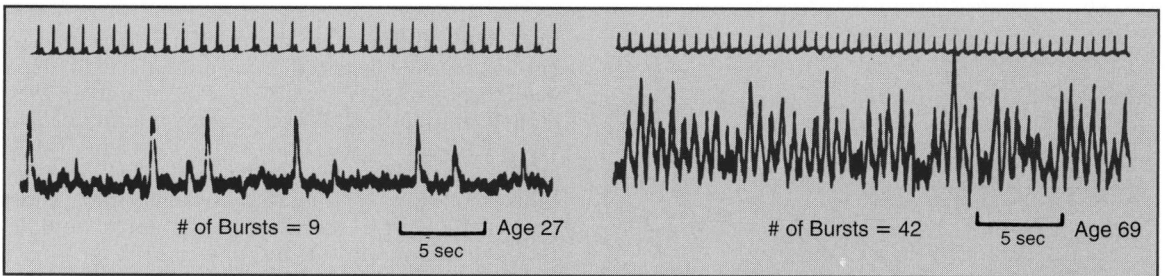

FIGURE 13–4. Representative tracings of the electrocardiograms *(upper tracings)* and mean voltage neuro-grams of muscle sympathetic nerve activity *(lower tracings)* in a normal subject *(left)* and a patient with heart failure *(right)*. (Reproduced by permission from Leimbach, W. N., Walling, B. G., Victor, R. G., et al.: Direct evidence from intraneural recordings for increased central sympathetic outflow in patients with heart failure. Circulation 73:913, 1986. Copyright 1986 American Heart Association.)

this redistribution of peripheral blood flow. Neurograms obtained from adrenergic nerves to the limbs display an increased traffic in heart failure (Fig. 13–4).[9] In patients with moderately severe heart failure, in whom the cardiac output at rest is normal, abnormal vasoconstriction occurs when an additional burden (such as exercise, fever, or anemia) is imposed on the circulation and the cardiac output does not rise normally to meet the peripheral demands. As cardiac performance declines, left ventricular output is ultimately redistributed, even at rest.[10–13] This redistribution maintains the delivery of oxygen to vital organs such as the brain and heart, while blood flow to less crucial areas, such as the skin, skeletal muscle, and kidney, is reduced.[14,15] This underperfusion of skeletal muscle leads to anaerobic metabolism,[16] lactic acidosis, an excess oxygen debt, weakness, and fatigue. Occasionally, serious complications can result from the redistribution of cardiac output and the resulting regional reductions of blood flow. These include marked sodium and nitrogen retention as a consequence of diminished renal perfusion (see Chap. 62) and, very rarely, gangrene of the tips of the phalanges and mesenteric infarction.

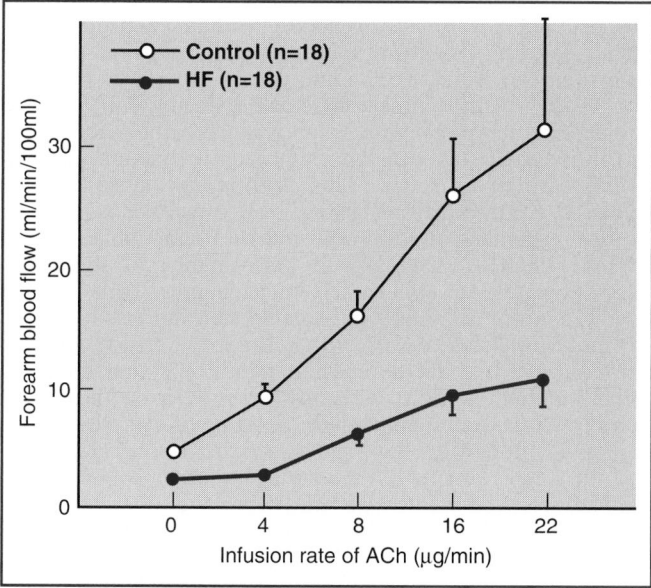

FIGURE 13–5. Responses of forearm blood flow (FBF) to acetylcholine in patients with heart failure (HF) (●) and in control subjects (○). The FBF at rest and during infusion of acetylcholine (ACh) was less in patients with heart failure than in control subjects. The magnitudes of the increases in FBF in response to ACh were less in patients with heart failure than in control subjects. In contrast, the responses to sodium nitroprusside were comparable. (Reproduced by permission from Hirooka, Y., Imaizumi, T., Tagawa, T., et al.: Effects of L-arginine on impaired acetylcholine-induced and ischemic vasodilation of the forearm in patients with heart failure. Circulation 90:658, 1994. Copyright 1994 American Heart Association.)

ENDOTHELIAL DYSFUNCTION. Both ischemia and exercise-induced vasodilation in the extremities are attenuated in patients with heart failure.[17] This attenuation is related in part to endothelial dysfunction (see p. 1166). The response of blood flow to infused acetylcholine and methacholine, endothelium-dependent vasodilators, is reduced in heart failure (Fig. 13–5). The vasodilator response can be restored by the administration of L-arginine, a precursor of endothelium-derived nitric oxide.[18,19] These findings suggest that defective endothelial function contributes to the impaired vasodilator capacity in heart failure. The mechanisms potentially responsible include impaired endothelial cell receptor function, deficiency of L-arginine substrate, abnormal expression of nitric oxide synthase, and the impaired release or rapid degradation of the endothelium-derived relaxing factor, nitric oxide.[19] In addition to abnormalities in endothelial vasodilator function, the release by the endothelium of the vasoconstrictor endothelin is augmented (see p. 415).

CHANGES IN THE VASCULAR WALL. The sodium content of the vascular wall is increased in heart failure, and this contributes to the stiffening, thickening, and compression of blood vessel walls, which raises vascular resistance and also prevents normal vasodilation during exercise.[12] The veins in the extremities of patients with heart failure are also constricted by the activity of the adrenergic nervous system as well as by circulating venoconstrictors (norepinephrine and angiotensin II). This venoconstriction results in displacement of blood to the heart and lungs.

2,3-DIPHOSPHOGLYCERATE. A progressive decline in the affinity of hemoglobin for oxygen due to an increase in 2,3-diphosphoglycerate (DPG) also occurs in heart failure.[20] The rightward shift in the oxygen-hemoglobin dissociation curve represents a compensatory mechanism that facilitates oxygen transport; the increased DPG, tissue acidosis, and the slowed circulation characteristic of heart failure act synergistically to maintain the delivery of oxygen to the metabolizing tissues in the face of a reduced cardiac output.

CONTRACTILITY OF HYPERTROPHIED AND FAILING MYOCARDIUM

When an excessive pressure or volume load is imposed on the ventricle, myocardial hypertrophy develops, providing one of the aforementioned key compensatory mechanisms that permits the ventricle to sustain an increased load.[2,4,21] However, as described below, a ventricle subjected to an abnormally elevated load for a prolonged period may fail to maintain compensation despite the presence of ventricular hypertrophy, and pump failure may ultimately occur.

ISOLATED MUSCLE. Cardiac muscle isolated from animals in which the heart had been subjected to a controlled stress has been studied by many investigators. One convenient

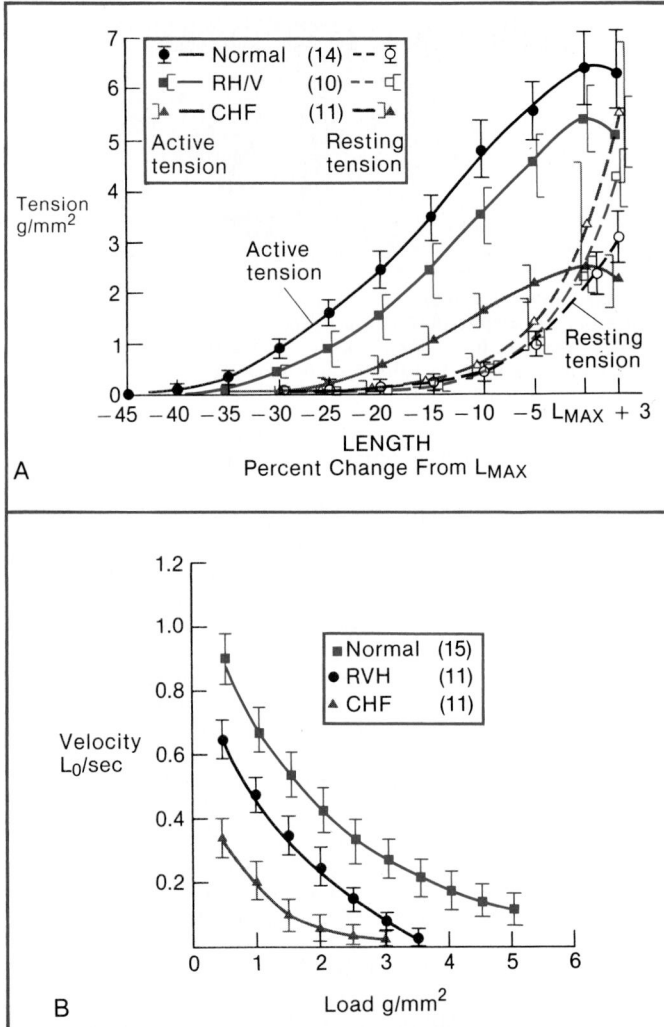

FIGURE 13–6. *A,* Relation between muscle length and tension of papillary muscles from normal (circles), hypertrophied (squares), and failing (triangles) right ventricles. Open symbols = resting tension; filled symbols = actively developed tension. Tension is corrected for cross-sectional area (g/mm²). Numbers in parentheses = number of animals. *B,* Force-velocity relations of the three groups of cat papillary muscles. Average values ± SEM are given for each point. Velocity has been corrected to muscle lengths per second (L_0/sec). (Reproduced by permission from Spann, J. F., Jr., Buccino, R. A., Sonnenblick, E. H., and Braunwald, E.: Contractile state of cardiac muscle obtained from cats with experimentally produced ventricular hypertrophy and heart failure. Circ. Res. *21:*341, 1967. Copyright 1967 American Heart Association.)

experimental model of ventricular pressure overload is the cat (or ferret) with pulmonary artery constriction. Papillary muscles are then removed from the right ventricles in which either hypertrophy or overt failure has developed, and the excised muscles are studied in vitro.[22,23] Both right ventricular hypertrophy and failure reduce the maximum velocity of (unloaded) shortening ($\dot{V}_{max}$) of excised muscle below the values observed in muscles obtained from normal cats. These changes are more marked in animals in which heart failure has been present than in those with hypertrophy alone (Fig. 13–6). Because the depression of myocardial contractility is evident in vitro, when the muscle's physical and chemical milieu is controlled, it is considered to be *intrinsic,* and not the result of any humoral or neural stimuli or abnormal loading conditions that are often present in vivo. The depression of contractility in hypertrophied myocardium is less marked or even absent when the stress is imposed slowly and when the measurements are made during a stable phase of the ventricular response to overload.[24]

The findings summarized above are, in general, consonant with those of a number of other investigations on cardiac muscle isolated from animals with experimentally produced pressure overload. For example, the trabeculae carnae or papillary muscles removed from the left ventricles of rats with left ventricular hypertrophy secondary to aortic constriction or renovascular hypertension also exhibit depression of the velocity of isotonic shortening and prolongation of duration of the action potential, of isometric contraction, and of the time-to-peak tension, even when the development of isometric tension is normal.[25] The force and rate of force development are also depressed in isometrically contracting myocardium obtained from hearts with totally different forms of heart failure (e.g., Syrian hamsters with hereditary cardiomyopathy), as well as papillary muscles removed from the left ventricles of patients with heart failure due to chronic valvular disease.[26] In contrast to the depressed performance of cardiac muscle removed from pressure-overloaded hearts, contractility has been found to be normal in papillary muscles removed from cats with a volume overload resulting from an experimentally produced atrial septal defect.[27]

In nonfailing myocardium, the force of contraction and rate of tension development rise with increased stimulation frequency, the so-called *positive force-frequency relationship* (Fig. 12–28, p. 380). However, there is evidence of an abnormal (negative) force-frequency relationship in failing human myocardium.[28] Gwathmey et al. showed in myocardium obtained from failing human hearts that pacing-induced tachycardia results in calcium accumulation.[29] These observations provide a potential explanation for the further deterioration of cardiac function that occurs with tachycardia in patients with heart failure and possibly for the beneficial effects of slowing the heart rate with beta blockade (see p. 486) or digitalis.

Structural Changes. There are a number of structural features of hypertrophied human myocytes (Fig. 13–7).[30] These include abnormal Z-band patterns, multiple intercalated discs, and prominent collagen fibrils connecting adjacent myocardial cells. Nuclei are enlarged and lobulated and contain well-developed nucleoli; there is an abundance of ribosomes, presumably reflecting enhanced protein synthesis. However, electron microscopic studies of myocardium removed from overloaded, dilated hearts fixed at the elevated filling pressures that existed during life have revealed sarcomere lengths averaging 2.2 µm—no longer than those at the apex of the length/active tension curve of normal cardiac muscle.[31] This finding indicates that the depressed contractility of failing heart muscle is *not* due to the disengagement of actin and myosin filaments.

INTACT HEARTS. Changes in performance of the intact heart subjected to abnormal hemodynamic loads are, in general, similar to those in isolated cardiac tissue. Thus, the right ventricles of cats with pulmonary artery constriction exhibit a marked depression paralleling that observed in the isolated papillary muscles removed from these ventricles.[32] When compared with normal values, the active tension developed by the right ventricle at equivalent end-diastolic fiber lengths is markedly reduced in cats with heart failure produced by pressure overload.

Immediately following the imposition of a volume overload (such as the opening of a large arteriovenous fistula), the contractility of the ventricle—as reflected in the end-systolic stress-circumference relationship—may actually increase, perhaps as a consequence of adrenergic stimulation. However, it then declines, while overall hemodynamic performance, i.e., cardiac work, is sustained.[33] Later in the course of a large volume overload, overt clinical heart failure develops, accompanied by increases in left ventricular end-diastolic volume and in the ratio of left ventricular weight to body weight and by depressed indices of left ventricular contractility[34,35] (see Chap. 14). As the ventricle fails, it moves to the right along a depressed performance (function) curve, so that it requires an abnormally elevated end-diastolic volume (and often an elevation of end-diastolic pressure as well) to generate a level of tension equal to that achieved by the normal heart at a normal end-diastolic volume (Fig. 13–1).

MYOCARDIAL HYPERTROPHY

PATTERNS OF VENTRICULAR HYPERTROPHY. The development of ventricular hypertrophy constitutes one of the principal mechanisms by which the heart compensates for an increased load.[36] One of the early cellular changes that occurs after a stimulus for hypertrophy is applied is the synthesis of mitochondria; presumably the expanded mitochondrial mass provides the high-energy phosphates required to meet the increased energy demands of the hypertrophied cell. This is accompanied by an expansion of the myofibrillar mass (Fig. 13–7). Myocytes isolated from patients with heart failure are longer than normal myocytes[37,38] (Fig. 13–8). After the neonatal period, the increase in myocardial mass is associated with a proportional increase in the size of individual cells, i.e., hypertrophy, without any increase in the number of cells (or a minimal increase), i.e., without hyperplasia.[2] These changes within the myocyte are accompanied by the laying down of interstitial collagen.[39]

There is evidence that hemodynamic overload reactivates growth factors present in the embryonic heart but dormant in the normal adult heart (Fig. 13–9). These reactivated growth factors accelerate protein synthesis.[3] Current understanding of the fundamental mechanisms responsible for hypertrophy is described on pages 747 to 748.

Grossman et al. examined systolic and diastolic wall stresses in normal subjects and in patients with chronic pressure- and volume-overloaded left ventricles who were compensated and not in heart failure.[40] Left ventricular mass was increased approximately equally in both the pressure- and volume-overloaded groups. There was a substantial increase in wall thickness in the pressure-overloaded ventricles but only a mild increase in wall thickness in the volume-overloaded ventricles (Fig. 13–10). The latter was just sufficient to counterbalance the increased radius, so that the ratio of wall thickness to radius remained normal for the patients with volume-overload hypertrophy. This ratio was substantially increased in patients with pressure-overload hypertrophy, in whom there was disproportionate thickening of the ventricular wall. These observations are consistent with those of other investigators, who have indicated that myocardial hypertrophy develops in a manner that maintains systolic stress within normal limits.[41–43] Thus, when the primary stimulus to hypertrophy is pressure overload, the resultant acute increase in systolic wall stress leads to parallel replication of myofibrils, thickening of individual myocytes,[44] and concentric hypertrophy. The wall thickening is usually sufficient to maintain a normal level of systolic stress (Fig. 13–11). When the primary stimulus is ventricular volume overload, increased diastolic wall stress leads to replication of sarcomeres in series, elongation of myocytes, and ventricular dilatation. This, in turn, results in a modest increase in systolic stress[45] (by the Laplace relationship), which causes proportional wall thickening that returns systolic stress toward normal. Thus, in compensated subjects, both volume and pressure overload alter ventricular geometry and wall thickness, so that systolic stress does not change greatly.

Left ventricular wall thickness is a crucial determinant of ventricular performance in patients with pressure-overload hypertrophy due to aortic stenosis or hypertension. Impaired performance in such patients may be secondary to inadequate hypertrophy leading to increased wall stress (afterload), which in turn may be responsible for inadequate

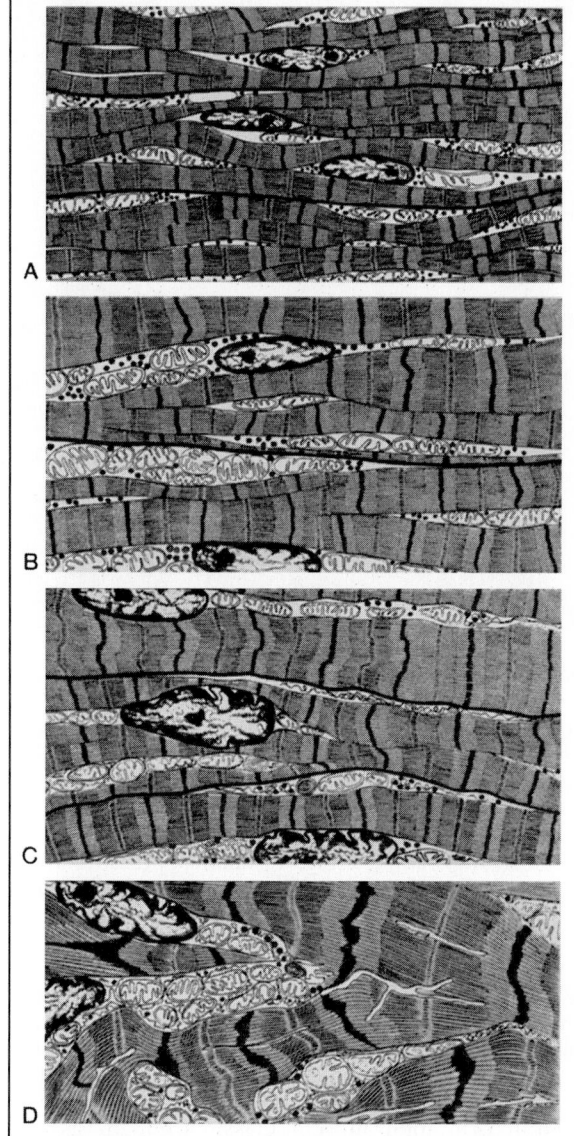

FIGURE 13–7. The early stage of cardiac hypertrophy *(A)* is characterized morphologically by increases in the number of myofibrils and mitochondria as well as enlargement of mitochondria and nuclei. Muscle cells are larger than normal, but cellular organization is largely preserved. At a more advanced stage of hypertrophy *(B)*, preferential increases in the size or number of specific organelles, such as mitochondria, as well as irregular addition of new contractile elements in localized areas of the cell, result in subtle abnormalities of cellular organization and contour. Adjacent cells may vary in their degree of enlargement. Cells subjected to longstanding hypertrophy *(C)* show more obvious disruptions in cellular organization, such as markedly enlarged nuclei with highly lobulated membranes, which displace adjacent myofibrils and cause breakdown of normal Z-band registration. The early preferential increase in mitochondria is supplanted by a predominance by volume of myofibrils. The late stage of hypertrophy *(D)* is characterized by loss of contractile elements with marked disruption of Z bands, severe disruption of the normal parallel arrangement of the sarcomeres, deposition of fibrous tissue, and dilation and increased tortuosity of T tubules. (From Ferrans, V. J.: Morphology of the heart in hypertrophy. Hosp. Pract. *18:*69, 1983. © 1983 The McGraw-Hill Companies, Inc.)

muscle shortening. This condition has been termed "afterload-mismatch" by Ross.[46] His group found that when the aorta in conscious dogs was suddenly constricted, left ventricular systolic pressure rose, the left ventricle dilated, and the left ventricular wall thinned; this was associated with a large increase in wall stress and a reciprocal reduction in the extent and velocity of shortening.[47] During the next few weeks the left ventricle became hypertrophied and left ventricular wall stress and shortening both returned toward

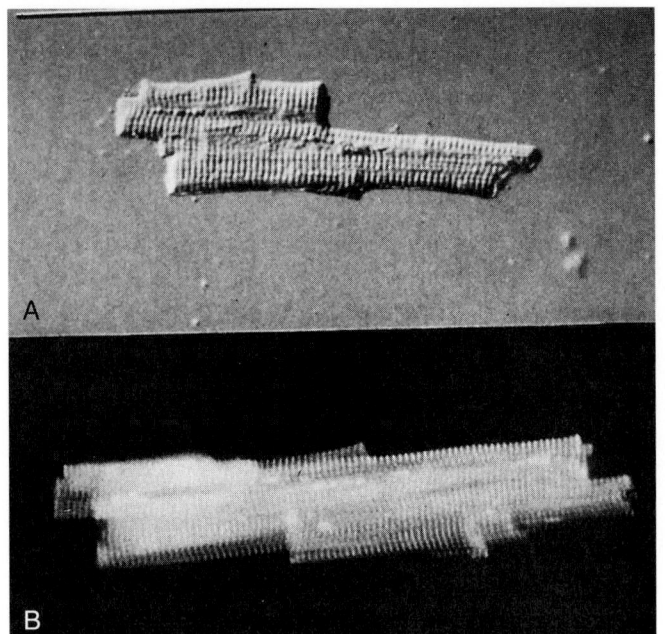

FIGURE 13–8. Isolated cardiac myocytes obtained from human left ventricular myocardium. *A,* Myocyte from a normal heart (bar = 100 μm). *B,* A hypertrophied myocyte from the left ventricle of a patient with ischemic cardiomyopathy, viewed at the same magnification as in *A.* This myocyte is longer than the normal myocyte. The myocytes have been stained with rhodamine-phalloidin for visualization of the sarcomere structure. In the myocyte from the failing heart, there has been addition of sarcomeres. These are otherwise organized in a normal pattern. (Modified by permission from Gerdes, A. M., et al.: Structural remodeling of cardiac myocytes in patients with ischemic cardiomyopathy. Circulation *86:*426, 1992. Copyright 1992 American Heart Association.)

normal. When the constriction was suddenly released, wall stress declined and shortening became supernormal.

Prolonged athletic training causes a moderate increase in myocardial mass.[48] Isotonic exercise, such as long-distance running or swimming, resembles volume overload and causes an increase in left ventricular diastolic volume, with only mild thickening of the wall. Isometric exercise, such as weightlifting or wrestling, resembles pressure overload and causes an increase in wall thickness. Neither form of hypertrophy appears to be deleterious in the absence of heart disease and rapidly disappears when training is discontinued.

DEVELOPMENT OF HEART FAILURE. When the ventricle is stressed, by either a pressure or a volume overload, the initial response is an increase in sarcomere length, so that the overlap between myofilaments becomes optimal, i.e., approximately 2.2 μm (see p. 360). This is followed by an increase in the total muscle mass, although, as already noted, the pattern of hypertrophy differs depending on whether the stress is a pressure load or a volume load (see p. 399).

When the hemodynamic overload is severe, myocardial contractility becomes depressed. In its mildest form, this depression is manifested by a reduction in the velocity of shortening of unloaded myocardium ($\dot{V}_{max}$) (Fig. 13–6) or by a reduction in the rate of force development during isometric contraction,[22] but by little if any reduction in the development of maximal isometric force or in the extent of shortening of afterloaded isotonic contractions. As myocardial contractility becomes further depressed, a more extensive reduction in $\dot{V}_{max}$ occurs, now accompanied by a decline in isometric force development and shortening. At this point, circulatory compensation may still be provided by cardiac dilation and an increase in muscle mass, which tend to maintain wall stress at normal levels. Although cardiac output and stroke volume remain normal in the

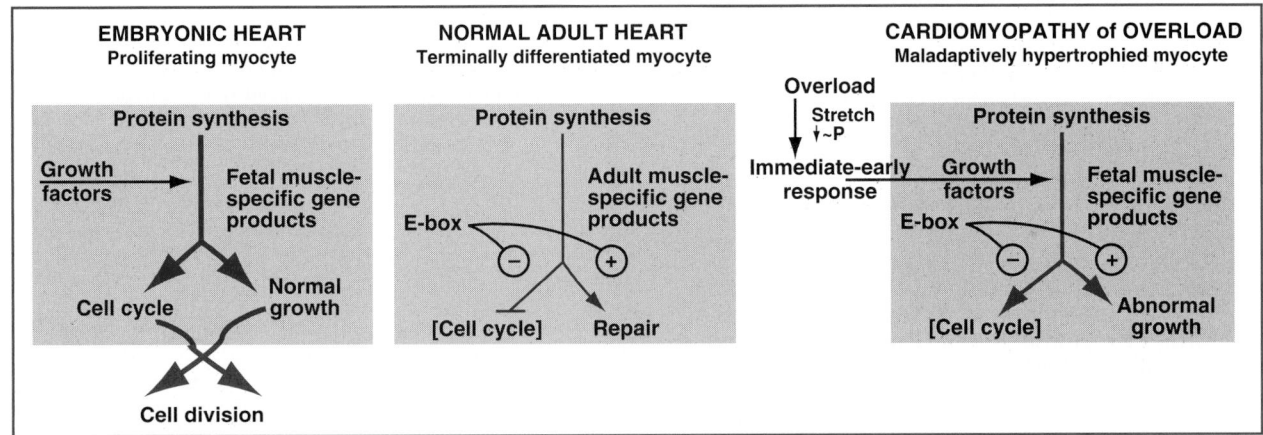

FIGURE 13–9. Overall growth pattern in the proliferating myocytes of the embryonic heart, the terminally differentiated myocytes of the normal adult heart, and the maladaptively hypertrophied myocytes of the failing heart. *Left,* In the embryonic heart, growth factors stimulate synthesis of fetal-specific gene products that, because protein synthesis is matched to active cell cycling, lead to normal cell division. *Center,* Withdrawal of growth factors and binding of myogenic factors to the E box (a DNA sequence found in muscle-specific genes) in the terminally differentiated cells of the normal adult heart slows protein synthesis, inhibits the cell cycle, and favors the synthesis of adult muscle-specific gene products. *Right,* Overloading of the adult heart initiates an immediate-early gene response that reactivates growth factor stimulation; this, in turn, accelerates protein synthesis and favors the expression of fetal muscle-specific gene products. However, because the cell cycle remains blocked, the overloaded heart undergoes an unnatural growth response which may lead to myocardial cell death. (From Katz, A. M.: The cardiomyopathy of overload: An unnatural growth response in the hypertrophied heart. Ann. Intern. Med. *121:*363, 1994.)

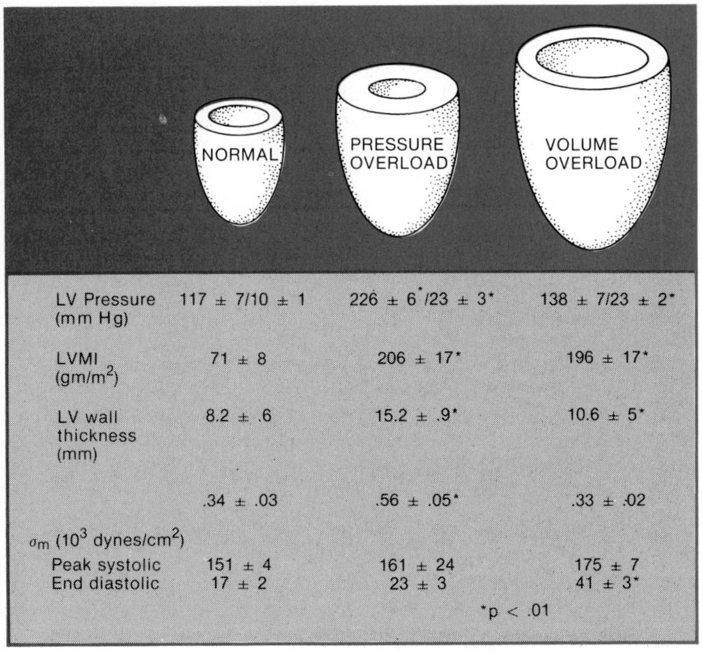

FIGURE 13–10. Mean values for left ventricular (LV) pressure, mass index (LVMI), left ventricular wall thickness, the ratio of wall thickness to radius (h/R), and peak systolic and end-diastolic meridional wall stress in patients with normal (6 subjects), pressure-overloaded (6 subjects), and volume-overloaded (18 subjects) ventricles. Although mass is increased similarly in both pressure- and volume-overloaded groups, the increase is accomplished primarily by wall thickening in the pressure-overloaded group. The h/R ratio is normal in volume-overload hypertrophy, indicating a "magnification" type of growth. In pressure overload, concentric hypertrophy is quantified by the increase in h/R. Patients were compensated with respect to heart failure, and peak systolic tension (σ_m) was not statistically different from normal. However, end-diastolic stress was consistently elevated in the volume-overloaded group. See text for details. (Reproduced from Grossman, W., et al.: Wall stress and patterns of hypertrophy in the human left ventricle. J. Clin. Invest. 56:56, 1975, by copyright permission of the American Society for Clinical Investigation.)

TABLE 13–2 THREE STAGES IN THE RESPONSE TO A SUDDEN HEMODYNAMIC OVERLOAD

Stage 1: (Days) Transient breakdown
Circulatory: Acute heart failure; pulmonary congestion, low output
Cardiac: Acute left ventricular dilatation, early hypertrophy
Myocardial: Increased content of mitochondria relative to myofibrils

Stage 2: (Weeks) Stable hyperfunction
Circulatory: Improved pulmonary congestion and cardiac output
Cardiac: Established hypertrophy
Myocardial: Increased content of myofibrils relative to mitochondria

Stage 3: (Months) Exhaustion and progressive cardiosclerosis
Circulatory: Progressive left ventricular failure
Cardiac: Further hypertrophy with progressive fibrosis
Myocardial: Cell death

From Katz, A. M.: Energy requirements of contraction and relaxation: Implications of inotropic stimulation of the failing heart. In Just, H., Holubarsch, C., and Scholz, H. (eds.): Inotropic Stimulation and Myocardial Energetics. New York, Springer-Verlag, 1989, p. 49.

compensatory phase sets in as the ventricle hypertrophies, and the contractile function returns to approximately normal levels. Mitochondria proliferate, and myofibrils are laid down in parallel and sarcomeres in series so that both the length and cross-sectional diameter of myocytes is increased[44] (Fig. 13–7). Later, alterations in cellular organization take place. In what Meerson has termed the "exhaustion" phase several events take place: (1) there is lysis of myofibrils, (2) lysosomes increase in number (presumably to digest worn-out cell constituents), (3) the sarcoplasmic reticulum becomes distorted,[30] (4) the surface densities of the key tubular system are reduced, and (5) fibrous tissue takes the place of cardiac cells.[50] In addition, capillary density and coronary reserve, as reflected in the increase in coronary blood flow during adenosine infusion (see p. 289), become reduced.[51] The resulting ischemia, most severe in the subendocardium (Fig. 36–15, p. 1170), may contribute further to the impairment of cardiac function. Myocyte function then deteriorates (see p. 1179), and overt heart failure occurs.

MYOCYTE NECROSIS. This is an important component of the transition to heart failure. Myocyte necrosis may be localized, as in myocardial infarction, which affects the ventricle in a manner analogous to a volume overload, with an increase both in diameter and length of the remaining cells. Necrosis may be diffuse, as in ischemic cardiomyopathy[36] or idiopathic dilated cardiomyopathy, or as in myocardium damaged by toxic agents such as daunorubicin (see p. 1800) or by myocarditis. Regardless of the cause of

resting state, the ejection fraction at rest, as well as the maximal cardiac output that can be attained during stress, decline. As contractility falls further, overt congestive heart failure, reflected in a depression of cardiac output and work and/or an elevation of ventricular end-diastolic volume and pressure at rest, supervenes.

TRANSITION FROM HYPERTROPHY TO HEART FAILURE. As described by Meerson[49] (Table 13–2), immediately upon imposition of a large pressure load, the increase in work performed by the ventricle exceeds the augmentation of cardiac mass and the heart dilates. As a consequence, a

FIGURE 13–11. The normal (N) relationship between LV wall thickness (h) and chamber radius (r) is shown (first panel). An acute increase in systolic pressure (acute load) causes an increase in systolic wall stress, which can be approximated by the equation P × r/h, where P is LV systolic pressure. Diastolic wall stress is also increased when there is chamber dilatation or when diastolic pressure is elevated (second panel). If sufficient compensatory hypertrophy occurs, the increase in ventricular wall thickness may normalize the systolic and diastolic wall stresses (third panel). However, if additional chamber dilatation occurs or the increase in wall thickness is insufficient, systolic and diastolic wall stresses remain abnormally elevated. In this situation, further chamber dilatation may occur in association with hemodynamic failure (fourth panel). (From Thaik, C. M., and Colucci, W. S.: Molecular and cellular events in myocardial hypertrophy and failure. In Colucci, W. S. (ed.): Heart Failure: Cardiac Function and Dysfunction, Atlas of Heart Diseases. Vol. 4. St. Louis, Mosby-Year Book, 1995, pp. 4.1–4.15.)

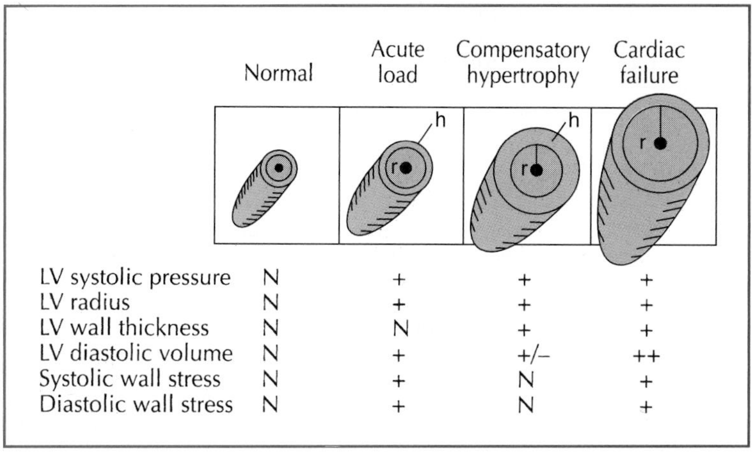

myocyte death, the load on the remaining cells rises and leads to reactive hypertrophy, which may impair further the function of these myocytes. This may be responsible for a vicious circle.

Drop-out of individual myocytes has been observed in the senescent rat[52] and human heart (Chap. 50). Olivetti et al. reported a loss of an average of 38 million nuclei per year in aging people without cardiovascular disease. This loss in myocyte number was accompanied by a reciprocal increase in myocyte cell volume per nucleus, averaging 110 μm^3 per year, thereby preserving ventricular wall thickness.[53] This process may contribute to the development of cardiac dysfunction and, when there is an additional stress such as hypertension, to heart failure in the elderly (see Chap. 50).

Myocardial overload, regardless of cause, can lead to heart failure as a consequence of afterload mismatch, i.e., inadequate hypertrophy. A marked increase in wall stress (afterload) may cause ventricular dilatation, which causes a further increased wall stress, in turn reducing myocardial fiber shortening, leading to further dilatation, and creating a vicious circle.[54] However, excess afterload may also cause *intrinsic* myocardial contractility to decline. Thus, Aoyagi et al.[55] studied an animal model of pressure overload hypertrophy produced by gradually tightening a hydraulic constrictor around the ascending aorta. A depression of myocardial contractility, as assessed by *load-independent* contractility indices, occurred (Fig. 13–12). They concluded that the cardiac dysfunction in this model was not due to insufficient hypertrophy causing afterload mismatch but to a depression of the myocardium's *intrinsic* contractility. Impaired myocardial contractility has also been observed in patients with hypertension and fully compensatory ventricular hypertrophy, normal myocardial stress, and apparently normal pump function. Such patients have displayed reduction of intramural myocardial shortening, as determined by spatial modulation of magnetization, using magnetic resonance imaging techniques[56]; this reduction

indicates a depression of myocardial contractility in the presence of apparently normal loading conditions.

The transition from pressure overload hypertrophy to heart failure in the rat with aortic stenosis can be delayed by means of inhibition of angiotensin-converting enzyme, indicating that the renin-angiotensin system contributes to this transition (see p. 413).[57] There is experimental evidence that impaired coronary reserve and inadequate subendocardial blood flow contribute to the transition as well. Thus, Vatner et al. have demonstrated a diminished response of endocardial blood flow to adenosine and exercise-induced vasodilation in dogs with pressure overload hypertrophy.[58] This is caused in part by hypertrophy and in part by an exercise-induced increase in left ventricular subendocardial wall stress. The reduced subendocardial perfusion in turn may cause subendocardial ischemic injury and replacement fibrosis, which impair both systolic and diastolic function, accelerating the development of heart failure (Fig. 36–15, p. 1170).

PATHOPHYSIOLOGY OF DIASTOLIC HEART FAILURE

(See also pp. 447 and 503)

Alterations in Diastolic Properties

Approximately one-third of patients with congestive heart failure have dominant diastolic heart failure, which may be defined as pulmonary (or systemic) venous congestion, and the symptoms consequent thereto, in the presence of normal or almost normal systolic function.[59-61] Another third have impairment of both systolic and diastolic function, and the remainder primarily disordered systolic function.

ALTERED VENTRICULAR RELAXATION. While two aspects of the heart's diastolic characteristics, i.e., relaxation and wall stiffness, are often considered together, they actually describe two different properties. Relaxation (inactivation of contraction) is a dynamic process that begins at the termination of contraction and occurs during isovolumetric relaxation and early ventricular filling (Fig. 13–13A; see also

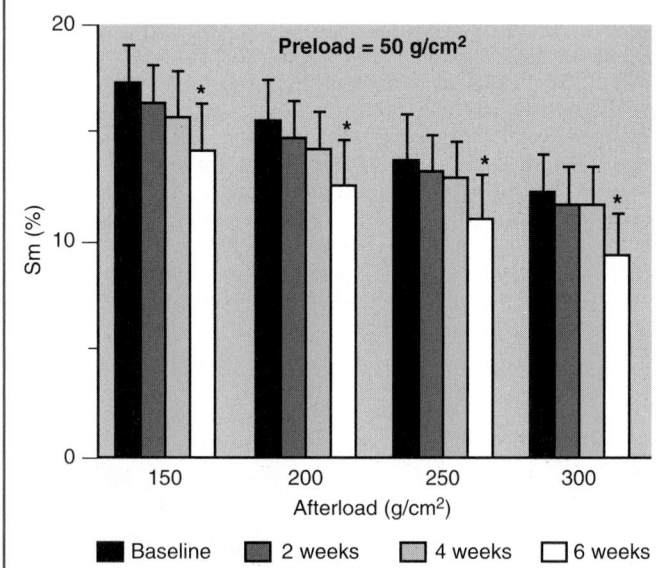

FIGURE 13–12. Time course of myocardial contractility following gradual imposition of a pressure load. Sm indicates midwall shortening at common preload of 50 g/cm^2 and various afterloads. Significant depression of myocardial contractility was detected (*P < .05) at the sixth week of the aortic constriction. (Reproduced by permission from Aoyagi, T., Fujii, A. M., Flanagan, M. F., et al.: Transition from compensated hypertrophy to intrinsic myocardial dysfunction during development of left ventricular pressure-overload hypertrophy in conscious sheep. Systolic dysfunction precedes diastolic dysfunction. Circulation **88**:2415, 1993. Copyright 1993 American Heart Association.)

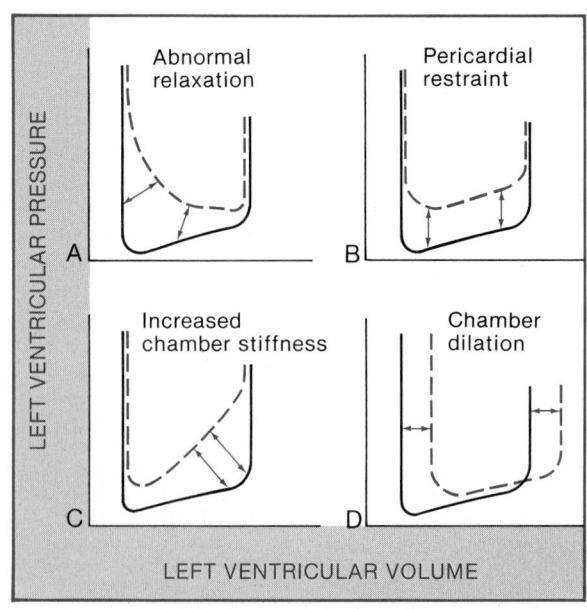

FIGURE 13–13. Mechanisms that cause diastolic dysfunction. Only the bottom half of the pressure-volume loop is depicted. Solid lines represent normal subjects; dashed lines represent patients with diastolic dysfunction. (Reproduced by permission from Zile, M. R.: Diastolic dysfunction: Detection, consequences, and treatment. Part 2: Diagnosis and treatment of diastolic function. Mod. Concepts Cardiovasc. Dis. **59**:1, 1990. Copyright 1990 American Heart Association.)

TABLE 13–3 CALCIUM HOMEOSTASIS IN FAILING HUMAN MYOCARDIUM

INTRACELLULAR CALCIUM LEVELS
Basal (diastolic) ↑
Peak (systolic) ↑
Rate of fall with diastole ↓

CALCIUM-HANDLING PROTEINS AND/OR mRNA LEVELS
SR Ca^{++}-ATPase ↓
Phospholamban ↓
Ca^{++} release channel ↓
Voltage-dependent Ca^{++} channels ↓
Na$^+$/Ca^{++} exchanger ↑
Calsequestrin ↔

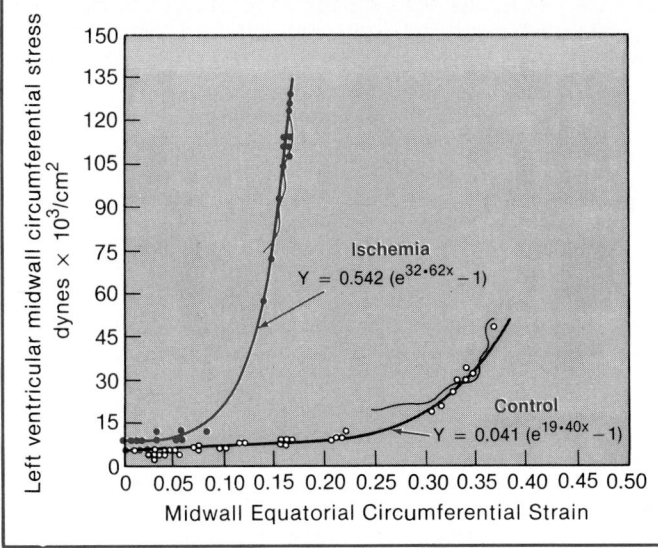

FIGURE 13–14. Diastolic pressure-strain and stress-strain relationships constructed from observations during control period and during ischemia. (Reproduced by permission from Visner, M. S., et al.: Effects of global ischemia on the diastolic properties of the left ventricle in the conscious dog. *Circulation 71:*616, 1985. Copyright 1985 American Heart Association.)

Fig. 12–32, p. 384). The rate of ventricular relaxation is controlled primarily by the uptake of Ca^{++} by the sarcoplasmic reticulum, but also by the efflux of Ca^{++} from the myocyte. These processes are regulated by the sarcoplasmic reticulum calcium ATPase, as well as by sarcolemmal calcium pumps (pp. 369 and 405, Table 13–3). Because these Ca^{++} movements are against concentration gradients, they are energy-consuming. Therefore, ischemia-induced ATP depletion interferes with these processes and slows myocardial relaxation. On the other hand, beta-adrenergic receptor stimulation, by increasing cyclic AMP and cyclic AMP–dependent protein kinase activity, causes the phosphorylation of phospholamban (see p. 368), which accelerates Ca^{++} uptake by the sarcoplasmic reticulum and thereby enhances relaxation.

An acute increase in ventricular afterload has also been shown to slow myocardial relaxation.[62] Thus, when pressure overload is applied (before compensatory hypertrophy has normalized afterload), ventricular relaxation is slowed. Myocardium isolated from patients with hypertrophic cardiomyopathy[63] and from ferrets with pressure-overload hypertrophy[64] exhibits a prolonged calcium transient (i.e., a prolonged elevation of myoplasmic Ca^{++}), associated with a prolonged tension decay, findings consistent with delayed uptake of Ca^{++} by the sarcoplasmic reticulum.

ALTERED VENTRICULAR FILLING. During early ventricular filling the myocardium normally lengthens rapidly and homogeneously. Regional variation in the onset, rate, and extent of myocardial lengthening is referred to as *ventricular heterogeneity,* or *diastolic asynergy;* temporal dispersion of relaxation, with some fibers commencing to lengthen later than others, is referred to as *asynchrony.*[65,66] Both diastolic asynergy and asynchrony interfere with early diastolic filling. In contrast to these early diastolic events, myocardial *elasticity,* i.e., the change in muscle length for a change in force, ventricular *compliance,* i.e., the change in ventricular volume for a given change in pressure, and ventricular *stiffness,* the inverse of compliance, are generally measured in the relaxed ventricle at end-diastole.

These diastolic properties of the ventricle are described by its curvilinear pressure-volume relation (Figs. 12–32, p. 384; 13–13; and 14–1, p. 422). The slope of a tangent to this curvilinear relation (dP/dv) defines the chamber compliance at any level of filling pressure. An increase in chamber stiffness may occur secondary to any one or a combination of these three mechanisms: (1) A rise in filling pressure,[67] i.e., movement of the ventricle up along its pressure-volume (stress-strain) curve to a steeper portion (Fig. 14–20, p. 435). This may occur in conditions such as volume overload secondary to acute valvular regurgitation and in acute left ventricular failure due to myocarditis. (2) A shift to a steeper ventricular pressure-volume (Fig. 13–13*C*) or stress-strain curve. This results most commonly from an increase in ventricular mass and wall thickness. Thus, while hypertrophy constitutes a principal compensatory mechanism to sustain systolic emptying of the overloaded ventricle, it may simultaneously interfere with the ventricle's diastolic properties and impair ventricular fill-

ing. This shift to a steeper pressure-volume curve can also be caused by an increase in *intrinsic* myocardial stiffness (the stiffness of a unit of the cardiac wall regardless of the total mass or thickness of the myocardium), as occurs with disorders in which there is myocardial infiltration (e.g., amyloidosis), endomyocardial fibrosis, or myocardial ischemia (Fig. 13–14). (3) A parallel upward displacement of the diastolic pressure-volume curve, generally referred to as a *decrease in ventricular distensibility,* usually caused by extrinsic compression of the ventricles (Fig. 13–13*B*).

Chronic Changes in Ventricular Diastolic Pressure-Volume Relationships

The compliance of the left ventricle, reflected in the end-diastolic pressure-volume relationship, is altered in a variety of cardiac disorders (p. 447). Substantial shifts in the diastolic pressure-volume curve of the left ventricle can be demonstrated during sustained volume overload.[68] For example, dogs with large chronic arteriovenous fistulas exhibit a rightward displacement of the entire diastolic pressure-volume curve, whereby ventricular volume is greater at any end-diastolic pressure but the slope of this curve is steeper, indicating increased chamber stiffness.[69] Patients with severe volume overloading due to chronic aortic and/or mitral regurgitation demonstrate similar shifts of the diastolic left ventricular pressure-volume relationship. Similar changes frequently occur in patients with dilated or ischemic cardiomyopathy or following large transmural myocardial infarction (see below).

In contrast, concentric left ventricular hypertrophy, as occurs in aortic stenosis, hypertension, and hypertrophic cardiomyopathy, shifts the pressure-volume relation of the ventricle to the left along its volume axis so that at any diastolic volume ventricular diastolic pressure is abnormally elevated[70–72] (Figs. 13–13*C* and 15–1, p. 447). In contrast to the changes in the diastolic properties of the ventricular *chamber,* the stiffness of *each unit of myocardium* may or may not be altered in the presence of myocardial hypertrophy secondary to pressure overload.[73]

In the presence of concentric left ventricular hypertrophy, there is an inverse relationship between the thickness of the posterior wall of the ventricle and its peak

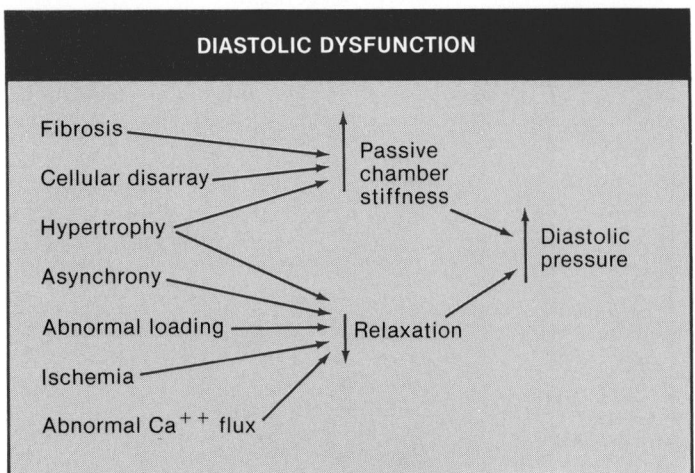

DIASTOLIC DYSFUNCTION

FIGURE 13–15. Factors responsible for diastolic dysfunction and increased left ventricular diastolic pressure. (From Gaasch, W. H., and Izzi, G.: Clinical diagnosis and management of left ventricular diastolic dysfunction. *In* Hori, M., Suga, H., Baan, J., and Yellin, E. L. [eds.]: Cardiac Mechanics and Function in the Normal and Diseased Heart. New York, Springer-Verlag, 1989, p. 296.)

thinning rate during early diastole[74]; a higher-than-normal diastolic ventricular pressure is required to fill the hypertrophied ventricle. Patients with hypertension have demonstrated slowing of ventricular filling by radionuclide angiography[75] and echocardiography, even when systolic function is normal.[76]

ISCHEMIC HEART DISEASE. Marked changes in the diastolic properties of the left ventricle can occur in the presence of ischemic heart disease (see p. 1194). First, as already pointed out, acute myocardial ischemia slows ventricular relaxation (Fig. 13–13A) and increases myocardial wall stiffness[77,78] (Figs. 13–14 and 13–15). Myocardial infarction causes more complex changes in ventricular pressure-volume relationships, depending on the size of the infarct and the time following infarction at which the measurements are made. Infarcted muscle tested very early exhibits reduced stiffness.[79–81] Subsequently, the development of myocardial contracture, interstitial edema, fibrocellular infiltration, and scar contribute to stiffening of the necrotic tissue and thereby to increased chamber stiffness, with a steeper ventricular pressure-volume curve (a greater increase in pressure for any increase in volume).[82] Later still, in the case of large infarcts, left ventricular remodeling and dilatation cause a rightward displacement of the pressure-volume curve,[83] resembling that observed in volume overload. The subendocardial ischemia that is characteristic of severe concentric hypertrophy (even in the presence of a normal coronary circulation) intensifies the failure of relaxation,[58,84] and when coronary artery obstruction accompanies severe hypertrophy, this abnormality may be particularly severe.[83] Tachycardia, by reducing the duration of diastole and thereby intensifying ischemia, exaggerates this diastolic abnormality and may raise ventricular diastolic pressure even while reducing diastolic ventricular volume, whereas bradycardia has the opposite effect. Successful treatment of ischemia improves diastolic relaxation and lowers ventricular diastolic and pulmonary venous pressures, thereby reducing dyspnea.

CARDIOMYOPATHY AND PERICARDIAL DISEASE. The restrictive cardiomyopathies, especially those such as amyloid heart disease with intracardiac infiltration (see p. 1427), the transplanted heart during rejection, and endomyocardial fibrosis (see p. 1433), all are characterized by upward and leftward displacement of the diastolic pressure-volume relation, with a higher pressure at any volume and a greater increase in diastolic pressure for any increase in volume. Pericardial tamponade and constrictive pericarditis also change the apparent diastolic properties of the heart. Early

filling is unimpaired because the myocardium is normal. However, filling is abruptly halted in mid-diastole by the constricted or tamponading pericardium, which imposes its mechanical properties on those of the ventricle in the latter half of diastole (Fig. 13–13B; Fig. 43–20, p. 1503).

ROLE OF COLLAGEN. The diastolic properties of the ventricle are determined not only by its myocytes but also by the coronary vessels, nerves, and interstitial connective tissue, consisting of fibroblasts, and types I and III fibrillar collagen.[39,85,86] The latter provide struts along which the myocytes are aligned. Branches of collagen fibers course at right angles to connect and align muscle bundles. Weber has pointed out that the diastolic properties of the ventricle are influenced profoundly by the quantity of collagen relative to myocytes, as well as by its elastic properties and its physical disposition.[85] The messenger RNA for types I and III collagen that is present in fibroblasts increases markedly after aortic banding in experimental animals,[87] and the left ventricular concentration of collagen is increased in experimentally induced chronic pressure overload hypertrophy,[39] as well as in patients with hypertension. Less information is available on the role of collagen in volume overload hypertrophy; however, the increase in diastolic stiffness sometimes seen in this condition has been associated with increased cross-linking of types I and III collagens.[88]

CELLULAR AND MOLECULAR MECHANISMS OF MYOCARDIAL DYSFUNCTION

Important changes at the cellular and molecular levels have been identified in hypertrophied and failing myocardium. Functional abnormalities in excitation-contraction coupling, contractile protein function, and energetics have been identified in failing animal and human myocardium, and at the molecular level alterations have been observed in the expression of several proteins that are central to normal myocardial structure and function.[89] There is strong evidence from in vitro and animal studies to suggest that these molecular and cellular events are secondary to both mechanical forces and a variety of neuronal, endocrine, and autocrine/paracrine mediators that act on the myocardium. Some of the responses are adaptive and sustain cardiac function. Others are maladaptive. It is not clear which or whether any of these are *responsible* for the impaired myocardial function of heart failure, or play contributory roles, or simply accompany the heart failure state as "epiphenomena."[90]

Excitation-Contraction Coupling and the Role of Ca++

(See also p. 366 and Table 13–3, p. 403)

Ca++ plays a central role in the regulation of myocardial contraction and relaxation.[91] Hypocalcemia, secondary to hypoparathyroidism and a variety of other conditions, can cause heart failure that is responsive to the infusion of calcium.[92,93] Elevation of serum ionized Ca++ has been shown to augment contractility in patients with renal failure undergoing dialysis[94] and in patients with severe heart failure secondary to cardiomyopathy who have downregulation of beta-adrenergic receptors.[95]

Myocardium obtained at the time of cardiac transplantation from patients with end-stage heart failure exhibits abnormal prolongation of the action potential and developed force, and impaired relaxation.[29] Observations using the Ca++ indicator aequorin in whole myocardium have shown that these alterations in electrical and contractile properties are associated with a prolonged elevation of the intracellular Ca++ transient during relaxation.[29] Likewise, in myocytes obtained from patients with end-stage heart failure, the action potential is prolonged. The intracellular Ca++

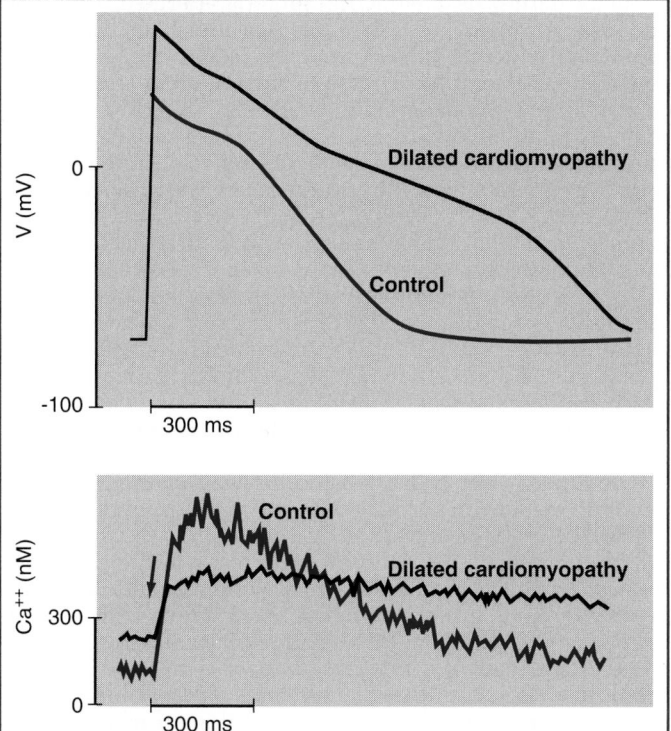

FIGURE 13–16. Abnormal action potential and intracellular calcium transient in failing cardiac myocytes. *Top panel,* The action potential recorded in a myocyte isolated from the heart of a patient with dilated cardiomyopathy is markedly prolonged, as compared to that in a myocyte from a normal heart (control). Such abnormalities could contribute to both the generation of arrhythmias and abnormal diastolic relaxation. *Bottom panel,* The intracellular calcium transient measured with the fluorescent calcium indicator fura-2 are also markedly abnormal in myocytes isolated from the myocardium of patients with dilated cardiomyopathy. As compared to a normal myocyte (control), the myocyte from a patient with dilated cardiomyopathy shows an attenuated rise with depolarization *(arrow)* and a markedly delayed return to baseline. These abnormalities reflect the altered expression or function of key calcium handling proteins (e.g., Ca++-ATPase) and likely contribute to the abnormal action potential illustrated in Panel A. (Modified by permission from Beuckelmann, D. J., Nabauer, M., and Erdmann, E.: Intracellular calcium handling in isolated ventricular myocytes from patients with terminal heart failure. Circulation *85*:1046, 1992. Copyright 1992 American Heart Association.)

transient, as assessed by the fluorescent indicator fura-2, demonstrates a blunted rise with depolarization reflecting a slower delivery of Ca++ to the contractile apparatus (causing slower activation) and a slowed rate of fall during repolarization (causing slowed relaxation) (Fig. 13–16).[96] These two abnormalities can explain both systolic and diastolic dysfunction.

Additional evidence of abnormal myocardial Ca++ handling is provided by the observation that there is a reduction in the amount of tension-independent heat produced in myocardium from patients with heart failure.[97] Tension-independent heat, which is believed to reflect the energy expended for Ca++ transport, can be used to estimate the amount of Ca++ cycled per heartbeat.[98] With this approach, it was shown that Ca++ cycling is reduced by approximately 50 per cent in failing human myocardium.[97]

Excitation-contraction coupling can also be assessed by examination of the force-frequency response. As already pointed out (see p. 398), in normal myocardium, contractile force increases with increasing rates of stimulation, whereas in myocardium obtained from patients with end-stage heart failure the force-frequency response is markedly attenuated.[99] A similar phenomenon is observed in patients with heart failure studied at the time of catheterization.[99a] In patients with normal ventricular function, left ventricular contractility (as measured by +dP/dt or the end-systolic

pressure-volume ratio) increases progressively as heart rate is increased by atrial pacing. By comparison, in patients with severe heart failure there is little or no increase in either contractile index.

The intracellular concentration of Ca++ is regulated by several enzymes and channels that are located in the sarcolemma, sarcoplasmic reticulum (SR), and mitochondria[91] (Chap. 12). Evidence is accumulating that the expression and/or function of a number of these proteins may be altered in hypertrophied and failing myocardium[100] (Table 13–3).

SARCOPLASMIC RETICULUM Ca++-ATPase. Ca++ reuptake by the SR is mediated primarily by the ATP-dependent enzyme Ca++-ATPase (SERCA2).[100] The activity of SERCA2 is inhibited by the associated protein, phospholamban,[100–102] and this inhibition is relieved by cyclic AMP–mediated phosphorylation of phospholamban (e.g., by beta-adrenergic receptor stimulation) thereby resulting in increased Ca++ reuptake into the SR and the acceleration of diastolic relaxation. The reuptake of Ca++ by the SR is also important for normal systolic function, which requires that ample SR Ca++ be available for release during systole to mediate contraction.[100]

Although these observations remain controversial, reports have indicated that the levels of SERCA2[103–105] and phospholamban[104–106] mRNA and SERCA2 protein[105] are reduced in myocardium obtained from patients with end-stage heart failure. In one study, the decrease in the level of SERCA2 mRNA was inversely related to the level of atrial natriuretic factor mRNA (Fig. 13–17), suggesting that the reduced expression of this adult muscle-specific protein is coupled to the reexpression of a fetal gene program.[104] These observations are consistent with several studies that have demonstrated a reduction in SR Ca++ reuptake in animal models of heart failure[107–109] and some[110] but not all[111] studies in patients with heart failure. In mice deficient in phospholamban due to targeted gene ablation, there is a marked increase in basal myocardial contractility and a loss of both the contractile and relaxant effects of beta-adrenergic stimulation.[102] It is therefore possible that a decrease in phospholamban activity is an adaptive response to the decrease in SERCA2 activity.

THE Ca++ RELEASE CHANNEL. The Ca++ release channel (CRC), located on the SR, mediates the release of Ca++ from the SR into the myoplasm during systole.[91] Studies in failing human myocardium have shown decreases in the

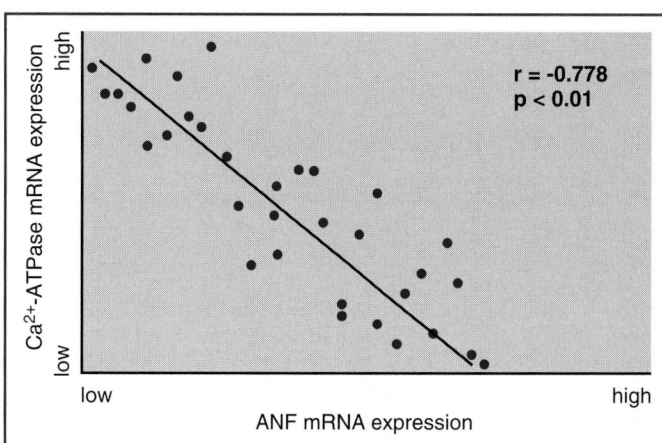

FIGURE 13–17. Inverse relationship between the mRNA levels for the fetal gene atrial natriuretic factor (ANF) and the adult muscle-specific gene encoding Ca++-ATPase in ventricular myocardium obtained from patients with various degrees of myocardial failure. The reexpression of a fetal gene program is typical of hypertrophied and failing myocardium. (Modified by permission from Arai, M., Matsui, H., and Periasamy, M.: Sarcoplasmic reticulum gene expression in cardiac hypertrophy and heart failure. Circ. Res. *74*:555, 1994. Copyright 1994 American Heart Association.)

mRNA level for the CRC. In one study, the mRNA level for CRC was reduced in patients with ischemic cardiomyopathy but not those with dilated cardiomyopathy.[112] In another study, the level of CRC mRNA was decreased in patients with heart failure of both causes.[104]

VOLTAGE-DEPENDENT Ca⁺⁺ CHANNEL. The mRNA and protein levels of the voltage-dependent Ca^{++} channel also have been shown to be decreased in failing human myocardium obtained from patients with both ischemic heart disease and dilated cardiomyopathy.[113]

Na⁺/Ca⁺⁺ EXCHANGER. The Na^+/Ca^{++} exchanger is the major route by which Ca^{++} is removed from the cardiac myocyte and can account for approximately 20 per cent of the removal of Ca^{++} from the cytoplasm during diastole.[105] The mRNA and protein levels of the Na^+/Ca^{++} exchanger were found to be increased in myocardium obtained from patients with heart failure due to both ischemic and idiopathic dilated cardiomyopathy, and correlated inversely with the decrease in SERCA2 mRNA levels.[105] This augmentation in Na^+/Ca^{++} exchange activity might be a compensatory response to the reduction in Ca^{++} reuptake caused by a decrease in SERCA2. Although this would facilitate diastolic Ca^{++} removal, it might do so at the expense of increased arrhythmogenicity, because this Ca^{++} efflux is associated with an influx of Na^+ that can prolong depolarization and cause afterdepolarizations.

CALSEQUESTRIN. This is the major protein in the SR that binds Ca^{++} and thereby serves a storage function. Several studies have found calsequestrin mRNA levels to be unchanged in failing human myocardium.[104,111,113]

Contractile Apparatus

The fraction of cell volume composed of myofibrils is initially increased in animal models of pressure-induced hypertrophy.[34,114] Patients with aortic stenosis without heart failure exhibit a normal fraction of myofibrils per cell, whereas those with left ventricular failure show a significant reduction in cell volume occupied by myofibrils, suggesting that this reduction in the quantity of the contractile machinery may play a role in the development of cardiac decompensation.[115] In end-stage heart failure in the human, electron microscopic observations likewise show a reduction of ventricular myofibrillar protein.[116]

REDUCTION OF MYOSIN ATPase. Considerable data suggest that qualitative, as well as quantitative, alterations of contractile proteins occur in heart failure. First, the finding that the reduced velocity of contraction of failing myocardium occurs in chemically skinned ventricular fibers suggests that this change reflects intrinsic alterations in the contractile apparatus. Early studies showed that the activity of myofibrillar ATPase is reduced in the hearts of patients who died of heart failure[117,118] and in dogs with naturally occurring heart failure.[119] Furthermore, reductions in the activities of myofibrillar ATPase, actomyosin ATPase, or myosin ATPase have been demonstrated in heart failure induced in cats by pulmonary artery constriction,[120] in guinea pigs with constriction of the ascending aorta,[121] in dogs with constriction of the pulmonary artery or aorta,[122] and in rats with renovascular hypertension.[123] These depressions of enzymatic activity could occur if an altered subunit of the myosin molecule, i.e., the portion of the molecule responsible for the ATPase activity, were produced in the overloaded heart and reduced contractility by lowering the rate of interaction between actin and myosin filaments. A reduction in the Mg^{++}-ATPase activity (which expresses the response of myofibrils to Ca^{++}) has been demonstrated in myofibrils obtained from patients with end-stage heart failure at the time of transplantation and in less sick patients undergoing valve replacement.[124]

MYOSIN ISOFORM CHANGES. Animal studies have indicated that when the adult heart hypertrophies, fetal and neonatal forms of contractile proteins (termed isoforms) and other proteins (such as atrial natriuretic peptide) reappear, signifying reexpression of the genes for these fetal and neonatal isoforms. Thus, hemodynamic overload leads to enhanced overall protein synthesis,[3] but it alters the proteins qualitatively, i.e., it leads to the synthesis of protein isoforms that were present during fetal and neonatal life when protein synthesis in the heart was also rapid.[124a] Altered isoforms of cardiac proteins may arise from the expression of different members of a multigene family or from the assembly of the same gene in a different pattern. In rodents the predominant myosin heavy chain (MHC) is the "fast" V_1 isoform (high ATPase activity, encoded by the alpha-MHC gene). With pressure-induced hypertrophy or myocardial failure following myocardial infarction in the rat, there is the reexpression of the "slow" V_3 isoform (low ATPase activity, encoded by the beta-MHC gene), and deinduction of the V_1 isoform.[125-129]

Although a shift in MHC isoforms would provide an attractive explanation for the reduction in myofibrillar ATPase activity observed in failing human myocardium, the predominant MHC isoform in humans is the slower V_3 isoform (encoded by the beta-MHC gene). In failing human myocardium, as in normal myocardium, alpha-MHC mRNA is not detectable; beta MHC and alpha cardiac actin are reduced and correlate inversely with the increase in atrial natriuretic factor mRNA level; and alpha-skeletal actin mRNA, which is expressed in normal human myocardium, is unchanged.[104] These observations are consistent with a general decrease in contractile protein-expression; however, they make it unlikely that a shift in myosin isoforms is responsible for the observed decrease in myosin ATPase activity. It remains possible that functional alterations in myosin and/or actin may be present, and it has been reported that there is a reduction in the number of cells containing alpha-MHC in failing human myocardium.[130]

ALTERED REGULATORY PROTEINS. Another possible cause of a decrease in contractile protein function is an alteration in the expression and/or activity of regulatory proteins. In animals with experimental heart failure, there are changes in the myosin light chain and the troponin-tropomyosin complex.[131,132] Changes in myosin light-chain isoforms have been observed in the atria and ventricles of patients sub-

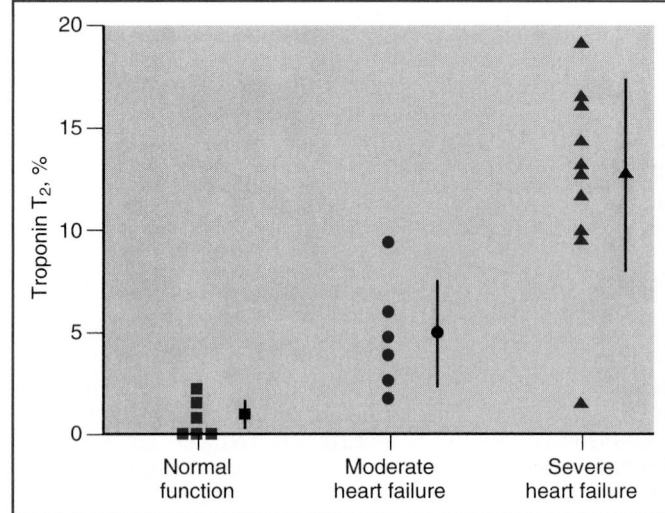

FIGURE 13–18. Increased expression in failing human myocardium of the troponin-T_2 isoform of troponin-T, a component of the tropomyosin complex which regulates the interaction of actin and myosin. Changes in the expression of troponin-T, or other regulatory proteins (e.g., myosin light chains), could contribute to altered contractile protein function in such patients. (Modified from Anderson, P. A. W., Malouf, N. N., Oakeley, A. E., et al.: Troponin T isoform expression in the normal and failing human left ventricle: A correlation with myofibrillar ATPase activity. Basic Res. Cardiol. *87*:175, 1992.)

jected to increased mechanical stress,[133] and the expression of troponin-T, a component of the troponin complex that regulates the interaction of myosin and actin, was found to be altered in failing human myocardium.[134] In normal myocardium, troponin-T is expressed as a single isoform (T_1), which accounts for approximately 98 per cent of the troponin-T. In myocardium from patients with end-stage heart failure, a second isoform (T_2) was expressed at increased levels, and its level of expression was related to the severity of heart failure (Fig. 13–18).[134] The functional significance of these changes in the expression of regulatory proteins is not known. However, these observations suggest that changes in myosin activity could be due to changes in regulatory proteins and need not reflect alterations in the contractile proteins themselves.

Myocardial Energetics

Heart failure frequently occurs in the presence of adequate myocardial perfusion, oxygen, and substrate. In early studies, measurement of coronary blood flow utilizing coronary sinus catheterization, both in humans and in dogs with chronic heart failure, showed that the coronary blood flow per gram of myocardium did not differ significantly from normal.[135] Several preparations of failing heart muscle were shown to require less oxygen than does normal muscle. When contractility is acutely depressed, myocardial oxygen consumption of the intact ventricle also declines.[136] Similarly, patients with chronic impairment of left ventricular performance and reduction of the velocity of myocardial fiber shortening exhibit reduction of coronary blood flow and myocardial oxygen consumption per unit of muscle.[137] Marked reductions in myocardial oxygen consumption have been described in the Syrian hamster with hereditary cardiomyopathy.[138] Papillary muscles removed from cats with pressure overload–induced right ventricular hypertrophy exhibit a depression of both contractility and oxygen consumption per unit of tension development.[23] These lowered energy needs of the failing heart may serve a protective function, reducing the likelihood of the exacerbation of heart failure by an imbalance between energy supply and demand.

MYOCARDIAL ENERGY PRODUCTION. Considerable dispute has centered on the question of whether or not mitochondrial oxidative phosphorylation, i.e., energy production, is abnormal in heart failure. Early studies indicated that electron transport and the tightness of respiratory control are normal in mitochondria obtained from failing human hearts[139] and cat hearts with experimental heart failure produced by pressure overload.[140] On the other hand, in one study in which mitochondria from the hearts of patients with end-stage dilated cardiomyopathy were studied, a reduction in cytochrome-a content and in cytochrome-dependent enzyme activity was reported.[141] The cytochromes are located in the inner mitochondrial membrane and are constituents of the respiratory chain that couples oxidation to the synthesis of chemical energy. Mitochondria obtained from failing human cardiac muscle have also shown reduced oxygen consumption during active phosphorylation and reduced rates of NADH-linked respiratory activity.[141] These and other observations have led to the thesis that myocardial failure in the setting of hemodynamic overload may be related to an inability of the energy-producing system, i.e., the mitochondria, to keep pace with the needs of the contractile apparatus.

The nucleotide-transporting protein located on the inner mitochondrial membrane, the so-called ADP-ATP carrier, has been identified as an autoantigen in viral myocarditis and dilated cardiomyopathy. In guinea pigs immunized to this carrier protein, both myocardial oxygen consumption and cardiac work fell.[142] These findings are compatible with the hypothesis that the impaired cardiac performance in some cases of myocarditis (and dilated cardiomyopathy) may be secondary to an imbalance between energy delivery and demand.

MYOCARDIAL ENERGY RESERVES. In compensated hypertrophy, observations on myocardial ATP concentration have shown no consistent change.[143] However, in myocardium from dogs with myocardial failure due to rapid pacing or chronic ischemia and from humans with end-stage cardiomyopathy, total creatine kinase activity and the concentrations of phosphocreatine and creatine are decreased.[143–145] These observations have led to the hypothesis that myocardial failure may be the consequence of a decreased energy reserve.[143] The measurement of creatine kinase flux provides a sensitive measure of myocardial energy reserves and may detect abnormalities in the absence of changes in ATP and phosphocreatine concentrations. By studying high-energy flux in vivo using nuclear magnetic resonance technology, it was demonstrated that creatine kinase activity is markedly reduced in the myopathic Syrian hamster.[146] This abnormality was almost completely corrected by treatment with the converting enzyme inhibitor enalapril. The mechanism responsible for a decrease in creatine kinase activity is not understood but is associated with alterations in the isoform of creatine kinase. In failing myocardium, there is a decrease in the adult (MM) isoform and an increase or no change in the fetal isoform (MB).[143]

One unusual form of heart failure that is primarily related to a reduction of myocardial energy stores is that due to phosphate deficiency. Chronic hypophosphatemia induced by dietary means is associated with reversible depression of myocardial performance in isolated muscle as well as in the intact heart of animals and humans, presumably as a consequence of reduced ATP stores.[147,148]

NEUROHORMONAL, AUTOCRINE, AND PARACRINE ADJUSTMENTS

A complex series of neurohormonal changes takes place consequent to the two principal hemodynamic alterations in heart failure: reduction of cardiac output and atrial hypertension (Fig. 13–19). Many of these neurohormonal changes occur in response to the inadequate arterial volume characteristic of systolic heart failure. In the early stages of acute systolic failure, these changes—heightened adrenergic drive, activation of the renin-angiotensin-aldosterone axis, and the augmented release of vasopressin and endothelin—are truly compensatory and act to maintain perfusion to vital organs and to expand the inadequate arterial blood volume. However, each of these mechanisms may be thought of as a "double-edged sword." As heart failure becomes chronic, several of these compensatory mechanisms can cause undesirable effects such as excessive vasoconstriction, increased afterload, excessive retention of salt and water, electrolyte abnormalities, and arrhythmias (Table 13–1). In contrast, other responses, such as the release of atrial natriuretic peptide (ANP) in response to atrial distention, may oppose these adverse effects by causing vasodilation and increased excretion of salt and water.

A variety of mediators are involved in control of the cardiovascular system in heart failure. Some are circulating hormones (endocrine effect). Some act on neighboring cells of another type (paracrine effect) or on the cell of origin (autocrine effect).[149] These include peptides that primarily act locally in the vicinity of their production, such as endothelin, peptide growth factors (e.g., transforming growth factor-alpha), and inflammatory cytokines (e.g., interleukin-1 beta and tumor necrosis factor-alpha). These and other local mediators act in concert with the autonomic nervous system and circulating hormones to modulate cardiovascular organ function. In addition, many if not all of these mediators have effects on the growth of cardiovascular tis-

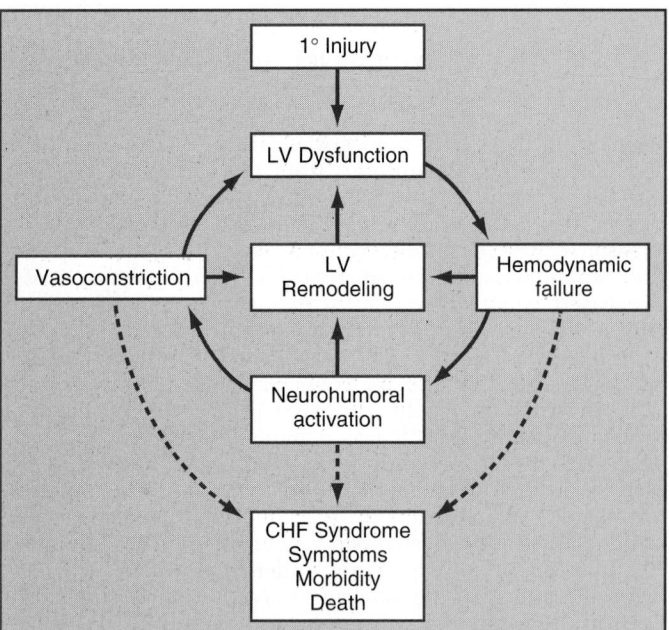

FIGURE 13–19. Schematic illustrating the proposed relationship between primary myocardial injury and secondary events which contribute to the clinical syndrome of heart failure and progression of the underlying myocardial disease. According to this thesis, hemodynamic and neurohormonal consequences of the initial myocardial injury result in both acute impairment of ventricular function due to increased ventricular afterload and chronic progression of disease due to ventricular remodeling.

sues and may thereby play an important role in the "remodeling" of myocardium and vasculature.

Autonomic Nervous System

INCREASED SYMPATHETIC ACTIVITY (see Fig. 13–2, p. 395). Measurements of the concentration of the adrenergic norepinephrine (NE) in arterial blood provide an index of the activity of this system, which is crucial to the normal regulation of cardiac performance. At rest, in patients with advanced heart failure, the circulating NE concentration is much higher, generally two to three times the level found in normal subjects,[150–153] and is accompanied by elevation of circulating dopamine and sometimes by epinephrine as well; the latter reflects increased adrenomedullary activity. Measurement of 24-hour urinary NE excretion also reveals marked elevations in patients with heart failure.[152] In the prevention arm of the SOLVD study (see p. 495), plasma NE was significantly elevated, even in asymptomatic patients, and was further elevated in patients with symptomatic heart failure (Fig. 13–20).[154] During comparable levels of exercise, much greater elevations in circulating NE occur in patients with heart failure than in normal subjects, presumably reflecting greater activation of the adrenergic nervous system during exercise in these patients.[155–157]

Elevation of Circulating Norepinephrine. The elevation of circulating NE may result from a combination of increased release of NE from adrenergic nerve endings and its consequent "spillover" into plasma,[158,159] as well as reduced uptake of NE by adrenergic nerve endings.[160] Patients with heart failure demonstrate increased adrenergic

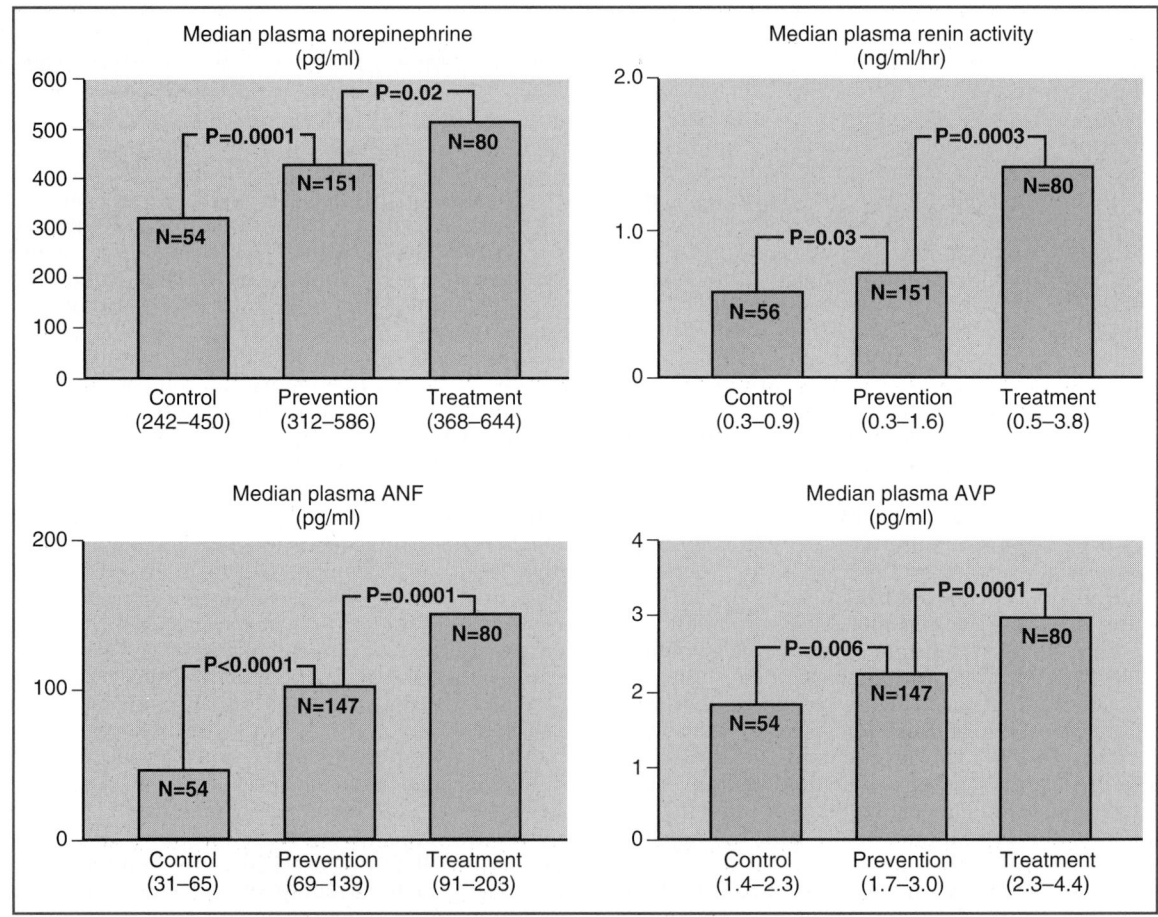

FIGURE 13–20. Activation of neurohormonal systems in patients with heart failure. In patients studied in the SOLVD trials, plasma norepinephrine, renin activity, atrial natriuretic factor (ANF), and arginine vasopressin (AVP) were elevated in patients with symptomatic heart failure enrolled in the treatment trial, and also, albeit to a lesser degree, in asymptomatic patients enrolled in the prevention trial. (Modified by permission from Francis, G. S., Benedict, C., Johnstone, D. E., et al.: Comparison of neuroendocrine activation in patients with left ventricular dysfunction with and without congestive heart failure. A substudy of the studies of left ventricular dysfunction (SOLVD). Circulation 82:1724, 1990. Copyright 1990 American Heart Association.)

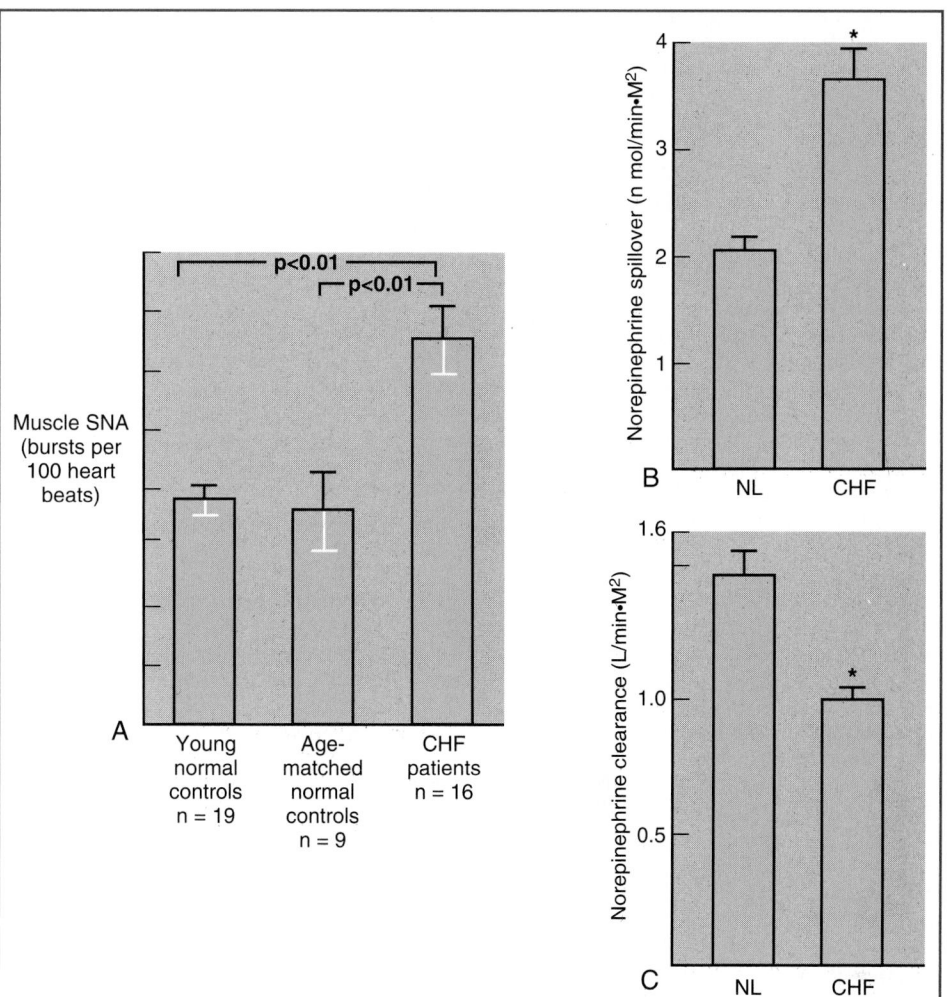

FIGURE 13–21. Activation of the sympathetic nervous system in heart failure. There is an increased rate of sympathetic nerve activity (SNA), as measured by the rate of nerve firing in the peroneal nerve, in patients with heart failure (Panel A). Studies of the clearance of plasma norepinephrine in normal (NL) subjects and patients with heart failure (CHF) indicate that both increased spillover (Panel B) and decreased clearance (Panel C) contribute to the higher norepinephrine levels observed in patients with heart failure. (Panel A modified from Leimbach, W. N., Jr., Wallin, G., Victor, R. G., et al.: Direct evidence from intrarenal recordings for increased central sympathetic outflow in patients with heart failure. Circulation 73:913, 1986. Copyright 1986 American Heart Association. Panels B and C modified from Davis, D., et al.: Abnormalities in systemic norepinephrine kinetics in human congestive heart failure. Am. J. Physiol. 254:E760, 1988.)

nerve outflow, as measured by microneurography of the peroneal nerve (Fig. 13–4), and the level of nerve activity correlates with the concentration of plasma NE (Fig. 13–21).[161] The level of adrenergic nerve activity also correlates directly with the levels of left and right ventricular filling pressures.[161] While the normal heart usually extracts NE, in patients with heart failure the coronary sinus NE level exceeds the arterial level, indicating increased adrenergic activation of the heart.[158] Drugs such as the alpha$_2$-agonist guanabenz (which reduces adrenergic nerve impulse traffic) and bromocriptine (a presynaptic dopamine-2 agonist[162]) reduce plasma NE, indicating that presynaptic control of adrenergic nervous activity is intact in patients with heart failure.[151] It has been suggested that treatment with such agents might be useful in interrupting the vicious circle already referred to.[162]

The extent of elevation of plasma NE concentration that occurs in patients with heart failure correlates directly with the severity of the left ventricular dysfunction,[150] as reflected in the height of the pulmonary capillary wedge pressure and depression of the cardiac index,[151,153] and with cardiac mortality.[163] The augmented adrenergic outflow from the central nervous system in patients with heart failure may trigger ventricular tachycardia or even sudden cardiac death, particularly in the presence of myocardial ischemia. However, it is not clear whether the elevated levels of circulating NE in patients who subsequently die of heart failure are causally related to death as a consequence of their vasoconstrictor, arrhythmogenic, or other actions or whether they represent an "epiphenomenon" that merely reflects the severity of the underlying heart failure.

In addition to activation of beta-adrenergic receptors in the heart, the heightened activity of the adrenergic nervous system leads to stimulation of myocardial alpha$_1$-adrenergic receptors, which elicits a modest positive inotropic effect.[164] Stimulation of myocardial alpha$_1$-adrenergic receptors may also cause myocyte hypertrophy, changes in phenotype characterized by the reexpression of a fetal gene program,[165] and the induction of peptide growth factors.[166] Alpha$_1$-adrenergic receptors are of low density in the human heart; however, in contrast to beta$_1$-adrenergic receptors, which are downregulated, alpha$_1$-adrenergic receptors appear to be unchanged in number in failing human myocardium.[167]

CARDIAC NOREPINEPHRINE DEPLETION. The concentration of NE in atrial[152] and ventricular tissue[26] removed at operation from patients with heart failure is extremely low. In patients, it has been reported that cardiac NE content determined from endomyocardial biopsies correlates directly with the ejection fraction and inversely with plasma epinephrine concentration.[168] NE concentrations are also markedly depressed in the ventricles of dogs with right ventricular failure produced by the creation of pulmonary stenosis and tricuspid regurgitation.[170] Local cardiac NE stores do not appear to play any role in the intrinsic contractile state of cardiac muscle. Thus, no differences were found in the length-tension or force-velocity relationships displayed by papillary muscles removed from normal cats and from cats with NE depletion produced by chronic cardiac denervation or reserpine pretreatment.[170] However, the reduction in cardiac NE stores represents a depletion of the adrenergic neurotransmitter in adrenergic nerve endings, and as a consequence the response to activation of the sympathetic nervous system is blunted[171] (Fig. 13–2, p. 395).

The mechanism responsible for cardiac NE depletion in severe heart failure is not clear; it may be an "exhaustion" phenomenon from the prolonged adrenergic activation of the cardiac adrenergic nerves in heart failure. Reductions in the activity of tyrosine hydroxylase,[172] which catalyzes the rate-limiting step in the biosynthesis of NE, and in the rate at which noradrenergic vesicles can take up dopamine[173] have also been incriminated. In patients with cardiomyopathy, [^{131}I]-labeled metaiodobenzylguanidine (MTBG), a radiopharmaceutical that is taken up by adrenergic nerve endings, is not taken up normally.[174] The technique based on this observation may provide a noninvasive approach to assessing disturbances in adrenergic function in heart failure.

ABNORMAL BAROREFLEX CONTROL IN HEART FAILURE. Increased adrenergic activity in heart failure is due, in part, to abnormal baroreflex control of adrenergic outflow from the central nervous system (Fig. 13–3). In dogs with experimental heart failure, carotid occlusion elicits a blunted reflex response of heart rate, arterial pressure, and vascular resistance.[175,176] The possibility of defective adrenergic control of heart rate in patients with heart failure has been studied by observing the reflex hemodynamic responses to stimuli such as upright tilt and vasodilator-induced hypotension.[177–181]

An inappropriately depressed increase in heart rate in humans with heart failure was observed when arterial pressure was reduced through administration of vasodilators.[182] While the changes in mean arterial pressure observed in response to the vasodilators were similar in patients with heart failure and in control subjects, the changes in heart rate after vasodilators correlated significantly with the changes in concentration of circulating NE and with the sum of circulating NE and epinephrine. In normal individuals, both heart rate and catecholamine concentrations rose, whereas in patients with heart failure, in whom resting catecholamine levels were already increased, cardiac acceleration was blunted, and catecholamine concentration failed to rise normally. Similarly, during upright tilt there is a blunting of the normal increases in plasma NE, forearm vascular resistance, and hepatic vascular resistance in patients with heart failure.[117,178] Some patients with heart failure exhibit a major reduction in arterial pressure during tilting, analogous to what is observed in idiopathic orthostatic hypotension.[179] In such patients, not surprisingly, exercise capacity in the upright position is markedly reduced.[183] Further evidence for impairment of baroreflex control of the systemic circulation comes from investigations in which lower body negative pressure fails to cause normal reflex augmentation of forearm vascular resistance.[180]

Atrial Stretch Receptors. Abnormal baroreflex control also contributes to the reduced ability of patients with heart failure to excrete salt and water. Under normal circumstances, elevated left atrial pressure stimulates atrial stretch receptors. The increased activity of both myelinated and nonmyelinated (C-fiber) afferents[184] inhibits the release of ADH, thereby increasing water excretion, which in turn reduces plasma volume and would act to restore left atrial pressure to normal. In addition, enhanced left atrial stretch receptor activation depresses renal efferent sympathetic nerve activity and increases renal blood flow and glomerular filtration rate, thereby enhancing the ability of the kidney to reduce plasma volume.

With continued stimulation as occurs in heart failure, there is desensitization of atrial (and arterial) baroreceptors. Zucker et al. observed that the decreased sensitivity of left atrial stretch receptors in dogs with heart failure is the result of cardiac dilatation and alterations in atrial compliance and is reversible following reversal of heart failure.[185,186] This resetting of atrial receptors may be responsible for the inappropriately high plasma ADH levels in heart failure[187] and may contribute to the renal vasoconstriction, peripheral edema, ascites, and hyponatremia characteristic of chronic severe heart failure. With chronic heart failure and its attendant cardiac distention and decreased sensitivity of cardiac receptors, the reflex inhibition of adrenergic activity disappears. The adrenergic drive to the peripheral vascular bed and the adrenal medulla is enhanced, contributing to the sodium retention, tachycardia, and the vasoconstricted state characteristic of heart failure.

There is evidence that abnormal baroreflex control is associated with increased activity of Na^+, K^+-ATPase in the baroreceptors.[188] Digitalis glycosides can partially correct the blunted baroreceptor responsiveness in patients with heart failure.[180] This effect of digitalis is apparently due to a direct action on one or more components of the baroreflex pathway rather than to an improvement in hemodynamic function, because a similar effect is not seen when hemodynamic function is acutely improved by infusion of the beta-adrenergic agonist dobutamine.[180] This thesis is also supported by the observation that, in dogs with pacing-induced heart failure, the selective perfusion of the carotid sinus with ouabain corrected abnormal baroreflex function.[188] This ability of digitalis to correct baroreflex function and thereby suppress adrenergic nerve activity may play a significant role in its clinical efficacy (see Chap. 16). The abnormal baroreflex response in patients with heart failure is usually corrected by cardiac transplantation,[189] indicating that it is a secondary manifestation (not a cause) of heart failure.

ADRENERGIC CONTROL OF THE SPLANCHNIC AND RENAL CIRCULATIONS. Substantial changes also occur in heart failure in the function of the adrenergic nerves that innervate splanchnic and renal vessels.[190,191] Adrenergically mediated vasoconstriction normally occurs in the vessels supplying the splanchnic viscera and kidneys during exercise. However, it has been shown that exercise induces a much more marked reduction in mesenteric blood flow and elevation of mesenteric vascular resistance in dogs with heart failure produced experimentally by inducing tricuspid regurgitation and constriction of the pulmonary artery than in normal dogs.[192] Similar changes during exercise were observed in other major visceral vascular beds, such as the renal bed. Evidence that this intense vasoconstriction during exercise is mediated by the adrenergic nervous system is provided by observations on dogs with experimentally produced heart failure in which one kidney was denervated. Blood flow through the normal kidney declined precipitously during exercise, and calculated renal vascular resistance increased markedly. In contrast, little change in renal blood flow and calculated renal vascular resistance occurred in the denervated kidney.[192] This intensive visceral vasoconstriction during exercise helps to divert the limited cardiac output to exercising muscle but, conversely, may contribute to hypoperfusion of the gut and kidneys.

Beta-Adrenergic Receptor–G Protein– Adenylate Cyclase Pathway

BETA-ADRENERGIC RECEPTORS. Ventricles obtained from patients with heart failure demonstrate a marked reduction in beta-adrenergic receptor density, isoproterenol-mediated adenylate cyclase stimulation, and the contractile response to beta-adrenergic agonists (Table 13–4).[193] It is generally believed that the downregulation of beta-adrenergic receptors is mediated by increased levels of NE in the vicinity of the receptor. In patients with right ventricular failure secondary to primary pulmonary hypertension, beta$_1$-adrenergic receptors are downregulated in the right ventricle but not in the normally functioning left ventricle,[194] suggesting that beta-adrenergic receptor downregulation is due to a local chamber-specific mechanism, presumably an increase in local NE concentrations. In patients with dilated cardiomyopathy, this reduction in receptor density is proportional to the severity of heart failure[195] and involves primarily beta$_1$, but not beta$_2$, receptors, thus reducing the ratio of beta$_1$ to beta$_2$ receptors (Fig. 13–22A).[196] The beta$_2$ receptor, although not downregulated, becomes partially

TABLE 13–4 ALTERATIONS IN THE BETA-ADRENERGIC RECEPTOR PATHWAY IN FAILING HUMAN MYOCARDIUM

CONTRACTILE RESPONSES TO VARIOUS AGONISTS (COMPARED WITH NORMAL MYOCARDIUM)
Calcium $\leftrightarrow$
Forskolin $\leftrightarrow$
β_2-adrenergic agonist $\leftrightarrow/\downarrow$
β_1-adrenergic agonist $\downarrow \downarrow$

COMPONENTS OF THE β-AR/ADENYLATE CYCLASE PATHWAY (COMPARED WITH NORMAL MYOCARDIUM)
Number of β_1-AR/mRNA $\downarrow \downarrow/\downarrow \downarrow$
Number of β_2-AR/mRNA $\leftrightarrow/\leftrightarrow$
G_i activity/mRNA $\uparrow/\leftrightarrow$
G_s activity/mRNA $\leftrightarrow/\leftrightarrow$
βARK activity/mRNA $\uparrow \uparrow/\uparrow \uparrow$

$\leftrightarrow$ = no change.

"uncoupled" from its effector enzyme (adenylate cyclase),[197] producing a similar effect.

The relative roles of beta-adrenergic receptor downregulation versus receptor uncoupling may depend on the cause of heart failure. In myocardium obtained from patients with heart failure secondary to ischemic heart disease, there is a relatively greater degree of receptor desensitization than in myocardium from patients with ischemic cardiomyopathy.[198] This observation, together with apparent differences in the regulation of G-protein function (discussed below), has led to the suggestion that there are differences in the behavior of the beta-adrenergic receptor G-protein complex in these forms of heart failure. The beneficial hemodynamic effects of chronic therapy with the beta-adrenergic antagonist bucindolol were significantly better in patients with idiopathic rather than ischemic cardiomyopathy,[199] suggesting that such differences in pathophysiology may also have therapeutic implications.

In myocardium from patients with heart failure the level of beta$_1$-adrenergic receptor mRNA is decreased, indicating that downregulation of beta$_1$-adrenergic receptors is mediated, at least in part, by a decrease in receptor synthesis, whereas the level of beta$_2$-adrenergic receptor mRNA is unchanged (Fig. 13–22A).[202] In addition, there are increases in the expression of beta-adrenergic receptor kinase (BARK) and its mRNA level in failing human myocardium (Fig. 13–22B).[203] BARK is an enzyme that phosphorylates both beta$_1$- and beta$_2$-adrenergic receptors and thereby plays a central role in uncoupling of the receptor from its G protein.[203] Increased BARK activity may therefore contribute to the uncoupling of both beta$_1$- and beta$_2$-adrenergic receptors in patients with heart failure.

Downregulation of beta$_1$ receptors in patients with heart failure may be reversed by the administration of metoprolol, a relatively specific beta$_1$ antagonist. The long-term clinical benefit of beta blockade in heart failure (see p. 486) has been reported to be associated with both a restoration of myocardial beta receptor density and the contractile response to administered catecholamines.[204]

G PROTEINS AND ADENYLATE CYCLASE. G proteins play a crucial role in coupling receptors, including beta-adrenergic

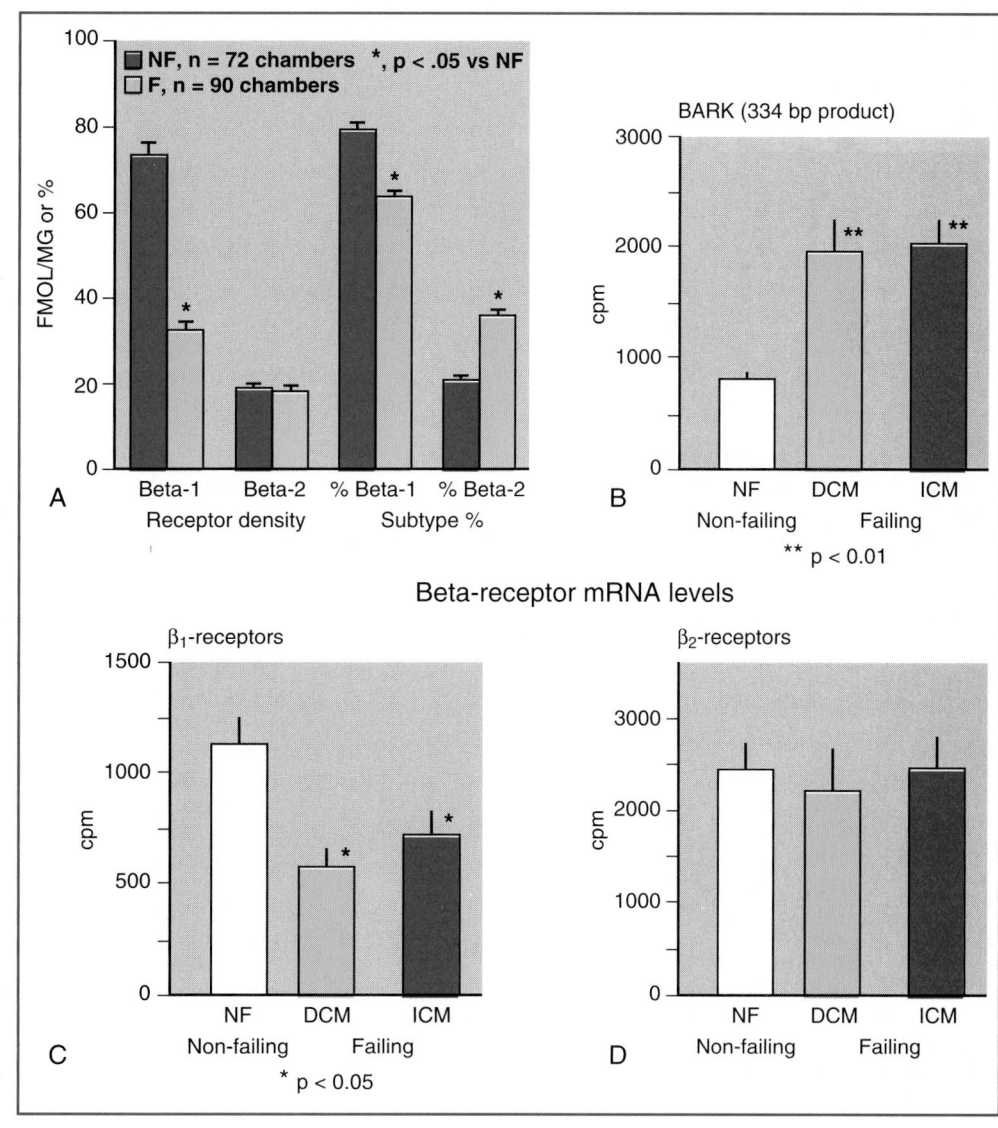

FIGURE 13–22. Downregulation of beta-adrenergic receptors in myocardium from patients with heart failure. Although human ventricular myocardium expresses both beta$_1$- and beta$_2$-adrenergic receptor subtypes, only the beta$_1$ subtype is significantly downregulated in failing myocardium *(Panel A).* Downregulation of beta$_1$ receptors is associated with upregulation of beta-adrenergic receptor kinase (BARK), an enzyme which phosphorylates beta-adrenergic receptors and thereby contributes to their uncoupling from second messenger pathways *(Panel B).* In addition, the mRNA level for beta$_1$-, but not beta$_2$-, adrenergic receptors is decreased in failing human myocardium *(Panels C and D).* NF = non-failure; F = congestive heart failure; DCM = dilated cardiomyopathy; ICM = ischemic cardiomyopathy. (Data from Bristow, M. R.: Changes in myocardial and vascular receptors in heart failure. J. Am. Coll. Cardiol. *22:*61A, 1993, and Ungerer, M., Bohm, M., Elce, J. S., et al.: Altered expression of beta-adrenergic receptor kinase and beta$_1$-adrenergic receptors in the failing human heart. Circulation *87:*454, 1993. Copyright 1993 American Heart Association.)

receptors, to effector enzymes such as adenylate cyclase (see p. 376). Cardiac cells contain at least two types of G proteins: (1) G_s, which mediates the stimulation of adenylate cyclase (and thereby causes a rise in intracellular cyclic AMP, which in turn stimulates Ca^{++} influx into the myocyte through Ca^{++} channels in the sarcolemma and accelerates the uptake of Ca^{++} by the sarcoplasmic reticulum); and (2) G_i, which mediates the inhibition of adenylate cyclase and has the opposite effect on the movements of Ca^{++}.

Heart failure caused by dilated cardiomyopathy is associated with an increase in G_i activity and protein level in heart muscle,[205,206] which may be accompanied by a reduction in the activity of adenylate cyclase.[207] The mechanism responsible for the increase in G_i activity is not known. The level of G_i assessed by Western blotting is increased in myocardium from patients with idiopathic dilated cardiomyopathy but not from those with ischemic heart disease, suggesting that alterations in G protein function are related to the cause of heart failure.[208] The mRNA levels of G_i are not increased in myocardium of patients with heart failure,[209] further suggesting that the increase in G_i activity reflects events at the post-transcriptional level. A reduction in the function of G_s has been reported in the Syrian hamster with dilated cardiomyopathy,[210] but G_s appears normal in failing human myocardium.[205] Overall, heart failure is characterized by an increase in the ratio of $G_i : G_s$.[206,209]

The functional consequences of an increase in G_i activity remain to be established. Although an increase in G_i activity could suppress adenylate cyclase activity and thereby depress basal and beta-adrenergic receptor–stimulated responses, the responses to muscarinic agonists and adenosine, which act via G_i to inhibit adenylate cyclase, are not altered in myocardium from patients with dilated cardiomyopathy.[208]

ADRENERGIC SUPPORT OF THE FAILING HEART. The importance of the adrenergic nervous system in maintaining ventricular contractility when myocardial function is depressed in heart failure is demonstrated by the effects of adrenergic blockade. Acute pharmacological blockade of the adrenergic nervous system may cause intensification of heart failure as well as sodium and water retention.[202,211,212] The acute administration of beta blockers to patients with heart failure results in reductions in both systolic and diastolic myocardial function[213] associated with falls in cardiac output and arterial pressure, and increased filling pressures.[214] Despite the long-term salutary effects of beta-blocker therapy in patients with heart failure (see p. 486), caution should be exercised in using these agents, particularly at the initiation of therapy.

Because of the depletion of cardiac NE stores and the changes in the postsynaptic beta-adrenoceptor pathway, the capacity of the myocardium to produce cyclic AMP is diminished, sometimes profoundly, in patients with heart failure.[193,215] As a consequence, the failing heart loses an important compensatory mechanism. In patients with heart failure, downregulation of postsynaptic beta-adrenoceptors in the sinoatrial node contributes to the attenuated chronotropic response to exercise.[157] Likewise, the positive inotropic response to an intracoronary infusion of the beta-adrenergic agonist dobutamine is markedly reduced in patients with heart failure.[216] The degree of attenuation of both the chronotropic and positive inotropic responses to adrenergic stimulation are correlated with the level of baseline adrenergic activation as reflected by the concentration of plasma norepinephrine (Fig. 13–23).[157,216] An important therapeutic consequence of the alterations of the beta-adrenergic pathway described above is that the positive inotropic response to beta-adrenoceptor agonists, and to a lesser extent to phosphodiesterase inhibitors, is markedly reduced

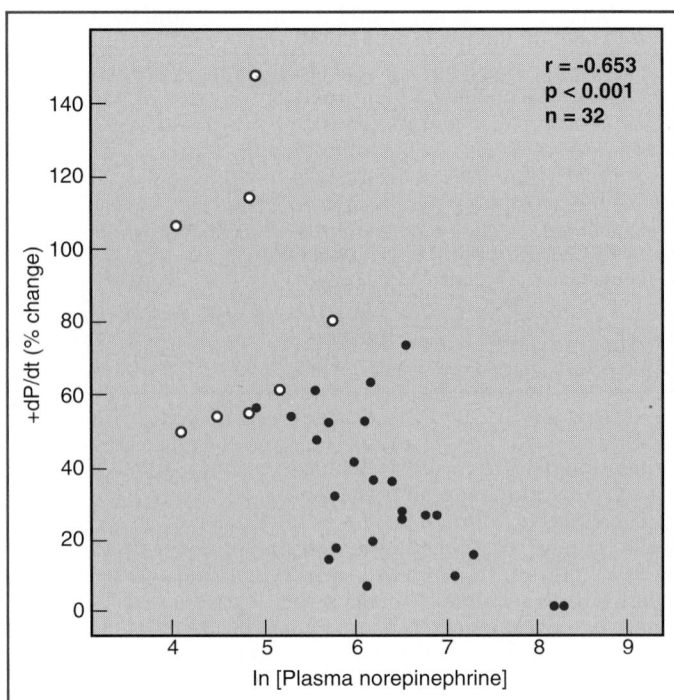

FIGURE 13–23. Relationship between plasma norepinephrine concentration and myocardial beta-adrenergic responsiveness. The positive inotropic response to an intracoronary infusion of the beta-adrenergic agonist dobutamine, as measured by an increase in +dP/dt, was inversely related to the resting level of the logarithm (ln) plasma norepinephrine in patients with heart failure (*solid circles*) or normal ventricular function (*open circles*). (Reproduced from Colucci, W. S., Denniss, A. R., Leatherman, G. F., et al.: Intracoronary infusion of dobutamine to patients with and without severe congestive heart failure. Dose-response relationships, correlation with circulating catecholamines, and effect of phosphodiesterase inhibition. J. Clin. Invest. *81*:1103, 1988, by copyright permission of the American Society for Clinical Investigation.)

in myocardium obtained from patients with end-stage heart failure.[215]

ADVERSE EFFECTS OF ADRENERGIC STIMULATION. Although increased adrenergic activity may play a compensatory role over the short term, chronic adrenergic activation may be deleterious by increasing afterload, precipitating cardiac arrhythmias, and perhaps by exerting toxic and direct receptor-mediated effects on the failing myocardium. Thus, it has been postulated that in heart failure there may be a positive feedback loop causing a vicious circle (Fig. 13–19). According to this concept, heart failure activates the adrenergic nervous system (as well as activating the renin-angiotensin system and stimulating the release of vasopressin and endothelin); this causes increases in preload and afterload that intensify heart failure.

Increased adrenergic nerve activity may also affect the growth and phenotype of the myocardium due to the direct effects of NE on alpha- and beta-adrenergic receptors located on several cell types, including cardiac myocytes, vascular smooth muscle cells, endothelial cells, and fibroblasts. NE, acting on alpha$_1$-adrenergic receptors, induces growth of both cardiac myocytes[165,217,218] and vascular smooth muscle cells.[219] In cardiac myocytes, this effect is associated with the reappearance of fetal genes and fetal isoforms of proteins involved in the development of contractile force, the regulation of myocardial energetics, and excitation-contraction coupling.[89] In addition, NE, acting on both alpha$_1$-adrenergic and beta-adrenergic receptors located on cardiac myocytes and fibroblasts,[166,220] can induce the expression of a variety of peptide growth factors that have been shown to have important effects on the growth and phenotype of myocytes and fibroblasts.[221]

Parasympathetic Function in Heart Failure

Cardiac enlargement, with or without heart failure, is associated with marked disturbances of parasympathetic as well as sympathetic function.[222] The parasympathetic restraint on sinoatrial node automaticity is markedly reduced in patients with heart failure (Fig. 13–3), who exhibit less heart rate slowing for any given elevation of systemic arterial pressure than do normal subjects. The sensitivity of the baroreceptor reflex to an increase in pressure has also been shown to be significantly reduced in dogs with heart failure.[175] Measurements of heart rate variability, which indirectly reflect autonomic nervous system function, indicate that parasympathetic activity in patients with heart failure is abnormal both at rest and in response to exercise.[223]

Abnormal parasympathetic function may also be altered at the level of the peripheral nerve and the postsynaptic receptor. Cardiomyopathic hamster hearts display a reduction in the activity of choline acetyltransferase, an enzyme that provides an estimate of the density of parasympathetic innervation,[224] and there is evidence that the density of high-affinity muscarinic receptors is reduced in the hearts of dogs with experimental heart failure.[225]

Renin-Angiotensin System
(See also pp. 819–820)

In low cardiac output states, there is activation of the renin-angiotensin system (RAS), which operates in concert with the activated adrenergic nervous–adrenal medullary system to maintain arterial pressure. These two compensatory systems are clearly coupled; stimulation of beta$_1$-adrenoceptors in the juxtaglomerular apparatus of the kidneys as a consequence of heightened adrenergic drive is a principal mechanism responsible for the release of renin in acute heart failure. Activation of the baroreceptors in the renal vascular bed by a reduction of renal blood flow is also responsible for the release of renin, and in patients with severe chronic heart failure following salt restriction and diuretic treatment, reduction of the sodium presented to the macula densa contributes to the release of renin. Elevated plasma renin activity is a common, although not universal, finding in heart failure.[151,154,226,227] In the SOLVD study, plasma angiotensin II was significantly elevated even in asymptomatic patients and was further elevated in patients with symptomatic heart failure (Fig. 13–20).[154]

Angiotensin II is a potent peripheral vasoconstrictor and contributes, along with increased adrenergic activity, to the excessive elevation of systemic vascular resistance and the vicious circle already referred to (see p. 402) in patients with heart failure. Angiotensin II also enhances the adrenergic nervous system's release of NE. Aldosterone has potent sodium-retaining properties. Therefore, it is not surprising that interruption of the renin-angiotensin-aldosterone axis by means of an angiotensin-converting enzyme inhibitor reduces system vascular resistance, diminishes afterload, and thereby elevates cardiac output in heart failure. In some patients, these compounds also exert a mild diuretic action, presumably by lowering the angiotensin II-stimulated production of aldosterone.

TISSUE RENIN ANGIOTENSIN SYSTEM (RAS). The major portion (90 to 99 per cent) of angiotensin-converting enzyme (ACE) in the body is found in tissues, and only 1 to 10 per cent is found in the circulation.[228,229] All of the necessary components of the RAS (Fig. 13–24) are likewise present in several organs and tissues, including the vasculature, heart, and kidneys. In myocardium from animals with experimental myocardial hypertrophy or failure, there is increased expression of ACE[230,231] and angiotensinogen,[232] the substrate for angiotensin I production by renin. It has been suggested that the tissue RAS may be activated during compensated heart failure at a time when activity of the circulating system can be relatively normal (Fig. 13–25).[228]

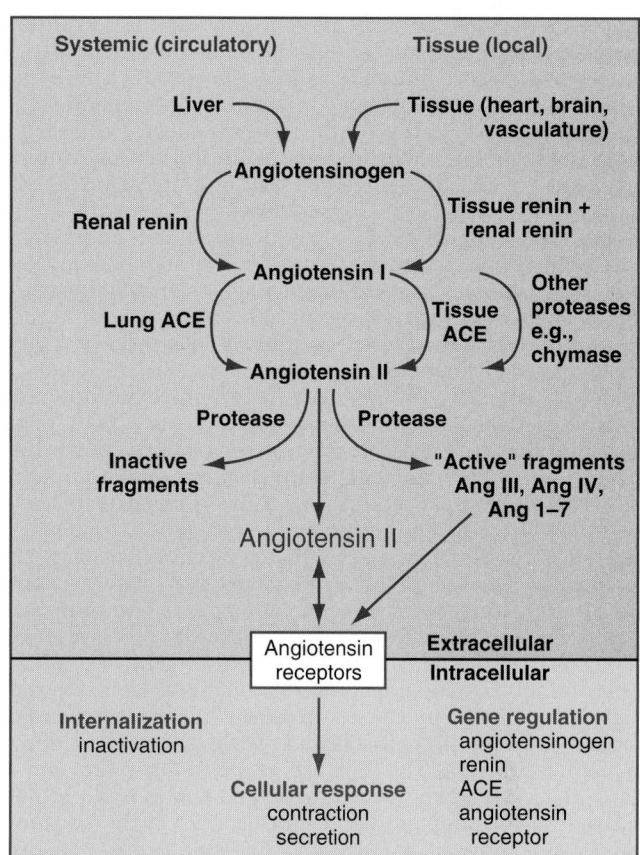

FIGURE 13–24. The systemic and tissue components of the renin-angiotensin system. Several tissues, including myocardium, vasculature, kidney, and brain, have the capacity to generate angiotensin II independent of the circulating renin-angiotensin system. Angiotensin II produced at the tissue level may play an important role in the pathophysiology of heart failure. (Modified from Timmermans, P. B., Wong, P. C., Chiu, A. T., et al.: Angiotensin II receptors and angiotensin II receptor antagonists. Pharmacol. Rev. *45:*205, 1993.)

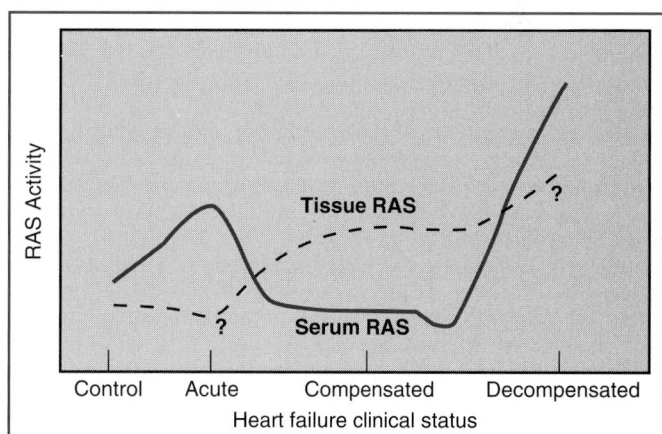

FIGURE 13–25. Relative roles of the circulating and tissue renin-angiotensin systems postulated in patients with heart failure. The tissue system may have alternative pathways for the production of angiotensin II that do not depend on converting enzyme (e.g., chymase), and which therefore are not suppressed by converting enzyme inhibitors. It has been proposed that activation of the tissue renin-angiotensin system may follow a different time course than that of the circulating system, particularly during the compensated phase of heart failure when the circulating renin-angiotensin system may be relatively quiescent and during treatment with converting enzyme inhibitors which may increase the activity of the tissue system by elevating circulating renin levels. (Modified from Dzau, V. J.: Tissue renin-angiotensin system in myocardial hypertrophy and failure. Arch. Intern. Med. *153:*937, 1993.)

and there is evidence that the activities of the tissue and circulating RAS systems can be regulated differentially in animals with heart failure.[233] The tissue production of angiotensin II may also occur by a pathway not dependent on ACE (the chymase pathway). It has been suggested that this pathway may be of major importance in the myocardium,[234] particularly when the levels of renin and angiotensin I are increased by the use of ACE inhibitors.

ANGIOTENSIN RECEPTORS. The predominant angiotensin receptor subtype in the vasculature is the angiotensin$_1$ subtype.[235] In human myocardium it appears that both angiotensin$_1$ and angiotensin$_2$ receptor subtypes are present, and the angiotensin$_2$ receptor predominates in a ratio of 2:1.[236] The number of angiotensin$_1$ and angiotensin$_2$ receptors is normal in patients with moderate heart failure but downregulated in patients with end-stage heart failure.[237] Downregulation of angiotensin receptors has been observed in myocardium from patients with both ischemic and idiopathic dilated cardiomyopathy and associated with a decrease in the mRNA level for the receptor.

Several observations suggest that a direct effect of angiotensin on cardiac angiotensin receptors may play a central role in modifying the structure and function of the myocardium in patients with heart failure by acting on a variety of cell types to promote cell growth and alter gene expression. In cardiac myocytes and fibroblasts obtained from the neonatal rat, angiotensin caused myocyte hypertrophy and fibroblast proliferation associated with the induction of mRNA for several early response genes (c-*fos*, c-*jun*, *jun B*, *Egr-1*, and c-*myc*), angiotensinogen and the peptide growth factor, transforming growth factor-beta$_1$.[238,239] In addition, angiotensin induced mRNA for the fetal genes encoding atrial natriuretic factor and alpha-skeletal actin in myocytes.[238] Because these observations were made in cultured cells, they indicate that angiotensin can exert important effects on the growth and phenotype of cardiac cells, independent of changes in loading conditions on the heart.

Arginine Vasopressin

Arginine vasopressin (AVP) is a pituitary hormone that plays a central role in the regulation of free water clearance and plasma osmolality. Circulating AVP is elevated in many patients with heart failure,[240] even after correction for plasma osmolality. Patients with acute heart failure secondary to massive myocardial infarction may have particularly elevated levels,[241] which are usually associated with elevated concentrations of catecholamines and renin. The plasma AVP concentration was significantly elevated in asymptomatic patients in the prevention arm of the SOLVD study and was elevated further in patients with symptomatic heart failure (Fig. 13–20).[154]

Control of circulating AVP concentration is abnormal in patients with heart failure who fail to show the normal reduction of AVP with a reduction of osmolality.[242] This may contribute to their inadequate ability to excrete free water and hence to the plasma hypoosmolarity in some patients with heart failure. Decreased sensitivity of atrial stretch receptors, which normally inhibit AVP release with atrial distention, may contribute to the elevation of circulating AVP.[243] In addition, patients with heart failure exhibit failure of the normal suppression of AVP following administration of ethanol[244] as well as failure of the normal augmentation of circulating AVP in response to orthostatic stress.[245]

Two types of AVP receptors (V$_1$ and V$_2$) have been identified in a variety of tissues. In dogs with pacing-induced heart failure, the selective inhibition of V$_1$ receptors increased cardiac output without affecting electrolytes or hormone levels.[245] In contrast, inhibition of V$_2$ receptors increased serum sodium concentration, plasma renin activity, and plasma AVP levels but did not affect hemodynamics.

When the two inhibitors were combined, the hemodynamic effects were potentiated. These results suggest that, in addition to regulating free water clearance through the V$_2$ receptor, in heart failure AVP may contribute to systemic vasoconstriction through the V$_1$ receptor.

Natriuretic Peptides

Three natriuretic peptides—atrial natriuretic peptide (ANP), brain natriuretic peptide (BNP), and C-natriuretic peptide (CNP)—have been identified in humans.[246] ANP is stored mainly in the right atrium and released in response to an increase in atrial distending pressure. This peptide causes vasodilation and natriuresis and counteracts the water-retaining effects of the adrenergic, renin-angiotensin, and AVP systems. BNP is stored mainly in cardiac ventricular myocardium and may be responsive—albeit less so than ANP—to changes in ventricular filling pressures.[247] BNP has a high level of homology with ANP at the structural level and, like ANP, causes natriuresis and vasodilation. CNP is located primarily in the vasculature. Although the physiological role of CNP is not yet clarified, it appears that it may play an important regulatory role in juxtaposition to the RAS system. At least three receptors for natriuretic peptides (A, B, and C) have been identified.[246] The A and B receptors mediate the vasodilatory and natriuretic effects of the peptides. The C type receptor appears to act primarily as a clearance receptor, which along with neutral endopeptidase, regulates available levels of the peptides.

Circulating levels of both ANP and BNP are elevated in the plasma of patients with heart failure.[248,249] In normal human hearts, ANP predominates in the atria, where there is also a low level of expression of BNP and CNP. In patients with heart failure, the atrial content of ANP is unchanged, and the contents of BNP and CNP increase 10-fold and 2- to 3-fold, respectively.[249] In the SOLVD study, the level of plasma ANP was elevated even in asymptomatic patients and was further elevated in patients with symptoms (Fig. 13–20).[154] Although the atrial peptides are present only in very low levels in normal ventricular myocardium, in patients with heart failure all three peptides are markedly elevated,[249] and ventricular production contributes significantly to the circulating levels.[250] The secretion of ANP and BNP appears to be regulated mainly by wall tension. The N-terminal of the ANP free-hormone (N-terminal pro-ANP) has a longer half-life and greater stability than ANP and has been shown to be a powerful and independent predictor of cardiovascular mortality and the development of heart failure.[251] ANP levels normalize following cardiac transplantation.[252]

The hemodynamic and natriuretic responses to an infusion of ANP are attenuated in patients and experimental animals with heart failure.[253,254] However, studies using an ANP receptor antagonist in dogs with pacing-induced heart failure showed that, despite attenuated hemodynamic and renal effects, the peptide continues to exert an important suppressive effect on the activity of the RAS and NE levels.[255]

One approach that attempts to capitalize on the beneficial effects of the natriuretic peptides is to inhibit their degradation through the use of neutral endopeptidase inhibitors. The infusion of the endopeptidase inhibitor candoxatrilat into patients with heart failure mimics the action of infused ANP; it causes a reduction in left and right heart filling pressures associated with suppression of plasma NE levels and a transient reduction in plasma vasopressin, aldosterone, and renin activity.[256] In addition to the beneficial effect of natriuretic peptides on neurohormones, renal function, and hemodynamics, there is evidence that the natriuretic peptides may directly inhibit myocyte and vascular smooth muscle hypertrophy and interstitial fibrosis.[257-259]

Endothelin

Endothelin is a potent peptide vasoconstrictor released by endothelial cells throughout the circulation.[260] Three endothelin peptides (endothelin-1, endothelin-2, and endothelin-3) have been identified, all of which are potent constrictors. At least two subtypes of endothelin receptors (types A and B) have been recognized. The release of endothelin from endothelial cells in vitro can be enhanced by several vasoactive agents (e.g., NE, angiotensin II, thrombin) and cytokines (e.g., transforming growth factor-beta and interleukin-1 beta).

Several reports have documented an increase in circulating levels of endothelin-1 in patients with heart failure.[261–264] Plasma endothelin correlates directly with pulmonary artery pressures and, in particular, the pulmonary vascular resistance and the resistance ratio of pulmonary vascular resistance to systemic resistance. This has led to the suggestion that endothelin plays a pathophysiological role in mediating pulmonary hypertension in patients with heart failure.[261,263]

In normal subjects, plasma endothelin levels increase with orthostatic stress. However, in heart failure patients, endothelin levels are already elevated and show no further increase with orthostatic stress, similar to the pattern of response seen with a variety of other vasoconstrictor substances, including angiotensin and NE.[262] Plasma endothelin levels have been shown to be increased in patients with acute myocardial infarction and to correlate with the Killip class in these patients.[264]

Antagonists of endothelin receptors are available and have been used to demonstrate the physiological effects of endothelin. When administered to rats with heart failure following myocardial infarction, the endothelin antagonist bosentan, which blocks both endothelin$_A$ and endothelin$_B$ receptors, significantly decreased arterial pressure and had an additive effect to that of an ACE inhibitor.[265] In cultured cardiac myocytes, endothelin induces cellular hypertrophy associated with the induction of fetal genes.[266,267] In rats with pressure overload–induced hypertrophy caused by aortic banding, administration of the endothelin$_A$ receptor antagonist BQ123 transiently inhibited myocyte hypertrophy and prevented fetal gene induction.[268] These observations suggest that endothelin receptor antagonists may be of value in both the acute and chronic treatment of patients with heart failure.

Cytokines

Several peptide mediators, including peptide growth factors and inflammatory cytokines, can have important effects on the myocardium and vasculature and appear to be involved in heart failure. Peptide growth factors can induce growth and modulate gene expression in cardiac myocytes, vascular smooth muscle cells, endothelial cells, and fibroblasts.[228] Several peptide growth factors have been shown to cause hypertrophy associated with the expression of fetal genes.[228] Peptide growth factors can be expressed by several cell types in the heart, including cardiac myocytes[166] and fibroblasts,[227] and there is increased expression of peptide growth factors in response to hemodynamic overload and NE. Increased levels of transforming growth factor-beta$_1$ have been observed in the myocardium in response to myocardial infarction in the rat.[269] These observations suggest that peptide growth factors may play a central role in mediating the changes in myocardial structure and function that occur in heart failure.

The circulating levels of the inflammatory cytokine, tumor necrosis factor-alpha (TNF-alpha) are increased in patients with heart failure.[270,271] TNF-alpha can induce immediate myocardial dysfunction and has been shown to attenuate intracellular calcium transients in vitro.[272–274] The

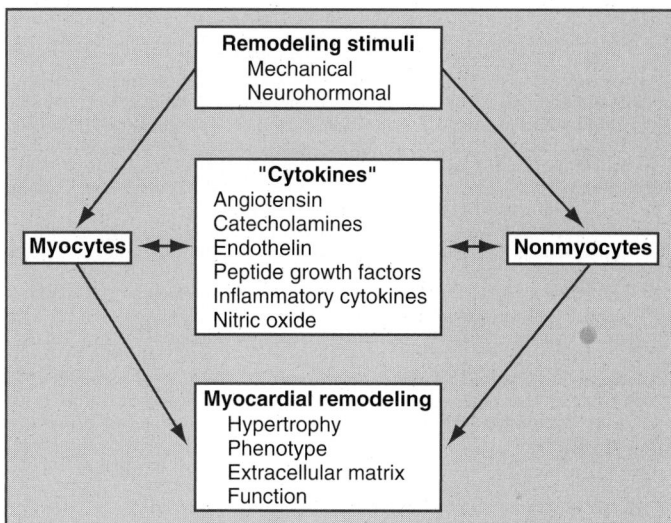

FIGURE 13–26. Central role of cell-to-cell interactions in myocardial remodeling. Both myocytes and nonmyocytes (e.g., fibroblasts, endothelial cells, vascular smooth muscle cells) in the myocardium produce a number of intercellular mediators, many of which are cytokines, that may act on neighboring cells in an autocrine or paracrine manner and thereby play a central role in modulating changes in the structure and function of the myocardium.

inflammatory cytokine, interleukin-1 beta, has been shown to induce myocyte hypertrophy in vitro,[275,276] and can induce the expression of nitric oxide synthase (NOS), resulting in increased levels of nitric oxide.[277] Nitric oxide has been shown to attenuate the positive inotropic response to a beta-adrenergic agonist in cardiac myocytes.[278,279] In normal subjects, the intracoronary infusion of nitroprusside, a nitric oxide donor, improved left ventricular distensibility,[280] whereas inhibition of nitric oxide synthesis by the intracoronary infusion of an NOS inhibitor potentiated the positive inotropic response to dobutamine in patients with left ventricular dysfunction.[281]

The role of inflammatory cytokines and nitric oxide in the pathophysiology of heart failure remains to be determined. The inflammatory cytokines may contribute to the myocardial depression that occurs in patients with inflammatory processes such as myocarditis, sepsis, and transplantation rejection. However, it also appears that inflammatory cytokines may play a role in patients without obvious inflammatory processes, such as those with ischemic and idiopathic dilated cardiomyopathy.[272] Cytokines may exert long-term effects on the remodeling of myocardial and vascular tissue and thereby contribute to the pathophysiology of chronic heart failure (Fig. 13–26). It is of interest that vesnarinone, an oral agent that appears to improve survival in patients with heart failure (see p. 485), has been shown to decrease the plasma levels of inflammatory cytokines.[282]

REFERENCES

ADAPTIVE MECHANISMS

1. Braunwald, E., Mock, M. B., and Watson, J. (eds.): Congestive Heart Failure: Current Research and Clinical Applications. New York, Grune and Stratton, 1982, 384 pp.
2. Katz, A. M.: Cardiomyopathy of overload: A major determinant of prognosis in congestive heart failure. N. Engl. J. Med. 322:100, 1990.
3. Katz, A. M.: The cardiomyopathy of overload: An unnatural growth response in the hypertrophied heart. Ann. Int. Med. 121:363, 1994.
4. Braunwald, E., Ross, J., Jr., and Sonnenblick, E. H.: Mechanisms of Contraction of the Normal and Failing Heart. 2nd ed. Boston, Little, Brown and Co., 1976, 417 pp.
5. Jennings, G. L., and Esler, M. D.: Circulatory regulation at rest and exercise and the functional assessment of patients with congestive heart failure. Circulation 81(Suppl II):5, 1990.
6. Anand, I. S., Ferrari, R., Kalra, G. S., et al.: Studies of body water and sodium, renal function, hemodynamic indexes, and plasma hormones in untreated congestive heart failure. Circulation 80:299, 1989.

7. Ross, J., Jr., and Braunwald, E.: Studies on Starling's law of the heart. IX. The effects of impeding venous return on performance of the normal and failing human left ventricle. Circulation 30:719, 1964.

8. Floras, J. S.: Clinical aspects of sympathetic activation and parasympathetic withdrawal in heart failure. J. Am. Coll. Cardiol. 22:72A, 1993.

9. Leimbach, W. N., Wallin, B. G., Victor, R. G., et al.: Direct evidence from intraneural recordings for increased central sympathetic outflow in patients with heart failure. Circulation 73:913, 1986.

10. Vanhoutte, P. M.: Adjustments in the peripheral circulation in chronic heart failure. Eur. Heart J. 4(Suppl. A):67, 1983.

11. Higgins, C. B., Vatner, S. F., Braunwald, E., et al.: Alterations in regional hemodynamics in experimental heart failure in conscious dogs. Trans. Assoc. Am. Physicians 85:267, 1972.

12. Zelis, R., Mason, D. T., and Braunwald, E.: A comparison of the effects of vasodilator stimuli on peripheral resistance vessels in normal subjects and in patients with congestive heart failure. J. Clin. Invest. 47:960, 1968.

13. Zelis, R., Mason, D. T., and Braunwald, E.: Partition of blood flow to the cutaneous and muscular beds of the forearm at rest and during leg exercise in normal subjects and in patients with heart failure. Circ. Res. 24:799, 1969.

14. Zelis, R., Sinoway, L. I., Musch, T. I., et al.: Regional blood flow in congestive heart failure. Concept of compensatory mechanisms with short and long term constants. Am. J. Cardiol. 62:2E, 1988.

15. Wilson, J. R., Mancini, D. M., McCully, K., et al.: Noninvasive detection of skeletal muscle underperfusion with near-infrared spectroscopy in patients with heart failure. Circulation 80:1668, 1989.

16. Mancini, D. M., Coyle, E., Coggan, A., et al.: Contribution of intrinsic skeletal muscle changes to 31P NMR skeletal muscle metabolic abnormalities in patients with chronic heart failure. Circulation 80:1338, 1989.

17. Wilson, J. R., and Mancini, D. M.: Factors contributing to the exercise limitation of heart failure. J. Am. Coll. Cardiol. 22(Suppl. A):93a, 1993.

18. Kubo, S. H., Rector, T. S., Bank, A. J., et al.: Endothelium-dependent vasodilatation is attenuated in patients with heart failure. Circulation 84:1589, 1991.

19. Hirooka, Y., Imaizumi, T., Tagawa, T., et al.: Effects of L-arginine on impaired acetylcholine-induced and ischemic vasodilation of the forearm in patients with heart failure. Circulation 90:658, 1994.

20. Woodson, R. D., Torrance, J. D., Shappell, S. D., and Lenfant, C.: The effect of cardiac diseases on hemoglobin-oxygen binding. J. Clin. Invest. 49:1349, 1970.

CONTRACTILITY OF HYPERTROPHIED AND FAILING MYOCARDIUM

21. Krayenbuehl, H. P., Hess, O. M., Schneider, J., and Turina, M.: Physiologic or pathologic hypertrophy. Eur. Heart J. 4(Suppl. A):29, 1983.

22. Spann, J. F., Jr., Buccino, R. A., Sonnenblick, E. H., and Braunwald, E.: Contractile state of cardiac muscle obtained from cats with experimentally produced ventricular hypertrophy and heart failure. Circ. Res. 21:341, 1967.

23. Cooper, G., IV, Tomanek, R. J., Ehrhardt, J. D., and Marcus, M. L.: Chronic progressive pressure overload of the cat right ventricle. Circ. Res. 48:488, 1981.

24. Crozatier, B., and Hittinger, L.: Mechanical adaptation to chronic pressure overload. Eur. Heart J. 9:E-7, 1988.

25. Capasso, J. M., Aronson, R. S., and Sonnenblick, E. H.: Reversible alterations in excitation-contraction coupling during myocardial hypertrophy in rat papillary muscle. Circ. Res. 51:189, 1982.

26. Chidsey, C. A., Sonnenblick, E. H., Morrow, A. G., and Braunwald, E.: Norepinephrine stores and contractile force of papillary muscle from the failing human heart. Circulation 33:43, 1966.

27. Cooper, G., IV, Puga, F., Zujko, K. J., et al.: Normal myocardial function and energetics in volume-overload hypertrophy in the cat. Circ. Res. 32:140, 1973.

28. Schwinger, R. H., Boh, M., Muller-Ehrnsen, J., et al.: Effect of inotropic stimulation on the negative force-frequency relationship in the failing human heart. Circulation 88:2267, 1993.

29. Gwathmey, J. K., Copelas, L., MacKinnon, R., et al.: Abnormal intracellular calcium handling in myocardium from patients with end-stage heart failure. Circ. Res. 61:70, 1987.

30. Dalen, H., Saetersdal, T., and Odegarden, S.: Some ultrastructural features of the myocardial cells in the hypertrophied human papillary muscle. Virchows Arch. A. 410:281, 1987.

31. Ross, J., Jr., Sonnenblick, E. H., Taylor, R. R., and Covell, J. W.: Diastolic geometry and sarcomere length in the chronically dilated canine left ventricle. Circ. Res. 28:49, 1971.

32. Spann, J. F., Jr., Covell, J. W., Eckberg, D. L., et al.: Contractile performance of the hypertrophied and chronically failing cat ventricle. Am. J. Physiol. 223:1150, 1972.

33. Alyono, D., Ring, W. S., Anderson, M. R., and Anderson, R. W.: Left ventricular adaptation to volume overload from large aortocaval fistula. Surgery 96:360, 1984.

34. Legault, D., Rouleau, J. L., Juneau, C., et al.: Functional and morphological characteristics of compensated and decompensated cardiac hypertrophy in dogs with chronic infrarenal aortocaval fistulas. Circ. Res. 66:846, 1990.

35. Carabello, B. A., Nakano, K., Corin, W., et al.: Left ventricular function in experimental volume overload hypertrophy. Am. J. Physiol. 256:H974, 1989.

MYOCARDIAL HYPERTROPHY

36. Cohn, J. N.: Structural basis for heart failure. Ventricular remodeling and its pharmacological inhibition. Circulation 91:2504, 1995.

37. Beltrami, C. A., Finato, N., Rocco, M., et al.: Structural basis of end-stage failure in ischemic cardiomyopathy in humans. Circulation 89:151, 1994.

38. Zak, R.: Cardiac hypertrophy: Biochemical and cellular relationships. Hosp. Pract. 18:85, 1983.

39. Weber, K. T., Nanicki, J. S., Schroff, S. G., Pick, R., et al.: Collagen remodeling of the pressure-overloaded, hypertrophied nonhuman primate myocardium. Circ. Res. 62:757, 1988.

40. Grossman, W., Jones, D., and McLaurin, L. P.: Wall stress and patterns of hypertrophy in the human left ventricle. J. Clin. Invest. 56:56, 1975.

41. Gunther, S., and Grossman, W.: Determinants of ventricular function in pressure overload hypertrophy in man. Circulation 59:679, 1979.

42. Donner, R., Carabello, B. A., Black, I., and Spann, J. F.: Left ventricular wall stress in compensated aortic stenosis in children. Am. J. Cardiol. 51:946, 1983.

43. Spann, J. F., Bove, A. A., Natarajean, G., and Kreulen, T.: Ventricular performance, pump function and compensatory mechanisms in patients with aortic stenosis. Circulation 82:2075, 1990.

44. Anversa, P., Ricci, R., and Olivetti, G.: Quantitative structural analyses of the myocardium during physiologic growth and induced cardiac hypertrophy: A review. J. Am. Coll. Cardiol. 7:1140, 1986.

45. Hayashida, W., Kumada, T., Nohara, R., et al.: Left ventricular regional wall stress in dilated cardiomyopathy. Circulation 82:2075, 1990.

46. Ross, J., Jr.: Afterload mismatch and preload reserve: A conceptual framework for the analysis of ventricular function. Prog. Cardiovasc. Dis. 18:255, 1976.

47. Sasayama, S., Ross, J., Jr., Franklin, D., et al.: Adaptations of the left ventricle to chronic pressure overload. Circ. Res. 38:172, 1976.

48. Pelliccia, A., Maron, B. J., Spataro, A., et al.: The upper limit of physiologic cardiac hypertrophy in highly trained elite athletes. N. Engl. J. Med. 324:295, 1991.

49. Meerson, F. Z.: The myocardium in hyperfunction, hypertrophy, and heart failure. Circ. Res. 25(Suppl. 2):1, 1969.

50. Ferrans, V. J.: Morphology of the heart in hypertrophy. Hosp. Pract. 18:67, 1983.

51. Breisch, E. A., White, F. C., and Bloor, C. M.: Myocardial characteristics of pressure overload hypertrophy: A structural and functional study. Lab. Invest. 51:333, 1984.

52. Anversa, P., Palackal, T., Sonnenblick, E. H., et al.: Myocyte cell loss and myocyte cellular hyperplasia in the hypertrophied aging rat heart. Circ. Res. 67:871, 1990.

53. Olivetti, G., Melissari, M., Capasso, J. M., and Anversa, B.: Cardiomyopathy of the aging human heart: Myocyte loss and reactive cellular hypertrophy. Circ. Res. 68:1560, 1991.

54. Pouleur, H. G., Konstam, M. A., Udelson, J. E., and Rousseau, M. F.: Changes in ventricular volume wall thickness and wall stress during progression of left ventricular dysfunction. J. Am. Coll. Cardiol. 224(Suppl. 4A):43a, 1993.

55. Aoyagi, T., Fujii, A. M., Flanagan, M. F., et al.: Transition from compensated hypertrophy to intrinsic myocardial dysfunction during development of left ventricular pressure-overload hypertrophy in conscious sheep. Systolic dysfunction precedes diastolic dysfunction. Circulation 88:2415, 1993.

56. Palmon, L. C., Reichek, N., Yeon, S. B., et al.: Intramural myocardial shortening in hypertensive left ventricular hypertrophy with normal pump function. Circulation 89:122, 1994.

57. Weinberg, E. O., Schoen, F. J., George, D., et al.: Angiotensin-converting enzyme inhibition prolongs survival and modifies the transition to heart failure in rats with pressure overload hypertrophy due to ascending aortic stenosis. Circulation 90:1410, 1994.

58. Vatner, S. F., and Hittinger, L.: Coronary vascular mechanisms involved in decompensation from hypertrophy to heart failure. J. Am. Coll. Cardiol. 224(Suppl. 4A):34a, 1993.

PATHOPHYSIOLOGY OF DIASTOLIC HEART FAILURE

59. Lenihan, D. J., Gerson, M. C., Hoit, B. D., et al.: Mechanisms, diagnosis and treatment of diastolic heart failure. Am. Heart J. 130:153, 1995.

60. Soufer, R., Wohlgelernter, D., Vita, N. A., et al.: Intact systolic left ventricular function in clinical congestive heart failure. Am. J. Cardiol. 55:1032, 1985.

61. Grossman, W.: Diastolic dysfunction in congestive heart failure. N. Engl. J. Med. 325:1557, 1991.

62. Brutsaert, D. L., Rademakers, F. E., and Sys, S. U.: Triple control of relaxation: Implications in cardiac disease. Circulation 69:190, 1984.

63. Gwathmey, J. K., Warren, S. E., Briggs, G. M., et al.: Diastolic dysfunction in hypertrophic cardiomyopathy; effect on active force generation during systole. J. Clin. Invest. 87:1023, 1991.

64. Gwathmey, J. K., and Morgan, J. P.: Altered calcium handling in experimental pressure-overload hypertrophy in the ferret. Circ. Res. 57:836, 1985.

65. Heyndrickx, G. R., and Paulus, W. J.: Effect of asynchrony on left ventricular relaxation. Circulation 81(Suppl. III):41, 1990.

66. Bonow, R. O.: Regional left ventricular nonuniformity: Effects of left ventricular diastolic function in ischemic heart disease, hypertrophic cardiomyopathy, and the normal heart. Circulation 81(Suppl. III):54, 1990.

67. Gaasch, W. H., Levine, H. J., Quinnes, M. A., and Alexander, J. K.: Left ventricular compliance: Mechanisms and clinical implications. Am. J. Cardiol. *38*:645, 1976.

68. Corin, W. J., Murakami, T., Monrad, E. S., et al.: Left ventricular passive diastolic properties in chronic mitral regurgitation. Circulation *83*:797, 1991.

69. McCullagh, W. H., Covell, J. W., and Ross, J., Jr.: Left ventricular dilatation and diastolic compliance changes during chronic volume overloading. Circulation *45*:943, 1972.

70. Lecarpentier, Y., Waldenstrom, A., Clergue, M., et al.: Major alterations in relaxation during cardiac hypertrophy induced by aortic stenosis in guinea pig. Circ. Res. *61*:107, 1987.

71. Warren, S. E., Coh, L. H., Schoen, F. J., et al.: Advanced diastolic heart failure in familial hypertrophic cardiomyopathy managed with cardiac transplantation. J. Appl. Cardiol. *3*:415, 1988.

72. Douglas, P. S., Berko, B., Lesh, M., and Reichek, N.: Alterations in diastolic function in response to progressive left ventricular hypertrophy. J. Am. Coll. Cardiol. *13*:461, 1989.

73. Williams, J. F., Jr., Potter, R. D., Hern, D. L., et al.: Hydroxyproline and passive stiffness of pressure-induced hypertrophied kitten myocardium. J. Clin. Invest. *89*:309, 1982.

74. Fifer, M. A., Bourne, K. M., Colan, S. D., and Lorell, B. H.: Early diastolic left ventricular function in children and adults with aortic stenosis. J. Am. Coll. Cardiol. *5*:1147, 1985.

75. Smith, V. E., Schulman, P., Karimeddini, M. K., et al.: Rapid ventricular filling in left ventricular hypertrophy. II. Pathologic hypertrophy. J. Am. Coll. Cardiol. *5*:869, 1985.

76. Papademetriou, V., Gottdiener, J. S., Fletcher, R. D., and Freis, E. D.: Echocardiographic assessment by computer-assisted analysis of diastolic left ventricular function and hypertrophy in borderline or mild systemic hypertension. Am. J. Cardiol. *56*:546, 1985.

77. Serizawa, T., Carabello, B. A., and Grossman, W.: Effect of pacing induced ischemia on left ventricular diastolic pressure-volume relations in dogs with coronary stenosis. Circ. Res. *46*:430, 1980.

78. Hess, O. M., Osakada, G., Lavelle, J. F., et al.: Diastolic myocardial wall stiffness and ventricular relaxation during partial and complete coronary occlusions in the conscious dog. Circ. Res. *52*:387, 1983.

79. Forrester, J., Diamond, C., Parmley, W. W., and Swan, H. J. C.: Early increase in left ventricular compliance following myocardial infarction. J. Clin. Invest. *51*:598, 1972.

80. Pirzada, F. A., Ekong, E. A., Vokonas, P. S., et al.: Experimental myocardial infarction. XIII. Sequential changes in left ventricular pressure-length relations in the acute phase. Circulation *53*:970, 1976.

81. Farhi, E. R., Canty, J. J., and Klocke, F. J.: Effects of graded reductions in coronary perfusion pressure on the diastolic pressure-segment length relation and the rate of isovolumic relaxation in the resulting conscious dog. Circulation *80*:1458, 1989.

82. Diamond, C., and Forrester, J. S.: Effect of coronary artery disease and acute myocardial infarction on left ventricular compliance in man. Circulation *45*:11, 1972.

83. Fletcher, P. J., Pfeffer, J. M., Pfeffer, M. A., and Braunwald, E.: Left ventricular diastolic pressure-volume relations in rats with healed myocardial infarction. Effects on systolic function. Circ. Res. *49*:618, 1981.

84. Vatner, S. F., Shannon, R., and Hittinger, L.: Reduced subendocardial coronary reserve: A potential mechanism for impaired diastolic function in the hypertrophied and failing heart. Circulation *81*(Suppl. III):8, 1990.

85. Weber, K. T., Jalil, J. E., Janicki, J. S., and Pick, R.: Myocardial collagen remodeling in pressure overload hypertrophy. Am. J. Hypertens. *2*:931, 1989.

86. Weber, K. T., Pick, R., Silver, M. A., et al.: Fibrillar collagen and remodeling of dilated canine left ventricle. Circulation *82*:1387, 1990.

87. Iimoto, D. S., Covell, J. W., and Harper, E.: Increase in cross-linking of Type I and Type III collagens associated with volume-overloaded hypertrophy. Circ. Res. *63*:399, 1988.

88. Chapman, D., Weber, K. T., and Eghbali, M.: Regulation of fibrillar collagen Types I and III and basement membrane Type IV collagen gene expression in pressure-overloaded rat myocardium. Circ. Res. *67*:787, 1990.

CELLULAR AND MOLECULAR MECHANISMS OF MYOCARDIAL DYSFUNCTION

89. Thaik, C. M., and Colucci, W. S.: Molecular and cellular events in myocardial hypertrophy and failure. *In* Braunwald, E. (ed.): Atlas of Heart Diseases. Heart Failure: Cardiac Function and Dysfunction. Vol. IV. Colucci, W. S. (volume ed.). St. Louis, Mosby-Year Book, 1995, p 4.2.

90. Mann, D. L., Urabe, Y., Kent, R. L., et al.: Cellular versus myocardial basis for the contractile dysfunction of hypertrophied myocardium. Circ. Res. *68*:402, 1991.

91. Morgan, J. P.: Abnormal intracellular modulation of calcium as a major cause of cardiac contractile dysfunction. N. Engl. J. Med. *325*:625, 1991.

92. Connor, T. B., Rosen, B. L., Blaustein, M. P., et al.: Hypocalcemia precipitating congestive heart failure. N. Engl. J. Med. *307*:869, 1982.

93. Levine, S. N., and Rheams, C. N.: Hypocalcemic heart failure. Am. J. Med. *78*:1033, 1985.

94. Henrich, W. L., Hunt, J. M., and Nixon, J. V.: Increased ionized calcium and left ventricular contractility during hemodialysis. N. Engl. J. Med. *310*:19, 1984.

95. Ginsburg, R., Esserman, L. J., and Bristow, M. R.: Myocardial performance and extracellular ionized calcium in a severely failing human heart. Ann. Intern. Med. *98*:603, 1983.

96. Beuckelmann, D. J., Nabauer, M., and Erdmann, E.: Intracellular calcium handling in isolated ventricular myocytes from patients with terminal heart failure. Circulation *85*:1046, 1992.

97. Hasenfuss, G., Mulieri, L. A., Leavitt, B. J., et al.: Alteration of contractile function and excitation-contraction coupling in dilated cardiomyopathy. Circ. Res. *70*:1225, 1992.

98. Hasenfuss, G., Mulieri, L. A., Blanchard, E. M., et al.: Energetics of isometric force development in control and volume-overload human myocardium: Comparison with animal species. Circ. Res. *68*:836, 1991.

99. Mulieri, L. A., Hasenfuss, G., Leavitt, B., Allen, P. D., and Alpert, N. R.: Altered myocardial force–frequency relation in human heart failure. Circulation *85*:1743, 1992.

99a. Feldman, M. D., Alderman, J. D., Aroesty, J. M., et al.: Depression of systolic and diastolic myocardial reserve during atrial pacing tachycardia in patients with dilated cardiomyopathy. J. Clin. Invest. *82*:1661, 1988.

100. Arai, M., Matsui, H., and Periasamy, M.: Sarcoplasmic reticulum gene expression in cardiac hypertrophy and heart failure. Circ. Res. *74*:555, 1994.

101. Sham, J. S. K., Jones, L. R., and Morad, M.: Phospholamban mediates the beta adrenergic–enhanced Ca^{2+} uptake in mammalian ventricular myocytes. Am. J. Physiol. *261*:H1344, 1991.

102. Luo, W., Grupp, I. L., Harrer, J., et al.: Targeted ablation of the phospholamban gene is associated with markedly enhanced myocardial contractility and loss of beta-agonist stimulation. Circ. Res. *75*:401, 1994.

103. Mercadier, J.-J., Lompre, A.-M., Duc, P., et al.: Altered sarcoplasmic reticulum Ca^{2+}-ATPase gene expression in the human ventricle during end-stage heart failure. J. Clin. Invest. *85*:305, 1990.

104. Arai, M., Alpert, N. R., MacLennan, D. H., et al.: Alterations in sarcoplasmic reticulum gene expression in human heart failure. A possible mechanism for alterations in systolic and diastolic properties of the failing myocardium. Circ. Res. *72*:463, 1993.

105. Studer, R., Reinecke, H., Bilger, J., et al.: Gene expression of the cardiac Na^+-Ca^{2+} exchanger in end-stage human heart failure. Circ. Res. *75*:443, 1994.

106. Feldman, A. M., Ray, P. E., Silan, C. M., et al.: Selective gene expression in failing human heart. Quantification of steady-state levels of messenger RNA in endomyocardial biopsies using the polymerase chain reaction. Circulation *83*:1866, 1991.

107. Sordahl, L. A., McCollum, W. B., Wood, W. G., and Schwartz, A.: Mitochondria and sarcoplasmic reticulum function in cardiac hypertrophy and failure. Am. J. Physiol. *224*:497, 1973.

108. Ito, Y., Suko, J., and Chidsey, A. A.: Intracellular calcium and myocardial contractility: V. Calcium uptake of sarcoplasmic reticulum fractions in hypertrophied and failing rabbit hearts. J. Mol. Cell. Cardiol. *6*:237, 1974.

109. Whitmer, J. T., Kumar, P., and Solaro, R. J.: Calcium transport properties of cardiac sarcoplasmic reticulum from cardiomyopathic Syrian hamsters (BIO 53.58 and 14.6): Evidence for a quantitative defect in dilated myopathic hearts not evident in hypertrophic hearts. Circ. Res. *62*:81, 1988.

110. Limas, C. J., Olivari, M.-T., Goldenberg, I. F., et al.: Calcium uptake by cardiac sarcoplasmic reticulum in human dilated cardiomyopathy. Cardiovasc. Res. *21*:601, 1987.

111. Movsesian, M. A., Karimi, M., Green, K., and Jones, L. R.: Ca^{2+}-transporting ATPase, phospholamban, and calsequestrin levels in nonfailing and failing human myocardium. Circulation *90*:653, 1994.

112. Brillantes, A.-M., Allen, P., Takahasi, T., et al.: Differences in cardiac calcium release channel (ryanodine receptor) expression in myocardium from patients with end-stage heart failure caused by ischemic versus dilated cardiomyopathy. Circ. Res. *71*:18, 1992.

113. Takahashi, T., Allen, P. D., Lacro, R. V., et al.: Expression of dihydropyridine receptor (Ca^{2+} channel) and calsequestrin genes in the myocardium of patients with end-stage heart failure. J. Clin. Invest. *90*:927, 1992.

114. Page, E., and McCallister, L. P.: Quantitative electron microscopic description of heart muscle cells. Application to normal, hypertrophied and thyroxin-stimulated hearts. Am. J. Cardiol. *31*:172, 1973.

115. Schwarz, F., Schaper, J., Kittstein, D., et al.: Reduced volume fraction of myofibrils in myocardium of patients with decompensated pressure overload. Circulation *63*:1299, 1981.

116. Hammond, E. H., Anderson, J. L., and Menlove, R. L.: Prognostic significance of myofilament loss in patients with idiopathic cardiomyopathy determined by electron microscopy. J. Am. Coll. Cardiol. *7*:204A, 1986.

117. Alpert, N. R., and Gordon, M. S.: Myofibrillar adenosine triphosphate activity in congestive failure. Am. J. Physiol. *202*:940, 1962.

118. Gordon, M. S., and Brown, A. L.: Myofibrillar adenosine triphosphate activity of human heart tissue and congestive failure: Effects of ouabain and calcium. Circ. Res. *19*:534, 1966.

119. Luchi, R. J., Dritcher, E. M., and Thyrum, P. T.: Reduced cardiac myosin adenosine triphosphate activity in dogs with spontaneously occurring heart failure. Circ. Res. *24*:513, 1969.

120. Chandler, B. M., Sonnenblick, E. H., Spann, J. R., Jr., and Pool, P. E.: Association of depressed myofibrillar adenosine triphosphatase and reduced contractility in experimental heart failure. Circ. Res. *21*:717, 1967.

121. Draper, M., Taylor, N., and Alpert, N. R.: Alteration in contractile protein in hypertrophied guinea pig hearts. *In* Alpert, N. (ed.): Cardiac Hypertrophy. New York, Academic Press, 1971, p. 315.

122. Wikman–Coffelt, J., Kamiyama, T., Salel, A. F., and Mason, D. T.: Differential responses of canine myosin ATPase activity and tissue gases in the pressure-overloaded ventricle dependent upon degree of obstruction—mild versus severe pulmonic and aortic stenosis. *In* Kobayashi, T., Yoshio, I., and Rona, G. (eds.): Recent Advances in Studies on Cardiac Structure and Metabolism. Vol. 12. Cardiac Adaption. Baltimore, University Park Press, 1978, p. 367.

123. Scheuer, J., Malhotra, A., Hirsch, C., et al.: Physiologic cardiac hypertrophy corrects contractile protein abnormalities associated with pathologic hypertrophy in rats. J. Clin. Invest. 70:1300, 1983.

124. Solaro, R. J., Powers, F. M., Gao, L., and Gwathmey, J. K.: Control of myofilament activation in heart failure. Circulation 87:VII–38, 1993.

124a. Kitsis, R. N., and Scheuer, J.: Functional significance of alterations in cardiac contractile protein isoforms. Clin. Cardiol. 19:9, 1996.

125. Walsh, R. A., Henkel, R., and Robbins, J.: Cardiac myosin heavy- and light-chain gene expression in hypertrophy and heart failure. Heart Failure 6:238, 1991.

126. Gorza, L., Pauletto, P., Pessina, A. C., et al.: Isomyosin distribution in normal and pressure-overloaded rat ventricular myocardium. An immunohistochemical study. Circ. Res. 49:1003, 1981.

127. Geenen, D. L., Malhotra, A., Scheuer, J.: Ventricular function and contractile proteins in the infarcted rat heart exposed to chronic pressure overload. Am. J. Physiol. 256:H745, 1989.

128. Scheuer, J.: Cardiac contractile proteins and congestive heart failure. J. Appl. Cardiol. 4:407, 1989.

129. Bugaisky, L. B., Anderson, P. G., Hall, R. S., and Bishop, S. P.: Differences in myosin isoform expression in the subepicardial and subendocardial myocardium during cardiac hypertrophy in the rat. Circ. Res. 66:1127, 1990.

130. Bouvagnet, P., Mairhofer, H., Leger, J. O. C., et al.: Distribution of pattern of myosin in normal and diseased human ventricular myocardium. Basic Res. Cardiol. 84:91, 1989.

131. Malhotra, A., and Scheuer, J.: Troponin-tropomyosin dysfunction in cardiomyopathy. Circulation 78:179, 1988.

132. Malhotra, A.: Regulatory proteins in hamster cardiomyopathy. Circ. Res. 66:1302, 1990.

133. Walsh, R. A., Henkel, R., and Robbins, J.: Cardiac myosin heavy- and light-chain gene expression in hypertrophy and heart disease. Heart Failure 6:238, 1991.

134. Anderson, P. A. W., Malouf, N. N., Oakeley, A. E., et al.: Troponin T isoform expression in the normal and failing human left ventricle: A correlation with myofibrillar ATPase activity. Basic Res. Cardiol. 87:175, 1992.

135. Bing, R. L.: The biochemical basis of myocardial failure. Hosp. Pract. 18:93, 1983.

136. Graham, T. P., Jr., Ross, J., Jr., and Covell, J. W.: Myocardial oxygen consumption in acute experimental cardiac depression. Circ. Res. 21:123, 1967.

137. Henry, P. D., Eckberg, D., Gault, J. H., and Ross, J., Jr.: Depressed inotropic state and reduced myocardial oxygen consumption in the human heart. Am. J. Cardiol. 31:300, 1973.

138. Sievers, R., Parmley, W. W., James, T., and Coffelt-Wilman, J.: Energy levels at systole vs. diastole in normal hamster hearts vs. myopathic hamster hearts. Circ. Res. 53:759, 1983.

139. Chidsey, C. A., Weinbach, E. C., Pool, P. E., and Morrow, A. G.: Biochemical studies of energy production in the failing human heart. J. Clin. Invest. 45:40, 1966.

140. Sobel, B. E., Spann, J. F., Jr., Pool, P. E., et al.: Normal oxidative phosphorylation in mitochondria from the failing heart. Circ. Res. 21:355, 1967.

141. Buchwald, A., Till, H., Unterberg, C., et al.: Alterations of the mitochondrial respiratory chain in human dilated cardiomyopathy. Eur. Heart J. 11:509, 1990.

142. Schulze, K., Becker, B. F., Schauer, R., and Schultheiss, H. P.: Antibodies to ADP-ATP carrier—an autoantigen in myocarditis and dilated cardiomyopathy—impair cardiac function. Circulation 81:959, 1990.

143. Ingwall, J. S.: Is cardiac failure a consequence of decreased energy reserve? Circulation 87:VII–58, 1993.

144. Conway, M. A., Allis, J., Ouwerkerk, R., et al.: Detection of low phosphocreatine to ATP ratio in failing hypertrophied human myocardium by ^{31}P magnetic resonance spectroscopy. Lancet 338:973, 1991.

145. Hardy, C. J., Weiss, R. G., Bottomley, P. A., and Gerstenblith, G.: Altered myocardial high-energy phosphate metabolites in patients with dilated cardiomyopathy. Am. Heart J. 122:795, 1991.

146. Nascimben, L., Friedrich, J., Liao, R., et al.: Enalapril treatment increases cardiac performance and energy reserve via the creatine kinase reaction in myocardium of Syrian myopathic hamsters with advanced heart failure. Circulation 91:1824, 1995.

147. Capasso, J. M., Aronson, R. S., Strobeck, J. E., and Sonnenblick, E. H.: Effects of experimental phosphate deficiency on action potential characteristics and contractile performance of rat myocardium. Cardiovasc. Res. 16:71, 1982.

148. Davis, S. V., Olichwier, K. K., and Chakko, S. C.: Reversible depression of myocardial performance in hypophosphatemia. Am. J. Med. Sci. 295:183, 1988.

149. Dzau, V. J.: Autocrine and paracrine mechanisms in the pathophysiology of heart failure. Am. J. Cardiol. 70:4C, 1992.

150. Thomas, J. A., and Marks, B. H.: Plasma norepinephrine in congestive heart failure. Am. J. Cardiol. 41:233, 1978.

151. Francis, G. S., Goldsmith, S. R., Levine, T. B., et al.: The neurohumoral axis in congestive heart failure. Ann. Intern. Med. 101:370, 1984.

152. Chidsey, C. A., Braunwald, E., and Morrow, A. G.: Catecholamine excretion and cardiac stores of norepinephrine in congestive heart failure. Am. J. Med. 39:442, 1965.

153. Viquerat, C. E., Daly, P., Swedberg, K., et al.: Endogenous catecholamine levels in chronic heart failure. A Relation to the severity of hemodynamic abnormalities. Am. J. Med. 78:455, 1985.

154. Francis, G. S., Benedict, C., Johnstone, D. E., et al.: Comparison of neuroendocrine activation in patients with left ventricular dysfunction with and without congestive heart failure. A substudy of the studies of left ventricular dysfunction (SOLVD). Circulation 82:1724, 1990.

155. Chidsey, C. A., Harrison, D. C., and Braunwald, E.: Augmentation of plasma norepinephrine response to exercise in patients with congestive heart failure. N. Engl. J. Med. 267:650, 1962.

156. Francis, G. S., Goldsmith, S. R., Ziesche, S., et al.: Relative attenuation of sympathetic drive during exercise in patients with congestive heart failure. J. Am. Coll. Cardiol. 5:832, 1985.

157. Colucci, W. S., Ribeiro, J. P., Rocco, M. B., et al.: Impaired chronotropic response to exercise in patients with congestive heart failure. Role of postsynaptic beta-adrenergic desensitization. Circulation 80:314, 1989.

158. Rose, C. P., Burgess, J. H., and Cousineau, D.: Tracer norepinephrine kinetics in coronary circulation of patients with heart failure secondary to chronic pressure and volume overload. J. Clin. Invest. 76:1740, 1985.

159. Hasking, G. J., Esler, M. D., Jennings, G. L., et al.: Norepinephrine spillover to plasma in patients with congestive heart failure: Evidence of increased overall and cardiorenal sympathetic nervous activity. Circulation 73:615, 1986.

160. Liang, C.-S., Fan, T.-H. M., Sullebarger, J. T., and Sakamoto, S.: Decreased adrenergic neuronal uptake activity in experimental right heart failure. A chamber-specific contributor to beta-adrenoceptor downregulation. J. Clin. Invest. 84:1267, 1989.

161. Leimbach, W. N., Jr., Wallin, G., Victor, R. G., et al.: Direct evidence from intrarenal recordings for increased central sympathetic outflow in patients with heart failure. Circulation 73:913, 1986.

162. Francis, G. S., Parks, R., and Cohn, J. N.: The effects of bromocriptine in patients with congestive heart failure. Am. Heart J. 106:100, 1983.

163. Cohn, J. N., Levine, T. B., Olivari, M. T., et al.: Plasma norepinephrine as a guide to prognosis in patients with chronic congestive heart failure. N. Engl. J. Med. 311:819, 1984.

164. Landzberg, J. S., Parker, J. D., Gauthier, D. F., and Colucci, W. S.: Effects of myocardial alpha$_1$-adrenergic receptor stimulation and blockade on contractility in humans. Circulation 84:1608, 1991.

165. Bisphoric, N. H., Simpson, P. C., and Ordahl, C. P.: Induction of the skeletal alpha-actin gene in alpha$_1$-adrenoreceptor-mediated hypertrophy of rat cardiac myocytes. J. Clin. Invest. 80:1194, 1987.

166. Takahashi, N., Calderone, A., Izzo, N. J., Jr., et al.: Hypertrophic stimuli induce transforming growth factor-beta$_1$ expression in rat ventricular myocytes. J. Clin. Invest. 94:1470, 1994.

167. Bristow, M. R., Minobe, W., Rasmussen, R., et al.: Alpha$_1$ adrenergic receptors in the nonfailing and failing human heart. J. Pharmacol. Exp. Ther. 247:1039, 1988.

168. Schoffer, J., Tews, A., Langes, K., et al.: Relationship between myocardial norepinephrine content and left ventricular function—an endomyocardial biopsy study. Eur. Heart J. 8:748, 1987.

169. Chidsey, C. A., Kaiser, G. A., Sonnenblick, E. H., and Braunwald, E.: Cardiac norepinephrine stores in experimental heart failure. J. Clin. Invest. 43:2386, 1964.

170. Spann, J. F., Jr., Sonnenblick, E. H., Cooper, T., and Braunwald, E.: Cardiac norepinephrine stores and the contractile state of heart muscle. Circ. Res. 19:317, 1966.

171. Covell, J. W., Chidsey, C. A., and Braunwald, E.: Reduction of the cardiac response to postganglionic sympathetic nerve stimulation in experimental heart failure. Circ. Res. 19:51, 1966.

172. Pool, P. E., Covell, J. W., Levitt, M., et al.: Reduction of cardiac tyrosine hydroxylase activity in experimental congestive heart failure. Its role in depletion of cardiac norepinephrine stores. Circ. Res. 20:349, 1967.

173. Sole, M. J.: Alterations in sympathetic and parasympathetic neurotransmitter activity: *In* Braunwald, E., Mock, M. B., and Watson, J. (eds.): Congestive Heart Failure: Current Research and Clinical Applications. New York, Grune and Stratton, 1982, p. 101.

174. Henderson, E. B., Kahn, J. K., Dorbett, J. R., et al.: Abnormal I-123 Metaoidobenzylguanidine myocardial washout and distribution may reflect myocardial adrenergic derangement in patients with congestive cardiomyopathy. Circulation 78:1192, 1988.

175. Higgins, C. B., Vatner, S. F., Eckberg, D. L., and Braunwald, E.: Alterations in the baroreceptor reflex in conscious dogs with heart failure. J. Clin. Invest. 51:715, 1972.

176. White, C. W.: Reversibility of abnormal arterial baroreflex control of heart rate in heart failure. Am. J. Physiol. 241:H778, 1981.

177. Levine, T. B., Francis, G. S., Goldsmith, S. R., and Cohn, J. N.: The neurohumoral and hemodynamic response to orthostatic tilt in patients with congestive heart failure. Circulation 67:1070, 1983.

178. Goldsmith, S. R., Francis, G. S., Levine, T. B., and Cohn, J. N.: Regional blood flow response to orthostasis in patients with congestive heart failure. J. Am. Coll. Cardiol. 1:1391, 1983.

179. Kubo, S. H., and Cody, R. J.: Circulatory autoregulation in chronic congestive heart failure: Responses to head-up tilt in 41 patients. Am. J. Cardiol. 52:512, 1983.

180. Ferguson, D. W., Abboud, F. M., and Mark, A. L.: Selective impairment of baroreflex-mediated vasoconstrictor responses in patients with ventricular dysfunction. Circulation 69:451, 1984.

181. Marin-Neto, J. A., Pintya, A. O., Gallo, L., Jr., and Maciel, B. C.: Abnormal baroreflex control of heart rate in decompensated congestive heart failure and reversal after compensation. Am. J. Cardiol. 67:604, 1991.

182. Levine, T. B., Olivari, T., and Cohn, J. N.: Dissociation of the responses of the renin-angiotensin system and sympathetic nervous system to a vasodilator stimulus in congestive heart failure. Int. J. Cardiol. 12:165, 1986.

183. Stone, G. W., Kubo, S. H., and Cody, R. J.: Adverse influence of baroreceptor dysfunction on upright exercise in congestive heart failure. Am. J. Med. 80:799, 1986.

184. Thoren, P., and Ricksten, S.-E.: Cardiac C-fiber endings in cardiovascular control under normal and pathophysiological conditions. In Abboud, F. M., Fozzard, H. A., Gilmore, J. P., and Reis, D. J. (eds.): Disturbances in Neurogenic Control of the Circulation. Bethesda, MD, Am. Physiol. Soc., 1981, p. 17.

185. Zucker, I. H., Earle, A. M., and Gilmore, J. P.: The mechanism of adaptation of left atrial stretch receptors in dogs with chronic congestive heart failure. J. Clin. Invest. 60:323, 1977.

186. Zucker, I. H., Earle, A. M., and Gilmore, J. P.: Changes in the sensitivity of left atrial receptors following reversal of heart failure. Am. J. Physiol. 237:H555, 1979.

187. Riegger, G. A. J., Leibau, G., and Kocksiek, K.: Antidiuretic hormone in congestive heart failure. Am. J. Med. 72:49, 1982.

188. Wang, W., Chen, J.-S., and Zucker, I. H.: Carotid sinus baroreceptor sensitivity in experimental heart failure. Circulation 81:1959, 1990.

189. Ellenbogen, K. A., Mohanty, P. K., Szentpetery, S., and Thames, M. D.: Arterial baroreflex abnormalities in heart failure. Reversal after orthotopic cardiac transplantation. Circulation 79:51, 1989.

190. Leier, C. V., Binkley, P. F., and Cody, R. J.: Alpha-adrenergic component of the sympathetic nervous system in congestive heart failure. Circulation 82:168, 1990.

191. Kubo, S. H., Rector, T. S., Heifets, S. M., and Cohn, J. N.: Alpha$_2$-receptor–mediated vasoconstriction in patients with congestive heart failure. Circulation 80:1660, 1989.

192. Higgins, C. B., Vatner, S. F., Millard, R. W., et al.: Alterations in regional hemodynamics in experimental heart failure in conscious dogs. Trans. Assoc. Am. Physicians 85:267, 1972.

193. Bristow, M. R.: Changes in myocardial and vascular receptors in heart failure. J. Am. Coll. Cardiol. 22:61A, 1993.

194. Bristow, M. R., Minobe, W., Rasmussen, R., et al.: Beta-adrenergic neuroeffector abnormalities in the failing human heart are produced by local rather than systemic mechanisms. J. Clin. Invest. 89:803, 1992.

195. Fowler, M. B., Laser, J. A., Hopkins, G. L., et al.: Assessment of the beta-adrenergic receptor pathway in the intact failing human heart. Circulation 74:1290, 1986.

196. Bristow, M. R., Ginsburg, R., Umans, V., et al.: Beta$_1$- and beta$_2$-adrenergic–receptor subpopulations in nonfailing and failing human ventricular myocardium: Coupling of both receptor subtypes to muscle contraction and selective beta$_1$-receptor downregulation in heart failure. Circ. Res. 59:297, 1986.

197. Bristow, M. R., Hershberger, R. E., Port, J. D., and Rasmussen, R.: Beta$_1$- and beta$_2$-adrenergic receptor–mediated adenylate cyclase stimulation in nonfailing and failing human ventricular myocardium. Mol. Pharmacol. 35:295, 1989.

198. Bristow, M. R., Anderson, F. L., Port, J. D., et al.: Differences in beta-adrenergic neuroeffector mechanisms in ischemic versus idiopathic dilated cardiomyopathy. Circulation 84:1024, 1991.

199. Woodley, S. L., Gilbert, E. M., Anderson, J. L., et al.: Beta-blockade with bucindolol in heart failure caused by ischemic versus idiopathic dilated cardiomyopathy. Circulation 84:2426, 1991.

200. Ungerer, M., Bohm, M., Elce, J. S., et al.: Altered expression of beta-adrenergic receptor kinase and beta$_1$-adrenergic receptors in the failing human heart. Circulation 87:454, 1990.

201. Bristow, M. R., Minobe, W. A., Raynolds, M. V., et al.: Reduced beta-1 receptor messenger RNA abundance in the failing human heart. J. Clin. Invest. 92:2737, 1993.

202. Gaffney, T. E., and Braunwald, E.: Importance of the adrenergic nervous system in the support of circulatory function in patients with congestive heart failure. Am. J. Med. 34:320, 1963.

203. Hausdorff, W. P., Caron, M. G., and Lefkowitz, R. J.: Turning off the signal: Desensitization of beta-adrenergic receptor function. FASEB J. 4:2881, 1990.

204. Heilbrunn, S. M., Shah, P., Bristow, M. R., et al.: Increased beta-receptor density and improved hemodynamic response to catecholamine stimulation during long-term metoprolol therapy in heart failure from dilated cardiomyopathy. Circulation 79:483, 1989.

205. Feldman, A. M., Gates, A. E., Veazey, W. B., et al.: Increase of the 40,000-mol wt pertussis toxin substrate (G protein) in the failing human heart. J. Clin. Invest. 82:189, 1988.

206. Neumann, J., Schmitz, W., Scholz, H., et al.: Increase in myocardial G$_i$ proteins in heart failure. Lancet 22:936, 1988.

207. Denniss, A. R., Marsh, J. D., Quigg, R. J., et al.: Beta-adrenergic receptor number and adenylate cyclase function in denervated transplanted and cardiomyopathic human hearts. Circulation 79:1028, 1989.

208. Böhm, M., Gierschik, P., Jakobs, K.-H., et al.: Increase of G$_i$ in human hearts with dilated but not ischemic cardiomyopathy. Circulation 82:1249, 1990.

209. Feldman, A. M., Ray, P. E., and Bristow, M. R.: Expression of alpha-subunits of G proteins in failing human heart: A reappraisal utilizing quantitative polymerase chain reaction. J. Mol. Cell. Cardiol. 23:1355, 1991.

210. Feldman, A. M., Tena, R. G., Kessler, P. D., et al.: Diminished beta-adrenergic responsiveness and cardiac dilatation in hearts of myopathic Syrian hamsters (BIO 53,58) are associated with a function abnormality of the G stimulatory protein. Circulation 81:1341, 1990.

211. Epstein, S. E., and Braunwald, E.: The effect of beta-adrenergic blockade on patterns of urinary sodium excretion: Studies in normal subjects and in patients with heart disease. Ann. Intern. Med. 75:20, 1966.

212. Vogel, J. H. K., and Chidsey, C. A.: Cardiac adrenergic activity in experimental heart failure assessed with beta-receptor blockade. Am. J. Cardiol. 24:198, 1969.

213. Haber, H. L., Simek, C. L., Gimple, L. W., et al.: Why do patients with congestive heart failure tolerate the initiation of beta blocker therapy? Circulation 88:1610, 1993.

214. Hjalmarson, A., and Waagstein, F.: Use of beta blockers in the treatment of dilated cardiomyopathy. In Gwathmey, J. D., Briggs, G. M., and Allen, P. D. (eds.): Heart Failure. Basic Science and Clinical Aspects. Marcel Dekker, New York, 1993, p. 223.

215. Feldman, M. D., Copelas, L., Gwathmey, J. K., et al.: Deficient production of cyclic AMP: Pharmacologic evidence of an important cause of contractile dysfunction in patients with end-stage heart failure. Circulation 75:331, 1987.

216. Colucci, W. S., Denniss, A. R., Leatherman, G. F., et al.: Intracoronary infusion of dobutamine to patients with and without severe congestive heart failure. Dose-response relationships, correlation with circulating catecholamines, and effect of phosphodiesterase inhibition. J. Clin. Invest. 81:1103, 1988.

217. Simpson, P., and McGrath, A.: Norepinephrine-stimulated hypertrophy of cultured rat myocardial cells is an alpha$_1$-adrenergic response. J. Clin. Invest. 72:732, 1983.

218. Iwaki, K., Sukhatme, V. P., Shubeita, H. E., and Chien, K. R.: α- and β-adrenergic stimulation induces distinct patterns of immediate early gene expression in neonatal rat myocardial cells. J. Biol. Chem. 265:13809, 1990.

219. Nakaki, T., Nakayama, M., Yamamoto, S., and Kato, R.: α$_1$-Adrenergic stimulation and beta$_2$-adrenergic inhibition of DNA synthesis in vascular smooth muscle cells. Molec. Pharmacol. 37:30, 1990.

220. Long, C. S., Hartogensis, W. E., and Simpson, P. C.: Beta-adrenergic stimulation of cardiac non-myocytes augments the growth-promoting activity of non-myocyte conditioned medium. J. Mol. Cell. Cardiol. 25:915, 1993.

221. Schneider, M. D., and Parker, T. G.: Cardiac myocytes as targets for the action of peptide growth factors. Circulation 81:1443, 1990.

222. Eckberg, D. L., Drabinsky, M., and Braunwald, E.: Defective cardiac parasympathetic control in patients with heart disease. N. Engl. J. Med. 285:877, 1971.

223. Arai, Y., Saul, J. P., Albrecht, P., et al.: Modulation of cardiac autonomic activity during and immediately after exercise. Am. J. Physiol. 256:H132, 1989.

224. Roskoski, R., Jr., Schmid, P. G., Mayer, H. E., and Abboud, F. M.: In vitro acetylcholine biosynthesis in normal and failing guinea pig hearts. Circ. Res. 36:547, 1975.

225. Vatner, D. E., Lee, D. L., Schwarz, K. R., et al.: Impaired cardiac muscarinic receptor function in dogs with heart failure. J. Clin. Invest. 81:1836, 1988.

226. Levine, T. B., Francis, G. S., Goldsmith, S. R., et al.: Activity of the sympathetic nervous system and renin-angiotensin system assessed by plasma hormone levels and their relation to hemodynamic abnormalities in congestive heart failure. Am. J. Cardiol. 49:1659, 1982.

227. Kluger, J., Cody, R. J., and Laragh, J. H.: The contributions of sympathetic tone and the renin-angiotensin system to severe chronic congestive heart failure. Response to specific inhibitors (prazosin and captopril). Am. J. Cardiol. 49:1667, 1982.

228. Dzau, V. J.: Tissue renin-angiotensin system in myocardial hypertrophy and failure. Arch. Int. Med. 153:937, 1993.

229. Dzau, V. J., and Re, R.: Tissue angiotensin system in cardiovascular medicine. A paradigm shift? Circulation 89:493, 1994.

230. Hirsch, A. T., Talsness, C. E., Schunkert, H., et al.: Tissue-specific activation of cardiac angiotensin converting enzyme in experimental heart failure. Circ. Res. 69:475, 1991.

231. Schunkert, H., Dzau, V. J., Tang, S. S., et al.: Increased rat cardiac angiotensin converting enzyme activity and mRNA expression in pressure overload left ventricular hypertrophy. Effects on coronary resistance, contractility, and relaxation. J. Clin. Invest. 86:1913, 1990.

232. Lindpaintner, K., Lu, W., Niedermajer, N., et al.: Selective activation of cardiac angiotensinogen gene expression in post-infarction ventricular remodeling in the rat. J. Mol. Cell. Cardiol. 25:133, 1993.

233. Huang, H., Arnal, J.-F., Llorens-Cortes, C., et al.: Discrepancy between plasma and lung angiotensin-converting enzyme activity in experimental congestive heart failure. A novel aspect of endothelium dysfunction. Circ. Res. 75:454, 1994.

234. Urata, H., Healy, B., Stewart, R. W., et al.: Angiotensin II-forming pathways in normal and failing human hearts. Circ. Res. *66*:883, 1990.

235. Timmermans, P. B., Wong, P. C., Chiu, A. T., et al.: Angiotensin II receptors and angiotensin II receptor antagonists. Pharmacol. Rev. *45*:205, 1993.

236. Regitz-Zagrosek, V., Friedel, N., Heymann, A., et al.: Regulation, chamber localization, and subtype distribution of angiotensin II receptors in human hearts. Circulation *91*:1461, 1995.

237. Nozawa, Y., Haruno, A., Oda, N., et al.: Angiotensin II receptor subtypes in bovine and human ventricular myocardium. J. Pharmacol. Exp. Ther. *270*:566, 1994.

238. Sadoshima, J.-I., and Izumo, S.: Molecular characterization of angiotensin II-induced hypertrophy of cardiac myocytes and hyperplasia of cardiac fibroblasts. Critical role of the AT_1 receptor subtype. Circ. Res. *73*:413, 1993.

239. Crawford, D. C., Chobanian, A. V., and Brecher, P.: Angiotensin II induces fibronectin expression associated with cardiac fibrosis in the rat. Circ. Res. *74*:727, 1994.

240. Goldsmith, S. R., Francis, G. S., and Cowley, A. W.: Arginine vasopressin and the renal response to water loading in congestive heart failure. Am. J. Cardiol. *58*:295, 1986.

241. Schaller, M.-D., Nussberger, J., Feihl, F., et al.: Clinical and hemodynamic correlates of elevated plasma arginine vasopressin after acute myocardial infarction. Am. J. Cardiol. *60*:1178, 1987.

242. Goldsmith, S. R.: Control of arginine vasopressin and congestive heart failure. Am. J. Cardiol. *71*:629, 1993.

243. Greenberg, T. T., Richmond, W. H., Stocking, R. A., et al.: Impaired atrial receptor responses in dogs with heart failure due to tricuspid insufficiency and pulmonary artery stenosis. Circ. Res. *32*:424, 1973.

244. Goldsmith, S. R., and Dodge, D.: Response of plasma vasopressin to ethanol in congestive heart failure. Am. J. Cardiol. *55*:1354, 1985.

245. Naitoh, M., Suzuki, H., Murakami, M., et al.: Effects of oral AVP receptor antagonists OPC-21268 and OPC-31260 on congestive heart failure in conscious dogs. Am. J. Physiol. *267*:H2245, 1994.

246. Struthers, A. D.: Ten years of natriuretic peptide research: A new dawn for their diagnostic and therapeutic use? Br. Med. J. *308*:1615, 1994.

247. Moe, G. W., Grima, E. A., Wong, N. L., et al.: Dual natriuretic peptide system in experimental heart failure. J. Am. Coll. Cardiol. *22*:891, 1993.

248. Yoshimura, M., Yasue, H., Okumura, K., et al.: Different secretion patterns of atrial natriuretic peptide and brain natriuretic peptide in patients with congestive heart failure. Circulation *87*:464, 1993.

249. Wei, C. M., Heublein, D. M., Perrella, M. A., et al.: Natriuretic peptide system in human heart failure. Circulation *88*:1004, 1993.

250. Yasue, H., Yoshimura, M., Sumida, H., et al.: Localization and mechanism of secretion of B-type natriuretic peptide in comparison with those of A-type natriuretic peptide in normal subjects and patients with heart failure. Circulation *90*:195, 1994.

251. Hall, C., Rouleau, J. L., Moye, L., et al.: N-terminal proatrial natriuretic factor. An independent predictor of long-term prognosis after myocardial infarction. Circulation *89*:1934, 1994.

252. Weston, M. W., Cintron, G. B., Giordano, A. T., and Vesely, D. L.: Normalization of circulating atrial natriuretic peptides in cardiac transplant recipients. Am. Heart J. *127*:129, 1994.

253. Cody, R. J., Atlas, S. A., Laragh, J. H., et al.: Atrial natriuretic factor in normal subjects and heart failure patients: Plasma levels and renal, hormonal, and hemodynamic responses to peptide infusion. J. Clin. Invest. *78*:1362, 1986.

254. Kohzuki, M., Hodsman, G. P., and Johnston, C. I.: Attenuated response to atrial natriuretic peptide in rats with myocardial infarction. Am. J. Physiol. *256*:H533, 1989.

255. Wada, A., Tsutamoto, T., Matsuda, Y., and Kinoshita, M.: Cardiorenal and neurohumoral effects of endogenous atrial natriuretic peptide in dogs with severe congestive heart failure using a specific antagonist for guanylate cyclase-coupled receptors. Circulation *89*:2232, 1994.

256. Münzel, T., Kurz, S., Holtz, J., et al.: Neurohormonal inhibition and hemodynamic unloading during prolonged inhibition of ANF degradation in patients with severe chronic heart failure. Circulation *86*:1089, 1992.

257. Calderone, A., Takahashi, N., Thaik, C. M., and Colucci, W. S.: Atrial natriuretic factor and cyclic guanosine monophosphate modulate cardiac myocyte growth and phenotype. Circulation *90*(Suppl. I):I-317, 1994.

258. Itoh, H., Pratt, R. E., and Dzau, V. J.: Atrial natriuretic polypeptide inhibits hypertrophy of vascular smooth cells. J. Clin. Invest. *86*:1690, 1990.

259. Cao, L., and Gardner, D. G.: Natriuretic peptides inhibit DNA synthesis in cardiac fibroblasts. Hypertension *25*:227, 1995.

260. Yanagisawa, M., Kurihara, H., Kimura, S., et al.: A novel potent vasoconstrictor peptide produced by vascular endothelial cells. Nature *332*:411, 1988.

261. Cody, R. J., Haas, G. J., Binkley, P. F., Capers, Q., and Kelley, R.: Plasma endothelin correlates with the extent of pulmonary hypertension in patients with chronic congestive heart failure. Circulation *85*:504, 1992.

262. Stewart, D. J., Cernacek, P., Costello, K. B., and Rouleau, J. L.: Elevated endothelin-1 in heart failure and loss of normal response to postural change. Circulation *85*:510, 1992.

263. Tsutamoto, T., Wada, A., Maeda, Y., et al.: Relation between endothelin-1 spillover in the lungs and pulmonary vascular resistance in patients with chronic heart failure. J. Am. Coll. Cardiol. *23*:1427, 1994.

264. Tomoda, H.: Plasma endothelin-1 in acute myocardial infarction with heart failure. Am. Heart J. *125*:667, 1993.

265. Teerlink, J. R., Loffler, B. M., Hess, P., et al.: Role of endothelin in the maintenance of blood pressure in conscious rats with chronic heart failure. Acute effects of the endothelin receptor antagonist Ro 47-0203 (bosentan). Circulation *90*:2510, 1994.

266. Shubeita, H. E., McDonough, P. M., Harris, A. N., et al.: Endothelin induction of inositol phospholipid hydrolysis, sarcomere assembly, and cardiac gene expression in ventricular myocytes. A paracrine mechanism for myocardial cell hypertrophy. J. Biol. Chem. *265*:20555, 1990.

267. Ito, H., Hirata, Y., Hiroe, M., et al.: Endothelin-1 induces hypertrophy with enhanced expression of muscle-specific genes in cultured neonatal rat cardiomyocytes. Circ. Res. *69*:209, 1991.

268. Ito, H., Hiroe, M., Hirata, Y., et al.: Endothelin ET_A receptor antagonist blocks cardiac hypertrophy provoked by hemodynamic overload. Circulation *89*:2198, 1994.

269. Casscells, W., Bazoberry, F., Speir, E., et al.: Transforming growth factor-beta1 in normal heart and in myocardial infarction. Ann. NY Acad. Sci. *593*:148, 1990.

270. Levine, B., Kalman, J., Mayer, L., Fillit, H. M., and Packer, M.: Elevated circulating levels of tumor necrosis factor in severe chronic heart failure. N. Engl. J. Med. *323*:236, 1990.

271. McMurray, J., Abdullah, I., Dargie, H. J., and Shapiro, D.: Increased concentrations of tumor necrosis factor in "cachectic" patients with severe chronic heart failure. Br. Heart J. *66*:356, 1991.

272. Mann, D. L., and Young, J. B.: Basic mechanisms in congestive heart failure. Recognizing the role of proinflammatory cytokines. Chest *105*:897, 1994.

273. Finkel, M. S., Oddis, C. V., Jacob, T. D., et al.: Negative inotropic effects of cytokines on the heart mediated by nitric oxide. Science *257*:387, 1992.

274. Yokoyama, T., Vaca, L., Rossen, R. D., et al.: Cellular basis for the negative inotropic effects of tumor necrosis factor-alpha in the adult mammalian heart. J. Clin. Invest. *92*:2303, 1993.

275. Thaik, C. M., Calderone, A., Takahashi, N., and Colucci, W. S.: Interleukin-1 beta modulates the growth and phenotype of neonatal rat cardiac myocytes. J. Clin. Invest. *96*:1093, 1995.

276. Palmer, J. N., Hartogensis, W. E., Patten, M., Fortuin, F. D., and Long, C. S.: Interleukin-1 beta induces cardiac myocyte growth but inhibits cardiac fibroblast proliferation in culture. J. Clin. Invest. *95*:2555, 1995.

277. Tsujino, M., Hirata, Y., Imai, T., et al.: Induction of nitric oxide synthase gene by interleukin-1 beta in cultured rat cardiocytes. Circulation *90*:375, 1994.

278. Balligand, J.-L., Kelly, R. A., Marsden, P. A., Smith, T. W., and Michel, T.: Control of cardiac muscle cell function by an endogenous nitric oxide signaling system. Proc. Natl. Acad. Sci. *90*:347, 1993.

279. Hare, J. M., and Colucci, W. S.: Role of nitric oxide in the regulation of myocardial function. Prog. Cardiovasc. Dis. *38*:1, 1995.

280. Paulus, W. J., Vantrimpont, P. J., and Shah, A. M.: Acute effects of nitric oxide on left ventricular relaxation and diastolic distensibility in humans. Assessment by bicoronary sodium nitroprusside infusion. Circulation *89*:2070, 1994.

281. Hare, J. M., Loh, E., Creager, M. A., and Colucci, W. S.: Nitric oxide inhibits the positive inotropic response to beta-adrenergic stimulation in humans with left ventricular dysfunction. Circulation *92*:2198, 1995.

282. Matsumori, A., Shioi, T., Yamada, T., et al.: Vesnarinone, a new inotropic agent, inhibits cytokine production by stimulated human blood from patients with heart failure. Circulation *89*:955, 1994.

Chapter 14
Assessment of Cardiac Function

WILLIAM C. LITTLE, EUGENE BRAUNWALD

THEORETICAL CONSIDERATIONS

Reasons to Focus on Left Ventricle

The cardiovascular system supplies the tissues with oxygen and metabolic substrates and removes carbon dioxide and other products of metabolism. This requires the integration of all of its components (venous circulation, right heart, pulmonary vascular system, left heart, arterial circulation, and blood). Most (but not all) circulatory dysfunction of cardiac origin in adults is due to abnormalities of the left heart. Thus the clinical evaluation of cardiac function predominantly involves assessment of the performance of the left ventricle.

Levels of Integration: Myocardium, Pump, Cardiac Output

The performance of the left ventricle as a pump depends on the contraction of the sarcomeres in the myocardium as well as the configuration of the left ventricular chamber and loading conditions. Ultimately the interaction of the left ventricle, the other cardiac chambers, and the arterial, pulmonary, and venous circulations results in the cardiac output. Thus, cardiac function can be evaluated at several levels of integration: (1) myocardial function, (2) chamber (usually left ventricular) pump performance, and (3) integrated cardiac output. It is important to recognize at which level of integration cardiac function is being evaluated. For example, changes in cardiac output or the level of left ventricular pump function can result from many factors and do not merely reflect myocardial contractility.[1] Thus, measurement of cardiac output alone provides a limited and insensitive assessment of ventricular function or of myocardial contractility. Furthermore, evaluation of left ventricular pump function alone cannot assess the adequacy of cardiac output or the level of myocardial contractility.

Factors Controlling Myocardial Function

As described in Chapter 13, myocardial shortening is determined by four factors: (1) preload, (2) afterload, (3) contractility, (4) and heart rate and cardiac rhythm. *Preload* is proportional to the stretch of the myocardium prior to stimulation and reflects the initial sarcomere length. Within the physiological range, the greater the preload the stronger the contraction and the greater the extent of shortening. *Afterload* is the load that the myocardium must bear to contract; the greater the afterload the less the amount of shortening. *Myocardial contractility* refers to a fundamental property of cardiac tissue reflecting the level of activation, and the formation and cycling of the cross bridges between actin and myosin filaments (Fig. 12–5, p. 365). At constant preload and afterload, increased contractility results in a greater extent and velocity of shortening. The final deter-

minants of cardiac function are the *heart rate* and *rhythm*. Within wide limits, with increasing rate there is enhancement of contractility (positive force-frequency relation). These factors (preload, afterload, contractility, rate, and rhythm) represent a simplification of the fundamental processes, since at the level of the sarcomere, load, contractility, and frequency are interrelated.[2,3]

Left Ventricle in Pressure-Volume Plane: Transformation of Myocardial to Pump Function

The transformation of myocardial function to left ventricular pump function can be understood by plotting the cardiac cycle in the pressure-volume plane.

LEFT VENTRICULAR PRESSURE-VOLUME LOOP. The relationship between left ventricular pressure and volume in a normal ejecting beat is shown in Figure 14–1. Contraction of the left ventricular myocardium begins at end diastole. The energy of the contraction is first utilized to increase ventricular pressure to the level of aortic diastolic pressure without a change in volume as the aortic and mitral valves are closed. When left ventricular pressure exceeds aortic pressure, the aortic valve opens. Myocardial fibers shorten as blood is ejected through the open aortic valve, and ventricular volume decreases. After the contraction reaches its peak at end systole, the myocardial fibers begin to relax, and when left ventricular pressure falls below aortic pressure, the aortic valve closes and cardiac ejection stops. Then, as the ventricle relaxes, ventricular pressure declines rapidly. With opening of the mitral valve, left ventricular filling begins, and the left ventricular pressure-volume loop is completed.

When cardiac ejection is prevented in an experimental preparation, peak isovolumetric left ventricular pressure increases as diastolic pressure increases, describing a straight line in the physiological range.[4,5] This is the end-systolic pressure-volume relation (ESPVR). Similarly, the upper left corner of the pressure-volume loops of variably loaded beats, denoted as end systole in Figure 14–1, fall close to isovolumetric ESPVR. The slope of this line, end-systolic elastance, termed E_{ES}, has units of pressure per volume and denotes the maximum stiffness or *elastance* of the left ventricle. The slope and position of the ESPVR respond to changes in myocardial contractile state. An increase in contractility increases the slope of the ESPVR, shifting the line toward the left in the physiological range. Conversely, the ESPVR flattens and shifts to the right when there is depressed myocardial contractile function. Thus the position and slope of the ESPVR can be used to measure contractile state (see below).

421

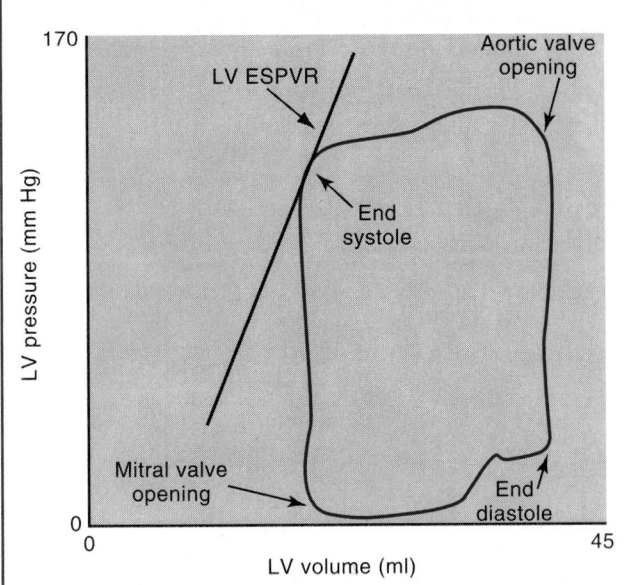

FIGURE 14–1. A left ventricular (LV) pressure-volume loop describing one cardiac cycle. At end diastole the mitral valve closes. The left ventricle is a closed chamber as the pressure increases without a change in volume during isovolumetric contraction. When left ventricular pressure exceeds aortic pressure, the aortic valve opens. During left ventricular ejection, left ventricular volume falls. Aortic valve closure occurs near the time of end systole. Following aortic valve closure, left ventricular pressure falls without a change in left ventricular volume until left ventricular pressure falls below left atrial pressure and mitral valve opening occurs. During diastole left ventricular volume increases, completing the cardiac cycle. End systole falls on the left ventricular end-systolic pressure-volume relation (ESPVR). (Data from Little, W. C., and Cheng, C. P.: Left ventricular-arterial coupling in conscious dogs. *Am. J. Physiol.* 261:H70, 1991.)

The effects on left ventricular performance of altering preload, afterload, and contractility are readily described in the left ventricular pressure-volume plane. In the intact circulation, alteration of any of these three determinants of left ventricular performance elicits a prompt compensatory response that modifies the other two factors and heart rate. However, it is useful to analyze the effect of a change in each of these parameters, assuming for illustrative purposes that the other two factors remain constant.

An acute increase in afterload results in a greater proportion of the contractile energy being utilized to develop pressure so there is less myocardial shortening (Fig. 14–2). As a consequence, emptying is impaired, causing reduced stroke volume and decreased ejection fraction. Thus, increased afterload can decrease left ventricular systolic emptying in the absence of any depression of myocardial con-

tractility. An increase in preload (increased end-diastolic volume), if it occurs without a change in end-systolic pressure, results in a larger stroke volume as the ventricle ejects to a similar end-systolic volume. A primary increase in myocardial contractility effects a steeper ESPVR. If preload and afterload remain constant, this brings about an increase in stroke volume.

MEASUREMENT OF KEY VARIABLES

Pressures

The intracardiac, arterial, and venous pressures are important variables used in assessing cardiac function. These pressures have been traditionally measured using fluid-filled catheters (see p. 423). Arterial pressure can be obtained noninvasively by sphygmomanometry. Recently, Doppler echocardiographic techniques have allowed noninvasive estimation of some intracardiac pressures.

TECHNICAL CONSIDERATIONS. Intracardiac pressures can be measured through a fluid-filled catheter connected to a strain-gauge manometer. If the system is carefully flushed to eliminate air bubbles, it has a flat frequency response from 0 to about 10 Hz.[6,7] These fluid-filled systems typically have a resonant frequency of approximately 15 Hz. Thus, catheter systems can accurately measure pressures when the waveform is not rapidly varying (Fig. 14–3). For example, venous pressures and late diastolic and late systolic ventricular and aortic pressures can be accurately measured. However, a fluid-filled catheter system cannot accurately determine rapidly changing pressures as occur during left ventricular isovolumetric contraction and relaxation. During a rapid change in pressure, the fluid-filled system initially lags behind the true pressure. After the transient, the fluid-filled system overshoots and may resonate. These effects can be minimized, but not entirely prevented, by optimal damping. Therefore the time derivative of left ventricular pressure (dP/dt) or the time constant of the isovolumetric fall in left ventricular pressure cannot be accurately determined from a fluid-filled catheter system.

Catheters tipped with a micromanometer provide a flat frequency response to above 100 Hz. Thus a micromanometer can accurately measure cardiac pressures throughout the cardiac cycle. Micromanometers are required to measure left ventricle dP/dt and determine the time constant of the isovolumetric decline in left ventricular pressure. Accurate pressure measurement with a micromanometer requires careful attention to calibration, drift, zeroing, and hydrostatic pressure gradients.[7a]

NONINVASIVE PRESSURE MEASUREMENT. Cuff sphygmomanometry (see p. 20) accurately measures arterial systolic and diastolic pressures. The combination of computer-controlled cuff inflation gated by the electrocardiogram with

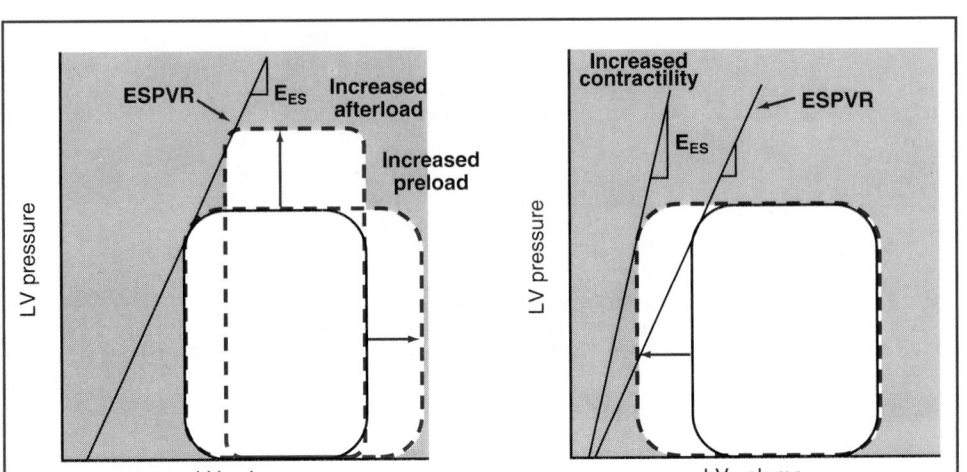

FIGURE 14–2. The responses of the left ventricle to increased afterload, increased preload, and increased contractility are shown in the pressure-volume plane. ESPVR = end-systolic pressure-volume relation; E_{ES} = the slope of the end-systolic pressure-volume relation. See text for discussion.

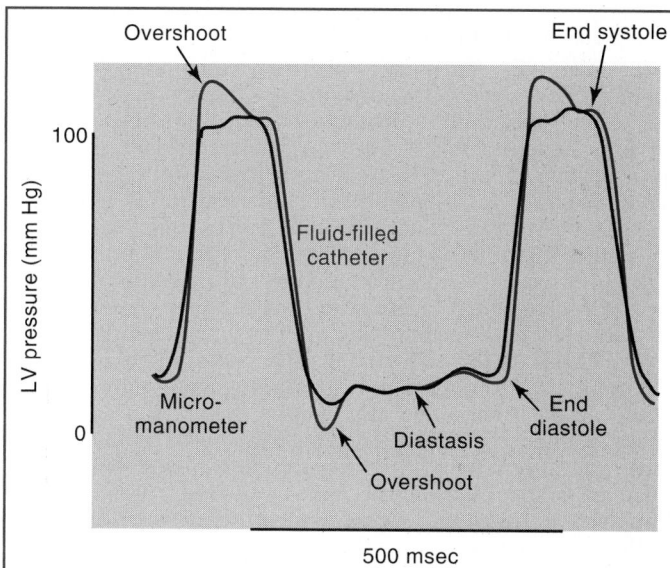

FIGURE 14–3. Recording of left ventricular pressure from a fluid-filled catheter and a micromanometer catheter. The recording with the fluid-filled catheter is delayed slightly relative to the recording with the micromanometer. During portions of the cardiac cycle when left ventricular pressure is not rapidly changing (diastasis, end diastole, end systole) the pressures recorded through the two systems are nearly identical. When pressure is rapidly increasing or decreasing, the pressure recorded through the fluid-filled catheter initially lags behind the micromanometer pressure and then overshoots. (Recording courtesy of Dr. Che-Ping Cheng, Bowman Gray School of Medicine of Wake Forest University.)

Doppler measurements of brachial arterial flow provides a quantitative measure of the entire arterial waveform.[8]

Doppler echocardiography can determine the velocity (v) of systolic regurgitant jet across the tricuspid, mitral, or aortic valves (see p. 56). Using the modified Bernoulli equation ($\Delta P = 4v^2$), the pressure gradient (ΔP) responsible for the regurgitant jet can be calculated. This can be used to estimate the time course of right and left ventricular systolic pressures.[9–11]

PULMONARY CAPILLARY WEDGE PRESSURE. The diastolic pressure that distends the left ventricle and determines left ventricular preload is the left ventricular end-diastolic pressure. This is measured at the relative nadir of left ventricular pressure that occurs after the *a* wave produced by atrial contraction. In the absence of mitral stenosis, left atrial and left ventricular pressures are equal during the mid-diastolic period (diastasis) and at end diastole. Because the pulmonary venous pressure approximates left atrial pressure in most circumstances, the mean pulmonary capillary wedge pressure provides a clinically useful estimate of mean left atrial pressure and the left ventricular filling pressure (see p. 421). The waveform of the pulmonary capillary wedge pressure also approximates the phasic left atrial wave pressure. However, the peak *a* and *v* waves in the pulmonary capillary wedge pressure are damped and delayed relative to the left atrial pressure.[12] Accurate recording of pulmonary wedge pressures requires correct positioning of the catheter tip in the true wedge position to avoid recording a damped pulmonary arterial pressure.[13] Failure to correct for the phase delay or mistaking a damped pulmonary arterial pressure for the wedge pressure may result in overestimating left atrial pressure.[14]

Ventricular Volume

Angiographic techniques, described below, provide the most widely accepted means of measuring ventricular chamber volumes and segmental wall motion. They allow calculation of the extent and velocity of wall shortening and assessment of regional wall motion. When they are combined with measurements of intraventricular pressure

and wall thickness, wall tension can be calculated and both ventricular systolic and diastolic stiffness can be determined. Although noninvasive techniques are now widely used in the assessment of ventricular dimensions and volumes, their application to the assessment of cardiac function is based on the earlier work using ventricular angiography, which remains a benchmark for these measurements.

QUANTITATIVE ANGIOCARDIOGRAPHY. The left ventricle is outlined most clearly by direct injection of contrast material into the ventricular cavity. In patients with severe aortic regurgitation the contrast material may be injected into the aorta, with the resultant reflux outlining the left ventricular cavity. Digital subtraction angiography utilizing injections into a peripheral vein, pulmonary artery, or left ventricle also may be used to define the left ventricle.[15,16]

Unless the effects of premature contractions and of the resultant postextrasystolic potentiation (see p. 380) are to be examined, ventricular irritability should be avoided during injection of the contrast material. Contact should be avoided between the tip of the catheter and the myocardium and a multiholed catheter used to diminish the impact of the jet of contrast agent striking the endocardium. If premature contractions are induced, the premature contraction itself and the postpremature beats may exhibit marked changes in cardiac function. The premature ventricular contraction also may induce mitral and/or tricuspid regurgitation. However, because the contrast material usually is injected within 3 or 4 sec and filming is carried out for 5 to 8 sec, one or two cardiac cycles usually are available for analysis, even if a single premature contraction occurs at the beginning of the injection.

Injection of the contrast agent does not begin to produce hemodynamic changes (except for premature beats) until about the sixth beat after injection.[17] The hyperosmolarity produced by the contrast agent increases the blood volume, which begins to increase preload and heart rate within 30 sec of the injection, an effect that may persist for as long as 2 hours. Regular contrast agents (so-called ionic agents, such as meglumine diatrizoate [see p. 245]) depress contractility directly. However, newer nonionic agents minimize these adverse effects and may be safer for patients with marked elevations of left ventricular end-diastolic pressures (> 25 mm Hg) or depressed cardiac function.[18] Digital subtraction techniques also are useful, since they allow the injection of much smaller quantities of contrast agent and still provide excellent resolution.[15]

In calculation of ventricular volumes or dimensions from angiograms, it is essential to take into account and apply appropriate correction factors for magnification as well as for distortion resulting from nonparallel X-ray beams (pincushion distortion).[19,20] To apply these correction factors, care must be exercised to determine with accuracy the tube-to-patient and tube-to-film distances.

THE CONDUCTANCE CATHETER

The conductance technique provides a useful method to measure left ventricular volume on-line in the cardiac catheterization laboratory, avoiding the problems associated with multiple injections of contrast agent.[21] In this technique, a multielectrode catheter is passed across the aortic valve, and the tip is advanced to the apex of the left ventricle. An electric field is generated (20 kHz, 0.03 mA RMS current) in the left ventricle between electrodes positioned at the top of the catheter in the apex and just above the aortic valve (Fig. 14–4). Sensing electrodes that are evenly distributed along the catheter are used to measure the potential produced by the current.

From these measurements, the *resistance* (and its inverse— *conductance*) between electrode pairs spanning the long axis of the left ventricle is calculated. The conductances from the electrode pairs are summed and converted to volume using a signal conditioner, assuming that all the current flows through blood in the left ventricular chamber. An uncorrected volume of the ventricle (V_M) at any time (t) is proportional to the sum of the measured conductances (G_M) and calculated as:

$$V_M(t) = L^2 \rho G_M(t)$$

where L is the distance between sensing electrodes, and ρ is the resistivity of blood, which is inversely related to conductivity.[21]

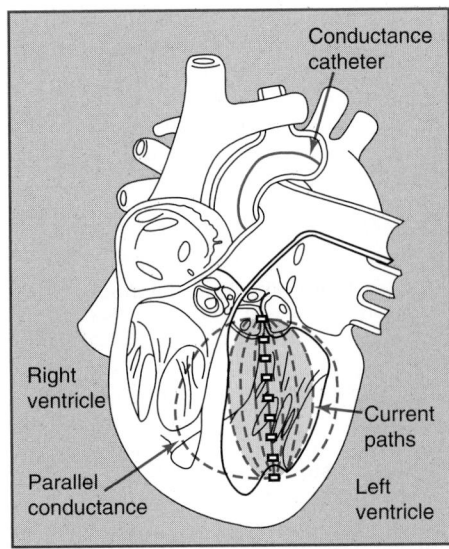

FIGURE 14–4. Measurement of left ventricular volume using a conductance catheter. A multielectrode catheter is passed retrograde across the aortic valve and positioned along the long axis of the left ventricle with the tip in the apex. A current is induced between the electrode in the tip of the left ventricle and an electrode positioned in the aorta above the aortic valve. Most of the current travels within the left ventricle. Thus the conductance of current between electrode pairs is proportional to the volume of blood in that portion of the ventricle. Some current may also travel through the right ventricle and left ventricular walls. These current paths outside the left ventricle contribute to the parallel conductance.

Most of the induced current flows through the blood in the left ventricular cavity. However, some current travels through the left ventricular wall, the right ventricle, and the pericardium. These other paths contribute to the total measured conductance. This is termed the *parallel conductance*, G_P, and produces a volume offset, V_c, equal to:

$$V_c = (L^2 \rho) G_P$$

Thus the left ventricular volume corrected for parallel conductance is given by:

$$V(t) = (1/\alpha)(V_M(t) - \alpha V_c)$$

where α is a unitless constant, V is left ventricular volume corrected for parallel conductance volume, and αV_c is the volume correction because of parallel conductance. Usually α is assumed to be 1.0. Baan et al.[21] developed a technique to calculate V_c by transiently altering blood conductivity within the left ventricle without actually changing left ventricular volume or ejection fraction. In this technique, hypertonic saline (5 ml 20% NaCl) is injected into the pulmonary artery, causing a transient increase in measured volume, V_M.

The calculation of parallel conductance by the saline method assumes that V_c remains constant and that ejection fraction does not change. The line characterizing the relation between the end-diastolic (ED) and end-systolic (ES) V_M is computed. This line is extrapolated to the point where end-diastolic and end-systolic V_M are equal. This point is equal to V_c because any V_M arising from parallel conductance is outside the left ventricle. Baan et al.,[21] Burkhoff et al.,[22] and Kass et al.[23] have evaluated this approach in the isolated heart and open-chest anesthetized dogs and have found that the saline method accurately measured parallel conductance (V_c). An alternate method to determine V_c is to subtract absolute left ventricular volume measured by quantitative angiography from the uncorrected volume measured by conductance.

The conductance catheter can be used to determine stroke volume accurately over a wide range of physiological values.[21,24,25] Determination of absolute left ventricular volumes under steady-state conditions, when α and V_c are nearly constant, is also feasible using the conductance catheter and the saline method of calculating parallel conductance volume. However, because of volume-dependent changes in α and V_c, the conductance catheter may not provide absolute volume measurements when volume varies over a wide range.[26,27] Particularly, analysis of ESPVRs over a range of volumes using the conductance catheter may underestimate the absolute slope because of volume-dependent changes in α and V_c. However, the direction and magnitude of changes in inotropic state are accurately measured by the conductance catheter.[27] In addition, the effect of maneuvers or pharmacological interventions on the ESPVR measured over similar volume ranges can be accurately compared in a single subject.[28] However, comparisons over markedly different volume ranges in a subject may be inaccurate. The recent development

of a dual-field stimulation technique may help minimize these technical problems with the conductance catheter.[29]

NONINVASIVE METHODS. Cardiac catheterization and quantitative selective angiography are the standard tools for evaluating the function of the heart, but these invasive procedures have some risk and are not suitable for repeated application in the same patient. Therefore investigators have searched for reliable noninvasive methods of assessing cardiac volume. Such methods are needed particularly for detecting serial changes in cardiac function and in evaluating both acute and chronic effects of interventions such as pharmacological agents and cardiac operations. Discussed elsewhere in this book are the four principal noninvasive methods for assessing cardiac performance: echocardiography (see p. 64), radionuclide angiography (see p. 300), ultrafast computed tomography (CT) (see p. 336), and gated magnetic resonance imaging (MRI) (see p. 329). All of these are alternatives to contrast angiography for measurement of ventricular volumes and/or dimensions and therefore permit the noninvasive estimation of ejection phase indices (see below). Other than in patients with obstruction to left ventricular outflow, wall stress (afterload) can be estimated from a combination of systemic arterial pressure, ventricular radius, and wall thickness. All four noninvasive imaging methods allow estimation of ventricular systolic and diastolic volumes and both global and regional ejection fractions (EFs).

LEFT VENTRICULAR VOLUME. The area-length method developed by Dodge and Sheehan is the most accepted technique for calculating left ventricular volume (Fig. 14–5).[20] In each of two orthogonal projections, the longest length (L) of the ventricular chamber, i.e., from the apex to the root of the aortic valve, is measured, and the diameter (D) of the ventricle is calculated from the formula D = 4A/L, where A = area of left ventricular cavity determined by planimetry. Ordinarily this calculation is made for images exposed in both 30-degree right anterior oblique (RAO) and 60-degree left anterior oblique (LAO) projections. The shape of the left ventricle usually resembles a prolate ellipsoid with one major and two minor diameters.[20,30] With use of this assumption, left ventricular volume is calculated from the formula:

$$V = \frac{8}{3\pi} \cdot \frac{A_{RAO} - A_{LAO}}{L_{min}}$$

where L_{min} is the shorter L in the RAO or LAO projection.

The actual ventricular volume is determined from the calculated volume using a regression formula that takes into account the volume occupied by the papillary muscles and chordae tendineae within the ventricular chamber as well as corrections for distortion of X-ray beams. Studies based on human autopsy specimens as well as on models and ventricular casts have proved the accuracy of this approach.[31]

Biplane angiographic methods are superior to single-plane methods for the calculation of left ventricular volumes. However, in patients without serious regional wall motion disorders, ventricular aneurysm, or distortion of the ventricular cavity, ventricular volume can be obtained by utilizing the RAO projection. Assuming that the two diameters (D) of the left ventricle are equal, ventricular volume is calculated from the formula:

$$V = L \cdot D^2 \cdot CF^3 \cdot \pi/6$$

where CF represents a one-dimensional correction factor.[31] Standardization of the degree of obliquity—usually 30-degree RAO and 60-degree LAO—is required for application of any particular correction factor in the calculation of ventricular volume. A close correlation has been found between left ventricular volume determined in the RAO projection and true cardiac volume; however, the overestimation of true volume is greater than with the biplane oblique volume method, and appropriate corrections must be made.[32,33]

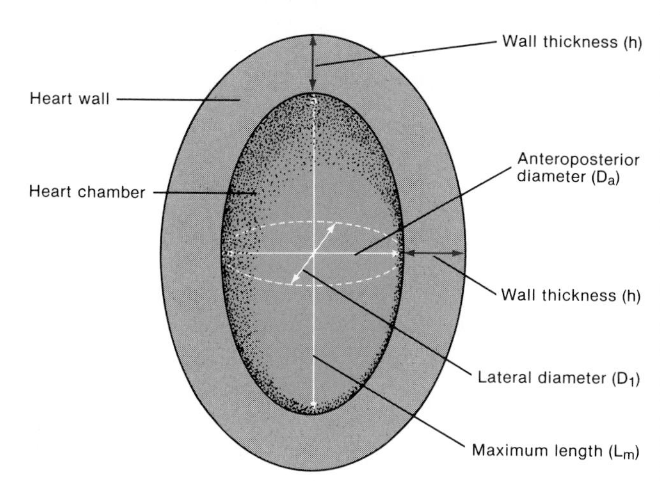

Volume of Chamber $V = \frac{4}{3}\pi\frac{D_a}{2} \times \frac{D_l}{2} \times \frac{L_m}{2}$

Adjusted Volume of Chamber $V' = 0.928V - 3.8$ ml

Volume of the Heart
(Chamber and Wall)

$V_{c+w} = \frac{4}{3}\pi(\frac{D_a}{2} + h) \times (\frac{D_l}{2} + h) \times (\frac{L_m}{2} + h)$

Weight of the Left Ventricle =
Left Ventricular Wall Volume ($V_{c+w} - V'$) × Muscle Specific Gravity (1.050)

FIGURE 14–5. A method to calculate left ventricular volume by means of quantitative angiocardiography. Margins of the projected image of the left ventricular chamber are traced, and maximum length is measured in the anteroposterior and lateral views. Minor axes are derived from the planimetered areas of the chamber in both views; all dimensions are corrected to allow for distortion caused by nonparallel X-rays. Left ventricular volumes are calculated using the formula for the volume of an ellipsoid, since (with regression-equation adjustment) this has given results that tally closely with directly measured ventricular volume. To determine left ventricular mass, volume of the ventricular chamber is subtracted from volume of chamber plus wall; multiplying wall volume by the specific gravity of cardiac muscle converts volume to heart weight or mass. (From Dodge, H. T.: Hemodynamic aspects of cardiac failure. *In* Braunwald, E. [ed.]: The Myocardium: Failure and Infarction. New York, HP Publishing Co., 1974, p. 70. Reproduced by permission of the McGraw-Hill Co. Illustration by Bunji Tagawa.)

The normal left ventricular end-diastolic volume averages 70 ± 20 (SD) ml/m² (Table 14–1).[33,34] Left ventricular performance ordinarily is considered to be depressed when ventricular end-diastolic volume is clearly elevated (i.e., >110 ml/m², or >2 SDs above the normal mean) and total stroke volume and/or cardiac index and work are either

reduced or within normal limits, while heart rate and arterial pressure are normal.

Left ventricular stroke volume (SV) is the quantity of blood ejected with each beat and is the difference between end-diastolic volume (EDV) and end-systolic volume (ESV). The normal SV is 45 ± 13 ml/m² (Table 14–1). The cardiac output is equal to the product of the SV and heart rate. In the absence of valvular regurgitation or intracardiac shunt, the angiographic SV should correlate closely with an independent measurement of SV (cardiac output/heart rate) using the Fick or thermodilution method. In the presence of valvular regurgitation or a shunt, the total SV determined by angiocardiography is greater than the effective forward SV determined by the Fick or indicator dilution method. The difference between the two represents the regurgitant (or shunt) flow per cardiac cycle.

Ejection Fraction (EF). This is the ratio between SV and EDV (SV/EDV). In the presence of valvular regurgitation, the total SV ejected by the ventricle, i.e., the sum of forward and regurgitant volumes, is used in this calculation. The regurgitant fraction (RF) is the ratio of regurgitant flow per beat to the total left ventricular SV:

$$RF = \frac{SV\ total - SV\ forward}{SV\ total},$$

where SV total is determined by angiography and SV forward by the Fick or indicator dilution method. When mitral and aortic regurgitation coexist, the regurgitant fraction reflects the sum of the two regurgitant volumes and does not distinguish between them. It is important to recognize that there are errors in measuring both total SV and forward SV. These errors may summate in the calculation of the regurgitant volume and the regurgitant fraction. Thus it is difficult to determine these parameters with accuracy.

LEFT VENTRICULAR MASS. Although left ventricular mass is usually calculated using echocardiography, it also can be determined by angiocardiography. Wall thickness, h, measured along the free lateral wall of the left ventricle just below the equator at end diastole (best measured on the AP or RAO projection), is added to the major and minor semiaxis to obtain the sum of volumes of the chamber and wall. This volume minus the chamber volume equals the volume of the wall. The product of wall volume and the specific gravity of heart muscle (1.050) equals left ventricular mass.[34] A simplifying assumption in this method, which introduces some inaccuracy, is that left ventricular wall thickness is uniform around the entire left ventricular cavity. However, this method has been validated by postmortem studies comparing actual and projected left ventricular weights.[33]

Left ventricular mass can be determined by two-dimensional echocardiography using several techniques.[35,36] In

TABLE 14–1   LEFT VENTRICULAR VOLUME DATA

GROUP	NO. OF PATIENTS	END-DIASTOLIC VOLUME (ml/m²)	STROKE VOLUME (ml/m²)	MASS (gm/m²)	EJECTION FRACTION
Normal*	—	70 ± 20.0	45 ± 13.0	92 ± 16.0	0.67 ± 0.08
AS	14	84 ± 22.9	44 ± 10.1	172 ± 32.7	0.56 ± 0.17
AR	22	193 ± 55.4	92 ± 30.9	223 ± 73.0	0.56 ± 0.13
AS and AR	13	138 ± 36.5	75 ± 19.1	231 ± 56.9	0.53 ± 0.10
MS	37	83 ± 21.2	43 ± 11.9	98 ± 24.1	0.57 ± 0.14
MR	29	160 ± 53.1	87 ± 21.3	166 ± 49.9	0.47 ± 0.10
MS and MR	29	106 ± 34.4	58 ± 14.7	119 ± 27.8	0.57 ± 0.12
A and M combined	45	130 ± 55.8	69 ± 25.5	156 ± 55.9	0.55 ± 0.12
Myocardial disease	15	199 ± 75.7	44 ± 14.5	145 ± 27.6	0.25 ± 0.09

From Dodge, H. T., and Baxley, W. A.: Left ventricular volume and mass and their significance in heart disease. Am. J. Cardiol. 23:528, 1969.

* Normal values from Kennedy, J. W., et al.: Quantitative angiocardiography. The normal left ventricle in man. Circulation 34:272, 1966.

AS = aortic valve stenosis with peak systolic pressure gradient >30 mm Hg; AR = aortic valve insufficiency with regurgitant flow >30 ml/beat; MS = mitral valve area <1.5 sq cm; MR = mitral valve regurgitant flow >20 ml/beat; A and M combined = combined aortic and mitral valve disease; Myocardial disease = primary cardiomyopathy or myocardial disease secondary to coronary atherosclerosis.

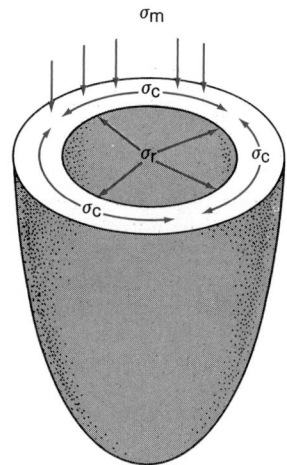

FIGURE 14–6. Circumferential (σ_c), meridional (σ_m), and radial (σ_r) components of left ventricular wall stress from an ellipsoid model. The three components of wall stress are mutually perpendicular. (From Fifer, M.A., and Grossman, W.: Measurement of ventricular volumes, ejection fraction, mass, and wall stress. In Grossman, W. [ed.]: Cardiac Catheterization and Angiography. 3rd ed. Philadelphia, Lea and Febiger, 1986, p. 293. Reproduced by permission.)

one of these, left ventricular mass is calculated as the difference between total ventricular volume (estimated from the product of the epicardial left ventricular length and the area of the left ventricle in the short axis) and the volume of the left ventricular cavity. This method has been validated against directly measured ventricular mass.[37] Echocardiographically determined left ventricular mass is an important prognostic factor.[38–40] Computed tomography and magnetic resonance imaging also are useful methods to measure left ventricular mass accurately.

Left ventricular wall thickness normally averages 10.9 ± 2.0 (SD) mm and left ventricular mass, 92 ± 16 gm/m² (Table 14–1).[31,34] Chronic cardiac dilatation secondary to volume overload or primary myocardial disease increases left ventricular mass, as does chronic pressure overload. Hypertrophy caused by pressure overload (such as aortic stenosis) is characterized by increased muscle mass resulting from augmentation of wall thickness with little change in ventricular chamber volume (concentric hypertrophy) (Table 14–1). In contrast, hypertrophy caused by volume overload or by primary myocardial disease is characterized by increased muscle mass resulting from ventricular dilatation, with only a slight increase in wall thickness (eccentric hypertrophy) (Table 14–1).

LEFT VENTRICULAR FORCES. The forces acting on the myocardial fibers within the ventricular wall can be calculated from the dimensions of the left ventricular cavity, wall thickness, and intraventricular pressure. Tension (force/cm) is defined as the force acting on a hypothetical slit in the ventricular wall that would tend to pull its edges apart. According to Laplace's law, tension is the product of the intraventricular pressure and radius. Wall stress (σ) is the force or tension per unit of cross-sectional area of the ventricular wall. Wall stress may be considered to act in three directions—circumferential, meridional, and radial (Fig. 14–6). The calculation of stress requires assumptions concerning the shape and configuration of the ventricle.[41,42] Circumferential wall stress, the strongest force generated within the ventricular wall, can be approximated as:

$$CWS = \frac{(P \cdot b)}{h}\left(1 - \frac{h}{2b}\right)\left(1 - \frac{hb}{2a^2}\right)$$

where CWS = circumferential wall stress in dynes per square centimeter × 10³; P = left ventricular pressure in dynes per square centimeter; a and b are major and minor semiaxes (i.e., half the longest lengths), respectively, in centimeters; and h = left ventricular wall thickness in

square centimeters.[7] Meridional wall stress (MWS) can be approximated as:

$$MWS = \frac{P \cdot r}{2h(1 + h/2r)}$$

where r is the internal radius of the ventricle in centimeters.[43]

Simultaneous recording of left ventricular dimensions (by angiography) and intraventricular pressure recorded with a high-fidelity micromanometer allows calculation of left ventricular tension and stress throughout the cardiac cycle (Fig. 14–7). A simpler method of analyzing the instantaneous left ventricular tension throughout the cardiac cycle consists of recording left ventricular pressure simultaneously with left ventricular diameter across the minor axis of the left ventricle determined by echocardiography. This combination of measurements provides the data necessary to calculate ventricular circumferential fiber shortening (at either the endocardium or the midwall) and midwall circumferential stress, using minor modifications of the equations presented above.[44] However, the use of echocardiography—especially M-mode—for these calculations is based on the assumption of uniform wall motion. This assumption is reasonable only in conditions that affect left ventricular function relatively uniformly, such as dilated cardiomyopathy or aortic or mitral regurgitation. These assumptions are not correct when there is regional left ventricular dysfunction.

During isovolumetric contraction, left ventricular wall

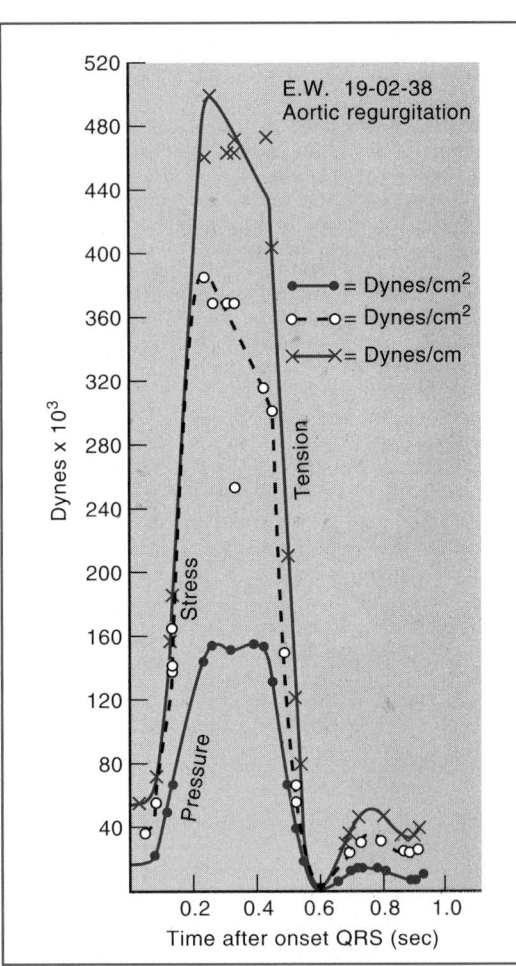

FIGURE 14–7. Sequential changes in left ventricular tension, stress, and pressure are shown throughout the cardiac cycle in a patient with aortic regurgitation. Note that tension and stress decline during ejection, although left ventricular pressure is maintained. (Reproduced with permission from Rackley, C. E.: Quantitative evaluation of left ventricular function by radiographic techniques. Circulation 54:862, 1976. Copyright 1976 the American Heart Association.)

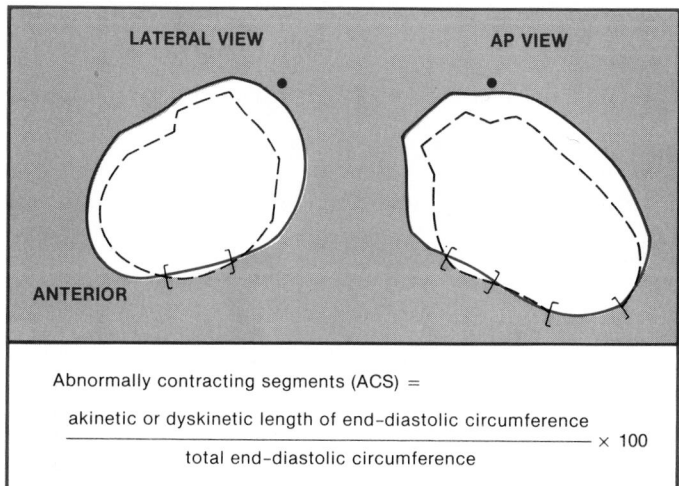

Abnormally contracting segments (ACS) =

$$\frac{\text{akinetic or dyskinetic length of end-diastolic circumference}}{\text{total end-diastolic circumference}} \times 100$$

FIGURE 14–8. Systolic *(dashed)* and diastolic *(solid)* lateral and anteroposterior (AP) contrast left ventriculograms are superimposed with a central marker as a reference point. The abnormally contracting segments are enclosed by the brackets on the diastolic silhouette. (Reproduced with permission from Rackley, C. E.: Quantitative evaluation of left ventricular function by radiographic techniques. Circulation *54:*862, 1976. Copyright 1976 the American Heart Association.)

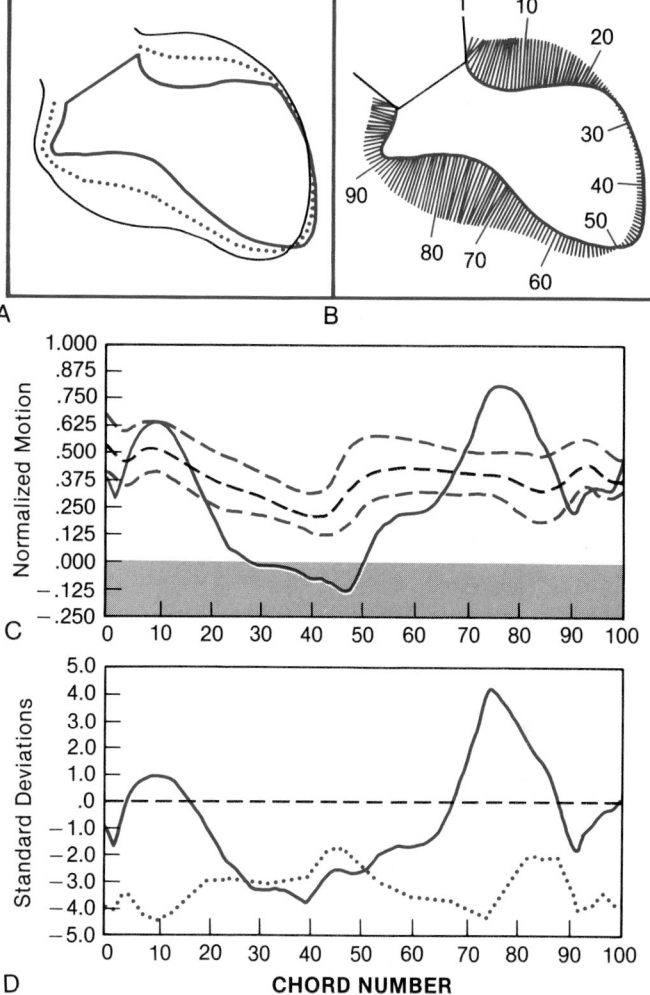

FIGURE 14–9. Center line method of left ventricular regional wall motion analysis. *A,* A center line is constructed midway between the end-diastolic and end-systolic endocardial contours. *B,* Motion is measured along 100 chords constructed perpendicular to the center line. *C,* Motion at each chord is normalized by the end-diastolic perimeter length to yield a shortening fraction. The contraction pattern ± SD measured in a normal population is plotted with a dashed line. *D,* The patient's wall motion is plotted in units of standard deviation (SD) from the normal mean *(dotted line).* Wall motion abnormality in the central infarct region, peripheral infarct region, and noninfarct region is calculated by averaging the motion of chords lying within these regions. (From Kennedy, J. W., and Sheehan, F. H.: Ventriculography. *In* Pepine, C. J., Hill, J. A., and Lambert, C. R. [eds.]: Diagnostic and Therapeutic Cardiac Catheterization. Baltimore, Williams and Wilkins, 1989, p. 171. Reproduced by permission.)

tension and stress rise rapidly as the ventricle contracts without decreasing the chamber volume. During ejection, as the left ventricular cavity decreases in size and wall thickness increases, the stress and tension decline even though pressure is maintained (Fig. 14–7).

REGIONAL VENTRICULAR WALL MOTION. Ischemic heart disease may produce focal, regional abnormalities of contraction. Hyperkinesis of normal areas may compensate for impaired function of an abnormal region, leaving global left ventricular function normal or only minimally depressed. Thus, assessment of regional wall motion is more sensitive in detecting ventricular dysfunction in such patients than analysis of global ventricular function.

Regional wall motion can be assessed with a variety of methods, including contrast angiography.[45] Marked focal abnormalities of contraction can be appreciated by visual inspection of cineventriculograms; segments of abnormal ventricular contraction can be localized by superimposing end-diastolic and end-systolic outlines of the left ventricular cavity. Akinesis is present when a portion of each of the two silhouettes shares a common line; dyskinesis is present when the end-systolic silhouette extends outside the end-diastolic silhouette. The abnormally contracting segments (both akinetic and dyskinetic) may be expressed simply as percentages of the total end-diastolic circumference (Fig. 14–8). Hypokinesis (focal decreases in the extent of contraction) as well as asynchrony (abnormalities of timing of contraction) are less severe disturbances of contraction. Analysis of wall motion from multiple cineframes and automated border detection may be necessary for the detection of these more subtle abnormalities.[46] By use of such techniques it is apparent that focal hypokinesis and abnormalities of timing of segmental wall motion cannot be readily detected by visual inspection of cineangiograms, and that they are relatively common disturbances, especially in ischemic heart disease.

The Center Line Method. Sheehan et al.[47,48] developed a technique in which end-diastolic and end-systolic endocardial contours are traced from a normal sinus beat (Fig. 14–9). A center line is drawn midway between the end-systolic and end-diastolic silhouettes (Fig. 14–9); 100 chords are then constructed perpendicular to this center line. The length of each chord is determined, and after appropriate corrections for ventricular size, it is then compared with that for a group of normal subjects expressed in units of standard deviation from the normal mean.

RIGHT VENTRICULAR AND ATRIAL VOLUME. The shape of the right ventricle is much more complex than the shape of the left ventricle. Thus the prolate ellipsoid that is a useful model to calculate left ventricular volume is not appropriate for the right ventricle.[49] One method is to consider the right ventricle as a pyramid with a triangular base.[50] An alternate approach is to calculate right ventricular volume using Simpson's rule.

The shapes of the atria are less complex than those of the right ventricle. Thus, the atrial volumes can be calculated assuming an ellipsoidal geometry.[51]

ASSESSMENT OF LEFT VENTRICULAR MYOCARDIAL FUNCTION

The factors that determine myocardial function (preload, afterload, contractility, heart rate, and rhythm) can be estimated from left ventricular pressure and volume.

Left ventricular preload can be assessed from the left ventricular filling pressure, the left ventricular end-diastolic volume, or left ventricular end-diastolic stress.[52,53] The pressure distending the ventricle immediately prior to contraction is the end-diastolic pressure. In the absence of disease of the mitral valve this is equivalent to the pressure in the left atrium at this time (the post *a*-wave or *z*-point pressure). When there is a vigorous atrial contraction, the end-diastolic pressure is substantially higher than the mean left atrial pressure. It is important to recognize that the amount of pulmonary congestion is related to the mean pulmonary capillary (or left atrial) pressure, while the end-diastolic volume is determined by the left ventricular end-diastolic pressure.[52] In the absence of pulmonary vascular disease, mean pulmonary capillary wedge pressure approximates the pulmonary artery diastolic pressure. In the presence of a tall *v* wave, the mean atrial pressure (and mean pulmonary capillary edge pressure) may exceed the ventricular end-diastolic pressure.[54,55]

The left ventricular preload depends on the end-diastolic volume produced by the distending pressure of the ventricle. Since interventions that alter end-diastolic pressure may also alter the relation between end-diastolic volume and pressure, changes in end-diastolic pressure do not always represent changes in end-diastolic volume or changes in end-diastolic fiber stretch.[56,57]

Afterload

Following aortic valve opening the ventricle ejects into the arterial circulation. Thus, in the simplest sense the systolic pressure represents the afterload opposing left ventricular ejection. However, arterial systolic pressure is not a pure measure of left ventricular afterload.[58] The tension in the ventricular wall that the sarcomeres must overcome to shorten is related not only to the systolic pressure but also to the cavity size through the Laplace relation. Thus, at similar systolic pressures a larger ventricle will have greater wall tension than a smaller ventricle. Furthermore, the arterial systolic pressure depends not only on the characteristics of the arterial circulation but also on the pumping performance of the left ventricle. The more vigorous the left ventricular contraction, the greater the volume ejected and the higher the systolic pressure. Thus, left ventricular systolic function and left ventricular afterload are interrelated.

The steady-state arterial load opposing left ventricular ejection can be quantified as the peripheral vascular resistance.[59] This is calculated as the cardiac output divided by the mean arterial pressure minus the mean venous pressure (see p. 439). Because mean venous pressure is very low relative to mean arterial pressure, it is frequently neglected in this calculation. The peripheral vascular resistance provides only steady-state information concerning the relation between flow and pressure in the arterial system. In fact, the left ventricular ejection is pulsatile and there are pulsatile elements to the arterial load that increase in importance with tachycardia, aging, and peripheral vascular disease.[60,61]

The full relation between flow and arterial pressure can be evaluated in the frequency domain as the *arterial input impedance*.[62-64] Calculation of the input impedance spectrum requires the high-fidelity measurement of aortic pressure and flow at the same point. The impedance spectrum consists of a magnitude and phase at each frequency. The magnitude of the impedance at a given frequency is the ratio of a sinusoidally varying pressure and related flow at that frequency. Since arterial pressure and flow do not vary sinusoidally, the Fourier transformation is used to mathematically describe the aortic pressure and flow as a combination of a fundamental sine wave (at the heart rate) and a series of harmonic waves. The impedance spectrum is then calculated as the ratio of the pressure to flow at each frequency. Figure 14–10 provides an example of such an impedance spectrum. Although the impedance spectrum contains all the information concerning the relation between pulsatile flow and pressure in the arterial circulation, its clinical usefulness is limited by the difficulty in obtaining the appropriate measurement and the calculations.

Evaluation of the interaction of the left ventricle and the arterial system requires that they be described in similar terms. Description of the arterial system in the frequency domain does not easily allow this coupling to be assessed because the left ventricle is difficult to describe in these terms. Because the left ventricle can be evaluated in the pressure-volume plane, Sunagawa et al.[65] proposed that the arterial system be evaluated in an analogous manner. In this analysis, the arterial system is described by the relation between the stroke volume and end-systolic pressure (Fig. 14–11). The higher the stroke volume, the greater the end-systolic pressure. The slope of this relation represents the effective arterial end-systolic elastance (E_A). If it is assumed that this relation passes through the origin, then E_A can be calculated as the ratio of end-systolic pressure to stroke volume. As shown in Figure 14–11, this can be plotted on the left ventricular pressure-volume loop. End systole occurs at the intersection of the arterial and ventricular relations. The production of stroke work is maximum when the E_{ES} and E_A are approximately equal.[66]

Under usual conditions, E_A, the slope of the arterial end-systolic pressure stroke volume relation, can be approximated by the product of the peripheral vascular resistance and the heart rate.[67] In older hypertensive patients, E_A may exceed peripheral vascular resistance times heart rate. However, E_A can be accurately estimated over a wide range

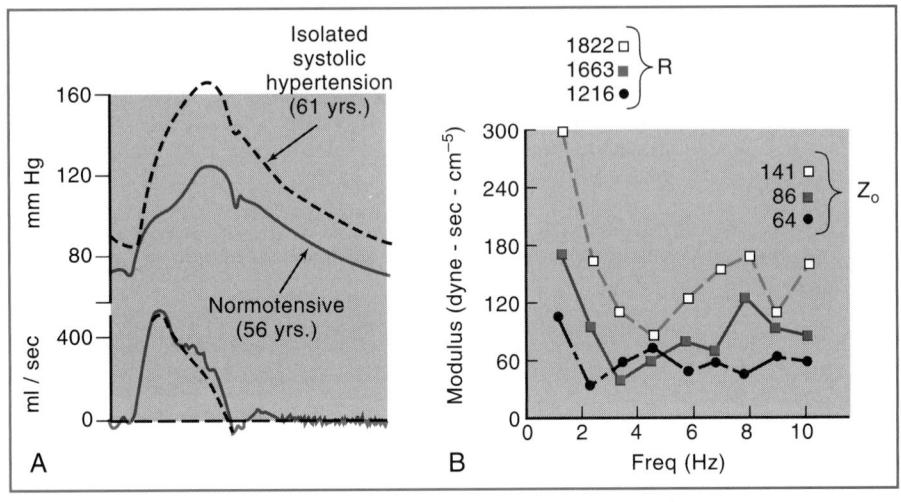

FIGURE 14–10. *A,* Recordings of ascending aortic pressure and flow, and *B,* the resulting aortic input impedance spectra from a 56-year-old normotensive subject *(solid colored lines/ closed boxes)* and a 61-year-old subject with isolated systolic hypertension *(broken lines/ open boxes),* with an impedance spectrum from a young (28 years) normotensive subject *(solid dots),* shown for comparison. Peripheral vascular resistance (**R**), impedance moduli of the first harmonic, and characteristic impedance (Z_0) were all higher in the subject with isolated systolic hypertension. Also, the impedance moduli minimum was shifted to a higher frequency in the subject with isolated systolic hypertension. Freq = frequency. (From Nichols, W. W., Nicolini, F. A., and Pepine, C. J.: Determinants of isolated systolic hypertension in the elderly. J. Hypertension *10*[Suppl. 6]:S73, 1992. Reproduced by permission of Current Science Ltd.)

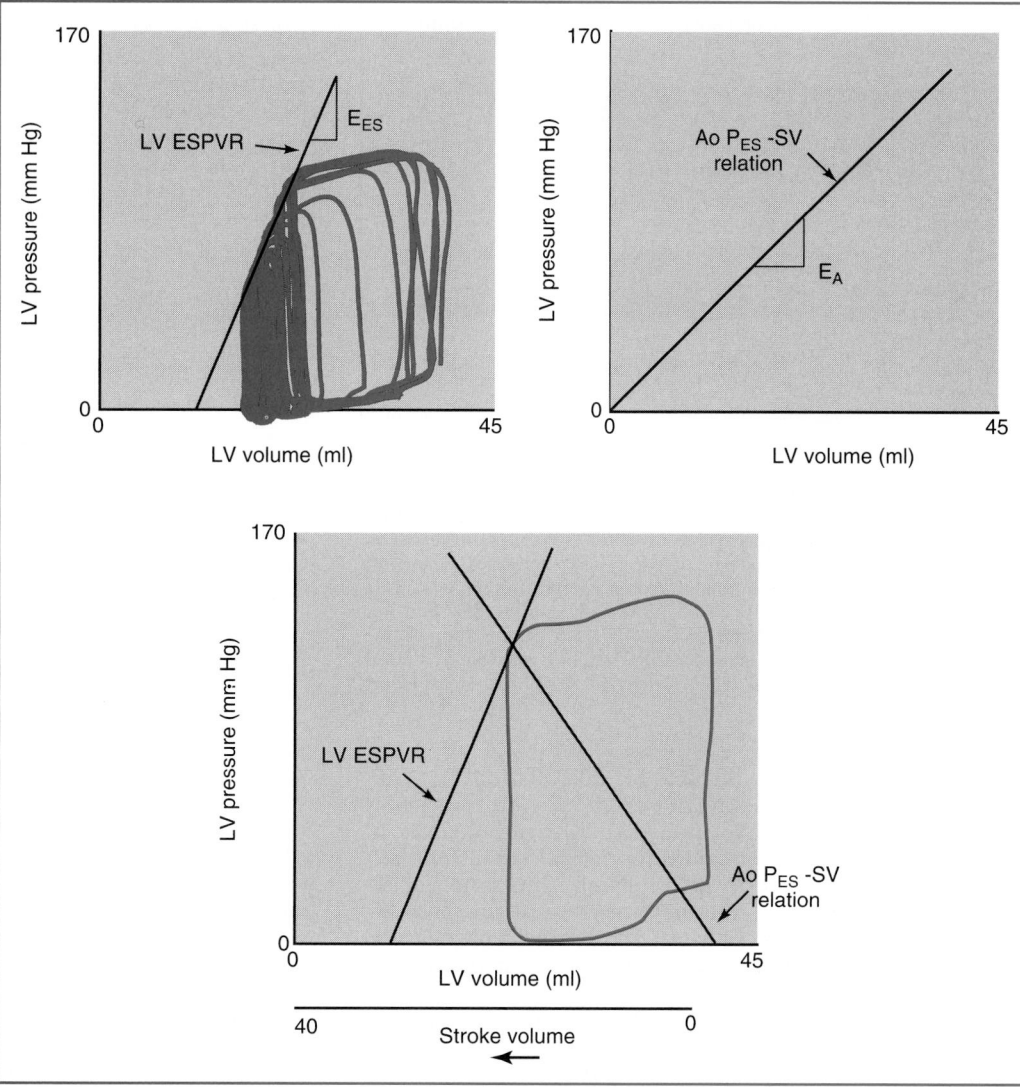

FIGURE 14–11. Left ventricular–arterial coupling assessed in the pressure-volume plane. The left ventricular (LV) end-systolic pressure-volume relation (ESPVR) is used to describe left ventricular systolic performance. In the upper left panel, pressure-volume loops for variably loaded beats are shown with the upper left corner of each beat falling on the end-systolic pressure-volume relation. In the upper right panel, the arterial circulation is described as a relation between stroke volume (SV) and end-systolic pressure. The slope of this relation represents the effective end-systolic arterial elastance (E_A). In the lower panel, the left ventricular ESPVR and the aortic end-systolic pressure-volume relation (A_oP_{ES}-V_{SV}) are plotted on the same axis. End systole occurs at the intersection of the two relations. Thus, description of the arterial circulation in terms of the aortic P_{ES}-SV relation allows understanding of the coupling between the left ventricle and arterial circulation. (Redrawn from Little, W. C., and Cheng, C. P.: Left ventricular–arterial coupling in conscious dogs. Am. J. Physiol. *261*:H70, 1991. Reproduced by permission of the American Physiological Society.)

of conditions from arterial systolic (P_{SYS}) and diastolic pressures (P_{diast}) as: $(2 \cdot P_{SYS} + P_{dias})/3$ divided by the SV.[67]

Contractility

In isolated cardiac muscle or in the isolated heart, loading can be readily controlled and the effects of an intervention on the strength, extent, and velocity of muscle shortening indicate its effect on contractility (Fig. 12–8, p. 366). It is more difficult to make analogous measurements in patients in whom preload, afterload, or both may be abnormal and cannot be readily controlled. Many drugs that affect myocardial contractility also act on the arterial and/or venous beds, thereby altering cardiac loading. Furthermore, in patients with valvular heart disease, it is necessary to evaluate the level of myocardial contractility despite the marked alterations in loading conditions. These considerations have led to the search for methods of evaluating cardiac function that go beyond analysis of the pumping function of the ventricle and provide an assessment of contractility. A number of indices of contractility have been proposed and investigated empirically. Unfortunately, there is no absolute measure of myocardial contractility, i.e., there is no gold standard with which these indices can be compared. Furthermore, at the sarcomere level, contractility and load are interrelated and thus not independent variables.[2,3]

Many indices have been proposed as measures of left ventricular contractile function[23,68] (Table 14–2). These can be divided into isovolumetric phase indices, ejection phase indices, and measures derived from left ventricular pressure-volume relations.

TABLE 14–2 EVALUATION OF LEFT VENTRICULAR SYSTOLIC PERFORMANCE: NORMAL VALUES FOR SOME ISOVOLUMETRIC AND EJECTION PHASE INDICES

CONTRACTILITY INDICES		NORMAL VALUES (MEAN ± S.D.)
ISOVOLUMETRIC PHASE INDICES		
Maximum dP/dt		1610 ± 290 mm Hg/sec
		1670 ± 320 mm Hg/sec
		1661 ± 323 mm Hg/sec
Maximum (dP/dt)/P)		44 ± 8.4 sec^{-1}
VPM or peak $\left[\dfrac{dP/dt}{28P}\right]$		1.47 ± 0.19 ML/sec
dP/dt/DP at DP = 40 mm Hg		37.6 ± 12.2 sec^{-1}
EJECTION PHASE INDICES		
LVSW		81 ± 23 gm-m
LVSWI		53 ± 22 gm-m/M^2
		41 ± 12 gm-m/M^2
EF	angio:	0.72 ± 0.08
MNSER	angio:	3.32 ± 0.84 EDV/sec
	echo:	2.29 ± 0.30 EDV/sec
Mean V_{CF}	angio:	1.83 ± 0.56 ED circ/sec
		1.50 ± 0.27 ED circ/sec
	echo:	1.09 ± 0.12 ED circ/sec

From Grossman, W.: Evaluation of systolic and diastolic function of the myocardium. *In* Grossman, W., and Baim, D. S. (eds.): Cardiac Catheterization, Angiography and Intervention. Philadelphia, Lea and Febiger, 1991, p. 326.

dP/dt = rate of rise of left ventricular (LV) pressure; DP = developed LV pressure; EF = ejection fraction; MNSER = mean normalized systolic ejection rate; ML = muscle lengths; ED = end-diastolic; V = volume; circ = circumference.

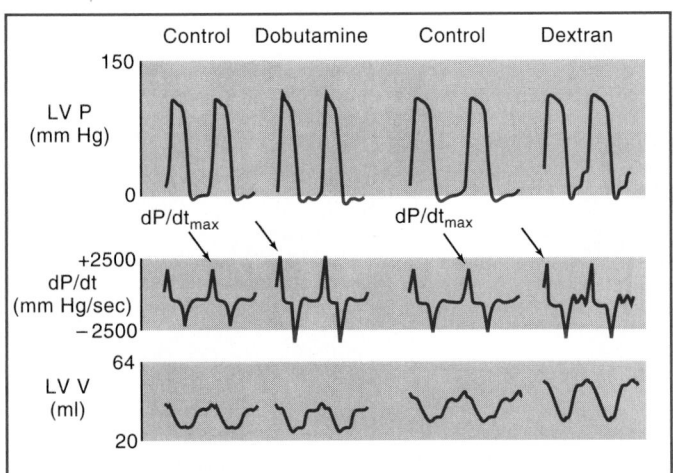

FIGURE 14–12. Recording of left ventricular pressure (LVP), the rate of change of left ventricular pressure (dp/dt), and left ventricular volume (LV V). The maximum value of dP/dt (dP/dt$_{max}$) increases in response to dobutamine; however, dP/dt$_{max}$ also increases when left ventricular end-diastolic volume is increased by infusing dextran. This demonstrates the sensitivity of dP/dt$_{max}$ to both contractility and left ventricular end-diastolic volume (preload). (Data from Little, W. C.: The left ventricular dP/dt$_{max}$-end-diastolic volume relation in closed chest dogs. Circ. Res. **56:**808, 1985. Copyright 1985 American Heart Association.)

ISOVOLUMETRIC PHASE INDICES OF CONTRACTILITY. Ventricular dP/dt. The maximum rate of rise of ventricular pressure (dP/dt$_{max}$) is highly sensitive to acute changes in contractility (Fig. 14–12).[69–71] Under normal conditions dP/dt$_{max}$ occurs before aortic valve opening; thus it is not affected by steady-state alterations in aortic pressure.[72] However, dP/dt$_{max}$ may be delayed until after aortic valve opening in patients with severe left ventricular depression or marked arterial vasodilation with very low aortic diastolic pressures. In the absence of these conditions, dP/dt$_{max}$ can be considered to be relatively independent of afterload. However, dP/dt$_{max}$ is very sensitive to changes in preload.[69,71] This preload sensitivity is greater in ventricles with enhanced contractility and reduced in depressed ventricles.[71] A change in dP/dt$_{max}$ without a change in preload or with an opposite change in preload indicates an alteration in contractility. Another difficulty with the use of dP/dt$_{max}$ as an index of contractility is that it can be altered by ventricular hypertrophy. This difficulty can be surmounted, however, by calculating the peak rate of stress development (dσ/dt).[73]

Although dP/dt$_{max}$ correlates with contractility, the wide variation between individuals and the marked preload dependence decrease its usefulness for assessing *basal* contractility. Instead, dP/dt$_{max}$ is more useful in assessing *directional* changes in contractility during acute interventions when used in combination with a measure of left ventricular preload. For example, dP/dt$_{max}$ increases during exercise,[73] with tachycardia,[74] and after administration of inotropic agents.[75]

V$_{max}$. V$_{max}$ is the maximum velocity of shortening of the unloaded contractile elements (CEs). It was originally proposed as a measure of myocardial contractility that is independent of preload or afterload. However, there are theoretical and practical limitations to the calculation of CE V$_{max}$ in isolated muscle, and even more so in the intact heart.[76] Because of the theoretical problems and practical difficulties in calculating V$_{max}$, it is no longer used as a clinical measure of contractility.

Relation Between dP/dt and Developed Pressure. Some of the difficulties involving the calculation of V$_{max}$ can be partially avoided by the selection of certain points on the curve relating dP/dt to DP, the developed left ventricular pressure (i.e., left ventricular pressure minus end-diastolic pressure). The dP/dt at a DP of 40 mm Hg, a level of pressure that almost always occurs before the opening of the aortic valve, is commonly used. dP/dt at a DP of 40 mm Hg and the maximum dP/dt/DP are useful for assessing directional changes in contractility, since it is unaffected by changes in afterload and less sensitive to changes in preload than dP/dt$_{max}$.[77–79]

EJECTION PHASE INDICES. The extent of left ventricular ejection can be measured as the stroke volume, ejection fraction, or fractional shortening, and the rate of ejection quantified as the mean and peak velocity of shortening (V$_{CF}$). All of these measurements are influenced by both contractility and load.[80] The marked preload dependence of the stroke volume is minimized by dividing by the end-diastolic volume producing the EF. However, the EF remains highly sensitive to changes in afterload, so it is best to consider it a measure of systolic performance and not a pure measure of contractility (see below).

The afterload dependence of the ejection fraction or measures of the left ventricular shortening can be minimized using concepts derived from the myocardial force-velocity relation of isolated cardiac muscle (Fig. 14–13). For example, the relation between fractional myocardial fiber shortening (determined noninvasively) and left ventricular end-systolic stress (obtained in the basal state), sometimes supplemented by the measurements made during a pharmacologically altered afterload, provides a useful and practical framework for assessing the basal level of ventricular contractility.[81–86] Similarly, the relation between end-systolic stress and mean V$_{CF}$ at various levels of wall stress is relatively preload independent and incorporates afterload. Thus, changes in the relation between the extent (or velocity) of myocardial wall shortening and the simultaneous ventricular wall stress reflect acute changes in contractility. For example, augmentation of (V$_{CF}$) at a constant wall stress signifies improvement of contractility. The relation between end-systolic wall stress and left ventricular fractional shortening of V$_{CF}$ can also provide assessment of the basal level of contractility. This relation is particularly

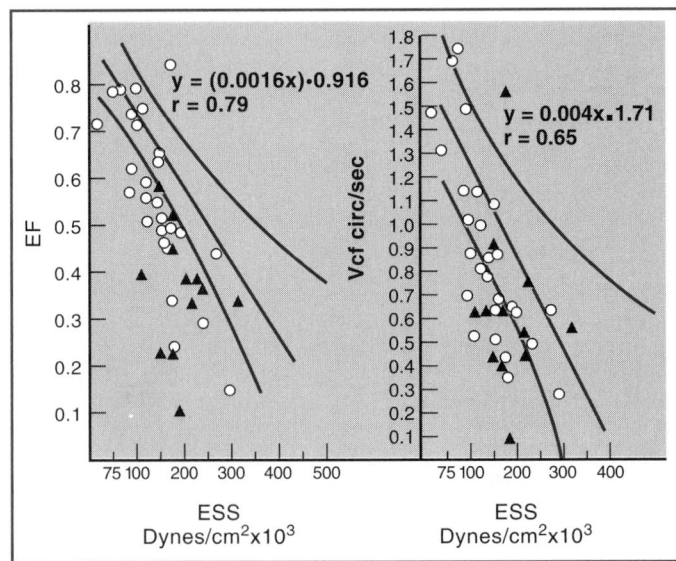

FIGURE 14–13. The ejection fraction (EF)–end-systolic stress (ESS) relationship is shown on the *left* and the mean velocity of circumferential fiber shortening (Vcf)–end-systolic stress relationship is shown on the *right*. In this example, data from patients with valvular heart disease are compared to observations from normal subjects (95 per cent confidence limits are shown for the normal relation). Those patients who fell down and to the left of the normal limits demonstrated reduced ejection performance for any given level of afterload suggesting impaired contractility. (From Carabello, B. A., Williams, H., Gash, A. K., et al.: Hemodynamic predictors of outcome in patients undergoing valve replacement. Circulation **74:**1309, 1986. Copyright 1986 American Heart Association.)

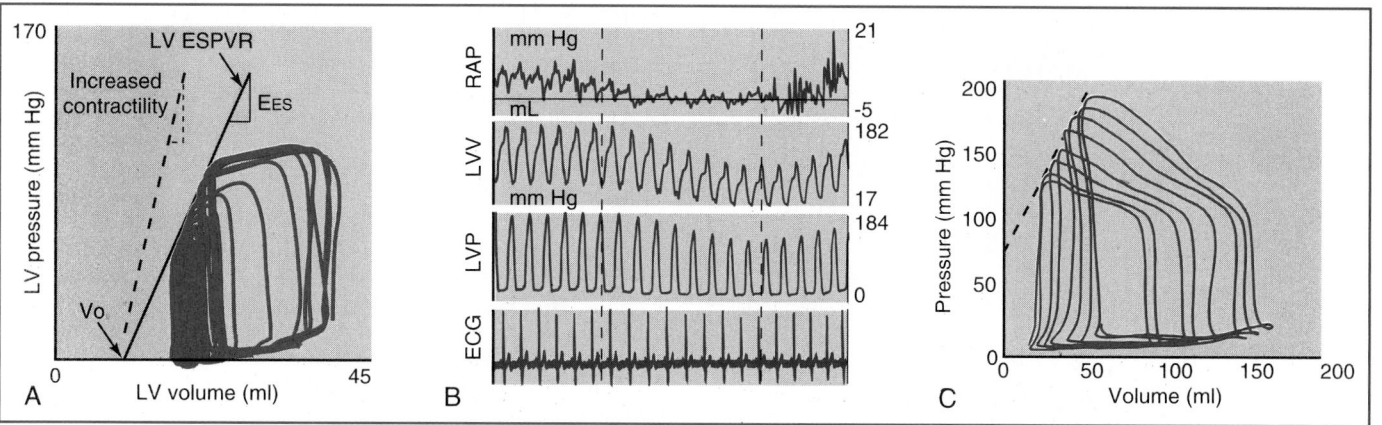

FIGURE 14–14. *A,* Variably loaded pressure-volume loops produced by caval occlusion in a conscious experimental animal. End systole occurs at the upper left corner of the pressure-volume loops. The end-systolic points of the variably loaded beats fall along a single relation, the left ventricular end-systolic pressure-volume relation (LV ESPVR). Within the physiological range, this relation is approximated by a straight line. The line can be described in terms of its slope (E_{ES}) and volume axis intercept (V_0). Note that the volume axis intercept results from extrapolation of the line outside the range of end-systolic pressures in which data can be acquired.

An increase in contractile state, produced by infusing dobutamine, shifts the left ventricular end-systolic pressure-volume relation toward the left while increasing the slope (E_{ES}). (Data from Little, W. C., Cheng, C. P., Mumma, M., et al.: Comparison of measures of left ventricular contractile performance derived from pressure-volume loops in conscious dogs. Circulation *80*:1378, 1989. Reproduced by permission of the American Heart Association, Inc.)

B, Recording of right atrial pressure (RAP), left ventricular volume (LVV) measured with the conductance catheter, and left ventricular pressure (LVP) in a patient during transient balloon occlusion of the inferior vena cava. These variably loaded beats are shown in the pressure-volume plane on the right *(C).* The upper left corner of these loops defines the left ventricular end-systolic pressure-volume relation *(dotted line).* (From Kass, D. A.: Clinical ventricular pathophysiology: A pressure-volume view. *In* Warltier, D. C.: Ventricular Function. Baltimore, Williams and Wilkins, 1995, p. 111. Reproduced by permission of the Society of Cardiovascular Anesthesiologists.)

useful in patients who have a reduced EF, because it distinguishes between reduced myocardial shortening due to excessive afterload and that due to depressed myocardial contractility.[87]

Because the $V_{CF} - \sigma_{ES}$ relation during a single beat is not defined by parallel straight lines, it may not be accurately defined from measurements made at a single loading condition.[88]

PRESSURE-VOLUME RELATIONS. As discussed above, consideration of the left ventricle in the pressure-volume plane provides a powerful method to understand left ventricular performance.[5,89–91] The generation of variably loaded beats allows determination of several relations that provide information concerning left ventricular contractility and systolic performance. The variably loaded beats can be produced by transient balloon occlusion of the inferior vena cava.[23,91,92] An alternate approach is to generate a range of loading conditions using graded infusions of vasoactive agents, such as methoxamine and nitroprusside.[93,94]

Left Ventricular ESPVR. The upper left corner of variably loaded pressure-volume loops defines the left ventricular end-systolic pressure-volume relation (Fig. 14–14). In the physiological range, this relation can be approximated as a straight line and can therefore be described with a slope (E_{ES}) and volume axis intercept (V_0), i.e., $P_{ES} = E_{ES}(V_{ES} - V_0)$.[89,95] E_{ES} has dimensions of pressure/volume (units of mm Hg/ml). This represents the end-systolic stiffness of the left ventricle and indicates how sensitive ejection is to increases in afterload (as reflected in the end-systolic pressure). With enhanced contractility, E_{ES} increases. The volume axis intercept (V_0) of the ESPVR has been referred to as the *dead volume* of the ventricle. This is the volume at which the left ventricle would generate no pressure. This volume intercept cannot be directly measured clinically. Instead it must be determined by extrapolation and thus is subject to significant errors.[89,95,96] In many clinical studies the extrapolated V_0 is negative, which is a physiological impossibility. This indicates the

difficulties involved in accurately determining V_0 in clinical studies.[89]

The position of the ESPVR on the volume axis at the operating pressure (e.g., the end-systolic volume associated with an end-systolic pressure of 100 mm Hg) indicates the extent of contraction. Global increases in contractility, such as the infusion of dobutamine, both increase E_{ES} and shift the ESPVR to the left in the physiological range.[89,95] Thus, at a constant afterload (i.e., constant left ventricular end-systolic pressure) the left ventricle with enhanced contractility ejects to a lower volume and is less sensitive to changes in systolic pressure. Global decreases in contractility produce the opposite effect. Thus, E_{ES} and the position of the ESPVR in the physiological range provide load-insensitive measures of contractility.[89,95]

Regional left ventricular dysfunction resulting from coronary artery occlusion produces a nearly parallel rightward shift of the left ventricular ESPVR in the physiological range with little change in the E_{ES}[97,98] (Fig. 14–15). A similar parallel shift of the ESPVR occurs when the normal activation sequence of the left ventricle is altered by pacing.[99]

An echocardiographically determined left ventricular end-systolic dimension or cross-sectional area can be used as a surrogate for left ventricular volume in the left ventricular end-systolic pressure-volume relation provided that there is no segmental wall motion abnormality.[100] Automated echocardiographic border detection makes it possible to determine pressure-area relations on-line.[101]

There are practical and theoretical difficulties in using the ESPVR as a clinical measure of left ventricular contractility. First, to define accurately the ESPVR, a wide range of loading conditions must be obtained. Such alterations in load may induce reflexly mediated changes in heart rate and left ventricular contractility. In addition, arterial vasoconstriction and vasodilation produce parallel shifts of the left ventricular ESPVR.[102,103] Thus, the interventions required to define the ESPVR accurately may themselves

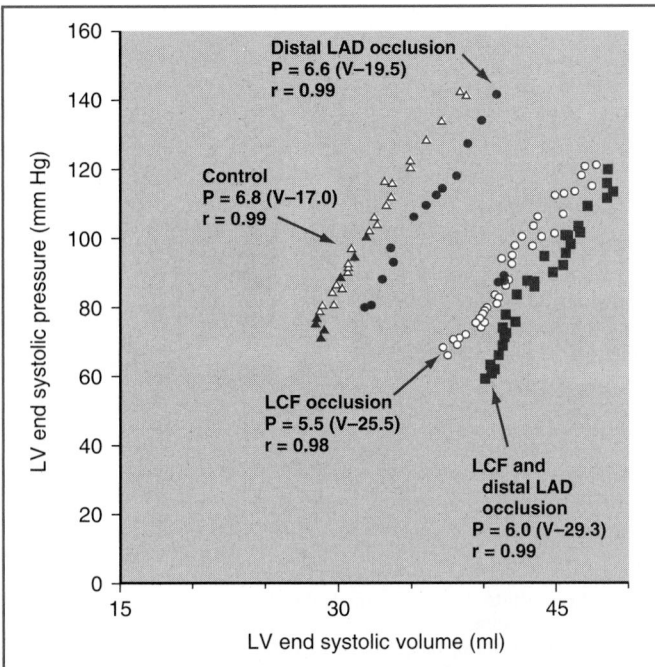

FIGURE 14–15. Left ventricular (LV) end-systolic pressure-volume (P-V) relations from a conscious experimental animal during a control period and after occlusion of the distal left anterior descending coronary artery (LAD), the proximal left circumflex coronary artery (LCF), and both the distal left anterior descending coronary artery and proximal left circumflex coronary artery. Progressively larger amounts of regional ischemia produce greater parallel leftward shifts of the end-systolic pressure-volume relations. (From Little, W. C., and O'Rourke, R. A.: Effect of regional ischemia on the left ventricular end-systolic pressure-volume relation in chronically instrumented dogs. Reproduced by permission of the American College of Cardiology.) J. Am. Coll. Cardiol. 5:297, 1985.

alter the relation, confounding the ability to define the ESPVR with precision in clinical studies.

A second difficulty in evaluating the ESPVR is the determination of the timing of end systole, defined as the upper left corner of the pressure-volume loop. This may not correspond exactly to aortic valve closure or the time of maximum ventricular elastance. This difference may be accentuated when there is reduced impedance to left ventricular ejection, as occurs in mitral regurgitation.[104]

A third difficulty is that because the slope of the ESPVR depends on the size of the ventricle, it is not possible to define a normal range for E_{ES}. Attempts to correct for ventricular size have not been uniformly successful. However, this does not prevent E_{ES} from differentiating patients with normal from those with abnormal left ventricular contractile function.[105] One method of correcting for differences in LV size is to evaluate the LV in the stress-strain plane.[106] In this analysis the LV end-systolic stress-strain relation is analogous to the ESPVR except that it has been normalized for wall thickness and chamber size and configuration.

If V_0 is assumed to be small, E_{ES} can be approximated by the ratio of LV systolic pressure to end-systolic volume (P_{ES}/V_{ES}).[89,107] This approach has the advantage of avoiding the need to evaluate multiply loaded beats and can be performed noninvasively. However, the P_{ES}/V_{ES} ratio is subject to significant errors in estimating E_{ES} when V_0 is large, and is not a sensitive measure of contractile performance.

Despite the theoretical and practical limitations to the clinical evaluation of contractility using the ESPVR, left ventricular pressure-volume analysis provides a powerful tool to help understand the interaction of contractile state and load to produce ventricular performance (Fig. 14–16).

Other Pressure-Volume Relations. Two other relations can be derived from variably loaded pressure-volume

loops: the dP/dt_{max}–end-diastolic volume (V_{ED}) relation and the SW-V_{ED} relation (Fig. 14–17).

During caval occlusion, dP/dt_{max} and V_{ED} are linearly related.[71] The slope of the relation (dE/dt_{max}) represents the maximum rate of change of left ventricular elastance during contraction and is very sensitive to contractile state.[71] Thus, this resting $dP/dt_{max} - V_{ED}$ relation accounts for the preload dependence of dP/dt_{max}, which increases when contractile state is augmented. Although it is very sensitive to changes in contractile state, the $dP/dt_{max} - V_{ED}$ relation has several limitations. First, dP/dt_{max} is more variable than P_{ES}, and this relation is less stable than the ESPVR.[108] Second, the $dP/dt_{max} - V_{ED}$ relation saturates at volumes only slightly above the operating point.[109] Thus this relation can be defined only by preload reduction and not by pharmacologically produced increases in load.

Stroke work (SW) is the external work performed by the left ventricle and is calculated as the area of the pressure-volume loop. It can be approximated as the product of stroke volume and mean arterial pressure. Thus, SW integrates the two determinants of tissue perfusion: flow and pressure.[65] During caval occlusions, SW and V_{ED} are linearly related. SW is insensitive to arterial load in the physiological range; thus the SW-V_{ED} relation is afterload independent under these conditions.[66,110,111] In response to an increase in contractile state the slope of this relation, termed *preload recruitable stroke work* (PRSW), increases. Thus, PRSW has been proposed as a load-independent measure of contractile state.[112] However, the SW-V_{ED} relation is not only determined by contractile state, it also can be altered by changes in the diastolic left ventricular pressure-volume relation.[108] For example, the diastolic pressure-volume relation can be altered under some circumstances without a change in the ESPVR.[113] This would alter the LV SW-V_{ED} relation and PRSW. Although importantly influenced by contractility, the SW-V_{ED} relation is best considered as a measure of integrated pump function (see below).

The SW-V_{ED} relation has several important advantages.[108] First, because SW integrates pressure and volume throughout the cardiac cycle, it is free of noise and is remarkably stable. Second, during reductions in preload as produced by caval occlusion, both determinants of SW (stroke volume and end-systolic pressure) decline, producing a wide range of SW values. This wide range of data increases the statistical precision with which the SW-V_{ED} relation can be defined. Finally, because the slope (PRSW) has dimensions of pressure, it therefore is independent of left ventricle cavity size.

PRELOAD ADJUSTED POWER. The power generated by the left ventricle can be calculated as the product of aortic flow and pressure. The maximum power (PWR_{max}) responds to changes in contractile state, is insensitive to changes in the arterial circulation, and is linearly related to the square of V_{ED} (V_{ED}^2) in the physiological range.[114] Thus, PWR_{max}/V_{ED}^2 may provide a preload-independent measure of contractility. PWR_{max}/V_{ED}^2 can be determined noninvasively using nuclear techniques or Doppler echocardiography to determine aortic flow, and measuring arterial pressure using indirect means.[115]

LEFT VENTRICULAR PUMP FUNCTION

The contraction of individual sarcomeres is integrated into the myocardial shortening that ultimately is expressed as the pumping function of the left ventricle. The left heart can be analyzed as a pump with an input (the pulmonary venous or mean left atrial pressure) and an output (which in simplest terms is the cardiac output = stroke volume × heart rate). The relationship between the input and output is the ventricular function curve or the Frank-Starling rela-

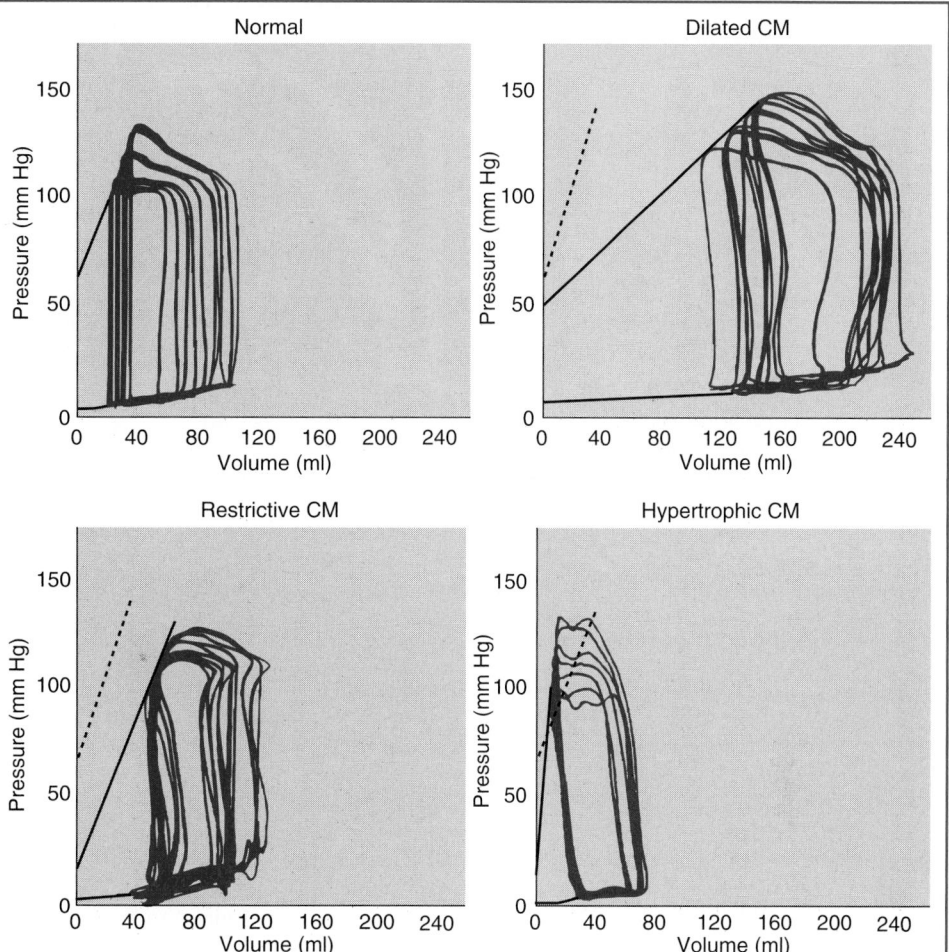

FIGURE 14–16. Variably loaded pressure-volume loops used to define the left ventricular end-systolic pressure-volume relations in four patients: *A,* normal ventricle; *B,* dilated cardiomyopathy (CM); *C,* restrictive heart disease; *D,* hypertrophic cardiomyopathy. (From Kass, D. A.: Clinical ventricular pathophysiology: A pressure-volume view. *In* Warltier, D. C.: Ventricular Function. Baltimore, Williams and Wilkins, 1995, p. 111. Reproduced by permission of the Society of Cardiovascular Anesthesiologists.)

tionship[116,117] (Figs. 14–18 and 14–19). In this relationship the output can be considered to be the SV, cardiac output, or the SW.

A family of Frank-Starling curves reflects the response of the pump performance of the ventricle to a spectrum of contractile states, and the position of a given curve provides a description of ventricular contractility. Movement along a single curve represents the operation of the Frank-Starling principle, which indicates that SV, cardiac output, or SW varies with preload. By contrast, upward or downward displacement of the curve represents a positive or negative inotropic effect, i.e., augmentation or depression

of contractility, respectively (Fig. 14–18). However, it is important to recognize that in an intact patient or animal the standard ventricular function curve represents a complex interaction of preload, afterload, and contractility.

The pump performance of the left ventricle depends on its ability to fill (diastolic performance) and to empty (systolic performance) (Fig. 14–19). The SV is equal to the product of the end-diastolic volume and the effective ejection fraction. Thus the generation of stroke volume depends on the conversion of the filling pressure to end-diastolic volume (diastolic performance) and on the effective ejection fraction (systolic performance).[53]

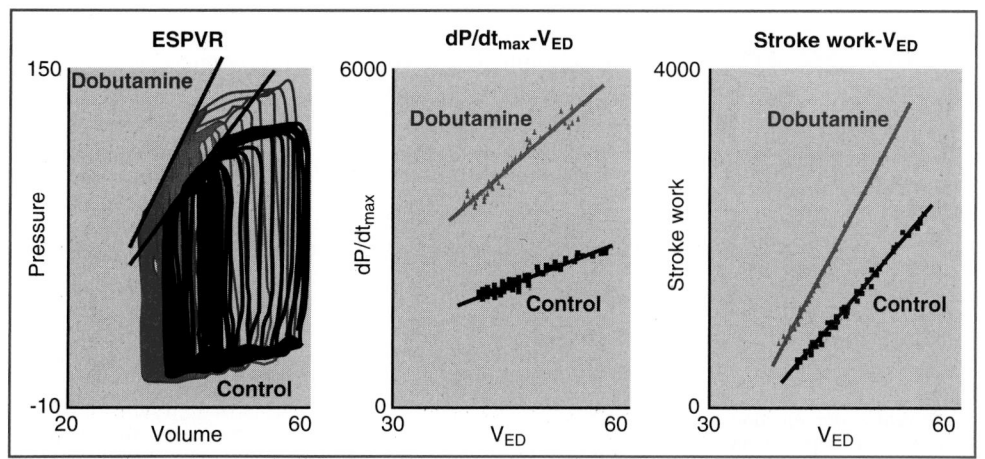

FIGURE 14–17. Three relations describing left ventricular contractile performance derived from variably loaded pressure-volume loops: the left ventricular end-systolic pressure-volume relation (ESPVR); the relation between dP/dt_{max} and end-diastolic volume (V_{ED}); and the relation between stroke work and V_{ED}. All three relations can be approximated by a straight line within the range of data generated by transient caval occlusion. Each relation is shifted toward the left with an increase in slope in response to increase in contractile state produced by dobutamine. (Reproduced with permission from Little, W. C., Cheng, C. P., Mumma, M., et al.: Comparison of measures of left ventricular contractile performance derived from pressure-volume loops in conscious dogs. Circulation *80:*1378, 1989. Copyright 1989 the American Heart Association.)

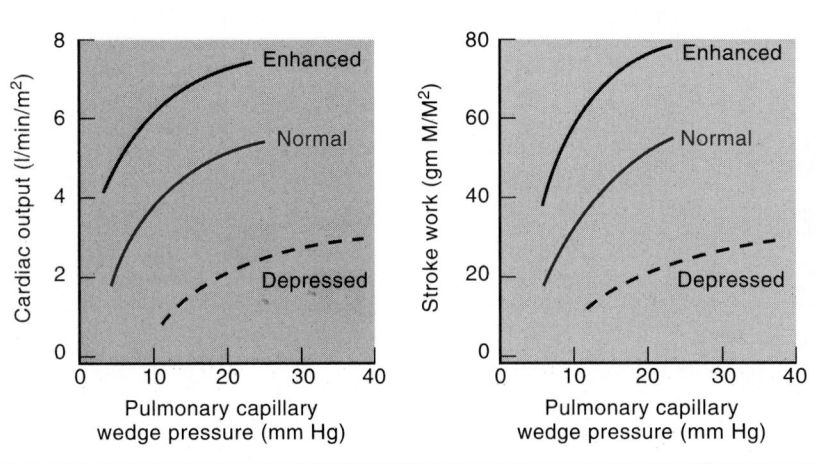

FIGURE 14–18. The Starling relationship. With increasing left ventricular filling pressure measured by the pulmonary capillary wedge pressure (reflecting the pulmonary venous pressure), there is an increase in cardiac output and stroke work. The positions of the curves are influenced by the contractile state of the left ventricle. An enhancement of contractile state shifts the curves upward while a depression produces a downward shift.

Systolic Performance

Left ventricular systolic performance is the ability of the left ventricle to empty. Because myocardial contractility is an important determinant of the left ventricle's systolic performance, systolic performance and contractility are frequently considered to be interchangeable. However, they are not the same because the systolic performance of the left ventricle is also importantly influenced by load and ventricular configuration. Thus it is possible to have abnormal systolic performance despite normal contractility when left ventricular afterload is excessive. Alternatively, left ventricular systolic performance may be nearly normal despite decreased myocardial contractility if left ventricular afterload is low, as occurs in some patients with mitral regurgitation.

Left ventricular systolic performance can be quantified as the left ventricular emptying fraction or ejection fraction (EF). In the presence of a left-sided valvular regurgitant lesion (mitral regurgitation or aortic regurgitation), or left-to-right shunt (ventricular septal defect or patent ductus arteriosus), the left ventricular stroke volume may be high, while the forward stroke volume (stroke volume minus re-gurgitant volume or shunt volume), which contributes to useful cardiac output, is lower. Accordingly, we define the *effective ejection fraction* as the forward stroke volume divided by end-diastolic volume.[53,118] The effective EF is a useful means to quantify systolic function because it represents the functional emptying of the left ventricle and is relatively independent of left ventricular end-diastolic volume over the clinically relevant range. An operational definition of systolic dysfunction is an effective EF of less than 50 per cent.[27,118] When defined in this manner, systolic left ventricular dysfunction may result from impaired myocardial function, increased left ventricular afterload, and/or structural abnormalities of the left heart.

The forward SV is equal to the product of the effective ejection fraction and the end-diastolic volume (Fig. 14–19). If left ventricular contractile state and arterial properties remain constant as end-diastolic volume increases, the EF stays constant or increases slightly.[80] Thus an increase in the end-diastolic volume will allow for a normal forward SV despite a reduced effective EF.

Diastolic Performance (See also p. 383)

For the left ventricle to function as a pump, it must not only empty but also fill. The left atrial (and pulmonary venous) pressure is the source pressure for left ventricular filling. Thus, normal left ventricular diastolic function can be defined as filling of the left ventricle sufficient to produce a cardiac output commensurate with the body's needs with a normal mean pulmonary venous pressure that does not exceed 12 mm Hg.[52]

A patient with systolic dysfunction (reduced effective ejection fraction) requires a larger end-diastolic volume to produce an adequate stroke volume and cardiac output. The achievement of a higher left ventricular end-diastolic volume without abnormally high pulmonary venous pressure, secondary to rightward displacement of the left ventricular diastolic pressure-volume curve (from curve B to curve A in Figure 14–20), can compensate for impaired systolic performance. However, more often the greater end-diastolic volume requires elevation of left ventricular diastolic, left atrial, and pulmonary venous pressures. Thus, systolic dysfunction is the most common cause of elevation of left ventricular diastolic pressure.

Diastolic dysfunction also occurs in the absence of systolic dysfunction and may be due to obstruction of left ventricular filling, impaired left ventricular distensibility, or external compression of the left ventricle.[53,119–122] A common cause of such primary diastolic dysfunction is altered diastolic distensibility. In the pressure-volume plane, this is represented by a leftward and upward shift of the end-diastolic pressure-volume relation (EDPVR) (Fig. 14–20). When this occurs, significantly higher pressures

---

Pulmonary venous
pressure

Input

Filling		Emptying		
ED volume	x	EF$_{effective}$	=	Stroke volume
LV Distensibility		Contractility		
Relaxation		Afterload		x
Left atrium		Preload		Heart
Mitral valve		Structure		rate
Pericardium				
Diastolic function		Systolic function		

Output

Cardiac output

FIGURE 14–19. Left ventricular pump performance. The input is considered to be the pulmonary venous pressure and the output the cardiac output. The stroke volume is equal to the product of the end-diastolic volume (ED) and the effective left ventricular ejection fraction (EF). Thus, the generation of the stroke volume depends on the conversion of the filling pressure to end-diastolic volume (diastolic performance) and on the effective ejection fraction (systolic performance).

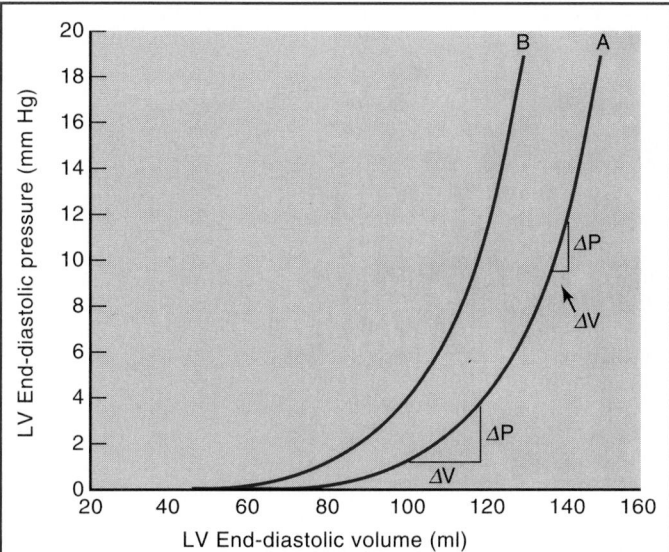

FIGURE 14-20. The slope of the LV end-diastolic pressure-volume relation indicates the passive chamber stiffness. Since the relation is exponential in shape, the slope ($\Delta P/\Delta V$) increases as the end-diastolic pressure increases. A shift of the curve from A to B indicates that a higher LV pressure will be required to distend the LV to a similar volume, indicating that the ventricle is less distensible. (From Little, W. C., and Downes, T. R.: Clinical evaluation of left ventricular diastolic performance. Prog. Cardiovasc. Dis. *32*(4):273, 1990. Reproduced by permission.)

are required to distend the left ventricle to achieve the same end-diastolic volume. If the shift in the EDPVR is severe enough, filling of the left ventricle to the level sufficient to produce a normal stroke volume can be achieved only with elevated pulmonary venous pressure that will be associated with pulmonary congestion. Thus, an alteration in diastolic distensibility may produce pulmonary congestion and congestive heart failure in the absence of systolic dysfunction.[119,120,122,123]

Evaluation of Diastolic Performance

The indices of diastolic function can be organized into three groups: measures of isovolumetric relaxation, indices of passive left ventricular characteristics derived from the diastolic left ventricular pressure-volume relations, and measurements of the pattern of left ventricular diastolic filling, which are obtained from Doppler echocardiography or radionuclide angiography.[52,124,125]

ISOVOLUMETRIC RELAXATION. Isovolumetric relaxation can be quantified by measuring its duration or by describing the time course of the fall in left ventricular pressure. The duration of isovolumetric relaxation, or the time from aortic valve closure to mitral valve opening, can be measured by M-mode echocardiography. A similar interval, the time from aortic valve closure to the onset of mitral valve flow, can be measured by combining phonocardiography and Doppler echocardiography. Unfortunately, the duration of isovolumetric relaxation depends not only on the rate of left ventricular relaxation but also on the difference in pressures between the aorta at the time of aortic valve closure and the left atrium at mitral valve opening.[126] Thus, the duration of isovolumetric relaxation can be increased by an elevation of aortic pressure or decreased by an elevation of left atrial pressure. The time from minimum left ventricular volume to peak left ventricular filling rate can be measured using radionuclear angiography.[125] Because this time interval spans both isovolumetric relaxation and part of early filling, the interpretation is even more complicated than the duration of isovolumetric relaxation alone.

The time course of isovolumetric pressure decline has been quantitatively described by the peak rate of pressure fall (dP/dt_{min}) and the time constant of an exponential fit of

the time course of isovolumetric pressure decline. Each of these requires the measurement of left ventricular pressure using a micromanometer. dP/dt_{min} is strongly influenced by the pressure at the time of aortic valve closure and is not a good measure of the rate of isovolumetric relaxation.

After aortic valve closure, left ventricular pressure declines in an exponential manner during isovolumetric relaxation[127] (Fig. 14-21). The rate of pressure decline can be quantified by the time constant of the exponential decline. The time constant (τ) is increased by processes such as ischemia or other causes of myocardial depression that slow ventricular relaxation.[128,129] It is shortened by acceleration of the rate of active relaxation, as caused by an increase in heart rate or sympathetic stimulation. The time constant of isovolumetric pressure decline can also be altered by changes in loading conditions. An increase in arterial pressure or end-diastolic volume can increase the time constant, although changes in the preload at a constant arterial pressure may have less effect.[129,130]

Calculation of the time constant of left ventricular isovolumetric pressure decline has several technical limitations. Data are analyzed from the time of minimum dP/dt to a pressure 5 or 10 mm Hg above end-diastolic pressure. Even if pressure is measured every 2 msec, there are only a limited number of data points. This contributes to a large beat-to-beat variability of τ.[131]

If mitral in-flow is prevented, left ventricular pressure will decline to subatmospheric levels. Thus, it has been suggested that the data should be fit to an exponential function with an asymptote (P_B):

$$P(t) = P_o e^{-t/\tau} + P_B.$$

This is usually done by differentiating both sides and then using the linear least squares technique to fit the equation:

$$dP(t)/dt = -(1/\tau)(P - P_B)$$

The normal range of values of τ calculated using this method is 37 to 67 msec.[132]

The use of an asymptote to calculate τ is particularly important when the external pressure of the left ventricle may be changing.[133] However, τ determined from a nonfilling beat in an experimental animal in which the full

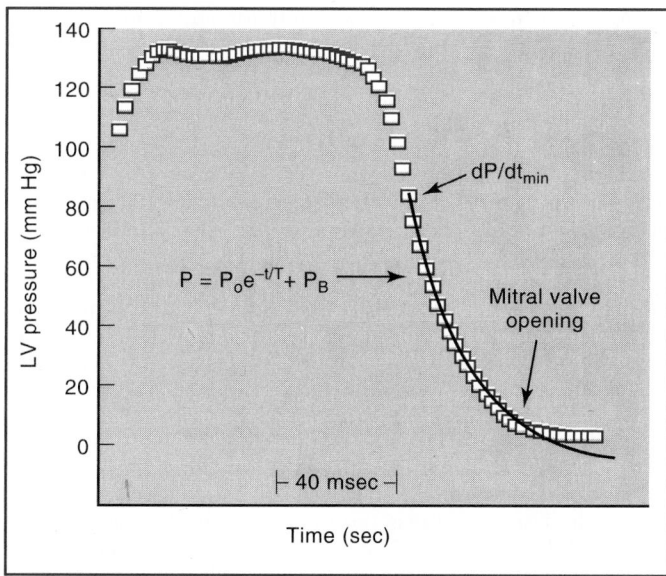

FIGURE 14-21. LV pressure measured at 2-msec intervals using a micromanometer. The LV pressure from the time of minimum dP/dt (dP/dt_{min}) to mitral valve opening is described by an exponential relation (*solid line*). After mitral valve opening, LV pressure deviates from the exponential line. $P_o + P_b$ = pressure (P) at dP/dt_{max}; t = time; T = time constant of relaxation; P_B = baseline pressure. (From Little, W. C., and Downes, T. R.: Clinical evaluation of left ventricular diastolic performance. Prog. Cardiovasc. Dis. *32*(4):273, 1990. Reproduced by permission.)

time course of left ventricular relaxation is available correlates most closely with τ calculated from a normal beat without the use of an asymptote (i.e., $P = P_o e^{-t/\tau}$).[134] To avoid the computational properties of nonlinear fitting in the calculation on τ without an asymptote, the relation is linearized using a natural logarithm transformation to result in:

$$\ln P = \ln P_o - {}^t/_\tau$$

The data are then fit to this equation using the linear least squares technique to determine τ. When calculated using this method, the normal range of values for τ is 28 to 45 msec.[132]

Recently, the time course of LV pressure during isovolumetric relaxation has been characterized using noninvasive Doppler measurement of the velocity of a regurgitant jet across the mitral or aortic valve.[10,11,135] In this method the modified Bernoulli equation is used to approximate LV pressure during isovolumetric relaxation allowing calculation of the maximum rate of left ventricular pressure decline and the exponential time constant.

PASSIVE DIASTOLIC CHARACTERISTICS OF THE LEFT VENTRICLE. The passive characteristics of the left ventricle can be described as the diastolic pressure-volume relation.[119,120,129] Optimally the passive left ventricular diastolic pressure-volume relation should be constructed from points that are obtained after relaxation is complete and at slow filling rates, so that viscous effects are not present.[129,136] Practically, this can be approximated using points obtained late in diastole, when relaxation is assumed to be complete, or from variously loaded beats at end diastole. However, it is important to correct for the effect of respiratory changes in intrathoracic pressure.

The slope of the end-diastolic pressure-volume relation is the *chamber stiffness*. Since the pressure-volume relation is nonlinear, the chamber stiffness depends on the point on the curve in which it is measured; stiffness increases with increasing volume (Fig. 14–20). Several techniques have been proposed to correct for this effect by normalizing chamber stiffness. One approach is to approximate the pressure-volume relation by an exponential function.[137] Another technique is to compare the chamber stiffness at a common pressure or volume. However, the analysis of chamber stiffness does not account for shifts in the pressure-volume relation that can occur from the alteration of load, diseases, or pharmacological agents.[56,57,129,136] The position of the diastolic pressure-volume relation indicates the distensibility of the left ventricle, an upward shift indicating a less distensible ventricle.[119]

The *diastolic pressure-volume* relation represents the net passive characteristics of the left ventricular chamber. To derive information concerning the properties of the myocardium alone, the effects of wall thickness, ventricular configuration, size, and external pressure must be removed.[138] This can be accomplished by deriving the myocardial stress-strain relation from the chamber transmural pressure-volume relation. In contrast to the slope of the pressure-volume relation that assesses the amount of ventricular chamber distention under pressure, the stress-strain relation represents the resistance of the myocardium to stretch when subjected to stress. Thus, it should not be influenced by the configuration of the left ventricle. However, calculation of stress requires the use of a geometrical model of the left ventricle, and calculation of strain requires assumption of the unstressed left ventricular volume. In addition to these potential theoretical limitations, these calculations require accurate measurements over a wide range of left ventricular pressures and volumes. Measurements made during rapid filling may be inappropriately influenced by active myocardial relaxation and viscoelastic effects. Observations during diastasis and atrial systole do not have this problem, but they may not supply a wide enough range of data points. The theoretical problems and the technical difficulties in determining myocardial stress-strain relations have limited their clinical application.

PATTERNS OF LEFT VENTRICULAR DIASTOLIC FILLING. Recently there has been interest in assessing quantified diastolic left ventricular performance by analyzing the pattern of left ventricular filling. Such information can be obtained by determining the left ventricular volume or dimension throughout the cardiac cycle, using contrast or radionuclide angiography, M-mode or two-dimensional echocardiography, or by measuring the left ventricular in-flow velocity using a Doppler determination of mitral valve flow velocities. The most widely used methods today are radionuclide angiography[125] and Doppler mitral valve flow-velocity determination[52,124,139–142] (see Fig. 4–37, p. 72).

Mechanisms of Diastolic Filling. To understand the significance of the patterns of left ventricular filling, it is important to consider the mechanisms of normal left ventricular filling.[142,143] The events surrounding normal left ventricular filling are shown in Figure 14–22. From the time of aortic valve closure until mitral valve opening, the left ventricle is normally a closed chamber with a constant volume. Myocardial relaxation begins in the latter part of systole and causes a steep, exponential fall in intraventricular pressure as elastic elements of the left ventricle that compressed and twisted during ejection are allowed to recoil. Although no filling occurs during isovolumetric relax-

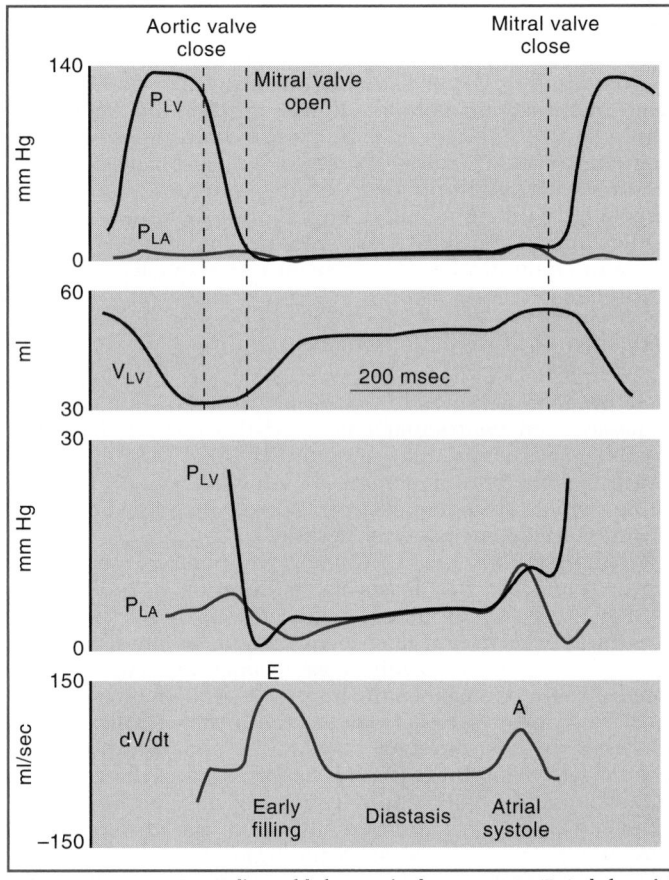

FIGURE 14–22. Recording of left ventricular pressure (P_{LV}), left atrial pressure (P_{LA}), left ventricular volume (V_{LV}), and the rate of change of left ventricular volume (dV/dt), which indicates the rate of left ventricular filling. Left ventricular filling occurs early in diastole and during atrial systole in response to pressure gradient from the left atrium to the left ventricle. The early diastolic pressure gradient is generated as left ventricular pressure falls below left atrial pressure and the late diastolic gradient is generated as atrial contraction increases left atrial pressure above left ventricular pressure. (Data from Cheng, C. P., Freeman, G. L., Santamore, W. P., et al.: Effect of loading conditions, contractile state and heart rate on early diastolic left ventricular filling in conscious dogs. Circ. Res. 66:814, 1990. Copyright 1990 American Heart Association.)

ation, the processes that determine the rate of decline of the isovolumetric pressure influence ventricular filling following opening of the mitral valve.[134,144] For the first 30 to 40 msec after mitral valve opening, decline of left ventricular wall tension is normally rapid enough to cause left ventricular pressure to fall, despite a substantial increase in left ventricular volume.[143] This fall in left ventricular pressure produces a pressure gradient that accelerates blood from the left atrium into the left ventricle, resulting in rapid early diastolic filling. The rate of early left ventricular filling is determined by the mitral valve pressure gradient (left atrial pressure–left ventricular pressure).[134,143,145] Although peak filling occurs after the peak pressure gradient, the two are closely related. Two major factors (myocardial relaxation and LA pressure) determine the early diastolic mitral valve pressure gradient and the rate of left ventricular filling. Under normal circumstances more than two-thirds of the stroke volume enters the left ventricle during early diastole.

After filling of the left ventricle begins, the mitral valve pressure gradient decreases and then transiently reverses. This occurs because left ventricular relaxation is nearing completion and the flow of blood from the left atrium fills the left ventricle, raising the left ventricular pressure while lowering the left atrial pressure. This reversed mitral valve pressure gradient decelerates and then stops the rapid flow of blood into the left ventricle early in diastole. The pressures in the left atrium and left ventricle equilibrate as mitral flow nearly ceases; thus, little left ventricular filling occurs during the midportion of diastole, termed *diastasis*.

Atrial contraction increases atrial pressure late in diastole producing a left atrium–to–left ventricle pressure gradient that again propels blood into the left ventricle. Following atrial systole, as the LA relaxes, its pressure decreases below left ventricular pressure, causing the mitral valve to begin closing.[146] The onset of ventricular systole produces a rapid increase in left ventricular pressure that seals the mitral valve and ends diastole.

Normal Pattern of Left Ventricular Filling. The normal pattern of left ventricular filling is characterized by rapid filling early in diastole with some additional filling during atrial contraction. This normal filling pattern can be quantified by measuring the peak early diastolic filling rate or mitral flow velocity (E), the integral of the early diastole filling or flow velocity, and the peak filling rate or mitral flow velocity during atrial contraction (A).[52,134,139–142] The relative contribution of early and late (atrial) filling is commonly expressed as the E/A ratio. Normally the E/A ratio is greater than 1. The time required for deceleration of the early diastolic flow (t_{dec}) and the rate of this deceleration (E/t_{dec}) are two other important parameters of the filling pattern. A variety of other measures have also been proposed. Table 14–3 contains a list of the ranges of normal values for these measures of left ventricular filling. The wide range of normal values is probably caused by variations in the technique of performing the observations, which are both operator and equipment sensitive. Furthermore, the measures can be altered by many physiological factors.

Abnormal Patterns of Left Ventricular Filling. The normal pattern of left ventricular filling is altered in many patients with cardiac disease.[52,124,139–141,147–149] By means of Doppler mitral flow velocity, three abnormal patterns (in the absence of mitral stenosis) have been identified indicating progressively greater impairment of diastolic function (Fig. 14–23).

The first abnormal pattern of filling has been termed *delayed relaxation*.[140,150] In this pattern there is reduced peak rate and amount of early left ventricular filling, and the relative importance of atrial filling is enhanced. This results in a reversed E/A ratio of less than 1 (i.e., E < A). The reduced peak rate of early filling is due to a decreased early diastolic left atrial–to–left ventricular pressure gra-

TABLE 14–3 PARAMETERS OF LEFT VENTRICULAR DIASTOLIC FILLING MEASURED BY DOPPLER ECHOCARDIOGRAPHY

Peak E	79 ± 26 cm/sec
Peak A	48 ± 22 cm/sec
E/A	1.7 ± 0.6
E Deceleration time	184 ± 24 msec
E Deceleration rate	5.6 ± 2.7 m/sec²
Isovolumetric relaxation time	74 ± 26 msec
Peak pulmonary venous AR wave	19 ± 4 cm/sec

Adapted from Little, W. C., and Downes, T. R.: Clinical evaluation of left ventricular diastolic performance. Prog. Cardiovasc. Dis. *32*(4):273, 1990.

dient, resulting from a slowed rate of left ventricular relaxation[151] (Fig. 14–24). A delayed relaxation pattern can be seen in patients with left ventricular hypertrophy, arterial hypertension, and coronary artery disease and in normal elderly subjects. In many of these patients, mean left atrial pressure is within the normal range at rest and the patients are asymptomatic.[52] In this situation the vigorous atrial contraction compensates for the reduced early filling due to impaired left ventricular relaxation while maintaining a normal mean left atrial pressure.

A second pattern of abnormal filling has been termed *pseudonormalized*.[140] This pattern, in which the E/A ratio is greater than 1 (as occurs in normal persons), is seen in patients with more severe impairment of diastolic performance than the pattern of delayed relaxation. The pseudonormalized pattern is due to restoration of the normal early diastolic left ventricular pressure gradient due to an increase in left atrial pressure that compensates for the slowed rate of left ventricular relaxation[151] (Fig. 14–24). The pseudonormalized pattern of filling is distinguished from normal by a more rapid rate of early diastolic flow deceleration and faster deceleration time (< 150 msec). The deceleration time is proportional to the inverse of the square root of the left ventricular chamber stiffness.[151,152] Thus, the faster deceleration time indicates increased left ventricular diastolic chamber stiffness.

A third abnormal pattern of left ventricular filling indicating a severe diastolic abnormality has been termed the *restrictive pattern*.[140,150] In this pattern the early filling is increased above the control level and greatly exceeds the filling that occurs during atrial contraction, and the E/A ratio is usually greater than 2. In fact, there may be little or

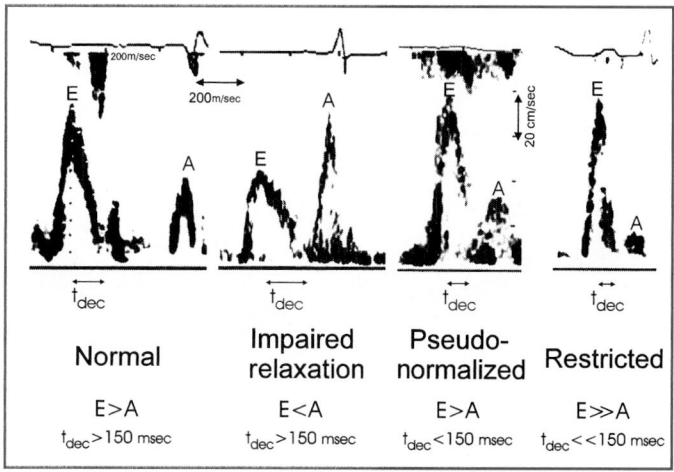

FIGURE 14–23. Patterns of left ventricular filling as recorded by diastolic Doppler mitral flow velocities. In the normal pattern there is a large E wave and a small A wave. There are three abnormal patterns of mitral filling representing progressively worsening left ventricular diastolic performance. With "delayed relaxation" the E wave is less than the A wave. The left ventricular deceleration (t_{dec}) is normal or prolonged. In the "pseudonormalized" pattern the E wave is larger than the A wave; however, t_{dec} is shortened. In the restricted filling pattern E is much larger than A with a very short t_{dec}.

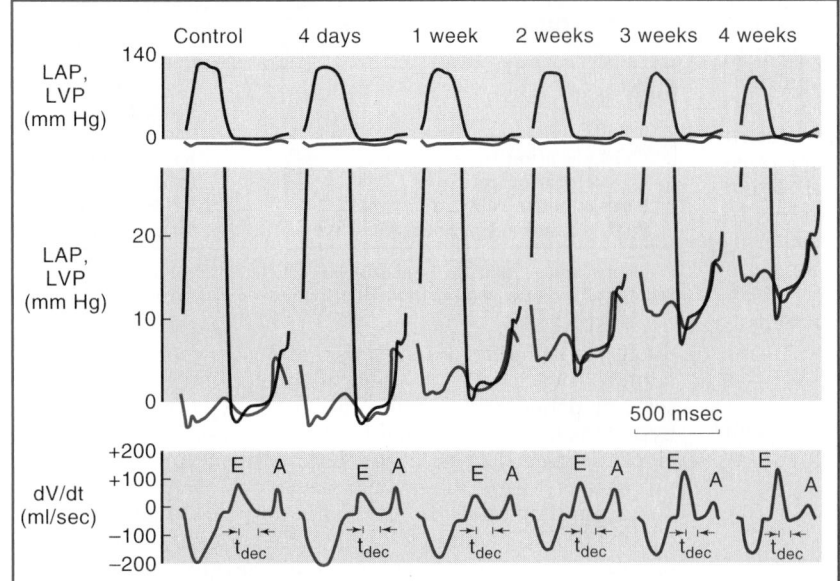

FIGURE 14–24. Recordings of left ventricular (LVP) and left atrial pressures (LAP) and the rate of change of left ventricular volume (dV/dt) during control and serially during the development of pacing-induced heart failure in an experimental animal. During control there is a normal filling pattern with E (early diastolic filling) larger than A (diastolic filling during atrial systole). At 4 days a pattern of "delayed relaxation" has developed with a small E and large A. This occurs in response to a slowing of the rate of left ventricular relaxation and a smaller pressure gradient from the left atrium to the left ventricle early in diastole. As heart failure subsequently worsened, left atrial pressure increased. This ultimately resulted in a pattern of "pseudonormalization" at 2 to 3 weeks and a pattern of "restricted filling" at 4 weeks. The increased early filling (E) occurring during these patterns was associated with increases in the early diastolic left atrial to left ventricular pressure gradient produced by the marked increase in left atrial pressure. (From Ohno, M., Cheng, C. P., and Little, W. C.: Mechanism of altered patterns of left ventricular filling during the development of congestive heart failure. Circulation 89:2241, 1994. Copyright 1994 American Heart Association.)

no filling during atrial contraction. The deceleration time is much less than 150 msec. This pattern is seen in patients with severe diastolic dysfunction and pulmonary congestion. The enhanced early filling in the restrictive pattern results from markedly elevated LA pressure that more than offsets the slowing of left ventricular relaxation.[151] In this situation, in which left ventricular stiffness is increased, the early flow deceleration time is very short, and the deceleration rate of early flow is rapid. The restrictive filling pattern is seen in patients with severe pulmonary congestion,[153] constrictive pericarditis,[154] and restrictive cardiomyopathies such as cardiac amyloidosis.[155]

The three abnormal patterns of left ventricular filling represent a continuum of increasing severity of diastolic abnormalities. The pattern of delayed relaxation may be observed in asymptomatic patients with only impaired diastolic reserve, while the pseudonormalized and restrictive patterns occur in patients with progressively more severe diastolic dysfunction who almost always have pulmonary congestion.

Pulmonary Venous Flow Patterns. The pattern of blood flow in the pulmonary veins provides additional information on diastolic filling.[124,150,156,157] The velocity of pulmonary venous flow can be measured by transthoracic Doppler in some patients and by transesophageal Doppler in most patients. The pulmonary venous flow velocity has three waves (Fig. 14–25): (1) the S wave, indicating antegrade flow into the left atrium during ventricular systole, (2) the D wave, indicating antegrade flow early in diastole just following the peak of the E wave mitral valve flow, and (3) the AR wave of retrograde flow out of the left atrium during atrial systole. The S and D waves correspond to the x and y descents in the left atrial pressure, while the pulmonary venous AR wave corresponds to the left atrial a wave. When left ventricular end-diastolic stiffness is increased, the AR wave is augmented and prolonged, unless atrial systolic failure or atrial fibrillation is present. Thus, pseudonormalized and restricted mitral flow patterns are associated with large, prolonged AR waves with a peak flow velocity > 35 cm/sec.[150]

Assessment of Right Ventricular Performance

Although most attention in adult cardiology is appropriately focused on the performance of the left ventricle, the right ventricle may be an important contributor to cardiac dysfunction.[158] The concepts of preload, afterload, and contractility and most of the methods of evaluating left ventricular performance are also applicable to the right ventricle. The ejection of the thin-walled right ventricle is more sensitive to increases in afterload than is the left ventricle. Right ventricular dilatation in response to increased afterload is limited by the tethering of the right ventricle to the much thicker left ventricle and the limitations imposed by the pericardium. With increased afterload the thin-walled right ventricle dilates, causing functional tricuspid regurgitation.[159] Right ventricular performance can be importantly influenced by the presence and severity of such regurgitation.

Right ventricular volume and ejection fraction can be measured using echocardiography, radionuclear techniques, and angiography. In addition, right ventricular stroke volume and ejection fraction can be monitored on-line using the thermodilution technique[160–162] (p. 191). This is performed by injecting a bolus of cold saline solution into the right atrium, while the temperature in the pulmonary artery is recorded using a rapidly responding thermistor mounted on a catheter. This technique, which allows serial measurements, is convenient, reproducible, and reasonably accurate.

The right ventricular end-systolic pressure-volume relation can be determined with a manometer-tipped catheter in the right ventricle and either an impedance catheter or a radionuclide ventriculogram to provide simultaneous measurements of right ventricular volume while varying right ventricular load.[163,164] The right ventricular ESPVR behaves

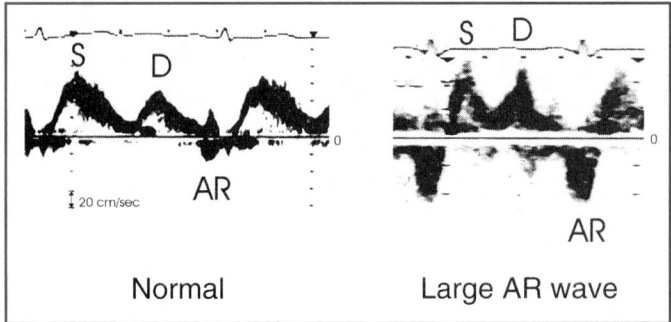

FIGURE 14–25. On the left is a normal pulmonary venous flow pattern recorded using transesophageal echocardiography. The S and D waves indicating flow into the left atrium are shown. There is a small atrial AR wave of retrograde flow out of the left atrium during atrial systole. On the right is an abnormal pulmonary venous flow pattern recorded in a patient with severe left ventricular hypertrophy. There is a large, prolonged AR wave with a peak velocity of more than 40 cm/sec. (Recordings courtesy of Dr. Abdel-Mohsen Nomeir of Bowman Gray School of Medicine of Wake Forest University.)

in a similar manner as the left ventricular ESPVR discussed above. The right ventricular ESPVR is linear in the physiological range and is shifted upward and leftward by the positive inotropic agent dobutamine.

INTEGRATED CARDIOVASCULAR PERFORMANCE

Cardiac Output (see p. 191)

The integrated pumping function of the cardiovascular system results ultimately in the cardiac output. The cardiac output can be measured using indicator dilution techniques, as described above. An alternate method to measure cardiac output is to use the Fick principle. Oxygen consumption is measured, or much less accurately assumed from the patient's height, weight, and age using a standard nomogram. The oxygen difference from the pulmonary artery to arterial circulation ($A - \dot{V}_{O_2}$ difference) is measured. Then the cardiac output is calculated as:

$$\text{Cardiac Output} = \frac{O_2 \text{ Consumption}}{A - \dot{V}_{O_2} \text{ Difference}}$$

The cardiac output is usually corrected for body size and expressed as the cardiac index, i.e., the cardiac output per square meter of body surface area. The normal range for the cardiac index, in the basal (resting) state in the supine position is wide, between 2.5 and 4.2 liters/min/m². The wide normal range makes it possible for cardiac output to decline by almost 40 per cent and still remain within the normal limits. Thus, a cardiac index of less than 2.5 liters/min/m² usually represents a marked disturbance of cardiovascular performance and is almost always clinically apparent. Although the resting cardiac output (or index) is insensitive in detecting mild to moderate cardiac impairment, it provides a valuable measure of the integrated function of the cardiovascular system, especially in critically ill patients.

Arteriovenous Oxygen Difference

The most crucial function of the cardiovascular system is to supply the tissues with oxygen. This requires the integrated action of the heart, circulation, lungs, and the peripheral metabolism[165] (Fig. 14–26). As defined by the Fick principle, the oxygen delivered to the body is the product of the cardiac output and the difference in oxygen content of the arterial blood and the mixed venous blood ($A - \dot{V}_{O_2}$ difference). Under normal circumstances at rest, adequate oxygen supply to the tissues is produced with a $A - \dot{V}_{O_2}$ difference of 40 ± 10 ml O_2/liter. With nearly fully oxygenated arterial blood (>98 per cent saturation) and normal

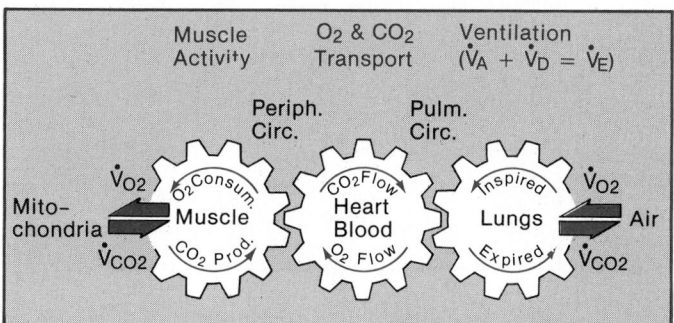

FIGURE 14–26. Interaction of physiological mechanisms coupling external to cellular respiration. Central role of circulation explains why cardiovascular diseases cause abnormalities in O_2 transport and O_2 uptake kinetics. O_2 consumption (O_2 consum.); CO_2 production (CO_2 prod.); alveolar ventilation ($\dot{V}_A$); physiological dead space ventilation ($\dot{V}_D$); expired ventilation ($\dot{V}_E$); O_2 uptake ($\dot{V}_{O_2}$); CO_2 output ($\dot{V}_{CO_2}$). (From Wasserman, K.: Measures of functional capacity in patients with heart failure. Circulation 81(Suppl. 2):1, 1990. Reproduced by permission of the American Heart Association, Inc.)

439

Ch 14

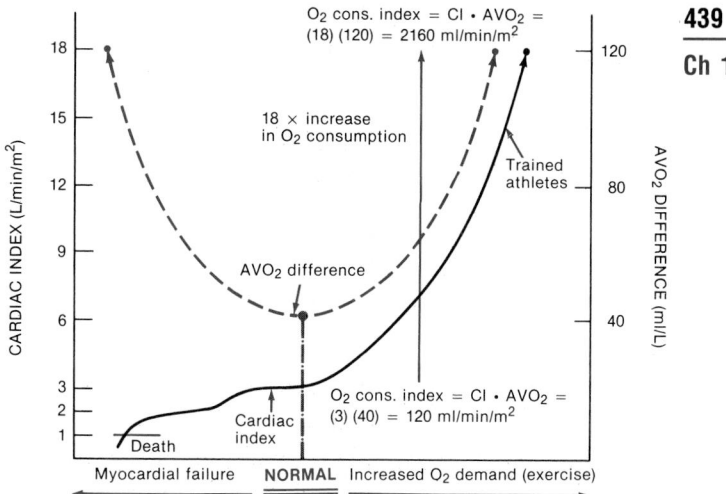

FIGURE 14–27. Relation between arteriovenous oxygen (AVO$_2$) difference (broken line) and cardiac index (solid curve) in normal subjects at rest (center) and during exercise (right), and in the patient with progressively worsening myocardial failure (left). (From Grossman, W.: Blood flow measurement: The cardiac output. In Grossman, W., and Baim, D. S.: Cardiac Catheterization, Angiography and Intervention. 4th ed. Philadelphia, Lea and Febiger, 1991, p. 106. Reproduced by permission.)

hemoglobin concentration and O_2-carrying capacity, the normal $A - \dot{V}_{O_2}$ difference is achieved with a mixed venous O_2 saturation of >70 per cent. If the cardiac output is inadequate the tissues extract more O_2, and the $A - \dot{V}_{O_2}$ difference increases. In this situation mixed venous O_2 saturation falls (Fig. 14–27). Thus, a normal mixed venous oxygen saturation (>70 per cent) indicates that the cardiac output is adequate to meet the body's demands.[166,167]

Reduced mixed venous O_2 saturation may result from an abnormality of cardiovascular function that is limiting the cardiac output, a deficiency in the O_2-carrying capacity of the blood, or pulmonary disease. When the ability to widen the $A - \dot{V}_{O_2}$ difference and increase oxygen extraction is exhausted, anaerobic metabolism produces lactate, and venous lactate levels rise precipitously.[168]

It should be noted that the myocardium extracts oxygen nearly maximally from blood at rest. Thus, the coronary sinus oxygen saturation is low (<40 per cent), and the myocardium cannot use an increase in oxygen extraction as a compensatory mechanism for inadequate coronary flow.

During exercise the body's oxygen consumption increases dramatically. This increased need is met by a combination of an increase in cardiac output and widening of the $A - \dot{V}_{O_2}$ difference.[169] For example, during very strenuous exercise, the oxygen consumption increases up to 18-fold. This is accomplished by a 6-fold increase in cardiac output (from 3 to 18 liters/min/m²) and a 3-fold increase in the $A - \dot{V}_{O_2}$ difference (from 40 to 120 ml/liter), with the mixed venous O_2 saturation decreasing from 75 to 25 per cent.

Cardiopulmonary Exercise Testing
(See also p. 153)

The integrated performance of the cardiovascular and pulmonary systems is evaluated by cardiopulmonary exercise testing.

A systematic approach to cardiopulmonary exercise testing requires the noninvasive assessment of total oxygen uptake ($\dot{V}_{O_2}$) and carbon dioxide production ($\dot{V}_{CO_2}$), while progressively increasing isotonic exercise is carried out on a treadmill or bicycle ergometer.[170–175] End-tidal O_2 and CO_2 concentrations and ventilation are measured continuously, allowing the monitoring of $\dot{V}_{O_2}$ and $\dot{V}_{CO_2}$ on a breath-by-breath basis. This permits determination of (1) the maximal oxygen uptake ($\dot{V}_{O_{2max}}$, or aerobic capacity),

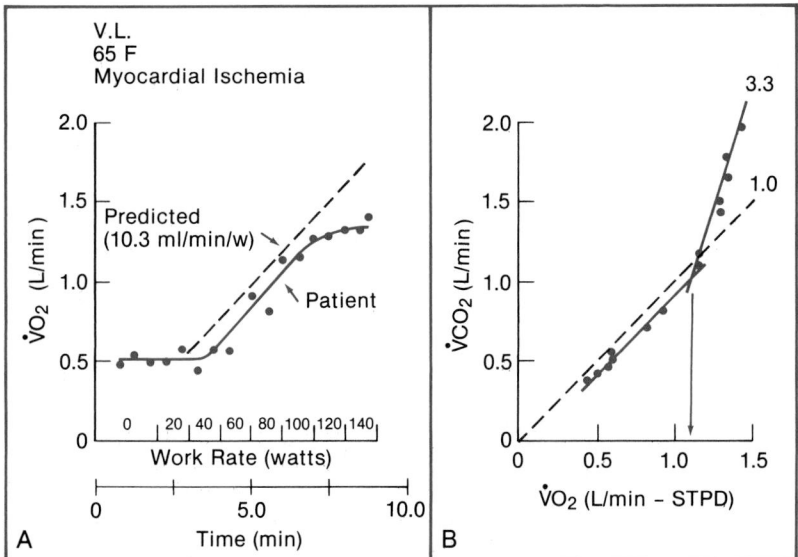

FIGURE 14–28. O_2 uptake ($\dot{V}_{O_2}$) plotted as the function of work rate *(panel A)* and CO_2 output ($\dot{V}_{CO_2}$) as function of $\dot{V}_{O_2}$ (V-slope plot) *(panel B)* of 64-year-old patient with shortness of breath at high altitude and ST-segment changes consistent with myocardial ischemia at 120 W cycle ergometer exercise, but without pain. Because of flattened $\dot{V}_{O_2}$ response *(panel A)* but continued steep rise in $\dot{V}_{O_2}$ above anaerobic threshold, the upper-component slope of $\dot{V}_{CO_2}$-$\dot{V}_{O_2}$ plot *(panel B)* is pathologically steep. Steep upper-component slope with a value of 3.3 suggests an exceptionally high rate of lactate release during exercise. Slope of 1 is drawn in *panel B* to provide visualization of steepening in the $\dot{V}_{CO_2}$-$\dot{V}_{O_2}$ plot reflecting the start of HCO_3 buffering of lactic acid. (From Wasserman, K., Beaver, W. L., and Whipp, B. J.: Gas exchange theory and the lactic acidosis (anaerobic) threshold. Circulation *81*(Suppl. 2):14, 1990. Copyright 1990 American Heart Association.)

defined as the value achieved when $\dot{V}_{O_2}$ remains stable despite an increase in the intensity of exercise (Figs. 14–28 and 5–1, p. 154), and (2) the anaerobic threshold. The latter is reached during the course of progressive exercise when the O_2 available to the tissues becomes inadequate. At this point, energy is generated inefficiently by anaerobic metabolism, a process producing lactate, which is buffered by bicarbonate, leading to increased production of CO_2. This can be recognized by a rise in $\dot{V}_{CO_2}$ that exceeds the rise in $\dot{V}_{O_2}$ producing a rise in the respiratory quotient (R), i.e., the ratio $\dot{V}_{CO_2}/\dot{V}_{O_2}$ (Fig. 14–28).

The anaerobic threshold indicates the maximum level of physical activity and O_2 uptake at which the cardiopulmonary system is able to provide sufficient O_2 to maintain aerobic metabolism in skeletal muscle. These two endpoints—the $\dot{V}_{O_2max}$ and the anaerobic threshold—can be determined objectively and are not affected by the bias of patient or examiner, which may limit the value of exercise tests. Although exercise capacity correlates with maximal $\dot{V}_{O_2}$, these correlations are not good enough to allow the former to serve as a substitute for the latter. The reproducibility of $\dot{V}_{O_2max}$ and the anaerobic threshold, when measured days or weeks apart in subjects whose condition has not changed, is excellent.[171,176] Normal values of $\dot{V}_{O_2max}$ and of the anaerobic threshold decline with age after 20 years and are higher in men than in women. Functional capacity has been conveniently categorized into five classes by Weber and his associates (A to E)[171]; impairment in group E is so severe that the patients cannot (or should not) exercise (Table 14–4).

The $\dot{V}_{O_2max}$ is a function of both the maximal cardiac output and the maximal extracton of O_2 by the tissues (maximal A – V[O_2]). The latter does not vary systematically in patients of various classes and usually exceeds 70 per cent at $\dot{V}_{O_2max}$. Therefore, $\dot{V}_{O_2max}$ reflects the maximum

cardiac output, which is a far more sensitive measurement than is the resting cardiac output in discriminating among patients in different degrees of cardiac disability.

Cardiopulmonary exercise testing is of clinical value in objectively assessing exercise tolerance and functional capacity, in evaluating the possible causes of exertional dyspnea and fatigue, in determining the severity of disability, in following its progress, and in assessing the response to therapy.[172,177] Impairment of pulmonary and/or musculoskeletal function can interfere with oxygen uptake during exertion. Therefore, in a patient with a reduced $\dot{V}_{O_2max}$ and clinical manifestations of lung disease, pulmonary function should be evaluated.[178]

When $\dot{V}_{O_2max}$ is reduced and arterial O_2 saturation declines during exercise, it is probably due to pulmonary dysfunction. Conversely, cardiac dysfunction can be recog-

TABLE 14–4 FUNCTIONAL IMPAIRMENT IN AEROBIC CAPACITY AND ANAEROBIC THRESHOLD AS MEASURED DURING INCREMENTAL EXERCISE TESTING

CLASS	DEGREE OF IMPAIRMENT	$\dot{V}_{O_2}$ MAX (ml/min/kg)	ANAEROBIC THRESHOLD (ml/min/kg)
A	Mild to none	>20	>14
B	Mild to moderate	16 to 20	11 to 14
C	Moderate to severe	10 to 16	8 to 11
D	Severe	6 to 10	5 to 8
E	Very severe	<6	≤ 4

From Weber, K. T., Janicki, J. S., and McElroy, P. A.: Cardiopulmonary exercise (CPX) testing. *In* Weber, K. T., and Janicki, J. S. (eds.): Cardiopulmonary Exercise Testing. Philadelphia, W. B. Saunders Co., 1986, p. 153.

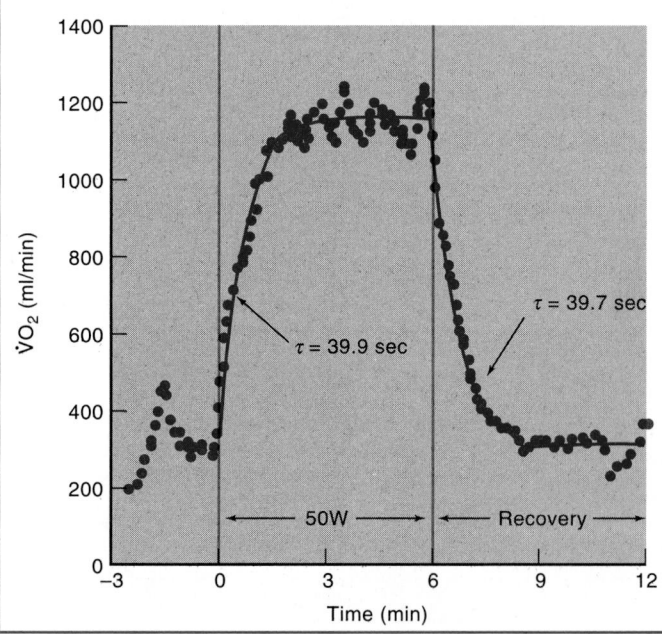

FIGURE 14–29. Plot of changes in oxygen uptake ($\dot{V}_{O_2}$) during 50 watts of constant work rate exercise and during recovery, along with the computer-derived line of the best fit to a single exponential model of the $\dot{V}_{O_2}$ response, for a representative normal subject. τ—time constant of upslope and downslope of $\dot{V}_{O_2}$. (From Koike, A., Yajima, T., Adachi, H., et al.: Evaluation of exercise capacity using submaximal exercise at a constant work rate in patients with cardiovascular disease. Circulation *91*:1719, 1995. Copyright 1995 American Heart Association.)

Angiography and Intervention. Philadelphia, Lea and Febiger, 1991, p. 47.

441

Ch 14

nized as the cause of reduced $\dot{V}_{O_{2max}}$ by measuring pulmonary capillary wedge pressure together with arterial pressure, cardiac output, and gas exchange at each stage of exercise. A triple-lumen balloon flotation thermodilution catheter can be used conveniently to make these measurements. As pump function deteriorates, wedge pressure rises and cardiac output declines at peak exercise.

A limitation of cardiopulmonary exercise testing is that many patients with heart disease, particularly ischemic heart disease, often do not attain a level of exercise in which $\dot{V}_{O_2}$ remains stable despite further increase in the intensity of exercise. The peak $\dot{V}_{O_2}$ they achieve is not the same as $\dot{V}_{O_{2max}}$, which by definition fails to rise despite a further increase in the intensity of exercise. Unlike $\dot{V}_{O_{2max}}$, peak $\dot{V}_{O_2}$ partially depends on the motivations of the patient and is subject to examiner bias.[179] On the other hand, the anaerobic threshold, which requires a lower level of activity than the $\dot{V}_{O_{2max}}$, can be more readily determined in patients with cardiac dysfunction and is quite reproducible.[176,180] Alterations in the anaerobic threshold reflect changes in the underlying condition.

The response of $\dot{V}_{O_2}$ to the onset and recovery from constant steady-state exercise is an alternate method of assessing exercise capacity (Fig. 14–29).[181] The time constant of the increase in $\dot{V}_{O_2}$ at the start of exercise is similar to the time constant of the fall in $\dot{V}_{O_2}$ after exercise (normal = 49 ± 10 sec). In patients with cardiovascular disease, this time constant is lengthened and inversely correlates with peak $\dot{V}_{O_2}$ and maximum work. The measurement of the time constant does not require the subject's maximum effort and may provide a useful measure of exercise capacity in patients with mild to moderate cardiovascular impairment.

REFERENCES

1. Braunwald, E.: On the difference between the heart's output and its contractile state (Editorial). Circulation 43:171, 1971.
2. Ter Keurs, H. E., Buex, J. J., de Tombe, P. P., et al.: The effect of sarcomere length and Ca^{++} on force and velocity of shortening in cardiac muscle. Adv. Exp. Med. Biol. 226:581, 1988.
3. de Tombe, P. P., and Little, W. C.: Inotropic effects of ejection are myocardial properties. Am. J. Physiol. 266:H1202, 1994.
4. Suga, H., Kitabatake, A., and Sagawa, K.: End-systolic pressure determines stroke volume from fixed end-diastolic volume in the isolated canine left ventricle under a constant contractile state. Circ. Res. 44:238, 1979.
5. Sagawa, K., Maughan, L., Suga, H., and Sunagawa, K.: Cardiac Contraction and the Pressure-Volume Relationship. New York, Oxford University Press, Inc. 1988.

MEASUREMENT OF KEY VARIABLES

6. Hipkins, S. F., Rutten, A. J., and Runciman, W. B.: Experimental analysis of catheter-manometer systems: In vitro and In vivo. Anesthesiology 71:893, 1989.
7. Grossman, W.: Pressure measurement. In Grossman, W., and Baim, D. S. (eds.): Cardiac Catheterization, Angiography, and Intervention. Philadelphia, Lea and Febiger, 1991, p. 123.
7a. Courtois, M., Fattal, P. G., Kovacs, S. J., Jr., et al.: Anatomically and physiologically based reference level for measurement of intracardiac pressures. Circulation 92:1994, 1995.
8. Sharir, T., Marmor, A., Ting, C. T., et al.: Validation of a method for noninvasive measurement of central arterial pressure. Hypertension 21:74, 1993.
9. Bargiggia, G. S., Bertucci, C., Recusani, F., et al.: A new method for estimating left ventricular dP/dt by continuous wave Doppler echocardiography: Validation studies at cardiac catheterization. Circulation 80:1287, 1989.
10. Nishimura, R. A., Schwartz, R. S., Tajik, A. J., and Holmes, D. R., Jr.: Noninvasive measurement of rate of left ventricular relaxation by Doppler echocardiography: Validation with simultaneous cardiac catheterization. Circulation 88:146, 1993.
11. Yamamoto, K., Masuyama, T., Doi, Y., et al.: Noninvasive assessment of left ventricular relaxation using continuous-wave Doppler aortic regurgitant velocity curve: Its comparative value to the mitral regurgitation method. Circulation 91:192, 1995.
12. Lange, R. A., Moore, D. M., Jr., Cigarroa, R. G., and Hillis, L. D.: Use of pulmonary capillary wedge pressure to assess severity of mitral stenosis: Is true left atrial pressure needed in this condition? J. Am. Coll. Cardiol. 13:825, 1989.
13. Grossman, W.: Cardiac catheterization by direct exposure of artery and vein. In Grossman, W., and Baim, D. S. (eds.): Cardiac Catheterization,
14. Schoenfeld, M. H., Palacios, I. F., Hutter, A. M., Jr., et al.: Underestimation of prosthetic mitral valve areas: Role of transseptal catheterization in avoiding unnecessary repeat mitral valve surgery. J. Am. Coll. Cardiol. 5:1387, 1985.
15. Tobis, J., Nalcioglu, O., Seibert, A., et al.: Measurement of left ventricular ejection fraction by videodensitometric analysis of digital subtraction angiograms. Am. J. Cardiol. 52:871, 1983.
16. Kronenberg, M. W., Price, R. R., Smith, C. W., et al.: Evaluation of left ventricular performance using digital subtraction angiography. Am. J. Cardiol. 51:837, 1983.
17. Vine, D. L., Hegg, T. D., Dodge, H. T., et al.: Immediate effect of contrast medium injection of left ventricular volumes and ejection fraction. Circulation 56:379, 1977.
18. Brogan, W. C., III, Hillis, L. D., and Lange, R. A.: Contrast agents for cardiac catheterization: Conceptions and misconceptions. Am. Heart J. 122:1129, 1991.
19. Rackley, C. E., and Hood, W. P., Jr.: Quantitative angiographic evaluation and pathophysiological mechanisms in valvular heart disease. Prog. Cardiovasc. Dis. 15:427, 1973.
20. Dodge, H. T., and Sheehan, F. H.: Quantitative contrast angiography for assessment of ventricular performance in heart disease. J. Am. Coll. Cardiol. 1:73, 1983.
21. Baan, J., Van der Velde, E. T., Van Dijk, A. D., et al.: Ventricular volume measured from intracardiac dimensions with impedance catheter: Theoretical and experimental aspects. Cardiovascular System Dynamics: Models and Measurements. New York, Plenum Press, 1992, p. 569.
22. Burkhoff, D., Van der Velde, E., Kass, D., et al.: Accuracy of volume measurement by conductance catheter in isolated, ejecting canine hearts. Circulation 72:440, 1984.
23. Kass, D. A., Yamazaki, T., Burkhoff, D., et al.: Determination of left ventricular end-systolic pressure-volume relationships by the conductance (volume) catheter technique. Circulation 73:586, 1986.
24. Kass, D. A., Midei, M., Graves, W., et al.: Use of a conductance (volume) catheter and transient inferior vena caval occlusion for rapid determination of pressure-volume relationships in man. Cathet. Cardiovasc. Diagn. 15:192, 1988.
25. Ferguson, J. J., Miller, M. J., Sahagian, P., et al.: Effects of respiration and vasodilation on venous volume in animals and man, as measured with an impedance catheter. Cathet. Cardiovasc. Diagn. 16:25, 1989.
26. Boltwood, C., Jr., Appleyard, R., and Glantz, S.: Parallel conductance of LV depends on end-systolic volume. Circulation 80:1360, 1989.
27. Applegate, R. J., Cheng, C. P., and Little, W. C.: Simultaneous conductance catheter and dimension assessment of left ventricle volume in the intact animal. Circulation 81:638, 1990.
28. Glantz, S. A., Boltwood, C. M., Jr., Appleyard, R. F., et al.: Volume conductance catheter. Circulation 81:703, 1990.
29. Steendijk, P., Van der Velde, E. T., and Baan, J.: Left ventricular stroke volume by single and dual excitation of conductance catheter in dogs. Am. J. Physiol. 264:2198, 1993.
30. Herman, H. J., and Bartle, S. H.: Left ventricular volumes by angiocardiography: Comparison of methods and simplification of techniques. Cardiovasc. Res. 2:404, 1968.
31. Rackley, C. E.: Quantitative evaluation of left ventricular function by radiographic techniques. Circulation 54:862, 1976.
32. Wynne, J., Green, L. H., Mann, T., et al.: Estimation of left ventricular volumes in man from biplane cineangiograms filmed in oblique projections. Am. J. Cardiol. 41:726, 1978.
33. Fifer, M. A., and Grossman, W.: Measurement of ventricular volumes, ejection fraction, mass and wall stress. In Grossman, E., and Baim, D. S. (eds.): Cardiac Catheterization, Angiography and Intervention. Philadelphia, Lea and Febiger, 1991, p. 300.
34. Dodge, H. T.: Hemodynamic aspects of cardiac failure. In Braunwald, E. (ed.): The Myocardium: Failure and Infarction. New York, HP Publishing Co., 1974, p. 70.
35. Schiller, N. B., Shah, P. M., Crawford, M., et al.: Recommendations for quantitation of the left ventricle by two-dimensional echocardiography. J. Am. Soc. Echocardiogr. 2:358, 1989.
36. Collins, H. W., Kronenberg, M. W., and Byrd, B. F., III: Reproducibility of left ventricular mass measurements by two-dimensional and m-mode echocardiography. J. Am. Coll. Cardiol. 14:672, 1989.
37. Reichek, N., Helak, J., Plappert, T., et al.: Validation of left ventricular mass estimates from clinical two-dimensional echocardiography: Initial results. Circulation 67:348, 1983.
38. Bikkina, M., Levy, D., Evans, J. C., et al.: Left ventricular mass and risk of stroke in an elderly cohort: The Framingham Heart Study. JAMA 272:33, 1994.
39. Krumholz, H. M., Larson, M., and Levy, D.: Prognosis of left ventricular geometric patterns in the Framingham Heart Study. J. Am. Coll. Cardiol. 25:879, 1995.
40. Devereux, R. B.: Left ventricular geometry, pathophysiology and prognosis. J. Am. Coll. Cardiol. 25:885, 1995.
41. Regen, D. M., Anversa, P., and Capasso, J. M.: Segmental calculation of left ventricular wall stresses. Am. J. Physiol. 264:H1411, 1993.
42. Regen, D. M.: Calculation of left ventricular wall stress. Circ. Res. 67:245, 1990.
43. Grossman, W., Jones, D., and McLaurin, L. P.: Wall stress and patterns of hypertrophy in the human left ventricle. J. Clin. Invest. 56:56, 1974.
44. Peterson, K. L.: Instantaneous force-velocity-length relations of the left

ventricle: Methods, limitations and applications in humans. *In* Fishman, A. P. (ed.): Heart Failure. Washington, D.C., Hemisphere Publishing Co., 1978, p. 121.

45. Pomerantsev, E. V., Stertzer, S. H., and Shaw, R. E.: Quantitative left ventriculography: Methods of assessment of the regional contractility. J. Invas. Cardiol. *7*:11, 1995.

46. Dodge, H. T., Stewart, D. K., and Frimer, M.: Implications of shape, stress and wall dynamics in clinical heart disease. *In* Fishman, A. P. (ed.): Heart Failure. Washington, D. C., Hemisphere Publishing Co., 1978, p. 43.

47. Sheehan, F. H., Dodge, H. T., Mathey, D. G., et al.: IEEE Comput. Cardiol. 1982, p. 9.

48. Sheehan, F. H., Stewart, D. K., Dodge, H. T., et al.: Variability in the measurement of regional left ventricular wall motion from contrast angiograms. Circulation *68*:550, 1983.

49. Kass, D. A.: Measuring right ventricular volumes. Am. J. Physiol. *254*:H619, 1988.

50. Sandler, H., and Dodge, H. T.: Angiographic methods for determination of left ventricular geometry and volume. *In* Mirsky, I., Ghista, D. N., and Sandler, H. (eds.): Cardiac Mechanics: Physiological, Clinical and Mathematical Considerations. New York, John Wiley and Sons, 1974.

51. Hoit, B. D., Shao, Y., McMannis, K., et al.: Determination of left atrial volume using sonomicrometry: A cast validation study. Am. J. Physiol. *264*:H1011, 1993.

ASSESSMENT OF LEFT VENTRICULAR FUNCTION

52. Little, W. C., and Downes, T. R.: Clinical evaluation of left ventricular diastolic performance. Prog. Cardiovasc. Dis. *32*:273, 1990.

53. Applegate, R. J., and Little, W. C.: Systolic and diastolic left ventricular function. Prog. Cardiol. *4*:63, 1991.

54. Downes, T. R., Hackshaw, B. T., Kahl, F. R., et al.: Frequency of large "V" waves in the pulmonary artery wedge pressure in ventricular septal defect of acquired (during acute myocardial infarction) or congenital origin. Am. J. Cardiol. *60*:415, 1987.

55. Snyder, R. W., II, Glamann, D. B., Lange, R. A., et al.: Predictive value of prominent pulmonary arterial wedge V waves in assessing the presence and severity of mitral regurgitation. Am. J. Cardiol. *73*:568, 1994.

56. Glantz, S. A., and Parmley, W.: Factors which affect the diastolic pressure-volume curve. Circ. Res. *42*:171, 1978.

57. Glantz, S. A.: Computing indices of diastolic stiffness has been counterproductive. Fed. Proc. *39*:162, 1980.

58. Noordergraaf, A., and Melbin, J.: Ventricular afterload: A succinct yet comprehensive definition (Editorial). Am. Heart J. *95*:545, 1978.

59. Grossman, W.: Clinical measurement of vascular resistance and assessment of vasodilator drugs. *In* Grossman, W., and Baim, D. S. (eds.): Cardiac Catheterization, Angiography and Intervention. Philadelphia, Lea and Febiger, 1991, p. 143.

60. O'Rourke, M. F.: Steady and pulsatile energy losses in the systemic circulation under normal conditions and in simulated arterial disease. Cardiovasc. Res. *1*:313, 1967.

61. Nichols, W. W., Nicolini, F. A., and Pepine, C. J.: Determinants of isolated systolic hypertension in the elderly. J Hypertension *10*:S73, 1992.

62. Nichols, W. W., Conti, C. R., Walker, W. E., and Milnor, W. R.: Input impedance of the systemic circulation in man. Circ. Res. *40*:451, 1977.

63. Nichols, W. W., and O'Rourke, M. F.: McDonald's Blood Flow in Arteries. London, Arnold, 1990.

64. O'Rourke, M. F., and Brunner, H. R.: Introduction to arterial compliance and function. J. Hypertension *10*:S3, 1992.

65. Sunagawa, K., Maughan, W. L., and Sagawa, K.: Optimal arterial resistance for the maximal stroke work studied in isolated canine left ventricle. Circ. Res. *56*:586, 1985.

66. Little, W. C., and Cheng, C. P.: Left ventricular-arterial coupling in conscious dogs. Am. J. Physiol. *261*:H70, 1991.

67. Kelly, R. P., Ting, C. T., Yang, T. M., et al.: Effective arterial elastance as index of arterial vascular load in humans. Circulation *86*:513, 1991.

68. Carabello, B. A.: Clinical assessment of systolic dysfunction. ACC Curr. J. Rev. Jan/Feb:25, 1994.

69. Gleason, W. L., and Braunwald, E.: Studies on the first derivative of the ventricular pressure pulse in man. J. Clin. Invest. *41*:80, 1962.

70. Krayenbuehl, H. P., Rutishauser, W., Wirz, P., et al.: High-fidelity left ventricular pressure measurements for the assessment of cardiac contractility in man. Am. J. Cardiol. *31*:415, 1973.

71. Little, W. C.: The left ventricular dP/dt_{max}-end-diastolic volume relation in closed chest dogs. Circ. Res. *56*:808, 1985.

72. Burns, J. W., Covell, J. W., and Ross, J., Jr.: Mechanics of isotonic left ventricular contractions. Am. J. Physiol. *224*:725, 1973.

73. Fifer, M. A., Gunther, S., Grossman, W., et al.: Myocardial contractile function in aortic stenosis as determined from the rate of stress development during isovolumic stress. Am. J. Cardiol. *44*:1318, 1979.

74. Feldman, M. D., Alderman, J. D., Aroesty, J. M., et al.: Depression of systolic and diastolic myocardial reserve during atrial pacing tachycardia in patients with dilated cardiomyopathy. J. Clin. Invest. *82*:1661, 1988.

75. Mason, D. T., and Braunwald, E.: Studies on digitalis. IX: Effects of ouabain on the nonfailing human heart. J. Clin. Invest. *42*:1105, 1963.

76. Ross, J., Jr., and Sobel, B. E.: Regulation of cardiac contraction. Ann. Rev. Physiol. *34*:47, 1972.

77. Mason, D. T., Braunwald, E., Covell, J. W., et al.: Assessment of cardiac contractility: The relation between the rate of pressure rise and ventricular pressure during isovolumic systole. Circulation *44*:47, 1971.

78. Davidson, D. M., Covell, J. W., Malloch, C. I., and Rosse, J., Jr.: Factors influencing indices of left ventricular contractility in the conscious dog. Cardiovasc. Res. *8*:299, 1974.

79. Quinones, M. A., Gaasch, W. H., and Alexander, J. K.: Influence of acute changes in preload, afterload, contractile state and heart rate on ejection and isovolumic indices of myocardial contractility in man. Circulation *53*:293, 1976.

80. Kass, A., Maughan, W. L., Guo, A. M., et al.: Comparative influence of load versus inotropic states on indexes of ventricular contractility: Experimental and theoretical analysis based on pressure-volume relationships. Circulation *76*:1422, 1987.

81. Carabello, B. A., Mee, R., Collins, J. J., Jr., et al.: Contractile function in chronic gradually developing subcoronary aortic stenosis. Am. J. Physiol. *240*:H80, 1981.

82. Borow, K. M., Henderson, I. C., Neumann, A., et al.: Assessment of left ventricular contractility in patients receiving doxorubicin. Ann. Intern. Med. *99*:750, 1983.

83. Colan, S. D., Borow, K. M., and Neumann, A.: Left ventricular end-systolic wall stress-velocity of fiber shortening relation: A load independent index of myocardial contractility. J. Am. Coll. Cardiol. *4*:715, 1984.

84. Wisenbaugh, T., Booth, D., DeMaria, A., et al.: Relationship of contractile state to ejection performance in patients with chronic aortic valve disease. Circulation *73*:47, 1986.

85. Mirsky, I., Corin, W. J., Murakami, T., et al.: Correction for preload in assessment of myocardial contractility in aortic and mitral valve disease: Application of the concept of systolic myocardial stiffness. Circulation *78*:68, 1988.

86. Lang, R. M., Fellner, S. K., Neumann, A., et al.: Left ventricular contractility varies directly with blood ionized calcium. Ann. Intern. Med. *108*:524, 1988.

87. Borow, K. M., Neumann, A., Marcus, R. H., et al.: Effects of simultaneous alterations in preload and afterload on measurements of left ventricular contractility in patients with dilated cardiomyopathy: Comparisons of ejection phase, isovolumetric and end-systolic force-velocity indexes. J. Am. Coll. Cardiol. *20*:787, 1992.

88. Banerjee, A., Brook, M. M., Klautz, R. J. M., and Teitel, D. F.: Nonlinearity of the left ventricular end-systolic wall stress-velocity of fiber shortening relation in young pigs: A potential pitfall in its use as a single-beat index of contractility. J. Am. Coll. Cardiol. *23*:514, 1994.

89. Kass, D. A., and Maughan, W. L.: From "Emax" to pressure-volume relations: A broader view. Circulation *77*:1203, 1988.

90. Little, W. C., and Cheng, C. P.: Left ventricular systolic and diastolic performance. *In* Warltier, D. C. (ed.): Ventricular Function. Baltimore, Williams and Wilkins, 1995, p. 111.

91. Kass, D. A.: Clinical ventricular pathophysiology: A pressure-volume view. *In* Warltier, D.C. (ed.): Ventricular Function. Baltimore, Williams and Wilkins, 1995, p. 131.

92. Kass, D. A., Grayson, R., and Marino, P.: Pressure-volume analysis as a method for quantifying simultaneous drug (amrinone) effects on arterial load and contractile state in vivo. J. Am. Coll. Cardiol. *16*:726, 1990.

93. Starling, M. R.: Left ventricular-arterial coupling relations in the normal human heart. Am. Heart J. *125*:1659, 1993.

94. Starling, M. R., Kirsh, M. M., Montgomery, D. G., and Gross, M. D.: Impaired left ventricular contractile function in patients with long-term mitral regurgitation and normal ejection fraction. J. Am. Coll. Cardiol. *22*:239, 1993.

95. Little, W. C., Cheng, C. P., Peterson, T., and Vinten-Johansen, J.: Response of the left ventricular end-systolic pressure-volume relation in conscious dogs to a wide range of contractile states. Circulation *78*:736, 1988.

96. Kass, D. A., Beyar, R., Lankford, E., et al.: Influence of contractile state on curvilinearity of in situ end-systolic pressure-volume relations. Circulation *79*:167, 1989.

97. Little, W. C., and O'Rourke, R. A.: Effect of regional ischemia on the left ventricular end-systolic pressure-volume relationship in chronically instrumented dogs. J. Am. Coll. Cardiol. *5*:297, 1985.

98. Kass, D. A., Marino, P., Maughan, W. L., and Sagawa, K.: Determinants of end-systolic pressure-volume relations during acute regional ischemia in situ. Circulation *80*:1783, 1989.

99. Park, R. D., Little, W. C., and O'Rourke, R. A.: Effect of alteration of the left ventricular activation sequence on the left ventricular end-systolic pressure-volume relation in closed-chest dogs. Circ. Res. *57*:706, 1986.

100. Little, W. C., Freeman, G. L., and O'Rourke, R. A.: Simultaneous determination of left ventricular end-systolic pressure-volume and pressure-dimension relationships in closed-chest dogs. Circulation *71*:1301, 1985.

101. Gorcsan, J., III, Romand, J. A., Mandarino, W. A., et al.: Assessment of left ventricular performance by on-line pressure-area relations using echocardiographic automated border detection. J. Am. Coll. Cardiol. *23*:242, 1994.

102. Sodums, M. T., Badke, F. R., Starling, M. R., et al.: Evaluation of left ventricular contractile performance utilizing end-systolic pressure-volume relationships in conscious dogs. Circ. Res. *54*:731, 1984.

103. Freeman, G. L., Little, W. C., and O'Rourke, R. A.: Effect of vasoactive agents on the left ventricular end-systolic pressure-volume relation in closed-chest dogs. Circulation *74*:1107, 1986.

104. Brickner, M. E., and Starling, M. R.: Dissociation of end systole from end ejection in patients with long-term mitral regurgitation. Circulation *81*:1277, 1990.

105. Hsia, H. H., and Starling, M. R.: Is standardization of left ventricular chamber elastance necessary? Circulation 81:1826, 1990.

106. Nakano, K., Sugawara, M., Ishihara, K., et al.: Myocardial stiffness derived from end-systolic wall stress and logarithm of reciprocal of wall thickness. Contractility index independent of ventricular size. Circulation 82:1352, 1990.

107. Pirwitz, M. J., Lange, R. A., Willard, J. E., et al.: Use of the left ventricular peak systolic pressure/end-systolic volume ratio to predict symptomatic improvement with valve replacement in patients with aortic regurgitation and enlarged end-systolic volume. J. Am. Coll. Cardiol. 24:1672, 1994.

108. Little, W. C., Cheng, C. P., Mumma, M., et al.: Comparison of measures of left ventricular contractile performance from pressure-volume loops in conscious dogs. Circulation 80:1378, 1989.

109. Noda, T., Cheng, C. P., de Tombe, P. P., and Little, W. C.: Curvilinearity of the left ventricular end-systolic pressure-volume and dP/dt$_{max}$-end diastolic volume relations. Am. J. Physiol. 265:H910, 1993.

110. Little, W. C., and Cheng, C. P.: Effect of exercise on left ventricular-arterial coupling assessed in the pressure-volume plane. Am. J. Physiol. 264:H1629, 1993.

111. de Tombe, P. P., Jones, S., Burkhoff, D., et al.: Ventricular stroke work and efficiency both remain nearly optimal despite altered vascular loading. Am. J. Physiol. 264:H1817, 1993.

112. Glower, D. D., Spratt, J. A., Snow, N. D., et al.: Linearity of the Frank-Starling relationship in the intact heart: The concept of preload recruitable stroke work. Circulation 71:994, 1985.

113. Zile, M. R., Izzi, G., and Gaasch, W. H.: Left ventricular diastolic dysfunction limits use of maximum systolic elastance as an index of contractile function. Circulation 83:674, 1991.

114. Kass, D. A., and Beyar, R.: Evaluation of contractile state by maximal ventricular power divided by the square of end-diastolic volume. Circulation 84:1698, 1991.

115. Sharir, T., Feldman, M. D., Haber, H., et al.: Ventricular systolic assessment in patients with dilated cardiomyopathy by preload-adjusted maximal power. Validation and noninvasive application. Circulation 89:2045, 1994.

LEFT VENTRICULAR PUMP FUNCTION

116. Starling, E. H.: Linacre Lecture on the Law of the Heart (1915). London, Longmans, 1918.

117. Sarnoff, S. J., and Mitchell, J. H.: Control of function of heart. In Hamilton, W. F., and Dow, P. (eds.): Handbook of Physiology. Washington, D. C., American Physiological Society, 1962, p. 489.

118. Little, W. C., and Applegate, R. J.: Congestive heart failure: Systolic and diastolic function. J. Cardiothor. Vasc. Anesth. 7(Suppl. 2):2, 1993.

119. Grossman, W.: Diastolic dysfunction in congestive heart failure. N. Engl. J. Med. 325:1557, 1991.

120. Litwin, S. E., and Grossman, W.: Diastolic dysfunction as a cause of heart failure. J. Am. Coll. Cardiol. 22:49A, 1993.

121. Brutsaert, D., Sys, S. U., and Gillebert, T. C.: Diastolic failure: Pathophysiology and therapeutic implications. J. Am. Coll. Cardiol. 22:318, 1993.

122. Gaasch, W. H.: Diagnosis and treatment of heart failure based on left ventricular systolic or diastolic dysfunction. JAMA 271:1276, 1994.

123. Kitzman, D. W., Higginbotham, M. B., Cobb, F. R., et al.: Exercise intolerance in patients with heart failure and preserved left ventricular systolic function: Failure of the Frank-Starling mechanism. J. Am. Coll. Cardiol. 17:1065, 1991.

124. Thomas, J. D., and Klein, A.: Doppler-echocardiographic evaluation of diastolic function. In Skorton, D. J. (eds.): Marcus Cardiac Imaging. Philadelphia, W. B. Saunders Co. 1996.

125. Bonow, R. O.: Radionuclide angiographic evaluation of left ventricular diastolic function. Circulation 84:1208, 1991.

126. Myreng, Y., and Smiseth, O. A.: Assessment of left ventricular relaxation by Doppler echocardiography: Comparison of isovolumic relaxation time and transmitral flow velocities with time constant of isovolumic relaxation. Circulation 81:260, 1990.

127. Weiss, J. L., Frederiksen, J. W., and Weisfeldt, M. L.: Hemodynamic determinants of the time-course of fall in canine left ventricular pressure. J. Clin. Invest. 58:751, 1976.

128. Eichhorn, E. J., Willard, J. E., Alvarez, L., et al.: Are contraction and relaxation coupled in patients with and without congestive heart failure? Circulation 85:2326, 1993.

129. Gilbert, J. C., and Glantz, S. A.: Determinants of left ventricular filling and of the diastolic pressure-volume relations. Circ. Res. 64:827, 1989.

130. Gaasch, W. H., Carroll, J. D., Blaustein, A. S., and Bing, O. H. L.: Myocardial relaxation: Effects of preload on the time course of isovolumic relaxation. Circulation 73:1037, 1986.

131. Freeman, G. L., Prabhu, S. D., Widman, L. E., and Colston, J. T.: An analysis of variability of left ventricular pressure decay. Am. J. Physiol. 264:H262, 1993.

132. Grossman, W.: Evaluation of systolic and diastolic function of the myocardium. In Grossman, W., and Baim, D. S. (eds.): Cardiac Catheterization, Angiography and Intervention. Philadelphia, Lea and Febiger, 1991, p. 319.

133. Frais, M. A., Bergman, D. W., Kingma, I., et al.: The dependence of the time constant of left ventricular isovolumic relaxation (Tau) on pericardial pressure. Circulation 81:1071, 1990.

134. Yellin, E. L., Nikolic, S., and Frater, R. W. M.: Left ventricular filling dynamics and diastolic function. Prog. Cardiovasc. Dis. 32:247, 1990.

135. Chen, C., Rodriguez, L., Guerrero, J. L., et al.: Noninvasive estimation of the instantaneous first derivative of left ventricular pressure using continuous-wave Doppler echocardiography. Circulation 83:2101, 1991.

136. Mirsky, I.: Assessment of diastolic function: Suggested methods and future considerations. Circulation 69:836, 1984.

137. Kennish, A., Yellin, E., and Frater, R. W.: Dynamic stiffness profiles in the left ventricle. J. Appl. Physiol. 39:665, 1975.

138. Mirsky, I., and Pasipoularides, A.: Clinical assessment of diastolic function. Prog. Cardiovasc. Dis. 32:291, 1990.

139. Keren, A., and Popp, R. L.: Assignment of patients into the classification of cardiomyopathies. Circulation 86:1622, 1992.

140. Appleton, C. P.: Doppler assessment of left ventricular diastolic function: The refinements continue. J. Am. Coll. Cardiol. 21:1697, 1993.

141. Pai, R. G., and Shah, P. M.: Echo-Doppler evaluation of left ventricular diastolic function. ACC Curr. J. Rev. 30, 1994.

142. Little, W. C., and Cheng, C. P.: Modulation of diastolic dysfunction in the intact heart. In Lorell, B. H., and Grossman, W. (eds.): Diastolic Relaxation of the Heart. Boston, Kluwer Academic Publishers, 1994, p. 167.

143. Cheng, C. P., Freeman, G. L., Santamore, W. P., et al.: Effect of loading conditions, contractile state, and heart rate on early diastolic left ventricular filling in conscious dogs. Circ. Res. 66:814, 1990.

144. Little, W. C.: Enhanced load dependence of relaxation in heart failure: Clinical implications. Circulation 85:2326, 1992.

145. Courtois, M., Mechem, C. J., Barzilai, B., et al.: Delineation of determinants of left ventricular early filling: Saline versus blood infusion. Circulation 90:2041, 1994.

146. Little, R. C.: The mechanism of closure of the mitral valve: A continuing controversy. Circulation 59:615, 1979.

147. Nishimura, R. A., Abel, M. D., Hatle, L. K., et al.: Significance of Doppler indices of diastolic filling of the left ventricle: Comparison with invasive hemodynamics in a canine model. Am. Heart J. 118:1248, 1989.

148. Kono, T., Sabbah, H. N., Rosman, H., et al.: Left atrial contribution to ventricular filling during the course of evolving heart failure. Circulation 86:1317, 1992.

149. Little, W. C., Kitzman, D., and Cheng, C. P.: Patterns of left ventricular filling indicating diastolic dysfunction: What is their importance? Choices Cardiol. (in press).

150. Appleton, C. P., and Hatle, L. K.: The natural history of left ventricular filling abnormalities: Assessment by two-dimensional and Doppler echocardiography. Echocardiography 9:437, 1992.

151. Ohno, M., Cheng, C. P., and Little, W. C.: Mechanism of altered patterns of left ventricular filling during the development of congestive heart failure. Circulation 89:2241, 1994.

152. Little, W. C., Ohno, M., Kitzman, D. W., et al.: Determination of left ventricular chamber stiffness from the time for deceleration of early left ventricular filling. Circulation 92:1933, 1995.

153. Pinamonti, B., Di Lenardo, A., Sinagra, G., and Camerini, F.: Restrictive left ventricular filling pattern in dilated cardiomyopathy assessed by Doppler echocardiography; clinical, echocardiographic and hemodynamic correlations and prognostic implications. J. Am. Coll. Cardiol. 22:808, 1993.

154. Oh, J. K., Hatle, L. K., Seward, J. B., et al.: Diagnostic role of Doppler echocardiography in constrictive pericarditis. J. Am. Coll. Cardiol. 23:154, 1994.

155. Klein, A. L., Hatle, L. K., Taliercio, C. P., et al.: Prognostic significance of Doppler measures of diastolic function in cardiac amyloidosis. A Doppler echocardiographic study. Circulation 83:808, 1991.

156. Klein, A. L., and Tajik, A. J.: Doppler assessment of pulmonary venous flow in healthy subjects and in patients with heart disease. J. Am. Soc. Echocardiogr. 4:379, 1991.

157. Basnight, M. A., Gonzalez, M. S., Kershenovich, S. C., and Appleton, C. P.: Pulmonary venous flow velocity: Relation to hemodynamics, mitral flow velocity and left atrial volume, and ejection fraction. J. Am. Soc. Echocardiol. 4:547, 1991.

158. Dell'Italia, L. J.: The right ventricle: Anatomy, physiology, and clinical importance. Curr. Probl. Cardiol. 16:653, 1991.

159. Morrison, D. A., Ovitt, T., Hammermeister, K. E., and Stoval, J. R.: Functional tricuspid regurgitation and right ventricular dysfunction in pulmonary hypertension. Am. J. Cardiol. 62:108, 1988.

160. Voelker, W., Gruber, H. P., Ickrath, O., et al.: Determination of right ventricular ejection fraction by thermodilution technique—a comparison to biplane cineventriculography. Intensive Care Med. 14:461, 1988.

161. Hurford, W. E., Zapol, W. M.: The right ventricle and critical illness: A review of anatomy, physiology, and clinical evaluation of its function. Intensive Care Med. 14:448, 1988.

162. Spinale, F. G., Smith, A. C., Carabello, B. A., and Crawford, F. A.: Right ventricular function computed by thermodilution and ventriculography: A comparison of methods. J Thorac. Cardiovasc. Surg. 99:141, 1990.

163. Brown, K. A., and Ditchey, R. V.: Human right ventricular end-systolic pressure-volume relation defined by maximal elastance. Circulation 78:81, 1988.

164. Yamaguchi, S., Tsuiki, K., Miyawaki, H., et al.: Effect of left ventricular volume on right ventricular end-systolic pressure-volume relations: Resetting of regional preload in right ventricular free wall. Circ. Res. 65:623, 1989.

165. Dell'Italia, L. J., Freeman, G. L., and Gaasch, W. H.: Cardiac function and functional capacity: Implications for the failing heart. Curr. Probl. Cardiol. 18:705, 1993.

166. Sumimoto, S., Sugiura, T., Tarumi, N., and Taniguchi, H.: Mixed venous oxygen saturation as a guide to tissue oxygenation and prognosis in patients with acute myocardial infarction. Am. Heart J. 122:27, 1991.

167. Inomata, S., Nishikawa, T., and Taguchi, M.: Continuous monitoring of mixed venous oxygen saturation for detecting alterations in cardiac output after discontinuation of cardiopulmonary bypass. Br. J. Anaesth. 72:11, 1994.

168. Koike, A., Wasserman, K., Taniguchi, K., et al.: Critical capillary oxygen partial pressure and lactate threshold in patients with cardiovascular disease. J. Am. Coll. Cardiol. 23:1644, 1994.

169. Grossman, W.: Blood flow measurement: The cardiac output. In Grossman, W., and Baim, D. S. (eds.): Cardiac Catheterization, Angiography and Intervention. Philadelphia, Lea and Febiger, 1990, p. 105.

170. Weber, K. T., and Janicki, J. S.: Lactate production during maximal and submaximal exercise in patients with chronic heart failure. J. Am. Coll. Cardiol. 6:717, 1985.

171. Weber, K. T., Janicki, J. S., and McElroy, P. A.: Cardiopulmonary Exercise Testing. Philadelphia, W. B. Saunders Co., 1986.

172. Wasserman, K.: Measures of functional capacity in patients with heart failure. Circulation 81(Suppl. 2):1, 1990.

173. Swedberg, K., and Gundersen, T.: The role of exercise testing in heart failure. J Cardiovasc. Pharmacol. 22:S13, 1993.

174. Swedberg, K.: Exercise testing in heart failure: A critical review. Drugs 47:14, 1994.

175. Weisman, I. M., and Zeballos, R. J.: An integrated approach to the interpretation of cardiopulmonary exercise testing. Clin. Chest Med. 15:421, 1994.

176. Simonton, C. A., Higginbotham, M. B., and Cobb, F. R.: The ventilatory threshold: Quantitative analysis of reproducibility and relation to arterial lactate concentration in normal subjects and in patients with chronic congestive heart failure. Am. J. Cardiol. 62:100, 1988.

177. Poole-Wilson, P. A.: Exercise as a means of assessing heart failure and its response to treatment. Cardiology 76:347, 1989.

178. Franciosa, J. A., Baker, B. J., and Seth, L.: Pulmonary versus systemic hemodynamics in determining exercise capacity of patients with chronic left ventricular failure. Am. Heart J. 110:807, 1985.

179. Jennings, G. L., and Esler, M. D.: Circulatory regulation at rest and exercise and the functional assessment of patients with congestive heart failure. Circulation 81(Suppl. 2):5, 1990.

180. Sullivan, M. J., Cobb, F. R.: The anaerobic threshold in chronic heart failure: Relation to blood lactate, ventilatory basis, reproducibility, and response of exercise training. Circulation 81(Suppl. 2):47, 1990.

181. Koike, A., Yajima, T., Adachi, H., et al.: Evaluation of exercise capacity using submaximal exercise at a constant work rate in patients with cardiovascular disease. Circulation 91:1719, 1995.

Chapter 15

Clinical Aspects of Heart Failure: High-Output Heart Failure; Pulmonary Edema

EUGENE BRAUNWALD, WILSON S. COLUCCI, WILLIAM GROSSMAN

Heart failure is a principal complication of virtually all forms of heart disease. A panel of the National Heart, Lung and Blood Institute described this condition as follows: "Heart failure occurs when an abnormality of cardiac function causes the heart to fail to pump blood at a rate required by the metabolizing tissues or when the heart can do so only with an elevated filling pressure. The heart's inability to pump a sufficient amount of blood to meet the needs of the body tissues may be due to insufficient or defective cardiac filling and/or impaired contraction and emptying. Compensatory mechanisms increase blood volume and raise cardiac filling pressures, heart rate, and cardiac muscle mass to maintain the heart's pumping function and cause redistribution of blood flow. Eventually, however, despite these compensatory mechanisms, the ability of the heart to contract and relax declines progressively, and the heart failure worsens."[1]

An alternative definition, which focuses more on the clinical consequences of heart failure, has been offered by Packer as follows: "Congestive heart failure represents a complex clinical syndrome characterized by abnormalities of left ventricular function and neurohormonal regulation,

which are accompanied by effort intolerance, fluid retention, and reduced longevity."[2] Included in these two definitions is a wide spectrum of clinicophysiological states, ranging from the rapid impairment of pumping function (occurring when, for example, a massive myocardial infarction, tachyarrhythmia, or bradyarrhythmia develops suddenly) to the gradual but progressive impairment of myocardial function, observed at first only during stress occurring in a patient whose heart sustains a pressure or volume overload for a prolonged period. Congestive heart failure is a relatively common disorder; it has been estimated that 2 million persons in the United States are being treated for heart failure and that there are 400,000 new cases each year.[3]

The clinical manifestations of heart failure vary enormously and depend on a variety of factors, including the age of the patient, the extent and rate at which cardiac performance becomes impaired, and the ventricle initially involved in the disease process.[4] A broad spectrum of severity of impairment of cardiac function is ordinarily included within the definition of heart failure, ranging from the mildest, which is manifest clinically only during stress, to the most advanced form, in which cardiac pump function is unable to sustain life without external support.

Useful criteria for the diagnosis of heart failure emerged from the Framingham study[5,6] (Table 15–1).

TABLE 15–1   FRAMINGHAM CRITERIA FOR CONGESTIVE HEART FAILURE

MAJOR CRITERIA
Paroxysmal nocturnal dyspnea or orthopnea
Neck-vein distention
Rales
Cardiomegaly
Acute pulmonary edema
S_3 gallop
Increased venous pressure >16 cm H_2O
Circulation time >25 sec
Hepatojugular reflux

MINOR CRITERIA
Ankle edema
Night cough
Dyspnea on exertion
Hepatomegaly
Pleural effusion
Vital capacity decrease 1/3 from maximum
Tachycardia (rate of >120/min)

MAJOR OR MINOR CRITERION
Weight loss >4.5 kg in 5 days in response to treatment

For establishing a definite diagnosis of congestive heart failure in this study, two major or one major and two minor criteria had to be present concurrently.

From McKee, P. A., Castelli, W. P., McNamara, P. M., and Kannel, W. B.: The natural history of congestive heart failure, the Framingham Study. N. Engl. J. Med. 285:1441, 1971. Copyright Massachusetts Medical Society.

FORMS OF HEART FAILURE

Forward vs. Backward Heart Failure

The clinical manifestations of heart failure arise as a consequence of inadequate cardiac output and/or damming up of blood behind one or both ventricles. These two principal mechanisms are the basis of the so-called forward and backward pressure theories of heart failure. The *backward failure hypothesis,* first proposed in 1832 by James Hope, contends that when the ventricle fails to discharge its contents, blood accumulates and pressure rises in the atrium and the venous system emptying into it.[7] There is substantial physiological evidence in favor of this theory. As discussed on page 398, the inability of cardiac muscle to shorten against a load alters the relationship between ventricular end-systolic pressure and volume so that end-systolic (residual) volume rises. The following sequence then occurs that at first maintains cardiac output at a normal level: (1) ventricular end-diastolic volume and pressure increase; (2) the volume and pressure rise in the atrium behind the failing ventricle; (3) the atrium contracts more vigorously (a manifestation of Starling's law, operating on the atrium)[8]; (4) the pressure in the venous and capillary beds behind (upstream to) the failing ventricle rises; and (5) transudation of fluid from the capillary bed into the interstitial space (pulmonary or systemic) increases. Many of the symptoms characteristic of heart failure can be traced to this sequence of events and the resultant increase in fluid in the interstitial spaces of the lungs, liver, subcutaneous tissues, and serous cavities.

Cardiac output in the resting (basal) state is a relatively *insensitive* index of cardiac function (see p. 439). In many patients, the entire sequence of events outlined above may transpire while cardiac output *at rest* is still within normal limits. Indeed, the backward pressure theory of heart failure reflects one of the principal compensatory mechanisms in heart failure, i.e., the operation of Starling's law of the heart (see p. 378), in which distention of the ventricle helps to maintain cardiac output. The failing ventricle operates on an ascending, albeit depressed and flattened, function curve,[9] and the augmented ventricular end-diastolic volume and pressure characteristic of heart failure must be regarded as aiding in the maintenance of cardiac output. When this compensatory mechanism is interfered with (e.g., by means of dietary sodium restriction and treatment with diuretics), the patient may be less symptomatic owing to loss of extracellular fluid volume, with its accompanying reduction in congestion of the lungs, liver, and lower extremities. However, at the same time, cardiac output may decline,[10] and symptoms secondary to a reduction of cardiac output, such as fatigue, may actually intensify. Thus, although many of the clinical manifestations of heart failure are secondary to excessive retention of extracellular fluid, the elevation of ventricular preload associated with this excess fluid constitutes an important adaptive mechanism.

An important extension of the backward failure theory is the development of right ventricular failure as a consequence of left ventricular failure. According to this concept, the elevation of left ventricular diastolic, left atrial, and pulmonary venous pressures results in backward transmission of pressure and leads to pulmonary hypertension, which ultimately causes right ventricular failure. Often, pulmonary vasoconstriction plays a part in this form of pulmonary hypertension as well (see p. 780).

Eighty years after publication of Hope's work, Mackenzie proposed the *forward failure hypothesis*, which relates clinical manifestations of heart failure to inadequate delivery of blood into the arterial system.[11] According to this hypothesis, the principal clinical manifestations of heart failure are due to reduced cardiac output, which results in diminished perfusion of vital organs, including the brain, leading to mental confusion; skeletal muscles, leading to weakness; and kidneys, leading to sodium and water retention through a series of complex mechanisms[12] (Chap. 62). This retention of sodium and water, in turn, augments extracellular fluid volume and ultimately leads to symptoms of heart failure which are caused by congestion of organs and tissues.

Although these two seemingly opposing views concerning the pathogenesis of heart failure led to lively controversy during the first half of this century, it no longer seems fruitful to make a rigid distinction between backward and forward heart failure, since *both* mechanisms appear to operate in the majority of patients with *chronic* heart failure.[13] Exceptions may occur, however, and some patients, particularly those with *acute* decompensation, develop relatively pure forms of forward or backward failure.

For instance, a massive myocardial infarction may result in either (1) forward failure with a marked reduction of left ventricular output and cardiogenic shock (see p. 1238) and clinical manifestations secondary to impaired perfusion (e.g., hypotension, mental confusion, oliguria), or (2) backward failure with a transient inequality of output between the two ventricles, resulting in acute pulmonary edema. More commonly, patients with large myocardial infarctions develop a combination of forward and backward failure, with symptoms resulting from both inadequate cardiac output and pulmonary congestion. Early in the course of acute myocardial infarction, patients may succumb long before renal retention of salt and water can occur. However, if the patients survive the acute insult, expansion of the extracellular fluid volume and manifestations resulting therefrom usually occur.

RIGHT-SIDED VS. LEFT-SIDED HEART FAILURE

Implicit in the backward failure theory is the idea that fluid localizes behind the specific cardiac chamber that is *initially* affected. Thus, symptoms secondary to pulmonary congestion initially predominate in patients with left ventricular infarction, hypertension, and aortic and mitral valve disease; i.e., they manifest *left heart failure*. With time, however, fluid accumulation becomes generalized, and ankle edema, congestive hepatomegaly, ascites, and pleural effusion occur (i.e., the patients later exhibit *right heart failure* as well). Less commonly, prolonged right ventricular failure with massive accumulation of extracellular fluid may be associated with dyspnea, particularly when the patient is in the supine position and when large pleural effusions are present.

FLUID RETENTION IN HEART FAILURE. There is general agreement that fluid retention in heart failure is caused ultimately in part by reduction in glomerular filtration rate and in part by activation of the renin-angiotensin-aldosterone system. Reduced cardiac output is associated with a lowered glomerular filtration rate and an increased elaboration of renin, which, through the activation of angiotensin, results in the release of aldosterone (see p. 413). The combination of impaired hepatic function, owing to hepatic venous congestion, and reduced hepatic blood flow interferes with the metabolism of aldosterone,[12] further raising its plasma concentration and augmenting the retention of sodium and water.

As already noted, cardiac output (and glomerular filtration rate) may be normal in many patients with heart failure, particularly when they are at rest. However, during stress, such as physical exercise or fever, the cardiac output fails to rise normally, the glomerular filtration rate declines, and the renal mechanisms for salt and water retention described above come into play. In addition, ventricular filling pressure, and therefore pressures in the atrium and systemic veins behind (upstream to) the ventricle, may be normal at rest, only to rise abnormally during the stress. This, in turn, may cause transudation and symptoms of tissue congestion (pulmonary in the case of the left ventricle and systemic in the case of the right) during exercise. For this reason, simple rest may induce diuresis and relieve symptoms in many patients with mild heart failure.

ACUTE VS. CHRONIC HEART FAILURE

The clinical manifestations of heart failure depend importantly on the *rate* at which the syndrome develops and specifically on whether sufficient time has elapsed for compensatory mechanisms to become operative and for fluid to accumulate in the interstitial space (Table 15–2). For example, when a previously normal individual suddenly develops a serious anatomical or functional abnormality of the heart (such as massive myocardial infarction, heart block with a very slow ventricular rate [<35/min], a tachyarrhythmia with a very rapid rate [>180/min], rupture of a valve secondary to infective endocarditis, or

TABLE 15–2   COMPARISONS OF ACUTE VS CHRONIC HEART FAILURE

FEATURE	ACUTE HEART FAILURE	DECOMPENSATED CHRONIC HEART FAILURE	CHRONIC HEART FAILURE
Symptom severity	Marked	Marked	Mild to moderate
Pulmonary edema	Frequent	Frequent	Rare
Peripheral edema	Rare	Frequent	Frequent
Weight gain	None to mild	Frequent	Frequent
Whole-body fluid volume load	No change or mild increase	Markedly increased	Increased
Cardiomegaly	Uncommon	Usual	Common
Ventricular systolic function	Hypo-, normo-, or hypercontractile	Reduced	Reduced
Wall stress	Elevated	Markedly elevated	Elevated
Activation of sympathetic nervous system	Marked	Marked	Mild to marked
Activation of renin-angiotensin-aldosterone axis	Often increased	Marked	Mild to marked
Reparable, remedial causative lesion(s)	Common	Occasional	Occasional

Clinical and pathophysiological characteristics of the two major categories of unstable heart failure (acute heart failure and decompensated chronic heart failure) are compared with those of chronic heart failure.

From Leier, C. V.: Unstable heart failure. *In* Colucci, W. S. (ed.): Heart Failure: Cardiac Function and Dysfunction. *In* Braunwald, E. (Series ed.): Atlas of Heart Diseases, Vol. 4: Philadelphia, Current Medicine, 1995, pp. 9.1–9.15.

occlusion of a large segment of the pulmonary vascular bed by a pulmonary embolus), a marked, sudden reduction in cardiac output with symptoms due to inadequate organ perfusion and/or acute congestion of the venous bed behind the affected ventricle will occur. If the same anatomical abnormality develops gradually, or if the patient survives the acute insult, a number of adaptive mechanisms become operational, especially cardiac hypertrophy, and these allow the patient to adjust to and tolerate not only the anatomical abnormality but also a reduction in cardiac output with less difficulty. Frequently, the important clinical manifestations of chronic heart failure secondary to tissue congestion may be suppressed by dietary sodium restriction and diuretics. Cardiac function may not have been improved, and such patients still are in "heart failure," albeit with fewer clinical manifestations thereof. Under these circumstances, an acute event such as an infection, an arrhythmia, or discontinuation of therapy may precipitate manifestations of acute heart failure.

LOW-OUTPUT VS. HIGH-OUTPUT HEART FAILURE

Low cardiac output at rest, or in milder cases only during exertion and other stresses, characterizes heart failure occurring in most forms of heart disease (i.e., congenital, valvular, rheumatic, hypertensive, coronary, and cardiomyopathic). A variety of high-output states, including thyrotoxicosis, arteriovenous fistulas, beriberi, Paget's disease of bone, anemia, and pregnancy (discussed later in this chapter), may lead to heart failure as well. Low-output heart failure is characterized by clinical evidence of impairment of the peripheral circulation, with systemic vasoconstriction and cold, pale, and sometimes cyanotic extremities; in advanced forms of low-output failure, as the stroke volume declines, the pulse pressure narrows.[14] In contrast, in high-output heart failure (see pp. 460 to 462), the extremities are usually warm and flushed, and the pulse pressure is widened or at least normal.

The ability of the heart to deliver the quantity of oxygen required by the metabolizing tissues is reflected in the arterial–mixed venous

oxygen difference, which is abnormally widened (i.e., >5.0 ml/liter in the resting state) in patients with low-output heart failure. This difference may be normal or even reduced in high-output states, owing to elevation of the mixed venous oxygen saturation by the admixture of blood that has been shunted away from metabolizing tissues. However, regardless of the absolute level of the arterial–mixed venous oxygen, this difference still exceeds the level that existed *before* the development of heart failure, and cardiac output, regardless of its absolute level, is lower than it had been before the development of heart failure.

Systolic vs. Diastolic Heart Failure
(See also p. 403)

Implicit in the physiological definition of heart failure (inability to pump an adequate volume of blood and/or to do so only from an abnormally elevated filling pressure) is that heart failure can be caused by an abnormality in systolic function leading to a defect in the expulsion of blood (i.e., *systolic heart failure*), or by an abnormality in diastolic function leading to a defect in ventricular filling (i.e., *diastolic heart failure*) (Fig. 15–1). The former is the more familiar, classic heart failure in which an impaired inotropic state is responsible. Less familiar, but perhaps just as important, is diastolic heart failure, in which the ability of the ventricle(s) to accept blood is impaired.[15,16] This may be due to slowed or incomplete ventricular relaxation which may be transient, as occurs in acute ischemia, or sustained, as in concentric myocardial hypertrophy or re-

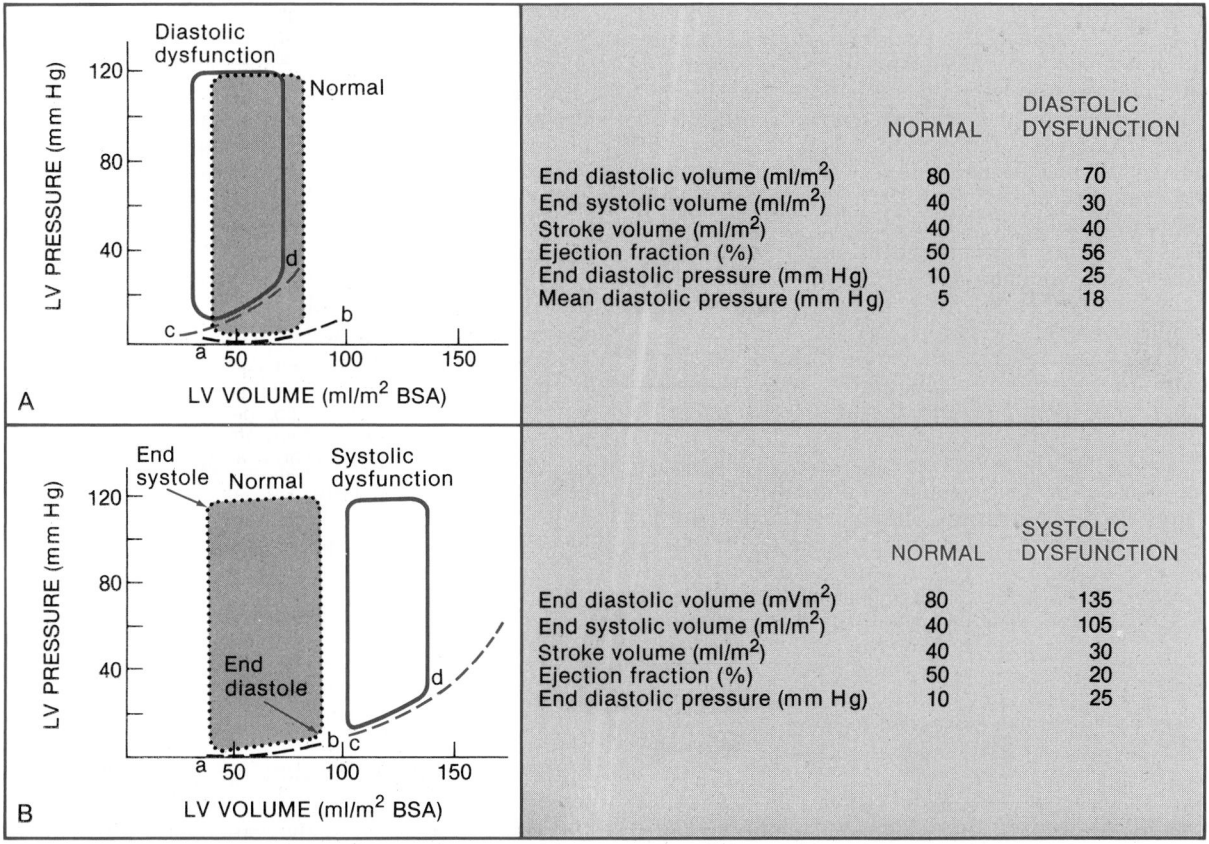

FIGURE 15–1. *A,* Schematic of a pressure-volume loop from a normal subject (dotted line) and a patient with diastolic dysfunction (solid line). Dashed lines represent the diastolic pressure-volume relation. Isolated diastolic dysfunction is characterized by a shift in pressure-volume loop to the left. Contractile performance is normal (normal or increased ejection fraction, normal or slightly decreased stroke volume). However, LV pressures throughout diastole are increased; at a common diastolic volume = 70 ml/m². LV diastolic pressure is 25 mm Hg in the patient with diastolic failure compared with a diastolic pressure of 5 mm Hg in normal subject. Thus, diastolic dysfunction increases modulus of chamber stiffness. LV, left ventricular. *B,* Schematic of pressure-volume loop from a normal subject (dotted line) and a patient with systolic dysfunction (solid line). Dashed line represents diastolic pressure-volume relation. Systolic dysfunction is characterized by displacement of pressure-volume loop to the right. Despite compensatory dilation, stroke volume or ejection fraction remains low. LV diastolic pressures are increased as a result of large LV volume. LV, left ventricular. (From Zile, M. R.: Diastolic dysfunction: Detection, consequences, and treatment: 2. Diagnosis and treatment of diastolic dysfunction. Mod. Concepts Cardiovasc. Dis. *59:*1, 1990.)

TABLE 15–3 SYSTOLIC VS. DIASTOLIC DYSFUNCTION IN HEART FAILURE

PARAMETERS	SYSTOLIC	DIASTOLIC	PARAMETERS	SYSTOLIC	DIASTOLIC
History			**Chest Roentgenogram**		
Coronary heart disease	++++	+	Cardiomegaly	+++	+
Hypertension	++	++++	Pulmonary congestion	+++	+++
Diabetes	+++	+	**Electrocardiograms**		
Valvular heart disease	++++	−	Low voltage	+++	−
Paroxysmal dyspnea	++	+++	Left ventricular hypertrophy	++	++++
Physical Examination			Q waves	++	+
Cardiomegaly	+++	+	**Echocardiograms**		
Soft heart sounds	++++	+	Low ejection fraction	++++	−
S₃ gallop	+++	+	Left ventricular dilation	++	−
S₄ gallop	+	+++	Left ventricular hypertrophy	++	++++
Hypertension	++	++++			
Mitral regurgitation	+++	+			
Rales	++	++			
Edema	+++	+			
Jugular venous distention	+++	+			

Certain aspects of the history and physical examination *(panel A)*, along with clinical measurements *(panel B)*, help to distinguish diastolic problems from those more often associated with systolic failure. Patients with hypertensive heart disease, for example, particularly severe left ventricular hypertrophy, often experience heart failure because of diastolic dysfunction. *Plus signs* indicate "suggestive" (the number reflects relative weight). *Minus signs* indicate "not very suggestive."

From Young, J. B.: Assessment of Heart Failure. *In* Colucci, W. S. (ed.): Heart Failure: Cardiac Function and Dysfunction. *In* Braunwald, E. (Series ed.): Atlas of Heart Diseases, Vol. 4: Philadelphia, Current Medicine, 1995, pp. 7.1–7.20.

strictive cardiomyopathy secondary to infiltrative conditions such as amyloidosis. The principal clinical manifestations of systolic failure result from an inadequate forward cardiac output, while the major consequences of diastolic failure relate to elevation of the ventricular filling pressure and the high venous pressure upstream to the ventricle, causing pulmonic and/or systemic congestion.

There are many examples of pure systolic or diastolic heart failure. Examples of the former are patients with acute massive pulmonary embolism or dilated cardiomyopathy, while examples of the latter are patients with hypertrophic cardiomyopathy or subendocardial fibrosis. However, in many patients, systolic and diastolic heart failure coexist. The most common form of heart failure, that caused by coronary atherosclerosis, is an example of combined systolic and diastolic failure. In this condition, systolic failure is caused by both the chronic loss of contracting myocardium secondary to myocardial necrosis resulting from previous infarction and the acute loss of myocardial contractility induced by a transient episode of ischemia. Diastolic failure is due to the ventricle's reduced compliance caused by replacement of normal, distensible myocardium with nondistensible fibrous scar tissue and by the acute reduction of diastolic distensibility of reversibly injured myocardium during a transient episode of ischemia. A number of clinical features and laboratory findings characterize these two forms of heart failure (Table 15–3).

CAUSES OF HEART FAILURE

From a clinical viewpoint, it is useful to classify the causes of heart failure into three broad categories: (1) *underlying causes,* comprising the structural abnormalities—congenital or acquired—that affect the peripheral and coronary vessels, pericardium, myocardium, or cardiac valves and lead to the increased hemodynamic burden or myocardial or coronary insufficiency responsible for heart failure; (2) *fundamental causes,* comprising the biochemical and physiological mechanisms through which either an increased hemodynamic burden or a reduction in oxygen delivery to the myocardium results in impairment of myocardial contraction (Chap. 13); and (3) *precipitating causes,* including the specific causes or incidents that precipitate

heart failure in 50 to 90 per cent of episodes of clinical heart failure.

It is helpful for the clinician to identify both the underlying and the precipitating causes of heart failure. Appropriate management of the underlying heart disease (e.g., surgical correction of a congenital defect or an acquired valvular abnormality or pharmacological management of hypertension) may prevent the development or recurrence of heart failure. Similarly, treatment of a precipitating cause such as an infection with fever will often terminate an episode of heart failure and may be life-saving. More important, *prevention* of a precipitating cause can prevent heart failure.

Overt heart failure may, of course, also be precipitated if there is progression of the underlying heart disease. A previously stable, compensated patient may develop heart failure that is apparent clinically for the first time when the intrinsic process has advanced to a critical point, such as with progressive obliteration of the pulmonary vascular bed in a patient with cor pulmonale or further narrowing of a stenotic aortic valve. Alternatively, decompensation may occur as a result of failure or exhaustion of the compensatory mechanisms but without any change in the load on the heart in patients with persistent severe pressure or volume overload.

Precipitating Causes of Heart Failure

In one study of 101 patients admitted to an inner city municipal hospital with the diagnosis of heart failure, precipitating factors could be identified in 93 per cent[17] (Table 15–4).

INAPPROPRIATE REDUCTION OF THERAPY. Perhaps the most common cause of decompensation in a previously compensated patient with heart failure is inappropriate reduction in the intensity of treatment—be it dietary sodium restriction, reduced physical activity, a drug regimen, or, most commonly, a combination of these measures. Many patients with serious underlying heart disease, regardless of whether they previously experienced heart failure, may be relatively asymptomatic for as long as they carefully adhere to their treatment regimen. Dietary excesses of sodium, incurred frequently on vacations or holidays or during an illness of the spouse responsible for preparing the patient's meals, are frequent causes of sudden cardiac decompensation. Careful and repeated instruction of the patient is a

TABLE 15–4 PRECIPITATING FACTORS IN CHRONIC HEART FAILURE

PRECIPITANT	NO. OF PATIENTS
Lack of compliance	64
With diet	22
With drugs	6
With both (diet and drugs)	37
Uncontrolled hypertension	44
Cardiac arrhythmias	29
Atrial fibrillation	20
Atrial flutter	7
Multifocal atrial tachycardia	1
Ventricular tachycardia	1
Environmental factors	19
Inadequate therapy	17
Pulmonary infection	12
Emotional stress	7
Administration of inappropriate medications or fluid overload	4
Myocardial infarction	6
Endocrine disorders (thyrotoxicosis)	1

Adapted from Ghali, J. K., Kadakia, S., Cooper, R., and Ferlinz, J.: Precipitating factors leading to decompensation of heart failure: Traits among urban blacks. Arch. Intern. Med. *148*:2013, 1988.

simple yet effective measure to prevent this common clinical problem.

ARRHYTHMIAS (see also Chap. 22). Cardiac arrhythmias are far more common in patients with underlying structural heart disease than in normal subjects and commonly precipitate or intensify heart failure. The development of arrhythmias may precipitate heart failure through several mechanisms: (1) *Tachyarrhythmias,* most commonly atrial fibrillation (Table 15–4), reduce the time available for ventricular filling. When there is already an impairment of ventricular filling, as in mitral stenosis, or reduced ventricular compliance (diastolic failure; see below), tachycardia will raise atrial pressure and reduce cardiac output further. In addition, tachyarrhythmias increase myocardial oxygen demands and, in a patient with obstructive coronary artery disease, may induce or intensify myocardial ischemia, which, in turn, impairs both cardiac relaxation and systolic function, thereby raising left atrial and pulmonary capillary pressure further and causing symptoms secondary to pulmonary congestion. (2) *Marked bradycardia* in a patient with underlying heart disease usually depresses cardiac output, since stroke volume may already be maximal and cannot rise further to maintain cardiac output. (3) *Dissociation between atrial and ventricular contraction,* which occurs in many arrhythmias, results in loss of the atrial booster pump mechanism, which impairs ventricular filling, lowers cardiac output, and raises atrial pressure.[18] This loss is particularly deleterious in patients with impaired ventricular filling due to concentric cardiac hypertrophy (e.g., in systemic hypertension, aortic stenosis, and hypertrophic cardiomyopathy). (4) *Abnormal intraventricular conduction,* which occurs in many arrhythmias such as ventricular tachycardia, impairs myocardial performance because of loss of the normal synchronicity of ventricular contraction. In addition to precipitating heart failure, arrhythmias—sometimes fatal—may be *caused* by heart failure.

SYSTEMIC INFECTION. Although patients with congestive heart failure are particularly susceptible to pulmonary infections, presumably because of the diminished ability of congested lungs to expel respiratory secretions, *any* infection may precipitate cardiac failure. The mechanisms include increased total metabolism as a consequence of fever, discomfort, and cough, which increase the hemodynamic

burden on the heart; the accompanying sinus tachycardia, secondary to fever and discomfort, plays an additional adverse role.

PULMONARY EMBOLISM (see also Chap. 46). Patients with congestive heart failure, particularly when confined to bed, are at high risk of developing pulmonary emboli. Such emboli may increase the hemodynamic burden on the right ventricle by elevating right ventricular systolic pressure further and may cause fever, tachypnea, and tachycardia, the deleterious effects of which have already been discussed.

PHYSICAL, ENVIRONMENTAL, AND EMOTIONAL EXCESSES. Intense, prolonged exertion or severe fatigue, such as may result from prolonged travel or emotional crises, and a severe climatic change, such as to a hot, humid environment, are relatively common precipitants of cardiac decompensation.

CARDIAC INFECTION AND INFLAMMATION. Myocarditis owing to a recurrence of acute rheumatic fever (Chap. 55) or to infective endocarditis (Chap. 33) or as a consequence of a variety of allergic inflammatory or infectious processes (including viral myocarditis) (Chap. 41) may impair myocardial function directly and exacerbate existing heart disease. The anemia, fever, and tachycardia that frequently accompany these processes are also deleterious. In patients with infective endocarditis, additional valvular damage also may precipitate cardiac decompensation.

DEVELOPMENT OF AN UNRELATED ILLNESS. Heart failure may be precipitated in patients with compensated heart disease when an unrelated illness develops. For example, the development of renal disease may impair further the ability of patients with heart failure to excrete sodium and thus may intensify the accumulation of fluid. Similarly, blood transfusion or the administration of sodium-containing fluid after a noncardiac operation may result in sudden heart failure in patients with underlying heart disease. Prostatic obstruction in the elderly male, parenchymal liver disease, and the administration of corticosteroids or estrogens with sodium-retaining properties also may precipitate heart failure in patients with underlying heart disease.

ADMINISTRATION OF CARDIAC DEPRESSANTS OR SALT-RETAINING DRUGS. A number of drugs depress myocardial function; among these are alcohol, beta-adrenoceptor blocking agents, many antiarrhythmic agents, verapamil, and antineoplastic drugs such as doxorubicin (Adriamycin) and cyclophosphamide (Chap. 42). Others, such as estrogens, androgens, glucocorticoids, and nonsteroidal antiinflammatory agents, may cause salt and water retention. Any of these drugs, when administered to a patient with heart disease, can precipitate or aggravate heart failure.

HIGH-OUTPUT STATES. Acute heart failure may be precipitated in patients with underlying heart disease, such as valvular heart disease, who develop one of the hyperkinetic circulatory states, such as pregnancy (see pp. 460 to 462).

DEVELOPMENT OF A SECOND FORM OF HEART DISEASE. Patients with one form of heart disease often remain compensated until they develop a second form. For example, a patient with chronic hypertension and left ventricular hypertrophy but without left ventricular failure may be asymptomatic until a myocardial infarction (which may be silent) develops and precipitates heart failure.

It is essential to search for these precipitating causes systematically in all patients with congestive heart failure, since lack of recognition or treatment or both may be responsible for otherwise refractory heart failure. In most instances, they can be treated effectively, after which appropriate measures should be instituted to avoid recurrence. When a precipitating cause of heart failure can be identified, it generally signifies a better prognosis than when a similar degree of heart failure is due simply to progression of the underlying cardiac disease.

Respiratory Distress

Breathlessness, a cardinal manifestation of left ventricular failure, may present with progressively increasing severity as (1) exertional dyspnea, (2) orthopnea, (3) paroxysmal nocturnal dyspnea, (4) dyspnea at rest, and (5) acute pulmonary edema.

EXERTIONAL DYSPNEA (see also p. 2). The principal difference between exertional dyspnea in normal subjects and in patients with heart failure is the degree of activity necessary to induce the symptom.[19] Indeed, as heart failure first develops, exertional dyspnea may simply appear to be an aggravation of the breathlessness that occurs in normal subjects during activity. An effort should be made to ascertain whether or not a *change* in the extent of exertion which causes dyspnea has actually occurred. As left ventricular failure advances, the intensity of exercise resulting in breathlessness declines progressively. However, there is no close correlation between subjective exercise capacity and objective measures of left ventricular performance at rest in patients with heart failure.[20] Exertional dyspnea may be absent in patients who are sedentary for a variety of reasons, such as habit, severe angina, intermittent claudication, or a noncardiovascular condition (e.g., crippling arthritis).

ORTHOPNEA. This symptom may be defined as dyspnea that develops in the recumbent position and is relieved by elevation of the head with pillows. Again, as in the case of exertional dyspnea, it is a *change* in the number of pillows required that is important. In the recumbent position there is reduced pooling of fluid in the lower extremities and abdomen; blood is displaced from the extrathoracic to the thoracic compartment. The failing left ventricle, operating on the flat portion of its depressed Starling curve (Fig. 14–18, p. 434), cannot accept and pump out the extra volume of blood delivered to it by the competent right ventricle without dilating, and pulmonary venous and capillary pressures rise further, causing interstitial pulmonary edema, reduced pulmonary compliance, increased airway resistance, and dyspnea. In contrast to paroxysmal nocturnal dyspnea (see below), orthopnea occurs rapidly, often within a minute or two of assuming recumbency, and develops when the patient is awake. It is a nonspecific symptom and may occur in any condition in which vital capacity is low; marked ascites, whatever its etiology, is an important cause of orthopnea.

The patient with orthopnea generally elevates his or her head and chest on several pillows to prevent nocturnal breathlessness and the development of paroxysmal nocturnal dyspnea (see below). In advanced left ventricular failure, orthopnea may be so severe that the patient cannot lie down and must spend the night in the sitting position. Often such patients are observed sitting at the side of the bed, slumped over a bedside table.

Cough may be caused by pulmonary congestion, occurs under the same circumstances as dyspnea (i.e., during exertion or recumbency), and is relieved by treatment of heart failure. Thus a nonproductive cough in patients with heart failure is often a "dyspnea equivalent," whereas a cough on recumbency may be considered an "orthopnea equivalent." Patients with severe chronic obstructive lung disease sometimes complain of orthopnea. *Trepopnea* is a rare form of orthopnea limited to one lateral decubitus position. It has been attributed to distortions of the great vessels in one position but not in the other.

PAROXYSMAL NOCTURNAL DYSPNEA. Attacks of paroxysmal dyspnea usually occur at night. The patient awakens, often quite suddenly, and with a feeling of severe anxiety and suffocation, sits bolt upright and gasps for breath. Bronchospasm, which may be caused by congestion of the bronchial mucosa and by interstitial pulmonary edema compressing the small bronchi, increases ventilatory difficulty and the work of breathing and is a common complicating factor of paroxysmal nocturnal dyspnea. The commonly associated wheezing is responsible for the alternate name of this condition, *cardiac asthma*. In contrast to orthopnea, which may be relieved immediately by sitting upright at the side of the bed with the legs dependent, attacks of paroxysmal nocturnal dyspnea may require 30 minutes or longer in this position for relief. Episodes of paroxysmal nocturnal dyspnea may be so frightening that the patient may be afraid to go back to sleep, even after the symptoms have abated.

The reason for the common occurrence of these episodes at night is not clear, but it seems likely that the combination of (1) the slow resorption of interstitial fluid from the dependent portion of the body and the resultant expansion of thoracic blood volume, (2) sudden elevation of thoracic blood volume and of the diaphragm which occurs immediately on assuming recumbency (as described above for orthopnea), (3) reduced adrenergic support of left ventricular function during sleep, and (4) normal nocturnal depression of the respiratory center all play major roles.

MECHANISMS OF DYSPNEA (Table 15-5)

Increased awareness of respiration or difficulty in breathing is commonly associated with pulmonary capillary hypertension caused by an elevation of left atrial or left ventricular filling pressure.[19] Patients with left ventricular failure typically exhibit a restrictive ventilatory defect, characterized by a reduction of vital capacity as a consequence of the replacement of the air in the lungs with blood or interstitial fluid or both. Consequently, the lungs become stiffer, air trapping occurs because of earlier than normal closure of dependent airways,[21] and the work of breathing is increased because higher intrapleural pressures are needed to distend the stiff lungs.[22] Tidal volume is reduced, and respiratory frequency rises in a compensatory fashion. Engorgement of blood vessels may reduce the caliber of the peripheral airways, increasing airway resistance. In addition, there are alterations in the distribution of ventilation and perfusion, resulting in widened alveolar-arterial differences for oxygen, hypoxemia, and an increased ratio of dead space to tidal volume. Thus, dyspnea (during exertion or at rest) and orthopnea are clinical expressions of pulmonary venous and capillary congestion. Paroxysmal nocturnal dyspnea reflects the presence of primarily *interstitial* edema, whereas pulmonary edema, in which there is transudation and expectoration of blood-tinged fluid (see p. 462), is often a manifestation of *alveolar* edema.

Whatever abnormalities in mechanics and gas exchange function of the lung that exist at rest are aggravated during exercise (and sometimes during recumbency) when pulmonary venous and capillary pressures rise further. Transudation of fluid from the intravascular to the extravascular space results in greater stiffening of the lungs, an augmentation in the work of breathing, and increased resistance to air flow.[23] There is an increased ventilatory drive, as a consequence of the stimulation of stretch receptors in the pulmonary vessels and interstitium, as well as a result of hypoxemia and metabolic acidosis. The increased work of breathing, combined with a low cardiac output and resulting impaired perfusion of the respiratory muscles, causes fatigue[21] and ultimately the sensation of dyspnea.

Dyspnea occurs whenever the work of respiration is excessive. Increased force generation is required for the respiratory muscles to move a given volume of air if the compliance of the lungs is reduced

TABLE 15–5   MECHANISMS OF DYSPNEA IN HEART FAILURE

1. **DECREASED PULMONARY FUNCTION**
   Decreased compliance
   Increased airway resistance

2. **INCREASED VENTILATORY DRIVE**
   Hypoxemia- ↑PCW
   V/Q mismatching- ↑PCW, ↓CO
   ↑CO_2 production- ↓CO-lactic acidosis

3. **RESPIRATORY MUSCLE DYSFUNCTION**
   Decreased strength
   Decreased endurance
   Ischemia

Abbreviations: PCW, mean pulmonary capillary wedge pressure; V/Q, ventilation/perfusion; CO, cardiac output; CO_2, carbon dioxide production.
From Mancini, D. M.: Pulmonary factors limiting exercise capacity in patients with heart failure. Prog. Cardiovasc. Dis. 37:347, 1995.

or the resistance to air flow is increased[22,23]; both of these changes occur in left heart failure. Dyspnea at rest also may occur in the late stages of heart failure when the combination of very low cardiac output, hypoxemia, and acidosis conspires to reduce the delivery of oxygen to the respiratory muscle.[24] Dyspnea may occur *without* pulmonary congestion in patients with right ventricular failure, a fixed low cardiac output, and/or a right-to-left shunt.

Differentiation Between Cardiac and Pulmonary Dyspnea

In most patients with dyspnea there is obvious clinical evidence of disease of either the heart *or* the lungs, but in some the differentiation between cardiac and pulmonary dyspnea may be difficult.[19] Like patients with heart failure, those with chronic obstructive lung disease also may waken at night with dyspnea, but this is usually associated with sputum production; the dyspnea is relieved after patients rid themselves of secretions by coughing rather than specifically by sitting up. When the dyspnea arises after a history of intensified cough and expectoration, it is usually primarily pulmonary in origin. *Acute cardiac asthma* (paroxysmal nocturnal dyspnea with prominent wheezing) usually occurs in patients who have obvious clinical evidence of heart disease and may be further differentiated from acute bronchial asthma by diaphoresis and bubblier airway sounds and the more common occurrence of cyanosis.

The difficulty in distinguishing between cardiac and pulmonary dyspnea may be compounded by the coexistence of diseases involving both organ systems. Thus, patients with a history of chronic bronchitis or asthma who develop left ventricular failure tend to develop particularly severe bronchoconstriction and wheezing in association with bouts of paroxysmal nocturnal dyspnea and pulmonary edema. Airway obstruction and dyspnea that respond to bronchodilators or smoking cessation favor a pulmonary origin of the dyspnea, while the response of these manifestations to diuretics supports heart failure as the cause of dyspnea.

PULMONARY FUNCTION TESTING. This testing should be carried out in patients in whom the etiology of dyspnea is unclear despite detailed clinical evaluation. The results may be helpful in determining whether dyspnea is produced by heart disease, lung disease, a combination of the two, or neither.

The major alterations in pulmonary function tests in congestive heart failure are reductions of vital capacity, total lung capacity, pulmonary diffusion capacity at rest and particularly during exercise, and pulmonary compliance; resistance to air flow is moderately increased; residual volume and functional residual volume are normal. Often there is hyperventilation at rest and during exercise, an increase in dead space, and some abnormalities of ventilation-perfusion relations with slight reductions in arterial P_{CO_2} and P_{O_2}. With pulmonary capillary hypertension, pulmonary compliance decreases and there is air trapping because of earlier than normal closure of dependent airways. The airway resistance rises,[25] as does the work of breathing.

Rarely, it may be difficult to differentiate among cardiac dyspnea, dyspnea based on *malingering,* and dyspnea caused by an *anxiety neurosis.* Careful observation for the appearance of effortless or irregular respiration during exercise testing often helps to identify the patient in whom dyspnea is related to the latter two noncardiac causes. Patients whose anxiety neurosis focuses on the heart may exhibit sighing respiration and difficulty in taking a deep breath as well as dyspnea at rest. Their breathing patterns are not rapid and shallow, as in cardiac dyspnea. Rarely a "therapeutic test" is helpful, and amelioration of dyspnea, accompanied by a weight loss exceeding 2 kg induced by administration of a diuretic, supports a cardiac origin for the dyspnea. Conversely, failure of these measures to achieve weight reduction in excess of 2 kg and to diminish dyspnea weighs heavily against a cardiac origin.

MECHANISMS OF EXERCISE INCOMPETENCE. A nearly universal manifestation of heart failure is a reduction in exercise capacity. Although exercise capacity may be limited for a variety of reasons in patients with heart failure, the most common causes are the development of dyspnea due to pulmonary vascular congestion and the failure of the cardiovascular system to provide sufficient blood flow to exercising muscles. The latter reflects primarily an inadequate cardiac output response to exercise due to reductions in stroke volume and heart rate.[26,27] In addition to the impaired central hemodynamic response to exercise, a number of other factors may contribute to reduced exercise capacity in patients with heart failure, including an attenuated peripheral vascular response,[28-30] abnormal skeletal muscle metabolism,[31] deconditioning of skeletal and respiratory muscles,[32,33] and patient anxiety related to the development of exertional symptoms. The importance of these additional factors is emphasized by the observation that the improvement in exercise capacity that occurs with long-term pharmacological therapy (e.g., converting enzyme inhibitors) requires weeks to develop and is dissociated temporally from the acute improvement in hemodynamics that occurs with the initiation of therapy. There is evidence that the judicious use of cardiac rehabilitation can improve functional capacity in patients with heart failure,[34,35] possibly by improving peripheral muscle blood flow, promoting skeletal muscle conditioning, and improving psychological outlook (Chap. 40).

Exercise Testing

(See also Chap. 5 and p. 439)

MAXIMAL EXERCISE CAPACITY. Exercise stress testing may be an exceedingly useful adjunct in the *clinical assessment* of patients with suspected or known heart failure.[36,37] With use of a cycle ergometer or treadmill with a progressively increasing load, the maximum level of exercise which can be achieved can be determined; the latter correlates closely with the total oxygen uptake ($\dot{V}_{O_2}$). Close observation of the patient during an exercise test may disclose obvious difficulty in breathing at a low level of exercise (or the opposite). Thus this simple test may be considered to be an extension of the clinical examination.

A more formal assessment in which $\dot{V}_{O_2}$ is measured at each stage of exercise, or preferably in which $\dot{V}_{O_2}$ and $\dot{V}_{CO_2}$ are measured continuously, allows determination of maximum $\dot{V}_{O_2}$ and the anaerobic threshold (i.e., the point during the exercise test at which the respiratory quotient rises as a consequence of the production of excess lactate)[25] (Figs. 5–1, p. 154, and 5–2, p. 156, and Fig. 14–29, p. 440). When a progressive exercise test is carried out until (1) $\dot{V}_{O_2}$ fails to rise with further increases in activity or (2) the patient is limited by severe dyspnea and/or fatigue, a $\dot{V}_{O_2}$ less than 25 mg/kg/min represents a reduction of maximum $\dot{V}_{O_2}$. When this reduction is caused by a cardiac abnormality (rather than by pulmonary disease, anemia, peripheral vascular disease, skeletal muscle deformity, marked obesity, severe deconditioning, or malingering), it may be used to classify the severity of heart failure, to follow the progress of the patient, and to assess the efficacy of therapeutic maneuvers.[36-38]

SUBMAXIMAL EXERCISE CAPACITY. Because usual daily activities generally require much less than maximal exercise capacity,[39-41] the measurement of submaximal exercise capacity may provide information that is complementary to that provided by maximum exercise testing. In contrast to maximal exercise capacity, which reflects the adequacy of the central hemodynamic response, the ability to sustain a submaximal exercise effort may reflect abnormalities in the regulation of peripheral blood flow and at the level of the skeletal musculature. There is no consensus as to the optimal way of measuring submaximal exercise capacity. In the

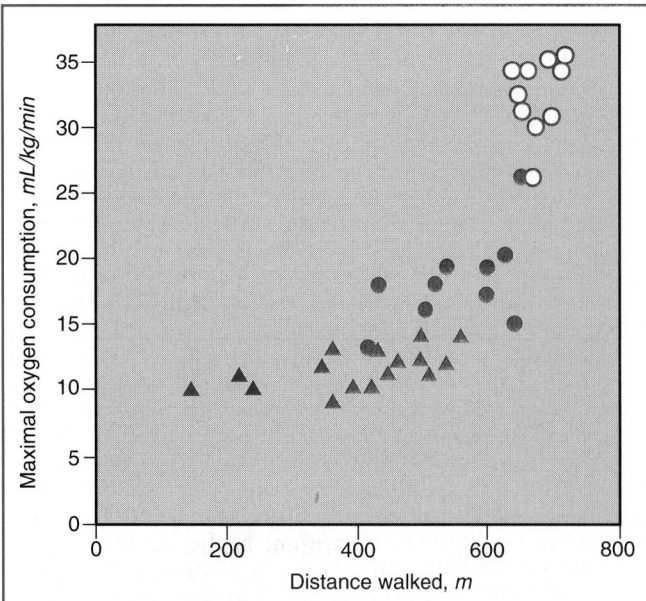

FIGURE 15–2. Relationship between the distance walked in 6 minutes and the peak V̇O₂ in patients with mild (New York Heart Association functional Class II) symptoms of heart failure (triangles), moderate symptoms (NYHA Class III) (filled circles), and normal subjects (open circles) (× 21). Because the 6-minute walk test involves only a submaximal exercise effort, it may be sensitive to changes in exercise function in the work range that is relevant to normal daily activities. (Adapted from Lipkin, D. P., et al.: Six minute walking test for assessing exercise capacity in chronic heart failure. BMJ *292*:653, 1986.)

exercise laboratory, submaximal exercise capacity can be assessed by measuring the duration of exercise at a constant workload that is generally chosen to be at or below the anaerobic threshold for the patient. A rough approximation of the submaximal exercise capacity can be obtained by measuring the distance walked in a fixed period of time. The "6-minute walk test," most common of the fixed-time tests, measures the distance walked on level ground in 6 minutes.[42–44] In this test, the patient is asked to walk in a level corridor as far as he or she can in 6 minutes. The patient can slow down or even stop, may be given a carefully controlled level of encouragement, and is told when 3 and 5 minutes have elapsed. The 6-minute walk test and other similar submaximal tests are being evaluated in clinical trials to determine if they are capable of detecting a therapeutic response. They appear to be predictive of maximal oxygen consumption (Fig. 15–2). Another form of submaximal exercise test measures the distance walked on a self-powered treadmill.[45]

Other Symptoms

FATIGUE AND WEAKNESS. These symptoms, often accompanied by a feeling of heaviness in the limbs, are generally related to poor perfusion of the skeletal muscles in patients with a lowered cardiac output. They may be associated with impaired vasodilation and altered metabolism in skeletal muscle.[24] Fatigue and weakness, of course, are notoriously nonspecific and may be caused by a variety of noncardiopulmonary diseases as well as by neurasthenia; they may be caused by sodium depletion, hypovolemia, or both, as a consequence of excessive treatment with diuretics and restriction of dietary sodium. Beta-adrenoreceptor blockers also may cause fatigue.

URINARY SYMPTOMS. *Nocturia* may occur relatively early in the course of heart failure. Urine formation is suppressed during the day when the patient is upright and active; this is due, at least in part, to a redistribution of blood flow away from the kidneys during activity.[46] When the patient rests in the recumbent position at night, the

deficit in cardiac output in relation to oxygen demand is reduced, renal vasoconstriction diminishes, and urine formation increases. Nocturia may be troublesome in that it prevents the patient with heart failure from obtaining much-needed rest. The diurnal pattern of urine flow characteristic of heart failure contrasts sharply with that existing in renal failure, in which urine formation occurs at a reasonably constant rate, both day and night. *Oliguria* is a sign of late cardiac failure and is related to the suppression of urine formation as a consequence of severely reduced cardiac output.

CEREBRAL SYMPTOMS. Confusion, impairment of memory, anxiety, headache, insomnia, bad dreams or nightmares, and rarely, psychosis with disorientation, delirium, and even hallucinations may occur in elderly patients with advanced heart failure, particularly in those with accompanying cerebral arteriosclerosis.

SYMPTOMS OF PREDOMINANT RIGHT HEART FAILURE. Breathlessness is not as prominent in isolated right ventricular failure as it is in left heart failure because pulmonary congestion is usually absent. Indeed, when a patient with mitral stenosis or left ventricular failure develops right ventricular failure, the more severe forms of dyspnea (i.e., paroxysmal nocturnal dyspnea and episodic pulmonary edema) tend to diminish in frequency and intensity. This reduction results from an inability of the right ventricle to augment its output, which prevents the temporary imbalance between blood flow into and out of the pulmonary vascular bed. On the other hand, when cardiac output becomes markedly reduced in patients with terminal right heart failure, as may occur in isolated right ventricular infarction and in the late stages of primary pulmonary hypertension and of pulmonary thromboembolic disease, severe dyspnea (air hunger) may occur, presumably as a consequence of the reduced cardiac output, poor perfusion of respiratory muscles, hypoxemia, and metabolic acidosis. In addition, dyspnea may be a prominent symptom in some patients with right ventricular failure and anasarca, hydrothorax, and ascites as a consequence of lung compression; such patients may even have orthopnea.

Congestive hepatomegaly may produce discomfort, generally described as a dull ache or heaviness, in the right upper quadrant or epigastrium. This discomfort, which is caused by stretching of the hepatic capsule, may be severe when the liver enlarges rapidly, as in acute right heart failure. In contrast, chronic, slowly developing hepatic enlargement is generally painless. Other gastrointestinal symptoms, including anorexia, nausea, bloating, a sense of fullness after meals, and constipation, occur owing to congestion of the liver and gastrointestinal tract. In severe, preterminal heart failure, inadequate bowel perfusion can cause abdominal pain, distention, and bloody stools. Nausea, anorexia, and emesis also may be due to cardiac drugs, particularly digitalis (see p. 484).

Functional Classification

A classification of patients with heart disease based on the relation between symptoms and the amount of effort required to provoke them has been developed by the New York Heart Association.[47] Although there are obvious limitations to assigning numerical values to subjective findings, this classification is nonetheless useful in comparing groups of patients as well as the same patient at different times.

Class I—*No limitation:* Ordinary physical activity does not cause undue fatigue, dyspnea, or palpitation.

Class II—*Slight limitation of physical activity:* Such patients are comfortable at rest. Ordinary physical activity results in fatigue, palpitation, dyspnea, or angina.

Class III—*Marked limitation of physical activity:* Although patients are comfortable at rest, less than ordinary activity will lead to symptoms.

Class IV—*Inability to carry on any physical activity without discomfort:* Symptoms of congestive failure are present even at rest. With any physical activity, increased discomfort is experienced.

As discussed on page 13, the accuracy and reproducibility of this classification are limited. To overcome these limitations, Goldman et al. have developed a useful classification based on the estimated metabolic cost of various activities[48] (Table 1–7, p. 12).

QUALITY OF LIFE. A good "quality of life" implies the ability to live as one wants, free of physical, social, emotional, and economic limitations. Heart failure can have an enormous deleterious impact on the quality of life. Although a number of questionnaires are available to assess quality of life, the Minnesota Living with Heart Failure (MLHF) questionnaire was designed specifically for use in these patients[49–51] (Fig. 15–3). It consists of 21 brief questions, each of which is answered on a scale of 0 to 5. Eight questions have a strong relationship to the symptoms of dyspnea and fatigue and are referred to as *physical dimension measures*. Five other questions that are strongly related to emotional issues are referred to as *emotional dimension measures*. The test is self-administered and takes only 5 to 10 minutes to complete. For each question, the patient selects a number from 0 to 5. Zero indicates that heart failure had no effect, and 5 indicates a very large effect. Although such questionnaires have little role in routine clinical management of patients, they have provided valuable information in research settings by allowing the response to various therapies to be quantified.

Physical Findings

GENERAL APPEARANCE. Patients with mild or moderate heart failure appear to be in no distress after a few minutes of rest. However, they may be obviously dyspneic during and immediately after moderate activity. Patients with left ventricular failure may become uncomfortable if they lie flat without elevation of the head for more than a few minutes. Those with severe heart failure appear anxious and may exhibit signs of air hunger in this position. Patients with heart failure of recent onset appear acutely ill but are ordinarily well nourished, whereas those with chronic cardiac failure often appear malnourished and sometimes even cachectic. Chronic, marked elevation of systemic venous pressure may produce exophthalmos and severe tricuspid regurgitation and may lead to visible systolic pulsation of the eyes[52] and of the neck veins. Cyanosis, icterus, and a malar flush may be evident in patients with severe heart failure.

In mild or moderately severe heart failure, stroke volume is normal at rest; in severe heart failure, it is reduced, and this is reflected in a diminished pulse pressure and dusky discoloration of the skin. With very severe failure, particularly if cardiac output has declined acutely, systolic arterial pressure may be reduced. The pulse may be rapid, weak, and thready. The proportional pulse pressure (pulse pressure/systolic pressure) correlates reasonably well with cardiac output. In one study,[14] when it was less than 25 per cent, it usually reflected a cardiac index of less than 2.2 liters/min/m².

EVIDENCE OF INCREASED ADRENERGIC ACTIVITY. Increased activity of the adrenergic nervous system is an important accompaniment of heart failure. It is responsible for a number of physical signs, including peripheral vasoconstriction, which is manifested as pallor and coldness of the extremities and cyanosis of the digits. There may be diaphoresis with sinus tachycardia, loss of normal sinus rhythm, and obvious distention of the peripheral veins secondary to venoconstriction. Diastolic arterial pressure may be slightly elevated.

PULMONARY RALES. Moist rales result from the transuda-

tion into the alveoli of fluid, which then moves into the airways. Rales heard over the lung bases are characteristic of congestive heart failure of at least moderate severity. In acute pulmonary edema, coarse, bubbling rales and wheezes are heard over both lung fields and are accompanied by the expectoration of frothy, blood-tinged sputum (see p. 464). However, the absence of rales by no means excludes considerable elevation of pulmonary capillary pressure. With congestion of the bronchial mucosa, excessive bronchial secretions or bronchospasm or both may give rise to rhonchi and wheezes. Rales are usually heard at both lung bases, but if unilateral, they occur more commonly on the right side. When rales are audible *only* over the left lung in a patient with heart failure, they may signify the presence of pulmonary embolism to that lung.

SYSTEMIC VENOUS HYPERTENSION (see also p. 18). This can be detected more readily by inspection of the jugular veins, which provides a useful index of right atrial pressure.[53,54] The upper limit of normal of the jugular venous pressure is approximately 4 cm above the sternal angle when the patient is examined at a 45-degree angle. When tricuspid regurgitation is present, the *v* wave and *y* descent are most prominent; however, with impedance to right ventricular filling (tricuspid stenosis) or right ventricular emptying (pulmonary hypertension, pulmonic stenosis), the *a* wave is most prominent. The jugular venous pressure normally declines on exertion, but in patients with heart failure (and in those with constrictive pericarditis; see p. 1496) it rises, a finding known as *Kussmaul's sign.* Rarely, venous pressure may be so high that the peripheral veins on the dorsum of the hands or in the temporal region are dilated.

HEPATOJUGULAR REFLUX (see also p. 19). In patients with mild right heart failure, the jugular venous pressure may be normal at rest but rises to abnormal levels with compression of the right upper quadrant, a sign known as the *hepatojugular reflux.* To elicit this sign, the right upper quadrant should be compressed firmly, gradually, and continuously for 1 minute while the veins of the neck are observed. The patient should be advised to avoid straining, holding the breath, or carrying out a Valsalva maneuver. A positive test (i.e., expansion of the jugular veins during and immediately after compression) usually reflects the combination of a congested abdomen and inability of the right side of the heart to accept or reject the transiently increased venous return. Thus a positive abdominojugular reflux is helpful in differentiating hepatic enlargement caused by heart failure from that caused by other conditions.

CONGESTIVE HEPATOMEGALY. The liver often enlarges *before* overt edema develops, and it may remain so even after other symptoms of right-sided heart failure have disappeared. Inspection of the abdomen may reveal epigastric fullness and, on percussion, dullness in the right upper quadrant. If hepatomegaly has occurred rapidly and relatively recently, the liver is usually tender, owing to stretching of its capsule. In longstanding heart failure this tenderness disappears, even though the liver remains enlarged.

In patients with tricuspid regurgitation, the prominent right atrial *v* wave may be transmitted to the liver, which pulsates during systole. A prominent presystolic pulsation in the liver owing to an enlarged right atrial *a* wave can occur in tricuspid stenosis, constrictive pericarditis, restrictive cardiomyopathy involving the right ventricle, pulmonary hypertension, and pulmonic stenosis.

EDEMA. Although a cardinal manifestation of congestive heart failure, edema does not correlate well with the level of systemic venous pressure. In patients with chronic left ventricular failure and a low cardiac output, extracellular fluid volume may be sufficiently expanded to cause edema in the presence of only slight elevations of systemic venous pressure. A substantial gain of extracellular fluid volume, a minimum of 5 liters in adults, must usually take place

---

LIVING WITH HEART FAILURE QUESTIONNAIRE

These questions concern how your heart failure (heart condition) has prevented you from living as you wanted during the last month. The items listed below describe different ways some people are affected. If you are sure an item does not apply to you or is not related to your heart failure then circle 0 (No) and go on to the next item. If an item does apply to you, then circle the number rating how much it prevented you from living as you wanted. Remember to think about ONLY THE LAST MONTH.

DID YOUR HEART FAILURE PREVENT YOU FROM LIVING AS YOU WANTED DURING THE LAST MONTH BY:	NO	VERY LITTLE				VERY MUCH
1. causing swelling in your ankles, legs, etc?	0	1	2	3	4	5
2. making you sit or lie down to rest during the day?	0	1	2	3	4	5
3. making your walking about or climbing stairs difficult?	0	1	2	3	4	5
4. making your working around the house or yard difficult?	0	1	2	3	4	5
5. making your going places away from home difficult?	0	1	2	3	4	5
6. making your sleeping well at night difficult?	0	1	2	3	4	5
7. making your relating to or doing things with your friends or family difficult?	0	1	2	3	4	5
8. making your working to earn a living difficult?	0	1	2	3	4	5
9. making your recreational pastimes, sports or hobbies difficult?	0	1	2	3	4	5
10. making your sexual activities difficult?	0	1	2	3	4	5
11. making you eat less of the foods you like?	0	1	2	3	4	5
12. making you short of breath?	0	1	2	3	4	5
13. making you tired, fatigued, or low on energy?	0	1	2	3	4	5
14. making you stay in a hospital?	0	1	2	3	4	5
15. costing you money for medical care?	0	1	2	3	4	5
16. giving you side effects from medications?	0	1	2	3	4	5
17. making you feel you are a burden to your family or friends?	0	1	2	3	4	5
18. making you feel a loss of self-control in your life?	0	1	2	3	4	5
19. making you worry?	0	1	2	3	4	5
20. making it difficult for you to concentrate or remember things?	0	1	2	3	4	5
21. making you feel depressed?	0	1	2	3	4	5

FIGURE 15–3. The Minnesota Living with Heart Failure questionnaire. Improvement in quality of life is one of two primary goals of therapy (prolonged survival being the other). This measure of quality of life, which has been used in many investigations of treatments for heart failure, defines quality of life as living as one wants with minimal limitations secondary to heart failure and its treatment. Physical, social, emotional, and economic limitations are included. Patients self-administer the questions after listening to a standard set of instructions. The score is the sum of the responses for all 21 questions. Eight questions including dyspnea and fatigue are highly interrelated and their sum is called the *physical dimension*. Similarly, five interrelated questions comprise an *emotional dimension*. (Adapted from Rector, T. S., and Cohn, J. N.: Assessment of patient outcome with the Minnesota Living with Heart Failure questionnaire: Reliability and validity during a randomized, double-blind, placebo controlled trial of pimobendan. Am. Heart J. *124*:1017, 1992.)

before peripheral edema is manifested. Therefore, edema may develop over a number of days and may not be present initially in patients with acute heart failure and marked systemic venous hypertension.

Edema is usually symmetrical, pitting, and generally occurs first in the dependent portions of the body, where the systemic venous pressure rises to its highest levels.

Accordingly, cardiac edema in ambulatory patients is usually first noted in the feet or ankles at the end of the day and generally resolves after a night's rest. In bedridden patients it is most commonly found over the sacrum. Facial edema seldom appears in adults with heart failure but may occur in infants and young children. Late in the course of heart failure, edema may become massive and generalized (anasarca). Longstanding edema results in pigmentation, reddening, and induration of the skin of the lower extremities, usually the dorsum of the feet and the pretibial areas.

HYDROTHORAX (PLEURAL EFFUSION). Because the pleural veins drain into both the systemic and the pulmonary venous beds, hydrothorax is observed most commonly in patients with hypertension involving both venous systems, but it also may occur when there is marked elevation of pressure in either venous bed. An increase in capillary permeability probably also plays a role in the pathogenesis of cardiac hydrothorax, since the protein content of the pleural fluid may be significantly greater (2 to 3 gm/dl) than that found in edema fluid (0.5 gm/dl). Hydrothorax is usually bilateral, but when unilateral it is usually confined to the right side of the chest. When hydrothorax develops, dyspnea usually intensifies, owing to a further reduction in vital capacity. Although the excess fluid in hydrothorax is usually resorbed as heart failure improves, sometimes interlobar effusions persist.

ASCITES. This finding occurs in patients with increased pressure in the hepatic veins and in the veins draining the peritoneum. Ascites usually reflects longstanding systemic venous hypertension. In patients with organic tricuspid valve disease and chronic constrictive pericarditis, ascites may be more prominent than subcutaneous edema. As in the case of hydrothorax, there is increased capillary permeability because the protein content is similar to that of hepatic lymph (i.e., four to six times that of edema fluid). Protein-losing enteropathy may occur in patients with visceral congestion,[55] and the resultant reduced plasma oncotic pressure may lower the threshold for the development of ascites.

Cardiac Findings

The presence of cardiac disease is usually readily evident on clinical examination of patients with congestive heart failure.

CARDIOMEGALY. This finding is nonspecific and occurs in the majority of patients with chronic heart failure. Notable exceptions are heart failure associated with chronic constrictive pericarditis, restrictive cardiomyopathy, and a variety of acute insults such as acute myocardial infarction, the sudden development of tachyarrhythmias or bradyarrhythmias, or rupture of a valve or chordae tendineae; in such circumstances heart failure may develop before the heart has had a chance to enlarge.

GALLOP SOUNDS. Protodiastolic sounds, generally emanating from the left ventricle (but occasionally from the right) and occurring 0.13 to 0.16 seconds after the second heart sound, are common findings in healthy children and young adults. Such physiological sounds are seldom audible in healthy persons after age 40 but occur in patients of all ages with heart failure and are referred to as *protodiastolic*, or S_3, *gallops*. In older adults they generally signify the presence of heart failure (see p. 35). In patients with mitral or tricuspid regurgitation or left-to-right shunts, rapid (torrential) flow into the ventricle in early diastole contributes to the generation of an S_3 (see p. 35), but under these conditions this sound is *not* to be interpreted as signifying the presence of heart failure. Thus, a protodiastolic gallop sound is an excellent sign of heart failure when other causes, such as a physiological S_3 occurring in a healthy child or young adult, constrictive pericarditis, mitral and tricuspid regurgitation, or a left-to-right shunt, can be excluded.

PULSUS ALTERNANS (see also p. 22). This sign is characterized by a regular rhythm with alternating strong and weak ventricular contractions. It should be distinguished from the alternation of strong and weak beats that occurs in pulsus bigeminus, in which the weak beat follows the strong beat by a shorter time interval than the strong beat follows the weak, whereas in pulsus alternans they are equally spaced or the weak beat is slightly closer to the succeeding than to

the preceding beat. Severe pulsus alternans may be detected either by palpation of the peripheral pulses (the femoral more readily than the brachial, radial, or carotid) or by sphygmomanometry. As the cuff is slowly deflated, only alternate beats are audible for a variable number of millimeters of mercury below the systolic level, depending on the severity of the alternans, and then all beats are heard. Rarely, the weak beat is so small that the aortic valve is not opened, and this results in an apparent halving of the pulse rate, a condition referred to as *total alternans*. Pulsus alternans may be accompanied by alternation in the intensity of the heart sounds and of existing heart murmurs.

Pulsus alternans occurs most commonly in heart failure secondary to increased resistance to left ventricular ejection, as occurs in systemic hypertension and aortic stenosis, as well as in coronary atherosclerosis and dilated cardiomyopathy. It is usually associated with a ventricular protodiastolic gallop sound (S_3), signifies advanced myocardial disease, and often disappears with treatment of heart failure. In patients with heart failure, pulsus alternans often can be elicited by reduction in systemic venous return, as occurs with assumption of the erect posture or application of venous tourniquets, and it is reduced by an increase in venous return, as in recumbency or with exercise. Pulsus alternans tends to be present during tachycardia and is often initiated by a premature beat.

Pulsus alternans is attributed to an alternation in the stroke volume ejected by the left ventricle[56] and, ultimately, to a deletion in the number of contracting cells in every other cycle, presumably owing to incomplete recovery. Alternans is almost always concordant in the two sides of the circulation; i.e., the strong and weak beats occur simultaneously in the two ventricles. Rarely, pulsus alternans is accompanied by *electrical alternans*; however, the latter condition is usually not due to mechanical alternans but to alternating positions of the heart within the fluid-filled pericardial sac (Fig. 3–103, p. 93).

ACCENTUATION OF P_2 AND SYSTOLIC MURMURS. With the development of left ventricular failure, pulmonary artery pressure rises and P_2 becomes accentuated—often louder than A_2—and more widely transmitted. As left ventricular failure improves, P_2 becomes softer. *Systolic murmurs* are common in heart failure owing to the relative mitral or tricuspid regurgitation that may occur secondary to ventricular dilatation. Often these murmurs diminish or disappear when compensation is restored.

FEVER. A low-grade temperature ($<38°C$), which results from cutaneous vasoconstriction and therefore impairment of heat loss, may occur in severe heart failure; fever usually subsides when compensation is restored. Greater elevations of temperature usually signify the presence of an infection, pulmonary infarction, or infective endocarditis.

CARDIAC CACHEXIA. Longstanding, severe congestive heart failure, particularly of the right ventricle, may lead to anorexia, owing to hepatic and intestinal congestion and sometimes to digitalis intoxication. Occasionally, there is impaired intestinal absorption of fat[57] and rarely protein-losing enteropathy.[55] Patients with heart failure also may exhibit increased total metabolism secondary to (1) an augmentation of myocardial oxygen consumption, as occurs in patients with aortic stenosis and hypertension, (2) excessive work of breathing, (3) low-grade fever, and (4) elevated levels of circulating tumor necrosis factor.[58] This cytokine is produced by monocytes and causes cachexia and anorexia. The combination of reduced caloric intake and increased caloric expenditure, however produced, may lead to a reduction of tissue mass and, in severe cases, to cardiac cachexia.[59,60] In some patients the cachexia may be severe enough to suggest the presence of disseminated malignant disease. In others, the loss of lean body mass may be masked by the accumulation of edema. There is evidence that inflammatory cytokines, including tumor necrosis factor-alpha, may depress myocardial contractility,[61–63] modulate the growth and phenotype of various cells in the myocardium,[64] and contribute to cardiac cachexia.

CHEYNE-STOKES RESPIRATION. Also known as *periodic* or *cyclic respiration*, Cheyne-Stokes respiration is characterized by the combination of depression in the sensitivity of the respiratory center to carbon dioxide and left ventricular failure.[65,66] During the apneic phase, arterial PO_2 falls and PCO_2 rises; this combination excites the depressed respiratory center, resulting in hyperventilation and, subsequently, hypocapnia, followed by another period of apnea. The principal causes of depression of the respiratory center in patients with Cheyne-Stokes respiration are cerebral lesions such as cerebral arteriosclerosis, stroke, or head injury. These causes are often exaggerated by sleep, barbiturates, and narcotics, all of which further depress the sensitivity of the respiratory center. Left ventricular failure, which prolongs the circulation time from the lung to the brain, results in a sluggish response of the system and is responsible for the oscillations between apnea and hyperpnea and prevents return to a steady state of ventilation and blood gases. Usually patients are not aware of Cheyne-Stokes respiration. However, it can be readily observed in a sleeping patient, or a history can be elicited from the patient's bed partner. Cheyne-Stokes respiration may contribute to daytime sleepiness in such patients,[67] and occasionally the patient with heart failure awakens at night with dyspnea precipitated by Cheyne-Stokes respiration.[68] Ventilatory oscillations also may occur during exercise and appear to reflect oscillations in the circulation.[69]

LUNGS. In patients who have died of left ventricular failure, the lungs are enlarged, firm, and dark and may be filled with bloody fluid. With longstanding pulmonary congestion, they are brown with deposition of hemosiderin and usually do not seep edema fluid. On microscopic examination, the capillaries are engorged, and there is thickening of the alveolar septa as well as extravasation of large mononuclear cells containing red blood cells or hemosiderin granules or both.[70] Often the pulmonary vessels show medial hypertrophy and intimal hyperplasia.

LIVER. In acute right heart failure, the liver is enlarged, firm, and filled with fluid. On microscopic examination, the central hepatic veins and sinusoids are dilated.[71,72] With longstanding right heart failure, the liver returns to normal size, subsequently atrophies, and becomes "nutmeg" in appearance as a consequence of the dark red areas of central venous congestion and the lighter, fatty area in the periphery of the lobule. Cardiac cirrhosis is characterized by central lobular necrosis and atrophy as well as extensive fibrous retraction; sometimes there is sclerosis of the hepatic veins. Because cardiac cirrhosis is a function of the level of hepatic venous pressure and the duration of its elevation, it is not surprising that it occurs most commonly in patients with chronic constrictive pericarditis and organic tricuspid valve disease and in children after a Fontan procedure for tricuspid atresia (see p. 933),[73,74] who often have prolonged elevation of systemic venous pressure. In patients with left ventricular failure, central hepatic necrosis without evidence of passive congestion may be present.[75,76]

Liver biopsies in patients with acute heart failure exhibiting fulminant hepatic failure show replacement of hepatocytes by red blood cells. Presumably, the hypoxia caused by hypoperfusion produces hepatocyte necrosis[77,78]; erythrocytes may then enter the space of Disse between damaged endothelial cells. These changes resulting from acute heart failure may be transient if there is hemodynamic recovery.

OTHER VISCERA. Patients with chronic hepatic venous hypertension develop portal hypertension that results in congestive splenomegaly. On microscopic examination, the spleen shows dilatation of the sinusoids and fibrosis, and there is chronic passive congestion of the pancreas and of the veins and capillaries of the gastrointestinal tract. Rarely, intense mesenteric vasoconstriction without thrombotic or embolic occlusion of a mesenteric artery may lead to a hemorrhagic, nonbacterial enterocolitis, with hemorrhagic necrosis.

Chronic venous congestion also occurs in the kidney and brain, with dilation and engorgement of the capillaries. Small infarcts are frequently observed in the spleen and kidneys of patients with longstanding atrial fibrillation.

Laboratory Findings

Proteinuria and a high urine specific gravity are common findings in heart failure. Blood urea nitrogen and creatinine levels are often moderately elevated secondary to reductions in renal blood flow and glomerular filtration rate[12] (prerenal azotemia). The erythrocyte sedimentation rate is usually quite low, presumably secondary to impaired fibrinogen synthesis and resultant decreased fibrinogen concentrations.

SERUM ELECTROLYTES. Serum electrolyte values are generally normal in patients with mild or moderate heart failure before treatment. However, in severe heart failure, prolonged, rigid sodium restriction, coupled with intensive diuretic therapy as well as the inability to excrete water, may lead to dilutional hyponatremia, which occurs because of substantial expansion of extracellular fluid volume and a normal or increased level of total body sodium. It may be accompanied by, and presumably is caused in part by, elevated concentrations of circulating vasopressin.[79] Serum potassium levels are usually normal, although the prolonged administration of kaliuretic diuretics, such as the thiazides or loop diuretics, may result in hypokalemia (see p. 849). Hyperkalemia may occur in patients with severe heart failure[80] who show marked reductions in glomerular filtration rate and inadequate delivery of sodium to the distal tubular sodium-potassium exchange sites, particularly if such patients are also receiving potassium-retaining diuretics and/or converting enzyme.

LIVER FUNCTION TESTS. Congestive hepatomegaly and cardiac cirrhosis are often associated with impaired hepatic function, characterized by abnormal values of aspartate aminotransferase (AST), alanine aminotransferase (ALT), lactic dehydrogenase (LDH), and other liver enzymes.[81,82]

Hyperbilirubinemia, secondary to an increase in both the directly and indirectly reacting bilirubins, is common, and in severe cases of acute (right or left) ventricular failure, frank jaundice may occur. *Acute* hepatic venous congestion can result in severe jaundice with a bilirubin level as high as 15 to 20 mg/dl, elevation of AST to more than 10 times the upper limit of normal, and elevation of the serum alkaline phosphatase level, as well as prolongation of the prothrombin time. Both the clinical and the laboratory pictures may resemble viral hepatitis, but the impairment of hepatic function is rapidly ameliorated by successful treatment of heart failure. In patients with longstanding cardiac cirrhosis, albumin synthesis may be impaired, with resultant hypoalbuminemia, intensifying the accumulation of fluid. Hepatic hypoglycemia, fulminant hepatic failure, and hepatic coma are uncommon, late, and sometimes terminal complications of cardiac cirrhosis. In general, disturbances of hepatic function are frequent when right atrial pressure rises above 10 mm Hg and cardiac index declines below 1.5/min/m^2.[82]

VENOUS PRESSURE. This can be conveniently measured with a spinal fluid manometer with the patient in the recumbent position and the arm abducted. The baseline for the measurement should be 5 cm below the sternal angle (i.e., the estimated position of the right atrium). The venous pressure is often elevated (i.e., >12 cm H$_2$O) at rest, but in mild or borderline cases it may be normal at rest but rises with hepatic compression or during exercise.

THE VALSALVA MANEUVER. Performance of this maneuver—forced expiration against a closed glottis—is helpful in the diagnosis of heart failure.[83,84] The test has been standardized as follows: The patient is asked to blow against an aneroid manometer and maintain a pressure of 40 mm Hg for 30 seconds. During the Valsalva maneuver, intrathoracic pressure rises, venous return to the heart diminishes, stroke volume falls, and venous pressure rises. Arterial pressure tracings normally show four distinct phases: (1) an initial rise in arterial pressure, which represents transmission to the periphery of the increased intrathoracic pressure; (2) with continuation of the strain and the accompanying reduction of venous return, reductions in systolic, diastolic, and pulse pressures accompanied by a reflex increase in heart rate; (3) on release of the strain, a sudden drop of arterial pressure equivalent to the fall in intrathoracic pressure; and (4) an overshoot of arterial pressure to above control levels, with a wide pulse pressure and bradycardia due to the combination of the inrush into the heart of blood that had been dammed up in the venous bed and reflex vasoconstriction and tachycardia secondary to the low perfusion pressure of the carotid and baroreceptors during phase 3.

In heart failure, phase 1 and 3 are normal; that is, there is normal transmission of the elevated intrathoracic pressure into the arterial tree during phase 1 and sudden loss of this with the release of the strain during phase 3. However, because the heart operates on the flat portion of its Starling curve (Fig. 13–2, p. 395), the impedance of venous return during phase 2 does not affect stroke volume. Therefore, the baroreceptor reflex is not activated, and there is no overshoot on release of the strain. This results in a "square-wave" appearance of the tracing. The abnormal blood pressure response is associated with "pseudonormalization" of the transmitral filling velocity pattern observed by Doppler echocardiography.

Although the Valsalva maneuver can be recorded most accurately through an indwelling needle, careful palpation of the pulse in normal individuals allows detection of phases 2 and 4 and their absence and slowing of the pulse in phase 4.[85] An automated device which monitors the arterial pulse in a finger has been used to detect an abnormal Valsalva response.[86]

The Chest Roentgenogram
(See also Chap. 7, pp. 228 to 229)

Two principal features of the chest roentgenogram are useful in the patient with congestive heart failure.

The *size and shape of the cardiac silhouette* provide important information concerning the precise nature of the underlying heart disease. Both the cardiothoracic ratio (Fig. 7–24, p. 220) and the heart volume determined on the plain film[87] are relatively specific but insensitive indicators of increased left ventricular end-diastolic volume.

In the presence of normal pulmonary capillary and venous pressure in the erect position, the lung bases are better perfused than the apices, and the vessels supplying the lower lobes are significantly larger than are those supplying the upper lobes.[88] With elevation of left atrial, pulmonary venous, and capillary pressures, interstitial and

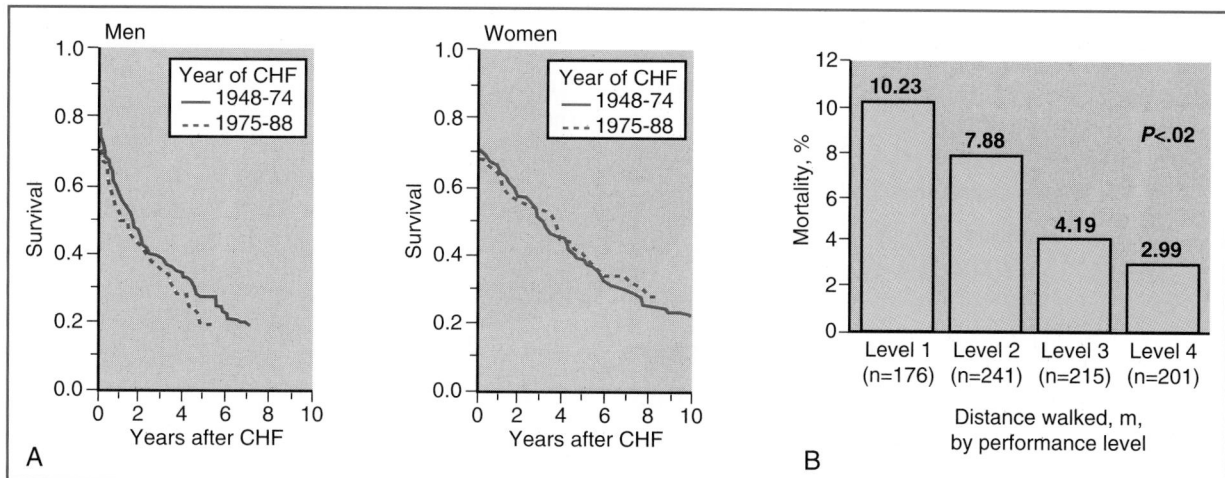

FIGURE 15–4. *A,* Graphs show age-adjusted survival rates after congestive heart failure (CHF) by calendar year of first diagnosis of CHF for men and women developing CHF during the calendar years 1948–1988. (From Ho, K. K. L., et al.: Survival after the onset of congestive heart failure in Framingham Heart Study subjects. Circulation *88*:107–115, 1993.) *B,* Mortality (%) as a function of performance level (base on distance walked). Mortality decreased as performance on the 6-minute walk test improved. (From Bittner, V., et al.: Prediction of mortality and morbidity with a 6-minute walk test in patients with left ventricular dysfunction. JAMA *270*:1702–1707, 1993. Copyright 1993 American Medical Association.)

perivascular edema develops and is most prominent at the lung bases because hydrostatic pressure is greater there. When pulmonary capillary pressure is slightly elevated, i.e., approximately 13 to 17 mm Hg,[89] the resultant compression of pulmonary vessels in the lower lobes causes equalization in size of the vessels at the apices and bases. With greater pressure elevation (approximately 18 to 23 mm Hg), actual pulmonary vascular redistribution occurs (i.e., further constriction of vessels leading to the lower lobes and dilatation of vessels leading to the upper lobes). When pulmonary capillary pressures exceed approximately 20 to 25 mm Hg, interstitial pulmonary edema occurs. This may be of several varieties: (1) *septal,* producing Kerley's lines (i.e., sharp, linear densities of interlobular interstitial edema) (p. 220); (2) *perivascular,* producing loss of sharpness of the central and peripheral vessels; and (3) *subpleural,* producing spindle-shaped accumulations of fluid between the lung and adjacent pleural surface. When pulmonary capillary pressure exceeds 25 mm Hg, alveolar edema, with a cloudlike appearance and concentration of the fluid around the hili in a "butterfly" pattern, and large pleural effusions may occur (Fig. 7–23, p. 219). With elevation of systemic venous pressure, the azygos vein and superior vena cava may enlarge.[90]

PROGNOSIS

SURVIVAL. Survival is reduced in patients with heart failure, which accounts for a substantial portion of all deaths from cardiovascular diseases. The Framingham Heart Study found that between the years of 1948 and 1988, patients with a diagnosis of heart failure had a median survival of 3.2 years for males and 5.4 years for females,[91] despite the fact that the patients with the poorest prognosis, i.e., those dying within 90 days of the diagnosis, were excluded from the analysis (Fig. 15–4A).

A large number of factors have been found to correlate with mortality in patients with congestive heart failure due to dilated cardiomyopathy (Table 15–6).[92] These fall into four major categories:

1. **Clinical.** In general, the presence of coronary artery disease as the etiology of heart failure, the presence of an audible S_3, low pulse and systolic arterial pressures, a high New York Heart Association Class, reduced exercise capacity, male gender (Figs. 15–4B and 15–5A), and the severity

TABLE 15–6 FACTORS AFFECTING SURVIVAL IN PATIENTS WITH CONGESTIVE HEART FAILURE

1. CLINICAL
   Coronary artery disease etiology
   New York Heart Association Class
   Exercise capacity
   Heart rate at rest
   Systolic arterial pressure
   Pulse pressure
   S_3

2. HEMODYNAMIC
   LV ejection fraction
   RV ejection fraction
   LV stroke work index
   LV filling pressure
   Right atrial pressure
   Maximal O_2 uptake
   LV systolic pressure
   Mean arterial pressure
   Cardiac index
   Systemic vascular resistance

3. BIOCHEMICAL
   Plasma norepinephrine
   Plasma renin
   Plasma vasopressin
   Plasma atrial natriuretic peptide
   Serum sodium
   Serum potassium
   Total potassium stores
   Serum magnesium

4. ELECTROPHYSIOLOGICAL
   Frequent ventricular asystole
   Complex ventricular arrhythmias
   Ventricular tachycardia
   Atrial fibrillation/flutter

Modified from Cohn, J. N., and Rector, T. S.: Prognosis of congestive heart failure and predictors of mortality. Am. J. Cardiol. *62*:25A, 1988.

of symptoms (Fig. 15–6) have each been shown to be associated with a high mortality. When the NYHA Class is integrated with the maximal O_2 consumption determined during exercise, the mortality is 20 per cent per year in patients in Class III with a $\dot{V}O_{2\,max}$ of 10 to 15 ml/kg/min and rises to 60 per cent in patients in Class IV with a $\dot{V}O_{2\,max}$ of less than 10 ml/kg/min.[93–95] The distance walked in 6 minutes predicted both morbidity and mortality in the SOLVD trial[96] (Fig. 15–4B).

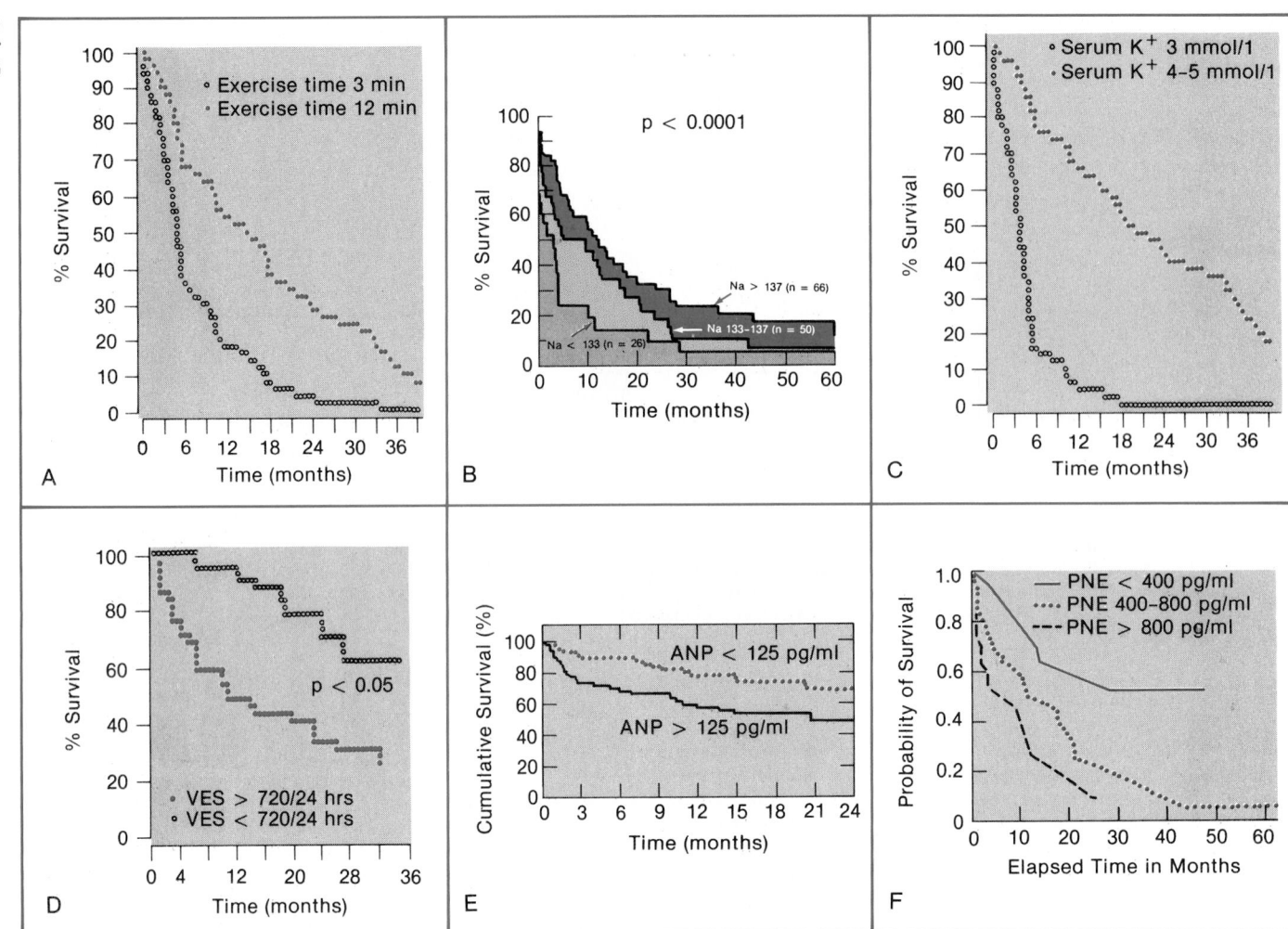

FIGURE 15–5. *A*, Estimated survival curve for patients with a short or a long exercise time in the modified Bruce protocol. Values were chosen arbitrarily. Patients had other important prognostic factors fixed at median values and were assumed to have coronary artery disease but not to be taking amiodarone. (From Cleland, J. G. F., Dargie, H. J., and Ford, I.: Mortality in heart failure: Clinical variables of prognostic value. Br. Heart J. *58*:572, 1987.) *B*, Kaplan-Meier analysis showing cumulative rates of survival in patients with severe chronic heart failure stratified into three groups based on pretreatment serum sodium concentration. Hyponatremic patients fared significantly worse than patients with a normal serum sodium concentration (p < .0001, Mantel-Cox). (From Packer, M., et al.: Role of neurohormonal mechanisms in determining survival in patients with severe chronic heart failure. Circulation *75* (Suppl. 4):80, 92, 1987, by permission of the American Heart Association, Inc.) *C*, Estimated survival curve for patients with a high or a low initial mean serum concentration of potassium. Values were chosen arbitrarily. Patients had other important prognostic factors fixed at median values and were assumed to have coronary artery disease but not to be taking amiodarone. (From Cleland, J. G. F., Dargie, H. J., and Ford, I.: Mortality in heart failure: Clinical variables of prognostic value. Br. Heart J. *58*:572, 1987.)

D, Relation between ventricular arrhythmia and survival in heart failure. VES = ventricular ectopic activity. (From Dargie, H. J., et al.: Relation of arrhythmias and electrolyte abnormalities to survival in patients with severe chronic heart failure. Circulation *75*:98, 1987, by permission of the American Heart Association, Inc.) *E*, Kaplan-Meier analysis of cumulative rates of survival in patients with heart failure stratified into two groups on the basis of median plasma concentration of atrial natriuretic peptide (ANP) (125 pg/ml). From Gottlieb, S. S., et al.: Prognostic importance of atrial natriuretic peptide in patients with chronic heart failure. Reprinted with permission from the American College of Cardiology. J. Am. Coll. Cardiol. *13*:1534, 1989.) *F*, Life-table analysis of survival, according to Tercile, based on level of plasma norepinephrine (PNE). Group 1 (<400 pg/ml) contained 27 patients, group 2 (400 to 800 pg/ml) 49 patients, and group 3 (>800 pg/ml) 30 patients. The probability of survival in each group was significantly different from the probabilities in the other two groups. (From Cohn, J. N., et al.: Plasma norepinephrine as a guide to prognosis in patients with chronic congestive heart failure. N. Engl. J. Med. *311*:822, 1984. Copyright Massachusetts Medical Society.)

2. **Hemodynamic.** Variables such as cardiac index, stroke work index, left ventricular cavity size, and both left and right ventricular ejection fraction[97–99] (Fig. 15–7) have been shown to correlate directly with survival in patients with heart failure, while systemic vascular resistance and heart rate correlate inversely. Combinations of hemodynamic abnormalities, such as depression of stroke work associated with elevation of filling pressure and systemic vascular resistance, are associated with a poor prognosis.[96]

3. **Biochemical.** The observation that there is activation of the neurohormonal axis in heart failure has prompted examination of the relations between a variety of biochemical measurements and clinical outcome. Strong inverse correlations have been reported between survival and plasma norepinephrine (Fig. 15–5*F*),[2,92,100–102] plasma renin,[92,102–104] vasopressin,[104] and atrial natriuretic peptide concentrations[105] (Fig. 15–5*E*). The concentrations of these substances reflect the severity of the underlying impair-

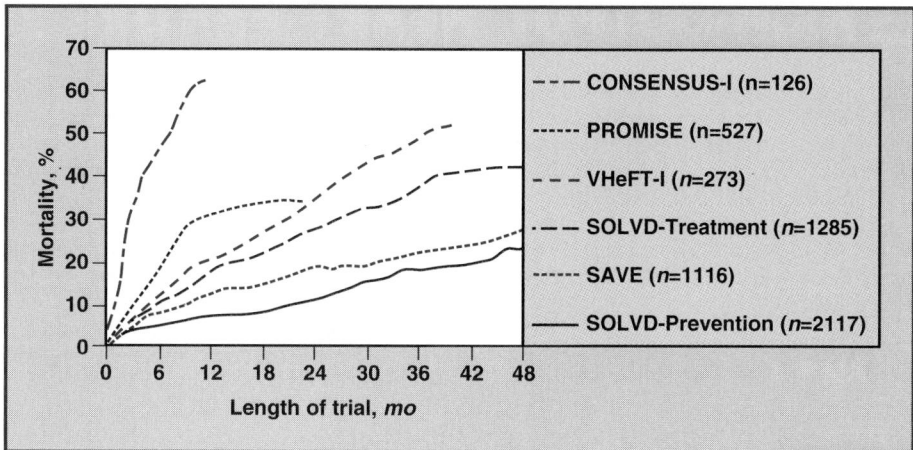

FIGURE 15-6. Based on data from several contemporary clinical trials which included placebo-treated groups, it can be estimated that the 1-year mortality is on the order of 50 to 60 per cent in patients with New York Heart Association (NYHA) functional Class IV symptoms, 15 to 30 per cent in patients with class II-III symptoms, and 5 to 10 per cent in asymptomatic patients with left ventricular dysfunction ($\times 46$-$\times 51$). Patients in CONSENSUS I were in NYHA Class IV treated with digitalis and diuretics; patients in SOLVD (prevention) and SAVE had reduced LV ejection fractions (< 35 and < 40 per cent, respectively) but no or mild limitation (NYHA Classes I and II). Patients in PROMISE, SOLD (treatment) and VHEFT I were in moderate failure (NYHA Classes II or III). (From Young, J. B.: Assessment of Heart Failure. *In* Colucci, W. S. (ed.): Heart Failure: Cardiac Function and Dysfunction. *In* Braunwald, E. (Series ed.): Atlas of Heart Disease. vol. 4. Philadelphia, Current Medicine, 1995, pp. 7.1-7.20.)

ment of circulatory function. In addition, some of these substances per se may exert adverse hemodynamic effects; norepinephrine, angiotensin II (the consequence of increasing renin concentration), and arginine vasopressin are potent vasoconstrictors, augmenting ventricular afterload and thereby reducing the shortening of myocardial fibers. Furthermore, they may be directly responsible for adverse bio-

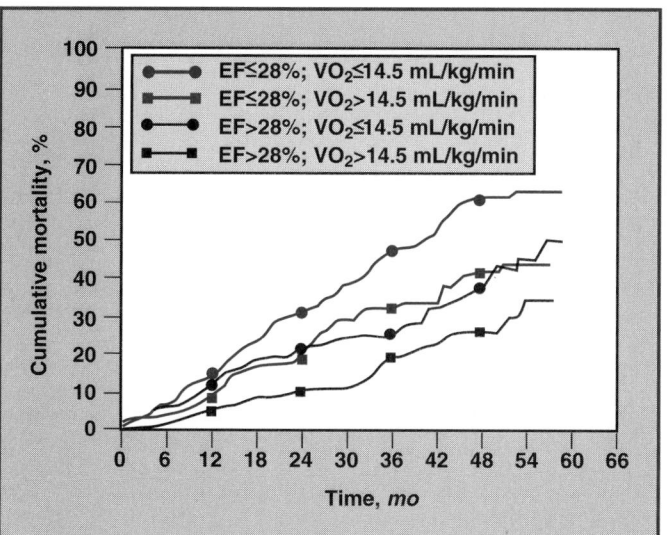

FIGURE 15-7. In a multivariate analysis of survival in the V-HEFT studies, the left ventricular ejection fraction (LVEF) and the peak oxygen consumption (peak $\dot{V}O_2$) were found to have independent prognostic value ($\times 45$). An LVEF < 0.28 and a peak $\dot{V}O_2 < 14.5$ ml/kg/min each predicted a poor survival, and the finding of both predicted a worse survival than if only one or the other were present. (From Rector, T. S., Cohn, J. N.: Prognosis, use of prognostic variables, and assessment of therapeutic responses. *In* Colucci, W. S. (ed.): Heart Failure: Cardiac Function and Dysfunction. *In* Braunwald, E. (Series ed.): Atlas of Heart Diseases, Vol. 4. Philadelphia, Current Medicine, 1995, pp. 8.1-8.10. Adapted from Cohn, J. N., et al.: Ejection fraction, peak exercise oxygen consumption, cardiothoracic ratio, ventricular arrhythmias, and plasma norepinephrine as determinants of prognosis in heart failure. Circulation *87*(Suppl. VI):5, 1993. Copyright 1993 American Heart Association.)

chemical effects on the myocardium. For example, the elevated norepinephrine concentration may be directly responsible for ventricular tachyarrhythmias,[100] as may the hypokalemia (Fig. 15-5C) and reduction of total body potassium stores resulting from the activation of the renin-angiotensin-aldosterone axis (and the administration of potassium-losing diuretics).[106] Hyponatremia also correlates well with high mortality[104] (Fig. 15-5B), but it is likely that this variable reflects activation of the renin-angiotensin-aldosterone axis; hyponatremic patients appear to be especially helped by angiotensin-converting enzyme inhibitors (see p. 494).

In most studies, the aforementioned variables have been assessed in a univariate manner, i.e., independently of one another, and there is still disagreement regarding whether each provides *independent* prognostic information. However, Cohn and Rector have shown that while ventricular function, as expressed in ejection fraction, appears to have the most profound effect on survival in patients with advanced heart failure, exercise tolerance (as reflected in peak O_2 consumption during a progressive exercise test) and activation of the sympathetic nervous system (as reflected in the plasma norepinephrine concentration) *each* provided important independent information.[92]

4. **Electrophysiological.** Death in patients with severe congestive heart failure occurs either by progressive pump failure or, in as many as one-half of all patients, suddenly and unexpectedly, presumably from an arrhythmia. When present, a variety of arrhythmias—especially frequent ventricular extrasystoles (Fig. 15-5D), ventricular tachyarrhythmias, left intraventricular conduction defects, as well as atrial flutter and fibrillation[92]—have been shown to be predictors of mortality. What is not yet clear is whether these arrhythmias are simply indicators of the severity of left ventricular dysfunction or whether they are responsible for and trigger fatal arrhythmias.[2] While there is some evidence that ventricular arrhythmias confer independent adverse prognostic effects,[100] routine treatment of patients with heart failure–associated arrhythmias with antiarrhythmic drugs has not yet been shown to exert a protective effect and reduce mortality. It has been speculated that repletion of potassium and magnesium stores will modify favorably the outcome in these patients.[2]

Although high-cardiac output states by themselves are seldom responsible for heart failure, their development in the presence of underlying heart disease often precipitates heart failure.[107] In these conditions, which are often characterized by arteriovenous shunting, the requirements of the peripheral tissues for oxygen can be satisfied only by an increase in cardiac output. While the normal heart is capable of augmenting its output on a long-term basis, this may not be true of the diseased heart.

Anemia
(See also p. 1786)

HISTORY. Chronic anemia in the absence of underlying heart disease produces surprisingly few symptoms, which may consist of easy fatigability, mild exertional dyspnea, and occasionally palpitations and cardiac awareness. Anemia, even when severe, rarely causes heart failure or angina pectoris, and when these are present, it is likely that the high cardiac output is superimposed on some specific cardiac abnormality, such as valvular or ischemic heart disease.

PHYSICAL EXAMINATION. The anemic patient generally has a pale, "pasty" appearance; in persons of color, the finding of paleness of the conjunctivae, mucous membranes, and palmar creases is helpful. Arterial pulses are bounding, "pistol shot" sounds can be heard over the femoral arteries (Duroziez's sign), and subungual capillary pulsations (Quincke's pulse) are present, as in patients with aortic regurgitation. A medium-pitched, midsystolic murmur along the left sternal border, generally Grade 1/6 to 3/6 in intensity (seldom accompanied by a thrill), is common. Heart sounds are accentuated, and the pulmonic component of the second heart sound may be particularly prominent in patients with sickle cell anemia and pulmonary hypertension; in such patients, a right ventricular lift can usually be palpated. A mid-diastolic flow murmur secondary to augmented blood flow across the mitral orifice, holosystolic murmurs resulting from tricuspid and mitral regurgitation secondary to ventricular dilatation, and rarely, diastolic murmurs resulting from aortic and pulmonic valve incompetence secondary to dilatation of these vessels may be heard. A protodiastolic gallop sound (S_3) frequently is audible at the cardiac apex. Jugular venous distention is uncommon, and although peripheral edema and hepatomegaly are occasionally present, they may be due not only to heart failure but also to accompanying abnormalities such as hypoproteinemia and nutritional deficiency.

Laboratory findings in patients with severe chronic anemia without underlying heart disease usually include mild to moderate cardiomegaly on the chest roentgenogram. The electrocardiogram usually does not show any specific changes but may show T-wave inversions in lateral precordial leads. The echocardiogram generally shows a modest and symmetrical increase in the size of all chambers, with large systolic excursions of the septal and posterior left ventricular walls. These findings are superimposed on those resulting from the underlying heart disease. Hematological and blood chemical findings reflect the specific type of anemia present.

MANAGEMENT OF HIGH-OUTPUT FAILURE DUE TO ANEMIA. Treatment of heart failure associated with severe anemia should be specific for the anemia (e.g., iron, folate, vitamin B_{12}, and so forth). When congestive heart failure is present, diuretics and cardiac glycosides are advisable, although some believe that the latter drugs are not helpful in this condition.

When both heart failure and anemia are severe, treatment must be carried out on an urgent basis and presents a difficult challenge. On the other hand, correction of the anemia is desirable to increase oxygen delivery to metabolizing tissues and thereby decrease the need for a sustained high cardiac output. On the other hand, a too-rapid expansion of the blood volume could intensify the manifestations of heart failure, and an increase in hematocrit will potentially depress cardiac output because of increased blood viscosity. The diagnostic steps for determining the etiology of the anemia should be taken immediately (e.g., blood drawn for serum iron, folate, and vitamin B_{12} measurements). The patient should be placed at bed rest and given supplementary oxygen. *Packed red blood cells* should then be transfused slowly (250 to 500 ml/24 hr), preceded or accompanied by vigorous diuretic therapy (e.g., furosemide, 40 mg intravenously immediately followed by 40 mg orally every 8 hours), and the patient should be observed closely for the development or exacerbation of dyspnea and pulmonary rales so that the transfusion can be discontinued immediately to avoid precipitating pulmonary edema. Vasodilator therapy is seldom helpful, since impedance to left ventricular emptying is already markedly reduced in most cases.

Systemic Arteriovenous Fistulas

Systemic arteriovenous fistulas may be congenital or acquired; the latter are either post-traumatic or iatrogenic. Increased cardiac output associated with such fistulas depends on the size of the communication and the magnitude of the resultant reduction in systemic vascular resistance.

The *physical findings* depend on the underlying disease and the location and size of the shunt. In general, a widened pulse pressure, brisk carotid and peripheral arterial pulsations, and mild tachycardia are present. *Branham's sign* (also called *Nicaladoni-Branham's sign*), which consists of slowing of the heart after manual compression of the fistula,[108,109] is present in the majority of cases; this maneuver also raises arterial and lowers venous pressure. It appears to result from the operation of a cardioaccelerator reflex with both afferent and efferent pathways in the vagus nerves.[110]

The skin overlying the fistula is warmer than normal, and a continuous "machinery" murmur and thrill are usually present over the lesion. Third and fourth heart sounds are commonly heard, as well as a precordial midsystolic murmur secondary to increased cardiac output. The electrocardiographic changes of left ventricular hypertrophy are often seen. Rarely, the fistula may become infected, leading to bacterial endarteritis.

ACQUIRED ARTERIOVENOUS FISTULAS. Acquired arteriovenous fistulas occur most frequently after such injuries as gunshot wounds and stab wounds and may involve any part of the body, most frequently the thigh.[111] Blood flow in the affected limb distal to the fistula diminishes after the creation of the fistula but then returns to normal and often increases with the passage of time. As a consequence, the affected limb is usually larger than its opposite member, and the overlying skin is warmer; cellulitis, venostasis, edema, and dermatitis with pigmentation frequently occur, in part as a consequence of chronically elevated venous pressure. Surgical repair or excision is generally advisable in fistulas that develop after gunshot wounds or trauma.

A rare form of acquired arteriovenous fistula results from spontaneous rupture of an aortic aneurysm into the inferior vena cava. This usually produces an enormous arteriovenous shunt and rapidly progressive left ventricular failure. On physical examination, a pulsating mass can be readily palpated superficially in the abdomen, and a continuous bruit is audible.

Massive fistulas may be associated with Wilms' tumors of the kidney, and these have been reported to cause high-output cardiac failure in children.[112]

High-output congestive heart failure resulting from the arteriovenous shunts surgically constructed for vascular access in patients undergoing long-term hemodialysis is not uncommon.[113,114] Cardiac outputs as high as 10 liters/min/m^2, which decrease substantially during temporary occlusion of the shunt, have been found in such patients. These values undoubtedly also reflect the chronic anemia present in many of these patients, but it is clear that it is the added hemodynamic burden imposed by the shunt that precipitates heart failure in patients who had previously tolerated chronic anemia without apparent impairment of cardiac function. It is usually possible to revise or band the fistula to reduce it to the appropriate size for dialysis without compromising cardiac function.[115]

CONGENITAL ARTERIOVENOUS FISTULAS. Congenital arteriovenous fistulas result from arrest of the normal embryonic development of the vascular system and are structurally similar to embryonic capillary networks. They range from barely noticeable strawberry birthmarks to enormous clusters of engorged vascular channels that may deform an entire extremity. Most frequently, the vessels of the lower extremities are involved.[116] When fistulas are large, patients generally complain of disfigurement as well as swelling and pain in the limb. On examination, erythema and cyanosis are usually apparent, as are venous varices, a continuous murmur, and thrill. Physical examination shows hemangiomatous changes associated with venous distention, deformity, and increased limb length. The fistulous connection may involve any vascular bed, including an internal mammary artery–pulmonary artery connection. *Left heart failure* occurs, particularly in patients with larger lesions that involve the pelvis as well as the extremities.[117,118] Angiography is useful in confirming the diagnosis and in determining the physical extent of the anomaly.

Surgical excision is the ideal treatment,[119] but in many instances the lesions are not sufficiently localized to permit this.[120] The results of ligation and excision have been unsatisfactory in the majority of cases, since the congenital arteriovenous communications are usually not confined to a single anatomical segment or to a circumscribed anatomical region. Complete cure of these lesions is possible in only a few instances. Embolization of Gelfoam pellets delivered through a catheter has been reported to obliterate multiple systemic arteriovenous fistulas and thereby diminish high-output heart failure.[119]

Hereditary Hemorrhagic Telangiectasia. Also known as *Osler-Weber-Rendu disease*, this condition may be associated with arteriovenous fistulas, particularly in the lungs and liver; the latter condition can produce a hyperkinetic circulation,[120–122] with heart failure as well as hepatomegaly with abdominal bruits. Because of the presence of oxygenated blood in the inferior vena cava and right atrium, this condition may be misdiagnosed as atrial septal defect.

The congenital arteriovenous communications resulting from *hemangioendothelioma of the liver* are commonly associated with marked increases in cardiac output, sometimes as high as 10 liters/min/m^2, and congestive heart failure.[123] These lesions, which are extremely difficult to treat surgically, may be quite large, increase in size with time, and lead to heart failure even in infancy. They are often associated with sizable cutaneous hemangiomas, which should alert the clinician to the possibility of their presence.

Hyperthyroidism
(See also p. 1891)

The principal findings on the physical examination of the cardiovascular system are tachycardia, a widened pulse pressure, brisk carotid and peripheral arterial pulsations, a hyperkinetic cardiac apex, and loud first heart sound. A midsystolic murmur along the left sternal border, secondary to increased flow is common; occasionally this murmur has an unusual scratchy component (the so-called Means-Lerman scratch) thought to be due to the rubbing together of normal pleural and pericardial surfaces as a consequence of hyperkinetic heart action. Rarely, systolic murmurs of mitral and tricuspid regurgitation, presumably secondary to papillary muscle dysfunction, may occur.

In patients with hyperthyroidism without heart disease, the *chest roentgenogram* is usually normal, although the *echocardiogram* may show increased left ventricular wall thickness and chamber dimensions and a normal or increased ejection fraction and velocity of shortening.[124] The *electrocardiogram* often shows widespread but nonspecific ST-segment elevation and upward coving, with terminal T-wave inversion in about one-fourth of patients and shortening of the Q-T interval.[125] Atrial fibrillation may occur and often is associated with an unusually rapid ventricular response (i.e., 170 to 220 beats/min). There is relative resistance to slowing of the ventricular rate with digitalis.[126] Spontaneous reversion to sinus rhythm is common when euthyroidism is restored.

As in many other high-output states, the hyperkinetic state of hyperthyroidism does not usually lead to heart failure in the absence of underlying cardiac or coronary artery disease; the normal heart appears capable of tolerating the burden imposed by hyperthyroidism simply by means of dilatation and hypertrophy. A rare exception is the development of heart failure in patients with neonatal thyrotoxicosis without underlying heart disease.[127] However, when the elevated flow load of hyperthyroidism is superimposed on a reduced cardiovascular reserve (i.e., asymptomatic or only mildly symptomatic heart disease), congestive heart failure is likely to ensue. Similarly, in patients with obstructive coronary artery disease who are asymptomatic or who have only mild evidence of ischemia in the euthyroid state, the demand for increased coronary blood flow with hyperthyroidism frequently leads to an exacerbation of angina.

MANAGEMENT. Beta-adrenoceptor blockade may be both helpful and harmful in patients with thyrotoxic heart disease and heart failure. Although it may be beneficial by lowering the ventricular rate, particularly by prolonging the refractory period of the atrioventricular conduction system in patients with atrial fibrillation, it also may diminish myocardial contractility by blocking the adrenergic support of the heart. Therefore, it must be administered cautiously to the patient with thyrotoxic heart disease and heart failure and only after treatment with a digitalis glycoside, with the patient at rest and under careful observation. The initial dose should be small (e.g., propranolol, 0.5 mg intravenously or 10 mg orally), and the patient should be observed after the administration to be sure that heart failure is not intensified.

It is particularly important to recognize *apathetic hyperthyroidism*, a condition in the elderly in which the usual clinical manifestations of thyrotoxicosis, such as palpitations, tachycardia, and moist skin, are not present. In such patients, the first clinical signs of hyperthyroidism may be unexplained heart failure, an exacerbation of angina pectoris, or unexplained atrial fibrillation, usually but not always with a rapid ventricular rate.

Beriberi Heart Disease

PATHOGENESIS AND CLINICAL CONSIDERATIONS
(Table 15–7)

This condition is due to severe thiamine deficiency persisting for at least 3 months. Clinical beriberi is found most frequently in the Far East, although even in that part of the world it is far less prevalent now than in the past. It occurs predominantly in those individuals whose staple diet consists of polished rice, which is deficient in thiamine but high in carbohydrates. The presence of thiamine in the enriched flour used in white bread has virtually eradicated this disease in the United States and western Europe, where beriberi is found most commonly in diet faddists and alcoholics. Like polished rice, alcohol is low in vitamin B_1 but has a high carbohydrate content. In the West, alcoholics become thiamine deficient not only because of a low intake of the vitamin but also because they eat "junk" foods or drink large quantities of beer. The high carbohydrate content of these foods leads to a greater requirement for thiamine.

Patients in Asia present with edema ("wet beriberi"), general malaise, and fatigue. The elevation of cardiac output[128–132] is presumably secondary to the reduced systemic vascular resistance and augmented venous return.

TABLE 15–7   DIAGNOSTIC CRITERIA FOR BERIBERI HEART DISEASE

CLINICAL FEATURES
Dependent edema
Low peripheral vascular resistance: decreased minimum blood pressure and increased pulse pressure
Hyperkinetic circulatory state: midsystolic murmur and third heart sound
Enlarged heart
T-wave changes (inverted, diphasic, depressed) on electrocardiogram
Peripheral neuritis
Dietary deficiency for at least 3 months or chronic alcoholism
PRESENCE OF THIAMINE DEFICIENCY
Decrease in blood thiamine concentration
Decrease in erythrocyte transketolase activity
Increase in TPP effect
IMPROVEMENT AFTER ADEQUATE THIAMINE THERAPY

From Kawai, C., and Nakamura, Y.: The heart in nutritional deficiencies. *In* Abelmann, W. H. (ed.): Cardiomyopathies, Myocarditis, and Pericardial Disease. *In* Braunwald, E. (Series ed.): Atlas of Heart Diseases, Vol. 2: Philadelphia, Current Medicine, 1995, pp. 7.1–7.18.

PHYSICAL FINDINGS. In most cases in Western countries these are of the high-output state and usually of severe generalized malnutrition and vitamin deficiency. Evidence of peripheral neuropathy with sensory and motor deficits is common (so-called dry beriberi), as is the presence of nutritional cirrhosis characterized by paresthesias of the extremities, absence of decreased knee and ankle jerks, painful glossitis, the anemia of combined iron and folate deficiency, and hyperkeratinized skin lesions.

Beriberi heart disease[131–136] is characterized by evidence of biventricular failure, sinus rhythm, and marked edema (so-called wet beriberi). There is arteriolar vasodilatation, and the cutaneous vessels may be dilated, or in later cases with congestive heart failure, they may be constricted. Therefore, the absence of warm hands does not exclude the diagnosis of beriberi. A third heart sound and an apical systolic murmur are heard almost invariably, and there is a wide pulse pressure characteristic of the hyperkinetic state.

ELECTROCARDIOGRAM. This characteristically exhibits low voltage of the QRS complex, prolongation of the Q-T interval, and low voltage or inversion of T waves. The chest roentgenogram usually shows biventricular enlargement, pulmonary congestion, and pleural effusions. In alcoholics with beriberi heart disease, the left ventricular ejection fraction and peak left ventricular dP/dt are usually reduced.[131] The role played by alcoholic cardiomyopathy (see p. 1412) in this hemodynamic picture is not clear. The cardiac output falls, and the peripheral resistance rises acutely when thiamine is administered in the catheterization laboratory.[132]

Laboratory diagnosis can be made by demonstration of increased serum pyruvate and lactate levels in the presence of a low red blood cell transketolase level.[137] The thiamine concentration may be determined in biological fluids to confirm the diagnosis.[138–140]

At *postmortem examination,* the heart usually shows simple dilation without other changes. On microscopic examination, there is sometimes edema and hydropic degeneration of the muscle fibers. Nonspecific but abnormal histological and electron microscopic changes have been found in cardiac biopsy specimens.

Heart failure may develop explosively in beriberi, and some patients succumb to the illness within 48 hours of the onset of symptoms. *Shoshin beriberi,* seen most frequently in Asia and Africa,[133,134] is a fulminating form of the disease[141] characterized by hypotension, tachycardia, and lactic acidosis; if left untreated, the patients die of pulmonary edema. Thus, since the course of the disease may advance rapidly, treatment must be begun immediately once the diagnosis has been established. In the Western world, this fulminant form of the disease is uncommon.

TREATMENT. Akbarian and coworkers have reported careful hemodynamic studies which suggest that vasomotor depression or paralysis may be responsible for the depressed vascular resistance.[130] They studied four patients in whom ethanol excess was responsible for the thiamine deficiency. All had increased heart rate and cardiac output (averaging 6 liters/min/m²) and reduced arterial–mixed venous oxygen difference and systemic vascular resistance. Right and left ventricular filling pressures and blood volume were also elevated.

Patients with beriberi heart disease fail to respond adequately to digitalis and diuretics alone. However, improvement after the administration of thiamine (up to 100 mg intravenously followed by 25 mg per day orally for 1 to 2 weeks) may be dramatic. Marked diuresis, decrease in heart rate and size, and clearing of pulmonary congestion may occur within 12 to 48 hours.[130,141,142] However, the acute reversal of the vasodilation induced by correction of the deficiency may cause the unprepared left ventricle to go into low-output failure. Therefore, patients should receive a glycoside and diuretic therapy along with thiamine.

Latent thiamine deficiency may occur in conditions such as alcoholic cardiomyopathy and in other forms of refractory congestive heart failure. The possibility of thiamine deficiency should be considered in many patients with heart failure of obscure origin, and patients with heart failure from other causes could develop superimposed beriberi heart disease unless adequate thiamine intake is maintained.

Paget's Disease

PATHOGENESIS. Paget's disease of bone is an asymmetrical process characterized by extremely rapid bone formation and resorption of the involved areas. Because of the increased vascularity of bone affected by Paget's disease, it has been assumed that this high flow occurred through the involved bone. However, it appears that the additional blood flow through an affected, resting limb passes through the *cutaneous tissue* overlying the involved bone, possibly secondary to local heat production resulting from the increased metabolic activity of affected bone.[143]

CLINICAL FINDINGS. These are a function of the extent of the disease and the specific bones involved. Involvement of at least 15 per cent of the skeleton by Paget's disease in an active stage, accompanied by a high alkaline phosphatase level, is necessary before a clinically significant augmentation of cardiac output is observed.

Such a high-output state may be well tolerated for years with the patient remaining asymptomatic. However, if a specific cardiac disorder (e.g., valvular disease, coronary stenosis) is present, the combination may cause rapid clinical deterioration.

The cardiovascular findings are not distinguishable from those in other conditions with high-output states. However, metastatic calcifications are characteristic. If they involve the heart, they may lead to sclerosis and calcification of the valve rings, with extension into the interventricular septum, and may produce abnormalities of atrioventricular or interventricular conduction.

Other Causes of High-Cardiac Output Failure

FIBROUS DYSPLASIA (ALBRIGHT SYNDROME). This condition, in which there is proliferation of fibrous tissue in bone, also may be associated with an elevated cardiac output, especially when multiple bones are involved.[144,145]

MULTIPLE MYELOMA. High-output heart failure also has been described in this condition.[146] The mechanism is not clear; it may be due to an associated anemia and/or hyperperfusion of the neoplastic tissue.

High-cardiac output failure also occurs in pregnancy (Chap. 59), renal disease, especially glomerulonephritis (Chap. 62), cor pulmonale (Chap. 43), polycythemia vera (Chap. 56), the carcinoid syndrome (Chap. 42), and obesity (Chap. 35).

PULMONARY EDEMA

Mechanism of Pulmonary Edema

ALVEOLAR-CAPILLARY MEMBRANE. Pulmonary edema develops when the movement of liquid from the blood to the interstitial space, and in some instances to the alveoli, exceeds the return of liquid to the blood and its drainage through the lymphatics.[147] The barrier between pulmonary capillaries and alveolar gas, the alveolar-capillary membrane, consists of three anatomical layers with distinct structural characteristics: (1) cytoplasmic projections of the capillary endothelial cells that join to form a continuous cytoplasmic tube; (2) the interstitial space, which varies in thickness and may contain connective tissue fibrils, fibroblasts, and macrophages between the capillary endothelium and the alveolar epithelium, terminal bronchioles, small arteries and veins, and lymphatic channels; and (3) the lining of the alveolar wall, which is continuous with the bronchial epithelium and is composed predominantly of large squamous cells (Type I) with thin cytoplasmic projections. There is normally a continuous exchange of liquid, colloid, and solutes between the vascular bed and interstitium.[148,149] A pathological state exists only when there is an increase in the net flux of liquid, colloid, and solutes from the vasculature into the interstitial space. Experimental studies have confirmed that the basic principles outlined in the classic Starling equation apply to the lung as well as to the systemic circulation.

$$\dot{Q}_{(iv-int)} = K_f[(P_{iv} - P_{int}) - \sigma_f(\Pi_{iv} - \Pi_{int})]$$

where

$\dot{Q}$ = net rate of transudation (flow of liquid from blood vessels to interstitial space)

P_{int} = interstitial hydrostatic pressures

P_{iv} = intravascular hydrostatic pressures

Π_{int} = interstitial colloid osmotic pressure

Π_{iv} = intravascular colloid osmotic pressure

σ_f = reflection coefficient for proteins

K_f = hydraulic conductance.

LYMPHATICS. These vessels serve to remove solutes, colloid, and liquid derived from the blood vessels. Because of a more negative pressure in the peribronchial and perivascular interstitial space and the increased compliance of this nonalveolar interstitium, liquid is more likely to increase here once the pumping capacity of the lymphatic channels is exceeded. As a consequence of the development of interstitial edema, small airways and blood vessels may become compressed.

The lymphatics play a key role in removing liquid from the interstitial space, and if the pumping capacity of the lymphatic channels is exceeded, edema will occur. It has been estimated that an average 70-kg person at rest has a Q_{lymph} of approximately 20 ml per hour,[150] and experimentally, lymph flow rates of up to 10 times control values have been reported. Thus it is possible that lymphatic pumping capacity can be as much as 200 ml per hour in an average-sized adult. With chronic elevations of left atrial pressure, the pulmonary lymphatic system hypertrophies and is able to transport greater quantities of capillary filtrate, thereby protecting the lungs from edema. Thus sudden marked increase in pulmonary capillary pressure can be rapidly fatal in a patient not preconditioned by growth of the lymphatic drainage system. The same hemodynamic abnormality may be well tolerated in the presence of well-developed lymphatics.

SEQUENCE OF FLUID ACCUMULATION DURING PULMONARY EDEMA.

Whether initiated by an imbalance of Starling forces or by primary damage to the various components of the alveolar-capillary membranes, the sequence of liquid exchange and accumulation in the lungs is the same, and it can be represented as three stages. In *stage 1*, there is an increase in mass transfer of liquid and colloid from blood capillaries through the interstitium. Despite the increased filtration, there is no measurable increase in interstitial volume because there is an equal increase in lymphatic outflow. *Stage 2* occurs when the filtered load from the pulmonary capillaries is sufficiently large that the pumping capacity of the lymphatics is approached or exceeded, and liquid and colloid begin to accumulate in the more compliant interstitial compartment surrounding bronchioles, arterioles, and venules. In *stage 3*, further increments in filtered load exceed the volume limits of the loose interstitial spaces, causing distention of the less compliant interstitial space of the alveolar-capillary septum and resulting in alveolar flooding.

GRAVITY DEPENDENCE OF PULMONARY EDEMA.

Since blood is more dense than gas-containing lung, the effects of gravity are much greater on the distribution of blood flow than on the distribution of tissue forces in the lung. From apex to base, the effective perfusion pressure of the pulmonary circulation (P_{pa}) increases by approximately 1.00 cm H_2O/cm vertical distance, whereas pleural pressures (P_{pl}) increase by only 0.25 cm H_2O/cm vertical distance.[151] Pulmonary capillaries (or alveolar vessels) are exposed to alveolar pressure (P_{alv}), which does not vary from apex to base. In contrast, pulmonary arteries, arterioles, veins, and venules (extraalveolar vessels) are exposed to pleural pressure, which does vary from apex to base. The consequences of these differences in forces on ventilation-perfusion relationships are described as three zones (Fig. 15–8). In *zone 1* (apex), pulmonary arterial pressure is less than alveolar pressure, and thus blood flow is strikingly diminished.[152] In *zone 2* (midlung), arterial pressure exceeds alveolar pressure, which in turn exceeds venous pressure. In *zone 3* (base), venous pressure exceeds alveolar pressure, resulting in distention of collapsible capillaries. Mean intravascular pressures are greatest in this zone; hence, with elevations of venous pressure or with disruption of alveolar-capillary membranes, edema formation is both more rapid and greatest here. It is only in this zone that the usual calculation of pulmonary vascular resistance is valid, and it is the only zone in which a valid pulmonary capillary wedge pressure measurement can be obtained.

In normal, erect humans, perfusion is greater in the basilar lung regions than in the apical ones. Deviation from this gravity-dependent pattern has been called *vascular redistri-*bution, a relative reduction in perfusion of the bases with a relative increase in apical perfusion. This phenomenon is most likely due to compression of the lumina of basilar vessels secondary to the greater and more rapid formation of edema at the lung bases and the tendency for extravascular liquid formed elsewhere to gravitate toward the bases. The situation with chronic elevations of left atrial pressure, as in mitral stenosis or chronic congestive heart failure, should be contrasted with that of acute pulmonary edema. Clinical experience with such chronic conditions suggests that redistribution of blood flow does occur, but with minimal or no evidence of interstitial edema and often in the absence of alveolar edema.

Classification of Pulmonary Edema

The two most common forms of pulmonary edema are those initiated by an imbalance of Starling forces and those initiated by disruption of one or more components of the alveolar-capillary membrane (Table 15–8).[153–156] Less often, lymphatic insufficiency can be involved as a predisposing, if not initiating, factor in the genesis of edema. Although the initiating or primary mechanism may be clearly identifi-

TABLE 15–8 CLASSIFICATION OF PULMONARY EDEMA BASED ON INITIATING MECHANISM

I. IMBALANCE OF STARLING FORCES
  A. Increased pulmonary capillary pressure
    1. Increased pulmonary venous pressure without left ventricular failure (e.g., mitral stenosis)
    2. Increased pulmonary venous pressure secondary to left ventricular failure
    3. Increased pulmonary capillary pressure secondary to increased pulmonary arterial pressure (so-called overperfusion pulmonary edema)*
  B. Decreased plasma oncotic pressure: Hypoalbuminemia secondary to renal, hepatic, protein-losing enteropathic, or dermatological disease or nutritional causes†
  C. Increased negativity of interstitial pressure
    1. Rapid removal of pneumothorax with large applied negative pressures (unilateral)
    2. Large negative pleural pressures due to acute airway obstruction along with increased end-expiratory volumes (asthma)*
  D. Increased interstitial oncotic pressure: No known clinical or experimental example

II. ALTERED ALVEOLAR-CAPILLARY MEMBRANE PERMEABILITY (ADULT RESPIRATORY DISTRESS SYNDROME)
  A. Infectious pneumonia—bacterial, viral, parasitic
  B. Inhaled toxins (e.g., phosgene, ozone, chlorine, Teflon fumes, nitrogen dioxide, smoke)
  C. Circulating foreign substances (e.g., snake venom, bacterial endotoxins, alloxan,‡ alpha-naphthyl thiourea‡)
  D. Aspiration of acidic gastric contents
  E. Acute radiation pneumonitis
  F. Endogenous vasoactive substances (e.g., histamine, kinins*)
  G. Disseminated intravascular coagulation
  H. Immunological—hypersensitivity pneumonitis, drugs (nitrofurantoin), leukoagglutinins
  I. Shock lung in association with nonthoracic trauma
  J. Acute hemorrhagic pancreatitis

III. LYMPHATIC INSUFFICIENCY
  A. Post-lung transplant
  B. Lymphangitic carcinomatosis
  C. Fibrosing lymphangitis (e.g., silicosis)

IV. UNKNOWN OR INCOMPLETELY UNDERSTOOD
  A. High-altitude pulmonary edema
  B. Neurogenic pulmonary edema
  C. Narcotic overdose
  D. Pulmonary embolism
  E. Eclampsia
  F. Post-cardioversion
  G. Post-anesthesia
  H. Post-cardiopulmonary bypass

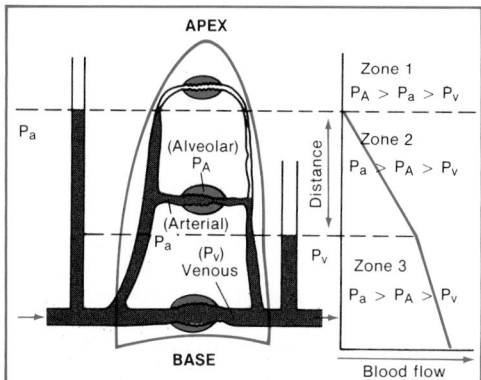

FIGURE 15–8. Schematic representation of the gravity-dependent, apex-to-base distribution of pulmonary blood flow in an upright lung. Pulmonary artery pressure (P_a) and pulmonary venous pressure (P_v) increase on a hydrostatic basis as the base is approached. Alveolar pressure (P_A) is constant with vertical distance. (The three zones are described at length in the text.)

* Not certain to exist as a clinical entity. † Not certain that this, as a single factor, leads to clinical pulmonary edema. ‡ Predominantly an experimental technique.

able, multiple factors come into play during the development of edema, and irrespective of the initiating event, the stage of alveolar flooding is characterized to some degree by disruption of the alveolar-capillary membrane.

IMBALANCE OF STARLING FORCES

INCREASED PULMONARY CAPILLARY PRESSURE. Pulmonary edema will occur only when the pulmonary capillary pressure rises to values exceeding the plasma colloid osmotic pressure, which is approximately 28 mm Hg in the human. Since the normal pulmonary capillary pressure is about 8 mm Hg, there is a substantial margin of safety in the development of pulmonary edema.[150] Although pulmonary capillary wedge pressures must be abnormally high to increase the flow of interstitial liquid, at a time when edema is clearly present, these pressures may not correlate with the severity of pulmonary edema.[157] In fact, pulmonary capillary wedge pressures may have returned to normal at a time when there is still considerable pulmonary edema, since time is required for removal of both interstitial and alveolar edema. Other factors obscure the relationship between the severity of edema and measured pulmonary capillary pressures in addition to slower rates of removal after edema has collected. The rate of increase in lung liquid at any given elevation of capillary pressure is related to the functional capacity of lymphatics,[158] which may vary from patient to patient, and to variations in interstitial oncotic and hydrostatic pressures.

HYPOALBUMINEMIA. Pulmonary edema does not develop with hypoalbuminemia alone. However, hypoalbuminemia may alter the fluid conductivity of the interstitial gel so that liquid moves more easily between capillaries and lymphatics to add to the lymphatic safety factor.[159] Thus there must be, in addition to hypoalbuminemia, some elevations of pulmonary capillary pressure, but only small increases are necessary before pulmonary edema ensues. Indeed, in such patients, only moderate fluid overload can precipitate overt pulmonary edema in the absence of left ventricular failure.

INCREASED NEGATIVE INTERSTITIAL PRESSURE. When this is due to rapid removal of pleural air for relief of a pneumothorax, it may be associated with pulmonary edema. Usually, the pneumothorax has been present for several hours to days, allowing time for alterations in surfactant so that large negative pressures are necessary to open collapsed alveoli.[160] In this instance, the edema is unilateral and is most often only a radiographic finding with few clinical findings.

PRIMARY ALVEOLAR-CAPILLARY MEMBRANE DAMAGE

Many diverse medical and surgical conditions are associated with pulmonary edema that appears to be due not to primary alteration in Starling forces but rather to damage of the alveolar-capillary membrane (Table 15–8). These conditions include acute pulmonary infections and pulmonary effects of gram-negative septicemia and nonthoracic trauma as well as any condition associated with disseminated intravascular coagulation.[153,154,161–163] Despite the diversity of underlying causes, once diffuse alveolar-capillary injury has occurred, the pathophysiological and clinical sequence of events is quite similar in most patients. Because of the resemblance of the clinical picture to that seen with respiratory distress of the neonate, these conditions have been referred to as the *adult respiratory distress syndrome* (ARDS).

Direct evidence for increased capillary permeability has come mainly from experimental studies in which pulmonary edema has been produced by endotoxin infusion,[164] hemorrhagic shock,[165] infusion of oleic acid,[166,167] alloxan, thiourea, phorbol myristate acetate, complement fragments, cobra venom factor,[167–171] freebase cocaine smoking,[172] and inhalation of high concentrations of oxygen[173] or toxic gases, such as phosgene,[174] ozone,[175] and nitrogen dioxide.[176] It is probable, though not yet proved, that increased permeability of the alveolar-capillary membrane is an initiating event in most of the cases designated as ARDS.

Cardiogenic Pulmonary Edema

CLINICAL MANIFESTATIONS. During Stage 1, the distention and recruitment of small pulmonary vessels may actually improve gas exchange in the lung and augment slightly the diffusing capacity for carbon monoxide.[177] It is doubtful that any symptoms, except for exertional dyspnea, accompany these abnormalities, and physical findings in the lungs would be scarce except for mild inspiratory rales due to opening of closed airways. With progression to Stage 2, interstitial edema attributable to increased liquid in the loose interstitial space contiguous with the perivascular tissue of larger vessels may cause a loss of the normally sharp radiographic definition of pulmonary vascular markings, haziness and loss of demarcation of hilar shadows, and thickening of interlobular septa (Kerley B lines) (Fig. 7–35, p. 226). Competition for space between vessels, airways,

and increased liquid within the loose interstitial space may compromise small airway lumina, particularly in the dependent portions of the lungs, and there may be reflex bronchoconstriction.[177] A mismatch exists between ventilation and perfusion that results in hypoxemia and more wasted ventilation. Indeed, in the setting of acute myocardial infarction, the degree of hypoxemia correlates with the degree of elevation of the pulmonary capillary wedge pressure.[178] Tachypnea is a frequent finding with interstitial edema and has been attributed to stimulation by the edema of interstitial J-type receptors or to stretch receptors in the interstitium rather than to hypoxemia, which is rarely of sufficient magnitude to stimulate breathing.[179] There are few changes in the standard spirometric indices.

With the onset of alveolar flooding, or Stage 3 edema, gas exchange is quite abnormal, with severe hypoxemia and often hypocapnia. Alveolar flooding can proceed to such a degree that many large airways are filled with blood-tinged foam that can be expectorated. Vital capacity and other lung volumes are markedly reduced. A right-to-left intrapulmonary shunt develops as a consequence of perfusion of the flooded alveoli. Although hypocapnia is the rule, hypercapnia with acute respiratory acidemia can occur in more severe cases. It is in such instances that morphine, with its well-known respiratory depressant effects, should be used with caution.

DIAGNOSIS. Acute cardiogenic pulmonary edema is the most dramatic symptom of left heart failure. Impaired left ventricular systolic and/or diastolic function, mitral stenosis, or whatever cause of elevated left atrial and pulmonary capillary pressures leading to cardiogenic pulmonary edema interferes with oxygen transfer in the lungs and, in turn, depresses arterial oxygen tension. Simultaneously, the sensation of suffocation and oppression in the chest intensifies the patient's fright, elevates heart rate and blood pressure, and further restricts ventricular filling. The increased discomfort and work of breathing place an additional load on the heart, and cardiac function becomes depressed further by the hypoxia. If this vicious circle is not interrupted, it may lead rapidly to death.

Acute cardiogenic pulmonary edema differs from orthopnea and paroxysmal nocturnal dyspnea in the more rapid and extreme development of pulmonary capillary hypertension. Acute pulmonary edema is a terrifying experience for the patient and often the bystander as well. Usually extreme breathlessness develops suddenly, and the patient becomes extremely anxious, coughs, and expectorates pink, frothy liquid, causing him or her to feel as if he or she is literally drowning. The patient sits bolt upright, or may stand, exhibits air hunger, and may thrash about. The respiratory rate is elevated, the alae nasi are dilated, and there is inspiratory retraction of the intercostal spaces and supraclavicular fossae that reflects the large negative intrapleural pressures required for inspiration. The patient often grasps the sides of the bed in order to allow use of the accessory muscles of respiration. Respiration is noisy, with loud inspiratory and expiratory gurgling sounds that are often easily audible across the room. Sweating is profuse, and the skin is usually cold, ashen, and cyanotic, reflecting low cardiac output and increased sympathetic drive.

On auscultation, the lungs are noisy, with rhonchi, wheezes, and moist and fine crepitant rales that appear at first over the lung bases but then extend upward to the apices as the condition worsens. Cardiac auscultation may be difficult because of the respiratory sounds, but a third heart sound and an accentuated pulmonic component of the second heart sound are frequently present.

The patient may suffer from intense precordial pain if the pulmonary edema is secondary to acute myocardial infarction. Unless cardiogenic shock is present, arterial pressure is usually elevated above the patient's normal level as a result of excitement and sympathetic vasoconstriction. Because of the presence of this systemic hypertension, it may be suspected (inappropriately) that the pulmonary edema is due to hypertensive heart disease. However, it should be noted that the latter condition is now quite rare, and if arterial pressure is elevated, examination of the fundi will usually indicate whether or not hypertensive heart disease is actually present.

DIFFERENTIATION FROM BRONCHIAL ASTHMA. It may be difficult to differentiate severe bronchial asthma from acute pulmonary edema, since both conditions may be associated with extreme dyspnea, pulsus paradoxus, demands for an upright posture, and diffuse wheezes that interfere with cardiac auscultation. In bronchial asthma, there is most often a history of previous similar episodes, and the patient is frequently aware of the diagnosis. During the acute attack, the asthmatic patient does not usually sweat profusely, and arterial hypoxemia, although present, is not usually of sufficient magnitude to produce cyanosis. In addition, the chest is hyperexpanded and hyperresonant, and use of accessory muscles is most prominent during respiration. The wheezes are more high-pitched and musical than in pulmonary edema, and other adventitious sounds such as rhonchi and rales are less prominent in asthma.

The patient with acute cardiogenic pulmonary edema most often perspires profusely and is frequently cyanotic owing to desaturation of arterial blood and decreased cutaneous blood flow. The chest is often dull to percussion, there is no hyperexpansion, accessory muscle use is less prominent than in asthma, and moist, bubbly rales and rhonchi are heard in addition to wheezes. As the patient recovers, the radiological appearance of pulmonary edema usually resolves more slowly than the elevated pulmonary capillary wedge pressure.

PULMONARY ARTERY WEDGE PRESSURE MEASUREMENTS. Measurement of pulmonary artery wedge pressure by means of a Swan-Ganz catheter may be critical to the differentiation between pulmonary edema secondary to an imbalance of Starling forces, i.e., cardiogenic pulmonary edema, and that secondary to alterations of the alveolar-capillary membrane. Specifically, a pulmonary capillary wedge or pulmonary artery diastolic pressure exceeding 25 mm Hg in a patient without previous pulmonary capillary pressure elevation (or exceeding 30 mm Hg in a patient with chronic pulmonary capillary pressure elevation) and with the clinical features of pulmonary edema strongly suggests that the edema is cardiogenic in origin.

Following effective treatment of the pulmonary edema, patients are often restored rapidly to the condition that existed before the attack, although they usually feel exhausted; between attacks of pulmonary edema, there may be few symptoms or signs of heart failure.

ADULT RESPIRATORY DISTRESS SYNDROME (ARDS)

There are many similarities between ARDS from diverse etiologies and the respiratory distress syndrome seen in infants, which is due only to immaturity of the surfactant system. Although surfactant deficiency cannot be assigned a primary role in the pathogenesis of ARDS, there are many data to support the idea that changes in the properties of surfactant are added to the initial impairment and serve to perpetuate pulmonary dysfunction. Impairment of surfactant has been shown to occur with cardiogenic pulmonary edema, exposure to various plasma constituents,[180] and high concentrations of oxygen[181] and in association with systemic hypotension.[182] Closely related to the pulmonary edema in the ARDS is that which is commonly associated with all forms of shock—the so-called *shock lung*.

POLYMORPHONUCLEAR LEUKOCYTES. Experimental and clinical data strongly imply a major role for interaction of polymorphonuclear leukocytes in the blood and circulating or cellular chemotactic macromolecules for the initiation, perpetuation, or amplification of lung injury leading to most forms of ARDS. Chemotaxins in the circulating blood (e.g., the fifth component of complement, C5a) or from alveolar macrophages can recruit polymorphonuclear leukocytes, cause them to adhere to the pulmonary capillary endothelium, and activate them to produce several toxic substances that alter alveolar-capillary membrane permeability or cause circulatory changes or both.

MONOCYTIC CELLS. Circulating monocytes and lymphocytes, tissue macrophages, and phagocytic cells along the vascular endothelium

(reticuloendothelial cells) appear to play an important pathogenic and/or amplification role in ARDS. Upon being stimulated with several agents (e.g., endotoxin, these cells release cytokines, including interleukin-1 (IL-1), interleukin-6 (IL-6), and tumor necrosis factor (TNF), which may play a role in ARDS.

PLATELETS. Although it has not been possible to ascribe a major pathogenetic role to platelets, a secondary role seems probable. Nonetheless, heterologous platelet transfusions given to patients with ARDS and thrombocytopenia have no adverse effects on the extent or degree of lung injury.

LYMPHATIC DYSFUNCTION. It is not known whether alterations in lymphatic function, alone, ever account for pulmonary edema. However, lymphatic flow is impaired following endotoxin infusion in sheep.[183] Cessation of lymphatic pumping would be expected to result in a net gain of interstitial liquid, and this may leave a clinical counterpart of pulmonary edema following anesthesia or sedative drug overdose. More important, the paralytic effect following endotoxin infusion suggests that lymphatic dysfunction may play a significant role in lung injury.

COMBINATIONS OF MECHANISMS. In certain clinical settings, typified by gram-negative sepsis, several mechanisms combine to increase pulmonary edema. In addition to the mechanisms already discussed, endotoxin may release cytokines from reticuloendothelial cells and oxidant and arachidonic acid metabolites from polymorphonuclear leukocytes. These or other factors may depress cardiac function and thereby further contribute to edema formation.

Pulmonary Edema of Unknown Pathogenesis

HIGH-ALTITUDE PULMONARY EDEMA (HAPE). Victims of this disorder are usually persons mostly in their teens or early twenties who have quickly ascended to altitudes in excess of 2500 m and who then engage in strenuous physical exercise at that altitude before they have become acclimated.[184–188] Estimates place the incidence at 6.4 clinically apparent cases per 100 exposure to high altitude in persons less than 21 years of age and 0.4 cases per 100 exposures in those older than 21 years. The pathogenesis is shown in Figure 15–9. Gradual ascent, allowing time for acclimatization, and limiting physical exertion upon more rapid ascent are thought to be preventive. Usually within one day of ascent, affected patients complain of cough, dyspnea, and, in some cases, chest pain in association with tachycardia, bilateral rales, and cyanosis accompanied by radiographic evidence of discrete patches of pulmonary infiltrate.

Reversal of this syndrome is both rapid (less than 48 hours) and certain either by returning the patient to a lower altitude and/or by administering a high inspiratory concentration of oxygen. Sleeping below 2500 m, gradual acclimatization, and avoidance of heavy exertion for the first 2 or 3 days at high altitude appear to be preventive.

NEUROGENIC PULMONARY EDEMA. Central nervous system disorders ranging from head trauma to grand mal seizures can be associated with acute pulmonary edema (without detectable left ventricular disease.[189] The current idea is that sympathetic overactivity produces shifts of blood volume from the systemic to the pulmonary circulation, with secondary elevations of left atrial and pulmonary capillary pressures. Thus, an imbalance of Starling forces may be the basis for this form of pulmonary edema, although capillary pressure quickly returns to normal after the acute and transitory sympathetic discharge. It should be emphasized that although sympatholytics prevent neurogenic pulmonary edema, they appear to have no place in the treatment of this syndrome, since it appears that pulmonary capillary pressures have returned to near normal by the time the syndrome is diagnosed.

NARCOTIC OVERDOSE PULMONARY EDEMA. Acute pulmonary edema is a well-recognized sequela of heroin overdose.[190] Because of the illicit traffic in this drug, which is given by the intravenous route, the syndrome was initially thought to be due to injected impurities rather than to the heroin itself. However, since oral methadone and dextra-propoxyphene also can be associated with pulmonary edema,[191,192] the syndrome cannot be attributed entirely to injected impurities. The fact that edema fluid contains protein concentrations nearly identical to those found in

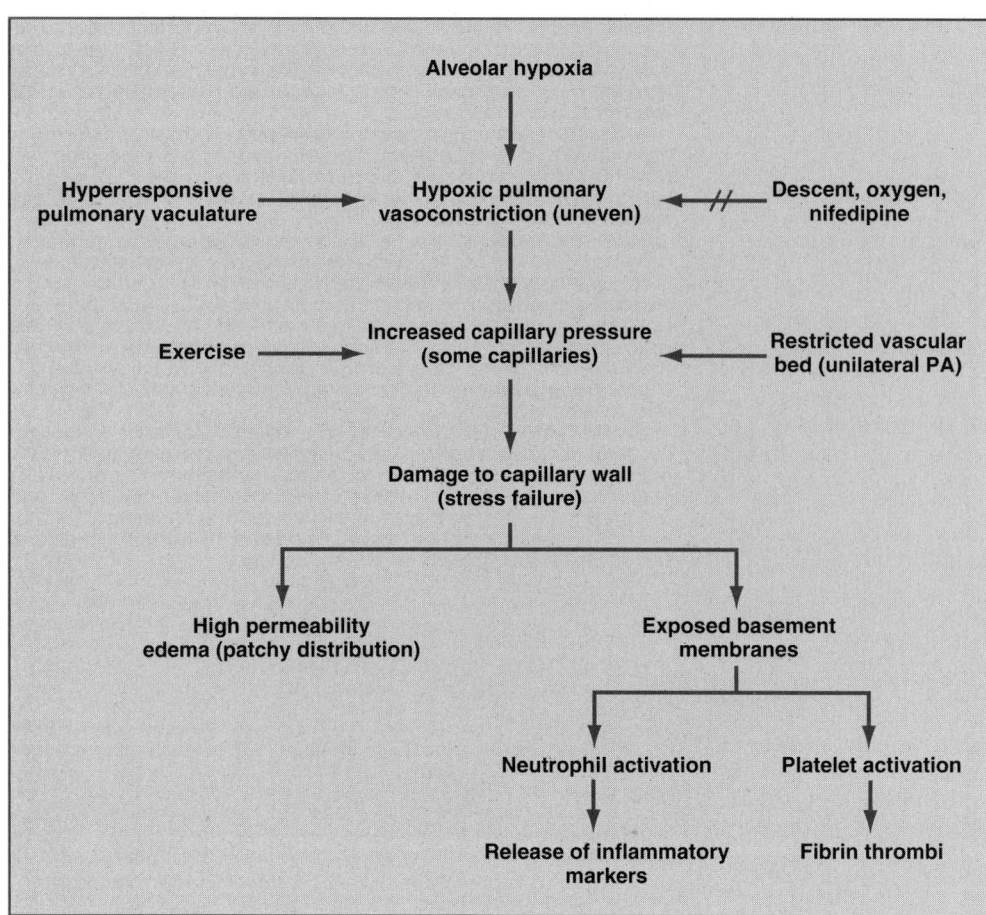

FIGURE 15–9. Diagram to show the sequence of events in the pathogenesis of HAPE. (From West, J. B., and Mathieu-Costello, O.: High-altitude pulmonary edema is caused by stress failure of pulmonary capillaries. Int. J. Sports Med. *13*:S54–S57, 1992.)

plasma,[193] and that pulmonary capillary wedge pressures, when measured, are normal,[194] argues for an alveolar-capillary membrane leak as the initiating cause. In animal experiments, histamine has been shown to be released in the lung after both heroin and morphine administration[195] and might play a role in this syndrome by increasing vascular permeability.

PULMONARY EMBOLISM (Chap. 46). Acute pulmonary edema in association with either a massive embolus or multiple smaller emboli has been well described and most often attributed to concomitant left ventricular dysfunction due to a combination of hypoxemia and encroachment of the interventricular septum on the left ventricular cavity. Although this sequence is quite likely to be applicable in the case of massive embolism, the mechanism of pulmonary edema in the case of microemboli has not been established. There are data to suggest, in the latter instance, that an increase in permeability of the alveolar-capillary membrane occurs.[162]

ECLAMPSIA (see p. 1852). Acute pulmonary edema frequently complicates eclampsia.[196] Multiple factors such as cerebral dysfunction with massive sympathetic discharge, left ventricular dysfunction secondary to acute systemic hypertension, hypervolemia, hypoalbuminemia (secondary to renal losses), and disseminated intravascular coagulation probably play a role in the pathogenesis.

POST-CARDIOVERSION. Although pulmonary edema has been documented to occur after cardioversion,[197] the mechanism is poorly understood. Ineffective left atrial function immediately following cardioversion has been suggested as a contributing factor, yet left ventricular dysfunction and neurogenic mechanisms are also possible.

POST-ANESTHESIA. In previously healthy subjects, pulmonary edema has been found in the early post-anesthesia period without a clear relationship to fluid overload or any subsequent evidence of left ventricular disease. The basis for this disorder is unknown, but it is tempting to invoke some role for temporary lymphatic dysfunction under anesthesia.

POST-CARDIOPULMONARY BYPASS. Although all patients who undergo cardiopulmonary bypass obviously have significant heart disease, the development of edema has been associated with normal left atrial pressures.[198,199] Alterations of surfactant due to prolonged collapse of the lung during the procedure, with subsequent need to apply high negative intrapleural pressures for reexpansion, and release of toxic substances have been suggested as mechanisms. Some data suggest that anaphylactic reactions to fresh frozen plasma may account for some episodes.[198] THe matter is far from settled, but the syndrome is fortunately rare.

Differential Diagnosis of Pulmonary Edema

The differentiation between the two principal forms of pulmonary edema, i.e., cardiogenic (hemodynamic) and noncardiogenic (caused by alterations in the pulmonary

TABLE 15–9 INITIAL DIFFERENTIATION OF CARDIOGENIC FROM NONCARDIOGENIC PULMONARY EDEMA

CARDIAC PULMONARY EDEMA	NONCARDIAC PULMONARY EDEMA
History	
Acute cardiac event	Acute cardiac event is uncommon in immediate history (but possible!)
	Underlying disease? (Table 15–1)
Clinical Examination	
Low-flow state = cool periphery	Usually high flow state = warm periphery
S₃ gallop/cardiomegaly	Bounding pulses
Jugular venous distention	No gallop
Crackles (wet)	No jugular venous distention
	Crackles (dry)
	Evidence of underlying disease (e.g., peritonitis)
Laboratory Tests	
ECG, ischemia/infarct?	ECG, usually normal
CXR, perihilar distribution	CXR, peripheral distribution
Cardiac enzymes may be ↑	Cardiac enzymes usually normal
PCWP >18 mm Hg	PCWP <18 mm Hg
Intrapulmonary shunting: small	Intrapulmonary shunting: large
Edema fluid/serum protein <0.5	Edema fluid/serum protein >0.7

From Sibbald, W. J., Cunningham, D. R., and Chin, D. N.: Noncardiac or cardiac pulmonary edema? A practical approach to clinical differentiation in critically ill patients. Chest *84*:460, 1983.

capillary membrane), usually can be made through assessment of the clinical context in which it occurs and through examination and consideration of the clinical data as shown in Table 15–9. Although this approach suggests an either/or situation, this may not be the case in reality. For example, sudden and large increases in intravascular pressure may disrupt the capillary and alveolar membranes leading to interstitial edema and alveolar loading with macromolecules that produce an edema liquid more compatible with noncardiogenic causes. Thus, a primary hemodynamic event can cause an alveolar-capillary membrane leak. Furthermore, high, normal, or only mild elevations in capillary hydrostatic pressures in the presence of alveolar capillary damage can cause an increase in the rate and extent of edema formation. Hence hemodynamic factors can and do play a role in increasing and perpetuating increased permeability.

REFERENCES

1. Report of the Task Force on Research in Heart Failure. National Heart, Lung and Blood Institute, 1994.
2. Packer, M.: Survival in patients with chronic heart failure and its potential modification by drug therapy. In Cohn, J. N. (ed.): Drug Treatment of Heart Failure, 2nd ed. Secaucus, N. J., ATC International, 1988, p. 273.
3. Kannel, W. B.: Epidemiologic aspects of heart failure. In Weber, K. T. (ed.): Heart Failure: Current Concepts and Management. Cardiology Clinics Series 7/1. Philadelphia, W. B. Saunders Co, 1989.
4. Braunwald, E., Mock, M. B., and Watson, J. (eds.): Congestive Heart Failure. Current Research and Clinical Applications. Orlando, Grune and Stratton, 1982.
5. McKee, P. A., Castell, W. P., McNamara, P. M., and Kannel, W. B.: The natural history of congestive heart failure, the Framingham Study. N. Engl. J. Med. 285:1441, 1971.
6. Marantz, P. R., Tobin, J. N., Wassertheil-Smoller, S., et al.: The relationship between left ventricular systolic function and congestive heart failure diagnosed by clinical criteria. Circulation 77:607, 1988.

FORMS AND CAUSES OF HEART FAILURE

7. Hope, J. A.: Treatise on the Diseases of the Heart and Great Vessels. London, Williams-Kidd, 1832.
8. Williams, J. F., Jr., Sonnenblick, E. H., and Braunwald, E.: Determinants of atrial contractile force in intact heart. Am. J. Physiol. 209:1061, 1965.
9. Ross, J., Jr., and Braunwald, E.: Studies on Starling's law of the heart. IX. The effects of impeding venous return on performance of the normal and failing human left ventricle. Circulation 30:719, 1964.
10. Stampfer, M., Epstein, S. E., Beiser, G. D., and Braunwald, E.: Hemodynamic effects of diuresis at rest and during intense upright exercise in patients with impaired cardiac function. Circulation 37:900, 1968.
11. Mackenzie, J.: Disease of the Heart, 3rd ed. London, Oxford University Press, 1913.
12. Moe, G. W., Legault, L., and Skorecki, K. L.: Control of extracellular fluid volume and pathophysiology of edema formation. In Brenner, B. M., and Rector, F. C., Jr. (eds.): The Kidney. 4th ed. Philadelphia, W. B. Saunders Company, 1991, pp. 623–676.
13. Braunwald, E.: The Pathogenesis of heart failure: Then and now. Medicine 70:68, 1991.
14. Stevenson, L. W., and Perloff, J. K.: The limited reliability of physical signs for estimating hemodynamics in chronic heart failure. JAMA 261:884, 1989.
15. Iriarte, M., Murga, N., Sagastagoitia, D., et al.: Congestive heart failure from left ventricular diastolic dysfunction in systemic hypertension. Am. J. Cardiol. 71:308, 1993.
16. Gaasch, W. H.: Diagnosis and treatment of heart failure based on left ventricular systolic or diastolic dysfunction. JAMA 271:1278, 1994.
17. Ghali, J. K., Kadakia, S., Cooper, R., and Ferlinz, J.: Precipitating factors leading to decompensation of heart failure: Traits among urban blacks. Arch. Intern. Med. 148:2013, 1988.
18. Braunwald, E., and Frahm, C. J.: Studies on Starling's law of the heart: IV. Observations on the hemodynamic functions of the left atrium in man. Circulation 24:633, 1961.

SYMPTOMS AND PROGNOSIS IN HEART FAILURE

19. Manning, H. L., and Schwartzstein, R. M.: Mechanisms of Disease: Pathophysiology of Dyspnea. N. Engl. J. Med. 333:1547, 1995.
20. Geltman, E. M.: Mild heart failure: Diagnosis and treatment. Am. Heart J. 118:1277, 1989.
21. Collins, J. V., Clark, T. J. H., and Brown, D. J.: Airway function in healthy subjects and in patients with left heart disease. Clin. Sci. Molec. Med. 49:217, 1975.
22. Macklem, P. T.: Respiratory muscles: The vital pump. Chest 78:753, 1980.
23. Fishman, A. P., and Ledlie, J. F.: Dyspnea. Bull. Eur. Physiopathol. Resp. 15:789, 1979.
24. Poole-Wilson, P. A., and Buller, N. P.: Causes of symptoms in chronic congestive heart failure and implications for treatment. Am. J. Cardiol. 62:31A, 1988.
25. Petermann, W., Barth, J., and Entzian, P.: Heart failure and airway obstruction. Int. J. Cardiol. 17:207, 1987.
26. Weber, K., Kinasewitz G., Janicki, J., and Fishman, A.: Oxygen utilization and ventilation during exercise in patients with chronic cardiac failure. Circulation 65:1213, 1982.
27. Colucci, W. S., Ribeiro, J. P., Rocco, M. B., et al.: Impaired chronotropic response to exercise in patients with congestive heart failure: Role of postsynaptic beta-adrenergic desensitization. Circulation 80:314, 1989.
28. Kubo, S. H., Rector, T., Bank, A., and Heifetz, S.: Endothelium-dependent vasodilation is attenuated in patients with heart failure. Circulation 84:1589, 1991.
29. Nakamura, M., Ishikawa, M., Funakoshi, T., et al.: Attenuated endothelium-dependent peripheral vasodilation and clinical characteristics in patients with chronic heart failure. Am. Heart J. 128:1164, 1994.
30. Kraemer, M. D., Kubo, S. H., Rector, T. S., et al.: Pulmonary and peripheral vascular factors are important determinants of peak exercise oxygen uptake in patients with heart failure. J. Am. Coll. Cardiol. 21:641, 1993.
31. Mancini, D. M., Walter, G., Reichek, N., et al.: Contribution of skeletal muscle atrophy to exercise intolerance and altered muscle metabolism in heart failure. Circulation 85:1364, 1992.
32. Mancini, D. M., Wilson, J. R., Bolinger, L., et al.: In vivo magnetic resonance spectroscopy measurement of deoxymyoglobin during exercise in patients with heart failure: Demonstration of abnormal muscle metabolism despite adequate oxygenation. Circulation 90:500, 1994.
33. Mancini, D. M., Henson, D., LaManca, J., and Levine, S.: Evidence of reduced respiratory muscle endurance in patients with heart failure. J. Am. Coll. Cardiol. 24:972, 1994.
34. Sullivan, M., Higginbotham, M., and Cobb, F.: Exercise training in patients with severe left ventricular dysfunction: Hemodynamic and metabolic benefits. Circulation 78:506, 1988.
35. Coats, A. J., Adamopoulos, S., Raddaelli, A., et al.: Controlled trial of physical training in chronic heart failure. Exercise performance, hemodynamics, ventilation, and autonomic function. Circulation 85:2119, 1992.
36. Weber, K. T., and Janicki, J. S.: Cardiopulmonary Exercise Testing. Philadelphia, W. B. Saunders Company, 1986.
37. Smith, R. F., Johnson, G., Ziesche, S., et al: Functional capacity in heart failure: Comparison of methods for assessment and their relation to other indexes of heart failure. The V-HeFT VA Cooperative Studies Group. Circulation 87:VI88, 1993.
38. Wasserman, D.: Dyspnea on exertion: Is it the heart or the lungs? JAMA 248:2042, 1982.
39. Oka, R. K., Stotts, N. A., Dae, M. W., et al.: Daily physical activity levels in congestive heart failure. Am. J. Cardiol. 71:921, 1993.
40. Cross, A. M., Jr., and Higginbotham, M. B.: Oxygen deficit during exercise testing in heart failure. Relation to submaximal exercise tolerance. Chest 107:904, 1995.
41. Francis, G. S., and Rector, T. S.: Maximal exercise tolerance as a therapeutic end point in heart failure—Are we relying on the right measure? (Editorial) Am. J. Cardiol. 73:304, 1994.
42. Lipkin, D. P., Bayliss, J., and Poole-Wilson, P. A.: The ability of a submaximal exercise test to predict maximal exercise capacity in patients with heart failure. Eur. Heart J. 6:829, 1985.
43. Guyatt, G. H., Sullivan, J. J., Thompson, P. J., et al.: The 6-minute walk: A new measure of exercise capacity in patients with chronic heart failure. Can. Med. Assoc. J. 132:919, 1985.
44. Lipkin, P., Scriven, A. J., Crake, T., and Poole-Wilson, P. A.: Six-minute walking test for assessing exercise capacity in chronic heart failure. Br. Med. J. 292:653, 1986.
45. Sparrow, J., Parameshwar, J., and Poole-Wilson, P. A.: Assessment of functional capacity in chronic heart failure: Time-limited exercise on a self-powered treadmill. Br. Heart J. 71:391, 1994.
46. Higgins, C. B., Vatner, S. F., Franklin, D., and Braunwald, E.: Effects of experimentally produced heart failure on the peripheral vascular response to severe exercise in conscious dogs. Circ. Res. 31:186, 1972.
47. Criteria Committee, New York Heart Association, Inc.: Diseases of the Heart and Blood Vessels. Nomenclature and Criteria for Diagnosis. 6th ed. Boston, Little, Brown and Co., 1964, p. 114.
48. Goldman, L., Hasimoto, B., Cook, E. F., and Loscalzo, A.: Comparative reproducibility and validity of symptoms for assessing cardiovascular functional class. Advantages of a new specific activity scale. Circulation 64:1227, 1981.
49. Rector, T. S., Kubo, S. H., and Cohn, J. N.: Patients' self-assessment of their congestive heart failure: Content, reliability and validity of a new measure. The Minnesota Living with Heart Failure questionnaire. In Heart Failure, Vol. 3. 1987, p 198.
50. Rector, T. S., and Cohn, J. N.: Assessment of patient outcome with the Minnesota Living with Heart Failure questionnaire: Reliability and validity during a randomized, double-blind, placebo-controlled trial of pimobendan. Am. Heart J. 124:1017, 1992.
51. Rector, T. S., Kubo, S. H., and Cohn, J. N.: Validity of the Minnesota Living with Heart Failure questionnaire as a measure of therapeutic response to enalapril or placebo. Am. J. Cardiol. 71:1106, 1993.
52. Earnest, D. L., and Hurst, J. W.: Exophthalmos, stare and increase in

intraocular pressure and systolic propulsion of the eyeballs due to congestive heart failure. Am. J. Cardiol. 26:351, 1970.

53. Chakko, S., Woska, D., Martinez, H., et al.: Clinical, radiographic, and hemodynamic correlations in chronic congestive heart failure: Conflicting results may lead to inappropriate care. Am. J. Med. 90:353, 1991.

54. Butman, S. M., Ewy, G. A., Standen, J. R., et al.: Bedside cardiovascular examination in patients with severe chronic heart failure: Importance of rest or inducible jugular venous distension. J. Am. Coll. Cardiol. 22:968, 1993.

55. Strober, W., Cohen, L. S., Waldmann, T. A., and Braunwald, E.: Tricuspid regurgitation: A newly recognized cause of protein-losing enteropathy, lymphocytopenia and immunologic deficiency. Am. J. Med. 44:842, 1968.

56. Gleason, W. L., and Braunwald, E.: Studies on Starling's law of the heart: VI. Relationships between left ventricular end-diastolic volume and stroke volume in man with observations on the mechanism of pulsus alternans. Circulation 25:841, 1962.

57. Berkowitz, D., Croll, M. N., and Likoff, W.: Malabsorption as a complication of congestive heart failure. Am. J. Cardiol. 11:43, 1963.

58. Levine, B., Kalman, J., Mayer, L., et al.: Elevated circulating levels of tumor necrosis factor in severe chronic heart failure. N. Engl. J. Med. 323:236, 1990.

59. Carr, J. G., Stevenson, L. W., Walden, J. A., and Heber, D.: Prevalence and hemodynamic correlates of malnutrition in severe congestive heart failure secondary to ischemic or idiopathic dilated cardiomyopathy. Am. J. Cardiol. 63:709, 1989.

60. Pittman, J., and Cohen, P.: The pathogenesis of cardiac cachexia. N. Engl. J. Med. 27:403, 1964.

61. Finkel, M. S., Oddis, C. V., Jacob, T. D., et al.: Negative inotropic effects of cytokines on the heart mediated by nitric oxide. Science 257:387, 1992.

62. Yokoyama, T., Vaca, L., Rossen, R. D., et al.: Cellular basis for the negative inotropic effects of tumor necrosis factor-alpha in the adult mammalian heart. J. Clin. Invest. 92:2303, 1993.

63. Mann, D. L., and Young, J. B.: Basic mechanisms in congestive heart failure: Recognizing the role of proinflammatory cytokines. Chest 105:897, 1994.

64. Thaik, C. M., Calderone, A., Takahashi, N., and Colucci, W. S.: Interleukin-1 beta modulates the growth and phenotype of rat cardiac myocytes. J. Clin. Invest. 96:1093, 1995.

65. Lange, R. L., and Hecht, H. H.: The mechanism of Cheyne-Stokes respiration. J. Clin. Invest. 41:42, 1962.

66. Hanly, P., Zuberi, N., and Gray, R.: Pathogenesis of Cheyne-Stokes respiration in patients with congestive heart failure. Relationship to arterial Pco$_2$. Chest 104:1079, 1993.

67. Hanly, P., and Zuberi-Khokhar, N.: Daytime sleepiness in patients with congestive heart failure and Cheyne-Stokes respiration. Chest 107:952, 1995.

68. Rees, P. J., and Clark, T. J. H.: Paroxysmal nocturnal dyspnoea and periodic respiration. Lancet 2:1315, 1979.

69. Ben-Dov, I., Sietsema, K. E., Casaburi, R., and Wasserman, K.: Evidence that circulatory oscillations accompany ventilatory oscillations during exercise in patients with heart failure. Am. Rev. Respir. Dis. 145:776, 1992.

70. Friedman-Mor, Z., Chalon, J., Turndorf, H., and Orkin, L. R.: Cardiac index and incidence of heart failure cells. Arch. Pathol. Lab. Med. 102:418, 1978.

71. Wolke, A. M., Brooks, K. M., and Schaffner, F.: The liver in congestive heart failure. Primary Cardiol. 8:130, 1982.

72. Blasco, V. V.: Features of hepatic involvement in congestive heart failure. Cardiovasc. Rev. Rep. 4:963, 1983.

73. Lemmer, J. H., Coran, A. G., Behrendt, D. M., et al.: Liver fibrosis (cardiac cirrhosis) five years after modified Fontan operation for tricuspid atresia. J. Thorac. Cardiovasc. Surg. 86:757, 1983.

74. Matsuda, H., Covino, E., Hirose, H., et al.: Acute liver dysfunction after modified Fontan operation for complex cardiac lesions. J. Thorac. Cardiovasc. Surg. 96:219, 1988.

75. Mace, S., Borkat, G., and Liebman, J.: Hepatic dysfunction and cardiovascular abnormalities: Occurrence in infants, children and young adults. Am. J. Dis. Child. 139:60, 1985.

76. Kanel, G. C., Ucci, A. A., Kaplan, M. M., and Wolfe, H. J.: A distinctive perivenular hepatic lesion associated with heart failure. Am. J. Clin. Pathol. 73:235, 1980.

77. Nouel, O., Henrion, J., Bernuau, J., et al.: Fulminant hepatic failure due to transient circulatory failure in patients with chronic heart disease. Dig. Dis. Sci. 25:49, 1980.

78. Jenkins, J. G., Lynn, A. M., Wood, A. E., et al.: Acute hepatic failure following cardiac operation in children. J. Thorac. Cardiovasc. Surg. 84:865, 1982.

79. Szatalowicz, V. L., Arnold, P. E., Chaimovitz, C., et al.: Radioimmunoassay of plasma arginine vasopressin in hyponatremic patients with congestive heart failure. N. Engl. J. Med. 305:263, 1981.

80. Chakko, S. C., Frutchey, J., and Gheorghiade, M.: Life-threatening hyperkalemia in severe heart failure. Am. Heart J. 117:1083, 1989.

81. Kaplan, M. M.: Liver dysfunction secondary to congestive heart failure. Practical Cardiol. 6:39, 1980.

82. Kubo, S. H., Walter, B. A., John, D. H. A., et al.: Liver function abnormalities in chronic heart failure: Influence of systemic hemodynamics. Arch. Intern. Med. 147:1227, 1987.

83. Gorlin, R., Knowles, J. H., and Storey, C. F.: The Valsalva maneuver as

a test of cardiac function. Pathologic physiology and clinical significance. Am. J. Med. 22:197, 1957.

84. Schmidt, D. E., and Shah, P. K.: Accurate detection of elevated left ventricular filling pressure by a simplified bedside application of the Valsalva maneuver. Am. J. Cardiol. 71:462, 1993.

85. Elisberg, E. I.: Heart rate response to the Valsalva maneuver as a test of circulatory integrity. JAMA 186:200, 1963.

86. McIntyre, K. M., Vita, J. A., Lambrew, C. T., et al.: A noninvasive method of predicting pulmonary-capillary wedge pressure. N. Engl. J. Med. 327:1715, 1992.

87. Baron, M. G.: Radiological and angiographic examination of the heart. In Braunwald, E. (ed.): Heart Disease. 3rd ed. Philadelphia, W. B. Saunders Company, 1988, p. 148.

88. Chakko, S., Woska, D., Martinez, H., et al.: Clinical, radiographic, and hemodynamic correlations in chronic congestive heart failure: Conflicting results may lead to inappropriate care. Am. J. Med. 90:353, 1991.

89. Evaluating the radiographic assessment of pulmonary venous hypertension in chronic heart disease. AJR 142:877, 1984.

90. Daves, M. L.: Cardiac Roentgenology. Chicago, Year Book Medical Publishers, 1981, pp. 78–86.

PROGNOSIS

91. Ho, K. K., Anderson, K. M., Kannel, W. B., et al.: Survival after the onset of congestive heart failure in Framingham Heart Study subjects. Circulation 88:107, 1993.

92. Cohn, J. N., and Rector, T. S.: Prognosis of congestive heart failure and predictors of mortality. Am. J. Cardiol. 62:25A, 1988.

93. Sziachic, J., et al.: Correlates and prognostic implications of exercise capacity in chronic congestive heart failure. Am. J. Cardiol. 55:1037, 1986.

94. Rahimtoola, S. H.: The pharmacologic treatment of chronic congestive heart failure. Circulation 80:693, 1989.

95. Murali, S., and Thompson, M. E.: Pathophysiology and drug therapy in congestive heart failure. Cardiology 7:41, 1990.

96. Gradman, A., Deedwania, P., Cody, R., et al.: Predictors of total mortality and sudden death in mild to moderate heart failure. J. Am. Coll. Cardiol. 14:564, 1989.

97. Lee, T. H., Hamilton, M. A., Stevenson, L. W., et al.: Impact of left ventricular cavity size on survival in advanced heart failure. Am. J. Cardiol. 72:672, 1993.

98. Di Salvo, T. G., Mathier, M., Semigran, M. J., and Dec, G. W.: Preserved right ventricular ejection fraction predicts exercise capacity and survival in advanced heart failure. J. Am. Coll. Cardiol. 25:1143, 1995.

99. Parameshwar, J., Keegan, J., Sparrow, J., et al.: Predictors of prognosis in severe heart failure. Am. Heart J. 123:421, 1992.

100. Cleland, J. G. F., and Dargie, H. J.: Arrhythmias, catecholamines and electrolyte. Am. J. Cardiol. 62:55A, 1988.

101. Cleland, J. G. F., Dargie, H. J., and Ford, I.: Mortality in heart failure: Clinical variables of prognostic value. Br. Heart J. 58:572, 1987.

102. Francis, G. S., Cohn, J. N., Johnson, G., et al.: Plasma norepinephrine, plasma renin activity, and congestive heart failure. Relations to survival and the effects of therapy in V-HeFT II. The V-HeFT VA Cooperative Studies Group. Circulation 87:VI40, 1993.

103. Packer, M., Gottlieb, S. S., and Blum, M. A.: Immediate and long-term pathophysiologic mechanisms underlying the genesis of sudden cardiac death in patients with congestive heart failure. Am. J. Med. 82(Suppl. 3a):4, 1987.

104. Packer, M., Lee, W. H., Kessler, P. D., et al.: Role of neurohormonal mechanisms in determining survival in patients with severe chronic heart failure. Circulation 75:(Suppl. 4)80, 1987.

105. Gottlieb, S. S., Kukin, M. L., Ahern, D., and Packer, M.: Prognostic importance of atrial natriuretic peptide in patients with chronic heart failure. J. Am. Coll. Cardiol. 13:1534, 1989.

106. Packer, M.: Potential role of potassium as a determinant of morbidity and mortality in patients with systemic hypertension and congestive heart failure. Am. J. Cardiol. 65:45E, 1990.

107. Hyperdynamic States. In Fowler, N. O.: Diagnosis of Heart Disease. New York, Springer-Verlag, 1991, pp. 389–399.

HIGH OUTPUT HEART FAILURE

108. Nicoladoni, C.: Phlebarteriectasie der rechten oberen Extermitat. Arch. Klin. Chir. 18:252, 1875.

109. Branham, H. H.: Aneurysmal varix of the femoral artery and vein following a gunshot wound. Int. J. Surg. 3:250, 1890.

110. Gupta, P. D., and Singh, M.: Neural mechanism underlying tachycardia induced by non-hypotensive A-V shunt. Am. J. Physiol. 236:H35, 1979.

111. Dorney, E. R.: Peripheral AV fistula of fifty-seven years' duration with refractory heart failure. Am. Heart J. 54:778, 1957.

112. Sanyal, S. K., Saldivar, V., Coburn, T. P., et al.: Hyperdynamic heart failure due to A-V fistula associated with Wilms' tumor. Pediatrics 57:564, 1976.

113. Ingram, C. W., Satler, L. F., and Rackley, C. E.: Progressive heart failure secondary to a high output state. Chest 92:1117, 1987.

114. Fee, H. J., Levisman, J., Doud, R. B., and Golding, A. L.: High output congestive failure from femoral arteriovenous shunts for vascular access. Ann. Surg. 183:321, 1976.

115. Anderson, C. B., Codd, J. R., Graff, R. A., et al.: Cardiac failure and upper extremity arteriovenous dialysis fistulas. Arch. Intern. Med. 136:292, 1976.

116. Szilagyi, D. E., Smith, R. F., Elliott, J. P., and Hageman, J. H.: Congenital arteriovenous anomalies of the limbs. Arch. Surg. *111*:423, 1976.

117. Becker, D. G., Fish, C. R., and Juergen, S. J. L.: Arteriovenous fistulas of the female pelvis. Obstet. Gynecol. *31*:799, 1968.

118. Price, A. C., Coran, A. G., and Mattern, A. L.: Hemangioendothelioma of the pelvis: A cause of cardiac failure in the newborn. N. Engl. J. Med. *286*:647, 1972.

119. Coel, M. N., and Alksne, J. F.: Embolization to diminish high output failure secondary to systemic angiomatosis (Ullman's syndrome). Vasc. Surg. *12*:336, 1978.

120. Vaksmann, G., Rey, C., Marache, P., et al.: Severe congestive heart failure in newborns due to giant cutaneous hemangiomas. Am. J. Cardiol. *60*:392, 1987.

121. Gong, B., Baken, L. A., Julian, T. M., and Kubo, S. H.: High-output heart failure due to hepatic arteriovenous fistula during pregnancy: A case report. Obstet. Gynecol. *72*:440, 1988.

122. Baranda, M. M., Perez, M., DeAndres, J., et al.: High-output congestive heart failure as first manifestation of Osler-Weber-Rendu disease. J. Vasc. Dis. *35*:568, 1984.

123. Zavota, L., Bini, F., Carano, N., et al.: Hepatic hemangiomatosis with congestive cardiac failure and development into a cholestatic hepatopathy. Pediatr. Med. Chir. *6*:621, 1984.

124. Lewis, B. S., Ehrenfelk, E. N., Lewis, N., and Gotsman, M. S.: Echocardiographic left ventricular function in thyrotoxicosis. Am. Heart J. *97*:460, 1979.

125. Hoffman, I., and Lowrey, R. D.: The electrocardiogram in thyrotoxicosis. Am. J. Cardiol. *8*:893, 1960.

126. Braunwald, E., Mason, D. T., and Ross, J., Jr.: Studies of the cardiocirculatory actions of digitalis. Medicine *44*:233, 1965.

127. Shapiro, S., Steiner, M., and Dimich, I.: Congestive heart failure in neonatal thyrotoxicosis. A curable cause of heart failure in the newborn. Clin. Pediatr. *14*:1155, 1975.

128. Weiss, S., and Wilkinson, R. W.: The nature of the cardiovascular disturbances in nutritional deficiency states (beriberi). Ann. Intern. Med. *11*:104, 1937.

129. Burwell, C. S., and Dexter, L.: Beriberi heart disease. Trans. Assoc. Am. Physicians *60*:59, 1947.

130. Akbarian, M., Yankopoulos, N. A., and Abelmann, W. H.: Hemodynamic studies in beriberi heart disease. Am. J. Med. *41*:197, 1966.

131. Ayzenberg, O., Silber, M. H., and Bortz, D.: Beriberi heart disease. A case report describing the hemodynamic features. S. Afr. Med. J. *68*:263, 1985.

132. Akram, H., Maslowski, A. H., Smith, B. L., and Nichols, M. G.: The haemodynamic, histopathological and hormonal features of alcoholic beriberi. Q. J. Med. *50*:359, 1981.

133. Naidoo, D. P.: Beriberi heart disease in Durban. S. Afr. Med. J. *72*:241, 1987.

134. Naidoo, D. P., Rawat, R., Dyer, R. B., et al.: Cardiac beriberi: A report of four cases. S. Afr. Med. J. *72*:283, 1987.

135. Carson, P.: Alcoholic cardiac beriberi. Br. Med. J. *284*:1817, 1982.

136. Cardiovascular beriberi (editorial). Lancet *1*:1287, 1982.

137. Akbarian, M., and Dreyfus, P. M.: Blood trans-ketolase activity in beriberi heart disease. JAMA *203*:23, 1968.

138. Baker, H., quoted in Sauberlich, H. E.: Biochemical alterations in thiamine deficiency—their interpretation. Am. J. Clin. Nutr. *20*:543, 1967.

139. Brin, M.: Erythrocyte transketolase in early thiamine deficiency. Ann. N. Y. Acad. Sci. *98*:528, 1962.

140. Baker, H., and Frank, O.: Clinical Vitaminology: Methods and Interpretation. New York, Wiley Interscience, 1968.

141. Jeffrey, F. E., and Abelmann, W. H.: Recovery of proved Shoshin beriberi. Am. J. Med. *50*:123, 1971.

142. Whittemore, R., and Caddell, J. L.: Metabolic and nutritional diseases. *In* Moss, A. J., et al. (eds.): Heart Disease in Infants, Children and Adolescents. 2nd ed. Baltimore, Williams and Wilkins Co., 1977, pp. 590 and 591.

143. Heistad, D. D., Abboud, F. M., Schmid, P. G., et al.: Regulation of blood flow in Paget's disease of the bone. J. Clin. Invest. *55*:69, 1975.

144. Rutishauser, E., Veyrat, R., and Rouiller, C.: La vascularization de l'os pagé tique, étude anatomo-pathologique. Presse Méd. *62*:654, 1954.

145. Lequime, J., and Denolin, H.: Circulatory dynamics in osteitis deformans. Circulation *12*:215, 1955.

146. McBride, W., Jackman, J. D., Jr., Gammon, R. S., and Willerson, J. T.: High-output cardiac failure in patients with multiple myeloma. N. Engl. J. Med. *319*:1651, 1988.

PULMONARY EDEMA

147. Harris, P., and Heath, D.: Pulmonary edema. *In* The Human Pulmonary Circulation. 3rd ed. New York, Churchill Livingstone, 1986, pp. 373–383.

148. Guyton, A. C., Parker, J. C., Taylor, A. E., et al.: Forces governing water movement in the lung. *In* Fishman, A. P., and Renkin, E. M. (eds.): Pulmonary Edema. Bethesda, American Physiological Society, 1979, p. 70.

149. Guyton, A. C.: Textbook of Medical Physiology. 7th ed. Philadelphia, W. B. Saunders Company, 1986, p. 372.

150. Staub, N. C.: Pulmonary edema due to increased microvascular permeability to fluid and protein. Circ. Res. *43*:143, 1978.

151. Agostoni, E.: Mechanics of the pleural space. Physiol. Rev. *52*:57, 1972.

152. Dollery, C. T., Heimberg, P., and Hugh-Jones, P.: Relationships between blood flow and clearance rate of radioactive carbon dioxide and oxygen in normal and oedematous lungs. J. Physiol. (London) *162*:93, 1962.

153. Bernard, G. R., and Brigham, K. L.: Pulmonary edema. Pathophysiologic mechanisms and new approaches to therapy. Chest *89*:594, 1986.

154. Snapper, J. R., and Brigham, K. L.: Pulmonary edema. Hosp. Pract. *21*:87, 1986.

155. Sprung, C. L., Rackow, E. C., Fein, I. A., et al.: The spectrum of pulmonary edema: Differentiation of cardiogenic, intermediate, and noncardiogenic forms of pulmonary edema. Ann. Rev. Respir. Dis. *124*:718, 1981.

156. West, J. B., and Mathieu-Costello, O.: Pulmonary edema and hemorrhage: Recent advances. *In* Potchen, E. J., Grainger, R. G., and Greene, R. (eds.): *Pulmonary Radiology.* Philadelphia, W. B. Saunders Company, 1993, p. 125.

157. Minnear, F. L., Barie, P. S., and Malik, A. B.: Effects of large, transient increases in pulmonary vascular pressures on lung fluid balance. J. Appl. Physiol. *55*:983, 1983.

158. Cross, C. E., Shaver, J. A., Wilson, R. J., and Robin, E. D.: Mitral stenosis and pulmonary fibrosis: Special reference to pulmonary edema and lung lymphatic function. Arch. Intern. Med. *125*:248, 1970.

159. Kramer, G. C., Harms, B. A., Gunther, R. A., et al.: The effects of hypoproteinemia on blood-to-lymph fluid transport in sheep lung. Circ. Res. *49*:1173, 1981.

160. Mahfood, S., Hix, W. R., Aaron, B. L., et al.: Reexpansion pulmonary edema. Ann. Thorac. Surg. *45*:340, 1988.

161. Malik, A. B., and Staub, N. C. (eds.): Mechanisms of Lung Microvascular Injury. New York, New York Academy of Sciences, 1982.

162. Staub, N. C.: Pulmonary edema due to increased microvascular permeability. Ann. Rev. Med. *32*:291, 1981.

163. Carlson, R. W., Schaeffer, R. C., Jr., Puri, V. K., et al.: Hypovolemia and permeability pulmonary edema associated with anaphylaxis. Crit. Care Med. *9*:883, 1981.

164. Snell, J. D., Jr., and Ramsey, L. H.: Pulmonary edema as a result of endotoxemia. Am. J. Physiol. *217*:170, 1969.

165. Ratliff, N. B., Wilson, J. W., Horckel, D. B., and Martin, A. M., Jr.: The lung in hemorrhagic shock. II. Observations on alveolar and vascular ultrastructure. Am. J. Pathol. *58*:353, 1970.

166. Henning, R. J., Heyman, V., Alcover, I., and Romeo, S.: Cardiopulmonary effects of oleic acid-induced pulmonary edema and mechanical ventilation. Anesth. Analg. *65*:925, 1986.

167. Glauser, F. L., Fairman, R. P., Miller, J. E., and Falls, R. K.: Indomethacin blunts ethchloryne induced pulmonary hypertension but not pulmonary edema. J. Appl. Physiol. *53*:563, 1982.

168. Havill, A. M., Gee, M. H., Washburne, J. D., et al.: Alpha naphthyl thiourea produces dose dependent lung vascular injury in sheep. Am. J. Physiol. *243*:505, 1982.

169. Weinberg, P. F., Mathey, M. A., Webster, R. O., et al.: Biologically active products of complement in acute lung injury in patients with sepsis syndrome. Am. Rev. Resp. Dis. *130*:791, 1984.

170. Rinaldo, J. E., Dauber, G. H., Christman, J., and Rogers, R. M.: Neutrophil alveolitis endotoxemia. Am. Rev. Respir. Dis. *130*:1065, 1984.

171. Biermann, G. J., Dockey, B. F., and Thrall, R. S.: Polymorphonuclear leukocyte participation in acute oleic acid induced lung injury. Am. Rev. Respir. Dis. *128*:845, 1983.

172. Kline, J. N., and Hirasuna, J. D.: Pulmonary edema after freebase cocaine smoking—not due to an adulterant. Chest *97*:1009, 1990.

173. Kapanci, Y., Weibel, E. R., Kaplan, H. P., and Robinson, P. V. M.: Pathogenesis and reversibility of the pulmonary lesions of oxygen toxicity in monkey. II. Ultrastructural and morphometric studies. Lab. Invest. *20*:101, 1969.

174. Cameron, G. R., and Courtice, F. C.: The production and removal of oedema fluid in the lungs after exposure to carbonyl chloride (phosgene). J. Physiol. (London) *105*:175, 1946.

175. Bils, R. F.: Ultrastructural alterations of alveolar tissue of mice. III. Ozone. Arch. Environ. Health *20*:468, 1970.

176. Sherwin, R. P., and Richters, V.: Lung capillary permeability: nitrogen dioxide exposure and leakage of tritiated serum. Arch. Intern. Med. *128*:61, 1971.

177. Murray, J. F.: The lungs and heart failure. Hosp. Prac. *20*:55, 1985.

178. Fillmore, S. J., Giumaraes, A. C., Scheidt, S. S., and Killip, T.: Blood gas changes and pulmonary hemodynamics following acute myocardial infarction. Circulation *45*:583, 1972.

179. Szidon, J. P., Pietra, G. G., and Fishman, A. P.: The alveolar-capillary membrane and pulmonary edema. N. Engl. J. Med. *286*:1200, 1972.

180. Said, S. I., Avery, M. E., Davis, R. K., et al.: Pulmonary surface activity in induced pulmonary edema. J. Clin. Invest. *44*:458, 1965.

181. Miller, W. W., Waldhausen, J. A., and Rashkind, W. J.: Comparison of oxygen poisoning of the lung in cyanotic and acyanotic dogs. N. Engl. J. Med. *282*:943, 1970.

182. Henry, J. H.: The effect of shock on pulmonary alveolar surfactant: Its role in refractory respiratory insufficiency of the critically ill or severely injured patient. J. Trauma *8*:756, 1968.

183. Elias, R. M., and Johnston, M. G.: Modulation of lymphatic pumping by lymph borne factors after endotoxin administration in sheep. J. Appl. Physiol. *68*:199, 1990.

184. Schoene, R. B., Hackett, P. H., Henderson, W. R., et al.: High-altitude pulmonary edema. Characteristics of lung lavage fluid. JAMA *256*:63, 1986.

185. Naeije, R., Melot, C., and Lejeune, P.: Hypoxic pulmonary vasoconstriction and high altitude pulmonary edema. Am. Rev. Respir. Dis. *134*:332, 1986.

186. Sophocles, A. M., Jr.: High-altitude pulmonary edema in Vail, Colorado, 1975–1982. West. J. Med. *144*:569, 1986.

187. Lockhart, A., and Saiag, B.: Altitude and the human pulmonary circulation. Clin. Sci. *60*:599, 1981.

188. West, J. B., and Mathieu-Costello, O.: High altitude pulmonary edema is caused by stress failure of pulmonary capillaries. Int. J. Sports Med. *13*:S54, 1992.

189. Yabumoto, M., Kuriyama, T., Iwamoto, M., and Kinoshita, T.: Neurogenic pulmonary edema associated with ruptured intracranial aneurysm: Case report. Neurosurgery *19*:300, 1986.

190. Steinberg, A. D., and Karliner, J. S.: The clinical spectrum of heroin pulmonary edema. Arch. Intern. Med. *122*:122, 1968.

191. Fraser, D. W.: Methadone overdose: Illicit use of pharmaceutically prepared narcotics. JAMA *217*:1387, 1971.

192. Bogartz, L. J., and Miller, W. C.: Pulmonary edema associated with propoxyphene intoxication. JAMA *215*:259, 1971.

193. Katz, S., Aberman, A., Frand, U. I., et al.: Heroin pulmonary edema: Evidence for increased pulmonary capillary permeability. Am. Rev. Respir. Dis. *106*:472, 1972.

194. Gopinathan, K., Saroja, D., Spears, J. R., et al.: Hemodynamic studies in heroin induced acute pulmonary edema. Circulation *42*(Suppl. 3):44, 1970.

195. Brashear, R. E., Kelly, M. T., and White, A. C.: Elevated plasma histamine after heroin and morphine. J. Lab. Clin. Med. *83*:451, 1974.

196. Rovinsky, J. J., and Guttmacher, A. F.: Medical, Surgical, and Gynecologic Complications of Pregnancy. 2nd ed. Baltimore, Williams and Wilkins Co., 1965.

197. Goldbaum, T. S., Bacos, J. M., and Lindsay, J., Jr.: Pulmonary edema following conversion of tachyarrhythmia. Chest *89*:465, 1986.

198. Hashim, S. E., Kay, H. R., Hammond, G. L., et al.: Noncardiac pulmonary edema after cardiopulmonary bypass. Am. J. Surg. *147*:560, 1984.

199. Culliford, A. T., Thomas, S., and Spencer, F. C.: Fulminating noncardiogenic pulmonary edema: A newly recognized hazard during cardiac operations. J. Thorac. Cardiovasc. Surg. *80*:868, 1980.

ACKNOWLEDGEMENT

Dr. Roland H. Ingram and one of the authors of this chapter (E.B.) co-authored a chapter entitled "Pulmonary Edema: Cardiogenic and Non-cardiogenic" in the first four editions of this textbook. Portions of that chapter were updated, revised, and added to the present chapter. Dr. Ingram's important contributions to the present chapter are gratefully acknowledged.

Chapter 16
Drugs Used in the Treatment of Heart Failure

RALPH A. KELLY, THOMAS W. SMITH

VASODILATORS

The rationale for the use of vasodilators grew out of experience with parenteral sympatholytic agents and nitroprusside in patients with severe heart failure.[1] Studies of vasodilators demonstrated that they were well tolerated and effective in improving symptoms. The effectiveness of the isosorbide dinitrate–hydralazine combination[2] and of angiotensin-converting enzyme (ACE) inhibitors in reducing mortality in heart failure was demonstrated in several prospective randomized controlled trials in the 1980's (see Chap. 17, p. 495).[3] Table 16–1 lists those vasodilators commonly employed or under active investigation for the treatment of heart failure.

Vasodilators, as a class, reverse several of the characteristic physiological adaptations that accompany the development of heart failure (Fig. 16–1). These neurohumoral and physiological responses resemble, in some respects, those that accompany a fall in blood pressure due to hypovolemia. These include tachycardia and venous and arterial vasoconstriction, with shunting of blood toward the thorax and brain and away from the splanchnic, renal, and other peripheral vascular beds.[4] Although these responses provide a clear evolutionary advantage for survival with dehydration or following blood loss, they are maladaptive and deleterious in chronic heart failure.

Renin-Angiotensin System Antagonists

RENIN-ANGIOTENSIN SYSTEMS. The importance of the renin-angiotensin system (RAS) in the pathophysiology of heart failure (see p. 413) has been underscored by the effectiveness of antagonists of this system in improving symptoms and in reducing mortality in this syndrome. Classically, this system has been viewed as a renin-angiotensin-aldosterone axis, the activity of which is determined by the rate of renin released into the systemic circulation from the juxtaglomerular apparatus in the glomerular afferent arterioles.[5] With the advent of highly specific and sensitive technologies for the detection and cellular localization of components of the renin-angiotensin system, such as autoradiography with radiolabeled ACE inhibitors, sensitive radioimmunoassay, in situ hybridization, quantitative polymerase chain reaction, and transgenic animal technology, it is now recognized that many "local" or "tissue" RAS exist throughout the vasculature and in parenchymal cells of most, if not all, organs.[5-9] Within the cellular components of blood vessels, for example, de novo synthesis and secretion of angiotensin II (Ang II) from aortic endothelial cells in vitro was described a decade ago by Kifor

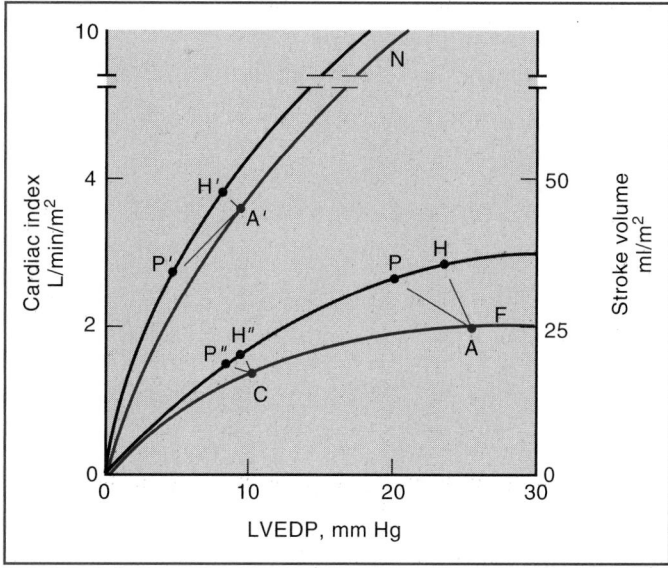

FIGURE 16–1. Effects of various vasodilators on the relationship between left ventricular end-diastolic pressure (LVEDP) and cardiac index or stroke volume in normal (N) and failing (F) hearts. "H" represents hydralazine or any other pure arterial vasodilator. It produces only a minimal increase in cardiac index in normal subjects (A′ → H′) or in patients with heart failure with a normal LVEDP (C → H″). In contrast, it elevates output in the patient with heart failure and elevated LVEDP (A → H). "C" represents a balanced vasodilator, such as sodium nitroprusside or captopril. It reduces filling pressure in all patients, elevates cardiac output in patients with heart failure and elevated LVEDP (A → C), lowers cardiac output in normal subjects (A′ → C′), and has little effect on cardiac output in heart failure patients with normal filling pressures (C → C″).

and Dzau,[10] and more recent evidence suggests that locally released Ang II acts within the vascular wall as a paracrine signalling peptide to promote the proliferation as well as the contraction of vascular smooth muscle cells.[5,11,12] Within the kidney, as well as within other organs classically associated with the renin-angiotensin-aldosterone axis, such as the adrenal cortex, all components of the classic systemic RAS (i.e., renin, angiotensinogen, and ACE) can be found, suggesting that the activity of Ang II within each of these tissues is largely, if not exclusively, determined by its local synthesis, activation, and release.

ANGIOTENSIN RECEPTORS. Two classes of Ang II receptors have been described to date, AT1 and AT2, both of which bind Ang II with roughly equal affinities and both of which are widely distributed in many tissues in a developmental and cell type–specific manner.[5,13-15] AT1 receptors are GTP-binding protein-linked integral membrane pro-

TABLE 16–1 VASODILATOR DRUGS USED IN THE TREATMENT OF HEART FAILURE

DRUG	MECHANISM	PRELOAD REDUCTION	AFTERLOAD REDUCTION	USUAL DOSE
RENIN-ANGIOTENSIN SYSTEM ANTAGONISTS				
Captopril	Inhibition of renal systemic and tissue generation of angiotensin II by ACE; decreased metabolism of bradykinin	++	++	6.25–50 mg p.o. q8h
Enalapril		++	++	2.5–10 mg p.o. q12h
Enalaprilat				0.5–2.0 mg IV q12h
Quinapril		++	++	10–80 mg p.o. q.d.
Lisinopril		++	++	2.5–20 mg p.o. q12–24h
Ramipril		++	++	1.25–5 mg p.o. q.d.
Losartan	Blockade of angiotensin II (AT$_1$) receptors	++	++	25–50 mg q12h
NITROVASODILATORS				
				0.2–10 μg/kg/min IV
Nitroglycerin	Nitric oxide donors	+++	+	5–6 mg transdermal
Isosorbide Dinitrate		+++	+	10–60 mg q.i.d.
Nitroprusside		+++	+++	0.1–3 μg/kg/min IV
DIRECT VASODILATORS				
Hydralazine	Unclear	+	+++	10–100 p.o. q6h
Nicorandil*	Increased K$^+$ channel conductance and other mechanisms	++	+++	Not determined
Minoxidil		+	+++	5–10 mg q.d.
Diazoxide		+	+++	1–3 mg/kg q4–24h
CALCIUM CHANNEL BLOCKING DRUGS				
Nifedipine	Inhibition of L-type voltage-sensitive Ca^{++} channels	+	+++	10–30 mg p.o. t.i.d.
Amlodipine		+	+++	5–10 mg p.o. q.d.
Felodipine		+	+++	5–10 mg p.o. q.d.
PHOSPHODIESTERASE INHIBITORS				
Amrinone	Inhibition of type III cAMP phosphodiesterase(s) and other mechanisms	++	++	0.5 mg/kg, then 2–20 μg/kg/min IV
Milrinone		++	++	50 μg/kg, then 0.25–1 μg/kg/min IV
Vesnarinone*				Not determined
SYMPATHOMIMETICS				
Dobutamine	Myocardial and vascular beta-adrenergic agonist	+	++	2–20 μg/kg/min
Dopamine	Selective renal arterial vasodilation	–	– –	≤ 2 μg/kg/min
SYMPATHOLYTICS				
Prazosin (and other quinazoline derivatives)	Alpha$_1$-adrenergic receptor antagonist	+++	++	1–5 mg p.o. q12h
Phentolamine	Nonselective alpha-adrenergic blockade	++	++	0.5–1.0 mg/min I.V.
Labetalol	Beta-adrenergic and alpha$_1$-adrenergic blockade	+	++	100–400 mg b.i.d.
Carvedilol*		+	++	12.5–50 mg p.o. b.i.d.
Bucindolol*	Additional mechanisms	+	++	6.25–100 mg p.o. b.i.d.

* Investigational and not approved by the US Food and Drug Administration at the time of this writing.

Adapted from Kelly, R. A., and Smith, T. W.: The pharmacologic treatment of heart failure. *In* Hardman, J. G., Limbird, L. (eds.): Goodman & Gilman's Pharmacologic Basis of Therapeutics, 9th ed. New York, McGraw Hill Book Co., 1996. © 1996 the McGraw-Hill Companies, Inc.

teins with seven transmembrane-spanning domains that bind the diphenylimidazole derivative losartan.[13] The AT2 receptor is also a seven transmembrane-spanning domain receptor, although the cellular signalling pathways initiated by Ang II binding at this receptor are not clear at this time. Two groups have independently reported that the ratio of AT2 to AT1 receptors is 2:1 in normal human myocardium.[16,17] The number of Ang II receptors has been reported to be decreased by over 50 per cent in myocardial tissue obtained from patients with end-stage heart failure, with no change in the ratio of AT2 to AT1 receptors.[16] The present limited literature on the molecular pharmacology of angiotensin receptors in human heart failure is now likely to expand rapidly with the identification of specific receptor subtypes.

CARDIOVASCULAR ACTIONS OF ANGIOTENSINS

Despite the fact that the molecular components of the renin-angiotensin-aldosterone axis have been known for decades and that specific angiotensin and aldosterone antagonists have been available for over 20 years, the recognition that angiotensins appear to play a major role in vascular and cardiac cell biology and pharmacology has occurred only relatively recently. Several recent reviews and editorials have focused on possible direct or indirect effects of angiotensins on vascular and myocardial remodeling and improved myocardial energetics among other mechanisms.[18,19]

VASOCONSTRICTION. Angiotensins have direct vasoconstrictor activity in vascular smooth muscle. In addition, Ang II enhances the activity of the sympathetic nervous system by several mechanisms, including blockade of norepinephrine reuptake and facilitation of norepinephrine release. In normal subjects, a significant proportion of peripheral arterial vasoconstriction to an Ang II infusion is mediated by the local release of norepinephrine.[20,21] In addition, angiotensins have direct effects on coagulation and fibrinolytic pathways and on vascular smooth muscle proliferation.[22,23]

INOTROPY. A positive inotropic effect of Ang II, mediated by AT1 receptors, has been demonstrated in atrial and ventricular muscle strips in several species, including normal human myocardium, although it is not clear how relevant this is to human physiology.[17,24–26] Experiments in animal models of cardiac hypertrophy have suggested that an activated intracardiac RAS plays a role in mediating a decrease in ventricular compliance.[27–30]

CELLULAR PROLIFERATION. In vitro, Ang II is known to induce activation of signalling pathways that lead to cellular proliferation of fibroblasts isolated from cardiac muscle and that contribute to the increased fibrosis characteristic of some forms of cardiac hypertrophy and cardiomyopathy.[31–33] Ang II can induce hypertrophic growth of neonatal ventricular myocytes in vitro and may do so in vivo as well by potentiating the activity of the sympathetic nervous system and the release of norepinephrine, which is known to induce myocyte hypertrophy in vitro by acting through α_1-adrenergic receptors.[34–36] These two actions of Ang II, in addition to its arterial and venous vasoconstrictor properties, probably contribute importantly to the remodeling that occurs in surviving ventricular muscle following myocardial infarction, first documented by observations in rats with experimental myocardial infarction in the early 1980's with the ACE inhibitor captopril and since replicated in other species.[19,37,38]

RAS ANTAGONISTS. In addition to inhibition of intracardiac RAS, renin-angiotensin antagonists, by virtue of their vasodilating activity, also reduce intracavity pressures and diminish wall stress, thereby decreasing myocardial oxygen demand. They also inhibit Ang II stimulation of aldosterone release, which reduces intravascular volume and preload and may have direct actions on the extent of interstitial collagen deposition in the heart.[39] ACE inhibitors have also been shown to decrease sympathetic nervous system activity and improve parasympathetic nervous system tone, which could result in reduced electrophysiological instability in infarcted or cardiomyopathic muscle.[40]

RENAL ACTIONS OF ANGIOTENSIN II AND RAS ANTAGONISTS. In addition to the above diverse actions, RAS antagonists also exhibit beneficial pharmacological effects on sodium homeostasis in heart failure. This is due to the important role of angiotensin II in the regulation of intrarenal hemodynamics, glomerular filtration, and tubular resorption of solute and water in the kidney. Angiotensin II regulates glomerular efferent arteriolar tone, a major determinant of the filtration fraction—that is, the fraction of renal plasma flow that crosses the glomerular membrane and passes into the proximal tubule. Intrarenal Angiotensin II activity, in the absence of a marked decline in renal blood flow or perfusion pressure, increases filtration fraction, leading to increased solute resorption in the proximal tubule (Fig. 16–2). Angiotensin II also appears to have additional direct effects on renal tubular epithelial cell salt and water resorption. Angiotensin II induces the release of aldosterone from the adrenal cortex, increasing sodium resorption in the distal nephron (see p. 413). Finally, ACE inhibitors inhibit the intrarenal metabolism of bradykinin and increase intrarenal levels of this natriuretic autacoid.[6]

Although the unique intrarenal actions of renin-angiotensin system antagonists among vasodilators provide a pharmacological advantage for this class of drugs, there is an important caveat. Owing to their selective effects on efferent arteriolar tone, renin-angiotensin antagonists, unlike other vasodilators, limit the kidney's ability to autoregulate glomerular perfusion pressure and thereby maintain glomerular filtration. This may be particularly important in patients with a marginal cardiac output or blood pressure and can result in a decline in the glomerular filtration rate (GFR), resulting in an increase in serum creatinine levels. In the first *Cooperative North Scandinavian Enalapril Survival Study* (CONSENSUS I), in which the efficacy of enalapril was compared with placebo in patients with severe (NYHA class III and IV) heart failure, the serum creatinine increased by a factor of 2 or greater in 11 per cent of 123 patients compared with 3 per cent in the placebo group.[41] The maximal increase in serum creatinine correlated inversely with mean arterial pressure. Patients on higher daily doses of a Na,K,2Cl symport inhibitor (e.g., furosemide) were at a slightly higher risk for a significant elevation in serum creatinine.[42]

The factors associated with a decline in renal function in heart failure in patients receiving an ACE inhibitor are listed in Table 16–2. It should be noted that most patients in the CONSENSUS I trial tolerated enalapril well, and the serum creatinine in fact fell in 24 per cent

TABLE 16–2 ACE INHIBITORS AND RENAL DYSFUNCTION IN HEART FAILURE

FACTORS FAVORING DETERIORATION IN RENAL FUNCTION
Na⁺ depletion or poor renal perfusion
  Large doses of diuretics
  Increased urea/creatinine ratio
  Mean arterial pressure < 80 mm Hg
Evidence of maximal neurohumoral activation
  Presence of hyponatremia secondary to AVP activation
Interruption of counterregulatory mechanisms
  Coadministration of prostaglandin inhibitors
  Presence of adrenergic dysfunction (e.g., diabetes mellitus)

FACTORS FAVORING IMPROVEMENT IN RENAL FUNCTION
Maintenance of Na⁺ balance
  Reduction in diuretic dosage
  Increase in sodium intake
  Mean arterial pressure > 80 mm Hg
Minimal neurohumoral activation
Intact counterregulatory mechanisms

From Miller, J. A., Tobe, S. W., and Skorecki, K. L.: Control of extracellular fluid volume and the pathophysiology of edema. *In* Brenner, B. M., and Rector, F. C. (eds.): The Kidney, 5th ed. Philadelphia, W.B. Saunders Company, 1995.

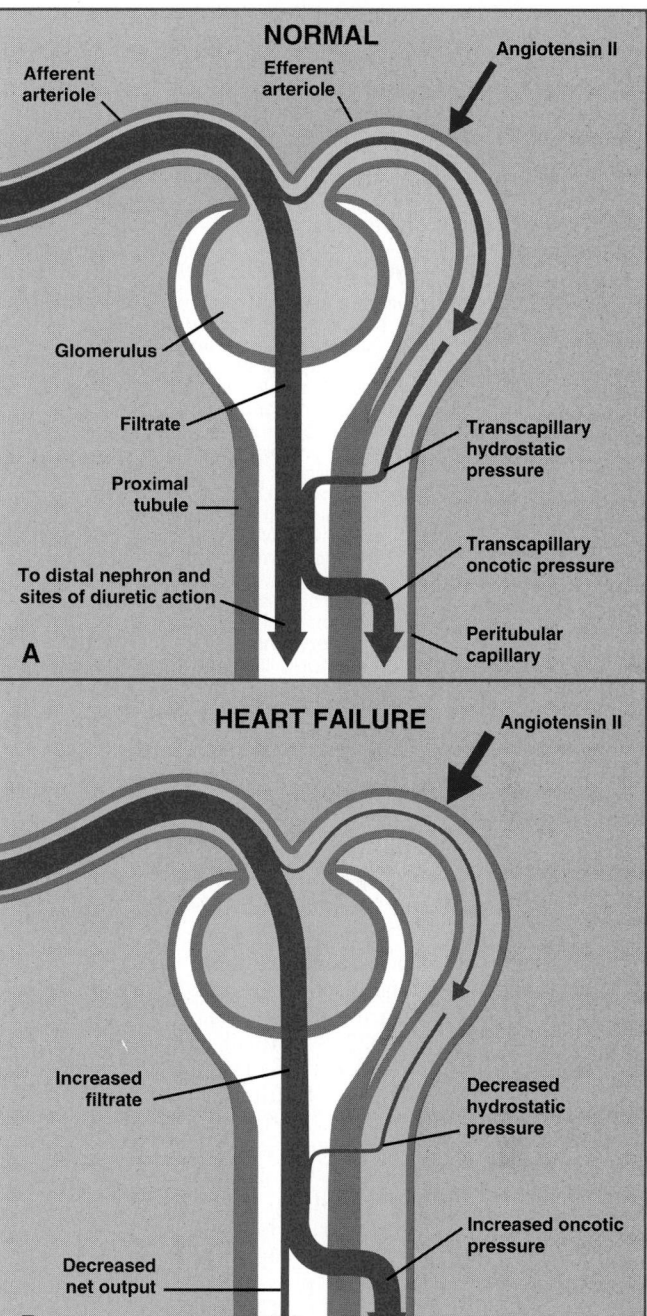

FIGURE 16–2. Renal function in the normal and heart failure states. Compared with normal glomerular function *(A)*, heart failure *(B)* is characterized by an increase in filtration fraction. This causes a fall in transcapillary hydrostatic pressure and increases oncotic pressure and thus promotes heightened solute and water reabsorption in the proximal tubule. This increase in filtration fraction is in large part mediated by increased constriction of the efferent arteriole by local intrarenal generation of angiotensin II. Renin angiotensin system antagonists can decrease the filtration fraction by causing relatively selective dilation of the efferent arteriole. (Adapted from Smith, T. W. and Kelly, R. A.: Therapeutic strategies for congestive heart failure in the 1990's. Hosp Pract 26:127, 1991. © 1991 The McGraw-Hill Companies, Inc.)

of patients.[41] This has generally been the experience in most of the later trials involving ACE inhibitors, reviewed in Chapter 17, in which patients on average had less severe heart failure than those in the CONSENSUS I trial. In the arm of the SOLVD trial that examined symptomatic patients with heart failure, approximately 11 per cent of patients receiving enalapril had an increase in serum creatinine above 2 mg/dl compared with 8 per cent receiving placebo.[43] In the GISSI-3 trial, there was a small but significantly increased risk of renal dysfunction at 6 weeks in patients randomized to receive lisinopril who had normal renal function at the entry of study (0.6 per cent for lisinopril versus 0.3 per cent among controls).[44] A similar small, but statistically significant, increase in the incidence of moderate renal dysfunction was observed in the ISIS-4 trial with captopril (1.1 per cent for captopril versus 0.6 per cent with placebo).[45]

An increase in serum creatinine need not require discontinuation of an ACE inhibitor, particularly if the decline in urea or creatinine clearance does not lead to symptoms and urinary sodium excretion with or without diuretics does not decrease. More than a doubling of the serum creatinine should lead to a reduction in the ACE inhibitor dose or to a substitution with another class of vasodilator, provided that arterial perfusion pressure remains adequate. ACE inhibitors have been shown to improve or slow the decline in renal function in some patients with primary renal pathology.[46,47]

ANGIOTENSIN-CONVERTING ENZYME INHIBITORS

Ondetti has recently provided a personal history of the synthesis of the first orally bioavailable ACE inhibitor.[48] A synthetic nonapeptide analog, teprotide, was first studied in normal volunteers in the early 1970's, and its efficacy in the treatment of hypertension and heart failure was documented in several small trials. This agent was not orally bioavailable and remained investigational. Then, based on the observation that benzylsuccinic acid derivatives such as succinyl-L-proline were potent inhibitors of carboxyl peptidase A (ACE is a carboxyl peptidase), Ondetti and colleagues synthesized 3-mercaptopropanoyl-L-proline. This compound was 3000 times more potent as an ACE inhibitor than succinyl-L-proline, and its α-methyl analogue—given the generic name captopril—was well absorbed orally.

All orally active ACE inhibitors currently available fall into three general categories: (1) those with a sulfhydryl group that binds to the zinc moiety in ACE, including captopril and zofenapril*; (2) those in which the carboxyl group in the original succinyl-L-proline molecule was designed to bind the zinc moiety, and these include the majority of ACE inhibitors, including enalapril, lisinopril, ramipril, cilazapril, quinapril, and others; and (3) proline derivatives in which a phosphinic acid group is used to bind to the zinc moiety, of which fosinopril is the prototype. Several of these drugs are inactive esters or pro-drugs, such as zofenapril, enalapril, and fosinapril, and must be de-esterified to the active drug in vivo.

TISSUE ACTIONS OF ACE INHIBITORS. When tissue ACE levels are measured directly, significant differences have been noted in the extent of ACE inhibition in a given tissue or organ among ACE inhibitors, and specific tissues or organs exhibit different degrees of ACE inhibition to the same ACE inhibitor.[49–51] These differences in ACE activity and physiological responsiveness among members of the same class of RAS antagonists are probably due to the accessibility of active drug to cellular sites of Ang II generation within a given tissue. The clinical importance of these differences in the site and extent of accumulation of specific ACE inhibitors requires additional investigation. ACE inhibitors also effectively inhibit the systemic renin-angiotensin-aldosterone axis by preventing the conversion of angiotensin I to angiotensin II in the circulation.

CLINICAL USE. It is advisable to begin therapy for heart failure with an ACE inhibitor at low doses of a relatively short-acting drug (e.g., 6.25 mg captopril or 2.5 mg enalapril). An abrupt fall in blood pressure occasionally occurs following an initial dose of an ACE inhibitor, particularly in patients with depletion of this intravascular volume. This response is often unpredictable, and therefore caution is recommended when beginning these drugs in any patient who has significant left ventricular dysfunction or who has received large doses of diuretics.[52–54] Unacceptable hypotension can usually be reversed by intravascular volume expansion.

Few consistent and clinically important pharmacokinetic drug interactions exist between the ACE inhibitors and most other class of drugs that would be administered to patients with heart failure.[55] There is no consistent evidence for an important interaction between any ACE inhibitor and digoxin. Because most ACE inhibitors are cleared primarily by the kidney, a reduction in dose and/or increase in dosing interval may be necessary in patients with renal impairment. *Cough* is a relatively frequent side effect of ACE inhibitors that may develop after weeks or even months of therapy (see also p. 497). *Angioedema* is a rare but potentially life-threatening side effect of these drugs.

---

* Not approved by the US Food and Drug Administration at the time of this writing.

ACE inhibitors are contraindicated in pregnancy because of drug-induced malformations of the kidney.

ANGIOTENSIN II RECEPTOR ANTAGONISTS. Although peptide Ang II antagonists such as saralasin (also a partial agonist) have been available for decades for experimental use, orally bioavailable angiotensin receptor antagonists have only recently become available.[13] The first of these to undergo dose-ranging and safety trials in humans with heart failure is the AT1-selective antagonist losartan. Despite its specificity for only one class of Ang II receptors (i.e., AT1) and the lack of bradykinin-potentiating activity that is characteristic of ACE inhibitors, losartan's spectrum of activity appears to be very similar to that of the ACE inhibitors,[56,57] although experience with patients in heart failure is limited to date. As with ACE inhibitors, there was no reflex tachycardia associated with the decline in blood pressure and no evidence of tolerance to the drug's hemodynamic effects over a 12-week period in one study.[57] In larger trials of losartan in the treatment of primary hypertension, there has been no increased frequency of cough associated with its use.

RENIN INHIBITORS. The pharmaceutical industry also has developed a number of agents that inhibit the enzymatic activity of renin, all of which are investigational at this time. The most promising of these are the transition state analogues of the peptide sequence at the renin cleavage site on angiotensinogen.[58,59] The data available to date do *not* suggest that either AT1 receptor antagonists or renin inhibitors have a spectrum of activity in heart failure that is importantly different from those of the ACE inhibitors. However, these agents may play an important role in the management of patients who cannot tolerate ACE inhibitors because of cough or angioedema.

Nitrovasodilators

The cellular mechanisms by which nitrovasodilators lead to the relaxation of vascular smooth muscle have become apparent only in the past decade despite the fact that these drugs are among the oldest vasodilators in clinical practice. It is now understood that these drugs mimic the activity of nitric oxide and its congeners. These are autocrine and paracrine signalling autacoids that are formed in endothelial and smooth muscle cells throughout the vasculature, as well as in many other cell types, including cardiac muscle cells.[60–63] Nitrogen oxides were originally identified as the bioactive factor(s) responsible for endothelium-dependent relaxation of blood vessels.[64] Their primary mechanism of action in vascular smooth muscle cells is probably based on their ability to bind to a heme moiety in soluble guanylate cyclase, resulting in an increase in intracellular cGMP. The pharmacological activity of each of the nitrovasodilators depends upon their biotransformation into nitrogen oxides within the blood and vascular tissues.[65]

Nitroprusside

Nitroprusside is an effective venous and arterial vasodilator and acts to reduce both ventricular preload and afterload. Owing to the fact that it is quickly metabolized to cyanide and nitric oxide, its onset of action is rapid and upward titration can usually be achieved expeditiously to achieve an optimal and predictable hemodynamic effect. For these reasons, nitroprusside is commonly used in intensive care settings for management of acutely decompensated heart failure when blood pressure is adequate to maintain cerebral, coronary, and renal perfusion. Ventricular filling pressures are rapidly reduced by an increase in venous compliance, resulting in a redistribution of blood volume from central (thoracic) to peripheral veins, particularly the splanchnic vasculature.[66]

Nitroprusside is among the most effective afterload-reducing agents due to its spectrum of vasodilating activity on different vascular beds. It reduces systemic vascular resistance, increases aortic wall compliance, and, at optimal doses, improves ventricular-vascular coupling. Nitroprusside also decreases pulmonary vascular resistance, and improves other components of right ventricular afterload, including the amplitude and timing of reflected pressure waves during ejection.

Hydrocyanic acid and cyanide are byproducts of the biotransformation of nitroprusside. Cyanide toxicity is uncommon, however, because cyanide is rapidly metabolized by the liver to thiocyanate, which is cleared by the kidney. Thiocyanate and/or cyanide toxicity may occur in the presence of hepatic or renal failure, and following prolonged infusions of nitroprusside in patients with marginal cardiac output or passive congestion of the liver. Thiocyanate toxicity, which is more common in patients with renal insufficiency, should be suspected in any patient receiving this drug who has unexplained abdominal pain, mental status changes, or convulsions. Clinical manifestations of cyanide toxicity are more subtle in onset and are usually manifested by a decline in cardiac output accompanied by a metabolic acidosis due to accumulation of lactic acid.

Organic Nitrates and Molsidomine*

Owing to their relatively selective vasodilating effects on the epicardial coronary vasculature, the organic nitrates (nitroglycerin, isosorbide dinitrate, and isosorbide mononitrate) may improve systolic and diastolic ventricular function by improving coronary flow in patients with an ischemic cardiomyopathy, in addition to their activity in reducing ventricular filling pressures, wall stress, and oxygen consumption (see p. 497).[68] In acute myocardial infarction, however, the effect of the routine use of nitrovasodilators on mortality remains controversial (see p. 1211).[45,69]

The experience with newer nitrovasodilators, including isosorbide mononitrate and molsidomine in the treatment of heart failure, is limited compared with their use in the treatment of angina. Molsidomine given intravenously or orally is effective in reducing systemic vascular resistance, pulmonary capillary wedge pressure, and right atrial pressure.[70] Tolerance to the arteriolar and venular vasodilating effects of this drug does develop, although its extent and time course may differ from tolerance associated with organic nitrates. The spectrum of activity of 5-isosorbide mononitrate would not be expected to differ from that of isosorbide dinitrate in heart failure.

TOLERANCE TO NITROVASODILATORS IN HEART FAILURE. The rapid development of tolerance to the venous and arteriolar vasodilating effects of the nitrovasodilators has been known for over a century. The reader is referred to recent comprehensive reviews[71-73] and page 1304. Although nitrate tolerance is well documented, the mechanism(s) responsible is not clearly understood. It is likely that several mechanisms contribute to decreased responsiveness to nitrovasodilators with time, and that the importance of the relative contribution of each potential mechanism differs with the specific drug employed, the underlying disease (heart failure versus angina), and among specific vascular beds.[74-76]

Most of the data on the efficacy of intermittent or eccentric nitroglycerin dosing protocols have been obtained in patients with angina rather than chronic congestive failure symptoms.[77,78] Nevertheless, it seems prudent to recommend a daily nitrate-free interval in patients on chronic doses of isosorbide dinitrate, which can usually be achieved by providing the last dose of isosorbide dinitrate in the early evening.

Hydralazine

Although its cellular mechanism of action remains poorly understood, hydralazine is an effective antihypertensive drug (see p. 498), particularly when combined with other agents that blunt compensatory increases in sympathetic tone and salt and water retention. In heart failure, hydralazine reduces right and left ventricular afterload by reducing systemic as well as pulmonary artery input impedance and vascular resistance. Unless symptomatic hypotension occurs, this is usually accompanied only by minor reflex increases in sympathetic nervous system ac-

tivity. These hemodynamic changes result in an augmentation of forward stroke volume and a reduction in ventricular systolic wall stress and in the regurgitant fraction in mitral insufficiency.

Hydralazine is effective in reducing renal vascular resistance and in increasing renal blood flow to a greater degree than most other vasodilators. Therefore, hydralazine may be the vasodilator of choice in heart failure patients with renal dysfunction who cannot tolerate an ACE inhibitor. Hydralazine has minimal effects on venous capacitance and therefore is most effective when combined with agents with venodilating activity (e.g., organic nitrates).

Side effects that may necessitate dose adjustment or withdrawal of hydralazine are common. The most common complaints—headache and dizziness—also may be due to nitrates that are usually administered concurrently with hydralazine. Often, with time, the symptoms diminish or respond to a reduction in dose.

Hydralazine metabolism is mediated primarily by hepatic acetylation, although many additional potential metabolic pathways have been described.[79] Therefore, patients with a "slow acetylater" phenotype have a prolonged elimination half-life of the drug. At the usual doses and dosing intervals of hydralazine, these patients are at greater risk of developing arthritis or other components of a lupus-like syndrome.

Calcium Channel Antagonists

Although all four classes of calcium channel antagonists now available (i.e., phenylalkylamine [e.g., verapamil], benzothiazepenes [e.g., diltiazem], diarylaminopropylamines [e.g., bepridil], and "first-generation" dihydropyridines [e.g., nifedipine, nimodipine, nitredipine]) are effective vasodilators (see also pp. 616 and 855), none has been shown to produce sustained improvement in symptoms in heart failure patients with predominant systolic ventricular dysfunction. Indeed, these drugs appear to worsen symptoms and may actually increase mortality in patients with systolic dysfunction. This includes patients with heart failure due to ischemic disease.[80] The reason for these adverse effects of calcium channel blockers in heart failure is unclear. It may be related to the known negative inotropic effects of these drugs, to reflex neurohumoral activation, or to a combination of these and other effects.

So-called second-generation calcium channel antagonists of the dihydropyridine class, particularly amlodopine and felodipine, appear to have fewer negative inotropic effects than earlier drugs, and are currently being evaluated in randomized prospective trials to determine their effects on both symptoms and mortality in heart failure patients already receiving standard medical management.[81,82]

K+ CHANNEL ACTIVATORS

Despite the well-known role of outward K+ currents in initiating repolarization and in the maintenance of membrane potential in most cell types, the molecular characterization of individual K+ channel proteins has occurred only recently.[83] They comprise diverse families of integral plasma membrane proteins, the K+ conductances of which are specific to each family and are regulated by a number of factors including changes in transmembrane voltage, intracellular Ca++ activity, and intracellular ATP levels, among other mechanisms.[83-85] The distribution of K+ channel isoforms is tissue- and cell type–specific, permitting the possibility of relatively selective tissue pharmacological activity of drugs acting on a specific family of K+ channels. In vascular smooth muscle, increased outward K+ conductance causes cellular hyperpolarization and decreased Ca++ entry, resulting in vasorelaxation.[85] Diazoxide and minoxidil, classic direct-acting vasodilators, are now known to act at K+ channels.

Nicorandil,* pinacidil,* and cromakalin* are representative of a new class of K+ channel activators that exhibit a unique spectrum of activity among vasodilator drugs. Like minoxidil, nicorandil is primarily an arteriolar vasodilator, but it is also effective in dilating epicardial coronary arteries and in reducing preload in experimental animals and patients with heart failure.[86,87] Nicorandil, pinacidil, and cromakalin have been tested in humans, primarily for hypertension and angina, and are effective and relatively well tolerated with fewer adverse effects than older direct vasodilators of this class.

---

* Not approved by the US Food and Drug Administration at the time of this writing.

The experience to date with these agents in patients with heart failure has been less extensive. Unlike nitrovasodilators, tolerance has not been observed to the antianginal effect of nicorandil or the drug's ability to cause a sustained reduction in left ventricular filling pressures.[88] As with any novel class of vasodilators, the utility of nicorandil, and of other K+ channel activators under development in the drug treatment of heart failure, must await the design and completion of large controlled efficacy and survival trials.

DIURETICS

The importance of diuretics in the treatment of the syndrome of congestive heart failure relates to the central role of the kidney as the target organ of many of the neurohumoral and hemodynamic changes that occur in response to a failing myocardium[89-92] (see also Chap. 62). Diuretics do not influence the natural history of the underlying heart disease responsible for the decline in cardiac output. However, they can improve symptoms of heart failure by acting directly on solute and water reabsorption by the kidney and may slow the progression of cardiac chamber dilation by reducing ventricular filling pressures (i.e., preload; Fig. 16–3).

Renal Adaptations in Heart Failure

The increase in salt and water retention by the kidney in heart failure is due to characteristic alterations in intrarenal hemodynamics that occur in response to a decline in cardiac output, in addition to the activation of the sympathetic nervous system and of several hormonal as well as locally acting peptide and nonpeptide signalling pathways. A decrease in cardiac output, with or without an increase in intrapulmonary vascular pressures and decreased arterial oxygen saturation, results in an increase in peripheral and intrarenal vascular resistance, in the activation of intrarenal and other tissue renin-angiotensin systems, and in the release of arginine vasopressin (i.e., AVP, antidiuretic hormone). Increased adrenal cortical angiotensin II activity promotes aldosterone synthesis and release while increased intra-atrial and intraventricular pressures promote the release of atrial natriuretic peptide (ANP) and brain natriuretic peptide (BNP) from cardiac muscle.

INTRARENAL HEMODYNAMICS IN HEART FAILURE (See also Chap. 62). The changes in intrarenal hemodynamics that occur in early heart failure result in preservation of the GFR despite a decline in cardiac output and renal blood flow.[89,91] Although increases in sympathetic nervous system activity and local intrarenal release of angiotensin II act to increase resistance in both the afferent and efferent arterioles, this preservation of GFR is due in large part to a greater increase in efferent than in afferent arteriolar tone (Fig. 16–2). This results in an increase in the fraction of renal plasma flow that is filtered by the kidney (i.e., the filtration fraction). The increased filtration fraction also leads to an increase in hydrostatic pressure in the proximal tubule relative to the peritubular capillaries which, in addition to the increase in colloid osmotic pressure in this portion of the nephron, favors the reuptake of solute and water from the proximal tubule.[93]

In addition to their importance in mediating the increased renal salt and water resorption in heart failure, these characteristic alterations in glomerular hemodynamics are often importantly affected by several classes of drugs used in the treatment of heart failure. The kidney's ability to autoregulate and sustain GFR despite a falling cardiac output in worsening heart failure is compromised by any drug that lowers mean arterial pressure. Therefore, GFR may fall despite an increase in cardiac output following administration of some vasodilators. The importance of efferent arteriolar tone to the maintenance of GFR in heart failure also means that administration of renin-angiotensin

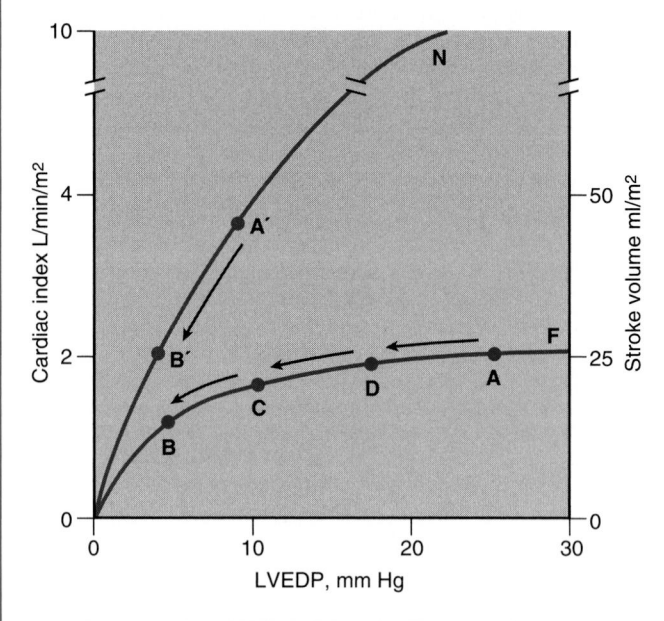

FIGURE 16–3. Effect of a venodilator (e.g., isosorbide dinitrate) or of diuretic therapy in a normal (N) subject (A' → B') and in a patient with heart failure (F) and markedly elevated left ventricular filling pressures (A → D), moderately elevated filling pressures (D → C), and normal filling pressures (C → B). In heart failure, a clinically significant decline in cardiac output usually does not occur until the LVEDP is below 10 mm Hg.

system antagonists, including ACE inhibitors, could cause a decline in GFR in some patients despite an increase in cardiac output.

Mechanisms of Action

There are a number of classification schemes for diuretics based on their mechanism of action, their anatomical locus of action in the nephron, and the form of diuresis they elicit. Because the specific ion transport proteins that are the molecular targets for all the diuretics in common clinical use for the treatment of congestive heart failure recently have been identified and their amino acid sequence and intrarenal distribution characterized, a new classification of these drugs based on their molecular pharmacology has been advocated.[94] This classification scheme, rather than molecular structure (e.g., "thiazide" diuretic), site of action (e.g., "loop" diuretic), or efficacy and clinical outcome (e.g., "high-ceiling" diuretic and "potassium-sparing" diuretic) is employed in this chapter as well as the more traditional nomenclature. Diuretics currently available in the United States are listed in Table 16–3.

Diuretic Classes

OSMOTIC DIURETICS AND CARBONIC ANHYDRASE INHIBITORS. Mannitol, as an inert extracellular osmotic agent, increases the extracellular fluid volume; consequently, the drug is contraindicated in patients with decompensated congestive heart failure. Inducing a metabolic acidosis with a carbonic anhydrase inhibitor may be of use in edematous patients with hypochloremic metabolic alkalosis due to long-term use of loop diuretics, particularly if the acid-base status of these patients is complicated by hypercarbia.

INHIBITORS OF THE Na+,K+,2Cl SYMPORT (LOOP DIURETICS). These agents, traditionally classified as loop or high-ceiling diuretics, including furosemide, bumetanide, ethacrynic acid, and torsemide, have been known for over 10 years to reversibly inhibit a Na,K,2Cl symporter (cotransporter) when applied to the luminal membranes of epithe-

TABLE 16-3 DIURETICS: ACTION, DOSAGE, AND DRUG INTERACTIONS   477

Ch 16

DIURETIC	BRAND NAME	PRINCIPAL SITE AND MECHANISM OF ACTION	EFFECTS ON URINARY ELECTROLYTES	EFFECTS ON BLOOD ELECTROLYTES AND ACID-BASE BALANCE	EXTRARENAL EFFECTS	USUAL DOSAGE*	DRUG INTERACTIONS
OSMOTIC DIURETICS							
Mannitol	Osmitrol	Proximal tubule (primarily)	↑Na⁺ ↑Cl⁻ ↑H₂O	↑Extracellular volume transiently	↓Intracranial pressure	50–200 gm/d	May enhance loop diuretic effectiveness by maintaining GFR
Glycerol	Glyrol				↓Intraocular pressure	1–1.5 gm/kg	
CARBONIC ANHYDRASE INHIBITORS							
Acetazolamide	Diamox	Proximal tubule	↑Na⁺ ↑K⁺ ↑HCO₃⁻	Metabolic acidosis	↑Ventilatory drive	250–500 mg/d	May be useful in alkalemia due to other diuretics
Dichlorphenamide	Doranide	Carbonic anhydrase inhibition			↓Intraocular pressure	10–20 mg/d	
Methazolamide	Neptazane					25–100 mg/d	
Na,K,2Cl SYMPORT INHIBITORS (LOOP DIURETICS)							
Furosemide	Lasix	Thick ascending limb of loop of Henle: Inhibition of Na/K/2Cl symport	↑Na⁺	Hypochloremic alkalosis	*Acute:*	20–1000 mg/d	Tubular secretion delayed by competing organic acids (renal failure) and some drugs
Bumetanide	Bumex		↑Cl⁻	↑HCO₃ ↓K⁺, ↓Na⁺ ↓Cl⁻, ↓Mg⁺⁺ ↑Uric acid	↑Venous capacitance	0.5–20 mg/d	
Piretanide†	Arelix Diumax Tauliz				↑Systemic vascular resitance *Chronic:* ↓Cardiac preload	6–20 mg/d	Effectiveness reduced by prostaglandin inhibitors
Ethacrynic acid	Edecrin				Ototoxicity	50–200 mg/d	Additive ototoxicity with aminoglycosides
Torsemide	Demadex					2.5–200 mg/d	Longer duration of action than furosemide
Na, Cl SYMPORT INHIBITORS (THIAZIDE AND THIAZIDE-LIKE DIURETICS)							
Chlorothiazide	Diuril	Distal tubule: Inhibit NaCl symport	↑Na⁺	↓Na⁺, particularly in elderly patients	↑Glucose ↑LDL/triglycerides (may be dose related)	50–100 mg	Efficacy reduced by prostaglandin inhibitors
Hydrochlorothiazide	Hydridiuril		↑Cl⁻			25–50 mg/d	
Trichlormethiazide	Metahydrin		↑K⁺			2–8 mg/d	Reduces renal clearance of lithium
Chlorthalidone	Hygroton		↑Mg⁺⁺	↓Cl, ↑HCO₃⁻ (mild alkalosis) ↑Uric acid ↑Ca⁺⁺ ↓K⁺, ↓Mg⁺⁺		25–100 mg/d	Additive effect on NaCl and K⁺ excretion with loop diuretics
Metolazone	Zaroxolyn		↓Ca⁺⁺			5–10 mg/d	
Hydroflumethiazide	Diucardin Saluron					25–200 mg/d	
Polythiazide	Renese					1–4 mg/d	
Quinethazone	Hydromox					50–100 mg/d	
Methyclothiazide	Enduron Aquatensen					2.5–10 mg/d	
Benzthiazide	Aquatag Exna					50–200 mg/d	
Bendroflumethiazide	Naturetin				Extrarenal effects less marked with indapamide	2.5–30 mg/d	
Indapamide	Lozol	Vasodilator				2.5–5 mg/d	
EPITHELIAL Na⁺ CHANNEL INHIBITORS (POTASSIUM-SPARING DIURETICS)							
Triamterene	Dyrenium	Collecting duct Inhibit apical membrane Na⁺ conductance	↑HCO₃⁻	↓GFR; metabolic acidosis ↑Mg⁺⁺		100–300 mg/d	Useful with K⁺ wasting diuretics; may induce hyperkalemia with ACE inhibitors
Amiloride	Midamor					5–10 mg/d	
TYPE I MINERALOCORTICOID RECEPTOR ANTAGONIST (POTASSIUM-SPARING DIURETICS)							
Spironolactone	Aldactone	Collecting duct: Aldosterone antagonists	↓K⁺ ↑Na⁺ ↑Cl	↑K⁺, particularly in patients	Gynecomastia	2 mg/d	Useful adjunct to therapy with K⁺ wasting diuretics
Canrenone						24 mg/d	

* Dosages are p.o.
† Not yet licensed for use in the United States.

lial cells of the thick ascending limb of the loop of Henle.[95] Inhibition of this symporter results in marked increases in the fractional excretion of Na⁺ and Cl⁻ and indirectly in the fractional excretion of Ca⁺⁺ and Mg⁺⁺. By inhibiting the concentration of solute within the medullary interstitium, these drugs also reduce the driving force for water resorption in the collecting duct, regardless of the presence of AVP, resulting in the production of urine that is nearly isotonic with that of plasma at the height of the diuresis. The delivery of large amounts of Na⁺ and fluid to the distal nephron increases both K⁺ and H⁺ secretion, a process that is accelerated by aldosterone.

The Na,K,2Cl symport inhibitors (loop diuretics) also exhibit several characteristic effects on intracardiac pressures and on systemic hemodynamics. An increase in venous capacitance and a lowering of pulmonary capillary wedge pressure within minutes of a bolus infusion of intravenous furosemide (0.5 to 1.0 mg/kg) have been well documented in patients with congestive symptoms following an acute myocardial infarction or with valvular heart disease.[96] All of the rapid hemodynamic actions of the loop diuretics are attenuated in patients with chronic congestive heart failure.

INHIBITORS OF THE Na⁺,Cl⁻ SYMPORTER (THIAZIDE CLASS DIURETICS). Despite being the focus of intensive research by renal pharmacology and physiology laboratories for several decades, the site of action of thiazide diuretics within the distal convoluted tubule has only recently been identified as the Na⁺,Cl⁻ symporter of the distal convoluted tubule.[97] This symporter (or related isoforms) is also present on cells within the vasculature and many cell types within other organs and tissues and may contribute to some of the other actions of these agents.

By blocking solute uptake in the distal convoluted tubule, Na^+/Cl^- symport inhibitors (thiazide class diuretics) prevent maximal dilution of the urine and decrease the kidney's ability to increase free water clearance. Thiazides increase Ca^{++} resorption in the distal nephron by several mechanisms, occasionally resulting in a small increase in the serum Ca^{++} concentration. In contrast, Mg^{++} resorption is diminished and hypomagnesemia may occur with prolonged use. Increased delivery of NaCl and fluid into the collecting duct directly enhances K^+ and H^+ secretion by this segment of the nephron and may lead to clinically important hypokalemia.

INHIBITORS OF EPITHELIAL Na$^+$ CHANNELS (POTASSIUM-SPARING DIURETICS). The apical (luminal) membranes of principal cells of the late distal convoluted tubule and the cortical collecting duct contain Na^+-selective channels that permit sodium entry from within the tubular lumen that is driven by the electrochemical gradient established by the Na,K-ATPase in the basolateral membranes of these cells.[98] Na^+ conductance by these channels is inhibited by amiloride and by triamterene, which subsequently diminish the electrochemical potential for K^+ secretion into the urine. Thus, these agents, along with mineralocorticoid inhibitors (below), are commonly referred to as "potassium-sparing" diuretics. Neither drug is effective in achieving a net negative Na^+ balance in heart failure when given alone.

INHIBITORS OF TYPE I MINERALOCORTICOID/GLUCOCORTICOID RECEPTORS (POTASSIUM-SPARING DIURETICS). Spironolactone and its active metabolites canrenone and potassium canrenoate bind to intracellular receptors that belong to a superfamily of cytosolic steroid receptor proteins. Upon ligand binding, these proteins translocate to the cell nucleus where they bind to specific DNA sequences and regulate the transcription and synthesis of a number of gene products, including apical membrane Na^+ channels, H,K-ATPase, and Na^+,K^+-ATPase, among others.[99,100] The spironolactone-bound type I receptor complex is inactive and diminishes K^+ and H^+ secretion by this portion of the nephron, particularly in patients with high plasma aldosterone levels, as in heart failure.[101] Hyperkalemia and, unusually, a metabolic acidosis, may result from the use of these drugs.

VASOPRESSIN ANTAGONISTS. Increased levels of circulating arginine vasopressin contribute to the increased systemic vascular resistance and positive solute and water balance in patients with advanced heart failure.[102] Classically, vasopressin receptors have been divided into V_1 and V_2 receptor subtypes, which exhibit different ligand-binding specificities. V_2 receptors are found largely in distal nephron segments within the kidney.[102] V_2-selective receptor antagonists inhibit recruitment of aquaporin-CD (aquaporin-2) water channels,[103,104] amiloride-sensitive Na^+ channels, and urea transporters into the apical membranes of collecting duct epithelial cells.

Orally bioavailable V_2-specific antagonists have been developed that induce in humans a marked increase in free water clearance and modest increases in Na^+, Cl^-, and urea clearance with no change in K^+ secretion.[105] Although the pharmacology of these drugs will undoubtedly prove to be complex in patients with heart failure, most of whom will be receiving other vasodilators and natriuretic drugs, these agents, all of which are currently investigational, are likely to be valuable adjuncts to the contemporary treatment of heart failure.

NATRIURETIC PEPTIDES. The contribution of the natriuretic peptides—ANP, BNP, and related proteins, including urodilatin and fragments of the proANP protein—in the physiological adaptations that accompany heart failure, and their potential role as drugs in the pharmacotherapy of this syndrome, have been the subject of intensive research over the past decade[106,107] (see also p. 414). Infusions of ANP have been shown to cause afferent arteriolar dilation and efferent arteriolar constriction, resulting in an increase in GFR.[106]

Even when infused at concentrations that do not affect GFR, ANP induces a natriuresis by inhibiting the resorptive capacity of the proximal tubular epithelium, largely by inhibiting the actions of locally acting antinatriuretic agents such as angiotensin II and by augmenting the activity of intrarenal dopamine. In the distal nephron, natriuretic peptides decrease Na^+ influx from the tubular lumen through amiloride-sensitive epithelial Na^+ channels.

The result is a natriuresis with minimal effect on urinary potassium excretion.

Although these natriuretic peptides appear to have a favorable pharmacological profile in heart failure, their practical utility so far has been disappointing owing to their short biological half-life and the development of pharmacological tolerance, as well as undesirable hemodynamic effects, including symptomatic hypotension and bradycardia, and these agents remain investigational. There is little evidence for any clinically significant direct effect on ventricular function.[108] Receptor-mediated clearance pathways and metabolism by the zinc metallopeptidase neutral endopeptidase (NEP) comprise the two predominant mechanisms for natriuretic peptide inactivation and removal and are the target of new pharmaceutical strategies to lengthen the biological half-life of endogenous and exogenously infused natriuretic peptides.

Diuretic Resistance

Inhibitors of the Na,K,2Cl symport (loop diuretics) are the only diuretics that are effective as single agents in moderate and advanced heart failure due to the magnitude of their maximal ("ceiling") natriuretic effect and to the fact that the natriuretic effect of more distally acting drugs is limited by the increased resorption of solute and water in proximal nephron segments in heart failure (Fig. 16–4). The effectiveness of even the loop diuretics usually decreases with worsening heart failure, however. Although the absolute bioavailability of these drugs is not decreased in heart failure, their rate of absorption may be delayed, resulting in inadequate peak drug levels within the tubular lumen of the ascending loop of Henle to induce a maximal natriuresis.[109,110] Switching to an intravenous formulation obviates this problem (Table 16–4). Continuous intravenous infusions of loop diuretics may be particularly effective in some patients by providing continuously high intraluminal drug levels. Adding a second diuretic that acts at a site distal to the loop of Henle (e.g., Na,Cl symport inhibitors [thiazide class diuretics]) is also often effective, although rapid intravascular volume depletion and large K^+ losses can occur.

There is a shift of the sigmoid-shaped curve describing the relationship between the log of the diuretic concentration in the tubular lumen and its natriuretic effect in heart failure, as well as a lower maximal effect (Fig. 16–4).[109-111] This shift in the diuretic dose-response relationship has been termed "diuretic resistance" and is usually due to several contributing factors. Diuretic resistance should be distinguished from "diuretic adaptation" or the "braking" phenomenon that is observed even in normal subjects

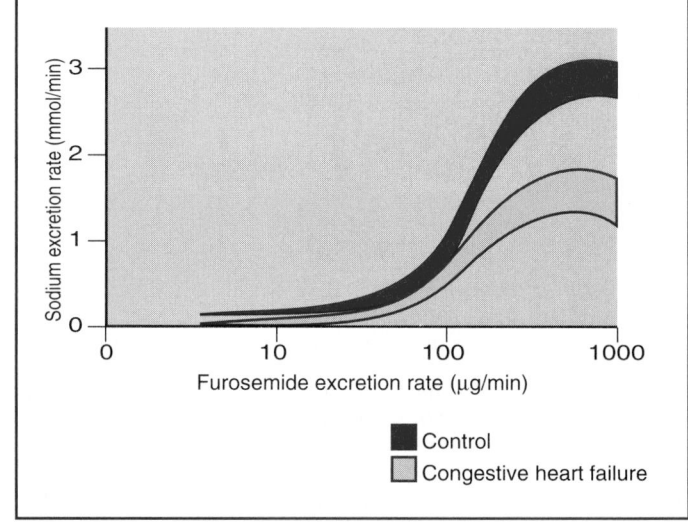

FIGURE 16–4. The relationship between urinary rate of excretion of furosemide and of sodium in normal subjects and in patients with congestive heart failure is shown. (Adapted from Knauf, H., and Matschler, E.: Functional state of the nephron and diuretic dose-response rationale for low dose combination therapy. *Cardiology* **84**(Suppl. 2):18, 1994.)

TABLE 16–4   MAXIMALLY EFFECTIVE ("CEILING") DOSES OF Na,K,2Cl SYMPORT INHIBITORS (LOOP DIURETICS)

	IV BOLUS DOSE (MG)		
	Furosemide	Bumetanide	Torsemide
Normal subjects	40	1	15–20
Congestive heart failure (normal GFR)	80–120	2–3	20–30
Renal insufficiency			
Moderate	80	3	60
Severe	200	10	200

GFR = glomerular filtration rate.
Adapted from Brater, D.C.: Diuretic resistance: Mechanisms and therapeutic strategies. Cardiology 84(Suppl 2):57–67, 1994.

given multiple doses of a short-acting loop diuretic.[112] Diuretic-induced alterations in intrarenal hemodynamics, due to tubuloglomerular feedback and increased sympathetic-nerve activity, among other possible mechanisms, result in avid renal sodium retention by all nephron segments as intraluminal drug levels decline. This is now known to be due in part to hypertrophy of the tubular epithelium distal to the site of action of the loop diuretics, increasing the solute resorptive capacity of the kidney, as well as other adaptive mechanisms.[109,112,113]

The cause of apparent resistance to diuretics in patients who had achieved initially an acceptable natriuretic response and weight loss may be multifactorial. In the absence of an abrupt decline in cardiac or renal function, and if patient noncompliance with either the drug regimen or dietary salt restriction can be excluded, then the usual reason for diuretic resistance is the concurrent administration of other drugs. All nonsteroidal anti-inflammatory drugs (NSAIDs), including aspirin, can diminish diuretic efficacy. Most commonly, increasing doses of vasodilators, with or without a marked decline in intravascular volume due to concomitant diuretic therapy, is the cause of diuretic resistance.

It is often difficult to distinguish clinically between intravascular volume depletion following aggressive diuretic and vasodilator therapy and a decrease in cardiac output due to primary cardiac failure, although a more marked decline in urea clearance than in creatinine clearance suggests intravascular volume depletion. Pulmonary arterial and venous or left atrial pressure monitoring may be required to make this distinction. In addition, all vasodilators commonly employed as afterload-reducing agents in heart failure dilate a number of central and peripheral vascular beds, directing blood flow away from the kidney. Therefore, renal blood flow may be reduced despite a moderate increase in cardiac output, resulting in a decline in diuretic effectiveness.

Acid-Base and Electrolyte Disorders in Heart Failure: Complications of Diuretic Therapy

POTASSIUM HOMEOSTASIS.   All of the diuretics discussed in this chapter, with the possible exception of V_2 vasopressin receptor antagonists, affect renal potassium handling.[112] In patients with congestive heart failure, both hypokalemia due to potassium-wasting diuretics and hyperkalemia due to potassium supplements administered with a potassium-sparing diuretic or a renin-angiotensin system antagonist may contribute to morbidity and mortality. Renal potassium losses due to diuretic use can be exacerbated by the hyperaldosteronism characteristic of patients with untreated heart failure and by the persistent chloride depletion and metabolic alkalosis that follows chronic use of loop diuretics. Long-term infusion of heparin, conversely, reduces aldosterone synthesis and may cause hyperkalemia, particularly in patients with insulin-dependent diabetes

and in patients receiving potassium replacement and/or potassium-sparing drugs.

Despite the absence of conclusive data to determine whether routine administration of potassium supplements and/or potassium-sparing diuretics reduces serious morbidity or mortality in the treatment of patients with either primary hypertension or congestive heart failure, the standard of care, as represented by recent editorials and review articles on this topic, recommends that the serum K^+ be maintained between 3.5 and 5.0 mEq/liter.[114–116] This recommendation stems from the concern that alone among the major class of drugs used in the treatment of heart failure, the efficacy and safety of routine diuretic use has not been subjected to the rigors of prospective, randomized, and placebo-controlled clinical trials.[117,118] With the recognition that such trials would be practically impossible for all but asymptomatic patients with ventricular dysfunction, guidelines for potassium replacement and the other potential metabolic consequences of diuretic therapy must be established based on limited and potentially biased data.[119] Despite this limitation, the majority of the data that are available, much of it obtained from retrospective or subgroup analysis of clinical trials evaluating diuretic use in hypertension, is reassuring.[119–123] In addition to hypokalemia, it should also be emphasized that hyperkalemia also is a cause of morbidity in heart failure patients. Potassium supplements may not be necessary in patients receiving an ACE inhibitor with a diuretic. Automatic, "sliding-scale" prescriptions for potassium supplementation in hospitalized patients should not be used owing to the risk of severe hyperkalemia and cardiac arrhythmias.

HYPOMAGNESEMIA.   Unlike urinary excretion of calcium, which is enhanced only by loop diuretics in volume-replete subjects, urinary magnesium wasting occurs with both thiazide and loop diuretics (although predominantly the latter), although not with potassium-sparing diuretics.[124,125] Magnesium deficiency is more commonly detected in patients with poor dietary magnesium intake (e.g., the elderly) and increased renal magnesium wasting due to diuretics as well as in patients with a history of a lengthy exposure to other drugs that exacerbate renal magnesium loss, including most commonly ethyl alcohol, but also cyclosporine, cisplatin, amphotericin B, and certain aminoglycoside antibiotics, including gentamicin and tobramycin.[124–126]

As emphasized by Leier et al.[114] and by Davies and Fraser,[127] despite a large and growing literature focusing on the importance of hypomagnesemia in diuretic use in heart failure, the absence of consistent use of a reliable test for magnesium deficiency and the reporting of data from poorly controlled, small, and statistically underpowered trials, have done little more than to further confuse this issue.

Unfortunately, the serum magnesium does not correlate well with other measures for determining magnesium homeostasis, as would be expected for this divalent cation that is largely bound to intracellular buffers or to bone (31 per cent and 67 per cent, respectively, of total body magnesium) with only approximately 1 per cent in the extracellular space. Although skeletal and cardiac muscle biopsies and/or measurements of free or total magnesium in circulating mononuclear cells are more reliable than serum magnesium levels, these measures are not readily available. The magnesium loading test is a reliable indicator of magnesium wasting in chronic malabsorption or renal magnesium losses due to intrinsic tubular defects. Nevertheless, the test requires careful patient compliance and has not been validated in the case of diuretic use. Newer techniques that measure either free or total magnesium in peripheral blood leukocytes are sufficiently sensitive and appear to be reliable indicators of total body magnesium depletion but are not yet widely available.

These issues notwithstanding, serial measurements of serum magnesium in a given patient reflect changes in total body magnesium homeostasis. For the clinician, a high index of suspicion (for example, a cachectic, elderly congestive heart failure patient receiving chronic loop diuretic therapy) coupled with a low normal serum magnesium level is sufficient to warrant beginning magnesium replacement therapy. If the total urinary magnesium excretion is less than 1 mEq/day (in the absence of diuretics), this also strongly increases the likelihood of significant magnesium depletion.

For the treatment of documented magnesium deficiency, which usually is found with concomitant potassium deficiency, enteric-coated $MgCl_2$ tablets, up to 32 mEq/day, may be safely given for a period of several months. Both epithelial Na^+ channel inhibitors and aldosterone receptor antagonists (potassium-sparing diuretics) reduce renal magnesium wasting caused by loop diuretics. By virtue of their antialdosterone activity, renin-angiotensin system antagonists also decrease diuretic-induced magnesium losses.

HYPONATREMIA.   This is a common complication of diuretic therapy in patients with congestive heart failure. The origin of hyponatremia in these patients is multifactorial and includes diuretic-induced defects in renal diluting ability, inappropriately high vasopressin levels due to a reduced cardiac output, and elevated intracerebral angiotensin II levels, leading to excessive thirst. Hyponatremic patients tend to have a high plasma renin activity, elevated plasma norepinephrine and epinephrine levels, and reduced renal plasma flow compared with nonhyponatremic (≥ 135 mEq/liter) patients. Mild hyponatremia (between 120 and 135 mEq/liter) generally responds to fluid restriction below urinary and insensible losses, usually less than 1500 ml/day, coupled with moderate (not severe) salt restriction. More severe hyponatremia (< 120 mEq/liter) should be treated more rapidly but cautiously, with a combination of a loop diuretic and administration of 0.9 per cent NaCl (or, rarely, 3 per cent NaCl) administered intravenously. This may require concomitant monitoring of cardiac filling pressures. Administration of a loop diuretic transiently diminishes the kidney's ability to sustain a hypertonic medullary interstitium, thereby diminishing water reabsorption in the collecting duct. This results in a diuresis that is approximately isotonic with the patient's own plasma. Combined therapy with an ACE inhibitor and a loop diuretic may often result in improved control of hyponatremia in heart failure patients.

ACID-BASE DISTURBANCES. Because diuretics are commonly used in patients who may have multiple metabolic and respiratory acid-base problems, the contribution of diuretics to the clinical problem requires careful analysis. Of importance is the assessment of intravascular volume status; this may require invasive hemodynamic monitoring, particularly in edematous heart failure patients continuously treated with diuretics who display signs and symptoms of intravascular volume depletion and who have a hypochloremic metabolic alkalosis. Severe intravascular volume depletion with a marked hypochloremic alkalosis may require the administration of intravenous saline, with concurrent potassium and magnesium supplementation. Carbonic anhydrase inhibitors in relatively small doses (e.g., acetazolamide, 250 mg twice daily) may gradually reverse the metabolic alkalosis if a saline infusion is contraindicated, although potassium and magnesium repletion is still required.

ADVERSE EFFECTS OF DIURETIC THERAPY

CARBOHYDRATE INTOLERANCE. For many years, Na,Cl symport inhibitors (thiazide class diuretics) have been known to induce a mild form of carbohydrate intolerance, with the development of the typical clinical pattern of adult-onset diabetes in those individuals genetically predisposed to this disease. Ketoacidosis is rare in these patients, although nonketotic hyperosmolar coma may develop in volume-depleted type II diabetics receiving Na,Cl symport inhibitors. Although the development of clinically important diabetes may be unusual, it is now clear that some degree of insulin resistance can be documented in many patients receiving drugs of this diuretic class. Repletion of potassium losses has been shown to improve carbohydrate tolerance in more severely potassium-depleted patients.

HYPERLIPIDEMIA. Since the early 1980's, studies on the drug therapy of hypertension have documented an unfavorable effect of thiazide class diuretics on plasma lipid levels. Low-dose thiazide diuretic therapy had less impact on serum lipids than high doses as determined in a metaanalysis that examined the safety and efficacy of antihypertensive drugs, but the hyperlipidemic effect persisted, particularly in African-Americans and in men.[128] Nevertheless, advocates for the thiazide class diuretics, noting their proven efficacy and minimal side effect profile, particularly in older patients, and relative safety and low cost, question whether the modest changes in total cholesterol, triglyceride levels, and/or LDL-cholesterol of, at most, 1 to 5 per cent using low-dose diuretics, are of clinical importance.[118–122,129] Also, alpha₁-antagonists such as prazosin or terazosin (which have additive antihypertensive effects when prescribed with thiazide diuretics), as well as ACE inhibitors, appear to minimize or reverse the hyperlipidemic effects of the thiazides, whereas beta-adrenergic antagonists do not.

Diuretics and Renal Insufficiency

Many patients with congestive heart failure manifest some degree of renal insufficiency as a consequence of hy-

pertensive glomerulosclerosis and/or atherosclerotic disease.[130] The pharmacokinetics of many drugs in common use in cardiovascular medicine are affected by a decline in renal function.[131] Renal dysfunction necessarily results in a decline in efficacy of diuretics. The loop diuretics remain the most effective class of diuretics in chronic renal failure, although their effectiveness is diminished by both pharmacokinetic and pharmacodynamic mechanisms. One useful approach to establishing an effective dose of a loop diuretic in congestive heart failure patients with chronic renal failure is to double the intravenous dose successively (i.e., from 40 mg furosemide, 1 mg bumetanide, or 20 mg torsemide intravenously) until a plateau is reached in NaCl excretion and urine volume (Table 16–4). Further increases in dose do not yield any greater immediate diuresis, although the duration of the natriuretic effect may be extended. The frequency of oral dosing can usually be diminished because of the prolonged elimination half-life of these drugs in chronic renal failure.

EXTRACORPOREAL ULTRAFILTRATION

In refractory heart failure, extracorporeal ultrafiltration has a place as a useful and relatively safe mechanism for removing fluid and electrolytes in a controlled fashion, whether or not there is underlying renal insufficiency.[132,133] Ultrafiltration also usually avoids the adverse hemodynamic effects of hemodialysis that can be difficult to manage in patients with heart failure and underlying ischemic heart disease. Ultrafiltration is far less effective in relieving symptoms attributable to uremia per se than is hemodialysis but is very effective in removing solutes and water.

Concurrent invasive hemodynamic monitoring is desirable, especially in unstable patients. Careful monitoring of plasma electrolytes and the hematocrit, which should not exceed 50 per cent, is required. Replacement electrolyte solutions are usually not necessary unless removal of intravascular volume has been excessive, or a specific electrolyte defect is being corrected (e.g., hyponatremia or hypokalemia). An improved response to diuretics has been reported following ultrafiltration, an effect that might be due to an improved cardiac output and reduced intracardiac filling pressures with a subsequent decline in the neurohumoral sodium-retaining signals to the kidney.

CARDIAC GLYCOSIDES

The chemical structure of this venerable class of drugs includes a steroid nucleus containing an unsaturated lactone at the C_{17} position and one or more glycosidic residues at C_3. Examples are found in a large number of plants and several toad species, typically serving as a venom or toxin that alters the future behavior of predators. William Withering's 1785 monograph contains the first comprehensive description of digitalis glycosides in the treatment of congestive heart failure.[134] This treatise describes the therapeutic efficacy and toxicities of the leaves of the common foxglove plant, *Digitalis purpurea*. Other digitalis glycosides are derived from the leaves of *Digitalis lanata* (digitoxin and digoxin), and from the seeds of *Strophanthus gratus* (ouabain). "Digitalis glycoside" and "cardiac glycoside" are often used interchangeably, although "cardiac glycoside" is the more inclusive term and "digitalis glycoside" should be reserved for compounds derived from *Digitalis* species. Digoxin is now the most commonly prescribed cardiac glycoside owing to its convenient pharmacokinetics, alternative routes of administration, and the widespread availability of serum drug level measurements. Both deslanoside, a rapidly acting agent available only for parenteral use, and digitoxin continue to be marketed in the United States.

Mechanisms of Action

INHIBITION OF MONOVALENT CATION ACTIVE TRANSPORT. All cardiac glycosides are potent and selective inhibitors of the active transport of Na^+ and K^+ across cell membranes. These drugs bind to specific high-affinity sites on the extracytoplasmic face of the alpha subunit of Na^+,K^+-ATPase, the enzymatic equivalent of the cellular "sodium pump."[135] The affinity of the alpha subunit for cardiac glycosides varies among species and among the three known mammalian alpha subunit isoforms, each of which is encoded by a separate gene.

The presence of the ouabain binding site on the alpha subunit of Na^+,K^+-ATPase has led to speculation that endogenous ouabain-like hormones or locally acting substances might exist that would serve as a regulatory ligand for the enzyme.[136] We have suggested the alternative possibility that the evolutionary persistence of the ouabain binding site could be due to a requirement for a specific amino acid sequence and conformation of the enzyme necessary for successful ion translocation, but which has also provided a target for evolutionary selection favoring certain plants and toads by serving as a means of poisoning animal predators.[137,138] There is evidence from site-directed mutagenesis studies that the affinity of Na^+,K^+-ATPase for cardiac glycosides is determined by the amino acid composition of the first transmembrane domain and the extracellular domain between the first and second (i.e., H_1 and H_2) transmembrane domains, and also the extracellular loop between the H_7 and H_8 transmembrane domains.[139]

Cardiac glycoside binding to and inhibition of the Na^+,K^+-ATPase sodium pump is reversible and entropically driven. Under physiological conditions these drugs bind preferentially to the enzyme following phosphorylation of a beta-aspartate on the cytoplasmic face of the alpha subunit, thus stabilizing this "E_2P" conformation.[135] Extracellular K^+ promotes dephosphorylation at this site as a step in this cation's active transport into the cytosol, accompanied by a decrease in the cardiac glycoside–binding affinity of the enzyme. This presumably explains why increased extracellular K^+ tends to reverse some manifestations of digitalis toxicity.

POSITIVE INOTROPIC EFFECT. For over 70 years cardiac glycosides have been known to increase the velocity and extent of shortening of cardiac muscle, resulting in a shift upward and to the left of the ventricular function (Frank-Starling) curve relating stroke work to filling volume or pressure. This occurs in normal as well as failing myocardium and in atrial as well as ventricular muscle. The effect appears to be sustained for periods of weeks or months without evidence of desensitization or tolerance.[140] This positive inotropic effect is due to an increase in the availability of cytosolic Ca^{++} during systole, thus increasing the velocity and extent of sarcomere shortening. This increase in intracellular Ca^{++} is a consequence of cardiac glycoside–induced inhibition of the sarcolemmal Na^+,K^+-ATPase.

Na^+ and Ca^{++} ions enter the cardiac muscle cell during each cycle of depolarization, contraction, and repolarization (Fig. 16–5 and Fig. 12–14, p. 370). Following activation of the fast Na^+ channel and the consequent depolarization, Ca^{++} enters the cell via the L-type Ca^{++} channel and triggers the release of additional Ca^{++} into the cytosol from the sarcoplasmic reticulum (SR). During repolarization and relaxation, Ca^{++} is again sequestered in the SR by a Ca^{++}-ATPase and is also extruded from the cell by the Na^+-Ca^{++} exchanger and by a sarcolemmal Ca^{++}-ATPase. Because the capacity of the Na^+-Ca^{++} exchanger to extrude Ca^{++} from the cell depends on the intracellular Na^+ activity, binding of a cardiac glycoside to the sarcolemmal Na^+,K^+-ATPase and inhibition of sodium pump activity reduces the rate of active Na^+ extrusion and cytosolic Na^+ content rises. This reduces the transmembrane Na^+ gradient driving the extrusion of intracellular Ca^{++} and more Ca^{++} is taken up by the SR and is available to activate contraction during the subsequent cell depolarization cycle. Evidence supporting this mechanism is available from studies using radionuclide tracers, cation-selective microelectrodes, and intracellular aequorin or ion-sensitive fluorescent dyes. Widespread acceptance of this mechanism of action awaited demonstration that small changes in intracellular Na^+ activity are accompanied by substantial increases in developed tension.[135,141]

ACTIONS ON VASCULAR SMOOTH MUSCLE. Alterations in peripheral arteriolar vascular smooth muscle Na^+-Ca^{++} exchange induced by cardiac glycosides have also been implicated as a mechanism by which these drugs could directly increase vascular tone and systemic vascular resistance, a rationale also promoted to link an endogenous circulating "digoxin-like" hormone to the pathogenesis of hypertension. Although this effect may occur transiently in normal humans following rapid increases in blood levels with bolus doses, no evidence exists that cardiac glycosides in the standard doses employed clinically affect blood pressure directly or "sensitize" the vasculature to endogenous or exogenous vasoconstrictors.[142] Indeed, as discussed below, digoxin administered chronically to patients with heart failure may decrease peripheral vascular resistance by decreasing centrally mediated sympathetic nervous system tone.

CARDIAC ENERGETICS. The immediate positive inotropic effect of cardiac glycosides, measured either in the intact heart in a conscious dog model or in isometrically contracting papillary muscle strips, is achieved with remarkable energy transfer efficiency and little oxygen wasting.[143,144] When compared with a beta-adrenergic agonist or a

FIGURE 16–5. Selected components regulating cellular calcium homeostasis in cardiac myocytes. Structures on the left side of the diagram depict pathways of transmembrane calcium entry. From the upper left, the L-type calcium channel, a voltage-sensitive protein complex, carries the slow inward calcium current during phase 2 of the cardiac action potential and provides the pulse of intracellular calcium that triggers calcium-induced release of a larger amount of activator calcium from stores in the sarcoplasmic reticulum (SR). The arrow indicates the principal direction of ion movement when the channel is activated. Depolarization of the cell, activating this voltage-sensitive calcium channel, occurs by opening of the fast sodium channel (not shown).

In the center of the diagram is shown the SR with its ATP-driven calcium pump on the left and the calcium release channel on the right. On the right side of the diagram are shown the pathways for calcium extrusion across the sarcolemmal membrane, including the Ca-ATP-ase that pumps calcium from cardiac cells against a large electrochemical gradient and helps to maintain the low levels of free intracellular calcium that prevail during diastole. The Na^+-Ca^{2+} exchanger extrudes calcium from the cell in exchange for Na^+ entry under conditions of normal diastolic repolarization of the cell and constitutes the main route of Ca^{2+} extrusion. Arrows or concentrations shown in color denote pathways that increase or decrease in magnitude in the presence of cardiac glycosides.

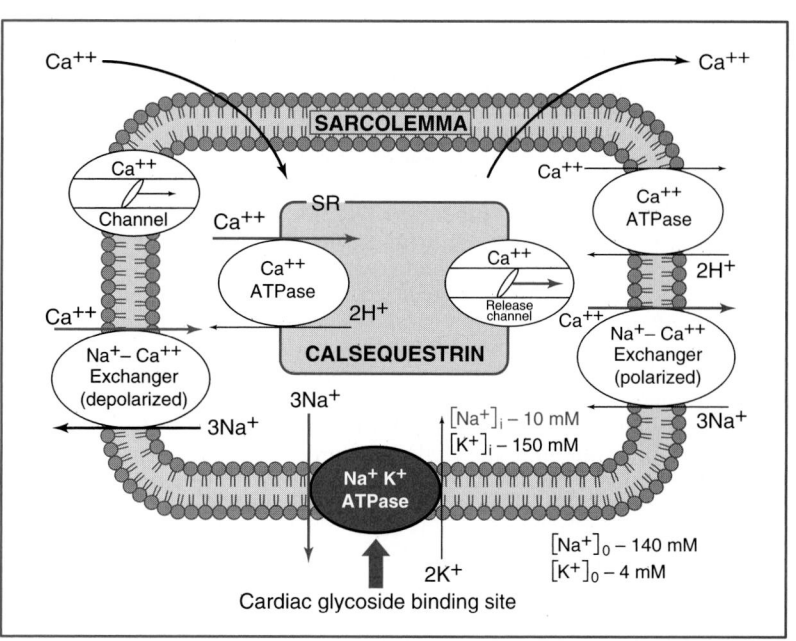

cAMP phosphodiesterase inhibitor, ouabain caused no significant change for the same degree of tension development in the tension-time integral per unit initial heat, an index of the economy of isometric contraction in an isolated muscle preparation.[144]

With chronic administration of cardiac glycosides, it has been argued that the increase in cardiac output that accompanies the positive inotropic effect would eventually lead to reduced oxygen consumption as ventricular chamber size and pressures decline and wall stress diminishes. These new data indicate that, even in the short term, cardiac glycosides provide a moderate and metabolically efficient inotropic effect. This is an important consideration in patients with ischemic cardiomyopathies. Excessive increases in intracellular Ca^{++} are believed to contribute to cardiac glycoside toxicity when Ca^{++} overload results in spontaneous cycles of Ca^{++} release and reuptake. This may lead to Ca^{++}-induced activation of inward Ca^{++} current, resulting in transient late depolarizations (afterdepolarizations) that may be accompanied by after contractions and likely contribute to toxic electrophysiological effects.

OTHER INOTROPIC MECHANISMS. Other mechanisms that may contribute to the inotropic actions of cardiac glycosides include increased cytosolic Ca^{++} acting as a positive feedback signal to increase Ca^{++} entry through sarcolemmal L-type Ca^{++} channels. Cardiac glycosides have also been reported to increase Ca^{++}-triggered Ca^{++} release via cardiac (but not skeletal) muscle SR Ca^{++} release channels in isolated SR vesicles due to an increased probability of channel openings (not increased single channel conductance) when cardiac glycosides in nanomolar concentrations were present at the cytosolic face of oriented SR vesicle preparations inserted into planar lipid membranes.[145] Finally, experimental evidence indicates that cardiac glycosides may facilitate the release of norepinephrine from postganglionic receptor nerves through a Ca^{++}-dependent exocytotic process and inhibit norepinephrine reuptake, effects that could contribute to the drug's positive inotropic effect.[146]

REGULATION OF SYMPATHETIC NERVOUS SYSTEM ACTIVITY. Heart failure is often accompanied by an increase in sympathetic nervous system activity due, in part, to a reduction in the sensitivity of the arterial baroreflex response to blood pressure. This results in a decline in tonic baroreflex suppression of central nervous system–directed sympathetic activity. This loss of sensitivity of the normal baroreflex arc also appears to contribute to the sustained elevation in plasma norepinephrine, renin, and vasopressin levels characteristic of heart failure.

Mason et al.[147] observed that intravenous ouabain increased mean arterial pressure, forearm vascular resistance, and venous tone in normal human subjects, probably due to direct but transient effects on vascular smooth muscle (see above). In contrast, patients with heart failure responded with a decline in heart rate and other effects that were consistent with enhanced baroreflex responsiveness. Direct effects of cardiac glycosides on carotid baroreflex responsiveness to changes in carotid sinus pressure have been reported in isolated baroreceptor preparations from animals with experimentally induced heart failure.[148] Ferguson et al.[149] further demonstrated in patients with moderate to severe heart failure that infusion of deslanoside increased forearm blood flow and cardiac index and decreased heart rate, concomitant with a marked decrease in skeletal muscle sympathetic nerve activity measured as an indicator of centrally mediated sympathetic nervous system.

In an uncontrolled prospective study of 26 ambulatory patients with minimal to moderate (NYHA class I to III) heart failure, plasma norepinephrine levels declined significantly and analyses of heart rate variability before and after chronic therapy with digoxin revealed an increase in parasympathetic nervous system activity, consistent with decreased central sympathetic nervous system drive.[150]

Additional central and peripheral autonomic nervous system effects can be elicited by cardiac glycosides and include fatigue, malaise, abnormal dreams, anorexia, abdominal pain, and an enhanced respiratory drive to hypoxia. Psychiatric side effects of digitalis administration are uncommon with contemporary formulations and doses of these drugs.[151]

ELECTROPHYSIOLOGICAL ACTIONS (see also p. 500). Atrial and ventricular muscle and specialized cardiac pacemaker and conduction fibers differ in their responses and sensitivity to cardiac glycosides. These responses represent the sum of the direct effects on cardiac cells added to indirect,

neurally mediated effects. At usual therapeutic serum concentrations (1.0 to 1.5 ng/ml), digoxin usually decreases automaticity and increases maximal diastolic resting membrane potential in atrial and atrioventricular (AV) nodal cells owing to augmented vagal tone and decreased sympathetic nervous system activity. This is accompanied by a prolongation of the effective refractory period and decreased AV nodal conduction velocity. At higher digoxin levels or in the presence of underlying disease, this may cause sinus bradycardia or arrest, prolongation of AV conduction, or heart block.

At toxic levels cardiac glycosides can increase sympathetic nervous system activity, potentially contributing to the generation of arrhythmias. Increased intracellular Ca^{++} loading and increased sympathetic tone both contribute to an increased rate of spontaneous (phase 4) diastolic depolarization and also to delayed afterdepolarizations (Fig. 16–5) that may reach threshold and generate propagated action potentials. The combination of increased automaticity and depressed conduction in the His-Purkinje network predisposes to arrhythmias, including ventricular tachycardia and fibrillation.

Pharmacokinetics and Dosing of Digoxin

The half-life for digoxin elimination of 36 to 48 hours in patients with normal or near-normal renal function permits once-a-day dosing. In the absence of loading doses, near steady-state blood levels are achieved in four to five half-lives, or about 1 week after initiation of maintenance therapy if normal renal function is present. Digoxin is largely excreted unchanged, with a clearance rate proportional to the GFR, resulting in the excretion of approximately one-third of body stores daily. In patients with heart failure and reduced cardiac reserve, increased cardiac output and renal blood flow in response to treatment with vasodilators or sympathomimetic agents may increase renal digoxin clearance, necessitating dosage adjustment. Digoxin is not removed effectively by peritoneal dialysis or hemodialysis because of its large (4 to 7 liter/kg) volume of distribution. The principal body reservoir is skeletal muscle and not adipose tissue. Accordingly, dosing should be based on estimated lean body mass. Neonates and infants tolerate and may require higher doses of digoxin for an equivalent therapeutic effect than older children or adults. Digoxin crosses the placenta and drug levels in maternal and umbilical vein blood are similar.

TABLE 16–5 FACTORS THAT ALTER PATIENT SENSITIVITY TO CARDIAC GLYCOSIDES

Serum electrolyte and acid-base disturbances
  ↑ Hypokalemia
  ↑ Hypomagnesemia
  ↑ Hypercalcemia
  ↑ Acidosis (typically respiratory)
  ↓ Hyperkalemia (may provoke AV block, however)

Thyroid status
  ↑ Hypothyroidism
  ↓ Hyperthyroidism

Underlying heart disease
  ↑ Ischemic cardiomyopathy
  ↑ Amyloid cardiomyopathy

Autonomic nervous system activity
  ↓ High sympathetic nervous system activity (but may exacerbate digoxin-induced arrhythmias)
  ↑ High parasympathetic (vagal) activity

Abnormal renal function
  Decreases digoxin clearance
  Decreases digoxin volume of distribution

Drug interactions (see Table 16–6)

Arrows indicate increased (↑) or decreased (↓) sensitivity to toxic effects of cardiac glycosides.

TABLE 16-6 DRUG INTERACTIONS WITH DIGOXIN

483

Ch 16

DRUG	MECHANISM	DIRECTION AND MAGNITUDE OF CHANGE IN BLOOD LEVEL	SUGGESTED CLINICAL MANAGEMENT
Cholestyramine, kaolin-pectin, neomycin, sulfasalazine	Decrease absorption	↓ 25%	Give 8 hr before digoxin, or use solution or gel form of digoxin
Antacids	Unclear	↓ 25%	Temporal dispersion of doses
Bran	Decreases absorption	↓ 25%	Temporal dispersion of doses
Propafenone, quinidine, verapamil, amiodarone	Decrease renal digoxin clearance, volume of distribution, or both	↑ 70–100%	Decrease digoxin by 50% and monitor serum digoxin levels as necessary
Thyroxine	Increases volume of distribution and renal clearance	Variable decreases in digoxin blood levels	Monitor serum digoxin levels
Erythromycin, omeprazole, tetracycline	Increase digoxin absorption	↑ 40–100%	Monitor serum digoxin levels
Albuterol	Increase volume of distribution	↓ 30%	Monitor serum digoxin levels
Captopril, diltiazem, nifedipine, nitrendipine	Variable moderate decrease in digoxin clearance and/or volume of distribution	Variable increase in blood levels	Monitor serum digoxin levels
Cyclosporine	May decrease renal function, and indirectly if renal function is impaired	Variable increase in blood levels	Monitor serum digoxin levels more frequently
Beta-blockers, verapamil, diltiazem, flecainide, disopyramide, bepridil	↓ SA or atrioventricular junctional conduction or automaticity		Monitor ECG for evidence of SA or AV block
Kaliuretic diuretics	Decreased serum and tissue K⁺ increases automaticity and promotes inhibition of Na, K-ATPase by digoxin		Monitor ECG for arrhythmias consistent with digoxin toxicity
Sympathomimetic drugs	Increase automaticity		Monitor ECG for arrhythmia
Verapamil, diltiazem, beta-adrenergic blocking agents	Diminish cardiac contractile state		Discontinue or lower dose of Ca⁺⁺ channel or beta-adrenergic antagonist

Current tablet preparations of digoxin average 70 to 80 per cent oral bioavailability, with elixir and encapsulated gel preparations approaching 90 to 100 per cent. Parenteral digoxin is available for intravenous use. Loading or maintenance doses can be given by intravenous injection, which should be carried out over at least 15 minutes to avoid vasoconstrictor responses to more rapid injection. Intramuscular digoxin is absorbed unpredictably, causes local pain, and is not recommended.

THERAPEUTIC DRUG MONITORING. Nomograms are available for estimating loading and maintenance doses of digoxin but are not widely used because of variability in individual patient responsiveness to cardiac glycosides and the ready availability in most clinical settings of serum digoxin concentration assays. Various clinical conditions and drug interactions that can alter digoxin's pharmacokinetics (Tables 16–5 and 16–6) are also reflected in the serum digoxin level. Reduced thyroid and renal function both decrease the volume of distribution of digoxin, necessitating downward adjustments in loading and maintenance doses. Hypochlorhydria (i.e., gastric pH > 7), which is common in elderly patients and patients receiving histamine H_2 receptor antagonists or gastric H^+,K^+-ATPase inhibitors, reduces gastric metabolism of digoxin and the nonrenal clearance of the drug.[152] This may lead to higher steady-state blood levels in these patients with reduced renal function, particularly in the elderly.

Table 16–5 lists disease states and alterations in plasma and tissue electrolytes that can change patient susceptibility to toxicity at any given dose or serum level of the drug. Both hypokalemia and hypercalcemia can independently increase ventricular automaticity and lower the threshold for digoxin-induced cardiac arrhythmias. Hypomagnesemia may also contribute to arrhythmias with digoxin. Hyperkalemia may exacerbate digoxin-induced conduction disorders and cause high-grade AV nodal block.

Studies using noninvasive indices of ventricular function suggest a nonlinear relation between the serum digoxin concentration and the observed inotropic effect, with the majority of the increase in contractility occurring by the time steady-state levels around 1.8 nmol/liter (1.4 ng/ml) are reached (Fig. 16–6). The relation of serum digoxin level to therapeutic effect is less clear in the control of the ventricular rate among patients with atrial fibrillation. The effectiveness of cardiac glycosides given as single agents in controlling ventricular rate during exercise is limited at doses and serum levels in the usual therapeutic range.

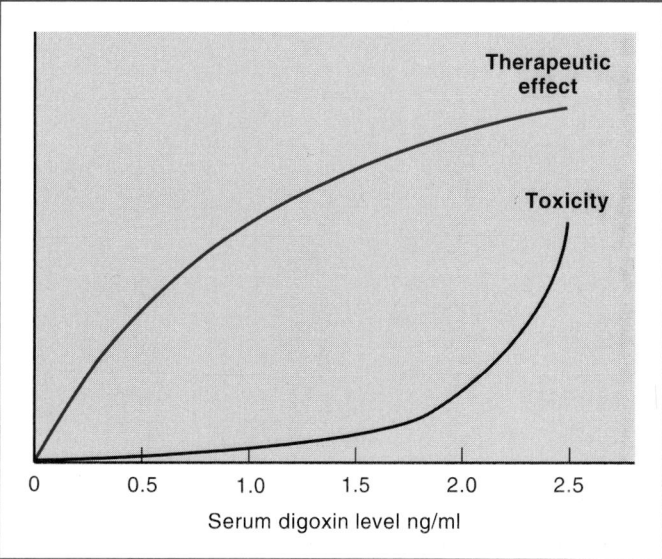

FIGURE 16–6. Schematic illustration of relationship between the therapeutic and toxic effects of digoxin and the serum digoxin level. Above a level of 1.8 nmol/L (1.5 ng/ml), there are minimal additional therapeutic effects and a substantial increase in the frequency of toxicity. (From Lewis, R. P.: Digitalis. *In* Leier, C. V. (ed.): Cardiotonic Drugs: A Clinical Survey. New York, Marcel Dekker, 1987, p. 85.)

Overt digitalis toxicity tends to emerge at two- to three-fold higher serum concentrations than the target 1.8 nmol/liter, but it must always be remembered that a substantial overlap of serum levels exists among patients exhibiting symptoms and signs of toxicity and those with no clinical evidence of intoxication. If ready access to serum digoxin assays is available, a reasonable approach to the initiation of therapy is to begin at 0.125 to 0.375 mg/day, depending on lean body mass and estimated creatinine clearance, and to measure a serum digoxin level 1 week later with careful monitoring of clinical status in the interim. Patients with impaired renal function will not yet have reached steady state and need to be monitored closely until four to five clearance half-lives have elapsed (as long as 3 weeks). Oral or intravenous loading with digoxin, although generally safe, is rarely necessary as other safer and more effective drugs exist for short-term inotropic support or for initial treatment of supraventricular arrhythmias.

Blood samples for serum digoxin level measurement should be taken at least 6 to 8 hours following the last digoxin dose. Serum level monitoring is justified in patients with substantially altered drug clearance rates or volumes of distribution (e.g., very old, debilitated, or very obese patients). Adequacy of digoxin dosing and risk of toxicity in a given patient should never be based on a single isolated serum digoxin concentration measurement.[153]

DIGITOXIN, OUABAIN, AND DESLANOSIDE. Digitoxin is the principal native cardiac glycoside present in digitalis leaf. It is the least polar and most slowly excreted of all available cardiac glycosides. Oral bioavailability approaches 100 per cent and is less affected by malabsorption syndromes than is digoxin. Unlike digoxin, digitoxin is about 97 per cent bound to albumin in normal plasma and is extensively metabolized in the liver with minimal renal clearance of the native glycoside. Displacement of digitoxin from plasma protein by some drugs, including warfarin, can occur but rarely results in clinically important changes in serum levels at usual digitoxin doses. The elimination half-life is 4 to 6 days irrespective of renal function, resulting in a stable steady-state level of drug 3 to 4 weeks after initiation of a daily maintenance dose. Therapeutic serum or plasma concentrations are about 10-fold higher than those of digoxin owing to serum protein binding.

Ouabain undergoes predominantly renal clearance, although some gastrointestinal excretion does occur, with an elimination half-life of 18 to 24 hours in normal subjects. Deslanoside also is cleared primarily by the kidney. The plasma half-life is similar to that of digoxin, permitting once-daily maintenance dosing.

DIGITALIS TOXICITY. Although the incidence and severity of digitalis intoxication are decreasing,[154,155] vigilance for this important complication of therapy is essential. Disturbances of cardiac impulse formation, conduction, or both are the hallmarks of digitalis toxicity. Among the common electrocardiographic manifestations are ectopic beats of AV junctional or ventricular origin, first-degree atrioventricular block, an excessively slow ventricular rate response to atrial fibrillation, or an accelerated AV junctional pacemaker. These manifestations may require only a dosage adjustment and monitoring as clinically appropriate. Sinus bradycardia, sinoatrial arrest or exit block, and second- or third-degree atrioventricular conduction delay often respond to atropine, but temporary ventricular pacing is sometimes necessary and should be available. Potassium administration is often useful for atrial, AV junctional, or ventricular ectopic rhythms, even when the serum potassium is in the normal range, unless high-grade atrioventricular block is also present. Magnesium may be useful in patients with atrial fibrillation and an accessory pathway in whom digoxin administration has facilitated a rapid accessory pathway–mediated ventricular response. Lidocaine or phenytoin, which in conventional doses have minimal effects on atrioventricular conduction, are useful in the management of worsening ventricular arrhythmias that threaten hemodynamic compromise. Electrical cardioversion can precipitate severe rhythm disturbances in patients with overt digitalis toxicity, and should be used with particular caution.

ANTIDIGOXIN IMMUNOTHERAPY. Potentially life-threatening digoxin or digitoxin toxicity can be reversed by antidigoxin immunotherapy. Purified Fab fragments from digoxin-specific antisera are available at most poison control centers and larger hospitals in North American and Europe. The smaller (molecular weight 50,000) Fab fragments have a larger volume of distribution, more rapid onset of action, and more rapid clearance as well as reduced immunogenicity than does intact IgG.[156] Clinical experience in adults and children has established the effectiveness and safety of antidigoxin Fab in treating life-threatening digoxin toxicity, including cases of massive ingestion with suicidal intent.[157] Doses of Fab are calculated on the basis of a simple formula based on either the estimated dose of drug ingested or the total body digoxin burden and are administered intravenously in saline over 30 to 60 minutes. Recrudescent digoxin toxicity is unusual but can occur 24 to 48 hours after Fab administration in patients with normal renal function, or later in patients with renal impairment.[156–158] The efficacy and cost-effectiveness of less than complete neutralizing doses of digoxin-specific Fab fragments for suspected or moderate cases of digoxin toxicity need further assessment.

PHOSPHODIESTERASE INHIBITORS

Agents such as theophylline, 3-isobutyl-l-methyl xanthine (IBMX), and caffeine have long been recognized as nonspecific cGMP and cAMP phosphodiesterase (PDE) inhibitors. PDE use in heart failure, however, awaited the 1980's when a number of PDE isoenzyme subclass-specific inhibitors became available. The isoenzyme classification scheme initially devised by Beavo and Reifsnyder[159] now includes at least seven distinct but related gene families based on known cDNA sequences. Tissue and cell-specific PDE isoenzyme distribution, as well as subcellular localization and links to specific cGMP- and cAMP-dependent signalling pathways, are increasingly being recognized.[160,161] There are important differences in expression of specific classes of PDE inhibitors in the same tissue among species and in the same species during development.[162] Any specificity of selective inhibitors for most PDE isoenzymes exists only within a relatively narrow concentration range, with increasingly nonspecific inhibition at higher concentrations.

AMRINONE AND MILRINONE. Parenteral formulations of amrinone and milrinone are approved for short-term support of the circulation in advanced heart failure. Although both drugs have excellent oral bioavailability, longer-term prospective trials of oral formulations of these agents showed a high incidence of side effects, exhibited minimal long-term efficacy, and in the doses used caused increased mortality in heart failure patients.[163–165] Both agents are bipyridine derivatives and relatively selective inhibitors of the low K_m cGMP-inhibited, cAMP PDE (type III) group. Both cause vasodilation with a consequent fall in systemic vascular resistance, and they are powerful positive inotropic agents; they increase contractile force and velocity of relaxation of cardiac muscle.

Amrinone or milrinone is often used in combination with other oral or intravenous drugs for short-term treatment of patients with severe heart failure due to systolic right or left ventricular dysfunction. These drugs are commonly employed as adjuvant therapy with a sympathomimetic amine, usually dobutamine, for circulatory support following cardiopulmonary bypass, or as alternative therapy for hospitalized patients who have developed tolerance to dobutamine.[165–167] Although both dobutamine and the bipyridines increased intracellular cAMP and are positively inotropic, there are important differences. Only dobutamine, for example, consistently decreased both diastolic left ventricular filling pressures and volume, whereas a type III PDE inhibitor caused only a decrease in diastolic filling pressure.[168,169]

Both drugs are initiated by an intravenous loading dose followed by a continuous infusion. For amrinone this is typically a 0.5 to 0.75 mg/kg bolus infusion over 2 to 3 minutes and then 2 to 20 μg/kg/min. Milrinone is about 10-fold more potent, with a typical loading dose of 50 μg/kg over 10 minutes and an infusion rate from 0.25 to 1.0 μg/kg/min. Half-lives of amrinone and milrinone clearance are 4 to 5 hours and 2 to 3 hours, respectively, and are approximately doubled in patients with advanced heart failure. Clinically significant thrombocytopenia is reported in about 10 per cent of patients receiving amrinone but is rare with milrinone. Because of its greater selectively for PDE III isoenzymes, shorter half-life, and fewer side effects, milrinone is the agent of choice among currently available PDE inhibitors for short-term parenteral inotropic support in severe heart failure.

VESNARINONE.* This orally active positive inotropic agent with vasodilator activity appears to act via multiple mechanisms. In addition to relatively selective inhibition of an isoform of a type III cAMP PDE present in human myocardial and kidney tissue, vesnarinone also affects sarcolemmal membrane voltage-activated sodium and potassium channels. This could contribute to the drug's positive inotropic action as well as exerting electrophysiological effects. The net effect is a decrease in heart rate and prolongation of action potential duration, opposite to the results observed with other class III PDE inhibitors.

Vesnarinone has also been reported to decrease production by lymphocytes of some inflammatory cytokines and exhibits viricidal activity in experimental animals and in vitro models.[170] Neutropenia (absolute granulocyte count <1000 mm³) is the most common important side effect of vesnarinone. The incidence in trials of vesnarinone in Europe and the United States has been approximately 3 per cent and several patients have died. The average daily dose of patients developing neutropenia was 60 mg/day and always occurred within the first 1 to 5 months of treatment.[171] Human recombinant granulocyte colony-stimulating factor (G-CSF) has been employed successfully in the treatment of severe neutropenia due to vesnarinone. Initially promising safety and efficacy data have been reported in heart failure patients for vesnarinone,[172] and trials are also underway for the related compound OPC-18790.*[173]

CALCIUM-SENSITIZING DRUGS

The classification of drugs as calcium-sensitizing agents refers to their ability to shift the relationship between the intracellular calcium concentration and the rate and extent of force development, producing increased force generation at any given intracellular calcium concentration. A calcium-sensitizing action of a drug can be detected and quantitated using several approaches; for example, force development in vitro over a range of Ca^{++} concentrations can be measured in skinned cardiac muscle fibers that have been made permeable to Ca^{++} using detergents. These drugs tend to be more energy efficient in generating increased force than agents that increase intracellular cAMP levels. This may prove advantageous in patients with heart failure due to an ischemic cardiomyopathy in whom cardiac ATP production is limited by O_2 delivery. However, these drugs may also adversely affect ventricular relaxation during diastole, an effect that depends on how Ca^{++}-sensitization is achieved and on which additional cardiovascular actions each drug may have.

PIMOBENDAN* AND SULMAZOLE.* Pimobendan and sulmazole have undergone extensive clinical testing in patients with heart failure.[174] Both inhibit type III cAMP PDEs and, like milrinone, are vasodilators. Unlike milrinone, these drugs also act as calcium sensitizers at clinically relevant concentrations. Pimobendan increased exercise tolerance and improved symptoms and quality of life in patients with heart failure in a series of relatively small prospective controlled trials.[175-177] However, these drugs, like milrinone, decreased survival in heart failure patients.

SIMENDAN* AND LEVOSIMENDAN.* Simendan is a type III PDE inhibitor that, like pimobendan, has also been shown to have Ca^{++}-sensitizing activity. This activity of racemic simendan was found to be due to its levo enantiomer, levosimendan, which is currently undergoing clinical testing. The cellular mechanisms by which levosimendan causes calcium sensitization are unknown, but recent data indicate that the drugs bind to a hydrophobic pocket on cardiac troponin C.[178]

---

* Not approved by the US Food and Drug Administration at the time of this writing.

In experimental animals, levosimendan decreased systemic vascular resistance and left ventricular end-diastolic pressure and increased myocardial contractility in a dose-dependent manner.[179,180] Importantly, the time constant of isovolumic relaxation and maximum segment lengthening velocity ($-dp/dt_{max}$) did not change significantly over a range of levosimendan concentrations.[180] This apparent lack of an effect on diastolic relaxation would not be predicted on the basis of the drug's Ca^{++}-sensitizing activity and may be due to its activity as a type III cAMP PDE inhibitor. Whether similar effects will be apparent in humans with heart failure is the subject of ongoing studies.

ADRENERGIC AND DOPAMINERGIC AGONISTS

A thorough grasp of the pharmacology of the peripheral adrenergic and dopaminergic signalling systems is essential to understanding the rationale for drug therapy of heart failure. Evidence for a generalized activation of the sympathetic nervous system in heart failure is reviewed on page 482. The reader is also referred to comprehensive reviews of the basic molecular pharmacology of G protein–linked receptors.[181-183]

A diminished cellular response to repeated or continuous administration of a drug or endogenous agonist is termed "desensitization" and represents a programmed response of the cell that typically involves several levels in the signal transduction sequence for that ligand. Desensitization for a given signalling pathway may be initiated by specific ligand-receptor signalling ("homologous desensitization") or by other endogenous agonists or drugs acting through different receptor pathways ("heterologous desensitization"). Desensitization of the beta-adrenergic signalling pathway has been the most extensively studied in heart failure[184-190] and is discussed on page 502.

DOBUTAMINE. This sympathomimetic amine is available for clinical use as a racemic mixture that stimulates both beta$_1$- and beta$_2$-adrenergic receptor subtypes and either binds but does not activate alpha-adrenergic receptors ([+] enantiomer) or stimulates alpha$_1$ and alpha$_2$ receptor subtypes ([−] enantiomer). Lower doses resulting in a clear positive inotropic effect in humans exert a predominant beta$_1$-adrenergic effect, while alpha-adrenergic agonist effects of the (−) enantiomer in the vasculature and myocardium appear to be blocked by the alpha receptor antagonist effect of the (+) enantiomer. Dobutamine does not stimulate dopaminergic receptors and unlike dopamine does not selectively alter renal blood flow (see below).

Racemic dobutamine also acts as a vasodilator to reduce aortic impedance and systemic vascular resistance, thus reducing afterload and improving ventricular-vascular coupling by reducing aortic impedance.[191-193] In contrast, dopamine may either have no effect or increase ventricular afterload by increasing systemic vascular resistance and by causing more rapid return of reflected aortic pressure waves, depending on the infusion rate of the drug. Therefore, dobutamine is preferable to dopamine for most patients with advanced heart failure who have not responded adequately to oral or intravenous vasodilators, digoxin, and diuretics.[193,194] Dobutamine infusions are initiated at 2 μg/kg/min and are titrated up according to a patient's hemodynamic response (usually not higher than 20 μg/kg/min; dosing is based on estimated lean body weight).

The importance of the vascular effects of dobutamine have been demonstrated by experiments in animals with an artificial (Jarvik 7) heart.[192] Even in the presence of a mechanical heart, dobutamine increased cardiac output by 10 to 15 per cent and decreased systemic vascular resistance. Interestingly, dobutamine also decreased venous capacitance and increased right atrial pressure, possibly owing to the alpha$_1$-adrenergic agonism of the (−) enantiomer. These experiments also demonstrated that the (+) enantiomer ("D-dobutamine") was responsible for the racemic drug's effects on aortic input impedance, wave reflectance, and systemic vascular resistance. These favorable actions on left ventricular afterload are also responsible for the reduction in functional mitral regurgitation often observed with dobutamine infusions in patients with large dilated ventricles and high left ventricular end-diastolic pressure.[195] Dobutamine also causes a decline in pulmonary vascular resistance that is present regardless of chronic background vasodilator therapy with organic nitrates, hydralazine, or captopril.

DOPAMINE. This endogenous catecholamine evokes vasodilatory responses by direct stimulation of dopaminergic D_1/D_5 postsynaptic as well as D_2 presynaptic receptors in the peripheral vasculature and on the luminal and basolateral membranes of renal tubular cells, particularly in the proximal tubule.[196] It causes relatively selective vasodilation of splanchnic and renal arterial beds at doses less than or equal to 2 μg/kg/min. This action may be useful in promoting renal blood flow and maintaining GFR in patients who become refractory to diuretics. At intermediate (2 to 10 μg/kg/min) infusion rates, dopamine enhances norepinephrine release from vascular sympathetic neurons, resulting in increased beta-adrenergic receptor activation in the heart. In patients with advanced heart failure, who often have depletion of intracardiac norepinephrine stores, dopamine may be a less effective positive inotropic drug than other direct-acting inotropes. At higher infusion rates (5 to 20 μg/kg/min) peripheral vasoconstriction occurs due to direct alpha-adrenergic receptor stimulation. Increases in systemic vascular resistance are common even at intermediate infusion rates. Tachycardia tends to be more pronounced than with dobutamine and may worsen systolic and diastolic function in patients with ischemic cardiomyopathies. Dose ranges noted above are based on estimated lean body weight rather than actual patient weight. Emergence of unexplained tachycardia or arrhythmias in a patient receiving "renal range" dopamine should raise the suspicion of an inappropriately high dopamine infusion rate.

DOPEXAMINE.* Dopexamine is a synthetic sympathomimetic agent designed as a dopamine analog for intravenous use that has a 60-fold higher affinity for beta$_2$ receptors than dopamine. Like dobutamine, dopexamine reduces pulmonary and systemic vascular resistance and has a positive inotropic effect at infusion rates of 0.25 μg/kg/min or higher.[197] Although dopexamine offers a hemodynamic profile that is intermediate between those of dobutamine and dopamine, no compelling evidence exists that this drug offers any important clinical advantages over the two older drugs.

ORAL DOPAMINE AGONISTS. Several orally bioavailable analogs of dopamine have been developed, including levodopa, fenoldopam,* and ibopamine.* Following absorption, ibopamine is converted into N-methyldopamine (epinine) and over 2 to 6 hours causes a gradual reduction in pulmonary and systemic vascular resistance.[198] Its use has been advocated in weaning patients off intravenous sympathomimetics while awaiting heart transplant.[199]

BETA-ADRENERGIC ANTAGONISTS

The development of intravenous and oral formulations of beta-adrenergic *agonists* for the support of the circulation in heart failure due to systolic ventricular dysfunction was based on the seemingly reasonable rationale that these drugs would improve contractile function and diastolic relaxation, much like endogenous catecholamines. However, results from clinical trials have indicated that beta-adrenergic agonists are not useful in the management of chronic heart failure and, except for temporary circulatory support in hospitalized patients, may actually be detrimental. In contrast, an increasing body of evidence indicates that beta-adrenergic *antagonists* improve symptoms, exercise tolerance, hemodynamics, and perhaps mortality in heart failure patients. Despite clinical and experimental animal data that these drugs have an initial negative inotropic effect and can worsen ventricular function, the introduction of beta-adrenergic antagonists in the treatment of heart failure has been based largely on empirical evidence from small observational studies.

---

* Not approved by the US Food and Drug Administration at the time of this writing.

PHARMACOLOGICAL CONSIDERATIONS (see also pp. 502 and 612). Beta-adrenergic antagonists are identified by their affinity for binding to beta-adrenergic receptors, which is sufficiently high to antagonize the binding of endogenous agonists (i.e., norepinephrine and epinephrine) at blood and tissue concentrations that do not cause other undesirable effects. Historically, these agents have been classified according to their relative selectivity for the beta$_1$- or beta$_2$-adrenergic receptors, their ability to bind other adrenergic receptors (usually alpha receptors), and their interactions with other molecular targets at clinically relevant doses (e.g., the K^+ channel antagonist activity of the [+]enantiomer of sotalol). In addition, many beta-adrenergic antagonists are characterized by their ability not only to prevent the binding of endogenous catecholamines but also to act as weak agonists (i.e., intrinsic sympathomimetic activity, or ISA), and also by chemical characteristics of the compound itself (e.g., lipophilicity) that determine the tissue distribution, oral bioavailability, and clearance mechanism(s) of each compound (Table 16–7).

This classification scheme recently has been made more complex with new evidence on the nature of drug binding to beta-adrenergic receptors. Although there has been evidence that cell-surface receptors linked to G protein signalling pathways might be capable of adapting an "active" conformation that initiates signal transduction even in the absence of agonist, conclusive proof has required the availability of experimental models in which the actions of endogenous catecholamines could be discounted or eliminated and which could exhibit an easily quantifiable biological signal. It is now known that the beta$_2$-adrenergic receptor appears to exist in equilibrium between two conformations, an inactive conformation (R) and an active conformation (R*). True agonists bind selectively to the R* conformation, stabilizing it and shifting the equilibrium toward the active signalling conformation, whereas "inverse agonists" favor the inactive conformation, shifting receptor equilibrium toward the conformation that does not initiate downstream signalling.[200,201] Neutral antagonists favor both conformations approximately equally, whereas partial agonists (i.e., beta-adrenergic antagonists with ISA) shift the binding equilibrium moderately toward the R* conformation.

Owing to their much higher affinities for the beta receptor than the endogenous catecholamines, all beta-adrenergic antagonists, regardless of whether they are "inverse agonists," neutral antagonists, or exhibit ISA, block the action of the endogenous catecholamines in vivo. Although the relevance of the distinction between neutral antagonists and drugs that exhibit inverse agonism for clinical cardiovascular pharmacology is not yet well defined, the acceptance of this model has broad implications for rational drug design beyond beta-adrenergic agonists and antagonists and is likely to be relevant to other G protein–coupled receptors.[201] Preliminary clinical data suggest that the distinction among agents with partial agonist, neutral antagonist, and inverse agonist properties also has clinical relevance.[202]

BETA BLOCKERS IN THE TREATMENT OF HEART FAILURE. In the 1970's, Waagstein and associates at the University of Göteberg in Sweden reported that the beta blockers alprenolol, metoprolol, and practolol improved symptoms and ventricular function over a period of several months in patients with mild to severe heart failure due to idiopathic dilated cardiomyopathy.[203] Although a number of smaller trials, many of which were not controlled, in the 1980's tended to support these observations, none was sufficiently large to provide definitive evidence regarding improvement in symptoms or exercise tolerance, or to have the statistical power to detect a change in mortality.[204–206]

Despite this accumulating evidence in support of the efficacy of long-term therapy with beta blockers in some patients with heart failure at the beginning of the 1990's, enthusiasm for this class of agents was clearly muted compared with that for ACE inhibitors and the promise of new classes of vasodilators and inotropic agents. This skepticism was reinforced by the early termination of the Xamoterol in Severe Heart Failure study, a beta-adrenergic antagonist with significant ISA properties, due to excess mortality in patients receiving active drug.[207,208] In addition, there has been no clear consensus as to why beta-adrenergic antagonists should be beneficial in heart failure. As reviewed by Bristow,[209] the characteristic downregulation of postsynaptic beta$_1$-adrenergic receptor in cardiac muscle

TABLE 16–7 PHARMACODYNAMIC PROPERTIES OF β-ADRENERGIC ANTAGONISTS

GENERIC NAME	PROPRIETARY NAME(S)	ADRENERGIC RECEPTOR SELECTIVITY	PARTIAL AGONISM (ISA)	INVERSE AGONISM‡	LIPID SOLUBILITY	VASODILATOR ACTIVITY	OTHER ACTIONS
Acebutol	Sectral	$+\beta_1$	+		+	+	
Atenolol	Tenormin	$+\beta_1$	0		0	0	
Betaxolol	Kerlone	$+\beta_1$	0		0		
Bevantolol*	—	$++\beta_1$	0		++	+	
Bisoprolol	Zebeta	$++\beta_1$	0		+	0	
Bucindolol*		$\beta_1\beta_2$	0		0	++	"Direct" vasodilator
Carteolol	Cartrol	$\beta_1\beta_2$	++		0	0	
Carvedilol	—	$(+)\beta_1, \alpha_1$	0	+	+	++	
Celiprolol*		$+\beta_1$	+		0	+	
Esmolol	Brevibloc	$+\beta_1$	0		0	+	
Labetalol	Trandate, Normodyne	$\beta_1, \beta_2\alpha_1$	0		++	++	
Metoprolol	Lopressor	$+\beta_1$	0	++	++	0	
Nadolol	Corgard	β_1, β_2	0		0	0	
Nebivelol*		$+\beta_1$	0		0	+	"Direct" vasodilator
Oxprenolol*	Trasicor	$\beta_1\beta_2$	++		+	0	
Penbutolol	Levatol	$\beta_1\beta_2$	++		+++	0	
Pindolol	Visken	$\beta_1\beta_2$	++		0		
Propranolol	Inderal	$\beta_1\beta_2$	0	++	+++	0	
Sotalol	Betapace	$\beta_1\beta_2$	0		0	0	Class III antiarrhythmic
Timolol	Blocadren	$\beta_1\beta_2$	0	+++	0	0	

ISA = Intrinsic sympathomimetic activity; + = mild effect; ++ = moderate effect; +++ = marked effect.

* Not approved by the US Food and Drug Administration at the time of this writing.

‡ Inverse agonism—the ability to bind and stabilize the inactive conformation of G protein–linked receptors—has not been well defined for beta-adrenergic antagonists to date in the context of human cardiovascular pharmacology. Adapted from Antman, E. M., and Kelly, R. A.: Pharmacological therapy of cardiac arrhythmias. *In* Antman, E. M., and Rutherford, J. D. (eds): Coronary Care Medicine: A Practical Approach. Norwell, MA, Kluwer Academic Press, 1996.

and moderate uncoupling of beta$_2$-adrenergic receptors could be viewed as an adaptive response of cardiac muscle that was designed to minimize the potential toxicity of high levels of catecholamines. However, this adaptation also compromises the ability of the heart to respond to appropriate increases in adrenergic tone, as with exercise.

The results of clinical trials in the 1990's (see p. 503), have tended to support the efficacy of these drugs in heart failure, although the mechanism(s) is not clear. It is not yet known, for example, whether long-term administration of beta-adrenergic antagonists increases beta receptor number in humans. Other mechanisms also may be operative that could increase the extent of activation of adenylate cyclase by endogenous beta-adrenergic agonists.[210] Thus, chronic beta-adrenergic antagonist administration could result in changes at a number of levels in the adrenergic signalling cascade that would favor improved cardiac function. There also is evidence that the favorable actions of these drugs in heart failure may be due to improved ventricular-arterial coupling, due in part to a decline in heart rate, but also a decrease in peak left ventricular end-systolic pressure and arterial elastance that reduces afterload.[211] Also, patients with idiopathic dilated cardiomyopathy receiving metoprolol had an increase in myocardial lactate extraction with exercise, suggesting either reduced ischemia and/or more efficient oxygen utilization.[212] Metoprolol also significantly decreased myocardial oxygen consumption and improved metabolic efficiency in patients undergoing acute atrial pacing studies both on the initiation of therapy and with long-term dosing (i.e., 3 months).[213] Beta-adrenergic antagonists may also reduce the incidence of sudden death due to primary ventricular arrhythmias, although this remains to be proven in heart failure. Detectable improvements in ventricular function usually are not apparent for a minimum of 1 to 3 months, and longer-term structural changes such as a decline in ventricular volume or mass may take 12 to 18 months (Fig. 16–7).[214]

Beta-adrenergic antagonists with vasodilator activity are also being evaluated for use in heart failure. *Labetalol,* a nonselective beta$_1$- and beta$_2$-antagonist that also blocks alpha$_1$ receptors and is already licensed in the United States for the treatment of hypertension, has been favorably evaluated in small trials of heart failure patients. *Carvedi-*

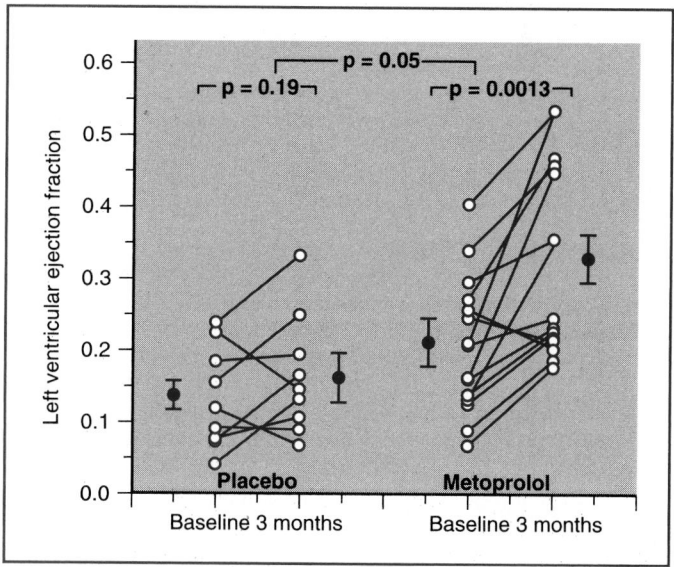

FIGURE 16–7. Changes in left ventricular ejection fraction between baseline and 3 months for placebo and metoprolol groups in patients with dilated cardiomyopathy. A significant increase in ejection fraction was seen only in the metoprolol group. Vertical bars are group mean value and standard error. (From Eichorn, E. J., Heesch, C. M. Barnett, J. H., et al.: Effect of metoprolol on myocardial function and energetics in patients with nonischemic dilated cardiomyopathy: A randomized, double-blind, placebo-controlled study. Reprinted with permission from the American College of Cardiology. J. Am. Coll. Cardiol. *24*:1310, 1994.)

*lol,** like labetolol, exhibits both alpha$_1$ and beta receptor antagonism with no partial agonist (ISA) activity, but modest beta$_1$ selectivity and an elimination half-life (2 to 8 hours) that permits once or twice daily dosing.[215,216] *Bucindolol** is a nonselective beta antagonist that is also a vasodilator, due to a mechanism other than alpha-adrenergic blockade in the vasculature.[217]

---

* Not approved by the US Food and Drug Administration at the time of this writing.

Carvedilol and bucindolol appear to be well tolerated in small trials of patients with both idiopathic and ischemic cardiomyopathies, and several preliminary reports support their efficacy in improving left ventricular ejection fraction, submaximal exercise tolerance, and symptoms. In a published report of 40 patients with idiopathic dilated cardiomyopathy randomized to receive either placebo or carvedilol (target dose, 25 mg twice a day) with background therapy of digoxin, diuretics, and an ACE inhibitor, carvedilol after 4 months improved symptoms, submaximal exercise capacity, and left ventricular ejection fraction (from 0.20 to 0.30) and decreased pulmonary artery wedge pressure.[218] Although pulmonary artery pressures and systemic vascular resistance both declined significantly after the first dose of carvedilol, resting pulmonary artery pressures and systemic vascular resistances declined little, if at all, upon readministration of the drug after several months of exposure. This suggests development of tolerance with time to the alpha$_1$ antagonist effects of this agent, an effect noted with chronic labetolol administration as well.

No clear consensus exists as yet on which of the pharmacological activities of beta-adrenergic antagonists listed in Table 16–7 are necessary or desirable in the treatment of heart failure. Nevertheless, the alpha$_1$ vasodilatory activity of carvedilol and the "direct" vasodilating action of bucindolol may make early upward dose titration of these drugs better tolerated than beta-adrenergic antagonists without vasodilator activity.

REFERENCES

VASODILATORS

1. Cohn, J. N., and Franciosa, J. A.: Vasodilator therapy of cardiac failure. N. Engl. J. Med. 297:27, 1977.
2. Cohn, J. N., Archibald, D. G., Ziesche, S., et al.: Effect of vasodilator therapy on mortality in chronic congestive heart failure: Results of a Veterans Administration Cooperative Study. N. Engl. J. Med. 314:1547, 1986.
3. CONSENSUS Trial Study Group: Effects of enalapril on mortality in severe congestive heart failure: Results of the Cooperative North Scandinavian Enalapril Survival Group (CONSENSUS). N. Engl. J. Med. 316:1429, 1987.
4. Wang, S. Y., Manyari, D. E., Scott-Douglas, N., et al.: Splanchnic venous pressure-volume relation during experimental acute ischemic heart failure: Differential effects of hydralazine, enalaprilat, and nitroglycerin. Circulation 91:1205, 1995.
5. Griendling, K. K., Murphy, T. J., and Alexander, R. W.: Molecular biology of the renin-angiotensin system. Circulation 87:1816, 1993.
6. Linz, W., Wiemer, G., Gohlke, P., et al.: Contribution of kinins to the cardiovascular actions of angiotensin-converting enzyme inhibitors. Pharmacol. Rev. 47:25, 1995.
7. Paul, M., Wagner, J., and Dzau, V. J.: Gene expression of the renin-angiotensin system in human tissues: Quantitative analysis by the polymerase chain reaction. J. Clin. Invest. 91:2058, 1993.
8. Yang, G., Merrill, D. C., Thompson, M. W., et al.: Functional expression of the human angiotensinogen gene in transgenic mice. J. Biol. Chem. 269:32497, 1994.
9. Dzau, V. J., and Re, R.: Tissue angiotensin system in cardiovascular medicine: A paradigm shift? Circulation 89:493, 1994.
10. Kifor, I., and Dzau, V. J.: Endothelial renin-angiotensin pathways: Evidence for intracellular synthesis and secretion of angiotensins. Circ. Res. 60:422, 1987.
11. Morishita, R., Gibbons, G. H., Ellison, K. E., et al.: Evidence for direct local effect of angiotensin in vascular hypertrophy: In vivo gene transfer of angiotensin converting enzyme. J. Clin. Invest. 94:978, 1994.
12. Lee, M. A., Bohm, M., Paul, M., et al.: Tissue renin-angiotensin systems: Their role in cardiovascular disease. Circulation 87:IV-7, 1993.
13. Smith, R. D., Chiu, A. T., Wong, P. C., et al.: Pharmacology of nonpeptide angiotensin II receptor antagonists. Annu. Rev. Pharmacol. Toxicol. 32:135, 1992.
14. Timmermans, P., and Smith, R. D.: Angiotensin II receptor subtypes: Selective antagonists and functional correlates. Eur. Heart J. 15:79, 1994.
15. Marrero, M. B., Schieffer, B., Paxton, W. G., et al.: Direct stimulation of Jak/STAT pathway by the angiotensin II AT$_1$ receptor. Nature 375:247, 1995.
16. Regitz-Zagrosek, V., Friedel, N., Heymann, A., et al.: Regulation, chamber localization, and subtype distribution of angiotensin II receptors in human hearts. Circulation 91:1461, 1995.
17. Holubarsch, C., Schmidt-Schweda, S., Knorr, A., et al.: Functional significance of angiotensin receptors in human myocardium: Significant differences between atrial and ventricular myocardium. Eur. Heart J. 15:88, 1994.
18. Lonn, E. M., Yusuf, S., Jha, P., et al.: Emerging role of angiotensin-converting enzyme inhibitors in cardiac and vascular protection. Circulation 90:2056, 1994.
19. Cohn, J. N.: Structural basis for heart failure: Ventricular remodeling and its pharmacological inhibition. Circulation 91:2504, 1995.
20. Goldsmith, S. R., Hasking, G. J., and Miller, E.: Angiotensin II and sympathetic activity in patients with congestive heart failure. J. Am. Coll. Cardiol. 21:1107, 1993.
21. Lyons, D., Webster, J., and Benjamin, N.: Angiotensin II: Adrenergic sympathetic constrictor action in humans. Circulation 91:1457, 1995.
22. Vaughn, D. E., Lazos, S. A., and Tong, K.: Angiotensin II regulates the expression of plasminogen activator inhibitor-1 in cultured endothelial cells: A potential link between the renin-angiotensin system and thrombosis. J. Clin. Invest. 95:995, 1995.
23. Feener, E. P., Northrup, J. M., Aiello, L. P., et al.: Angiotensin II induces plasminogen activator inhibitor-1 and -2 expression in vascular endothelial and smooth muscle cells. J. Clin. Invest. 95:1353, 1995.
24. Ishihata, A., and Endo, M.: Pharmacological characteristics of the positive inotropic effect of angiotensin II in the rabbit ventricular myocardium. Br. J. Pharmacol. 108:999, 1993.
25. Holubarsch, C., Hasenfuss, G., Schmidt-Schweda, S., et al.: Angiotensin I and II exert inotropic effects in atrial but not in ventricular human myocardium. Circulation 88:1228, 1993.
26. Moravec, C. S., Schluchter, M. D., Paranaudi, L., et al.: Inotropic effects of angiotensin II and human cardiac muscle in vitro. Circulation 82:1973, 1990.
27. Weinberg, E. O., Schoen, F. J., George, D., et al.: Angiotensin-converting enzyme inhibition prolongs survival and modifies the transition to heart failure in rats with pressure overload hypertrophy due to ascending aortic stenosis. Circulation 90:1410, 1994.
28. Friedrich, S. P., Lorell, B. H., Rousseau, M. F., et al.: Intracardiac angiotensin-converting enzyme inhibition improves diastolic function in patients with left ventricular hypertrophy due to aortic stenosis. Circulation 90:2761, 1994.
29. Hayashida, W., van Eyll, C., Rousseau, M. F., et al.: Regional remodeling and nonuniform changes in diastolic function in patients with left ventricular dysfunction: Modification by long-term enalapril treatment. J. Am. Coll. Cardiol. 22:1403, 1993.
30. Pouleur, H., Rousseau, M. F., van Eyll, C., et al.: Effects of long-term enalapril therapy on left ventricular diastolic properties in patients with depressed ejection fraction. Circulation 88:481, 1993.
31. Matsubara, H., Kanasaki, M., Murasawa, S., et al.: Differential gene expression and regulation of angiotensin II receptor subtypes in rat cardiac fibroblasts and cardiomyocytes in culture. J. Clin. Invest. 93:1592, 1994.
32. Schorb, W., Peeler, T. C., Madigan, N. N., et al.: Angiotensin II–induced protein tyrosine phosphorylation in neonatal rat cardiac fibroblasts. J. Biol. Chem. 269:19626, 1994.
33. Crabos, M., Roth, M., Hahn, A. W. A., et al.: Characterization of angiotensin II receptors in cultured adult rat cardiac fibroblasts: Coupling to signaling systems and gene expression. J. Clin. Invest. 93:2372, 1994.
34. Waspe, L. E., Ordahl, C. P., and Simpson, P. C.: The cardiac β-myosin heavy chain isogene is induced selectively in α$_1$-adrenergic receptor-stimulated hypertrophy of cultured rat heart myocytes. J. Clin. Invest. 85:1206, 1990.
35. Schunkert, H., Sadoshima, J.-I., Cornelius, T., et al.: Angiotensin II–induced growth responses in isolated adult rat hearts: Evidence for load-independent induction of cardiac protein synthesis by angiotensin II. Circ. Res. 76:489, 1995.
36. LaMorte, V. J., Thorburn, J., Absher, D., et al.: G$_q$- and ras-dependent pathways mediate hypertrophy of neonatal rat ventricular myocytes following α$_1$-adrenergic stimulation. J. Biol. Chem. 269:13490, 1994.
37. Pfeffer, J. M., Pfeffer, M. A., Mirsky, I., et al.: Regression of left ventricular hypertrophy and prevention of left ventricular dysfunction by captopril in the spontaneously hypertensive rat. Proc. Natl. Acad. Sci. U.S.A. 79:3310, 1992.
38. Jufsurr, V. I., Khan, M. I., Jugdutt, S. J., et al.: Effect of enalapril on ventricular remodeling and function during healing after anterior myocardial infarction in the dog. Circulation 91:802, 1995.
39. Weber, K. T., and Brilla, C. G.: Pathological hypertrophy and cardiac interstitium. Circulation 83:1849, 1991.
40. Binkley, P. F., Haas, G. J., Starling, R. C., et al.: Sustained augmentation of parasympathetic tone with angiotensin converting enzyme inhibition in patients with congestive heart failure. J. Am. Coll. Cardiol. 21:655, 1993.
41. Ljungman, S., Kjekshus, J., and Swedberg, K., for the CONSENSUS Group: Renal function in severe congestive heart failure during treatment with enalapril (the Cooperative North Scandinavian Enalapril Survival Study [CONSENSUS] Trial). Am. J. Cardiol. 70:479, 1992.
42. Mandal, A. K., Markert, R. J., Saklayen, M. G., et al.: Diuretics potentiate angiotensin converting enzyme inhibitor–induced acute renal failure. Clin. Nephrol. 42:170, 1994.
43. SOLVD Investigators: Effect of enalapril on survival in patients with reduced left ventricular ejection fractions and congestive heart failure. N. Engl. J. Med. 325:293, 1991.
44. Gruppo Italiano per lo Studio della Sopravvivenza nell'Infarto Miocardico, GISSI-3 Investigators: Effects of lisinopril and transdermal glyceryl trinitrate singly and together on 6-week mortality and ventricular function after acute myocardial infarction. Lancet 343:1115, 1994.
45. ISIS-4 (Fourth International Study of Infarct Survival) Collaborative Group: ISIS-4: A randomized factorial trial assessing early oral capto-

pril, oral mononitrate, and intravenous magnesium sulphate in 58,050 patients with suspected acute myocardial infarction. Lancet *345:*669, 1995.

46. Lewis, E. J., Hunsicker, I. G., Bain, R. P., et al.: The effect of angiotensin-converting-enzyme inhibition on diabetic nephropathy. N. Engl. J. Med. *329:*1456, 1993.

47. Keilani, T., Schlueter, M., and Batlle, D.: Selected aspects of ACE inhibitor therapy for patients with renal disease: Impact on proteinuria, lipids and potassium. J. Clin. Pharmacol. *35:*87, 1995.

48. Ondetti, M. A.: From peptides to peptidases: A chronicle of drug discovery. Annu. Rev. Pharmacol. Toxicol. *34:*1, 1994.

49. Zusman, R. M.: Fosinopril and cardiac performance. Rev. Contemp. Pharmacother. *4:*25, 1993.

50. Cushman, D. W., Wang, W. L., Fung, W. C., et al.: Differentiation of angiotensin converting enzyme inhibitors by their selective inhibition of ACE in physiologically important target organs. Am. J. Hypertens. *2:*294, 1989.

51. Zusman, R. M.: Angiotensin-converting enzyme inhibitors: More different than alike? Focus on cardiac performance. Am. J. Cardiol. *72:*25H, 1993.

52. Kostis, J. B., Shelton, B. J., Yusuf, S., et al.: Tolerability of enalapril initiation by patients with left ventricular dysfunction: Results of the medication challenge phase of the studies of left ventricular dysfunction. Am. Heart J. *128:*358, 1994.

53. Lang, R. M., DiBianco, R., Broderick, G. T., et al.: First-dose effects of enalapril 2.5 mg and captopril 6.25 mg in patients with heart failure: A double-blind, randomized, multicenter study. Am. Heart J. *128:*551, 1994.

54. Reid, J. L., MacFadyen, R. J., Squire, I. B., et al.: Blood pressure response to the first dose of angiotensin-converting enzyme inhibitors in congestive heart failure. Am. J. Cardiol. *71:*57E, 1993.

55. Shionoiri, H.: Pharmacokinetic drug interactions with ACE inhibitors. Clin. Pharamcokinet. *25:*20, 1993.

56. Sweet, C. S., and Rucinska, E. J.: Losartan in heart failure: Preclinical experiences and initial clinical outcomes. Eur. Heart J. *15:*139, 1994.

57. Crozier, I., Ikram, H., Awan, N., et al.: Losartan in heart failure: Hemodynamic effects and tolerability. Circulation *91:*691, 1995.

58. Wood, J. M., Cumin, F., and Maibaum, J.: Pharmacology of renin inhibitors and their application to the treatment of hypertension. Pharmacol. Ther. *61:*325, 1994.

59. Frishman, W. H., Fozailoff, A., Lin, C., et al.: Renin inhibition: A new approach to cardiovascular therapy. J. Clin. Pharmacol. *34:*873, 1994.

60. Stamler, J. S.: Redox signaling: Nitrosylation and related target interactions of nitric oxide. Cell *78:*931, 1994.

61. Nathan, C., and Xie, Q.-W.: Nitric oxide synthases: Roles, tolls, and controls. Cell *78:*915, 1994.

62. Balligand, J.-L., Kobzik, L., Han, X., et al.: Nitric oxide–dependent parasympathetic signalling in cardiac myocytes is due to activation of type III (constitutive endothelial) NO synthase. J. Biol. Chem. *270:*14582, 1995.

63. Hare, J. M., Loh, E., Creager, M. A., and Colucci, W. S.: Nitric oxide inhibits the positive inotropic response to β-adrenergic stimulation in humans with left ventricular dysfunction. Circulation *92:*2198, 1995.

64. Furchgott, R. F., and Zawadzki, J. V.: The obligatory role of endothelial cells in the relaxation of arterial smooth muscle by acetylcholine. Nature *288:*373, 1980.

65. Harrison, D. G., and Bates, J. N.: The nitrovasodilators: New ideas about old drugs. Circulation *87:*1461, 1993.

66. Risoe, C., Simonsen, S., Rootwelt, K., et al.: Nitroprusside and regional vascular capacitance in patients with severe congestive heart failure. Circulation *85:*997, 1992.

67. Heesch, C. M., Hatfield, B. A., Marcoux, L., et al.: Predictors of pressure and stroke volume response to afterload reduction with nitroprusside in patients with congestive heart failure secondary to idiopathic dilated cardiomyopathy. Am. J. Cardiol. *74:*951, 1994.

68. Fallen, E. L., Nahmias, C., Scheffel, A., et al.: Redistribution of myocardial blood flow with topical nitroglycerin in patients with coronary artery disease. Circulation *91:*1381, 1995.

69. European Study of Prevention of Infarct with Molsidomine (ESPRIM) Group: The ESPRIM trial: Short-term treatment of acute myocardial infarction with molsidomine. Lancet *344:*91, 1994.

70. Unger, P., Vachiery, J.-L., de Canniere, D., et al.: Comparison of the hemodynamic responses to molsidomine and isosorbide dinitrate in congestive heart failure. Am. Heart J. *128:*557, 1994.

71. Elkayam, U.: Tolerance to organic nitrates: Evidence, mechanisms, clinical relevance, and strategies for prevention. Ann. Intern. Med. *114:*667, 1991.

72. Mangione, N. J., and Glasser, S. P.: Phenomenon of nitrate tolerance. Am. Heart J. *128:*137, 1994.

73. Dupuis, J.: Nitrates in congestive heart failure. Cardiovasc. Drugs Ther. *8:*501, 1994.

74. Ignarro, L., Edwards, J., Gruetter, D. Y., et al.: Possible involvement of S-nitrosothiols in the activation of guanylate cyclase by nitrous compounds. FEBS Lett. *110:*275, 1980.

75. Mehra, A., Shotan, A., Ostrzega, E., et al.: Potentiation of isosorbide dinitrate effects with N-acetylcysteine in patients with chronic heart failure. Circulation *89:*2595, 1994.

76. Munzel, T., Sayegh, H., Freeman, B. A., et al.: Evidence for enhanced vascular superoxide anion production in nitrate tolerance. A novel mechanism underlying tolerance and cross-tolerance. J. Clin. Invest. *95:*187, 1995.

77. Parker, J. D., Parker, A. B., Farrell, B., et al.: Intermittent transdermal nitroglycerin therapy. Decreased anginal threshold during the nitrate-free interval. Circulation *91:*973, 1995.

78. Parker, J. O., Amies, M. H., Hawkinson, R. W., et al.: Intermittent transdermal nitroglycerin therapy in angina pectoris. Clinically effective without tolerance or rebound. Circulation *91:*1368, 1995.

79. Hofstra, A. H.: Metabolism of hydralazine: Relevance to drug-induced lupus. Drug Metab. Rev. *26:*485, 1994.

80. Elkayam, U., Shotan, A., Mehra, A., et al.: Calcium channel blockers in the heart. J. Am. Coll. Cardiol. *22:*139A, 1993.

81. Conti, C. R.: Use of calcium antagonists to treat heart failure. Clin. Cardiol. *17:*101, 1994.

82. Little, W. C., and Cheng, C.-P.: Vascular versus myocardial effects of calcium antagonists. Drugs *47:*41, 1994.

83. Kukuljan, M., Labarca, P., and Latorre, R.: Molecular determinants of ion conduction and inactivation in K$^+$ channels. Am. J. Physiol. *268:*C535, 1995.

84. Philipson, D. H., and Steiner, D. F.: Pas de deux or more: The sulfonylurea receptor and K$^+$ channels. Science *268:*372, 1995.

85. Nelson, M. T., and Quayle, J. M.: Physiological roles and properties of potassium channels in arterial smooth muscle. Am. J. Physiol. *268:*C799, 1995.

86. Kukovetz, W. R., Holzmann, S., and Poch, G.: Molecular mechanisms of the action of nicorandil. J. Cardiovasc. Pharmacol. *20:*S1, 1992.

87. Kato, K.: Hemodynamic and clinical effects of an intravenous potassium channel opener—a review. Eur. Heart J. *14:*40, 1993.

88. Tsutamoto, T., Kinoshita, M., Nakae, I., et al.: Absence of hemodynamic tolerance to nicorandil in patients with severe congestive heart failure. Am. Heart J. *127:*866, 1994.

DIURETICS

89. Awazu, M., and Ichikawa, I.: Alterations in renal function in experimental congestive heart failure. Semin. Nephrol. *14:*401, 1994.

90. Rouse, D., and Suki, W. N.: Effects of neural and humoral agents on the renal tubules in congestive heart failure. Sem. Nephrol. *14:*412, 1994.

91. Miller, J. A., Tobe, S. W., and Skorecki, K. L.: Control of extracellular fluid volume and the pathophysiology of edema. In Brenner, B. M., and Rector, F. C. (eds.): The Kidney. 5th ed. Philadelphia, W. B. Saunders Company, 1996.

92. Young, J. B., and Pratt, C. M.: Hemodynamic and hormonal alterations in patients with heart failure: Toward a contemporary definition of heart failure. Sem. Nephrol. *14:*427, 1994.

93. Maddox, D. A., and Brenner, B. M.: Glomerular ultrafiltration. In Brenner, B. M., and Rector, F. C. (eds.): The Kidney. 5th ed. Philadelphia, W. B. Saunders Company, 1996.

94. Jackson, E. K.: Diuretics and other agents employed in the mobilization of edema fluid. In Hardman, J. G., Limbird, L. (eds.): Goodman & Gilman's The Pharmacological Basis of Therapeutics, 9th ed. New York, McGraw-Hill Book Co., 1996.

95. Haas, M.: The Na-K-Cl cotransporters. Am. J. Physiol. *267:*C869, 1994.

96. Raftery, E. B.: Hemodynamic effects of diuretics in heart failure. Br. Heart J. *72:*44, 1994.

97. Gamba, G., Saltzberg, S. N., Lombardi, M., et al.: Primary structure and functional expression of a cDNA encoding the thiazide-sensitive, electroneutral sodium-chloride cotransporter. Proc. Natl. Acad. Sci. U.S.A. *90:*2749, 1993.

98. Palmer, L. G.: Epithelial Na channels and their kin. News Physiol. Sci. *10:*61, 1995.

99. Funder, J. W.: Mineralocorticoids, glucocorticoids, receptors and response elements. Science *259:*1132, 1993.

100. Funder, J. W.: Aldosterone action. Annu. Rev. Physiol. *55:*115, 1993.

101. Weber, K. T., and Villarreal, D.: Aldosterone and antialdosterone therapy in congestive heart failure. Am. J. Cardiol. *71:*3A, 1993.

102. Jackson, E. K.: Vasopressin and other agents affecting the renal conservation of water. In Hardman, J. G., Limbird, L. (eds.): Goodman & Gilman's The Pharmacological Basis of Therapeutics, 9th ed. New York, McGraw-Hill Book Co., 1996.

103. Nielsen, S., Chou, C.-L., Marples, D., et al.: Vasopressin increases water permeability of kidney collecting duct by inducing translocation of aquaporin-CD water channels to plasma membrane. Proc. Natl. Acad. Sci. *92:*1013, 1995.

104. Knoers, N. V. A., and van Os, C. H.: The clinical importance of the urinary excretion of aquaporin-2. N. Engl. J. Med. *332:*1575, 1995.

105. Ohnishi, A., Orita, Y., Takagi, N., et al.: Aquaretic effect of a potent, orally active, nonpeptide V$_2$ antagonist in men. J. Pharmacol. Exp. Therap. *272:*546, 1995.

106. Gunning, M. E., Ingelfinger, J. R., King, A. J., et al.: Vasoactive peptides and the kidney. In Brenner, B. M., and Rector, F. C. (eds.): The Kidney, 5th ed. Philadelphia, W. B. Saunders Company, 1996.

107. Deutsch, A., Frishman, W. H., Sukenik, D., et al.: Atrial natriuretic peptide and its potential role in pharmacotherapy. J. Clin. Pharmacol. *34:*1133, 1994.

108. Semigran, M. J., Aroney, C. N., Herrmann, H. C., et al.: Effects of atrial natriuretic peptide on myocardial contractile and diastolic function in patients with heart failure. J. Am. Coll. Cardiol. *20:*98, 1992.

109. Brater, D. C.: Diuretic resistance: Mechanisms and therapeutic strategies. Cardiology *84:*57, 1994.

110. Brater, D. C.: Pharmacokinetics of loop diuretics in congestive heart failure. Br. Heart J. *72:*S40, 1994.

111. Knauf, H., and Mutschler, E.: Functional state of the nephron and diuretic dose-response-rationale for low-dose combination therapy. Cardiology 84:18, 1994.

112. Wilcox, C. S.: Diuretics. In Brenner, B. M., and Rector, F. C. (eds.): The Kidney, 5th ed. Philadelphia, W. B. Saunders Company, 1995.

113. Ellison, D. H.: The physiologic basis of diuretic synergism: Its role in treating diuretic resistance. Ann. Intern. Med. 114:886, 1991.

114. Leier, C. V., Dei Cas, L., and Metra, M.: Clinical relevance and management of the major electrolyte abnormalities in congestive heart failure: Hyponatremia, hypokalemia, and hypomagnesemia. Am. Heart J. 128:564, 1994.

115. Bigger, J. T., Jr.: Diuretic therapy, hypertension, and cardiac arrest. N. Engl. J. Med. 330:1899, 1994.

116. Siscovick, D. S., Raghunathan, T. E., Psaty, B. M., et al.: Diuretic therapy for hypertension and the risk of primary cardiac arrest. N. Engl. J. Med. 330:1852, 1994.

117. Siegel, D., Hulley, S. B., Black, D. M., et al.: Diuretics, serum and intracellular electrolyte levels, and ventricular arrhythmias in hypertensive men. JAMA 267:1083, 1992.

118. Cody, R. J.: Clinical trials of diuretic therapy in heart failure: Research directions and clinical considerations. J. Am. Coll. Cardiol. 22:165A, 1993.

119. Hampton, J. R.: Results of clinical trials with diuretics in heart failure. Br. Heart J. 72:S68, 1994.

120. Ramsay, L. E., Yeo, W. W., and Jackson, P. R.: Metabolic effects of diuretics. Cardiology 84:48, 1994.

121. Moser, M.: Effect of diuretics on morbidity and mortality in the treatment of hypertension. Cardiology 84:27, 1994.

122. Silke, B.: Diuretic induced changes in symptoms and quality of life. Br. Heart J. 72:S57, 1994.

123. Freis, E. D.: The efficacy and safety of diuretics in treating hypertension. Ann. Intern. Med. 122:223, 1995.

124. Dorup, I.: Magnesium and potassium deficiency, its diagnosis, occurrence, and treatment in diuretic therapy and its consequences for growth, protein synthesis and growth factors. Acta Physiol. Scand. 150:7, 1994.

125. Arsenian, M. A.: Magnesium and cardiovascular disease. Prog. Cardiovasc. Dis. 35:271, 1993.

126. Al-Ghamdi, S. M. G., Cameron, E. C., and Sutton, R. A. L.: Magnesium deficiency: Pathophysiologic and clinical overview. Am. J. Kidney Dis. 24:737, 1994.

127. Davies, D. L., and Fraser, R.: Do diuretics cause magnesium deficiency? Br. J. Clin. Pharmacol. 36:1, 1993.

128. Materson, B. J., Reda, D. J., Cushman, W. C., et al.: Single-drug therapy for hypertension in men. A comparison of six antihypertensive agents with placebo. N. Engl. J. Med. 328:914, 1993.

129. Kasiske, B. L., Ma, J. Z., Kalil, R. S. N., et al.: Effects of antihypertensive therapy on serum lipids. Ann. Intern. Med. 122:133, 1995.

130. Lajoie, G., Laszik, Z., Nadasdy, T., et al.: The renal-cardiac connection: Renal parenchymal alterations in patients with heart disease. Sem. Nephrol. 14:441, 1994.

131. Shuler, C., Golper, T. A., and Bennett, W. M.: Prescribing drugs in renal disease. In Brenner, B. M., and Rector, F. C. (eds.): The Kidney, 5th ed. Philadelphia, W. B. Saunders Company, 1996.

132. Kaplan, A. A.: Ultrafiltration in the treatment of congestive heart failure. Heart Failure 10:192, 1994.

133. Agostoni, P., Marenzi, G., Lauri, G., et al.: Sustained improvement in functional capacity after removal of body fluid with isolated ultrafiltration in chronic cardiac insufficiency: Failure of furosemide to provide the same result. Am. J. Med. 96:191, 1994.

134. Withering, W.: An account of the foxglove and some of its medical uses, with practical remarks on dropsy, and other diseases. In Willius, F. A., and Keys, T. E., (eds.): Classics of Cardiology. New York, Dover, 1:231, 1941.

135. Eisner, D. A., and Smith, T. W.: The Na-K pump and its effectors in cardiac muscle. In Fozzard, H. A., Haber, E., Katz, A. M., et al.: (eds.): The Heart and Cardiovascular System. New York, Raven Press, 1992.

136. Blaustein, M. P.: Physiological effects of endogenous ouabain: Control of intracellular Ca^{2+} stores and cell responsiveness. Am. J. Physiol. 264:C1367, 1993.

137. Kelly, R. A., and Smith, T. W.: The search for the endogenous digitalis: An alternative hypothesis. Am. J. Physiol. 256:C937, 1989.

138. Kelly, R. A., and Smith, T. W.: Endogenous cardiac glycosides. Adv. Pharmacol. 25:263, 1994.

139. Lingrel, J. B., Van Huysse, J., O'Brien, W., et al.: Structure-function studies of the Na,K-ATPase. Kidney Int. 45:S32, 1994.

140. Schmidt, T. A., Allen, P. D., Colucci, W. S., et al.: No adaptation to digitalization as evaluated by digitalis receptor (Na,K-ATPase) quantification in explanted hearts from donors without heart disease and from digitalized recipients with end-stage heart failure. Am. J. Cardiol. 70:110, 1992.

141. Harrison, S. M., McCall, E., and Boyett, M. R.: The relationship between contraction and intracellular sodium in rat and guinea-pig ventricular myocytes. J. Physiol. (London) 449:517, 1992.

142. Pidgeon, G. B., Richards, A. M., Nicholls, M. G., et al.: Effect of ouabain on pressor responsiveness in normal man. Am. J. Physiol. 267:E642, 1994.

143. Lucke, J. C., Elbeery, J. R., Koutlas, T. C., et al.: Effects of cardiac glycosides on myocardial function and energetics in conscious dogs. Am. J. Physiol. 267:H2042, 1994.

144. Holubarsch, C., Hasenfuss, G., Just, H., et al.: Positive inotropism and myocardial energetics: Influence of β receptor agonist stimulation, phosphodiesterase inhibition, and ouabain. Cardiovasc. Res. 28:994, 1994.

145. McGarry, S. J., and Williams, A. J.: Digoxin activates sarcoplasmic reticulum Ca^{2+} release channels: A possible role in cardiac inotropy. Br. J. Pharmacol. 108:1043, 1993.

146. Kranzhofer, R., Haass, M., Kurz, T., et al.: Effect of digitalis glycosides on norepinephrine release in the heart. Dual mechanisms of action. Circ. Res. 68:1628, 1991.

147. Mason, D. T., Braunwald, E., Karsh, R. B., et al.: Studies on digitalis. X. Effects of ouabain on forearm vascular resistance and venous tone in normal subjects and in patients in heart failure. J. Clin. Invest. 43:532, 1964.

148. Wang, W., Chen, J.-S., and Zucker, I. H.: Carotid sinus baroreceptor sensitivity in experimental heart failure. Circulation 81:1959, 1990.

149. Ferguson, D. W., Berg, W. J., Sanders, J. S., et al.: Sympathoinhibitory responses to digitalis glycosides in heart failure patients. Direct evidence from sympathetic neural recordings. Circulation 80:65, 1989.

150. Krum, H., Bigger, J. T., Jr., Goldsmith, R. L., et al.: Effect of long-term digoxin therapy on autonomic function in patients with chronic heart failure. J. Am. Coll. Cardiol. 25:289, 1995.

151. Patten, S. B., and Love, E. J.: Neuropsychiatric adverse drug reactions: Passive reports to Health and Welfare Canada's adverse drug reaction database (1965-Present). Intl. J. Psychiat. Med. 24:45, 1994.

152. Hui, J., Geraets, D. R., Chandrasekaran, A., et al.: Digoxin disposition in elderly humans with hypochlorhydria. J. Clin. Pharmacol. 34:734, 1994.

153. Kelly, R. A., and Smith, T. W.: Use and misuse of digitalis blood levels. Heart Dis. Stroke 1:117, 1992.

154. Mahdyoon, H., Battilana, G., Rosman, H., et al.: The evolving pattern of digoxin intoxication: Observations at a large urban hospital from 1980 to 1988. Am. Heart J. 120:1189, 1990.

155. Kelly, R. A., and Smith, T. W.: Recognition and management of digitalis toxicity. Am. J. Cardiol. 69:108G, 1992.

156. Kelly, R. A., and Smith, T. W.: Antibody therapies for drug overdose. In Austen, K. F., Burakoff, S. J., Rosen, F. S., et al. (eds.): Therapeutic Immunology. Cambridge, Blackwell Scientific, 1996.

157. Bosse, G. M., and Pope, T. M.: Recurrent digoxin overdose and treatment with digoxin-specific Fab antibody fragments. J. Emerg. Med. 12:179, 1994.

158. Clark, R. F., and Barton, E. D.: Pitfalls in the administration of digoxin-specific Fab fragments. J. Emerg. Med. 12:233, 1994.

159. Beavo, J. A., and Reifsnyder, D. H.: Primary sequence of cyclic nucleotide phosphodiesterase isozymes and the design of selective inhibitors. Trends Pharmacol. Sci. 11:150, 1990.

160. Nicholson, C. D., Challiss, R. A. J., and Shahid, M.: Differential modulation of tissue function and therapeutic potential of selective inhibitors of cyclic nucleotide phosphodiesterase isoenzymes. Trends Pharmacol. Sci. 12:19, 1991.

161. Bode, D. C., Kanter, J. R., and Brunton, L. L.: Cellular distribution of phosphodiesterase isoforms in rat cardiac tissue. Circ. Res. 68:1070, 1991.

162. Beavo, J. A.: cGMP inhibition of heart phosphodiesterase: Is it clinically relevant? J. Clin. Invest. 95:444, 1995.

163. Packer, M., Carver, J. R., Rodeheffer, R. J., et al.: Effect of oral milrinone on mortality in severe chronic heart failure. N. Engl. J. Med. 325:1468, 1991.

164. Packer, M.: The development of positive inotropic agents for chronic heart failure; How have we gone astray? J. Am. Coll. Cardiol. 22:119A, 1993.

165. Nony, P., Boissel, J.-P., Lievre, M., et al.: Evaluation of the effect of phosphodiesterase inhibitors on mortality in chronic heart failure patients. Eur. J. Clin. Pharmacol. 46:191, 1994.

166. Cheng, D. C. H., Asokumar, B., and Nakagawa, T.: Amrinone therapy for severe pulmonary hypertension and biventricular failure after complicated valvular heart surgery. Chest 104:1618, 1993.

167. Wynands, J. E.: The role of amrinone in treating heart failure during and after coronary artery surgery supported by cardiopulmonary bypass. J. Cardiac Surg. 9:453, 1994.

168. Installe, E., DeCoster, P., Gonzalez, M., et al.: Comparison between the positive inotropic effects of enoximone, a cardiac phosphodiesterase III inhibitor, and dobutamine in patients with moderate to severe congestive heart failure. Eur. Heart J. 12:985, 1991.

169. Nagata, K., Iwase, M., Sobue, T., et al.: Differential effects of dobutamine and a phosphodiesterase inhibitor on early diastolic filling in patients with congestive heart failure. J. Am. Coll. Cardiol. 25:295, 1995.

170. Matsui, S., Matsumori, A., Matoba, Y., et al.: Treatment of virus-induced myocardial injury with a novel immunomodulating agent, vesnarinone. Suppression of natural killer cell activity and tumor necrosis factor-α production. J. Clin. Invest. 94:1212, 1994.

171. Bertolet, B. D., White, B. G., and Pepine, C. J.: Neutropenia occurring during treatment with vesnarinone (OPC-8212). Am. J. Cardiol. 74:968, 1994.

172. Feldman, A. M., Bristow, M. R., Parmley, W. W., et al.: Effects of vesnarinone on morbidity and mortality in patients with heart failure. N. Engl. J. Med. 329:149, 1993.

173. Hoit, B. D., Burwig, S., Eppert, D., et al.: Effects of a novel inotropic agent (OPC-18790) on systolic and diastolic function in patients with severe heart failure. Am. Heart J. 128:1156, 1994.

174. Hagemeijer, F.: Calcium sensitization with pimobendan: Pharmacology,

hemodynamic improvement, and sudden death in patients with chronic congestive heart failure. Eur. Heart J. *14*:551, 1993.

175. Rector, T. S., and Cohn, J. N.: Assessment of patient outcome with the Minnesota Living with Heart Failure Questionnaire: Reliability and validity during a randomized, double-blind, placebo-controlled trial of pimobendan. Am. Heart J. *124*:1017, 1992.

176. Kubo, S. H., Gollub, S., Bourge, R., et al., for the Pimobendan Multicenter Research Group: Beneficial effects of pimobendan on exercise tolerance and quality of life in patients with heart failure. Results of a multicenter trial. Circulation *85*:942, 1992.

177. Remme, W. J., Krayenbuhl, H. P., Baumann, G., et al., for the Pimobendan-Enalapril Study Group: Long-term efficacy and safety of pimobendan in moderate heart failure. A double-blind parallel 6-month comparison with enalapril. Eur. Heart J. *15*:947, 1994.

178. Pollesello, P., Ovaska, M., Kaivola, J., et al.: Binding of a new Ca^{2+} sensitizer, levosimendan, to recombinant human cardiac troponin C. A molecular modelling, fluorescence probe, and protein nuclear magnetic resonance study. J. Biol. Chem. *269*:28584, 1994.

179. Rump, A. F. E., Acar, D., and Klaus, W.: A quantitative comparison of functional and anti-ischemic effects of the phosphodiesterase-inhibitors, amrinone, milrinone and levosimendan in rabbit isolated hearts. Br. J. Pharmacol. *112*:757, 1994.

180. Pagel, P. S., Harkin, C. P., Hettrick, D. A., et al.: Levosimendan (OR-1259), a myofilament calcium sensitizer, enhances myocardial contractility but does not alter isovolumic relaxation in conscious and anesthetized dogs. Anesthesiology *81*:974, 1994.

ADRENERGIC AGONISTS

181. Neer, E. J.: Heterotrimeric G proteins: Organizers of transmembrane signals. Cell *80*:249, 1995.

182. Clapham, D. E., and Neer, E. J.: New roles for G protein $\beta\gamma$ dimers in transmembrane signaling. Nature *365*:403, 1993.

183. Hoffman, B. R., and Lefkowitz, R. J.: Catecholamines, sympathomimetic drugs, and adrenergic receptor antagonists. *In* Hardman, J. G., Limbard, L. (eds.): Goodman & Gilman's The Pharmacological Basis of Therapeutics, 9th ed. New York, McGraw-Hill Book Co., 1996.

184. Muntz, K. H., Zhao, M., and Miller, J. C.: Downregulation of myocardial β-adrenergic receptors. Receptor subtype selectivity. Circ. Res. *74*:369, 1994.

185. Bristow, M. R., Minobe, W. A., Raynolds, M. V., et al.: Reduced β_1 receptor messenger RNA abundance in the failing human heart. J. Clin. Invest. *92*:2737, 1993.

186. Bristow, M. R.: Changes in myocardial and vascular receptors in heart failure. J. Am. Coll. Cardiol. *22*:61A, 1993.

187. Insel, P. A.: β-Adrenergic receptors in heart failure. J. Clin. Invest. *92*:2563, 1993.

188. Gurevich, V. V., Dion, S. B., Onorato, J. J., et al.: Arrestin interactions with G protein-coupled receptors. Direct binding studies of wild type and mutant arrestins with rhodopsin, beta₂-adrenergic, and m2 muscarinic cholinergic receptors. J. Biol. Chem. *270*:720, 1995.

189. Harding, S. E., Brown, L. A., Wynne, D. G., et al.: Mechanisms of β adrenoceptor desensitization in the failing human heart. Cardiovasc. Res. *28*:1451, 1994.

190. Hershberger, R. E.: Beta-adrenergic receptor agonists and antagonists in heart failure. *In* Hosenpud, J. D., and Greenberg, B. H. (eds.): Congestive Heart Failure. New York, Springer-Verlag, 1994, p. 454.

191. Binkley, P. F., VanFossen, D. V., Nunziata, E., et al.: Influence of positive inotropic therapy on pulsatile hydraulic load and ventricular-vascular coupling in congestive heart failure. J. Am. Coll. Cardiol. *15*:1127, 1990.

192. Binkley, P. F., Murray, K. D., Watson, K. M., et al.: Dobutamine increases cardiac output of total artificial heart. Implications for vascular contribution of inotropic agents to augmented ventricular function. Circulation *84*:1210, 1991.

193. Leier, C. V.: Current status of non-digitalis positive inotropic drugs. Am. J. Cardiol. *69*:120G, 1992.

194. Good, J., Frost, G., Oakley, C. M., et al.: The renal effects of dopamine and dobutamine in stable chronic heart failure. Postgrad. Med. J. *68*:S7, 1992.

195. Keren, G., Laniado, S., Sonnenblick, E. H., et al.: Dynamics of functional mitral regurgitation during dobutamine therapy in patients with severe congestive heart failure. A Doppler echocardiographic study. Am. Heart J. *118*:748, 1989.

196. Lokhandwala, M. F., and Amenta, F.: Anatomical distribution and function of dopamine receptors in the kidney. FASEB J. *5*:3023, 1991.

197. MacGregor, D. A., Butterworth, J. F., IV, Zaloga, G. P., et al.: Hemodynamic and renal effects of dopexamine and dobutamine in patients with reduced cardiac output following coronary artery bypass grafting. Chest *106*:835, 1994.

198. Leier, C. V., Hua Ren, J., Huss, P., et al.: The hemodynamic effects of ibopamine, a dopamine congener, in patients with congestive heart failure. Pharmacotherapy *6*:35, 1988.

199. Kleber, F. X., Sabin, G. V., Thyroff-Friesinger, U., et al.: Ibopamine as a valuable adjunct and substitute for dopamine in bridging therapy before heart transplantation. Cardiology *81*:121, 1992.

BETA-ADRENERGIC ANTAGONISTS

200. Bond, R. A., Leff, P., Johnson, T. D., et al.: Physiological effects of inverse agonists in transgenic mice with myocardial overexpression of the β_2-adrenoceptor. Nature *374*:272, 1995.

201. Black, J. W., and Shankley, N. P.: Inverse agonists exposed. Nature *374*:214, 1995.

202. Lowes, B. D., Chidiac, P., Olsen, S., et al.: Clinical relevance of inverse agonism and guanine nucleotide modulatable binding properties of β-adrenergic receptor blocking agents. Circulation *90*:I-543, 1994.

203. Waagstein, F., Hjalmarson, A., Varnauskas, E., et al.: Effect of chronic beta-adrenergic receptor blockade in congestive cardiomyopathy. Br. Heart J. *37*:1022, 1975.

204. Swedberg, K.: Initial experience with beta blockers in dilated cardiomyopathy. Am. J. Cardiol. *71*:30C, 1993.

205. Ikram, H., Fitzpatrick, D., and Crozier, I. G.: Therapeutic controversies with use of beta-adrenoceptor blockade in heart failure. Am. J. Cardiol. *71*:54C, 1993.

206. Doughty, R. N., MacMahon, S., and Sharpe, N.: Beta-blockers in heart failure: Promising or proved? J. Am. Coll. Cardiol. *23*:814, 1994.

207. The German and Austrian Xamoterol Study Group: Double-blind placebo-controlled comparison of digoxin and xamoterol in chronic heart failure. Lancet *1*:489, 1988.

208. The Xamoterol in Severe Heart Failure Study Group: Xamoterol in severe heart failure. Lancet *336*:1, 1990.

209. Bristow, M. R.: Pathophysiologic and pharmacologic rationales for clinical management of chronic heart failure with beta-blocking agents. Am. J. Cardiol. *21*:12C, 1993.

210. Ping, P., Gelzer-Bell, Roth, D. A., et al.: Reduced β-adrenergic activation decreases G-protein expression and β-adrenergic receptor kinase activity in porcine heart. J. Clin. Invest. *95*:1271, 1995.

211. Andersson, B., Hamm, C., Persson, S., et al.: Improved exercise hemodynamic status in dilated cardiomyopathy after beta-adrenergic blockade treatment. J. Am. Coll. Cardiol. *23*:1397, 1994.

212. Eichhorn, E. J., Heesch, C. M., Barnett, J. H., et al.: Effect of metoprolol on myocardial function and energetics in patients with nonischemic dilated cardiomyopathy: A randomized, double-blind, placebo-controlled study. J. Am. Coll. Cardiol. *24*:1310, 1994.

213. Heesch, C. M., Marcoux, L., Hatfield, B., et al.: Hemodynamic and energetic comparison of bucindolol and metoprolol for the treatment of congestive heart failure. Am. J. Cardiol. *75*:360, 1995.

214. Hall, S. A., Cigarroa, C. G., Marcoux, L., et al.: Time course of improvement in left ventricular function, mass and geometry in patients with congestive heart failure treated with beta-adrenergic blockade. J. Am. Coll. Cardiol. *25*:1154, 1995.

215. Fowler, M. B.: Beta-blockers in heart failure: Potential of carvedilol. J. Human Hypertens. *7*:S62, 1993.

216. Krum, H., Sackner-Bernstein, J. D., Goldsmith, R. L., et al.: Double-blind, placebo-controlled study of the long-term efficacy of carvedilol in patients with severe chronic heart failure. Circulation *92*:1499, 1995.

217. Bristow, M. R., O'Connell, J. B., Gilbert, E. M., et al., for the Bucindolol Investigators: Dose-response of chronic β-blocker treatment in heart failure from either idiopathic dilated or ischemic cardiomyopathy. Circulation *89*:1632, 1994.

218. Metra, M., Nardi, M., Giubbini, R., et al.: Effects of short- and long-term carvedilol administration on rest and exercise hemodynamic variables, exercise capacity and clinical conditions in patients with idiopathic dilated cardiomyopathy. J. Am. Coll. Cardiol. *24*:1678, 1994.

Chapter 17
Management of Heart Failure
THOMAS W. SMITH, RALPH A. KELLY, LYNNE WARNER STEVENSON, EUGENE BRAUNWALD

THERAPEUTIC STRATEGY FOR MANAGEMENT OF HEART FAILURE

The goals of therapy in patients with heart failure are to improve quality and length of life and to prevent progression of the syndrome. The relative importance of these goals and the design of therapy for each patient vary according to the clinical stage of heart failure (Fig. 17–1). Evidence for improvement in survival with medical therapy has now been shown for each stage from asymptomatic left ventricular dysfunction to severely symptomatic heart failure. Quality of life has been more difficult to assess, but objective measurement of functional capacity has shown improvement with therapy that is more dramatic as the severity of symptoms increases. The impact of therapy to reduce progression of disease, however, as measured by left-ventricular dimensions and ejection fraction, is most apparent before severe disease develops.

Table 17–1 classifies specific therapeutic targets in heart failure (HF) and the intensity with which they are pursued according to symptoms or functional class. The management of heart failure has three principal components: the removal or amelioration of the underlying cause, the re-moval of the precipitating cause, and the control of the heart failure state.

REMOVAL OF THE UNDERLYING CAUSE. All patients with heart failure should undergo evaluation for treatable causes of this condition. This includes the improvement of coronary blood flow through catheter-based intervention or coronary bypass surgery and repair of structural abnormalities such as congenital heart defects, valvular lesions, or left-ventricular aneurysms. When symptoms, such as dyspnea on exertion or orthopnea, are due to impairment of ventricular relaxation rather than diminished systolic contraction, specific measures may be indicated to reduce left ventricular hypertrophy or myocardial ischemia.

RECOGNITION AND REMOVAL OF PRECIPITATING CAUSES (see also p. 448). The recognition, prompt treatment, and, whenever possible, prevention of the specific entities that cause or exacerbate heart failure, such as infections, arrhythmias, and pulmonary emboli, are crucial to the successful management of heart failure. Excessive intake of alcohol, incessant tachycardia, or thyroid disease can serve as primary causes of heart failure and secondary causes of clinical deterioration in patients with heart failure due to other conditions such as chronic valvular or coronary artery disease.

General Approach to the Patient with Established Heart Failure

A condition as complex and variable as heart failure cannot be treated according to a simple formula; however, useful treatment guidelines have been developed[1] (i.e., pp. 1985 to 1989). Effective management depends not only on an appreciation of the nature of the underlying condition, but also on the tempo of progression; the presence of associated illnesses; the patient's age, occupation, personality, life style, family setting, and ability and motivation to cooperate with treatment; and, importantly, response to the therapeutic measures. The course of heart failure is rarely smoothly progressive; rather it is usually punctuated by a series of abrupt downward steps due to acute decompensation, generally as a consequence of one of the precipitating causes described on page 448 (see Fig. 17–1). When the precipitating cause has been removed and treatment has been intensified, the patient's previous condition may be restored. In other patients there are long periods—many months or even years—when the course is stable without any discernible deterioration.

After potentially reversible factors are addressed, the therapeutic regimen is designed according to the clinical stage (see Table 17–1), usually classified according to the New York Heart Association class (see p. 452). Most clinical studies addressing the efficacy of various interventions

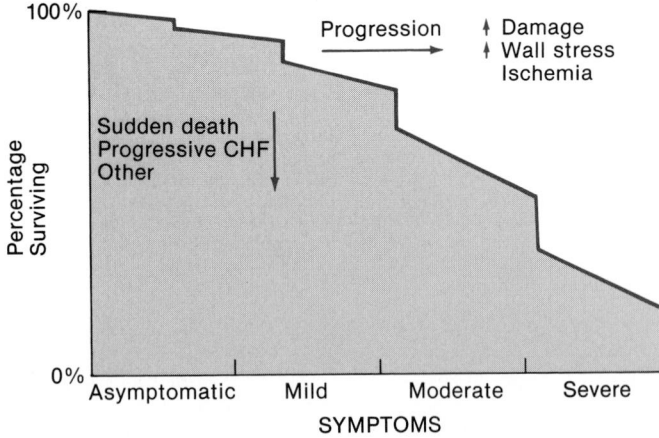

FIGURE 17–1. The natural history of congestive heart failure (CHF) is illustrated schematically. CHF usually progresses over time (either gradually or abruptly) from asymptomatic left ventricular dysfunction to severe CHF, as indicated on the horizontal axis. The mechanism of progression varies. The vertical axis indicates the proportion of patients surviving. Although mortality rates accelerate as CHF worsens, sudden death may occur at any stage (shown by the abrupt decreases in survival rate). Other deaths occur from progressive CHF and a variety of complications. (From Cheitlin, M. D. [ed.]: Dilemmas in Clinical Cardiology. Philadelphia, F.A. Davis, 1990, p. 256; with permission.)

TABLE 17–1 TARGETS OF THERAPY FOR HEART FAILURE

PATIENT DESCRIPTION		SYMPTOMS	MORTALITY		DISEASE PROGRESSION
Class			Progressive Heart Failure	Unexpected	
I	Asymptomatic			++	+++
II	Mildly symptomatic *(with vigorous activity)*	(+)	(+)	++	++
III	Moderately to severely symptomatic *(with routine activity)*	++	++	+	+
IV	Decompensated *(bed and chair)*	+++	+++	+	(+)

+++ Very strong target for therapy.   +   Probable target.
++ Strong target.   (+)   Possible target.

have described the heart failure in the populations under study as "asymptomatic" (NYHA Class I), "mild-to-moderate" (Classes II and III), or "severe (Class IV)." Once believed to be a hopeless condition, heart failure at every stage has now been shown to be influenced favorably by judicious intervention. Although much emphasis is still placed on the limited prognosis of patients with overt congestive heart failure, the current therapeutic armamentarium, carefully tailored to the individual patient, can yield good results even in severely symptomatic patients, as indicated by the ability of many patients to achieve functional capacity similar to that after transplantation. Two-year survival equivalent to that of cardiac transplantation can be achieved in many patients previously thought to have "end-stage heart failure" refractory to medical therapy.

The clinical features of heart failure reflect both the hemodynamic abnormalities and the disturbances of neurohormonal regulation that precede and may hasten the onset of symptoms. Therapy is initially directed at limitation of neurohormonal activation and broadened to address hemodynamic abnormalities as they become sufficiently severe to cause symptoms, first during activity and ultimately at rest.

Asymptomatic Patients with Ventricular Dysfunction

In asymptomatic patients (that is, patients with impaired cardiac function, NYHA Class I), therapy focuses on prevention of progression of disease (Fig. 17–2). Angiotensin-converting enzyme (ACE) inhibitors have been shown to diminish ventricular dilation in patients with symptomatic left-ventricular dysfunction who have suffered myocardial infarction, and they are useful in such patients because they delay the development of heart failure.[1a] Extended follow-up has shown that this therapy eventually translates into improved survival.[2–4] Recent trials have also demonstrated that ACE inhibitors reduce or delay the onset of congestive heart failure in asymptomatic patients with compromised ejection fractions from multiple causes.[5] Emphasis should also be placed on the reduction of factors that could hasten progression of disease such as hypertension, obesity, excessive use of alcohol, and, in the case of coronary artery disease, the risk factors for atherosclerosis. It is prudent to moderate salt intake in order to delay the onset of fluid retention that will lead to increased intracardiac filling pressures and eventually to congestive symptoms. The impact of digoxin is not well defined in these patients, who might derive benefit from the suppression of sympathetic tone caused by this drug but would be at some risk of developing arrhythmias.

Symptomatic Heart Failure

The cardinal symptoms of heart failure reflect the hemodynamic abnormalities of elevated filling pressures and reduced cardiac output that occur first with major exertion (Class II), then during routine activity (Class III), and ultimately at rest (Class IV). Less commonly, symptoms may relate to arrhythmias or embolic events associated with

heart failure. As patients progress through cycles of compensation and decompensation, a consistent approach to clinical assessment, as described in detail in Chapter 15, provides the continuity necessary to optimize hemodynamic status and minimize symptoms.

Patients who describe symptoms of dyspnea and fatigue only with major exertion (NY Heart Association Class II) often demonstrate normal resting hemodynamics but reduced maximal oxygen uptake (see Ch. 5 and Fig. 14–26, p. 439), maximal cardiac output, and elevated intracardiac filling pressures during peak exercise. The distinction between this group and asymptomatic patients is frequently the result of differences in levels of activity and perception of fatigue. These patients should, in the absence of contraindications or side effects, receive ACE inhibitors to prevent progression of disease; therapy in this setting is designed primarily to reduce future risk rather than to improve clinical status. Although severe volume depletion should be avoided at the time that ACE inhibition is initiated, salt restriction is part of the regimen for these patients, consisting first of avoiding added salt then avoiding foods prepared with salt such as canned foods and processed foods. Levels of exertion that cause severe fatigue should be avoided, but patients should be encouraged to continue regular aerobic activity at a level that they can easily tolerate. Isometric exercise, associated with increases

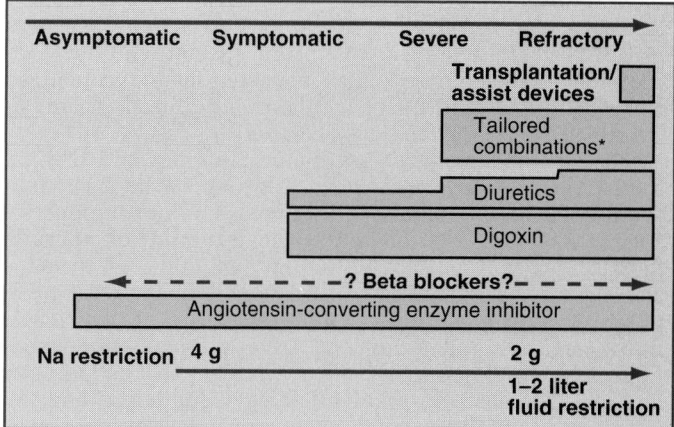

FIGURE 17–2. Escalation of therapy for left ventricular dysfunction in relation to the severity of symptoms and hemodynamic decompensation. Angiotensin-converting enzyme (ACE) inhibition has been demonstrated to improve prognosis for patients at all levels of heart failure. Digoxin decreases symptoms of heart failure once they have developed. It is not yet known which patients may benefit from beta-adrenergic blocking agents. Cardiac transplantation or implantable ventricular assist devices are considered only for a very small population with heart failure refractory to all other therapies.

*The term tailored combinations refers to the use of additional vasodilators (usually in combination with an ACE inhibitor) and, when necessary, short-term hemodynamic monitoring and use of intravenous nitroprusside, or dobutamine.

in peripheral resistance rather than the beneficial decreases during aerobic exercise, is generally proscribed.

SYMPTOMATIC TREATMENT. The general strategy in treating symptomatic heart failure is to use relatively simple means and then progressively stricter and more aggressive measures if clinical manifestations of heart failure persist or recur. An hour of supine rest in the afternoon frequently reduces overall fatigue. Depending on the level of symptoms and the physical demands of employment, some patients will need to restrict their hours or retire from work as symptoms become more severe. Initial symptoms can in many cases be treated with ACE inhibitors, which should be increased to target doses (Table 16–1, p. 472) or instituted if not previously prescribed. In addition to reducing progression of disease, ACE inhibitors help to address hemodynamic abnormalities through complex interactions involving inhibition of angiotensin II generation and aldosterone release, reducing sympathetic tone and thirst, and increasing bradykinin and prostaglandin levels.

Patients developing evidence of congestion despite adequate degrees of ACE inhibition and salt restriction should begin therapy with a *diuretic*. Although thiazide diuretics may restore fluid balance initially, many patients progress to need a loop diuretic. Patients with more advanced heart failure who are already on large doses of loop diuretics often respond to the addition of metolazone or a thiazide (see p. 477).

There is evidence of benefit from the use of *digoxin* in patients with symptomatic heart failure due to predominant systolic dysfunction, in whom ejection fraction and exercise capacity are improved, while rehospitalizations are decreased (see p. 501). Whether or not digoxin also improves survival in this population should be known after completion of the Digoxin Investigators Group (DIG) trial. A routine of regular exercise should continue.

Both the ACE inhibitors and the combination of hydralazine and isosorbide dinitrate have been shown to improve functional capacity and survival in mild-to-moderate heart failure.[4–7] Although ACE inhibitors offer additional survival benefits, the combination of hydralazine and isosorbide dinitrate represents a good alternative for the patient who cannot tolerate ACE inhibitors owing to cough, renal dysfunction, rash, angioneurotic edema, or other side effects. When symptoms and evidence of congestion persist during therapy with ACE inhibitors, the patient who is already receiving high doses of these agents (150 mg/day of captopril or 20 mg/day of enalapril) or the patient who develops symptomatic hypotension may benefit from individualized combinations of multiple vasodilator and diuretic agents as described below for refractory heart failure (see p. 507).

Careful adjustment of vasodilator, diuretic, and digoxin therapy can render the majority of patients with heart failure free from clinical evidence of congestion or hypoperfusion at rest. Relief of congestion usually improves not only the resting symptoms but also the symptoms of dyspnea and fatigue during minimal exertion. Patients with heart failure and severe fatigue *without* elevation of ventricular filling pressure often do not derive symptomatic benefit from additional modifications of a regimen that already includes standard doses of effective vasodilators and digoxin. Some patients with severe exertional dyspnea will derive benefit from the addition of oral nitrates (including a nitrate-free interval) to the baseline regimen or the use of prophylactic sublingual isosorbide dinitrate immediately before exertion.

When hypoperfusion becomes clinically evident (Table 17–2), outpatient therapy of symptomatic congestion is usually insufficient to achieve the patient's optimal condition. The cautious alterations in diuretic and vasodilator doses that are feasible in an outpatient setting usually have little effect or may precipitate hypotension and renal dysfunction. The presence of frequent angina or symptomatic ventricular arrhythmias should lower the threshold for hos-

TABLE 17–2 CONDITIONS THAT MAY WARRANT HEMODYNAMIC MONITORING

Hypoperfusion suspected from:
 Narrow pulse pressure
 Cool extremities
 Mental obtundation
 Declining renal function with volume overload
 Marked hyponatremia

Congestion in the presence of:
 Angina or other evidence of active ischemia
 Hemodynamically significant arrhythmias
 Persistent systematic hypotension during ACEI therapy
 Baseline renal impairment
 Severe intrinsic pulmonary disease

Persistent congestion despite all of the following:
 Salt and fluid restriction
 High-dose loop diuretics
 Metolazone or a thiazide

Evaluation for heart transplantation for advanced heart failure

pital admission to adjust hemodynamic status (see Table 17–2). Hypotension, hyponatremia, and azotemia further identify patients who may be particularly difficult to stabilize without extensive redesign of the medical regimen. Unsuccessful attempts to address congestion and hypoperfusion simultaneously in the outpatient setting may lead to the erroneous conclusion that heart failure has become refractory to medical therapy. Similarly, repeated relapses after admissions for brief inotropic and diuretic infusions may indicate the need to redesign oral therapy during hemodynamic monitoring. Thus, these patients may be considered as refractory to outpatient management. Their treatment is discussed on page 507.

VASODILATORS

A convenient framework in which to address the principles of vasodilator therapy include the concepts of preload and afterload reduction. Although this discussion focuses on heart failure due to predominant left-ventricular dysfunction, the general principles of vasodilator therapy are applicable to failure of either or both ventricles. There will be differences, however, in the specific drugs or other forms of therapy that can be used. For example, inhaled nitric oxide may effectively reduce pulmonary vascular resistance, whereas hydralazine reduces systemic vascular resistance. Nitroprusside decreases both pulmonary and systemic vascular resistance.

PRELOAD REDUCTION. Increases in heart rate as well as in diastolic intraventricular volume and pressure compensate for a decline in ventricular systolic performance. The relationship between ventricular filling pressures and cardiac stroke work is the familiar Frank-Starling curve (see p. 378) and is shown in Figure 17–3. In more advanced heart failure, there is often little augmentation of stroke volume with increasing filling pressures, and the transmission of increased pressure into the pulmonary and systemic venous beds produces edema and congestive symptoms.

These hemodynamic adaptations are often accompanied by worsening myocardial energy metabolism due to an increase in systolic and diastolic ventricular wall stress. They also result in a decrease in coronary blood flow, even in the absence of coronary artery disease, owing to the increase in heart rate, decline in mean arterial pressure, and increase in intracavitary and right atrial pressures. Therefore, agents that reduce ventricular filling pressures by selectively decreasing intravascular volume (e.g., diuretics) or by increasing venous capacitance (e.g., predominantly venous vasodilators such as nitrates) reduce pulmonary venous congestion with minimal effects on stroke volume and cardiac output.

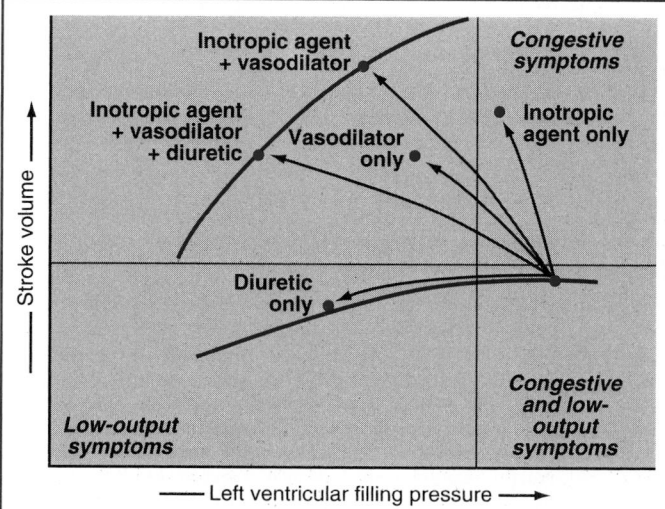

FIGURE 17–3. Frank-Starling ventricular function curves in heart failure due to systolic dysfunction. Predicted hemodynamic effects and consequent impact on symptoms of positive inotropic agents (e.g., digoxin), a balanced vasodilator (e.g., captopril), or a diuretic (e.g., furosemide) alone or in combination, in a patient with mild ventricular systolic dysfunction *(upper curve)* or severe ventricular systolic dysfunction *(lower curve)*. (Modified from: Smith, T. W., and Kelly, R. A.: Therapeutic strategies for CHF in the 1990's. Hosp. Pract. **26**:127, 1991. © 1991, The McGraw-Hill Companies, Inc.)

Preload reduction clearly improves symptoms due to systolic ventricular dysfunction and may also benefit patients with congestive symptoms due to impaired diastolic function (reduced compliance) (see p. 402). It should be kept in mind, however, that patients with diastolic dysfunction due to poorly compliant, hypertrophied ventricles may require elevated end-diastolic filling pressures to support an adequate forward stroke volume. In critical aortic stenosis, for example, a large decrease in preload may markedly reduce cardiac output, and therefore vasodilators and diuretics should be administered cautiously to these patients.

AFTERLOAD REDUCTION. Afterload, the sum of forces opposing ventricular emptying during systole, includes aortic and aortic outflow tract (including valvular) impedance and systemic vascular resistance. Afterload is also affected by the volume of blood in the ventricle at the initiation of systole and by ventricular-vascular coupling (i.e., the harmonics of reflected arterial pressure waves during systole). Hypertrophy of cardiac muscle is a physiological response to an increase in afterload and initially tends to preserve ventricular systolic function (Fig. 13–7, p. 399). A reduction in ventricular wall stress during systole, whether achieved by corrective surgery, intra-aortic balloon counterpulsation, or vasodilator drugs, results in improved systolic contractile function. The lowering of afterload improves forward stroke volume (Fig. 17–4) and reduces the regurgitant fraction due to functional mitral regurgitation, a common complicating factor in patients with enlarged left ventricles and severe heart failure secondary to systolic dysfunction.

Vasodilators are often classified as either predominantly "arteriolar" (afterload reducing) or predominantly "venous" (preload reducing), although many vasodilators exhibit activity in both vascular beds. The arteriolar vasodilator hydralazine, for example, may have little or no effect on venous capacitance despite causing a significant reduction in systemic vascular resistance. Nitroglycerin, a predominantly venous vasodilator, at lower doses may cause a pronounced increase in venous capacitance with little effect on the systemic arterial vasculature. The hemodynamic effects of vasodilators in current use are listed in Table 16–1, page 472. Nitroprusside is among the most effective afterload reducing agents because, in addition to reducing sys-

temic vascular resistance, it increases aortic wall compliance and improves ventricular-vascular coupling. Direct intrarenal effects of several classes of these drugs, such as hydralazine and ACE inhibitors, may also prove effective in preserving renal blood flow and in promoting the effectiveness of diuretics.

Renin-Angiotensin System Antagonists
Survival Trials of ACE Inhibitors in Heart Failure

A number of well-designed prospective trials have demonstrated that ACE inhibitors improve survival in patients with overt heart failure due to systolic ventricular dysfunction regardless of the etiology or severity of symptoms. The COoperative Northern Scandinavian ENalapril SUrvival Study (CONSENSUS-1)[3] demonstrated a 40 per cent reduction in mortality at 6 months in patients with severe heart failure already treated with digoxin, diuretics, and other vasodilators, who were randomized to enalapril rather than placebo (Fig. 17–5). This finding, combined with those of smaller trials, convincingly demonstrates that ACE inhibitors improve survival of patients with severe heart failure (i.e., patients who were symptomatic at rest). Subsequent trials have examined the question of whether the much larger population of patients with left ventricular systolic dysfunction who have mild or moderate heart failure or who are asymptomatic also receive a survival benefit. The "treatment" arm of the Studies on Left Ventricular Dysfunction[4] (SOLVD) trial that randomized patients with symptomatic mild-to-moderate heart failure with left ventricular ejection fractions less than 35 per cent who received either enalapril or placebo reported a statistically significant 16 per cent reduction in overall mortality in the enalapril-treated group. Although the "prevention" arm of this trial that examined asymptomatic patients with a simi-

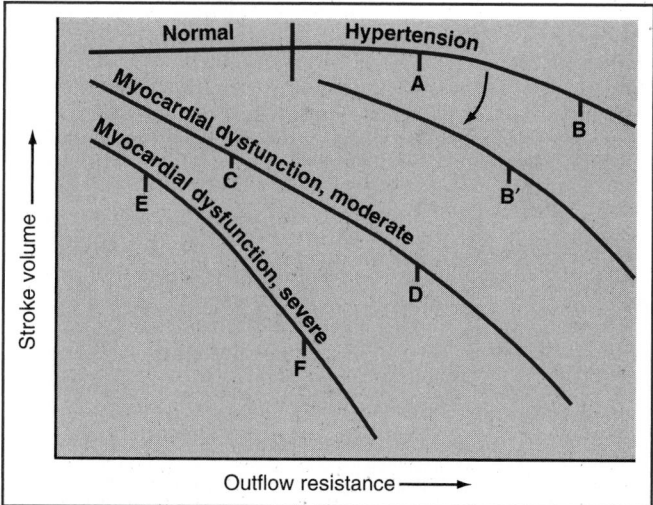

FIGURE 17–4. Relation of left ventricular stroke volume to systemic outflow resistance in normal and diseased hearts. A family of curves may be described, depending on the severity of the myocardial disease. If cardiac function is normal, a rise in resistance results in hypertension, as cardiac output remains fairly constant. Heart failure in a hypertensive patient could be shown by a move to either point B, a high resistance with normal function, or point B', which represents a shift to a slightly depressed ventricular function curve. When myocardial dysfunction is more severe, as shown by the lower two curves, blood pressure is no longer directly determined by resistance, as stroke volume and resistance are inversely related. Consequently, arterial pressure may be similar at points E and F despite marked differences in cardiac output and resistance. It is also apparent that a reduction in outflow resistance will not affect significantly the stroke volume of the normal ventricle. However, it can produce a marked increase in the stroke volume on the failing ventricle (F → E). (From Cohn, J. N., and Franciosa, J. A.: Vasodilator therapy of cardiac failure. N. Engl. J. Med. **297**:27, 1977. Copyright 1977 Massachusetts Medical Society.)

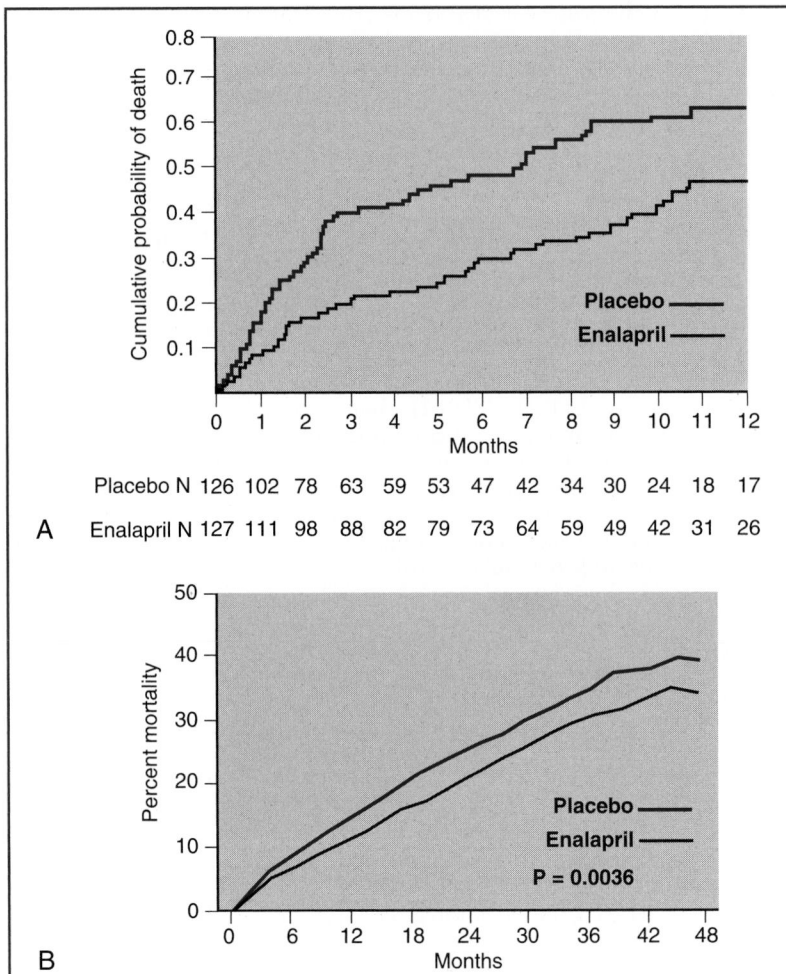

FIGURE 17–5. *A*, Cumulative probability of death in the placebo and enalapril groups in the CONSENSUS trial and *B*, in the SOLVD trial. (*A*, Reprinted from CONSENSUS Trial Study Group: Effects of enalapril on mortality in severe congestive heart failure: Results of the Cooperative North Scandinavian Enalapril Survival Study [CONSENSUS]. N. Engl. J. Med. *316*:1429, 1987, with permission. *B*, From SOLVD Investigators: Effect of enalapril on survival in patients with reduced left ventricular ejection fractions and congestive heart failure. N. Engl. J. Med. *325*:293, 1991. Copyright 1991 Massachusetts Medical Society.)

lar degree of left ventricular dysfunction failed to demonstrate a statistically significant reduction in mortality among enalapril-treated patients,[5] there was a significant (29 per cent) reduction in the combined endpoints of development of symptomatic heart failure and death due to any cause.

The second Veterans Administration Cooperative Vasodilator Heart Failure Trial[6] (V-HeFT-II) showed a small but clear survival benefit in patients with mild-to-moderate heart failure who had been randomized to receive enalapril rather than the combination of hydralazine and isosorbide dinitrate. A smaller randomized trial comparing captopril to hydralazine isosorbide dinitrate in patients with moderate-to-severe heart failure also demonstrated a significant survival advantage in patients receiving ACE inhibitors.[7]

The Survival And Ventricular Enlargement (SAVE) trial[8,9] studied patients with recent myocardial infarctions and ejection fractions of 40 per cent or less, but without overt heart failure, and showed a 20 per cent reduction in mortality and a 36 per cent reduction in the rate of progression to severe heart failure in the captopril-treated group after 48 months of follow-up. Both the SOLVD[10] and the SAVE trials[11] demonstrated that enalapril and captopril, respectively, markedly reduced or prevented the increases in left ventricular end-diastolic and end-systolic volumes and decline in ejection fraction observed in patients randomized to receive placebo. The Acute Infarction Ramipril Efficacy (AIRE) trial[12] had a study design similar to that of the SAVE trial, except that it randomized only patients who manifested clinical evidence of heart failure to either ramipril or placebo. There was a significant (27 per cent) reduction in mortality in the ACE inhibitor-treated group that was apparent within 30 days of treatment (unlike SAVE, in which the survival curves did not diverge until 1 year).

The Trandelopril Cardiac Evaluation (TRACE) trial studied patients with severe left-ventricular dysfunction 3 to 7 days following myocardial infarction and reported a 20 per cent reduction in mortality.[13] Taken together, these trials indicate that ACE inhibitors prolong survival in a broad spectrum of patients with myocardial infarction and heart failure, ranging from those who are asymptomatic with ventricular dysfunction to those who have symptomatic heart failure but are normotensive and hemodynamically stable. The role of ACE inhibitors in the early treatment of patients with acute myocardial infarction is discussed in Chapter 37.

DOSES OF ACE INHIBITORS. There is no precisely defined relationship between dosage and long-term clinical effectiveness of these drugs.[2,14] The target dosages of an ACE inhibitor in several large prospective trials in which a positive effect was demonstrated on mortality as well as other endpoints were 50 mg of captopril three times daily,[8] 10 mg of enalapril twice daily,[6] 10 mg of lisinopril once daily,[15] 5 mg of ramipril twice daily,[12] or 30 mg of zofenopril twice daily.[16] Higher dosages are often used in the treatment of hypertension, but it is unclear whether increasing the dosage beyond that used in these trials will necessarily result in additional benefit.[14] Upward dosage titration may be prudent if a patient's blood pressure remains above a target level and may be of benefit in selected patients with significant functional mitral regurgitation. Despite the evidence for a class effect with these drugs, Pitt[14] has argued persuasively that it may be unwise to assume that all ACE inhibitors are equal or that dosages other than those shown to improve mortality in controlled clinical trials can be relied on to exert the demonstrated effects. Adding a second vasodilator (e.g., hydralazine, with or without nitrates) has been advocated by some investigators[17] in patients with advanced heart failure. However, this approach has not yet been evaluated in controlled clinical survival trials.

Yusuf et al.[18] and Lonn et al.,[19] in an overview of several clinical trials, have noted that ACE inhibitors appear to be reducing mortality by more than one mechanism. The most important reason for a reduction in mortality was a decrease in the rate of progression to worsening heart failure due in part to the direct hemodynamic effects of these drugs on ventricular remodeling and progressive dilation. However, both the SOLVD[4,5] and SAVE trials[8,9] also documented a reduction in acute myocardial infarction, an effect that could be due to improved myocardial energetics (due to decreased ventricular wall stress), prevention of myocardial hypertrophy, or a number of other mechanisms that are the subject of active investigation.

COST-BENEFIT RATIO. Paul et al.[20] have analyzed the cost-per-year of life extended of ACE inhibitors and combined hydralazine isosorbide dinitrate therapy for heart failure based on data from the SOLVD[4,5] and V-HeFT II[6] trials. Based on a decision analytic model, they estimated that enalapril added to standard heart failure therapy cost approximately $9700 per year of life extended (compared to $25,000 per year of life saved for the treatment of moderate hypertension), a cost that is well within the accepted range for many medical therapies. Although the combination of hydralazine and isosorbide dinitrate was more cost-effective than enalapril, the survival advantage with ACE inhibitors is significantly higher, and the cost differential will disappear as generic ACE inhibitors become available.

QUALITY OF LIFE. Despite the clear gains in survival, the impact of ACE inhibitors on quality of life measures, when compared to placebo or to other classes of vasodilators, has been less consistent. A marginal improvement in self-assessment of quality of life was observed in symptomatic patients randomized to receive enalapril in the SOLVD treatment trial.[21] However, there was no difference between symptomatic patients receiving enalapril and placebo in the SOLVD prevention trial or between patients with mild heart failure receiving either quinapril or placebo.[22] Quality of life measures were also not different in patients with more advanced heart failure randomized to receive either enalapril or the combination of hydralazine and isosorbide dinitrate in VeHeFT-II.[23] These data indicate that vasodilators probably have little impact on quality of life measures in patients with asymptomatic or mild heart failure (i.e., NYHA Class I or II), and that ACE inhibitors offer little or no advantage over other effective vasodilators in patients with more severe heart failure insofar as quality of life is concerned.

ACE Inhibitors and Valvular Regurgitation

The efficacy of ACE inhibitors in the treatment of chronic mitral or aortic regurgitation has been directly evaluated in a small number of studies (Chap. 32). Many patients with advanced heart failure secondary to ventricular systolic dysfunction have functional mitral regurgitation on the basis of dilation of the left ventricle and mitral valve ring. While treatment of mitral regurgitation with hydralazine or sodium nitroprusside is successful in short-term treatment, intravenous nitroprusside is impractical as chronic therapy, and hydralazine, when given alone, must be used at relatively high doses that often are associated with adverse effects. Intravenous enalapril has been shown to reduce the volume of regurgitant flow and to increase cardiac index significantly in patients with severe functional mitral regurgitation.[24] Captopril has been demonstrated to reduce functional mitral regurgitation in patients with heart failure and ischemic cardiomyopathy; significant improvements in stroke volume, systemic vascular resistance, left atrial size, and a daily activity status index were present in patients receiving 100 mg/day of captopril.[25] These findings, when combined with results of the SAVE study[8,11] and the SOLVD treatment trial[4,10] demonstrate that

progressive left ventricular dilation, which is associated with functional mitral regurgitation, can often be reduced by ACE inhibitors and that these drugs are effective in the chronic management of this complication of left ventricular dysfunction.

Although less well documented, ACE inhibitors may also be of benefit in the medical management of left ventricular dysfunction secondary to aortic regurgitation. Enalapril (20 mg twice a day) was more effective than hydralazine in reducing left ventricular dimensions and left ventricular mass index in patients with mild-to-severe acute regurgitation.[26] Similar results were observed with quinapril (20 mg/day).[27]

FIRST-DOSE EFFECTS

It is advisable to begin therapy with an ACE inhibitor at low doses of a relatively short-acting drug (e.g., 6.25 mg of captopril or 2.5 mg of enalapril). An abrupt fall in blood pressure occasionally occurs following an initial dose of an ACE inhibitor, particularly in patients with depletion of intravascular volume. This response is often unpredictable; therefore, caution is recommended when beginning these drugs in any patient with significant left ventricular dysfunction, especially those who have received large doses of diuretics. Unacceptable hypotension can usually be reversed by intravascular volume expansion, although this is obviously not ideal in patients with heart failure.

The maximal hypotensive response to an initial oral dose of captopril occurs 1 to 2 hours after dosing, whereas the maximal response to oral enalapril occurs 4 to 6 hours after dosing. Among patients with left ventricular dysfunction without heart failure who, shortly after myocardial infarction, were given 12.5 mg of captopril in the SAVE trial, 5 per cent experienced dizziness, although the number of patients withdrawn from the trial owing to this symptom was not different from that of patients receiving placebo. Among patients in the SOLVD trials begun on 2.5 mg of enalapril, only 1.3 per cent experienced unacceptable side effects, most commonly symptoms of hypotension. In comparing the first-dose effects of enalapril (2.5 mg), captopril (6.25 mg), and quinapril (2.5 mg) in patients with mild-to-moderate heart failure, each drug dropped blood pressure to a comparable degree, although with a more rapid time course in the case of captopril.[28-31] Only approximately 4 per cent of patients experienced mild and transient side effects.

This favorable experience with oral captopril, enalapril, and quinapril may not be directly transferable to other ACE inhibitors owing to differences in the rate of activation of prodrugs and other pharmacokinetic considerations. For example, intravenous infusion of 1.5 mg of enalaprilat leads to a much more rapid decline in arterial pressure than oral enalapril, causing a 15 to 20 per cent decline in mean arterial pressure within 60 minutes that typically persists for 4 to 6 hours.[32]

It is reasonable to initiate ACE inhibitor therapy in patients with chronic left ventricular dysfunction with those drugs for which extensive pharmacokinetic data exist in this patient population. (As of this writing, these include captopril, enalapril, lisinopril, and ramipril.) With careful observation of blood pressure, serum electrolytes, and serum creatinine levels, ACE inhibitor doses are customarily titrated upward over several days in hospitalized patients or a few weeks in ambulatory patients.

ACE INHIBITORS AND COUGH

Cough is an annoying side effect occurring in up to 5 per cent of patients on long-term therapy with ACE inhibitors.[33,34] The mechanism is unclear, but it is presumed to be due to inhibition of the metabolism of bradykinin and to substance P and inflammatory neuropeptides in the lung.[35] Patients with underlying structural lung disease or asthma are not at increased risk for this adverse effect. Cough often appears only after weeks or months of ACE inhibitor therapy, explaining why shorter prospective trials of these drugs reported a relatively low incidence of cough (i.e., 0.5 per cent in GISSI-3).[15] Approximately 3 per cent of patients in the SAVE study receiving active drug had to be withdrawn owing to cough compared with 1 per cent receiving placebo.[8] This symptom usually disappears within several days but may persist for up to 2 weeks after discontinuing the drug. Although switching to a different ACE inhibitor is rarely effective, some patients respond to a reduction in dosage.[34] Angiotensin receptor antagonists may be the best alternative for most patients with intractable cough. Inhaled sodium cromoglycate (40 mg/day in divided doses) has proved effective in reducing the frequency of cough in short-term trials.[36]

Nitrovasodilators

Nitrovasodilators have a well-established role in the management of heart failure (p. 474). Intravenous sodium nitroprusside (nitroprusside) is particularly useful in patients with advanced heart failure characterized by a reduced cardiac output and a high left ventricular filling pressure and systemic vascular resistance.[37,38] Although mean arterial pressure may be slightly reduced in these patients, most will respond to judicious administration of intravenous nitroprusside with a larger increase in stroke volume than patients with less severe ventricular dysfunction (see Fig. 17–4).[39] Forward stroke volume is often further enhanced by decreased "functional" mitral regurgitation as systemic vascular resistance and ventricular-filling pressures and volumes decrease; as a consequence, systemic arterial pressure can usually be sustained.[37] With continuous hemodynamic monitoring of right atrial, pulmonary capillary wedge, and systemic arterial pressures, sodium nitroprusside is often used as an initial strategy in the "tailored" medical management of advanced heart failure discussed on pages 508 to 509. The initial infusion rate is typically 0.3 μg/kg/min and is titrated upward depending on hemodynamic response. Cyanide and/or thiocyanate toxicities may be observed at infusion rates above 1.5 μg/kg/min.

As with most vasodilators, the most common adverse effect of nitroprusside is hypotension. The redistribution of blood flow from central organs to peripheral vascular beds may limit or prevent an increase in renal blood flow despite an increase in cardiac output. Nitroprusside-induced nonselective pulmonary arteriolar vasodilation may improve right ventricular function but also may worsen ventilation–perfusion mismatches in patients with advanced chronic obstructive pulmonary disease or large pleural effusions.[39] Coronary arteriolar dilation may reduce perfusion pressure to myocardium supplied by partially occluded vessels, creating a "coronary steal" in patients with heart failure and severe fixed obstructions in epicardial coronary arteries. This may account for an increase in the frequency of angina in response to nitroprusside in some patients with an ischemic cardiomyopathy despite a favorable hemodynamic response. An organic nitrate and hydralazine or an ACE inhibitor should then be substituted.

OTHER ORGANIC NITRATES. Despite its limited effects on systemic vascular resistance and the problem of pharmacological tolerance, isosorbide dinitrate has been shown to be more effective than placebo in improving capacity for exercise and in reducing symptoms when administered chronically to patients with heart failure. Isosorbide dinitrate has been shown to increase the clinical effectiveness of other vasodilators such as hydralazine, resulting in a sustained improvement in hemodynamics that exceeded that of either drug given alone. At a dose of 40 mg four times daily in combination with hydralazine, isosorbide dinitrate reduced overall mortality compared either to placebo or to the alpha$_1$-adrenergic receptor antagonist prazosin in the V-HeFT-I trial carried out in patients with mild-to-moderate heart failure concurrently treated with digoxin and diuretics.[40]

Hydralazine

As already mentioned, the combination of hydralazine (200 to 300 mg/day) and isosorbide dinitrate (120 to 160 mg/day) increased survival compared with placebo in V-HeFT I[40] but was less effective than enalapril in reducing mortality in heart failure patients in the V-HeFT II trial.[6] In another prospective trial comparing hydralazine with an ACE inhibitor, the Hydralazine versus ACE Inhibition with Captopril on Mortality in Advanced Heart Failure, or "Hy-C" study,[7] patients receiving captopril had a greater survival advantage than those receiving hydralazine (23 per cent cause mortality on captopril compared with 43 per cent on hydralazine at 8 months). However, hydralazine—with or without nitrates—may provide additional hemodynamic improvement for patients already being treated with conventional doses of an ACE inhibitor, digoxin, and di-

uretics,[17,41] although this has not yet been tested rigorously in clinical trials.

As with the ACE inhibitors, the most appropriate dosage of hydralazine has not been determined in heart failure. A target dosage of 300 mg daily was employed in the V-HeFT[14,40] trials and, in combination with isosorbide dinitrate, was documented to have a positive impact on survival. Although additional hemodynamic benefit may be demonstrable at higher dosages (the average dose of hydralazine in the Hy-C trial was 410 mg/day[7]), this has not been shown to translate into prolonged survival when compared to an ACE inhibitor.

DIURETICS

(See also pp. 849 to 851)

Unlike all other classes of drugs commonly employed in the treatment of heart failure, there have been no controlled prospective clinical trials designed to test the efficacy and safety of diuretics in the contemporary medical management of heart failure.[41a] Although recent evidence from studies of diuretic use in hypertension is reassuring regarding the safety of these drugs, these data cannot be directly applied to patients with heart failure.[42–45a] In our view, diuretics should not be used as first-line agents in the treatment of asymptomatic or mild heart failure (NYHA Class I and early Class II). Diuretics should be used periodically if signs or symptoms of heart failure persist or worsen on an optimal medical regimen of vasodilators and moderate salt restriction, with or without digoxin.

In patients with moderately severe heart failure (NYHA Class III), daily administration of loop diuretics will usually be necessary. Thiazide diuretics are usually ineffective as single agents in advanced heart failure. Potassium-sparing diuretics, particularly spironolactone or amiloride, or oral potassium (KCl) supplements, are often useful to prevent hypokalemia in patients on a daily loop diuretic regimen. However, their routine use is probably not necessary in patients receiving an ACE inhibitor and may be dangerous in patients with reduced renal function (i.e., a serum creatinine over 2 mg/dl).[46]

For patients with severe decompensated heart failure (NHYA Class IV), more aggressive use of loop diuretics alone or in combination with thiazide diuretics is warranted in the context of a tailored medical management approach to advanced heart failure. Sufficiently high doses of a loop diuretic need to be employed to exceed the threshold drug concentration within the renal tubular lumen needed to initiate and sustain a natriuresis. As in renal failure, this threshold response can be achieved by successive doubling of the intravenous dose until an adequate natriuretic response is achieved (Table 16–4, p. 479). For most patients with advanced heart failure, more than one "threshold" dose of a loop diuretic will be necessary each day to maintain a net negative sodium balance during the initial phase of a hospitalization. Adding a distally acting diuretic such as a thiazide is also effective but often is complicated by large urinary potassium losses. For a more detailed description of the metabolic complications of diuretic use in heart failure, see Chapter 16.

An alternative strategy in hospitalized patients is to administer the same daily parenteral dose of a loop diuretic by a continuous intravenous infusion.[47] This will lead to a sustained natriuresis due to the continual presence of high drug levels within the tubular lumen. This approach requires the use of a constant infusion pump but permits more precise control over the natriuretic effect. It also diminishes the potential for a too-rapid decline in intravascular volume and hypotension as well as the risk of ototoxicity in patients given large bolus intravenous doses of loop diuretics. A typical continuous furosemide infusion is initiated with a 20- to 40-mg intravenous loading dose as a bolus injection followed by a continuous infusion of 5 mg/hr, for a patient who had been receiving 200 mg of oral furosemide (or 100 mg intravenously) per day in divided doses.

USE OF DIURETICS IN THE ELDERLY. The age of patients with heart failure is increasing progressively. Elderly patients present special problems with diuretic use. In general, absorption of oral agents is delayed and renal clearance rates are lower in the elderly, thus slowing delivery of active drug to its renal tubular site of action. The decline in renal function that naturally occurs with aging diminishes the effectiveness of the thiazide diuretics earlier than the loop diuretics, since the thiazide diuretics are virtually ineffective at creatinine clearance rates below 30 to 40 ml/min. Epithelial Na^+ channel inhibitors (potassium-sparing diuretics), such as amiloride, also lose effectiveness as natriuretic agents in this range of creatinine clearance rate, although their potassium-sparing effects may be maintained. The elderly also have decreased baroreceptor responsiveness; reduced cerebral, renal, coronary, and splanchnic blood flow; and a tendency to electrolyte depletion.[48]

Elderly patients with congestive heart failure, with or without concomitant hypertension, often require multiple daily doses of a loop diuretic, often necessitating potassium and magnesium replacement.[48] Another important problem for which the elderly are probably at greater risk is hyponatremia. Although hyponatremia can occur with any diuretic, whether or not congestive heart failure is present, the longer-acting thiazide diuretics, alone or in combination with a potassium-sparing diuretic, appear to pose an unusually high risk. The decline in serum sodium is often exacerbated by poor dietary sodium and excessive free water intake and an inability to increase free water clearance (i.e., to dilute the urine appropriately), in part because of diuretic-induced hypovolemia. Hyponatremia may occur insidiously over weeks in the elderly and may be unassociated with any change in serum potassium levels. Mild confusion may go unnoticed in the elderly, but can rapidly degenerate into dementia, convulsions, and coma, even at serum sodium values near 130 mEq/liter, particularly if the fall in serum sodium has been rapid. Long-term administration of a loop diuretic may also lead to significant degrees of calcium depletion. Consequently, calcium supplements are recommended in elderly patients receiving these drugs. Magnesium losses, which occur with both thiazide and loop diuretics, may need to be replaced to increase serum ionized calcium and potassium levels (see Chap. 16).

DIGITALIS

Cardiac glycosides are of potential value in most patients with symptoms and signs of systolic heart failure secondary to ischemic, valvular, hypertensive, or congenital heart disease; dilated cardiomyopathies; and cor pulmonale. Improvement of depressed myocardial contractility by glycosides increases cardiac output, promotes diuresis, and reduces the filling pressure of the failing ventricle(s), with the consequent reduction of pulmonary vascular congestion and central venous pressure.

Digitalis is of no demonstrable benefit in isolated mitral stenosis with normal sinus rhythm unless right ventricular failure has supervened, or in patients with constrictive pericarditis except when there is invasion of the myocardium. There is no evidence that patients with left ventricular hypertrophy, normal left ventricular ejection fraction, and symptoms related to elevated filling pressures benefit from digitalis. Hypertrophic obstructive cardiomyopathy represents another condition in which digitalis is often of little

value and may actually be deleterious because it can increase left ventricular outflow obstruction by augmenting the contractility of the hypertrophic outflow tract segment. In the later stages of hypertrophic cardiomyopathy, in which ventricular dilation and congestive problems occasionally predominate over obstructive hemodynamics, cardiac glycosides may be beneficial.

Evidence of Clinical Efficacy

It is widely accepted that cardiac glycosides are of benefit in the treatment of patients with heart failure accompanied by atrial fibrillation or atrial flutter and a rapid ventricular response. Since the turn of the century, however, there has been ongoing controversy surrounding the efficacy of cardiac glycosides in the treatment of patients with heart failure who are in sinus rhythm.[49] Several small observational trials in ambulatory patients with mild-to-moderate heart failure in sinus rhythm in the 1970's and early 1980's questioned the effectiveness of digoxin. However, during the past decade, the results of several randomized controlled trials support the use of digoxin when administered either alone or with vasodilators to patients with heart failure due to predominant systolic dysfunction. Although some of these trials were designed to test the safety and efficacy of a new therapeutic agent in the treatment of heart failure rather than to verify the effectiveness of digoxin, a prospective, randomized placebo group crossover design was typically included that permitted an independent assessment of the effectiveness of digoxin in each trial.[50,51]

The PROVED (Prospective Randomized Study of Ventricular Failure and Efficacy of Digoxin)[52] and RADIANCE (Randomized Assessment of Digoxin on Inhibition of ANgiotensin-Converting Enzyme)[53] trials are two prospective multicenter placebo-controlled trials that examined the effects of withdrawal of digoxin in patients with stable mild-to-moderate heart failure (i.e., New York Heart Association Classes II and III) and systolic ventricular dysfunction (left ventricular ejection fraction ≤ 0.35). All patients studied were in normal sinus rhythm. The target serum digoxin concentration in both studies during the baseline run-in phase was 0.7 to 2.0 ng/ml, with an average digoxin dose of 0.38 mg/day. Patients in the RADIANCE trial also received concurrent therapy with an ACE inhibitor. When patients were randomly assigned to either continue active digoxin therapy or to withdraw from active therapy and receive a matching placebo, 40 per cent of patients in the PROVED trial and 28 per cent of patients in the RADIANCE trial who received placebo noted a significant worsening of heart failure symptoms compared to 20 per cent and 6 per cent, respectively, in patients who continued to receive active drug (Fig. 17–6). This absolute risk reduction of 20 per cent in digoxin-treated patients constituted a substantial treatment effect.[54] Maximal treadmill exercise tolerance also declined significantly in patients withdrawn from digoxin in both trials, despite continuation of other medical therapies for heart failure, including ACE inhibitor therapy in RADIANCE.[53]

In the Dutch Ibopamine Multicenter Trial (DIMT), which was designed to test the efficacy of ibopamine (see p. 486) in ambulatory patients with heart failure with mild-to-moderate congestive heart failure compared to patients receiving digoxin or placebo, digoxin also significantly increased exercise time at 6 months, prevented clinical deterioration, and reduced plasma norepinephrine concentrations.[55]

These trials did not have the statistical power to detect an effect of digoxin therapy on the survival of patients with heart failure, an endpoint for which efficacy had already been established for the use of selected vasodilators in heart failure. The effect of digoxin on survival in both idiopathic dilated and ischemic cardiomyopathies was the pri-

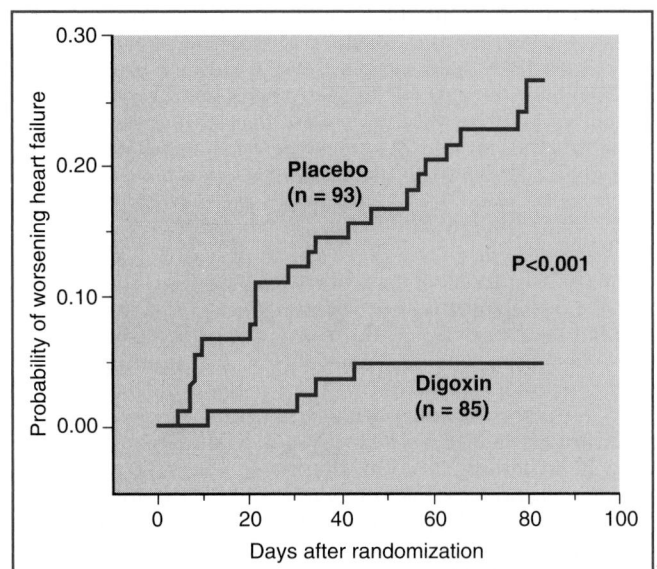

FIGURE 17–6. Kaplan-Meier analysis of the cumulative probability of worsening heart failure in patients continuing to receive digoxin and those switched to placebo. The patients in the placebo group had a higher risk of worsening heart failure throughout the 12-week study (relative risk, 5.9; 95 per cent confidence interval, 2.1 to 17.2; $P < 0.001$). (From Packer, M., Gheorghiade, M., Young, J. B., et al.: Withdrawal of digoxin from patients with chronic heart failure treated with angiotensin-converting enzyme inhibitors. N. Engl. J. Med. 329:1, 1993. Copyright Massachusetts Medical Society, with permission.)

mary endpoint for the multicenter National Insitutes of Health and Veterans Affairs Cooperative Studies Program-sponsored Digoxin Investigators' Group (DIG) trial, which enrolled 6800 patients with left ventricular ejection fractions of 45 per cent or lower, and who were receiving an ACE inhibitor (if tolerated) and diuretic. These patients and an additional group of 988 with a history of heart failure but with ejection fractions above 45 per cent were randomized to receive either digoxin or placebo.[56,57]

Follow-up at 3 to 5 years (mean 37 months) demonstrated no net impact on all-cause or cardiovascular mortality, with a lower incidence of mortality from progressive heart failure in the patients receiving digitalis being offset by an increased risk of presumed arrhythmia deaths. There was a substantial favorable effect of digoxin on the combined endpoint of death or hospitalization due to progressive heart failure. Treating 1000 patients with digoxin prevented 67 deaths or hospitalizations from worsening heart failure, while increasing risk of death or hospitalization from presumed arrhythmia for 15 patients.

Therapeutic Endpoints

The clinical use of cardiac glycosides is complicated by the absence of a readily measurable therapeutic endpoint except in atrial flutter or fibrillation, the lack of a reliable means to predict individual cardiac responses, and the difficulty in defining proximity to toxicity. The optimal dose of digitalis is not necessarily the largest dose that can be tolerated without the emergence of overt toxicity. The ratio of toxic to therapeutic effect for cardiac glycosides is small, and the availability of other measures of treating heart failure, particularly potent oral diuretics and vasodilators, usually obviates balancing therapy at the edge of toxicity. Electrocardiographic ST-segment and T-wave changes and slowing of sinus tachycardia are of little value in gauging the adequacy of digitalis dosage.

In patients with atrial flutter or fibrillation, control of the ventricular response provides a relatively straightforward endpoint, but digoxin alone does not provide adequate control of rate during exertion in many patients; ancillary use of a beta-adrenergic blocking agent, calcium channel blocker (verapamil or diltiazem), or amiodarone is often needed.

When congestive heart failure is the indication for use of digitalis, it is helpful to remember that positive inotropy is a graded response that is appreciable at dosages well short of "maximally tolerated doses." Available data suggest that further inotropic benefit may not occur clinically beyond serum digoxin levels in the range of 1.5 ng/ml. Improved autonomic balance with reduced sympathetic and enhanced vagal tone may occur at still lower serum levels, and it is our usual practice to target serum levels to the 1.0-ng/ml range. Oral maintenance doses predicted to produce a given serum digoxin concentration vary widely with renal function and lean body mass, as discussed on page 482. Carotid sinus massage can provide useful bedside clues to impending digitalis excess; for example, rhythm disorders such as second-degree atrioventricular block, accelerated atrioventricular junctional rhythm, and ventricular premature beats or bigeminy may emerge in response to carotid sinus stimulation before they occur spontaneously.[58]

Individual Sensitivity to Digitalis

A number of factors influencing individual sensitivity to cardiac glycosides are listed in Table 16–5, page 482.

Electrolyte and Acid-Base Disturbances

Disturbances of potassium homeostasis clearly influence the action of digitalis.[59] Myocardial concentrations of digoxin tend to decrease with increasing serum potassium concentration. Furthermore, hypokalemia has primary arrhythmogenic effects, both decreasing the effective refractory period of Purkinje cells and shortening the coupling interval for ventricular premature beats. Depression of atrioventricular nodal conduction can occur with both digitalis excess and either a very low or extremely high level of serum potassium.[60] Diuretics, catecholamines, insulin or carbohydrate loading, renal disease, and acid-base disturbances must all be considered as potential causes of clinically significant alterations in potassium homeostasis, which can in turn importantly affect the response to cardiac glycosides.

Administration of magnesium suppresses digitalis-induced arrhythmias, whereas hypomagnesemia appears to predispose to digitalis toxicity.[59,61] There is some evidence that the digitalis-induced potassium efflux from the myocardium is reduced by magnesium.[59] Magnesium depletion may become clinically important with the long-term administration of diuretic agents[61–63] and with gastrointestinal disease, diabetes mellitus, or poor nutritional states. Moreover, in patients with congestive heart failure, significant depletion of total body magnesium stores may occur owing to prolonged secondary aldosteronism.[61,64,65] Although the clinical importance of magnesium depletion in digitalis therapy remains unresolved, it deserves consideration in cases of suspected digitalis toxicity. Poor or no correlation was found between serum and tissue magnesium in patients with heart failure, leaving unsolved the problem of clinical assessment of magnesium stores.[64–68]

Type and Severity of Underlying Heart Disease

The effects of digitalis on the heart are modified by the type and severity of the underlying heart disease. This is dramatically demonstrated in otherwise healthy subjects who ingest massive doses of digitalis. Toxicity in such situations is frequently manifested by progressively impaired atrioventricular conduction or by sinoatrial exit block, rather than enhanced automaticity and ventricular ectopic activity as seen in patients with underlying heart disease.[69,70] In many patients with ischemic, myocardial, or valvular heart disease, the effects of digitalis are superimposed on an electrophysiologically unstable condition with preexisting abnormalities of impulse formation and conduction. The more severe and advanced the heart disease, the more likely the occurrence of focal ischemia, myocardial fibrosis, and ventricular dilation with stretching of the Purkinje fibers and resultant tendency toward increased automaticity. The observation that digitalis toxicity is particularly common in patients with amyloidosis involving the heart may be accounted for, at least in part, by digoxin binding by amyloid fibrils.[71]

CORONARY ARTERY DISEASE. Changes in myocardial oxygen consumption produced by digitalis are the net result of two opposing effects of the drug: a potential reduction in wall tension and an increase in contractility.[72] The increase in consumption of oxygen in response to digitalis in the normal heart results from increased velocity of contraction with little change in wall tension. In the failing heart, decreased consumption of oxygen typically occurs in response to cardiac glycosides and can be explained by a decrease in left ventricular end-diastolic pressure and volume and, consequently, on the basis of the Laplace relation, a decline in intramyocardial tension.

These considerations are of clinical importance when a decision must be made on whether to use digitalis in patients with coronary artery disease. Angina pectoris has been observed to improve after digitalization in patients with heart failure but occasionally to worsen in those who are well compensated. In patients with angina pectoris without heart failure, ouabain improved the depressed myocardial performance noted on exercise.[73] Despite these beneficial effects on left ventricular performance, there was no consistent alteration in exercise tolerance or the pressure-rate product at which angina occurred. Improved myocardial perfusion judged by means of thallium-201 scans was found in response to maintenance doses of digoxin in patients with coronary artery disease and left ventricular dysfunction.[74] The combination of a beta blocker and digoxin appears to be beneficial in patients with angina pectoris and abnormal ventricular function.[75] As a general rule, digoxin should be considered for use in patients with ischemic heart disease in the presence of atrial fibrillation or atrial flutter with a rapid ventricular response and in patients with symptomatic heart failure due to predominant systolic dysfunction who remain symptomatic on appropriate doses of an ACE inhibitor and diuretic.

ACUTE MYOCARDIAL INFARCTION (see also p. 1245). There is little to be gained from administration of digitalis to patients who have infarction uncomplicated by evidence of heart failure. There is limited clinical documentation of its value in cardiogenic shock, except in the management of supraventricular arrhythmias. Small increases in cardiac index and stroke work, as well as a reduction in left ventricular end-diastolic pressure, have been observed after digitalization of patients with left ventricular failure following myocardial infarction.[76] Although ouabain did not alter cardiac output in another series of patients with acute myocardial infarction,[77] it caused significant improvement in other indices of left ventricular performance such as end-diastolic pressure and stroke work. However, these hemodynamic changes have not been shown to be accompanied by improved survival.

Although the issue has been long debated, there appears to be no convincing evidence for an increased incidence of arrhythmias complicating digitalization in patients with acute infarction (when serum levels do not exceed the conventional therapeutic range).[78] The clearest indication for digitalis after acute myocardial infarction is in the treatment of atrial fibrillation with a rapid ventricular rate. Electrical cardioversion may be preferred in the treatment of other supraventricular tachyarrhythmias.[79]

Thus, current evidence indicates that digitalis has no well-defined role in the management of myocardial infarction without heart failure or supraventricular tachyarrhythmias. Insofar as the long-term management of patients with myocardial infarction is concerned, ACE inhibitor therapy is considered first-line therapy for left ventricular dysfunction and heart failure, followed by diuretics. Digitalis is

indicated in the subgroup of patients with chronic congestive heart failure and a dilated left ventricle.

We recommend a three-part approach: (1) careful consideration whether any treatment of ventricular dysfunction is needed, (2) consideration of alternatives to digoxin therapy, and (3) restriction of digoxin use to the subgroup of patients with chronic congestive heart failure and systolic dysfunction who remain symptomatic on diuretics and an ACE inhibitor or other appropriate vasodilator regimen.

ADVANCED AGE. The diminished glomerular filtration rate in the elderly leads to a prolonged half-life and increased serum levels of digoxin and an increased probability of toxicity on a given dosage regimen. Advanced age is frequently associated with other factors that increase the likelihood of digitalis intoxication, including more severe heart disease; impairment of pulmonary, renal, and neurological function; and an increased number of concurrent medications.

RENAL FAILURE. The marked diminution of glomerular filtration rate with renal failure prolongs the half-life of digoxin and thus increases serum digoxin levels. Toxicity can be avoided by careful and frequent adjustments of dosage to correlate with the level of renal function present. Less predictably, dialysis can cause at least a transient decrease in serum potassium that increases the tendency toward digitalis-induced arrhythmias. Depending on the magnesium content of the dialysate and the use of magnesium-containing antacids, there may be significant aberrations of serum magnesium levels in patients undergoing dialysis. The minimum dose of digoxin that yields a serum digoxin level of about 1.0 ng/ml should be used in patients on dialysis, which is characterized by extreme fluctuations in fluid and electrolyte balance.

THYROID DISEASE. In hypothyroid patients the serum digoxin half-life is consistently prolonged, whereas in those with hyperthyroidism, serum digoxin levels tend to be decreased.[80] An increased distribution space for digoxin may exist in hyperthyroid patients. This is of interest in light of two experimental findings; the first is the demonstration of higher levels of Na$^+$, K$^+$-ATPase activity in the myocardium of hyperthyroid animals.[81] The second is increased tolerance to cardiac glycosides in heart cells grown in culture in the presence of high thyroid hormone concentrations, associated with an increased number of Na$^+$, K$^+$-ATPase sites and enhanced monovalent cation transport capacity.[82] Thus, the apparent resistance or sensitivity to digitalis in thyroid disease probably depends on changes in target organ responsiveness as well as on the pharmacokinetics of digoxin. Oral maintenance doses should be monitored with steady-state serum level measurements, and ventricular rate control in hyperthyroid patients with atrial fibrillation should be sought using approaches other than "pushing" digoxin to potentially toxic levels (e.g., additional use of beta blockers or verapamil).

PULMONARY DISEASE. Ventricular ectopic activity consistent with digitalis toxicity frequently occurs in patients with respiratory disease who are receiving digitalis.[83] However, respiratory failure and hypoxemia frequently provoke arrhythmias indistinguishable from those associated with an excess of digitalis. A total population of 931 patients admitted consecutively to a medical service and studied prospectively demonstrated an increased incidence of rhythm disturbance consistent with digitalis toxicity among the subset of patients with acute or chronic lung disease.[84] Excessive sensitivity to digitalis in patients with pulmonary disease generally correlates with overt cor pulmonale, hypercapnia, and hypoxemia. Thus, patients with a variety of pulmonary diseases may be sensitive to the arrhythmogenic effects of digitalis at relatively low serum concentrations.

DIGITALIS TOXICITY. Mechanisms, clinical manifestations, and treatment of digitalis toxicity are considered on page 484.

The pharmacology of these drugs is discussed on pages 485 to 486.

DOBUTAMINE. In patients with heart failure refractory to conventional oral medications, intravenous infusions of dobutamine up to several days in duration are usually well tolerated, although pharmacological tolerance generally limits long-term use. Dobutamine is typically initiated at 2 to 3 μg/kg/min without a loading dose and may be titrated according to symptoms and diuretic responsiveness or toward a hemodynamic target.[84a] Systemic arterial pressure may increase, remain constant, or decline depending on the extent of vasodilation and changes in cardiac output. Heart rate may fall after several hours if cardiac output is significantly increased and central sympathetic tone declines, although sinus tachycardia and supraventricular arrhythmias may also occur. Use of a flow-directed catheter to monitor pulmonary capillary wedge pressure as well as cardiac output allows more effective use of dobutamine alone or in conjunction with other vasodilators and diuretics.

The maximal effective dose of dobutamine depends on the individual patient. Teboul et al.[85] observed that in patients with severe heart failure, increasing the rate of infusion of dobutamine above 10 μg/kg/min resulted in no further increase in mixed venous oxygen saturation but was accompanied by a significant increase in myocardial oxygen consumption and could therefore be detrimental.

Outpatient therapy with dobutamine, administered continuously by a portable infusion pump through a central venous catheter, has been used successfully in patients with advanced heart failure and symptoms refractory to other drugs.[86–89] Although this approach has been useful in maintaining an acceptable functional status in some patients, it has not gained widespread clinical acceptance largely due to concern regarding its safety and the development of tolerance to a fixed-dose infusion rate. There have been no prospective controlled studies of this form of therapy for severe heart failure and no clear criteria have been established to identify those patients who, for reasons of safety, should be excluded from continuous dobutamine therapy.[86]

Intermittent use of dobutamine in a monitored setting may be appropriate for selected patients in order to minimize the development of tolerance. Periodic withdrawal of this synthetic sympathomimetic may prevent or diminish the onset of tolerance, although this strategy also has not been tested for efficacy or safety in patients with heart failure by prospective randomized clinical trials. Patients who become tolerant to dobutamine on continuous infusions may benefit from a Class III cAMP phosphodiesterase inhibitor (e.g., milrinone) for several days, after which dobutamine can be reinstituted.[90] Weaning patients from intravenous sympathomimetic agents is often difficult and may require aggressive use of vasodilators with continuous hemodynamic monitoring, as well as digoxin and diuretics (see p. 483).

DOPAMINE. The pharmacodynamic spectrum of activity of dobutamine is superior to that of dopamine for most patients with advanced heart failure, as discussed in Chapter 16. Therefore, dopamine is no longer a first-line agent for use in patients with decompensated congestive heart failure. There is also increasing debate regarding whether low-dose or "renal range" dopamine improves renal function and diuretic effectiveness in patients with heart failure and a depressed cardiac output.[91,92] There are no controlled trials that demonstrate the efficacy and safety of "renal range" dopamine infusions in patients with heart failure and declining renal function receiving vasodilators. Indeed, recent data from surgical intensive care patients do not support the contention that "renal range" dopamine is useful in preserving renal function or promoting a significant natriuresis in humans.[93–95]

Dopamine dosing must be based on an estimate of lean body weight and dosing based on actual body weight in heart failure patients may lead to toxic drug levels. As tachycardia and arrhythmias are frequent complications of dopamine administration in patients with heart failure, even if a correct dosing algorithm is used, this drug should only be used temporarily in hypotensive, decompensated patients with heart failure until other measures (e.g., an intra-aortic balloon pump) can be instituted.

OTHER PHARMACOLOGICAL AGENTS

Newer Inotropic Agents

PHOSPHODIESTERASE INHIBITORS. Development of *oral* formulations of phosphodiesterase (PDE) inhibitors for treatment of chronic heart failure has been deterred by the premature termination of the Prospective Randomized Milrinone Survival Evaluation (PROMISE) trial,[96] which showed a 53 per cent increase in mortality in patients with NYHA Class IV heart failure receiving milrinone. Unfavorable results were also evident in a smaller trial that compared oral milrinone to digoxin or placebo.[97] Sustained hemodynamic improvement was lacking in the milrinone group, and the incidence of adverse events, particularly cardiac arrhythmias, was greater.

Amrinone and milrinone are available for short-term circulatory support in patients with decompensated cardiac failure and following cardiac surgery. Milrinone, which is approximately tenfold more potent and has a shorter half life than amrinone, is also associated with a reduced risk of thrombocytopenia and therefore is the preferred drug in these patient groups. Milrinone, following a loading dose of 50 μg/kg and initiation of a maintenance infusion of between 0.25 to 1.0 μg/kg/min, acts both to reduce systemic vascular resistance and to increase cardiac contractility.[97a] As with all agents that mimic the activity of beta-adrenergic agonists, milrinone also accelerates the rate of relaxation of the heart (i.e., a positive lusitropic effect). Milrinone (or amrinone) may be used temporarily in decompensated hospitalized patients who have developed tolerance to dobutamine or, with dobutamine, as a bridge to transplantation or insertion of a ventricular assist device in end-stage heart failure.

VESNARINONE (see p. 485). Vesnarinone appeared to decrease mortality in one large placebo-controlled trial.[98] Patients on standard therapy for mild to moderately severe heart failure were randomized to placebo or vesnarinone at 60 mg or 120 mg/day. An increase in mortality in patients receiving the larger dose of active drug caused the early termination of that arm of the trial. The lower dose of 60 mg/day of vesnarinone, however, was associated with a greater than 50 per cent reduction in mortality at 12 weeks compared to placebo. Symptoms of heart failure and quality of life also improved in the 60-mg/day vesnarinone group, consistent with prior smaller trials.[98] Results of additional clinical trials in progress are awaited with interest.

Beta-Adrenergic Blocking Agents

The rationale for this approach is considered on pages 411 and 486. The Metoprolol in Dilated Cardiomyopathy (MDC) trial[99] compared metoprolol to placebo in patients with mild to moderate (Class II and III) heart failure due to an idiopathic dilated cardiomyopathy and an ejection fraction averaging 22 per cent who were already receiving optimal medical management, including an ACE inhibitor. Metoprolol therapy was initiated as a test dose of 5 mg. The target dose was 100 to 150 mg/day achieved over 7 weeks, and the mean dose of those on active drug was 108 mg at 3

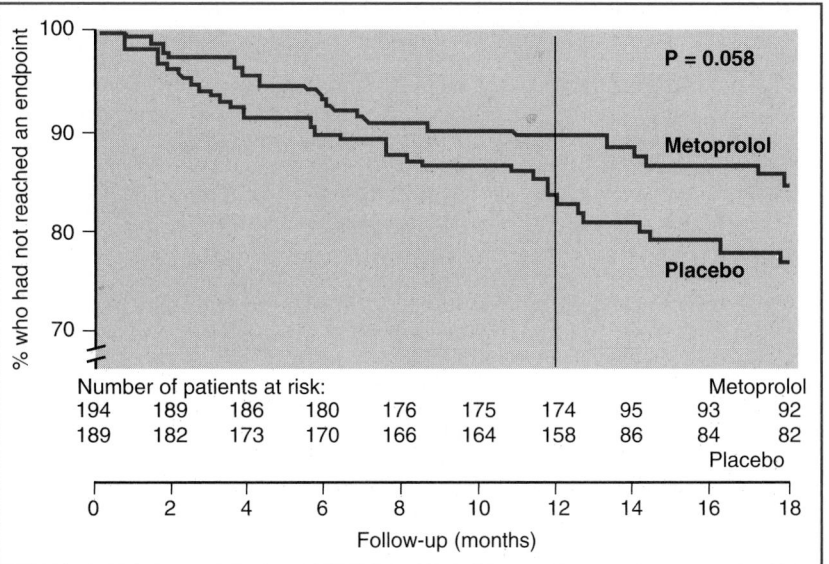

FIGURE 17–7. Percentage of patients who had not reached a primary endpoint (i.e., death or need for cardiac transplantation) in the metoprolol in dilated cardiomyopathy (MDC) trial. Although there was no difference in mortality between patients randomized to receive metoprolol or placebo, there was a significant reduction in the number of patients who required listing for cardiac transplantation (i.e., 19 in the placebo group versus two in the metoprolol group; $P < 0.001$). (From Waagstein, F., et al: Beneficial effects of metoprolol in idiopathic dilated cardiomyopathy. Lancet 342:1441, 1993. © by The Lancet Ltd.)

months. Although there was no difference in mortality after 12 months of follow-up, the number of patients requiring hospitalization for worsening heart failure or listing for cardiac transplantation was significantly less in the metoprolol group (Fig. 17–7). Over 12 months, ejection fraction improved significantly more in patients receiving metoprolol (0.22 to 0.34) than patients receiving placebo (0.22 to 0.28).[99]

The Cardiac Insufficiency BIsoprolol Study (CIBIS)[100] examined the effects of this beta$_1$-selective antagonist in 641 patients with heart failure and NYHA Class III functional status, due to either an ischemic or a primary dilated cardiomyopathy. As in the MDC trial, mortality was not reduced, but functional status improved, and the incidence of clinical decompensation due to worsening heart failure declined. Eichhorn and Hjalmarson[101] have suggested that this trial was underpowered to detect a decrease in mortality. Interestingly, bisoprolol reduced mortality significantly in patients with idiopathic dilated cardiomyopathy, supporting the results of the MDC trial[99] but did not do so in patients with ischemic cardiomyopathy.

Fisher et al., on the other hand, have reported that both the functional status and the need for hospitalizations due to worsening heart failure were improved in patients with ischemic heart disease and an ejection fraction below 40 per cent who were randomized to receive metoprolol compared to placebo[102]; ejection fraction also improved significantly. Bucindolol, a nonselective beta-adrenergic antagonist with vasodilating activity, was superior to placebo in improving symptoms, NYHA functional class, and ejection fraction in patients with idiopathic cardiomyopathy over a 2-year follow-up period.[103,104] Maximal exercise tolerance declined on the highest dose of bucindolol, consistent with a decline in maximal heart rate achieved during active drug therapy from 150 beats/min on placebo to 110 beats/min.[105] However, there was a trend toward an improvement in submaximal exercise tolerance, which may be a more reliable indicator of functional status for patients receiving drug therapy for heart failure.[103,105] High-dose bucindolol (200 mg/day) significantly improved ejection fraction in patients with ischemic cardiomyopathy as well: results consistent with the report by Fisher et al. with metoprolol.[102] Preliminary reports of a large (1052 patients) multicenter, placebo-controlled trial of carvedilol, a nonselective beta-adrenergic antagonist with alpha-adrenergic antagonist (vasodilating) activity, has demonstrated a clear survival benefit as well as improved exercise tolerance for patients with mild as well as more severe (NYHA Class II-IV) symptoms of heart failure.[105a] Unlike previous trials of beta-

antagonists in heart failure, a two-thirds reduction in mortality was identified in patients with ischemic as well as with idiopathic cardiomyopathies. While these data strongly support the use of beta-adrenergic agonists in most patients with heart failure, considerable care must be exercised both in the selection of patients and in the initiation of therapy, during which heart failure symptoms are often exacerbated. In another, smaller trial of carvedilol of heart failure, for example, 37 per cent of patients with advanced heart failure developed increasing dyspnea and fluid retention during initiation of low-dose therapy.[105b]

Thus, despite the lack of an understanding of underlying mechanisms, available evidence supports a potential role for beta-adrenergic antagonists in the treatment of patients with symptomatic heart failure. In all reported studies, which were conducted by investigators with substantial experience in the management of heart failure, the initial doses were low (e.g., 5-mg test doses for metoprolol, followed by 10 mg/day) and were slowly titrated upward over at least 4 to 6 weeks. Although this approach appears promising, as of this writing it is investigational, and beta blockers have not been approved by the U.S. Food and Drug Administration for the treatment of heart failure. A large-scale trial of bucindolol, the BEST trial, will further test this therapy on survival of patients with heart failure.

HEART FAILURE WITH PREDOMINANT DIASTOLIC VENTRICULAR DYSFUNCTION

The pathophysiology and assessment of diastolic dysfunction have been considered on pages 402, 434, and 447. The various abnormalities leading to diastolic dysfunction, shown in Figure 13–13, p. 402, stiffen the ventricles during diastole and/or diminish their rate of relaxation, elevating ventricular diastolic pressure and causing pulmonary and/or systemic venous congestion. The therapeutic approach to diastolic dysfunction has two major components.[106] The first involves attempts to reverse the heart's abnormal diastolic properties; the second is directed toward reducing filling pressure and thereby venous congestion (Table 17–3).

Examples of the first approach include pericardiectomy for constrictive pericarditis, the relief of ventricular systolic overload, and the subsequent regression of ventricular hypertrophy. Efforts to achieve such regression involve the aggressive control of hypertension and the relief of valvular, supravalvular, and subvalvular obstruction to ventricu-

TABLE 17-3 TREATMENT OF DIASTOLIC DYSFUNCTION

GOAL OF TREATMENT	METHOD OF TREATMENT
Produce hypertrophy progression:	Antihypertensive therapy Surgery (e.g., AVR for aortic stenosis)
Improve ventricular relaxation:	Systolic unloading Ischemia treatment Calcium channel blockers (?)
Prevent/treat ischemia:	Beta-adrenergic blockers Calcium channel blockers Nitrates Coronary bypass or angioplasty

Reduce venous pressure:	CBV decreased
	Diuretics
	Salt restriction
	Venodilation
	   Nitrates
	   ACE inhibitors
	   Morphine
	   Tourniquets

Decrease heart rate:	Digoxin in atrial fibrillation Beta-adrenergic blockers Verapamil, diltiazem
Maintain atrial contraction:	Cardioversion of atrial fibrillation Sequential AV pacing

AVR = aortic valve replacement; CBV = central blood volume.

Modified from Levine, H. J., and Gaasch, W. H.: Clinical recognition and treatment of diastolic dysfunction and heart failure. In Gaasch, W. H., and LeWinter, M. M. (eds.): Left Ventricular Diastolic Dysfunction and Heart Failure. Philadelphia, Lea and Febiger, 1994, p. 445.

lar outflow by operation[107] or balloon dilatation. There is some evidence that ACE inhibitors and aldosterone antagonists slow, arrest, or perhaps even reverse myocardial fibrosis in the presence of systolic overload,[108] and these agents might be useful in the management of diastolic dysfunction in such patients. The rapid relief of acute myocardial ischemia is often effective when diastolic dysfunction is secondary to this condition. Nitroglycerin, anti-ischemic agents (beta blockers and calcium antagonists), thrombolysis, mechanical revascularization, or a combination of these measures may be used, depending on the specific clinical circumstance. Calcium antagonists (see p. 1425), especially verapamil, have been shown to accelerate ventricular relaxation in patients with hypertrophic cardiomyopathy[109,110] and have been reported to be useful in the treatment of diastolic dysfunction characteristic of this condition (see p. 403).

Ventricular filling pressure and secondary venous congestion may be reduced by restriction of sodium intake and the administration of diuretics and venodilators. Even in the absence of myocardial ischemia, nitrates, by reducing preload, are useful in the management of diastolic ventricular dysfunction and in the treatment and prevention of consequent severe pulmonary congestion. Nitroglycerin may be administered intravenously or sublingually in emergency situations, and long-acting nitrates, such as isosorbide dinitrate, are often effective in the long term. In the long-term management of patients with diastolic dysfunction, however, excessive preload reduction should be avoided, because these patients often require higher-than-normal filling pressures to maintain an adequate stroke volume.

The maintenance of normal heart rate and rhythm is of critical importance in patients with predominant diastolic dysfunction. Tachycardia, whatever the underlying mechanism, must be controlled, thereby increasing the fraction of each cardiac cycle available for ventricular filling. Maintenance of sinus rhythm with synchronized atrioventricular sequential pacing may be critical in permitting atrial augmentation of ventricular filling, thereby raising ventricular

filling pressure. Digoxin has no established place in the management of patients with predominant diastolic dysfunction and a well-preserved ventricular ejection fraction, and could, in principle, have an adverse effect in this group.

SUDDEN DEATH AND ARRHYTHMIAS

Sudden death accounts for 30 to 70 per cent of all deaths in patients with heart failure.[111] Sudden death increases in absolute frequency with the clinical severity of disease. Its relative importance, however, is substantial in patients with less advanced disease.[111] The incidence of sudden death ranges from 2 to 3 per cent yearly in patients with asymptomatic left-ventricular dysfunction[5,8] to 7 to 20 per cent yearly in patients with severe heart failure.[3,7] Death may occur unexpectedly in patients with heart failure for whom therapy has allowed the maintenance of good quality of life. The incidence of sudden death appears to be lower during therapy with ACE inhibitors.[6,7]

The multiple underlying causes of sudden death in this population have confounded attempts to predict or prevent it (Table 17–4). Sudden death can be caused not only by ventricular tachyarrhythmias, but also by bradyarrhythmias, which accounted for almost half of unexpected cardiac arrests in a series of ambulatory patients hospitalized during evaluation for cardiac transplantation.[112] Both tachyarrhythmias and bradyarrhythmias may occur without obvious underlying cause or result from another acute event such as myocardial infarction or pulmonary embolism.[112]

Substrate for Arrhythmias

The ventricular hypertrophy that commonly accompanies heart failure is associated with a variety of electrophysiological abnormalities that may enhance the potential for arrhythmias.[113–116] Prolonged duration of the action potential, slow impulse propagation, and heterogeneous recovery following depolarization facilitate reentry. Patchy interstitial fibrosis may decrease electrical coupling and slow impulse propagation between myocytes, establishing further the substrate for microreentrant ventricular arrhythmias.

Patients with heart failure consequent to previous myocardial infarctions have focal sites of fibrosis and adjacent

**TABLE 17-4 CAUSES OF SUDDEN DEATH
IN HEART FAILURE**

UNDERLYING CAUSE	RHYTHM OBSERVED
Acute myocardial ischemia or infarction (coronary artery disease or embolus)	VT (usually polymorphic) or VF, bradycardia, EMD
Pulmonary embolism	Bradycardia, EMD
Embolic or hemorrhagic stroke	Bradycardia, polymorphic VT
Drugs prolonging QT interval	Polymorphic VT
Electrolyte depletion (potassium, magnesium)	Polymorphic VT
Hyperkalemia	Bradycardia Apparent VT*
Exaggerated vagal reflexes?	Sinus bradycardia Complete heart block

Primary arrhythmia
  Ventricular tachyarrhythmias
  Conduction system disease
	
	VT, VF
	Sinus bradycardia
	Complete heart block

EMD = electromechanical dissociation; VF = ventricular fibrillation; VT = ventricular tachycardia.

* Rhythms during hyperkalemia are frequently diagnosed as ventricular tachycardia. These may also be "sinoventricular rhythms" in which the prolonged conduction causes absence of apparent atrial activity and marked widening of the QRS complex.

Adapted from Stevenson, W. G., Stevenson, L. W., Middlekauff, H. R., and Saxon, L. A.: Sudden death prevention in patients with advanced ventricular dysfunction. Circulation 88:2953, 1993.

viable myocardium that may foster the occurrence of conduction block and macro-reentry arrhythmias, manifested usually as monomorphic ventricular tachycardia. Focal ischemia more commonly causes polymorphic ventricular tachycardia.

Ventricular hypertrophy and the accompanying abnormalities in intracellular calcium handling confer increased susceptibility to triggered activity from early afterdepolarizations, which in animal models have been strongly linked to polymorphic ventricular tachycardia (torsades de pointes).[114] Stretch of myocytes, as occurs in heart failure (Chap. 13), can also produce afterdepolarizations; animal models demonstrate increased susceptibility to ventricular fibrillation when intraventricular pressures are increased.[116]

Abnormalities of autonomic nervous system function in heart failure may also be arrhythmogenic. Increased beta-adrenergic stimulation augments intracellular calcium and increases delayed afterdepolarizations,[117] whereas alpha-adrenergic stimulation may promote early afterdepolarizations by prolonging action potential duration.[118] Sympathetic stimulation may cause heterogeneous changes in conduction and refractoriness, which predispose to reentrant ventricular arrhythmias. Reduced resting vagal tone also increases susceptibility to ventricular tachyarrhythmias. Abnormal autonomic balance may also predispose to sudden vasodepressor responses manifested as bradycardiac arrests. Depletion of potassium and magnesium during diuretic therapy has been associated with increased susceptibility to early afterdepolarizations and torsades de pointes.[119] Hypokalemia may specifically increase the risk of ventricular fibrillation during myocardial ischemia. Hyperkalemia causes slowing of conduction, which can lead to reentrant arrhythmias in addition to the more commonly recognized suppression of sinus and atrioventricular node function.

Approach to Ventricular Arrhythmias

EVALUATION OF CARDIAC ARREST SURVIVORS
(see also Chap. 24). Among patients who have been resuscitated from ventricular fibrillation or ventricular tachycardia, those with left ventricular ejection fractions below 30 per cent have higher risk of recurrent sudden death than do patients with better ventricular function.[120,121] Once heart failure is severe, however, a history of prior cardiac arrest may not itself augur a worse outcome. One study of potential transplant candidates receiving selected antiarrhythmic therapy or an implantable defibrillator after previous resuscitation from cardiac arrest attributed to ventricular tachycardia or fibrillation showed a 17 per cent risk of sudden death during the next year, which was identical to the risk for potential candidates without such a history.[122]

The current diagnostic approach to cardiac arrest survivors with heart failure usually includes 24-hour electrocardiographic monitoring, exercise testing, and electrophysiological study to identify the responsible arrhythmia, which is often ventricular tachycardia but can be bradycardia due to conduction-system disease. Electrolyte abnormalities and active ischemia should also be sought as potential causes or contributing factors. Inducibility of ventricular tachycardia is more common in the patient with previous myocardial infarction than in the patient with nonischemic cardiomyopathy.[123] When ventricular tachycardia is inducible in patients with heart failure secondary to nonischemic cardiomyopathy, it may originate from bundle branch reentry in as many as a third of cases,[124] particularly if there is evidence of conduction system disease on the resting electrocardiogram. This type of ventricular tachycardia is particularly amenable to radiofrequency ablation techniques[125] (see Chap. 21).

Patients in whom ventricular tachycardia can be induced following cardiac arrest have a 15 to 50 per cent risk of recurrent cardiac arrest during the next 2 to 3 years during therapy with antiarrhythmic drugs. This risk includes both

the risk of the underlying arrhythmia and the proarrhythmic risk of the drugs used to suppress arrhythmias. The choice of drug is often determined by efficacy of suppression of arrhythmia during serial electrophysiological testing. Amiodarone, however, may often be clinically effective despite continued inducibility of arrhythmias by programmed stimulation.[126] Cardiac arrest survivors with poor ventricular function in whom a cause cannot be found have a 30 per cent risk of recurrent arrest during the next 1 to 3 years.[120,127,128] Cardiac arrests attributed to factors such as hypoxia during pulmonary edema or torsades de pointes during antiarrhythmic drug therapy may identify patients at subsequent high risk despite the apparently transitory nature of the inciting cause. In one study of "secondary arrests" in advanced heart failure, the risk of sudden death was 39 per cent over the following year despite attempts to remove precipitating factors.[122]

PREVENTION OF RECURRENT VENTRICULAR TACHYARRHYTHMIAS. The risks of antiarrhythmic drug therapy are increased in patients with heart failure. With the exception of quinidine and amiodarone, most commonly used antiarrhythmic drugs depress contractility.[129] Heart failure was exacerbated by antiarrhythmic drug therapy in 3.8 per cent of patients enrolled in drug trials, most commonly in those with left ventricular ejection fractions below 25 per cent.[130] This observation is consistent with the finding that exacerbation of arrhythmias by drug therapy also occurs more commonly in patients with depressed ventricular function.[131] In the Cardiac Arrhythmia Suppression Trial (see p. 609), in patients with depressed ventricular function after myocardial infarction, the Type I agents flecainide, encainide, and moricizine suppressed ventricular ectopy but increased mortality.[132] Increased mortality has been suggested from other heart failure populations treated with Type I antiarrhythmic agents.[133] Thus, these drugs should be avoided when possible in patients with heart failure. Management objectives should include maintenance of potassium and magnesium balance and avoidance of noncardiac drugs such as phenothiazines or erythromycin that are known to cause Q-T prolongation.

Of currently available antiarrhythmic drugs, amiodarone appears to have the greatest potential to reduce sudden death in heart failure. Even in the presence of advanced heart failure, it is hemodynamically well tolerated and may actually improve ejection fraction.[134] Amiodarone has been reported to improve survival after myocardial infarction[135] and has been suggested to improve survival in the GESICA trial of severe heart failure[136,136a] (Fig. 17-8). The side effects of pulmonary and hepatic toxicity increase progressively over time (see p. 614) but are more easily accepted in a population with a 5-year survival of less than 50 per cent. In the absence of contraindications, amiodarone is generally the antiarrhythmic drug of choice for therapy of ventricular arrhythmias or atrial arrhythmias in patients with severe heart failure. In the absence of clinically significant arrhythmias, the role of amiodarone has not yet been clearly established.[136,137]

Unlike monomorphic ventricular tachycardia, polymorphic tachycardia usually cannot be reproduced with electrophysiological testing. It may result from ischemia or from factors that prolong the Q-T interval. A history of torsades de pointes in heart failure is associated with increased subsequent sudden death.[122] Although rarely incriminated as a primary cause of torsades de pointes, amiodarone may increase the risk of sudden death in patients with heart failure with a previous history of arrhythmias in the setting of Q-T prolongation.[138]

Implantable cardioverter debrillators offer a nonpharmacological approach for prevention of cardiac arrest due to ventricular arrhythmias[125] (see p. 621). The development of transvenous devices has markedly decreased the morbidity and mortality associated with implantation even in patients with severe heart failure, although induction and termina-

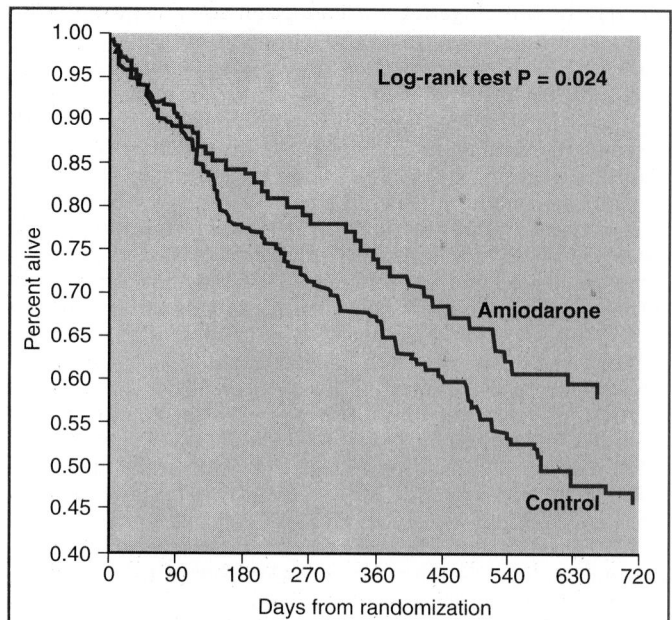

Log-rank test P = 0.024

Amiodarone

Control

FIGURE 17-8. GESICA trial. Actuarial survival of patients with severe heart failure randomized to treatment with amiodarone (300 mg daily after loading dose of 600 mg daily for 14 days) or no treatment in addition to digitalis, diuretics, and, in most cases, ACE inhibitors. Reduction in mortality appeared to result equally from a decrease in sudden death and a decrease in death from progressive heart failure. (From Doval, H. C., Nul, D. R., Grancelli, H. O., et al.: Randomized trial of low-dose amiodarone in severe congestive heart failure. Lancet 344:493, 1994.)

tion of ventricular tachyarrhythmias necessary to test the device may be poorly tolerated by patients with severe hemodynamic decompensation. Although effective in the majority of cases, these devices occasionally fail to defibrillate successfully, a problem that may be slightly more common in the population with heart failure. It should be emphasized that these devices do not prevent arrhythmias, and the discharges of the device may cause marked discomfort, the anticipation of which may severely limit activity in patients with frequent ventricular arrhythmias. Although these devices appear effective in reducing sudden death,[121] they have not yet been shown to reduce overall mortality in heart failure. Indeed, they may simply change the mode of death from arrhythmia to pump failure. At present, and pending the results of ongoing studies, there is no consensus regarding the relative efficacy of the use of amiodarone versus automatic implanted cardioverter defibrillators (AICDs) in patients with heart failure and symptomatic ventricular arrhythmias. Either would constitute a reasonable first choice, although most clinicians with extensive experience would proceed to placement of an AICD if events recur on amiodarone.

SYNCOPE. Loss of consciousness in a patient with depressed ventricular function warrants careful investigation (see p. 872). A history of such an episode, which occurs in up to 12 per cent of patients with heart failure, should not be casually attributed to fatigue or medications. In up to a third of cases, electrophysiological investigation may reveal ventricular tachycardia that requires specific therapy with drugs or devices. Implantation of a pacemaker may be indicated in patients found to have severe impairment of sinus or atrioventricular node function resulting from coronary artery disease or from cardiomyopathy of various causes. Syncope without obvious cause may represent an impaired ability to maintain adequate perfusion in response to stress, for which there is currently no specific therapy. In patients with advanced heart failure, a history of syncope was associated with a 45 per cent risk of sudden death at 1 year, whether or not a specific cause was identified.[139]

ASYMPTOMATIC VENTRICULAR ECTOPY AND NONSUSTAINED VENTRICULAR TACHYCARDIA. Ambulatory electrocardiographic monitoring reveals premature ventricular complexes in over 90 per cent of patients with heart failure, and nonsustained ventricular tachycardia (three or more consecutive beats) in up to 60 per cent.[125,140] In patients after myocardial infarction, frequent ventricular premature beats and nonsustained ventricular tachycardia are associated with more depressed left ventricular function, but the risk of sudden death with premature beats is increased independently of ejection fraction.[141] In contrast, patients with these asymptomatic arrhythmias in the presence of symptomatic heart failure due either to ischemic or nonischemic cardiomyopathy have a higher total mortality but not necessarily a higher risk of sudden death.[140] The ability to induce ventricular tachycardia in patients after myocardial infarction correlates with subsequent mortality.[142] In patients with heart failure, however, the ability to induce ventricular tachycardia with programmed ventricular stimulation did not predict subsequent sudden death.[123]

As with CAST, the postinfarction trial (see p. 600), suppression of asymptomatic ventricular arrhythmias with Type I antiarrhythmic agents not only fails to reduce mortality, but actually increases it.[132] Amiodarone, which is highly effective for suppression of ventricular ectopy and nonsustained ventricular tachycardia, does not worsen and may improve survival in heart failure patients.[136] The benefit shown from amiodarone, however, has been equal in groups with and without nonsustained ventricular tachycardia, and reduction was seen both in sudden death and heart failure endpoints.[136] There is currently no information that indicates a specific benefit from arrhythmia suppression in the absence of symptomatic ventricular arrhythmias.

ATRIAL FIBRILLATION. This arrhythmia, which occurs in approximately 20 per cent of patients with heart failure, has been associated with increased mortality in some[143] but not in all[144] studies of heart failure. Chronic atrial fibrillation in the presence of major left-ventricular dysfunction conferred a 16 per cent annual incidence of stroke, increasing to 20 per cent if the left atrial diameter was more than 2.5 cm/m^2.[133] This risk is decreased by anticoagulant therapy. In addition to the risk of emboli, atrial fibrillation decreases ventricular filling in heart failure, both through loss of the atrial booster pump and through reduction of filling time when the ventricular response is rapid. The regulation of the heart rate response to exercise is impaired in atrial fibrillation, and improved following successful cardioversion to sinus rhythm.[145] Digoxin is usually inadequate for the control of exercise heart rate response, which frequently increases to over 150 beats/min with minimal activity in patients with heart failure, even when the heart rate appears to be adequately controlled at rest. This degree of tachycardia may exacerbate ischemia and/or left ventricular dysfunction. Conversion to sinus rhythm has often been associated with improvement in symptoms and exercise capacity and at times in dramatic improvement in ejection fraction, which may deteriorate again with recurrence of atrial fibrillation.[146]

The risk of emboli, excessive ventricular rates, and possibly increased mortality mandate vigorous attempts to restore sinus rhythm in patients with heart failure, even when initial attempts have failed. Quinidine may maintain sinus rhythm in up to 50 per cent of patients.[133,147] However, concern has been raised based on data from meta-analyses and the Stroke Prevention in Atrial Fibrillation trial, indicating that quinidine may be associated with an up to threefold higher mortality.[133,147] Amiodarone has facilitated conversion to sinus rhythm in 80 per cent of patients with atrial fibrillation and heart failure, and sinus rhythm is maintained at a year in approximately 60 per cent of patients.[145] Amiodarone is generally preferred to quinidine both for efficacy and safety in patients with heart failure.

When sinus rhythm cannot be maintained, rate control is facilitated by amiodarone, usually combined with digoxin. Calcium antagonists may be deleterious, and the use of beta-blocking agents in this setting remains investigational. When pharmacological therapy is not tolerated or is inadequate to maintain adequate rate control, electrical ablation of the atrioventricular junction with placement of a rate-responsive ventricular pacemaker should be considered.[148]

REFRACTORY HEART FAILURE

Heart failure is usually considered to be refractory to medical therapy when severe symptoms persist despite therapy with ACE inhibitors and/or other vasodilators, as well as diuretics, and digoxin. Marked improvement can, however, frequently be achieved after further evaluation and intensification of therapy, which includes patient education as well as an individualized regimen of drugs, diet, and the judicious use of exercise.

The first step in dealing with a patient considered to be in refractory heart failure is to step back and take a fresh look to determine whether other conditions are responsible for the symptoms attributed to heart failure.

1. Could digitalis intoxication be present? Digitalis toxicity can occur despite a serum glycoside level in the usual therapeutic range and can cause fatigue, lethargy, and anorexia that may mimic refractory heart failure.

2. Are the symptoms due to electrolyte imbalance, such as hypokalemic alkalosis or hyponatremia, which may have developed as a consequence of excessive diuresis and restriction of sodium intake?

3. Could the patient with established heart disease be suffering from an unrelated illness such as occult neoplasm, viral hepatitis, or hepatic cirrhosis?

4. Has the patient been treated for predominant systolic dysfunction when the underlying pathophysiology is actually predominant diastolic dysfunction?

As in the initial evaluation of heart failure, heart failure that has become apparently refractory merits close evaluation for potentially reversible factors that could have precipitated or exacerbated circulatory decompensation. These include the following:

1. Could the patient be "cheating" on the restricted sodium diet or drinking excessive volumes of liquids?

2. Is the patient not complying with the medication schedule prescribed despite protestations to the contrary? A "pill count" is often helpful in determining compliance.

3. Is the patient receiving optimal doses of cardiac glycosides? Prescribed digoxin doses in the conventional range do not exclude the possibility of noncompliance or inadequate absorption. Benefit may derive from checking the serum digoxin concentration and adjusting the dose to maintain a steady-state serum level in the 1.0-ng/ml range without precipitating signs or symptoms of toxicity.

4. Could the patient be suffering from unrecognized pulmonary embolism (see Chap. 46)? This condition occurs frequently in heart failure, is often silent, and may be manifested only by slight tachycardia, anxiety, tachypnea, and intensification of heart failure. Dense areas on the chest roentgenogram may make it difficult or impossible to interpret lung scans, and a pulmonary angiogram may be required to establish the diagnosis. Although this procedure is not without risk, a positive result may lead to treatment with anticoagulants and/or interruption of the inferior vena cava that could prevent further emboli and prove to be life saving.

5. Could pulmonary infection be present? Pneumonitis, a frequent complication of left ventricular failure, may be difficult to recognize in patients with chronic congestive heart failure who often have increased interstitial markings

on the chest roentgenogram and pulmonary rales on clinical examination. Is the suspicion of pulmonary infection high enough to warrant sputum culture and consideration of a course of antibiotics?

6. Could hyperthyroidism or infective endocarditis be present? Thyrotoxicosis (often apathetic in the elderly) and infective endocarditis may not have typical clinical manifestations in the presence of heart failure, but they can lead to refractory heart failure. Should thyroid function studies and/or multiple blood cultures be obtained?

7. Could alcohol, a potent myocardial depressant, be playing a role? In addition to producing cardiomyopathy (see p. 1412), alcohol can contribute to heart failure even when it is not the primary cause, but when its use is superimposed on some other form of heart disease.

8. Has the combination of ACE inhibition, other vasodilators, intensive diuretic therapy, and sodium restriction caused hypovolemia, low cardiac output, and hypotension?

9. Does the patient have inappropriate bradycardia due to sinus node dysfunction or atrioventricular block that could be corrected by means of a pacemaker? Could AV sequential pacing restore atrial augmentation of ventricular stroke volume?

10. Is the patient receiving any medications with salt-retaining effects, such as corticosteroids, estrogens, or nonsteroidal anti-inflammatory drugs, or drugs with undesired negative inotropic actions such as disopyramide or calcium antagonists?

11. Could therapy with vasodilators or other agents be responsible for an increased tendency to retention of salt and water that has not been adequately addressed by diuretic therapy?

12. Have the initial favorable hemodynamic effects of any drug in the regimen waned during long-term therapy (e.g., the development of nitrate tolerance)?

13. Can any aspect of therapy be intensified without producing adverse effects?

Management

If, after attention to these factors, patients are still in refractory heart failure, therapies that may initially have been considered to carry unacceptable risks for a stable patient may warrant reconsideration. For example, resection of a large ventricular aneurysm might have been deferred initially owing to high surgical risk in an otherwise stable patient, but reconsideration might be in order when the response to medical therapy wanes. Similar consideration may apply to patients with known multivessel coronary artery disease[149,150] or advanced valvular heart disease and poor left ventricular function. Other forms of surgically correctable heart failure that are not readily recognized on clinical examination include cardiac tumors (see Chap. 42), and constrictive pericarditis without calcification (see Chap. 43). Such conditions should be considered and excluded if possible. When other correctable factors have been addressed, a hemodynamic profile should be obtained and the potential for improvement with readjustment of loading conditions should be assessed.

Hemodynamic Goals

The dominant symptoms of severe heart failure usually reflect marked elevations in intracardiac filling pressures. Hospitalization for intravenous diuretics or brief infusions of inotropic agents facilitate fluid loss to achieve comfort at rest but often leave the patient just below the threshold for visceral congestion or pulmonary edema. Reversal of this cycle of decongestion and recongestion often requires more aggressive reduction of filling pressures. In severe heart failure, preload and afterload are interdependent.[151] Reduction of systemic vascular resistance (afterload) also reduces ventricular filling pressures (preload). Diuresis to reduce preload typically reduces the afterload faced by the ventricle. Therapy of severe persistent congestion requires careful adjustment of both vasodilator and diuretic therapy.

Reduction of intracardiac filling pressures has frequently been limited by concern that cardiac output will become further compromised. Cardiac output is closely related to filling pressures in the normal heart and in acute myocardial infarction.[152] In the chronically dilated ventricle, however, elevations in filling pressures can increase wall stress, compromise subendocardial perfusion, and worsen mitral regurgitation so that cardiac output actually decreases. Maximal stroke volumes are often achieved when the pulmonary capillary wedge pressures approach the normal range[153] (Fig. 17–9). In an average-sized adult, systemic vascular resistances of 1000 to 1200 dynes-sec-cm^{-5} are generally adequate for an optimal cardiac output while maintaining a systolic arterial pressure of at least 80 mm Hg. Most of the improvement in stroke volume with optimization of loading conditions in patients with severe heart failure results from a decrease in mitral regurgitant volume.[154] Similar considerations regarding tricuspid regurgitation apply to the right ventricle, in addition to which right ventricular contractility may actually improve acutely with the reduction of pulmonary vascular resistance. The level of right ventricular compensation determines the minimal levels of right atrial pressure, which may be below 5 mm Hg in some patients with left ventricular failure but in others cannot be reduced below 10 mm Hg owing to irreversible right ventricular dysfunction. Recognition of the importance of reducing filling pressures and secondary valvular regurgitation has led to the hemodynamic goals for refractory heart failure shown in Table 17–5.

Indications for Tailored Therapy with Hemodynamic Monitoring

In patients with severely symptomatic heart failure or with clinical evidence of hypoperfusion and/or congestion despite careful empiric adjustment of therapy (see Table 17–2), the insertion of a multilumen flotation catheter into the pulmonary artery often facilitates management. Right atrial and pulmonary artery pressures can be followed simultaneously, with intermittent brief inflation of a balloon-tipped distal end to obtain pulmonary capillary wedge pressures as an estimate of left ventricular filling pressures. Cardiac output is measured using temperature dilution be-

TABLE 17–5 PRINCIPLES OF HEART FAILURE MANAGEMENT BASED ON HEMODYNAMIC MONITORING

1. Measurement of baseline hemodynamics
2. Intravenous nitroprusside and diuretics tailored to hemodynamic goals:
   Pulmonary capillary wedge pressure ≤ 15 mm Hg
   Systemic vascular resistance ≤ 1000-1200 dynes-sec-cm^{-5}
   Right atrial pressure ≤ 7 mm Hg
   Systolic blood pressure ≥ 80 mm Hg
3. Above hemodynamic goals achieved by 24 to 48 hours
4. Titration of high-dose oral vasodilators as nitroprusside weaned:
   ACE inhibitor, isosorbide dinitrate
   Addition or substitution of hydralazine, if necessary
5. Monitored ambulation and diuretic adjustment for 24 to 48 hours
6. Maintenance of digoxin levels at 1.0 to 1.5 ng/ml if no contraindication
7. Detailed patient education including salt and fluid restriction
8. Flexible outpatient diuretic regimen including occasional metolazone
9. Progressive walking or other exercise program
10. Vigilant follow-up

ACE = angiotensin-converting enzyme.

tween the right atrial port and pulmonary artery thermistor. This hemodynamic monitoring allows simultaneous optimization of filling pressures and systemic vascular resistance. This is often achieved first by the use of short-acting intravenous agents, such as nitroprusside or dobutamine, to reestablish a baseline of compensation upon which an oral regimen can then be imposed.[155–157] Nitroprusside is generally effective when the systemic vascular resistance is elevated. Dobutamine or dopamine may be required when the systemic vascular resistance is normal or low. Intravenous diuretics are administered concomitantly, guided in large part by the right atrial pressure and the presence of hepatomegaly or edema.

The advantages of hemodynamic monitoring include the ability to alter both systemic vascular resistance and filling pressures simultaneously and safely. In the patient with a severely impaired left ventricle, refractory congestion often cannot be relieved by diuretics until the systemic vascular resistance is also effectively reduced. Intravenous nitroprusside is usually effective for improving hemodynamics in patients in whom the systemic vascular resistance is severely elevated and filling pressures are high, even in the presence of low systemic blood pressure.[156] Intravenous nitroprusside can be initiated at 20 μg/min (not per kilogram) titrating up to 200 to 300 μg/min as needed to reduce the systemic vascular resistance. Less commonly, the use of dobutamine may be required to improve cardiac output sufficiently to initiate vasodilation and diuresis.

Optimal hemodynamics are usually achieved within 48 hours of the aggressive institution of intravenous medications (see Table 17–5). Adjustment of oral vasodilators is performed under continuous hemodynamic monitoring, with oral diuretic doses estimated once the patient is considered to be euvolemic. Tailoring of therapy has allowed hospital discharge for almost 90 per cent of patients initially considered to be refractory to oral medical therapy. The sustained benefit of this approach has been demonstrated in terms of hemodynamic status, reduction of mitral regurgitation, freedom from congestive symptoms, improved exercise capacity, and reduced rehospitalizations.[155,158] Close outpatient supervision demonstrates clinical stability at one month in 60 to 70 per cent of patients undergoing tailored therapy for refractory heart failure, most of whom have been referred initially as potential candidates for transplantation.[159] As outlined in the

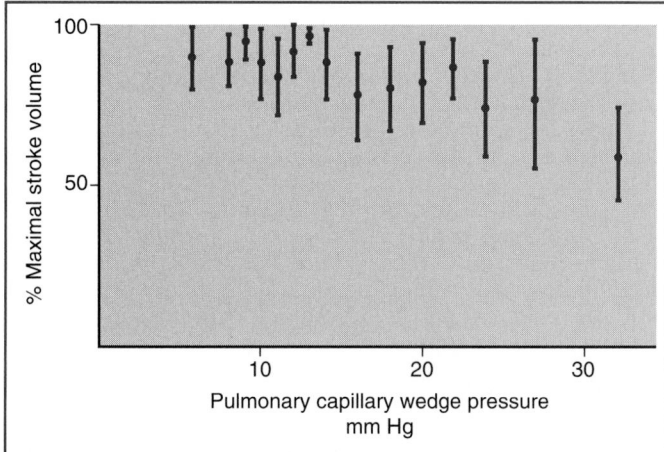

FIGURE 17–9. **Maintenance of stroke volume with decreasing pulmonary capillary wedge pressures in 25 patients with advanced heart failure (average left-ventricular ejection fraction 18 per cent) presenting with clinical decompensation (initial average pulmonary capillary wedge pressure 31 ± 5 mm Hg, cardiac index 1.9 ± 4 liters/min/m²). For each patient, the highest stroke volume measured was compared with that achieved with each pulmonary capillary wedge pressure achieved during therapy with intravenous nitroprusside and diuretics. (From Stevenson, L. W., and Tillisch, J. H.: Maintenance of cardiac output with normal filling pressures in dilated heart failure. Circulation 74:1303, 1986; with permission.)**

Bethesda guidelines for evaluation for cardiac transplantation: "Patients should not be considered to have *refractory* hemodynamic decompensation until therapy with intravenous followed by oral vasodilators and diuretic agents has been pursued using continuous hemodynamic monitoring to approach hemodynamic goals."[160]

Additional Considerations

The indications for anticoagulation in heart failure remain controversial (see p. 1988). In patients with Class II and III heart failure from the V-HeFT II trial,[6] the incidence of embolic events was 2.1/100 patient years, with 12 per cent of patients receiving anticoagulants. In ambulatory Class III and IV patients awaiting transplantation, the incidence was 3 per cent over an average follow-up of 301 days, with 37 per cent of patients receiving anticoagulation.[164] Anticoagulation is uniformly recommended in heart failure accompanied by atrial fibrillation or a history of embolic events, and considered in the presence of a mobile intracardiac thrombus. The risk/benefit ratio of anticoagulation for other patients with heart failure is unlikely to be defined in a randomized trial due to the low incidence of endpoints.

High-dose loop diuretics such as furosemide, bumetamide, and torsemide, with or without additional diuretics acting more distally (such as metolazone), may be used in patients with refractory heart failure. Ultrafiltration may be considered in patients with late-stage heart failure resistant to conventional treatment (see p. 480). Cheyne-Stokes respiration with severe sleep hypoxemia occurs relatively commonly in advanced heart failure. Supplemental oxygen therapy at night reduces Cheyne-Stokes respiration, correcting hypoxemia, and improves sleep by reducing arousals caused by the hyperpneic phase of the Cheyne-Stokes cycle.[161] Continuous positive airway pressure (CPAP) has been advocated as well in this setting.[162,163] In patients who do not have evidence of resting congestion but remain severely limited, a careful trial of exercise training may improve peak functional capacity by 20 per cent and lengthen submaximal exercise duration.[164]

Reestablishment of hemodynamic compensation with intravenous dobutamine and/or nitroprusside therapy often allows the reintroduction of ACE inhibitors that are not tolerated when angiotensin II is necessary to support arterial pressure in patients with a failing circulation. As oral vasodilators are substituted for intravenous agents after recompensation, the doses necessary to provide optimal loading conditions can be defined. Some patients, typically those with severe hyponatremia, develop symptomatic hypotension with very small (3 mg) doses of captopril, whereas others require doses as high as 100 mg every 6 hours. Patients who have not been stable on single vasodilators frequently demonstrate better hemodynamic responses to combination therapy, which may include nitrates and hydralazine in addition to or in place of ACE inhibitors.[7] Therapy can best be adjusted to meet the hemodynamic goals using agents with relatively rapid onset and short duration of action. Longer-acting inotrope vasodilators, such as milrinone or amrinone, may occasionally be necessary for prolonged intravenous support but patients are not easily weaned from these during titration of oral vasodilators. For similar reasons, captopril is the easiest drug to titrate acutely but can often be exchanged for longer-acting ACE inhibitors after patients have demonstrated stability at home.

SELECTION OF CANDIDATES FOR CARDIAC TRANSPLANTATION

(See also Chap. 18)

As the results of cardiac transplantation have improved to offer over 60 per cent survival after 6 years,[165] the pool of potential candidates has expanded to include patients with less immediate compromise and patients with conditions such as diabetes, who would once have been considered to have an absolute contraindication. At the same time, however, advances in medical therapy and revascularization procedures have challenged previous assumptions about when heart failure becomes "end-stage," allowing many patients once thought to need transplantation to maintain good quality of life without it, at least for a period of time. Current selection practice focuses on the identification of patients who truly have no option except transplantation and the selection of those patients who are most likely to derive major benefit in terms of both quality of life and survival.

INDICATIONS. Heart failure is the primary indication for cardiac transplantation. After potentially reversible factors, including myocardial ischemia, have been addressed, and the medical regimen has been optimized, the potential candidate for transplantation is evaluated in terms of an estimated 1-year mortality, which should generally exceed 25 to 50 per cent without transplantation.[166] The limitation of donor supply and of life span after transplantation require that indications for transplantation include a clearly improved early prognosis with transplantation.

Presentation with New York Heart Association Class IV symptoms is no longer sufficient indication for cardiac transplantation, as many patients respond favorably to redesign of their medical regimen during their evaluation for transplantation. Patients requiring continuing or repeated hospitalization to maintain hemodynamic compensation despite optimal medical management are considered to meet indications for transplantation without other functional assessment and are evaluated primarily for contraindications. The challenge is to identify from the population of ambulatory patients with heart failure those in greatest need of transplantation. Although survival of patients with severe heart failure on optimal management has improved, almost one-half of patients discharged after initial evaluation with Class IV symptoms will come to urgent transplantation or death within the next 2 years.[167] A left ventricular ejection fraction of 20 to 25 per cent was at one time also considered to be necessary and sufficient indication for transplantation. However, many patients with such values may exhibit a stable course when receiving optimal medical management.

Peak oxygen consumption ($\dot{V}_{O_2}$) in the ambulatory heart failure population (Fig. 5–21, p. 172) does provide a useful predictor of both mortality with heart failure and functional benefit from cardiac transplantation.[168] Measured through a mouthpiece and gas analyzer during bicycle or treadmill exercise, the peak $\dot{V}_{O_2}$ reflects cardiac reserve, integrative circulatory response, and the degree of peripheral muscle conditioning or deconditioning. Synthesis of several large experiences[166–168] yields a consensus that a peak $\dot{V}_{O_2}$ less than 10 to 12 ml/kg/min (the level required for walking and light household activity) confers a particularly poor prognosis, with 1-year mortality in the range of 50 per cent. Peak $\dot{V}_{O_2}$ exceeding 16 to 18 ml/kg/min (almost adequate for jogging) identifies a group of patients with a 2-year survival of over 80 per cent. This then leaves a middle group with a peak $\dot{V}_{O_2}$ of 12 to 16 ml/kg/min within which decisions regarding transplantation must be further refined by other factors, as well as by the patient's preference. For this intermediate group, the decision to proceed to transplantation must take into account the needs and resources of the individual patient. For example, although survival benefits from transplantation are predicted, many patients are not willing to accept the burdens of immunosuppression, biopsies, and intensive medical follow-up unless accompanied by a substantial improvement in the quality of life.

Quantification of functional capacity using peak $\dot{V}_{O_2}$ not only provides a valuable prognostic index but also allows

TABLE 17–6 SUMMARY OF GENERAL RECOMMENDATIONS: BETHESDA CONFERENCE ON CARDIAC TRANSPLANTATION

Functional status should not be assessed until patients have undergone aggressive therapy with combinations of vasodilators and diuretic agents. "Therapy should be adjusted until clinical congestion has been resolved or until further therapy has been repeatedly limited by severe hypotension (generally systolic blood pressure < 80 mm Hg) or marked azotemia. Patients should not be considered to have *refractory* hemodynamic decompensation until therapy with intravenous followed by oral vasodilators and diuretic agents has been pursued using continuous hemodynamic monitoring to approach hemodynamic goals."

SELECTION CRITERIA FOR BENEFITS FROM TRANSPLANTATION

I. Accepted Indications for Transplantation
  1. Peak $\dot{V}_{O_2}$ < 10 ml/kg/min with achievement of anaerobic metabolism
  2. Severe ischemia consistently limiting routine activity not amenable to bypass surgery or angioplasty
  3. Recurrent symptomatic ventricular arrhythmias refractory to all accepted therapeutic modalities

II. Probable Indications for Cardiac Transplantation
  1. Peak $\dot{V}_{O_2}$ < 14 mg/kg/min and major limitation of the patient's daily activities
  2. Recurrent unstable ischemia not amenable to bypass or angioplasty
  3. Instability of fluid balance/renal function not due to patient noncompliance with regimen of weight monitoring, flexible use of diuretic drugs and salt restriction

III. Inadequate Indications for Transplantation
  1. Ejection fraction ≤ 20 per cent
  2. History of functional Class III or IV symptoms of heart failure
  3. Previous ventricular arrhythmias
  4. Peak $\dot{V}_{O_2}$ > 15 m/kg/min without other indications

From Mudge, G. H., Goldstein, S., Addonizio, L. J., et al.: Cardiac transplantation: Recipient guidelines/prioritization. Reprinted with permission from the American College of Cardiology. J. Am. Coll. Cardiol. *22*:21, 1993.

comparison between pretransplant heart failure status and posttransplant status in recipients. Although the left ventricular ejection fraction is usually normal after transplantation, cardiac reserve is markedly limited. Many other factors, such as hypertension and the systemic effects of corti-

costeroids, also impair physical capacity. Most cardiac transplant recipients achieve a peak $\dot{V}_{O_2}$ in the range of 15 to 18 ml/kg/min, or 50 to 70 per cent of predicted, which is similar to that achieved by many patients with stable heart failure.[159] For comparison, the average healthy middle-aged man has a predicted maximal oxygen consumption of 25 to 35 ml/kg/min.

Considering both survival and functional benefits, very low peak $\dot{V}_{O_2}$ (≤ 10 ml/kg/min) is sufficient indication for transplantation in a patient on optimal therapy without contraindications (Table 17–6). Patients with higher peak oxygen consumption may still need transplantation for conditions such as recurrent severe myocardial ischemia not amenable to revascularization or refractory symptomatic ventricular arrhythmias. Although heart failure leading to cardiac transplantation is usually secondary to ischemic or idiopathic cardiomyopathy with a dilated left ventricle and depressed ejection fraction, these are neither necessary nor sufficient indications. Patients in New York Heart Association Class IV with restrictive cardiomyopathy, in which the left ventricle is minimally dilated and the ejection fraction is 30 to 40 per cent may be candidates for transplantation. Hypertrophic cardiomyopathy rarely requires transplantation when still in the hypercontractile stage during which drug therapy, pacemaker therapy, and other surgical options should be used. In the small percentage of patients in whom hypertrophic cardiomyopathy has become "burned out," congestive symptoms and exercise intolerance may become severe with only modest reductions in left ventricular ejection fraction.

CONTRAINDICATIONS (see Table 18–1, p. 516).

THE WAITING LIST FOR TRANSPLANTATION. The waiting list for cardiac transplantation continues to lengthen, as more than twice as many patients are listed monthly in the United States than actually receive donor hearts.[169] In 1984, there were 37 centers performing cardiac transplantation in the United States. The average waiting time was 6 weeks, and each center could identify the candidate in the greatest need when a donor heart became available. In 1994, there were 151 programs competing for donor hearts in the United States, which are distributed through the United Network of Organ Sharing (UNOS) according to priority and to time on the list.[170] In the United States, priority (Status I) is accorded first to hospitalized patients requiring

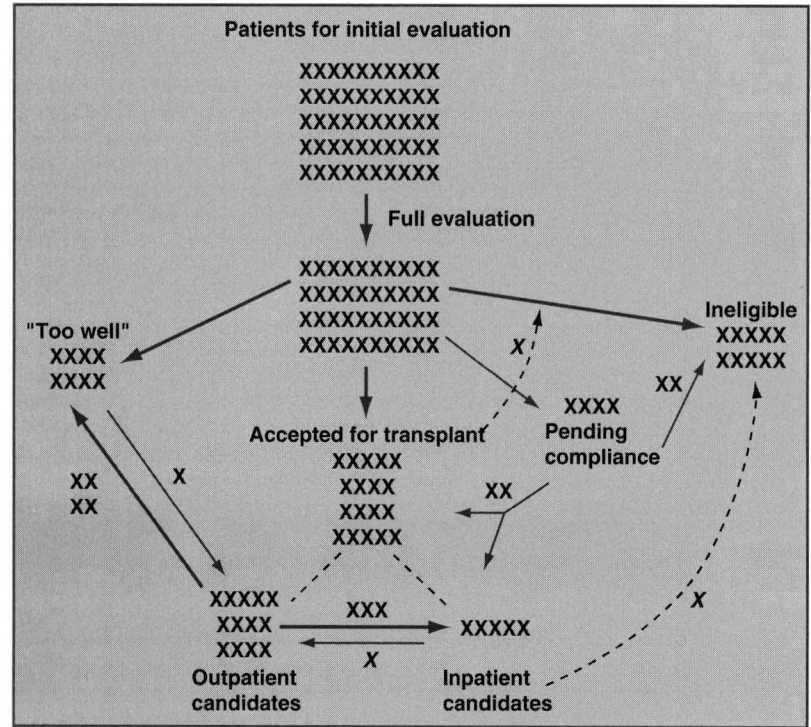

FIGURE 17–10. Diagram demonstrating dynamic nature of candidacy for transplantation. Patients may be "too well" at initial referral or as a result of improvement while on the waiting list. Accepted candidates may deteriorate from outpatient to critical status. One of the benefits of a combined heart failure transplant treatment and education program is the opportunity for ongoing assessment of compliance with a heart failure regimen that frequently allows eventual acceptance of patients previously considered ineligible due to noncompliance. Density of x's gives a semiquantitative estimate of patient flow.

TABLE 17–7 CRITERIA FOR CLINICAL STABILITY IN CANDIDATES AWAITING TRANSPLANTATION

Clinical Criteria
1. **Stable fluid balance without orthopnea, elevated jugular venous pressure, or other evidence of congestion on the flexible diuretic regimen**
2. **Stable blood pressure with systolic pressure $\geq$ 80 mm Hg**
3. **Stable serum sodium concentration and renal function**
4. **Absence of symptomatic ventricular arrhythmias**
5. **Absence of frequent angina**
6. **Absence of severe drug side effects**
7. **Stable or improving activity level without dyspnea during self-care or 1 block exertion**

Exercise Criteria (if initial peak $\dot{V}_{O_2} <$ 14 ml/kg/min)
1. **Improvement in peak oxygen consumption of $\geq$ 2 ml/kg/min**
2. **Peak oxygen consumption $\geq$ 12 ml/kg/min**

assist devices or intravenous inotropic therapy in intensive care units. All other patients are Status II, except in some regions in which variances exist allowing intermediate priority among hospitalized patients. Currently, over half of all transplanted hearts are distributed to hospitalized patients.

The average waiting time for patients at home is currently over 18 months and continues to lengthen. Sudden death occurs in 10 to 20 per cent of patients on the waiting list during this time.[111–112] A slightly higher proportion develop deterioration of cardiac function sufficient to require continued hospitalization until transplantation. Hospitalization may be indicated either to prevent imminent death or deterioration that would significantly increase perioperative mortality from transplantation. The approach to the hospitalized candidate with refractory heart failure includes hemodynamic monitoring to optimize supportive therapy as outlined above. Prolonged infusions of dobutamine, dopamine, or phosphodiesterase inhibitors may support patients in the hospital or occasionally at home, until transplantation. The need for more potent agents such as epinephrine should raise consideration of mechanical support devices as a bridge to transplantation (see pp. 517 and 538).

Clinical improvement may also occur while patients are on a waiting list. The highest risk of death is in the first 6 months after listing, after which some factors causing deterioration before referral may resolve and the benefits of optimized medical therapy may be realized. Ambulatory patients on the waiting list require periodic reevaluation, during which both clinical stability and functional capacity are assessed (Table 17–7). Up to 30 per cent of ambulatory transplant candidates may later meet criteria for stability and leave the active waiting list, with subsequent 2-year survival and exercise performance equivalent to that after cardiac transplantation.[171] Candidacy for transplantation is increasingly considered to be a dynamic state (Fig. 17–10).

Although cardiac transplantation was greeted in 1968 as a solution to the problem of end-stage heart failure,[172] the inevitable disparity between the donor supply and demand severely limits the application of this procedure. Implantable left ventricular devices (Chap. 19) provide not only bridges but eventually alternatives to transplantation and may thus lead to major revision of current criteria for selection and reevaluation of candidates for transplantation.

REFERENCES

THERAPEUTIC STRATEGY FOR MANAGEMENT OF HEART FAILURE

1. Williams, J. F., Jr., Bristow, M. R., Fowler, M. B., et al.: Guidelines for the evaluation and management of heart failure. Report of the American College of Cardiology/American Heart Association Task Force on Practical Guidelines (Committee on Evaluation and Management of Heart Failure). J. Am. Coll. Cardiol. 26:1376, 1995.
1a. Cohn, J. N.: Structural basis for heart failure. Ventricular remodeling and its pharmacological inhibition. Circulation 91:2504, 1995.
2. Pfeffer, M. A.: ACE inhibition in acute myocardial infarction. N. Engl. J. Med. 332:118, 1995.
3. CONSENSUS Trial Study Group: Effects of enalapril on mortality in severe congestive heart failure. Results of the Cooperative North Scandinavian Enalapril Survival Group (CONSENSUS). N. Engl. J. Med. 316:1429, 1987.
4. SOLVD Investigators: Effect of enalapril on survival in patients with reduced left ventricular ejection fractions and congestive heart failure. N. Engl. J. Med. 325:293, 1991.

VASODILATORS

5. SOLVD Investigators: Effect of enalapril on mortality and the development of heart failure in asymptomatic patients with reduced ventricular ejection fractions. N. Engl. J. Med. 327:685, 1992.
6. Cohn, J. N., Johnson, G., Ziesche, S., et al.: A comparison of enalapril with hydralazine-isosorbide dinitrate in the treatment of chronic congestive heart failure. N. Engl. J. Med. 325:303, 1991.
7. Fonarow, G. C., Chelimsky-Fallick, C., Stevenson, L. W., et al.: Effect of direct vasodilation with hydralazine versus angiotensin-converting enzyme inhibition with captopril on mortality in advanced heart failure: The Hy-C trial. J. Am. Coll. Cardiol. 19:842, 1992.
8. Pfeffer, M. A., Braunwald, E., Moye, L. A., et al.: Effect of captopril on mortality and morbidity in patients with left ventricular dysfunction after myocardial infarction. N. Engl. J. Med. 327:669, 1992.
9. Rutherford, J. D., Pfeffer, M. A., Moye, L. A., et al.: Effects of captopril on ischemic events after myocardial infarction. Results of the survival and ventricular enlargement trial. Circulation 90:1731, 1994.
10. Konstam, M. A., Rousseau, M. F., Kronenberg, M. W., et al.: Effects of the angiotensin converting enzyme inhibitor enalapril on the long-term progression of left ventricular dysfunction in patients with heart failure. Circulation 86:431, 1992.
11. St. John Sutton, M., Pfeffer, M. A., Plappert, T., et al.: Quantitative two-dimensional echocardiographic measurements are major predictors of adverse cardiovascular events after acute myocardial infarction. The protective effects of captopril. Circulation 89:68, 1994.
12. Acute Infarction Ramipril Efficacy (AIRE) Study Investigators: Effect of ramipril on mortality and morbidity of survivors of acute myocardial infarction with clinical evidence of heart failure. Lancet 342:821, 1993.
13. Kober, L., Torp-Pedersen, C., Carlsen, C., et al.: A clinical trial of the ACE inhibitor trandolapril in patients with left ventricular dysfunction after myocardial infarction. N. Engl. J. Med. 333:1670, 1995.
14. Pitt, B.: Use of "xapril" in patients with chronic heart failure. A paradigm or epitaph for our times? Circulation 90:1550, 1994.
15. Gruppo Italiano per lo Studio della Sopravvivenza nell'Infarto Miocardico. GISSI-3 Investigators: Effects of lisinopril and transdermal glyceryl trinitrate singly and together on 6-week mortality and ventricular function after acute myocardial infarction. Lancet 343:1115, 1994.
16. Ambrosioni, E., Borghi, C., and Magnani, B., for the Survival of Myocardial Infarction Long-Term Evaluation (SMILE) Study Investigators: The effect of the angiotensin-converting-enzyme inhibitor zofenopril on mortality and morbidity after anterior myocardial infarction. N. Engl. J. Med. 332:80, 1995.
17. Cohn, J. N.: Treatment of infarct related heart failure: Vasodilators other than ACE inhibitors. Cardiovasc. Drug Ther. 8:119, 1994.
18. Yusuf, S., Garg, R., and McConachie, D.: Effect of angiotensin-converting enzyme inhibitors in left ventricular dysfunction: Results of the studies of left ventricular dysfunction in the context of other similar trials. J. Cardiovasc. Pharmacol. 22:S28, 1993.
19. Lonn, E. M., Yusuf, S., Jha, P., et al.: Emerging role of angiotensin-converting enzyme inhibitors in cardiac and vascular protection. Circulation 90:2056, 1994.
20. Paul, S. D., Kuntz, K. M., Eagle, K. A., et al.: Costs and effectiveness of enzyme inhibition in patients with heart failure. Arch. Intern. Med. 154:1143, 1994.
21. Rogers, W. J., Johnstone, D. E., Yusuf, S., et al.: Quality of life among 5025 patients with left ventricular dysfunction randomized between placebo and enalapril: The studies of left ventricular dysfunction. J. Am. Coll. Cardiol. 23:393, 1994.
22. Northridge, D. B., Rose, E., Raftery, E. D., et al.: A multicentre, double-blind, placebo-controlled trial of quinapril in mild, chronic heart failure. Eur. Heart J. 14:403, 1993.
23. Rector, T. S., Johnson, G., Dunkman, W. B., for the V-HeFT VA Cooperative Studies Group: Evaluation by patients with heart failure of the effects of enalapril compared with hydralazine plus isosorbide dinitrate on quality of life. Circulation 87 (Suppl. VI):71, 1993.
24. Varriale, P., David, W., and Chryssos, B. E.: Hemodynamic response to intravenous enalaprilat in patients with severe congestive heart failure and mitral regurgitation. Clin. Cardiol. 16:235, 1993.
25. Seneviratne, B., Moore, G. A., and West, P. D.: Effect of captopril on functional mitral regurgitation in dilated heart failure: A randomized double blind placebo controlled trial. Br. Heart J. 72:63, 1994.
26. Lin, M., Chiang, H.-T., Lin, S.-L., et al.: Vasodilator therapy in chronic asymptomatic aortic regurgitation: Enalapril versus hydralazine therapy. J. Am. Coll. Cardiol. 24:1046, 1994.
27. Schon, H. R.: Hemodynamic and morphologic changes after long-term angiotensin converting enzyme inhibition in patients with chronic valvular regurgitation. J. Hypertens. 12:95, 1994.
28. Kostis, J. B., Shelton, B. J., Yusuf, S., et al.: Tolerability of enalapril initiation by patients with left ventricular dysfunction: Results of the

medication challenge phase of the studies of left ventricular dysfunction. Am. Heart J. *128:*358, 1994.

29. Lang, R. M., DiBianco, R., Broderick, G. T., et al.: First-dose effects of enalapril 2.5 mg and captopril 6.25 mg in patients with heart failure: A double-blind, randomized, multicenter study. Am. Heart J. *128:*551, 1994.

30. Squire, I. B., MacFadyen, R. J., Lees, K. R., et al.: Hemodynamic response and pharmacokinetics after the first dose of quinapril in patients with congestive heart failure. Br. J. Clin. Pharmacol. *38:*117, 1994.

31. Nussberger, J., Fleck, E., Bahrmann, H., et al.: Dose-related effects of ACE inhibition in man: Quinapril in patients with moderate congestive heart failure. Eur. Heart J. *15:*113, 1994.

32. Reid, J. L., MacFadyen, R. J., Squire, I. B., and Lees, K. R.: Blood pressure response to the first dose of angiotensin-converting enzyme inhibitors in congestive heart failure. Am. J. Cardiol. *71:*57, 1993.

33. Israili, Z. H., and Hall, W. D.: Cough and angioneurotic edema associated with angiotensin-converting enzyme inhibitor therapy. Ann. Intern. Med. *117:*234, 1992.

34. Ravid, D., Lishner, M., Lang, R., and Ravid, M.: Angiotensin-converting enzyme inhibitors and cough: A prospective evaluation in hypertension and in congestive heart failure. J. Clin. Pharmacol. *34:*1116, 1994.

35. Andersson, R. G. G., and Persson, K.: ACE inhibitors and their influence on inflammation, bronchial reactivity and cough. Eur. Heart J. *15:*52, 1994.

36. Hargreaves, M. R., and Benson, M. K.: Inhaled sodium cromoglycate in angiotensin-converting enzyme inhibitor cough. Lancet *345:*13, 1995.

37. Heesch, C. M., Hatfield, B. A., Marcoux, L., and Eichhorn, E. J.: Predictors of pressure and stroke volume response to afterload reduction with nitroprusside in patients with congestive heart failure secondary to idiopathic dilated cardiomyopathy. Am. J. Cardiol. *74:*1941, 1994.

38. Risoe, C., Simonsen, S., Rootwelt, K., et al.: Nitroprusside and regional vascular capacitance in patients with severe congestive heart failure. Circulation *85:*997, 1992.

39. Haas, G. J., and Leier, C. V.: Vasodilators. *In* Hosenpud, J. D., and Greenberg, G. H. (eds.): Congestive Heart Failure. New York, Springer-Verlag, 1994, p. 400.

40. Cohn, J. N., Archibald, D. G., Ziesche, S., et al.: Effect of vasodilator therapy on mortality in chronic congestive heart failure. Results of a Veterans Administration Cooperative Study. N. Engl. J. Med. *314:*1547, 1986.

41. Massie, B. M., Packer, M., Hanlon, J. T., and Combs, D. T.: Hemodynamic responses to combined therapy with captopril and hydralazine in patients with severe heart failure. J. Am. Coll. Cardiol. *2:*338, 1983.

DIURETICS

41a. Cody, R. J.: Clinical trials of diuretic therapy in heart failure: Research directions and clinical considerations. J. Am. Coll. Cardiol. *22:*165A, 1993.

42. Bigger, J. T., Jr.: Diuretic therapy, hypertension, and cardiac arrest. N. Engl. J. Med. *330:*1899, 1994.

43. Siscovick, D. S., Raghunathan, T. E., Psaty, B. M., et al.: Diuretic therapy for hypertension and the risk of primary cardiac arrest. N. Engl. J. Med. *330:*1852, 1994.

44. Silke, B.: Diuretic induced changes in symptoms and quality of life. Br. Heart J. *72:*57, 1994.

45. Freis, E. D.: The efficacy and safety of diuretics in treating hypertension. Ann. Intern. Med. *122:*223, 1995.

45a. Jackson, E. K.: Diuretics. *In* Hardman, J. G., et al. (eds.): Goodman & Gilman's: The pharmacological basis of therapeutics. 9th ed. New York, McGraw-Hill, 1996, pp. 199–248.

46. Leier, C. V., Dei Cas, L., and Metra, M.: Clinical relevance and management of the major electrolyte abnormalities in congestive heart failure: Hyponatremia, hypokalemia, and hypomagnesemia. Am. Heart J. *128:*564, 1994.

47. Lahav, M., Regev, A., Ra'anani, P., and Theodor, E.: Intermittent administration of furosemide vs continuous infusion preceded by a loading dose for congestive heart failure. Chest *102:*725, 1992.

48. McMurray, J., and McDevitt, D. G.: Treatment of heart failure in the elderly. Br. Med. Bull. *46:*202, 1990.

DIGITALIS

49. Christian, H. A.: Digitalis effects in chronic cardiac cases with regular rhythm in contrast to auricular fibrillation. Med. Clin. North Am. *5:*117, 1922.

50. Kelly, R. A., and Smith, T. W.: Digoxin in heart failure: Implications of recent trials. J. Am. Coll. Cardiol. *22:*107, 1993.

51. Tauke, J., Goldstein, S., and Gheorghiade, M.: Digoxin for chronic heart failure: A review of the randomized controlled trials with special attention to the PROVED and RADIANCE trials. Prog. Cardiovasc. Dis. *37:*49, 1994.

52. Uretsky, B. F., Young, J. B., Shahidi, F. E., et al.: Randomized study assessing the effect of digoxin withdrawal in patients with mild to moderate chronic congestive heart failure: Results of the PROVED trial. J. Am. Coll. Cardiol. *22:*955, 1993.

53. Packer, M., Gheorghiade, M., Young, J. B., et al.: Withdrawal of digoxin from patients with chronic heart failure treated with angiotensin-converting enzyme inhibitors. N. Engl. J. Med. *329:*1, 1993.

54. Smith, T. W.: Digoxin in heart failure. N. Engl. J. Med. *329:*51, 1993.

55. van Veldhuisen, K. J., Man in 'T Veld, A. J., Dunselman, H. J., et al.: Double-blind placebo-controlled study of ibopamine in patients with mild to moderate heart failure: Results of the Dutch Ibopamine Multicenter Trial (DIMT). J. Am. Coll. Cardiol. *22:*1564, 1993.

56. Yusuf, S., Garg, R., Held, P., et al.: Need for a large randomized trial to evaluate the effects of digitalis on morbidity and mortality in congestive heart failure. Am. J. Cardiol. *69:*64, 1992.

57. Digoxin Investigators' Group: The effect of digoxin on mortality and hospitalizations in patients with heart failure. Presentation at the 45th Annual Scientific Sessions, American College of Cardiology, Orlando, FL, March, 1996.

58. Lown, B., and Levine, S. A.: The carotid sinus: Clinical value of its stimulation. Circulation *23:*766, 1961.

59. Kelly, R. A.: Cardiac glycosides and congestive heart failure. Am. J. Cardiol. *65:*33, 1990.

60. Friedman, P. L.: Therapeutic and toxic electrophysiologic effects of cardiac glycosides. *In* Smith, T. W. (ed.): Digitalis Glycosides. Orlando, Grune & Stratton, 1985, p. 29.

61. Seelig, M.: Cardiovascular consequences of magnesium deficiency and loss: Pathogenesis, prevalence and manifestations: Magnesium and chloride loss in refractory potassium repletion. Am. J. Cardiol. *63:*4, 1989.

62. Cronin, R. E.: Magnesium disorders. *In* Kokko, J. P., and Tannen, R. L. (eds.): Fluids and Electrolytes. 2nd ed. Philadelphia, W. B. Saunders Company, 1990, p. 631.

63. Dorup, I., Skajaa, K., Clausen, T., and Kjeldsen, K.: Reduced concentrations of potassium, magnesium, and sodium-potassium pumps in human skeletal muscle during treatment with diuretics. Br. Med. J. *296:*455, 1988.

64. Gottlieb, S. S., Baruch, L., Kukin, M. L., et al.: Prognostic importance of the serum magnesium concentration in patients with congestive heart failure. J. Am. Coll. Cardiol. *16:*827, 1990.

65. Ralston, M. A., Murnane, M. R., Unverferth, D. V., and Leier, C. V.: Serum and tissue magnesium concentrations in patients with heart failure and serious ventricular arrhythmias. Ann. Intern. Med. *113:*841, 1990.

66. Gottlieb, S. S.: Importance of magnesium in congestive heart failure. Am. J. Cardiol. *63:*39, 1989.

67. Leier, C. V., Dei Cas, L., and Metra, M.: Clinical relevance and management of the major electrolyte abnormalities in congestive heart failure: Hyponatremia, hypokalemia, and hypomagnesemia. Am. Heart J. *128:*564, 1994.

68. Davies, D. L., and Fraser, R.: Do diuretics cause magnesium deficiency? Br. J. Clin. Pharmacol. *36:*1, 1993.

69. Smith, T. W., and Willerson, J. T.: Suicidal and accidental digoxin ingestion: Report of five cases with serum digoxin level correlations. Circulation *44:*29, 1971.

70. Smith, T. W., Butler, V. P., Jr., Haber, E., et al.: Treatment of life-threatening digitalis intoxication with digoxin-specific Fab fragments: Experience in 26 cases. N. Engl. J. Med. *307:*1357, 1982.

71. Rubinow, A., Skinner, M., and Cohen, A. S.: Digoxin sensitivity in amyloid cardiomyopathy. Circulation *63:*1285, 1981.

72. Braunwald, E.: 13th Bowditch Lecture. The determinants of myocardial oxygen consumption. The Physiologist *12:*65, 1969.

73. Glancy, D. L., Higgs, L. M., O'Brien, K. P., and Epstein, S. E.: Effects of ouabain on the left ventricular response to exercise in patients with angina pectoris. Circulation *43:*45, 1971.

74. Vogel, R., Kirch, D., LeFree, M., et al.: Effects of digitalis on resting and isometric exercise myocardial perfusion in patients with coronary artery disease and left ventricular dysfunction. Circulation *56:*355, 1977.

75. Crawford, M. H., LeWinter, M. M., O'Rourke, R. A., et al.: Combined propranolol and digoxin therapy in angina pectoris. Ann. Intern. Med. *83:*449, 1975.

76. Ratshin, R. A., Rackley, C. E., and Russell, R. O., Jr.: Hemodynamic evaluation of left ventricular function in shock complicating myocardial infarction. Circulation *45:*127, 1972.

77. Rahimtoola, S. H., Sinno, M. Z., Chuquimia, R., et al.: Effects of ouabain on impaired left ventricular function in acute myocardial infarction. N. Engl. J. Med. *287:*527, 1972.

78. Rahimtoola, S. H., and Gunnar, R. M.: Digitalis in acute myocardial infarction: Help or hazard? Ann. Intern. Med. *82:*234, 1975.

79. Selzer, A.: The use of digitalis in acute myocardial infarction. Prog. Cardiovasc. Dis. *10:*518, 1968.

80. Croxson, M. S., and Ibbertson, H. K.: Serum digoxin in patients with thyroid disease. Br. Med. J. *3:*566, 1975.

81. Curfman, G. D., Crowley, W. F., and Smith, T. W.: Thyroid-induced alterations in myocardial sodium- and potassium-activated adenosine triphosphatase, monovalent cation active transport, and cardiac glycoside binding. J. Clin. Invest. *59:*586, 1977.

82. Kim, D., and Smith, T. W.: Effects of thyroid hormone on sodium pump sites, sodium content, and contractile responses to cardiac glycosides in cultured chick ventricular cells. J. Clin. Invest. *74:*1481, 1984.

83. Green, L. H., and Smith, T. W.: The use of digitalis in patients with pulmonary disease. Ann. Intern. Med. *87:*459, 1977.

84. Beller, G. A., Smith, T. W., Abelmann, W. H., et al.: Digitalis intoxication: Prospective clinical study with serum level correlations. N. Engl. J. Med. *284:*989, 1971.

84a. Hoffman, B. B., and Lefkowitz, R. J.: Catecholamines, sympathomimetic drugs, and adrenergic receptor antagonists. *In* Hardman, J. G., et al.

(eds.): Goodman & Gilman's: The pharmacological basis of therapeutics. 9th ed. New York: McGraw-Hill, 1996, pp. 685–714.

INTRAVENOUS SYMPATHOMIMETIC AGENTS

85. Teboul, J.-L., Graini, L., Boujdaria, F., et al.: Cardiac index vs oxygen-derived parameters for rational use of dobutamine in patients with congestive heart failure. Chest 103:81, 1993.

86. Sacher, H. L., Sacher, M. L., Landau, S. W., et al.: Outpatient dobutamine therapy: The rhyme and the riddle. J. Clin. Pharmacol. 32:141, 1992.

87. Miller, L. W.: Outpatient dobutamine for refractory congestive heart failure: Advantages, techniques, and results. J. Heart Lung Transplant. 10:482, 1991.

88. DeBroux, E., Lagace, G., Dumont, L., and Chartrand, C.: Efficacy of dobutamine in the failing transplanted heart. J. Heart Lung Transplant. 11:1133, 1992.

89. Levy, D. K., Schwartz, J. M., Frishman, W. H., et al.: Ischemic hepatitis in a patient with congestive cardiomyopathy: An innovative approach to therapy using intravenous dobutamine. J. Clin. Pharmacol. 34:270, 1994.

90. Thuillez, Ch., Richard, Ch., Teboul, J. L., et al.: Arterial hemodynamics and cardiac effects of enoximone, dobutamine, and their combination in severe heart failure. Am. Heart J. 125:799, 1993.

91. Vendegna, T. R., and Anderson, R. J.: Are dopamine and/or dobutamine renoprotective in intensive care unit patients? Crit. Care Med. 22:1893, 1994.

92. Thompson, B. T., and Cockrill, B. A.: Renal-dose dopamine: A siren song? Lancet 344:7, 1994.

93. Duke, G. J., Briedis, J. H., and Weaver, R. A.: Renal support in critically ill patients: Low-dose dopamine or low-dose dobutamine? Crit. Care Med. 22:1919, 1994.

94. Flancbaum, L., Choban, P. S., and Dasta, J. F.: Quantitative effects of low-dose dopamine on urine output in oliguric surgical intensive care unit patients. Crit. Care Med. 22:61, 1994.

95. Baldwin, L., Henderson, A., and Hickman, P.: Effect of postoperative low-dose dopamine on renal function after elective major vascular surgery. Ann. Intern. Med. 120:744, 1994.

NEWER INOTROPIC AGENTS

96. Packer, M.: The development of positive inotropic agents for chronic heart failure: How have we gone astray? J. Am. Coll. Cardiol. 22:119, 1993.

97. DiBianco, R., Shabetai, R., Kostik, W., et al.: A comparison of oral milrinone, digoxin, and their combination in the treatment of patients with chronic heart failure. N. Engl. J. Med. 320:677, 1989.

97a. Karlsberg, R. P., DeWood, M. A., DeMaria, A. N., et al.: Comparative efficacy of short-term intravenous infusions of milrinone and dobutamine in acute congestive heart failure following acute myocardial infarction. Clin. Cardiol. 19:21, 1996.

98. Feldman, A. M., Bristow, M. R., Parmley, W. W., et al.: Effects of vesnarinone on morbidity and mortality in patients with heart failure. N. Engl. J. Med. 329:149, 1993.

BETA-ADRENERGIC ANTAGONISTS

99. Waagstein, F., Bristow, M. R., Swedberg, K., et al.: Beneficial effects of metoprolol in idiopathic dilated cardiomyopathy. Lancet 342:1441, 1993.

100. CIBIS Investigators and Committees: A randomized trial of β-blockade in heart failure. The Cardiac Insufficiency Bisoprolol Study (CIBIS). Circulation 90:1765, 1994.

101. Eichhorn, E. J., and Hjalmarson, A.: β-Blocker treatment for chronic heart failure. The frog prince. Circulation 90:2153, 1994.

102. Fisher, M. L., Gottlieb, S. S., Plotnick, G. D., et al.: Beneficial effects of metoprolol in heart failure associated with coronary artery disease: A randomized trial. J. Am. Coll. Cardiol. 23:943, 1994.

103. Hjalmarson, A., and Waagstein, F.: The role of β-blockers in the treatment of cardiomyopathy and ischemic heart disease. Drugs 47:31, 1994.

104. Woodley, S. L., Gilbert, E. M., and Anderson, J. L.: β-Blockade with bucindolol in heart failure due to ischemic vs idiopathic dilated cardiomyopathy. Circulation 84:2426, 1991.

105. Bristow, M. R., O'Connell, J. B., Gilbert, E. M., et al., for the Bucindolol Investigators: Dose-response of chronic β-blocker treatment in heart failure from either idiopathic dilated or ischemic cardiomyopathy. Circulation 89:1632, 1994.

105a. Packer, M., Bristow, M., and Cohn, J. N.: Effect of carvedilol on the survival of patients with chronic heart failure. Circulation 92(Suppl. I):142, 1995.

105b. Krum, H., Sackner-Bernstein, J. D., Goldsmith, R. L., et al.: Double-blind placebo-controlled study of the long-term efficacy of carvedilol in patients with severe chronic heart failure. Circulation 92:1499, 1995.

HEART FAILURE WITH PREDOMINANT DIASTOLIC VENTRICULAR DYSFUNCTION

106. Levine, H. J., and Gaasch, W. H.: Clinical recognition and treatment of diastolic dysfunction and heart failure. In Gaasch, W. H., and LeWinter,

M. M. (eds.): Left Ventricular Diastolic Dysfunction and Heart Failure. Philadelphia: Lea and Febiger, 1994, p. 445.

107. Villari, B., Vasalli, G., Monrad, E. S., Chiariello, M., Turina, M., and Hess, O. M.: Normalization of diastolic dysfunction in aortic stenosis late after valve replacement. Circulation 91:2353, 1995.

108. Brilla, C. G., Janicki, J. S., and Weber, K. T.: Cardioreparative effects of lisinopril in rats with genetic hypertension and left ventricular hypertrophy. Circulation 83:1771, 1991.

109. Bonow, R. O., Frederick, T. M., Bacharach, S. L., et al.: Atrial systole and left ventricular filling in hypertrophic cardiomyopathy: Effect of verapamil. Am. J. Cardiol. 51:1386, 1983.

110. Gilligan, D. M., Chan, W. L., Joshi, J., et al.: A double-blind, placebo-controlled crossover trial of nadolol and verapamil in mild and moderately symptomatic hypertrophic cardiomyopathy. J. Am. Coll. Cardiol. 21:1672, 1993.

SUDDEN DEATH AND ARRHYTHMIAS

111. Stevenson, W. G., Stevenson, L. W., Middlekauff, H. R., and Saxon, L. A.: Sudden death prevention in patients with advanced ventricular dysfunction. Circulation 88:2953, 1993.

112. Luu, M., Stevenson, W. G., Stevenson, L. W., et al.: Diverse mechanisms of unexpected cardiac arrest in advanced heart failure. Circulation 80:1675, 1989.

113. Aronson, R. S.: Mechanisms of arrhythmias in ventricular hypertrophy. J. Cardiovasc. Electrophysiol. 14:1735, 1991.

114. Charpentier, F., Baudet, S., and Le Marec, H.: Triggered activity as a possible mechanism for arrhythmias to ventricular hypertrophy. PACE Pacing Clin. Electrophysiol. 14:1735, 1991.

115. Calkins, H., Maughan, L., Wiseman, H. F., et al.: Effect of acute volume load on refractoriness and arrhythmia development in isolated chronically infarcted canine hearts. Circulation 79:687, 1989.

116. Franz, M. R., Cima, R., Wang, D., et al.: Electrophysiological effects of myocardial stretch and mechanical determinants of stretch-activated arrhythmias. Circulation 86:968, 1992.

117. Lubbe, W. F., Podzuweit, T., and Opie, L. H.: Potential arrhythmogenic role of cyclic adenosine monophosphate (AMP) and systolic calcium overload: Implications for prophylactic effects of beta-blockers in myocardial infarction and proarrhythmic effects of phosphodiesterase inhibitors. J. Am. Coll. Cardiol. 19:1622, 1992.

118. Ben-David, J., and Zipes, D. Alpha-adrenoceptor stimulation and blockade modulates cesium-induced early afterdepolarizations and ventricular tachyarrhythmias in dogs. Circulation 82:225, 1990.

119. Gettes, L. S.: Electrolyte abnormalities underlying lethal ventricular arrhythmias. Circulation 85(Suppl. 1):I-70, 1992.

120. Wilber, D., Garan, H., Finkelstein, D., et al.: Out-of-hospital cardiac arrest: Use of electrophysiologic testing in the prediction of long-term outcome. N. Engl. J. Med. 318:19, 1988.

121. Kim, S. G., Fisher, J. D., Choue, C. W., et al.: Influence of left ventricular function on outcome of patients treated with implantable defibrillators. Circulation 85:1304, 1992.

122. Stevenson, W. G., Middlekauff, H. M., Stevenson, L. W., et al.: Significance of aborted cardiac arrest and sustained ventricular tachycardia in patients referred for treatment therapy of advanced heart failure. Am. Heart J. 124:123, 1992.

123. Stevenson, W. G., Stevenson, L. W., Weiss, J., and Tillisch, J. H.: Inducible ventricular arrhythmias and sudden death during vasodilator therapy of severe heart failure. Am. Heart J. 116:1447, 1988.

124. Canceres, J., Jazayeri, M., McKinnie, J., et al.: Sustained bundle branch re-entry as a mechanism of clinical tachycardia. Circulation 79:256, 1989.

125. Stevenson, W. G., Middlekauff, H. R., and Saxon, L. A.: Ventricular arrhythmias in heart failure. In Zipes D. P., and Jalife J., (eds.): Cardiac Electrophysiology: From Cell to Bedside. Philadelphia, W. B. Saunders Company, 1994, p. 848.

126. Horowitz, L. N., Greenspan, A. M., Spielman, S. R., et al.: Usefulness of electrophysiologic testing in evaluation of amiodarone therapy for sustained ventricular tachyarrhythmias associated with coronary heart disease. Am. J. Cardiol. 55:367, 1985.

127. Weinberg, B. A., Miles, W. M., Klein, L. S., et al.: Five-year follow-up of 589 patients treated with amiodarone. Am. Heart J. 125:109, 1993.

128. Sager, P. T., Choudhary, R., Leon, C., et al.: The long-term prognosis of patients with out-of-hospital cardiac arrest but no inducible ventricular tachycardia. Am. Heart J. 120:1334, 1990.

129. Gottlieb, S. S., Kukin, M. L., Medina, N., et al.: Comparative hemodynamic effects of procainamides tocainide and encainide in severe chronic heart failure. Circulation 81:860, 1990.

130. Ravid, S., Podrid, P. J., Lampert, S., et al.: Congestive heart failure induced by six of the newer antiarrhythmic drugs. J. Am. Coll. Cardiol. 14:1289, 1989.

131. Stanton, M. S., Prystowsky, E. N., Fineberg, N. A., et al.: Arrhythmogenic effects of antiarrhythmic drugs: A study of 506 patients treated for ventricular tachycardia or fibrillation. J. Am. Coll. Cardiol. 14:209, 1989.

132. The Cardiac Arrhythmia Suppression Trial (CAST) Investigators: CAST mortality and morbidity. Treatment versus placebo. N. Engl. J. Med. 324:781, 1991.

133. Flaker, G. C., Blackshear, J. L., McBride, R., et al.: Predictors of thromboembolism in atrial fibrillation: Clinical features of patients at risk. The Stroke Prevention in Atrial Fibrillation Investigators. Ann. Intern. Med. 116:2, 1992.

134. Hamer, A. W. F., Arkles, L. B., and Johns, J. A.: Beneficial effects of low dose amiodarone in patients with congestive heart failure: A placebo-controlled trial. J. Am. Coll. Cardiol. *14*:1768, 1989.

135. Pfisterer, M., Kiowski, W., Burckhardt, D., et al.: Beneficial effect of amiodarone on cardiac mortality in patients with asymptomatic complex ventricular arrhythmias after acute myocardial infarction and preserved, but not impaired left ventricular function. Am. J. Cardiol. *69*:1399, 1992.

136. Doval, H. C., Nul, D. R., Grancelli, H. O., et al.: Randomized trial of low-dose amiodarone in severe congestive heart failure. Lancet *344*:493, 1994.

136a. Hammill, S. C., and Packer, D. L.: Amiodarone in congestive heart failure unraveling the GESICA and CHF-STATE differences. Heart *75*:6, 1996.

137. Singh, S. N., Fletcher, R. D., Fisher, S. G., et al.: Amiodarone in patients with congestive heart failure and asymptomatic ventricular arrhythmia. N. Engl. J. Med. *333*:77, 1995.

138. Middlekauff, H. R., Stevenson, W. G., Saxon, L. A., and Stevenson, L. W.: Amiodarone and torsades de pointes in patients with advanced heart failure. Am. J. Cardiol. *76*:499, 1995.

139. Middlekauff, H. R., Stevenson, W. G., Stevenson, L. W., and Saxon, L. A.: Syncope in advanced heart failure: High sudden death regardless of etiology. J. Am. Coll. Cardiol. *21*:110, 1993.

140. Cohn, J. N., Johnson, G. R., Shabetai, R., et al.: Ejection fraction, peak exercise oxygen consumption, cardiothoracic ratio, ventricular arrhythmias, and plasma norepinephrine as determinants of prognosis in heart failure. Circulation *87*:5, 1993.

141. Hallstrom, A. P., Bigger, J. T., Doen, D., et al.: Prognostic significance of ventricular premature depolarizations measured 1 year after myocardial infarction in patients with early postinfarction asymptomatic ventricular arrhythmia. J. Am. Coll. Cardiol. *20*:259, 1992.

142. Bourke, J. P., Richards, D. A. B., Ross, D. L., et al.: Routine programmed electrical stimulation in survivors of acute myocardial infarction for prediction of spontaneous ventricular tachyarrhythmias during follow-up results, optimal stimulation protocol and cost-effective screening. J. Am. Coll. Cardiol. *18*:780, 1991.

143. Middlekauff, H. R., Stevenson, W. G., and Stevenson, L. W.: Prognostic significance of atrial fibrillation in advanced heart failure: A study of 390 patients. Circulation *84*:40, 1991.

144. Carson, P. E., Johnson, G. R., Dunkman, W. B., et al.: The influence of atrial fibrillation on prognosis in mild to moderate heart failure. Circulation *87*:VI-102, 1993.

145. Middlekauff, H. R., Wiener, I., and Stevenson, W. G.: Low-dose amiodarone for atrial fibrillation. Am. J. Cardiol. *72*:75, 1993.

146. Grogan, M., Smith, H. C., Gersh, B. J., and Wood, D. W.: Left ventricular dysfunction due to atrial fibrillation in patients initially believed to have idiopathic dilated cardiomyopathy. Am. J. Cardiol. *69*:1570, 1992.

147. Coplen, S. E., Antman, E. M., Berlin, J. A., et al.: Efficacy and safety of quinidine therapy for maintenance of sinus rhythm after cardioversion. Circulation *82*:1106, 1990.

148. Heinz, G., Siostrzonek, P., Kreiner, G., et al.: Improvement in left ventricular systolic function after successful radiofrequency His bundle ablation for drug refractory, chronic atrial fibrillation and recurrent atrial flutter. Am. J. Cardiol. *69*:489, 1992.

REFRACTORY HEART FAILURE

149. Elefteriades, J. A., Tolis, G., Levi, E., et al.: Coronary artery bypass grafting in severe left ventricular dysfunction: Excellent survival with improved ejection fraction and functional state. J. Am. Coll. Cardiol. *22*:1411, 1993.

150. Louie, H. W., Laks, H., Milgalter, E., et al.: Ischemic cardiomyopathy: Criteria for coronary revascularization and cardiac transplantation. Circulation *84*(Suppl. III):290, 1991.

151. Lang, R. M., Borow, K. M., Neumann, A., and Janzen, D.: Systemic vascular resistance: An unreliable index of left ventricular afterload. Circulation *74*:1114, 1989.

152. Forrester, J. S., Diamond, G., Chatterjee, K., and Swan, H. J. C.: Medical therapy of acute myocardial infarction by application of hemodynamic subsets. N. Engl. J. Med. *295*(24):1356, 1976.

153. Stevenson, L. W., and Tillisch, J. H.: Maintenance of cardiac output with normal filling pressures in dilated heart failure. Circulation *74*:1303, 1986.

154. Stevenson, L. W., Brunken, R. C., Belil, D., et al.: Afterload reduction with vasodilators and diuretics decreases mitral valve regurgitation during upright exercise in advanced heart failure. J. Am. Coll. Cardiol. *15*:174, 1990.

155. Stevenson, L. W.: Tailored therapy before transplantation for treatment of advanced heart failure: Effective use of vasodilators and diuretics. J. Heart Lung Transplant. *10*(3):468, 1991.

156. Guiha, N. H., Cohn, J. N., Mikulic, E., et al.: Treatment of refractory heart failure with infusion of nitroprusside. N. Engl. J. Med. *291*:587, 1974.

157. Pierpont, G. L., and Francis, G. S.: Medical management of terminal cardiomyopathy. Heart Transplant. *2*(1):18, 1982.

158. Fonarow, G. C., Stevenson, L. W., Walden, J. A., et al.: Impact of a comprehensive management program on the hospitalization rate for patients with advanced heart failure. J. Am. Coll. Cardiol. *25*:264, 1995.

159. Stevenson, L. W., Siestsema, K., Tillisch, J. H., et al.: Exercise capacity for survivors of cardiac transplantation or sustained medical therapy for stable heart failure. Circulation *81*:78, 1990.

160. Mudge, G. H., Goldstein, S., Addonizio, L. J., et al.: Cardiac transplantation: Recipient guidelines/prioritization. J. Am. Coll. Cardiol. *22*:21, 1993.

161. Hanly, P. J., Millnar, T. W., Steljes, D. G., et al.: The effect of oxygen on respiration and sleep in patients with congestive heart failure. Ann. Intern. Med. *111*:777, 1989.

162. Naughton, M. T., Liu, P. P., Benard, D. C., et al.: Treatment of congestive heart failure and Cheyne-Stokes respiration during sleep by CPAP. Am. J. Respir. Crit. Care Med. *152*:92, 1995.

163. Naughton, M. T., Rahman, A., Hara, K., et al.: Effect of CPAP on intrathoracic and left ventricular transmural pressures in patients with congestive heart failure. Circulation *91*:1725, 1995.

164. Sullivan, M. J., Higginbotham, M. B., and Cobb, F. R.: Exercise training in patients with chronic heart failure delays ventilatory anaerobic threshold and improves submaximal exercise performance. Circulation *79*:324, 1989.

164a. Natterson, P. D., Stevenson, W. G., Saxon, L. A., et al.: Risk of arterial embolization in 224 patients awaiting cardiac transplantation. Am. Heart J. *129*:564, 1995.

165. Hosenpud, J. D., Novick, R. J., Breen, T. J., and Daily, O. P.: The registry of the International Society for Heart and Lung Transplantation: Eleventh official report—1994. J. Heart Lung Transplant. *13*:561, 1994.

166. Kaye, M. P.: Registry of the International Society for Heart and Lung Transplantation: Tenth official report—1993. J. Heart Lung Transplant. *12*:541, 1993.

167. Stevenson, L. W., Couper, G., Natterson, B. J., et al.: Target heart failure population for new therapies. Circulation *92*:II-174, 1995.

168. Mancini, D. M., Eisen, H., Kussmaul, W., et al.: Value of peak exercise oxygen consumption for optimal timing of cardiac transplantation in ambulatory patients with heart failure. Circulation *83*:778, 1991.

169. Stevenson, L. W., Warner, S. L., Steimle, A. E., et al.: The impending crisis awaiting cardiac transplantation: Modeling a solution based on selection. Circulation *89*:450, 1994.

170. McManus, R. P., O'Hair, D. P., Beitzinger, J. M., et al.: Patients who die awaiting heart transplantation. J. Heart Lung Transplant. *12*:159, 1993.

171. Stevenson, L. W., Steimle, A. E., Fonarow, G., et al.: Improvement in exercise capacity of candidates awaiting heart transplantation. J. Am. Coll. Cardiol. *25*:163, 1995.

172. Moore, F. D. (Chairman): Fifth Bethesda Conference Report: Cardiac and other organ transplantation. Am. J. Cardiol. *22*:896, 1968.

Chapter 18
Heart and Heart-Lung Transplantation

MARK G. PERLROTH, BRUCE A. REITZ

Although cardiac transplantation in humans was first carried out in 1967, it is only since the early 1980's that it has been established as an accepted treatment for end-stage heart disease. The advances in immunosuppression and transplant management that have made this possible also have led to successful heart-lung and lung transplantation, which are continuing to evolve. The increasingly widespread application of thoracic organ transplantation has brought this therapy to many centers around the world and to an ever-increasing patient population.

The Registry of the International Society for Heart Transplantation in 1994 listed a cumulative total of more than 30,200 cardiac transplant procedures performed in 257 transplant centers.[1] The recent expansion of heart transplantation is emphasized by the fact that before 1980, fewer than 360 transplantations had been performed. The management philosophies and strategies discussed in this chapter are based in part on the experience of the Johns Hopkins Hospital and the Stanford University teams, and have been reviewed elsewhere.[2]

HISTORY

There are several mentions of heart transplantation in ancient Chinese mythology and biblical reference, but not until the pioneering work of Alexis Carrel at the beginning of the 20th century did surgeons have the ability to transplant organs such as the heart.[3] In a number of imaginative experiments, Carrel demonstrated that a heart could be transplanted and resume functioning in the new host. Not only did Carrel transplant hearts but he also suggested and performed the en bloc transplantation of heart and lungs,[4] both of these procedures being heterotopic transplants into the necks of recipient dogs.

With the advent of techniques for successful cardiac surgery in the 1950's, major attention was finally directed to the problem of transplantation of the heart in the chest in the normal, or orthotopic, position. The current most commonly used surgical technique for heart transplantation originated with the work of Lower and Shumway in 1959.[5] A number of important questions about transplants, including protocols for immunosuppression,[6] correlation of the surface electrocardiogram with allograft rejection,[7] and reversal of these changes with augmented immunosuppression, were subjects of early laboratory study. Despite this prior laboratory work, many were surprised when the first human heart transplant was performed by Christian Barnard in Capetown, South Africa in December 1967.[8] This transplant initiated a great amount of interest at other centers around the world, with 170 transplants by 65 surgical teams between December 1967 and March 1971. The one-year survival was only 15 per cent, and because of this, enthusiasm for heart transplantation rapidly waned by the end of 1971.

Only at Stanford University and the Medical College of Virginia did surgical teams continue with programs in heart transplantation. Working virtually alone through the decade of the 1970's, these investigators refined recipient selection criteria,[9] saw the development of the transvenous endomyocardial biopsy for diagnosing rejection,[10] developed rabbit antithymocyte globulin as an effective treatment of acute rejection,[11] and defined many of the late post-transplant complications and management principles.[12]

IMMUNOSUPPRESSIVE THERAPY. Widespread application of heart transplantation depended on the development of better immunosuppressive therapy (see pp. 522–523). This goal was reached with the discovery that cyclosporin A (cyclosporine), a novel cyclic undecapeptide of fungal origin, could selectively block the effect of interleukin-2 (IL-2) in stimulating T cells.[13–19]

Heart and lung transplantation has been extended to a large number of additional recipients, including neonates with hypoplastic left heart syndrome, the elderly (age 60 to 70), and patients with primary lung disease, such as emphysema and cystic fibrosis.

ORGANIZATION OF A TRANSPLANT PROGRAM

In 1994, there were 257 centers performing cardiac transplantation worldwide. Experience has shown that a successful program depends on both institutional commitment and participation of multiple professional groups within the institution that must work together in caring for the patient. Careful attention to detail in organizing a transplant program is crucial in obtaining and sustaining good outcomes in transplant patients.

The development of an effective cardiac transplant program requires careful organization and cooperation from both clinical and nonclinical personnel. Some but not all states require a certificate of need to initiate a new program of heart transplantation. The National Organ Transplantation Act of 1984 established certain minimum criteria for transplant programs to enroll in the nationwide computerized matching system.[20] To encourage excellent patient care and to discourage transplantation in centers with suboptimal results, the act established the United Network for Organ Sharing (UNOS), with membership limited to those centers that perform a minimum of 12 transplant procedures per year and that obtain a one-year survival rate of at least 70 per cent. In addition to these performance criteria, the center must have adequate operating room facilities and trained physicians and nursing personnel and be a participating member in a local organ procurement organization. The program must have established protocols and procedures for the selection of patients, the evaluation and distribution of donor organs, postoperative management, and long-term follow-up. Both surgeons and physicians involved in the care of the patient must meet certain criteria in terms of training and prior experience. The ability of an individual center to obtain funding from Medicare depends on similar criteria.[21]

RECIPIENT SELECTION

With improved outcomes in both quality of life and percentage of patients surviving, cardiac transplantation has become accepted therapy for many patients with end-stage heart disease. A fairly rigid selection process is required in order to obtain excellent results in individual patients. Although in recent years there has been a tendency to relax these criteria in an effort to extend the benefits of transplantation to a larger number of patients, this has heightened the problem of donor scarcity. The number of potential recipients rises exponentially with an extension of the upper age accepted, as shown in Figure 18–1. The diagnoses of patients undergoing heart transplantation are listed in Figure 18–2. The most frequent indications are

515

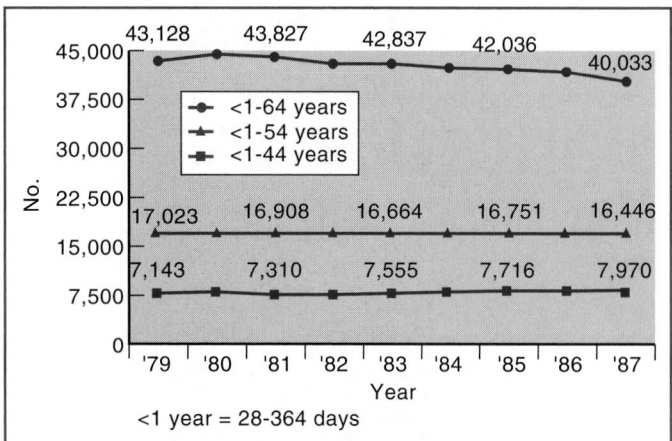

FIGURE 18–1. The need for heart transplantation in the United States, 1979 to 1987. (From O'Connell J. B., Gunnar, R. M., Evans, R. W., et al.: Task Force 1: Organization of Heart Transplantation in the U.S. J. Am. Coll. Cardiol. *22*(1):9, 1993. Reprinted with permission from the American College of Cardiology.)

TABLE 18–1 CONTRAINDICATIONS TO HEART TRANSPLANTATION

Advanced age (> 70 years)
Irreversible hepatic, renal, or pulmonary dysfunction
Severe peripheral vascular or cerebrovascular disease
Insulin-requiring diabetes mellitus with end-organ damage
Active infection
Recent cancer with uncertain status
Psychiatric illness, poor medical compliance
Systemic disease that would significantly limit survival or rehabilitation
Pulmonary hypertension with pulmonary vascular resistance > 6 Wood units or 3 Wood units after treatment with vasodilators

equally divided between ischemic heart disease and cardiomyopathy. Contraindications (Table 18–1) vary somewhat by program. (See also pp. 509–511.)

An important aspect of evaluation is a comprehensive psychosocial evaluation by a clinical social worker or psychologist. The ability of the patient to follow a complex medical regimen is extremely important, as is the family support necessary to help the patient through multiple medical procedures and evaluations and to maintain the essential medical regimen after transplantation.

All conventional medical or surgical therapies should be used before consideration of transplantation. Evaluation might reasonably include endomyocardial biopsy to rule out other treatable causes of cardiomyopathy, especially for patients without ischemic heart disease. Occasionally, unsuspected sarcoidosis or myocarditis is detected that might respond favorably to an alternative therapy, and some patients with recurrent life-threatening arrhythmias may be best treated initially by placement of an automatic implantable cardiac defibrillator.

Although it may be easy to identify the most severely ill patients with a poor prognosis for six-month survival, there is a large group of patients with symptomatic cardiomyopathy and ominous objective findings (ejection fraction < 20 per cent, stroke volume ≤ 40 ml, severe ventricular arrhythmias) for whom timing may be somewhat difficult. A further consideration may be the quality of life, which is a judgment of the patient and the physicians caring for the patient. This comes into play in patients with intractable angina and coronary vessels that cannot be bypassed.

UPPER AGE LIMIT. One of the most controversial aspects of patient selection is the upper age limit for cardiac transplantation. The initial Stanford University criteria considered an upper age limit of 50 years. This was modified to include patients older than 55 and then up to age 60 during the era of improving results because of cyclosporine therapy in the early 1980's. Sufficient additional experience has now been reported in patients over age 55 to indicate that a strict chronological age criterion is not appropriate.[22–24] Older people can undergo transplantation with good expectation of survival and improvement in quality of life, although these patients should be optimal in every other respect. Some evidence has been reported suggesting that older patients may experience less rejection than younger patients.[25] The additional relative contraindication of diabetes or other systemic disease, such as chronic pulmonary disease, probably would eliminate most patients over 60 as potential candidates.

PULMONARY VASCULAR DISEASE. This is an important consideration. Orthotopic cardiac transplantation requires that the pulmonary vascular resistance be low, so that the normal right ventricle of the donor heart can adequately support the recipient's circulation after transplantation. A great deal of controversy has developed over the optimal measure of pulmonary vascular resistance. Most programs use the measurement of the traditional Wood unit, and limit the value to ≤ 6 units at rest or < 3 with maximal vasodilation. Other centers use the pulmonary vascular resistance index (Wood units × body surface area) or transpulmonary pressure gradient (mean pulmonary artery pressure minus mean pulmonary capillary wedge pressure) ≤ 15 mm Hg.[26] Whatever measure of resistance is used, in those patients with values toward the upper limits, it is imperative to demonstrate in the catheterization laboratory that the resistance can be manipulated with either oxygen or vasodilators with or without inotropic agents.[27] If the pulmonary vascular resistance measurements remain elevated, strong consideration should be given to either heterotopic cardiac transplantation, which leaves the recipient's heart intact, or heart-lung transplantation. Because patients may remain on a waiting list for more than six months, repeat cardiac catheterization may be necessary semiannually to determine if the pulmonary vascular resistance has increased. Significantly elevated pulmonary vascular resistance and right heart failure remain problems after orthotopic cardiac transplantation and are major causes of early postoperative mortality.

CLINICAL CONSIDERATIONS. Ultimately, the selection of a candidate for heart transplantation results from a clinical assessment that a patient free of established contraindications (see Table 18–1) suffers severe cardiac disability refractory to expert management. The pathophysiology usually encompasses congestive heart failure but is occasionally dominated by recurrent lethal arrhythmias or intolerable ischemic symptoms. Reliance solely on a low (< 20 per cent) ejection fraction has become less reliable

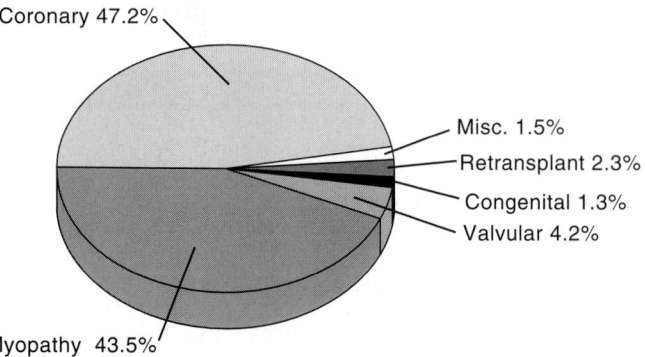

FIGURE 18–2. Adult heart transplantation indications. (From Hosenpud, J. D., Novick, R. J., Breen, T. J., and Daily, O. P.: The Registry of the International Society for Heart and Lung Transplantation: Eleventh Official Report—1994*. J. Heart Lung Transplant. *13*(4):561, 1994. Reprinted with permission from Mosby-Year Book, Inc.)

since the introduction of aggressive vasodilator therapy. Some patients with extensive left ventricular dysfunction are remarkably symptom-free, and subgroups can experience one-year survivals of more than 60 per cent.[28] The success and acceptance of heart transplantation has encouraged enlistment of less severely ill candidates for this procedure to such an extent that expected survival has increased from almost none at 6 months to 50 per cent at 2 years.[29]

PEAK $\dot{V}O_2$. The measurement of peak oxygen consumption ($\dot{V}O_2$; ml/kg/min) (Figs. 5–1, p. 155, 5–2, p. 156, 14–29, p. 440) has been a useful supplementary criterion for the selection of recipients and the timing of transplantation.[30,31] Maximal exercise performance exceeding 14 ml/kg/min predicted a 1-year survival of greater than 90 per cent. The worst outlook was for those patients whose peak $\dot{V}O_2$ was < 10 ml/kg/min, and they, if otherwise acceptable, should be recommended for cardiac transplantation. Those with intermediate values require additional evaluation based on disability, quality of life, and age.

COEXISTING DISEASES. Patients with involvement of other organs that precluded selection in the past, but that now respond to transplantation, may be considered candidates for *dual organ transplantation*. In addition to heart-lung, these include heart-kidney (notably for retransplantation of heart transplant recipients who have developed cyclosporine nephrotoxicity) and heart-liver (for homozygous familial hypercholesterolemia). Dual organ candidacy does not change a patient's status or position on the waiting list, but when patients become eligible for a heart or liver based on standard criteria, the second required organ may be allocated from the same donor.[32] The ethical dilemma of improving one life instead of two remains unresolved.

Patients with infective endocarditis (without metastatic infection) and patients with malignancy without evidence of recurrence (often with anthracycline cardiomyopathy) have successfully received heart transplants. Systemic amyloidosis, because of its frequent multiorgan involvement as well as documented recurrence in the allograft, remains an unlikely condition for transplantation at most centers.

Inevitably, all programs exercise some subjectivity in the selection process determined by the prior experience of the transplant team with the many clinical, physiological, and social variables involved. Although the evaluation of potential candidates for cardiac transplantation is difficult, these established criteria have led to certain predictable outcomes in terms of quality of life and actuarial survival. Deviations from these protocols usually produce less favorable results. As with any medical or surgical procedure, the final decision ultimately rests with the patient, in accordance with the concept of informed consent.

MANAGEMENT OF PATIENTS AWAITING TRANSPLANTATION

Because there are a number of patients awaiting transplantation at any point in time, their management is important. The UNOS patient waiting list for needed organs in August 1994 totaled 2892 patients awaiting heart transplantation and 214 United States patients awaiting heart-lung transplantation.[33] Because the current yearly number of procedures performed is about 2100, a number of awaiting recipients will not survive to receive a needed organ. Most centers experience between 20 and 30 per cent mortality of patients on the waiting list. United States heart-lung transplants, after peaking at 74 in 1988, have declined to approximately 50 to 60 per year, while lung transplants have steadily risen to an annual rate of more than 500.[34]

The management of end-stage congestive heart failure is described in Chapter 17. Although digitalis remains the only generally available oral inotropic agent, the use of intravenous low-dose dopa-

mine or dobutamine has been a helpful tool for managing some of these patients.[35] Combined with brief hospitalizations for hemodynamic monitoring to optimize vasodilators, diuretics, and intravenous inotropes, patients will often sustain improvement lasting for weeks or even months. The use of anticoagulants as prophylaxis against systemic or pulmonary thromboembolism is practiced routinely at some centers.

MECHANICAL DEVICES FOR BRIDGING. Patients in whom conventional medical therapy fails may require intraaortic balloon counterpulsation or possibly a mechanical assist device for bridging to transplantation[36-38] (see Chap. 19). Growing experience has demonstrated that for short-term bridging, up to one week, the use of a centrifugal pump similar to types used during routine cardiac surgery can be effective. For longer-term mechanical support, ventricular assist devices have been successful. The use of the totally implantable heart has resulted in poor bridging to transplantation, with multiple complications owing to infections and/or thromboemboli.[39] Two long-term mechanical assist devices have been evaluated in multicenter studies, the Novacor and the ThermoCardiosystems, Inc. (TCI) HeartMate. Each was tested in approximately 100 patients for periods of up to a year or more. The Novacor required systemic anticoagulation, whereas the TCI did not. Thromboembolic complications were uncommon in both. Approximately 60 per cent of patients so treated went on to cardiac transplantation; of these, 85 to 89 per cent survived.[40]

Even before development of such sophisticated devices, the intraaortic balloon pump was and continues to be used successfully for this purpose. The first successful use of these mechanical devices occurred in 1984 for the left ventricular assist pump and in 1985 for a total artificial heart. Subsequently, more than 1000 patients have received one or the other device, and more than 500 have subsequently undergone cardiac transplantation. A recent review reported that 69 per cent of patients in whom the device was inserted as a bridge to transplantation ultimately underwent the transplant, with 95 per cent of these patients being discharged from the hospital. The one- and two-year survival estimates for patients requiring only univentricular mechanical support were equivalent to those of patients having isolated orthotopic cardiac transplantation alone. It is now accepted that ventricular assist devices are able to provide reasonable and safe circulatory support in patients dying of cardiac failure and have the potential to resuscitate and rehabilitate patients prior to undergoing cardiac transplantation.[41]

Once selected, patients are categorized on the basis of size, ABO blood group, time on the waiting list, and clinical status. The latter consists of two classes: In adults, status I comprises patients in an intensive care unit receiving parenteral inotropic drugs or mechanical support (i.e., ventilator, intraaortic balloon pump, or ventricular assist device). It does not automatically include patients with an intracardiac defibrillator or those who require continuous infusions of antiarrhythmic drugs. Status II comprises all other patients. Separate waiting lists are maintained for the two status classes.

Patients are "de-listed" if they improve or if they suffer complications (e.g., cerebral or pulmonary embolism) or superimposed illnesses (e.g., infections, gastrointestinal bleeding), which increase the risk of surgery and immunosuppression or which compromise rehabilitation or survival. They are reactivated when clinically appropriate.

EVALUATION AND MANAGEMENT OF THE HEART DONOR

The factor limiting the number of heart transplants performed is the availability of donor organs. Thus, it is imperative to obtain as high a percentage of potential donor organs as possible by increasing the donation rate and also to consider all donor organs that might possibly be suitable for transplantation. The cardiologist frequently is asked to take part in the donor evaluation process, so that the adequate function of the graft can be predicted before transplantation.

Brain death has been accepted as the legal definition of death throughout the United States.[42] The diagnosis should not involve physicians caring for the potential candidate, and it requires the absence of hypothermia (core temperature $> 32.5°C$) or drugs capable of altering neurological or neuromuscular function.[43]

The specific neurological catastrophe that has resulted in brain death may include blunt traumatic injury to the head, intracranial hemorrhage, or penetrating traumatic injury. The characteristics of cardiac donors are listed in Table 18–2. Until fairly recently, heart and heart-lung transplant donor criteria were very selective. The upper age limit was usually 35 years of age, and there were a number of other

TABLE 18–2   CAUSES OF DEATH IN DONORS* FOR HEART TRANSPLANT PROCEDURES IN THE JOHNS HOPKINS SERIES (JULY 1983–JUNE 1990)

CAUSE OF DEATH	NO. DONORS
Head trauma	68
Gunshot wound	21
Cerebrovascular accident	23
Asphyxiation	5
Brain tumor	1
Liver failure	1
Heart-lung recipient	1

* Age, 24 years mean (0.7–47); sex, 92 males/28 females.

criteria.[44] With the need to increase the number of transplants, these criteria have been modified.[45,46] Most centers evaluate any potential donor up to as high as 55 years of age. Especially with the older or suboptimal donor, a careful cardiac history must be obtained from the next of kin and adequate cardiac function ensured, including potential evaluation with coronary arteriography for men older than 45 or women older than 55. The use of "on the operating table" coronary arteriography has been suggested because of the logistic requirements for performing coronary arteriography in a brain-dead patient.[47] Alternatively, simple inspection of the graft with palpation of the coronary arteries at the time of harvesting has been used by some groups to determine the presence of significant atherosclerosis. Sweeney and colleagues have reported on the use of hearts from donors who did not meet the standard criteria.[45] Recipients received grafts from older donors (> age 40) or from patients with a history of prolonged cardiac arrest or septicemia. Their results indicate that selective use of such donors is possible with reasonable outcomes. Hearts from older donors should, whenever possible, be reserved for older recipients because of inherent loss of function with age.

The evaluation of potential donors includes obtaining adequate background data, a physical examination, a 12-lead electrocardiogram, and an echocardiogram. Brain death and increased intracranial pressure often result in nonspecific ST- and T-wave changes. These also may be seen with hypothermia. The echocardiogram has assumed an even greater role in recent years in evaluating cardiac function. This evaluation should be done at a time when dosages of intravenous inotropic agents have been lowered to as low as is compatible with adequate blood pressure and cardiac output, and after adequate fluid resuscitation.

Current matching criteria of donors and recipients include only ABO compatibility and appropriate size match. A prospective specific cross-match between donor and recipient is performed only when recipients have been identified who have more than 5 per cent of reactivity when evaluated against a panel of random donors. When heart transplantation is performed across the ABO blood barrier, there is a significant risk of hyperacute rejection.[48]

With respect to size, fairly wide limits are acceptable, although donors who weigh less than 80 per cent of the recipient's weight should not be accepted for those patients who have higher levels of pulmonary vascular resistance. Similarly, hearts with ischemic times over two hours should be avoided in this situation.

Signs in patients with brain death usually are unstable and close attention is required to fluid balance, owing to diabetes insipidus. This necessitates monitoring of central venous pressure and adequate fluid resuscitation, administration of vasopressin, and replacement of fluid lost through urine output. If hypotension occurs despite adequate volume replacement, a vasopressor is infused. Dopamine is the standard inotropic agent used, but some donors will be better maintained on an alpha-adrenergic agent.

Donor evaluation currently also includes various serology results. These are for human immunodeficiency virus (HIV), hepatitis B antigen, cytomegalovirus (CMV), and toxoplasmosis. The finding of HIV antibody rules out a potential donor, and the presence of CMV antibody may disqualify a potential heart-lung donor for a CMV-negative recipient at some centers. UNOS guidelines suggest deferring organ donors who have received human pituitary-derived growth hormone.[49] Present consensus also excludes donors with carbon monoxide-hemoglobin levels above 20 per cent, arterial oxygen saturation less than 80 per cent, previous myocardial infarction, or severe coronary or structural heart disease. The presence of metastatic malignancy is also an exclusion at many centers, although those with primary brain tumors and skin cancers may be excepted. Relative contraindications include sepsis, prolonged (>6 hours) severe (<60 mm Hg) hypotension, noncritical coronary disease, hepatitis B surface antigen or hepatitis C antibodies (unless the organs are destined for recipients with the same serology), multiple resuscitations, severe left ventricular hypertrophy, or the need for inotropic support (dopamine >20 μg/kg/min) for 24 hours.[42]

Distant procurement of the heart and heart-lung for transplantation is now routine in almost all transplant centers.[50] The technique for heart preservation remains quite simple, with cold crystalloid or blood cardioplegia infusion combined with topical cold for extended preservation. Average ischemic times are between 3 and 4 hours, with excellent function in most cases. Data from the Registry of the International Society for Heart Transplantation show some relation between ischemic time and survival, although most experienced centers see no particular relation for up to 6 hours of ischemia.[51] Although laboratory work has shown satisfactory preservation using various techniques for up to 24 hours of ischemia, these have not been clinically applied.[52] The longest ex vivo preservation of the human heart has been 16 hours, but the heart was implanted heterotopically, so it did not supply all of the recipient's cardiac output immediately.[53]

Techniques for distant heart-lung procurement and preservation of isolated lung grafts include flush solutions in the pulmonary artery with potent pulmonary vasodilators,[54] the use of cold blood for flush,[55] placing the donor on cardiopulmonary bypass,[56] and the use of an autoperfusing heart-lung preparation for maintaining the organs at normothermia in a working state.[57] Again, distant procurement is limited to 6 hours or less, with most procurements having an ischemic period between 3 and 4 hours.

This length of allowable ischemic time has usually kept procurement between centers of not more than 1000 miles distance. The tendency to use donor organs within the local region also has limited times.

Allocation of organs begins with Status I patients in ever-widening zones. It is offered first to candidates in the local Organ Procurement Organization (OPO), then to patients within a 500-mile and then 1000-mile radius. If no recipient is found, the process is repeated for the Status II list.[58]

Regional organ procurement organizations (OPO) are available to assist doctors and hospitals with all medical and legal considerations involved in organ donation. Their telephone numbers (800 listings) have been listed by location.[58a]

OPERATIVE TECHNIQUE

The current technique for orthotopic heart transplantation was described in 1960 by Lower and Shumway.[5] The method involves retaining a large portion of the posterior wall of the right and left atrium in the recipient and implanting the donor heart with relatively long suture lines in the atria, together with direct end-to-end anastomoses of the aorta and the pulmonary artery. Modification of this technique with venous anastomoses at the level of the cavae and the pulmonary veins permits a more physiological atrial contribution to ventricular filling and causes less distortion of the mitral and tricuspid annuli, with less tendency to atrioventricular valve regurgitation; however, the long-term clinical advantage of this innovation remains

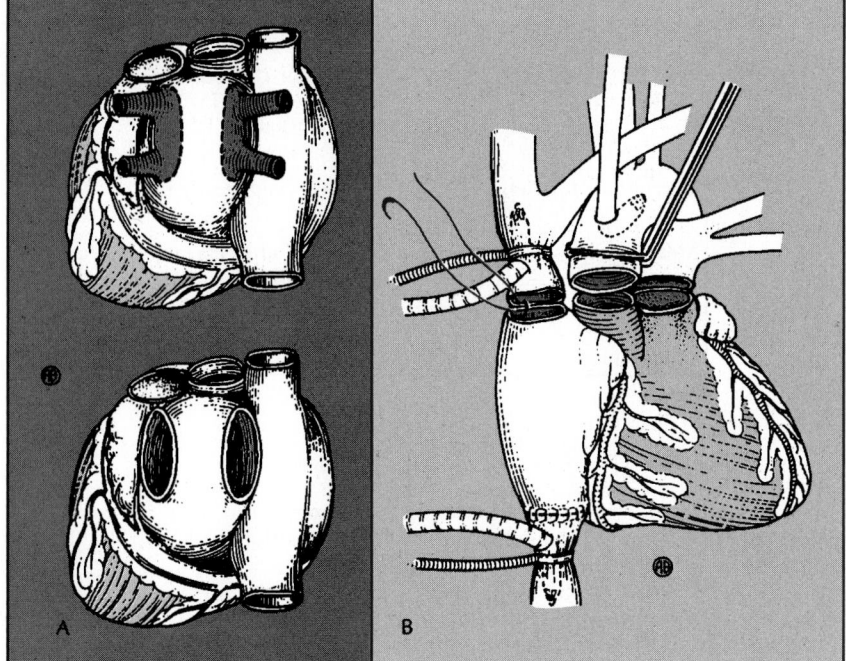

FIGURE 18–3. Total heart replacement by pulmonary venous anastomoses on right or left and caval anastomosis at the superior and inferior vena cava. Aorta and pulmonary artery attached as in the previous bi-atrial transplantation technique.

uncertain. No differences in patient survival can be demonstrated. The technique is illustrated in Figure 18–3.[59–61]

The operation is performed by way of a median sternotomy incision, with routine cannulation of the aorta and both venae cavae. Cardiopulmonary bypass is usually performed with moderate hypothermia of between 28° and 30°C. The implantation procedure usually requires from 45 to 60 minutes, and after careful attention to de-airing maneuvers and resuscitation of the heart, cardiopulmonary bypass is weaned. After placement of temporary pacing wires and chest drainage catheters, the incision is routinely closed.

RIGHT VENTRICULAR FAILURE. Because the pulmonary vascular resistance of the recipient may be elevated, acute right ventricular failure is a frequent cause of early morbidity and mortality. The normal donor right ventricle may be unable to meet the elevated resistance, and there is a high degree of both pulmonary and tricuspid valve insufficiency in the early post-transplant period.[62] This problem may be exacerbated by a relatively long ischemic time or by a donor heart somewhat smaller than that of the recipient. Isoproterenol is often routinely given for its chronotropic and inotropic effects, as well as for its beneficial lowering of pulmonary vascular resistance. Armitage and associates reported that elevated pulmonary vascular resistance could be successfully treated with an infusion of prostaglandin E_1.[63] Inhaled nitric oxide has also been utilized successfully.[64,65] Support of the transplanted heart with a right ventricular assist device helps overcome this early postoperative problem.[66]

Multiple types of congenital anomalies have been dealt with during cardiac transplantation. For example, absence of the right superior vena cava or persistent left superior vena cava can easily be accommodated.[67] Corrected transposition of the great vessels requires extra length of the donor aorta and pulmonary artery.[68]

HETEROTOPIC HEART TRANSPLANTATION. For certain rather limited indications, cardiac transplantation can be performed as a heterotopic graft. This procedure was first described by Demikhov[69] and in the early experimental work performed by McGough and colleagues.[70] It was introduced into clinical practice by Barnard in 1974, with the placement of a heterotopic heart in the right lower thorax, and the donor heart anastomosed in parallel with the retained recipient heart.[71] In cases in which the pulmonary vascular resistance remains severely elevated, the recipient's right heart can continue to function while the left heart is bypassed with the transplant.[71a] Other indications include a patient with a relatively small donor heart, a donor heart with a long ischemic time and anticipated poor early function, and a patient who has a reversible type of heart disease in which the graft may be removed when the native heart recovers. Heterotopic transplants account for about 2.5 per cent of the cardiac transplants currently performed. The operative technique includes left atrial-to-left atrial anastomosis, aorta-to-aorta anastomosis, superior vena cava-to-right atrium, and pulmonary artery-to-pulmonary artery connection.

Early Postoperative Recovery

Much of the early postoperative management is similar to that of other patients recovering from cardiac surgical procedures. Strict isolation precautions are no longer considered mandatory. The patient is weaned from the ventilator and from inotropic drugs, as tolerated. Early mobilization and use of physical therapy are begun as soon as tolerated.

The most important feature of early management is the institution of the immunosuppressive regimen, which will be continued throughout the patient's lifetime. Numerous protocols exist for maintenance immunosuppression, and they are continually changing. Most patients receive cyclosporine in combination with several other medications. Currently, the most common protocol involves triple-drug therapy of cyclosporine, azathioprine, and prednisone. They are usually given in higher doses in the early post-transplant period, with weaning to lower and less toxic levels for chronic administration. A typical protocol for immunosuppression is shown in Table 18–3. At the Stanford University Hospital, patients are given 500 mg of methylprednisolone intraoperatively. Postoperatively, patients receive cyclosporine at 6 to 8 mg/kg/day in divided doses, depending on serum levels and renal function, and intravenous methylprednisolone. After the third dose of methylprednisolone, oral prednisone is begun in doses of 1 mg/kg of body weight and is tapered to 0.4 mg/kg over 2 weeks. Azathioprine is given at about 2 mg/kg and is lowered if the white blood cell count falls below 4000/mm³.

The demonstration of certain advantages has popularized prophylactic induction therapy,[72] although randomized trials have revealed no significant differences in total number of rejection episodes, infections, or serum creatinine levels.[73] The Utah transplant group showed that the monoclonal antibody directed against the CD3 (helper) lymphocyte (Orthoclone, OKT3) results in excellent early renal function and almost a complete absence of early acute rejection, allowing the patient to recover from the surgical procedure and begin rehabilitation. There is a low incidence of sensitization against the mouse monoclonal antibody, so early prophylactic administration does not preclude later use of OKT3 for treatment of acute rejection, if necessary.[74] Detection of circulating antibody of OKT3 at titers >1:1000 in previously treated patients predicts a poor response. An alternative anti–T-cell antibody preparation should then be selected.

Chronic maintenance immunosuppression usually consists of either cyclosporine, azathioprine, and prednisone or cyclosporine and azathioprine alone. Withdrawal or marked reduction of corticosteroids is of particular benefit in diabetics and in the presence of severe osteoporosis or aseptic necrosis of bone. In children, a corticosteroid-free

TABLE 18-3 IMMUNOSUPPRESSION FOR HEART TRANSPLANTATION PROTOCOLS

| DRUG | POSTOPERATIVE | |
	Early	Late
Cyclosporine	6–10 mg/kg/day PO* *or* 0.5–2 mg/kg/day IV	3–6 mg/kg/PO†
or		
Tacrolimus (FK506)	0.15–0.30 mg/kg/day PO	0.15–0.30 mg/kg/day PO†
Methylprednisolone	500 mg IV after cardiopulmonary bypass 125 mg q8h × 3	
Prednisone	1 mg/kg/day PO tapered to 0.4 mg/kg	0.1–0.2 mg/kg/day PO
Azathioprine	2 mg/kg/day PO‡	1–2 mg/kg/day PO

* Omit if preoperative serum creatinine level is greater than 1.5 mg/dl and use IV.
† Or as modified by blood levels.
‡ Omit if white blood count < 4000/mm³.

regimen permits normal axial growth and prevents the development of the cushingoid features and acne which contribute to noncompliance in adolescents.[75]

Detection of Rejection

Detection and treatment of allograft rejection remain perhaps the most crucial aspects of transplant management. The most reliable and frequent technique to assess allograft rejection is the endomyocardial biopsy. Other less invasive techniques have relied on the detection of activated circulating lymphoblasts,[76] changes in the appearance of the heart by echocardiography[77] or in the voltage of the electrocardiogram,[78] and experimental techniques looking at the energy state of the myocardium by nuclear magnetic resonance (NMR) spectroscopy.[79]

NONINVASIVE TECHNIQUES

Imaging techniques rely on demonstration of myocardial depression as a result of injury from the rejection process. Myocyte necrosis is a relatively late manifestation of rejection, emphasizing the need for more sensitive and specific early signs.

In 1965, Lower and associates noted a consistent drop in the summed values of electrocardiographic voltage, coincident with rejection in 20 untreated dogs with heart transplants.[7] Later, electrocardiographic monitoring was used for patients treated with prednisone and azathioprine and found to be helpful. A decrease in the summed QRS voltage by 20 per cent was thought to be indicative of rejection.[80] However, a number of other conditions influence the QRS voltage, including myocardial and pulmonary edema, pulmonary infiltrates owing to a variety of causes, and pericardial effusion. Furthermore, cyclosporine-treated patients have less cardiac tissue edema, and thus the standard electrocardiogram is less sensitive. A directly implanted epicardial electrode with a telemetry monitoring system for following heart transplant patients' electrocardiograms has been successfully used by the Berlin transplant group, but it has not been widely adopted because of the need to implant electrodes and to maintain equipment for telemetry.[81,82]

ECHOCARDIOGRAPHY. This can aid in diagnosing rejection episodes. Dubroff and others have shown that there is an increase in left ventricular wall thickness during episodes of cardiac rejection.[77] Further studies have shown that this is a relatively insensitive technique. The appearance of rejection can be correlated with a decrease in the isovolumetric relaxation time[83]; however, the use of diastolic parameters is complicated by changes in heart rate between measurements, as well as by the unsynchronized hemodynamic contribution of the recipient atrial remnant. Thus, changes associated with rejection are an increase in posterior wall thickness, an increase in left ventricular mass, and a decrease in diastolic compliance. Unfortunately, most of these changes are indicative of advanced stages of rejection and therefore have limited usefulness. Echocardiograms are currently obtained as baseline studies early after transplantation and are correlated with those obtained during moderate or severe rejection to assess left ventricular performance during treatment and to ensure that left ventricular function is stable or improving. Patients' echocardiograms are recorded on their own individual tapes, which allows easy review and increases the sensitivity of Doppler echocardiographic studies for identifying subtle changes in ventricular performance.

RADIONUCLIDE TESTS. Among radionuclide tests, *technetium-99m pyrophosphate scintigraphy* (see p. 278) is a sensitive and specific indication of myocardial injury caused by ischemia. With increasingly severe cardiac rejection, there is a progressive increase in myocardial

uptake in laboratory animals.[84] Other studies with thallium-201 or indium-111 have suggested some usefulness in experimental laboratory studies, but none of the nuclear scans are used clinically on a routine basis.[85]

Antimyosin antibodies (see p. 296), which are monoclonal Fab fragments directed against myosin, can be used to evaluate myosin exposure during the cell death associated with cardiac rejection.[86]

Nuclear magnetic resonance spectroscopy is a recent noninvasive technique for evaluating tissue biochemical characteristics. In rejecting dog and human hearts, there is a decline in phosphocreatine detected by NMR spectroscopy during the course of allograft rejection. The ratio of phosphocreatine to inorganic phosphorus declines, and these changes occur 24 to 48 hours before the appearance of myocyte necrosis on endomyocardial biopsies.[79] Although these techniques hold promise for a less invasive measure and would be particularly helpful in pediatric recipients, a low-cost, sensitive, and reliable technique has yet to be developed.

Other investigators have examined urinary byproducts of cellular degradation, such as urinary *thromboxane* B_2[87] and *putrescine*; however, these studies show minimal changes in cyclosporine-treated patients, and the techniques are not widely used.

Measurement of lymphocyte subsets has been a potentially attractive method for detecting rejection. In general, these techniques have not been sensitive or specific.[88] Recipients of heart and heart-lung transplants were followed for one year but demonstrated no reproducible correlation of CD4 to CD8 ratios with rejection episodes. These lymphocyte subsets were found to be affected more by viral infections than by rejection episodes.

Endomyocardial Biopsy

With the inadequacy of these noninvasive tests, the endomyocardial biopsy remains the standard method for the detection of rejection and its effective treatment with augmented immunosuppression. The technique was introduced for cardiac transplantation by Caves and associates in 1973.[89] The relatively diffuse interstitial infiltrate associated with rejection makes it possible for the focal biopsy to be a good reflection of events throughout the myocardium.[90] Although the endomyocardial biopsy is an invasive procedure, it seems relatively well-tolerated and can be performed in a sequential manner. Complications are usually mild, and include pneumothoraces, transient rhythm disturbances, and a rare instance of myocardial perforation or tricuspid regurgitation due to chordal interruption. Because it is a percutaneous and transvenous technique, there is no operative incision and only local anesthetic is required with minimal discomfort. The procedure is rapidly performed, usually through the right internal jugular vein, and can be repeated on many occasions through the same access site. It can also be placed from the left jugular vein or from the subclavian vein, and from the femoral veins, as shown in Figure 18–4. Fluoroscopy is usually used, although some operators prefer echocardiography for bioptome guidance.

To get an adequate sample for examination, four to six biopsy specimens are taken at each examination.[90] A typical post-transplant biopsy schedule is shown in Table 18–4. Patients who demonstrate allograft rejection are treated with an appropriate immunosuppressive regimen (see

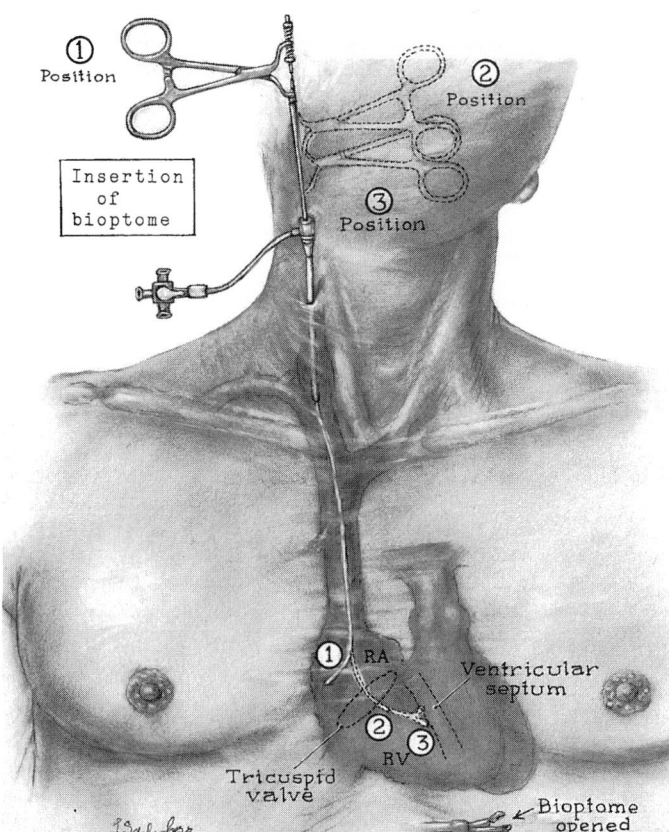

FIGURE 18–4. Positioning of the bioptome for endomyocardial biopsy. 1. Bioptome is inserted with the tip pointed toward the lateral wall of the right atrium. 2. At the level of the mid-right atrium, the bioptome is rotated anteriorly about 180° and is advanced through the tricuspid valve apparatus toward the right ventricle. 3. The bioptome is advanced to the interventricular septum with the jaws opened. (From Baughman, K. L.: History and current techniques of endomyocardial biopsy. *In* Baumgartner, W. A., Reitz, B. A., and Achuff, S. A. [eds.]: Heart and Heart-Lung Transplantation. Philadelphia, W.B. Saunders Company, 1990.)

below) and repeat endomyocardial biopsy is performed again after an interval of 10 to 14 days. The effect of treatment during this time is usually followed by echocardiographic and clinical assessment.

The variety and significance of the observed histological changes in cardiac allografts have now been reasonably well-defined. Multiple grading systems have been advocated by different transplant groups, but recently the International Society for Heart and Lung Transplantation has adopted uniform criteria.[91] The tissue fragments are embedded together in a single block, processed, and sectioned. Most biopsies are assessed using standard hematoxylin and eosin stains, but other special stains may be useful for additional information, such as the amount of collagen present or identification of specific subtypes of infiltrating lymphocytes.

The most important feature of most post-transplant biopsies is the detection of lymphocyte infiltration and the presence of myocyte necrosis. The continuum of histologi-

TABLE 18–4 RECOMMENDED FREQUENCY OF ENDOMYOCARDIAL BIOPSY FOR ROUTINE MONITORING OF HEART TRANSPLANT REJECTION*

TIME AFTER TRANSPLANT	INTERVAL	NO. BIOPSIES
0–4 weeks	Every week	4
4–8 weeks	Every 2 weeks	2
8–16 weeks	Every month	2
6 months to indefinite	Every 3 months	

* Rebiopsy if indeterminate and 10 days after conclusion of rejection treatment.

cal findings from a normal biopsy to one showing severe acute rejection will include a variety of subtle findings, which are listed in Table 18–5. Figure 18–5 shows examples of acute rejection of varying grades.

A certain number of confusing histopathological changes can be seen in some biopsy specimens and be unrelated to rejection. For example, in specimens taken early after transplantation, there may be necrotic myocytes undergoing macrophagic removal because of ischemia at the time of the transplant procedure itself. Necrosis may also be secondary to infectious agents, such as CMV and toxoplasmosis. Oc-

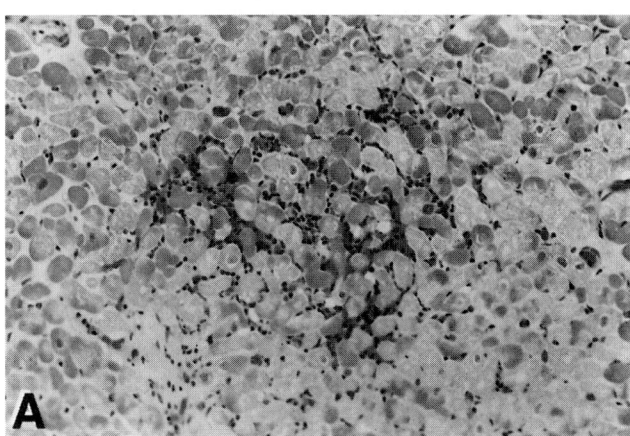

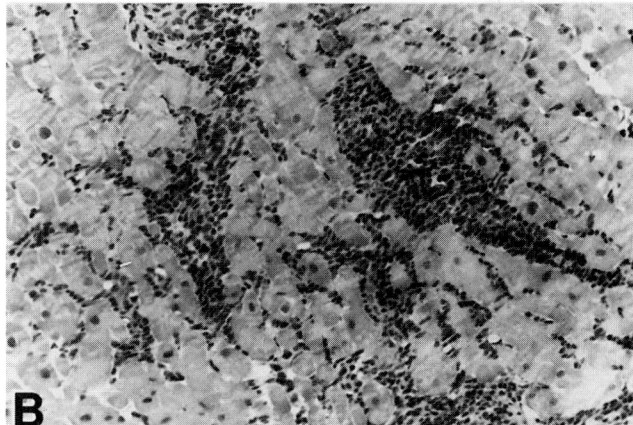

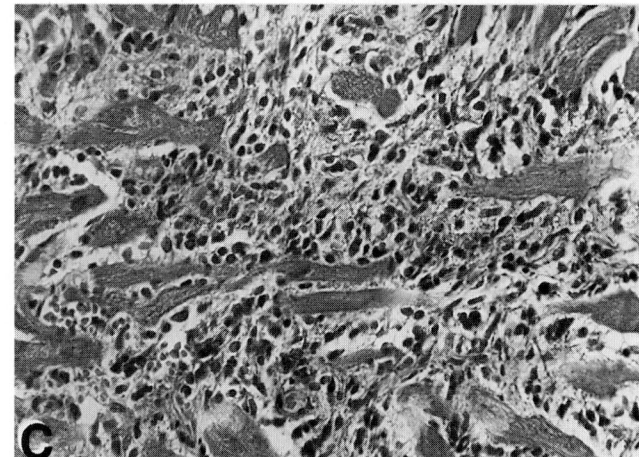

FIGURE 18–5. Composite photomicrograph showing different stages of acute cardiac rejection: *A,* Shows mild acute rejection, with a sparse interstitial lymphocytic infiltrate (Grade 1B, ISHLT) (Hematoxylin and eosin, original magnification × 200). *B,* Shows moderate acute rejection with islands of lymphocytes replacing myocardial tissue (Grade 3A, ISHLT) (Hematoxylin and eosin, original magnification × 200). *C,* Shows severe acute rejection with marked myocyte damage and a mixed inflammatory infiltrate (Grade 4, ISHLT) (Hematoxylin and eosin, original magnification × 300). (Courtesy of Margaret Billingham, M. D.)

TABLE 18–5 STANDARDIZED CARDIAC BIOPSY GRADING (ISHLT SCALE)

GRADE	FINDINGS
0	No rejection
1	1A = focal (perivascular or interstitial) infiltrate without necrosis
	1B = diffuse but sparse infiltrate without necrosis
2	One focus only with aggressive infiltration and/or focal myocyte damage
3	3A = multifocal aggressive infiltrates and/or myocyte damage
	3B = diffuse inflammatory process with necrosis
4	Diffuse aggressive polymorphous infiltrate, ± edema, ± hemorrhage, ± vasculitis, with necrosis

ISHLT = International Society for Heart and Lung Transplantation.
Modified from Miller, L.W., Schlant, R.C., Kobashigawa J., et al.: Task Force 5: Complications. J. Am. Coll. Cardiol. *22*(1):43, 1993. Reprinted with permission from the American College of Cardiology.

casional infections with these agents have been first diagnosed by the endomyocardial biopsy. Perhaps the most frequent abnormality is a biopsy taken from a previous biopsy site that may contain contraction bands and evidence of inflammation and collagen formation as a result of healing of the previous biopsy site. The findings associated with previous biopsy site histology are described in more detail elsewhere.[92]

In addition to classical cell-mediated rejection, occasional cases of hyperacute rejection due to preformed circulating antibodies from prior transfusion, pregnancy, or ABO incompatibility may occur within hours of surgery and require prompt retransplantation. In established allografts, vascular damage in the absence of lymphocytic infiltration has been accompanied by deposition of complement and IgG on endothelial cells that are swollen or disrupted.[93] The specificity of these findings remains somewhat controversial;[93a] however, when they are accompanied by clinical deterioration, treatment with an augmented immunosuppressive regimen and plasmapheresis has been used successfully.[94]

Treatment of Acute Rejection

Immunosuppression to prevent allograft rejection begins at the time of the transplant procedure and continues throughout the life of the recipient. Although a number of strategies are being developed to enhance the induction of immunosuppression and to maximize the potential for developing tolerance in the recipient, virtually every patient probably experiences some acute allograft rejection during the first post-transplant year. The balance between effective immunosuppression and excess immunosuppression with multiple opportunistic infections requires careful tailoring of the immunosuppressive therapy to the specific needs of the individual recipient. Although a number of new immunosuppressive agents will probably become available in the next few years, as of this writing acute rejection episodes are treated by a relatively small number of standard therapies.

The highest incidence of acute rejection occurs within the first 3 months after transplantation. Of patients receiving standard triple-drug therapy that includes cyclosporine, azathioprine, and prednisone, the authors found that 84 per cent have at least one episode of rejection during the first 3 months. After 3 months, the incidence of rejection diminishes significantly to about one episode per patient-year. Those patients with a relatively good match between donor and recipient, and who do not experience rejection within the first 3 months, usually have a lower incidence of late rejection. Recent combined data from 25 institutions covering 911 patients receiving their first heart transplant were more favorable, with 40 per cent of patients free of rejection at one year. There was a higher likelihood of rejection associated with younger recipients and female donors.[95]

The timing and severity of rejection episodes dictate the appropriate therapy. A representative algorithm for treatment is shown in Figure 18–6. Episodes that occur within the first 3 months or that are moderate to severe are best treated by pulse therapy with methylprednisolone. Methylprednisolone sodium succinate is administered intravenously at a dose of 1000 mg/day for 3 consecutive days. Rejection that occurs later than one month may be treated by augmenting oral steroid intake to 100 mg of prednisone per day for 3 consecutive days, tapered gradually back to a baseline over 2 weeks. Several studies have demonstrated that an equivalent oral dose of prednisone may be as effective as intravenous methylprednisolone in early acute rejection.[96] In children or small adults, the dosage of methylprednisolone and prednisone should be decreased proportionate to body size.

SEVERE REJECTION. Because of the side effects of increased corticosteroid therapy, the patient should be carefully monitored for infections, increased fluid retention, glucose intolerance, and psychological or mood changes. When prednisone treatment is ineffective or in particularly severe cases of rejection associated with hemodynamic changes, more aggressive therapy is given. The use of ATGAM (horse anti-thymocyte globulin), rabbit ATG, or OKT3 monoclonal antibody constitutes rescue therapy after unsuccessful use of prednisone or methylprednisolone. Unfortunately, the availability of commercial preparations of ATGAM is limited. Similarly, the availability of rabbit ATG preparations is erratic because such preparations are not commercially available and require special local arrange-

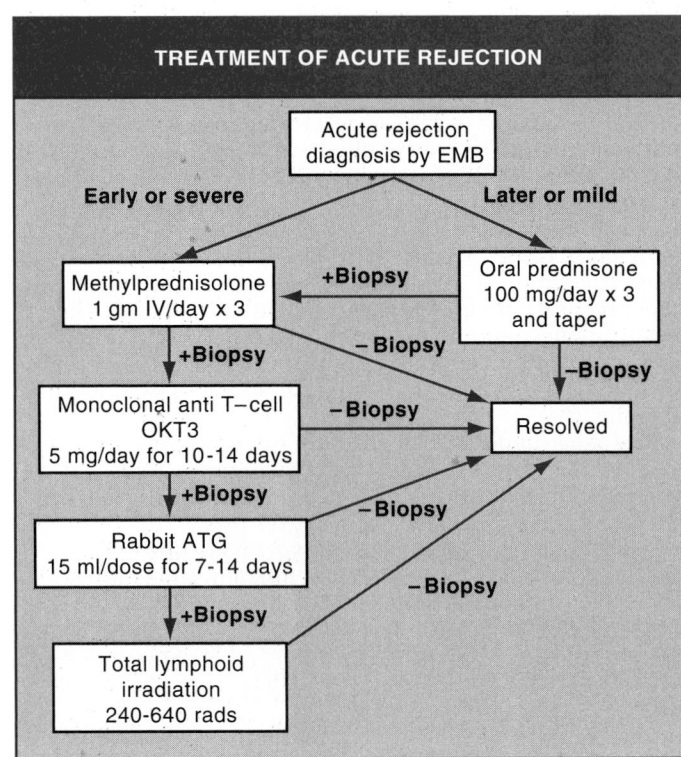

FIGURE 18–6. Algorithm for treating acute allograft rejection. EMB = endomyocardial biopsy; ATG = antithymocyte globulin.

ments for preparation. Consequently, OKT3 therapy is probably the most frequent type of rescue therapy being used, and is an effective treatment for most resistant rejection episodes.[97] Treatment with OKT3 is costly ($3,000 for a 10-day course). Because it stimulates the CD3 receptors to which it binds, it releases lymphokines, and initial doses may cause hypotension, fever, bronchospasm, diarrhea, or sterile meningitis. For these reasons, patients are transferred to acute care settings and pretreated with antihistamines, acetaminophen, and intravenous corticosteroids.

MILD REJECTION. Additional strategies for treatment of early or mild rejection have been advocated. Kobashigawa and associates treated patients with mild acute rejection with increases in oral cyclosporine, treating 40 episodes in 28 patients.[98] In their study of those patients with an actual increase in serum cyclosporine levels, 90 per cent had no progression of rejection or clearing of rejection, whereas 37 per cent of those who had no increase in levels progressed with more evidence of acute rejection requiring treatment. An alternative approach is simply to observe the patient in cases of grade IA or IB rejection and rebiopsy in 2 weeks, since almost two-thirds of patients with stable cyclosporine levels reverted to normal spontaneously. Olsen and coworkers from the University of Utah reported using methotrexate in the treatment of persistent low-grade rejection.[99] Methotrexate was given three times a week for an average of 8 weeks to 16 patients. All rejections were reversed, and the dose of prednisone could be reduced. Although there were no infections, azathioprine dosage had to be reduced in 10 patients because of leukopenia. Methotrexate has also been advocated for recurrent acute, as well as refractory, rejection in doses up to 15 mg/week.[100]

PERSISTENT OR RECURRENT REJECTION. For patients with persistent recurrent rejection episodes despite multiple courses of conventional therapy, Hunt and colleagues at Stanford[101] and Kirklin's group at Alabama[102] have supported the use of total lymphoid irradiation (TLI). It was administered according to standard protocols. Total doses varied from 240 to 1200 cGy (rads) over 5 to 10 weeks and were adjusted in response to leukopenia and thrombocytopenia. Measurement of absolute T-cell counts may also be helpful. Azathioprine should be discontinued or diminished during TLI. The frequency of rejection episodes eventually fell to 5 per cent of the pretreatment rate.

NEW IMMUNOSUPPRESSIVE AGENTS

TACROLIMUS (FK-506). The introduction of cyclosporine in the early 1980's was the stimulus for the tremendous growth in heart transplantation. Attention has subsequently focused on a variety of other agents, which also have selective effects and which may have a different side effect profile. The first of these new agents to be introduced into clinical practice is the macrolide antibiotic compound tacrolimus (FK-506), identified by the Fujisawa Company of Japan[103] and now approved by the Food and Drug Administration. This compound is produced by *Streptomyces tsukubaensis*. It appears to be about 100 times more effective per unit dose than cyclosporine. It too interacts with cyclophilin and binds calcineurin, preventing helper cell amplification by blocking IL-2 synthesis.[16]

Only 25 per cent of the oral dose is absorbed, and, like cyclosporine, it is metabolized by the hepatic P450 cytochrome system and then excreted in the bile. Drugs influencing the P450 system may alter clearance of tacrolimus. Adverse effects include nephrotoxicity, gastrointestinal disturbances, neurotoxicity, hyperglycemia, headache, and hypertension.[19,104] Preliminary experience in thoracic transplantation suggests that it has a definite role in both primary and rescue therapy.[105,106]

MYCOPHENOLATE MOFETIL. This immunosuppressant is now FDA-approved. It is a pro-drug, which is converted in vivo to mycophenolic acid, which interferes with the synthesis of guanosine. This purine is essential for the production of DNA, as well as cell surface glycoprotein adhesion molecules by both B and T cells. Nonimmune cells utilize the salvage pathway for guanosine synthesis and are therefore relatively insensitive to mycophenolate. Because its site of action differs from that of cyclosporine and tacrolimus, it may be synergistic with them in both acute and chronic rejection.[107] Side effects are primarily limited to gastrointestinal distress, but renal function seems unaffected.[108]

RAPAMYCIN. This investigative compound of fungal origin also binds to the FK-binding protein; however, its mode of action is not

linked to calcineurin. Instead, it interferes with the action of growth factors on T cells. It selectively targets only those cells responsive to IL-2 and similar lymphokines and does not inhibit the replication of other rapidly dividing cells. Its mechanism complements that of cyclosporine and tacrolimus.[107] The availability of multiple agents for selective immunosuppression will almost certainly enhance the early and late acceptance of cardiac allografts, minimize toxicities, and increase the safety of cardiac transplantation.

Infection After Cardiac Transplantation

In most centers, infectious complications are the most common cause of death after transplantation. Despite the fact that more effective immunosuppressive therapy has reduced the incidence and severity of infections, they still remain a major problem.[109] The overall incidence of infections ranges from 41 to 71 per cent in various series, and multiple infections are frequent. In a multicenter analysis of 814 consecutive patients undergoing primary heart transplantation between 1990 and 1991, approximately half suffered acute infection at 6 months. This rose to almost two-thirds by one year.[110]

With the extensive experience now available from both kidney, liver, and heart transplant recipients, certain typical infection patterns can be described. Infections in the first postoperative month tend to involve bacterial pathogens encountered in surgical patients in general. Infections in the time from 1 to 4 months after surgery usually involve opportunistic pathogens, especially CMV. After this period, a mixture of both conventional and opportunistic infections is found.

In contradistinction to renal transplant recipients, cardiac recipients must receive somewhat higher levels of pharmacological immunosuppression, which cannot be significantly reduced at the time of infectious complications. This emphasizes the need for early diagnosis and aggressive therapy for any type of infection.

The role of immunization in preventing post-transplant infections is too often overlooked. If given before the institution of immunosuppressive regimens, immunization is more likely to be successful. Pretransplant inoculation with pneumococcal and hepatitis B vaccines, boosters for DPT, and, for young people not previously immunized, MMR and polio vaccines are recommended. Since these last two are live virus vaccines, they should be avoided by patients (and immediate family members) after transplantation when immunosuppression may enhance their virulence. The regular use of influenza vaccine every two years is controversial but has been advocated for HIV-infected patients, and may be useful in transplant patients as well.

EARLY INFECTION. Infections in the first month after transplantation are commonly bacterial and most frequently pulmonary. This is especially true for patients with lung transplants, in addition to heart. Typically, nosocomial organisms, such as *Legionella, Staphylococcus epidermidis, Pseudomonas aeruginosa, Proteus, Klebsiella,* and *Escherichia coli,* are encountered. The incidence of significant mediastinitis is between 0.4 and 4.5 per cent in heart transplant recipients. Treatment includes prolonged courses of antibiotics, debridement of devitalized bone, and the use of vascularized muscle flaps for subsequent wound closure. Other typical causes of early postoperative infection, such as urinary tract infections, bacteremias, and pneumonia, should be suspected. The clinical diagnosis of pneumonia is made on the basis of typical clinical features, including cough, fever, sputum production, and chest radiographs showing a new pulmonary infiltrate. An aggressive approach to early diagnosis is recommended. This may include bronchoscopy with washings and culture. The results of these cultures will determine specific antibiotic therapy, but early broad-spectrum coverage started immediately after obtaining appropriate cultures is recommended.

LATE INFECTION. Late post-transplant infections are more diverse. These are frequently of the opportunistic variety, including viruses (CMV, Herpes), *Pneumocystis carinii* (PCP), and fungi (e.g., *Candida* and *Aspergillus*), as well as more exotic varieties. Occasionally, *Nocardia* or *Toxoplasma gondii* are encountered. The variety of late post-transplant pneumonias may vary from center to center, depending on local prevalences and the use of prophylactic treatments. For example, in some series, *Pneumocystis carinii* is the most common late pulmonary infection, whereas in other series it is absent. The regular prophylactic administration of trimethoprim-sulfamethoxazole (TMP-SMZ) three times per week on a long-term basis is now routinely recommended by most transplant programs to prevent PCP and *Toxoplasma* infection (or if TMP-SMZ is not tolerated, monthly pentamidine aerosol inhalation for PCP prophylaxis).[111]

CYTOMEGALOVIRUS INFECTION. CMV infection is the most frequent and important viral infection in transplant recipients, with an incidence in cardiac recipients of between 73 and 100 per cent.[112,113] It is the single most frequent infecting organism, accounting for 26 per cent of all infections in a large cooperative study.[110] This can be minimized in CMV-negative patients by the use of CMV-negative blood products, but a CMV-positive donor will almost invariably transmit infection. It may be detected in some patients only by seroconversion or, if they are seropositive preoperatively, by a rise in IgG titers or the appearance of an IgM antibody. Some infections remain subclinical. When clinical disease is present, it may present as leukopenia, pneumonia, gastroenteritis, hepatitis, or retinitis in varying combinations. Of these, pneumonia is the most lethal (13 per cent mortality), while retinitis is the most refractory and requires indefinite maintenance therapy. Most cases are responsive to ganciclovir (DHPG) or foscarnet. The addition of hyperimmune globulin has further improved therapeutic outcome and decreased mortality, particularly from CMV pneumonia. Although seronegative recipients who accept allografts from CMV-positive donors are the most vulnerable, prior seropositivity does not offer protection from infection (15 per cent disease frequency) and late reactivation, reflecting the persistence of this member of the Herpesvirus family, may occur.

Unfortunately, diagnostic tests are not always positive. Viral cultures may be negative in the presence of infection, and serological responses may be diminished due to immunosuppression. The recent addition of polymerase chain reaction (PCR) technology for the detection of CMV viremia has added a more sensitive diagnostic method, but greater experience is needed before it becomes the standard.[114] Because of these limitations, CMV should always be suspected in the event of unexplained fevers, gastroenteritis, or culture-negative interstitial pneumonitis. Endoscopy with biopsy may establish the diagnosis promptly in these latter cases.[114a] Early prophylaxis with ganciclovir in the setting of positive CMV graft into a negative recipient includes the use of ganciclovir and hyperimmune globulin for 6 to 8 weeks post-transplant. Prophylaxis against CMV infection decreased the incidence of CMV disease in recipients who were seropositive pretransplant, but not in those who were seronegative.[115]

The importance of CMV infection cannot be overemphasized because of its relation to the development of late graft atherosclerosis. The availability of newer antiviral treatments may help to minimize the complications of this particular infection in the future.

FUNGAL INFECTIONS. Although less common than viral and bacterial infections, fungal infections are more serious, less responsive to therapy, and more likely to be lethal. (*Pneumocystis carinii*, originally thought to be a protozoan, has now been reclassified as fungus by ribosomal DNA analysis.[116]) *Candida* and *Aspergillus* are the most commonly encountered pathogens. Treatment with imidazoles is often effective for *Candida* and coccidioidomycosis, but their use may raise cyclosporine levels. Infections of vital organs usually require amphotericin B and flucytosine, which compromise renal function and potentiate leukopenia, respectively.

Toxoplasmosis is uncommon but responds to pyrimethamine.[117]

OTHER COMPLICATIONS OF IMMUNOSUPPRESSION

The cardiologist following cardiac transplant patients should be aware of the multiple complications of the immunosuppressive drugs. All of the commonly used drugs increase the risk of infection and are also associated with neoplasia.[118]

CYCLOSPORINE TOXICITY. Cyclosporine is associated with a number of complications. The most clinically significant effect of cyclosporine involves the kidneys. Almost all patient groups receiving cyclosporine have a fall in creatinine clearance, an increase in serum creatinine level, and hypertension.[119,120] Histopathological changes after chronic administration are found in the proximal convoluted tubule and in the distal tubules and consist of vacuolization of cells, epithelial swelling, hydropic degeneration, and necrosis. Increasing clinical and experimental evidence exists that cyclosporine produces a derangement in the prostaglandin system in the renal tubules. Indomethacin exacerbates renal dysfunction after cyclosporine administration.

Cyclosporine may act by increasing urinary thromboxane B_2 levels in a dose-dependent manner, with local vasoconstriction, platelet aggregation, and release of platelet-produced thromboxane. This may explain the development of hypertension, renal ischemia, and the dysfunction that is seen clinically, although azotemia and hypertension are occasionally independent of one another.[121] Acute elevation of cyclosporine to three to four times customary maintenance levels may cause acute oliguria and rapid decline in renal function. This is probably due to vasoconstriction and is promptly reversible with adjustment of dosage or removal of drugs hindering cyclosporine catabolism. Chronic interstitial fibrosis and nephron loss is common but is usually stable. It may be intermittently exacerbated by nephrotoxins used for therapy (e.g., amphotericin B, nonsteroidal anti-inflammatory drugs) or diagnosis (radiocontrast agents).

Early after transplant, many patients have oliguria. Thus, many transplant groups restrict the use of cyclosporine to continuous intravenous administration with careful control of circulating levels during the early post-transplant period, or omit cyclosporine altogether and use induction therapy with OKT3 until serum creatinine is normal and the patient has recovered from the effects of cardiopulmonary bypass.[120,122,123]

Hepatotoxicity, although uncommon, is usually acute and secondary to exceptionally high levels of cyclosporine. It is evidenced by an increase in bilirubin and by increases in serum liver enzymes. There are no characteristic cellular pathological alterations except for centrilobular fatty changes. The hepatotoxicity is dose-related and reverts to normal after the dose of cyclosporine is lowered or eliminated. In general, hepatotoxicity is uncommon after cardiac transplantation, and, so far, no long-term sequelae of cyclosporine on liver function have been reported.

Neurotoxic reactions are manifested by a fine tremor, paresthesias, and occasionally seizures. Most of these events are dose-related and reversible. Other unusual side effects include the development of hirsutism or hypertrichosis, observed in almost all patients who receive cyclosporine. These effects tend to regress as the dosage of cyclosporine is lowered. Similarly, gingival hyperplasia has been observed. A combination of cyclosporine and nifedipine has resulted in an increased rate of gingival hyperplasia (51 per cent) when compared with cyclosporine alone (8 per cent).[124] Because cyclosporine is metabolized almost exclusively by the liver, hepatic dysfunction can cause abrupt elevations of blood levels of cyclosporine, precipitating renal dysfunction. Many commonly used compounds can influence the hepatic P450 cytochrome system, which is responsible for cyclosporine catabolism. Drugs that raise cyclosporine levels include the antimicrobials erythromycin, doxycycline, imipenem, cilastatin, ticarcillin, norfloxacin, ketoconazole, and itraconazole; the calcium channel blockers diltiazem, verapamil, nifedipine, and nicardipine; hormone products such as danazol, androgens, estradiol, and oral contraceptives, as well as other commonly utilized medications such as cimetidine, ranitidine, warfarin, acetazolamide, metoclopramide, and amiodarone. (Diltiazem and ketoconazole have been used adjunctively to lower the consumption and cost of cyclosporine maintenance.[125])

Conversely, a drop in circulating cyclosporine levels, with the danger of causing rejection, may be precipitated by omeprazole, by the antibiotics rifampin and nafcillin, and by the anticonvulsants phenytoin, carbamazepine, valproic acid, primidone, and methsuximide.[126,127] The use of lovastatin to control hypercholesterolemia in patients on cyclosporine has rarely been associated with rhabdomyolysis.[128]

CORTICOSTEROID TOXICITY. Perhaps the most troublesome side effects of immunosuppressive therapy are associated with long-term administration of corticosteroids. In patients who require relatively high doses of steroids, these can be especially severe and include adrenal cortical atrophy, cushingoid appearance, cataracts, skin fragility, severe osteoporosis, peptic ulcers, aseptic necrosis of bone, weight gain, psychiatric effects, diabetes, elevated serum lipid levels, and heightened susceptibility to infection of all types. In children, axial growth may be impaired. Perhaps the major advance in transplantation will come when corticosteroid therapy can be completely eliminated, a strategy under investigation.[129]

AZATHIOPRINE TOXICITY. The major morbidity of long-term azathioprine administration is bone marrow suppression. Severe granulocytopenia has resulted from inadvertent coadministration of allopurinol for the treatment of CyA-induced hyperuricemia and gout and has been life-threatening. Azathioprine also causes hepatotoxicity in some patients, which may be so severe that the drug must be discontinued with substitution of an alkylating agent, such as cyclophosphamide.

NEOPLASMS IN IMMUNOSUPPRESSED CARDIAC TRANSPLANT RECIPIENTS

Cancer is an unfortunate consequence of chronic immunosuppression.[118] In general, transplant recipients have a threefold increase in the incidence of various cancers when compared with age-matched controls. Some specific cancers are more than 100 times more frequent in immunosuppressed patients than in the general population. For all tumors, the average time of appearance of the cancer after transplantation is 58 months, although some tumors may characteristically appear at other intervals. Cardiac transplant recipients have a somewhat higher incidence of cancer than do renal transplant patients, perhaps because of the higher levels of immunosuppression. The most common tumors among transplant patients are those of the skin and lips, non-Hodgkin's lymphomas, Kaposi's sarcomas, and uterine, cervical, vulval, and perineal neoplasms.[118] The frequency of common adenocarcinomas, such as those of breast, lung, prostate, and colon, does not exceed that of the general population.[130]

Perhaps the most important neoplasms are the lymphoproliferative tumors that occur early after transplantation, more frequently in younger recipients. Most of these tumors are thought to be the result of Epstein-Barr viral infection and consist of B-cell proliferation unchecked because of T-cell suppression or depletion.[131] The recurrent use of OKT3 has been identified as a risk factor in some programs,[132] but this has not been confirmed by others.[133] Approximately 15 per cent are of T-cell origin, and some of these also carry EBV markers.[130,134]

The tumors typically arise in extranodal sites, such as lung, gut, or central nervous system. Treatment has included diminishing immunosuppression, adding antiviral therapy with acyclovir or ganciclovir,[135] and irradiation or surgical removal for monofocal tumor. Closer surveillance by cardiac echocardiography and biopsy is essential during this period. If rejection occurs or if the tumor is refractory, additional therapy with alpha-interferon, chemotherapy, and monoclonal B cell antibodies have been employed with success.[136] Roughly one-third of patients will respond, and recurrence is uncommon.

Graft Atherosclerosis

The major long-term problem after cardiac transplantation, assuming greater importance as the number of survivors increases, is the development of significant coronary artery disease in the transplanted heart. Graft atherosclerosis was first observed by Thomson in 1969 in the first long-term survivor reported from South Africa.[137] Nineteen months after transplantation for ischemic cardiomyopathy, the patient died with extensive coronary artery disease. A variety of reports show an incidence of between 20 and 50 per cent at 5 years.[138–142]

With the advent of protocols using cyclosporine for immunosuppression, there has been no significant decline in the incidence of this disease.[143]

Graft atherosclerosis has been observed as an incidental finding at autopsy as early as 3 months after transplantation. Significant coronary disease may produce arrhythmias, myocardial infarction, sudden death, or impaired left ventricular function with congestive heart failure.[144] Angina pectoris is extremely rare because the cardiac allograft remains essentially denervated, although a patient has been reported who had angina pectoris in the presence of coronary artery disease.[145] The disease tends to be rather diffuse and concentric, and coronary angiograms must be closely inspected and compared with previous studies to appreciate the reduction in coronary diameter. The recent introduction of intravascular ultrasound to assess thickness and composition of the coronary arterial wall, as well as precise measurement of lumen diameter, has demonstrated the presence of disease which was not visible angiographically (Fig. 18–7A). Definite intimal thickening was present in one-quarter of patients at Stanford at 1 year and its preva-

lence increased to approximately 80 per cent at 5 years post-transplant. Calcification was uncommon (<10 per cent) up to 5 years, but approached 25 per cent at 6 to 10 years and 50 per cent at 11 to 15 years.[146]

Noninvasive stress imaging with thallium and sestaMIBI scans has been generally disappointing, probably because of the diffuse nature of the vascular lesion.

PATHOGENESIS. The cause of graft atherosclerosis remains controversial and is probably multifactorial.[147] Vascular endothelium is known to be immunologically active, and similar vascular changes are seen late after kidney and liver transplantation. The early stages of cardiac allograft rejection are characterized by lymphocytic perivascular infiltration, and vasculitis frequently is a prominent part of moderate to severe allograft rejection. Vascular changes with deposition of immunoglobulin, complement, and fibrin have been demonstrated both in patients and in animals. Platelet-derived growth factor producing activation and aggregation of platelets, as well as proliferation of mononuclear cells, has been demonstrated to occur during acute rejection. These data strongly support a complex immune mechanism for the development of graft atherosclerosis. Histological features of graft arteriopathy demonstrate extensive concentric intimal proliferation (Fig. 18–8) with hyperplasia of smooth muscle and lipid-laden macrophages.[148] Grossly, the vessels show diffuse disease extending symmetrically into distal branches with few collateral vessels. Proximal stenoses occur rarely.[149] Angiography may not be sensitive enough to show this disease (Fig. 18–7B).

RISK FACTORS. Several clinical studies have attempted to identify risk factors. In the most comprehensive report of patients treated with prednisone and azathioprine, significant clinical factors were donor age over 35, incompatibility at HLA-A1 and A2 loci, and serum triglyceride concentration greater than 280 mg/dl.[150] Lipoprotein(a) concentration in one study was more than three times higher in patients with angiographic coronary disease than in those with normal angiograms.[151] In other reports, which include experience with cyclosporine, the development of graft atherosclerosis was correlated with two or more rejection episodes, but not with lipid levels or donor age.[138]

Cytomegalovirus (CMV) Infection. Several reports emphasize the possible role of CMV infection in atherogenesis in general[152] and graft atherosclerosis in particular. In a review of 301 cardiac transplant recipients during the cyclosporine era, the Stanford group divided patients into two groups based on freedom from CMV infection.[153] Two hundred and ten patients were included in this group and 91 patients in the CMV infection group. The incidence of graft rejection was significantly higher in the CMV infection group and, using angiographic criteria or autopsy examination, graft atherosclerosis was also found to be significantly more severe. Intimal proliferation has been linked to the inactivation of p53 (a tumor suppressor) by CMV, permitting enhanced proliferation of smooth muscle cells.[154] Actuarial 5-year survival in the CMV infection–free group was 68.3 per cent, compared with only 32.2 per cent for the CMV infection group. Data from Johns Hopkins Hospital indicate that the presence of CMV infection and donor age were the two factors in a multifactorial analysis that correlated with the development of graft atherosclerosis.

In addition to measures to limit CMV, strategies have been directed toward limiting the amount of steroid administered. Hypercholesterolemia is a known risk factor for the development of coronary artery disease in general, and the use of prednisone[155] and cyclosporine[156] is correlated with elevated serum cholesterol levels in cardiac transplant recipients.

PREVENTION. Most centers use some preventive measures in the hope of reducing the incidence of graft atherosclerosis. These include modification of known risk factors,

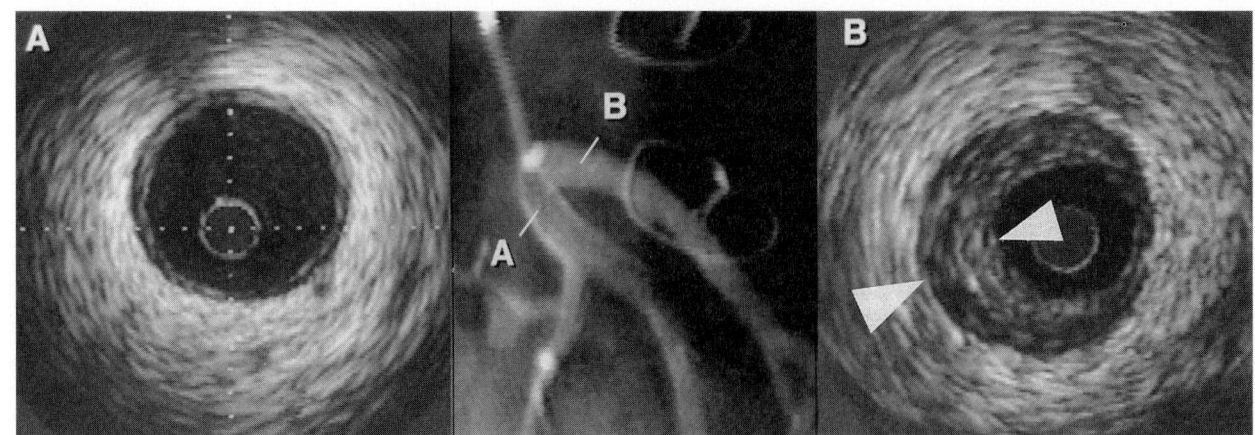

FIGURE 18–7. *A,* Intravascular ultrasound of the left anterior descending coronary artery in a transplant patient at the site shown at A in the middle panel depicting the coronary angiogram. *B,* Intravascular ultrasound in the proximal circumflex coronary artery at the point marked in the coronary angiogram in the central panel at B. Arrows show thickened intima. (Courtesy of Peter Fitzgerald, M.D.)

maintenance of ideal body weight through dietary restriction, reduced intake of cholesterol and saturated fats, the use of lipid-lowering agents such as pravastatin,[156a] cessation of smoking, regular exercise, and the use of an antiplatelet agent such as low-dose aspirin. The addition of diltiazem to the post-transplant regimen has retarded progression of allograft coronary disease, and its cyclosporine-sparing effect has also reduced costs.[157]

TREATMENT. The existence of more discrete proximal lesions has been treated by percutaneous transluminal coronary angioplasty in some cases, and even coronary artery bypass grafting has been reported.[158–161] However, retransplantation is the major alternative once diffuse graft atherosclerosis develops. The results of retransplantation are less good than for the primary procedure, with a reported patient survival rate of approximately 48 per cent at one year (n = 449) reported by the International Society for Heart and Lung Transplantation. Uncontrolled rejection and an interval of less than 6 months between operation and the need for pretransplant mechanical support were listed as risk factors.[162]

Late Follow-up

The late follow-up of cardiac transplant recipients requires a coordinated and systematic approach. The drug regimen for late follow-up is shown in Table 18–6. The

TABLE 18–6   DRUG REGIMEN FOR LONG-TERM RECIPIENT

Prednisone 0.1–0.2 mg/kg/day
Cyclosporine 3–6 mg/kg/day
Diltiazem 120–240 mg/kg/day
Sulfamethoxazole-trimethoprim b.i.d. 3 days/week
Azathioprine 1–2 mg/kg/day
Miscellaneous
Furosemide
Potassium supplements
Antacids
Aspirin
Additional antihypertensives p.r.n.

two leading causes of early morbidity and mortality are rejection and infection. Later surveillance should focus also on graft atherosclerosis and cancer. The frequency and timing of transplant follow-up visits are determined by the general condition of the patient and the time after transplant. Endomyocardial biopsy remains a necessity and is performed every 3 to 4 months indefinitely. The authors currently recommend performing coronary arteriography on a yearly basis, although some programs alternate this with noninvasive studies of myocardial function or ischemia.

In addition to the objective laboratory data, a detailed interval history and physical examination are important to detect other complicating illnesses at an early stage. Patients may minimize new symptoms, and the physician

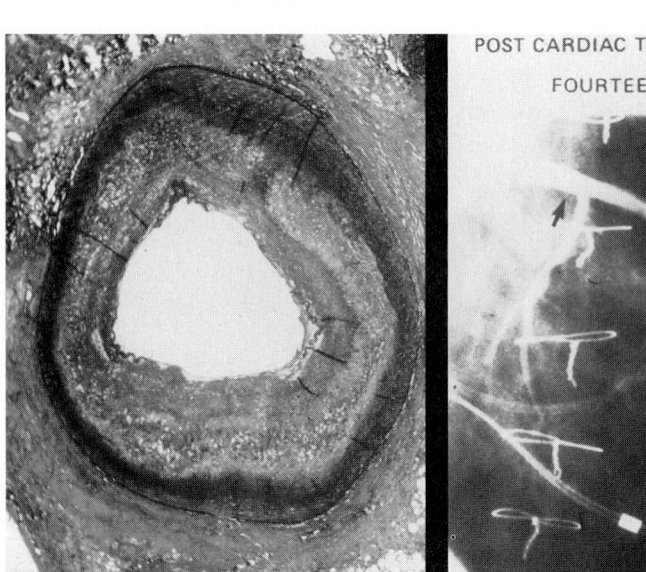

FIGURE 18–8. *A,* Histologic section of left main coronary artery showing concentric atheromatous plaque composed of a fibrous cap overlying a basal layer of extracellular and intracellular lipid. (Original magnification ×15.) *B,* Coronary arteriogram performed 4 days prior to death, 14 months after transplantation. (From Johnson, D. E., Alderman, E. L., Schroeder, J. S. et al.: Transplant coronary artery disease: Histopathologic correlations with angiographic morphology. J. Am. Coll. Cardiol. *17:*449, 1991. Reprinted with permission from the American College of Cardiology.)

must be constantly alert to the possibility of an occult, but potentially life-threatening, infectious complication. A detailed inquiry into all medications that the patient is taking should be performed to avoid errors of omission, dosage misunderstanding, or unexplained additions that might alter the metabolism or excretion of immunosuppressive drugs, potentially causing rejection (e.g., rifampin), nephropathy (e.g., erythromycin), or bone marrow suppression (e.g., allopurinol). A sampling of other late problems routinely encountered includes aseptic necrosis of bone, azotemia, cataracts, cholelithiasis, gout, heart failure, herpes zoster, impotence, obesity, rejection, vertebral compression fractures, and an assortment of skin lesions. A typical drug regimen for the long-term recipient is listed in Table 18–6.

Survival Expectations

Long-term survival and complete rehabilitation can be attained by most patients currently undergoing heart transplantation. Several studies have attempted to define the rehabilitation potential of surviving patients. In a reported series of 56 patients at Stanford, 51 (91 per cent) were classified as successfully rehabilitated; however, only 26 out of 51 patients (46 per cent of the total) returned to full-time work.[163] This may reflect planned early retirement, unwillingness to give up disability and insurance benefits, or the employer's resistance to hiring someone with a chronic disorder, rather than any physical limitation. In another study, 90 per cent of surviving patients were judged to be in a functional New York Heart Association Class I.[164] In a study by Lough and associates, a measure of life satisfaction demonstrated that 89 per cent of recipients rated their quality of life as good to excellent[165] and 86 per cent thought that they led "normal lives."[166]

Simple survival statistics, as reported by the International Society for Heart and Lung Transplantation, indicate a one-year actuarial survival of slightly greater than 80 per cent.[1,166] Individual programs may report survivals up to 90 to 95 per cent at one year. The current data from the International Society are shown in Figure 18–9. Survival was somewhat lower in patients below the age of 5 and above 65.[167] Other factors that may play a role in marginally decreasing survival are longer donor ischemic time, older donor age, and non-O blood type.[168] The probability of lethal rejection within 2 years was 5 per cent when three to six HLA mismatches were present.[169]

Physiology of the Transplanted Heart

The transplanted heart remains largely,[170] but not entirely,[171] denervated throughout the life of the recipient. A variety of studies document the cardiac response to exercise or stress, which is less than normal but adequate for almost all activities (Fig. 18–10).[172–174] The heart rate accelerates slowly during the first stages of exercise, accompanied by an immediate increase in filling pressures as a result of augmented venous return from exercising muscles and decreased compliance. The latter may result from rejection, arteriopathy, arterial hypertension, small donor heart size, or cyclosporine. Atrial contribution to end-diastolic filling is compromised by the dissociation between host and donor atrial contractions. The mid-atrial anastomosis may partially deform the atrioventricular annuli, leading to mitral and tricuspid regurgitation. In the absence of hypertension or rejection, ventricular ejection fractions are normal to high.[175,176]

The effect of denervation is to isolate the heart from anatomically mediated reflexes while enhancing its sensitivity to circulating norepinephrine. The resting heart rate is generally higher due to absence of vagal tone. Respiratory sinus arrhythmia and carotid reflex bradycardia are absent. The more gradual increase of heart rate with exercise parallels the rise in circulating catecholamines, which also leads to an increase in the inotropic state of the myocardium. With augmented venous return and higher filling pressures, the stroke volume increases, contributing to the necessary increase in cardiac output during exercise.

Cardiac denervation results in an increase in beta-adrenergic receptor density.[177] In laboratory animals, denervation results in an increased responsiveness to noradrenaline and isoproterenol. This supersensitivity appears to be due both to upregulation of beta receptors and to a loss of norepinephrine uptake in postganglionic sympathetic neurones. In a study by Borow and associates, the heart

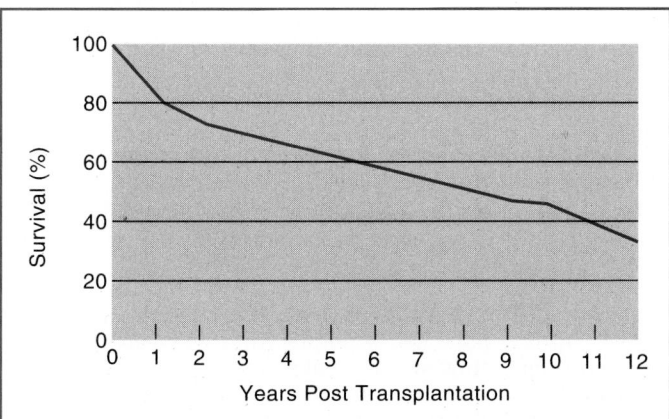

FIGURE 18–9. Heart transplantation actuarial survival for all patients reported to the Registry of the International Society for Heart Transplantation from 1975 to 1993. (From Hosenpud, J. D., Novick, R. J., Breen, T. J., and Daily, O. P.: The Registry of the International Society for Heart and Lung Transplantation: Eleventh Official Report —1994. J. Heart Lung Transplant. 13(4):561, 1994. Reprinted with permission from Mosby-Year Book, Inc.)

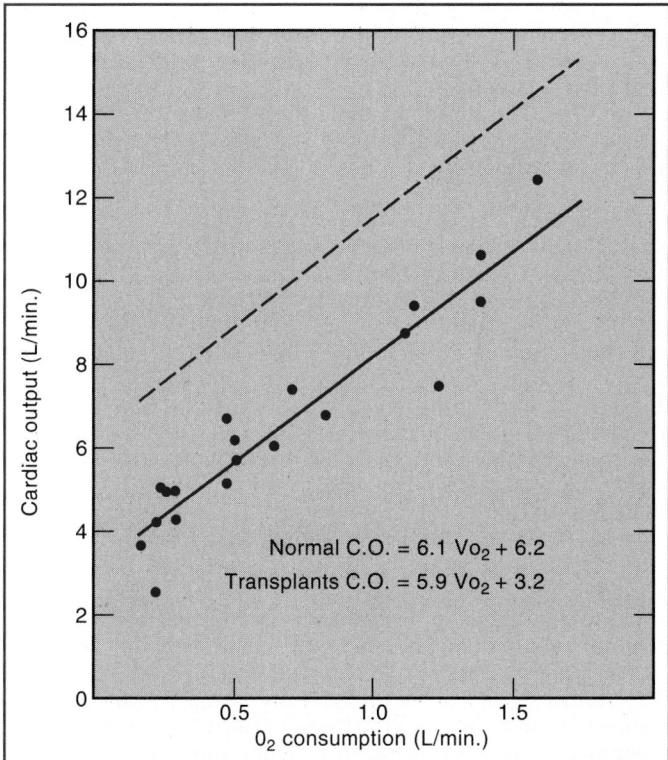

Normal C.O. = 6.1 Vo$_2$ + 6.2
Transplants C.O. = 5.9 Vo$_2$ + 3.2

FIGURE 18–10. The relationship between cardiac output (C.O.) and oxygen consumption in seven patients one year after cardiac transplantation (dots and solid line), and in 27 normal subjects age 14 to 41 (dashed line). (From Hosenpud, J. D., Novick, R. J., Breen, T. J., and Daily, O. P.: The Registry of the International Society for Heart and Lung Transplantation: Eleventh Official Report—1994. J. Heart Lung Transplant. 13(4):561, 1994. Reprinted with permission from Mosby-Year Book, Inc.)

rate response to dobutamine was compared with that of normal subjects pretreated with atropine and found to be greater in the transplanted group.[178] In other studies, infusions of isoproterenol produced a greater increase in heart rate than in normal controls.[179] This slight supersensitivity of the chronically denervated heart may be important in maintaining the necessary inotropic and chronotropic response to exercise and other stresses. All of the mechanisms underlying this supersensitivity have not been fully defined. Denervation of the allograft also blunts systemic responses to volume changes. Failure to reduce sympathetic tone during hypervolemia may contribute to hypertension and persistence of edema,[180] while blunted rate response to hypovolemia may predispose to orthostatic hypotension.

Arrhythmias are uncommon. Sinus node dysfunction occurs in 10 to 20 per cent of patients in the immediate perioperative period but is readily repaired in most cases with theophylline.[181] When this fails, permanent pacing may be necessary.

Pronounced sinus tachycardia (>120) at rest in an afebrile patient without obvious cause suggests physiological distress and warrants a search for hypovolemia, hypoglycemia, rejection, silent myocardial infarction, pulmonary emboli, adrenal insufficiency, tamponade, or abdominal catastrophe masked by corticosteroids.

Atrial arrhythmias—particularly atrial flutter—may signal rejection and are a sufficient indication for heart biopsy. Ventricular arrhythmias are uncommon except with ischemic disease or severe rejection. Ventricular fibrillation is often refractory to resuscitation.

With respect to the coronary circulation, it has been shown that coronary vasodilator reserve of the transplanted heart is normal in the absence of rejection, hypertrophy, or regional wall motion abnormalities. During periods of acute rejection, coronary flow reserve is impaired.

Cost Considerations

The cost of care has been divided into pretransplantation, evaluation and candidacy, transplantation, and posttransplantation by Evans.[182] Pretransplantation costs derive from the care needs of patients with end-stage heart disease and are multiplied by the steadily increasing time spent on waiting lists, which reached a median in 1993 of 208 days (22 per cent waited 6 to 12 months and 42 per cent waited more than a year).[183] Depending on the need for hospitalization, intensive care, or mechanical support, such costs easily exceed $100,000. These costs are considerably higher for Status 1 patients.[183a]

The cost of candidacy, including catheterization, myocardial biopsy, social service evaluation, special studies,[184] and professional fees totals between $10,000 to $20,000.

The median charge for a heart transplant in 1993 dollars was $123,000, with a median length of hospital stay of 23 days (range 1 to 554). The charge, when separated into its components, was distributed as follows: hospital charges $84,000, donor organ acquisition $17,000, surgeons' fees $13,000, and other professional fees $9000. The extremes for these figures varied by factors of 5 to 10.[182] Charges for the entire first year have been estimated at $209,000. Yearly follow-up thereafter, including angiography and regular biopsies (three to four/year), probably exceeds $15,000, with immunosuppressive drugs alone costing $4000 to $6000 annually.[185]

The increasing numbers of patients on waiting lists, the longer waiting periods, the growing proportion of Status 1 patients,[183a] the increased survival after surgery, and steady inflation guarantee continued increases in the total expenditure for each patient undergoing heart transplantation. Fortunately, there has been widespread acceptance of this burden, and, as early as 1985, the majority of private insurers[186] and, by 1990, 78 per cent of state Medicaid programs[187] covered heart transplantation. Medicare also pays for care at designated centers which meet Federal operational criteria.[21]

Reimbursement is usually less than 80 per cent of charges and long-term medication costs are not always recovered.[187] Insurance contracts that pay ongoing costs only when linked to claims of continued disability necessarily inhibit return to work.

Heart Transplantation in Children

Although the total number of heart transplant procedures has remained relatively constant since 1988, the number of children undergoing heart transplantation is increasing yearly. Approximately 320 patients under the age of 18 years received a heart transplant in 1993, with over 100 being younger than 1 year of age. The most common indication for heart transplantation in children has been cardiomyopathy, although congenital heart disease is rapidly increasing as an indication. The largest segment of children having transplant for congenital defects are those less than 1 year of age who frequently have hypoplastic left heart syndrome.

Various other indications have included severe Ebstein's anomaly, single ventricle, and tricuspid and pulmonary atresia with coronary artery sinusoids. Other patients with previous palliative operations may develop cardiomyopathy or late tricuspid valve insufficiency, which makes them inappropriate candidates for further palliative operations.[188]

The use of heart transplantation for this indication was pioneered by Bailey, who initially began with a xenograft procedure using a donor baboon.[189] Human heart donors subsequently have been utilized, although the availability of donors is limited.[190] The longest surviving pediatric heart transplant patient is just over 17 years. A one-year survival of about 85 per cent has been reported, with excellent early growth and development.[191] There is some evidence that rejection complications are less frequent in children in whom transplant occurs before one month of age. After that time, rejection is clearly common and appears to be no less than in adult patients.

A major drawback to transplantation in children is the need for invasive endomyocardial biopsy to monitor the function of the transplanted heart. Because of these difficulties, Bailey and coworkers have advocated using clinical signs together with echocardiography as a means of diagnosing rejection episodes. Rejection in neonatal patients may be associated with fever, fussiness, and difficulty feeding, together with thickening of the left ventricular free wall on echocardiogram and slight depression of function. There has not been a good study of concomitant endomyocardial biopsy and of clinical events such as these to prove the utility of this approach. The lack of careful monitoring and treatment of rejection may result in an increased incidence of graft coronary artery disease in these patients, but the frequency of this complication has yet to be determined in the neonatal transplants.

With continual improvements in immunosuppression, the consequence of long-term administration of these drugs may be lessened, and the need for retransplantation later in life may also be alleviated. These issues, together with limited donor resources, remain the major stumbling blocks to more widespread use of transplantation in infants and children.

Retransplantation

An important consideration in cardiac transplantation is the question of retransplantation. The major indications are (1) the development of graft coronary atherosclerosis, (2) treatment of severe acute early rejection, and (3) treatment of early acute right heart failure. All of these patient groups are less desirable potential recipients than are primary transplant candidates, either because of chronic immunosuppression or the circumstances surrounding early graft failure.

These patients should meet the same standard criteria as initial candidates. These include a lack of evidence of systemic infection, no other irreversible major organ system failure, and the potential for adequate rehabilitation. Recipients should be screened for the presence of pre-existing cytotoxic antibodies. If a sufficient percentage is determined against a panel of random donor cells, a specific cross-match will be required for the retransplantation procedure.

A variety of reports have demonstrated that the survival of retransplant procedures is less than for primary procedures. Survival has been reported from between 0 and 75 per cent, depending on the center, the number of patients treated, and the indication for retransplantation.[192,193] In the largest report, 63 patients underwent 66 retransplantations out of 792 total procedures at the Stanford University Medical Center. Seventeen patients were treated for early rejection and 37 patients for development of coronary artery disease. Causes of death were similar to those for other transplant recipients, and survival was 55 ± 8 per cent at one year. A major determinant of patient survival was a

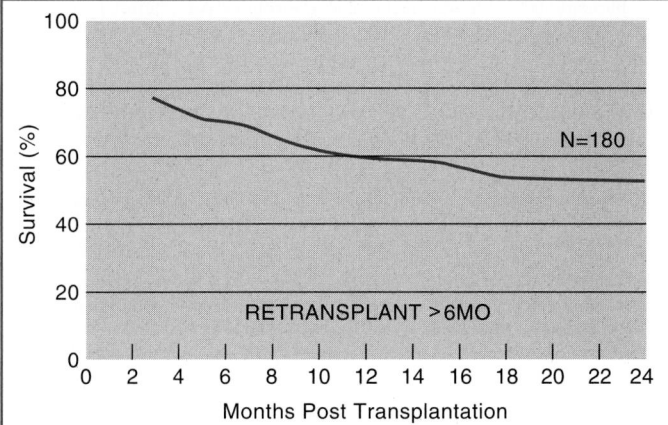

FIGURE 18–11. Actuarial survival for patients undergoing heart retransplantation reported to the Registry of the International Society for Heart Transplantation. (From Hosenpud, J. D., Novick, R. J., Breen, T. J., and Daily, O. P.: The Registry of the International Society for Heart and Lung Transplantation: Eleventh Official Report—1994. J. Heart Lung Transplant. 13(4):561, 1994. Reprinted with permission from Mosby-Year Book, Inc.)

serum creatinine level of less than 2.0 mg/dl.[194] The actuarial survival of patients undergoing retransplant procedures reported to the Registry of the International Society for Heart and Lung Transplantation is shown in Figure 18–11. One-year survival in this group of 180 patients retransplanted after 6 months was 60 per cent. (Survival was 40 per cent for earlier retransplantation.)

HEART AND LUNG TRANSPLANTATION

Transplantation of the entire cardiopulmonary axis was accomplished experimentally even before orthotopic heart transplantation.[69,195] Despite early experimental attempts, it was a difficult clinical endeavor because of problems inherent with lung transplantation. The rather diffuse and nonspecific immunosuppression available before cyclosporine therapy led to major problems with pulmonary infections and delayed healing of the trachea or bronchus, such that no truly therapeutic and extended lung transplant had been reported.[196] The availability of cyclosporine-based protocols led to success in primate allografts in the laboratory[197] and then a clinical series initiated at Stanford Uni-

versity Medical Center. The first reported therapeutic success in heart-lung transplantation was reported in 1981.[18]

The indications for heart-lung transplantation initially were severe pulmonary vascular disease, either primary or secondary to congenital heart disease. Later, heart-lung transplantation was extended to patients with a variety of diffuse pulmonary diseases, such as emphysema, lymphangioleiomyomatosis, diffuse pulmonary atriovenous fistulas, and cystic fibrosis.[198,199] Long-term survival figures for heart-lung transplantation (Fig. 18–12) are not as favorable as for heart transplantation (Fig. 18–9).

Single Lung Transplantation

Based on work with cyclosporine-based immunosuppressive protocols, single lung transplantation has been reported for interstitial pulmonary fibrosis[200] and double lung transplantation for emphysema and cystic fibrosis, among other indications.[201] Lung transplantation currently is undergoing a widespread renaissance with ever-increasing survival expectations. A number of centers are offering lung transplant procedures, and the availability of organ donors is also improving with an increasing awareness of the value and success of lung transplantation.

Current data show that the most frequent indication for single lung transplantation is interstitial pulmonary fibrosis, with the second indication being emphysema (Fig. 18–13). More diffuse pulmonary diseases are being treated by either bilateral single lung transplantation, en bloc double lung transplantation, or heart-lung transplantation in which the recipient's relatively normal heart is used as a donor for a second recipient (the "domino donor" procedure).[202,203]

INDICATIONS. Patient selection for lung transplantation follows the guidelines for heart transplants. Most patients over age 60 are excluded, as are patients who are ventilator-dependent or who have irreversible hepatic or renal disease, insulin-dependent diabetes, or a history of cancer or other systemic disease that might limit rehabilitation. Chronic pulmonary disease is somewhat difficult to gauge for potential timing of transplantation, but patients who are severely oxygen-dependent and demonstrate a course of clinical deterioration should be considered. A good indication of disability suggesting the need for transplant is a marked decrease in oxygen saturation with exercise.

THE DONOR LUNGS. Potential donors for lung transplant procedures must be infection-free, have good pulmonary gas exchange, lack a significant smoking history, and have a lung volume similar to or less than that of the intended recipient. Lung volumes can be judged by measurements on the chest film or by the lung volume determined by standard tables based on weight and height, comparing them with ideal similar measurements of lung volume for the intended recipient. In bilateral lung transplants, the volume of donor lungs should be the same or less than that of the intended recipient, although larger lungs in single lung transplantation can be placed on the left side, where the diaphragm has the potential to descend because of the absence of the liver under the left hemidiaphragm. Infection remains a major consideration, since this is the greatest source of morbidity and mortality. The presence of CMV in the donor

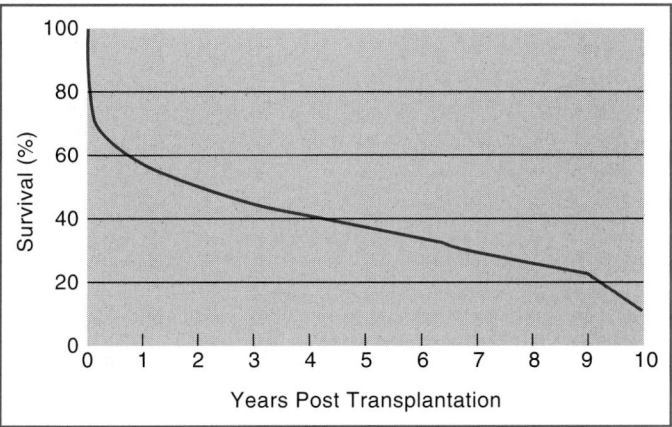

FIGURE 18–12. Survival of patients receiving heart-lung transplants, as reported to the Registry for the International Society for Heart Transplantation. (From Hosenpud, J. D., Novick, R. J., Breen, T. J., and Daily, O. P.: The Registry of the International Society for Heart and Lung Transplantation: Eleventh Official Report—1994. J. Heart Lung Transplant. 13(4):561, 1994. Reprinted with permission from Mosby-Year Book, Inc.)

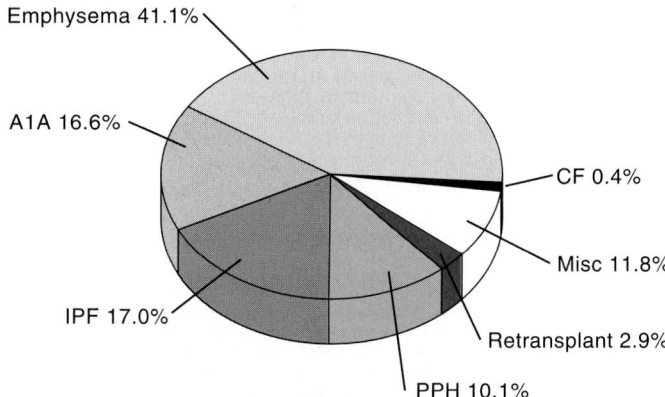

FIGURE 18–13. The indications for adult single lung transplantation. PPH = primary pulmonary hypertension, IPF = idiopathic pulmonary fibrosis, CF = cystic fibrosis, A1A = alpha₁-antitrypsin deficiency. (From Hosenpud, J. D., Novick, R. J., Breen, T. J., and Daily, O. P.: The Registry of the International Society for Heart and Lung Transplantation: Eleventh Official Report—1994. J. Heart Lung Transplant. 13(4):561, 1994. Reprinted with permission from Mosby-Year Book, Inc.)

when transplanted into a CMV negative recipient has resulted in significant morbidity.[204-206] Other donor-transmitted pathogens are frequent, as well.

PREVENTION OF REJECTION. Immunosuppression protocols are similar to those for cardiac transplantation, with the exception that prednisone is often omitted for the first several weeks due to its effect on retardation of bronchial healing. Induction therapy with polyclonal ATG preparations or monoclonal OKT3 prophylaxis is advocated by some groups to allow for a rejection-free interval without the use of steroids. Ultimately, most patients are maintained on triple-drug therapy, which has been shown to correlate with better long-term survival and a reduced incidence of bronchiolitis obliterans.[207]

The diagnosis of rejection remains somewhat imprecise and is based in large degree on clinical grounds. The use of fiberoptic bronchoscopy with transbronchial parenchymal lung biopsy has been most successful in following recipients.[208] Transbronchial biopsy can usually differentiate infection from rejection. It is performed in a prospective surveillance manner, as well as for specific indications. When used for specific indications, it usually gives a higher percentage of positive results, which are about equally divided between the diagnosis of infection or rejection.[209,210] When cardiac biopsies and transbronchial biopsies are compared, pulmonary and cardiac rejection were present synchronously on six occasions and asynchronously on 16 occasions (nine pulmonary and seven cardiac). Thus, cardiac biopsy alone is insufficient to follow the heart-lung transplant patient.

Early acute pulmonary rejection usually is manifested by an interstitial infiltrate, a decrease in lung volume and in pulmonary compliance, a low-grade fever, cough, and a feeling of breathlessness. These changes can all be rapidly reversed by using intravenous methylprednisolone, usually 1 gram intravenously daily for 3 days. It is not uncommon for recipients to undergo two or three rejection episodes in the first month after transplantation. Later, more chronic episodes of rejection may present without a pulmonary infiltrate on x-ray film, and long-term follow-up requires careful attention to pulmonary function testing. Patients frequently use a home spirometer to check for expiratory indices, such as the forced expiratory volume at 1 second, which will show a decline as a consequence of chronic rejection. When suspected, these changes need to be followed up by transbronchial parenchymal biopsy or augmented immunosuppression to preserve pulmonary function as much as possible.

OTHER COMPLICATIONS. *Infection* is an important complication of lung transplantation. The absence of cough reflex in the denervated lung surely contributes to a frequency of pulmonary infection at least three times more frequent than that of heart transplant recipients, and is the major cause of death in long-term surviving patients.[211] The transplanted lung may have deficiencies in lymphatic drainage, especially early after transplant, and ciliary function may be depressed. Patients frequently develop chronic bronchitis and may lack bronchus-associated lymphatic tissue as a result of chronic rejection.[212]

The late development of *bronchiolitis obliterans* limits the results in long-term surviving patients.[209-213] The incidence was reported as high as 50 per cent from the initial Stanford series, and is 20 to 30 per cent in most recent reports. The causes are almost certainly immunological; there is a demonstrated higher incidence in patients with a poor human leukocyte antigen match and in patients treated with a two-drug protocol, as compared with a three-drug protocol. Bronchiolitis obliterans is partially reversed or arrested by an aggressive increase in immunosuppression. This complication has been reported to occur both after isolated single lung and double lung transplantation, as well as after heart-lung transplantation.[214]

The therapeutic potential of lung transplant procedures is readily apparent. Patients are able to exercise without oxygen, to have a much greater feeling of well-being, and to resume active lifestyles. Late pulmonary function is usually quite satisfactory. Most reports show a progressive improvement in pulmonary function over time, and gas exchange and ventilation are essentially normal at 1 and 2 years.[215] Continuing improvement in immunosuppressive protocols will certainly lead to an even more reliable and safer long-term result in such patients.[216]

REFERENCES

1. Hosenpud, J. D., Novick, R. J., and Breen, T. J., et al.: The Registry of the International Society for Heart and Lung Transplantation: Eleventh Official Report—1994. J. Heart Lung Transplant. *13*:561, 1994.
2. Baumgartner, W. A., Reitz, B. A., and Achuff, S. A.: Heart and Heart-Lung Transplantation. Philadelphia, W.B. Saunders Company, 1990.
3. Carrel, A., and Guthrie, C. C.: The transplantation of veins and organs. Am. J. Med. *10*:1101, 1905.
4. Carrel, A.: The surgery of blood vessels. Johns Hopkins Hosp. Bull. *18*:18, 1907.
5. Lower, R. R., and Shumway, N. E.: Studies on the orthotopic homotransplantation of the canine heart. Surg. Forum *11*:18, 1960.
6. Lower, R. R., Dong, E., and Shumway, N. E.: Long-term survival of cardiac homografts. Surgery *58*:110, 1965.
7. Lower, R. R., Dong, E., and Shumway, N. E.: Suppression of rejection crises in the cardiac homograft. Ann. Thorac. Surg. *1*:645, 1965.
8. Barnard, C. N.: A human cardiac transplant: An interim report of a successful operation performed at Groote Shuur Hospital, Capetown. S. Afr. Med. J. *41*:1271, 1967.
9. Griepp, R. B., Stinson, E. B., and Dong, E., et al.: Determinants of operative risk in human heart transplantation. Am. J. Surg. *122*:192, 1971.
10. Caves, P. K., Stinson, E. B., and Billingham, M. E., et al.: Percutaneous endomyocardial biopsy in human heart recipients. Ann. Thorac. Surg. *16*:325, 1973.
11. Bieber, C. P., Griepp, R. B., and Oyer, P. E., et al.: Use of rabbit antithymocyte globulin in cardiac transplantation: Relationship of serum clearance rates in clinical outcomes. Transplantation *22*:478, 1976.
12. Baumgartner, W. A., Reitz, B. A., and Oyer, P. E., et al.: Cardiac homotransplantation. Curr. Probl. Surg. *16*:24, 1979.
13. Kostakis, A. J., White, D. J. G., and Calne, R. Y.: Prolongation of the rat heart allograft survival by cyclosporine-A. IRCS Med. Sci. *5*:280, 1977.
14. Borel, J. F.: The history of cyclosporine-A and its significance. In White, D. J. G. (ed.): Cyclosporine-A: Proceedings of an International Conference on Cyclosporin-A. New York, Elsevier North Holland, Inc., 1982.
15. Calne, R. Y., Rolles, K., and White, D. J. G., et al.: Cyclosporin-A initially as the only immunosuppressant in 34 recipients of cadaveric organs: Thirty-two kidneys, two pancreases, two livers. Lancet *2*:1033, 1979.
16. Schreiber, S. L., and Crabtree, G. R.: The mechanism of action of cyclosporin A and FK506. Immunol. Today *13*:136, 1992.
17. Oyer, P. E., Stinson, E. B., and Jamieson, S. W., et al.: Cyclosporine in cardiac transplantation: A two and a half year follow-up. Transplant. Proc. *15*:2546, 1983.
18. Reitz, B. A., Wallwork, J. L., and Hunt, S. A., et al.: Heart-lung transplantation: Successful therapy for patients with pulmonary vascular disease. N. Engl. J. Med. *306*:557, 1982.
19. Abramowicz, M. (ed.): Medical Letter *36*:82, 1994.
20. Annas, G. J.: Regulating the introduction of heart and liver transplantation. Am. J. Public Health *75*:93, 1985.
21. Medicare Program: Criteria for Medicare coverage of heart transplants. Fed. Reg. *52*:10935, 1987.
22. Miller, L. W., Vitale-Noedel, N., Pennington, D. G., et al.: Heart transplantation in patients over age 55 years. J. Heart Transplant. *7*:254, 1988.
23. Olivari, M. T., Antolick, A., Kaye, M. P., et al.: Heart transplantation in elderly patients. J. Heart Transplant. *7*:258, 1988.
24. Loebe, M., Schueler, S., Warnecke, H., et al.: The effect of older age on the outcome of heart transplantation. J. Heart Transplant. *8*:107, 1989.
25. Renlund, D. G., Gilbert, E. M., O'Connell, J. B., et al.: Age-associated decline in cardiac allograft rejection. Am. J. Med. *83*:391, 1987.
26. Murali, S., Uretsky, B. F., Reddy, P. S., et al.: The use of transpulmonary pressure gradient in the selection of cardiac transplantation candidates. J. Am. Coll. Cardiol. *11*:45, 1988.
27. Deeb, G. M., Bolling, S. F., Guynn, T. P., et al.: Amrinone versus conventional therapy in pulmonary hypertensive patients awaiting cardiac transplantation. Ann. Thorac. Surg. *48*:665, 1989.
28. Stevenson, L. W., Tillisch, J. H., Hamilton, M., Luu, M., et al.: Importance of hemodynamic response to therapy in predicting survival with ejection fraction ≤20% secondary to ischemic or non-ischemic dilated cardiomyopathy. Am. J. Cardiol. *66*:1348, 1990.
29. Stevenson, L. W., Dracup, K. A., and Tilliach, J. H.: Efficacy of medical therapy tailored for severe congestive heart failure in patients transferred for urgent cardiac transplantation. Am. J. Cardiol. *58*:1046, 1988.
30. Mancini, D. M., Eisen, H., Kussmaul, W., et al.: Value of peak exercise oxygen consumption for optimal timing of cardiac transplantation in ambulatory patients with heart failure. Circulation *83*:778, 1991.
31. Kermani, M., Stevenson, L. W., Chelimsky-Fallick, C., et al.: Importance of serial exercise testing after evaluation for cardiac transplantation. J. Heart Lung Transplant. *11*:191, 1992.
32. UNOS 1994 Annual Report of the U.S. Scientific Registry of Transplant Recipients and the Organ Procurement and Transplantation Network. Transplant Data: 1988–1993. U.N.O.S., Richmond, Va, and the Division of Organ Transplantation, Bureau of Health Resources Development, Health Resources and Services Administration, and Services Administration, U.S. Department of Health and Human Services, Bethesda, Md., L-7.
33. UNOS Update. 11:30–31, June 1995.
34. UNOS Update. 11:50–53, March 1995.
35. Applefeld, M. M., Newman, K. A., Grove, W. R., et al.: Intermittent, continuous outpatient dobutamine infusion in the management of congestive heart failure. Am. J. Cardiol. *51*:455, 1983.
36. Miller, C. A., Pae, W. E., and Pierce, W. S.: Combined registry for the clinical use of mechanical ventricular assist pumps and the total artificial heart in conjunction with heart transplantation: 4th official report—1989. J. Heart Transplant. *9*:453, 1990.
37. Shumway, S. J., and Bolman, R. M., III: Cardiac transplantation and ventricular assist devices. Curr. Opin. Cardiol. *6*:269, 1991.
38. Farrar, D. J., Hill, J. D., Gray, L. A., et al.: Heterotopic prosthetic ventricles as a bridge to cardiac transplantation: A multi-center study in 29 patients. N. Engl. J. Med. *318*:33, 1988.
39. Griffith, B. P., Kormos, R. L., Hardesty, R. L., et al.: The artificial heart: Infection-related morbidity and its effect on transplantation. Ann. Thorac. Surg. *45*:409, 1988.
40. Costanzo-Nordin, M. R., Cooper, D. K. C., Jessup, M., et al.: 24th Bethesda Conference: Cardiac Transplantation, Report Task Force 6: Future Developments. J. Am. Coll. Cardiol. *22*:54, 1993.

41. Pae, W. E.: Ventricular assist devices and total artificial hearts: A combined registry experience. Ann. Thorac. Surg. 55:295, 1993.

42. Baldwin, J. C., Anderson, J. L., Boucek, M. M., et al.: 24th Bethesda Conference: Cardiac Transplantation, Report Task Force 2: Donor Guidelines. J. Am. Coll. Cardiol. 22:15, 1993.

43. Presidential Commission for the Study of Ethical Problems in Medicine and Biomedical and Behavioral Research. Guidelines for the determination of death. JAMA 246:2184, 1981.

44. Griepp, R. B., Stinson, E. B., Clark, D. A., et al.: The cardiac donor. Surg. Gynecol. Obstet. 133:792, 1971.

45. Sweeney, M. S., Lammermeier, D. E., Frazier, O. H., et al.: Extension of donor criteria in cardiac transplantation: Surgical risk vs. supply-side economics. Ann. Thorac. Surg. 50:7, 1990.

46. Schueler, S., Warneke, H., Leob, E. M., et al.: Extended donor age in cardiac transplantation. Circulation 3:133, 1989.

47. Robicsek, F., Masters, T. N., Thomley, A. M., et al.: Bench coronary cineangiography. J. Thorac. Cardiovasc. Surg. 103:490, 1992.

48. Cooper, D. K. C., Human, P. A., Rose, A. G., et al.: Can cardiac allografts and xenografts be transplanted against the ABO blood group barrier? Transplant. Proc. 21:549, 1989.

49. UNOS 1994 Annual Report of the U.S. Scientific Registry of Transplant Recipients and the Organ Procurement and Transplantation Network. Transplant Data: 1988–1993. U.N.O.S., Richmond, Va, and the Division of Organ Transplantation, Bureau of Health Resources Development, Health Resources and Services Administration, U.S. Department of Health and Human Services, Bethesda, Md., L-8.

50. Baumgartner, W. A.: Evaluation and management of the heart donor. In Baumgartner, W. A., Reitz, B. A., and Achuff, S. A. (eds.): Heart and Heart-Lung Transplantation. Philadelphia, W. B. Saunders Company, 1990, p. 86.

51. Kaye, M. P.: The Registry of the International Society for Heart Transplantation: Fourth Official Report—1987. J. Heart Transplant. 6:63, 1987.

52. Yacoub, M., Mancad, P., and Ledingham, S.: Donor procurement and surgical techniques for cardiac transplantation. Semin. Thorac. Cardiovasc. Surg. 2:153, 1990.

53. Wicomb, W. N., Cooper, D. K. C., Novitsky, D., et al.: Cardiac transplantation following storage of the donor heart by a portable hypothermic perfusion system. Ann. Thorac. Surg. 37:243, 1984.

54. Baldwin, J. C., Frist, W. H., Starkey, T. D., et al.: Distant graft procurement for combined heart and lung transplantation using pulmonary artery flush and simple topical hypothermia for graft preservation. Ann. Thorac. Surg. 43:670, 1987.

55. Wallwork, J., Jones, K., Cavarocchi, N., et al.: Distant procurement of organs for clinical heart-lung transplantation using a single flush technique. Transplantation 44:654, 1987.

56. Hardesty, R. L., and Griffith, B. P.: Autoperfusion of the heart and lungs for preservation during distant procurement. J. Thorac. Cardiovasc. Surg. 93:11, 1987.

57. Baumgartner, W. A., Williams, G. M., Fraser, C. D., et al.: Cardiopulmonary bypass with profound hypothermia: An optimal preservation method for multi-organ procurement. Transplantation 47:123, 1989.

58. UNOS 1994 Annual Report of the U.S. Scientific Registry of Transplant Recipients and the Organ Procurement and Transplantation Network. Transplant Data: 1988–1993. U.N.O.S., Richmond, Va, and the Division of Organ Transplantation, Bureau of Health Resources Development, Health Resources and Services Administration, U.S. Department of Health and Human Services, Bethesda, Md., R-43.

58a. Abramowicz, M.: Medical Letter 37:61, 1995.

59. Dreyfus, G., Jebaara, V., Mihaileanu, S., and Carpentier, A.: Total orthotopic heart transplantation: An alternative to the standard technique. Ann. Thorac. Surg. 52:1181, 1991.

60. Kendall, S., Ciulli, F., Mullin, S. P., et al.: Total orthotopic heart transplantation: An alternative to the standard technique (Letter). Ann. Thorac. Surg. 54:187, 1992.

61. Rees, A. P., Milani, R. V., Lavie, C. J., et al.: Valvular regurgitation and right-sided cardiac pressures in heart transplant recipients by complete Doppler and color flow evaluation. Chest 104:82, 1993.

62. Bhatia, S. J. S., Kirshenbaum, J. M., Shemin, R. J., et al.: Time course of resolution of pulmonary hypertension and right ventricular remodeling after orthotopic cardiac transplantation. Circulation 76:819, 1987.

63. Armitage, J. M., Hardesty, R. L., and Griffith, B. P.: Prostaglandin E$_1$: An effective treatment of right heart failure after orthotopic heart transplantation. J. Heart Transplant. 6:348, 1987.

64. Girard, C., Durand, P. G., Vedrinne, C., et al.: Inhaled nitric oxide for right ventricular failure after heart transplantation. J. Cardiothorac. Vasc. Anesth. 7:481, 1993.

65. Foubert, L., Latimer, R., Oduro, A., et al.: Use of inhaled nitrous oxide to reduce pulmonary hypertension after heart transplantation. J. Cardiothorac. Vasc. Anesth. 7:640, 1993.

66. Fonger, J. D., Borkon, A. M., Baumgartner, W. A., et al.: Acute right ventricular failure following heart transplantation. Improvement with prostaglandin E$_1$ and right ventricular assist. J. Heart Transplant. 5:317, 1986.

67. McGriffin, D. C., and Carp, R. B.: Cardiac transplantation in a patient with a persistent left superior vena cava and an absent right superior vena cava. J. Heart Transplant. 3:115, 1984.

68. Reitz, B. A., Jamieson, S. W., Gaudiani, V. A., et al.: Method for cardiac transplantation in corrected transposition of the great arteries. J. Cardiovasc. Surg. (Torino) 23:293, 1982.

69. Demikhov, V. P.: Experimental Transplantation of Vital Organs. New York, Consultants Bureau, 1962.

70. McGough, E. C., Brener, P. L., and Reemstma, K.: The parallel heart studies of intrathoracic auxiliary cardiac transplants. Surgery 60:153, 1966.

71. Barnard, C. N., Losman, J. G.: Left ventricular bypass. S. Afr. Med. J. 49:303, 1985.

71a. Cochrane, A. D., Adams, D. H., Radley-Smith, R., et al.: Heterotopic heart transplantation for elevated pulmonary vascular resistance in pediatric patients. J. Heart Lung Transplant. 14:296, 1995.

72. Renlund, D. G., O'Connell, J. B., and Bristow, M. R.: Early rejection prophylaxis in heart transplantation: Is cytolytic therapy necessary? J. Heart Transplant. 8:191, 1989.

73. Kobashigawa, J. A., Stevenson, L. W., Brownfield, E., et al.: Does short-course induction with OKT3 improve outcome after heart transplantation? A randomized trial. J. Heart Lung Transplant. 12:205, 1993.

74. First, M. R., Schroeder, T. J., Hurtubise, P. E., et al.: Successful retreatment of allograft rejection with OKT3. J. Transplant. 47:88, 1989.

75. Livi, U., Luciani, G. B., Boffa, G. M., et al.: Clinical results of steroid-induction immunosuppression after heart transplantation. Ann. Thorac. Surg. 55:1160, 1993.

76. Reichenspurner, H., Ertel, W., Hammer, C., et al.: Immunologic monitoring of heart transplant patients under cyclosporine immunosuppression. Transplant. Proc. 16:1251, 1984.

77. Dubroff, J. M., Clark, M. B., Wong, C. Y. H., et al.: Changes in left ventricular mass associated with the onset of acute rejection after cardiac transplantation. J. Heart Transplant. 3:105, 1984.

78. Haberl, R., Weber, M., Reichenspurner, H., et al.: Frequency analysis of the surface electrocardiogram for recognition of acute rejection after orthotopic cardiac transplantation in man. Circulation 76:101, 1987.

79. Fraser, C. D., Jr., Chacko, V. P., Jacobus, W. E., et al.: Evidence of 31p nuclear magnetic resonance studies of cardiac allografts that early rejection is characterized by reversible biochemical changes. Transplantation 48:1068, 1989.

80. Griepp, R. B., Stinson, E. B., Dong, E., Jr., et al.: Acute rejection of the allografted human heart: Diagnosis and treatment. Ann. Thorac. Surg. 12:1113, 1971.

81. Warnecke, H., Muller, J., Cohnert, T., et al.: Clinical heart transplantation without routine endomyocardial biopsy. J. Heart Lung Transplant. 11:1093, 1992.

82. Muller, J., Warnecke, H., Spiegelsberger, S., et al.: Reliable noninvasive rejection diagnosis after heart transplantation in childhood. J. Heart Lung Transplant. 12:189, 1993.

83. Valentine, H. A., Fowler, M. B., Hunt, S. A., et al.: Changes in Doppler echocardiographic indexes of left ventricular function as potential markers of acute cardiac rejection. Circulation 76(Suppl. 5):V-86, 1987.

84. Golitsin, A., Pinedo, J. I., Cienfuegos, J. A., et al.: Thallium-201 uptake: A useful method for assessing heart transplantation. Transplant. Proc. 16:1262, 1984.

85. McKillop, J. H., McDougall, I. R., Goris, M. L., et al.: Failure to diagnose cardiac transplant rejection with Tc-99m-pyp images. Clin. Nucl. Med. 6:375, 1981.

86. Hesse, B., Mortensen, S. A., Folke, M., et al.: Ability of antimyosin scintigraphy monitoring to exclude acute rejection during the first year after heart transplantation. J. Heart Lung Transplant. 14:23, 1995.

87. Foegh, M. L., Khirabadi, B. S., Shapiro, R., et al.: Monitoring of rat heart allograft rejection by urinary thromboxane. Transplant. Proc. 16:1606, 1984.

88. O'Toole, C. M., Maher, P., Spiegelhalter, D., et al.: "Rejection or Infection" predictive value of T-cell subset ratio before and after heart transplantation. Heart Transplant. 4:518, 1985.

89. Caves, P. K., Billingham, M. E., Schultz, W. P., et al.: Transvenous biopsy from canine orthotopic heart allografts. Am. Heart J. 85:525, 1973.

90. Billingham, M. E.: The pathology of transplanted hearts. Semin. Thorac. Cardiovasc. Surg. 2:233, 1990.

91. Billingham, M. E., Cary, N. R., Hammond, M. E., et al.: A working formulation for the standardization of nomenclature in the diagnosis of heart and lung rejection: Heart Rejection Study Group. J. Heart Transplant. 9:587, 1990.

92. Hutchins, G. M.: The pathology of heart transplantation. In Baumgartner, W. A., Reitz, B. A., and Achuff, S. A. (eds.): Heart and Heart-Lung Transplantation. Philadelphia, W.B. Saunders Company, 1990, p. 183.

93. Normann, S. J., Salomon, D. R., Leelachaikul, P., et al.: Acute vascular rejection of the coronary arteries in human heart transplantation: Pathology and correlations with immunosuppression and cytomegalovirus infection. J. Heart Lung Transplant. 10:674, 1991.

93a. Lones, M. A., Czer, L. S. C., Trento, A., et al.: Clinical-pathologic features of humoral rejection in cardiac allografts: A study in 81 consecutive patients. J. Heart Lung Transplant. 14:151, 1995.

94. Czerska, B., Hobbs, R. E., James, K. B., et al.: Clinical manifestation of acute vascular rejection in cardiac transplant recipients. J. Heart Lung Transplant. 14:S46, 1995.

95. Kobashigawa, J. A., Kirklin, J. K., Naftel, D. C., et al.: Pretransplantation risk factors for acute rejection after heart transplantation: A multi-institutional study. The Transplant Cardiologists Research Database Group. J. Heart Lung Transplant. 12:355, 1993.

96. Michler, R. E., Smith, C. R., Drusin, R. E., et al.: Reversal of cardiac transplant rejection without massive immunosuppression. Circulation 74:III-68, 1986.

97. Haverty, T. P., Sanders, M., and Sheahan, M.: OKT$_3$ treatment of cardiac allograft rejection. J. Heart Lung Transplant. *12*:591, 1993.

98. Kobashigawa, J., Stevenson, L. W., Moriguchi, J., et al.: Randomized study of high-dose oral cyclosporine therapy for mild acute cardiac rejection. J. Heart Transplant. *8*:53, 1989.

99. Olsen, S. L., O'Connell, J. B., Bristow, M. R., et al.: Methotrexate in the treatment of persistent cardiac allograft rejection. J. Heart Transplant. *8*(abstr):96, 1989.

100. Bourge, R. C., Kirklin, J. K., White-Williams, C., et al.: Methotrexate pulse therapy in the treatment of recurrent acute heart rejection. J. Heart Lung Transplant. *11*:1116, 1992.

101. Hunt, S., Strober, S., Hoppe, R., et al.: Use of total lymphoid irradiation for therapy of intractable cardiac allograft rejection. J. Heart Transplant. *8*(abstr):104, 1989.

102. Salter, M. M., Kirklin, J. K., Bourge, R. C., et al.: Total lymphoid irradiation in the treatment of early or recurrent heart rejection. J. Heart Lung Transplant. *11*:902, 1992.

103. Todo, S., Fung, J. J., Demetris, A. J., et al.: Early trials with FK506 as primary treatment in liver transplantation. Transplant. Proc. *22*:13, 1990.

104. Peters, D. H., Fitton, A., Plosker, G. L., et al.: Tacrolimus. A review of its pharmacology and therapeutic potential in hepatic and renal transplantation. Drugs *46*:746, 1993.

105. Armitage, J. M., Kormos, R. L., Fung, J., et al.: Preliminary experience with FK506 in thoracic transplantation. Transplantation *52*:164, 1991.

106. Griffith, B. P., Bando, K., Hardesty, R. L., et al.: A prospective randomized trial of FK506 versus cyclosporine after human pulmonary transplantation. Transplantation *57*:848, 1994.

107. Morris, R. E.: New small molecule immunosuppressants for transplantation: Review of essential concepts. J. Heart Lung Transplant. *12*:S275, 1993.

108. Kirklin, J. K., Bourge, R. C., Naftel, D. C., et al.: Treatment of recurrent heart rejection with mycophenolate mofetil (RS-61443): Initial clinical experience. J. Heart Lung Transplant. *13*:444, 1994.

109. Horn, J. E., and Bartlett, J. G.: Infectious complications following heart transplantation. *In* Baumgartner, W. A., Reitz, B. A., and Achuff, S. A. (eds.): Heart and Heart-Lung Transplantation. Philadelphia, W.B. Saunders Company, 1990, p. 220.

110. Miller, L. W., Naftel, D. C., Bourge, R. C., et al.: Infection after heart transplantation: A multi-international study. Cardiac Transplant Research Database Group. J. Heart Lung Transplant. *13*:381, 1994.

111. Fox, B. C., Sollinger, H. W., Belzer, F. O., et al.: Prospective randomized double-blind study of trimethoprim-sulfamethoxazole for prophylaxis of infection in renal transplantation: Clinical efficacy, absorption of trimethoprim-sulfamethoxazole, effects of microflora, and the cost-benefit of prophylaxis. Am. J. Med. *89*:225, 1990.

112. Dummer, J. S., Gardy, A., Poorsattar, A., et al.: Early infections in kidney, heart, and liver transplant recipients on cyclosporine. Transplantation *36*:259, 1983.

113. Onorato, I. M., Morens, D. M., Martone, W. J., et al.: Epidemiology of cytomegaloviral infections: Recommendations for prevention and control. Rev. Infect. Dis. *7*:479, 1985.

114. Wolf, D. G., and Spector, S. A.: Early diagnosis of CMV disease in transplant recipients by DNA amplification in plasma. Transplantation *56*:330, 1993.

114a. Macdonald, P. S., Keogh, A. M., Marshman, D., et al.: A double-blind placebo-controlled trial of low-dose ganciclovir to prevent cytomegalovirus disease after heart transplantation. J. Heart Lung Transplant. *14*:32, 1995.

115. Merigan, T. C., Renlund, D. G., Keay, S., et al.: A controlled trial of ganciclovir to prevent cytomegalovirus disease after heart transplantation. N. Engl. J. Med. *326*:1182, 1992.

116. Edman, J. C., Kovacs, J. A., Strand, M., et al.: Ribosomal RNA sequence shows *Pneumocystis carinii* to be a member of the fungi. Nature *334*:519, 1988.

117. Holliman, R. E., Johnson, J. D., Adams, S., et al.: Toxoplasmosis and heart transplantation. J. Heart Transplant. *10*:608, 1991.

118. Penn, I., and Brunson, M. E.: Cancers after cyclosporine therapy. Transplant. Proc. *20*:85, 1988.

119. Myers, B. D., Ross, J., Newton, L., et al.: Cyclosporine-associated chronic nephropathy. N. Engl. J. Med. *311*:699, 1984.

120. McGiffin, D. C., Kirklin, J. K., and Naftel, D. C.: Acute renal failure after heart transplantation and cyclosporine therapy. J. Heart Transplant. *4*:396, 1985.

121. Luke, R. G.: Mechanisms of cyclosporine-induced hypertension. Am. J. Hypertens. *4*:468, 1991.

122. Renlund, D. G., O'Connell, J. B., Gilbert, E. M., et al.: A prospective comparison of murine monoclonal CD-3 antibody-based and equine antithymocyte globulin-based rejection prophylaxis in cardiac transplantation: Decreased rejection and less corticosteroid use with OKT$_3$. Transplantation *47*:599, 1989.

123. Copeland, J. G., Emery, R. W., Levinson, M. M., et al.: Cyclosporine: An immunosuppressive panacea? J. Thorac. Cardiovasc. Surg. *91*:26, 1986.

124. Slavin, J., and Taylor, J.: Cyclosporine, nifedipine, and gingival hyperplasia. Lancet *2*:739, 1987.

125. Patton, P. R., Brunson, M. E., Pfaff, W. W., et al.: A preliminary report of diltiazem and ketoconazole: Their cyclosporine-sparing effect and impact on transplant outcome. Transplantation *57*:889, 1994.

126. Cockburn, I. T., and Krupp, P.: An appraisal of drug interactions with Sandimmune. Transplant. Proc. *21*:385, 1989.

127. Henricsson, S., Lindholm, A., and Aravoglou, M.: Cyclosporine metabolism in human liver microsomes and its inhibition by other drugs. Pharmacol. Toxicol. *66*:49, 1990.

128. East, C., Alivizato, P. A., Grundy, S. M., et al.: Rhabdomyolysis in patients receiving lovastatin after cardiac transplantation (letter). N. Engl. J. Med. *318*:47, 1988.

129. Olivari, M-T., Jessen, M. E., Baldwin, B. J., et al.: Triple-drug immunosuppression with steroid discontinuation by six months after heart transplantation. J. Heart Lung Transplant. *14*:127, 1995.

130. Penn, I.: Tumors after renal and cardiac transplantation. Hematol. Oncol. Clin. North Am. *7*:431, 1993.

131. Hanto, D. W., Frizzera, G., Gajl-Peczalska, K. J., et al.: Epstein-Barr virus, immunodeficiency, and B-cell lymphoproliferation. Transplantation *39*:461, 1985.

132. Swinnen, L. J., Costanzo-Nordin, M. R., Fisher, S. G., et al.: Increased incidence of lymphoproliferative disorder after immunosuppression with monoclonal antibody OKT$_3$ in cardiac transplant recipients. N. Engl. J. Med. *323*:1723, 1990.

133. Miller, L. W., Schlant, R. C., Kobashigawa, J., et al.: 24th Bethesda Conference: Cardiac Transplantation, Report Task Force 5: Complications. J. Am. Coll. Cardiol. *22*:41, 1993.

134. van Gorp, J., Dornewaard, H., Verdonck, L. F., et al.: Post-transplant T-cell lymphoma. Cancer *73*:3064, 1994.

135. Oettle, H., Wilborn, F., Schmidt, C. A., et al.: Treatment with ganciclovir and Ig for acute Epstein-Barr infection after allogenic bone marrow transplantation (letter). Blood *82*:2257, 1993.

136. Benkerrou, M. D., Durandy, A., and Fischer, A.: Therapy for transplant-related lymphoproliferative diseases. Hematol. Oncol. Clin. North Am. *7*:467, 1993.

137. Thomson, J. G.: Production of severe atheroma in a transplanted human heart. Lancet *2*:1088, 1969.

138. Billingham, M. E.: Cardiac transplant atherosclerosis. Transplant. Proc. *19* (Suppl. 5):19, 1987.

139. Hess, M. L., Hastillo, A., Thompson, J. A., et al.: Lipid mediators in organ transplantation: Does cyclosporine accelerate coronary atherosclerosis? Transplant. Proc. *19* (Suppl. 5):71, 1987.

140. Uretsky, B. F., Murali, S., Reedy, S., et al.: Development of coronary artery disease in cardiac transplant patients receiving immunosuppressive therapy with cyclosporine and prednisone. Circulation *76*:827, 1987.

141. Nitkin, R. S., and Schroeder, J. S.: Accelerated coronary artery disease risk in heart transplant patients. J. Am. Coll. Cardiol. *5* (Suppl. II):535, 1985.

142. Johnson, D. E., Alderman, E. L., Schroeder, J. S., et al.: Transplant coronary artery disease: Histopathologic correlations with angiographic morphology. J. Am. Coll. Cardiol. *17*:449, 1991.

143. Grattan, M. T., Moreno-Cabral, C. E., Starnes, V. A., et al.: Eight-year results of cyclosporine-treated patients with cardiac transplants. J. Thorac. Cardiovasc. Surg. *99*:500, 1990.

144. Gao, S. Z., Schroeder, J. S., Hunt, S. A., et al.: Myocardial infarction in cardiac transplant recipients: A clinicopathologic correlation. Am. J. Cardiol. *64*:1093, 1989.

145. Banner, N. R., and Yacoub, M. H.: Physiology of the orthotopic cardiac transplant recipient. Semin. Thorac. Cardiovasc. Surg. *2*:259, 1990.

146. Rickenbacher, P. R., Pinto, F. J., Chenzbraun, A., et al.: Incidence and severity of transplant coronary artery disease early and up to 15 years after transplantation, as detected by intravascular ultrasound. J. Am. Coll. Cardiol. *25*:171, 1995.

147. Gao, S., Hunt, S. A., and Schroeder, J. S.: Accelerated transplant coronary artery disease. Semin. Thorac. Cardiovasc. Surg. *2*:241, 1990.

148. Billingham, M. E.: Graft coronary disease: The lesions and the patients. Transplant. Proc. *21*:3665, 1989.

149. Gao, S.-Z., Alderman, E. A., Schroeder, J. S., et al.: Accelerated coronary vascular disease in the heart transplant patient: Coronary arteriographic findings. J. Am. Coll. Cardiol. *12*:334, 1988.

150. Bieber, C. P., Hunt, S. A., Schwinn, D. A., et al.: Complications in long-term survivors of cardiac transplantation. Transplant. Proc. *13*:207, 1981.

151. Barbir, M., Kushwaha, S., Hunt, B., et al.: Lipoprotein(a) and accelerated coronary artery disease in cardiac transplant patients. Lancet *340*:(8834)1500, 1992.

152. Melnick, J. L., Adam, E., and DeBakey, M. E.: Possible role of cytomegalovirus in atherogenesis. JAMA *263*:2204, 1990.

153. Grattan, M. T., Moreno-Cabral, C. E., Starnes, V. A., et al.: Cytomegalovirus infection is associated with cardiac allograft rejection and atherosclerosis. JAMA *261*:3561, 1989.

154. Speir, E., Modali, R., Huang, E. S., et al.: Potential role of human cytomegalovirus and P53 interaction in coronary restenosis. Science *265*:391, 1994.

155. Butman, S. M.: Hyperlipidemia after cardiac transplantation: Be aware and possibly wary of drug therapy for lowering of serum lipids. Am. Heart J. *121*:1585, 1991.

156. Superko, H. R., Haskell, W. L., and DiRicco, C. D.: Lipoprotein and hepatic lipase activity and high-density lipoprotein subclasses after cardiac transplantation. Am. J. Cardiol. *66*:1131, 1990.

156a. Kobashigawa, J. A., Katznelson, S., Laks, H., et al.: Effect of pravastatin on outcomes after cardiac transplantation. N. Engl. J. Med. *333*:621, 1995.

157. Schroeder, J. S., Gao, S.-Z., Alderman, E. A., et al.: A preliminary study of diltiazem in the prevention of coronary artery disease in heart transplant recipients. N. Engl. J. Med. *328*:164, 1993.

158. Vetrovec, G. W., Cowley, M. J., Newton, C. M., et al.: Applications of

percutaneous transluminal coronary angioplasty in cardiac transplantation: Preliminary results in 5 patients. Circulation *78*(Suppl. III):83, 1988.

159. Copeland, J. G., Butman, S. M., and Cethi, G.: Successful coronary artery bypass grafting for high-risk left main coronary artery atherosclerosis after cardiac transplantation. Ann. Thorac. Surg. *49*:106, 1990.

160. Halle, A. A., DiSciascio, G., Massin, E. K., et al.: Coronary angioplasty, atherectomy and bypass surgery in cardiac transplant recipients. J. Am. Coll. Cardiol. *26*:120, 1995.

161. Dunning, J. J., Kendall, S. W., Mullins, P. A., et al.: Coronary artery bypass grafting nine years after cardiac transplantation. Ann. Thorac. Surg. *54*:571, 1992.

162. Karawande, S. V., Ensley, R. D., Renlund, D. G., et al.: Cardiac retransplantation: A viable option? The Registry of the International Society for Heart and Lung Transplantation. Ann. Thorac. Surg. *54*:840, 1992.

163. Christopherson, L. K., Griepp, R. B., and Stinson, E. B.: Rehabilitation after heart transplantation. JAMA *236*:2082, 1976.

164. Hunt, S. A., Rider, A. K., Stinson, E. B., et al.: Does cardiac transplantation prolong life and improve its quality? Cardiovasc. Surg. *54*:56, 1975.

165. Lough, M. E., Lindsey, A. M., and Shinn, J. A., et al.: Life satisfaction following heart transplantation. J. Heart Transplant. *4*:446, 1985.

166. UNOS 1994 Annual Report of the U.S. Scientific Registry of Transplant Recipients and the Organ Procurement and Transplantation Network. Transplant Data: 1988–1993. U.N.O.S., Richmond, Va, and the Division of Organ Transplantation, Bureau of Health Resources Development, Health Resources and Services Administration, U.S. Department of Health and Human Services, Bethesda, Md., VII-9.

167. UNOS. Annual Report of the U.S. Scientific Registry for Organ Transplantation and the Organ Procurement and Transplantation Network. U.S. Department of Health and Human Services, 1990.

168. O'Connell, J. B., Gunnar, R. M., Evans, R. W., et al.: 24th Bethesda Conference: Cardiac Transplantation. Task Force 1. Organization of Heart Transplantation in the U.S. J. Am. Coll. Cardiol. *22*:8, 1993.

169. Jarcho, J., Naftel, D. C., Shroyer, T. W., et al.: Influence of HLA mismatch on rejection after heart transplantation: A multi-institutional study. J. Heart Lung Transplant. *13*:583, 1994.

170. Mason, J. W., and Harrison, D. C.: Electrophysiology and electropharmacology of the transplanted human heart. *In* Narula OS (ed.): Cardiac Arrhythmias: Electrophysiology, Diagnosis, Management. Baltimore, Williams and Wilkins, 1979, p. 66.

171. Burke, M. N., McGinn, A. L., Homans, D. C., et al.: Evidence for functional sympathetic reinnervation of left ventricle and coronary arteries after orthotopic cardiac transplantation in humans. Circulation *91*:72, 1995.

172. Banner, N. R., Lloyd, M. H., Hamilton, R. D., et al.: Cardiopulmonary response to dynamic exercise after heart and combined heart-lung transplantation. Br. Heart J. *61*:215, 1989.

173. Kavanagh, T., Yacoub, M. H., Mertens, D. J., et al.: Cardiorespiratory responses to exercise training after orthotopic cardiac transplantation. Circulation *77*:162, 1988.

174. von Scheidt, W., Neudert, J., Erdmann, E., et al.: Contractility of the transplanted, denervated human heart. Am. Heart J. *121*:1480, 1991.

175. Uretsky, B. F.: Physiology of the transplanted heart. Cardiovascular Clin. *20*:23, 1990.

176. Verani, M. S., George, S. E., Leon, C. A., et al.: Systolic and diastolic ventricular performance at rest and during exercise in heart transplant recipients. J. Heart Transplant. *7*:145, 1988.

177. Naurie, K. G., Bristow, M. R., and Reitz, B. A.: Increased beta adrenergic receptor density in an experimental model of cardiac transplantation. J. Thorac. Cardiovasc. Surg. *86*:195, 1983.

178. Borow, K. M., Neumann, A. A., Arensman, F. W., et al.: Cardiac and peripheral vascular responses to adrenoceptor stimulation and blockage after cardiac transplantation. J. Am. Coll. Cardiol. *14*:1229, 1989.

179. Yusuf, S., Theodoropoulos, S., Mathias, C. J., et al.: Increased sensitivity of the denervated transplanted human heart to isoprenaline both before and after beta-adrenergic blockade. Circulation *75*:696, 1987.

180. Scherrer, U., Vissing, S. F., Morgan, B. J., et al.: Cyclosporine induced sympathetic activation and hypertension after heart transplantation. N. Engl. J. Med. *323*:693, 1990.

181. Redmond, J. M., Zehr, K. J., Gillinov, M. A., et al.: Use of theophylline for treatment of prolonged sinus node dysfunction in human orthotopic heart transplantation. J. Heart Lung Transplant. *12*(1 Pt 1):133, 1993.

182. Evans, R. W.: Measuring the costs of heart transplantation. Primary Cardiol. *20*:48, 1994.

183. UNOS 1994 Annual Report of the U.S. Scientific Registry of Transplant Recipients and the Organ Procurement and Transplantation Network. Transplant Data: 1988–1993. U.N.O.S., Richmond, Va, and the Division of Organ Transplantation, Bureau of Health Resources Development, Health Resources and Services Administration, U.S. Department of Health and Human Services, Bethesda, Md., F-29.

183a. Votapka, T. V., Swartz, M. T., Reedy, J. E., et al.: Heart transplantation charges: Status 1 versus Status 2 patients. J. Heart Lung Transplant. *14*:366, 1995.

184. Mudge, G. H., Goldstein, S., Addonizio, I. J., et al.: 24th Bethesda Conference: Cardiac Transplantation. Task Force 3: Recipient guidelines/prioritization. J. Am. Coll. Cardiol. *22*:21, 1993.

185. Evans, R. W.: Social, economic, and insurance issues in heart transplantation. *In* O'Connell, J. B., and Kaye, M. P., (eds.) Intrathoracic Transplantation 2000. Austin, Tx: RG Landes *1*:17, 1993.

186. Evans, R. W.: Cost-effectiveness of transplantation. Surg. Clin. North Am. *66*(3):603, 1986.

187. Evans, R. W.: Executive summary: The National Cooperative Transplantation Study: BHARC-100-91-020. Seattle, Battelle-Seattle Research Center, June 1991.

188. Cameron, D. E., and Gardner, T. J.: Heart transplantation in children. *In* Baumgartner, W. A., Reitz, B. A., and Achuff, S. A. (eds.): Heart and Heart-Lung Transplantation. Philadelphia, W.B. Saunders Company, 1990, p. 293.

189. Bailey, L. L., Nehlsen-Cannarella, S. L., Concepcion, W., et al.: Baboon to human cardiac xenotransplantation in a neonate. JAMA *254*:3321, 1985.

190. Boucek, M. M., Kanakriyeh, M. S., Mathis, C. M., et al.: Cardiac transplantation in infancy: Donors and recipients. J. Pediatr. *116*:171, 1990.

191. Bernstein, D., Baum, D., Hunt, S., Miller, J., Reitz, B., and Stinson, E. B.: Long-term (> 5-year) survivors of pediatric heart transplantation. J. Heart Lung Transplant (*in press*).

192. Watson, D. C., Reitz, B. A., Oyer, P. E., et al.: Sequential orthotopic heart transplantation in man. Transplantation *30*:401, 1980.

193. Novitsky, D., Cooper, D. K. C., Brink, J. G., et al.: Sequential second and third transplants in patients with heterotopic heart allografts. Clin. Transplant. *1*:57, 1987.

194. Smith, J. A., Ribakove, G. H., Hunt, S. A., Miller, J., Stinson, E. B., Oyer, P. E., Robbins, R. C., Shumway, N. E., and Reitz, B. A.: Cardiac retransplantation: The 25-year experience at a single institution. J. Heart Lung Transplant (*in press*).

195. Neptune, W. B., Cookson, B. A., Bailey, C. P., et al.: Complete homologous heart transplantation. Arch. Surg. *66*:174, 1953.

196. Veith, F. J.: Lung transplantation. Surg. Clin. North Am. *58*:357, 1978.

197. Reitz, B. A., Burton, N. A., Jamieson, S. W., et al.: Heart and lung transplantation, autotransplantation, and allotransplantation in primates with extended survival. J. Thorac. Cardiovasc. Surg. *80*:360, 1980.

198. Wellens, F., Estenne, M., deFrancquen, P., et al.: Combined heart-lung transplantation for terminal pulmonary lymphangioleiomatosis. J. Thorac. Cardiovasc. Surg. *89*:872, 1985.

199. Jones, D. K., Higgenbottam, T. W., and Wallwork, J.: Long-term survival after heart-lung transplantation in cystic fibrosis. Chest *93*:644, 1988.

200. Toronto Lung Transplant Group: Experience with single lung transplantation for pulmonary fibrosis. JAMA *259*:2258, 1988.

201. Cooper, J. D., Patterson, G. A., Grosman, R., et al.: Double lung transplant for advanced chronic obstructive lung disease. Am. Rev. Respir. Dis. *139*:303, 1989.

202. Baumgartner, W. A., Traill, T. A., Cameron, D. E., et al.: Unique aspects of heart and lung transplantation exhibited in the "domino-donor" operation. JAMA *261*:3121, 1989.

203. Yacoub, M. H., Banner, N. R., Khaghani, A., et al.: Heart-lung transplantation for cystic fibrosis and subsequent domino heart transplantation. J. Heart Transplant. *9*:459, 1990.

204. Burke, C. M., Glanville, A. R., Macoviak, J. A., et al.: The spectrum of cytomegalovirus infection following human heart-lung transplantation. J. Heart Transplant. *5*:267, 1986.

205. Dummer, J. S., White, L. T., Monto, H. O., et al.: Morbidity of cytomegalovirus infection in recipients of heart or heart-lung transplant who received cyclosporine. J. Infect. Dis. *152*:1182, 1985.

206. Hutter, J. A., Scott, J. P., Wreghitt, T., et al.: The importance of cytomegalovirus in heart-lung transplantation. Chest *95*:627, 1989.

207. McCarthy, P. M., Starnes, V. A., Theodore, J., et al.: Improved survival after heart-lung transplantation. J. Thorac. Cardiovasc. Surg. *99*:54, 1990.

208. Higgenbottam, T., Stewart, S., Penketh, A., et al.: Transbronchial lung biopsy for the diagnosis of rejection in heart-lung transplant patients. Transplantation *46*:532, 1988.

209. Starnes, V. A., Theodore, J., Oyer, P. E., et al.: Pulmonary infiltrates after heart-lung transplantation: Evaluation by serial transbronchial biopsies. J. Thorac. Cardiovasc. Surg. *98*:945, 1989.

210. Starnes, V. A., Theodore, J., Oyer, P. E., et al.: Evaluation of heart-lung transplant recipients with prospective, serial, transbronchial biopsies in pulmonary function studies. J. Thorac. Cardiovasc. Surg. *98*:683, 1989.

211. Dummer, J. S., Montero, C. G., Griffith, B. P., et al.: Infections in heart-lung recipients. Transplantation *41*:725, 1986.

212. Ren, H., Hruban, R. H., Baumgartner, W. A., et al.: Hemorrhagic infarction of hilar lymph nodes associated with combined heart-lung transplantation. J. Thorac. Cardiovasc. Surg. *99*:861, 1990.

213. Allen, M. D., Burke, C. M., McGregor, C. G. A., et al.: Steroid-responsive bronchiolitis after human heart-lung transplantation. J. Thorac. Cardiovasc. Surg. *92*:449, 1986.

214. LoCicero, J., Robinson, P. G., Fisher, M.: Chronic rejection in single lung transplantation manifested by obliterative bronchiolitis. J. Thorac. Cardiovasc. Surg. *99*:1059, 1990.

215. Theodore, J., Morris, A. J., Burke, C. M., et al.: Cardiopulmonary function at maximum tolerable constant work rate exercise following human heart-lung transplantation. Chest *92*:433, 1987.

216. Davis, R. D., and Pasque, M. K.: Pulmonary transplantation. Ann. Surg. *221*(1):14, 1995.

Chapter 19
Assisted Circulation and the Mechanical Heart

WAYNE E. RICHENBACHER, WILLIAM S. PIERCE

Four hundred thousand new cases of congestive heart failure are diagnosed in the United States annually.[1] According to the Framingham Heart Study, the 5-year mortality rate for patients with congestive heart failure was 75 per cent in men and 62 per cent in women.[2] Standard medical and surgical therapies benefit only a small percentage of patients with ventricular dysfunction. Potential cardiac transplant recipients with hemodynamic instability may receive temporary mechanical circulatory support as a bridge to cardiac transplantation. Best estimates suggest that 17,000 to 66,000 patients in the United States may benefit from a permanent implantable blood pump each year.[3] Once they are perfected, not only will mechanical blood pumps be immediately accessible but they will ultimately provide a cost-effective alternative to cardiac transplantation or long-term medical treatment of patients in New York Heart Association (NYHA) functional Classes III and IV.[4]

Another population of patients who would benefit from mechanical circulatory support are individuals with reversible ventricular dysfunction. Two to 6 per cent of patients who undergo an open heart operation develop postcardiotomy cardiogenic shock.[5] Aggressive medical management, including intraaortic balloon (IAB) counterpulsation, allows 75 to 85 per cent of these patients to be weaned from cardiopulmonary bypass. Thus, approximately 1 per cent of patients who undergo an open heart procedure would benefit from interval support with a mechanical blood pump.

Patients with cardiovascular disease in whom hemodynamic deterioration is evident first receive conventional medical therapy. Conventional management is directed toward correction of any electrolyte or acid-base imbalance, hypoxemia, rhythm disturbance, or hypovolemic state. Cardiogenic shock, as defined in Table 19–1, is next treated with inotropic and, if systemic blood pressure permits, afterload-reducing agents. Patients who manifest ongoing hemodynamic instability, and who fulfill the selection criteria outlined in Table 19–2, may qualify for an advanced form of mechanical circulatory support.

Mechanical circulatory support devices can be roughly divided into three major groups. The IAB is a readily available, catheter-mounted intravascular device designed to improve the balance between myocardial oxygen supply and demand while increasing systemic perfusion to a modest degree. The ventricular assist device (VAD) is a blood pump that is designed to assist or replace the function of either the right or left ventricle. A right VAD will support the pulmonary circulation, while a left VAD provides systemic perfusion, in the absence of right or left ventricular ejection, respectively. Implantable VADs are positioned intracorporeally—in the anterior abdominal wall or within a body cavity other than the pericardium. Extracorporeal

VADs may be located in a paracorporeal position, along the patient's anterior abdominal wall, or externally, at the patient's bedside. Two VADs have received Food and Drug Administration (FDA) approval for clinical use, although access to the majority of these devices is controlled by clinical trials as of this writing. The total artificial heart (TAH) is an orthotopically positioned cardiac replacement device. The pneumatic TAH is used infrequently, and only with FDA approval, as a mechanical bridge to cardiac transplantation. Completely implantable electric artificial hearts have been successfully implanted in experimental animals but are not expected to reach the clinical arena until the year 2000.

HISTORY

Extracorporeal counterpulsation was introduced by Clauss and co-workers in 1961.[6] The concept was modified by Moulopoulos and colleagues who described an intravascular counterpulsation balloon in 1962.[7] The first successful clinical application of balloon counterpulsation was reported by Kantrowitz et al. in 1968.[8] IAB insertion originally required a surgical procedure. In 1980, Bregman and Casarella described percutaneous IAB insertion utilizing a sheath and dilators.[9] The IAB is now a standard form of therapy for a variety of patients with cardiovascular disease. In 1993, nearly 100,000 IABs were inserted in the United States alone.[10]

The dawn of complete, clinical mechanical circulatory support occurred on May 6, 1953 when Gibbon successfully closed a secundum atrial septal defect in a patient supported with cardiopulmonary bypass.[11] The majority of patients with ventricular dysfunction, however, do not require pulmonary support with an in-line oxygenator. Roller-pump left ventricular assistance using atrial transseptal uptake and femoral arterial return was introduced by Dennis et al. in 1962.[12] Subsequently, DeBakey successfully employed left atrial to aortic bypass in patients who could not be weaned from cardiopulmonary bypass.[13] By the late 1970's, a variety of intracorporeal and extracorporeal mechanical blood pumps were being tested for both "support to weaning"[14] and "bridge to transplant"[15] indications. Patient selection and hemodynamic criteria were developed, and cannulation techniques, blood-biomaterial interactions, and control strategies evaluated. During the 1980's patient management was refined and clinical results improved. Advances in myocardial preservation resulted in fewer blood pumps being required for postcardiotomy cardiogenic shock. However, a disparity in the ratio of cardiac donors to recipients increased the need for long-term circulatory support in patients requiring a bridge to cardiac transplantation. Results in this patient population proved gratifying, with survival statistics approaching those achieved with conventional cardiac transplantation.[16] The early 1990's have seen research efforts focus on the development of implantable VADs suitable for permanent implantation in patients with end-stage cardiomyopathy.

While IAB and VAD development were in their infancy, investigators also initiated laboratory efforts to develop a cardiac replacement device. In 1958, Akutsu and Kolff described an experiment in which a pneumatic TAH was implanted in a dog.[17] By the mid 1960's, Kolff and Nosé had achieved 24-hour survival with sac-type hearts implanted in calves.[18] By the end of the decade, survival times approached 3 to 5 days.[19] Experimental animals with TAHs have now lived for up to 1 year. The TAH entered the clinical arena in 1969 when Cooley and associates introduced the concept of staged cardiac replacement.[20] DeVries and coworkers were the first to implant a TAH as a permanent cardiac replacement.[21]

TABLE 19–1   DEFINITION OF CARDIOGENIC SHOCK

Cardiac output index	< 1.8 liters/min/m²
Systolic blood pressure	< 90 mm Hg
Left or right atrial pressure	> 20 mm Hg
Urine output	< 20 ml/hr
Systemic vascular resistance	> 2100 dynes-sec/cm⁵

INTRAAORTIC BALLOON COUNTERPULSATION

The design and function of the IAB have not changed substantially during the past three decades. The IAB is an intravascular catheter-mounted counterpulsation device with a balloon volume between 30 and 50 ml. A central lumen allows passage of the balloon catheter over a small-diameter guidewire and subsequent monitoring of central aortic blood pressure. The IAB is attached to a small bed-side console and triggered to the patient's arterial pressure curve or electrocardiogram. The shuttle gas is helium, as its viscosity allows rapid balloon inflation and deflation, which facilitates counterpulsation in patients with tachyarrhythmias.

The IAB is positioned in the descending thoracic aorta and set to inflate at the dicrotic notch of the arterial pressure waveform when monitoring the aortic pressure (Fig. 19–1). The diastolic rise in aortic root pressure augments coronary blood flow and myocardial oxygen supply. The increase in systemic perfusion may be less than 0.5 liter/min. The IAB is deflated during the isovolumetric phase of left ventricular contraction. The reduction in the afterload component of cardiac work decreases peak left ventricular pressure and myocardial oxygen consumption. The net effect is a favorable shift in the myocardial oxygen supply/demand ratio, with a small increase in systemic perfusion.

Indications and Results of Clinical Use

Traditional indications for IAB counterpulsation include refractory cardiogenic shock following cardiac surgery or an acute myocardial infarction (see p. 1239). The latter indication includes patients suffering from primary pump failure in addition to those with mechanical complications, such as acute mitral regurgitation or a postinfarction ventricular septal defect.

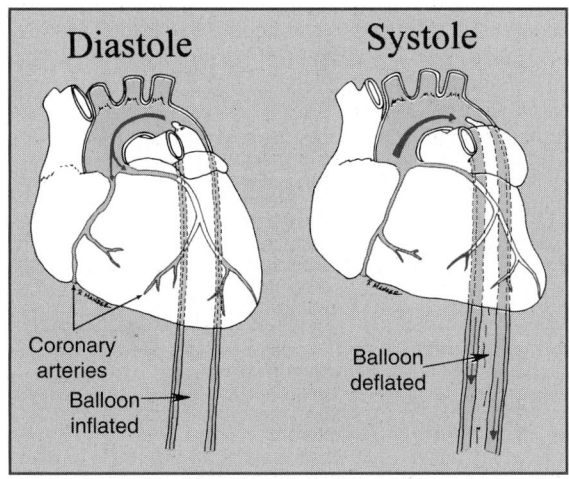

FIGURE 19–1. The intraaortic balloon is inserted via the common femoral artery and positioned in the descending thoracic aorta. The tip is located just distal to the left subclavian artery. The balloon is inflated during cardiac diastole, thereby increasing coronary artery perfusion. Left ventricular afterload is decreased as the balloon is deflated during cardiac systole. Proper balloon timing improves the ratio between myocardial oxygen supply and demand. (Courtesy of Arrow International, Inc. Redrawn by Richard Manzer.)

Seventy-five per cent of patients with an acute myocardial infarction who develop cardiogenic shock not amenable to conventional medical therapy will improve hemodynamically with IAB counterpulsation.[22] Outcome, however, is largely determined by the underlying coronary artery pathology. Patients with operable disease who undergo prompt revascularization achieve an early survival rate as high as 93 per cent.[23] Patients who develop a mechanical complication following an acute myocardial infarction are best managed with IAB counterpulsation, urgent cardiac catheterization, and immediate surgical repair. IAB counterpulsation will reduce the left-to-right shunt and maintain coronary perfusion in patients with a postinfarction *ventricular septal defect* (see p. 1243). Hospital mortality in patients managed with an IAB and urgent operation is 20 per cent to 27 per cent.[24] Patients with postinfarction *mitral regurgitation* secondary to papillary muscle dysfunction or rupture also benefit from IAB insertion (see p. 1243). IAB counterpulsation will increase coronary perfusion and reduce ischemic ventricular dysfunction, mitral regurgitation, and the pulmonary capillary wedge pressure. Outcome is related to the extent of cardiac dysfunction with surgical mortality approaching 55 per cent.[25]

Refractory *postcardiotomy cardiogenic shock* is related to preoperative left ventricular dysfunction, inadequate myocardial preservation, intraoperative myocardial infarction, prolonged cardiopulmonary bypass, and ischemic times, or technical difficulties with the conduct of the operation. With maximal medical support and IAB counterpulsation, survival rates average 52 to 66 per cent.[26]

An additional group of patients in cardiogenic shock who benefit from IAB counterpulsation are approved *cardiac transplant recipients* with hemodynamic decompensation before a donor heart becomes available (see p. 1239). The rationale for IAB counterpulsation in this clinical setting is to maintain systemic perfusion and preserve end-organ function until cardiac transplantation occurs. One-year actuarial survival in patients who require IAB counterpulsation prior to cardiac transplantation is 72 to 77 per cent.[27,28]

More recently the indications for IAB support have been expanded to include patients who do not fulfill hemodynamic selection criteria but who suffer from *unstable angina* or *malignant ventricular tachyarrhythmias*. Although nonrandomized trials suggest that IAB counterpulsation and subsequent myocardial revascularization may be of some benefit in patients with preinfarction angina,[29] aggressive preoperative medical management and judicious use of a cardiac anesthetic may eliminate the need for an IAB with equally good results. The role of IAB counterpulsation in patients with postinfarction angina is equally controversial.[30] In general, IAB support is reserved for patients with deteriorating hemodynamics or ongoing ischemia, as evidenced by rest pain or electrocardiographic changes in the region of the infarct, before myocardial revascularization.

TABLE 19–2   MECHANICAL CIRCULATORY SUPPORT SELECTION CRITERIA

Patient fulfills hemodynamic criteria (Table 19–1)
Maximal inotropic support and IAB counterpulsation
Exclude patient if:
Blood urea nitrogen > 100 mg/dl
Serum creatinine > 5.0 mg/dl
Chronic lung disease
Chronic liver disease
Metastatic cancer
Sepsis
Neurological deficit
Technically incomplete cardiac operative procedure (if postcardiotomy cardiogenic shock)
Age > 60 yr (if bridge to transplant)

IAB = Intraaortic balloon.

IAB counterpulsation may be beneficial in patients with *ventricular tachyarrhythmias,* particularly when these abnormalities are related to ischemia.[31] Ectopic impulses originate in the ischemic area surrounding an infarct zone, and the IAB may reduce the frequency of such arrhythmias by increasing myocardial perfusion and oxygenation in the ischemic zone. The role of perioperative IAB counterpulsation in hemodynamically stable patients with left main coronary artery disease or severe left ventricular dysfunction, and in high-risk patients undergoing a general surgical procedure, is less well defined.

Absolute contraindications to IAB counterpulsation include aortic insufficiency and aortic dissection. Contraindications to IAB insertion via the femoral arterial route include the presence of an abdominal aortic aneurysm or severe calcific aortoiliac or femoral arterial disease. The percutaneous insertion technique should not be employed in a patient who has a recent groin incision with violation of the subcutaneous tissue at the proposed puncture site.

INSERTION TECHNIQUE

The IAB is most commonly inserted in a percutaneous fashion via the common femoral artery.[32] Preinsertion evaluation of the patient's femoral arterial and pedal pulses facilitates rapid recognition of limb ischemia following balloon insertion. With the use of strict aseptic technique the femoral artery is accessed by means of the Seldinger approach. The femoral arterial puncture should occur below the inguinal ligament, to avoid a transperitoneal puncture, and above the profunda femoris artery, to reduce the potential for superficial femoral arterial cannulation.

The common femoral artery is dilated and the final dilator and sheath advanced over a J wire into the descending thoracic aorta. The final dilator is withdrawn and the IAB inserted into the introducer sheath. The radiopaque tip of the IAB is positioned just distal to the left subclavian artery. The balloon is unwound, purged, connected to the bedside console, and pulsed. Proper augmentation is best accomplished with the IAB synchronized 1:2 with the patient's arterial pressure trace. Once inflation and deflation times are determined, augmentation is set at 1:1. Postinsertion anticoagulation is usually accomplished with low molecular weight (10 per cent) dextran (20 ml/hr). Prophylactic heparin sodium administration is recommended in patients who have not had surgical intervention.

Alternatively the IAB may be inserted into the femoral artery using an open technique. The femoral artery is exposed and a 5-cm segment of an 8- to 10-mm diameter vascular graft anastomosed, at a 45-degree angle, to the common femoral artery. The IAB is passed through the vascular graft into the artery and positioned as already described. The IAB is fixed in position by tying umbilical tapes around the vascular graft.

When an abdominal aortic aneurysm or severe peripheral vascular disease precludes femoral arterial insertion, the IAB may be inserted directly into the ascending aorta or transverse arch.[33] Access is obtained through a median sternotomy, usually at the time of cardiotomy. The balloon is inserted through a vascular graft in a manner identical to that described in the open femoral arterial technique. The balloon is advanced across the transverse arch into the descending thoracic aorta. Alternatively, the IAB can simply be inserted through two, concentric pursestring sutures.

When greater patient mobility is desired, the IAB may be inserted into the subclavian or iliac artery.[34,35] These insertion sites are particularly applicable when long-term IAB support is anticipated, as in patients who require a mechanical bridge to cardiac transplantation. In the authors' opinion, however, hemodynamically unstable potential cardiac transplant recipients are best managed with a brief trial of IAB counterpulsation using the femoral arterial approach. If the patient's condition fails to improve within 48 to 72 hours, VAD implantation should be considered.

REMOVAL TECHNIQUE

As the patient's hemodynamic status improves, balloon augmentation is serially decreased. If the patient tolerates augmentation of every fourth to eighth heartbeat (1:4 to 1:8), the IAB can be safely withdrawn.[32] Balloon inflation is discontinued and the balloon aspirated to ensure deflation is complete. The balloon is withdrawn into the sheath. Manual pressure is applied to the femoral artery distal to the insertion site, and the balloon and insertion sheath withdrawn as a single unit. Blood is permitted to eject from the insertion site for one or two heart beats to clear any thrombotic debris from the vascular space. Pressure is then applied to the insertion site: manually for 30 minutes and with a sandbag for an additional 8 hours. One should make certain that the limb is adequately perfused during IAB removal. Withdrawal of an IAB inserted by the open technique requires surgical groin exploration, balloon and vascular graft removal, and femoral artery repair, usually with a vein patch. Open removal is also recommended when there has been high (proximal) percutane-

ous insertion, in morbidly obese patients, and in patients who develop limb ischemia following percutaneous insertion.

Balloons inserted into the ascending aorta can be removed under local anesthesia if the side arm graft is brought into the subcutaneous space.[36] The authors of this chapter, however, recommend repeat sternotomy with direct visualization of the insertion site.

COMPLICATIONS OF IAB USE

The complication rate from IAB counterpulsation varies from 6 to 46 per cent.[37] Major complications, including limb ischemia necessitating thrombectomy or amputation, aortic dissection, aortoiliac laceration or perforation, and deep wound infection requiring debridement, occur in 4 to 17 per cent of patients. Major complications lead to an additional operative procedure, prolonged hospitalization, long-term morbidity, or death. Minor complications, including bleeding at the insertion site, superficial wound infections, asymptomatic loss of peripheral pulse, or lymphocele, occur in 7 to 42 per cent of patients. Minor complications are usually self-limited or resolve following IAB removal.

The most common complications related to femoral IAB use are vascular.[37-39] Vascular complication rates vary from 6 to 24 per cent, and are usually related to the initial insertion procedure rather than the presence of the IAB within the vascular space. Risk factors for developing a major vascular complication following femoral IAB insertion include diabetes mellitus, systemic hypertension, female gender, and peripheral vascular disease. Interestingly, percutaneous IAB insertion has a major vascular complication rate similar to IAB insertion using an open surgical technique.[40,41] The risk of vascular complications associated with percutaneous insertion is related to the possibility of superficial, rather than common, femoral arterial cannulation and the potential for intimal disruption at the time of arterial cannulation.

LEG ISCHEMIA. This is the most common vascular complication of femoral IAB insertion, occurring in 5 to 19 per cent of patients.[37-39] When a patient develops leg ischemia following femoral IAB insertion, the IAB should be removed. Persistent ischemia following IAB removal requires emergent femoral arterial exploration, thrombectomy, and patch angioplasty. Balloon-dependent patients with limb ischemia benefit from moving the IAB to the contralateral leg or a femoral-femoral crossover graft.[42] Modified IABs, intended for sheathless insertion, may reduce the incidence of leg ischemia, particularly in patients with small femoral arteries.

Aortic dissection occurs in fewer than 5 per cent of patients[37]; however, the majority of patients who develop this complication do not survive. Aortic dissection occurs at the time of femoral IAB insertion and is managed by IAB removal. The incidence of aortic dissection may be reduced by using a guidewire and fluoroscopy and avoiding excessive force during IAB insertion.

The complication rate of transthoracic IAB counterpulsation is 0 to 13 per cent.[33,37] Complications associated with IAB insertion in the ascending aorta include side arm graft infection with mediastinitis, coronary artery or arch vessel embolization, and inability to close the sternum secondary to mechanical tamponade.

THE VENTRICULAR ASSIST DEVICE

Unlike the IAB that is designed to improve the ratio between myocardial oxygen supply and demand while supporting systemic perfusion to only a modest degree, the VAD is designed to effectively unload either the right or left ventricle while completely supporting the pulmonary or systemic circulation. The term *VAD* describes any of a variety of mechanical blood pumps employed singly to replace the function of either the right or left ventricle. Two blood pumps can be utilized for biventricular support. For right ventricular assistance, blood is withdrawn from the right atrium and returned to the main pulmonary artery. For left ventricular assistance, blood is withdrawn from either the left atrium or the apex of the left ventricle. The blood passes through the left VAD and is returned to the ascending aorta.

There is a wealth of information in the literature regarding the advantages and disadvantages of left atrial versus left ventricular inflow (with respect to the VAD) cannulation.[43,44] In general, left atrial inflow cannulation is technically easier to perform and may employ cannulas readily available to any open heart surgical team; however, it is thought to provide incomplete ventricular decompression. Left ventricular inflow cannulation requires a custom-designed cannula but provides very effective left ventricular decompression. The reduction in myocardial oxygen de-

TABLE 19-3   COMPARISON OF VENTRICULAR ASSIST PUMPS

VAD TYPE	ADVANTAGE	DISADVANTAGE
Roller	Readily available Simple to use Inexpensive	Flow limitation Blood trauma Tubing spallation Nonpulsatile Systemic anticoagulation Short-term use Constant supervision required
Centrifugal	Readily available Simple to use Relatively inexpensive Blood handling characteristics	Nonpulsatile Systemic anticoagulation Constant supervision required Not FDA approved as a VAD
Pulsatile	No blood trauma +/− anticoagulation Pulsatile flow Minimal supervision required Patient mobility	Expensive

VAD = Ventricular assist device; FDA = Food and Drug Administration.

mand is offset by the fact that left ventricular apical cannulation damages the myocardium, an important consideration in a patient with marginal ventricular function. A left ventricular apex cannula is, however, ideally suited to patients who receive mechanical circulatory support as a bridge to cardiac transplantation. In this patient population, ventricular recovery is not expected, and the apical cannula is removed in its entirety at the time of recipient cardiectomy.

REGULATORY AFFAIRS

To better understand the enormous amount of effort that has been expended developing mechanical blood pumps, and limitations imposed on clinicians who desire access to a VAD, it is important to become familiar with the process by which medical devices are evaluated and approved for clinical use.[45,46] In the United States the Medical Device Amendment of 1976 amended the Federal Food, Drug and Cosmetic Act to require the FDA to approve clinical investigation of new medical devices and to approve new medical devices before they could be sold for general use. To prove that a new medical device is both safe and effective, the device must be the subject of a carefully controlled clinical trial.

An investigator/manufacturer first conducts extensive in vitro device testing followed by in vivo animal experimentation. The data derived from the preclinical evaluation are submitted to the FDA along with results, if any, from foreign clinical trials. The investigator must also submit a formal clinical protocol and informed consent material that have been approved by the Institutional Review Board at the site of the proposed clinical trial. If the application for clinical investigation of the device is deemed satisfactory by the FDA, an Investigational Device Exemption (IDE) is granted to the investigator. It is expected that the clinical protocol will answer specific questions concerning the proposed indications and contraindications for use of the device.

Because of the inordinate expense of device research and development, and the cost incurred during the conduct of a clinical trial (under an approved IDE), most investigators have an industrial partner. Assuming that the clinical trial shows the device to be safe and effective for a well-defined set of indications, the next step is to seek approval from the FDA for commercial sale of the device. In general, the industrial partner will submit a Pre Market Approval (PMA) request to the FDA. The focus of the PMA application is to provide more extensive durability testing, an important consideration in devices intended for long-term clinical use.

Durability testing is most often accomplished by accelerated in vitro experimentation, frequently performed under conditions more severe than those experienced when the device is in actual clinical use. Approval of a PMA by the FDA allows the manufacturer to release the medical device for commercial sale.

Description of Devices

Mechanical blood pumps capable of replacing the function of a single ventricle can be divided into four categories. The advantages and disadvantages of each category of blood pump are summarized in Table 19-3. Representative members of each class of VAD are listed in Table 19-4. Specific design features and functional characteristics of each VAD are described below. Specific details regarding implantation and explanation technique are described in the section entitled Management Considerations.

ROLLER PUMP. The roller pump employs cannulas, tubing, and a roller head, all of which are readily available to any cardiac surgeon.[47,48] The inflow and outflow cannulas employed for roller pump ventricular assistance are the same as those employed for cardiopulmonary bypass in any open heart operation. The cannulas are connected to a length of $\frac{3}{8}$ inch ID medical grade silicone rubber tubing. The tubing is placed in the roller head and forward flow imparted to blood by the rotating, occlusive rollers. Cannula and tubing size frequently limit total blood flow, while the occlusive roller head is responsible for hemolysis and trauma to formed blood elements, in addition to tubing spallation and fatigue.[49,50] The system provides nonpulsatile flow, requires that the patient be fully anticoagulated, and is not pressure limited, which demands that the drive unit receive constant supervision. A fall in atrial pressure can lead to air embolism as air is drawn into the atrium around the atrial cannula. A sudden obstruction to VAD

TABLE 19-4   REPRESENTATIVE MEMBERS OF EACH VAD TYPE

VAD TYPE	NAME	MANUFACTURER
Roller	Roller	Many
Centrifugal	Bio-Pump Delphin Isoflow	Medtronic Bio-Medicus, Inc. Sarns, Inc./3M Aries Medical/St. Jude
Pulsatile (Pneumatic)	BVS 5000 Bi-ventricular Support System HeartMate 1000 IP LVAS Thoratec VAD System	Abiomed, Inc. ThermoCardiosystems, Inc. Thoratec Laboratories Corp.
Pulsatile (Electric)	Novacor N-100 HeartMate 1000 VE LVAS Penn State	Novacor Medical Division, Baxter Healthcare Corp. ThermoCardiosystems, Inc. Arrow International, Inc.

VAD = Ventricular assist device.

outflow can result in rapid system pressurization and tubing disruption. The roller pump is capable of providing right or left ventricular support, and two pumps can be employed for biventricular support. The limitations preclude use of this system beyond a few hours or days.

CENTRIFUGAL PUMPS. Centrifugal pumps are also simple to use and readily available to most cardiac surgeons (Fig. 19–2A).[51,52] Standard cardiopulmonary bypass atrial and arterial cannulas are connected to the centrifugal head by short lengths of medical grade polyvinylchloride tubing. Unlike the roller head, however, the centrifugal head imparts forward flow to blood by creating a vortex with a rapidly spinning series of cones or impeller blades that are located within the rigid pump housing (Fig. 19–2B). The nonocclusive pump head reportedly has better blood handling characteristics than a roller head, and the system is pressure limited, virtually eliminating the potential for air embolus or tubing disruption.[49,53] Centrifugal blood pumps provide nonpulsatile blood flow and require full systemic anticoagulation and constant driver supervision.[54] The pump can provide left or right heart support, or two pumps can be used for biventricular assistance.

Centrifugal pumps entered the clinical arena prior to the

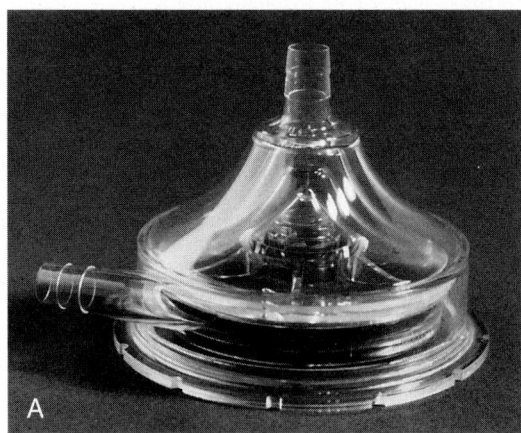

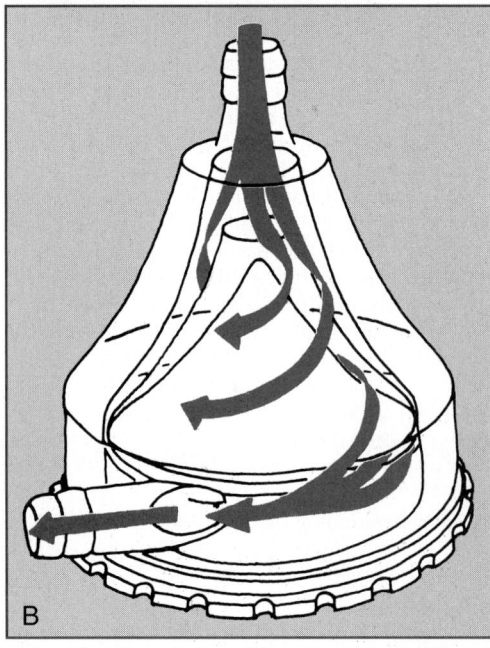

FIGURE 19–2. The Bio-Pump centrifugal pump. *A,* This extracorporeal blood pump can be used for either right or left ventricular assistance. Two pumps can be used for biventricular assistance. *B,* The Bio-Pump centrifugal blood pump imparts forward flow to blood by creating a vortex with a rapidly spinning series of cones. (Courtesy of Medtronic Bio-Medicus, Inc.)

Medical Device Amendment of 1976. However, centrifugal blood pumps are considered a Class III medical device, subject to the constraints imposed by this amendment to the Federal Food, Drug and Cosmetic Act. Currently, centrifugal blood pumps are approved only for up to 6 hours of use, suitable for cardiopulmonary bypass, but not for short-term temporary ventricular assistance. Recently a coalition of centrifugal blood pump manufacturers formed the Health Industries Manufacturers Task Force to petition the FDA to reclassify centrifugal blood pumps as a Class II medical device, thereby removing the time constraints for ventricular support. This down-class petition is based upon the proven track record of centrifugal blood pumps in providing safe and effective ventricular assistance in non-FDA-approved clinical experience.

Pneumatic Pulsatile Blood Pumps

Complex air-driven pulsatile VADs are considerably more expensive than either roller or centrifugal pumps and until recently were available only to centers participating in a clinical trial. These devices produce pulsatile flow with no trauma to formed blood elements. Furthermore, integral sophisticated control systems are largely self-regulating, and beyond the first few days following device insertion minimal supervision is required. As drive units become more refined and portable drivers are developed, patient mobility and life style have improved dramatically.

ABIOMED BVS 5000 BIVENTRICULAR SUPPORT SYSTEM. This system received PMA approval from the FDA in 1992 for treatment of patients with postcardiotomy cardiogenic shock (Fig. 19–3).[55–57] The BVS 5000 (Abiomed, Inc., Danvers, MA) is an external dual-chamber device that is capable of providing short-term univentricular or biventricular circulatory support. Each chamber contains a 100-ml polyurethane blood sac. Trileaflet polyurethane valves are located at the inlet and outlet side of the ventricular chamber. The atrial chamber fills passively throughout pump systole and diastole, while the ventricular chamber is intermittently pulsed with air from the drive console. Custom-designed cannulas provide right or left atrial inflow. The distal portion of the outlet cannula is a coated vascular prosthesis that is anastomosed to either the pulmonary artery or aorta. The cannulas traverse the skin subcostally. The drive unit functions asynchronously with respect to the patient's native cardiac rhythm. The control system maintains a constant 80-ml stroke volume by automatically adjusting the duration of pump systole and diastole in response to changes in preload and afterload.

THE HEARTMATE 1000 IP LVAS. This system received PMA approval from the FDA in 1994 for use as a mechanical bridge to cardiac transplantation (Fig. 19–4).[58–60] This implantable blood pump (ThermoCardiosystems, Inc., Woburn, MA) is connected to an external drive unit by a percutaneous air drive line. The titanium VAD housing contains a flexible segmented polyurethane diaphragm that is bonded to a rigid pusher plate. The unique, textured blood-containing surface promotes the formation of a stable neointima.[61] Patients do not require systemic anticoagulation and instead receive only antiplatelet agents. Intermittent air pulses from the external drive console actuate the pusher-plate diaphragm and eject blood from the VAD housing. The pump has a maximum stroke volume of 83 ml and a maximum pump output of 11 liters/min. Valved conduits containing 25-mm porcine valves are located at the inlet and outlet ports of the VAD housing. The VAD is designed only for left ventricular support, withdrawing blood from the left ventricular apex. Blood is returned to the ascending aorta. The device was originally designed to be implanted in the left upper quadrant of the patient's abdomen. However, in selected patients the device may be positioned preperitoneally, in the abdominal wall.[62] When the blood pump is placed in a preperitoneal position, the potential visceral complications associated

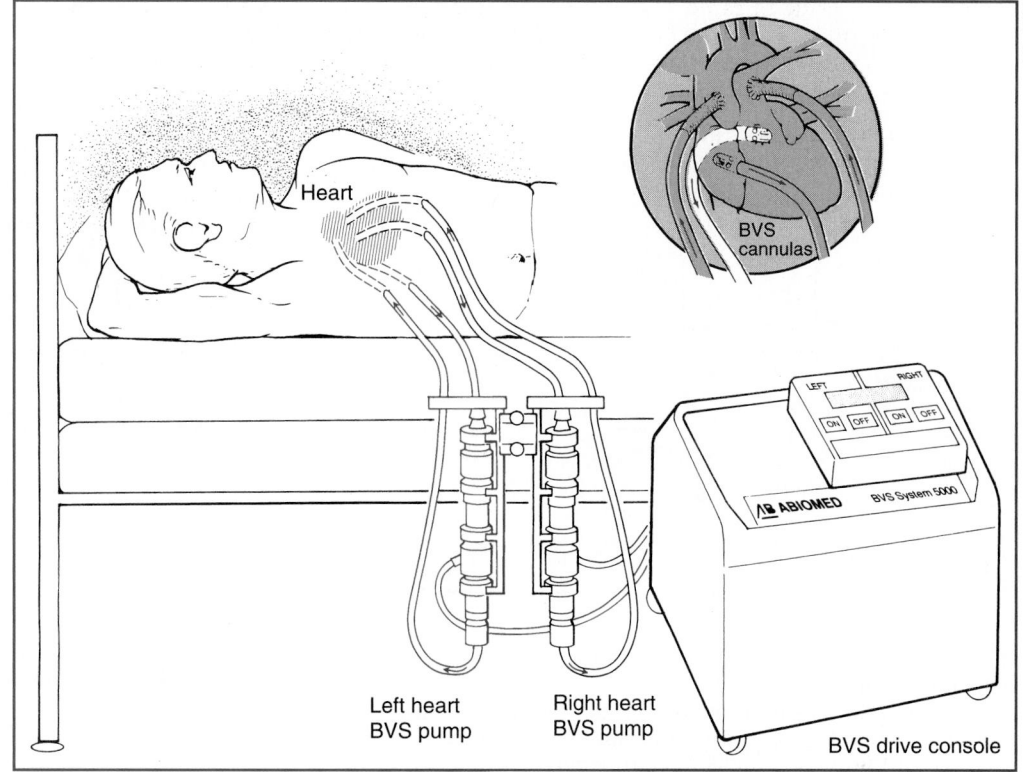

FIGURE 19–3. The Abiomed BVS 5000 Bi-ventricular Support System can support either right or left ventricular function. The system is simple in design and relatively inexpensive by pulsatile blood pump standards. The dual chamber, gravity-fed device restricts patient mobility more than implantable pulsatile blood pumps, but is ideally suited for use in postcardiotomy cardiogenic shock patients in whom the duration of support is less than 1 week. (From Shook, B.J.: The Abiomed BVS 5000 Bi-ventricular Support System. System description and clinical summary. Cardiac Surgery State of the Art Reviews 7:309, 1993. Reproduced with permission.)

with peritoneal implantation are avoided. The drive console runs on standard alternating current, as well as internal rechargeable batteries. The batteries provide up to 40 minutes of support. The control system allows the VAD to function in a fixed rate or pump-on-full mode. The latter is a rate-responsive mode in which the VAD is automatically pulsed when the pump chamber is 90 per cent filled.

PIERCE-DONACHY SYSTEMS. The prototypical pneumatic, pulsatile VAD, and the device that has probably seen the largest US clinical experience, is the Thoratec Ventricular Assist Device (Thoratec Laboratories Corp., Berkeley, CA) based on the Pierce-Donachy design (Fig. 19–5).[63–65] In 1994 the Circulatory System Devices Advisory Panel to the FDA recommended approval of this paracorporeal blood pump as

a bridge to cardiac transplantation; in 1995 the FDA granted full commercial approval. This versatile blood pump can be used for right, left, or biventricular assistance (Fig. 19–6). In the case of left ventricular assistance, custom-designed cannulas allow blood to be withdrawn from either the left atrium or the apex of the left ventricle. The blood pump consists of a machined polysulfone housing that contains a polyurethane blood sac and Sorin monostrut inlet and outlet valves (Sorin Biomedical, Inc., Irvine, CA). Patients are maintained on sodium warfarin. The blood pump has a stroke volume of 65 ml with a dynamic ejection fraction of approximately 0.75. Air pulses from the

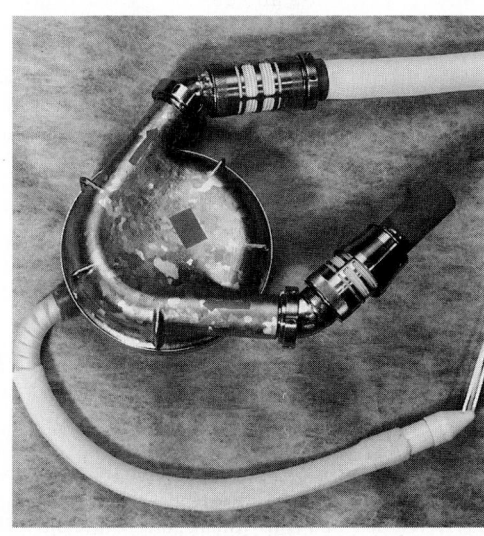

FIGURE 19–4. The implantable HeartMate 1000 IP LVAS blood pump has a percutaneous air drive line located at the bottom of this photograph. The short left ventricular apex inlet conduit, at right, and the outlet conduit at the top of this photograph, contain bioprosthetic valves that ensure a unidirectional flow of blood through the blood pump. The vascular graft on the outlet conduit is cut to length and sutured to the ascending aorta. (Courtesy of ThermoCardiosystems, Inc.)

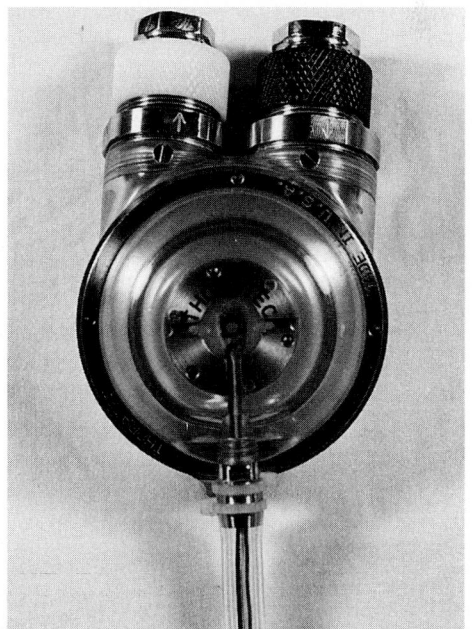

FIGURE 19–5. The paracorporeal Thoratec blood pump is positioned on the patient's anterior abdominal wall. The inlet and outlet cannulas (not shown) traverse the skin subcostally. The air drive line is located at the bottom of this photograph. The device can be used for either right or left heart support. Two devices can be used to provide biventricular assistance. (Courtesy of Thoratec Laboratories, Corp.)

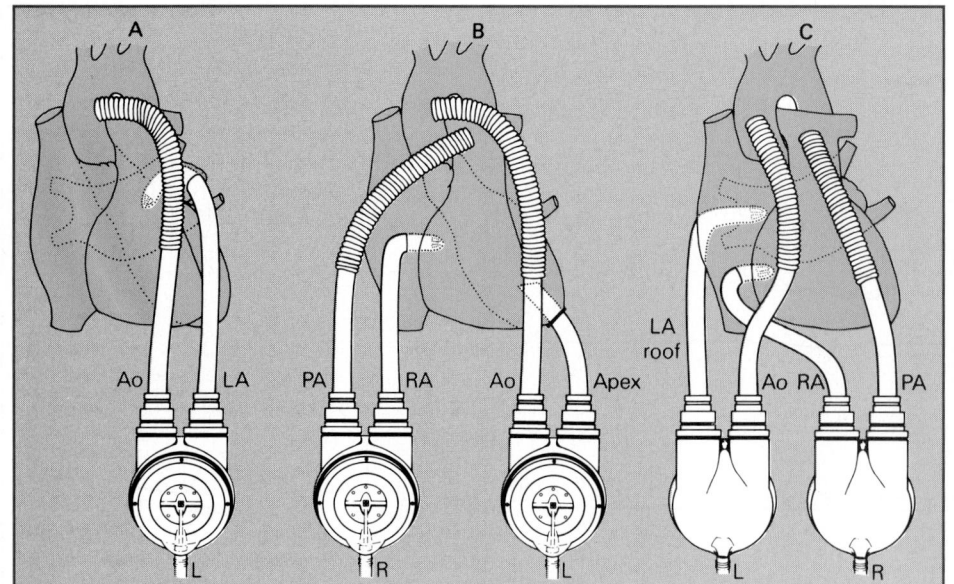

FIGURE 19–6. Cannulation configurations for the Thoratec ventricular assist device. *A,* Left atrial appendage to aortic left ventricular assistance. *B,* Left ventricular apex to aortic, and right atrium to main pulmonary artery biventricular assistance. *C,* Biventricular assistance where the left ventricular assist device inflow cannula is inserted into the left atrium via the right superior pulmonary vein. (*L* = left, *R* = right, *LA* = left atrium, *Ao* = aorta, *RA* = right atrium, *PA* = pulmonary artery. (From Farrar, D. J., Hill, J. O., Gray, L. A., Jr., et al.: Heterotopic prosthetic ventricles as a bridge to cardiac transplantation: A multicenter study in 29 patients. N. Engl. J. Med. *318*:333, 1988. Copyright Massachusetts Medical Society.)

drive unit intermittently compress the flexible blood sac ejecting blood from the VAD housing. The control system allows the device to function in one of three modes: a manual fixed-rate mode, a synchronized mode in which the R wave of the patient's electrocardiogram serves as an electronic trigger, and an asynchronous full-to-empty mode in which the VAD enters systole each time the blood sac fills. The last mode maximizes cardiac output by allowing the VAD pump rate to be determined by preload.

Electric Pulsatile Blood Pumps

The electric VAD will ultimately be completely implantable and capable of providing years of left ventricular support. These devices provide left-ventricular-apex to aortic flow and are not designed for right ventricular assistance. In addition to a mechanical blood pump, the electric VAD system will have an implantable controller and back-up battery. An external, portable battery pack will serve as the primary power source. The external battery pack will be carried in a shoulder bag and transfer energy to the implantable controller and blood pump using transcutaneous energy transmission.[66] Energy will be passed from an external primary coil located on the surface of the skin to a subcutaneous secondary coil by inductive coupling. There will be no break in the integument, eliminating the potential for an ascending drive line infection. The internal, rechargeable battery will allow brief periods of entirely tether-free VAD function. As these systems will be completely sealed, air displaced from the blood pump housing during diastole will move to an implanted reservoir known as a compliance chamber.[67] As the final technological barriers to the development of implantable electric VADs are overcome, these systems will be permanently implanted in patients with unreconstructable coronary artery disease or end stage cardiomyopathy not amenable to cardiac transplantation.

NOVACOR N-100 LEFT VENTRICULAR ASSIST SYSTEM. This system contains a polyurethane blood sac that is compressed by dual symmetrically opposed pusher plates.[68] In this system (Novacor Medical Division, Baxter Healthcare Corp., Oakland, CA), the pump is actuated by a spring-decoupled solenoid energy converter. The blood pump and energy converter are contained within a lightweight housing that is implanted in a preperitoneal position in the left upper quadrant of the patient's abdomen.[69] The inflow conduit and outflow conduit each contains a bioprosthetic pericardial valve. Patients require full anticoagulation with sodium warfarin.

The Novacor blood pump has a maximum stroke volume of 67 ml. The tethered configuration, the subject of an ongoing clinical trial that began in 1984, employs a percutaneous vented tube containing power and control wires.[68] The external console-based controller typ-

ically allows the device to function in a fill-rate trigger mode that provides synchronized counterpulsation to the native heart. Recently the clinical trial protocol was amended to allow testing of the wearable microprocessor-based controller.[70,71] The compact controller and rechargeable batteries are worn as a belt or carried in a "camera bag" and can support the blood pump for up to 7 hours.

HEARTMATE 1000 VE LVAS. This system (ThermoCardiosystems, Inc., Woburn, MA) utilizes a blood pump similar to that employed in the pneumatically powered ventricular assist system produced by the same manufacturer.[72,73] In the vented electric version, however, the

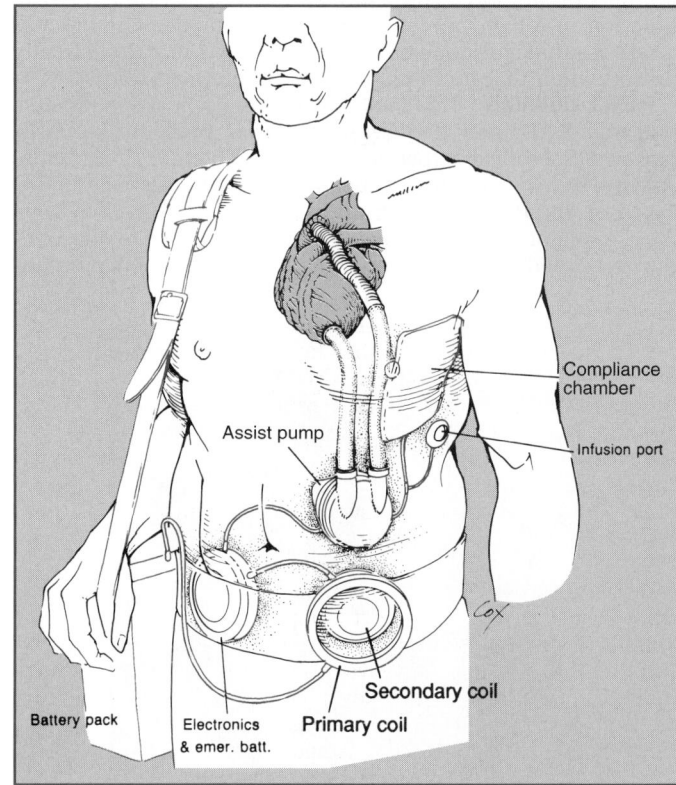

FIGURE 19–7. The completely implantable electric ventricular assist system being developed at Pennsylvania State University. The blood pump and energy converter are located preperitoneally in the patient's left upper quadrant. The implantable control system and rechargeable back-up battery are powered by an external battery pack. Energy passes from the superficial primary coil to the subcutaneous secondary coil using inductive coupling. Air displaced from the blood pump housing during diastole will enter the intrathoracic compliance chamber. Air that diffuses out of the compliance chamber over time is replenished using the subcutaneous infusion port.

TABLE 19–5   RESULTS OF CENTRIFUGAL BLOOD PUMP SUPPORT FOR POSTCARDIOTOMY CARDIOGENIC SHOCK

AUTHOR	DEVICE	NO. PATIENTS	WEANED (%)	SURVIVED (%)
Golding[78]	Bio-Pump	79	49 (62)	20 (25)
Lee[77]	Bio-Pump	28	N/A	9 (32)
Noon[79]*	Bio-Pump	89	42 (47)	19 (21)
Killen[76]	Bio-Pump	41	17 (41)	8 (20)
Curtis[52]	Delphin	60	23 (38)	12 (20)
Registry[5]	Centrifugal	559	254 (45)	143 (26)

* Includes 61 postcardiotomy patients.

diaphragm pusher-plate mechanism is pulsed by a low-speed high-torque motor. The percutaneous electrical leads connect the blood pump to the external controller and batteries. The rechargeable batteries are carried in a shoulder holster, or the device may be connected to a stationary control console. The clinical trial of the VE LVAS began in 1991, with selected patients managed in an outpatient setting.[73]

PENNSYLVANIA STATE UNIVERSITY SYSTEM.   The completely implantable sealed system being developed at Pennsylvania State University contains a segmented polyurethane blood sac enclosed in a rigid polysulfone housing (Fig. 19–7).[74,75] Björk-Shiley inlet and outlet valves provide unidirectional blood flow. The blood sac is compressed by a pusher plate driven by a brushless direct current motor. Air displaced from the pump housing during VAD diastole is managed by a polyurethane compliance chamber.[67] Control electronics and a 30-minute battery pack are contained in an implantable cannister that receives power from a subcutaneous energy transmission coil. The external battery pack carried by the patient transfers energy to the implanted coil using transcutaneous energy transmission.[66] The device has a stroke volume of 62 ml and can pump up to 8.5 liters/min. The controller adjusts the VAD beat rate in response to physiologic conditions, ensuring that the blood pump functions in a full-to-empty mode.

The Penn State electric VAD has run continuously for more than one year on a mock circulatory system.[74] The system has provided circulatory support for more than one week in 26 Holstein calves. The average duration of support was 62 days; the longest nearly 8 months.

Indications and Results of Clinical Use

POSTCARDIOTOMY CARDIOGENIC SHOCK.   The original indication for VAD support was postcardiotomy cardiogenic shock. One per cent of patients cannot be removed from cardiopulmonary bypass despite maximum medical therapy and IAB counterpulsation.[76,77] These patients are considered potential candidates for VAD insertion. The goal of mechanical circulatory support in this clinical setting is to alter the balance between myocardial oxygen supply and demand to create a milieu that favors myocardial recovery. At the same time, systemic perfusion is maintained. The endpoint in this situation is a return of ventricular function, with the expectation that following a few days of mechanical circulatory support the VAD(s) could be removed.

Reports describing the use of roller pumps to support patients with postcardiotomy ventricular dysfunction are dated and are mentioned primarily out of historical interest. In 1985, Litwak and associates reported the use of roller pump left-atrial-to-aortic-bypass in 27 patients who could not be weaned from cardiopulmonary bypass.[47] Eighteen patients (67 per cent) were separated from the device, and nine patients (33 per cent) were discharged from the hospital. Seven of the nine patients were alive and well at the time of the report, the longest survivor having been

observed for more than a decade. Also in 1985, Rose and coworkers described left-atrial-to-aortic bypass in 46 patients with refractory postoperative cardiac failure.[48] Twenty-one patients (46 per cent) were weaned from the device. Five patients died within 90 days of device removal, with two additional deaths occurring 4 months and 4 years postoperatively. Of the 16 long-term survivors, who were observed for 6 to 54 months, 14 had excellent cardiac function, with 13 patients being in NYHA functional Class I or II. These excellent results, reported more than a decade ago, compare favorably with recent reports using more advanced forms of mechanical blood pumps.

The results achieved with centrifugal blood pump support for postcardiotomy cardiogenic shock are summarized in Table 19–5. The Combined Registry for the Clinical Use of Mechanical Ventricular Assist Devices and the Total Artificial Heart was developed in 1988 under the auspices of the International Society for Heart Transplantation and the American Society for Artificial Internal Organs.[5] Investigators from 70 centers worldwide voluntarily submit data to this registry. Although the registry gathers data from patients who receive support with either a centrifugal or pulsatile VAD, only patients who received centrifugal blood pump support are recorded in Table 19–5.

To summarize lessons learned from the use of centrifugal blood pumps in the management of postcardiotomy cardiogenic shock: Approximately 58 per cent of patients require left ventricular assistance alone, 15 per cent require right ventricular assistance alone, and 27 per cent require biventricular assistance.[52,76–79] The duration of support is brief, varying between 1.7 and 3.6 days.[52,76–78] In general, lower survival is associated with biventricular failure,[78] renal failure,[78] and age over 64 years.[76] Registry data show no significant difference in weaning from support or hospital discharge rates between the groups of patients supported with a pneumatic pulsatile device and those supported with a nonpulsatile centrifugal blood pump.[5] The Registry combines data from patients supported with centrifugal and pulsatile blood pumps, but supports the conclusion that advanced age (greater than 70 years) negatively affects patient survival.

Paracorporeal pulsatile VADs are ideally suited to provide circulatory support for patients with postcardiotomy cardiogenic shock, as they are designed to provide either left or right ventricular assistance, and they do not require left ventricular apex cannulation for left heart support. Results achieved with pulsatile blood pump support for postcardiotomy cardiogenic shock are summarized in Table 19–6 and are similar to those achieved with centrifugal blood pumps. Approximately 49 per cent of patients re-

TABLE 19–6   RESULTS OF PULSATILE VAD SUPPORT FOR POSTCARDIOTOMY CARDIOGENIC SHOCK

AUTHOR	DEVICE	NO. PATIENTS	WEANED (%)	SURVIVED (%)
Gray and Champsauer[55]	Abiomed BVS 5000	211	87 (41)	N/A
Guyton[56]	Abiomed BVS 5000	31	17 (55)	9 (29)
Pennington[80]	Thoratec	30	15 (50)	11 (37)
Farrar[81]	Thoratec	123	47 (38)	27 (22)
Registry[5]	Pneumatic	272	117 (43)	57 (21)

VAD = Ventricular assist device.

TABLE 19–7   RESULTS OF VAD SUPPORT AS A BRIDGE TO CARDIAC TRANSPLANTATION

AUTHOR	DEVICE	NO. PATIENTS	TRANSPLANTED (%)	SURVIVED (%)
McBride[83]	Centrifugal	77	56 (73)	36 (47)
Gray and Champsauer[55]	Abiomed BVS 5000	94	66 (70)	39 (41)
Hill[84]	Thoratec	300	187/287 (65)	159/287 (55)
Kormos[85]	Novacor N-100	43	30 (70)	28 (65)
Myers and Macris[60]*	Heartmate 1000 IP	39	21/33 (64)	19/33 (58)
Burton[59]	Heartmate 1000 IP	11	9 (82)	9 (82)

VAD = Ventricular assist device.
* Includes 7 VE LVAS patients.

quire left ventricular assistance alone, 7 per cent require right ventricular assistance alone, and 44 per cent require biventricular assistance.[55,56,80,81] The mean duration of support varied between 3.6 days and 4 days.[55,80] Survival was negatively influenced by presupport cardiac arrest events,[56] myocardial infarction, and renal failure.[80] Although an overall salvage rate of 25 per cent seems low, it must be understood that without mechanical circulatory support patients with refractory postcardiotomy cardiogenic shock would die. More importantly, 82 per cent of Registry patients who survived to hospital discharge were alive at 2 years (including both centrifugal and pulsatile blood pump patients)[5]; 86 per cent of those patients were in NYHA functional Class I or II.

ADJUNCT TO CARDIAC TRANSPLANTATION. With the introduction of cyclosporine-based immunosuppressive regimens and the resurgence of interest in cardiac transplantation in the early 1980's, a second patient population was identified who could potentially benefit from mechanical ventricular assistance. The number of patients with end-stage cardiomyopathy quickly exceeded the number of donor hearts available. The list of approved cardiac transplant candidates grew, and the time a patient spent waiting for a donor heart increased. In 1993, 3775 potential cardiac transplant recipients were listed with the United Network for Organ Sharing (UNOS).[82] During the same year, 730 potential cardiac transplant recipients died while on the UNOS waiting list.[82] Cardiac transplant recipients in whom there is hemodynamic decompensation before availability of a donor heart are potential candidates for VAD implantation. The role of mechanical circulatory support in this clinical setting would be to maintain systemic perfusion and end-organ function until a donor heart was available.[83] The recipient's heart and VAD would be removed at the time of cardiac transplantation.

Results of mechanical blood pump support as a bridge to cardiac transplantation are summarized in Table 19–7. Although the time a cardiac transplant candidate will wait for a suitable donor heart varies with status, blood type, and weight, the average waiting time is a number of months and can be as long as 1 to 2 years. The average duration of support for the series summarized in Table 19–7 varied between 23 and 98 days.[55,59,60,84,85] Pulsatile devices, and in particular implantable VADs, are designed to provide long-term support; 54 per cent of patients who receive support with a pulsatile device survive to hospital discharge following cardiac transplantation.[55,59,60,84,85] Some would question the wisdom of allocating hearts to this critically ill patient population, when the 1-year survival following conventional heart transplantation now exceeds 80 per cent.[86] Interestingly, 87 per cent of patients who receive VAD support, and are successfully transplanted, will survive to hospital discharge.[59,60,84,85] Thereafter, the clinical course of patients requiring interim circulatory support prior to cardiac transplantation parallels the course of patients who undergo conventional cardiac transplantation. All VAD patients are in NYHA functional Class IV at the time of implantation. Following transplantation the majority of patients return to NYHA functional Class I.[58] One- and two-year actuarial survival following transplantation averages 80 to 100 per cent.[60,84,85]

The benefits of an extended period of VAD support are well defined. Patients undergo vigorous nutritional and physical rehabilitation.[87] Exercise tolerance and end-organ dysfunction improve.[88–90] The vented electric version of the ThermoCardiosystems HeartMate has recently entered a clinical trial.[73] Although this device is still intended to serve as a bridge to cardiac transplantation, the protocol was amended to allow patients enrolled in this trial to be discharged from the hospital. The first four patients have been able to manage the system at home without assistance from medical or engineering personnel. Tether-free device function in an outpatient setting represents a dramatic improvement in quality of life[91,92] and health care economics.[3]

Mechanical circulatory support has been employed in two additional subpopulations of patients requiring cardiac transplantation—both following donor heart implantation. According to the Registry, 40 patients have been treated with circulatory support during a rejection episode complicated by hemodynamic compromise.[93] Only 23 patients (58 per cent) underwent a second cardiac transplant. Eight of the 23 patients (35 per cent) were discharged from the hospital. This represents an absolute salvage rate of 20 per cent. Sixty-eight other post-transplant patients suffered from presumed reversible cardiogenic shock unrelated to rejection.[93] VAD support in this patient population resulted in an absolute salvage rate of 19 per cent, statistically *equal* to the survival rate when ventricular assistance was employed in patients with postcardiotomy cardiogenic shock after other types of procedures.

ACUTE MYOCARDIAL INFARCTION. Patients in cardiogenic shock following acute myocardial infarction treated with mechanical circulatory support alone have a mortality rate of 80 per cent, the same as patients treated medically.[94] However, ventricular assistance may stabilize the patient's condition to allow cardiac catheterization and emergent revascularization. Mortality in certain subsets of patients may be reduced to 40 per cent.[94] Poor results with this patient population, however, leave the role for mechanical circulatory support in this clinical setting less well defined.

Complications Associated with VAD Use

Hemorrhage occurs in 27 to 87 per cent of patients who require mechanical ventricular assistance[5,76–78,83,95] and is related to hematologic abnormalities associated with prolonged cardiopulmonary bypass in postcardiotomy cardiogenic shock patients, and to platelet activation and disseminated intravascular coagulation secondary to blood-biomaterial interaction.[96] Stasis of blood within the blood pump and inadequate anticoagulation, however, may lead to thrombus deposition.[97] Thromboembolic complications occur in 9 to 44 per cent of patients,[5,76,78,83] although device-related thromboembolic events in patients supported with the HeartMate occur infrequently.[58,60,61,98] Multisystem organ failure is usually related to preimplantation end-organ hypoperfusion, but may be exacerbated by postimplantation low-flow states. Significant renal and hepatic dysfunction occur in 15 to 47 per cent of patients.[5,76,78,83,95] The degree to which pre-existing end-organ dysfunction is reversible is unknown. Following left VAD insertion, systemic hypoperfusion is most often related to right ventricular failure and inadequate left VAD filling.[99,100] Rapid recognition of profound right ventricular dysfunction and implantation of a right VAD may reduce the incidence of this lethal complication. Infection occurs in 7 to 25 per cent of patients and is attributable to prolonged hospitalization, indwelling lines and catheters, and percutaneous cannulas or drive lines.[5,76,77,83,95,101]

In a group of 965 patients supported with an external VAD for postcardiotomy cardiogenic shock, univariant analysis indicated that bleeding, renal and biventricular failure, systemic arterial desaturation secondary to an unrecognized patent foramen ovale, and inadequate cardiac output were associated with inability to wean a patient from mechanical circulatory support regardless of type of VAD employed.[93] From 27 to 45 per cent of patients who require a VAD as a bridge to cardiac transplantation develop a complication that precludes subsequent heart transplant.[102] Stepwise logistic regression analysis of data gathered from 544 patients who received mechanical circulatory support in conjunction with cardiac transplantation indicated, in decreasing order of importance, that bleeding, neurologic events, and biventricular and renal failure had a significant negative effect on future cardiac transplantation.[93]

Management Considerations

POSTCARDIOTOMY CARDIOGENIC SHOCK. Patients who have preexisting ventricular dysfunction and who are at risk for intractable heart failure following an open heart procedure have a femoral arterial line placed before initiation of cardiopulmonary bypass. The presence of a femoral arterial line facilitates subsequent IAB insertion. Selected patients also undergo a cursory pretransplant evaluation. Of 965 postcardiotomy cardiogenic shock patients reported to the Registry for Mechanical Circulatory Support, 43 patients (4.5 per cent) were activated as potential cardiac transplant recipients when they developed device dependency and had no contraindication to transplant.[5]

Upon completion of the cardiac operation, acid-base balance and electrolyte abnormalities are corrected. A functional cardiac rhythm is restored utilizing temporary cardiac pacing, if necessary. A patient is considered a candidate for VAD insertion when he or she fulfills the hemodynamic criteria outlined in Table 19–1, has no contraindication to VAD insertion as outlined in Table 19–2, and cannot be weaned from cardiopulmonary bypass despite moderate inotropic support[103] and IAB counterpulsation. It is imperative that operative decision-making be performed rapidly, and VAD insertion undertaken expeditiously, to avoid the complications associated with prolonged cardiopulmonary bypass time.[104]

Standard cardiopulmonary bypass cannulas are employed for roller or centrifugal VAD support.[105] Custom-designed cannulas are utilized with pulsatile VADs. For left ventricular assistance, left atrial cannulation is preferred, as myocardium is spared, and decannulation following a return of ventricular function can be performed without cardiopulmonary bypass (see Fig. 19–6). With a left VAD in place, cardiopulmonary bypass is discontinued. Simultaneous monitoring of left and right atrial pressures aids in the distinction among inflow cannula obstruction, hypovole-

mia, and right ventricular failure, should left VAD filling be less than satisfactory (Table 19–8). Right ventricular failure can be managed with judicious volume loading and intravenous isoproterenol hydrochloride or prostaglandin E_1. Intractable right heart failure mandates insertion of a right VAD. The goal is to achieve a cardiac index >2.2 liters/min/m². The IAB may be left in place to impart a degree of pulsatility to nonpulsatile roller or centrifugal left ventricular assistance. To avoid septic complications, however, the IAB is usually withdrawn in the immediate postoperative period.

Postoperatively, abnormal coagulation studies are aggressively corrected with protamine sulfate and blood product administration. When mediastinal tube drainage slows, anticoagulation is effected with continuous intravenous administration of heparin sodium. Sodium warfarin is not usually employed as the time course for ventricular recovery is measured in days. Various weaning protocols have been employed.[47,106] In general, ventricular support is periodically decreased to assess a patient's native ventricular function. This can be accomplished with Swan-Ganz catheter measurements of cardiac output, or observations of wall motion using transesophageal echocardiography,[107] or radionuclide imaging.[108] When ventricular recovery is complete, the patient is returned to the operating room for device explantation. Management is conventional thereafter.

BRIDGE TO CARDIAC TRANSPLANTATION. To be considered for mechanical circulatory support before cardiac transplantation, patients must not only fulfill VAD selection criteria but must also meet cardiac transplant selection and exclusion criteria (Chap. 18). When investigators were bound by clinical trial protocols, VAD implantation was often performed as a salvage procedure on an urgent or emergent basis. In the authors' opinion, prospective transplant recipients whose condition deteriorates to the point where they require an IAB should be considered for VAD insertion in the next 48 to 72 hours. VAD implantation can be accomplished on a semi-elective basis and the patient rehabilitated, rather than endure a prolonged debilitating intensive care unit admission.

Pulsatile devices are most frequently employed in this clinical setting. Implantation techniques are highly specialized, but well documented.[62,69,106] Cardiopulmonary bypass times are often brief, but postoperative bleeding can be troublesome. Consideration should be given to the use of aprotinin.[109] However, sensitization to aprotinin does occur; it may be prudent to use aminocaproic acid at the first operation, reserving aprotinin for VAD explantation and cardiac transplantation. Management of right ventricular failure in the presence of a pulsatile VAD can be problematic. Should a right VAD be necessary, device selection is limited. The versatile Thoratec device can be employed for either right- or left-sided support.[64] If an implantable device is employed on the left, right ventricular support can be provided only with a hybrid pump configuration utilizing a paracorporeal Thoratec VAD or nonpulsatile blood pump.

Postoperatively the patient should be rapidly extubated and all invasive monitoring lines removed as soon as medically allowed, to avoid nosocomial infection.[101] Fastidious cannula–drive line care will delay tract colonization.[110]

TABLE 19–8 HEMODYNAMIC STATUS DURING MECHANICAL LEFT VENTRICULAR ASSISTANCE

CVP (mm Hg)	LAP (mm Hg)	SYSTOLIC AoP (mm Hg)	CI (liters/min/m²)	DIAGNOSIS
15–20	< 15	> 90	> 2.0	Satisfactory pumping
< 15	< 15	< 90	< 2.0	Hypovolemia
15–20	> 20	< 90	< 2.0	Inlet cannula obstruction
> 20	< 15	< 90	< 2.0	Right ventricular failure

CVP = Central venous pressure; LAP = left atrial pressure; AoP = aortic pressure; CI = cardiac output index.

Blood transfusions should be minimized and only leukode-pleted blood administered. Interval panel reactive antibody determinations will detect the presence of preformed anti-bodies to human lymphocyte antigens and determine the need for a prospective crossmatch with the cardiac donor. Aggressive nutritional and physical rehabilitation will pre-pare the patient for the subsequent cardiac transplant.[87,92] It is probably wise to delay cardiac transplantation for 2 to 4 weeks following VAD insertion to allow time for end-organ recovery.[89,90] The VAD is explanted at the time of recipient cardiectomy.

TOTAL ARTIFICIAL HEART

The total artificial heart (TAH) is a biventricular device capable of supporting both the pulmonary and systemic circulations. It is implanted within the patient's pericar-dium (orthotopic position) in a manner very similar to donor heart implantation at the time of cardiac transplanta-tion. The TAH must be compact and possess a control system capable of balancing the output of the two pros-thetic ventricles, while varying cardiac output with physio-logic need.

Pneumatic Total Artificial Heart

At least 11 different TAHs have been employed clinically worldwide (Fig. 19–8).[111] All possess similar design charac-teristics. Each prosthetic ventricle contains a flexible blood sac that is housed in a rigid case. Air pulses, generated by a bedside drive unit, are transmitted through small-diame-ter percutaneous drive lines and periodically compress the flexible blood sacs. Inlet and outlet valves ensure a unidi-rectional flow of blood through the prosthetic ventricle. Cardiac output and output balance between the ventricles are achieved with a sophisticated control system. A manual fixed-rate control system functions using the Starling mechanism. The prosthetic ventricles completely empty during systole, but heart rate and diastolic fill time are modified to limit diastolic filling. Any increase in preload

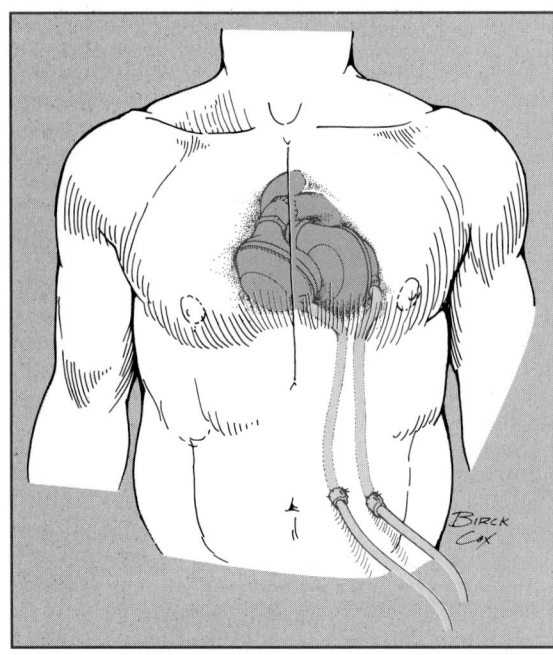

FIGURE 19–8. The pneumatic artificial heart is a biventricular de-vice that is positioned within the patient's pericardium. Small-diame-ter percutaneous drive lines traverse the skin in the left subcostal region. (From Richenbacher, W. E., Pennock, J. L., Pae, W. E., and Pierce, W. S.: Artificial heart implantation for end-stage cardiac dis-ease. J. Cardiovasc. Surg. 1:3, 1986.)

results in more complete ventricular filling, a higher stroke volume, and increased cardiac output. An automatic con-trol system employs two negative feedback servomecha-nisms.[112] The left ventricle pumps a full stroke with each beat, varying the rate to maintain systemic pressure within normal limits. The right ventricular beat rate varies to maintain a left atrial pressure of 5 to 12 mm Hg.

TAH implantation is carried out using cardiopulmonary bypass, with bicaval venous and aortic cannulation.[113,114] The patient's heart is excised by transecting the great ves-sels just distal to the semilunar valves, and the atria along the atrioventricular groove. Prosthetic atrial cuffs are su-tured to the atrial remnants. Vascular grafts are anasto-mosed to the aorta and pulmonary artery. The prosthetic ventricles are attached to the atrial cuffs and outlet grafts with snap-on quick connects or a threaded union nut. The ventricles are de-aired, pumping initiated, and cardiopul-monary bypass discontinued.

The pneumatic TAH has been employed extensively as a mechanical bridge to transplantation. Patient selection cri-teria are identical to those outlined in the VAD section. The sole exception is patient size. Patients must weigh at least 150 pounds and have an adequate anteroposterior thoracic dimension to avoid atrial compression and inflow obstruction at the time of sternal closure.[115] A recent Regis-try report includes 189 patients who received TAH support as a bridge to cardiac transplantation[93]: 135 patients (71.4 per cent) underwent transplantation and 67 patients (49.6 per cent) were discharged from the hospital. Transplanta-tion rates were statistically equal regardless of whether the patient was supported with a right or left VAD, two VADs, or the TAH.[93] However, there was a highly statistically sig-nificant difference in outcome, with the best outcome ob-tained with univentricular support and least favorable out-come with the TAH. The only pneumatic TAH still employed as a bridge to transplantation under an investiga-tional device exemption in the United States is the Cardio-West (Jarvik) Artificial Heart (CardioWest, Tucson, AZ).[116] Between January 1990 and December 1994, the CardioWest TAH was implanted in 49 patients.[116] Follow-up was avail-able in 46 patients, 17 (37 per cent) of whom were long-term survivors following cardiac transplantation.

Of historical interest, four patients received the Jarvik-7-100 TAH under an FDA-approved protocol, as a permanent form of circulatory replacement.[117] The longest-term survi-vor lived for 620 days, and all four patients succumbed to hematological, thromboembolic, and infectious complica-tions. Currently, infectious complications secondary to per-cutaneous drive lines, and life style issues related to the requisite bulky external drive unit, preclude the use of pneumatic TAHs as a permanent form of circulatory sup-port. Although the TAH can provide safe and effective he-modynamic support to a patient before transplant, the TAH is more expensive and technically more difficult to implant than a VAD. Furthermore, univentricular support will suf-fice in the majority of patients who require a mechanical bridge to cardiac transplantation. In the authors' opinion, transplant recipients in whom there is hemodynamic de-compensation prior to cardiac transplantation are best served by VAD insertion. The TAH, if available, should be reserved for selected patients with a postinfarction ventric-ular septal defect, valvular heart disease, or intractable ar-rhythmias.

Electric Total Artificial Heart

When available for clinical use, the electric TAH will serve as a readily available cardiac replacement for patients with irreparable acute or chronic heart failure. The electric TAH is being designed for permanent use and, as such, will be completely implantable. Size constraints represent the most significant hurdle to device development. Two blood pumps are located within the pericardium, and un-

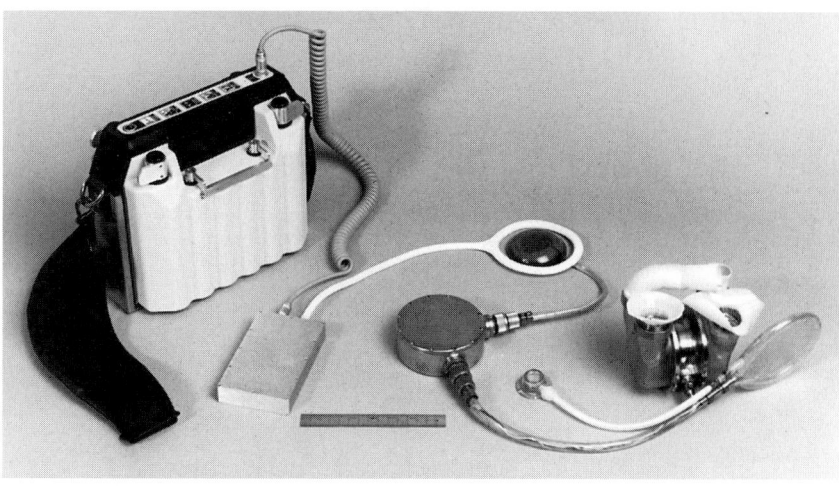

FIGURE 19–9. The electric motor-driven artificial heart being developed at Pennsylvania State University. Components from *left* to *right*: portable external electronics and battery pack with superficial primary transcutaneous energy transmission coil *(white ring)*, circular can containing control electronics and back-up battery connected to the subcutaneous secondary transcutaneous energy transmission coil (beneath the white primary coil), subcutaneous access port, artificial heart containing two prosthetic ventricles, and interposed energy converter, compliance chamber.

like the pneumatic TAH that employs a separate external drive unit for each ventricle, the electric TAH uses a single implantable energy converter to drive both ventricles, greatly increasing the complexity of device control. The electric TAH has a minimum energy requirement of 14 watts. Implantable batteries cannot provide the power required. Thus, currently available electric TAHs will rely on an external power source and transcutaneous energy transmission, with a small rechargeable implantable back-up battery capable of serving as a power source for 30 to 60 minutes. In the future, higher-energy density batteries may reduce or eliminate the need for a primary external power source altogether.[118,119]

Three research teams consisting of both a medical and industrial partner are currently developing an electric TAH under a contract program established by the National Heart, Lung, and Blood Institute in 1988.[120] The Abiomed/Texas Heart Institute TAH (Abiomed, Inc., Danvers, MA) is an electrohydraulically actuated device capable of providing cardiac output in excess of 10 liters/min.[121] An atrial flow balancing chamber is used to control the left-right blood flow balance.[122] Animal implantation has begun only recently, with survival exceeding 3 months.[123]

The Cleveland Clinic Foundation/Nimbus TAH (Nimbus, Inc., Rancho Cordova, CA) employs an electrohydraulic energy converter[124] and biolized blood contacting surface.[125] The device has been implanted in 12 calves for up to 120 days.[125] Two embolic events were attributed to fungal infections in the outlet grafts, while the gelatin-coated pump surfaces were clean despite nonuse of anticoagulants or antiplatelet agents postoperatively.

The Pennsylvania State University/Sarns (Sarns/3M Health Care, Ann Arbor, MI) TAH employs a dual pusher plate roller screw energy converter (Fig. 19–9).[126] Left-right output balance is achieved with an implanted control algorithm that adjusts the left-pump diastolic fill time and speed of systole, to just barely allow complete left pump filling while maximizing pump rate.[112] The device, in its current design, has been implanted in 14 calves with survival times exceeding 3 months.[126] The investigators are prepared to embark on long-term device durability testing using a mock circulatory loop.[127] At the current rate of development, the electric TAH is expected to enter a clinical trial within the next 5 to 10 years.

Acknowledgment

The authors gratefully acknowledge the assistance of Phyllis B. Jones in the preparation of this manuscript.

REFERENCES

1. Gillum, R. F.: Epidemiology of heart failure in the United States. Am. Heart J. *126:*1042, 1993.

2. Ho, K. K. L., Anderson, K. M., Kannel, W. B., et al.: Survival after the onset of congestive heart failure in Framingham Heart Study subjects. Circulation *88:*107, 1993.

3. Poirier, V.: The economic burden of artificial hearts. *In* Nosé, Y., Kjellstrand, C., and Ivanovich, P. (eds.): Progress in Artificial Organs—1985. Cleveland, ISAO Press, 1986, p. 96.

4. Frazier, O. H.: Ventricular assistance: A perspective on the future. Heart Failure *10:*259, 1995.

5. Pae, W. E., Jr., Miller, C. A., Matthews, Y., and Pierce, W. S.: Ventricular assist devices for postcardiotomy cardiogenic shock. J. Thorac. Cardiovasc. Surg. *104:*541, 1992.

6. Clauss, R. H., Birtwell, W. C., Albertal, G., et al.: Assisted circulation: I. The arterial counterpulsator. J. Thorac. Cardiovasc. Surg. *41:*447, 1961.

7. Moulopoulos, S. D., Topaz, S., and Kolff, W. J.: Diastolic balloon pumping (with carbon dioxide) in the aorta—A mechanical assistance to the failing circulation. Am. Heart J. *63:*669, 1992.

8. Kantrowitz, A., Tjonneland, S., Freed, P. S., et al.: Initial clinical experience with intraaortic balloon pumping in cardiogenic shock. JAMA *203:*135, 1968.

9. Bregman, D., and Casarella, W. J.: Percutaneous intraaortic balloon pumping: Initial clinical experience. Ann. Thorac. Surg. *29:*153, 1980.

10. U.S.A. Market for Diagnostic and Interventional Catheters and Allied Vascular Devices. D & MD Reports. Southborough, International Business Communications, Inc., 1994, Exhibit #6–16, pp. 6–48.

11. Gibbon, J. H., Jr.: Application of a mechanical heart and lung apparatus to cardiac surgery. Minn. Med. *37:*171, 1954.

12. Dennis, C., Carlens, E., Senning, A., et al.: Clinical use of a cannula for left heart bypass without thoracotomy: Experimental protection against fibrillation by left heart bypass. Ann. Surg. *156:*623, 1962.

13. DeBakey, M. E.: Left ventricular bypass pump for cardiac assistance. Clinical experience. Am. J. Cardiol. *27:*3, 1971.

14. Pierce, W. S., Parr, G. V. S., Myers, J. L., et al.: Ventricular-assist pumping in patients with cardiogenic shock after cardiac operations. N. Engl. J. Med. *305:*1606, 1981.

15. Normal, J. C., Cooley, D. A., Kahan, B. D., et al.: Total support of the circulation of a patient with post-cardiotomy stone-heart syndrome by a partial artificial heart (ALVAD) for 5 days followed by heart and kidney transplantation. Lancet *1:*1125, 1978.

16. Reedy, J. E., Pennington, D. G., Miller, L. W., et al.: Status I heart transplant patients: Conventional versus ventricular assist device support. J. Heart Lung Transplant. *11:*246, 1992.

17. Akutsu, T., and Kolff, W. J.: Permanent substitutes for valves and hearts. Trans. Am. Soc. Artif. Intern. Organs *4:*230, 1958.

18. Nosé Y., Topaz, S., SenGupta, A., et al.: Artificial hearts inside the pericardial sac in calves. Trans. Am. Soc. Artif. Intern. Organs. *11:*255, 1965.

19. Klain, M., Mrava, G. L., Tajima, K., et al.: Can we achieve over 100 hours' survival with a total mechanical heart? Trans. Am. Soc. Artif. Intern. Organ. *17:*437, 1971.

20. Cooley, D. A., Liotta, D., Hallman, G. L., et al.: Orthotopic cardiac prosthesis for two-staged cardiac replacement. Am. J. Cardiol. *24:*723, 1969.

21. Joyce, L. D., DeBries, W. C., Hastings, W. L., et al.: Response of the human body to the first permanent implant of the Jarvik-7 total artificial heart. Trans. Am. Soc. Artif. Intern. Organs *29:*81, 1983.

INTRAAORTIC BALLOON COUNTERPULSATION

22. Pae, W. E., Jr., and Pierce, W. S.: Intra-aortic balloon counterpulsation, ventricular assist pumping, and the artificial heart. *In* Baue, A. E., Geha, A. S., Hammond, G. L., et al. (eds.): Glenn's Thoracic and Cardiovascular Surgery. East Norwalk, Conn., Appleton and Lange, 1991, p. 1585.

23. Allen, B. S., Rosenkranz, E., Buckberg, G. D., et al.: Studies on prolonged acute regional ischemia: VI. Myocardial infarction with left ventricular power failure: A medical/surgical emergency requiring urgent revascularization with maximal protection of remote muscle. J. Thorac. Cardiovasc. Surg. *98:*691, 1989.

24. Komeda, M., Fremes, S. E., and David, T. E.: Surgical repair of postinfarction ventricular septal defect. Circulation 82:IV-243, 1990.

25. Tepe, N. A., and Edmunds, L. H., Jr.: Operation for acute postinfarction mitral insufficiency and cardiogenic shock. J. Thorac. Cardiovasc. Surg. 89:525, 1985.

26. Naunheim, K. S., Swartz, M. T., Pennington, D. G., et al.: Intraaortic balloon pumping in patients requiring cardiac operations. Risk analysis and long-term follow-up. J. Thorac. Cardiovasc. Surg. 104:1654, 1992.

27. Peric, M., Frazier, O. H., Macris, M., and Radovancevic, B.: Intra-aortic balloon pump as a bridge to transplantation. J. Heart Transplant. 5:380, 1986.

28. Birovljev, S., Radovancevic, B., Burnett, C. M., et al.: Heart transplantation after mechanical circulatory support: Four years' experience. J. Heart Lung Transplant. 11:240, 1992.

29. Levine, F. H., Gold, H. K., Leinbach, R. C., et al.: Management of acute myocardial ischemia with intraaortic balloon pumping and coronary bypass surgery. Circulation 58:(suppl. I):69, 1978.

30. Bardet, J., Rigaud, M., Kahn, J. C., et al.: Treatment of post-myocardial infarction angina by intra-aortic balloon pumping and emergency revascularization. J. Thorac. Cardiovasc. Surg. 74:299, 1977.

31. Hanson, E. C., Levine, F. H., Kay, H. R., et al.: Control of postinfarction ventricular irritability with the intraaortic balloon pump. Circulation 62:(Suppl. I):130, 1980.

32. Bregman, D., and Kaskel, P.: Advances in percutaneous intra-aortic balloon pumping. Crit. Care Clin. 2:221, 1986.

33. McGeehin, W., Sheikh, F., Donahoo, J. S., et al.: Transthoracic intraaortic balloon pump support: Experience in 39 patients. Ann. Thorac. Surg. 44:26, 1987.

34. Rubenstein, R. B., and Karhade, N.V.: Supraclavicular subclavian technique of intra-aortic balloon insertion. J. Vasc. Surg. 1:577, 1984.

35. Buchanan, S. A., Langenburg, S. E., Mauney, M. C., et al.: Ambulatory intraaortic balloon counterpulsation. Ann. Thorac. Surg. 58:1547, 1994.

36. Krause, A. H., Jr., Bigelow, J. C., and Page, U. S.: Transthoracic intraaortic balloon cannulation to avoid repeat sternotomy for removal. Ann. Thorac. Surg. 21:562, 1976.

37. Richenbacher, W. E., and Pierce, W. S.: Management of complications of intraaortic balloon counterpulsation. In Waldhausen, J. A., and Orringer, M. B. (eds.): Complications in Cardiothoracic Surgery. St. Louis, Mosby-Year Book, Inc., 1991, p. 97.

38. Iverson, L. I. G., Herfindahl, G., Ecker, R. R., et al.: Vascular complications of intraaortic balloon counterpulsation. Am. J. Surg. 154:99, 1987.

39. Gottlieb, S. O., Brinker, J. A., Borkon, A. M., et al.: Identification of patients at high risk for complications of intraoartic balloon counterpulsation: A multivariate risk factor analysis. Am. J. Cardiol. 53:1135, 1984.

40. Shahian, D. M., Neptune, W. B., Ellis, F. H., Jr., and Maggs, P. R.: Intraaortic balloon pump morbidity: A comparative analysis of risk factors between percutaneous and surgical techniques. Ann. Thorac. Surg. 36:644, 1983.

41. Gol, M. K., Bayazit, M., Emir, M., et al.: Vascular complications related to percutaneous insertion of intraaortic balloon pumps. Ann. Thorac. Surg. 58:1476, 1994.

42. Friedell, M. L., Alpert, J., Parsonnet, V., et al.: Femorofemoral grafts for lower limb ischemia caused by intra-aortic balloon pump. J. Vasc. Surg. 5:180, 1987.

THE VENTRICULAR ASSIST DEVICE

43. Lohmann, D. P., Swartz, M. T., Pennington, D. G., et al.: Left ventricular versus left atrial cannulation for the Thoratec ventricular assist device. Trans. Am. Soc. Artif. Intern. Organs 36:M545, 1990.

44. Cohen, D. J., Kress, D. C., Swanson, D. K., et al.: Effect of cannulation site on the primary determinants of myocardial oxygen consumption during left heart bypass. J. Surg. Res. 47:159, 1989.

45. Rahmoeller, G. A.: FDA requirements for clinical approval of left ventricular assist devices. In Attar, S. (ed.): New Developments in Cardiac Assist Devices. New York, Praeger Publishers, 1985, p. 36.

46. Kessler, D. A.: Hastings lecture, December 10, 1993, Rockville, Maryland, USA. Artif. Organs 18:718, 1994.

47. Litwak, R. S., Koffsky, R. M., Jurado, R. A., et al.: A decade of experience with a left heart assist device in patients undergoing open intracardiac operation. World J. Surg. 9:18, 1985.

48. Rose, D. M., Laschinger, J., Grossi, E., et al.: Experimental and clinical results with a simplified left heart assist device for treatment of profound left ventricular dysfunction. World J. Surg. 9:11, 1985.

49. Oku, T., Harasaki, H., Smith, W., and Nosé, Y.: Hemolysis: A comparative study of four nonpulsatile pumps. Trans. Am. Soc. Artif. Intern. Organs 34:500, 1988.

50. Noon, G. P., Kane, L. E., Feldman, L., et al.: Reduction of blood trauma in roller pumps for long-term perfusion. World J. Surg. 9:65, 1985.

51. Magovern, G. J., Jr.: The Biopump and postoperative circulatory support. Ann. Thorac. Surg. 55:245, 1993.

52. Curtis, J. J.: Centrifugal mechanical assist for postcardiotomy ventricular failure. Semin. Thorac. Cardiovasc. Surg. 6:140, 1994.

53. Nishinaka, T., Nishida, H., Endo, M., and Koyanagi, H.: Less platelet damage in the curved vane centrifugal pump: A comparative study with the roller pump in open heart surgery. Artif. Organs 18:687, 1994.

54. Morin, B. J., and Riley, J. B.: Thrombus formation in centrifugal pumps. J. Extra-Corporeal Technol. 24:20, 1992.

55. Gray, L. A., Jr., and Champsaur, G. G.: The BVS 5000 biventricular assist device. The worldwide registry experience. ASAIO H 40:M460, 1994.

56. Guyton, R. A., Schonberger, J. P. A. M., Everts, P. A. M., et al.: Postcardiotomy shock: Clinical evaluation of the BVS 5000 biventricular support system. Ann. Thorac. Surg. 56:346, 1993.

57. Shook, B. J.: The Abiomed BVS 5000 biventricular support system. System description and clinical summary. Cardiac Surgery: State of the Art Reviews 7:309, 1993.

58. Frazier, O. H., Rose, E. A., Macmanus, Q., et al.: Multicenter clinical evaluation of the HeartMate 1000 IP left ventricular assist device. Ann. Thorac. Surg. 53:1080, 1992.

59. Burton, N. A., Lefrak, E. A., Macmanus, Q., et al.: A reliable bridge to cardiac transplantation: The TCI left ventricular assist device. Ann. Thorac. Surg. 55:1425, 1993.

60. Myers, T. J., and Macris, M. P.: Clinical experience with the HeartMate left ventricular assist device. Heart Failure 10:247, 1995.

61. Rose, E. A., Levin, H. R., Oz, M. C., et al.: Artificial circulatory support with textured interior surfaces. A counterintuitive approach to minimizing thromboembolism. Circulation 90:II-87, 1994.

62. McCarthy, P. M., Wang, N., and Vargo, R.: Preperitoneal insertion of the HeartMate 1000 IP implantable left ventricular assist device. Ann. Thorac. Surg. 57:634, 1994.

63. Farrar, D. J., Lawson, J. H., Litwak, P., and Cedarwall, G.: Thoratec VAD system as a bridge to heart transplantation. J. Heart Transplant. 9:415, 1990.

64. Farrar, D. J., and Hill, J. D.: Univentricular and biventricular Thoratec VAD support as a bridge to transplantation. Ann. Thorac. Surg. 55:276, 1993.

65. Holman, W. L., Bourge, R. C., McGiffin, D. C., and Kirklin, J. K.: Ventricular assist: Experience with a pulsatile heterotopic device. Semin. Thorac. Cardiovasc. Surg. 6:147, 1994.

66. Weiss, W. J., Rosenberg, G., Snyder, A. J., et al.: In vivo performance of a transcutaneous energy transmission system with the Penn State motor driven ventricular assist device. Trans. Am. Soc. Artif. Intern. Organs 35:284, 1989.

67. Wisman, C. B., Rosenberg, G., Weiss, W. J., et al.: Development and successful application of an intrathoracic compliance chamber for the implantable electric motor-driven ventricular-assist pump. Surg. Forum 34:253, 1983.

68. Starnes, V. A., Oyer, P. E., Portner, P. M., et al.: Isolated left ventricular assist as bridge to cardiac transplantation. J. Thorac. Cardiovasc. Surg. 96:62, 1988.

69. Pennington, D. G., McBride, L. R., and Swartz, M. T.: Implantation technique for the Novacor left ventricular assist system. J. Thorac. Cardiovasc. Surg. 108:604, 1994.

70. Loisance, D. Y., Deleuze, P. H., Mazzucotelli, J. P., et al.: Clinical implantation of the wearable Baxter Novacor ventricular assist system. Ann. Thorac. Surg. 58:551, 1994.

71. Miller, P. J., Billich, T. J., LaForge, D. H., et al.: Initial clinical experience with a wearable controller for the Novacor left ventricular assist system. ASAIO J. 40:M465, 1994.

72. Frazier, O. H.: Chronic left ventricular support with a vented electric assist device. Ann. Thorac. Surg. 55:273, 1993.

73. Myers, T. J., Dasse, K. A., Macris, M. P., et al.: Use of a left ventricular assist device in an outpatient setting. ASAIO J. 40:M471, 1994.

74. Pierce, W. S., Snyder, A. J., Rosenberg, G., et al.: A long-term ventricular assist system. J. Thorac. Cardiovasc. Surg. 105:520, 1993.

75. Weiss, W. J., Rosenberg, G., Snyder, A., et al.: Results of in vivo testing of a completely implanted ventricular assist device. Proceedings, Cardiovascular Science and Technology Conference. Arlington, Association for the Advancement of Medical Instrumentation, 1993, p. 154.

76. Killen, D. A., Piehler, J. M., Borkon, A. M., and Reed, W. A.: Bio-Medicus ventricular assist device for salvage of cardiac surgical patients. Ann. Thorac. Surg. 52:230, 1991.

77. Lee, W. A., Gillinov, A. M., Cameron, D. E., et al.: Centrifugal ventricular assist device for support of the failing heart after cardiac surgery. Crit. Care Med. 21:1186, 1993.

78. Golding, L. A. R., Crouch, R. D., Stewart, R. W., et al.: Postcardiotomy centrifugal mechanical ventricular support. Ann. Thorac. Surg. 54:1059, 1992.

79. Noon, G. P.: Bio-Medicus ventricular assistance. Ann. Thorac. Surg. 52:180, 1991.

80. Pennington, D. G., McBride, L. W., Swartz, M. T., et al.: Use of the Pierce-Donachy ventricular assist device in patients with cardiogenic shock after cardiac operations. Ann. Thorac. Surg. 47:130, 1989.

81. FDA panel recommends approval. Thoratec's Heartbeat 8.3:6, 1994.

82. United Network for Organ Sharing: Personal communication. 1995.

83. McBride, L. R.: Bridging to cardiac transplantation with external ventricular assist devices. Semin. Thorac. Cardiovasc. Surg. 6:169, 1994.

84. Hill, J. D., Farrar, D. J., and Thoratec VAD Principal Investigators: Multicenter clinical results with the Thoratec VAD system as a bridge to cardiac transplant. Proceedings, ASAIO Cardiovascular Science and Technology Conference. Boca Raton, The American Society for Artificial Internal Organs, 1994, p. 41.

85. Kormos, R. L., Pham, S. M., Hattler, B. G., and Griffith, B. P.: Evolution of bridge to cardiac transplantation from intermediate inpatient use to chronic outpatient care. Proceedings, ASAIO Cardiovascular Science and Technology Conference. Boca Raton, The American Society for Artificial Internal Organs, 1994, p. 41.

86. United Network for Organ Sharing. 1994 center specific report: Heart data. Overall survival rates. UNOS Update 11:24, 1995.

87. Vega, J. D., Poindexter, S. M., Radovancevic, B., et al.: Nutritional assessment of patients with extended left ventricular assist device support. Trans. Am. Soc. Artif. Intern. Organs *36*:M555, 1990.

88. Levin, H. R., Chen, J. M., Oz, M. C., et al.: Potential of left ventricular assist devices as outpatient therapy while awaiting transplantation. Ann. Thorac. Surg. *58*:1515, 1994.

89. Farrar, D. J., and Hill, J. D.: Recovery of major organ function in patients awaiting heart transplantation with Thoratec ventricular assist devices. J. Heart Lung Transplant. *13*:1125, 1994.

90. Burnett, C. M., Duncan, J. M., Frazier, O. H., et al.: Improved multiorgan function after prolonged univentricular support. Ann. Thorac. Surg. *55*:65, 1993.

91. Dew, M. A., Kormos, R. L., Roth, L. H., et al.: Life quality in the era of bridging to cardiac transplantation. Bridge patients in an outpatient setting. ASAIO J. *39*:145, 1993.

92. Kormos, R. L., Murali, S., Dew, M. A., et al.: Chronic mechanical circulatory support: Rehabilitation, low morbidity, and superior survival. Ann. Thorac. Surg. *57*:51, 1994.

93. Pae, W. E., Jr.: Ventricular assist devices and total artificial hearts: A combined registry experience. Ann. Thorac. Surg. *55*:295, 1993.

94. Moritz, A., and Wolner, E.: Circulatory support with shock due to acute myocardial infarction. Ann. Thorac. Surg. *55*:238, 1993.

95. Oaks, T. E., Pae, W. E., Jr., Miller, C. A., and Pierce, W. S.: Combined registry for the clinical use of mechanical ventricular assist pumps and the total artificial heart in conjunction with heart transplantation. Fifth official report—1990. J. Heart Lung Transplant. *10*:621, 1991.

96. Bick, R. L.: Hemostasis defects associated with cardiac surgery, prosthetic devices, and other extracorporeal circuits. Semin. Thromb. Hemostas. *11*:249, 1985.

97. Copeland, J. G., III, Frazier, O. H., McBride, L. R., et al.: Panel II. Anticoagulation. Ann. Thorac. Surg. *55*:213, 1993.

98. McCarthy, P. M., James, K. B., Savage, R. M., et al.: Implantable left ventricular assist device. Approaching an alternative for end-stage heart failure. Circulation *90*(Suppl. II):83, 1994.

99. Fukuda, S., Takano, H., Taenaka, Y., et al.: Chronic effect of left ventricular assist pumping on right ventricular function. Trans. Am. Soc. Artif. Intern. Organs *34*:712, 1988.

100. Elbeery, J. R., Owen, C. H., Savitt, M. A., et al.: Effects of the left ventricular assist device on right ventricular function. J. Thorac. Cardiovasc. Surg. *99*:809, 1990.

101. Hill, J. D., Griffith, B. P., Meli, M., and Didisheim, P.: Panel III. Infections-prophylaxis and treatment. Ann. Thorac. Surg. *55*:217, 1993.

102. Richenbacher, W. E., and Pierce, W. S.: Management of complications of mechanical circulatory assistance. *In* Waldhausen, J. A., and Orringer, M. B. (eds.): Complications in Cardiothoracic Surgery. St. Louis, Mosby-Year Book, Inc., 1991, p. 103.

103. Emery, R. W., and Joyce, L. D.: Directions in cardiac assistance. J. Card. Surg. *6*:400, 1991.

104. Anstadt, M. P., Tedder, M., Hegde, S. S., et al.: Intraoperative timing may provide criteria for use of post-cardiotomy ventricular assist devices. ASAIO J. *38*:M147, 1992.

105. Magovern, G. J., Jr., Wampler, R. W., Joyce, L. D., and Wareing, T. H.: Nonpulsatile circulatory support: Techniques of insertion. Ann. Thorac. Surg. *55*:266, 1993.

106. Aufiero, T. X., and Pae, W. E., Jr.: Extracorporeal pneumatic ventricular assistance for postcardiotomy cardiogenic shock. Cardiac Surgery: State of the Art Reviews *7*:277, 1993.

107. Barzilai, B., Davila-Roman, V. G., Eaton, M. H., et al.: Transesophageal echocardiography predicts successful withdrawal of ventricular assist devices. J. Thorac. Cardiovasc. Surg. *104*:1410, 1992.

108. Sekela, M. E., Verani, M. S., and Noon, G. P.: Comparison of hemodynamics and ejection fraction during left heart bypass. Ann. Thorac. Surg. *51*:804, 1991.

109. Pae, W. E., Jr., Aufiero, T. X., Weldner, P. W., et al.: Aprotinin therapy for insertion of ventricular assist devices for staged heart transplantation. J. Heart Lung Transplant. *13*:811, 1994.

110. Hravnak, M., George, E., and Kormos, R. L.: Management of chronic left ventricular assist device percutaneous lead insertion sites. J. Heart Lung Transplant. *12*:856, 1993.

THE ARTIFICIAL HEART

111. Johnson, K. E., Prieto, M., Joyce, L. D., et al.: World experience with total artificial heart (TAH) implantation: A registry report. *In* Cardiovascular Science and Technology: Basic and Applied, II. Boston, Oxymoron Press, 1990, p. 32.

112. Snyder, A. J., Rosenberg, G., and Pierce, W. S.: Noninvasive control of cardiac output for alternately ejecting dual-pusherplate pumps. Artif. Organs *16*:189, 1992.

113. Richenbacher, W. E., Pennock J. L., Pae, W. E., Jr., and Pierce, W. S.: Artificial heart implantation for end-stage cardiac disease. J. Card. Surg. *1*:3, 1986.

114. DeVries, W. C.: Surgical technique for implantation of the Jarvik-7-100 total artificial heart. JAMA *259*:875, 1988.

115. Jarvik, R. K., DeVries, W. C., Semb, B. K. H., et al.: Surgical positioning of the Jarvik-7 artificial heart. J. Heart Transplant. *5*:184, 1986.

116. Arabia, F. A., Rosado, L. J., Sethi, G. K., et al.: CardioWest (Jarvik) artificial heart. Proceedings, ASAIO Cardiovascular Science and Technology Conference. Boca Raton, The American Society for Artificial Internal Organs, 1994, p. 42.

117. DeVries, W. C.: The permanent artificial heart. Four case reports. JAMA *259*:849, 1988.

118. Eisenberg, M.: High energy nickel-zinc batteries for LVAD applications. *In* Cardiovascular Science and Technology: Basic and Applied, II. Boston, Oxymoron Press, 1990, p. 273.

119. MacLean, G. K., Aiken, P. A., Adams, W. A., and Mussivand, T.: Comparison of rechargeable lithium and nickel/cadmium battery cells for implantable circulatory support devices. Artif. Organs *18*:331, 1994.

120. Sapirstein, J. S., Pae, W. E., Jr., Rosenberg, G., and Pierce, W. S.: The development of permanent circulatory support systems. Semin. Thorac. Cardiovasc. Surg. *6*:188, 1994.

121. Parnis, S. M., Yu, L. S., Ochs, B. D., et al.: Chronic in vivo evaluation of an electrohydraulic total artificial heart. ASAIO J. *40*:M489, 1994.

122. Kung, R. T. V., Yu, L. S., Ochs, B., et al.: An atrial hydraulic shunt in a total artificial heart. A balance mechanism for the bronchial shunt. ASAIO J. *39*:M213, 1993.

123. Kung, R. T. V., Yu, L. S., Ochs, B. D., et al.: Progress in the Abiomed total artificial heart. Proceedings, ASAIO Cardiovascular Science and Technology Conference. Boca Raton, The American Society for Artificial Internal Organs, 1994, p. 38.

124. Massiello, A., Kiraly, R., Butler, K., et al.: The Cleveland Clinic–Nimbus total artificial heart. Design and in vitro function. J. Thorac. Cardiovasc. Surg. *108*:412, 1994.

125. Harasaki, H., Fukamachi, K., Massiello, A., et al.: Progress in Cleveland Clinic–Nimbus total artificial heart development. ASAIO J. *40*:M494, 1994.

126. Snyder, A. J., Rosenberg, G., Weiss, W. J., et al. In vivo testing of a completely implanted total artificial heart system. ASAIO J. *39*:M177, 1993.

127. Weiss, W. J., Rosenberg, G., Snyder, A. J., et al.: Design improvements to the completely implantable Penn State total artificial heart. Proceedings, ASAIO Cardiovascular Science and Technology Conference. Boca Raton, The American Society for Artificial Organs, 1994, p. 38.

Chapter 20
Genesis of Cardiac Arrhythmias: Electrophysiological Considerations

DOUGLAS P. ZIPES

ANATOMY OF THE CARDIAC CONDUCTION SYSTEM

Sinus Node

In humans, the sinus node is a spindle-shaped structure composed of a fibrous tissue matrix with closely packed cells. It is 10 to 20 mm long, 2 to 3 mm wide, and thick, tending to narrow caudally toward the inferior vena cava. It lies less than 1 mm from the epicardial surface, laterally in the right atrial sulcus terminalis, at the junction of the superior vena cava and right atrium (Figs. 20–1 and 20–2). The artery supplying the sinus node branches from the right (55 to 60 per cent of the time) or the left circumflex (40 to 45 per cent) coronary artery, approaching the node from a clockwise or counterclockwise direction around the superior vena caval–right atrial junction.

CELLULAR STRUCTURE. Cell types in the sinus node include nodal cells, transitional cells, and atrial muscle cells. *Nodal cells,* also called "P cells," thought to be the source of normal impulse formation, are small (5 to 10 μm), ovoid, primitive-appearing cells with relatively few organelles, mitochondria, and myofibrils. They are grouped in elongated clusters located centrally in the sinus node. No transverse tubular system exists. Contact between nodal cells appears to occur via nexus connections.

TRANSITIONAL CELLS. Also known as "T cells," these are elongated cells intermediate in size and complexity between nodal cells and atrial muscle cells. T cells near nodal cells have simple intercellular connections, while more fully developed intercalated discs exist between T cells and atrial myocardium. Since nodal cells make contact only with each other or T cells, the latter may provide the only functional pathway for distribution of the sinus impulse formed in the nodal cells to the rest of the atrial myocardium.

ATRIAL MYOCARDIAL CELLS. These cells extend as peninsulas into the nodal boundaries, with overlapping zones of sinus and atrial cells most prominent on the nodal surface that abuts the crista terminalis.

GAP JUNCTIONS. Gap junctional channels (see p. 555) formed by connexin 45, 43, and 40, depending on the species and tissue type, electrically couple sinus node cells and probably account for their synchronized electrical activity.[1–3] Relative paucity and small size of gap junctions may account for slow conduction in the sinus node.[3] Few gap junctions may be required for frequency entrainment.[4] Although most gap junctions contain connexin 40, 43, and 45, the sinus and AV nodes are virtually devoid of connexin 43 but contain connexin 40 and connexin 45.[5–7] Abnormalities can cause arrhythmias.[8]

FUNCTION. Very probably no single cell in the sinus node serves as the pacemaker. Rather, sinus nodal cells function as electrically cou-

pled oscillators, discharging synchronously because of mutual entrainment. Thus, faster-discharging cells are slowed by cells firing more slowly, while they themselves are sped so that a "democratically derived" discharge rate occurs.[9] In humans, sinus rhythm may result from impulse origin at widely separated sites, creating two or three individual wavefronts that merge to form a single widely disseminated wavefront.[10] Modulated parasystole can occur.[9]

INNERVATION. The sinus node is richly innervated with postganglionic adrenergic and cholinergic nerve terminals.[11–16] Discrete vagal efferent pathways innervate both the sinus and atrioventricular (AV) regions of the dog and nonhuman primate. The concentration of norepinephrine is two to four times higher in atrial than in ventricular tissue in canine and guinea pig hearts. Although the sinus nodal region contains amounts of norepinephrine equivalent to those in other parts of the right atrium, acetylcholine, acetylcholinesterase, and choline acetyltransferase (the enzyme necessary for the synthesis of acetylcholine) have all been found in greatest concentration in the sinus node, with the next highest concentration in the right and then the left atrium. The concentration of acetylcholine in the ventricles is only 20 to 50 per cent of that in the atria.

Vagal stimulation, by releasing acetylcholine, slows sinus nodal discharge rate and prolongs intranodal conduction time, at times to the point of sinus nodal exit block. Acetylcholine increases and norepinephrine decreases refractoriness in the center of the sinus node. Adrenergic stimulation speeds sinus discharge rate. The phase (timing) in the cardiac cycle at which vagal discharge occurs and the background sympathetic tone importantly influence vagal effects on sinus rate and conduction (see below). Negative chronotropic effects of acetylcholine are due to inhibition of the hyperpolarization-activated pacemaker current i_f,[17–21] probably mediated by a G protein (see p. 372). Acetylcholine also activates the muscarinic m_2 receptor in the pacemaker cell, which in turn activates a specific G protein (G_K) that activates the K channel [I_K(Ach)], which also modulates discharge rate.[22] The m_2 receptor also inhibits adenylate cyclase via G_i to antagonize adrenergic effects on the sinus node. After cessation of vagal stimulation, sinus nodal automatically may accelerate transiently (postvagal tachycardia).

Internodal and Intraatrial Conduction

Whether impulses travel from the sinus to the AV node over preferentially conducting pathways has been contested. Anatomical evidence has been interpreted to indicate the presence of three intraatrial pathways. The *anterior internodal pathway* begins at the anterior margin of the sinus node and curves anteriorly around the superior vena cava to enter the anterior interatrial band, called *Bachmann's bundle.* This band continues to the left atrium, with the anterior internodal pathway entering the superior margin of the AV node. *Bachmann's bundle* is a large muscle bundle that appears to conduct the cardiac impulse preferentially from right to left atrium. The *middle interno-*

dal tract begins at the superior and posterior margins of the sinus node and travels behind the superior vena cava to the crest of the interatrial septum, descending in the interatrial septum to the superior margin of the AV node. The *posterior internodal tract* starts at the posterior margin of the sinus node and travels posteriorly around the superior vena cava and along the crista terminalis to the eustachian ridge and then into the interatrial septum above the coronary sinus, joining the posterior portion of the AV node. Some fibers from all three tracts bypass the crest of the AV node and enter its more distal segment. These groups of internodal tissue are best referred to as *internodal atrial myocardium*, not tracts, because they do not appear to be histologically discrete specialized tracts, only plain atrial myocardium.

The basis for specialized tracts stems from finding cell types in the atrium that differ electrophysiologically and anatomically, but it is not clear that these different cells are responsible for more rapid conduction velocity. Also, differential sensitivity of atrial fibers to potassium, giving rise to an apparent sinoventricular rhythm[23] (i.e., impulse propagation from the sinus node to the ventricle without activating atrial myocardium), and activation changes following localized surgical lesions designed to interrupt discrete pathways provide further functional data to support the presence of specialized tracts. However, the *weight of evidence does not support the presence of specialized internodal tracts resembling the bundle branches, i.e., discrete histologically identifiable tracts of tissue.*

Preferential internodal conduction, i.e., more rapid conduction velocity between the nodes in some parts of the atrium compared with other parts, does exist and may be due to fiber orientation, size, geometry, or other factors rather than to specialized tracts located between the nodes. Importantly, the atrial anterosuperior and posteroinferior inputs or approaches to the AV node may be the anatomical substrates comprising the fast and anterograde slow pathways of AV nodal reentry, the upper end of the retrograde fast pathway being located at the apex of Koch's triangle, near the His bundle, and the upper end of the anterograde pathway being located near the coronary sinus os.[24-26]

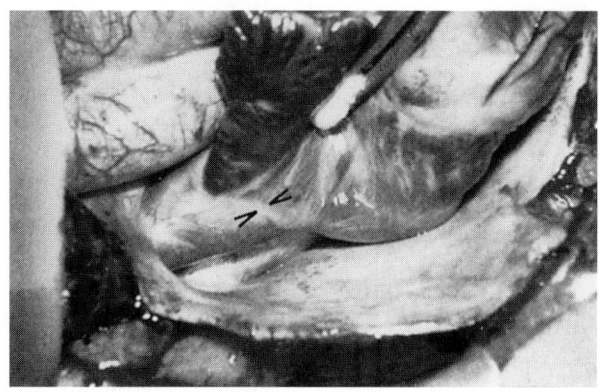

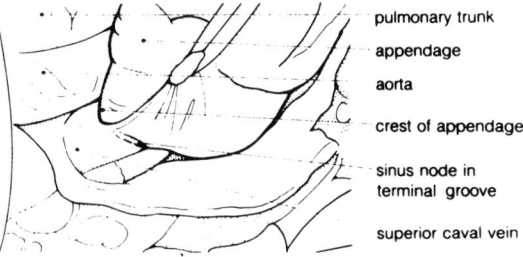

pulmonary trunk

appendage

aorta

crest of appendage

sinus node in terminal groove

superior caval vein

FIGURE 20–1. The human sinus node. This photograph, taken in the operating room, shows the location of the normal cigar-shaped sinus node along the lateral border of the terminal groove at the superior vena cava–atrial junction (arrowheads). (From Anderson, R. H., Wilcox, B. R., and Becker, A. E.: Anatomy of the normal heart. *In* Hurst, J. W., Anderson, R. H., Becker, A. E., and Wilcox, B. R. [eds.]: Atlas of the Heart. New York, Gower Medical Publishing, 1988, p. 1.2.)

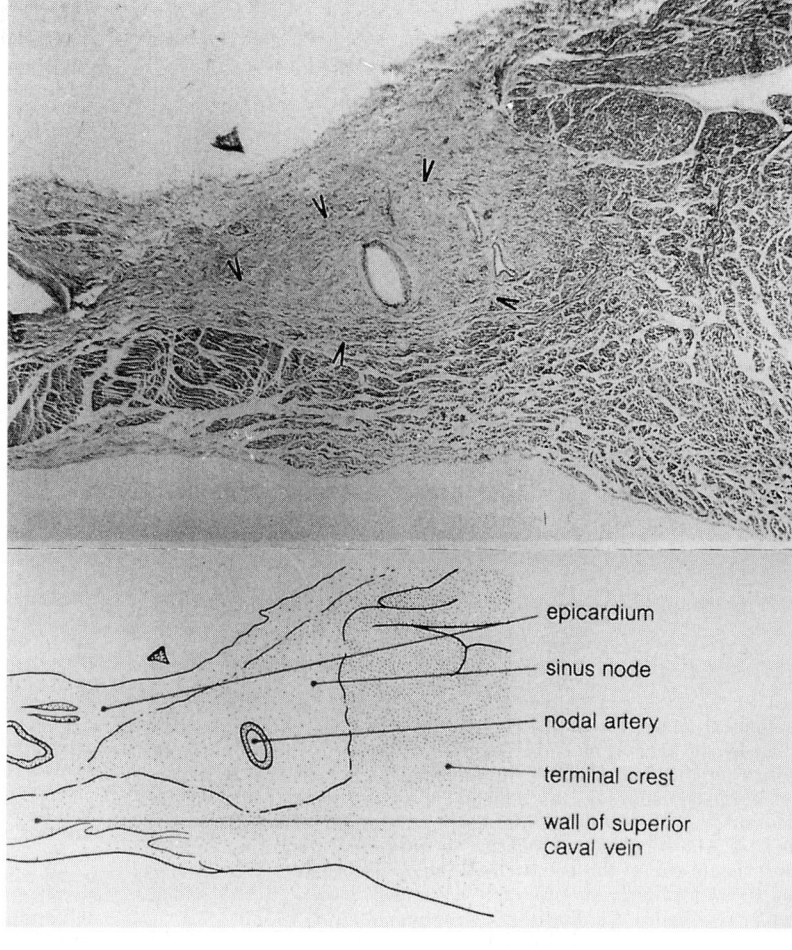

FIGURE 20–2. Histological section taken at right angles to the cigar-shaped sinus node shows how, in short axis, the node is a wedge-shaped structure located between the wall of the superior vena cava and the terminal crest. Discrete boundaries between the sinus node and atrial muscle are noted (arrowheads). The node is penetrated by the sinus nodal artery. (From Anderson, R. H., Wilcox, B. R., and Becker, A. E.: Anatomy of the normal heart. *In* Hurst, J. W., Anderson, R. H., Becker, A. E., and Wilcox, B. R. [eds.]: Atlas of the Heart. New York, Gower Medical Publishing, 1988, p. 1.2.)

epicardium

sinus node

nodal artery

terminal crest

wall of superior caval vein

The Atrioventricular Junctional Area and Intraventricular Conduction System

The normal AV junctional area (Figs. 20–3 and 20–4) can be divided into distinct regions: transitional cell zone, also called nodal approaches; compact portion, or the AV node itself; and the penetrating part of the AV bundle (His bundle), which continues as a nonbranching portion.

TRANSITIONAL CELL ZONE. In the rabbit AV node, the transitional cells or nodal approaches are located in posterior, superficial, and deep groups of cells. They differ histologically from atrial myocardium and connect the latter with the compact portion of the AV node. Some fibers may pass from the posterior internodal tract to the distal portion of the AV node or His bundle and provide the anatomical substrate for conduction to bypass AV nodal slowing. How-

ever, the importance of this structure is unclear (see p. 574).

THE AV NODE. The compact portion of the AV node is a superficial structure, lying just beneath the right atrial endocardium, anterior to the ostium of the coronary sinus, and directly above the insertion of the sepal leaflet of the tricuspid valve. It is at the apex of a triangle formed by the tricuspid annulus and the tendon of Todaro, which originates in the central fibrous body and passes posteriorly through the atrial septum to continue with the eustachian valve[24,25,27,28] (Figs. 20–3 and 20–4). The compact portion of the AV node is divided from and becomes the penetrating portion of the His bundle at the point where it enters the central fibrous body. In 85 to 90 per cent of human hearts, the arterial supply to the AV node is a branch from the right coronary artery that originates at the posterior intersection of the AV and interventricular grooves (crux). A branch of the circumflex coronary artery provides the AV nodal artery in the remaining hearts. Fibers in the lower part of the AV node may exhibit automatic impulse formation.

THE BUNDLE OF HIS, OR PENETRATING PORTION OF THE AV BUNDLE. This connects with the distal part of the compact AV node and perforates the central fibrous body, continuing through the annulus fibrosis, where it is called the nonbranching portion as it penetrates the membranous septum (Fig. 20–4). Proximal cells of the penetrating portion are heterogeneous, resembling those of the compact AV node, while distal cells are similar to cells in the proximal bundle branches. Connective tissue of the central fibrous body and membranous septum encloses the penetrating portion of the AV bundle, which may send out extensions into the central fibrous body.[24,25,27,28] However, large well-formed fasciculoventricular connections between the penetrating portion of the AV bundle and the ventricular septal crest are rarely found in adult hearts. Branches from the anterior and posterior descending coronary arteries supply the upper muscular interventricular septum with blood, making the conduction system at this site more impervious to ischemic damage unless the ischemia is extensive.

THE BUNDLE BRANCHES, OR BRANCHING PORTION OF THE AV BUNDLE. These structures begin at the superior margin of the muscular interventricular septum, immediately beneath the membranous septum, with the cells of the left bundle branch cascading downward as a continuous sheet onto the septum beneath the noncoronary aortic cusp (Fig. 20–5). The AV bundle then may give off other left bundle branches, sometimes constituting a true bifascicular system with an anterosuperior branch, in other hearts giving rise to a group of central fibers, and in still others appearing more as a network without a clear division into a fascicular system. The right bundle branch continues intramyocardially as an unbranched extension of the AV bundle down the right side of the interventricular septum to the apex of the right ventricle and base of the anterior papillary muscle. In some human hearts, the His bundle traverses the right interventricular crest, giving rise to a right-sided narrow stem origin of the left bundle branch. The anatomy of the left bundle branch system may be variable and may not conform to a constant bifascicular division. However, the concept of a trifascicular system remains useful to both the electrocardiographer and the clinician (Fig. 20–5).

TERMINAL PURKINJE FIBERS. These fibers connect with the ends of the bundle branches to form interweaving networks on the endocardial surface of both ventricles that transmit the cardiac impulse almost simultaneously to the entire right and left ventricular endocardium. Purkinje fibers tend to be less concentrated at the base of the ventricle and at the papillary muscle tips. They penetrate the myocardium for varying distances depending on the animal species; in humans, they apparently penetrate only the inner third of the endocardium, while in the pig they almost reach the epicardium. Such variations could influence changes produced by myocardial ischemia, for example, since Purkinje fibers appear more resistant to ischemia than are ordinary myocardial fibers.

CELLULAR COMPOSITION OF THE AV JUNCTIONAL AREA. Transitional cells in the rabbit are elongated, smaller than atrial cells, stain more palely, and are separated by numerous strands of connective tissue. They merge at the entrance of the compact portion of the AV node, where the cells are small and spherical, not separated by muscle or connective tissue, and have very few nexuses. They interweave in interconnecting whorls of fasciculi. The AV node is divided, based on electrophysiological characteristics, into AN, N, and NH regions[29] (Fig. 20–6).

In the rabbit, the AN region corresponds to the transitional cell groups of the posterior portion of the node, the NH region to the anterior portion of the bundle of lower nodal cells, and the N region to the small enclosed node where transitional cells merge with mid-nodal cells. *Dead-end pathways*—groups of cells that form an apparent electrophysiological cul-de-sac that does not contribute to overall conduction in the node—are also found at several sites. Cells in

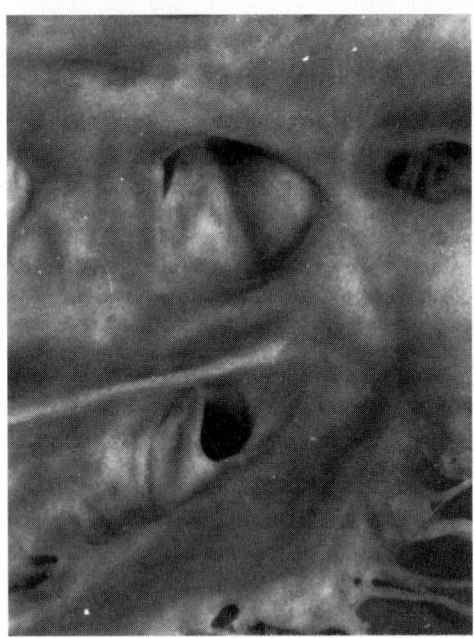

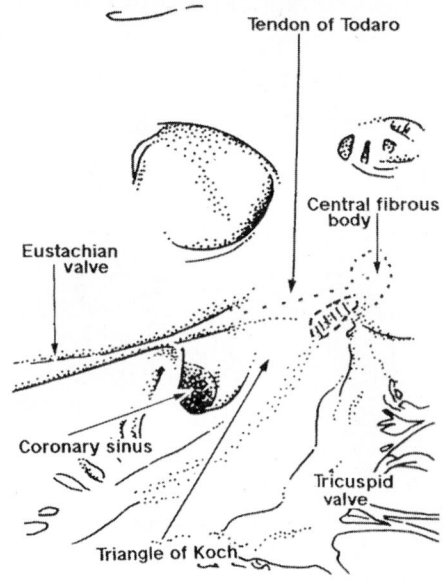

Tendon of Todaro

Central fibrous body

Eustachian valve

Coronary sinus

Tricuspid valve

Triangle of Koch

FIGURE 20–3. A photograph of a normal human heart showing the anatomical landmarks of the triangle of Koch. This triangle is delimited by the tendon of Todaro superiorly, which is the fibrous commissure of the flap guarding the openings of the inferior vena cava and coronary sinus, by the attachment of the septal leaflet of the tricuspid valve inferiorly and by the mouth of the coronary sinus at the base. The stippled area adjacent to the central fibrous body is the approximate site of the compact AV node. (From Janse, M. J., Anderson, R. H., McGuire, M. A., et al.: "AV nodal" reentry: I. "AV nodal" reentry revisited. J. Cardiovasc. Electrophysiol. 4:561, 1993.)

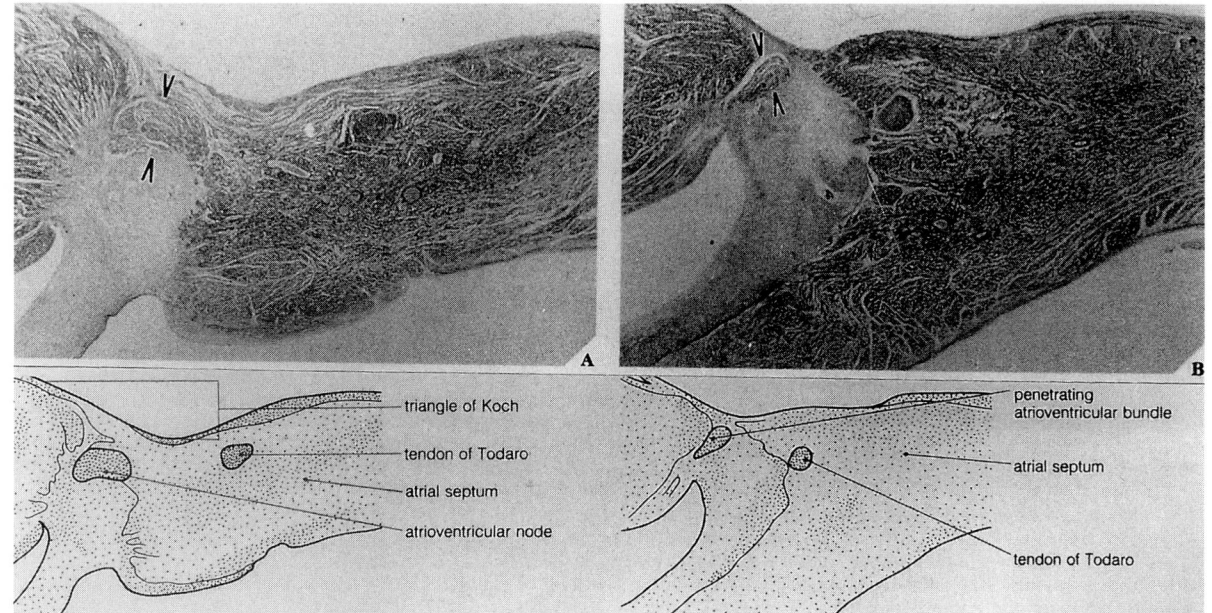

FIGURE 20–4. Sections through the atrioventricular junction show the position of the atrioventricular node (arrowhead) within the triangle of Koch *(A)* and the penetrating atrioventricular bundle of His (arrowheads) within the central fibrous body *(B)*. (From Anderson, R. H., Wilcox, B. R., and Becker, A. E.: Anatomy of the normal heart. *In* Hurst, J. W., Anderson, R. H., Becker, A. E., and Wilcox, B. R. [eds.]: Atlas of the Heart. New York, Gower Medical Publishing, 1988, p. 1.2.)

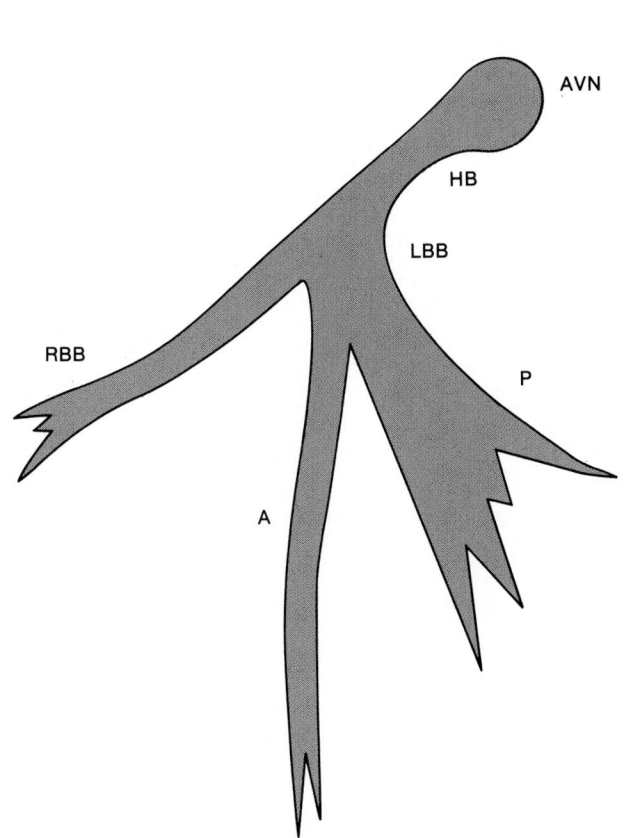

FIGURE 20–5. Schematic representation of the trifascicular bundle branch system. AVN, atrioventricular node; HB, His bundle; LBB, main left bundle branch; A, anterosuperior fascicle of the left bundle; P, posteroinferior fascicle of the left bundle branch; RBB, right bundle branch. (Modified from Rosenbaum, M. B., Elizari, M. V., and Lazzari, J. O.: The Hemiblocks. Oldsmar, FL, Tampa Tracings, 1970, cover illustration.)

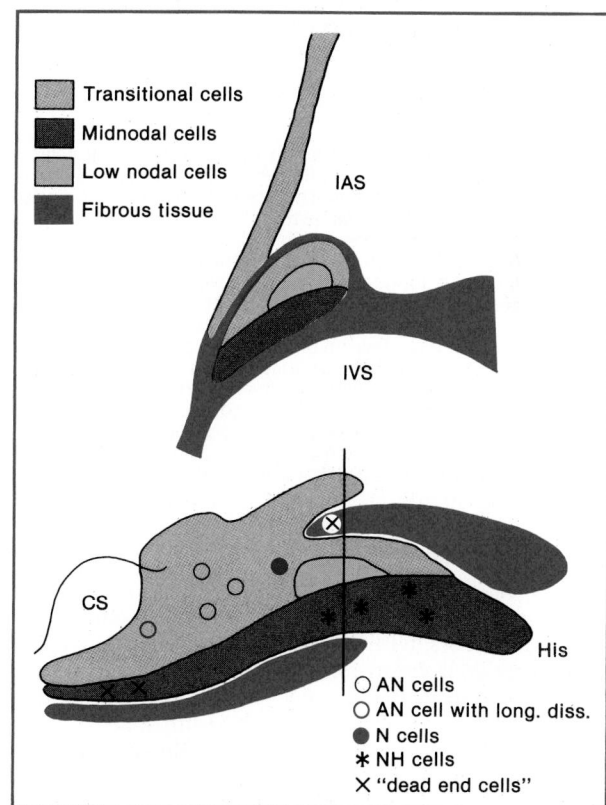

FIGURE 20–6. Diagram showing distribution of morphologically different cell types in AV node. *Upper panel,* Transverse section showing trilaminar appearance of the interior part of the node. The level of sectioning is indicated by the vertical dark line in the lower panel. *Lower panel,* Diagram of the AV node indicating the different sites identified histologically after recording typical action potentials. (From Janse, M. J., et al.: Electrophysiology and structure of the atrioventricular node of the isolated rabbit heart. *In* Wellens, J. H. H., et al. [eds.]: The Conduction System of the Heart. Philadelphia, Lea and Febiger, 1976, p. 296.)

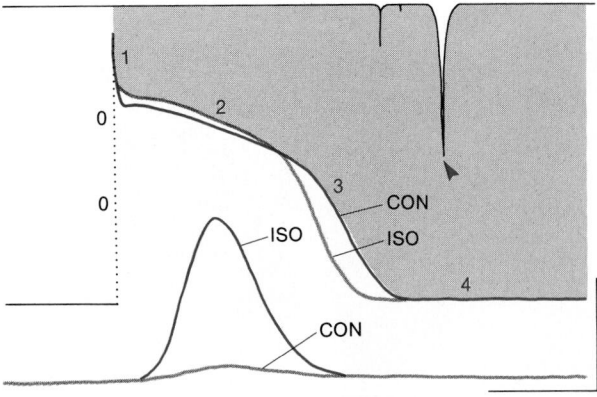

FIGURE 20–7. Recordings of canine Purkinje fiber action potential and developed tension before and during isoproterenol administration. Tracings from above downward show upstroke velocity of phase 0 (V_{max}, arrowhead), action potential configuration of Purkinje fiber, and developed tension in the Purkinje fiber bundle during control (CON) and after exposure to isoproterenol (ISO, 0.1 ml/10^{-5} M, added directly to the tissue bath). The five phases of the action potential are indicated by the large numerals. The short horizontal line to the left with a zero near the peak of the action potential indicates the zero voltage potential. Vertical calibration: 400 V/sec for V_{max}/sec, 50 mV for action potential amplitude, and 400 mg for the developed tension, respectively. Horizontal calibration: 4 msec for the upper record and 100 msec for the middle and lower records. (V = volts; mV = millivolts; msec = milliseconds.) Isoproterenol increased plateau height of the action potential and developed tension and decreased action potential duration during the terminal phase of repolarization, without significantly affecting resting membrane potential or phase 0. (From Gilmour, R. F., Jr., and Zipes, D. P.: Basic electrophysiology of the slow inward current. *In* Antman, E., and Stone, P. [eds.]: Calcium Blocking Agents in the Treatment of Cardiovascular Disorders. Mt. Kisco, N.Y., Futura, 1983, pp. 1–37.)

the penetrating bundle remain similar to compact AV nodal cells. In the dog, P cells, similar to those found in the sinus node, and several types of transitional cells have been noted and related to the automaticity and conduction properties of the AV node.[24,25]

Purkinje cells are found in the His bundle and bundle branches, cover much of the endocardium of both ventricles, and align to form multicellular bundles in longitudinal strands separated by collagen. They are large, clear cells (10 to 30 μm in diameter, 20 to 50 μm long) with loosely arrayed mitochondria distributed between few linearly aligned myofibrils that have few myofilaments. Round nuclei occupy the center of the cell. Although conduction of the cardiac impulse appears to be their major function, free-running Purkinje fibers, sometimes called *false tendons*, which are composed of many Purkinje cells in a series, are capable of contraction (Fig. 20–7). Extensive lateral and end-to-end gap junctions, made up primarily of connexin 43, apparently transform the individual Purkinje cells into functioning like a cable.[3,6,7,30]

Innervation of AV Node and His Bundle

PATHWAYS OF INNERVATION. The AV node and His bundle region are innervated by a rich supply of cholinergic and adrenergic fibers with a density exceeding that found in the ventricular myocardium. Ganglia, nerve fibers, and nerve nets lie close to the AV node. Parasympathetic nerves to the AV node region enter the canine heart at the junction of the inferior vena cava and the inferior left atrium, adjacent to the coronary sinus entrance. Nerves in direct contact with AV nodal fibers have been noted, along with agranular and granular vesicular processes, presumably representing cholinergic and adrenergic processes. Acetylcholine release may be concentrated around the N region of the AV node.[13–15]

In general, autonomic neural input to the heart exhibits some degree of "sidedness," with the right sympathetic and vagal nerves affecting the sinus node more than the AV node and the left sympathetic and vagal nerves affecting the AV node more than the sinus node. The distribution of the neural input to the sinus and AV nodes is complex because of substantial overlapping innervation. Despite the overlap, specific branches of the vagal and sympathetic nerves

can be shown to innervate certain regions preferentially, and sympathetic or vagal nerves to the sinus node can be interrupted discretely without affecting AV nodal innervation. Similarly, vagal or sympathetic neural input to the AV node can be interrupted without affecting sinus innervation. Supersensitivity to acetylcholine follows vagal denervation. Stimulation of the right stellate ganglion produces sinus tachycardia with less effect on AV nodal conduction, while stimulation of the left stellate ganglion generally produces a shift in the sinus pacemaker to an ectopic site and consistently shortens AV nodal conduction time and refractoriness but inconsistently speeds the sinus nodal discharge rate. Stimulation of the right cervical vagus nerve primarily slows the sinus nodal discharge rate, while stimulation of the left vagus primarily prolongs AV nodal conduction time and refractoriness when "sidedness" is present. While neither sympathetic nor vagal stimulation affects normal conduction in the His bundle, either can affect abnormal AV conduction.

Most efferent sympathetic impulses reach the canine ventricles over the ansae subclaviae, branches from the stellate ganglia. Sympathetic nerves then synapse primarily in the caudal cervical ganglia and form individual cardiac nerves that innervate relatively localized parts of the ventricles. On the right side, the major route to the heart is the recurrent cardiac nerve, and on the left, the ventrolateral cardiac nerve. In general, the right sympathetic chain shortens refractoriness primarily of the anterior portion of the ventricles, while the left affects primarily the posterior surface of the ventricles, although overlapping areas of distribution occur.

The intraventricular route of sympathetic nerves generally follows coronary arteries. Functional data suggest that afferent and efferent sympathetic nerves travel in the superficial layers of the epicardium and dive to innervate the endocardium, and anatomical observations support this conclusion. Vagal fibers travel intramurally or subendocardially, rising to the epicardium at the AV groove[13–15,31] (Fig. 20–8).

EFFECTS OF VAGAL STIMULATION. The vagus modulates cardiac sympathetic activity at prejunctional and postjunctional sites by regulating the amount of norepinephrine released and by inhibiting cyclic AMP-induced phosphorylation of cardiac proteins such as phospholamban.[22] The latter inhibition occurs at more than one level in the series of reactions comprising the adenylate cyclase, cyclic AMP–dependent, protein kinase system. Neuropeptides released from nerve fibers of both autonomic limbs also modulate autonomic responses. For example, neuropeptide Y released from sympathetic nerve terminals inhibits cardiac vagal effects.[11,12]

Tonic vagal stimulation produces a greater absolute reduction in sinus rate in the presence of tonic background sympathetic stimulation, a sympathetic-parasympathetic interaction termed *accentuated antagonism*. In contrast, changes in AV conduction during concomitant sympathetic and vagal stimulation are essentially the *algebraic sum* of the individual AV conduction responses to tonic vagal and sympathetic stimulation alone. Cardiac responses to brief vagal bursts begin after a short latency and dissipate quickly; in contrast, cardiac responses to sympathetic stimulation commence and dissipate slowly. The rapid onset and offset of responses to vagal stimulation allow for dynamic beat-to-beat vagal modulation of heart rate and AV conduction, whereas the slow temporal response to sympathetic stimulation precludes any beat-to-beat regulation by sympathetic activity. Periodic vagal bursting (as may occur each time a systolic pressure wave arrives at the baroreceptor regions in the aortic and carotid sinuses) induces phasic changes in sinus cycle length and can entrain the sinus node to discharge faster or slower at periods that are identical to those of the vagal burst. In a similar phasic manner, vagal bursts prolong AV nodal conduction time and are influenced by background levels of sympathetic tone. Because the peak vagal effects on sinus rate and AV nodal conduction occur at different times in the cardiac cycle, a brief vagal burst can slow the sinus rate without affecting AV nodal conduction or can prolong AV nodal conduction time and not slow the sinus rate.[9,11,12]

EFFECTS OF SYMPATHETIC STIMULATION. Stimulation of sympathetic ganglia shortens the refractory period equally in the epicardium and underlying endocardium of the left ventricular free wall, although dispersion of recovery properties occurs, i.e., different degrees of shortening of refractoriness occur when measured at different epicardial sites. Nonuniform distribution of norepinephrine may, in part, contribute to some of the nonuniform electrophysiological effects, since the ventricular content of norepinephrine is greater at the base than at the apex of the heart, with greater distribution to muscle than to Purkinje fibers. Afferent vagal activity appears to be greater in the posterior ventricular myocardium. This may account for the vagomimetic effects of inferior myocardial infarction.[13–15]

The vagi exert minimal but measurable effects on ven-

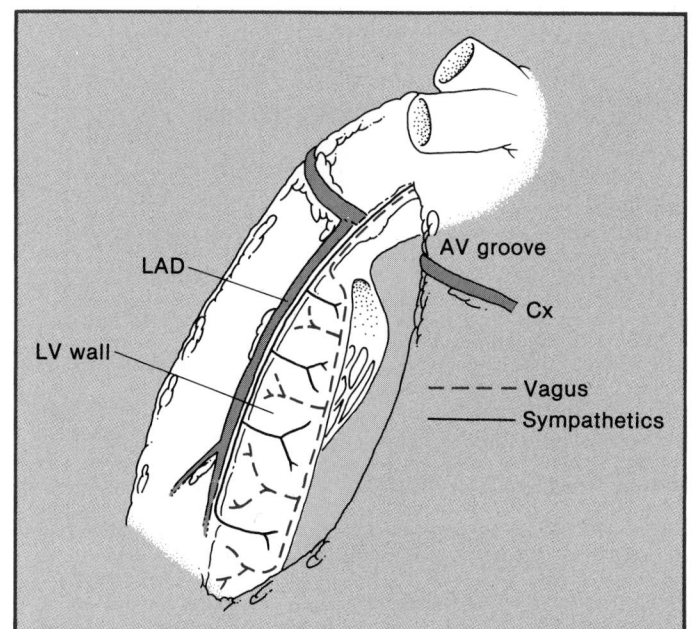 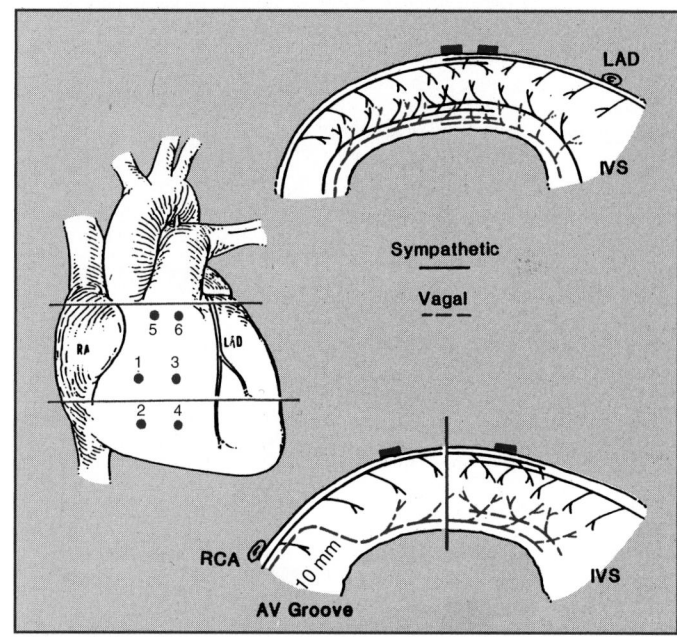

FIGURE 20–8. *Left panel,* Intraventricular route of sympathetic and vagal nerves to the left ventricle. *Right panel,* Schematic of the transverse views of the right ventricular wall showing functional pathways of efferent sympathetic and vagal nerves. *Top right,* Transverse view of the RV outflow tract at the upper horizontal line on the left. *Bottom right,* Transverse view of the anterolateral wall at the lower horizontal line on the left. Vertical solid line indicates center of RV anterolateral wall. Closed circles indicate positions of plunge electrodes labeled 1–6. IVS, interventricular septum; LAD, left anterior descending coronary artery; RCA, right coronary artery; RA, right atrium. (Reproduced with permission from Ito, M., and Zipes, D. P.: Efferent sympathetic and vagal innervation of the canine right ventricle. Circulation *90:*1459, 1994. Copyright 1994 American Heart Association.)

tricular tissue, decreasing the strength of myocardial contraction and prolonging refractoriness. Under some circumstances, acetylcholine can cause a positive inotropic effect. It is now clear that the vagus (acetylcholine) can exert direct effects on some types of ventricular fibers, as well as exert indirect effects by modulating sympathetic influences.[14,32]

ARRHYTHMIAS AND THE AUTONOMIC NERVOUS SYSTEM. Alterations in vagal and sympathetic innervation can influence the development of arrhythmias.[14,32] Damage to nerves extrinsic to the heart, such as the stellate ganglia, as well as to intrinsic cardiac nerves from diseases that may affect nerves primarily, e.g., viral infections, or secondarily, from diseases that cause cardiac damage, may produce cardioneuropathy. Such neural changes may create electrical instability via a variety of electrophysiological mechanisms. For example, myocardial infarction can interrupt afferent and efferent neural transmission and create areas of sympathetic supersensitivity that may be conducive to the development of arrhythmias.[13,14]

BASIC ELECTROPHYSIOLOGICAL PRINCIPLES

Cell Membrane (Sarcolemma)
(See also p. 369)

The cell membrane constitutes a bilayer boundary of phospholipid molecules[33] (Fig. 20–9). The tail end of the phospholipid molecules is nonpolar and hydrophobic, pointing toward the center of the membrane, while the head end is polar and hydrophilic, pointing toward the outer and inner layers of the membrane, in contact with the aqueous extracellular and intracellular environment. The sarcolemma, particularly the hydrophobic core, provides a high-resistance, insulated wrapping around the cell that exhibits selective permeability to ions—a property responsible for creating an electrical potential across the cell membrane. Ions are positively (cations) or negatively

(anions) charged atoms such as Na^+, K^+, Ca^{++}, or Cl^- and other molecules whose movement inside the cell or across the cell membrane creates a flow of current that generates signals in excitable membranes.

At rest, the resistance to ion flow is greater across the cell membrane than in the cytoplasm of the cell interior. The cell membrane has openings called *channels* that span the cell membrane and serve as conduits through which ions move. The different protein or phospholipoprotein channels are selective, favoring passage of one ion over another. In contrast to the membrane lipids that act primarily as inert barriers, membrane proteins appear to be responsible for most of the known biological activities of membranes. Some kinds of channels open as a result of a neurotransmitter binding to their extracellular site and are called *receptor-operated channels*. Others open in response to a voltage change and are called *voltage-operated channels*. Gates, influenced by the electric field and by time, control ion movement through the channels and, when opened or closed, permit or prevent ion travel. Drugs can bind to sites within the channel and prevent ion passage. Sodium[34–37] and calcium[38–50] membrane channels cycle through three states during each action potential that include the closed or resting state, the open or activation state, and the closed or inactivation state (Fig. 20–10). Voltage-dependent ion channels are glycosylated proteins. Each subunit of these channels contains four covalently linked domains (except for potassium channels) designated I to IV (Fig. 20–9, *left*), and each domain contains six alpha-helical transmembrane segments designated S_1 to S_6 (Fig. 20–9, *right*). S_4 is thought to represent the m gate (see p. 558), and the cytoplasmic loop connecting the S_6 transmembrane segment of domain III to the S_1 segment of domain IV may be to the h gate.[35]

In addition to the channels, pumps and carriers (e.g., Na-K pump, which is blocked by digitalis [see p. 499], Ca^{++} pump, Na/Ca countertransport system, Na/H exchanger), receptors (e.g., α, β, muscarinic, and purinergic), and cytoplasmic regulators of second messengers (e.g., cyc-

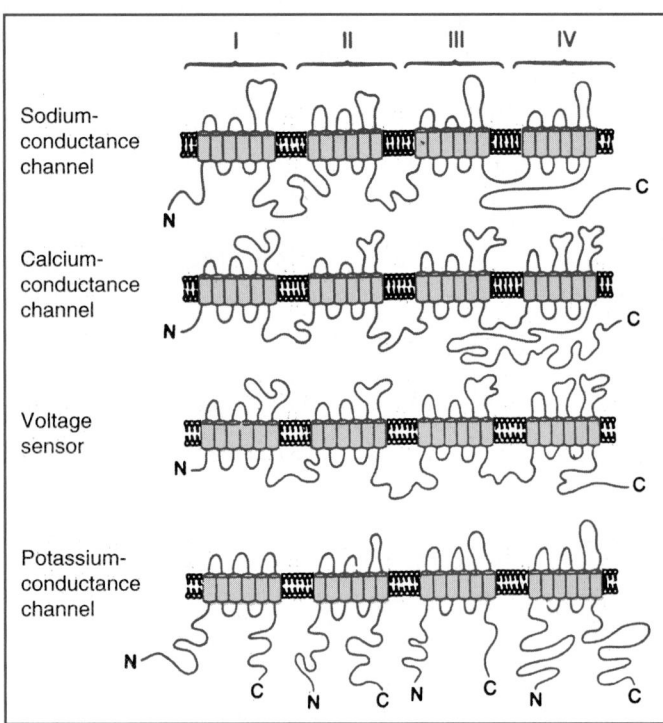

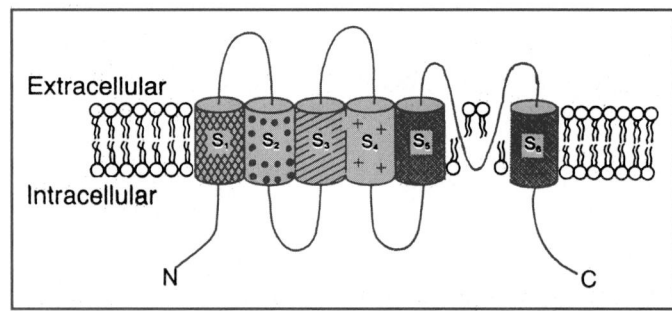

FIGURE 20–9. *Left panel,* Four members of the family of ion-channel proteins. The major subunits of the calcium and sodium channels are tetramers made up of four covalently linked domains that are numbered I–IV. The voltage sensor that initiates contraction in the depolarized mammalian skeletal muscle resembles the calcium channel but is smaller, because it lacks the portion of the C-terminal amino acid sequence present in the calcium channel. Potassium channels also contain four domains, but unlike calcium and sodium channels, the domains are not covalently linked. *Right panel,* An ion channel domain. The ion channels shown on the left are tetramers made up of four domains, each of which contains six alpha-helical transmembrane segments. The S_4 segment, which is rich in positively charged amino acids, is believed to open the channel in response to membrane depolarization. The transmembrane segments S_5 and S_6, along with the intervening peptide chain, probably surround the pore through which ions cross the lipid barrier in the core of the membrane bilayer. (Modified from Katz, A. M.: Molecular biology in cardiology, a paradigmatic shift. J. Mol. Cell. Cardiol. *20:*355, 1988.)

lic AMP–phosphodiesterase) influence electrophysiological function.[51] Some protein complexes penetrate only the outer cell membrane and may serve as receptor sites for neurotransmitters and hormones, while others, such as the adenylate cyclase system, protrude through the inner cell membrane and may be involved in various enzymatic activities. Protein molecules protruding through the entire cell membrane, such as the Na-K pump, may help regulate ionic fluxes. The Na-K pump requires adenosine triphosphate (ATP) to extrude intracellular Na against its concentration and electrical gradients and to move K intracellularly, against its concentration gradient, resulting in high concentrations of K inside and of Na outside the cell (Table 20–1).

INTERCALATED DISCS

The cell membranes of some types of adjacent cells form close margins called *intercalated discs.* Three types of specialized junctions make up each intercalated disc. The macula adherens or desmosome and fascia adherens form the areas of strong adhesions between cells and may provide a linkage for the transfer of mechanical energy from one cell to the next. The *nexus,* also called *tight* or *gap junction,* is a region in the intercalated disc where cells are in functional contact with each other. Membranes at these junctions are separated by only about 10 to 20 Å and are connected by a series of hexagonally packed subunit bridges. Gap junctions provide low-resistance electrical coupling between adjacent cells by establishing aqueous pores that directly link the cytoplasms of these adjacent cells. The gap junctions allow movement of ions and perhaps of small molecules between cells, linking interiors of adjacent cells.

The gap junctions permit a multicellular structure such as the heart to function electrically like an orderly, synchronized, interconnected unit and are probably responsible in part for the fact that conduction in the myocardium is *anisotropic;* i.e., its anatomical and biophysical properties vary according to the direction in which they are measured. Usually, conduction velocity is two to three times faster longitudinally, i.e., in the direction of the long axis of the fiber, than it is

FIGURE 20–10. Three states through which ion channels cycle.

**CLOSED
Resting**

(Recovery)   (Activation)

**CLOSED
Inactive**   (Inactivation)   **OPEN
Activated**

TABLE 20–1 INTRACELLULAR AND EXTRACELLULAR ION CONCENTRATIONS IN CARDIAC MUSCLE

ION	EXTRACELLULAR CONCENTRATION	INTRACELLULAR CONCENTRATION	RATIO OF EXTRACELLULAR TO INTRACELLULAR CONCENTRATION	E_i
Na	145 mM	15 mM	9.7	+60 mV
K	4 mM	150 mM	0.027	−94 mV
Cl	120 mM	5 mM	24	−83 mV
Ca	2 mM	10^{-7} M	2×10^4	+129 mV

E_i = equilibrium potential for a particular ion.

Although intracellular Ca content is about 2 mM, most of this is bound or sequestered in intracellular organelles (mitochondria and sarcoplasmic reticulum). For the same reason, the actual free Na concentration may be less. Intracellular Cl concentration depends on the average membrane potential, if Cl is passively distributed, and therefore on heart rate.

From Sperelakis, N.: Origin of the cardiac resting potential. *In* Berne, R. M., et al. (eds.): Handbook of Physiology, The Cardiovascular System, Bethesda, Md., American Physiological Society, 1979, p. 193.

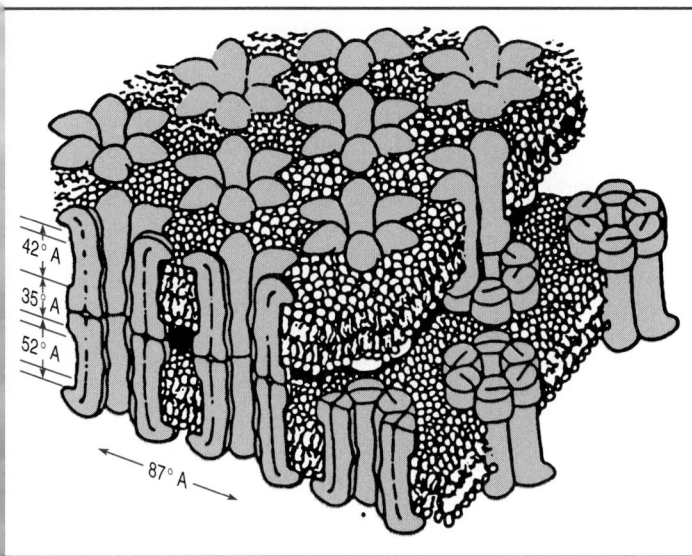

FIGURE 20–11. A model of the structure of a gap junction based on results of x-ray diffraction studies. Individual channels are composed of paired hexamers that travel in the membranes of adjacent cells and adjoin in the extracellular gap to form an aqueous pore that provides continuity of the cytoplasm of the two cells. (From Saffitz, J. E.: Cell-to-cell communication in the heart. Cardiol. Rev. *3*:86, 1995.)

transversely, i.e., in the direction perpendicular to this long axis. Resistivity is lower longitudinally than transversely. Interestingly, the safety factor for propagation is greater transversely than horizontally. Conduction delay or block occurs more commonly in the longitudinal direction than it does transversely. Because of anisotropy, propagation is discontinuous and can be a cause of reentry.

Gap junctions also may provide "biochemical coupling" that might permit cell-to-cell movement of ATP on other high-energy phosphates. Gap junctions also can change their electrical resistance. When intracellular calcium rises, as in myocardial infarction, the gap junction may close to help "seal off" the effects of injured from noninjured cells. Acidosis increases and alkalosis decreases gap junctional resistance. Increased gap junctional resistance tends to slow the rate of action potential propagation, a condition that could lead to conduction delay or block.[3,6–8,52–56]

Connexins are the proteins that form the intercellular channels of gap junctions. An individual channel (connexin) is created by two hemichannels, each located in the plasma membrane of adjacent cells, that are composed of six integral membrane protein subunits (connexins) that surround an aqueous pore, creating a transmembrane channel (Fig. 20–11). Connexin 43, a 43-kDa polypeptide, is the most abundant cardiac connexin, with connexin 40 and 45 found in smaller amounts. Gap junctions in the distal His bundle and proximal bundle branches have large amounts of connexin 40 and 43. Atrial gap junctions have large amounts of all three connexins, while ventricular gap junctions have large amounts of connexin 43 and 45 and much less connexin 40 (see p. 548).[3,6]

Phases of the Cardiac Action Potential

The cardiac transmembrane potential consists of five phases: phase 0—the upstroke or rapid depolarization; phase 1—early rapid repolarization; phase 2—plateau; phase 3—final rapid repolarization; and phase 4—resting membrane potential and diastolic depolarization (see Fig. 20–7). These phases are the result of passive ion fluxes moving down electrochemical gradients established by active ion pumps and exchange mechanisms. Each ion moves primarily through its own ion-specific channel. Impulses spread from one cell to the next without requiring neural input. The transplanted heart dramatically demonstrates this fact. The following discussion will explain the electrogenesis of each of these phases. For in-depth coverage, the reader is referred to other reference sources.[57,58]

Phase 4—The Resting Membrane Potential

Intracellular electrical activity can be recorded by inserting a glass microelectrode with a tip diameter less than 0.5 μm into a single cell. The electrode produces minimal damage, its entry point apparently being sealed by the cell. The transmembrane potential is recorded using this electrode in reference to an extracellular ground electrode placed in the tissue bath near the cell membrane and represents the potential difference between intracellular and extracellular voltages (Fig. 20–12, *left*). A variety of other techniques, including voltage and patch clamp procedures, can be used to study the passage of individual ionic species across specific channels in the cell membrane (Figs. 20–12, 20–13, and 20–14).

Intracellular potential during electrical quiescence in diastole is -50 to -95 mV, depending on the cell type (Table 20–2). This means that the inside of the cell is 50 to 95 mV negative relative to the outside of the cell owing to the distribution of ions such as K^+, Na^+, Cl^-, and Ca^{++} across the cell membrane.

K^+ is the major ion determining the resting potential.[59–65] During diastole, the cell membrane is quite permeable to K^+ and relatively impermeable to Na^+. Because of the Na-K pump, which pumps Na^+ out of the cell against its electrochemical gradient and simultaneously pumps K^+ into the cell against its chemical gradient, intracellular K^+ concentration remains high and intracellular Na^+ concentration remains low. This pump, fueled by an Na^+, K^+-ATPase enzyme that hydrolyzes ATP for energy, is bound to the membrane. It requires both Na^+ and K^+ to function and can transport three Na^+ ions outward for two K^+ ions inward. Therefore, the pump can be electrogenic, generating a net outward movement of positive charges. The rate of Na^+-K^+ pumping to maintain the same ionic gradients must increase as heart rate increases, since the cell gains a slight amount of Na^+ and loses a slight amount of K^+ with each depolarization. Cardiac glycosides block this pump.

THE NERNST EQUATION. Little Na^+, despite its concentration gradient, can diffuse into the cell, owing to the relative impermeability to Na^+ of the polarized cell membrane. However, K^+ can diffuse freely out of the cell down its concentration gradient and does so, removing with it a positive charge and leaving the inside of the cell more negative. Negative intracellular charges, presumably due to large polyvalent ions such as proteins, do not cross the membrane and help maintain intracellular negativity. K^+ continues to leave the cell until the forces driving it down its concentration gradient are balanced by the negative intracellular electrical charges that attract K^+ back into the cell. The transmembrane voltage at which the electrical

TABLE 20–2 PROPERTIES OF TRANSMEMBRANE POTENTIALS IN MAMMALIAN HEARTS

	SINUS NODAL CELL	ATRIAL MUSCLE CELL	AV NODAL CELL	PURKINJE FIBER	VENTRICULAR MUSCLE CELL
Resting potential (mV)	-50 to -60	-80 to -90	-60 to -70	-90 to -95	-80 to -90
Action potential					
Amplitude (mV)	60 to 70	110 to 120	70 to 80	120	110 to 120
Overshoot (mV)	0 to 10	30	5 to 15	30	30
Duration (msec)	100 to 300	100 to 300	100 to 300	300 to 500	200 to 300
Vmax (V/S)	1 to 10	100 to 200	5 to 15	500 to 700	100 to 200
Propagation velocity (M/sec)	<0.05	0.3 to 0.4	0.1	2 to 3	0.3 to 0.4
Fiber diameter (μm)	5 to 10	10 to 15	5 to 10	100	10 to 16

Modified from Sperelakis, N.: Origin of the cardiac resting potential. *In* Berne, R. M., Sperelakis, N., and Geiger, S. R. (eds.): Handbook of Physiology, The Cardiovascular System, Bethesda, Md., American Physiological Society, 1979, p. 190.

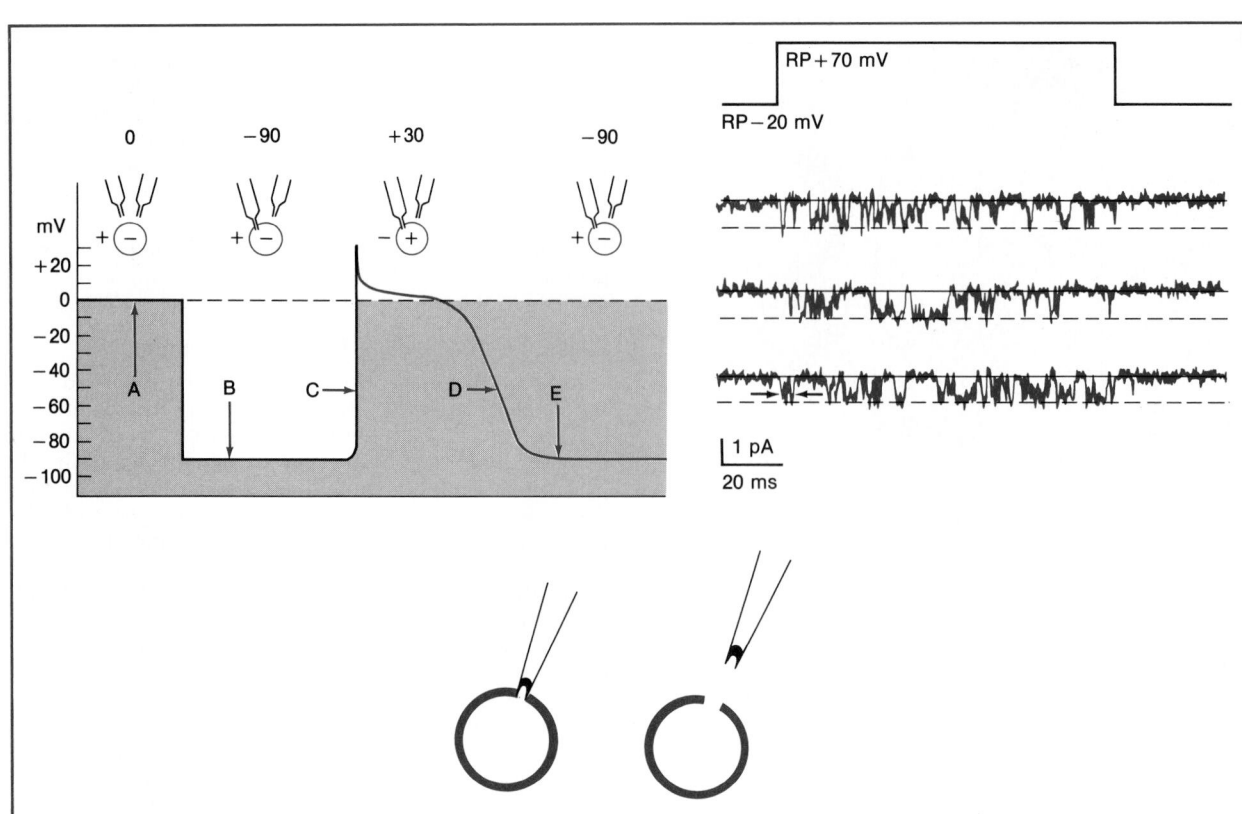

FIGURE 20–12. *Left,* A demonstration of action potentials recorded during impalement of a cardiac cell. The upper row of diagrams shows a cell (circle), two microelectrodes, and stages during impalement of the cell and its activation and recovery. *A,* Both microelectrodes are extracellular, and no difference in potential exists between them (0 potential). The environment inside the cell is negative and the outside is positive, since the cell is polarized. *B,* One microelectrode has pierced the cell membrane to record the intracellular resting membrane potential, which is − 90 mV with respect to the outside of the cell. *C,* The cell has depolarized and the upstroke of the action potential is recorded. At its peak voltage, the inside of the cell is about + 30 mV with respect to the outside of the cell. *D,* Phase of repolarization, returning the membrane to its former resting potential *(E)* (From Cranefield, P. F.: The Conduction of the Cardiac Impulse. Mt. Kisco, N.Y., Futura, 1975.)

Right, Calcium channel recording. A portion or patch of the sarcolemmal membrane from a single guinea pig ventricular muscle cell is sucked up into a micropipette to record the opening and closing of single calcium channels. The pipette is filled with 110 mM Ba^{++}. The Ba^{++} crosses the membrane through the calcium channel when it opens and generates a current, recorded as the large downward pulses that reach the interrupted line (first in the bottom tracing). The solid line indicates average baseline current while the interrupted line (about 1 pA) indicates average single channel current. The channel stays open for brief but varied durations and then closes (upward deflection back to solid line, second). Three sequentially obtained current records are shown. Resting membrane potential (RP) was near − 60 mV by addition of 10 mM [K]o. The RP was then reduced by 20 mV (RP − 20 mV) and virtually no Ca^{++} channel openings occurred. When RP was made 70 mV more positive (RP + 70 mV) Ca^{++} channel activity was generated. (Square wave-shaped tracing at very top indicates RP changes). Thus, this figure illustrates opening and closing of single calcium channels when the RP is reduced to the range at which the slow inward current functions. (From Tsien, R.: Excitable tissues: The heart. *In* Andreoli, T. E., et al. [eds.]: Physiology of Membrane Disorders. New York, Plenum Press, 1986, p. 478.)

Bottom insert shows micropipette technique used to study single channels in a portion of the membrane still attached to the cell *(left).* Membrane studied after being detached from the rest of the cell *(right).*

gradient is equal and opposite to the concentration gradient so that the algebraic sum of these two passive forces equals zero, is the K^+ electrochemical equilibrium potential E_k, and is described by the *Nernst equation:*

$$E_k = \frac{RT}{F} \ln \frac{[K^+]_o}{[K^+]_i} \qquad (1)$$

where R is the gas constant, T is the absolute temperature, F is the Faraday number, ln is the logarithm to the base e, $[K^+]_o$ is the extracellular K^+ concentration, and $[K^+]_i$ is the intracellular K^+ concentration.[57,58]

Solving this equation predicts a transmembrane voltage of about − 96 mV in cardiac muscle, which is very near the observed voltages. However, certain factors make the equation an approximation. Because the $[K^+]_o/[K^+]_i$ ratio primarily determines transmembrane voltage, the cell membrane is said to behave as a K^+ electrode during diastole and more closely follows the values predicted by the Nernst equation at $[K^+]_o$ greater than 10 mM. When $[K^+]_o$ is reduced, membrane permeability to K^+ also decreases, the small inward movement of Na^+, negligible at high $[K^+]_o$, becomes more important, and the actual resting membrane voltage becomes less than that predicted by the Nernst equation for a K^+ electrode. The difference between predicted and observed voltages increases as $[K^+]_o$ is reduced further.

The contribution of the minimal inward movement of Na^+ to the resting membrane potential can be incorporated into an equation called the *Goldman constant-field equation* and is a slight modification of the Nernst equation. If one assumes that the membrane is permeable to only Na^+ and K^+, the resting membrane potential (V_r) would be

$$V_r = \frac{RT}{F} \ln \frac{[K^+]_o + P_{Na}/P_K [Na]_o}{[K^+]_i + P_{Na}/P_K [Na]_i} \qquad (2)$$

where P_{Na}/P_K is the ratio of the sodium to the potassium permeability coefficient of the cell membrane, $[Na]_o$ is the extracellular sodium concentration, and $[Na]_i$ is the intracellular sodium concentration. The equation can be modified further to include the minimal contributions of other ions.

Calcium contributes little to the resting membrane potential, although changes in Ca concentration can affect the permeability of the cell membrane to other ions. An increase in $[Ca]_i$ increases potassium conductance. Ca^{++} is handled by several mechanisms, including uptake by the sarcoplasmic reticulum. Also, there appears to be a passive transsarcolemmal Ca^{++}-Na^+ exchange reaction. This exchange depends in part on maintenance of the Na^+ concentration gradient by the Na^+-K^+ pump. Under normal conditions, one internal Ca^{++} ion is probably exchanged for three or more external Na^+ ions. Na^+-Ca^{++}

exchange generates a current across the cell membrane. Under some pathological conditions or drug actions when [Na+]i is abnormally high, external Ca++ may be exchanged for internal Na+. Cells that gain Na+, in general, gain Ca++—a reaction important to the genesis of some digitalis-induced arrhythmias. The role of Ca++ is further considered on page 366.

Phase 0—Upstroke or Rapid Depolarization

A stimulus delivered to excitable tissue evokes an action potential characterized by a sudden voltage change due to transient depolarization followed by repolarization. The action potential is conducted throughout the heart and is responsible for initiating each "heartbeat." Electrical changes of the action potential follow a relatively fixed time and voltage relationship that differs according to specific cell types (Figs. 20–13, 20–14, and 20–15). In nerve, the entire process takes several milliseconds, while action potentials in cardiac fibers last several hundred milliseconds. Normally, the action potential is independent of the size of the depolarizing stimulus, if the latter exceeds a certain threshold potential. Small subthreshold depolarizing stimuli depolarize the membrane in proportion to the strength of the stimulus. However, once the stimulus is sufficiently intense to reduce membrane potential to a threshold value in the range of -70 to -65 mV for normal Purkinje fibers, more intense stimuli do not produce larger action potential responses, and an "all-or-none" response results. In contrast, hyperpolarizing pulses, i.e., stimuli that render the membrane potential more negative, elicit a response proportional to the strength of the stimulus.

MECHANISM OF PHASE 0. The upstroke of the cardiac ac-

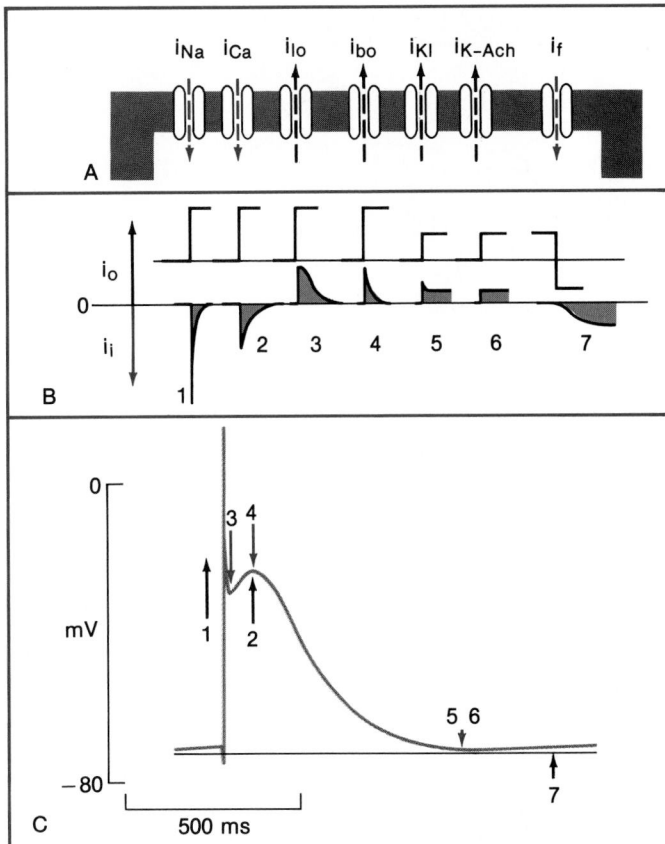

FIGURE 20–14. Schematic diagram of ionic channels *(A)* and corresponding transmembrane currents *(B)* presently known in human atrial myocardium and their influences on development of cellular action potential *(C)*. A, Currents crossing different channels under normal conditions are either inward (downward arrows) and therefore depolarize the membrane or outward (upward arrows) and therefore repolarize the membrane. i_{Na}, sodium current; i_{ca}, calcium current; i_{lo} and i_{bo}, long-lasting and brief transient potassium currents; i_{K1}, background potassium current; i_{K-ACh}, potassium current flowing through muscarinic cholinergic receptor channels; i_f, pacemaker current carried by both sodium and potassium ions. B, Time course of different transmembrane ionic currents (hatched areas) occurring when the membrane is submitted to rectangular (top traces) depolarizing pulses (1–6) or repolarizing pulses (7). Currents i_{Ki} and i_{K-ACh} are shown here as outward currents, but because of the inward rectification, they are much smaller in the outward than in the inward direction. i_o, outward current; i_i, inward current. C, 1–7 correspond to the currents shown in *A* and *B*, and arrows indicate effect of each ionic current on the action potential; upward arrows, depolarizing effect; downward arrows, repolarizing or hyperpolarizing effects. (From Coraboeuf, E., and Escande, D.: Ionic currents in the human myocardium. NIPS 5:28, 1990.)

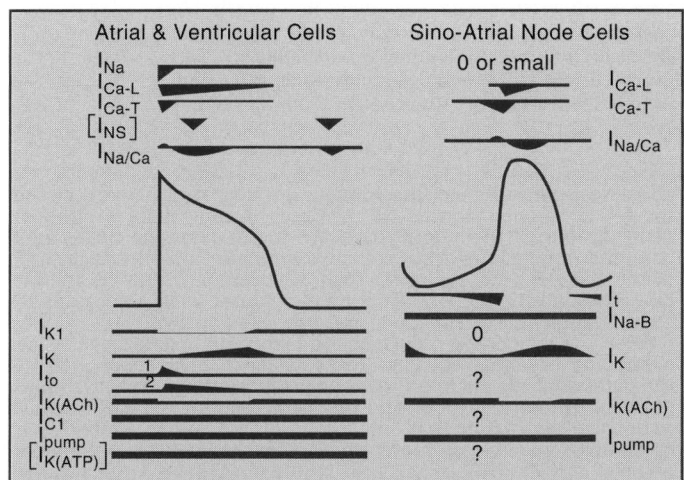

FIGURE 20–13. Currents and channels involved in generating the resting and action potential. The time course of a stylized action potential of atrial and ventricular cells is shown on the left and of sinoatrial node cells on the right. Above and below are the various channels and pumps that contribute the currents underlying the electrical events. See Table 20–3 for identification of the symbols and description of the channels or currents. Where possible, the approximate time courses of the currents associated with the channels or pumps are shown symbolically without effort to represent their magnitudes relative to each other. I_K incorporates at least two currents, I_{K-R} and I_{K-S}. There appears to be an ultrarapid component as well, designated I_{K-UR}.

The heavy bars for I_{Cl}, I_{pump}, and $I_{K(ATP)}$ only indicate the presence of these channels or pump, without implying magnitude of currents, since that would vary with physiological and pathophysiological conditions. The channels identified by brackets (I_{NS} and $I_{K(ATP)}$) imply that they are active only under pathological conditions. For the sinoatrial node cells, I_{Na} and I_{K1} are small or absent. Question marks indicate that experimental evidence is not yet available to determine the presence of these channels in sinoatrial cell membranes. Although it is likely that other ionic current mechanisms exist, they are not shown here because their roles in electrogenesis are not sufficiently well defined. (From Members of the Sicilian Gambit: Antiarrhythmic Therapy: A Pathophysiologic Approach. Mt. Kisco, N.Y., Futura, 1994, p. 13.)

tion potential in atrial and ventricular muscle and His-Purkinje fibers is due to a sudden increase in membrane conductance to Na+. An externally applied stimulus or a spontaneously generated local membrane circuit current in advance of a propagating action potential depolarizes a sufficiently large area of membrane at a sufficiently rapid rate to open the Na+ channels and depolarize the membrane further. When the membrane voltage reaches threshold, Na+ rushes through ion-specific channels into the cell, down its electrochemical gradient—i.e., Na+ is "drawn" into the cell by the low [Na+]i and the negatively charged intracellular environment. The excited membrane no longer behaves like a K+ electrode, i.e., exclusively permeable to K+, but more closely approximates an Na+ electrode, and the membrane moves toward the Na+ equilibrium potential.

The rate at which depolarization occurs during phase 0, i.e., the maximum rate of change of voltage over time, is indicated by the expression dV/dt$_{max}$ or V̇$_{max}$ (Table 20–2), which is a reasonable ap-

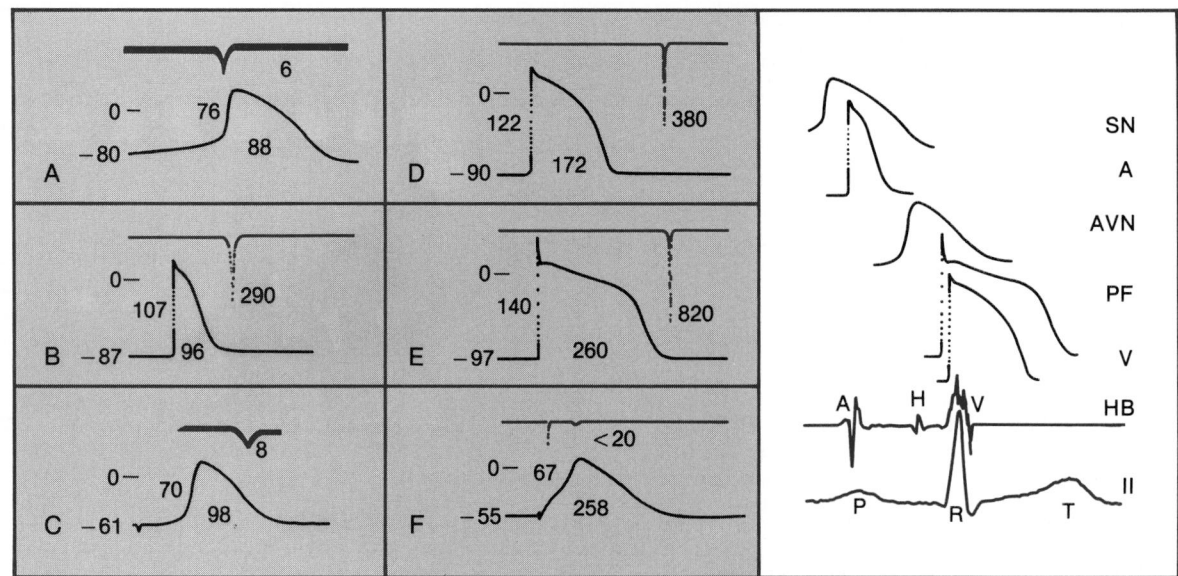

FIGURE 20–15. Action potentials recorded from different tissues in the heart *(left)*, remounted along with a His bundle recording and scalar ECG from a patient *(right)* to illustrate the timing during a single cardiac cycle. In panels *A* to *F*, the top tracing is dV/dt of phase 0 and the second tracing is the action potential. For each panel, the numbers (from left to right) indicate maximum diastolic potential (mV), action potential amplitude (mV), action potential duration at 90 per cent of repolarization (msec), and $\dot{V}_{max}$ of phase 0 (V/sec). Zero potential is indicated by the short horizontal line next to the zero on the upper left of each action potential. *A*, Rabbit sinoatrial node; *B*, canine atrial muscle; *C*, rabbit atrioventricular node; *D*, canine ventricular muscle; *E*, canine Purkinje fiber; *F*, diseased human ventricle. Note that the action potentials recorded in *A*, *C*, and *F* have reduced resting membrane potentials, amplitudes, and $\dot{V}_{max}$ compared with the other action potentials. In the *right panel*, SN = sinus nodal potential; A = atrial muscle potential; AVN = atrioventricular nodal potential; PF = Purkinje fiber potential; V = ventricular muscle potential; HB = His bundle recording; II = lead II. Horizontal calibration on the left: 50 msec for *A* and *C*, 100 msec for *B*, *D*, *E*, and *F*; 200 msec on the right. Vertical calibration on the left: 50 mV. Horizontal calibration on the right: 200 msec. (Modified from Gilmour, R. F., Jr., and Zipes, D. P.: Basic electrophysiology of the slow inward current. *In* Antman, E., and Stone, P. H. [eds.]: Calcium Blocking Agents in the Treatment of Cardiovascular Disorders. Mt. Kisco, N.Y., Futura, 1983, pp. 1–37.)

proximation of the rate and magnitude of Na$^+$ entry into the cell and a determinant of conduction velocity for the propagated action potential. The transient increase in sodium conductance lasts 1 to 2 msec. The action potential, or more properly the Na$^+$ current (I_{Na}), is said to be regenerative; that is, intracellular movement of a little Na$^+$ depolarizes the membrane more, which increases conductance to Na$^+$ more, which allows more Na$^+$ to enter, and so on. As this is occurring, however, [Na$^+$]$_i$ and positive intracellular charges increase and reduce the driving force for Na$^+$. When the equilibrium potential for Na$^+$ (E_{Na}) is reached, Na$^+$ no longer enters the cell, i.e., when the driving force acting on the ion to enter the cell balances the driving force acting on the ion to exit the cell, no current will flow. In addition, Na$^+$ conductance is time dependent so that when the membrane spends some time at voltages less negative than the resting potential, Na$^+$ conductance decreases. Therefore, an intervention that reduces membrane potential for a time—but not to threshold—partially inactivates Na$^+$ channels, and if threshold is now achieved, the magnitude and rate of Na$^+$ influx are reduced.

In cardiac Purkinje fibers and to a lesser extent in ventricular muscle, two different populations of Na$^+$ channels, or two different modes of operation of the same Na$^+$ channel, exist. One is responsible for the brief Na$^+$ current of phase 0, while the other, which is longer lasting, participates in the action potential plateau. Tetrodotoxin (TTX) and local anesthetics block both types of channels, diminishing the rate of rise of phase 0 and shortening action potential duration.[35] Further, there may be a background Na$^+$ current (I_{Na-B}) through a voltage-independent channel in sinus nodal cells that contributes to pacemaker behavior.[66]

At this point, several concepts need to be expanded. Ohm's law states that voltage equals current times resistance. The term *conductance* (g) is the inverse or reciprocal of resistance and is related to the ease with which ions can cross the cell membrane when driven by a potential difference across the membrane. As resistance of the membrane to passage of an ion increases, conductance decreases. Membrane permeability or conductance of the Na$^+$ channel during phase 0 is regulated hypothetically by two types of gates, the m gate and the h gate, which modulate Na ion passage through the channel (Fig. 20–16).

THE GATED SYSTEM—A HYPOTHETICAL MODEL. In this hypothetical model, three m (activation) gates and one h (inactivation) gate can be considered to be lined up in series in the membrane Na$^+$ channel (Fig. 20–16), with the m gate on the extracellular side and the h gate on the intracellular side of the membrane. When the membrane is in a resting polarized state, the m gates are almost completely closed, the h gate is open, and no Na$^+$ can cross the membrane. Although depolarization of the membrane opens the m gates and closes the h gate, the m gates open faster than the h gate closes, i.e., activation of the channel proceeds faster than inactivation can occur, and Na$^+$ flows through the Na$^+$ channel for about 1 msec while both gates are open simultaneously (Fig. 20–16, *left panel*, red arrow).

When the membrane repolarizes to fairly high negative values, i.e., membrane potential becomes more negative than about −60 mV, the gates shut rapidly, the h gate opens more slowly (reactivation or recovery from inactivation), and the membrane is once again capable of depolarization. Until that time, the cell is absolutely refractory; i.e., no stimulus, regardless of intensity, can activate the cell. If the membrane is activated a second time before reaching a large negative value, all the h gates have not yet reopened so that the maximum number of Na$^+$ channels that can open is reduced. The resulting action potential will have reduced $\dot{V}_{max}$, amplitude, duration, and conduction velocity. The state of the gates at any time depends on the membrane potential and the length of time the potential has been maintained.[35]

A sequence of positively charged amino acids has been identified as the activation (m) gate that opens the channel in response to depolarization, while an intracellular peptide loop is the inactivation (h) gate. When it dangles free, ions can move in or out of the channel. When the protein ball plugs the mouth of the pore, ion flow stops and inactivation results[37] (Fig. 20–17).

Using this model, the amount of current (I) generated by a specific ion (I_i) equals the membrane conductance for the ion (g_i) multiplied by the driving force for that ion. The driving force is the difference between the actual membrane voltage (V_m) and the equilibrium potential for that ion (E_i). Thus

$$I_i = g_i (V_m - E_i)$$

Conductance can be determined by rearranging the equation:

$$g_i = I_i (V_m - E_i)$$

The equations indicate that the current flow is voltage dependent; i.e., as the voltage of the membrane (V_m) changes relative to the equilibrium potential (E_i), the electrical driving force for an ion ($V_m - E_i$) changes and so does the current. The relationship between membrane voltage (V_m) at the time of depolarization and I_{Na}, measured in terms of $\dot{V}_{max}$ (maximum rate of rise of phase 0), is indicated by the so-called membrane responsiveness curve. When depolarization occurs at reduced membrane potentials, it results in decreased I_{Na} and $\dot{V}_{max}$.

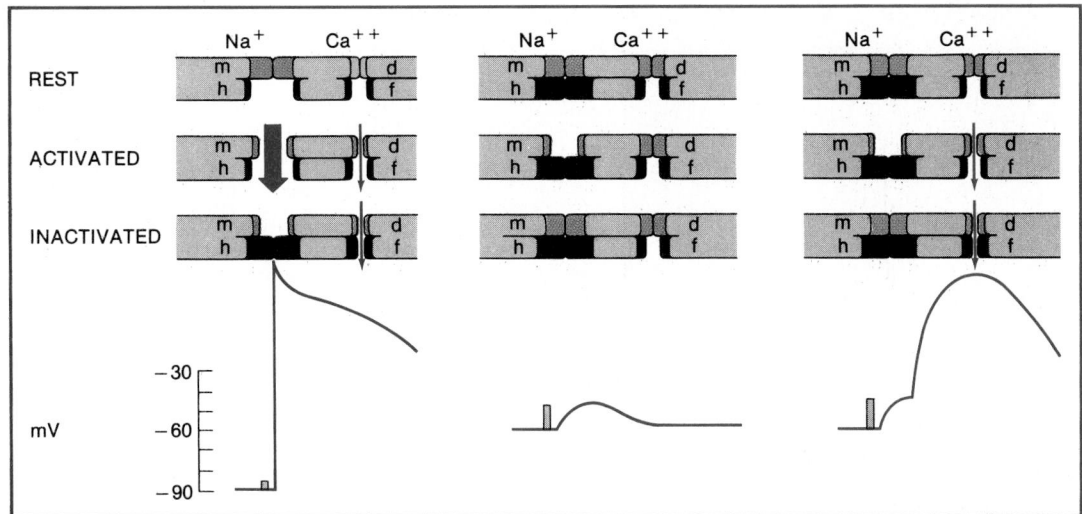

FIGURE 20–16. Schematic representation of membrane channels for rapid and slow inward currents at resting membrane potential *(top row)*, during the activated state *(middle row)*, and during the inactivated state *(bottom row)*. Vertically separated panels depict fibers with a normal resting potential of −90 mV *(left)*, with resting membrane potential reduced to less than −60 mV *(middle)*, and after stimulation of the cell with catecholamines *(right)*. The activation (m) and inactivation (h) gates of the fast channel and the activation (d) and inactivation (f) gates of the slow channel are depicted.

During the resting state *(left panel)*, the activation gates of both channels are closed while the inactivation gates are open. When the cell is stimulated, the m gates of the fast channel open, and for a brief period of time, the open m gates and h gates allow inward sodium current to flow, depolarize the cell, and produce its upstroke. The action potential is depicted below. The h gates then close the channel and inactivate sodium conductance. When the upstroke of the action potential exceeds the threshold for activation of the slow inward current, the d gates open, allowing ingress of the slow inward current that contributes to the plateau phase of the action potential. The f gates of the slow channel close more slowly than the h gates. Although the slow inward channel remains open longer than does the fast channel, less total current flows.

When the resting membrane potential is reduced below −60 mV by increasing $[K]_o$ from 4.0 to 14.0 mm *(middle panel)*, the cell depolarizes to −60 mV and the fast channel becomes inactivated because the h gates remain closed. Even though the m gate may open during activation, the amount of sodium current is too small to elicit an action potential. The inactivation gates of the slow channel (f gates) are only partially closed, and when the cell is excited after addition of catecholamine *(right panel)*, the d gates open and permit flow of a slow inward current that causes a slow-response action potential. This action potential resembles those in panels A, C, and F of Figure 20–15. (Reproduced by permission from Wit, A. L., and Bigger, J. T., Jr.: Possible electrophysiological mechanisms for lethal arrhythmias accompanying myocardial ischemia and infarction. Circulation 52 (Suppl. 3):96, 1975. Copyright 1975 American Heart Association.)

Membrane voltage also may regulate current flow by altering the status of the channel gates, thereby altering conductance. For the Na^+ channel,

$$gi_{Na} = \bar{g}_{Na}\ m^3h$$

where gi_{Na} is the conductance of the Na^+ channel at a given voltage, $\bar{g}_{Na}$ is the maximum possible conductance of the channel, m^3 represents the status of the activation gate (m = 1, the gate is open; m = 0, the gate is closed), and h represents the status of the inactivation gate (h = 1, gate open; h = 0, gate closed). Since the opening and closing of the gates are voltage and time dependent, the conductance of the channel (g) will be some fraction of the maximum possible conductance ($\bar{g}_{Na}$), depending on membrane voltage and the period during which the membrane has been at that voltage. $\dot{V}_{max}$ in Purkinje fibers approximates the Na^+ current. The state of the channel influences the effects of drugs (Fig. 20–18; see also Chap. 21).

UPSTROKE OF THE ACTION POTENTIAL. In normal atrial and ventricular muscle and in the fibers in the His-Purkinje system, action potentials have very rapid upstrokes with a large $\dot{V}_{max}$ and are called *fast responses*. Action potentials in the normal sinus and atrioventricular (AV) nodes have very slow upstrokes with a reduced $\dot{V}_{max}$ and are called *slow responses*[30] (Fig. 20–15 and Table 20–3). Upstrokes of "slow responses" are mediated by a slow inward, predominantly Ca^{++} current (I_{Ca}) rather than the fast inward I_{Na} (Table 20–4). These potentials received the name *slow response* because the time required for activation and inactivation of the slow inward current (I_{si}) is approximately an order of magnitude slower than that for the fast inward Na^+ current (I_{Na}). Recovery from inactivation also takes longer. Calcium entry and $[Ca^{++}]_i$ help promote inactivation. Thus the slow channel opens (activation gates d) and closes (inactivation gates f) more slowly than the fast channel, remains open for a longer time, and requires more time following a stimulus to be reactivated (see Fig. 20–16). In fact, recovery of excitability outlasts full restoration of maximum diastolic potential. This means that even though the membrane potential has returned to normal, the cell has not recovered excitability completely because the latter depends on elapse of a certain amount of time (i.e., is time

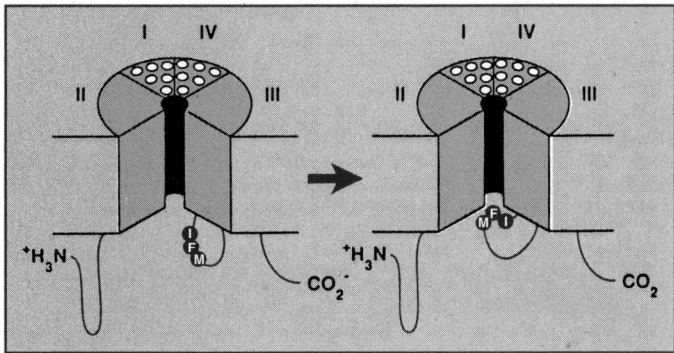

FIGURE 20–17. Mechanism of inactivation of sodium channels. The hinged-lid mechanism of sodium channel inactivation is illustrated. The intracellular loop connecting domains III and IV of the sodium channel is depicted as forming a hinged lid. The critical residue (Phe 1489 F) is shown as occluding the intracellular mouth of the pore. (From Catteral, W. A.: Molecular analysis of voltage gated sodium channels in the heart and other tissues. *In* Zipes, D. P., and Jalife, J. [eds.]: Cardiac Electrophysiology: From Cell to Bedside. 2nd ed. Philadelphia, W. B. Saunders Company, 1994, p. 1.)

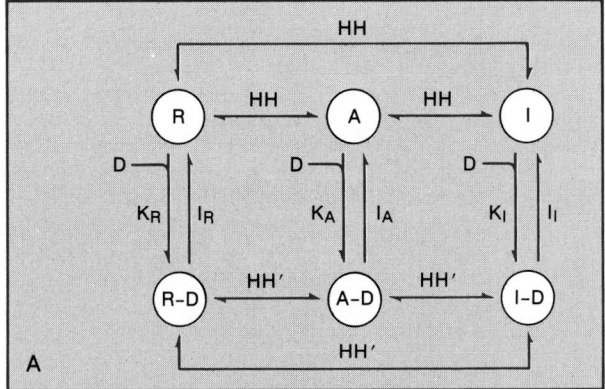

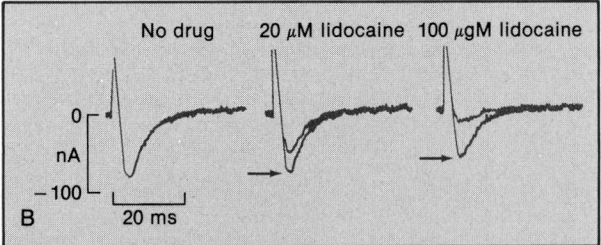

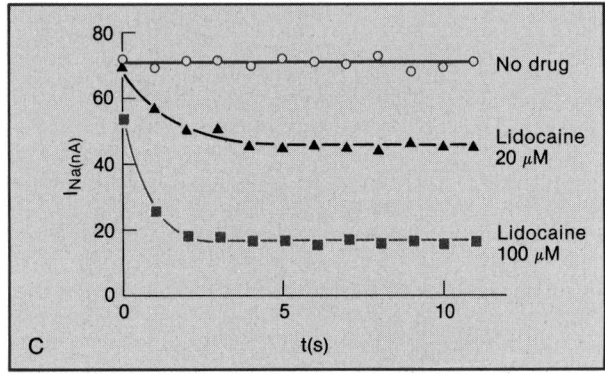

FIGURE 20–18. Interaction between sodium channels and lidocaine. *A,* Schematic of the modulated receptor hypothesis is presented. Sodium channel gating is represented by transitions between a resting state (R), an open state (A), and an inactivated state (I). The rate constants for binding and unbinding of drug to the channel (k's, I's) depend on the gating state. The presence of bound drug alters the gating transitions from their normal kinetics (HH for Hodgkin-Huxley) to modified kinetics (HH'). Application of this hypothesis explains why some drugs affect cardiac electrophysiological properties according to different channel states, e.g., depolarized or repolarized conditions. (Reproduced with permission from Hondeghem, L. M., and Katzung, B. G.: Antiarrhythmic agents: The modulated receptor mechanism of action of sodium and calcium-blocking drugs. Annu. Rev. Pharmacol. Toxicol. *24:*387, © 1984 by Annual Reviews Inc.).

B, An example of use dependent block of I_{Na} by lidocaine is demonstrated. I_{Na} was measured (nA) during trains of 500 msec pulses when the cell was depolarized from a holding potential of -105 mV to -35 mV at 1 Hz following a period of rest. The traces show membrane currents associated with the 1st and 12th pulses superimposed, and the graph *(C)* plots measured I_{Na} amplitudes for each of the 12 pulses. Lidocaine exerted relatively little effect on the first inward current signal following the rest period (arrows, *B*), but it substantially reduced peak I_{Na} following repetitive depolarizations. Lidocaine exerted a greater effect at the higher concentration. This figure illustrates that lidocaine blocks the sodium channel and reduces I_{Na} to a greater degree after repeated depolarizations of the cell compared with the first depolarization when the cell has been resting (use-dependence). (From Bean, B. P., Cohen, C. J., and Tsien, R. W.: Lidocaine block of cardiac sodium channels. J. Gen. Physiol. *81:*613, 1983.)

dependent) and not just on recovery of a particular membrane potential (i.e., voltage dependence).

Calcium channels are much more selective for Ca^{++} than sodium channels are for Na^+. Selectivity results from the presence of binding sites for which the permeant ions must compete, and under physiological conditions, more than 90 per cent of the inward current through the calcium channel is carried by Ca^{++}. Other divalent cations such as barium and strontium also can carry I_{si}. The magnitude of I_{si} is determined by the probability of calcium channel opening (P), the current through an open channel (i), and the number of channels (N): $I_{si} = N \cdot P \cdot i$. There are estimated to be 1 to 10 functional Ca^{++} channels/μM^2 surface area. At 3 mM $[Ca^{++}]_o$ and a membrane potential of 0 mV, i approximates 0.05 pA.

The threshold for activation of I_{si}, i.e., the voltage the cell must reach to "turn on" the slow inward current, is about -30 to -40 mV. In fast-response type fibers, I_{si} is normally activated during phase 0 by the regenerative depolarization caused by the fast sodium current. Current flows through both fast and slow channels during the latter part of the action potential upstroke. However, I_{si} is much smaller than the peak Na^+ current and therefore contributes little to the action potential until the fast Na^+ current is inactivated, after completion of phase 0. Thus, I_{si} affects mainly the plateau of action potentials recorded in atrial and ventricular muscle and His-Purkinje fibers. When the fast Na^+ current inactivates rapidly, such as in frog ventricle, I_{si} may contribute noticeably to the peak of phase 0. In addition, I_{si} can be activated and may play a prominent role in partially depolarized cells in which the fast Na^+

channels have been inactivated, if conditions are appropriate for slow-channel activation.

At least two types of calcium currents exist: a slowly inactivating high-threshold dihydropyridine-sensitive current (slow or L current, I_{Ca-L}) and a fast inactivating low-threshold dihydropyridine-insensitive current (fast or T current, I_{Ca-T}). I_{Ca-L} produces repolarization and propagation in sinus and AV nodal cells and contributes to the plateau, triggering calcium release from the sarcoplasmic reticulum in atrial, ventricular, and His-Purkinje cells. Calcium channel blockers block this channel, which is strongly modulated by neurotransmitters. I_{Ca-T} is activated at thresholds intermediate between I_{Na} and I_{Ca-L} and probably contributes inward current to the later stages of phase 4 depolarizations in the sinus node and His-Purkinje cells.[41,43–50]

Other significant differences exist between the fast and slow channels (Table 20–4). Drugs that elevate cyclic AMP levels such as beta-adrenoceptor agonists, phosphodiesterase inhibitors such as theophylline, and the lipid-soluble derivative of cyclic AMP, dibutyryl cyclic AMP, increase I_{Ca-L}. The beta-adrenoceptor agonist, binding to specific sarcolemmal receptors, facilitates the dissociation of two subunits of a regulatory protein (G protein, p. 372), one of which (G_s) activates adenylate cyclase and thus increases intracellular levels of cyclic AMP. The latter binds to a regulatory subunit of a cyclic AMP–dependent protein kinase that promotes phosphorylation of specific membrane proteins controlling the permeability of the slow channel. This putative conformational change in the channel increases the magnitude of the current or the conductance to the ion, presumably by increasing the amount of time the individual channels are open, without increasing the total number of calcium channels. The probability of channel opening increases.

The alpha subunit of the regulatory protein G_s can activate Ca channels directly. Acetylcholine reduces I_{Ca-L} by decreasing adenylate cyclase activity. However, acetylcholine stimulates cGMP accumula-

TABLE 20–3   CARDIAC CURRENTS

561

Ch 20

INWARD CURRENTS

I_{Na}	Fast inward current carried by Na^+ through a voltage-activated sodium channel.
I_{Na-B}	Proposed background Na^+ current through a voltage-independent channel in sinus nodal cells.
I_{Ca-L}	L-type (long-lasting) calcium current blocked by verapamil, diltiazem, and dihydropyridines, produces depolarization and propagation in SA and AV nodal cells, and contributes to the plateau of atrial, His-Purkinje, and ventricular cells; may induce early afterdepolarizations and calcium overload that could induce delayed afterdepolarizations.
I_{Ca-T}	T-type (transient) calcium current, may contribute inward current to the later stages of phase 4 depolarization in SA nodal and His-Purkinje cells.
I_f	Inward current carried by Na^+ and K^+ that is activated by polarization to negative membrane potentials in SA and AV nodal cells and His-Purkinje cells, generating phase 4 depolarization; increases the rate of impulse initiation in pacemaker cells.
I_{NS}	Inward current carried by Na^+ and, under some conditions, activated by Ca^{++} release from the sarcoplasmic reticulum during intracellular Ca^{++} overload, contributes to delayed afterdepolarizations; also can be the I_{T1}, the transient inward current.

OUTWARD CURRENTS

I_{K1}	K^+ current responsible for maintaining resting potential near the K^+ equilibrium potential in atrial, AV nodal, His-Purkinje, and ventricular cells; also called the inward rectifier.
I_K	K^+ current carried through voltage-gated channels; also called delayed rectifier; major current causing repolarization; enhancement shortens repolarization while blockade lengthens it. This current is subdivided into a current with rapid activation and inactivation kinetics (I_{K-R}), a current with ultrarapid kinetics (I_{K-UR}), and a current with slow kinetics (I_{K-S}).
I_{to}	K^+ current turns on rapidly after depolarization and then inactivates; one type is voltage activated and modulated by neurotransmitters; the other type is activated by intracellular Ca^{++}.
$I_{K(ACh)}$	K^+ current whose channel is activated by the muscarinic (M_2) receptor via GTP regulatory (G) protein signal transduction; particularly important in SA and AV nodal cells and in atrial cells, where it can produce significant hyperpolarization, and in atrium, where it produces marked shortening of repolarization; appears identical to the channel opened by purinergic (adenosine) receptor and also designated $I_{K(Ado)}$.
$I_{K(ATP)}$	K^+ channel blocked by ATP and strongly activated during hypoxia and ischemia when intracellular ATP concentration falls; may contribute to shortening of action potential duration during ischemia.
I_{Cl}	Cl^- current increased by adrenergic stimulation, contributing to repolarization.
$I_{K(Ca)}$	K^+ current carried through a channel that is activated by intracellular Ca^{++}, accelerating repolarization in calcium-overloaded heart.
$I_{K(Na)}$	K^+ current activated by high cytosolic sodium concentrations and may promote repolarization in sodium overloaded heart.
I_{Arach}	Current activated by arachidonic acid and other fatty acids, especially in acid pH, for example, when these metabolites are liberated during ischemia.

PUMPS

Na-K	Blocked by digitalis; generates small outward $I_{Na-K pump}$ current; when fully operative, $3Na^+$ leave and $2K^+$ enter the cell.
Ca	Found in sarcoplasmic reticulum; ATP-dependent.

CARRIERS

Na/Ca	Countertransport system in sarcolemma and mitochondria; generates $I_{Na/Ca}$ by exchanging $1Ca^{++}$ for $3Na^+$; may contribute to generation of delayed afterdepolarizations during Ca^{++} overload.
Na/H	Exchanger blocked by amiloride.
Na/K/Cl	Cotransporter blocked by amiloride.
Cl/HCO_3	Exchanger.

tion. cGMP has negligible effects on the basal I_{Ca-L} but decreases I_{Ca-L} that has been elevated by beta-adrenoceptor agonists. This effect is mediated by cyclic AMP hydrolysis via a cGMP-stimulated cyclic nucleotide phosphodiesterase.[22]

DIFFERENCES BETWEEN CHANNELS. Fast and slow channels can be differentiated on the basis of their pharmacological sensitivity. Drugs that block the slow channel with a *fair* degree of specificity include verapamil, nifedipine, diltiazem, D-600 (a methoxy derivative of verapamil), and compounds such as manganese, lanthanum, nickel, and cobalt. Antiarrhythmic agents such as lidocaine, quinidine, procainamide, and disopyramide (see Chap. 21) affect the fast channel and not the slow channel. The puffer fish poison tetrodotoxin (TTX), which is too toxic to be used clinically, blocks the fast channel with considerable specificity (Table 20–4).

While fast-response action potentials are characteristic of atrial and ventricular muscle and His-Purkinje tissue, slow-response type action potentials are found in the normal sinus and AV nodes and many kinds of diseased tissue (Table 20–4). Normal action potentials recorded from the sinus node and the N region of the AV node have a reduced resting membrane potential, action potential amplitude, overshoot, upstroke, and conduction velocity compared with action potentials in muscle or Purkinje fibers (Fig. 20–15).

Slow-channel blockers, but not TTX, suppress sinus and AV nodal action potentials. The prolonged time for reactivation of the I_{Ca-L} probably accounts for the fact that sinus and AV nodal cells remain refractory longer than the time it takes for full voltage repolarization to occur. Thus premature stimulation immediately after the membrane potential reaches full repolarization leads to action potentials with reduced amplitudes and upstroke velocities. Therefore, slow conduction and prolonged refractoriness are characteristic features of nodal cells. These cells also have a reduced "safety factor for conduction," which means that the stimulating efficacy of the propagating impulse is low and conduction block occurs easily. Membranes of

nodal cells probably do have Na channels that are inactivated by the relatively depolarized range of potentials over which activity takes place. Hyperpolarization exposes a fast TTX-sensitive sodium current in nodal cells.

INWARD CURRENTS. Thus I_{Na} and I_{Ca} represent two important inward currents. Another important inward current is I_f, also called the *pacemaker current.*[17-21] This current is activated by hyperpolarization and is carried by Na^+ and K^+. It generates phase 4 diastolic depolarization in the sinus node. I_f activation is the major mechanism by which beta-adrenergic and cholinergic neurotransmitters regulate the cardiac rhythm under physiologic conditions (see p. 63). Catecholamines increase the probability of channel opening, with no change in single channel amplitude, and increase the discharge rate, with cholinergic action, in general, having an opposite effect.

A variety of manipulations, including those which block or inactivate I_{Na} (such as administration of TTX or depolarization of the cell membrane with K^+), combined with those that increase I_{Ca-L} (such as administration of Ca^{++} or catecholamines), or those that decrease the outward potassium currents (such as barium), can transform a fast-channel–dependent fiber (e.g., a Purkinje fiber) to a slow-channel–dependent fiber. Whether these artificial in vitro alterations have clinical relevance is not known, but it is possible that myocardial ischemia or infarction, for example, can produce this transformation (Fig. 20–15F).

The electrophysiological changes accompanying *acute* myocardial ischemia may represent a depressed form of a fast response in the center of the ischemic zone and a slow response in the border area.[67] Probable slow-response activity has been shown in myocardium resected from patients undergoing surgery for recurrent ventricular tachyarrhythmias (Fig. 20–19). Whether and how slow responses play a role in the genesis of ventricular arrhythmias in these patients has not been established. I_{Na} is another inward current gated by [Ca^{++}] that contributes to delayed afterdepolarizations (Table 20–3).

TABLE 20–4 CHARACTERISTICS OF FAST AND SLOW INWARD CURRENTS IN CARDIAC TISSUE

	FAST	SLOW
Primary charge carrier	NA	Ca (Na)
Activation threshold	−70 to −55 mV	−55 to −30 mV
Magnitude	1 to 30 μA	0.1 to 3.0 μA
Time constant of		
Activation	<1 msec	10 to 20 msec
Inactivation	<1 msec	50 to 500 msec
Inhibitors	Tetrodotoxin, local anesthetics, sustained depolarization at <−40 mV	Verapamil, D-600, nifedipine, diltiazem, Mn, Co, Ni, La
Resting membrane potential	−80 to −95 mV	−40 to −70 mV
Conduction velocity	0.3 to 3.0 M/sec	0.01 to 0.10 M/sec
Rate of rise ($\dot{V}_{max}$) of action potential upstroke	200 to 1000 V/sec	1 to 10 V/sec
Action potential amplitude	100 to 130 mV	35 to 75 mV
Response to stimulus	All-or-none	Affected by characteristics of stimulus
Recovery of excitability	Prompt, ends with repolarization	Delayed, outlasts full repolarization
Safety factor for conduction	High	Low
Major current of action potential upstroke in the following:		
SA node	−	+
Atrial myocardium	+	−
AV node (N region)	−	+
His-Purkinje system	+	−
Ventricular myocardium	+	−
Neurotransmitter influence		
Beta-adrenergic	−	↑ ↑
Alpha-adrenergic	−	
Muscarinic cholinergic	−	↓ In atrium ↓ In ventricle

Phase 1—Early Rapid Repolarization

Following phase 0, the membrane repolarizes rapidly and transiently to near 0 mV, partly owing to inactivation of I_{Na} or activation of a transient outward current carried mostly by K ions. I_{to},[65] a K⁺ current (Table 20–3), turns on rapidly after depolarization and then inactivates. One type of I_{to} is activated by $[Ca^{++}]_i$, and the other is voltage activated and modulated by neurotransmitter. I_{to} can modulate action potential duration and is nonuniformly distributed, being found in subepicardial but not subendocardial ventricular muscle cells. M cells are in a uniform subepicardial sheet and have repolarization characteristics similar to Purkinje fibers. They have sparse I_{k-s} and may be important in the development of early afterdepolarizations and torsades de pointes[68-70] (see p. 566). They may be responsible for the U wave in the electrocardiogram (ECG). Cl⁻ moving intracellularly through a Cl channel also may affect the plateau. Beta-adrenoceptor stimulation via cyclic AMP–dependent protein kinase, activation of adenylate cyclase, and histamine activate the chloride current.[71] The increase in intra-

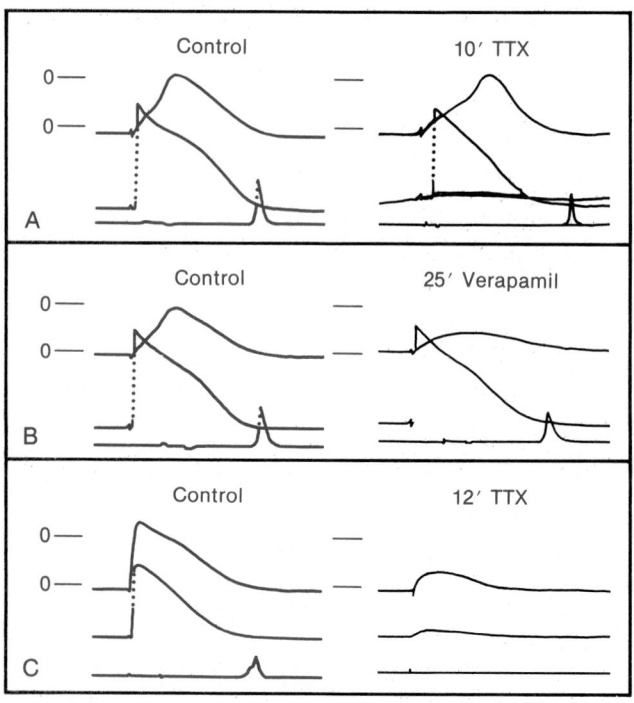

FIGURE 20–19. Effects of tetrodotoxin (TTX) and verapamil on action potentials in diseased human ventricle, removed from a patient at the time of endocardial resection for recurrent ventricular tachycardia. A, Action potentials and upstroke velocity recordings from an abnormal cell (upper action potential recording) and a relatively normal cell (lower action potential recording) before (left) and after (right) exposure to TTX for 10 minutes. V_{max} for the lower cell is shown in the bottom tracing. TTX produced activation delay and intermittent conduction block in the normal cell but had little effect on the action potential of the abnormal cell (right panel). Two consecutive cycles are superimposed in the right panel. B, After washout of TTX, the same two cells were exposed to verapamil for 25 minutes. Verapamil reduced both the action potential and the amplitude of the abnormal cell without affecting its resting membrane potential and slightly reduced both the action potential amplitude and V_{max} in the normal cell (right panel). C, Effects of TTX on a different specimen of myocardium from the same patient. Control recordings are shown on the left. In these cells, TTX markedly reduced action potential amplitude and $\dot{V}_{max}$ (right panel), while verapamil only slightly reduced action potential amplitude (not shown). (From Gilmour, R. F., Jr., et al.: Cellular electrophysiological abnormalities of diseased human ventricular myocardium. Am. J. Cardiol. 51:137, 1983.)

cellular negative ions reduces the positive membrane voltage, and the membrane potential returns to near 0 mV, from which the plateau, or phase 2, arises. Sometimes a slight transient depolarization follows phase 1 repolarization. Phase 1 is well defined and separated from phase 2 in Purkinje fibers and some muscle fibers.

Phase 2—Plateau

During the plateau phase, which may last several hundred milliseconds, membrane conductance to all ions falls to rather low values. Potassium conductance (g_K) falls almost immediately upon depolarization, in spite of the large electrochemical gradient for K^+, owing to "inward-going rectification." *Rectification* simply means voltage dependence of membrane resistance. Inward-going rectification means that when the membrane depolarizes, it passes inward current more easily than it passes outward current, or in this instance, K^+ can enter the cell more easily than it can exit, and therefore, despite multiple important outward K^+ currents and a large electrochemical gradient, g_K is low and few K^+ ions leave the cell. Sodium conductance (g_{Na}) is low because of inactivation of sodium channels. Minor contributions to repolarization include a small inward Cl^- flux and electrogenic Na^+-K^+ exchange, pumping out 3 Na^+ in exchange for 2 K^+. The Na^+-K^+ exchange does not turn on and off with each single action potential but restores the ionic gradient over a cumulative time period. I_{Ca-L}, active during the plateau, supplies a small (compared with I_{Na}) inward current and balances these outward currents, and membrane voltage remains near zero for more than 100 msec. An inward Na^+ current, mentioned earlier, is blocked by tetrodotoxin, and also contributes to the plateau.

Phase 3—Final Rapid Repolarization

In this portion of the action potential, repolarization proceeds rapidly, owing at least in part to two currents: time-dependent inactivation of I_{Ca-L}, so that intracellular movement of positive charges decreases, and activation of an outward K^+ current (called the *delayed rectifier* or I_K, the major current-causing repolarization) (Table 20-3), so that extracellular movement of positive charges increases. The net membrane current becomes more outward, and the membrane potential shifts in a negative direction. As repolarization continues, g_K increases, and these repolarization changes self-perpetuate in a regenerative manner.

Phase 4—Diastolic Depolarization
(See also p. 557)

Under normal conditions, the membrane potential of atrial and ventricular muscle cells remains steady throughout diastole. I_{K1} is the current responsible for maintaining

the resting potential near the K^+ equilibrium potential in atrial, AV nodal, His-Purkinje, and ventricular cells. I_{K1} is the inward rectifier, shutting off during depolarization. It is absent in sinus nodal cells. In other fibers found in certain parts of the atria, in the muscle of the mitral and tricuspid valves, in His-Purkinje fibers, and in the sinus node and distal portion of the AV node, the resting membrane potential does not remain constant in diastole but gradually depolarizes (Fig. 20-15A). If a propagating impulse does not depolarize the cell or group of cells, it may reach threshold by itself and produce a spontaneous action potential. The property possessed by spontaneously discharging cells is called *phase 4 diastolic depolarization;* when it leads to initiation of action potentials, automaticity results. The discharge rate of the sinus node normally exceeds the discharge rate of other potentially automatic pacemaker sites and thus maintains dominance of the cardiac rhythm. Discharge rate of the sinus node is more sensitive to the effects of norepinephrine and acetylcholine than is the discharge rate of ventricular muscle cells (Fig. 20-20). Normal or abnormal automaticity at other sites can discharge at rates faster than the sinus nodal discharge rate and can usurp control of the cardiac rhythm for one cycle or many.

Normal Automaticity

The ionic basis of automaticity is explained by a net gain in intracellular positive charges during diastole. Contributing to this change is a voltage-dependent channel activated by potentials negative to -50 to -60 mV, i.e., a hyperpolarization-activated inward pacemaker current. At this potential an inward current called I_f becomes activated and is carried by a channel relatively nonselective for monovalent cations. Hyperpolarization increases its rate of activation, and at -70 mV, the time constant ranges from 2 to 4 sec. I_f probably underlies the slow diastolic depolarization that occurs between -90 and -60 mV in Purkinje fibers. Although either K^+ or Na^+ can serve as ion transporters, I_f carries largely Na^+ at the more negative intracellular voltages. Extracellular K^+ ions activate I_f, but $[Na^+]_o$ does not influence its conductance.[17-21]

AUTOMATICITY IN SINUS NODAL CELLS. At the reduced membrane potentials of sinus nodal cells, I_f contributes only about 20 per cent of the pacemaker current, and automaticity is primarily dependent on I_K and I_{Ca-L}. However, sinus nodal cells exhibit significant I_f current if they are hyperpolarized in the range of -50 to -100 mV. Conversely, I_K in normally polarized Purkinje fibers adds little to the pacemaker current. The decay of I_K, together with the presence of an unidentified background inward current, and I_{Ca-L} are the essential processes governing the rate of

FIGURE 20-20. Effects of different doses of ACh on spontaneous activity in single SA node cell. *A-D,* Activity in the control Tyrode solution *(C)* is compared with that in the presence of 0.01, 0.1, 1.0, and 10 μM ACh, respectively. Each concentration of ACh was perfused for about 20 sec. Note that slowing occurred with 0.01 and 0.1 μM ACh and that the cell ceased to beat at higher concentrations, at which point hyperpolarization of the maximum diastolic depolarization also clearly appeared. (From DiFrancisco, D.: Current i_f and the neuronal modulation of heart rate. *In* Zipes, D. P., and Jalife, J. [eds.]: Cardiac Electrophysiology. From Cell to Bedside. Philadelphia, W. B. Saunders Company, 1990.)

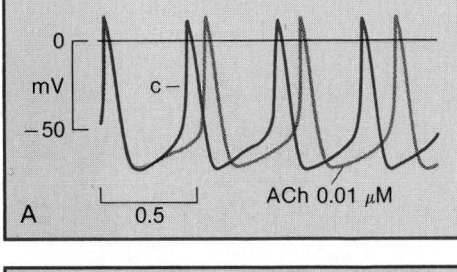

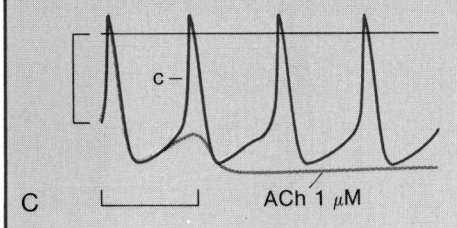

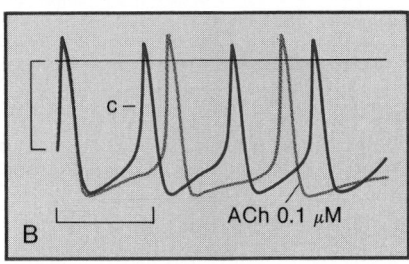

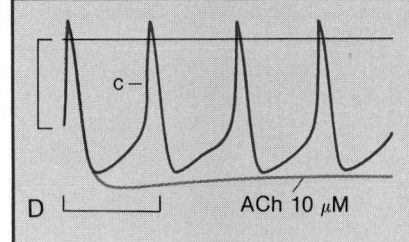

pacemaker depolarization in sinus and AV nodal cells and in Purkinje fibers whose membrane potential has been depolarized to voltages largely positive to the activation range of I_f.[72]

Sinus nodal discharge rate maintains dominance over latent pacemaker sites because it depolarizes more rapidly and because of the mechanism called *overdrive suppression*, a phenomenon characterized by prolonged suppression of normal pacemakers in proportion to the duration and rate of stimulation by a more rapidly discharging pacemaker. The mechanism may relate to active Na extrusion during the more rapid rate that maintains diastolic depolarization of latent pacemakers at a level more negative than the threshold potential for automatic discharge.

The rate of sinus nodal discharge can be varied by several mechanisms in response to autonomic or other influences. The pacemaker locus can shift within or outside the sinus node to cells discharging faster or more slowly. If the pacemaker site remains the same, alterations in the slope of the diastolic depolarization, maximum diastolic potential, or threshold potential can speed or slow the discharge rate (Fig. 20–20). For example, if the slope of diastolic depolarization steepens, and if the resting membrane potential becomes less negative or the threshold potential more negative (within limits), discharge rate increases. Opposite changes slow the discharge rate.

Passive Membrane Electrical Properties

We have just discussed many of the features of active membrane properties. In addition, it is important to be aware of some features of the passive membrane properties, such as membrane resistance, capacitance, and cable properties.[35,57] The important difference between the active and passive states is that the active system responds out of proportion to the applied stimulus and thereby adds energy to the electrical system; the passive system responds proportionately to the size of the stimulus and does not add energy.

Although the cardiac cell membrane is resistant to current flow, it also has capacitive properties, which means it behaves like a battery and can store charges of opposite sign on its two sides: an excess of negative charges inside the membrane balanced by equivalent positive charges outside the membrane. These resistive and capacitive properties cause the membrane to take a certain amount of time to respond to an applied stimulus, rather than responding instantly, because the charges across the capacitive membrane must be altered first. A subthreshold rectangular-shaped current pulse applied to the membrane produces a slowly rising and decaying membrane-voltage change rather than a rectangular voltage change. A value called the *time constant of the membrane* reflects this property and is the time taken by the membrane voltage to reach 63 per cent of its final value after application of a steady current.

When aligned end to end, cardiac cells, particularly the His-Purkinje system, behave like a long cable in which current flows more easily inside the cell and to the adjacent cell across the gap junction than it does across the cell membrane to the outside. When current is injected at a point, most of it flows along the cell, but some leaks out. Because of this loss of current, the voltage change of a cell at a site distant from the point of applied current is less than the change in membrane voltage where the stimulus was given. A measure of this property of a cable is called the space or length constant λ; it is the distance along the cable from the point of stimulation that the voltage at steady state is 1/e (37 per cent) of its value at the point of introduction.

Restated, λ describes how far current flows before leaking passively across the surface membrane to a value about one-third its initial value. This distance is normally about 2 mm for Purkinje fibers, 0.5 mm for the sinus node, and 0.8 mm for ventricular muscle fibers. λ is about 10 times the length of an individual cell. As an example, if e is about 2.7 and a hyperpolarizing current pulse in a Purkinje fiber produces a membrane-voltage change of 15 mV at the site of current injection, the membrane potential change one space constant (2 mm) away would be 15/2.7 = 5.5 mV.

Since the current loop in any circuit must be closed, current must flow back to its point of origin. Local circuit currents pass across gap junctions between cells and exit across the sarcolemmal membrane to close the loop and complete the circuit. Inward excitation currents in one area (carried by Na+ in most regions) flow intracellularly along the length of the tissue (carried mostly by K+), escape across the membrane, and flow extracellularly in a longitudinal direction. The outside local circuit current is the current recorded in an electrocardiogram. Through these local circuit currents the transmembrane potential of each cell influences the transmembrane potential of its neighbor because of the passive flow of current from one segment of the fiber to another across the low-resistance gap junctions.

If two cells having different resting membrane potentials are coupled to one another, the resting potentials of each cell will equalize; i.e., one cell will depolarize and the other will hyperpolarize. This "electrotonic" influence of neighboring cells on each other is determined chiefly by the length constant of the fiber and is due to the passive spread of current.

As discussed earlier, the speed of conduction depends on active membrane properties such as the magnitude of the Na+ current, a measure of which is $\dot{V}_{max}$. Passive membrane properties also contribute to conduction velocity and include excitability threshold, which influences the capability of cells adjacent to the one that has been discharged to reach threshold; the intracellular resistance of the cell, which is determined by the free ions in the cytoplasm, the resistance of the gap junction, and the cross-sectional area of the cell. Direction of propagation is crucial due to the influence of anisotropy, as mentioned earlier.

Loss of Membrane Potential and Arrhythmia Development

Most acquired abnormalities of cardiac muscle or specialized fibers that result in arrhythmias produce a loss of membrane potential; i.e., maximum diastolic potential becomes less negative. This change should be viewed as a symptom of an underlying abnormality, analogous to fever or jaundice, rather than a diagnostic category in and of itself, because both the ionic changes resulting in cellular depolarization and the more fundamental biochemical or metabolic abnormalities responsible for the ionic alterations are probably multicausal. Cellular depolarization can result from elevated $[K^+]_o$ or decreased $[K^+]_i$, an increase in membrane permeability to Na+ (P_{Na} increases), or a decrease in membrane permeability to K+ (P_K decreases). Reference to Equation 2 (see p. 556) illustrates that these changes alone or in combination make V_r less negative.

Normal cells perfused by an abnormal milieu (e.g., hyperkalemia), abnormal cells perfused by a normal milieu (e.g., healed myocardial infarction), or abnormal cells perfused by an abnormal milieu (e.g., acute myocardial ischemia and infarction) may exist alone or in combination to reduce resting membrane voltage. Each of these changes can have one or more biochemical or metabolic causes. For example, acute myocardial ischemia results in decreased $[K^+]_i$[73–75] and increased $[K^+]_o$, norepinephrine release, and acidosis that may be related to an increase in intracellular Ca^{++} and Ca-induced membrane oscillations and accumulation of amphipathic lipid metabolites and oxygen-free radicals. All these changes can contribute to the development of abnormal electrophysiological environment and arrhythmias during ischemia and reperfusion. Knowledge of these changes may provide insight into therapy that actually reverses basic defects and restores membrane potential or other abnormalities to normal.

EFFECTS OF REDUCED RESTING POTENTIAL. The reduced resting membrane potential alters depolarization and repolarization phases of the cardiac action potential. For example, partial membrane depolarization prevents complete recovery from inactivation (h gate) of the rapid Na+ channel. This reduces the number of available Na+ channels for depolarization and decreases the magnitude of the rapid Na+ current during phase 0. The subsequent reduction in $\dot{V}_{max}$ and action potential amplitude prolongs conduction time of the propagated impulse, at times to the point of block.

Action potentials with upstrokes dependent on the rapid Na+ current flowing through partially inactivated Na+ channels are called *depressed fast responses* (Fig. 20–19C). Their contours often resemble, and may be difficult to distinguish from, slow responses, in which upstrokes are due to I_{Ca-L} (Fig. 20–15F). Membrane depolarization to levels of −60 to −70 mV may inactivate half the Na+ channels, while depolarization to −50 mV or less may inactivate all the Na+ channels. At membrane potentials positive to −50 mV, I_{Ca-L} can be activated to generate phase 0 if conditions are appropriate. These action potential changes are

TABLE 20–5 MECHANISMS OF ARRHYTHMOGENESIS **565**

Ch 20

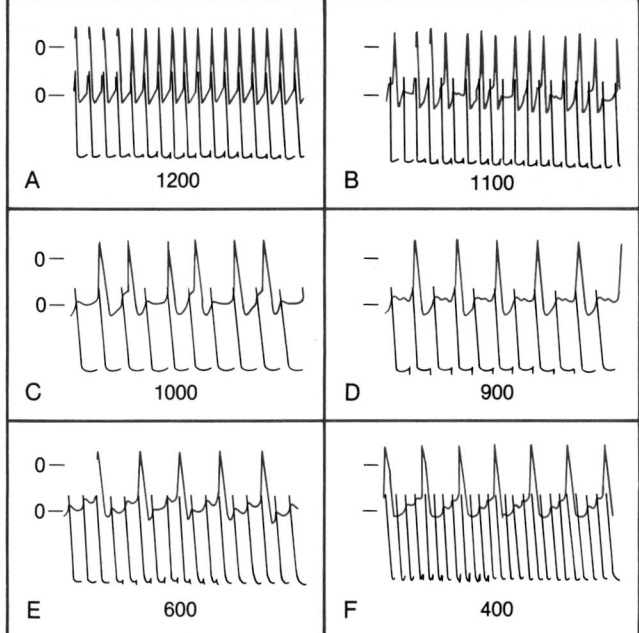

FIGURE 20–21. Rate-dependent conduction from the normal zone into the abnormal zone. When the pacing cycle length in the normal zone was shortened from 1200 to 400 msec *(panels A to F)*, increasing degrees of entrance block into the abnormal area occurred, progressing from 1:1 conduction at a cycle length of 1200 msec, to 4:3 conduction at 1100 msec, 3:2 conduction at 1000 msec, 2:1 conduction at 900 msec, 3:1 conduction at 600 msec, and 4:1 conduction at 400 msec. Pacing the abnormal zone (not shown) resulted in block to the normal zone (unidirectional propagation). Vertical calibration: 50 mV. Horizontal calibration: 4 sec in *A* and *B* and 2 sec in *C* to *F*. (From Gilmour, R. F., Jr., et al.: Cellular electrophysiologic abnormalities of diseased human ventricular myocardium. Am. J. Cardiol. *51*:137, 1983.)

TABLE 20–5   MECHANISMS OF ARRHYTHMOGENESIS

I. DISORDERS OF IMPULSE FORMATION
  A. Automaticity
    1. Normal automaticity
      a. Experimental examples—Normal in vivo or in vitro sinus node, Purkinje fibers, others
      b. Clinical examples—Sinus tachycardia or bradycardia inappropriate for the clinical situation, possibly ventricular parasystole
    2. Abnormal automaticity
      a. Experimental example—Depolarization-induced automaticity in Purkinje fibers or ventricular muscle
      b. Clinical example—Possibly accelerated ventricular rhythms after myocardial infarction
  B. Triggered Activity
    1. Early afterdepolarizations (EADs)
      a. Experimental examples—EADs produced by barium, hypoxia, high concentrations of catecholamines, drugs such as sotalol, N-acetylprocainamide, cesium
      b. Clinical examples—Possibly idiopathic and acquired long Q-T syndromes and associated ventricular arrhythmias
    2. Delayed afterdepolarizations (DADs)
      a. Experimental example—DADs produced in Purkinje fibers by digitalis
      b. Clinical example—Possibly some digitalis-induced arrhythmias

II. DISORDERS OF IMPULSE CONDUCTION
  A. Block
    1. Bidirectional or unidirectional without reentry
      a. Experimental example—SA, AV, bundle branch, Purkinje-muscle, others
      b. Clinical example—SA, AV, bundle branch, others
    2. Unidirectional block with reentry
      a. Experimental examples—AV node, Purkinje-muscle junction, infarcted myocardium, others
      b. Clinical examples—Reciprocating tachycardia in WPW syndrome, AV nodal reentry, VT due to bundle branch reentry, others
    3. Reflection
      a. Experimental example—Purkinje fiber with area of inexcitability
      b. Clinical example—Unknown

III. COMBINED DISORDERS
  A. Interactions between automatic foci
    1. Experimental examples—Depolarizing or hyperpolarizing subthreshold stimuli speed or slow automatic discharge rate
    2. Clinical examples—Modulated parasystole
  B. Interactions between automaticity and conduction
    1. Experimental examples—Deceleration-dependent block, overdrive suppression of conduction, entrance and exit block
    2. Clinical examples—Similar to experimental

likely to be heterogeneous with unequal degrees if Na+ inactivation that create areas with minimally reduced velocity, more severely depressed zones, and areas of complete block. These uneven changes are propitious for the development of arrhythmias (Fig. 20–21).

In these cells with reduced membrane potential, refractoriness may outlast voltage recovery of the action potential; i.e., the cell may still be refractory or partially refractory after the resting membrane potential returns to its most negative value. Further, if block of the cardiac impulse occurs in a fairly localized area without significant slowing of conduction proximal to the site of block, cells in this proximal zone exhibit short action potentials and refractory periods because unexcited cells distal to the block (still in a polarized state) electrotonically speed recovery in cells proximal to the site of block.

If conduction slows gradually proximal to the site of block, the duration of these action potentials and their refractory periods may be prolonged. Some cells may exhibit abnormal electrophysiological properties even though they have a relatively normal resting membrane potential.

MECHANISMS OF ARRHYTHMOGENESIS

(Table 20–5)

The mechanisms responsible for cardiac arrhythmias are generally divided into categories of disorders of impulse formation, disorders of impulse conduction, or combinations of both.[58,76–79] It is important to realize, however, that our present diagnostic tools do not permit unequivocal determination of the electrophysiological mechanisms responsible for most clinically occurring arrhythmias or their ionic bases. This is especially true for ventricular arrhyth-

mias. It is very difficult to separate reentry from automaticity clinically. At best, one can postulate that a particular arrhythmia is "most consistent with" or "best explained by" one or the other electrophysiological mechanism. Some tachyarrhythmias can be started by one mechanism and perpetuated by another. For example, premature ventricular depolarization due to abnormal automaticity can precipitate an episode of ventricular tachycardia sustained by reentry. An episode of tachycardia due to one mechanism can precipitate another episode due to a different mechanism.[80]

Disorders of Impulse Formation

This category is defined as inappropriate discharge rate of the normal pacemaker, the sinus node (e.g., sinus rates too fast or too slow for the physiological needs of the patient), or discharge of an ectopic pacemaker that controls the atrial or ventricular rhythm. Pacemaker discharge from ectopic sites, often called *latent* or *subsidiary pacemakers,* can occur in fibers located in several parts of the atria, the coronary sinus, atrioventricular valves, portions of the AV junction, and the His-Purkinje system. Ordinarily kept from reaching the level of threshold potential because of overdrive suppression by the more rapidly firing sinus node or electrotonic depression from contiguous fibers, ectopic pacemaker activity at one of these latent sites can become manifest when sinus nodal discharge rate slows or block occurs at some level between the sinus node and the ectopic pacemaker site, permitting *escape* of the latent pacemaker at the latter's normal discharge rate. A clinical example would be sinus bradycardia to a rate of 45 beats/min that permits an AV junctional escape complex to occur at a rate of 50 beats/min.

Alternatively, the discharge rate of the latent pacemaker can speed up inappropriately and usurp control of the cardiac rhythm from the sinus node that has been discharging at a normal rate. A clinical example would be interruption of normal sinus rhythm by a premature ventricular complex or a burst of ventricular tachycardia. It is important to remember that such disorders of impulse formation can be due to a speeding or slowing of a *normal* pacemaker mechanism (e.g., phase 4 diastolic depolarization that is ionically normal for the sinus node or for an ectopic site such as a Purkinje fiber but occurs inappropriately fast or slow) or due to an ionically *abnormal* pacemaker mechanism.

The patient with persistent sinus tachycardia at rest or sinus bradycardia during exertion exhibits inappropriate sinus nodal discharge rates, but the ionic mechanisms responsible for sinus nodal discharge may still be normal, although the kinetics or magnitude of the currents may be altered. Conversely, when a patient experiences ventricular tachycardia during an acute myocardial infarction, ionic mechanisms ordinarily not involved in formation of spontaneous impulses for this fiber type may be operative to generate this tachycardia. For example, although pacemaker activity generally is not found in ordinary working myocardium, the effects of myocardial infarction perhaps can depolarize these cells to membrane potentials at which inactivation of I_K and activation of I_{Ca-L} cause automatic discharge. Recent experimental evidence suggests that some areas of the ventricle during *acute* myocardial ischemia can enhance, while others suppress, automaticity and afterdepolarizations.[67] Areas of conduction block that may produce entrance block to the automatic focus can protect it from the effects of overdrive suppression and favor the development of automatic discharge. Because the maximum rate that can be achieved by adrenergic stimulation of normal automaticity is generally less than 200 beats/min, it is likely that episodes of faster tachycardia are not due to enhanced normal automaticity.

ABNORMAL AUTOMATICITY. Mechanisms responsible for *normal* automaticity were described earlier (see p. 563). *Abnormal* automaticity can arise from cells that have reduced maximum diastolic potentials, often at membrane potentials positive to −50 mV, when I_K and I_{Ca-L} may be operative.

Automaticity at membrane potentials more negative than −70 mV may be due to I_f. When the membrane potential is between −50 and −70 mV, the cell may be quiescent. Electrotonic effects from surrounding normally polarized or more depolarized myocardium will influence the development of automaticity. Abnormal automaticity has been found in Purkinje fibers removed from dogs subjected to myocardial infarction, in rat myocardium damaged by epinephrine, in human atrial samples, and in ventricular myocardial specimens from patients undergoing aneurysmectomy and endocardial resection for recurrent ventricular tachyarrhythmias.

Abnormal automaticity can be produced in normal muscle or Purkinje fibers by appropriate interventions such as current passage that reduces diastolic potential. Automatic discharge rate speeds up with progressive depolarization, while hyperpolarizing pulses slow the spontaneous firing. Other interventions, such as barium administration, produce automaticity during which action potentials are similar to those produced by current passage. Both may be due to I_K and

I_{Ca-L}. It is possible that partial depolarization and failure to reach normal maximal diastolic potential can induce automatic discharge in most if not all cardiac fibers. Although this type of spontaneous automatic activity has been found in human atrial and ventricular fibers, its relation to the genesis of clinical arrhythmias has not been established.

Rhythms due to automaticity may be slow atrial, junctional and ventricular escape rhythms, certain types of atrial tachycardias (such as those produced by digitalis), accelerated junctional (nonparoxysmal junctional tachycardia), and idioventricular rhythms and parasystole (see Chap. 22).

Triggered Activity

Automaticity is the property of a fiber to initiate an impulse *spontaneously*, without need for prior stimulation, so that electrical quiescence does not occur. *Triggered activity* is initiated by afterdepolarizations that are depolarizing oscillations in membrane voltage induced by one or more preceding action potentials. Thus triggered activity is pacemaker activity that results *consequent* to a preceding impulse or series of impulses, without which electrical quiescence occurs (Figs. 20–22 and 20–23). This is not an automatic self-generating mechanism, and the term *triggered automaticity* is therefore contradictory. These depolarizations can occur before (Fig. 20–22) or after (Fig. 20–23) full repolarization of the fiber and are best termed *early afterdepolarizations* (EADs)[81–94] when they arise from a reduced level of membrane potential during phases 2 (type 1) and 3 (type 2) of the cardiac action potential and *late* or *delayed afterdepolarizations* (DADs) when they occur after completion of repolarization (phase 4) generally at a more negative membrane potential than from which EADs arise[95] (Table 20–6). All afterdepolarizations may not reach threshold potential, but if they do, they can trigger another afterdepolarization and thus self-perpetuate.

Early Afterdepolarizations (EADS)

A variety of interventions, each of which results in an increase in intracellular positivity, can cause EADs.[81–85] EADs may be responsible for the lengthened repolarization time and ventricular tachyarrhythmias in several clinical situations, such as the acquired and congenital forms of the long Q-T syndrome.[86–94] Left ansae subclaviae stimulation (Fig. 20–24) increases the amplitude of cesium-induced EADs in dogs and the prevalence of ventricular tachyarrhythmias more than does right ansae subclaviae stimulation. This is possibly because of a greater quantitative effect that the left stellate ganglion exerts on the left ventricle compared with the right stellate ganglion.

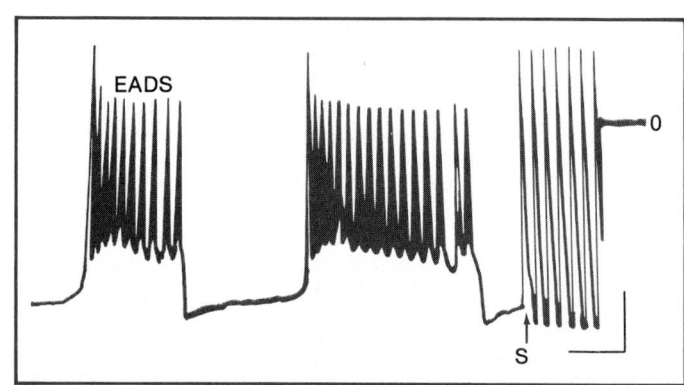

FIGURE 20–22. Early afterdepolarizations (EADs). Early afterdepolarizations occur spontaneously in an isolated canine cardiac Purkinje fiber when exposed to reduced extracellular potassium concentration. Note spontaneous phase four diastolic depolarization is present. In the initial two action potentials, a series of spontaneous depolarizations (EADs) result before the membrane returns to its maximum diastolic potential. Following the second series of EADs, pacing is begun (S) and normal action potentials follow. Horizontal calibration bar = 5 seconds, vertical bar = 25 mV. (From Kovacs, R. J., Bailey, J. C., and Zipes, D. P.: Mechanisms of cardiac arrhythmias. *In* Parmley, W. W., et al. [eds.]: Cardiology. Philadelphia, J. B. Lippincott, 1989.)

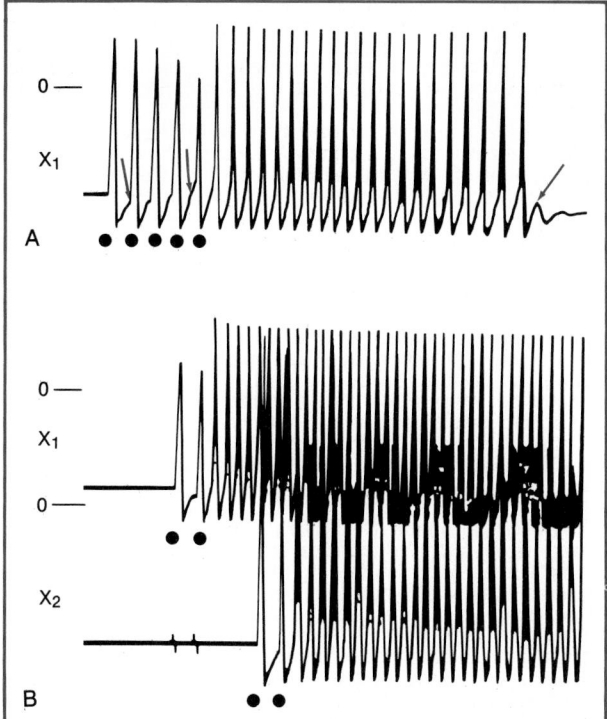

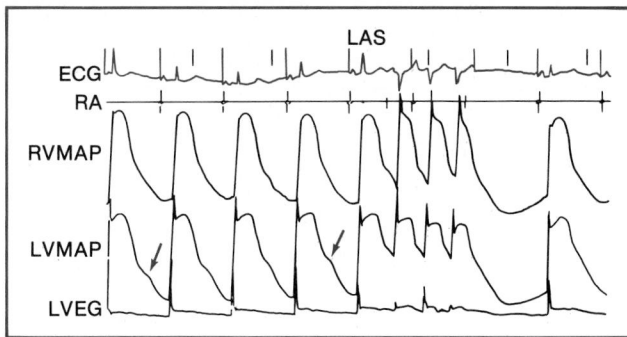

FIGURE 20–24. Following cesium administration during left ansae subclaviae stimulation (LAS), early afterdepolarizations increase in amplitude (arrows), culminating in a short run of nonsustained ventricular tachycardia. RVMAP, right ventricular monophasic action potential recording; LVMAP, left ventricular monophasic action potential recording; LVEG, left ventricular electrograms; time lines, one second. (Reproduced by permission from Ben-David, J., and Zipes, D. P.: Differential response to right and left stellate stimulation of early afterdepolarizations and ventricular tachycardia in the dog. Circulation 78:1241, 1988. Copyright 1988 American Heart Association.)

FIGURE 20–23. Triggered sustained rhythmic activity and delayed afterdepolarizations in diseased human ventricle. *A,* Spontaneous activity triggered by a series of driven action potentials (indicated by the dots) at a recording site X1. Note the gradual increase in size of the delayed afterdepolarizations (arrows) until the afterdepolarizations reaches threshold and maintains sustained rhythmic activity after cessation of pacing. The sustained rhythmic activity finally terminates when the last afterdepolarization fails to reach threshold (arrow). *B,* Initiation of triggered activity by intracellular current injection (indicated by dots beneath the respective action potential recordings) at sites X1 and X2, which lie along the same trabeculum. Although sites X1 and X2 were only about 4 mm apart, triggered sustained rhythmic activity from one site did not propagate to the other site, indicating complete dissociation between these two sites. For current pulses, cycle length = 2000 msec; pulse duration = 10 msec; pulse intensity = 200 na. Vertical calibration: 50 mV. Horizontal calibration: 10 sec. (From Gilmour, R. F., Jr., et al.: Cellular electrophysiological abnormalities of diseased human ventricular myocardium. Am. J. Cardiol. 51:137, 1983.)

Patients with the idiopathic congenital long Q-T syndrome may have a myocardial defect in repolarization, e.g., involving an outward potassium current or an inward slow calcium current, rather than "sympathetic imbalance."[90,91,93,94] Sympathetic stimulation, primarily left, could periodically increase the EAD amplitude to provoke ventricular tachyarrhythmias (Fig. 20–24). Alpha-adrenoceptor stimulation also increases the amplitude of cesium-induced EADs and the prevalence of ventricular tachyarrhythmias, both of which are suppressed

by magnesium. Alpha-adrenoceptor blockade may be helpful in suppressing arrhythmias in some of these patients (see Chap. 22).

The ionic basis of EADs is unclear but may be via the L-type calcium channel.[81,82,85,95–98] EADs that arise at voltages close to the plateau (phase 2) appear to result from time- and voltage-dependent reactivation of L-type Ca^{++} channels. Lengthening action potential by a variety of ways allows development of this type of EAD. They may occur preferentially in Purkinje cells and M cells of ventricular myocardium.[83] EADs that arise at voltages negative to the action potential plateau appear to have separable time- and voltage-dependent properties, and the mechanism is uncertain. Short coupling intervals and rapid rates suppress EADs.

In patients with the acquired long Q-T syndrome and torsades de pointes due to drugs such as quinidine, N-acetyl procainamide, erythromycin,[99] and some class III antiarrhythmic agents, EADs also may be responsible. Such drugs easily elicit EADs experimentally and clinically, while magnesium suppresses them (Figs. 20–25 and 20–26). It is possible that multiple drugs can cause summating effects to provoke EADs and torsades de pointes in patients.[100] The potassium channel activators pinacidil and chromakalim can eliminate EADs.

Delayed Afterdepolarizations (DADs)

DADs and triggered activity have been demonstrated in Purkinje fibers, specialized atrial fibers and ventricular muscle fibers exposed to digitalis preparations, normal Purkinje fibers exposed to Na-free superfusates from the endocardium of the intact heart, ventricular myocardial cells,[101] and endocardial preparations 1 day after a myocardial infarction. When fibers in the rabbit, canine, simian, and human mitral valves and in the canine tricuspid valve and coronary sinus are superfused with norepinephrine, they exhibit the capacity for sustained triggered rhythmic activity. It has been produced by palmitoyl carnitine in isolated ventricular myocytes.[102]

Triggered activity due to DADs also has been noted in diseased human atrial and ventricular fibers (Fig. 20–23) studied in vitro. Left stellate ganglion stimulation can elicit DADs in canine ventricles. In vivo, atrial and ventricular arrhythmias apparently due to triggered activity have been reported in the dog and possibly in humans. It is tempting to ascribe certain clinical arrhythmias to DADs, such as some arrhythmias precipitated by digitalis. The accelerated idioventricular rhythm one day after experimental canine myocardial infarction may be due to DADs, and some evidence suggests that certain ventricular tachycardias, such as that arising in the right ventricular outflow tract, may be due to DADs,[103] while other data suggest that EADs[104] are responsible.

IONIC BASIS OF DELAYED AFTERDEPOLARIZATIONS. DADs appear to be caused by a transient inward current (I_{Ti}) that is small or absent under normal physiological conditions. When intracellular calcium overload occurs,[97,98,102] as during extensive sympathetic stimulation,[101] high $[Ca^{++}]_o$, or after large doses of digitalis, oscillatory release of Ca^{++} from the sarcoplasmic reticulum activates a nonselective cation channel (or an electrogenic Na^{+}-Ca^{++} exchange). This results in a transient inward current, carried primarily by Na^{+}, that generates the DAD. Drugs that block the diastolic Ca^{++} transient, by reducing Ca^{++} overload (e.g., Ca^{++} channel blockers, beta receptor blockers) or by inhibiting Ca^{++} release from the sarcoplasmic reticulum (caffeine, ryanodine), inhibit the DAD. Drugs that reduce the Na^{+} current also reduce $[Na^{+}]_i$ (tetrodotoxin, lidocaine, phenytoin), relieve the Ca^{++} overload, and also can abolish DADs.

TABLE 20–6 DETERMINANTS OF THE AMPLITUDE OF AFTERDEPOLARIZATIONS

INTERVENTION	EFFECT ON AMPLITUDE OF EADs	EFFECT ON AMPLITUDE OF DADs
Long cycles (basic and premature)	↑	↓
Long action potential duration	↑	↑
Reduced membrane potential	↑	↓
Na channel blockers	No effect	↓
Ca channel blockers	↓	↓
Catecholamines	↑	↑

↑ Increase amplitude
↓ Decrease amplitude
EADs = Early afterdepolarizations
DADs = Delayed afterdepolarizations

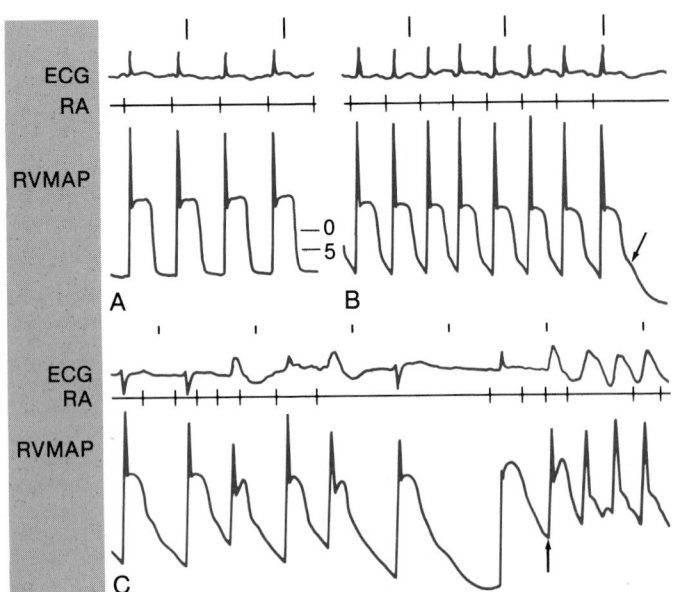

FIGURE 20–25. Induction of early afterdepolarizations in the dog by cesium chloride. Monophasic action potentials recorded from the right ventricle (RVMAP) initially show uniform contour with rapid upstroke, plateau, smooth continuous repolarization, and isoelectric interval for the resting potential (*panel A, control*). A prominent early afterdepolarization is apparent several seconds after cesium administration (*panel B, arrow*). *Panel C* shows development of premature ventricular complexes and long-short RR cycle grouping, culminating in the onset of ventricular tachycardia. A particularly prominent early afterdepolarization (arrow) follows a QRS complex that terminates the long cycle. Paper speed, 50 mm per second; time lines, one second intervals; ECG, electrocardiogram lead II; RA, right atrial electrogram; RVMAP, monophasic action potentials recorded from the apex of the right ventricle. Numbers in millivolts. (Reproduced by permission from Baillie, D. S., Inoue, H., Kaseda, S., et al.: Magnesium suppresses early depolarizations and ventricular tachyarrhythmias induced in dogs by cesium. Circulation 77:1395, 1989. Copyright 1989 American Heart Association.)

DADs due to *digitalis toxicity* (see p. 484) behave differently from DADs due to catecholamines. Catecholamine-induced triggering often slows slightly after initiation, then regularizes, but slows still further prior to termination, without a progressive increase in maximum diastolic potential. A subthreshold DAD often follows termination of

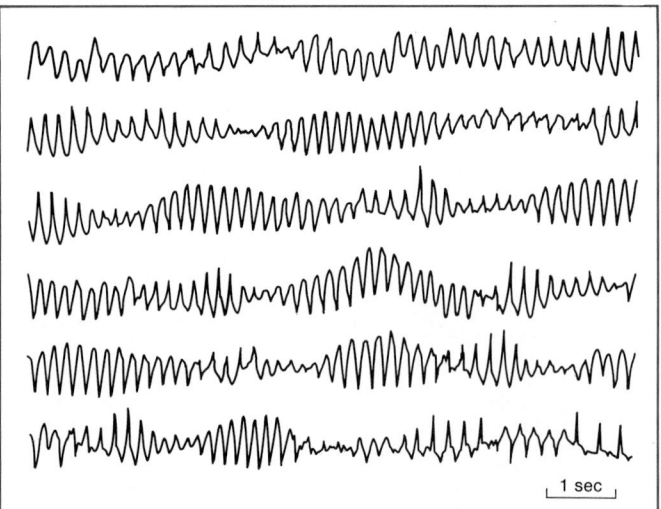

FIGURE 20–26. Torsades de pointes. Ventricular tachycardia initiated in Figure 20–25 continued, with varying morphology characteristic of torsades de points. Continuous recording of lead II. (Reproduced by permission from Zipes, D. P., and Ben-David, J.: Autonomic neural modulation of cardiac rhythm: 2. Mechanisms and examples. Mod. Concepts Cardiovasc. Dis. 57:47, 1988. Copyright 1988 American Heart Association.)

TABLE 20–7 EFFECTS OF ELECTRICAL STIMULATION ON AUTOMATICITY AND TRIGGERED ACTIVITY

	NORMAL AUTOMATICITY	EADs	DADs
Suppressed by overdrive pacing	Yes	Not usually	Not usually
Terminated by premature stimulation	Not usually	Not usually	Usually

EADs = early afterdepolarizations; DADs = delayed afterdepolarizations

triggered activity. Spontaneous termination may be due, in part, to an increase in the rate of electrogenic sodium extrusion. Termination of digitalis-induced triggering is often characterized by speeding of the rate, decrease in action potential amplitude, and decrease in membrane potential, possibly due to $[Na^+]_i$ or $[Ca^{++}]_i$ accumulation.

Short coupling intervals or pacing at rates more rapid than the triggered activity rate (overdrive pacing) increases the amplitude and shortens the cycle length of the DAD following cessation of pacing (overdrive acceleration) rather than suppressing and delaying the escape rate of the afterdepolarization, as in normal automatic mechanisms (Table 20–7). Premature stimulation exerts a similar effect; the shorter the premature interval, the larger the amplitude and shorter the escape interval of the triggered event.

The clinical implication might be that tachyarrhythmias due to DAD-triggered activity may not be suppressed easily or, indeed, may be precipitated by rapid rates, either spontaneous (such as a sinus tachycardia) or pacing induced. Finally, because a single premature stimulus can both initiate and terminate triggered activity, differentiation from reentry (see below) becomes quite difficult. The response to overdrive pacing may help separate triggered arrhythmias from reentrant ones.

Parasystole
(See also p. 693)

Classically, parasystole has been likened to the function of a fixed-rate asynchronously discharging pacemaker: Its timing is not altered by the dominant rhythm, it produces depolarization when the myocardium is excitable, and the intervals between discharges are multiples of a basic interval.[105] Complete *entrance block*, constant or intermittent, insulates and protects the parasystolic focus from surrounding electrical events and accounts for such behavior. Occasionally, the focus may exhibit *exit block*, during which it may fail to depolarize excitable myocardium. In fact, the dominant cardiac rhythm may modulate parasystolic discharge to speed up or slow down its rate. Experimental simulations of parasystole demonstrate that the discharge rate of an isolated, "protected" focus can be modulated by electrotonic interactions with the dominant rhythm across an area of depressed excitability. Brief subthreshold depolarizations induced during the first half of the cardiac cycle of a spontaneously discharging pacemaker will delay the subsequent discharge, while similar depolarizations induced in the second half of the cardiac cycle will accelerate it (Fig. 20–27).

The ionic basis for these rate changes is not totally established, but it is probable that early depolarizing stimuli reactivate outward potassium currents and retard repolarization, while late stimuli contribute depolarizing current that enables the cell to reach threshold more quickly. Early hyperpolarizing subthreshold stimuli accelerate, while late hyperpolarizing stimuli retard discharge. Similar examples have been noted in human ventricular tissue, and interactions may be predicted according to the general rules of biological oscillators. Numerous clinical examples have been published to support these experimental observations.

DISORDERS OF IMPULSE CONDUCTION

Conduction delay and block[106] can result in bradyarrhythmias or tachyarrhythmias, the former when the propagating impulse blocks and is followed by asystole or a slow escape rhythm and the latter when the delay and block produce reentrant excitation (see below). Various factors,

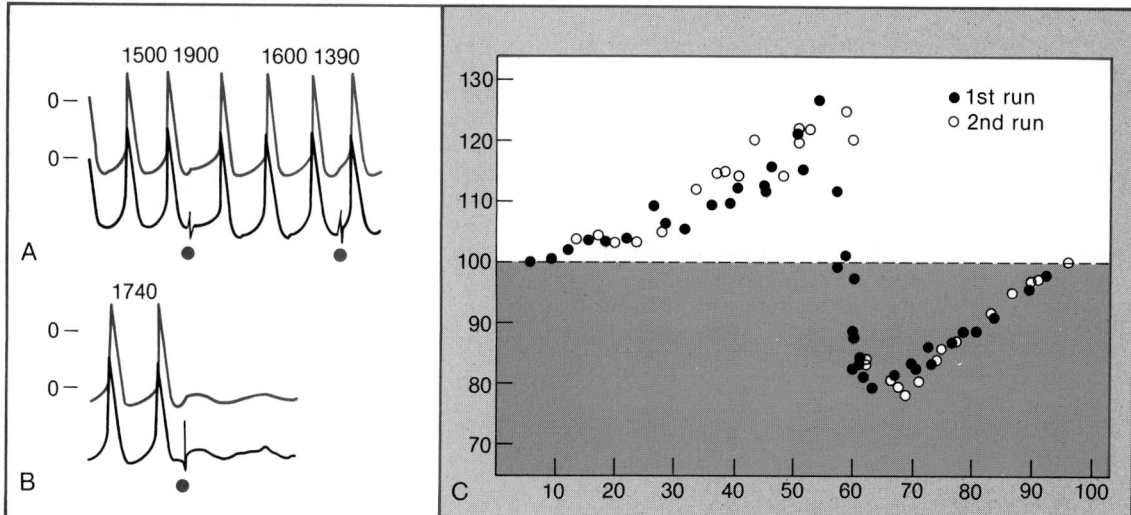

FIGURE 20–27. *Left,* Modulation of pacemaker activity by subthreshold current pulses in diseased human ventricle. *Panel A,* Two recording sites along the same trabeculum in a spontaneously active preparation. Current pulses (indicated by the dots) of 30 msec duration were injected through the lower microelectrode at various times. The interval between the spontaneous action potentials is given in milliseconds above each cycle. Injection of a subthreshold current pulse through the lower microelectrode relatively early in the spontaneous cycle (about 680 msec after initiation of the rapid portion of the preceding action potential upstroke) produced a subthreshold depolarization in the upper recording and delayed the next spontaneous discharge by 400 msec to 1900 msec. This response curve would fall in the first half of the curve indicated in panel C. The current pulse of the same intensity and duration delivered later in the spontaneous cycle (950 msec after the preceding upstroke) accelerated the next discharge by 210 msec to 1390 msec, relative to the previous two action potentials. The response to this current injection falls in the second half of the graph depicted in panel C.

Panel B, A stimulus at a precise interval in the cardiac cycle (called the singular point, in this example, 930 msec after the preceding action potential upstroke) abolishes pacemaker activity. (From Gilmour, R. F., Jr., et al.: Cellular electrophysiological abnormalities of diseased human ventricular myocardium. Am. J. Cardiol. *51:*137, 1983.) *Panel C,* Phase response curves from experimental data obtained in canine Purkinje fibers in a manner similar to the human experiment shown in panels A and B. Two different runs are shown. Ordinate: Percentage increase or decrease in the spontaneous cycle length of the "parasystolic focus" (control cycle length equals 100 per cent), Abscissa: Percentage of the "parasystolic focus" spontaneous cycle length during which stimulation was performed. The spontaneous cycle length was maximally prolonged (by 26 per cent) or shortened (by 20 per cent) by subthreshold depolarizations that entered the "parasystolic focus" after approximately 50 and 60 per cent of cycle had elapsed, respectively. Very similar curves can be plotted for patients with parasystole (for example, see Figures 9 and 10 from Zipes, D. P.: Plenary lecture. Cardiac electrophysiology: Promises and contributions. J. Am. Coll. Cardiol. *13:*1329, 1989). (Reproduced by permission from Jalife, J., and Moe, G. K.: Effect of electronic potentials on pacemaker activity of canine Purkinje fibers and relation to parasystole. Circ. Res. *39:*801, 1976. Copyright 1976 American Heart Association.)

involving both active and passive membrane properties, determine the conduction velocity of an impulse and whether or not conduction is successful. Among these factors are the stimulating efficacy of the propagating impulse, which is related to the amplitude and rate of rise of phase 0, the excitability of the tissue into which the impulse conducts, and the geometry of the tissue.

DECELERATION-DEPENDENT BLOCK. Diastolic depolarization has been suggested as a cause of conduction block at slow rates, so-called bradycardia or deceleration-dependent block (see p. 126). Yet excitability *increases* as the membrane depolarizes until about −70 mV, despite a reduction in action potential amplitude and $\dot{V}_{max}$. Evidently depolarization-induced inactivation of fast Na^+ channels is offset by other factors such as reduction in the difference between membrane potential and threshold potential. A more probable explanation of deceleration-dependent block is the reduction in action potential amplitude and excitability at long diastolic intervals. Rapid pacing also can produce overdrive suppression of conduction, with a similar mechanism related to the depression of action potential amplitude and excitability.

PHASE 3 OR TACHYCARDIA-DEPENDENT BLOCK. More commonly, impulses block at rapid rates or short cycle lengths, due to incomplete recovery of refractoriness, because of incomplete time- or voltage-dependent recovery of excitability (see p. 125). For example, this is the usual mechanism responsible for a nonconducted premature P wave or one that conducts with functional bundle branch block.

DECREMENTAL CONDUCTION. This term is used commonly in the clinical literature but often is misapplied to describe any Wenckebach-like conduction block, i.e., responses similar to block in the AV node during which progressive conduction delay precedes the nonconducted impulse. Correctly used, *decremental conduction* refers to the situation in which the properties of the fiber change along its length so that the action potential loses its efficacy as a stimulus to excite the fiber ahead of it. Thus the stimulating efficacy of the propagating action potential diminishes progressively, possibly as a result of its decreasing amplitude and $\dot{V}_{max}$.

Reentry

Electrical activity during each normal cardiac cycle begins in the sinus node and continues until the entire heart has been activated. Each cell becomes activated in turn, and the cardiac impulse dies out when all fibers have been discharged and are completely refractory. During this absolute refractory period, the cardiac impulse has "no place to go." It must be extinguished and restarted by the next sinus impulse. If, however, a group of fibers not activated during the initial wave of depolarization recovers excitability in time to be discharged before the impulse dies out, they may serve as a link to reexcite areas that were just discharged and have now recovered from the initial depolarization. Such a process is given various names, all meaning approximately the same thing: reentry, reentrant excitation, circus movement, reciprocal or echo beat, or reciprocating tachycardia.

ANATOMICAL REENTRY. The earliest studies on reentry were with models that had anatomically defined separate pathways in which it could be shown that there was (1) an area of unidirectional block, (2) recirculation of the impulse to its point of origin, and (3) elimination of the arrhythmia by cutting the pathway. In models with anatomi-

cally defined pathways, because the two (or more) pathways have different electrophysiological properties, e.g., a refractory period longer in one pathway than the other, the impulse (1) blocks in one pathway (site A in Fig. 20–28A) and (2) propagates slowly in the adjacent pathway (serpentine arrow, D to C, Fig. 20–28A). If conduction in this alternative route is sufficiently depressed, the slowly propagating impulse excites tissue beyond the blocked pathway (horizontal lined area in Fig. 20–28A) and returns in a reversed direction along the pathway initially blocked (B to A in Fig. 20–28A) to (3) reexcite tissue proximal to the site of block (A to D in Fig. 20–28A).

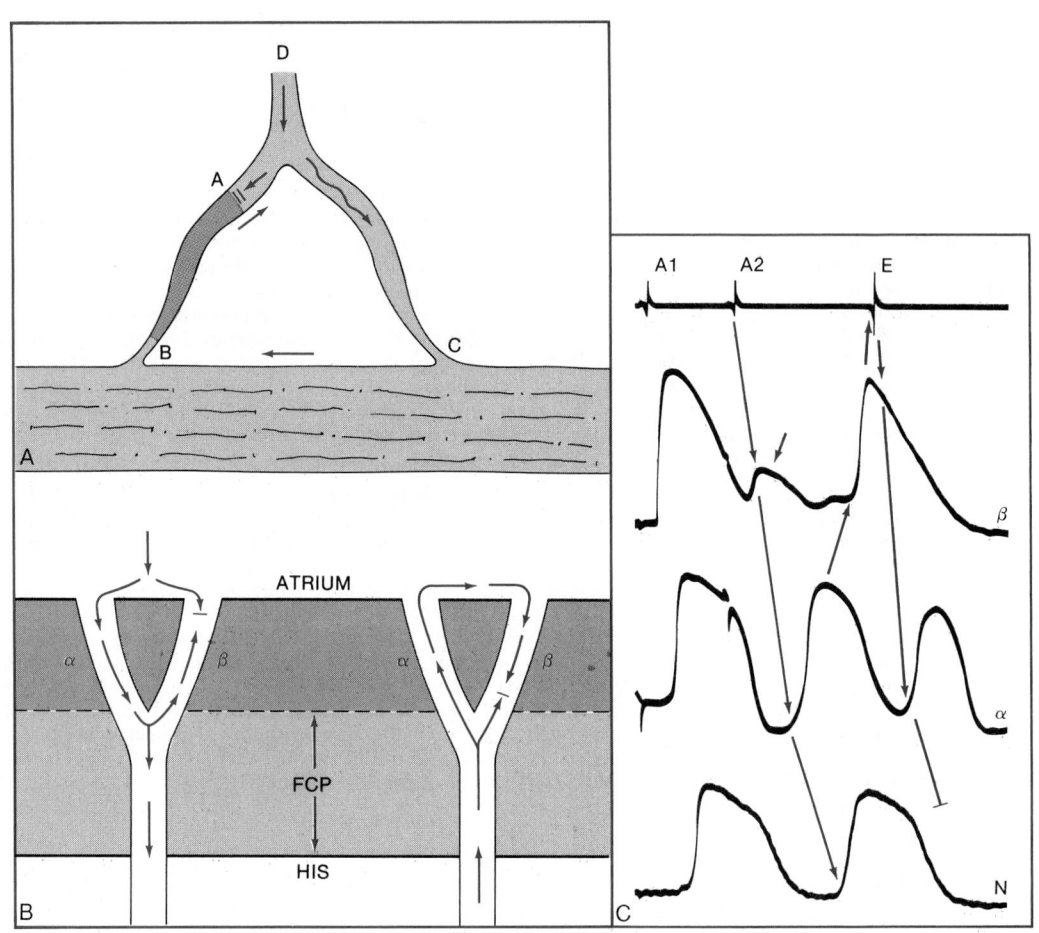

FIGURE 20–28. *Top left, A,* A diagram of reentry published by Schmitt and Erlanger in 1928. A Purkinje fiber (D) divides into two pathways (B and C), both of which join ventricular muscle. It is assumed that the original impulse travels down D, blocks in its anterograde direction at site A (arrow followed by double bar), but continues slowly down C (serpentine arrow) to excite ventricular muscle. The impulse then reenters the Purkinje twig at B and retrogradely excites A and D. If the impulse continues to propagate through D to the ventricular myocardium and elicits ventricular depolarization, a reentrant ventricular extrasystole results. Continued reentry of this type would produce ventricular tachycardia.

Bottom left, B, Atrial echoes. Schematic representation of intranodal dissociation responsible for an atrial echo *(left diagram).* A premature atrial response fails to penetrate the beta pathway, which exhibits unidirectional block, but propagates anterogradely through the alpha pathway. Once the final common pathway (FCP) is engaged, the impulse may return to the atrium via the now recovered beta pathway to produce an atrial echo. The neighboring *(right)* diagram illustrates the pattern of propagation during generation of a ventricular echo. A premature response in the His bundle traverses the final common pathway, encounters a refractory beta pathway (unidirectional block), reaches the atrium over the alpha pathway, and returns through a now recovered beta pathway to produce a ventricular echo.

Right, C, Actual recordings from the atrium (top tracing), cells impaled in the beta region (second tracing), alpha region (third tracing), and N portion of the AV node (bottom tracing) in an isolated rabbit preparation. The basic response to A_1 activated both alpha and beta pathways and the N cell (first tier of action potentials). The premature atrial response, A_2, caused only a local response in the beta cell (heavy arrow), was delayed in transmission to the alpha cell, and was further delayed in propagation to the N cell. Following the alpha response, a retrograde spontaneous response occurred in the beta cell and propagated to the atrium (E). This atrial response represents an atrial echo. The echo returned to stimulate the alpha cell but was not propagated to the N cell. It is important that while intranodal reentry has been shown to occur within the rabbit AV node, AV nodal reentry in humans probably occurs over extranodal pathways. (Reproduced by permission from Mendez, C., and Moe, G. K.: Demonstrations of a dual AV nodal conduction system in the isolated rabbit heart. Circ. Res. *19:*378, 1966. Copyright 1966 American Heart Association.)

For reentry of this type to occur, the time for conduction within the depressed but unblocked area and for excitation of the distal segments must exceed the refractory period of the initially blocked pathway (A in Fig. 20–28A) and the tissue proximal to the site of block (D in Fig. 20–28A). Stated another way, continuous reentry requires the anatomical length of the circuit traveled to equal or exceed the reentrant wavelength. The latter is equal to mean conduction velocity of the impulse multiplied by the longest refractory period of the elements in the circuit.

CONDITIONS FOR REENTRY. The length of the pathway is fixed and determined by the anatomy. Conditions that depress conduction velocity or abbreviate the refractory period will promote the development of reentry in this model, while prolonging refractoriness and speeding conduction velocity can hinder it. For example, if conduction velocity (0.30 m/sec) and refractoriness (350 m/sec) for ventricular muscle were normal, a pathway of 105 mm (0.30 m/sec × 0.35 sec) would be necessary for reentry to occur. However, under certain conditions, conduction velocity in ventricular muscle and Purkinje fibers can be very slow (0.03 m/sec), and if refractoriness is not greatly prolonged (600 msec), a pathway of only 18 mm (0.03 m/sec × 0.60 sec) may be necessary. Such reentry frequently exhibits an excitable gap, i.e., a time interval between the end of refractoriness from one cycle and beginning of depolarization in the next, when tissue in the circuit is excitable. This results because the wavelength of the reentrant circuit is less than the pathway length. Electrical stimulation during this time period can invade the reentrant circuit and reset its timing or terminate the tachycardia.

Rapid pacing can entrain the tachycardia, i.e., continuously reset it by entering the circuit and propagating around it in the same way as the reentrant impulse, increasing the tachycardia rate to the pacing rate without terminating the tachycardia. In reentrant circuits with an excitable gap, conduction velocity determines the revolution time of the impulse around the circuit and hence the rate of the tachycardia. Prolongation of refractoriness, unless it is great enough to eliminate the excitable gap and make the impulse propagate in relatively refractory tissue, will not influence the revolution time around the circuit or the rate of the tachycardia. Anatomical reentry occurs in patients with the Wolff-Parkinson-White syndrome, AV nodal reentry, in some atrial flutters, and in some ventricular tachycardias.

FUNCTIONAL REENTRY. Functional reentry lacks confining anatomical boundaries and can occur in contiguous fibers that exhibit functionally different electrophysiological properties. This depends on heterogeneous electrophysiological properties of cardiac muscle caused by local differences in the transmembrane action potentials. Dispersion of excitability and/or refractoriness, as well as anisotropic distributions of intercellular resistances, permits initiation and maintenance of reentry.[107–109]

Leading Circle Reentry. Leading circle reentry, important in atrial fibrillation, is reentrant excitation during which the reentrant circuit propagates around a functionally refractory core and follows a course along fibers that have a shorter refractory period, blocking in one direction in fibers with a longer refractory period (Fig. 20–29).

The pathway length of a functional circuit is determined by the smallest circuit in which the leading wavefront is just able to excite tissue ahead that is still relatively refractory. If these parameters change, the size of the circuit may change also, altering the rate of the tachycardia. Shorter wavelengths may predispose to fibrillation. No or a very short excitable gap exists, and the duration of the refractory period of the tissue in the circuit primarily determines the cycle length of the tachycardia because the stimulating efficacy of the head of the next impulse is just sufficient to excite the relatively refractory tissue in the wake of the preceding impulse. Propagating impulses originating outside the circuit cannot easily enter the circuit to reset, entrain, or terminate the reentry.[110]

Theoretically, drugs that prolong refractoriness and do not delay conduction would slow tachycardia due to the leading circle mechanism and not affect tachycardia with an excitable gap until the prolongation of refractoriness exceeded the duration of the excitable gap. Drugs that pri-

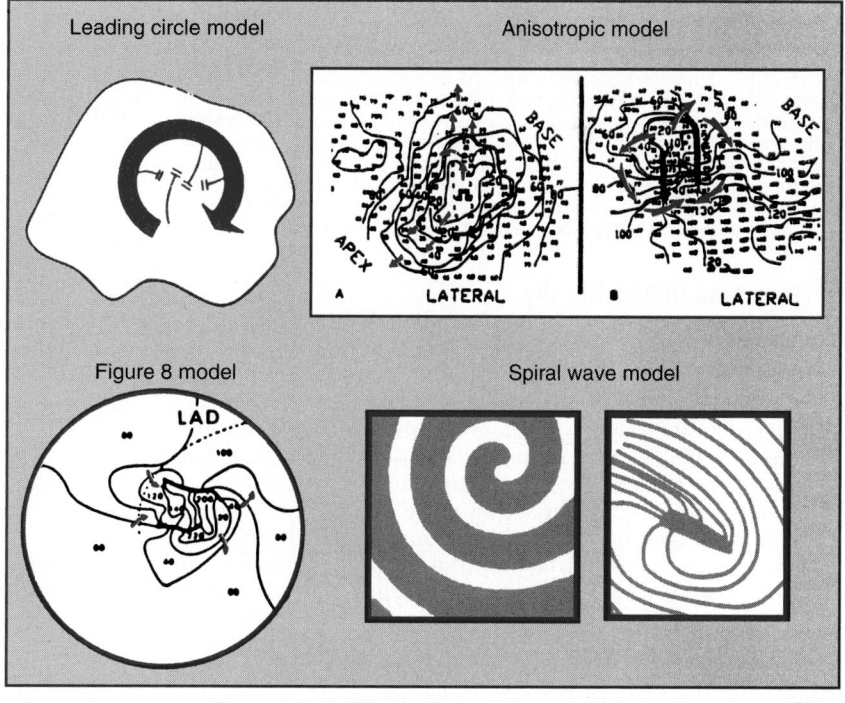

FIGURE 20–29. **Functional models of reentry.** *Leading circle model*, a diagrammatic representation of the leading circle model of reentry in isolated left atrium of the rabbit. The central area is activated by converging centripetal wavelets. (Reproduced with permission from Allessie, M. A., Bonke, F. I. M., and Schopman, F. J. G.: Circus movement in rabbit atrial muscle as a mechanism of tachycardia: III. The "leading circle" concept: A new model of circus movement in cardiac tissue without the involvement of an anatomical obstacle. Circ. Res. *41:*9, 1977. Copyright 1977 American Heart Association.)

Figure-of-8 model, activation map (in 20-msec isochrones) of a figure-of-8 circuit in the surviving epicardial layer of a dog 4 days after ligation of the left anterior descending coronary artery (LAD). The circuit consists of clockwise and counterclockwise wavefronts around two functional arcs of block that coalesce into a central common front that usually represents the slow zone of the circuit. (From El-Sherif, N.: The figure 8 model of reentrant excitation in the canine post-infarction heart. *In* Zipes, D. P., and Jalife, J. [eds.]: Cardiac Electrophysiology and Arrhythmias. New York, Grune and Stratton, 1985, p. 363.)

Anisotropic model, showing stimulation from the center of a multiple electrode array (at the pulse symbol, *A*) on the epicardial border zone of a 4-day-old canine infarct, producing an elliptical pattern of activation characteristic of conduction in an anisotropic medium. Arrows indicate the direction of the fast axes of conduction and the longitudinal orientation of the myocardial fibers. *B*, activation map of a reentrant circuit on the epicardial border obtained with the same electrode array during sustained ventricular tachycardia in the same heart. Arrows indicate the sequence of isochrones and thus the direction of movement of activation. (From Wit, A. L., and Janse, M. J. J.: The Ventricular Arrhythmias of Ischemia and Infarction: Electrophysiological Mechanisms. Mt. Kisco, N.Y., Futura, 1992.)

Spiral wave model, activation map of spiral wave activity in a thin slice of isolated ventricular muscle from a sheep heart *(right panel)*. Isochrone lines were drawn from raw data by overlaying transparent paper on snapshots of video images during spiral wave activity *(left panel, not from same experiment)*. Each line represents consecutive positions of the activation front recorded every 16.6 msec. (From Krinsky, V. I., et al.: Proc. R. Soc. Lond. [A] *437:*645, 1992.) (Entire figure modified from El-Sherif, N.: Reentrant mechanisms in ventricular arrhythmias. *In* Zipes, D. P., and Jalife, J. [eds.]: Cardiac Electrophysiology: From Cell to Bedside. Philadelphia, W. B. Saunders Company, 1994, p. 567.)

marily slow conduction would have major effects on tachycardia with an excitable gap and not on tachycardias due to the leading circle concept. Mixed circuits with both anatomical and functional pathways obfuscate these differences.

Random Reentry. Random reentry, also important in atrial fibrillation, occurs when the reentry propagates continuously and randomly, reexciting areas that were excited shortly before by another wavelet.

Anisotropic Reentry. Anisotropic reentry is due to the structural features responsible for variations in conduction velocity and time course of repolarization, such as concentration of gap junctions at the ends rather than on the side of cells, that can result in block and slowed conduction causing reentry[99] (Fig. 20–29). Even in normal cardiac tissue showing normal transmembrane potentials and uniform refractory periods, conduction can block in the direction parallel to the long axis of fiber orientation, propagate slowly in the direction transverse to the long axis of fiber orientation, and reenter the area of block. Spatial differences in refractoriness may not be necessary for reentry to occur. Such anisotropic reentry has been shown in atrial and ventricular muscle and may be responsible for ventricular tachycardia in epicardial muscle surviving myocardial infarction. An excitable gap may be present.[109]

Figure-of-Eight Reentry. This is reentry consisting of clockwise and counterclockwise wavefronts around two functional arcs of block that coalesce into a central common front commonly representing the slow zone of the circuit. Such reentry has been shown in both atrial and ventricular muscle[107] (Fig. 20–29).

Spiral Wave Reentry. Spiral waves of excitation have been demonstrated in cardiac muscle and represent a two-dimensional form of reentry; in three dimensions, spiral waves may be represented by scroll waves. Spiral waves may be stationary when the shape, size, and location of the arc remain unchanged throughout the episode; drifting, when the arc migrates away from its site of origin; or anchoring, when the drifting core becomes anchored to some small obstacle, such as a blood vessel. One can speculate that a stationary spiral wave could be responsible for a monomorphic tachycardia, a drifting spiral wave responsible for rhythm with changing contours such as torsades de pointes, and an anchoring spiral wave responsible for the transition from a polymorphic to a monomorphic tachycardia[110a–112] (Fig. 20–29).

REFLECTION. This can be considered a special subclass of reentry. As in reentry, an area of conduction delay is required, and the total time for the impulse to leave and return to its site of origin must exceed the refractory period of the proximal segment.

Reflection differs from reentry in that the impulse does not require a circuit but appears to travel along the *same* pathway in both directions. The impulse travels in one direction and meets an area of impaired conduction where active transmission pauses. Electrotonically, the impulse spans the zone of impairment, activates the distal segment, and returns electrotonically across the zone of impaired conduction to reexcite the proximal segment. A single reflection could cause a coupled premature complex, while continued reflection back and forth across an inexcitable zone could cause a tachycardia.

Tachycardias Due to Reentry

Reentry is probably the cause of many tachyarrhythmias, including various kinds of supraventricular and ventricular tachycardias, flutter, and fibrillation. However, in complex preparations, such as large pieces of tissue in vitro or the intact heart, it becomes much more difficult to prove unequivocally that reentry exists. In addition, many other factors, such as stretch, autonomic stimulation, and a host of modulating influences can act on these electrophysiological mechanisms, obscuring the cause of many arrhythmias. Initiation or termination of tachycardia by pacing stimuli, the demonstration of electrical activity bridging diastole, fixed coupling, and a variety of other clinically used techniques such as entrainment and resetting curves, while consistent with reentry, do not constitute absolute proof of its existence. The most compelling evidence probably is provided by entrainment.[113]

ATRIAL FLUTTER (see also p. 652). Reentry is the most likely cause of the usual form of atrial flutter, with the reentrant circuit confined to the right atrium, where it travels counterclockwise, in a caudocranial direction in the interatrial septum and in a craniocaudal direction in the right atrial free wall.[113–123] An area of slow conduction is present in the posterolateral to posteromedial inferior right atrium with a central area of block that can include an anatomical (inferior vena cava) and functional component.

It is possible that several different reentrant circuits exist in patients with atrial flutter. However, this area of slow conduction is rather constant and represents the site of successful ablation of atrial flutter. It is also important in the conversion of atrial flutter to fibrillation.[117] Double potentials can be recorded from this area, with each one reflecting activation on either side of the block.[121] Ventricular activation can modulate the atrial flutter rate, probably through mechanotechnical coupling, and atrial volume changes.[123,124] Ablation results are consistent with a macroreentry circuit.[125–132]

ATRIAL AND VENTRICULAR FIBRILLATION (see also pp. 654 and 686). A critical mass of myocardium appears to be required to maintain fibrillation. Ventricular myocardium cut into small pieces ceases fibrillating when the pieces reach a critically small size. Partitioning the atrium into small segments presents atrial fibrillation, a concept that has led to a corrective surgical[133,134] and ablation[135,135a,b] procedure (see p. 621).

Ventricles of small animals stop fibrillating spontaneously, while this seldom occurs in the canine or human heart. In the canine ventricle, the left ventricular free wall and septum appear to be required as a critical mass to maintain fibrillation, since, if they are depolarized, the right ventricle stops fibrillating spontaneously. Fibrillation in the atrial appendage stops when it is clamped off from the rest of the atria in which fibrillation is induced by rapid atrial pacing and vagal stimulation. These observations support Moe's hypothesis that multiple wavelets of reentry, influenced by the mass of the tissue, refractory periods, and conduction velocity, maintain fibrillation.[110,136] These factors determine the number of wavelets present and the likelihood of continuation of fibrillation. One or more wavelets propagating in different directions characterize pacing-induced atrial fibrillation in humans.

Intraatrial reentry of the leading circle type appears responsible for multiple wavelets and has a short excitable gap.[110,136] Rapid pacing can regionally entrain portions of the atria but cannot terminate atrial fibrillation.[137,138] New-onset atrial fibrillation shortens atrial refractory period within 24 hours and can facilitate maintenance of atrial fibrillation. Atrial fibrillation begets atrial fibrillation and cellular adaptive changes result.[139,140,140a] Some patients may have rapidly discharging foci that maintain fibrillation.[141] Autonomic influences may be important in some patients.[142]

SINUS REENTRY (see also p. 649). The sinus node shares with the AV node electrophysiological features such as the potential for *dissociation of conduction;* i.e., an impulse can conduct in some nodal fibers but not in others, permitting reentry to occur.[143] The reentrant circuit may be located entirely within the sinus node or involve both the sinus node and atrium. Supraventricular tachycardias due to sinus node reentry generally may be less symptomatic than other supraventricular tachycardias because of slower rates. Ablation of the sinus node may be necessary in an occasional refractory tachycardia.[144]

ATRIAL REENTRY (see also p. 656). Reentry within the atrium, unrelated to the sinus node, may be a cause of supraventricular tachycardia in humans.[145–150] Atrial reentry appears to be less frequently encountered than other types of supraventricular tachycardia.[148] It has been shown to be due to reentry,[145,150] automaticity,[151] and afterdepolarizations causing triggered activity. There does not appear to be a relationship between the site of origin and mechanism. Adenosine has been used to probe for mechanism.[147] Distinguishing atrial tachycardia due to automaticity from atrial tachycardia sustained by reentry over quite small areas, i.e., microreentry of the leading circle type, is difficult. Multiple foci can be present.[152]

AV NODAL REENTRY (AVNR) (see also p. 661). Longitudinal dissociation of the AV node into two or more pathways has been demonstrated in animal studies.[153] For example, microelectrode studies on isolated rabbit AV nodal preparations reveal that cells in the upper portion of the AV node can be dissociated during propagation of premature stimuli so that one group of cells, called *alpha,* can discharge in response to a premature stimulus at a time when another group of cells, called *beta,* fails to discharge. The impulse can then propagate to the middle and lower portions of the AV node and turn around (without needing to activate the His bundle) to reexcite the beta group of cells and produce an atrial echo (Fig. 20–28B) or sustained tachycardia.

Dual AV nodal pathways also have been supported by finding that an impulse traveling from ventricle to atrium, if timed properly, can reach the atrium at the same time that another impulse is traveling from atrium to ventricle (Fig. 20–30). For this event to occur, the impulses traveling in opposite directions without colliding must be conducting in different AV nodal pathways. Another convincing fact is the finding of two ventricular responses to a single atrial depolarization or of two atrial responses to a single ventricular depolarization, due to simultaneous transmission over both the slow and fast AV nodal pathways.[154,155] Finally, the onset of AVNR is consistent with dual AV nodal pathways.[156–164]

Usually, a premature atrial response that can block anterogradely in one AV nodal pathway which conducts more rapidly (fast pathway, or beta pathway in Fig. 20–28B), but has a longer refractory period than a second pathway (slow pathway, or alpha pathway in Fig. 20–28B). The premature atrial response travels to the ventricle over the slow (alpha) pathway, prolonging the A-H interval, and back to the atrium over the fast (beta) pathway, with a short H-A interval, so-called slow-fast AVNR. Less commonly, the slow pathway has a long refractory period, and the premature atrial response can block anterogradely in the slow pathway and travel in the fast pathway, using the slow pathway retrogradely; this is called the uncommon form of AVNR, so-called fast-slow AVNR. Finally, some patients can have both anterograde and retrograde conduction over slowly conducting AV nodal fibers, so-called slow-slow AVNR.[164,165] Some patients may have more than two pathways. The nodal anatomic structure in patients with AVNR appears to be normal.[166,167]

LOCATION OF AV NODAL PATHWAYS. While the presence of dual AV nodal pathways in AVNR is indisputable,[23–25] the question is, Where are they located—intranodal and due to longitudinal dissociation or extranodal, involving separate atrial inputs into the AV node? The results from radiofrequency (RF) catheter ablation,[168–182] as well as surgery,[183–187] to treat patients with AVNR leaves little doubt that the

fast and slow pathways have their origins well outside the limits of the compact portion of the AV node and, at the point they are interrupted, are composed of ordinary working atrial myocardium. While low[168] and high[26] amplitude potentials have been recorded in the posteroinferior right atrium, the evidence[187] suggests that these potentials may be due to local atrial activity and serve as markers of the posterior septal space rather than representing depolarizations of the slow pathway or its connections.

LH (low followed by high) frequency potentials are caused by asynchronous activation of muscle bundles above and below the coronary sinus orifice, while HL (high followed by low) frequency potentials are caused by asynchronous activation of atrial cells and a band of nodal-type cells that may represent the substrate of the slow pathway.[185,186] Thus, the slow and fast pathways are likely to be atrionodal approaches or connections rather than discreet intranodal pathways.

During the common form of AVNR, anterograde conduction occurs over a posteroinferior atrial approach, or "slow" pathway, whose upper end is located posteroinferiorly to the AV node, toward the coronary sinus orifice. RF lesions in this area eliminate AVNR by selectively affecting conduction over the slow pathway. The lower end of this pathway enters the compact portion of the AV node, where the impulse is able to "turn around" and retrogradely enter the "fast" or anterosuperior atrial approach, whose upper end inserts at the apex of Koch's triangle near the His bundle. This pathway also can be selectively ablated (Fig. 20–31).

During sinus rhythm, anterograde conduction probably occurs over the anterosuperior atrial approaches. A premature atrial impulse can block in this pathway, because of its longer refractory period, and now conduct anterogradely over the posteroinferior approaches, causing the "jump" in

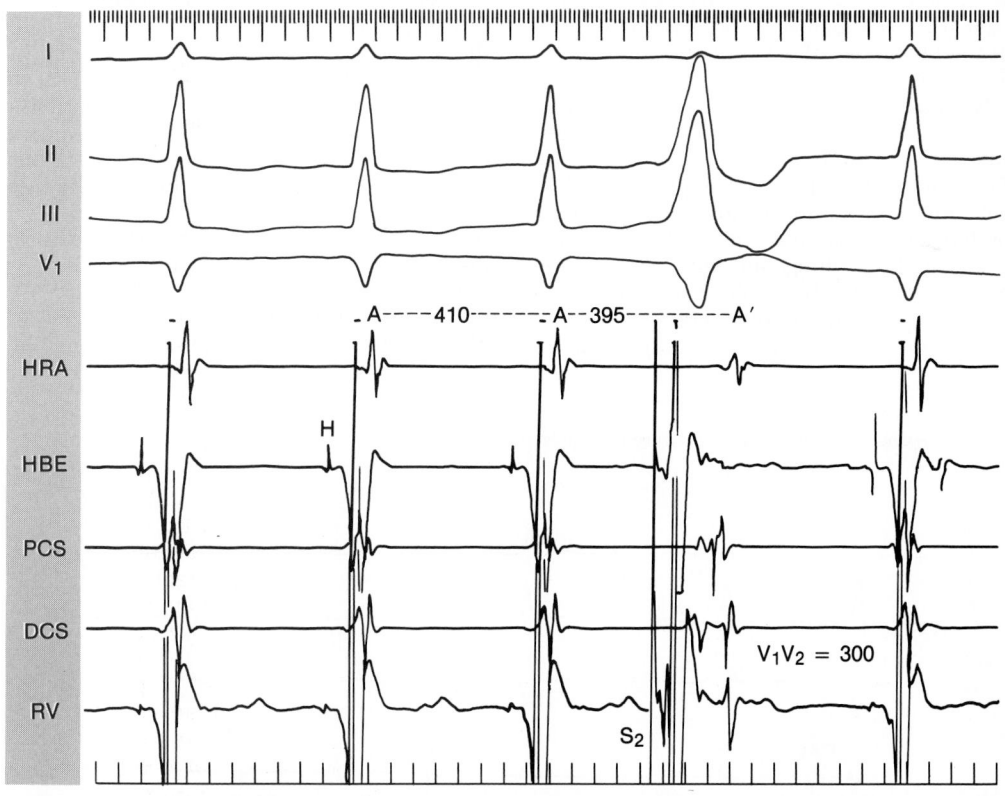

FIGURE 20–30. Atrial preexcitation during AV nodal reentry. AV nodal reentrant tachycardia is present with a cycle length of 410 msec. A premature ventricular complex (S2) from the right ventricular outflow tract with a coupling interval of 300 msec is introduced during the tachycardia before His is activated and penetrates the AV node retrogradely to shorten the AA interval to 395 msec. Shorter V1V2 intervals decreased the AA interval to 355 msec. Dual AV nodal pathways best explain how two impulses can travel in opposite directions in the AV node, i.e., the impulse from the tachycardia traveling anterogradely and the impulse from premature ventricular stimulation traveling retrogradely and not collide. Surface leads I, II, III, V1 are displayed along with high right atrial (HRA), His bundle (HBE), proximal coronary sinus (PCS), distal coronary sinus (DCS), and right ventricular (RV) electrograms. Numbers indicated in msec. Premature ventricular stimulus indicated by S2. His bundle activation indicated by H and atrial activation indicated by A. Large time 50 msec, small time 10 msec. (Reproduced with permission from Miles, W. M., Yee, R., Klein, G., et al.: The preexcitation index: An aid in determining the mechanism of supraventricular tachycardia and localizing accessory pathways. Circulation 74:493, 1986. Copyright 1986 American Heart Association.)

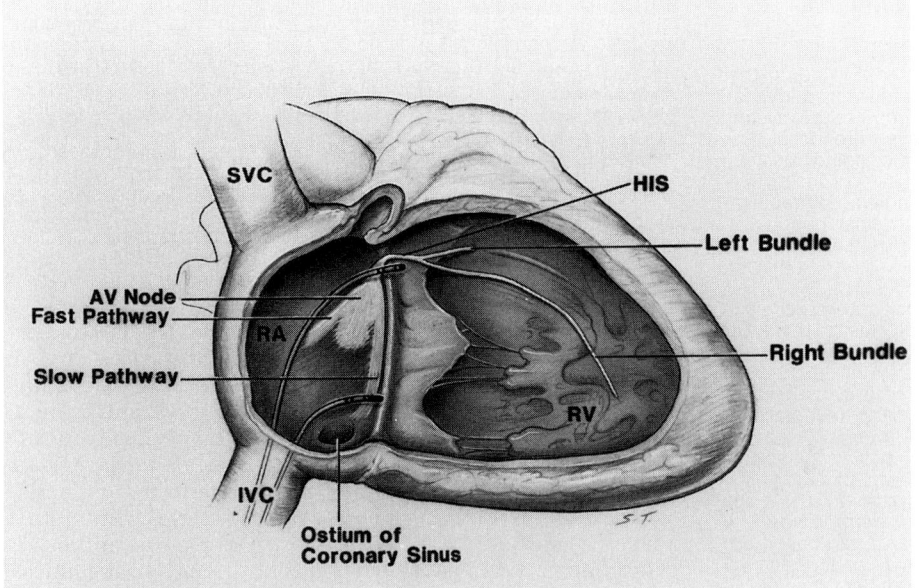

FIGURE 20–31. Schematic diagram of atrial approaches to the AV node that constitute the fast and slow pathways. AV node and pathways greatly enlarged for graphic purposes. Lower catheter lies posteroinferiorly over the slow pathway, while the upper catheter lies anterosuperiorly over the His bundle. SVC, superior vena cava; RA, right atrium; IVC, inferior vena cava; and RV, right ventricle.

the AH interval. At this point AVNR can occur. In the uncommon form of AVNR, anterograde conduction occurs over the fast pathway and retrograde conduction over the slow pathway, and in the slow-slow form, over two slow pathways.

In patients who have dual AV nodal physiology, both pathways exhibit electrophysiological responses in the anterograde direction characteristic of AV nodal fibers. However, the electrophysiological features of the pathway conducting retrogradely during the tachycardia differ from those of either anterogradely conducting pathways, in response not only to atrial or ventricular pacing but also to various drugs.[188] For example, drugs such as procainamide prolong conduction time in the retrogradely conducting, but not in either anterogradely conducting, pathway. Also, pacing at short cycle lengths prolongs anterograde, but not retrograde, AV nodal conduction time. Yet verapamil prolongs retrograde AV nodal conduction time, consistent with an effect on nodal fibers. The area of slow conduction in

AVNR is located in the same region as the area of slow conduction in atrial flutter.[189]

While it is clear that activation of the ventricle is not necessary for AVNR (Fig. 20–32) and activation of the His bundle is also probably not required in some patients, the necessary role of atrial participation in the reentrant circuit is still debated.[156,157,163] The obligatory role of the atrium in the reentry is implicit in the diagram in Figure 20–28B. Figure 20–33 is an example of *apparent* dissociation of the atrium with uninterrupted continuation of the supraventricular tachycardia, leading to the conclusion that the atrium may *not* be a necessary part of the reentrant circuit in humans. However, data refuting the role of the atrium as a necessary link in the reentrant pathway must be obtained from studies in which both atria are carefully mapped for the presence of localized atrial activity, particularly near the upper AV node.

PREEXCITATION SYNDROME (see also p. 667). Atrioventricular reentry is the mechanism responsible for about 80 per

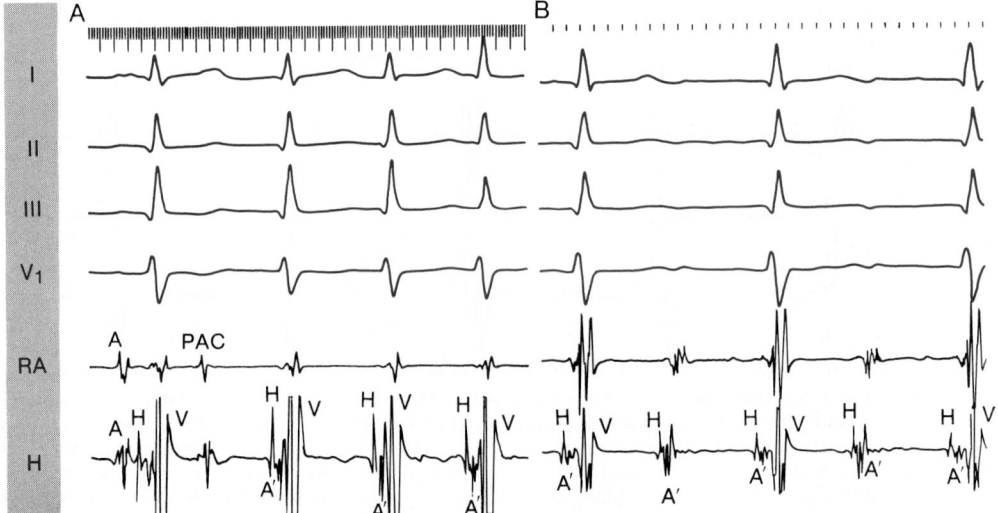

FIGURE 20–32. His-Purkinje block during AV nodal reentry. In panel *A*, a spontaneous premature atrial complex (PAC) is followed by PR (AH) prolongation and the initiation of AV nodal reentry. Retrograde atrial activation (A') occurs simultaneously with the onset of the QRS complex. In panel *B*, 2:1 block distal to the His bundle recording site is present, with continuation of the AV nodal reentry, indicating that activation of the ventricle is not required for perpetuation of the tachycardia. Such an event could not occur during reciprocating tachycardia utilizing an accessory atrioventricular connection in the Wolff-Parkinson-White syndrome. Conventions as in Figure 20–30.

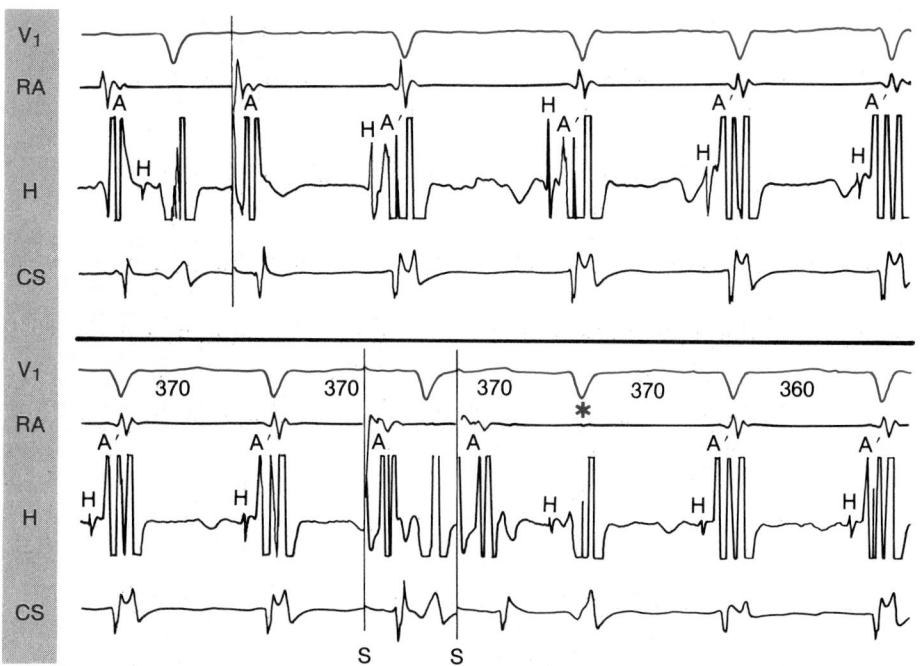

FIGURE 20–33. Dissociation of atria from ventricles without interrupting AV nodal reentrant supraventricular tachycardia. During sinus rhythm, a single premature atrial complex (S, *top panel*) was conducted with AV nodal delay (prolonged A-H interval) and initiated an AV nodal reentrant supraventricular tachycardia. Note that retrograde atrial activation (A′) occurred prior to onset of the QRS complex. Two premature atrial stimuli (S-S, *bottom panel*) captured the atria on both occasions without altering the regular cycle length of the AV nodal reentrant supraventricular tachycardia. Note that the QRS complex marked by an asterisk has no accompanying atrial complex, suggesting that atrial participation in the reentrant circuit was not required. V₁ = scalar lead; RA = right atrial electrogram; H = His bundle electgrogram; CS = coronary sinus electrogram.

cent of the tachycardias related to an accessory pathway.[190] In fact, the bundle described by Kent[191,192] was used to explain a reentrant mechanism for paroxysmal tachycardia even before the preexcitation syndrome was ever described in humans.

In most patients who have reciprocating tachycardias associated with the Wolff-Parkinson-White syndrome, the accessory pathway conducts more rapidly than does the normal AV node but takes a longer time to recover excitability; i.e., the anterograde refractory period of the accessory pathway exceeds that of the AV node at long cycles.[193,194] Consequently, a premature atrial complex that occurs sufficiently early blocks anterogradely in the accessory pathway and continues to the ventricle over the normal AV node and His bundle. After the ventricles have been excited, the impulse is able to enter the accessory pathway retrogradely and return to the atrium. A continuous conduction loop of this kind establishes the circuit for the tachycardia. The usual (orthodromic) activation wave during such a reciprocating tachycardia in a patient with an accessory pathway occurs in this manner: anterogradely over the normal AV node–His-Purkinje system and retrogradely over the accessory pathway, resulting in a normal QRS complex (Fig. 20–34).

Because the circuit requires both atria and ventricles, the term *supraventricular tachycardia* is not precisely correct, and the tachycardia is more accurately called *atrioventricular reciprocating tachycardia* (AVRT). The reentrant loop can be interrupted by ablation of the normal AV node–His bundle pathway *or* the accessory pathway.[195–204] Occasionally, the activation wave travels in a reverse (antidromic) direction to the ventricles over the accessory pathway and to the atria retrogradely up the AV node.[193,194] Two accessory pathways may form the circuit in some patients with antidromic AVRT. In some patients, the accessory pathway can be capable only of retrograde conduction ("concealed"), but the circuit and mechanism of AVRT remain the same. Less commonly, the accessory pathway can con-

duct only anterogradely. The pathway can be localized by analysis of the scalar ECG.[205–209,209a] Patients can have atrial fibrillation as well as AVRT.[210]

Unusual accessory pathways with AV nodal–like electrophysiological properties, nodofascicular or nodoventricular fibers, can constitute the circuit for reciprocating tachycardias in patients who have some form of the Wolff-Parkinson-White syndrome. Tachycardia in patients with nodoventricular fibers can be due to reentry using these fibers as the anterograde pathway and the His-Purkinje fibers and a portion of the AV node retrogradely.[194,195] In the Lown-Ganong-Levine syndrome (short P-R interval and normal QRS complex), conduction over a James fiber that connects atrium to the distal portion of the AV node and His bundle has been *proposed,* although little functional evidence to support the presence of this entity has been published, except in a rare patient with an unusual atrio–His connection (see p. 672).

VENTRICULAR TACHYCARDIA DUE TO REENTRY (see also p. 667). Reentry in the ventricle, both anatomical and functional, as a cause of sustained ventricular tachycardia has been supported by many animal[211–218] and clinical[219–222] studies (Fig. 20–29). Reentry in ventricular muscle, with or without contribution from specialized tissue, is responsible for many or most ventricular tachycardias in patients with ischemic heart disease. The area of microreentry appears to be quite small, and only uncommonly is a macroreentry found around the infarct scar. Surviving myocardial tissue (Fig. 20–35) separated by connective tissue provides serpentine routes of activation traversing infarcted areas that can establish reentry pathways. Bundle branch reentry can cause sustained ventricular tachycardia, particularly in patients with dilated cardiomyopathy.[221,223]

Both figure-of-eight[215] (Fig. 20–29) and single-circle[219] (Fig. 20–36) reentrant loops have been described, circulating around an area of functional block in a manner consistent with the leading circle hypothesis or conducting slowly across an apparent area of block created by anisotropy.[213]

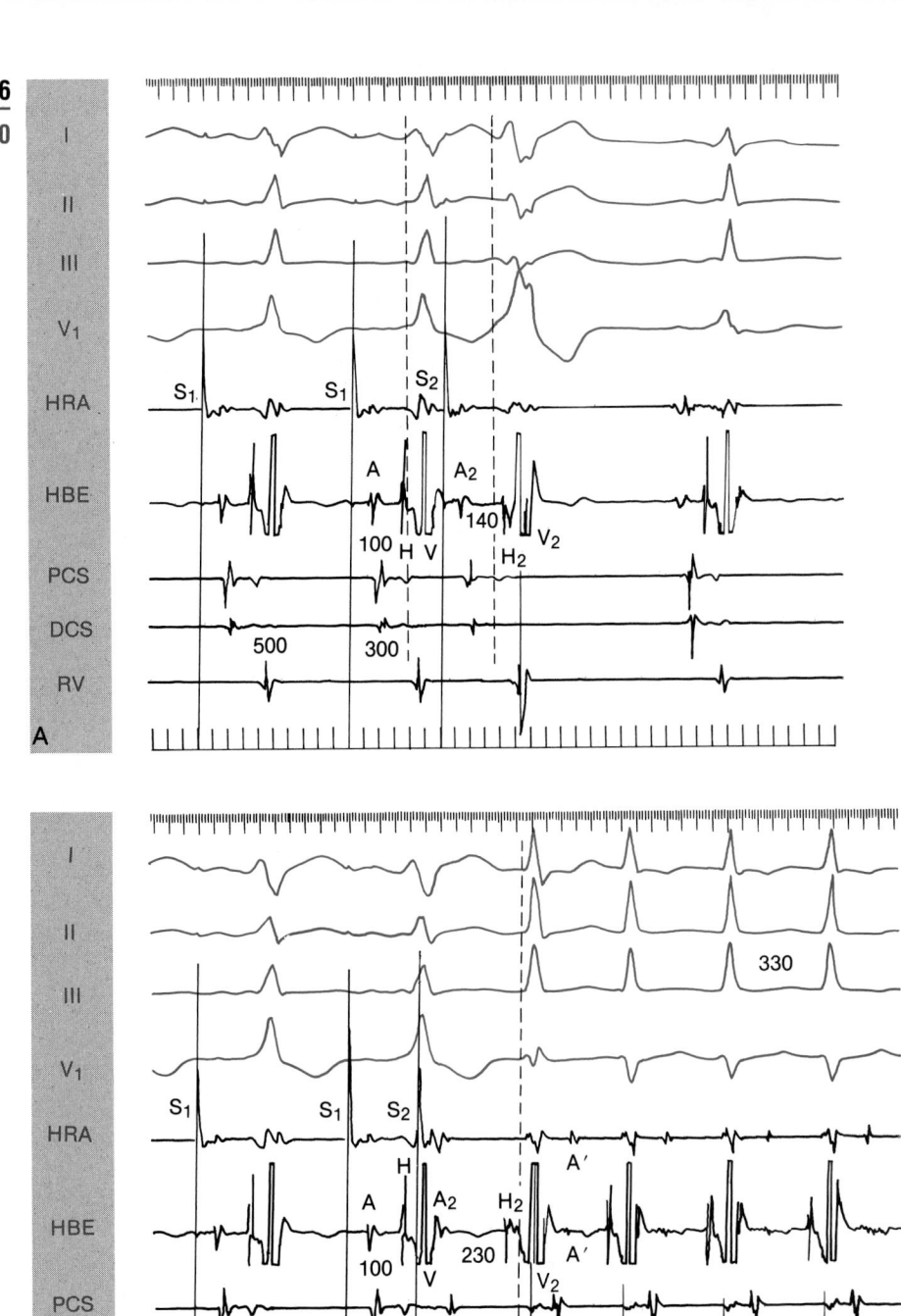

FIGURE 20–34. *A*, Wolff-Parkinson-White syndrome. Following high right atrial pacing at a cycle length of 500 msec (S_1-S_1), premature stimulation at a coupling interval of 300 msec (S_1-S_2) produces physiological delay in AV nodal conduction resulting in an increase in the AH interval from 100 to 140 msec but no delay in the AV interval. Consequently, activation of the His bundle occurs following activation of the QRS complex (second interrupted line) and the QRS complex becomes more anomalous in appearance due to increased ventricular activation over the accessory pathway. I, II, III, and V_1 and scalar leads. HRA, high right atrium; HBE, His bundle electrogram; PCS, proximal coronary sinus electrogram; DCS, distal coronary sinus electrogram; RV, right ventricular electrogram. Time lines 50 and 10 msec intervals. S_1, stimulus of the drive train; S_2, premature stimulus. A, H V, atrial His bundle, and ventricular activation during the drive train. A_2, H_2, V_2, atrial His bundle, and ventricular activation during the premature stimulus.

B, Induction of reciprocating atrioventricular tachycardia. Premature stimulation at a coupling interval of 230 msec prolongs the AH interval to 230 msec and results in anterograde block in the accessory pathway and normalization of the QRS complex (slight functional aberrancy in the nature of incomplete right bundle branch block occurs). Note that H2 precedes the onset of the QRS complex (interrupted line). Following V_2, the atria are excited retrogradely (A') beginning in the distal coronary sinus, then followed by atrial activation in leads recording from the proximal coronary sinus, His bundle, and high right atrium. A supraventricular tachycardia is initiated at a cycle length of 330 msec. Conventions as in panel A. (From Zipes, D. P., Mahomed, Y., King, R. D., et al.: Wolff-Parkinson-White syndrome: Cryosurgical treatment. *Indiana Med. 89:*432, 1986.)

When intramural myocardium survives, it may form part of the reentrant loop. Structural discontinuities that separate muscle bundles, owing to naturally occurring myocardial fiber orientation and anisotropic conduction as well as to collagen matrices formed from the fibrosis after a myocardial infarction, establish the basis for slowed conduction, fragmented electrograms, and continuous electrical activity that can lead to reentry. After the infarction, action potential recordings from surviving cells return to normal, suggesting that depressed activity in these cells does not account for the slowed conduction. However, ventricular myocardium resected from humans with recurrent ventricular tachycardia demonstrates abnormal action potentials, suggesting that causes of depressed conduction in humans may be multifactorial (Figs. 20–21 and 20–23). During acute ischemia, a variety of factors, including elevated $[K]_o$ and reduced pH, combine to create depressed action poten-

tials in ischemic cells that retards conduction and can lead to reentry.[67,213,222]

Ventricular Tachycardias Due to Nonreentrant Mechanisms

In some instances of ventricular tachycardias related to coronary artery disease, but especially in patients without coronary artery disease, nonreentrant mechanisms are important causes of ventricular tachycardias. Experimentally, nonreentrant forms of ventricular tachycardia appear to cause 25 per cent of acute ischemic-induced ventricular tachycardias and 75 per cent of ventricular tachycardias due to reperfusion; rapidly firing nonreentrant foci are responsible for the transition to ventricular fibrillation.[224,224a] Nonreentrant mechanisms also can cause ventricular tachycardias clinically. However, in many patients, the mechanism of the ventricular tachycardia remains unknown.[225]

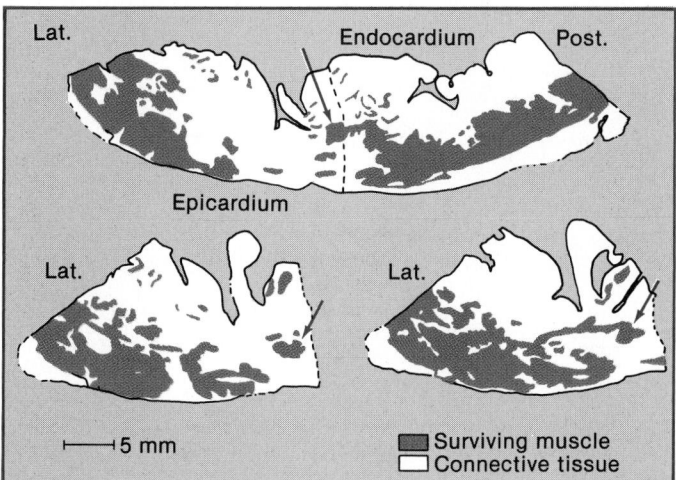

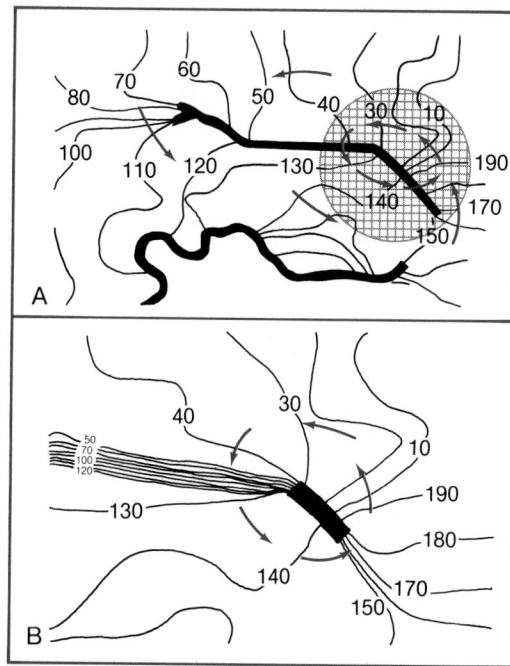

FIGURE 20–35. *Top panel* iş a schematic drawing illustrating left ventricular myocardial sections of a human heart studied electrophysiologically and histologically after removal for cardiac transplant. Dark areas mark surviving cardiac tissue, while light areas point to fibrotic and fatty tissue. Note the irregularity of the surviving cardiac tissue interspersed with fibrotic tissue. Lower two panels are schematic drawings of sections from the lateral left ventricular wall 500 *(left)* and 1000 *(right)* μm, respectively, beneath the level of those shown in the top panel. Note that bulge of viable tissue at the left of the surviving posterior wall (arrow in the top panel) becomes isolated in the *lower left panel* (arrow). In the *lower right panel,* this isolated area merges with the bulk of surviving tissue in the lateral wall (arrow). (From deBakken, J. M. T., Coronel, R., Tisserons, S., et al.: Ventricular tachycardia in the infarcted Langendorff-perfused human heart: Role of the arrangement of surviving cardiac fibers. J. Am. Coll. Cardiol. 15:1594, 1990. Reprinted with permission from the American College of Cardiology.)

FIGURE 20–36. Model of anisotropic reentry in the epicardial border zone. *A,* The activation map of the single reentrant circuit is shown. The large arrows point out the general activation pattern; activation appears to occur around a long line of block. However, parallel isochrones adjacent to the line (isochrones 130 and 140) suggest that activation is also occurring across the line, resulting in the smaller circuit shown by the small arrows. *B,* This circuit is shown enlarged. Rapid activation occurs parallel to the long axis of the fiber orientation (isochrones 10–40 and at 130–150), whereas very slow activation (closely bunched isochrones 50–120) occurs transverse to fiber orientation in the circuit. The dark black rectangle is an area of either functional or anatomical block that forms the fulcrum of the circuit. (From Wit, A. L., and Dillon, S. M.: Anisotropic reentry. *In* Zipes, D. P., and Jalife, J. [eds.]: Cardiac Electrophysiology. From Cell to Bedside. Philadelphia, W. B. Saunders Company, 1990.)

TRIGGERED ACTIVITY. Early afterdepolarizations and triggered activity may be responsible for torsade de pointes.[226] A group of probably nonreentrant ventricular tachycardias occurring in the absence of structural heart disease can be initiated and terminated by programmed stimulation. They are catecholamine dependent and are terminated by Valsalva, adenosine, and verapamil. These ventricular tachycardias are generally but not exclusively located in the right ventricular outflow tract and may be due to triggered activity, possibly delayed afterdepolarizations that are cyclic AMP dependent.[96,103,227–229] Early afterdepolarizations have been recorded in this tachycardia as well.[104] Left ventricular fascicular tachycardias can be suppressed by verapamil but generally not adenosine,[229] and some may be due to triggered activity[230] and others due to reentry.[231] Adenosine can be a useful pharmacological probe to uncover arrhythmias dependent on adenylyl cyclase,[103] which is inhibited by the regulatory protein G_i;[232] adenosine can suppress some left ventricular tachycardias as well.[233] Early afterdepolarizations may not necessarily be the cause of reperfusion arrhythmias.[233a]

AUTOMATICITY. Automatic discharge can be responsible for some ventricular tachycardias[234,235] and does not appear to be suppressed by adenosine.[103] Unless invasive studies are undertaken, mechanisms of ventricular tachycardias can only be conjectured.[236–238]

APPROACH TO THE DIAGNOSIS OF CARDIAC ARRHYTHMIAS

It is important to remember that the physician evaluates a *patient* who has a rhythm disturbance and does not evaluate a rhythm disturbance in isolation.[239] Some arrhythmias are hazardous to the patient regardless of the clinical setting, while others are hazardous *because* of the clinical setting. Evaluation of the patient begins with a careful his-

tory[240] and physical examination and should usually progress from the simplest to the most complex test, from the least invasive and safest to the most invasive and risky, and from the least expensive out-of-hospital evaluations to those which require hospitalization and sophisticated, costly procedures. Occasionally, depending on the clinical circumstances, the physician may wish to proceed directly to a high-risk, expensive procedure, such as an electrophysiological study, prior to obtaining a 24-hour ECG recording.

Patients with cardiac rhythm disturbances may present with a variety of complaints, but commonly symptoms such as palpitations, syncope, presyncope, or congestive heart failure cause them to seek a physician's help. Their awareness of regular or irregular cardiac rhythm varies greatly. Some patients perceive slight variations in their heart rhythm with uncommon accuracy, while others are oblivious even to sustained episodes of ventricular tachycardia; still others complain of palpitations when they actually have regular sinus rhythm. The following tests can be used to evaluate patients who have cardiac arrhythmias.

Exercise Testing
(See also Chap. 5)

Exercise can induce various types of supraventricular and ventricular tachyarrhythmias and, uncommonly, bradyarrhythmias.[241–246] About one-third of normal subjects develop ventricular ectopy in response to exercise testing. Ectopy is more likely to occur at faster heart rates, usually in the form of occasional premature ventricular complexes (PVCs) of constant morphology, or even pairs of PVCs, and is often not reproducible from one stress test to the next.

Three to six beats of nonsustained ventricular tachycardia can occur in normal patients, especially the elderly, and its occurrence does not establish the existence of ischemic or other forms of heart disease or predict increased cardiovascular morbidity or mortality. Supraventricular premature complexes are often more common during exercise than at rest and increase in frequency with age; their occurrence does not suggest the presence of structural heart disease.

Approximately 50 per cent of patients who have coronary artery disease develop PVCs in response to exercise testing. Ventricular ectopy appears in these patients at lower heart rates (less than 130 beats/min) than in the normal population and often occurs in the early recovery period as well. In one study, exercise reproduced sustained ventricular tachycardia (VT) or ventricular fibrillation (VF) in only 11 per cent of patients with spontaneous VT or VF late after myocardial infarction,[243] but those who had it experienced a worse outcome. The relation of exercise to ventricular arrhythmia in patients with structurally normal hearts has no prognostic implications.[244] Stress testing with Holter monitoring has been used to assess antiarrhythmic drug efficacy.[247–249]

Patients who have symptoms consistent with an arrhythmia induced by exercise (e.g., syncope, sustained palpitation) should be considered for stress testing. Stress testing may be indicated to uncover more complex grades of ventricular arrhythmia, to provoke supraventricular arrhythmias, to determine the relationship of the arrhythmia to activity, to aid in choosing antiarrhythmic therapy and uncovering proarrhythmic responses, and possibly to provide some insight into the mechanism of the tachycardia. The test can be performed safely[245] and appears more sensitive than a standard 12-lead resting ECG to detect ventricular ectopy. However, prolonged ambulatory recording is more sensitive than exercise testing in detecting ventricular ectopy. Since either technique may uncover serious arrhythmias that the other technique misses, both examinations may be indicated for selected patients.

Long-Term Electrocardiographic Recording

Prolonged ECG recording in patients engaged in normal daily activities is the most useful noninvasive method to document and quantitate frequency and complexity of arrhythmia, correlate arrhythmia with the patient's symptoms, and evaluate the effect of antiarrhythmic therapy on spontaneous arrhythmia. For example, recording normal sinus rhythm during the patient's typical symptomatic episode effectively excludes cardiac arrhythmia as a cause. In addition, some recorders can document alterations in QRS, ST, and T contours (Fig. 20–37).

Several modes of recordings are available[250]: (1) A recording can be continuous. If a tape recorder is used, every beat is recorded and is available for analysis. A real-time analysis device also can be used. (2) A recording can be patient activated. This is useful if the patient is able to perceive symptoms of the arrhythmia and activate the recorder. (3) A recording can be arrhythmia (event) activated. This is an effective mode, but it depends on the accuracy and reliability of the device's arrhythmia-detection algorithm. Many implantable pacemakers and defibrillators have the capability of long-term ECG (and device function) recording, and there is a recording device that can actually be implanted subcutaneously for long-term monitoring.

Transmitters that send an electrocardiographic signal transtelephonically to a receiver unit can be used to transmit on-line or stored electrocardiographic information. This device may be indicated when the rhythm disturbance is sufficiently infrequent and short lasting that continuous ECG recording is impractical. The arrhythmia must be of sufficient duration to permit real-time actual transmission or for storage and later transmission. It must not be associated with syncope or other symptoms that prevent the

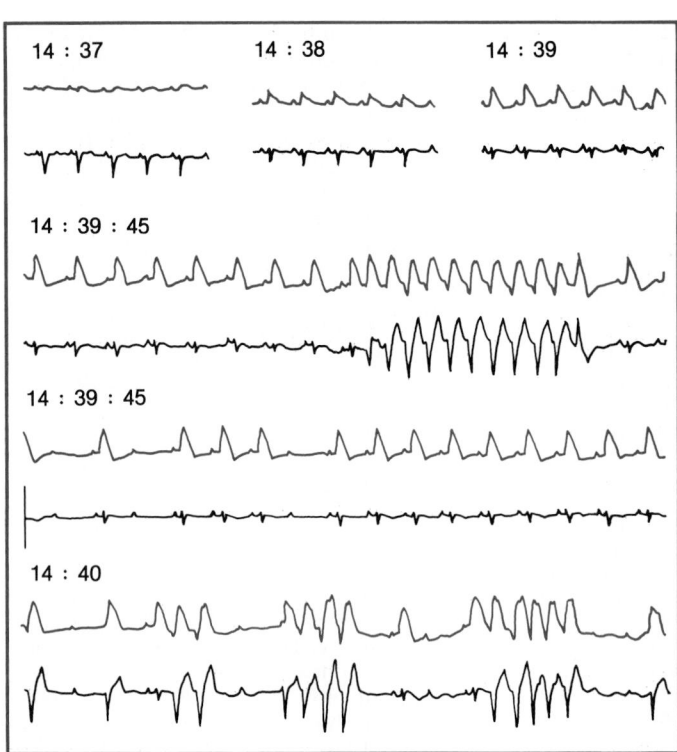

FIGURE 20–37. Long-term ECG recording in a patient with atypical angina. The top channel reflects an inferior lead while the bottom channel records an anterior lead. Note progressive ST-segment elevation in the inferior lead, eventually resembling a monophasic action potential. Bursts of nonsustained ventricular tachycardia result. Then, sinus slowing and Wenckebach AV block occur from a vasodepressor reflex response elicited by ischemia of the inferior myocardial wall, or possibly caused by ischemia of the sinus and AV nodes. In the bottom tracing, both AV block and ventricular arrhythmias are apparent. Numbers indicate time, e.g., 2:37 P.M. (Tracing of a patient of D. A. Chilson, M.D.)

patient from transmitting or recording, or the patient must have another individual available to record the event. A disadvantage is that this approach relies on the patient's perception of a cardiac rhythm disturbance, and many patients may be unaware of significant or serious bradyarrhythmias and tachyarrhythmias. In addition, the technique requires access to a receiver 24 hours a day. Such an approach can be adapted for continuous monitoring. Home monitoring systems, presently not widely available, operate in a fashion similar to telemetry monitoring in a hospital, but transmit ECG data over telephone lines.

HOLTER MONITORING. Continuous ECG tape recorders represent the traditional Holter "monitor" and typically record on tape two ECG channels for 24 hours. Interpretative accuracy of long-term tape recordings varies with the system used, but most computers that scan the tapes are sufficiently accurate to meet clinical needs. All systems can potentially record more information than the physician needs or can assimilate.[251] So long as the system detects important episodes of ectopic activity, ventricular tachycardia, or asystolic intervals and semiquantitates these abnormalities, the physician probably receives all the clinical information that is needed. Approximately 25 to 50 per cent of patients experience a complaint during a 24-hour recording, caused by an arrhythmia in 2 to 15 per cent.

Significant rhythm disturbances are fairly uncommon in healthy young persons. However, sinus bradycardia with heart rates of 35 to 40 beats/min, sinus arrhythmia with pauses exceeding 3 sec, sinoatrial exit block, Wenckebach second-degree AV block (often during sleep), a wandering atrial pacemaker, junctional escape complexes, and premature atrial complexes (PACs) and PVCs are not necessarily abnormal. Frequent and complex atrial and ventricular rhythm disturbances are less commonly observed, however, and type II second-degree AV conduction disturbances are not recorded in normal patients. Elderly patients may have a greater prevalence of arrhythmias, some of which may be responsible for neurological symptoms. The long-term prognosis in asymptomatic healthy subjects with frequent and complex PVCs resembles that of the healthy U.S. population without an increased risk of death.

A majority of patients who have ischemic heart disease, particularly those after myocardial infarction, exhibit PVCs when monitored for periods of 6 to 24 hours[252,253] (p. 675). The frequency of PVCs progressively increases over the first several weeks, decreasing at about 6 months after infarction. Frequent and complex PVCs are an independent risk factor and are associated with a two- to fivefold increased risk of cardiac or sudden death in patients after myocardial infarction. Recent evidence from the Cardiac Arrhythmia Suppression Trial (CAST) raises the possibility that the ventricular ectopy may be a *marker* identifying the patient at risk rather than being *causally related* to sudden death, since PVC suppression with flecainide, encainide, or moricizine was associated with increased mortality compared with placebo. Thus the PVC may be an *innocent bystander,* unrelated to the tachyarrhythmia producing sudden death. Although the mechanism responsible for the drug-induced exacerbation of mortality is not clear, it may relate to an increase in ischemia-produced conduction delay due to sodium channel blocking drugs.

Holter recordings have been used to determine antiarrhythmic drug efficacy. In one study, Holter recordings led to predictions of antiarrhythmic drug efficacy more often than did electrophysiological testing in patients with sustained ventricular tachyarrhythmias, and there was no significant difference in the success of drug therapy as selected by the two methods.[247] The study also found sotalol to be the most efficacious of the seven antiarrhythmic drugs tested.[248] The beneficial results of noninvasive compared with invasive assessment of drug efficacy in this study have been challenged.[254,255]

Long-term ECG recording also has exposed potentially serious arrhythmias and complex ventricular ectopy in patients with left ventricular hypertrophy,[256] in those with mitral valve prolapse (see p. 1033), in those who have otherwise unexplained syncope (Chap. 22) or transient vague cerebrovascular symptoms, and in those with conduction disturbances, sinus node dysfunction, the bradycardia-tachycardia syndrome, the Wolff-Parkinson-White syndrome, Q-T dispersion,[257] pacemaker malfunction, and after thrombolytic therapy.[258,259] It has shown that asymptomatic atrial fibrillation occurs far more often than symptomatic atrial fibrillation in patients with that arrhythmia.[260]

HEART RATE VARIABILITY. Heart rate variability is used to evaluate vagal and sympathetic influences on the heart and to identify patients at risk for a cardiovascular event or death.[261-269] Frequency domain analysis resolves parasympathetic and sympathetic influences better than does time domain analysis, but both types of spectral analyses are useful. R-R variability predicts all-cause mortality as well as does left ventricular ejection fraction or nonsustained VT in patients after myocardial infarction[270-274] and can be added to other measures of risk to enhance prediction accuracy.[275-283] Perceived high- and low-frequency components of R-R interval variability suggest that both vagal and sympathetic activities, respectively, are at physiological levels. However, reduced R-R interval variability, the marker of increased risk,[284] merely indicates loss or reduction of the physiological periodic fluctuations, which can be due to many different influences, and cannot necessarily be interpreted to represent a particular shift in autonomic modulation.[284a]

T-WAVE ALTERNANS. Beat-to-beat alternation in the amplitude and/or morphology of the ECG measurement of repolarization, the ST segment and T wave, has been found in conditions favoring the development of ventricular tachyarrhythmias such as ischemia[285-289] and long Q-T interval syndrome,[32,290-292] and in patients with ventricular arrhythmias.[288,289] The electrophysiological basis of the alternation is not known and may vary with different disease states. T-wave alternans may represent a fundamental marker of an electrically unstable myocardium prone to developing VT or VF, and as such, ST-T wave analysis for alternans may be useful in the future as a method to stratify risk patients.

Invasive Electrophysiological Studies

An invasive electrophysiological procedure involves introducing multipolar catheter electrodes into the venous and/or arterial system, positioning the electrodes at various intracardiac sites to record electrical activity from portions of the atria or ventricles, from the region of the His bundle, bundle branches, accessory pathways, and other structures, and stimulating the atria, ventricles, or other sites electrically. Such studies are performed *diagnostically* to provide information on the type of rhythm disturbance and insight into its electrophysiological mechanism; *therapeutically* to terminate a tachycardia by electrical stimulation or electroshock, to evaluate effects of therapy by determining whether a particular intervention modifies or prevents electrical induction of a tachycardia or whether an electrical device properly senses and terminates an induced tachyarrhythmia, and to ablate myocardium involved in the tachycardia. Finally, these tests have been used *prognostically* to identify patients at risk for sudden cardiac death. The study may be helpful in patients who have AV block, intraventricular conduction disturbance, sinus node dysfunction, tachycardia, and unexplained syncope or palpitations.[293]

False-negative responses—not finding a particular electrical abnormality known to be present—as well as false-positive ones—induction of a nonclinical arrhythmia—may complicate interpretation of the results, as may lack of reproducibility. Altered autonomic tone in a supine patient undergoing study, hemodynamic or ischemic influences, changing anatomy (e.g., new infarction) after the study, day-to-day variability, and the fact that the test employs an artificial "trigger" (electrical stimulation) to induce the arrhythmia are several of many factors that may explain the disparity between test results and spontaneous clinical occurrences. Overall, these studies are quite safe when performed by skilled clinical electrophysiologists.

AV Block
(See also pp. 687–692)

In patients with AV block, the site of block usually dictates the clinical course of the patient and whether or not a pacemaker is needed.[106] Generally, the site of AV block can be determined from an analysis of the scalar ECG. When the site of block cannot be determined from such an analysis, and when knowing the site of block is imperative for patient management, an invasive electrophysiological study is indicated. Candidates include symptomatic patients in whom His-Purkinje block is suspected but not established and patients with AV block treated with a pacemaker who continue to be symptomatic, to search for a causal ventricular tachyarrhythmia. Possible candidates are those with second- or third-degree AV block in whom knowledge of the site of block or its mechanism may help direct therapy or assess prognosis, and patients suspected of having concealed His extrasystoles (Fig. 20–38). Patients with block in the His-Purkinje system more commonly become symptomatic because of periods of bradycardia or asystole and require pacemaker implantation than do patients who have AV nodal block.[294] Wenckebach (type I) AV block in older patients may have clinical implications similar to type II AV block.

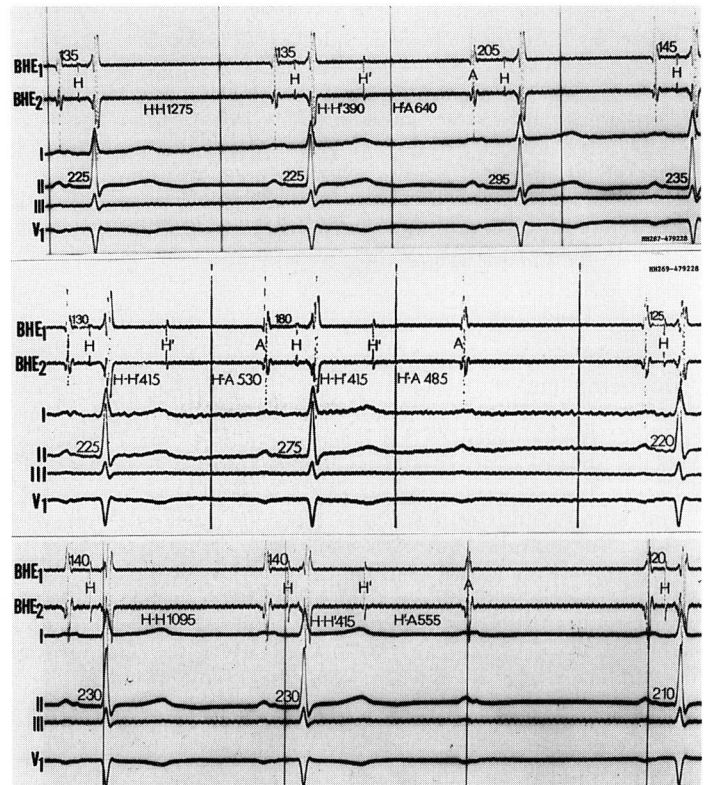

FIGURE 20–38. Concealed discharge from the bundle of His mimicking first-degree *(top)*, type I *(middle)*, and type II *(bottom)* second-degree AV block. Numbers are in milliseconds. Time lines are one second. (Magnification differs in the three panels.) Numbers in the bipolar His electrogram (BHE₁) indicate A-H intervals; the H-V interval is constant. Numbers in lead II indicate the P-R interval. H-H = interval between His responses in normal conducted cycles. H-H′ = interval between the last normal His discharge and the premature His discharge. H′ − A = interval between the premature His depolarization and the next normal sinus-initiated atrial discharge. H′ invaded the AV node and lengthened the A-H interval or produced AV nodal block of the next atrial depolarization. (From Bonner, A. J., and Zipes, D. P.: Lidocaine and His bundle extrasystoles. His bundle discharge conducted normally, conducted with functional right or left branch block, or blocked entirely (concealed). Arch. Intern. Med. *136:*700, 1976. Copyright 1976 American Medical Association.)

Intraventricular Conduction Disturbance

For patients with an intraventricular conduction disturbance, an electrophysiological study provides information on the duration of the H-V interval, which can be prolonged with a normal P-R interval or normal with a prolonged P-R interval. A prolonged H-V interval (> 55 msec) is associated with a greater likelihood of developing trifascicular block (but the rate of progression is slow, 2 to 3 per cent annually), having structural disease, and higher mortality. Finding very long H-V intervals (> 80 to 90 msec) identifies patients at increased risk of developing AV block. The H-V interval has a high specificity (about 80 per cent) but low sensitivity (about 66 per cent) for predicting the development of complete AV block. During the study, atrial pacing is used to uncover abnormal His-Purkinje conduction.[295] A positive response is provocation of distal His block during 1:1 AV nodal conduction. Once again, sensitivity is low but specificity is high. Functional His-Purkinje block due to normal His-Purkinje refractoriness is not a positive response. Drug infusion, such as with procainamide or ajmaline, sometimes exposes abnormal His-Purkinje conduction. Ajmaline can cause arrhythmias and should be used cautiously.

An electrophysiological study is indicated in the patient with symptoms (syncope or presyncope) that appear to be related to a bradyarrhythmia or tachyarrhythmia when no other cause of symptoms is found. For many of these patients, ventricular *tachyarrhythmias* rather than AV block might be the cause of their symptoms.[296]

Sinus Nodal Dysfunction

The demonstration of slow sinus rates, sinus exit block, or sinus pauses temporally related to symptoms suggests a causal relationship and usually obviates further diagnostic studies.[297–301] Carotid sinus pressure that results in complete cardiac asystole or AV block with the patient's usual symptoms exposes the presence of a hypersensitive carotid sinus reflex (see p. 647). Carotid sinus massage must be done cautiously. Rarely, carotid sinus massage can precipitate a stroke. Neurohumoral agents, adenosine,[302] or stress testing can be employed to evaluate effects of autonomic tone on sinus node automaticity and sinoatrial conduction time. Electrophysiological studies should be considered in patients who have symptoms attributable to bradycardia or asystole, such as presyncope or syncope, and for whom noninvasive approaches have provided no explanation for the symptoms.[303]

SINUS NODE RECOVERY TIME (SNRT). This technique can be a useful test to evaluate sinus node function. The interval between the last paced high right atrial response and the first spontaneous (sinus) high right atrial response after termination of pacing is measured to determine the *sinus node recovery time* (SNRT). Because the spontaneous sinus rate influences the SNRT, the value is corrected by subtracting the spontaneous sinus node cycle length (prior to pacing) from the sinus recovery time (CSNRT) (Fig. 20–39). Normal CSNRT values are generally less than 525 msec. Prolonged CSNRT has been found in patients suspected of having sinus node dysfunction. Direct recordings of sinus node electrogram have documented that SNRT is influenced by prolongation of sinoatrial conduction time, as well as by changes in sinus nodal automaticity, especially in the first beat after cessation of pacing. After cessation of pacing, the first return sinus cycle can be normal and can be followed by secondary pauses (Fig. 20–39). Secondary pauses appear to be more common in patients whose sinus node dysfunction is caused by sinoatrial exit block. Sinoatrial exit block can cause some sinus pauses. It is important to evaluate AV nodal and His-Purkinje function in patients with sinus node dysfunction, since many also exhibit impaired AV conduction.

SINOATRIAL CONDUCTION TIME (SACT). This time can be estimated, based on the assumptions that (1) conduction times into and out of the sinus node are equal, (2) no depression of sinus node automaticity occurs, and (3) the pacemaker site does not shift following premature stimulation. These assumptions may be erroneous, particularly in patients with sinus nodal dysfunction; SACT can be measured directly with extracellular electrodes placed in the region of the sinus node and correlates well with the CSACT measured indirectly in patients with normal sinus node function. The sensitivity of the SACT and SNRT tests

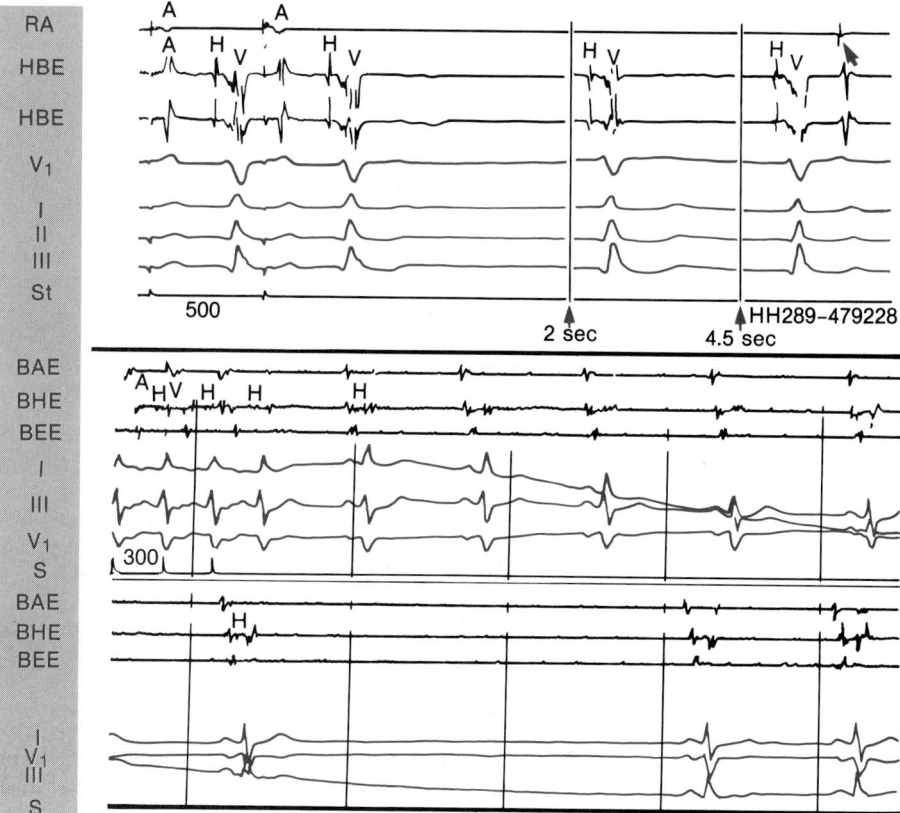

FIGURE 20–39. Abnormal response of sinus node to overdrive pacing. *Top,* After 30 sec of right atrial pacing at a cycle length of 500 msec, sinus nodal discharge is suppressed for more than 8 sec. (Sections of 2 sec and 4.5 sec removed for mounting.) *Bottom,* Right atrial pacing at a cycle length of 300 msec was followed by initial P waves occurring at an appropriate rate. The rate then slowed progressively, with P-P prolongation reaching 3 seconds and reproducing the patient's symptoms. Continuous recording; time lines = 1 sec. RA and BAE = bipolar right atrial electrogram; HBE and BHE = bi-polar His electrogram; BEE = bipolar esophageal electrogram; I, II, III, and V = scalar leads; St and S = stimulus. (Modified from Zipes, D. P., and Noble, R. J.: Assessment of electrical abnormalities. *In* Hurst, J. W. [ed.]: The Heart. 5th ed. New York, McGraw-Hill Book Co., 1982, pp. 333–357.)

is only about 50 per cent for each test alone and about 65 per cent when combined. The specificity, when combined, is about 88 per cent, with a low predictive value. Thus, if they are abnormal, the likelihood of the patient having sinus nodal dysfunction is great. However, if they are normal, that does not exclude the possibility of sinus node disease. Candidates for invasive electrophysiological study are symptomatic patients in whom sinus node dysfunction has not been established as a cause of the symptoms. Potential candidates are those requiring pacemakers to determine the pacing modality, patients with sinus node dysfunction to determine the mechanism and response to therapy, and patients in whom other causes of symptoms, e.g., tachyarrhythmias, are to be excluded.

Tachycardia

In patients with tachycardias, an electrophysiological study may be used to diagnose the arrhythmia, determine and deliver therapy, determine anatomical site(s) involved in the tachycardia, identify patients at high risk for developing serious arrhythmias, and gain insights into mechanisms responsible for the arrhythmia. The study can differentiate aberrant supraventricular conduction from ventricular tachyarrhythmias.[304] Since the electrocardiographic manifestations of ventricular tachycardia can be mimicked by aberrantly conducted supraventricular tachycardia, exceptions exist to the criteria that help to differentiate supraventricular tachyarrhythmias with abnormal QRS complexes from ventricular tachyarrhythmias.[237]

A *supraventricular tachycardia* is recognized electrophysiologically by the presence of an H-V interval equaling or exceeding that recorded during normal sinus rhythm (Fig. 20–40). In contrast, during *ventricular tachycardia,* the H-V interval is shorter than normal, or more commonly, the His deflection cannot be recorded clearly. Only two situations exist when a consistently short H-V interval occurs: during retrograde activation of the His bundle from activation originating in the ventricle, i.e., ventricular premature complex or tachycardia (see p. 677), or during conduction over an accessory pathway (preexcitation syndrome; see p. 667). Atrial pacing at rates exceeding the tachycardia rate

can demonstrate ventricular origin of the wide QRS tachycardia by producing fusion and capture beats and normalization of the H-V interval (Fig. 20–41). The only ventricular tachycardia that exhibits an H-V interval resembling the normal sinus H-V interval is bundle branch reentry (see p. 686), but His activation will be in the retrograde direction.

INDICATIONS FOR TACHYCARDIA. An electrophysiological study should be considered (1) in patients who have symptomatic, recurrent, or drug-resistant supraventricular or ventricular tachyarrhythmias to help select optimal therapy; (2) in patients with tachyarrhythmias occurring too infrequently to permit adequate diagnostic or therapeutic assessment; (3) to differentiate supraventricular tachycardia and aberrant conduction from ventricular tachycardia; (4) whenever nonpharmacological therapy such as the use of electrical devices, catheter ablation, or surgery is contemplated; and (5) in patients surviving an episode of cardiac arrest occurring ≥ 48 hours after an acute myocardial infarction or without evidence of an acute Q-wave myocardial infarction. Electrophysiological studies are generally *not* indicated in patients with the long Q-T syndrome and torsades de pointes, although recent information about early afterdepolarizations (see p. 566) may make such studies useful in the future.

The process of initiation and termination of supraventricular or ventricular tachycardia with programmed electrical stimulation to test the potential efficacy of pharmacological, electrical, or surgical therapy represents an important application of electrophysiological studies in patients with tachycardia. Arrhythmia-free survival is higher among patients in whom a drug prevents electrical reinduction of a sustained monomorphic ventricular tachycardia that was induced during the predrug control state. Among patients in whom ventricular tachycardia remains inducible, characteristics of the induced arrhythmia predict features of future recurrences. When the tachycardia and its hemodynamic response are not altered, an adverse risk for recurrence and mortality is predicted. When the tachycardia cycle length prolongs more than 100 msec and stable hemodynamics result, mortality improves.

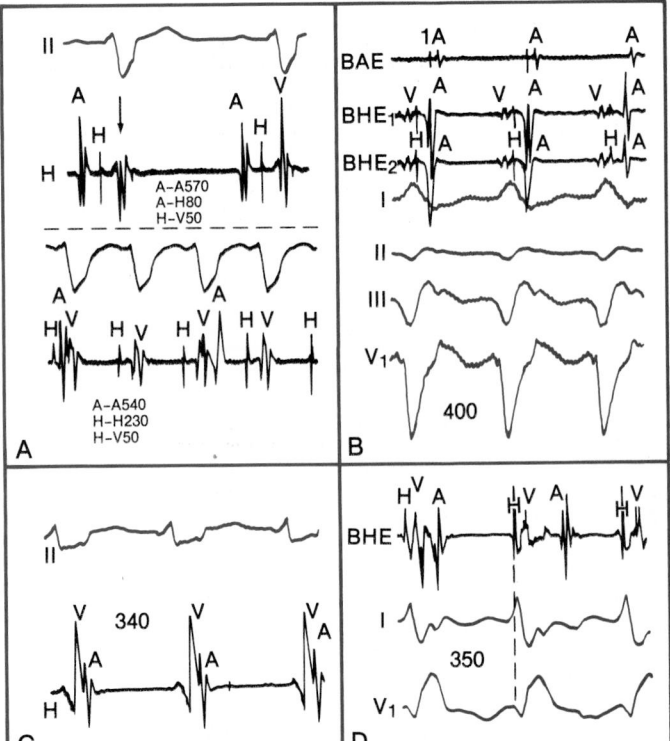

FIGURE 20–40. His bundle recording in four different patients with tachycardias. *A,* The top portion of the tracing shows His bundle recording during sinus rhythm. The H-V interval is 50 msec. The bottom portion shows His bundle recording during tachycardia. Since the QRS complex and H-V interval are the same as those recorded during sinus rhythm, this is a supraventricular tachycardia. Of note is the fact that the atria discharged at a rate that was different from (not a multiple of) the ventricular rate. Thus AV dissociation is present during this supraventricular tachycardia. *B,* His bundle activity occurred after the onset of the QRS complex, during ventricular tachycardia. (WPW had been excluded.) The R-P interval remained constant, and the atria were captured retrogradely from the ventricles. Thus AV dissociation is not present during this ventricular tachycardia. *C,* His bundle activity was not recorded despite careful exploration of the His bundle area with the catheter electrode tip. This most likely represents ventricular tachycardia with 1:1 retrograde atrial capture, but the diagnosis cannot be as clear as in panels *B* and *D.* In panel *D,* His bundle activity (interrupted line) preceded the onset of ventricular septal depolarization but followed the onset of the QRS complex. Thus this must be ventricular tachycardia. Retrograde (VA) Wenckebach conduction (not shown in its entirety) also was present. (From Zipes, D. P., et al.: Clinical electrophysiology and electrocardiography. *In* Willerson, J. T., and Sanders, C. A. [eds.]: Clinical Cardiology. New York, Grune and Stratton, 1977, pp. 235–248.)

Determination of drug efficacy based on results from long-term ECG recordings may be insufficient to predict a patient's therapeutic response when a low frequency of spontaneous ventricular arrhythmias are present. However, recently two studies have concluded that noninvasive assessment of drug efficacy testing beta blockers[305] and amiodarone[306] may be superior to the results of programmed electrical stimulation using conventional antiarrhythmic agents. Another controlled randomized study comparing invasive and noninvasive assessments of conventional drugs[248] found both techniques to be equivalent.[247] As of this writing both invasive and noninvasive methods should be considered appropriate approaches for guiding drug therapy.

Patients with Unexplained Syncope
(See p. 868)

The three common arrhythmic causes of syncope include sinus node dysfunction, tachyarrhythmias, and AV block. Of the three, tachyarrhythmias are most reliably initiated in

the electrophysiology laboratory, followed by sinus node abnormalities and then His-Purkinje block.[307]

The cause of syncope goes undetected in up to 50 per cent of patients, depending in part on the extent of the evaluation. A careful, accurately performed history and physical examination begin the evaluation,[239] followed by noninvasive tests, including a 12-lead and 24-hour ECG recording, and can lead to a diagnosis in half or more of the patients.[307–311] The 1-year mortality is about 6 per cent in patients with unknown cause, 1 to 12 per cent in patients with noncardiovascular causes, but 19 to 30 per cent in patients with cardiovascular causes. The incidence of sudden death is also higher in patients with a cardiovascular cause of syncope. A small percentage (< 5 per cent) of patients develop an arrhythmia coincident with syncope or presyncope during a 24-hour ECG recording, while a large percentage (15 per cent) have symptoms without an arrhythmia, excluding an arrhythmic cause. Prolonged ECG monitoring with patient-activated transtelephonic event recorders that have memory loops may increase the yield. Signal averaging (see p. 583) has a high sensitivity (about 75 per cent) and specificity (about 90 per cent) for predicting patients with syncope in whom ventricular tachycardia can be induced at electrophysiological study.[312] Tilt table testing[313–315,315a] and stress testing[316] can be useful in some patients, as can long-term ECG recordings.[317]

The electrophysiological study helps explain the cause of syncope or palpitations when it induces an arrhythmia that replicates the patient's symptoms. Syncopal patients with a nondiagnostic electrophysiological study have a low incidence of sudden death and 80 per cent remission rate. In those with recurrent syncope, the test is falsely negative in ≥ 20 per cent, due to failure to find AV block or sinus node dysfunction.

Syncopal patients considered for electrophysiological study are those whose spells remain undiagnosed despite general, neurological, and noninvasive cardiac evaluation, particularly if the patient has structural heart disease. The diagnostic yield is about 70 per cent in that group but only about 12 per cent in patients without structural heart disease. Prevention of syncope is economically important.[318] Mortality and incidence of sudden cardiac death are mainly determined by the presence of underlying heart disease.[319] Therapy of a putative cause found during electrophysiological testing prevents recurrence of syncope in about 80 per cent of patients. At times, empiric pacing is justified.

Palpitations

An electrophysiological study is indicated in patients with palpitations[240,320,321] who have had a pulse rate that medical personnel documented to be inappropriately rapid without electrocardiographic recording or in those suspected of having clinically significant palpitations without ECG documentation.

In patients with syncope or palpitation, the sensitivity of the electrophysiological test may be very low but may be increased at the expense of specificity. For example, more aggressive pacing techniques (e.g., using three or four premature stimuli), administration of drugs (e.g., isoproterenol), or left ventricular pacing can increase the success rate of ventricular tachycardia induction, but by precipitating nonclinical ventricular tachyarrhythmias such as nonsustained polymorphic or monomorphic ventricular tachycardia or ventricular fibrillation. Similarly, aggressive techniques during atrial pacing can induce nonspecific episodes of atrial flutter or atrial fibrillation. A diagnostic dilemma arises when the patient's clinical, symptom-producing arrhythmia is one of these nonspecific arrhythmias that can be produced in the normal patient who has no arrhythmia. Induction of *sustained* supraventricular (e.g., AV nodal reentry, AV reciprocating tachycardia) or monomorphic ventricular tachycardia in patients who are not subject

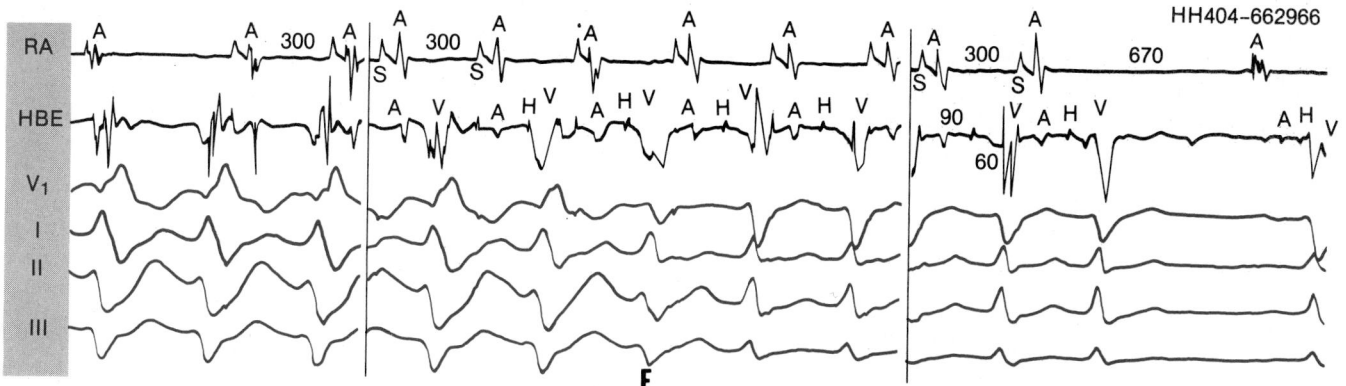

FIGURE 20–41. Termination of ventricular tachycardia by rapid atrial pacing. Ventricular tachycardia (*left panel*) with AV dissociation became captured by rapid atrial pacing (200 bpm) (*middle panel*) and was terminated after cessation of atrial pacing (*right panel*). Note fusion beat (F) in the midportion of panel 2 and normalization of the H-V interval. (From Foster, P. R., and Zipes, D. P.: Pacing and cardiac arrhythmias. *In* Mandel, W. J. [ed.]: Cardiac Arrhythmias: Their Mechanisms, Diagnosis and Management. Philadelphia, J. B. Lippincott, 1980, pp. 605–624.)

to the spontaneous development of the tachycardia appears to be uncommon and provides important information that the induced tachyarrhythmia may be clinically significant and responsible for the patient's symptoms. Generally, other abnormalities such as prolonged sinus pauses following overdrive atrial pacing or His-Purkinje AV block are not induced in patients who do not or may not experience these abnormalities spontaneously. Induction of these arrhythmias has a high degree of specificity.

Complications of Electrophysiological Studies

The risks of undergoing only an electrophysiological study are small. Adding therapeutic maneuvers, e.g., ablation, to the procedure increases the incidence of complications. In a European survey[322] published in 1993 based on 4398 patients reported from 68 institutions, procedure-related complications ranged from 3.2 to 8 per cent. Five deaths occurred within the perioperative period of the ablation. In an NASPE survey[323] of 164 hospitals reporting in 1994 on over 10,000 patients who received RF ablation, complications ranged from 1 to 3 per cent, with procedure-related deaths about 0.2 per cent. The improvement in the complication rate probably reflects the learning curve for RF ablation.

OTHER DIAGNOSTIC ELECTROCARDIOGRAPHIC TECHNIQUES

ESOPHAGEAL ELECTROCARDIOGRAPHY. Esophageal electrocardiography is a useful noninvasive technique to diagnose arrhythmias.[324,325] The esophagus is adjacent to the posterior atria, and an electrode inserted into the esophagus can record atrial potentials. Bipolar recording is superior to unipolar recording. In addition, atrial and occasionally ventricular pacing can be performed via a catheter electrode inserted into the esophagus, and initiation and termination of tachycardias can be accomplished. Optimal electrode position for pacing correlates with patient height and is within about 1 cm of the site at which the maximum amplitude of the atrial electrogram is recorded. No serious immediate complications of transesophageal pacing have been reported. A capsule electrode that is easily swallowed has been used to record continuous atrial electrograms from the esophagus.

The esophageal atrial electrogram is useful to differentiate supraventricular tachycardia with aberrancy from ventricular tachycardia (see p. 677) and to define the mechanism of supraventricular tachycardias. For example, if atrial and ventricular depolarization occur simultaneously during a narrow QRS tachycardia, reentry utilizing an ac-

cessory AV pathway (Wolff-Parkinson-White) can be excluded, and AV nodal reentry is the most likely mechanism for the tachycardia (see p. 661).

BODY SURFACE MAPPING. Isopotential body surface maps are used to provide a complete picture of the effects of the currents from the heart on the body surface. The potential distributions are represented by contour lines of equal potential, and each distribution is displayed instant by instant throughout activation or recovery, or both.[327–329]

Body surface maps have been used clinically to localize and size areas of myocardial ischemia, localize ectopic foci or accessory pathways, differentiate aberrant supraventricular conduction from ventricular origin, recognize the patient prone to developing arrhythmias, and possibly understand the mechanisms involved.[330–337] Although these procedures are of interest, their clinical utility has not yet been established.

DIRECT CARDIAC MAPPING: RECORDING POTENTIALS DIRECTLY FROM THE HEART. Cardiac mapping is a method whereby potentials recorded directly from the heart are spatially depicted as a function of time in an integrated manner. The location of recording electrodes (epicardial, intramural, or endocardial) and the recording mode used (unipolar versus bipolar) as well as the method of display (isopotential versus isochrone maps) depend upon the problem under consideration. Special electrodes can record monophasic action potentials.[338]

Direct cardiac mapping via catheter electrodes or at the time of cardiac surgery can be used to identify and localize the site of rhythm disturbances in patients with supraventricular and ventricular tachyarrhythmias for electrical or surgical ablation, isolation, or resection, such as accessory pathways associated with the Wolff-Parkinson-White syndrome, the slow pathway in AV nodal reentry, and VT circuits, or to delineate the anatomical course of the His bundle to avoid injury during open-heart surgery. These approaches are discussed in greater detail in Chap. 21 under nonpharmacological approaches and in Chap. 22 under the individual arrhythmias.

SIGNAL-AVERAGING TECHNIQUES. Signal averaging is a method that improves signal-to-noise ratio when signals are recurrent and the noise is random.[339] In conjunction with appropriate filtering and other methods of noise reduction, signal averaging can detect cardiac signals of a few microvolts in amplitude, reducing noise amplitude, such as muscle potentials that are typically 5 to 25 μV, to less than 1 μV. With this method, electrical potentials generated by the sinus and AV nodes, His bundle, and bundle branches are detectable at the body surface.

Signal averaging has been applied clinically most often to detect late ventricular potentials of 1 to 25 μV, which

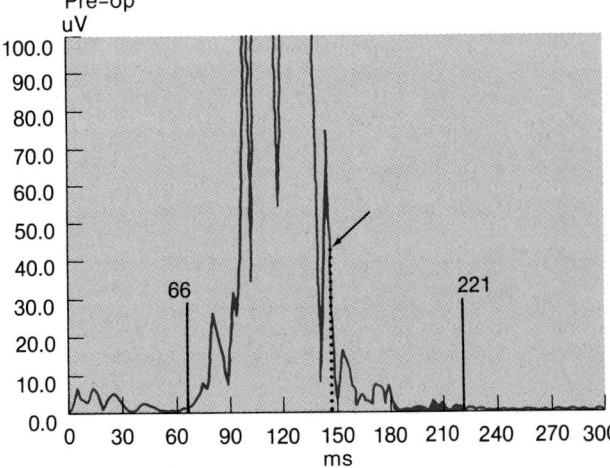

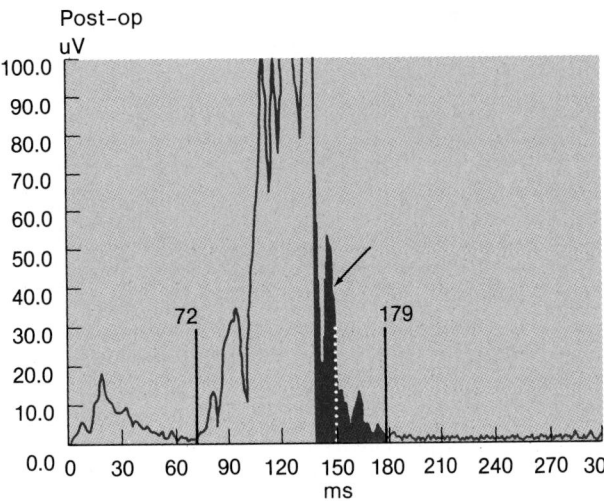

FIGURE 20–42. Signal-averaged ECG showing the presence of prolonged QRS duration due to late potentials (dark filled components in the terminal portion of the complex) present preoperatively but not postoperatively. RMS, root mean square (in mV); IN, integral of wave form delineated by the onset and offset markers; LAS, low amplitude signal. MN, mean value in the terminal QRS. Arrow indicates the 40 mV mark, after which the presence of low amplitude signals is determined. Scale = number of mV per notch.

are microvolt waveforms continuous with the QRS complex, probably corresponding to delayed and fragmented conduction in the ventricle[340–343] (Fig. 20–42). Criteria for late potentials are (1) filtered QRS complex duration > 114 to 120 msec, (2) < 20 μV of signal in the last 40 msec of the filtered QRS complex, and (3) the terminal filtered QRS complex remains below 40 μV for longer than 39 msec. These late potentials have been recorded in 70 to 90 per cent of patients with sustained and inducible ventricular tachycardia after myocardial infarction, in only 0 to 6 per cent of normal volunteers, and in 7 to 15 per cent of patients after myocardial infarction who do not have ventricular tachycardia. Late potentials can be detected as early as 3 hours after the onset of chest pain and increase in prevalence in the first week after infarction and may disappear in some patients after 1 year. If not present initially, late potentials usually do not appear later. Early use of thrombolytic agents may reduce the prevalence of late potentials after coronary occlusion.

Late potentials also have been recorded in patients with ventricular tachycardia not related to ischemia, such as dilated cardiomyopathies. Successful surgical resection of the ventricular tachycardia can eliminate late potentials but is not necessary to cause tachycardia suppression. Antiarrhythmic drug therapy, on the other hand, decreases the amplitude of the late potentials without abolishing them. Late potentials after myocardial infarction are an independent risk factor that identifies patients prone to develop ventricular tachycardia and can be combined with other data such as ejection fraction, spontaneous ventricular ectopy on a 24-hour ECG recording, or response to stress testing to recognize with high sensitivity and specificity patients at risk for ventricular tachycardia or sudden cardiac death. It also can be used to identify patients with

nonsustained ventricular tachycardia or syncope who may develop sustained ventricular tachycardia at electrophysiological study.

The high-pass filtering used to record late potentials meeting the criteria just noted is called *time domain analysis* because the filter output corresponds in time with the input signal. Since late potentials are high-frequency signals, Fourier transform can be applied to extract high-frequency content from the signal-averaged ECG, called *frequency domain analysis*. Some but not all data suggest that frequency domain analysis provides useful information not available in the time domain analysis. The preferable alternative has not been determined.

UPRIGHT TILT TESTING (see also p. 870). The tilt test is used to identify patients who have a vasodepressor and/or a cardioinhibitory response as a cause of syncope.[344,345] Patients are positioned on a tilt table in the supine position and are tilted upright to a maximum of 60 to 80 degrees for 20 to 45 minutes, or longer if necessary. Isoproterenol,[346–348] a bolus or an infusion, may provoke syncope in patients asymptomatic after initial upright tilt testing or after just several minutes of tilt to shorten the time of the test necessary to produce a positive response. An initial intravenous isoproterenol dose of 2 μg can be increased in 2-μg steps until symptoms occur or a maximum of 8 μg is given. Isoproterenol induces a vasodepressor response in upright susceptible patients generally consisting of a decrease in heart rate and blood pressure along with near syncope or syncope. Intravenous edrophonium,[349] nitroglycerin,[344] and esmolol[350] withdrawal have been used. Atropine can block the early bradycardia but not the hypotension. Beta blockers[351,352] can inhibit the latter. Tilt test results are positive in two-thirds to three-quarters of patients susceptible to neurally mediated syncope, are repro-

TABLE 20–8   CLASSIFICATION OF HEART RATE AND HEMODYNAMIC RESPONSES TO HEAD-UP TILT TABLE TESTING

Type I: Mixed

Heart rate rises initially and then falls, but the ventricular rate does not fall to less than 40 beats/min or falls to 40 beats/min for less than 10 seconds with or without asystole for less than 3 seconds.

Blood pressure rises initially and then falls before heart rate falls.

Type IIA: Cardioinhibitory

Heart rate rises initially and then falls to a ventricular rate of less than 40 beats/min for greater than 10 seconds, or asystole occurs for greater than 3 seconds.

Blood pressure rises initially and then falls before heart rate falls.

Type IIB: Cardioinhibitory

Heart rate rises initially and then falls to a ventricular rate of less than 40 beats/min for more than 10 seconds, or asystole occurs for more than 3 seconds.

Blood pressure rises initially and only falls to hypotensive levels less than 80 mm Hg systolic at or after onset of rapid and severe heart rate fall.

Type III: Pure vasodepressor

Heart rate rises progressively and does not fall more than 10 per cent from peak at time of syncope.

Blood pressure falls to cause syncope.

---

ducible in about 80 per cent,[353–356] but have a 10 to 15 per cent false-positive response rate. Positive can be divided into mixed, cardioinhibitory, and vasodepressor categories[357] (Table 20–8). Therapy with beta blockers,[351,352] disopyramide,[358] and theophylline has been tried.

Mechanism. Vasodepressor reactions, which are thought to be caused by activation of unmyelinated left ventricular vagal C fibers, can be excited by a variety of substances, including increased left ventricular pressure. Stimulation of C fibers from vigorous left ventricular contraction on an empty cavity reduces efferent sympathetic tone while increasing efferent vagal tone, possibly producing vasodepression and paradoxic bradycardia. Isoproterenol increases left ventricular contractility while reducing left ventricular volume. A passive upright tilt exaggerates these responses because the tilt also reduces venous return and prevents isoproterenol from increasing cardiac output. Some patients may experience profound bradycardia while others may have a prominent vasodepressor component (Table 20–8).

BARORECEPTOR REFLEX SENSITIVITY TESTING. Acute blood pressure elevation triggers a baroreceptor reflex that augments vagal "tone" to the heart and slows the sinus rate. The increase in sinus cycle length per mm Hg increase is a measure of the sensitivity of the baroreceptor reflex (BRS) and identifies patients susceptible to developing VT and VF.[32] The mechanism of the redirection in BRS is not known. However, this test may be useful to identify patients at risk for developing a serious ventricular arrhythmia after myocardial infarction.

REFERENCES

ANATOMY OF THE CARDIAC CONDUCTION SYSTEM

1. Trabka-Janik, E., Coombs, W., Lemanski, L. F., et al.: Immunohistochemical focalization of gap junction protein channels in hamster sinoatrial node in correlation with electrophysiologic mapping of the pacemaker region. J. Cardiovasc. Electrophysiol. 5:125, 1994.
2. Opthof, T.: Gap junctions in the sinoatrial node: Immunohistochemical focalization and correlation with activation pattern. J. Cardiovasc. Electrophysiol. 5:138, 1994.
3. Saffitz, J. E.: Cell-to-cell communication in the heart. Cardiol. Rev. 3:86, 1995.
4. Cai, D., Winslow, R. L., and Noble, D.: Effects of gap junction conductance on dynamics of the sinoatrial node cells: T-cell and large scale network models. IEEE Trans. Biomed. Eng. 41:217, 1994.
5. Davis, L. M., Kanter, H. L., Beyer, E. C., et al.: Distinct gap junction protein phenotypes in cardiac tissues with disparate conduction properties. J. Am. Coll. Cardiol. 24:1124, 1994.
6. Beyer, E. C., Veenstra, R. D., Kanter, H. L., et al.: Molecular structure and patterns of expression of cardiac gap junction proteins. In Zipes, D. P., and Jalife, J. (eds.): Cardiac Electrophysiology: From Cell to Bedside. 2nd ed. Philadelphia, W. B. Saunders Company, 1994, p. 31.
7. Pressler, M. L., Munster, P. N., and Haung, X.: Gap junction distribution in the heart: Functional relevance. In Zipes, D. P., and Jalife, J.

(eds.): Cardiac Electrophysiology: From Cell to Bedside. 2nd ed. Philadelphia, W. B. Saunders Company, 1994, p. 144.
8. Severs, N. J.: Pathophysiology of gap junctions in heart disease. J. Cardiovasc. Electrophysiol. 5:462, 1994.
9. Anumonwo, J. M. B., and Jalife, J.: Cellular and subcellular mechanisms of pacemaker activity initiation and synchronization in the heart. In Zipes, D. P., and Jalife, J. (eds.): Cardiac Electrophysiology: From Cell to Bedside. 2nd ed. Philadelphia, W. B. Saunders Company, 1994, p. 151.
10. Schuessler, R. B., Boineau, J. P., Bromberg, B. I., et al.: Normal and abnormal activation of the atrium. In Zipes, D. P., and Jalife, J. (eds.): Cardiac Electrophysiology: From Cell to Bedside. 2nd ed. Philadelphia, W. B. Saunders Company, 1994, p. 543.
11. Pappano, A. J.: Modulation of the heart beat by the vagus nerve. In Zipes, D. P., and Jalife, J. (eds.): Cardiac Electrophysiology: From Cell to Bedside. 2nd ed. Philadelphia, W. B. Saunders Company, 1994, p. 411.
12. Levy, M. N.: Time dependency of the autonomic interactions that regulate heart rate and rhythms. In Zipes, D. P., and Jalife, J. (eds.): Cardiac Electrophysiology: From Cell to Bedside. 2nd ed. Philadelphia, W. B. Saunders Company, 1994, p. 454.
13. Mitrani, R. D., and Zipes, D. P.: Clinical neurocardiology: Arrhythmias. In Ardell, J. L., and Armour, J. A. (eds.): Neurocardiology. Oxford, England, Oxford University Press, 1994, pp. 365–395.
14. Zipes, D. P.: Autonomic modulation of cardiac arrhythmias. In Zipes, D. P., and Jalife, J. (eds.): Cardiac Electrophysiology: From Cell to Bedside. 2nd ed. Philadelphia, W. B. Saunders Company, 1994, p. 441.
15. Elvan, A., and Zipes, D. P.: Functional anatomy of autonomic innervation of the atria. In Waldo, A., and Touboul, P. (eds.): Recent Advances in Atrial Flutter. Mt. Kisco, N. Y., Futura (in press).
16. Levy, M. N., and Schwartz, P. J. (eds.): Vagal Control of the Heart: Experimental Basis and Clinical Implications. Mt. Kisco, N. Y., Futura, 1994.
17. DiFrancesco, D.: A contribution of the hyperpolarization-activated current (I_f) to the generation of spontaneous activity in rabbit sinoatrial node myocytes. J. Physiol. 434:23, 1991.
18. DiFrancesco, D., and Tortora, P.: Direct activation of cardiac pacemaker channels by intracellular cyclic AMP. Nature 351:145, 1991.
19. DiFrancesco, D., and Zaza, A.: The cardiac pacemaker current I_f. J. Cardiovasc. Electrophysiol. 3:334, 1992.
20. DiFrancesco, D.: Pacemaker mechanisms in cardiac tissue. Annu. Rev. Physiol. 55:451, 1993.
21. DiFrancesco, D., Mangoni, M., and Maccaferri, G.: The pacemaker current in cardiac cells. In Zipes, D. P., and Jalife, J. (eds.): Cardiac Electrophysiology: From Cell to Bedside. 2nd ed. Philadelphia, W. B. Saunders Company, 1994, p. 96.
22. Kuarmby, L. M., and Hartzell, H. C.: Molecular biology of G proteins and their role in cardiac excitability. In Zipes, D. P., and Jalife, J. (eds.): Cardiac Electrophysiology: From Cell to Bedside. 2nd ed. Philadelphia, W. B. Saunders Company, 1994, p. 38.
23. Racker, D. K.: Transmission and reentrant activity in the sinoventricular conducting system and in the circumferential lamina of the tricuspid valve. J. Cardiovasc. Electrophysiol. 4:513, 1993.
24. Janse, M. J., Anderson, R. H., McGuire, M. A., et al.: "AV nodal" reentry: 1. "AV nodal" reentry revisited. J. Cardiovasc. Electrophysiol. 4:561, 1993.
25. McGuire, M. A., Janse, M. J., and Ross, D. L.: "AV nodal" reentry: 2. AV nodal, AV junctional or atrial nodal reentry? J. Cardiovasc. Electrophysiol. 4:573, 1993.
26. Jackman, W. M., Beckman, K. J., McClelland, J. H., et al.: Treatment of supraventricular tachycardia due to atrioventricular nodal reentry by radiofrequency ablation of slow-pathway conduction. N. Engl. J. Med. 327:313, 1992.

27. Ho, S. Y., McComb, J. M., Scott, C. D., et al.: Morphology of the cardiac conduction system in patients with electrophysiologically proven dual atrioventricular nodal pathways. J. Cardiovasc. Electrophysiol. *4*:504, 1993.

28. Ho, S. Y., Kilpatrick, L., Kanai, T., et al.: The architecture of the atrioventricular conduction axis in dogs compared to humans: Its significance to ablation of the atrioventricular nodal approaches. J. Cardiovasc. Electrophysiol. *6*:26, 1995.

29. Paes de Carvalho, A., and de Almeida, D. F.: Spread of activity through the atrioventricular node. Circ. Res. *8*:801, 1960.

30. Jongsma, H. J., and Rook, M. B.: Morphology and electrophysiology of cardiac gap junction channels. *In* Zipes, D. P., and Jalife, J. (eds.): Cardiac Electrophysiology: From Cell to Bedside. 2nd ed. Philadelphia, W. B. Saunders Company, 1994, p. 115.

31. Ito, M., and Zipes, D. P.: Efferent sympathetic and vagal innervation of the canine right ventricle. Circulation *90*:1459, 1994.

32. DeFerrari, G. M., Vanoli, E., and Schwartz, P. J.: Cardiac vagal activity, myocardial ischemia, and sudden death. *In* Zipes, D. P., and Jalife, J. (eds.): Cardiac Electrophysiology: From Cell to Bedside. 2nd ed. Philadelphia, W. B. Saunders Company, 1994, p. 422.

33. Spooner, P. M., and Brown, A. M.: Ion Channels in the Cardiovascular System. Mt. Kisco, N. Y., Futura, 1994.

BASIC ELECTROPHYSIOLOGICAL PRINCIPLES

34. Grant, A. O.: Evolving concepts of cardiac sodium channel function. J. Cardiovasc. Electrophysiol. *1*:53, 1990.

35. Katz, A. M.: Cardiac ion channels. N. Engl. J. Med. *328*:1244, 1993.

36. Hanck, D. A.: Biophysics of sodium channels. *In* Zipes, D. P., and Jalife, J. (eds.): Cardiac Electrophysiology: From Cell to Bedside. 2nd ed. Philadelphia, W. B. Saunders Company, 1994, p. 65.

37. Catterall, W. A.: Molecular analysis of voltage gated sodium channels in the heart and other tissues. *In* Zipes, D. P., and Jalife, J. (eds.): Cardiac Electrophysiology: From Cell to Bedside. 2nd ed. Philadelphia, W. B. Saunders Company, 1994, p. 1.

38. Marban, E., and O'Rourke, B.: Calcium channels: Structure, function and regulation. *In* Zipes, D. P., and Jalife, J. (eds.): Cardiac Electrophysiology: From Cell to Bedside. 2nd ed. Philadelphia, W. B. Saunders Company, 1994, p. 11.

39. Alvarez, J., and Vassort, G.: Cardiac T-type Ca current: Pharmacology and emphasis on its roles in cardiac tissues. J. Cardiovasc. Electrophysiol. *5*:376, 1994.

40. Borgatta, L., Watras, J., Katz, A. M., et al.: Regional differences in calcium-release channels from heart. Proc. Natl. Acad. Sci. U.S.A. *88*:2486, 1991.

41. January, C. T., Cunningham, P. M., and Zhou, Z.: Pharmacology of L- and T-type calcium channels in the heart. *In* Zipes, D. P., and Jalife, J. (eds.): Cardiac Electrophysiology: From Cell to Bedside. 2nd ed. Philadelphia, W. B. Saunders Company, 1994, p. 269.

42. Campbell, D. L., Rasmusson, R. L., Comer, M. B., et al.: The cardiac calcium-independent transient outward potassium current: Kinetics, molecular properties and role in ventricular repolarizations. *In* Zipes, D. P., and Jalife, J. (eds.): Cardiac Electrophysiology: From Cell to Bedside. 2nd ed. Philadelphia, W. B. Saunders Company, 1995, p. 83.

43. Rose, W. C., Balke, C. W., Wier, W. G., et al.: Macroscopic and unitary properties of physiological ion flux through L-type Ca channels in guinea-pig heart cells. J. Physiol. *456*:267, 1992.

44. Tang, S., Mikala, G., Bahinski, A., et al.: Molecular focalization of ion selectivity sites within the pore of a human cardiac L-type calcium channel. J. Biol. Chem. *286*:13026, 1993.

45. Clapham, D. E.: Control of intracellular calcium. *In* Zipes, D. P., and Jalife, J. (eds.): Cardiac Electrophysiology: From Cell to Bedside. 2nd ed. Philadelphia, W. B. Saunders Company, 1994, p. 127.

46. Hartzell, H. C., and Buchatelle-Gourdon, I.: Structure and neuromodulation of cardiac calcium channels. J. Cardiovasc. Electrophysiol. *3*:567, 1992.

47. Cohen, N. M., and Lederer, W. J.: Calcium current in single human cardiac myocytes. J. Cardiovasc. Electrophysiol. *4*:422, 1993.

48. Ming, Z., Nordin, C., and Aronson, R. S.: Role of L-type calcium channel window current in generating current-induced early afterdepolarizations. J. Cardiovasc. Electrophysiol. *5*:323, 1994.

49. Singh, B. N., Wellens, H. J. J., and Hiraoka, M. (eds.): Electropharmacological Control of Cardiac Arrhythmias. To Delay Conduction or Prolong Refractoriness? Edited by Mt. Kisco, N. Y., Futura, 1994.

50. Vassort, G., and Alvarez, J.: Cardiac T-type calcium current: Pharmacology and roles in cardiac tissues. J. Cardiovasc. Electrophysiol. *5*:376, 1994.

51. Members of the Sicilian Gambit: Antiarrhythmic Therapy: A Pathophysiologic Approach. Mt. Kisco, N. Y., Futura, 1994.

52. Pressler, M. L., and Rardon, D. P.: Molecular basis for arrhythmias: Role of two nonsarcolemmal ion channels. J. Cardiovasc. Electrophysiol. *1*:464, 1990.

53. Veenstra, R. D.: Physiological modulation of cardiac gap junction channels. J. Cardiovasc. Electrophysiol. *1*:168, 1990.

54. Brink, P. R.: Gap junction channels and cell-to-cell messengers in myocardium. J. Cardiovasc. Electrophysiol. *2*:360, 1991.

55. Shenasa, M., Borggrefe, M., and Breithardt, G. (eds.): Cardiac Mapping. Mt. Kisco, N. Y., Futura, 1993.

56. Delmar, M., Liu, S., and Morley, G. E.: Toward a moleculum model for the pH regulation of intercellular communication in the heart. *In* Zipes,

D. P., and Jalife, J. (eds.): Cardiac Electrophysiology: From Cell to Bedside. 2nd ed. Philadelphia, W. B. Saunders Company, 1994, p. 135.

57. Fozzard, H. A., Haber, E., Jennings, R. B., Katz, A. M., and Morgan, H. E.: The Heart and Cardiovascular System. New York, Raven Press, 1991.

58. Zipes, D. P., and Jalife, J. (eds.): Cardiac Electrophysiology: From Cell to Bedside. 2nd ed. Philadelphia, W. B. Saunders Company, 1994.

59. Carmeliet, E.: Potassium channels in cardiac cells. Cardiovasc. Drugs Ther. *6*:305, 1992.

60. Tamkun, M. M., Bennett, T. B., and Snyder, S. D. J.: Cloning and expression of human cardiac potassium channels. *In* Zipes, D. P., and Jalife, J. (eds.): Cardiac Electrophysiology: From Cell to Bedside. 2nd ed. Philadelphia, W. B. Saunders Company, 1994, p. 21.

61. Lazdunski, M.: Potassium channels: Structure-function relationships, diversity and pharmacology. Cardiovasc. Drugs Ther. *6*:313, 1992.

62. Kass, R. S.: Delayed potassium channels in the heart: Cellular molecular and regulatory properties. *In* Zipes, D. P., and Jalife, J. (eds.): Cardiac Electrophysiology: From Cell to Bedside. 2nd ed. Philadelphia, W. B. Saunders Company, 1994, p. 74.

63. Joho, R. H.: Toward a molecular understanding of voltage-gaited potassium channels. J. Cardiovasc. Electrophysiol. *3*:589, 1992.

64. Delmar, M.: Role of potassium currents on cell excitability in cardiac ventricular myocytes. J. Cardiovasc. Electrophysiol. *3*:474, 1992.

65. Nabauer, M., Beuckelmann, D. J., and Erdmann, E.: Characteristics of transient outward current in human ventricular myocytes from patients with terminal heart failure. Circ. Res. *73*:386, 1993.

66. Hagiwara, N., Irisawa, H., Kasanuki, H., et al.: Background inward current sensitive to sodium ion in the sinoatrial node of rabbit heart. J. Physiol. (Lond.) (*in press*).

67. Fleet, W. F., Johnson, T. A., Cascio, W. E., et al.: Marked activation delay caused by ischemia initiated after regional K^+ elevation in in situ pig hearts. Circulation *90*:3009, 1994.

68. Sicouri, S., Fish, J., and Antzelevitch, C.: Distribution of M cells in the canine ventricle. J. Cardiovasc. Electrophysiol. *5*:824, 1994.

69. Antzelevitch, C., Sicouri, S., Lukas, A., et al.: Regional differences in the electrophysiology of ventricular cells: Physiological and clinical implications. *In* Zipes, D. P., and Jalife, J. (eds.): Cardiac Electrophysiology: From Cell to Bedside. 2nd ed. Philadelphia, W. B. Saunders Company, 1994, p. 228.

70. Antzelevitch, C., and Sicouri, S.: Clinical relevance of cardiac arrhythmias generated by afterdepolarizations: The role of M cells in the generation of U waves, triggered activity and torsade de point. J. Am. Coll. Cardiol. *23*:259, 1994.

71. Harvey, R. D., and Hume, J. R.: Histamine activates the chloride current in cardiac ventricular myocytes. J. Cardiovasc. Electrophysiol. *1*:309, 1990.

72. Irisawa, H., and Hagiwara, N.: Ionic current in sinoatrial node cells. J. Cardiovasc. Electrophysiol. *2*:531, 1991.

73. Cohen, N. M., Lederer, W. J., and Nichols, C. G.: Activation of ATP-sensitive potassium channels underlies contractile failure in single human cardiac myocytes during complete metabolic inhibition. J. Cardiovasc. Electrophysiol. *3*:56, 1992.

74. Lederer, W. J., and Nichols, C. G.: Regulation and function of adenosine triphosphate-sensitive potassium channels in the cardiovascular system. *In* Zipes, D. P., and Jalife, J. (eds.): Cardiac Electrophysiology: From Cell to Bedside. 2nd ed. Philadelphia, W. B. Saunders Company, 1994, p. 103.

75. Ho, K., Nichols, C. G., Lederer, W. J., et al.: Cloning and expression of an inwardly rectifying ATP-regulated potassium channel. Nature *362*:31, 1993.

MECHANISMS OF ARRHYTHMOGENESIS

76. Wit, A. L., and Janse, M. J. (eds.): The Ventricular Arrhythmias of Ischemia and Infarction: Electrophysiological Mechanisms. Mt. Kisco, N. Y., Futura, 1993.

77. Akhtar, M., Myerburg, R. J., and Ruskin, J. N. (eds.): Sudden Cardiac Death: Prevalence, Mechanisms, and Approaches to Diagnosis and Management. Baltimore, Williams & Wilkins, 1994.

78. Josephson, M. E.: Clinical Cardiac Electrophysiology: Techniques and Interpretations. 2nd ed. Philadelphia, Lea and Febiger, 1993.

79. Podrid, P. J., and Kowey, P. R.: Cardiac Arrhythmia: Mechanisms, Diagnosis, and Management. Baltimore, Williams & Wilkins, 1995.

80. Zipes, D. P., Miles, W. M., and Klein, L. S.: Assessment of the patient with a cardiac arrhythmia. *In* Zipes, D. P., and Jalife, J. (eds.): Cardiac Electrophysiology: From Cell to Bedside. 2nd ed. Philadelphia, W. B. Saunders Company, 1994, p. 1009.

81. El-Sherif, N., and Craelius, W.: Early afterdepolarizations and arrhythmogenesis. J. Cardiovasc. Electrophysiol. *1*:145, 1990.

82. January, C. T., and Shorofsky, S.: Early afterdepolarizations: Newer insights into cellular mechanisms. J. Cardiovasc. Electrophysiol. *1*:161, 1990.

83. Sicouri, S., and Antzelevitch, C.: Drug-induced afterdepolarizations and triggered activity occur in a discreet subpopulation of ventricular muscle cells (M cells) in the canine heart: Quinidine and digitalis. J. Cardiovasc. Electrophysiol. *4*:48, 1993.

84. Boutjdir, M., Restivo, M., Wei, Y., et al.: Early afterdepolarization formation in cardiac myocytes: Analysis of phase plane patterns, action potential and membrane currents. J. Cardiovasc. Electrophysiol. *5*:609, 1994.

85. Rozanski, G. J., and Witt, R. C.: Alterations in repolarization of cardiac Purkinje fibers recovering from ischemic-like conditions: Genesis of early afterdepolarizations. J. Cardiovasc. Electrophysiol. 4:134, 1993.

86. Jackman, W. M., Szabo, B., Friday, K. J., et al.: Ventricular tachyarrhythmias related to early afterdepolarization and triggered firing: Relationship to QT interval prolongation and potential therapeutic role for calcium channel blocking agents. J. Cardiovasc. Electrophysiol. 1:170, 1990.

87. Zipes, D. P.: Monophasic action potentials in the diagnosis of triggered arrhythmia. Prog. Cardiovasc. Dis. 33:385, 1991.

88. Zipes, D. P.: The long QT syndrome: A Rosetta stone for sympathetic related arrhythmias (Editorial). Circulation 84: 1414, 1991.

89. Ben-David, J., and Zipes, D. P.: Torsades de pointes and proarrhythmia. Lancet 341:1578, 1993.

90. Schwartz, P. J., Locati, E. H., Napolitano, C., et al.: The long QT syndrome. In Zipes, D. P., and Jalife, J. (eds.): Cardiac Electrophysiology: From Cell to Bedside. 2nd ed. Philadelphia, W. B. Saunders Company, 1994, p. 788.

91. Zhou, J., Zheng, L., Liu, W., et al.: Early afterdepolarizations in the familial long QTU syndrome. J. Cardiovasc. Electrophysiol. 3:431, 1992.

92. Aaronson, R. S.: Mechanisms of arrhythmias in ventricular hypertrophy. J. Cardiovasc. Electrophysiol. 2:249, 1991.

93. Krause, P. C., Rardon, D. P., Miles, W. M., et al.: Characteristics of Ca^{2+}-activated K^+ channels isolated from the left ventricle of a patient with idiopathic long QT syndrome. Am. Heart J. 126:1134, 1993.

94. Shimizu, W., Ohe, T., Kurita, T., et al.: Epinephrine-induced ventricular premature complexes due to early afterdepolarizations and effects of verapamil and propanolol in a patient with congenital long QT syndrome. J. Cardiovasc. Electrophysiol. 5:438, 1994.

95. Ming, Z., Aronson, R., and Nordin, C.: Mechanism of current-induced early afterdepolarizations in guinea pig ventricular myocytes. Am. J. Physiol. 267:H1419, 1994.

96. Furukawa, T., Bassett, A. L., Furukawa, N., et al.: The ionic mechanism of reperfusion-induced early afterdepolarizations in feline left ventricular hypertrophy. J. Clin. Invest. 91:1521, 1993.

97. Luo, Z. H., and Rudy, Y.: A dynamic model of the cardiac ventricular action potential: II. Afterdepolarizations, triggered activity and potentiations. Circ. Res. 74:1097, 1994.

98. Luo, Z. H., and Rudy, Y.: A dynamic model of the cardiac ventricular action potential: I. Simulations of ionic currents and concentration changes. Circ. Res. 74:1071, 1994.

99. Rubart, M., Pressler, M. L., Pride, H. P., and Zipes, D. P.: Electrophysiological mechanisms in a canine model of erythromycin-associated long QT syndrome. Circulation 88:1832, 1993.

100. Zipes, D. P.: Unwitting exposure to risk (Editorial). Cardiol. Rev. 1:1, 1993.

101. Marchi, S., Szabo, B., and Lazzara, R.: Adrenergic induction of delayed afterdepolarizations in ventricular myocardial cells: Beta induction and alpha modulation. J. Cardiovasc. Electrophysiol. 2:476, 1991.

102. Wu, J., and Corr, P. B.: Palmitoyl carnitine modifies sodium currents and induces transient inward current in ventricular myocytes. Am. J. Physiol. 266:H1034, 1994.

103. Lerman, B. B.: Response of nonreentrant catecholamine-mediated ventricular tachycardia to endogenous adenosine and acetylcholine: Evidence for myocardial receptor-mediated effects. Circulation 87:382, 1993.

104. Nakagawa, H., Mukai, J., Nagata, K., et al.: Early afterdepolarizations in a patient with idiopathic monomorphic right ventricular tachycardia. PACE 16:2067, 1993.

105. Castellanos, A., Saoubi, N., Moleiro, F., et al.: Parasystole. In Zipes, D. P., and Jalife, J. (eds.): Cardiac Electrophysiology: From Cell to Bedside. 2nd ed. Philadelphia, W. B. Saunders Company, 1994, p. 942.

DISORDERS OF IMPULSE CONDUCTION

106. Rardon, D. P., Miles, W. M., Mitrani, R. D., et al.: Atrioventricular block and dissociation. In Zipes, D. P., and Jalife, J. (eds.): Cardiac Electrophysiology: From Cell to Bedside. 2nd ed. Philadelphia, W. B. Saunders Company, 1994, p. 935.

107. El-Sherif, N.: Reentrant mechanisms in ventricular arrhythmias. In Zipes, D. P., and Jalife, J. (eds.): Cardiac Electrophysiology: From Cell to Bedside. 2nd ed. Philadelphia, W. B. Saunders Company, 1994, p. 567.

108. Janse, M. J., and Opthof, T.: Mechanisms of ischemia induced arrhythmias. In Zipes, D. P., and Jalife, J. (eds.): Cardiac Electrophysiology: From Cell to Bedside. 2nd ed. Philadelphia, W. B. Saunders Company, 1994, p. 489.

109. Wit, A. L., Dillon, S. M., and Coromilas, J.: Anisotropic reentry as a cause of ventricular tachyarrhythmias in myocardial infarction. In Zipes, D. P., and Jalife, J. (eds.): Cardiac Electrophysiology: From Cell to Bedside. 2nd ed. Philadelphia, W. B. Saunders Company, 1994, p. 511.

110. Allessie, M. A.: Reentrant mechanisms underlying atrial fibrillation. In Zipes, D. P., and Jalife, J. (eds.): Cardiac Electrophysiology: From Cell to Bedside. 2nd ed. Philadelphia, W. B. Saunders Company, 1994, p. 562.

110a. Winfree, A. T.: Theory of spirals. In Zipes, D. P., and Jalife, J. (eds.): Cardiac Electrophysiology: From Cell to Bedside. 2nd ed. Philadelphia, W. B. Saunders Company, 1994, p. 279.

111. Pertsov, A. M., and Jalife, J.: Three-dimensional vortex-like reentry. In Zipes, D. P., and Jalife, J. (eds.): Cardiac Electrophysiology: From Cell to Bedside. 2nd ed. Philadelphia, W. B. Saunders Company, 1994, p. 403.

112. Davidenko, J. M.: Spiral waves in the heart: Experimental demonstration of a theory. In Zipes, D. P., and Jalife, J. (eds.): Cardiac Electrophysiology: From Cell to Bedside. 2nd ed. Philadelphia, W. B. Saunders Company, 1994, p. 478.

113. Waldo, A. L.: Atrial flutter: Mechanisms, clinical features, and management. In Zipes, D. P., and Jalife, J. (eds.): Cardiac Electrophysiology: From Cell to Bedside. 2nd ed. Philadelphia, W. B. Saunders Company, 1994, p. 666.

114. Schoels, W., Offner, B., Brachmann, J., et al.: Circus movement atrial flutter in the canine sterile pericarditis model: Relation of characteristics of the surface electrocardiogram and conduction properties of the reentrant pathway. J. Am. Coll. Cardiol. 23:799, 1994.

115. Ortiz, J., Nozaki, A., Shimizu, A., et al.: Mechanism of interruption of atrial flutter by moricizine: Electrophysiological and multiplexing studies in the canine sterile pericarditis model of atrial flutter. Circulation 89:2860, 1994.

116. Cosio, F. G., Lopez, G. M., Arribas, F., et al.: Mechanisms of entrainment of human common flutter studied with multiple endocardial recordings. Circulation 89:2117, 1994.

117. Lammers, W. J. E. P., Ravelli, F., Disertori, M., et al.: Variations in human atrial flutter cycle length induced by ventricular beats: Evidence of a reentrant circuit with a partially excitable gap. J. Cardiovasc. Electrophysiol. 2:375, 1991.

118. Ravelli, F., Disertori, M., Cozzi, F., et al.: Ventricular beats induce variations in cycle length of rapid (type II) atrial flutter in humans: Evidence of leading circle reentry. Circulation 89:2107, 1994.

119. Ortiz, J., Niwano, S., Abe, H., et al.: Mapping the conversion of atrial flutter to atrial fibrillation and atrial fibrillation to atrial flutter. Insights into mechanisms. Circ. Res. 74:882, 1994.

120. Pinto, J. M., Graziano, J. N., and Boyden, T. A.: Endocardial mapping of reentry around an anatomical barrier in the canine right atrium: Observations during the action of the class IC agent, flecainide. J. Cardiovasc. Electrophysiol. 4:672, 1993.

121. Shimizu, A., Nozaki, A., Rudy, Y., et al.: Characterization of double potentials in a functionally determined reentrant circuit: Multiplexing studies during interruption of atrial flutter in the canine pericarditis model. J. Am. Coll. Cardiol. 22:2022, 1993.

122. Scholes, W., Kuebler, W., Yang, H., et al.: A unified functional/anatomic substrate for circus movement atrial flutter: Activation and refractory patterns in the canine right atrial enlargement model. J. Am. Coll. Cardiol. 21:73, 1993.

123. Waxman, M. B., Yao, L., Cameron, D. A., et al.: Effects of posture, Valsalva maneuver and respiration on atrial flutter rate: An effect mediated through cardiac volume. J. Am. Coll. Cardiol. 17:1545, 1991.

124. Waxman, M. B., Kirsh, J. A., Yao, L., et al.: Slowing of the atrial flutter rate during 1:1 atrioventricular conduction in humans and dogs: An effect mediated through atrial pressure and volume. J. Cardiovasc. Electrophysiol. 3:544, 1992.

125. Lesh, M. D., VanHare, G. F., Epstein, L. M., et al.: Radiofrequency catheter ablation of atrial arrhythmias: Results and mechanisms. Circulation 89:1074, 1994.

126. Epstein, L. M., Chiesa, N., Wong, M. N., et al.: Radiofrequency catheter ablation in the treatment of supraventricular tachycardia in the elderly. J. Am. Coll. Cardiol. 23:1356, 1994.

127. Toboul, T., Saoudi, N., Atallah, G., et al.: Catheter ablation for atrial flutter: Current concepts and results. J. Cardiovasc. Electrophysiol. 3:641, 1992.

128. Calkins, H., Leon, A. R., Deam, A. G., et al.: Catheter ablation of atrial flutter using radiofrequency energy. Am. J. Cardiol. 73:353, 1994.

129. Isber, N., Restivo, M., Gough, W. B., et al.: Circus movement atrial flutter in the canine sterile pericarditis model: Cryothermal termination from the epicardial site of the slow zone of the reentrant circuit. Circulation 87:1649, 1993.

130. Cosio, F. G., Lopez-Gil, M., Giocolea, A., et al.: Radiofrequency ablation of the inferior vena cava-tricuspid valve isthmus in common atrial flutter. Am. J. Cardiol. 71:705, 1993.

131. Interian, A., Jr., Cox, M. M., Jimenez, R. A., et al.: A shared pathway in atrioventricular nodal reentrant tachycardia and atrial flutter: Implications for pathophysiology and therapy. Am. J. Cardiol. 71:297, 1993.

132. Feld, G. K., Fleck, R. P., Chen, P. S., et al.: Radiofrequency catheter ablation for the treatment of human type I atrial flutter: Identification of a critical zone in the reentrant circuit by endocardial mapping techniques. Circulation 86:1233, 1992.

133. Cox, J. L., Boineau, J. P., and Schuessler, R. D.: A review of surgery for atrial fibrillation. J. Cardiovasc. Electrophysiol. 2:541, 1991.

134. Cox, J. L., Boineau, J. P., Schuessler, R. B., et al.: Five-year experience with the maze procedure for atrial fibrillation. Ann. Thorac. Surg. 56:814, 1993.

135. Elvan, A., Pride, H. B., Eble, J. N., and Zipes, D. P.: Radiofrequency catheter ablation of the atria reduces the inducibility and duration of atrial fibrillation in dogs. Circulation 91:2235, 1995.

135a. Haissaguerre, M., Gencel, L., Fischer, B., et al.: Successful catheter ablation of atrial fibrillation. J. Cardiovasc. Electrophysiol. 5:1045, 1994.

135b. Swartz, J. F., Pellersels, G., Silvers, J., et al.: Catheter-based curative approach to atrial fibrillation in humans. Circulation (in press).

136. Konings, K. T., Kirchhof, C. J., Smeets, J. R., et al.: High-density mapping of electrically induced atrial fibrillation in humans. Circulation *89*:1665, 1994.

137. Kirchhof, C. J., Chorro, F., Scheffer, G. J., et al.: Regional entrainment of atrial fibrillation studied by high-resolution mapping in open-chest dogs. Circulation *88*:736, 1993.

138. Allessie, M. A., Kirchhof, C. J., Scheffer, G. J., et al.: Regional control of atrial fibrillation by rapid pacing in conscious dogs. Circulation *84*:1689, 1991.

139. Wijffels, M., Dorland, R., Kirchhof, C. J., et al.: What causes electrical remodeling of the atria due to atrial fibrillation? Circulation *90* (Suppl. 4):I-41 (Abs.), 1994.

140. Borgers, M., Ausma, J., Wijffels, M., et al.: Atrial fibrillation in the goat: A model for chronic hibernating myocardium. Circulation *90* (Suppl. 4):I-467 (Abs.), 1994.

140a. Wijffels, M. C. E. F., Kirchof, C. J. H. J., Dorland, R., et al.: Atrial fibrillation begets atrial fibrillation. Circulation *92*:1954, 1995.

141. Haissaguerre, M., Marcus, F. I., Fischer, B., et al.: Radiofrequency catheter ablation in unusual mechanisms of atrial fibrillation: Report of three cases. J. Cardiovasc. Electrophysiol. *9*:743, 1994.

142. Coumel, T.: Paroxysmal atrial fibrillation: A disorder of autonomic tone? Eur. Heart J. *15* (Suppl. A):9, 1994.

143. Naccarelli, G. V., Shih, H. T., and Jalal, S.: Sinus node reentry and atrial tachycardias. *In* Zipes, D. P., and Jalife, J. (eds.): Cardiac Electrophysiology: From Cell to Bedside. 2nd ed. Philadelphia, W. B. Saunders Company, 1994, p. 607.

144. Sperry, R. E., Ellenbogen, K. A., Wood, M. A., et al.: Radiofrequency catheter ablation of sinus node reentrant tachycardia. PACE *16*:2202, 1993.

145. Haines, D. E., and DiMarco, J. P.: Sustained intraatrial reentrant tachycardia: Clinical, electrocardiographic and electrophysiologic characteristics and long-term follow-up. J. Am. Coll. Cardiol. *15*:1345, 1990.

146. Chen, S. A., Chiang, C. E., Yang, C. J., et al.: Sustained atrial tachycardia in adult patients: Electrophysiological characteristics, pharmacological response, possible mechanisms, and effects of radiofrequency ablation. Circulation *90*:1262, 1994.

147. Engelstein, E. D., Lippman, N., Stein, K. M., et al.: Mechanism specific effects of adenosine on atrial tachycardia. Circulation *89*:2645, 1994.

148. Wellens, H. J. J.: Atrial tachycardia: How important is the mechanism? Circulation *90*:1576, 1994.

149. Chen, S. A., Chiang, C. E., Yang, C. J., et al.: Radiofrequency catheter ablation of sustained intra-atrial reentrant tachycardia in adult patients: Identification of electrophysiological characteristics and endocardial mapping techniques. Circulation *88*:578, 1993.

150. Kay, G. N., Chong, F., Epstein, A. E., et al.: Radiofrequency ablation for treatment of primary atrial tachycardias. J. Am. Coll. Cardiol. *21*:901, 1993.

151. DeBakker, J. M. T., Hauer, R. N. W., Bakker, P. F. A., et al.: Abnormal automaticity as mechanism of atrial tachycardia in the human heart—Electrophysiologic and histologic correlation: A case report. J. Cardiovasc. Electrophysiol. *5*:335, 1994.

152. Garson, A., Jr., Gillette, P. C., Moak, J. P., et al.: Supraventricular tachycardia due to multiple atrial ectopic foci: A relatively common problem. J. Cardiovasc. Electrophysiol. *1*:132, 1990.

153. Watanabe, Y., and Watanabe, M.: Impulse formulation and conduction of excitation in the atrioventricular node. J. Cardiovasc. Electrophysiol. *5*:517, 1994.

154. Kalbfleisch, S. J., Strickberger, S. A., Hummel, J. D., et al.: Double retrograde atrial response after radiofrequency ablation of typical AV nodal reentrant tachycardia. J. Cardiovasc. Electrophysiol. *4*:695, 1993.

155. Sakurada, H., Sakamoto, M., Hiyoshi, Y., et al.: Double ventricular responses to a single atrial depolarization in a patient with dual AV nodal pathways. PACE *15*:28, 1992.

156. Akhtar, M., Jazayeri, M. R., Sra, J., et al.: Atrioventricular nodal reentry: Clinical, electrophysiological and therapeutic considerations. Circulation *88*:282, 1993.

157. Josephson, M. E., and Miller, J. M.: Atrioventricular nodal reentry: Evidence supporting an intranodal location. PACE *16*:599, 1993.

158. Elizari, M. V., Sanchez, R. A., and Chiale, T. A.: Manifest fast and slow pathway conduction patterns and reentry in a patient with dual AV nodal physiology. J. Cardiovasc. Electrophysiol. *2*:98, 1991.

159. Ward, D. E., and Garratt, C. J.: The substrate for atrioventricular "nodal" reentrant tachycardia: Is there a "third pathway"? J. Cardiovasc. Electrophysiol. *4*:62, 1993.

160. Jazayeri, M. R., Sra, J. S., Deshpande, S. S., et al.: Electrophysiologic spectrum of atrioventricular nodal behavior in patients with atrioventricular nodal reentrant tachycardia undergoing selective fast or slow pathway ablation. J. Cardiovasc. Electrophysiol. *4*:99, 1993.

161. Perry, J. C., and Garson, A., Jr.: Complexities of junctional tachycardias. J. Cardiovasc. Electrophysiol. *4*:224, 1993.

162. Billette, J., and Nattel, S.: Dynamic behavior of the atrioventricular node: A functional model of interaction between recovery, facilitation, and fatigue. J. Cardiovasc. Electrophysiol. *5*:90, 1994.

163. Spach, M. S., and Josephson, M. E.: Initiating reentry: The role of nonuniform anisotropy in small circuits. J. Cardiovasc. Electrophysiol. *5*:182, 1994.

164. Jackman, W. M., Nakagawa, H., Heidbuchel, H., et al.: Three forms of atrioventricular nodal (junctional) reentrant tachycardia: Differential diagnosis, electrophysiological characteristics, and implications for anatomy of the reentrant circuit. *In* Zipes, D. P., and Jalife, J. (eds.): Cardiac Electrophysiology: From Cell to Bedside. 2nd ed. Philadelphia, W. B. Saunders Company, 1994, p. 620.

165. Silka, M. J., Kron, J., Park, J. K., et al.: Atypical forms of supraventricular tachycardia due to atrioventricular node reentry in children after radiofrequency modification of slow pathway conduction. J. Am. Coll. Cardiol. *23*:1363, 1994.

166. Yen, S., McComb, J. M., Scott, C. B., et al.: Morphology of the cardiac conduction system in patients with electrophysiologically proven dual atrioventricular nodal pathways. J. Cardiovasc. Electrophysiol. *4*:504, 1993.

167. McGuire, M. A., Yip, A. S., Robotin, M., et al.: Surgical procedure for the cure of atrioventricular junctional (AV node) reentrant tachycardia: Anatomic and electrophysiologic effects of dissection of the anterior atrionodal connections in a canine model. J. Am. Coll. Cardiol. *24*:784, 1994.

168. Haissaguerre, M., Gaita, F., Fischer, B., et al.: Elimination of atrioventricular nodal reentrant tachycardia using discreet slow potentials to guide applicaiton of radiofrequency energy. Circulation *85*:2162, 1992.

169. Langberg, J. J.: Radiofrequency catheter ablation of AV nodal reentry: The anterior approach. PACE *16*:615, 1993.

170. Lee, M. A., Morady, F., Kadish, A., et al.: Catheter modification of the atrioventricular junction with radiofrequency energy for control of atrioventricular nodal reentry tachycardia. Circulation *83*:827, 1991.

171. Gursoy, S., Schluter, M., and Kuck, K. H.: Radiofrequency current catheter ablation for control of supraventricular arrhythmias. J. Cardiovasc. Electrophysiol. *4*:194, 1993.

172. Kay, G. N., Epstein, A. E., Dailey, S. M., et al.: Role of radiofrequency ablation in the management of supraventricular arrhythmias: Experience in 760 consecutive patients. J. Cardiovasc. Electrophysiol. *4*:371, 1993.

173. Miles, W. M., Hubbard, J. E., Zipes, D. P., et al.: Elimination of AV nodal reentrant tachycardia with 2:1 VA block by posteroseptal ablation. J. Cardiovasc. Electrophysiol. *5*:510, 1994.

174. Strickberger, S. A., Daoud, E., Niebauer, M., et al.: Effects of partial and complete ablation of the slow pathway on fast pathway properties in patients with atrioventricular nodal reentrant tachycardia. J. Cardiovasc. Electrophysiol. *5*:645, 1994.

175. Baker, J. H., II, Plumb, V. J., Epstein, A. E., et al.: Predictors of recurrent atrioventricular nodal reentry after selective slow pathway ablation. Am. J. Cardiol. *73*:765, 1994.

176. Natale, A., Wathen, M., Wolfe, K., et al.: Comparative atrioventricular node properties after radiofrequency ablation and operative therapy of atrioventricular node reentry. PACE *16*:971, 1993.

177. Jazayeri, M. R., Hempe, S. L., Sra, J. S., et al.: Selective transcatheter ablation of the fast and slow pathways using radiofrequency energy in patients with atrioventricular nodal reentrant tachycardia. Circulation *85*:1318, 1992.

178. Natale, A., Kline, G., Yee, R., et al.: Shortening of fast pathway refractoriness after slow pathway ablation: Effects of autonomic blockade. Circulation *89*:1103, 1994.

179. Mitrani, R. D., Klein, L. S., Hackett, F. K., et al.: Radiofrequency ablation for atrioventricular node reentrant tachycardia: Comparison between fast (anterior) and slow (posterior) pathway ablation. J. Am. Coll. Cardiol. *21*:432, 1993.

180. Wu, D., Yeh, S. J., Wang, C. C., et al.: Nature of dual atrioventricular node pathways and the tachycardia circuit as defined by radiofrequency ablation technique. J. Am. Coll. Cardiol. *20*:884, 1992.

181. Langberg, J. J., Kim, Y. N., Goyal, R., et al.: Conversion of typical to atypical atrioventricular nodal reentrant tachycardia after radiofrequency catheter modification of the atrioventricular junction. Am. J. Cardiol. *69*:503, 1992.

182. Kalbfleisch, S. J., and Morady, F.: Catheter ablation of atrioventricular nodal reentrant tachycardia. *In* Zipes, D. P., and Jalife, J. (eds.): Cardiac Electrophysiology: From Cell to Bedside. 2nd ed. Philadelphia, W. B. Saunders Company, 1994, p. 1477.

183. Mahomed, Y., King, R. D., Zipes, D. P., et al.: Surgery for atrioventricular node reentry tachycardia: Results with surgical skeletonization of the atrioventricular node and discreet perinodal cryosurgery. J. Thorac. Cardiovasc. Surg. *104*:1035, 1992.

184. Mahomed, Y.: Surgery for atrioventricular nodal reentrant tachycardia. *In* Zipes, D. P., and Jalife, J. (eds.): Cardiac Electrophysiology: From Cell to Bedside. 2nd ed. Philadelphia, W. B. Saunders Company, 1994, p. 1577.

185. DeBakker, J. M., Coronel, R., McGuire, M. A., et al.: Slow potentials in the atrioventricular junctional area of patients operated on for atrioventricular node tachycardias and in isolated hearts. J. Am. Coll. Cardiol. *23*:709, 1994.

186. McGuire, M. A., DeBakker, J. M., Vermeulen, J. T., et al.: Origin and significance of double potentials near the atrioventricular node: Correlation of extracellular potentials, intracellular potentials and histology. Circulation *89*:2351, 1994.

187. McGuire, M. A., Bourke, J. P., Robotin, M. C., et al.: HIgh resolution mapping of Koch's triangle using 60 electrodes in humans with atrioventricular junctional (AV nodal) reentrant tachycardia. Circulation *88*:2315, 1993.

188. Philippon, F., Plumb, V. J., and Kay, G. N.: Differential effect of esmolol on the fast and slow AV nodal pathways in patients with AV nodal reentrant tachycardia. J. Cardiovasc. Electrophysiol. *5*:810, 1994.

189. Kalbfleisch, S. J., El-Atassi, R., Calkins, H., et al.: Associations between atrioventricular node reentrant tachycardia and inducible atrial flutter. J. Am. Coll. Cardiol. *22*:80, 1993.

190. Munger, T. M., Packer, D. L., Hammill, S. C., et al.: A population study of the natural history of Wolff-Parkinson-White syndrome in Olmsted County, Minnesota, 1953–1989. Circulation 87:866, 1993.

191. Kent, A. F. S.: Researches on the structure and function of mammalian heart. J. Physiol. 14:233, 1893.

192. Kent, A. F. S.: Observation on the auriculo-ventricular junction of the mammalian heart. Q. J. Exp. Physiol. 7:193, 1913.

193. Packer, D. L., and Prystowsky, E. N.: Anatomical and physiological substrate for antidromic reciprocating tachycardia. In Zipes, D. P., and Jalife, J. (eds.): Cardiac Electrophysiology: From Cell to Bedside. 2nd ed. Philadelphia, W. B. Saunders Company, 1994, p. 655.

194. Miles, W. M., Klein, L. S., Rardon, D. P., et al.: Atrioventricular reentry and variants: Mechanisms, clinical features, and management. In Zipes, D. P., and Jalife, J. (eds.): Cardiac Electrophysiology: From Cell to Bedside. 2nd ed. Philadelphia, W. B. Saunders Company, 1994, p. 638.

195. Haissaguerre, M., Clementy, J., and Warin, J. F.: Catheter ablation of atrioventricular reentrant tachycardias. In Zipes, D. P., and Jalife, J. (eds.): Cardiac Electrophysiology: From Cell to Bedside. 2nd ed. Philadelphia, W. B. Saunders Company, 1994, p. 1487.

196. Guiraudon, G. M., Guiraudon, C. M., Klein, G. J., et al.: Operation for the Wolff-Parkinson-White syndrome in the catheter ablation era. Ann. Thorac. Surg. 57:1084, 1994.

197. Ferguson, T. B., Jr., and Cox, J. L.: Surgery for atrial fibrillation. In Zipes, D. P., and Jalife, J. (eds.): Cardiac Electrophysiology: From Cell to Bedside. 2nd ed. Philadelphia, W. B. Saunders Company, 1994, p. 1563.

198. Guiraudon, G. M., Klein, G. J., Yee, R., et al.: Surgery for the Wolff-Parkinson-White syndrome. In Zipes, D. P., and Jalife, J. (eds.): Cardiac Electrophysiology: From Cell to Bedside. 2nd ed. Philadelphia, W. B. Saunders Company, 1994, p. 1553.

199. Jackman, W. M., Wang, W., Friday, K., et al.: Catheter ablation of accessory atrioventricular pathways (Wolff-Parkinson-White syndrome) by radiofrequency current. N. Engl. J. Med. 324:1605, 1991.

200. Calkins, H., Souza, J., El-Atassi, R., et al.: Diagnosis and cure of the Wolff-Parkinson-White syndrome of paroxysmal supraventricular tachycardias during a simple electrophysiologic test. N. Engl. J. Med. 324:1612, 1991.

201. Misaki, T., Watanabe, G., Iwa, T., et al.: Surgical treatment of Wolff-Parkinson-White syndrome in infants and children. Ann. Thorac. Surg. 58:103, 1994.

202. Chen, S. A., Cheng, C. C., Chiang, C. E., et al.: Radiofrequency ablation in a patient with tachycardia incorporating triple free wall accessory pathways and atrioventricular nodal reentrant tachycardia. Am. Heart J. 127:1656, 1994.

203. Chen, S. A., Chiang, C. E., Yang, C. J., et al.: Accessory pathway and atrioventricular node reentrant tachycardia in elderly patients: Clinical features, electrophysiologic characteristics and results of radiofrequency ablation. J. Am. Coll. Cardiol. 23:702, 1994.

204. Yeh, S. J., Wang, C. C., Wen, M. S., et al.: Characteristics and radiofrequency ablation therapy of intermediate septal accessory pathway. Am. J. Cardiol. 73:50, 1994.

205. Xie, B., Heald, S. C., Bashir, Y., et al.: Localization of accessory pathways from the 12-lead electrocardiogram using a new algorithm. Am. J. Cardiol. 74:161, 1994.

206. Damle, R. S., Choe, W., Kanaan, N. M., et al.: Atrial and accessory pathway activation direction in patients with orthodromic supraventricular tachycardia: Insights from vector mapping. J. Am. Coll. Cardiol. 23:684, 1994.

207. Rodriguez, L. M., Smeets, J. L., deChillou, C., et al.: The 12-lead electrocardiogram in mid-septal, anteroseptal, posteroseptal and right free wall accessory pathways. Am. J. Cardiol. 72:1274, 1993.

208. Young, C., Lauer, M. R., Liem, L. B., et al.: A characteristic electrocardiographic pattern indicative of manifest left-sided posterior septal/paraseptal accessory atrioventricular connections. Am. J. Cardiol. 72:471, 1993.

209. deChillou, C., Rodriguez, L. M., Schlapfer, J., et al.: Clinical characteristics and electrophysiologic properties of atrioventricular accessory pathways: Importance of the accessory pathway location. J. Am. Coll. Cardiol. 20:666, 1992.

209a. Fitzpatrick, A.: The ECG in Wolff-Parkinson-White syndrome. PACE 18:1469, 1995.

210. Clair, W. K., Wilkinson, W. E., McCarthy, E. A., et al.: Spontaneous occurrence of symptomatic paroxysmal atrial fibrillation and paroxysmal supraventricular tachycardia in untreated patients. Circulation 87:1114, 1993.

211. Davidenko, J. M.: Spiral waves in the heart: Experimental demonstration of a theory. In Zipes, D. P., and Jalife, J. (eds.): Cardiac Electrophysiology: From Cell to Bedside. 2nd ed. Philadelphia, W. B. Saunders Company, 1994, p. 478.

212. Janse, M. J., and Opthof, T.: Mechanisms of ischemia-induced arrhythmias. In Zipes, D. P., and Jalife, J. (eds.): Cardiac Electrophysiology: From Cell to Bedside. 2nd ed. Philadelphia, W. B. Saunders Company, 1994, p. 489.

213. Wit, A. L., Dillon, S. M., and Coromilas, J.: Anisotropic reentry as a cause of ventricular tachyarrhythmias in myocardial infarction. In Zipes, D. P., and Jalife, J. (eds.): Cardiac Electrophysiology: From Cell to Bedside. 2nd ed. Philadelphia, W. B. Saunders Company, 1994, p. 511.

214. Witkowski, F. X., Penkoske, P. A., and Kavanagh, K. M.: Activation patterns during ventricular fibrillation. In Zipes, D. P., and Jalife, J. (eds.):

Cardiac Electrophysiology: From Cell to Bedside. 2nd ed. Philadelphia, W. B. Saunders Company, 1994, p. 539.

215. El-Sherif, N.: Reentrant mechanisms in ventricular arrhythmias. In Zipes, D. P., and Jalife, J. (eds.): Cardiac Electrophysiology: From Cell to Bedside. 2nd ed. Philadelphia, W. B. Saunders Company, 1994, p. 567.

216. Watanabe, M., and Gilmour, R. F., Jr.: Dynamics of reentry in a ring-like Purkinje-muscle preparation. In Zipes, D. P., and Jalife, J. (eds.): Cardiac Electrophysiology: From Cell to Bedside. 2nd ed. Philadelphia, W. B. Saunders Company, 1994, p. 583.

217. Davidenko, J. M.: Spiral wave activity: A possible common mechanism for polymorphic and monomorphic ventricular tachycardias. J. Cardiovasc. Electrophysiol. 4:730, 1993.

218. Dillon, S. M., Coromilas, J., Waldecker, B., et al.: Effects of overdrive stimulation on functional reentrant circuits causing ventricular tachycardia in the canine heart: Mechanisms for resumption or alteration of tachycardia. J. Cardiovasc. Electrophysiol. 4:393, 1993.

219. Callans, D. J., and Josephson, M. E.: Ventricular tachycardias in the setting of coronary artery disease. In Zipes, D. P., and Jalife, J. (eds.): Cardiac Electrophysiology: From Cell to Bedside. 2nd ed. Philadelphia, W. B. Saunders Company, 1994, p. 732.

220. Marchlinski, F. E., Schwartzman, D., Gottlieb, C. D., et al.: Electrical events associated with arrhythmia initiation and stimulation techniques for arrhythmia prevention. In Zipes, D. P., and Jalife, J. (eds.): Cardiac Electrophysiology: From Cell to Bedside. 2nd ed. Philadelphia, W. B. Saunders Company, 1994, p. 863.

221. Blanck, Z., Sra, J., Dhala, A., et al.: Bundle branch reentry: Mechanisms, diagnosis, and treatment. In Zipes, D. P., and Jalife, J. (eds.): Cardiac Electrophysiology: From Cell to Bedside. 2nd ed. Philadelphia, W. B. Saunders Company, 1994, p. 878.

222. Gettes, L. S., Cascio, W. E., and Sanders, W. E.: Mechanisms of sudden cardiac death. In Zipes, D. P., and Jalife, J. (eds.): Cardiac Electrophysiology: From Cell to Bedside. 2nd ed. Philadelphia, W. B. Saunders Company, 1994, p. 527.

223. Blanck, Z., Dahla, A., Desphande, S., et al.: Bundle branch reentrant ventricular tachycardia: Cumulative experience in 48 patients. J. Cardiovasc. Electrophysiol. 4:253, 1993.

224. Pogwizd, S. M., and Corr, P.: The contribution of nonreentrant mechanisms to malignant ventricular arrhythmias. Basic Res. Cardiol. 87 (Suppl. 2):115, 1992.

224a. Pogwizd, S. M.: Nonreentrant mechanisms underlying spontaneous ventricular arrhythmias in a model of nonischemic heart failure in rabbits. Circulation 92:1034, 1995.

225. Belhassen, B., and Viskin, S.: Idiopathic ventricular tachycardia and fibrillation. J. Cardiovasc. Electrophysiol. 4:356, 1993.

226. Ben-David, J., Zipes, D. P., Ayers, G. M., et al.: Canine left ventricular hypertrophy predisposes to ventricular tachycardia induction by phase II early afterdepolarizations after administration of BAY K 8644. J. Am. Coll. Cardiol. 20:1576, 1992.

227. Wilber, D. J., Baerman, J., Olshansky, B., et al.: Adenosine-sensitive ventricular tachycardia: Clinical characteristics and response to catheter ablation. Circulation 87:126, 1993.

228. Kobayashi, Y., Kikushima, S., Tanno, K., et al.: Sustained left ventricular tachycardia terminated by dipyridamole: Cyclic AMP-mediated triggered activity as a possible mechanism. PACE 17:377, 1994.

229. Griffith, M. J., Garratt, C. J., Rowland, E., et al.: Effects of intravenous adenosine on verapamil-sensitive idiopathic ventricular tachycardia. Am. J. Cardiol. 73:759, 1994.

230. Gonzalez, R. P., Scheinman, M. N., Lesh, M. D., et al.: Clinical and electrophysiologic spectrum of fascicular tachycardias. Am. Heart J. 128:146, 1994.

231. Lauer, M. R., Liem, L. D., Young, C., et al.: Cellular and clinical electrophysiology of verapamil-sensitive ventricular tachycardias. J. Cardiovasc. Electrophysiol. 3:500, 1992.

232. Priori, S. G., Napolitano, C., and Schwartz, P. J.: Cardiac receptor activation and arrhythmogenesis. Eur. Heart J. 14 (Suppl. E):20, 1993.

233. DeLacey, W. A., Nath, S., Haines, D. E., et al.: Adenosine and verapamil-sensitive ventricular tachycardia originating from the left ventricle: Radiofrequency catheter ablation. PACE 15:2240, 1992.

233a. Vera, Z., Pride, H. P., and Zipes, D. P.: Reperfusion arrhythmias: Role of early afterdepolarizations studied by monophasic action potential recordings in the intact canine heart during autonomically denervated and stimulated states. J. Cardiovasc. Electrophysiol. 6:532, 1995.

234. Tai, Y. T., Lau, C. P., Fong, P. C., et al.: Incessant automatic ventricular tachycardia complicating acute coxsackie B myocarditis. Cardiology 80:339, 1992.

235. James, T. N.: Congenital disorders of cardiac rhythm and conduction. J. Cardiovasc. Electrophysiol. 4:702, 1993.

236. Leenhardt, A., Coumel, P., and Slama, R.: Torsades de pointes. J. Cardiovasc. Electrophysiol. 3:281, 1992.

237. Miller, J. M.: The many manifestations of ventricular tachycardia. J. Cardiovasc. Electrophysiol. 3:88, 1992.

238. Morady, F.: Further insight into mechanisms of ventricular tachycardia from the clinical electrophysiology laboratory. J. Cardiovasc. Electrophysiol. 2:207, 1991.

APPROACH TO THE DIAGNOSIS OF CARDIAC ARRHYTHMIAS

239. Zipes, D. P., Miles, W. M., and Klein, L. S.: Assessment of the patient with a cardiac arrhythmia. In Zipes, D. P., and Jalife, J. (eds.): Cardiac

Electrophysiology: From Cell to Bedside. 2nd ed. Philadelphia, W. B. Saunders Company, 1994, p. 1009.

240. Barsky, A. J., Cleary, P. D., Barnett, M. C., et al.: The accuracy of symptom reporting by patients complaining of palpitations. Am. J. Med. 97:214, 1994.

241. Sung, R. J., and Lauer, M. R.: Exercise-induced cardiac arrhythmias. In Zipes, D. P., and Jalife, J. (eds.): Cardiac Electrophysiology: From Cell to Bedside. 2nd ed. Philadelphia, W. B. Saunders Company, 1994, p. 1013.

242. Kobayashi, S., Yoshida, K., Nishimura, M., et al.: Paradoxical bradycardia during exercise and hypoxic exposure: The possible direct effect of hypoxia on sinoatrial node activity in humans. Chest 102:1893, 1992.

243. O'Hara, G. E., Brugada, P., Rodriguez, L. M., et al.: Incidence, pathophysiology and prognosis of exercise-induced sustained ventricular tachycardia associated with healed myocardial infarction. Am. J. Cardiol. 70:875, 1992.

244. Mont, L., Seixas, T., Brugada, P., et al.: Clinical and electrophysiologic characteristics of exercise-related idiopathic ventricular tachycardia. Am. J. Cardiol. 68:897, 1991.

245. Yang, J. C., Wesley, R. C., Jr., and Froelicher, Z. F.: Ventricular tachycardia during routine treadmill testing: Risk and prognosis. Arch. Intern. Med. 151:349, 1991.

246. Tuininga, Y. S., Orijns, H. J., Wiesfeld, A. C., et al.: Electrocardiographic patterns relative to initiating mechanisms of exercise-induced ventricular tachycardia. Am. Heart J. 126:359, 1993.

247. Mason, J. W.: A comparison of electrophysiologic testing with Holter monitoring to predict antiarrhythmic-drug efficacy for ventricular tachyarrhythmias: Electrophysiologic study versus electrocardiographic monitoring. N. Engl. J. Med. 329:445, 1993.

248. Mason, J. W.: A comparison of seven antiarrhythmic drugs in patients with ventricular arrhythmias: Electrophysiologic study versus electrocardiographic monitoring. N. Engl. J. Med. 329:452, 1993.

249. Wever, E. F., Hauer, R. N., Oomen, A., et al.: Unfavorable outcome in patients with primary electrical disease who survived an episode of ventricular fibrillation. Circulation 88:1021, 1993.

250. Kennedy, H. L.: Ambulatory (Holter) electrocardiography recordings. In Zipes, D. P., and Jalife, J. (eds.): Cardiac Electrophysiology: From Cell to Bedside. 2nd ed. Philadelphia, W. B. Saunders Company, 1994, p. 1024.

251. Kotar, S. L., and Gessler, J. E.: Full-disclosure monitoring: A concept that will change the way arrhythmias are detected and interpreted in the hospitalized patient. Heart Lung 22:482, 1993.

252. Manolio, T. A., Furberg, C. D., Rautaharju, T. M., et al.: Cardiac arrhythmias on 24-h ambulatory electrocardiography in older women and men: The Cardiovascular Health Study. J. Am. Coll. Cardiol. 23:916, 1994.

253. Marino, P., Nidasio, G., Golia, G., et al.: Frequency of predischarge ventricular arrhythmias in post myocardial infarction patients depends on residual left ventricular pump performance and is independent of the occurrence of acute reperfusion. The GISSI-2 investigators. J. Am. Coll. Cardiol. 23:290, 1994.

254. Lazzara, R.: Results of Holter ECG guided therapy for ventricular arrhythmias: The ESVEM trial. PACE 17:473, 1994.

255. Wyse, D. G., and Mitchell, B.: Selection of antiarrhythmic therapy: ESVEM in focus and in context. Cardiol. Rev. 2:291, 1994.

256. Bikkina, M., Larson, M. G., and Levy, D.: Asymptomatic ventricular arrhythmias and mortality risk in subjects with left ventricular hypertrophy. J. Am. Coll. Cardiol. 22:1111, 1993.

257. Statters, D. J., Malik, M., Ward, D. E., et al.: QT dispersion: Problems in methodology and clinical significance. J. Cardiovasc. Electrophysiol. 5:672, 1994.

258. Berger, P. B., Ruocco, N. A., Ryan, T. J., et al.: Incidence and significance of ventricular tachycardia and fibrillation in the absence of hypotension or heart failure in acute myocardial infarction treated with recombinant tissue-type plasminogen activator: Results from the Thrombolysis in Myocardial Infarction (TIMI) phase II trial. J. Am. Coll. Cardiol. 22:1773, 1993.

259. Maggioni, A. P., Zuanetti, G., Franzosi, M. G., et al.: Prevalence and prognostic significance of ventricular arrhythmias after acute myocardial infarction in the fibrinolytic era. Circulation 87:312, 1993.

260. Page, R. L., Wilkinson, W. E., Clair, W. K., et al.: Asymptomatic arrhythmias in patients with symptomatic paroxysmal atrial fibrillation and paroxysmal supraventricular tachycardia. Circulation 89:224, 1994.

261. Hohnloser, S. H., Klingenheben, T., vandeLoo, A., et al.: Reflex versus tonic vagal activity as a prognostic parameter in patients with sustained ventricular tachycardia or ventricular fibrillation. Circulation 89:1068, 1994.

262. Fei, L., Anderson, M. H., Katritsis, D., et al.: Decreased heart rate variability in survivors of sudden cardiac death not associated with coronary artery disease. Br. Heart J. 71:16, 1994.

263. Moise, N. S., Meyers-Wallen, V., Flohive, W. J., et al.: Inherited ventricular arrhythmias and sudden death in German Shepherd dogs. J. Am. Coll. Cardiol. 24:233, 1994.

264. Vybiral, T., Glaeser, D. H., Goldberger, A. L., et al.: Conventional heart rate variability analysis of ambulatory electrocardiographic recordings fails to predict imminent ventricular fibrillation. J. Am. Coll. Cardiol. 22:557, 1993.

265. Stein, K. M., Borer, J. S., Hochriter, C., et al.: Prognostic value and physiological correlates of heart rate variability in chronic severe mitral regurgitation. Circulation 88:127, 1993.

266. Huikuri, H. V., Valkama, J. D., Airaksinen, K. E., et al.: Frequency domain measures of heart rate variability before the onset of nonsustained and sustained ventricular tachycardia in patients with coronary artery disease. Circulation 84:1220, 1993.

267. Bigger, J. T.: Spectral analysis of R-R variability to evaluate autonomic physiology and pharmacology and to predict cardiovascular outcomes in humans. In Zipes, D. P., and Jalife, J. (eds.): Cardiac Electrophysiology: From Cell to Bedside. 2nd ed. Philadelphia, W. B. Saunders Company, 1994, p. 1151.

268. Coumel, P., Maison-Blanche, P., and Catuli, D.: Heart rate and heart rate variability in normal young adults. J. Cardiovasc. Electrophysiol. 5:899, 1994.

269. Malliani, A., Lombardi, F., Pagani, M., et al.: Power spectral analysis of cardiovascular variability in patients at risk for sudden cardiac death. J. Cardiovasc. Electrophysiol. 5:274, 1994.

270. Yarnold, P. R., Soltysik, R. C., and Martin, G. J.: Heart rate variability and susceptibility for sudden cardiac death: An example of multivariable optimal discriminate analysis. Stat. Med. 13:1015, 1994.

271. Sandrone, G., Mortara, A., Torzillo, D., et al.: Effects of beta blockers (atenolol or metoprolol) on heart rate variability after acute myocardial infarction. Am. J. Cardiol. 74:340, 1994.

272. Odemuyiwa, O., Poloniecki, J., Malik, M., et al.: Temporal influences on the prediction of post infarction mortality by heart rate variability: A comparison with the left ventricular ejection fraction. Br. Heart J. 71:521, 1994.

273. Zabel, M., Klingenheben, T., and Hohnloser, S. H.: Changes in autonomic tone following thrombolytic therapy for acute myocardial infarction: Assessment by analysis of heart rate variability. J. Cardiovasc. Electrophysiol. 5:211, 1994.

274. Niemela, M. J., Airaksinen, K. E., and Huikuri, H. V.: Effect of beta-blockade on heart rate variability in patients with coronary artery disease. J. Am. Coll. Cardiol. 23:1370, 1994.

275. Adamson, P. B., Huang, M. H., Vanoli, et al.: Unexpected interaction between beta-adrenergic blockade and heart rate variability before and after myocardial infarction: A longitudinal study in dogs at high and low risk for sudden death. Circulation 90:976, 1994.

276. Moser, M., Lehofer, M., Sedminek, A., et al.: Heart rate variability as a prognostic tool in cardiology: A contribution to the problem from a theoretical point of view. Circulation 90:1078, 1994.

277. Huikuri, H. V., Niemela, M. J., Ojala, S., et al.: Circadian rhythms of frequency domain measures of heart rate variability in healthy subjects and patients with coronary artery disease: Effects of arousal and upright posture. Circulation 90:121, 1994.

278. McClements, B. M., and Adgey, A. A.: Value of signal-averaged electrocardiography, radionuclide ventriculography, Holter monitoring and clinical variables for prediction of arrhythmic events in survivors of acute myocardial infarction in the thrombolytic era. J. Am. Coll. Cardiol. 21:1419, 1993.

279. Mortara, A., LaRovere, M. T., Signorini, M. G., et al.: Can power spectral analysis of heart rate variability identify a high risk subgroup of congestive heart failure patients with excessive sympathetic activation? A pilot study before and after heart transplantation. Br. Heart J. 71:422, 1994.

280. Goldberger, J. J., Ahmed, M. W., Parker, M. A., et al.: Dissociation of heart rate variability from parasympathetic tone. Am. J. Physiol. 266:H2152, 1994.

281. Fei, L., Keeling, P. J., Gill, J. S., et al.: Heart rate variability and its relation to ventricular arrhythmias in congestive heart failure. Br. Heart J. 71:322, 1994.

282. Griffin, M. P., Scollan, D. F., and Moorman, J. R.: The dynamic range of neonatal heart rate variability. J. Cardiovasc. Electrophysiol. 5:112, 1994.

283. Bootsma, M., Swenne, C. A., vanBolhuis, H. H., et al.: Heart rate and heart rate variability as indexes of sympathovagal balance. Am. J. Physiol. 266:H1565, 1994.

284. Tsuji, H., Venditti, F. J., Jr., Manders, E. S., et al.: Reduced heart rate variability and mortality risk in an elderly cohort: The Framingham Heart Study. Circulation 90:878, 1994.

284a. Malik, M., and Camm, A. J.: Components of heart rate variability: What they really mean and what we really measure. Am. J. Cardiol. 72:821, 1993.

285. Nearing, B. D., Huang, A. H., and Verrier, R. L.: Dynamic tracking of cardiac vulnerability by complex demodulation of the T wave. Science 252:437, 1991.

286. Verrier, R. L., and Nearing, B. B.: Electrophysiologic basis for T wave alternans as an index of vulnerability to ventricular fibrillation. J. Cardiovasc. Electrophysiol. 5:445, 1994.

287. Verrier, R. L., and Nearing, B. D.: T wave alternans as a harbinger of ischemia-induced sudden cardiac death. In Zipes, D. P., and Jalife, J. (eds.): Cardiac Electrophysiology: From Cell to Bedside. 2nd ed. Philadelphia, W. B. Saunders Company, 1994, p. 467.

288. Rosenbaum, D. S., He, B., and Cohen, R. J.: New approaches for evaluating cardiac electrical activity: Repolarization alternans and body surface Laplacian imaging. In Zipes, D. P., and Jalife, J. (eds.): Cardiac Electrophysiology: From Cell to Bedside. 2nd ed. Philadelphia, W. B. Saunders Company, 1994, p. 1187.

289. Rosenbaum, D. S., Jackson, L. E., Smith, J. M., et al.: Electrical alternans and vulnerability to ventricular arrhythmias. N. Engl. J. Med. 330:235, 1994.

290. Zareba, W., Moss, A. J., leCessie, S., et al.: T wave alternans in idiopathic long QT syndrome. J. Am. Coll. Cardiol. 23:1541, 1994.

291. Kanemoto, N., Goto, Y., Iwasaki, M., et al.: Torsades de pointes in patients with electrical alternans of T-U wave without change in QRS complex. Jpn. Circ. J. *56*:551, 1992.

292. Kothari, S. S., Patel, T., and Patel, T. K.: T-U wave alternans: A case report and review of the literature. Jpn. Heart J. *32*:843, 1991.

293. Zipes, D. P., DiMarco, J., Gillette, P., et al.: Guidelines to perform electrophysiologic studies. Circulation *92*:673, 1995.

294. Behar, S., Zissman, E., Zion, M., et al.: Prognostic significance of second-degree atrioventricular block in inferior wall acute myocardial infarction. SPRINT Study Group. Am. J. Coll. Cardiol. *72*:831, 1993.

295. Chiale, T. A., Sanchez, R. A., Franco, D. A., et al.: Overdrive prolongation of refractoriness and fatigue in the early stages of human bundle branch disease. J. Am. Coll. Cardiol. *23*:724, 1994.

296. Brugada, P., and Brugada, J.: Right bundle branch block, persistent ST segment elevation and sudden cardiac death: A distinct clinical and electrocardiographic syndrome. J. Am. Coll. Cardiol. *20*:1391, 1992.

297. Benditt, D. G., Sakaguchi, S., Goldstein, M. A., et al.: Sinus node dysfunction: Pathology, clinical features, evaluation, and treatment. *In* Zipes, D. P., and Jalife, J. (eds.): Cardiac Electrophysiology: From Cell to Bedside. 2nd ed. Philadelphia, W. B. Saunders Company, 1994, p. 1215.

298. deMarneffe, M., Gregoire, J. M., Waterschoot, P., et al.: The sinus node function: Normal and pathological. Eur. Heart J. *14*:649, 1993.

299. Lee, W. J., Wu, M. H., Young, M. L., et al.: Sinus node dysfunction in children. Acta Paediatr. Scand. *33*:159, 1992.

300. Asseman, P., Berzin, B., Desry, D., et al.: Postextrasystolic sinoatrial exit block in human sick sinus syndrome: Demonstration by direct recording of sinus node electrograms. Am. Heart J. *122*:1633, 1991.

301. Marcus, B., Gillette, P. C., and Garson, A., Jr.: Electrophysiologic evaluation of sinus node dysfunction in postoperative children and young adults utilizing combined autonomic blockade. Clin. Cardiol. *14*:33, 1991.

302. Resh, W., Feuer, J., and Wesley, R. C., Jr.: Intravenous adenosine: A noninvasive diagnostic test for sick sinus syndrome. PACE *15*:2068, 1992.

303. Wu, D. L., Yeh, S. J., Lin, F. C., et al.: Sinus automaticity and sinoatrial conduction in severe symptomatic sick sinus syndrome. J. Am. Coll. Cardiol. *19*:355, 1992.

304. Suyama, A. C., Sunagawa, K., Sugimachi, M., et al.: Differentiation between aberrant ventricular conduction and ventricular ectopy in atrial fibrillation using RR intervals scattergram. Circulation *88*:2307, 1993.

305. Steinbeck, G., Andersen, D., Bach, P., et al.: Comparison of electrophysiologically guided antiarrhythmic therapy with beta-blocker therapy in patients with symptomatic sustained ventricular tachyarrhythmias. N. Engl. J. Med. *327*:987, 1992.

306. CASCADE Investigators: Randomized antiarrhythmic drug therapy in survivors of cardiac arrest (the CASCADE Study). Am. J. Cardiol. *72*:280, 1993.

307. Brooks, R., and Ruskin, J.: Evaluation of the patient with unexplained syncope. *In* Zipes, D. P., and Jalife, J. (eds.): Cardiac Electrophysiology: From Cell to Bedside. 2nd ed. Philadelphia, W. B. Saunders Company, 1994, p. 1247.

308. Lerman-Sagie, T., Lerman, T., Mukamel, M., et al.: A prospective evaluation of pediatric patients with syncope. Clin. Pediatr. *33*:67, 1994.

309. Strieper, M. J., Auld, D. O., Hulse, J. E., et al.: Evaluation of recurrent pediatric syncope: Role of tilt table testing. Pediatrics *93*:660, 1994.

310. Kapoor, W. N.: Evaluation and management of the patient with syncope. J. A. M. A. *268*:2553, 1992.

311. Wilmshurst, T. T., Willicombe, P. R., and Webb-Peploe, M. M.: Effect of aortic valve replacement on syncope in patients with aortic stenosis. Br. Heart J. *70*:542, 1993.

312. Steinberg, J. S., Prystowsky, E., Freedman, R. A., et al.: Use of the signal-averaged electrocardiogram for predicting inducible ventricular tachycardia in patients with unexplained syncope: Relation to clinical variables in a multi-variate analysis. J. Am. Coll. Cardiol. *23*:99, 1994.

313. Sneddon, J. F., Counihan, P. J., Bashir, Y., et al.: Assessment of autonomic function in patients with neurally mediated syncope: Augmented cardiopulmonary baroreceptor responses to graded orthostatic stress. J. Am. Coll. Cardiol. *21*:1193, 1993.

314. Gilligan, D. M., Nihoyannopoulos, P., Chan, W. L., et al.: Investigation of a hemodynamic basis for syncope in hypertrophic cardiomyopathy: Use of head-up tilt test. Circulation *85*:2140, 1992.

315. Balaji, S., Oslizlok, P. C., Allen, M. C., et al.: Neurocardiogenic syncope in children with a normal heart. J. Am. Coll. Cardiol. *23*:779, 1994.

315a. Sutton, R., and Petersen, M. E. V.: The clinical spectrum of neurocardiogenic syncope. J. Cardiovasc. Electrophysiol. *6*:569, 1995.

316. Dilsizian, V., Bonow, R. O., Epstein, S. E., et al.: Myocardial ischemia detected by thallium scintigraphy is frequently related to cardiac arrest and syncope in young patients with hypertrophic cardiomyopathy. J. Am. Coll. Cardiol. *22*:796, 1993.

317. Aronow, W. S., Mercando, A. D., and Epstein, S.: Prevalence of arrhythmias detected by 24-hour ambulatory electrocardiography and value of antiarrhythmic therapy in elderly patients with unexplained syncope. Am. J. Cardiol. *70*:408, 1992.

318. Calkins, H., Byrne, M., and El-atassi, R.: The economic burden of unrecognized vasodepressor syncope. Am. J. Med. *95*:473, 1993.

319. Middlekauff, H. R., Stevenson, W. G., Stevenson, L. W., et al.: Syncope in advanced heart failure: High risk of sudden death regardless of origin of syncope. J. Am. Coll. Cardiol. *21*:110, 1993.

320. Brugada, P., Gursoy, S., Brugada, J., et al.: Investigation of palpitations. Lancet *341*:1254, 1993.

321. Biffi, A., Ammirati, F., Caselli, G., et al.: Usefulness of transesophageal pacing during exercise for evaluating palpitations in professional athletes. Am. J. Cardiol. *72*:922, 1993.

322. Hindricks, G., on behalf of the Multicenter European Radiofrequency Survey (MERFS) Investigators of the Working Group on Arrhythmias of the European Society of Cardiology: The Multicenter European Radiofrequency Survey (MERFS): Complications of radiofrequency catheter ablation of arrhythmias. Eur. Heart J. *14*:1644, 1993.

323. Scheinman, M. M.: Patterns of catheter ablation practice in the United States: Results of the 1992 NASPE Survey. PACE *17*:873, 1994.

OTHER DIAGNOSTIC ELECTROCARDIOGRAPHIC TECHNIQUES

324. Katz, A., Guetta, V., and Ovsyshcher, I. A.: Transesophageal electrocardiography using a temporary pacing balloon-tipped electrode in acute cardiac care. Ann. Emerg. Med. *20*:961, 1991.

325. Klein, L. S., Miles, W. M., Rardon, D. P., et al.: Transesophageal recording. *In* Zipes, D. P., and Jalife, J. (eds.): Cardiac Electrophysiology: From Cell to Bedside. 2nd ed. Philadelphia, W. B. Saunders Company, 1994, p. 1112.

327. Flowers, N. C., and Horan, L. G.: Body surface potential mapping. *In* Zipes, D. P., and Jalife, J. (eds.): Cardiac Electrophysiology: From Cell to Bedside. 2nd ed. Philadelphia, W. B. Saunders Company, 1994, p. 1049.

328. Franzone, P. C., Guerri, L., and Taccardi, B.: Spread of excitation in a myocardial volume: simulation studies in a model of anisotropic ventricular muscle activated by point stimulation. J. Cardiovasc. Electrophysiol. *4*:144, 1993.

329. Franzone, P. C., Guerri, L., and Taccardi, B.: Potential distributions generated by point stimulation in a myocardial volume: Simulation studies in a model of anisotropic ventricular muscle. J. Cardiovasc. Electrophysiol. *4*:438, 1993.

330. Green, L. S., Lux, R. L., Ershler, P. R., et al.: Resolution of pace mapping stimulus site separation using body surface potentials. Circulation *90*:462, 1994.

331. SippensGroenewegen, A., Spekhorst, H., vanHemel, N. M., et al.: Localization of the site of origin of post infarction ventricular tachycardia by endocardial pace mapping: Body surface mapping compared with a 12-lead electrocardiogram. Circulation *88*:2290, 1993.

332. DeAmbroggi, L., and Santambrogio, C.: Clinical use of body surface potential mapping in cardiac arrhythmias. Physiol. Res. *42*:137, 1993.

333. He, B., Kirby, D. A., Mullen, T. J., et al.: Body surface Laplacian mapping of cardiac excitation in intact pigs. PACE *16*:1017, 1993.

334. Dubuc, M., Nadeau, R., Tremblay, G., et al.: Pace mapping using body surface potential maps to guide catheter ablation of accessory pathways in patients with Wolff-Parkinson-White syndrome. Circulation *87*:135, 1993.

335. SippensGroenewegen, A., Spekhorst, H., vanHemel, N. M., et al.: Body surface mapping of ectopic left ventricular activation: QRS spectrum in patients with prior myocardial infarction. Circ. Res. *71*:1361, 1992.

336. Mitchell, L. B., Hubley-Koszey, C. L., Smith, E. R., et al.: Electrocardiographic body surface mapping in patients with ventricular tachycardia: Assessment of utility in the identification of effective pharmacologic therapy. Circulation *86*:383, 1992.

337. Liebeman, J., Zeno, J. A., Olshansky, B., et al.: Electrocardiographic body surface potential mapping in the Wolff-Parkinson-White syndrome: Noninvasive determination of the ventricular insertion sites of accessory atrioventricular connections. Circulation *83*:886, 1991.

338. Franz, M. R.: Bridging the gap between basic and clinical electrophysiology: What can be learned from monophasic action potential recordings? J. Cardiovasc. Electrophysiol. *5*:699, 1994.

339. Simson, M. B.: Signal-averaged electrocardiography. *In* Zipes, D. P., and Jalife, J. (eds.): Cardiac Electrophysiology: From Cell to Bedside. 2nd ed. Philadelphia, W. B. Saunders Company, 1994, p. 1038.

340. Shenasa, M., Fetsch, T., Martinez-Rubio, A., et al.: Signal averaging in patients with coronary artery disease: How helpful is it? J. Cardiovasc. Electrophysiol. *4*:609, 1993.

341. Berbari, E. J., Lander, P., Geselowitz, D. B., et al.: Identifying the end of ventricular activation: Body surface late potentials versus electrogram measurements in a canine infarction model. J. Cardiovasc. Electrophysiol. *5*:28, 1994.

342. Jordaens, L., Schoenfeld, P., Demeester, C., et al.: Late potentials and ejection fraction at hospital discharge: Prognostic value in thrombolyzed and non-thrombolyzed patients. A preliminary report. Acta Cardiol. *46*:531, 1991.

343. Kremers, M. S., Hsia, H., Wells, P., et al.: Diastolic potentials recorded by surface electrocardiographic signal averaging during sustained ventricular tachycardia: Possible origin from the reentrant circuit. PACE *14*:1000, 1991.

344. Benditt, D. G., Lurie, K. G., Adler, S. W., et al.: Rationale and methodology of head-up tilt table testing for evaluation of neurally mediated (cardioneurogenic) syncope. *In* Zipes, D. P., and Jalife, J. (eds.): Cardiac Electrophysiology: From Cell to Bedside. 2nd ed. Philadelphia, W. B. Saunders Company, 1994, p. 1115.

345. Kapoor, W. N., Smith, M. A., and Miller, N. L.: Upright tilt testing in evaluating syncope: A comprehensive literature review. Am. J. Med. *97*:78, 1994.

346. Tonnessen, G. E., Haft, J. I., Fulton, J., et al.: The value of tilt table testing with isoproterenol in determining therapy in adults with syn-

cope and presyncope of unexplained origin. Arch. Intern. Med. *154:*1613, 1994.

347. Sra, J. S., Murphy, V., Natale, A., et al.: Circulatory and catecholamine changes during head-up tilt testing in neurocardiogenic (vasovagal) syncope. Am. J. Cardiol. *73:*33, 1994.

348. Sheldon, R.: Evaluation of single-stage isoproterenol-tilt table test in patients with syncope. J. Am. Coll. Cardiol. *22:*114, 1993.

349. Lurie, K. G., Dutton, J., Mangat, R., et al.: Evaluation of edrophonium as a provocative agent for vasovagal syncope during head-up tilt-table testing. Am. J. Cardiol. *72:*1286, 1993.

350. Ovadia, M., and Thoele, D.: Tilt testing with esmolol withdrawal for the evaluation of syncope in the young. Circulation *89:*228, 1994.

351. Leor, J., Rotstein, Z., Vered, Z., et al.: Absence of tachycardia during tilt test predicts failure of beta-blocker therapy in patients with neurocardiogenic syncope. Am. Heart J. *127:*1539, 1994.

352. O'Marcaigh, A. S., MacLellan-Tobert, S. G., and Porter, C. J.: Tilt-table testing and oral metoprolol therapy in young patients with unexplained syncope. Pediatrics *93:*278, 1994.

353. Blanc, J. J., Mansourati, J., Maheu, B., et al.: Reproducibility of a posi-tive passive upright tilt test at 7-day interval in patients with syncope. Am. J. Cardiol. *72:*469, 1993.

354. Brooks, R., Ruskin, J. N., Powell, A. C., et al.: Prospective evaluation of day-to-day reproducibility of upright tilt-table testing in unexplained syncope. Am. J. Cardiol. *71:*1289, 1993.

355. deBuitlier, M., Grogan, E. W., Jr., Picone, M. F., et al.: Immediate repro-ducibility of the tilt-table test in adults with unexplained syncope. Am. J. Cardiol. *71:*304, 1993.

356. Chen, X. C., Chen, M. Y., Remole, S., et al.: Reproducibility of head-up tilt-table testing for eliciting susceptibility to neurally mediated syncope in patients without structural heart disease. Am. J. Cardiol. *69:*755, 1992.

357. Sutton, R., and Petersen, M.E.V.: The clinical spectrum of neurocardiogenic syncope. J. Cardiovasc. Electrophysiol. *6:*569, 1995.

358. Morillo, C. A., Leitch, J. W., Yee, R., et al.: A placebo-controlled trial of intravenous and oral disopyramide for prevention of neurally mediated syncope induced by head-up tilt. J. Am. Coll. Cardiol. *22:*1843, 1993.

Chapter 21
Management of Cardiac Arrhythmias:
Pharmacological, Electrical, and Surgical Techniques

DOUGLAS P. ZIPES

━━━━━━━━ PHARMACOLOGICAL THERAPY ━━━━━━━━

PRINCIPLES OF CLINICAL PHARMACOKINETICS

Pharmacological treatment of a patient with a cardiac arrhythmia has as its primary objective to reach an effective and well-tolerated plasma drug concentration as rapidly as possible and to maintain this concentration for as long as required without producing adverse effects. In many but not all situations and not with all drugs, plasma concentration after equilibration correlates with the pharmacodynamic as well as adverse effects of the drug. Therapeutic serum concentrations for the most important available antiarrhythmic agents are listed in Table 21–1 and are based on concentrations of drugs that exert therapeutic effects on often benign arrhythmias such as premature ventricular complexes (PVCs), without adverse effects in a majority of patients. However, the therapeutic concentration for any individual patient is the amount of drug required *for that patient* to suppress or terminate the specific cardiac arrhythmia requiring treatment without producing adverse effects.

For a specific patient, one must consider the response both of the patient and of the arrhythmia to the drug; the actual plasma concentration of the drug is often of secondary importance. Low drug concentrations can exert a therapeutic or toxic effect in some patients, while drug concentrations higher than the normal range may be needed and tolerated in another patient. In some patients, measured plasma concentrations can be useful to establish concentrations needed for prophylaxis, to judge the sensitivity or resistance of the arrhythmia to the drug, and to evaluate symptoms that suggest drug toxicity. Plasma concentrations also can be used to determine the effects of changing physiological states on drug concentrations, establish drug compliance or abuse, search for drug interactions that affect the pharmacokinetics, and establish the importance of physiologically active metabolites of the parent compound.[1,2] Active metabolites may be suspected when the clinical effect of the drug outlasts the therapeutic serum concentration of

the parent compound or when results immediately following intravenous drug administration differ from those after oral administration of the drug.

Normally, because antiarrhythmic agents have a narrow toxic-therapeutic relationship, important complications of therapy can result from amounts of drug that only slightly exceed the amount necessary to produce beneficial effects; lesser concentrations are often subtherapeutic. It is obvious that careful dosing with these agents is essential to maintain adequate but nontoxic amounts of drug in the body, a task facilitated by understanding drug pharmacokinetics.[3–5] The latter consists of a quantitative assessment of drug dose-concentration factors, including drug absorption, distribution, metabolism, and excretion. Alterations in the rate of any of these processes can account for significant intra- and interpatient variations in plasma concentrations. In addition, changes in the functional status of any of the organs involved, e.g., the heart, liver, or kidneys, can significantly alter dose requirements in a given patient. The latter concerns a study of pharmacodynamics, or drug concentration-response issues.[2,6]

ABSORPTION

Drug absorption from the intestinal tract occurs for most drugs with a half-life of absorption in the range of 20 to 30 minutes. Completeness of absorption can vary between 50 and over 90 per cent, depending on the drug, with most absorption occurring in the small intestine. Different preparations of the same drug can undergo different rates of absorption in the same patient because the tablet preparations have different dissolution rates. Thus different brands of drug may not result in the same serum concentration. By altering the properties of the tablet, a slow-release form of a drug ordinarily rapidly absorbed and metabolized, such as procainamide, can be developed. Large amounts of some orally administered drugs, such as propranolol or verapamil, are transformed to inactive metabolites in the liver before they reach the systemic circulation—the so-called first-pass hepatic effect.[5] For such an agent, much more drug must be administered orally than intravenously to achieve the same physiological effect.

ABSORPTION ABNORMALITIES. Disease states and other factors can alter the rate and completeness of drug absorption. For example, heart failure can cause mucosal edema of the gut and impair the

593

TABLE 21-1 DOSAGE AND THERAPEUTIC SERUM CONCENTRATIONS FOR ANTIARRHYTHMIC AGENTS

DRUG	USUAL DOSE RANGES			
	Intravenous (mg)		Oral (mg)	
	Loading	*Maintenance*	*Loading*	*Maintenance*
Quinidine	6 to 10 mg/kg at 0.3 to 0.5 mg/kg/min	600 to 1000	300 to600 q6h	
Procainamide	6 to 13 mg/kg at 0.2 to 0.5 mg/kg/min	2 to 6 mg/min	500 to 1000	350 to 1000 q3–6h
Disopyramide	1 to 2 mg/kg over 15–45 min*	1 mg/kg/h		100 to 400 q6–8h
Lidocaine	1 to 3 mg/kg at 20 to 50 mg/min	1 to 4 mg/min	N/A	N/A
Mexiletine	500 mg*	0.5 to 1.0 gm/24 h	400 to 600	150 to 300 q6–8h
Tocainide	750 mg*		400 to 600	400 to 600 q8–12h
Phenytoin	100 mg q5min for ≤ 1000 mg		1000	100 to 400 q12–24h
Flecainide	2 mg/kg*	100 to 200 q12h		
Propafenone	1 to 2 mg/kg		600 to 900	150 to 300 q8–12h
Moricizine			300	100 to 400 q8h
Propranolol	0.25 to 0.5 mg, q5min for ≤ 0.15 to 0.20 mg/kg			10 to 200 q6–8h
Amiodarone	15mg/kg for 10 min, 1 mg/kg for 360 min, 0.5 mg/kg there-after		800 to 1600 q.d. for 1 to 3 weeks	200 to 400 q.d.
Bretylium	5 to 10 mg/kg at 1 to 2 mg/kg/ min	½ to 2 mg/min	N/A	4 mg/kg/day†
Verapamil	10 mg over 1 to 2 min	0.005 mg/kg/min		80 to 120 q6–8h
Adenosine	6–12 mg (rapidly)		N/A	N/A
Sotalol			N/A	80 mg q12h to start incrementing grad-ually to 320 mg/ day as needed

* Investigational; IV.
† Investigational only.

absorption of orally administered drugs, as can decreased intestinal blood flow. Renal or hepatic hypoperfusion can reduce drug elimination and metabolism. Reduced volume of distribution and impaired

TABLE 21-2 KNOWN INFLUENCE OF DISEASE STATES AND OTHER CONDITIONS ON ANTIARRHYTHMIC DRUG PHARMACOKINETICS

DISEASE OR CONDITION	EFFECTS
Congestive heart failure	Reduced clearance of: lidocaine procainamide flecainide Reduced volume of distribution of: lidocaine
Liver disease	Reduced clearance of: lidocaine disopyramide phenytoin propranolol
Renal disease	Reduced clearance of: disopyramide procainamide bretylium tocainide flecainide Altered protein binding (with usually unchanged drug requirements) of: phenytoin
Post-myocardial infarction	Reduced clearance of: procainamide Altered protein binding of: lidocaine quinidine
Prolonged administration	Reduced clearance of: lidocaine
Obesity	Increased volume of distribution of: lidocaine

From Roden, D.: New concepts in antiarrhythmic drug pharmacokinetics. Progr. Cardiol. *15*:19, 1987.

clearance can increase elimination half-life, requiring a reduction in loading and maintenance doses (Table 21-2). Malabsorption syndromes, concomitant use of other drugs, or changes in gut motility or flora caused by diarrheal states, antibiotics, or the use of cathartics can alter absorption. Since most antiarrhythmic agents are basic compounds, they are ionized and poorly absorbed at normal gastric pH, and some drugs can decompose at gastric pH. Conditions that delay gastric emptying increase the absorption lag phase between ingestion of these drugs and their arrival in the small intestine, where most absorption takes place, and therefore can decrease absorption. In patients with severe hypotension, shock, or cardiac arrest, impaired tissue perfusion prevents reliable absorption of intramuscularly administered agents; these patients should receive all medications by the intravenous (IV) route.

BIOAVAILABILITY

The rate of drug absorption, determined by the time required to achieve maximum plasma concentration, and the fraction of drug absorbed influence the drug's *bioavailability*, which is a measure of the amount of drug that reaches the systemic circulation intact. Bioavailability of a drug is influenced by factors such as pill dissolution, metabolism by gut mucosa, hepatic metabolism and binding, and absorption. It is a most important property of the drug. Absorption is thus only one component affecting bioavailability.

The fraction of an orally administered drug reaching the systemic circulation intact, or *systemic availability*, can be calculated (assuming equal clearances for IV and oral forms of drug) by comparing the areas under the plasma concentration curve achieved with oral and intravenous administrations using the following relationship. Systemic availability equals the area under the plasma concentration curve following oral administration divided by the area under the plasma concentration curve following IV administration times 100 (assuming equal IV and oral doses).

DRUG DISTRIBUTION

Most antiarrhythmic drugs in the therapeutic range are eliminated according to *first-order kinetics*, which means that the amount of drug eliminated per unit of time is directly proportional to the amount (or concentration) of drug in the body. More drug in the body results in more drug excreted by the kidneys or metabolized by the liver so that the *fraction* of drug eliminated per unit of time remains constant regardless of the amount of drug in the body. For example, one-half the drug may be eliminated in 6 hours whether the total amount of drug in the body is 4 gm or 10 gm, resulting in

TIME TO PEAK PLASMA CONCENTRATION (ORAL) (h)	EFFECTIVE SERUM OR PLASMA CONCENTRATION (μg/ml)	ELIMINATION HALF-LIFE (h)	BIOAVAILABILITY (%)	MAJOR ROUTE OF ELIMINATION
1.5 to 3.0	3 to 6	5 to 9	60 to 80	Liver
1	4 to 10	3 to 5	70 to 85	Kidneys
1 to 2	2 to 5	8 to 9	80 to 90	Kidneys
N/A	1 to 5	1 to 2	N/A	Liver
2 to 4	0.75 to 2	10 to 17	90	Liver
0.5 to 2	4 to 10	11	90	Liver
8 to 12	10 to 20	18 to 36	50 to 70	Liver
3 to 4	0.2 to 1.0	20	95	Liver
1 to 3	0.2 to 3.0	5 to 8	25 to 75	Liver
	0.1			
4	1 to 2.5	50 days	35 to 65	Liver
	0.5 to 1.5	8 to 14	25	Kidneys
2 to 4	0.04 to 0.90	3 to 6	20 to 50	Liver
1 to 2	0.10 to 0.15	3 to 8	10 to 35	Liver
2.5 to 4	2.5	12	90 to 100	Kidneys

Note: Results presented may vary according to doses, disease state, and IV or oral administration.

elimination of 2 gm in the first example and 5 gm in the second. As a consequence, the elimination half-life, or time required to eliminate half the body load (or to halve the plasma concentration) of such a drug, is constant and independent of the total-body load. The following discussion will assume first-order kinetics unless otherwise stated. (*Zero-order kinetics* indicates that the reaction occurs at a constant, usually maximal, rate and cannot increase further despite increased drug concentrations. Such nonlinear or saturable kinetics can occur at high concentrations of a drug that at usual concentrations exhibits first-order kinetics.[2])

The One-Compartment Model

Generally, two models, a *one-compartment open model* and a *two-compartment open model*, are used with relative accuracy to describe and predict serum concentrations at a given time for a variety of dose regimens. Even though these models are oversimplified representations of drug disposition, they provide guidelines for choosing loading doses and maintenance dose schedules for a given patient. In the one-compartment open model, drugs are considered to enter and to be eliminated from a single homogeneous unit that represents the entire body. Drugs entering the compartment are considered to be distributed immediately throughout the compartment, making the concentration of the drug equal to the amount of drug in the compartment divided by the volume of the compartment. The latter equals the amount of the drug in the compartment divided by the drug concentration.

In reality, a one-compartment open model is not entirely appropriate because a certain amount of time is needed to distribute the drug throughout the volume of the compartment. However, the one-compartment model predicts plasma concentration as a function of time and dose if distribution is significantly faster than the rate of administration or of excretion, which is the case for many antiarrhythmic drugs.

The Two-Compartment Model

If the rate of drug administration is rapid in relation to drug distribution (e.g., intravenous administration), a two-compartment open model more accurately predicts drug concentrations (Fig. 21-1). In this model the drug enters the system by the central compartment and can leave the system only by distribution into a peripheral compartment or elimination from the central compartment. The central compartment, in dynamic equilibrium with the more slowly equilibrating peripheral compartment, is assumed to consist of the blood volume and extracellular fluid of highly perfused tissues such as heart, lungs, kidneys, and liver, while the peripheral compartment, acting as a reservoir, consists of less well perfused tissue such as muscle, skin, and adipose tissue. The first-order rate constants $K_{1\rightarrow2}$ and $K_{2\rightarrow1}$ determine the rate of transfer of drug between the central and peripheral compartments or vice versa, with Ke representing the overall elimination rate constant. Ke relates the sum of all methods of irreversible drug elimination from the central compartment to the concentration of drug in that compartment (Fig. 21-1).

For antiarrhythmic drugs, the peripheral compartment is generally larger than the central compartment. The concepts of distribution

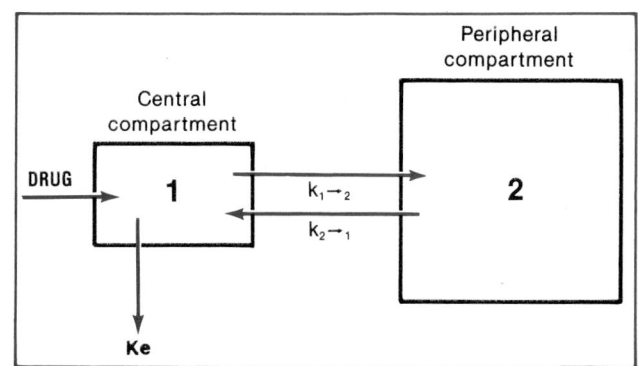

FIGURE 21-1. Two-compartment open model. A smaller central compartment into which drug is administered and from which it is eliminated (Ke) connects in dynamic equilibrium with a larger peripheral compartment.

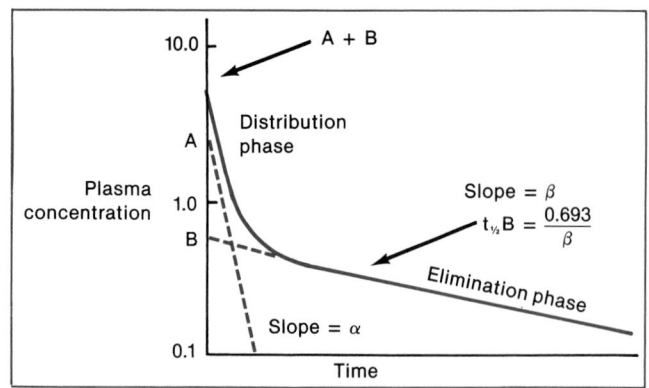

FIGURE 21–2. Schematic diagram of the semilogarithmic plot of drug plasma concentration as a function of time following rapid intravenous injection, according to the principles outlined for a two-compartment open model. (From Gibaldi, M., and Perrier, D.: Drugs and the pharmaceutical sciences. *In* Pharmacokinetics, Vol. 1. New York, Marcel Dekker, 1975.)

terized by rapidly falling plasma drug concentrations due to distribution between the central compartment and the peripheral compartment, and a second phase (beta, or elimination, phase) of slower decline in plasma drug concentration, representing primarily elimination of drugs from the central compartment (Fig. 21–2). *Alpha* is often referred to as the *rate constant for distribution* and *beta* as the *rate constant for elimination.* During the latter beta phase, when the drug is in distribution equilibrium, serum concentrations correlate with the pharmacological effects of the drug. The distribution of quinidine is shown in Figure 21–3.

VOLUME OF DISTRIBUTION. The extent of extravascular distribution of a drug is obtained by measuring the apparent *volume of distribution,* which is the hypothetical volume into which a dose of drug would have to be diluted to give the observed plasma concentration. It is determined by the dose administered divided by the plasma concentration at time 0. The latter equals the sum of A and B on the logarithmic plasma concentration axis obtained by extrapolating the alpha and beta phases back to 0 time (Fig. 21–2). It is also calculated by dividing the systemic clearance of the drug by beta, the rate constant of elimination. A large volume of distribution indicates a wide distribution and extensive tissue uptake of the drug and often exceeds by several times the actual amount of total-body water. The large volume of distribution for most antiarrhythmic agents indicates that they are present in higher concentrations in some tissues than in the plasma. The volume of distribution is dependent on the relative serum and tissue binding characteristics of the drug and can be constricted in some patients, such as those with renal failure, during which a change in serum protein or tissue binding can occur. Quinidine decreases the volume of distribution of digoxin, probably as a result of a decrease in tissue binding of digoxin.

DRUG METABOLISM AND EXCRETION. Approximately 97 per cent of the dose of any drug is removed from the body in a time equal to five half-lives. *Serum elimination half-life* is defined as the time interval for 50 per cent of the drug present in the body at the beginning of the interval to be eliminated. After one half-life, 50 per cent of the drug remains in the body (assuming no further drug is administered), after two half-lives 25 per cent remains, after three half-lives 12.5 per cent remains, and so forth. Half-life is determined from the relation-

volumes and drug movement are more complex in the two-compartment open model than in the one-compartment open model. The two-compartment model may behave similarly to the one-compartment model when drugs are infused slowly or given orally and K_1 approximates K_2, but pronounced differences exist when injections are given rapidly.

DISTRIBUTION AND ELIMINATION PHASES. Following administration of drugs for which the kinetics are described by a two-compartment model, the curve of plasma drug concentration demonstrates two distinct phases: an early phase (alpha, or distribution, phase), charac-

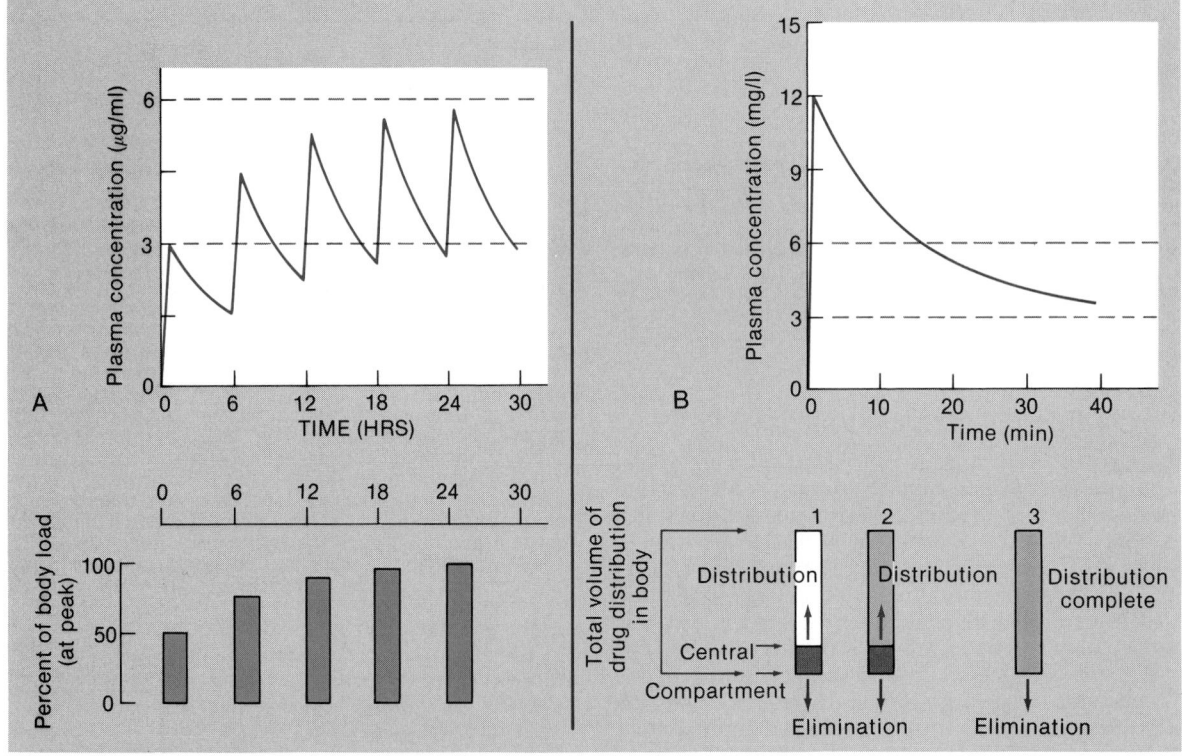

FIGURE 21–3. *A,* Changes in plasma concentration over time after beginning treatment with quinidine. *Top,* Quinidine plasma concentration over time, with the dashed line indicating the therapeutic range. *Bottom,* The hatched bars represent the body load immediately after each dose of quinidine, expressed as a percentage of the load after a dose when a steady state has been achieved. Quinidine is administered every 6 hours (the half-life in this case). Four half-lives, or 24 hours, are required to achieve a body load of quinidine that exceeds 90 per cent of the load at steady state. *B, Top,* Plasma concentrations produced by administering a full intravenous loading dose of quinidine as a bolus, with the therapeutic range shown by a dashed line. *Bottom,* The numbered vertical boxes indicate the volume of distribution of quinidine. Just after the drug is given, it is dissolved only in the small central compartment, as in box 1, and very high peak concentrations are achieved (in the toxic range). The drug then distributes throughout the rest of the body. Distribution has a half-life of about 8 minutes and is complete by 30 minutes (box 3). Quinidine concentration is now in the therapeutic range, and further decreases in plasma concentration are due solely to drug elimination. (From Nattel, S., and Zipes, D. P.: Clinical pharmacology of old and new antiarrhythmic drugs. Cardiovasc. Clin. *11*:221, 1980.)

ship t½ = 0.693/beta for a two-compartment model (Fig. 21–2). Since changes in drug distribution influence elimination half-life, the equation can be rewritten as t½ = 0.693 × volume of distribution/total-body clearance.

DRUG CLEARANCE. This is analogous to renal clearance and is the volume of blood totally cleared of drug per unit of time. It is the sum of the clearances for each process by which the drug is eliminated and can be calculated from the relationship: clearance = dose of the drug/area under the plasma concentration time curve (AUC). Expressed differently, clearance equals volume of distribution × beta, or volume of distribution × 0.693/half-life. A larger volume of distribution increases the elimination half-life at a given clearance. The larger volume of distribution of antiarrhythmic drugs accounts for the relatively long half-life despite their high clearance rates. Quinidine prolongs digitoxin's half-life by decreasing total-body clearance. Clearance of drugs with high extraction ratios strongly depends on blood flow to the organ from which they are eliminated, such as propranolol, verapamil, or lidocaine in the liver. For antiarrhythmic drugs that have a high renal extraction ratio, such as procainamide and quinidine, reduction of renal flow decreases their clearance.

ELIMINATION HALF-LIFE. Function of the organ system that eliminates a given drug from the body determines the elimination half-life. Primary routes of elimination are hepatic metabolism and renal clearance. The kidneys can remove unchanged drug or metabolites. For drugs rapidly metabolized in the liver, hepatic blood flow limits the rate of drug elimination. Disorders that reduce liver blood flow (e.g., low cardiac output, hepatic disease with portacaval shunting) markedly slow the elimination of such drugs. Drugs with a short half-life are convenient to use by intravenous infusion but not by chronic oral dosing, since the short half-life requires frequent oral doses to maintain a fairly constant plasma concentration. Generally, maintenance dosing involves giving a certain amount of the drug at a time interval that equals the elimination half-life. However, with drugs that have very long half-lives, such as 12 hours, this can result in excessive peak values shortly after administration and consequent side effects. Maintaining constant plasma concentrations is necessary because of the narrow toxic-therapeutic ratios exhibited by antiarrhythmic agents.

Some drugs have active metabolites with half-lives considerably longer than the parent compound, allowing dosing intervals to be more widely spaced than those predicted by the half-life of the parent drug. Procainamide (see p. 603) has an active metabolite, N-acetylprocainamide (NAPA), that is eliminated unchanged by the kidneys and can accumulate in high concentrations in patients with renal disease. The rate and extent of metabolism of the same drug can vary greatly from patient to patient owing to a variety of factors, including environment, genetics, age, disease states, and influence of other drugs given concomitantly. A genetically controlled acetyltransferase enzyme system influences the metabolism of some drugs making about half the American population "rapid" and half "slow acetylators." Rapid acetylators metabolize a greater proportion of a drug dose than do slow acetylators, who may require less drug to achieve any desired serum level or pharmacological effect. Also, rapid acetylators may be more prone to develop reactions from the metabolites of drugs or are less likely to develop side effects from the parent compound for a constant drug dose.

DRUG BINDING

Drugs exist in plasma both in the free form and bound to plasma proteins. Only free drug is capable of distributing into tissues and exerting a pharmacological action. Some drugs, e.g., verapamil, sotalol, and disopyramide, have optical isomers, with different potencies and effects. Virtually all assays for drug concentration in the blood measure *both* free and protein-bound drug. For antiarrhythmic drugs, the fraction of drug that is bound varies greatly among the different agents but is fairly constant for individual drugs over the clinically relevant range of plasma concentrations with the exception of phenytoin, lidocaine, propafenone, and disopyramide. With these drugs, binding sites become saturated at high concentrations, and therefore, a doubling of total drug concentration represents more than a doubling of unbound drug. Total plasma concentrations of a given drug generally correlate well with its clinical effects, and it has not been necessary to develop assays to measure free drug concentrations for antiarrhythmic agents. Some drugs, such as quinidine and lidocaine, bind to an α1-glycoprotein that increases in acute disease states such as myocardial infarction, which may decrease the concentration of free drug.

When a constant dose of a drug is administered repeatedly (orally or parenterally) at a constant dosing interval, accumulation occurs until drug concentration approaches a constant steady-state level, at which time the rate of drug administration equals the rate of drug elimination. The time it takes to reach steady state is a function of the half-life of the drug; 94 per cent of steady state is achieved after four half-lives and 99 per cent after seven half-lives. A drug with a long half-life takes longer to reach steady state than does one with a short half-life. The average steady-

state concentration of a drug equals the fraction of the dose absorbed (F) × the maintenance dose (dose$_m$) divided by the total-body clearance (Cl$_s$) × the dosing interval (τ).

Average steady-state concentration

$$= \frac{F \times \text{dose}_m}{Cl_s \times \tau} = \frac{F \times \text{dose}_m t½}{0.693 \times V_{d\tau}}$$

If the drug is given intravenously,

$$\text{Steady-state concentration} = \frac{\text{infusion rate}}{Cl_s} = \frac{\text{infusion rate } t½}{0.693 \, V_d}$$

Finally, it is important to stress that drug pharmacokinetics may differ in normal healthy volunteers compared with patients who have a variety of illnesses. Therefore, information derived from patients as well as normal subjects must be considered when one is planning dosing regimens.

GENERAL CONSIDERATIONS REGARDING ANTIARRHYTHMIC DRUGS

Most of the available antiarrhythmic drugs (Table 21–1) can be classified according to whether they exert blocking actions predominantly on sodium, potassium, or calcium channels and whether they block beta-adrenoceptors.[6,7] The commonly used Vaughan Williams classification is limited because it is based on the electrophysiological effects exerted by an arbitrary concentration of the drug, generally on normal cardiac tissue. Actually, the actions of these drugs are quite complex and depend on tissue type, species, the degree of acute or chronic damage, heart rate, membrane potential, the ionic composition of the extracellular milieu, and other factors (Table 21–2). Many drugs exhibit actions that belong in multiple categories or operate indirectly, such as by altering hemodynamics, myocardial metabolism, or autonomic neural transmission. Some drugs have active metabolites that exert different effects from the parent compound. Not all drugs in the same class have identical effects, e.g., bretylium, sotalol, and amiodarone are dramatically different, while some drugs in different classes have overlapping actions, e.g., class IA and IC drugs. In vitro studies on healthy fibers usually establish the properties of antiarrhythmic agents rather than their antiarrhythmic properties.

Despite these limitations, the Vaughan Williams classification[8] is widely known and provides a useful communication shorthand. It is listed here, but the reader is cautioned that drug actions are more complex than depicted by the classification. A more realistic view of antiarrhythmic agents is provided by the "Sicilian gambit."[9,10] This approach to drug classification is an attempt to identify the mechanisms of a particular arrhythmia, determine the vulnerable parameter of the arrhythmia most susceptible to modification, define the target most likely to affect the vulnerable parameter, and then select a drug that will modify the target. This concept provides a framework in which to consider antiarrhythmic drugs (Table 21–3 and 21–4).

DRUG CLASSIFICATION. According to the Vaughan Williams classification, *class I* drugs block the fast sodium channel. They, in turn, may be divided into three subgroups:

Class IA. Drugs that reduce $\dot{V}_{max}$ and prolong action potential duration: quinidine, procainamide, disopyramide; kinetics of onset and offset in blocking the Na$^+$ channel are of intermediate rapidity (< 5 sec).

Class IB. Drugs that do not reduce $\dot{V}_{max}$ and that shorten action potential duration: mexiletine, phenytoin, and lidocaine; fast onset and offset kinetics (< 500 msec).

TABLE 21–3 CLASSIFICATION OF DRUG ACTIONS ON ARRHYTHMIAS BASED ON MODIFICATION OF VULNERABLE PARAMETER

ARRHYTHMIA	MECHANISMS	VULNERABLE PARAMETER	DRUGS
	Automaticity (a) Enhanced normal		
Inappropriate sinus tachycardia Some idiopathic ventricular tachycardias		Phase 4 depolarization (decrease)	β-adrenergic blocking agents Na^+-channel blocking agents
	(b) Abnormal		
Atrial tachycardia		Maximal diastolic potential (hyperpolarization) or	M_2-agonist
		Phase 4 depolarization (decrease)	Ca^{++}- or Na^+-channel blocking agents M_2 agonists
Accelerated idioventricular rhythms		Phase 4 depolarization (decrease)	Ca^{++}- or Na^+-channel blocking agents
	Triggered activity (a) EAD		
Torsades de pointes		Action potential duration (shorten) or	β-agonists; vagolytic agents (increase rate)
		EAD (suppress)	Ca^{++}-channel blocking agents; Mg^{++}; β-adrenergic blockers
	(b) DAD		
Digitalis-induced arrhythmias		Calcium overload (unload) or	Ca^{++}-channel blocking agents
		DAD (suppress)	Na^+-channel blocking agents
Certain autonomically mediated ventricular tachycardias		Calcium overload (unload) or	β-adrenergic blocking agents
		DAD (suppress)	Ca^{++}-channel blocking agents, adenosine
	Reentry (Na^+ channel-dependent) (a) Long excitable gap		
Atrial flutter type I		Conduction and excitability (depress)	Na^+-channel blocking agents (except lidocaine, mexiletine, tocainide)
Circus movement tachycardia in WPW		Conduction and excitability (depress)	Na^+-channel blocking agents (except lidocaine, mexiletine, tocainide)
Sustained monomorphic ventricular tachycardia		Conduction and excitability (depress)	Na^+-channel blocking agents
	(b) Short excitable gap		
Atrial flutter type II		Refractory period (prolong)	K^+-channel blockers
Atrial fibrillation		Refractory period (prolong)	K^+-channel blockers
Circus movement tachycardia in WPW		Refractory period (prolong)	Amiodarone, sotalol
Polymorphic and sustained monomorphic ventricular tachycardia		Refractory period (prolong)	Quinidine, procainamide, disopyramide
Bundle branch reentry		Refractory period (prolong)	Quinidine, procainamide, disopyramide, bretylium
Ventricular fibrillation		Refractory period (prolong)	
	Reentry (Ca^{++}-channel-dependent)		
AV nodal reentrant tachycardia		Conduction and excitability (depress)	Ca^+-channel blocking agents
Circus movement tachycardia in WPW		Conduction and excitability (depress)	Ca^+-channel blocking agents
Verapamil-sensitive ventricular tachycardia		Conduction and excitability (depress)	Ca^+-channel blocking agents

Reproduced with permission from Task Force of the Working Group on Arrhythmias of the European Society of Cardiology: The Sicilian gambit. A new approach to the classification of antiarrhythmic drugs based on their actions on arrhythmogenic mechanisms. Circulation *84*:1831, 1991. Copyright 1991, American Heart Association.

Class IC. Drugs that reduce $\dot{V}_{max}$, primarily slow conduction, and can prolong refractoriness minimally: flecainide, propafenone, and probably moricizine; slow onset and offset kinetics (10 to 20 sec).

Class II drugs block beta-adrenergic receptors and include propranolol, timolol, metoprolol, and others (Table 38–7, p. 1307).

Class III drugs block potassium channels and prolong repolarization. They include sotalol, amiodarone, bretylium, and N-acetylprocainamide.

Class IV drugs block the slow calcium channel and include verapamil, diltiazem, nifedipine, and others.

A recently proposed model suggests that antiarrhythmic drugs cross the cell membrane and interact with receptors in the membrane channels when the latter are in the rested, activated, or inactivated state (Table 20–1) and that each of these interactions is characterized by a different association and dissociation rate constant (Figs. 20–10, p. 554 and 20–16, p. 559). Such interactions are voltage- and time-dependent. Transitions among rested, activated, and inactivated states are governed by standard Hodgkin-Huxley–type equations. When the drug is bound (associated) to a receptor site at or very close to the ionic channel (the drug probably does not actually plug the channel), the latter cannot conduct, even in the activated state.

USE-DEPENDENCE. Some drugs exert greater inhibitory effects on the upstroke of the action potential at more rapid rates of stimulation and after longer periods of stimulation, a characteristic called *use-dependence*. Use-dependence

TABLE 21–4 ACTIONS OF ANTIARRHYTHMIC DRUGS   **599**

Ch 21

DRUG	CHANNELS NA Fast	Med	Slow	Ca	K	I_f	RECEPTORS α	β	M₂	P	PUMPS Na-K ATPase	CLINICAL EFFECTS Left ventricular function	Sinus Rate	Extra-cardiac	ECG EFFECTS P-R interval	QRS width	J-T interval
Lidocaine	○											→	→	◎			↓
Mexiletine	○											→	→	◎			↓
Tocainide	○											→	→	●			↓
Moricizine	❶											↓	→	○		↑	
Procainamide		Ⓐ			◎							↓	→	●	↑	↑	↑
Disopyramide		Ⓐ			◎				○			↓	→	◎	↑↓	↑	↑
Quinidine		Ⓐ			◎		○		○			→	↑	◎	↑↓	↑	↑
Propafenone		Ⓐ						◎				↓	↓	○	↑	↑	
Flecainide			Ⓐ		○							↓	→	○	↑	↑	
Encainide			Ⓐ									↓	→	○	↑	↑	↑
Bepridil	○			●	◎							?	↓	○			↑
Verapamil	○			●			◎					↓	↓	○	↑		↑
Diltiazem				◎								↓	↓	○	↑		
Bretylium					●		▱	▱				→	↓	○			↑
Sotalol					●			●				↓	↓	○	↑		↑
Amiodarone	○			○	●		◎	◎				→	↓	●	↑		↑
Alinidine					◎	●						?	↓	●			
Nadolol								●				↓	↓	○	↑		
Propranolol	○							●				↓	↓	○	↑		
Atropine									●			→	→	◎	↓		
Adenosine										□		?	↓	○	↓		
Digoxin										□	●	↑	↓	●	↑		↓

Relative potency of block: ○ Low ◎ Moderate ● High	A = Activated state blocker
□ = Agonist ▱ = Agonist/Antagonist	I = Inactivated state blocker

From Schwartz, P. J., and Zaza, A.: Eur. Heart J. *13*:26, 1992. Copyright © 1992 reproduced by permission of the publisher W.B. Saunders Company Limited.

means that depression of $\dot{V}_{max}$ is greater after the channel has been "used," i.e., after action potential depolarization rather than after a rest period. It is possible that this use-dependence results from preferential interaction of the antiarrhythmic drug with either the open or the inactive channel and little interaction with the resting channels of the unstimulated cell. Agents in class IB exhibit fast kinetics of onset and offset or use-dependent block of the fast channel; that is, they bind and dissociate quickly from the receptors. Class IC drugs have slow kinetics, and class IA drugs are intermediate. With increased time spent in diastole (slower rate), a greater proportion of receptors become drug-free, and the drug exerts less effect. Cells with reduced membrane potentials recover more slowly from drug actions than cells with more negative membrane potentials (Fig. 20–15, p. 558).

REVERSE DRUG DEPENDENCE. Some drugs exert greater effects at slow rates than at fast rates. This is particularly true for drugs that lengthen repolarization. The Q-T interval becomes prolonged more at slow than fast rates. This is opposite to what the ideal antiarrhythmic agent would do, since prolongation of refractoriness should be increased at fast rates so as to interrupt or prevent a tachycardia and should be maximal at slow rates to avoid precipitating torsades de pointes.[11]

MECHANISMS OF ARRHYTHMIA SUPPRESSION. Given the fact that enhanced automaticity, triggered activity, or reentry can cause cardiac arrhythmias (see Chap. 20), mechanisms by which antiarrhythmic agents suppress arrhythmias can be postulated.[9,10] Antiarrhythmic agents can slow the spontaneous discharge frequency of an automatic pacemaker by depressing the slope of diastolic depolarization, shifting the threshold voltage toward zero, or hyperpolarizing the resting membrane potential. Mechanisms by which

different drugs suppress normal or abnormal automaticity may not be the same. In general, however, most antiarrhythmic agents in therapeutic doses depress the automatic firing rate of spontaneously discharging ectopic sites while minimally affecting the discharge rate of the normal sinus node. Slow-channel blockers like verapamil, beta blockers like propranolol, and some antiarrhythmic agents like amiodarone also depress spontaneous discharge of the normal sinus node, while drugs that exert vagolytic effects, such as disopyramide or quinidine, can increase the sinus discharge rate. Drugs can also suppress early or delayed afterdepolarizations (see pp. 566 and 567) and eliminate triggered arrhythmias due to these mechanisms.

As mentioned earlier (see p. 571), reentry depends critically on the timing interrelationships between refractoriness and conduction velocity, the presence of unidirectional block in one of the pathways, and other factors that influence refractoriness and conduction, such as excitability. An antiarrhythmic agent can stop reentry that is already present or prevent it from starting if the drug improves or depresses conduction. For example, *improved conduction* can (1) eliminate the unidirectional block so that reentry cannot begin or (2) facilitate conduction in the reentrant loop so that the returning wavefront reenters too quickly, encroaches on fibers still refractory, and becomes extinguished. A drug that *depresses conduction* can transform the unidirectional block to bidirectional block and thus terminate reentry or prevent it from occurring by creating an area of complete block in the reentrant pathway. Conversely, a drug that slows conduction without producing block or lengthening refractoriness significantly can promote reentry. Finally, most antiarrhythmic agents share the ability to prolong refractoriness relative to their effects on action potential duration; i.e., the ratio of effective refractory period to action potential duration exceeds 1.0. If a drug *prolongs refractoriness* of fibers in the reentrant pathway, the pathway may not recover excitability in time to be depolarized by the reentering impulse, and the reentrant propagation ceases. The different types of reentry (see pp. 571 and 572) influence the effects and effectiveness of a drug.

When one is discussing any of the properties of a drug, it is important that the situation and/or model from which conclusions are drawn be defined with care. Electrophysiological, hemodynamic, autonomic, pharmacokinetic, and adverse effects all may differ in normal subjects compared with patients, in normal tissue compared with abnormal tissue, in muscle compared with specialized fibers, and in different species.

STEREOSELECTIVITY. Drug interactions with a channel, receptor, or enzyme may depend on the three-dimensional geometry of the drug.[12] Many drugs have stereoisomers, molecules with the same atomic composition but different spatial arrangement, that can influence drug effects, metabolism, binding, clearance, and excretion. Most drugs are prescribed as 50/50 mixtures of their two forms (racemates), which may make 50 per cent of the dose ineffective for some drugs. Except for timolol, virtually all beta blockers are racemates. d-Propranolol exerts antiarrhythmic actions unrelated to beta-adrenoceptor blockade, while l-propranolol blocks the beta receptor. Both enantiomers (mirror images) of sotalol block the potassium channel to prolong action potential duration and suppress arrhythmias equally, but d-sotalol does not block the beta-adrenoceptor. Racemic propafenone exhibits beta-blocking actions due to the S-enantiomer. Other drugs with notable stereoselective differences include disopyramide with one form (S [+]) prolonging repolarization and having greater antiarrhythmic effects than R (−), which shortens repolarization. The latter form has less anticholinergic effects. The (−) enantiomer of verapamil exerts much more negative inotropic and dromotropic effects than does the (+) form and may have more potent antiarrhythmic actions. Stereoselectivity affects sodium channel blocking drugs less than it affects beta-adrenoceptor, potassium, and calcium blockers.

DRUG METABOLITES. Drug metabolites may add to or alter the effects of the parent compound by exerting similar actions, competing with the parent compound, or mediating drug toxicity. Quinidine has at least four active metabolites, but none with a potency exceeding the parent drug and none preliminarily implicated in causing torsades de pointes. About 50 per cent of procainamide is metabolized to NAPA. Only the parent drug blocks cardiac sodium channels and slows impulse propagation in the His-Purkinje system. NAPA prolongs repolarization and is a less effective antiarrhythmic drug but competes with procainamide for renal tubular secretory sites and can increase the parent's elimination half-life. Lidocaine's metabolite can compete with lidocaine for sodium channels and partially reverse block produced by lidocaine.

Genetically determined metabolic pathways account for many of the differences in patients' responses to some drugs. The genetically determined activity of hepatic *N*-acetyltransferase regulates the development of antinuclear antibodies and development of the lupus syndrome in response to procainamide. Slow acetylator phenotypes appear more prone to develop lupus than do rapid acetylators.[13–15] About 7 per cent of white and black subjects lack debrisoquin 4-hydroxylase. This enzyme is needed to metabolize debrisoquin (an antihypertensive drug) and propafenone, to hydroxylate several beta blockers, and to biotransform flecainide. The gene coding for this enzyme (termed $P450_{dbl}$) is on human chromosome 22. Lack of this enzyme reduces metabolism of the parent compound, leading to increased plasma concentrations of the parent drug and reduced concentrations of metabolites. Quinidine in low doses can inhibit this enzyme and thereby alter concentrations of the drugs and metabolites given in combination that are affected by the $P450_{dbl}$ enzyme, such as propafenone or flecainide. Understanding stereoselectivity and pharmacogenetics can provide major clues to understanding differences in drug efficacy and toxicity from one patient to the next. Cimetidine and ranitidine also affect drug metabolism,

probably by inhibiting hepatic P450-metabolizing enzymes (Table 21–5).

SIDE EFFECTS. Antiarrhythmic drugs produce one group of side effects that relate to excessive dosage and plasma concentrations, resulting in both noncardiac (e.g., neurological defects) and cardiac (e.g., heart failure, some arrhythmias) toxicity, and another group of side effects unrelated to plasma concentrations, termed *idiopathic*. Examples of the latter include procainamide-induced lupus syndrome, amiodarone-induced pulmonary toxicity (although a recent publication relates maintenance dose to this side effect), and some arrhythmias such as quinidine-induced torsades de pointes.

PROARRHYTHMIA. Drug-induced or drug-aggravated cardiac arrhythmias (proarrhythmia) are a major clinical problem.[16–21] Electrophysiological mechanisms probably relate to prolongation of repolarization, the development of early afterdepolarizations to cause torsades de pointes,[22–31] and alterations in reentry pathways[32] to initiate or sustain ventricular tachyarrhythmias. Proarrhythmic events can occur in as many as 5 to 10 per cent of patients. Heart failure increases proarrhythmic risk. Patients with atrial fibrillation treated with antiarrhythmic agents had a 4.7 relative risk of cardiac death if they had a history of heart failure compared with patients not so treated who had a 3.7 relative risk of arrhythmic death. Patients without a history of congestive heart failure had no increased risk of cardiac mortality during antiarrhythmic drug treatment.[33] Reduced left ventricular function, treatment with digitalis and diuretics, and longer pretreatment Q-T interval characterize patients who develop drug-induced ventricular fibrillation. The more commonly known proarrhythmic events occur within several days of beginning drug therapy or changing dosage and are represented by such developments as incessant ventricular tachycardia, long Q-T syndrome, and torsades de pointes. However, in the Cardiac Arrhythmia Suppression Trial (CAST),[34–36] encainide and flecainide reduced spontaneous ventricular arrhythmias but were associated with a total mortality of 7.7 versus 3.0 per cent in the group receiving placebo. Deaths were equally distributed throughout the treatment period, raising the im-

TABLE 21–5 PHARMACOKINETIC INTERACTIONS OF ANTIARRHYTHMIC DRUGS

AGENTS	EFFECTS
Phenytoin Phenobarbital Rifampin	Increase clearance of: quinidine disopyramide mexiletine digitoxin
Cimetidine	Reduces clearance of: quinidine lidocaine procainamide flecainide moricizine
Amiodarone	Reduces clearance of: warfarin phenytoin quinidine procainamide digoxin
Digoxin	Clearance reduced by: quinidine verapamil amiodarone Volume of distribution reduced by: quinidine
Lidocaine	Clearance reduced by: propranolol cimetidine

From Roden, D.: New concepts in antiarrhythmic drug pharmacokinetics. Progr. Cardiol. *15*:19, 1987.

portant consideration that another kind of proarrhythmic response can occur some time after the beginning of drug therapy. Such late proarrhythmic effects may relate to drug-induced exacerbation of regional myocardial conduction delay due to ischemia and heterogeneous drug concentrations that may promote reentry. Moricizine also increased mortality, leading to termination of CAST II.[34-36]

CLASS IA ANTIARRHYTHMIC AGENTS

Quinidine

Quinidine and quinine are isometric alkaloids isolated from the cinchona bark.[37] Although quinidine shares the antimalarial, antipyretic, and vagolytic actions of quinine, the latter lacks the significant electrophysiological and antiarrhythmic effects of quinidine.

ELECTROPHYSIOLOGICAL ACTIONS (Tables 21–6 and 21–7). Quinidine exerts little effect on automaticity of the isolated or denervated normal sinus node but suppresses automaticity in normal Purkinje fibers, especially in ectopic pacemakers, by decreasing the slope of phase 4 diastolic depolarization and shifting threshold voltage toward zero. In patients with the sick sinus syndrome, quinidine can depress sinus nodal automaticity. It does not affect abnormal automaticity in depolarized Purkinje fibers. Quinidine produces early afterdepolarizations in experimental preparations and in humans, which may be responsible for torsades de pointes.[22-31] Because of its significant anticholinergic effect and reflex sympathetic stimulation resulting from alpha-adrenergic blockade that causes peripheral vasodilation, quinidine can increase sinus nodal discharge rate and can improve atrioventricular (AV) nodal conduction in the innervated heart in vivo. Direct myocardial effects can prolong AV nodal and His-Purkinje conduction times and refractoriness in the accessory pathway. Quinidine prolongs the duration of action potential of atrial and ventricular muscle and Purkinje fibers slightly (quinine shortens it) while also prolonging the effective refractory period without significantly changing resting membrane potential. Prolongation of repolarization is more prominent at slow heart rates (reverse use dependence)[38,39] owing to block of I_K.[40] Action potential amplitude, overshoot, and $\dot{V}_{max}$ of phase 0 are reduced, more so during ischemia, hypoxia, and in depolarized fibers, especially at fast rates. The open channel has a high affinity for quinidine, resulting in block of a fraction of sodium channels with each action potential upstroke.[41] The time for unblocking by IA drugs (about 4 sec) is slower than for IB drugs but faster than for IC drugs. For the duration of the plateau of the action potential (inactivated state) or in depolarized fibers, the rate of unblocking is slow, proceeding much faster in polarized fibers. Therefore, faster rates result in more block of sodium channels and less unblocking because of a lesser percentage of time spent in a polarized state (use-dependence). Isoproterenol can modulate the effects of quinidine on reentrant circuits in humans.[42]

HEMODYNAMIC EFFECTS. Quinidine decreases peripheral vascular resistance and can cause significant hypotension because of its alpha-adrenergic receptor blocking effects. Concomitant administration of vasodilators can exaggerate the potential for hypotension. In some patients, quinidine can increase cardiac output, possibly by reducing afterload and preload. No significant direct myocardial depressant action occurs unless large doses are given rapidly, intravenously. Most of the adverse effects of intravenous quinidine are probably the result of excessive vasodilation.

PHARMACOKINETICS (Table 21–1). Although orally administered quinidine sulfate and quinidine gluconate exhibit similar degrees of systemic availability, plasma quinidine concentrations peak at about 90 minutes after oral administration of quinidine sulfate and at 3 to 4 hours after oral administration of quinidine gluconate. Intramuscular quinidine produces a higher and an earlier peak plasma concentration but results in incomplete absorption and tissue necrosis. Quinidine may be given intravenously if it is infused slowly. Approximately 80 per cent of plasma quinidine is protein-bound, especially to α1-acid glycoprotein, which increases in heart failure. Both the liver and the kidneys remove quinidine, and dose adjustments may be made according to the creatinine clearance.[43,44] Metabolism is via the P450 cytochrome system. Approximately 20 per cent is excreted unchanged in the urine. Because congestive heart failure, hepatic disease, or poor renal function can reduce quinidine elimination and increase plasma concentration, dosage probably should be reduced and the drug given cautiously to patients with these disorders while serum quinidine concentration is monitored. Elimi-

TABLE 21–6 IN VIVO ELECTROPHYSIOLOGICAL CHARACTERISTICS OF ANTIARRHYTHMIC DRUGS

DRUG	ELECTROCARDIOGRAPHIC INTERVALS						ELECTROPHYSIOLOGICAL INTERVALS				
	Sinus Rate	P-R	QRS	Q-T	A-H	H-V	ERP AVN	ERP HPS	ERP A	ERP V	ERP AP
Quinidine	0 ↑	↓ 0 ↑	↑	↑	↓ 0 ↑	↑	0 ↑	↑	↑	↑	↑
Procainamide	0	0 ↑	↑	↑	0 ↑	↑	0 ↑	↑	↑	↑	↑
Disopyramide	0 ↑	↓ 0 ↑	↑	↑	↓ 0 ↑	↑	↑ 0	↑	↑	↑	↑
Lidocaine	0	0	0	0 ↓	0 ↓	0 ↑	0 ↓	0 ↑	0	0	0
Mexiletine	0	0	0	0 ↓	0 ↑	0 ↑	0 ↑	0 ↑	0	0	0
Tocainide	0	0	0	0 ↓	0	0	0	0	0	0	0
Phenytoin	0	0	0	0 ↓	0 ↓	0	0 ↓	↓	0	0	0
Moricizine	0 ↓	0 ↑	0 ↑	0	↑	↑	0	0	0 ↑	0 ↑	↑
Flecainide	0 ↓	↑	↑	0 ↑	↑	↑	↑	↑	↑	↑	↑
Propafenone	0 ↓	↑	↑	0 ↑	↑	↑	0 ↑	0 ↑	0 ↑	↑	↑
Amiodarone	↓	0 ↑	↑	↑	↑	↑	↑	↑	↑	↑	↑
Bretylium	↑ 0 ↓	0	0	0 ↑			0	↑	↑	↑	0
Propranolol	↓	0 ↑	0	0 ↓	0	0	↑	0	0	0	0 ↑
Verapamil	0 ↓	↑	0	0	↑	0	↑	0	0	0	0 ↑
Adenosine	↓ then ↑	↑	0	0	↑	0	↑	0	↓	0	0 ↓
Sotalol	↓	0 ↑	0	↑	↑	0	↑	↑	↑	↑	↑

Results presented may vary according to tissue type, experimental conditions, and drug concentration. ↑ = increase; ↓ = decrease; 0 = no change; 0 ↑ or 0 ↓ = slight inconsistent increase or decrease. A = atrium; AVN = AV node; HPS = His-Purkinje system; V = ventricle; AP = accessory pathway (WPW); ERP = effective refractory period—longest S_1–S_2 interval at which S_2 fails to produce a response.

TABLE 21-7 IN VITRO ELECTROPHYSIOLOGICAL CHARACTERISTICS OF ANTIARRHYTHMIC DRUGS

DRUG	APA	APD	dV/dt	MDP	ERP	CONDUCTION VELOCITY	PF PHASE 4	SINUS NODAL AUTOMATICITY
Quinidine	↓	↑	↓	0	↑	↓	↓	0
Procainamide	↓	↑	↓	0	↑	↓	↓	0
Disopyramide	↓	↑	↓	0	↑	↓	↓	↑ 0 ↓
Lidocaine	0 ↓	↓	0 ↓	0	↓	0 ↓	↓	0
Mexiletine	0	↓	0 ↓	0	↓	↓	↓	0
Tocainide	0	↓	0 ↓	0	↓	↓	0	↓
Phenytoin	0	↓	↑ 0 ↓	0	↓	0	↓	0
Moricizine	↓	↓	↓	0	↓	↓	0	0
Flecainide	↓	0 ↑	↓	0	↑	↓ ↓	↓	0
Propafenone	↓	0 ↑	↓	0	↑	↓ ↓	↓	0
Propranolol	0 ↓	0 ↓	0 ↓	0	↓	0	↓ *	↓
Amiodarone	0	↑	0 ↓	0	↑	↓	↓	↓
Bretylium	0	↑	0	0	↑	0	0 ↓ *	0 ↓
Verapamil	0	↓	0	0	0	0	↓ *	↓
Adenosine	0	0	0	0	0	0	0	↓
Sotalol	0 ↓	↑	0 ↓	0	↑	0	0 ↓	↓

* With a background of sympathetic activity.

APA = action potential amplitude; APD = action potential duration; dV/dt = rate of rise of action potential; MDP = maximum diastolic potential; ERP = effective refractory period; PF = Purkinje fibers.

nation half-life is 5 to 8 hours after oral administration. Quinidine can increase plasma concentrations of flecainide by inhibiting the P450 enzyme system.[12]

DOSAGE AND ADMINISTRATION (Table 21–1). The usual oral dose of quinidine sulfate for an adult is 300 to 600 mg four times daily, which results in a steady-state level within about 24 hours. A loading dose of 600 to 1000 mg produces an earlier effective concentration. Similar doses of quinidine gluconate are used intramuscularly, while the intravenous dose of quinidine gluconate is about 10 mg/kg given at a rate of about 0.5 mg/kg/min as blood pressure and electrocardiographic (ECG) parameters are checked frequently. Oral doses of the gluconate are about 30 per cent greater than those of sulfate. Important interactions with other drugs occur (Table 21–2).

INDICATIONS. Quinidine is a versatile antiarrhythmic agent, useful for treating premature supraventricular and ventricular complexes and sustained tachyarrhythmias. It may prevent spontaneous recurrences or electrical induction of AV nodal reentrant tachycardia by prolonging atrial and ventricular refractoriness and depressing conduction in the retrograde fast pathway. In patients with the Wolff-Parkinson-White syndrome, quinidine prolongs the effective refractory period of the accessory pathway and, by so doing, can prevent reciprocating tachycardias and slow the ventricular response from conduction over the accessory pathway during atrial flutter or atrial fibrillation. Quinidine and other antiarrhythmic agents also can prevent recurrences of tachycardia by suppressing the "trigger," i.e., the premature atrial or ventricular complex that initiates a sustained tachycardia.

Quinidine successfully terminates atrial flutter or atrial fibrillation in about 10 to 20 per cent of patients, with higher success rates if the arrhythmia is of more recent onset and if the atria are not enlarged. Before quinidine is administered to these patients, the ventricular response should be slowed sufficiently with digitalis, propranolol, or verapamil, since quinidine-induced slowing of the atrial flutter rate—e.g., over the range of 300 to 200 beats/min—plus its vagolytic effect on AV nodal conduction may convert a 2:1 atrioventricular response (two atrial impulses for each QRS complex) to a 1:1 atrioventricular response, with an *increase* in the ventricular rate. Before elective cardioversion of patients with atrial fibrillation, quinidine probably should be given for 1 to 2 days, since this regimen restores sinus rhythm in some patients, thus obviating the need for direct-current cardioversion, and helps maintain sinus rhythm once it is achieved. A metaanalysis of six studies testing the effects of quinidine versus control in maintaining sinus rhythm in patients with atrial fibrillation

showed that quinidine-treated patients remained in sinus rhythm longer than did the control group but had an increased total mortality over the same period. This important conclusion needs to be verified in a controlled, prospective study.

Quinidine has prevented sudden death in some patients resuscitated after out-of-hospital cardiac arrest and may be combined with other antiarrhythmic agents for increased efficacy in suppressing ventricular tachyarrhythmias. No published data from controlled, randomized studies indicate improved survival in quinidine-treated patients after myocardial infarction (Fig. 21–5). Cardiac arrest can occur despite quinidine therapy.[45,46] Because it crosses the placenta, quinidine can be used to treat arrhythmias in the fetus.

ADVERSE EFFECTS. The most common adverse effects of chronic oral quinidine therapy are gastrointestinal, including nausea, vomiting, diarrhea, abdominal pain, and anorexia. Gastrointestinal side effects may be milder with the gluconate form. Central nervous system toxicity includes tinnitus, hearing loss, visual disturbances, confusion, delirium, and psychosis. *Cinchonism* is the term usually applied to these side effects. Allergic reactions may be manifested as rash, fever, immune-mediated thrombocytopenia, hemolytic anemia, and rarely, anaphylaxis. Thrombocytopenia is due to the presence of antibodies to quinidine-platelet complexes, causing platelets to agglutinate and lyse. In patients receiving oral anticoagulants, quinidine may cause bleeding. Side effects may preclude long-term administration of quinidine in 30 to 40 per cent of patients.

Quinidine can slow cardiac conduction, sometimes to the point of block, manifested as prolongation of the QRS duration or sinoatrial (SA) or AV nodal conduction disturbances. Quinidine-induced cardiac toxicity can be treated with molar sodium lactate. Quinidine can prolong the Q-T interval and cause torsades de pointes in 1 to 3 per cent of patients.[19–30]

Quinidine may produce syncope in 0.5 to 2.0 per cent of patients, most often the result of a self-terminating episode of torsades de pointes (see pp. 684 and 767). Torsades de pointes may be due to the development of early afterdepolarizations, as noted above. Quinidine prolongs the Q-T interval in most patients, whether or not ventricular arrhythmias occur, but significant Q-T prolongation (Q-T interval of 500 to 600 msec) is often a characteristic of quinidine syncope. Many of these patients are also receiving digitalis or diuretics. Syncope is unrelated to plasma concentrations of quinidine or duration of therapy. Hypokalemia often is a prominent feature. Therapy for quinidine syncope requires immediate discontinuation of the drug and avoidance of

DRUG	MEMBRANE RESPONSIVENESS	ET	VFT	CONTRACTILITY	SLOW INWARD CURRENT	AUTONOMIC NERVOUS SYSTEM	LOCAL ANESTHETIC EFFECT
Quinidine	↓	↑	↑	0	0	Antivagal; alpha blocker	Yes
Procainamide	↓	↑	↑	0	0	Slight antivagal	Yes
Disopyramide	↓	↑	↑	↓	0	Central: antivagal, antisympathetic	Yes
Lidocaine	0 ↓	0 ↑	↑	0	0	0	Yes
Mexiletine	↓	↑	↑	↓	0	0	Yes
Tocainide	↓	↑	↑	0	0	0	Yes
Phenytoin	0 ↑	0		0	0	0	No
Moricizine	↓	↑	0		0	0	No
Flecainide	↓			↓	0	0	Yes
Propafenone	↓	↑	↑	↓	May inhibit	Antisympathetic	Yes
Propranolol	↓			↓ ↑	0 ↓	Antisympathetic	No
Amiodarone	0	0	↑	0 ↑	0	Antisympathetic	Yes
Bretylium	0 ↑	0	0 ↑	↓	0	Antisympathetic	Yes
Verapamil	0	0	0	↓	Inhibit	? Block alpha receptors; enhance vagal	Yes
Adenosine	0	0	0	0	May inhibit	Vagomimetic	No
Sotalol	0 ↓	0	0	↓	0 ↓	Antisympathetic	No

ET = excitability threshold; VFT = ventricular fibrillation threshold.

other drugs that have similar pharmacological effects, such as disopyramide, since cross-sensitivity exists in some patients. Magnesium given intravenously (2 gm over 1 to 2 min, followed by an infusion of 3 to 20 mg/min) is probably the initial drug treatment of choice. Atrial or ventricular pacing can be used to suppress the ventricular tachyarrhythmia and may act by suppressing afterdepolarizations. For some patients, drugs that do not prolong the Q-T interval, such as lidocaine or phenytoin, can be tried. When pacing is not available, isoproterenol can be given *with caution.*

Drugs that induce hepatic enzyme production, such as phenobarbital and phenytoin, can shorten the duration of quinidine's action by increasing its rate of elimination. Quinidine may elevate serum digoxin and digitoxin concentrations by decreasing total-body clearance of digitoxin and by decreasing the clearance, volume of distribution, and affinity of tissue receptors for digoxin (see p. 499).

Procainamide

ELECTROPHYSIOLOGICAL ACTIONS (Tables 21–6 and 21–7). The cardiac actions of procainamide on automaticity, conduction, excitability, and membrane responsiveness resemble those of quinidine. Procainamide predominantly blocks the inactivated state of I_{Na}. It also blocks I_K and $I_{K ATP}$.[47] Like quinidine, procainamide usually prolongs the effective refractory period (ERP) more than it prolongs the action potential duration (APD) and thus prevents early responses from occurring, arising from less negative resting potentials that might conduct slowly or block and cause an arrhythmia. Compared with disopyramide and quinidine, procainamide exerts the least anticholinergic effects but does produce more local anesthetic effects than quinidine. It does not affect normal sinus nodal automaticity. In vitro, procainamide decreases abnormal automaticity, with less effect on triggered activity or catecholamine-enhanced normal automaticity.

The electrophysiogical effects of NAPA,[48] procainamide's major metabolite, differ from those of the parent compound. NAPA (10 to 40 mg/liter) does not suppress the rate of phase 4 diastolic depolarization of Purkinje fibers and does not alter resting membrane potential, action potential amplitude, or $\dot{V}_{max}$ of phase 0 of the action potential of Purkinje fibers or ventricular muscle. However, NAPA, a K+ channel blocker, exerts a class III action and prolongs the action potential duration of ventricular muscle and Purkinje fibers in a dose-dependent manner. Toxic doses produce early afterdepolarizations, triggered activity, and ventricular tachyarrhythmias, including torsades de pointes.

Procainamide appears to exert greater electrophysiological effects than NAPA.

HEMODYNAMIC EFFECTS. Procainamide can depress myocardial contractility in high doses. It does not produce alpha blockade but can result in peripheral vasodilation, possibly via antisympathetic effects on brain or spinal cord that can impair cardiovascular reflexes.[49]

PHARMACOKINETICS (Table 21–1). Oral administration produces peak plasma concentration in about 1 hour. Absorption may be reduced in the first week after myocardial infarction. Approximately 80 per cent of oral procainamide is bioavailable, with 20 per cent bound to serum proteins. The overall elimination half-life for procainamide is 3 to 5 hours, with 50 to 60 per cent of the drug eliminated by the kidney and 10 to 30 per cent eliminated by hepatic metabolism. A prolonged-release form of procainamide given every 6 hours provides steady-state plasma levels of the drug equivalent to an equal total daily dose of short-acting procainamide given every 3 hours.

The drug is acetylated to NAPA, which is excreted almost exclusively by the kidneys. As renal function decreases and in patients with heart failure, procainamide levels—and particularly NAPA levels—increase and, because of the risk of serious cardiotoxicity, need to be carefully monitored in such situations. NAPA has an elimination half-life of 7 to 8 hours but exceeds 10 hours if high doses are used. Small amounts of procainamide are present in patients receiving NAPA because of deacetylation. Increased age, congestive heart failure, and reduced creatinine clearance lower the procainamide clearance and necessitate reduced dosage.

DOSAGE AND ADMINISTRATION (Table 21–1). Procainamide can be given by the oral, intravenous, or intramuscular route to achieve plasma concentrations that produce an antiarrhythmic effect in the range of 4 to 10 μg/ml. Occasionally, plasma concentrations exceeding 10 μg/ml have been required, but the probability of adverse effects generally precludes long-term administration at these higher plasma concentrations. Several intravenous regimens have been used to administer procainamide. Twenty-five to 50 mg can be given over a 1-minute period and then repeated every 5 minutes until the arrhythmia is controlled, hypotension results, or the QRS complex is prolonged more than 50 per cent. Doses of 10 to 15 mg/kg at 50 mg/min are commonly used during electrophysiological testing.[50,51] Using this method, plasma concentration falls rapidly during the first 15 minutes after the loading dose, with parallel effects on refractoriness and conduction. A constant-rate intravenous infusion of procainamide can be given at a dose of 2 to 6 mg/min. The upper limits regarding total IV dose are flexible and range between 1000 and 2000 mg depending on the patient's response.

Oral administration of procainamide requires a 3- to 4-hour dosing interval at a total daily dose of 2 to 6 gm, with a steady state reached within 1 day. When a loading dose is used, it should be twice the maintenance dose. Frequent dosing is required because of the short elimination half-life in normal subjects. For the prolonged-release form of procainamide, dosing is at 6-hour intervals. While a longer half-life may be seen in some cardiac patients, allowing longer intervals between drug administration, this needs to be documented for the individual patient. Procainamide is well absorbed after intramuscular injection, with virtually 100 per cent of the dose bioavailable.

INDICATIONS. Procainamide is used to treat both supraventricular and ventricular arrhythmias in a manner comparable with that of quinidine.[52] Although both drugs have similar electrophysiological actions, either drug can effectively suppress a supraventricular or ventricular arrhythmia that is resistant to the other drug.

Procainamide can be used to convert atrial fibrillation of recent onset to sinus rhythm.[53] As with quinidine, prior treatment with digitalis, propranolol, or verapamil is recommended to prevent acceleration of the ventricular response following procainamide therapy. In patients with paroxysmal supraventricular tachycardia, procainamide can inhibit the induction of sustained AV nodal reentrant tachycardia as a result of selective depression of retrograde AV nodal conduction in the fast pathway. Procainamide can block conduction in the accessory pathway of patients with the Wolff-Parkinson-White syndrome and is particularly useful in patients with atrial fibrillation and a rapid ventricular response due to conduction over the accessory pathway (see p. 655). Whether it can be used intravenously to identify those patients who have a short anterograde effective refractory period is not resolved. It can produce His-Purkinje block (see p. 750).

Procainamide is more effective than lidocaine in preventing the induction of ventricular tachycardia by programmed stimulation[54] and in acutely terminating sustained ventricular tachycardia. The electrophysiological response to procainamide given intravenously appears to predict the response to the drug given orally. Patients with ejection fractions ≥40 per cent whose ventricular tachycardia procainamide renders noninducible have a high likelihood of responding to the drug given orally. High doses, 500 to 1000 mg orally every 4 hours, resulting in a plasma concentration exceeding 10.0 μg/ml, may be necessary to suppress ventricular tachycardia in some patients. Most consistently, procainamide slows the rate of the induced ventricular tachycardia, a change correlated with the increase in QRS duration. Adding amiodarone to procainamide slows the ventricular tachycardia cycle length further but increases the noninducibility success rate only slightly. Procainamide appears to affect preferentially the reentrant circuit of the ventricular tachycardia compared with other areas of myocardium. The antiarrhythmic response to procainamide does not predict the response to NAPA.

ADVERSE EFFECTS. Multiple adverse noncardiac effects have been reported with procainamide administration and include skin rashes, myalgias, digital vasculitis, and Raynaud's phenomenon. Fever and agranulocytosis may be due to hypersensitivity reactions, and white blood cell and differential blood counts should be performed at regular intervals. Gastrointestinal side effects are less frequent than with quinidine, and adverse central nervous system side effects are less frequent than with lidocaine. Procainamide can cause giddiness, psychosis, hallucinations, and depression. Toxic concentrations of procainamide can diminish myocardial performance and promote hypotension. A variety of conduction disturbances or ventricular tachyarrhythmias[55] can occur similar to those produced by quinidine,

including prolonged Q-T syndrome and polymorphous ventricular tachycardia. NAPA also can induce Q-T prolongation and torsades de pointes. In the absence of sinus node disease, procainamide does not adversely affect sinus node function. In patients with sinus dysfunction, procainamide tends to prolong corrected sinus node recovery time and can worsen symptoms in some patients who have the bradycardia-tachycardia syndrome. Procainamide does not increase the serum digoxin concentration.

Arthralgia, fever, pleuropericarditis, hepatomegaly, and hemorrhagic pericardial effusion with tamponade have been described in a systemic lupus erythematosus (SLE)–like syndrome. The syndrome can occur more frequently and earlier in patients who are "slow acetylators" of procainamide and is influenced by genetic factors.[13] The aromatic amino group on procainamide appears important for induction of SLE syndrome, since acetylating this amino group to form NAPA appears to block the SLE-inducing effect. Sixty to 70 per cent of patients who receive procainamide on a chronic basis develop antinuclear antibodies, with clinical symptoms in 20 to 30 per cent, but this is reversible when procainamide is stopped. When symptoms occur, SLE cell preparations are often positive. Positive serological tests are not necessarily a reason to discontinue drug therapy; however, the development of symptoms or a positive anti-DNA antibody is, except for patients whose life-threatening arrhythmia is controlled only by procainamide. Steroid administration in these patients may eliminate the symptoms. In contrast to naturally occurring SLE, the brain and kidney are spared, and there is no predilection for females.

Disopyramide

Disopyramide has been approved in the United States for oral but not intravenous administration to treat patients with ventricular arrhythmias.

ELECTROPHYSIOLOGICAL ACTIONS (Tables 21–6 and 21–7). Although structurally different from quinidine and procainamide, disopyramide produces similar electrophysiological effects in vitro. It causes use-dependent block of I_{Na} and non-use-dependent block of I_K.[40] Along with quinidine, low concentrations tend to prolong action potential duration and induce early afterdepolarizations (EADs) just as do higher concentrations.[31] Disopyramide also inhibits $I_{K ATP}$.[47] It decreases the slope of phase 4 diastolic depolarization in Purkinje fibers, produces a rate-dependent depression of $\dot{V}_{max}$ of phase 0, prolongs the effective refractory period more than it prolongs the action potential duration, lengthens conduction time in normal and depolarized Purkinje fibers, and does not affect calcium-dependent action potentials, except possibly at very high concentrations, or suppress late potentials in the signal-averaged ECG. Disopyramide, like procainamide, reduces the differences in action potential duration between normal and infarcted tissue by lengthening the action potential of normal cells more than it lengthens the action potential of cells from infarcted regions of the heart.

Stereochemical properties influence the effects of disopyramide. Racemic (clinically used) and (+)-disopyramide prolong canine Purkinje fiber action potential, while (−)-disopyramide shortens it. The (+) isomer exerts approximately three times more vagolytic effects than does the (−) isomer. Disopyramide, as a muscarinic blocker, can speed the sinus nodal discharge rate and shorten AV nodal conduction time and refractoriness when the nodes are restrained by cholinergic influences. Disopyramide also can slow the sinus nodal discharge rate by a direct action when given in high concentration and can significantly depress sinus nodal activity in patients with sinus node dysfunction. Disopyramide exerts greater anticholinergic effects than quinidine and does not appear to affect alpha- or beta-adrenoceptors.

Atrial and ventricular refractory periods increase, as do conduction time and refractoriness of the accessory pathway in patients with the Wolff-Parkinson-White syndrome. Disopyramide's effect on AV nodal conduction and refractoriness in vivo is not consistent. Disopyramide prolongs His-Purkinje conduction time, but infra-His block results infrequently. Disopyramide can be administered safely to patients who have first degree AV block and narrow QRS complexes.

HEMODYNAMIC EFFECTS. Disopyramide administered intravenously reduces systemic blood pressure and cardiac and stroke index and increases right atrial pressures and total peripheral resistance. Profound hemodynamic deterioration can occur, and patients who have abnormal ventricular function tolerate the negative inotropic effects of IV and oral disopyramide quite poorly. In these patients, the drug should be used with extreme caution or not at all.

PHARMACOKINETICS (Table 21–1). Disopyramide is 80 to 90 per cent absorbed, with a mean elimination half-life of 8 to 9 hours in healthy volunteers but almost 10 hours in patients with heart failure and sometimes longer in some patients with ventricular arrhythmias. Total-body clearance and volume of distribution decrease in patients, and mean serum concentration is higher than reported in normal subjects. Renal insufficiency prolongs the elimination time. Thus, in patients who have renal, hepatic, or cardiac insufficiency, loading and maintenance doses need to be reduced. Peak blood levels after oral administration result in 1 to 2 hours, and bioavailability exceeds 80 per cent. The fraction of disopyramide bound to serum protein varies inversely with the total plasma concentration of the drug but may be more stable (30 to 40 per cent) at clinically relevant concentrations of 3 μg/ml. It is bound to α1-acid glycoprotein and passes through the placenta. About half an oral dose is recovered unchanged in the urine, with about 30 per cent as the mono-N-dealkylated metabolite. The metabolites appear to exert less effect than the parent compound. Erythromycin inhibits its metabolism.[56]

DOSAGE AND ADMINISTRATION (Table 21–1). Doses are generally 100 to 200 mg orally every 6 hours with a range of 400 to 1200 mg/day. A controlled-release preparation can be given as 200 to 300 mg every 12 hours. The intravenous (investigational) dose is 1 to 2 mg/kg as an initial bolus given over 5 to 10 minutes, which may be followed by an infusion of 1 mg/kg/h.

INDICATIONS. Disopyramide appears comparable to quinidine and procainamide in reducing the frequency of premature ventricular complexes and effectively preventing recurrence of ventricular tachycardia in selected patients. Disopyramide has been combined with other drugs such as mexiletine to treat patients who do not respond or only partially respond to one drug.

Disopyramide terminates and prevents recurrent episodes of paroxysmal supraventricular tachycardia due to AV and AV nodal reentry. It prolongs the anterograde and retrograde refractory period of the accessory pathway in patients with the Wolff-Parkinson-White syndrome, helps prevent recurrence of atrial fibrillation after successful cardioversion as effectively as quinidine, and may terminate atrial flutter. In treating patients with atrial fibrillation, and particularly atrial flutter, the ventricular rate must be controlled prior to administering disopyramide, or the atrial rate may decrease sufficiently, aided by the vagolytic effects of disopyramide, to create 1:1 conduction during atrial flutter. Disopyramide may be useful in preventing inducible and spontaneous neurally mediated syncope.

ADVERSE EFFECTS. Three categories of adverse effects follow disopyramide administration. The most common relates to the drug's potent parasympatholytic properties and includes urinary hesitancy or retention, constipation, blurred vision, closed-angle glaucoma, and dry mouth. Symptoms may be minimized by concomitant administration of pyridostigmine. Second, disopyramide can produce ventricular tachyarrhythmias that are commonly associated

with Q-T prolongation and torsades de pointes. Some patients can have "cross-sensitivity" to both quinidine and disopyramide and develop torsades de pointes while receiving either drug. When drug-induced torsades de pointes occurs, agents that prolong the Q-T interval should be used very cautiously or not at all. Finally, disopyramide can reduce contractility of the normal ventricle, but the depression of ventricular function is much more pronounced in patients with preexisting ventricular failure. Occasionally, cardiovascular collapse can result.

CLASS IB ANTIARRHYTHMIC AGENTS

Lidocaine

ELECTROPHYSIOLOGICAL ACTIONS (Tables 21–6 and 21–7). Lidocaine blocks I_{Na}, predominantly in the open or possibly inactivated state.[57] It has rapid onset and offset kinetics and does not affect normal sinus nodal automaticity but does depress both normal and abnormal forms of automaticity, as well as early and late afterdepolarizations in Purkinje fibers in vitro. Lidocaine exhibits only a modest depressant effect on $\dot{V}_{max}$ and has no effect on maximal diastolic potential of normal muscle and specialized tissue in concentrations of about 1.5 μg/ml. However, faster rates of stimulation, reduced pH,[58] increased extracellular K^+ concentration, and reduced membrane potential—all changes that can result from ischemia—increase the ability of lidocaine to block I_{Na}. Lidocaine reduces the magnitude of the transient inward current responsible for some forms of afterdepolarizations. Intracellular calcium activity may be reduced because of the sodium-calcium exchange mechanism. Lidocaine can convert areas of unidirectional block into bidirectional block during ischemia and prevent development of ventricular fibrillation by preventing fragmentation of organized large wavefronts into heterogeneous wavelets. Lidocaine may be arrhythmogenic if it depresses conduction but not to the point of bidirectional block, but this does not appear to be an important clinical problem.

Lidocaine, except in very high concentrations, does *not* affect slow-channel-dependent action potentials despite its moderate suppression of the slow inward current. In fact, its depressant effect on electrical potentials from ischemic myocardium supports the notion that these ischemic potentials are depressed fast responses rather than slow responses. Lidocaine significantly reduces the action potential duration and the effective refractory period of Purkinje fibers and ventricular muscle due to blocking of tetrodotoxin-sensitive sodium channels, and decreasing entry of sodium into the cell. It has little effect on atrial fibers and does not affect conduction in accessory pathways. In some in vitro preparations, lidocaine can improve conduction by hyperpolarizing tissues depolarized as a result of stretch or low external potassium concentration.

In vivo, lidocaine has a minimal effect on automaticity or conduction except in unusual circumstances. Patients with preexisting sinus nodal dysfunction, abnormal His-Purkinje conduction, or junctional or ventricular escape rhythms may develop depressed automaticity or conduction. Part of its effects may be to inhibit cardiac sympathetic nerve activity.

HEMODYNAMIC EFFECTS. Clinically significant adverse hemodynamic effects are rarely noted at usual drug concentrations unless left ventricular function is severely impaired.

PHARMACOKINETICS (Table 21–1). Lidocaine is used only parenterally because oral administration results in extensive first-pass hepatic metabolism and unpredictable, low plasma levels with excessive metabolites that can produce toxicity. Hepatic metabolism of lidocaine depends greatly on hepatic blood flow, so clearance of this drug almost equals (and can be approximated by) measurements of this flow. Severe hepatic disease or reduced hepatic blood flow, as in heart failure or shock, can markedly decrease the rate of lidocaine metabolism. Beta-adrenoceptor blockers can decrease hepatic blood flow and increase lidocaine serum concentration. Prolonged infusion can reduce lidocaine clearance. Its elimination half-life averages about 1 to 2 hours in normal subjects, more than 4 hours in patients after relatively uncomplicated myocardial infarction, more than 10 hours in patients after myocardial infarction complicated by cardiac failure, and even longer in the presence of cardiogenic shock. Maintenance doses should be reduced by one-third to one-half for patients with low cardiac output. Lidocaine is 50 to 80 per cent protein-bound and binds to α1-acid glycoprotein, which may increase in heart failure and myocardial infarction. Intravenous infusions should be discontinued as far in advance of electrophysiological studies as possible to avoid residual lidocaine effects. A two-compartment model accurately predicts serum concentrations.[59]

DOSAGE AND ADMINISTRATION (Table 21–1). Although lidocaine can be given intramuscularly, the intravenous route is most commonly used (Fig. 21–4). Intramuscular lidocaine is given in doses of 4 to 5 mg/kg (250 to 350 mg), resulting in effective serum levels at about 15 minutes and lasting for about 90 minutes. Intravenously, lidocaine is given as an initial bolus of 1 to 2 mg/kg of body weight at a rate of approximately 20 to 50 mg/min, with a second injection of one-half the initial dose 20 to 40 minutes later. Patients treated with an initial bolus followed by a maintenance infusion may experience transient subtherapeutic plasma concentrations at 30 to 120 minutes after initiation of therapy. A second bolus of about 0.5 mg/kg without increasing the maintenance infusion rate reestablishes therapeutic serum concentrations.

If recurrence of arrhythmia appears after a steady state

has been achieved (e.g., 6 to 10 hours after starting therapy), a similar bolus should be given and the maintenance infusion rate increased. Increasing the maintenance infusion rate alone without an additional bolus results in a very slow increase in plasma lidocaine concentrations, reaching a new plateau in over 6 hours (four elimination half-lives), and is therefore not recommended. Another recommended intravenous dosing is 1.5 mg/kg initially and 0.8 mg/kg at 8-minute intervals for three doses. Doses are reduced by about 50 per cent for patients with heart failure.

If the initial bolus of lidocaine is ineffective, up to two more boluses of 1 mg/kg may be administered at 5-minute intervals. Patients who require more than one bolus to achieve a therapeutic effect have arrhythmias that respond only to higher lidocaine plasma concentrations, and a greater maintenance dose may be necessary to sustain these higher concentrations. Patients requiring only a single initial bolus of lidocaine should probably receive a maintenance infusion of 30 μg/kg/min, while those requiring two or three boluses may need infusions at 40 to 50 μg/kg/min.

Loading doses also may be administered by rapid infusion, and a constant-rate intravenous infusion may be used to maintain an effective concentration. Maintenance infusion rates in the range of 1 to 4 mg/min produce steady-state plasma levels of 1 to 5 μg/ml in patients with uncomplicated myocardial infarction, but these rates must be reduced during heart failure or shock because of concomitant reduced hepatic blood flow. A loading dose of approximately 75 mg followed by an initial infusion rate of 5.33 mg/min that declines exponentially to 2 mg/min with a half-life of 25 min also has been recommended.

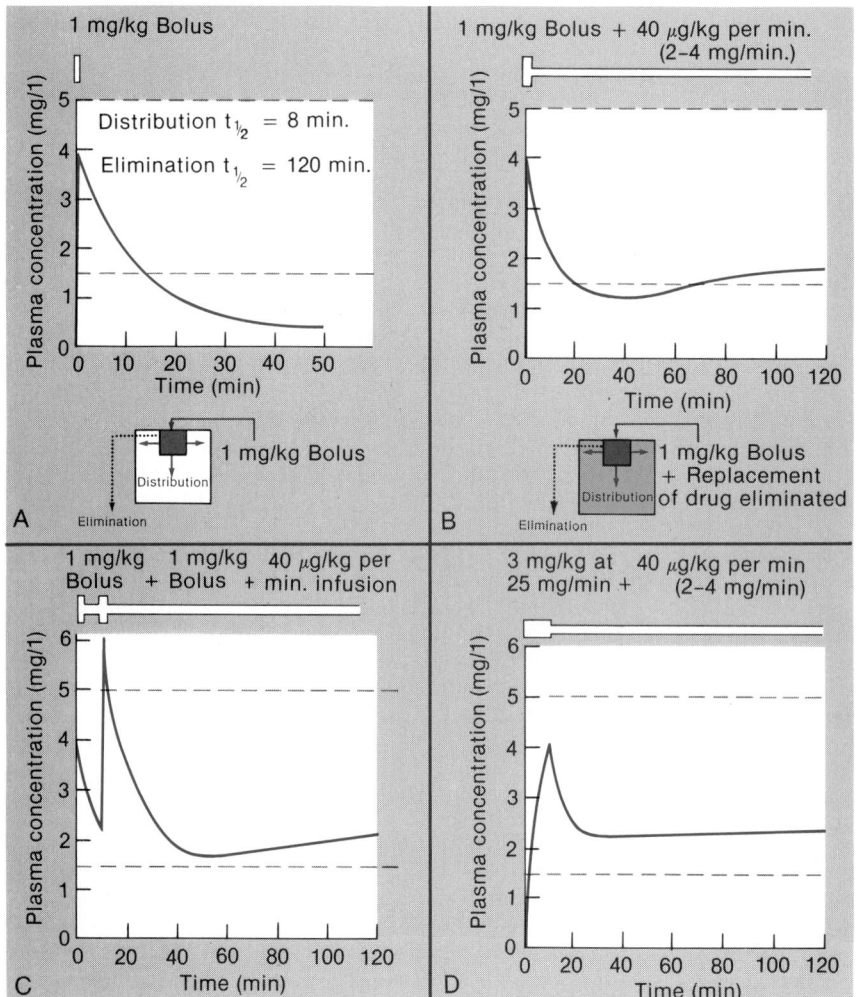

FIGURE 21–4. *A, Top,* Plasma concentrations after a bolus of lidocaine, with the therapeutic range indicated by a dashed line. *Bottom,* The disposition of the drug in the body, with the larger box indicating the total volume of distribution and the smaller box the central compartment. The bolus initially produces therapeutic lidocaine concentrations in the small central compartment. Rapid distribution of the drug to the rest of the body produces subtherapeutic concentrations within 15 minutes. *B,* Lidocaine is administered by an initial bolus as in *A,* with a maintenance infusion begun just after the bolus. The maintenance infusion replaces drug eliminated from the body, but drug is also lost from the central compartment by distribution, which is more rapid than elimination. As a result, plasma concentrations decrease transiently. In this instance, lidocaine concentration is subtherapeutic between 30 and 70 minutes after initiation of therapy. *C,* Subtherapeutic lidocaine concentrations after an initial bolus (as in *B*) can be prevented by giving a second lidocaine bolus 10 minutes after the first. A maintenance infusion should be started after the second bolus rather than after the first, as shown here. This will prevent excessive lidocaine concentrations after the second bolus. *D,* An alternative method to produce therapeutic lidocaine concentrations rapidly. This illustration indicates plasma concentrations after the administration of a loading dose of lidocaine given over 10 minutes. A maintenance infusion is begun after the loading dose has been given. (From Nattel, S., and Zipes, D. P.: Clinical pharmacology of old and new antiarrhythmic drugs. Cardiovasc. Clin. *11*:221, 1980.)

INDICATIONS. Lidocaine demonstrates efficacy against ventricular arrhythmias of diverse etiology, the ability to achieve effective plasma concentrations rapidly, and a fairly wide toxic-to-therapeutic ratio with a low incidence of hemodynamic complications and other side effects. However, its first-pass hepatic effect precludes oral use, and it is generally ineffective against supraventricular arrhythmias. In patients with the Wolff-Parkinson-White syndrome, for whom the effective refractory period of the accessory pathway is relatively short, lidocaine generally has no significant effect and may even accelerate the ventricular response during atrial fibrillation.

Lidocaine is used primarily for patients with acute myocardial infarction[60,61] or recurrent ventricular tachyarrhythmias. It has been effective in patients resuscitated from out-of-hospital ventricular fibrillation[62] and in patients after coronary revascularization.[63] Lidocaine prophylaxis in patients with acute myocardial infarction is controversial. However, most data suggest that the benefits of prophylactic lidocaine therapy in reducing the incidence of ventricular fibrillation in hospitalized patients who have had acute myocardial infarction have not been clearly established[60,61] (see p. 1248). Drug-induced side effects and a possible increase in the risk of developing asystole lead to the conclusion that prophylaxis is probably not indicated for all patients. Subcutaneous lidocaine can affect inducibility of ventricular arrhythmias by programed electrical stimulation.[64]

ADVERSE EFFECTS. The most commonly reported adverse effects of lidocaine are dose-related manifestations of central nervous system toxicity: dizziness, paresthesias, confusion, delirium, stupor, coma, and seizures.[65] Occasional sinus node depression and His-Purkinje block have been reported. In patients with atrial tachyarrhythmias, ventricular rate acceleration has been noted. Rarely, lidocaine can cause malignant hyperthermia.[66] Both lidocaine and procainamide can elevate defibrillation thresholds.[67]

Mexiletine

Mexiletine, a local anesthetic congener of lidocaine with anticonvulsant properties, is used for oral treatment of patients with symptomatic ventricular arrhythmias.

ELECTROPHYSIOLOGICAL ACTIONS (Table 21–6 and 21–7). Mexiletine is similar to lidocaine in many of its electrophysiological actions. In vitro, mexiletine shortens the duration of the action potential and refractory period of Purkinje fibers and to a lesser extent of ventricular muscle. It depresses $\dot{V}_{max}$ of phase 0 by blocking I_{Na}, especially at faster rates, and depresses automaticity of Purkinje fibers but not of the normal sinus node. Its onset and offset kinetics are rapid. Hypoxia or ischemia can increase its effects on $\dot{V}_{max}$.

Mexiletine can result in severe bradycardia and abnormal sinus nodal recovery time in patients with sinus node disease but not in patients with a normal sinus node. It does not affect AV nodal conduction and can depress His-Purkinje conduction, but not greatly, unless conduction was abnormal initially. Mexiletine does not appear to affect the refractory period of human atrial and ventricular muscle. The duration of the Q-T interval does not increase. Because of its rate-dependent effects, theoretically, mexiletine might be expected to suppress closely coupled rather than late coupled ventricular extrasystoles or faster tachycardias.

HEMODYNAMIC EFFECTS. Mexiletine exerts no major hemodynamic effects. It does not depress myocardial performance when given orally, although intravenous administration can produce hypotension.

PHARMACOKINETICS. Mexiletine has been reported to be rapidly and almost completely absorbed after oral ingestion by volunteers, with peak plasma concentrations attained in 2 to 4 hours. Elimination half-life in healthy subjects is approximately 10 hours and in patients after myocardial

infarction, 17 hours. Therapeutic plasma levels of 1 to 2 μg/ml are maintained by oral doses of 200 to 300 mg every 6 to 8 hours. Absorption with less than 10 per cent first-pass hepatic effect occurs in the upper small intestine and is delayed and incomplete in patients who have myocardial infarction and in patients receiving narcotic analgesics, antacids, or atropine-like drugs that retard gastric emptying. Bioavailability of orally administered mexiletine is approximately 90 per cent, and about 70 per cent of the drug is protein-bound. The apparent volume of distribution is large, reflecting extensive tissue uptake. Normally, mexiletine is eliminated metabolically by the liver, with less than 10 per cent excreted unchanged in the urine. Doses probably should be reduced in patients with cirrhosis and those with left ventricular failure. Renal clearance of mexiletine decreases as urinary pH increases. Known metabolites exert no electrophysiological effects. Metabolism can be increased by phenytoin, phenobarbital, and rifampin and reduced by cimetidine. It is influenced by the genotype for the CYP206 gene.[3]

DOSAGE AND ADMINISTRATION. Recommended starting dose is 200 mg orally every 8 hours when rapid arrhythmia control is not essential. Doses may be increased or decreased by 50 to 100 mg every 2 to 3 days and are better tolerated when given with food. Total daily dose should not exceed 1200 mg. In some patients, administration every 12 hours can be effective. For rapid loading, 400 mg followed in 8 hours by a 200-mg dose is suggested.

INDICATIONS. Mexiletine is an effective antiarrhythmic agent for treating patients with both acute and chronic ventricular tachyarrhythmias but not with supraventricular tachycardias. Success rates vary from 6 to 60 per cent and can be increased in some patients if mexiletine is combined with other drugs such as procainamide, beta blockers, quinidine, disopyramide, or amiodarone. Most studies show no clear superiority of mexiletine over other class I agents. In the Electrophysiologic Study Versus Electrocardiographic Monitoring (ESVEM) investigation, sotalol was more effective than mexiletine.[68,69] It may be very useful in children with congenital heart disease and serious ventricular arrhythmias. In treating patients with a long Q-T interval, mexiletine probably would be safer than drugs such as quinidine that increase the Q-T interval further. It does not appear to alter the prognosis of patients with inducible ventricular tachyarrhythmias after myocardial infarction. It may be effectively combined with propafenone.[70,71] Mexiletine does not alter late potentials.[72]

ADVERSE EFFECTS. Thirty to 40 per cent of patients may require a change in dose or discontinuation of mexiletine therapy as a result of adverse effects, including tremor, dysarthria, dizziness, paresthesia, diplopia, nystagmus, mental confusion, anxiety, nausea, vomiting, and dyspepsia. Cardiovascular side effects are seen most often after intravenous dosing and include hypotension, bradycardia, and exacerbation of arrhythmia. Adverse effects of mexiletine appear to be dose-related, and toxic effects occur at plasma concentrations only slightly higher than therapeutic levels. Therefore, effective use of this antiarrhythmic drug requires careful titration of dose and monitoring of plasma concentration. Lidocaine should be avoided, or dose reduced, in patients also receiving lidocaine congeners like mexiletine.[73]

Tocainide

Tocainide is a primary amine analog of lidocaine that lacks two ethyl groups; this characteristic protects it from first-pass hepatic elimination and makes it effective orally.

ELECTROPHYSIOLOGICAL AND HEMODYNAMIC ACTIONS (Tables 21–6 and 21–7). Electrophysiological effects are virtually the same as those exerted by lidocaine and mexiletine. It has a small negative inotropic effect and increases peripheral vascular resistance slightly. Oral administration in patients after myocardial infarction does not appear to affect hemodynamic compensation adversely.

PHARMACOKINETICS. Bioavailability of tocainide is almost 100 per cent. The drug is rapidly and completely absorbed, yielding peak plasma concentrations 0.5 to 2 hours after oral ingestion. Approximately 40 per cent is excreted unchanged in the urine. Protein binding is 10 to 50 per cent, and there are no known active metabolites. Enantiomers may be more effective than the racemic mixture. Mean elimination half-life is 11 hours in normal volunteers, possibly longer in patients. There appears to be no pharmacokinetic interaction with other drugs, but caution must be used when combining drugs because of additive antiarrhythmic effects.

DOSAGE AND ADMINISTRATION. Oral regimens of 400 to 600 mg every 8 hours produce therapeutic plasma concentrations of 4 to 10 μg/ml. Dosing increases should not be made more often than every 3 or 4 days. Twice-daily doses can be tried in patients who respond to dosing three times a day. Doses should be reduced in patients with heart failure, or liver or renal disease.

INDICATIONS. Although tocainide effectively reduces the frequency of premature ventricular complexes, it has been less effective in preventing chronic recurrent ventricular tachycardia–ventricular fibrillation because of inefficacy and side effects. Tocainide and mexiletine may be acceptable choices for patients with ventricular arrhythmias in whom the Q-T interval is prolonged.

ADVERSE EFFECTS. Adverse effects are dose-related, similar to those produced by lidocaine, and include nausea, vomiting, anorexia, tremulousness, memory impairment, skin rash, sweating, paresthesia, diplopia, dizziness, anxiety, and tinnitus. Dosing with meals may reduce side effects, possibly by reducing peak serum concentrations of the drug. Occasionally, tocainide may produce pulmonary fibrosis or induce or aggravate ventricular arrhythmias. Hematological disorders including agranulocytosis, bone marrow depression, leukopenia, hypoplastic anemia, and thrombocytopenia have been reported with an estimated incidence of 0.18 per cent and may seriously limit the use of tocainide.[74]

Phenytoin (Diphenylhydantoin)

Phenytoin was employed originally to treat seizure disorders. Its value as an antiarrhythmic agent remains limited.

ELECTROPHYSIOLOGICAL ACTIONS (Tables 21–6 and 21–7). Therapeutic concentrations of phenytoin do not alter the discharge rate of rabbit sinus nodal tissue but may depress normal automaticity in cardiac Purkinje fibers in vitro or spontaneous ventricular rate in vivo. Phenytoin effectively abolishes abnormal automaticity caused by digitalis-induced delayed afterdepolarizations in cardiac Purkinje fibers and suppresses certain digitalis-induced arrhythmias in humans. Similar to lidocaine, phenytoin abbreviates Purkinje fiber action potential duration more than it shortens the effective refractory period, thus increasing the ratio of effective refractory period to action potential duration. Phenytoin can cause depolarized cells to repolarize by increasing potassium conductance and, in so doing, may increase the $\dot{V}_{max}$ of phase 0 in Purkinje fibers, particularly when these are depressed by digitalis.

The rate of rise of action potentials initiated early in the relative refractory period is increased, as is membrane responsiveness, possibly reducing the chance for impaired conduction and block. Phenytoin may slow conduction at high potassium concentrations but minimally affects sinus discharge rate and AV conduction in humans. As with other class IB agents, it has little effect on $\dot{V}_{max}$ in normally polarized fibers at slow rates and shows use dependence and rapid kinetics for onset and termination of effects.

Some of phenytoin's antiarrhythmic effects may be neurally mediated, since phenytoin may reduce the increase in impulse traffic in cardiac sympathetic nerves caused by ouabain toxicity and protect against some arrhythmias when it is injected into the central nervous system. The drug also may modulate vagal efferent activity centrally. It has no peripheral cholinergic or beta-adrenergic blocking actions.

Phenytoin exerts minimal *hemodynamic effects*.

PHARMACOKINETICS (Table 21–7). The pharmacokinetics of phenytoin are less than ideal. Absorption following oral administration is incomplete and varies with the brand of drug. Plasma concentrations peak 8 to 12 hours after an oral dose. Ninety per cent of the drug is protein-bound. Phenytoin has limited solubility at physiological pH,

and intramuscular administration is associated with pain, muscle necrosis, sterile abscesses, and variable absorption. Therapeutic serum concentrations of phenytoin (10 to 20 μg/ml) are similar for treating both cardiac arrhythmias and epilepsy. Lower concentrations can suppress certain digitalis-induced arrhythmias or other arrhythmias when decreased plasma protein binding occurs (as in uremia), since a larger fraction of drug is free and pharmacologically active.

METABOLISM. Over 90 per cent of a dose is hydroxylated in the liver to presumably inactive compounds. Some families have a genetically determined inability to hydroxylate phenytoin, while others have a higher than usual capability for hydroxylation. Elimination half-time is about 24 hours and can be slowed in the presence of liver disease or when phenytoin is administered concomitantly with drugs such as phenylbutazone, dicumarol, isoniazid, chloramphenicol, and phenothiazines that compete with phenytoin for hepatic enzymes (Table 21–2). Because of the large number of medications that can increase or decrease phenytoin levels during chronic therapy, phenytoin plasma concentration should be determined frequently when changes are made in other medications. In some patients, maintenance dose regimens of phenytoin are difficult to predict because the enzyme system that metabolizes phenytoin becomes saturated at plasma concentrations within the therapeutic range. The half-life then increases with increasing phenytoin load. Above the saturation point, phenytoin elimination follows zero-order kinetics, so only a fixed amount of drug is eliminated per unit time. These concentration-dependent kinetics for elimination can cause unexpected toxicity, since disproportionately large changes in plasma concentration can follow dose increases.

DOSAGE AND ADMINISTRATION (Table 21–7). To achieve therapeutic plasma concentration rapidly, 100 mg of phenytoin should be administered intravenously every 5 minutes until the arrhythmia is controlled, about 1 gm has been given, or adverse side effects result. Generally, 700 to 1000 mg will control the arrhythmia. A large central vein should be used to avoid pain and development of phlebitis produced by the severely alkalotic (pH 11.0) vehicle in which phenytoin is dissolved. Orally, phenytoin is given as a loading dose of approximately 1000 mg the first day, 500 mg on the second and third days, and 400 mg daily thereafter. All maintenance doses can be given once or twice daily, depending on the brand, because of the long half-life of elimination.

INDICATIONS. Phenytoin has been used successfully to treat atrial and ventricular arrhythmias caused by digitalis toxicity but is much less effective in treating ventricular arrhythmias in patients with ischemic heart disease or with atrial arrhythmias not due to digitalis toxicity. The drug has been somewhat more successful in treating ventricular arrhythmias associated with general anesthesia and cardiac surgery. It can be tried in patients with the long Q-T syndrome.

ADVERSE EFFECTS. The most common manifestations of phenytoin toxicity are central nervous system effects of nystagmus, ataxia, drowsiness, stupor, and coma. Progression of such symptoms can be correlated with increases in plasma drug concentration. Neurological signs, such as nystagmus on lateral gaze, develop at plasma drug levels of about 20 μg/ml. Nausea, epigastric pain, and anorexia are also relatively common effects of phenytoin. Long-term administration can result in hyperglycemia, hypocalcemia, skin rashes, megaloblastic anemia, gingival hypertrophy, lymph node hyperplasia (a syndrome resembling malignant lymphoma), peripheral neuropathy, pneumonitis,[75] and drug-induced systemic lupus erythematosus. Birth defects also can result.[76,77]

CLASS IC ANTIARRHYTHMIC AGENTS

Flecainide

Flecainide is approved by the FDA for the treatment of patients with life-threatening ventricular arrhythmias.

ELECTROPHYSIOLOGICAL ACTIONS. Flecainide exhibits marked use-dependent depressant effects on the rapid sodium channel,[78] decreasing $\dot{V}_{max}$ with slow onset and offset kinetics. Drug dissociation from the sodium channel is very slow, with time constants of 10 to 30 sec (compared with 4 to 8 sec for quinidine and <1 second for lidocaine). Marked drug effects occur at physiological heart rates. Flecainide shortens the duration of Purkinje fiber action potential but prolongs it in ventricular muscle, actions that, depending on the circumstances, could enhance or reduce electrical heterogeneity and create or suppress arrhythmias. Flecainide profoundly slows conduction in all cardiac fibers and, in high concentrations, inhibits the slow channel. Conduction time in the atria, ventricles, AV node, and His-Purkinje system is prolonged. It can terminate experimental atrial reentry by causing conduction block in the reentry pathway[79–81] and eliminate atrial tachycardia by producing exit block from the focus.[82] Flecainide also can promote reentry.[83] Minimal increases in atrial or ventricular refractoriness or in the Q-T interval result. Anterograde and retrograde refractoriness in accessory pathways can increase significantly in a use-dependent fashion.[84] Normal sinus node function remains unchanged, but abnormal sinus node discharge may be depressed. Pacing thresholds are increased.

HEMODYNAMIC EFFECTS. Flecainide depresses cardiac performance, particularly in patients with compromised myocardial function. Left ventricular ejection fraction decreases after oral (single dose of 200 to 250 mg) or intravenous (1 mg) administration. Caution is warranted, particularly in patients with a history of heart failure. Flecainide should be used cautiously, if at all, in patients with severely compromised cardiac function.

PHARMACOKINETICS. Flecainide is at least 90 per cent absorbed with peak plasma concentrations in 3 to 4 hours. Elimination half-life in patients with ventricular arrhythmias is 20 hours, 85 per cent of the drug being excreted unchanged or as an inactive metabolite in urine. Two major metabolites exert fewer effects than the parent drug. Rate of elimination is slower in patients with renal disease and heart failure, and doses should be reduced in these situations. Therapeutic plasma concentrations range from 0.2 to 1.0 μg/ml. About 40 per cent of the drug is protein-bound. Increases in serum concentrations of digoxin (15 to 25 per cent) and propranolol (30 per cent) result during coadministration with flecainide. Propranolol, quinidine, and amiodarone may increase flecainide serum concentrations. Five to 7 days of dosing may be required to reach steady-state in some patients.

DOSAGE AND ADMINISTRATION. Starting dose is 100 mg every 12 hours, increased in increments of 50 mg twice daily, no sooner than every 3 to 4 days, until efficacy is achieved, an adverse effect is noted, or to a maximum of 400 mg/day. Cardiac rhythm and QRS duration should be monitored.

INDICATIONS. Flecainide is indicated for the treatment of life-threatening ventricular tachyarrhythmias.[85,86] Therapy should begin in the hospital while the ECG is being monitored because of the high incidence of proarrhythmic events (see below). Serum concentration should not exceed 1.0 μg/ml. Flecainide is particularly effective, more so than quinidine, in almost totally suppressing premature ventricular complexes and short runs of nonsustained ventricular tachycardia, although the importance of such a response on the subsequent outcome of the patient has not been established. As with other class I antiarrhythmic drugs, there are no data from controlled studies to indicate that the drug favorably affects survival or sudden cardiac death. Flecainide prevents electrical induction of ventricular tachyarrhythmias in a small percentage of patients (10 to 30 per cent) and eliminates recurrence of life-threatening ventricular tachyarrhythmias in about 40 per cent. However, it produces a use-dependent prolongation of ventricular tachycardia cycle length that improves hemodynamic tolerance.[86]

Flecainide may be very useful in a variety of supraventricular tachycardias,[87-90] such as atrial flutter[91] and atrial fibrillation,[87,92-94] in Wolff-Parkinson-White syndrome,[95] and for atrial tachycardia.[96] Flecainide may be more effective than procainamide in the acute termination of atrial fibrillation.[87] It is important to slow the ventricular rate before treating with flecainide to avoid 1:1 conduction.[97] Isoproterenol can reverse some of these effects. Flecainide has been used to treat fetal arrhythmias[98,99] and arrhythmias in children.[100] It may increase defibrillation thresholds.[101]

ADVERSE EFFECTS. Proarrhythmic effects are one of the most important adverse effects of flecainide. Its marked slowing of conduction precludes its use in patients with second degree AV block without a pacemaker and warrants

cautious administration in patients with intraventricular conduction disorders. Aggravation of existing ventricular arrhythmias or onset of new ventricular arrhythmias can occur in 5 to 30 per cent of patients, the increased percentage in patients with preexisting sustained ventricular tachycardia, cardiac decompensation, and higher doses of the drug. Failure of the flecainide-related arrhythmia to respond to therapy, including electrical cardioversion-defibrillation, may result in a mortality as high as 10 per cent in patients who develop proarrhythmic events. Negative inotropic effects can cause or worsen heart failure. Patients with sinus node dysfunction may experience sinus arrest, and those with pacemakers may develop an increase in pacing threshold. In the Cardiac Arrhythmia Suppression Trial, patients treated with flecainide had 5.1 per cent mortality or nonfatal cardiac arrest compared with 2.3 per cent in the placebo group over 10 months.[34] Mortality was highest in those with non-Q-wave infarction, frequent premature ventricular complexes, and faster heart rates, raising the possibility of drug interaction with ischemia and electrical instability.[35,102,103] Exercise can amplify the conduction slowing in the ventricle produced by flecainide and in some cases can precipitate a proarrhythmic response. Therefore, exercise testing has been recommended to screen for proarrhythmia. Central nervous system complaints, including confusion and irritability, represent the most frequent noncardiac adverse effect.

Propafenone

Propafenone has been approved by the FDA for treatment of patients with life-threatening ventricular tachyarrhythmias.

ELECTROPHYSIOLOGICAL ACTIONS (Tables 21–6 and 21–7). Propafenone blocks the fast sodium current in a use-dependent manner, as well as at rest, in Purkinje fibers and to a lesser degree in ventricular muscle. Use-dependent effects contribute to its ability to terminate experimental atrial fibrillation.[104] The dissociation constant is slow, like that of flecainide. Effects are greater in ischemic than normal tissue and at reduced membrane potentials. Propafenone decreases excitability and suppresses spontaneous automaticity and triggered activity. It terminates experimental ventricular tachycardia by producing conduction block or by collision of the impulse with an echo wave.[105] Effects on action potential duration are variable in that guinea pig action potential duration is shortened, while rabbit action potential duration is prolonged. Although ventricular refractoriness increases, conduction slowing is the major effect. The active metabolites of propafenone exert important actions, reducing $\dot{V}_{max}$, action potential amplitude, and duration in canine Purkinje fibers. In contrast to propafenone and the N-depropylpropafenone metabolite, the 5-hydroxy-propafenone metabolite suppressed ventricular tachycardia in the postinfarct canine model. Propafenone depresses sinus nodal automaticity. In patients, the A-H, H-V, P-R, and QRS intervals increase, as do refractory periods of the atria, ventricles, AV node, and accessory pathways. The corrected Q-T interval increases only as a function of increased QRS duration.

HEMODYNAMIC EFFECTS. Propafenone and 5-hydroxypropafenone exhibit negative inotropic properties at high concentrations in vitro, and large doses depress left ventricular function in vivo.[106] In patients with ejection fractions exceeding 40 per cent, the negative inotropic effects are well tolerated, but patients with preexisting left ventricular dysfunction and congestive heart failure may have symptomatic worsening of their hemodynamic status.

PHARMACOKINETICS. With more than 95 per cent of the drug absorbed, propafenone's maximum plasma concentration occurs in 2 to 3 hours. Systemic bioavailability is dose-dependent and ranges from 3 to 40 per cent due to variable presystemic clearance. Bioavailability increases as the dose increases, and plasma concentration is therefore nonlinear. A threefold increase in dosage (300 to 900 mg/day) results in a tenfold increase in plasma concentration, presumably due to saturation of hepatic metabolic mechanisms. Propafenone is 97 per cent bound to α1-acid glycoprotein with an elimination half-life of 5 to 8 hours. Maximum therapeutic effects occur at serum concentrations of 0.2 to 1.5 μg/ml. Marked interpatient variability of pharmacokinetics and pharmacodynamics may be due to genetically determined differences in metabolism. About 93 per cent of the population are extensive metabolizers and exhibit shorter elimination half-lives (5 to 6 hours), lower plasma concentrations of the parent compound, and higher concentrations of metabolites. Poor metabolizers, due to diminished capacity of the microsomal cytochrome P450 enzyme system in the liver (see earlier), exhibit an elimination half-life of 15 to 20 hours for the parent compound and virtually no 5-hydroxypropafenone.[3] Low-dose quinidine may inhibit the metabolism of propafenone, and stereoselectivity may be important with the (+)-enantiomer, providing nonspecific beta-adrenergic receptor blockade approximately 2.5 to 5 per cent the potency of propranolol. Poor metabolizers have a greater beta-adrenergic receptor blocking effect than extensive metabolizers. Since plasma propafenone concentrations may be 50 times or more propranolol levels, these beta-blocking properties may be relevant.[107] Propafenone also blocks the slow calcium channel to a degree about 100 times less than verapamil.

DOSAGE AND ADMINISTRATION. Most patients respond to oral doses of 150 to 300 mg every 8 hours, not exceeding 1200 mg/day. Doses are similar for both patients of both phenotypes. Concomitant food administration increases bioavailability, as does hepatic dysfunction. No good correlation between plasma propafenone concentration and arrhythmia suppression has been shown. Doses should not be increased more often than every 3 to 4 days. Propafenone increases plasma concentrations of warfarin, digoxin, and metoprolol.

INDICATIONS. Propafenone is indicated for the treatment of life-threatening ventricular tachyarrhythmias and effectively suppresses spontaneous premature ventricular complexes[108] and nonsustained and sustained ventricular tachycardia.[109] Spontaneous sinus rate during exercise is reduced. Although propafenone has not been approved by the FDA for treatment of patients with supraventricular tachycardias, the drug is effective in patients with atrial tachycardia,[109,110] AV nodal reentry, AV reentry,[111] and atrial flutter[112] or fibrillation.[108,113–116] It has been used effectively in the pediatric age group.[117–120] Propafenone increases the pacing threshold[121,122] but minimally affects the defibrillation threshold. Propafenoul is associated with a higher mortality in cardiac arrest survivors compared with an implantable defibrillator.[124] Sotalol was less effective than propafenone in the ESVEM trial.[68] Propafenone has been combined effectively with mexiletine.[70,71]

ADVERSE EFFECTS. Minor noncardiac effects occur in about 15 per cent of patients, with dizziness, disturbances in taste, and blurred vision the most common and gastrointestinal side effects next. Exacerbation of bronchospastic lung disease can occur. Cardiovascular side effects occur in 10 to 15 per cent of patients, including conduction abnormalities such as AV block, sinus node depression, and worsening of heart failure. Proarrhythmic responses, more often in patients with a history of sustained ventricular tachycardia and decreased ejection fractions, appear less commonly than with flecainide and may be in the range of 5 per cent. The applicability of data from the Cardiac Arrhythmic Suppression Trial about flecainide to propafenone is not clear, but limiting propafenone's application in a manner similar to other IC drugs seems prudent at present until more information is available. Its beta-blocking actions may make it different, however.[107]

Moricizine HCl (Ethmozine)

Moricizine HCl is a phenothiazine derivative used for treatment of patients with ventricular tachyarrhythmias. It was formerly discussed as a IB antiarrhythmic drug because it shortens Purkinje fiber action potential. However, the intensity of its effect on the Na^+ channel is more like that of a IA antiarrhythmic drug, while the time constants for onset and offset resemble those of class IC agents.

ELECTROPHYSIOLOGICAL ACTIONS. Moricizine decreases I_{Na} predominantly in the inactivated state, with a resultant decrease in $\dot{V}_{max}$ of phase 0, action potential amplitude, and action potential duration in canine cardiac Purkinje fibers (Tables 21–6 and 21–7). Maximum diastolic potential is not changed. Moricizine blocks I_{Ca-L} and I_K and prolongs AV nodal and His-Purkinje conduction time and QRS duration. The J-T interval shortens slightly, while the Q-T$_c$ prolongs <5 per cent due to QRS prolongation. Ventricular refractoriness prolongs slightly with no consistent atrial change. No alterations in sinus node automaticity result. In vitro, moricizine slows spontaneous automaticity in normal Purkinje fibers and suppresses abnormal automaticity arising from depolarized fibers and delayed afterdepolarizations. It terminates experimental flutter by causing block in the area of slow conduction.[126] Moricizine decreases R-R interval variability, which does not predict mortality.[127] Moricizine minimally raises the defibrillation threshold.[128]

HEMODYNAMIC EFFECTS. Moricizine exerts minimal effects on cardiac performance in patients with impaired left ventricular function. Exercise tolerance and ejection fraction do not change. A small but consistent increase in blood pressure and heart rate results. An occasional patient with significant left ventricular dysfunction may have worsening of heart failure.

PHARMACOKINETICS. Following oral ingestion, moricizine undergoes extensive first-pass metabolism resulting in absolute bioavailability of 35 to 40 per cent. Peak plasma concentrations are reached in 0.5 to 2 hours and later if the drug is taken after meals. Extent of absorption is not changed. Proportionality exists between dose and plasma concentrations in the therapeutic range. Protein binding is 95 per cent to α1-acid glycoprotein and albumin. Antiarrhythmic and electrophysiological actions do not relate to plasma concentrations or to any identified metabolite, of which there are more than 20. At least two metabolites are pharmacologically active but are in small concentrations. Moricizine induces its own metabolism,[129] and plasma concentrations decrease with multiple dosing. Plasma elimination half-life is 1.5 to 3.5 hours, with slightly more than half the drug excreted in the feces and slightly less than half excreted in the urine.

DOSAGE AND ADMINISTRATION. The usual adult dose is 600 to 900 mg/day, given every 8 hours in three equally divided doses. Increments of 150 mg/day at 3-day intervals can be tried. Some patients may be treated every 12 hours. Dose reductions in patients with hepatic or neural disease, AV conduction disturbances, or sick sinus syndrome without a pacemaker and with significant congestive heart failure should be observed.

INDICATIONS. Moricizine exerts an efficacy that is about comparable with those of quinidine and disopyramide.[130] It is less effective in preventing ventricular tachycardia initiation at electrophysiological study and may have proarrhythmic effects. It caused an increase in mortality compared with placebo during initial treatment of patients who had symptomatic or minimally symptomatic ventricular arrhythmias after myocardial infarction[35,134] (see p. 677). Risk was greater in patients taking diuretics.[36]

ADVERSE EFFECTS. Usually the drug is well tolerated. Noncardiac adverse effects primarily involve the nervous system and include tremor, mood changes, headache, vertigo, nystagmus, and dizziness. Gastrointestinal side effects include nausea, vomiting, and diarrhea. Worsening of congestive heart failure is uncommon but can happen. Proarrhythmic effects have been reported in about 3 to 15 per cent of patients[135,136] and appear to be more common in patients with severe ventricular arrhythmias. Advancing age increases the susceptibility to adverse effects.[137]

CLASS II ANTIARRHYTHMIC AGENTS

Beta-Adrenoceptor Blocking Agents

Although many beta-adrenoceptor blockings drugs have been approved for use in the United States (see Table 21–8), acebutolol (PVCs), esmolol (SVT), metoprolol (post-myocardial infarction), atenolol (post-myocardial infarction), propranolol (post-myocardial infarction, SVT, ventricular tachycardia [VT]), and timolol (post-myocardial infarction) have been approved to treat arrhythmias or to prevent sudden death after myocardial infarction.[138] While it is generally considered that no beta blocker offers distinct advantages over the others and that, when titrated to

TABLE 21–8 PHARMACODYNAMIC PROPERTIES OF BETA-ADRENOCEPTOR BLOCKING DRUGS

DRUG	β_2-BLOCKADE POTENCY RATIO (PROPRANOLOL = 1.0)	RELATIVE β_2-SELECTIVITY	INTRINSIC SYMPATHOMIMETIC ACTIVITY	CLASS I ACTIVITY
Acebutolol	0.3	+	+	+
Atenolol	1.0	++	0	0
Bevantolol	0.3	++	0	0
Bisoprolol	10.3	++	0	0
Bucindolol*		0	+	0
Carteolol	10.0	0	+	0
Carvedilol†	10.0	0	0	++
Celiprolol‡	9.4	+	+	0
Dilevalol§	1.0	0	+	0
Esmolol	0.02	++	0	0
Labetalol*	0.3	0	+	0
Metoprolol	1.0	++	0	0
Nadolol	1.0	0	0	0
Oxprenolol	0.5–1.0	0	+	+
Penbutolol	1.0	0	+	0
Pindolol	6.0	0	++	+
Propranolol	1.0	0	0	++
Sotalol¶	0.3	0	0	0
Timolol	6.0	0	0	0

* Bucinodolol and labetalol have additional α_1-adrenergic blocking activity and direct vasodilatory actions (β_2-agonism).
† Carvedilol has additional α_1-adrenergic blocking activity without peripheral β_2-agonism.
‡ Celiprolol may have additional peripheral α_2-adrenergic blocking activity at high doses.
§ Dilevalol is an isomer of labetalol adrenergic with peripheral β_2-agonism but no α_1-blocking activity.
¶ Sotalol has an additional type of antiarrhythmic activity.
Adapted from Duran, A., and Myerburg, R. J.: In Singh, B. N., et al. (eds.): Cardiovascular Pharmacology and Therapeutics. New York, Churchill Livingstone, 1994, pp. 665–674.

the proper dose, all can be used effectively to treat cardiac arrhythmias, hypertension, or other disorders, differences in pharmacokinetic or pharmacodynamic properties that confer safety, reduce adverse effects, or affect dosing intervals or drug interactions influence the choice of agent. Also, some beta blockers such as sotalol exert unique actions.

Beta receptors can be separated into those that affect predominantly the heart (beta$_1$) or the bronchi and those that affect predominantly blood vessels (beta$_2$). In low doses, selective beta blockers can block beta$_1$ receptors more than they block beta$_2$ receptors and might be preferable for treating patients with pulmonary or peripheral vascular diseases. In high doses, the selective beta$_1$ blockers also block beta$_2$ receptors.

Some beta blockers exert intrinsic sympathomimetic activity; i.e., they slightly activate the beta receptor. These drugs appear to be as efficacious as beta blockers without intrinsic sympathomimetic actions and may cause less slowing of heart rate at rest and less prolongation of AV nodal conduction time. They have been shown to induce less depression of left ventricular function than beta blockers without intrinsic sympathomimetic activity. Only nonselective beta blockers without intrinsic sympathomimetic activity have been demonstrated to reduce mortality in patients after myocardial infarction[138a] (Fig. 21–5).

The following discussion will concentrate on the use of propranolol as a prototypical antiarrhythmic agent.

ELECTROPHYSIOLOGICAL ACTIONS. Beta blockers exert an electrophysiological action by competitively inhibiting catecholamine binding at beta-adrenoceptor sites, an effect almost entirely due to the (−) levorotatory stereoisomer, or by their quinidine-like or direct membrane-stabilizing action (Tables 21–6 and 21–7). The latter is a local anesthetic effect that depresses I_{Na} and membrane responsiveness in cardiac Purkinje fibers, occurs at concentrations generally 10 times that necessary to produce beta blockade, and most likely plays an insignificant antiarrhythmic role. Thus major effects of beta blockers will take place in cells most actively stimulated by adrenergic actions. At beta-blocking concentrations, propranolol slows spontaneous automaticity in the sinus node or in Purkinje fibers that are being stimulated by adrenergic tone, producing block of I_f. Beta

blockers also block I_{Ca-L} stimulated by beta-agonists. In the absence of adrenergic stimulation, only high concentrations of propranolol slow normal automaticity in Purkinje fibers, probably by a direct membrane action.

Concentrations that cause beta-receptor blockade but no local anesthetic effects do not alter the normal resting membrane potential, maximum diastolic potential amplitude, $\dot{V}_{max}$, repolarization, or refractoriness of atrial, Purkinje, or ventricular muscle cells when these tissues are not being superfused with catecholamines. However, in the presence of isoproterenol, a pure beta-receptor stimulator, beta blockers reverse isoproterenol's accelerating effects on repolarization; in the presence of norepinephrine, beta blockade permits unopposed alpha-adrenoceptor stimulation to prolong action potential duration in Purkinje fibers.

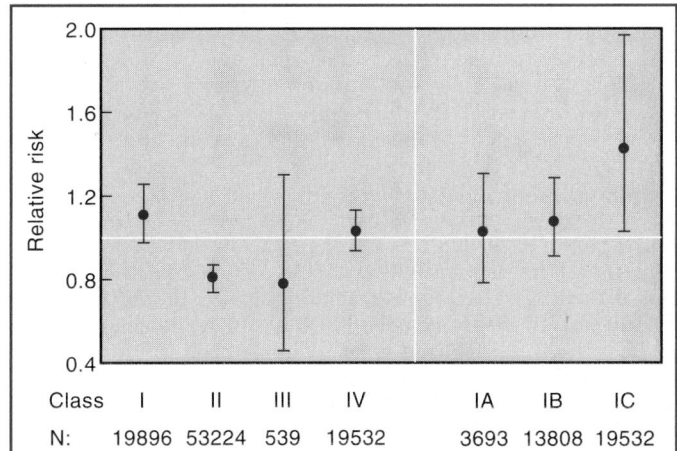

FIGURE 21–5. Meta-analytical data from randomized clinical trials of antiarrhythmic drugs in survivors of acute myocardial infarction. The relative risk is compared with placebo therapy (mean and 95 per cent confidence interval) for death during therapy with various electrophysiological classes of compounds. Class IA agents, particularly IC, increase mortality, while beta blockers and class III agents (essentially amiodarone) decrease mortality. (Data from Teo, K. K., and Yusuf, S. In Singh, B. N., et al. [eds.]: Cardiovascular Pharmacology and Therapeutics. New York, Churchill-Livingstone, 1994, pp. 631–643.)

Propranolol (2×10^{-6} M) reduces the amplitude of digitalis-induced delayed afterdepolarizations and suppresses triggered activity in Purkinje fibers.

Propranolol upregulates beta adrenoceptors in part by externalizing receptors from a light vesicle fraction to the sarcolemma. Beta blockers do not blunt heart rate variability in dogs after myocardial infarction.[139]

Concentrations exceeding 3 μg/ml are required to depress $\dot{V}_{max}$ action potential amplitude, membrane responsiveness, and conduction in normal atrial, ventricular, and Purkinje fibers without altering resting membrane potential. These effects probably result from depression of I_{Na}. Propranolol shortens the action potential duration of Purkinje fibers and, to a lesser extent, of atrial and ventricular muscle fibers. Long-term administration of propranolol may lengthen action potential duration. Similar to the effects of lidocaine, acceleration of repolarization of Purkinje fibers is most marked in areas of the ventricular conduction system in which the action potential duration is greatest. The reduction in refractory period is not as great as the reduction in action potential duration (effective refractory period duration/action potential duration >1.0). At least one beta blocker, sotalol, markedly increases the time course of repolarization in Purkinje fibers and ventricular muscles (see p. 615). Smaller doses of propranolol are required to prevent sympathetically induced shortening of ventricular refractoriness than are required to prevent sympathetically induced sinus acceleration.

Propranolol slows the sinus discharge rate in humans by 10 to 20 per cent, while severe bradycardia occasionally results if the heart is particularly dependent on sympathetic tone or if sinus node dysfunction is present. The slowing is probably due to beta blockade because D-propranolol does not significantly slow the sinus discharge rate in doses comparable to the racemic mixture. The P-R interval lengthens, as do AV nodal conduction time and effective and functional refractory periods (if the heart rate is maintained constant), but refractoriness and conduction in the normal His-Purkinje system remain unchanged even after high doses of propranolol. Therefore, therapeutic doses of propranolol in humans do not exert a direct depressant or "quinidine-like" action but influence cardiac electrophysiology via a beta-blocking action. Beta blockers do not affect conduction in normal ventricular muscle, as evidenced by their lack of effect on the QRS complex, and they insignificantly prolong the right ventricular effective refractory period and uncorrected Q-T interval.

Because administration of beta blockers that do not have direct membrane action prevents many arrhythmias resulting from activation of the autonomic nervous system, it is thought that the beta-blocking action is responsible for their antiarrhythmic effects.[140–144] However, the possible importance of direct membrane effect of some of these drugs cannot be discounted totally because beta blockers with direct membrane actions can affect transmembrane potentials of diseased cardiac fibers at much lower concentrations than are needed to affect normal fibers directly. However, indirect actions on arrhythmogenic effects of ischemia are probably quite important. Beta blockers reduce myocardial injury during experimental cardiopulmonary resuscitation.[145]

HEMODYNAMIC EFFECTS. Beta blockers exert negative inotropic effects and can precipitate or worsen heart failure. By blocking beta receptors, these drugs may cause peripheral vasoconstriction and exacerbate coronary artery spasm in some patients.

PHARMACOKINETICS (Table 21–1). Although various types of beta blockers exert similar pharmacological effects, their pharmacokinetics differ substantially. Propranolol is almost 100 per cent absorbed, but the effects of first-pass hepatic metabolism reduce bioavailability to about 30 per cent and produce significant interpatient variability of plasma concentration for a given dose. Reduction in hepatic blood flow, as in patients with heart failure, decreases the hepatic extraction of propranolol, and in these patients propranolol may further decrease its own elimination rate by reducing cardiac output and hepatic blood flow. Beta blockers eliminated by the kidney tend to have longer half-lives and exhibit less interpatient variability of drug concentration than do those beta blockers metabolized by the liver.

DOSAGE AND ADMINISTRATION (Table 21–7). The appropriate dose of propranolol is best determined by a measure of the patient's physiological response, such as changes in resting heart rate or in the prevention of exercise-induced tachycardia, since wide individual differences exist between the observed physiological effect and plasma concentration. For example, intravenous dosing is best achieved by titrating the dose to a clinical effect, beginning with doses of 0.25 to 0.50 mg, increasing to 1.0 mg if necessary, and administering doses every 5 minutes until either a desired effect or toxicity is produced or a total of 0.15 to 0.20 mg/kg has been given. In many instances, the short-acting effects of esmolol are preferred. Orally, propranolol is given in four divided doses, usually ranging from 40 to 160 mg a day to more than 1 gm a day. A once-daily long-acting propranolol preparation is available. Generally, if one agent in adequate doses proves to be ineffective, other beta blockers will be ineffective also.

INDICATIONS. Arrhythmias associated with thyrotoxicosis, pheochromocytoma, and anesthesia with cyclopropane or halothane, or arrhythmias largely due to excessive cardiac adrenergic stimulation, such as those initiated by exercise or emotion, often respond to propranolol therapy. Beta-blocking drugs usually do not convert chronic atrial flutter or atrial fibrillation to normal sinus rhythm but may do so if the arrhythmia is of recent onset. The rate of the atrial flutter/fibrillation is not changed, but the ventricular response decreases because beta blockade prolongs AV nodal conduction time and refractoriness. Esmolol combined with digoxin has been useful.[146] In the absence of heart failure, beta blockers can be more effective than digoxin to control the rate.[147] For reentrant supraventricular tachycardias using the AV node as one of the reentrant pathways, such as AV nodal reentrant tachycardia[148,149] and orthodromic reciprocating tachycardias in Wolff-Parkinson-White syndrome or inappropriate sinus tachycardia,[150,151] or for sinus reentrant tachycardia, propranolol may slow or terminate the tachycardia and be used prophylactically to prevent a recurrence. Combining propranolol with digitalis, quinidine, or a variety of other agents may be effective when propranolol as a single agent fails. *Metoprolol* and *esmolol* may be useful in patients with multifocal atrial tachycardia.[152]

Propranolol may be effective for digitalis-induced arrhythmias such as atrial tachycardia, nonparoxysmal AV junctional tachycardia, premature ventricular complexes, or ventricular tachycardia. If a significant degree of AV block is present during a digitalis-induced arrhythmia, lidocaine or phenytoin may be preferable to propranolol. Propranolol also may be useful to treat ventricular arrhythmias associated with the prolonged Q-T interval syndrome[153–155] and with mitral valve prolapse. For patients with ischemic heart disease, propranolol generally does not prevent episodes of chronic recurrent monomorphic ventricular tachycardia that occur in the absence of acute ischemia but may be effective in some patients, usually at a beta-blocking concentration. It is well accepted that propranolol, timolol, and metoprolol reduce the incidence of overall death and sudden cardiac death after myocardial infarction[156–158] (Fig. 21–5). The mechanism of this reduction in mortality is not entirely clear and may relate to reduction in the extent of ischemic drainage, autonomic effects, a direct antiarrhythmic effect, or combinations of these factors. Beta blockers may have been protective against proarrhythmic responses in CAST[159] and may be more effective in some patients than electrophysiologically guided antiarrhythmic drug therapy[160] for ventricular tachyarrhythmias. Labetalol has been used for ventricular arrhythmias in eclampsia.[161]

Labetalol is an alpha$_1$- and beta-blocking drug. *Esmolol* is an ultra-short-acting (elimination half-life 9 min) cardioselective beta-adrenoceptor blocker useful for the rapid control of the ventricular rate in patients with atrial flutter/fibrillation.[162] Its withdrawal has been used in tilt-table testing.[163]

ADVERSE EFFECTS. Adverse cardiovascular effects from propranolol include unacceptable hypotension, bradycardia, and congestive heart failure. The bradycardia may be due to sinus bradycardia or AV block. Sudden withdrawal of propranolol in patients with angina pectoris can precipitate or worsen angina and cardiac arrhythmias and cause an acute myocardial infarction, possibly owing to heightened sensitivity to beta-agonists caused by previous beta blockade (upregulation). Heightened sensitivity may begin several days after cessation of propranolol therapy and may last 5 or 6 days. Other adverse effects of propranolol include worsening of asthma or chronic obstructive pulmonary disease, intermittent claudication, Raynaud's phenomenon, mental depression, increased risk of hypoglycemia among insulin-dependent diabetic patients, easy fatigability, disturbingly vivid dreams or insomnia, and impaired sexual function.

CLASS III ANTIARRHYTHMIC AGENTS

Amiodarone

Amiodarone is a benzofuran derivative approved by the FDA for the treatment of patients with life-threatening ventricular tachyarrhythmias when other drugs are ineffective or are not tolerated.

ELECTROPHYSIOLOGICAL ACTIONS (Tables 21–6 and 21–7). When chronically given orally, amiodarone prolongs action potential duration and refractoriness of all cardiac fibers without affecting resting membrane potential. When acute effects are evaluated, amiodarone and its metabolite, desethylamiodarone, prolong the action potential duration of ventricular muscle but shorten the action potential duration of Purkinje fibers. Injected into the sinus and AV nodal arteries, amiodarone reduces sinus and junctional discharge rates and prolongs AV nodal conduction time. It decreases the slope of diastolic depolarization of the sinus node and markedly depresses $\dot{V}_{max}$ in guinea pig papillary muscle in a rate- or use-dependent manner. Such depression of $\dot{V}_{max}$ is caused by blocking of inactivated sodium channels, an effect that is accentuated by depolarized and reduced by hyperpolarized membrane potentials. Amiodarone also inhibits depolarization-induced automaticity. Amiodarone depresses conduction at fast rates more than at slow rates (use or frequency dependence),[164–166] not only by depressing $\dot{V}_{max}$ but also by increasing resistance to passive current flow. It does not prolong repolarization more at slow than fast rates (does not exert reverse use or frequency dependence) but does exert time-dependent effects on refractoriness, which may in part explain the low incidence of torsades de pointes and high efficacy.[164,165]

Desethylamiodarone has relatively greater effects on fast-channel tissue and probably contributes importantly to antiarrhythmic efficacy. The delay to build up adequate concentrations of this metabolite may explain in part the delay in amiodarone's antiarrhythmic action.

In vivo, amiodarone noncompetitively antagonizes alpha and beta receptors and blocks conversion of thyroxine (T_4) to triiodothyronine (T_3), which may account for some of its electrophysiological effects. Amiodarone exhibits slow-channel blocking effects, and chronic oral therapy slows the spontaneous sinus nodal discharge rate in anesthetized dogs even after pretreatment with propranolol and atropine. With oral administration it prolongs the Q-T interval,

at times changing the contour of the T wave and producing U waves, and slows the sinus rate by 20 to 30 per cent.

Effective refractory periods of all cardiac tissues are prolonged. His-Purkinje conduction time increases and QRS duration lengthens, especially at fast rates. Amiodarone given intravenously modestly prolongs the refractory period of atrial and ventricular muscle. P-R interval and AV nodal conduction time lengthen. The duration of the QRS complex lengthens at increased rates but less than after oral amiodarone. Thus, far less increase in prolongation of conduction time (except for the AV node), duration of repolarization, and refractoriness occurs after intravenous administration compared with the oral route. Considering these actions, it is clear that amiodarone has class I (blocks I_{Na}), class II (antiadrenergic), and class IV (blocks I_{Ca-L}) actions, in addition to class III effects (blocks I_K). Amiodarone's actions approximate those of a theoretically ideal drug that exhibits use-dependence of Na^+ channels with fast diastolic recovery from block and use-dependent prolongation of action potential duration. It does not increase[167] and may decrease[168] Q-T dispersion. Catecholamines can partially reverse some of the effects of amiodarone.[164,169]

HEMODYNAMIC EFFECTS. Amiodarone is a peripheral and coronary vasodilator. When administered intravenously in doses of 2.5 to 10 mg/kg, amiodarone decreases heart rate, systemic vascular resistance, left ventricular contractile force, and left ventricular dP/dt. Left ventricular output may increase. Oral doses of amiodarone sufficient to control cardiac arrhythmias do not depress left ventricular ejection fraction, even in patients with reduced ejection fractions measured by radionuclide ventriculography. However, because antiadrenergic actions of amiodarone may block I_{si} to some degree, and because it does exert some negative inotropic action, it should be given cautiously, particularly intravenously, to patients with marginal cardiac compensation.

PHARMACOKINETICS. Amiodarone is slowly, variably, and incompletely absorbed, with systemic bioavailability of 35 to 65 per cent. Plasma concentrations peak 3 to 7 hours after a single oral dose. There is minimal first-pass effect, indicating little hepatic extraction. Elimination is by hepatic excretion into bile with some enterohepatic recirculation. Extensive hepatic metabolism occurs with desethylamiodarone as a major metabolite. The plasma concentration ratio of parent to metabolite is 3:2. Both extensively accumulate in liver, lung, fat, "blue" skin, and other tissues. Myocardium develops a concentration 10 to 50 times that found in the plasma. Plasma clearance of amiodarone is low, and renal excretion negligible. Doses need not be reduced in patients with renal disease. Amiodarone and desethylamiodarone are not dialyzable. Volume of distribution is large but variable, averaging 60 liters/kg. Amiodarone is highly protein-bound (96 per cent), crosses the placenta (10 to 50 per cent), and is found in breast milk.

The onset of action after intravenous administration generally is within several hours. Following oral administration, the onset of action may require 2 to 3 days, often 1 to 3 weeks, and, on occasion, even longer. Loading doses reduce this time interval. Plasma concentrations relate well to oral doses during chronic treatment, averaging about 0.5 μg/ml for each 100 mg/day at doses between 100 and 600 mg/day. Elimination half-life is multiphasic with an initial 50 per cent reduction in plasma concentration 3 to 10 days after cessation of drug ingestion (probably representing elimination from well-perfused tissues) followed by a terminal half-life of 26 to 107 days (mean 53 days), with most patients in the 40- to 55-day range. To achieve steady state without a loading dose takes about 265 days. Interpatient variability of these pharmacokinetic parameters mandates close monitoring of the patient. Therapeutic serum concentrations range from 1 to 2.5 μg/ml. Greater suppression of arrhythmias may occur up to 3.5 μg/ml, but the risk of side effects increases.

DOSAGE AND ADMINISTRATION. An optimal dosing schedule for all patients has not been achieved.[170–173] One recommended approach is to treat with 800 to 1600 mg daily for 1 to 3 weeks,[174] reduced to 800 mg daily for the next 2 to 4 weeks, then 600 mg daily for 4 to 8 weeks, and finally, after 2 to 3 months of treatment, a maintenance dose of 400 mg or less per day. Maintenance drug can be given once or twice daily and should be titrated to the *lowest effective dose* to minimize the occurrence of side effects.[175] Doses as low as 100 mg/day can be effective in some patients.[176] Regimens must be individualized for a given patient and clinical situation. Amiodarone may be administered intravenously[177] to achieve more rapid loading and effect in emergencies at initial doses of 15 mg/min for 10 minutes, followed by 1 mg/min for 6 hours, and then 0.5 mg/min for the remaining 18 hours and for the next several days, as necessary. Supplemental infusions of 150 mg over 10 minutes can be used for breakthrough VT or ventricular fibrillation (VF). IV infusions have been continued safely for 2 to 3 weeks. Patients with depressed ejection fractions should receive intravenous amiodarone with great caution because of hypotension. High-dose oral loading (800 to 2000 mg two or three times a day to maintain trough serum concentrations of 2 to 3 μg/ml) may suppress ventricular arrhythmias in 1 to 2 days.

INDICATIONS. Amiodarone has been used to suppress a wide spectrum of supraventricular and ventricular tachyarrhythmias in utero,[178,179] in adults,[175] and in children,[180,181] including AV nodal and AV entry, junctional tachycardia,[182] atrial flutter and fibrillation,[183–188] ventricular tachycardia and ventricular fibrillation associated with coronary artery disease,[189–192] and hypertrophic cardiomyopathy. Success rates vary widely depending on patient population,[193] arrhythmia, underlying heart disease, length of follow-up, definition and determination of success, and other factors. In general, however, amidarone's efficacy equals or exceeds that of all other antiarrhythmic agents and may be in the range of 60 to 80 per cent for most supraventricular tachyarrhythmias (including those associated with the Wolff-Parkinson-White syndrome) and 40 to 60 per cent for ventricular tachyarrhythmias. Amiodarone may be useful in improving survival in patients with hypertrophic cardiomyopathy, asymptomatic ventricular arrhythmias after myocardial infarction, and ventricular tachyarrhythmia after resuscitation.

Patients who have an internal cardioverter-defibrillator receive fewer shocks if they are treated with amiodarone compared with conventional drugs.[194] Amiodarone may facilitate defibrillation experimentally[195] but increases the electrical defibrillation threshold.[196,197] Because of its long half-life and the difficulty involved in starting another antiarrhythmic drug (while not knowing if amiodarone's effects are still present), as well as its side effects profile, amiodarone is generally among the last antiarrhythmic agents tried.

A number of prospective, randomized, controlled trials with amiodarone have been performed recently.[191,198] They have demonstrated the superiority of amiodarone over placebo[199–201] and metoprolol[202] on mortality in patients after myocardial infarction, documented an effect not different from placebo in patients with congestive heart failure in one study,[203] showed a benefit in another,[204] and found a greater improvement in mortality in patients resuscitated from ventricular fibrillation compared with conventional drugs.[205,206] Several studies are in progress, including the European Myocardial Infarction Amiodarone Trial (EMIAT)[207] that compares amiodarone with placebo in patients with reduced left ventricular function after myocardial infarction, the Canadian Amiodarone Myocardial Infarction Arrhythmia Trial (CAMIAT),[208] similar to EMIAT in patients with ventricular ectopy, and trials comparing amiodarone with implantable defibrillators.[137,209,210]

Some controversy exists regarding the ability to predict effectiveness of amiodarone in patients with ventricular tachyarrhythmias. Clinical assessment, suppression of spontaneous ventricular arrhythmias as documented by 24-hour ECG recordings, and response to electrophysiological testing have served as endpoints to judge therapy. In the patient with a history of sustained ventricular tachycardia or fibrillation and minimal spontaneous ventricular arrhythmias in between symptomatic episodes, an invasive electrophysiological study is indicated to judge drug efficacy. The answer to when, after amiodarone therapy is started, such a study should be done is still not entirely resolved but probably should be 1 week or longer. In the 10 to 40 per cent of patients whose electrically induced clinical ventricular tachyarrhythmias become no longer inducible while they are receiving amiodarone, the chances for a spontaneous recurrence of the arrhythmias are low while the patients are taking amiodarone, probably less than 5 to 10 per cent at 1 year. For those patients whose ventricular tachyarrhythmias are still inducible, the recurrence rate is 40 to 50 per cent at 1 year. However, in this latter group, greater difficulty in inducing the arrhythmias may predict a less likely possibility of a recurrence.

Patients' hemodynamic responses to the induced arrhythmia also may predict how they tolerate a spontaneous recurrence. Amiodarone slows the ventricular tachycardia,[211,212] but it is important to remember that the supine patient in the electrophysiology laboratory may tolerate the same tachycardia better than when in an erect position. The arrhythmia's response to sotalol may predict its response to amiodarone.[213] An ejection fraction ≥ 0.4 may predict a good response to amiodarone in patients with ventricular tachycardia or ventricular fibrillation.[214]

Because of the serious nature of the arrhythmias being treated, the unusual pharmacokinetics of the drug, and its adverse effects (see below), amiodarone therapy should be started with the patient hospitalized and monitored for several days to a week. Combining other antiarrhythmic agents with amiodarone may improve efficacy in some patients.[215,216]

ADVERSE EFFECTS. Adverse effects are reported by about 75 per cent of patients treated with amiodarone for 5 years but compel stopping the drug in 18 to 37 per cent. The most frequent side effects requiring drug discontinuation involve pulmonary and gastrointestinal complaints.[175] Most adverse effects are reversible with dose reduction or cessation of treatment. Adverse effects become more frequent when therapy is continued long term. Of the noncardiac adverse reactions, pulmonary toxicity is the most serious; in one study it occurred between 6 days and 60 months of treatment in 33 of 573 patients, with 3 deaths. The mechanism is unclear but may relate to a hypersensitivity reaction and/or widespread phospholipidosis. Dyspnea, nonproductive cough, and fever are common symptoms, with rales, hypoxia, a positive gallium scan, reduced diffusion capacity,[217] and radiographic evidence of pulmonary infiltrates noted. Amiodarone must be discontinued if such pulmonary inflammatory changes occur. Steroids can be tried, but no controlled studies have been done to support their use. A 10 per cent mortality in patients with pulmonary inflammatory changes results, often in patients with unrecognized pulmonary involvement that is allowed to progress. Chest roentgenograms at 3-month intervals for the first year and then twice a year for several years have been recommended. At maintenance doses less than 300 mg daily, pulmonary toxicity is uncommon. Advanced age, high drug maintenance dose, and reduced predrug diffusion capacity (DL$_{co}$) are risk factors for developing pulmonary toxicity. An unchanged DL$_{co}$ volume may be a negative predictor of pulmonary toxicity.

Although asymptomatic elevations of liver enzymes are found in most patients, the drug is not stopped unless values exceed two or three times normal in a patient with initially abnormal values. Cirrhosis occurs uncommonly but may be fatal. Neurological dysfunction, photosensitivity (perhaps minimized by sunscreens), bluish skin discoloration, corneal microdeposits (in almost 100 per cent of adults receiving the drug more than 6 months), gastroenterological disturbances, and hyperthyroidism[218,219] (1 to 2 per cent) or hypothyroidism (2 to 4 per cent) can occur. Amiodarone appears to inhibit the peripheral conversion of T_4 to T_3 so that chemical changes result, characterized by a slight increase in T_4, reverse T_3 and thyroid-stimulating hormone (TSH), and a slight decrease in T_3. Reverse T_3 concentration has been used as an index of drug efficacy. During hypothyroidism, TSH increases greatly while T_3 increases in hyperthyroidism.

Cardiac side effects include symptomatic bradycardias in about 2 per cent, aggravation of ventricular tachyarrhythmias (with occasional development of torsades de pointes) in 1 to 2 per cent,[220] possibly higher in women,[221] and worsening of congestive heart failure in 2 per cent. Possibly due to interactions with anesthetics, complications after open-heart surgery have been noted by some,[222] but not all,[223] investigators, including pulmonary dysfunction, hypotension, hepatic dysfunction, and low cardiac output.

Important interactions with other drugs occur, and when given concomitantly with amiodarone, the dose of warfarin, digoxin, and other antiarrhythmic drugs should be reduced by one-third to one-half and the patient watched closely. Drugs with synergistic actions, such as beta blockers or calcium channel blockers, must be given cautiously.

Bretylium Tosylate

Bretylium is a quaternary ammonium compound that is approved by the FDA for parenteral use only in patients with life-threatening ventricular tachyarrhythmias.

ELECTROPHYSIOLOGICAL ACTIONS (Tables 21–6 and 21–7). Bretylium is selectively concentrated in sympathetic ganglia and their postganglionic adrenergic nerve terminals. After initially *causing* norepinephrine release, bretylium *prevents* norepinephrine release by depressing sympathetic nerve terminal excitability without depressing pre- or postganglionic sympathetic nerve conduction, impairing conduction across sympathetic ganglia, depleting the adrenergic neuron of norepinephrine, or decreasing the responsiveness of adrenergic receptors. It produces a state resembling chemical sympathectomy. During chronic bretylium treatment, the beta-adrenergic responses to circulating catecholamines are increased. The initial release of catecholamines results in several transient electrophysiological responses such as an increase in the discharge rates of the isolated perfused sinus node and of in vitro Purkinje fibers, often making quiescent fibers automatic.

Bretylium initially increases conduction velocity and excitability and decreases refractoriness in the rabbit atrium, and partially depolarized fibers may hyperpolarize. Pretreatment with reserpine or propranolol prevents these early changes. Initial catecholamine release can aggravate some arrhythmias, such as those caused by digitalis excess or myocardial infarction. Prolonged drug administration lengthens the duration of the action potential and refractoriness of atrial and ventricular muscle and Purkinje fibers, possibly by blocking one or more repolarizing potassium currents. The ratio of effective refractory period to action potential duration does not change, nor do membrane responsiveness and conduction velocity. Bretylium exerts little effect on diastolic excitability but increases ventricular fibrillation thresholds in some studies[224,225] but not others.[226] It is not clear whether the chemical sympathectomy-like state alone or together with other actions exerts the antifibrillatory effect. Reduced disparity between action potential duration and refractory period in regions of normal and infarcted myocardium may account for some of its antifibrillatory effects. Bretylium has no effect on vagal reflexes and does not alter the responsiveness of cholinergic receptors in the heart.

HEMODYNAMIC EFFECTS. Bretylium does not depress myocardial contractility. After an initial increase in blood pressure, the drug can cause significant hypotension by blocking the efferent limb of the baroceptor reflex. Hypotension results most commonly when patients are sitting or standing but also can occur in the supine position in seriously ill patients. Bretylium reduces the extent of the vasoconstriction and tachycardia reflexes during standing. Orthostatic hypotension can persist for several days after the drug has been discontinued.

PHARMACOKINETICS (Table 21–1). Bretylium is effective orally as well as parenterally, but it is absorbed poorly and erratically from the gastrointestinal tract. Bioavailability may be less than 50 per cent, and elimination is almost exclusively by renal excretion without significant metabolism or active metabolites being recognized. Elimination half-life is 5 to 10 hours but with fairly wide variability. Doses should be reduced in patients with renal insufficiency. In survivors of ventricular tachycardia or ventricular fibrillation, bretylium had an elimination half-life of 13.5 hours following single intravenous dosing, which was similar to previous results in normal subjects. Renal clearance accounted for virtually all elimination. Onset of action after intravenous administration occurs within several minutes, but full antiarrhythmic effects may not be seen for 30 minutes to 2 hours.

DOSAGE AND ADMINISTRATION (Table 21–1). Bretylium can be given intravenously in doses of 5 to 10 mg/kg of body weight diluted in 50 to 100 ml of 5 per cent dextrose in water and administered over 10 to 20 minutes or more quickly in a life-threatening state. This dose can be repeated in 1 to 2 hours if the arrhythmia persists. The total daily dose probably should not exceed 30 mg/kg. A similar initial dose, but undiluted, can be given intramuscularly. The maintenance intravenous dose is 0.5 to 2.0 mg/min. Intramuscular injection during cardiopulmonary resuscitation from cardiac arrest and in shock states should be avoided because of unreliable absorption during reduced tissue perfusion. In this situation, bretylium should be given intravenously.

INDICATIONS. Bretylium is used in patients who are in an intensive care setting and who have life-threatening recurrent ventricular tachyarrhythmias that have not responded to other antiarrhythmic drugs. Bretylium has been effective in treating some patients with drug-resistant tachyarrhythmias and in treating victims of out-of-hospital ventricular fibrillation.

ADVERSE EFFECTS. Hypotension, most prominently orthostatic but also supine, appears to be the most significant side effect and can be prevented with tricyclic drugs such as protriptyline. Transient hypertension, increased sinus rate, and worsening of arrhythmias, often those due to digitalis excess or ischemia, may follow initial drug administration and may be due to initial release of catecholamines. Bretylium should be used cautiously or not at all in patients who have a relatively fixed cardiac output, such as those with severe aortic stenosis. Vasodilators or diuretics can enhance these hypotensive effects. Nausea and vomiting can occur following parenteral administration. Parotid pain primarily during meals commonly occurs after 2 to 4 months of oral therapy and is associated with increased salivation without parotid swelling or inflammation.

Sotalol

Sotalol is a nonspecific beta-adrenoceptor blocker without intrinsic sympathomimetic activity that prolongs repolarization. It was approved in 1992 by the FDA to treat patients with life-threatening ventricular tachyarrhythmias.[191,227]

ELECTROPHYSIOLOGICAL ACTIONS. Both d- and l-isomers

have similar effects on prolonging repolarization, while the l-isomer is responsible for virtually all the beta-blocking activity. Sotalol does not block alpha adrenoceptors and does not block the sodium channel (no membrane-stabilizing effects) but does prolong atrial and ventricular repolarization times[228] by reducing I_K thus prolonging the plateau of the action potential. Action potential prolongation is greater at slower rates (reverse use dependence). Resting membrane potential, action potential amplitude, and $\dot{V}_{max}$ are not significantly altered. Sotalol prolongs atrial and ventricular refractoriness, A-H and Q-T intervals, and sinus cycle length. It narrows the excitable gap in reentrant ventricular tachycardia.[229]

HEMODYNAMICS. Sotalol exerts a negative inotropic effect only through its beta-blocking action. It can increase the strength of contraction by prolonging repolarization, which will occur maximally at slow heart rates. In patients with reduced cardiac function, sotalol can cause a decrease in cardiac index, an increase in filling pressure, and overt heart failure. Therefore, it must be used cautiously in patients with marginal cardiac compensation but appears to be well tolerated in patients with normal cardiac function.[230-232]

PHARMACOKINETICS. Sotalol is completely absorbed and not metabolized, making it 90 to 100 per cent bioavailable. It is not bound to plasma proteins, is excreted unchanged primarily by the kidneys, and has an elimination half-life of 10 to 15 hours. The plasma concentrations occur 2.5 to 4.0 hours after oral ingestion, with steady state attained after five or six doses. Effective antiarrhythmic plasma concentration is in the range of 2.5 μg/ml. There is very little intersubject variability in plasma levels. Over the dose range of 160 to 640 mg, sotalol displays dose proportionality with plasma concentration. The dose must be reduced in patients with renal disease. The beta-blocking effect is half maximal at 80 mg/day and maximal at $\geq$ 320 mg/day. Significant beta-blocking action occurs at 160 mg/day.

DOSAGE. The typical oral dose is 80 to 160 mg every 12 hours, allowing 2 to 3 days between dose adjustments to attain steady state and monitor the ECG for arrhythmias and Q-T prolongation. Doses exceeding 320 mg/day can be used in patients when the potential benefits outweigh the risk of proarrhythmia.

INDICATIONS. Approved only to treat patients with ventricular tachyarrhythmias,[233-235] sotalol is also useful to prevent recurrence of a wide variety of supraventricular tachycardias, including atrial flutter and fibrillation,[236,237] atrial tachycardia, AV nodal reentry, and AV reentry. It also shows the ventricular response to atrial tachyarrhythmias.[238] It appears to be more effective than conventional antiarrhythmic drugs and comparable with amiodarone in treating patients with ventricular tachyarrhythmias.[68] Sotalol has been shown to be superior to lidocaine for acute termination of sustained ventricular tachycardia[239] and is useful in patients with arrhythmogenic right ventricular dysplasia.[240] It can prolong the duration of late potentials.[241] Sotalol may be effective in pediatric patients.[242] It may reduce the defibrillation threshold.[196]

ADVERSE EFFECTS. Proarrhythmia is the most serious adverse effect. Overall, new or worsened ventricular tachyarrhythmias occur in about 4 per cent, and this response is due to torsades de pointes in about 2.5 per cent. The incidence of torsades de pointes increases to 4 per cent in patients with a history of sustained ventricular tachycardia and is dose related, reportedly only 1.6 per cent at 320 mg/day but 4.4 per cent at 480 mg/day.[243] Other adverse effects commonly seen with other beta blockers also apply to sotalol. Sotalol should be used with caution or not at all in combination with other drugs that prolong the Q-T interval. However, such combinations have been used successfully.[244]

CLASS IV ANTIARRHYTHMIC AGENTS

The Calcium Channel Antagonists: Verapamil and Diltiazem

Verapamil, a synthetic papaverine derivative, is the prototype of a class of drugs that block the slow calcium channel and reduce I_{Ca-L} in cardiac muscle. *Diltiazem* has electrophysiological actions similar to those of verapamil.[138] *Nifedipine* (see p. 1308) exhibits minimal electrophysiological effects at clinically used doses and will not be discussed here.

ELECTROPHYSIOLOGICAL ACTIONS (Tables 21–6 and 21–7). By blocking the slow inward current in all cardiac fibers, verapamil reduces the plateau height of the action potential, slightly shortens muscle action potential, and slightly prolongs total Purkinje fiber action potential. It does not appreciably affect the action potential amplitude, $\dot{V}_{max}$ of phase 0, or resting membrane voltage in cells that have fast-response characteristics due to I_{Na} (atrial and ventricular muscle, the His-Purkinje system). Verapamil suppresses slow responses elicited by a variety of experimental methods as well as triggered sustained rhythmic activity and early and late afterdepolarizations (see pp. 566 to 567). Verapamil and other slow-channel blockers suppress electrical activity in the normal sinus and AV nodes in concentrations that do not suppress action potentials of fast-channel-dependent cells. Verapamil depresses the slope of diastolic depolarization in sinus nodal cells, $\dot{V}_{max}$ of phase 0, maximum diastolic potential, and action potential amplitude in the sinus and AV nodal cells and prolongs conduction time and the effective and functional refractory periods of the AV node. The AV nodal blocking effects of verapamil and diltiazem[245] are more apparent at faster rates of stimulation (use-dependence) and in depolarized fibers (voltage-dependence). Verapamil slows the activation and delays recovery from inactivation of the slow channel. Unbinding of the drug from its receptor occurs more rapidly in tissue that is hyperpolarized.

Verapamil does exert some local anesthetic activity because the dextrorotatory stereoisomer of the clinically used racemic mixture exerts slight blocking effects on I_{Na}. The levorotatory stereoisomer blocks the slow inward current carried by calcium, as well as other ions, traveling through the slow channel. Verapamil does not modify calcium uptake, binding, or exchange by cardiac microsomes, nor does it affect calcium-activated ATPase. Verapamil does not block beta receptors and may block alpha receptors and potentiate vagal effects on the AV node. Verapamil also may cause other effects that indirectly alter cardiac electrophysiology, such as decreasing platelet adhesiveness or reducing the extent of myocardial ischemia.

In vivo, both in experimental animals and in humans, verapamil prolongs conduction time through the AV node (the A-H interval) without affecting the P-A, H-V, or QRS interval and lengthens the anterograde and retrograde functional and effective refractory periods of the AV node. Spontaneous sinus rate may decrease slightly, an event only partially reversed by atropine. More commonly, the sinus rate does not change significantly in vivo because verapamil causes peripheral vasodilation, transient hypotension, and reflex sympathetic stimulation that mitigates any direct slowing effect verapamil may exert on the sinus node. If verapamil is given to a patient who is also receiving a beta blocker, the sinus nodal discharge rate may slow because reflex sympathetic stimulation is blocked. Verapamil does not exert a direct effect on atrial or ventricular refractoriness or on anterograde or retrograde properties of accessory pathways. However, reflex sympathetic stimulation may increase the ventricular response over the accessory pathway during atrial fibrillation in patients with the Wolff-Parkinson-White syndrome.

HEMODYNAMIC EFFECTS. Since verapamil interferes with excitation-contraction coupling, it inhibits vascular smooth muscle contraction and causes marked vasodilation in coronary and other peripheral vascular beds. Propranolol does not block the vasodilation produced by verapamil. Reflex sympathetic effects may reduce in vivo the marked negative inotropic action of verapamil on isolated cardiac muscle, but direct myocardial depressant effects of verapamil may predominate when the drug is given in high doses. In patients with well-preserved left ventricular function, combined therapy with propranolol and verapamil appears to be well tolerated, but beta blockade can accentuate the hemodynamic depressant effects produced by oral verapamil. Patients who have reduced left ventricular function may not tolerate the combined blockade of beta receptors and of slow channels, and the combined use of verapamil and propranolol in these patients must be undertaken cautiously or not at all. Verapamil decreases myocardial oxygen demand while decreasing coronary vascular resistance and reduces the extent of ischemic damage in experimental preparations. Such changes may be antiarrhythmic. Diltiazem also reduces ventricular arrhythmias during coronary occlusion in the dog, possibly by preventing calcium overload. In a hamster model of hereditary cardiomyopathy, verapamil prevents progression of the disease and the secondary heart failure.

Peak alterations in hemodynamic variables occur 3 to 5 minutes after completion of the verapamil injection, the major effects being dissipated within 10 minutes. Mean arterial pressure decreases and left ventricular end-diastolic pressure increases; systemic resistance decreases and left ventricular dP/dt max decreases. Heart rate, cardiac index, left ventricular minute work, and mean pulmonary artery pressure do not change significantly. Thus afterload reduction produced by verapamil significantly minimizes its negative inotropic action so that cardiac index may not be reduced. In addition, when verapamil slows the ventricular rate in a patient with a tachycardia, cardiac slowing also may improve hemodynamics. Nevertheless, caution should be exercised when giving verapamil to patients with severe myocardial depression or those receiving beta blockers or disopyramide because hemodynamic deterioration may progress in some patients.

PHARMACOKINETICS (Table 21-1). Following single oral doses of verapamil, measurable prolongation of AV nodal conduction time occurs in 30 minutes and lasts 4 to 6 hours. After intravenous administration, AV nodal conduction delay occurs within 1 to 2 minutes, and A-H interval prolongation is still detectable after 6 hours. Effective plasma concentrations necessary to terminate supraventricular tachycardia are in the range of 125 ng/ml following doses of 0.075 to 0.150 mg/kg. After oral administration, absorption is almost complete, but an overall bioavailability of 20 to 35 per cent suggests substantial first-pass metabolism in the liver, particularly of the l-isomer. The elimination half-life of verapamil is 3 to 7 hours, with up to 70 per cent of the drug excreted by the kidneys. Norverapamil is a major metabolite that may contribute to verapamil's electrophysiological actions. Serum protein binding is approximately 90 per cent. With diltiazem, percentage of heart rate reduction in atrial fibrillation relates to plasma concentration.[246]

DOSAGE AND ADMINISTRATION (Table 21-1). The most commonly used intravenous dose is 10 mg infused over 1 to 2 minutes while cardiac rhythm and blood pressure are monitored. A second injection of equal dose may be given 30 minutes later. The initial effect achieved with the first bolus injection, such as slowing of the ventricular response during atrial fibrillation, may be maintained by a continuous infusion of the drug at a rate of 0.005 mg/kg/min. The oral dose is 240 to 480 mg/day in divided doses. Diltiazem is given intravenously at a dose of 0.25 mg/kg as a bolus

over 2 minutes, with a second dose in 15 minutes if necessary. Orally, doses must be adjusted to the patient's needs with a 120- to 360-mg range. Various long-acting preparations exist for verapamil and diltiazem.

INDICATIONS. After simple vagal maneuvers have been tried and adenosine given, intravenous verapamil or diltiazem[247] is the next treatment of choice for terminating sustained sinus nodal reentry, AV nodal reentry, or orthodromic AV reciprocating tachycardia associated with the Wolff-Parkinson-White syndrome. Verapamil is as effective as adenosine for termination of these arrhythmias.[248] Verapamil should definitely be tried prior to attempting termination by digitalis administration, pacing, electrical direct-current cardioversion, or acute blood pressure elevation with vasopressors. Verapamil and diltiazem terminate 60 to more than 90 per cent of episodes of paroxysmal supraventricular tachycardias within several minutes. Verapamil may be of use in some fetal supraventricular tachycardias as well. Although intravenous verapamil has been given along with intravenous propranolol, this combination should be used only with great caution.

Verapamil and diltiazem decrease the ventricular response over the AV node during atrial fibrillation or atrial flutter, possibly converting a small number of episodes to sinus rhythm, particularly if the atrial flutter or fibrillation is of recent onset.[126] Some patients who exhibit atrial flutter may develop atrial fibrillation following verapamil administration. Quinidine, flecainide, and esmolol appear to be more effective than verapamil in establishing and maintaining sinus rhythm in patients with atrial fibrillation. As noted earlier, in patients with atrial fibrillation associated with the Wolff-Parkinson-White syndrome, intravenous verapamil may *accelerate* the ventricular response, and therefore, the intravenous route is contraindicated in this situation. Verapamil can terminate some atrial tachycardias. Even though verapamil terminates a left septal ventricular tachycardia,[249] hemodynamic collapse can occur if intravenous verapamil is given to patients with the more common forms of ventricular tachycardia. *A general rule to avoid complications, however, is to not give intravenous verapamil to any patient with wide-QRS tachycardia unless one is absolutely certain of the nature of the tachycardia and its response to verapamil.*

Orally, verapamil or diltiazem may prevent the recurrence of AV nodal reentrant and orthodromic AV reciprocating tachycardias[247,248,250] associated with the Wolff-Parkinson-White syndrome as well as help maintain a decreased ventricular response during atrial flutter or atrial fibrillation in patients without an accessory pathway.[251-253] In this regard, the effectiveness of verapamil appears to be enhanced when given concomitantly with quinidine, and diltiazem when given with digoxin.[254] Verapamil generally has not been effective in treating patients who have recurrent ventricular tachyarrhythmias, although it may suppress some forms of ventricular tachycardia such as a left septal ventricular tachycardia,[249,254a,255-258] as noted above. It may be useful in about two-thirds of patients with idiopathic ventricular tachycardia that has a left bundle branch block morphology,[254a] in patients with hypertrophic cardiomyopathy who have experienced cardiac arrest,[259] in patients with a short-coupled variant of torsades de pointes,[260] in patients with right ventricular dysplasia,[240] and in patients with ventricular arrhythmias due to coronary artery spasm.[261] While data from animal models suggest that verapamil may be useful in reducing or preventing ventricular arrhythmias due to acute myocardial ischemia, calcium antagonists have not been shown to reduce mortality or prevent sudden cardiac death in patients after acute myocardial infarction, except for diltiazem in patients with non-Q-wave infarctions. Verapamil abolishes the wall motion abnormality found in patients with the long Q-T syndrome.[262]

ADVERSE EFFECTS. Verapamil must be used cautiously in patients with significant hemodynamic impairment or in those receiving beta blockers, as previously noted. Hypotension, bradycardia, AV block, and asystole are more likely to occur when the drug is given to patients who are already receiving beta-blocking agents. Hemodynamic collapse has been noted in infants, and verapamil should be used cautiously in patients less than 1 year old. Verapamil also should be used with caution in patients with sinus node abnormalities, since marked depression of sinus nodal function or asystole can result in some of these patients. Isoproterenol, calcium, glucagon infusion, dopamine, or atropine (which may be only partially effective) or temporary pacing may be necessary to counteract some of the adverse effects of verapamil. Isoproterenol may be more effective for treating bradyarrhythmias and calcium for treating hemodynamic dysfunction secondary to verapamil. AV nodal depression is common in overdoses.[263] Contraindications to the use of verapamil and diltiazem include the presence of advanced heart failure, second or third degree AV block without a pacemaker in place, atrial fibrillation and anterograde conduction over an accessory pathway, significant sinus node dysfunction, most ventricular tachycardias, cardiogenic shock, and other hypotensive states. While the drugs probably should not be used in patients with manifest heart failure, if the latter is due to one of the supraventricular tachyarrhythmias noted earlier, verapamil or diltiazem may restore sinus rhythm or significantly decrease the ventricular rate, leading to hemodynamic improvement. Finally, it is important to note that verapamil can decrease the excretion of digoxin by about 30 per cent. Hepatotoxicity may occur on occasion.

OTHER ANTIARRHYTHMIC AGENTS

Adenosine

Adenosine is an endogenous nucleoside present throughout the body and has been approved by the FDA to treat patients with supraventricular tachycardias.[264]

ELECTROPHYSIOLOGICAL ACTIONS (Tables 21–6 and 21–7). Adenosine interacts with A_1 receptors present on the extracellular surface of cardiac cells, activating K^+ channels ($I_{K\ Ach}$, $I_{K\ Ado}$) in a fashion similar to that produced by acetylcholine. The increase in K^+ conductance shortens atrial action potential duration, hyperpolarizes the membrane potential, and decreases atrial contractility. Similar changes occur in the sinus and AV nodes. In contrast to these direct effects mediated through guanine nucleotide regulatory proteins G_i and G_o, adenosine antagonizes catecholamine-stimulated adenylate cyclase to decrease cyclic AMP accumulation and to decrease I_{Ca-L} and the pacemaker current i_f in sinus nodal cells. $\dot{V}_{max}$ is reduced. Shifts in pacemaker site within the sinus node and sinus exit block may occur. Reflex-mediated sinus tachycardia can follow adenosine administration. In the N region of the AV node, conduction is depressed, along with decreases in action potential amplitude, duration, and $\dot{V}_{max}$. Adenosine slows the sinus rate in humans, which is followed by a reflex increase in sinus discharge. Transient prolongation of the A-H interval results, often with transient first, second, or third degree AV nodal block. Delay in AV nodal conduction is rate-dependent.[265] His-Purkinje conduction is generally not directly affected. Adenosine does not affect conduction in normal accessory pathways. Conduction may be blocked in accessory pathways that have long conduction times or decremental conduction properties. Patients with heart transplants exhibit a supersensitive response to adenosine.[266] Adenosine may mediate the phenomenon of preconditioning ischemia.[264]

PHARMACOKINETICS. Adenosine is removed from the extracellular space by washout, enzymatically by degradation to inosine, by phosphorylation to AMP, or by reuptake into cells via a nucleoside transport system. The vascular endothelium and the formed blood elements contain these elimination systems that result in very rapid clearance of adenosine from the circulation. Elimination half-life is 1 to 6 seconds. Most of adenosine's effects are produced during its first passage through the circulation. Important drug interactions occur. Methyl xanthines are competitive antagonists, and therapeutic concentrations of theophylline totally block the exogeneous adenosine effect. Dipyridamole is a nucleoside transport blocker that blocks reuptake of adenosine, delaying its clearance from the circulation or interstitial space and potentiating its effect. Smaller adenosine doses should be used in patients receiving dipyridamole.

DOSAGE AND ADMINISTRATION. To terminate tachycardia, a bolus of adenosine is injected intravenously rapidly into a central vein (if possible) at doses of 6 to 12 mg. When given into a central vein, and in patients after heart transplantation, or in patients receiving dipyridamole, the initial dose should be reduced to 3 mg.[267] Transient sinus slowing or AV nodal block results.

INDICATIONS. Adenosine has become the drug of first choice to terminate acutely a supraventricular tachycardia such as AV junctional tachycardias[268] or AV nodal or AV reentry.[269–273] It is useful in pediatric patients[274,275] and to judge the effectiveness of ablation of accessory pathways.[276] Adenosine can produce AV block or terminate atrial tachycardias[277,278] and sinus node reentry. It results in transient AV block during atrial flutter or fibrillation. Adenosine terminates a group of ventricular tachycardias whose maintenance depends on adrenergic drive, most often located in the right ventricular outflow tract, but found at other sites as well.[256,279–281] Adenosine has less potential than verapamil for lowering the blood pressure should tachycardia persist after injection.

Doses as low as 2.5 mg terminate some tachycardias; doses of 12 mg or less terminate 92 per cent of supraventricular tachycardias, usually within 30 seconds. Successful termination rates with adenosine are comparable with those achieved with verapamil. Because of its effectiveness and extremely short duration of action, adenosine is preferable to verapamil in most instances, particularly in patients who previously have received intravenous beta-adrenoceptor blockers, in those having poorly compensated heart failure or severe hypotension, and in neonates. Verapamil might be chosen first in patients receiving drugs, such as theophylline, known to interfere with adenosine's actions or metabolism, in patients with active bronchoconstriction, and in those with inadequate venous access. Adenosine produces transient AV nodal block in patients with atrial flutter, atrial fibrillation, and some types of atrial tachycardia, facilitating the diagnosis by exposing the atrial rhythm.

Adenosine may be useful to help differentiate wide-QRS tachycardias,[281] since it terminates many supraventricular tachycardias with aberrancy or reveals the underlying atrial mechanism, and it does not block conduction over the accessory pathway or terminate most ventricular tachycardias. Adenosine does terminate some ventricular tachycardias, and therefore tachycardia termination is not completely diagnostic for a supraventricular tachycardia.[282] This agent may predispose to the development of atrial fibrillation and possibly can increase the ventricular response in patients with atrial fibrillation conducting over an accessory pathway. Adenosine also may be useful in differentiating conduction over the AV node versus an accessory pathway during ablative procedures designed to interrupt the accessory pathway. Endogenously released adenosine may be important in ischemia and hypoxia-induced AV nodal block and in postdefibrillation bradyarrhythmias.

ADVERSE EFFECTS. Transient side effects occur in almost 40 per cent of patients with supraventricular tachycardia given adenosine and are most commonly flushing, dyspnea, and chest pressure. These symptoms are fleeting, generally less than 1 minute, and are well tolerated. Premature ventricular complexes, transient sinus bradycardia, sinus arrest, and AV block are common when a supraventricular tachycardia abruptly terminates. Induction of atrial fibrillation can be problematic in patients with the Wolff-Parkinson-White syndrome or rapid AV conduction.[283,284]

ELECTRICAL THERAPY OF CARDIAC ARRHYTHMIAS

DIRECT-CURRENT CARDIOVERSION

Electrical cardioversion offers obvious advantages over drug therapy in terminating tachycardia. Under conditions optimal for close supervision and monitoring, a precisely regulated "dose" of electricity can restore sinus rhythm immediately and safely. The distinction between supraventricular and ventricular tachyarrhythmias—crucial to the proper medical management of arrhythmias—becomes less significant, and the time-consuming titration of drugs with potential side effects is abolished.[285]

MECHANISMS. Electrical cardioversion appears to terminate most effectively those tachycardias presumed to be due to reentry, such as atrial flutter and atrial fibrillation, AV nodal reentry, reciprocating tachycardias associated with Wolff-Parkinson-White syndrome, most forms of ventricular tachycardia, ventricular flutter, and ventricular fibrillation. The electrical shock, by depolarizing all excitable myocardium, and possibly by prolonging refractoriness, interrupts reentrant circuits, discharges foci, and establishes electrical homogeneity that terminates reentry. The mechanism by which a shock successfully terminates ventricular fibrillation has not been completely explained. If the precipitating factors are no longer present, interrupting the tachyarrhythmia for only the brief time produced by the shock may prevent its return for long duration even though the anatomical and electrophysiological substrates required for the tachycardia are still present.

Tachycardias thought to be due to disorders of impulse formation (automaticity) include parasystole, some forms of atrial tachycardia, nonparoxysmal AV junctional tachycardia, and accelerated idioventricular rhythms. An attempt to cardiovert these tachycardias electrically is not indicated in most instances. It has not been established whether the shock can terminate tachycardias due to enhanced automaticity or triggered activity.

TECHNIQUE. Prior to elective cardioversion, a careful physical examination, including palpation of all pulses, should be performed. A 12-lead electrocardiogram is obtained before and after cardioversion, as well as a rhythm strip during the electroshock. The patient, who should be informed completely about what to expect, is in a fasting state and "metabolically balanced," i.e., blood gases, pH, and electrolytes should be normal with no evidence of drug toxicity. Withholding digitalis for several days before elective cardioversion in patients without clinical evidence of digitalis toxicity is not necessary. Maintenance antiarrhythmic drug administration 1 to 2 days before electrical cardioversion of patients with atrial fibrillation may revert some patients to sinus rhythm, may help prevent recurrence of atrial fibrillation once sinus rhythm is restored, and may help determine patient tolerance to the drug.

Self-adhesive pads applied in the standard apex-anterior or apex-posterior paddle positions have transthoracic impedances similar to paddles and are very useful in elective cardioversions or other situations in which there is time for their application, such as at the start of an electrophysiological study.[286] Paddles 12 to 13 cm in diameter can be used to deliver maximum current to the heart, but the benefits of these paddles as compared with those of 8 to 9 cm diameter have not been clearly established. Larger paddles may distribute the intracardiac current over a wider area and may reduce shock-induced myocardial necrosis.

A synchronized shock, i.e., one delivered during the QRS complex, is used for all cardioversions except for very rapid ventricular tachyarrhythmias, such as ventricular flutter or fibrillation. Recent data suggest that for internal cardioversion, shocks delivered late in the QRS complex during ventricular tachycardia are more effective and have a lower risk of acceleration than those delivered near QRS onset.[287] Because myocardial damage increases directly with increases in applied energy, the minimum effective energy should be used. Therefore, shocks are "titrated" when the clinical situation permits. Except for atrial fibrillation, shocks in the range of 25 to 50 joules successfully terminate most supraventricular tachycardias and should be tried initially. If unsuccessful, a second shock of higher energy can be delivered. The starting level to terminate atrial fibrillation should probably be 50 to 100 joules. Intracardiac defibrillation can be tried if external cardioversion fails.[288–290] For patients with stable ventricular tachycardia, starting levels in the range of 25 to 50 joules can be employed. If there is some urgency to terminate the tachyarrhythmia, one can begin with higher energies. To terminate ventricular fibrillation, 200 to 400 joules generally are used, although much lower energies (<100 joules) terminate ventricular fibrillation when the shock is delivered at the *very onset* of the arrhythmia, using adhesive pads in the electrophysiology laboratory, for example. Research in new waveforms will likely improve defibrillation capabilities.[291–294]

During elective cardioversion, a short-acting barbiturate such as methohexital or an amnesic such as diazepam or midazolam can be used. A physician skilled in airway management should be in attendance, an intravenous route should be established, and all equipment necessary for emergency resuscitation should be immediately accessible. Before cardioversion, 100 per cent oxygen may be administered for 5 to 15 minutes and is continued throughout the procedure. Manual ventilation of the patient may be necessary to avoid hypoxia during periods of deepest sleep.

INDICATIONS. As a rule, any tachycardia that produces hypotension, congestive heart failure, or angina and does not respond promptly to medical management should be terminated electrically. Very rapid ventricular rates in patients with atrial fibrillation and the Wolff-Parkinson-White syndrome are often best treated by electrical cardioversion. In almost all instances, the patient's hemodynamic status improves after cardioversion. An occasional patient may develop hypotension, reduced cardiac output, or congestive heart failure following the shock. This may be related to complications of the cardioversion, such as embolic events, myocardial depression resulting from the anesthetic agent or the shock itself,[295,296] hypoxia, lack of restoration of left atrial contraction despite return of electrical atrial systole,[297] or post-shock arrhythmias. Direct-current countershock of digitalis-induced tachyarrhythmias is contraindicated.

Favorable candidates for electrical cardioversion of atrial fibrillation include those patients who (1) have symptomatic atrial fibrillation of less than 12 months' duration and derive significant hemodynamic benefits from sinus rhythm, (2) have embolic episodes, (3) continue to have atrial fibrillation after the precipitating cause has been removed (e.g., following treatment of thyrotoxicosis), and (4) have a rapid ventricular rate that is difficult to slow.

Unfavorable candidates include patients with (1) digitalis toxicity, (2) no symptoms and a well-controlled ventricular rate without therapy, (3) sinus node dysfunction and various unstable supraventricular tachyarrhythmias or bradyarrhythmias (often the bradycardia-tachycardia syndrome) who finally develop and maintain atrial fibrillation (which in essence represents a "cure" of the sick sinus syndrome), (4) little or no benefit from normal sinus rhythm who promptly revert to atrial fibrillation after cardioversion despite drug therapy, (5) a large left atrium and longstanding atrial fibrillation, (6) infrequent episodes of atrial fibrillation that revert spontaneously to sinus rhythm, (7) no mechanical atrial systole after the return of electrical atrial systole, (8) atrial fibrillation and advanced heart block, (9) cardiac surgery planned in the near future, and (10) antiarrhythmic drug intolerance. Atrial fibrillation is likely to recur after cardioversion in patients who have significant chronic obstructive lung disease, congestive heart failure, mitral valve disease (particularly mitral regurgitation), atrial fibrillation longer than 1 year, and an enlarged left atrium.

In patients with atrial flutter, slowing the ventricular rate by administering digitalis or terminating the flutter with an antiarrhythmic agent may be difficult, so electrical cardioversion is often the initial treatment of choice. For the patient with other types of supraventricular tachycardia, electrical cardioversion may be employed when (1) vagal maneuvers or simple medical management (e.g., intravenous adenosine and verapamil) has failed to terminate the tachycardia and (2) the clinical setting indicates that fairly prompt restoration of sinus rhythm is desirable because of hemodynamic decompensation or electrophysiological consequences of the tachycardia. Similarly, in patients with ventricular tachycardia, the hemodynamic and electrophysiological consequences of the arrhythmias determine the need and urgency for direct-current cardioversion (see p. 680). Electrical countershock is the *initial* treatment of choice for ventricular flutter or ventricular fibrillation.[285,298,299] Speed is essential.

If, after the first shock, reversion to sinus rhythm does not occur, a higher energy level should be tried. When transient ventricular arrhythmias result after an unsuccessful shock, a bolus of lidocaine can be given prior to delivering a shock at the next energy level. If sinus rhythm returns only transiently and is promptly supplanted by the tachycardia, a repeat shock can be tried, depending on the tachyarrhythmia being treated and its consequences. Administration of an antiarrhythmic agent intravenously may be useful prior to delivering the next cardioversion shock. After cardioversion, the patient should be monitored at least until full consciousness has been restored and preferably for several hours thereafter.

RESULTS. Cardioversion restores sinus rhythm in 70 to 95 per cent of patients depending on the type of tachyarrhythmia. However, sinus rhythm remains after 12 months in less than one-third to one-half the patients with chronic atrial fibrillation. Thus, maintenance of sinus rhythm, once established, is the difficult problem, not the immediate termination of the tachycardia, and depends on the particular arrhythmia, the presence of underlying heart disease, and the response to antiarrhythmic drug therapy. Atrial size decreases following termination of atrial fibrillation and restoration of sinus rhythm,[300,301] and functional capacity improves.[302–304]

COMPLICATIONS. Arrhythmias induced by the cardioversion generally are caused by inadequate synchronization, with the shock occurring during the ST segment or T wave. Occasionally, a properly synchronized shock can produce ventricular fibrillation (Fig. 21–6). Post-shock arrhythmias usually are transient and do not require therapy. Embolic episodes are reported to occur in 1 to 3 per cent of the patients converted from atrial fibrillation to sinus rhythm. Prior anticoagulation for 2 to 3 weeks should be considered for patients who have no contraindication to such therapy and have atrial fibrillation present for longer than 2 to 3 days. This is particularly true for those who are at high risk for emboli, such as those with mitral stenosis and atrial fibrillation of recent onset, a history of recent or recurrent emboli, a prosthetic mitral valve, enlarged heart (including left atrial enlargement), or congestive heart failure. Anticoagulation with warfarin for several weeks afterward is recommended. Importantly, exclusion of left atrial thrombus by transesophageal echocardiography does not preclude embolism after cardioversion of atrial fibrillation.[305–308] Atrial thrombi may be present in patients with nonfibrillation atrial tachyarrhythmias and congenital heart disease.[309]

Although direct-current shock has been demonstrated in animals to cause cardiac injury, studies in humans indicate that elevations of myocardial enzymes after cardioversion are not common. ST-segment elevation can occur with elective direct-current cardioversion, although cardiac enzymes and myocardial scintigraphy may be unremarkable. A decrease in serum K^+ and Mg^{++} can occur after cardioversion of ventricular tachycardia.[310]

Cardioversion of ventricular tachycardia also can be achieved by a chest thump. Its mechanism of termination probably relates to a mechanically induced premature atrial or ventricular complex that interrupts a tachycardia. The thump cannot be timed very well and is probably only effective when delivered during a nonrefractory part of the cardiac cycle. Care must therefore be taken, because the thump can alter a ventricular tachycardia and possibly induce ventricular flutter or fibrillation if it occurs during the vulnerable period of the T wave.

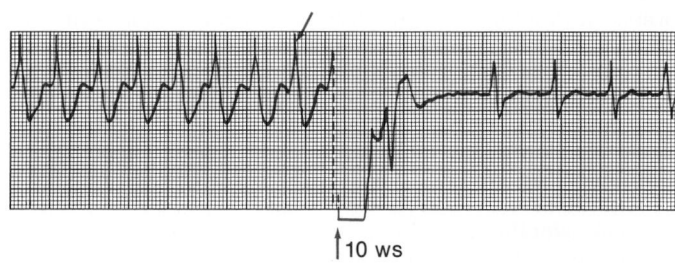

↑10 ws

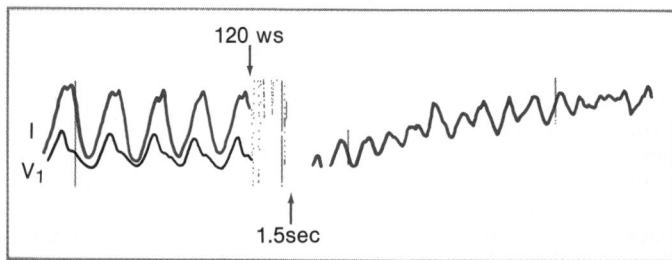

FIGURE 21–6. *Top,* A synchronized shock (note synchronization marks in the apex of the QRS complex [↓]) during ventricular tachycardia is followed by a single repetitive ventricular response and then normal sinus rhythm. *Bottom,* A shock synchronized to the terminal portion of the QRS complex in a patient with atrial fibrillation and conduction to the ventricle over an accessory pathway (WPW syndrome) results in ventricular fibrillation that was promptly terminated by a 400 joule shock. Recording was lost for 1.5 sec (↑) owing to baseline drift after the shock.

IMPLANTABLE ELECTRICAL DEVICES FOR TREATMENT OF CARDIAC ARRHYTHMIAS

Implantable devices that monitor the cardiac rhythm and can deliver competing pacing stimuli and low- and high-energy shocks have been used effectively in selected patients and are discussed fully in Chapter 23.

ABLATION THERAPY OF CARDIAC ARRHYTHMIAS

Ablation Therapy

The purpose of catheter ablation is to destroy myocardial tissue by delivering electrical energy over electrodes on a catheter placed next to an area of the endocardium integrally related to the onset and/or maintenance of the arrhythmia. Lasers, cryothermy, and microwave energy sources have been used, but not commonly. RF catheter ablation (Fig. 21–7) has largely replaced the DC shock. RF energy is delivered from an external generator and destroys tissue by controlled heat production (Fig. 21–8).

Radiofrequency Catheter Ablation of Accessory Pathways

LOCATION OF PATHWAYS. The safety, efficacy, and cost-effectiveness of RF catheter ablation of an accessory atrioventricular pathway[311–314] have made ablation the treatment of choice in most adult and many pediatric patients who have AV reentrant tachycardia[315] or atrial flutter/fibrillation associated with a rapid ventricular response over the accessory pathway.[316–319] However, the fact that the lesion size, when RF energy is delivered to an immature heart, can increase as the heart grows makes the long-term outlook for ablation less certain in the very young.[320–324] RF energy has replaced DC shock as the optimal energy source.[325–327]

An electrophysiological study is performed initially, to determine that the accessory pathway is part of the tachycardia circuit and to locate the optimal site for ablation. Pathways can be located in the right or left free wall or septum of the heart (Fig. 21–9). Septal accessory pathways are classified as anteroseptal, midseptal, and posteroseptal.[328–331] Parahissian pathways can be distinguished from anteroseptal pathways.[329] Midseptal locations are true septal pathways, while those classified as antero-

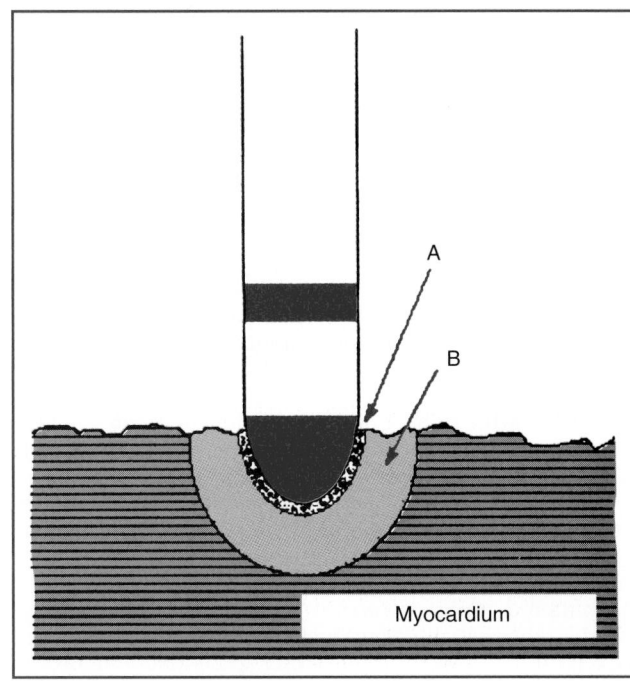

FIGURE 21–8. Mechanism of heating during radiofrequency catheter ablation. Because current density drops off rapidly as a function of distance from the electrode surface, only a small shell of myocardium adjacent to the distal electrode *(A)* is heated directly. The major portion of the lesion *(B)* is produced by conduction of heat away from the electrode-tissue interface into surrounding tissue. (From Langberg, J. J., and Leon, A.: Energy sources for catheter ablation. *In* Zipes, D. P., and Jalife, J. [eds.]: Cardiac Electrophysiology: From Cell to Bedside. 2nd ed. Philadelphia, W. B. Saunders Company, 1994, pp. 1434–1441.)

septal generally have no septal connection but are located anteriorly along the central fibrous body or the right fibrous trigone at the right anterior free wall. Pathways classified as posteroseptal are located posterior to the central fibrous body within the pyramidal space. Anteroseptal pathways are found near the His bundle, and accessory pathway activation potential as well as a His bundle potential can be recorded simultaneously from a catheter placed at the His bundle region. Midseptal pathways are classified as right midseptal if an accessory pathway potential is recorded through a catheter located in an area bounded anteriorly by the tip electrode of the His bundle catheter and posteriorly by the coronary sinus ostium. For left midseptal pathways, the accessory pathway potential recording catheter is

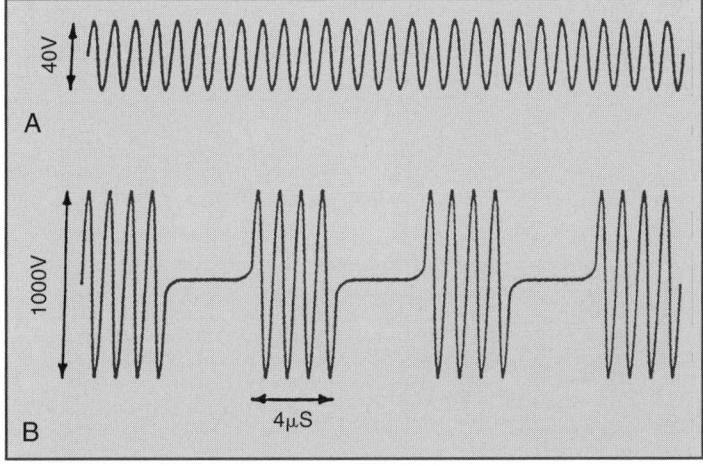

FIGURE 21–7. Comparison of output waveforms used for radiofrequency catheter ablation *(A)* and electrosurgical cutting *(B)*. Resistive heating during ablation is produced by a relatively low voltage (40 to 70 V) delivered in a continuous unmodulated fashion. The brief, high-voltage pulses used during electrosurgery promote arcing and coagulum formation. (From Kalbfleisch, S. J., and Langberg, J. J.: Catheter ablation with radiofrequency energy: biophysical aspects and clinical applications. J. Cardiovasc. Electrophysiol. 3:173, 1992.)

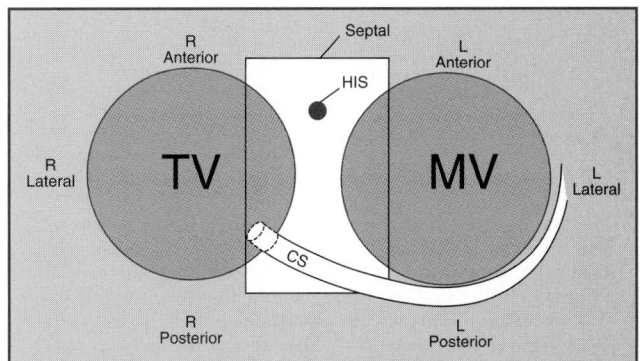

FIGURE 21–9. Schematic of free wall accessory pathway locations around the mitral and tricuspid annuli as visualized in the left anterior oblique projection. TV = tricuspid valve; MV = mitral valve; CS = coronary sinus; and His = His bundle. (From Miles, W. M., Zipes, D. P., and Klein, L. S.: Ablation of free wall accessory pathways. *In* Zipes, D. P. [ed.]: Catheter Ablation of Arrhythmias. Armonk, N.Y., Futura Publishing Company, 1994, pp. 211–230.)

placed at the left side of the septum within a similar region. Right posteroseptal pathways insert along the tricuspid ring in the immediate vicinity of the coronary sinus ostium, while left posteroseptal pathways are close to the terminal portion of the coronary sinus and may be located at a subepicardial site around the proximal coronary sinus, within a middle cardiac vein, or subendocardially along the ventricular aspect of the mitral annulus. Pathways at all locations and in all age groups can be ablated successfully.[332,333] Multiple pathways are present in about 5 per cent of patients.[334,335] Epicardial locations may be more easily approached from within the coronary sinus.[336] Conduction block after ablation usually occurs between the local atrial electrogram and the accessory pathway potential.[337]

ABLATION SITE. The optimal ablation site can be found by direct recordings of the accessory pathway (Fig. 21–10). The ventricular insertion site can be determined by finding the site of the earliest onset of the ventricular electrogram in relation to the onset of the delta wave, while the atrial insertion site can be found by locating the region of the shortest ventriculoatrial interval. Other helpful guidelines are unfiltered unipolar recordings that register a QS wave and the shortest AV conduction time during maximal preexcitation. A major ventricular potential synchronous with the onset of the delta wave can be a target site in left-sided preexcitation, while earlier ventricular excitation in relation to the delta wave is to be found for right-sided preexcitation. Reproducible mechanical inhibition of accessory pathway conduction[338] and subthreshold stimulation[339] also have been used to determine the optimal site. Accidental catheter trauma should be avoided, however.[340] Intracardiac echocardiography can be helpful at times.[341,342]

Accessory pathways often cross the left atrioventricular groove obliquely, with the atrial insertion site located closer to the ostium of the coronary sinus.[343] Therefore, a retrograde accessory pathway potential is recorded proximally close to the atrial potential at the atrial insertion site of the accessory pathway and recorded distally close to the ventricular potential at the ventricular insertion site. Consequently, the earliest site of retrograde atrial activation and the earliest site of anterograde ventricular activation are not directly across the AV groove from each other.

Thus, if ablation of the accessory pathway is from the atrial aspect of the mitral annulus, the site of earliest atrial activation is the optimal site for ablation, while if the ventricular aspect of the mitral annulus is the ablation target, the site of earliest ventricular activation would be the optimal position. Identification of the earliest site of atrial activation is usually performed during orthodromic atrioventricular reentrant tachycardia (AVRT).

. Successful ablation sites should exhibit stable fluoroscopic and electrical characteristics. During orthodromic AVRT, the interval between the onset of ventricular activation in any lead and local atrial activation is usually 70 to 90 msec at the successful ablation site. When thermistor-tipped ablation catheters are used, a stable rise in catheter tip temperature is a helpful adjunct to insure catheter stability and adequate catheter-tissue contact. In such an instance, the tip temperature generally exceeds 50°C.[344] The retrograde transaortic and transseptal approaches have been used with equal success to ablate accessory pathways located on the left side of the heart.[345,346] Routine electrophysiological study performed weeks after the ablation procedure is generally not indicated but should be considered in patients who have recurrent delta wave or symptoms of tachycardia.[347,348]

Patients with atriofascicular accessory pathways have connections consisting of a proximal portion responsible for conduction delay and decremental conduction properties and a long distal segment located along the endocardial surface of the right ventricular free wall that has electrophysiological properties similar to the right bundle branch. The distal end of the right atriofascicular accessory pathway can insert into the apical region of the right ventricular free wall close to the distal right bundle branch or can actually fuse with the latter.[349] Right atriofascicular accessory pathways actually may represent a duplication of the AV conduction system and can be localized for ablation by recording potentials from the rapidly conducting distal component extending from the tricuspid annulus to the apical region of the right ventricular free wall.[350] Ablation attempts should be performed more proximally to avoid inadvertently ablating the distal right bundle branch, which could actually be proarrhythmic and create incessant tachycardia by lengthening the reentrant circuit.[351–353]

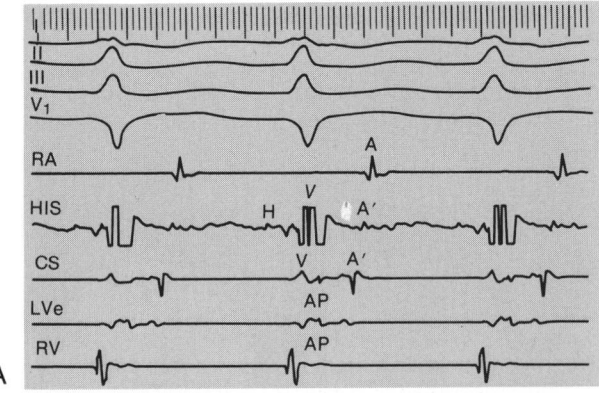

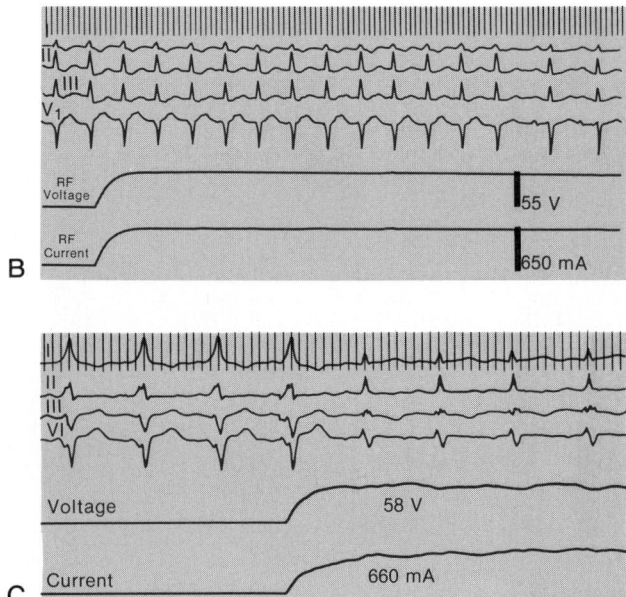

FIGURE 21–10. *A* and *B*, Radiofrequency (RF) ablation of a left free-wall accessory pathway. *A*, Depicts atrioventricular reentrant tachycardia with anterograde conduction over the normal pathway and retrograde conduction over the left free-wall accessory pathway. The electrodes in the coronary sinus (CS) record activation over the accessory pathway (AP), which is apposed by the catheter positioned in the left ventricular endocardium (LV$_e$). *B*, RF energy is delivered during the tachycardia and produces termination after 3.8 seconds. The delta wave has disappeared and tachycardia can no longer be initiated (not shown). Conventions as in Figure 21–11. *C*, Radiofrequency catheter ablation of a right free-wall accessory pathway. Elimination of accessory pathway conduction almost immediately after delivery of radiofrequency energy indicates that the catheter is positioned virtually on the accessory pathway and best insures a successful ablation. Leads I, II, III, V scalar recordings. (From Zipes, D. P., et al.: Nonpharmacologic therapy: Can it replace antiarrhythmic drug therapy? J. Cardiovasc. Electrophysiol. 2:S255, 1991.)

INDICATIONS. Ablation of accessory pathways is indicated in patients with symptomatic AV reentrant tachycardia that is drug resistant or when the patient is drug intolerant or does not desire long-term drug therapy. It is also indicated in patients with atrial fibrillation (or other atrial tachyarrhythmias) and a rapid ventricular response via accessory pathway when the tachycardia is drug resistant or when the patient is drug intolerant or does not desire long-term drug therapy. Other candidates might include patients with AVRT or atrial fibrillation with rapid ventricular rates identified during electrophysiological study of another arrhythmia; asymptomatic patients with ventricular preexcitation whose livelihood, profession, and important activities, insurability, mental well-being, or the public safety would be affected by spontaneous tachyarrhythmias or by the presence of the electrocardiographic abnormality; patients with atrial fibrillation and a controlled ventricular response via the accessory pathway; and patients with a family history of sudden cardiac death.[354]

RESULTS. From the results of a NASPE survey,[355] successful ablation of left free wall accessory pathways was obtained in 2312 of 2527 (91 per cent) patients; for septal accessory pathways, 1115 of 1279 (87 per cent); and for right free wall accessory pathways, 585 of 715 (82 per cent). Significant complications were reported in 94 of 4521 patients (2.1 per cent) and there were 13 procedure-related deaths in 4521 patients studies (0.2 per cent). In Europe, the complication rate was 4.4 per cent, with 3 deaths in 2222 patients.[356]

Radiofrequency Catheter Modification of the AV Node for AV Nodal Reentrant Tachycardias (AVNRT)

FAST-PATHWAY ABLATION. Ablation can be performed to eliminate conduction in the fast pathway or the slow pathway.[357–368] Ablation of the latter is preferred because the complication of heart block is minimized, patients with slow-slow reentry can be effectively treated and residual 1° AV block is avoided. Nevertheless, for fast-pathway ablation, the electrode tip is positioned along the AV node–His bundle axis in the anterosuperior portion of the tricuspid annulus. The catheter is gradually withdrawn until the atrial electrogram amplitude equals or exceeds that of the ventricular electrogram and the His bundle recording is either absent or extremely small (< 0.05 mV). During energy delivery, the ECG is monitored for PR prolongation and/or the occurrence of AV block. If accelerated junctional rhythm is noted during delivery of RF energy, the atrium can be paced at a faster rate to ensure integrity of AV conduction. The initial RF pulse is delivered at 15 to 20 watts for 10 to 15 seconds and gradually increased. Endpoints are P-R prolongation, elimination of retrograde fast-pathway conduction, and noninducibility of AVNRT. An alternative approach is to apply RF current at the site of earliest retrograde atrial activation during tachycardia. RF current should be discontinued if the P-R interval prolongs by more than 50 per cent or if AV block results.[357,358]

The major electrophysiological effects of fast-pathway ablation are elimination or marked attenuation of ventriculo-atrial conduction, an increase in the A-H interval, and elimination of dual AV nodal physiology (Fig. 21–11). Titrating the energy may reduce the risk of complete AV block, which is the most important complication associated with ablation of the fast pathway. If it is going to occur, complete AV block usually occurs during the ablation procedure, but some episodes have occurred 24 hours or more after the procedure, possibly as a result of the extension of the RF lesion over time. Tachycardia recurrence rate after successful fast-pathway ablation is approximately 10 to 15 per cent.[357,358]

SLOW-PATHWAY ABLATION. The slow pathway can be located by mapping along the posteromedial tricuspid annulus close to the coronary sinus os. Electrogram recordings

IU1071660B

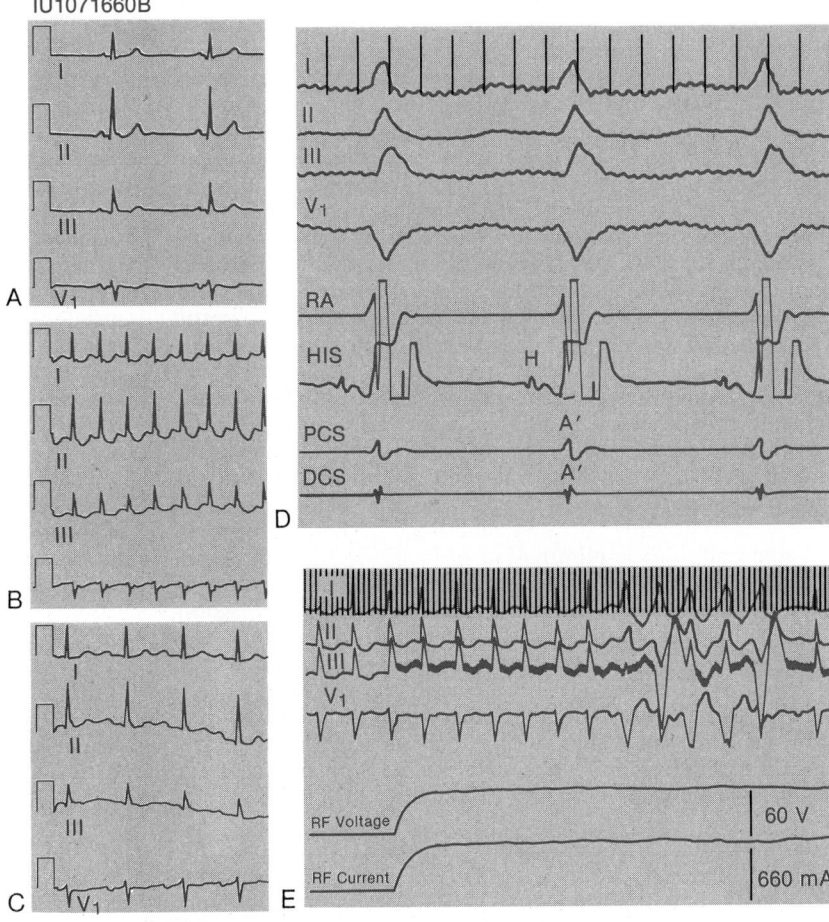

FIGURE 21–11. Radiofrequency (RF) AV nodal modification for AV nodal reentrant tachycardia. Panel A, Normal sinus rhythm. Panel B, AV nodal reentrant tachycardia. Panel C, Normal sinus rhythm following AV nodal ablation. Note prolonged P-R interval. Panel D, AV nodal reentrant tachycardia with intracavitary recordings. Note virtually simultaneous activation of atria and ventricles, consistent with AV nodal reentrant tachycardia. Panel E, Radiofrequency ablation with catheter placed in the anterior region of the AV node producing selective ablation of the anterogradely conducting fast pathway. Leads I, II, III, and V₁, scalar recordings. RA, right atrial electrogram; His, His bundle electrogram; PCS, electrogram recorded from the proximal electrodes of the coronary sinus catheter; DCS, electrogram recorded from the distal electrode of the coronary sinus catheter. Large time lines 50 msec; small time lines 10 msec. Vertical bars, calibration for RF voltage and current. Square wave for ECG = 1 mV, 200 msec.

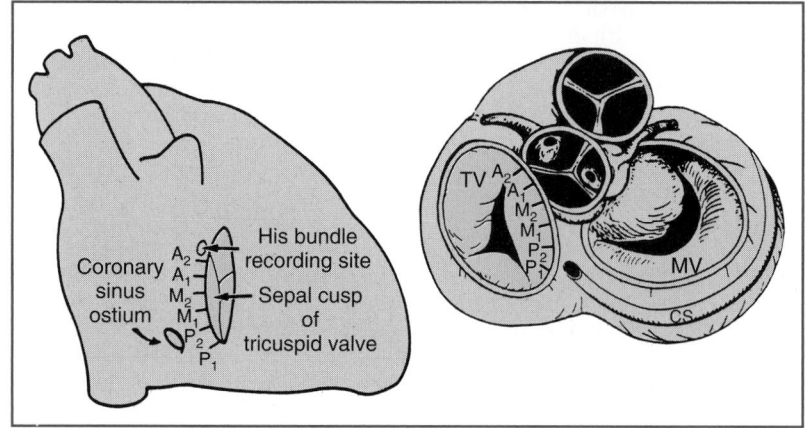

FIGURE 21–12. Radiographic and anatomical correlation during selective modification of the AV node. Schematic representations of right anterior oblique *(left)* and left anterior oblique *(right)* views. The most posterior location (P₁) is initially targeted for selective slow pathway ablation. Depending on the response, the catheter can be advanced progressively to a more anterior location (from P₁ to P₂ and then to M₁ and M₂). TV = tricuspid valve; MV = mitral valve; CS = coronary sinus. (Reproduced with permission from Akhtar, M., Jazayeri, M. R., Sra, J. S., et al.: Atrioventricular nodal reentry: Clinical, electrophysiologic and therapeutic considerations. Circulation *88:*282, 1993. Copyright 1993 American Heart Association.)

are obtained with an atrial-to-ventricular electrogram ratio of less than 0.5 and either a multicomponent atrial electrogram or a recording of possible slow-pathway potential.[362,362a] In the anatomical approach,[357,363] target sites are selected fluoroscopically by dividing the level of the coronary sinus os and the His bundle electrogram recording position into six anatomical regions (Fig. 21–12). Serial RF lesions are created in each region starting at the most posterior site and progressing to the more anterior locus. Finally, the slow pathway can be localized during ventricular pacing. The success rate with the anatomical or electrogram mapping approach is equivalent, and most often, combinations of both are used, yielding success rates approaching 100 per cent with less than 1 per cent chance of complete heart block.

Slow-pathway ablation results in an increase in the anterograde AV block cycle length and AV nodal effective refractory period without a change in the A-H interval or retrograde conduction properties of the AV node (see Chap. 22). Approximately 40 per cent of patients may have evidence of residual slow-pathway function after successful elimination of sustained AVNRT, usually manifested as persistent dual AV nodal physiology and single AV nodal echos during atrial extrastimulation. The endpoint for slow-pathway ablation is the elimination of sustained AVNRT both with and without an infusion of isoproterenol.[359,365,367]

AVNRT recurs in about 5 per cent of patients after slow-pathway ablation. In some patients, the effective refractory period of the fast pathway decreases after slow-pathway ablation, possibly due to electrotonic interaction between the two pathways.[369,370] Atypical forms of reentry can result following ablation,[371] as can apparent parasympathetic denervation, resulting in inappropriate sinus tachycardia.[372]

At present, the fast-pathway approach is appropriate when the slow-pathway approach has been found unsuccessful and perhaps in some patients in whom the induction of AVNRT is not reproducible, because fast-pathway ablation provides a reliable endpoint of P-R prolongation, in contrast to slow-pathway ablation, for which the only reliable endpoint is elimination of tachycardia. Ablation of the slow pathway is a safe and effective means for treating atypical AVNRT. In patients with AVNRT undergoing slow-pathway ablation, junctional ectopy during application of RF energy is a sensitive but nonspecific marker of successful ablation,[373–375] occurring in longer bursts at effective target sites than at ineffective sites. VA conduction should be expected during the junctional ectopy, and poor VA conduction or actual block is a predictor of AV block in patients undergoing RF ablation of the slow pathway.

INDICATIONS. Radiofrequency catheter ablation for AV nodal reentrant tachycardia can be considered in patients with symptomatic sustained AVNRT that is drug resistant or when the patient is drug intolerant or does not desire long-term drug treatment. The procedure also can be considered in patients with sustained AVNRT identified during electrophysiological study or catheter ablation of another arrhythmia or when finding dual AV nodal pathway physiology and atrial echos but without AVNRT during electrophysiological study in a patient suspected to have AVNRT clinically.[354]

RESULTS. Results of the NASPE survey indicate that 3052 patients had slow-pathway ablation with a 96 per cent reported success rate, while 255 had fast-pathway ablation that was successful in 229 (90 per cent). Significant complications occurred in 0.96 per cent, but no procedure-related deaths were reported.[355] In Europe, the complication rate was 8.0 per cent, mostly due to AV block following fast-pathway ablation, and there were no deaths in 815 patients.[356]

Radiofrequency Catheter Ablation of Atrial Tachycardia, Sinus Node Reentry/Inappropriate Sinus Tachycardia, and Atrial Flutter

Atrial arrhythmias amenable to catheter ablation include atrial tachycardias that are automatic or reentrant,[376–379] sinus node reentry,[380] incessant/inappropriate sinus tachycardia, junctional tachycardias,[381] and typical and atypical atrial flutter.[382–384] Activation mapping is used to determine the site of the atrial tachycardia by recording the earliest onset of local activation. Ten to 15 per cent of patients may have multiple atrial foci. Sites tend to cluster near the pulmonary veins in the left atrium and the mouths of the atrial appendages and along the crista terminalis on the right. Reentrant atrial tachycardia appears to occur more commonly in the setting of structural heart disease, specifically following prior atrial surgery. The region of slow conduction is not in a constant anatomical location but varies from patient to patient depending on the operation performed. Therefore, careful review of operative reports and electrophysiological mapping is essential. The atriotomy scar often plays an important role in the genesis of the tachycardia. When the sinus node area is to be ablated, it can be identified anatomically as well as electrophysiologically, and ablation lesions are usually placed between the superior vena cava and crista terminalis.

Understanding the reentrant pathway for typical atrial flutter (negative sawtooth waves in leads II, III, and aV_f at a rate of about 300/min) has been essential to developing an ablation approach. Reentry in the right atrium, with the left atrium passively activated, constitutes the mechanism of typical atrial flutter with a caudocranial activation along the right atrial septum and a craniocaudal activation of the right atrial free wall. A zone of slow conduction in the low right atrium, typically bounded by the tricuspid annulus, the inferior vena cava, and the coronary sinus, exists in the

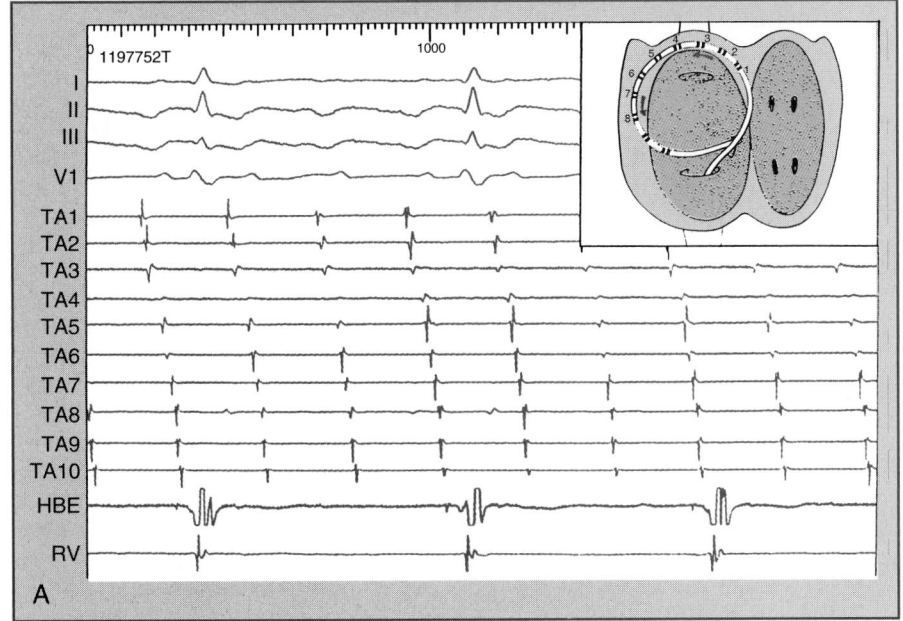

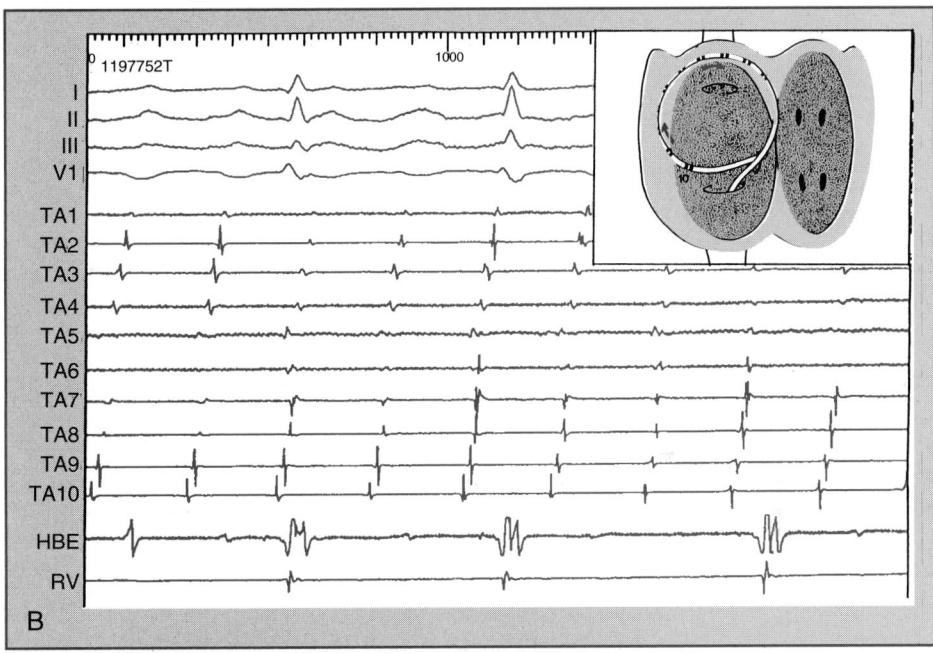

FIGURE 21–13. Atrial flutter. Panel *A* records typical atrial flutter, with negative flutter waves in leads II and III. The insert *(upper right)* is a schematic of the right and left atria. A catheter has been inserted through the inferior vena cava and loops around the right atrium. Electrodes 1 to 10 are marked and correspond to electrogram recordings TA1 to TA10. Note that the atrial activation sequence proceeds in a counterclockwise direction from TA1 to TA10, cephalad up the septum and caudally down the right atrial free wall. HBE = His bundle electrogram; RV = right ventricular electrogram; I, II, III, and V₁ = scalar recordings. *B,* Atypical atrial flutter in the same patient, with flutter waves positive in leads II and III. Recordings as in panel *A.* Note that the activation sequence travels in a clockwise direction in this example from the same patient. (Figure prepared by L. Brick Rigden, M.D.)

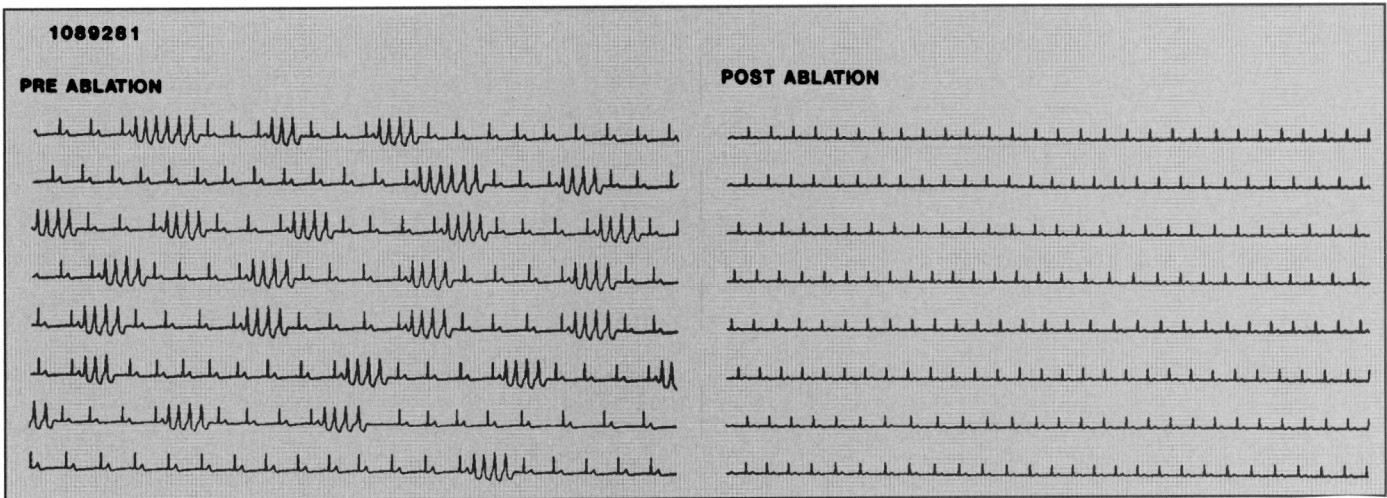

FIGURE 21–14. Recordings from a patient with ventricular tachycardia arising from the right ventricular outflow tract. Before the ablation procedure, frequent runs of symptomatic nonsustained ventricular tachycardia were recorded *(top half)*. After ablation, all spontaneous episodes of ventricular tachycardia were eliminated *(bottom half)*. (From Klein, L. S., Miles, W. M., and Zipes, D. P.: Ablation of idiopathic ventricular tachycardia and bundle branch reentry. *In* Zipes, D. P. [ed.]: Catheter Ablation of Arrhythmias. Armonk, N.Y., Futura Publishing Company, 1994, pp. 259–276.)

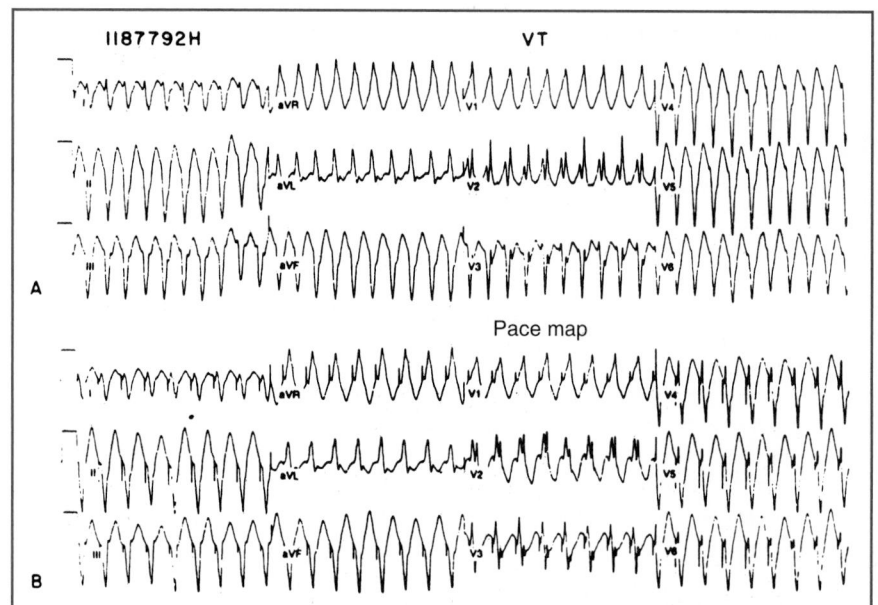

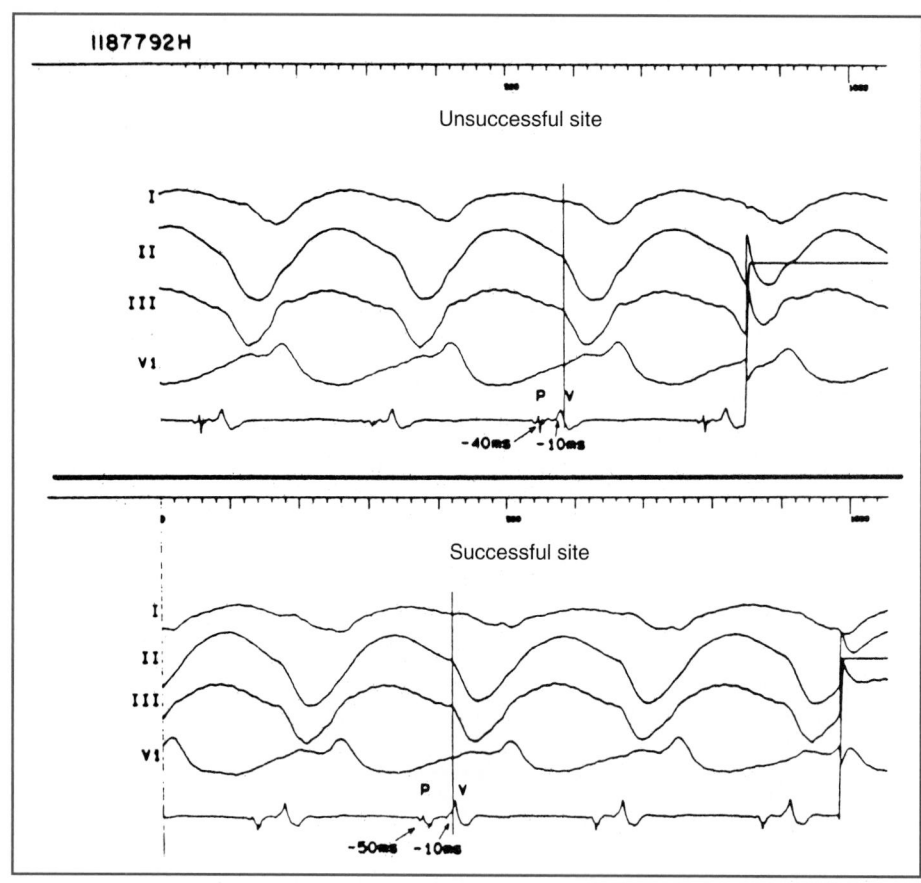

FIGURE 21–15. *Top panel,* Scalar ECG from a patient with verapamil-sensitive VT having the morphology of a right bundle branch block with extreme left axis deviation before (A) and during (B) pacing. *Bottom,* Left ventricular pacing at electrophysiological study exactly replicated the spontaneous ventricular tachycardia. *Bottom panel,* Intracardiac recordings from the same patient as in panel A. Four surface leads are shown along with an intracardiac recording from the distal poles of an ablation catheter positioned in the left ventricle. Recordings from the ablation catheter show a ventricular electrogram ($\dot{V}$) and a Purkinje potential (P). Ablation, delivered at the vertical line at the right, failed to eliminate the ventricular tachycardia in the top panel but did so in the bottom panel. Note that the timing of the ventricular electrogram to the onset of the QRS complex during VT (vertical line) is the same at both successful and unsuccessful ablation sites, but the Purkinje potential is recorded earlier from the site at which VT was ultimately eliminated.

region of the slow pathway.[385–387] Placing an ablation lesion across the zone of slow conduction abolishes the atrial flutter. This can be accomplished near the entrance of the slow zone in the low posterolateral right atrium, at the midpoint of the slow zone in the posterior right atrium, or near the exit at the posteromedial right atrium. Lesions can be guided anatomically or electrophysiologically. Atypical atrial flutter may be more difficult to ablate and has a clockwise rotation, cephalad up the right atrial free wall and caudad down the septum, with upright flutter waves in the inferior leads (Fig. 21–13).

INDICATIONS. Candidates for RF catheter ablation include patients with atrial tachycardia, sinus node reentry, inappropriate sinus tachycardia, or atrial flutter that is drug resistant, those who are drug intolerant, or those who do not desire long-term drug therapy.[354]

RESULTS. From the U.S. NASPE survey, 371 patients underwent ablation for atrial tachycardia and atrial flutter

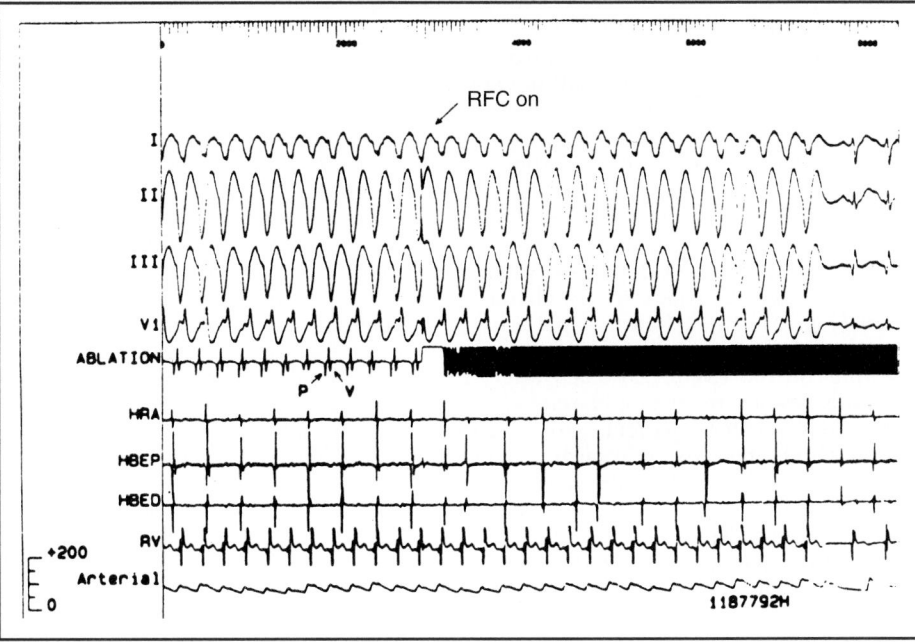

FIGURE 21–15. *Continued* The elimination of ventricular tachycardia by radiofrequency current delivered to the site at which the earliest Purkinje potential was identified. Ventricular tachycardia stopped spontaneously 4.7 seconds after the onset of RF energy and was no longer inducible. (Reproduced with permission from Klein, L. S., Miles, W. M., and Zipes, D. P.: Ablation of idiopathic ventricular tachycardia and bundle branch reentry. *In* Zipes, D. P. [ed.]: Catheter Ablation of Arrhythmias. Armonk, N.Y., Futura Publishing Company, 1994, pp. 259–276.)

with a success rate of 75 per cent and three significant complications (0.8 per cent) with no deaths.[355] The complication rate was 5 per cent in the European survey, and there were no deaths in 141 patients.[356]

Radiofrequency Catheter Ablation of Atrial Fibrillation

Although surgical procedures involving incision and isolation of atrial myocardium have been devised to eliminate atrial fibrillation, and their feasibility demonstrated catheter techniques for eliminating atrial fibrillation are in the relatively early stage of development, but preliminary success has been reported.[388–392]

Ablation and Modification of Atrioventricular Conduction for Atrial Tachyarrhythmias

To achieve RF catheter ablation of AV conduction, a catheter is placed across the tricuspid valve and positioned to record the largest His bundle electrogram associated with the largest atrial electrogram. RF energy is applied until complete AV block is achieved and is continued for an additional 30 seconds. If no change in AV conduction is observed after 60 seconds of RF ablation, the catheter is repositioned and the attempt is repeated. Patients who fail conventional RF ablation attempts from the right ventricle can undergo an attempt from the left ventricle with a catheter positioned along the posterior interventricular septum to record a large sharp His bundle electrogram. Energy is applied between the catheter electrode and the skin patch or between catheters in the left and right ventricles. Success rates approach 100 per cent in most studies today, with recurrence of AV conduction in less than 5 per cent.[393] Improved left ventricular function can result.[394]

More recently, the AV junction has been modified to slow the ventricular rate without producing complete AV block by ablating in the region of the slow pathway, as described under AV nodal modification for AV nodal reentry. Success rates for slowing the ventricular response vary but this procedure can be tried prior to producing complete AV block.[395–397]

INDICATIONS. Ablation and modification of atrioventricular conduction can be considered in (1) patients with symptomatic atrial tachyarrhythmias who have inadequately controlled ventricular rates unless primary ablation of the atrial tachyarrhythmia is possible, (2) similar patients when drugs are not tolerated or the patient does not wish to take them, even though the ventricular rate can be controlled, (3) patients with symptomatic nonparoxysmal junctional tachycardia that is drug resistant or by whom drugs are not tolerated or are not desired, (4) patients resuscitated from sudden cardiac death due to atrial flutter or atrial fibrillation with a rapid ventricular response in the absence of an accessory pathway, and (5) patients with a dual-chamber pacemaker and a pacemaker-mediated tachycardia that cannot be treated effectively by drugs or by reprograming the pacemaker.[354]

RESULTS. Results from the U.S. survey indicated that the procedure was successful in producing complete AV block in 95 per cent of 1600 patients, with significant complications occurring in 21 (1.3 per cent) and 2 procedure-related deaths (0.1 per cent).[355] In Europe, the complication rate was 3.2 per cent, and there was 1 death in 900 patients.[356]

Radiofrequency Catheter Ablation of Ventricular Tachycardia

In general, the success rate for ablation of ventricular tachycardias is lower than for AV nodal or AV reentry.[398–410] This may be related to the fact that this procedure is often a last-ditch effort in patients with drug-resistant ventricular tachycardias but also relates to very difficult mapping and ablation requirements in the thick-walled ventricles. Further, the ventricular tachycardia must be reproducibly inducible, monomorphic, sustained, and hemodynamically stable so that the patient can tolerate the ventricular tachycardia during the procedure. Also, the origin of the ventricular tachycardia must be fairly circumscribed and endocardially situated. Very rapid ventricular tachycardias, polymorphic ventricular tachycardias, and infrequent nonsustained episodes are not amenable to this form of therapy at this time.[398,399]

Radiofrequency catheter ablation of ventricular tachycardia must be divided into idiopathic ventricular tachycardia that occurs in patients with essentially normal hearts,[399,402–404,406,408,410] ventricular tachycardia that occurs in a variety of disease settings but without coronary artery disease, and ventricular tachycardia in patients with coronary artery disease.[398,400,405,407,409] In the first group, the ventricular tachycardias occur most commonly in the right ventricular outflow tract (Fig. 21–14) and less often in the inflow tract. Left ventricular tachycardias are characteristically septal in origin (Fig. 21–15). Abnormal patterns of sympathetic innervation may be present.[411] Ventricular tachycardias in abnormal hearts without coronary artery disease can be due to bundle branch reentry, a characteristic of dilated cardiomyopathies. In these patients, ablation of the right bundle branch eliminates the tachycardia.[412] Ventricular tachycardia can occur in right ventricular dysplasia, hypertrophic cardiomyopathy, and a host of other noncoronary disease problems (see p. 679).

Activation mapping[401,407] and pace mapping are effective in patients with idiopathic ventricular tachycardias to locate the site of origin of the ventricular tachycardia. Purkinje potentials (Fig. 21–15) can be recorded in some patients with left ventricular tachycardias.[399,406] Pace mapping involves stimulation of various ventricular sites to initiate a QRS contour that duplicates the QRS contour of the spontaneous ventricular tachycardia, thus establishing the apparent site of origin of the arrhythmia. This technique is limited by several methodological problems but may be useful when the tachycardia cannot be initiated and when a 12-lead ECG has been obtained during the spontaneous ventricular tachycardia. Localization of the site of origin of ventricular tachycardia in patients with coronary artery disease is more difficult than in patients with structurally normal hearts because of the altered anatomy and electrophysiology. Pace mapping is not as helpful as it is for idiopathic ventricular tachycardia. Further, reentry circuits can sometimes be large and resistant to the relatively small lesions produced by RF catheter ablation. Finding the area of slow conduction used as part of the reentrant circuit is helpful, since ablation at this site has a good chance of eliminating the tachycardia.

In patients without structural heart disease, only a single ventricular tachycardia is usually present, and catheter ablation of that ventricular tachycardia is curative. In patients with extensive structural heart disease, especially those with prior myocardial infarction, multiple ventricular tachycardias are often present. Catheter ablation of a single ventricular tachycardia in such patients may only be palliative and may not eliminate the need for further antiarrhythmic therapy.

INDICATIONS. Patients considered for RF catheter ablation of ventricular tachycardia are those with symptomatic sustained monomorphic ventricular tachycardia when the tachycardia is drug resistant, when the patient is drug intolerant, or when the patient does not desire long-term drug therapy; patients with bundle branch reentrant ventricular tachycardia; and patients with sustained monomorphic ventricular tachycardia and an implantable cardioverter-defibrillator who are receiving multiple shocks not manageable by reprograming or concomitant drug therapy. Occasionally, nonsustained ventricular tachycardia or even severely symptomatic premature ventricular complexes can be eliminated by RF catheter ablation.[354]

RESULTS. In the U.S. NASPE survey, 429 patients underwent ablation with an overall success rate of 71 per cent. In 224 patients with structurally normal hearts, the success rate was 85 per cent. The success rate was 54 per cent in 115 patients with ventricular tachycardia due to ischemic heart disease and 61 per cent in 90 patients with idiopathic cardiomyopathy. There were 13 significant complications (3.0 per cent) and, interestingly, considering the nature of the disease, no procedure-related deaths.[355] The complication rate was 7.5 per cent in the European survey, and there was 1 death in 320 patients.[356]

Chemical Ablation

Chemical ablation with alcohol or phenol of an area of myocardium involved in a tachycardia has been used to create AV block in patients not responding to catheter ablation and to eliminate atrial and ventricular tachycardias.[413,414] Excessive myocardial necrosis is the major complication, and alcohol ablation should be considered only when other ablative approaches fail or cannot be done.

SURGICAL THERAPY OF TACHYARRHYTHMIAS

The objectives of a surgical approach to treating a tachycardia are to excise, isolate, or interrupt tissue in the heart critical for the initiation, maintenance, or propagation of the tachycardia while preserving or even improving myocardial function. In addition to a direct surgical approach to the arrhythmia, indirect approaches such as aneurysmectomy, coronary artery bypass grafting, and relief of valvular regurgitation or stenosis can be useful in selected patients by improving cardiac hemodynamics and myocardial blood flow. Cardiac sympathectomy alters adrenergic influences on the heart and has been effective in some patients, particularly those who have recurrent ventricular tachycardia with the long Q-T syndrome.

Supraventricular Tachycardias

Surgical procedures[415–420] exist for patients (adults and children) with atrial tachycardias,[420] atrial flutter, AV nodal reentry,[416] and AV reentry,[417,421,422] (Fig. 21–16). Radiofrequency (RF) catheter ablation adequately treats the majority of these patients except for those with atrial fibrillation. Therefore, RF catheter ablation has replaced direct surgical intervention except for the occasional patient in whom RF catheter ablation fails or who is having concomitant cardiovascular surgery. In some instances, a prior attempt at RF catheter ablation complicates surgery by obliterating the normal tissue planes that exist in the AV groove of the heart or by rendering tissues too friable. Occasionally, pa-

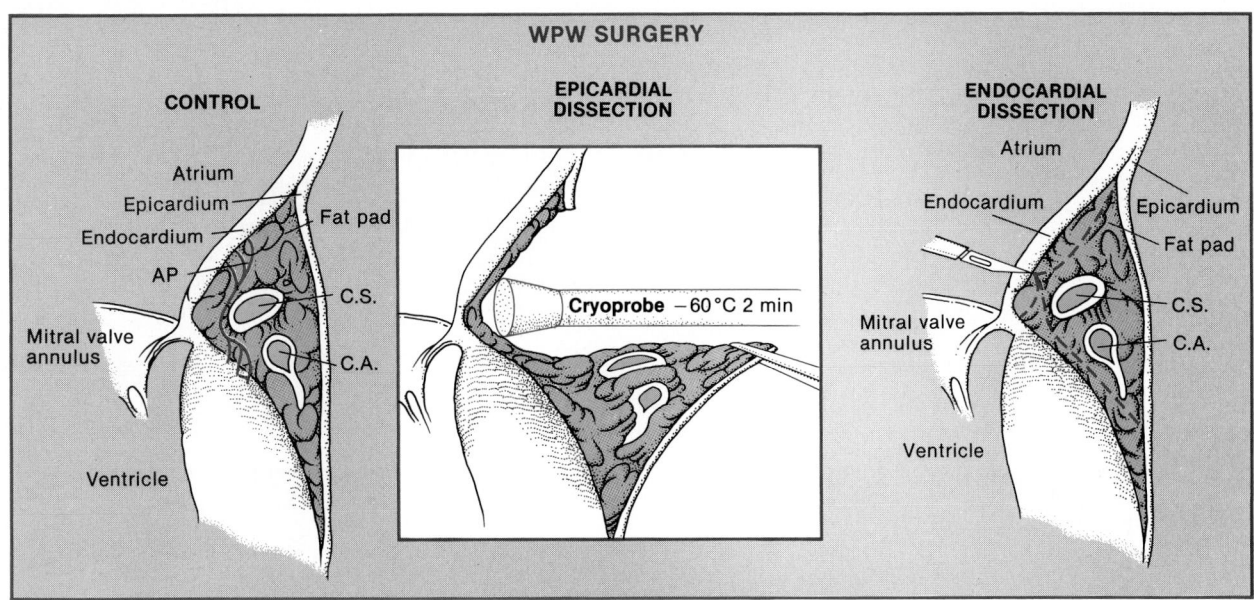

FIGURE 21–16. Schematic diagram showing the two approaches for surgical interruption of the accessory pathway. The left panel depicts the left atrioventricular groove and its vascular contents, the coronary sinus (C.S.) and circumflex coronary artery (C.A.). Multiple accessory pathways (AP) course through the fat pad. The middle panel shows the epicardial dissection approach while the right panel exhibits the endocardial dissection. Both approaches clear out the fat pad and interrupt any accessory pathways. (From Zipes, D.P.: Cardiac electrophysiology: promises and contributions. Reprinted by permission of the American College of Cardiology. J. Am. Coll. Cardiol. *13*:1329, 1989.)

tients with atrial tachycardias have multiple foci that require surgical intervention.[420]

The Maze procedure,[418,423] developed to treat patients with atrial fibrillation (see p. 656), eliminates the arrhythmia by reducing atrial tissue mass to a size at any instant in time too small to perpetuate the reentrant circuits responsible for atrial fibrillation. It forces atrial activation to proceed along a surgically determined pathway, thus maintaining sinus rhythm with AV nodal conduction. The Maze procedure permits organized electrical depolarization of the atria, restores atrial transport function, and in so doing decreases the risk of thromboembolism. Maintenance of sinus rhythm more than 3 months after the procedure approaches 100 per cent, although 30 to 40 per cent of patients require pacemakers because of chronotropic incompetence of the sinus node. The advent of minimally invasive endoscopic and endovascular techniques may make it possible to perform an equivalent of the Maze procedure without thoracotomy in the future.

Ventricular Tachycardia

In contrast to patients with supraventricular arrhythmias, candidates for surgical therapy of ventricular arrhythmias often have severe left ventricular dysfunction, generally caused by coronary artery disease. The etiology of the underlying heart disease influences the type of surgery performed. Candidates are patients with drug-resistant, symptomatic recurrent ventricular tachyarrhythmias who, ideally, have a localized abnormality, scar, or aneurysm with good left ventricular function. Poorer surgical results are obtained in patients with a history of congestive heart failure and left ventricular dysfunction.

Ischemic Heart Disease

In almost all patients who have ventricular tachycardia associated with ischemic heart disease, the arrhythmia, regardless of its configuration on the surface ECG, arises in the left ventricle or on the left ventricular side of the interventricular septum. The contour of the ventricular tachycardia can change from a right bundle branch block to a left bundle branch block pattern without a change in the

1earliest activation site, suggesting that the left ventricular site of origin remains the same, often near the septum, but its exit pathway is altered.

Indirect surgical approaches, including cardiac thoracic sympathectomy, coronary artery bypass grafting (CABG), and ventricular aneurysm or infarct resection with or without CABG, have been successful in about 60 per cent of reported cases. Coronary artery bypass grafting as a primary therapeutic approach generally has been limited to patients who experience ventricular tachycardia during ischemia

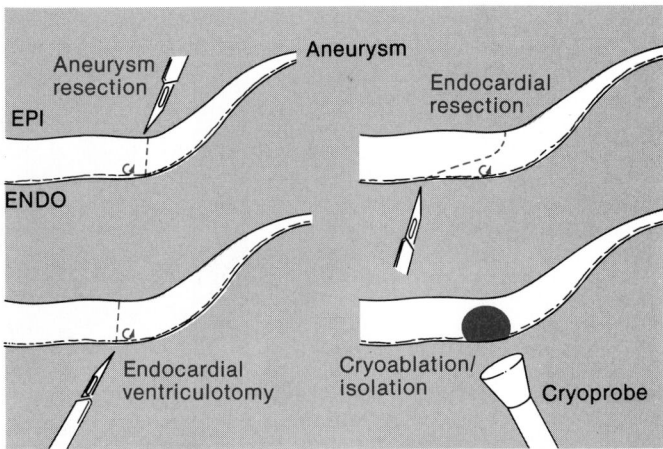

FIGURE 21–17. Schematic diagram showing the surgical approaches to ventricular tachycardia surgery in a patient with a left ventricular aneurysm. In the top left, the aneurysm is resected but the area of ventricular tachycardia origin remains (small circle with arrow) and tachycardia can recur. Bottom left panel demonstrates the technique for endocardial encircling ventriculotomy, no longer used. A nontransmural incision is made, which isolates the area of arrhythmia development. Top right panel demonstrates the method for endocardial resection. The aneurysm and a strip of endocardium containing the tachycardia focus are removed. Bottom right panel demonstrates cryoablation of the ventricular tachycardia focus. (From Zipes, D. P.: Cardiac electrophysiology: promises and contributions. Reprinted by permission of the American College of Cardiology. J. Am. Coll. Cardiol. *13*:1329, 1989.)

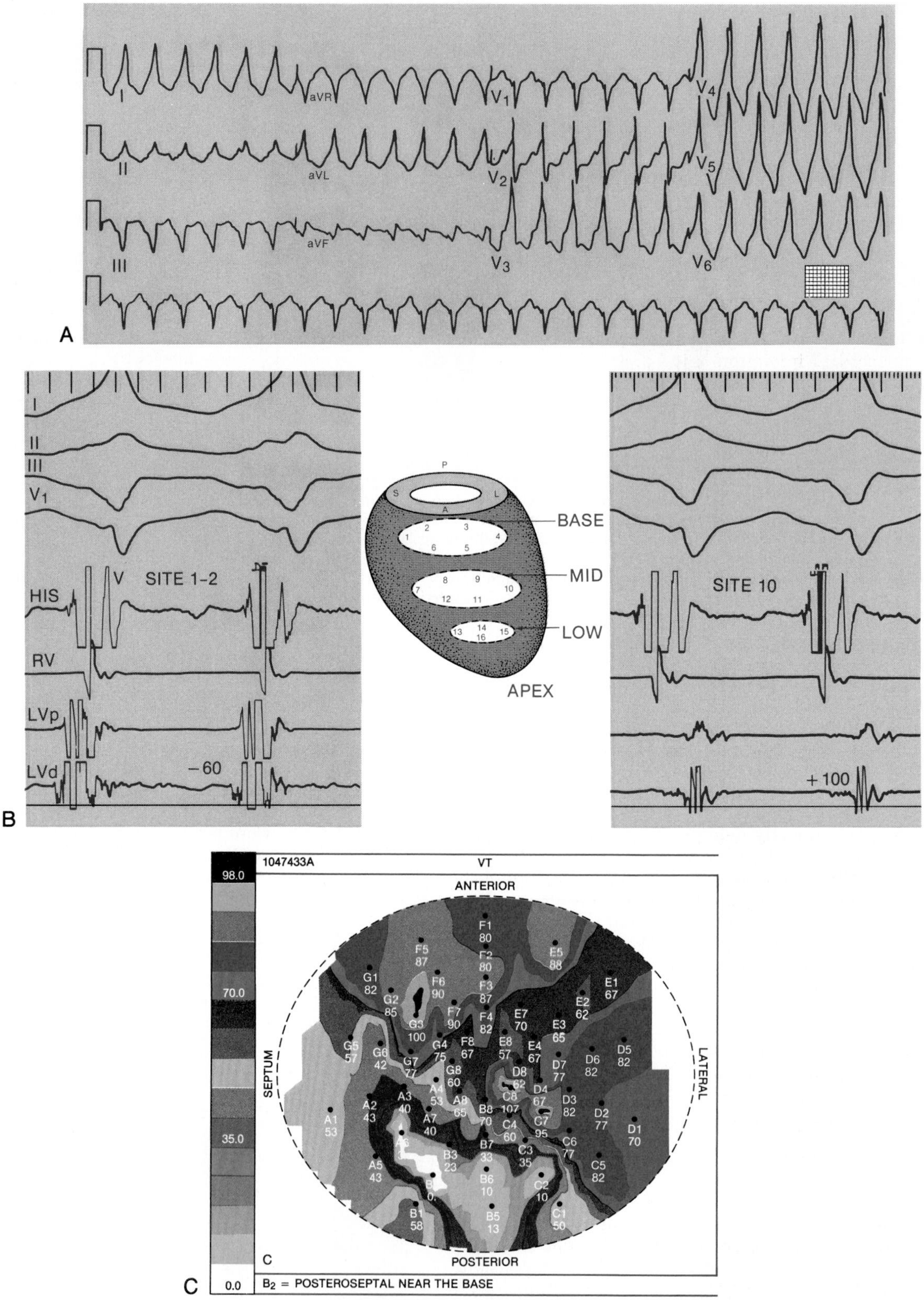

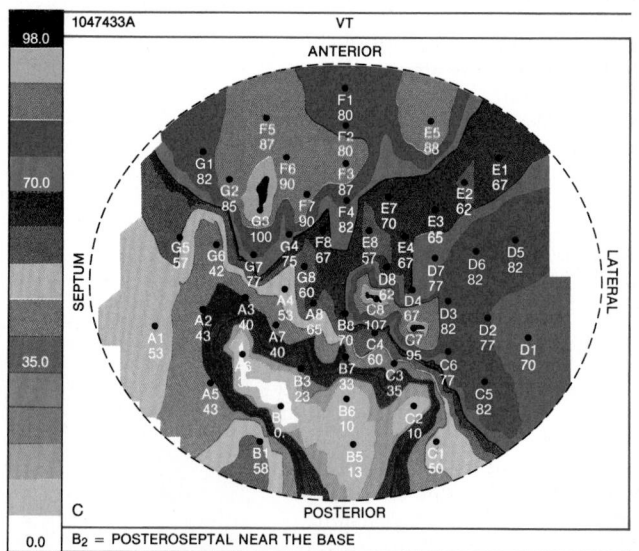

FIGURE 21–18. Mapping of a ventricular tachycardia. *A*, The 12-lead ECG demonstrates a ventricular tachycardia with a normal axis and left bundle branch block contour. *B*, A left ventricular catheter placed in the posteroseptal region of the left ventricle (positions 1, 2 in the schematic insert) records electrical activity from the distal electrodes of the left ventricular catheter (LVd) 60 msec in advance of the onset of the QRS complex. This illustrates that the tip of the catheter is close to the "origin" of the ventricular tachycardia. Electrical activity in the proximal left ventricular electrodes (LVp) and in the right ventricular recording (RV) is quite late (left panel). In the right panel, electrical activity recorded at site 10 in the midlateral left ventricle occurs well after the onset of the QRS complex, indicating that it is far from the origin of the tachycardia. *C*, At the time of surgery, a balloon studded with electrodes was inflated in the left ventricle and recorded an isopotential map that confirmed the origin of the ventricular tachycardia at a posteroseptal position in the left ventricle. (Schematic in *B* reproduced with permission from Dusman, R. E., et al.: Electrophysiological directed endocardial resection and cryoablation in the treatment of ventricular tachyarrhythmias. Indiana Med. *81:*242, 1988.)

but can be useful in patients with coronary disease resuscitated from sudden death who have no inducible arrhythmias at electrophysiological study. Patients with sustained monomorphic ventricular tachycardia or only polymorphic ventricular tachycardia or ventricular fibrillation uncommonly have their arrhythmia affected by coronary bypass surgery, although the latter can reduce the frequency of the arrhythmic episodes in some patients and prevent new ischemic events.

SURGICAL TECHNIQUES. Generally two types of direct surgical procedures are used: resection and ablation (Fig. 21–17). The *encircling endocardial ventriculotomy* (EEV) involving a transmural ventriculotomy to isolate areas of endocardial fibrosis that are recognized visually is no longer employed. The rationale for *endocardial resection* is based on animal and clinical data indicating that arrhythmias after myocardial infarction arise mostly in the subendocardial borders between normal and infarcted tissue. Endocardial resection involves peeling off a layer of endocardium, often in the rim of an aneurysm, that has been demonstrated by means of mapping procedures to be the site of earliest activation recorded during the ventricular tachycardia (Fig. 21–18). Some ventricular tachycardias can arise from the epicardium. Tachycardias arising from the base of the papillary muscles are cryoablated. Cryoablation also can be used to isolate areas of the ventricle that cannot be resected and is often combined with resection. *Laser approaches* are experimental but appear promising.

RESULTS. For ventricular tachyarrhythmias, operative mortality ranges from 6 to 23 per cent, with success rates defined as absence of recurrence of spontaneous ventricular arrhythmias ranging from 59 to 98 per cent. In experienced centers, operative mortality may be as low as 5 per cent in stable patients undergoing elective procedures, with 85 to 95 per cent of survivors free of inducible or spontaneous ventricular tachyarrhythmias. Recurrence rates range from 2 to 38 per cent. Postoperative survival is strongly influenced by the degree of left ventricular dysfunction. Patients with less favorable anatomy who are poor surgical candidates and who fail drug treatment are generally considered for an implantable cardioverter-defibrillator. By no longer having to operate on these patients, surgeons have improved the overall operative mortality.[419,424]

Operative mortality for nonthoracotomy implantable cardioverter-defibrillator (ICD) implantation is less than 1 per cent, with an annual sudden cardiac death mortality rate of less than 1 per cent.[425] Nevertheless, the latter patients are obligated to a lifetime of ICD therapy, which, naturally, does not prevent the arrhythmia but only terminates it after its onset. Some experts recommend surgery for patients with ventricular tachycardia who have discrete aneurysms that are amenable to intraoperative mapping and resection because such patients have a very high probability for cure of their arrhythmia.[426]

Electrophysiological Studies

PREOPERATIVE ELECTROPHYSIOLOGICAL STUDY. This involves induction of the ventricular tachycardia and electrophysiological mapping to pinpoint the area to be resected. A resolution of 4 to 8 cm^2 of ventricular endocardium is probably achieved, although more accurate anatomical localization of the mapping electrode tip in the ventricle may be possible. Tachycardias that are too rapid, short in duration, or polymorphic cannot be mapped accurately unless multiple catheters or a multielectrode array is used. Administering a drug such as procainamide may slow the ventricular tachycardia and transform a nonsustained pleomorphic ventricular tachycardia into a sustained ventricular tachycardia of uniform contour that can be mapped.

INTRAOPERATIVE VENTRICULAR MAPPING. Electrophysiological mapping is also performed at the time of surgery, with the operator using a handheld probe or an electrode array coupled with on-line computer techniques that instantaneously provide an activation map cycle by cycle. The sequence of activation during ventricular tachycardia can be plotted and the area of earliest activation determined (Fig. 21–18).

During ventricular tachycardia, the origin of the arrhythmia is generally ascribed to electrical activity recorded 25 to 50 msec in advance of the QRS complex. However, that is an arbitrary value, and it is quite clear that such activity can be late following the preceding cycle or early in advance of the next cycle. In addition, when such activity is recorded well after termination of the QRS complex, it becomes important to determine whether the deflections represent depolarization or repolarization. Potentials recorded prior to the onset of the surface QRS complex suggest that the origin of the tachycardia is nearby. When the earliest recordable electrical activity occurs with the onset of the QRS complex, the site of origin may be in the interventricular septum.

It is important to emphasize that the area of earliest recorded electrical activity during ventricular tachycardia may not actually represent the site of origin of the tachycardia, since the latter may originate several centimeters away, e.g., in a small scarred area, and be conducted very slowly until it reaches more normally excitable tissue where it exits the endocardium and generates a recordable extracellular complex. However, this area of early activation is probably closely related to the origin of the tachycardia which, based on present state of knowledge and results from surgery, warrants surgical intervention at that site. Finding an area of "continuous electrical activity" does not necessarily mean that reentry is present or that this is the origin of the tachycardia, since similar activity can be produced by automatically discharging foci, by recording slowly propagating, overlapping, or fragmented wavefronts from several areas, or by recording repolarization activity. However, it is likely that the origin of the tachycardia is close to the area of continuous electrical activity. In some patients, intramural mapping using a plunge needle electrode can be useful, particularly if the origin of the tachycardia is not located in the subendocardium.

Acknowledgments

Some of the illustrations were taken from studies performed by William M. Miles and Lawrence S. Klein.

REFERENCES

CLINICAL PHARMACOKINETICS

1. Follath, F.: The utility of serum drug level monitoring during therapy with class III antiarrhythmic agents. J. Cardiovasc. Pharmacol. *20* (Suppl. II):S41, 1992.
2. Roden, D. M., and Murray, K. T.: Pharmacokinetics, pharmacodynamics, and pharmacogenetics. *In* Zipes, D. P., and Jalife, J. (eds.): Cardiac Electrophysiology: From Cell to Bedside. 2nd ed. Philadelphia, W. B. Saunders Company, 1994, pp. 1289–1296.
3. Buchert, E., and Woosley, R. L.: Clinical implications of variable antiarrhythmic drug metabolism. Pharmacogenetics *2*:2, 1992.
4. Roden, D. M.: Are pharmacokinetics helpful for the clinician? J. Cardiovasc. Electrophysiol. *2*:S178, 1991.
5. Lalka, D., Griffith, R. K., and Cronenberger, C. L.: The hepatic first-pass metabolism of problematic drugs. J. Clin. Pharmacol. *33*:657, 1993.
6. Stanton, M. S.: Class I antiarrhythmic drugs: Quinidine, procainamide, disopyramide, lidocaine, mexiletine, tocainide, phenytoin, moricizine, flecainide, propafenone. *In* Zipes, D. P., and Jalife, J. (eds.): Cardiac Electrophysiology: From Cell to Bedside. 2nd ed. Philadelphia, W. B. Saunders Company, 1994, pp. 1296–1317.
7. Nattel, S.: Antiarrhythmic drug classifications: A critical appraisal of their history, present status and clinical relevance. Drugs *41*:672, 1991.
8. Vaughan Williams, E. M.: The relevance of cellular to clinical electrophysiology in classifying antiarrhythmic actions. J. Cardiovasc. Pharmacol. *20* (Suppl. 2):S1, 1992.
9. Rosen, M. R., Strauss, H. C., and Janse, M. J.: The classification of antiarrhythmic drugs. *In* Zipes, D. P., and Jalife, J. (eds.): Cardiac Electrophysiology: From Cell to Bedside. 2nd ed. Philadelphia, W. B. Saunders Company, 1994, pp. 1277–1286.
10. Members of the Sicilian Gambit: Antiarrhythmic Therapy: A Pathophysiologic Approach. Armonk, N.Y., Futura Publishing Company, 1994.
11. Sadanaga, T., Ogawa, S., Okada, Y., et al.: Clinical evaluation of the use-dependent QRS prolongation and the reverse use-dependent QT prolongation of class I and class III antiarrhythmic agents and their value in predicting efficacy. Am. Heart J. *126*:114, 1993.
12. Birgersdotter, U. M., Wong, W., Turgeon, J., et al.: Stereoselective genetically determined interaction between chronic flecainide and quinidine in patients with arrhythmias. Br. J. Clin. Pharmacol. *33*:275, 1992.
13. Adams, L. E., Baldrkishnan, K., Roberts, S. M., et al.: Genetic, immunologic and biotransformation studies of patients on procainamide. Lupus *2*:89, 1993.
14. Danielly, J., DeJong, R., Radke-Mitchell, L. C., et al.: Procainamide-associated blood dyscrasias. Am. J. Cardiol. *74*:1179, 1994.
15. Skaer, T. L.: Medication-induced systemic lupus erythematosus. Clin. Ther. *14*:496, 1992.
16. Falk, R. H.: Proarrhythmia in patients treated for atrial fibrillation or flutter. Ann. Intern. Med. *117*:141, 1992.
17. Kidwell, G. A.: Drug-induced ventricular proarrhythmia. Cardiovasc. Clin. *22*:317, 1992.
18. Patterson, E., Szabo, B., Scherlag, B. J., et al.: Arrhythmogenic effects of antiarrhythmic drugs. *In* Zipes, D. P., and Jalife, J. (eds.): Cardiac Elec-

trophysiology: From Cell to Bedside. 2nd ed. Philadelphia, W. B. Saunders Company, 1994, pp. 496–511.

19. Benditt, D. G., Bailin, S., Remole, S., et al.: Proarrhythmia: Recognition of patients at risk. J. Cardiovasc. Electrophysiol. *2*:S221, 1991.
20. Bhein, S., Muller, M., Gerwin, R., et al.: Comparative study on the proarrhythmic effects of some antiarrhythmic agents. Circulation *87*:617, 1993.
21. Morganroth, J.: Early and late proarrhythmia from antiarrhythmic drug therapy. Cardiovasc. Drugs Ther. *6*:11, 1992.
22. Ben-David, J., and Zipes, D. P.: Torsades de pointes and proarrhythmia. Lancet *341*(8860):1578, 1993.
23. Roden, D. M.: Torsade de pointes. Clin. Cardiol. *16*:683, 1993.
24. Lazzara, R.: Antiarrhythmic drugs and torsade de pointes. Eur. Heart J. *14* (Suppl. H):88, 1993.
25. Roden, D. M.: Early after-depolarizations and torsade de pointes: Implications for the control of cardiac arrhythmias by prolonging repolarization. Eur. Heart J. *14* (Suppl. H):56, 1993.
26. Banai, S., and Tzivoni, D.: Drug therapy for torsade de pointes. J. Cardiovasc. Electrophysiol. *4*:206, 1993.
27. Weissenburger, J., Davy, J. M., and Chezalviel, F.: Experimental models of torsades de pointes. Fund. Clin. Pharmacol. *7*:29, 1993.
28. Lazzara, R.: Mechanistic and clinical aspects of acquired long QT syndromes. Ann. N.Y. Acad. Sci. *644*:48, 1992.
29. Sicouri, S., and Antzelevitch, C.: Drug-induced afterdepolarizations and triggered activity occur in a discreet subpopulation of ventricular muscle cells (M cells) in the canine heart: Quinidine and digitalis. J. Cardiovasc. Electrophysiol. *4*:48, 1993.
30. Faber, T. S., Zehender, M., Van de Loo, A., et al.: Torsade de pointes complicating drug treatment of low-malignant forms of arrhythmia: Four case reports. Clin. Cardiol. *17*:197, 1994.
31. Wyse, K. R., Ye, V., and Campbell, T. J.: Action potential prolongation exhibits simple dose-dependence for sotalol, but reverse dose-dependence for quinidine and disopyramide: Implications for proarrhythmia due to triggered activity. J. Cardiovasc. Pharmacol. *21*:316, 1993.
32. Fast, V. G., and Pertsov, A. M.: Shift and termination of functional reentry in isolated ventricular preparations with quinidine-induced inhomogeneity in refractory period. J. Cardiovasc. Electrophysiol. *3*:255, 1992.
33. Flaker, G. C., Blackshear, J. L., McBride, R., et al.: Antiarrhythmic drug therapy and cardiac mortality in atrial fibrillation. The Stroke Prevention in Atrial Fibrillation Investigators. J. Am. Coll. Cardiol. *20*:527, 1992.
34. Epstein, A. E., Halstrom, A. P., Rogers, W. J., et al.: Mortality following ventricular arrhythmia suppression by encainide, flecainide and moricizine after myocardial infarction: The original design concept of the Cardiac Arrhythmia Suppression Trial (CAST). JAMA *270*:2451, 1993.
35. Cardiac Arrhythmia Suppression Trial II Investigators: Effect of the antiarrhythmic agent moricizine on survival after myocardial infarction. N. Engl. J. Med. *327*:227, 1992.
36. Anderson, J. L., Platia, E. V., Hallstrom A., et al.: Interaction of baseline characteristics with the hazard of encainide, flecainide and moricizine therapy in patients with myocardial infarction. A possible explanation for increased mortality in the Cardiac Arrhythmia Suppression Trial (CAST). Circulation *90*:2843, 1994.

CLASS IA AGENTS

37. Levy, S., and Azoulay, S.: Stories about the origin of quinquina and quinidine. J. Cardiovasc. Electrophysiol. *5*:635, 1994.
38. Cappato, R., Alboni, P., Codeca, L., et al.: Direct and autonomically mediated effects of oral quinidine on RR/QT relation after an abrupt increase in heart rate. J. Am. Coll. Cardiol. *22*:99, 1993.
39. Hondeghem, L. M.: Ideal antiarrhythmic agents: Chemical defibrillators. J. Cardiovasc. Electrophysiol. *2*:S169, 1991.
40. Carmeliet, E.: Use-dependent block of the delayed K⁺ current in rabbit ventricular myocytes. Cardiovasc. Drugs Ther. *7* (Suppl. 3):599, 1993.
41. Grant, A. O., and Wendt, D. J.: Blockade of ion channels by antiarrhythmic drugs. J. Cardiovasc. Electrophysiol. *2*:S153, 1991.
42. Markel, M. L., Miles, W. M., Luck, J. C., et al.: Differential effects of isoproterenol on sustained ventricular tachycardia before and during procainamide and quinidine antiarrhythmic drug therapy. Circulation *87*:783, 1993.
43. Allen, N. M.: Relationship between serum quinidine concentration and quinidine dosage. Pharmacol. Ther. *12*:189, 1992.
44. Packer, M.: Hemodynamic consequences of antiarrhythmic drug therapy in patients with chronic heart failure. J. Cardiovasc. Electrophysiol. *2*:S240, 1991.
45. Hook, B. G., Rosenthal, M. E., Marchlinski, F. E., et al.: Results of electrophysiological testing and long-term follow-up in patients sustaining cardiac arrest only while receiving type IA antiarrhythmic agents. PACE *15*:324, 1992.
46. Sager, P. T., Pearlmutter, R. A., Rosenfeld, L. E., et al.: Antiarrhythmic drug exacerbation of ventricular tachycardia inducibility during electrophysiologic study. Am. Heart J. *123*:926, 1992.
47. Wu, B., Sato, T., Kiyosue, T., et al.: Blockade of two, four-dinotrophenol induced ATP sensitive potassium currents in guinea pig ventricular myocytes by class I antiarrhythmic drugs. Cardiovasc. Res. *26*:1095, 1992.
48. Kar, P. M., Kellner, K., Ing, T. S., et al.: Combined high-efficiency he-

modialysis and charcoal hemoperfusion in severe N-acetylprocainamide intoxication. Am. J. Kidney Dis. *20*:403, 1992.
49. Dibner-Dunlap, M. E., Cohen, M. D., Yuih, S. N., et al.: Procainamide inhibits sympathetic nerve activity in rabbits. J. Lab. Clin. Med. *119*:211, 1992.
50. Grimm, W., Cho, J.-G., and Marchlinski, F. E.: Effects of incremental doses of procainamide in patients with sustained uniform ventricular tachycardia. J. Cardiovasc. Electrophysiol. *5*:313, 1994.
51. Brautigam, R. T., Porter, S., and Kutalek, S. P.: The effects of programmed ventricular stimulation on plasma procainamide levels: An experimental model. J. Clin. Pharmacol. *34*:184, 1994.
52. Ellenbogen, K. A., Wood, M. A., and Stambler, B. S.: Procainamide: A perspective on its value and danger. Heart Dis. Stroke *2*:493, 1993.
53. Edvardsson, N.: Comparison of class I and class III action in atrial fibrillation. Eur. Heart J. *14* (Suppl. H):62, 1993.
54. Kudenchuk, P. J., Halperin, B., Kron, J., et al.: Serial electropharmacologic studies in patients with ischemic heart disease and sustained ventricular tachyarrhythmias: When is drug testing sufficient. Am. J. Cardiol. *72*:1400, 1993.
55. Steinberg, J. S., Sahar, B. I., Rosenbaum, M., et al.: Proarrhythmic effects of procainamide and tocainide in a canine infarction model. J. Cardiovasc. Pharmacol. *19*:52, 1992.
56. Echizen, H., Kawasaki, H., Chiba, K., et al.: A potent inhibitory effect of erythromycin and other macrolide antibiotics on the mono-N-dealkylation metabolism of disopyramide with human liver microsomes. J. Pharmacol. Exp. Ther. *264*:1425, 1993.

CLASS IB AGENTS

57. Chahine, M., Chen, L. Q, Barchi, R. L., et al.: Lidocaine block of human heart sodium channels expressed in *Zenopus* oocytes. J. Mol. Cell Cardiol. *24*:1231, 1992.
58. Ye, V. Z., Wyse, K. R., and Campbell, T. J.: Lidocaine shows greater selective depression of depolarized and acidotic myocardium than propafenone: Possible implications for proarrhythmia. J. Cardiovasc. Pharmacol. *21*:47, 1993.
59. Destache, C. J., Hilleman, D. E., Mohiuddin, S. J., et al.: Predictive performance of Bayesian and nonlinear least-squares regression programs for lidocaine. Ther. Drug Monit. *14*:286, 1992.
60. Nattel, S., and Arenal, A.: Antiarrhythmic prophylaxis after acute myocardial infarction: Is lidocaine still useful? Drugs *45*:9, 1993.
61. Jaffe, A. S.: Prophylatic lidocaine for suspected acute myocardial infarction? Heart Dis. Stroke *1*:179, 1992.
62. Jaffe, A. S.: The use of antiarrhythmics in advanced cardiac life support. Ann. Emerg. Med. *22*:307, 1993.
63. Johnson, R. G., Goldberger, A. L., Thurer, R. L., et al.: Lidocaine prophylaxis in coronary revascularization patients: A randomized, prospective trial. Ann. Thorac. Surg. *55*:1180, 1993.
64. Buckles, D. S., Ick, B., and Gillette, P. C.: Subcutaneous lidocaine affects inducibility in programmed electrophysiology testing in children: A follow-up study. Am. Heart J. *124*:1241, 1992.
65. McCaughey, W.: Adverse effects of local anesthetics. Drug Saf. *7*:178, 1992.
66. Tatsukawa, H., Okuda, J., Kondoh, M., et al.: Malignant hyperthermia caused by intravenous lidocaine for ventricular arrhythmia. Ann. Intern. Med. *31*:1069, 1992.
67. Echt, D. S., Gremillion, S. T., Lee, J. T., et al.: Effects of procainamide and lidocaine on defibrillation energy requirements in patients receiving implantable cardioverter defibrillator devices. J. Cardiovasc. Electrophysiol. *5*:752, 1994.
68. Mason, J. W.: A comparison of seven antiarrhythmic drugs in patients with ventricular tachyarrhythmias: Electrophysiologic Study Versus Electrocardiographic Monitoring investigators. N. Engl. J. Med. *329*:452, 1993.
69. Lazzara, R.: Results of Holter ECG guided therapy for ventricular arrhythmias: The ESVEM trial. PACE *17*:473, 1994.
70. Takanaka, C., Nonokawa, M., Machii, T., et al.: Mexiletine and propafenone: A comparative study of monotherapy, low and full dose combination therapy. PACE *15*:2130, 1992.
71. Yeung-Lai-Wah, J. A., Murdock, C. J., Boone, J., et al.: Propafenone-mexiletine combination for the treatment of sustained ventricular tachycardia. J. Am. Coll. Cardiol. *20*:547, 1992.
72. Lombardi, F., Finocciaro, M. L., DallaVecchia, L., et al.: Effects of mexiletine, propafenone and flecainide on signal-averaged electrocardiogram. Eur. Heart J. *13*:517, 1992.
73. Geraets, D. R., Scott, S. D., and Ballew, K. A.: Toxicity potential of oral lidocaine in a patient receiving mexiletine. Ann. Pharmacol. Ther. *26*:1380, 1992.
74. Gelfand, M. S., Yunus, F., and White, F. L.: Bone marrow granulomas, fever, pancytopenia, and lupus-like syndrome due to tocainide. South. Med. J. *87*:839, 1994.
75. Kahn, A. S., Dadparvar, S., Brown, S. J., et al.: The role of gallium-67-citrate in the detection of phenytoin-induced pneumonitis. J. Nucl. Med. *35*:471, 1994.
76. Danielson, M. K., Danielson, B. R., Marchner, H., et al.: Histopathological and hemodynamic studies supporting hypoxia and vascular disruption as explanation to phenytoin teratogenicity. Teratology *46*:485, 1992.
77. Lindhout, D., and Omtzigt, J. G.: Pregnancy and the risk of teratogenicity. Epilepsia 33 (Suppl. 4):S41, 1992.

78. Wang, Z., Fremini, B., and Nattel, S.: Mechanism of flecainide's rate-dependent actions on action potential duration in canine atrial tissue. J. Pharmacol. Exp. Ther. 267:575, 1993.

79. Yamashita, T., Inoue, H., Nozaki, A., et al.: Role of anisotropy in determining the selective action of antiarrhythmics in atrial fluttter in the dog. Cardiovasc. Res. 26:244, 1992.

80. Crijns, H. J., deLangen, C. D., Grandjean, J. G., et al.: Sustained atrial flutter around the tricuspid valve in pigs: Differentiation of procainamide (class IA) from flecainide (class IC) and their rate-dependent effects. J. Cardiovasc. Pharmacol. 21:462, 1993.

81. Pinto, J. M., Graziano, J. N., and Boyden, P. A.: Endocardial mapping of reentry around an anatomical barrier in the canine right atrium: Observations during the action of the class IC agent, flecainide. J. Cardiovasc. Electrophysiol. 4:672, 1993.

82. Windle, J. R., Witt, R. C., and Rozanski, G. J.: Effects of flecainide on ectopic atrial automaticity and conduction. Circulation 88:1878, 1993.

83. Krishnan, S. C., and Antzelevitch, C.: Flecainide-induced arrhythmia in canine ventricular epicardium. Phase II reentry? Circulation 87:562, 1993.

84. Goldberger, J., Helmy, I., Katzung, B., et al.: Use-dependent properties of flecainide acetate in accessory atrioventricular pathways. Am. J. Cardiol. 73:43, 1994.

85. Gill, J. S., Mehta, D., Ward, D. E., et al.: Efficacy of flecainide, sotalol and verapamil in the treatment of right ventricular tachycardia in patients without overt cardiac abnormality. Br. Heart J. 68:392, 1992.

86. Kidwell, G. A., Greenspon, A. J., Greenberg, R. M., et al.: Use-dependent prolongation of ventricular tachycardia cycle length by type I antiarrhythmic drugs in humans. Circulation 87:118, 1993.

87. Madrid, A. H., Moro, C., Marin-Huerta, E., et al.: Comparison of flecainide and procainamide in conversion of atrial fibrillation. Eur. Heart J. 14:1127, 1993.

88. Hohnloser, S. H., and Zabel, M.: Short- and long-term efficacy and safety of flecainide acetate for supraventricular arrhythmias. Am. J. Cardiol. 70:3A, 1992.

89. A symposium: Use of flecainide for the treatment of supraventricular arrhythmias. Am. J. Cardiol. 70:1A, 1992.

90. Anderson, J. L., Platt, M. L., Guarnier, I. T., et al.: Flecainide acetate for paroxysmal supraventricular tachyarrhythmias: The flecainide supraventricular tachycardia study group. Am. J. Cardiol. 74:578, 1994.

91. Balaji, S., Johnson, T. B., Sade, R. M., et al.: Management of atrial flutter after the Fontan procedure. J. Am. Coll. Cardiol. 23:1209, 1994.

92. Lau, C. P., Leung, W. H., and Wong, C. K.: A randomized double-blind crossover study comparing the efficacy and tolerability of flecainide and quinidine in the control of patients with symptomatic paroxysmal atrial fibrillation. Am. Heart J. 124:645, 1992.

93. Grey, E., and Silverman, D. I.: Efficacy of type IC antiarrhythmic agents for treatment of resistant atrial fibrillation. PACE 16:2235, 1993.

94. LeClercq, J. F., Chouty, F., Denjoy, I., et al.: Flecainide in quinidine-resistant atrial fibrillation. Am. J. Cardiol. 70:62A, 1992.

95. Auricchio, A.: Reversible protective effect of propafenone or flecainide during atrial fibrillation in patients with an accessory atrioventricular connection. Am. Heart J. 124:932, 1992.

96. vonBernuth, G., Engelhardt, W., Kramer, H. H., et al.: Atrial automatic tachycardia in infancy and childhood. Eur. Heart J. 13:1410, 1992.

97. Ahsan, A., Aldridge, R., and Bowes, R.: 1:1 Atrioventricular conduction in atrial flutter with digoxin and flecainide. Int. J. Cardiol. 39:88, 1993.

98. vanEngelen, A. D., Weijtens, O., Brenner, J. I., et al.: Management outcome and follow-up of fetal tachycardia. J. Am. Coll. Cardiol. 24:1371, 1994.

99. Ito, S., Magee, L., and Smallhorn, J.: Drug therapy for fetal arrhythmias. Clin. Perinatol. 21:543, 1994.

100. Perry, J. C., and Garson, A., Jr.: Flecainide acetate for treatment of tachyarrhythmias in children: Review of world literature on efficacy, safety and dosing. Am. Heart J. 124:1614, 1992.

101. Manz, M., Jung, W., and Luderitz, B.: Interactions between drugs and devices: Experimental and clinical studies. Am. Heart J. 127:978, 1994.

102. Stramba-Badiale, M., Lazzarotti, M., Facchini, M., et al.: Malignant arrhythmias and acute myocardial ischemia: Interaction between flecainide and the autonomic nervous system. Am. Heart J. 128:973, 1994.

103. Sadanaga, T., and Ogawa, S.: Ischemia enhances use-dependent sodium channel blockade by pilsicainide, a class IC antiarrhythmic agent. J. Am. Coll. Cardiol. 23:1378, 1994.

104. Wang, J., Bourne, G. W., Wang, Z., et al.: Comparative mechanisms of antiarrhythmic drug action in experimental atrial fibrillation: Importance of use-dependent effects on refractoriness. Circulation 88:1030, 1993.

105. Brugada, J., Boersma, L., Abdollah, H., et al.: Echo-wave termination of ventricular tachycardia: A common mechanism of termination of reentrant arrhythmias by various pharmacological interventions. Circulation 85:1879, 1992.

106. Santinelli, V., Arnese, M., Oppo, I., et al.: Effects of flecainide and propafenone on systolic performance in subjects with normal cardiac function. Chest 103:1068, 1993.

107. Lombardi, F., Torzillo, D., Sandrone, G., et al.: Beta-blocking effect of propafenone based on spectral analysis of heart rate variability. Am. J. Cardiol. 70:1028, 1992.

108. Zehender, M., Hohnloser, S., Geibel, A., et al.: Short-term and long-term treatment with propafenone: Determinance of arrhythmia suppression, persistence of efficacy, arrhythmogenesis, and side effects in patients with symptoms. Br. Heart J. 67:491, 1992.

109. Bryson, H. M., Palmer, K. J., Langtry, H. D., et al.: Propafenone: A reappraisal of its pharmacology, pharmacokinetics and therapeutic use in cardiac arrhythmias. Drugs 45:85, 1993.

110. Paul, T., Reimer, A., Janousek, J., et al.: Efficacy and safety of propafenone in congenital junctional ectopic tachycardia. J. Am. Coll. Cardiol. 20:911, 1992.

111. Furlanello, F., Guarnerio, M., Inama, G., et al.: Long-term follow-up of patients with inducible supraventricular tachycardia treated with flecainide or propafenone: Therapy guided by transesophageal electropharmacologic testing. Am. J. Cardiol. 70:19A, 1992.

112. Balaji, S., Johnson, T. B., Sade, R. M., et al.: Management of atrial flutter after Fontan procedure. J. Am. Coll. Cardiol. 23:1209, 1994.

113. Kingma, J. H., and Suttorp, M. J.: Acute pharmacologic conversion of atrial fibrillation and flutter: The role of flecainide, propafenone and verapamil. Am. J. Cardiol. 70:56A, 1992.

114. Capucci, A., Boriani, G., Boto, G. L., et al.: Conversion of recent-onset atrial fibrillation by a single or loading dose of propafenone or flecainide. Am. J. Cardiol. 74:503, 1994.

115. Reimold, S. C., Cantillon, C. O., Friedman, P. L., et al.: Propafenone versus sotalol for suppression of recurrent symptomatic atrial fibrillation. Am. J. Cardiol. 71:558, 1993.

116. Gentili, C., Giordano, F., Alois, A., et al.: Efficacy of intravenous propafenone in acute atrial fibrillation complicating open-heart surgery. Am. Heart J. 123:1225, 1992.

117. Paul, T., and Janousek, J.: New antiarrhythmic drugs in pediatric use: Propafenone. Pediatr. Cardiol. 15:190, 1994.

118. Heusch, A., Kramer, H. H., Krogmann, O. N., et al.: Clinical experience with propafenone for cardiac arrhythmias in the young. Eur. Heart J. 15:1050, 1994.

119. Janousek, J., Paul, T., Reimer, A., et al.: Usefulness of propafenone for supraventricular arrhythmias in infants and children. Am. J. Cardiol. 72:294, 1993.

120. Vignati, G., Mauri, L., and Figini, A.: The use of propafenone in the treatment of tachyarrhythmias in children. Eur. Heart J. 14:546, 1993.

121. Cornacchia, D., Fabbri, M., Maresta, A., et al.: Effect of steroid eluting versus conventional electrodes on propafenone induced rise in chronic ventricular pacing threshold. PACE 16:2279, 1993.

122. Bianconi, L., Boccadamo, R., Toscano, S., et al.: Effects of oral propafenone therapy on chronic myocardial pacing threshold. PACE 15:148, 1992.

123. Natale, A., Montenero, A. S., Bombardieri, G., et al.: Effects of acute and prolonged administration of propafenone on internal defibrillation in the pig. Am. Heart J. 124:104, 1992.

124. Siebels, J., and Kuck, K. H.: Implantable cardioverter defibrillator compared with antiarrhythmic drug treatment in cardiac arrest survivors (The Cardiac Arrest Study, Hamburg). Am. Heart J. 127:1139, 1994.

125. Yamane, T., Sunami, A., Sawanobori, T., et al.: Use-dependent block of Ca^{2+} current by moricizine in guinea-pig ventricular myocytes: A possible ionic mechanism of action potential shortening. Br. J. Pharmacol. 108:812, 1993.

126. Ortiz, J., Nozaki, A., Shimizu, A., et al.: Mechanism of interruption of atrial flutter by moricizine: Electrophysiological and multiplexing studies in the canine sterile pericarditis model of atrial flutter. Circulation 89:2860, 1994.

127. Bigger, J. T., Jr., Rolnitzky, L. M., Steinman, R. C., et al.: Predicting mortality after myocardial infarction from the response of RR variability to antiarrhythmic drug therapy. J. Am. Coll. Cardiol. 23:733, 1994.

128. Ujhelyi, M. R., O'Rangers, E. A., Kluger, J., et al.: Defibrillation energy requirements during moricizine and moricizine-lidocaine therapy. J. Cardiovasc. Pharmacol. 20:932, 1992.

129. Benedek, I. H., Davidson, A. F., and Pieniaszek, H. J., Jr.: Enzyme induction by moricizine: Time course and extent in healthy subjects. J. Clin. Pharmacol. 34:167, 1994.

130. Clyne, C. A., Estes, N. A., III, and Wang, P. J.: Moricizine. N. Engl. J. Med. 327:255, 1992.

131. Damle, R., Levine, J., Matos, J., et al.: Efficacy and risks of moricizine in inducible sustained ventricular tachycardia. Ann. Intern. Med. 116:375, 1992.

132. Powell, A. C., Gold, M. R., Brooks, R., et al.: Electrophysiologic response to moricizine in patients with sustained venricular arrhythmias. Ann. Intern. Med. 116:382, 1992.

133. Bhandari, A. K., Lerman, R., Erlich, S., et al.: Electrophysiological evaluation of moricizine in patients with sustained ventricular tachyarrhythmias: Low efficacy and high incidence of proarrhythmia. PACE 16:1853, 1993.

134. Greene, H. L., Roden, D. M., Katz, R. J., et al.: The Cardiac Arrhythmia Suppression Trial: First CAST then CAST-II. J. Am. Coll. Cardiol. 19:894, 1992.

135. Nazari, J., Bauman, J., Pham, T., et al.: Exercise induced fatal sinusoidal ventricular tachycardia secondary to moricizine. PACE 15:1421, 1992.

136. Tschaidse, O., Graboys, T. B., Lown, B., et al.: The prevalence of proarrhythmic events during moricizine therapy. Am. Heart J. 124:912, 1992.

137. Akiyama, T., Pawitan, Y., Campbell, W. B., et al.: Effects of advancing age on the efficacy and side effects of antiarrhythmic drugs in post-myocardial infarction patients with ventricular arrhythmias: The CAST Investigators. J. Am. Geriatr. Soc. 40:666, 1992.

138. Singh, B. N.: Beta-blockers and calcium channel blockers as antiarrhythmic drugs. In Zipes, D. P., and Jalife, J. (eds.): Cardiac Electrophysiology: From Cell to Bedside. 2nd ed. Philadelphia, W. B., Saunders Company, 1994, pp. 1317–1330.

138a. Kendall, M. J., Lynch, K. P., and Hjalmarson, A.: β-Blockers and sudden cardiac death. Ann. Intern. Med. 123:358, 1995.

139. Adamson, P. B., Huang, M. H., Vanolie, E., et al.: Unexpected interaction between beta-adrenergic blockade and heart rate variability before and after myocardial infarction: A longitudinal study in dogs at high and low risk for sudden death. Circulation 90:976, 1994.

140. Patel, J., Lee, W., Fusilli, L., et al.: Anti-arrhythmic efficacy of beta-adrenergic blockade during acute ischemia in the myocardium with scar. Am. J. Med. Sci. 307:259, 1994.

141. Lubbe, W. F., Todzuweit, T., and Opie, L. H.: Potential arrhythmogenic role of cyclic adenosine monophosphate (AMP) and cytosolic calcium overload: Implications for prophylactic effects of beta-blockers in myocardial infarction and proarrhythmic effects of phosphodiesterase inhibitors. J. Am. Coll. Cardiol. 19:1622, 1992.

142. Krishnan, S., and Levy, M. N.: Effects of coronary artery occlusion and reperfusion on the idioventricular rate in anesthetized dogs. J. Am. Coll. Cardiol. 23:1484, 1994.

143. Aronow, W. S., Ahn, C., Mercando, A. D., et al.: Decrease in mortality by propranolol in patients with heart disease and complex ventricular arrhythmias is more an anti-ischemic than an antiarrhythmic effect. Am. J. Cardiol. 74:613, 1994.

144. Hopson, J. R., and Martins, J. B.: Hemodynamic and reflex sympathetic control of transmural activation and rate of ventricular tachycardia in ischemic and hypertrophic ventricular myocardium of the dog. Circulation 86:618, 1992.

145. Ditchey, R. V., Rubio-Perez, A., and Slinker, B. K.: Beta-adrenergic blockade reduces myocardial injury during experimental cardiopulmonary resuscitation. J. Am. Coll. Cardiol. 24:804, 1994.

146. Shettigar, U. R., Toole, J. G., and Appunn, D. O.: Combined use of esmolol and digoxin in the acute treatment of atrial fibrillation or flutter. Am. Heart J. 126: 368, 1993.

147. Sarter, D. H., and Marchlinski, F. E.: Redefining the role of digoxin in the treatment of atrial fibrillation. Am. J. Cardiol. 69:71G, 1992.

148. Natale, A., Klein, G., Yee, R., et al.: Shortening of fast pathway refractoriness after slow pathway ablation: Effects of autonomic blockade. Circulation 89:1003, 1994.

149. Elvas, L., Gursoy, S., Brugada, J., et al.: Atrioventricular nodal reentrant tachycardia: A review. Can. J. Cardiol. 10:342, 1994.

150. Skeberis, V., Simonis, F., Tsakonas, K., et al.: Inappropriate sinus tachycardia following radiofrequency ablation of AV nodal tachycardia: Incidence and clinical significance. PACE 17:924, 1994.

151. Morillo, C. A., Klein, G. J., Thakur, R. K., et al.: Mechanism of "inappropriate" sinus tachycardia: Role of sympathovagal balance. Circulation 90:873, 1994.

152. Hill, G. A., and Owens, S. D.: Esmolol in the treatment of multifocal atrial tachycardia. Chest 101:1726, 1992.

153. Garson, A., Jr., Dick, M., II, Fournier, A., et al.: The long QT syndrome in children. An international study of 287 patients. Circulation 87:1866, 1993.

154. Malfatto, G., Beria, G., Sala, S., et al.: Quantitative analysis of T wave abnormalities and their prognostic implications in the idiopathic long QT syndrome. J. Am. Coll. Cardiol. 23:296, 1994.

155. Moss, A. J., and Robinson, J.: Clinical features of the idiopathic long QT syndrome. Circulation 85 (Suppl. 1):1140, 1992.

156. Hjalmarson, Å.: Empiric therapy with beta-blockers. PACE 17:460, 1994.

157. Sweeney, M. O., Moss, A. J., and Eberly, S.: Instantaneous cardiac death in the posthospital period after acute myocardial infarction. Am. J. Cardiol. 70:1375, 1992.

158. Pitt, B.: The role of beta-adrenergic blocking agents in preventing sudden cardiac death. Circulation 85 (Suppl. 1):1107, 1992.

159. Kennedy, H. L., Brooks, A. H., Bergstrand, R., et al.: Beta-blocker therapy in the Cardiac Arrhythmia Suppression Trial: CAST Investigators. Am. J. Cardiol. 74:674, 1994.

160. Steinbeck, G., Andresen, D., Bach, P., et al.: A comparison of electrophysiologically guided antiarrhythmic drug therapy with beta-blocker therapy in patients with symptomatic sustained ventricular tachyarrhythmias. N. Engl. J. Med. 327:987, 1992.

161. Bhorat, I. E., Naidoo, D. P., Rout, C. C., et al.: Malignant ventricular arrhythmias in eclampsia: A comparison of labetalol with dihydralazine. Am. J. Obstet. Gynecol. 168:1292, 1993.

162. Ko, W. J., and Chu, S. H.: A new dosing regimen for esmolol to treat supraventricular tachyarrhythmia in Chinese patients. J. Am. Coll. Cardiol. 23:302, 1994.

163. Ovadia, M., and Thoele, D.: Esmolol tilt testing with esmolol withdrawal for the evaluation of syncope in the young. Circulation 89:228, 1994.

CLASS III AGENTS

164. Sager, P. T., Follmer, C., Uppal, P., et al.: The effects of beta-adrenergic stimulation on the frequency-dependent electrophysiologic actions of amiodarone and sematilide in humans. Circulation 90:1811, 1994.

165. Sager, P. T., Uppal, P., Follmer, C., et al.: Frequency-dependent electrophysiologic effects of amiodarone in humans. Circulation 88:1063, 1993.

166. Chiamvimonvat, N., Mitchell, L. B., Gillis, A. M., et al.: Use-dependent electrophysiologic effects of amiodarone in coronary artery disease and inducible ventricular tachycardia. Am. J. Cardiol. 70:598, 1992.

167. Hii, J. T., Wyse, B. G., Gillis, A. M., et al.: Precordial QT interval dispersion as a marker of torsade de pointes: Disparate effects of class IA antiarrhythmic drugs and amiodarone. Circulation 86:1376, 1992.

168. Cui, G., Sen, L., Sager, P., et al.: Effects of amiodarone, sematilide, and sotalol on QT dispersion. Am. J. Cardiol. 74:896, 1994.

169. Calkins, H., Sousa, J., el-Atassi, R., et al.: Reversal of antiarrhythmic drug effects by epinephrine: Quinidine versus amiodarone. J. Am. Coll. Cardiol. 19:347, 1992.

170. Kalbfleisch, S. J., Williamson, B., Man, K. C., et al.: Prospective, randomized comparison of conventional and high dose loading regimens of amiodarone in the treatment of ventricular tachycardia. J. Am. Coll. Cardiol. 22:1723, 1993.

171. Summitt, J., Morady, F., and Kadish, A.: A comparison of standard and high-dose regimens for the initiation of amiodarone therapy. Am. Heart J. 124:366, 1992.

172. Kim, S. G., Mannino, M. M., Chou, R., et al.: Rapid suppression of spontaneous ventricular arrhythmias during oral amiodarone loading. Ann. Intern. Med. 117:197, 1992.

173. Evans, S. J., Myers, M., Zaher, C., et al.: High dose oral amiodarone loading: Electrophysiologic effects and clinical tolerance. J. Am. Coll. Cardiol. 19:169, 1992.

174. Russo, A. M., Beauregard, L. M., and Waxman, H. L.: Oral amiodarone loading for the rapid treatment of frequent refractory sustained ventricular arrhythmias associated with coronary artery disease. Am. J. Cardiol. 72:1395, 1993.

175. Weinberg, B. A., Miles, W. M., Klein, L. S., et al.: Five-year follow-up of 589 patients treated with amiodarone. Am. Heart J. 125:109, 1993.

176. Mahmarian, J. J., Smart, F. W., Moye, L. A., et al.: Exploring the minimal dose of amiodarone with antiarrhythmic and hemodynamic activity. Am. J. Cardiol. 74:681, 1994.

177. Perry, J. C., Knilans, T. K., Marlow, D., et al.: Inravenous amiodarone for life-threatening tachyarrhythmias in children and young adults. J. Am. Coll. Cardiol. 22:95, 1993.

178. Flack, N. J., Zosmer, N., Bennet, P. R., et al.: Amiodarone given by three routes to terminate fetal atrial flutter associated with severe hydrops. Obstet. Gynecol. 82:714, 1994.

179. Azancot-Benisty, A., Jacqz-Aigrain, E., Guirgis, N. M., et al.: Clinical and pharmacologic study of fetal supraventricular tachyarrhythmias. J. Pediatr. 121:608, 1992.

180. Shuler, C. O., Case, C. L., and Gillette, P. C.: Efficacy and safety of amiodarone in infants. Am. Heart J. 125:430, 1993.

181. Figa, F. H., Gow, R. M., Hamilton, R. M., et al.: Clinical efficacy and safety of intravenous amiodarone in infants and children. Am. J. Cardiol. 74:573, 1994.

182. Raja, P., Hawker, R. E., Chaikitpinyo, A., et al.: Amiodarone management of junctional ectopic tachycardia after cardiac surgery in children. Br. Heart J. 72:261, 1994.

183. Disch, D. L., Greenberg, M. L., and Holzberger, P. T.: Managing chronic atrial fibrillation: A Markov decision analysis comparing warfarin, quinidine and low-dose amiodarone. Ann. Intern. Med. 120:449, 1994.

184. Skoularigis, J., Rothlisberger, C., Skudicky, D., et al.: Effectiveness of amiodarone and electrical cardioversion for chronic rheumatic atrial fibrillation after mitral valve surgery. Am. J. Cardiol. 72:423, 1992.

185. Estes, N. A., III: Evolving strategies for the management of atrial fibrillation: The role of amiodarone. JAMA 267:3332, 1992.

186. Gosselink, A. T., Crijns, H. J., VanGelder, I. C., et al.: Low-dose amiodarone for maintenance of sinus rhythm after cardioversion of atrial fibrillation or flutter. JAMA 267:3289, 1992.

187. Zehender, M., Hohnloser, S., Muller, B., et al.: Effects of amiodarone versus quinidine and verapamil in patients with chronic atrial fibrillation: Results of a comparative study and 2-year follow-up. J. Am. Coll. Cardiol. 19:1054, 1992.

188. Middlekauff, H. R., Wiener, I., and Stevenson, W. G.: Low-dose amiodarone for atrial fibrillation. Am. J. Cardiol. 72:75F, 1993.

189. Butler, J., Harriss, D. R., Sinclair, M., et al.: Amiodarone prophylaxis for tachycardias after coronary artery surgery: A randomized double-blind placebo control trial. Br. Heart J. 70:56, 1993.

190. Roden, D. M.: Current status of class III antiarrhythmic drug therapy. Am. J. Cardiol. 72:44B, 1993.

191. Nora, M., and Zipes, D. P.: Empiric use of amiodarone and sotalol. Am. J. Cardiol. 72:62F, 1993.

192. Singh, B. N.: Controlling cardiac arrhythmias by lengthening repolarization: Historical overview. Am. J. Cardiol. 72:18F, 1993.

193. Stevenson, W. G., Stevenson, L. W., Middlekauff, H. R., et al.: Sudden death prevention in patients with advanced ventricular dysfunction. Circulation 88:2953, 1993.

194. Dolack, G. L.: Clinical predictors of implantable cardioverter-defibrillator shocks (results of the CASCADE trial). Cardiac Arrest in Seattle, Conventional versus Amiodarone Drug Evaluation. Am. J. Cardiol. 73:237, 1994.

195. Anastasiou-Nana, M. I., Nanas, J. N., Nanas, S. N., et al.: Effects of amiodarone on refractory ventricular fibrillation in acute myocardial infarction: Experimental study. J. Am. Coll. Cardiol. 23:253, 1994.

196. Dorian, P., and Newman, D.: Effect of sotalol on ventricular fibrillation and defibrillation in humans. Am. J. Cardiol. 72:72A, 1993.

197. Jung, W., Manz, M., Pizzulli, L., et al.: Effects of chronic amiodarone therapy on defibrillation threshold. Am. J. Cardiol. 70:1023, 1992.

198. Nademanee, K., Singh, B. N., Stevenson, W. G., et al.: Amiodarone in post-MI patients. Circulation 88:264, 1993

199. Ceremuzynski, L.: Secondary prevention after myocardial infarction with class III antiarrhythmic drugs. Am. J. Cardiol. 72:82F, 1993.

200. Pfisterer, M. E., Kiowski, W., Brunner, H., et al.: Long-term benefit of one-year amiodarone treatment for persistent complex ventricular arrhythmias after myocardial infarction. Circulation 87:309, 1993.

201. Zarenbski, D. G., Nolan, P. E., Jr., Slack, M. K., et al.: Empiric long-term amiodarone prophylaxis following a myocardial infarction. A meta-analysis. Arch. Intern. Med. 153:2661, 1993.

202. Navarro-Lopez, F., Cosin, J., Marrugat, J., et al.: Comparison of the effects of amiodarone versus metoprolol on the frequency of ventricular arrhythmias and on mortality after acute myocardial infarction: Spanish study on sudden death. Am. J. Cardiol. 72:1243, 1993.

203. Singh, S. N., Fletcher, R. D., Fisher, S., et al.: Amiodarone in patients with congestive heart failure and symptomatic arrhythmia. N. Engl. J. Med. 333:77, 1995.

204. Doval, H. C., Nul, D. R., Grancelli, H. O., et al.: Randomized trial of low-dose amiodarone in severe congestive heart failure: Grupo de Estudio de la Sobrevida en la Insuficiencia Cardiaca en Argentina (GESICA). Lancet 344:493, 1994.

205. Greene, H. L.: The CASCADE Study: Randomized antiarrhythmic drug therapy in survivors of cardiac arrest in Seattle. CASCADE Investigators. Am. J. Cardiol. 72:70F, 1993.

206. The CASCADE Investigators: Randomized antiarrhythmic drug therapy in survivors of cardiac arrest (The CASCADE Study). Am. J. Cardiol. 72:280, 1993.

207. Camm, A. J., Julian, D., Janse, G., et al.: The European Myocardial Infarct Amiodarone Trial (EMIAT). EMIAT Investigators. Am. J. Cardiol. 72:95F, 1993.

208. Cairns, J. A., Connolly, S. J., Roberts, R., et al.: Canadian Amiodarone Myocardial Infarction Arrhythmia Trial (CAMIAT): Rationale and protocol. CAMIAT Investigators. Am. J. Cardiol. 72:87F, 1993.

209. Connolly, S. J., Gent, M., Roberts, R. S., et al.: Canadian Implantable Defibrillator Study (CIDS): Study design and organization. CIDS Co-investigators. Am. J. Cardiol. 72:103F, 1993.

210. AVID Investigators: Antiarrhythmics Versus Implantable Defibrillators (AVID): Rationale, design and methods. Am. J. Cardiol. 75:470, 1995.

211. Man, K. C., Williamson, B. D., Niebauer, M., et al.: Electrophysiologic effects of sotalol and amiodarone in patients with sustained monomorphic ventricular tachycardia. Am. J. Cardiol. 74:1119, 1994.

212. Pastor, A., Almendral, J. M., Arenal, A., et al.: Comparison of electrophysiologic effects of quinidine and amiodarone in sustained ventricular tachyarrhythmias associated with coronary artery disease. Am. J. Cardiol. 72:1389, 1993.

213. Martinez-Rubio, A., Shenasa, M., Chen, X., et al.: Response to sotalol predicts the response to amiodarone during serial drug testing in patients with sustained ventricular tachycardia and coronary artery disease. Am. J. Cardiol. 73:357, 1994.

214. Olson, P. J., Woelfel, A., Simpson, R. J., Jr., et al.: Stratification of sudden death risk in patients receiving long-term amiodarone treatment for sustained ventricular tachycardia or ventricular fibrillation. Am. J. Cardiol. 71:823, 1993.

215. Kerin, N. Z., Ansari-Leesar, M., Faitel, K., et al.: The effectiveness and safety of the simultaneous administration of quinidine and amiodarone in the conversion of chronic atrial fibrillation. Am. Heart J. 125:1017, 1993.

216. Bashir, Y., Paul, V. E., Griffith, M. J., et al.: A prospective study of the efficacy and safety of adjuvant metoprolol and xamoterol in combination with amiodarone for resistant ventricular tachycardia associated with impaired left ventricular function. Am. Heart J. 124:1233, 1992.

217. Ulrik, C. S., Backer, V., Aldershvile, J., et al.: Serial pulmonary function tests in patients treated with low-dose amiodarone. Am. Heart J. 123:1550, 1992.

218. Davies, P. H., Franklyn, J. A., and Sheppard, M. C.: Treatment of amiodarone induced thyrotoxicosis with carbimazole alone and continuation of amiodarone. B.M.J. 305:224, 1992.

219. Trip, M. D., Duren, D. R., and Wiersinga, W. M.: Two cases of amiodarone-induced thyrotoxicosis successfully treated with a short course of antithyroid drugs while amiodarone was continued. Br. Heart J. 72:266, 1994.

220. Hohnloser, S. H., Klingenheben, T., and Singh, B. N.: Amiodarone-associated proarrhythmic effects: A review with special reference to torsade de pointes tachycardia. Ann. Intern. Med. 121:529, 1994.

221. Makkar, R. R., Fromm, B. S., Steinman, R. T., et al.: Female gender as a risk factor for torsades de pointes associated with cardiovascular drugs. JAMA 270:2590, 1993.

222. Mickleborough, L. L., Maruyiama, H., Mohamed, S., et al.: Are patients receiving amiodarone at increased risk for cardiac operations? Ann. Thorac. Surg. 58:622, 1994.

223. Chelimsky-Fallick, C., Middlekauff, H. R., Stevenson, W. G., et al.: Amiodarone therapy does not compromise subsequent heart transplantation. J. Am. Coll. Cardiol. 20:1556, 1992.

224. Quesada, A., Sanchis, J., Charro, F. J., et al.: Changes in canine ventricular fibrillation threshold induced by verapamil, flecainide and bretylium. Eur. Heart J. 14:712, 1993.

225. Usui, M., Inoue, H., Saihara, S., et al.: Antifibrillatory effects of class III antiarrhythmic drugs: Comparative study with flecainide. J. Cardiovasc. Pharmacol. 21:376, 1993.

226. Jones, D. L., Kim, Y. H., Natale, A., et al.: Bretylium decreases and verapamil increases defibrillation threshold in pigs. PACE 17:1380, 1994.

227. Hohnloser, S. H., and Woosley, R. L.: Sotalol. N. Engl. J. Med. 331:31, 1994.

228. Singh, B. N.: Electrophysiologic basis for the antiarrhythmic actions of sotalol and comparison with other agents. Am. J. Cardiol. 72:8A, 1993.

229. Reiter, M. J., Zetelaki, Z., Kirchhof, C. J., et al.: Interaction of acute ventricular dilation and d-sotalol during sustained reentrant ventricular tachycardia around a fixed obstacle. Circulation 89:423, 1994.

230. Alboni, P., Razzolini, R., Scarfo, S., et al.: Hemodynamic effects of oral sotalol during both sinus rhythm and atrial fibrillation. J. Am. Coll. Cardiol. 22:1373, 1993.

231. Winters, S. L., Kukin, M. K., Tee, E., et al.: Effects of oral sotalol on systemic hemodynamics and programmed electrical stimulation in patients with ventricular arrhythmias and structural heart disease. Am. J. Cardiol. 72:38A, 1993.

232. Hohnloser, S. H., Zabel, M., Krause, T., et al.: Short- and long-term antiarrhythmic and hemodynamic effects of d,l-sotalol in patients with symptomatic ventricular arrhythmias. Am. Heart J. 123:1220, 1992.

233. Kehoe, R. F., MacNeil, D. J., Zheutlin, T. A., et al.: Safety and efficacy of oral sotalol for sustained ventricular tachyarrhythmias refractory to other antiarrhythmic agents. Am. J. Cardiol. 72:56A, 1993.

234. Young, G. D., Kerr, C. R., Mohama, R., et al.: Efficacy of sotalol guided by programmed electrical stimulation for sustained ventricular arrhythmias secondary to coronary artery disease. Am. J. Cardiol. 73:677, 1994.

235. Sotalol in life-threatening ventricular arrhythmias: An unique class III antiarrhythmic. Symposium proceedings. Am. J. Cardiol. 72:1A, 1993.

236. Wang, J., Bourne, G. W., Wang, Z., et al.: Comparative mechanisms of antiarrhythmic drug action in experimental atrial fibrillation. Importance of use-dependent effects on refractoriness. Circulation 88:1030, 1993.

237. Wang, J., Feng, J., and Nattel, S.: Class III antiarrhythmic drug action in experimental atrial fibrillation: Differences in reverse use dependence and effectiveness between d-sotalol and the new antiarrhythmic drug ambasilide. Circulation 90:2032, 1994.

238. Brodsky, M., Saini, R., Bellinger, R., et al.: Comparative effects of the combination of digoxin and dl-sotalol therapy versus digoxin monotherapy for control of ventricular response in chronic atrial fibrillation. Am. Heart J. 127:572, 1994.

239. Ho, D. S., Zecchin, R. P., Richards, D. A., et al.: Double-blind trial of lignocaine versus sotalol for acute termination of spontaneous sustained ventricular tachycardia. Lancet 344:18, 1994.

240. Wichter, T., Borggrefe, M., Haverkamp, W., et al.: Efficacy of antiarrhythmic drugs in patients with arrhythmogenic right ventricular disease: Results in patients with inducible and noninducible ventricular tachycardia. Circulation 86:29, 1992.

241. Freedman, R. A., Karagounis, L. A., and Steinberg, J. S.: Effects of sotalol on the signal-averaged electrocardiogram in patients with sustained ventricular tachycardia: Relation to suppression of inducibility and changes in tachycardia cycle length. J. Am. Coll. Cardiol. 20:1213, 1992.

242. Maragnes, P., Tipple, M., and Fournier, A.: Effectiveness of oral sotalol for treatment of pediatric arrhythmias. Am. J. Cardiol. 69:751, 1992.

243. MacNeil, D. J., Davies, R. O., and Beitchman, D.: Clinical safety profile of sotalol in the treatment of arrhythmias. Am. J. Cardiol. 72:44A, 1993.

244. Dorian, P., Newman, D., Berman, N., et al.: Sotalol and type IA drugs in combination prevent recurrence of sustained ventricular tachycardia. J. Am. Cardiol. 22:106, 1993.

CLASS IV AGENTS

245. Talajic, M., Lemery, R., Roy, D., et al.: Rate-dependent effects of diltiazem on human atrioventricular nodal properties. Circulation 86:870, 1992.

246. Dias, V. C., Weir, S. J., and Ellenbogen, K. A.: Pharmacokinetics and pharmacodynamics of intravenous diltiazem in patients with atrial fibrillation or atrial flutter. Circulation 86:1421, 1992.

247. Dougherty, A. H., Jackman, W. M., Naccarelli, G. V., et al.: Acute conversion of paroxysmal supraventricular tachycardia with intravenous diltiazem. IV Diltiazem Study Group. Am. J. Cardiol. 70:587, 1992.

248. Hood, M. A., and Smith, W. M.: Adenosine versus verapamil in the treatment of supraventricular tachycardia: A randomized double-crossover trial. Am. Heart J. 123:1543, 1992.

249. Ohe, T., Aihara, N., Kamakura, S., et al.: Long-term outcome of verapamil-sensitive sustained left ventricular tachycardia in patients without structural heart disease. J. Am. Coll. Cardiol. 25:54, 1995.

250. Lai, W. T., Voon, W. C., Yen, H. W., et al.: Comparison of the electrophysiologic effects of oral sustained-release and intravenous verapamil in patients with paroxysmal supraventricular tachycardia. Am. J. Cardiol. 71:405, 1993.

251. Ellenbogen, K. A.: Role of calcium antagonists for heart rate control in atrial fibrillation. Am. J. Cardiol. 69:36B, 1992.

252. Ellenbogen, K. A., Dias, V. C., and Cardello, F. P.: Safety and efficacy of intravenous diltiazem in atrial fibrillation or atrial flutter. Am. J. Cardiol. 75:45, 1995.

253. Goldenberg, I. F., Lewis, W. R., Dias, V. C., et al.: Intravenous diltiazem for the treatment of patients with atrial fibrillation or flutter and moderate to severe congestive heart failure. Am. J. Cardiol. 74:884, 1994.

254. Koh, K. K., Kwan, K. S., Park, H. B., et al.: Efficacy and safety of digoxin alone and in combination with low-dose diltiazem or betaxolol

to control ventricular rate in chronic atrial fibrillation. Am. J. Cardiol. 75:88, 1995.

254a. Gill, J. S., Blaszyk, K., Ward, D. E., et al.: Verapamil for the suppression of idiopathic ventricular tachycardia of left bundle branch block-like morphology. Am. Heart J. 126:1126, 1993.

255. Griffith, M. J., Garrett, C. J., Rowland, E., et al.: Effects of intravenous adenosine on verapamil-sensitive idiopathic ventricular tachycardia. Am. J. Cardiol. 73:759, 1994.

256. Wen, M. S., Yeh, S. J., Wang C. C., et al.: Radiofrequency ablation therapy in idiopathic left ventricular tachycardia with no obvious structural heart disease. Circulation 89:1690, 1994.

257. Nakagawa, H., Beckman, K. J., McClelland, J. H., et al.: Radiofrequency catheter ablation of idiopathic left ventricular tachycardia guided by a Purkinje potential. Circulation 88:2607, 1993.

258. Bhadha, K., Marchlinski, F. E., and Iskandrian, A. S.: Ventricular tachycardia in patients without structural heart disease. Am. Heart J. 126:1194, 1993.

259. Dilsizian, V., Bonow, R. O., Epstein, S. E., et al.: Myocardial ischemia detected by thallium scintigraphy is frequently related to cardiac arrest and syncope in young patients with hypertrophic cardiomyopathy. J. Am. Coll. Cardiol. 22:796, 1993.

260. Leenhardt, A., Glaser, E., Burguera, M., et al.: Short-coupled variant of torsade de pointes: A new electrocardiographic entity in the spectrum of idiopathic ventricular tachyarrhythmias. Circulation 89:206, 1994.

261. Myerburg, R. J., Kessler, K. M., Mallon, S. M., et al.: Life-threatening ventricular arrhythmias in patients with silent myocardial ischemia due to coronary artery spasm. N. Engl. J. Med. 326:1451, 1992.

262. DeFerrari, G. M., Mador, F., Beria, G., et al.: Effect of calcium channel block on the wall motion abnormality of the idiopathic long QT syndrome. Circulation 89:2126, 1994.

263. Ramoska, E. A., Spiller, H. A., Winter, M., et al.: A 1-year evaluation of calcium channel blocker overdoses: Toxicity and treatment. Ann. Emerg. Med. 22:196, 1993.

OTHER ANTIARRHYTHMIC AGENTS

264. DiMarco, J. P.: Adenosine. In Zipes, D. P., and Jalife, J. (eds.): Cardiac Electrophysiology: From Cell to Bedside. 2nd ed. Philadelphia, W. B. Saunders Company, 1994, pp. 1336–1344.

265. Nayebpour, M., Billette, J., Amellal, F., et al.: Effects of adenosine on rate-dependent atrioventricular nodal function: Potential roles in tachycardia termination and physiological regulation. Circulation 88:2632, 1993.

266. O'Nuanin, S., Jennison, S., Bashir, Y., et al.: Effects of adenosine on atrial repolarization in the transplanted human heart. Am. J. Cardiol. 71:248, 1993.

267. McIntosh-Yellin, N. L., Drew, B. J., and Scheinman, M. M.: Safety and efficacy of central intravenous bolus administration of adenosine for termination of supraventricular tachycardia. J. Am. Coll. Cardiol. 22:741, 1993.

268. Scheinman, M. M., Gonzalez, R. P., Cooper, M. W., et al.: Clinical and electrophysiologic features and role of catheter ablation techniques in adult patients with automatic atrioventricular junctional tachycardia. Am. J. Cardiol. 74:565, 1994

269. Akhtar, M., Jazayeri, M. R., Sra, J., et al.: Atrioventricular nodal reentry: Clinical, electrophysiological and therapeutic considerations. Circulation 88:282, 1993.

270. Lauer, M. R., Young, C., Liem, L. B., et al.: Efficacy of adenosine in terminating catecholamine-dependent supraventricular tachycardia. Am. J. Cardiol. 73:38, 1994.

271. Klein, L. S., Hackett, F. K., Zipes D. P., et al.: Radiofrequency catheter ablation of Mahaim fibers at the tricuspid annulus. Circulation 87:738, 1993.

272. Li, H. G., Morillo, C. A., Zardini, M., et al.: Effect of adenosine or adenosine triphosphate on antidromic tachycardia. J. Am. Coll. Cardiol. 24:728, 1994.

273. Garratt, C. J., O'Nunain, S., Griffith, M. J., et al.: Effects of intravenous adenosine in patients with preexcited junctional tachycardias: Therapeutic efficacy and incidence of proarrhythmic events. Am. J. Cardiol. 74:401, 1994.

274. Ralston, M. A., Knilans, T. K., Hannon, D. W., et al.: Use of adenosine for diagnosis and treatment of tachyarrhythmias in pediatric patients. J. Pediatr. 124:139, 1994.

275. Reyes, G., Stanton, R., and Galvis, A. G.: Adenosine in the treatment of paroxysmal supraventricular tachycardia in children. Ann. Emerg. Med. 21:1499, 1992.

276. Keim, S., Curtis, A. B., Belardinelli, L., et al.: Adenosine-induced atrioventricular block: A rapid and reliable method to assess surgical and radiofrequency catheter ablation of accessory atrioventricular pathways. J. Am. Coll. Cardiol. 19:1005, 1992.

277. Chen, S. A., Chiang, C. E., Yang, C. J., et al.: Sustained atrial tachycardia in adult patients: Electrophysiological characteristics, pharmacological response, possible mechanisms, and effective radiofrequency ablation. Circulation 90:1262, 1994.

278. Engelstein, E. D., Lippman, N., Stein, K. M., et al.: Mechanism-specific effects of adenosine on atrial tachycardia. Circulation 89:2645, 1994.

279. Griffith, M. J., Garratt, C. J., Rowland, E., et al.: Effects of intravenous adenosine on verapamil-sensitive idiopathic ventricular tachycardia. Am. J. Cardiol. 73:759, 1994.

280. Lerman, B. B.: Response of nonreentrant catecholamine-mediated ventricular tachycardia to endogenous adenosine and acetylcholine. Evi-

dence for myocardial receptor-mediated effects. Circulation 87:382, 1993.

281. Wilber, D. J., Baerman, J., Olshansky, B., et al.: Adenosine-sensitive ventricular tachycardia. Clinical characteristics and response to catheter ablation. Circulation 87:126, 1993.

282. Crosson, J. E., Etheridge, S. P., Milstein, S., et al.: Therapeutic and diagnostic utility of adenosine during tachycardia evaluation in children. Am. J. Cardiol. 74:155, 1994.

283. Cowell, R. T., Paul, V. E., and Ilsley, C. D.: Hemodynamic deterioration after treatment with adenosine. Br. Heart J. 71:569, 1994.

284. Exner, D. V., Muzigka, T., and Gillis, A. M.: Proarrhythmia in patients with the Wolff-Parkinson-White syndrome after standard doses of intravenous adenosine. Ann. Intern. Med. 122:351, 1995.

ELECTRICAL THERAPY OF CARDIAC ARRHYTHMIAS

285. Kerber, R. E.: External direct current cardioversion-defibrillation. In Zipes, D. P., and Jalife, T. (eds.): Cardiac Electrophysiology: From Cell to Bedside. 2nd ed. Philadelphia, W. B. Saunders Company, 1994, pp. 1360–1365.

286. Ewy, G. A.: The optimal technique for electrical cardioversion of atrial fibrillation. Clin. Cardiol. 17:79, 1994.

287. Li, H. G., Yee, R., Mehra, R., et al.: Effect of shock timing on efficacy and safety of internal cardioversion for ventricular tachycardia. J. Am. Coll. Cardiol. 24:703, 1994.

288. Alt, E., Schmitt, C., Ammer, R., et al.: Initial experience with intracardiac atrial defibrillation in patients with chronic atrial fibrillation. PACE 17:1067, 1994.

289. Wharton, J. M., and Johnson, F. E.: Catheter based atrial defibrillation. PACE 17:1058, 1994.

290. Levy, S., and Richard, P.: Is there any indication for an intracardiac defibrillator for the treatment of atrial fibrillation? J. Cardiovasc. Electrophysiol. 5:982, 1994.

291. Kerber, R. E., Spencer, K. T., Kallok, M. J., et al.: Overlapping sequential pulses: A new waveform for transthoracic defibrillation. Circulation 89:2369, 1994.

292. Hillsley, R. E., Wharton, J. M., Cates, A. W., et al.: Why do some patients have high defibrillation thresholds at defibrillator implantation? Answers from basic research. PACE 17:222, 1994.

293. Blanchard, S. M., and Ideker, R. E.: Mechanisms of electrical defibrillation: Impact of new experimental defibrillator waveforms. Am. Heart J. 127:970, 1994.

294. Hoch, D. H., Batsford, W. P., Greenberg, S. M., et al.: Double sequential external shocks for refractory ventricular fibrillation. J. Am. Coll. Cardiol. 23:1141, 1994.

295. Grimm, R. A., Stewart, W. J., Maloney, J. D., et al.: Impact of electrical cardioversion for atrial fibrillation on left atrial appendage function and spontaneous echo contrast: Characterization by simultaneous transesophageal echocardiograhy. J. Am. Coll. Cardiol. 22:1359, 1993.

296. Ito, M., Pride, H. P., and Zipes, D. P.: Defibrillating shocks delivered to the heart heterogeneously impair efferent sympathetic responsiveness. Circulation 88:2661, 1993.

297. Manning, W. J., Silverman, D. I., Katz, S. E., et al.: Impaired left atrial mechanical function after cardioversion: Relation to duration of atrial fibrillation. J. Am. Coll. Cardiol. 23:1535, 1994.

298. Schneider, T., Mauer, D., Diehl, P., et al.: Early defibrillation by emergency physicians or emergency medical technicians? A controlled, prospective multi-center study. Resuscitation 27:297, 1994.

299. Ekstrom, L., Herlitz, J., Wennerblom, D., et al.: Survival after cardiac arrest outside hospital over a 12-year period in Gothenburg. Resuscitation 27:181, 1994.

300. Welikovitch, L., Lafreniere, G., Burggraf, G. W., et al.: Change in atrial volume following restoration of sinus rhythm in patients with atrial fibrillation: A prospective echocardiographic study. Can. J. Cardiol. 10:993, 1994.

301. Gosselink, A. T., Crijns, H. J., Hamer, H. P., et al.: Changes in left and right atrial size after cardioversion of atrial fibrillation: Role of mitral valve disease. J. Am. Coll. Cardiol. 22:1666, 1993.

302. Shite, J., Yokota, Y., and Yokoyama, M.: Heterogeneity and time course of improvement in cardiac function after cardioversion in chronic atrial fibrillation: Assessment of serial echocardiographic indices. Br. Heart J. 70:154, 1993.

303. VanGelder, I. C., Orijns, H. J., Blanksma, P. K., et al.: Time course of hemodynamic changes and improvement of exercise tolerance after cardioversion of chronic atrial fibrillation unassociated with cardiac valve disease. Am. J. Cardiol. 72:560, 1993.

304. Gosselink, A. T., Orijns, H. J., VandenBerg, M. P., et al.: Functional capacity before and after cardioversion of atrial fibrillation: A controlled study. Br. Heart J. 72:161, 1994.

305. Missault, L., Jordaens, L., Gheeraert, P., et al.: Embolic stroke after an anticoagulated cardioversion despite prior exclusion of atrial thrombi by transesophageal echocardiography. Eur. Heart J. 15:1279, 1994.

306. Black, I. W., Fatkin, D., Sagar, K. B., et al.: Exclusion of atrial thrombus by transesophageal echocardiography does not preclude embolism after cardioversion of atrial fibrillation: A multicenter study. Circulation 89:2509, 1994.

307. Fatkin, D., Kurchar, D. L., Thorburn, C. W., et al.: Transesophageal echocardiography before and during direct current cardioversion of atrial fibrillation: Evidence of atrial stunning as a mechanism of thromboembolic complications. J. Am. Coll. Cardiol. 23:307, 1994.

308. Grimm, R. A., Stewart, W. J., Black, I. W., et al.: Should all patients undergo transesophageal echocardiography before electrical cardioversion of atrial fibrillation? J. Am. Coll. Cardiol. 23:533, 1994.

309. Feltes, T. F., and Friedman, R. A.: Transesophageal echocardiographic detection of atrial thrombi in patients with nonfibrillation atrial tachyarrhythmias and congenital heart disease. J. Am. Coll. Cardiol. 24:1365, 1994.

310. Salerno, D. M., Katz, A., Dunbar, D. N., et al.: Serum electrolytes and catecholamines after cardioversion from ventricular tachycardia and atrial fibrillation. PACE 16:1862, 1993.

ABLATION THERAPY

311. Catheter ablation for cardiac arrhythmias: Clinical applications, personnel and facilities. American College of Cardiology Cardiovascular Technology Assessment Committee. J. Am. Coll. Cardiol. 24:828, 1994.

312. Manolis, A. S., Wang, P. J., and Estes, N. A., III: Radiofrequency catheter ablation for cardiac tachyarrhythmias. Ann. Intern. Med. 121:452–461, 1994.

313. Zipes, D. P. (ed.): Catheter Ablation of Arrhythmias. Armonk, N.Y., Futura Publishing Company, 1994.

313a. Jackman, W. M., Wang, X., Friday, K. J., et al.: Catheter ablation of accessory atrioventricular pathways (Wolff-Parkinson-White syndrome) by radiofrequency current. N. Engl. J. Med. 324:1605, 1991.

313b. Calkins, H., Sousa, J., el-Atassi, R., et al.: Diagnosis and cure of the Wolff-Parkinson-White syndrome or paroxysmal supraventricular tachycardias during a single electrophysiologic test. N. Engl. J. Med. 324:1612, 1991.

314. Haissaguerre, M., Gaita, F., Marcus, F. I., et al.: Radiofrequency catheter ablation of accessory pathways: A contemporary review. J. Cardiovasc. Elecrophysiol. 5:532, 1994.

315. Haissaguerre, M., Clementy, J., and Warin, J. F.: Catheter ablation of atrioventricular reentrant tachycardias. In Zipes, D. P., and Jalife, J. (eds.): Cardiac Electrophysiology: From Cell to Bedside. 2nd ed. Philadelphia, W. B. Saunders Company, 1994, pp. 1487–1499.

316. Miles, W. M., Zipes, D. P., and Klein, L. S.: Ablation of free wall accessory pathways. In Zipes, D. P. (ed.): Catheter Ablation of Arrhythmias. Armonk, N.Y., Futura Publishing Company, 1994, pp. 211–230.

317. Kuck, K., Schleuter, M., Cappato, R., et al.: Ablation of septal accessory pathways. In Zipes, D. P. (ed.): Catheter Ablation of Arrhythmias. Armonk, N.Y., Futura Publishing Company, 1994, pp. 231–257.

318. Ganz, L. I., and Friedman, P. L.: Supraventricular tachycardia. N. Engl. J. Med. 332:162, 1995.

319. Thakur, R. K., Klein, G. K., and Yee, R.: Radiofrequency catheter ablation in patients with Wolff-Parkinson-White syndrome. Can. Med. Assoc. J. 151:771, 1994.

320. Park, J. K., Halperin, B. D., McAnulty, J. H., et al.: Comparison of radiofrequency catheter ablation procedures in children, adolescents and adults and the impact of accessory pathway location. Am. J. Cardiol. 74:786, 1994.

321. Sreeram, N., Smeets, J. L., Pulles-Heintzberger, C. F., et al.: Radiofrequency catheter ablation of accessory atrioventricular pathways in children and young adults. Br. Heart J. 70:160, 1993.

322. Saul, J. P., Hulse, J. E., Papagiannis, J., et al.: Late enlargement of radiofrequency lesions in infant lambs: Implications for ablation procedures in small children. Circulation 90:492, 1994.

323. Kugler, J. D., Danford, D. A., Deal, B. J., et al.: Radiofrequency catheter ablation for tachyarrhythmias in children and adolescents: The Pediatric Electrophysiology Society. N. Engl. J. Med. 330: 1481, 1994.

324. vanHare, G. F., Witherell, C. L., and Lesh, M. D.: Follow-up of radiofrequency catheter ablation in children: Results in 100 consecutive patients. J. Am. Coll. Cardiol. 23:1651, 1994.

325. Nath, S., Whayne, J. G., Kaul, S., et al.: Effects of radiofrequency catheter ablation on regional myocardial blood flow: Possible mechanism for late electrophysiological outcome. Circulation 89:2667, 1994.

326. Nath, S., Redick, J. A., Whayne, J. G., et al.: Ultrastructural observations in the myocardium beyond the reach of an acute coagulation necrosis following radiofrequency catheter ablation. J. Cardiovasc. Electrophysiol. 5:838, 1994.

327. Nath, S., DiMarco, J. P., and Haines, D. E.: Basic aspects of radiofrequency catheter ablation. J. Cardiovasc. Electrophysiol. 5:863, 1994.

328. Xie, B., Heald, S. C., Bashir, Y., et al.: Radiofrequency catheter ablation of septal accessory atrioventricular pathways. Br. Heart J. 72:281, 1994.

329. Haissaguerre, M., Marcus, F., Poquet, F., et al.: Electrocardiographic characteristics and catheter ablation of parahissian accessory pathways. Circulation 90:1124, 1994.

330. Scheinman, M. M., Wang, Y. S., vanHare, G. F., et al.: Electrocardiographic and electrophysiologic characteristics of anterior, midseptal and right anterior free wall accessory pathways. J. Am. Coll. Cardiol. 20:1220, 1992.

331. Dhala, A. A., Deshpande, S. S., Bremner, S., et al.: Transcatheter ablation of posteroseptal accessory pathways using a venous approach and radiofrequency energy. Circulation 90:1799, 1994.

332. Epstein, L. M., Chiesa, N., Wong, M. N., et al.: Radiofrequency catheter ablation in the treatment of supraventricular tachycardia in the elderly. J. Am. Coll. Cardiol. 23:1356, 1994.

333. Chen, S. A., Chiang, C. E., Yang, C. J., et al.: Accessory pathway and atrioventricular node reentrant tachycardia in elderly patients: Clinical features, electrophysiologic characteristics and results of radiofrequency ablation. J. Am. Coll. Cardiol. 23:702, 1994.

334. Cappato, R., Schluter, M., Mont, L., et al.: Anatomic, electrical, and mechanical factors affecting bipolar endocardial electrograms: Impact on catheter ablation of manifest left free-wall accessory pathways. Circulation 90:884, 1994.

335. Shih, H. T., Miles, W. M., Klein, L. S., et al.: Multiple accessory pathways in the permanent form of junctional reciprocating tachycardia. Am. J. Cardiol. 73:361, 1994.

336. Langberg, J. J., Man, K. C., Varperian, V. R., et al.: Recognition and catheter ablation of subepicardial accessory pathways. J. Am. Coll. Cardiol. 22:1100, 1993.

337. Calkins, H., Mann, C., Kalbfleisch, S., et al.: Site of accessory pathway block after radiofrequency catheter ablation in patients with the Wolff-Parkinson-White syndrome. J. Cardiovasc. Electrophysiol. 5:20, 1994.

338. Cappato, R., Schluter, M., Weiss, C., et al.: Catheter-induced mechanical conduction block of right-sided accessory fibers with Mahaim-type preexcitation to guide radiofrequency ablation. Circulation 90:282, 1994.

339. Willems, S., Hendricks, G., Shenasa, M., et al.: Termination of orthodromic tachycardia using direct current sub-threshold stimulation in patients with concealed accessory pathways. Eur. Heart J. 14(Abs.):294, 1993.

340. Chiang, C. E., Chen, S. A., Wu, T. J., et al.: Incidence, significance, and pharmacological responses of catheter-induced mechanical trauma in patients receiving radiofrequency ablation for supraventricular tachycardias. Circulation 90:1847, 1994.

341. Chu, E., Kalman, J. M., Kwasman, M. A., et al.: Intracardiac echocardiography during radiofrequency catheter ablation of cardiac arrhythmias in humans. J. Am. Coll. Cardiol. 24:1351, 1994.

342. Chu, E., Fitzpatrick, A. P., Chin, M. C., et al.: Radiofrequency catheter ablation guided by intracardiac echocardiography. Circulation 89:1301, 1994.

343. Damle, R. S., Choe, W., Kanaan, N. M., et al.: Atrial and accessory pathway activation direction in patients with orthodromic supraventricular tachycardia: Insights from vector mapping. J. Am. Coll. Cardiol. 23:684, 1994.

344. Calkins, H., Prystowsky, E., Carlson, M., et al.: Temperature monitoring during radiofrequency catheter ablation procedures using a closed loop control. Atakar Multicenter Investigators Group. Circulation 90:1279, 1994

345. Lesh, M. D., vanHare, G. F., Scheinman, M. M., et al.: Comparison of the retrograde and transseptal methods for ablation of left freewall accessory pathways. J. Am. Coll. Cardiol. 22:542, 1993.

346. Deshpande, S. S., Bremner, S., Sra, J. S., et al.: Ablation of left free-wall accessory pathways using radiofrequency energy at the atrial insertion site: Transseptal versus transaortic approach. J. Cardiovasc. Electrophysiol. 5:219, 1994.

347. Wagshal, A. B., Pires, L. A., and Young, P. G.: Usefulness of follow-up electrophysiologic study and event monitoring after successful radiofrequency catheter ablation of supraventricular tachycardia. Am. J. Cardiol. 75:50, 1995.

348. Chen, S. A., Chiang, C. E., Yang, C. J., et al.: Usefulness of serial follow-up electrophysiologic studies in predicting late outcome of radiofrequency ablation for accessory pathways and atrioventricular nodal reentrant tachycardia. Am. Heart J. 126:619, 1993.

349. Jackman, W. M., McClelland, J. H., Nakagawa, H., et al.: Ablation of right atriofascicular (Mahaim) accessory pathways. In Zipes, D. P. (ed.): Catheter Ablation of Arrhythmias. Armonk, N.Y., Futura Publishing Company, 1994, pp. 187–210.

350. McClelland, J. H., Wang, X., Beckman, K. J., et al.: Radiofrequency catheter ablation of right atrial fascicular (Mahaim) accessory pathways guided by accessory pathway activation potentials. Circulation 89:2655, 1994.

351. Klein, L. S., Hackett, F. K., Zipes, D. P., and Miles, W. M.: Radiofrequency catheter ablation of "Mahaim fibers" at the tricuspid annulus. Circulation 87:738, 1993.

352. Li, H. G., Klein, G. K., Thakur, R. K., et al.: Radiofrequency ablation of decremental accessory pathways mimicking nodal ventricular conduction. Am. J. Cardiol. 74:829, 1994.

353. Grogin, H. R., Lee, R. J., Kwasman, M., et al.: Radiofrequency catheter ablation of atriofascicular and nodoventricular Mahaim tracts. Circulation 90:272, 1994.

354. Zipes, D. P., DiMarco, J. P., Gillette, P. C., et al.: ACC/AHA guidelines for clinical intracardiac electrophysiologic procedures. Circulation 92:673, 1995; J. Am. Coll. Cardiol. 26:555, 1995; J. Cardiovasc. Electrophysiol. 6:652, 1995.

355. Scheinman, M. M.: Patterns of catheter ablation practice in the United States: Results of the 1992 NASPE survey. PACE 17:873, 1994.

356. Hindricks, G., on behalf of the Multicentre European Radiofrequency Survey (MERFS) Investigators of the Working Group on Arrhythmias of the European Society of Cardiology: The Multicentre European Radiofrequency Survey (MERFS): Complications of radiofrequency catheter ablation of arrhythmias. Eur. Heart J. 14:1644, 1993.

357. Deshpande, S., Jazayeri, M., Dahla, A., et al.: Selective transcatheter modification of the atrioventricular node. In Zipes, D. P. (ed.): Catheter Ablation of Arrhythmias. Armonk, N.Y., Futura Publishing Company, 1994, pp. 151–186.

357a. Jackman, W., Beckman, K. J., McClelland, J. H., et al.: Treatment of supraventricular tachycardia due to atrioventricular nodal reentry by radiofrequency catheter ablation of the slow-pathway conduction. N. Engl. J. Med. 327:313, 1992.

358. Kalbfleisch, S. J., and Morady, F.: Catheter ablation of atrioventricular nodal reentrant tachycardia. *In* Zipes, D. P., and Jalife, J. (eds.): Cardiac Electrophysiology: From Cell to Bedside. 2nd ed. Philadelphia, W. B. Saunders Company, 1994, pp. 1477–1487.

359. Manolis, A. S., Wang, P. J., and Estes, N. A. M., III: Radiofrequency ablation of slow pathway in patients with atrioventricular nodal reentrant tachycardia: Do arrhythmia recurrences correlate with persistent slow pathway conduction or site of successful ablation? Circulation 90:2815, 1994.

360. Dhala, A., Bremner, S., Deshpande, S., et al.: Efficacy and safety of atrioventricular nodal modification for atrioventricular nodal reentrant tachycardia in the pediatric population. Am. Heart J. 128:903, 1994.

361. Sra, J. S., Jazayeri, M. R., Blanck, Z., et al.: Slow pathway ablation in patients with atrioventricular node reentrant tachycardia and a prolonged PR interval. J. Am. Coll. Cardiol. 24:1064, 1994.

362. DeBakker, J. N., Coronel, R., McGuire, M. A., et al.: Slow potentials in the atrioventricular junctional area of patients operated on for atrioventricular node tachycardias and in isolated porcine hearts. J. Am. Coll. Cardiol. 23:709, 1994.

362a. McGuire, M. A., deBakker, J. M., Vermeulen, J. T., et al.: Origin and significance of double potentials near the atrioventricular node. Correlation of extracellular potentials, intracellular potentials and histology. Circulation 89:2351, 1994.

363. Kalbfleisch, S. J., Strickberger, S. A., Williamson, B., et al.: Randomized comparison of anatomic and electrogram mapping approaches to ablation of the slow pathway of atrioventricular node reentrant tachycardia. J. Am. Coll. Cardiol. 23:716, 1994.

364. Li, H. G., Klein, G. J., Stites, H. W., et al.: Elimination of slow pathway conduction: An accurate indicator of clinical success after radiofrequency atrioventricular node modification. J. Am. Coll. Cardiol. 22:1849, 1993.

365. Lindsay, B. D., Chung, M. K., Gamache, M. C., et al.: Therapeutic endpoints for the treatment of atrioventricular node reentrant tachycardia by catheter-guided radiofrequency current. J. Am. Coll. Cardiol. 22:733, 1993.

366. Langberg, J. J., Leon, A., Borganelli, M., et al.: A randomized, prospective comparison of anterior and posterior approaches to radiofrequency catheter ablation of atrioventricular nodal reentry tachycardia. Circulation 87:1551, 1993.

367. Mitrani, R. D., Klein, L. S., Hackett, F. K., et al.: Radiofrequency ablation for atrioventricular node reentrant tachycardia: Comparison between fast (anterior) and slow (posterior) pathway ablation. J. Am. Coll. Cardiol. 21:432, 1993.

368. Miles, W. M., Hubbard, J. E., Zipes, D. P., et al.: Elimination of AV nodal reentrant tachycardia with 2:1 VA block by posteroseptal ablation. J. Cardiovasc. Electrophysiol. 5:510, 1994.

369. Strickberger, S. A., Daoud, E., Niebauer, M., et al.: Effects of partial and complete ablation of the slow pathway on fast pathway properties in patients with atrioventricular nodal reentrant tachycardia. J. Cardiovasc. Electrophysiol. 5:645, 1994.

370. Natale, A., Klein, G., and Yee, R.: Shortening of fast pathway refractoriness after slow pathway ablation: Effects of autonomic blockade. Circulation 89:1103, 1994.

371. Silka, M. J., Kron, J., Park, J. K., et al.: Atypical forms of supraventricular tachycardia due to atrioventricular node reentry in children after radiofrequency modification of slow pathway conduction. J. Am. Coll. Cardiol. 23:1363, 1994.

372. Kocovic, D. Z., Harada, T., Shea, J. B., et al.: Alterations of heart rate and of heart rate variability after radiofrequency catheter ablation of supraventricular tachycardia. Circulation 88:1671, 1993.

373. Alison, J. F., Yeung-Lai-Wah, J. A., Schulzer, M., et al.: Characterization of junctional rhythm after atrioventricular node ablation. Circulation 91:84, 1995.

374. Gentzer, J. H., Goyal, R., Williamson, B. D., et al.: Analysis of junctional ectopy during radiofrequency ablation of the slow pathway in patients with atrioventricular nodal reentrant tachycardia. Circulation 90:2820, 1994.

375. Thakur, R. K., Klein, G. J., Yee, R., et al.: Junctional tachycardia: A useful marker during radiofrequency ablation for atrioventricular node reentrant tachycardia. J. Am. Coll. Cardiol. 22:1706, 1993.

376. Chen, S. A., Chiang, C. E., Yang, C. J., et al.: Sustained atrial tachycardia in adult patients: Electrophysiological characteristics, pharmacological response, possible mechanisms, and effects of radiofrequency ablation. Circulation 90:1262, 1994.

377. Lesh, M. D., vanHare, G. F., Epstein, L. M., et al.: Radiofrequency catheter ablation of atrial arrhythmias: Results and mechanisms. Circulation 89:1074, 1994.

378. Tracy, C. M., Swartz, J. F., Fletcher, R. D., et al.: Radiofrequency catheter ablation of ectopic atrial tachycardia using paced activation sequence mapping. J. Am. Coll. Cardiol. 21:910, 1993.

379. Kay, G. N., Chong, F., Epstein, A. E., et al.: Radiofrequency ablation for treatment of primary atrial tachycardias. J. Am. Coll. Cardiol. 21:901, 1993.

380. Sanders, W. E., Jr., Sorrentino, R. A., Greenfield, R. A., et al.: Catheter ablation of sinoatrial node reentrant tachycardia. J. Am. Coll. Cardiol. 23:926, 1994.

381. Scheinman, M. M., Gonzalez, R. P., Cooper, M. W., et al.: Clinical and electrophysiologic features and role of catheter ablation techniques in adult patients with automatic atrioventricular junctional tachycardia. Am. J. Cardiol. 74:565, 1994.

382. Kirkorian, G., Mancada, E., Chevalier, P., et al.: Radiofrequency ablation of atrial flutter: Efficacy of an anatomically guided approach. Circulation 90:2804, 1994.

383. Calkins, H., Leon, A. R., Dean, A. G., et al.: Catheter ablation of atrial flutter using radiofrequency energy. Am. J. Cardiol. 73:353, 1994.

384. Cosio, F. G., Lopez, G. M., Goicholea, A., et al.: Radiofrequency ablation of the inferior vena cava-tricuspid valve isthmus in common atrial flutter. Am. J. Cardiol. 71:705, 1993.

385. Kalbfleisch, S. J., el-Atassi, R., Calkins, H., et al.: Association between atrioventricular node reentrant tachycardia and inducible atrial flutter. J. Am. Coll. Cardiol. 22:80 1993.

386. Interian, A., Jr., Cox, M. M., Jimenez, R. A., et al.: A shared pathway in atrioventricular nodal reentrant tachycardia and atrial flutter: Implications for pathophysiology and therapy. Am. J. Cardiol. 71:297, 1993.

387. Olshansky, B., Okumura, K., Hess, P. G., et al.: Demonstration of an area of slow conduction in human atrial flutter. J. Am. Coll. Cardiol. 16:1639, 1990.

388. Haissaguerre, M., Marcus, F. I., Fischer, B., et al.: Radiofrequency catheter ablation in unusual mechanisms of atrial fibrillation: Report of three cases. J. Cardiovasc. Electrophysiol. 5:743, 1994.

389. Haissaguerre, M., Gencel, L., Fischer, B., et al.: Successful catheter ablation of atrial fibrillation. J. Cardiovasc. Electrophysiol. 5:1045, 1994.

390. Swartz, J. F., Pellersels, G., Silvers, J., et al.: Catheter-based curative approach to atrial fibrillation in humans. Circulation 90 (Suppl. 1): I335, 1994.

391. Elvan, A., Pride, H. P., Eble, J. N., et al.: Radiofrequency catheter ablation of the atria reduces the inducibility and duration of atrial fibrillation in dogs. Circulation 91:2235, 1995.

392. Morillo, C. A., Klein, G. J., Jones, D. L., et al.: Chronic rapid atrial pacing: Structural, functional and electrophysiological characteristics of a new model of sustained atrial fibrillation. Circulation 91:1588, 1995.

393. Olgin, J., and Scheinman, M.: Catheter ablation of the atrioventricular node for treatment of supraventricular tachyarrhythmias. *In* Zipes, D. P., and Jalife, J. (eds.): Cardiac Electrophysiology: From Cell to Bedside. 2nd ed. Philadelphia, W. B. Saunders Company, 1994, pp. 1453–1460.

394. Rodriguez, L. M., Smeets, J. L., Xie, B., et al.: Improvement in left ventricular function by ablation of atrioventricular nodal conduction in selected patients with lone atrial fibrillation. Am. J. Cardiol. 72:1137, 1993.

395. Feld, G. K., Fleck, R. P., Fujimura, O., et al.: Control of rapid ventricular response by radiofrequency catheter modification of the atrioventricular node in patients with medically refractory atrial fibrillation. Circulation 90:2299, 1994.

396. DellaBella, P., Carbucicchio, C., Tondo, C., et al.: Modulation of atrioventricular conduction by ablation of the slow atrioventricular node pathway in patients with drug-refractory atrial fibrillation or flutter. J. Am. Coll. Cardiol. 25:39, 1995.

397. Williamson, B. D., Man, K. C., Daoud, E., et al.: Radiofrequency catheter modification of atrioventricular conduction to control the ventricular rate during atrial fibrillation. N. Engl. J. Med. 331:910, 1994.

398. Borggrefe, M., Chen, X., Hindricks, G., et al.: Catheter ablation of ventricular tachycardia in patients with coronary heart disease. *In* Zipes, D. P., and Jalife, J. (eds.): Cardiac Electrophysiology: From Cell to Bedside. 2nd ed. Philadelphia, W. B. Saunders Company, 1994, pp. 1502–1517.

399. Klein L. S., Miles, W. M., Mitrani, R. D., et al.: Ablation of ventricular tachycardia in patients with structurally normal hearts. *In* Zipes, D. P., and Jalife, J. (eds.): Cardiac Electrophysiology: From Cell to Bedside. 2nd ed. Philadelphia, W. B. Saunders Company, 1994, pp. 1518–1523.

400. Gonska, B. D., Cao, K., Schauman, N. A., et al.: Catheter ablation of ventricular tachycardia in 136 patients with coronary artery disease: Results and longterm follow-up. J. Am. Coll. Cardiol. 24:1506, 1994.

401. Davis, L. M., Cooper, M. W., Johnson, D. C., et al.: Simultaneous 60-electrode mapping of ventricular tachycardia using percutaneous catheters. J. Am. Coll. Cardiol. 24:709, 1994.

402. Gill, J. S., deBelder, M., and Ward, D. E.: Right ventricular outflow tract ventricular tachycardia associated with an aneurysmal malformation: Use of transesophageal echocardiography during low-energy direct-current ablation. Am. Heart J. 128:620, 1994.

403. Coggins, D. L., Lee, R. J., Sweeney, J., et al.: Radiofrequency catheter ablation as a cure for idiopathic tachycardia of both left and right ventricular origin. J. Am. Coll. Cardiol. 23:1333, 1994.

404. Wen, M. S., Yeh, S. J., Wang, C. C., et al.: Radiofrequency ablation therapy in idiopathic left ventricular tachycardia with no obvious structural heart disease. Circulation 89:1690, 1994.

405. Kim, Y. H., Sosa-Suarez, G., Trouton, T. G., et al.: Treatment of ventricular tachycardia by transcatheter radiofrequency ablation in patients with ischemic heart disease. Circulation 89:1094, 1994.

406. Nakagawa, H., Beckman, K. J., McClelland, J. H., et al.: Radiofrequency catheter ablation of idiopathic left ventricular tachycardia guided by a Purkinje potential. Circulation 88:2607, 1993.

407. Stevenson, W. G., Kahn, H., Sager, P., et al.: Identification of reentry circuit sites during catheter mapping and radiofrequency ablation of ventricular tachycardia late after myocardial infarction. Circulation 88:1647, 1993.

408. Calkins, H., Kalbfleisch, S. J., el-Atassi, R., et al.: Relation between efficacy of radiofrequency catheter ablation and site of origin of idiopathic ventricular tachycardia. Am. J. Cardiol. 71:827, 1993.

409. Morady, F., Harvey, M., and Kalbfleisch, S. J.: Radiofrequency catheter

ablation of ventricular tachycardia in patients with coronary artery disease. Circulation 87:363, 1993.

410. Kottkamp, H, Chen, X., Hindricks, G., et al.: Radiofrequency catheter ablation of idiopathic left ventricular tachycardia: Further evidence for microreentry as the underlying mechanism. J. Cardiovasc. Electrophysiol. 5:268, 1994.

411. Mitrani, R. D., Klein, L. S., Miles, W. M., et al.: Regional cardiac sympathetic denervation in patients with ventricular tachycardia in the absence of coronary artery disease. J. Am. Coll. Cardiol. 22:1344, 1993.

412. Blanck, Z., Dhala, A., Deshpande, S., et al.: Bundle branch reentrant ventricular tachycardia: Cumulative experience in 48 patients. J. Cardiovasc. Electrophysiol. 4:253, 1993.

413. Haines, D. E., Verow, A. F., Sinusas, A. J., et al.: Intracoronary ethanol ablation in swine: Characterization of myocardial injury in target and remote vascular beds. J. Cardiovasc. Electrophysiol. 5:41, 1994.

414. Haines, D. E.: Chemical ablative therapy for arrhythmias. In Zipes, D. P., and Jalife, J. (eds.): Cardiac Electrophysiology: From Cell to Bedside. 2nd ed. Philadelphia, W. B. Saunders Company, 1994, pp. 1537–1546.

SURGICAL THERAPY

415. Crawford, F. A., Jr., and Gillette, P. C.: Surgical treatment of cardiac dysrhythmias in infants and children. Ann. Thorac. Surg. 58:1262, 1994.

416. Mahomed, Y.: Surgery for atrioventricular nodal reentrant tachycardia. In Zipes, D. P., and Jalife, J. (eds.): Cardiac Electrophysiology: From Cell to Bedside. 2nd ed. Philadelphia, W. B. Saunders Company, 1994, pp. 1577–1583.

417. Guiraudon, G. M., Klein, G. J., Yee, R., et al.: Surgery for the Wolff-Parkinson-White syndrome. In Zipes, D. P., and Jalife, J. (eds.): Cardiac Electrophysiology: From Cell to Bedside. 2nd ed. Philadelphia, W. B. Saunders Company, 1994, pp. 1553–1563.

418. Ferguson, T. B., Jr., and Cox, J. L.: Surgery for atrial fibrillation. In Zipes, D. P., and Jalife, J. (eds.): Cardiac Electrophysiology: From Cell to Bedside. 2nd ed. Philadelphia, W. B. Saunders Company, 1994, pp. 1563–1576.

419. Lawrie, G. M., and Pacifico, A.: Surgery for ventricular tachycardia. In Zipes, D. P., and Jalife, J. (eds.): Cardiac Electrophysiology: From Cell to Bedside. 2nd ed. Philadelphia, W. B. Saunders Company, 1994, pp. 1547–1552.

420. Ferguson, T. B., Jr.: The future of arrhythmia surgery. J. Cardiovasc. Electrophysiol. 5:621, 1994.

421. Misaki, T., Watanabe, G., Iwa, T., et al.: Surgical treatment of Wolff-Parkinson-White syndrome in infants and children. Ann. Thorac. Surg. 58:103, 1994.

422. Guiraudon, G. M., Guiraudon, C. M., Klein, G. J., et al.: Operation for the Wolff-Parkinson-White syndrome in the catheter ablation era. Ann. Thorac. Surg. 57:1084, 1994.

423. Cox, J. L., Boineau, J. P., Schuessler, R. B., et al.: Five-year experience with the Maze procedure for atrial fibrillation. Ann. Thorac. Surg. 56:814, 1993.

424. DiMarco, J. P.: Management of sudden cardiac death survivors. Role of surgical and catheter ablation. Circulation 85 (Suppl. I):I125, 1992.

425. Zipes, D. P., Roberts, D., for the PCD Investigators: Results of the World Wide Study of the Implantable Pacemaker, Cardioverter, Defibrillator: A comparison of epicardial and endocardial lead systems. Circulation 92:59, 1995.

426. Ferguson, T. B., Jr., Smith, J. M., Cox, J. L., et al.: Direct operation versus ICD therapy for ischemic ventricular tachycardia. Ann. Thorac. Surg. 58:1291, 1994.

Chapter 22
Specific Arrhythmias: Diagnosis and Treatment

DOUGLAS P. ZIPES

DIAGNOSTIC AND THERAPEUTIC CONSIDERATIONS

History

The initial evaluation of the patient suspected of having a cardiac arrhythmia begins with a careful history, specifically questioning the patient regarding the presence of palpitations, syncope, spells of lightheadedness, chest pain, or symptoms of congestive heart failure. Palpitations,[1] an awareness of the heartbeat (see p. 9), may result from irregularities in cardiac rate or rhythm or a change in contractility of the heart. Some patients are able to reproduce this sensation by tapping their hand on their chest, knee, or a table top in a fashion similar to the perceived palpitation or recognize a cadence tapped out by a physician. Such a maneuver can help establish the rate and rhythm of the arrhythmia, narrowing it to a particular rate range, a regular or irregular arrhythmia, or one in which a regular rhythm is interrupted by premature beats. The latter often are perceived only upon the contraction that ends the pause that follows the premature beat. The patient may feel as if the heart has stopped for a moment. A rapid, irregular tapping can suggest the ventricular response to atrial fibrillation, while a rapid, regular tapping can suggest an atrioventricular (AV) nodal reentrant supraventricular tachycardia, for example, particularly in a young person, or ventricular tachycardia in an older person. Information regarding the nature of onset and termination of the rhythm disturbance is particularly important. Knowing the rate of the arrhythmia is crucial, and a brief demonstration by the physician of how to determine heart rate can yield important dividends. The patient, and sometimes a close relative, should be instructed in how to count the pulse.

Answers by the patient to key questions can provide clues to the type of rhythm disturbance, particularly if the physician has some additional information, such as physical findings and a 12-lead electrocardiogram. For example, a young adult with presyncope, normal physical findings, and electrocardiographic changes indicating Wolff-Parkinson-White (WPW) syndrome (see p. 667) should be asked whether the palpitations are regular or irregular, how fast they are, and how they start and stop. If the tachycardia is regular, with a rate of approximately 200 beats per minute, and of sudden onset and termination, it is likely that the patient is experiencing an AV reciprocating tachycardia (see p. 669); on the other hand, if the rhythm is irregular, the patient may have atrial fibrillation, a potentially more serious arrhythmia in the presence of WPW syndrome. In an older patient with presyncope, especially with a history of myocardial infarction, the physician should suspect ventricular tachycardia (see p. 675) if the ventricular rate is rapid and AV heart block (see p. 684) or sinus nodal disease (see p. 648) if the rate is slow. The ventricular rhythm can be regular or irregular. Premature atrial or ventricular beats, perceived as dropped or skipped beats by the patient, are probably the most common cause of palpitations.

The physician should inquire about circumstances that can trigger the arrhythmia, such as emotionally upsetting events, ingestion of caffeine-containing beverages, cigarette smoking, exercise, excessive alcohol intake, or gastrointestinal problems (Fig. 22–1). A careful diet and drug history can be useful, for example, in revealing that the patient develops palpitations only after using a nasal decongestant that contains a sympathomimetic vasoconstrictor or that the patient has been exposed to "street" drugs such as cocaine. States conducive to the genesis of arrhythmias should be considered, such as thyrotoxicosis, pericarditis, mitral valve prolapse, hypokalemia secondary to diuretics, and so forth. Family history can be helpful. A variety of familial disorders can result in arrhythmias, including myotonic dystrophy, Duchenne muscular dystrophy (see p. 1865), and dilated cardiomyopathy (see p. 1407). Congenital conduction system disorders can result in sudden death.

Physical Examination

In addition to recording cardiac rate and rhythm, a number of physical findings can be helpful. For example, findings accompanying AV dissociation (see p. 692) include variable peak systolic blood pressure as the atria alter their contribution to ventricular filling, variable intensity of the first heart sound as the P-R interval changes despite a regular ventricular rhythm, intermittent cannon *a* waves in the jugular venous pulse as atrial contraction occurs against closed AV valves, and apparent "intermittent" gallop sounds when atrial systole occurs at various times of the cardiac cycle. The *venous pulse* provides a window through which to judge atrial and ventricular rates and relative timing relationships. It is of interest that Wenckebach first noted the two types of second degree AV block that bear his name (see p. 689) by recording the jugular phlebogram before the electrocardiogram was available.

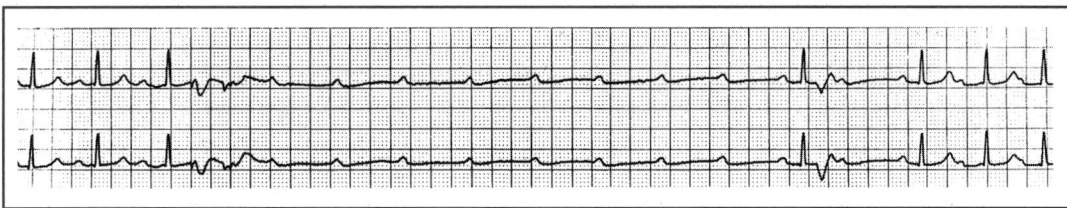

FIGURE 22–1. Transient AV block. This monitor lead recording demonstrates transient AV block during a period of nausea and vomiting, most probably due to excessive vagal stimulation.

Examining the *second heart sound* can be helpful (p. 32). A paradoxically split second heart sound can occur during a QRS complex with a left bundle branch block contour that results from ventricular tachycardia or supraventricular tachycardia with aberration. A widely split second heart sound that does not become single during expiration can accompany right bundle branch block. Unfortunately, similar physical findings occur with different cardiac arrhythmias. For example, progressive diminution of the intensity of the first heart sound results as the P-R interval lengthens, which can occur during AV dissociation when the atrial rate exceeds the ventricular rate or during Wenckebach second degree AV block. Similarly, constant cannon *a* waves can occur with 1:1 atrioventricular relationships during ventricular or supraventricular tachycardia. Since AV dissociation can occur (uncommonly) during a supraventricular tachycardia and VA association can occur during a ventricular tachycardia, the clues provided by physical findings can be only suggestive.

CAROTID SINUS MASSAGE. The response to carotid sinus massage or the Valsalva maneuver provides important diagnostic information by increasing vagal tone and primarily slowing the rate of sinus nodal discharge and prolonging AV nodal conduction time and refractoriness. Sinus tachycardia slows gradually during carotid massage and then returns to the previous rate when massage is discontinued; AV nodal reentry and AV reciprocating tachycardias that involve the AV node in one of its pathways can slow slightly, terminate abruptly, or not change; and ventricular response to atrial flutter, atrial fibrillation, and some atrial tachycardias usually decreases (Table 22–1). Rarely, carotid sinus massage terminates a ventricular tachycardia.

To perform carotid massage, the patient is placed in a supine position, with the neck hyperextended and the head turned away from the side being tested, the sternocleidomastoid muscles relaxed or gently pushed out of the way, and the carotid impulse felt at the angle of the jaw. The carotid bifurcation is touched gently initially with the palmar portion of the fingertips to detect hypersensitive responses. Then, if no change in cardiac rhythm occurs, pressure is applied more firmly for approximately 5 seconds, first on one side and then on the other (*never on both sides simultaneously*) with a gentle rotating massaging motion. External pressure stimulates baroreceptors in the carotid sinus to trigger a reflex increase in vagal activity and sympathetic withdrawal. Responses can occur with right-sided massage and not left, or vice versa, so each side should be tested separately. Generally, the maximal response occurs with the first massage if repeated attempts are performed at short intervals. Some risk is associated with carotid sinus massage, particularly in older patients, and cerebral emboli can occur.[2] Before massage, the carotid artery should be auscultated so that massage is not performed in patients who have carotid bruits indicative of carotid arterial disease.

Electrocardiography

The ECG remains the most important and definitive single noninvasive diagnostic test. Initially, a 12-lead electrocardiogram is recorded, and a long recording employing the lead that shows distinct P waves is obtained for proper analysis. If P waves are not clearly visible, atrial activity can be recorded by placing the right and left arm leads in various chest positions to discern P waves (so-called Lewis leads) using esophageal electrodes or intracavitary right atrial leads. An echocardiogram showing atrial contraction can be helpful.

Each arrhythmia must be approached in a systematic manner to answer the following questions: Are P waves present? What are the atrial and ventricular rates? Are they identical? Are the P-P and R-R intervals regular or irregular? If irregular, is it a consistent, repeating irregularity? Is there a P wave related to each ventricular complex? Does the P wave precede or follow the QRS complex? Is the resultant P-R or R-P interval constant? Is the R-P interval long and the P-R interval short, or vice versa? Are all P waves and QRS complexes identical and normal in contour? To determine the significance of changes in P-wave or QRS contour, or amplitude, one must know the lead being recorded. Are P, P-R, QRS, and Q-T durations normal? Considering the clinical setting, what is the significance of the arrhythmia? Should it be treated and, if so, how? For supraventricular tachycardias with a normal QRS complex, a branching decision tree may be useful.

THE LADDER DIAGRAM. This is employed to depict depolarization and conduction schematically. Straight or slightly slanting lines drawn on a tiered framework beneath an ECG trace represent electrical events occurring in the various cardiac structures (Fig. 22–2*A* and *B*). Since the ECG and therefore the ladder diagram represent electrical activity against a time base, conduction is indicated by the lines of the ladder diagram sloping in a left-to-right direction. A less steep line depicts slower conduction. A short bar drawn perpendicular to a sloping line represents blocked conduction (Fig. 22–2*C*). Activity originating in an ectopic site such as the ventricle is indicated in another tier drawn beneath the ventricular tier. In general, atrial, AV junctional, or ventricular activity is diagrammed to begin in that particular tier. It is important to remember that sinus nodal discharge and conduction and, under certain circumstances, AV junctional discharge and conduction can only be assumed; their activity is not recorded on scalar ECG.

ELECTROPHYSIOLOGICAL STUDY. When this study is indicated, it is performed by introducing multipolar catheter electrodes into the vascular system and positioning them in various parts of the heart. The catheters are used to record local electrical activity and to stimulate the heart. Multiple leads are recorded simultaneously, usually at a paper speed of 50 to 100 mm/sec. (Standard ECGs generally are recorded at a paper speed of 25 mm/sec.) Because of the rapid recording speed, intervals or complexes of normal duration may appear prolonged. An electrode positioned across the septal leaflet of the tricuspid valve records His bundle activity as well as low right atrial activity and high ventricular septal depolarization. Occasionally, a right bundle branch deflection also can be recorded. Three basic measurements are made using the ECG and the His bundle catheter recording: the P-A, A-H, and H-V intervals (Fig. 22–2*D*). The *P-A interval* is the time between the onset of the P wave in the surface tracing (which generally slightly precedes the onset of the high right atrial recording) and the low right atrial deflection, recorded in the His lead.

TABLE 22–1   ARRHYTHMIA CHARACTERISTICS*

TYPE OF ARRHYTHMIA	P WAVES Rate (bpm)	P WAVES Rhythm	P WAVES Contour	QRS COMPLEXES Rate	QRS COMPLEXES Rhythm	QRS COMPLEXES Contour
Sinus rhythm	60 to 100	Regular**	Normal	60 to 100	Regular	Normal
Sinus bradycardia	<60	Regular	Normal	<60	Regular	Normal
Sinus tachycardia	100 to 180	Regular	May be peaked	100 to 180	Regular	Normal
AV nodal reentry	150 to 250	Very regular except at onset and termination	Retrograde; difficult to see; lost in QRS complex	150 to 250	Very regular except at onset and termination	Normal
Atrial flutter	250 to 350	Regular	Sawtooth	75 to 175	Generally regular in absence of drugs or disease	Normal
Atrial fibrillation	400 to 600	Grossly irregular	Baseline undulation, no P waves	100 to 160	Grossly irregular	Normal
Atrial tachycardia with block	150 to 250	Regular; may be irregular	Abnormal	75 to 200	Generally regular in absence of drugs or disease	Normal
AV junctional rhythm	40 to 100‡	Regular	Normal	40 to 60	Fairly regular	Normal
Reciprocating tachycardias using an accessory (WPW) pathway	150 to 250	Very regular except at onset and termination	Retrograde; difficult to see; follow the QRS complex	150 to 250	Very regular except at onset and termination	Normal
Nonparoxysmal AV junctional tachycardia	60 to 100‡	Regular	Normal	70 to 130	Fairly regular	Normal
Ventricular tachycardia	60 to 100‡	Regular	Normal	110 to 250	Fairly regular; may be irregular	Abnormal, >0.12 second
Accelerated idioventricular rhythm	60 to 100‡	Regular	Normal	50 to 110	Fairly regular; may be irregular	Abnormal, >0.12 second
Ventricular flutter	60 to 100‡	Regular	Normal; difficult to see	150 to 300	Regular	Sine wave
Ventricular fibrillation	60 to 100‡	Regular	Normal; difficult to see	400 to 600	Grossly irregular	Baseline undulations; no QRS complexes
First degree AV block	60 to 100¶	Regular	Normal	60 to 100	Regular	Normal
Type I second degree AV block	60 to 100¶	Regular	Normal	30 to 100	Irregular‖	Normal
Type II second degree AV block	60 to 100¶	Regular	Normal	30 to 100	Irregular‖	Abnormal, >0.12 second
Complete AV block	60 to 100‡	Regular	Normal	<40	Fairly regular	Abnormal, >0.12 second
Right bundle branch block	60 to 100	Regular	Normal	60 to 100	Regular	Abnormal, >0.12 second
Left bundle branch block	60 to 100	Regular	Normal	60 to 100	Regular	Abnormal, >0.12 second

* In an effort to summarize these arrhythmias in a tabular form, generalizations have to be made. For example, response to carotid sinus massage may be slightly different from what is listed. Acute therapy to terminate a tachycardia may be different from chronic therapy to prevent a recurrence. Some of the exceptions are indicated in the footnotes; the reader is referred to the text for a complete discussion.

** P waves initiated by sinus node discharge may not be precisely regular because of sinus arrhythmia.

† Often, carotid sinus massage fails to slow a sinus tachycardia.

‡ Any independent atrial arrhythmia may exist or the atria may be captured retrogradely.

§ Constant if atria are captured retrogradely.

¶ Atrial rhythm and rate may vary, depending on whether sinus bradycardia or tachycardia, etc., is the atrial mechanism.

‖ Regular or constant if block is unchanging.

Modified from Zipes, D. P.: Arrhythmias. *In* Andreoli, K., et al. (eds): Comprehensive Cardiac Care. 6th ed. St. Louis, C. V. Mosby, 1987.

This interval reflects intraatrial conduction and has not proved to be of much clinical value.

The A-H Interval. This is timed from the onset of the first rapid deflection recorded in the atrial electrogram (A) in the His bundle lead to the beginning of the His (H) deflection. Since the low right atrium and His bundle anatomically delineate the boundaries of the AV node, the A-H interval closely approximates AV nodal conduction time. The A-H interval is affected by various interventions: atropine and isoproterenol shorten the A-H interval, while vagal maneuvers, digitalis, propranolol, verapamil, adenosine, and rapid or premature atrial pacing lengthen it. Normal range for the A-H interval is 55 to 130 msec, depending on heart rate, autonomic tone, and other factors.

The H-V Interval. This is the time from the beginning of the H deflection to the earliest onset of ventricular depolarization recorded in *any* lead. This interval represents conduction from the His bundle through the bundle

VENTRICULAR RESPONSE TO CAROTID SINUS MASSAGE	P WAVES — PHYSICAL EXAMINATION			QRS COMPLEXES
	Intensity of S_1	Splitting of S_2	*a* Waves	Treatment
Gradual slowing and return to former rate	Constant	Normal	Normal	None
Gradual slowing and return to former rate	Constant	Normal	Normal	None, unless symptomatic; atropine
Gradual slowing† and return to former rate	Constant	Normal	Normal	None, unless symptomatic; treat underlying disease
Abrupt slowing caused by termination of tachycardia, or no effect	Constant	Normal	Constant cannon *a* waves	Vagal stimulation, adenosine, verapamil, digitalis, propranolol, DC shock, pacing
Abrupt slowing and return to former rate; flutter remains	Constant; variable if AV block changing	Normal	Flutter waves	DC shock, digitalis, quinidine, propranolol, verapamil, adenosine
Slowing; gross irregularity remains	Variable	Normal	No *a* waves	Digitalis, quinidine, DC shock, verapamil, adenosine
Abrupt slowing and return to normal rate; tachycardia remains	Constant; variable if AV block changing	Normal	More *a* waves than *c-v* waves	Stop digitalis if toxic; digitalis if not toxic; possibly verapamil
None; may be slight slowing	Variable§	Normal	Intermittent cannon waves§	None, unless symptomatic; atropine
Abrupt slowing caused by termination of tachycardia, or no effect	Constant but decreased	Normal	Constant cannon waves	(See AV nodal reentry above)
None, may be slight slowing	Variable§	Normal	Intermittent cannon waves§	None, unless symptomatic; stop digitalis if toxic
None	Variable§	Abnormal	Intermittent cannon waves§	Lidocaine, procainamide, DC shock, quinidine, amiodarone
None	Variable§	Abnormal	Intermittent cannon waves§	None, unless symptomatic; lidocaine, atropine
None	Soft or absent	Soft or absent	Cannon waves	DC shock
None	None	None	Cannon waves	DC shock
Gradual slowing caused by sinus slowing	Constant, diminished	Normal	Normal	None
Slowing caused by sinus slowing and an increase in AV block	Cyclic decrease then increase after pause	Normal	Normal; increasing *a-c* interval; *a* waves without *c* waves	None, unless symptomatic; atropine
Gradual slowing caused by sinus slowing	Constant	Abnormal	Normal; constant *a-c* interval; *a* waves without *c* waves	Pacemaker
None	Variable§	Abnormal	Intermittent cannon waves§	Pacemaker
Gradual slowing and return to former rate	Constant	Wide	Normal	None
Gradual slowing and return to former rate	Constant	Paradoxical	Normal	None

branch–Purkinje system to the point of ventricular muscle activation and is usually constant—between 30 and 55 msec—regardless of heart rate or autonomic tone. Other intervals are discussed under the individual tachycardias.

CONSEQUENCES OF ARRHYTHMIAS. The ventricular rate and duration of an arrhythmia, its site of origin, and the cardiovascular status of the patient primarily determine the electrophysiological and hemodynamic consequences of a particular rhythm disturbance. Electrophysiological consequences, often influenced by the presence of underlying heart disease such as acute myocardial infarction, include the development of serious arrhythmias as a result of rapid or slow rates, initiation of sustained arrhythmias by premature systoles, or the progression of rhythms such as ventricular tachycardia to ventricular fibrillation. Extremes of heart rate or loss of the atrial contribution to ventricular filling can alter circulatory dynamics. Rapid rates greatly shorten the diastolic filling time, and particularly in diseased hearts, the increased heart rate can fail to compensate for the reduced stroke output; as a consequence, arterial pressure, cardiac output, and coronary blood flow decline. Arrhythmias that prevent sequential AV contraction mitigate the hemodynamic benefits of the atrial booster pump, whereas atrial fibrillation causes complete loss of atrial contraction and can reduce cardiac output. Chronic tachycardias can cause cardiac dilation and heart failure from a tachycardia-induced cardiomyopathy.

Management

The therapeutic approach to a patient with a cardiac arrhythmia begins with an accurate electrocardiographic *interpretation* of the arrhythmia and continues with determination of the *cause* of the arrhythmia (if possible), the

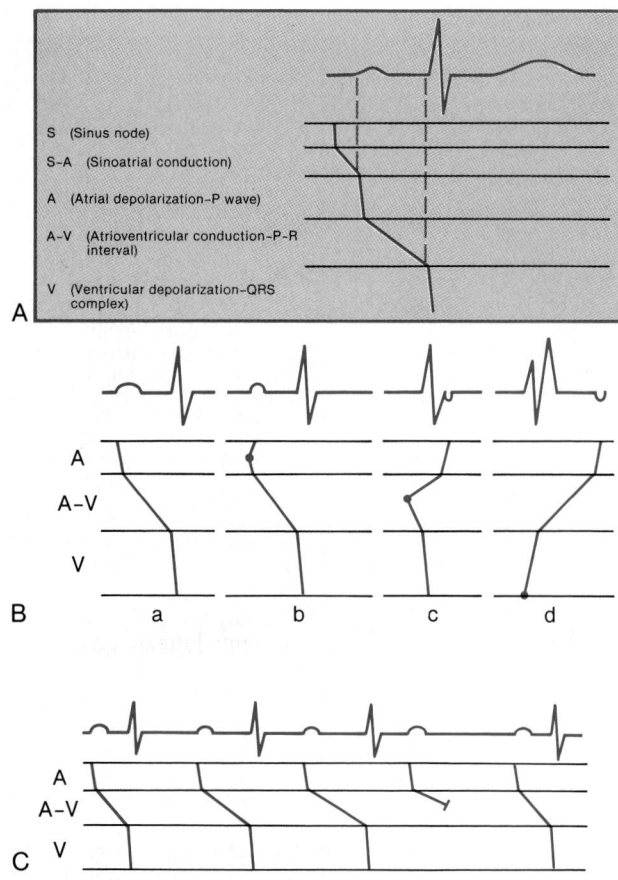

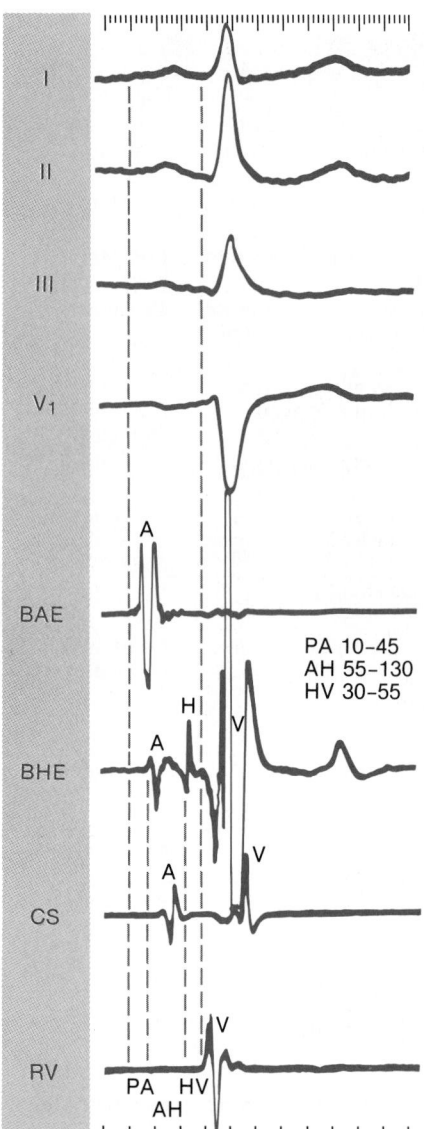

FIGURE 22–2. *A,* Ladder diagram. Straight or slightly sloping lines beginning with the P wave and QRS complex indicate atrial and ventricular depolarization. The instants at which the sinus node discharges and the duration of sinoatrial conduction cannot be measured in the surface ECG and are therefore assumed. The sloping line connecting A and V, delimited by the interrupted lines, represents AV conduction.

B, Normal and ectopic beats. a = Normal sinus rhythm; b = ectopic atrial beat; c = AV junctional beat; d = ventricular ectopic beats. All are drawn with appropriate ladder diagrams beneath (T waves omitted). Retrograde atrial conduction is inscribed for the latter two beats. As with the sinus node, the exact discharge time of the AV junctional focus and conduction time from that point to the ventricles and atria are assumed.

C, Second degree Wenckebach type I AV block. The P-R interval lengthens progressively until finally the fourth P wave fails to reach the ventricles. As the P-R interval is prolonged, note decreasing slope of the line representing AV conduction and the small line perpendicular to the fourth sloping line indicating that the P wave is blocked. (*A* to *C* reproduced with permission from Zipes, D. P., and Fisch, C.: ECG Analysis: 1. Introduction. Premature ventricular complexes. Arch. Intern. Med. *128:*140, 1971. Copyright American Medical Association.)

D, A single cardiac cycle showing the intervals measured during an electrophysiological study. In this and in similar subsequent figures, BAE indicates bipolar atrial electrogram recording high right atrial activity; BHE indicates the bipolar His electrogram recording low right atrial activity (A), His bundle activity (H), and ventricular septal activity (V); CS indicates bipolar electrogram recording of left atrial activity in coronary sinus lead; RV indicates right ventricular electrogram recording right ventricular activity; I = lead I; II = lead II; III = lead III; V₁ = lead V₁; PA = interval representing intraatrial conduction time; AH = interval representing AV nodal conduction time; HV = interval representing His-Purkinje conduction time. All values are in milliseconds. Normal values for P-A, A-H, and H-V intervals are given at the upper right. Paper speed = 100 mm/sec unless otherwise stated. Interrupted lines demarcate the various intervals. Note the normal sequence of atrial activation recorded with this technique: high right atrial activity (BAE) precedes low right atrial activity recorded in the BHE lead, which precedes left atrial activity recorded in the CS lead. Large time lines = 50 msec. Small time lines = 10 msec.

nature of the underlying *heart disease* (if any), and the *consequences* of the arrhythmias in the individual patient. Thus one does not treat arrhythmias as isolated events without having knowledge of the entire clinical situation. *Patients* who have arrhythmias, rather than the arrhythmias themselves, are treated.

When a patient develops a tachyarrhythmia, slowing the ventricular rate is the initial and often most important therapeutic maneuver. Therapy can differ radically for the same arrhythmia in two different patients because the consequences of tachycardia in individual patients differ. For example, a supraventricular tachycardia at a rate of 200 beats/min can produce few or no symptoms in a healthy young adult and therefore requires little or no therapy because it is usually self-limited. The same arrhythmia can

precipitate pulmonary edema in a patient with mitral stenosis, syncope in a patient with aortic stenosis, shock in a patient with acute myocardial infarction, or hemiparesis in a patient with cerebrovascular disease. In these situations, the tachycardia requires prompt electrical conversion.

The *cause* of the arrhythmia can influence therapy greatly. Electrolyte imbalance (potassium, magnesium, calcium), acidosis or alkalosis, hypoxemia, and many drugs can produce rhythm disturbances, and their identification and treatment can abolish or prevent these arrhythmias. Because heart failure can cause arrhythmias, treatment of this condition with digitalis, diuretics, or vasodilators can suppress some of the arrhythmias that accompany cardiac decompensation. Similarly, arrhythmias secondary to hypotension may respond to leg elevation or vasopressor therapy. Mild sedation or reassurance can be successful in treating some arrhythmias related to emotional stress. Precipitating or contributing disease states such as myocarditis, infection, hypokalemia, anemia, and thyroid disorders should be sought and treated when possible. Since therapy always involves some risk, one must be sure—particularly as the therapeutic regimen escalates—that the risks of *not* treating the arrhythmia continue to outweigh the risks of therapy with potentially hazardous antiarrhythmic measures.

INDIVIDUAL CARDIAC ARRHYTHMIAS

SINUS NODAL DISTURBANCES

NORMAL SINUS RHYTHM

Normal sinus rhythm is arbitrarily limited to impulse formation beginning in the sinus node at frequencies between 60 and 100 beats/min. A range of 50 to 90 beats/min has been suggested recently.[3] Infants and children generally have faster heart rates than do adults, both at rest and during exercise. The P wave is upright in leads I, II, and aV_f and negative in lead aV_r, with a vector in the frontal plane between 0 and +90 degrees. In the horizontal plane, the P vector is directed anteriorly and slightly leftward and therefore can be negative in leads V_1 and V_2 but positive in V_3 to V_6. The P-R interval exceeds 120 msec and can vary slightly with rate. If the pacemaker site shifts, a change in the morphology of the P wave can occur. The rate of sinus rhythm varies significantly and depends on many factors, including age, sex, and physical activity.

The sinus nodal discharge rate responds readily to autonomic stimuli and depends on the effect of the two opposing autonomic influences. Steady vagal stimulation decreases the spontaneous sinus nodal discharge rate and predominates over steady sympathetic stimulation, which increases the spontaneous sinus nodal discharge rate. Single or brief bursts of vagal stimulation can speed, slow, or entrain sinus nodal discharge. A given vagal stimulus produces a greater absolute reduction in heart rate when the basal heart rate has been increased by sympathetic stimulation, a phenomenon known as *accentuated antagonism.*

SINUS TACHYCARDIA

ELECTROCARDIOGRAPHIC RECOGNITION (Fig. 22–3A). *Tachycardia* in the adult is defined as a rate exceeding 100 beats/min. During sinus tachycardia, the sinus node exhibits a discharge frequency between 100 and 180 beats/min, but it may be higher with extreme exertion. The maximum heart rate achieved during strenuous physical activity decreases with age from near 200 beats/min to less than 140 beats/min. Sinus tachycardia generally has a gradual onset and termination. The P-P interval can vary slightly from cycle to cycle. P waves have a normal contour but can develop a larger amplitude and become peaked. They appear before each QRS complex with a stable P-R interval unless concomitant AV block ensues.

Accelerated phase 4 diastolic depolarization of sinus nodal cells generally is responsible for sinus tachycardia. Rate changes can result from a shift in pacemaker cells to a different locus within the sinus node. Carotid sinus massage and Valsalva or other vagal maneuvers gradually slow a sinus tachycardia, which then accelerates to its previous rate upon cessation of enhanced vagal tone. More rapid sinus rates can fail to slow in response to a vagal maneuver.

CLINICAL FEATURES. Sinus tachycardia is common in infancy and early childhood and is the normal reaction to a variety of physiological or pathophysiological stresses such as fever, hypotension, thyrotoxicosis, anemia, anxiety, exertion, hypovolemia, pulmonary emboli, myocardial ischemia, congestive heart failure, or shock. It can occur during REM sleep[4] and can be an adverse prognostic sign after heart transplantation.[5] Drugs, such as atropine, catecholamines,[6] thyroid medications,[7] alcohol, nicotine, or caffeine, or inflammation can produce sinus tachycardia. Persistent sinus tachycardia can be a manifestation of heart failure.

In patients with mitral stenosis or severe ischemic heart disease, sinus tachycardia can result in a reduced cardiac output or angina or can precipitate another arrhythmia, in part related to the abbreviated ventricular filling time and compromised coronary blood flow. Sinus tachycardia can be a cause of inappropriate defibrillator discharge.[8] *Chronic inappropriate sinus tachycardia* has been described in otherwise healthy persons, possibly owing to increased automaticity of the sinus node or an automatic atrial focus located near the sinus node.[9] The abnormality can result from a defect in either sympathetic or vagal nerve control of sinoatrial automaticity, or there can be an abnormality of the intrinsic heart rate.[10] It has been noted following radiofrequency catheter ablation of AV nodal tachycardia.[11-13]

MANAGEMENT. This should focus on the *cause* of the sinus tachycardia. Elimination of tobacco, alcohol, coffee, tea, or other stimulants, such as the sympathomimetic agents in nose drops, may be helpful. Drugs such as propranolol or verapamil or fluid replacement in a hypovolemic patient or fever reduction in a febrile patient can be used to help slow the sinus nodal discharge rate. Treatment of inappropriate sinus tachycardia requires beta blockers, calcium channel blockers, or digitalis, alone or in combination. In severe cases, sinus node radiofrequency[14] or surgical[15] ablation may be indicated. Occlusion of the sinus node artery has been attempted as treatment.[16]

SINUS BRADYCARDIA

ELECTROCARDIOGRAPHIC RECOGNITION (Fig. 22–3B). Sinus bradycardia exists in the adult when the sinus node discharges at a rate less than 60 beats/min. P waves have a normal contour and occur before each QRS complex with a constant P-R interval exceeding 120 msec

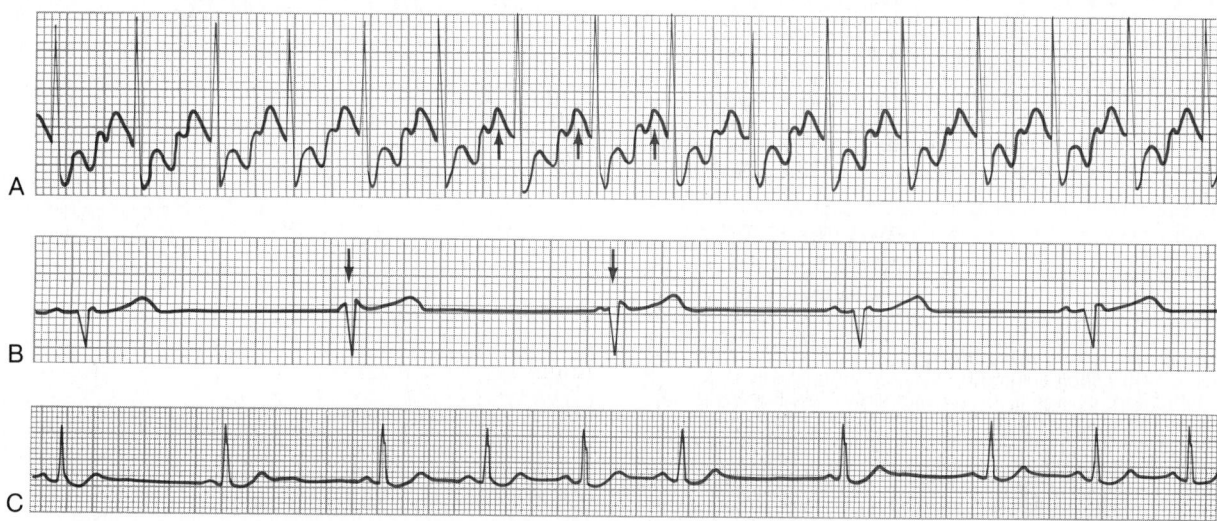

FIGURE 22–3. *A,* Sinus tachycardia (150 beats/min) in a patient during acute myocardial ischemia; note ST-segment depression. P waves are indicated by arrows. *B,* Sinus bradycardia at a rate of 40 to 48 beats/min. The second and third QRS complexes (arrows) represent junctional escape beats. Note P waves at onset of QRS complex. *C,* Nonrespiratory sinus arrhythmia occurring as a consequence of digitalis toxicity. Monitor leads.

unless concomitant AV block is present. Sinus arrhythmia often coexists.

CLINICAL FEATURES. Sinus bradycardia can result from excessive vagal or decreased sympathetic tone as well as from anatomical changes in the sinus node (see Sick Sinus Syndrome, p. 648). Sinus bradycardia frequently occurs in healthy young adults, particularly well-trained athletes (who also can have tachyarrhythmias), and decreases in prevalence with advancing age. It may be present in patients with anorexia nervosa[17] and following cardiac transplantation.[18] During sleep, the normal heart rate can fall to 35 to 40 beats/min, especially in adolescents and young adults, with marked sinus arrhythmia sometimes producing pauses of 2 seconds or longer. Eye surgery, coronary arteriography, meningitis, intracranial tumors, increased intracranial pressure, cervical and mediastinal tumors, and certain disease states such as severe hypoxia, Chagas' disease,[19] myxedema, hypothermia, fibrodegenerative changes, convalescence from some infections, gram-negative sepsis, and mental depression can produce sinus bradycardia. Obstructive jaundice is considered to cause sinus bradycardia, but the evidence is not clear. Sinus bradycardia also occurs during vomiting or vasovagal syncope (see p. 863) and can be produced by carotid sinus stimulation or by administration of parasympathomimetic drugs, lithium, amiodarone, beta-adrenoceptor blocking drugs, clonidine, propafenone, or calcium-antagonists. Conjunctival instillation of beta blockers for glaucoma can produce sinus or AV nodal abnormalities.

In most instances, sinus bradycardia is a benign arrhythmia and actually can be beneficial by producing a longer period of diastole and increasing ventricular filling time. It can be associated with syncope due to an abnormal reflex.[20] Sinus bradycardia occurs in 10 to 15 per cent of patients with acute myocardial infarction and may be even more prevalent when patients are seen in the early hours of infarction. Unless accompanied by hemodynamic decompensation or arrhythmias, sinus bradycardia generally is associated with a more favorable outcome following myocardial infarction than is the presence of sinus tachycardia. It usually is transient and occurs more commonly during inferior than anterior myocardial infarction; it has been noted during reperfusion with thrombolytic agents. Bradycardia following resuscitation from cardiac arrest is associated with a poor prognosis.

MANAGEMENT. Treatment of sinus bradycardia per se is usually not necessary. For example, if the patient with an acute myocardial infarction is asymptomatic, it is probably best not to speed up the sinus rate. If cardiac output is inadequate or if arrhythmias are associated with the slow rate, atropine (0.5 mg IV as an initial dose, repeated if necessary) is usually effective. Lower doses of atropine, particularly when given subcutaneously or intramuscularly, can exert an initial parasympathomimetic effect, possibly via a central action. Ephedrine, hydralazine, or theophylline can be useful in managing some patients with symptomatic sinus bradycardia. These drugs should be given with caution so as not to "overshoot" and produce too rapid a rate. In some patients who experience congestive heart failure or symptoms of low cardiac output as a result of chronic sinus bradycardia, electrical pacing may be needed. Atrial pacing is usually preferable to ventricular pacing in order to preserve sequential atrioventricular contraction and is preferable to drug therapy for long-term management of sinus bradycardia. As a general rule, no available drugs increase the heart rate reliably and safely over long periods without important side effects.

SINUS ARRHYTHMIA

Sinus arrhythmia (Fig. 22–3C) is characterized by a phasic variation in sinus cycle length during which the maximum sinus cycle length minus minimum sinus cycle length exceeds 120 msec or the maximum sinus cycle length minus minimum sinus cycle length divided by the minimum sinus cycle length exceeds 10 per cent. It is the most frequent form of arrhythmia and is considered to be a normal event. P-wave morphology usually does not vary, and the P-R interval exceeds 120 msec and remains unchanged, since the focus of discharge remains relatively fixed within the sinus node. Occasionally, the pacemaker focus can wander within the sinus node, or its exit to the atrium may change, producing P waves of slightly different contour (but not retrograde) and a slightly changing P-R interval that exceeds 120 msec.

Sinus arrhythmia commonly occurs in the young, especially with slower heart rates or following enhanced vagal tone, such as after the administration of digitalis or morphine, and decreases with age or with autonomic dysfunction, such as diabetic neuropathy. Sinus arrhythmia appears in two basic forms. In the *respiratory* form, the P-P interval cyclically shortens during inspiration, primarily as a result of reflex inhibition of vagal tone, and slows during expiration; breath-holding eliminates the cycle-length variation. Efferent vagal effects alone have been suggested as responsible for respiratory sinus arrhythmias. *Nonrespiratory* sinus arrhythmia is characterized by a phasic variation in P-P interval unrelated to the respiratory cycle and may be the result of digitalis intoxication. Loss of sinus rhythm variability is a risk factor for sudden cardiac death (see p. 750). Loss of sinus arrhythmia can occur in patients with acute intracranial lesions.[21]

Symptoms produced by sinus arrhythmia are uncommon, but on occasion, if the pauses between beats are excessively long, palpitations or dizziness may result. Marked sinus arrhythmia can produce a sinus pause sufficiently long to produce syncope if not accompanied by an escape rhythm.

Treatment is usually unnecessary. Increasing the heart rate by exercise or drugs generally abolishes sinus arrhythmia. Symptomatic individuals may experience relief from palpitations with sedatives, tranquilizers, atropine, ephedrine, or isoproterenol administration, as in the treatment of sinus bradycardia.

VENTRICULOPHASIC SINUS ARRHYTHMIA. This arrhythmia occurs when the ventricular rate is slow. The most common example occurs during complete AV block, when P-P cycles that contain a QRS complex are shorter than P-P cycles without a QRS complex. Similar lengthening can be present in the P-P cycle that follows a premature ventricular complex with a compensatory pause. Alterations in the P-P interval are probably due to the influence of the autonomic nervous system responding to changes in ventricular stroke volume.

Sinus Pause or Sinus Arrest

Sinus pause or sinus arrest (Fig. 22–4) is recognized by a pause in the sinus rhythm. The P-P interval delimiting the pause does not equal a multiple of the basic P-P interval. Differentiation of sinus arrest, which is thought to be due to a slowing or cessation of spontaneous sinus nodal automaticity and therefore a disorder of impulse formation, from sinoatrial exit block (see below) in patients with sinus arrhythmia can be quite difficult without direct recordings of sinus node discharge.[22,23]

Failure of sinus nodal discharge results in absence of atrial depolarization and in periods of ventricular asystole if escape beats initiated by latent pacemakers do not occur (Fig. 22–4). Involvement of the sinus node by acute myocardial infarction,[24] degenerative fibrotic changes, effects of digitalis toxicity, stroke, or excessive vagal tone all can produce sinus arrest. Transient sinus arrest may have no clinical significance by itself if latent pacemakers promptly escape to prevent ventricular asystole or the genesis of other arrhythmias precipitated by the slow rates. Sinus arrest and AV block have been demonstrated in as many as 30 per cent of patients with sleep apnea.[25]

Treatment is as outlined above for sinus bradycardia. In patients who have a chronic form of sinus node disease characterized by marked sinus bradycardia or sinus arrest, permanent pacing is often necessary.

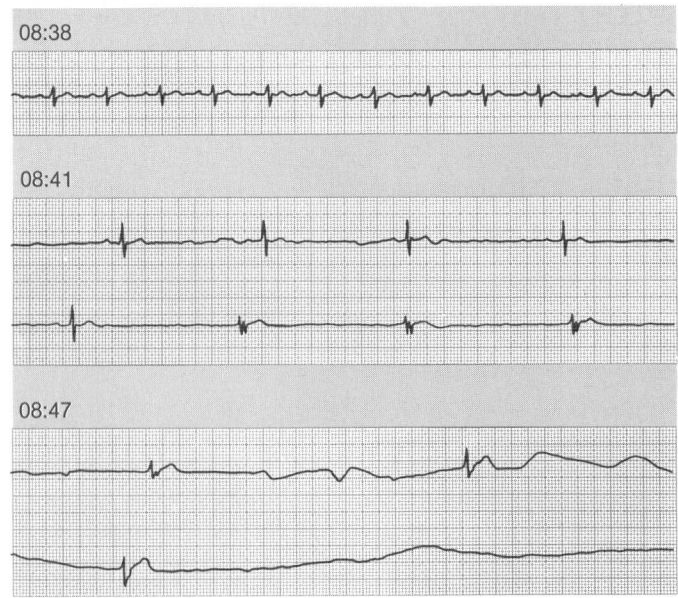

FIGURE 22–4. Sinus arrest. The patient had a long-term ECG recorder connected when he died suddenly due to cardiac standstill. The rhythms demonstrate progressive sinus bradycardia and sinus arrest at 08:41. The rhythm then becomes a ventricular escape rhythm which progressively slows and finally ceases at 08:47. Monitor lead. Double ECG strips are continuous recordings.

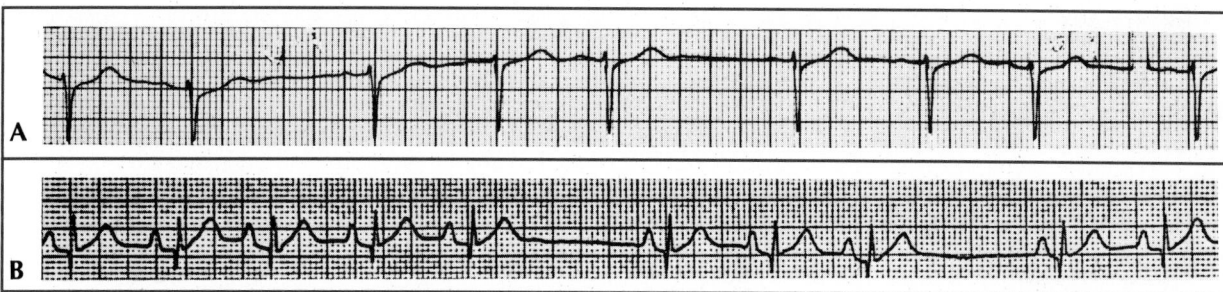

FIGURE 22–5. Sinus nodal exit block. *A,* Type I SA nodal exit block has the following features: the P-P interval shortens from the first to the second cycle in each grouping, followed by a pause. The duration of the pause is less than twice the shortest cycle length, and the cycle after the pause exceeds the cycle before the pause. The P-R interval is normal and constant. Lead V₁. *B,* The P-P interval varies slightly because of sinus arrhythmia. Two pauses in sinus nodal activity occur, equalling twice the basic P-P interval and are consistent with type II 2:1 SA nodal exit block. The P-R interval is normal and constant. Lead III.

Sinoatrial (SA) Exit Block

This arrhythmia is recognized electrocardiographically by a pause due to the absence of the normally expected P wave[23,26] (Fig. 22–5). The duration of the pause is a multiple of the basic P-P interval. SA exit block is due to a conduction disturbance during which an impulse formed within the sinus node fails to depolarize the atria or does so with delay[27] (Fig. 22–6). An interval without P waves that equals approximately two, three, or four times the normal P-P cycle characterizes type II second degree SA exit block. During type I (Wenckebach) second degree SA exit block, the P-P interval progressively shortens prior to the pause, and the duration of the pause is less than two P-P cycles. (See p. 689 and Fig. 22–52, p. 689, for further discussion of Wenckebach intervals.) First degree SA exit block cannot be recognized electrocardiographically because SA nodal discharge is not recorded. Third degree SA exit block can present as complete absence of P waves and is difficult to diagnose with certainty without sinus node electrograms.

Excessive vagal stimulation, acute myocarditis, infarction, or fibrosis involving the atrium as well as drugs such as quinidine, procainamide, or digitalis can produce SA exit block. SA exit block is usually transient. It may be of no clinical importance except to prompt a search for the underlying cause. Occasionally, syncope can result if the

SA block is prolonged and unaccompanied by an escape rhythm. SA exit block can occur in well-trained athletes[28] and can be a factor in sick sinus syndrome.[27]

Therapy for patients who have symptomatic SA exit block is as outlined for sinus bradycardia.

Wandering Pacemaker

This variant of sinus arrhythmia involves the passive transfer of the dominant pacemaker focus from the sinus node to latent pacemakers that have the next highest degree of automaticity located in other atrial sites or in AV junctional tissue. Thus only one pacemaker at a time controls the rhythm, in sharp contrast to AV dissociation (see p. 692). As with other forms of sinus arrhythmia, the change occurs in a gradual fashion over the duration of several beats. The ECG (Fig. 22–7) displays a cyclical increase in R-R interval, a P-R interval that gradually shortens and can become less than 120 msec, and a change in the P-wave contour, which becomes negative in lead I or II (depending on the site of discharge) or is lost within the QRS complex. Generally, these changes occur in reverse as the pacemaker shifts back to the sinus node. Rarely, the rate may remain unchanged during these P-wave transitions.

Wandering pacemaker is a normal phenomenon that often occurs in the very young and particularly in athletes, presumably because of augmented vagal tone. Persistence of an AV junctional rhythm for long periods of time, however, may indicate underlying heart disease. *Treatment* is usually not indicated but, if necessary, is the same as that for sinus bradycardia (see above).

Hypersensitive Carotid Sinus Syndrome
(See also p. 865)

ELECTROCARDIOGRAPHIC RECOGNITION (Fig. 22–8). This condition is characterized most frequently by ventricular asystole due to cessation of atrial activity from sinus arrest or SA exit block. AV block is observed less frequently, probably in part because the absence of atrial activity due to sinus arrest precludes the manifestations of AV block. However, if an atrial pacemaker maintained an atrial rhythm during the episodes, a higher prevalence of AV block probably would be noted. In symptomatic patients, AV junctional or ventricular escapes generally do not occur or are present at very slow rates, suggesting that heightened vagal tone and sympathetic withdrawal can suppress subsidiary pacemakers located in the ventricles as well as supraventricular structures.

CLINICAL FEATURES. Two types of hypersensitive carotid sinus responses are noted. *Cardioinhibitory* carotid sinus hypersensitivity is generally defined as ventricular asystole exceeding 3 seconds during carotid sinus stimulation, although normal limits have not been carefully established. In fact, asystole exceeding 3 seconds during carotid

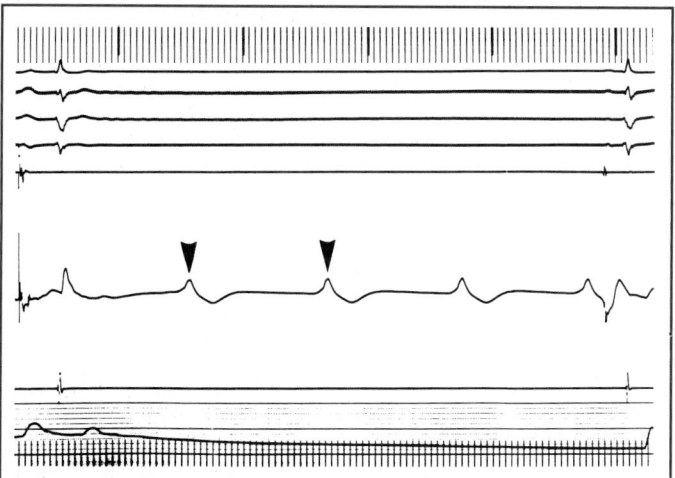

FIGURE 22–6. Sinus node exit block. Following a period of atrial pacing (only the last paced cycle is shown), the patient developed sinus node exit block. The tracing demonstrates sinus node potentials (arrowheads), recorded with a catheter electrode, not conducting to the atrium until the last complex. Recordings are leads I, II, III, and V₁, right atrial recording, sinus node recording, and right ventricular apical recording. The bottom tracing is femoral artery blood pressure.

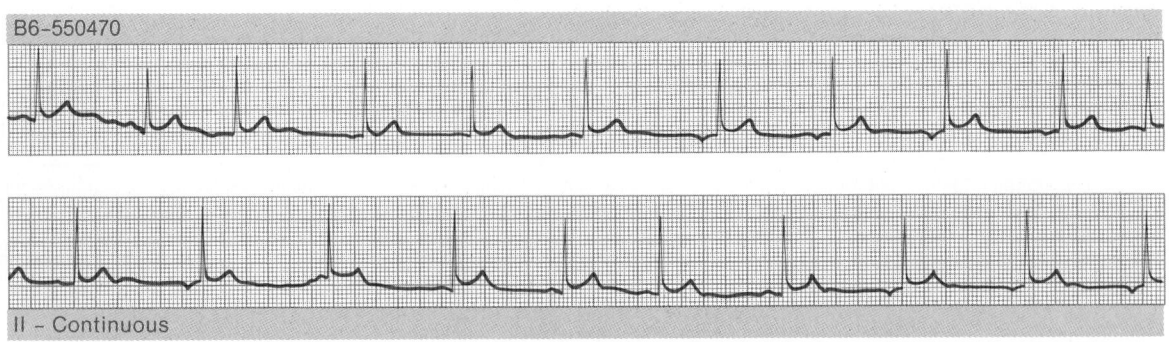

B6-550470

II – Continuous

FIGURE 22–7. Wandering atrial pacemaker. As the heart rate slows, the P waves become inverted and then gradually revert toward normal when the heart rate speeds up again. The P-R interval shortens to 0.14 sec with the inverted P wave and is 0.16 sec with the upright P wave. This phasic variation in cycle length with varying P-wave contour suggests a shift in pacemaker site and is characteristic of wandering atrial pacemaker.

sinus massage is not common but can occur in asymptomatic subjects (Fig. 22–8). *Vasodepressor* carotid sinus hypersensitivity is generally defined as a decrease in systolic blood pressure of 50 mm Hg or more without associated cardiac slowing or a decrease in systolic blood pressure exceeding 30 mm Hg when the patient's symptoms are reproduced.

Even if a hyperactive carotid sinus reflex is elicited in patients, particularly in older patients who complain of syncope or presyncope, the hyperactive reflex elicited with carotid sinus massage may not necessarily be responsible for these symptoms. Direct pressure or extension on the carotid sinus from head turning, neck tension, and tight collars also can be a source of syncope by reducing blood flow through the cerebral arteries.

Hypersensitive carotid sinus reflex is most commonly associated with coronary artery disease. The mechanism responsible for hypersensitive carotid sinus reflex is not known, but possibilities include a high level of resting vagal tone, hyperresponsiveness to acetylcholine, excessive release of acetylcholine, baroreflex hypersensitivity, inadequate cholinesterase activity to metabolize the acetylcholine released, and concomitant sympathetic abnormality. Carotid sinus receptors, autonomic centers of the brain stem, and the afferent limb of the reflex have all been incriminated.

MANAGEMENT. Atropine abolishes cardioinhibitory carotid sinus hypersensitivity. However, the majority of symptomatic patients require pacemaker implantation. It must be stressed that because AV block can occur during the periods of hypersensitive carotid reflex, some form of *ventricular* pacing, with or without atrial pacing, is generally required. Atropine and pacing do not prevent the decrease in systemic blood pressure in the vasodepressor form of carotid sinus hypersensitivity,[29] which may result from inhibition of sympathetic vasoconstrictor nerves and possibly activation of cholinergic sympathetic vasodilator fibers. Combinations of vasodepressor and cardioinhibitory types can occur, and vasodepression can account for continued syncope after pacemaker implantation in some patients. Patients who have a hyperactive carotid sinus reflex that does not cause symptoms require no treatment. Drugs such as digitalis, alpha-methyldopa, clonidine, and propranolol can enhance the response to

carotid sinus massage and be responsible for symptoms in some patients. Severe vasodepressor or mixed vasodepressor and cardioinhibitory responses may require treatment with either radiation therapy or surgical denervation of the carotid sinus. Elastic support hose and sodium-retaining drugs may be helpful in patients with vasodepressor responses.

Sick Sinus Syndrome

This term is applied to a syndrome encompassing a number of sinus nodal abnormalities[23] that include (1) persistent spontaneous sinus bradycardia not caused by drugs and inappropriate for the physiological circumstance, (2) sinus arrest or exit block,[26,27,30] (3) combinations of SA and AV conduction disturbances, or (4) alternation of paroxysms of rapid regular or irregular atrial tachyarrhythmias and periods of slow atrial and ventricular rates (bradycardia-tachycardia syndrome, Fig. 22–9). More than one of these conditions can be recorded in the same patient on different occasions, and often their mechanisms can be shown to be causally interrelated and combined with an abnormal state of AV conduction or automaticity.

More than one pathophysiological mechanism can produce the clinical manifestations of sick sinus syndrome. The spontaneous clinical arrhythmia and the response to electrophysiological testing (see Chap. 20) depend on the underlying mechanism of sinus nodal dysfunction. Patients who have sinus node disease can be categorized as having intrinsic sinus node disease unrelated to autonomic abnormalities or combinations of intrinsic and autonomic abnormalities. Symptomatic patients with sinus pauses and/or

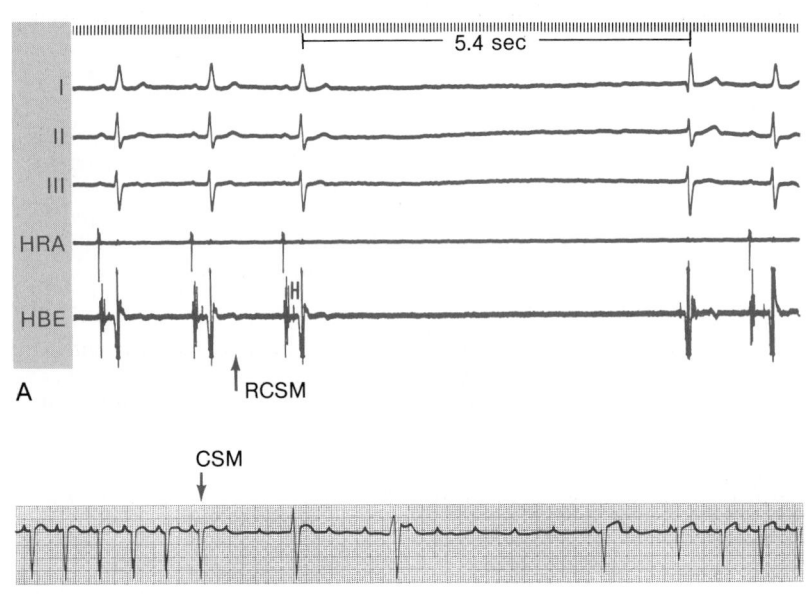

FIGURE 22–8. *A,* Right carotid sinus massage (arrow, RCSM) results in sinus arrest and a ventricular escape beat (probably fascicular) 5.4 sec later. Sinus discharge then resumes. *B,* (Monitor lead) carotid sinus massage (see arrow, CSM) results in slight sinus slowing but, more importantly, advanced AV block. Obviously, an atrial pacemaker without ventricular pacing would be inappropriate for this patient.

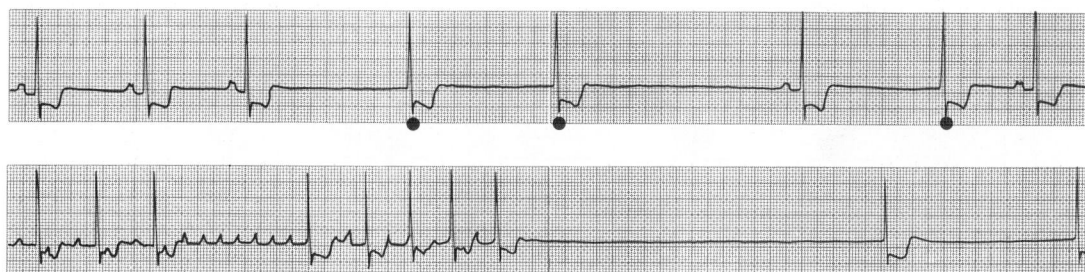

FIGURE 22–9. Sick sinus syndrome with bradycardia-tachycardia. Intermittent sinus arrest is apparent with junctional escape beats at irregular intervals (filled circles, *top*). In the bottom panel of this continuous monitor lead recording, a short episode of atrial flutter is followed by almost 5 sec of asystole before a junctional escape rhythm resumes. The patient became presyncopal at this point.

SA exit block frequently show abnormal responses on electrophysiological testing and can have a relatively high incidence of atrial fibrillation[31] and/or embolic episodes.[32] In children, sinus node dysfunction most commonly occurs in those with congenital or acquired heart disease, particularly following corrective cardiac surgery.[33–35] A familial disorder has been suggested. However, sick sinus syndrome can occur in the absence of other cardiac abnormalities. The course of the disease is frequently intermittent and unpredictable, influenced by the severity of the underlying heart disease. Excessive physical training can heighten vagal tone and produce syncope related to sinus bradycardia or AV conduction abnormalities in otherwise normal individuals.

The anatomical basis of sick sinus syndrome can involve total or subtotal destruction of the sinus node, areas of nodal-atrial discontinuity, inflammatory or degenerative changes of the nerves and ganglia surrounding the node, and pathological changes in the atrial wall. Fibrosis and fatty infiltration occur, and the sclerodegenerative processes generally involve the sinus node and the AV node or the bundle of His and its branches or distal subdivisions.[36] Occlusion of the sinus node artery may be important.[37]

MANAGEMENT. For patients with sick sinus syndrome, treatment depends on the basic rhythm problem but generally involves permanent pacemaker implantation when symptoms are manifested[38] (see Chap. 23). DDD pacing may be preferable.[39] Theophylline has been used.[40] Pacing for the bradycardia combined with drug therapy to treat the tachycardia is required in those with the bradycardia-tachycardia syndrome. In these patients, drug therapy without pacing can aggravate the bradycardia. Digitalis and other drugs that can affect sinus discharge should be used cautiously in patients with sick sinus syndrome without a pacemaker. Beta blockers with intrinsic sympathetic activity may help prevent bradycardia.[41] Prolonged sinoatrial conduction time or sinus nodal recovery time at electrophysiological study in the absence of symptoms is not an indication for prophylactic pacing, since therapy is directed toward control of symptoms. Adenosine has been suggested as a noninvasive test of sinus node function.[42,43]

SINUS NODAL REENTRY TACHYCARDIA

The rate of sinus nodal reentrant tachycardia varies from 80 to 200 beats/min but is generally slower than the other forms of supraventricular tachycardia, with an average rate of 130 to 140 beats/min[44] (Fig. 22–10) (see also p. 581). Electrocardiographically, P waves are identical or very similar to the sinus P-wave morphologically; the P-R interval is related to the tachycardia rate, but generally the R-P interval is long, with a shorter P-R interval (Fig. 22–11D). AV block can occur without affecting the tachycardia, and vagal maneuvers can slow and then abruptly terminate the tachycardia. Electrophysiologically, the tachycardia can be initiated and terminated by premature atrial and, uncommonly, premature ventricular stimulation (Fig. 22–10). Initiation of sinus nodal reentry does not depend on a critical degree of intraatrial or AV nodal conduction delay, and the atrial activation sequence is the same as during sinus rhythm. AV nodal Wenckebach block during the tachycardia is common. The development of bundle branch block does not affect the cycle length or P-R interval during tachycardia. Prolongation of AV nodal conduction time or development of AV nodal block can occur prior to termination of the tachycardia but does not affect the sinus nodal reentry.

Sinus nodal reentry may account for 5 to 10 per cent of cases of supraventricular tachycardia. It occurs in all age groups, without sex predilection. Patients may be slightly older and have a higher incidence of heart disease than patients with supraventricular tachycardia due to other mechanisms. Many may not seek medical attention because the relatively slow rate of the tachycardia does not result in serious symptoms. On the other hand, sinus nodal reentry may be responsible for apparent "anxiety-related sinus tachycardia" in some patients. Drugs such as propranolol, verapamil, and digitalis may be effective in terminating and preventing recurrences of sinus node reentrant tachycardia. Surgery or radiofrequency catheter ablation[45] to destroy all or part of the sinus node is occasionally necessary.

FIGURE 22–10. Sinus node reentry. Following three spontaneous sinus-initiated beats, premature stimulation of the high right atrium (S_2, S_3) initiates a sustained tachycardia at a cycle length of 450 msec that has the identical high-low atrial activation sequence characteristic of sinus node discharge. This is sinus node reentry. Leads I, II, III, and V_1 are scalar leads; HRA, high right atrial electrogram; HBE, His bundle electrogram; RV, right ventricular electrogram. Numbers in milliseconds. A, atrial electrogram; H, His electrogram; V, ventricular electrogram.

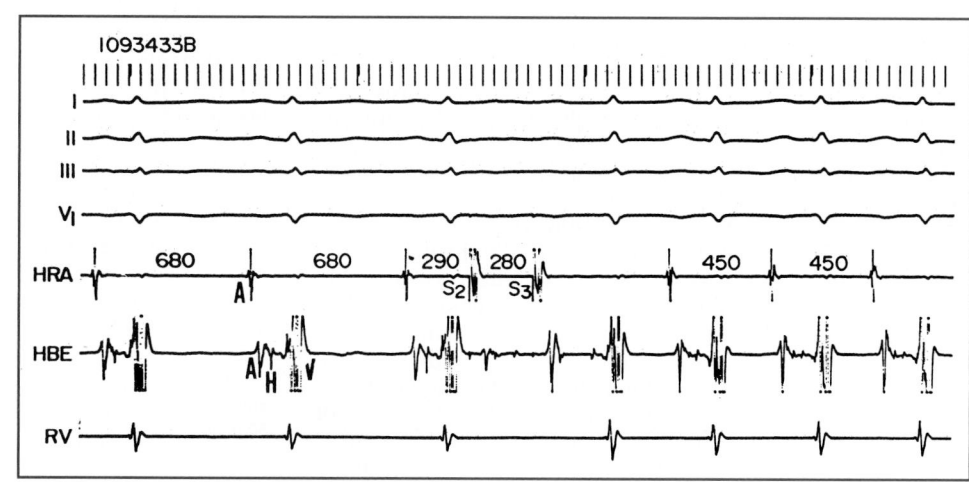

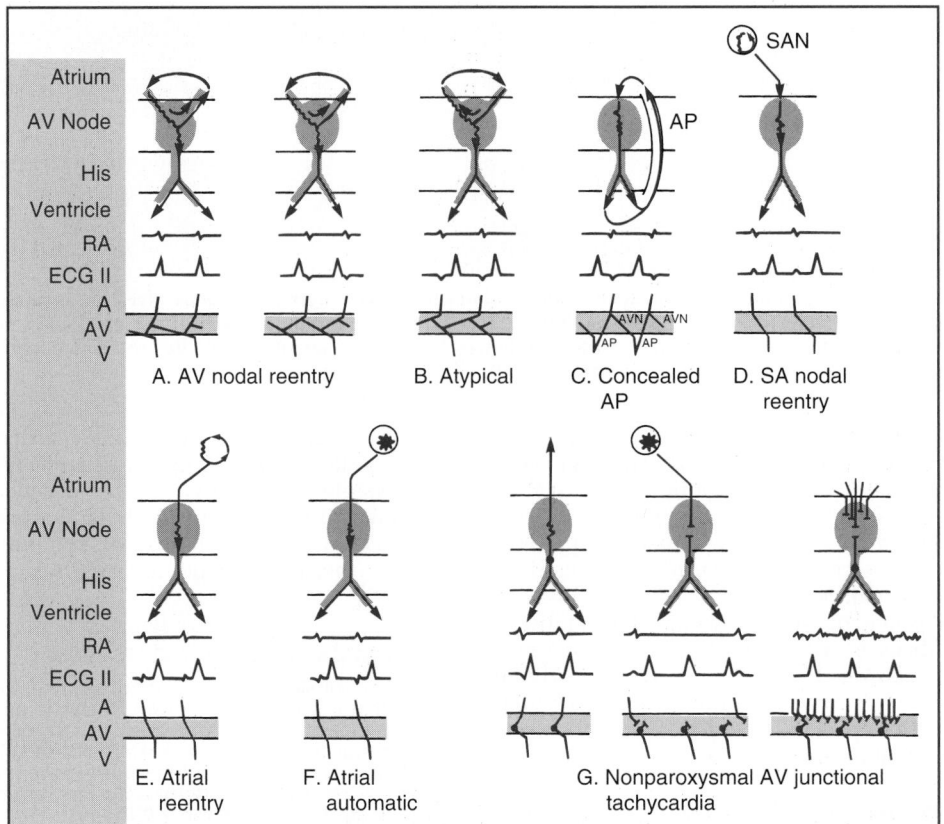

FIGURE 22–11. Diagrammatic representation of various tachycardias. In the top portion of each example, a schematic of the presumed anatomical pathways is drawn; in the bottom half, the ECG presentation and the explanatory ladder diagram are depicted. *A,* AV nodal reentry. In the left example, reentrant excitation is drawn with retrograde atrial activity occurring simultaneously with ventricular activity owing to anterograde conduction over the slow AV nodal pathway (SP) and retrograde conduction over the fast AV nodal pathway (FP). In the right example, atrial activity occurs slightly later than ventricular activity, owing to retrograde conduction delay. *B,* Atypical AV nodal reentry due to anterograde conduction over a fast AV nodal pathway and retrograde conduction over a slow AV nodal pathway. *C,* Concealed accessory pathway. Reciprocating tachycardia is due to anterograde conduction over the AV node and retrograde conduction over the accessory pathway. Retrograde P waves occur after the QRS complex. *D,* Sinus nodal reentry. The tachycardia is due to reentry within the sinus node, which then conducts to the rest of the heart. *E,* Atrial reentry. Tachycardia is due to reentry within the atrium, which then conducts to the rest of the heart. *F,* Automatic atrial tachycardia. Tachycardia is due to automatic discharge in the atrium, which then conducts to the rest of the heart; it is difficult to distinguish from atrial reentry. *G,* Nonparoxysmal AV junctional tachycardia. Various presentations of this tachycardia are depicted with retrograde atrial capture, AV dissociation with the sinus node in control of the atria, and AV dissociation with atrial fibrillation.

DISTURBANCES OF ATRIAL RHYTHM

Premature Atrial Complexes

Premature complexes are among the most common causes of an irregular pulse. They can originate from any area in the heart—most frequently from the ventricles, less often from the atria and from the AV junctional area, and rarely from the sinus node. Although premature complexes arise commonly in normal hearts, they are more often associated with structural heart disease and increase in frequency with age.

ELECTROCARDIOGRAPHIC RECOGNITION (Fig. 22–12). The diagnosis of premature atrial complexes is indicated on the ECG by a premature P wave with a P-R interval exceeding 120 msec (except in WPW syndrome, in which the P-R interval is usually less than 120 msec). Although the contour of the premature P wave can resemble that of the normal sinus P wave, it generally differs. While variations in the basic sinus rate at times can make the diagnosis of prematurity difficult, differences in the contour of the P waves are usually apparent and indicate a different focus of origin. When a premature atrial complex occurs early in

diastole, conduction may not be completely normal. The AV junction may still be refractory from the preceding beat and prevent propagation of the impulse (blocked or nonconducted premature atrial complex, Fig. 22–12*A*) or cause conduction to be slowed (premature atrial complex with a prolonged P-R interval). As a general rule, the R-P interval is inversely related to the P-R interval; thus a short R-P interval produced by an early premature atrial complex occurring close to the preceding QRS complex is followed by a long P-R interval. When premature atrial complexes occur early in the cardiac cycle, the premature P waves can be difficult to discern because they are superimposed on T waves. Careful examination of tracings from several leads may be necessary before the premature atrial complex is recognized as a slight deformity of the T wave. Often such premature atrial complexes block before reaching the ventricle and can be misinterpreted as a sinus pause or sinus exit block (Fig. 22–12*A*).

The length of the pause following any premature complex or series of premature complexes is determined by the interaction of several factors. If the premature atrial complex occurs when the sinus node and perinodal tissue are not refractory, the impulse can conduct into the sinus node, discharge it prematurely, and cause the next sinus cycle to begin from that time. The interval between the

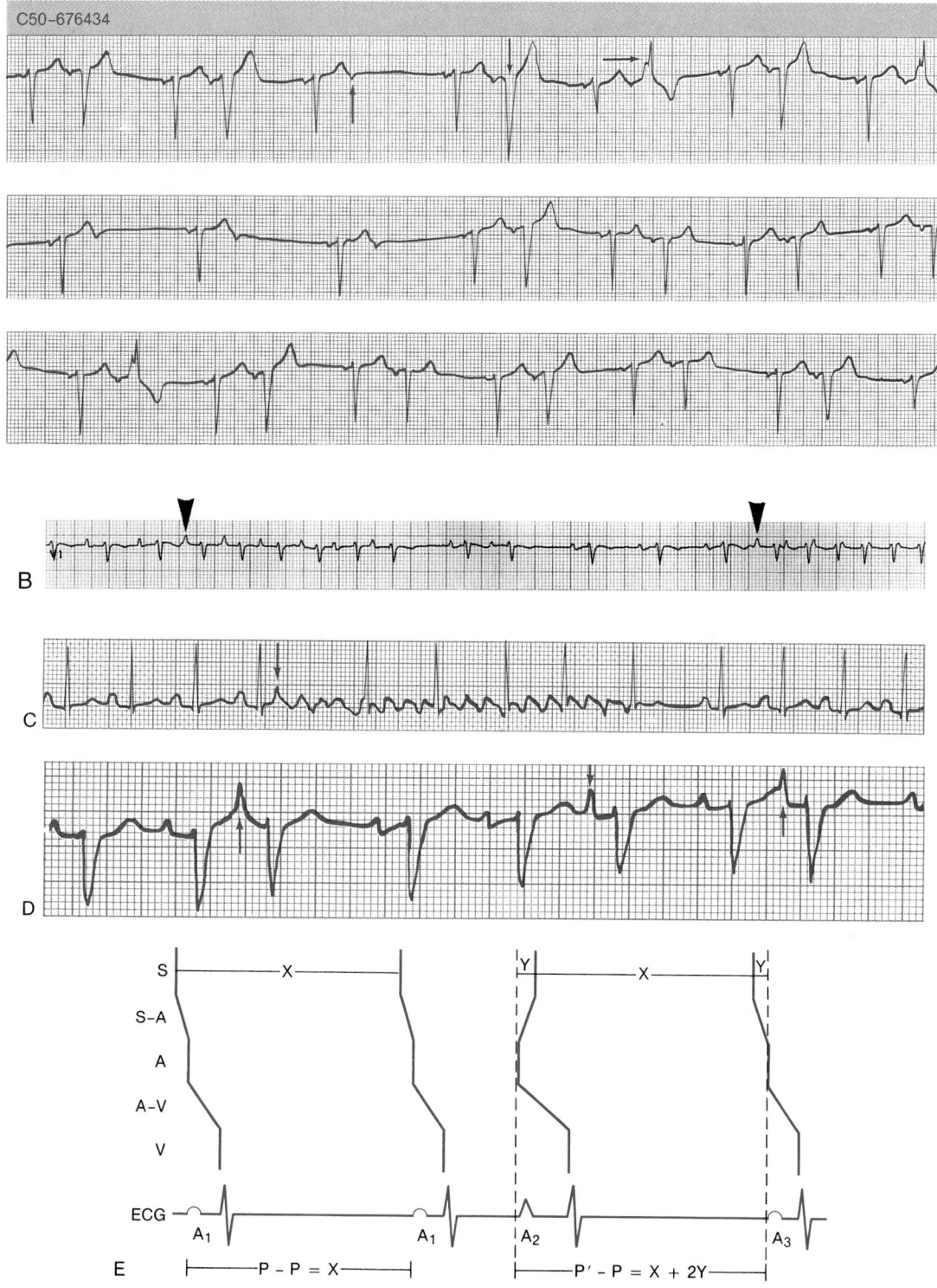

FIGURE 22–12. *A,* Premature atrial complexes that block entirely or conduct with functional right or functional left bundle branch block. Depending on preceding cycle length and coupling interval of the premature atrial complex, the latter blocks entirely in the AV node (↑) or conducts with functional left bundle branch block (↓) or functional right bundle branch block (→).

B, Premature atrial complex on the left (arrowhead) initiates AV nodal reentry that is due to reentry anterogradely and retrogradely over two slow AV nodal pathways, producing a retrograde P wave midway in the cardiac cycle. On the right, a premature atrial complex initiates AV nodal reentry due to anterograde conduction over the slow pathway and retrograde conduction over the fast pathway (Fig. 22–11*A*), producing a retrograde P wave in the terminal portion of the QRS complex, simulating an R prime.

C and D, A premature atrial complex (↓) initiating a short run of atrial flutter (*C*) and a premature atrial complex (↑) depressing the return of the next sinus nodal discharge (*D*). A slightly later premature atrial complex (↓) in *D* does not depress sinus nodal automaticity. Panels *B–D,* Monitor leads.

E, Diagrammatic example of effects of a premature atrial complex. Sinus interval (A₁-A₁) equals X. Third P wave represents premature atrial complex (A₂) that reaches and discharges SA node, causing the next sinus cycle to begin at that time. Therefore, the P'-P (A₂-A₃) equals X + 2Y msec, assuming no depression of SA nodal automaticity. (Modified from Zipes, D. P., and Fisch, C.: Premature atrial contraction. Arch. Intern. Med. *128:*453, 1971.)

two normal P waves flanking a premature atrial complex that has reset the timing of the basic sinus rhythm is less than twice the normal P-P interval, and the pause after the premature atrial complex is said to be "noncompensatory." Referring to Figure 22–12E, reset (noncompensatory pause) occurs when A_1-A_2 interval + A_2-A_3 interval is less than two times the A_1-A_1 interval, and A_2-A_3 interval is greater than A_1-A_1 interval. The interval between the premature atrial complex (A_2) and the following sinus-initiated P wave (A_3) exceeds one sinus cycle but is less than "fully compensatory" (see below), because the A_2-A_3 interval is lengthened by the time it takes the ectopic atrial impulse to conduct to the sinus node and depolarize it and then for the sinus impulse to return to the atrium. These factors lengthen the return cycle, i.e., the interval between the premature atrial complex (A_2) and the following sinus-initiated P wave (A_3) (Fig. 22–12E). Premature discharge of the sinus node by an early premature atrial complex can temporarily depress sinus nodal automatic activity, causing the sinus node to beat more slowly initially (Fig. 22–12D). Often when this happens the interval between the A_3 and the next sinus-initiated P wave exceeds the A_1-A_1 interval.

Less commonly, the premature atrial complex encounters a refractory sinus node or perinodal tissue, in which case the timing of the basic sinus rhythm is not altered, since the sinus node is not reset by the premature atrial complex, and the interval between the two normal, sinus-initiated P waves flanking the premature atrial complex is twice the normal P-P interval. The interval following this premature atrial discharge is said to be a "full compensatory pause," i.e., of sufficient duration so that the P-P interval bounding the premature atrial complex is twice the normal P-P interval. However, sinus arrhythmia can lengthen or shorten this pause. Rarely, an *interpolated premature atrial* complex may occur. In this case, the pause after the premature atrial complex is very short, and the interval bounded by the normal sinus-initiated P waves on each side of the premature atrial complex is only slightly longer than or equals one normal P-P cycle length. The interpolated premature atrial complex fails to affect the sinus nodal pacemaker, and the sinus impulse following the premature atrial complex is conducted to the ventricles, often with a slightly lengthened P-R interval. An interpolated premature complex of any type represents the only type of premature systole that does not actually replace the normally conducted beat. Premature atrial complexes can originate in the sinus node and are identified by premature P waves that have a contour identical to the normal sinus P wave. The cycle after the premature sinus complex equals or is slightly shorter than the basic sinus cycle. Premature sinus complexes are not commonly recognized.

On occasion, when the AV node has had sufficient time to repolarize and conduct without delay, the supraventricular QRS complex initiated by the premature atrial complex can be aberrant in configuration because the His-Purkinje system or ventricular muscle has *not* completely repolarized and conducts with functional delay or block (Fig. 22–12A). It is important to remember that the refractory period of cardiac fibers is related directly to cycle length. (In the adult, the AV nodal effective refractory period is prolonged at shorter cycle lengths.) A slow heart rate (long cycle length) produces a longer His-Purkinje refractory period than does a faster heart rate. As a consequence, a premature atrial complex that follows a long R-R interval (long refractory period) can result in functional bundle branch block (aberrant ventricular conduction). Since the right bundle branch at long cycles has a longer refractory period than the left bundle branch, aberration with a right bundle branch block pattern at slow rates occurs more commonly than aberration with a left bundle branch block pattern. At shorter cycles, the refractory period of the left bundle branch exceeds that of the right bundle branch, and a left bundle branch block pattern may be more likely to occur.

CLINICAL FEATURES. Premature atrial complexes can occur in a variety of situations, e.g., during infection, inflammation, or myocardial ischemia, or they can be provoked by a variety of medications, by tension states, or by tobacco, alcohol, or caffeine. Premature atrial complexes can precipitate or presage the occurrence of sustained supraventricular (Fig. 24–12B and C) and rarely ventricular tachyarrhythmias.

MANAGEMENT. Premature atrial complexes generally do not require therapy.[46] In symptomatic patients or when the premature atrial complexes precipitate tachycardias, treatment with digitalis, a beta blocker, or a calcium antagonist can be tried.

Atrial Flutter
(See also p. 572)

ELECTROCARDIOGRAPHIC RECOGNITION. The atrial rate during typical (sometimes called *type I*) atrial flutter is usually 250 to 350 beats/min, although class IA and IC antiarrhythmic drugs and amiodarone can reduce the rate to the range of 200 beats/min. If this occurs, the ventricles can respond in a 1:1 fashion to the slower atrial rate. Ordinarily, the atrial rate is about 300 beats/min, and in untreated patients the ventricular rate is half the atrial rate, i.e., 150 beats/min (Fig. 22–13A). A significantly slower ventricular rate (in the absence of drugs) suggests abnormal AV conduction. In children, in patients with the preexcitation syndrome (see p. 667), occasionally in patients with hyperthyroidism, and in those whose AV nodes conduct rapidly, atrial flutter can conduct to the ventricle in a 1:1 fashion, producing a ventricular rate of 300 beats/min. The rate in atypical (sometimes called *type II*) flutter, is 350 to 450 beats/min. Reentry is probably responsible for most atrial flutters.[47]

In typical atrial flutter, the ECG reveals identically recurring regular sawtooth flutter waves (Figs. 22–12C and 22–13B) and evidence of continual electrical activity (lack of an isoelectric interval between flutter waves), often best visualized in leads II, III, aV_f, or V_1 (Fig. 22–14). The flutter waves for (type I) typical atrial flutter are inverted (negative) in these leads because of a counterclockwise reentrant pathway, and sometimes they are upright (positive) when the reentrant loop is clockwise (see Chap. 20). If the AV conduction ratio remains constant, the ventricular rhythm will be regular; if the ratio of conducted beats varies (usually the result of a Wenckebach AV block), the ventricular rhythm will be irregular. Alternation between 2:1 and 4:1 AV conduction often occurs and may be due to two levels of block—2:1 high in the AV node and 3:2 lower down. The irregular ventricular response is frequently due to Wenckebach periodicity. Recurrent alternation of short and long ventricular intervals can be due to concealed conduction (see p. 693). Various degrees of penetration into the AV junction by the flutter impulses also can influence AV conduction. The ratio of flutter waves to conducted ventricular complexes most often is an even number (e.g., 2:1, 4:1, and so on). Impure flutter (flutter-fibrillation, or "flutter"), occurring at a rate faster than pure flutter, shows variability in the contour and spacing of the flutter waves and in some instances can represent dissimilar atrial rhythms, i.e., fibrillation in one atrium and a slower, more regular rhythm resembling atrial flutter in the opposite atrium. Prolonged atrial conduction time has been found to be a predisposing factor for the development of atrial flutter.

CLINICAL FEATURES. Atrial flutter is less common than atrial fibrillation. Paroxysmal atrial flutter can occur in patients without structural heart disease, while chronic (persistent) atrial flutter is usually associated with underlying heart disease such as rheumatic or ischemic heart disease or cardiomyopathy. It can occur as a result of atrial dilation from septal defects, pulmonary emboli, mitral or tricuspid valve stenosis or regurgitation, or chronic ventricular failure. Toxic and metabolic conditions that affect the heart, such as thyrotoxicosis, alcoholism, and pericarditis, can cause atrial flutter. Occasionally, it can be congenital or follow surgery for congenital heart disease,[48] or even occur in utero.[49,50] Atrial flutter tends to be unstable, reverting to sinus rhythm or degenerating into atrial fibrillation. Less commonly, the atria can continue to flutter for months or years. In atrial flutter, the atria contract, which may, in part, account for fewer systemic emboli than in atrial fibrillation. In children, continued episodes of atrial flutter are associated with an increased possibility of sudden death.

Atrial flutter usually responds to carotid sinus massage with a decrease in ventricular rate in stepwise multiples, returning in a reverse manner to the former ventricular rate at the termination of carotid massage (Fig. 22–13A). Very rarely, sinus rhythm follows carotid sinus massage. Exercise, by enhancing sympathetic or lessening parasympathetic tone, can reduce the AV conduction delay and produce a doubling of the ventricular rate.

Physical examination may reveal rapid flutter waves in

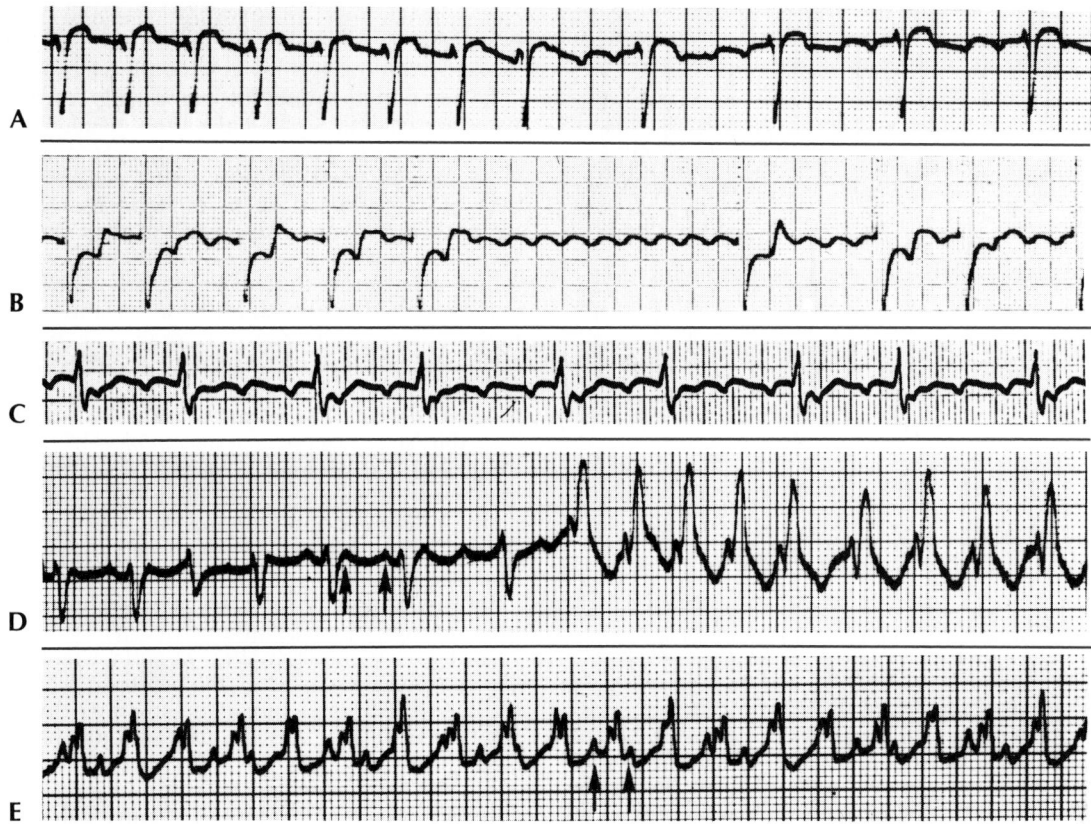

FIGURE 22–13. Various manifestations of atrial flutter. *A,* Atrial flutter at a rate of 300 beats/min conducts to ventricles with 2:1 block. In the midportion of the tracing, carotid sinus massage converts the block to 4:1 and the ventricular rate slows to 75 beats/min. *B,* Carotid sinus massage produces a transient period of AV block clearly revealing the flutter waves. *C,* Quinidine has slowed the atrial flutter rate to approximately 188 beats/min. The block is variable. *D,* Wide QRS complexes with an RSR′ configuration in V$_1$ begin after a short cycle that follows a long cycle in the midportion of the ECG strip. This represents functional right bundle branch block. Arrows indicate flutter waves. *E,* The QRS complexes are 0.12 sec in duration and have a regular interval at a rate of 200 beats/min. Atrial activity is also regular at a rate of 300 beats/min and independent from the ventricular activity (arrows). Thus atrial flutter is present with a probable ventricular tachycardia, an example of complete AV dissociation. Monitor leads in *A, B, C,* and *E.*

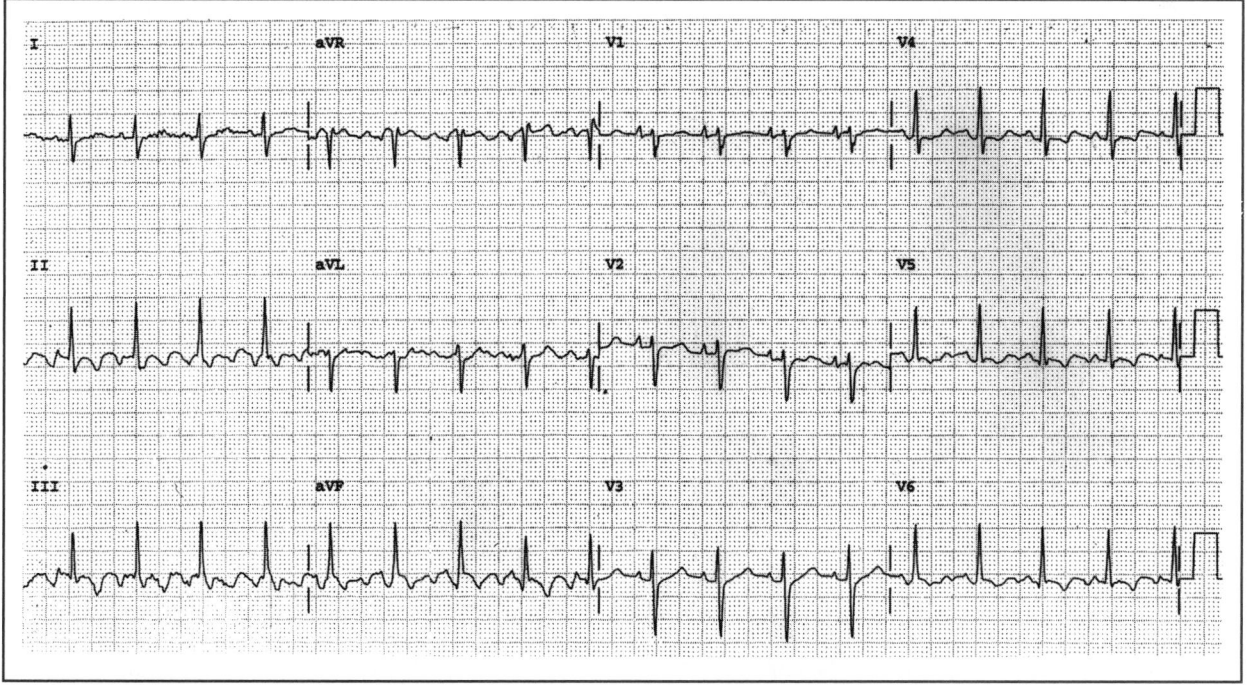

FIGURE 22–14. Simultaneous atrial flutter and sinus rhythm. In this patient with a heart transplant, the recipient atrium exhibits atrial flutter, best seen in leads II, III and aV$_f$, while the donor atrium exhibits sinus rhythm (best seen in the chest leads). (Tracing courtesy of Sharon Hunt.)

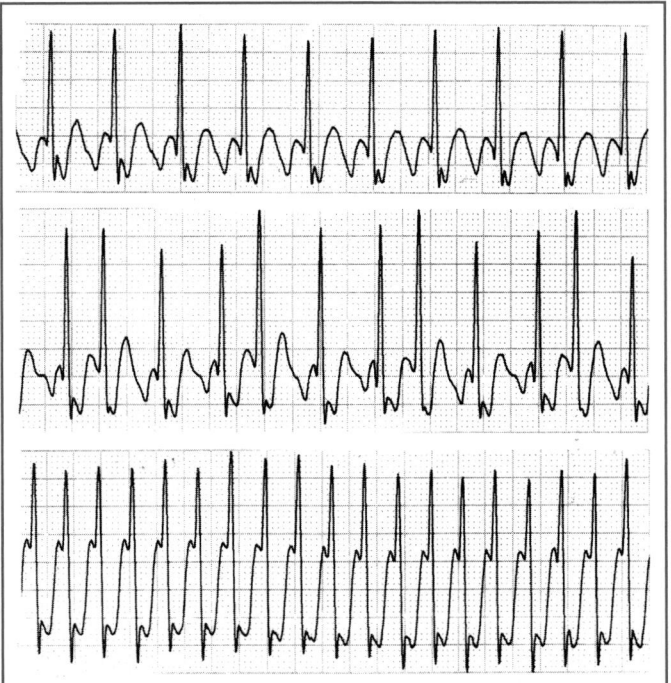

FIGURE 22–15. Atrial flutter with 1:1 conduction caused by flecainide. In the top panel, atrial flutter occurs with 2:1 conduction. In the middle panel, 2:1 conduction alternates with 3:2 conduction. In the bottom panel, flecainide has been started and the atrial flutter rate slows, resulting in 1:1 conduction.

the jugular venous pulse. If the relationship of flutter waves to conducted QRS complexes remains constant, the first heart sound will have a constant intensity. Occasionally, sounds caused by atrial contraction can be auscultated.

MANAGEMENT. Synchronous direct-current (DC) cardioversion (see p. 619) is commonly the initial treatment of choice for atrial flutter, since cardioversion promptly and effectively restores sinus rhythm, often requiring relatively low energies (<50 joules). If the electrical shock results in atrial fibrillation, a second shock at a higher energy level is used to restore sinus rhythm or, depending on the clinical circumstances, the atrial fibrillation can be left untreated. The latter can revert to atrial flutter or sinus rhythm. If the patient cannot be electrically cardioverted or if electrical cardioversion is contraindicated—for example, after large amounts of digitalis are administered—*rapid atrial pacing* with a catheter in the esophagus[51] or the right atrium can terminate type I (but not type II) atrial flutter effectively in most patients, producing sinus rhythm or atrial fibrillation with a slowing of the ventricular rate and concomitant clinical improvement.[52–54]

Verapamil (see p. 616), given as an initial bolus of 5 to 10 mg IV, followed by a constant infusion at a rate of 5 μg/kg/min, or *diltiazem*, 0.25 mg/kg, to slow the ventricular response, can be tried. Calcium antagonists can restore sinus rhythm in patients with atrial flutter of recent onset but less commonly terminate chronic atrial flutter. *Adenosine* produces transient AV block and can be used to reveal flutter waves if the diagnosis of the arrhythmias is in doubt. It generally will not terminate the atrial flutter and

can provoke atrial fibrillation.[55] Esmolol, a beta-adrenergic blocker with a 9-min elimination half-life, can be used in doses of 200 μg/kg/min to slow the ventricular rate.[56]

If the flutter cannot be electrically cardioverted, terminated by pacing, or slowed by the preceding drugs, a *short-acting digitalis preparation* (such as digoxin or deslanoside) can be tried alone or with a calcium antagonist or beta blocker. The dose of digitalis necessary to slow the ventricular response varies and at times can result in toxic levels because it is often difficult to slow the ventricular rate during atrial flutter. Frequently, atrial fibrillation develops after digitalis administration and can revert to normal sinus rhythm upon withdrawal of digitalis; occasionally, normal sinus rhythm may occur without intervening atrial fibrillation. Intravenous amiodarone has been shown to slow the ventricular rate as effectively as digoxin.[57]

If the atrial flutter persists, class IA or IC drugs (see Chap. 20) can be tried to restore sinus rhythm and to prevent a recurrence of atrial flutter.[58] Amiodarone, also, especially in low doses of 200 mg/day, can prevent recurrences. Side effects of these drugs, especially proarrhythmic responses, must be carefully considered and are dealt with at length in Chapter 21. Sometimes treatment of the underlying disorder, such as thyrotoxicosis, is necessary to effect conversion to sinus rhythm. In certain instances, atrial flutter can continue, and if the ventricular rate can be controlled with drugs, conversion to sinus rhythm may not be indicated. Class I and III drugs should be discontinued if flutter remains.

It is important to reemphasize that class I or III drugs should *not* be used unless the ventricular rate during atrial flutter has been *slowed* with digitalis or a calcium antagonist or beta-blocking drug.[59] Because of the vagolytic action of quinidine, procainamide, and disopyramide (see Chap. 21), but primarily because of the ability of class I drugs to slow the flutter rate, AV conduction can be *facilitated* sufficiently to result in a 1:1 ventricular response to the atrial flutter (Fig. 22–15).

Prevention of recurrent atrial flutter is often difficult to achieve but should be approached as outlined for the prevention of paroxysmal supraventricular tachycardia due to AV nodal reentry (see p. 661). If recurrences cannot be prevented, therapy is directed toward controlling the ventricular rate when the flutter does recur, with digitalis alone or combined with beta blockers or calcium antagonists. The risks of emboli in type I atrial flutter appear to be low, presumably because the atria contract, and therefore anticoagulation is usually not necessary.[60] However, carefully controlled studies are lacking. Radiofrequency catheter ablation (see p. 624) can eliminate typical atrial flutter with a success rate of about 75 to 90 per cent.[61–70]

Atrial Fibrillation
(See also p. 627)

ELECTROCARDIOGRAPHIC RECOGNITION (Fig. 22–16). This arrhythmia is characterized by wavelets propagating in different directions,[71] causing disorganized atrial depolarizations without effective atrial contraction.[72–74] Electrical activity of the atrium can be detected electrocardiographically as small irregular baseline undulations of variable amplitude and morphology, called f waves, at a rate of 350 to 600 beats/min. At times, small, fine, rapid f waves can occur and are detectable only by right atrial leads or by

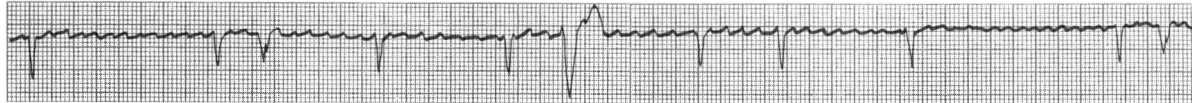

FIGURE 22–16. Atrial fibrillation with ventricular extrasystoles following the longer pauses (monitor lead). Fibrillatory waves are quite obvious. When the ventricular cycle lengths prolong, ventricular extrasystoles result. This phenomenon has been called the "rule of bigeminy."

intracavitary or esophageal electrodes. The ventricular response is grossly irregular ("irregularly irregular") and, in the untreated patient with normal AV conduction, is usually between 100 and 160 beats/min. In patients with the WPW syndrome (see p. 667), the ventricular rate during atrial fibrillation at times can exceed 300 beats/min and lead to ventricular fibrillation. Atrial fibrillation should be suspected when the ECG shows supraventricular complexes at an irregular rhythm and no obvious P waves. The recognizable f waves probably do not represent total atrial activity but depict only the larger vectors generated by the multiple wavelets of depolarization that occur at any given moment.

Each recorded f wave is not conducted through the AV junction, so a rapid ventricular response comparable with the atrial rate does not occur. Many atrial impulses are canceled, owing to a collision of wavefronts, or are blocked in the AV junction without reaching the ventricles (i.e., concealed conduction [see p. 693]), which accounts for the irregular ventricular rhythm. The refractory period and conductivity of the AV node are determinants of the ventricular rate. When the ventricular rate is very rapid or very slow, it may appear to be more regular. Even though the conversion of atrial fibrillation to atrial flutter is accompanied by slowing of the atrial rate, an increase in the ventricular response can result, since more atrial impulses are transmitted to the ventricle because of less concealed conduction. Also, it is easier to slow the ventricular rate during atrial fibrillation than during atrial flutter with drugs such as digitalis, calcium antagonists, and beta blockers, because the increased concealed conduction makes it easier to produce AV block.

It has been suggested that transmission of impulses across the AV node during atrial fibrillation occurs electrotonically and that the distal portion of the AV node behaves as a pacemaker, producing the ventricular rhythm during atrial fibrillation.[74a] This postulate has not been proven.[75]

CLINICAL FEATURES. Atrial fibrillation is a common arrhythmia, found in 1 per cent of persons older than 60 years to more than 5 per cent in patients over 69 years old.[76] The overall chance of atrial fibrillation developing over 2 decades in patients more than 30 years old, according to Framingham data, is 2 per cent. Estimates are that 1 to 1.5 million Americans have atrial fibrillation, occurring more commonly in men than in women.[77] In one study[78] of men and women 65 years or older, atrial fibrillation had a prevalence of 9.1 per cent in those with clinical cardiovascular disease, 4.6 per cent in those with subclinical cardiovascular disease, and 1.6 per cent in those without cardiovascular disease. A history of congestive heart failure, valvular heart disease and stroke, left atrial enlargement, abnormal mitral or aortic valve function, treated systemic hypertension, and advanced age was independently associated with the prevalence of atrial fibrillation. Four important aspects of atrial fibrillation are etiology, control of the ventricular rate, prevention of recurrences, and prevention of thromboembolic episodes. Occult or manifest thyrotoxicosis should be considered in patients with recent-onset atrial fibrillation.[79,80] Atrial fibrillation can be intermittent or chronic and may be influenced by autonomic activity.[81] Atrial fibrillation, whether it is persistent or intermittent, is a predictor of stroke. Symptoms as a result of atrial fibrillation are determined by multiple factors, including the underlying cardiac status, the rapid ventricular rate, and loss of atrial contraction.

Physical findings include a slight variation in the intensity of the first heart sound, absence of *a* waves in the jugular venous pulse, and an irregularly irregular ventricular rhythm. Often, with fast ventricular rates, a significant pulse deficit appears, during which the auscultated or palpated apical rate is faster than the rate palpated at the wrist (pulse deficit) because each contraction is not sufficiently

strong to open the aortic valve or to transmit an arterial pressure wave through the peripheral artery. If the ventricular rhythm becomes regular in patients with atrial fibrillation, conversion to sinus rhythm, atrial tachycardia, atrial flutter with a constant ratio of conducted beats, or development of junctional or ventricular tachycardia should be suspected.

EMBOLIZATION AND ANTICOAGULATION (see also Ch. 48). In addition to hemodynamic alterations, the risk of systemic emboli, probably arising in the left atrial cavity or appendage due to circulatory stasis, is an important consideration. Nonvalvular atrial fibrillation is the most common cardiac disease associated with cerebral embolism. In fact, almost half of cardiogenic emboli in the United States occur in patients with nonvalvular atrial fibrillation. The risk of stroke in patients with nonvalvular atrial fibrillation is 5 to 7 times greater than in controls without atrial fibrillation. Overall, 20 to 25 per cent of ischemic strokes are due to cardiogenic emboli.

Many studies have evaluated the risk of stroke in patients with nonvalvular atrial fibrillation and the benefits of anticoagulation and antiplatelet therapy.[82–91] Certain patients with atrial fibrillation appear at higher risk of emboli.[92] For example, patients with mitral stenosis and atrial fibrillation have a 4 to 6 per cent incidence of embolism per year. Risk factors that predict stroke in patients with nonvalvular atrial fibrillation include a history of previous stroke or transient ischemic attack (relative risk 22.5), diabetes (relative risk 1.7), history of hypertension (relative risk 1.6), and increasing age (relative risk 1.4 for each decade). Patients with any of these risk factors have an annual stroke risk of at least 4 per cent if untreated. Patients whose only stroke risk factor is congestive heart failure or coronary artery disease have stroke rates approximately three times higher than do patients without any risk factors.[93] Left ventricular dysfunction and a left atrial size greater than 2.5 cm/m^2 on echocardiographic examination are associated with thromboembolism. Patients younger than age 60 who have a normal echocardiogram and no risk factors have an extremely low risk for stroke (1 per cent per year).[94]

Patients younger than age 65 with no risk factors have an annual rate of stroke of 1 per cent. Therefore, the risk of stroke in patients with *lone atrial fibrillation,* i.e., idiopathic atrial fibrillation in the absence of any structural heart disease or any of the above risk factors, is quite low.

The annual rate of stroke for the unanticoagulated control group in five large anticoagulation trials[95] was 4.5 per cent and was reduced to 1.4 per cent (68 per cent risk reduction) for the warfarin-treated group (60 per cent risk reduction in men; 84 per cent risk reduction in women). Aspirin, 325 mg per day, produced a risk reduction of 44 per cent. The annual rate of major hemorrhage was 1 per cent for the control group, 1 per cent for the aspirin group, and 1.3 per cent for the warfarin group. There was no difference in stroke risk when patients with paroxysmal (intermittent) atrial fibrillation were compared with those with constant (chronic) atrial fibrillation. Anticoagulation therapy was approximately 50 per cent more effective than aspirin therapy for prevention of ischemic stroke in atrial fibrillation patients. Risk factors for anticoagulant-associated intracranial hemorrhage included excessive anticoagulation and poorly controlled hypertension. Elderly individuals were at increased risk for anticoagulant-associated brain hemorrhage, especially if overanticoagulated.[95]

From these and other data, it appears that individuals less than 60 years of age without any clinical risk factors (lone atrial fibrillation) do not require antithrombotic therapy for stroke prevention because of their low risk. The stroke rate is also low (about 2 per cent per year) in patients with lone atrial fibrillation between the ages of 60 and 75 years. These patients appear to be adequately protected from stroke with aspirin therapy. In very elderly (over 75 years of age) patients with atrial fibrillation, anticoagulation should be used with caution and carefully monitored because of the potential increased risk of intracranial hemorrhage. Despite this, elderly patients with atrial fibrillation are still likely to benefit from anticoagulation because they are at particularly high stroke risk.[96] Food[97] and drugs such as antibiotics and antiarrhythmics (e.g., amiodarone) can influence the effects of warfarin (see p. 615).

The following recommendations for antithrombotic therapy can be made[93,96]: Any patient with atrial fibrillation who has risk factors for stroke (prior stroke or transient ischemic attack, significant valvular heart disease, hypertension, diabetes, age greater than 75 years, left atrial enlargement, coronary artery disease, or congestive heart failure) should be treated with warfarin anticoagulation to achieve an INR of 2.0 to 3.0 for stroke prevention if the individual is a good candidate for oral anticoagulation. Patients with contraindications to anticoagulation and unreliable individuals should be considered for aspirin treatment. Patients with atrial fibrillation who do not have any of the preceding risk factors have a low stroke risk (2 per cent per year or less) and can be protected from stroke with aspirin. In patients over the age of 75 years, anticoagulation should be used with caution and monitored carefully to keep the INR less than 3.0 because of the risk of intracranial hemorrhage.[98–103]

The risk of embolism following cardioversion to sinus rhythm in patients with atrial fibrillation varies from 0 to 7 per cent, depending on the underlying risk factors. Patients at high risk are those with prior embolism, a mechanical valve prosthesis, or mitral stenosis. Low-risk patients are those younger than age 60 without underlying heart disease. The high-risk group should receive chronic anticoagulation (see below), whether or not they will undergo cardioversion, while anticoagulation may not be necessary in the low-risk group. Patients not in the low-risk group with atrial fibrillation longer in duration than 2 days should receive warfarin to achieve an INR of 2.0 to 3.0 for 3 weeks before elective cardioversion and for 3 to 4 weeks after reversion to sinus rhythm.[104] Anticoagulation with heparin has been recommended for emergency cardioversion. Risk stratification with transesophageal echocardiography may be useful,[105] but the absence of a left atrial thrombus on echocardiography is not necessarily assurance that the patient will not have an embolus at or after cardioversion.[106,107]

It is important to emphasize that these suggestions must be individualized for a given patient. For example, patients at risk of trauma by virtue of occupation, participation in sports, and episodes of dizziness or syncope are at increased risk of bleeding if given anticoagulants and probably should not receive warfarin. Patients should be warned about taking any new drugs, e.g., nonsteroidal antiinflammatory agents, if they are receiving warfarin.

For patients with intermittent atrial fibrillation, guidelines are unclear. A reasonable approach would be to treat them according to the recommendations noted above, particularly if recurrences are frequent.

MANAGEMENT. The atria are often abnormal in patients with atrial fibrillation, showing increased conduction time or enlargement. Maintenance of sinus rhythm after cardioversion is influenced by the duration of atrial fibrillation and, in some adults, atrial dilatation. Animal studies[73,108–110a] indicate that atrial fibrillation begets atrial fibrillation; the longer the patient has atrial fibrillation, the greater is the likelihood that it will remain.

The patient with atrial fibrillation discovered for the first time should be evaluated for a precipitating cause, such as thyrotoxicosis, mitral stenosis, pulmonary emboli, or pericarditis. The patient's clinical status determines initial therapy, the objectives being to slow the ventricular rate

and to restore atrial systole. If the sudden onset of atrial fibrillation with a rapid ventricular rate results in acute cardiovascular decompensation, electrical cardioversion is the initial treatment of choice. High-energy shock over a right atrial catheter can be successful when transthoracic shocks fail. Atrial contraction may not return immediately after restoration of electrical systole, and clinical improvement may be delayed.[111,112] DC cardioversion establishes normal sinus rhythm in over 90 per cent of patients, but sinus rhythm remains for 12 months in only 30 to 50 per cent. Patients with atrial fibrillation of less than 12 months' duration have a greater chance of maintaining sinus rhythm after cardioversion. In the absence of decompensation, the patient can be treated with drugs such as digitalis, beta blockers, or calcium antagonists to maintain a resting apical rate of 60 to 80 beats/min that does not exceed 100 beats/min after slight exercise.[113] The combined use of digitalis and a beta blocker[56] or calcium antagonist can be helpful in slowing the ventricular rate. Digitalis may be more effective if associated left ventricular dysfunction is present; without this, a beta blocker may be preferable to control the ventricular rate.[114] Clonidine has been used to slow the rate.[115]

Classes IA, IC,[116] and III (amiodarone, sotalol[117]) agents can be used to terminate acute-onset atrial fibrillation and prevent recurrences of atrial fibrillation.[58] No one drug, with the possible exception of amiodarone,[99] appears clearly superior, and selection is often based on side effect profile and risk of proarrhythmia.[118–120] These drugs increase the likelihood of maintaining sinus rhythm from about 30 to 50 per cent to 50 to 70 per cent of patients per year after cardioversion. However, whether it is preferable to allow atrial fibrillation to continue with just rate control has not been established.[121] Before electrical cardioversion, an antiarrhythmic agent is often administered for a few days to help prevent relapse of atrial fibrillation, as well as to convert some patients to sinus rhythm.[122] Rapid atrial pacing will not terminate atrial fibrillation.[108,123] In some patients with frequent recurrence and rapid ventricular rates not controlled by drugs, AV node modification[124] or interruption by radiofrequency catheter ablation and implantation of a rate-adaptive VVI (VVIR) pacemaker can be acceptable therapy[125,126] (see Chap. 23). Whenever possible, atrial or dual-chamber pacing is preferable, since the incidence of atrial fibrillation and stroke is reduced compared with VVI pacing. Application of the maze procedure,[127] the atrial compartment operation,[128] and new ablation approaches have been used to eliminate atrial fibrillation[129–132] (see p. 628). An atrial defibrillator also has received interest recently (see Chap. 23).[133–135] Atrial or dual-chamber pacing may reduce recurrence of atrial fibrillation in some patients who have intermittent episodes.[136]

Many elderly patients tolerate atrial fibrillation well without therapy because the ventricular rate is slow as a result of concomitant AV nodal disease. These patients often have associated sick sinus syndrome, and the development of atrial fibrillation represents a cure of sorts. Such patients may demonstrate serious supraventricular and ventricular arrhythmias or asystole after cardioversion, so the likelihood of establishing and maintaining sinus rhythm should be weighed against the risks of cardioversion or other forms of therapy.

Atrial Tachycardias

ELECTROCARDIOGRAPHIC RECOGNITION (Fig. 22–17). Atrial tachycardia has an atrial rate of generally 150 to 200 beats/min with a P-wave contour different from that of the sinus P wave. P waves are usually in the second half of the tachycardia cycle (long R-P/short P-R tachycardia).[44] When the tachycardia is due to digitalis excess, the atrial rate can increase gradually as the digitalis is continued (a similar

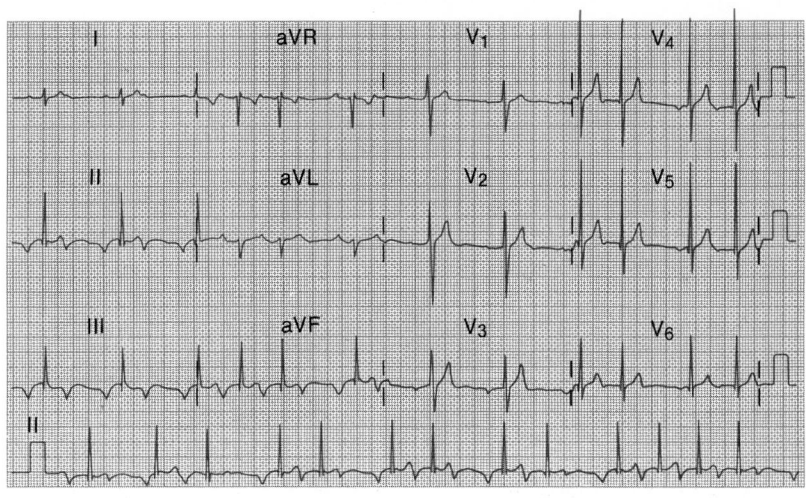

FIGURE 22–17. Atrial tachycardia. This 12-lead ECG and rhythm strip (*bottom*) demonstrate an atrial tachycardia at a cycle length of approximately 520 msec. Conduction varies between 3:2 and 2:1. Note the negative P waves in leads 2, 3, and aVF and, when consecutive P waves conduct, that the R-P interval exceeds the P-R interval. Note also that the tachycardia persists despite the development of AV block, an important finding that excludes the participation of an atrioventricular accessory pathway and sharply differentiates this tachycardia from the one shown in Figure 22–34, p. 673.

response can occur in nonparoxysmal AV junctional tachycardia); this increase may be associated with gradual prolongation of the P-R interval. If the atrial rate is not excessive and AV conduction is not significantly depressed by the digitalis, each P wave may conduct to the ventricles. As the atrial rate increases and AV conduction becomes impaired, Wenckebach (Mobitz type I) second degree AV block (see p. 689) can ensue. This is sometimes called *atrial tachycardia with block.* Frequently, other manifestations of digitalis excess, such as premature ventricular complexes, are present. In nearly half the cases of atrial tachycardia with block, the atrial rate is irregular. Characteristic isoelectric intervals between P waves, in contrast to atrial flutter, are usually present in all leads. However, at rapid atrial rates, the distinction between atrial tachycardia with block and atrial flutter can be difficult. Analysis of P-wave configuration during tachycardia indicates that a positive or biphasic P wave in aVL predicts a right atrial focus, whereas a positive P wave in V_1 predicts a left atrial focus.

CLINICAL FEATURES. Atrial tachycardia occurs most commonly in patients with significant structural heart disease, such as coronary artery disease, with or without myocardial infarction, cor pulmonale, or digitalis intoxication. Potassium depletion can precipitate the arrhythmia in patients taking digitalis. The signs, symptoms, and prognosis are usually related to underlying cardiovascular status.

Physical findings include a variable rhythm and intensity of the first heart sound, owing to the varying AV block and P-R interval. An excessive number of *a* waves may be seen in the jugular venous pulse. Carotid sinus massage increases the degree of AV block by slowing the ventricular rate in a stepwise fashion without terminating the tachycardia, as in atrial flutter. It should be performed cautiously in patients who have digitalis toxicity because serious ventricular arrhythmias can result.

MANAGEMENT. Atrial tachycardia with block in a patient not receiving digitalis is treated in a manner similar to other atrial tachyarrhythmias. Depending on the clinical situation, digitalis, a beta blocker, or a calcium channel blocker can be administered to slow the ventricular rate, and then if atrial tachycardia remains, class IA, IC, or III drugs can be added. Ablation procedures can be tried, including surgical isolation and radiofrequency catheter ablation[62,137,138] (see p. 621). Tachycardias can recur at a different site following a successful ablation attempt. If atrial tachycardia appears in a patient receiving digitalis, the drug initially should be assumed to be responsible for the arrthythmia. Therapy includes cessation of digitalis and administration of potassium chloride orally or intravenously if serum $[K^+]$ is not abnormally elevated or a drug such as lidocaine, propranolol, and phenytoin while cardiac

rhythm is monitored. Often, the ventricular response is not excessively fast, and simply withholding digitalis is all that is necessary.

Mechanisms: Automatic Atrial Tachycardia

Three types of atrial tachycardias have been distinguished experimentally: automatic, triggered, and reentrant atrial tachycardia. The characteristics of automatic and reentrant tachycardias will be discussed separately. Entrainment, resetting curve patterns in response to overdrive pacing,[139] and recording monophasic action potentials can be used to help distinguish one mechanism from the other.[140,141] Adenosine has been used to distinguish mechanisms.[142] However, there are no clear clinical distinctions between tachycardias of different mechanisms.

ELECTROCARDIOGRAPHIC FEATURES (Fig. 22–11F). Automatic atrial tachycardia is characterized electrocardiographically by a supraventricular tachycardia that generally accelerates after its initiation, with heart rates less than 200 beats/min. The P-wave contour differs from the sinus P wave, the P-R interval is influenced directly by the tachycardia rate, and AV block can exist without affecting the tachycardia; i.e., it continues uninterrupted. Vagal maneuvers generally do not terminate the tachycardia, even though they can produce AV nodal block. Thus pharmacological or physiological maneuvers that selectively result in AV block do not affect the automatic focus nor does the development of bundle branch block alter the P-R or R-P interval unless it is associated with prolongation of the H-V interval.

Initiation of tachycardia with premature atrial stimulation is generally not possible but is independent of intra-atrial or AV nodal conduction delay when it occurs. The atrial activation sequence usually differs from a sinus-initiated P wave, and the A-H interval is related to the tachycardia rate. The first P wave of the tachycardia is the same as the subsequent P waves of the tachycardia in contrast to most forms of reentrant supraventricular tachycardias, in which the initial and subsequent P waves differ.[143] Usually the tachycardia cannot be terminated by pacing, although it can exhibit overdrive suppression. The introduction of premature atrial complexes during tachycardia merely resets the timing of the tachycardia. It is very difficult to differentiate this mechanism from microreentry, using the leading-circle concept (see p. 571).

CLINICAL FEATURES. Many supraventricular tachycardias associated with AV block are probably due to automatic atrial tachycardia,[143] including atrial tachycardia due to digitalis intoxication (Fig. 22–17). Automatic atrial tachycardia occurs in all age groups and is seen in settings of myocardial infarction, chronic lung disease (especially with acute infection), acute alcohol ingestion, and a variety of

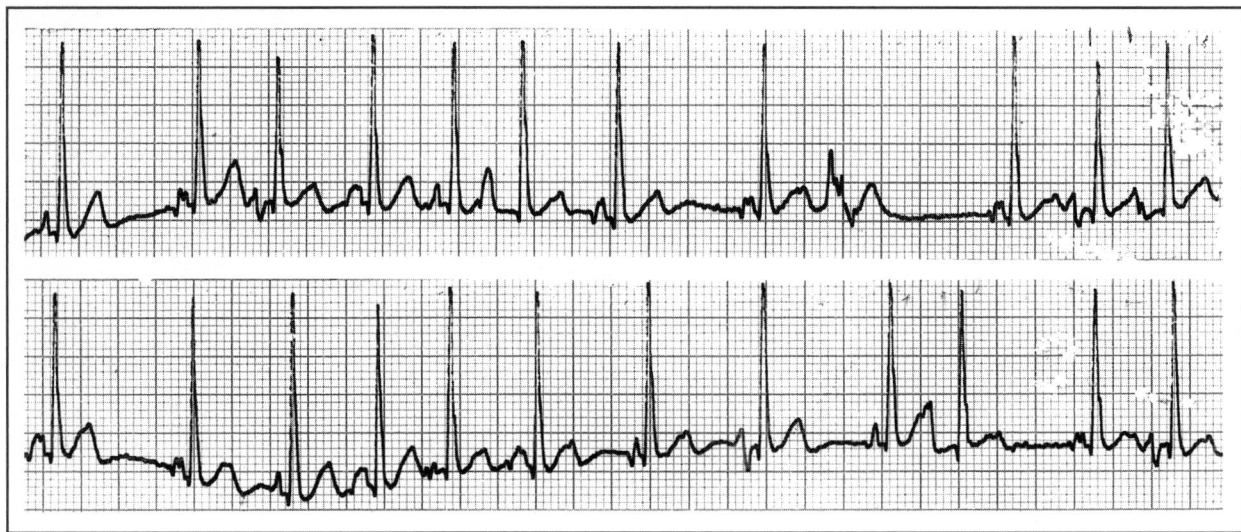

FIGURE 22–18. Chaotic (multifocal) atrial tachycardia. Premature atrial complexes occur at varying cycle lengths and with differing contours.

metabolic derangements. Abnormal histology can be present.[143] Differentiation from other tachycardias such as sinus nodal reentry (if the P waves of the automatic atrial tachycardia resemble the sinus-initiated P waves), atrial reentry (particularly if caused by microreentry), and some other mechanisms can be difficult.

Management is as discussed under atrial tachycardia due to digitalis.

Mechansims: Atrial Tachycardia Due to Reentry

ELECTROCARDIOGRAPHIC RECOGNITION (Fig. 22–11*E*). This arrhythmia presents electrocardiographically with a P wave that has a contour different from the sinus P wave, a P-R interval influenced directly by the tachycardia rate, and the ability to develop AV block without interrupting the tachycardia. Reentry can exist around a surgical scar, anatomical defect, or atriotomy incision.[62] Electrophysiologically, initiation of the tachycardia occurs with premature stimulation during the atrial relative refractory period, resulting in a critical degree of intraatrial conduction delay, an atrial activation sequence different from that which occurs during sinus rhythm, and an AV nodal conduction time related to the tachycardia rate. Vagal maneuvers generally do not terminate the tachycardia and can produce AV block.

CLINICAL FEATURES. The relative infrequency of published reports suggests that atrial reentry is not a commonly recognized cause of supraventricular tachycardia. The tachycardia can be started and stopped by an atrial extrastimulus. Spontaneous termination can be either sudden, with progressive slowing, or with alternating long-short cycle lengths.

Chaotic Atrial Tachycardia

Chaotic (sometimes called *multifocal*) atrial tachycardia is characterized by atrial rates between 100 and 130 beats/min, with marked variation in P-wave morphology and totally irregular P-P intervals (Figs. 22–18). Generally, at least three P-wave contours are noted, with most P waves conducted to the ventricles. This tachycardia occurs commonly in older patients with chronic obstructive pulmonary disease and congestive heart failure and may eventually develop into atrial fibrillation. Digitalis appears to be an unusual cause, while theophylline administration has been implicated. Chaotic atrial tachycardia can occur in childhood.

MANAGEMENT. This is primarily directed toward the underlying disease. Antiarrhythmic agents are often ineffective in slowing either the rate of the atrial tachycardia or the ventricular response. Beta-adrenoreceptor blockers should be avoided in patients with bronchospastic pulmonary disease but can be effective if tolerated. Verapamil and amiodarone have been useful. Potassium and magnesium replacement may suppress the tachycardia.

AV Junctional Rhythm Disturbances

AV Junctional Escape Beats

MECHANISM. Automatic fibers that are prevented from initiating depolarization by a pacemaker such as the sinus node, which possesses a more rapid rate of firing, are called *latent pacemakers*. Such latent pacemakers are found in some parts of the atrium, in the AV node–His bundle area, in the right and left bundle branches, and in the Purkinje system. Under usual conditions, automatic fibers are *not* found in atrial or ventricular myocardium. It is possible that the N region of the AV node is automatic, at least in some species, but is kept suppressed by neighboring atrial tissue. A latent pacemaker can become the dominant pacemaker by default or usurpation, i.e., by passive or active mechanisms. A decrease in the number of impulses arriving at a latent pacemaker site, the result of slowing of the sinus node or interruption of the propagation of the normal impulse anywhere along its course, allows the latent pacemaker to escape and initiate depolarization passively, by default. An increase in the discharge rate of a latent pacemaker can capture pacemaker control actively, by usurpation. As will be seen, the implication of the two different mechanisms of ectopic impulse formation is important therapeutically.

ELECTROCARDIOGRAPHIC RECOGNITION. An AV junctional escape beat occurs when the rate of impulse formation of the primary pacemaker, generally the sinus node, becomes less than that of the AV junctional region or when impulses from the primary pacemaker do not penetrate to the region of the escape focus and allow the AV junctional focus to reach threshold and discharge. The interval from the last normally conducted beat to the AV junctional escape beat is a measure of the initial discharge rate of the AV junctional focus and generally corresponds to a rate of 35 to 60 beats/min (Fig. 22–3*B*). Although an AV junctional escape rhythm is usually fairly regular, intervals between subsequent escape beats after the initial escape beat can gradually shorten as the rate of discharge of the escape focus increases, the so-called *rhythm of development* or *warm-up phenomenon*.

The electrocardiogram displays pauses longer than the normal P-P interval, interrupted by a QRS complex of supraventricular configuration with absent, retrograde, fusion, or sinus P waves that do not conduct to the ventricle. If P waves precede the QRS, they have a P-R interval generally less than 0.12 sec. The exact site of impulse formation (i.e., AN, N, or NH regions; low atrium; or His bundle) is not known and may differ from patient to patient and be influenced by the cause of the arrhythmia.

Treatment, if any, lies in increasing the discharge rate of the higher pacemakers and improving AV conduction and can require pacing. Frequently, no treatment is necessary.

Premature AV Junctional Complexes

Premature AV junctional complexes are characterized by an impulse that arises prematurely in the AV junction (the exact site—i.e., AN, N, or NH regions; low atrium; or His bundle—is not known and may vary from patient to patient) and that attempts conduction in

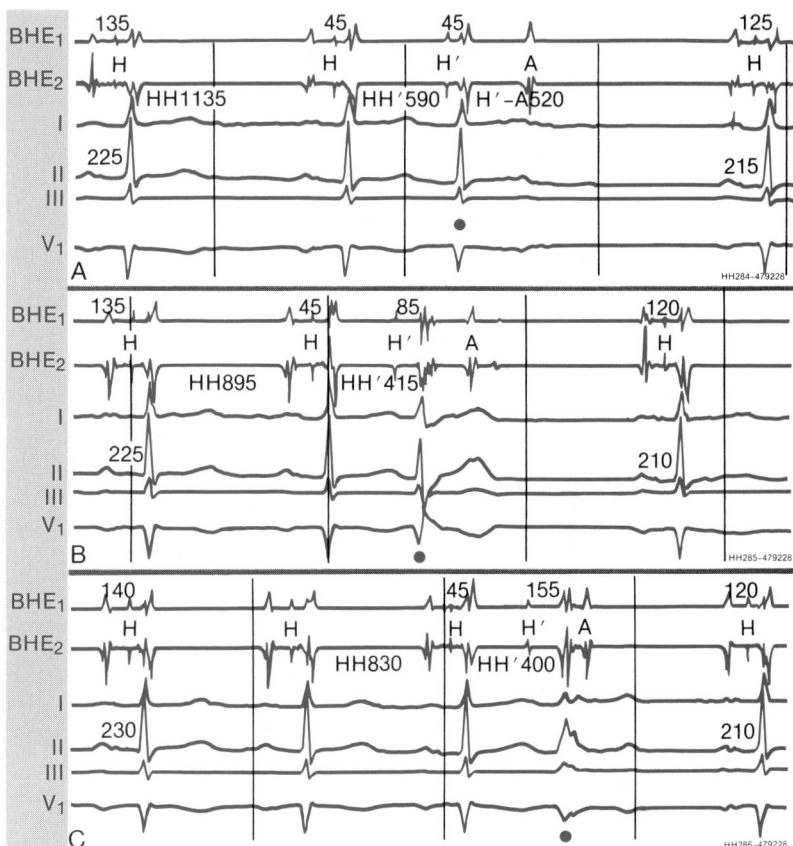

FIGURE 22–19. Premature AV junctional complexes arising in or near the bundle of His (H') conduct normally (A) or with (B) functional right or (C) functional left bundle branch block. The filled circles indicate the premature junctional complex. Anterograde conduction of the premature junctional (H') discharges depends on the coupling interval between the last normal His discharge (H) and H-H' interval and the spontaneous cycle length (H-H) that preceded H'. When H' follows a shorter preceding cycle length and occurs at longer coupling intervals, a normal QRS complex results. As the preceding H-H cycle lengthens or as the H-H' interval shortens, a zone of functional right bundle branch block occurs, followed by a zone of functional left bundle branch block. Not shown are premature His discharges that fail to conduct entirely. Numbers in milliseconds. Time lines = 1 sec in each panel. (Magnification is not the same in all three panels.) (From Bonner, A. J., and Zipes, D. P.: Lidocaine and His bundle extrasystoles. His bundle discharge conducted normally, conducted with functional right or left bundle branch block, or blocked entirely [concealed]. Arch. Intern. Med. *136*:700, 1976. Copyright American Medical Association.)

anterograde and retrograde directions. If unimpeded in its course, the impulse discharges the atrium to produce a premature retrograde P wave and a premature QRS complex with a supraventricular contour. The retrograde P wave can occur before, during, or after the QRS complex. Alterations in conduction time can influence the P-R or R-P relationships without a change in the site of origin of the impulse. Premature AV junctional complexes that conduct aberrantly are difficult to distinguish from premature ventricular complexes using the scalar ECG (Fig. 22–19).

Treatment of premature AV junctional complexes is generally not necessary. However, since they may arise distal to the AV node, they can occur early in the cardiac cycle and can initiate a ventricular tachyarrhythmia in some instances. Under these circumstances therapy is approached as for premature ventricular complexes (see p. 675).

AV Junctional Rhythm

If the AV junctional escape beats continue for a period of time, the rhythm is called an *AV junctional rhythm* (Fig. 22–20). Since the inherent rate of the AV junctional tissue is 35 to 60 beats/min, the AV junctional tissue can assume the role of the dominant pacemaker at this rate only by passive default of the sinus pacemaker. The ECG displays a normally conducted QRS complex, which can conduct retrogradely to the atrium or can occur independently of atrial discharge, producing AV dissociation (see p. 692).

An AV junctional escape rhythm can be a normal phenomenon in response to the effects of vagal tone, or it can occur during pathological sinus bradycardia or heart block. The escape beat or rhythm serves as a safety mechanism to prevent the occurrence of ventricular asystole. *Physical findings* vary depending on the P-QRS relationship. Large *a* waves in the jugular venous pulse and a loud, soft, or changing intensity of the first heart sound may be present if atrial contraction occurs when the tricuspid valve is shut.

Therapy is discussed under AV junctional escape beats (see above).

Nonparoxysmal AV Junctional Tachycardia

ELECTROCARDIOGRAPHIC RECOGNITION (Figs. 22–21 and 22–22). To usurp dominant pacemaker status, the AV junctional tissue must exhibit enhanced discharge rate such

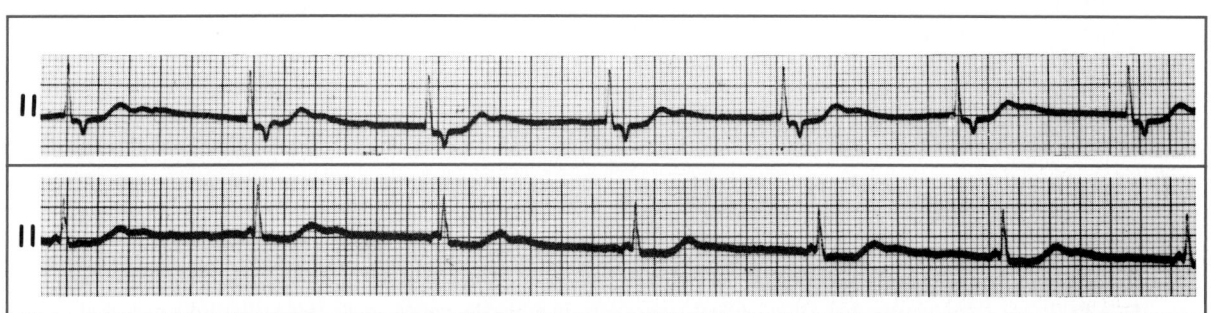

FIGURE 22–20. AV junctional rhythm. *Top,* AV junctional discharge occurs fairly regularly at a rate of approximately 50 beats/min. Retrograde atrial activity follows each junctional discharge. *Bottom,* Recording made on a different day in the same patient; the AV junctional rate is slightly more variable, and retrograde P waves precede the onset of the QRS complex. The positive terminal portion of the P wave gives the appearance of AV dissociation, which was not present.

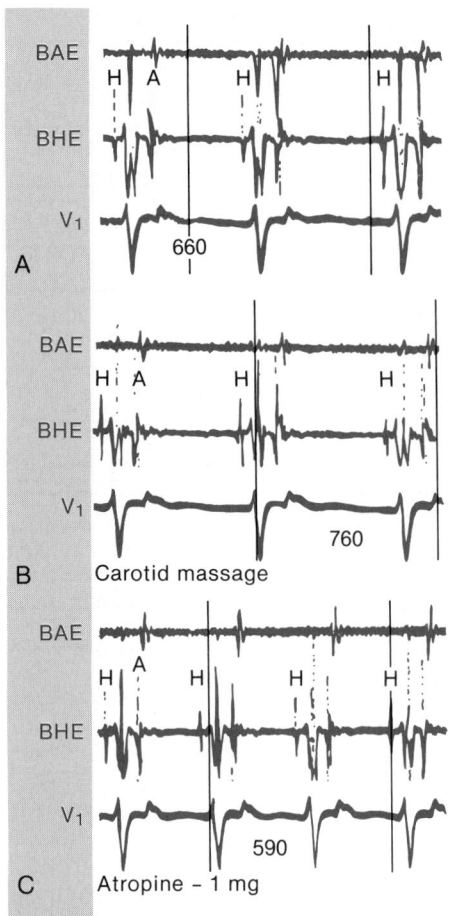

FIGURE 22–21. Nonparoxysmal AV junctional tachycardia. *A,* Control; *B,* response to carotid sinus massage; *C,* response to atropine, 1 mg intravenously. Note that His bundle depolarization is the earliest recordable electrical activity in each cycle. The atria are depolarized retrogradely (low right atrial activity recorded in BHE precedes high right atrial activity recorded in BAE). Note also that carotid sinus massage slows the junctional discharge rate while atropine speeds it up. From these tracings alone one could not distinguish the rhythm from some other types of supraventricular tachycardias. However, onset and termination of this tachycardia were typical of nonparoxysmal AV junctional tachycardia.

as during nonparoxysmal AV junctional tachycardia. The tachycardia is usually of gradual onset and termination, hence the modifier *nonparoxysmal.* On occasion, nonparoxysmal AV junctional tachycardia can become manifest abruptly because of slowing of the dominant pacemaker that may then allow sudden capture and control of the rhythm by the AV junctional focus.

Nonparoxysmal AV junctional tachycardia is recognized by a QRS of supraventricular configuration at a fairly regular rate of 70 to 130 beats/min but can be faster. Accepted terminology assigns the label of tachycardia to rates exceeding 100 beats/min. The term *nonparoxysmal AV junctional tachycardia,* although not entirely correct when the rate is 70 to 100 beats/min, has generally been accepted, since rates exceeding 60 beats/min represent in effect a tachycardia for the AV junctional tissue. Enhanced vagal tone can slow while vagolytic agents can speed up the discharge rate. Although retrograde activation of the atria can occur, the atria commonly are controlled by an independent sinus, atrial, or on occasion a second AV junctional focus resulting in AV dissociation (Fig. 22–11*G*). The electrocardiographic diagnosis can be complicated by the presence of entrance and exit blocks at the AV junctional tissue level and incomplete forms of AV dissociation.

The cause of this arrhythmia probably is *accelerated automatic discharge* in or near the His bundle. It is possible that nonparoxysmal AV junctional tachycardia originates in atrial fibers without recognition of the latter's role from analysis of the scalar ECG or on intracardiac electrograms, unless a careful search is made. Wenckebach periods can occur (Fig. 3–50, color plate 2), but the presence of exit block has not yet been demonstrated by His bundle recording in humans, and the block can be in the AV node with the origin of the nonparoxysmal AV junctional tachycardia proximal to the site of the His bundle recording.

CLINICAL FEATURES. Nonparoxysmal AV junctional tachycardia occurs most commonly in patients with underlying heart disease, such as inferior infarction or myocarditis (often the result of acute rheumatic fever), or after open-heart surgery.[144–146] An important cause is excessive digitalis, which also can produce the ECG manifestations of varying degrees of exit block (usually Wenckebach type) from the accelerated AV junctional focus. Junctional tachycardia occurs commonly during radiofrequency catheter ab-

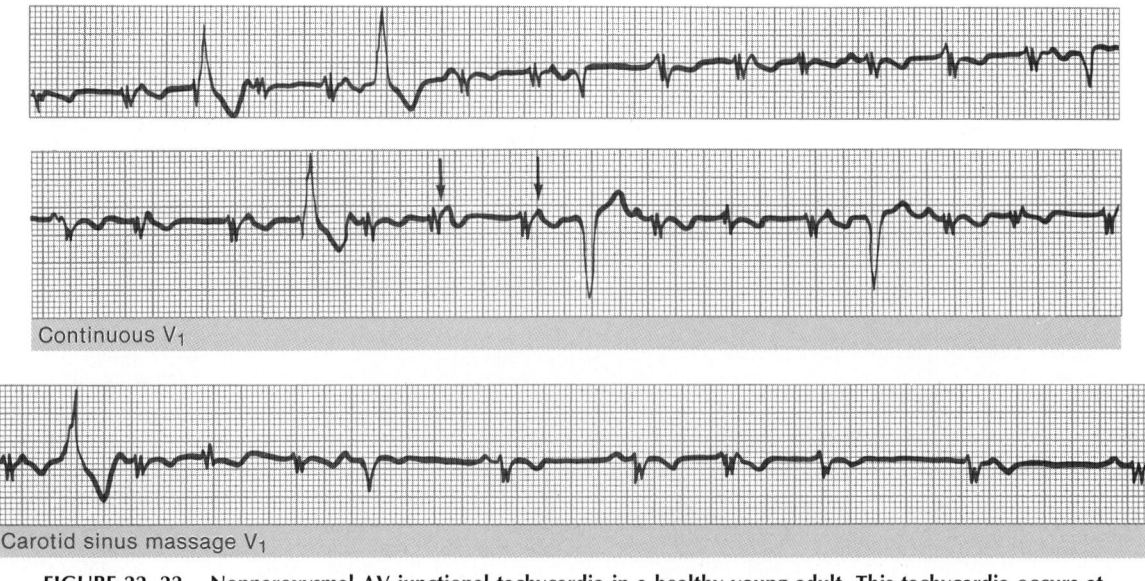

FIGURE 22–22. Nonparoxysmal AV junctional tachycardia in a healthy young adult. This tachycardia occurs at a fairly regular interval ("W-shaped" complexes) and is interrupted intermittently with sinus captures that produce functional right and left bundle branch block. Two P waves are indicated by arrows. The junctional discharge rate is approximately 120 beats/min (cycle length = 500 msec) and the rhythm irregular, sometimes shortened by sinus captures or delayed by concealed conduction that resets and displaces the junctional focus. In the bottom panel, carotid sinus massage slows the junctional as well as the sinus discharge rate.

lation of the slow pathway[147] (see p. 623). Nonparoxysmal AV junctional tachycardia can occur in otherwise healthy individuals without symptoms (Fig. 22–22) or can be a serious and difficult-to-control tachycardia, occasionally chronic, rapid, and long-lasting. It can occur congenitally in infants or children, with a relatively high mortality.[148,149]

The clinical features vary depending on the rate of the arrhythmia and the underlying etiology and severity of heart disease. As in most arrhythmias, the physical signs are determined by the relationship of the P wave to the QRS complex and the rate of atrial and ventricular discharge. The first heart sound can therefore be constant or varying, and cannon *a* waves may or may not occur in the jugular venous pulse.

The ventricular rhythm can be regular or irregular, often in a constant fashion. It is especially important to recognize slowing and regularization of the ventricular rhythm in a patient with atrial fibrillation as being caused by nonparoxysmal AV junctional tachycardia and as a possible early sign of *digitalis intoxication* (see p. 484). Initially, during atrial fibrillation, the regular ventricular rhythm can result from an AV junctional escape rhythm because the depressed AV conduction caused by digitalis blocks the passage of impulses from the fibrillating atria (Fig. 22–11G). As digitalis administration is continued, the ventricular rate can then speed because of increased discharge of the AV junctional pacemaker but can still be regular. Further digitalis administration can produce a rate that is slow and irregular because of varying degrees of AV junctional exit block. The rhythm can be misdiagnosed as resumption of conduction from the fibrillating atria. The rate then can increase further because of development of a ventricular tachycardia.

MANAGEMENT. Therapy is directed toward the underlying etiological factor and functional support of the cardiovascular system. If the rhythm is regular, the cardiovascular status is not compromised, and if the patient is not taking digitalis, digitalis administration could be considered. Electrical cardioversion can be tried if necessary and if digitalis toxicity is excluded; theoretically, however, if the nonparoxysmal AV junctional tachycardia is due to enhanced automaticity, cardioversion may be ineffective. If the patient tolerates the arrhythmia well, careful monitoring and attention to the underlying heart disease are usually all that are required in the adult. The arrhythmia usually will abate spontaneously. If digitalis toxicity is the cause, the drug must be stopped, and potassium, lidocaine, phenytoin, or propranolol administered. Drug therapy includes agents from classes IA, IC, and III.[144,148–150] Catheter ablation of the junctional site can be effective.[151–154]

Tachycardias Involving the AV Junction

Much confusion exists regarding the nomenclature of tachycardias characterized by a supraventricular QRS complex, a regular R-R interval, and no evidence of ventricular preexcitation. Because it is now apparent that a variety of electrophysiological mechanisms can account for these tachycardias (Fig. 22–11), the nonspecific term *paroxysmal supraventricular tachycardia* (PSVT) has been proposed to encompass the entire group. This term may be inappropriate because tachycardias in patients with accessory pathways (see below) are no more supraventricular than they are ventricular in origin, since they may require participation of both the atria and the ventricles in the reentrant pathway, and they exhibit a QRS complex of normal contour and duration only because anterograde conduction occurs over the normal AV node–His bundle pathways (Fig. 22–11C). If conduction over the reentrant pathway reverses direction and travels in an "antidromic" direction—i.e., to the ventricles over the accessory pathway and to the atria over the AV node–His bundle—the QRS com-

plex exhibits a prolonged duration, although the tachycardia is basically the same. The term *reciprocating tachycardia* has been offered as a substitute for paroxysmal supraventricular tachycardia, but use of such a term presumes the mechanism of the tachycardia to be reentrant (which is probably the case for many supraventricular tachycardias). Reciprocating tachycardia is probably the mechanism of many ventricular tachycardias as well. Thus no universally acceptable nomenclature exists for these tachycardias. In this chapter, descriptive titles, although cumbersome, will be used for the sake of clarity. In addition, the mechanism of reentry will be assumed operative when the weight of evidence supports its presence even though unequivocal proof is lacking.

Atrioventricular (AV) Nodal Reentrant Tachycardia

ELECTROCARDIOGRAPHIC RECOGNITION. Reentrant tachycardia in the AV node is characterized by a tachycardia with a QRS complex of supraventricular origin, with sudden onset and termination generally at rates between 150 and 250 beats/min (commonly 180 to 200 beats/min in adults) and with a regular rhythm. Uncommonly, the rate may be as low as 110 beats/min and occasionally, especially in children, may exceed 250. Unless functional aberrant ventricular conduction or a previous conduction defect exists, the QRS complex is normal in contour and duration. P waves are generally buried in the QRS complex. AV nodal reentry recorded at the onset begins abruptly, usually following a premature atrial complex that conducts with a prolonged P-R interval (see Figs. 22–11A and 22–11B and Figs. 20–28 through 20–33), pp. 570 through 575. The abrupt termination, usually with a retrograde P wave, is sometimes followed by a brief period of asystole or bradycardia. The R-R interval can shorten over the course of the first few beats at the onset or lengthen during the last few beats preceding termination of the tachycardia. Variation in cycle length is usually caused by variation in anterograde AV nodal conduction time. Cycle-length and/or QRS alternans can occur, usually when the rate is very fast. Carotid sinus massage can slow the tachycardia slightly prior to its termination or, if termination does not occur, can produce only slight slowing of the tachycardia.

ELECTROPHYSIOLOGICAL FEATURES

An atrial complex that conducts with a critical prolongation of AV nodal conduction time generally precipitates AV nodal reentry (see Figs. 22–23, 22–24, and 22–25). Premature ventricular stimulation also can induce AV nodal reentry in about one-third of patients. Data from radiofrequency catheter ablation results[157,158] and mapping[159–162] support the presence of separate atrial inputs into the AV node, the fast and slow pathways,[155,156] to explain this tachycardia (see Chap. 20). In Figure 20–31 (p. 574), and Figure 22–11A and B (p. 650), the atria are shown as a necessary link between the fast and slow pathways. In most examples, the retrograde P wave occurs at the onset of the QRS complex, clearly excluding the possibility of an accessory pathway. If an accessory pathway in the ventricle were part of the tachycardia circuit, the ventricles would have to be activated anterogradely before the accessory pathway could be activated retrogradely and depolarize the atria, placing the retrograde P wave no earlier than during the ST segment (see Preexcitation Syndrome, p. 667).

In approximately 30 per cent of instances, atrial activation begins at the end of, or just after, the QRS complex, giving rise to a discrete P wave on the surface ECG (often appearing as a nubbin of an R' in V₁) (Fig. 22–11A), while in the majority of patients P waves are not seen, since they are buried within the inscription of the QRS complex. In the most common variety of AV nodal reentrant tachycardia, the V-A interval (i.e., interval between onset of QRS and onset of atrial activity) is less than 50 per cent of the R-R interval, and the ratio of A-V to V-A interval exceeds 1.0. Most of these patients during tachycardia have a V-A minimum value of ≤61 msec measured to the earliest recorded atrial activity and of ≤95 msec measured to atrial activity recorded in the high right atrial electrogram. These V-A intervals are longer in patients with tachycardia related to accessory pathways as well as in atypical forms of AV nodal reentry (Fig. 22–11B).

SLOW AND FAST PATHWAYS. In the majority of patients, anterograde conduction occurs to the ventricle over the slow (alpha) pathway and retrograde conduction over the fast (beta) pathway (see Fig. 20–28B and Fig. 22–11A and B). To initiate tachycardia, an

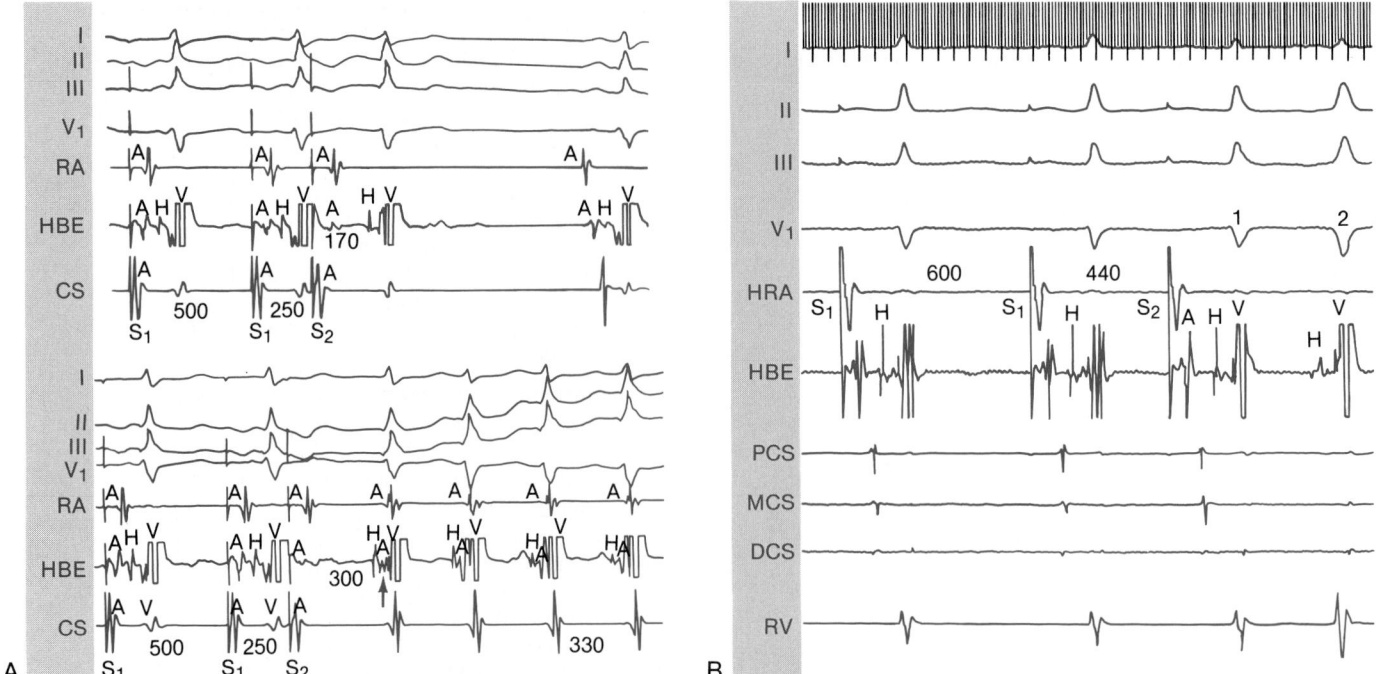

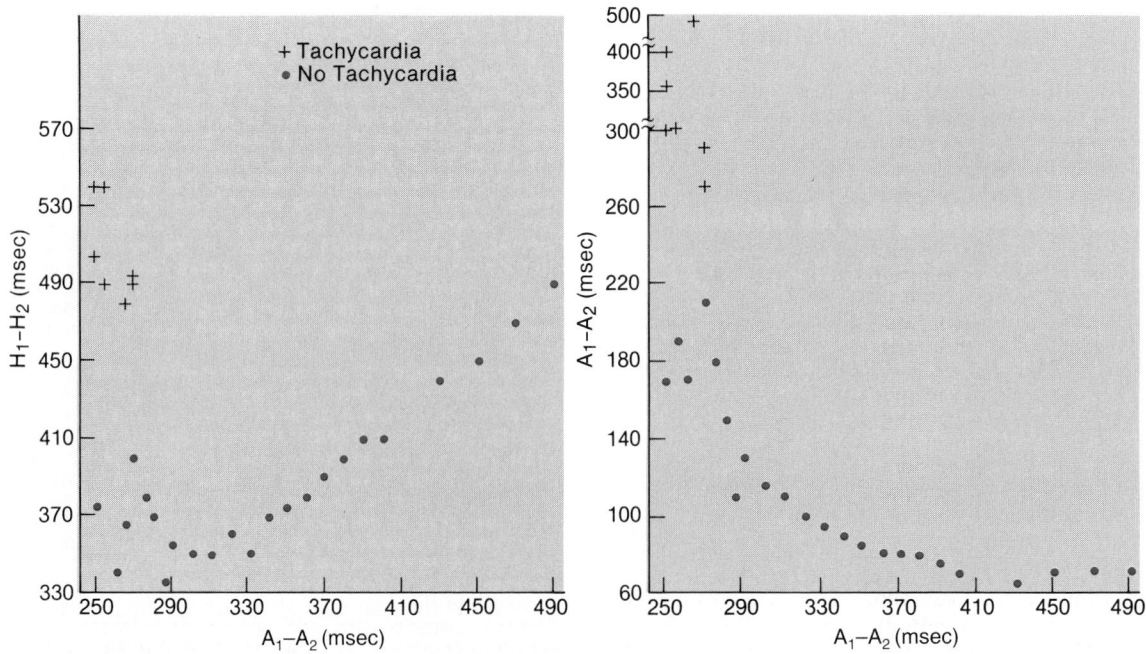

FIGURE 22–23. *A*, Initiation of AV nodal reentrant tachycardia in a patient with dual atrioventricular nodal pathways. Upper and lower panels show the last two paced beats of a train of stimuli delivered to the coronary sinus at a pacing cycle length of 500 msec. The results of premature atrial stimulation at an S$_1$-S$_2$ interval of 250 msec on two occasions are shown. In the upper panel, S$_2$ was conducted to the ventricle with an A-H interval of 170 msec and then was followed by a sinus beat. In the lower panel, S$_2$ was conducted with an A-H interval of 300 msec and initiated AV nodal reentry. Note that the retrograde atrial activity occurs (arrow) prior to the onset of ventricular septal depolarization and is superimposed on the QRS complex. Retrograde atrial activity begins first in the low right atrium (HBE lead) and then progresses to the high right atrium (RA) and coronary sinus (CS) recordings.

B, Two QRS complexes in response to a single atrial premature complex. Following a basic train of S$_1$ stimuli at 600 msec, an S$_2$ at 440 msec is introduced. The first QRS complex in response to S$_2$ occurs following a short (95 msec) A-H interval due to anterograde conduction over the fast AV nodal pathway. The first QRS complex is labeled number 1 (in lead V$_1$). The second QRS complex in response to the S$_2$ stimulus (labeled number 2) follows a long A-H interval (430 msec) due to anterograde conduction over the slow AV nodal pathway.

FIGURE 22–24. H$_1$-H$_2$ intervals *(left)* and A$_2$-H$_2$ intervals *(right)* at various A$_1$-A$_2$ intervals. Discontinuous AV nodal curve. At a critical A$_1$-A$_2$ interval the H$_1$-H$_2$ interval and the A$_1$-H$_2$ intervals increase markedly. At the break in the curves, AV nodal reentrant tachycardia is initiated.

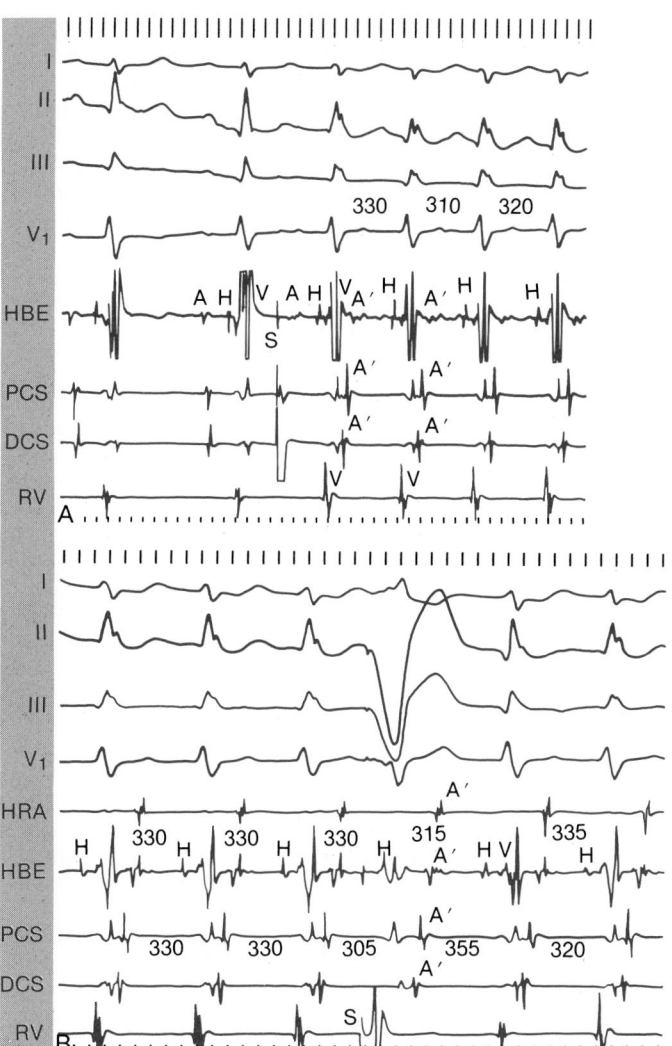

FIGURE 22–25. Atrial preexcitation during atrioventricular reciprocating tachycardia (AVRT) in a patient with a concealed accessory pathway. No evidence of an accessory pathway conduction is present in the two sinus-initiated beats shown in panel *A*. A premature stimulus in the coronary sinus (S) precipitates a supraventricular tachycardia at a cycle length of approximately 330 msec. The retrograde atrial activation sequence begins first in the distal coronary sinus (A', DCS), followed by activation recorded in the proximal coronary sinus (PCS), low right atrium (HBE), and then high right atrium (not shown). The QRS complex is normal and identical to the sinus-initiated QRS complex. (The terminal portion is slightly deformed by the superimposition of the retrograde atrial recording.) Note that the R-P interval is short and the P-R interval is long. The shortest V-A interval exceeds 65 msec, consistent with conduction over a retrogradely conducting atrioventricular pathway.

In panel *B*, premature ventricular stimulation at a time when the His bundle is still refractory from anterograde activation during tachycardia shortens the A-A interval from 330 to 305 msec without a change in the retrograde atrial activation sequence. (Note that no change occurs in the H-H interval when the right ventricular stimulus, S, is delivered. H-H intervals are in msec in HBE lead.) Thus the ventricular stimulus, despite His bundle refractoriness, still reaches the atrium and produces an identical retrograde atrial activation sequence. The only way this can be explained is via conduction over a retrogradely conducting accessory pathway. Therefore, the patient has a concealed accessory pathway with the Wolff-Parkinson-White syndrome.

---

atrial complex blocks in the fast pathway anterogradely, travels to the ventricle over the slow pathway, and returns to the atrium over the previously blocked fast pathway. The proximal and distal final pathways for this circus movement appear to be located within the AV node so that, as currently conceived, the circus movement occurs over the two atrial approaches and the AV node (Fig. 22–11*A* and *B*). The reentrant loop for typical AV nodal reentry is anterograde slow AV nodal pathway → final distal common pathway (probably distal AV

node) → retrograde fast AV nodal pathway → atrial myocardium. In atypical AV node reentry, the reentry occurs in an opposite direction.[163] In some patients, the His bundle may be incorporated in the reentrant circuit. Less commonly, the reentry pathway can be over two slow pathways, so-called slow-slow AV node reentry (Fig. 22–12*B*). Some data are consistent with intranodal activity.[164]

The cycle length of the tachycardia generally depends on how well the slow pathway conducts, because the fast pathway usually exhibits excellent capability for retrograde conduction and has the shorter refractory period in the retrograde direction. Therefore, conduction time in the anterograde slow pathway is a major determinant of the cycle length of the tachycardia.

THE DUAL PATHWAY CONCEPT. The evidence supporting the dual pathway concept derives from several observations, the most compelling of which is that radiofrequency catheter ablation of *either* the slow pathway or the fast pathway eliminates AV nodal reentry without eliminating AV nodal conduction. Other observations provide supporting proof. For example, in these patients, a plot of the A_1-A_2 versus the A_2-H_2 or A_1-A_2 versus the H_1-H_2 intervals shows a discontinuous curve (Fig. 22–24). The explanation is that at a crucial A_1-A_2 interval the impulse suddenly blocks in the fast pathway and conducts with delay over the slow pathway, with sudden prolongation of the A_2-H_2 (or H_1-H_2) interval. Generally, the A-H interval increases at least 50 msec with only a 10- to 20-msec decrease in the coupling interval of the premature atrial complex. Less commonly, dual pathways may be manifested by different P-R or A-H intervals during sinus rhythm or at identical paced rates or by a sudden jump in the A-H interval during atrial pacing at a constant cycle length. Two QRS complexes in response to one P wave provide additional evidence[165] (Fig. 22–23*B*).

Some patients with AV nodal reentry may not have discontinuous refractory period curves, and some patients who do not have AV nodal reentry can exhibit discontinuous refractory curves. In the latter patients, dual AV nodal pathways can be a benign finding. Many of these patients also exhibit discontinuous curves retrogradely. Similar mechanisms of tachycardia can occur in children. Triple AV nodal pathways can be demonstrated in occasional patients. Virtually irrefutable proof of dual AV nodal pathways is the simultaneous propagation in opposite directions of two AV nodal wavefronts without collision (Fig. 20–30, p. 573) or the production of two QRS complexes from one P wave (Fig. 22–23*B*) or two P waves from one QRS complex.[166]

In fewer than 5 to 10 per cent of patients with AV nodal reentry, anterograde conduction proceeds over the fast pathway and retrograde conduction over the slow pathway (termed the *unusual form* of AV nodal reentry or atypical AV node reentry), producing a long V-A interval and a relatively short A-V interval[156–163] (generally A-V/V-A < 0.75; Fig. 22–11*B*). Finally, it is possible to have tachycardias that use either the anterograde slow or fast pathways and conduct retrogradely over an accessory pathway (see below).

The ventricles are not needed to maintain AV nodal reentry in humans, and spontaneous AV block has been noted on occasion, particularly at the onset of the arrhythmia. Such block can take place in the AV node distal to the reentry circuit, between the AV node and bundle of His, within the bundle of His, or distal to it[167] (see Fig. 20–32, p. 574). Rarely, the block can be located between the reentry circuit in the AV node and the atrium. Most commonly, when block appears, it is below the bundle of His. Termination of the tachycardia generally results from block in the anterogradely conducting slow pathway ("weak link") so that a retrograde atrial response is not followed by a His or ventricular response.

RETROGRADE ATRIAL ACTIVATION. The sequence of retrograde atrial activation is normal during AV nodal reentrant supraventricular tachycardia. This means that the earliest site of atrial activation during retrograde conduction over the fast pathway is recorded in the His bundle electrogram followed by electrograms recorded from the os of the coronary sinus and then spreading to depolarize the rest of the right and left atria. During retrograde conduction over the slow pathway in the atypical type of AV nodal reentry, atrial activation recorded in the proximal coronary sinus precedes atrial activation recorded in the low right atrium, suggesting that the slow and fast pathways can enter the atria at slightly different positions. Mapping at the time of surgery confirms this conclusion. Functional bundle branch block during AV nodal reentrant tachycardia does not modify the tachycardia significantly.

CLINICAL FEATURES. AV nodal reentry commonly occurs in patients who have no structural heart disease. Symptoms frequently accompany the tachycardia and range from feelings of palpitations,[168] nervousness, and anxiety to angina, heart failure, syncope, or shock depending on the duration and rate of the tachycardia and the presence of structural heart disease. Tachycardia can cause syncope because of the rapid ventricular rate, reduced cardiac output, and cerebral circulation or because of asystole when the tachycardia terminates, owing to tachycardia-induced depression of sinus node automaticity. The prognosis for patients without heart disease is usually good.

Hemodynamic consequences of supraventricular tachyarrhythmias in patients with normal ventricular function are due primarily to a marked decrease in left ventricular end-diastolic and stroke volumes with an increase in ejection rate and cardiac output without a significant change in ejection fraction as heart rate is increased and the atrial contribution to ventricular filling is lost. Heart disease or tachycardia can reduce the ejection fraction. Initial hypotension during tachycardia can evoke a sympathetic response that increases blood pressure and in turn causes a rise in vagal tone that can terminate the tachycardia.

MANAGEMENT

THE ACUTE ATTACK (Table 22-2). This depends on the underlying heart disease, how well the tachycardia is tolerated, and the natural history of previous attacks in the individual patient. For some patients, rest, reassurance, and sedation may be all that are required to abort an attack. Vagal maneuvers, including carotid sinus massage, Valsalva and Mueller maneuvers, gagging, and occasionally exposure of the face to ice water serve as the first line of therapy. These maneuvers may slightly slow the tachycardia rate, which then may speed up to the original rate following cessation of the attempt, or may terminate it. Vagal maneuvers should be tried *again* after each pharmacological approach. Digitalis, calcium antagonists, beta-adrenoceptor blockers, and adenosine normally depress conduction in the anterogradely conducting slow AV nodal pathway, while class IA and IC drugs depress conduction in the retrogradely conducting fast pathway.

Adenosine (see p. 619), 6 to 12 mg given rapidly IV, is the initial drug of choice.[169] *Verapamil* (see p. 616), 5 to 10 mg IV, or diltiazem, 0.25 to 0.35 mg/kg IV, terminates AV nodal reentry successfully in about 2 minutes in about 90 per cent of instances and is given when simple vagal maneuvers and adenosine fail.

Cholinergic drugs, such as *edrophonium chloride* (Tensilon), a short-acting cholinesterase inhibitor, can terminate AV nodal reentry when administered initially at a trial dose of 3 to 5 mg IV. If unsuccessful, a dose of 10 mg IV may be given. Edrophonium is infrequently needed. Similarly, *intravenous digitalis* administration is usually not necessary to terminate AV nodal reentry. If digitalis is used, digoxin can be given, 0.5 to 1.0 mg IV over 10 to 15 min, followed by 0.25 mg every 2 to 4 hours, with a total dose less than 1.5 mg within any 24-hour period. *Oral digitalis* administration to terminate an acute attack is generally not indicated. Vagal maneuvers that were ineffective previously can terminate the tachycardia following digitalis administration and therefore should be repeated.

If a beta-adrenoceptor antagonist is selected, esmolol (50 to 200 μg/kg/min) would seem preferable because of its shorter duration of action. *Propranolol* can be tried. Recommended IV dosing is best achieved by titrating the dose to the clinical effect, begun with doses of 0.25 to 0.5 mg, increasing to 1.0 mg if necessary, and administering doses every 5 minutes until either a desired effect or toxicity is produced or a total of 0.15 to 0.2 mg/kg is given. Beta-

adrenoceptor blockers must be used cautiously, if at all, in patients with heart failure, chronic lung disease, or a history of asthma because its beta-adrenoceptor blocking action depresses myocardial contractility and can produce bronchospasm. Digitalis, calcium antagonists, beta blockers, and adenosine normally depress conduction in the anterogradely conducting slow pathway, whereas class 1A and 1C drugs depress conduction in the retrogradely conducting fast pathway.

DC CARDIOVERSION. Before digitalis or a beta blocker is administered, it is advisable to reassess the clinical status of the patient and consider whether DC cardioversion may be advisable. DC shock administered to patients who have received excessive amounts of digitalis can be dangerous and can result in serious postshock ventricular arrhythmias (see p. 621). Particularly if signs or symptoms of cardiac decompensation occur, DC electrical shock should be considered early. DC shock, synchronized to the QRS complex to avoid precipitating ventricular fibrillation, successfully terminates AV nodal reentry with energies in the range of 10 to 50 joules; higher energies can be required in some instances (see p. 623).

In the event that digitalis has been given in large doses and DC shock is contraindicated, competitive *atrial* or *ventricular pacing* can restore sinus rhythm. In some instances, esophageal pacing can be useful (see p. 705).

Class IA, IC, and III drugs are usually not required to terminate AV nodal reentry. Unless contraindicated, DC cardioversion generally should be employed before using these agents, which are more often administered to prevent recurrences.

Pressor drugs can terminate AV nodal reentry by inducting reflex vagal stimulation mediated by baroreceptors in the carotid sinus and aorta when the systolic blood pressure is acutely elevated to levels of about 180 mm Hg. One of the following drugs, diluted in 5 to 10 ml of 5 per cent dextrose and water, can be given over 1 to 3 minutes: phenylephrine (Neo-Synephrine), 0.5 to 1.0 mg; methoxamine (Vasoxyl), 3 to 5 mg; or metaraminol (Aramine), 0.5 to 2.0 mg. Pressor drugs should be used cautiously or not at all in the elderly and in patients who have structural heart disease, significant hypertension, hyperthyroidism, or acute myocardial infarction. This potentially dangerous and almost always uncomfortable mode of therapy is rarely needed unless the patient is also hypotensive.

PREVENTION OF RECURRENCES. Initially, one must decide whether the frequency and severity of the attacks warrant long-term therapy. If the attacks of paroxysmal tachycardia are infrequent, well tolerated, short lasting, and either terminate spontaneously or are easily terminated by the patient, no prophylactic therapy may be necessary. If the attacks are sufficiently frequent and/or long lasting to necessitate therapy, the patient can be treated with drugs empirically or on the basis of serial electrophysiological testing. If empirical testing is desirable, digitalis, a long-acting calcium antagonist, or long-acting beta-adrenoceptor blocker is a reasonable initial choice. The clinical situation and potential contraindications, e.g., beta blockers in an asthmatic, usually dictate the selection. If digitalis is used, rapid oral digitalization can be accomplished in 24 to 36 hours with digoxin at an initial dose of 1.0 to 1.5 mg, followed by 0.25 to 0.5 mg every 6 hours for a total dose of 2.0 to 3.0 mg. A less rapid oral regimen digitalizes in 2 to 3 days with an initial dose of 0.75 to 1.0 mg, followed by 0.25 to 0.50 mg every 12 hours for a total dose of 2.0 to 3.0 mg. Alternatively, digoxin administered as a maintenance dose of 0.125 to 0.500 mg achieves digitalization in about 1 week.

Sustained-release verapamil in the range of 240 mg per day, long-acting diltiazem 60 to 120 mg twice daily, or long-acting propranolol in doses of 80 to 120 mg per day can be tried. If these drugs are ineffective taken singly, combinations can be tested.

TABLE 22-2 DRUGS THAT SLOW CONDUCTION IN, AND PROLONG REFRACTORINESS OF, ACCESSORY PATHWAY AND AV NODE

AFFECTED TISSUE	DRUGS
Accessory pathway	Class IA
AV node	Class II Class IV Adenosine Digitalis
Both	Class IC Class III (amiodarone)

Because it is preferable to *cure* the patient of the tachycardia rather than to use potentially toxic drugs to suppress it or to implant an antitachycardia device that only terminates the tachycardia after its onset (Chap. 23), radiofrequency catheter ablation should be considered early in the management of patients with symptomatic recurrent episodes of AV node reentry. For patients who do not wish to take drugs, are drug intolerant, or in whom drugs are ineffective, radiofrequency catheter ablation is the treatment of choice.[170,171] It should be considered before long-term therapy with class IA, IC, or III antiarrhythmic drugs. Ablation has replaced surgery[162,172,173] in virtually all instances.[70,174-183]

Reentry Over a Retrogradely Conducting (Concealed) Accessory Pathway

ELECTROCARDIOGRAPHIC RECOGNITION (Fig. 22–25). The presence of an accessory pathway that conducts unidirectionally from the ventricle to the atrium but not in the reverse direction is not apparent by analysis of the scalar ECG during sinus rhythm because the ventricle is not preexcited.[184,185] Therefore, the ECG manifestations of the Wolff-Parkinson-White (WPW) syndrome are absent, and the accessory pathway is said to be "concealed." Since the mechanism responsible for most tachycardias in patients who have the WPW syndrome is macroreentry caused by anterograde conduction over the AV node–His bundle pathway and retrograde conduction over an accessory pathway, the latter, even if it only conducts retrogradely, can still participate in the reentrant circuit to cause an *AV reciprocating* tachycardia. Electrocardiographically, a tachycardia due to this mechanism can be *suspected* when the QRS complex is normal and the retrograde P wave occurs *after* completion of the QRS complex, in the ST segment, or early in the T wave (Fig. 22–11C).

MECHANISMS. The cause of unidirectional propagation is not clear and can relate to multiple factors. During sinus rhythm, the atrial impulse probably enters the accessory pathway but blocks near the ventricular insertion site with both right- and left-sided concealed accessory pathways. During functional block in patients with anterograde conduction over accessory pathways, block occurs near the ventricular insertion site most commonly with left-sided pathways but more often near the atrial insertion site with right-sided accessory pathways.

The P wave follows the QRS complex during tachycardia because the ventricle must be activated before the propagating impulse can enter the accessory pathway and excite the atria retrogradely. Therefore, the retrograde P wave must occur after ventricular excitation, in contrast to AV nodal reentry, in which the atria usually are excited during ventricular activation (Fig. 22–11A). Also, the contour of the retrograde P wave can differ from the usual retrograde P wave, since the atria may be activated eccentrically, i.e., in a manner other than the normal retrograde activation sequence, which starts at the low right atrial septum as in AV nodal reentry. This occurs because the concealed accessory pathway in most instances is left-sided, i.e., inserts into the left atrium, making the left atrium the first site of retrograde atrial activation and causing the retrograde P wave to be negative in lead I (Fig. 22–25).

Finally, since the tachycardia circuit involves the ventricles, if functional bundle branch block occurs in the same ventricle in which the accessory pathway is located, the V-A interval and cycle length of the tachycardia can become longer (see Fig. 22–30B). This important change ensues because the bundle branch block lengthens the reentrant circuit (see Preexcitation Syndrome). For example, the normal activation sequence for a reciprocating tachycardia circuit with a left-sided accessory pathway without functional bundle branch block progresses from atrium → AV node–His bundle → right and left ventricles → accessory pathway → atrium. However, during functional left bundle branch block, for example, the tachycardia circuit travels from atrium → AV node–His bundle → right ventricle → septum → left ventricle → accessory pathway → atrium. This increase in the V-A interval provides definitive proof that the ventricle and accessory pathway are part of the reentry circuit. The additional time required for the impulse to travel across the septum from the right to the left ventricle before reaching the accessory pathway and atrium lengthens the V-A interval, which lengthens the cycle length of the tachycardia by an equal amount, assuming no other changes in conduction times occur within the circuit. Thus lengthening of the tachycardia cycle length by more than 35 msec during ipsilateral functional bundle branch block is diagnostic of a free wall accessory

pathway if the lengthening can be shown to be due to V-A prolongation only and not to prolongation of the H-V interval (which can develop with the appearance of bundle branch block). In an occasional patient, the increase in cycle length due to prolongation of VA conduction can be nullified by a simultaneous decrease in the P-R (A-H) interval.

The presence of ipsilateral bundle branch block can facilitate reentry and cause an incessant AV reentrant tachycardia.[186] Functional bundle branch block in the ventricle contralateral to the accessory pathway does not lengthen the tachycardia cycle if the H-V interval does not lengthen.

Septal Accessory Pathway. An exception to these observations occurs in the patient with a concealed septal accessory pathway (see Preexcitation Syndrome, p. 667). First, retrograde atrial activation is normal because it occurs retrogradely up the septum. Second, the V-A interval and the cycle length of the tachycardia increase 25 msec or less with the development of ipsilateral functional bundle branch block.

Functional bundle branch block, particularly functional left bundle branch block, during tachycardia occurs more commonly in patients who have an accessory pathway than in those with AV nodal reentry, possibly because in the latter, slow pathway anterograde conduction allows for longer recovery time of the His-Purkinje system, while in tachycardias associated with accessory pathways, anterograde conduction over the AV node may be more rapid. Functional left bundle branch block can occur more commonly during rapid tachycardias, perhaps because the refractory period of the right bundle branch appears to be shorter than that of the left bundle branch at short cycle lengths. Premature right ventricular stimulation that starts an AV reciprocating tachycardia is more likely to induce functional left bundle branch block than is premature atrial stimulation.

Vagal maneuvers, by acting predominantly on the AV node, produce a response on AV reentry similar to AV nodal reentry, and the tachycardia can transiently slow and sometimes terminate. Generally, termination occurs in the anterograde direction so that the last retrograde P wave fails to conduct to the ventricle.

ELECTROPHYSIOLOGICAL FEATURES. Electrophysiological criteria supporting the diagnosis of tachycardia involving reentry over a concealed accessory pathway include the fact that initiation of tachycardia depends on a critical degree of atrioventricular delay (necessary to allow time for the accessory pathway to recover excitability so that it can conduct retrogradely), but the delay can be in the AV node or His-Purkinje system; i.e., a critical degree of A-H delay is not necessary. Occasionally, a tachycardia can start with little or no measurable lengthening of AV nodal or His-Purkinje conduction time. The AV nodal refractory period curve is smooth, in contrast to the discontinuous curve found in many patients with AV nodal reentry. Dual AV nodal pathways occasionally can be noted as a concomitant but unrelated finding.

DIAGNOSIS OF ACCESSORY PATHWAYS. This can be accomplished by demonstrating that during ventricular pacing, premature ventricular stimulation activates the atria before retrograde depolarization of the His bundle, indicating that the impulse reached the atria before it depolarized the His bundle and must have traveled a different pathway to do so. Also, if the ventricles can be stimulated prematurely during tachycardia at a time when the His bundle is refractory, and the impulse still conducts to the atrium, this indicates that retrograde propagation traveled to the atrium over a pathway other than the bundle of His (Fig. 22–25B). If the premature ventricular complex depolarizes the atria without lengthening of the V-A interval and with the same retrograde atrial activation sequence, one assumes that the stimulation site (i.e., ventricle) is within the reentrant circuit without intervening His-Purkinje or AV nodal tissue that might increase the V-A interval and therefore the A-A interval. In addition, if a premature ventricular complex delivered at a time when the His bundle is refractory terminates the tachycardia without activating the atria retrogradely, it most likely invaded, and blocked in, an accessory pathway.

The V-A interval (a measurement of conduction over the accessory pathway) generally is constant over a wide range of ventricular paced rates and coupling intervals of premature ventricular complexes as well as during the tachycardia in the absence of aberration. Similar short V-A intervals can be observed in some patients during AV nodal reentry, but if the VA conduction time or R-P interval is the same during tachycardia *and* ventricular pacing at comparable rates, an accessory pathway is almost certainly present. The V-A interval is usually less than 50 per cent of the R-R interval. The tachycardia can be easily initiated following premature ventricular stimulation that conducts retrogradely in the accessory pathway but blocks in the AV node or His bundle. Atria and ventricles are required components of the macroreentrant circuit, and therefore continuation of the tachycardia in the presence of AV or VA block excludes an accessory atrioventricular pathway as part of the reentrant circuit.

CLINICAL FEATURES. The presence of concealed accessory pathways is estimated to account for about 30 per cent of patients with apparent supraventricular tachycardia referred for electrophysiological evaluation. The great majority of these accessory pathways are located between the left ventricle and left atrium and in the posteroseptal area, less

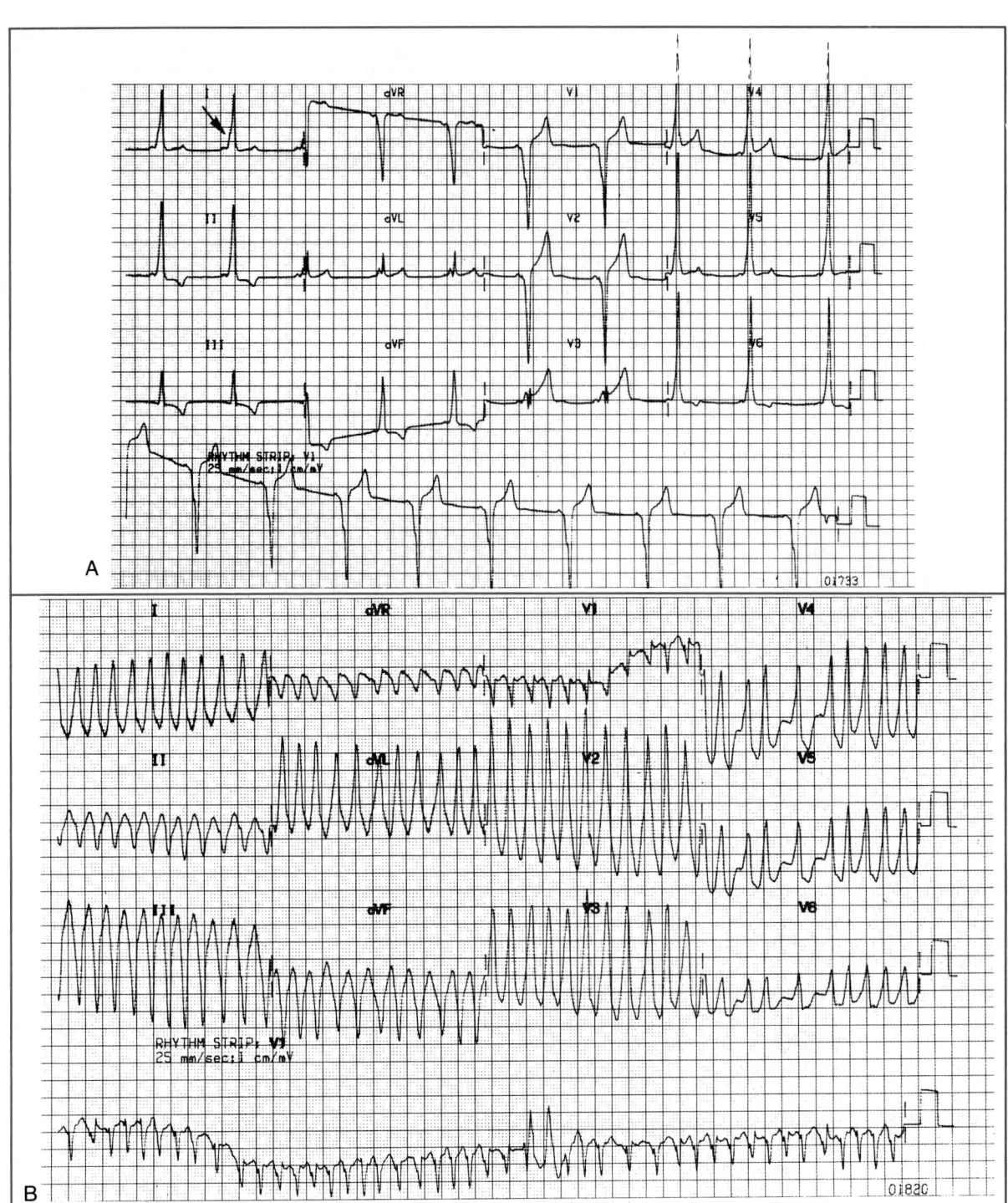

FIGURE 22–26. *A,* Right anteroseptal accessory pathway. The 12-lead ECG characteristically exhibits a normal to inferior axis. The delta wave is negative in V_1 and V_2, upright in leads I, II, aV_l, and aV_f, isoelectric in lead III, and negative in aV_r. Location verified at surgery. Arrow indicates delta wave (lead I).

B, Right posteroseptal accessory pathway. Negative delta waves in leads II, III, and AVF, upright in I and AVL, localize this pathway to the posteroseptal region. The negative delta wave in V_1 with sharp transition to an upright delta wave in V_2 pinpoint it to the right posteroseptal area. Atrial fibrillation is present. Location verified at surgery.

commonly between the right ventricle and right atrium. It is important to be aware of a concealed accessory pathway as a possible cause for apparently "routine" supraventricular tachycardia, since the therapeutic response at times may not follow the usual guidelines. The tachycardia rates tend to be somewhat faster than those occurring in AV nodal reentry (≥ 200 beats/min), but a great deal of overlap exists between the two groups.

Paroxysmal supraventricular tachycardia can be followed by polyuria after termination due to atrial dilatation and release of atrionatriuretic factor. Syncope can occur because the rapid ventricular rate fails to provide adequate cerebral circulation or because the tachyarrhythmia depresses the sinus pacemaker, causing a period of asystole when the tachyarrhythmia terminates. Physical examination reveals an unvarying, regular ventricular rhythm with constant intensity of the first heart sound. The jugular venous pressure can be elevated, but the waveform generally remains constant.

MANAGEMENT. The therapeutic approach to terminate

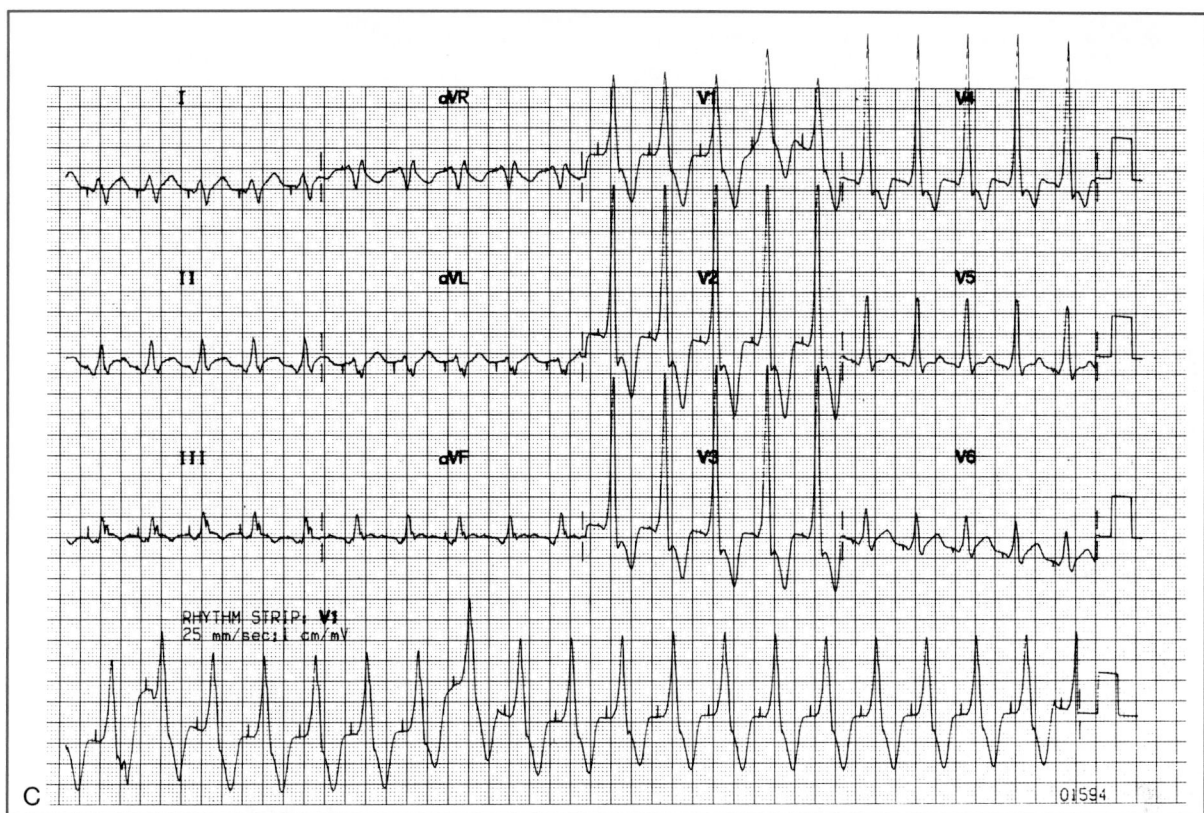

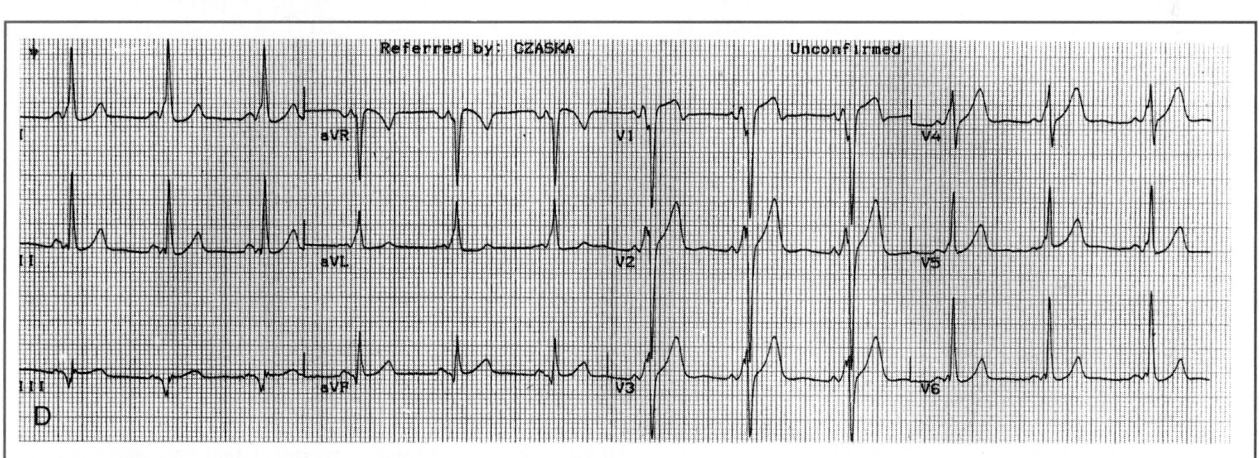

FIGURE 22–26 *Continued C,* Left lateral accessory pathway. Positive delta wave in the anterior precordial leads and in leads II, III, and AVF, positive or isoelectric in lead I and AVL, and isoelectric or negative in V₅ and V₆ are typical of a left lateral accessory pathway. Rapid coronary sinus pacing (450 msec cycle length) was used to enhance preexcitation (negative P wave I, II, III, aVf, V₃₋₆). Location verified at surgery.

D, Right free wall accessory pathway. Predominantly negative delta wave in V₁ and axis more leftward than in panel *A* indicate the presence of a right free wall accessory pathway.

Illustration continued on following page

this form of tachycardia acutely is as outlined for AV nodal reentry (see p. 664). It is necessary to achieve block of a single impulse from atrium to ventricle or ventricle to atrium. Generally, the most successful method is to produce transient AV nodal block; therefore, vagal maneuvers, IV adenosine, verapamil or diltiazem, digitalis, and beta blockers are acceptable choices. Radiofrequency catheter ablation and conventional antiarrhythmic agents that prolong activation time or refractory period in the accessory pathway need to be considered for chronic prophylactic therapy, similar to that discussed for reciprocating tachycardias associated with the preexcitation syndrome. Radiofrequency catheter ablation is curative, has low risk, and should be considered early for symptomatic patients[70,184,185,187–189] (see p. 621). The presence of atrial

fibrillation in patients with a *concealed accessory pathway* should not be a greater therapeutic challenge than in patients who do not have such a pathway, because anterograde AV conduction occurs only over the AV node and not over an accessory pathway. Intravenous verapamil and digitalis are not contraindicated. However, it must be remembered that under some circumstances, such as catecholamine stimulation, anterograde conduction in the apparently concealed accessory pathway can occur.

Preexcitation Syndrome

ELECTROCARDIOGRAPHIC RECOGNITION (Fig. 22–26). Preexcitation or the Wolff-Parkinson-White electrocardiographic abnormality occurs when the atrial impulse activates the

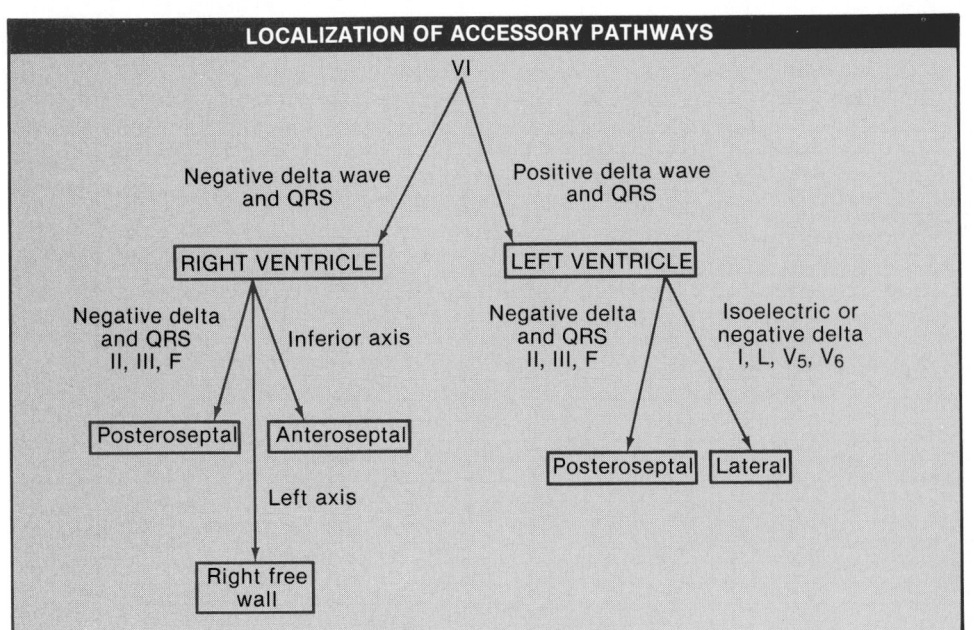

LOCALIZATION OF ACCESSORY PATHWAYS

FIGURE 22–26 *Continued E*, Logic diagram to determine location of accessory pathways. Begin with analysis of V_1 to determine whether the delta wave and the QRS complex are negative or positive. That establishes the ventricle in which the accessory pathway is located. Next, determine whether the delta wave and QRS complex are negative in leads II, III and AVF. If so, then the accessory pathway is located in a posteroseptal position. If the accessory pathway is located in the right ventricle, an inferior axis indicates an anteroseptal location while left axis indicates a right free wall location. If the accessory pathway is located in the left ventricle, an isoelectric or negative delta wave and QRS complex in leads I, aVI, V_5, and V_6 indicate a left lateral (free wall) location.

whole or some part of the ventricle, or the ventricular impulse activates the whole or some part of the atrium, earlier than would be expected if the impulse traveled by way of the normal specialized conduction system only.[184,185] This is caused by muscular connections composed of working myocardial fibers that exist outside the specialized conducting tissue and connect the atrium and ventricle, bypassing AV nodal conduction delay. They are named *accessory atrioventricular pathways* or connections, commonly called *Kent bundles,* and are responsible for the most common variety of preexcitation (incidentally noted in other species such as monkeys, dogs, and cats). The term *syndrome* is attached to this disorder when tachyarrhythmias due to the accessory pathway occur. Three basic features typify the ECG abnormalities of patients with the usual form of WPW conduction caused by an AV connection: (1) P-R interval less than 120 msec during sinus rhythm, (2) QRS complex duration exceeding 120 msec with a slurred, slowly rising onset of the QRS in some leads (delta wave) and usually a normal terminal QRS portion, and (3) secondary ST-T wave changes that are generally directed opposite to the major delta and QRS vectors. Analysis of the scalar ECG can be used to localize the accessory pathway[190,191] (Fig. 22–26D). Body surface mapping can be useful.[192]

In the *Wolff-Parkinson-White* (WPW) *syndrome,* the most common tachycardia is characterized by a normal QRS, a regular rhythm, ventricular rates of 150 to 250 beats/min

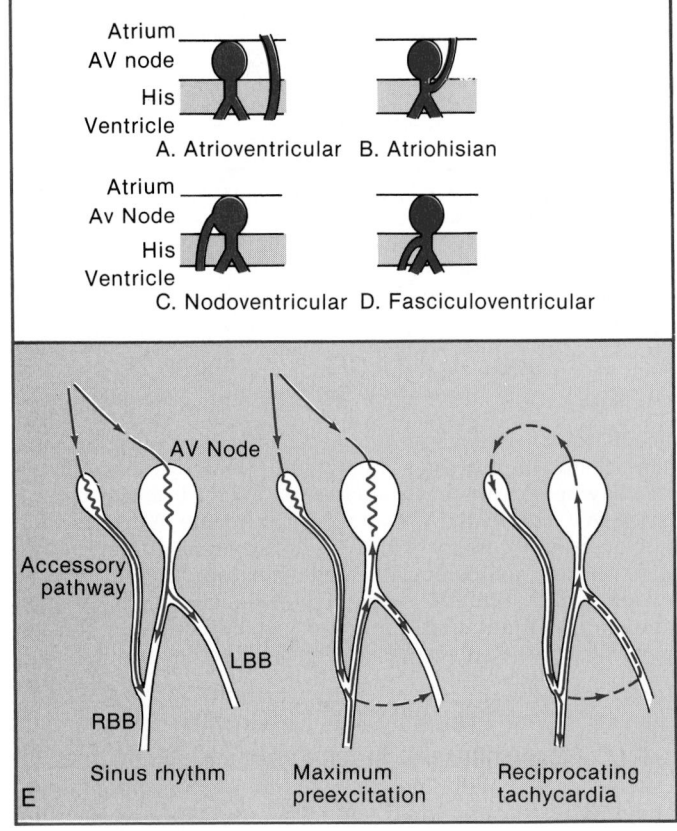

FIGURE 22–27. Schematic representation of accessory pathways. Panel A demonstrates the "usual" atrioventricular accessory pathway giving rise to most clinical presentations of tachycardia associated with Wolff-Parkinson-White syndrome. Panel B illustrates the very uncommon atriohisian accessory pathway. If the LGL syndrome exists, it would have this type of anatomy which has been demonstrated on occasion histopathologically. Panel C, nodoventricular pathways, original concept, in which anterograde conduction travels down the accessory pathway with retrograde conduction in the bundle branch–His bundle–AV node (see below). Panel D demonstrates the fasciculoventricular connections, not thought to play an important role in the genesis of tachycardias. Panel E illustrates the current concept of nodoventricular accessory pathway in which the accessory pathway is an atrioventricular communication with AV nodal–like properties. Sinus rhythm results in a fusion QRS complex, as in the usual form of WPW shown in panel A. Maximum preexcitation results in ventricular activation over the accessory pathway and the His bundle is activated retrogradely. During reciprocating tachycardia, anterograde conduction occurs over the accessory pathway with retrograde conduction over the normal pathway. (Panel E reproduced with permission from Benditt, D. G., and Milstein, S.: Nodoventricular accessory connection: A misnomer or a structural/functional spectrum. J. Cardiovasc. Electrophys. *1*:231, 1990.)

(generally faster than AV nodal reentry), and sudden onset and termination, behaving in most respects like the tachycardia described for conduction utilizing a concealed pathway (see p. 665). The major difference between the two is the capacity for anterograde conduction over the accessory pathway during atrial flutter or atrial fibrillation (see below).

Variants

A variety of other anatomical substrates exist that provide the basis for different ECG manifestations of several variations of the preexcitation syndrome[184] (Fig. 22–27). Fibers from atrium to His bundle bypassing the physiological delay of the AV node are called *atriohisian tracts* (Fig. 22–27B) and are associated with a short P-R interval and a normal QRS complex. Although demonstrated anatomically (see below), the electrophysiological significance of these tracts in the genesis of tachycardias with a short P-R interval and a normal QRS complex (Lown-Ganong-Levine, or LGL, syndrome) remains to be established. Indeed, evidence does *not* support the presence of a specific LGL syndrome comprising a short P-R interval, normal QRS complex, and tachycardias related to an atriohisian bypass tract.

Two varieties of Mahaim fibers include those passing from the AV node to the ventricle, called *nodoventricular fibers* (or nodofascicular if the insertion is into the right bundle branch rather than ventricular muscle (Fig. 22–27C), and those arising in the His bundle or bundle branches and inserting in the ventricular myocardium, called *fasciculoventricular fibers* (Fig. 22–27D). For nodoventricular connections, the P-R interval may be normal or short, and the QRS complex is a fusion beat. Nodoventricular connections can be involved in tachycardias, but fasciculoventricular pathways generally are not.

In patients who have an atriohisian tract, theoretically, the QRS complex would remain normal and the short A-H interval fixed or show very little increase during atrial pacing at more rapid rates. The author has found this response to be uncommon. Rapid atrial pacing in patients who have nodoventricular or nodofascicular connections shortens the H-V interval and widens the QRS complex, producing a left bundle branch block contour, but in contrast to the situation in patients who have an atrioventricular connection (Fig. 22–28), the A-V interval also lengthens. In patients who have fasciculoventricular connections, the H-V interval remains short and the QRS complex unchanged and anomalous during rapid atrial pacing.

ATRIOFASCICULAR ACCESSORY PATHWAYS. These fibers almost always represent a duplication of the AV node and the distal conducting system and are located in the right

ventricular free wall. The apical end lies close to the lateral tricuspid annulus and conducts slowly, with AV node–like properties. After a long course, the distal portion of these fibers, which conducts rapidly, inserts into the distal right bundle branch or the apical region of the right ventricle.[184,193] No preexcitation is generally apparent during sinus rhythm but can be exposed by premature right atrial stimulation. The absence of retrograde conduction in these pathways produces only an antidromic AV reentry tachycardia ("preexcited" tachycardia) characterized by anterograde conduction over the accessory pathway and retrograde conduction over the right bundle branch–His bundle–AV node, making the atrium a necessary part of the circuit. The preexcited tachycardia has a left bundle branch block pattern, long A-V interval (due to the long conduction time over the accessory pathway), and short V-A interval. Right bundle branch block can be proarrhythmic by increasing the length of the tachycardia circuit (V-A interval prolongs due to delay in retrograde activation of the His bundle), and the tachycardia can become incessant.[184,193]

ELECTROPHYSIOLOGICAL FEATURES OF PREEXCITATION (Figs. 22–27 to 22–36; see also p. 665). If the Kent bundle accessory pathway is capable of anterograde conduction, two parallel routes of AV conduction are possible, one subject to physiological delay over the AV node and the other passing directly without delay from atrium to ventricle. This produces the typical QRS complex that is a fusion beat, due to depolarization of the ventricle in part by the wavefront traveling over the accessory pathway and in part by the wavefront traveling over the normal AV node–His bundle route. The delta wave represents ventricular activation from input over the accessory pathway. The extent of contribution to ventricular depolarization by the wavefront over each route depends on their relative activation times. If AV nodal conduction delay occurs, for example, because of a rapid atrial pacing rate or premature atrial complex, more of the ventricle becomes activated over the accessory pathway, and the QRS complex becomes more anomalous in contour. Total activation of the ventricle over the accessory pathway can occur if the AV nodal conduction delay is sufficiently long. In contrast, if the accessory pathway is relatively far from the sinus node, for example, a left lateral accessory pathway, or if AV nodal conduction time is relatively short, more of the ventricle may be activated by conduction over the normal pathway (Fig. 22–28). The normal fusion beat during sinus rhythm has a short H-V interval, or His bundle activation actually begins after the onset of ventricular depolarization, because part of the atrial impulse bypasses the AV node and activates the ventricle early, at a time when the atrial impulse traveling the nor-

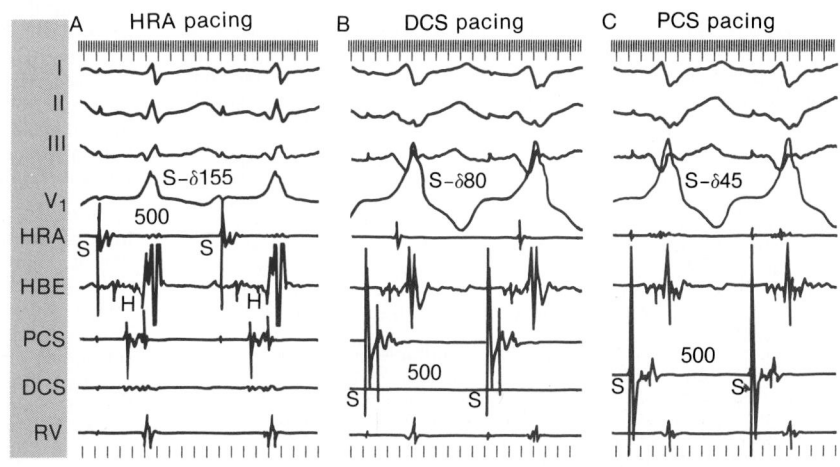

FIGURE 22–28. Atrial pacing at different atrial sites illustrating different conduction over the accessory pathway. In panel A, high right atrial pacing at a cycle length of 500 msec produces anomalous activation of the ventricle (note upright QRS complex in V_1) and a stimulus-delta interval of 155 msec. This indicates that the time from the onset of the stimulus to the beginning of the QRS complex is relatively long because the stimulus is delivered at a fairly large distance from the accessory pathway. Note that the His bundle activation (H) occurs at about the onset of the QRS complex. In panel B atrial pacing occurs through the distal coronary sinus electrode (DCS). At the same pacing cycle length, DCS pacing results in more anomalous ventricular activation and a shorter stimulus-delta interval (80 msec). His bundle activation is now buried within the inscription of the ventricular electrogram in the HBE lead. Panel C, Pacing from the proximal coronary sinus electrode (PCS) results in the shortest stimulus-delta interval (45 msec) indicating that the pacing stimulus is being delivered very close to the atrial insertion of the accessory pathway, which is located in the left posteroseptal region of the atrioventricular groove.

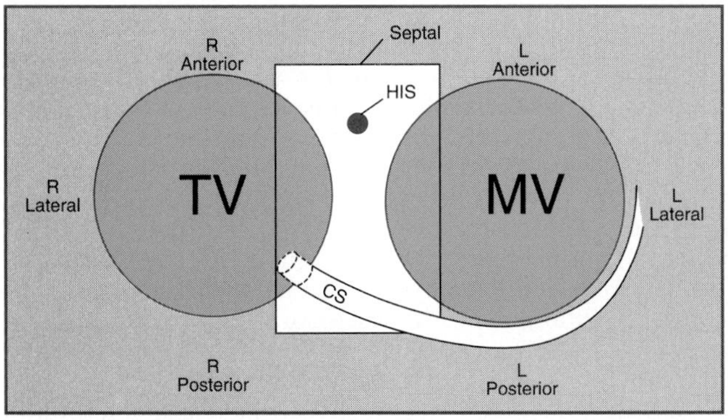

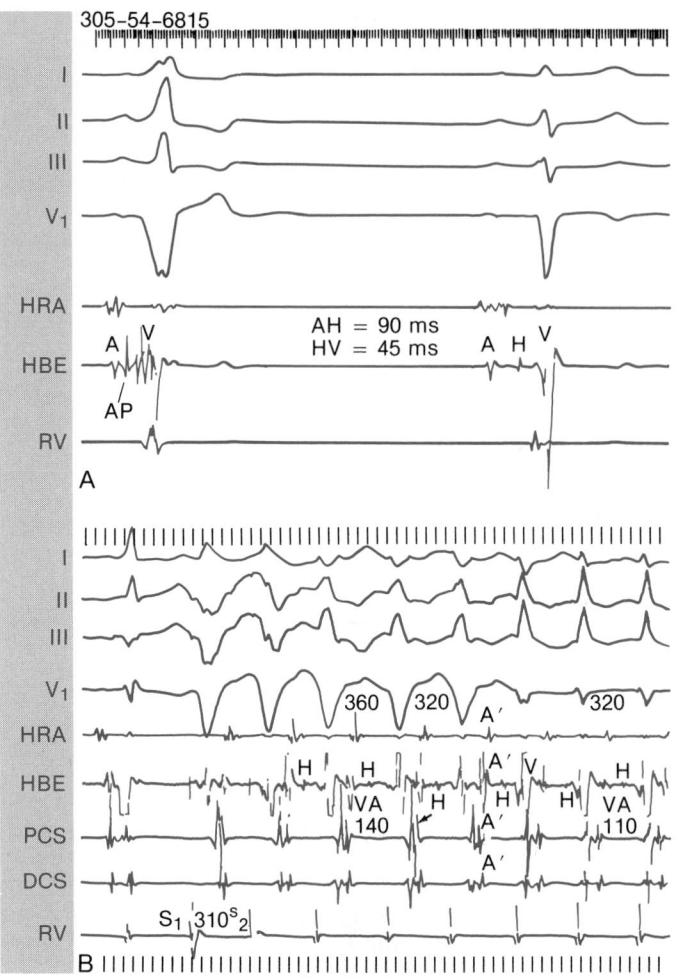

FIGURE 22–29. Schematic representation of the tricuspid (TV) and mitral (MV) valves, and the position of the coronary sinus (CS). This figure indicates the quadrants in which accessory pathways can be located. (Reproduced with permission from Miles, W. M., Zipes, D. P., and Klein, L. S.: Ablation of free wall accessory pathways. *In* Zipes, D. P. [eds.]: Catheter Ablation of Arrhythmias. Armonk, N.Y., Futura, 1994, p. 212.)

mal route just reaches the His bundle. This finding of a short or negative H-V interval occurs *only* during conduction over an accessory pathway or from retrograde His activation during a complex originating in the ventricle, such as a ventricular tachycardia.

Pacing the atrium at rapid rates, at premature intervals, or from a site close to the atrial insertion of the Kent bundle accentuates the anomalous activation of the ventricles and shortens the H-V interval even more (His activation may become buried in the ventricular electrogram, as in Fig. 22–28B). The position of the accessory pathway can be determined by a careful analysis of the spatial direction of the delta wave in the 12-lead ECG in maximally preexcited beats[190,191] (Figs. 22–26 and 22–29). T-wave abnormalities can occur after disappearance of preexcitation with orientation of the T wave according to the site of preexcitation (T-wave memory). A variety of electrical (Fig. 22–30), radionuclide, and echocardiographic techniques can be used to localize the insertion site of the accessory pathway (Chap. 21). The location of the pathway may be associated with specific electrophysiological responses.[194]

KENT BUNDLE CONDUCTION. Even though the Kent bundle conducts more rapidly than does the AV node (conduction velocity is faster in the accessory pathway), the Kent bundle usually has a longer refractory period during long cycle lengths (e.g., sinus rhythm)—i.e., it takes longer for the accessory pathway to recover excitability than it does for the AV node. Consequently, a premature atrial complex can occur sufficiently early to block anterogradely in the accessory pathway and conduct to the ventricle only over the normal AV node–His bundle (Figs. 22–31A,B and 20–34). The resultant H-V interval and the QRS complex become normal. Such an event can initiate the most common type of reciprocating tachycardia, which is characterized by anterograde conduction over the normal pathway and retrograde conduction over the accessory pathway *(orthodromic AV reciprocating tachycardia)* (Figs. 22–31 and 20–34). The accessory pathway, blocking in an anterograde direction, recovers excitability in time to be activated following the QRS complex, in a retrograde direction, completing the reentrant loop.

Much less commonly, patients can have tachycardias called *antidromic* tachycardias during which anterograde conduction occurs over the accessory pathway and retrograde conduction over the AV node. The resultant QRS complex is abnormal owing to total ventricular activation over the accessory pathway (Figs. 22–31C and 22–32). In both tachycardias, the accessory pathway is an obligatory part of the reentrant circuit. In patients with bidirectional conduction over the accessory pathway, different fibers may be used anterogradely and retrogradely.

Five to ten per cent of patients have multiple accessory pathways often suggested by various ECG clues, and on occasion, tachycardia can be due to a reentrant loop conducting anterogradely over one accessory pathway and retrogradely over the other. Interestingly, 15 to 20 per cent of patients may exhibit AV nodal echoes or AV nodal reentry after interruption of the accessory pathway.

PERMANENT FORM OF AV JUNCTIONAL RECIPROCATING TACHYCARDIA (PJRT). An incessant form of supraventricular tachycardia has been recognized that generally occurs with a long R-P interval that ex-

ceeds the P-R interval (Figs. 22–33 and 22–34). Usually, a posteroseptal accessory pathway (most often right ventricular but other locations as well[194a]) that conducts very slowly, possibly due to a long and tortuous route, appears responsible. Tachycardia is maintained by anterograde AV nodal conduction and retrograde conduction over the accessory pathway (Fig. 22–31D). While anterograde conduction over this pathway has been demonstrated, the long anterograde conduction time over the accessory pathway ordinarily prevents ECG manifestations of accessory pathway conduction during sinus rhythm. Therefore, during sinus rhythm, the QRS is prolonged from conduction over this accessory pathway only when conduction times

FIGURE 22–30. *A,* Recording of depolarization of an accessory pathway (AP) with a catheter electrode. The first QRS complex illustrates conduction over the accessory pathway (AP). In the scalar ECG a short P-R interval and delta wave (best seen in leads I and V_1) are apparent. His bundle activation is buried within the ventricular complex. In the following complex, conduction has blocked over the accessory pathway and a normal QRS complex results. His bundle activation clearly precedes the onset of ventricular depolarization by 45 msec. The A-H interval for this complex is 90 msec. (From Prystowsky, E. N., Browne, K. F., and Zipes, D. P.: Intracardiac recording by catheter electrode of accessory pathway depolarization. Reprinted with permission from the American College of Cardiology. J. Am. Coll. Cardiol. 1:468, 1983.)

B, Influence of functional ipsilateral bundle branch block on the V-A interval during an atrioventricular reciprocating tachycardia (AVRT). Partial preexcitation can be noted in the sinus-initiated complex (first complex). Two premature ventricular stimuli (S_1, S_2) initiate a sustained supraventricular tachycardia that persists with a left bundle branch block for several complexes, finally reverting to normal. The retrograde atrial activation sequence is recorded first in the proximal coronary sinus lead (arrow, PCS), then in the distal coronary sinus lead (DCS) and low right atrium (HBE) and then high right atrium (HRA). During the functional bundle branch block, the V-A interval in the PCS lead is 140 msec, shortening to 110 msec when the QRS complex reverts to normal. Such behavior is characteristic of a left-sided accessory pathway with prolongation of the reentrant pathway by the functional left bundle branch block.

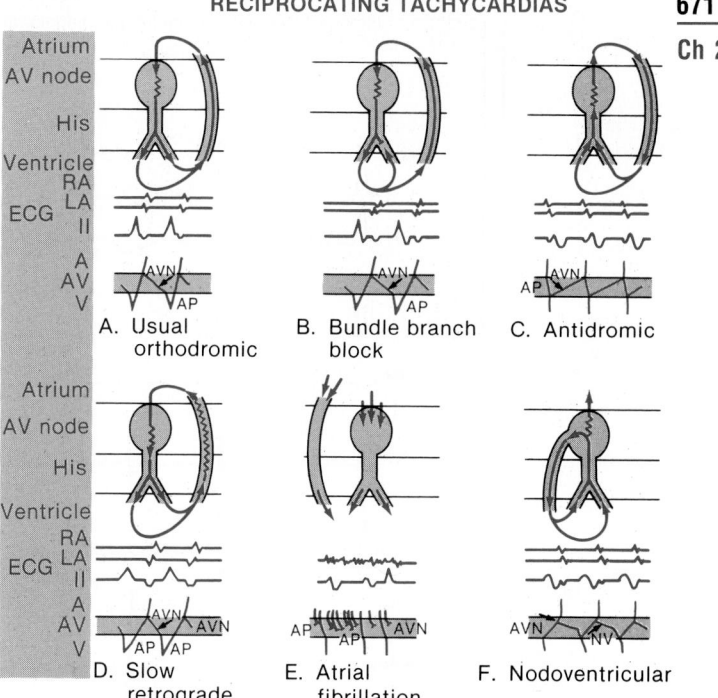

FIGURE 22–31. Schematic diagram of tachycardias associated with accessory pathways. Format as in Figure 22–11. *A*, Orthodromic tachycardia with anterograde conduction over the AV node–His bundle route and retrograde conduction over the accessory pathway (left-sided for this example as depicted by LA activation preceding RA activation). *B*, Orthodromic tachycardia and ipsilateral functional bundle branch block. *C*, Antidromic tachycardia with anterograde conduction over the accessory pathway and retrograde conduction over the AV node–His bundle. *D*, Orthodromic tachycardia with a slowly conducting accessory pathway. *E*, Atrial fibrillation with the accessory pathway as a bystander. *F*, Anterograde conduction over a portion of the AV node and a nodoventricular pathway and retrograde conduction over the AV node.

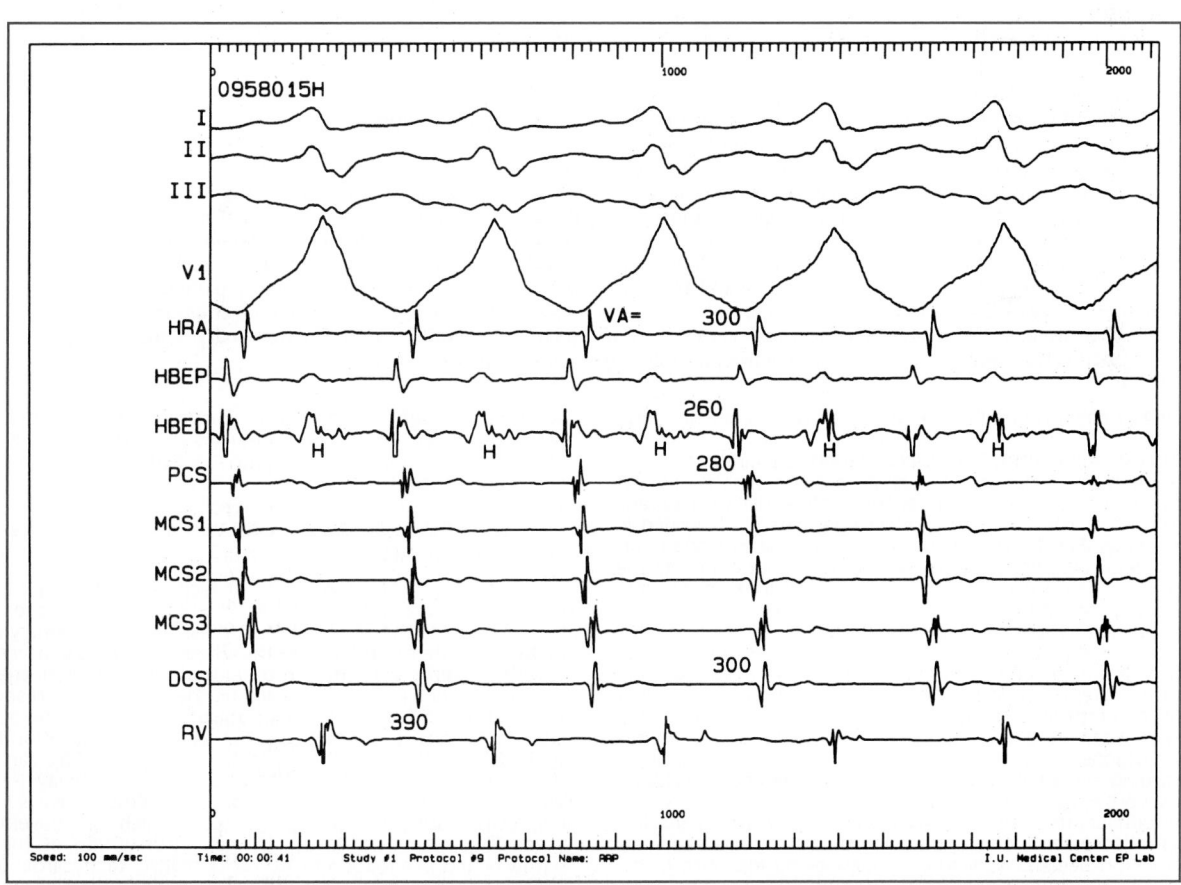

FIGURE 22–32.   Antidromic atrioventricular reciprocating tachycardia. Tachycardia in this example is due to anterograde conduction over the accessory pathway (note the abnormal QRS complex of a left posterior accessory pathway) and a normal retrograde atrial activation sequence (beginning first in the HBED lead) due to retrograde conduction over the atrioventricular node. Tachycardia cycle length is 390 msec, with a VA interval of 300 msec measured in the high right atrial lead, 260 msec in the distal His lead and 280 msec in the proximal coronary sinus lead. I, II, III, and V₁ are scalar leads; HRA, high right atrial electrogram; HBEP and HBED leads are His bundle electrogram proximal and distal, respectively; PCS, proximal coronary sinus; MCS1-3, midcoronary sinus leads; DCS, distal coronary sinus lead; RV, right ventricular electrogram.

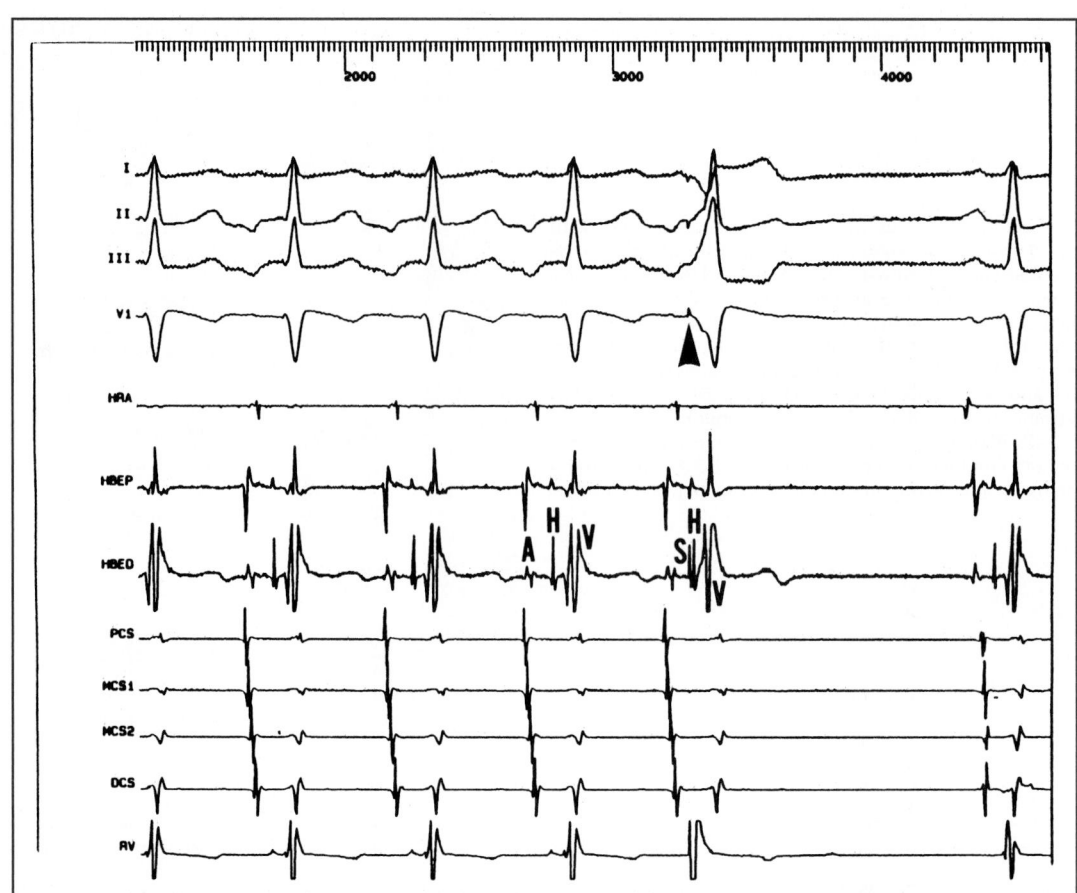

FIGURE 22–33. Termination of the permanent form of AV junctional reciprocating tachycardia (PJRT). In the left portion of this example, PJRT is present. The atrial activation sequence is indistinguishable from atypical AV nodal reentry and atrial tachycardia originating in the low right atrium. The response to premature stimulation(s) identifies the tachycardia as PJRT. Premature ventricular stimulation (arrowhead) occurs at a time when the His bundle is refractory from depolarization during the tachycardia (second labeled H). Therefore, premature ventricular stimulation cannot enter the AV node. Further, premature ventricular stimulation does not reach the atrium. Yet premature ventricular stimulation terminates the tachycardia. This can only be explained by the premature ventricular complex invading and blocking in a retrogradely conducting accessory pathway. I, II, III, and V$_1$ are scalar ECG leads; HRA, high right atrial electrogram; HBEP, HBED, His bundle electrogram proximal and distal, respectively; PCS, proximal coronary sinus electrogram; MCS1, MCS2, midcoronary sinus electrograms; DCS, distal coronary sinus electrograms; RV, right ventricular electrogram.

through the AV node–His bundle exceed those in the accessory pathway.[184,185]

RECOGNITION OF ACCESSORY PATHWAYS. When retrograde atrial activation during tachycardia occurs over an accessory pathway that connects the left atrium to the left ventricle, the earliest retrograde activity is recorded from a left atrial electrode usually positioned in the coronary sinus (Fig. 22–25). When retrograde atrial activation during tachycardia occurs over an accessory pathway that connects the right ventricle to the right atrium, the earliest retrograde atrial activity generally is recorded from a lateral right atrial electrode. Participation of a septal accessory pathway creates earliest retrograde atrial activation in the low right atrium situated near the septum, anterior or posterior, depending on the insertion site. These mapping techniques with catheter electrodes and at the time of surgery (see p. 583) provide accurate assessments of the position of the accessory pathway, which can be anywhere in the AV groove except in the intervalvular trigone between the mitral valve and the aortic valve annuli. Recording electrical activity directly from the accessory pathway obviously provides precise localization (Fig. 22–30A).

It may be difficult to distinguish AV nodal reentry from participation of a septal accessory connection using the retrograde sequence of atrial activation because activation sequences during both tachycardias are similar. Other approaches to demonstrate retrograde atrial activation over the accessory pathway must be tried and can be accomplished by inducing premature ventricular complexes during tachycardia to determine whether retrograde atrial excitation can occur from the ventricle at a time when the His bundle is refractory (Fig. 22–25B). Since ventriculoatrial conduction cannot occur over the normal conduction system because the His bundle is refractory, an accessory pathway must be present for the atria to become excited and is most likely participating in the tachycardia circuit. No patient with a reciprocating tachycardia due to an accessory AV pathway has a V-A interval of less than 70 msec measured from the onset of ventricular depolarization to the onset of the earliest atrial activity recorded on an esophageal lead or of less than 95 msec when mea-

sured to the high right atrium. In contrast, in the majority of patients with reentry in the AV node, intervals from the onset of ventricular activity to the earliest onset of atrial activity recorded in the esophageal lead are less than 70 msec.

OTHER FORMS OF TACHYCARDIA IN PATIENTS WITH WPW SYNDROME

Patients can have other types of tachycardia during which the accessory pathway is a "bystander," i.e., uninvolved in the mechanism responsible for the tachycardia, such as AV nodal reentry or an atrial tachycardia that conducts to the ventricle over the accessory pathway. In patients with atrial flutter or atrial fibrillation, the accessory pathway is not a requisite part of the mechanism responsible for tachycardia, and the flutter or fibrillation occurs in the atrium unrelated to the accessory pathway (Fig. 22–31E). Propagation to the ventricle during atrial flutter or atrial fibrillation therefore can occur over the normal AV node–His bundle or accessory pathway. Patients with WPW syndrome who have atrial fibrillation almost always have inducible reciprocating tachycardias as well, which can develop into the atrial fibrillation (Fig. 22–35). In fact, interruption of the accessory pathway and elimination of AV reciprocating tachycardia usually prevent recurrence of the atrial fibrillation. Atrial fibrillation presents a potentially serious risk because of the possibility for very rapid conduction over the accessory pathway. At more rapid rates, the refractory period of the accessory pathway can shorten significantly and permit an extremely rapid ventricular response during atrial flutter or atrial fibrillation (Figs. 22–26B and 22–30) that can lead to ventricular fibrillation. The rapid ventricular response can exceed the ability of the ventricle to follow in an organized manner, resulting in fragmented, disorganized ventricular activation and hypotension, and can lead to ventricular fibrillation (Fig. 22–36). Alternatively, supraventricular discharge bypassing AV nodal delay can activate the ventricle during the vulnerable period of the antecedent T wave and precipitate ventricular fibrillation. Patients who have had ventricular fibrilla-

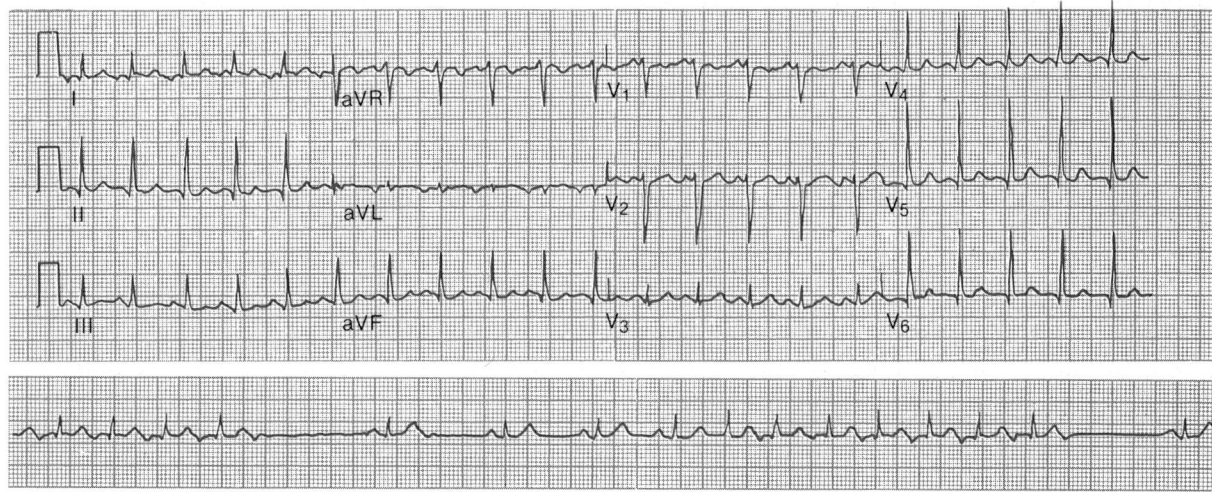

FIGURE 22-34. Permanent form of junctional reciprocating tachycardia (PJRT) in a patient with a left-sided accessory pathway. The 12-lead ECG demonstrates a long R-P interval–short PR interval tachycardia, which, in contrast to the usual form of PJRT, exhibits negative P waves in leads I and aVL. The rhythm strips below (lead I) indicate that whenever a nonconducted P wave occurs, the tachycardia always terminates, only to begin again after several sinus beats. This is in marked contrast to Figure 22-13, in which the tachycardia continues despite nonconducted P waves.

tion have ventricular cycle lengths during atrial fibrillation in the range of 200 msec or less.

Patients with preexcitation syndrome can have other causes of tachycardia such as AV nodal reentry, sometimes with dual AV nodal curves, sinus nodal reentry, or even ventricular tachycardia unrelated to the accessory pathway. Some accessory pathways can conduct anterogradely only, and others retrogradely only. If the pathway conducts only anterogradely, it cannot participate in the usual form of reciprocating tachycardia (Fig. 22-31A). It can, however, participate in antidromic tachycardia (Fig. 22-31C) as well as conduct to the ventricle during atrial flutter or atrial fibrillation (Fig. 22-31E). Some data suggest that the accessory pathway demonstrates automatic activity, which could conceivably be responsible for some instances of tachycardia.

"WIDE QRS TACHYCARDIAS." In patients with the preexcitation syndrome, so-called wide QRS tachycardias can be due to multiple mechanisms, including sinus or atrial tachycardias, AV nodal reentry, atrial flutter or fibrillation with anterograde conduction over the accessory pathway; orthodromic reciprocating tachycardia with functional or preexisting bundle branch block; antidromic reciprocating tachycardia; reciprocating tachycardia with anterograde conduction over one accessory pathway and retrograde conduction over a second one; tachycardias using Mahaim fibers; or ventricular tachycardia.[195]

CLINICAL FEATURES. The reported incidence of preexcitation syndrome depends on large measure on the population studied, varying from 0.1 to 3.0 per thousand in apparently healthy subjects, with an average of about 1.5 per thousand. The incidence of the electrocardiographic pattern of WPW conduction in 22,500 healthy aviation personnel was 0.25 per cent with a prevalence of documented tachyarrhythmias of 1.8 per cent. Left free wall accessory pathways are most common, followed in frequency by posteroseptal, right free wall, and anteroseptal locations. WPW syndrome is found in all age groups, from fetal and neonatal periods to the elderly, and in identical twins. The prevalence is higher in males and decreases with age, apparently due to loss of preexcitation. The majority of adults with preexcitation syndrome have normal hearts, although a variety of acquired and congenital cardiac defects have been reported, including Ebstein's anomaly,[196] mitral valve prolapse,[197] and cardiomyopathies. Patients with Ebstein's anomaly (see p. 934) often have multiple accessory pathways, right-sided either in the posterior septum or posterolateral wall, with preexcitation localized to the atrialized ventricle. They often have reciprocating tachycardia with a long V-A interval and a right bundle branch block morphology.

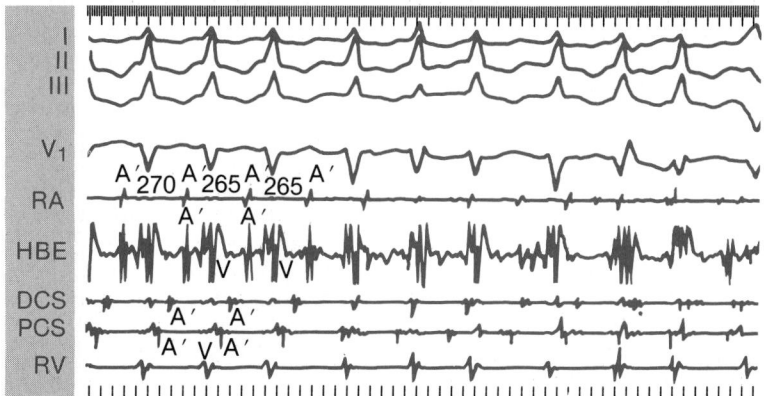

FIGURE 22-35. AV reciprocating tachycardia disorganizing into atrial fibrillation. During sustained atrioventricular reciprocating tachycardia at a cycle length of approximately 265 msec, retrograde atrial activation sequence began first in the right paraseptal region (not shown in this example; location proven at surgery) and was then recorded in the proximal coronary sinus electrogram, followed by atrial activity in the distal coronary sinus, in the low right atrium recorded in the His bundle lead and then in the high right atrium. Spontaneously, the atrial activation sequence becomes irregular (after the last A') and atrial fibrillation begins. Note that the last QRS complex reflects conduction over the accessory pathway. Such a transformation occurred repeatedly in this patient and was associated with a quickening of the ventricular rate. Atrial fibrillation did not recur following surgical interruption of the accessory pathway.

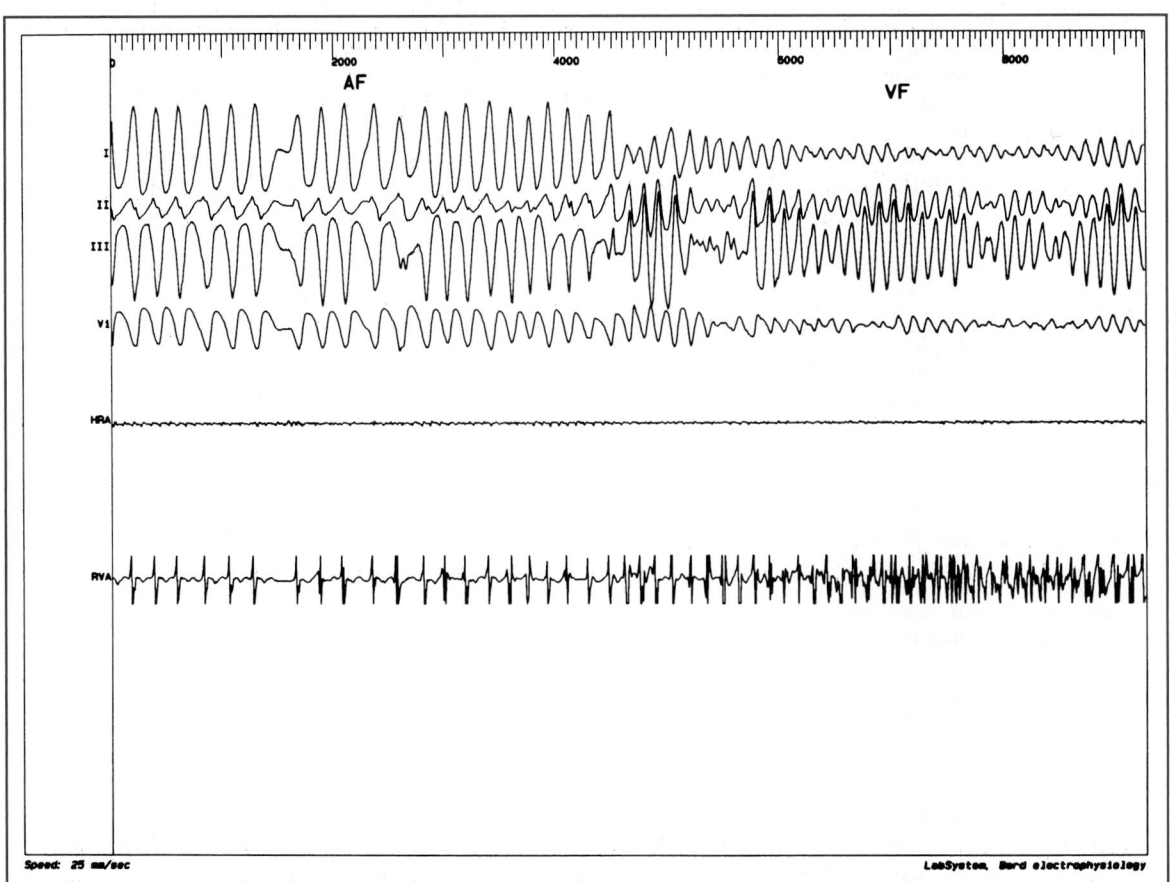

FIGURE 22–36. Atrial fibrillation becoming ventricular fibrillation. In the left portion of this panel, the ECG demonstrates atrial fibrillation with conduction over an accessory pathway producing a rapid ventricular response, at times in excess of 350 beats/min. In the midportion of the tracing, ventricular fibrillation develops. I, II, III, and V_1 are scalar ECG leads; HRA, high right atrial electrogram; RVA, right ventricular apex electrogram; AF, atrial fibrillation; VF, ventricular fibrillation.

The frequency of paroxysmal tachycardia apparently increases with age, from 10 per 100 patients with WPW syndrome in a 20- to 39-year age group to 36 per 100 in patients more than 60 years old. Approximately 80 per cent of patients with tachycardia have a reciprocating tachycardia, 15 to 30 per cent have atrial fibrillation, and 5 per cent atrial flutter. Ventricular tachycardia occurs uncommonly. The anomalous complexes can mask or mimic myocardial infarction (see p. 135), bundle branch block, or ventricular hypertrophy, and the presence of the preexcitation syndrome can call attention to an associated cardiac defect. The prognosis is excellent in patients without tachycardia or an associated cardiac anomaly. For most patients with recurrent tachycardia the prognosis is good, but sudden death occurs rarely,[198] with an estimated frequency of <0.1 per cent.[199]

It is very likely that an accessory pathway is congenital, although its manifestations can be detected in later years and appear to be "acquired." Relatives of patients with preexcitation, particularly those with multiple pathways, have an increased prevalence of preexcitation, suggesting a hereditary mode of acquisition. Some children and adults can lose their tendency to develop tachyarrhythmias as they grow older, possibly owing to fibrotic or other changes at the site of the accessory pathway insertion. Pathways can lose their ability to conduct anterogradely. Tachycardia beginning in infancy can disappear but frequently recurs. Tachycardia still present after age 5 years persists in 75 per cent of patients, regardless of accessory pathway location. Intermittent preexcitation during sinus rhythm and abrupt loss of conduction over the accessory pathway after intravenous ajmaline or procainamide and with exercise suggest that the refractory period of the accessory pathway is long and that the patient is not at risk of developing a rapid

ventricular rate should atrial flutter or fibrillation develop. These approaches are relatively specific, but not very sensitive, with a low positive predictive accuracy. Exceptions to these safeguards can occur.

TREATMENT. Patients with ventricular preexcitation who have only the electrocardiographic abnormality, without tachyarrhythmias, do not require electrophysiological evaluation or therapy. However, for the patient with frequent episodes of symptomatic tachyarrhythmias, therapy should be initiated.

Three therapeutic options exist: electrical (see p. 619) or surgical (see p. 628) ablation and pharmacological therapy. Drugs are chosen to prolong conduction time and/or refractoriness in the AV node, the accessory pathway, or both to prevent rapid rates from occurring. If successful, this would prevent maintenance of an AV reciprocating tachycardia or a rapid ventricular response to atrial flutter or atrial fibrillation. Some drugs might suppress premature complexes that precipitate the arrhythmias.

Adenosine, verapamil, propranolol, and digitalis all prolong conduction time and refractoriness in the AV node. Verapamil and propranolol do not directly affect conduction in the accessory pathway, while digitalis has had variable effects. Because digitalis has been reported to shorten refractoriness in the accessory pathway and speed the ventricular response in some patients with atrial fibrillation, it is advisable *not* to use digitalis as a single drug in patients with the WPW syndrome who have or may develop atrial flutter or atrial fibrillation. Since many patients can develop atrial fibrillation *during* the reciprocating tachycardia (Fig. 22–35), this caveat probably applies to *all* patients who have tachycardia and WPW syndrome. Rather, drugs that prolong the refractory period in the accessory pathway such as class IA and IC drugs (Chap. 21) should be used.

Class IC[200,201] drugs, amiodarone[202], and sotalol can affect both the AV node and the accessory pathway. Lidocaine does not prolong refactoriness of the accessory pathway in patients whose effective refractory period is ≤ 300 msec. Verapamil and IV lidocaine can *increase* the ventricular rate during atrial fibrillation in patients with the WPW syndrome. Intravenous verapamil can precipitate *ventricular fibrillation* when given to a patient with the WPW syndrome who has a rapid ventricular rate during atrial fibrillation. This does not appear to happen with *oral* verapamil. Catecholamines can expose WPW syndromes, shorten the refractory period of the accessory pathway, and reverse the effects of some antiarrhythmic drugs.[203]

Termination of an Acute Episode. Termination of the acute episode of reciprocating tachycardia, suspected electrocardiographically from a normal QRS complex, regular R-R intervals, a rate of about 200 beats/min, and a retrograde P wave in the ST segment, should be approached as for AV nodal reentry. After vagal maneuvers, adenosine followed by intravenous verapamil or diltiazem is the initial treatment of choice. It is important to note that atrial fibrillation can occur after drug administration, particularly adenosine, with a rapid ventricular response. An external cardioverter-defibrillator should be immediately available if necessary. For atrial flutter or fibrillation, the latter suspected from an anomalous QRS complex and grossly irregular R-R intervals (Figs. 22–26B and 22–35), drugs that prolong refractoriness in the accessory pathway, often coupled with drugs that prolong AV nodal refractoriness (e.g., procainamide and propranolol), must be used. In many patients, particularly those with a very rapid ventricular response and any signs of hemodynamic impairment, electrical cardioversion is the *initial* treatment of choice.

Prevention. For long-term therapy to prevent a recurrence, it is not always possible to predict which drugs may be most effective for an individual patient. Some drugs actually can increase the frequency of episodes of reciprocating tachycardia by prolonging the duration of anterograde and not retrograde refractory periods of the accessory pathway, thereby making it easier for a premature atrial complex to block anterogradely in the accessory pathway and initiate tachycardia. Oral administration of two drugs, such as quinidine and propranolol or procainamide and verapamil, to decrease conduction capabilities in both limbs of the reentrant circuit can be beneficial. Class IC drugs, amiodarone, or sotalol, which prolong refractoriness in both the accessory pathway and the AV node, can be effective.[204,205] Depending on the clinical situation, empirical drug trials or serial electrophysiological drug testing can be employed to determine optimal drug therapy for patients with reciprocating tachycardia. For patients who have atrial fibrillation with a rapid ventricular response, induction of atrial fibrillation while the patient is receiving therapy is essential to be certain that the ventricular rate is controlled. Patients who have accessory pathways with very short refractory periods may be poor candidates for drug therapy, since the refractory periods may be prolonged insignificantly in response to the standard agents.

Electrical or Surgical Ablation (see Chap. 21). Radio-frequency catheter ablation of the accessory pathway is advisable for patients with frequent symptomatic arrhythmias that are not fully controlled by drugs, in patients who are drug intolerant, or in those who do not wish to take drugs. This option should be considered early in the course of therapy of the symptomatic patient because of its high success rate and low frequency of complications and potential cost-effectiveness.[63,65,70,206–208] Rarely, surgical interruption of the accessory pathway may be necessary[209,210] (see p. 631).

Summary of Supraventricular Tachycardias

Electrocardiographic clues are often present that permit differentiation among the various supraventricular tachy-

TABLE 22–3 SUPRAVENTRICULAR TACHYCARDIAS **675**

Ch 22

SHORT R-P/LONG P-R	LONG R-P/SHORT P-R
AV node reentry	Atrial tachycardia
AV reentry	Sinus node reentry
	Atypical AV node reentry
	AVRT with a slowly conducting accessory pathway (e.g., PJRT)

cardias. P waves during tachycardia identical to sinus P waves and occurring with a long R-P interval and a short P-R interval are most likely due to sinus nodal reentry. Retrograde (inverted in II, III, and aV_f) P waves generally represent reentry involving the AV junction, either AV nodal reentry or reciprocating tachycardia using a paraseptal accessory pathway. Tachycardia without manifest P waves is probably due to AV nodal reentry (P waves buried in QRS), while a tachycardia with an R-P interval exceeding 60 to 70 msec may be due to an accessory pathway. AV dissociation or AV block during tachycardia excludes the presence of a functioning AV accessory pathway and makes AV nodal reentry less likely. Multiple tachycardias can occur at different times in the same patient. QRS alternans, thought to be a feature of AV reciprocating tachycardia, is more likely a rapid rate–related phenomenon, independent of the tachycardia mechanism. RP-PR relationships (Table 22–3) help differentiate supraventricular tachycardias.

VENTRICULAR RHYTHM DISTURBANCES

Premature Ventricular Complexes

ELECTROCARDIOGRAPHIC RECOGNITION. A premature ventricular complex is characterized by the premature occurrence of a QRS complex that is bizarre in shape and has a duration usually exceeding the dominant QRS complex, generally greater than 120 msec. The T wave is commonly large and opposite in direction to the major deflection of the QRS. The QRS complex is not preceded by a premature P wave but can be preceded by a nonconducted sinus P wave occurring at its expected time. The diagnosis of a premature ventricular complex can never be made with unequivocal certainty from the scalar electrocardiogram, since a supraventricular beat or rhythm can mimic the manifestations of ventricular arrhythmia (Figs. 22–19 and 22–37). Retrograde transmission to the atria from the premature ventricular complex occurs fairly frequently but is often obscured by the distorted QRS complex and T wave. If the retrograde impulse discharges and resects the sinus node prematurely, it produces a pause that is not fully compensatory. More commonly, the sinus node and atria are not discharged prematurely by the retrograde impulse, since interference of impulses frequently occurs at the AV junction (see p. 692), establishing a collision between the anterograde impulse conducted from the sinus node and the retrograde impulse conducted from the premature ventricular complex. Therefore, a fully compensatory pause usually follows a premature ventricular complex: the R-R interval produced by the two sinus-initiated QRS complexes on either side of the premature complex equals twice the normally conducted R-R interval. The premature ventricular complex may not produce any pause and may therefore be interpolated (Fig. 22–37E), or it may produce a postponed compensatory pause when an interpolated premature complex causes P-R prolongation of the first postextrasystolic beat to such a degree that the P wave of the second postextrasystolic beat occurs at a very short R-P interval and is therefore blocked.[211]

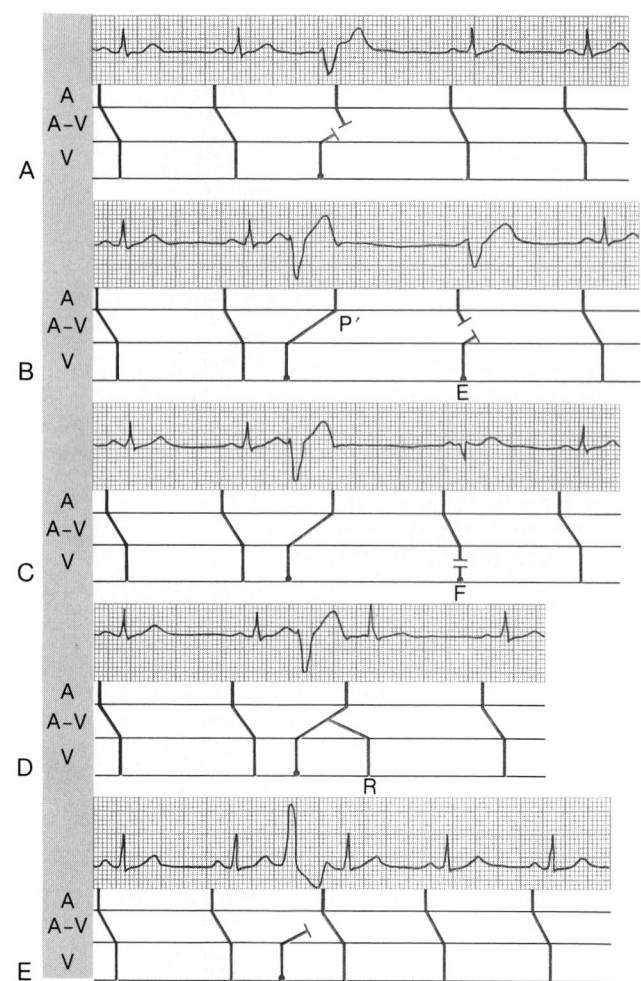

FIGURE 22–37. Premature ventricular complexes. *A* to *D* were recorded in the same patient. *A,* A late premature ventricular complex results in a compensatory pause. *B,* A slower sinus rate and a slightly earlier premature complex results in retrograde atrial excitation (P'). The sinus node is reset, producing a noncompensatory pause. Before the sinus-initiated P wave that follows the retrograde P wave can conduct to the ventricle, a ventricular escape (E) occurs. *C,* Events are similar to those in *B* except that a ventricular fusion beat (F) results following the premature ventricular complex owing to a slightly faster sinus rate. *D,* The impulse propagating retrogradely to the atrium reverses its direction after a delay and returns to reexcite the ventricles (R) to produce a ventricular echo. *E,* An interpolated premature ventricular complex is followed by a slightly prolonged P-R interval of the sinus-initiated beat. Lead II.

Interference within the ventricle can result in *ventricular fusion beats* (see p. 712) due to the simultaneous activation of the ventricle by two foci, one of them from the supraventricular impulse and the other from the premature ventricular complex. On occasion, a fusion beat can be narrower than the dominant sinus beat. This occurs when a right bundle branch block pattern of a premature ventricular complex arising in the left ventricle fuses with the sinus-initiated complex conducting through the AV junction or when the ventricle with a left bundle branch block pattern is paced artificially, producing a narrow ventricular fusion beat between the paced and the sinus-conducted beats. Narrow premature ventricular complexes also have been explained as originating at a point equidistant from

each ventricle in the ventricular septum and by arising high in the fascicular system. Whether a compensatory or noncompensatory pause, retrograde atrial excitation, or an interpolated complex, fusion complex, or echo beat occurs (Fig. 22–37), it is merely a function of how the AV junction conducts and the timing of the events taking place.

The term *bigeminy* refers to pairs of complexes and indicates a normal and premature complex; *trigeminy* indicates a premature complex following two normal beats; a premature complex following three normal beats is called *quadrigeminy;* and so on. Two successive premature ventricular complexes are termed a *pair* or a *couplet,* while three successive premature ventricular complexes are called a *triplet.* Arbitrarily, three or more successive premature ventricular complexes are termed *ventricular tachycardia.* Premature ventricular complexes can have different contours and often are called *multifocal* (Fig. 22–38). More properly they should be called "multiform," "polymorphic," or "pleomorphic," since it is not known whether multiple foci are discharging or whether conduction of the impulse originating from one site is merely changing.

Premature ventricular complexes can exhibit fixed or variable coupling; i.e., the interval between the normal QRS complex and the premature ventricular complex can be relatively stable or variable. Fixed coupling can be due to reentry, triggered activity (see p. 566), or other mechanisms. Variable coupling can be due to parasystole[212] (see p. 693), to changing conduction in a reentrant circuit, or to changing discharge rates of triggered activity. Usually, it is difficult to determine the precise mechanism responsible for the premature ventricular complex based on either constant or variable coupling intervals. Focal mechanism can be important, without macroreentry.[213]

CLINICAL FEATURES. The prevalence of premature complexes increases with age and is associated with male sex and reduced serum potassium concentration.[214] They are more frequent in the morning in patients after myocardial infarction, but this circadian variation is absent in patients with severe left ventricular dysfunction.[215] Symptoms of palpitations or discomfort in the neck or chest can result because of the greater-than-normal contractile force of the postextrasystolic beat or the feeling that the heart has stopped during the long pause after the premature complex. Long runs of frequent premature ventricular complexes in patients with heart disease can produce angina or hypotension. Frequent interpolated premature ventricular complexes actually represent a doubling of the heart rate and can compromise the patient's hemodynamic status. Activity that increases the heart rate can decrease the patient's awareness of the premature systole or reduce their number. Exercise can increase the number of premature complexes in some patients. Premature systoles can be quite uncomfortable in patients who have aortic regurgitation because of the large stroke volume. Sleep is usually associated with a decrease in the frequency of ventricular arrhythmias, but some patients can experience an increase.

Premature ventricular complexes occur in association with a variety of stimuli and can be produced by direct mechanical, electrical, and chemical stimulation of the myocardium. Often they are noted in patients with left ventricular false tendons, during infection, in ischemic or inflamed myocardium, and during hypoxia, anesthesia, or surgery. They can be provoked by a variety of medications, by electrolyte imbalance, by tension states, by myocardial stretch,[216,217] and by excessive use of tobacco, caffeine, or

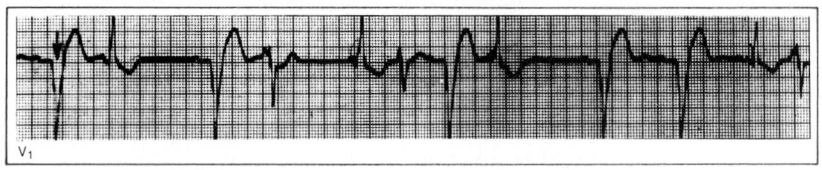

FIGURE 22–38. Multiform premature ventricular complexes. The normally conducted QRS complexes exhibit a left bundle branch block contour (arrow) and are followed by premature ventricular complexes with three different morphologies.

alcohol. Both central and peripheral autonomic stimulation have profound effects on heart rate, which can produce or suppress premature complexes. Almost 20 per cent of patients recovering from acute myocardial infarction treated by fibrinolytic drugs have more than 10 premature ventricular complexes per hour.[218] Increased premature ventricular complexes during anitarrhythmic drug titration in the CAST study predicted patients at increased risk of arrhythmic death despite antiarrhythmic drug treatment.[219]

Physical examination reveals the presence of a premature beat followed by a pause that is longer than normal. A fully compensatory pause can be distinguished from one that is not fully compensatory, since the former does not change the timing of the basic rhythm. The premature beat is often accompanied by a decrease in intensity of the heart sounds, often with auscultation of just the first heart sound, which can be sharp and snapping, and a decreased or absent peripheral (e.g., radial) pulse. The relationship of atrial to ventricular systole determines the presence of normal *a* waves or giant *a* waves in the jugular venous pulse, and the length of the P-R interval determines the intensity of the first heart sound. The second heart sound can be abnormally split, depending on the origin of the ventricular complex.

The importance of premature ventricular complexes varies depending on the clinical setting. In the absence of underlying heart disease, the presence of premature ventricular complexes usually has no impact on longevity or limitation of activity; antiarrhythmic drugs are not indicated.[220,221] The patient should be reassured if he or she is symptomatic (see Chap. 20, Exercise Testing and Long-Term ECG Recording). In men without apparent coronary disease, the incidental detection of ventricular arrthymias is associated with a twofold increase in risk for all-cause mortality and myocardial infarction or death due to coronary disease.[222] However, it has not been demonstrated that premature ventricular systoles or complex ventricular arrhythmias play a *precipitating* role in the genesis of sudden death in these patients, and the arrhythmias may simply be a marker of heart disease. Results from electrophysiologic testing suggest that patients with premature ventricular complexes who do not have ventricular tachycardia induced at electrophysiological study have a low incidence of subsequent sudden death. Antiarrhythmic therapy given to suppress the premature ventricular systoles or complex ventricular arrhythmias has not been shown to reduce the incidence of sudden death in such apparently healthy men.

In patients suffering from acute myocardial infarction, premature ventricular complexes considered to presage the onset of ventricular fibrillation, such as those occurring close to the preceding T wave, more than five or six per minute, bigeminal or multiform complexes, or those occurring in salvoes of two, three, or more, do not occur in about half the patients who develop ventricular fibrillation, and about half of those patients who have these premature ventricular complexes do not develop ventricular fibrillation. Thus these premature ventricular complexes are not particularly helpful prognostically. The presence of one[223] to more than ten ventricular extrasystoles per hour[224] can identify patients at increased risk of developing ventricular tachycardia or sudden cardiac death after myocardial infarction.[225]

MANAGEMENT. Both fast and slow heart rates can provoke the development of premature ventricular complexes. Premature ventricular complexes accompanying slow ventricular rates can be abolished by increasing the basic rate with atropine or isoproterenol or by pacing, whereas slowing the heart rate in some patients with sinus tachycardia can eradicate premature ventricular complexes. In the hospitalized patient, intravenous lidocaine (see p. 605) is generally the initial treatment of choice to suppress premature ventricular complexes. If maximum dosages of lidocaine are unsuccessful, then procainamide given intravenously

can be tried. Quinidine can be given intravenously slowly and cautiously. Propranolol can be tried if the other drugs have been unsuccessful. Intravenous magnesium can be useful.[226] For long-term oral maintenance, a variety of class I,[205] II,[227] and III[202,228] drugs can be useful, to prevent ventricular tachycardia. Class IC drugs seem particularly successful in suppressing premature ventricular complexes, but flecainide and moricizine have been shown to increase mortality in patients treated after myocardial infarction.[229] Amiodarone[202,230–234] can be quite effective. Athletes with structural heart disease and ventricular extrasystoles who are in high-risk groups can participate in low-intensity sports only.[46] In patients with isolated systolic hypertension, chlorthalidone in doses that are effective in decreasing stroke and cardiovascular event rates do not increase the frequency of ventricular extrasystole.[235] Thrombolysis therapy does not influence the frequency of ventricular extrasystoles,[236] which are related to residual left ventricular pump performance after myocardial infarction.[237] Low levels of serum potassium and magnesium are associated with higher prevalence rates of ventricular arrhythmias.[238] Metroprolol and diltiazem but not enalapril or hydrochlorothiazide reduce premature ventricular complexes in patients with hypertension.[239]

Ventricular Tachycardia

ELECTROCARDIOGRAPHIC RECOGNITION. Ventricular tachycardia arises distal to the bifurcation of the His bundle, in the specialized conduction system, in ventricular muscle, or in combinations of both tissue types.[240] The mechanisms include disorders of impulse formation and conduction considered earlier (Chap. 20). Autonomic modulation can be important. The electrocardiographic diagnosis of ventricular tachycardia is suggested by the occurrence of a series of three or more consecutive, bizarrely shaped premature ventricular complexes whose duration exceeds 120 msec, with the ST-T vector pointing opposite to the major QRS deflection. The R-R interval can be exceedingly regular or can vary. Patients can have ventricular tachycardias with multiple morphologies originating at the same or closely adjacent sites, probably with different exit paths. Others have multiple sites of origin. Atrial activity can be independent of ventricular activity (AV dissociation, p. 692), or the atria can be depolarized by the ventricles retrogradely (VA association). Depending on the particular type of ventricular tachycardia, the rates range from 70 to 250 beats/min, and the onset can be paroxysmal (sudden) or nonparoxysmal. QRS contours during the ventricular tachycardia can be unchanging (uniform, monomorphic), can vary randomly (multiform, polymorphic, or pleomorphic), can vary in a more or less repetitive manner (torsades de pointes), can vary in alternate complexes (bidirectional ventricular tachycardia), or can vary in a stable but changing contour (i.e., right bundle branch contour changing to left bundle branch contour). Ventricular tachycardia can be sustained, defined arbitrarily as lasting longer than 30 sec or requiring termination because of hemodynamic collapse, or nonsustained, when it stops spontaneously in less than 30 sec. Most commonly, very premature stimulation is required to initiate ventricular tachycardia electrically, while late coupled ventricular complexes usually initiate its spontaneous onset[240] (Fig. 22–39).

Making the electrocardiographic distinction between supraventricular tachycardia with aberration and ventricular tachycardia can be difficult at times, since features of both arrhythmias overlap, and under certain circumstances a supraventricular tachycardia can mimic the criteria established for ventricular tachycardia.[241–243] Ventricular complexes with a bizarre or prolonged configuration indicate only that conduction through the ventricle is abnormal, and such complexes can occur in supraventricular rhythms due to preexisting bundle branch block, aberrant conduc-

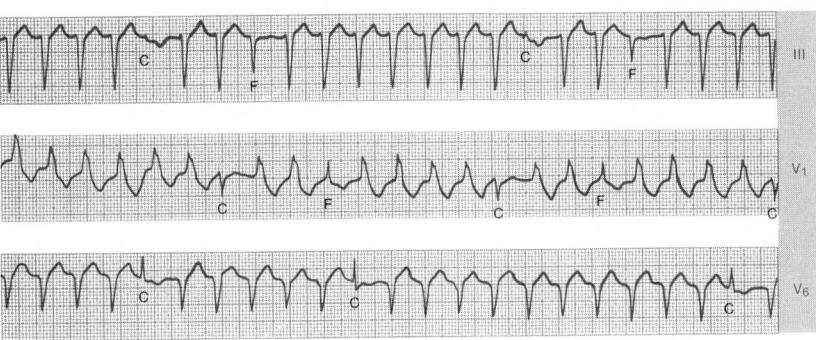

FIGURE 22–39. Fusion and capture beats during a ventricular tachycardia. The QRS complex is prolonged, and the R-R interval is regular except for occasional capture beats (C) that have a normal contour and are slightly premature. Complexes intermediate in contour represent fusion beats (F). Thus, even though atrial activity is not clearly apparent, AV dissociation is present during a ventricular tachycardia and produces intermittent capture and fusion beats.

tion during incomplete recovery of repolarization, conduction over accessory pathways, and several other conditions. These complexes do not necessarily indicate the origin of impulse formation or the reason for the abnormal conduction. Conversely, ectopic beats originating in the ventricle uncommonly can have a fairly normal duration and shape. However, it is important to emphasize that ventricular tachycardia is the most common cause of a wide QRS complex tachycardia. A past history of myocardial infarction makes the diagnosis even more likely.

During the course of a tachycardia characterized by widespread, bizarre QRS complexes, the presence of fusion beats and capture beats provides maximum support for the diagnosis of ventricular tachycardia (Table 22–4). *Fusion beats* indicate activation of the ventricle from two different foci, implying that one of the foci had a ventricular origin. *Capture* of the ventricle by the supraventricular rhythm with a normal configuration of the captured QRS complex at an interval shorter than the tachycardia in question indicates that the impulse has a supraventricular origin (Fig. 22–39). Atrioventricular dissociation (see p. 692) has long been considered a hallmark of ventricular tachycardia. However, retrograde VA conduction to the atria from ventricular beats occur in at least 25 per cent of patients, and therefore, ventricular tachycardia may not exhibit AV dissociation. Atrioventricular dissociation can occur uncommonly during supraventricular tachycardias. Even if a P wave appears to be related to each QRS complex, it is at times difficult to determine whether the P wave is conducted anterogradely to the next QRS complex (i.e., supraventricular tachycardia with aberrancy and a long P-R interval) or retrogradely from the preceding QRS complex (i.e., a ventricular tachycardia). As a general rule, however, AV dissociation during a wide QRS tachycardia is strong presumptive evidence that the tachycardia is of ventricular origin.

DIFFERENTIATION BETWEEN VENTRICULAR AND SUPRAVENTRICULAR TACHYCARDIA. Some electrocardiographic features characterizing supraventricular arrhythmia with aberrancy are (1) consistent onset of the tachycardia with a premature P wave, (2) a very short R-P interval (≤ 0.1 sec) often requiring an esophageal recording to visualize the P waves, (3) a QRS configuration the same as that which occurs from known supraventricular conduction at similar rates, (4) P-wave and QRS rate and rhythm linked to suggest that ventricular activation depends on atrial discharge (e.g., AV Wenckebach block), and (5) slowing or termination of the tachycardia by vagal maneuvers.

Analysis of specific QRS contours also can be helpful in diagnosing ventricular tachycardia and localizing its site of origin. For example, QRS contours suggesting a ventricular tachycardia include the left-axis deviation in the frontal plane and a QRS duration exceeding 140 msec with a QRS of normal duration during sinus rhythm. During ventricular tachycardia with a right bundle branch block appearance, (1) the QRS complex is monophasic or biphasic in V_1 with an initial deflection different from sinus-initiated QRS complex, (2) the amplitude of the R wave in V_1 exceeds the R′, and (3) small R and large S wave or a QS pattern in V_6 may be present. With a ventricular tachycardia having a left bundle branch block contour, (1) the axis can be rightward with negative deflections deeper in V_1 than in V_6, (2) a broad prolonged (> 40 msec) R wave in V_1, and (3) a small Q–large R-wave or QS pattern in V_6 can exist. A QRS complex that is similar in V_1 through V_6, either all negative or all positive, favors a ventricular origin as does the presence of 2:1 ventriculoatrial block. (An upright QRS complex in V_1 through V_6 also can occur due to conduction over a left-sided accessory pathway.) Supraventricular beats with aberration often have a triphasic pattern in V_1, an initial vector of the abnormal complex similar to that of the normally conducted beats, and a wide QRS complex that terminates a short cycle length that follows a long cycle (long-short cycle sequence). During atrial fibrillation, fixed coupling, short coupling intervals, a long pause after the abnormal beat, and runs of bigeminy rather than a consecutive series of abnormal complexes all favor ventricular origin of the premature complex rather than supraventricular origin with aberration. A grossly irregular, wide QRS tachycardia with ventricular rates exceeding 200 beats/min should raise the question of atrial fibrillation with conduction over an accessory pathway (Figs. 22–6B and 22–30). In the presence of preexisting bundle branch block, a wide QRS tachycardia with a contour different from that which occurred during sinus rhythm is most likely a ventricular tachycardia. Exceptions exist to all the aforementioned criteria, especially in patients who have preexisting conduction disturbances or preexcitation syndrome; when in doubt, one must rely on sound clinical judgment, considering the ECG as only one of several helpful ancillary tests.

Termination of a tachycardia by triggering vagal reflexes is considered diagnostic of supraventricular tachycardias. However, ventricular tachycardia rarely can be stopped in a similar manner.

ELECTROPHYSIOLOGICAL FEATURES. Electrophysiologically, ventricular tachycardia can be distinguished by a short or negative H-V interval (i.e., H begins after the onset of ventricular depolarization) because of retrograde activa-

TABLE 22–4 MAJOR FEATURES IN THE DIFFERENTIAL DIAGNOSIS OF WIDE QRS BEATS VERSUS TACHYCARDIA

SUPPORTS SVT	SUPPORTS VT
Slowing or termination by ↑ vagal tone	Fusion beats
Onset with premature P wave	Capture beats
RP interval ≤ 100 msec	AV dissociation
P and QRS rate and rhythm linked to suggest ventricular activation depends on atrial discharge, e.g., 2:1 AV block	P and QRS rate and rhythm linked to suggest atrial activation depends on ventricular discharge, e.g., 2:1 VA block
RSR′ V_1	
Long-short cycle sequence	"Compensatory" pause
	Left axis deviation; QRS duration > 140 msec
	Specific QRS contours (see text)

SVT = supraventricular tachycardia; VT = ventricular tachycardia.

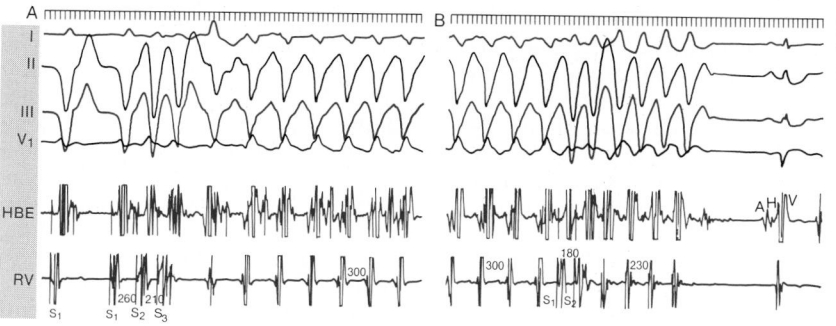

FIGURE 22–40. Initiation and termination of ventricular tachycardia using programed ventricular stimulation. The last two ventricular-paced beats at a cycle length of 600 msec are shown in panel A. A premature stimulus (S_2) at an S_1-S_2 interval of 260 msec and another premature stimulus (S_3) at a cycle length of 210 msec initiate a sustained monomorphic ventricular tachycardia at a cycle length of 300 msec. Two premature ventricular stimuli (S_1-S_2) in panel B create an unstable ventricular tachycardia which persists for several beats at a shorter cycle length (230 msec) and then terminates, followed by sinus rhythm.

tion from the ventricles (see Fig. 20–40, p. 582). His bundle deflections usually are not apparent during ventricular tachycardia because they are obscured by simultaneous ventricular septal depolarization or because of inadequate catheter position. The latter must be determined during supraventricular rhythm before the onset or after the termination of ventricular tachycardia (Fig. 22–40). His bundle deflections dissociated from ventricular activation are diagnostic, with rare exception. Ventricular tachycardia can produce QRS complexes of narrow duration and of short H-V interval, most likely when the site of origin is close to the His bundle in the fascicles.

Successful electrical induction of ventricular tachycardia by premature stimulation of the ventricle (Fig. 22–40) depends on the characteristics of the ventricular tachycardia and the anatomical substrate. Patients with sustained, hemodynamically stable ventricular tachycardia and ventricular tachycardia due to chronic coronary artery disease have monomorphic ventricular tachycardia induced (>90 per cent) more frequently than patients who present with nonsustained ventricular tachycardia, ventricular tachycardia due to noncoronary-related causes or acute ischemia, and cardiac arrest (40 to 75 per cent).[244] In general, it is more difficult to induce ventricular tachycardia with late premature ventricular stimuli compared with early premature stimuli, during sinus rhythm compared with ventricular pacing, and with one premature stimulus compared with two or three.[245] The specificity of ventricular tachycardia induction using more than two premature ventricular stimuli begins to decrease (while the sensitivity increases), and nonsustained polymorphic ventricular tachycardia or ventricular fibrillation can be induced in patients who have no history of ventricular tachycardia. Of patients who present with stable ventricular tachycardia who have inducible sustained monomorphic ventricular tachycardia, the latter is induced in about 25 per cent with single extra stimuli, 50 per cent with double extrastimuli, and 25 per cent with triple extrastimuli.[246] A recent study suggests that using a single basic cycle length of 400 msec and up to four extrastimuli can be an adequate induction technique.[247] Occasionally, ventricular tachycardia can be initiated only from the left ventricle or from specific sites in the right ventricle. Multiple premature stimuli reduce the need for left ventricular stimulation. Drugs such as isoproterenol, various antiarrhythmic agents, and alcohol can facilitate the induction of ventricular tachycardia. Coughing during ventricular tachycardia that causes hypotension can help to maintain blood pressure.

Termination by pacing depends significantly on the rate of the ventricular tachycardia and the site of pacing.[248] Slower ventricular tachycardias are terminated more easily and with fewer stimuli than are more rapid ones. An increasing number of stimuli are required to terminate more rapid ventricular tachycardias, which increases the risks of pacing-induced acceleration of the ventricular tachycardia. Subthreshold stimulation and transthoracic stimulation can terminate ventricular tachycardia. Atrial pacing, at times, also can induce and terminate ventricular tachycardia (see Fig. 20–41, p. 583).

CLINICAL FEATURES. Symptoms occurring during ventric-

ular tachycardia depend on the ventricular rate, duration of tachycardia, the presence and extent of the underlying heart disease and peripheral vascular disease. Ventricular tachycardia can be in the form of short, asymptomatic, nonsustained episodes,[249] sustained, hemodynamically stable events, generally occurring at slower rates or in otherwise normal hearts, or unstable runs, often degenerating into ventricular fibrillation. Some patients who have nonsustained ventricular tachycardias initially, later develop sustained episodes or ventricular fibrillation.[246] The location of impulse formation and therefore the way in which the depolarization wave spreads across the myocardium also can be important. Physical findings depend in part on the P-to-QRS relationship. If atrial activity is dissociated from the ventricular contractions, the findings of AV dissociation (see p. 692) are present. If the atria are captured retrogradely, regularly occurring cannon *a* waves appear when atrial and ventricular contractions occur simultaneously and the signs of AV dissociation are absent.

More than half the patients treated for symptomatic recurrent ventricular tachycardia have ischemic heart disease. The next biggest group has cardiomyopathy (both congestive[250–252] and hypertrophic[253–255]) with lesser percentages divided among those with primary electrical disease,[256] mitral valve prolapse,[257] valvular heart disease, congenital heart disease,[258] and miscellaneous causes. Left ventricular hypertrophy can lead to ventricular arrhythmias.[259,260] Coronary artery spasm can cause transient myocardial ischemia with severe ventricular arrhythmias (during ischemia as well as during the apparent reperfusion period) in some patients.[244] Complex ventricular arrhythmias can occur *after* coronary artery bypass grafting. In patients resuscitated from sudden cardiac death (Chap. 24), the majority (75 per cent) have severe coronary artery disease, and ventricular tachyarrhythmias can be induced by premature ventricular stimulation in approximately 75 per cent. When ventricular tachycardia occurs in the ambulatory patient, it is uncommonly induced by R-on-T premature ventricular complexes (see Ventricular Fibrillation, p. 686). Patients who have sustained ventricular tachycardia are more likely to have reduced ejection fraction, slowed ventricular conduction and electrogram abnormalities, left ventricular aneurysm, abnormal signal-averaged ECGs, and previous myocardial infarction than are patients who have ventricular fibrillation, indicating different electrophysiological and anatomical substances. When sustained ventricular tachycardia can be induced electrically, patients who present with cardiac arrest have faster rates than do patients who present with ventricular tachycardia. Cycle length of induced ventricular tachycardia correlates with whether the patient presents with cardiac arrest or sustained ventricular tachycardia.[246] Young patients also can suffer cardiac arrest from ventricular tachycardia or ventricular fibrillation, and persistent electrical inducibility of arrhythmias in these patients connotes a poor prognosis. In patients with coronary artery disease, sustained ventricular tachycardia displays a circadian variation, with peak frequency in the morning.[261]

Many approaches have been used to assess prognosis in patients with ventricular arrhythmias. Reduced baroreceptor sensitivity and heart period variability apparently due to reduced vagal activity may indicate an increased risk of ventricular tachycardia or sudden cardiac death.[262,263] The presence of nonsustained ventricular tachycardia after myocardial infarction often presages sudden cardiac death. Findings of reduced left ventricular function, spontaneous ventricular arrhythmias, late potentials on signal-averaged ECG,[264] Q-T interval dispersion,[265,266] and inducible sustained ventricular tachyarrhythmias at electrophysiological study all carry increased risk, further exaggerated when two or more of these features are present in the same patient. Also, clinical presentation of cardiac arrest during the first spontaneous episode of ventricular arrhythmia identifies patients at increased risk. Ventricular fibrillation is more likely to occur earlier than sustained ventricular tachycardia in patients after myocardial infarction. Electrophysiological testing can be used to stratify patients according to risk and to help guide therapy in cardiac arrest survivors and patients with sustained or nonsustained ventricular tachycardia, unexplained syncope after myocardial infarction, and cardiomyopathy.

MANAGEMENT. The most important decision involves whether or not to treat. Because reduction in sudden death with antiarrhythmic drug therapy (excluding beta blockers and perhaps amiodarone[202,267]) has not been demonstrated in controlled studies, therapy of asymptomatic patients should, in general, be discouraged. Treatment is reserved for prevention or reduction of symptoms produced by sustained and at times nonsustained ventricular tachyarrhythmias; it can be divided into approaches used to terminate sustained ventricular tachycardia and to prevent recurrences.

Termination of Sustained Ventricular Tachycardia. Ventricular tachycardia that does not cause hemodynamic decompression can be treated medically to achieve acute termination by administering intravenous lidocaine or procainamide, followed by an infusion of the successful drug. Lidocaine is often ineffective[232]; sotalol[268,269] and procainamide appear to be superior. Although quinidine can be used intravenously, great caution is needed because of hypotension. Amiodarone is effective intravenously.[270–274a]

If the arrhythmia does not respond to medical therapy, electrical DC cardioversion can be employed. Ventricular tachycardia that precipitates hypotension, shock, angina, or congestive heart failure or symptoms of cerebral hypoperfusion should be treated *promptly* with DC cardioversion (see p. 619). Very low energies can terminate ventricular tachycardia, beginning with a synchronized shock of 10 to 50 joules. Digitalis-induced ventricular tachycardia is best treated pharmacologically. After conversion of the arrhythmia to a normal rhythm, it is essential to institute measures to prevent a recurrence.

Striking the patient's chest, sometimes called "thumpversion" (see p. 762), can terminate ventricular tachycardia by mechanically inducing a premature ventricular complex that presumably interrupts the reentrant pathway necessary to support it. Chest stimulation at the time of the vulnerable period during the arrhythmia can accelerate the ventricular tachycardia or possibly provoke ventricular fibrillation.

In patients with recurrent ventricular tachycardia, competitive ventricular pacing via a pacing catheter inserted into the right ventricle or transcutaneously can be used. This procedure incurs the risk of accelerating the ventricular tachycardia to ventricular flutter or ventricular fibrillation. Synchronized cardioversion via a catheter electrode in the ventricle can be performed. Intermittent ventricular tachycardia, interrupted by several supraventricular beats, is generally best treated pharmacologically.

A search for reversible conditions contributing to the initiation and maintenance of ventricular tachycardia should be made and the conditions corrected if possible. For example, ventricular tachycardia related to ischemia, hypo-

tension, or hypokalemia at times can be terminated by antianginal treatment, vasopressors, or potassium, respectively. Correction of heart failure can reduce the frequency of ventricular arrhythmias.[252] Slow ventricular rates that are caused by sinus bradycardia or AV block can permit the occurrence of premature ventricular complexes and ventricular tachyarrhythmias that can be corrected by administering atropine, by temporary isoproterenol administration, or by transvenous pacing. Supraventricular tachycardia can initiate ventricular tachyarrhythmias and should be prevented if possible.

Prevention of Recurrences. This is generally more difficult than is terminating the acute episode, and there is no "right" drug to choose. Often, because of similar levels of efficacy, drugs are selected on the basis of potential side effects, e.g., avoiding procainamide for long-term therapy because of the development of drug-induced lupus, avoiding flecainide and disopyramide in patients with reduced left ventricular function, not giving disopyramide to patients with prostate enlargement, and withholding flecainide and moricizine from patients after myocardial infarction. Positive attributes of drugs are helpful. For example, class IB drugs might be chosen early for a patient whose Q-T interval is prolonged. Moricizine, sotalol,[269,275,276] and propafenone are well tolerated by patients and have minimal side effects, allowing for an early choice. One group of patients may have a unique form of ventricular tachycardia that may be precipitated by physical activity and is mediated or triggered by catecholamines and cyclic AMP and is suppressed by adenosine, vagal maneuvers, beta-adrenoceptor blockade, and verapamil[277,278] (see p. 616). Verapamil can be effective in some other types of ventricular tachycardia. Verapamil-sensitive ventricular tachycardias often have a right bundle branch block morphology with left-axis deviation, often arise in the left ventricular septum in patients without structure heart disease, and are precipitated when critical heart rates are achieved (see p. 683). Usually, however, verapamil is not effective in the vast majority of patients with ventricular tachycardia. Although amiodarone is very effective, side effects can limit its use.[202,267] While propranolol reduces sudden death after myocardial infarction, it does not do so to a greater degree in patients with complex ventricular arrhythmias. This suggests that it may be effective via an anti-ischemic mechanism.

When single drugs fail, combinations of drugs with different mechanisms of action can be successful, allowing use of low doses of both agents rather than high or toxic doses of one drug. Most of the combinations represent empirical trials, but I generally attempt to combine drugs to which the patient has exhibited a partial therapeutic response. Evaluating the effectiveness of drug therapy is often difficult. Whether serial drug testing by electrophysiological methods is preferable to the use of endpoints obtained by electrocardiographic methods is unsettled, and both invasive and noninvasive techniques should be considered appropriate for guiding drug selection.[70] One recent study suggests that a noninvasive assessment is less expensive.[239]

Different thresholds for arrhythmic suppression can exist. For example, the serum concentration of procainamide necessary to suppress spontaneous ventricular tachycardia can be lower than the concentration necessary to achieve a significant suppression of premature ventricular complexes.

Ventricular or *atrial pacing*, combined with antiarrhythmic agents if necessary, can be tried, but generally, unless the ventricular tachycardia is initiated by significant bradycardia, such as ventricular rates less than 40 due to complete AV block, attempts at "overdrive" pacing are ineffective over the long term.

Implantable devices that pace, cardiovert, and defibrillate,[280–284] surgery,[285–293] and ablation[294–299] techniques are used frequently in patients for whom drugs are ineffective or not tolerated due to side effects (see Chaps. 21 and 23). Revascularization procedures can be beneficial in selected patients.

Specific Types of Ventricular Tachycardia

A number of fairly specific types of ventricular tachycardia have been identified, related either to a constellation of distinctive electrocardiographic and electrophysiological features or to a specific set of clinical events. While our understanding of electrophysiological mechanisms responsible for clinically occurring ventricular tachycardias is still naive, being able to identify different kinds of ventricular tachycardias is the first step toward understanding their mechanisms.

ARRHYTHMOGENIC RIGHT VENTRICULAR DYSPLASIA. These patients present with ventricular tachycardia that generally has a left bundle branch block contour, often with right-axis deviation, with T waves inverted over the right precordial leads[300] (Fig. 22–41A). The ventricular tachycardia may be due to reentry.[301] Supraventricular arrhythmias also

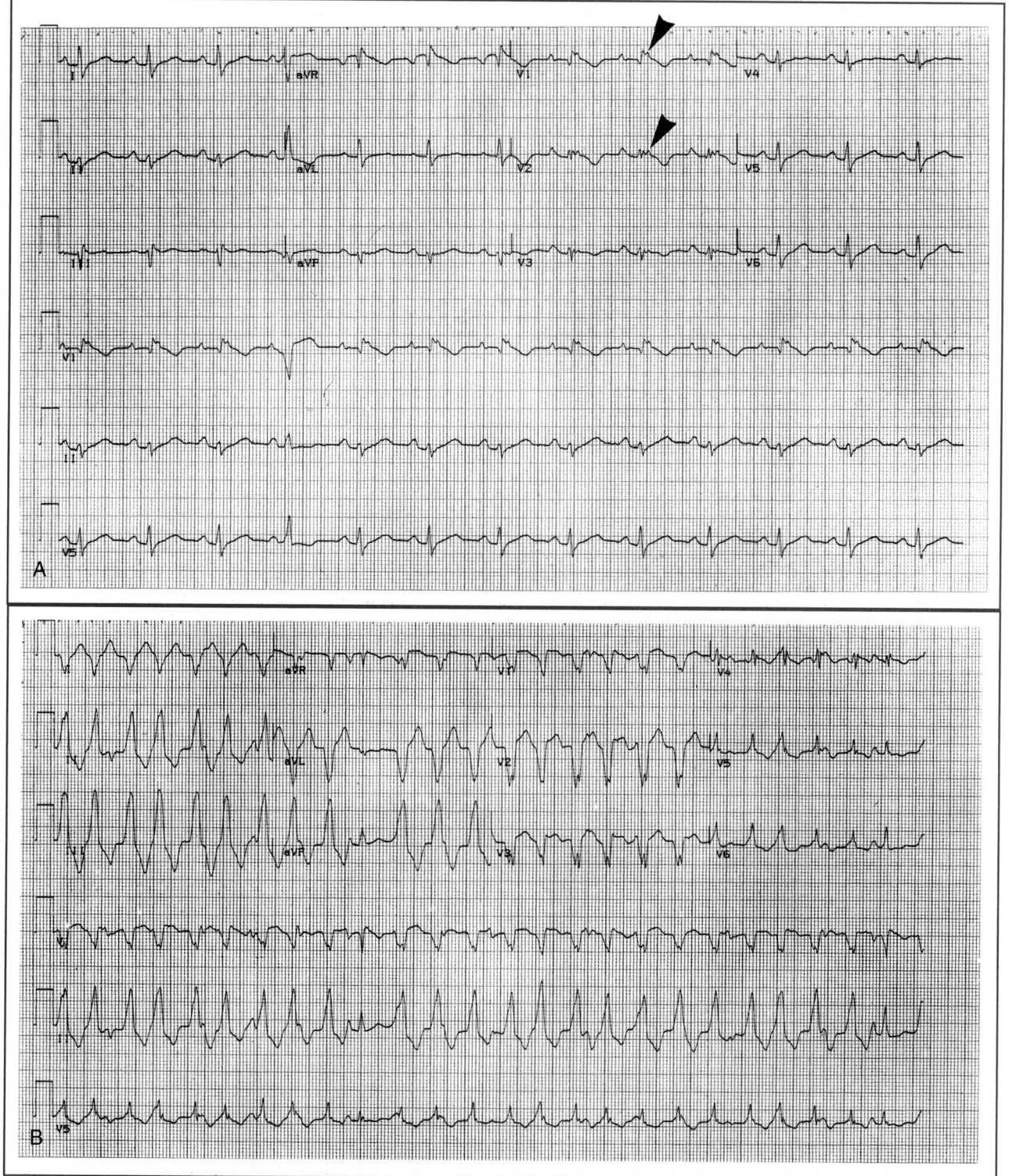

FIGURE 22–41. *A,* Normal sinus rhythm in a patient with arrhythmogenic right ventricular dysplasia. The arrowheads point to late right ventricular activation called an *epsilon wave. B,* Ventricular tachycardia in the same patient with right ventricular dysplasia.

can occur, and exercise can induce the ventricular tachycardia in some patients.

Arrhythmogenic right ventricular dysplasia is due to a type of cardiomyopathy,[302] possibly familial in some patients,[303] with hypokinetic areas involving the wall of the right ventricle. In the familial form, the genetic abnormality has been mapped to an unknown gene[303a] on chromosome 14. It can be an important cause of ventricular arrhythmias in children and young adults with an apparently normal heart, as well as in older patients. Initial presentation can be subtle.[304] Right heart failure or asymptomatic right ventricular enlargement can be present with normal pulmonary vasculature. Males predominate, and all patients usually show an abnormal right ventricle by echocardiography,[305] computed tomography,[306] right ventricular angiography, or magnetic resonance imaging.[307,308] Sympathetic innervation appears to be abnormal.[309] ECG during sinus rhythm exhibits complete or incomplete right bundle branch block.[310] Signal-averaged ECG is abnormal.[311,312] Although the conventional pharmacological approaches to therapy may be appropriate, surgical manipulations have been successful in some of these patients,[289,290,313] as has been implantable defibrillator therapy.[314] Radiofrequency catheter ablation can be tried.

TETRALOGY OF FALLOT (see also pp. 929 and 968). Chronic serious ventricular arrhythmias can occur in patients some years after repair of *tetralogy of Fallot.*[258] Sustained ventricular tachycardia after repair can be caused by reentry at the site of previous operation in the right ventricular outflow tract and can be cured by resection[292] or catheter ablation[315,316] of this area. The signal-averaged ECG can be abnormal.[317] Decreased cardiac output can occur during ventricular tachycardia and residual right ventricular outflow obstruction, leading to ventricular fibrillation.[318]

CARDIOMYOPATHIES (see also Ch. 41)

Dilated Cardiomyopathy (see also p. 1407). Both dilated and hypertrophic cardiomyopathies can be associated with ventricular tachycardias and an increased risk of sudden cardiac death. The use of the signal-averaged ECG in identifying patients with dilated cardiomyopathy at risk for sudden death is controversial, with positive[319] and negative[320,321] results. Induction of ventricular tachycardia by programed stimulation[322] does not appear to identify high-risk patients,[250,323] while Q-T dispersion may.[265] Because it is difficult to predict patients at risk of sudden death or those who might respond favorably to an antiarrhythmic drug, implantable cardioverter-defibrillators have been advocated for the patient with life-threatening ventricular arrhythmias and dilated cardiomyopathy.[324,325] Bundle branch reentry may be the basis of some ventricular tachycardias in this population and can be treated by ablating the right bundle branch.[326–328] Asymptomatic ventricular arrhythmias are common.[329]

Hypertrophic Cardiomyopathy (see also p. 1414). The risk of sudden death in patients with hypertrophic cardiomyopathy is increased by the presence of syncope, family history of sudden death in first-degree relatives, or the presence of nonsustained ventricular tachycardia on 24-hour ECG recordings.[255,330] Asymptomatic or mildly symptomatic patients with brief and infrequent episodes of nonsustained ventricular tachycardia have a low mortality.[331] Results of electrophysiological testing can help identify patients at increased risk of ventricular arrhythmias and sudden death.[332,333] Triggering events such as supraventricular tachycardia and atrial fibrillation[334] and ischemia[335] may be important. Amiodarone has been useful in some patients with mildly symptomatic, nonsustained ventricular tachycardia[330,336] but not in patients with nonarrhythmic problems.[337] Q-T dispersion is increased in those with ventricular arrhythmias and sudden death.[338] DDD pacing has been useful to reduce the outflow gradient, and its role in affecting ventricular arrhythmia is being evaluated.

MITRAL VALVE PROLAPSE (see also p. 1029). Patients with mitral valve prolapse[257] frequently have ventricular arrhythmias, although a causal relationship is not clearly established between the arrhythmia and the mitral valve prolapse. The prognosis for most patients appears good, although sudden death can occur.[339]

IDIOPATHIC VENTRICULAR TACHYARRHYTHMIAS. *Idiopathic ventricular fibrillation* may occur in about 1 per cent of cases of out-of-hospital ventricular fibrillation, affecting mostly men and those in middle

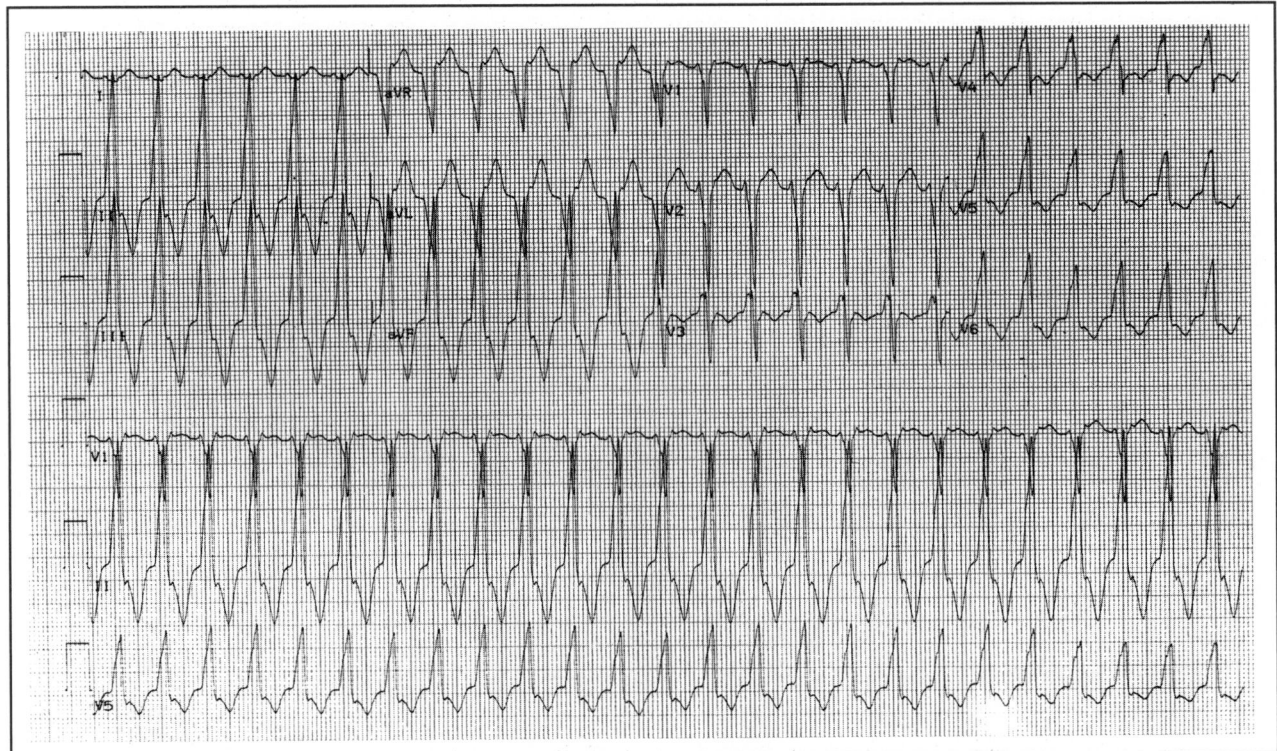

FIGURE 22–42. Ventricular tachycardia originating from the right ventricular outflow tract. This tachycardia is characterized by a left bundle branch block contour in V$_1$ and an inferior axis.

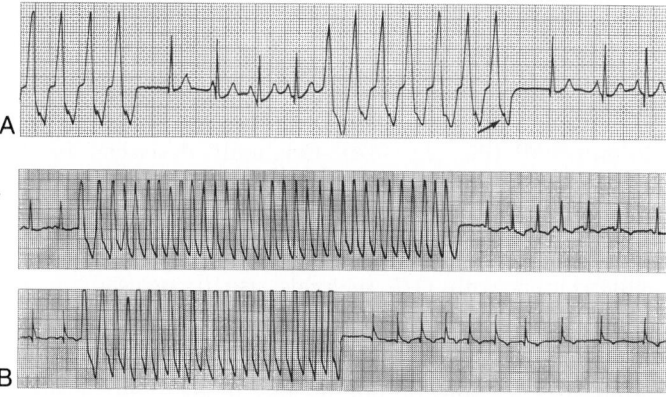

FIGURE 22-43. Panel *A*, Repetitive monomorphic ventricular tachycardia. Short episodes of a monomorphic ventricular tachycardia at a rate of 160 beats/min repeatedly interrupt the normal sinus rhythm. Retrograde atrial capture probably occurs (arrow points to the deflection in the ST segment) and the retrograde P wave of the last complex of the repetitive monomorphic ventricular tachycardia conducts over the normal pathway to produce a normal contour QRS complex. In panel *B*, short runs of a very rapid (260 beats/min) ventricular tachycardia of uniform contour occur. They probably provoke a compensatory sympathetic response because each is followed by a brief period of sinus tachycardia. The sinus pacemaker appears unstable as changes in P-wave morphology result.

---

age.[340] Cardiovascular evaluation is normal except for the arrhythmia. Monomorphic ventricular tachycardia is rarely induced at electrophysiological study. The natural history is incompletely known, but recurrences are not uncommon.[341,342] Antiarrhythmic drugs and implantable defibrillators[343] are useful therapeutic choices. Some patients may have right bundle branch block and ST-segment elevation.[344,345] It is important in this entity, as well as in patients with idiopathic ventricular tachycardias (see below), to remember that the arrhythmia at times may be an early manifestation of a developing cardiomyopathy, at least in some of the patients.

Idiopathic ventricular tachycardias with monomorphic contours can be divided into at least three types. Two types, paroxysmal ventricular tachycardia and repetitive monomorphic ventricular tachycardia,[346] appear to originate from the region of the right ventricular outflow tract (Figs. 22–42 and 22–43). Right ventricular outflow tract ventricular tachycardias have a characteristic ECG appearance of left bundle branch block contour in V_1 and an inferior axis in the frontal plane. Vagal maneuvers, including adenosine,[347] terminate the ventricular tachycardia, while exercise, stress, isoproterenol infusion, and rapid or premature stimulation can initiate or perpetuate the tachycardia. Beta blockers and verapamil[348] can suppress this tachycardia as well. The responsible mechanism may be cyclic adenosine monophosphate–triggered activity due to early[349] or delayed[350] afterdepolarizations. The paroxysmal form is exercise or stress induced, while the repetitive monomorphic type occurs at rest with sinus beats interposed between runs of nonsustained ventricular tachycardia that may be precipitated by transient increases in sympathetic activity unrelated to exertion.[350] The prognosis for most patients is quite good. Radiofrequency catheter ablation effectively eliminates this focal tachycardia in symptomatic patients.[351] In others, antiarrhythmic drugs can be effective.[352] An anatomic abnormality in the outflow tract of the right ventricle has been recognized in some patients.[353,354] In a small number of patients, the tachycardia seems to arise in the inflow tract or apex of the right ventricle.[351]

A *left septal ventricular tachycardia* has been described as arising in the left posterior septum, often preceded by a fascicular potential,[355] and is sometimes called a *fascicular tachycardia* (Fig. 22–44). Entrainment has been demonstrated, suggesting reentry as a cause of some of the tachycardias.[356] Verapamil[277,278] or dilitiazem[357] suppresses this tachycardia, while adenosine does so only rarely.[358–360] The response to verapamil suggests that the slow inward current may be important, possibly in a reentrant circuit or via delayed afterdepolarizations. Several mechanisms may be operative, and the group may not be homogeneous.[361] Oral verapamil is not as effective as intravenous verapamil. Once initiated, the tachycardia is paroxysmal and sustained. It can be started by rapid atrial or ventricular pacing and sometimes by exercise or isoproterenol. Generally, the prognosis is good.[277,278] Radiofrequency catheter ablation is effective in symptomatic patients.[297,351,355] Late potentials have been reported in one-third of patients.[362]

Sudden unexplained nocturnal death syndrome (SUNDS) occurs in apparently healthy young Southeast Asians, sometimes associated with nightmares. Thiamine deficiency has been suggested.[362a]

Accelerated Idioventricular Rhythm

ELECTROCARDIOGRAPHIC RECOGNITION.

The ventricular rate, commonly between 60 and 110 beats/min, usually

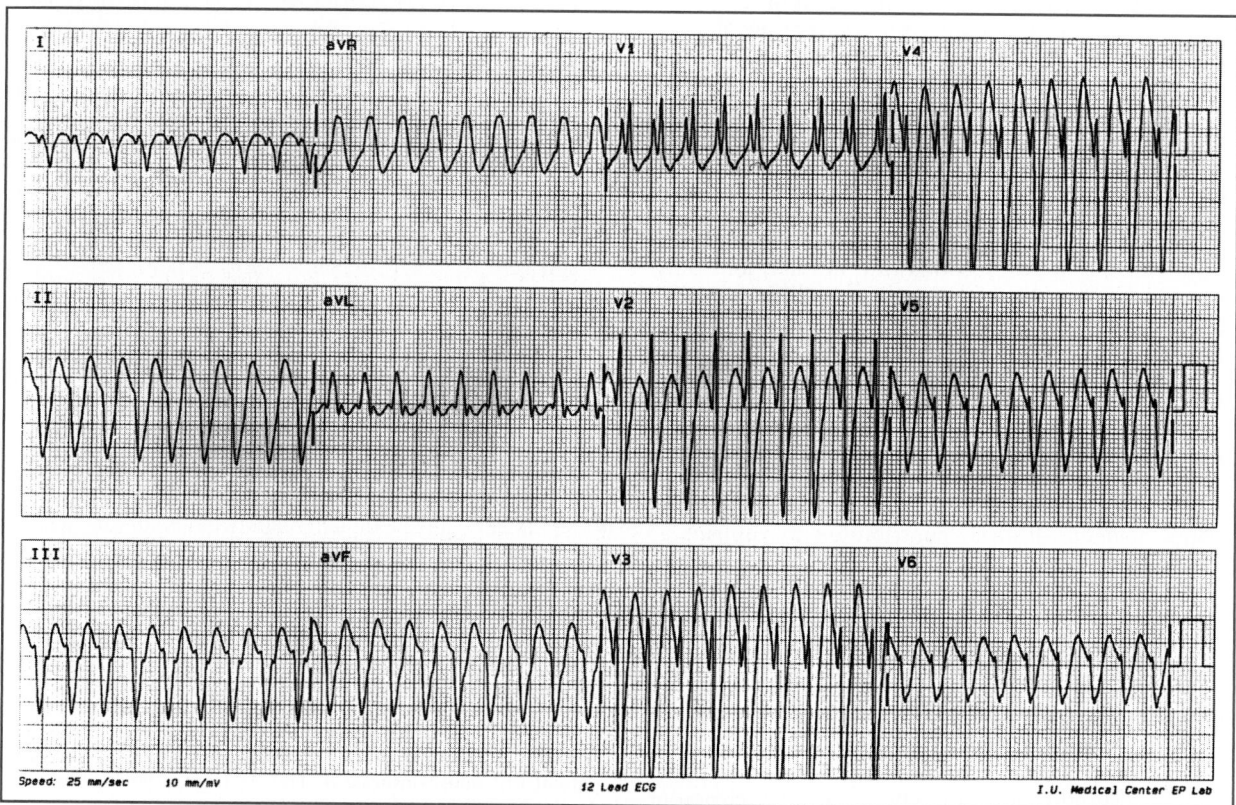

Speed: 25 mm/sec   10 mm/mV   12 Lead ECG   I.U. Medical Center EP Lab

FIGURE 22–44. Left septal ventricular tachycardia. This tachycardia is characterized by a right bundle branch block contour. In this instance, the axis was rightward. The site of the ventricular tachycardia was established to be in the left posterior septum by electrophysiological mapping and ablation.

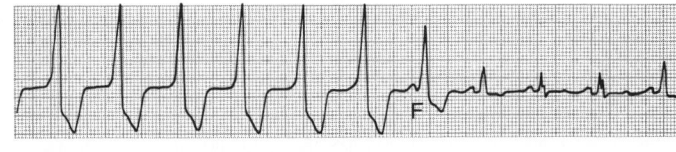

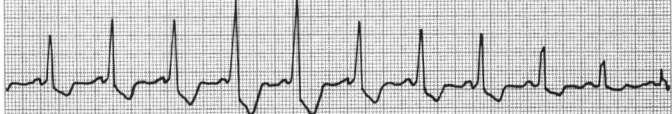

FIGURE 22–45. **Accelerated idioventricular rhythm. In this continuous monitor-lead recording, an accelerated idioventricular rhythm competes with the sinus rhythm. Wide QRS complexes at a rate of 90 beats/min fuse (F) with the sinus rhythm, which takes control briefly, generating the narrow QRS complexes, and then yields once again to the accelerated idioventricular rhythm as the P waves move "in and out" of the QRS complex. This example of isorhythmic AV dissociation may be due to hemodynamic modulation of the sinus rate via the autonomic nervous system.**

hovers within 10 beats of the sinus rate so that control of the cardiac rhythm is passed back and forth between these two competing pacemaker sites.[363] Consequently, fusion beats often occur at the onset and termination of the arrhythmia as the pacemakers vie for control of ventricular depolarization (Fig. 22–45). Because of the slow rate, capture beats are common. The onset of this arrhythmia is generally gradual (nonparoxysmal) and occurs when the rate of the ventricular tachycardia exceeds the sinus rate because of sinus slowing or SA or AV block. The ectopic mechanism also can begin after a premature ventricular complex, or the ectopic ventricular focus can simply accelerate sufficiently to overtake the sinus rhythm. The slow rate and nonparoxysmal onset avoid the problems initiated by excitation during the vulnerable period, and consequently, precipitation of more rapid ventricular arrhythmias is rarely seen. Termination of the rhythm generally occurs gradually as the dominant sinus rhythm accelerates or as the ectopic ventricular rhythm decelerates. The ventricular rhythm can be regular or irregular and occasionally can show sudden doubling, suggesting the presence of exit block. Many characteristics incriminate enhanced automaticity as the responsible mechanism.

The arrhythmia occurs as a rule in patients who have heart disease, e.g., those with acute myocardial infarction or with digitalis toxicity. It is transient and intermittent, with episodes lasting a few seconds to a minute, and does not appear to affect seriously the patient's clinical course or the prognosis. It commonly occurs at the moment of reperfusion of a previously occluded coronary artery,[364] and it can be found during resuscitation.[365]

MANAGEMENT. Suppressive therapy rarely is necessary because the ventricular rate is generally less than 100 beats/min. The following conditions exist during which therapy may be considered: (1) when AV dissociation results in loss of sequential AV contraction and with it the hemodynamic benefits of atrial contribution to ventricular filling, (2) when accelerated idioventricular rhythm occurs together with a more rapid ventricular tachycardia, (3) when accelerated idioventricular rhythm begins with a premature ventricular complex that has a short coupling interval, which causes discharge in the vulnerable period of the preceding T wave, (4) when the ventricular rate is too rapid and produces symptoms, and (5) if ventricular fibrillation develops as a result of the accelerated idioventricular rhythm. This last event appears to be fairly rare. Therapy, when indicated, should be as already noted for ventricular tachycardia. Often simply increasing the sinus rate with atropine or atrial pacing suppresses the accelerated idioventricular rhythm.

Torsades de Pointes

ELECTROCARDIOGRAPHIC RECOGNITION. The term *torsades de pointes* refers to a ventricular tachycardia characterized by QRS complexes of changing amplitude that appear to twist around the isoelectric line and occur at rates of 200 to 250/min[366–368] (Fig. 22–46A). Originally described in the setting of bradycardia due to complete heart block,[369] the term *torsades de pointes* is usually used to connote a *syndrome*, not simply an ECG description of the QRS complex of the tachycardia, characterized by prolonged ventricular repolarization with Q-T intervals usually exceeding 500 msec. The U wave also can become prominent, but its role in this syndrome and in the long Q-T syndrome is not clear. Long-short R-R cycle sequences commonly precede the onset of torsades de pointes due to acquired causes.[370] Relatively late premature ventricular complexes can discharge during the termination of the long T wave, precipitating successive bursts of ventricular tachycardia during which the peaks of the QRS complexes appear successively on one side and then on the other or the isoelectric baseline, giving the typical twisting appearance with continuous and progressive changes in QRS contour and amplitude.[371] Recently, a tachycardia resembling torsades de pointes has been described in which the Q-T interval is normal, and premature ventricular complexes with short coupling intervals initiate the tachycardia.[372] Torsades de

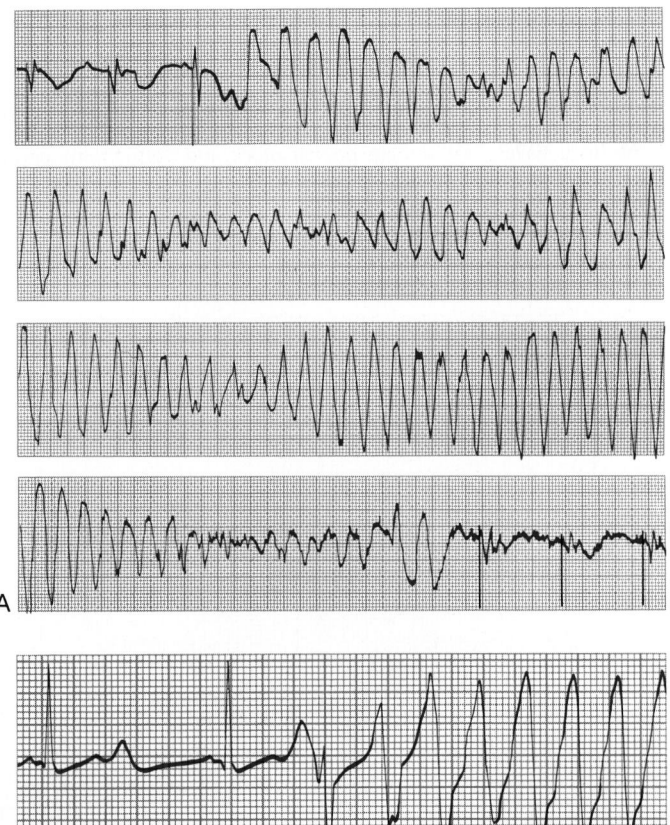

FIGURE 22–46. **Torsades de pointes. *A,* Continuous-recording monitor lead. A demand ventricular pacemaker (VVI) had been implanted because of type II second degree AV block. After treatment with amiodarone for recurrent ventricular tachycardia, the Q-T interval became prolonged (about 640 msec during paced beats), and the patient developed episodes of torsades de pointes. In this recording, the tachycardia spontaneously terminates and a paced ventricular rhythm is restored. Motion artifact is noted at the end of the recording as the patient lost consciousness. *B,* Tracing from a young boy with a congenital long Q-T syndrome. The Q-TU interval in the sinus beats is at least 600 msec. Note TU wave alternans in the first and second complexes. A late premature complex occurring in the downslope of the TU wave initiates an episode of ventricular tachycardia.**

pointes can terminate with progressive prolongation of cycle lengths and larger and more distinctly formed QRS complexes, ending with a return to the basal rhythm, a period of ventricular standstill, a new attack of torsades de pointes, or ventricular fibrillation.

Ventricular tachycardia that is similar morphologically to torsades de pointes and occurs in patients *without* Q-T prolongation, whether spontaneous or electrically induced, generally should be classified as polymorphic ventricular tachycardia, not as torsades de pointes. The distinction has important therapeutic implications (see below).

ELECTROPHYSIOLOGICAL FEATURES. Electrophysiological mechanisms responsible for torsades de pointes are not completely understood.[373,374] Most data suggest that early afterdepolarizations (see Fig. 20–22, p. 566) are responsible for both the long Q-T and the torsades de pointes or at least its initiation.[375–377] Perpetuation may be due to triggered activity, reentry due to dispersion of repolarization[378] produced by the early afterdepolarizations, or abnormal automaticity. Two out-of-phase discharging foci have been shown experimentally to produce a tachycardia similar to torsades de pointes, as have drifting rotors[379] (see p. 1378).

CLINICAL FEATURES. While many predisposing factors have been cited, the most common causes are congenital, severe bradycardia, potassium depletion, and use of class IA and some IC drugs. Clinical features depend on whether the torsades de pointes is due to the acquired or congenital (idiopathic) long Q-T syndrome (see below). Symptoms from the tachycardia depend on its rate and duration, as with other ventricular tachycardias, and range from palpitations to syncope and death. Females, perhaps because of a longer Q-T interval, are at greater risk for developing torsades de pointes than are males.[380]

MANAGEMENT. The approach to ventricular tachycardia with a polymorphic pattern depends on whether or not it occurs in the setting of a prolonged Q-T interval. For this practical reason and because the mechanism of the tachycardia can differ depending on whether or not a long Q-T interval is present, it is important to restrict the definition of torsades de pointes to the typical polymorphic ventricular tachycardia in the setting of a long Q-T and/or U wave in the basal complexes. In all patients with torsades de pointes, administration of class IA, possibly some class IC, and class III antiarrhythmic agents (amiodarone and sotalol) can increase the abnormal Q-T interval and worsen the arrhythmia. Intravenous magnesium is the initial treatment of choice for torsades de pointes due to an acquired cause,[281,282] followed by temporary ventricular or atrial pacing. Isoproterenol, given cautiously because it can exacerbate the arrhythmia, can be used until pacing is instituted. Lidocaine, mexiletine, or phenytoin can be tried. Potassium channel openers may be useful.[383–385] The cause of the long Q-T should be determined and corrected if possible. When the Q-T interval is normal, polymorphic ventricular tachycardia *resembling* torsades de pointes is diagnosed, and standard antiarrhythmic drugs can be given. In borderline cases, the clinical context may help determine whether treatment should be initiated with antiarrhythmic drugs. Torsades de pointes due to the congenital long Q-T interval syndrome is treated with beta blockade, surgical sympathetic interruption, pacing, and implantable defibrillators (see below). ECGs taken on close relatives can help secure the diagnosis of long Q-T syndrome in borderline cases.

Long Q-T Syndrome

ELECTROCARDIOGRAPHIC RECOGNITION (Fig. 22–46*B*). The upper limit for the duration of the normal Q-T interval *corrected* for heart rate (Q-Tc) is often given as 0.44 sec. However, the normal corrected Q-T interval actually may be longer, 0.46 for men and 0.47 for women, with a normal range ± 15 per cent of the mean value.[386] The nature of the

U-wave abnormality and its relationship to the long Q-T syndrome are not clear. M cells may be responsible for the U wave (see p. 562).[387] The probable risk of developing life-threatening ventricular arrhythmias in patients with the idiopathic long Q-T syndrome is exponentially related to the length of the Q-Tc interval.[386] T-wave "humps" in the ECG suggest the presence of the long Q-T syndrome[388] and may be caused by early afterdepolarizations.[389] A point score system has been suggested to aid in the diagnosis.[390] Two-to-one AV block (because of the long repolarization time) and T-wave alternans can occur.[391,392]

CLINICAL FEATURES. The long Q-T syndrome can be divided into idiopathic (congenital) and acquired forms.[368] The idiopathic form is a familial disorder (see p. 951) that can be associated with sensorineural deafness (Jervell and Lange-Nielsen syndrome, autosomal recessive) or normal hearing (Romano-Ward syndrome, autosomal dominant). A nonfamilial form with normal hearing has been called the sporadic form.

The hypothesis that the idiopathic long Q-T syndrome results from a preponderance of left sympathetic tone has been replaced by genetic information linking the disorder in different families to sites in chromosomes 3p21–24, 4, 7q35–36, and 11p15.5,[393–399] and recently establishing two genes, HERG on chromosome 7, a putative potassium gene,[400] and SCN5A on chromosome 3,[401] the cardiac sodium gene, as potential causes.[401a] Clear evidence for genetic heterogeneity exists (see p. 750) and can be responsible for different shaped T waves. Chromosome 3 abnormality is associated with the longest Q-Tc durations and delay in onset of the T wave, while chromosome 7 abnormality results in T waves of low amplitude.[401b,401c] Thus it is likely that an intrinsic cardiac repolarization abnormality gives rise to early afterdepolarizations that prolong the Q-T interval and produce torsades de pointes. The acquired form has a long Q-T interval caused by various drugs such as quinidine, procainamide, N-acetylprocainamide, sotalol,[402] amiodarone, disopyramide,[403] phenothiazines, or tricyclic antidepressants; nonsedating antihistamines such as astemizole and terfenedine,[404–406] whose actions can be exacerbated by drugs affecting their metabolism such as ketoconazoles; drugs such as erythromycin,[407–409] pentamidine,[410,411] and some antimalarials; electrolyte abnormalities such as hypokalemia and hypomagnesemia; the results of a liquid protein diet and starvation; central nervous system lesions; significant bradyarrhythmias; cardiac ganglionitis; mitral valve prolapse; and probucol.[412]

Patients with congenital long Q-T syndrome can present with syncope, at times misdiagnosed as epilepsy,[413,414,414a] due to ventricular tachycardias that are often caused by torsades de pointes. Sudden death can occur in this group of patients, and it occurs in 9 per cent of pediatric patients without preceding symptoms.[414,415] It is obvious that in some the ventricular arrhythmia becomes sustained and probably results in ventricular fibrillation. Patients with idiopathic long Q-T syndrome who are at increased risk for sudden death include those with family members who died suddenly at an early age and those who have experienced syncope. They commonly develop ventricular tachyarrhythmias during periods of adrenergic stimulation such as fright or exertion. Syndactyly has been described recently in some patients with the idiopathic form.[416] Stress testing can prolong the Q-T interval and produce T-wave alternans, the latter indicative of electrical instability.[417] Electrocardiograms should be obtained for all family members when the propositus presents with symptoms. Patients should undergo prolonged ECG recording,[418,419] with various stresses designed to evoke ventricular arrhythmias, such as auditory stimuli, psychological stress, cold pressor stimulation, and exercise. The Valsalva maneuver can lengthen the Q-T interval and cause T-wave alternans and ventricular tachycardia in patients who have prolonged Q-T syndromes. Catecholamines[420,421,421a] can be infused in some patients, but this challenge must be performed cautiously, with resuscitative equipment along with alpha and beta antagonists close at hand. Stellate ganglion stimulation and blockade have been useful to provoke or abolish arrhythmias. Premature ventricular stimulation electrically generally does not induce arrhythmias in this syndrome. Patients with the acquired form commonly develop torsades de pointes during periods of bradycardia or after a long pause in the R-R interval, while those with the idiopathic form can have a sinus tachycardia preceding the ventricular arrhythmia. Competitive sports are generally contraindicated for patients with the congenital long Q-T syndrome.[46] An interesting contractile abnormality has been described in patients with the idiopathic long Q-T syndrome that is abolished by verapamil.[422] Cardiac sympathetic innervation appears to be normal,[423] although this is not completely resolved.[424]

Recently, a dog colony with sudden death and ventricular tachyarrhythmias, apparently due to early afterdepolarizations with a normal Q-T interval, has been described.[425,425a] In humans with normal Q-T intervals, ventricular tachyarrhythmias resembling torsades de pointes also have been noted.[426]

MANAGEMENT. For patients who have the idiopathic long Q-T syndrome but do not have syncope, complex ventricular arrhythmias, or a family history of sudden cardiac death, no therapy is recommended. In asymptomatic patients with complex ventricular arrhythmias or a family history of early sudden cardiac death, beta-adrenoceptor blockers at maximally tolerated doses are recommended. In patients with syncope, beta blockers at maximally tolerated doses, perhaps combined with a class IB antiarrhythmic drug, are suggested. For patients who continue to have syncope despite maximum drug therapy, left-sided cervicothoracic sympathetic ganglionectomy that interrupts the stellate ganglion and the first three or four thoracic ganglia may be helpful, and permanent pacing[427] also has been used. Implantation of a cardioverter-defibrillator seems advisable in patients who have syncope despite sympathetic interruption[368,428] (Chap. 23). For patients with the acquired form and torsades de pointes, IV magnesium and atrial or ventricular pacing are initial choices. Class IB antiarrhythmic drugs or isoproterenol (cautiously) to increase heart rate can be tried. Avoidance of precipitating drugs is mandatory. Potassium channel activating drugs such as pinacidil and cromakalim may be useful[383–385] in both forms of long Q-T syndrome. Interventions that reduce Q-T dispersion may be beneficial.[427]

BIDIRECTIONAL VENTRICULAR TACHYCARDIA

This is an uncommon type of ventricular tachycardia characterized by QRS complexes with a right bundle branch block pattern, alternating polarity in the frontal plane from −60 to −90 degrees to +120 to +130 degrees, and a regular rhythm. The ventricular rate is between 140 and 200 beats/min. Although the mechanism and site of origin of this tachycardia have remained somewhat controversial, most evidence supports a ventricular origin.

Bidirectional ventricular tachycardia is usually but not exclusively a manifestation of digitalis excess, typically in older patients and in those with severe myocardial disease. When the tachycardia is due to digitalis, the extent of toxicity is often advanced, with a poor prognosis.

Drugs useful to treat digitalis toxicity such as lidocaine, potassium, phenytoin, and propranolol should be considered if excessive digitalis administration is suspected. Otherwise, the usual therapeutic approach to ventricular tachycardia (see p. 680) is recommended.

BUNDLE BRANCH REENTRANT VENTRICULAR TACHYCARDIA

Ventricular tachycardia due to bundle branch reentry is characterized by a QRS morphology determined by the circuit established over the bundle branches or fascicles. Retrograde conduction over the left bundle branch system and anterograde conduction over the right bundle branch create a QRS complex with a left bundle branch block contour and constitute the most common form. The frontal plane axis may be about +30 degrees. Conduction in the opposite direction produces a right bundle branch block contour. Reentry also can occur over the anterior and posterior fascicles. Electrophysiologically, bundle branch reentrant complexes are started after a critical S_2-H_2 or S_3-H_3 delay. The H-V interval of the bundle branch reentrant complex equals or exceeds the H-V interval of the spontaneous normally conducted QRS complex.

Bundle branch reentry is a form of monomorphic sustained ventricular tachycardia usually seen in patients with structural heart disease, such as dilated cardiomyopathy. During follow-up, congestive heart failure is the most common cause of death in this population.[430,431] Myocardial ventricular tachycardias also can be present. Uncommonly, bundle branch reentry can occur in the absence of myocardial disease.[430,431]

The therapeutic approach is as for other types of ventricular tachycardia, except that creation of bundle branch block interrupts the reentry circuit and can eliminate the tachycardia.[294]

Ventricular Flutter and Fibrillation
(See also Chap. 24)

ELECTROCARDIOGRAPHIC RECOGNITION. These arrhythmias represent severe derangements of the heartbeat that usually terminate fatally within 3 to 5 minutes unless corrective measures are undertaken promptly. Ventricular flutter presents as a sine wave in appearance: regular large oscillations occurring at a rate of 150 to 300/min (usually about 200) (Fig. 22–47A). The distinction between rapid ventricular tachycardia and ventricular flutter can be difficult and is usually of academic interest only. Hemodynamic collapse is present with both. Ventricular fibrillation is recognized by the presence of irregular undulations of varying contour and amplitude (Fig. 22–47B). Distinct QRS complexes, ST segments, and T waves are absent. Fine-amplitude fibrillatory waves (<0.2 mV) are present with prolonged ventricular fibrillation. These five waves identify patients with worse survival rates, and are sometimes confused with asystole.[432]

MECHANISMS. Ventricular fibrillation occurs in a variety of clinical situations, most commonly associated with coronary artery disease and as a terminal event. Intracellular calcium accumulation,[433] action

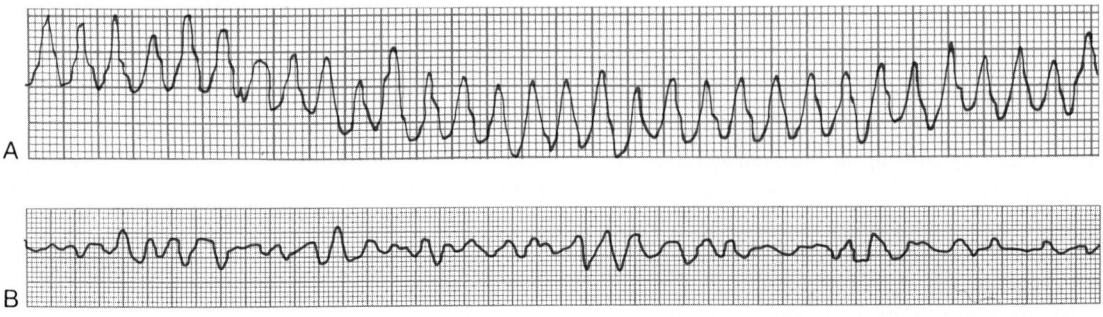

FIGURE 22–47. Ventricular flutter and ventricular fibrillation. *A,* The sine wave appearance of the complexes occurring at a rate of 300 beats/min is characteristic of ventricular flutter. *B,* The irregular undulating baseline typifies ventricular fibrillation.

of free radicals, metabolic alterations, and autonomic modulation are some important influences on development of ventricular fibrillation during ischemia. Thrombolytic agents reduce the incidence of ventricular arrhythmias[433a] and of inducible ventricular tachycardia after myocardial infarction. Cardiovascular events, including sudden cardiac death due to ventricular fibrillation, but not asystole,[434] occur most frequently in the morning and may be related to increased platelet aggregability. Aspirin reduces this mortality. Ventricular fibrillation can occur during antiarrhythmic drug administration, hypoxia, ischemia, atrial fibrillation and very rapid ventricular rates in the preexcitation syndrome (see p. 667) after electrical shock administered during cardioversion (see p. 619) or accidentally by improperly grounded equipment, and during competitive ventricular pacing to terminate ventricular tachycardia.

CLINICAL FEATURES. Ventricular flutter or ventricular fibrillation results in faintness, followed by loss of consciousness, seizures, apnea, and eventually, if the rhythm continues untreated, death. The blood pressure is unobtainable, and heart sounds are usually absent. The atria can continue to beat at an independent rhythm for a time or in response to impulses from the fibrillating ventricles. Eventually, electrical activity of the heart ceases.

In patients resuscitated from out-of-hospital cardiac arrest, 75 per cent have ventricular fibrillation. Bradycardia and asystole can occur in 15 to 25 per cent of these patients and is associated with a worse prognosis than is ventricular fibrillation. Ventricular tachycardia commonly precedes the onset of ventricular fibrillation, although frequently no consistent premonitory patterns emerge. Heart rate variability may be decreased.[435,436]

While 75 per cent of resuscitated patients exhibit significant coronary artery disease, only 20 to 30 per cent develop acute transmural myocardial infarction. In one study,[437] 73 per cent had recent thrombosis. Those who do *not* develop a myocardial infarction have an increased recurrence rate for sudden cardiac death or nonfatal ventricular fibrillation. Patients who have ventricular fibrillation and acute myocardial infarction have a recurrence rate at 1 year of 2 per cent. In the past 20 years, there appears to have been an overall decrease in the incidence of sudden cardiac death, parallel to the decrease in death from coronary heart disease. In some studies, patients at risk for sudden cardiac death have ischemia, reduced left ventricular function, 10 or more premature ventricular complexes per hour, spontaneous and induced ventricular tachycardia, hypertension and left ventricular hypertrophy, obesity, and elevated cholesterol levels; smoking, male sex, increased age, and excess alcohol consumption also predispose to sudden cardiac death.

Predictors of death for resuscitated patients include reduced ejection fraction,[438,439] abnormal wall motion, history of congestive heart failure, history of myocardial infarction but no acute event, and the presence of ventricular arrhythmias. Patients discharged after an anterior myocardial infarction complicated by ventricular fibrillation appear to represent a subgroup at high risk of sudden death. Ventricular fibrillation can occur in infants, young people, athletes, persons without known structural heart disease,[440,441] and in unexplained syndromes. Survival chances for the elderly are reasonable if ventricular tachycardia/fibrillation is the presenting rhythm. Severe bradycardia or asystole bodes a reduced survival rate for most patients. Transcutaneous pacing does not seem to be helpful.[442] Persons in lower socioeconomic strata are at greater risk for cardiac mortality and are less likely to survive an episode of out-of-hospital cardiac arrest.[443]

MANAGEMENT (see also pp. 619 and 731). *Immediate* nonsynchronized DC electrical shock using 200 to 400 joules is mandatory treatment for ventricular fibrillation and for ventricular flutter that has caused loss of consciousness. Cardiopulmonary resuscitation is employed only until defibrillation equipment is readied. *Time should not be wasted with cardiopulmonary resuscitation maneuvers if electrical defibrillation can be done promptly.* Defibrillation requires fewer joules if done early. If the circulation is markedly inadequate despite return to sinus rhythm, closed-chest massage with artificial ventilation as needed should be instituted. The use of anesthesia during electrical shock obviously is dictated by the patient's condition and is generally not required. After conversion of the arrhythmia to a normal rhythm, it is essential to monitor the rhythm continuously and to institute measures to prevent a recurrence.

Metabolic acidosis quickly follows cardiovascular collapse. If the arrhythmia is terminated within 30 to 60 seconds, significant acidosis does not occur. The use of sodium bicarbonate to reverse the acidosis may be necessary, but its efficacy is presently being reevaluated (see p. 766). Intravenous calcium generally is recommended only for situations characterized by hypocalcemia, hyperkalemia, calcium-antagonist overdose, and possibly electromechanical dissociation.

In this short period of time, artificial ventilation by means of a tightly fitting rubber face mask and an Ambu bag is quite satisfactory and eliminates the delay attending intubation by inexperienced personnel. If such a mask and bag are not available, mouth-to-mouth or mouth-to-nose resuscitation is indicated. It is important to reemphasize that there should be *no delay in instituting electrical shock.* If the patient is not monitored and it cannot be established whether asystole or ventricular fibrillation caused the cardiovascular collapse, the electrical shock should be administered *without* wasting precious seconds attempting to obtain an electrocardiogram. The DC shock may cause the asystolic heart to begin discharging and also termi-

nate ventricular fibrillation, if the latter is present. Lidocaine administration may be associated with asystole.

A search for conditions contributing to the initiation of ventricular flutter or fibrillation should be made and the conditions corrected, if possible. Initial medical approaches to prevent a recurrence of ventricular fibrillation include intravenous administration of lidocaine, bretylium, procainamide, or amiodarone. Ventricular fibrillation rarely terminates spontaneously, and death results unless countermeasures are instituted immediately. Subsequent therapy is necessary to prevent a recurrence. Antiischemic approaches are useful in selected patients.[444] Catheter ablation techniques are useful in only well-tolerated monomorphic ventricular arrhythmias.[445]

HEART BLOCK

Heart block is a disturbance of impulse conduction that can be permanent or transient owing to anatomical or functional impairment. It must be distinguished from *interference*, a normal phenomenon that is a disturbance of impulse conduction caused by physiological refractoriness due to inexcitability from a preceding impulse. Either interference or block can occur at any site where impulses are conducted, but they are recognized most commonly between the sinus node and atrium (SA block), between the atria and ventricles (AV block), within the atria (intra-atrial block), or within the ventricles (intraventricular block). During AV block, the block can occur in the AV node, His bundle, or bundle branches. In some instances of bundle branch block the impulse may only be delayed and not completely blocked in the bundle branch, yet the resulting QRS complex may be indistinguishable from a QRS complex generated by complete bundle branch block.

The conduction disturbance is classified by severity in three categories. During *first degree heart block,* conduction time is prolonged but all impulses are conducted. *Second degree heart block* occurs in two forms: Mobitz type I (Wenckebach) and type II. Type I heart block is characterized by a progressive lengthening of the conduction time until an impulse is not conducted. Type II heart block denotes occasional or repetitive sudden block of conduction of an impulse without prior measurable lengthening of conduction time. When no impulses are conducted, *complete* or *third degree block* is present. The degree of block may depend in part on the direction of impulse propagation. For unknown reasons, normal retrograde conduction can occur in the presence of advanced anterograde AV block. The reverse also can occur. Some electrocardiographers use the term *advanced heart block* to indicate blockage of two or more consecutive impulses.[445a]

Certain features of type I second degree block deserve special emphasis because when actual conduction times are not apparent in the electrocardiogram, e.g., during SA, junctional, or ventricular exit block (Fig. 22–48), type I conduction disturbance can be difficult to recognize. During typical type I block, the increment in conduction time is greatest in the second beat of the Wenckebach group, and the absolute *increase* in conduction time *decreases* progressively over subsequent beats. These two features serve to establish the characteristics of classic Wenckebach group beating: (1) the interval between successive beats progressively decreases, although the conduction time increases (but by a decreasing function), (2) the duration of the pause produced by the nonconducted impulse is less than twice the interval preceding the blocked impulse (which is usually the shortest interval), and (3) the cycle following the nonconducted beat (beginning the Wenckebach group) is longer than the cycle preceding the blocked impulse. Although much emphasis has been placed on this characteristic grouping of cycles, primarily to be able to diagnose Wenckebach exit block, this typical grouping occurs in fewer than 50 per cent of patients who have type I Wenckebach AV nodal block.

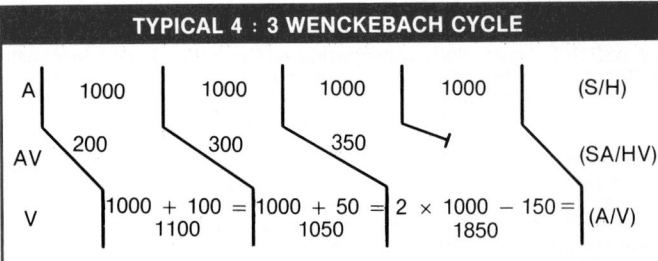

TYPICAL 4 : 3 WENCKEBACH CYCLE

A	1000	1000	1000	1000	(S/H)
AV	200	300	350		(SA/HV)
V	1000 + 100 = 1100	1000 + 50 = 1050	2 × 1000 − 150 = 1850		(A/V)

FIGURE 22–48. Typical 4:3 Wenckebach cycle. P waves ("A" tier) occur at a cycle length of 1000 msec. The P-R interval ("A-V" tier) is 200 msec for the first beat and generates a ventricular response ("V" tier). The P-R interval increases by 100 msec in the next complex, resulting in an R-R interval of 1100 msec (1000 + 100). The increment in the P-R interval is only 50 msec for the third cycle, and the P-R interval becomes 350 msec. The R-R interval shortens to 1050 msec (1000 + 50). The next P wave blocks, creating an R-R interval that is less than twice the P-P interval by an amount equal to the increments in the P-R interval. Thus, the Wenckebach features explained in the text can be found in this diagram. If the increment in the P-R interval of the last conducted complex *increased* rather than decreased (e.g., 150 msec rather than 50 msec) then the last R-R interval before the block would increase (1150 msec) rather than decrease and thus become an example of atypical Wenckebach (Fig. 22–43).

If this were a Wenckebach exit block from the sinus node to the atrium, the sinus node cycle length (S) would be 1000 msec, and the S-A interval would increase from 200 to 300 to 350 msec, culminating in block. These events would be inapparent in the scalar ECG. However, the P-P interval in the ECG would shorten from 1100 to 1050 msec and finally there would be a pause of 1850 msec (A) (Fig. 22–4). If this were a junctional rhythm arising from the His bundle and conducting to the ventricle, the junctional rhythm cycle length would be 1000 msec (H), and the H-V interval would progressively lengthen from 200 to 300 to 350 msec, while the R-R interval would decrease from 1100 to 1050 msec and then increase to 1850 msec (V). The only clue to the Wenckebach exit block would be the cycle length changes in the ventricular rhythm.

Differences in these cycle-length patterns can result from changes in pacemaker rate (e.g., sinus arrhythmia), in neurogenic control of conduction, and in the increment of conduction delay. For example, if the P-R increment in the last cycle *increases,* the R-R cycle of the last conducted beat can lengthen rather than shorten. In addition, since the last conducted beat is often at a critical state of conduction, it can become blocked, producing a 5:3 or 3:1 conduction ratio instead of a 5:4 or 3:2 ratio. During a 3:2 Wenckebach structure, the duration of the cycle following the nonconducted beat will be the same as the duration of the cycle preceding the nonconducted beat.

Atrioventricular (AV) Block

AV block exists when the atrial impulse is conducted with delay or is not conducted at all to the ventricle at a time when the AV junction is not physiologically refractory.

FIRST DEGREE AV BLOCK. During first degree AV block, every atrial impulse conducts to the ventricles, producing a regular ventricular rate, but the P-R interval exceeds 0.20 sec in the adult. P-R intervals as long as 1.0 sec have been noted and at times can exceed the P-P interval, a phenomenon known as "skipped" P waves. Clinically important P-R interval prolongation can result from conduction delay in the AV node (A-H interval), in the His-Purkinje system (H-V interval), or at both sites. Equally delayed conduction over both bundle branches uncommonly can produce P-R prolongation without significant QRS complex aberration. Occasionally, intraatrial conduction delay can result in P-R prolongation. If the QRS complex in the scalar ECG is normal in contour and duration, the AV delay almost always resides in the AV node, rarely within the His bundle itself.

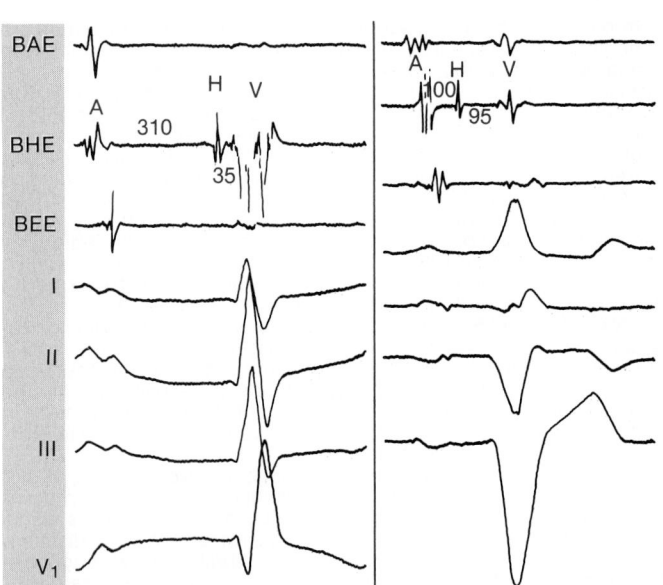

FIGURE 22–49. First degree AV block. One complex during sinus rhythm is shown. The P-R interval in the left panel measured 370 msec (P-A = 25 msec; A-H = 310 msec; H-V = 35 msec) during a right bundle branch block. Conduction delay in the AV node causes the first degree AV block. In the panel on the right, the P-R interval is 230 msec (P-A = 35 msec; A-H = 100 msec; H-V = 95 msec) during a left bundle branch block. The conduction delay in the His-Purkinje system causes the first degree AV block.

If the QRS complex shows a bundle branch block pattern, conduction delay may be within the AV node and/or His-Purkinje system (Fig. 22–49). In this latter instance, His bundle electrocardiography is necessary to localize the site of conduction delay. Acceleration of the atrial rate or enhancement of vagal tone by carotid massage can cause first degree AV nodal block to progress to type I second degree AV block. Conversely, type I second degree AV nodal block can revert to first degree block with deceleration of the sinus rate.

SECOND DEGREE AV BLOCK (Figs. 22–48, 22–50, and 22–51). The block of some atrial impulses conducted to the ventricle at a time when physiological interference is not involved constitutes second degree AV block. The nonconducted P wave can be intermittent or frequent, at regular or irregular intervals, and can be preceded by fixed or lengthening P-R intervals. A distinguishing feature is that conducted P waves relate to the QRS complex with recurring P-R intervals; i.e., the association of P with QRS is not random. Wenckebach and Hay, by analyzing the *a-c* and *v* waves in the jugular venous pulse, described two types of second degree AV block. After the introduction of the electrocardiograph, Mobitz classified them as type I and type II. Electrocardiographically, typical type I second degree AV block is characterized by progressive P-R prolongation culminating in a nonconducted P wave (Figs. 22–50 and 22–51), while in type II second degree AV block, the P-R interval remains constant prior to the blocked P wave (Fig.

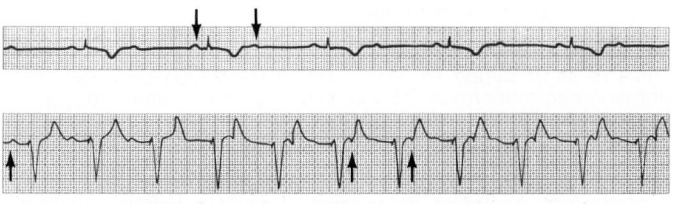

FIGURE 22–50. Unidirectional block. *Top,* During spontaneous sinus rhythm at a rate of 68 beats/min, 2:1 anterograde AV conduction occurs. In the bottom ECG, during ventricular pacing at a rate of 70 beats/min, 1:1 retrograde conduction is seen. P waves are indicated by arrows.

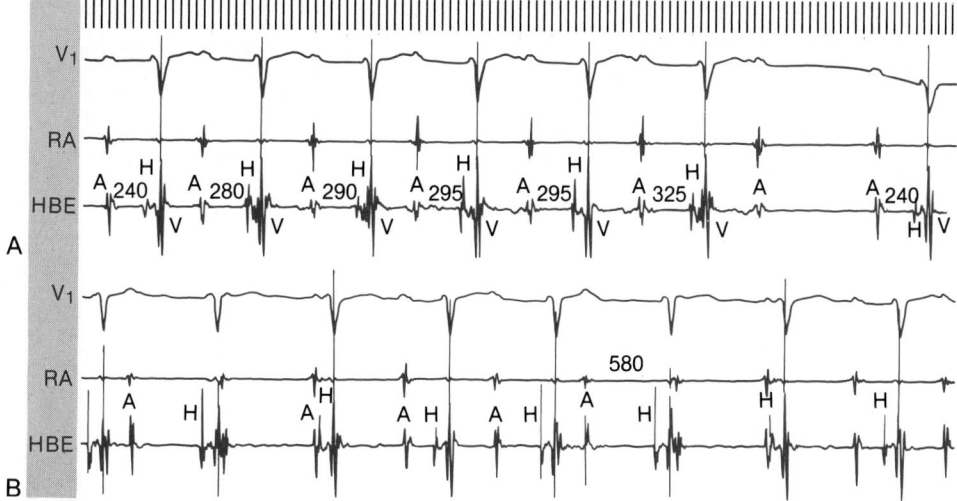

FIGURE 22–51. Type I (Wenckebach) atrioventricular nodal block (panel A). During spontaneous sinus rhythm, progressive P-R prolongation occurs, culminating in a nonconducted P wave. From the His bundle recording (HBE), it is apparent that the conduction delay and subsequent block occurs within the AV node. Since the increment in conduction delay does not consistently decrease, the R-R intervals do not reflect the classic Wenckebach structure diagrammed in Figure 22–42. Panel B was recorded 5 min following 0.6 mg IV atropine. Atropine has had its predominant effect on sinus and junctional automaticity at this time, with little improvement in AV conduction. Consequently, more P waves are blocked and AV dissociation, due to a combination of AV block and enhanced junctional discharge rate, is present. At 8 min (not shown), when atropine finally improved AV conduction, 1:1 atrioventricular conduction occurred.

22–52A). In both instances the AV block is intermittent and generally repetitive and can block several P waves in a row. Often, the eponyms *Mobitz type I* and *Mobitz type II* are applied to the two types of block, while the term *Wenckebach block* refers to type I block only. Wenckebach block in the His-Purkinje system in a patient with a bundle branch block can resemble AV nodal Wenckebach block very closely (Fig. 22–52B).

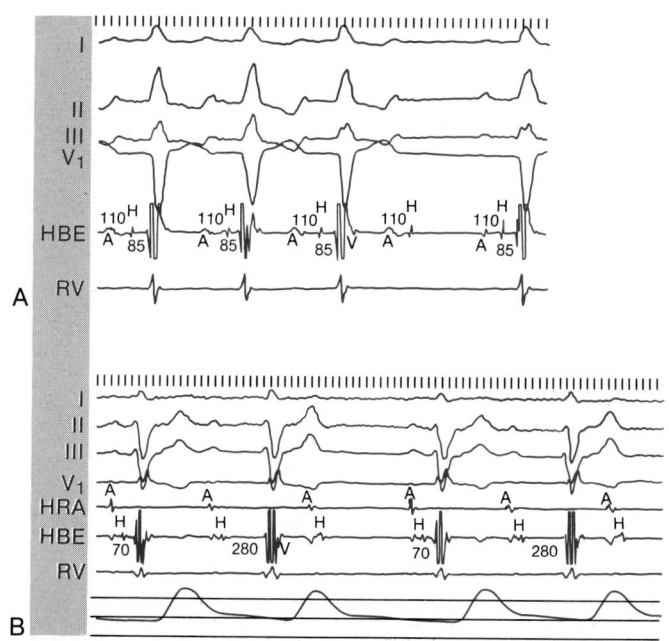

FIGURE 22–52. Type II AV block. *A,* Sudden development of His-Purkinje block is apparent. The A-H and H-V intervals remain constant, as does the P-R interval. Left bundle branch block is present. *B,* Wenckebach AV block in the His-Purkinje system. The QRS complex exhibits a right bundle branch block morphology. However, note that the second QRS complex in the 3:2 conduction exhibits a slightly different contour from the first QRS complex, particularly in V₁. This is the clue that the Wenckebach AV block might be in the His-Purkinje system. The HV interval increases from 70 msec to 280 msec, and then block distal to His results.

Although it has been suggested that type I and type II AV block are different manifestations of the same electrophysiological mechanism, differing only quantitatively in the size of the increments, clinically separating second degree AV block into type I and type II serves a useful function, and in most instances, the differentiation can be made easily and reliably from the surface ECG. Type II AV block often antedates the development of Adams-Stokes syncope and complete AV block, while type I AV block with a normal QRS complex is generally more benign and does not progress to more advanced forms of AV conduction disturbance. In older people, type I AV block with or without bundle branch block has been associated with a clinical picture similar to that in type II AV block.

In the patient with an acute myocardial infarction, type I AV block usually accompanies inferior infarction (perhaps more often if a right ventricular infarction also occurs), is transient, and does not require temporary pacing, whereas type II AV block occurs in the setting of an acute anterior myocardial infarction, can require temporary or permanent pacing, and is associated with a high rate of mortality, generally due to pump failure.[446] A high degree of AV block can occur in patients with acute inferior myocardial infarction and is associated with more myocardial damage and a higher mortality rate compared with those without AV block.

While type I conduction disturbance is ubiquitous and can occur in any cardiac tissue in vivo, as well as in vitro, the site of block for the usual forms of second degree AV block can be judged from the surface ECG with sufficient reliability to permit clinical decisions without requiring invasive electrophysiological studies in most instances. Type I AV block with a normal QRS complex almost always takes place at the level of the AV node, proximal to the His bundle. An exception is the uncommon patient with type I intrahisian block. Type II AV block, particularly in association with a bundle branch block, is localized to the His-Purkinje system. Type I AV block in a patient with a bundle branch block can be due to block in the AV node or in the His-Purkinje system. Type II AV block in a patient with a normal QRS complex can be due to intrahisian AV block, but the block is likely to be type I AV nodal block, which exhibits small increments in AV conduction time.

The preceding generalizations encompass the vast majority of patients who present with second degree AV block. However, certain caveats must be heeded to avoid misdiagnosis because of subtle ECG changes or exceptions:

1. The 2:1 AV block can be a form of type I or type II AV block (Fig. 22–53). If the QRS complex is normal, the block is more likely to be type I, located in the AV node, and one should search for a transition of the 2:1 block to 3:2 block, during which the P-R interval lengthens in the second cardiac cycle. If a bundle branch block is present, the block can be located either in the AV node or in the His-Purkinje system.

2. AV block can occur simultaneously at two or more levels and can cause difficulty in distinguishing between types I and II.[447]

3. If the atrial rate varies, it can alter conduction times and cause type I AV block to stimulate type II or change type II AV block into type I.[448] For example, if the shortest atrial cycle length that just achieved 1:1 AV nodal conduction at a constant P-R interval is decreased by as little as 10 or 20 msec, the P wave of the shortened cycle can block at the level of the AV node without an apparent increase in the antecedent P-R interval. Apparent type II AV block in the His-Purkinje system can be converted to type I in the His-Purkinje system in some patients by increasing the atrial rate.

4. Concealed premature His depolarizations can create electrocardiographic patterns that simulate type I or type II AV block (see Fig. 20–38, p. 580).

5. Abrupt, transient alterations in autonomic tone can cause sudden block of one or more P waves without altering the P-R interval of the conducted P wave before or after block. Thus apparent type II AV block would be produced at the AV node. Clinically, a burst of vagal tone usually lengthens the P-P interval as well as producing AV block.

6. The response of the AV block to autonomic changes either spontaneous or induced to distinguish type I from type II AV block, can be misleading. Although vagal stimulation generally increases and vagolytic agents decrease the extent of type I AV block, such conclusions are based on the assumption that the intervention acts primarily on the AV node and fail to consider rate changes. For example, atropine can minimally improve conduction in the AV node and markedly increase the sinus rate, resulting in an *increase* in AV nodal-conduction time and the degree of AV block as a result of the faster atrial rate (Fig. 22–51*B*). Conversely, if an increase in vagal tone minimally prolongs AV conduction time but greatly slows the heart rate, the net effect on type I AV block may be to improve conduction. In general, however, carotid sinus massage improves and atropine worsens AV conduction in patients with His-Purkinje block, while the opposite results are to be expected in patients who have AV nodal block. These two interventions can help differentiate the site of block without invasive study, although damaged His-Purkinje tissue may be influenced by changes in autonomic tone.

7. During type I AV block with high ratios of conducted beats, the increment in P-R interval can be quite small, suggesting type II AV block if only the last few P-R intervals before the blocked P wave are measured. By comparing the P-R interval of the first beat in the long Wenckebach cycle with that of the beats immediately preceding the blocked P wave, the increment in AV conduction becomes readily apparent.

8. The classic AV Wenckebach structure depends on a stable atrial rate and a maximal increment in AV conduction time for the second P-R interval of the Wenckebach cycle, with a progressive decrease in subsequent beats. Unstable or unusual alterations in the increment of AV conduction time or in the atrial rate, often seen with long Wenckebach cycles, result in atypical forms of type I AV block in which the last R-R interval can lengthen because the P-R increment *increases;* these are common.

9. Finally, it is important to remember that the P-R interval in the scalar ECG is made up of conduction through the atrium, the AV node, and the His-Purkinje system. An increment in HV conduction, for example, can be masked in the scalar ECG by a reduction in the A-H interval, and the resulting P-R interval will not reflect the entire increment in His-Purkinje conduction time. Very long P-R intervals (>200 msec) are more likely to result from AV nodal conduction delay (and block), with or without concomitant His-Purkinje conduction delay, although an H-V interval of 350 msec is quite possible.

First degree and type I second degree AV block can occur in normal healthy children, and Wenckebach AV block can be a normal phenomenon in well-trained athletes, probably related to an increase in resting vagal tone. Occasionally, progressive worsening of the Wenckebach AV conduction disorder can result so that the athlete becomes symptomatic and has to decondition. In patients who have chronic second degree AV nodal block (proximal to the His bundle)

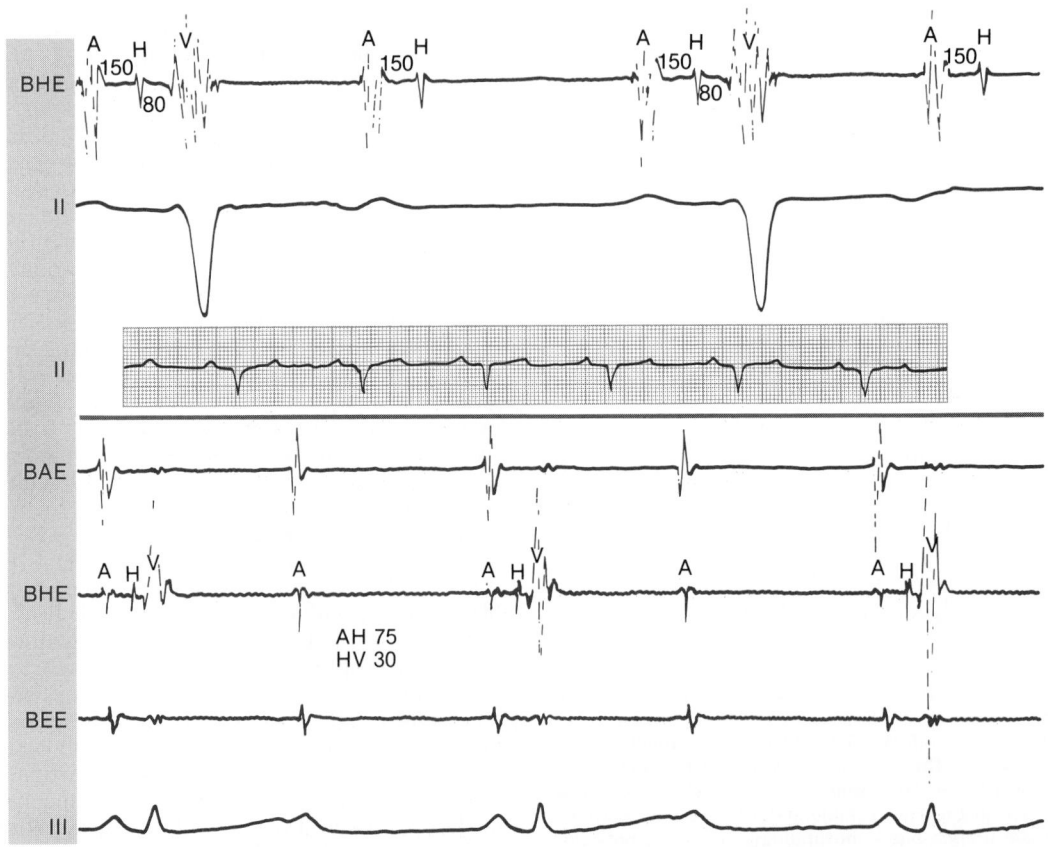

FIGURE 22–53. 2:1 AV block proximal and distal to the His bundle deflection in two different patients. *Top*, 2:1 AV block seen in the scalar ECG occurs distal to the His bundle recording site in a patient with right bundle branch block and anterior hemiblock. The A-H interval (150 msec) and H-V interval (80 msec) are both prolonged. *Bottom*, 2:1 AV block occurs proximal to the bundle of His in a patient with a normal QRS complex. The A-H interval (75 msec) and the H-V interval (30 msec) remain constant and normal.

without structural heart disease, the course is relatively benign (except in older age groups), while in those who have structural heart disease the prognosis is poor and related to underlying heart disease. *Advanced AV block* indicates block of two or more consecutive P waves.

Complete AV Block

ELECTROCARDIOGRAPHIC RECOGNITION. Complete AV block occurs when no atrial activity conducts to the ventricles, and therefore, the atria and ventricles are controlled by independent pacemakers. Thus, complete AV block is one type of complete AV dissociation (see p. 692). The atrial pacemaker can be sinus or ectopic (tachycardia, flutter, or fibrillation) or can result from an AV junctional focus occurring above the block with retrograde atrial conduction. The ventricular focus is usually located just below the region of block, which can be above or below the His bundle bifurcation. Sites of ventricular pacemaker activity that are in, or closer to, the His bundle appear to be more stable and can produce a faster escape rate than those located more distally in the ventricular conduction system. The ventricular rate in acquired complete heart block is less than 40 beats/min but can be faster in congenital complete AV block. The ventricular rhythm, usually regular, can vary owing to premature ventricular complexes, a shift in the pacemaker site, an irregularly discharging pacemaker focus, or autonomic influences.

CLINICAL FEATURES. Complete AV block can result from block at the level of the AV node (usually congenital) (Fig. 22–54), within the bundle of His, or distal to it in the Purkinje system (usually acquired) (Fig. 22–55). Block proximal to the His bundle generally exhibits normal QRS complexes and rates of 40 to 60 beats/min because the

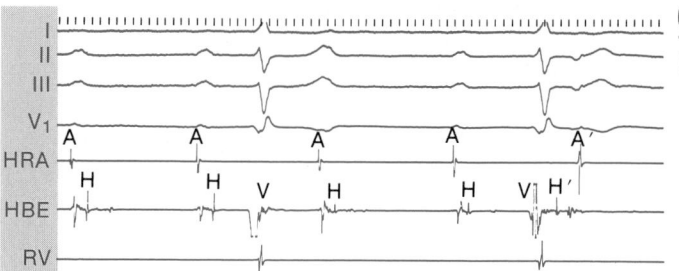

FIGURE 22–55. Complete anterograde AV block with retrograde VA conduction. All the sinus P waves block distal to His, consistent with acquired complete AV block. The ventricles escape at a cycle length of approximately 1800 msec (33 beats/min) and are not preceded by His bundle activation. The ventricular escape rhythm produces a QRS contour with left axis deviation and right bundle branch block, possibly due to impulse origin in the posterior fascicle of the left bundle branch. Of interest is the fact that the second ventricular escape beat conducts retrogradely through His (H') and to the atrium (note the low-high atrial activation sequence and the negative P wave in leads II and III). The first ventricular complex does not conduct retrogradely, probably because the His bundle is still refractory from the immediately atrial impulse.

escape focus that controls the ventricle arises in or near the His bundle. In complete AV nodal block, the P wave is not followed by a His deflection, but each ventricular complex is preceded by a His deflection (Fig. 22–54). His bundle electrocardiography can be useful to differentiate AV nodal from intrahisian block, since the latter may carry a more serious prognosis than the former. Intrahisian block is recognized infrequently without invasive studies. In patients with AV nodal block, atropine usually speeds both the atrial and the ventricular rates. Exercise can reduce the extent of AV nodal block. Acquired complete AV block occurs most commonly distal to the bundle of His owing to trifascicular conduction disturbance. Each P wave is followed by a His deflection, and the ventricular escape complexes are not preceded by a His deflection (Fig. 22–55). The QRS complex is abnormal, and the ventricular rate is usually less than 40 beats/min.

Unusual forms such as paroxysmal AV block or AV block following a period of rapid ventricular rate can occur. Paroxysmal AV block in some instances can be due to hyperresponsiveness of the AV node to vagotonic reflexes. Surgery, electrolyte disturbances, myoendocarditis,[449] tumors, Chagas' disease, rheumatoid nodules, calcific aortic stenosis, myxedema, polymyositis, infiltrative processes (such as amyloid, sarcoid, or scleroderma), and an almost endless assortment of common and unusual conditions can produce AV block. In the adult, drug toxicity, coronary disease, and degenerative processes appear to be the most common causes of AV heart block. The degenerative process produces partial or complete anatomical or electrical disruption within the AV nodal region, the AV bundle, or both bundle branches. Rapid rates can sometimes be followed by block, an event known as *overdrive suppression* of conduction. This form of block may be important as a cause of paroxysmal AV block after cessation of a tachycardia.

AV Block in Children. In children, the most common cause of AV block is congenital (Chap. 29). Under such circumstances, the AV block can be an isolated finding or associated with other lesions. Connective tissue disease (see p. 1667) and the presence of anti–Rh_0 negative antibodies in maternal sera of patients with congenital complete AV block raise the possibility that placentally transmitted antibodies play a role in some instances.[450–452] Anatomical disruption between the atrial musculature and peripheral parts of the conduction system and nodoventricular discontinuity are two common histological findings. Children are most often asymptomatic; however, some develop symptoms that require pacemaker implantation. Mortality from

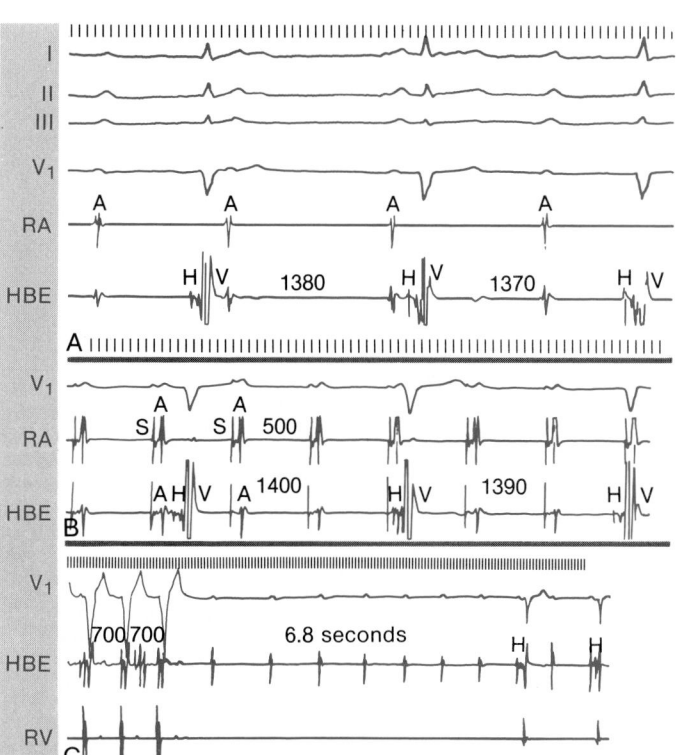

FIGURE 22–54. Congenital third degree AV block. In panel *A*, complete AV nodal block is apparent. No P wave is followed by a His bundle potential, while each ventricular depolarization is preceded by a His bundle potential. In panel *B*, atrial pacing (cycle length 500 msec) fails to alter cycle length of the functional rhythm. Still, no P wave is followed by a His bundle potential. In panel *C*, after 30 sec of ventricular pacing (cycle length 700 msec), suppression of the junctional focus results for almost 7 sec (overdrive suppression of automaticity; see Chapter 20).

congenital AV block is highest in the neonatal period, is much lower during childhood and adolescence, and increases slowly later in life. Adams-Stokes attacks can occur in patients with congenital heart block at any age. It is difficult to predict the prognosis in the individual patient. A persistent heart rate at rest of 50 beats/min or less correlates with the incidence of syncope, and extreme bradycardia can contribute to the frequency of Adams-Stokes attacks in children with congenital complete AV block. The site of block may not distinguish symptomatic children who have congenital or surgically induced complete heart block from those without symptoms. Prolonged recovery times of escape foci following rapid pacing (Fig. 22–54C) (see discussion of sinus node recovery time, p. 648) slow heart rates on 24-hour ECG recordings, and the occurrence of paroxysmal tachycardias may be predisposing factors to the development of symptoms.

CLINICAL FEATURES. Many of the signs of AV block are evidenced at the bedside. First degree AV block can be recognized by a long *a-c* wave interval in the jugular venous pulse and by diminished intensity of the first heart sound as the P-R interval lengthens. In type I second degree AV block, the heart rate may increase imperceptibly with gradually diminishing intensity of the first heart sound, widening of the *a-c* interval, terminated by a pause, and an *a* wave not followed by a *v* wave. Intermittent ventricular pauses and *a* waves in the neck not followed by *v* waves characterize type II AV block. The first heart sound maintains a constant intensity. In complete AV block, the findings are the same as those in AV dissociation (see below).

Significant clinical manifestations of first and second degree AV block usually consist of palpitations or subjective feelings of the heart "missing a beat." Persistent 2:1 AV block can produce symptoms of chronic bradycardia. Complete AV block can be accompanied by signs and symptoms of reduced cardiac output, syncope or presyncope, angina, or palpitations due to ventricular tachyarrhythmias. It can occur in twins.[453]

MANAGEMENT. As discussed in Chapter 23, drugs cannot be relied on to increase the heart rate for more than several hours to several days in patients with symptomatic heart block without producing significant side effects. Therefore, temporary or permanent pacemaker insertion is indicated in patients with symptomatic bradyarrhythmias.[454] Long-

term pacing can alter cardiac function.[455] For short-term therapy when the block is likely to be evanescent but still requires treatment or until adequate pacing therapy can be established, vagolytic agents such as atropine are useful for patients who have AV nodal disturbances, while catecholamines such as isoproterenol can be used transiently to treat patients who have heart block at any site (see treatment for Sinus Bradycardia, above). Isoproterenol should be used with extreme caution or not at all in patients who have acute myocardial infarction. The use of transcutaneous pacing is preferable.

Atrioventricular (AV) Dissociation

CLASSIFICATION. As the term indicates, dissociated or independent beating of atria and ventricles defines AV dissociation. AV dissociation is never a *primary* disturbance of rhythm but is a "symptom" of an underlying rhythm disturbance produced by one of three causes or a combination of causes (Fig. 22–56) that prevent the normal transmission of impulses from atrium to ventricle, as follows:

1. Slowing of the dominant pacemaker of the heart (usually the sinus node), which allows escape of a subsidiary or latent pacemaker. AV dissociation by *default* of the primary pacemaker to a subsidiary one in this manner is often a normal phenomenon. It may occur during sinus arrhythmia or sinus bradycardia, permitting an independent AV junction rhythm to arise (Fig. 22–3B).

2. Acceleration of a latent pacemaker that *usurps* control of the ventricles. Abnormally enhanced discharge rate of a usually slower subsidiary pacemaker is pathological and commonly occurs during nonparoxysmal AV junctional tachycardia or ventricular tachycardia without retrograde atrial capture (see Figs. 22–22 and 22–39).

3. Block, generally at the AV junction, that prevents impulses formed at a normal rate in a dominant pacemaker from reaching the ventricles and allows the ventricles to beat under the control of a subsidiary pacemaker. Junctional or ventricular escape rhythm during AV block, without retrograde atrial capture, is a common example in which block gives rise to AV dissociation. It is important to remember that complete AV block is *not* synonymous with complete AV dissociation; patients who have complete AV block have complete AV dissociation, but patients who

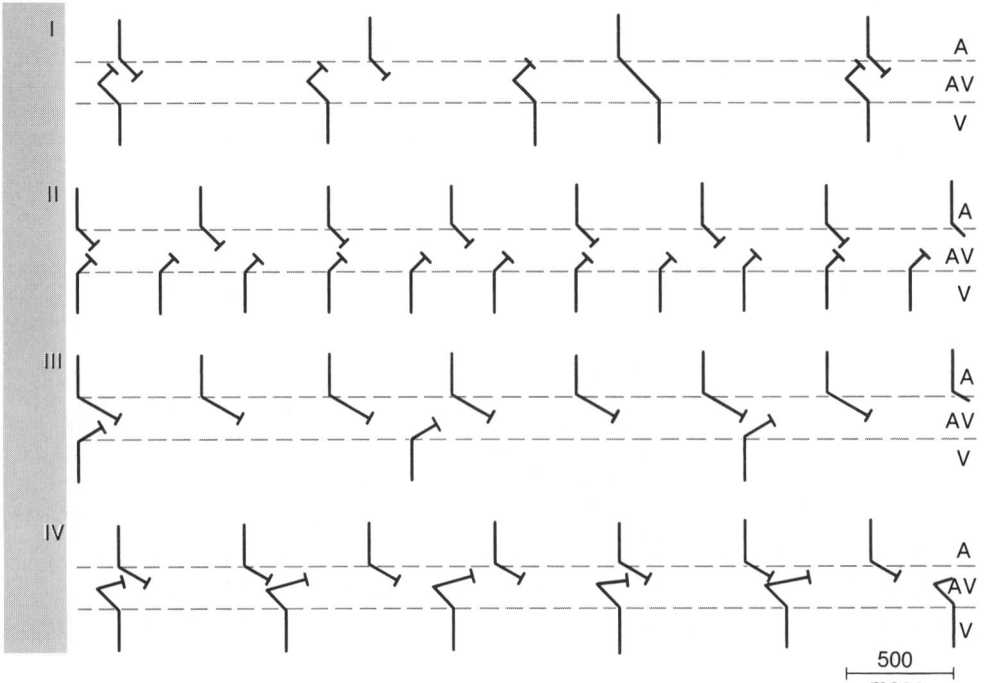

FIGURE 22–56. Diagrammatic illustration of the causes of AV dissociation. A sinus bradycardia that allows the escape of an AV junctional rhythm which does not capture the atria retrogradely illustrates cause I (top panel). Intermittent sinus captures occur (third P wave) to produce incomplete AV dissociation (see Fig. 22–3B). For cause II, a ventricular tachycardia without retrograde atrial capture produces complete AV dissociation (see Figs. 22–22 and 22–39). As the third cause, complete AV block with a ventricular escape rhythm is diagrammed (see Figs. 22–54 and 22–55). The combination of causes II and III is shown in panel IV, representing a nonparoxysmal AV junctional tachycardia and some degree of AV block.

500
msec

have complete AV dissociation may or may not have complete AV block (see Figs. 22–54 and 22–55).

4. A combination of causes. For example, when digitalis excess results in the production of nonparoxysmal AV junctional tachycardia associated with SA or AV block.

MECHANISMS. With this classification in mind, it is important to emphasize that the term *AV dissociation* is *not* a diagnosis and is analogous to the term *jaundice* or *fever.* One must state that "AV dissociation is present *due to . . .*" and then give the cause. The accelerated rate of a slower, normally subsidiary pacemaker or the slower rate of a faster, normally dominant pacemaker that prevents conduction due to physiological collision and mutual extinction of opposing wavefronts (interference) or the manifestations of AV block are the basic disturbances producing AV dissociation. The atria in all these cases beat independently from the ventricles, under control of the sinus node or ectopic atrial or AV junctional pacemakers, and can exhibit any type of supraventricular rhythms. If a single pacemaker establishes control of both atria and ventricles for one beat (capture) or a series of beats (sinus rhythm, AV junctional rhythm with retrograde atrial capture, ventricular tachycardia with retrograde atrial capture, and so forth), AV dissociation is abolished for that period. Conversely, as stated above, whenever the atria and ventricles fail to respond to a single impulse for one beat (premature ventricular complex without retrograde capture of the atrium) or a series of beats (ventricular tachycardia without retrograde atrial capture), AV dissociation exists for that period. The interruption of AV dissociation by one or a series of beats under the control of one pacemaker, either anterogradely or retrogradely, indicates that the AV dissociation is incomplete. Complete or incomplete dissociation also can occur in association with all forms of AV block. Commonly, when AV dissociation occurs as a result of AV block, the atrial rate exceeds the ventricular rate. For example, a subsidiary pacemaker with a rate of 40 beats/min can escape in the presence of a 2:1 AV block when the atrial rate is 78. If the AV block is bidirectional, AV dissociation results.

ELECTROCARDIOGRAPHIC AND CLINICAL FEATURES. The electrocardiogram demonstrates the independence of P waves and QRS complexes. The P-wave morphology depends on the rhythm controlling the atria (sinus, atrial tachycardia, junctional, flutter, or fibrillation). During complete AV dissociation, both the QRS complex and the P waves appear regularly spaced without a fixed temporal relationship to each other. When the dissociation is incomplete, a QRS complex of supraventricular contour occurs early and is preceded by a P wave at a P-R interval exceeding 0.12 sec and within a conductable range. This indicates ventricular capture by the supraventricular focus. Similarly, a premature P wave with a retrograde morphology and a conductable R-P interval may indicate retrograde atrial capture by the subsidiary focus.

The physical findings include a variable intensity of the first heart sound as the P-R interval changes, atrial sounds, and *a* waves in the jugular venous pulse lacking a consistent relationship to ventricular contraction. Intermittent large (cannon) *a* waves may be seen in the jugular venous pulse when atrial and ventricular contractions occur simultaneously. The second heart sound can split normally or paradoxically, depending on the manner of ventricular activation. A premature beat representing a ventricular capture can interrupt a regular heart rhythm. When the ventricular rate exceeds the atrial rate, a cyclic increase in intensity of the first heart sound is produced as the P-R interval shortens, climaxed by a very loud sound (bruit de canon). This intense sound is followed by a sudden reduction in intensity of the first heart sound and the appearance of giant *a* waves as the P-R interval shortens and P waves "march through" the cardiac cycle.

MANAGEMENT. This is directed toward the underlying heart disease and precipitating cause. The individual components *producing the AV dissociation*—not the AV dissociation per se—determine the specific type of antiarrhythmic approaches. Therapy ranges from pacemaker insertion in a patient who has AV dissociation due to complete AV block to antiarrhythmic drug administration in a patient who has AV dissociation due to a ventricular tachycardia.

OTHER ELECTROPHYSIOLOGICAL ABNORMALITIES LEADING TO CARDIAC ARRHYTHMIAS

SUPERNORMAL CONDUCTION AND EXCITATION

SUPERNORMAL CONDUCTION. This is the term applied to situations characterized by conduction that is better than expected but generally not as good as normal.[456–459] The phenomenon almost always occurs when conduction is depressed but can be present in normal cardiac tissues as well. It generally occurs when conduction takes place during the relative refractory period of the preceding complex (Fig. 22–57). The electrophysiological basis can relate, in some examples, to supernormal excitability (see below) but probably to other mechanisms as well. Supernormal conduction commonly has been invoked to explain AV (most probably His-Purkinje rather than AV nodal) conduction that is more rapid than expected or AV conduction that results when AV block is expected.

SUPERNORMAL EXCITATION. This phenomenon results when a stimulus, normally subthreshold, occurs during the supernormal period of recovery of the preceding complex and produces a propagated response. Stimuli occurring earlier or later fail to produce a propagated response. Demonstrated in vitro in Purkinje fibers but not ventricular muscle, supernormal excitation occurs during phase 3 of the cardiac action potential when the membrane potential, closer to threshold at the end of repolarization, requires less current to produce a propagated response. A similar phenomenon occurs during phase 4 diastolic depolarization or during afterdepolarizations that reduce the membrane potential closer to threshold. The phenomenon is most easily recognized when a nonsensing pacemaker, failing because of battery exhaustion and reduced output, produces a propagated response only when discharge falls during a specific time period in a cardiac cycle (Fig. 22–58). Similar phenomena probably occur spontaneously with "weak" automatic foci, but the recognition of these events clinically is difficult and often speculative.

CONCEALED CONDUCTION

Concealed conduction describes the phenomenon during which impulses penetrate an area of the conduction tissue, the AV node commonly but other areas as well, without emerging.[460] Since the transmission of the impulse is concealed, i.e., electrically silent in the standard electrocardiogram, concealed conduction becomes manifested only by its *effects* on the conduction and/or formation of subsequent impulses.[461] The most common example follows a premature ventricular complex. Partial retrograde penetration of the AV node by the premature ventricular complex is *deduced* because the following sinus-initiated P wave blocks to produce a compensatory pause (Fig. 22–59) or conducts with a longer P-R interval if the premature ventricular complex is interpolated. The slower ventricular response when the atrial rate increases from atrial flutter to atrial fibrillation is due to a greater number of atrial impulses blocking (conducting into, without emerging) in the AV node and is a manifestation of concealed conduction.[462] Concealed conduction occurs in WPW syndrome and can be manifested by unidirectional block anterogradely or retrogradely in an accessory pathway[463] (see p. 665). Concealed junctional extrasystoles (Fig. 20–38, p. 580) can create electrocardiographic manifestations of apparent AV block. Strict confirmation of concealed conduction should be the demonstration of conduction, such as in the form of conducted junctional extrasystoles (Fig. 22–19, p. 659).

PARASYSTOLE (Fig. 22–60)

This refers to a cardiac arrhythmia characterized electrocardiographically by (1) varying coupling interval between the ectopic (parasystolic) complex and the dominant (generally, sinus-initiated) complex, (2) a common minimal time interval between interectopic intervals, with the longer interectopic intervals being multiples of this minimal interval, (3) fusion complexes, and (4) the presence of the parasystolic impulse whenever the cardiac chamber is excitable. Parasystole with exit block is suspected when the parasystolic discharge focus fails to appear even though cardiac tissue is excitable. The analogy commonly invoked to represent parasystole is the behavior of a fixed-rate nonsensing (VOO) pacemaker (Chap. 23). Parasystole can occur in the sinus and AV nodes, atrium and ventricle, and AV junction. The parasystolic mechanism presumably results from the regular discharge of an automatic focus that is independent of, and protected from, discharge by the dominant cardiac rhythm. A

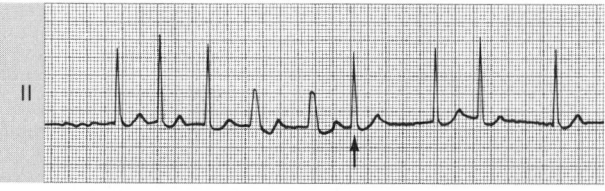

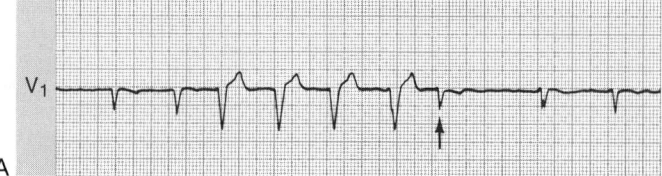

A

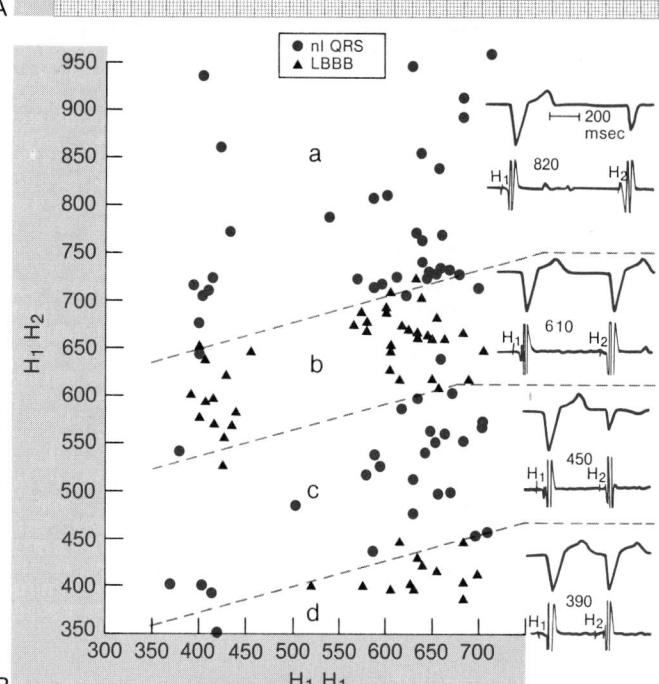

B

FIGURE 22–57. Supernormal conduction. Panel *A* illustrates atrial fibrillation with long-short R-R cycle sequences giving rise to QRS complexes conducted with a functional left bundle branch block. In each example, however, a shorter R-R cycle length is terminated by a normal QRS complex (arrow), an example of supernormal conduction.

Panel *B* shows a graph of the intervals and illustrative recordings during an electrophysiological study of the patient whose ECG is shown in panel *A*. The H-V interval of the complexes conducted with a left bundle branch block morphology is 45 msec, while the H-V interval of those conducted with a normal morphology is 35 msec. The graph indicates the premature interval (H_1-H_2, ordinate) plotted against the preceding cycle length (H_1-H_1, abscissa). All H_1-H_1 intervals were taken from complexes with a left bundle branch block morphology. Normal complexes are represented by filled circles and left bundle branch block contours by filled triangles. Four zones of conduction are identified, and illustrated by the four examples to the right. The longest H_1-H_2 intervals are followed by a normal intraventricular conduction (zone A), while at shorter intervals, left bundle branch block occurs (zone B). When the H_1-H_2 interval shortens further, normal intraventricular conduction returns and the H-V intervals shorten to 35 msec (zone C, supernormal conduction). At the shortest H_1-H_2 interval, left bundle branch block again appears (zone D). (From Miles, W. M., Prystowsky, E. N., Heger, J. J., and Zipes, D. P.: Evaluation of the patient with wide QRS tachycardia. Med. Clin. North Am. *68*:1015, 1984.)

FIGURE 22–58. Supernormal excitation. Panels *A* and *B* represent noncontiguous portions of a continuous ECG recording with a middle segment removed (dotted line). The patient presented with a bipolar pacemaker that had exceeded end-of-life and was no longer consistently producing ventricular depolarization (small negative deflections indicated by the upright arrow). A temporary pacemaker was implanted and set at a fixed rate (asynchronous, V00). These large deflections are indicated by the inverted arrow. The numbers in msec indicate the interval between the onset of the QRS complex and the following subthreshold pacemaker stimulus. At intervals of 370 msec (beginning, panel *A*) and 490 msec (end, panel *B*), the subthreshold stimulus fails to produce a propagated ventricular response. However, at intervals between 380 and 480 msec, ventricular depolarizations result (filled circles). Thus the period of supernormal excitation is 100 msec duration, from 380 to 480 msec after the onset of the QRS complex.

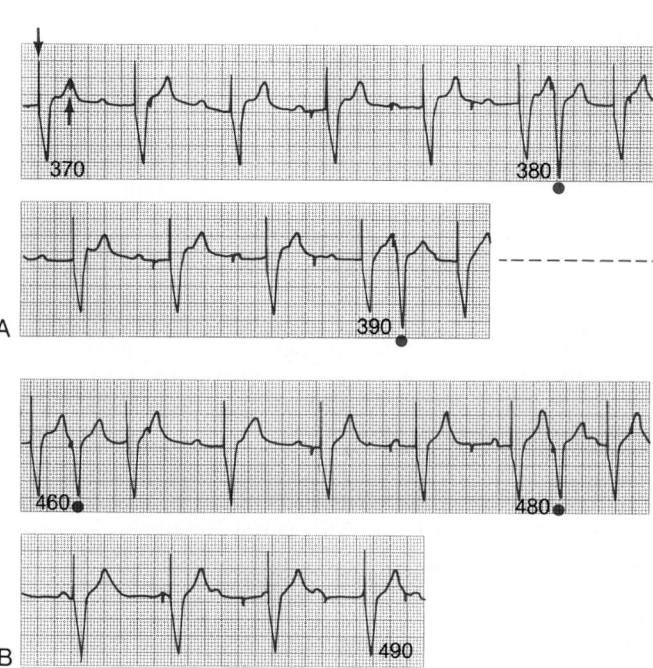

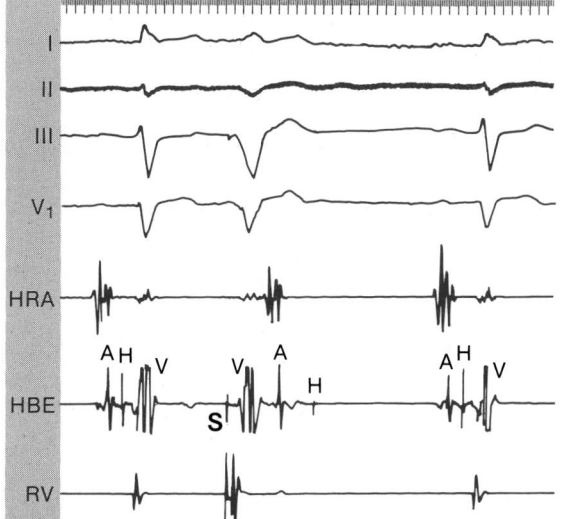

plexes without intervening beats. Phase response curves can be generated. Fixed coupling between the dominant and parasystolic rhythms can occur due to a variety of mechanisms, including entrainment. It is possible that modulated parasystole in the presence of supernormal excitability can trigger ventricular fibrillation.

FIGURE 22-59. Concealed conduction. Following the first normally conducted sinus-initiated complex, a premature ventricular complex is stimulated (S). The next spontaneous sinus-initiated P wave blocks to produce a fully compensatory pause. The third sinus-initiated P wave conducts normally. From the His bundle recording it is obvious that the nonconducted sinus beat blocks distal to the His bundle recording site. Note that the A-H interval of the nonconducted sinus P wave beat is prolonged, suggesting that the premature ventricular complex retrogradely activated His and invaded the AV node, making it partially refractory to the next sinus beat. Since retrograde conduction into the AV node is not recorded, and can only be surmised on the basis of the increase in the following A-H interval, it is an example of concealed conduction. Further, since retrograde His and AV node activation by the premature ventricular complex would not be apparent in the scalar ECG but is responsible for the compensatory pause, the blocked P wave is an example of concealed conduction.

Acknowledgments

The author thanks William M. Miles, M.D., and Lawrence S. Klein, M.D., for critical comments and Joan Zipes and Robin Reid for secretarial assistance.

REFERENCES

1. Barsky, A. J., Cleary, P. D., Barnett, M. C., et al.: The accuracy of symptom reporting by patients complaining of palpitations. Am. J. Med. 97:214, 1994.
2. Munro, N. C., McIntosh, S., Lawson, J., et al.: Incidence of complications after carotid sinus massage in older patients with syncope. J. Am. Geriatr. Soc. 42:1248, 1994.

SINUS NODAL DISTURBANCES

3. Spodick, D. H.: Normal sinus heart rate: Sinus tachycardia and sinus bradycardia redefined. Am. Heart J. 124:1119, 1992.
4. Dickerson, L. W., Huang, A. H., Thurnher, M. M., et al.: Relationship between coronary hemodynamic changes and the phasic events of rapid eye movement sleep. Sleep 16:1550, 1993.
5. Scott, C. D., McComb, J. M., and Dark, J. H.: Heart rate and late mortality in cardiac transplant recipients. Eur. Heart J. 14:530, 1993.
6. Tsai, J., Chern, T. L., Hu, S. C., et al.: The clinical implication of theophylline intoxication in the emergency department. Hum. Exp. Toxicol. 13:651, 1994.
7. Sills, I. N.: Hyperthyroidism. Pediatr. Rev. 15:417, 1994.
8. Johnson, N. J., and Marchlinski, F. E.: Arrhythmias induced by device antitachycardia therapy due to diagnostic nonspecificity. J. Am. Coll. Cardiol. 18:1418, 1991.
9. Gelb, B. D., and Garson, A., Jr.: Noninvasive discrimination of right atrial ectopic tachycardia from sinus tachycardia in dilated cardiomyopathy. Am. Heart J. 120:886, 1990.
10. Morillo, C. A., Klein, G. J., Thakur, R. K., et al.: Mechanism of "inappropriate" sinus tachycardia: Role of sympathovagal balance. Circulation 90:873, 1994.
11. Skeberis, V., Simonis, F., Tsakonas, K., et al.: Inappropriate sinus tachycardia following radiofrequency ablation of AV nodal tachycardia: Incidence and clinical significance. PACE 17:924, 1994.
12. Kocovic, D. Z., Harada, T., Shea, J. B., et al.: Alterations of heart rate and of heart rate variability after radiofrequency catheter ablation of supraventricular tachycardia: Delineation of parasympathetic pathways in the human heart. Circulation 88:1671, 1993.
13. Ehlert, F. A., Goldberger, J. J., Brooks, R., et al.: Persistent inappropriate sinus tachycardia after radiofrequency current catheter modification of the atrioventricular node. Am. J. Cardiol. 69:1092, 1992.
14. Waspe, L. E., Chien, W. W., Merillat, J. C., et al.: Sinus node modification using radiofrequency current in a patient with persistent inappropriate sinus tachycardia. PACE 17:1569, 1994.
15. Hendry, P. J., Packer, D. L., Anstadt, M. P., et al.: Surgical treatment of automatic atrial tachycardias. Ann. Thorac. Surg. 42:253, 1990.
16. DePaola, A. A. G., Horowitz, L. N., Vattimo, A. C., et al.: Sinus node artery occlusion for treatment of chronic nonparoxysmal sinus tachycardia. Am. J. Cardiol. 70:128, 1992.
17. Kollai, M., Bonyhay, I., Jokkel, G., et al.: Cardiac vagal hyperactivity in adolescent anorexia nervosa. Eur. Heart J. 15:1113, 1994.
18. Scott, C. D., Dark, J. H., and McComb, J. M.: Sinus node function after cardiac transplantation. J. Am. Coll. Cardiol. 24:1334, 1994.
19. Caeiro, T., and Iosa, D.: Chronic Chagas' disease: Possible mechanism of sinus bradycardia. Can. J. Cardiol. 10:765, 1994.
20. Alboni, T., Menozzi, C., Brignole, M., et al.: An abnormal neuroreflex plays a role in causing syncope in sinus bradycardia. J. Am. Coll. Cardiol. 22:1130, 1993.
21. Frank, J. I., Ropper, A. H., and Zuniga, G.: Acute intracranial lesions and respiratory sinus arrhythmia. Arch. Neurol. 49:1200, 1992.
22. Sneddon, J. F., and Camm, A. J.: Sinus node disease: Current concepts in diagnosis and therapy. Drugs. 44:728, 1992.
23. Benditt, D. G., Sakaguchi, S., Goldstein, M. A., et al.: Sinus node dysfunction: Pathophysiology, clinical features, evaluation and treatment. In Zipes, D. P., and Jalife, J. (eds.): Cardiac Electrophysiology: From Cell to Bedside. 2nd ed. Philadelphia, W. B. Saunders Company, 1994, p. 1215.
24. Kyrickidis, M., Barbetseas, J., Antonopoulos, A., et al.: Early atrial arrhythmias in acute myocardial infarction: Role of the sinus node artery. Chest 101:944, 1992.
25. Becker, H., Brandenburg, U., Peter, J. H., et al.: Reversal of sinus arrest and atrioventricular conduction block in patients with sleep apnea during nasal continuous positive airway pressure. Am. J. Respir. Crit. Care Med. 151:215, 1995.
26. Fisch, C.: Electrocardiographic manifestations of exit block. In Zipes, D.P., and Jalife, J. (eds.): Cardiac Electrophysiology: From Cell to Bedside. 2nd ed. Philadelphia, W. B. Saunders Company, 1994, p. 955.

number of mechanisms have been postulated to explain the apparent protection enjoyed by the parasystolic rhythm.[464]

These "classic" definitions of parasystole now need to be modified because it has been well established that the dominant sinus beats can modulate the discharge rate of the parasystolic rhythm despite entrance block. Thus wide variations in the modulated parasystolic cycle may occur. The "true" or unmodulated parasystolic cycle length can be determined by finding two consecutive parasystolic com-

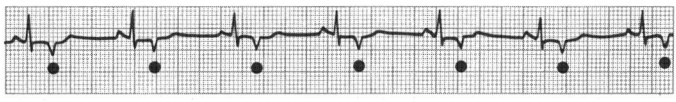

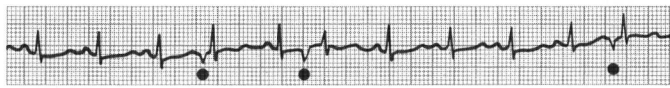

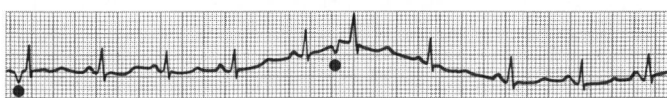

FIGURE 22-60. Atrial parasystole. *Top panel,* The atrial parasystolic impulses (filled circles under the negative P waves) are present at a fixed coupling interval to the dominant sinus rhythm. The reason for the fixed coupling is as follows: Each time the parasystolic impulse depolarizes the atrium, it also discharges the sinus node. Diastolic depolarization in the sinus node begins at that point (reset) and results in the following sinus P wave (positive P wave). Thus the constant parasystolic discharge rate (interectopic interval approximately 960 msec), resetting of the sinus node, and constant phase 4 diastolic depolarization in the sinus node combine to result in fixed coupling. *Middle and bottom panels,* The sinus discharge rate is slightly faster. It is no longer discharged by the parasystolic impulse which is still occurring at approximately 960 msec (slightly longer interval in the bottom tracing). Variable coupling, the usual presentation of parasystole, results. Lead II.

27. Wu, D. L., Yeh, S. J., Lin, F. C., et al.: Sinus automaticity and sinoatrial conduction in severe symptomatic sick sinus syndrome. J. Am. Coll. Cardiol. *19*:355, 1992.

28. Bjornstad, H., Storstein, L., Meen, H. D., et al.: Ambulatory electrocardiographic findings in top athletes, athletic students and controlled subjects. Cardiology *84*:42, 1994.

29. Benditt, D. G., Petersen, M., Lurie, K. G., et al.: Cardiac pacing for prevention of recurrent vasovagal syncope. Ann. Intern. Med. *122*:204, 1995.

30. Asseman, P., Berzin, B., Desry, D., et al.: Postextrasystolic sinoatrial exit block in human sick sinus syndrome: Demonstration by direct recording of sinus node electrograms. Am. Heart J. *122*:1633, 1991.

31. Centurion, O. A., Fukatani, M., Konoe, A., et al.: Different distribution of abnormal endocardial electrograms within the right atrium in patients with sick sinus syndrome. Br. Heart J. *68*:596, 1992.

32. Sgarbossa, E. B., Pinski, S. L., Maloney, J. D., et al.: Chronic atrial fibrillation and stroke in paced patients with sick sinus syndrome: Relevance of clinical characteristics and pacing modalities. Circulation *88*:1045, 1993.

33. Marcus, B., Gillette, P. C., and Garson, A., Jr.: Electrophysiologic evaluation of sinus node dysfunction in postoperative children and young adults utilizing combined autonomic blockade. Clin. Cardiol. *14*:33, 1991.

34. Matthys, D., and Verhaaren, H.: Exercise-induced bradycardia after Mustard repair for complete transposition. Int. J. Cardiol. *36*:126, 1992.

35. Lee, W. J., Wu, M. H., Young, M. L., et al.: Sinus node dysfunction in children. Acta Paediatr. Sin. *33*:159, 1992.

36. Bharati, S., and Lev, M.: The pathologic changes in the conduction system beyond the age of 90. Am. Heart J. *124*:486, 1992.

37. Alboni, P., Baggioni, G. F., Scarfo, S., et al.: Role of sinus node artery disease in sick sinus syndrome in inferior wall acute myocardial infarction. Am. J. Cardiol. *67*:1180, 1991.

38. Haywood, G. A., Katritsis, D., Ward, J., et al.: Atrial adaptive rate pacing in sick sinus syndrome: Effects on exercise capacity and arrhythmias. Br. Heart J. *69*:174, 1993.

39. Hesselson, A. B., Parsonnet, V., Bernstein, A. D., et al.: Deleterious effects of long-term single-chamber ventricular pacing in patients with sick sinus syndrome: The hidden benefits of dual-chamber pacing. J. Am. Coll. Cardiol. *19*:1542, 1992.

40. Saito, D., Matsubara, K., Yamanari, H., et al.: Effects of oral theophylline on sick sinus syndrome. J. Am. Coll. Cardiol. *21*:1199, 1993.

41. Strickberger, S. A., Fish, R. D., Lamas, G. A., et al.: Comparison of the effects of propanolol versus pindolol on sinus rate and pacing frequency in sick sinus syndrome. Am. J. Cardiol. *71*:53, 1993.

42. Resh, W., Feuer, J., and Wesley, R. C., Jr.: Intravenous adenosine: A noninvasive diagnostic test for sick sinus syndrome. PACE *15*:2068, 1992.

43. Saito, D., Yamanari, H., Matsubara, K., et al.: Intravenous injection of adenosine triphosphate for assessing sinus node dysfunction in patients with sick sinus syndrome. Arzneimittelforschung *43*:1313, 1993.

44. Naccarelli, G. V., Shih, H., and Jalal, S.: Sinus node reentry and atrial tachycardias. *In* Zipes, D. P., and Jalife, J. (eds.): Cardiac Electrophysiology: From Cell to Bedside. 2nd ed. Philadelphia, W. B. Saunders Company, 1994, p. 607.

44a. Tang, C. W., Scheinman, M. M., Van Hare, G. F., et al.: Use of P wave configuration during atrial tachycardia to predict site of origin. J. Am. Coll. Cardiol. *26*:1315, 1995.

45. Sperry, R. E., Ellenbogen, K. A., Wood, M. A., et al.: Radiofrequency catheter ablation of sinus node reentrant tachycardia. PACE *16*:2202, 1993.

DISTURBANCES OF ATRIAL RHYTHM

46. Zipes, D. P., and Garson, A., Jr.: Twenty-sixth Bethesda Conference: Recommendation for determining eligibility for competition in athletes with cardiovascular abnormalities. Task force 6: Arrhythmias. J. Am. Coll. Cardiol. *24*:892, 1994.

47. Waldo, A. L.: Atrial flutter: Mechanisms, clinical features and management. *In* Zipes, D. P., and Jalife, J. (eds.): Cardiac Electrophysiology: From Cell to Bedside. 2nd ed. Philadelphia, W. B. Saunders Company, 1994, p. 666.

48. Balaji, S., Johnson, T. B., Sade, R. M., et al.: Management of atrial flutter after the Fontan procedure. J. Am. Coll. Cardiol. *23*:1209, 1994.

49. Flack, N. J., Zosmer, N., Bennett, P. R., et al.: Amiodarone given by three routes to terminate fetal atrial flutter associated with severe hydrops. Obstet. Gynecol. *82* (4 Pt. 2, Suppl.):714, 1993.

50. Chang, J. S., Chen, V. C., Tsai, C. H., et al.: Successful conversion of fetal atrial flutter with digoxin: Report of one case. Acta Paediatr. Sin. *35*:229, 1994.

51. Tucker, K. J., and Wilson, C.: A comparison of transesophageal atrial pacing and direct current cardioversion for the termination of atrial flutter: A prospective randomized clinical trial. Br. Heart J. *69*:530, 1993.

52. Yoshitake, N., Tanoiri, T., Nomoto, J., et al.: Patterns of interruption of atrial flutter induced by rapid atrial pacing. Jpn. Circ. J. *58*:181, 1990.

53. Baeriswyl, G., Zimmerman, M., and Adamec, R.: Efficacy of rapid atrial pacing for conversion of atrial flutter in medically treated patients. Clin. Cardiol. *17*:246, 1994.

54. Cosio, F. G., Lopez-Gill, M., Arribas, F., et al.: Mechanisms of entrain-

ment of human common flutter studied with multiple endocardial recordings. Circulation *89*:2117, 1994.

55. Botteron, G. W., and Smith, J. M.: Spatial and temporal inhomogeneity of adenosine's effect on atrial refractoriness in humans: Using atrial fibrillation to probe atrial refractoriness. J. Cardiovasc. Electrophysiol. *5*:477, 1994.

56. Shettigar, U. R., Toole, J. G., and Appunn, A. O.: Combined use of esmolol and digoxin in the acute treatment of atrial fibrillation or flutter. Am. Heart J. *126*:368, 1993.

57. Cochrane, A. D., Siddins, M., Rosenfeldt, F. L., et al.: A comparison of amiodarone and digoxin for treatment of supraventricular arrhythmias after cardiac surgery. Eur. J. Cardiothorac. Surg. *8*:194, 1994.

58. Crijns, H. J., VanGelder, I. C., and Lie, K. I.: Benefits and risks of antiarrhythmic drug therapy after DC electrical cardioversion of atrial fibrillation or flutter. Eur. Heart J. *15* (Suppl. A):17, 1994.

59. Till, J. A., Baxendall, M., and Benetar, A.: Acceleration of the ventricular response to atrial flutter by amiodarone in an infant with Wolff-Parkinson-White syndrome. Br. Heart J. *70*:84, 1993.

60. Santiago, D., Warshofsky, M., LiMandri, G., et al.: Left atrial appendage function and thrombus formation in atrial fibrillation-flutter: A transesophageal echocardiographic study. J. Am. Coll. Cardiol. *24*:159, 1994.

61. American College of Cardiology Cardiovascular Technology Assessment Committee: Catheter ablation for cardiac arrhythmias: Clinical applications, personnel and facilities. J. Am. Coll. Cardiol. *24*:828, 1994.

62. Lesh, M. D., and VanHare, G. F.: Status of ablation in patients with atrial tachycardia and atrial flutter. PACE *17*:1026, 1994.

63. Scheinman, M. M.: Patterns of catheter ablation practice in the United States: Results of the 1992 NASPE survey. North American Society of Pacing and Electrophysiology. PACE *17*:873, 1994.

64. Epstein, L. M., Chiesa, N., Wong, M. N., et al.: Radiofrequency catheter ablation in the treatment of supraventricular tachycardia in the elderly. J. Am. Coll. Cardiol. *23*:1356, 1994.

65. Hindricks, G.: The Multicenter European Radiofrequency Survey (MERFS): Complications of radiofrequency catheter ablation of arrhythmias. The Multicenter European Radiofrequency Survey (MERFS) Investigators of the Working Group on Arrhythmias of the European Society of Cardiology. Eur. Heart J. *14*:1644, 1993.

66. Lesh, M. D., VanHare, G. F., Epstein, L. M., et al.: Radiofrequency catheter ablation of atrial arrhythmias: Results and mechanisms. Circulation *89*:1074, 1994.

67. Calkins, H., Leon, A. R., Deam, A. G., et al.: Catheter ablation of atrial flutter using radiofrequency energy. Am. J. Cardiol. *73*:353, 1994.

68. Kay, G. N., Epstein, A. E., Dailey, S. M., et al.: Role of radiofrequency ablation in the management of supraventricular arrhythmias: Experience in 760 consecutive patients. J. Cardiovasc. Electrophysiol. *4*:371, 1993.

69. Olshansky, B., Wilber, D. J., and Hariman, R. J.: Atrial flutter: Update on the mechanism and treatment. PACE *15*:2308, 1992.

70. Zipes, D. P., DiMarco, J. P., Gillette, P. C., et al.: AHA/ACC guidelines for clinical intracardiac electrophysiologic procedures. Circulation *92*:673, 1995.

71. Konings, K. T., Kirchhof, C. J., Smeets, J. R., et al.: High-density mapping of electrically induced atrial fibrillation in humans. Circulation *89*:1665, 1994.

72. Ruffy, R.: Atrial fibrillation. *In* Zipes, D. P., and Jalife, J. (eds.): Cardiac Electrophysiology: From Cell to Bedside. 2nd ed. Philadelphia, W. B. Saunders Company, 1994, p. 682.

73. Allessie, M. A.: Reentrant mechanisms underlying atrial fibrillation. *In* Zipes, D. P., and Jalife, J. (eds.): Cardiac Electrophysiology: From Cell to Bedside. 2nd ed. Philadelphia, W. B. Saunders Company, 1994, p. 562.

74. Falk, R. H., and Podrid, P. J. (eds.): Atrial Fibrillation: Mechanisms and Management. New York, Raven Press, 1992.

74a. Meijler, F. L., Wittkampf, F. H., Brennen, K. R., et al.: Electrocardiogram of the humpback whale (Megaptera novaengliae), with specific reference to atrioventricular transmission and ventricular excitation. J. Am. Coll. Cardiol. *20*:475, 1992.

75. Watanabe, Y., and Watanabe, M.: Impulse formation and conduction of excitation in the atrioventricular node. J. Cardiovasc. Electrophysiol. *5*:517, 1994.

76. The National Heart Lung and Blood Institute Working Group on Atrial Fibrillation: Atrial fibrillation: Current understandings and research imperatives. J. Am. Coll. Cardiol. *22*:1830, 1993.

77. Domanski, M. J.: The epidemiology of atrial fibrillation. Coronary Artery Dis. *6*:95, 1995.

78. Furberg, C. D., Psaty, B. M., Manolio, T. A., et al.: Prevalence of atrial fibrillation in elderly subjects (The Cardiovascular Health Study). Am. J. Cardiol. *74*:236, 1994.

79. Sawin, C. T., Geller, A., Wolf, P. A., et al.: Low serum thyrotropin concentrations as a risk factor for atrial fibrillation in older persons. N. Engl. J. Med. *331*:1249, 1994.

80. Woeber, K. A.: Thyrotoxicosis and the heart. N. Engl. J. Med. *327*:94, 1992.

81. Coumel, P.: Paroxysmal atrial fibrillation: A disorder of autonomic tone. Eur. Heart J. *15* (Suppl. A):9, 1994.

82. Warfarin versus aspirin for prevention of thromboembolism in atrial fibrillation: Stroke Prevention in Atrial Fibrillation II. Lancet *343*:687, 1994.

83. EAFT (European Atrial Fibrillation Trial) Study Group: Secondary prevention in non-rheumatic atrial fibrillation after transient ischemic attack or minor stroke. Lancet *342*:1255, 1993.

84. Ezekowitz, M. D., Bridgers, S. L., James, K. E., et al.: Warfarin in the prevention of stroke associated with nonrheumatic atrial fibrillation. N. Engl. J. Med. *327*:1406, 1992.

85. Connolly, S. J., Laupacis, A., Gent, M., et al.: Canadian Atrial Fibrillation Anti-Coagulation (CAFA) Study. J. Am. Coll. Cardiol. *18*:349, 1991.

86. The Boston Area Anticoagulation Trial for Atrial Fibrillation Investigators: The effect of low-dose warfarin on the risk of stroke in patients with nonrheumatic atrial fibrillation. N. Engl. J. Med *323*:1505, 1990.

87. Stroke Prevention in Atrial Fibrillation Study Group Investigators: Preliminary report of the Stroke Prevention in Atrial Fibrillation Study. N. Engl. J. Med *322*:863, 1990.

88. Petersen, P., Boisen, G., Godtfredsen, J., et al.: Placebo-controlled, randomized trial of warfarin and aspirin for prevention of thromboembolic complications in chronic atrial fibrillation. The Copenhagen AFASAK Study. Lancet *1*:175, 1989.

89. Stroke Prevention in Atrial Fibrillation Investigators: Stroke Prevention in Atrial Fibrillation Study: Final results. Circulation *84*:527, 1991.

90. The Stroke Prevention in Atrial Fibrillation Investigators: Predictors of thromboembolism in atrial fibrillation: I. Clinical features of patients at risk. Ann. Intern. Med. *116*:1, 1992.

91. The Stroke Prevention in Atrial Fibrillation Investigators: Predictors of thromboembolism in atrial fibrillation: II. Echocardiographic features of patients at risk. Ann. Intern. Med. *116*:6, 1992.

92. Chimowitz, M. I., DeGeorgia, M. A., Poole, R. M., et al.: Left atrial spontaneous echo contrast is highly associated with previous stroke in patients with atrial fibrillation or mitral stenosis. Stroke *25*:1295, 1994.

93. Albers, G. W.: Atrial fibrillation and stroke: Three new studies, three remaining questions. Arch. Intern. Med. *154*:1443, 1994.

94. Matchar, D. B., McCrory, D. C., Barnett, H. J., et al.: Medical treatment for stroke prevention. Ann. Intern. Med. *121*:41, 1994.

95. Risk factors for stroke and efficacy of antithrombotic therapy in atrial fibrillation: Analysis of pooled data from five randomized controlled trials. Atrial Fibrillation Investigators: Atrial Fibrillation, Aspirin, Anticoagulation Study; Boston Area Anticoagulation Trial for Atrial Fibrillation Study; Canadian Atrial Fibrillation Anticoagulation Study; Stroke Prevention in Atrial Fibrillation Study; Veterans Affairs Stroke Prevention in Nonrheumatic Atrial Fibrillation Study. Arch. Intern. Med. *154*:1449, 1994.

96. Albers, G. W., and Hirsh, J.: Anticoagulation/platelet inhibition for atrial fibrillation. Coronary Artery Dis. *6*:129, 1995.

97. Wells, T. S., Holbrook, A. M., Crowther, N. R., et al.: Interactions of warfarin with drugs and food. Ann. Intern. Med. *121*:676, 1994.

98. Guidelines for medical treatment for stroke prevention. Ann. Intern. Med. *121*:54, 1994.

99. Disch, D. L., Greenberg, M. L., Holzberger, P. T., et al.: Managing chronic atrial fibrillation: A Markov decision analysis comparing warfarin, quinidine and low-dose amiodarone. Ann. Intern. Med. *120*:449, 1994.

100. Fuster, V., Dyken, M. L., Vokonas, P. S., et al.: Aspirin as a therapeutic agent in cardiovascular disease. Circulation *87*:659, 1993.

101. Patrono, C.: Aspirin as an antiplatelet drug. N. Engl. J. Med. *330*:1287, 1994.

102. Pritchett, E. L. C.: Management of atrial fibrillation. N. Engl. J. Med. *326*:1264, 1992.

103. Hirsh, J.: Oral anticoagulant drugs. N. Engl. J. Med. *324*:1865, 1991.

104. Laupacis, A., Albers, G. W., Dunn, M., et al.: Antithrombotic therapy in atrial fibrillation. Chest *102*:426S, 1992.

105. Leung, D. Y., Black, I. W., Cranney, G. B., et al.: Prognostic implications of left atrial spontaneous echo contrast in nonvalvular atrial fibrillation. J. Am. Coll. Cardiol. *24*:755, 1994.

106. Black, I. W., Fatkin, D., Sagar, K. B., et al.: Exclusion of atrial thrombus by transesophageal echocardiography does not preclude embolism after cardioversion of atrial fibrillation: A multicenter study. Circulation *89*:2509, 1994.

107. Manning, W. J., Silverman, D. I., and Gordon, S. P. F.: Cardioversion from atrial fibrillation without prolonged anticoagulation with use of transesophageal echocardiography to exclude the presence of atrial thrombi. N. Engl. J. Med. *328*:750, 1993.

108. Allessie, M. A., Wijffels, M. C., and Kirchhof, C. J.: Experimental models of arrhythmias: Toys or truth? Eur. Heart J. *15* (Suppl. A):2, 1994.

109. Janse, M. J.: Electrophysiology of atrial fibrillation. Coronary Artery Dis. *6*:101, 1995.

110. Morillo, C. A., Klein, G. J., Jones, D. L., et al.: Chronic rapid atrial pacing: Structural, functional, and electrophysiological characteristics of a new model of sustained atrial fibrillation. Circulation *91*:1588, 1995.

110a. Wijffels, M. C. E. F., Kirchhef, C. J. H. J., Dorland, R., et al.: Atrial fibrillation begets atrial fibrillation: A study in awake chronically instrumented goats. Circulation *92*:1954, 1995.

111. Shite, J., Yokota, Y., and Yokoyama, M.: Heterogeneity and time course of improvement in cardiac function after cardioversion of chronic atrial fibrillation: Assessment of serial echocardiographic indices. Br. Heart J. *70*:154, 1993.

112. Manning, W. J., Silverman, D. I., and Katz, S. E.: Impaired left atrial mechanical function after cardioversion: Relation to the duration of atrial fibrillation. J. Am. Coll. Cardiol. *23*:1535, 1994.

113. Lundstrom, T., Moor, E., and Ryden, L.: Differential effects of xamoterol and verapamil on ventricular rate regulation in patients with chronic atrial fibrillation. Am. Heart J. *124*:917, 1992.

114. Sarter, B. H., and Marchlinski, F. E.: Redefining the role of digoxin in the treatment of atrial fibrillation. Am. J. Cardiol. *69*:71G, 1992.

115. Roth, A., Kaluski, E., Felner, S., et al.: Clonidine for patients with rapid atrial fibrillation. Ann. Intern. Med. *116*:388, 1992.

116. Weiner, P., Ganam, R., Ganem, R., et al.: Clinical course of recent-onset atrial fibrillation treated with oral propafenone. Chest *105*:1013, 1994.

117. Ruffy, R.: Sotalol. J. Cardiovasc. Electrophysiol. *4*:81, 1993.

118. Falk, R. H.: Proarrhythmia in patients treated for atrial fibrillation or flutter. Ann. Intern. Med. *117*:141, 1992.

119. Hohnloser, S. H., Klingenhaben, T., and Singh, B. N.: Amiodarone-associated proarrhythmic effects: A review with special reference to torsades de pointes tachycardia. Ann. Intern. Med. *121*:529, 1994.

120. Roden, D. M.: Risks and benefits of antiarrhythmic therapy. N. Engl. J. Med. *331*:785, 1994.

121. Sopher, M., and Camm, A. J.: Therapy for atrial fibrillation: Control of the ventricular response and prevention of recurrence. Coronary Artery Dis. *6*:105, 1995.

122. Fujiki, A., Yoshida, S., Tani, M., et al.: Efficacy of class IA antiarrhythmic drugs in converting atrial fibrillation unassociated with organic heart disease and their relation to atrial electrophysiologic characteristics. Am. J. Cardiol. *74*:282, 1994.

123. Kirchhof, C., Charro, F., Scheffer, G. J., et al.: Regional entrainment of atrial fibrillation studied by high-resolution mapping in open-chest dogs. Circulation *88*:736, 1993.

124. Williamson, B. D., Man, K. C., Daoud, E., et al.: Radiofrequency catheter modification of atrioventricular conduction to control the ventricular rate during atrial fibrillation. N. Engl. J. Med. *331*:910, 1994.

125. Brignole, M., Gianfranchi, L., Menozzi, C., et al.: Influence of atrioventricular junction radiofrequency ablation in patients with chronic atrial fibrillation and flutter on quality of life and cardiac performance. Am. J. Cardiol. *74*:242, 1964.

126. Harvey, M. N., and Morady, F.: Radiofrequency catheter ablation for atrial fibrillation. Coronary Artery Dis. *6*:114, 1995.

127. Ferguson, T. B., Jr.: Surgery for atrial fibrillation. Coronary Artery Dis. *6*:120, 1995.

128. Shyu, K. G., Cheng, J. J., Chen, J. J., et al.: Recovery of atrial function after atrial compartment operation for chronic atrial fibrillation in mitral valve disease. J. Am. Coll. Cardiol. *24*:392, 1994.

129. Haissaguerre, M., Marcus, F. I., Fischer, B., et al.: Radiofrequency catheter ablation in unusual mechanisms of atrial fibrillation: Report of three cases. J. Cardiovasc. Electrophysiol. *5*:743, 1994.

130. Haissaguerre, M., Gencel, L., Fischer, B., et al.: Successful catheter ablation of atrial fibrillation. J. Cardiovasc. Electrophysiol. *5*:1045, 1994.

131. Swartz, J. F., Pollersels, G., Silvers, J., et al.: A catheter-based curative approach to atrial fibrillation in humans. Circulation *90* (Suppl. I):(Abs.):1335, 1994.

132. Elvan, A., Pride, H. P., Eble, J. N., et al.: Radiofrequency catheter ablation of the atria reduces the inducibility and duration of atrial fibrillation in dogs. Circulation *91*:2235, 1995.

133. Keane, B., Boyd, E., Anderson, D., et al.: Comparison of biphasic and monophasic waveforms in epicardial atrial defibrillation. J. Am. Coll. Cardiol. *24*:171, 1994.

134. Benditt, B. G., Dunbar, B., Fetter, J., et al.: Low-energy transvenous cardioversion defibrillation of atrial tachyarrhythmias in the canine: An assessment of electrode configurations and monophasic pulse sequencing. Am. Heart J. *127*:994, 1994.

135. Ayers, G. M., Alferness, C. A., Ilina, M., et al.: Ventricular proarrhythmic effects of ventricular cycle length and shock strength in a sheep model of transvenous atrial defibrillation. Circulation *89*:413, 1994.

136. Pollak, A., and Falk, R. H.: Pacemaker therapy in patients with atrial fibrillation. Am. Heart J. *125*:824, 1993.

137. Kay, G. N., Chong, F., Epstein, A. E., et al.: Radiofrequency ablation for treatment of primary atrial tachycardias. J. Am. Coll. Cardiol. *21*:901, 1993.

138. Chen, S. A., Chiang, C. E., Yang, C. J., et al.: Radiofrequency catheter ablation of intraatrial reentrant tachycardia in adult patients: Identification of electrophysiological characteristics and endocardial mapping techniques. Circulation *88*:578, 1993.

139. Kadish, A. H., and Morady, F.: The response of paroxysmal supraventricular tachycardia to overdrive atrial and ventricular pacing: Can it help determine the tachycardia mechanism? J. Cardiovasc. Electrophysiol. *4*:239, 1993.

140. Case, C. L., and Gillette, P. C.: Automatic atrial and junctional tachycardias in the pediatric patient: Strategies for diagnosis and management. PACE *16*:1323, 1993.

141. Chen, S. A., Chiang, C. E., Yang, C. J., et al.: Sustained atrial tachycardia in adult patients: Electrophysiological characteristics, pharmacological response, possible mechanisms and effects of radiofrequency ablation. Circulation *90*:1262, 1994.

142. Engelstein, E. D., Littman, N., Stein, K. M., et al.: Mechanism-specific effects of adenosine on atrial tachycardia. Circulation *89*:2645, 1994.

143. DeBakker, J. M. T., Hauer, R. N. W., Bakker, P. F. A., et al.: Abnormal automaticity as mechanism of atrial tachycardia in the human heart—Electrophysiologic and histologic correlation: A case report. J. Cardiovasc. Electrophysiol. *5*:335, 1994.

144. Raja, T., Hawker, R. E., Chaikitpinyo, A., et al.: Amiodarone management of junctional ectopic tachycardia after cardiac surgery in children. Br. Heart J. 72:261, 1994.

145. Till, J. A., Ho, S. Y., and Rowland, E.: Histopathological findings in three children with His bundle tachycardia occurring subsequent to cardiac surgery. Eur. Heart J. 13:709, 1992.

146. Braunstein, P. W., Jr., Sade, R. M., and Gillette, P. C.: Life-threatening postoperative junctional ectopic tachycardia. Ann. Thorac. Surg. 53:726, 1992.

147. Gentzer, J. H., Goyal, R., Williamson, B. D., et al.: Analysis of junctional ectopy during radiofrequency ablation of the slow pathway in patients with atrioventricular nodal reentrant tachycardia. Circulation 90:2820, 1994.

148. Heusch, A., Kramer, H. H., Krogmann, O. N., et al.: Clinical experience with propafenone for cardiac arrhythmias in the young. Eur. Heart J. 15:1050, 1994.

149. Case, C. L., and Gillette, P. C.: Automatic atrial and junctional tachycardias in the pediatric patient: Strategies for diagnosis and management. PACE 16:1323, 1993.

150. Paul, T., Reimer, A., Janousek, J., et al.: Efficacy and safety of propafenone in congenital junctional ectopic tachycardia. J. Am. Coll. Cardiol. 20:911, 1992.

151. Scheinman, M. M., Gonzalez, R. P., Cooper, M. W., et al.: Clinical and electrophysiologic features and role of catheter ablation techniques in adult patients with automatic atrioventricular junctional tachycardia. Am. J. Cardiol. 74:565, 1994.

152. Gonzalez, R. V., and Scheinman, M. M.: Paroxysmal junctional and fascicular tachycardia in adults: Clinical presentation course and therapy. In Zipes, D. P., and Jalife, J. (eds.): Cardiac Electrophysiology: From Cell to Bedside. 2nd ed. Philadelphia, W. B. Saunders Company, 1994, p. 691.

153. Kuck, K. H., and Schluter, M.: Junctional tachycardia and the role of catheter ablation. Lancet 341:1386, 1993.

154. Ehlert, F. A., Goldberger, J. J., Deal, B. J., et al.: Successful radiofrequency energy ablation of automatic junctional tachycardia preserving normal atrioventricular nodal conduction. PACE 16:54, 1993.

155. Akhtar, M., Jazayeri, M. R., Sra, J., et al.: Atrioventricular nodal reentry. Clinical, electrophysiological, and therapeutic considerations. Circulation 88:282, 1993.

156. Jackman, W. M., Nakagawa, H., and Heidbuchel, H.: Three forms of atrioventricular nodal (junctional) reentrant tachycardia: Differential diagnosis, electrophysiological characteristics, and implications for anatomy of the reentrant circuit. In Zipes, D. P., and Jalife, J. (eds.): Cardiac Electrophysiology: From Cell to Bedside. 2nd ed. Philadelphia, W. B. Saunders Company, 1994, p. 620.

157. Gamache, M. C., Bharati, S., Lev, M., et al.: Histopathological study following catheter guided radiofrequency current ablation of the slow pathway in a patient with atrioventricular nodal reentrant tachycardia. PACE 17:247, 1994.

158. Langberg, J. J.: Radiofrequency catheter ablation of AV nodal reentry: The anterior approach. PACE 16:615, 1993.

159. DeBakker, J. M., Coronel, R., McGuire, M. A., et al.: Slow potentials in the atrioventricular junctional area of patients operated on for atrioventricular node tachycardias and in isolated porcine hearts. J. Am. Coll. Cardiol. 23:709, 1994.

160. Janse, M. J., Anderson, R. H., McGuire, M. A., et al.: AV nodal reentry: I. AV nodal reentry revisited. J. Cardiovasc. Electrophysiol. 4:561, 1993.

161. McGuire, M. A., Janse, M. J., and Ross, D. L.: AV nodal reentry: II. AV nodal, AV junctional or atrial nodal reentry? J. Cardiovasc. Electrophysiol. 4:573, 1993.

162. McGuire, M. A., Yit, A. S., Robotin, M., et al.: Surgical procedure for the cure of atrioventricular junctional (AV node) reentrant tachycardia: Anatomic and electrophysiologic effects of dissection of the anterior atrial nodal connections in a canine model. J. Am. Coll. Cardiol. 24:784, 1994.

163. Silka, M. J., Kron, J., Park, J. K., et al.: Atypical forms of supraventricular tachycardia due to atrioventricular node reentry in children after radiofrequency modification of slow pathway conduction. J. Am. Coll. Cardiol. 23:1363, 1994.

164. Josephson, M. E., and Miller, J. M.: Atrioventricular nodal reentry: Evidence supporting an intranodal location. PACE 16:599, 1993.

165. Suzuki, F., Tanaka, K., Ishihara, N., et al.: Double ventricular responses during extrastimulation of atrioventricular nodal reentrant tachycardia. Eur. Heart J. 15:285, 1994.

166. Kalbfleisch, S. J., Strickberger, S. A., Hummel, J. D., et al.: Double retrograde atrial response after radiofrequency ablation of typical AV nodal reentrant tachycardia. J. Cardiovasc. Electrophysiol. 4:695, 1993.

167. Abe, H., Ohkita, T., Fujita, M., et al.: Atrioventricular (AV) nodal reentry associated with 2:1 infra-His conduction block during tachycardia in a patient with AV nodal triple pathways. Jpn. Heart J. 35:241, 1994.

168. Gursoy, S., Steurer, G., Brugada, J., et al.: Brief report: The hemodynamic mechanism of pounding in the neck in atrioventricular nodal reentrant tachycardia. N. Engl. J. Med. 327:772, 1992.

169. Nayebpour, M., Billette, J., Amellal, F., et al.: Effects of adenosine on rate-dependent atrioventricular nodal function: Potential roles in tachycardia termination and physiological regulation. Circulation 88:2632, 1993.

170. Jackman, W. M., Beckman, K. J., McClelland, J. H., et al.: Treatment of supraventricular tachycardia due to atrioventricular nodal reentry by radiofrequency catheter ablation of the slow-pathway conduction. N. Engl. J. Med. 327:313, 1992.

171. Lee, M. A., Morady, F., Kadish, A., et al.: Catheter modification of the atrioventricular junction with radiofrequency energy for control of atrioventricular nodal reentrant tachycardia. Circulation 83:827, 1991.

172. Mahomed, Y., King, R. D., Zipes, D. P., et al.: Surgery for atrioventricular node reentry tachycardia: Results with surgical skeletonization of the atrioventricular node and discrete perinodal cryosurgery. J. Thorac. Cardiovasc. Surg. 104:1035, 1992.

173. McGuire, M. A., Bourke, J. P., Robotin, M. C., et al.: High resolution mapping of Koch's triangle using 60 electrodes in humans with atrioventricular junctional (AV nodal) reentrant tachycardia. Circulation 88:2315, 1993.

174. Mitrani, R. D., Klein, L. S., Hackett, F. K., et al.: Radiofrequency ablation for atrioventricular node reentrant tachycardia: Comparison between fast (anterior) and slow (posterior) pathway ablation. J. Am. Coll. Cardiol. 21:432, 1993.

175. Miles, W. M., Hubbard, J. E., Zipes, D. P., et al.: Elimination of AV nodal reentrant tachycardia with 2:1 VA block by posteroseptal ablation. J. Cardiovasc. Electrophysiol. 5:510, 1994.

176. Kalbfleisch, S. J., and Morady, F.: Catheter ablation of atrioventricular nodal reentrant tachycardia. In Zipes, D. P., and Jalife, J. (eds.): Cardiac Electrophysiology: From Cell to Bedside. 2nd ed. Philadelphia, W. B. Saunders Company, 1994, p. 1477.

177. Baker, J. H., II, Plumb, V. J., Epstein, A. E., et al.: Predictors of recurrent atrioventricular nodal reentry after selective slow pathway ablation. Am. J. Cardiol. 73:765, 1994.

178. Kay, G. N., Epstein, A. E., Dailey, S. M., et al.: Role of radiofrequency ablation in the management of supraventricular arrhythmias: Experience in 760 consecutive patients. J. Cardiovasc. Electrophysiol. 4:371, 1993.

179. Jazayeri, M. R., Sra, J. S., Deshpande, S. S., et al.: Electrophysiologic spectrum of atrioventricular nodal behavior in patients with atrioventricular nodal reentrant tachycardia undergoing selective fast or slow pathway ablation. J. Cardiovasc. Electrophysiol. 4:99, 1993.

180. Gursoy, S., Schluter, M., and Kuck, K. H.: Radiofrequency current catheter ablation for control of supraventricular arrhythmias. J. Cardiovasc. Electrophysiol. 4:194, 1993.

181. Li, H. G., Klein, G. J., Stites, H. W., et al.: Elimination of slow pathway conduction: An accurate indicator of clinical success after radiofrequency atrioventricular node modification. J. Am. Coll. Cardiol. 22:1849, 1993.

182. Lindsay, D. D., Chung, M. K., Gamache, M. C., et al.: Therapeutic endpoints for the treatment of atrioventricular node reentrant tachycardia by catheter-guided radiofrequency current. J. Am. Coll. Cardiol. 22:733, 1993.

183. Wu, D., Yeh, S. J., Wang, C. C., et al.: A simple technique for selective radiofrequency ablation of the slow pathway in atrioventricular node reentrant tachycardia. J. Am. Coll. Cardiol. 21:1612, 1993.

184. Miles, W. M., Klein, L. S., Rardon, D. P., et al.: Atrioventricular reentry and variants: Mechanisms, clinical features, and management. In Zipes, D.P., and Jalife, J. (eds.): Cardiac Electrophysiology: From Cell to Bedside. 2nd ed. Philadelphia, W. B. Saunders Company, 1994, p. 638.

185. Yee, R., Klein, G. J., and Guiraudon, G. M.: The Wolff-Parkinson-White syndrome. In Zipes, D. P., and Jalife, J. (eds.): Cardiac Electrophysiology: From Cell to Bedside. 2nd ed. Philadelphia, W. B. Saunders Company, 1994, p. 1199.

186. Stanke, A., Storti, C., DePonti, R., et al.: Spontaneous incessant AV reentrant tachycardia related to left bundle branch block and concealed left-sided accessory AV pathway. J. Cardiovasc. Electrophysiol. 5:777, 1994.

187. Calkins, H., Langberg, J., Sousa, J., et al.: Radiofrequency catheter ablation of accessory atrioventricular connections in 250 patients. Abbreviated therapeutic approach to Wolff-Parkinson-White syndrome. Circulation 85:1337, 1992.

188. Kuck, K. H., Schluter, M., and Gursoy, S.: Preservation of atrioventricular nodal conduction during radiofrequency current catheter ablation of midseptal accessory pathways. Circulation 86:1743, 1992.

189. Bashir, Y., Heald, S. C., O'Nunain, S., et al.: Radiofrequency current delivery by way of a bipolar tricuspid annulus-mitral annulus electrode configuration for ablation of posteroseptal accessory pathways. J. Am. Coll. Cardiol. 22:550, 1993.

190. Xie, B., Heald, S. C., Bashir, Y., et al.: Localization of accessory pathways from the 12-lead electrocardiogram using a new algorithm. Am. J. Cardiol. 74:161, 1994.

191. Rodriguez, L. M., Smeets, J. L., deChillou, C., et al.: The 12-lead electrocardiogram in midseptal, anteroseptal, posteroseptal and right free wall accessory pathways. Am. J. Cardiol. 72:1274, 1994.

192. Dubuc, M., Nadeau, R., Tremblay, G., et al.: Pace mapping using body surface potential maps to guide catheter ablation of accessory pathways in patients with Wolff-Parkinson-White syndrome. Circulation 87:135, 1993.

193. Jackman, W. M., McClelland, J. H., Nakagawa, H., et al.: Ablation of right atriofascicular (Mahaim) accessory pathways. In Zipes, D. P. (ed.): Catheter Ablation of Arrhythmias. Armonk, N.Y., Futura, 1994, p. 187.

194. deChillou, C., Rodriguez, L. M., Schlapfer, J., et al.: Clinical characteristics and electrophysiologic properties of atrioventricular accessory pathways: Importance of the accessory pathway location. J. Am. Coll. Cardiol. 20:666, 1992.

194a. Shih, H. T., Miles, W. M., Klein, L. S., et al.: Multiple accessory pathways in the permanent forms of junctional reciprocating tachycardia. Am. J. Cardiol. 73:361, 1994.

195. Wienecke, M., Case, C., Buckles, D., et al.: Inducible ventricular tachyarrhythmia in children with Wolff-Parkinson-White syndrome. Am. J. Cardiol. 73:396, 1994.

196. Pressley, J. C., Wharton, J. M., Tang, A. S., et al.: Effect of Ebstein's anomaly on short- and long-term outcome of surgically treated patients with Wolff-Parkinson-White syndrome. Circulation 86:1147, 1992.

197. Rechavia, E., Mager, A., Birnbaum, Y., et al.: Mitral valve prolapse, sick sinus and Wolff-Parkinson-White syndromes: Interrelationships with respect to sudden cardiac death. Isr. J. Med. Sci. 29:654, 1993.

198. Munger, T. M., Packer, D. L., Hammill, S. C., et al.: A population study of the natural history of Wolff-Parkinson-White syndrome in Olmstead County, Minnesota, 1953–1989. Circulation 87:866, 1993.

199. Zardini, M., Yee, R., Thakur, R. K., et al.: Risk of sudden arrhythmic death in the Wolff-Parkinson-White syndrome: Current perspectives. PACE 17:966, 1994.

200. Camm, A. J., Katritsis, D., and Nunain, S. O.: Effects of flecainide on atrial electrophysiology in the Wolff-Parkinson-White syndrome. Am. J. Cardiol. 70:33A, 1992.

201. Crozier, I.: Flecainide in the Wolff-Parkinson-White syndrome. Am. J. Cardiol. 70:26A, 1992.

202. Podrid, P. J.: Amiodarone. Ann. Intern. Med. 122:689, 1995.

203. Manolis, A. S., Katsaros, C., and Kokkinos, D. V.: Electrophysiological and electropharmacological studies in preexcitation syndromes: Results with propafenone therapy and isoproterenol infusion testing. Eur. Heart J. 13:1489, 1992.

204. Auricchio, A.: Reversible protective effect of propafenone or flecainide during atrial fibrillation in patients with an accessory atrioventricular connection. Am. Heart J. 124:932, 1992.

205. Stanton, M. S.: Class I antiarrhythmic drugs: Quinidine, procainamide, disopyramide, lidocaine, mexiletine, tocainide, phenytoin, moricizine, flecainide, propafenone. In Zipes, D. P., and Jalife, J. (eds.): Cardiac Electrophysiology: From Cell to Bedside. 2nd ed. Philadelphia, W. B. Saunders Company, 1994, p. 1296.

206. Haissaguerre, M., Clementy, J., and Warin, J. F.: Catheter ablation of atrioventricular reentrant tachycardias. In Zipes, D. P., and Jalife, J. (eds.): Cardiac Electrophysiology: From Cell to Bedside. 2nd ed. Philadelphia, W. B. Saunders Company, 1994, p. 1487.

207. Hogenhuis, W., Stevens, S. K., Wang, P., et al.: Cost-effectiveness of radiofrequency ablation compared with other strategies in Wolff-Parkinson-White syndrome. Circulation 88:11437, 1993.

208. Kalbfleisch, S. J., el-Atassi, R., Calkins, H., et al.: Safety, feasibility and cost of outpatient radiofrequency catheter ablation of accessory atrioventricular connections. J. Am. Coll. Cardiol. 21:567, 1993.

209. Guiraudon, G. M., Klein, G. J., Yee, R., et al.: Surgery for the Wolff-Parkinson-White syndrome. In Zipes, D. P., and Jalife, J. (eds.): Cardiac Electrophysiology: From Cell to Bedside. 2nd ed. Philadelphia, W. B. Saunders Company, 1994, p. 1553.

210. Guiraudon, G. M., Guiraudon, C. M., Klein, G. J., et al.: Operation for the Wolff-Parkinson-White syndrome in the catheter ablation era. Ann. Thorac. Surg. 57:1084, 1994.

VENTRICULAR RHYTHM DISTURBANCES

211. Wang, K., and Hodges, M.: The premature ventricular complex as a diagnostic aid. Ann. Intern. Med. 117:766, 1992.

212. Murakawa, Y., Inoue, H., Koide, T., et al.: Reappraisal of the coupling interval of ventricular extrasystoles as an index of ectopic mechanisms. Br. Heart J. 68:589, 1992.

213. Pogwizd, S. M.: Focal mechanisms underlying ventricular tachycardia during prolonged ischemic cardiomyopathy. Circulation 90:1441, 1994.

214. Kostis, J. B., Allen, R., Berkson, D. M., et al.: Correlates of ventricular ectopic activity in isolated systolic hypertension. SHEP Cooperative Research Group. Am. Heart J. 127:112, 1994.

215. Gillis, A. M., Peters, R. W., Mitchell, L. B., et al.: Effects of left ventricular dysfunction on the circadian variation of ventricular premature complexes in healed myocardial infarction. Am. J. Cardiol. 69:1009, 1992.

216. Franz, M. R., Cima, R., Wang, D., et al.: Electrophysiological effects of myocardial stretch and mechanical determinants of stretch-activated arrhythmias. Circulation 86:968, 1992.

217. Wang, Z., Taylor, L. K., Denney, W. D., et al.: Initiation of ventricular extrasystoles by myocardial stretch in chronically dilated and failing canine left ventricle. Circulation 90:2022, 1994.

218. Maggioni, A. P., Zuanetti, G., Franzosi, M. G., et al.: Prevalence and prognostic significance of ventricular arrhythmias after acute myocardial infarction in the fibrinolytic area. GISSI-2 results. Circulation 87:312, 1993.

219. Wyse, D. G., Morganroth, J., Ledingham, R., et al.: New insights into the definition and meaning of proarrhythmia from initiation of antiarrhythmic drug therapy from the Cardiac Arrhythmia Suppression Trial and its private study. The CAST Investigators. J. Am. Coll. Cardiol. 23:1130, 1994.

220. Fleg, J. L., and Kennedy, H. L.: Long-term prognostic significance of ambulatory electrocardiographic findings in apparently healthy subjects greater than or equal to 60 years of age. Am. J. Cardiol. 70:748, 1992.

221. Kennedy, H. L.: Ambulatory (Holter) electrocardiography recordings. In Zipes, D. P., and Jalife, J. (eds.): Cardiac Electrophysiology: From Cell to Bedside. 2nd ed. Philadelphia, W. B. Saunders Company, 1994, p. 1024.

222. Bikkina, M., Larson, M. G., and Levy, D.: Prognostic implications of asymptomatic ventricular arrhythmias: The Framingham Heart Study. Ann. Intern. Med. 117:990, 1992.

223. Wilson, A. C., and Kostis, J. B.: The prognostic significance of very low frequency ventricular activity in survivors of acute myocardial infarction. The BHAT Study Group. Chest 102:732, 1992.

224. Odemuyiwa, O., Farrell, T. G., Malik, M., et al.: Influence of age on the relation between heart rate variability, left ventricular ejection fraction, frequency of ventricular extrasystoles, and sudden death after myocardial infarction. Br. Heart J. 67:387, 1992.

225. Hallstrom, A. P., Bigger, J. T., Jr., Roden, D., et al.: Prognostic significance of ventricular premature depolarizations measured one year after myocardial infarction in patients with early post infarction asymptomatic ventricular arrhythmia. J. Am. Coll. Cardiol. 20:259, 1992.

226. Sueta, C. A., Clarke, S. W., Dunlop, S. H., et al.: Effect of acute magnesium administration on the frequency of ventricular arrhythmia in patients with heart failure. Circulation 89:660, 1994.

227. Singh, B. N.: Beta-blockers and calcium channel blockers as anti-arrhythmic drugs. In Zipes, D. P., and Jalife, J. (eds.): Cardiac Electrophysiology: From Cell to Bedside. 2nd ed. Philadelphia, W. B. Saunders Company, 1994, p. 1317.

228. Hondeghem, L. M.: Class III agents: Amiodarone, bretylium and sotalol. In Zipes, D. P., and Jalife, J. (eds.): Cardiac Electrophysiology: From Cell to Bedside. 2nd ed. Philadelphia, W. B. Saunders Company, 1994, p. 1330.

229. The Cardiac Arrhythmia Suppression Trial II Investigators: Effect of the antiarrhythmic agent moricizine on survival after myocardial infarction. N. Engl. J. Med. 327:227, 1992.

230. Navarro-Lopez, F., Kosin, J., Marrugat, J., et al.: Comparison of the effects of amiodarone versus metoprolol on the frequency of ventricular arrhythmias and on mortality after acute myocardial infarction. SSSD Investigators. Spanish Study on Sudden Death. Am. J. Cardiol. 72:1243, 1993.

231. Zarembski, D. G., Nolan, P. E., Jr., Slack, M. K., et al.: Empiric long-term amiodarone prophylaxis following myocardial infarction: A metaanalysis. Arch. Intern. Med. 153:2661, 1993.

232. Nasir, N., Jr., Taylor, A., Doyle, T. K., et al.: Evaluation of intravenous lidocaine for the termination of sustained monomorphic ventricular tachycardia in patients with coronary artery disease with or without healed myocardial infarction. Am. J. Cardiol. 74:1183, 1994.

233. Nasir, N., Jr., Doyle, T. K., Wheeler, S. H., et al.: Usefulness of Holter monitoring in predicting efficacy of amiodarone therapy for sustained ventricular tachycardia associated with coronary artery disease. Am. J. Cardiol. 73:554, 1994.

234. Man, K. C., Williamson, B. D., Niebauer, M., et al.: Electrophysiologic effects of sotalol and amiodarone in patients with sustained monomorphic ventricular tachycardia. Am. J. Cardiol. 74:1119, 1994.

235. Kostis, J. B., Lacy, C. R., Hall, W. D., et al.: The effect of chlorthalidone on ventricular ectopic activity in patients with isolated systolic hypertension. The SHEP Study Group. Am. J. Cardiol. 74:464, 1994.

236. Dorian, P., Langer, A., Morgan, C., et al.: Importance of ST-segment depression as a determinant of ventricular premature complex frequency after thrombolysis for acute myocardial infarction. Tissue Plasminogen Activator: Toronto (TPAT) Study Group. Am. J. Cardiol. 74:419, 1994.

237. Marino, P., Nidasio, G., Golia, G., et al.: Frequency of predischarge ventricular arrhythmias in post myocardial infarction patients depends on residual left ventricular pump performance and is independent of the occurrence of acute reperfusion. The GISSI-2 Investigators. J. Am. Coll. Cardiol. 23:290, 1994.

238. Tsuji, H., Venditti, F. J., Jr., Evans, J. C., et al.: The associations of levels of serum potassium and magnesium with ventricular premature complexes. The Framingham Heart Study. Am. J. Cardiol. 74:232, 1994.

239. Papademetriou, V., Narayan, P., and Kokkinos, P.: Effects of diltiazem, metoprolol, enalapril, and hydrochlorothiazide on frequency of ventricular premature complexes. Am. J. Cardiol. 73:242, 1994.

240. Shenasa, M., Borggrefe, M., Haverkamp, W., et al.: Ventricular tachycardia. Lancet 341(8859):512, 1993.

241. Griffith, M. J., Garratt, C. J., Mounsey, P., et al.: Ventricular tachycardia as default diagnosis in broad complex tachycardia. Lancet 343(8894):386, 1994.

242. Miller, J. M.: Recognition of ventricular tachycardia. In Zipes, D. P., and Jalife, J. (eds.): Cardiac Electrophysiology: From Cell to Bedside. 2nd ed. Philadelphia, W. B. Saunders Company, 1994, p. 990.

243. Jazayeri, M. R., and Akhtar, M.: Wide QRS complex tachycardia: Electrophysiological mechanisms and electrocardiographic features. In Zipes, D. P., and Jalife, J. (eds.): Cardiac Electrophysiology: From Cell to Bedside. Philadelphia, W. B. Saunders Company, 1994, p. 977.

244. Myerburg, R. J., Kessler, K. M., Kimura, S., et al.: Life-threatening ventricular arrhythmias: The link between epidemiology and pathophysiology. In Zipes, D. P., and Jalife, J. (eds.): Cardiac Electrophysiology: From Cell to Bedside. 2nd ed. Philadelphia, W. B. Saunders Company, 1994, p. 723.

700

245. Hummel, J. D., Strickberger, S. A., Daoud, E., et al.: Results and efficiency of programmed ventricular stimulation with four extrastimuli compared with one, two and three extrastimuli. Circulation 90:2827, 1994.

246. Cossú, S. F., and Buxton, A. E.: The clinical spectrum of ventricular tachyarrhythmias in patients with coronary artery disease: Relationship between clinical and electrophysiologic characteristics in patients with nonsustained ventricular tachycardia and cardiac arrest. Cardiol. Rev. 3:240, 1995.

247. Ho, D. S., Cooper, M. J., Richards, D. A., et al.: Comparison of number of extrastimuli versus change in basic cycle length for induction of ventricular tachycardia by programmed ventricular stimulation. J. Am. Coll. Cardiol. 22:1711, 1993.

248. Callans, D. J., and Josephson, M. E.: Ventricular tachycardias in the setting of coronary artery disease. In Zipes, D. P., and Jalife, J. (eds.): Cardiac Electrophysiology: From Cell to Bedside. 2nd ed. Philadelphia, W. B. Saunders Company, 1994, p. 732.

249. Mitra, R. L., and Buxton, A. E.: The clinical significance of nonsustained ventricular tachycardia. J. Cardiovasc. Electrophysiol. 4:490, 1993.

250. Turitto, G., Ahuja, R. K., Caref, E. B., et al.: Risk stratification for arrhythmic events in patients with nonischemic dilated cardiomyopathy and nonsustained ventricular tachycardia: Role of programmed ventricular stimulation and the signal-averaged electrocardiogram. J. Am. Coll. Cardiol. 24:1523, 1994.

251. Roelke, M., and Ruskin, J. N.: Dilated cardiomyopathy: Ventricular arrhythmias and sudden death. In Zipes, D. P., and Jalife, J. (eds.): Cardiac Electrophysiology: From Cell to Bedside. 2nd ed. Philadelphia, W. B. Saunders Company, 1994, p. 744.

252. Stevenson, W. G., Middlekauff, H. R., and Saxon, L. A.: Ventricular arrhythmias in heart failure. In Zipes, D. P., and Jalife, J. (eds.): Cardiac Electrophysiology: From Cell to Bedside. 2nd ed. Philadelphia, W. B. Saunders Company, 1994, p. 848.

253. Spirito, P., Rapezzi, C., Autore, C., et al.: Prognosis of asymptomatic patients with hypertrophic cardiomyopathy and nonsustained ventricular tachycardia. Circulation 90:2743, 1994.

254. Dilsizian, V., Bonow, R. O., Epstein, S. E., et al.: Myocardial ischemia detected by thallium scintigraphy is frequently related to cardiac arrest and syncope in young patients with hypertrophic cardiomyopathy. J. Am. Coll. Cardiol. 22:796, 1993.

255. Fananapazir, L., McAreavy, D., and Epstein, N. D.: Hypertrophic cardiomyopathy. In Zipes, D. P., and Jalife, J. (eds.): Cardiac Electrophysiology: From Cell to Bedside. 2nd ed. Philadelphia, W. B. Saunders Company, 1994, p. 769.

256. Wellens, H. J. J., Rodriguez, L. M., and Smeets, J. L.: Ventricular tachycardia in structurally normal hearts. In Zipes, D. P., and Jalife, J. (eds.): Cardiac Electrophysiology: From Cell to Bedside. 2nd ed. Philadelphia, W. B. Saunders Company, 1994, p. 780.

257. Hauer, R. N. W., and Wilde, A. A. W.: Mitral valve prolapse. In Zipes, D. P., and Jalife, J. (eds.): Cardiac Electrophysiology: From Cell to Bedside. 2nd ed. Philadelphia, W. B. Saunders Company, 1994, p. 833.

258. Perry, J. C., and Garson, A., Jr.: Arrhythmias following surgery for congenital heart disease. In Zipes, D. P., and Jalife, J. (eds.): Cardiac Electrophysiology: From Cell to Bedside. 2nd ed. Philadelphia, W. B. Saunders Company, 1994, p. 838.

259. Rials, S. J., Wu, Y., Ford, N., et al.: Effect of left ventricular hypertrophy in its regression on ventricular electrophysiology and vulnerability to inducible arrhythmia in the feline heart. Circulation 91:426, 1995.

260. Ben-David, J., Zipes, D. P., Ayers, G. M., et al.: Canine left ventricular hypertrophy predisposes to ventricular tachycardia induction by phase-II early afterdepolarizations after administration of BAY K 8644. J. Am. Coll. Cardiol. 20:1576, 1992.

261. Lampert, R., Rosenfeld, L., Batsford, W., et al.: Circadian variation of sustained ventricular tachycardia in patients with coronary artery disease and implantable cardioverter-defibrillators. Circulation 90:241, 1994.

262. Fei, L., Satters, D. J., Hnatkova, K., et al.: Change of autonomic influence on the heart immediately before the onset of spontaneous idiopathic ventricular tachycardia. J. Am. Coll. Cardiol. 24:1515, 1994.

263. Hohnloser, S. H., Klingenheben, T., vandeLoo, A., et al.: Reflex versus tonic vagal activity as a prognostic parameter in patients with sustained ventricular tachycardia or ventricular fibrillation. Circulation 89:1068, 1994.

264. Elami, A., Merin, G., Flugelman, M. Y., et al.: Usefulness of late potentials on the immediate postoperative signal-averaged electrocardiogram in predicting ventricular tachyarrhythmias early after isolated coronary artery bypass grafting. Am. J. Cardiol. 74:33, 1994.

265. Pye, M., Quinn, A. C., and Cobbe, S. M.: QT interval dispersion: A non-invasive marker of susceptibility to arrhythmia in patients with sustained ventricular arrhythmias? Br. Heart J. 71:511, 1994.

266. Hingham, P. D., Furniss, S. S., and Campbell, R. W.: QT dispersion and components of the AT interval in ischemia and infarction. Br. Heart J. 73:32, 1995.

267. Nora, M., and Zipes, D. P.: Empiric use of amiodarone and sotalol. Am. J. Cardiol. 72:62F, 1993.

268. Ho, D. S., Zecchin, R. P., Richards, D. A., et al.: Double-blind trial of lignocaine versus sotalol for acute termination of spontaneous sustained ventricular tachycardia. Lancet 344(8914):18, 1994.

269. Sotalol in life-threatening ventricular arrhythmias: A unique class III antiarrhythmic. Symposium proceedings. Am. J. Cardiol. 72:1A, 1993.

270. Perry, J. C., Knilans, T. K., Marlow, D., et al.: Intravenous amiodarone for life-threatening tachyarrhythmias in children and young adults. J. Am. Coll. Cardiol. 22:95, 1993.

271. Wolfe, C. L., Nibley, C., Bhandari, A., et al.: Polymorphous ventricular tachycardia associated with acute myocardial infarction. Circulation 84:1543, 1991.

272. Nalos, P. C., Ismail, Y., Pappas, J. M., et al.: Intravenous amiodarone for short-term treatment of refractory ventricular tachycardia or fibrillation. Am. Heart J. 122:1629, 1991.

273. Kowey, P. R., Mirinchak, R. A., Rials, S. J., et al.: Electrophysiologic testing in patients who respond acutely to intravenous amiodarone for incessant ventricular tachyarrhythmias. Am. Heart J. 125:1628, 1993.

274. Figa, F. H., Gow, R. M., Hamilton, R. M., et al.: Clinical efficacy and safety of intravenous amiodarone in infants and children. Am. J. Cardiol. 74:573, 1994.

274a. Scheinman, M. M.: Parenteral antiarrhythmic drug therapy in ventricular tachycardia / ventricular fibrillation: Evolving role of class III agents—focus on amiodarone. J. Cardiovasc. Electrophysiol. 6(Part 2):914, 1995.

275. Hohnloser, S. H., and Woosley, R. L.: Sotalol. N. Engl. J. Med. 331:31, 1994.

276. Young, G. D., Kerr, C. R., Mohama, R., et al.: Efficacy of sotalol guided by programmed electrical stimulation for sustained ventricular arrhythmias secondary to coronary artery disease. Am. J. Cardiol. 73:677, 1994.

277. Ohe, T., Aihara, N., Kamakura, S., et al.: Long-term outcome of verapamil-sensitive sustained left ventricular tachycardia in patients without structural heart disease. J. Am. Coll. Cardiol. 25:54, 1995.

278. Sung, R. J., Lauer, M. R., and Lai, W. T.: Verapamil-responsive ventricular tachycardia: Adenosine sensitivity and role of catecholamines. In Zipes, D. P., and Jalife, J. (eds.): Cardiac Electrophysiology: From Cell to Bedside. 2nd ed. Philadelphia, W. B. Saunders Company, 1994, p. 907.

279. Omoigui, N. A., Marcus, F. I., Mason, J. W., et al.: Cost of initial therapy in the Electrophysiological Study Versus ECG Monitoring Trial (ESVEM). Circulation 91:1070, 1995.

280. Kudenchuk, P. J., Bardy, G. H., Dolack, G. L., et al.: Efficacy of a single-lead unipolar transvenous defibrillator compared with a system employing an additional coronary sinus electrode: A prospective, randomized study. Circulation 89:2641, 1994.

281. Choue, C. W., Kim, S. G., Fischer, J. D., et al.: Comparison of defibrillator therapy and other therapeutic modalities for sustained ventricular tachycardia or ventricular fibrillation associated with coronary artery disease. Am. J. Cardiol. 73:1075, 1994.

282. Strickberger, S. A., Hummel, J. D., Daoud, E., et al.: Implantation by electrophysiologists of 100 consecutive cardioverter defibrillators with nonthoracotomy lead systems. Circulation 90:868, 1994.

283. Sweeney, M. O., and Ruskin, J. N.: Mortality benefits and the implantable cardioverter-defibrillator. Circulation 89:1851, 1994.

284. Zipes, D. P., Roberts, D., for the PCD Investigators: Results of the world wide study of the implantable pacemaker, cardioverter defibrillator: A comparison of epicardial and endocardial lead systems. Circulation 92:59, 1995.

285. Ferguson, T. D., Jr., Smith, J. M., Cox, J. L., et al.: Direct operation versus ICD therapy for ischemic ventricular tachycardia. Ann. Thorac. Surg. 58:1291, 1994.

286. Crawford, F. A., Jr., and Gillette, P. C.: Surgical treatment of cardiac dysrhythmias in infants and children. Ann. Thorac. Surg. 58:1262, 1994.

287. Guiraudon, G. M., Thakur, R. K., Klein, G. J., et al.: Encircling endocardial cryoablation for ventricular tachycardia after myocardial infarction: Experience with 33 patients. Am. Heart J. 128:982, 1994.

288. Morris, J. J., Rastogi, A., Stanton, M. S., et al.: Operation for ventricular tachyarrhythmias: Refining current treatment strategies. Ann. Thorac. Surg. 58:1490, 1994.

289. Misaki, T., Watanabe, G., Iwa, T., et al.: Surgical treatment of arrhythmogenic right ventricular dysplasia: Long-term outcome. Ann. Thorac. Surg. 58:1380, 1994.

290. Misaki, T., Watanabe, G., Iwa, T., et al.: Surgical treatment of arrhythmogenic right ventricular dysplasia: Long-term outcome. Ann. Thorac. Surg. 58:1380, 1994.

291. Rokkas, C. K., Nitta, T., Schuessler, R. B., et al.: Human ventricular tachycardia: Precise intraoperative localization with potential distribution mapping. Ann. Thorac. Surg. 57:1628, 1994.

292. Misaki, T., Tsubota, M., Watanabe, G., et al.: Surgical treatment of ventricular tachycardia after surgical repair of tetralogy of Fallot: Relation between intraoperative mapping and histological findings. Circulation 90:264, 1994.

293. Lee, R., Mitchell, J. B., Garan, H., et al.: Operation for recurrent ventricular tachycardia: Predictors of short- and long-term efficacy. J. Thorac. Cardiovasc. Surg. 107:732, 1994.

294. Klein, L. S., and Miles, W. M.: Ablative therapy for ventricular arrhythmias. Prog. Cardiovasc. Dis. 37:225, 1995.

295. Gonska, D. D., Cao, K., Schaumann, A., et al.: Catheter ablation of ventricular tachycardia in 136 patients with coronary artery disease: Results and long-term follow-up. J. Am. Coll. Cardiol. 24:1506, 1994.

296. Blanck, Z., Dhala, A., Deshpande, S., et al.: Catheter ablation of ventricular tachycardia. Am. Heart J. 127:1126, 1994.

297. Wen, M. S., Yeh, S. J., Wang, C. C., et al.: Radiofrequency ablation therapy in idiopathic left ventricular tachycardia with no obvious structural heart disease. Circulation 89:1690, 1994.

298. Borggrefe, M., Chen, X., Hindricks, W., et al.: Catheter ablation of ventricular tachycardia in patients with coronary heart disease. In Zipes, D. P., and Jalife, J. (eds.): Cardiac Electrophysiology: From Cell to Bedside. Philadelphia, W. B. Saunders Company, 1994, p. 1502.

299. Klein, L. S., Miles, W. M., Mitrani, R. D., et al.: Ablation of ventricular tachycardia in patients with structurally normal hearts. In Zipes, D. P., and Jalife, J. (eds.): Cardiac Electrophysiology: From Cell to Bedside. Philadelphia, W. B. Saunders Company, 1994, p. 1518.

300. Fontaine, G., Fontaliran, F., Lascault, G., et al.: Arrhythmogenic right ventricular dysplasia. In Zipes, D. P., and Jalife, J. (eds.): Cardiac Electrophysiology: From Cell to Bedside. Philadelphia, W. B. Saunders Company, 1994, p. 754.

301. Yamabe, H., Okumura, K., Tsuchiya, T., et al.: Demonstration of entrainment and presence of slow conduction during ventricular tachycardia in arrhythmogenic right ventricular dysplasia. PACE 17:172, 1994.

302. Lee, A. H., Morgan, J. M., and Gallagher, P. J.: Arrhythmogenic right ventricular cardiomyopathy. J. Pathol. 171:157, 1993.

303. Solenthaler, M., Ritter, M., Candinas, R., et al.: Arrhythmogenic right ventricular dysplasia in identical twins. Am. J. Cardiol. 74:303, 1994.

303a. Rampazzo, A., Nava, A., Danieli, G. A., et al.: The gene for arrhythmogenic right ventricular cardiomyopathy maps to chromosome 14q23-q24. Hum. Mol. Genet. 3:959, 1994.

304. Mehta, D., Davies, M. J., Ward, D. E., et al.: Ventricular tachycardias of right ventricular origin: Markers of subclinical right ventricular disease. Am. Heart J. 127:360, 1994.

305. Rolov, M. V., Brodsky, M. A., Allen, B. J., et al.: Spectrum of right heart involvement in patients with ventricular tachycardia unrelated to coronary artery disease or left ventricular dysfunction. Am. Heart J. 126:1348, 1993.

306. Hamada, S., Tamamiya, M., Ohe, T., et al.: Arrhythmogenic right ventricular dysplasia: Evaluation with electron-beam CT. Radiology 187:723, 1993.

307. Auffermann, W., Wichter, T., Breithardt, G., et al.: Arrhythmogenic right ventricular disease: MR imaging versus angiography. A.J.R. 161:549, 1993.

308. Blake, L. M., Scheinman, M. M., and Higgins, C. B.: MR features of arrhythmogenic right ventricular dysplasia. A.J.R. 162:809, 1994.

309. Wichter, T., Hendricks, G., Lerch, H., et al.: Regional myocardial sympathetic dysinnervation in arrhythmogenic right ventricular cardiomyopathy. An analysis using ^{123}I-meta-iodobenzylguanidine scintigraphy. Circulation 89:667, 1994.

310. Metzger, J. T., deChillou, C., Cherieax, E., et al.: Value of the 12-lead electrocardiogram in arrhythmogenic right ventricular dysplasia, and absence of correlation with echocardiographic findings. Am. J. Cardiol. 72:964, 1993.

311. Kinoshita, O., Kamakura, S., Ohe, T., et al.: Frequency analysis of signal-averaged electrocardiogram in patients with right ventricular tachycardia. J. Am. Coll. Cardiol. 20:1230, 1992.

312. Kinoshita, O., Fontaine, G., Rosas, F., et al.: Optimal high-pass filter settings of the signal-averaged electrocardiogram in patients with arrhythmogenic right ventricular dysplasia. Am. J. Cardiol. 74:1074, 1994.

313. McLay, J. S., Norris, A., Campbell, R. W., et al.: Arrhythmogenic right ventricular dysplasia: An uncommon cause of ventricular tachycardia in young and old? Br. Heart J. 69:158, 1993.

314. Breithardt, G., Wichter, T., Haverkamp, W., et al.: Implantable cardioverter defibrillator therapy in patients with arrhythmogenic right ventricular cardiomyopathy, long QT syndrome or no structural heart disease. Am. Heart J. 127:1151, 1994.

315. Burton, M. E., and Leon, A. R.: Radiofrequency catheter ablation of right ventricular outflow tract tachycardia late after complete repair of tetralogy of Fallot using the pace mapping technique. PACE 16:2319, 1993.

316. Biblo, L. A., and Carlson, M. D.: Transcatheter radiofrequency ablation of ventricular tachycardia following surgical correction of tetralogy of Fallot. PACE 17:1556, 1994.

317. Matsuoka, S., Akita, H., Hayabuchi, Y., et al.: Abnormal signal averaged ECG after surgical repair of tetralogy of Fallot: A combined analysis in the time and frequency domain. Jpn. Circ. J. 57:841, 1993.

318. Dreyer, W. J., Paridon, S. M., Fisher, D. J., et al.: Rapid ventricular pacing in dogs with right ventricular outflow tract obstruction: Insights into a mechanism of sudden death in postoperative tetralogy of Fallot. J. Am. Coll. Cardiol. 21:1731, 1993.

319. Mancini, D. M., Wong, K. L., and Simson, M. B.: Prognostic value of an abnormal signal-averaged electrocardiogram in patients with nonischemic congestive cardiomyopathy. Circulation 87:1083, 1993.

320. Keeling, P. J., Kulakowski, T., Yi, G., et al.: Usefulness of signal-averaged electrocardiogram in idiopathic dilated cardiomyopathy for identifying patients with ventricular arrhythmias. Am. J. Cardiol. 72:78, 1993.

321. Turitto, G., Ahuja, R. K., Bekheit, S., et al.: Incidence and prediction of induced ventricular tachyarrhythmias in idiopathic dilated cardiomyopathy. Am. J. Cardiol. 73:770, 1994.

322. Marchlinski, F. E., Schwartzman, D., Gottlieb, C. D., et al.: Electrical events associated with arrhythmia initiation and stimulation techniques for arrhythmia prevention. In Zipes, D. P., and Jalife, J. (eds.): Cardiac Electrophysiology: From Cell to Bedside. Philadelphia, W. B. Saunders Company, 1994, p. 863.

323. Chen, X., Shenasa, M., Borggrefe, M., et al.: Role of programmed ventricular stimulation in patients with idiopathic dilated cardiomyopathy and documented sustained ventricular tachyarrhythmias: Inducibility and prognostic value in 102 patients. Eur. Heart J. 15:76, 1994.

324. Borggrefe, M., Chen, X., Martinez-Rubio, A., et al.: The role of implantable cardioverter defibrillators in dilated cardiomyopathy. Am. Heart J. 127:1145, 1994.

325. Lessmeier, T. J., Lehmann, M. H., Steinman, R. T., et al.: Outcome with implantable cardioverter-defibrillator therapy for survivors of ventricular fibrillation secondary to idiopathic dilated cardiomyopathy or coronary artery disease without myocardial infarction. Am. J. Cardiol. 72:911, 1993.

326. Blanck, Z., Deshpande, S., Mohammad, R., et al.: Catheter ablation of the left bundle branch for the treatment of sustained bundle branch reentrant ventricular tachycardia. J. Cardiovasc. Electrophysiol. 6:40, 1995.

327. Blanck, Z., Sra, J., Dhala, A., et al.: Bundle branch reentry: Mechanisms, diagnosis and treatment. In Zipes, D. P., and Jalife, J. (eds.): Cardiac Electrophysiology: From Cell to Bedside. Philadelphia, W. B. Saunders Company, 1994, p. 878.

328. Callans, D. J., Schwartzman, D., Gottlieb, C. B., et al.: Insights into the electrophysiology of ventricular tachycardia gained by the catheter ablation experience: Learning while burning. J. Cardiovasc. Electrophysiol. 5:877, 1994.

329. Larsen, L., Markham, J., and Haffajee, C. I.: Sudden death in idiopathic dilated cardiomyopathy: Role of ventricular arrhythmias. PACE 16:1051, 1993.

330. McKenna, W. J., Sadoul, N., Slade, A. K., et al.: The prognostic significance of nonsustained ventricular tachycardia in hypertrophic cardiomyopathy. Circulation 90:3115, 1994.

331. Spirito, P., Rapezzi, C., Autore, C., et al.: Prognosis of asymptomatic patients with hypertrophic cardiomyopathy and nonsustained ventricular tachycardia. Circulation 90:2743, 1994.

332. Fananapazir, L., Chang, A. C., Epstein, S. E., et al.: Prognostic determinants in hypertrophic cardiomyopathy: Prospective evaluation of a therapeutic strategy based on clinical, Holter, hemodynamic, and electrophysiological findings. Circulation 86:730, 1992.

333. Saumarez, R. C., Camm, A. J., Panagos, A., et al.: Ventricular fibrillation in hypertrophic cardiomyopathy is associated with increased fractionation of paced right ventricular electrograms. Circulation 86:467, 1992.

334. Shakespeare, C. F., Keeling, P. J., Slade, A. K., et al.: Arrhythmias and hypertrophic cardiomyopathy. Arch. Mal. Coeur Vaiss 87:31, 1992.

335. Dilsizian, V., Bonow, R. O., Epstein, S. E., et al.: Myocardial ischemia detected by thallium scintigraphy is frequently related to cardiac arrest and syncope in young patients with hypertrophic cardiomyopathy. J. Am. Coll. Cardiol. 22:796, 1993.

336. Stewart, J. T., and McKenna, W. J.: Management of arrhythmias in hypertrophic cardiomyopathy. Cardiovasc. Drugs. Ther. 8:95, 1994.

337. Almendral, J. M., Ormaetxe, J., and Martinez-Alday, J. D.: Treatment of ventricular arrhythmias in patients with hypertrophic cardiomyopathy. Eur. Heart J. 14 (Suppl. J):71, 1993.

338. Buja, G., Miroelli, M., Turrini, P., et al.: Comparison of QT dispersion in hypertrophic cardiomyopathy between patients with and without ventricular arrhythmias and sudden death. Am. J. Cardiol. 72:973, 1993.

339. Vohra, J., Sathe, S., Warren, R., et al.: Malignant ventricular arrhythmias in patients with mitral valve prolapse and mild mitral regurgitation. PACE 16:387, 1993.

340. Belhassen, B., and Viskin, S.: Idiopathic ventricular tachycardia and fibrillation. J. Cardiovasc. Electrophysiol. 4:356, 1993.

341. Tung, R. T., Shen, W. K., Hammill, S. C., et al.: Idiopathic ventricular fibrillation in out-of-hospital cardiac arrest survivors. PACE 17:1405, 1994.

342. Almendral, J., Ormaetxe, J., and Delcan, J. L.: Idiopathic ventricular tachycardia and fibrillation: Incidence, prognosis and therapy. PACE 15:627, 1992.

343. Masrani, K., Cowley, C., Bekheit, S., et al.: Recurrent syncope for over a decade due to idiopathic ventricular fibrillation. Chest 106:1601, 1994.

344. Sumiyoshi, M., Nakata, Y., Hisaoka, T., et al.: A case of idiopathic ventricular fibrillation with incomplete right bundle branch block and persistent ST segment elevation. Jpn. Heart J. 34:661, 1993.

345. Brugada, P., and Brugada, J.: Right bundle branch block, persistent ST segment elevation and sudden cardiac death: A distinct clinical and electrocardiographic syndrome. J. Am. Coll. Cardiol. 20:1391, 1992.

346. Katritsis, D. G., Jaswinder, S. G., and Camm, A. J.: Repetitive monomorphic ventricular tachycardia. In Zipes, D. P., and Jalife, J. (eds.): Cardiac Electrophysiology: From Cell to Bedside. 2nd ed. Philadelphia, W. B. Saunders Company, 1994, p. 900.

347. Lerman, B. B.: Response of nonreentrant catecholamine-mediated ventricular tachycardia to endogenous adenosine and acetylcholine: Evidence of myocardial receptor-mediated effects. Circulation 87:382, 1993.

348. Gill, J. S., Mehta, D., Ward, D. E., et al.: Efficacy of flecainide, sotalol, and verapamil in the treatment of right ventricular tachycardia in patients without overt cardiac abnormality. Br. Heart J. 68:392, 1992.

349. Nakagawa, H., Mukai, J., Nagata, K., et al.: Early afterdepolarizations in a patient with idiopathic monomorphic right ventricular tachycardia. PACE 16:2067, 1993.

350. Lerman, B. B., Stein, K., Engelstein, E. D., et al.: Mechanism of repetitive monomorphic ventricular tachycardia. Circulation 92:421, 1995.

351. Klein, L. S., Miles, W. M., Mitrani, R. D., et al.: Catheter ablation of ventricular tachycardia. In Smith, T. W., Antman, E. M., Bittl, J. A., Colucci, W. S., Gotto, A. M., Loscalzo, J., Williams, G. H., and Zipes, D. P. (eds.): Cardiovascular Therapeutics. Philadelphia, W. B. Saunders Company, 1996.

352. Gill, J. S., Blaszyk, K., Ward, D. E., et al.: Verapamil for the suppression of idiopathic ventricular tachycardia of left bundle branch block-like morphology. Am. Heart J. 126:1126, 1993.

353. Carlson, M. D., White, R. D., Trohman, R. G., et al.: Right ventricular outflow tract ventricular tachycardia: Detection of previously unrecognized anatomic abnormalities using cine magnetic resonance imaging. J. Am. Coll. Cardiol. 24:720, 1994.

354. Gill, J. S., DeBelder, M., and Ward, D. E.: Right ventricular outflow tract ventricular tachycardia associated with an aneurysmal malformation: Use of transesophageal echocardiography during low-energy direct-current ablation. Am. Heart J. 128:620, 1994.

355. Nakagawa, H., Beckman, K. J., McClelland, J. H., et al.: Radiofrequency catheter ablation of idiopathic left ventricular tachycardia guided by a Purkinje potential. Circulation 88:2607, 1993.

356. Kottkamp, H., Chen, X., Hindricks, G., et al.: Radiofrequency catheter ablation of idiopathic left ventricular tachycardia: Further evidence for microreentry as the underlying mechanism. J. Cardiovasc. Electrophysiol. 5:268, 1994.

357. Gill, J. S., Ward, D. E., and Camm, A. J.: Comparison of verapamil and diltiazem in the suppression of idiopathic ventricular tachycardia. PACE 15:2122, 1992.

358. DeLacey, W. A., Nath, S., Haines, D. E., et al.: Adenosine and verapamil-sensitive ventricular tachycardia originating from the left ventricle: Radiofrequency catheter ablation. PACE 15:2240, 1992.

359. Kobayashi, Y., Kikushima, S., Tanno, K., et al.: Sustained left ventricular tachycardia terminated by dipyridamole: Cyclic AMP-mediated triggered activity as a possible mechanism. PACE 17:377, 1994.

360. Griffith, M. J., Garratt, C. J., and Rowland, E.: Effects of intravenous adenosine on verapamil-sensitive idiopathic ventricular tachycardia. Am. J. Cardiol. 73:759, 1994.

361. Gonzalez, R. P., Scheinman, M. M., Lesh, M. D., et al.: Clinical and electrophysiologic spectrum of fascicular tachycardias. Am. Heart J. 128:147, 1994.

362. Gaita, F., Giustetto, C., Leclercq, J. F., et al.: Idiopathic verapamil-responsive left ventricular tachycardia: Clinical characteristics and long-term follow-up of 33 patients. Eur. Heart J. 15:1252, 1994.

362a. Munger, R. G., and Booton, E. A.: Thiamine and sudden death in sleep of South-East Asian refugees. Lancet 335:1154, 1990.

363. Grimm, W., and Marchlinski, F. E.: Accelerated idioventricular rhythm, bidirectional ventricular tachycardia. In Zipes, D. P., and Jalife, J. (eds.): Cardiac Electrophysiology: From Cell to Bedside. 2nd ed. Philadelphia, W. B. Saunders Company, 1994, p. 920.

364. Zipes, D. P.: Unwitting exposure to risk (Editorial). Cardiol. Rev. 1:1, 1993.

365. Pepe, P. E., Levine, R. L., Fromm, R. E., Jr., et al.: Cardiac arrest presenting with rhythms other than ventricular fibrillation: Contribution of resuscitative efforts toward total survivorship. Crit. Care Med. 21:1838, 1993.

366. Roden, D. M.: Torsade de pointes. Clin. Cardiol. 16:683, 1993.

367. Ben-David, J., and Zipes, D. P.: Torsades de pointes and proarrhythmia. Lancet 341:1578, 1993.

368. Schwartz, P. J., Locati, E. H., Napolitano, C., et al.: The long QT syndrome. In Zipes, D. P., and Jalife, J. (eds.): Cardiac Electrophysiology: From Cell to Bedside. Philadelphia, W. B. Saunders Company, 1994, p. 788.

369. Fontaine, G.: A new look at torsades de pointes. Ann. N.Y. Acad. Sci. 644:157, 1992.

370. Kurita, T., Ohe, T., Marui, N., et al.: Bradycardia-induced abnormal QT prolongation in patients with complete atrioventricular block with torsades de pointes. Am. J. Cardiol. 69:628, 1992.

371. Haverkamp, W., Shenasa, M., Borggrefe, M., et al.: Torsades de pointes. In Zipes, D. P., and Jalife, J. (eds.): Cardiac Electrophysiology: From Cell to Bedside. 2nd ed. Philadelphia, W. B. Saunders Company, 1994, p. 885.

372. Leenhardt, A., Glaser, E., Burguera, M., et al.: Short-coupled variant of torsade de pointes: A new electrocardiographic entity in the spectrum of idiopathic ventricular tachyarrhythmias. Circulation 89:206, 1994.

373. Napolitano, C., Priori, S. G., and Schwartz, P. J.: Torsade de pointes: Mechanisms and management. Drugs 47:51, 1994.

374. Tan, H. L., Hou, C. J. Y., Lauer, M. R., et al.: Electrophysiologic mechanisms of the long QT interval syndromes and torsade de pointes. Ann. Intern. Med. 122:701, 1995.

375. Miwa, S., Inoue, T., and Yokoyama, M.: Monophasic action potentials in patients with torsades de pointes. Jpn. Circ. J. 58:248, 1994.

376. Roden, D. M.: Early after-depolarizations and torsade de pointes: Implications for the control of cardiac arrhythmias by prolonging repolarization. Eur. Heart J. 14 (Suppl. H):56, 1993.

377. Weissenburger, J., Davy, J. M., and Chezalviel, F.: Experimental models of torsades de pointes. Fund. Clin. Pharmacol. 7:29, 1993.

378. Hii, J. T., Wyse, D. G., Gillis, A. M., et al.: Precordial QT interval dispersion as a marker of torsade de pointes: Disparate effects of class IA antiarrhythmic drugs and amiodarone. Circulation 86:1376, 1992.

379. Pertsov, A. M., and Jalife, J.: Three-dimensional vortex-like reentry. In Zipes, D. P., and Jalife, J. (eds.): Cardiac Electrophysiology: From Cell to Bedside. 2nd ed. Philadelphia, W. B. Saunders Company, 1994, p. 403.

380. Makkar, R. R., Fromm, B. S., Steinman, R. T., et al.: Female gender as a risk factor for torsades de pointes associated with cardiovascular drugs. J.A.M.A. 270:2590, 1993.

381. Perticone, F., Ceravolo, R., DeNovara, G., et al.: New data on the antiarrhythmic value of magnesium treatment: Magnesium and ventricular arrhythmias. Magnet. Reson. 5:265, 1992.

382. Banai, S., and Tzivoni, D.: Drug therapy for torsade de pointes. J. Cardiovasc. Electrophysiol. 4:206, 1993.

383. Carlsson, L., Abrahamsson, C., and Drews, L.: Antiarrhythmic effects of potassium channel openers in rhythm abnormalities related to delayed repolarization. Circulation 85:1491, 1992.

384. Vos, M. A., Gorgels, A. P., Lipcsei, G. C., et al.: Mechanism-specific antiarrhythmic effects of the potassium channel activator levcromakalim against repolarization-dependent tachycardias. J. Cardiovasc. Electrophysiol. 5:731, 1994.

385. Sato, T., Yoshiki, H., Yamamoto, M., et al.: Early afterdepolarization abolished by potassium channel opener in a patient with idiopathic long QT syndrome. J. Cardiovasc. Electrophysiol. 6:279, 1995.

386. Moss, A. J.: Measurement of the QT interval and the risk associated with QTc interval prolongation: A review. Am. J. Cardiol. 72:23B, 1993.

387. Antzelevitch, C., and Sicouri, S.: Clinical relevance of cardiac arrhythmias generated by afterdepolarizations: Role of M cells in the generation of U waves, triggered activity and torsade de pointes. J. Am. Coll. Cardiol. 23:259, 1994.

388. Lehmann, M. H., Suzuki, F., Fromm, B. S., et al.: T wave humps as a potential electrocardiographic marker of the long QT syndrome. J. Am. Coll. Cardiol. 24:746, 1994.

389. Krause, P. C., Rardon, D. P., Miles, W. M., et al.: Characteristics of Ca^{2+}-activated K^+ channels isolated from the left ventricle of the patient with idiopathic long QT syndrome. Am. Heart J. 126:1134, 1993.

390. Schwartz, P. J., Moss, A. J., Vincent, G. M., et al.: Diagnostic criteria for the long QT syndrome: An update. Circulation 88:782, 1993.

391. Habbab, M. A., and El-Sherif, N.: TU alternans, long QTU and torsade de pointes: Clinical and experimental observations. PACE 15:916, 1992.

392. Rosenbaum, M. B., and Acunzo, R. S.: Pseudo 2:1 atrioventricular block and T wave alternans in the long QT syndromes. J. Am. Coll. Cardiol. 18:1363, 1991.

393. Keating, M.: Genetics of the long QT syndrome. J. Cardiovasc. Electrophysiol. 5:146, 1994.

394. Vincent, G. M.: Hypothesis for the molecular physiology of the Romano-Ward long QT syndrome. J. Am. Coll. Cardiol. 20:500, 1992.

395. Tanaka, T., Nakahara, K., Kato, N., et al.: Genetic linkage analyses of Romano-Ward syndrome (RWS) in 13 Japanese families. Hum. Genet. 94:380, 1994.

396. Weitkamp, L. R., Moss, A. J., Lewis, R. A., et al.: Analysis of HLA and disease susceptibility: Chromosome 6 genes and sex influence on long-QT phenotype. Am. J. Hum. Genet. 55:1230, 1994.

397. Towbin, J. A., Li, H., Taggart, R. T., et al.: Evidence of genetic heterogeneity in Romano-Ward long QT syndrome: Analysis of 23 families. Circulation 90:2635, 1994.

398. Desmyttere, S., Bonduelle, M., DeWolf, D., et al.: A case of term mors in utero in chromosome 11p linked long QT syndrome family. Genet. Couns. 5:289, 1994.

399. Jiang, C., Atkinson, D., Towbin, J. A., et al.: Two long QT syndrome loci map to chromosomes 3 and 7 with evidence for further heterogeneity. Nat. Genet. 8:141, 1994.

400. Curran, M. E., Splawski, I., Timothy, K. W., et al.: A molecular basis for cardiac arrhythmia: HERG mutations cause long QT syndrome. Cell 80:795, 1995.

401. Wang, Q., Shen, J., Splawski, I., et al.: SCN5A mutations associated with an inherited cardiac arrhythmia, long QT syndrome. Cell 80:805, 1995.

401a. Roden, D. M., George, A. L., Jr., and Bennett, P. B.: Recent advances in understanding the molecular mechanism of the long QT syndrome. J. Cardiovasc. Electrophysiol. 6:1023, 1995.

401b. Grace, A. A., and Chien, K. R.: Congenital long QT syndromes. Toward molecular dissection of arrhythmia substrates. Circulation 92:2786, 1995.

401c. Moss, A. J., Zareba, W., Benhorin, J., et al.: ECG T-wave patterns in genetically distinct forms of the hereditary long QT syndrome. Circulation 92:2929, 1995.

402. Vos, M. A., Verduyn, S. C., Gorgels, A. P., et al.: Reproducible induction of early afterdepolarizations and torsade de pointes arrhythmias by d-sotalol and pacing in dogs with chronic atrioventricular block. Circulation 91:864, 1995.

403. Lazzara, R.: Antiarrhythmic drugs and torsade de pointes. Eur. Heart J. 14 (Suppl. H):88, 1993.

404. Woosley, R. L., Chen, Y., Freiman, J. P., et al.: Mechanism of the cardiotoxic actions of terfenadine. JAMA 269:1532, 1993.

405. Smith, J.: Cardiovascular toxicity of antihistamines. Otolaryngol. Head Neck Surg. 111:348, 1994.

406. Herings, R. M., Stricker, B. H., Leufkens, H. G., et al.: Public health problems and the rapid estimation of the size of the population at risk:

Torsades de pointes and the use of terfenadine and astemizole in The Netherlands. Pharm. World Sci. *15*:212, 1993.

407. Brandriss, M. W., Richardson, W. S., and Barold, S. S.: Erythromycin-induced QT prolongation and polymorphic ventricular tachycardia (torsades de pointes): Case report and review. Clin. Infect. Dis. *18*:995, 1994.

408. Rubart, M., Pressler, M. L., Pride, H. P., et al.: Electrophysiological mechanisms in a canine model of erythromycin-associated long QT syndrome. Circulation *88*:1832, 1993.

409. Gitler, B., Berger, L. S., and Buffa, S. D.: Torsades de pointes induced by erythromycin. Chest *105*:368, 1994.

410. Mani, S., Kocheril, A. G., and Andriole, V. T.: Case report: Pentamidine and polymorphic ventricular tachycardia revisited. Am. J. Med. Sci. *305*:236, 1993.

411. Eisenhauer, M. D., Eliasson, A. H., Taylor, A. J., et al.: Incidence of cardiac arrhythmias during intravenous pentamidine therapy in HIV-infected patients. Chest *105*:389, 1994.

412. Tamura, M., Ueki, Y., Ohtsuka, E., et al.: Probucol-induced QT prolongation and syncope. Jpn. Circ. J. *58*:374, 1994.

413. Singh, B., al Shahwan, S. A., Habbab, M. A., et al.: Idiopathic long QT syndrome: Asking the right question. Lancet *341*:741, 1993.

414. Villain, E., Levy, M., Kachaner, J., et al.: Prolonged QT interval in neonates: Benign, transient, or prolonged risk of sudden death. Am. Heart J. *124*:194, 1992.

414a. Pacia, S. V., Devinsky, O., Luciano, D. J., et al.: The prolonged QT syndrome presenting as epilepsy: A report of two cases and literature review. Neurology *44*:1408, 1994.

415. Garson, A., Jr., Dick, M., II, Fournier, A., et al.: The long QT syndrome in children: An international study of 287 patients. Circulation *87*:1866, 1993.

416. Marks, M. L., Whisler, S. L., Clericuzio, C., et al.: A new form of long QT syndrome associated with syndactyly. J. Am. Coll. Cardiol. *25*:59, 1995.

417. Zareba, W., Moss, A. J., leCessie, S., et al.: T wave alternans in idiopathic long QT syndrome. J. Am. Coll. Cardiol. *23*:1541, 1994.

418. Buckingham, T. A., Bhutto, Z. R., Telfer, E. A., et al.: Differences in corrected QT intervals at minimal and maximal heart rate may identify patients at risk for torsades de pointes during treatment with antiarrhythmic drugs. J. Cardiovasc. Electrophysiol. *5*:408, 1994.

419. Eggeling, T., Osterhues, H. H., Hoeher, M., et al.: Value of Holter monitoring in patients with the long QT syndrome. Cardiology *81*:107, 1992.

420. Ohe, T., Kurita, T., Shimizu, W., et al.: Introduction of TU abnormalities in patients with torsades de pointes. Ann. N.Y. Acad. Sci. *644*:178, 1992.

421. Shimizu, W., Ohe, T., Kurita, T., et al.: Epinephrine-induced ventricular premature complexes due to early afterdepolarizations and effects of verapamil and propanolol in a patient with the congenital long QT syndrome. J. Cardiovasc. Electrophysiol. *5*:438, 1994.

421a. Shimizu, W., Ohe, T., Kurita, T., et al.: Effects of verapamil and propranolol on early afterdepolarizations and ventricular arrhythmias induced by epinephrine in congenital long QT syndrome. J. Am. Coll. Cardiol. *26*:1299, 1995.

422. DeFerrari, G. M., Nador, F., Beria, G., et al.: Effect of calcium channel block on the wall motion abnormality of the idiopathic long QT syndrome. Circulation *89*:2126, 1994.

423. Calkins, H., Lehmann, M. H., Allman, K., et al.: Scintigraphic pattern of regional cardiac sympathetic innervation in patients with familial long QT syndrome using positron emission tomography. Circulation *87*:1616, 1993.

424. Muller, K. D., Jakob, H., Neuzner, J., et al.: ^{123}I-metaiodobenzylguanidine scintigraphy in the detection of irregular regional sympathetic innervation in long QT syndrome. Eur. Heart J. *14*:316, 1993.

425. Moise, N. S., Meyers-Wallen, V., Flahive, W. J., et al.: Inherited ventricular arrhythmias and sudden death in German Shepherd dogs. J. Am. Coll. Cardiol. *24*:233, 1994.

425a. Moise, M. D., Moon, P. F., Flahive, W. J., et al.: Phenylprine-induced ventricular arrhythmias in dogs with inherited sudden death. J. Cardiovasc. Electrophysiol. (*In press*).

426. Leenhardt, A., Lucet, V., Denjoy, I., et al.: Catecholaminergic polymorphic ventricular tachycardia in children: A seven-year follow-up of 21 patients. Circulation *91*:1512, 1995.

427. Eldar, M., Griffin, J. C., VanHare, G. F., et al.: Combined use of beta-adrenergic blocking agents and long-term cardiac pacing for patients with the long QT syndrome. J. Am. Coll. Cardiol. *20*:830, 1992.

428. Moss, A. J., and Robinson, J.: Clinical features of the idiopathic long QT syndrome. Circulation *85* (Suppl. 1):1140, 1992.

429. Malfatto, G., Beria, G., Sala, S., et al.: Quantitative analysis of T wave abnormalities and their prognostic implications in the idiopathic long QT syndrome. J. Am. Coll. Cardiol. *23*:296, 1994.

430. Blanck, Z., Dhala, A., Deshpande, S., et al.: Bundle branch reentrant ventricular tachycardia: Cumulative experience in 48 patients. J. Cardiovasc. Electrophysiol. *4*:253, 1993.

431. Blanck, Z., Jazayeri, M., Dhala, A., et al.: Bundle branch reentry: A mechanism of ventricular tachycardia in the absence of myocardial or valvular dysfunction. J. Am. Coll. Cardiol. *22*:1718, 1993.

432. Epstein, A. E., and Ideker, R. E.: Ventricular fibrillation. *In* Zipes, D. P., and Jalife, J. (eds.): Cardiac Electrophysiology: From Cell to Bedside. 2nd ed. Philadelphia, W. B. Saunders Company, 1994, p. 927.

433. Lubbe, W. F., Podzweit, T., and Opie, L. H.: Potential arrhythmogenic role of cyclic adenosine monophosphate (AMP) and cytosolic calcium overload: Implications for prophylactic effects of beta-blockers in myocardial infarction and proarrhythmic effects of phosphodiesterase inhibitors. J. Am. Coll. Cardiol. *19*:1622, 1992.

433a. Tobe, T. J., deLangen, C. D., Crijns, H. J., et al.: Effects of streptokinase during acute myocardial infarction on the signal-averaged electrocardiogram and on the frequency of late arrhythmias. Am. J. Cardiol. *72*:647, 1993.

434. Arntz, H. R., Willich, S. N., Oeff, M., et al.: Circadian variation of sudden cardiac death reflects age-related variability in ventricular fibrillation. Circulation *88*:2284, 1993.

435. Fei, L., Anderson, M. H., Katritsis, D., et al.: Decreased heart rate variability in survivors of sudden cardiac death not associated with coronary artery disease. Br. Heart J. *71*:16, 1994.

436. Dougherty, C. M., and Burr, R. L.: Comparison of heart rate variability in survivors and nonsurvivors of sudden cardiac arrest. Am. J. Cardiol. *70*:441, 1992.

437. Davies, M. J.: Anatomic features in victims of sudden coronary death: Coronary artery pathology. Circulation *85* (Suppl. 1):119, 1992.

438. Rodriguez, L. M., Smeets, J., O'Hara, G. E., et al.: Incidence and timing of recurrences of sudden death and ventricular tachycardia during antiarrhythmic drug treatment after myocardial infarction. Am. J. Cardiol. *69*:1403, 1992.

439. Kim, S. G., Fisher, J. D., Choue, C. W., et al.: Influence of left ventricular function on outcome of patients treated with implantable defibrillators. Circulation *85*:1304, 1992.

440. Wever, E. F., Hauer, R. N., Oomen, A., et al.: Unfavorable outcome in patients with primary electrical disease who survived an episode of ventricular fibrillation. Circulation *88*:1021, 1993.

441. Meissner, M. D., Lehmann, M. H., Steinman, R. T., et al.: Ventricular fibrillation in patients without significant structural heart disease: A multicenter experience with implantable cardioverter-defibrillator therapy. J. Am. Coll. Cardiol. *21*:1406, 1993.

442. Cummins, R. O., Graves, J. R., Larsen, M. P., et al.: Out-of-hospital transcutaneous pacing by emergency medical technicians in patients with asystolic cardiac arrest. N. Engl. J. Med. *328*:1377, 1993.

443. Hallstrom, A., Boutin, P., and Cobb, L.: Socioeconomic status and prediction of ventricular fibrillation survival. Am. J. Public Health *83*:245, 1993.

444. Every, N. R., Fahrenbruch, C. E., Hallstrom, A. P., et al.: Influence of coronary bypass surgery on subsequent outcome of patients resuscitated from out of hospital cardiac arrest. J. Am. Coll. Cardiol. *19*:1435, 1992.

445. Kim, Y. H., Sosa-Suarez, G., Trouton, T. G., et al.: Treatment of ventricular tachycardia by transcatheter radiofrequency ablation in patients with ischemic heart disease. Circulation *89*:1094, 1994.

HEART BLOCK

445a. Rardon, D. P., Miles, W. M., Mitrani, R. D., et al.: Atrioventricular block and dissociation. *In* Zipes, D. P., and Jalife, J. (eds.): Cardiac Electrophysiology: From Cell to Bedside. 2nd ed. Philadelphia, W. B. Saunders Company, 1994, p. 935.

446. Behar, S., Zissman, E., Zion, M., et al.: Prognostic significance of second-degree atrioventricular block in inferior wall acute myocardial infarction. SPRINT Study Group. Am. J. Cardiol. *72*:831, 1993.

447. Castellanos, A., Cox, M. M., Fernandez, P. R., et al.: Mechanisms and dynamics of episodes of progression of 2:1 atrioventricular block in patients with documented 2-level conduction disturbances. Am. J. Cardiol. *70*:193, 1992.

448. Gonzalez, M. D., Scherlag, B. J., Mabo, P., et al.: Functional dissociation of cellular activation as a mechanism of Mobitz type II atrioventricular block. Circulation *87*:1389, 1993.

449. Terasaki, F., James, T. N., and Nakayama, Y.: Ultrastructural alterations of the conduction system in mice exhibiting sinus arrest or heart block during coxsackievirus B3 acute myocarditis. Am. Heart J. *123*:439, 1992.

450. Alexander, E., Buyon, J. P., and Provost, T. T.: Anti-Ro/SS-A antibodies in the pathophysiology of congenital heart block in neonatal lupus syndrome, an experimental model: In vitro electrophysiologic and immunocytochemical studies. Arthritis Rheum *35*:176, 1992.

451. Frohn-Mulder, I. M., Meilof, J. F., Szatmari, A., et al.: Clinical significance of maternal anti-Ro/SS-A antibodies in children with isolated heart block. J. Am. Coll. Cardiol. *23*:1677, 1994.

452. Julkunen, H., Kurki, T., Kaaja, R., et al.: Isolated congenital heart block: Long-term outcome of mothers and characterization of the immune response to SS-A/Ro and to SS-B/La. Arthritis Rheum *36*:1588, 1993.

453. Antretter, H., Dapunt, O. E., Robl, W., et al.: Third-degree atrioventricular block in adult identical twins. Lancet *343*:1576, 1994.

454. Shen, W. K., Hammill, S. C., Hayes, D. L., et al.: Long-term survival after pacemaker implantation for heart block in patients greater than or equal to 65 years. Am. J. Cardiol. *74*:560, 1994.

455. Lee, M. A., Dae, M. W., Langberg, J. J., et al.: Effects of long-term right ventricular apical pacing on left ventricular perfusion, innervation, function and histology. J. Am. Coll. Cardiol. *24*:225, 1994.

OTHER ELECTROPHYSIOLOGICAL ABNORMALITIES LEADING TO CARDIAC ARRHYTHMIAS

456. Oreto, G., Smeets, J. L., and Rodriguez, L. M.: Supernormal conduction in the left bundle branch. J. Cardiovasc. Electrophysiol. *5*:345, 1994.

457. Centurion, O. A., Isomoto, S., Shimizu, A., et al.: Supernormal atrial conduction and its relation to atrial vulnerability and atrial fibrillation in patients with sick sinus syndrome and paroxysmal atrial fibrillation. Am. Heart J. *128*:88, 1994.

458. Moore, E. N., Spear, J. F., and Fisch, C.: Supernormal conduction and excitability. J. Cardiovasc. Electrophysiol. *4*:320, 1993.

459. Chen, P. S., Wolf, P. L., Cha, Y. M., et al.: Effects of subendocardial ablation on anodal supernormal excitation and ventricular vulnerability in open-chest dogs. Circulation *87*:216, 1993.

460. Liu, Y., Zeng, W., Delmar, M., et al.: Ionic mechanisms of electrotonic inhibition and concealed conduction in rabbit atrioventricular nodal myocytes. Circulation *88*:1634, 1993.

461. Fisch, C.: Electrocardiographic manifestations of exit block, concealed conduction and "supernormal" conduction. *In* Zipes, D. P., and Jalife, J. (eds.): Cardiac Electrophysiology: From Cell to Bedside. 2nd ed. Philadelphia, W. B. Saunders Company, 1994, p. 955.

462. Fujiki, A., Mizumaki, K., and Tani, M.: Effects of diltiazem on concealed atrioventricular nodal conduction in relation to ventricular response during atrial fibrillation in anesthetized dogs. Am. Heart J. *125*:1284, 1993.

463. Martinez-Alday, J. D., Almendral, J., Arenal, A., et al.: Identification of concealed posteroseptal Kent pathways by comparison of ventriculoatrial intervals from apical and posterobasal right ventricular sites. Circulation *89*:1060, 1994.

464. Castellanos, A., Saoudi, N., Moleiro, F., et al.: Parasystole. *In* Zipes, D. P., and Jalife, J. (eds.): Cardiac Electrophysiology: From Cell to Bedside. 2nd ed. Philadelphia, W. B. Saunders Company, 1994, p. 942.

Chapter 23
Cardiac Pacemakers and Antiarrhythmic Devices

S. SERGE BAROLD, DOUGLAS P. ZIPES

Since the first pacemaker implantation in 1958, cardiac pacing has continued to grow so that presently more than 500,000 patients in the United States have pacemakers. Almost 400,000 pacemakers are implanted worldwide each year. In addition to pacemakers that treat bradyarrhythmias with the aim of restoring normal or near-normal hemodynamics at rest and exercise, electrical therapy of ventricular tachyarrhythmias with devices capable of pacing, cardioversion, and defibrillation has become very important.[1]

A pacemaker is a device that delivers battery-supplied electric stimuli over leads with electrodes in contact with the heart. Virtually all leads are inserted transvenously. There are two types of leads: (1) unipolar, with only one electrode in the heart (cathode) and the other on the pacemaker casing, and (2) bipolar, with two electrodes in the heart (the tip is usually the cathode). All leads serve as two-way conductors for delivery of electrical impulses to the heart and the detection of spontaneous electrical activity. Electronic circuitry regulates the timing and characteristics of the stimuli. The power source is a lithium-iodine battery that has a high-energy density (energy content/volume), low interval losses caused by self-discharge, and a long shelf life; it can be hermetically sealed to prevent ingress of body fluids. Importantly, the lithium-iodine battery has predictable characteristics that permit early warning of battery depletion. As the voltage drops near end of life, the pacing rate on magnet application declines as an indicator of the elective replacement time. For single-chamber pulse generators the expected life is 7 to 12 years and for dual-chamber pulse generators it is 5 to 10 years, depending on function and appropriate programming to conserve battery life.

PACEMAKER MODALITIES AND FUNCTION

Pacemakers are categorized with a basic three-letter identification code according to the site of the pacing electrodes and the mode of pacing[1a]: V = ventricle, A = atrium, D = dual (A and V), I = inhibited, T = triggered, and O = none. The first position denotes the chamber paced, and the second position indicates the chamber sensed. The third position indicates the response to sensing, if any, with I indicating an inhibited response (pacemaker discharge suppressed by a sensed signal), T indicating a triggered response (pacemaker discharge triggered by a sensed signal), and D indicating both inhibited and triggered functions. I and T responses reset the timing circuit controlling the pacemaker lower rate interval. Occasionally, the letter S is used for the first or second position to indicate that a single-chamber device is suitable for either atrial or ventricular pacing, depending on how the parameters are programmed. For most pacemakers, the first three positions contain all the information of practical importance. Fourth and fifth positions are available to describe additional functions; however, the letters are infrequently stated in practice except for R, which indicates a rate-adaptive pulse generator driven by a nonatrial sensor (Table 23–1).

Cardiac pacing can be performed to treat patients who have bradyarrhythmias and tachyarrhythmias. Temporary pacing is used when an arrhythmia is transient, and permanent pacing is used when an arrhythmia is likely to be recurrent or permanent.

TEMPORARY PACING

Temporary cardiac pacing can be accomplished transvenously, via the esophagus, transcutaneously, epicardially, and via a coronary artery. *Transvenous* pacing is usually done through percutaneous puncture of the internal jugular, subclavian, or femoral vein using balloon-tipped and semifloating catheters without fluoroscopy or stiffer catheters with fluoroscopy.[2,3] The (intracardiac) electrogram from the distal electrode identifies the location of the lead.[4] For atrial pacing, a preformed J-catheter is positioned in the right atrial appendage. Atrioventricular (AV) sequential pacing usually requires two leads. Single-lead atrial synchronous ventricular inhibited (VDD) pacing is feasible, but atrial pacing from floating electrodes requires further development.[5] VDD pacing also can be achieved with atrial sensing via an esophageal electrode.[6] An electrode in the *esophagus* uniformly achieves atrial pacing with a 10-msec stimulus. Pacing is relatively noninvasive, safe, and simple and can be useful to treat sinus bradycardia or arrest, to initiate and terminate some supraventricular tachycardias, and to provide overdrive suppression of ventricular tachyarrhythmias.[7–9] Current technology cannot provide reliable esophageal ventricular pacing.

Transcutaneous ventricular pacing is used during emergency treatment of asystole or severe bradycardia; it involves large-surface-area, high-impedance electrodes placed on the anterior and posterior chest walls, stimuli of long duration (20 to 40 msec), and high current (50 to 100 mA).[10–12] Barring terminal asystole from severe metabolic derangement, failure to pace is almost always due to incorrect electrode placement. Identification of ventricular capture requires a filtered electrocardiogram (ECG). Some patients cannot tolerate transcutaneous pacing because of severe pain from skeletal muscle stimulation despite analgesics. Transcutaneous pacing produces a hemodynamic response similar to that of transvenous ventricular pacing, **705**

TABLE 23-1   THE NASPE/BPEG GENERIC (NBG) PACEMAKER CODE

POSITION:	I	II	III	IV Programmability, Rate	V Antitachyarrhythmia
Category:	Chamber(s) Paced	Chamber(s) Sensed	Response to Sensing	Modulation	Function(s)
Letters:	0 = none A = atrium V = ventricle D = dual (A + V)	0 = none A = atrium V = ventricle D = dual (A + V)	0 = none T = triggered I = inhibited D = dual (T + I)	0 = none P = simple programmable M = multiprogrammable C = communicating R = rate modulation	0 = none P = pacing (antitachyarrhythmia) S = shock D = dual (P + S)
Manufacturers' designation only:	S = single (A or V)	S = single (A or V)			

Note: Positions I through III are used exclusively for antibradyarrhythmia function. NASPE = North American Society of Pacing and Electrophysiology; BPEG = British Pacing and Electrophysiology Group.

Modified with permission from Bernstein, A.D., Camm, A.J., Fletcher, R.D., et al.: The NASPE/BPEG Generic Pacemaker Code for antibradyarrhythmia and adaptive-rate pacing and antitachyarrhythmia devices. PACE *10*:794, 1987.

and demand pacing can be accomplished by sensing the surface QRS complex. Pacing can initiate and terminate many reentrant supraventricular and ventricular tachyarrhythmias.[13,14] Transcutaneous pacing may be useful when endocardial pacing is contraindicated and avoids some of the possible complications associated with temporary endocardial pacing such as infection, phlebitis, venous thrombosis, and perforation of the right ventricle. *Epicardial* pacing using ventricular and/or atrial pacing wires implanted at surgery is done in postoperative cardiac surgical patients, while pacing via a *coronary artery* (or the left ventricle) can be accomplished during percutaneous transluminal coronary angioplasty.[15,16]

INDICATIONS. Temporary pacing is indicated prophylactically in patients with a high risk of developing high-degree AV block, severe sinus node dysfunction, or asystole in acute myocardial infarction, after cardiac surgery, at times after cardioversion, during cardiac catheterization, and occasionally before implantation or replacement of a permanent pacemaker. Asymptomatic patients with bifascicular block who only undergo surgery with general anesthesia do not need prophylactic pacing. Pacing is also indicated when temporary bradycardia causes symptomatic, hemodynamic, or electrophysiological consequences as in acute myocardial infarction (discussed later), hyperkalemia, drug-induced bradycardia or toxicity (e.g., digitalis), bradycardia-dependent ventricular tachycardia, before implantation of a permanent pacemaker in a patient with unstable rhythm, and at times in myocarditis such as Lyme disease. Finally, rapid (burst) temporary pacing can be used to terminate tachycardias such as atrial flutter, AV nodal and AV reentry, and sustained monomorphic ventricular tachycardia (see p. 683). Atrial fibrillation, ventricular fibrillation, and very rapid ventricular tachycardias cannot be treated by pacing techniques. Cardioversion by transvenous leads designed for low energy delivery can terminate ventricular tachycardia, atrial flutter, and atrial fibrillation.[17] Pacing at relatively fast rates can prevent some ventricular tachycardias that are bradycardia-dependent or associated with Q-T prolongation and torsades de pointes. Less frequent uses include atrial pacing at a rate faster than a supraventricular tachycardia to increase the degree of AV block, synchronized atrial pacing to restore AV synchrony during incessant ventricular tachycardia, and coupled ventricular pacing with an early stimulus timed to provide an electrical but not a mechanical response to slow the effective rate.

TEMPORARY PACING IN ACUTE MYOCARDIAL INFARCTION (see also p. 1252). The role of temporary pacing in AV block during acute myocardial infarction is still controversial because the risk/benefit ratio is unclear. Death is generally not related directly to the conduction disturbance, and the prognosis depends more on the size of the myocardial infarction than on the degree of AV block. AV block in *inferior infarction* is almost always localized in the AV node

and is relatively benign. Inferior infarction does not cause narrow QRS type II second degree AV block.[18,19] Most hemodynamically stable patients with second degree AV block can be treated without pacing but require monitoring. Pacing is rarely necessary in hemodynamically stable patients with complete AV block and a ventricular rate around 40 to 45 per minute in the absence of ventricular arrhythmia. Temporary ventricular pacing is indicated in second or third degree AV block only in the presence of an excessively slow ventricular rate, ventricular arrhythmia, hypotension, signs of hypoperfusion, or congestive heart failure. Dual-chamber pacing may sometimes be required to improve hemodynamics, especially when there is right ventricular infarction.[20] *Right ventricular infarction* causes an acute increase in diastolic stiffness so that the right ventricle becomes far more dependent on preload and acts more or less as a passive conduit for the atrial pump. Right ventricular infarction can be associated with hypotension or shock, partly or entirely due to AV block and loss of AV synchrony. Ventricular pacing may not improve the hemodynamic state, but AV sequential pacing with restoration of AV synchrony can cause a dramatic increase in the blood pressure, cardiac output, and stroke volume.

The development of second or third degree AV block associated with bundle branch block during *anterior infarction* necessitates temporary pacing, but the mortality rate is nonetheless quite high because these conduction disturbances generally occur in patients with very large infarcts. Dual-chamber pacing should be used in pacemaker-dependent patients.[20] Prophylactic pacing traditionally has been recommended in the presence of new right bundle branch block with left-axis deviation (left anterior hemiblock), right bundle branch block with right-axis deviation (left posterior hemiblock), left bundle branch block with first degree AV block, and alternating right and left bundle branch block because these patients are at higher risk of suddenly developing high-degree AV block with catastrophic consequences. Vagally induced AV block with a narrow QRS complex (such as during vomiting) does not require pacing.

The role of pacing for *right bundle branch block* with a normal axis or *left bundle branch block* with a normal P-R interval is more controversial. Preexisting right or left bundle branch block is usually not an indication for temporary pacing. During prophylactic pacing in anterior infarction, the pacemaker can be turned off in some patients until needed to avoid ventricular fibrillation that may result from delivery of a stimulus in the vulnerable period if the pacemaker is not inhibited appropriately by spontaneous ventricular activity. Furthermore, continuous ventricular pacing can mask the development of transient second or third degree AV block, considered by many to be an indication for permanent pacing.

The advent of reliable external transcutaneous pacing has diminished the need in many patients for prophylactic temporary right ventricular pacing in acute myocardial infarction, an important consideration in patients treated with thrombolytic therapy and anticoagulants. Patients with anterior myocardial infarction and bifascicular block can be managed simply by application of large pacing electrodes on the chest and keeping an external pulse generator close by for transcutaneous pacing.

PERMANENT PACING

Indications for permanent pacing were published by a Joint Committee in the American College of Cardiology (ACC) and the American Heart Association (AHA) in 1984 and 1991.[21] The ACC/AHA document recognizes the fact that indications for permanent pacing in an individual patient may not always be clear-cut; however, they have been grouped according to the following classifications: Class I, conditions for which there is general agreement that permanent pacemakers should be implanted; Class II, conditions for which permanent pacemakers are used frequently but opinion diverges on whether they are necessary; and Class III, conditions for which there is general agreement that pacemakers are unnecessary. The ACC/AHA guidelines also indicate that in those patients being considered for pacemakers, decision making may be influenced by a number of additional factors. Despite their shortcomings,[22,23] the 1991 ACC/AHA guidelines provide a useful framework on which Table 23–2 is based (see also p. 1963).

AV Block

Type II second degree AV block is defined as the occurrence of a single nonconducted P wave associated with constant PR intervals before and after the blocked impulse, provided that the sinus rate or the P-P interval is constant and there are at least two consecutive conducted P waves (i.e., 3:2 AV block) to determine the behavior of the P-R interval.[22,24] The definitions of type I and type II second degree AV block are purely descriptive and do not refer to the site of block. However, type II AV block invariably occurs below the AV node, while type I AV block in the setting of a normal QRS complex generally occurs in the AV node. Although 2:1 AV block can occur in either the AV node or the His-Purkinje system, it cannot be classified into type I or type II. Advanced second degree AV block refers to 2:1, 3:1, or 4:1 AV block, and the like.

Although the meaning of bifascicular block is obvious, that of trifascicular block is not as simple.[22] In this respect, the ACC/AHA guidelines use the term *trifascicular block* rather loosely. The combination of bifascicular block (right bundle branch block + left anterior hemiblock, right bundle branch block + left posterior hemiblock or left bundle branch block) and first degree AV block on the surface electrocardiogram must not be designated as trifascicular block because the site of AV block can be either in the AV node or in the His-Purkinje system. Electrocardiographic documentation of trifascicular block during 1:1 AV conduction is rare and occurs usually in the presence of alternating right bundle branch block and left bundle branch block or fixed right bundle branch block with alternating left anterior hemiblock and left posterior hemiblock. In Table 23–2, left bundle branch block is bifascicular block, while right bundle branch block is described as bundle branch block rather than unifascicular block to avoid confusion with left anterior or left posterior hemiblock.

Before pacemaker implantation, reversible causes of AV block such as Lyme disease, athletic heart,[25] hypervagotonia, ischemia, and drug, metabolic, or electrolyte imbalance must be excluded. There is general (although not unanimous) agreement that permanent pacing is indicated

in asymptomatic patients with acquired complete AV block. It is also indicated in asymptomatic patients with alternating right and left bundle branch block and those with well-documented second degree AV block in the His-Purkinje system, often associated with bundle branch block, because symptoms usually develop in a relatively short time. His bundle recordings are often required to demonstrate the site of block (AV node or His-Purkinje system) in patients with bundle branch block and type I or advanced second degree AV block. Some symptomatic patients with marked first degree AV block may benefit from dual-chamber pacing with a more physiological AV interval.[26,27]

ACUTE MYOCARDIAL INFARCTION (see also p. 1252). Permanent pacing is rarely, if ever, indicated in AV block due to inferior infarction because it is almost always transient, occasionally lasting as long as 2 to 3 weeks. Pacing is not required in anterior infarction complicated by permanent bundle branch or bifascicular block but can be considered (although this is still controversial) to prevent sudden death from asystole in those patients who develop transient trifascicular block (second or third degree AV block) even though 1:1 AV conduction returns.

CONGENITAL AV BLOCK (see also p. 966). Permanent pacing in asymptomatic patients with congenital AV block is recommended if there is (1) a mean daytime junctional rate slower than 50/min, (2) no or little change in the junctional rate with physical activity, (3) long periods of asystole during sleep secondary to junctional exit block, (4) cardiomegaly, (5) depressed left ventricular function detected echocardiographically, and (6) electrocardiographic evidence of atrial enlargement. Pacing can be considered if the patient has a prolonged QRS complex (≥ 0.12 sec), frequent multiformed or repetitive ventricular ectopy, or Q-Tc > 0.45 sec.[28–30]

BUNDLE BRANCH BLOCK. Eighty per cent of patients with asymptomatic bundle branch block have associated heart disease, with coronary artery disease found in almost half. Half the deaths are sudden and are usually not due to bradycardia but rather to myocardial infarction or ventricular tachycardia. H-V interval prolongation is found in 40 to 50 per cent of patients with bundle branch block and bifascicular block. However, a prolonged H-V interval that is shorter than 100 msec generally is not predictive of future events such as syncope and death. Although the development of AV block is more frequent in patients with H-V interval prolongation (1 to 2 per cent per year), the low incidence militates against investigation or treatment of the asymptomatic patient.[30]

INDUCIBLE AV BLOCK. His-Purkinje block induced by atrial pacing, though an insensitive sign of conduction system disease, may constitute an indication for permanent pacing provided that functional infranodal block is excluded.[30] Exercise-induced AV block is an indication for pacing because it is almost always infranodal and most asymptomatic patients eventually develop serious problems.[30] Rarely, exercise-induced AV block is secondary to myocardial ischemia and does not require pacing unless ischemia cannot be alleviated.[31] The use of drugs such as ajmaline and procainamide that depress His-Purkinje conduction to provoke His-Purkinje block in susceptible patients is still controversial.[32,33]

BUNDLE BRANCH BLOCK AND SYNCOPE. In patients with bundle branch block and syncope, it is important to perform a complete electrophysiological study because sustained monomorphic ventricular tachycardia is the cause of symptoms in 20 to 30 per cent of patients.[30] An abnormal electrophysiological study including the induction of ventricular tachycardia is associated with a greater incidence of total and sudden death during follow-up, while a normal or nondiagnostic study correlates with a higher rate of symptomatic remission and a better prognosis with a low risk of dying from an arrhythmia. Obviously, a negative

TABLE 23-2 INDICATIONS FOR PERMANENT PACING

1. Acquired AV Block in Adults

Class I
A. Permanent or intermittent complete AV block at any anatomic level in the absence of reversible causes, regardless of symptoms.*†
B. Permanent or intermittent second degree AV block regardless of the type or the site of block, with symptomatic bradycardia.†
C. Permanent or intermittent asymptomatic type II second degree AV block.†‡
D. Asymptomatic type I or advanced second degree AV block at intra-His or infra-His levels.†‡
E. Exercise-induced second or complete AV block regardless of symptoms but without reversible ischemia.†
F. Atrial fibrillation, atrial flutter, or rare cases of supraventricular tachycardia with AV block and bradycardia associated with congestive heart failure or periods of asystole ≥3.0 sec or escape rate <40 beats/min or alternating tachycardia and bradycardia difficult to control pharmacologically. The bradycardia must be unrelated to drugs known to impair AV conduction.

Class II
Symptomatic first degree AV block improved by temporary dual-chamber pacing.

Class III
A. Asymptomatic first degree AV block.
B. Asymptomatic type I second degree AV block at the supra-His (AV node) level.

2. After Acute Myocardial Infarction

Class I
Persistent or transient second degree or complete AV block in the His-Purkinje system.

Class II
Persistent advanced or complete AV block at the AV node (longer than 16 days).

Class III
A. Transient AV conduction disturbances without intraventricular conduction defects.
B. Transient AV block in the presence of isolated left anterior hemiblock.
C. Acquired left anterior hemiblock, bundle branch block, or bifascicular block with or without first degree AV block, but in the absence of second degree or complete AV block.

3. Chronic Intraventricular Block

Class I
A. Bundle branch block or bifascicular block with second or complete AV block associated with symptomatic bradycardia.
B. Bundle branch block or bifascicular block with intermittent type II second degree AV block without symptoms (see section 1).
C. Bundle branch block or bifascicular block with infranodal block without symptoms: type I, advanced second degree, or complete AV block (see section 1).
D. Trifascicular block during 1:1 AV conduction regardless of symptoms such as (1) alternating left bundle branch block and right bundle branch block, (2) fixed right bundle branch block with alternating left anterior hemiblock and left posterior hemiblock.
E. Exercise-induced second or complete AV block regardless of symptoms, but without demonstrable ischemia as a cause of AV block.

Class II
A. Bundle branch block or bifascicular block with syncope that is not proved to be due to complete AV block but other possible causes of syncope are not identified.
B. Markedly prolonged HV (≥100 msec).
C. Pacing-induced infra-His block.

Class III
A. Hemiblock, bundle branch block, or bifascicular block without second degree or complete AV block or symptoms.
B. Hemiblock, bundle branch block, or bifascicular block with first degree AV block without symptoms.

---

study does not exclude transient bradycardia as a cause of syncope or the possibility of sudden death, although the risk is quite low, and recurrence of syncope does not correlate with a higher mortality or sudden death. An H-V interval ≥ 100 msec identifies patients with a higher risk of AV block who require pacing.[32] Pacing can be considered in patients who have an H-V between 70 and 100 msec and no identifiable cause for syncope.[33]

Sick Sinus Syndrome

About half of all pacemakers are used to treat sick sinus syndrome (see p. 648). A pacemaker should be implanted only when a causal relationship has been demonstrated between bradycardia and symptoms, which may be difficult to accomplish in elderly patients with vague symptoms. If in doubt about the need for pacing, it is usually safe to wait because arrhythmias associated with sick sinus syndrome rarely result in sudden cardiac death. In the bradycardia-tachycardia syndrome (Chap. 22), drugs alone may worsen the bradycardia; symptomatic patients are usually best managed by a combination of pacemaker and antiarrhythmic drugs.[34] When bradycardia is secondary to necessary drug therapy, e.g., beta blocker or amiodarone, a pacemaker can be used to treat the consequences of the drug. Permanent pacing should not be considered when there is transient bradycardia due to an increase in vagal tone or drug therapy that can be discontinued or reduced. In the sick sinus syndrome, pacing improves the quality of

life and facilitates treatment of supraventricular tachycardias exhibited by over a third of the patients. Most patients have structural heart disease, and single-chamber ventricular pacing (as opposed to atrial-based pacing, discussed later) is no longer recommended.

The role of prophylactic pacing in asymptomatic patients with ECG evidence of sick sinus syndrome has not been established. Asymptomatic patients should be followed closely, and drugs that depress sinus node function should be avoided. Two-second pauses are usually harmless. During sleep, the sinus rate normally may fall to 30/min and exhibit pauses of 3 sec. While it is often stated that sinus pauses are abnormal if they exceed 3 sec without intervening escape beats, the validity of such a conclusion has not been established; neither has the validity of permanent pacing in these asymptomatic patients.

Hypersensitive Carotid Sinus Syndrome and Neurally Mediated (Vasovagal) Syncope

HYPERSENSITIVE CAROTID SINUS SYNDROME. In the carotid sinus syndrome (see p. 865), patients with a predominant cardioinhibitory reflex response (slowing of sinus rate and/or prolongation of AV conduction with AV block) benefit from permanent pacing. The AAI mode is contraindicated, and the VVI mode generally is poorly tolerated. Most patients require dual-chamber pacing with the DDI or DDD mode, preferably with hysteresis (discussed later). In pre-

TABLE 23-2 INDICATIONS FOR PERMANENT PACING—*Continued* **709**

Ch 23

4. Sick Sinus Syndrome

Class I
  Sinus node dysfunction with documented symptomatic bradycardia. (In some patients this will occur as a consequence of long-term essential drug therapy of a type and dose for which there are no acceptable alternatives.)
Class II
  Sinus node dysfunction, occurring spontaneously or as a result of necessary drug therapy, with heart rate < 40 beats/min when a clear association between significant symptoms consistent with bradycardia and the actual presence of bradycardia has not been documented.
Class III
  A. Sinus node dysfunction in asymptomatic patients, including those in whom substantial sinus bradycardia (heart rate < 40 beats/min) is a consequence of long-term drug treatment.
  B. Sinus node dysfunction in patients in whom symptoms suggestive of bradycardia are clearly documented *not* to be associated with a slow heart rate.

5. Hypersensitive Carotid Sinus and Malignant Vasovagal Syndromes

Class I
  Recurrent syncope associated with clear, spontaneous events provoked by carotid sinus stimulation; minimal carotid sinus pressure induces asystole of > 3 sec duration in the absence of any medication that depresses the sinus node or AV conduction.
Class II
  A. Recurrent syncope without clear, provocative events and with a hypersensitive cardioinhibitory response.
  B. Syncope with associated bradycardia reproduced by a head-up tilt with or without isoproterenol or other forms of provocative maneuvers and in which a temporary pacemaker and a second provocative test can establish the likely benefits of a permanent pacemaker. Pacing should be considered only in patients refractory to drug therapy.
Class III
  A. A hyperactive cardioinhibitory response to carotid sinus stimulation in the absence of symptoms.
  B. Vague symptoms such as dizziness or lightheadedness, or both, with a hyperactive cardioinhibitory response to carotid sinus stimulation.
  C. Recurrent syncope, lightheadedness or dizziness in the absence of a cardioinhibitory response.

* Asymptomatic complete AV block, permanent or intermittent, at any anatomic site is a Class II indication in the 1991 ACC/AHA guidelines when the ventricular rate ≥ 40 beats/min in asymptomatic patients and a Class I indication when the ventricular rate < 40 beats/min or there is asystole ≥ 3 sec in asymptomatic patients. The 1991 ACC/AHA guidelines classify permanent or intermittent complete AV block at any level as a Class I indication when associated with (1) symptomatic bradycardia, (2) congestive heart failure, (3) conditions requiring therapy with drugs that suppress automacity.

† A number of conditions are listed in the 1991 ACC/AHA guidelines in both the section on acquired AV block and the sections on bifascicular and trifasicular block (chronic intraventricular block). The same format was adopted in this table to facilitate comparison with the ACC/AHA guidelines.

‡ Class II indication in the 1991 ACC/AHA guidelines.

Adapted from Dreifus, L. S., et al.: ACC/AHA guidelines for implantation of cardiac pacemakers and antiarrhythmia devices. Reprinted with permission from American College of Cardiology. J. Am. Coll. Cardiol. *18*:1, 1991.

dominant vasodepressor syncope, dual-chamber pacing may not abolish symptoms.[35-37]

NEURALLY MEDIATED SYNCOPE. *Neurally mediated syncope* refers to vasovagal syncope often reproducible by tilt-table testing. Pacing should not be first-line therapy because many patients respond to drug therapy with beta blockers or other agents. In drug-refractory patients who show a significant bradycardia component during syncope, dual-chamber pacing with hysteresis may prolong the time from onset of symptoms to loss of consciousness or may prevent syncope altogether. Pacing may permit a more gradual blood pressure decline during the attacks that would be perceived by the patient, who can then take appropriate protective measures (such as lying down, stopping car driving, and the like).[37-39] Thus pacing can be beneficial by retarding symptoms. The AAI, VVI, or VDD modes are contraindicated.[37-40]

Pacing Without Conduction System Disease

Dual-chamber pacing with a short A-V interval has emerged as effective therapy for many patients with obstructive hypertrophic cardiomyopathy and a resting or provocable left ventricular outflow tract gradient ≥ 30 mm Hg[41,42] (see p. 1426). Pacing produces apical preexcitation, and a favorable response is closely tied to optimization of the A-V interval to ensure pacing-induced ventricular depolarization at all times. Preliminary results of dual-chamber pacing with a short A-V interval in a small number of patients with end-stage idiopathic dilated cardiomyopathy are promising.[43] Such therapy presently remains investigational. The benefit of dual-chamber pacing with a short A-V interval in patients with congestive heart failure due to left ventricular systolic dysfunction (regardless of etiology) has not yet been determined. Permanent pacing combined with beta-blocker therapy appears highly effective in patients with the long Q-T syndrome (see p. 685) who do not respond to beta-blocker therapy alone and/or

cardiac sympathectomy. Pacing at a rate designed to normalize the Q-T interval provides adjunctive therapy because complete protection requires the implantation of an automatic defibrillator.[44] Finally, rapid atrial pacing in conjunction with drug therapy may benefit patients with drug-refractory orthostatic hypotension.[45,46]

METHODS OF PACEMAKER IMPLANTATION

Virtually all pacemakers are implanted transvenously under local anesthesia using either the cephalic vein exposed by cutdown or blind percutaneous puncture of the subclavian vein.[47-49] The pacemaker pocket is fashioned over the pectoralis major muscle. The cephalic vein is often of sufficient size to accept one or two pacing leads. If not, passage of a flexible guidewire followed by a standard subclavian vein introducer provides simple and direct access to the subclavian vein. Although blind percutaneous subclavian vein puncture is potentially more dangerous than insertion through the cephalic vein, in skilled hands it is remarkably safe. It reduces the time required for implantation, facilitates implanting two leads, reduces the need for surgical expertise (especially with peel-away sheaths), and has made the implantation of most sophisticated pacemakers a relatively simple surgical procedure.[50] Many of the complications (some lethal) of blind subclavian puncture, which include pneumothorax, subclavian arterial puncture with hemothorax, air embolism, hemopneumomediastinum, subcutaneous emphysema, nerve injury, and thoracic duct injury, are preventable. Leads inserted via medial subclavian puncture are susceptible to compression damage in the tight costoclavicular angle (subclavian crush).[49,51,52]

With contemporary transvenous leads, complications are related more to the skill and experience of the implanter and implantation technique than to lead design because all leads now possess good performance characteristics. Epicardial leads are used only if there is no venous access, in

TABLE 23–3   TECHNICAL ASPECTS OF PACEMAKER IMPLANTATION

1. Pacing threshold (also during cough and deep respiration) in terms of voltage and pulse width with matching external pacemaker. The voltage threshold at a single pulse width of 0.5 to 0.6 msec is usually sufficient.

2. Lead impedance at 5-V output and 0.5- to 0.6-msec pulse width.

3. Recording of atrial and ventricular electrograms: unipolar, bipolar (if applicable), morphology, amplitude and current of injury (ST-segment elevation associated with good contact) during normal and deep inspiration. The signal amplitude also can be measured with a PSA.

4. Determination of slew rate (dV/dt) if signal is small.

5. High-voltage pacing (10 V) to detect left diaphragmatic stimulation from ventricular electrode and right phrenic nerve–diaphragmatic stimulation from atrial electrode.

6. Blood pressure measurement during ventricular pacing to determine susceptibility to pacemaker syndrome.

7. Atrial and ventricular pacing to determine antegrade AV and retrograde VA conduction.

8. Interrogation and reprogramming of the pulse generator before implantation.

9. ECG recordings with and without magnet application to demonstrate atrial and/or ventricular pacing and normal atrial and/or ventricular sensing.

10. Chest x-ray immediately after implantation to exclude pneumothorax when applicable.

certain pediatric patients, or in patients undergoing open-heart surgery. Alternatively, endocardial leads can be introduced via a transatrial approach with a limited thoracotomy.[48,53] The operative techniques and intraoperative measurements necessary for safe and long-term pacing (Table 23–3) are straightforward compared with the technical knowledge required to understand the electrophysiology of pacing and follow-up of patients so as to make the best use of the important programmable functions.

Capture Thresholds, Sensing, and Leads

DETERMINATION OF THE PACING THRESHOLD

This is crucial to optimize pacemaker longevity and is determined at the time of implantation using an external testing device (pacing system analyzer, or PSA) with circuitry similar to that of the implantable pulse generator. Most implantable pulse generators are constant voltage sources; the leading edge of the voltage pulse remains constant regardless of the impedance (resistance). The threshold should be determined in volts at a given pulse width of 0.5 to 0.6 msec. To measure the threshold, the PSA is set at 5 V and pulse width 0.5 msec (usually the nominal parameters of an implantable device). The pacing rate is increased until consistent pacing capture is achieved. The voltage is then slowly reduced until loss of capture occurs outside the myocardial refractory period. The lowest voltage at a given pulse width capable of causing consistent capture outside the myocardial refractory period defines the stimulation threshold (Fig. 23–1). Ventricular capture near the pacing threshold may occur only when stimuli fall in the supernormal phase (Fig. 23–1).

The current delivered to the myocardium is determined by the impedance (resistance) according to Ohm's law. Normal lead impedance, ranging between 250 and 1000 ohms, typically is 500 to 700 ohms at the nominal output of 5 V. The relationship of threshold voltage and pulse width is not linear and establishes the strength-duration curve; the shorter the pulse width, the higher is the voltage threshold.

THE STRENGTH-DURATION CURVE (Fig. 23–2). This is steep, with a short pulse width, and becomes essentially flat at a pulse width exceeding 2 msec (rheobase). The acute ventricular pacing threshold should be ≤ 0.8 V at 0.5 msec, and the acute atrial pacing threshold should be ≤ 1.5 V at 0.5 msec. Lower values are often obtained. A high initial threshold value requires lead repositioning. The lowest threshold possible at implantation should be sought because ultimately it may determine the threshold at maturity and hence the voltage required for long-term pacing.

After implantation, the output of the pulse generator is usually left at 5 V and 0.5 msec or at a longer pulse width for the first 8 weeks. At 8 weeks, when the chronic threshold has been attained in most cases, the output voltage and pulse width should be programmed to

reduce current drain from the battery and yet maintain an adequate margin of safety. A low output voltage and/or short pulse width enhances battery longevity. The safety margin for capture is the amount by which the pulse generator voltage output exceeds the chronic threshold value at a given pulse duration and should be 1.75; i.e., the output voltage should be at least 1.75 times the chronic threshold voltage at the same pulse width.[50] In practice, a voltage safety margin of 2 is often used, so the output voltage is set at twice the chronic threshold voltage at the same pulse width. An output voltage exceeding 5 V should not be used routinely because of reduced pulse generator efficiency and longevity.

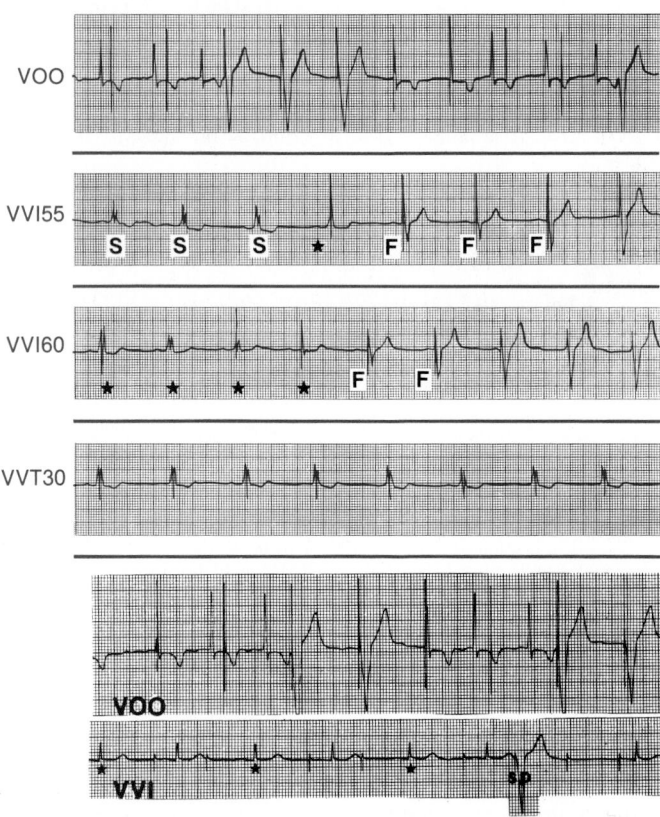

FIGURE 23–1.   VOO, VVI, and VVT pacing. *Top strip:* VOO pacing. The pacemaker competes with the spontaneous rhythm and stimuli capture the ventricle only beyond the myocardial refractory period.

Second strip: VVI pacemaker, rate = 55/min. The first three beats are sensed (S) and the 4th beat (star) is a ventricular pseudofusion beat. The 5th, 6th, and 7th complexes are ventricular fusion beats (F).

Third strip: VVI pacemaker, rate = 60/min. The first three beats (stars) are ventricular pseudofusion beats. The 4th beat (star) appears to be a ventricular pseudofusion beat because the initial QRS vector occurs just before the stimulus. The T wave of the 4th beat is identical to that of the previous beat, suggesting that depolarization was also identical, providing further proof for pseudofusion. The 5th and 6th complexes are ventricular fusion beats (F) while the last three beats are pure ventricular-paced beats.

Fourth strip: Same patient as in third strip. The pacemaker was programmed to the VVT mode, rate = 30/min. The pacemaker emits or triggers a ventricular stimulus immediately upon sensing each QRS complex. Thus, the stimulus marks the precise time of sensing the VVT mode. This may be correlated with the ventricular pseudofusion beats in the third strip where the first pseudofusion beat is deformed by a ventricular stimulus just before the R wave returns to baseline, i.e., just before sensing would have occurred as determined from the VVT mode in the 4th strip.

Bottom strip: VVI pacemaker with ineffectual stimuli but normal sensing. The high pacing threshold was close to the output of the pulse generator. The 3rd to the last stimulus captures the ventricle in the supernormal phase (SP) when the excitability threshold attains its lowest value. Spontaneous QRS complexes falling within the pacemaker refractory period (for sensing—350 ms after the stimulus) are not sensed; those beyond the pacemaker refractory period are sensed and recycle the pacemaker.

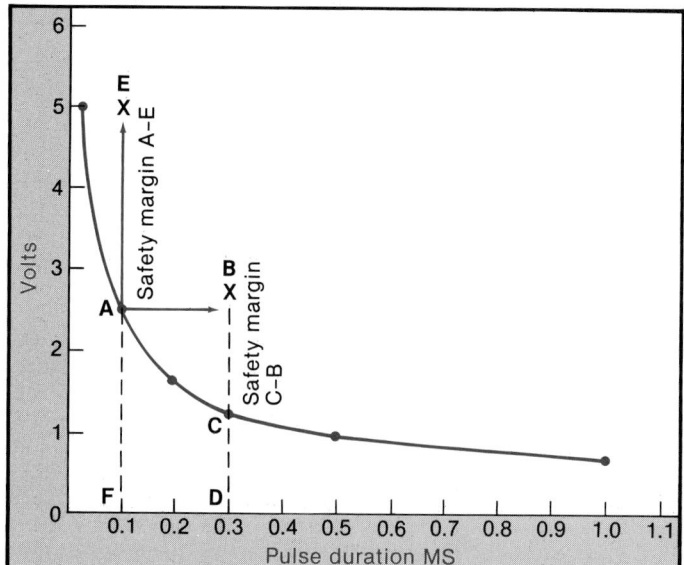

FIGURE 23–2. Strength-duration curve relating voltage and pulse width at the chronic pacing threshold. Values above the curve pace the heart while values below the curve fail to capture. The threshold for pacing at A is 2.5 V at a pulse width of 0.1 ms. Consequently, starting from the threshold at A, the output voltage of the pulse generator could be doubled to 5 V while the pulse width is kept constant at 0.1 ms, i.e, going to E. This would provide a voltage safety margin of EF/AF = 2. Alternatively, the output voltage could be left at 2.5 V and the pulse width increased to 0.3 ms to B. This would yield a voltage safety margin of BD/CD or slightly more than 2. The second option consumes less battery current and is to be preferred.

ADJUSTMENT OF PULSE WIDTH. If the pulse width is varied without a programmable voltage output, it should be adjusted to 3 times the value at threshold provided that the pulse width at threshold is ≤ 0.2 msec. Because of the configuration of the strength-duration curve, with a pulse width at threshold ≥ 0.3 msec, tripling the pulse width (keeping the voltage constant) may or may not provide a voltage safety margin of 2 and probably should not be used in pacemaker-dependent patients.

The relatively flat characteristic of the voltage strength-duration curve from 0.5 to 1.5 msec means that an increase in the pulse width alone in this range will not provide a sufficient margin of safety in terms of volts. Therefore, when the voltage at threshold requires a pulse width ≥ 0.4 to 0.5 msec, an adequate safety margin cannot be obtained by programming pulse width alone. With a threshold of 2.5 V/0.1 msec, the pulse generator could be programmed to 2.5 V/0.3 msec or 5 V/0.1 msec to provide a voltage safety factor of at least 2. However, pulse widths < 0.2 msec situated on the steep portion of the voltage strength-duration curve are not recommended because shifts of the curve in response to the vagaries of daily living become more pronounced, while fluctuations of pulse width (electronic jitter) cannot always be discounted at short pulse widths. In terms of battery current drain, multiplying the voltage output by 2 (keeping the pulse width constant) is equivalent to multiplying the pulse width by 4 (keeping the voltage constant). Consequently, if the pacemaker circuit is more efficient at 2.5 V than at 5 V, with a threshold of 2.5 V/0.2 msec, an output of 2.5 V/0.6 msec is preferable to 5.0 V/0.2 msec. With a voltage threshold of 2.5 V/0.3 msec, an output of 5.0 V/0.3 msec is usually recommended. With a relatively high chronic threshold exceeding 3 to 3.5 V at a pulse width of 0.5 msec at the time of pacemaker replacement or during follow-up, the output voltage should exceed 5 V. In this situation, use of a new lead or (less preferably) a pulse generator programmable to a high voltage (10 V) should be considered.

LEAD IMPEDANCE. In addition to testing thresholds, the integrity of new and old leads can be evaluated by determining the voltage threshold and lead impedance either directly or noninvasively by telemetry. Lead impedance normally remains constant or falls slightly over time. Lead fracture (with apposed ends) elevates both the voltage threshold and the lead impedance (> 1000 ohms), while with an insulation defect the voltage threshold may be low or normal and the lead impedance will be low (< 250 ohms). A high voltage threshold due to lead displacement or an excessive tissue reaction around the electrode (exit block) is associated with a normal lead impedance.

CHANGES IN THE PACING THRESHOLD. With conventional leads, this variable rises shortly after implantation because edema and inflammation separate the tip from the myocardium. Most of the threshold

increase appears to result from the formation of nonexcitable fibrous tissue around the electrode, increasing the effective size of the "virtual" electrode at the interface with the myocardium.[54,55] The threshold usually reaches its maximum value 10 to 20 days after implantation and stabilizes to about 2 to 4 times the acute value at 1 to 2 months. Small electrodes have lower initial thresholds and a greater proportional rise during the initial reaction, but the chronic threshold is lower than that of larger electrodes.

Threshold evolution sometimes takes longer than expected, and on rare occasions, the threshold continues to rise gradually with ultimate failure to capture. If there is no lead displacement, such failure to capture is often called *exit block;* this is a relatively rare complication. Exercise, sympathomimetic drugs, and glucocorticoids decrease the threshold, while food, sleep, insulin, ischemia, hypothyroidism, hyperkalemia, mineralocorticoids, and certain antiarrhythmic agents increase the threshold. Type 1C (see p. 608) antiarrhythmic drugs (especially flecainide),[56–58] toxic levels of Type 1A antiarrhythmic agents, and hyperkalemia may cause exit block.[59] Amiodarone has no important effect on the threshold.[59] Isoproterenol infusion or systemic steroids can be used to treat a high threshold temporarily until the underlying condition is corrected.

SENSING. A pacemaker senses the potential difference between the two electrodes used for pacing. In a bipolar system, the bipolar electrogram should be recorded to determine adequate electrode position for sensing. In a unipolar system, the unipolar electrogram is recorded from the tip electrode and closely reflects the cardiac signal because the anodal contribution from the pacemaker plate is generally negligible. The amplitude and slew rate (dV/dt) of the electrogram must exceed the sensitivity of the pulse generator to ensure reliable sensing.[55,60,61]

SIGNAL AMPLITUDE. The ventricular signal is often 6 to 15 mV, a range that exceeds the sensitivity threshold of a pulse generator. The ventricular electrogram should measure at least 5 to 6 mV and the atrial electrogram at least 1.5 to 2 mV. A signal with a gradual slope (lower slew rate) is more difficult to sense than is a sharp upstroke signal. Determination of the slew rate may be useful when the signal is low or borderline (3 to 5 mV for ventricular signals) but is not necessary if the amplitude of the signal is large. A low electrographic signal may require repositioning of the lead. Rarely, unipolar and bipolar ventricular electrograms are too small for sensing at nominal sensitivity because of chronic ischemia or cardiomyopathy. In this situation, a bipolar pulse generator programmable to a high sensitivity should be used.

Following initial lead placement, the ventricular electrogram from the tip electrode shows an initial current of injury (ST-segment elevation) that reflects good endocardial contact and disappears after a few days.[61] Over the long term, the amplitude of the QRS signal from conventional leads diminished slightly, but the slew rate can diminish further (about 40 per cent).[60,61] These changes normally are of no clinical importance for ventricular sensing but can be important in the case of smaller atrial signals, although studies with contemporary leads have documented the stability of the atrial signal chronically.[62]

LEAD DESIGN

New lead technology and design have improved bipolar leads sufficiently to eliminate the previous advantages of unipolar leads over bipolar leads. Generally, bipolar leads are preferred because of greater signal-to-noise ratio, less sensitivity to extraneous interference (especially skeletal myopotentials), less frequent crosstalk (atrial stimulus sensed by ventricular lead in a dual-chamber system), and avoidance of muscle stimulation occasionally seen at the anodal site of unipolar pulse generators.[60,63,64] Improvement in the design of lead fixation mechanisms has reduced the incidence of dislodgment to 0.5 to 1.5 per cent or less with ventricular leads and about 1 to 5 per cent with atrial leads. Adhering leads utilize either passive fixation with tines or fins to enhance entanglement in trabeculae or active fixation with myocardial penetration by grasping screws or small jaws. Tined and screw-in leads are the most popular and exhibit equally good performance. Active fixation leads are particularly useful in right ventricular dilatation, in tricuspid insufficiency, and when pacing of the right ventricular outflow tract is needed. Screw-in leads exhibit a decrease in the pacing threshold and an increase in signal amplitude in the first 30 minutes after implantation because of partial resolution of the initial local injury.

Contemporary electrodes have a small surface area that reduces stimulation thresholds because of a higher current density. Porous electrodes with a small surface area yield a low pacing threshold and yet provide a greater surface area for improved sensing. Steroid-eluting leads have a reservoir within the electrode tip that elutes a trace of dexamethasone directly at the electrode-tissue interface and reduces the local tissue reaction and the thickness of the fibrous capsule surrounding the tip electrode.[54,64–68] Steroid-eluting leads are associated with very low pacing thresholds and lack of initial peaking and excellent sensing with less chronic degradation of the endocardial signal,[55] and they have virtually eliminated so-called exit block with ineffectual pacemaker stimuli. Such leads permit low output pacing and conservation of battery life.[67]

TYPES OF PACEMAKERS

Single-Chamber Pacemakers

AOO AND VOO MODES. In the AOO and VOO modes, the pacemaker stimuli are generated at a fixed rate (asynchronously) with no relationship to the spontaneous rhythm. Stimuli capture the atrium or ventricle only when they fall outside the refractory period following spontaneous beats (Fig. 23–1). Ventricular fibrillation induced by a pacemaker stimulus falling in the ventricular vulnerable period is extremely rare unless myocardial ischemia or severe electrolyte abnormalities are present. AOO or VOO pacing is used only temporarily during pacemaker testing with application of the magnet or for competitive pacing to terminate some tachycardias.

VVI MODE. A VVI (ventricular demand) pacemaker prevents the ventricular rate from decreasing below a predetermined programmed level (Fig. 23–1). If the spontaneous rate decreases below the set rate, the pacemaker paces at a cycle length appropriate to maintain the preset rate. A faster spontaneous rate inhibits pacemaker discharge. The timing cycle (or internal clock) of a VVI pulse generator begins with either a sensed or a paced ventricular event. The initial portion of the cycle consists of a refractory period (usually 200 to 350 msec) during which the pulse generator is insensitive to any signals so as to avoid sensing its own stimulus, the paced or spontaneous QRS complex, T waves, and the decaying residual voltage at the electrode-myocardial interface. Beyond the pacemaker refractory period, a sensed spontaneous QRS complex inhibits the pacemaker, and its timing clock returns to the baseline; a new pacing style is initiated, and the output circuit remains inhibited for a period equal to the programmed pacemaker interval. If no spontaneous QRS complex is sensed, the timing cycle ends with the delivery of a ventricular stimulus, and a new cycle is started. The sensing function conserves battery capacity and prevents competition between the pacemaker and the intrinsic rhythm. VVI (or VVIR, p. 723) pacing is still the most common mode of pacing worldwide. A VVI pacemaker is simple, inexpensive, and reliable and has a small size and long life. However, its inability to maintain AV synchrony and provide an increased rate on exercise constitutes an important disadvantage.

AAI MODE. This (atrial demand) mode is similar to the VVI mode except that the pacemaker senses atrial electrical activity and paces the atrium (Fig. 23–3). AAI units must have a greater sensitivity than VVI units because the atrial electrogram is considerably smaller than the ventricular electrogram and the refractory period should be longer (400 msec) to avoid sensing the "far-field" ventricular electrogram via the atrial lead. AAI pacing is used for patients with sick sinus syndrome and intact AV conduction.

VVT MODE. In the VVT mode, upon sensing a spontaneous QRS complex, the pacemaker immediately discharges (rather than inhibits) its stimulus during the absolute refractory period of the ventricular myocardium (Fig. 23–1). If no QRS complex is sensed, the pacemaker delivers its impulse at the end of the interval corresponding to the programmed (lower) rate. The maximum pacing rate that

can be generated by continual sensing is either factory-set or programmable. The triggered mode can be used to activate discharge of an implanted pacemaker by the application of chest wall stimuli (generating signals for sensing) from an external pacemaker. In this way, appropriately timed stimuli to the chest wall can be used to initiate or terminate some tachycardias by triggering corresponding stimuli from the implanted pacemaker.

Intervals and Rates

Three pacemaker intervals are important. The *automatic interval* is the period between two consecutive stimuli during continuous pacing. The *escape interval* is measured from the onset of the sensed surface QRS complex (in a ventricular pacemaker) to the following stimulus and exceeds the automatic interval by a few milliseconds to almost the duration of the entire QRS complex, depending on when during the surface QRS complex the intracardiac electrogram is sensed by the pacemaker. A special magnet held over a pulse generator closes a magnetic reed switch that eliminates the sensing function with conversion to the AOO/VOO mode. The *magnet interval* varies according to the manufacturer and is generally shorter than the automatic interval so as to override the spontaneous rhythm. The magnetic interval is often used to assess battery status and lengthens with impending battery depletion.

Some pacemakers have a hysteresis interval; i.e., the escape interval is significantly longer than the automatic interval. Its purpose is to maintain sinus rhythm (and AV synchrony) by preventing the onset of pacing for as long as possible at a rate lower than the automatic rate of the pacemaker. However, hysteresis appears to have no advantage over a simple decrease in the pacing rate, and its advantages are more theoretical than real during single-chamber pacing.

Electrocardiogram During Pacing

Evaluation of the pacemaker stimulus recorded on digital ECG machines is meaningless because the recording circuitry distorts stimuli with striking changes in amplitude and polarity. The vector of the pacemaker stimulus in the frontal plane when recorded with an analog ECG machine correlates with lead position, and amplitude changes are meaningful. A change from small bipolar stimuli to large-amplitude spikes suggests an insulation defect, while spike attenuation of a unipolar stimulus in several ECG leads during held respiration suggests an increase in lead impedance due to a fracture or loose connection

FUSION AND PSEUDOFUSION BEATS. During ventricular pacing, ventricular fusion beats occur when the ventricles are activated simultaneously by a spontaneous depolarization and a paced impulse. A ventricular fusion beat is often narrower than a pure paced beat and can exhibit various morphologies depending on the relative contribution of the two foci to ventricular depolarization (Fig. 23–1). Pseudofusion beats consist of the superimposition of an ineffectual pacemaker spike on the spontaneous QRS complex originating from a single focus and represent a normal manifestation of VVI pacing. A large portion of the surface QRS complex may be inscribed before its intracardiac counterpart (electrogram) generates the necessary voltage (about 3 to 4 mV) capable of inhibiting a VVI pacemaker (Fig. 23–4). Therefore, a normally functioning VVI pacemaker can deliver its impulse within a spontaneous surface QRS complex (mimicking undersensing) before the pulse generator has the opportunity to sense the somewhat late intracardiac electrogram in the right ventricle.[69]

In a pseudofusion beat, the pacemaker stimulus occurs too late to cause true fusion because it falls within the absolute refractory period of the myocardium initiated by the spontaneous depolarization. In the presence of normal sensing, striking examples of pseudofusion beats with

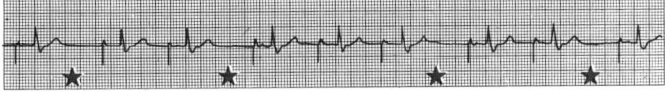

FIGURE 23–3. AAI pacemaker, rate = 70/min (automatic interval = 857 msec) and refractory period = 250 msec. There is intermittent prolongation of the interstimulus interval (stars) because the atrial lead senses the farfield QRS complex just beyond the 250 msec pacemaker refractory period. When the refractory period was programmed to 400 msec, the irregularity disappeared, with restoration of regular atrial pacing at a rate of 70/min.

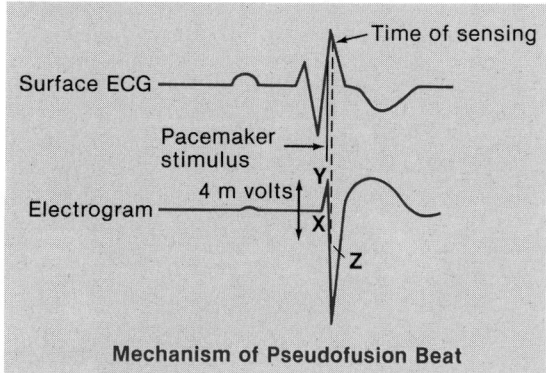

Mechanism of Pseudofusion Beat

FIGURE 23–4. Mechanism of pseudofusion beat. The surface ECG and the ventricular electrogram are recorded simultaneously. The electrogram generates the necessary intracardiac voltage to inhibit the pacemaker (yz assumed at 4 mV) at a point corresponding with the descending limb of the surface QRS complex in its second half (dotted line). Consequently, it is possible for a pacemaker stimulus to occur at the apex of the R deflection just before the dotted line (which depicts the time of sensing) because the ventricular electrogram has not yet generated the required voltage to reach the sensitivity of the pulse generator and inhibit it. (From Barold, S. S., Falkoff, M. D., Ong, L. S., and Heinle, R. A.: Electrocardiographic analysis of normal and abnormal pacemaker function. *In* Dreifus L. S. (ed): Pacemaker Therapy. Cardiovasc. Clin. Philadelphia, F. A. Davis, *14*:97, 1983.)

pacemaker stimuli occurring late within the QRS complex can be seen in right bundle branch block, left ventricular extrasystoles, and any condition causing delayed intraventricular conduction. True sensing failure must be excluded whenever pseudofusion beats are observed. Pacemaker spikes falling clearly after termination of the surface QRS complex indicate sensing failure. Atrial fusion and pseudofusion beats also can occur with atrial pacing but are more difficult to recognize in view of the smaller size of the P wave in the ECG.

RIGHT VENTRICULAR PACING. Right ventricular (RV) pacing produces a left bundle branch block (LBBB) pattern of depolarization. During RV pacing, paced beats usually exhibit a typical LBBB pattern in leads 1 and aV_l, but leads V_5 and V_6 sometimes show deep S waves because the main electrical forces may be moving away from the horizontal level where V_5 and V_6 are recorded. The mean electrical axis of the paced QRS complex in the frontal plane is oriented superiorly (more often in the left than in the right upper quadrant) because the sequence of activation travels from apex to base, away from the inferior leads. As the pacing electrode moves toward the RV outflow tract, activation travels simultaneously to the base superiorly and the apex inferiorly, and the mean axis of the paced QRS complex in the frontal plane may point to the left lower quadrant. RV outflow tract stimulation immediately below the pulmonary valve causes right-axis deviation of the paced QRS complex in the frontal plane because most of the activation travels from base to apex, but the pattern in the left precordial lead always remains that of LBBB. Paced beats from the RV outflow tract not uncommonly exhibit qR, QR, or Qr configuration leads 1 and aV_l, but the inferior leads show a dominant R wave. In this situation, the precordial leads do not exhibit Qr, qR, or QR complexes.

LEFT VENTRICULAR PACING. Epicardial or endocardial stimulation of the left ventricle produces late activation of the RV and therefore a right bundle branch block (RBBB) pattern.[70,71] Pacing from the distal coronary sinus produces the same pattern.

MYOCARDIAL INFARCTION. Because the QRS complex during RV pacing resembles that of spontaneous LBBB (except for the initial forces), the diagnosis of myocardial infarction often can be made during RV pacing by applying the criteria used in complete LBBB.[72] Ventricular fusion beats must be absent. Large unipolar stimuli can mask Q waves. An extensive anteroseptal myocardial infarction can cause a q wave in leads 1, aV_l, V_5 and V_6, producing a qR pattern following the stimulus (not to be confused with a normal QS pattern). Although the sensitivity of the qR change is low, its specificity approaches 100 per cent because it is never seen in leads V_5 and V_6 during uncomplicated pacing. A QR or Qr complex in leads II, III, and aV_f is also diagnostic of an inferior myocardial infarction. Also, an anterior myocardial infarction can be associated with late notching of the ascending limb of the QRS complex in the left precordial leads, indicating an extensive infarction.

During RV apical pacing, the inferior leads and the anterior leads (V_1 to V_3) often record secondary ST-segment elevation. ST-segment depression can occur as a normal finding in leads 1, aV_l, V_5, and V_6. Relatively stable ST-T-wave changes resembling primary abnormalities occasionally can be seen during uncomplicated RV pacing. Dis-

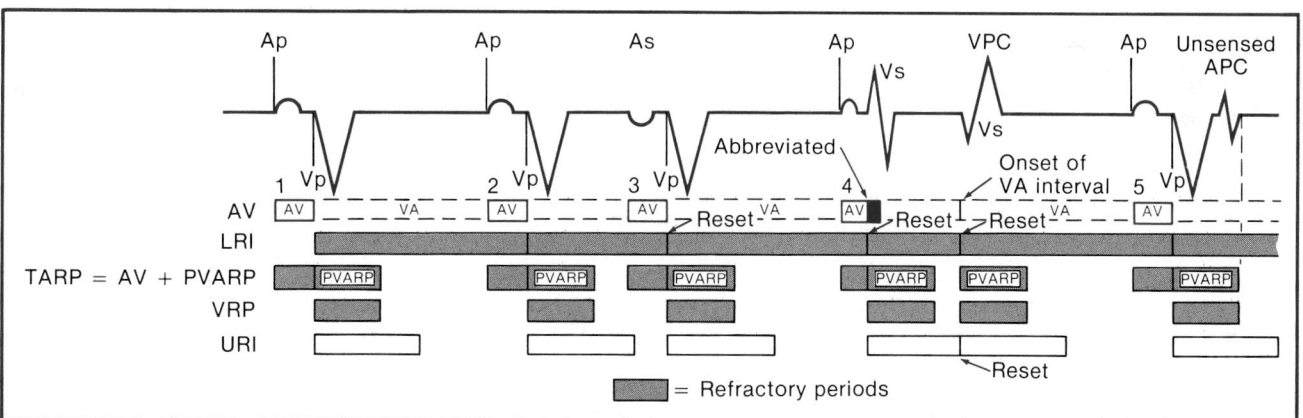

FIGURE 23–5. Diagram showing the function and timing intervals of a simple DDD pacemaker (with ventricular-based lower rate timing) consisting of only four fundamental intervals: lower rate interval = LRI; ventricular refractory period = VRP; atrioventricular delay = AV; postventricular atrial refractory period = PVARP. These provide two derived intervals: atrial escape interval (AEI or pacemaker VA interval) = LRI − AV, and total atrial refractory period (TARP) = AV + PVARP. Ap = atrial paced event; Vp = ventricular paced event; As = atrial sensed event; Vs = ventricular sensed event. Reset refers to the termination and reinitiation of a timing interval before it has timed out to its completion according to its programmed duration. Premature termination of the programmed AV delay by a ventricular sensed event (Vs) is indicated by its abbreviation. The upper rate interval (URI) is equal to the TARP. An atrial sensed event, As (third beat), initiates an A-V interval, terminating with a ventricular paced beat (Vp); As also aborts the AEI initiated by the second Vp. The third Vp resets the LRI and starts the PVARP, VRP, URI, AEI, and LRI. The fourth beat consists of an atrial paced beat (Ap) that terminates the AEI initiated by the third ventricular paced beat (Vp). The atrial paced beat (Ap) is followed by a sensed conducted QRS (Vs) that occurs before the expected release of Vp. Vs inhibits the release of Vp and the AV interval is abbreviated.

The QRS of the fourth beat sensed (Vs) initiates the AEI, LRI, PVARP, VRP, and URI. The fifth beat is a ventricular extrasystole (VPC) that initiates an AEI, PVARP, and VRP; it resets the LRI and URI. The last beat is followed by an atrial extrasystole (APC) unsensed by the atrial channel because it falls within the PVARP. Such a simple DDD pacemaker equipped with six timing cycles functions quite well provided that crosstalk (sensing of atrial stimulus by ventricular channel) does not occur.

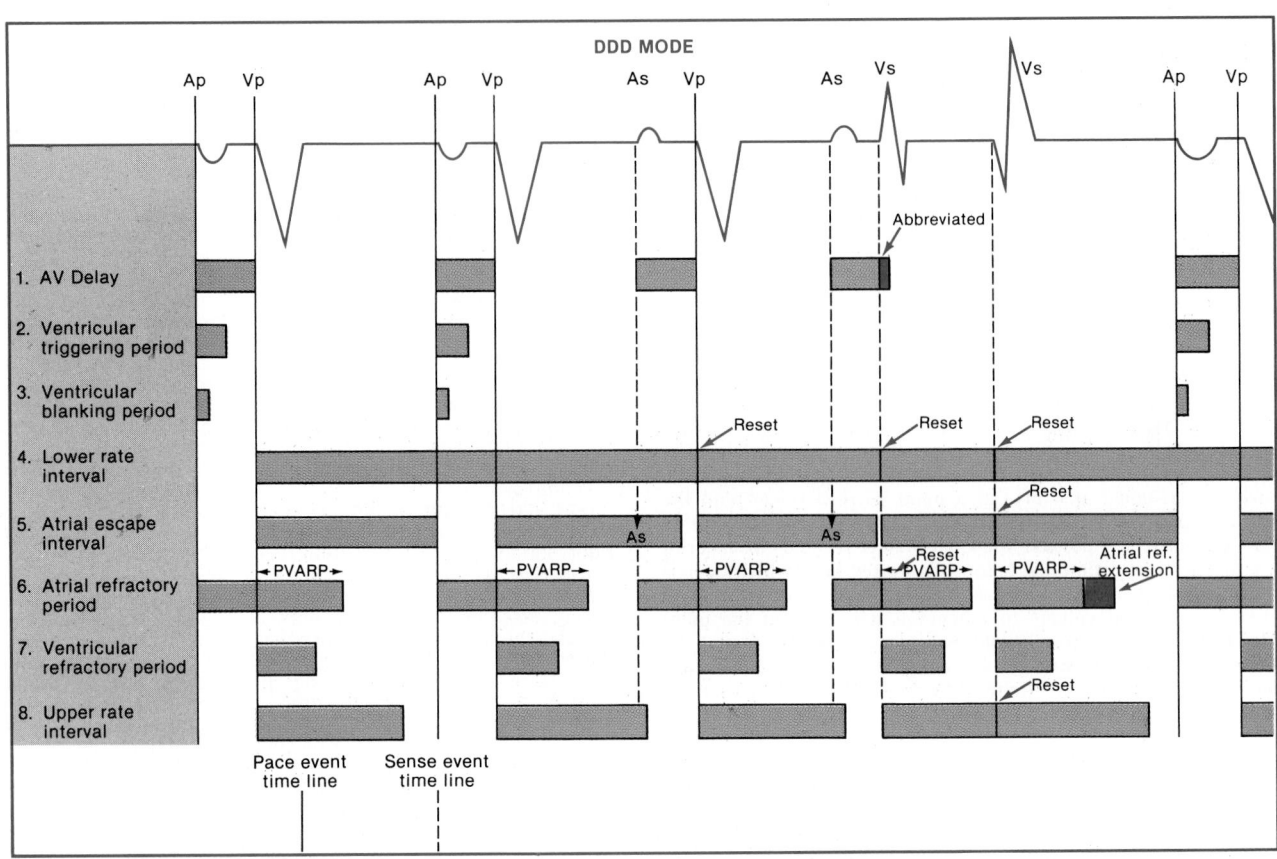

FIGURE 23–6. DDD mode. Diagrammatic representation of timing cycles. Ventricular triggering period = ventricular safety pacing. The second Vs (ventricular sensed event) is a ventricular extrasystole. The fourth A-V interval initiated by As (atrial sensed event) is abbreviated because the conducted QRS (Vs) occurs before the A-V interval has timed out. The postventricular atrial refractory (ref) period (PVARP) generated by the ventricular extrasystole is automatically extended by the atrial refractory period extension. (This design is based on the concept that most episodes of endless-loop tachycardia are initiated by a ventricular extrasystole with retrograde ventriculoatrial conduction.) The arrow pointing down within the atrial escape (pacemaker VA) interval indicates that an atrial sensed event (As) has taken place; the atrial escape interval actually terminates at this point, but the atrial escape interval is depicted in its entirety (as if As had not occurred) for the sake of clarity. The signal As inhibits release of the atrial stimulus otherwise expected at the completion of the atrial escape interval. Ap = atrial paced beat; Vp = ventricular paced beat; As = atrial sensed event; Vs = ventricular sensed event. The abbreviations and format used in this illustration are the same for Figs. 23–9 to 23–11 and 23–13. (From Barold, S. S., et al.: All dual-chamber pacemakers function in the DDD mode. Am. Heart J. *115*:1353, 1988.)

cordant T waves are of no diagnostic value. Sequential electrocardiograms are often needed to determine the significance of the ST–T-wave abnormalities.

ST–T-wave abnormalities occur more commonly in acute myocardial infarction than the qR pattern or QRS notching noted earlier. Pronounced primary ST-segment elevation with convex configuration clinches the diagnosis of myocardial infarction. When less obvious, the diagnosis becomes fairly certain only when the polarity of the T wave is opposite to that of the ST-segment elevation. ST-segment depression concordant with the QRS complex occasionally can occur in V_3 to V_6 during uncomplicated RV pacing and rarely in leads V_1 and V_2. Consequently, obvious ST-segment depression in leads V_1 and V_2 should be considered abnormal and indicative of anterior or inferior myocardial infarction (or ischemia). Inhibition of the pacemaker by chest wall stimulation or by reduction of the rate or output may allow the emergence of the spontaneous rhythm and reveal diagnostic Q waves. Continuous ventricular pacing per se can induce striking ST–T-wave abnormalities in the underlying spontaneous beats.[73]

Dual-Chamber Pacemakers

Types, Rates, and Intervals

TIMING INTERVALS. In the various types of dual-chamber pacemakers, the timing intervals are best understood by focusing first on the DDD mode. A DDD pulse generator paces and senses in both the atrium and the ventricle. Simple dual-chamber pacing modes are then derived by the removal of "building blocks" from the DDD mode and equalization of the various timing intervals.[69] These simpler pacing modes are important because a DDD pacemaker may

have to be downgraded for treatment of certain complications.

As in a standard VVI pacemaker, the ventricular channel of a DDD device requires two basic timing cycles: the lower rate interval and the ventricular refractory period. A simple DDD system consists of the VVI mode with an added atrial channel (Fig. 23–5). This arrangement necessitates two new intervals, an atrioventricular (A-V) interval (the electronic analog of the P-R interval) and an upper rate interval (equal to the pacemaker total atrial refractory period, discussed later), to control the response of the ventricular channel to sensed atrial activity and maintain 1:1 AV synchrony between the lower and upper rates (Fig. 23–5). The atrial escape interval is obtained by subtracting the programmed AV delay from the lower rate interval. The atrial escape interval starts with a ventricular paced or sensed event and terminates with the release of an atrial stimulus.

Most dual-chamber pulse generators are designed with ventricular-based (V-V) lower rate timing controlled by ventricular events and a constant atrial escape interval, as in all examples discussed in this chapter.[74] An atrial sensed event triggers a ventricular stimulus after the completion of the AV interval (provided that no ventricular sensed event occurs during the A-V interval) and inhibits release of the atrial stimulus expected at completion of the atrial escape interval. A ventricular sensed event beyond the A-V interval inhibits both the atrial and ventricular

FIGURE 23–7. Ventricular safety pacing during DDD pacing (ECG leads V_1, V_2, and V_3). **A,** In the absence of crosstalk, the first, fourth, and last A-V intervals are equal to the programmed value of 200 msec. Intermittent crosstalk (solid black circles) leads to activation of the ventricular safety pacing mechanism so that the A-V interval of the second, third, fifth, sixth, and seventh beats (solid black circles) is abbreviated to 110 msec. The marker channel below the ECG confirms the presence of crosstalk with ventricular sensing (Vs) of the atrial stimulus (Ap) within the ventricular safety pacing period but beyond the short ventricular blanking period initiated by Vp. The arrows point to Vp triggered at the end of the ventricular safety pacing period (110 msec after the release of Ap). In a DDD pulse generator with ventricular-based lower rate timing, activation of the ventricular safety pacing mechanism due to continual crosstalk leads to an increase in the pacing rate (although the atrial escape interval remains constant).

B, Activation of the ventricular safety pacing (VSP) mechanism of a DDD pulse generator by sensed ventricular extrasystoles. The ECG was recorded at double speed and double standardization. Lower-rate interval = 857 msec, A-V = 200 msec. The first and second ventricular extrasystoles (1 and 2) are sensed by the ventricular channel of the DDD pacemaker. The onset of these two ventricular extrasystoles is deformed by an atrial stimulus; the atrial stimulus occurs because the ventricular electrogram has not yet generated sufficient voltage for sensing by the ventricular channel to inhibit the atrial and ventricular channels. The mechanism is identical to that of ventricular pseudofusion beats (Fig. 23–4). This particular pseudofusion beat is created by events occurring in different chambers (atrial stimulus and spontaneous ventricular depolarization). The ventricular channel senses the ventricular electrogram of the first and second ventricular extrasystoles within the ventricular safety pacing period but beyond the short ventricular blanking period initiated by the atrial stimulus. The pacemaker therefore triggers a ventricular stimulus at the completion of the ventricular safety pacing period, producing an abbreviated A-V interval of 110 msec: the ventricular stimulus therefore falls at the end of the QRS complex (1 and 2). This ECG represents normal function of a DDD pacemaker with a ventricular safety pacing mechanism. The third ventricular extrasystole (3) is deformed by a ventricular stimulus delivered after the onset of the QRS deflection on the surface ECG, thereby producing a pseudofusion beat. The fourth ventricular extrasystole (4) is also sensed by the ventricular channel. Note that the preceding atrial stimulus occurs at the termination of the atrial escape interval (about 660 msec) and almost simultaneously with the onset of the QRS complex. The interval from Ap preceding the fourth ventricular extrasystole to the last Ap measures 770 to 780 msec. This interval indicates that the pacemaker senses the fourth ventricular extrasystole just beyond the ventricular safety pacing period of 110 msec initiated by the preceding Ap.

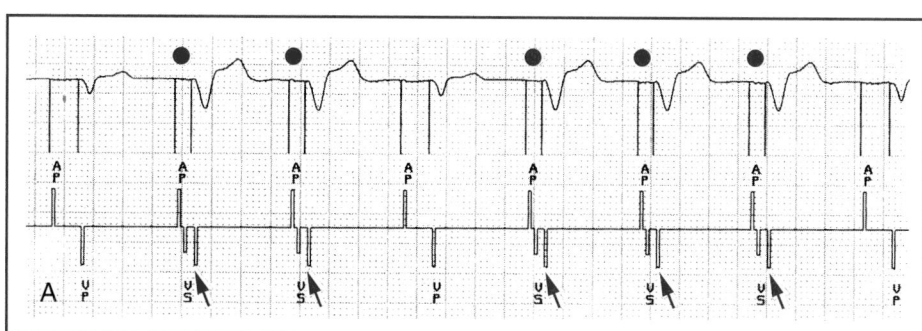

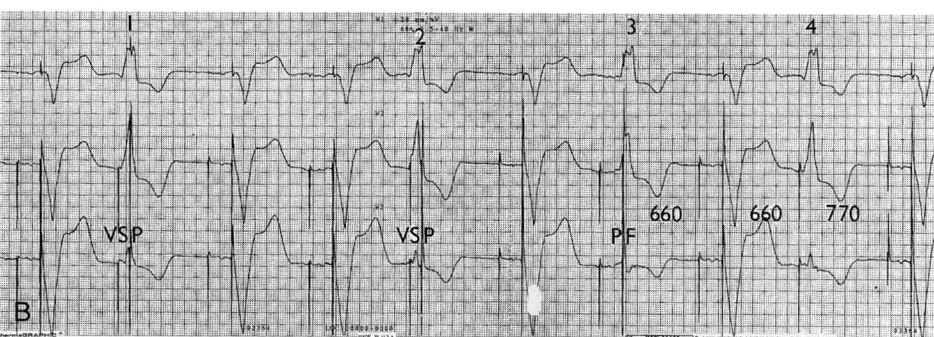

channels and initiates new lower rate and atrial escape intervals. An atrial paced or sensed event initiates the atrial refractory period because the atrial channel must remain refractory during the A-V interval to prevent initiation of a new A-V interval when one is already in progress.[69,75] The A-V interval must terminate with a paced or sensed ventricular event that continues the atrial refractory period. The second part, called the *postventricular atrial refractory period* (PVARP), must be programmed appropriately to prevent sensing of retrograde P waves due to ventriculoatrial (VA) conduction. The total atrial refractory period is equal to the sum of the AV delay and the PVARP.

In a simple DDD pulse generator, the upper rate interval is equal to the total atrial refractory period. The A-V interval, PVARP, and upper rate interval are interrelated according to the formula: upper rate (ppm) = 60/total atrial refractory period (sec). Consequently, a pacemaker with an upper rate of 120/min can sense atrial signals only 500 msec or longer apart.

LOWER RATE TIMING. Some pacemakers exhibit atrial-based lower rate timing in response to certain combinations of atrial and ventricular activity that make up the P-R or A-V interval. With atrial-based timing, the lower rate interval starts with an atrial sensed or paced event and terminates with a subsequent atrial paced event so that the atrial escape interval must vary to maintain constancy of the lower rate interval.[74]

CROSSTALK. Also known as *self-inhibition,* this refers to the inappropriate detection of the atrial stimulus by the ventricular channel.[69] Crosstalk depends on the amplitude of the atrial stimulus and the sensitivity of the ventricular channel and is less frequent with bipolar leads. Crosstalk often can be eliminated by reduction of the atrial output and/or ventricular sensitivity. The prevention of crosstalk also requires a ventricular blanking (refractory) period (10 to 60 msec) that starts coincidentally with the atrial stimulus[69] (Fig. 23–6). In some DDD pacemakers, the first part of the A-V interval (beyond the blanking period) initiated by an atrial stimulus contains an additional backup system known as *ventricular safety pacing* (VSP) (Fig. 23–6).

During the VSP interval (or its initial portion), any signal (atrial stimulus, QRS, and the like) sensed by the ventricular channel triggers a ventricular stimulus at the completion of the VSP period (usually lasting 100 to 120 msec from the atrial stimulus). Activation of the VSP mechanism produces characteristic abbreviation of the paced A-V interval (Fig. 23–7). Crosstalk without a VSP mechanism produces unexpected prolongation of the interval from the atrial stimulus to the succeeding spontaneous QRS complex (if any) to a value longer than the programmed A-V interval (Fig. 23–8). In patients without underlying spontaneous rhythm, crosstalk without a VSP mechanism can cause asystole (Fig. 23–8); however, with appropriate programming of the ventricular blanking period and the VSP mechanism, crosstalk is rarely a clinical problem.

UPPER RATE RESPONSE OF DDD PULSE GENERATORS. The programmed upper rate of a DDD pulse generator depends on the patient's activity level, age, left ventricular function, and the presence of coronary artery disease, atrial tachyarrhythmias, and retrograde VA conduction. The maximal rate of a DDD pacemaker can be defined by either the duration of the total atrial refractory period (causing fixed-ratio pacemaker AV block such as 2:1, 3:1, and so on) or a separate upper rate timing circuit causing Wenckebach-like AV block (6:5, 5:4, and so on).[69,75]

FIXED-RATIO AV BLOCK. This provides the simplest way of controlling the upper rate by programming the total atrial refractory period. The number of unsensed P waves depends on the atrial rate and where the P waves occur in the pacemaker cycle (Fig. 23–9). The A-V interval always remains constant. This response is often called 2:1 AV block. Actually, the paced ventricular rate will be exactly half the atrial rate or equal to the lower rate of the pacemaker, whichever is higher. An upper rate using fixed-ratio AV block only may be inappropriate in some patients, especially young and physically active individuals, because the sudden reduction of the ventricular rate with 2:1 AV block on exercise may be poorly tolerated.

WENCKEBACH UPPER RATE RESPONSE. This mode avoids sudden reduction of the paced ventricular rate and maintains some degree of AV synchrony. A Wenckebach response can occur only if the upper rate interval is programmed to a value longer than the total atrial refractory period (Fig. 23–10). Prolongation of the A-V interval (atrial

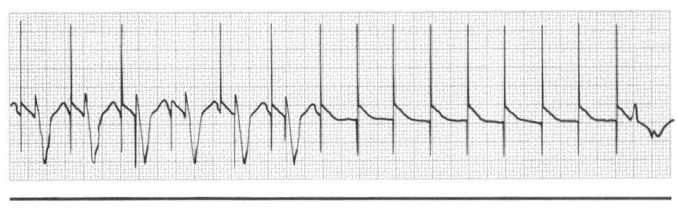

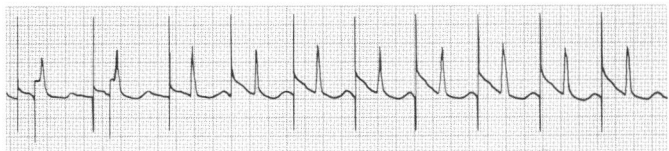

FIGURE 23–8. Crosstalk during DDD pacing without a ventricular safety pacing mechanism. *Top strip,* The lower rate was increased to test for crosstalk. Lower rate interval = 580 msec, AV = 170 msec. The interval between atrial stimuli on the right is shorter than the lower rate interval. Crosstalk causes an increase in the atrial pacing rate faster than the freerunning (lower) AV sequential rate on the left. Continual crosstalk causes prolonged ventricular asystole. *Bottom strip,* Crosstalk with AV conduction. Lower rate interval = 857 msec, AV interval = 200 msec. Crosstalk occurs with the third atrial stimulus and prolongs the interval between the atrial stimulus and the succeeding conducted QRS complex to a value longer than the programmed AV interval. The rate of atrial pacing increases because the sensed atrial stimulus by the ventricular channel initiates a new atrial escape interval just beyond termination of the ventricular blanking period. Consequently, the interval between two consecutive atrial stimuli becomes equal to the atrial escape interval of 657 msec (857–200) plus the duration of the ventricular blanking period (50 msec), providing a total of about 700 msec.

sensed, ventricular paced) occurs only when the upper rate interval > P-P interval > total atrial refractory period. With a progressive increase in atrial rate, when the P-P interval is less than or equal to the total atrial refractory period, the Wenckebach response switches to 2:1 fixed-ratio AV block.[69,75]

OTHER DUAL-CHAMBER PACING MODES

DVI MODE. The DVI mode can be considered as the DDD mode with the PVARP extending through the entire atrial escape interval.[69] No atrial sensing occurs because the total atrial refractory period extends through the entire lower rate interval. Asynchronous atrial

pacing can precipitate atrial fibrillation. Three types of DVI function are possible: uncommitted, partially committed, and committed. In the uncommitted DVI mode the ventricular channel can sense through the entire duration of the A-V interval, while in the partially committed DVI mode the ventricular channel can sense only beyond an initial ventricular blanking period. In contrast, a committed DVI pacemaker possesses a ventricular blanking period encompassing the entire A-V interval, making crosstalk impossible. In the committed DVI mode, AV sequential pacing occurs in an all-or-none manner; i.e., two sequential stimuli always occur together, while sensing spontaneous ventricular activity inhibits the release of both stimuli.

VDD MODE. The VDD mode functions like the DDD mode except

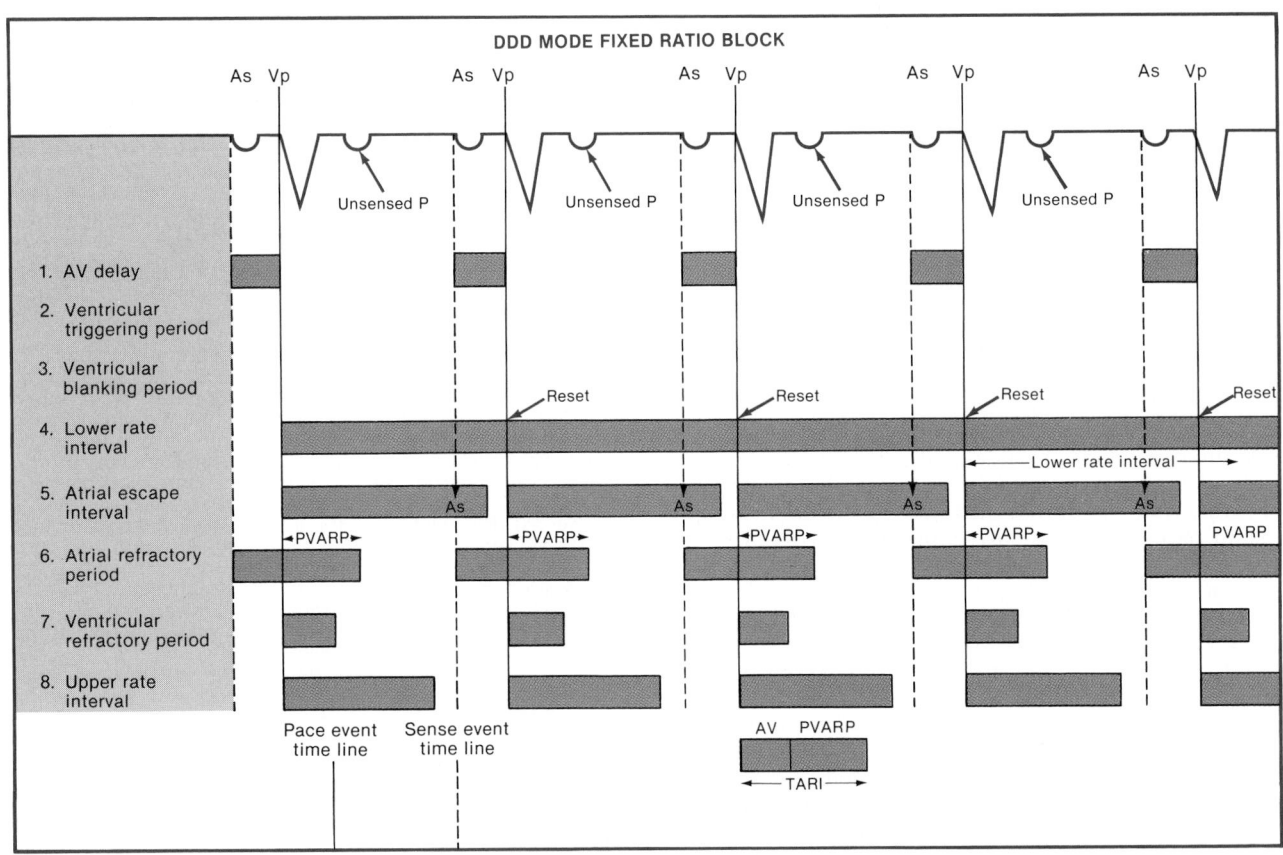

FIGURE 23–9. Upper rate response of DDD pacemaker with fixed-ratio AV block. The upper rate interval is longer than the total atrial refractory period (AV + postventricular atrial refractory period, or PVARP), and the P-P interval (As-As) is shorter than the total atrial refractory period (TARP). The arrow pointing down within the atrial escape (pacemaker VA) interval indicates that an atrial sensed event (As) has taken place; the atrial escape interval actually terminates at this point but the atrial escape interval is depicted in its entirety (as if As had not occurred) for the sake of clarity. Every second P wave falls within the PVARP and is unsensed. The AV interval remains constant. An upper rate response with fixed ratio pacemaker AV block occurs in two types of DDD pacemakers. (1) A device without a separately progammable upper rate interval in which the TARP is equal to the upper rate interval. (2) A device with a separately programmable upper rate interval (i.e., upper rate interval > TARP) only when the P-P interval < TARP as shown in this figure. In such a device, an upper rate response with pacemaker Wenckebach AV block can only occur when the P-P interval > TARP as shown in Figure 25–10. (From Barold, S. S.: Management of patients with dual chamber pulse generators: Central role of pacemaker atrial refractory period. Learning Center Highlights, Heart House, American College of Cardiology 5:[4], 8, 1990, with permission.) (See Fig. 23–6 for abbreviations.)

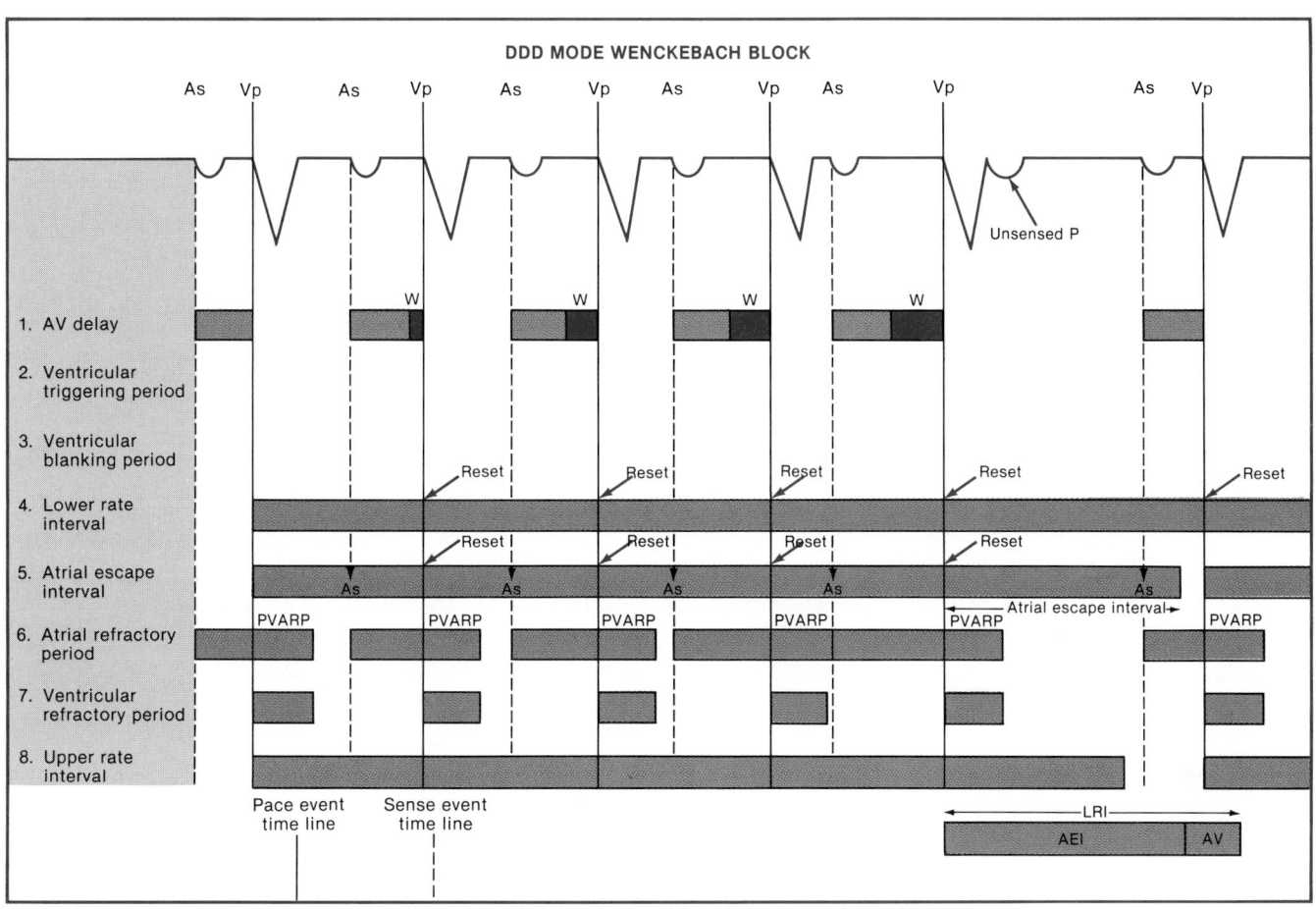

FIGURE 23–10. DDD mode. Upper rate response with pacemaker Wenckebach AV block. The upper rate interval is *longer* than the programmed total atrial refractory period, a mandatory prerequisite for a Wenckebach upper rate response. The P-P interval (As-As) is *longer* than the programmed total atrial refractory period. The As-Vp (atrial sensed–ventricular paced) interval lengthens by a varying period to conform to the upper rate interval. During the Wenckebach sequence, the pacemaker synchronizes a ventricular paced beat (Vp) to an atrial sensed event (As). Because the pacemaker cannot violate its programmed (ventricular) upper rate interval, the ventricular paced beat (Vp) can be released only at the completion of the upper rate interval. The AV delay (As-Vp) becomes progressively longer (than the programmed value) as the ventricular channel waits to deliver its ventricular stimulus (Vp) until the upper rate interval has timed out. The maximum prolongation of the AV delay (As-Vp) represents the difference between the upper rate interval and the total atrial refractory period. The As-Vp (atrial sensed–ventricular paced) interval lengthens during the pacemaker Wenckebach sequence as long as the As-As interval (P-P) remains longer than the total atrial refractory period. The sixth P wave falls within the postventricular atrial refractory period (PVARP) and is unsensed and thus not followed by a ventricular stimulus (Vp). A pause occurs and the Wenckebach cycle restarts. In the first four pacing cycles, the intervals between pacemaker stimuli (Vp-Vp) are constant and equal to the upper rate interval. When the P-P interval becomes shorter than the programmed total atrial refractory period, Wenckebach pacemaker AV block cannot occur and fixed ratio pacemaker AV block, e.g., 2:1, will supervene as in Figure 23–9. The arrow pointing down within the atrial escape interval (AEI) indicates that an atrial sensed event (As) has taken place; the atrial escape interval actually terminates at this point, but for the sake of clarity the atrial escape interval is depicted as if As had not occurred. LRI = lower rate interval. AEI = Atrial escape interval. (From Barold, S. S., et al.: All dual chamber pacemakers function in the DDD mode. Am. Heart J. *115*:1353, 1988.)

that the generated atrial stimulus is diverted internally rather than emitted.[69] Therefore, no atrial pacing occurs. The absence of the atrial stimulus eliminates the need for crosstalk intervals (Fig. 23–11). The omitted atrial stimulus nevertheless begins an "implied" A-V interval that must be refractory in its entirety so that in most contemporary designs a P wave occurring within the "implied" A-V interval is not sensed. Without sensed atrial activity, the VDD mode paces effectively in the VVI mode at the lower rate of the pacemaker.

DDI MODE. The DDI mode generally has been described as an improved DVI mode or a hybrid of the DVI and DDD modes. Sensing and pacing occur in both atrium and ventricle. The DDI mode is best considered as a DDD mode with identical upper and lower rate intervals (provided that the lower rate is controlled by ventricular events, i.e., V-V timing)[69] (Fig. 23–12). Atrial sensing occurs beyond the PVARP. An atrial sensed event initiates an A-V interval that terminates (as in the DDD mode) only at the completion of the upper rate interval (identical to the lower rate interval). Although atrial sensing occurs, the pacemaker cannot increase the ventricular pacing rate in response to a faster atrial rate, so ventricular pacing always occurs at the programmed lower rate. In other words, there is no atrial tracking. For this reason, the DDI mode is useful in patients with the sick sinus syndrome and paroxysmal atrial tachyarrhythmias. The DDI

mode provides atrial pacing and AV synchrony (in the absence of atrial tachyarrhythmias) with the potential of preventing atrial tachyarrhythmias by overdrive suppression.

During atrial tachyarrhythmia with continual atrial sensing, the DDI pacemaker simply paces the ventricle at its constant rate and becomes functionally identical to the VVI mode (Fig. 23–12). In patients with AV block and a sinus rate faster than the programmed pacing rate, the DDI mode produces an unfavorable hemodynamic situation identical to the VVI mode with AV dissociation (with occasional delivery of an atrial stimulus when the preceding P wave occurs in the PVARP).[76,77] The DDI mode has become less useful than in the past because a number of DDD or DDDR devices now respond to supraventricular tachyarrhythmias by automatic mode conversion to a slower, nonatrial tracking mode (VVI, VVIR, DDI, DDIR). Upon cessation of the arrhythmia, these devices revert to the DDD or DDDR mode with AV synchrony over a relatively broad range of atrial rates.[78,79]

RETROGRADE VA CONDUCTION AND ENDLESS-LOOP TACHYCARDIA. Endless-loop tachycardia (sometimes incorrectly called *pacemaker-mediated tachycardia*) is a well-known complication of dual-chamber pacing (VDD, DDD, or

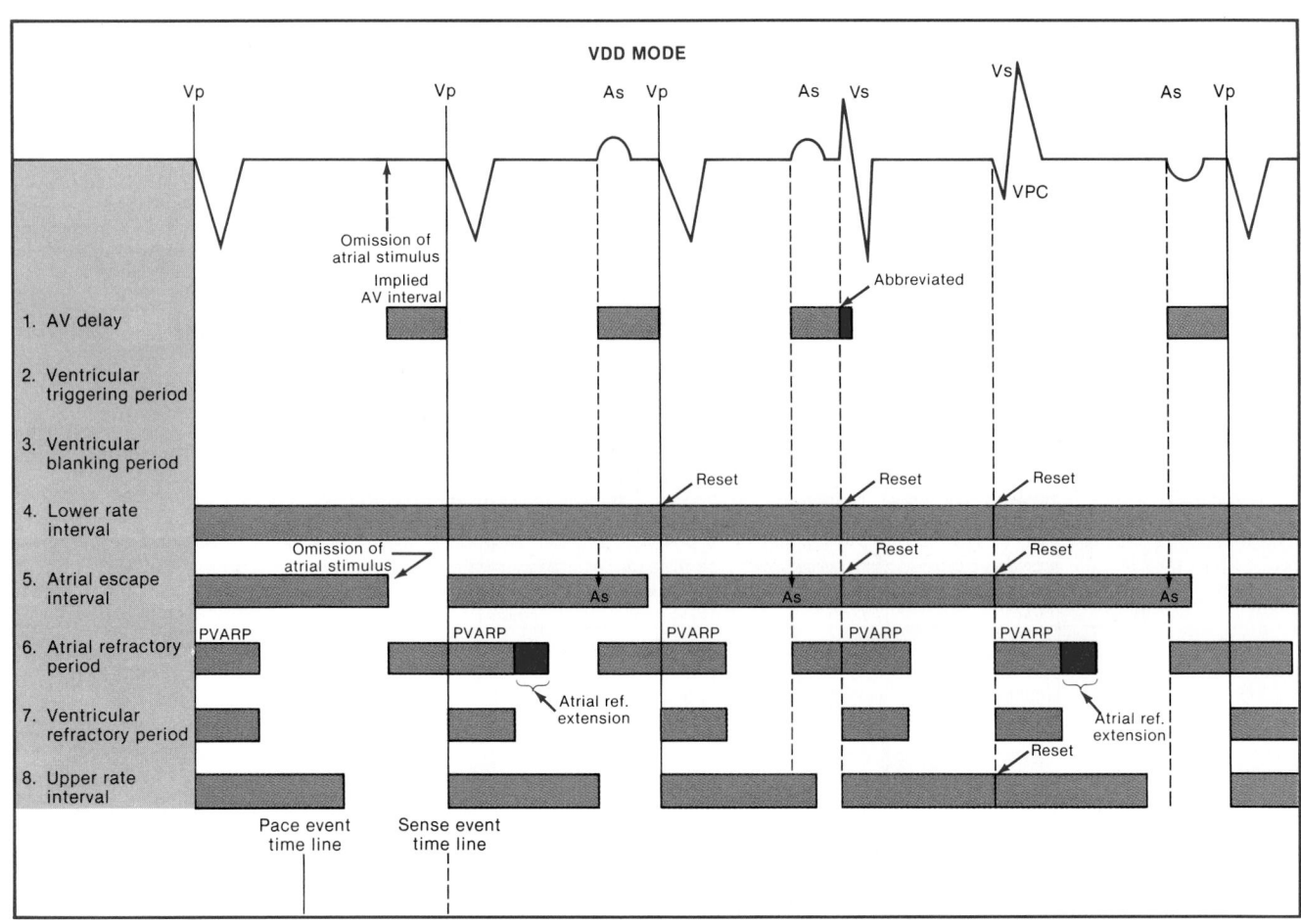

FIGURE 23-11. VDD mode. In the DDD mode, an atrial stimulus is released at the completion of the atrial escape interval whenever an atrial sensed event (As) or ventricular sensed event does not occur within the atrial escape interval. This atrial stimulus is omitted in the VDD mode. Nevertheless, the pulse generator initiates an implied AV interval with the same characteristics as in the DDD mode. In the first ventricular cycle (Vp-Vp) because the ventricular paced beat (Vp) terminating the implied AV interval is not preceded by an atrial paced beat or atrial sensed event (As), the post-ventricular atrial refractory period (PVARP) is automatically extended as occurs after a sensed ventricular extrasystole (depicted as VPC) (Fig. 23-6). Ventricular blanking and ventricular triggering (ventricular safety pacing) periods are not needed because there are no atrial stimuli in the VDD mode. In the absence of atrial sensed events (As), the pulse generator effectively paces in the VVI mode at the programmed lower rate interval (first cycle). The atrial escape interval terminates at the onset of the implied AV interval.

To promote AV synchrony for as long as possible, atrial sensing can occur in the implied AV interval of some contemporary dual chamber pacemakers functioning in the VDD mode. In such a situation, As (in the implied AV interval) initiates an entirely new AV interval so that the pacemaker releases Vp beyond the lower rate interval. The maximal extension of the lower rate interval by this response is equal to the programmed As-Vp interval. The arrow pointing down within the atrial escape interval indicates that an atrial sensed event (As) has taken place; the atrial escape interval actually terminates at this point, but for the sake of clarity it is depicted as if As had not occurred. (From Barold, S. S., et al.: All dual chamber pacemakers function in the DDD mode. Am. Heart J. *115:*1353, 1988.)

DDDR) and starts with sensing of a retrograde P wave usually linked to a ventricular extrasystole[69] (Fig. 23-13). Endless-loop tachycardia can be sustained or unsustained and often occurs at the programmed upper rate of the pacemaker. When the sum of the retrograde VA conduction time and the programmed A-V interval exceeds the upper rate interval, the tachycardia is slower than the programmed upper rate. Intact retrograde VA conduction occurs in approximately two-thirds or more of patients with sinus node dysfunction and in 15 to 35 per cent of patients with AV block. Thus 35 to 50 percent of all patients receiving dual-chamber pacemakers may be susceptible to endless-loop tachycardia. Absent retrograde VA conduction at the time of implantation or even later provides no guarantee of protection because a few patients may exhibit VA conduction subsequently, particularly during states of sympathetic stimulation. Rarely, VA conduction occurs only with exercise. Any condition capable of sepa-

rating the sinus P wave from the QRS complex, coupled with retrograde VA conduction, can initiate endless-loop tachycardia.[69,80] These include a ventricular extrasystole, loss of atrial capture, myopotential sensing by the atrial channel of unipolar devices, undersensing of sinus P waves (with preserved sensing of retrograde P waves), an excessively long A-V interval, and application and removal of the magnet.

Endless-loop tachycardia can be induced when the atrial output is programmed below the pacing threshold, PVARP is at its minimum value, and there is a lower rate above the spontaneous rate (Fig. 23-14). When atrial capture persists at the lowest output, endless-loop tachycardia can be induced by chest wall stimulation (delivered by a temporary pacemaker) provided that the external signals are sensed selectively by the atrial channel. Conversion to the asynchronous mode with the magnet over the pacemaker terminates endless-loop tachycardia with rare exceptions.

FIGURE 23–12. DDI pacing during atrial fibrillation. The DDI mode is equivalent to the DDD mode with identical lower rate interval and upper rate interval (provided there is ventricular-based lower rate timing). *Top,* ECG recorded simultaneously with event markers. *Bottom,* ECG recorded simultaneously with the telemetered atrial electrogram (AEGM). F = fusion beat; As = atrial sensed event; AR = atrial event detected in the postventricular atrial refractory period; Vp = ventricular paced event. Lower rate interval = 750 msec, A-V interval = 200 msec, postventricular atrial refractory period = 250 msec. Sensed events in the atrial refractory period (AR) do not initiate any timing cycles. Although the pacemaker senses atrial events (As), it does not track atrial activity so that ventricular pacing can occur only at the programmed lower rate of 80 beats/min. The As-Vp intervals are always longer than the programmed Ap-Vp interval, a characteristic feature of the DDI mode. There is intermittent sensing of the f

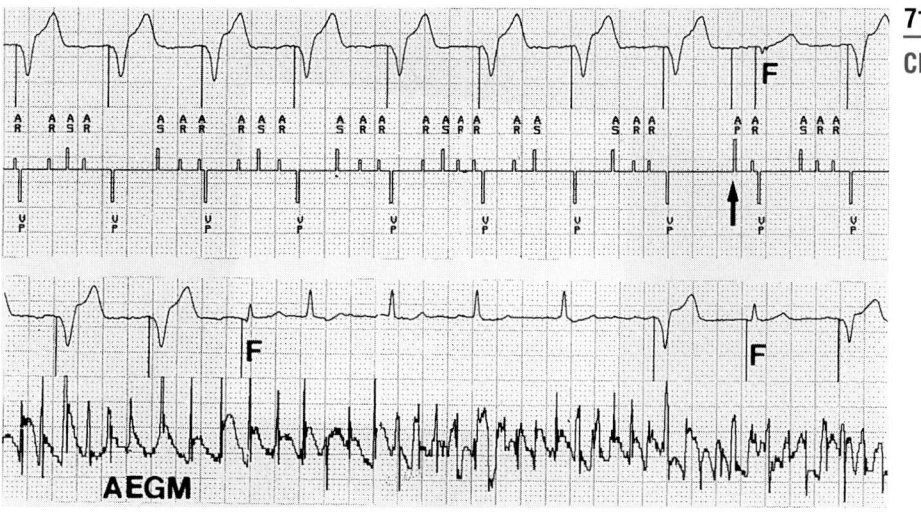

waves. The arrow points to a cycle where the pacemaker does not sense f waves and therefore releases Ap at the completion of the atrial escape interval. Except for this cycle, the ECG cannot be distinguished from VVI pacing.

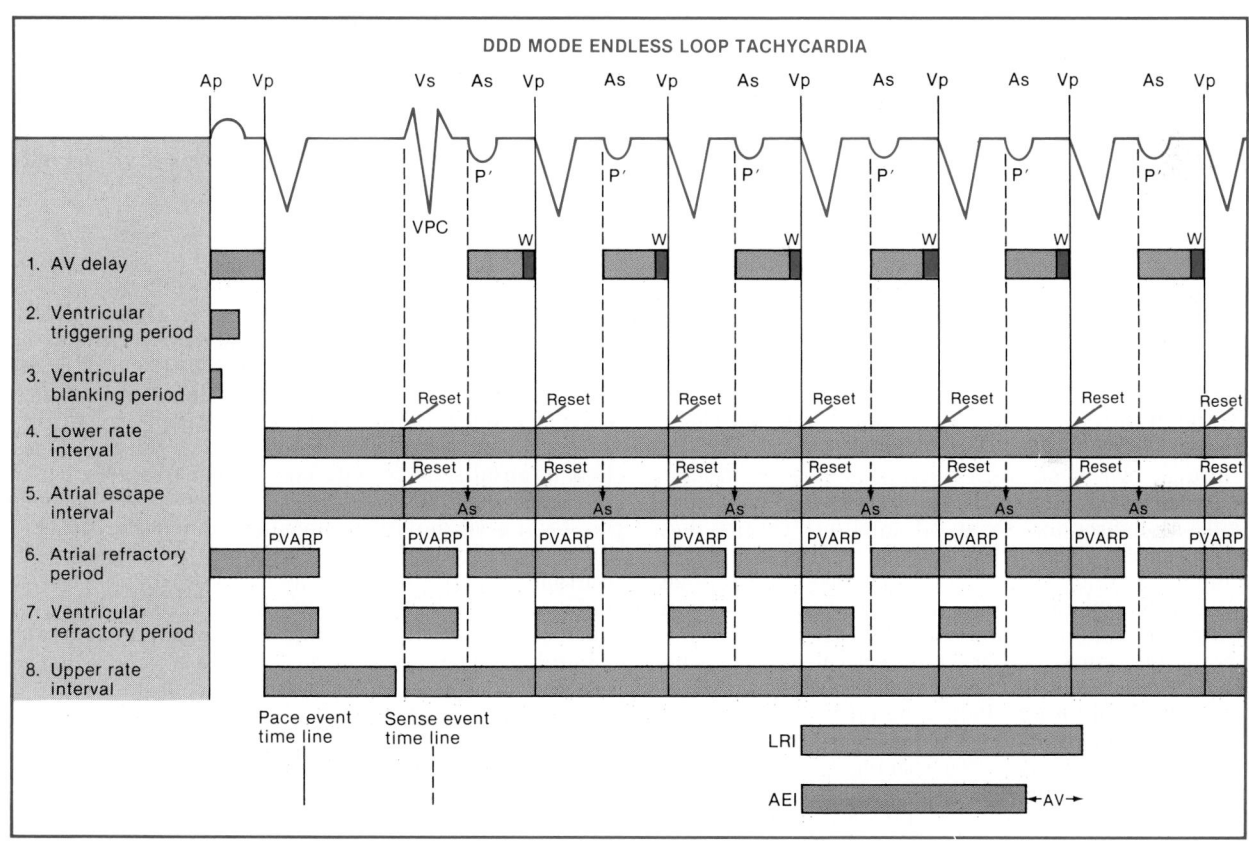

FIGURE 23–13. DDD mode. Endless loop (reentrant) tachycardia initiated by a ventricular extrasystole (VPC, second beat) with retrograde ventriculoatrial (VA) conduction (P′ or As). The atrial channel senses the retrograde P wave (P′) and a ventricular pacemaker stimulus (Vp) is issued after extension of the As-Vp (atrial sensed–ventricular paced) interval to conform to the supremacy of the upper rate interval (as in Fig. 23–10). The ventricular paced beat (Vp) generates another retrograde P wave, again sensed by the pulse generator outside its postventricular atrial refractory period (PVARP) and the process perpetuates itself. The pulse generator itself provides the anterograde limb of the macroreentrant process because it functions as an artificial AV junction. Retrograde VA conduction (P′) following a ventricular paced beat (Vp) provides the retrograde limb of the reentrant process. The cycle length of the endless loop tachycardia is equal to the upper rate interval. However, the cycle length of an endless loop tachycardia may occasionally be longer than the upper rate interval if retrograde VA conduction is prolonged. In this situation when the AV interval is *not* extended, the retrograde VA conduction time (as seen by the pacemaker) may be calculated by subtracting the AV interval from the cycle length of the tachycardia. Disruption of either the anterograde limb (by eliminating atrial sensing) or the retrograde limb (by eliminating retrograde VA conduction) terminates endless loop tachycardia. The arrow pointing down within the atrial escape interval indicates that an atrial sensed event (As) has taken place. Although the atrial escape interval actually terminates at this point, for the sake of clarity it is depicted as if As had not occurred. LRI = lower rate interval; AEI = atrial escape interval. (From Barold, S. S., et al.: All dual chamber pacemakers function in the DDD mode. Am. Heart J. *115:*1353, 1988.)

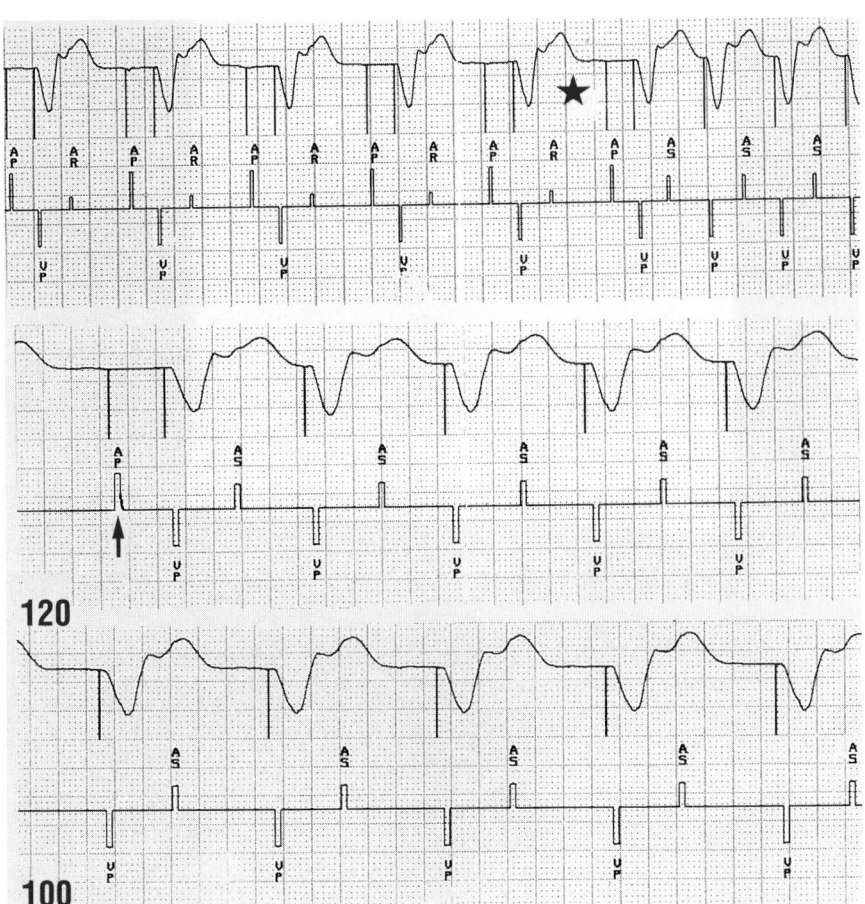

FIGURE 23–14. *Top,* DDD pacing with endless loop tachycardia. Lower rate interval = 857 msec, A-V = 200 msec after atrial pacing and 150 msec after atrial sensing, postventricular atrial refractory period (PVARP) = 300 msec; upper rate interval = 500 msec (120 beats/min). *Top,* Subthreshold atrial stimulation (Ap). Ventricular pacing causes retrograde VA conduction. On the left, the retrograde P waves fall within the PVARP and are unsensed. The PVARP was shortened to 200 msec at the star. The pacemaker then senses the retrograde P waves and initiates endless-loop tachycardia (recorded at a speed of 25 mm/sec).

Bottom, This panel (recorded at a speed of 50 mm/sec) also shows the initiation of endless-loop tachycardia by subthreshold atrial stimulation. The markers indicate that the retrograde VA time measures approximately 240 msec. The As-Vp interval is prolonged to conform to the upper rate interval, i.e., Vp-Vp interval = upper rate interval = 500 msec (120 beats/min). In the bottom panel (also recorded at 50 mm/sec), the upper rate interval was programmed to 600 msec (100 beats/min). The retrograde VA conduction time during endless-loop tachycardia remains constant at 240 msec, but the As-Vp interval lengthens further to conform to the upper rate interval, i.e., Vp-Vp interval = 600 msec. Endless-loop tachycardia was no longer induced by subthreshold atrial stimulation when the PVARP was again programmed to 300 msec, as in the top panel on the left.

To prevent endless-loop tachycardia, the PVARP should be programmed to 50 msec beyond the duration of retrograde VA conduction determined noninvasively by pacemaker programming. Other measures include a shorter A-V interval, differential discrimination of a larger anterograde P wave from smaller retrograde atrial depolarization, and activation of a special mechanism upon sensing a ventricular event (outside AV delay) that is interpreted as a ventricular extrasystole: synchronous atrial stimulation (to preempt retrograde atrial depolarization) or automatic PVARP extension for one cycle (Fig. 23–8). Some pacemakers possess an automatic tachycardia-terminating algorithm (e.g., omission of a ventricular stimulus, temporary PVARP prolongation, or shortening of a single A-V interval) activated when ventricular pacing occurs at designated rates (usually the programmed upper rate) for a certain duration.

TACHYCARDIA DURING DDD PACING. Various types of tachycardia can occur during DDD pacing.[80] The diagnosis is usually simple and facilitated by telemetry of event markers or electrograms (discussed later). Tachycardias other than endless-loop tachycardia return upon removal of the magnet. The magnet, by producing a slower rate in the DOO or VOO mode, permits identification of P or f waves. Programming to slow VVI pacing allows analysis of atrial activity. Atrial flutter or fibrillation can cause regular or irregular atrial and ventricular pacing due to intermittent lack of atrial sensing with consequent release of atrial stimuli. This response, coupled with periods of rapid ventricular pacing secondary to sensing rapid atrial activity, produces a chaotic pattern virtually diagnostic of atrial fibrillation or flutter (Fig 23–15). Tachycardia triggered by myopotentials sensed by the atrial channel of a unipolar device is easily reproducible with isometric exercise (Fig. 23–16).

Multiprogrammability

A programmable pulse generator is capable of noninvasive adjustment of its function so that an appropriate pacemaker "prescription" can be "written" by the physician. The available technology, which is reliable and cost-effective, is mandatory in modern pacemaker prac-

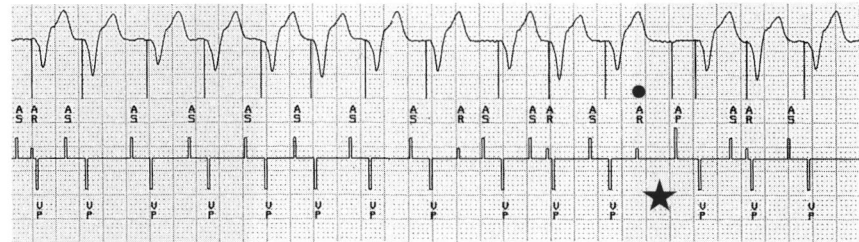

FIGURE 23–15. DDD pacing with atrial fibrillation causing rapid and irregular ventricular pacing. Lower rate interval = 750 msec, upper rate interval = 440 msec, As-Vp interval = 160 msec, Ap-Vp interval = 200 msec, PVARP = 250 msec. The constantly changing pattern of ventricular pacing is due to intermittent sensing of f waves. When the pacemaker fails to sense f waves beyond the PVARP, it delivers an atrial stimulus (Ap) at the completion of the atrial escape interval (star). This chaotic pattern is virtually diagnostic of atrial fibrillation or flutter during DDD pacing. AR = atrial sensing during the atrial refractory period. AR cannot initiate any timing cycles.

FIGURE 23–16. Unipolar DDD pacing with myopotential triggering induced by arm exercise. The atrial channel senses myopotentials, whereupon ventricular stimulation is delivered at an irregular and rapid rate, sometimes at the programmed upper rate of 140 beats/min (upper rate interval = approximately 430 msec). Lower rate interval = 857 msec, As-Vp interval = 150 msec, Ap-Vp interval = 150 msec, postventricular atrial refractory period = 250 msec. AR represents atrial sensing during the postventricular atrial refractory period. AR cannot initiate any timing intervals. Myopotential oversensing was eliminated by decreasing the sensitivity of the atrial channel without compromising P-wave sensing.

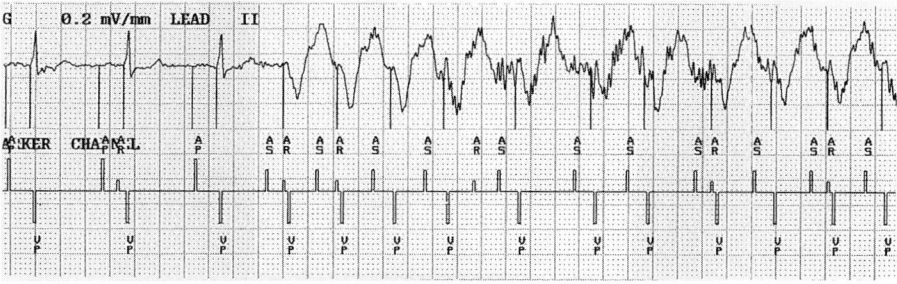

tice because it reduces the need for secondary interventions and increases device longevity by optimizing output. A program change should always be confirmed by telemetry to reduce the likelihood of error and should be entered in the patient's chart. Programmability after pacemaker implantation is often underutilized. It offers the opportunity to create an optimal pacing system for a specific clinical situation. Like chronic pharmacological therapy requiring dosage adjustment according to changing circumstances, pacemaker parameters appropriate at the time of implantation may cease to be adequate in the future and may need modification. Programmability has simplified troubleshooting many pacemaker problems and often obviates operative revision to treat many pacemaker complications (Table 23–4).

SINGLE-CHAMBER PACEMAKERS. The three most important parameters for single-chamber pacing are rate, output (voltage and pulse width), and sensitivity. The ability to program other parameters such as refractory period, mode, polarity, and hysteresis is also desirable in certain clinical circumstances.

Programming an increase in output may be necessary when the acute or chronic pacing threshold rises disproportionately. When the pacing threshold has stabilized several weeks after implantation, decreasing output is important to conserve battery life and increase longevity of the pulse generator. For most patients, the nominal output delivered by the pacemaker is excessive and wasteful. Reducing voltage rather than pulse width often minimizes or eliminates undesirable diaphragmatic pacing or muscle stimulation at the anodal site of normally functioning and positioned unipolar pacemakers (in the absence of insulation leak). Programming the output to subthreshold levels (or very low rate) permits study of the underlying rhythm.

The pacemaker should be programmed to be twice as sensitive as the value of the sensing threshold. This corresponds to a numerical setting at least half the threshold value. For example, if the sensitivity threshold, i.e., the lowest setting associated with regular sensing during deep inspiration, is 8 mV, the sensitivity value should be programmed to 4 mV. Oversensing the T wave and/or residual voltage at the electrode-myocardial interface (afterpotential) is easily remedied by decreasing the sensitivity (increasing the numerical value) and/or prolonging the refractory period. Oversensing myopotentials by a unipolar pacemaker requires reduction of sensitivity; however, if this is associated with undersensing the QRS, programming to the triggered (VVT, AAT) mode may be required.

DUAL-CHAMBER PACEMAKERS. The programming of DDD pacemakers requires special considerations. Most of the parameters in Table 23–4 must be programmed individually in each chamber. The PVARP must be programmed to prevent sensing retrograde P waves and the possibility of endless-loop tachycardia. Programming the ventricular blanking period may be desirable to prevent crosstalk. The upper rate (interval) must be programmed according to the patient's age, activity, retrograde VA conduction, nature of heart disease, and propensity to supraventricular tachycardia. Programming the sensor response of rate-adaptive pacemakers requires special care. The A-V interval should be programmed to obtain a maximum hemodynamic advantage.[81] Some pulse generators possess algorithms that shorten the A-V interval during exercise as the normal heart does. Electrical events on the right side of the heart must be translated into optimal timing of atrial and ventricular mechanical activity on the left side of the heart.[82-84]

It may be reasonable to start with an A-V interval of 100 to 150 msec after atrial sensing and to prolong the A-V interval after atrial

TABLE 23–4 MULTIPROGRAMMABILITY IN SINGLE-CHAMBER PACEMAKERS*

PARAMETER	VARIABILITY	PURPOSE
Rate	Increase	To optimize output, to overdrive or terminate tachyarrhythmias, to adapt pediatric needs, to test AV conduction with AAI pacemakers, to confirm atrial capture during AAI pacing by observing concomitant change in ventricular rate
	Decrease	To assess underlying rhythm and dependency status, to adjust rate below angina threshold, to allow emergence of normal sinus rhythm and preservation of atrial transport, to test sensing function
Output	Increase	To adapt to pacing threshold
	Decrease	To test threshold for pacing, to conserve battery longevity according to threshold for pacing, to reduce extracardiac stimulation (pectoral muscle, diaphragm), to assess underlying rhythm and dependency status
Sensitivity	Increase (reduction of numerical value)	To sense low electrographic signals (P and QRS)
	Decrease (increase of numerical value)	To test sensing threshold, to avoid T-wave or afterpotential sensing, to avoid sensing extracardiac signals, e.g., myopotentials
Refractory period	Increase	To minimize farfield QRS sensing (AAI pacing), to minimize T-wave sensing (VVI pacing), to minimize afterpotential sensing
	Decrease	To maximize QRS sensing (VVI pacing), to detect early premature ventricular complexes
Hysteresis		To delay onset of ventricular pacing to preserve atrial transport function
Polarity	Conversion to unipolar mode	To amplify the signal for sensing in the presence of a low bipolar electrogram, to compensate temporarily for lead fracture in the other electrode
	Conversion to bipolar mode	To decrease electromagnetic or myopotential interference, to evaluate oversensing, to eliminate extracardiac anodal stimulation
Mode	VVT/AAT	To perform noninvasive electrophysiologic study and to terminate reentrant tachycardias (chest wall stimulation with external pacemaker), to prevent inhibition of unipolar pacemaker by extracardiac interference, to evaluate oversensing by "marking" sensed signals
	VOO/AOO	To prevent inhibition of pacemaker by interference (usually as a temporary measure) when triggered mode is not available or is undesirable

* Also applicable to dual-chamber pacemakers when each channel is considered individually.

pacing by 50 msec to produce basically the same effective A-V interval as that initiated by atrial sensing.[85] Abnormal depolarization from ventricular pacing results in an altered contraction pattern that can decrease LV function.[81,86,87] Consequently, one should try initially to program an A-V interval that allows spontaneous AV conduction and native ventricular activation (associated with increased battery longevity).[88] However, an excessively long A-V interval can be counterproductive. The optimal A-V interval can vary considerably from patient to patient and depends on many factors, including LV compliance, LV filling pressure, atrial size and contractility, mitral valve function, heart rate, and variability of the interatrial conduction time.[83,88,89] The optimal A-V interval can change with time due to progressive delay in interatrial conduction or changes in LV function.[90] Two-dimensional and Doppler echocardiography can be useful to optimize the A-V interval at rest and on exercise.

Programming a dual-chamber pacemaker to different modes may be necessary to respond to changing circumstances or complications. Chronic atrial fibrillation is the most important cause of change in the pacing mode to VVI(R) pacing. About 85 to 90 per cent of DDD and DDDR pulse generators should remain in the original programmed mode at 5 years because of improved atrial sensitivity, better leads, and increasing experience.[81,91–93] In the absence of automatic mode conversion or fallback (to a slower rate), the DDI or DDIR mode is useful in patients with atrial chronotropic incompetence and paroxysmal supraventricular tachyarrhythmias.[76] The VDD mode may be useful in patients with relatively normal atrial response to activity when atrial pacing is not functioning appropriately owing to a high pacing threshold or atrial lead displacement. If the VDD mode is not available, the DDD mode can be used with the atrial output turned off or programmed to the lowest value for subthreshold stimulation.

HEMODYNAMICS OF CARDIAC PACING

In a normal subject, increase in cardiac output with exercise is provided by a rate increase (300 per cent) with only a modest contribution from the increased stroke volume (50 per cent). Advancing age changes the relative contributions; however, increase in heart rate at age 70 still provides approximately two-thirds of the total increase in cardiac output with maximum exercise. Although patients with fixed-frequency pacing (VVI) may tolerate loss of AV synchrony, their effort tolerance is limited because in them cardiac output increase relies solely on an increase in stroke volume. This limitation is worse in patients with severe LV dysfunction because their stroke volume is fixed, making an increase in cardiac output dependent solely on rate augmentation.[94]

In the normal heart, AV synchrony at rest contributes about 20 to 30 per cent of the cardiac output. In some patients with congestive heart failure, atrial systole may contribute little to the resting cardiac output because of a substantial increase in LV filling pressure. However, such patients should not be denied AV sequential pacing; medical therapy can improve their ventricular performance, reduce LV filling pressure, and restore their responsiveness to the benefits of atrial systole. AV synchrony is quite important in patients with LV diastolic dysfunction (and normal systolic function), contributing 30 to 40 per cent to end-diastolic volume and cardiac output at rest. Loss of AV synchrony in such patients leads to marked reduction in cardiac output and produces serious hemodynamic changes, including pulmonary venous congestion. Consequently, AV sequential pacing should be used in all patients with LV diastolic dysfunction (aortic stenosis, hypertrophic cardiomyopathy, and LV hypertrophy secondary to hypertension).

Most studies showing the negligible contribution of AV synchrony during relatively high levels of exercise were conducted predominantly in patients with AV block, normal LV function, and devices with a fixed A-V interval.[81,83,95–97] It seems that AV synchrony is important at lesser levels of exercise, particularly in patients with borderline heart failure, LV dysfunction, or decreased LV compliance. The P-R interval normally shortens on exercise (4 to 5 msec/10 beats/min). Pacemakers designed with a rate-adaptive automatic shortening of the A-V interval on exer-

cise are associated with better exercise performance, especially if exercise is begun with the optimal A-V interval determined at rest.[98–101]

Many studies have shown that during exercise an increase in the pacing rate provided by VVIR, VDD, DDD, or DDDR modes increases the cardiac output and duration of exercise more than does fixed-frequency VVI pacing.[81,89,94] In addition to superior hemodynamic effects, an increase in maximum oxygen consumption, reduced AV oxygen difference, and an increase in subjective well-being result.[81,89] The hemodynamic advantage is retained on an ongoing basis, because studies have shown no difference between acute and long-term results. Furthermore, rate-adaptive pacemakers actually may lead to improved LV function over time.[81,94]

Pacemaker Syndrome

Pacemaker syndrome is a clinical constellation of signs and symptoms produced by adverse hemodynamic and electrophysiological responses to pacing because of inadequate timing of atrial and ventricular contractions.[81,102–106] During VVI pacing, the pacemaker syndrome most commonly occurs in patients with normal or near-normal LV function and retrograde VA conduction. Early reports suggested that during VVI pacing, only 15 per cent of patients with preserved VA conduction develop symptoms suggestive of the pacemaker syndrome, with about half exhibiting its full-blown form. Its true incidence now seems higher because about two-thirds of patients with dual-chamber pulse generators prefer the dual-chamber mode to the VVI mode.[77,107–112] Thus the obvious cases during VVI pacing represent the tip of a much larger "iceberg" of cardiac dysfunction, often with subtle, unrecognized manifestations. Indeed, "asymptomatic" patients often feel better when their VVI pacemaker is upgraded to a DDD system, suggesting the existence of a "subclinical" pacemaker syndrome.[77]

The prominent symptoms of the pacemaker syndrome are due mostly to reduction in cardiac output, hypotension (more pronounced in the upright position), and higher ventricular filling pressures,[104,105] but many patients have subtle manifestations. Symptoms include orthostatic hypotension (especially in the first few seconds of ventricular pacing taking over from normal sinus rhythm), syncope or near syncope (due to reduction in cerebral flow), fatigue, exercise intolerance, lightheadedness, malaise, weakness, lethargy, dyspnea, induction of congestive heart failure, cough, patient awareness of beat-to-beat variations of cardiac response (from spontaneous to paced beats), neck pulsations or pressure sensation or fullness in the chest, neck, or head, headache, chest pain, impaired exercise capacity, and disturbed mentation. Many nonspecific symptoms similar to those of the pacemaker syndrome are common in the elderly and complicate the diagnosis. Physical examination may show cannon waves in the jugular venous pulse and palpable liver pulsations.

MECHANISM. Loss of AV synchrony can decrease cardiac output by 20 to 30 per cent at rest, but hemodynamic compromise in the pacemaker syndrome is more complex because retrograde VA conduction causes a "negative atrial kick" with more profound hemodynamic disadvantage than simple loss of AV synchrony. Atrial contraction against closed mitral and tricuspid AV valves causes systemic and pulmonary venous regurgitation and congestion (cannon *a* waves), sometimes leading to the development of congestive heart failure in previously compensated patients. In addition to the marked reduction in cardiac output, retrograde VA conduction leads to atrial distension and activation of stretch receptors that produce a reflex vasodepressor effect mediated by the autonomic nervous system.[104,105] Thus, in the face of hypotension due to low cardiac output, compensatory mechanisms that ordinarily increase the peripheral resistance become attenuated. In some cases involving profound hypotension there can even be a net reduction in peripheral resistance, and for this reason, concomitant treatment of congestive heart failure with vasodilators can precipitate the pacemaker syndrome during VVI pacing.

The relatively small group of patients who have pacemaker syndrome without VA conduction often exhibit venous cannon *a* waves that probably initiate the same hemodynamic disturbance as retrograde VA conduction. Patients intolerant of VVI or VVIR pacing demonstrate increased variability of anterograde Doppler-determined left atrial flow during VVI compared with DDD pacing.[113] The precise role of atrial natriuretic peptide in the genesis of the pacemaker syndrome is unclear. The high atrial natriuretic peptide level may be a marker of the pacemaker syndrome rather than contributing to its pathophysiology.[114,115]

Implantation of a VVIR pacemaker (see below) does not protect the patient from retrograde VA conduction and the pacemaker syndrome. It can develop on exercise when sinus rhythm gives way to ventricular pacing in patients with atrial chronotropic incompetence. On exercise, VA conduction can persist, or if absent at rest, it can occasionally appear with exercise under the influence of catecholamines. Atrial-based pacemakers (single-lead atrial and dual-chamber) also can produce the pacemaker syndrome at rest and/or exercise whenever inappropriate programming and/or selection of the pacing mode result in "inadequate timing of atrial and ventricular contractions."[103] If left atrial activation is delayed, the programmed A-V interval may not provide adequate time for effective left atrial systole before LV systole, and in extreme cases, left atrial systole may actually begin after the onset of LV systole.[85,88,116] Simultaneous atrial pacing from the right atrial appendage and coronary sinus can restore optimal timing of left atrial and left ventricular systole in patients with severe interatrial conduction delay.[117,118] In patients with complete AV block, the pacemaker syndrome can occur in the DDI mode secondary to AV dissociation whenever the sinus rate exceeds the programmed lower rate.

MANAGEMENT. The pacemaker syndrome due to VVI (VVIR) pacing is an iatrogenic condition[106] and can be eliminated by restoring AV synchrony either with atrial pacing alone (if AV conduction is normal) or dual-chamber

pacing with an appropriate AV delay. Occasionally, restoration of AV synchrony during VVI pacing can be achieved by reducing the pacing rate (or using hysteresis) to minimize competition with sinus rhythm. At the time of pacemaker implantation, the lack of a drop in blood pressure with VVI pacing does not eliminate the potential for pacemaker syndrome.

Rate-Adaptive Pacemakers

Atrial chronotropic incompetence is the inability to increase the heart rate to appropriate levels that satisfy body needs. Guidelines such as the inability to achieve a heart rate exceeding 70 per cent of the maximum heart rate predicted for a given level of metabolic demand and the inability to reach a heart rate of 100/min on exercise provide practical definitions of atrial chronotropic incompetence. Testing can be by treadmill or long-term ambulatory ECG recordings during walking or ordinary activities. About 40 per cent of patients with sick sinus syndrome exhibit varying degrees of atrial chronotropic incompetence.[119] It is also found in some patients with AV block. The rate of a pacemaker can be designed to respond to the activity of a biological parameter that varies in parallel with the need for greater cardiac output. Such a rate-responsive system is called *rate-modulated, rate-adaptive,* or *sensor-driven* and is designated by the letter R in the fourth position of the pacemaker code, e.g., VVIR is a rate-adaptive ventricular demand pacemaker and DDDR is a rate-adaptive DDD device (Fig. 23–17). The magnitude and rate of change of the sensor-driven response are programmable. The ideal sensor should be stable, reliable long-term, and easy to implant, program, and troubleshoot. It also should respond in direct proportion to metabolic demand, use a standard lead, consume little battery current, be autoprogrammable, respond quickly, and decelerate gradually at the end of exercise. No existing single sensor satisfies all of these criteria.

Types of Rate-Adaptive Pacemakers

Of the many sensors in clinical use or investigation[120–122] (Table 23–5), currently approved devices in the United States respond to activity, minute ventilation, or temperature.

ACTIVITY-SENSING PACEMAKERS. This is the most commonly used system. It employs a piezoelectric sensor bonded to the inner surface of the pacemaker to detect

TABLE 23–5 CATEGORIES OF SENSORS FOR RATE-ADAPTIVE PACING

FUNCTIONAL-ORGANIC SOURCE	SIGNAL	SENSOR/METHOD OF DETECTION
1. Activity	Vibration generated by body movement	Piezoelectric
	Horizontal motion	Piezoelectric or silicone integrated accelerometer-accelerometric
	Vertical motion	Encapsulated mercury droplet gravimetric acceleration
2. Respiration	Respiratory rate	Transthoracic impedance
	Minute ventilation	Transthoracic impedance
3. Evoked (paced) parameters	Paced ventricular repolarization (Q-T interval)	Electrogram
	Paced ventricular depolarization integral*	Calculates area under the paced ventricular deflection electrogram
4. Hemodynamic parameters	Right ventricular pressure (dP/dt)	Piezoelectric crystal on ventricular lead tip
	Preejection interval	Intracardiac impedance and electrogram—onset of ventricular signal to beginning of ejection (preejection interval)
	Right ventricular volume	Intracardiac impedance—peak to peak voltage amplitude (relative stroke volume)
	Rate of change in right ventricular volume (dV/dt)	Intracardiac impedance (relative contractility)
5. Central venous blood	Temperature	Thermistor, electrical
	H+ ion concentration	pH, electrical
	O₂ saturation	Reflectance of blood

* Withdrawn as a single-sensor system but incorporated with minute ventilation in a dual-sensor system.
Adapted from Benedek, Z. M., Gross, J., Furman, S: Rate-modulated pacemakers. The Newspaper of Cardiology, April 1993, with permission.

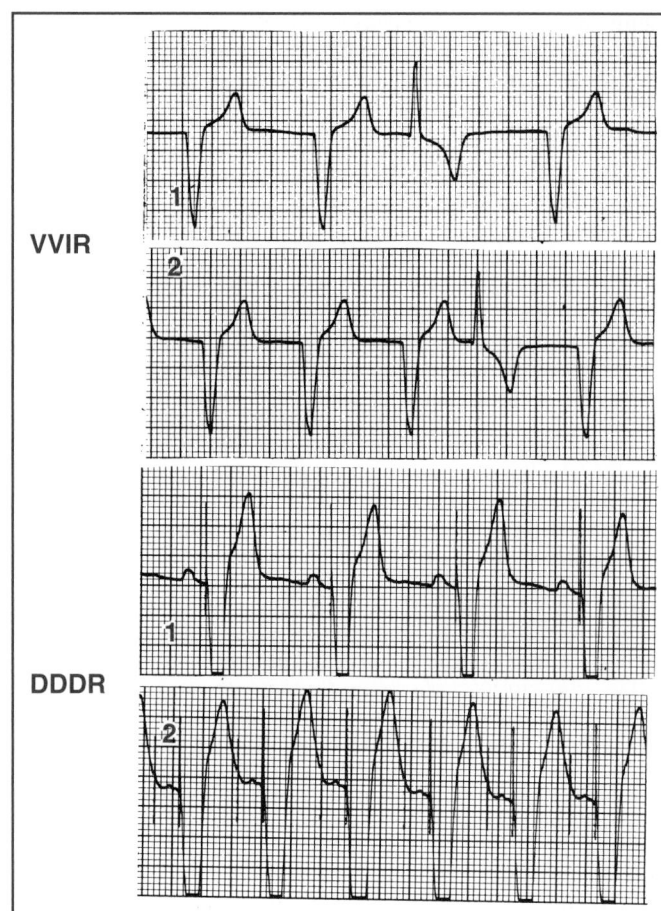

VVIR

DDDR

FIGURE 23–17.   Response of rate-adaptive VVIR and DDDR pacemakers to exercise. *Top,* VVIR. The tiny bipolar stimuli cannot be discerned. *Panel 1* shows pacing at the programmed lower rate interval (LRI) = 857 mscec (corresponding to a rate of 70/min). The third beat is a ventricular extrasystole sensed by the pacemaker. The escape interval is essentially equal to the automatic interval. *Panel 2* shows the response on exercise when the ventricular rate increases to about 88/min (sensor-driven interval = 680 msec) so that a sensed ventricular extrasystole now resets the pacemaker with an escape interval of about 680 ms. *Bottom panels,* DDDR. *Panel 1* shows DDD pacing with sensing of P waves (LRI = 1000 msec). In *panel 2* during exercise the AV sequential (Ap-Vp) pacing rate increases to 107/min (cycle length 560 msec). (Reproduced with permission from Barold, S. S., et al.: Pacing in the nineties: Technologic, hemodynamic and electrophysiologic considerations in the selection of the optimal mode of pacing. *In* Rackley, C. E. [ed.]: Challenges in Cardiology 1, Mt. Kisco, N.Y., Futura, 1992, p. 39.)

mechanical forces or vibrations (body movements but not myopotentials) that are transformed to electrical energy to control the pacing rate. The pacing rate is increased in proportion to the detected vibration. The sensor is nonmetabolic and therefore nonphysiological. It does not respond to an increase in metabolic demand such as with emotional stimuli that are unrelated to exercise. Nevertheless, it works well in practice. The system is simple, reliable, stable, easy to program, uses a standard lead, and exhibits a fast response to brief periods of exercise. The sensor is unaffected by drugs or disease. Its main advantage is the precise recognition of onset and end of exercise, an important characteristic in older patients who do not exercise much and do so primarily in short bursts of physical work such as walking or climbing stairs. Other sensor-driven systems that exhibit a delayed response at the onset of exercise and reach a maximum rate after the end of the exercise are less desirable for the elderly. Several disadvantages exist. Pacing rate plateaus after the initial increase despite continued exercise. The pacing rate depends on the type of activity and does not correlate with the level of exercise or the amount of work, particularly at high levels of exercise. Rate change does not occur during mental exercise, emotional stress, or isometric exercise. Physical pressure on the pacemaker such as lying on it can cause an inappropriate rate increase during sleep. Pacing rate may be slower when stairs are climbed compared with when they are descended. External vibrations such as occur when riding in a vehicle in rough terrain or in a train or a helicopter can increase the pacing rate. Generally, these aberrations are innocuous. To overcome the limitations of vibration-sensitive pacemakers, some manufacturers have replaced the activity sensor with an accelerometer (itself containing a piezoelectric crystal) integrated within the circuitry rather than on the inner surface of the device. Accelerometer-based pacemakers respond to changes (velocity) in motion (not deflections of the casing) and exhibit less susceptibility to environmental noise and more specificity than conventional activity sensors.[123–126]

OTHER TYPES OF SENSORS

RESPIRATORY-DEPENDENT PACEMAKER. The original system that measured only respiratory rate[127] has been supplanted by devices calculating minute ventilation volume (tidal volume × respiratory rate) derived from the transthoracic impedance. The system injects a small current between the pacemaker casing and the proximal electrode of a standard bipolar lead and determines impedance between the tip electrode and the pacemaker casing. The pacemaker ignores the impedance change related to stroke volume by appropriate filtering. The transthoracic impedance increases with inspiration and decreases with expiration, and its amplitude varies according to the tidal volume. The calculated minute ventilation volume (and the generated pacing rate) correlates closely with metabolic demand or workload. The system is highly physiological, reliable, and works well clinically.[128–130] Programming generally requires a treadmill stress test. Drawbacks include a delayed reaction to the onset and bursts of exercise (recently improved with new algorithms[131]), inappropriately fast rates after the end of exercise, additional battery current for sensor function that may reduce the life of the pulse generator, and excessive pacing rates in patients with tachypnea from congestive heart failure or other causes, as well as a response to swinging of the arms, shoulder movements, or coughing. Electrocautery can increase the sensor-driven rate to its upper limit.

TEMPERATURE-SENSING PACEMAKER. This pacemaker's operation is based on an increase in metabolic rate with activity that produces heat transported in the blood. A small thermistor totally incorporated into a special pacing lead can detect the rate of change of blood temperature (not the absolute value) in the right ventricle. A slow rise in central venous temperature as a result of fever, emotion, or high external temperature is generally disregarded by the pacemaker. A special algorithm compensates for the decrease in blood temperature at the onset of exercise as the cooler blood returns from the extremities. Temperature accurately reflects oxygen consumption in the middle and late stages of exercise. Thus, while central venous temperature correlates well with metabolic demand at high workloads, the rate response is insufficient at low workloads such as brief everyday activities because of the relatively slow and minimal increase in central venous temperature.[132] In some patients with congestive heart failure, a very gradual (slow) and prolonged temperature dip (due to sluggish flow of blood from extremities) early during exercise may cause a paradoxical drop in the pacing rate. Also, the heat-dissipation mechanism at the end of exercise is often impaired in patients with heart failure. The drawbacks of this system have made it far less popular than activity, minute ventilation, and Q-T sensors.

Q-T INTERVAL–SENSING PACEMAKER. This unipolar ventricular system operates on the principle that the Q-T interval shortens with physical exercise due to the release of catecholamines.[121,133–135] Mental stress also increases the pacing rate.[136] The Q-T system provides a stable, rugged sensor using a standard pacemaker lead. Its disadvantages include a relatively slow response, nonsustained rate changes, and some difficulty in ensuring reliable T-wave sensing, especially with chronic leads. Type 1A and 3 antiarrhythmic drugs and beta blockers may interfere with pacemaker response, while myocardial ischemia or infarction may cause an inappropriate increase in the pacing rate.

SENSOR COMBINATIONS. New generation devices utilize two non-atrial sensors to overcome the drawbacks (false-positive or false-negative response) of each sensor used alone. Data from the sensors are crosschecked to avoid an unphysiological response.[137–140] Activity sensors react quickly and, while nonspecific, are more suitable to determine the onset of exercise. An activity sensor can therefore be combined with another, more physiological but slower-reacting sensor. Such combinations include (1) activity and Q-T interval, (2) activity and minute ventilation volume, and (3) activity and temperature. The Q-T sensor is best suited for detection of increased catecholamine effect during emotional circumstances, but an increase in rate in this situation may constitute a disadvantage in some patients with heart disease. Experience with dual-sensor devices is limited, and their clinical superiority over single-sensor devices with refined algorithms and optimally programmed parameters has not yet been established. Some dual-sensor devices may not require more complex programming because they can adapt their rate response automatically by a process of "learning" according to memorized patterns of patient activity.[41]

PROGRAMMING RATE-ADAPTIVE PACEMAKERS. The rate-adaptive pulse generator should be programmed so that a casual 2- to 3-min walk increases the rate 10 to 25/min to about 90/min and a fast walk or stair climbing increases the rate 20 to 45/min to about 100 to 120/min.[142,143] Stress testing and Holter recordings can be useful to set appropriate functions, and telemetered paced-derived histograms can help assess rate response. Pacemaker function in elderly patients should be evaluated at low exercise loads to correspond with their activities of daily living and not with maximum exercise, which obviously represents an artificial situation. Overprogramming causes unpleasant palpitations with minimal effort. Very rapid rate increases and decreases generally should be avoided. Care should be taken that fast rates do not precipitate angina in patients with coronary artery disease, worsening of congestive heart failure, or hypotension in patients with cardiomyopathy or atrial or ventricular tachyarrhythmias.[144] In patients with bradycardia-tachycardia syndrome, the sensor-controlled upper rate of a DDDR device can be programmed to a faster value than the atrial controlled upper rate to prevent rapid paced ventricular rates from tracking of a supraventricular tachyarrhythmia.

EVOLVING SENSOR APPLICATIONS. These include (1) detection of unphysiological atrial rates (crosschecking) to activate a protective mechanism preventing rapid ventricular pacing as in automatic mode conversion, (2) automatic capture detection, e.g., presence or absence of a Q-T interval,[145,146] and (3) optimization of timing intervals such as AV delay or refractory periods to adjust the pacemaker to changing physiological circumstances.[140,147]

Selection of Pacing Mode

ATRIAL-BASED PACING. Atrial-based pacing is gaining popularity because atrial pacing and sensing are reliable on a long-term basis and atrial lead dislodgment is relatively rare. It can provide normal or near-normal hemodynamics at rest and on exercise with enhancement of quality of life and avoidance of pacemaker syndrome. Atrial and AV pacing are preferable to single-chamber ventricular pacing because they reduce the incidence of chronic (and perhaps paroxysmal) atrial fibrillation, particularly in patients with the bradycardia-tachycardia syndrome.[81,148–152] If supraventricular tachyarrhythmia recurs after pacemaker implantation, increasing the atrial pacing rate to 80/min may help. If not, antiarrhythmic drug therapy is indicated because poor arrhythmia control predisposes to systemic embolism. Atrial arrhythmias seem to respond better to antiarrhythmic agents in patients with atrial or dual-chamber pacemakers than in those with single-lead ventricular devices. Long-term anticoagulation should be strongly considered in pa-

tients with refractory paroxysmal atrial fibrillation (see p. 655). Atrial and AV pacing also decrease the risk of embolization and stroke, the incidence of congestive heart failure, and overall mortality,[81,148,151,153–158] especially in sick sinus patients older than 70 years.[148,151,154] Single-chamber ventricular pacing should therefore be avoided in most patients, especially those with sick sinus syndrome.

VVIR VERSUS DDD PACING. In patients with atrial chronotropic incompetence, maintenance of AV synchrony at rest in the DDD mode contributes more to quality of life than improved exercise tolerance in the VVIR mode.[159,160] Most patients spend their lives predominantly at rest, punctuated by relatively short periods of mild exercise during the course of the day when a moderate rate response would be clearly beneficial. In patients with complete AV block (normal atrial chronotropic function) and without significant LV dysfunction, VDD, DDD, and VVIR pacing provide almost the same degree of enhanced exercise performance.[95,161,162] Yet a substantial number of patients remain intolerant of VVIR pacing *at rest.*

VVIR VERSUS DDDR PACING. In patients with atrial chronotropic incompetence, the VVIR and DDDR modes are clearly superior to the DDD mode in terms of exercise performance because the sensor increases the pacing rate according to activity.[163,164] Many studies[98,112,165–169] (but not all[170,171]) of patients with atrial chronotropic incompetence and DDDR pulse generators have shown superior performance on exercise, improved sense of well-being, and patient preference of the DDDR mode compared with the VVIR mode. In some cases, patients describe a subjective improvement in their sense of well-being or quality of life and elimination of bothersome nonspecific symptoms when DDDR mode is used instead of the VVIR mode, even though the patients have no demonstrable objective improvement in functional exercise capacity.[112]

AAI AND AAIR PACING. In the United States, perhaps 1 per cent or less of patients requiring pacing receive a single-chamber atrial pacemaker. AAI and AAIR pacemakers are underutilized despite the wealth of information showing their superiority over VVI pacing in sick sinus patients without AV block.[62,149,150,172,173] The concern that patients with AAI (AAIR) pacemakers may develop AV block is largely unfounded. Second or third degree AV block has an annual incidence of about 1 per cent in carefully selected patients with AAI (AAIR) pacemakers, and its occurrence is rarely catastrophic and often related to drug therapy. Guidelines for selecting AAI or AAIR pacing include 1:1 AV conduction with atrial pacing to rates 120 to 140/min (despite its poor predictive value for the development of AV block), P-R interval ≤ 0.24 sec at rest, and absence of bundle branch block.[172–174] With careful patient selection, AAI or AAIR pacing could be used safely in probably 40 per cent of patients with sick sinus syndrome, and of these, about 40 per cent may require rate-adaptive devices (AAIR) because of atrial chronotropic incompetence.[94,119]

Individual Patient Considerations

When deciding the type of pacemaker to be used, the physician needs to determine whether the atrium can be paced and/or sensed, whether latent or overt AV block exists, and whether atrial chronotropic incompetence is present[175] (Fig. 23–18). The majority of patients with atria that can be paced and/or sensed should be considered for single-chamber atrial or dual-chamber pacing (AAI, AAIR, VDD, DDD, or DDDR) because VVI or VVIR pacing causes greater morbidity and mortality. Single-lead ventricular pacing should be reserved primarily for patients with chronic atrial fibrillation and AV block. A VVI pacemaker programmed to a low rate may be justified in the occasional patient with infrequent episodes of bradycardia. Replacement of a depleted VVI pacemaker with another VVI or VVIR unit is reasonable in many asymptomatic patients.

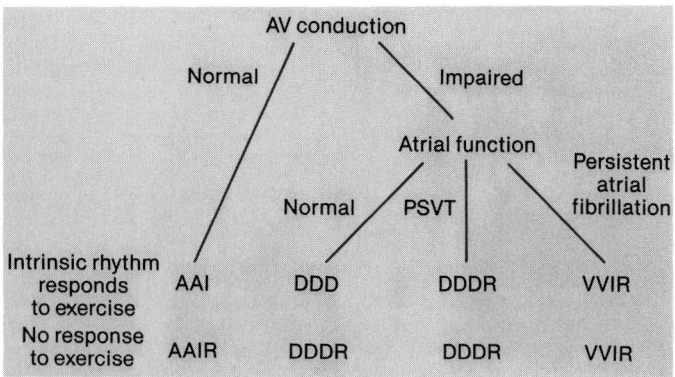

FIGURE 23–18. Algorithm for determining the optimal pacemaker mode for an individual patient. PSVT = paroxysmal supraventricular arrhythmias of all types including atrial fibrillation. A DDDR should be considered in patients with the bradycardia-tachycardia syndrome with intrinsic or drug-induced AV conduction delay to provide greater flexibility because (1) drug therapy of supraventricular tachyarrhythmias may further depress the atrial chronotropic response on exercise and (2) troublesome paroxysmal atrial tachyarrhythmias may necessitate programming to the DDIR mode or using a device with a fallback or automatic mode conversion mechanism to control the paced ventricular rate during supraventricular tachyarrhythmia. (From Griffin, J. C.: The optimal pacing mode for the individual patient: The role of DDDR. In Barold, S. S., and Mugica, J. [eds.]: New Perspectives in Cardiac Pacing 2, Mt. Kisco, N.Y., Futura, 1991, p. 325.)

Single-lead ventricular pacing is appropriate in patients who are incapacitated and inactive as well as those with a short life expectancy. VVIR does not improve survival when compared with the VVI mode.

It is important to assess what is best for the patient's level of activity, whether there is underlying coronary artery disease or LV dysfunction, what is affordable, what is the simplest system that will optimize hemodynamics, what is the natural history of the condition for which pacing is being used, and what is the impact of present and future drug therapy. Advanced age is not an indication for a simpler (and cheaper) VVI or VVIR system.[111,176,177] Active elderly patients benefit greatly from restoration of AV synchrony because the atrial contribution to cardiac output normally increases with advanced age. Dual-chamber pacemakers in the elderly appear cost-effective on a long-term basis by avoiding or reducing the complications associated with single-lead ventricular pacing.

Patients with angina pectoris generally tolerate DDD, DDDR, or VVIR modes better than the VVI mode, provided the upper rate is not excessively high. The increased MVO_2 related to rate increase on exercise is counterbalanced by the increase in MVO_2 during fixed-frequency VVI pacing, probably secondary to enhanced contractility (from increased sympathetic activity) and wall tension, which increase stroke volume.[178] The DDI or DDD mode with search hysteresis is preferred for carotid sinus hypersensitivity or neurally mediated syncope. For example, pacing might occur at a relatively fast rate of 100 beats/min when the spontaneous rate drops below a certain value such as 50 beats/min. After a given period of pacing, the pacemaker "searches" for the return of normal rhythm (>50 beats/min) by intermittent prolongation of one or more pacing intervals.[69] Pacing ceases if the spontaneous R-R interval is <1200 msec. This feature avoids continuation of pacing at 100 beats/min until it is inhibited by a spontaneous rhythm >100 beats/min, as with conventional hysteresis function. Patients with paroxysmal supraventricular tachyarrhythmias require a DDD or DDDR system with automatic mode conversion or fallback to slower paced ventricular rates to avoid tracking of unphysiological atrial rates. A single-lead VDD pacing system may provide a relatively simple and less expensive VDD/VVIR pacemaker for patients with AV block and normal atrial chronotropic function.[179–182]

Cost considerations aside, either a sensor-driven single-chamber or a sensor-driven dual-chamber pacemaker with extensive programmability of pacing modes would meet the needs of all patients given the high incidence of atrial chronotropic incompetence in the elderly and its progression or development over time.

COMPLICATIONS OF PACEMAKERS

Complications of venous entry, complications of lead placement and pocket formation, and electrical complications or pacemaker malfunction constitute three major groups of complications associated with permanent pacemaker implantation.

Complications of Lead Placement and Pocket Formation

Lead displacement can produce loss of pacing and/or sensing. Whereas myocardial perforation is rare with contemporary leads, it is more common with stiff temporary leads. Perforation may produce no symptoms or may cause intermittent or complete failure to pace and/or diaphragmatic pacing. A friction rub may be audible. If the lead has migrated to the left ventricle, paced beats can have a right bundle branch block contour in lead V_1. Echocardiography can be diagnostic. Although cardiac tamponade is rare, if it does occur, it is usually at the time of lead insertion and rarely after the first 24 hours; at this time, the lead may be withdrawn and safely repositioned under careful observation.

The incidence of symptomatic venous thrombosis is quite low despite the fact that contrast venography is abnormal in 30 to 45 per cent of patients, with total subclavian vein obstruction in 8 to 20 per cent. Subclavian venous obstruction probably occurs gradually, so the development of collaterals makes symptomatic obstruction rare. Should symptoms occur, treatment with anticoagulants is required for several weeks. Superior vena caval obstruction is a rare complication and has been treated successfully with thrombolytic agents, while superior vena caval stenosis has been treated successfully with balloon angioplasty alone or with stents.[183–186] Symptomatic pacemaker-related right atrial thrombus also can be treated with a thrombolytic agent.[187]

Contraction of the left diaphragm in synchrony with a paced stimulus can occur with or without lead perforation and is generally eliminated or minimized by programming the pacemaker output to a lower value. Contraction of the right diaphragm is due to phrenic nerve stimulation from a malpositioned right atrial electrode. Invariably, left intercostal muscle stimulation is due to lead perforation of the right ventricle. An insulation break causing a current leak either from the extravascular portion of the lead or the pulse generator can be associated with pectoral muscle twitching at or near the site of implantation. Some normally functioning unipolar pulse generators can cause pectoral muscle stimulation by the indifferent (anodal) plate without an insulation leak, particularly if the pacemaker has flipped over in a large pocket.

Twiddler's syndrome usually occurs when there is a relatively large pacemaker pocket and the patient repeatedly rotates the implanted pulse generator under the skin. The lead may retract from the heart to produce pacemaker failure. A pulse generator can erode through the skin or migrate, usually because of suboptimal implantation technique. Early infections are rare. *Staphylococcus aureus* is the most common offending organism in early infections, and *S. epidermidis* is most common in late infections. Transesophageal echocardiography may confirm vegetations related to a pacemaker lead.[188,189] The eradication of infection often requires removal of the entire pacing system, now feasible without thoracotomy with intravascular techniques that should be performed by an experienced operator because of the risk of bleeding, cardiac tamponade, and death.[190]

Pacemaker Malfunction

LOSS OF CAPTURE. The causes of loss of capture by visible pacemaker stimuli and pacemaker failure with no stimuli are listed in Table 23–6. Many of the abnormalities with visible stimuli are due to changes in the electrode-tissue interface that can be overcome by reprogramming or correcting any reversible metabolic or drug-related abnormalities[191] (Fig. 23–1). In some cases of chronic progressive increases in pacing threshold, lead replacement can be required. Absence of stimuli is often due to interruption of electric circuit with no current flow related to a broken electrode with intact insulation or less commonly due to pulse generator failure (battery component). Wire breakage is not always evident radiologically, while an insulation defect is not visible. A tight ligature on polyurethane leads can compress the insulation and spread the coil of wire without interfering with function, giving the appearance of a fracture (pseudofracture) radiologically.[192] A particular design feature without malfunction of one type of bifurcated bipolar lead resembles a pseudofracture.[192] Compression or distortion of the conductor coil identifies a point of stress on the lead.

ABNORMAL PACING RATE. A change in the pacing rate or erratic pacing can occur due to normal function (Table 23–7). Abnormal causes due to pacemaker malfunction are often found by exclusion. A constantly changing spike-to-spike interval during pacing often is caused by oversensing and/or a problem with the electrode rather than component failure. "Runaway pacemakers" with very rapid, life-threat-

TABLE 23–6 CAUSES OF LOSS OF CAPTURE BY VISIBLE PACEMAKER STIMULI AND LOSS OF PACING STIMULI

Loss of Capture

1. *Normal situation:* Stimuli in myocardial refractory period
2. *Electrode-tissue interface:* Early displacement or unstable position of pacing leads (most common cause); perforation (sometimes inapparent); malposition into coronary sinus or middle cardiac vein; elevated threshold (acute or chronic); inapparent displacement (exit block); subcutaneous emphysema (with loss of anodal contact of unipolar pacemakers), Twiddler's syndrome; myocardial infarction, elevation of pacing threshold after defibrillation or cardioversion; electrolyte abnormalities, e.g., hyperkalemia; drug toxicity, e.g., type 1A antiarrhythmic agents or drug effect, e.g., 1C antiarrhythmic agents (flecainide and propafenone)
3. *Electrode:* Fracture, short circuit, and insulation break
4. *Pulse generator:* Normally functioning pulse generator with inappropriate programming of output parameters, spontaneous pacemaker failure due to battery exhaustion or component failure, component failure from iatrogenic causes such as defibrillation, therapeutic radiation, and electrocautery

Loss of Pacing Stimuli

1. *Normal situation:* Total inhibition of pulse generator when the intrinsic rate is faster than the preset pacemaker rate.
2. *Hysteresis with normal function:* Escape interval > automatic interval
3. *Pseudomalfunction:* Overlooking tiny bipolar pacemaker stimuli in the ECG
4. *Lead:* Fracture, loose connection, or set screw problems
5. *Pulse generator:* Total battery depletion, component failure, sticky magnetic reed switch (application of magnet produces no effect). Subcutaneous emphysema (unipolar systems)
6. *Extreme electromagnetic interference*
7. *Oversensing* (signals originating from outside or inside the pulse generator)

TABLE 23–7 CAUSES OF CHANGES IN PACING RATE   727

Ch 23

Normal Function

1. Low programmed rate
2. Application of the magnet
3. Inaccurate speed of ECG machine drive
4. Apparent malfunction in special function pulse generators, e.g., triggered mode (AAT, VVT)
5. Reversion to interference rate (in response to electromagnetic or other signals) with either a faster or a slower rate than the spontaneous freerunning or magnet rate (according to manufacturer)

Abnormal Function

1. Battery failure (slowing of rate)
2. Runaway pacemaker: Spontaneous or due to therapeutic radiation or electrocautery
3. Component failure, e.g., erratic delivery of pacemaker stimuli; spontaneous or due to therapeutic radiation, electrocautery, or defibrillation
4. Permanent or temporary change in mode after therapeutic radiation, electrocautery, or defibrillation. If functionally reset from electromagnetic interference, the device can be reprogrammed to its original mode.
5. Phantom reprogramming (done without documentation), misprogramming
6. Oversensing

ening rates of stimulation are now rare but can still occur. At extremely rapid rates, stimulation is either ineffectual or can occur intermittently, producing bursts of tachycardia. This situation requires immediate disconnection and removal of the pacemaker.

UNDERSENSING. Low-amplitude electrograms and/or signals with a low slew rate (inappropriate frequency content) represent the most common cause of undersensing. An inadequate signal can be due to poor lead position at the time of implantation, lead displacement, or lead maturation with attenuation of a previously small but adequate electrogram. Lead dislodgment, low-amplitude signal from premature ventricular complexes, and myocardial infarction are common causes, often correctable by programming a higher sensitivity. Undersensing also can occur with component failure of a pulse generator, an abnormal (jammed) magnetic reed switch (that fails to restore sensing upon magnet removal), or inappropriate programming of sensitivity or refractory period. A DDD pacemaker will not sense an adequate ventricular signal falling within the blanking period designed to prevent crosstalk. Asynchronous pacing (noise mode) also can occur at a preset rate as a protective response to continually sensed interference. Insulation or wire fracture defects also can attenuate the effective electrogram detected by a pulse generator. Hyperkalemia, toxic effects of antiarrhythmic drugs (especially antiarrhythmic drugs in classes 1A and 1C) and cardioversion and defibrillation also can lead to transient undersensing. Oversensing of an extraneous signal that initiates a new refractory period can lead to undersensing if the electrogram falls within the refractory period initiated by the sensed extraneous event. Occasionally, oversensing can present only with undersensing when the relatively fast spontaneous rhythm precludes pacemaker pauses.

OVERSENSING. This is by far the most common cause of pacemaker pauses, i.e., failure of delivery of a ventricular pacemaker stimulus at the anticipated time according to the programmed automatic (escape) interval; its occurrence is confirmed by magnet-induced conversion to the asynchronous mode. Unwanted signals causing oversensing arise from several sources.[193] For example, atrial depolarization can be sensed during VVI pacing when the ventricular lead becomes displaced toward the RV inflow tract.

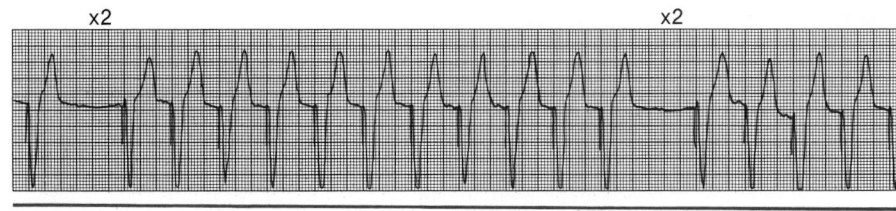

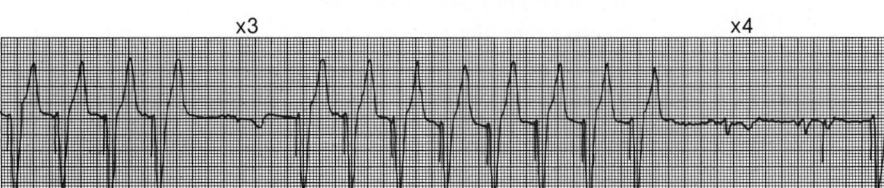

FIGURE 23–19. Electrocardiographic diagnosis of intermittent lead fracture or loose connection during VVI pacing. During spontaneous pacing an ECG (not shown) revealed intermittent pacemaker pauses of varying duration. The ECG shows asynchronous pacing at 100/min upon application of the magnet over the pulse generator. Wriggling the pulse generator in its pocket produces pauses that are exact multiples of the magnet interval (×2, ×3, and ×4) a response diagnostic of an intermittent electrode problem because it reflects the correct timing of a normally functioning pulse generator delivering its impulse into a transiently disrupted circuit with high impedance. (From Barold, S. S. et al.: Differential diagnosis of pacemaker pauses. *In* Barold S. S. [ed.]: Modern Cardiac Pacing. Mt. Kisco, NY, Futura Publishing Co., 1985, p. 592.)

Prevention of asystole requires magnet application or programming to the VOO or VVT mode. T-wave sensing often represents detection of the voltage at the electrode-myocardial interface generated by a pacemaker stimulus (discussed later) and the natural T wave and can be corrected by programming a lesser sensitivity and/or a longer pacemaker refractory period.

The pacing system itself can generate signals that are sensed and inhibit delivery of the pacemaker stimulus. For example, the electrode-tissue interface can act as a capacitor that generates voltage (polarization voltage or afterpotential) that is subsequently dissipated over a relatively long period. The decay of the "afterpotential" constitutes a time-changing voltage that can be sensed when the pacemaker refractory period terminates. Also, abrupt changes in resistance within a pacing system can produce corresponding voltage changes that generate signals often invisible on the surface ECG. Such "make-break," or false, signals can occur from loose connections, wire fractures with intermittent contact, short circuits, insulation defects, or the interaction of two pacemaker catheters lying side by side and touching each other within the heart.

Intermittent electrode problems, especially oversensing due to an intermittent fracture, constitute the "great imitator" in cardiac pacing and often cause a chaotic pattern of pacing. Indeed, erratic behavior with pauses of varying lengths suggests a defective lead system rather than pacemaker component malfunction. False signals tend to occur at random, producing inhibition of stimuli for relatively long and constantly changing periods. Magnet application eliminates only pauses caused by oversensing. The demonstration of pacemaker pauses that are exact multiples of the *magnet* interval during asynchronous pacing is virtually diagnostic of an intermittent wire fracture (or electrode problem) (Fig. 23–19). Sometimes this irregularity can be demonstrated only by wriggling the pacemaker in its pocket.

Oversensing skeletal muscle potentials (myopotential interference) remains the most common cause of pacemaker pauses and occurs almost invariably with unipolar pulse generators[194–196] (Fig. 23–20). Although myopotential interference can be demonstrated in as many as 50 per cent of patients with unipolar pulse generators, only 10 per cent report symptoms and require pacemaker reprogramming.[194] Oversensing of diaphragmatic potentials on deep inspiration is uncommon and associated with short pauses. The

incidence of myopotential interference has remained unchanged over the last 25 years because absolute discrimination between the cardiac electrogram and myopotentials is difficult. The problem will disappear as bipolar systems eventually replace unipolar ones. In the meantime, myopotential oversensing can be corrected by reducing the input sensitivity, converting to the triggered VVT (AAT) or VOO (AOO) mode, programming from unipolar to bipolar sensing, and rarely, pacemaker replacement. In the DDD mode, myopotential oversensing by the atrial channel can result in rapid paced ventricular rates.

INTERFERENCE

Transthoracic cardioversion or defibrillation delivers a large amount of energy to the heart. Circuitry designed to protect the pulse generator shunts energy to the lead. Contemporary pulse generators, especially unipolar systems, are more susceptible than in the past to disturbance from this type of electric discharge.[197,198] The shock can damage circuitry, with partial or complete destruction of the pulse generator, which can result in a runaway state, induction of end-of-life behavior, and reversible or irreversible alteration of the microprocessor program. It also can cause an acute, temporary (usual), or chronic increase in the pacing threshold, probably due to myocardial burns; undersensing abnormalities, usually temporary but sometimes lasting as long as 10 days; reprogramming to another mode, even with different parameters; and reset to the VOO or VVI mode (with change of polarity from bipolar to unipolar in some designs) in response to high-level interference. A reset pacemaker returns to normal when reprogrammed.

Similar problems can occur from discharge of an implanted cardioverter-defibrillator.[199] Patients with an implanted cardioverter-defibrillator (ICD) should receive a dedicated bipolar pacing system that can be reset only to the bipolar VVI or VOO mode because large unipolar stimuli can interfere with sensing of ventricular fibrillation by an ICD. While thermal electrical burns at the electrode-myocardial interface can theoretically precipitate ventricular fibrillation, this has not yet been clearly documented in humans with external shocks. Paddles or patches for cardioversion must be placed well away from the pacemaker along a line perpendicular to the axis of the ventricular lead inside the heart, as with anterior and posterior paddles.

ELECTROCAUTERY. This is the most common form of interference in the hospital environment.[198] Apart from the expected response during its application (temporary inhibition, reversion to asynchronous interference mode, or reset to the VVI or VOO mode as a normal response to high-intensity interference), electrical and thermal burns at the electrode-myocardial interface can cause ventricular fibrillation or chronic elevation of pacing thresholds. Damage to a pulse generator can result with permanent loss of output, runaway behavior, random failure, and reprogramming. Application of the magnet over the pulse generator or programming to an asynchronous mode may prevent oversensing but does not protect the pacemaker from irreversible malfunction. During electrocautery, patients must be managed according to a careful protocol, with pacemaker testing before and after the procedure. Radiofrequency catheter ablation of arrhythmias potentially can cause similar disturbances of pacemaker behavior and can produce upper-rate pacing in a minute ventilation–driven DDDR pacemaker.[198]

RADIATION THERAPY. This can damage pacemaker electronics and cause unpredictable transient or permanent malfunction including unaway behavior. The effect is cumulative and similar whether the dose is given at one time or spread over several treatments. Given a sufficiently high cumulative absorbed dose, all pulse generators will fail catastrophically.[199–202] Appropriate shielding of the pulse generator during radiation therapy is mandatory. Barring reset and other responses related to sensing electromagnetic interference, malfunc-

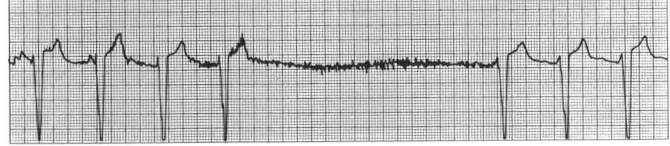

FIGURE 23–20. Prolonged inhibition of unipolar VVI pacemaker (rate = 70 ppm) from myopotential oversensing.

tion requires pacemaker replacement because long-term reliability becomes questionable.

MAGNETIC RESONANCE IMAGING (MRI). This can cause rapid pacing, inhibition, resetting of DDD pulse generators, and transient reed switch malfunction with asynchronous pacing. MRI is generally contraindicated in patients with pacemakers.[199,203,204] Serious malfunction with no output or rapid pacing may occur because pulsed energy from MRI can enter the lead by capacitive coupling and cause rapid ventricular pacing. Permanent component damage has not been reported. When an MRI is considered absolutely essential, it is reasonable to program the pacemaker to its lowest voltage and pulse width or to the OOO mode, provided the patient has an adequate underlying rhythm.[191]

Pacemaker Follow-up

Despite the reliability of modern pacemakers, a follow-up program is mandatory because complications are not uncommon and pacemaker failure is ultimately inevitable. Good follow-up should provide improved pacemaker longevity by appropriate programming and should identify impending pacemaker failure in most instances. The frequency and type of follow-up depend on the projected battery life, type, mode, and programming of pulse generators, the stability of pacing and sensing, the need for programming changes, the underlying rhythm (pacemaker dependency), travel logistics, and the use of alternative methods of follow-up such as the telephone.[205]

Transtelephonic pacemaker monitoring is the simplest method of pacemaker follow-up, and its main function is to detect changes in pacemaker rate as an indirect reflection of battery depletion.[205,206] Transtelephonic monitoring should complement and not replace comprehensive follow-up and is generally used to document satisfactory pacing function between visits. Transtelephonic monitoring usually is performed every 2 to 3 months until the first indication of battery depletion, when it may be performed once a month. The ECG is recorded with and without magnet placement. Free-running and magnet intervals and pulse width are measured. In dual-chamber pacemakers, rate and pulse widths are measured along with the A-V interval. Complex ECGs from DDD pulse generators transmitted by phone are often uninterpretable. As a rule, transtelephonic follow-up does not allow programming or transmission of telemetered data.

When the patient is discharged after pacemaker implantation, the pulse generator is programmed to optimize function during the expected physiological changes in the early phase. The patient should be seen about 2 weeks after implantation, when the operative site is also inspected. The pacing system is evaluated 2 months after implantation, when pacing and sensing thresholds have stabilized, and in virtually all patients, definitive programming can be performed for long-term function. Follow-up in the clinic should be done every 6 to 12 months for single-chamber and every 3 to 6 months for dual-chamber pacemakers. The complexity of contemporary pacemakers requires meticulous record keeping (Table 23–8). Periodic transtelephonic pacemaker monitoring should supplement these visits. More frequent follow-up can become necessary when impending battery depletion is detected.

Pacemaker follow-up requires equipment such as a multichannel ECG machine, magnet, digital counter for interval measurement, programmers, temporary pacemaker and chest electrodes for chest wall stimulation, Doppler echocardiography, long-term ECG recorders, closed-loop event recorders, and equipment for cardiopulmonary resuscitation. First, a 12-lead ECG is obtained with and without application of the magnet. Various intervals (lower rate, pulse width, and so on) are measured with an electronic counter. If telemetry is available, the pulse generator is interrogated to document initial pacemaker parameters. The following aspects of pacemaker function are then evaluated systematically.

Battery voltage can be evaluated directly by telemetry or

TABLE 23–8 DATA REQUIRED IN PACEMAKER CHART 729

Ch 23

Pacemaker data: Date(s) of implant(s), model and serial number of pacemaker lead(s), model and serial number of pulse generator

Data from implant: Indication, pacing threshold(s), sensing threshold(s), intracardiac electrograms, lead impedance(s), presence of retrograde ventriculoatrial (VA) conduction, presence of diaphragmatic or accessory muscle stimulation at 5- and 10-V output, chest x-ray soon after implantation

Technical specifications: Pacemaker behavior in the magnet mode, record of elective replacement indicator, magnet and/or freerunning rate, mode change, telemetered battery data (impedance and voltage)

Data from pacemaker clinic: Programmed parameters from time of implant and most recent changes, 12-lead ECG and long rhythm strips showing pacing and inhibition of pacing (if possible) to determine underlying rhythm (by programming very low output, OOO mode, low rate or with chest wall stimulation). Degree of pacemaker dependency. 12-lead ECG on application of the magnet. Rhythm strip of magnet mode for at least 1 min. Electronic rate intervals and pulse widths freerunning and upon application of the magnet before programming. Interrogation and printout of telemetry, e.g., memory or programmed and real-time data.

Systematic evaluation of pacing system: Atrial and/or ventricular pacing and sensing thresholds documented by rhythm strip. Retrograde ventriculoatrial conduction and propensity to endless loop tachycardia in dual chamber systems. Crosstalk in dual chamber systems. Myopotential interference (record best way of reproducing abnormality). Printouts showing pacemaker function when a parameter is programmed. Evaluation of atrial chronotropic response. Evaluation of sensor function with exercise protocols. Histograms or other data to demonstrate heart rate response in the rate-adaptive mode. Efficacy of rate-adaptive parameters. Response to onset and cessation of exercise. Doppler echocardiography to optimize AV interval (rest and exercise). Final telemetry printout at end of pacemaker evaluation and date. Check that any changes in parameters are intentional by comparing the final parameters with those obtained at the time of initial pacemaker interrogation.* Any discrepancy must be justified in the record.

Ancillary data: Symptoms and potential problems, e.g., accessory muscle stimulation. ECG with event marker recorders, telemetered electrogram and diagnostic diagrams. Holter recordings. Transtelephonic data. Special functions such as automatic PVARP extension, tachycardia terminating algorithms, automatic mode conversion, etc. Intolerance of VOO pacing on application of magnet.

* In one system an arrow points to a parameter when its final programmed value differs from the value at the initial interrogation.

indirectly. When it reaches a critical level, the elective replacement indicator (ERI) is activated, and the pacing rate in the free-running and/or magnet mode slows. This change can be gradual or stepwise (sudden). The ERI of some DDD pulse generators consists of reversion to a simpler VVI or VOO mode to reduce current drain from the battery. Approximately 6 months exist between activation of the ERI and the dangerous end-of-life state. Ventricular pacing is documented from the control ECG and the ECG after application of the magnet. Ventricular pacing threshold is best determined in the VVI mode (or DDD with short A-V interval to ensure ventricular capture) by programming voltage and/or pulse width until capture is lost. Ventricular sensing is also best confirmed in the VVI mode by reducing the pacing rate to allow the spontaneous rhythm to emerge. The ventricular sensing threshold can be determined by decreasing the ventricular sensitivity gradually until sensing failure occurs.

In patients with dual-chamber pacemakers, provided there is an underlying ventricular rhythm, using the AAI or AOO mode at various rates confirms atrial capture (Fig. 23–21). If a paced P wave is not visible with double stan-

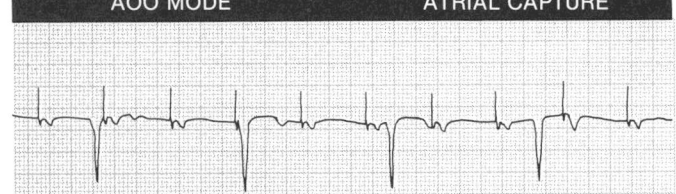

FIGURE 23–21. Determination of atrial capture in a patient with a DDD pulse generator and complete AV block. The pulse generator was first reprogrammed to the VVI mode and the rate was gradually decreased to 30/min, whereupon a ventricular escape rhythm at a rate of 45/min emerged. The pulse generator was then programmed to the AOO mode at a rapid rate. The atrial stimuli dissociated from the QRS complex demonstrate successful atrial capture. This maneuver is contraindicated in pacemaker-dependent patients.

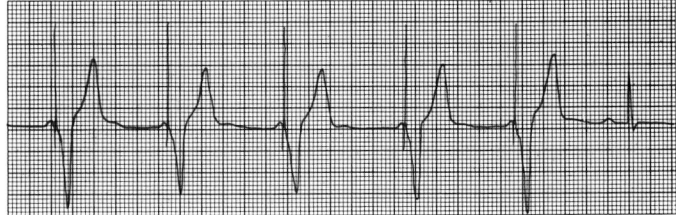

FIGURE 23–22. Semiquantitative assessment of atrial signal amplitude by programming the sensitivity of a DDD pulse generator. To demonstrate atrial sensing, the pulse generator was programmed to a lower rate of 50 ppm and AV = 50 msec. With an atrial sensitivity of 1.2 mV, all the P waves were sensed (not shown). At an atrial sensitivity of 1.6 mV, the tracing shows intermittent failure of atrial sensing (last P wave, i.e., if it had been sensed the ventricular stimulus would have occurred near the apex of the P wave). In this case, the lowest sensitivity (corresponding to the highest numerical value) causing consistent P wave sensing was 1.2 mV. Consequently, the atrial sensitivity should be programmed to 0.6 mV.

dardization of the ECG and/or lengthening of the A-V interval, echocardiography or esophageal electrocardiography can be used to document atrial systole. Alternatively, evaluation of atrial capture can be determined by competitive atrial pacing in the DVI mode at a slow rate. Evaluating atrial sensing is extremely important because atrial undersensing is one of the most common problems in DDD pacing. To evaluate atrial sensing, the pacemaker lower rate should be reduced below that of spontaneous atrial activity and the AV delay shortened to 50 to 100 msec to guarantee that any sensed P wave will trigger a ventricular stimulus. Atrial sensing can be assessed by decreasing the atrial sensitivity from the lowest numerical value (or most sensitive) to the highest numerical value (or least sensitive) until P wave tracking is lost (Fig. 23–22). The final programmed value should be double the atrial sensing threshold (half the numerical value). Telemetry, when available, provides proof of atrial sensing and its exact timing by transmitted event markers (Fig. 23–23). Random rather than sustained loss of atrial sensing is not uncommon in Holter recordings but rarely is of any clinical significance. Changes in body position, respiration, congestive heart failure, and exercise may alter the amplitude of the P-wave signal and affect atrial sensing.

Myopotential interference in unipolar pulse generators should be evaluated routinely with isometric exercise and 24-hour Holter recordings. In DDD pacing, myopotential interference can inhibit the ventricular channel (Fig. 23–20),

can increase the ventricular pacing rate when the atrial channel senses myopotentials (Fig. 23–16), can cause the pacemaker to revert to the asynchronous interference mode at a predetermined rate, and can activate the ventricular safety pacing mechanism.

Evaluating retrograde VA conduction is important in patients prone to development of endless-loop tachycardia. Susceptibility to crosstalk should be determined as previously discussed.

Telemetry is an indispensable feature of contemporary pulse generators and provides information on all programmed values as well as real-time or measured data on how the pacemaker is operating at the time of interrogation. These data include information on the output circuit, battery parameters, sensor activity for rate-adaptive pacemakers, event markers, and transmission of electrograms. Telemetered battery voltage and impedance correlate with battery depletion. Pacing impedance reflects lead integrity. Telemetry also provides diagnostic data about the interaction between the pulse generator and the patient over an extended period of time. Cumulative totals of sensed and paced events are useful in programming the pacemaker.

Advanced telemetry systems can memorize the occurrence and duration of certain arrhythmias and document

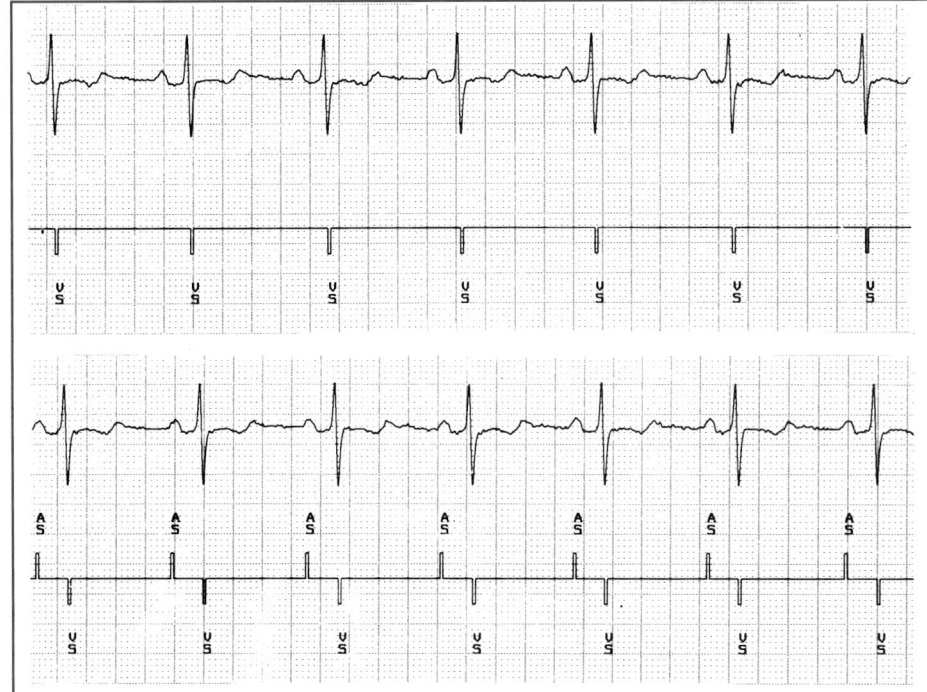

FIGURE 23–23. ECGs with annotated marker channel during DDD pacing. As = atrial sensed event; Vs = ventricular sensed event. Lower rate interval = 1200 msec, A-V delay = 200 msec after atrial sensing and atrial pacing, atrial escape interval = 1000 msec. *Top,* The marker channel shows appropriate inhibition of ventricular stimulation by sensed ventricular depolarizations (Vs). There is loss of atrial sensing because there are no markers consistent with atrial sensing. *Bottom,* The atrial sensitivity was increased and atrial sensing was restored. In the top panel the atrial stimulus is inhibited because the Vs-Vs interval is shorter than the atrial escape interval; i.e., Vs resets the atrial escape interval and the lower rate interval continually.

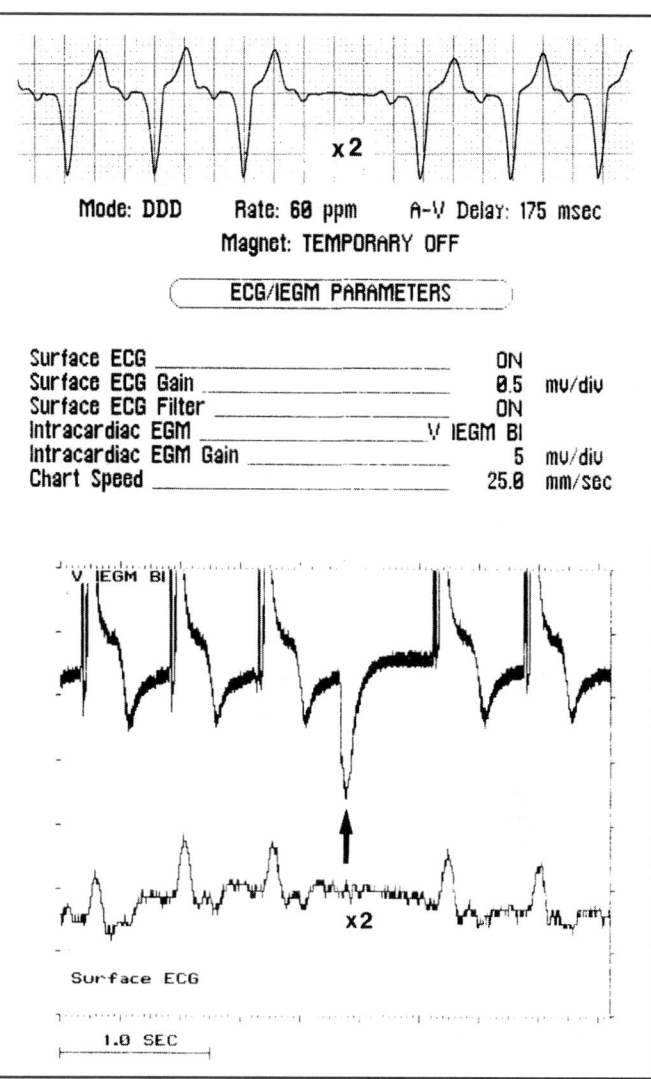

Mode: DDD   Rate: 60 ppm   A-V Delay: 175 msec

Magnet: TEMPORARY OFF

ECG/IEGM PARAMETERS

Surface ECG _____ ON

Surface ECG Gain _____ 0.5   mv/div

Surface ECG Filter _____ ON

Intracardiac EGM _____ V IEGM BI

Intracardiac EGM Gain _____ 5   mv/div

Chart Speed _____ 25.0   mm/sec

V IEGM BI

x2

Surface ECG

1.0 SEC

FIGURE 23–24. *Top,* DDD pacing with intermittent inhibition of the ventricular channel by false signals caused by defective lead insulation. The tiny bipolar stimuli are not discernible. A-V delay = 175 msec. The pacemaker senses the P wave and triggers an appropriate ventricular stimulus. Oversensing of a false signal from an intermittent insulation defect causes a pause (x2) exactly double the duration of the undisturbed Vp-Vp interval during 1:1 atrial tracking.

Bottom, Simultaneous recording of telemetered bipolar ventricular electrogram (V IEGM BI) and surface ECG. The ventricular electrogram registers a false signal (arrow) generated by the insulation defect. The signal measures approximately 10 mV. and is invisible on the surface ECG. The ventricular channel senses the false signal and inhibits the release of Vp. The prolonged Vp-Vp interval is an exact multiple of the atrial-driven Vp-Vp interval because timing of the P wave or sinus rhythm remains undisturbed. In contrast, during continual AV sequential (Ap-Vp) pacing (without magnet application), oversensing of a false signal produces pauses that are not multiples of the Vp-Vp interval because the timing of Ap (terminating the atrial escape interval) depends on the timing of the false signal that initiates the atrial escape interval. (Compare with Fig. 23–19.)

the time and duration of changes in pacemaker function such as automatic mode conversion in response to supraventricular tachyarrhythmias. Event markers depicting pacing and sensing are recorded simultaneously with the ECG and permit real-time evaluation of the pacing system and facilitate troubleshooting (Figs. 23–7A, 23–12, 23–14 to 23–16, and 23–23). Although the actual sensed signal cannot be identified, event markers indicate how the pacemaker interprets a specific paced or sensed event and provide precise representation of timing intervals. While the telemetered endocardial electrogram is generally less useful than event markers, it may demonstrate the nature of a malfunction caused by lead displacement or fracture, un-

dersensing due to a poor signal, or oversensing, especially when the nature of the signal cannot be determined from the ECG (Figs. 23–12 and 23–24). The telemetered atrial electrogram or atrial event markers can easily document the existence of retrograde VA conduction and its precise duration (Fig. 23–14). In the future, replay of stored electrograms will improve the diagnosis of arrhythmias and pacemaker malfunction.

Finally, long-term ECG recordings help to investigate pacemaker function and the significance of syncope, dizziness, and palpitations.[207] Syncope in pacemaker patients is often due to causes other than pacemaker malfunction.[207,208]

ELECTRICAL DEVICES
TO TREAT TACHYCARDIAS

Electric devices can be used to treat tachycardias by preventing the tachycardia onset or terminating the tachycardia after it has developed. Techniques to prevent tachycardia onset are applicable to a very small number of patients and include pacing at normal or increased rates to suppress bradycardia-dependent tachyarrhythmias such as torsades de pointes associated with a long Q-T syndrome (see p. 685). In the absence of bradycardia, an increase in pacing

rate rarely successfully suppresses refractory ventricular tachyarrhythmias chronically. Dual-chamber pacing with a short A-V interval can prevent some AV nodal or AV reciprocating tachycardias, and rapid continuous atrial pacing can be used to produce a fast atrial tachycardia with a high degree of AV block to override a slower atrial tachycardia associated with a faster ventricular rate, but ablative cures are preferable.

SUPRAVENTRICULAR TACHYCARDIA. Rapid pacing and/or premature stimulation can be used to terminate AV nodal and AV reciprocating tachycardias, atrial flutter, and some atrial tachycardias. Automatic tachycardia-terminating pacemakers are no longer popular for most patients with supraventricular tachycardias because ablation procedures can be curative (see p. 621). Only when drug therapy is ineffective or not tolerated and the patient has undergone an unsuccessful curative procedure or refuses to have it should an antitachycardia pacemaker be considered. Considering the fact that catheter ablative therapy and surgery successfully eliminate AV nodal and AV reentry in over 95 per cent of patients with a mortality close to zero, success rates of antitachycardia pacing are not impressive.

IMPLANTABLE CARDIOVERTER-DEFIBRILLATORS (ICDs)

Table 23–9 outlines the indications for ICD implantation. These guidelines are more liberal than those drawn up in 1991 by two separate task forces before the general availability of third-generation transvenous ICDs.[21,209] The efficacy of antitachycardia pacing for ventricular tachycardia (VT) termination by an easily implantable transvenous device with backup defibrillation has encouraged the use of ICDs often as first-line therapy for hemodynamically tolerated VT with or without antiarrhythmic agents. ICDs are powered by lithium silver vanadium pentoxide cells and have decreased in weight and volume from 250 to 280 gm (150 cm³) to 132 gm (83 cm³), and future devices will soon be 60 cm³.

While longevity varies depending on the use of the ICD in an individual patient, it is in the range of 4 to 5 years with the ability to deliver about 300 shocks. ICDs utilize a hierarchical approach to the treatment of VT with multiprogrammable tiered therapy (antitachycardia pacing, low-energy cardioversion, defibrillation, and backup VVI pacing) together with advanced diagnostic and telemetry function and the capability of testing therapy through noninvasive programmed stimulation by the induction of VT and ventricular fibrillation (VF)[210–212] (Fig. 23–25). The maximum output is usually delivered for defibrillation when synchronization of the shock is not necessary. Therapy can be programmed to escalate from pacing to low-energy synchronized cardioversion to high-energy defibrillation, depending on the arrhythmia and the patient's response. Energy of the shocks is programmable, generally 0.1 to 35 or 40 J. The number of consecutive cycles before tachycardia recognition is programmable, and therefore the time to respond with therapy, is variable. Charging to about 30 J takes 5 to 15 seconds (depending on circumstances). The number of times the device retries therapy is programmable. For VF, if the first shock fails, the device will recharge and deliver up to three to six additional shocks according to the manufacturer. In early "committed" ICDs, delivery of therapy occurred despite spontaneous termination of arrhythmia during capacitor charging. Such a response can cause unnecessary shocks that may occasionally induce VT or VF (device proarrhythmia). To prevent shocks for nonsustained arrhythmias, newer devices are "uncommitted." A "second look" confirms that the arrhythmia is still present during capacitor charging and immediately before the shock is to be delivered. A shock is therefore aborted if an arrhythmia terminates spontaneously.

ARRHYTHMIA SENSING. ICDs contain complex sensing circuitry that permits reliable sensing of small signals during VF without oversensing in normal sinus rhythm.[213,214] ICDs are biased for high detection sensitivity (rather than specificity). Most commonly, rate only (for a programmable duration) is used for VT and VF detection. Rate sensing

TABLE 23–9 INDICATIONS FOR ICDs

ICD Implantation Generally Indicated

1. Patients with hypotensive ventricular tachycardia (VT) or ventricular fibrillation (VF) not associated with acute ischemia/infarction, severe electrolyte imbalance, or drug toxicity in whom EP-guided therapy or ambulatory monitoring cannot be used to accurately predict efficacy of therapy (e.g., in patients in whom VT/VF is noninducible during EP testing, patients with nonischemic cardiomyopathy) and in patients who remain at high risk despite guided antiarrhythmic drug therapy (e.g., patients with severe left ventricular dysfunction).

2. VF or hypotensive VT with contraindications to drug or surgical therapy (including drug intolerance and noncompliance).

3. Persistently inducible clinically relevant VT or VF during EP testing despite drug therapy, corrective surgery, or catheter ablation.

4. Recurrent episodes of spontaneous VT or VF despite EP- or Holter-guided antiarrhythmic drug therapy.

5. Unexplained syncope in a patient with hypotensive VT inducible during EPS with characteristics 1, 2, or 3 above.

6. Highly symptomatic long Q-T interval syndromes despite medical therapy (with or without permanent pacemaker implantation).

ICD Implantation an Option but No Medical Consensus

1. Hypotensive VT or VF in a patient in whom serial drug testing is possible but ICD implantation is preferred over drug/ablative therapy.

2. Inducible nonclinical VT following drug, ablative, or surgical therapy in high-risk patients.

3. VT/VF apparently controlled by drug, surgical, or ablative therapy in a patient in whom the longterm efficacy of such treatment is unknown (e.g., hypertrophic cardiomyopathy).

ICD Implantation Generally Not Indicated

1. Frequent recurrent (e.g., daily) or incessant VT or VF.

2. VT or VF attributable to acute ischemia/infarction, severe electrolyte imbalance, drug toxicity or other reversible causes.

3. Recurrent syncope of undetermined etiology without inducible VT/VF during EP testing.

4. VF secondary to atrial fibrillation in the Wolff-Parkinson-White syndrome.

5. Hemodynamically significant VT/VF in a patient with limited life expectancy (< 6 months). This may include patients with Class IV heart failure who are not heart transplant candidates.

6. Surgical, medical, or psychiatric contraindications.

Reproduced with permission from Roelke, M., O'Nunain, S., Ruskin, J. N.: Implantable cardioverter-defibrillator: A clinician's guide to patient and device selection, The Newspaper of Cardiology, Sept/Oct 1994.

alone is quite sensitive but not specific because therapy can be delivered for supraventricular tachycardia when the rate exceeds the programmed upper rate cutoff (Fig. 23–26). Some ICDs possess a rate or interval *stability* criterion that defines how widely the R-R interval can vary and still be sensed as VT or VF. This feature improves device diagnosis of atrial fibrillation and can prevent unnecessary shocks.[215] A less helpful feature is the *sudden onset* criterion to differentiate the sudden onset of a high-rate VT from the more gradual increase in ventricular rate with sinus tachycardia. These and other measures to improve specificity must be used with care because they reduce the sensitivity of the detection algorithm.[216] Spurious shocks due to supraventricular tachyarrhythmias remain an important problem. Future ICDs will incorporate improved

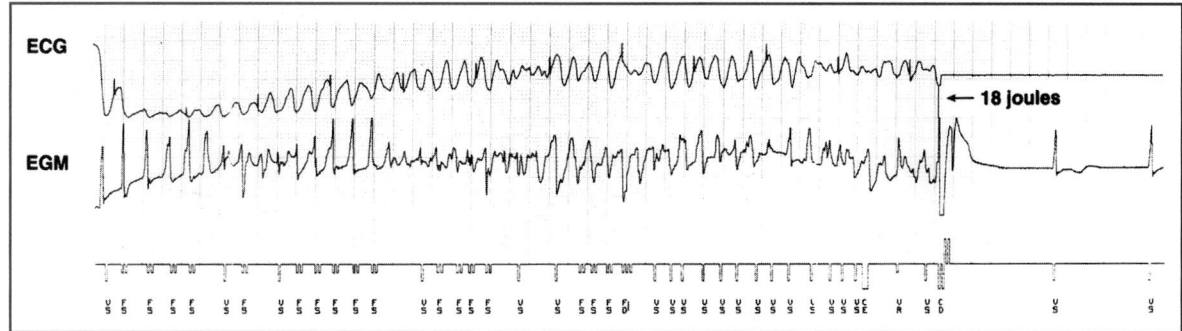

FIGURE 23–25. Termination of ventricular fibrillation by ICD. Scalar ECG and intracavitary electrogram record ventricular fibrillation. Marker channel senses fibrillation (FS) for most, but not all, impulses. Only 75 per cent of the intervals need to be counted for device diagnosis of ventricular fibrillation. Defibrillation (CD) is accomplished with an 18-J shock.

electrogram recognition and an atrial lead for better diagnosis of arrhythmias (also for atrial pacing and/or atrial defibrillation), and biosensors will provide on-line hemodynamic monitoring to better detect life-threatening arrhythmias.[217–219]

ICD Implantation

THORACOTOMY IMPLANTATION. ICDs were originally implanted by thoracotomy, now an outmoded approach. Two to three defibrillating patches were applied inside or outside the pericardium. Additional pacemaker electrodes were applied epicardially and less often transvenously. All leads were then tunneled subcutaneously to the device implanted in an abdominal pocket in the left upper quadrant.

NONTHORACOTOMY IMPLANTATION. Most ICDs are now implanted transvenously, and small devices can now be placed pectorally.[220] Transvenous systems generally utilize two relatively long intravascular spring or coil electrodes (with or without subcutaneous patches) for defibrillation. Earlier systems with a monophasic waveform were successful in 70 to 80 per cent of patients.[215,221–225] Contemporary devices with a biphasic waveform (reversal of shock polarity) are associated with a lower energy requirement for defibrillation and allow successful transvenous ICD implantation in virtually all patients[220,225–232] (including epicardial systems[233]). It is not known why a biphasic waveform is superior to a monophasic one for transvenous and epicardial defibrillation. There are presently three transvenous systems according to lead configuration: (1) single right ventricular (RV) lead (two spring electrodes, one in the RV and one in the superior vena cava, and a third tip electrode that participates in the pacing/sensing functions)[234]; (2) an RV lead (one spring electrode in the RV and distal electrodes that participate in the pacing/sensing functions) and a second lead (spring electrode) placed in the superior vena cava, right atrium, right atrial appendage, coronary sinus, or left inominate vein[215,221,235]; and (3) an RV lead as in (2), with an electrically "active" pacemaker titanium shell that obviates the need for a second spring electrode.[236,237] Subcutaneous patches can be used to provide a variety of configurations to lower the defibrillation threshold. Most monophasic systems require a tripolar lead arrangement with a subcutaneous patch (bidirectional shock).[215,221,238] The introduction of biphasic shock devices has greatly reduced the number of VF inductions during implantation and the need for subcutaneous patches, required in only 5 to 15 per cent of cases.[217,220,228,230,231,239,239a]

Careful testing at the time of implantation must establish adequate electrograms (voltage and slew rate) for sensing during sinus rhythm, VT, and VF, as well as appropriate pacing thresholds. The optimal pulse duration of the shock is calculated from the defibrillation impedance derived by delivering a low-energy test shock during the patient's normal rhythm. The lowest energy that consistently defibrillates (LED) is determined by inducing VF and delivering a test shock (usually starting with 15 to 20 J 10 to 15 sec after VF induction).[240,241] The LED should be at least 10 J less than the maximum output of the device.[223] As a rule, LED testing requires three consecutive successful shocks delivered at least 5 min apart. Even if the ICD is being used to treat VT alone, it must be shown to defibrillate as well. In contrast to the LED, the actual defibrillation threshold (DFT) is a more complex parameter that characterizes the probability of successful defibrillation (in the form of a dose-response sigmoid curve).[240,241] Precise DFT testing requires too many shocks to be practical clinically. Although it is strictly incorrect, the terms LED and DFT are often used interchangeably.

Antiarrhythmic drugs can alter the LED and DFT. Chronic amiodarone administration raises the DFT.[36,37] Class 1B agents (lidocaine and rarely mexiletine)[243,244] and class 1C agents (flecainide and moricizine)[245] also can increase the DFT. Animal data for propafenone are conflicting.[246,247] Propanolol (but not timolol) and verapamil increase DFT,[248–250] while class 1A agents have little effect. Sotalol decreases DFT.[244,251] Continuing efficacy of the ICD should be reevaluated whenever antiarrhythmic therapy is altered.

Antitachycardia Pacing and Low-Energy Synchronized Cardioversion

Rapid pacing often can terminate VT with a cycle length >250 msec.[252] Antitachycardia pacing (ATP) is best used in patients with hemodynamically stable VT with a cycle length equal to or more than 300 msec. ICDs can deliver a large number of ATP algorithms. A common method, adaptive burst pacing, starts with a cycle length shorter than that of the VT by a given percentage, usually 80 to 90 per cent. Pacing bursts can be fixed (constant cycle length) or autodecremental (ramp pacing), where each successive cycle in the burst is decremented[253,254] (Fig. 23–26). Both methods are commonly used and equally effective.[215,254–257] Other variations include a scanning function that introduces each burst with increasing prematurity and a program that adds a stimulus to each successive burst. All these therapies, number of stimuli in a burst, and the number of ATP attempts are programmable. The success of ATP increases in parallel with increase in VT cycle length.[256,257] ATP is successful in 60 to 90 per cent of carefully selected cases,[215,254,256–260] but the risk of acceleration or inducing VF ranges from 3 to 35 per cent and is inversely related to VT cycle length.[230,253,254,256–258,261]

The success and complications of low-energy synchronized cardioversion are similar to those of

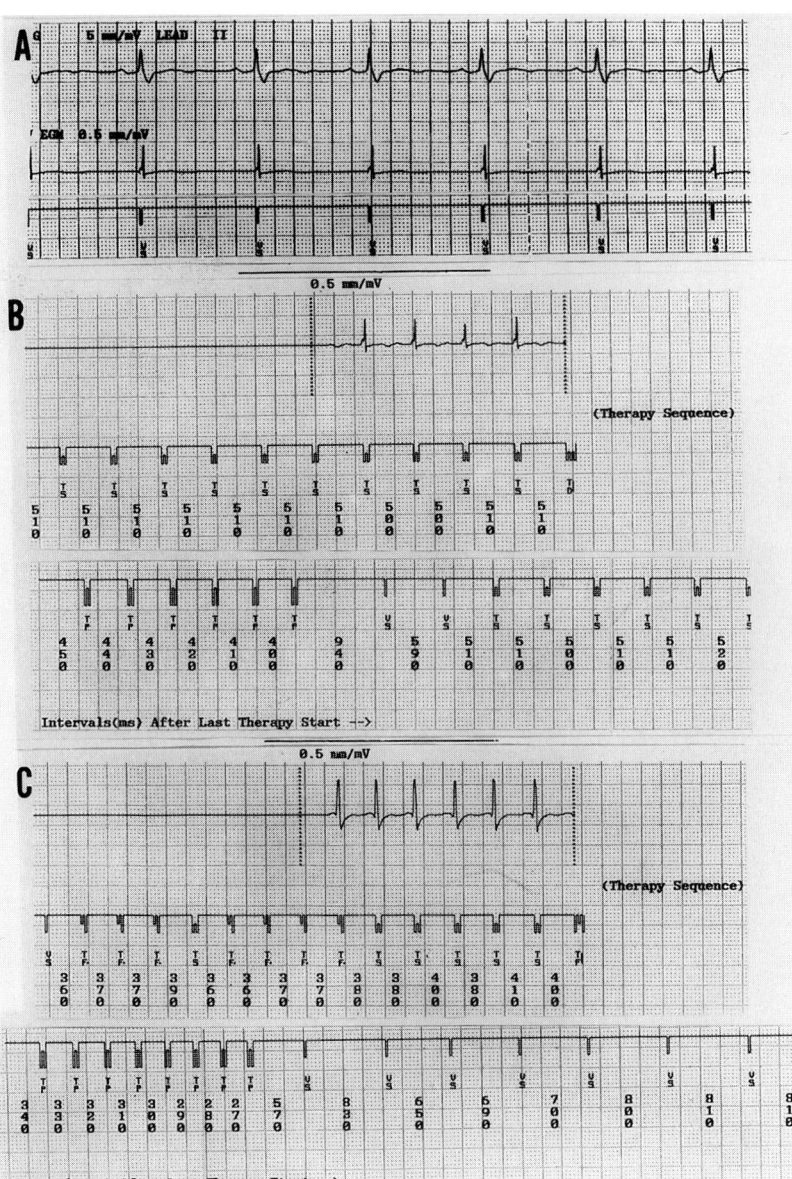

FIGURE 23–26. Electrogram recordings from a Medtronic Jewel ICD. Two different tachycardia zones were programmed for detection and therapy. In the top panel, (A) lead II is recorded simultaneously with the ventricular electrogram and an event channel that registers ventricular sensing (VS). In the middle panel (B), the contour of the ventricular electrogram is unchanged, indicating a supraventricular rhythm, but the rate is about 120/min. (Msec are given vertically beneath each cycle). This supraventricular tachycardia (probably a sinus tachycardia) falls in the tachycardia sensing zone, as indicated by the tachycardia sensing (TS) markings. When a sufficient number of cycles meet the criteria for tachycardia detection (TD), therapy in the form of rapid pacing at decreasing cycle lengths (450 to 400 msec) is delivered. Sinus tachycardia resumes after a pause of 940 msec. In the bottom panel, (C) the device detects a ventricular tachycardia (note electrogram change) that hovers between fast (TF) and slow (TS) ventricular tachycardia zones. Antitachycardia pacing at decreasing cycle lengths (340 to 270 msec) terminates the ventricular tachycardia, with restoration of a slower rhythm, probably sinus.

ATP.[218,253,256,257,260,262,263] Low-energy synchronized cardioversion sometimes works better than ATP. However, shocks of 0.5 to 3.0 J are generally painful and poorly tolerated, so low-energy synchronized cardioversion is often used as secondary therapy.[218] ATP saves the patient the discomfort of shock delivery and can lead to a significant reduction in the number of shocks. Both ATP and low-energy synchronized cardioversion must be carefully individualized. An ICD automatically switches to more aggressive therapy (including defibrillation) whenever it identifies failure of programmed therapy with ATP or low-energy synchronized cardioversion or when VT acceleration or VF occurs as a result of therapy.

COMPLICATIONS. The mortality of ICD implantation by thoracotomy is about 3 to 5 per cent and is less than 1 per cent when implanted transvenously.[264] The morbidity of the transvenous procedure is considerably less than that associated with thoracotomy. The complications of transvenous ICDs include those of venous access and pocket formation (as with pacemakers), infection, and lead problems such as perforation, displacement, fracture, or insulation breakdown, as well as migration or fracture, crinkling, and erosion of subcutaneous patches.[221,264–268] Other complications include high DFT, component or battery failure, inappropriate shocks for unsustained VT or sinus tachycardia or supraventricular tachyarrhythmias (that may precipitate VT or VF), undersensing, oversensing (T wave, signals from lead fracture or loose connection with or without myopotential oversensing, counting of non-ICD pacemaker stimuli), and the induction of atrial fibrillation by a shock.[222,269–272] Psychological complications are important and include the fear of painful shocks, anxiety, and depression that may respond to psychological counseling and rarely may lead to explantation.[273,274]

Follow-up

Acceptable ICD function, including its ability to defibrillate, is tested before the patient is discharged. After implantation, about half the patients require antiarrhythmic drug therapy to control sustained or nonsustained VT to avoid repeated device therapy. However, when an implanted ICD is in place, the number of drugs and dosages can be reduced to avoid side effects, with the knowledge that the ICD will adequately treat an occasional "breakthrough" tachycardia. Patients should be seen every 2 to 3 months, depending on individual responses. In older ICDs, the capacitors of the device needed periodic reformation (charged and discharged) for proper continuing function. Newer devices provide for automatic capacitor reformation at programmable intervals.

Periodic chest x-rays should be done in the first 6 months to detect transvenous lead and patch displacement. The DFT of transvenous systems can rise in the first 2 months, so DFT testing should be repeated at 2 months, especially in patients with a relatively high DFT at the time of implantation.[275,276] At the time of each visit, the device is investigated to determine the number and type of events, type of therapy delivered, and the patient's response. Event registers, stored intervals, and/or electrograms (from the sensing electrodes) allow retrospective validation of events that activate the ICD. The pacing and sensing functions are evaluated in the usual manner, together with determination of pacing lead impedance and recording of the ventricular electrogram. Unfortunately, at the time of follow-up, the high-voltage shock impedance (of the defibrillating leads) cannot be measured without delivery of a shock. The elective replacement time of the device is indicated by increase in battery voltage and an increase in the charge time. The majority of patients receive shocks during long-term follow-up.[277] The likelihood of appropriate shocks increases with decreasing left ventricular ejection fraction, inducible sustained VT before treatment, inducible sustained VT while on drug therapy, and the induction of VT by only one or two stimuli. Multiple ICD discharges, especially by devices with limited memory, usually require hospitalization for further investigation.

STORED ELECTROGRAMS. Replay of stored electrograms (and simultaneous display of event markers) provides data similar to Holter monitoring or an ECG loop recorder in that it allows review of device diagnosis of arrhythmias, triggering mechanism of arrhythmias, and response to therapy.[54,278–280] Significant changes in electrogram morphology allow differentiation of VT from supraventricular tachycardia in 93 per cent of cases[278] (Figs. 23–26 and 23–27). Electrogram analysis is also useful in troubleshooting and for management decisions to prevent the delivery of unnecessary shocks, e.g., spurious shocks from lead fracture (Fig. 23–28), and double counting of QRS and T wave.

The incidence of shocks for non-life-threatening rhythms is about 20 to 30 per cent, often due to atrial fibrillation.[260] Device reprogramming or antiarrhythmic drug therapy (beta blockers for sinus tachycardia and digitalis for atrial fibrillation) based on analysis of stored electrograms has led to a dramatic reduction of ICD response to non-VT rhythms.[279] Stored electrograms also can document abnormalities leading to aborted shocks in uncommitted ICDs. Stored electrograms have indicated that preceding symptoms are not always a reliable indicator of the arrhythmia that triggered ICD therapy. Some patients with rapid VT or even VF can receive appropriate therapy before the development of significant symptoms such as syncope.[281] Severe symptoms preceding a shock suggest VT or VF as the underlying rhythm.

Impact on Survival

It is generally accepted that the ICD reduces the incidence of sudden death to ≤1 to 2 per cent annually in high-risk patients.[264,282] The impact of ICD therapy on overall cardiovascular survival is uncertain because no controlled randomized trials comparing the ICD with other forms of therapy have been reported. Total mortality of ICD patients is high because of poor LV function, myocardial infarction, and congestive heart failure.[283–285] A number of large trials are underway to determine the effectiveness of drug therapy versus ICD and whether prophylactic ICD implantation might benefit patients with a high risk of sudden death.[286–296]

Future Directions

With the "active" system, the DFT is 24 J or less in 98 per cent of patients.[236] The system promises to be nearly as simple to implant as a VVI pacemaker, with profound implications for safety (low number of VF inductions), cost, reliability, and use. Pectoral implantation should increase lead longevity by avoiding the stress imposed on tunneled leads to the abdomen. This and elimination of subcutaneous patches and the use of a single incision will reduce complications, infection, and surgical implantation time to <1 hour. Local anesthesia with sedation will largely re-

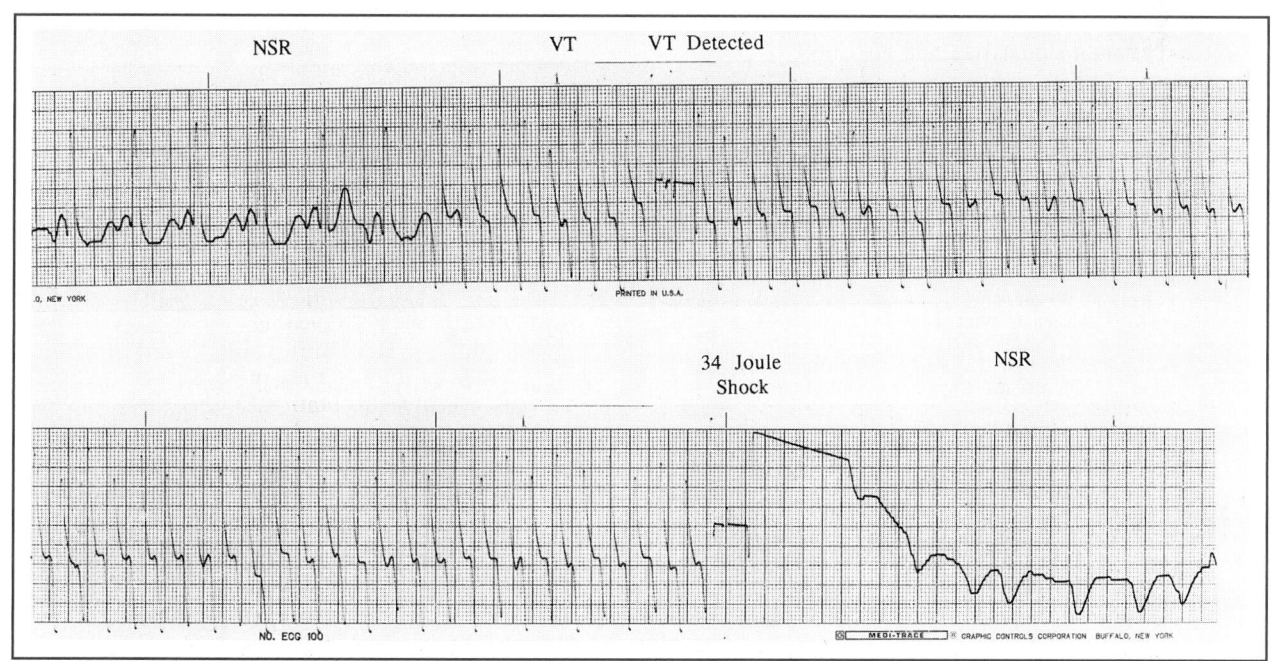

FIGURE 23–27. Intracavitary electrogram recordings from an AICD P2 Endotak demonstrating the transition from sinus rhythm (NSR, note negative P wave preceding each ventricular depolarization) to ventricular tachycardia (VT, note change in electrogram and loss of preceding P wave), prompting, in the lower tracing, a 34-J shock with restoration of sinus rhythm. This device uses an integrated bipolar sensing system from the distal tip electrode to the large right ventricular shocking coil, and is able to record P waves.

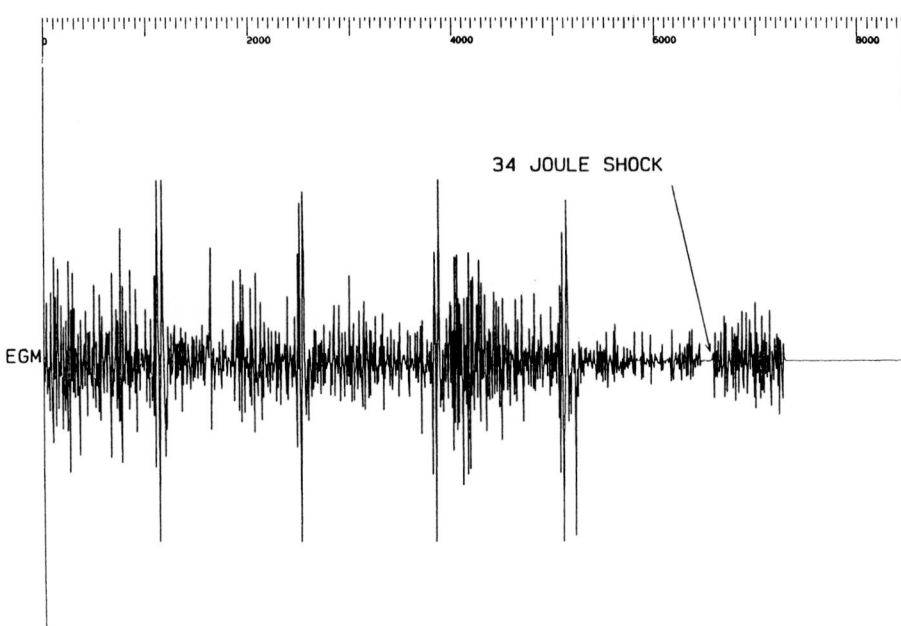

34 JOULE SHOCK

EGM

FIGURE 23–28. Electrogram recordings from a Cadence ICD demonstrating recording artifacts due to a lead insulation break. The ICD erroneously sensed these artifacts as ventricular depolarizations and delivered a 34-J shock.

place general anesthesia. These advances will further broaden the indications for ICDs. Future ICDs will be smaller (60 to 70 cm³), especially if more efficient waveforms and better leads permit a maximum output of 20 to 25 J. Leads of different design will be smaller, while new subcutaneous patch arrays will ensure transvenous implantation in 100 per cent of cases. The devices will incorporate dual-chamber pacing (now required in 5 to 15 per cent of patients[210]), improved sensing and diagnostic algorithms, and more memory with extended electrogram storage. Transtelephonic monitoring and programming will be available. Overall costs will drop because of brief hospitalizations, fewer complications, and the use of less sophisticated "shock-only devices" with backup VVI pacing in selected patients.

REFERENCES

PACEMAKER MODALITIES AND FUNCTION

1. Kusumoto, F. M., and Goldschlager, N.: Medical progress: Cardiac pacing. N. Engl. J. Med. *334:*89, 1996.
1a. Bernstein, A. D., Camm, A. J., Fletcher, R. D., et al.: The NASPE/BPEG generic pacemaker code for antibradyarrhythmia and adaptive-rate pacing and antitachyarrhythmia devices. PACE *10:*794, 1987.
2. Bartecchi, C. E.: Temporary pacing catheter electrodes. *In* Bartecchi, C. E., and Mann, D. E. (eds.): Temporary Cardiac Pacing. Chicago, Precept Press, 1990, p. 268.
3. Fitzpatrick, A., and Sutton, R.: A guide to temporary pacing. Br. Med. J. *304:*365, 1992.
4. Goldberger, J., Kruse, J., Ehlert, F. A., and Kadish, A.: Temporary transvenous pacemaker placement: What criteria constitute an adequate pacing site? Am. Heart J. *126:*488, 1993.
5. Bongiorni, M. G., and Bedendi, N.: Atrial stimulation by means of floating electrodes: A multicenter experience, The Multicenter Study Group. PACE *15:*1977, 1992.
6. Vrouchos, G. T., and Vardas, P. E.: Sensing through the esophagus for temporary atrial synchronous ventricular VDD pacing. PACE *14:*511, 1991.
7. Santini, M., Ansalone, G., Cacciatore, G., and Turitto, G.: Transesophageal pacing. PACE *13:*298, 1990.
8. Guarnerio, M., Furlanello, F., Vergara, G., et al.: Electropharmacological testing by transesophageal atrial pacing in inducible supraventricular tachyarrhythmias: A good approach for selection of long-term antiarrhythmic therapy. Eur. Heart J. *13:*763, 1992.
9. Biffi, A., Ammirati, F., Caselli, G., et al.: Usefulness of transesophageal pacing during exercise for evaluating palpitations in top-level athletes. Am. J. Cardiol. *72:*922, 1993.
10. Zoll, P. M.: Noninvasive cardiac stimulation revisited. PACE *13:*2014, 1990.
11. Luck, J. C., and Markel, M. L.: Clinical applications of external pacing: A renaissance? PACE *14:*1299, 1991.
12. Trigano, J. A., Birkui, P. J., and Mugica, J.: Noninvasive transcutaneous cardiac pacing: Modern instrumentation and new perspectives. PACE *15:*1937, 1992.
13. Grubb, B. P., Markel, M. L., Artman, S. E., et al.: Observations on induction and termination of paroxysmal supraventricular tachycardia by external pacing. PACE *15:*1944, 1992.
14. Grubb, B. P., Temesy-Armos, P., Hahn, H., and Elliott, L.: The use of external, noninvasive pacing for the termination of ventricular tachycardia in the emergency department setting. Ann. Emerg. Med. *21:*174, 1992.
15. de la Serna, F., Meier, B., Pande, A. K., et al.: Coronary and left ventricular pacing as standby in invasive cardiology. Cathet. Cardiovasc. Diagn. *25:*285, 1992.
16. Laird, J. R., Hull, R., Stajduhar, K. C., et al.: Transcoronary cardiac pacing during myocardial ischemia. Cathet. Cardiovasc. Diagn. *30:*162, 1993.
17. Lévy, S., Lauribe, P., Dolla, E., et al.: A randomized comparison of external and internal cardioversion of chronic atrial fibrillation. Circulation *86:*1415, 1992.
18. Barold, S. S.: Narrow QRS Mobitz type II second-degree AV block in acute myocardial infarction: True or false? Am. J. Cardiol. *67:*1291, 1991.
19. Behar, S., Zissman, E., Zion, M., et al.: Prognostic significance of second-degree block in inferior wall acute myocardial infarction. Am. J. Cardiol. *72:*831, 1993.
20. Murphy, P., Morton, P., Murtagh, J. G., et al.: Hemodynamic effects of different temporary pacing modes for the management of bradycardias complicating acute myocardial infarction. PACE *15:*381, 1992.
21. Dreifus, L. S., Fisch, C., Griffin, J. C., et al.: Guidelines for implantation of cardiac pacemakers and antiarrhythmia devices: A report of the American College of Cardiology/American Heart Association Task Force on Assessment of Diagnostic and Therapeutic Procedures (Committee on Pacemaker Implantation). J. Am. Coll. Cardiol. *18:*1, 1991.
22. Barold, S. S.: ACC/AHA guidelines for implantation of cardiac pacemakers: How accurate are the definitions of atrioventricular and intraventricular conduction blocks? PACE *16:*1221, 1993.
23. Barold, S. S.: Indications for permanent pacemakers: Comments on the 1991 ACC/AHA and BPEG guidelines. *In* Santini, M., Pistolese, M., and Alliegro, A. (eds.): Progress in Clinical Pacing 1992. Mt. Kisco, N.Y., Futura, 1993, p. 439.
24. Rardon, D. P., Miles, W. M., Mitrani, R. D., et al.: Atrioventricular block and dissociation. *In* Zipes, D. P., and Jalife, J. (eds.): Cardiac Electrophysiology: From Cell to Bedside. 2nd ed. Philadelphia, W. B. Saunders Company, 1995, p. 935.
25. Cooper, J. P., Fraser, A. G., and Penny, W. J.: Reversibility and benign recurrence of complete heart block in athletes. Int. J. Cardiol. *35:*118, 1992.
26. Kim, Y. H., O'Nunain, S., Trouton, T., et al.: Pseudo-pacemaker syndrome following inadvertent fast pathway ablation for atrioventricular nodal reentrant tachycardia. J. Cardiovasc. Electrophysiol. *4:*178, 1993.
27. Mabo, P., DePlace, C., Gras, D., et al.: Isolated first degree AV block: An indication for permanent DDD pacing. PACE *16*(Abs.):1123, 1993.
28. Odemuyiwa, O., and Camm, A. J.: Prophylactic pacing for prevention of sudden death in congenital complete heart block? PACE *15:*1526, 1992.
29. Solti, F., Szatmary, L., Vecsey, T., et al.: Congenital complete heart block associated with QT prolongation. Eur. Heart J. *13:*1080, 1992.
30. Barold, S. S., Falkoff, M. D., Ong, L. S., et al.: Atrioventricular block: New insights. *In* Barold, S. S., and Mugica, J. (eds.): New Perspectives in Cardiac Pacing 2. Mt. Kisco, N.Y., Futura, 1991, p. 23.

31. Coplan, N. L., Morales, M. C., Romanello, P., et al.: Exercise-induced atrioventricular block: Influence of myocardial ischemia. Chest *100:* 1728, 1991.

32. Gaggioli, G., Bottoni, N., Brignole, M., et al.: Progression to 2d and 3d grade atrioventricular block in patients after electrostimulation for bundle-branch block and syncope: A long-term study. G. Ital. Cardiol. *24:*409, 1994.

33. Bergfeldt, L., Edvardsson, N., Rosenqvist, M., et al.: Atrioventricular block progression in patients with bifascicular block assessed by repeated electrocardiography and a bradycardia-detecting pacemaker. Am. J. Cardiol. *74:*1129, 1994.

34. Sneddon, J. F., and Camm, A. J.: Sinus node disease: Current concepts in diagnosis and therapy. Drugs *44:*728, 1992.

35. Katritsis, D., Ward, D. E., and Camm, A. J.: Can we treat carotid sinus syndrome? PACE *14:*1367, 1991.

36. Benditt, D. G., Remole, S., Asso, A., et al.: Cardiac pacing for carotid sinus syndrome and vasovagal syncope. *In* Barold, S. S., and Mugica, J. (eds.): New Perspectives in Cardiac Pacing 3. Mt. Kisco, N.Y., Futura, 1993, p. 15.

37. Maloney, J. D., Jaeger, F. J., Rizo-Patron, C., and Zhu, D. W.: The role of pacing for the management of neurally mediated syncope: Carotid sinus syndrome and vasovagal syncope. Am. Heart J. *127:*1030, 1994.

38. Petersen, M. E., Chamberlain-Webber, R., Fitzpatrick, A. P., et al.: Permanent pacing for cardioinhibitory malignant vasovagal syndrome. Br. Heart J. *71:*274, 1994.

39. Benditt, D. G., Petersen, M., Lurie, K. G., et al.: Cardiac pacing for prevention of recurrent vasovagal syncope. Ann. Intern. Med. *122:*204, 1995.

40. Petersen, M. E., Price, D., Williams, T., et al.: Short AV interval VDD pacing does not prevent tilt induced vasovagal syncope in patients with cardioinhibitory vasovagal syndrome. PACE *17:*882, 1994.

41. Fananapazir, L., Epstein, N. D., Curiel, R. V., et al.: Long-term results of dual-chamber (DDD) pacing in obstructive hypertrophic cardiomyopathy: Evidence for progressive symptomatic and hemodynamic improvement and reduction of left ventricular hypertrophy. Circulation *90:*2731, 1994.

42. Jeanrenaud, X., Goy, J. J., and Kappenberger, L.: Effects of dual-chamber pacing in hypertrophic obstructive cardiomyopathy. Lancet *339:*1318, 1992.

43. Hochleitner, M., Hörtnagl, H., Hörtnagl, H., et al.: Long-term efficacy of physiologic dual chamber pacing in the treatment of end-stage idiopathic dilated cardiomyopathy. Am. J. Cardiol. *70:*1320, 1992.

44. Eldar, M., Griffin, J. C., VanHare, G. F., et al.: Combined use of beta-adrenergic blocking agents and long-term cardiac pacing for patients with the long QT syndrome. J. Am. Coll. Cardiol. *20:*830, 1992.

45. Weisman, P., Chin, M. T., and Moss, A. J.: Cardiac tachypacing for severe refractory orthostatic hypotension. Ann. Intern. Med. *16:*650, 1992.

46. Grubb, B. P., Wolfe, D. A., Samoil, D., et al.: Adaptive rate pacing controlled by right ventricular preejection interval for severe refractory orthostatic hypotension. PACE *16:*801, 1993.

METHODS OF PACEMAKER IMPLANTATION

47. Byrd, C. L.: Clinical experience with the extrathoracic introducer insertion technique. PACE *16:*1781, 1993.

48. Belott, P. H., and Reynolds, D. W.: Permanent pacemaker implantation. *In* Ellenbogen, K. A., Kay, G. N., and Wilkoff, B. L. (eds.): Clinical Cardiac Pacing. Philadelphia, W. B. Saunders Company, 1995, p. 447.

49. Magney, J. E., Staplin, D. H., Flynn, D. M., and Hunter, D. W.: A new approach to percutaneous subclavian venipuncture to avoid lead fracture or central venous catheter occlusion. PACE *16:*2133, 1993.

50. Hayes, D. L., Naccarelli, G. V., Furman, S., and Parsonnet, V.: Report of the NASPE policy conference training requirements for permanent pacemaker implantation and follow-up, North American Society of Pacing and Electrophysiology. PACE *17:*6, 1994.

51. Fyke, F. E., III.: Infraclavicular lead failure: Tarnish on a golden route. PACE *16:*445, 1993.

52. Jacobs, D. M., Fink, A. S., Miller, R. P., et al.: Anatomical and morphological evaluation of pacemaker lead compression. PACE *16:*434, 1993.

53. Hoyer, M. H., Beerman, L. B., Ettedgui, J. A., et al.: Transatrial lead placement for endocardial pacing in children. Ann. Thorac. Surg. *58:*97, 1994.

54. Stokes, K. B., and Kay, G. N.: Artificial electric cardiac stimulation. *In* Ellenbogen, K. A., Kay, G. N., and Wilkoff, B. L. (eds.): Clinical Cardiac Pacing. Philadelphia, W. B. Saunders Company, 1995, p. 3.

55. Kay, G. N.: Basic aspects of cardiac pacing. *In* Ellenbogen, K. A. (ed.): Cardiac Pacing. Boston, Blackwell Scientific, 1992, p. 32.

56. Soriano, J., Almendral, J., Arenal, A., et al.: Rate-dependent failure of ventricular capture in patients treated with oral propafenone. Eur. Heart J. *13:*269, 1992.

57. Bianconi, L., Boccadamo, R., Toscano, S., et al.: Effects of oral propafenone therapy on chronic myocardial pacing threshold. PACE *15:*148, 1992.

58. Cornacchia, D., Fabbri, M., Maresta, A., et al.: Effect of steroid eluting versus conventional electrodes on propafenone induced rise in chronic ventricular pacing threshold. PACE *16:*2279, 1993.

59. Barold, S. S., McVenes, R., and Stokes, K.: Effect of drugs on pacing threshold in man and in canines: Old and new facts. *In* Barold, S. S.,

and Mugica, J. (eds.): New Perspectives in Cardiac Pacing 3. Mt. Kisco, N.Y., Futura, 1993, p. 57.

60. Kay, G. N., and Ellenbogen, K. A.: Sensing. *In* Ellenbogen, K. A., Kay, G. N., and Wilkoff, B. L. (eds.): Clinical Cardiac Pacing. Philadelphia, W. B. Saunders Company, 1995, p. 38.

61. Furman, S.: Sensing and timing the cardiac electrogram. *In* Furman, S., Hayes, D. L., and Holmes, D. R., Jr. (eds.): A Practice of Cardiac Pacing. 3rd ed. Mt. Kisco, N.Y., Futura, 1993, p. 89.

62. Santini, M., Ansalone, G., Cacciatore, G., and Turitto, G.: Status of single chamber atrial pacing. *In* Barold, S. S., and Mugica, J. (eds.): New Perspectives in Cardiac Pacing 2. Mt. Kisco, N.Y., Futura, 1991, p. 273.

63. Hayes, D. L.: Pacemaker polarity configuration: What is best for the patient? PACE *15:*1099, 1992.

64. Mond, H. G., and Helland, J. R.: Engineering and clinical aspects of clinical leads. *In* Ellenbogen, K. A., Kay, G. N., and Wilkoff, B. L. (eds.): Clinical Cardiac Pacing. Philadelphia, W. B. Saunders Company, 1995, p. 69.

65. Mond, H., and Stokes, K.: The electrode-tissue interface: The revolutionary role of steroid elution. PACE *15:*95, 1992.

66. Rhoden, W. E., Llewellyn, M. J., Schofield, S. W., and Bennett, D. H.: Acute and chronic performance of a steroid eluting electrode for ventricular pacing. Int. J. Cardiol. *37:*209, 1992.

67. Stamato, N. J., O'Toole, M. F., Fetter, J. G., and Enger, E. L.: The safety and efficacy of chronic ventricular pacing at 1.6 volts using a steroid eluting lead. PACE *15:*248, 1992.

68. Gillis, A. M., Rothschild, J. M., Hillier, K., et al.: A randomized comparison of a bipolar steroid-eluting electrode and a bipolar microporous platinum electrode: Implications for long-term programming. PACE *16:*964, 1993.

TYPES OF PACEMAKERS

69. Barold, S. S.: Timing cycles and operational characteristics of pacemakers. *In* Ellenbogen, K. A., Kay, G. N., and Wilkoff, B. L. (eds.): Clinical Cardiac Pacing. Philadelphia, W. B. Saunders Company, 1995, p. 567.

70. Ghani, M., Thakur, R. K., Boughner, D., et al.: Malposition of transvenous pacing lead in the left ventricle. PACE *16:*1800, 1993.

71. Shmuely, H., Erdman, S., Strasberg, B., and Rosenfeld, J. B.: Seven years of left ventricular pacing due to malposition of pacing electrode. PACE *15:*369, 1992.

72. Barold, S. S., Falkoff, M. D., Ong, L. S., and Heinle, R. A.: Electrocardiographic diagnosis of myocardial infarction during ventricular pacing. Cardiol. Clin. *5:*403, 1987.

73. Fu, L., Imai, K., Okabe, A., et al.: A possible mechanism for pacemaker-induced T-wave changes. Eur. Heart J. *13:*1173, 1992.

74. Barold, S. S.: Ventricular- versus atrial-based lower rate timing in dual chamber pacemakers: Does it really matter? PACE *18:*83, 1995.

75. Furman, S.: Comprehension of pacemaker cycles. *In* Furman, S., Hayes, D. L., and Holmes, D. R., Jr. (eds.): A Practice of Cardiac Pacing. 3rd ed. Mt. Kisco, N.Y., Futura, 1993, p. 135.

76. Irwin, M., Harris, L., Cameron, D., et al.: DDI pacing: Indications, expectations, and follow-up. PACE *17:*274, 1994.

77. Sulke, N., Drisas, A., Bostock, J., et al.: "Subclinical" pacemaker syndrome: A randomized study of symptom free patients with ventricular demand (VVI) pacemakers upgraded to dual chamber devices. Br. Heart J. *67:*57, 1992.

78. Barold, S. S., and Mond, H. G.: Fallback responses of dual chamber (DDD and DDDR) pacemakers: A proposed classification. PACE *17:*1160, 1994.

79. Mond, H. G., and Barold, S. S.: Dual chamber rate adaptive pacing in patients with paroxysmal supraventricular tachyarrhythmias: Protective measures for rate control. PACE *16:*2168, 1993.

80. Barold, S. S., Falkoff, M. D., Ong, L. S., and Heinle, R. A.: Electrocardiography of contemporary DDD pacemakers: Basic concepts, upper rate response, retrograde ventriculoatrial conduction and differential diagnosis of pacemaker tachycardias. *In* Saksena, S., and Goldschlager, N. (eds.): Electrical Therapy for Cardiac Arrhythmias: Pacing, Antitachycardia Devices, Catheter Ablation. Philadelphia, W. B. Saunders Company, 1990, p. 225.

81. Barold, S. S.: The fourth decade of cardiac pacing: Hemodynamic, electrophysiological and clinical considerations in the selection of the optimal pacemaker. *In* Zipes, D. P., and Jalife, J. (eds.): Cardiac Electrophysiology: From Cell to Bedside. 2nd ed. Philadelphia, W. B. Saunders Company, 1995, p. 1366.

82. Chirife, R., Ortega, D. F., and Salazar, A. I.: Nonphysiological left heart AV intervals as a result of DDD and AAI "physiological" pacing. PACE *14:*1752, 1991.

83. Frielingsdorf, J., Gerber, A. E., and Hess, O. M.: Importance of maintained atrioventricular synchrony in patients with pacemakers. Eur. Heart J. *15:*1431, 1994.

84. Chirife, R.: Proposal of a method for automatic optimization of left heart atrioventricular interval applicable to DDD pacemakers. PACE *18:*49, 1995.

85. Camous, J. P., Raybaud, F., Dolisi, C., et al.: Interatrial conduction in patients undergoing AV stimulation: Effects of increasing right atrial stimulation rate. PACE *16:*2082, 1993.

86. Prinzen, F. W., Delhaas, T., Arts, T., and Reneman, R. S.: Asymmetrical changes in ventricular wall mass by asynchronous electrical activation of the heart. Adv. Exp. Med. Biol. *346:*257, 1993.

87. Lee, M. A., Dae, M. W., Langberg, J. J., et al.: Effects of long-term right ventricular apical pacing on left ventricular perfusion, innervation, function and histology. J. Am. Coll. Cardiol. 24:225, 1994.

88. Daubert, C., Ritter, P., Mabo, P., et al.: AV delay optimization in DDD and DDDR pacing. In Barold, S. S., and Mugica, J. (eds.): New Perspectives in Cardiac Pacing 3. Mt. Kisco, N.Y., Futura, 1993, p. 259.

89. Buckingham, T. A., Janosik, D. L., and Pearson, A. C.: Pacemaker hemodynamics: Clinical implications. Prog. Cardiovasc. Dis. 34:347, 1992.

90. Pierantozzi, A., Bocconcelli, P., and Sgarbi, E.: DDD pacemaker syndrome and atrial conduction time. PACE 17:374, 1994.

91. Benditt, D. G., Wilbert, L., Hansen, R., et al.: Late follow-up of dual-chamber rate-adaptive pacing. Am. J. Cardiol. 71:714, 1993.

92. Detollenaere, M., vanWassenhove, E., and Jordaens, L.: Atrial arrhythmias in dual chamber pacing and their influence on long-term mortality. PACE 15:1846, 1992.

93. Ray, S. G., Connelly, D. T., Hughes, M., et al.: Stability of the DDD pacing mode in patients 80 years of age and older. PACE 17:1218, 1994.

HEMODYNAMICS OF CARDIAC PACING

94. Maloney, J. D., Helguera, M. E., and Woscoboinik, J. R.: Physiology of rate-responsive pacing. Cardiol. Clin. 10:619, 1992.

95. Oldroyd, K. G., Rae, A., Carter, R., et al.: Double blind crossover comparison of the effects of dual chamber pacing (DDD) and ventricular rate adaptive (VVIR) pacing on neuroendocrine variables, exercise performance and symptoms in complete heart block. Br. Heart J. 65:188, 1991.

96. Griffin, J. C.: VVIR or DDDR: Does it matter? Clin. Cardiol. 14:257, 1991.

97. Janosik, D. L., and Labovitz, A. J.: Basic physiology of cardiac pacing. In Ellenbogen, K. A., Kay, G. N., and Wilkoff, B. L. (eds.): Clinical Cardiac Pacing. Philadelphia, W. B. Saunders Company, 1995, p. 367.

98. Sulke, A. N., Chambers, J. B., and Sowton, E.: The effect of atrio-ventricular delay programming in patients with DDDR pacemakers. Eur. Heart J. 13:464, 1992.

99. Mabo, P., Ritter, P., Varin, C., et al.: Intérêt d'un algorithme d'adaptation automatique du délai auriculo-ventriculaire à la fréquence atriale instantanée en stimulation cardiaque DDD. Arch. Mal. Coeur 85:1001, 1992.

100. Ritter, P. H., Vai, F., Bonnet, J. L., et al.: Rate adaptive atrio-ventricular delay improves cardio-pulmonary performance in patients implanted with a dual chamber pacemaker for complete heart block. Eur. J. Cardiac Pacing Electrophysiol. 1:31, 1991.

101. Potratz, J., Stierle, U., Djonlagic, H., et al.: The hemodynamic effect of a rate responsive AV delay in dual chamber pacing. PACE 16(Abs.):920, 1993.

102. Schüller, N., and Brandt, J.: The pacemaker syndrome: Old and new causes. Clin. Cardiol. 14:336, 1991.

103. Barold, S. S.: Pacemaker syndrome during atrial-based pacing. In Aubert, A. E., Ector, H., and Stroobandt, R. (eds.): Cardiac Pacing and Electrophysiology: A Bridge to the 21st Century. Dordrecht, Holland, Kluwer Academic Publishers, 1994, p. 251.

104. Ellenbogen, K. A., and Stambler, B. D.: Pacemaker syndrome. In Ellenbogen, K. A., Kay, G. N., and Wilkoff, B. L. (eds.): Clinical Cardiac Pacing. Philadelphia, W. B. Saunders Company, 1995, p. 419.

105. Ellenbogen, K. A., Wood, M. A., and Stambler, B.: Pacemaker syndrome: Clinical, hemodynamic and neurohumoral features. In Barold, S. S., and Mugica, J. (eds.): New Perspectives in Cardiac Pacing 3. Mt. Kisco, N.Y., Futura, 1993, p. 85.

106. Travill, C. M., and Sutton, R.: Pacemaker syndrome: An iatrogenic condition. Br. Heart J. 68:163, 1992.

107. Heldman, D., Mulvihill, D., Nguyen, H., et al.: True incidence of pacemaker syndrome. PACE 13:1742, 1990.

108. Rediker, D. E., Eagle, K. A., Homma, S., et al.: Clinical and hemodynamic comparison of VVI versus DDD pacing in patients with DDD pacemakers. Am. J. Cardiol. 63:323, 1988.

109. Linde-Edelstam, C., Nordlander, R., Pehrsson, K., and Rydén, L.: A double-blind study of submaximal exercise tolerance and variation in paced rate in atrial synchronous compared to activity sensor modulated ventricular pacing. PACE 15:905, 1992.

110. Linde, C.: Is atrioventricular synchronous pacing the superior treatment in patients with high degree atrioventricular block? Eur. J. Cardiac Pacing Electrophysiol. 3:42, 1993.

111. Channon, K. M., Hargreaves, M. R., Cripps, T. R., et al.: DDD vs. VVI pacing in patients aged over 75 years with complete heart block: A double-blind crossover comparison. Q. J. Med. 87:245, 1994.

112. Sulke, N., Chambers, J., Dritsas, A., and Sowton, E.: A randomized double-blind crossover comparison of four rate-responsive pacing modes. J. Am. Coll. Cardiol. 17:696, 1991.

113. Sulke, N., Chambers, J., and Sowton, E.: Variability of left atrial blood-flow predicts intolerance of ventricular demand pacing and may cause pacemaker syndrome. PACE 17:1149, 1994.

114. Theodorakis, G. N., Kremastinos, D. T., Markianos, M., et al.: Total sympathetic activity and natriuretic factor levels in VVI and DDD pacing with different atrioventricular delays during daily activity and exercise. Eur. Heart J. 13:1477, 1992.

115. Clemo, H. F., Baumgarten, C. M., Stambler, B. S., et al.: Atrial natriuretic factor: Implications for cardiac pacing and electrophysiology. PACE 17:70, 1994.

116. Grant, S. C. D., and Bennett, D. H.: Atrial latency in a dual chambered pacing system causing inappropriate sequence of cardiac chamber activation. PACE 15:116, 1992.

117. Daubert, C., Mabo, P., and Leclercq, C.: Physiologic pacing systems in patients with sick sinus syndrome. In Benditt, D. G. (ed.): Rate-Adaptive Pacing. Cambridge, MA, Blackwell Scientific Publications, 1993, p. 151.

118. Daubert, C., Mabo, P., Berder, V., et al.: Atrial tachyarrhythmias associated with high degree interatrial conduction block: Prevention by permanent atrial resynchronisation. Eur. J. Pacing Electrophysiol. 3:35, 1994.

119. Brandt, J., and Schüller, H.: Consideration for the selection of rate-adaptive single lead atrial (AAIR) pacing. In Barold, S. S., and Mugica, J. (eds.): New Perspectives in Cardiac Pacing 3. Mt. Kisco, N.Y., Futura, 1993, p. 349.

120. Katritsis, D., and Camm, A. J.: Adaptive-rate pacemakers: Comparison of sensors and clinical experience. Cardiol. Clin. 10:671, 1992.

121. Lau, C. P.: The range of sensors and algorithms used in rate adaptive cardiac pacing. PACE 15:1177, 1992.

122. Katritsis, D., Shakespeare, C. F., and Camm, A. J.: New and combined sensors for adaptive rate pacing. Clin. Cardiol. 16:240, 1993.

123. Lau, C. P., Tai, Y. T., Fong, P. C., et al.: Clinical experience with an activity sensing DDDR pacemaker using an accelerometer sensor. PACE 15:334, 1992.

124. Bacharach, D. W., Hilden, T. S., Millerhagen, J. O., et al.: Activity-based pacing: Comparison of a device using an accelerometer versus a piezoelectric crystal. PACE 15:188, 1992.

125. Charles, R. G., Heemels, J. P., and Westrum, B. L.: Accelerometer-based adaptive-rate pacing: A multicenter study, European EXCEL Study Group. PACE 16:418, 1993.

126. Alt, E., and Matula, M.: Comparison of two activity-controlled rate-adaptive pacing principles: Acceleration versus vibration. Cardiol. Clin. 10:635, 1992.

127. Santomauro, M., Fazio, S., Ferraro, S., et al.: Follow-up of a respiratory rate modulated pacemaker. PACE 15:17, 1992.

128. Nappholz, T., Maloney, J. D., and Kay, G. N.: Rate-adaptive pacing based on impedance derived minute ventilation. In Ellenbogen, K. A., Kay, G. N., and Wilkoff, B. L. (eds.): Clinical Cardiac Pacing. Philadelphia, W. B. Saunders Company, 1995, p. 219.

129. Li, H., Neubauer, S. A., and Hayes, D. L.: Follow-up of a minute ventilation rate adaptive pacemaker. PACE 15:1826, 1992.

130. Abrahamsen, A. M., Barvik, S., Aarsland, T., and Dickstein, K.: Rate responsive cardiac pacing using a minute ventilation sensor. PACE 16:1650, 1993.

131. Slade, A. K. B., Pee, S., Jones, S., et al.: New algorithms to increase initial rate response in a minute ventilation volume rate adaptive pacemaker. PACE 17:1960, 1994.

132. Sellers, T. D., Fearnot, N. E., and Smith, H. J.: Temperature controlled rate-adaptive pacing. In Ellenbogen, K. A., Kay, G. N., and Wilkoff, B. L. (eds.): Clinical Cardiac Pacing. Philadelphia, W. B. Saunders Company, 1995, p. 201.

133. Bellamy, C. M., Roberts, D. H., Hughes, S., and Charles, R. G.: Comparative evaluation of rate modulation in new generation evoked QT and activity sensing pacemaker. PACE 15:993, 1992.

134. Connelly, D. T., and Rickards, A. F.: The evoked QT interval. In Ellenbogen, K. A., Kay, G. N., and Wilkoff, B. L. (eds.): Clinical Cardiac Pacing. Philadelphia, W. B. Saunders Company, 1995, p. 250.

135. Connelly, D. T., and Rickards, A. F.: Rate-responsive pacing using electrographic parameters as sensors. Cardiol. Clin. 10:659, 1992.

136. Frais, M. A., Dowie, A., McEwen, A., et al.: Response of the QT-sensing, rate-adaptive ventricular pacemaker to mental stress. Am. Heart J. 126:1219, 1993.

137. Cowell, R., Morris-Thurgood, J., Paul, V., et al.: Are we being driven to two sensors? Clinical benefits of sensor cross-checking. PACE 16:1441, 1993.

138. Connelly, D. T.: Initial experience with a new single chamber, dual sensor rate responsive pacemaker, the Topaz Study Group. PACE 16:1833, 1993.

139. Provenier, F., vanAcker, R., Backers, J., et al.: Clinical observations with a dual sensor rate adaptive single chamber pacemaker. PACE 15:1821, 1992.

140. Benditt, D. G., Mianulli, M., Lurie, K., et al.: Multiple-sensor systems for physiologic cardiac pacing. Ann. Intern. Med. 121:960, 1994.

141. VanKrieken, F. M., Perrins, J. P., and Sigmund, M.: Clinical results of automatic slope adaptation in a dual sensor VVIR pacemaker. PACE 15:1815, 1992.

142. Provenier, F., and Jordaens, L.: Evaluation of six minute walking test in patients with single chamber rate responsive pacemakers. Br. Heart J. 72:192, 1994.

143. Hayes, D. L., VonFeldt, L., and Higano, S. T.: Standardized informal exercise testing for programming rate adaptive pacemakers. PACE 14:1772, 1991.

144. Lefroy, D. C., Crake, T., and Davies, D. W.: Ventricular tachycardia: An unusual pacemaker-mediated tachycardia. Br. Heart J. 71:481, 1994.

145. Alt, E., Kriegler, C., Fotuhi, P., et al.: Feasibility of using intracardiac impedance measurements for capture detection. PACE 15:1873, 1992.

146. Bolz, A., Hubmann, M., Hardt, R., et al.: Low polarization pacing lead for detecting the ventricular-evoked response. Med. Prog. Technol. 19:192, 1993.

147. Chirife, R., Ortega, D. F., and Salazar, A. I.: Feasibility of measuring relative right ventricular volumes and ejection fraction with implantable rhythm control devices. PACE 16:1673, 1993.

148. Santini, M., Alexidou, G., Ansalone, G., et al.: Relation of prognosis in sick sinus syndrome to age, conduction defect, and modes of permanent cardiac pacing. Am. J. Cardiol. 65:729, 1990.

149. Andersen, H. R., Thuesen, L., Bagger, J. P., et al.: Prospective randomized trial of atrial versus ventricular pacing in sick-sinus syndrome. Lancet 344:1523, 1994.

150. Barold, S. S., and Santini, M.: Natural history of sick sinus syndrome after pacemaker implantation. In Barold, S. S., and Mugica, J. (eds.): New Perspectives in Cardiac Pacing 3. Mt. Kisco, N.Y., Futura, 1993, p. 169.

151. Hesselson, A. B., Parsonnet, V., Bernstein, A. D., and Bonavita, G. J.: Deleterious effect of long-term single-chamber ventricular pacing in patients with sick sinus syndrome: The hidden benefits of dual chamber pacing. J. Am. Coll. Cardiol. 19:1542, 1992.

152. Sgarbossa, E. B., Pinski, S. L., Maloney, J. D., et al.: Chronic atrial fibrillation and stroke in paced patients with sick sinus syndrome: Relevance of clinical characteristics and pacing modalities. Circulation 88:1045, 1993.

153. Linde-Edelstam, C., Gullberg, B., Nordlander, R., et al.: Longevity in patients with high degree atrioventricular block paced in the atrial synchronous or the fixed-rate ventricular-inhibited mode. PACE 15:304, 1992.

154. Shen, W. K., Neubauer, S. A., Espinosa, R. E., et al.: Should age be a consideration in mode selection in permanent pacing? A survival analysis. J. Am. Coll. Cardiol. (Abs. Suppl.):13A, 1995.

155. Rosenqvist, M., Brandt, J., and Schüller, H.: Long-term pacing in sinus node disease: Effects of stimulation mode on cardiovascular morbidity and mortality. Am. Heart J. 116:16, 1988.

156. Witte, J., v. Knorre, G. H., Volkman, H. J., et al.: Survival rate in sinus syndrome patients: AAI/DDD versus VVI pacing. In Santini, M., Pistolese, M., and Alliegro, A. (eds.): Progress in Clinical Pacing 1992. Mt. Kisco, N.Y., Futura, 1993, p. 175.

157. Sethi, K. K., Mohan, J. C., and Khalilullah, M.: Pacing in sick sinus syndrome. PACE 16(Abs.):1543, 1993.

158. Lamas, G. A., Pashos, C. L., Normand, S. L. T., and McNeil, B. J.: Factors affecting 2-year survival in Medicare pacemaker patients. PACE 16(Abs.):919, 1993.

159. Lukl, J., Doupal, V., and Heinc, P.: Quality-of-life during DDD and dual sensor VVIR pacing. PACE 17:1844, 1994.

160. Lau, C. P., Tai, Y. T., Lee, P. W. E., et al.: Quality-of-life in DDDR pacing: Atrioventricular synchrony or rate adaptation? PACE 17:1838, 1994.

161. Menozzi, C., Brignole, M., Moracchini, P. V., et al.: Inpatient comparison between chronic VVIR and VDD pacing in patients affected by high degree AV block without heart failure. PACE 13:1816, 1990.

162. Lascault, G., Frank, R., Iwa, T., et al.: Comparison of DDD and "VVIR like" pacing during moderate exercise: Echo-Doppler study. Eur. Heart J. 13:914, 1992.

163. Jutzy, R. V., Isaeff, D. M., Bansal, R. C., et al.: Comparison of VVIR, DDD, and DDDR pacing. J. Electrophysiol. 3:194, 1989.

164. Batey, R., Sweesy, M. W., Scala, G., and Forney, R. C.: Comparison of low rate dual chamber pacing to activity responsive rate variable ventricular pacing. PACE 13:646, 1990.

165. Landzberg, J. S., Franklin, J. O., Mahawar, S. K., et al.: Benefits of physiologic atrioventricular synchronization for pacing with an exercise rate response. Am. J. Cardiol. 66:193, 1990.

166. Jutzy, R. V., Florio, J., Isaeff, D. M., et al.: Comparative evaluation of rate modulated dual chamber and VVIR pacing. PACE 13:1838, 1990.

167. Alagona, P., Jr., Batey, R., Sweesy, M., et al.: Improved exercise tolerance with dual chamber versus single chamber rate adaptive pacing. PACE 13:532, 1990.

168. Higano, S. T., and Hayes, D. L.: Hemodynamic importance of atrioventricular synchrony during low levels of exercise. PACE 13(Abs.):509, 1990.

169. Adornato, E., Bacca, F., Polimeni, R. M., and DeSeta, F.: Ventricular single chamber RR pacing in comparison to dual chamber RR pacing: Preliminary results of an Italian multicenter trial. PACE 16(Abs.):1147, 1993.

170. Lemke, B., Dryander, S. V., Jager, D., et al.: Aerobic capacity in rate modulated pacing. PACE 15:1914, 1992.

171. Windle, J., Plath, R., Eisenger, G., and Easley, A., Jr.: Effect of pacing mode in patients with left ventricular dysfunction. PACE 14(Abs.):684, 1991.

172. Brandt, J., Anderson, H., Fåhraeus, T., and Schüller, H.: Natural history of sinus node disease treated with atrial pacing in 213 patients: Implications for selection of stimulation mode. J. Am. Coll. Cardiol. 20:633, 1992.

173. Brandt, J., and Schüller, H.: Pacing for sinus node disease: A therapeutic rationale. Clin. Cardiol. 17:495, 1994.

174. Katritsis, D., and Camm, A. J.: AAI pacing mode: When is it indicated and how can it be achieved? Clin. Cardiol. 16:339, 1993.

175. Clarke, M., Sutton, R., Ward, D., et al.: Recommendations for pacemaker prescription for symptomatic bradycardia: Report of a working party of the British Pacing and Electrophysiology Group. Br. Heart J. 66:185, 1991.

176. Payne, G. E., and Skehan, J. D.: Issues in cardiac pacing: Can agism be justified? Br. Heart J. 72:102, 1994.

177. Bush, D. E., and Finucane, T. E.: Permanent cardiac pacemakers in the elderly. J. Am. Geriatr. Soc. 42:326, 1994.

178. Barold, S. S.: Cardiac pacing in special and complex situations: Indications and modes of stimulation. Cardiol. Clin. 10:573, 1992.

179. Sutton, R.: The second coming of VDD. Eur. J. Cardiac Pacing Electrophysiol. 1:225, 1992.

180. Antonioli, G. E., Ansani, L., Barbieri, D., et al.: Italian multicenter study on a single lead VDD pacing system using a narrow atrial dipole spacing. PACE 15:1890, 1992.

181. Lau, C. P., Tai, Y. T., Li, J. P., et al.: Initial clinical experience with a single pass VDDR pacing system. PACE 15:1894, 1992.

182. Varriale, P., and Chryssos, B. E.: Atrial sensing performance of the single-lead VDD pacemaker during exercise. J. Am. Coll. Cardiol. 22:1854, 1993.

COMPLICATIONS OF PACEMAKERS

183. Lindsay, H. S., Chennells, P. M., and Perrins, E. J.: Successful treatment by balloon venoplasty and stent insertion of obstruction of the superior vena cava by an endocardial pacemaker lead. Br. Heart J. 71:363, 1994.

184. Sunder, S. K., Ekong, E. A., Sivalingam, K., and Kumar, A.: Superior vena cava thrombosis due to pacing electrodes: Successful treatment with combined thrombolysis and angioplasty. Am. Heart J. 123:790, 1992.

185. Mazzetti, H., Dussaut, A., Tentori, C., et al.: Superior vena cava occlusion and/or syndrome related to pacemaker leads. Am. Heart J. 125:831, 1993.

186. Spittell, P. C., and Hayes, D. L.: Venous complications after insertion of a transvenous pacemaker. Mayo Clinic Proc. 67:258, 1992.

187. Cooper, C. J., Dweik, R., and Gabbay, S.: Treatment of pacemaker-associated right atrial thrombus with 2-hour rTPA infusion. Am. Heart J. 126:228, 1993.

188. Vilacosta, I., Zamorano, J., Camino, A., et al.: Infected transvenous permanent pacemakers: Role of transesophageal echocardiography. Am. Heart J. 125:904, 1993.

189. Vilacosta, I., Sarria, C., San Roman, J. A., et al.: Usefulness of transesophageal echocardiography for diagnosis of infected transvenous permanent pacemakers. Circulation 89:2684, 1994.

190. Smith, H. J., Fearnot, N. E., Byrd, C. L., et al.: Five-years experience with intravascular lead extraction. PACE 17:2016, 1994.

191. Hayes, D. L., and Vliestra, R. E.: Pacemaker malfunction. Ann. Intern. Med. 119:828, 1993.

192. Castle, L. W., and Cook, S.: Pacemaker radiography. In Ellenbogen, K. A., Kay, G. N., and Wilkoff, B. L. (eds.): Clinical Cardiac Pacing. Philadelphia, W. B. Saunders Company, 1995, p. 538.

193. Barold, S. S.: Oversensing by single-chamber pacemakers: Mechanisms, diagnosis, and treatment. Cardiol. Clin. 3:565, 1985.

194. Barold, S. S., Falkoff, M. D., Ong, L. S., and Heinle, R. A.: Interference in cardiac pacemakers: Endogenous sources. In El Sherif, N., and Samet, P. (eds.): Cardiac Pacing and Electrophysiology. 3rd ed. Philadelphia, W. B. Saunders Company, 1991, p. 634.

195. Gross, J. N., Platt, S., Ritacco, R., et al.: The clinical relevance of electromyopotential oversensing in current unipolar devices. PACE 15:2023, 1992.

196. Jain, P., Kaul, U., and Wasir, H. S.: Myopotential inhibition of unipolar demand pacemakers: Utility of provocative manoeuvres in assessment and management. Int. J. Cardiol. 34:33, 1992.

197. Altamura, G., Bianconi, L., LoBiano, F., et al.: Transthoracic DC shock may represent a serious hazard in pacemaker dependent patients. PACE 18:194, 1995.

198. van Gelder, B. M., Bracke, F. A., and el Gamal, M. I.: Upper rate pacing after radiofrequency catheter ablation in a minute ventilation rate adaptive DDD pacemaker. PACE 17:1437, 1994.

199. Barold, S. S., Falkoff, M. D., Ong, L. S., and Heinle, R. A.: Interference in cardiac pacemakers: Exogenous sources. In El Sherif, N., and Samet, P. (eds.): Cardiac Pacing and Electrophysiology. 3rd ed. Philadelphia, W. B. Saunders Company, 1991, p. 608.

200. Epstein, A. E., and Wilkoff, B. L.: Pacemaker-defibrillator interactions. In Ellenbogen, K. A., Kay, G. N., and Wilkoff, B. L. (eds.): Clinical Cardiac Pacing. Philadelphia, W. B. Saunders Company, 1995, p. 757.

201. Souliman, S. K., and Christie, J.: Pacemaker failure induced by radiotherapy. PACE 17:270, 1994.

202. Raitt, M. H., Stelzer, K. J., Laramore, G. E., et al.: Runaway pacemaker during high-energy neutron radiation therapy. Chest 106:955, 1994.

203. Lauck, G., vonSmekal, A., Jung, W., et al.: Influence of nuclear magnetic resonance imaging on software-controlled cardiac pacemakers. PACE 16(Abs.):1140, 1993.

204. Tobisch, R. J., Irnich, W., and Batz, L.: Electromagnetic compatibility of pacemakers and nuclear magnetic resonance imaging. PACE 16(Abs.):1140, 1993.

205. Bernstein, A. D., Irwin, M. E., Parsonnet, V., et al.: NASPE Policy Conference Report: Antibradycardia pacemaker follow-up: Effectiveness, needs and resources. PACE 17:1714, 1994.

206. Sweesy, W., Erickson, S. L., Crago, J. A., et al.: Analysis of the effectiveness of in-office and transtelephonic follow-up in terms of pacemaker system complications. PACE 17:2001, 1994.

207. Barold, S. S.: Evaluation of pacemaker function by Holter recordings. In Moss, A., and Stern, S. (eds.): Non-invasive electrocardiology. London, W. B. Saunders Company, 1996, p. 107.

208. Sgarbossa, E. B., Pinski, S. L., Jaeger, F. J., et al.: Incidence and predictors of syncope in paced patients with sick sinus syndrome. PACE *15:*2055, 1992.

ELECTRICAL DEVICES TO TREAT TACHYCARDIAS

209. Lehman, M. H., and Saksena, S.: Implantable cardioverter defibrillators in cardiovascular practice: Report of the Policy Conference of the North American Society of Pacing and Electrophysiology, NASPE Policy Conference Committee. PACE *14:*969, 1991.

210. Mitrani, R. D., Klein, L. S., Rardon, D. P., et al.: Current trends in the implantable cardioverter defibrillator. *In* Zipes, D. P., and Jalife, J. (eds.): Cardiac Electrophysiology: From Cell to Bedside. Philadelphia, W. B. Saunders Company, 1995, p. 1393.

211. Naccarelli, G. V.: Implantable cardioverter/defibrillator. *In* Willerson, J. T., and Cohn, J. N. (eds.): Cardiovascular Medicine. New York, Churchill-Livingstone, 1995, p. 1441.

212. Cannom, D. S.: Internal cardioverter-defibrillator: Newer technology and newer devices. *In* Podrid, P. J., and Kowey, P. R. (eds.): Cardiac Arrhythmia: Mechanisms, Diagnosis, and Treatment. Baltimore, Williams & Wilkins, 1995, p. 708.

213. Olson, W. H.: Tachyarrhythmia sensing and detection. *In* Singer, I. (ed.): Implantable Cardioverter-Defibrillator. Armonk, N.Y., Futura, 1994, p. 71.

214. Estes, N. A. M., III: Overview of the implantable cardioverter-defibrillator. *In* Estes, N. A. M., III, Manolis, A. S., and Wang, P. J. (eds.): Implantable Cardioverter-Defibrillator: A Comprehensive Textbook. New York, Marcel Dekker, 1994, p. 635.

215. Saksena, S., for the PCD Investigator Group: Clinical outcome of patients with malignant ventricular tachyarrhythmias and a multiprogrammable implantable cardioverter-defibrillator implanted with or without thoracotomy: An international multicenter study. J. Am. Coll. Cardiol. *23:*1521, 1994.

216. Swerdlow, C. D., Ahern, T., Chen, P. S., et al.: Underdetection of ventricular tachycardia by algorithms to enhance specificity in a tiered-therapy cardioverter-defibrillator. J. Am. Coll. Cardiol. *24:*416, 1994.

217. Luceri, R. M., Zilo, P., and the United States and Canadian Enguard Investigators: Initial clinical experience with a dual lead endocardial defibrillation system with atrial pace/sense capability. PACE *18:*163, 1995.

218. Saksena, S., Krol, R. B., and Kaushik, R. R.: Innovations in pulse generators and lead systems: Balancing complexity with clinical benefit and long-term results. Am. Heart J. *127:*1010, 1994.

219. Duffin, E. G., and Barold, S. S.: Implantable cardioverter-defibrillators: An overview and future directions. *In* Singer, I. (ed.): Implantable Cardioverter Defibrillator. Armonk, N.Y., Futura Publishing Co., 1994, p. 751.

220. Stanton, M. S., Hayes, D. L., Munger, T. M., et al.: Consistent subcutaneous prepectoral implantation of a new implantable cardioverter defibrillator. Mayo Clin. Proc. *69:*309, 1994.

221. Bardy, G. H., Hofer, B., Johnson, G., et al.: Implantable transvenous cardioverter-defibrillators. Circulation *87:*1152, 1993.

222. Brachmann, J., Sterns, L. D., Hilbel, T., et al.: Acute efficacy and chronic follow-up of patients with non-thoracotomy third generation implantable defibrillators. PACE *17:*499, 1994.

223. Brooks, R., Garan, H., Torchiana, D., et al.: Three-year outcome of a nonthoracotomy approach to cardioverter-defibrillator implantation in 198 consecutive patients. Am. J. Cardiol. *74:*1011, 1994.

224. Camunas, J., Mehta, D., Ip, J., et al.: Total pectoral implantation: A new technique for implantation of transvenous defibrillator lead systems and implantable cardioverter defibrillator. PACE *16:*380, 1993.

225. Natale, A., Sra, J., Axtell, K., et al.: Preliminary experience with a hybrid nonthoracotomy defibrillating system that includes a biphasic device: Comparison with a standard monophasic device using the same lead system. J. Am. Coll. Cardiol. *24:*406, 1994.

226. Neuzner, J., Pitschner, H. F., Huth, C., and Schlepper, M.: Effect of biphasic waveform pulse on endocardial defibrillation efficacy in humans. PACE *17:*207, 1994.

227. Marks, M. L., Johnson, G., Hofer, B. O., and Bardy, G. H.: Biphasic waveform defibrillation using a three-electrode transvenous lead system in humans. J. Cardiovasc. Electrophysiol. *5:*103, 1994.

228. Heuzner, J., for the European Ventak P₂ Investigator Group: Clinical experience with a new cardioverter defibrillator capable of biphasic waveform pulse and enhanced data storage: Results of a prospective multicenter study, European Ventak P₂ Investigator Group. PACE *17:*1243, 1994.

229. Wyse, D. G., Kavanagh, K. M., Gillis, A. M., et al.: Comparison of biphasic and monophasic shocks for defibrillation using a nonthoracotomy system. Am. J. Cardiol. *71:*197, 1993.

230. Trappe, H. J., Fieguth, H. G., Pfitzner, P., et al.: Epicardial and nonthoracotomy defibrillation lead systems combined with a cardioverter defibrillator. PACE *18:*127, 1995.

231. Manolis, A. S., Rastegar, H., Wang, P. J., and Estes, N. A., 3rd: Fully transvenous cardioverter defibrillators: Rare need for subcutaneous patch with two newer-generation systems. Am. Heart J. *128:*808, 1994.

232. Saksena, S., An, H., Mehra, R., et al.: Prospective comparison of biphasic and monophasic shocks for implantable cardioverter defibrillators using endocardial leads. Am. J. Cardiol. *70:*304, 1992.

233. Thakur, R. K., Souza, J. J., Troup, P. J., et al.: A direct comparison of

234. Manolis, A. S.: Implantable cardioverter-defibrillators lead systems. *In* Estes, N. A. M., III, Manolis, A. S., and Wang, P. J. (eds.): Implantable Cardioverter-Defibrillator: A Comprehensive Textbook. New York, Marcel Dekker, 1994, p. 607.

235. Accorti, P. R., Jr.: Lead technology. *In* Singer, I. (ed.): Implantable Cardioverter-Defibrillator. Armonk, N.Y., Futura, 1994, p. 179.

236. Bardy, G. H., Dolack, G. L., Kudenchuk, P. J., et al.: Prospective, randomized comparison in humans of a unipolar defibrillation system with that using an additional superior vena cava electrode. Circulation *89:*1090, 1994.

237. Raitt, M. H., and Bardy, G. H.: Advances in implantable cardioverter defibrillator therapy. Curr. Opin. Cardiol. *9:*23, 1994.

238. Saksena, S., DeGroot, P., Krol, R. B., et al.: Low-energy endocardial defibrillation using an axillary or a pectoral thoracic electrode location. Circulation *88:*2655, 1993.

239. Neuzner, J., Pitschner, H. F., and Steinmetz, F.: 100% successful implantation of nonthoracotomy lead systems with biphasic cardioverter/defibrillator: European multicenter results in 832 patients. PACE *17*(Abs.):760, 1994.

239a. Villacastin, J., Almendral, J., Arenal, A., et al.: Incidence and clinical significance of multiple consecutive, appropriate, high-energy discharges in patients with implanted cardioverter-defibrillators. Circulation *93:*753, 1996.

240. Jones, D. L.: The defibrillation threshold: A reliable method for rapid determination of defibrillation efficacy. *In* Estes, N. A. M., III, Manolis, A. S., and Wang, P. J. (eds.): Implantable Cardioverter-Defibrillator: A Comprehensive Textbook. New York, Marcel Dekker, 1994, p. 29.

241. Austin, E., and Singer, I.: Operative techniques for implantation and testing of implantable cardioverter-defibrillators. *In* Singer, I. (ed.): Implantable Cardioverter-Defibrillator. Armonk, N.Y., Futura, 1994, p. 327.

242. Jung, W., Manz, M., Pizzulli, L., et al.: Effects of chronic amiodarone therapy on defibrillation threshold. Am. J. Cardiol. *70:*1023, 1992.

243. Jung, W., Manz, M., Pfeiffer, D., et al.: Effects of antiarrhythmic drugs on epicardial defibrillation energy requirements and the rate of defibrillator discharge. PACE *16:*198, 1992.

244. Manz, M., Jung, W., and Lüderitz, B.: Interactions between drugs and devices: Experimental and clinical studies. Am. Heart J. *127:*978, 1994.

245. Avitall, B., Hare, J., Zander, G., et al.: Cardioversion, defibrillation, and overdrive pacing of ventricular arrhythmias: The effect of Moricizine in dogs with sustained monomorphic ventricular tachycardia. PACE *16:*2092, 1993.

246. Peters, W., Gang, E. S., Solrngen, S., et al.: Acute effects of intravenous propafenone on the internal ventricular defibrillation energy requirements in the anesthetized dog. J. Am. Coll. Cardiol. *17*(Abs.):129A, 1991.

247. Natale, A., Montenero, A. S., Bombardieri, G., et al.: Effects of acute and prolonged administration of propafenone on internal defibrillation in the pig. Am. Heart J. *124:*104, 1992.

248. Schrader, R., Brooks, M., and Echt, D. S.: Effects of verapamil and Bay K 8644 on defibrillation energy requirements in dogs. J. Cardiovasc. Pharmacol. *19:*839, 1992.

249. Jones, D. L., Klein, G. J., Guiraudon, G. M., et al.: Effects of lidocaine and verapamil on defibrillation in humans. J. Electrocardiol. *24:*299, 1991.

250. Barold, S. S.: Effect of drugs on defibrillation threshold. *In* Antonioli, G. E., Aubert, A. E., and Ector, H. (eds.): Pacemaker Leads 1991. Amsterdam, Elsevier, 1991, p. 59.

251. Dorian, P., and Newman, D.: Effect of sotalol on ventricular fibrillation and defibrillation in humans. Am. J. Cardiol. *72:*72A, 1993.

252. Akhtar, M., Jazayeri, M., Sra, J., et al.: Role of implantable cardioverter-defibrillator in the management of patients with ventricular tachycardia and ventricular fibrillation. *In* Akhtar, M., Myerburg, R. J., and Ruskin, J. N. (eds.): Sudden Cardiac Death: Prevalence, Mechanisms, and Approaches to Diagnosis and Management. Baltimore, Williams and Wilkins, 1994, p. 588.

253. Bardy, G. H., Poole, J. E., Kudenchuk, P. J., et al.: A prospective, randomized repeat-crossover comparison of antitachycardia pacing with low-energy cardioversion. Circulation *87:*1889, 1993.

254. Kantoch, M. J., Green, M. S., and Tang, A. S.: Randomized cross-over evaluation of two adaptive pacing algorithms for the termination of ventricular tachycardia. PACE *16:*1664, 1993.

255. Calkins, H., el-Atassi, R., Kalbfleisch, S., et al.: Comparison of fixed burst versus decremental burst pacing for termination of ventricular tachycardia. PACE *16:*26, 1993.

256. Estes, N. A., 3rd, Naugh, C. J., Wang, P. J., and Manolis, A. S.: Antitachycardia pacing and low-energy cardioversion for ventricular tachycardia termination: A clinical perspective. Am. Heart J. *127:*1038, 1994.

257. Hammill, S. C., Packer, D. L., Stanton, M. S., Fetter, J., and the Multicenter PCD Investigator Group: Termination and acceleration of ventricular tachycardia with autodecremental pacing, burst pacing and cardioversion in patients with an implantable cardioverter defibrillator. PACE *18:*3, 1995.

258. Heisel, A., Neuzner, J., Himmrich, E., et al.: Safety of antitachycardia pacing in patients with implantable cardioverter defibrillators and severely depressed left ventricular function. PACE *18:*137, 1995.

259. Rabinovich, R., Muratore, C., Iglesias, R., et al.: Results of delivered

therapy for VT or VF in patients with third-generation implantable cardioverter defibrillators. PACE 18:133, 1995.

260. Rankin, A. C., Zaim, S., Powell, A., et al.: Efficacy of a tiered therapy defibrillator system used to treat recurrent ventricular arrhythmias refractory to drugs. Br. Heart J. 70:61, 1993.

261. Callans, D. J., and Josephson, M. E.: Future developments in implantable cardioverter defibrillators: The optimal device. Progr. Cardiovasc. Dis. 36:227, 1993.

262. Nathan, A. W.: The role of cardioversion therapy in patients with implanted cardioverter defibrillators. Am. Heart J. 127:1046, 1994.

263. Lauer, M. R., Young, C., Liem, L. B., et al.: Ventricular fibrillation induced by low-energy shock from programmable implantable cardioverter-defibrillators in patients with coronary artery disease. Am. J. Cardiol. 73:559, 1994.

264. Zipes, D. P., Roberts, D., for the PCD Investigators: Results of the worldwide study of the implantable cardioverter-defibrillator: A comparison of epicardial and endocardial lead systems. Circulation 92:59, 1995.

265. Timmis, G. C.: The development of implantable cardioversion defibrillation systems: The clinical chronicle of defibrillation leads. Am. Heart J. 127:1003, 1994.

266. Fahy, G. J., Kleman, J. M., Wilkoff, B. L., et al.: Low incidence of lead related complications associated with nonthoracotomy implantable cardioverter defibrillator systems. PACE 18:172, 1995.

267. Pfeiffer, D., Jung, W., Fehske, W., et al.: Complications of pacemaker-defibrillator devices: Diagnosis and management. Am. Heart J. 127:1073, 1994.

268. Spratt, K. A., Blumenberg, E. A., Wood, C. A., et al.: Infections of implantable cardioverter defibrillators: Approach to management. Clin. Infect. Dis. 17:679, 1993.

269. Kelly, P. A., Mann, D. E., Damle, R. S., and Reiter, M. J.: Oversensing during ventricular pacing in patients with a third-generation implantable-cardioverter-defibrillator. J. Am. Coll. Cardiol. 23:1531, 1994.

270. Sandler, M. J., and Kutalek, S. P.: Inappropriate discharge by an implantable cardioverter defibrillator: Recognition of myopotential sensing using telemetered intracardiac electrograms. PACE 17:665, 1994.

271. Manz, M., Jung, W., Hogl, B., et al.: Atrial fibrillation following defibrillator discharge: Comparison of two lead systems. Eur. Heart J. 13(Suppl.):152A, 1992.

272. Jung, W., Mletzko, R., Hugl, B., et al.: Incidence of atrial tachyarrhythmias following shock delivery of implantable cardioverter/defibrillators. Circulation 84/4(Abs.):II-612, 1991.

273. Fricchione, G. L., Vlay, L. C., and Vlay, S. C.: Cardiac psychiatry and the management of malignant ventricular arrhythmias with the internal cardioverter-defibrillator. Am. Heart J. 128:1050, 1994.

274. Quill, T. E., Barold, S. S., and Sussman, B. L.: Discontinuing an implantable cardioverter defibrillator as a life sustaining treatment. Am. J. Cardiol. 74:205, 1994.

275. Venditti, F. J., Jr., Martin, D. T., Vassolas, G., and Bowen, S.: Rise in chronic defibrillation thresholds in nonthoracotomy implantable defibrillator. Circulation 89:216, 1994.

276. Hsia, H. H., Mitra, R. L., Flores, B. T., and Marchlinski, F. E.: Early postoperative increase in defibrillation threshold with nonthoracotomy system in humans. PACE 17:1166, 1994.

277. Tchou, P. J., Keim, S. G., Mehdirad, A. A., and Rist, K. E.: ICDs: Clinical outcome in the first decade. In Naccarelli, G. V., and Veltri, E. P. (eds.): Implantable Cardioverter-Defibrillators. Boston, Blackwell Scientific, 1993, p. 216.

278. Marchlinski, F. E., Gottlieb, C. D., Sarter, B., et al.: ICD data storage: Value in arrhythmia management. PACE 16:527, 1993.

279. Hook, B. G., Callans, D. F., Kleiman, R. B., et al.: Implantable cardioverter-defibrillator therapy in the absence of significant symptoms: Rhythm diagnosis and management aided by stored electrogram analysis. Circulation 87:1897, 1993.

280. Roelke, M., Garan, H., McGovern, B. A., and Ruskin, J. N.: Analysis of the initiation of spontaneous monomorphic ventricular tachycardia by stored intracardiac electrograms. J. Am. Coll. Cardiol. 23:117, 1994.

281. Grimm, W., Flores, B. F., and Marchlinski, F. E.: Symptoms and electrocardiographically documented rhythm preceding spontaneous shocks in patients with implantable cardioverter-defibrillator. Am. J. Cardiol. 71:1415, 1993.

282. Klein, L. S., Miles, W. M., and Zipes, D. P.: Antitachycardia devices: Realities and promises. J. Am. Coll. Cardiol. 18:1349, 1991.

283. Powell, A. C., Fuchs, T., Finkelstein, D. M., et al.: Influence of implantable cardioverter-defibrillators on the long-term prognosis of survivors of out-of-hospital cardiac arrest. Circulation 88:1083, 1993.

284. Grimm, W., Flores, B. T., and Marchlinski, F. E.: Shock occurrence and survival in 241 patients with implantable cardioverter-defibrillator therapy. Circulation 87:1880, 1993.

285. Sweeney, M. O., and Ruskin, J. N.: Mortality benefits and the implantable cardioverter-defibrillator. Circulation 89:1851, 1994.

286. Zipes, D. P.: Implantable cardioverter-defibrillator: Lifesaver or a device looking for a disease? Circulation 89:2934, 1994.

287. Zipes, D. P.: The implantable cardioverter defibrillator revolution continues. Mayo Clin. Proc. 69:395, 1994.

288. Kim, S. G., Fisher, J. D., and Furman, S.: Hypothetical death rates of patients with implantable defibrillators remain very hypothetical. Am. J. Cardiol. 72:1453, 1993.

289. Kim, S. G.: Implantable defibrillator therapy: Does it really prolong life? How can we prove it? Am. J. Cardiol. 71:1213, 1993.

290. Dorian, P., Connolly, S., and Yusuf, S.: The impact of left ventricular dysfunction on outcomes with the implantable defibrillator. Am. Heart J. 127:1159, 1994.

291. Bigger, J. T., Jr.: Prediction and prevention of sudden cardiac death. In Estes, N. A. M., III, Manolis, A. S., and Wang, P. J. (eds.): Implantable Cardioverter Defibrillator: A Comprehensive Textbook. New York, Marcel Dekker, 1994, p. 557.

292. Kim, S. G.: Impact of implantable cardioverter-defibrillator therapy on patient survival. Cardiol. Rev. 2:113, 1994.

293. O'Nunain, S., and Ruskin, J.: Cardiac arrest. Lancet 341:1641, 1993.

294. Moss, A. J.: Influence of the implantable cardioverter-defibrillator on survival: Retrospective studies and prospective trials. Progr. Cardiovasc. Dis. 36:85, 1993.

295. Kolettis, T. M., and Saksena, S.: Prophylactic implantable cardioverter defibrillator therapy in high-risk patients with coronary artery disease. Am. Heart J. 127:1164, 1994.

296. Zipes, D. P.: Are implantable cardioverter defibrillators better than conventional antiarrhythmic drugs for survivors of cardiac arrest? Circulation 91:2115, 1995.

Chapter 24
Cardiac Arrest and Sudden Cardiac Death

ROBERT J. MYERBURG, AGUSTIN CASTELLANOS

DEFINITION

Sudden cardiac death (SCD) is natural death due to cardiac causes, heralded by abrupt loss of consciousness within 1 hour of the onset of acute symptoms. Preexisting heart disease may or may not have been known to be present, but the time and mode of death are unexpected. This definition incorporates the key elements of "natural," "rapid," and "unexpected." It consolidates previous definitions which have conflicted,[1–20a] largely because the most useful operational definition of SCD differs for the clinician, the cardiovascular epidemiologist, the pathologist, and the scientist attempting to define pathophysiological mechanisms.

Four elements must be considered in the construction of a definition of SCD to satisfy medical, scientific, legal, and social considerations: (1) prodromes, (2) onset, (3) cardiac arrest, and (4) biological death (Fig. 24–1). Because the proximate cause of SCD is a disturbance of cardiovascular function, which is incompatible with maintaining consciousness because of abrupt loss of cerebral blood flow,

any definition must recognize the brief time interval between the onset of the mechanism directly responsible for cardiac arrest and the consequent loss of consciousness (Fig. 24–1C). The 1-hour definition, however, refers to the duration of the "terminal event" (Fig. 24–1B), which defines the interval between the onset of symptoms signalling the pathophysiological disturbance leading to cardiac arrest and the onset of the cardiac arrest itself (Fig. 24–1B and C).

Premonitory signs and symptoms, which may occur during the days or weeks before a cardiac arrest,[17] tend to be nonspecific for the impending event.[8] *Prodromes* (Fig. 24–1A), which may be more specific for an imminent cardiac arrest, are relatively abrupt changes that begin during an arbitrarily defined period of up to 24 hours before the cardiac arrest.[4,21] The fourth element, *biological death* (Fig. 24–1D), is an immediate consequence of the clinical cardiac arrest in the past, occurring within minutes. However, since the development of community-based intervention systems, and long-term life support systems, patients may

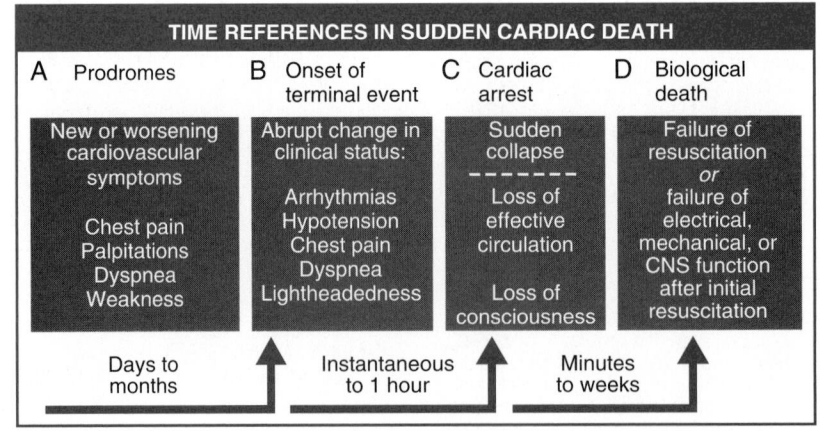

TIME REFERENCES IN SUDDEN CARDIAC DEATH			
A Prodromes	**B** Onset of terminal event	**C** Cardiac arrest	**D** Biological death
New or worsening cardiovascular symptoms Chest pain Palpitations Dyspnea Weakness	Abrupt change in clinical status: Arrhythmias Hypotension Chest pain Dyspnea Lightheadedness	Sudden collapse - - - - - - - Loss of effective circulation Loss of consciousness	Failure of resuscitation *or* failure of electrical, mechanical, or CNS function after initial resuscitation
Days to months	Instantaneous to 1 hour	Minutes to weeks	

FIGURE 24–1. Sudden cardiac death is viewed from four temporal perspectives: *(A)* prodromes, *(B)* onset of the terminal event, *(C)* cardiac arrest, and *(D)* progression to biological death. Individual variability of the components influence clinical expression: some victims experience no prodromes, with onset leading almost instantaneously to cardiac arrest; others may have an onset which lasts up to 1 hour before clinical arrest; some patients may live weeks after the cardiac arrest before progression to biological death if there has been irreversible brain damage and life-support systems are used. These modifying factors influence interpretation of the 1-hour definition. From the perspective of the clinician, the two most relevant factors are the onset of the terminal event *(B)* and the clinical cardiac arrest itself *(C)*. In contrast, legal and social considerations focus on the time of biological death *(D)*.

TABLE 24–1 DEFINITION OF TERMS RELATED TO SUDDEN CARDIAC DEATH

TERM	DEFINITION	QUALIFIERS OR EXCEPTIONS
Death	Irreversible cessation of all biological functions	None
Cardiac arrest	Abrupt cessation of cardiac pump function which may be reversible by a prompt intervention but will lead to death in its absence	Rare spontaneous reversions; likelihood of successful intervention relates to mechanism of arrest and clinical setting
Cardiovascular collapse	A (sudden) loss of effective blood flow due to cardiac and/or peripheral vascular factors which may revert spontaneously (e.g., vasodepressor syncope) or only with interventions (e.g., cardiac arrest)	Nonspecific term which includes cardiac arrest and its consequences and also events which characteristically revert spontaneously

now remain biologically alive for a long period of time after the onset of a pathophysiological process which has caused irreversible damage and will ultimately lead to death.[18–20,22] In this circumstance, the causative pathophysiological and clinical event is the cardiac arrest itself, rather than the factors responsible for the delayed biological death. However, in legal, forensic, and certain social circumstances, biological death must continue to be used as the absolute definition of death. Finally, the forensic pathologist studying *unwitnessed deaths* may use the definition of sudden death for a person known to be alive and functioning normally 24 hours before,[4] and this remains appropriate within its obvious limits because unwitnessed death cannot be ignored in their studies.[23] Thus the

generally accepted clinical-pathophysiological definition of up to 1 hour between onset of the terminal event and biological death requires qualifications for specific circumstances.

The development of community-based intervention systems also has led to inconsistencies in the use of terms considered absolute. *Death* is defined biologically, legally, and literally as an absolute and irreversible event. Thus SCD may be aborted, or a patient may survive cardiac arrest or cardiovascular collapse; however, survival after (sudden) death is a contradiction in terms. Table 24–1 provides definitions for events and terms related to the concept of SCD—death, cardiac arrest, and cardiovascular collapse.

EPIDEMIOLOGY AND CAUSES OF SUDDEN DEATH

EPIDEMIOLOGY

The worldwide incidence of SCD is difficult to estimate because it varies largely as a function of coronary heart disease prevalence in different countries.[24] Estimates for the United States range from 300,000 to nearly 400,000 SCDs annually,[25] the variation based in part on the definition of sudden death used in individual studies.[5,16] The most widely used estimate is 300,000 SCDs annually,[26] a figure which represents 50 per cent or more of all cardiovascular deaths in the United States.[24–28]

The influence of the temporal definition of SCD on epidemiological data[4] is demonstrated by a retrospective death certificate study in a large metropolitan area in the United States reported by Kuller et al.[4] When the temporal definition was restricted to death less than 2 hours after the onset of symptoms, 12 per cent of all natural deaths were sudden, and 88 per cent of the sudden natural deaths were due to cardiac causes. This estimate is similar to observations in a large prospective cohort study—the Framingham study—in which 13 per cent of all deaths observed during a 26-year period were "sudden," defined as death within 1 hour of the onset of symptoms.[29,30] In contrast to deaths occurring less than 2 hours after the onset of symptoms, the application of the 24-hour definition of sudden death to the data from Kuller et al.[4] increased the fraction of all natural deaths falling into the "sudden" category to 32 per cent but reduced the proportion of all sudden natural deaths which were cardiac deaths to 75 per cent.

Prospective studies demonstrate that about 50 per cent of all coronary heart disease deaths are sudden and unexpected, occurring shortly (instantaneous to 1 hour) after the onset of symptoms. In the prospective combined Albany-Framingham study of 4120 males, sudden deaths within 1 hour of an observed collapse were analyzed for a population of men dying between 45 and 74 years of age.[9] During a 16-year follow-up, there were 234 total coronary deaths/1000 population observed, of which 109 (47 per cent) were sudden and unexpected. Because coronary heart disease dominates sudden and total cardiac deaths in the United States, the fraction of total cardiac deaths which are sudden is similar to the fraction of coronary heart disease deaths which are sudden, although there does appear to be a geographical variation in the fraction of coronary deaths which are sudden.[31] This 50 per cent fraction may not apply to other nations or to subcultures which have a lower prevalence of coronary heart disease. It also is of interest that the recent decline in coronary heart

disease mortality in the United States[32] has not changed the fraction of coronary deaths that are sudden and unexpected,[33] even though there may be a decline in out-of-hospital deaths compared with emergency department deaths.[27]

POPULATION POOLS AND TIME-DEPENDENCE OF RISK

Two factors are of primary importance for identifying populations at risk and when considering strategies for primary prevention of SCD: (1) the size of denominators of population subgroups (Fig. 24–2A), and (2) time-dependence of risk (Fig. 24–2B).

POPULATION SUBGROUPS AND SCD. The more than 300,000 adult SCDs which occur annually in the United States can be viewed in terms of incidence in an unselected adult population. Because of the large denominator which this population pool represents, the overall incidence is 1 to 2/1000 population (0.1–0.2 per cent) per year. This large population base includes both those victims whose SCDs occur as a first cardiac event and those whose SCDs may be predicted with greater accuracy because they are included in higher-risk subgroups. Any intervention designed for the *general* population must, therefore, be applied to the 99/1000 who will not have an event to reach and possibly influence the 1/1000 who will. The cost and risk-to-benefit uncertainties limit the nature of such broadbased interventions and demand a higher resolution of risk identification. Figure 24–2A highlights this problem by expressing the incidence (per cent/year) of SCD among various subgroups and comparing the incidence figures to the total number of events which occur annually in each subgroup. By moving from the total adult population to a subgroup with high risk because of the presence of selected coronary risk factors, there may be a 10-fold or greater increase in the incidence of events annually, with the mag-

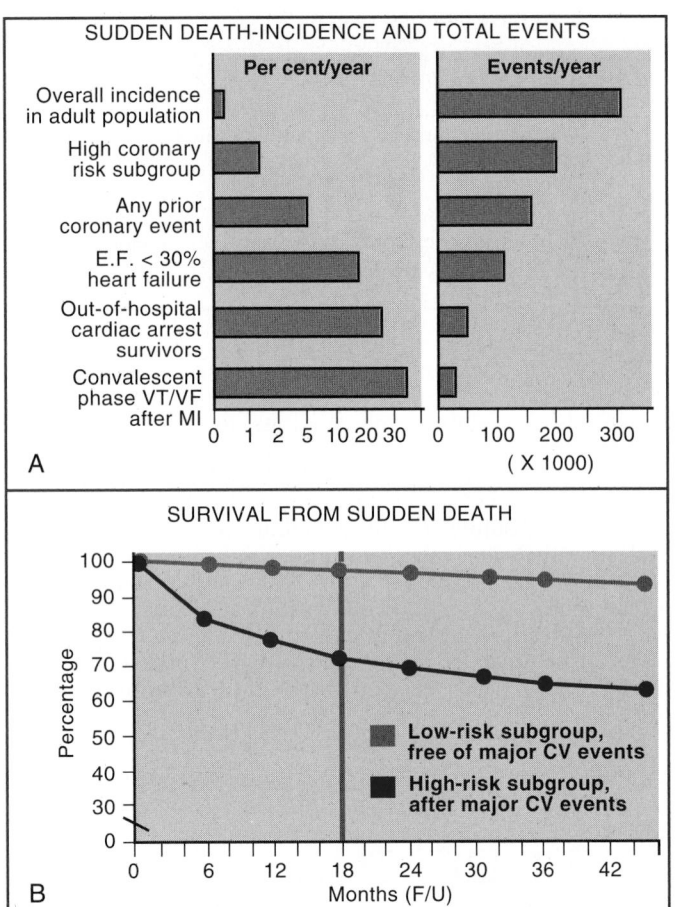

SUDDEN DEATH-INCIDENCE AND TOTAL EVENTS

A

SURVIVAL FROM SUDDEN DEATH

- Low-risk subgroup, free of major CV events
- High-risk subgroup, after major CV events

B

FIGURE 24–2. Impact of population pools and time-from-events on the clinical epidemiology of sudden cardiac death. The top panel *(A)* compares incidence and total numbers of sudden cardiac deaths in different subgroups; the lower panel *(B)* demonstrates time-dependence of risk for sudden death after major cardiovascular events.

In the top panel *(A)*, estimates of incidence figures (per cent/year) and the total number of events/year are shown for the overall adult population in the United States, and for increasingly higher-risk subgroups. The overall adult population has an estimated sudden death incidence of 0.1 to 0.2 per cent/year, accounting for a total number of events of more than 300,000/year. With the identification of increasingly powerful risk factors, the incidence *increases* progressively, but it is accomplished by a progressive *decrease* in the total number of patients identified. The inverse relation between incidence and total number of events occurs because of the progressively smaller denominator pool in the highest subgroup categories.

Successful interventions among larger population subgroups will require identification of specific markers to increase the ability to identify specific patients who will be at particularly high risk for a future event (*Note:* The horizontal axis for the incidence figures is not linear, and should be interpreted accordingly.)

In the lower panel *(B)*, idealized curves of survival from sudden death are shown for a population of patients with known cardiovascular disease but at low risk because of freedom from major cardiovascular (CV) events *(top curve)*, and for populations of patients who have survived a major cardiovascular event *(bottom curve)*. Attrition over time is accelerated in both absolute and relative terms for the initial 6 to 18 months after the major cardiovascular event. After the initial attrition, the slopes of the curves for the high-risk and low-risk populations parallel each other, highlighting both the early attrition and the attenuation of risk after 18 to 24 months.

These relations have been observed in diverse high-risk subgroups (cardiac arrest survivors, post-myocardial infarction patients with high-risk markers, recent onset of heart failure), and highlight the changing risk pattern as a function of time and the importance of the time dimension for recognition and intervention in strategies designed to alter outcome. (Modified from Myerburg, R. J., et al.: Sudden cardiac death: Structure, function and time-dependence of risk. Circulation *85*(Suppl. I):I-2, 1992. Copyright 1992 American Heart Association.)

nitude of increase dependent on the number of risk factors operating in the subgroup. The size of the denominator pool, however, remains very large, and implementation of interventions remains problematic, even at this heightened level of risk. Higher resolution is desirable and can be achieved by identification of more specific subgroups. The corresponding absolute number of deaths becomes progressively smaller as the subgroups become more focused (Fig. 24–2*A*), limiting the potential benefit of interventions to the much smaller subgroups.

TIME-DEPENDENCE OF RISK. Risk of SCD is not linear as a function of time after a change in cardiovascular status.[26,34,35] Survival curves after major cardiovascular events, which identify populations at high risk for both sudden and total cardiac death, usually demonstrate that the most rapid rate of attrition occurs during the first 6 to 18 months (Fig. 24–2*B*). Thus there is a time-dependence of risk which focuses the opportunity for effective intervention to the early period after a conditioning event. Curves that have these characteristics have been generated from among survivors of out-of-hospital cardiac arrest, new onset of heart failure, and unstable angina, and from high-risk subgroups of patients having recent myocardial infarction. *The addition of time as a dimension for measuring risk may increase the resolution within subgroups.*

AGE, HEREDITY, GENDER, AND RACE

AGE. There are two ages of peak incidence of sudden death: between birth and 6 months of age (the sudden infant death syndrome) and between 45 and 75 years of age.[3] In the adult population the *incidence* of sudden death owing to coronary heart disease increases as a function of advancing age,[33,36–38] in parallel with the age-related increase in incidence of total coronary heart disease deaths.[32] However, the *proportion* of deaths caused by coronary heart disease that are sudden and unexpected decreases with advancing age.[19,33,36–38] Kuller et al.[39] reported that 76 per cent of coronary heart disease deaths in the 20-to-39-year age group were sudden and unexpected, and the Framingham data demonstrated that 62 per cent of all coronary heart disease deaths were sudden in the 45-to-54 year age group in men. The proportion fell progressively to 58 per cent in the 55-to-64-year age group and to 42 per cent in the 65-to-74-year age group.[36,37] Age also influences the proportion of cardiovascular causes among all causes of natural sudden death in that the proportion of coronary deaths and of all cardiac causes of death which are sudden is highest in the younger age groups, whereas the fraction of total sudden natural deaths which are due to any cardiovascular cause is higher in the older age groups.[40] In their study of sudden death in children and young adults, Neuspiel and Kuller[40] reported that only 19 per cent of sudden natural deaths in children between 1 and 13 years of age were cardiac deaths; the proportion increased to 30 per cent in the 14-to-21-year age group. All of these studies of age factors used a 24-hour definition of sudden death.

HEREDITY. To the extent that SCD is an expression of underlying coronary heart disease, hereditary factors that contribute to coronary heart disease risk operate nonspecifically for the SCD syndrome.[41]

Among the less common causes of SCD, hereditary patterns have been reported for some specific syndromes. Such patterns are described for some forms of congenital and hereditary Q-T interval prolongation (see p. 951),[42] hypertrophic obstructive cardiomyopathy,[43] and familial SCD in children and young adults.[44] Although stable congenital conducting system abnormalities have a good prognosis,[45] progressive familial conducting system disease, which appears to have a hereditary pattern, carried an increased risk of SCD.[46] Familial sudden death associated with cardiac ganglionitis has been reported,[47] but an inheritance pattern has not been demonstrated in the reports to date. Linkage analyses in families with long Q-T interval syndromes have provided a major advance in the understanding of a genetic basis for one cause of sudden death (see p. 1667). Abnormalities on three different chromosomes (loci on chromosomes 11, 7, and 3) each associate with congenital long Q-T syndrome. Two of the three (on chromosomes 7 and 3) encode a membrane channel abnormality that can prolong repolarization.[48–50] This observation may provide a screening tool for individuals at risk, as well as the potential for specific therapeutic strategies.

GENDER. The SCD syndrome has a huge preponderance in males compared with females because of the protection females enjoy from coronary atherosclerosis before advanced years.[29,30,37] During the first 14 years of follow-up in the Framingham study, 59 of 66 (89 per cent) sudden unexpected coronary deaths (<1 hour) occurred in men.[8] The Framingham study at 20 years of follow-up demonstrated a 3.8-fold excess incidence of sudden coronary death in men compared with women.[37] This male/female ratio is similar to data recorded in three prospective studies of prehospital cardiac arrest in which the percentages of males observed were 75 per cent (mean age 63 years),[18] 85 per cent (mean age 60 years),[19] and 89 per cent (mean age 58 years),[51] respectively. In the study by Kuller et al.,[4] 75 per cent of all SCDs (using the 24-hour definition) in a 40-to-64-year-old population were in men. When the data in another study by Kuller et al. were analyzed for survival of less than 2 hours, the proportion of men increased to 80 per cent.[52] In the Framingham study[37] the excess risk in men peaked at 6.75:1 in the 55-to-64-year age group and then fell to 2.17:1 in the 65-to-74-year age group. Even though the overall risk is much lower in women, the classic coronary risk factors are expressed in them.[29,30,53,54] Cigarette smoking, diabetes, use of oral contraceptives,[55] and reduced vital capacity[30] are particularly strong factors.

RACE. A number of studies comparing racial differences and relative risk of SCD in whites and blacks with coronary heart disease in the United States have yielded conflicting and inconclusive data.[4,56,57] However, a recent large study from an urban area demonstrated excess risk of cardiac arrest and SCD in blacks compared with whites.[57] An excess was observed across all age groups, but the magnitude of excess risk among adults decreased with increasing age.

Data on the prevalence of coronary heart disease in Japanese men living in the United States have demonstrated that the low rates reported in those living in Japan tend to increase toward, but do not reach, levels observed in white men in the United States.[58] Thus, an interplay between race and environmental factors may be operative.

BIOLOGICAL RISK FACTORS AND SUDDEN DEATH

The known coronary risk factors cannot be used to distinguish the patients at risk for SCD from those at risk for other manifestations of coronary heart disease.[9] Using a multivariate analysis of selected risk factors (i.e., age, systolic blood pressure, heart rate, electrocardiographic abnormalities, vital capacity, relative weight, cigarette consumption, and serum cholesterol) from the population in the Framingham data, Kannel and Schatzkin[33] determined that 53 per cent of the SCDs in men and 42 per cent of those in women occurred among the 10 per cent of the population in the highest risk decile (Fig. 24–3). The comparison of risk factors in the victims of SCD with those in people who developed any manifestations of coronary artery disease did not provide useful patterns, by either univariate or multivariate analysis, to distinguish victims of SCD from the overall pool.[9] In addition, data from 19,946 patients in the Coronary Artery Surgery Study identified no angiographic or hemodynamic patterns that discriminated sudden from nonsudden cardiac deaths.[38]

Hypertension is a clearly established risk factor for coronary heart disease and also emerges as a highly significant risk factor for incidence of SCD.[9] However, there is no influence of increasing systolic blood pressure levels on the ratio of sudden deaths to total coronary heart disease

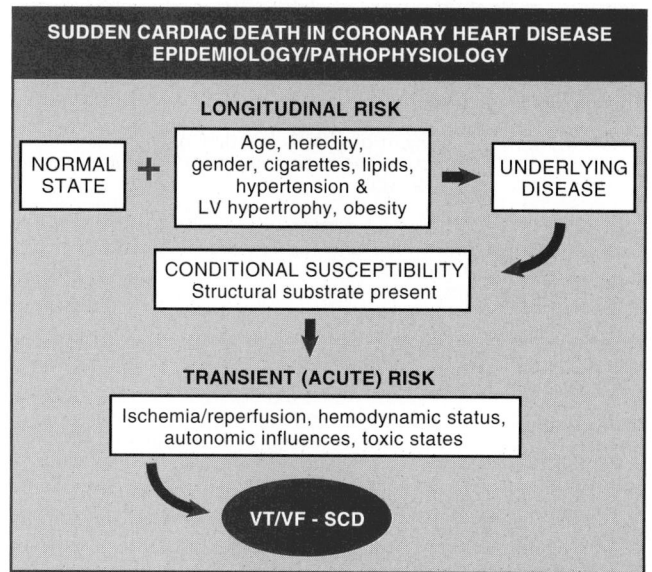

FIGURE 24–4. Epidemiology of SCD: conventional (conditioning) risk factors versus transient (triggering) risk factors. Conventional risk factors predict risk of the disease underlying SCD; transient risk factors predict risk of the pathophysiological event that initiates the fatal event. (Modified from Myerburg, R. J., Kessler, K. M., Kimura, S., et al.: Life-threatening ventricular arrhythmias: The link between epidemiology and pathophysiology. *In* Zipes, D. P., and Jalife, J. [eds.]: Cardiac Electrophysiology, 2nd ed. Philadelphia, W. B. Saunders Company, 1995.)

deaths.[36] No relationship has been observed between cholesterol concentration and the proportion of coronary deaths that were sudden.[37] Neither the electrocardiographic pattern of left ventricular hypertrophy nor nonspecific ST-T wave abnormalities influence the proportion of total coronary deaths that are sudden and unexpected[36]; *only intraventricular conduction abnormalities are suggestive of a disproportionate number of SCDs.*[37] A low vital capacity also suggests a disproportionate risk for sudden versus total coronary deaths.[37] This is of interest because such a relation was particularly striking in the analysis of data on women in the Framingham study who had died suddenly.[29,30] A high hematocrit also was predictive in women.[31]

The conventional risk factors used in most studies of SCD are the risk factors for coronary artery disease. The rationale is based upon two facts: (1) Coronary disease is the structural basis for 80 per cent of SCDs in the United States, and (2) the coronary risk factors are easy to identify because they tend to be present continuously over time (Fig. 24–4). However, risk factors specific for fatal arrhythmias are dynamic pathophysiological events and occur transiently.[59] Transient pathophysiological events are being modeled epidemiologically,[60] in an attempt to express and use them as clinical risk factors[61] for both profiling and intervention.[62]

LIFE STYLE AND PSYCHOSOCIAL FACTORS

LIFE STYLE. There is a strong association between *cigarette smoking* and all manifestations of coronary heart disease. The Framingham study demonstrates that cigarette smokers have a two- to threefold increase in sudden death risk in each decade of life at entry between 30 and 59 years, and that this is one of the few risk factors in which the proportion of coronary heart disease deaths that are sudden increases in association with the risk factor.[37] In addition, in a study of 310 survivors of out-of-hospital cardiac arrest, Hallstrom et al.[63] observed a 27 per cent incidence of recurrent cardiac arrest at 3 years in those who continued to smoke after their index event, compared with 19 per cent in those who stopped (P < .04). Obesity is a second factor which appears to influence the proportion of coronary deaths that occur suddenly.[30,37] With increasing relative weight, the percentage of coronary heart disease deaths that were sudden in the Framingham study increased linearly from a low of 39 per cent to a high of 70 per cent. Total coronary heart disease deaths increased with increasing relative weight as well.

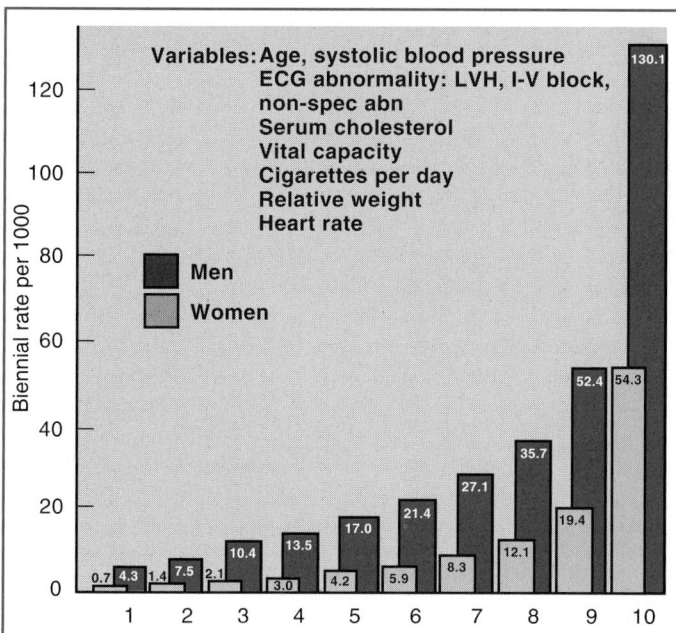

FIGURE 24–3. Risk of sudden death by decile of multivariant risk: 26-year follow-up, the Framingham Study. ECG = electrocardiographic; I-V = intraventricular; LVH = left ventricular hypertrophy; non-spec abn = nonspecific abnormality. (From Kannel, W. B., and Shatzkin, A.: Sudden death: Lessons from subsets in population studies. Reprinted by permission of the American College of Cardiology. J. Am. Coll. Cardiol. 5[Suppl. 6]:141B, 1985.)

Epidemiological observations suggest a relationship between *low levels of physical activity* and increased coronary heart disease death risk.[64] The Framingham study, however, showed an *insignificant* relationship between low levels of physical activity and incidence of sudden death but a high proportion of sudden to total cardiac deaths at higher levels of physical activity.[37] An association between acute physical exertion (especially in physically inactive individuals) and the onset of myocardial infarction has been suggested,[62] but it is not yet known if this also applies to SCD.

PSYCHOSOCIAL FACTORS. These appear to influence the risk for SCDs. Rahe and coworkers[65] recorded recent life changes in the realms of health, work, home and family, and personal and social factors, relating the magnitude of such changes to myocardial infarction and SCD. There was an association between significant elevations of life-change scores during the 6 months before a coronary event, and the association was particularly striking in victims of SCD. In a study of sudden death in women,[66] those who died suddenly were less often married, had fewer children, and had greater educational discrepancies with their spouses than did age-related controls living in the same neighborhood as the sudden death victims. A history of psychiatric treatment, cigarette smoking, and greater quantities of alcohol consumption than the controls also characterized the sudden death group.[66] Ruberman and coworkers reported on the influences of psychosocial factors on sudden and total death after myocardial infarction in 2320 male survivors of myocardial infarction.[67] Controlling for other major prognostic factors, including frequency of premature ventricular contractions, a greater than fourfold increase in risk of sudden and total deaths was predicted by *social isolation* and a *high level of life stress*. These psychosocial factors were inversely related to levels of education. In an earlier study, a more than threefold increase of sudden death risk during follow-up after myocardial infarction had been reported in men who had complex ventricular ectopy and low levels of education compared with better-educated men with the same arrhythmias.[68] Interestingly, there was no relation between educational level and recurrent myocardial infarction.

In a survey of life style, it was found that people with lower educational levels smoked more cigarettes, drank more alcohol, exercised less, and were more overweight.[69] The studies by Friedman and Rosenman[70] on the time-oriented, aggressive *type A personality* characteristics have suggested an increased incidence of all manifestations of coronary heart disease in such patients, including the incidence of sudden cardiac death. The validity of the discrimination of a high-risk subgroup based on type A personality characteristics has recently been challenged.[71]

FUNCTIONAL CLASSIFICATION AND SUDDEN DEATH. The Framingham study demonstrated a striking relation between functional classification and death during a 2-year follow-up period. However, the proportion of deaths that were sudden did not vary with functional classification, ranging from 50 to 57 per cent in all groups, ranging from those free of clinical heart disease to those in functional Class IV.[37]

Sudden Death and Previous Coronary Heart Disease

Although SCD is the first clinical manifestation of coronary heart disease in 20 to 25 per cent or more of all coronary heart disease patients,[9,16,23,26] a previous myocardial infarction can be identified in as many as 75 per cent of patients who die suddenly. The high incidence of both clinical and unrecognized prior myocardial infarction in victims of SCD has led to a search for predictors of SCD in survivors of myocardial infarction, as well as in patients

with other clinical manifestations of coronary heart disease.

LEFT VENTRICULAR EJECTION FRACTION IN CHRONIC ISCHEMIC HEART DISEASE. A marked depression of the left ventricular ejection fraction is the most powerful predictor of SCD in patients with chronic ischemic heart disease, as well as those whose SCD results from other causes (see below). Increased risk, independent of other risk factors, is measurable at ejection fractions greater than 40 per cent, but the greatest rate of change of risk is between 30 and 40 per cent.[72] An ejection fraction equal to or less than 30 per cent is the single most powerful predictor for SCD, but it has a low specificity. Low ejection fraction data parallel risk data based on arrhythmias, but ejection fraction remains an independent predictor.[72]

VENTRICULAR ECTOPY IN CHRONIC ISCHEMIC HEART DISEASE. Most forms of ventricular ectopic activity (premature ventricular contractions, PVCs) in the absence of heart disease[73] are prognostically benign. When present in people over the age of 30, however, PVCs select a subgroup with a higher probability of coronary artery disease and of SCD.[74] In addition, the occurrence of PVCs in survivors of myocardial infarction,[75] particularly if frequent and of complex forms such as multiform or repetitive PVCs,[72,76] predicts an increased risk of SCD on long-term follow-up. Most of these studies have identified both *frequency* and *forms* of ventricular ectopic activity as indicators of risk, but uniformity for such classifications is lacking.[77] Although most studies cite a frequency cutoff of 10 PVCs/hour as a threshold level for increased risk, some have identified frequency cutoffs in the range of 1 to 9 PVCs/hour, 10 PVCs/1000 sinus beats, and more than 20 PVCs/hour. Forms suggestive of high risk include multiform PVCs, bigeminy, short coupling intervals (R-on-T phenomenon), and salvos of three or more ectopic beats.[77] Several investigators have emphasized that the most powerful predictors among the various forms of PVCs are salvos of three or more complexes.[72,76,78]

Many of the reported studies have been based on a single ambulatory monitor sample recorded 1 week to several months after the onset of acute myocardial infarction, and the duration of the samples has ranged from 1 hour to 48 hours. Ruberman et al.[78] reported that repeated short-term (1-hour) ambulatory recordings at 6-month intervals beginning 1 month after myocardial infarction reestablished the increased risk imparted by complex forms of PVCs for the ensuing 3½-year interval, as long as complex forms remained on the interval recordings.

All early drug intervention studies were limited by design features which made interpretation of therapeutic efficacy (mortality reduction) impossible.[79] The results of the Cardiac Arrhythmia Suppression Trial (CAST) (see p. 1265), designed to test the hypothesis that PVC suppression by antiarrhythmic drugs alters risk of SCD after myocardial

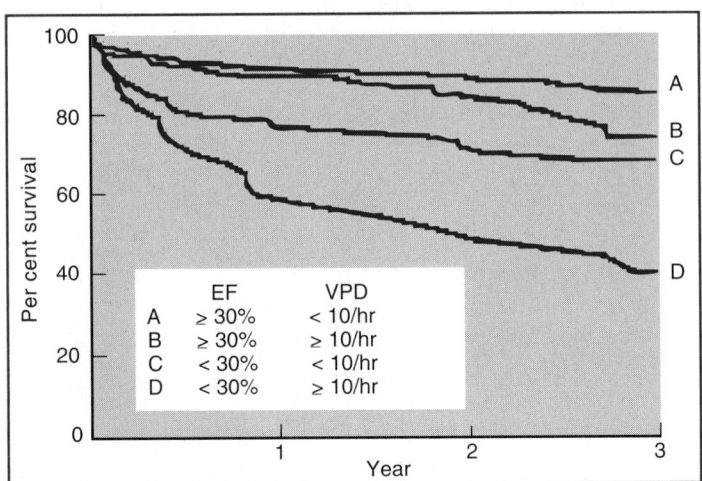

	EF	VPD
A	≥ 30%	< 10/hr
B	≥ 30%	≥ 10/hr
C	< 30%	< 10/hr
D	< 30%	≥ 10/hr

FIGURE 24-5. Survival during 3 years of follow-up after acute myocardial infarction as a function of left ventricular dysfunction (ejection fraction, EF) and ventricular arrhythmias (VPDs/hour as measured by Holter monitoring). The survival curves were calculated as Kaplan-Meier estimates. With higher PVC frequencies and lower ejection fractions, the mortality rates increase. The number of patients in groups A, B, C, and D were 536, 136, 80, and 37, respectively. (From Bigger, J. T.: Relation between left ventricular dysfunction and ventricular arrhythmias after myocardial infarction. Am. J. Cardiol. *57:*8B, 1986.)

infarction, were surprising for two reasons.[80] First, the death rate in the randomized placebo group was lower than expected, and second, the rate among patients in the encainide and flecainide arms exceeded control rates by more than three times. Thus, for these two Class IC drugs, treatment had an adverse effect for a population dominated by frequent single PVCs, and with a mean ejection fraction of about 40 per cent. Subgroup analysis demonstrated increased risk in the placebo group for patients with nonsustained ventricular tachycardia and with ejection fraction of 30 per cent or less, but excess risk in the treated group was still observed. The role of antiarrhythmic drugs for patients with the latter characteristics (ejection fraction less than 30 per cent and nonsustained ventricular tachycardia) requires prospective study, but CAST has shown that antiarrhythmics can have an adverse effect in lower-risk groups. In the continuation of CAST (CAST II), comparing moricizine with placebo and altering enrollment to favor patients with more advanced disease, no adverse effect (other than short-term proarrhythmic risk at initiation of therapy) was observed, but no long-term benefit emerged either.[81] Whether the conclusions from CAST and CAST II extend beyond the drugs studied or to other diseases remains to be learned.[82]

Left ventricular dysfunction is a major co-factor for the risk implied by chronic PVCs after myocardial infarction,[72] and complex forms of both PVCs and left ventricular dysfunction are independent predictors which exert lethal expressions most powerfully in different time periods after myocardial infarction. The risk of death indicated by post-myocardial infarction PVCs is therefore enhanced by the presence of left ventricular dysfunction (Fig. 24–5); the latter appears to exert its influence most strongly in the first 6 months after infarction.[72] Finally, there are data suggesting that the risk associated with post-infarction complex PVCs is higher in patients who have non-Q-wave infarctions than in those with transmural infarctions.[83]

Causes of Sudden Cardiac Death

Coronary heart disease and its consequences account for at least 80 per cent of SCDs in Western cultures. It also is the most common cause in many areas of the world in which the prevalence of coronary heart disease is lower. Despite the established relation between coronary heart disease and SCD,[18–20,34] a complete understanding of SCD requires recognition of other causes which, although less common and often quite rare (Table 24–2), may be recognizable before death, have therapeutic implications, and provide broad insight into the sudden death problem.

CORONARY ARTERY ABNORMALITIES. Although structural abnormalities of coronary arteries other than coronary atherosclerosis are infrequent causes of SCD, the relative risk of SCD may be quite high for specific abnormalities. Nonatherosclerotic coronary artery abnormalities include congenital lesions, coronary artery embolism, coronary arteritis, and mechanical abnormalities of the coronary arteries. Among the congenital lesions, *anomalous origin of a left coronary artery from the pulmonary artery* (see p. 909) is relatively common[84] and has a high death rate in childhood if not surgically treated.[85] The early risk for SCD is not excessively high,[84] but patients who survive to adulthood without surgical intervention are at risk.[85] Other forms of coronary AV fistulas are much less frequent and have a low incidence of SCD. *Anomalous origin of a left coronary artery from the right or noncoronary aortic sinus of Valsalva* (see p. 260) appears to have increased risk of SCD,[86–88] particularly when the anomalous artery passes between the aortic and the pulmonary artery roots. *Anomalous origin of the right coronary artery from the left sinus of Valsalva* also has been reported in association with SCD[86–88] but may not have the same risk as origin of the left coronary from the right sinus of Valsalva. Congenitally hypoplastic, stenotic, or atretic left coronary arteries are uncommon abnormalities which have a high risk of myocardial infarction but not of SCD.[84]

Embolism to the coronary arteries occurs most commonly in aortic valve endocarditis and from thrombotic material on diseased or prosthetic aortic or mitral valves.[89] Emboli also may originate from left ventricular mural thrombi or as a consequence of surgery or cardiac catheterization. Symptoms and signs of myocardial ischemia or infarction are the most common manifestations. In each of these cate-

gories SCD is a risk resulting from the electrophysiological consequences of the embolic ischemic event. Although embolism of platelet aggregates is a pathophysiological mechanism which has not clearly been demonstrated to be associated with SCD in clinical settings, some observations have focused attention on the feasibility of such a mechanism.

The *mucocutaneous lymph node syndrome* (Kawasaki's disease)[91] (see p. 994) carries a risk of SCD in association with coronary arteritis. Polyarteritis nodosa and related vasculitis syndromes (see p. 1783) can cause SCD presumably because of coronary arteritis,[92] as can coronary ostial stenosis in syphilitic aortitis[45] (see p. 1441). The latter has become a very rare manifestation of syphilis.[93]

Several types of mechanical obstruction to coronary arteries must be listed among causes of SCD. Coronary dissection, with or without dissection of the aorta, occurs in the Marfan syndrome[94] (see p. 1669) and has also been reported in the peripartum period of pregnancy.[95] Among the rare mechanical causes of SCD is prolapse of myxomatous polyps from the aortic valve into coronary ostia[96] as well as dissection or rupture of a sinus of Valsalva aneurysm, with involvement of the coronary ostia and proximal coronary arteries.[97] Finally, deep myocardial bridges over coronary arteries (see p. 258) have been reported in association with SCD occurring during strenuous exercise,[98] possibly due to dynamic mechanical obstruction.

Coronary artery spasm (see p. 1340) may cause serious arrhythmias and SCD[99–101] with or without concomitant coronary atherosclerotic lesions.[100] Painless myocardial ischemia, associated with either spasm or fixed lesions, may be a cause of heretofore unexplained sudden death.[101–103] Different patterns of silent ischemia (e.g., totally asymptomatic, post-myocardial infarction, and mixed silent/anginal pattern) may have different prognostic implications.[104]

VENTRICULAR HYPERTROPHY. Left ventricular hypertrophy is an independent risk factor for SCD,[6] accompanies many causes of SCD,[105] and may be a physiological contributor to mechanisms of potentially lethal arrhythmias.[105,106] The underlying states resulting in hypertrophy include hypertensive heart disease with or without atherosclerosis, valvular heart disease, obstructive and nonobstructive hypertrophic cardiomyopathy, primary pulmonary hypertension with right ventricular hypertrophy, and advanced right ventricular overload secondary to congenital heart disease. Each of these conditions is associated with risk of SCD, and it has been suggested that patients with severely hypertrophic ventricles are particularly susceptible to arrhythmic death.[105]

HYPERTROPHIC OBSTRUCTIVE CARDIOMYOPATHY (see p. 1414). Risk of SCD in hypertrophic obstructive cardiomyopathy was identified in the early clinical and hemodynamic studies of this entity.[107] Two subsequent large series have yielded similar data on the magnitude of this risk. Goodwin[108] observed 48 deaths, of which 36 (67 per cent) were sudden, among a cohort of 254 patients followed for a mean of 6 years, while Shah et al.[109] reported that 26 of 49 deaths (55 per cent) among 190 patients were sudden. Cardiac arrest survivors in this etiological group may have better long-term outcome than do survivors with other etiologies. In one report only 11/33 (33 per cent) had recurrent cardiac arrest or death during a mean follow-up of 7 years.[110]

Specific clinical markers have not been especially predictive of SCD in individual patients, although young age at onset,[108,111] strong family history,[43,108] and worsening symptoms[108] appear to indicate higher risk. In one study, however, 54 per cent of the sudden deaths occurred in patients without any functional limitations.[111] The mechanism of SCD in patients with hypertrophic obstructive cardiomyopathy was initially thought to involve outflow tract obstruction, possibly as a consequence of catecholamine stimulation, but more recent data have focused on lethal arrhythmias as the common mechanism of sudden death in this disease.[105,111–116] These studies have demonstrated a high prevalence of PVCs and nonsustained ventricular tachycardia on ambulatory monitoring,[112,114] or the inducibility of potentially lethal arrhythmias during programed electrical stimulation.[115,116] However, stable and asymptomatic nonsustained ventricular tachycardia has limited predictive power for SCD in these patients. Rapid and/or polymorphic symptomatic nonsustained tachycardias have better predictive power.

The question of whether the pathogenesis of the arrhythmias represents an interaction between electrophysiological and hemodynamic abnormalities or is a consequence of electrophysiological

I. CORONARY ARTERY ABNORMALITIES
  A. Coronary atherosclerosis
    1. Chronic ischemic heart disease with transient supply/demand imbalance—thrombosis, spasm, physical stress
    2. Acute myocardial infarction
    3. Chronic atherosclerosis with change in myocardial substrate
  B. Congenital abnormalities of coronary arteries
    1. Anomalous origin from pulmonary artery
    2. Other coronary AV fistula
    3. Origin of left coronary artery from right sinus of Valsalva
    4. Origin of right coronary artery from left sinus of Valsalva
    5. Hypoplastic or aplastic coronary arteries
    6. Coronary-intracardiac shunt
  C. Coronary artery embolism
    1. Aortic or mitral endocarditis
    2. Prosthetic aortic or mitral valves
    3. Abnormal native valves or LV mural thrombus
    4. Platelet embolism
  D. Coronary arteritis
    1. Polyarteritis nodosa, progressive systemic sclerosis, giant cell arteritis
    2. Mucocutaneous lymph node syndrome (Kawasaki's disease)
    3. Syphilitic coronary ostial stenosis
  E. Miscellaneous mechanical obstruction of coronary arteries
    1. Coronary artery dissection in Marfan syndrome
    2. Coronary artery dissection in pregnancy
    3. Prolapse of aortic valve myxomatous polyps into coronary ostia
    4. Dissection or rupture of sinus of Valsalva
  F. Functional obstruction of coronary arteries
    1. Coronary artery spasm with or without atherosclerosis
    2. Myocardial bridges
II. HYPERTROPHY OF VENTRICULAR MYOCARDIUM
  A. Left ventricular hypertrophy associated with coronary heart disease
  B. Hypertensive heart disease without significant coronary atherosclerosis
  C. Hypertrophic myocardium secondary to valvular heart disease
  D. Hypertrophic cardiomyopathy

    1. Obstructive
    2. Nonobstructive
  E. Primary or secondary pulmonary hypertension
    1. Advanced chronic right ventricular overload
    2. Pulmonary hypertension in pregnancy (highest risk peripartum)
III. MYOCARDIAL DISEASES AND HEART FAILURE
  A. Chronic congestive heart failure
    1. Ischemic cardiomyopathy
    2. Idiopathic congestive cardiomyopathy
    3. Alcoholic cardiomyopathy
    4. Hypertensive cardiomyopathy
    5. Post-myocarditis cardiomyopathy
    6. Postpartum cardiomyopathy
  B. Acute cardiac failure
    1. Massive acute myocardial infarction
    2. Acute myocarditis
    3. Acute alcoholic cardiac dysfunction
    4. Ball-valve embolism in aortic stenosis or prosthesis
    5. Mechanical disruptions of cardiac structures
      (a) Rupture of ventricular free wall
      (b) Disruption of mitral apparatus
        (1) Papillary muscle
        (2) Chordae tendineae
        (3) Leaflet
      (c) Rupture of interventricular septum
    6. Acute pulmonary edema in noncompliant ventricles
IV. INFLAMMATORY, INFILTRATIVE, NEOPLASTIC, AND DEGENERATIVE PROCESSES
  A. Acute viral myocarditis with or without ventricular dysfunction
  B. Myocarditis associated with the vasculitides
  C. Sarcoidosis
  D. Progressive systemic sclerosis
  E. Amyloidosis
  F. Hemochromatosis
  G. Idiopathic giant cell myocarditis
  H. Chagas' disease
  I. Cardiac ganglionitis
  J. Arrhythmogenic right ventricular dysplasia; right ventricular cardiomyopathy
  K. Neuromuscular diseases (e.g., muscular dystrophy, Friedreich's ataxia, myotonic dystrophy)
  L. Intramural tumors
    1. Primary
    2. Metastatic

derangement of hypertrophied muscle[105,106] is unanswered. The observation that patients with nonobstructive hypertrophic cardiomyopathy have high-risk arrhythmias and are at increased risk for SCD[112] suggests that an electrophysiological mechanism secondary to the hypertrophied muscle itself plays some role. Stafford and colleagues[117] reported exercise-related cardiac arrest in nonobstructive hypertrophic cardiomyopathy. Ventricular fibrillation (VF) was reproduced during electrophysiological testing after induction of atrial fibrillation with a rapid ventricular response. In athletes under 35 years of age, hypertrophic cardiomyopathy is the most common cause of SCD, in contrast to athletes over the age of 35, among whom ischemic heart disease is the most common cause.[87,88,118–120]

SUDDEN DEATH IN DILATED CARDIOMYOPATHY AND HEART FAILURE. The advent of therapeutic interventions which provide better long-term control of congestive heart failure has begun to improve long-term survival of such patients (see p. 493). However, the proportion of heart failure patients with stable hemodynamics who die suddenly appears to be increasing.[121] In reports to date, as many as 47 per cent of deaths in heart failure patients are categorized as SCDs, and the risk of SCD increases with deteriorating left ventricular function.[122] The mechanism (VT/VF versus bradyarrhythmias/asystole) appears to relate to cause—i.e., ischemic versus nonischemic.[122] Among patients with cardiomyopathy who have good functional capacity (Class I and II), total mortality risk is considerably better than for those with poor functional capacity (Class III and IV). However, the proportional risk of death being sudden and unexpected is higher in the better functional class group[123] (Fig. 24–6). In contrast, unexplained syncope has been ob-

served to be a powerful predictor of SCD in patients who are functional Class II or IV due to any etiology.[124] The actuarial 1-year probability of SCD was 45 per cent in this study.

The interaction between post-myocardial infarction ventricular arrhythmia and depressed ejection fraction in determining risk for SCD has been described.[72] The majority of studies addressing the relation between chronic congestive heart failure and SCD focused on patients with ischemic, idiopathic, and alcoholic congestive cardiomyopathy.[121,123,125–127] A chronic myopathic syndrome after myocarditis has been cited as an infrequent but well-documented cause of SCD.[128] Peripartum cardiomyopathy (see p. 1851) also may cause SCD.

Acute Heart Failure. All causes of acute cardiac failure, in the absence of prompt interventions, may result in SCD caused by either the circulatory failure itself or secondary arrhythmias. The electrophysiological mechanisms involved have been proposed to be related to acute stretching of myocardial fibers and/or the His-Purkinje system, with its experimentally demonstrated arrhythmogenic effect,[129] but the roles of neurohumoral mechanisms and acute electrolyte shifts have not been fully evaluated.[121] Among the causes of acute cardiac failure which are associated with SCD are massive acute myocardial infarction, acute myocarditis, acute alcoholic cardiac dysfunction, and a number of mechanical causes of heart failure such as massive pulmonary embolism, mechanical disruption of intracardiac

M. Obstructive intracavitary tumors
  1. Neoplastic
  2. Thrombotic
V. DISEASES OF THE CARDIAC VALVES
  A. Valvular aortic stenosis/insufficiency
  B. Mitral valve disruption
  C. Mitral valve prolapse
  D. Endocarditis
  E. Prosthetic valve dysfunction
VI. CONGENITAL HEART DISEASE
  A. Congenital aortic or pulmonic valve stenosis
  B. Right-to-left shunts with Eisenmenger's physiology
    1. Advanced disease
    2. During labor and delivery
  C. After surgical repair of congenital lesions, e.g., tetralogy of Fallot
VII. ELECTROPHYSIOLOGICAL ABNORMALITIES
  A. Abnormalities of the conducting system
    1. Fibrosis of the His-Purkinje system
      (a) Primary degeneration (Lenegre's disease)
      (b) Secondary to fibrosis and calcification of the "cardiac skeleton" (Lev's disease)
      (c) Post-viral conducting system fibrosis
      (d) Hereditary conducting system disease
    2. Anomalous pathways of conduction
  B. Prolonged Q-T interval syndrome
    1. Congenital
      (a) With deafness
      (b) Without deafness
    2. Acquired
      (a) Drug effect
        (1) Cardiac, antiarrhythmic
        (2) Noncardiac
      (b) Electrolyte abnormality
      (c) Toxic substances
      (d) Hypothermia
      (e) Central nervous system injury
  C. Ventricular fibrillation of unknown or uncertain cause
    1. Absence of identifiable structural or functional causes
      (a) "Idiopathic" ventricular fibrillation
      (b) Short-coupled torsades de pointes, polymorphic VT
      (c) Nonspecific (?) fibrofatty infiltration in previously healthy victim

  2. Sleep-death in Southeast Asians
    (a) Bangungut
    (b) Pokkuri
    (c) Nonlaitai
VIII. ELECTRICAL INSTABILITY RELATED TO NEURO-HUMORAL AND CENTRAL NERVOUS SYSTEM INFLUENCES
  A. Catecholamine-dependent lethal arrhythmias
  B. Central nervous system–related
    1. Psychic stress, emotional extremes
    2. Auditory-related
    3. "Voodoo" death in primitive cultures
    4. Diseases of the cardiac nerves
    5. Congenital Q-T interval prolongation
IX. SUDDEN INFANT DEATH SYNDROME AND SUDDEN DEATH IN CHILDREN
  A. Sudden infant death syndrome
    1. Immature respiratory control functions
    2. Susceptibility to lethal arrhythmias
    3. Congenital heart disease
    4. Myocarditis
  B. Sudden death in children
    1. Eisenmenger syndrome, aortic stenosis, hypertrophic cardiomyopathy, pulmonary atresia
    2. After corrective surgery for congenital heart disease
    3. Myocarditis
    4. No identified structural or functional cause
X. MISCELLANEOUS
  A. Sudden death during extreme physical activity
  B. Mechanical interference with venous return
    1. Acute cardiac tamponade
    2. Massive pulmonary embolism
    3. Acute intracardiac thrombosis
  C. Dissecting aneurysm of the aorta
  D. Toxic/metabolic disturbances
    1. Electrolyte disturbances
    2. Metabolic disturbances
    3. Proarrhythmic effects of antiarrhythmic drugs
    4. Proarrhythmic effects of noncardiac drugs
  E. Mimics of sudden cardiac death
    1. "Cafe coronary"
    2. Acute alcoholic states ("holiday heart")
    3. Acute asthmatic attacks
    4. Air or amniotic fluid embolism

---

structures secondary to infarction or infection, and ball-valve embolism in aortic or mitral stenosis (Table 24–2).

INFLAMMATORY, INFILTRATIVE, NEOPLASTIC, AND DEGENERATIVE DISEASES OF THE HEART. Almost all diseases in this category have been associated with SCD, with or without concomitant cardiac failure. Acute viral myocarditis with left ventricular dysfunction (see p. 1437) is commonly associated with cardiac arrhythmias, including potentially lethal arrhythmias. It is now recognized that serious ventricular arrhythmias or SCD can occur in myocarditis in the absence of clinical evidence of left ventricular dysfunction.[45,128,130] In a report of 19 SCDs among 1,606,167 previously screened US Air Force recruits, 8 of the 19 (42 per cent) had evidence of myocarditis (5 nonrheumatic, 3 rheumatic) at postmortem examination, and 15 (79 per cent) suffered their cardiac arrests during strenuous exertion.[131] Viral carditis also may cause damage isolated to the specialized conducting system and result in a propensity to arrhythmias; the rare association of this process with SCD has been reported.[132] The risk of potentially lethal arrhythmias is not limited to the acute phase of the disease.[128]

Myocardial involvement in collagen-vascular disorders, tumors, chronic granulomatous diseases, infiltrative disorders, and protozoan infestations varies widely, but in all instances SCD may be the initial or terminal manifestation of the disease process. Among the granulomatous diseases, *sarcoidosis* (see p. 1431) stands out because of the frequency of SCD associated with it. Roberts et al.[133] reported that SCD was the terminal event in 67 per cent of sarcoid heart disease deaths; the occurrence of SCD has been related to the extent of cardiac involvement.[134] In a report on the pathological findings in nine patients who died of *progressive systemic sclerosis*, (see p. 1781), eight who died suddenly had evidence of transient ischemia and reperfusion histologically, suggesting that this might represent Raynaud-like involvement of coronary vessels.[135] *Amyloidosis* of the heart (see p. 1421) may also cause sudden death. An incidence of 30 per cent has been reported[139]; diffuse involvement of ventricular muscle or of the specialized conducting system may be associated with SCD.

Arrhythmogenic Right Ventricular Dysplasia (see p. 681). This condition is associated with a high incidence of ventricular arrhythmias, particularly recurrent ventricular tachycardia.[136] Although symptomatic ventricular tachycardia has been well recognized in the syndrome for many years, the risk of SCD was unclear[136] and thought to be relatively low. However, isolated right ventricular *cardiomyopathy* has histopathological features similar to right ventricular dysplasia and may be a variant, or advanced form, of the same process. Right ventricular cardiomyopathy carries a high risk of SCD,[137,138] suggesting that selection may have influenced the perception in the past that risk of SCD was low in right ventricular displasia.

VALVULAR HEART DISEASE (see Chap. 32). Before the advent of surgery for valvular heart disease, *aortic stenosis* was one of the more common noncoronary causes of SCD. Campbell reported in 1968 that 44 of 70 (73 per cent) deaths in patients with aortic stenosis were sudden.[141] The advent of safe and effective procedures for aortic valve replacement has reduced the incidence of this cause of sudden death,[142] but patients with prosthetic or heterograft aortic valve replacements remain at some risk for SCD caused by arrhythmias, prosthetic valve dysfunction, or coexistent coronary heart disease.[143] SCD has been reported to be the second most common mode of death after valve replacement surgery, accounting for 62 of 298 deaths (21 per cent).[144] The incidence peaked 3 weeks after operation and then plateaued after 8 months. Nonetheless, the risk is appreciably lower than in those patients who had not had the advantage of valvular surgery in prior years. In another report analyzing outcome in patients receiving prosthetic

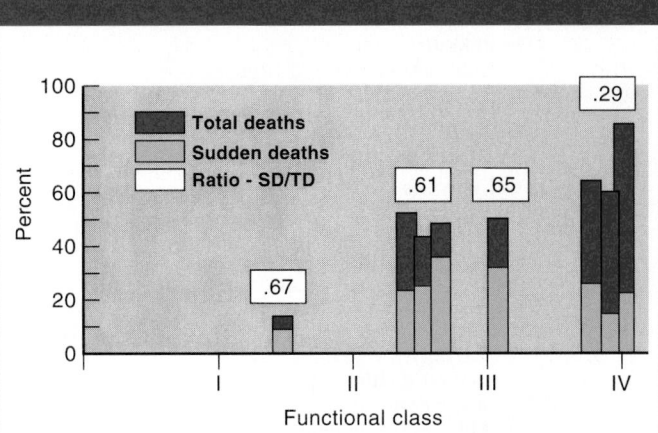

SUDDEN DEATH IN HEART FAILURE

FIGURE 24–6. Risk of sudden cardiac death related to functional classification in heart failure. The relative probability of death being sudden is higher in the patients with better functional capacity who are at lower total mortality risk. (Modified from Kjekshus, J.: Arrhythmia and mortality in congestive heart failure. Am. J. Cardiol. 65:42-I, 1990.)

valves for isolated severe aortic stenosis, SCD occurred at a rate of only 0.3 per cent/year and was responsible for only 18 per cent of late deaths.[145] A high incidence of ventricular arrhythmia has been observed during follow-up of patients with valve replacement,[145,146] especially in those who had aortic stenosis, multiple valve surgery, or cardiomegaly.[146] Sudden death during follow-up was associated with ventricular arrhythmias and thromboembolism. Hemodynamic variables were less predictive. Stenotic lesions of other valves imply much lower risk of SCD. Regurgitant lesions, particularly chronic aortic regurgitation and acute mitral regurgitation, may cause SCD, but the risk is also lower than with aortic stenosis.

Mitral valve prolapse (see p. 1029) is prevalent and associated with a high incidence of cardiac arrhythmias; however, the incidence of SCD is quite low.[147] This uncommon complication appears to correlate with nonspecific ST-T wave changes in the inferior leads on the ECG.[148] In data reviewed from 17 reported instances of SCD in mitral valve prolapse patients, these nonspecific ST-T wave changes were present in 6 of 8 who had had prior electrocardiograms.[149] An association with redundancy of mitral leaflets on echocardiogram also has been suggested.[150] Reported associations between Q-T interval prolongation or preexcitation and SCD in mitral prolapse syndrome are less consistent.[147]

Endocarditis of the aortic and mitral valves (see Chap. 33) may be associated with rapid death resulting from acute disruption of the valvular apparatus, coronary embolism, or abscesses of valvular rings or the septum; however, such deaths are rarely true sudden deaths as conventionally defined.

CONGENITAL HEART DISEASE. The congenital lesions most commonly associated with SCD are aortic stenosis (see p. 1035)[130,151,152] and communications between the left and right sides of the heart with the Eisenmenger physiology (see p. 799).[153] In the latter the risk of SCD is a function of pulmonary vascular disease severity; also, there is an extraordinarily high risk of maternal mortality during labor and delivery in the pregnant patient with Eisenmenger syndrome (see p. 975).[154] Potentially lethal arrhythmias and SCD have been described as late complications after surgical repair of complex congenital lesions, particularly tetralogy of Fallot (see p. 929), transposition of the great arteries, and atrioventricular canal.[155,156] These patients should be followed closely and treated aggressively when cardiac ar-

rhythmias are identified, although the late risk of SCD may not be as high as previously thought.[157]

ELECTROPHYSIOLOGICAL ABNORMALITIES. Acquired disease of the AV node and His-Purkinje system and the presence of accessory pathways of conduction are two groups of structural abnormalities of specialized conduction which may be associated with SCD. Epidemiological studies have suggested that intraventricular conduction disturbances in coronary heart disease are one of the few factors that may increase the proportion of SCD in coronary heart disease.[37] A specific clinical example is the risk of VF during the first 30 days after myocardial infarction in patients with anterior infarctions and bundle branch block. Lie et al.[158] reported that 47 per cent of patients who had late hospital VF had had anteroseptal infarcts with bundle branch block, and that these 14 were from a total pool of only 40 patients with the combination of bundle branch block and anterior myocardial infarction. Thus there was a 35 per cent incidence of VF in this subgroup, which represented only 4.1 per cent of a total of 966 myocardial infarctions. This risk persists for 6 weeks after the infarction and then abates.[159] AV block or intraventricular conduction abnormalities were found in 9 of 10 patients who had recurrent VF during hospitalization after resuscitation from prehospital cardiac arrest.[20]

Primary fibrosis (Lenegre's disease)[160] or secondary mechanical injury (Lev's disease)[161] of the His-Purkinje system is commonly associated with intraventricular conduction abnormalities and symptomatic AV block, and less commonly with SCD. The identification of people at risk and the efficacy of pacemakers for preventing SCD, rather than only ameliorating symptoms, have been the subjects of debate.[162,163] However, current prevailing thought is that survival may depend more on the nature and extent of the underlying disease than on the conduction disturbance itself.[164]

Patients with congenital AV block (see p. 966) or nonprogressive congenital intraventricular block usually have a low risk of SCD.[165] Progressive congenital intraventricular blocks predict a high risk,[165] as does the coexistence of structural congenital defects. A hereditary form has been reported in association with a familial propensity to SCD.[46,165]

The anomalous pathways of conduction, bundles of Kent in the Wolff-Parkinson-White syndrome, and Mahaim fibers, are commonly associated with nonlethal arrhythmias. However, when the anomalous pathways of conduction have short refractory periods, the occurrence of atrial fibrillation may allow the induction of VF during very rapid conduction across the bypass tract.[166] The incidence of SCD in patients with short refractory period bypass tracts is not yet known. Patients who have multiple pathways appear to be at higher risk of SCD,[166] as do patients with a familial pattern of anomalous pathways and premature SCD.[167]

Q-T Prolongation (see also pp. 685 and 1667). The prolonged Q-T interval syndrome is a functional abnormality, perhaps associated with neurogenic influences, that may cause lethal arrhythmias.[168] In the hereditary *congenital form* two varieties have been reported: those with autosomal recessive inheritance and associated deafness, the Jervell and Lange-Nielsen syndrome,[169] and those without deafness, the Romano-Ward syndrome.[42] Some patients have prolonged Q-T intervals throughout life without any manifest arrhythmias, whereas others are highly susceptible to symptomatic and potentially fatal ventricular arrhythmias, particularly the torsades de pointes form of ventricular tachycardia.[170] Patients at higher risk are characterized by deafness, female gender, syncope, and documented torsades depointes or prior ventricular fibrillation, and they require aggressive medical or surgical interventions.[171,172] Moreover, making an effort to identify relatives at risk is an important preventive measure, given the familial pattern of the entity. A recent major advance has been the identification of three specific genetic markers by linkage analyses[48-50] (see p. 1667).

The *acquired form* of prolonged Q-T interval may be due to drug idiosyncrasies (particularly antiarrhythmics and psychotropic drugs), electrolyte abnormalities, hypothermia, toxic substances, and central nervous system injury.[172] It also has been reported both in intensive weight reduction programs that involve the use of liquid protein diets[173] and in anorexia nervosa.[174] Lithium carbonate may prolong the Q-T interval and has been reported to be associated with an increased incidence of SCD in cancer patients with preexisting heart disease.[175] Drug interactions recently have been recognized as a mechanism of prolongation of the Q-T interval and torsades de pointes. For example, terfenadine (Seldane), which can prolong the Q-T interval, is normally converted by a hepatic P450 enzyme to a metabolite that retains antihistamine activity, but not Q-T prolonging effects. It may be arrhythmogenic when the hepatic enzyme is blocked by another substance, such as ketoconazole.[176] Acquired prolonged Q-T intervals usually carry a risk of serious arrhythmias and SCD, but the risk is abolished when the inciting factor is removed. In acquired prolonged Q-T syndrome, as in the congenital form, the torsades de pointes form of ventricular tachycardia is commonly the specific arrhythmia that triggers or degenerates into lethal VF.

ELECTRICAL INSTABILITY RESULTING FROM NEUROHUMORAL AND CENTRAL NERVOUS SYSTEM INFLUENCES. Catecholamine-dependent lethal arrhythmias in the absence of Q-T interval prolongation, with control by beta-adrenoceptor blocking agents, have been described.[177] Several central nervous system–related interactions with cardiac electrical stability have been suggested (see p. 1878). The hereditary forms of prolonged Q-T interval syndrome, discussed above, appear to have a relation to sympathetic nervous system imbalance.[168,178] Lown and coworkers identified psychic stress as a mediating factor for advanced cardiac arrhythmias and perhaps SCD.[179] Epidemiological data also suggest an association between behavioral abnormalities and the risk of SCD, particularly in women[67,68]; emotional

extremes have been suggested as a triggering mechanism for SCD.[3,180] Associations between auditory stimulation[130] and auditory auras[181] and SCD have been reported.[130] The auditory abnormalities in some forms of congenital Q-T prolongation have already been cited.[169]

A variant of torsades de pointes, characterized by short coupling intervals between a normal impulse and the initiating impulse, has been described (Fig. 24–7). It appears to have familial trends and to be related to alterations in autonomic nervous system activity. The 12-lead ECG demonstrates normal Q-T intervals; but ventricular fibrillation and sudden death are common.

The syndrome of "voodoo death" in developing countries has been studied extensively.[183,184] There appears to be an association between isolation from the tribe, a sense of hopelessness, severe bradyarrhythmias, and sudden death. With cultural changes in many of these areas, the syndrome has become less amenable to observation and study; however, there do remain pockets of cultural isolation in which the syndrome no doubt still exists.

SUDDEN INFANT DEATH SYNDROME AND SCD IN CHILDREN

The sudden infant death syndrome (SIDS) occurs between birth and 6 months of age, more commonly in males, and has an incidence of 0.1 to 0.3 per cent of live births.[185] Because of its abrupt nature, a cardiac mechanism has been suspected for many years,[186] but a variety of causes, with central respiratory dysfunction playing a major role, are considered likely.[187] Many cases of the sudden infant death syndrome are believed to represent a form of "sleep apnea" which, if prolonged, may lead to hypoxia, cyanosis, and cardiac arrhythmias. Experience with "near-misses" and the results of respiratory monitoring, in conjunction with the propensity of the syndrome to occur in premature infants, all suggest impaired central nervous system respiratory control reflexes, possibly owing to immaturity.[185,187-189] There has recently been interest, however, in the possibility of obstructive apnea as another mechanism.[187] Identification of individual infants at risk is difficult, but the risk does not persist beyond the first 6 months of life.

Despite the current focus on the respiratory mechanisms involved in the syndrome, their role has not yet been explicitly established. Furthermore, the question of whether or not an identifiable subset of infants who have apneic spells are particularly prone to genesis of cardiac arrhythmias remains conjectural.[188-190] A primary cardiac cause is still considered the basis of this syndrome in some victims.[186,190] Marino and Kane[191] observed either accessory pathways (two cases)

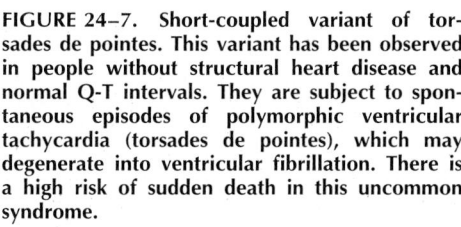

FIGURE 24–7. Short-coupled variant of torsades de pointes. This variant has been observed in people without structural heart disease and normal Q-T intervals. They are subject to spontaneous episodes of polymorphic ventricular tachycardia (torsades de pointes), which may degenerate into ventricular fibrillation. There is a high risk of sudden death in this uncommon syndrome.

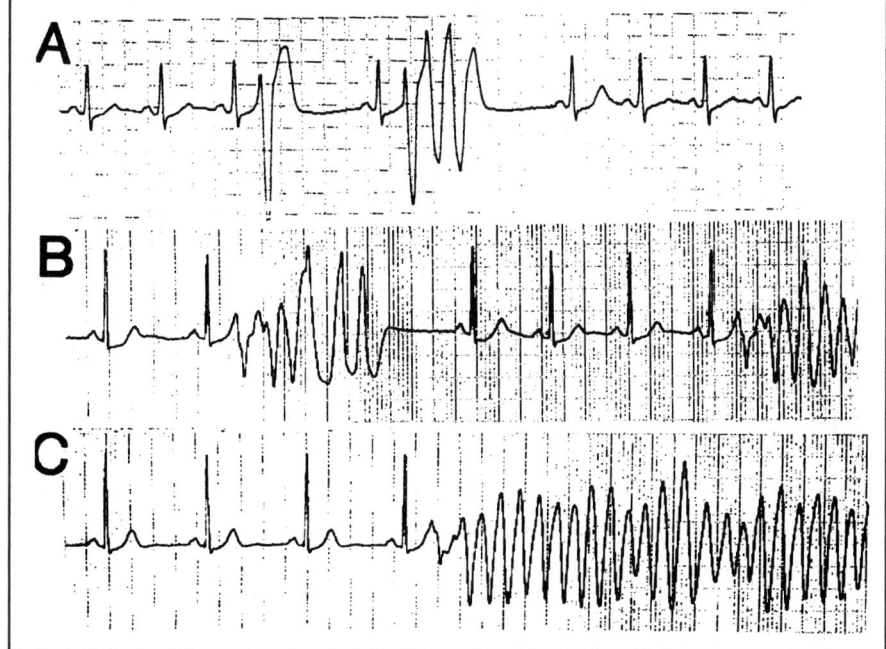

or dispersed or immature AV nodal or bundle branch cells in the annulus fibrosus (four cases) among a group of seven sudden infant death syndrome victims studied by detailed histopathology.

Sudden death in children beyond the age group at risk for SIDS often is associated with identifiable heart disease,[129,192] although one study identified cardiac causes in only 25 per cent of sudden natural death victims between the ages of 1 and 21 years.[40] About 25 per cent of SCDs in children occur in those who have undergone previous surgery for congenital cardiac disease. Of the remaining 75 per cent, more than one-half occur in children who have one of four lesions: congenital aortic stenosis, Eisenmenger syndrome, pulmonary stenosis or atresia, or obstructive hypertrophic cardiomyopathy.[192] Neuspiel and Kuller[40] observed 14 cases of myocarditis among 51 SCDs in children (27 per cent).

OTHER CAUSES OF SUDDEN DEATH

SCD in athletes during or after extreme physical activity is infrequent but receives a great deal of attention when it does occur. The special position of prominent athletes in society has created unusual, conflicting, and sometimes inconsistent attitudes in response to SCD risk in these individuals.[193] The majority of such individuals have a previously unrecognized cardiac abnormality, with hypertrophic cardiomyopathy with or without obstruction, valvular aortic stenosis, and occult coronary artery disease as the most common causes identified after death.[88,118–120,194,195] A surprisingly large fraction of people who died suddenly during exertion had unsuspected myocarditis, according to a report of a large cohort of US Air Force recruits.[131] A small group of such victims, however, have neither previously determined functional abnormality nor structural abnormalities at postmortem examination.[20,87,88,128,129]

There are rare instances of idiopathic VF causing SCD in the absence of any identifiable structural or functional abnormality of the heart.[196] Although long-term survival after a potentially fatal event appears to be good, some degree of risk appears to remain.[197] Limited data suggest that risk persists primarily in patients with subtle cardiac abnormalities, in contrast to patients who are truly normal.[198] In addition, these events tend to occur in young, otherwise healthy people. A specific variation of this syndrome has been observed in southeast Asians. Many years ago syndromes referred to as *Bangungut* in young Filipino males,[199] *Pokkuri* in young Japanese males,[200] and *Nonlaitai* in young Laotian males[201] were reported. In each there was a tendency for sudden death to occur during sleep, and at one time a toxic cause was suspected.[199,200] Documented cases have now

been reported in Laotians who came to the United States after the Vietnam war. The mechanism was identified to be ventricular fibrillation in some of these cases; in at least one instance electrophysiological study demonstrated inducible ventricular arrhythmia by programmed electrical stimulation.[202] Pathological examinations have revealed a high incidence of mild to significant cardiomegaly (14 of 18) and a variety of structural abnormalities of specialized conducting tissue.[203] The fact that these cases continue to occur in a new cultural setting suggests that there may be a hereditary predisposition.

There also are a number of noncardiac conditions which *mimic* SCD. These include the so-called *cafe coronary*,[204,205] in which food, usually an unchewed piece of meat, lodges in the oropharynx and causes an abrupt obstruction at the glottis. The classic description of a cafe coronary is sudden cyanosis and collapse in a restaurant, during a meal accompanied by lively conversation. The *holiday heart syndrome* is characterized by cardiac arrhythmias, most commonly atrial, and other cardiac abnormalities associated with acute alcoholic states.[206] It has not been determined whether potentially lethal arrhythmias occurring in such settings account for reported sudden deaths associated with acute alcoholic states.[3] *Massive pulmonary embolism* (Chap. 46) may cause acute cardiovascular collapse and sudden death; sudden death in severe acute asthmatic attacks, without prolonged deterioration of the patient's condition, is well recognized.[207] Air or amniotic fluid embolism at the time of labor and delivery may cause sudden death on rare occasions, with the clinical picture mimicking sudden cardiac death.[208] Peripartum air embolism caused by an unusual sexual practice has been reported as a cause of such sudden deaths.[209]

Proarrhythmic effects of antiarrhythmic drugs have received particular attention,[210] but psychotropic drugs, arrhythmogenic effects of toxic substances, and electrolyte disturbances—particularly hypokalemia, hypocalcemia, and hypomagnesemia—also have been implicated.[172] Classic proarrhythmia is an event which tends to appear within days after the initiation of antiarrhythmic therapy.[211] The pattern of SCD over time among patients treated with two of the drugs used in the Cardiac Arrhythmia Suppression Trial suggests a different pattern of proarrhythmic risk, likely caused by a different mechanism.[59,82] This form of risk appears to be a continuous function extending over 1 or more years of exposure.

Finally, a number of abnormalities that do not directly involve the heart may cause SCD or mimic it. These include aortic dissection (see p. 1564), acute cardiac tamponade (see p. 1503), and rapid exsanguination (see p. 1539).

PATHOLOGY AND PATHOPHYSIOLOGY

Pathological observations in SCD victims reflect the epidemiological and clinical preponderance of coronary heart disease as the major structural predisposing factor.[212] Liberthson and coworkers[213] reported that 81 per cent of 220 autopsied victims of SCD had significant coronary heart disease, defined as more than one coronary vessel with greater than 75 per cent stenosis as the primary pathological feature. At least one vessel with more than 75 per cent stenosis was found in 94 per cent of victims, acute coronary occlusion in 58 per cent, healed myocardial infarction in 44 per cent, and acute myocardial infarction in 27 per cent. These observations are consistent with many other studies of the frequency of coronary disease in sudden death victims. All of the other causes of SCD (Table 24–2) collectively account for no more than 10 to 20 per cent of cases, but they have provided a large base of enlightening pathological data.[45,128]

THE PATHOLOGY OF SUDDEN DEATH CAUSED BY CORONARY HEART DISEASE

THE CORONARY ARTERIES. Extensive atherosclerosis is the most common pathological finding in the coronary arteries of victims of SCD (Table 24–3). In postmortem examinations of 169 hearts, sites of 75 per cent or more stenosis were present in three or four major vessels in 61 per cent of the hearts studied; two vessels with at least 75 per cent stenosis were found in 15 per cent; and 24 per cent of the hearts had either single-vessel disease or no vessels having

lesions producing 75 per cent stenosis.[214] A distinctly higher proportion of hearts having three or four vessels with 75 per cent stenotic lesions was observed in white men (70 per cent) compared with white women (34 per cent). In contrast, 58 per cent of the hearts of both black men and black women had three or four vessels with 75 per cent or more stenoses. Consistent with clinical findings in survivors of out-of-hospital cardiac arrest,[20] there was no special predilection of disease distribution for any coronary artery, and there was no quantitative difference between proximal and distal distribution of disease.

Kuller et al.[52] pointed out that 90 per cent or greater narrowing of at least one coronary artery was found in 77 per cent of autopsied victims of sudden *coronary* death, compared with 8 per cent of victims of other causes of sudden death. Davies[45] reported that 61 per cent of patients dying suddenly because of coronary heart disease had three vessels with 75 per cent or more stenosis at any one point; an additional 18 (23 per cent) had two vessels with 75 per

TABLE 24–3 PATHOLOGICAL FINDINGS IN SUDDEN DEATH DUE TO CORONARY HEART DISEASE

THE CORONARY ARTERIES	VENTRICULAR MYOCARDIUM
A. Chronic atherosclerosis	A. Healed myocardial infarction
B. Acute lesions	B. Left ventricular hypertrophy
1. Plaque fissuring	C. Ventricular aneurysm
2. Platelet aggregates	D. Acute myocardial infarction
3. Organizing thrombus	
4. Coronary artery spasm	

cent or more stenosis. Among 100 age- and sex-matched controls who died of trauma or cerebral tumors, only 27 per cent had two- or three-vessel disease, and 52 per cent had no vessels with lesions of 75 per cent or more. In the same study the majority of sudden deaths caused by coronary heart disease were associated with at least one point of more than 85 per cent stenosis, and Davies suggested that this parameter provided the best discrimination between hearts of SCD victims and controls.

Several studies have demonstrated no specific pattern of distribution of coronary artery lesions which preselect for SCD. In a quantitative analysis comparing coronary artery narrowing at postmortem examination in SCD victims and controls, 36 per cent of the 5-mm segments of the coronary arteries from the SCD group had 76 to 100 per cent cross-sectional area reductions compared with 3 per cent in the controls.[215] An additional 34 per cent of the sections from the SCD group had 51 to 75 per cent reductions in cross-sectional areas. Only 7 per cent of the sections from the SCD patients had 0 to 25 per cent reductions in cross-sectional areas. The *distribution* of the lesions causing greater than 75 per cent narrowing was similar in the three major coronary arteries, but quantitative differences between proximal and distal halves of the vessels were inconsistent.[215] Similar conclusions resulted from pathological observations of out-of-hospital cardiac arrest victims who were not successfully resuscitated.[213] These studies indicate that extensive coronary artery disease is the pathological hallmark of SCDs caused by coronary heart disease and that no specific anatomical pattern of distribution of the disease preselects SCD victims.

The role of acute (active) *coronary artery* lesions, such as plaque fissuring, platelet aggregation, and thrombosis, in the onset of cardiac arrest leading to SCD, is becoming clarified.[216,217] In one study of 100 consecutive sudden coronary death victims, 44 per cent had major (more than 50 per cent luminal occlusion) recent coronary thrombi, 30 per cent had minor occlusive thrombi, and 21 per cent had plaque fissuring.[216] Only 5 per cent had no acute coronary artery changes; 65 per cent of the thrombi occurred at sites of preexisting high-grade stenoses, and an additional 19 per cent were found at sites of more than 50 per cent stenosis. In a subsequent study by the same investigators, 50/168 victims (30 per cent) had occlusive intraluminal coronary thrombi, and 73 (44 per cent) had mural intraluminal thrombi.[217] Single-vessel disease, acute infarction at postmortem examination, and prodromal symptoms were associated with the presence of thrombi.

An overview of the major studies on the incidence of acute thrombotic occlusions, in which the definition of sudden death ranges from 15 minutes to 24 hours, reveals wide variation in the reported frequency of recent coronary thrombosis in sudden death. It ranges from 15 to 64 per cent, but the majority of studies which used 6 hours or less as the definition of "sudden" had frequencies of less than 40 per cent.[212,213,216–219] Factors which confound the analysis of such data include relations between platelet aggregates and thrombus formation and the spontaneous lysis of clots.

Baba et al.[219] reported the presence of *organizing* thrombus in about 31 per cent of 121 sudden coronary heart disease deaths. They were commonly associated with sites of more than 75 per cent chronic obstruction and with concomitant acute lesions at the same sites, leading to the speculation that clinical events 5 to 7 days before death might create a substrate for fatal acute coronal events. *Coronary artery spasm*, an established cause of acute ischemia, also may cause SCD and is recognizable in rare instances at postmortem examination.[220]

THE MYOCARDIUM. Myocardial pathology in SCD caused by coronary heart disease reflects the extensive atherosclerosis which usually is present. Studies in victims of out-of-hospital SCD and from epidemiological sources both indi-

cate that healed myocardial infarction is a common finding in sudden coronary death victims, with most investigators reporting frequencies ranging from 40 to more than 70 per cent.[8,196,221,222] For example, Newman and coworkers[221,222] reported that 72 per cent of men in a 25-to-44-year age group who died suddenly (24 or fewer hours) with no previous clinical history of coronary heart disease had scars of large (63 per cent) or small (less than 1 cm cross-sectional area, 9 per cent) areas of healed myocardial necrosis. The incidence of acute myocardial infarction is considerably less, with cytopathological evidence of recent myocardial infarction averaging about 20 per cent. This estimate corresponds well with studies in out-of-hospital cardiac arrest survivors, who have an incidence of new myocardial infarction in the range of 20 to 30 per cent.

VENTRICULAR HYPERTROPHY. Myocardial hypertrophy may coexist and interact with acute or chronic ischemia but appears to confer an independent mortality risk.[223] There is not a close correlation between increased heart weight and severity of coronary heart disease in SCD victims[214]; heart weights are higher in SCD victims than in those with non–sudden death despite similar prevalence of history of hypertension before death.[8] Hypertrophy-associated mortality risk is also independent of left ventricular function and extent of coronary artery disease.[223] Anderson[105] suggests that left ventricular hypertrophy itself may be a predisposing factor to SCD. Experimental data also suggest increased susceptibility to potentially lethal ventricular arrhythmias in left ventricular hypertrophy with ischemia and reperfusion.[224] A study of massively enlarged hearts (i.e., weighing more than 1000 gm), however, did not indicate an excess incidence of SCD,[225] but the underlying pathology in that study was dominated by lesions that produce volume overload.

SPECIALIZED CONDUCTING SYSTEM IN SCD

Pathological data on the specialized conducting system of victims of SCD are relatively sparse. Lie[226] studied the specialized conducting system of 49 of 120 SCD patients with no previous history of coronary heart disease who died within 6 hours of onset of symptoms. Thirty-nine patients had acute myocardial infarction and 10 did not. Two patients with acute anteroseptal infarctions had hemorrhage and/or infarction involving the AV node and peripheral bundle branches. Luminal narrowing of the artery to the AV node was present in 50 per cent, but there were no thromboses of vessels to the specialized conducting system. Evidence of ischemic injury was present with an equal frequency in SCD[226] and myocardial infarction patients.[227]

Fibrosis of the specialized conducting system is a common but nonspecific endpoint of multiple causes. Although this process is associated with AV block or intraventricular conduction abnormalities, its role in SCD is uncertain. Lev's and Lenegre's diseases, ischemic injury caused by small-vessel disease, and numerous infiltrative or inflammatory processes all may result in such changes. In addition, active inflammatory processes such as myocarditis and infiltrative processes such as amyloidosis, scleroderma, hemochromatosis, and morbid obesity all may damage or destroy the AV node and/or bundle of His and result in AV block.[228]

Focal diseases such as sarcoidosis, Whipple's disease, and rheumatoid arthritis also may involve the conducting system. These various categories of conducting system disease have been considered as possible pathological substrates for SCD which may be overlooked because of the difficulty in doing careful postmortem examinations of the conducting system routinely.[228] Focal involvement of conducting tissue by tumors (especially mesothelioma of the AV node but also lymphoma, carcinoma, rhabdomyoma, and fibroma) also has been reported,[228] and rare cases of SCD have been associated with these lesions. It has been suggested that abnormal postnatal morphogenesis of the specialized conducting system may be a significant factor in some SCDs in infants and children.[228]

CARDIAC NERVES AND SCD

Diseases of cardiac nerves have been postulated to have a role in SCD.[229,230] Neural involvement may be the result of random damage to neural elements within the myocardium (i.e., "secondary" cardioneuropathy), or may be "primary," as in a selective cardiac viral neuropathy.[230] Secondary involvement may be a consequence of ischemic neural injury in coronary heart disease and has been postulated to result in autonomic destabilization, enhancing the propensity to arrhythmias. Some experimental data support this hypothesis, and a clinical technique for imaging cardiac neural fibers suggests a changing pattern over time after myocardial infarction.[231-234] Involvement of neural plexuses, with or without conducting system involvement, has been observed at necropsy in 54 per cent of patients who died within 24 hours of onset of myocardial infarction.[229] Specific causes for primary cardioneuropathies are less obvious. Viral, neurotoxic, and hereditary causes (e.g., progressive muscular dystrophy and Friedreich's ataxia) have been emphasized.

Disordered extrinsic neural involvement of the heart usually is considered to be functional, such as in prolonged Q-T interval syndrome. However, a primary role for neural dysfunction in hereditary long Q-T syndrome is open to question now that genetic abnormalities that alter specific membrane ion channels involved in repolarization processes have been demonstrated in a number of families (see p. 1667).[48-50] Nonetheless, stellate ganglion inflammation has been observed in some tissues removed surgically for symptomatic Q-T prolongation in hereditary Q-T syndrome[235] or after myocardial infarction.[236] The possible significance of such extrinsic cardiac neural involvement is not yet clear.[236]

MECHANISMS AND PATHOPHYSIOLOGY

The occurrence of potentially lethal tachyarrhythmias, or of severe bradyarrhythmia or asystole, is the end of a cascade of pathophysiological abnormalities which result from complex interactions between coronary vascular events, myocardial injury, variations in autonomic tone, and/or the metabolic and electrolyte state of the myocardium. There is no uniform hypothesis regarding mechanisms by which these elements interact to lead to the final pathway of lethal arrhythmias. However, Figure 24–8 shows a model of the pathophysiology of SCD, in which the central event is the initiation of a potentially fatal arrhythmia. The possibility of this event is increased by a variety of *structural abnormalities* and modulated by *functional variations.*[237]

Pathophysiological Mechanisms of Lethal Tachyarrhythmias

CORONARY ARTERY STRUCTURE AND FUNCTION. In that large majority of SCDs associated with coronary atherosclerosis, the distribution of chronic arterial narrowing has been well defined by pathological studies.[45,212,213] However, the specific mechanisms by which these lesions lead to potentially lethal disturbances of electrical stability are poorly understood. Steady-state reductions in regional myocardial blood flow, in the absence of superimposed acute lesions, may create a setting in which alterations in the metabolic or electrolyte state of the myocardium or neural fluctuations result in loss of electrical stability.[121] Increased myocardial oxygen demand with a fixed supply

may be the mechanism of exercise-induced arrhythmias and sudden death during intense physical activity in athletes or others whose heart disease had not previously become clinically manifested.[87,88,118-120,131,194,195,238] Vasoactive events leading to acute reduction in regional myocardial blood flow in the presence of a normal or previously compromised circulation constitute a common cause of transient ischemia, angina pectoris, arrhythmias, and perhaps SCD.[101-104] Coronary artery spasm or modulation of coronary collateral flow exposes the myocardium to the double hazard of transient ischemia and reperfusion (Fig. 24–9).[101,224,239] The mechanism of production of spasm is unclear, although sites of endothelial disease appear to predispose.[240] A role of the autonomic nervous system, particularly mechanisms related to alpha-adrenoceptor activity, has been suggested[241]; vagal activity also may be involved in the production of spasm,[242] possibly due to failure of acetylcholine to trigger release of nitrous oxide in areas of endothelial disease. However, neurogenic influences do not appear to be a sine qua non for the production of spasm. Vessel susceptibility and humoral factors, particularly those related to platelet activation and aggregation,[243] also appear to be important mechanisms.

Transition of stable atherosclerotic plaques to an "active" state because of endothelial damage, with plaque fissuring leading to platelet activation and aggregation followed by thrombosis, appears to contribute to mechanisms of SCD. In addition to initiating the thrombus, platelet activation produces a series of biochemical alterations which may enhance or retard susceptibility to VF by means of vasomotor modulation. Hammon and Oates studied the effects of thromboxane synthetase inhibitors[244] and demonstrated protection against the induction of experimental VF, presumably by blocking conversion of prostaglandin H_2 (PGH_2) to thromboxane A_2, which theoretically shunts accumulated PGH_2 to metabolic pathways that favor conversion to prostacyclin. Inhibition of cyclo-oxygenase by concurrent indomethacin administration gave further support to the hypothesis that PGH_2 shunting to other prostaglandin pathways might protect against VF by prostacyclin production. The possibility that inhibition of prostacyclin production might enhance the risk of VF[244] is supported by the finding from the Aspirin–Myocardial Infarction Study that the incidence of recurrent myocardial infarction was reduced by aspirin, but the relative and perhaps absolute numbers of SCD tended to increase.[245]

A number of pieces of indirect evidence support the possibility that more than the mechanical consequences to flow is involved in platelet-activated thrombosis of coro-

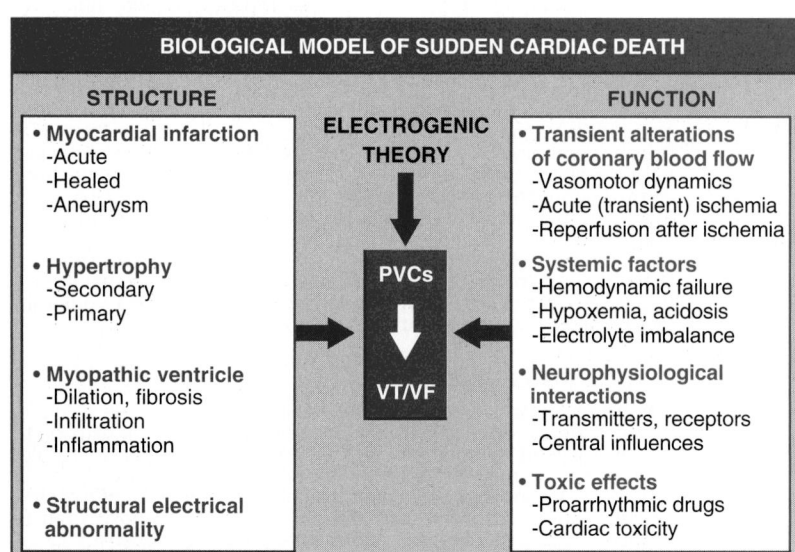

FIGURE 24–8. Biological model of sudden cardiac death. Structural cardiac abnormalities are commonly defined as the causative basis for SCD. However, functional alterations of the abnormal anatomic substrate usually are required to alter stability of the myocardium, permitting a potentially fatal arrhythmia to be initiated. In this conceptual model, short- or long-term structural abnormalities interact with functional modulations to influence the probability that premature ventricular contractions (PVCs) initiate ventricular tachycardia or fibrillation (VT/VF). (From Myerburg, R. J., et al.: A biological approach to sudden cardiac death: Structure, function, and cause. Am. J. Cardiol. *63:*1512, 1989.)

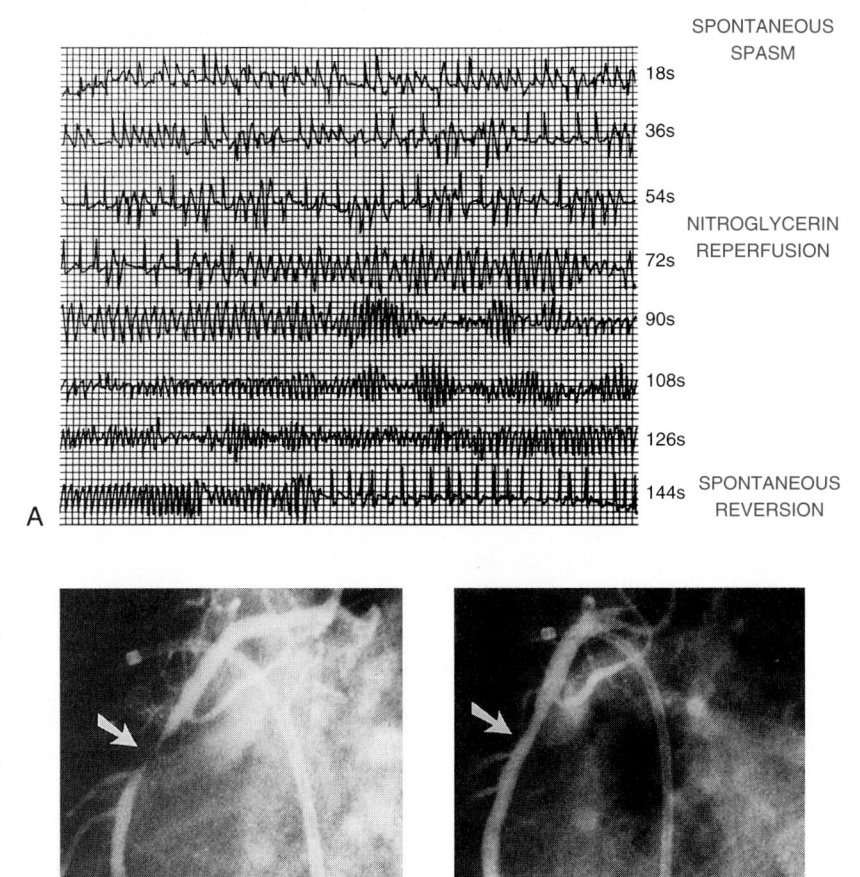

SPONTANEOUS
SPASM

18s

36s

54s

NITROGLYCERIN
REPERFUSION

72s

90s

108s

126s

144s

SPONTANEOUS
REVERSION

A

B

C

FIGURE 24–9. Life-threatening ventricular arrhythmias associated with acute myocardial ischemia due to coronary artery spasm and with reperfusion. *A,* Continuous lead II electrocardiographic monitor recording during ischemia [time 0 to 55 sec] due to spasm of the right coronary artery *(B).* There is an abrupt transition [time 56 sec to 72 sec] from repetitive ventricular ectopy to a rapid polymorphic, prefibrillatory tachyarrhythmia [time 80 sec to 130 sec] associated with nitroglycerin-induced reversal of the spasm *(C).*

nary arteries in SCD. Davies and Thomas[216] pointed out that 95 of 100 subjects who died suddenly (fewer than 6 hours after the onset of symptoms) had acute coronary thrombi, plaque fissuring, or both. This incidence was considerably higher than in many previous reports, but it is noteworthy that only 44 per cent of the patients had the largest thrombus occluding 51 per cent or more of the cross-sectional area of the involved vessel, and only 18 per cent of the patients had more than 75 per cent occlusion. This raises questions whether mechanical obstruction to flow was dominant, or whether the high incidence of nonoccluding thrombi simply reflected the state of activation of the platelets. The discrepancy between the relatively high incidence of acute thrombi in postmortem studies and the low incidence of evolution of new myocardial infarction among survivors of out-of-hospital VF[18–20,246] highlights this question. Spontaneous thrombolysis, a dominant role of spasm induced by platelet products, or a combination may explain this discrepancy.

ACUTE ISCHEMIA AND INITIATION OF LETHAL ARRHYTHMIAS. The onset of acute ischemia produces immediate electrical, mechanical, and biochemical dysfunction of cardiac muscle (Fig. 24–8). The specialized conducting tissue is more resistant to acute ischemia than is working myocardium, and therefore the electrophysiological consequences are less intense and delayed in onset in this tissue.[247] Experimental studies also have provided data on the long-term consequences of left ventricular hypertrophy and healed experimental myocardial infarction. Tissue exposed to chronic stress produced by long-term left ventricular pressure overload[248] and tissue which has healed after ischemic injury[249,250] both show lasting cellular electrophysiological abnormalities, including regional changes in trans-

membrane action potentials and refractory periods. Moreover, acute ischemic injury or acute myocardial infarction in the presence of healed myocardial infarction is more arrhythmogenic than is the same extent of acute ischemia in previously normal tissue.[250,251] In addition to the direct effect of ischemia on normal or previously abnormal tissue, it is possible that reperfusion after transient ischemia may cause lethal arrhythmias.[101,252,253] Reperfusion of ischemic areas may occur by three mechanisms: (1) spontaneous thrombolysis, (2) collateral flow from other coronary vascular beds to the ischemic bed, and (3) reversal of vasospasm. Some mechanisms of reperfusion-induced arrhythmogenesis appear to be related to the duration of ischemia prior to reperfusion.[253,254] Experimentally, there is a window of vulnerability beginning 5 to 10 minutes after the onset of ischemia and lasting up to 20 to 30 minutes.

ELECTROPHYSIOLOGICAL EFFECTS OF ACUTE ISCHEMIA. Within the first minutes after experimental coronary ligation there is a propensity to ventricular arrhythmias which abates after 30 minutes and reappears after several hours.[255] The initial 30 minutes of arrhythmias is divided into two periods, the first of which lasts for about 10 minutes and is presumably directly related to the initial ischemic injury. The second period (20 to 30 minutes) may be related either to reperfusion of ischemic areas or to the evolution of differing injury patterns in the epicardial and endocardial muscle. Multiple mechanisms of reperfusion arrhythmias have been observed experimentally.[224,256,257]

At the level of the myocyte, the immediate consequences of ischemia, which include loss of integrity of cell membranes with efflux of K^+, influx of Ca^{++}, acidosis, reduction of transmembrane resting potentials, and enhanced automaticity in some tissues, are followed by a separate series of changes during reperfusion. Those of particular current interest are the possible continued influx of Ca^{++} which may produce electrical instability,[253,258] responses to alpha- and/or beta-adrenoceptor stimulation,[233,234,259-261] and neurophysiologically induced afterdepolarization as triggering responses for Ca^{++}-dependent arrhythmias.[258,260] Other possible mechanisms studied experimentally include formation of superoxide radicals in reperfusion arrhythmias[262,263] and differential responses of endocardial and epicardial muscle activation times and refractory periods during ischemia or reperfusion.[256,264]

The importance of the myocardial response to the onset of ischemia has been emphasized, on the basis of the demonstration of dramatic cellular electrophysiological changes during the early period after coronary occlusion.[255,256,265] However, the state of the myocardium at the time of onset of ischemia is a critical additional factor. Tissue healed after previous injury appears to be more susceptible to the electrical destabilizing effects of acute ischemia, as is chronically hypertrophied muscle. Of more direct clinical relevance is the suggestion that K^+ depletion by diuretics and clinical hypokalemia may make ventricular myocardium more susceptible to potentially lethal arrhythmias.[266,267]

The association of metabolic and electrolyte abnormalities, as well as neurophysiological and neurohumoral changes,[268-271] with SCD emphasizes the importance of changes in the myocardial substrate in the propensity to lethal arrhythmias. Most direct among myocardial metabolic changes in response to ischemia are acute increase in interstitial K^+ levels to values exceeding 15 mM, a fall in tissue pH to below 6.0, changes in adrenoceptor activity, and alterations in autonomic nerve traffic,[129] all of which tend to create and maintain electrical instability, especially if regional in distribution. Other metabolic changes such as cyclic adenosine monophosphate elevation, accumulation of free fatty acids and their metabolites, formation of lysophosphoglycerides, and impaired myocardial glycolysis also have been suggested as myocardial destabilizing influences.[272]

Local myocardial and systemic influences integrate to establish operational mechanisms. Associations between systemic patterns of autonomic fluctuation are expressed as patterns of heart rate variability,[273,274] identifying subsets of patients at higher risk for SCD.

TRANSITION FROM MYOCARDIAL INSTABILITY TO LETHAL ARRHYTHMIAS. *The combination of a triggering event and a susceptible myocardium is evolving as a fundamental electrophysiological concept for the mechanism of initiation of potentially lethal arrhythmias* (Figs. 24–4 and 24–8). The endpoint of their interaction is disorganization of patterns of myocardial activation, usually by premature impulses (i.e., the "trigger"), into multiple uncoordinated reentrant pathways (i.e., ventricular fibrillation). Clinical,[77,275] experimental,[249,276] and pharmacological[276] data all suggest that triggering events and the myocardial instability permitting the evolution of lethal arrhythmias may be dissociated from one another. In the absence of myocardial vulnerability, many triggering events, such as frequent and complex PVCs, may be innocuous.[237]

The onset of ischemia is accompanied by abrupt reduction in transmembrane resting potential and amplitude and in duration of the action potential in the affected area,[265] with little change in remote areas. When ischemic cells depolarize to resting potentials less than -60 mV, they may become inexcitable and of little electrophysiological importance. As they are depolarizing to that range, however, or repolarizing as a consequence of reperfusion, the membranes pass through ranges of reduced excitability, upstroke velocity, and time courses of repolarization. These characteristics result in slow conduction and electrophysiological instability. These events that occur regionally in ischemic myocardium, adjacent to nonischemic tissue,

create a setting for the key elements of reentry—slow conduction and unidirectional block—which makes them vulnerable to reentrant arrhythmias. When premature impulses are generated in this environment, they may further alter the dispersion of recovery between ischemic tissue, chronically abnormal tissue, and normal cells,[250] ultimately leading to complete disorganization and VF. VF is probably not a consequence only of reentry.[129] Rapid-enhanced automaticity caused by ischemic injury to the specialized conducting tissue, or slow-channel–triggered activity in partially depolarized tissue, may result in rapid bursts of automatic activity which also could lead to failure of coordinated conduction and VF.

The dispersion of refractory periods produced by acute ischemia, which provides the substrate for reentrant tachycardias and VF, may be further enhanced by a healed ischemic injury. The time course of repolarization is lengthened after healing of ischemic injury[249,250] and shortened by acute ischemia.[250,253,265] The coexistence of the two appears to make the ventricle more susceptible to sustained arrhythmias in some experimental models.[250]

Bradyarrhythmias and Asystolic Arrest

The basic electrophysiological mechanism in this form of arrest is failure of normal subordinate automatic activity to assume pacemaking function of the heart in the absence of normal function of the sinus node and/or AV junction. Bradyarrhythmic and asystolic arrests are more common in severely diseased hearts and probably represent diffuse involvement of subendocardial Purkinje fibers. Systemic influences which increase extracellular K^+ concentration, such as anoxia, acidosis, shock, renal failure, trauma, and hypothermia, may result in partial depolarization of normal or already diseased pacemaker cells in the His-Purkinje system, with a decrease in the slope of spontaneous phase 4 depolarization and ultimate loss of automaticity.[277] These processes usually produce global dysfunction of automatic cell activity, in contrast to the regional dysfunction more common in acute ischemia. Functionally depressed automatic cells (e.g., owing to increased extracellular K^+ concentration) are more susceptible to overdrive suppression. Under these conditions, brief bursts of tachycardia may be followed by prolonged asystolic periods, with further depression of automaticity by the consequent acidosis and increased local K^+ concentration, or by changes in adrenergic tone. The ultimate consequence may be degeneration into VF or persistent asystole.

Pulseless Electrical Activity

Pulseless electrical activity, formerly called electromechanical dissociation (EMD), is separated into *primary* and *secondary* forms. The common denominator in both is continued electrical rhythmicity of the heart in the absence of effective mechanical function. The secondary form includes those causes which result from an abrupt cessation of cardiac venous return, such as massive pulmonary embolism, acute malfunction of prosthetic valves, exsanguination, and cardiac tamponade from hemopericardium. The primary form is the more familiar; in it none of these obvious mechanical factors are present, but ventricular muscle fails to produce an effective contraction despite continued electrical activity (i.e., *failure of electromechanical coupling*).[278] It usually occurs as an end-stage event in advanced heart disease, but it may occur in patients with acute ischemic events or, more commonly, after electrical resuscitation from a prolonged cardiac arrest. Although not thoroughly understood, it appears that diffuse disease, metabolic abnormalities, or global ischemia provides the pathophysiological substrate. The proximate mechanism for failure of electromechanical coupling may be abnormal intracellular Ca^{++} metabolism, intracellular acidosis, or perhaps adenosine triphosphate depletion.

Before the development of coronary care units, the in-hospital mortality owing to acute myocardial infarction was in the range of 25 to 30 per cent.[279] The current in-hospital mortality rate (see Chap. 37) is lower in large part because of prevention of in-hospital sudden deaths, now that acute potentially lethal arrhythmias in this setting are preventable or reversible.[280] However, the prior relationship between acute myocardial infarction and SCD in the hospitalized patient ingrained the concept of the association between the two, which was then extrapolated to the victims of out-of-hospital cardiac arrest. The advent of community-based emergency rescue systems generated cohorts of survivors of out-of-hospital cardiac arrest, and it soon became apparent that the majority of these cardiac arrests were, in fact, *not* associated with the evolution of a new transmural myocardial infarction.

Studies from Seattle[19] and from Miami[246] demonstrated that only a minority of survivors of out-of-hospital VF had clinical evidence indicating that a new transmural myocardial infarction was associated with the cardiac arrest. In the Seattle study, only one of five survivors had new transmural infarctions.[19] These studies led to the conclusion that in the majority of such patients, transient pathophysiological events were responsible for cardiac arrest. That this conclusion is reasonable and has clinical relevance is supported by the fact that the recurrence rate in survivors of out-of-hospital cardiac arrest is low in the subgroup of patients who had documentation of a new transmural myocardial infarction. It was found to be 30 per cent at 1 year and 45 per cent at 2 years in those survivors who did not have a new transmural myocardial infarction.[18,19] Recurrence rates decreased subsequently,[51] possibly owing in part to long-term interventions. However, it is not known whether this results from a change in the natural history, changes in preventive strategies for underlying disease, or long-term interventions for controlling arrhythmic risk.[26]

Clinical cardiac arrest and SCD are best described in the framework of the same four phases of the event used to establish definitions (Fig. 24–1): prodromes, onset of the terminal event, the cardiac arrest, and progression to biological death or survival.

Prodromal Symptoms

Patients risk for SCD may have prodromes such as chest pain, dyspnea, weakness or fatigue, palpitations, and a number of nonspecific complaints. Several epidemiological and clinical studies demonstrated that such symptoms may presage coronary events, particularly myocardial infarction and SCD,[8,52,281] and result in contact with the medical system weeks to months before SCD.

In a prospective study in Edinburgh, Scotland, however, only 12 per cent of victims of SCD had consulted a physician because of new or worsening angina pectoris during periods of up to 6 months before death.[282] In contrast, 33 per cent of myocardial infarction patients had consulted their physicians for this complaint. Nonetheless, 46 per cent of victims of SCD had seen a physician within 4 weeks before death, but three-fourths of them had sought medical help for complaints which appeared to be unrelated to the heart. Liberthson et al.,[18] in a study of patients successfully resuscitated after out-of-hospital cardiac arrest, noted that 28 per cent reported retrospectively that they had had new or changing angina pectoris or dyspnea in the 4 weeks before arrest, and that 31 per cent had seen a physician during this time but only 12 per cent because of these symptoms.

Patients who have chest pain as a prodrome to SCD appear to have a higher probability of intraluminal coronary thrombosis at postmortem examination.[217] Attempts to identify early prodromal symptoms which are more specific for the patient at risk for SCD have not yet

been successful. Fatigue has been a particularly common symptom in the days or weeks before SCD in a number of studies,[281] but this symptom is nonspecific. The symptoms that occur within the last hours or minutes before cardiac arrest are more specific for heart disease and may include symptoms of arrhythmias, ischemia, or heart failure.[21,283] Liberthson et al.[213] reported specific cardiac symptoms at a mean interval of about 3.8 hours before collapse in 24 per cent of victims of SCD. However, most studies have reported such symptoms even less commonly, particularly when victims whose deaths were instantaneous are included.[8]

Onset of the Terminal Event

The period of 1 hour or less between acute changes in cardiovascular status and the cardiac arrest itself, which has been defined as the "onset of the terminal event," is a subject about which there is limited information. Reports from ambulatory monitor recordings fortuitously obtained at the time of unexpected cardiac arrest indicate dynamic change in cardiac electrical activity during the minutes or hours before the onset of cardiac arrest.[284–286] These reports suggest that increasing heart rate and advancing grades of ventricular ectopy are common antecedents of VF. Although these recordings suggest transient electrophysiological destabilization of the myocardium, the extent to which these objective observations are paralleled by clinical symptoms is less well documented. SCDs caused by either arrhythmias or acute circulatory failure mechanisms involve a high incidence of acute myocardial disorders at the onset of the terminal event; such disorders are more likely to be ischemic when the death is due to arrhythmias and to be associated with low-output states or myocardial anoxia when the deaths are due to circulatory failure.[21,287]

Abrupt, unexpected loss of effective circulation may be caused by cardiac arrhythmias or mechanical disturbances, but the majority of such events that terminate in SCD are arrhythmic in origin. Hinkle and Thaler[287] classified cardiac deaths among 142 subjects who died during a follow-up of 5 to 10 years. Class I was labeled arrhythmic death and Class II was death caused by circulatory failure. The distinction between the two classes was based on whether circulatory failure preceded (Class II) or followed (Class I) the disappearance of the pulse. Among deaths which occurred less than 1 hour after the onset of the terminal illness, 93 per cent were due to arrhythmias; in addition, 90 per cent of deaths caused by heart disease were initiated by arrhythmic events rather than circulatory failure. Table 24–4 demonstrates that deaths caused by circulatory failure occurred predominantly in patients who could be identified as having terminal illnesses (95 per cent were comatose), were associated more fre-

TABLE 24–4 DIFFERENCES IN CLINICAL STATUS IMMEDIATELY BEFORE DEATH IN PATIENTS DYING OF ARRHYTHMIA AND CIRCULATORY FAILURE

CLINICAL STATUS IMMEDIATELY BEFORE DEATH	ARRHYTHMIC DEATHS (N = 82) (CLASS I)	CIRCULATORY FAILURE DEATHS (N = 59) (CLASS II)
Comatose	0/82 (0%)	56/59 (95%)
Standing or actively moving	39/82 (48%)	0/59 (0%)
Terminal arrhythmia		
• Ventricular fibrillation	15/18 (83%)	3/9 (33%)
• Asystole	3/18 (17%)	6/9 (67%)
Duration of terminal illness		
• <1 hour	53/82 (65%)	4/59 (7%)
• >24 hours	17/82 (21%)	48/59 (81%)
Nature of terminal illness		
• Acute cardiac events	80/82 (98%)	8/59 (14%)
• Noncardiac events	1/82 (1%)	51/59 (86%)

Data from Hinkle, L. E. and Thaler, H. T.: Clinical classification of cardiac deaths. Circulation 65:457, 1982.

quently with bradyarrhythmias than with VF as the terminal arrhythmias, and were dominated by noncardiac events as the terminal illness. In contrast, 98 per cent of the arrhythmic deaths were associated primarily with cardiac disorders.

Clinical Features of Cardiac Arrest

The cardiac arrest itself is characterized by abrupt loss of consciousness owing to lack of adequate cerebral blood flow. It is an event which uniformly leads to death in the absence of an active intervention, although spontaneous reversions occur rarely. The most common cardiac mechanism is VF, followed by bradyarrhythmias or asystole, and sustained VT.[20] Other, less frequent mechanisms include electromechanical dissociation, rupture of the ventricle,[288] cardiac tamponade, acute mechanical obstruction to flow, and acute disruption of a major blood vessel.[3,45,128]

The potential for successful resuscitation is a function of the setting in which cardiac arrest occurs, the mechanism of the arrest, and the underlying clinical status of the victim.[289] Closely related to the potential for successful resuscitation is the decision of whether or not to attempt to resuscitate.[290]

At present there are fewer low-risk patients with otherwise uncomplicated myocardial infarctions weighting in-hospital cardiac arrest statistics than previously.[288] Bedell and coworkers[291] reported that only 14 per cent of in-hospital CPR patients were discharged from the hospital alive, and that 20 per cent of these died within the ensuing 6 months. Although 41 per cent of the patients had suffered an acute myocardial infarction, 73 per cent had a history of congestive heart failure, and 20 per cent had had prior cardiac arrests. The mean age of 70 years (10 years older than the populations in several major prehospital cardiac arrest studies[18,19,51]) may have influenced the outcome statistics, but the patient population at risk for in-hospital cardiac arrest was heavily influenced by patients with high-risk complicated myocardial infarction or patients with other high-risk markers. Noncardiac clinical diagnoses were dominated by renal failure, pneumonia, sepsis, diabetes, and a history of cancer. The strong male preponderance consistently reported in out-of-hospital cardiac arrest studies is not present in in-hospital patients, but the better prognosis of ventricular tachycardia (VT) or VF mechanisms, compared with bradyarrhythmic or asystolic mechanisms, persists (27 per cent survival versus 8 per cent survival). However, the proportion of arrests which are due to in-hospital VT or VF is considerably less (33 per cent), with the combination of respiratory arrest, asystole, and electromechanical dissociation dominating the statistics (61 per cent).

The important risk factors for death after CPR are listed in Table 24–5. The facts that the fraction of out-of-hospital cardiac arrest survivors who are discharged from the hospital alive may now equal or exceed the fraction of in-hospital cardiac arrest victims who are discharged alive,[292] and that the postdischarge mortality rate for in-hospital cardiac arrest survivors is higher than that for out-of-hospital cardiac arrest survivors,[51,291,293] are telling clinical statistics. Not only do they emphasize the success of preventive mea-

TABLE 24–5 PREDICTORS OF MORTALITY AFTER IN-HOSPITAL CARDIOPULMONARY RESUSCITATION

BEFORE ARREST
Hypotension (systolic BP < 100 mm Hg)
Pneumonia
Renal failure (BUN > 50 mg/dl)
Cancer
Homebound life style

DURING ARREST
Arrest duration > 15 minutes
Intubation
Hypotension (systolic BP < 100 mm Hg)
Pneumonia
Homebound life style

AFTER RESUSCITATION
Coma
Need for pressors
Arrest duration > 15 minutes

Modified from Bedell, S. E., et al.: Survival after cardiopulmonary resuscitation in the hospital. N. Engl. J. Med. *309*:569, 1983. Copyright Massachusetts Medical Society.

sures for cardiac arrest in low-risk in-hospital patients, causing those statistics to be dominated by higher-risk patients, but they also emphasize the improvement in prehospital and in-hospital care of out-of-hospital cardiac arrest victims.[294]

Cardiac arrest associated with coronary heart disease in the hospitalized elderly patient has a similar outcome. Gulati et al.[295] reported that 14 of 52 (27 per cent) elderly patients (mean age 76 years) were successfully resuscitated, although only 9 (17 per cent) remained alive after 1 week. Similar outcome was observed in another report comparing patients younger and older than 70 years.[296] Coronary heart disease was the cause in 48 patients (92 per cent); 5 of 22 patients (23 per cent) with VF arrests survived and only 1 of 19 (5 per cent) with asystole survived.[295] Among those 70 years of age or older, survival to discharge from hospital after out-of-hospital cardiac arrest was lower (29 per cent) than among younger patients (47 per cent).[297] However, long-term neurological status, survival, and length of hospitalization were similar among older and younger patients.

Progression to Biological Death

The time course for progression from cardiac arrest to biological death relates to the mechanism of the cardiac arrest, the nature of the underlying disease process, and the delay between onset and resuscitative efforts. Unattended VF characteristically leads to the onset of irreversible brain damage within 4 to 6 minutes, and biological death follows within a matter of minutes. In large series, however, it has been demonstrated that a limited number of victims may remain biologically alive for longer periods and may be resuscitated after delays in excess of 8 minutes before beginning basic life support and in excess of 16 minutes before advanced life support.[298] Despite these exceptions, it is clear that the probability for a favorable outcome deteriorates rapidly as a function of time after unattended cardiac arrest. Younger patients with less severe cardiac disease and the absence of coexistent multisystem disease appear to have a higher probability of a favorable outcome after such delays. Irreversible injury of the central nervous system usually occurs before biological death, and the interval may extend to a period of weeks in those patients who are resuscitated during the temporal gap between brain damage and biological death (see Definition, p. 742). In-hospital cardiac arrest caused by VF is less likely to have a protracted course between the arrest and biological death, with patients either surviving after a prompt intervention or succumbing rapidly because of inability to stabilize cardiac rhythm or hemodynamics.[291]

Those patients whose cardiac arrest is due to sustained VT with cardiac output inadequate to maintain consciousness may remain in VT for considerably longer periods, with flow which is marginally sufficient to maintain viability. This allows a longer interval between the onset of cardiac arrest and the end of the period, which will allow successful resuscitation. The lives of such patients usually end in VF or an asystolic arrest if the VT is not actively or spontaneously reverted. Once the transition from VT to VF or to a bradyarrhythmia occurs, the subsequent course to biological death is similar to that in patients in whom VF or bradyarrhythmias are the initiating event.

The progression in patients with asystole or bradyarrhythmias as the initiating event is more rapid. Such patients, whether in an in-hospital[291] or out-of-hospital[20,299] environment, have a very poor prognosis because of advanced heart disease or coexistent multisystem disease. They tend to respond poorly to interventions, even if the heart is successfully paced.[300] Although a small subgroup of patients with bradyarrhythmias associated with electrolyte or pharmacological abnormalities may respond well to interventions, the majority progress rapidly to biological death.[299] The infrequent cardiac arrests caused by mechanical factors such as tamponade, structural disruption, and impedance to flow by major thromboembolic obstructions to right or left ventricular outflow are reversible only in those instances in which the mechanism is recognized and an intervention is feasible. The vast majority of these events lead to rapid biological death, although prompt relief of tamponade may save some lives.

Hospital Course of Survivors of Cardiac Arrest

The hospital course of survivors of cardiac arrest is characterized by an initial period of instability, followed by clinical features which are determined by the electrical and hemodynamic status of the patient, and the consequence of central nervous system injury occurring during the cardiac arrest.[20,22] The conditions of patients who are resuscitated immediately from *primary* VF associated with acute myocardial infarction usually stabilize promptly, and they require no special management after the early phase of the infarction (Chap. 37). The management after *secondary cardiac arrest in myocardial infarction* is dominated by the hemodynamic status of the patient. Among survivors of *out-of-hospital cardiac arrest,* the initial 24 to 48 hours of hospitalization are characterized by a tendency to ventricular arrhythmias, which usually respond well to antiarrhythmic therapy.[20,246,283] The overall rate of recurrent cardiac arrest is low, about 10 to 20 per cent, but the mortality rate in patients who have recurrent cardiac arrests is about 50 per cent.[18-20] Only 5 to 10 per cent of in-hospital deaths after prehospital resuscitation are due to recurrent cardiac arrhythmias.[20,22] Patients who have recurrent cardiac arrest have a high incidence of either new or preexisting AV or intraventricular conduction abnormalities.[20]

The most common causes of death in hospitalized survivors of out-of-hospital cardiac arrest are noncardiac events related to central nervous system injury suffered during the cardiac arrest itself. These include anoxic encephalopathy and sepsis related to prolonged intubation and hemodynamic monitoring lines.[20,22] Fifty-nine per cent of deaths during index hospitalization after prehospital resuscitation have been reported to be due to such causes.[20] It has been reported that 39 per cent of 457 consecutive patients in coma never awakened after admission to the hospital and died after a median survival of 3.5 days.[301] Two-thirds of the 61 per cent who awakened had no gross deficits, and an additional 21 per cent had persisting cognitive deficits only. Of the patients who did awaken, 25 per cent had done so by admission, 71 per cent by the first hospital day, and 92 per cent by the third day. A small number of patients awakened after prolonged hospitalization. Of the 206 hospital deaths (45 per cent of the 457 patients), 80 per cent had not awakened before death.

Cardiac causes of delayed death during hospitalization after out-of-hospital cardiac arrest are most commonly related to hemodynamic deterioration, which accounts for about one-third of deaths in-hospital.[20,22] Among all deaths, those that occurred within the first 48 hours of hospitalization usually were due to hemodynamic deterioration or arrhythmias, regardless of the neurological status; later deaths were related to neurological complications. Admission characteristics most predictive of subsequent awakening included motor response, pupillary light response, spontaneous eye movement, and blood sugar below 300 mg/dl.[302]

Clinical Profile of Survivors of Out-of-Hospital Cardiac Arrest

The clinical features of survivors of out-of-hospital cardiac arrest are heavily influenced by the type and extent of the underlying disease associated with the event. Causation is dominated by coronary heart disease, which accounts for approximately 80 per cent of out-of-hospital cardiac arrest in the United States[246] and is commonly extensive. The cardiomyopathies collectively account for another 10 to 15 per cent, with all other structural heart diseases, plus functional and toxic/environmental causes, accounting for the remainder (Table 24–2, p. 748).

Complex PVCs have been reported in the majority of survivors of prehospital cardiac arrest who had serial ambulatory monitor recordings.[246,303,304] These arrhythmias are difficult to suppress[303] and show trends to higher grades of ventricular ectopy in victims of recurrent cardiac arrest compared with long-term survivors.[51,304] Complex forms were strongly associated with a history of congestive heart failure or previous myocardial infarction. The strongest predictors of subsequent mortality were use of digitalis, elevated BUN, cerebrovascular accident, previous myocardial infarction, and age; however, the presence of complex PVCs or frequent ectopy (≥ 25 PVCs/hour) added strongly to risk.

LEFT VENTRICULAR FUNCTION. This is abnormal in the majority of survivors of out-of-hospital cardiac arrest, often severely so, but there is a wide variation, ranging from severe dysfunction to normal or near-normal measurements, with as many as 50 per cent ranging from normal to moderate dysfunction (Fig. 24–10).[51] The author found that the ejection fraction of those who died during follow-up was lower than that of the long-term survivors (38 versus 45 per cent, respectively).[20,51] From data reported in a number of large series, the mean ejection fraction has been in the range of 32 to 35 per cent. Patients who died of recurrent cardiac arrest had higher ejection fractions than those who died non-sudden cardiac deaths (43 versus 25 per cent). Ritchie et al.[305] reported on studies of left ventricular function by radionuclide techniques in 154 survivors of out-of-hospital VF, 91 of whom had both rest and exercise studies. The mean ejection fraction at rest was 40 per cent, with 20 per cent having values greater than 50 per cent. Only 3 of 91 patients (3 per cent) studied had a normal increase (>5 per cent) in ejection fraction during exertion; 18 per cent had normal resting wall motion. The ejection fraction at rest was the best predictor of death during follow-up.[305] Fifty per cent of survivors studied by cardiac catheterization and angiography had ejection fractions below 50 per cent, and 30 per cent had left ventricular end-diastolic pressures greater than 15 mm Hg[306]; in this study, ejection fraction and severity of wall motion abnormality correlated with risk of recurrent cardiac arrest.

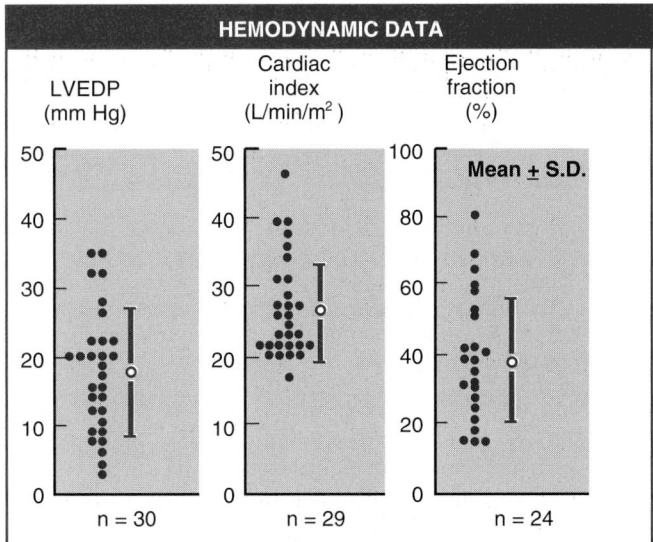

FIGURE 24–10. Hemodynamic data from prehospital cardiac arrest victims studied during initial post-arrest hospitalization, and the relation between ejection fraction (EF) at initial study and long-term outcome. These data indicate a broad range of cardiac function and a statistically insignificant difference between EF at entry in long-term survivors and in recurrent cardiac arrest victims. (From Myerburg, R. J., et al.: Clinical, electrophysiologic, and hemodynamic profile of patients resuscitated from prehospital cardiac arrest. Am. J. Med. 68:568, 1980.)

CORONARY ANGIOGRAPHY. Studies in survivors of out-of-hospital cardiac arrest have shown that as a group, this population tends to have extensive disease but no specific pattern of abnormalities. Moderate to severe stenosis of the left main coronary artery was present in only 8 per cent of the patients in one series,[306] and only 9 per cent in another,[20] frequencies not different from those in the overall population of coronary heart disease patients. Significant lesions in two or more vessels were present in 74 per cent of the patients who had any coronary lesions in one study,[20] and 94 per cent of the patients in another had 70 per cent or greater degrees of stenosis in one or more arteries.[306] Among patients who had recurrent cardiac arrests, the incidence of triple-vessel disease was higher than among those who did not.

EXERCISE TESTING. This is commonly used to evaluate the need for and response to antiischemic therapy in survivors of out-of-hospital cardiac arrest. The incidence of positive tests related to ischemia is relatively low, although termination of testing because of fatigue is common.[246,303,307] Mortality during follow-up was greater in patients who had angina or failure of a normal rise in systolic blood pressure occurring during exercise.[307]

ELECTROCARDIOGRAPHIC OBSERVATIONS. In survivors of out-of-hospital cardiac arrest these have proved of value only for discriminating risk of recurrence among those whose cardiac arrest was associated with new transmural myocardial infarction. Patients who develop documented new Q waves, in association with a clinical picture suggesting that an acute ischemic event began prior to the cardiac arrest itself, are at much lower risk for recurrence.[18,246,308] A higher incidence of repolarization abnormalities (ST-segment depression, flat T waves, prolonged $Q-T_c$) occurs in out-of-hospital cardiac arrest survivors than in post-myocardial infarction patients, and these might be markers for increased risk.[309]

Lower serum K^+ levels were observed in survivors of cardiac arrest than in patients with acute myocardial infarction or stable coronary heart disease.[310] The investigators concluded that this was a consequence of resuscitation interventions, rather than a preexisting state owing to chronic diuretic use. Low ionized Ca^{++} levels, with normal total calcium levels, also were observed during resuscitation from out-of-hospital cardiac arrest.[311] Higher resting lactate levels have been reported in out-of-hospital cardiac arrest survivors than in normal subjects.[312] Lactate levels correlated inversely with ejection fractions and directly with PVC frequency and complexity.

Studies from the early 1970's in both Miami[18] and Seattle[19] indicated that the risk of recurrent cardiac arrest in the first year after surviving an initial event was about 30 per cent and at 2 years was 45 per cent. Total mortality at 2 years was about 60 per cent in both studies. In both of these studies, less than half of the patients followed were being treated with long-term antiarrhythmic therapy; beta-adrenoceptor blocker therapy was in its infancy, and Ca^{++}-entry blockers were not yet available. Thus these figures appear to be as close to valid natural history figures as possible. However, they can serve only as historical control figures for current observations, and thus are of limited value, because the risk of recurrent cardiac arrest

likely is lower now than it was in the early 1970's.[313] Moreover, the risk of recurrent cardiac arrest/SCD appears to be lower for survivors with hypertrophic cardiomyopathy—about 33 per cent during a mean follow-up period of 7 years.[110] In a recent report of cardiac arrest survivors with and without successful medical and/or surgical antiarrhythmic endpoints, the 1-year recurrent cardiac arrest rate was 14.5 per cent and the 2-year cumulative rate was 21.1 per cent, with a clustering of events within the first 6 to 12 months (i.e., time-dependent risk) (Fig. 24–11).[314]

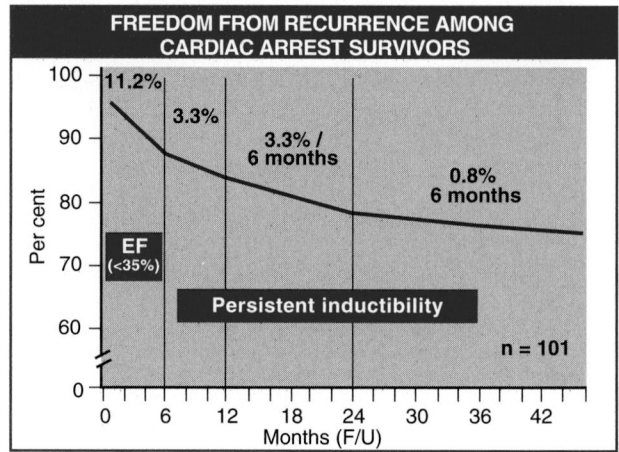

FIGURE 24–11. Time-dependence of recurrences among survivors of cardiac arrest. Actuarial analysis of occurrences among a population of 101 cardiac arrest survivors with coronary artery disease is demonstrated. The risk was highest in the first 6 months (11.2 per cent) and then fell to 3.3 per cent/6 months for the next three 6-month blocks. After 24 months the rate fell to 0.8 per cent/6 months. A low ejection fraction (EF) was the most powerful predictor of death during the first 6 months; subsequently, persistent inducibility during programmed stimulation, despite drug therapy or surgery, was the most powerful predictor. (Modified from Furukawa, T., et al.: Time-dependent risk of and predictors for cardiac arrest recurrence in survivors of out-of-hospital cardiac arrest with chronic coronary artery disease. Circulation *80*:599, 1989. The figure is reproduced from Myerburg, R. J., et al.: Sudden cardiac death: Structure, function and time-dependence of risk. Circulation *85*(Suppl. I):I-2, 1992. Copyright 1992 American Heart Association.)

MANObserved MANAGEMENT OF CARDIAC ARREST

COMMUNITY-BASED INTERVENTIONS

Systems for intervention in out-of-hospital cardiac arrest have their roots in the development of the coronary care unit (CCU) approach to the management of potentially lethal arrhythmias.[315] Previously, cardiac arrest in the setting of acute coronary events was almost uniformly fatal, wherever it occurred. With the confluence of the key elements of the CCU in the late 1950's and early 1960's (i.e., continuous monitoring, CPR, effective acute drug therapy, and electrical management of tachycardias, bradycardias, and VF), there was a dramatic reduction in the immediate in-hospital mortality from potentially lethal arrhythmias occurring in the course of acute coronary events.[316] The next step toward the development of community-based intervention for cardiac arrest was the concept of the mobile coronary care unit,[317] which was based on the rationale of providing a CCU environment during the high-risk prehospital phase of acute myocardial infarction. Only a small extension in concept in the late 1960's led to the development of community-based intervention systems designed to respond routinely to out-of-hospital cardiac arrests.

The systems as developed in the United States are largely

integrated into fire departments as emergency rescue systems. They employ paramedical personnel or emergency medical technicians trained in CPR and the use of telemetered monitoring equipment, defibrillators, and specific intravenous drug therapy. Although the initial out-of-hospital intervention experience in Miami and Seattle[18,19] reported in the early 1970's yielded only 14 and 10 per cent survivals to discharge, respectively, later data indicate that such systems are becoming increasingly effective in saving lives (Fig. 24–12).[292,308] By the mid-1970's, both had increased survival rates to about 25 per cent,[20,292] and by the early 1980's to 30 per cent or more.[292] Survival rates in these centers appear to have decreased since then, presumably because of the extension of rescue systems into less densely populated regions.[318]

Conversely, recent reports from very densely populated areas (i.e., Chicago and New York City) have provided disturbing outcomes data. The Chicago study reported that only 9 per cent of out-of-hospital cardiac arrest victims survived to be hospitalized and that only 2 per cent were discharged alive.[57] Moreover, outcomes in blacks were far worse than in whites (0.8 per cent versus 2.6 per cent). The fact that a large majority had bradyarrhythmias, asystole, or

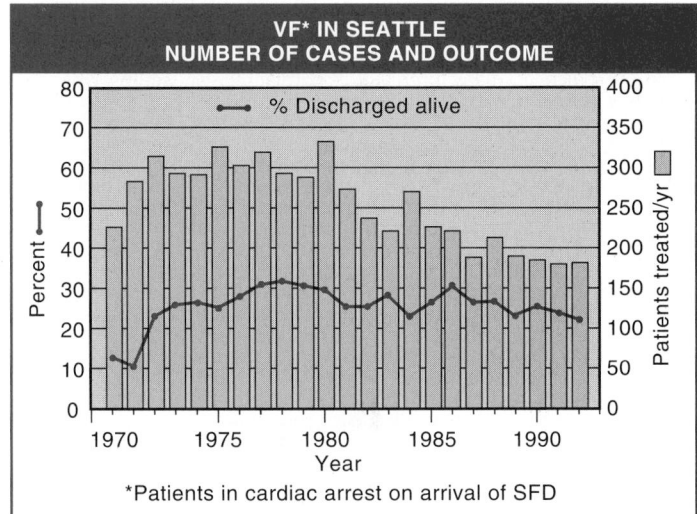

FIGURE 24–12. Annual number of emergency rescue responses to out-of-hospital cardiac arrest *(vertical bars)* and the percent of patients discharged alive *(solid line)*, from 1970 through 1992 in Seattle, Washington. Patients were in cardiac arrest when initially examined by emergency rescue personnel. (Courtesy of Leonard A. Cobb, M.D., Seattle, Washington.)

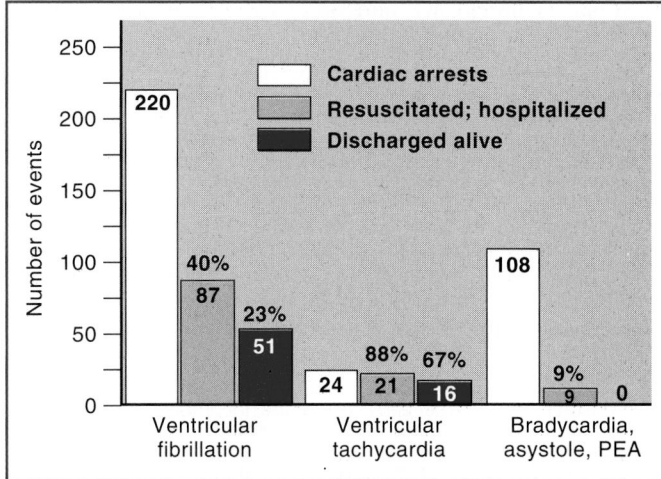

FIGURE 24–13. Survival after out-of-hospital cardiac arrest as function of the intial electrophysiological mechanism recorded by emergency rescue personnel. The mechanisms among 352 out-of-hospital cardiac arrest victims are separated into three categories: ventricular fibrillation (n = 220; 62 per cent), ventricular tachycardia (n = 24; 7 per cent), and bradycardia/asystole/pulseless electrical activity (PEA) (n = 108; 31 per cent). The white bars illustrate the total number of events in each category. The light-colored bars illustrate the number and per cent of patients who were initially resuscitated in the field and reached the hospital alive in each category, and the dark bars illustrate the percentage of total events in which patients were discharged from the hospital alive for each category. The data are derived from the Miami, Florida experience.[20]

pulseless electrical activity on initial emergency medical services contact suggests prolonged times between collapse and emergency medical services arrival and/or absent or ineffective bystander interventions. The New York City report indicated a survival-to-hospital-discharge rate of only 1.4 per cent.[319] Among those who had bystander CPR, the rate increased to 2.9 per cent, and bystander CPR plus VF as the initial rhythm yielded a further increase to 5.3 per cent. Finally, for those whose arrests occurred after emergency medical services arrival, the success rate increased further to 8.5 per cent. This trend, together with the fact that (as in Chicago) nontachyarrhythmic events constituted a majority, suggests that delays and breaks in the "chain of survival"[294] exert a major negative impact on emergency medical services results in densely populated areas.

IMPORTANCE OF ELECTRICAL MECHANISMS. The electrical mechanism of out-of-hospital cardiac arrest, as defined by the initial rhythm recorded by emergency rescue personnel, has a powerful impact on success of initial resuscitation and outcome, the latter measured in terms of patients discharged from the hospital alive. The subgroup of patients who are in sustained VT at the time of first contact, although the smallest group statistically, has the best outcome (Fig. 24–13). Eighty-eight per cent of patients in cardiac arrest due to VT were successfully resuscitated and admitted to the hospital alive, and 67 per cent were ultimately discharged alive.[20] However, this relatively low-risk group represents only 7 to 10 per cent of all cardiac arrests in studies reported to date. Because of the inherent time lag between collapse and initial recordings, it is possible that many more cardiac arrests begin as rapid sustained VT and degenerate into VF before arrival of emergency rescue personnel.

Patients who are in a bradyarrhythmia or asystole at initial contact have the worst prognosis; only 9 per cent of such patients in the Miami study were admitted to the hospital alive and none was discharged.[20] In a later experience there was some improvement in outcome, although the improvement was strictly limited to those patients in whom the initial bradyarrhythmia recorded was an idioventricular rhythm which responded promptly to chronotropic agents in the field.[299] Bradyarrhythmias also have adverse prognostic implications after defibrillation from VF in the field. Patients who were defibrillated to an initial heart rate less than 60 beats/min, regardless of the specific bradyarrhythmic mechanism, had a poor prognosis, with 95

per cent of such patients dying either before hospitalization or in the hospital (Fig. 24–14).[18] In contrast, an initial heart rate in excess of 100 beats/min yielded a 43 per cent rate of discharge from hospital, with only 17 per cent of such patients dying before hospitalization, and 40 per cent during hospitalization. Heart rates between 60 and 100 beats/min after defibrillation yield intermediate results.

The outcome in the largest group of patients, those in whom VF is the initial rhythm recorded, is intermediate

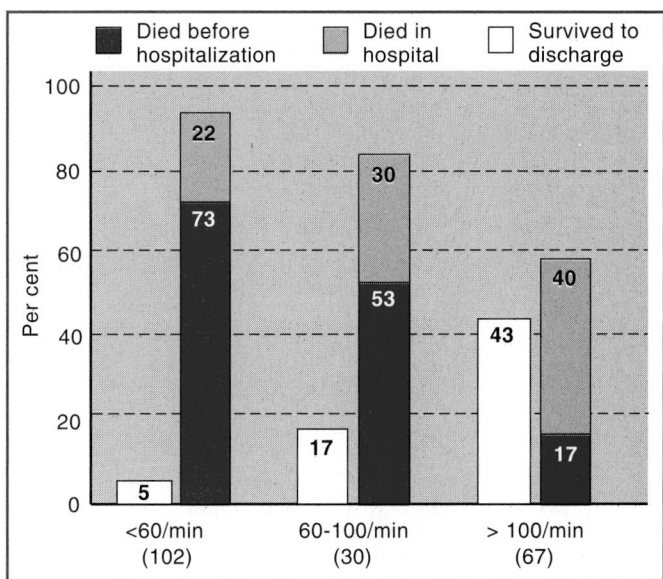

FIGURE 24–14. Prognostic implication of initial heart rate after prehospital defibrillation. Prehospital and in-hospital deaths and long-range survival (i.e., discharged survivors) are compared with the initial postdefibrillation heart rate: <60 beats/min, 60 to 100 beats/min, or >100 beats/min. Numbers in parentheses represent the number of patients in each group. (Modified from Liberthson, R. R., et al.: Prehospital ventricular fibrillation: Prognosis and follow-up course. Reprinted by permission of N. Engl. J. Med. 291:317, 1974. Copyright Massachusetts Medical Society.)

between sustained VT and bradyarrhythmia and asystole. Figure 24–13 demonstrates that 40 per cent of such patients were successfully resuscitated and admitted to the hospital alive, and 23 per cent were ultimately discharged alive.[20] More recent data indicate improvement in outcome. The proportion of each of the electrophysiological mechanisms responsible for cardiac arrest varied among the earlier reports, with VF ranging from 65 to greater than 90 per cent of the study populations, and bradyarrhythmia and asystole ranging from 10 to 30 per cent.[20,283,292,308] However, in recent reports from very densely populated metropolitan areas, the ratios of tachyarrhythmic to bradyarrhythmic/pulseless activity events were reversed, and outcomes were far worse.[57,319]

The factors which have contributed to improved outcome since the first observations in the early 1970's are incompletely understood. Both improved prehospital care and improvements in in-hospital technology and practices may contribute, as described in the "chain of survival" concept.[294] Of these two general factors, the influence of prehospital care has been studied in more detail. Eisenberg and co-workers[320] compared initial resuscitation and ultimate discharge alive in two subgroups of patients, those who had standard CPR continuously from the arrival of emergency rescue personnel through transport to an emergency department where defibrillation took place, and another group in whom paramedics or emergency rescue personnel trained to defibrillate were allowed to do so at the scene of the cardiac arrest. The standard CPR technique resulted in only 23 per cent of patients arriving at the hospital alive and 7 per cent discharged alive, in contrast to the immediate defibrillation group in which 53 per cent arrived at the hospital alive and 26 per cent were discharged alive. Subsequent data continue to support the concept that early defibrillation is a key element in improving survival rates (Fig. 24–15).[292,298] Immediate defibrillation by ambulance technicians is especially important in rural communities, where it yields a 19 per cent survival, compared with only 3 per cent from standard CPR.[318]

A second element in prehospital care which appears to contribute to outcome is the role of bystander CPR by laypeople awaiting the arrival of emergency rescue personnel. It has been reported that

although there was no significant difference in the percentage of patients successfully resuscitated and admitted to the hospital alive with (67 per cent) or without (61 per cent) bystander intervention, almost twice as many prehospital cardiac arrest victims were ultimately discharged alive when they had had bystander CPR (43 per cent) than when such support was not provided (22 per cent).[22] Central nervous system protection, expressed as early regaining of consciousness, appears to be the major protective element of bystander CPR.[22] The rationale for bystander intervention is further highlighted by the relation between time to defibrillation and survival, when analyzed as a function of time to initiation of basic CPR. It has been reported that more than 40 per cent of victims whose defibrillation and other advanced life support activities were instituted more than 8 minutes after collapse survived if basic CPR had been initiated less than 2 minutes after onset of the arrest. A delay of more than 5 minutes to basic CPR was associated with no survivors.[292]

The time from onset of cardiac arrest to advanced life support influences outcome statistics. Mayer[321] reported improved short-term (to hospital admission) and long-term (to hospital discharge) survival rates for prehospital VF victims with short paramedic response times compared with those with long response times. Improvement in both early neurological status and survival occurs in the patient defibrillated by first responders, even if they are minimally trained emergency technicians allowed to carry out defibrillation as part of basic life support, compared with outcomes associated with awaiting more highly trained paramedics.[322] Thus the time to defibrillation plays a central role in determining outcome in cardiac arrest caused by VF. The development and deployment of automatic external defibrillators (see p. 1252) in the community holds promise for progress in the future.[323] This technology is a natural extension of lay bystander CPR.

MANAGEMENT OF THE INDIVIDUAL PATIENT

Management of the cardiac arrest victim is divided into five elements: (1) initial assessment, (2) basic life support, (3) advanced life support and definitive resuscitative efforts, (4) post–cardiac arrest care, and (5) long-term management. The first of these can be applied by a broad population base, which includes physicians and nurses as well as paramedical personnel, emergency rescue technicians, and laypeople educated in bystander intervention. The requirements for specialized knowledge and skills become progressively more focused as the patient moves through post–cardiac arrest management and into long-term follow-up care.

Initial Assessment and Basic Life Support

This activity includes both diagnostic maneuvers and elementary interventions. The first action of the person(s) in attendance when an individual collapses unexpectedly must be *confirmation that collapse is due to (or suspected to be due to) a cardiac arrest*. A few seconds of observation for response to voice, respiratory movements, and skin color, and simultaneous palpation of major arteries for the presence or absence of a pulse, yield sufficient information to determine whether a life-threatening incident is in progress. Once suspected or confirmed, contact with an available emergency medical rescue system (911) should be an immediate priority.[324]

The absence of carotid or femoral pulse, particularly if confirmed by the absence of an audible heartbeat, is the primary diagnostic criterion and can be performed accurately by trained laypeople. Skin color may be pale or intensely cyanotic. Absence of respiratory efforts, or the presence of only agonal respiratory efforts, in conjunction with an absent pulse, is diagnostic of cardiac arrest; however, respiratory efforts may persist for a minute or more after the onset of the arrest. In contrast, absence of respiratory efforts or severe stridor with persistence of a pulse suggests a primary respiratory arrest which will lead to a cardiac arrest in a short time. In the latter circumstance, initial efforts should include exploration of the oropharynx in search of a foreign body and the Heimlich maneuver, particularly if this occurs in a setting in which aspiration is likely (e.g., restaurant death or "cafe coronary").[204,205]

THUMPVERSION. Once the diagnosis of a pulseless collapse (presumed cardiac arrest) is established, a blow to the

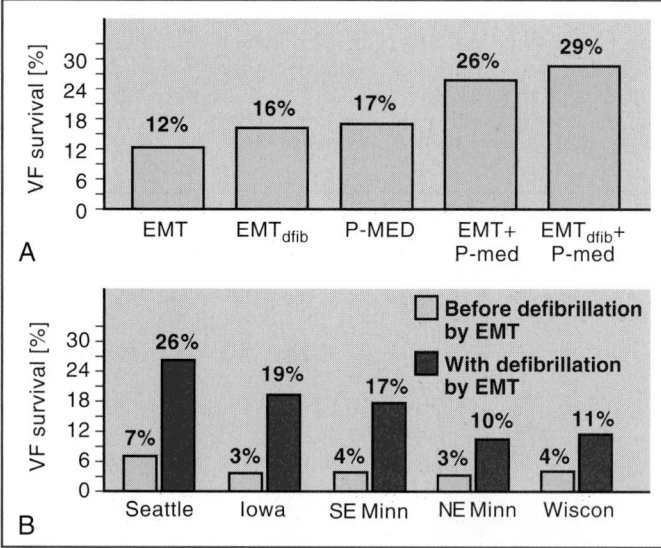

FIGURE 24–15. Impact of emergency rescue system design and immediate defibrillation on out-of-hospital cardiac arrest survival. *A,* Per cent survival to hospital discharge with rescue activities by standard emergency medical technician (EMT) trained in CPR, EMTs allowed to defibrillate immediately (EMT$_{dfib}$), initial response by paramedics (P-MED), two-tiered system with EMT and P-MED, and two-tiered system with EMT allowed to defibrillate if they are the first responders plus P-MED. Training of first-responders (EMT$_{dfib}$) and a two-tiered system have the best outcome. *B,* Comparison of outcomes observed in five geographic areas with EMT providing only CPR (dark color) versus EMT trained to defibrillate as first-responders (light color). In each group, there was a marked improvement in outcome when EMT personnel were trained and permitted to defibrillate. (Modified from Ornato, J. P., and Om, A.: Community experience in treating out-of-hospital cardiac arrest. *In* Akhtar, M., Myerburg, R. J., and Ruskin, J. N. [eds.]: Sudden Cardiac Death: Prevalence, Mechanisms and Approach to Diagnosis and Management. Baltimore, Williams & Wilkins, 1994, p. 450, with permission of the publisher.)

chest (precordial thump, "thumpversion"[325]) may be attempted by a properly trained rescuer. It has been recommended to be reserved as an advanced life support activity.[289] Caldwell and coworkers supported its use on the basis of a prospective study in 5000 patients.[325] In their study precordial thumps successfully reverted VF in 5 events, VT in 11, asystole in 2, and undefined cardiovascular collapse in 2 others in whom the electrical mechanism was unknown. In no instance was conversion of VT to VF observed. Because the latter is the only major concern of the precordial thump technique, and electrical activity can be initiated by mechanical stimulation in the asystolic heart,[326] the technique is considered optional for responding to a *pulseless* cardiac arrest in the absence of monitoring when a defibrillator is not immediately available. It should not be used unmonitored for the patient with a rapid tachycardia without complete loss of consciousness. For attempted thumpversion in cardiac arrest, one or two blows should be delivered firmly to the junction of the middle and lower thirds of the sternum from a height of 8 to 10 inches, but the effort should be abandoned if the patient does not immediately develop a spontaneous pulse and begin breathing. Another mechanical method, which requires that the patient is still conscious, is "cough-induced cardiac compression"[327] or "cough-version."[325] In the former a conscious act of forceful coughing by the patient in VF may support forward flow by cyclic increases in intrathoracic pressure[327]; the same act during sustained VT may cause conversion.[325,328]

THE ABCs OF CPR. The goal of this activity is to maintain viability of the central nervous system, heart, and other vital organs until definitive intervention can be achieved. The activities included within basic life support encompass both the initial responses outlined above and their natural flow into establishing ventilation and perfusion.[289] This range of activities can be carried out not only by professional and paraprofessional personnel, but also by trained emergency technicians and laypeople. Time is the key issue, and there should be no delay between the diagnosis and preparatory efforts in the initial response and the institution of basic life support.

AIRWAY. Clearing the airway is a critical step in preparing for successful resuscitation. This includes tilting the head backward and lifting the chin, in addition to seeking foreign bodies—including dentures—and removing them. The Heimlich maneuver should be performed if there is reason to suspect a foreign body lodged in the oropharynx. This entails wrapping the arms around the victim from the back and delivering a sharp thrust to the upper abdomen with a closed fist.[329] If it is not possible for the person in attendance to carry out the maneuver because of insufficient physical strength, mechanical dislodgment of the foreign body can sometimes be achieved by abdominal thrusts with the unconscious patient in a supine position. The Heimlich maneuver is not entirely benign: Ruptured abdominal viscera in the victim have been reported,[330] as has an instance in which the rescuer disrupted his own aortic root and died.[331]

If there is strong suspicion that respiratory arrest precipitated cardiac arrest, particularly in the presence of a mechanical airway obstruction, a second precordial thump should be delivered after the airway is cleared.

BREATHING. With the head properly placed and the oropharynx clear, mouth-to-mouth respiration can be initiated if no specific rescue equipment is available. To a large extent, the procedure used for establishing ventilation depends on the site at which the cardiac arrest occurs. A variety of devices are available, including plastic oropharyngeal airways, esophageal obturators, the masked AMBU bag, and endotracheal tubes. Intubation is the preferred procedure, but time should not be sacrificed even in the in-hospital setting while awaiting an endotracheal tube or a person trained to insert it quickly and properly. Thus, in the in-hospital setting, temporary support with AMBU bag ventilation is the usual method until endotracheal intubation can be carried out, and in the out-of-hospital setting mouth-to-mouth resuscitation is used while awaiting emergency rescue personnel. The effect of the acquired immunodeficiency syndrome and hepatitis B transmission on attitudes toward mouth-to-mouth resuscitation by bystanders and even professional personnel in hospitals is an area of concern,[289] but currently available data assessing risk of infection suggest that it is minimal.[332,333] The impact of this concern on attitudes toward, and outcomes of, resuscitative efforts has not been assessed.

Conventional CPR ventilatory techniques require that the lungs be inflated 10 to 12 times/minute whether one or two rescuers are present.[289] For one-rescuer resuscitation, a pause for ventilation (two breaths) is taken after every 15 chest compressions; for two rescuers, one breath is administered after every fifth compression. Techniques of CPR based on the hypothesis that increased intrathoracic pressure is the prime mover of blood, rather than cardiac compression itself,[334,335] have been evaluated; the cyclic ventilatory techniques are altered in these procedures (see below). However, clinical applicability is still not clarified.

CIRCULATION (Fig. 24–16). This element of basic life support is intended to maintain blood flow (i.e., circulation)

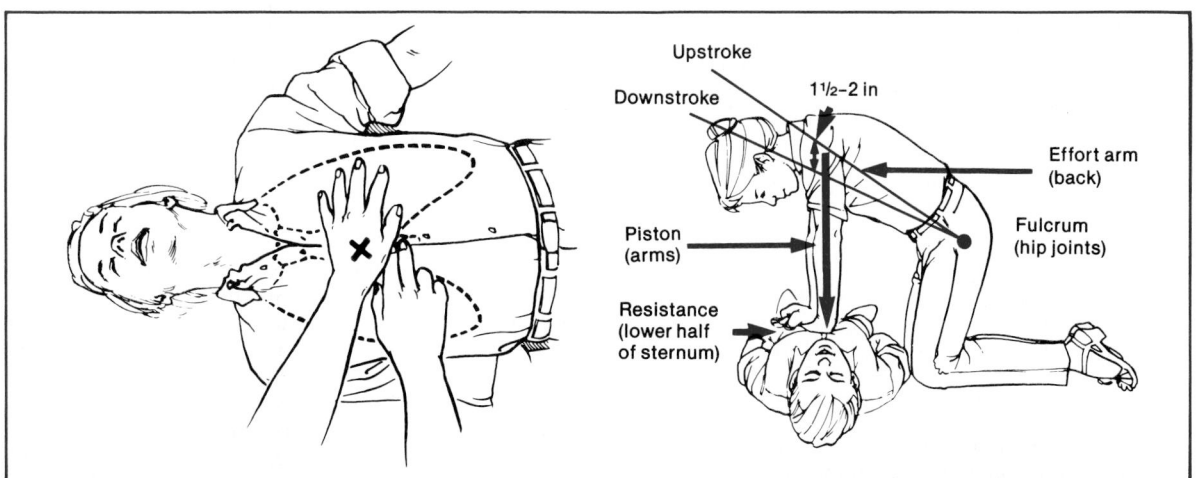

FIGURE 24–16. External chest compression. *Left,* Locating the correct hand position on the lower half of the sternum. *Right,* Proper position of the rescuer, with shoulders directly over the victim's sternum and elbows locked. (From Standards and guidelines for cardiopulmonary resuscitation [CPR] and emergency cardiac care [ECC]. JAMA 255:2906, 1986. Copyright 1986, the American Medical Association.)

TABLE 24–6 ADVANCED LIFE SUPPORT FOR CARDIAC ARREST VICTIMS

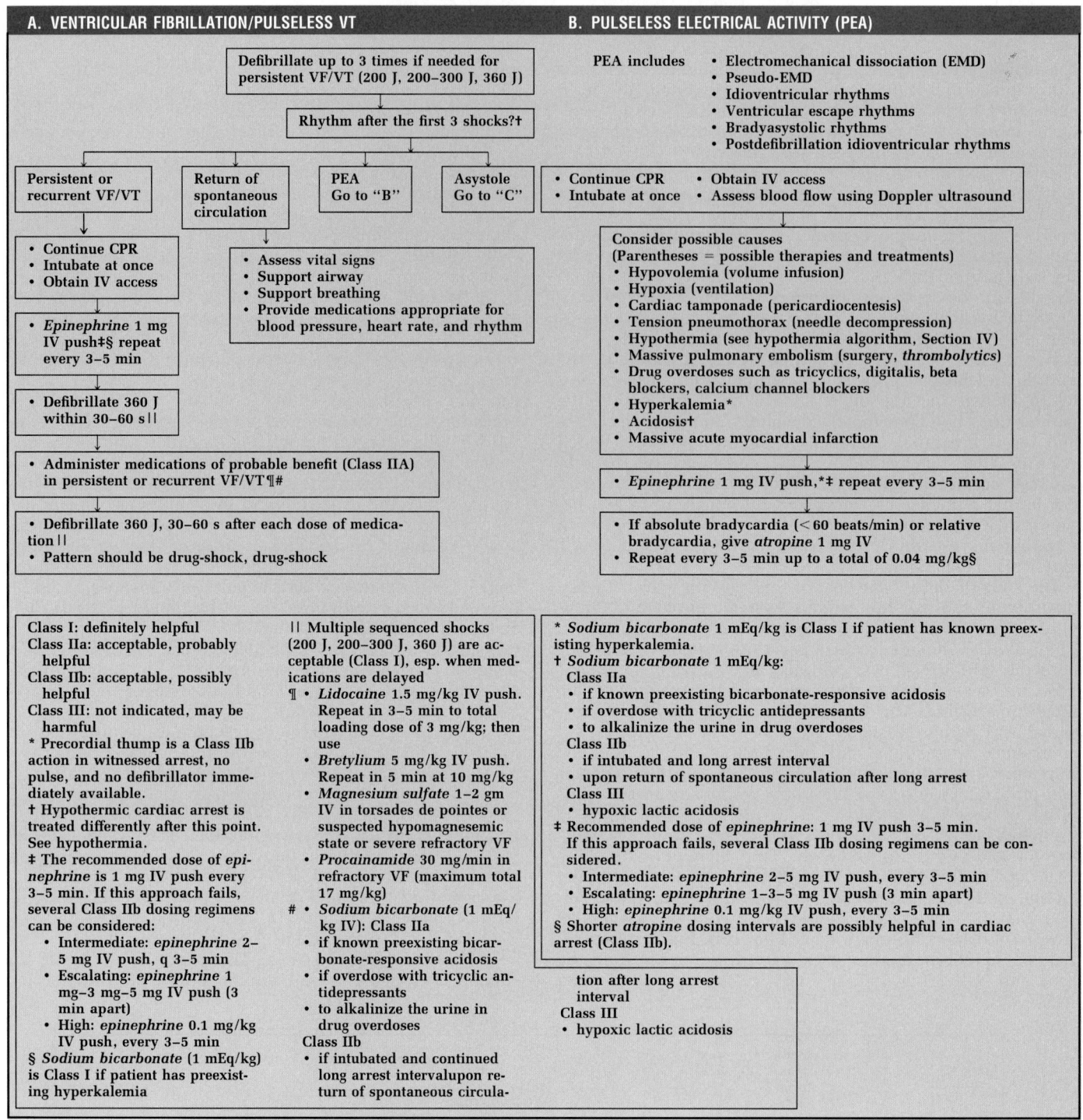

A. VENTRICULAR FIBRILLATION/PULSELESS VT

Defibrillate up to 3 times if needed for persistent VF/VT (200 J, 200–300 J, 360 J)

Rhythm after the first 3 shocks?†

- Persistent or recurrent VF/VT
- Return of spontaneous circulation
- PEA Go to "B"
- Asystole Go to "C"

- Continue CPR
- Intubate at once
- Obtain IV access

- *Epinephrine* 1 mg IV push‡§ repeat every 3–5 min

- Defibrillate 360 J within 30–60 s∥

- Assess vital signs
- Support airway
- Support breathing
- Provide medications appropriate for blood pressure, heart rate, and rhythm

- Administer medications of probable benefit (Class IIA) in persistent or recurrent VF/VT¶#

- Defibrillate 360 J, 30–60 s after each dose of medication∥
- Pattern should be drug-shock, drug-shock

B. PULSELESS ELECTRICAL ACTIVITY (PEA)

PEA includes
- Electromechanical dissociation (EMD)
- Pseudo-EMD
- Idioventricular rhythms
- Ventricular escape rhythms
- Bradyasystolic rhythms
- Postdefibrillation idioventricular rhythms

- Continue CPR
- Intubate at once
- Obtain IV access
- Assess blood flow using Doppler ultrasound

Consider possible causes
(Parentheses = possible therapies and treatments)
- Hypovolemia (volume infusion)
- Hypoxia (ventilation)
- Cardiac tamponade (pericardiocentesis)
- Tension pneumothorax (needle decompression)
- Hypothermia (see hypothermia algorithm, Section IV)
- Massive pulmonary embolism (surgery, *thrombolytics*)
- Drug overdoses such as tricyclics, digitalis, beta blockers, calcium channel blockers
- Hyperkalemia*
- Acidosis†
- Massive acute myocardial infarction

- *Epinephrine* 1 mg IV push,*‡ repeat every 3–5 min

- If absolute bradycardia (< 60 beats/min) or relative bradycardia, give *atropine* 1 mg IV
- Repeat every 3–5 min up to a total of 0.04 mg/kg§

Class I: definitely helpful
Class IIa: acceptable, probably helpful
Class IIb: acceptable, possibly helpful
Class III: not indicated, may be harmful
* Precordial thump is a Class IIb action in witnessed arrest, no pulse, and no defibrillator immediately available.
† Hypothermic cardiac arrest is treated differently after this point. See hypothermia.
‡ The recommended dose of *epinephrine* is 1 mg IV push every 3–5 min. If this approach fails, several Class IIb dosing regimens can be considered:
- Intermediate: *epinephrine* 2–5 mg IV push, q 3–5 min
- Escalating: *epinephrine* 1 mg–3 mg–5 mg IV push (3 min apart)
- High: *epinephrine* 0.1 mg/kg IV push, every 3–5 min
§ *Sodium bicarbonate* (1 mEq/kg) is Class I if patient has preexisting hyperkalemia

∥ Multiple sequenced shocks (200 J, 200–300 J, 360 J) are acceptable (Class I), esp. when medications are delayed
¶ • *Lidocaine* 1.5 mg/kg IV push. Repeat in 3–5 min to total loading dose of 3 mg/kg; then use
- *Bretylium* 5 mg/kg IV push. Repeat in 5 min at 10 mg/kg
- *Magnesium sulfate* 1–2 gm IV in torsades de pointes or suspected hypomagnesemic state or severe refractory VF
- *Procainamide* 30 mg/min in refractory VF (maximum total 17 mg/kg)
• *Sodium bicarbonate* (1 mEq/kg IV): Class IIa
- if known preexisting bicarbonate-responsive acidosis
- if overdose with tricyclic antidepressants
- to alkalinize the urine in drug overdoses
Class IIb
- if intubated and continued long arrest intervalupon return of spontaneous circula-

* *Sodium bicarbonate* 1 mEq/kg is Class I if patient has known preexisting hyperkalemia.
† *Sodium bicarbonate* 1 mEq/kg:
Class IIa
- if known preexisting bicarbonate-responsive acidosis
- if overdose with tricyclic antidepressants
- to alkalinize the urine in drug overdoses
Class IIb
- if intubated and long arrest interval
- upon return of spontaneous circulation after long arrest
Class III
- hypoxic lactic acidosis
‡ Recommended dose of *epinephrine*: 1 mg IV push 3–5 min. If this approach fails, several Class IIb dosing regimens can be considered.
- Intermediate: *epinephrine* 2–5 mg IV push, every 3–5 min
- Escalating: *epinephrine* 1–3–5 mg IV push (3 min apart)
- High: *epinephrine* 0.1 mg/kg IV push, every 3–5 min
§ Shorter *atropine* dosing intervals are possibly helpful in cardiac arrest (Class IIb).

tion after long arrest interval
Class III
- hypoxic lactic acidosis

Modified from Guidelines for cardiopulmonary resuscitation and emergency cardiac care. JAMA *268*:2171, 1992. Copyright 1992 American Medical Association.

until definitive steps can be taken. The rationale as originally developed was based on the hypothesis that chest compression allows the heart to maintain an externally driven pump function by sequential emptying and filling of its chambers, with competent valves favoring the forward direction of flow. In fact, the application of this technique has proved successful when used as recommended.[289] The palm of one hand is placed over the lower sternum and the heel of the other rests on the dorsum of the lower hand. The sternum is then depressed with the resuscitator's arms straight at the elbows to provide a less tiring and more forceful fulcrum at the junction of the shoulders and back (Fig. 24–16). Using this technique, sufficient force is applied to depress the sternum about 3 to 5 cm, with abrupt

relaxation, and the cycle is carried out at a rate of about 80 to 100 compressions/min.[289] Despite the fact that this conventional technique produces measurable carotid artery flow and a record of successful resuscitations, the absence of a pressure gradient across the heart in the presence of an extrathoracic arterial-venous pressure gradient has led to a concept that it is not cardiac compression per se, but rather a pumping action produced by pressure changes in the entire thoracic cavity that optimizes systemic blood flow during resuscitation.[334–337] Experimental work in which the chest is compressed during ventilations rather than between them (simultaneous compression-ventilation, SCV) demonstrates better extrathoracic arterial flow.[334,337,338] However, increased carotid artery flow does not necessarily

TABLE 24-6 ADVANCED LIFE SUPPORT FOR CARDIAC ARREST VICTIMS—*Continued*

C. ASYSTOLE/SEVERE BRADYCARDIA

- Continue CPR
- Intubate at once
- Obtain IV access
- Confirm asystole in more than one lead

↓

Consider possible causes
- Hypoxia
- Hyperkalemia
- Hypokalemia
- Preexisting acidosis
- Drug overdose
- Hypothermia

↓

Consider immediate transcutaneous pacing (TCP)*

↓

- *Epinephrine* 1 mg IV push,†‡ repeat every 3–5 min

↓

- *Atropine* 1 mg IV, repeat every 3–5 min up to a total of 0.04 mg/kg§ ||

↓

Consider
- Termination of efforts¶

---

* TCP is a Class IIb intervention. Lack of success may be due to delays in pacing. To be effective TCP must be performed early, simultaneously with drugs. Evidence does not support routine use of TCP for asystole.
† The recommended dose of *epinephrine* is 1 mg IV push every 3–5 min. If this approach fails, several Class IIb dosing regimens can be considered:
- Intermediate: *epinephrine* 2–5 mg IV push, every 3–5 min
- Escalating: *epinephrine* 1 mg–3 mg–5 mg IV push (3 min apart)
- High: *epinephrine* 0.1 mg/kg IV push, every 3–5 min
‡ *Sodium bicarbonate* 1 mEq/kg is Class I if patient has known preexisting hyperkalemia.

§ Shorter *atropine* dosing intervals are Class IIb in asystolic arrest.
|| *Sodium bicarbonate* 1 mEq/kg:
  Class IIa
  - if known preexisting bicarbonate-responsive acidosis
  - if overdose with tricyclic antidepressants
  - to alkalinize the urine in drug overdoses
  Class IIb
  - if intubated and continued long arrest interval
  - upon return of spontaneous circulation after long arrest interval
  Class III
  - hypoxic lactic acidosis
¶ If patient remains in asystole or other agonal rhythms after successful intubation and initial medications and no reversible causes are identified, consider termination of resuscitative efforts by a physician. Consider interval since arrest.

Advanced Life Support and Definitive Resuscitation

This next step in the sequence of resuscitative efforts is designed to achieve definitive support and stabilization of the patient.[289] The implementation of advanced life support does not indicate abrupt cessation of basic life support activities, but rather a transition from one level of activity to the next. In the past, advanced life support required judgments and technical skills which removed it from the realm of activity of lay bystanders and even emergency medical technicians, limiting these activities to specifically trained paramedical personnel, nurses, and physicians. With further education of emergency technicians, most community-based CPR programs now permit them to carry out advanced life support activities.[289,298,320] In addition, the development and testing of equipment—the automatic external defibrillator—which has the ability to sense and analyze air flow, sense cardiac electrical activity, and provide definitive electrical intervention[323,347] may provide a role for less highly trained rescue personnel (i.e., police, ambulance drivers) and perhaps even trained lay bystanders in advanced life support.

The general goals of advanced life support are to optimize ventilation, revert the cardiac rhythm to one which is hemodynamically effective, and maintain and support the restored circulation. Thus, during advanced life support, the patient (1) is intubated and well oxygenated, (2) is defibrillated, cardioverted, or paced, and (3) has an intravenous line established to deliver necessary medications. After intubation, the goal of ventilation is to reverse hypoxemia and not merely achieve a high alveolar pO_2. Thus oxygen rather than room air should be used to ventilate the patient; if possible, the arterial pO_2 should be monitored. Respirator support in hospital and AMBU bag by means of an endotracheal tube or face mask in the out-of-hospital setting usually are used.

DEFIBRILLATION-CARDIOVERSION (Table 24–6*A*). Rapid conversion to an effective cardiac electrical mechanism is a key step for successful resuscitation.[292,308] Delay should be minimal, even when conditions for CPR are optimal. When VF or a rapid VT is recognized on a monitor or by telemetry, defibrillation should be carried out immediately with a shock of 200 joules. Up to 90 per cent of VF victims weighing up to 90 kg can be successfully resuscitated with a 200-joule shock,[348] and a 300- or 360-joule shock may be used if this is not successful.[289] Failure of the initial shocks to successfully cardiovert to an effective rhythm is a poor prognostic sign.[289] After failure of three shocks up to a maximum of 360 joules of energy, CPR should be continued while the patient is intubated and intravenous access achieved. Epinephrine, 1 mg IV, is administered and followed by repeated defibrillation attempts at 360 joules. Epinephrine may be repeated at 3- to 5-minute intervals with defibrillator shocks in between. Simultaneously, the rescuer should focus on ventilation to correct the biochemistry of the blood, efforts which render the heart more likely to reestablish a stable rhythm (i.e., improved oxygenation, reversal of acidosis, and improvement of the underlying electrophysiological condition). Although adequate oxygenation of the blood is crucial in the immediate management of the metabolic acidosis of cardiac arrest, additional correction may be achieved if necessary by intravenous administration of sodium bicarbonate. This is recommended for circumstances of known or suspected preexisting bicarbonate-responsive causes of acidosis, certain drug overdoses, and prolonged resuscitation runs.[289] The more general role for bicarbonate during cardiac arrest has been questioned[349–351]; but in any circumstance, much less sodium bicarbonate than was previously recommended is adequate for treatment of acidosis in this setting.[352] Excessive quantities can be deleterious.[351,352] Although some investigators have questioned the use of sodium bicarbonate at all because

---

equate with improved cerebral perfusion,[335,339,340] and the reduction in coronary blood flow caused by elevated intrathoracic pressures by certain techniques[335,341] may be too high a price for the improved peripheral flow. In addition, a high thoracoabdominal gradient has been demonstrated during experimental SCV,[342] which could divert flow from the brain in the absence of concomitant abdominal binding. The comparative hemodynamics of models of conventional cardiac compression and techniques based on chest (thoracic) compression suggest that blood movement is based on both mechanisms in experimental[343] and clinical[344] studies. Based upon these observations, new mechanically assisted techniques for improving circulation during CPR are being evaluated.[344–346] More clinical studies are needed before establishing their general clinical applications.

risks of alkalosis, hypernatremia, and hyperosmolality may outweigh its benefits,[353] the circumstances cited may benefit from administration of 1 mEq/kg of sodium bicarbonate while CPR is being carried out. Up to 50 per cent of this dose may be repeated every 10 to 15 minutes during the course of CPR.[354] When possible, arterial pH, pO_2, and pCO_2 should be monitored during the resuscitation.

PHARMACOTHERAPY. For the patient who remains in VT or VF despite direct current (DC) cardioversion after epinephrine, electrical stability of the heart may be achieved by intravenous administration of antiarrhythmic agents during continued resuscitation. As a matter of routine, lidocaine is tried first as an IV bolus, at a dose of 1.0 to 1.5 mg/kg (p. 605), with the dose repeated in 3 to 5 minutes in those in whom resuscitation remains unsuccessful or unstable electrical activity persists. If a total loading dose of 3.0 mg/kg has failed to support successful defibrillation, bretylium tosylate,[355] 5 mg/kg IV, should be given next. It can be repeated 5 minutes later in a dose of 10 mg/kg. Continued failure is an indication for other intravenous antiarrhythmic drugs, such as *procainamide hydrochloride* (see p. 1248)[356] or IV amiodarone (see p. 1248).[357] Procainamide is administered as a 30 mg/min intravenous infusion, to a maximum of 17 mg/kg. Intravenous amiodarone (see p. 1248), given as a 150- to 500-mg bolus and a 10 mg/kg/day infusion, may also be effective for refractory VT and VF.[357] In patients in whom acute hyperkalemia is the triggering event for resistant VF, or who are hypocalcemic or toxic from Ca^{++}-entry blocking drugs, 10 per cent calcium gluconate, 5 to 20 ml infused at a rate of 2 to 4 ml/min, may be helpful.[289] Calcium should *not* be used routinely during resuscitation,[358] even though ionized Ca^{++} levels may be low during resuscitation from cardiac arrest.[311] Some resistant forms of polymorphic VT or torsades de pointes, rapid monomorphic VT or ventricular flutter (rate ≥260/min), or resistant VF may respond to intravenous beta-blocker therapy (propranolol, 1 mg IV boluses to a total dose of up to 15 to 20 mg; metoprolol, 5 mg IV, up to 20 mg) or intravenous $MgSO_4$, 1 to 2 gm IV given over 1 to 2 minutes.

BRADYARRHYTHMIC AND ASYSTOLIC ARREST; PULSELESS ELECTRICAL ACTIVITY (Table 24–6B and C). The approach to the patient with bradyarrhythmic or asystolic arrest, or pulseless electrical activity, differs from the approach to patients with tachyarrhythmic events (VT/VF). Once this form of cardiac arrest is recognized, efforts should focus first on gaining control of the cardiorespiratory status (i.e., continue CPR, intubate, and establish IV access), then reconfirming the rhythm (in two leads if possible), and finally on taking actions which are likely to favor the emergence of a stable spontaneous rhythm, or attempts should be made to pace the heart. Possible reversible causes, particularly for bradyarrhythmia and asystole, should be considered and excluded (or treated) promptly. These include hypovolemia, hypoxia, cardiac tamponade, tension pneumothorax, preexisting acidosis, drug overdose, hypothermia, and hyperkalemia. Epinephrine (1.0 mg IV every 3 to 5 minutes) and atropine, 1.0 to 2.0 mg intravenously, are commonly used in an attempt to elicit spontaneous electrical activity or increase the rate of a bradycardia. These have had only limited success, as have intravenous isoproterenol infusions in doses up to 15 to 20 μg/min. In the absence of an intravenous line, epinephrine (1 mg [i.e., 10 ml of a 1:10,000 solution]) may be given by the intracardiac route, but there is danger of coronary or myocardial laceration. Sodium bicarbonate, 1 mEq/kg, may be tried for known or strongly suspected preexisting hyperkalemia or bicarbonate-responsive acidosis.

Pacing of the bradyarrhythmic or asystolic heart has been limited in the past by the unavailability of personnel capable of carrying out such procedures at the scene of cardiac arrests. With the development of more effective external pacing systems in recent years,[359] the role of pacing and its

influence on outcome must now be reevaluated. Unfortunately all data to date suggest that the *asystolic* patient continues to have a very poor prognosis, despite new techniques.[291,299,360]

A recently published update on standards for CPR and emergency cardiac care[289] included a series of teaching algorithms to be used as guides to appropriate care. Table 24–6 provides the algorithms for VF and pulseless VT, asystole (or cardiac standstill), and pulseless electrical activity. These general guides are not to be interpreted as inclusive of all possible approaches or contingencies. The special circumstance of CPR in pregnant women requires additional attention to effects of drugs on the gravid uterus and the fetus, mechanical and physiological influences of pregnancy on efficacy of CPR, and risk of complications such as ruptured uterus and lacerated liver.[361]

STABILIZATION. As soon as electrical resuscitation from VT, VF, bradycardia, asystole, or pulseless electrical activity is achieved, the focus of attention shifts to maintaining a stable electrical and hemodynamic status. For electrical stability, a continuous infusion of an effective drug, based on observation during the cardiac arrest run, is commonly used. This may be lidocaine, 1 to 4 mg/min depending on size and clinical factors, or procainamide, 2 to 4 mg/min. Occasionally, a continuous infusion of propranolol or esmolol is used. Catecholamines are used in cardiac arrest not only in an attempt to achieve better electrical stability (e.g., conversion from fine to coarse VF, or increasing the rate of spontaneous contraction during bradyarrhythmias), but also for their inotropic and peripheral vascular effects. Epinephrine is the first choice among the catecholamines for use in cardiac arrest because it increases myocardial contractility, elevates perfusion pressure, may convert electromechanical dissociation to electromechanical coupling, and improves chances for defibrillation. Because of its adverse effects on renal and mesenteric flow, norepinephrine is a less desirable agent despite its inotropic effects. When the chronotropic effect of epinephrine is undesirable, dopamine or dobutamine is preferable to norepinephrine for inotropic effect. Isoproterenol may be used for the treatment of primary or postdefibrillation bradycardia when heart rate control is the primary goal of therapy intended to improve cardiac output. Calcium chloride, 2 to 4 mg/kg, is sometimes used in patients with pulseless electrical activity which persists after administration of catecholamines. The efficacy of this intervention is uncertain. Stimulation of alpha-adrenoceptors may be important during definitive resuscitative efforts.[362,363] For instance, the alpha-adrenoceptor stimulating effects of epinephrine and higher dosages of dopamine, producing elevation of aortic diastolic pressures by peripheral vasoconstriction[363] with increased cerebral[362] and myocardial flow,[362] have recently been reemphasized.[335,362] The importance of stimulating alpha-adrenoceptors in defibrillation in experimental VF also has been suggested.[363]

Post–Cardiac Arrest Care

For successfully resuscitated cardiac arrest victims, whether the event occurred in or out of hospital, post–cardiac arrest care includes admission to an intensive care unit and continuous monitoring for a minimum of 48 to 72 hours. Some elements of post-arrest management are common to all resuscitated patients, but prognosis and certain details of management are specific for the clinical setting in which the cardiac arrest occurred. The major management categories include (1) primary cardiac arrest in acute myocardial infarction, (2) secondary cardiac arrest in acute myocardial infarction, (3) cardiac arrest associated with noncardiac disorders, and (4) survival of out-of-hospital cardiac arrest.

PRIMARY CARDIAC ARREST IN ACUTE MYOCARDIAL INFARCTION (see also p. 1208). VF in the absence of preexisting hemodynamic complications (i.e., primary VF) currently is less common in hospitalized patients than the 15 to 20 per cent incidence which existed before availability of cardiac care units (CCUs). Early aggressive antiarrhythmic treatment is probably responsible,[364] and those events which do occur are almost always successfully reverted by prompt interventions in properly equipped emergency departments or CCUs.[365] After resuscitation, patients are often maintained on a lidocaine infusion at 2 to 4 mg/min. Antiarrhythmic support is usually discontinued after 24 hours if arrhythmias do not recur (see p. 1245). The occurrence of VF in the early phase of myocardial infarction is not an indication for long-term antiarrhythmic therapy.[366] Rapid VT producing the clinical picture of cardiac arrest in acute myocardial infarction is treated similarly; its intermediate and long-term implications are the same as those of VF. Cardiac arrest caused by bradyarrhythmias or asystole in acute inferior wall myocardial infarction, in the absence of primary hemodynamic consequences, is uncommon and may respond to either atropine or pacing. The prognosis is good, with no special long-term care required in most instances. Rarely, symptomatic bradyarrhythmias that require permanent pacemakers persist in survivors. In contrast to inferior myocardial infarction, bradyarrhythmic cardiac arrest associated with large anterior wall infarctions (and atrioventricular or intraventricular block) has a very poor prognosis (see p. 1250).

SECONDARY CARDIAC ARREST IN ACUTE MYOCARDIAL INFARCTION (see also p. 1233). This is defined as cardiac arrest occurring in association with, or as a result of, hemodynamic or mechanical dysfunction. The immediate mortality among patients in this setting ranges from 59 to 89 per cent, depending on severity of the hemodynamic abnormalities and size of the myocardial infarction.[367] Resuscitative efforts commonly fail in such patients, and when they are successful, the post–cardiac arrest management often is difficult. When secondary cardiac arrest occurs by the mechanisms of VT or VF, lidocaine in standard dosages is used, although the dose may have to be reduced in the presence of severe heart failure.[368] Other antiarrhythmics may have to be used in addition to or instead of lidocaine if complex arrhythmias persist or cardiac arrest recurs. The success of interventions and prevention of recurrent cardiac arrest relate closely to the outcome of managing the hemodynamic status. The incidence of cardiac arrest caused by bradyarrhythmias or asystole, or by electromechanical dissociation, is higher in the secondary form of cardiac arrest in acute myocardial infarction.[369] Such patients usually have large myocardial infarctions and major hemodynamic abnormalities and may be acidotic and hypoxemic. Even with aggressive therapy the prognosis after a bradyarrhythmic or asystolic arrest in such patients is very poor, and patients are resuscitated only rarely from electromechanical dissociation. All patients in circulatory failure at the onset of arrest are in a high-risk category, with only a 2 per cent survival rate among hypotensive patients in one study.[291]

CARDIAC ARREST AMONG IN-HOSPITAL PATIENTS WITH NONCARDIAC ABNORMALITIES. These patients fall into two major categories: (1) those with life-limiting diseases such as malignancies, sepsis, organ failure, end-stage pulmonary disease, and advanced central nervous system disease; and (2) those with acute toxic or proarrhythmic states which are potentially reversible. In the former category, the ratio of tachyarrhythmic to bradyarrhythmic cardiac arrest is low,[291] and the prognosis for surviving cardiac arrest is poor. Although the data may be somewhat skewed by the practice of assigning "do not resuscitate" orders to patients with end-stage disease, available data for attempted resuscitations show a poor outcome. Bedell et al.[291] reported that only 7 per cent of cancer patients, 3 per cent of renal failure patients, and no patients with sepsis or acute central nervous system disease were successfully resuscitated

and discharged from the hospital alive. For the few successfully resuscitated patients in these categories, post-arrest management is dictated by the underlying precipitating factors, such as transient hypoxia, electrolyte imbalances, and acidosis. Additional supportive cardiac care is directed to stabilizing hemodynamic, respiratory, and cardiac electrical states.

Most antiarrhythmic drugs (see Chap. 21),[170,172,210,211] a number of drugs used for noncardiac purposes,[172,175,176] and electrolyte disturbances may precipitate potentially lethal arrhythmias and cardiac arrest. Quinidine[370] and the other Class IA antiarrhythmic drugs, and the Class III drugs, are proarrhythmic by the generation of torsades de pointes, the Class IA drugs generally producing a dose-independent idiosyncratic response and the Class III, a dose-dependent adverse effect. The Class IC drugs rarely, if ever, cause torsades de pointes[371] but cause excess SCD risk in patients with recent myocardial infarction,[80] possibly by interacting with ischemia[372,373] or other transient risk factors.[374] Among other categories of drugs,[172,375] the phenothiazines, tricyclic antidepressants, lithium,[175] terfenadine,[176] pentamidine,[376] cocaine,[377] and cardiovascular drugs which are not antiarrhythmics—such as phenylamine and lidoflazine—are recognized causes. Beyond these, a broad array of pharmacological and pathophysiological/metabolic causes have been reported.[375] Hypokalemia, hypomagnesemia, and perhaps hypocalcemia are the electrolyte disturbances most closely associated with cardiac arrest. Acidosis and hypoxia may potentiate the vulnerability associated with electrolyte disturbances. Proarrhythmic effects may be foreshadowed by prolongation of the Q-T interval, although this electrocardiographic change is often not present.[173]

The torsades de pointes form of VT is a common manifestation of proarrhythmic effects of Class IA drugs. This arrhythmia usually is unstable and self-limiting and may terminate spontaneously, degenerate to VF, or evolve into a sustained VT. Cardiac arrest caused by this mechanism is managed by pacing, isoproterenol, and removal of the offending agent. Class IC drugs may cause a rapid, sinusoidal VT pattern, especially among patients with poor left ventricular function. This VT has a tendency to recur repetitively after cardioversion until the drug has begun to clear; this proarrhythmic form has been controlled by propranolol in some patients.[378]

When the patient's condition can be stabilized until the offending factor is removed (e.g., proarrhythmic drugs) or corrected (e.g., electrolyte imbalances, hypothermia), the prognosis is excellent. The recognition of torsades de pointes (see p. 684) and the identification of its risk by prolongation of the Q-T interval in association with the offending agent are helpful in managing these patients. No long-term prophylaxis is required in most patients. In contrast, beta-adrenoceptor blocking drugs or stellate ganglionectomy is required for long-term management of patients with the congenital form of Q-T interval prolongation who have been resuscitated after life-threatening arrhythmias.

POST–CARDIAC ARREST CARE IN SURVIVORS OF OUT-OF-HOSPITAL CARDIAC ARREST. The initial management of survivors of out-of-hospital cardiac arrest centers on stabilizing the cardiac electrical status, supporting hemodynamics, and providing supportive care for reversal of organ damage which has occurred as a consequence of the cardiac arrest. Frequent complex ventricular arrhythmias are common during the first 48 to 72 hours after resuscitation[20]; however, they often are manageable by conventional treatment. The risk of recurrent cardiac arrest is relatively low, and arrhythmias account for only 10 per cent of in-hospital deaths after successful prehospital resuscitation.[20,320] However, the mortality rate among those who do have recurrent cardiac arrest during the index hospitalization is 50 per cent. Antiarrhythmic therapy is used in an attempt to prevent recurrent cardiac arrest in patients who demonstrate residual electrophysiological instability and recurrent arrhythmia during the first 48 hours of post-arrest hospitalization. Lidocaine is the drug of choice for initial management, followed by intravenous procainamide or bretylium if initial drug therapy fails. Patients who have either preexisting or new atrioventricular or intraventricular conduction disturbances are at particularly high risk for recurrent cardiac arrest.[20] The routine use of temporary pacemakers has been evaluated in such patients but was not found to be useful for preventing early recurrent cardiac arrest. Invasive techniques for hemodynamic monitoring are used in unstable patients but not routinely for those who are stable on admission.

Respiratory support by conventional methods is used as necessary. During the convalescent period, attention to central nervous system status, including physical rehabilitation, is of primary importance to an optimal outcome. Bass[379] has recently summarized the neurological sequelae to cardiac arrest, including a review of various interventions. Preliminary data which suggested a beneficial effect of barbiturate loading for reversal of ischemic brain injury during and after cardiac arrest[380] have not been supported by a multicenter study of thiopental loading in comatose post-arrest patients[381] Management of other organ system injury (e.g., renal, hepatic), as well as early recognition and treatment of infectious complications, also contributes to ultimate survival.

LONG-TERM MANAGEMENT OF SURVIVORS OF OUT-OF-HOSPITAL CARDIAC ARREST. When the survivor of an out-of-hospital cardiac arrest has awakened and achieved electrical and hemodynamic stability, usually between 1 and 7 days after the event, decisions must be made regarding the nature and extent of the work-up required to establish a long-term management strategy. The goals of the work-up are to identify the specific etiological and triggering cause of the cardiac arrest[374] (if not already evident), clarify the functional status of the patient's cardiovascular system, and establish long-term therapeutic strategies. The extent of the work-up is largely dictated by the degree of central nervous system recovery and the factors already known to have contributed to the cardiac arrest. For instance, patients who have limited return of central nervous system function usually do not undergo extensive work-ups, and patients whose cardiac arrests were triggered by an acute transmural myocardial infarction have work-ups similar to those for other patients with acute myocardial infarction.

Survivors of out-of-hospital cardiac arrest not associated with acute myocardial infarction who have good return of neurological function undergo extensive diagnostic work-ups and carefully designed long-term therapy. The work-up normally includes cardiac catheterization with coronary angiography, an evaluation of functional significance of coronary lesions by stress-imaging techniques, determination of functional and hemodynamic status, and estimation of baseline susceptibility to life-threatening arrhythmias and of the expected response to long-term therapy.

GENERAL CARE. The general management of survivors of cardiac arrest is determined by the specific cause and the pathophysiology of the underlying process. For patients with ischemic heart disease (who constitute approximately 80 per cent of this population), control of episodes of myocardial ischemia, optimization of therapy for left ventricular dysfunction, and attention to general medical status are all addressed. Ischemic risk may be managed pharmacologically, surgically, or by catheter intervention techniques, depending on the anatomy and physiology of the disease process. Although there are limited data suggesting that coronary bypass surgery may improve the recurrence rate and total mortality rates after survival from out-of-hospital cardiac arrest,[382–384] no properly controlled prospective studies have validated this impression for either bypass surgery or angioplasty. Therefore, indications for surgery are limited to two groups of patients: (1) those who have a generally accepted indication for surgery[246] (including a documented ischemic mechanism for the cardiac arrest), and (2) those who meet specific criteria for surgery directed to arrhythmia control.[385]

Medical antiischemic therapy includes nitrates, beta-adrenoceptor blocking agents, and Ca^{2+}-entry blockers. Beta-adrenoceptors may have an antianginal effect and also influence the role of sympathetic nervous system activity on the genesis of potentially lethal arrhyth-

mias. Although no placebo-controlled data are available to define a benefit of beta-blockers or other medical antiischemic therapy for long-term survival after out-of-hospital cardiac arrest, Morady and colleagues[99] suggested that medical or surgical antiischemic therapy, rather than antiarrhythmic therapy, should be the primary approach to long-term management of the subgroup of prehospital cardiac arrest survivors in whom transient myocardial ischemia was the inciting factor. Moreover, in an uncontrolled observation comparing cardiac arrest survivors who had ever been on beta-blockers after the index event with those who had not received the drug, a significant improvement in long-term outcome was observed among those who had received beta-blockers.[386]

In a report from the Coronary Artery Surgery Study (CASS), Holmes et al.[387] compared sudden death rates in medically and surgically treated patients in the CASS registry. This study did not directly address the issue of surgery in survivors of out-of-hospital cardiac arrest, but there was a significant difference at 5 years, with a 98 per cent sudden death–free survival in the surgical group versus 94 per cent in the medical group (P < .0001). The differences were minimal in the groups with one- or two-vessel disease and no history of heart failure, but expanded to 91 and 69 per cent, respectively, in patients with three-vessel disease and a history of heart failure. The question of how to apply these data to indications for surgery for cardiac arrest survivors remains unanswered at this time. The problem is further confounded by the fact that assignment of the 13,476 analyzable patients to medical versus surgical groups was not randomized (i.e., it was based instead on clinical judgment). Further evaluation of the specific role of coronary surgery *after* out-of-hospital cardiac arrest is needed.

The long-term management of the consequences of left ventricular dysfunction by conventional means such as digitalis preparations and chronic diuretic use has been evaluated in several studies. Data from the Multiple Risk Factor Intervention Trial (MRFIT) suggested a higher mortality rate in the special intervention group,[388] presumably related to diuretic use and K^+ depletion, and other data regarding the relation between K^+ depletion and arrhythmias have focused attention on routine use of such drugs. Although the facts currently are far from conclusive,[266] use of diuretics should be accompanied by careful monitoring of electrolytes. Similar concerns have been raised in respect to digitalis use in high-risk patients after acute myocardial infarction.[389–392] The use of digoxin in survivors of prehospital cardiac arrest should be tailored to specific indications for left ventricular dysfunction.

PREVENTION OF RECURRENT CARDIAC ARREST

In a survivor of out-of-hospital cardiac arrest, the risk of recurrent cardiac arrest not associated with acute transmural myocardial infarction was 30 per cent at 1 year and 45 per cent at 2 years in the early 1970's.[18,19] Although it is not known whether this natural history risk is the same currently, it is generally believed that the risk of recurrence remains substantial (Fig. 24–17). Long-term therapeutic strategies intended to prevent recurrences of potentially lethal arrhythmias have been based on several medical approaches, on antiarrhythmic surgery, and on the use of implantable devices. Antiarrhythmic surgery evolved in parallel with programmed stimulation approaches to management, and most recently antitachycardiac and antifibrillatory devices have been developed for use in subgroups of these patients. A problem which impinges on all long-term strategies is the lack of a reliable current natural history denominator against which to compare the results of any intervention (Fig. 24–17).

LONG-TERM ANTIARRHYTHMIC THERAPY. The antiarrhythmic approach to long-term management of survivors of out-of-hospital cardiac arrest was based initially on two assumptions: (1) that the high frequency of chronic PVCs identified in cardiac arrest survivors constitutes a triggering mechanism for potentially lethal arrhythmias, and (2) that electrophysiological instability of the myocardium predisposing to potentially lethal arrhythmias can be modified by antiarrhythmic drugs.[275,303] Therapeutic strategies derived from these assumptions included endpoints identified by the ability to suppress induction of VT/VF by programmed electrical stimulation,[393,394] suppression of ambient arrhythmias on ambulatory monitors,[395,396] and by empiric therapy using amiodarone,[397,398] beta blockers,[386,399] or membrane-active antiarrhythmic drugs.[275,303,386]

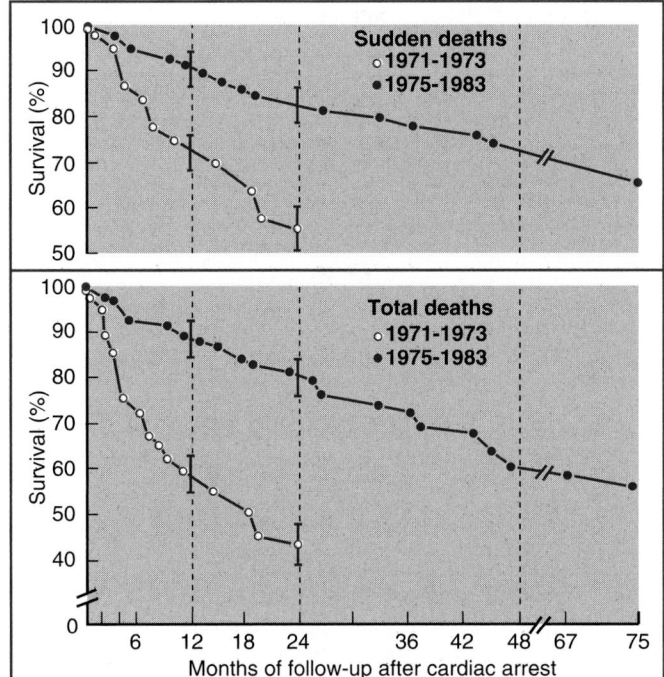

FIGURE 24–17. **Sudden deaths and total deaths in survivors of pre-hospital cardiac arrest during an 8-year follow-up period** *(closed circles),* **compared with 1970–1973 historical experience during the initial Miami studies** *(open circles).* **The more recent experience indicates a 67 per cent reduction in recurrent cardiac arrest rate in the first year of follow-up. Whether this was due to aggressive antiarrhythmic therapy or other factors in the patient populations or their management cannot be determined from comparison to historical controls. However, the 10 per cent 1-year mortality rate is similar to outcome with other forms of antiarrhythmic intervention in recent years. (From Myerburg, R. J., and Kessler, K. M.: Management of patients who survive cardiac arrest. Mod. Concepts Cardiovasc. Dis. 55:61, 1986.)**

One major limitation hovers over the interpretation of all antiarrhythmic drug studies in patients who have survived out-of-hospital cardiac arrest—namely, the lack of randomized, concurrent placebo-controlled studies. This limitation derives from the ethical consideration of withholding active therapy from patients known to be at high risk for recurrent cardiac arrest, when a drug could reasonably be expected to provide a benefit. The results of CAST,[80,81] and of other antiarrhythmic drug observations in out-of-hospital cardiac arrest survivors,[386] give reason to question this limitation, but no concurrent placebo-controlled data are currently forthcoming using any of the methods listed above. Accordingly, studies have been designed in which outcomes after suppression of inducibility by programmed electrical stimulation or suppression of "high-risk" ventricular ectopic activity on ambulatory monitoring, are compared with outcomes after failure of suppression. In another type of study design, one antiarrhythmic therapeutic strategy serves as a positive control for another (e.g., empiric amiodarone versus electrophysiologically guided antiarrhythmic therapy). Each of these approaches remains limited by the inability to identify a mortality benefit in a positively controlled study design.[26,400] Relative efficacy may be identified, but not an absolute mortality benefit.

PROGRAMMED ELECTRICAL STIMULATION. The use of programmed electrical stimulation (see p. 720) to identify benefit on the basis of suppression of inducibility by an antiarrhythmic drug gained early popularity for evaluating long-term therapy among survivors of out-of-hospital cardiac arrest.[393,394,401–406] It evolved as the preferred method of management, despite problems relative to sensitivity and specificity of the various pacing protocols[407] and concerns about the extent to which the myocardial status at the time of the programmed electrical stimulation study reflected

that present at the time of the clinical cardiac arrest. Imponderables such as the extent to which electrode catheter–stimulated extrasystoles mimic spontaneous PVCs, and the ischemic, autonomic, and biochemical status of the heart at the time of the study, may influence the data.[408] Nonetheless, among a series of six reports,[393,394,401–404] induction of sustained VT or VF at baseline study ranged from 31 to 79 per cent, and successful suppression of inducibility has ranged from 18 to 78 per cent. The mortality rate during follow-up on those patients in whom inducibility was suppressed by antiarrhythmic therapy ranged from 0 to 22 per cent (mean = 9 per cent), compared with the range of 22 to 78 per cent (mean = 43 per cent) in those patients in whom VT or VF was still inducible on any antiarrhythmic therapy.

The evaluation of these data is significantly influenced by definitions of inducibility and noninducibility, and also by the clinical features of the patient population in each of the studies, which varied considerably. In most reports VF or sustained VT could not be induced in 25 to 30 per cent of the patients. It is probable that differences are determined in part by the numbers of patients who have anatomically discrete versus ischemic substrates among various populations studied.[313] Careful attention to protocol details, anatomy of the disease processes, and definitions of inducibility may help to clarify these discrepancies in the future. For the present, however, 50 to 70 per cent of *unselected* survivors of cardiac arrest caused by VF or sustained VT can be anticipated to be inducible into sustained arrhythmias. For the subgroup with discrete ventricular aneurysms, more than 90 per cent may be inducible.[246,401] The clinical significance of induced VF, as opposed to a sustained VT or VF which evolves from an induced VT, is often difficult to interpret. Induced VF is commonly considered nonspecific when the induction protocol is aggressive and the patient has not had a clinical cardiac arrest. However, most accept it as a valid positive study in survivors of out-of-hospital cardiac arrest, especially when the protocol is less aggressive (e.g., double extrastimuli or triple extrastimuli in which coupling intervals are not excessively short) and the induction is reproducible.

Most investigators agree that inducibility into a *sustained* clinical arrhythmia provides an indication of risk and that its prevention is an endpoint for therapy, but the implications of induced *nonsustained* forms are more controversial. While it has been suggested that induction of nonsustained rhythms may indicate risk, it often is nonspecific if an aggressive protocol is used.[407] The use of the suppression of nonsustained arrhythmias as an endpoint of therapy is not considered valid. The significance of *noninducibility* at baseline electrophysiological stimulation testing in relation to risk and long-term management also is a controversial issue. Opinions have ranged from the conclusion that patients showing noninducibility are not electrophysiologically unstable and require no long-term antiarrhythmic therapy[99,393,404,414] to the other extreme that such patients remain at risk but do not provide an objective endpoint of therapy by this method, and therefore must be treated by other techniques.[51,246,303,395] Some patients in this category have had cardiac arrest clearly resulting from transient ischemia and require only antiischemic therapy.[99] In the 6 reports, 24-month mortality in patients who had noninducibility ranged from 3 to 38 per cent, higher than in patients in whom inducibility could be suppressed by antiarrhythmic therapy (average 9 per cent) but lower than in those in whom inducibility could not be suppressed (average 43 per cent). In one study, left ventricular ejection fraction discriminated high risk from low risk in noninducible patients; in another, reversible causes of the index event predicted noninducibility.[406,415] A recent report[416] demonstrated that patients in whom ventricular arrhythmias could not be induced were at risk for recurrent cardiac arrest, although the risk is lower than would be anticipated for patients in whom arrhythmias could be induced. There was a 12 per cent event rate at 24 months in the patient population reported. When patients with structural heart disease and low ejection fractions cannot be induced into VT or VF after cardiac arrest, it is generally agreed that high risk of recurrence persists.

AMBULATORY ELECTROCARDIOGRAPHIC MONITORING. The development of detailed methods of analysis of ambulatory monitor recordings[395] led some investigators to study suppressibility of ambient arrhythmias as a specific and individualized means of evaluating drug therapy. Graboys et al.[395] reported outcome in a group of 123 patients with advanced ambient ventricular arrhythmias who had survived one or more cardiac arrests. Suppression of specific forms of complex ventricular ectopy (then defined as three or more consecutive beats and early-cycle PVCs) identified on either ambulatory monitoring or exercise testing was accompanied by a significantly lower mortality rate compared with those in whom such suppression was not achieved. The mortality rate was more than 80 per cent at 3 years in patients whose complex forms could not be suppressed compared with a nearly 90 per cent survival among the patients in whom complex PVCs were suppressed. A subsequent report confirmed the original observation.[396]

Other investigators provided data suggesting the possibility that ambient arrhythmia suppression might be equivalent to suppression of inducible arrhythmias by programmed electrical stimulation in predicting outcome.[409–411] Moreover, analysis of the CAST data base also suggested an association between the ease of suppression of ambient ventricular arrhythmias and survival,[412] supporting the notion of a meaningful relationship between *suppressibility* of ambient arrhythmias and survival. Data from the Electrophysiologic Study versus Electrocardiographic Monitoring (ESVEM) trial[410] did demonstrate a benefit favoring outcome prediction by programmed stimulation compared with ambulatory monitoring techniques in coronary artery disease patients, most evident in the interval of the first 2 years of follow-up. For nonischemic diseases, the opposite was true. In another randomized trial comparing invasive and noninvasive techniques among patients who had symptomatic tachyarrhythmias, the invasive technique was superior in prevention of recurrences.[413] However, the qualifying arrhythmias were not restricted to cardiac arrests, and therefore the applicability to cardiac arrest survivors remains uncertain.

While a high fraction of patients will have successful suppression of the therapeutic targets using ambulatory monitor techniques compared to programmed electrical stimulation, more patients will have programmed electrical stimulation–inducible arrhythmias than ambient ectopy targets,[409–411] and programmed electrical stimulation still maintains preference as the method of choice for evaluating antiarrhythmic therapy. The question of whether *suppressibility* rather than *suppression* is the meaningful marker remains uncertain[412] for both techniques.

Finally, empiric antiarrhythmic therapy predominantly using amiodarone has been supported as having a relative benefit in several studies.[397,398] Whether it has an absolute mortality benefit can only be determined by placebo-controlled data, which are not available.

SURGICAL INTERVENTION

Direct antiarrhythmic surgical techniques (see p. 619) which were originally conceived for control of recurrent sustained VT, such as map-guided endocardial resection[417] and encircling endocardial ventriculotomy,[418] have largely yielded to the technology of intraoperative map-guided cryoablation techniques.[419] This approach is limited primarily to those patients who have inducible, hemodynamically stable sustained monomorphic VT during electrophysiological testing and are unresponsive to drug therapy and have suitable ventricular and coronary artery anatomy. While the outcome using this technique has been much better than that of previous techniques,[419] it has very little applicability to survivors of out-of-hospital cardiac arrest because the type of arrhythmia favoring this surgical approach

is infrequently observed among cardiac arrest survivors. The less specific antiarrhythmic surgical techniques used previously demonstrate less efficacy and higher mortality.

In contrast, coronary revascularization procedures have a clearly defined role for cardiac arrest survivors in whom an ischemic mechanism was responsible for the event and suitable surgical anatomy is present.[99,420]

Platia et al.[421] evaluated the concomitant use of ventricular endocardial resection with implantable defibrillators for patients with refractory ventricular arrhythmias. During a mean 25-month follow-up, 4 of 25 patients (16 per cent) had recurrent tachycardia which was successfully reverted by the device, but 1 patient died because the device malfunctioned. The practice of implanting cardioverter-defibrillator patches at the time of antiarrhythmic or antiischemic surgery in anticipation of a possible need at a later time based on results of postsurgical electrophysiological studies has now largely been abandoned because of the success of transvenous defibrillator lead systems.

IMPLANTABLE DEVICES (see Chap. 23)

The development of a reliable implantable cardioverter-defibrillator added a new dimension to the management of patients at high risk of cardiac arrest.[422] In their initial report,[423] Mirowski and coworkers evaluated the results in 52 patients who had survived an arrhythmic cardiac arrest plus at least one recurrence not associated with acute myocardial infarction. Other forms of preventive management had failed in all these patients, and the group had a mean of 3.9 cardiac arrests per patient. The analysis is complicated by the fact that concomitant cardiovascular surgical procedures were carried out in 15 patients, and about the same number had previous surgery, plus pacemaker implantation in 9. Although 12 of these 52 very high-risk patients died during a 14-month mean follow-up period, producing a 23 per cent 1-year total mortality rate, the 1-year sudden death rate was 8.5 per cent. Devices were triggered 62 times in 17 patients. Assuming death would have followed in these patients without the device, the total 1-year mortality rate would have been 48 per cent.

Subsequently, Echt and colleagues[424] reported their experience in 70 patients. Because 35 of their patients (50 per cent) had had no previous cardiac arrests (14 patients with uncontrollable recurrent ventricular tachycardia) or only 1 previous arrest (21 patients), this population may have been less "unstable" than Mirowski's group.[423] There was a mean of 1.9 ± 1.7 cardiac arrests/patient, 3.1 ± 2.3 arrhythmic episodes/patient, and 4.0 ± 2.1 drug failures/patient. During an average follow-up period of 8.9 months (range, 1 to 33 months), 37 patients (53 per cent) received one or more shocks. The 12-month total death rate was 10 per cent, the sudden death rate was less than 2 per cent, and the complication rate was acceptably low. Subsequent reports have confirmed that implantable cardioverter-defibrillators can achieve sudden death rates consistently less than 5 per cent at 1 year, and total death rates in the 10 to 20 per cent range, among populations who have high mortality risks, as predicted by mortality surrogates such as historical controls or time to first appropriate shock.[425–430]

The interpretation of the benefit of implantable defibrillator devices for automated intervention during onset of cardiac arrest, and for a mortality benefit, remain uncertain and debated.[400,431] While the studies cited above document the ability of implantable devices to successfully revert potentially fatal arrhythmias, the absence of placebo-controlled trials limits the ability to identify a true mortality benefit because of confounding factors such as competing risks for sudden and nonsudden death,[26] the degree to which appropriate shocks represent the interruption of an event that would have been fatal,[400] and the lack of ability of a positive control to determine mortality benefit of either or both interventions.[79] Despite these limitations, implantable defibrillator therapy has continued to increase its relative position among other forms of therapy for survivors of out-of-hospital cardiac arrest because of the issues of efficacy and safety of antiarrhythmic therapy cited earlier, and the limited applicability of antiarrhythmic surgical therapy. Issues that leave major questions unanswered and could affect the defibrillator approach for survivors of out-of-hospital cardiac arrest include relative benefit of amiodarone versus defibrillators, the role of beta blockers as antiadrenergic therapy, and the role of antiischemic surgical and medical therapy as definitive approaches.

A much larger issue, and one that has not yet been defined, is the use of implantable defibrillators among patients who are at high risk for cardiac arrest, but who have not yet had an event. A number of trials are under way to attempt to determine whether preventive defibrillator therapy is an effective means of preventing the first cardiac arrest. Many of the trials are studying cost efficacy in addition to medical efficacy. One of the more important strategies being tested is a comparison of defibrillator therapy versus empiric amiodarone therapy.

MANAGEMENT ALGORITHM

The options for diagnostic evaluation and long-term management of cardiac arrest survivors are complex, with specific problems unique both to patient subgroups and to the various therapeutic strategies. A two-tiered algorithm has been developed as a guide to management.[432] Management stage I (Fig. 24–18) addresses diagnostic evaluation and general management, and stage II (Fig. 24–19) is oriented to strategies specifically for control of potentially lethal arrhythmias. Endpoints of management are reached in stage I for those patients in whom cardiac arrest was precipitated by acute myocardial infarction, those who have some form of noncoronary heart disease or cardiac arrest clearly related to transient ischemia, and those who have cardiac arrest caused by proarrhythmic factors, such as adverse drug effect or electrolyte imbalances. Patients with life-limiting concurrent morbid states and those who have major post-arrest residual damage of the central nervous system also reach their management endpoints in stage I, without progressing to Stage II, except for the possible use of empiric therapy such as amiodarone.

Among the remainder, who constitute the majority of survivors and most commonly have chronic ischemic heart disease, electrophysiological stimulation studies should be performed (Fig. 24–19). In that subgroup of patients among whom sustained VT with or without degeneration to VF is inducible, a primary endpoint of therapy is prevention of inducibility by an appropriate antiarrhythmic agent or drug combination. The former practice of testing multiple antiarrhythmic drugs and drug combinations has largely been abandoned. Most Class I antiarrhythmic drugs have been effective in no more than 20 per cent of patients who have programmed electrical stimulation–inducible ventricular arrhythmias and up to 40 to 50 per cent of ambient arrhythmias evaluated by ambulatory monitoring. A possible exception is sotalol, which showed greater efficacy in one study.[411] The combination of limited short-term endpoint efficacy, uncertain long-term benefit (especially among patients with advanced heart disease[414]), and safety issues[80,81] has led to a trend away from the use of these drugs. Evaluation of beta-blocker therapy by programmed electrical stimulation in selected cardiac arrest survivors has been suggested.[433] The Class III drugs, including amiodarone, sotalol, and newly developing agents, are being evaluated.

Among those patients in whom the programmed electrical stimulation approach is not feasible because of noninducibility of sustained VT or VF, another objective approach should be used (Fig. 24–19). Some patients who have salvos or nonsustained VT on ambulatory monitoring may be treated with antiarrhythmic drugs in an attempt to suppress repetitive forms[395,409–411] or treated with amiodarone empirically.[397,398] If this is successful, it may be used as the endpoint of therapy.[409] Those patients who have neither inducibility by electrophysiological stimulation nor complex forms on ambulatory monitoring in conjunction with low (< 35 per cent) ejection fractions should receive implantable cardioverter-defibrillator devices[414,421,423,424] in lieu of empiric therapy.

Antiarrhythmic surgical intervention is preferred only in patients who have inducible and intraoperatively mappable VT that appears related to the cardiac arrest event and cannot be managed by antiarrhythmic drugs. The results of surgery in such patients have been encouraging.[385,419]

An implantable device is therapy of choice for an increasing number of cardiac arrest survivors.[434] Candidates include cardiac arrest survivors who fail endpoints for antiarrhythmic drug therapy, survivors who are not inducible into VT/VF and do not have a defined ischemic mechanism or do have an ejection fraction less than 35 per cent, and all patients who fall into either of the two previous

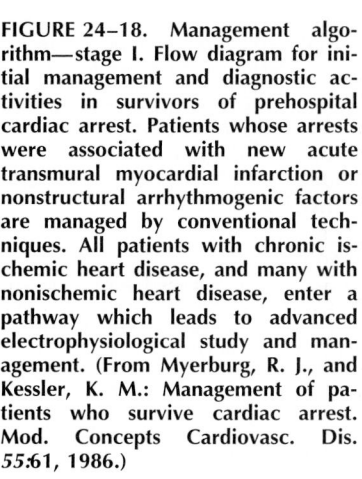

FIGURE 24–18. Management algorithm—stage I. Flow diagram for initial management and diagnostic activities in survivors of prehospital cardiac arrest. Patients whose arrests were associated with new acute transmural myocardial infarction or nonstructural arrhythmogenic factors are managed by conventional techniques. All patients with chronic ischemic heart disease, and many with nonischemic heart disease, enter a pathway which leads to advanced electrophysiological study and management. (From Myerburg, R. J., and Kessler, K. M.: Management of patients who survive cardiac arrest. Mod. Concepts Cardiovasc. Dis. 55:61, 1986.)

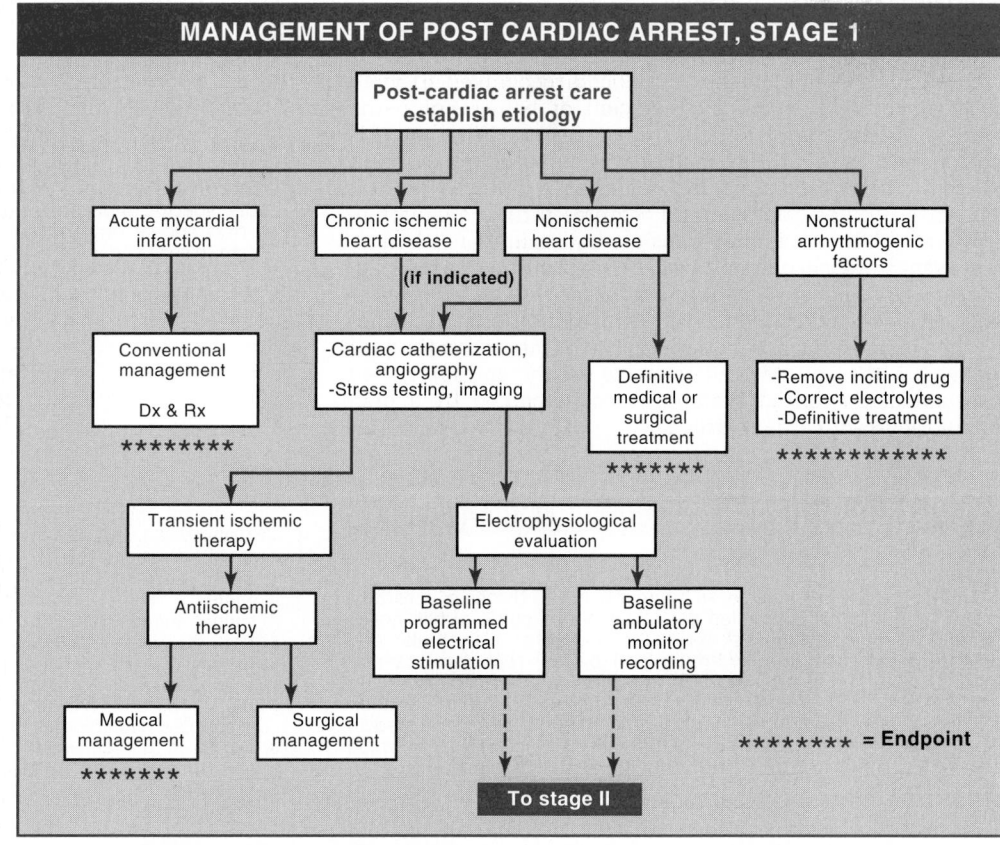

FIGURE 24–19. Management algorithm—stage II. Advanced electrophysiological evaluation of survivors of out-of-hospital cardiac arrest. Patients enter the programmed electrical stimulation (or ambulatory monitor) pathway and are initially evaluated by drug testing using this technique. If the heart is inducible into sustained VT or VF (with some limitations of interpretation for the latter), and drug testing results in successful prevention of inducibility, an acceptable endpoint of therapy has been achieved (****). If the arrhythmia remains inducible (failure by programmed stimulation), antiarrhythmic surgery or an implantable device is considered. If the heart is noninducible into an arrhythmia at baseline and the patient is at low risk for recurrence because of either (1) an identifiable and controllable ischemic mechanism, (2) reversible metabolic mechanisms, or (3) no more than moderate depression of ejection fraction, the patient may be managed by appropriate medical therapy.

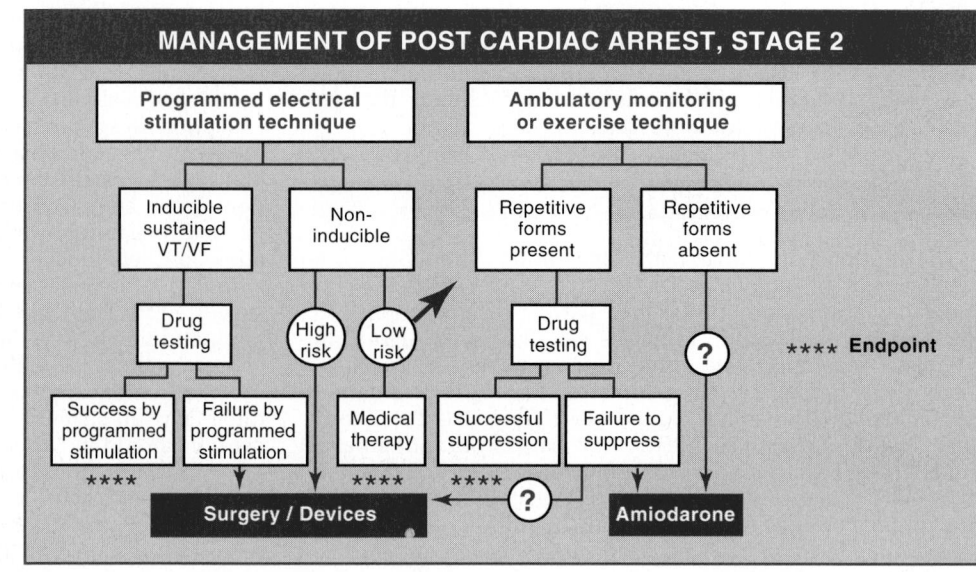

Ambulatory monitoring techniques are applicable if repetitive forms are present.

When programmed stimulation is not available or not applicable to an individual patient, the ambulatory monitoring or exercise techniques may be used. For drug testing, repetitive forms must be identified as the target arrhythmia and successful suppression by conventional drug therapy is considered an acceptable endpoint, perhaps equivalent to electrophysiological testing under some conditions.[409–411] Failure to suppress repetitive forms in high-risk patients should lead to considerations for implantable devices and possibly some forms of surgical intervention. Among others in this category, amiodarone is an acceptable therapeutic approach. If repetitive forms are absent and the patient is at high risk (e.g., very low EF), amiodarone or implantable devices are the therapies of choice. (From Myerburg, R. J., and Kessler, K. M.: Management of patients who survive cardiac arrest. Med. Concepts Cardiovasc. Dis. 55:61, 1986.)

categories and are not candidates for antiarrhythmic surgery. Moreover, despite the fact that there may be a statistical benefit for successful programmed electrical stimulation–guided antiarrhythmic therapy in cardiac arrest survivors with ejection fractions less than 30%,[406] the mortality rate in such patients remains substantial,[406,414] and such patients *may* have a better outcome with implantable-device therapy. However, it must be reiterated that mortality benefit for implantable defibrillators in this circumstance has not been proven.

When used according to defined indications, the recent statistics for each of the approaches outlined above are intriguing. Each method has now been recognized to yield a 1-year survival rate of 90 per cent or better, compared with the 70 per cent survival cited earlier. Whether this means that each of the methods is equally effective or whether some other uncontrolled factor is influencing outcome has not been defined and requires further evaluation. However, high risk is attendant on indiscriminate changes in pharmacological therapy which has been determined appropriate by any of the endpoints used. Swerdlow et al.[401] and Myerburg et al.,[51] using different therapeutic approaches, both have reported that arbitrary cessation, or changes in therapy without retesting for the endpoint used to establish the initial therapy, is accompanied by a high risk of recurrent cardiac arrest.

SUDDEN DEATH AND PUBLIC SAFETY

The unexpectedness of SCD has raised questions concerning secondary risk to the public created by people in the throes of a cardiac arrest. There are no controlled data available to guide public policy regarding people at high risk for potentially lethal arrhythmias and for abrupt incapacitation. Myerburg and Davis[435] reported observations on 1348 sudden deaths caused by coronary heart disease in people 65 years of age or less during a 7-year period in Dade County, Florida. One hundred one (7.5 per cent) of these deaths occurred in people who were engaged in activities at the time of death which were potentially hazardous to the public (e.g., 56 driving private automobiles or taxis, 15 driving trucks, 10 working at altitude, 2 piloting aircraft) and 122 (9.1 per cent) of the victims had occupations which could create potential hazards to others if an abrupt loss of consciousness had occurred while at work (e.g., 57 taxi and truck drivers,

8 aircraft pilots, 9 bus drivers, 9 policemen and firemen). There were no catastrophic events as a result of these cardiac arrests, only minor property damage in 19 and minor injuries in 5.

Levy et al.[436] reported a case of a bus driver with a strong history of coronary heart disease who caused the deaths of himself and several others, but they did not conclusively demonstrate that unexpected cardiac arrest was the proximate cause of the accident. Furthermore, Waller[437] studied an elderly population and demonstrated that cardiac disease alone was not responsible for a significant increase in accident risk: *senility*, or *senility plus cardiovascular disease, was much more important*. Several other studies also have led to the conclusion that risk to the public is small.[438] In specific reference to private automobile drivers, most of the data show that sudden death at the wheel usually involves enough of a prodrome to allow the driver to get to the roadside before losing consciousness.[435,438–440] A recent analysis of recurrent VT/VF events among cardiac arrest survivors suggested limitation of driving privileges for the first 8 months after the index event,[35] based on the clustering of recurrent event rates early after the index event.[34,35] Therefore, although there are likely to be isolated instances in which cardiac arrest causes public hazards in the future, the risk appears to be small, and because it is difficult to identify specific individuals at risk, sweeping restrictions to avoid such risks appear unwarranted. The exceptions are people with multisystem disease, particularly senility, and individual circumstances that require specific consideration, such as high-risk patients who have special responsibilities—school bus drivers, aircraft pilots, trainmen, and truck drivers.

REFERENCES

DEFINITION

1. Weiss, S.: Instantaneous "physiologic" death. N. Engl. J. Med. 223:793, 1940.
2. Spain, D. M., Bradess, V. A., and Mohr, C.: Coronary atherosclerosis as a cause of unexpected and unexplained death: An autopsy study from 1949–1959. JAMA 174:384, 1960.
3. Burch, G. E., and DePasquale, N. P.: Sudden, unexpected, natural death. Am. J. Med. Sci. 249:86, 1965.
4. Kuller, L., Lilienfeld, A., and Fisher, R.: An epidemiological study of sudden and unexpected deaths in adults. Medicine 46:341, 1967.
5. Paul, O., and Schatz, M.: On sudden death. Circulation 43:7, 1971.
6. Gordon, T., and Kannel, W. B.: Premature mortality from coronary heart disease. The Framingham Study. JAMA 215:1617, 1971.
7. Biorck, C., and Wikland, B.: Sudden death—what are we talking about? Circulation 45:256, 1972.
8. Friedman, M., Manwaring, J. H., Rosenman, R. H., et al.: Instantaneous and sudden deaths: Clinical and pathological differentiation in coronary artery disease. JAMA 225:1319, 1973.
9. Kannel, W. B., Doyle, J. T., McNamara, P. M., et al.: Precursors of sudden coronary death: Factors related to the incidence of sudden death. Circulation 51:606, 1975.

10. Helmers, C., Lundman, T., Maasing, R., and Wester, P. O.: Mortality pattern among initial survivors of acute myocardial infarction using a life-table technique. Acta Med. Scand. 200:469, 1976.

11. Mitchell, J. R. A., and Schwartz, C. J.: Arterial Disease. Oxford, Blackwell, 1965.

12. Ruberman, W., Weinblatt, E., Goldberg, J. D., et al.: Ventricular premature beats and mortality after myocardial infarction. N. Engl. J. Med. 297:750, 1977.

13. Myerburg, R. J.: Sudden death. J. Cont. Ed. Cardiol. 14:15, 1978.

14. Lovegrove, T., and Thompson, P.: The role of acute myocardial infarction in sudden cardiac death—a statistician's nightmare. Am. Heart J. 96:711, 1978.

15. Thomas, A. C., Davies, M. J., and Popple, A. W.: A pathologist's view of sudden cardiac death. In Kulbertus, H. E., and Wellens, H. J. J. (eds.): Sudden Death. The Hague, Netherlands, Martinus Nijhoff, 1980, pp. 34–48.

16. Goldstein, S.: The necessity of a uniform definition of sudden coronary death: Witnessed death within 1 hour of the onset of acute symptoms. Am. Heart J. 103:156, 1982.

17. Kuller, L. H.: Prodromata of sudden death and myocardial infarction. Adv. Cardiol. 25:61, 1978.

18. Liberthson, R. R., Nagel, E. L., Hirschman, J. C., and Nussenfeld, S. R.: Prehospital ventricular fibrillation: Prognosis and follow-up course. N. Engl. J. Med. 291:317, 1974.

19. Baum, R. S., Alvarez, H., and Cobb, L. A.: Survival after resuscitation from out-of-hospital ventricular fibrillation. Circulation 50:1231, 1974.

20. Myerburg, R. J., Conde, C. A., Sung, R. J., et al.: Clinical, electrophysiologic, and hemodynamic profile of patients resuscitated from prehospital cardiac arrest. Am. J. Med. 68:568, 1980.

20a. Sequeira, R. F., and Myerburg, R. J.: Sudden cardiac death. In Fuster, V., Ross, R., and Topol, E. J. (eds.): Atherosclerosis and coronary artery disease. Philadelphia, Lippincott-Raven Publishers, 1996, pp. 1031–1050.

21. Hinkle, L. E.: The immediate antecedents of sudden death. Acta Med. Scand. 210:207, 1981.

22. Thompson, R. G., Hallstrom, A. P., and Cobb, L. A.: Bystander-initiated cardiopulmonary resuscitation in the management of ventricular fibrillation. Ann. Intern. Med. 90:737, 1979.

23. Kuller, L. H.: Sudden death: Definition and epidemiologic considerations. Prog. Cardiovasc. Dis. 23:1, 1980.

EPIDEMIOLOGY AND CAUSES OF SUDDEN DEATH

24. Epstein, F. H., and Pisa, Z.: International comparisons in ischemic heart disease mortality. Proc. Conf. Decline in Coronary Heart Disease Mortality. DHEW, NIH Publication No. 79–1610, Washington, D.C., U.S. Government Printing Office, 1979, pp. 58–88.

25. Report of the Working Group on Arteriosclerosis of the National Heart, Lung, and Blood Institute (Volume 2): Patient Oriented Research—Fundamental and Applied, Sudden cardiac death. DHEW, NIH Publication No. 82–2035, Washington, D.C., U.S. Government Printing Office, 1981, pp. 114–122.

26. Myerburg, R. J., Kessler, K. M., and Castellanos, A.: Sudden cardiac death: Epidemiology, transient risk, and intervention assessment. Ann. Intern. Med. 119:1187, 1993.

27. Gillum, R. F.: Sudden coronary death in the United States; 1980–1985. Circulation 79:756, 1989.

28. Epstein, S. E., Quyyumi, A. A., and Bonow, R. O.: Sudden cardiac death without warning: Possible mechanisms and implications for screening asymptomatic populations. N. Engl. J. Med. 321:321, 1989.

29. Schatzkin, A., Cupples, L. A., Heeren, T., et al.: The epidemiology of sudden unexpected death: Risk factors for men and women in the Framingham Heart Study. Am. Heart J. 107:1300, 1984.

30. Schatzkin, A., Cupples, L. A., Heeren, T., et al.: Sudden death in the Framingham Heart Study: Differences in incidence and risk factors by sex and coronary disease status. Am. J. Epidemiol. 120:888, 1984.

31. Gillum, R. F.: Geographic variations in sudden coronary death. Am. Heart J. 119:380, 1990.

32. Rosenberg, H. M., and Klebbs, A. J.: Trends in cardiovascular mortality with a focus on ischemic heart disease: United States, 1950–1976. Proc. Conf. Decline in Coronary Heart Disease Mortality. DHEW, NIH Publication No. 79–1610, Washington, D.C., U.S. Government Printing Office, 1979, pp. 11–41.

33. Kannel, W. B., and Schatzkin, A.: Sudden death: Lessons from subsets in population studies. J. Am. Coll. Cardiol. 5(Suppl. 6):141B, 1985.

34. Myerburg, R. J., Kessler, K. M., Castellanos, A.: Sudden cardiac death: Structure, function, and time-dependence of risk. Circulation 85(Suppl. I):I-2, 1992.

35. Larsen, G. C., Stupey, M. R., Walance, C. G., et al.: Recurrent cardiac events in survivors of ventricular fibrillation or tachycardia: Implications for driving restrictions. JAMA 271:1335, 1994.

36. Doyle, J. T., Kannel, W. B., McNamara, P. M., et al.: Factors related to suddenness of death from coronary disease: Combined Albany-Framingham studies. Am. J. Cardiol. 37:1073, 1976.

37. Kannel, W. B., and Thomas, H. E.: Sudden coronary death: The Framingham study. Ann. N.Y. Acad. Sci. 382:3, 1982.

38. Holmes, D. R., Davis, K., Gersh, B. J., et al.: Rich factor profiles of patients with sudden cardiac death and death from other cardiac causes: A report from the Coronary Artery Surgery Study (CASS). J. Am. Coll. Cardiol. 13:524, 1989.

39. Kuller, L., Lilienfeld, A., and Fischer, R.: Sudden and unexpected deaths in young adults: An epidemiologic study. JAMA 198:158, 1966.

40. Neuspiel, D. R., and Kuller, L. H.: Sudden and unexpected natural death in childhood and adolescence. JAMA 254:1321, 1985.

41. Neufeld, H. N., and Goldbourt, V.: Coronary heart disease: Genetic aspects. Circulation 67:943, 1983.

42. Garza, L. A., Vick, R. L., Nora, J. J., and McNamara, D. G.: Heritable Q-T prolongation without deafness. Circulation 41:39, 1970.

43. Clark, C. E., Henry, W. L., and Epstein, S. E.: Familial prevalence and genetic transmission of idiopathic hypertrophic subaortic stenosis. N. Engl. J. Med. 289:709, 1973.

44. Green, J. R., Krovetz, M. J., Shanklin, D. R., et al.: Sudden unexpected death in three generations. Arch. Intern. Med. 124:359, 1969.

45. Davies, M. J.: Pathological view of sudden cardiac death. Br. Heart J. 45:88, 1981.

46. Brookfield, L., Bharati, S., Denes, P., et al.: Familial sudden death: Report of a case and review of the literature. Chest 94:989, 1988.

47. James, T. N., and MacLean, W. A. H.: Paroxysmal ventricular arrhythmias and familial sudden death associated with neural lesions in the heart. Chest 78:24, 1980.

48. Keating, M. T., Atkinson, D., Dunn, C., et al.: Linkage of a cardiac arrhythmia, the long QT syndrome, and the Harvey ras-1 gene. Science 252:704, 1991.

49. Curran, M. E., Splawski, I., Timothy, K. W., et al.: A molecular basis for cardiac arrhythmia; HERG mutations cause long QT syndrome. Cell 80:795, 1995.

50. Wang, O., Shen, J., Splawski, I., et al.: SCN5A mutations associated with an inherited cardiac arrhythmia, long QT syndrome. Cell 80:805, 1995.

51. Myerburg, R. J., Kessler, K. M., Estes, D., et al.: Long-term survival after prehospital cardiac arrest: Analysis of outcome during an 8-year study. Circulation 70:538, 1984.

52. Kuller, L., Cooper, M., and Perper, J.: Epidemiology of sudden death. Arch. Intern. Med. 129:714, 1972.

53. Krueger, D. E., Ellenberg, S. S., Bloom, S., et al.: Risk factors for fatal heart attack in young women. Am. J. Epidemiol. 113:357, 1981.

54. Wenger, N. K.: Coronary disease in women. Annu. Rev. Med. 36:285, 1985.

55. Jick, H., Dinan, B., Herman, R., and Rothman, K. J.: Myocardial infarction and other vascular diseases in young women: Role of estrogens and other factors. JAMA 240:2548, 1978.

56. Hagstrom, R. M., Federspiel, C. F., and Ho, Y. C.: Incidence of myocardial infarction and sudden death from coronary heart disease in Nashville, Tennessee. Circulation 44:884, 1971.

57. Becker, L. B., Han, B. H., Mayer, P. M., et al.: Racial differences in the incidence of cardiac arrest and subsequent survival. N. Engl. J. Med. 329:600, 1993.

58. Marmot, M. E., Syme, S. L., Kagan, A., et al.: Epidemiologic studies of coronary heart disease and stroke in Japanese men living in Japan, Hawaii, and California: Prevalence of coronary and hypertensive heart disease and associated risk factors. Am. J. Epidemiol. 102:514, 1975.

59. Myerburg, R. J., Kessler, K. M., Kimura, S., et al.: Life-threatening ventricular arrhythmias: The link between epidemiology and pathophysiology. In Zipes, D. P., and Jalife, J. (eds.): Cardiac Electrophysiology. 2nd ed. Philadelphia, W. B. Saunders Company, 1995, p. 723.

60. Maclure, M.: The case-crossover design: A method for studying transient effects on the risk of acute events. Am. J. Epidemiol. 33:144, 1991.

61. Muller, J. E., Tofler, G. H., and Stone, P. H.: Circadian variation and triggers of onset of acute cardiovascular disease. Circulation 79:733, 1989.

62. Mittleman, M. A., Maclure, M., Tofler, G. H., et al.: Triggering of acute myocardial infarction by heavy physical exertion: Protection against triggering by regular exertion. N. Engl. J. Med. 329:1677, 1993.

63. Hallstrom, A. P., Cobb, L. A., and Ray, R.: Smoking as a risk factor for recurrence of sudden cardiac arrest. N. Engl. J. Med. 314:271, 1986.

64. Paffenbarger, R. S., Hale, W. E., Brand, R. J., and Hyde, R. T.: Work energy level, personal characteristics, and fatal heart attack: A birth-cohort effect. Am. J. Epidemiol. 105:200, 1977.

65. Rahe, R. H., Romo, M., Bennett, L., and Siltman, P.: Recent life changes, myocardial infarction, and abrupt coronary death. Arch. Intern. J. 133:221, 1974.

66. Talbott, E., Kuller, L. H., Petre, K., and Perper, J.: Biologic and psychosocial risk factors of sudden death from coronary disease in white women. Am. J. Cardiol. 39:858, 1977.

67. Ruberman, W., Weinblatt, E., Goldberg, J. D., and Chaudhary, B. S.: Psychosocial influences on mortality after myocardial infarction. N. Engl. J. Med. 311:552, 1984.

68. Weinblatt, E., Ruberman, W., Goldberg, J. D., et al.: Relation of education to sudden death after myocardial infarction. N. Engl. J. Med. 299:60, 1978.

69. Lambert, C. A., Netherton, D. R., Finison, L. J., et al.: Risk factors and life style: A statewide health-interview survey. N. Engl. J. Med. 306:1048, 1982.

70. Friedman, M., and Rosenman, R. H.: Association of specific overt behavior pattern with blood and cardiovascular findings. JAMA 169:1286, 1959.

71. Shekelle, R. B., Gale, M., and Norosis, M.: Type A score (Jenkins Activity Survey) and risk of recurrent coronary heart disease in the aspirin-myocardial study. Am. J. Cardiol. 56:221, 1985.

72. Bigger, J. T., Fleiss, J. L., Kleiger, R., et al.: The relationships among ventricular arrhythmias, left ventricular dysfunction, and mortality in the 2 years after myocardial infarction. Circulation 69:250, 1984.

73. Kennedy, H. L., Whitlock, J. A., Sprague, M. K., et al.: Long-term follow-up of asymptomatic healthy subjects with frequent and complex ventricular ectopy. N. Engl. J. Med. 312:193, 1985.

74. Chiang, B. N., Perlman, L., Ostrander, L. D., and Epstein, F.: Relation of premature systole to coronary heart disease and sudden death in the Tecumseh epidemiologic study. Ann. Intern. Med. 70:1159, 1969.

75. Pratt, C. M., Theroux, P., Slymen, D., et al.: Spontaneous variability of ventricular arrhythmias in patients at increased risk for sudden death after acute myocardial infarction: Consecutive ambulatory electrocardiographic recordings of 88 patients. Am. J. Cardiol. 59:278, 1987.

76. Ruberman, W., Weinblatt, E., Goldberg, J. D., et al.: Ventricular premature complexes and sudden death after myocardial infarction. Circulation 64:297, 1981.

77. Myerburg, R. J., Kessler, K. M., Luceri, R. M., et al.: Classification of ventricular arrhythmias based on parallel hierarchies of frequency and form. Am. J. Cardiol. 54:1355, 1984.

78. Ruberman, W., Weinblatt, E., Frank, C. W., et al.: Repeated 1-hour electrocardiographic monitoring of survivors of myocardial infarction at 6-month intervals: Arrhythmia detection and relation to prognosis. Am. J. Cardiol. 47:1197, 1981.

79. Myerburg, R. J., Kessler, K. M., Chakko, S., et al.: Future evaluation of antiarrhythmic therapy. Am. Heart J. 127:1111, 1994.

80. Echt, D. S., Liebson, P. R., Mitchell, L. B., et al.: Mortality and morbidity in patients receiving encainide, flecainide, or placebo: The Cardiac Arrhythmia Suppression Trial. N. Engl. J. Med. 324:781, 1991.

81. The Cardiac Arrhythmia Suppression Trial II Investigators: Effect of the antiarrhythmic agent moricizine on survival after myocardial infarction. N. Engl. J. Med. 327:227, 1992.

82. Akhtar, M., Breithardt, G., Camm, A. J., et al.: CAST and beyond: Implications of the Cardiac Arrhythmia Suppression Trial. Circulation 81:1123, 1990.

83. Maisel, A. S., Scott, N., Gilpin, E., et al.: Complex ventricular arrhythmias in patients with Q wave versus non-Q wave myocardial infarction. Circulation 72:963, 1985.

84. Levin, D. C., Fellows, K. E., and Abrams, H. L.: Hemodynamically significant primary anomalies of the coronary arteries: Angiographic aspects. Circulation 58:25, 1978.

85. Harthorne, J. W., Scannell, J. G., and Dinsmore, R. E.: Anomalous origin of the left coronary artery: Remedial cause of sudden death in adults. N. Engl. J. Med. 275:660, 1966.

86. Roberts, W. C., Siegel, R. J., and Zipes, D. P.: Origin of the right coronary artery from the left sinus of Valsalva and its functional consequences: Analysis of 10 necropsy patients. Am. J. Cardiol. 49:863, 1982.

87. Maron, B. J., Epstein, S. E., and Roberts, W. C.: Causes of sudden death in competitive athletes. J. Am. Coll. Cardiol. 7:204, 1986.

88. Waller, B. F.: Exercise-related sudden death in young (age ≤ 30 years) and old (age > 30 years) conditioned subjects. In Wenger, N. K. (ed.): Exercise and the Heart, Philadelphia, F. A. Davis Co., 1985, pp. 9–73.

89. Roberts, W. C.: Coronary embolism: A review of causes, consequences, and diagnostic considerations. Cardiovasc. Med. 3:699, 1978.

90. El Maraghi, N., and Genton, E.: The relevance of platelet and fibrin thromboembolism of the coronary microcirculation, with special reference to sudden cardiac death. Circulation 62:936, 1980.

91. Kegel, S. M., Dorsey, T. J., Rowen, M., and Taylor, W. F.: Cardiac death in mucocutaneous lymph node syndrome. Am. J. Cardiol. 40:282, 1977.

92. Thiene, G., Valente, M., and Rossi, L.: Involvement of the cardiac conduction system in panarteritis nodosa. Am. Heart J. 95:716, 1978.

93. Heggveit, H. A.: Syphilitic aortitis—a clinicopathological autopsy of 100 cases. Circulation 29:346, 1964.

94. Roberts, W. C., and Honig, H. S.: The spectrum of cardiovascular disease in the Marfan syndrome. Am. Heart J. 104:115, 1982.

95. Shaver, P. J., Carrig, T. F., and Baker, W. P.: Postpartum coronary artery dissection. Br. Heart J. 40:83, 1978.

96. Harris, L. S., and Adelson, L.: Fatal coronary embolism from a myxomatous polyp of the aortic valve. An unusual cause of sudden death. Am. J. Clin. Pathol. 43:61, 1965.

97. Roberts, W. C.: Pathology of arterial aneurysms. In Bergan, J. J., and Yao, S. T. (eds.): Aneurysms, Diagnosis and Treatment. New York, Grune and Stratton, 1982, pp. 17–43.

98. Morales, A. R., Romanelli, R., and Boucek, R. J.: The mural left anterior descending coronary artery, strenuous exercise, and sudden death. Circulation 62:230, 1980.

99. Morady, F., DiCarlo, L., Winston, S., et al.: Clinical features and prognosis of patients with out-of-hospital cardiac arrest and a normal electrophysiologic study. J. Am. Coll. Cardiol. 4:39, 1984.

100. Nakamura, M., Takeshita, A., and Nose, Y.: Clinical characteristics associated with myocardial infarction, arrhythmias, and sudden death in patients with vasospastic angina. Circulation 75:1110, 1987.

101. Myerburg, R. J., Kessler, K. M., Mallon, S. M., et al.: Life-threatening ventricular arrhythmias in patients with silent myocardial ischemia due to coronary artery spasm. N. Engl. J. Med. 326:1451, 1992.

102. Sharma, B., Francis, G., Hodges, M., and Asinger, R.: Demonstration of exercise-induced ischemia without angina in patients who recover from out-of-hospital ventricular fibrillation. Am. J. Cardiol. 47(Abs.):445, 1981.

103. Maseri, A., Severi, S., and Marzullo, P.: Role of coronary arterial spasm in sudden coronary ischemic death. Ann. N.Y. Acad. Sci. 382:204, 1982.

104. Sheps, D. S., and Heiss, G.: Sudden death and silent myocardial ischemia. Am. Heart J. 117:177, 1989.

105. Anderson, K. P.: Sudden death, hypertension, and hypertrophy. J. Cardiovasc. Pharmacol. 6(Suppl. 3):S498, 1984.

106. Messerli, F. H., Ventura, H. O., Elizardi, D. J., et al.: Hypertension and sudden death: Increased ventricular ectopic activity in left ventricular hypertrophy. Am. J. Med. 77:18, 1984.

107. Braunwald, E., Morrow, A. G., Cornell, W. P., et al.: Idiopathic hypertrophic subaortic stenosis: Clinical, hemodynamic, and angiographic manifestations. Am. J. Med. 29:924, 1960.

108. Goodwin, J. F.: The frontiers of cardiomyopathy. Br. Heart J. 48:1, 1982.

109. Shah, P. M., Adelman, A. G., Wigle, E. D., et al.: The natural (and unnatural) history of hypertrophic obstructive cardiomyopathy. Circ. Res. 35(Suppl. 2):179, 1974.

110. Cecchi, F., Maron, B. J., and Epstein, S. E.: Long-term outcome of patients with hypertrophic cardiomyopathy successfully resuscitated after cardiac arrest. J. Am. Coll. Cardiol. 13:1283, 1989.

111. Maron, B. J., Roberts, W. C., and Epstein, S. E.: Sudden death in hypertrophic cardiomyopathy: A profile of 78 patients. Circulation 65:1388, 1982.

112. Savage, D. D., Seides, S. F., Maron, B. J., et al.: Prevalence of arrhythmias during 24-hour electrocardiographic monitoring and exercise testing in patients with obstructive and non-obstructive hypertrophic cardiomyopathy. Circulation 59:866, 1979.

113. Goodwin, J. F., and Krikler, D. M.: Arrhythmia as a cause of sudden death in hypertrophic cardiomyopathy. Lancet 2:937, 1976.

114. Maron, B. J., Savage, D. D., Wolfson, J. K., and Epstein, S. E.: Prognostic significance of 24 hour ambulatory electrocardiographic monitoring in patients with hypertrophic cardiomyopathy: A prospective study. Am. J. Cardiol. 48:252, 1981.

115. Fananapazir, L., and Epstein, S. E.: Hemodynamic and electrophysiologic evaluation of patients with hypertrophic cardiomyopathy surviving cardiac arrest. Am. J. Cardiol. 67:280, 1991.

116. Kowey, P. R., Eisenberg, R., and Engel, T. R.: Sustained arrhythmias in hypertrophic obstructive cardiomyopathy. N. Engl. J. Med. 310:156, 1984.

117. Stafford, W. J., Trohman, R. G., Bilsker, M., et al.: Cardiac arrest in an adolescent with atrial fibrillation and hypertrophic cardiomyopathy. J. Am. Coll. Cardiol. 7:701, 1986.

118. Maron, B. J., Epstein, S. E., and Roberts, W. C.: Hypertrophic cardiomyopathy: A common cause of sudden death in the young competitive athlete. Eur. Heart J. 4(Suppl. F):135, 1983.

119. Waller, B. F.: Sudden death in midlife. Cardiovasc. Med. 10:55, 1985.

120. Northcote, R. J., Flannigan, C., and Ballantyne, D.: Sudden death and vigorous exercise: A study of 60 deaths associated with squash. Br. Heart J. 55:198, 1986.

121. Packer, M.: Sudden unexpected death in patients with congestive heart failure: A second frontier. Circulation 72:681, 1985.

122. Stevenson, W. E., Stevenson, L. W., Middlekauff, H. R., et al.: Sudden death prevention in patients with advanced ventricular dysfunction. Circulation 88:2953, 1993.

123. Kjekshus, J.: Arrhythmia and mortality in congestive heart failure. Am. J. Cardiol. 65:42-I, 1990.

124. Middlekauff, H. R., Stevenson, W. G., Stevenson, L. W., et al.: Syncope in advanced heart failure: High sudden death risk regardless of syncope etiology. J. Am. Coll. Cardiol. 21:110, 1993.

125. Huang, S. K., Messer, J. V., and Denes, P.: Significance of ventricular tachycardia in idiopathic dilated cardiomyopathy: Observations in 35 patients. Am. J. Cardiol. 51:507, 1983.

126. Meinertz, T., Hoffmann, T., Kasper, W., et al.: Significance of ventricular arrhythmias in idiopathic dilated cardiomyopathy. Am. J. Cardiol. 53:902, 1984.

127. Poll, D. S., Marchinski, F. E., Buxton, A. E., et al.: Sustained ventricular tachycardia in patients with idiopathic dilated cardiomyopathy: Electrophysiologic testing and lack of response to antiarrhythmic drug therapy. Circulation 70:451, 1984.

128. Warren, J. V.: Unusual sudden death. Cardiol. Ser. 8(4):5, 1984.

129. Surawicz, B.: Ventricular fibrillation. J. Am. Coll. Cardiol. 51(Suppl. B):43, 1985.

130. Topaz, O., and Edwards, J. E.: Pathologic features of sudden death in children, adolescents, and young adults. Chest 87:476, 1985.

131. Phillips, M., Rabinowitz, M., Higgins, J. R., et al.: Sudden cardiac death in air force recruits. JAMA 256:2696, 1986.

132. Robboy, S. J.: Atrioventricular node inflammation: Mechanisms of sudden death in protracted meningococcemia. N. Engl. J. Med. 286:1091, 1972.

133. Roberts, W. C., McAllister, H. A., and Farrans, V. J.: Sarcoidosis of the heart: A clinicopathologic study of 35 necropsy patients (group I) and review of 78 previously described necropsy patients (group II). Am. J. Med. 63:86, 1977.

134. Silverman, K. J., Hutchins, G. M., and Bulkley, B. H.: Cardiac sarcoid: A clinicopathologic study of 84 unselected patients with systemic sarcoidosis. Circulation 58:1204, 1978.

135. Bulkley, B. H., Klacsman, P. G., and Hutchins, G. M.: Angina pectoris, myocardial infarction and sudden cardiac death with normal coronary arteries: A clinicopathologic study of nine patients with progressive systemic sclerosis. Am. Heart J. 95:563, 1978.

136. Marcus, F. L., Fontaine, G. H., Guiraudon, G., et al.: Right ventricular dysplasia: A report of 24 adult cases. Circulation 65:384, 1982.

137. Ibsen, H. H. W., Baandrup, U., and Simonsen, E. E.: Familial right ventricular dilated cardiomyopathy. Br. Heart J. *54*:156, 1985.

138. Thiene, G., Nava, A., Corrado, D., et al.: Right ventricular cardiomyopathy and sudden death in young people. N. Engl. J. Med. *318*:129, 1988.

139. Wright, J. R., and Calkins, E.: Clinical-pathologic differentiation of common amyloid syndromes. Medicine *60*:429, 1981.

140. Ridolfi, R. L., Bulkley, B. H., and Hutchins, G. M.: The conduction system in cardiac amyloidosis: Clinical and pathologic features of 23 patients. Am. J. Med. *62*:677, 1977.

141. Campbell, M.: Calcific aortic stenosis and congenital bicuspid aortic valves. Br. Heart J. *30*:606, 1968.

142. Smith, N., McAnulty, J. G., and Rahimtoola, S. H.: Severe aortic stenosis with impaired left ventricular function and clinical heart failure: Results of valve replacement. Circulation *58*:255, 1978.

143. Rahimtoola, S. H.: Valvular heart disease: A perspective. J. Am. Coll. Cardiol. *1*:199, 1983.

144. Blackstone, E. H., and Kirklin, J. W.: Death and other time-related events after valve replacement. Circulation *72*:753, 1985.

145. Gohlke-Barwolf, C., Peters, K., Petersen, J., et al.: Influence of aortic valve replacement on sudden death in patients with pure aortic stenosis. Eur. Heart J. *9*(Suppl. E):139, 1988.

146. Konishi, Y., Matsuda, K., Nishiwaki, N., et al.: Ventricular arrhythmias late after aortic and/or mitral valve replacement. Jpn. Cir. J. *49*:576, 1985.

147. Chesler, E., King, R. A., and Edwards, J. E.: The myxomatous mitral valve and sudden death. Circulation *67*:632, 1983.

148. Campbell, R. W. F., Godman, M. G., Fiddler, G. I., et al.: Ventricular arrhythmias in the syndrome of balloon deformity of mitral valve: Definition of possible high-risk group. Br. Heart J. *38*:1053, 1976.

149. Pocock, W. A., Bosman, C. K., Chesler, E., et al.: Sudden death in primary mitral valve prolapse. Am. Heart J. *107*:378, 1984.

150. Nishimura, R. A., McGoon, M. D., Shub, C., et al.: Echocardiographically documented mitral valve prolapse: Long-term follow-up of 237 patients. N. Engl. J. Med. *313*:1305, 1985.

151. Glew, R. H., Varghese, P. J., Krovetz, L. J., et al.: Sudden death in congenital aortic stenosis: A review of 8 cases with an evaluation of premonitory clinical features. Am. Heart J. *78*:615, 1969.

152. Hoffman, J. I. E.: The natural history of congenital isolated pulmonic and aortic stenosis. Annu. Rev. Med. *20*:15, 1969.

153. Young, D., and Marks, H.: Fate of the patient with the Eisenmenger syndrome. Am. J. Cardiol. *28*:658, 1971.

154. Jones, A. M., and Howitt, G.: Eisenmenger syndrome in pregnancy. Br. Med. J. *1*:1627, 1965.

155. Garson, A., Nihill, M. R., McNamara, D. G., and Cooley, D. A.: Status of the adult and adolescent after repair of tetralogy of Fallot. Circulation *59*:1232, 1979.

156. Gillette, P. C., Kugler, J. D., Garson, A., et al.: The mechanism of cardiac dysrhythmia after Mustard operation for transposition of the great arteries. Am. J. Cardiol. *45*:1225, 1980.

157. Murphy, J. G., Gersh, B. J., Mair, D. D., et al.: Long-term outcome in patients undergoing surgical repair of tetralogy of Fallot. N. Engl. J. Med. *329*:593, 1993.

158. Lie, K. I., Leim, K. L., Schuilenberg, R. M., et al.: Early identification of patients developing late in-hospital ventricular fibrillation after discharge from the coronary care unit. Am. J. Cardiol. *41*:674, 1978.

159. Hauer, R. N. W., Lie, K. I., Liem, K. L., and Durrer, D.: Long-term prognosis in patients with bundle branch block complicating acute anteroseptal infarction. Am. J. Cardiol. *49*:1581, 1982.

160. Lenegre, J.: The pathology of complete atrioventricular block. Prog. Cardiovasc. Dis. *6*:317, 1964.

161. Lev, M.: Anatomic basis for atrioventricular block. Am. J. Med. *37*:742, 1964.

162. Denes, P., Dhingra, R. C., Wu, D., et al.: Sudden death in patients with chronic bifascicular block. Arch. Intern. Med. *137*:1005, 1977.

163. McAnulty, J. H., Rahimtoola, S. H., Murphy, E. S., et al.: A prospective study of sudden death in "high risk" bundle branch block. N. Engl. J. Med. *299*:209, 1978.

164. McAnulty, J. H., Rahimtoola, S. H., Murphy, E., et al.: Natural history of "high-risk" bundle-branch block: Final report of a prospective study. N. Engl. J. Med. *307*:137, 1982.

165. Stephan, E.: Hereditary bundle branch system defect. Survey of a family with four affected generations. Am. Heart J. *95*:89, 1978.

166. Kline, G. J., Bashore, T. M., Sellers, T. D., et al.: Ventricular fibrillation in the Wolff-Parkinson-White syndrome. N. Engl. J. Med. *301*:1080, 1979.

167. Vidaillet, H. J., Pressley, J. C., Henke, E., et al.: Familial occurrence of accessory atrioventricular pathways (preexcitation syndrome). N. Engl. J. Med. *317*:65, 1987.

168. Schwartz, P. J., Periti, M., and Malliani, A.: The long Q-T syndrome. Am. Heart J. *89*:378, 1975.

169. Fraser, G. R., Froggatt, P., and James, T. N.: Congenital deafness associated with electrocardiographic abnormalities, fainting attacks and sudden death. Q. J. Med. *33*:362, 1964.

170. Smith, W. M., and Gallagher, J. J.: Les torsades de pointes. Ann. Intern. Med. *93*:578, 1980.

171. Moss, A. J., Schwartz, P. J., Crampton, R. S., et al.: The long-QT syndrome: A prospective international study. Circulation *71*:17, 1985.

172. Bhandari, A. K., and Scheinman, M.: The long QT syndrome. Mod. Concepts Cardiovasc. Dis. *54*:45, 1985.

173. Isner, J. M., Sours, H. E., Paris, A. L., et al.: Sudden, unexpected death in avid dieters using the liquid-protein-modified-fast diet: Observations in 17 patients and the role of the prolonged QT interval. Circulation *60*:1401, 1979.

174. Isner, J. M., Roberts, W. C., Heymsfield, S. B., and Yager, J.: Anorexia nervosa and sudden death. Ann. Intern. Med. *102*:49, 1985.

175. Lyman, G. H., Williams, C. C., Dinwoodie, W. R., and Schocken, D. D.: Sudden death in cancer patients receiving lithium. J. Clin. Oncol. *2*:1270, 1984.

176. Woosley, R. L., Chen, Y., Freiman, J. P., and Gillis, R. A.: Mechanism of cardiotoxic actions of terfenadine. JAMA *269*:1532, 1993.

177. Coumel, P., Rosengarten, M. D., Leclercq, J. F., and Attuel, P.: Role of sympathetic nervous system in nonischemic ventricular arrhythmias. Br. Heart J. *47*:137, 1982.

178. Schwartz, P. J.: The idiopathic long Q-T syndrome. Ann. Intern. Med. *99*:561, 1982.

179. Lown, B., DeSilva, R. A., and Lenson, R.: Role of psychologic stress and autonomic nervous system changes in provocation of ventricular premature complexes. Am. J. Cardiol. *41*:979, 1977.

180. Engel, G. L.: Psychologic stress, vasodepressor vasovagal syncope, and sudden death. Ann. Intern. Med. *89*:403, 1978.

181. Sheps, D. S., Conde, C. A., Mayorga-Cortes, A., et al.: Primary ventricular fibrillation: Some unusual features. Chest *72*:235, 1977.

182. Leenhardt, A., Glaser, E., Burguera, M., et al.: Short-coupled variant of *torsade de pointes*: A new electrocardiographic entity in the spectrum of idiopathic ventricular tachyarrhythmias. Circulation *89*:206, 1994.

183. Burrell, R. J. W.: The possible bearing of curse death and other factors in Bantu culture in the etiology of myocardial infarction. *In* James, T. N., and Keyes, J. W. (eds.): The Etiology of Myocardial Infarction. Boston, Little, Brown, 1963.

184. Cannon, W. B.: "Voodoo" death. Psychosom. Med., *19*:182, 1957.

185. Baba, N., Quattrochi, J. J., Reiner, C. B., et al.: Possible role of the brain stem in sudden infant death syndrome. JAMA *249*:2789, 1983.

186. Valdes-Dapena, M. A.: Sudden infant death syndrome: A review of the medical literature. Pediatrics *66*:597, 1980.

187. Valdes-Dapena, M. A.: Are some sudden crib deaths sudden cardiac deaths? J. Am. Coll. Cardiol. *5*(Suppl. B):113B, 1985.

188. Brooks, J. G.: Apnea of infancy and sudden infant death syndrome. Am. J. Dis. Child. *136*:1012, 1982.

189. Hodgman, J. E., Hoppenbrouwers, T., Geidel, S., et al.: Respiratory behavior in near-miss sudden infant death syndrome. Pediatrics *69*:785, 1982.

190. Southall, D. P., Richard, J. M., de Swiet, M., et al.: Identification of infants destined to die unexpectedly during infancy: Evaluation of predictive importance of prolonged apnea and disorders of cardiac rhythm or conduction. Br. Med. J. *286*:1092, 1983.

191. Marino, T. A., and Kane, B. M.: Cardiac atrioventricular junctional tissues in hearts from infants who died suddenly. J. Am. Coll. Cardiol. *5*:1178, 1985.

192. Lambert, E. C., Menon, V. A., Wagner, H. R., and Viad, P.: Sudden unexpected death from cardiovascular disease in children. Am. J. Cardiol. *34*:89, 1974.

193. Maron, B. J.: Sudden death in young athletes—lessions from the Hank Gathers affair. N. Engl. J. Med. *329*:55, 1993.

194. Roberts, W. C., and Maron, B. J.: Sudden death while playing professional football. Am. Heart J. *102*:1061, 1981.

195. Waller, B. F., Csere, R. S., Baker, W. P., and Roberts, W. C.: Running to death. Chest *79*:346, 1981.

196. Reichenbach, D. D., Moss, N. S., and Meyer, E.: Pathology of the heart in sudden cardiac death. Am. J. Cardiol. *39*:865, 1977.

197. Meissner, M. D., Lehmann, M. H., and Steinman, R. T.: Ventricular fibrillation in patients without significant structural heart disease: A multicenter experience with implantable cardioverter-defibrillator therapy. J. Am. Coll. Cardiol. *21*:1406, 1993.

198. Deal, B. J., Miller, S. W., Scagliotti, D., et al.: Ventricular tachycardia in a young population without overt heart disease. Circulation *73*:1111, 1986.

199. Aponte, C.: The enigma of "bangungut." Ann. Intern. Med. *52*:1259, 1960.

200. Sugai, M.: A pathologic study on sudden and unexpected death, especially on the cardiac death autopsied by medical examiners in Tokyo, Acute Pathol. Jpn. *9*:723, 1959.

201. Baron, R. C., Thacker, S. B., Gorelkin, L., et al.: Sudden death among Southeast Asian refugees: An unexplained nocturnal phenomenon. JAMA *250*:2947, 1983.

202. Otto, C. M., Tauxe, R. V., Cobb, L. A., et al.: Ventricular fibrillation causes sudden death in Southeast Asian immigrants. Ann. Intern. Med. *101*:45, 1984.

203. Kirschner, R. H., Eckner, F. A. A., and Baron, R. C.: The cardiac pathology of sudden, unexplained nocturnal death in Southeast Asian refugees. JAMA *256*:2700, 1986.

204. Haugen, R. K.: The cafe coronary: Sudden deaths in restaurants. JAMA *186*:142, 1963.

205. Eller, W. C., and Haugen, R. K.: Food asphyxiation—restaurant rescue. N. Engl. J. Med. *289*:81, 1973.

206. Ettinger, P. O., Wu, C. F., De La Cruz, C., et al.: Arrhythmias and the "holiday heart": Alcohol-associated cardiac rhythm disorders. Am. Heart J. *95*:555, 1978.

207. Benatar, S. R.: Fatal asthma. N. Engl. J. Med. *314*:243, 1986.

208. Morgan, M.: Amniotic fluid embolism. Anaesthesia *34*:20, 1979.

209. Aronson, M. E., and Nelson, P. K.: Fatal air embolism in pregnancy resulting from an unusual sexual act. Obstet. Gynecol. *30*:127, 1967.

210. Ruskin, J. N., McGovern, B., Garan, H., et al.: Antiarrhythmic drugs: A possible cause of out-of-hospital cardiac arrest. N. Engl. J. Med. *309*:1302, 1983.

211. Minardo, J. D., Heger, J. J., Miles, W. M., et al.: Clinical characteristics of patients with ventricular fibrillation during antiarrhythmia drug therapy. N. Engl. M. Med. *319*:257, 1988.

PATHOLOGY AND PATHOPHYSIOLOGY OF SUDDEN DEATH

212. Baroldi, G., Falzi, G., and Mariani, F.: Sudden coronary death: A postmortem study in 208 selected cases compared to 97 "control" subjects. Am. Heart J. *98*:20, 1979.

213. Liberthson, R. R., Nagel, E. L., Hirschman, J. C., et al.: Pathophysiologic observations in prehospital ventricular fibrillation and sudden cardiac death. Circulation *49*:790, 1974.

214. Perper, J. A., Kuller, L. H., Cooper, M.: Arteriosclerosis of coronary arteries in sudden, unexpected deaths. Circulation *52*(Suppl. 3):27, 1975.

215. Warnes, C. A., and Roberts, W. C.: Sudden coronary death: Relation of amount and distribution of coronary narrowing at necropsy to previous symptoms of myocardial ischemia, left ventricular scarring, and heart weight. Am. J. Cardiol. *54*:65, 1984.

216. Davies, M. J., and Thomas, A.: Thrombosis and acute coronary artery lesions in sudden cardiac ischemic death. N. Engl. J. Med. *310*:1137, 1984.

217. Davies, M. J., Bland, J. M., Hangartner, J. R. W., et al.: Factors influencing the presence or absence of acute coronary artery thrombi in sudden ischaemic death. Eur. Heart J. *10*:203, 1989.

218. Baroldi, G., Falzi, A., Mariani, F., and Baroldi, L. A.: Morphology, frequency, and significance of intramural arterial lesions in sudden coronary death. G. Ital. Cardiol. *10*:644, 1980.

219. Baba, N., Bashe, W. J., Jr., Keller, M. D., et al.: Pathology of atherosclerotic heart disease in sudden death. I. Organizing thrombus and acute coronary vessel lesions. Circulation *52*(Suppl. 3):53, 1975.

220. Roberts, W. C., Currey, R. C., Isner, J. M., et al.: Sudden death in Prinzmetal's angina with coronary spasm documented by angiography. Analysis of three necropsy patients. Am. J. Cardiol. *50*:203, 1982.

221. Newman, W. P., Strong, J. P., Johnson, W. D., et al.: Community pathology of atherosclerosis and coronary heart disease in New Orleans: Morphologic findings in young black and white men. Lab. Invest. *44*:496, 1981.

222. Newman, W. P., Tracy, R. E., Strong, J. P., et al.: Pathology of sudden cardiac death. Ann. N.Y. Acad. Sci. *382*:39, 1982.

223. Cooper, R. S., Simmons, B. E., Castaner, A., et al.: Left ventricular hypertrophy is associated with worse survival independent of ventricular function and number of coronary arteries severely narrowed. Am. J. Cardiol. *65*:441, 1990.

224. Furukawa, T., Bassett, A. L., Furukawa, N., et al.: The ionic mechanism of reperfusion-induced early afterdepolarizations in the feline left ventricular hypertrophy. J. Clin. Invest. *91*:1521, 1993.

225. Roberts, W. C., and Podolak, N. J.: The king of hearts: Analysis of 23 patients with hearts weighing 1,000 grams or more. Am. J. Cardiol. *55*:485, 1985.

226. Lie, J. T.: Histopathology of the conduction system in sudden death from coronary heart disease. Circulation *51*:446, 1975.

227. Lie, J. T., and Hunt, D.: The cardiac conduction system in acute myocardial infarction. Aust. N.Z. J. Med. *4*:331, 1974.

228. James, T. N.: Neural variations and pathologic changes in structure of the cardiac conduction system and their functional significance. J. Am. Coll. Cardiol. *5*(Suppl.):71B, 1985.

229. Rossi, L.: Pathologic changes in the cardiac conduction and nervous system in sudden coronary death. Ann. N.Y. Acad. Sci. *382*:50, 1982.

230. James, T. N.: Primary and secondary cardioneuropathies and their functional significance. J. Am. Coll. Cardiol. *2*:983, 1983.

231. Tuli, M., Minardo, J., Mock, B. H., et al.: SPECT with high purity I-123-MIBG after transmural myocardial infarction (TMI), demonstrating sympathetic denervation following reinnervation in a dog model. J. Nucl. Med. *28*:669, 1987.

232. Stanton, M. S., Tuli, M. M., Radtke, N. L., et al.: Regional sympathetic denervation after myocardial infarction in humans detected noninvasively using ¹²³I-metaiodobenzlguanidine (MIBG). J. Am. Coll. Cardiol. *14*:1519, 1989.

233. Barber, M. J., Mueller, T. M., Henry, D. P., et al.: Transmural myocardial infarction in the dog produces sympathectomy in non-infarcted myocardium. Circulation *67*:787, 1982.

234. Gaide, M. S., Myerburg, R. J., Kozlovskis, P. L., and Bassett, A. L.: Elevated sympathetic response of epicardium proximal to healed myocardial infarction. Am. J. Physiol. *14*:646, 1983.

235. Diederick, K., Djoniagic, H., Schreiner, W. B., and Bos, I.: Hereditares QT syndrom: ein weiterer Fall mit Grenzstrang Ganglionitis. Herz-Kreis *3*:149, 1982.

236. Rossi, L.: Cardioneuropathy and extracardiac neural disease. J. Am. Coll. Cardiol. *5*(Suppl.):66B, 1985.

237. Myerburg, R. J., Kessler, K. M., Bassett, A. L., and Castellanos, A.: A biological approach to sudden cardiac death: Structure, function, and cause. Am. J. Cardiol. *63*:1512, 1989.

238. Cobb, L. A., and Weaver, W. D.: Exercise: A risk for sudden death in patients with coronary heart disease. J. Am. Coll. Cardiol. *7*:215, 1986.

239. Schamroth, L.: Mechanism of lethal arrhythmias in sudden death. Possible role of vasospasm and release. Pract. Cardiol. *7*:105, 1981.

240. MacAlpin R. N.: Relation of coronary arterial spasm to sites of organic stenosis. Am. J. Cardiol. *46*:143, 1980.

241. Robertson, D., Robertson, R. M., Nies, A. S., et al.: Variant angina pectoris: Investigation of indexes of sympathetic nervous system function. Am. J. Cardiol. *43*:1080, 1979.

242. Endo, M., Hirosawa, K., Kaneko, N., et al.: Prinzmetal's variant angina. Coronary arteriogram and left ventriculogram during angina attack induced by methacholine, N. Engl. J. Med. *294*:252, 1976.

243. Buda, A. J., Fowles, R. E., Schroeder, J. S., et al.: Coronary artery spasm in the denervated transplanted human heart. A clue to underlying mechanisms. Am. J. Med. *70*:1144, 1981.

244. Hammon, J. W., and Oates, J. A.: Interaction of platelets with the vessel wall in the pathophysiology of sudden cardiac death. Circulation *73*:224, 1986.

245. Aspirin-Myocardial Infarction Study Research Group: A randomized controlled trial of aspirin in persons recovered from myocardial infarction. JAMA *243*:661, 1980.

246. Myerburg, R. J., Kessler, K. M., Zaman, L., et al.: Survivors of prehospital cardiac arrest. JAMA *247*:1485, 1982.

247. Cox, J. L., Daniel, T. M., and Boineau, J. P.: The electrophysiologic time-course of acute myocardial ischemia and the effects of early coronary artery reperfusion. Circulation *48*:971, 1973.

248. Cameron, J. S., Myerburg, R. J., Wong, S. S., et al.: Electrophysiologic consequences of chronic experimentally induced left ventricular pressure overload. J. Am. Coll. Cardiol. *2*:481, 1983.

249. Myerburg, R. J., Bassett, A. L., Epstein, K., et al.: Electrophysiologic effects of procainamide in acute and healed experimental ischemic injury of cat myocardium. Circ. Res. *50*:386, 1982.

250. Myerburg, R. J., Epstein, K., Gaide, M. S., et al.: Electrophysiologic consequences of experimental acute ischemia superimposed upon healed myocardial infarction in cats. Am. J. Cardiol. *49*:323, 1982.

251. Furukawa, T., Moroe, K., Mayrovitz, H. N., et al.: Arrhythmogenic effects of graded coronary blood flow reductions superimposed on prior myocardial infarction in dogs. Circulation *84*:368, 1991.

252. Kaplinsky, E., Ogawa, S., Michelson, E. L., and Dreifus, L. S.: Instantaneous and delayed arrhythmias after reperfusion of acutely ischemic myocardium: Evidence for multiple mechanisms. Circulation *63*:333, 1981.

253. Kimura, S., Bassett, A. L., Saoudi, N. C., et al.: Cellular electrophysiological changes and "arrhythmias" during experimental ischemia and reperfusion in isolated cat ventricular myocardium. J. Am. Coll. Cardiol. *7*:833, 1986.

254. Manning, A. S., and Hearse, D. J.: Reperfusion-induced arrhythmias: Mechanisms and prevention. J. Mol. Cell Cardiol. *16*:497, 1984.

255. Harris, A. S.: Delayed development of ventricular ectopic rhythms following experimental coronary occlusion. Circulation *1*:1318, 1950.

256. Kimura, S., Bassett, A. L., Kohya, T., et al.: Simultaneous recording of action potentials from endocardium and epicardium during ischemia in the isolated cat ventricle: Relation of temporal electrophysiological heterogeneities to arrhythmias. Circulation *74*:401, 1986.

257. Coronel, R., Wilms-Schopman, F. J. G., Opthof, T., et al.: Reperfusion arrhythmias in isolated perfused pig hearts: Inhomogeneities in extracellular potassium, ST and QT potentials, and transmembrane action potentials. Circ. Res. *71*:1131, 1992.

258. Sharma, A. D., Saffitz, J. E., Lee, B. L., et al.: Alpha adrenergic-mediated accumulation of calcium in reperfused myocardium. J. Clin. Invest. *72*:802, 1982.

259. Corr, P. B., Shayman, J. A., Kramer, J. B., and Kipnis, R. J.: Increased alpha-adrenergic receptors in ischemic cat myocardium. J. Clin. Invest. *67*:1232, 1981.

260. Sheridan, D. J., Penkoske, P. A., Sobel, B. E., and Corr, P. B.: Alpha-adrenergic contributions to dysrhythmia during myocardial ischemia and reperfusion in cats. J. Clin. Invest. *65*:161, 1980.

261. Schwartz, P. J., and Stone, H. L.: Left stellectomy in the prevention of ventricular fibrillation caused by acute myocardial ischemia in conscious dogs with anterior myocardial infarction. Circulation *62*:1256, 1980.

262. Gaudel, Y., and Duvelleroy, M.: Role of oxygen radicals in cardiac injury due to reoxygenation. J. Mol. Cell Cardiol. *16*:459, 1984:

263. Manning, A. S., Coltart, D. J., and Hearse, D. J.: Ischemia and reperfusion-induced arrhythmias in the rat: Effects of xanthine oxidase inhibition with allopurinol. Circ. Res. *55*:545, 1984.

264. Chilson, D. A., Peigh, P., Mahomed, Y., and Zipes, D. P.: Encircling endocardial ventriculotomy interrupts vagal-induced prolongation of endocardial and epicardial refractoriness in the dog. J. Am. Coll. Cardiol. *5*:290, 1985.

265. Janse, M. J., and Downer, E.: The effect of acute ischaemia on transmembrane potentials in the intact heart. Relation to re-entry mechanisms. *In* Kulbertus, H. E. (ed.): Re-entrant Arrhythmias. Lancaster, PA, MTP Press, 1977, pp. 195–209.

266. Kuller, L. H., Hulley, S. B., Cohen, J. D., and Neaton, J.: Unexpected effects of treating hypertension in men with electrocardiographic abnormalities: A critical analysis. Circulation *73*:114, 1986.

267. Struthers, A. D., Whitesmith, R., and Reid, J. L.: Prior thiazide diuretic treatment increases adrenaline-induced hypokalaemia. Lancet *1*:1358, 1983.

268. Skinner, J. E.: Regulation of cardiac vulnerability by the cerebral defense system. J. Am. Coll. Cardiol. *5*(Suppl. B):88, 1985.

269. Schwartz, P. J., Billman, G. E., and Stone, H. L.: Autonomic mechanisms in ventricular fibrillation induced by myocardial ischemia dur-

ing exercise in dogs with healed myocardial infarction. Circulation 69:790, 1984.

270. Verrier, R. L., and Hagestad, E. L.: Role of the autonomic neuron system in sudden death. In Josephson, M. E. (ed.): Sudden Cardiac Death. Philadelphia, F. A. Davis Co., 1985, pp. 41–63.

271. Schwartz, P. J., and Stone, H. L.: The role of autonomic nervous system in sudden coronary death. Ann. N.Y. Acad. Sci. 382:162, 1982.

272. Opie, L. H.: Products of myocardial ischemia and electrical instability of the heart. J. Am. Coll. Cardiol. 5(Suppl. B):162, 1985.

273. Huikuri, H. V., Linnaluoto, M. K., Seppanen, T., et al.: Circadian rhythm of heart rate variability in survivors of cardiac arrest. Am. J. Cardiol. 70:610, 1992.

274. Huikuri, H. V., Valkama, J. O., Airakainen, K. E., et al.: Frequency domain measures of heart rate variability before the onset of nonsustained and sustained ventricular tachycardia in patients with coronary artery disease. Circulation 87:1220, 1993.

275. Myerburg, R. J., Kessler, K. M., Kiem, I., et al.: The relationship between plasma levels of procainamide, suppression of premature ventricular contractions, and prevention of recurrent ventricular tachycardia. Circulation 64:280, 1981.

276. Task Force of the Working Group on Arrhythmias of the European Society of Cardiology: The Sicilian Gambit: A new approach to the classification of antiarrhythmic drugs based on their action on arrhythmogenic mechanisms. Circulation 84:1831, 1991.

277. Vassalle, M.: On the mechanisms underlying cardiac standstill: Factors determining success or failure of escape pacemakers in the heart. J. Am. Coll. Cardiol. 5(Suppl. B):35, 1985.

278. Fozzard, H. A.: Electromechanical dissociation and its possible role in sudden cardiac death. J. Am. Coll. Cardiol. 5(Suppl. B):31, 1985.

CLINICAL CHARACTERISTICS OF THE PATIENT WITH CARDIAC ARREST

279. Pell, S., and D'Alonzo, C. A.: Immediate mortality and five-year survival of employed men with a first myocardial infarction. N. Engl. J. Med. 270:915, 1964.

280. Kimball, J. J., and Killip, T.: Aggressive treatment of arrhythmias in acute myocardial infarction: Procedures and results. Prog. Cardiovasc. Dis. 10:483, 1968.

281. Feinlieb, M., Simon, A. B., Gillum, J. R., and Margolis, J. R.: Prodromal symptoms and signs of sudden death. Circulation 52(Suppl. 3):155, 1975.

282. Fulton, M., Lutz, W., Donald, K. W., et al.: Natural history of unstable angina. Lancet 1:860, 1972.

283. Goldstein, S., Landis, J. R., Leighton, R., et al.: Characteristics of the resuscitated out-of-hospital cardiac arrest victim with coronary heart disease. Circulation 64:977, 1981.

284. Nikolic, G., Bishop, R. L., and Singh, J. B.: Sudden death recorded during Holter monitoring. Circulation 66:218, 1982.

285. Pratt, C. M., Francis, M. J., Luck, J. C., et al.: Analysis of ambulatory electrocardiograms in 15 patients during spontaneous ventricular fibrillation with special reference to preceding arrhythmic events. J. Am. Coll. Cardiol. 2:789, 1983.

286. Bayes de Luna, A., Coumel, P., and Leclercq, J. F.: Ambulatory sudden death: Mechanisms of production of fatal arrhythmia on the basis of data from 157 cases. Am. Heart J. 117:151, 1989.

287. Hinkle, L. E., and Thaler, H. T.: Clinical classification of cardiac deaths. Circulation 65:457, 1982.

288. Bates, R. J., Beutler, S., Resnekov, L., and Anagnostopoulos, C. E.: Cardiac rupture: Challenge in diagnosis and management. Am. J. Cardiol. 40:429, 1977.

289. Emergency Cardiac Care Committee and Subcommittees, American Heart Association: Guidelines for cardiopulmonary resuscitation and emergency cardiac care. JAMA 268:2172, 1992.

290. Lo, B., and Steinbrook, R. L.: Deciding whether to resuscitate. Arch. Intern. Med. 143:1561, 1983.

291. Bedell, S. E., Delbanco, T. L., Cook, E. F., and Epstein, F. H.: Survival after cardiopulmonary resuscitation in the hospital. N. Engl. J. Med. 309:569, 1983.

292. Cobb, L. A., Weaver, W. D., and Fahrenbrush, C. E.: Community-based interventions for sudden cardiac death: Impact, limitations, and charges. Circulation 85(Suppl. I):I-98, 1992.

293. Goldstein, S., Landis, J. R., Leighton, R., et al.: Predictive survival models for resuscitated victims of out-of-hospital cardiac arrest with coronary heart disease. Circulation 71:873, 1985.

294. Cummins, R. O., Ornato, J. P., Thies, W. H., and Pepe, P. E.: Improving survival from sudden cardiac arrest: The "chain of survival" concept: A statement for heart professionals from the Advanced Cardiac Life Support Subcommittee and the Emergency Cardiac Care Committee, American Heart Association. Circulation 83:1832, 1991.

295. Gulati, R. S., Bhan, G. L., and Horan, M. A.: Cardiopulmonary resuscitation of old people. Lancet 2:267, 1983.

296. Taffet, G. E., Teasdale, T. A., and Luchi, R. J.: In-hospital cardiopulmonary resuscitation. JAMA 260:2069, 1988.

297. Tresch, D. D., Thakur, R. K., Hoffmann, R. G., et al.: Should the elderly be resuscitated following out-of-hospital cardiac arrest? Am. J. Med. 86:145, 1989.

298. Eisenberg, M. S., Bergner, L., and Hallstrom, A. P.: Cardiac resuscitation in the community: Importance of rapid provision and implications of program planning. JAMA 241:1905, 1979.

299. Myerburg, R. J., Estes, D., Zaman, L., et al.: Outcome of resuscitation from bradyarrhythmic or asystolic prehospital cardiac arrest. J. Am. Coll. Cardiol. 4:1118, 1984.

300. Jaggarao, N. S. V., Heber, M., Grainger, R., et al.: Use of an automated external defibrillator-pacemaker by ambulance staff. Lancet 2:73, 1982.

301. Longstreth, W. T., Inui, T. S., Cobb, L. A., and Copass, M. K.: Neurologic recovery after out-of-hospital cardiac arrest. Ann. Intern. Med. 98:588, 1983.

302. Longstreth, W. T., Diehr, P., and Inui, T. S.: Prediction of awakening after out-of-hospital cardiac arrest. N. Engl. J. Med. 308:1378, 1983.

303. Myerburg, R. J., Conde, C. A., Sheps, D. S., et al.: Antiarrhythmic drug therapy in survivors of prehospital cardiac arrest: Comparison of effects on chronic ventricular arrhythmias and on recurrent cardiac arrest. Circulation 59:855, 1979.

304. Weaver, W. D., Cobb, L. A., and Hallstrom, A. P.: Ambulatory arrhythmia in resuscitated victims of cardiac arrest. Circulation 66:212, 1982.

305. Ritchie, J. L., Hallstrom, A. P., Troubaugh, G. B., et al.: Out-of-hospital sudden coronary death: Rest and exercise radionuclide left ventricular function in survivors. Am. J. Cardiol. 55:645, 1985.

306. Weaver, W. D., Lorch, G. S., Alvarez, H. A., and Cobb, L. A.: Angiographic findings and prognostic indicators in patients resuscitated from sudden cardiac death. Circulation 54:895, 1976.

307. Weaver, W. D., Cobb, L. A., and Hallstrom, A. P.: Characteristics of survivors of exertion- and nonexertion-related cardiac arrest: Value of subsequent exercise testing. Am. J. Cardiol. 50:671, 1982.

308. Cobb, L. A., Werner, J. A., and Troubaugh, G. B.: Sudden cardiac death: I. A decade's experience with out-of-hospital resuscitation; and II. Outcome of resuscitation, management, and future directions. Mod. Concepts Cardiovasc. Dis. 49:31, 1980.

309. Haynes, R. E., Hallstrom, A. P., and Cobb, L. A.: Repolarization abnormalities in survivors of out-of-hospital ventricular fibrillation. Circulation 57:654, 1978.

310. Thompson, R. G., and Cobb, L. A.: Hypokalemia after resuscitation from out-of-hospital cardiac arrest. JAMA 248:2860, 1982.

311. Urban, P., Scheidegger, D., Buchmann, B., and Barth, D.: Cardiac arrest and blood ionized calcium levels. Ann. Intern. Med. 109:110, 1988.

312. Sheps, D. S., Conde, C., Cameron, B., et al.: Resting peripheral blood lactate elevation in survivors of prehospital cardiac arrest: Correlation with hemodynamic, electrophysiologic, and oxyhemoglobin dissociation indexes. Am. J. Cardiol. 44:1276, 1979.

313. Myerburg, R. J., Kessler, K. M., Zaman, L., et al.: Factors leading to decreasing mortality among patients resuscitated from out-of-hospital cardiac arrest. In Brugada, P., and Wellens, H. J. J. (eds.): Cardiac Arrhythmias: Where to Go from Here? Mt. Kisko, N.Y., Futura, 1987, pp. 505–525.

MANAGEMENT OF CARDIAC ARREST

314. Furukawa, T., Rozanski, J. J., Nogami, J., et al.: Time-dependent risk of and predictors for cardiac arrest recurrence in survivors of out-of-hospital cardiac arrest with chronic coronary artery disease. Circulation 80:599, 1989.

315. Goldman, L.: Coronary care units: A perspective on their epidemiologic impact. Int. J. Cardiol. 2:284, 1982.

316. Killip, T., and Kimball, J. T.: Treatment of myocardial infarction in a coronary care unit: A two-year experience with 250 patients. Am. J. Cardiol. 20:457, 1967.

317. Pantridge, J. F., and Adgey, A. A. J.: Pre-hospital coronary care. The mobile coronary care unit. Am. J. Cardiol. 24:666, 1969.

318. Stults, K. R., Brown, D. D., Schug, V. L., and Bean, J. A.: Prehospital defibrillation performed by emergency medical technicians in rural communities. N. Engl. J. Med. 310:219, 1984.

319. Lombardi, G., Gallagher, J., and Gennis, P.: Outcome of out-of-hospital cardiac arrest in New York City: The Pre-Hospital Arrest Survival Evaluation (PHASE) Study. JAMA 271:678, 1994.

320. Eisenberg, M. S., Copass, M. K., Hallstrom, A. P., et al.: Treatment of out-of-hospital cardiac arrests with rapid defibrillation by emergency medical technicians. N. Engl. J. Med. 302:1379, 1980.

321. Mayer, J. D.: Paramedic response time and survival from cardiac arrest. Soc. Sci. Med. 13D:267, 1979.

322. Weaver, W. D., Copass, M. K., Bufi, D., et al.: Improved neurologic recovery and survival after early defibrillation. Circulation 69:943, 1984.

323. Weaver, W. D., Hill, D., Fahrenbruch, C. E., et al.: Use of the automatic external defibrillator in the management of out-of-hospital cardiac arrest. N. Engl. J. Med. 318:661, 1988.

324. Stults, K. R.: Phone first. J. Emerg. Med. Serv. 12:28, 1987.

325. Caldwell, G., Miller, G., Quinn, E., et al.: Simple mechanical methods for cardioversion: Defense of the precordial thump and cough version. Br. Med. J. 291:627, 1985.

326. Lown, B., and Taylor, J.: "Thumpversion" (editorial). N. Engl. J. Med. 283:1223, 1970.

327. Criley, J. M., Blaufuss, A. N., and Kissel, J. L.: Cough-induced cardiac compression: Self-administered form of cardiopulmonary resuscitation. JAMA 263:1246, 1976.

328. Wei, J. Y., Greene, H. L., and Weisfeldt, M. L.: Cough-facilitated conversion of ventricular tachycardia. Am. J. Cardiol. 45:174, 1980.

329. Heimlich, H. J.: A life-saving maneuver to prevent food-choking. JAMA 234:398, 1975.

330. Visintine, R. E., and Baick, C. H.: Ruptured stomach after Heimlich maneuver. JAMA *234*:415, 1975.

331. Feldman, T., Mallon, S. M., Bolooki, H., et al.: Fatal acute aortic regurgitation in a person performing the Heimlich maneuver (letter). N. Engl. J. Med. *315*:1613, 1986.

332. Centers for Disease Control: Guidelines for prevention and transmission of human immunodeficiency virus and hepatitis B virus to health-care and public-safety workers. M.M.W.R. *38*(Suppl. 6):1, 1989.

333. Sande, M. A.: Transmission of AIDS: The case against casual contagion. N. Engl. J. Med. *314*:380, 1986.

334. Weisfeldt, M. L., and Chandra, N.: Physiology of cardiopulmonary resuscitation. Annu. Rev. Med. *32*:435, 1981.

335. Ewy, G. A.: Current status of cardiopulmonary resuscitation. Mod. Concepts Cardiac Dis. *53*:43, 1984.

336. Weisfeldt, M. L., Chandra, N., and Tsitlik, J. E.: Increased intrathoracic pressure—not direct heart compression—causes the rise in intrathoracic vascular pressures during CPR in dogs and pigs. Crit. Care Med. *9*:377, 1981.

337. Rudikoff, M. T., Maughan, W. L., Effrom, M., et al.: Mechanisms of blood flow during cardiopulmonary resuscitation. Circulation *61*:345, 1980.

338. Chandra, N., Rudikoff, M., and Weisfeldt, M. L.: Simultaneous chest compression and ventilation at high airway pressure during cardiopulmonary resuscitation. Lancet *1*:175, 1980.

339. Ditchey, R. V., and Lindenfeld, J.: Potential adverse effects of volume loading on perfusion of vital organs during closed-chest resuscitation. Circulation *69*:181, 1984.

340. Michael, J. R., Guerci, D., Koehler, R. C., et al.: Mechanisms by which epinephrine augments cerebral and myocardial perfusion during cardiopulmonary resuscitation in dogs. Circulation *69*:822, 1984.

341. Sanders, A. B., Ewy, G. A., Alferness, A., et al.: Failure of one method of simultaneous chest compression, ventilation, and abdominal binding during CPR. Crit. Care Med. *120*:509, 1982.

342. Ducas, J., Roussos, C. H., Karsaidis, C., and Magder, S.: Thoraco-abdominal mechanisms during resuscitation maneuvers. Chest *84*:446, 1983.

343. Guerci, A. D., Halperin, H. R., Beyar, R., et al.: Aortic diameter and pressure-flow sequence identify mechanism of blood flow during external chest compression in dogs. J. Am. Coll. Cardiol. *14*:790, 1989.

344. Paradis, N. A., Martin, G. B., Goetting, M. B., et al.: Simultaneous aortic, jugular, and right atrial pressures during cardiopulmonary resuscitation in humans: Insights into mechanisms. Circulation *80*:361, 1989.

345. Sack, J. B., Kesselbrenner, M. B., and Bregman, D.: Survival from in-hospital cardiac arrest with interposed abdominal counterpulsation during cardiopulmonary resuscitation. JAMA *267*:379, 1992.

346. Cohen, T. J., Turaker, K. G., Lurie, K. G., et al.: Active compression-decompression: A new method of cardiopulmonary resuscitation. JAMA *267*:2916, 1992.

347. Cummins, R. O., Eisenberg, M., Bergner, L., and Murray, J. A.: Sensitivity, accuracy, and safety of an automatic external defibrillator. Lancet *2*:318, 1984.

348. Gascho, J. A., Crampton, R. S., Cherwek, M. L., et al.: Determinants of ventricular defibrillation in adults. Circulation *60*:231, 1979.

349. Federiuk, C. S., Sanders, A. B., Kern, K. B., et al.: The effect of bicarbonate on resuscitation from cardiac arrest. Ann. Emerg. Med. *20*:1173, 1991.

350. Aufderheide, T. P., Martin, D. R., Olson, D. W., et al.: Prehospital bicarbonate use in cardiac arrest: A 3-year experience. Am. J. Emerg. Med. *10*:4, 1992.

351. Kette, F., Weil, M. H., and Gazmuri, R. J.: Buffer solutions may compromise cardiac resuscitation by reducing coronary perfusion pressure. JAMA *266*:2121, 1991.

352. Sodium bicarbonate in cardiac arrest (editorial). Lancet *1*:946, 1976.

353. Weil, M. H., Trevino, R. P., and Rackow, E. C.: Sodium bicarbonate during CPR: Does it help or hinder? Chest *88*:487, 1985.

354. White, R. D.: Cardiovascular pharmacology: Part I. *In* McIntyre, K. M., and Lewis, A. J. (eds.): Textbook of Advanced Life Support. Dallas, American Heart Association, Inc., 1983, pp. 99–114.

355. Haynes, R. E., Chinn, T. L., Copass, M. K., and Cobb, L. A.: Comparison of bretylium tosylate and lidocaine in the resuscitation of patients from out-of-hospital ventricular fibrillation: A randomized clinical trial. Am. J. Cardiol. *487*:353, 1981.

356. Giardina, E. G., Heissenbuttel, R. H., and Bigger, J. T.: Intermittent intravenous procainamide to treat ventricular arrhythmias. Correlation of plasma concentration with effect on arrhythmia, electrocardiogram, and blood pressure. Ann. Intern. Med. *78*:183, 1973.

357. Williams, M. L., Woelfel, A., Cascio, W. E., et al.: Intravenous amiodarone during prolonged resuscitation from cardiac arrest. Ann. Intern. Med. *110*:839, 1989.

358. Hughes, W. G., and Ruedy, J. R.: Should calcium be used in cardiac arrest? Am. J. Med. *81*:285, 1986.

359. Zoll, P. M., Zoll, R. H., Clinton, J. E., et al.: External non-invasive temporary cardiac pacing: Clinical trials. Circulation *71*:937, 1985.

360. Knowlton, A. A., and Falk, R. H.: External cardiac pacing during in hospital cardiac arrest. Am. J. Cardiol. *51*:1295, 1986.

361. Lee, R. V., Rogers, B. D., White, L. M., and Harvey, R. C.: Cardiopulmonary resuscitation of pregnant women. Am. J. Med. *81*:311, 1986.

362. Holmes, H. R., Babbs, C. F., Voorhees, W. D., et al.: Influence of adrenergic drugs upon vital organ perfusion during CPR. Crit. Care Med. *8*:137, 1980.

363. Yakaitis, R. W., Otto, C. W., and Blitt, C. D.: Relative importance of alpha and beta-adrenergic receptors during resuscitation. Crit. Care Med. *7*:293, 1979.

364. Wyman, M. G., and Hammersmith, L.: Comprehensive treatment plan for the prevention of primary ventricular fibrillation in acute myocardial infarction. Am. J. Cardiol. *33*:661, 1974.

365. Conley, M. J., McNeer, J. F., Lee, K. L., et al.: Cardiac arrest complicating acute myocardial infarction: Predictability and prognosis. Am. J. Cardiol. *39*:7, 1977.

366. Vismara, L. A., Amsterdam, B. A., and Mason, D. T.: Relation of ventricular arrhythmias in the late-hospital phase of acute myocardial infarction to sudden death after hospital discharge. Am. J. Med. *59*:6, 1975.

367. Robinson, J. S., Sloman, G., Mathew, T. H., and Goble, A. J.: Survival after resuscitation from cardiac arrest in acute myocardial infarction. Am. Heart J. *69*:740, 1965.

368. Thompson, P. D., Melmon, K. L., Richardson, J. A., et al.: Lidocaine pharmacokinetics in advanced heart failure, liver disease, and renal failure in humans. Ann. Intern. Med. *78*:499, 1973.

369. Norris, R. M., and Mercer, C. J.: Significance of idioventricular rhythms in acute myocardial infarction. Prog. Cardiovasc. Dis. *16*:455, 1974.

370. Selzer, A., and Wray, H. W.: Quinidine syncope: Paroxysmal ventricular fibrillation occurring during treatment of chronic atrial arrhythmias. Circulation *30*:17, 1964.

371. The Cardiac Arrhythmia Pilot Study (CAPS) Investigators: Effects of encainide, flecainide, imipramine, and moricizine on ventricular arrhythmias during the year after myocardial infarction: The CAPS. Am. J. Cardiol. *61*:501, 1988.

372. Nattel, S., Pedersen, D. H., and Zipes, D. P.: Alterations in regional myocardial distribution and arrhythmogenic effects of aprindine produced by coronary artery occlusion in the dog. Cardiovasc. Res. *15*:80, 1981.

373. Starmer, C. F., Lastra, A. A., Nesterenko, V. V., and Grant, A. O.: Proarrhythmic response to sodium channel blockade: Theoretical model and numerical experiments. Circulation *84*:1364, 1991.

374. Myerburg, R. J., Kessler, K. M., Kimura, S., Castellanos, A.: Sudden cardiac death: Future approaches based on identification and control of transient risk factors. J. Cardiovasc. Electrophysiol. *3*:626, 1992.

375. Haverkamp, W., Shenasa, M., Borggrefe, M., and Breithardt, G.: Torsade de pointes. *In* Zipes, D. P., and Jalife, J. (ed.): Cardiac Electrophysiology: From Cell to Bedside. 2nd ed. Philadelphia, W.B. Saunders Company, 1995, p. 885.

376. Wharton, J. M., Demopulus, P. A., and Goldschlager, N.: Torsade de pointes during administration of pentamidine isethionate. Am. J. Med. *83*:571, 1987.

377. Kimura, S., Bassett, A. L., Xi, H., and Myerburg, R. J.: Early afterdepolarizations and triggered activity produced by cocaine: A possible mechanism of cocaine arrhythmogenesis. Circulation *85*:2227, 1992.

378. Myerburg, R. J., Kessler, K. M., Cox, M. M., et al.: Reversal of proarrhythmic effects of flecainide acetate and encainide hydrochloride by propranolol. Circulation *80*:1571, 1989.

379. Bass, E.: Cardiopulmonary arrest: Pathophysiology and neurologic complications. Ann. Intern. Med. *103*:920, 1985.

380. Breivik, H., Safar, P., Sands, P., et al.: Clinical feasibility trials of barbiturate therapy after cardiac arrest. Crit. Care Med. *6*:228, 1978.

381. Brain Resuscitation Clinical Trial I Study Group: Randomized clinical study of thiopental loading in comatose survivors of cardiac arrest. N. Engl. J. Med. *314*:397, 1986.

382. Cobb, L. A., Hallstrom, A. P., Zia, M., et al.: Influence of coronary revascularization on recurrent sudden cardiac death syndrome. J. Am. Coll. Cardiol. *1*(Abs.):688, 1983.

383. Kron, I. L., Lerman, B. B., Haines, D. E., et al.: Coronary bypass grafting in patients with ventricular fibrillation. Ann. Thorac. Surg. *48*:85, 1989.

384. O'Rourke, R. A.: Role of myocardial revascularization in sudden cardiac death. Circulation *85*(Suppl. I):I-112, 1992.

385. Harken, A. H., Wetstein, L., and Josephson, M. E.: Mechanisms and surgical management of ventricular tachyarrhythmias. *In* Josephson, M. E. (ed.): Sudden Cardiac Death. Philadelphia, F. A. Davis Co., 1985, pp. 287–300.

386. Hallstrom, A. P., Cobb, L. A., Yu, B. H., et al.: An antiarrhythmic drug experience in 941 patients resuscitated from an initial cardiac arrest between 1970 and 1985. Am. J. Cardiol. *68*:1025, 1991.

387. Holmes, D. R., Davis, K. B., Mock, B. B., et al.: The effect of medical and surgical treatment on subsequent sudden cardiac death in patients with coronary artery disease: A report from the Coronary Artery Surgery Study. Circulation *73*:1254, 1986.

388. Multiple Risk Factor Intervention Trial Research Group: Baseline rest electrocardiographic abnormalities, antihypertensive treatment, and mortality in the Multiple Risk Factor Intervention Trial. Am. J. Cardiol. *55*:1, 1985.

389. Bigger, J. T., Fleiss, J. L., Rolnitzky, L. M., et al.: Effect of digitalis treatment on survival after acute myocardial infarction. Am. J. Cardiol. *55*:623, 1985.

390. Ryan, T. J., Bailey, K. R., McCabe, C. H., et al.: The effects of digitalis on survival in high risk patients with coronary artery disease. The Coronary Artery Surgery Study (CASS). Circulation *67*:735, 1983.

391. Madsen, E. G., Gilpin, E., Henning, H., et al.: Prognostic importance of digitalis after acute myocardial infarction. J. Am. Coll. Cardiol. *3*:681, 1984.

392. Muller, J. E., Turi, Z. G., Stone, P. H., et al.: Digoxin therapy and mortality after myocardial infarction: Experience in the MILIS study. N. Engl. J. Med. *314*:265, 1986.

393. Ruskin, J. N., DiMarco, J. P., and Garan, H.: Out-of-hospital cardiac arrest: Electrophysiologic observations and selection of long-term antiarrhythmic therapy. N. Engl. J. Med. *303:*607, 1980.

394. Josephson, M. E., Horowitz, L. N., Spielman, S. C., and Greenspan, A. M.: Electrophysiologic and hemodynamic studies in patients resuscitated from cardiac arrest. Am. J. Cardiol. *46:*948, 1980.

395. Graboys, T. B., Lown, B., Podrid, P. J., and DeSilva, R.: Long-term survival of patients with malignant ventricular arrhythmias treated with antiarrhythmic drugs. Am. J. Cardiol. *50:*437, 1982.

396. Lampert, S., Lown, B., Graboys, T. B., et al.: Determinants of survival in patients with malignant ventricular arrhythmia associated with coronary artery disease. Am. J. Cardiol. *61:*791, 1988.

397. Herre, J., Sauve, M. J., Malone, P., et al.: Long-term results of amiodarone therapy in patients with recurrent sustained ventricular tachycardia or ventricular fibrillation. J. Am. Coll. Cardiol. *13:*442, 1989.

398. The CASCADE Investigators: Randomized antiarrhythmic drug therapy in survivors of cardiac arrest (The CASCADE Study). Am. J. Cardiol. *72:*280, 1993.

399. Steinbeck, G., Andresen, S., Bach, P., et al.: A comparison of electrophysiologically guided antiarrhythmic drug therapy with beta-blocker therapy in patients with symptomatic sustained ventricular tachyarrhythmias. N. Engl. J. Med. *327:*987, 1992.

400. Connolly, S. J., and Yusuf, S.: Evaluation of the implantable cardioverter defibrillator in survivors of cardiac arrest: The need for randomized trials. Am. J. Cardiol. *69:*959, 1992.

401. Swerdlow, C. R., Winkle, R. A., and Mason, J. W.: Determinants of survival in patients with ventricular tachycardia. N. Engl. J. Med. *308:*1436, 1983.

402. Roy, D., Waxman, H. L., Kienzle, M. G., et al.: Clinical characteristics and long-term follow-up in 119 survivors of cardiac arrest: Relation to inducibility at electrophysiologic testing. Am. J. Cardiol. *52:*969, 1983.

403. Benditt, D. G., Benson, D. W., Jr., Klein, G. J., et al.: Prevention of recurrent sudden cardiac arrest: Role of provocative electropharmacologic testing. J. Am. Coll. Cardiol. *2:*418, 1983.

404. Morady, F., Scheinman, M. M., Hess, D. S., et al.: Electrophysiologic testing in the management of survivors of out-of-hospital cardiac arrest. Am. J. Cardiol. *51:*85, 1983.

405. Skale, B. T., Miles, W. M., Heger, J. J., et al.: Survivors of cardiac arrest: Prevention of recurrence by drug therapy as predicted by electrophysiologic testing or electrocardiographic monitoring. Am. J. Cardiol. *57:*113, 1986.

406. Wilbur, D. J., Garan, H., Finkelstein, D., et al.: Out-of-hospital cardiac arrest: Use of electrophysiological testing in the prediction of long-term outcome. N. Engl. J. Med. *318:*19, 1988.

407. Wellens, H. J. J., Brugada, P., and Stevenson, W. G.: Programmed electrical stimulation of the heart in patients with life-threatening ventricular arrhythmias: What is the significance of induced arrhythmias and what is the correct stimulation protocol? Circulation *72:*1, 1985.

408. Myerburg, R. J., and Zaman, L.: Indications for intracardiac electrophysiologic studies in survivors of prehospital cardiac arrest. Circulation *75:*151, 1987.

409. Kim, S. O., Seiden, S. W., Felder, S. D., et al.: Is programmed stimulation of value in predicting the long-term success of antiarrhythmic therapy for ventricular tachycardia? N. Engl. J. Med. *315:*356, 1986.

410. Mason, J. W., for The Electrophysiologic Study versus Electrocardiographic Monitoring Investigators: A comparison of electrophysiologic testing with Holter monitoring to predict antiarrhythmic-drug efficacy for ventricular tachyarrhythmias. N. Engl. J. Med. *329:*445, 1993.

411. The ESVEM Investigators: Determinants of predicted efficacy of antiarrhythmic drugs in The Electrophysiologic Study versus Electrocardiographic Monitoring Trial. Circulation *87:*323, 1993.

412. Goldstein, S., Brooks, M. M., Ledingham, R., et al.: The association between ease of suppression of ventricular arrhythmias and survival. Circulation *91:*79, 1995.

413. Mitchell, L. B., Duff, H. J., Manyeri, D. E., and Wyse, D. G.: Randomized clinical trial of invasive and non-invasive approaches to drug therapy of ventricular tachycardia. N. Engl. J. Med. *317:*1681, 1987.

414. Akhtar, M., Guran, H., Lehmann, M. H., and Troup, P. J.: Sudden cardiac death: Management of high-risk patients. Ann. Intern. Med. *114:*499, 1991.

415. Zheutlin, T. A., Steinman, R. T., Mattioni, T. A., and Kehoe, R. F.: Long-term arrhythmic outcome in survivors of ventricular fibrillation with absence of inducible ventricular tachycardia. Am. J. Cardiol. *62:*1213, 1988.

416. Crandall, B. G., Morris, C. D., Cutler, J. E., et al.: Implantable cardioverter-defibrillator therapy in survivors of out-of-hospital sudden cardiac death without inducible arrhythmias. J. Am. Coll. Cardiol. *21:*1186, 1993.

417. Josephson, M. E., Harken, A. H., and Horowitz, L. N.: Endocardial excision: A new surgical technique for the treatment of recurrent ventricular tachycardia. Circulation *60:*1430, 1979.

418. Guiradon, G., Gontaine, G., Frank, R., et al.: Encircling endocardial ventriculotomy: A new surgical treatment for life-threatening ventricular tachycardias resistant to medical treatment following myocardial infarction. Ann. Thorac. Surg. *26:*438, 1978.

419. Bolooki, H., Horowitz, M. D., Interian, A., et al.: Long-term surgical syndrome associated with cardiac dysfunction after myocardial infarction. Ann. Surg. *216:*333, 1992.

420. Kelly, P., Ruskin, J. N., Vlahakes, G. J., et al.: Surgical coronary revascularization in survivors of prehospital cardiac arrest. J. Am. Coll. Cardiol. *15:*267, 1990.

421. Platia, E. V., Griffith, L. S. C., Watkins, L., et al.: Treatment of malignant ventricular arrhythmias with endocardial resection and implantation of the automatic cardioverter-defibrillator. N. Engl. J. Med. *314:*213, 1986.

422. Mirowski, M., Reid, P. R., Mower, M. M., et al.: Termination of malignant ventricular arrhythmias with an implanted automatic defibrillator in human beings. N. Engl. J. Med. *303:*322, 1980.

423. Mirowski, M., Reid, P. R., Winkle, R. A., et al.: Mortality in patients with implanted automatic defibrillators. Ann. Intern. Med. *98:*585, 1983.

424. Echt, D. S., Armstrong, K., Schmidt, P., et al.: Clinical experience, complications, and survival in 70 patients with the automatic implantable cardioverter/defibrillator. Circulation *71:*289, 1985.

425. Kelly, P. A., Cannom, D. S., Garan, H., et al.: The automatic implantable defibrillator (AICD): Efficacy, complications and survival in patients with malignant ventricular arrhythmias. J. Am. Coll. Cardiol. *11:*1278, 1988.

426. Tchou, P. J., Kadri, N., Anderson, J., et al.: Automatic implantable cardioverter-defibrillators and survival of patients with left ventricular dysfunction and malignant ventricular arrhythmias. Ann. Intern. Med. *109:*529, 1988.

427. Fogoros, R. N., Elson, J. J., and Bonnet, C. A.: Actuarial incidence and pattern of occurrence of shocks following implantation of the automatic implantable cardioverter-defibrillator. PACE *12:*1465, 1989.

428. Myerburg, R. J., Luceri, R. M., Thurer, R., et al.: Time to first shock and clinical outcome in patients receiving automatic implantable cardioverter-defibrillators. J. Am. Coll. Cardiol. *14:*508, 1989.

429. Newman, D., Sauve, M. J., Herre, J., et al.: Survival after implantation of the cardioverter defibrillator. Am. J. Cardiol. *69:*899, 1992.

430. Siebels, J., Kuck, K.-H., and the CASH Investigators: Implantable cardioverter defibrillator compared with antiarrhythmic drug treatment in cardiac arrest survivors (the Cardiac Arrest Study, Hamburg). Am. Heart J. *127:*1139, 1994.

431. Kim, S. G., Fisher, J. D., Furman, S., et al.: Benefits of implantable defibrillators are overestimated by sudden death rates and better represented by the total arrhythmic death rate. J. Am. Coll. Cardiol. *17:*1587, 1991.

432. Myerburg, R. J., and Kessler, K. M.: Management of patients who survive cardiac arrest. Mod. Concepts Cardiovasc. Dis. *55:*61, 1986.

433. Huikuri, H. V., Cox, M., Interian, A., et al.: Efficacy of intravenous propranolol for significance of inducibility of ventricular tachyarrhythmias with different electrophysiological characteristics in coronary artery disease. Am. J. Cardiol. *64:*1305, 1989.

434. Lehmann, M. H., and Saksena, S., for the NASPE Policy Conference Committee: Implantable cardioverter defibrillators in cardiovascular practice: Report of the Policy Conference of the North American Society of Pacing and Electrophysiology. PACE *14:*969, 1991.

435. Myerburg, R. J., and Davis, J. H.: The medical ecology of public safety. I. Sudden death due to coronary heart disease. Am. Heart J. *68:*586, 1964.

436. Levy, R. I., De La Chapelle, C. E., and Richards, D. W.: Heart disease in drivers of public motor vehicles as a cause of highway accidents. JAMA *184:*143, 1963.

437. Waller, J. A.: Cardiovascular disease, aging, and traffic accidents. J. Chron. Dis. *20:*615, 1967.

438. Kerwin, A. J.: Sudden death while driving. Can. Med. Assoc. J. *131:*312, 1984.

439. Öström, M., and Eriksson, A.: Natural death while driving. J. Forensic Sci. *32:*988, 1987.

440. Christian, M. S.: Incidence and implications of natural deaths of road users. B.M.J. *297:*1021, 1988.

Chapter 25
Pulmonary Hypertension
STUART RICH, EUGENE BRAUNWALD, WILLIAM GROSSMAN

NORMAL PULMONARY CIRCULATION

During the passage of red blood cells through the lungs, hemoglobin is normally oxygenated to nearly full capacity and the blood is cleansed of much particulate matter and bacteria. The lungs, in addition to functioning as a blood oxygenator and filter, play a dominant role in achieving acid-base balance by excreting carbon dioxide, thereby helping to maintain an optimal blood pH.[1] Normally, the pulmonary vascular bed offers remarkably little resistance to flow. Pulmonary hypertension results from reductions in the caliber of the pulmonary vessels and/or increases in pulmonary blood flow.

PULMONARY BLOOD FLOW, PRESSURE, AND RESISTANCE

PULMONARY CIRCULATION IN THE NORMAL ADULT. *Pulmonary blood flow* refers to the volume of blood per unit of time that passes from the pulmonary artery through the capillary bed and into the pulmonary veins. However, it must be remembered that the lungs have a dual circulation and receive both systemic venous blood (the "pulmonary blood flow") through the pulmonary artery and arterial blood through the bronchial circulation. The bronchial arteries ramify normally into a capillary network drained by bronchial veins, some of which empty into the pulmonary veins, whereas the remainder empty into the systemic venous bed. Therefore, the bronchial circulation constitutes a physiological "right-to-left" shunt. The function of the bronchial circulation is to provide nutrition to the airways. Normally, blood flow through this system is quite low, amounting to approximately 1 per cent of cardiac output[2]; the resulting desaturation of left atrial blood is usually trivial. However, in some forms of pulmonary disease, e.g., severe bronchiectasis, and in the presence of many congenital cardiovascular malformations that cause cyanosis, the blood flow through the bronchial circulation can increase significantly, account for nearly 30 per cent of the left ventricular output,[3] and produce a significant right-to-left shunt. In pulmonary disease, significant right-to-left shunting through the bronchial circulation may also result in arterial desaturation. In cyanotic congenital heart disease, bronchial blood is not fully oxygenated; it may participate in gas exchange and improve systemic oxygenation.

The normal pulmonary artery pressure in a person living at sea level has a peak systolic value of 18 to 25 mm Hg, an end-diastolic value of 6 to 10 mm Hg, and a mean value ranging from 12 to 16 mm Hg (Chap. 6).* Definite pulmonary hypertension is present when pulmonary artery systolic and mean pressures exceed 30 and 20 mm Hg, respectively. The normal mean pulmonary venous pressure is 6 to 10 mm Hg; therefore, the normal arteriovenous pressure difference, which moves the entire cardiac output across the pulmonary vascular bed, ranges from 2 to 10 mm Hg. This small pressure gradient is all the more remarkable when one considers that to move the same amount of blood per minute through the systemic vascular bed a pressure differential of approximately 90 mm Hg (systemic arterial mean pressure minus right atrial mean pressure) is required.

Thus, the normal pulmonary vascular bed offers less than one-tenth the *resistance* to flow offered by the systemic bed. *Vascular resistance* is generally quantified, by analogy to Ohm's law, as the ratio of pressure drop (ΔP in mm Hg) to mean flow (Q in liters/min). The ratio is commonly multiplied by 79.9 (or 80 for simplification) to express the results in dynes-seconds-centimeters^{-5}. This conversion to metric units may be avoided, i.e., resistance may be expressed in units of mm Hg/liter/min, which are sometimes referred to as hybrid units, PRU (peripheral resistance units), or Wood units (after the English cardiologist Paul Wood). The calculated pulmonary vascular resistance in normal adults[4] is 67 ± 23 (S.D.) dynes-sec-cm^{-5}, or 1 Wood unit.

Vascular resistance reflects a composite of variables that includes, but is not limited to, the cross-sectional area of small muscular arteries and arterioles. Other determinants are blood viscosity, the total mass of lung tissue (i.e., resistance is higher in infants and children than in adults), proximal vascular obstruction (e.g., pulmonary coarctation, pulmonary embolism, peripheral pulmonic stenosis), and extramural compression of vessels (perivascular edema).

Because the pulmonary vascular bed contains considerable elastic tissue, the cross-sectional area of the bed varies directly with transmural pressure and flow. Therefore, pulmonary vascular resistance decreases passively with increases in flow. This fall in resistance results in part from the increase in the radius of distensible vessels secondary to increased flow. From a consideration of the Poiseuille relationship—in which $R = \Delta P/Q = 8\eta l/\pi r^4$, where R = resistance, ΔP = pressure drop, Q = flow, η = viscosity of fluid, and l and r = length and radius of the vessel, respectively—it is apparent that resistance can be effectively influenced by even small changes in the radius of the vessel. Recruitment of additional vascular channels also contributes to the fall in resistance that characterizes increased flow through the pulmonary circuit. This phenomenon is particularly prominent in the upright position, where vessels in the upper parts of the lungs are in a partially collapsed state owing to low hydrostatic pressure.

The reduction in resistance in a distensible vascular bed that occurs with increased flow has been offered as the explanation for the ab-

---

* All pressures discussed here are in reference to atmospheric pressure at the level of the heart. True transmural pressures are more physiologically meaningful, especially when pulmonary parenchymal disease is present, but these are rarely measured.

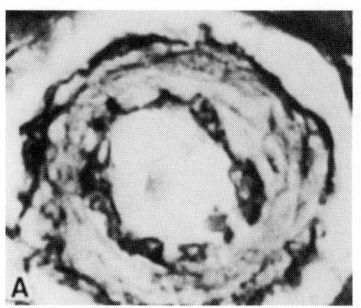 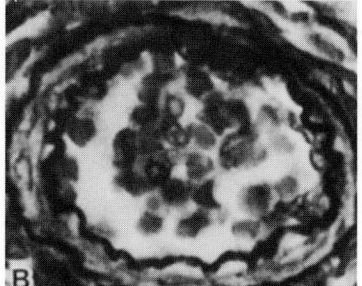 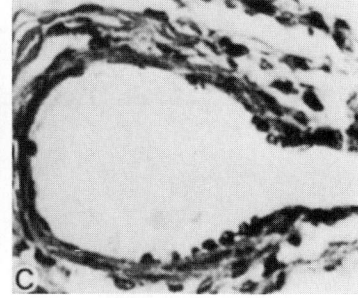

FIGURE 25–1. Changes in pulmonary arteries after birth. Comparison of relative medial thicknesses at birth *(A)*, at age 2 months *(B)*, and at age 7 months *(C)*. Elastic-van Gieson stain; magnification × 360; reduced 17 per cent. (From Petersen, R. C., and Edwards, W. D.: Pulmonary vascular disease in 57 necropsy cases of total anomalous pulmonary venous connections. Histopathology *7:*47, 1983, with permission of Blackwell Scientific Publications.)

sence of pulmonary hypertension in many patients with large left-to-right intracardiac shunts, particularly atrial septal defects. However, it must be pointed out that the increased distensibility of pulmonary vessels in such situations has developed over years and that this principle is not necessarily applicable to acute increase in pulmonary blood flow.[5] In this regard, the results of studies with unilateral occlusion of a pulmonary artery using a balloon catheter are relevant.[6] Acute increases in flow in the supine position were associated with increases in ∆P, so that vascular resistance of the lung (the slope of the line relating ∆P to flow) remained unchanged. In the upright position, however, blood vessels in the upper part of the lung usually are in a partially or fully collapsed state and with an increase in flow, these vessels may expand, thereby reducing vascular resistance.[5]

FETAL AND NEONATAL CIRCULATIONS (see also p. 1607). In the fetus, oxygenated blood enters the heart from the inferior vena cava and streams across the foramen ovale to the left atrium, left ventricle, ascending aorta, and cranial vessels. Desaturated blood returns from the superior vena cava and passes through the tricuspid valve into the right ventricle and pulmonary artery. Because the resistance of the pulmonary vascular bed in the collapsed fetal lung is extremely high, only 10 to 30 per cent of the total right ventricular output passes through the lungs, the remainder being shunted across the ductus arteriosus to the descending aorta and then back to the placenta. At birth, there is an abrupt change in the pulmonary circulation. With the first breath, expansion of the lungs and the abrupt rise in the Po₂ of blood lead to a release of pulmonary arteriolar vasoconstriction and a stretching and dilatation of muscular pulmonary arteries and arterioles, with a marked drop in vascular resistance.[7] This facilitates a large increase in pulmonary blood flow and raises left atrial volume and pressure. The latter closes the flap valve of the foramen ovale, so that interatrial right-to-left shunting ordinarily ceases within the first hour of life. Normally, the ductus arteriosus closes over the next 10 hours as a result of contraction of the thick smooth muscle bundles within its wall in response to a rising arterial oxygen tension and a change in the prostaglandin milieu.[8] Following the initial dramatic fall in pulmonary vascular resistance at birth, there is a continuous decline over the first few months of life associated with thinning of the media of muscular pulmonary arteries and arterioles until the normal adult pattern is achieved[29] (Fig. 25–1).

AGING AND THE PULMONARY CIRCULATION. Pulmonary artery pressure and pulmonary vascular resistance increase with advanced age, similar to increases that occur in systemic vascular resistance.[10–12] Reduced compliance of the pulmonary vascular bed secondary to intimal fibrosis or increased wall thickness in the muscular pulmonary arteries is a possible cause.[13] It is also possible that some of the changes in the pulmonary arteries relate to reduced compliance of left ventricular filling, which is passively reflected back on the pulmonary vascular bed.[14] The prevalence of mild pulmonary hypertension (mean pulmonary artery pressure ≥ 20 mm Hg) may be as high as 13 per cent in ages up to 45 years, and 28 per cent in ages up to 75 years.[15]

RESPONSE TO ANOXIA, DRUGS, AND NEURAL AND ENVIRONMENTAL FACTORS

HYPOXIA. It is well established that acute *hypoxia* elicits pulmonary vasoconstriction,[16,17] and there is general agreement that this response is part of a self-regulatory mechanism for adjusting capillary perfusion to alveolar ventilation. There appears to be an age dependency and a considerable species variability in the magnitude of this vasoconstrictor response, which is quite intense in cattle, intermediate in humans and the pig, and comparatively mild in dogs and sheep; hypoxic vasoconstriction is more

profound in the infant or young mammal than in the adult. Variability exists within a given species as well, and there is strong evidence for a genetic determination of individual reactivity to hypoxia in animals.[18]

The mechanism of the acute pulmonary vasoconstriction that occurs in response to hypoxia is uncertain (Fig. 25–2). There is some evidence that hypoxia-induced local release of histamine may play an important role, with pulmonary vasoconstriction secondary to stimulation of pulmonary vascular H_1-receptors (cf. discussion of histamine below). There has been considerable speculation about the role of vascular endothelium as a mediator of hypoxia-induced pulmonary vasoconstriction.[19] This is based on recent findings concerning the role of vascular endothelium in the regulation of vascular smooth muscle contraction and relaxation.[20–22] Balanced release of endothelial-derived relaxing factor (EDRF)[20] and of the vasoconstrictor peptide endothelin[22] by endothelial cells plays a critical role in regulation of tone in systemic vascular resistance vessels and may be of considerable importance in the pulmonary circulation as well.

Considerable evidence suggests a role for increased Ca^{++} entry into vascular smooth muscle mediating hypoxic pulmonary vasoconstriction.[24] The concentration of Ca^{++} in the vicinity of the contractile machinery represents a balance between the inflow and outflow across the cell membrane and intracellular release and uptake. Within the cell Ca^{++} can be mobilized from the sarcoplasmic reticulum, mitochondrial membrane, or inner aspect of the cell membrane.[25] Although most of the evidence favors an influx of Ca^{++} from extracellular fluid, the relative contribution of differential mobilization from intracellular stores is unsettled. The mechanism responsible for intracellular mobilization of Ca^{++} is also unclear.[26,27]

Changes in alveolar oxygenation affect the oxygenation of blood in small pulmonary arteries and arterioles by direct gaseous diffusion from the alveoli, respiratory bronchioles, and alveolar ducts in the pulmonary arterioles, even though the latter are "upstream" in relation to the alveoli. This fact, taken together with evidence for a reduction in pulmonary arterial blood volume during hypoxia,[28] supports the view that the small pulmonary arteries and arterioles are the main sites of vasoconstriction and increased resistance during hypoxia.[28,29] Although alveolar oxygen tension is a major physiological determinant of pulmonary arteriolar tone, a reduction in the oxygen tension in the mixed venous blood flowing through the small pulmonary arteries and arterioles may also lead to pulmonary arterial vasoconstriction.[30] *Acidemia* appears to potentiate the effects of hypoxemia, whereas alkalosis may be protective.[31]

NEURAL REGULATION. The media and adventitia of the large elastic pulmonary arteries and of the large pulmonary veins are supplied by nerve fibers that may influence the distensibility of these capacitance vessels.[2,10] Although *neural regulation* of pulmonary vascular resistance can be

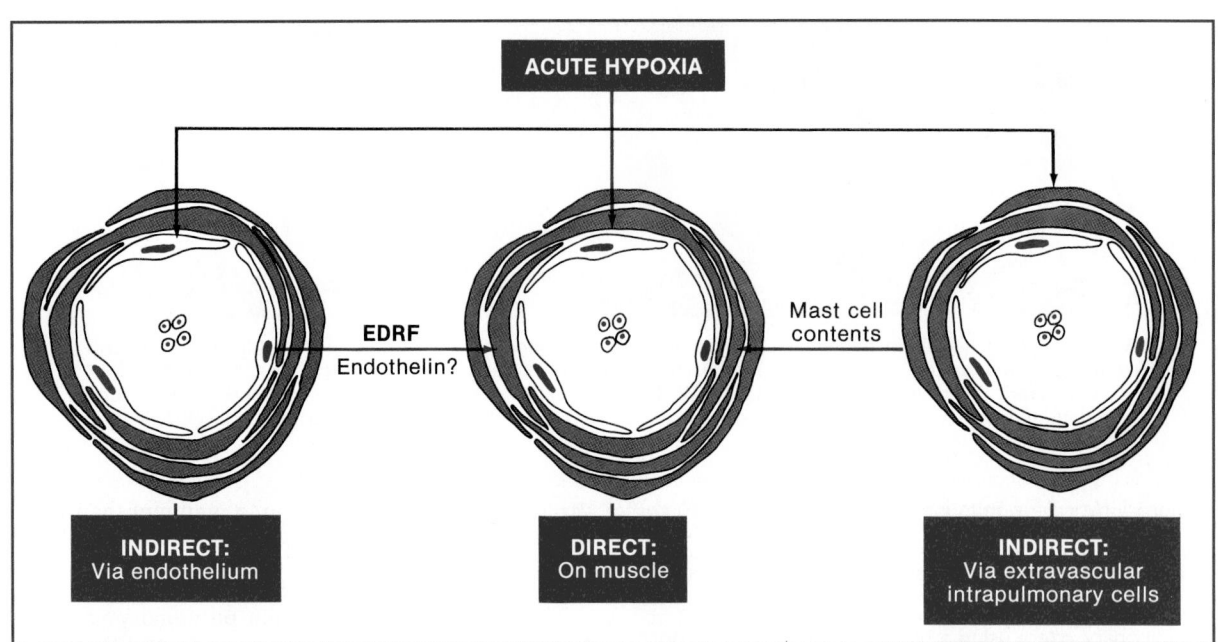

FIGURE 25–2. Possible mechanisms whereby acute hypoxia leads to pulmonary vasoconstriction. A small pulmonary artery can be affected in one of three ways: indirectly via the endothelium *(left)*, indirectly via extravascular cells in the lung *(right)*, or directly via an effect of hypoxia on vascular smooth muscle cells *(middle)*. (From Fishman, A. P.: The enigma of hypoxic pulmonary vasoconstriction. *In* Fishman, A. P. [ed.]: The Pulmonary Circulation: Normal and Abnormal. Philadelphia, University of Pennsylvania Press, 1990, pp. 109–129.)

demonstrated[32] and may be particularly important in fetal life, its importance in the normal human adult is uncertain. *Chemical and hormonal regulation* of pulmonary vascular resistance is a complex and as yet incompletely understood subject, with roles having been reported for catecholamines, acetylcholine, prostaglandins, histamine, bradykinin, serotonin, and angiotensin.[2,19,33–45] The exact site of action of these agents within the pulmonary vascular tree (i.e., arterioles, venules, capillaries, and so on) is uncertain at present.

DRUGS. Controversy exists concerning the effects of *alpha-adrenergic agonists* on the pulmonary vascular bed. Some studies have shown that norepinephrine causes increases in pulmonary arterial and wedge pressures with no change in pulmonary blood flow or pulmonary vascular resistance.[41] Evidence exists for alpha-adrenergic–mediated

constriction of small pulmonary arteries and veins induced by the stimulation of sympathetic nerves.[42]

Both the alpha-adrenergic blocking agent phentolamine and tolazoline (Priscoline), which also exhibits alpha-adrenergic blocking action, can lower pulmonary vascular resistance. *Beta-adrenergic stimulation* with isoproterenol has been shown repeatedly to cause pulmonary *vasodilatation*. In contrast, beta-adrenergic blockade does not produce any change in pulmonary vascular resistance, suggesting that there is no tonic activation of beta receptors for maintenance of the normal low pulmonary vascular resistance. *Acetylcholine* is also a potent relaxant of pulmonary arteries and arterioles[33] and transiently lowers pulmonary vascular resistance in patients with elevated pulmonary vascular resistance with a major reversible component. Whether this effect of acetylcholine is mediated by release

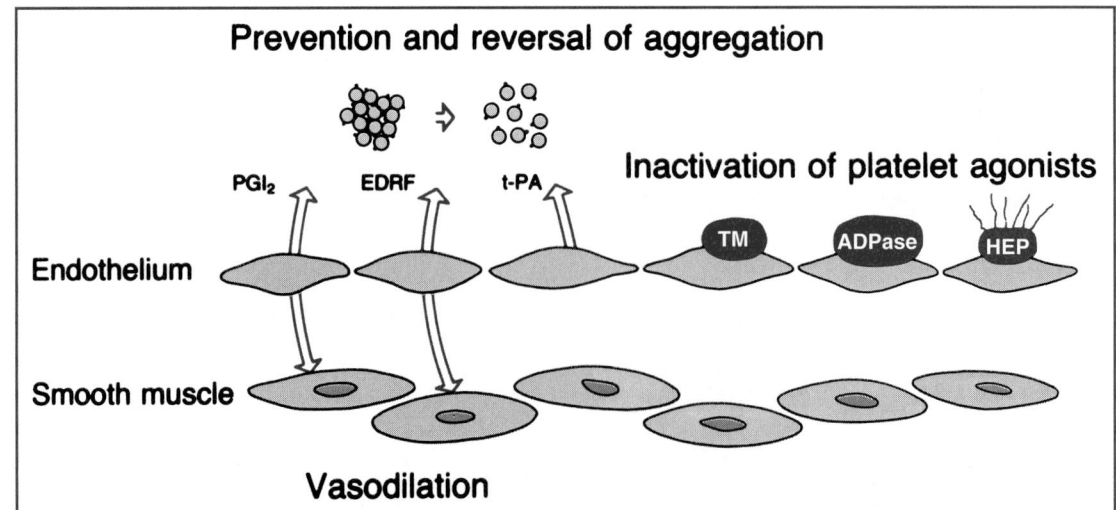

FIGURE 25–3. The vasoactive and anti-aggregatory properties of the normal vascular endothelium are illustrated. Endothelial cells both retain and release into the blood many substances that are anti-aggregatory and fibrinolytic. These include prostacyclin (PGI_2), endothelium-derived relaxing factor (EDRF), and tissue plasminogen activator (t-PA). Some endothelium-derived substances also diffuse from the endothelium to the vascular smooth muscle to produce vasodilation. (From Ware, J. A., and Heistadt, D. D.: Platelet-endothelium interactions. N. Engl. J. Med. *328:*628, 1993. Copyright Massachusetts Medical Society.)

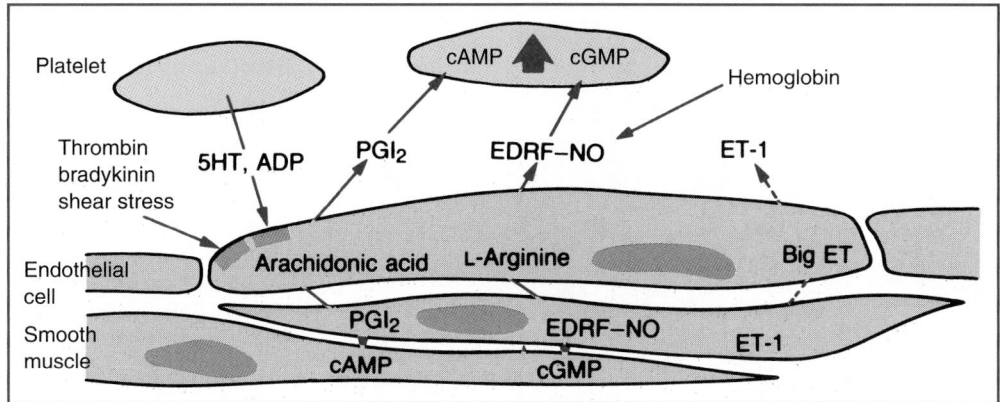

FIGURE 25–4. Generation of PGI$_2$, EDRF–nitric oxide (NO), and endothelin-1 (ET-1) in endothelial cells. Stimulation of receptors on the cells by serotonin or ADP released from platelets or by thrombin, bradykinin, or shear stress leads to the release of vasoactive mediators. Prostacyclin relaxes vascular smooth muscle and inhibits aggregation of platelets by increasing levels of cyclic AMP (cAMP). EDRF-NO relaxes vascular smooth muscle and inhibits platelet aggregation and adhesion, increasing levels of cyclic GMP (cGMP). The simultaneous increase in cAMP and cGMP inhibits platelet aggregation. (From Vane, J. R., Anggard, E. E., and Botting, R. M.: Regulatory functions of the vascular endothelium. N. Engl. J. Med. *323:*27, 1990. Copyright Massachusetts Medical Society.)

of EDRF from pulmonary vascular endothelium has not been determined.

Lung tissue is particularly active in the synthesis, metabolism, and release of a number of the *prostaglandins,* some of which may play a role in the regulation of pulmonary vascular resistance. Prostaglandins I$_2$ and E are active pulmonary vasodilators, whereas F$_2\alpha$ and A$_2$ are pulmonary vasoconstrictors.[34] Prostacyclin (PGI$_2$) is a powerful vasodilator that also inhibits platelet aggregation through activation of adenylate cyclase. Its metabolic half-life in the bloodstream is less than one circulation time with its metabolite 6-keto-prostaglandin F$_1\alpha$ having little biological activity.[35] A variety of drugs with diverse mechanisms of action are reported to encourage prostacyclin production and include calcium channel blockers, angiotensin-converting enzyme inhibitors, diuretics, and nitrates.[36] Physiologically, prostacyclin is a local hormone rather than a circulating one. The release of prostacyclin by endothelial cells causes relaxation of the underlying vascular smooth vessel and prevents platelet aggregation within the bloodstream. Because the biological actions of prostacyclin are the opposite from those of thromboxane, the balance between these two peptides appears to control the local environment within the vascular bed (Fig. 25–3).

The biological action of nitric oxide (EDRF), is quite similar to that of prostacyclin in that it relaxes vascular smooth muscle and potentially inhibits the aggregation and adhesions of platelets by raising platelet levels of cyclic GMP.[37,37a] The observation that activation of the same receptors or a change in membrane confirmation induced by shear stress leads to the release of both nitric oxide and prostacyclin suggests that these substances act in concert as

a common mechanism that defends the vascular endothelium[38,38a] (Fig. 25–4).

Histamine, a vasodilator in the systemic circulation, is primarily a vasoconstrictor in the pulmonary vascular bed. Because large doses of histamine receptor blockers or histamine depletors attenuate the hypoxia-induced pulmonary vasoconstrictor response, it has been suggested that histamine may actually be the chemical mediator of hypoxia-induced vasoconstriction in animals.[39,40] This suggestion is supported by the observation that the periarterial mast cells in the rat and guinea pig lung lose their granules and apparently release histamine during hypoxia.[29] However, other experimental findings are contradictory,[16] and as a consequence, the role of histamine in the regulation of the pulmonary circulation in humans remains unclear. *Serotonin* is a potent pulmonary vasoconstrictor in experimental animals but apparently has little or no effect in humans. *Angiotensin II,* generated in the lung by means of enzymatic conversion of angiotensin I, is thought to be a potent pulmonary vasoconstrictor.[29] However, its role in the normal regulation of pulmonary vascular resistance in humans is unknown.

HIGH ALTITUDE. Life at high altitudes is associated with pulmonary hypertension of variable severity, reflecting the range of reactivities of different persons to the pulmonary vasoconstrictive effect of hypoxia.[44] As discussed earlier, pulmonary arterial pressure normally declines rapidly following birth at sea level. However, the fall in pulmonary artery pressure of infants born at high altitude may be slower in onset and of lesser magnitude. Mean pulmonary arterial pressure in normal adults living 10,000 feet above sea level is approximately 25 mm Hg[45] and increases to over 50 mm Hg with exercise.

PRIMARY PULMONARY HYPERTENSION

Primary pulmonary hypertension (PPH) is the diagnosis given to patients with pulmonary hypertension of unexplained etiology, making it essentially a diagnosis of exclusion.[46] However, PPH has well-characterized clinical features that allow a diagnosis to be made with reasonable precision if an orderly evaluation of the heart and lungs is made in affected patients.[47] The actual incidence of PPH appears to be approximately two cases per million population, thus qualifying it as an orphan disease.[48]

ETIOLOGY

Although the precise cause of PPH is, by definition, unknown, recent developments in our understanding of vascular biology point to an abnormality in the pulmonary vascular endothelium. The normal pulmonary vascular endothelial cell maintains the vascular smooth muscle in a state of relaxation.[36] The findings of increased pulmonary

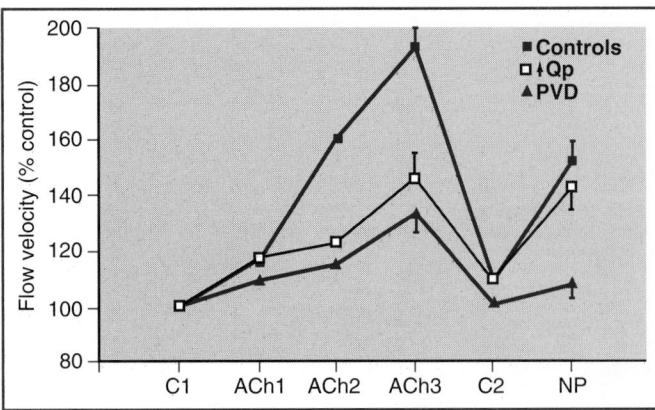

FIGURE 25–5. Relative effects of endothelium-dependent and independent vasodilators on injured pulmonary vessels. The vasodilator response to increasing doses of acetylcholine (ACh 1, 2, 3) and nitroprusside (NP) are shown in children with normal pulmonary vasculature, children with increased pulmonary blood flow but normal vasculature (↑ Qp), and children with pulmonary vascular disease (PVD). The response to acetylcholine, an endothelium-dependent vasodilator, is reduced in patients with increased pulmonary blood flow and pulmonary vascular disease, whereas the response to nitroprusside, an endothelium-independent vasodilator, is lost only in patients with pulmonary vascular disease. (Reproduced with permission from Celermajor, D. S., Cullen, S., and Deanfield, J. E.: Impairment of endothelium-dependent pulmonary artery relaxation in children with congenital heart disease and abnormal pulmonary hemodynamics. Circulation **87:**440, 1993. Copyright 1993 American Heart Association.)

vascular reactivity and vasoconstriction in patients with PPH suggest that a marked vasoconstrictive tendency underlies the development of PPH in predisposed individuals,[49] possibly as a result of loss of endothelial cell integrity[36] (Fig. 25–5) The autonomic nervous system has been considered a contributory factor in the development of PPH through stimulation of the pulmonary vascular bed by either neuronally released or circulating catecholamines. In some patients with PPH the response to vasodilators such as tolazoline, acetylcholine, or isoproterenol is a reduction in pulmonary artery pressure and pulmonary vascular

resistance,[50–52] which supports the notion that the autonomic nervous system is at least in part maintaining a role in the constant elevation of the pulmonary vascular resistance.

As in the systemic circulation (see p. 1164), vascular endothelial cells promote relaxation or contraction of adjacent smooth muscle cells via elaboration of endothelium-derived relaxing factor (EDRF) and endothelin, respectively[20,21] (Fig. 36–4, p. 1164). The secretion of EDRF by vascular endothelium, which serves to dampen or counter many direct vasoconstrictor influences, is lost with endothelial dysfunction that may result from a variety of causes (e.g., shear stress). Studies of vasodilators in pulmonary-hypertension demonstrate that responsiveness to endothelium-dependent vasodilating agents is impaired before response to endothelium-dependent vasodilators[53,54] (Fig. 25–5). This may reflect the underlying severity of vascular damage. Conversely, endothelin, a potent vasoconstrictor peptide, may also play an important role in the regulation of pulmonary vascular tone.[55] Its secretion may be enhanced in the presence of vasoconstriction or in the setting of platelet aggregation. Because it has a long half-life, subtle disturbances in production or release could lead to sustained vasoconstriction.[22] Recently, endothelin ETA receptor antagonists have been reported to reduce pulmonary artery pressure in experimental animals.[56] Given that the major resistance vessels in the pulmonary vascular bed are at the arteriolar level, diffuse arteriolar vasoconstriction could easily cause chronically sustained elevations in pulmonary vascular resistance, resulting in pulmonary hypertension. In postmortem examinations in PPH, the pulmonary vasculature is typified by severe medial hypertrophy,[57] consistent with the appearance of chronic sustained pulmonary vasoconstriction.

A striking feature of the pulmonary vasculature in patients with PPH is intimal proliferation, and in some vessels it causes virtually complete vascular occlusion[57,58] (Fig. 25–6). Several growth factors have been implicated in the development of this type of vascular pathology, which includes basic fibroblast growth factor from the endothelium[59] and platelet derived growth factor[60] and transform-

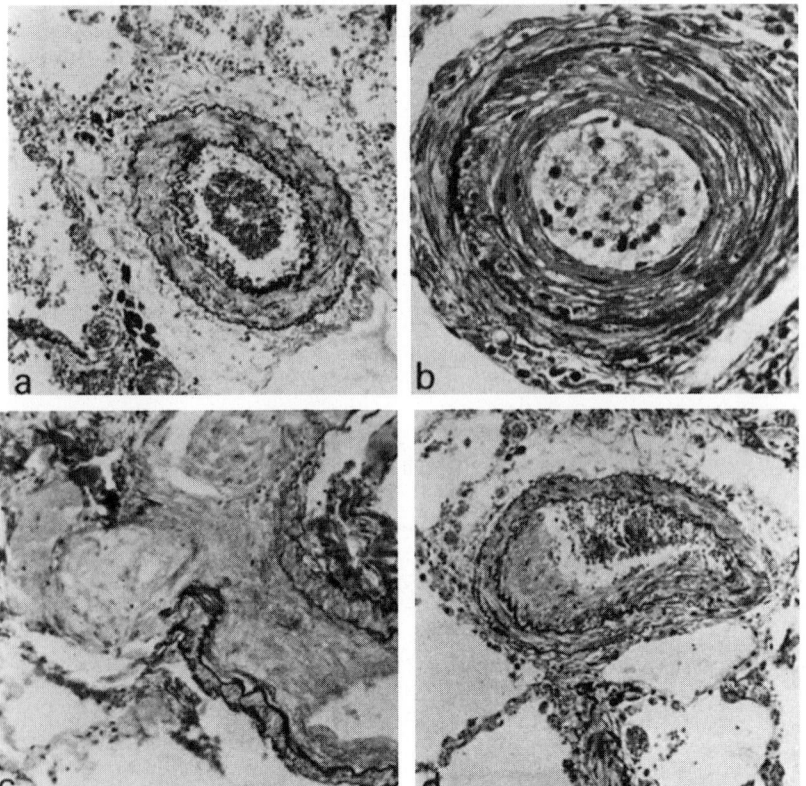

FIGURE 25–6. Photomicrographs of pulmonary arterial histologic lesions seen in clinically unexplained pulmonary hypertension. All slides were stained with Verhoeff-van Gieson stain. *A,* Medial hypertrophy (× 100). *B,* Concentric laminal intimal fibrosis—seen most often in association with plexiform lesion (× 200). *C,* Plexiform lesion demonstrating obstruction in the arterial lumen, aneurysmal dilatation, and proliferation of anastomosing vascular channels (× 200). *D,* Eccentric intimal fibrosis—often seen in association with organized microthrombi but also present in many patients with plexiform lesions (× 100). (Reproduced with permission from Palevsky, H. I., Schloo, B. L., Pietria, G. G., et al.: Primary pulmonary hypertension. Vascular structure, morphometry and responsiveness to vasodilator agents. Circulation **80:**1207, 1989. Copyright 1989 American Heart Association.)

ing growth factor-β[61] from platelets. Enhanced growth factor release, activation, and intracellular signaling may lead to smooth muscle cell proliferation and migration as well as extracellular matrix synthesis. Even advanced lesions show evidence of in situ activity of ongoing synthesis of connective tissue proteins such as elastin, collagen, and fibronectin.[62,63]

An equally important etiologic feature of PPH is the widespread development of thrombosis in situ of the small pulmonary arteries with resultant vascular obstruction.[57,58,64,65] Although it was once believed that recurrent, systemic venous microembolism could be an underlying mechanism in PPH,[46] this theory has been essentially rejected for lack of both animal and human data to support it as a clinical entity. Animal studies suggest that more than 22 million thromboemboli to the pulmonary arterioles would be required to raise the mean pulmonary artery pressure 5 mm Hg, yet no source of these emboli has ever been found in patients dying of PPH.[64] Various defects in coagulation, including abnormal platelet function and defective fibrinolysis, have been demonstrated in patients with PPH.[64,66–70] Increased production of biologically active von Willebrand factor in patients with PPH could predispose to platelet fibrin microthrombi,[71] and exposure of sub-endothelial cell surface structures due to injury may provide the substrate for ongoing vascular thrombosis in this condition.[72] Alterations of the normal physiological function of endothelial cells has been shown to create a local procoagulant environment[36] (Fig. 25–3).

Endothelial denudation results in platelet adherence to exposed tissue collagen, with release of platelet derived smooth muscle mitogens which also have vasoconstrictor properties. This process in turn leads to an inflammatory response and thrombosis, thereby narrowing the lumen of the pulmonary vessels. In a person who is susceptible—whether on a genetic or an acquired basis—intense vasoconstriction may lead to fibrinoid necrosis of the arteriolar wall and the development of plexiform lesions. Ultimately, the vessels are reduced in number, and the residua of these destroyed vessels can be seen histologically as "ghost vessels." Destruction of large numbers of pulmonary arterioles reduces the cross-sectional area of the pulmonary vascular bed, thus producing a permanent increase in pulmonary vascular resistance and fixed pulmonary hypertension. The latter, in turn, damages other blood vessels and initiates a vicious circle, with progressively rising pulmonary arterial pressure (Fig. 25–7).

An important emerging concept for the development of PPH is that patients with an underlying genetic predisposition develop the disease following exposure to specific stimuli, which serve as triggers. Predisposition to the development of pulmonary hypertension has been noted by the marked heterogeneity in responses of the pulmonary vasculature in a variety of disease states. Examples include the considerable variability among individuals to vasoconstrictive stimuli such as hypoxia or acidosis, which can produce marked pulmonary hypertension in one person and be essentially without effect in another.[44] The pulmonary arterial pressure response to hypoxia is particularly great in individuals with blood group A.[16] This variability in the responsiveness of the pulmonary vascular bed undoubtedly accounts for the fact that only a minority of individuals develop pulmonary edema on exposure to high altitude (see p. 462). Also, the severity of pulmonary hypertension and the level of pulmonary vascular resistance vary considerably among individuals with congenital heart

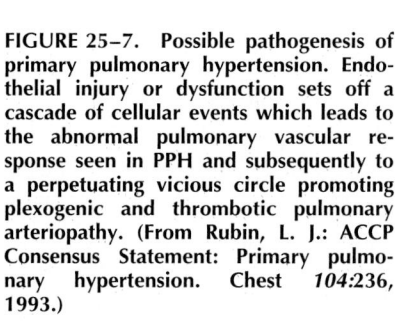

FIGURE 25–7. Possible pathogenesis of primary pulmonary hypertension. Endothelial injury or dysfunction sets off a cascade of cellular events which leads to the abnormal pulmonary vascular response seen in PPH and subsequently to a perpetuating vicious circle promoting plexogenic and thrombotic pulmonary arteriopathy. (From Rubin, L. J.: ACCP Consensus Statement: Primary pulmonary hypertension. Chest *104*:236, 1993.)

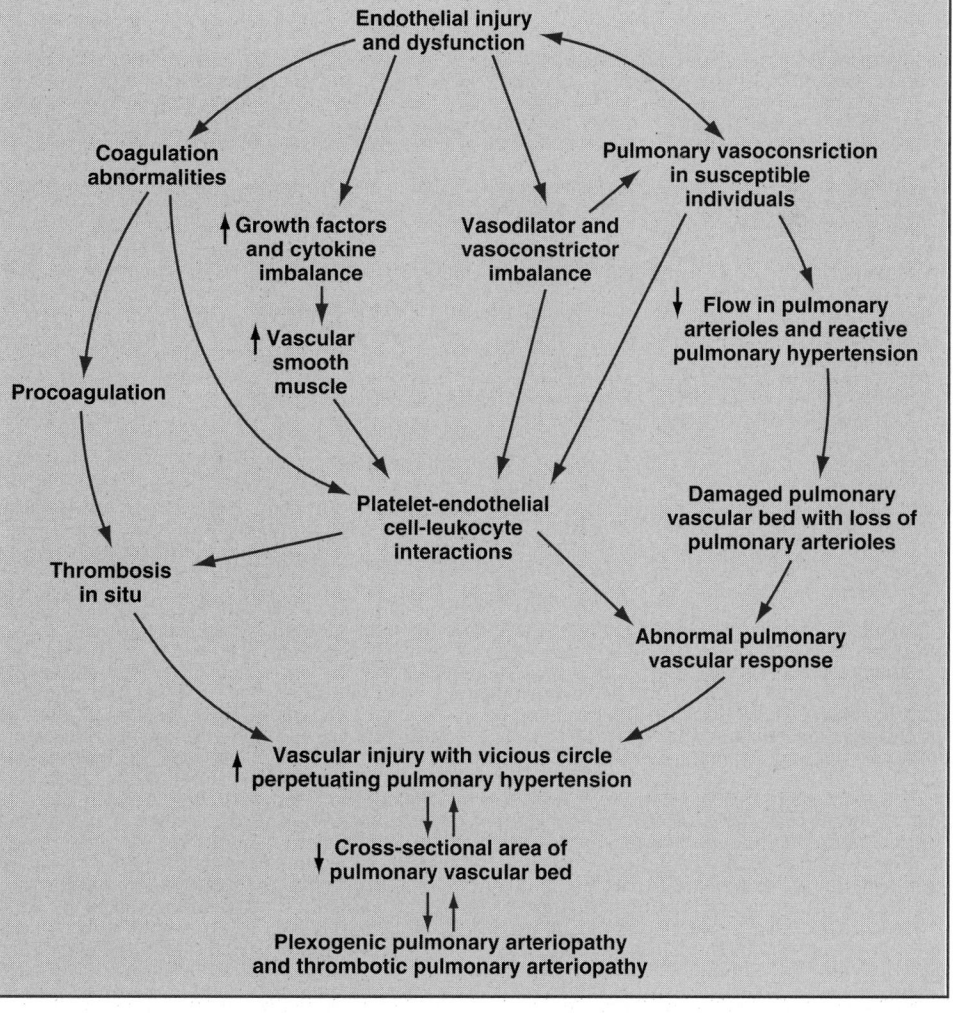

disease and comparably sized ventricular septal defects. Presumably there is a genetic basis for these differences in pulmonary vascular reactivity, just as there appears to be a genetic basis for the increased reactivity of the systemic vascular bed in essential systemic hypertension.

Specific Risk Factors in the Development of Pulmonary Hypertension

Although pulmonary hypertension can be the clear result of a disease process affecting the pulmonary parenchyma or vessels directly, a number of conditions have been identified that appear to be associated with the development of primary or unexplained pulmonary hypertension in which a clearly defined cause-and-effect relationship are lacking. Whereas risk factors for the development of PPH were once thought to be uncommon, a recent study suggests that it may be the rule rather than the exception.[48] Obesity,[48] portal hypertension,[73-82] anorexigens,[83-87] human immunodeficiency virus,[88-92] systemic hypertension,[93-96] and chronically increased pulmonary blood flow[97,98] have all been implicated as risk factors in the development of pulmonary hypertension. The translation into PPH may depend upon other clinical features such as the patient's age or gender at the time of disease expression. However, PPH should no longer be considered a constellation of distinct subtypes, but rather the expression of an entire spectrum of vascular responses to endothelial injury resulting in vasoconstriction and in situ thrombosis, with associated varying degrees of intimal proliferation.[64]

PORTAL HYPERTENSION

Pulmonary abnormalities have been commonly associated with the development of hepatic cirrhosis and portal hypertension. These include hypoxemia and intrapulmonary shunting,[73] portal-pulmonary shunting, impaired hypoxic pulmonary vasoconstriction,[73] and pulmonary hypertension.[74,78-82] Studies show that the liver plays an important role in regulating pulmonary vascular tone. Although the relative risk associated with the development of pulmonary hypertension in patients with portal hypertension is unknown, a large postmortem study from the Johns Hopkins Hospital showed that the prevalence of unexplained or pulmonary hypertension in patients with cirrhosis was 5.6 times higher than that of PPH alone.[74] There was early speculation that the mechanism related to recurrent thromboemboli originating from the portal vein which gain access to the pulmonary circulation via portal-systemic venous shunts, whereas others hypothesized that the development of pulmonary hypertension may be a result of the inability of cirrhotic livers to detoxify vasoactive substances normally absorbed from the gastrointestinal track and activated by the hepatic circulation.[83]

Elevated levels of tumor necrosis factor-α (TNF-α) have recently been reported in rats made portal-hypertensive by partial ligation of the portal vein.[75] TNF-α is a cytokine which, in addition to contributing to a hyperdynamic state, has been implicated in causing structural and metabolic damage to vascular endothelial cells.[76,77] Increased levels of platelet activating factor have also been reported in cirrhosis.

Patients who develop PPH in association with cirrhosis appear to be similar to patients without cirrhosis with the sole exception that they tend to have higher cardiac outputs and consequently lower calculated systemic and pulmonary vascular resistances, which are characteristic of the cirrhotic state.[78]

ANOREXIGENS

A marked increase in the incidence of PPH among the populations of Austria, Germany, and Switzerland in 1967, associated with the use of aminorex, suggested that in predisposed individuals aminorex could lead to the development of severe pulmonary vascular disease.[83] Aminorex has similarities to both adrenalin and ephedrine in its chemical structure and is a potent anorexigen. The influence of aminorex became apparent because of a marked increase in the number of patients with PPH admitted to hospitals between 1967 and 1973. The female to male incidence was 4.5 : 1 but may reflect the fact that aminorex was more often used by women than by men. The clinical features of pulmonary hypertension in affected patients were identical to those attributed to PPH. The mechanism by which aminorex may induce pulmonary hypertension has never been resolved, but the fact that it occurred in less than 1 per cent of patients exposed to the drug points to some underlying predisposition. Of note, however, is that the association occurred not only with aminorex but with other amphetamine-like agents as well.

More recently, PPH has been associated with the use of the appetite suppressants fenfluramine and dexfenfluramine.[84-87] A large series from France has shown an increased likelihood of developing pulmonary hypertension when exposed to these drugs, particularly for periods of greater than 3 months. Although they are known to decrease serotonin uptake, the mechanism by which they produce pulmonary hypertension remains unknown. As with aminorex, only a small percentage of the people exposed developed pulmonary hypertension. Whether or not the pulmonary hypertension is reversible upon discontinuation of usage remains unknown at this time.

HIV INFECTION

Over the past 5 years there have been reports of patients with HIV infection developing unexplained or primary pulmonary hypertension.[88-92] A series of 20 patients from France were recently reported,[91] but the majority of the them had a history of intravenous heroin abuse, raising the possibility of more than one risk factor contributing to the pulmonary hypertension. The patients with HIV tended to be younger, with less severe symptoms and lower values of pulmonary vascular resistance. However, in most other clinical parameters they were quite similar to patients with PPH. The mechanism by which HIV infection causes pulmonary hypertension is unclear, but it does not appear to be simply a phenomenon of immunodeficiency. Attempts to localize the HIV infection to the pulmonary vascular endothelium with electron microscopy, immunohistochemistry, DNA in situ hybridization, and polymerase chain reaction techniques have been unsuccessful.[92] The nonspecific finding of tuboreticular intracytoplasmic inclusions on electron microscopy suggests that the HIV virus may be related to PPH via some mediator such as interferon-α and β that is released from the HIV infection.[92]

SYSTEMIC HYPERTENSION

Systemic hypertension is two to three times more common in patients with PPH than in an age-matched population.[48] The underlying mechanisms related to the development of essential hypertension are quite diverse, but the possibility exists that in some patients the mechanism that increases systemic vascular resistance similarly affects the pulmonary vascular bed.[93,94] It has been suggested that neurohumoral factors may play a role[95] or that the pulmonary vasculature is hypercontractile and overreacts to sympathetic stimulation.[96] Given that essential hypertension is extremely common in the general population, other confounding factors likely contribute to the development of pulmonary hypertension in affected individuals.

INCREASED PULMONARY BLOOD FLOW

For many years the observation has been made that patients with atrial septal defect can develop PPH as an adult.[97] However, the incidence of this is extremely low, raising the possibility that they are two completely unrelated events. It is possible that chronically increased pulmonary blood flow may have effects on the pulmonary endothelium through some type of mechanical means that would cause perturbations in the integrity of the vascular wall and lead to the development of pulmonary vascular disease. Recently increased pulmonary blood flow from hyperthyroidism and beriberi have been reported to be associated with the development of unexplained pulmonary hypertension, suggesting that high pulmonary blood flow,[98] rather than mere coincidence, is the basis for the development of pulmonary hypertension in patients with pre-tricuspid shunts such as atrial septal defect or anomalous pulmonary venous drainage.

FAMILIAL PPH

A familial incidence of PPH in a minority of patients (approximately 6 per cent) has been documented.[46] The transmission in families is unpredictable, and incomplete penetrance, in which the gene is transmitted to affected progeny by individuals who manifest no evidence of disease, is a major confounding feature.[99-102] The vertical transmission in some families strongly suggests the action of a single dominant gene. Recently, genetic anticipation, by which there is worsening of the disease in subsequent generations manifest by an earlier age of onset, has been described.[103] Genetic anticipation has been described in several unrelated neurologic diseases, in which the molecular basis has been attributed to trinucleotide repeat expansion. It is hoped that newer methodology designed to detect single copies of large trinucleotide repeats may lead to the discovery of a gene responsible for familial PPH.

The clinical features of familial PPH are identical to those in patients with the sporadic form with the exception that it typically has an earlier diagnosis from the onset of symptoms, likely due to an increased awareness by the patient or family.[104] Survival also appears similar between the sporadic and familial forms, as an analysis of 36 familial PPH patients found few differences from 41 patients with the sporadic disease. Pathologically all of the characteristics of patients with PPH have been described, including plexogenic arteriopathy, thrombotic arteriopathy, pulmonary veno-occlusive disease, and even pulmonary capillary hemangiomatosis.

The prevalence of antinuclear antibodies in patients with PPH is considerably higher than in the population at large.[105] Some investigators have suggested that PPH may be a forme fruste of an underlying collagen vascular disease. Recently an association between PPH and the major histocompatibility complex has been described in children.[106] Specifically, increased frequencies of HLA-DR3, DRw52, and DQw2 as well as decreased DR5 have been reported. The familial clustering of these HLA antigens in four families with PPH raises the possibility of a susceptibility factor for PPH located near the major histocompatibility locus on chromosome 6p21.3.

PATHOLOGICAL FINDINGS

In 1973 the World Health Organization (WHO) characterized PPH as three distinct subsets: plexogenic arteriopathy, recurrent thromboembolism, and pulmonary veno-occlusive disease.[46] Since that time, however, several large pathology series of patients with PPH have allowed better characterization and understanding of the pathological changes that occur in these patients[57,107,108] (Table 25–1). A classification developed by Heath and Edwards for pulmonary vascular disease from congenital heart disease has been adapted to patients with PPH because of the striking similarities in many of these patients.[109] However, the Heath and Edwards classification implies a natural progression of pulmonary vascular changes not typical of the patients with PPH.

Pathological changes of PPH can be limited to the pulmonary arteriolar circulation or involve the capillaries, venules, and veins (Fig. 25–6). The most common vascular changes can be best characterized as a *hypertensive pulmonary arteriopathy*, which is present in 85 per cent of cases.[57] These changes involve medial hypertrophy of the arteries and arterioles, often in conjunction with other vascular changes. Isolated medial hypertrophy is uncommon, and when it exists it has been assumed to represent an early stage in the disease. The presence of a plexogenic pulmonary arteriopathy is the most common type of hypertensive arteriopathy seen in patients with PPH.[107] It is characterized by medial hypertrophy along with intimal proliferation and other complex lesions. The intimal proliferation may be concentric laminar intimal fibrosis, eccentric intimal fibrosis, or concentric nonlaminar intimal fibrosis. The frequency of these findings differs from case to case and within regions in the same lung of the same patient. In addition, plexiform and dilatation lesions, as well as a necrotizing arteritis, may be seen throughout the lungs. These lesions, however, are not pathognomonic for PPH but representative of a chronic, severe pulmonary hypertensive state.

The other major classification of vascular changes in PPH is a *thrombotic pulmonary arteriopathy*.[57] The typical features include medial hypertrophy of the arteries and arterioles with both eccentric and concentric nonlaminar intimal fibrosis. The presence of colander lesions, representing recanalized thrombi, is also typical. These lesions are believed to arise as a result of a primary in situ thrombosis of the small vascular arteries and not from recurrent pulmonary embolism.

On rare occasion a diffuse pulmonary arteritis with secondary thrombosis has been reported in patients with PPH, predominantly in children.[108,109] Although the association has not been reported in patients with underlying collagen vascular diseases, it may reflect the vascular response to a specific but not clearly identified risk factor.

PULMONARY VENO-OCCLUSIVE DISEASE

Pulmonary veno-occlusive disease is a rare form of PPH, observed in approximately 5 per cent of cases.[57,58] The histopathological diagnosis is based on the presence of obstructive eccentric fibrous intimal pads within the pulmonary veins and venules. There is often arterialization of the pulmonary veins with associated alveolar capillary congestion. Other changes of chronic pulmonary hypertension such as medial hypertrophy and muscularization of the arterioles with eccentric intimal fibrosis may also be present.[110] The pulmonary venous obstruction explains the increased pulmonary capillary wedge pressure described in patients in the late stages of the disease, and the increase in basilar bronchovascular markings described on the chest radiograph. These clinical findings, along with a perfusion lung showing diffuse, patchy nonsegmental abnormalities, is highly suggestive of the diagnosis on a clinical basis.[111]

PULMONARY CAPILLARY HEMANGIOMATOSIS

This extremely rare condition is characterized by proliferation of the thin-walled microvessels that infiltrate the peribronchial and perivascular interstitium and lung parenchyma.[112–114] On occasion it may be confused with pulmonary veno-occlusive disease. The lesions are often patchy and the proliferating vessels may form small nodules within the alveolar interstitial space. These thin-walled vessels

TABLE 25–1 HISTOPATHOLOGIC CLASSIFICATION OF PRIMARY PULMONARY VASCULAR DISEASE

PRESENT CLASSIFICATION	PREVIOUS CLASSIFICATION	CHARACTERISTIC HISTOPATHOLOGIC FEATURES*
Primary Pulmonary Arteriopathy with Plexiform lesions with or without thrombotic lesions	Plexogenic pulmonary arteriopathy	Plexiform lesions; medial hypertrophy, eccentric or concentric-laminar intimal proliferation and fibrosis, fibrinoid degeneration, arteritis, dilatation lesions, and thrombotic lesions
Thrombotic lesions	Thromboembolic pulmonary arteriopathy	Thrombi (fresh, organizing, or organized, and recanalized-collander lesions); varying degrees of medial hypertrophy; no plexiform lesions
Isolated medial hypertrophy	Plexogenic pulmonary arteriopathy	Medial hypertrophy; increase of medial muscle, muscular arteries, muscularization of nonmuscularized intra-acinar arteries; no appreciable intimal or luminal obstructive lesions
Intimal fibrosis and medial hypertrophy	Plexogenic pulmonary arteriopathy	Eccentric or concentric-laminar proliferation and fibrosis; varying degrees of medial hypertrophy; no thrombotic or plexiform lesions
Isolated arteritis	Plexogenic pulmonary arteriopathy	Active or healed arteritis limited to pulmonary arteries; varying degrees of medial hypertrophy, intimal fibrosis, and thrombotic lesions; no plexiform lesions
Pulmonary veno-occlusive disease	Pulmonary veno-occlusive disease	Intimal fibrosis and recanalized thrombi (collander lesions); pulmonary veins and venules; arterialized veins, capillary congestion, alveolar edema and siderophages, dilated lymphatics, pleural and septal edema and arterial medial hypertrophy, intimal fibrosis, and thrombotic lesions
Pulmonary capillary hemangiomatosis	—	Infiltrating thin-walled blood vessels widespread throughout pulmonary parenchyma, pleura, bronchi, and walls of pulmonary veins and arteries

* Medial hypertrophy may be accompanied by muscularization of arterioles.
From Pietra, G. G., Edwards, W. D., Kay, J. M., et al.: Histopathology of primary pulmonary hypertension: A qualitative and quantitative study of pulmonary blood vessels from 58 patients in the National Heart, Lung, and Blood Institute Primary Pulmonary Hypertension Registry. Circulation 80:1198, 1989. Copyright 1989 by American Heart Association.

are prone to bleeding and may be manifest clinically as overt hemoptysis in affected patients. The perfusion lung scan in these patients may show "hot spots" reflective of the local areas within the lung that have increased vascularity. These are typically seen at the lung periphery and can be confirmed by pulmonary angiography. The natural history of this form of PPH is not yet defined.

CLINICAL FEATURES

NATURAL HISTORY AND SYMPTOMATOLOGY. The most extensive study on the natural history of PPH was reported from the NIH Registry on Primary Pulmonary Hypertension from 1981 to 1987.[46] The study included the long-term follow-up of 194 patients in whom PPH was diagnosed by established clinical and hemodynamic criteria. Sixty-three per cent of the patients were female, with the mean age of 36 ± 15 years (range 1 to 81 years) at the time of diagnosis. The mean interval from the onset of symptoms to diagnosis was 2 years, and the most common presenting symptoms were dyspnea (60 per cent), fatigue (19 per cent), syncope or near syncope (13 per cent), and Raynaud's phenomenon (10 per cent). There was no ethnic differentiation, with 12.3 per cent being black and 2.3 per cent being Hispanic.

Syncope is a characteristic symptom of PPH, assumed to be due to a fixed cardiac output. A recent study on the systolic function and interactions of the left and right ventricles in patients with PPH revealed an increased right ventricular end-diastolic volume and reduced right ventricular ejection fraction, with a greater stroke volume than the left ventricle.[115] The mechanism for maintaining cardiac output with exercise was primarily through increased heart rate, as the stroke volume actually decreased. Right ventricular ejection fraction decreased with exercise, suggesting exercise-induced right ventricular failure. This is expected because pulmonary artery pressure increases with exercise in PPH. Left ventricular ejection fraction is maintained, however, but left ventricular end-diastolic volume decreases and left ventricular end-systolic volume becomes extremely small, suggesting that the left ventricle is shortening to its maximal extent. The fact that left ventricular end-diastolic and systolic volumes decreased, whereas right ventricular end-systolic and diastolic volumes remained unchanged, supports the concept that underfilling, and not external compression, accounts for the small left ventricular chamber size observed in PPH. Syncope occurs because of exercise-induced right ventricular failure whereby heart rate becomes the only mechanism by which to increase cardiac output, which has limited effectiveness.

On *physical examination* an increased pulmonic component of the second heart sound was the most common finding (93 per cent), with tricuspid regurgitation noted in 40 per cent and peripheral edema in 32 per cent. In 90 per cent of patients the chest radiograph revealed enlargement of the main pulmonary arteries, and the electrocardiogram revealed right ventricular hypertrophy in 87 per cent. The clinical profiles of these patients were remarkably similar to those in a previously reported retrospective study of 120 patients from the Mayo Clinic.[65] In the Mayo Clinic series, 75 per cent of the patients were women with a mean age of 34 years (range 3 to 64 years) and a mean interval from onset of symptoms to diagnosis of 1.9 years.

The NIH Registry also revealed that restrictive changes in pulmonary function testing and reduced diffusing capacity for carbon monoxide were very common, with the forced vital capacity approximately 80 per cent of predicted and the diffusing capacity 70 per cent of predicted. These changes, however, do not relate with any measure of severity of the pulmonary hypertension. An additional, virtually universal finding was mild to moderate hypoxemia (mean Po_2 72 ± 16 mm Hg), which is attributed to the effect of a low mixed venous oxygen from low cardiac output amplified by underlying ventilation-perfusion inequality.

The hemodynamic findings also suggested that the severity of the disease could be related to a rising right atrial pressure and falling cardiac index, both of which reflect underlying right ventricular dysfunction. The fact that the mean pulmonary artery pressure was similar in patients whose duration of symptoms was less than 1 year and those who were symptomatic for more than 3 years suggests that the pulmonary artery pressure rises to fairly high levels early in the course of the disease.

Univariate analysis from the Registry pointed to the mean right atrial pressure, mean pulmonary artery pressure, and cardiac index as well as the diffusing capacity from carbon monoxide as significantly related to mortality.[116] In addition, the New York Heart Association classification also has been shown to relate very strongly to survival (Fig. 25–8). Based on estimates obtained from the proportional hazards model, a regression equation was developed that describes the relation between these three hemodynamic variables and subsequent mortality.

$$P(t) = [(t)]A(x,y,z)$$
$$H(t) = [0.88 - 0.14t + 0.01t^2]$$
$$A(x,y,z) = e^{(0.007325x) + (0.0526y) - (0.3275z)}$$

Where p(t) = per cent survival at t years, t = number of years, x = mean pulmonary artery pressure, y = mean right atrial pressure, and z = cardiac index. This equation has since been validated in two subsequent studies,[117,118] suggesting that baseline hemodynamic characteristics are very predictive of outcome.

The most common cause of death in patients with PPH in the NIH Registry was progressive right heart failure (47 per cent). Sudden cardiac death (both witnessed and unwitnessed) occurred in 26 per cent. Of interest is that sudden cardiac death was limited to patients who were New York Heart Association Class IV, suggesting that it is a manifestation of end-stage disease rather than a phenomenon that occurs early or unpredictably in the clinical course of the disease. The remainder of the patients died of some other medical complication such as pneumonia or

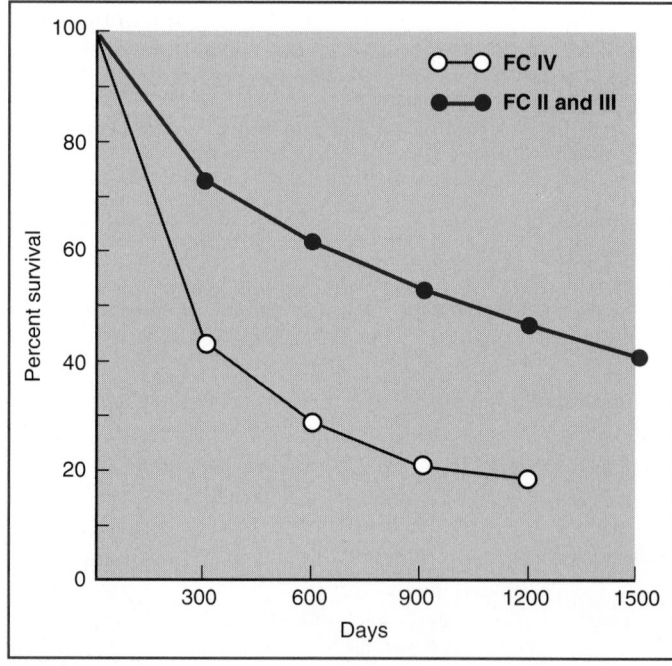

FIGURE 25–8. Five-year survival of patients enrolled in the NIH Registry on PPH based on New York Heart Association functional class. Survival of patients who were FC II and III was slightly greater than 3 years, whereas the mean survival of patients who were FC IV was approximately 6 months. (Adapted from D'Alonzo, G. E., Barst, R. G., Levy, P. S., et al.: Survival in patients with primary pulmonary hypertension: Results of a national prospective registry. Ann. Intern. Med. *115*:343, 1991.)

bleeding, suggesting that patients with PPH do not tolerate coexistent medical conditions well. In the Registry experience there were no deaths or sustained morbidity related to the diagnostic evaluation done at baseline assessment. It should be pointed out, however, that these were university centers with an established experience in the management of patients with PPH.

MECHANISMS FOR RIGHT VENTRICULAR FAILURE. It is presumed that right ventricular dysfunction in patients with chronic pulmonary hypertension is a result of chronic pressure overload and associated volume overload with the development of tricuspid regurgitation. However, animal studies suggest that right ventricular ischemia may also be a feature and potentially a very common one.[118-121] The mechanism of right ventricular failure in pulmonary hypertension is complex. The chronic pressure overload that induces right ventricular hypertrophy and reduced contractility has been shown to cause a reduction in coronary blood flow to the right ventricular myocardium, which can produce right ventricular ischemia, both acutely and chronically. This appears to be a result of a reduction in right ventricular coronary artery driving pressure. In an interesting animal study by Vlahakes et al.,[122] acute right ventricular failure due to right ventricular hypertension was overcome by increasing central aortic pressure, which resulted in increasing right ventricular coronary driving pressure. Murray and Vatner[123] reported that a moderate increase in aortic pressure was accompanied by a large increase in right ventricular myocardial perfusion only when the autonomic nervous system was blocked with an alpha blocker. As the symptom of angina associated with PPH is characteristic of myocardial ischemia, it likely represents ongoing ischemia due to this phenomenon.

The clinical course of patients with PPH can be highly variable. However, with the onset of overt right ventricular failure manifested by worsening symptoms and systemic venous congestion, patient survival is generally limited to approximately 6 months. Understanding the clinical course of patients with PPH is important especially when considering major interventional therapy such as organ transplantation.

PHYSICAL EXAMINATION. Findings are consistent with pulmonary hypertension and right ventricular pressure overload: a large *a* wave in the jugular venous pulse; a low-volume carotid arterial pulse with a normal upstroke; a left parasternal (right ventricular) heave; a systolic pulsation produced by a dilated, tense pulmonary artery in the second left interspace; an ejection click and flow murmur in the same area; a closely split second heart sound with a loud pulmonic component; and a fourth heart sound of right ventricular origin. Late in the course, signs of right ventricular failure (hepatomegaly, peripheral edema, and ascites) may be present. Patients with severe pulmonary hypertension may also have prominent *v* waves in the jug-

ular venous pulse, owing to tricuspid regurgitation; a third heart sound of right ventricular origin; a high-pitched early diastolic murmur of pulmonic regurgitation; and a holosystolic murmur of tricuspid regurgitation. Cyanosis is a late finding in PPH and may be worsened by a patent foramen ovale with right-to-left shunting. Other causes for cyanosis include a markedly reduced cardiac output with systemic vasoconstriction and ventilation-perfusion mismatches in the lung. Uncommonly, the left laryngeal nerve becomes paralyzed as a consequence of compression by a dilated pulmonary artery (Ortner's syndrome).[124]

LABORATORY FINDINGS

HEMATOLOGICAL AND CHEMICAL STUDIES. Results of these studies are usually normal in patients with PPH. If there is chronic arterial oxygen desaturation, polycythemia may be present. A number of investigators have reported hypercoagulable states, abnormal platelet function, defects in fibrinolysis, and other abnormalities of coagulation in patients with PPH.[66,69] Abnormal liver function tests can indicate right ventricular failure with resultant systemic venous hypertension.

ELECTROCARDIOGRAPHY. The electrocardiogram in PPH usually exhibits right atrial and right ventricular enlargement. A direct correlation between the amplitude of the R in V_1, the R/S ratio in V_1, and the level of pulmonary arterial pressure has been reported.[125]

ROENTGENOGRAPHY. Radiographic examination of the chest in patients with PPH shows enlargement of the main pulmonary artery and its major branches, with marked tapering of peripheral arteries.[126,127] The right ventricle and atrium may also be enlarged. Fluoroscopic examination may disclose exaggerated pulsations of secondary pulmonary arterial branches, reflecting an elevation in pulmonary arterial pulse pressure. However, in contrast to the plethoric peripheral lung fields in patients with left-to-right shunts, oligemia is noted in these lung regions in patients with PPH. It has been suggested that survival in PPH correlates inversely with the size of the main pulmonary artery[127]—a reasonable suggestion because the latter correlates with the height of the pulmonary arterial pressure. The diameter of the pulmonary artery may be determined from computed tomographic (CT) scans and used to estimate pulmonary artery pressures.[128]

PULMONARY FUNCTION TESTS. Pulmonary function tests typically show mild restriction with a reduced diffusion capacity for carbon monoxide (DL_{CO}) and hypoxemia with hypocapnea. Some patients have increased residual volumes and reduced maximum voluntary ventilation.

ECHOCARDIOGRAPHY. This usually demonstrates enlargement of the right atrium and ventricle, normal or small left

FIGURE 25–9. Perfusion lung scans in patients with pulmonary hypertension. *A*, Patient with primary pulmonary hypertension (PPH). *B*, Patient with pulmonary thromboembolism causing pulmonary hypertension (PTE). Both perfusion scans are abnormal. The scan on the patient with PPH shows a mottled distribution in a nonsegmental, nonanatomic manner. The scan on the patient with PTE reveals lobar, segmental, and subsegmental defects highly suggestive of an anatomic obstruction to pulmonary blood flow.

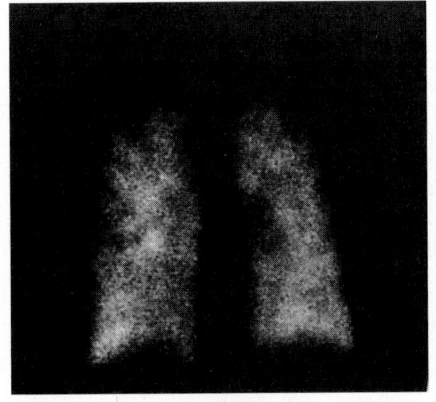
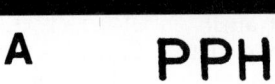
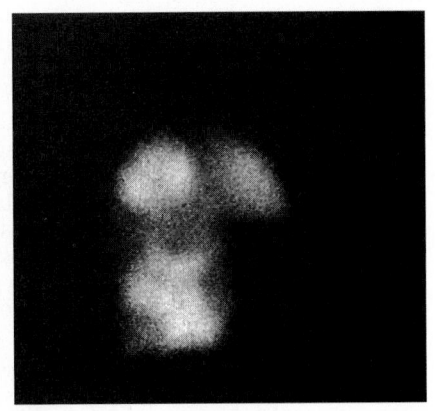

A PPH   **B PTE**

ventricular dimensions, and a thickened interventricular septum. The septal/posterior left ventricular wall ratio may be abnormally increased, as in hypertrophic obstructive cardiomyopathy, but the other echocardiographic signs characteristic of that condition are not present. Systolic prolapse of the mitral valve is frequently present, as is abnormal septal motion of the ventricular septum, due to chronic right ventricular pressure overload and reduced left ventricular filling.[129,130] Doppler echocardiographic evidence of right ventricular systolic hypertension may be obtained by measuring the velocity of the tricuspid regurgitant jet and using the Bernoulli formula (see p. 69). Doppler techniques have demonstrated left ventricular diastolic dysfunction with marked dependence on atrial contraction for ventricular filling.[130]

LUNG SCINTIGRAPHY. A perfusion lung scan is an essential component in making the correct diagnosis of PPH. It may reveal a relatively normal perfusion pattern or diffuse, patchy perfusion abnormalities.[131] The severity of the perfusion abnormality in lung scans does not parallel the hemodynamics, as serial lung scans performed in patients with PPH over time do not show progressive changes consistent with the patients' worsening clinical state.[131] A perfusion lung scan should help distinguish patients with PPH from those who have pulmonary hypertension secondary to chronic pulmonary thromboembolism[132] (Fig. 25–9). The risk associated with lung scans in PPH has been grossly overstated. The early literature reported three patients with pulmonary hypertension who died following lung scans, but it is not clear that the deaths were caused by the procedure. In the NIH Registry on PPH not one morbid clinical event was associated with the performance of lung scan in any of the patients with pulmonary hypertension.[46]

PULMONARY ANGIOGRAPHY. Pulmonary angiography is essential to establish the correct diagnosis in a patient with presumed PPH in whom the perfusion lung scan suggests segmental or lobar defects. Typically pulmonary angiography demonstrates large central pulmonary arteries with marked peripheral tapering. Postmortem arteriograms demonstrate the absence of "background haze" secondary to the loss of small, nonmuscular pulmonary arterioles[67] (Fig. 25–10). Although pulmonary angiography carries an increased risk in patients with PPH, it can be performed safely if adequate precautions are taken.[65] The NIH Registry contains no deaths or serious morbidity associated with pulmonary angiography.

Maintenance of adequate oxygenation by the administration of supplemental oxygen and the avoidance of vasovagal reactions (and rapid treatment of those that occur with intravenous atropine) should reduce the associated risk in this patient group. The placement of an arterial line for continuous arterial pressure monitoring is advised, and nonionic contrast agents appear to be better tolerated. Injections are preferably limited to the individual lungs or specific lobes to reduce the contrast load. Pulmonary wedge angiography, using a segmental angiographic technique with hand injection of small amounts of angiographic contrast through the terminal lumen of a balloon-flotation catheter while the balloon is inflated, is not a substitute for pulmonary angiography.

CARDIAC CATHETERIZATION. The diagnosis of PPH cannot be confirmed without cardiac catheterization (Table 25–2). Besides allowing the exclusion of other causes, it also establishes the severity of disease and allows the assessment of prognosis. By definition, patients with PPH should have a low or normal pulmonary capillary wedge pressure. Although it has often been stated that one may be unable to obtain an accurate wedge pressure in these patients, this is rarely the case in experienced hands.[133] However, when an increased wedge pressure is obtained, it must be correlated with left ventricular end-diastolic pressure and not attributed to a "falsely elevated" reading. It has been shown that left ventricular diastolic compliance becomes significantly

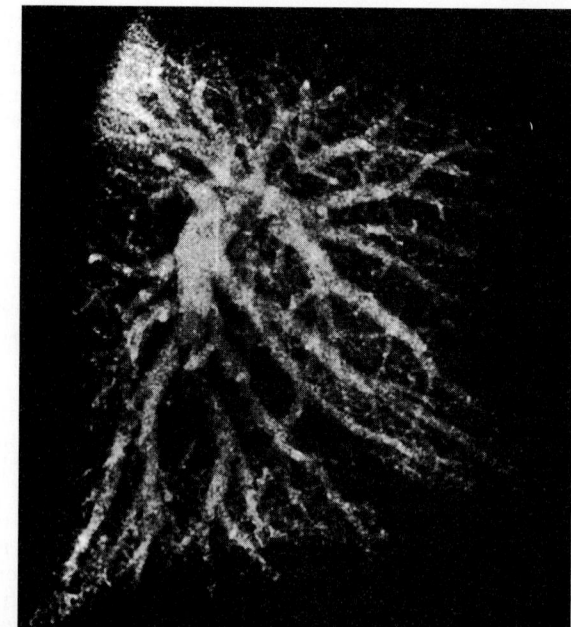

A

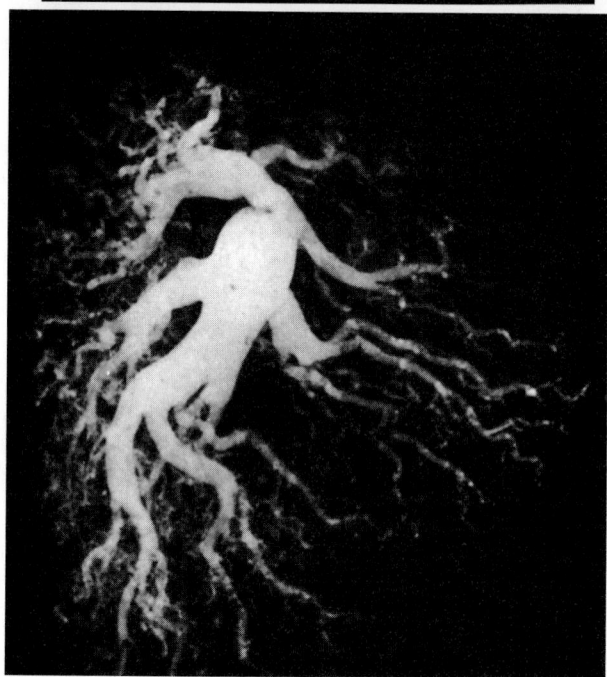

B

FIGURE 25–10. *A,* Postmortem pulmonary arteriogram of a normal lung in a 22-year-old man. The caliber of the pulmonary arteries tapers down gradually, and there is a rather dense background filling of vessels. *B,* Postmortem pulmonary arteriogram from an 18-year-old man with unexplained plexogenic pulmonary arteriopathy (primary pulmonary hypertension). The main branches are dilated. (From Wagenvoort, C. A., and Wagenvoort, N.: Pathology of Pulmonary Hypertension. New York, copyright 1977, reprinted by permission of John Wiley and Sons, Inc.)

impaired in PPH and parallels the severity of the disease; thus, pulmonary capillary wedge pressures tend to rise slightly in the late stages of PPH, although they rarely exceed 16 mm Hg.[134] The measurements of all right-sided pressures are properly made at expiration to avoid incorporating negative intrathoracic pressures.

It can be extremely difficult to pass a catheter into the pulmonary artery in patients with pulmonary hypertension owing to the tricuspid regurgitation, dilated right atrium and ventricle, and low cardiac output. The flow-directed thermodilution balloon catheters which are properly used also lack stiffness and can be difficult to place. A specific flow-directed thermodilution balloon catheter has been developed for patients with pulmonary hypertension (Ameri-

CONDITION	TEST APPLIED	FINDING
Congenital heart disease	Step-up in O_2 saturation in right heart Step-down in O_2 saturation in left heart Cardiac angiography	Left-to-right shunt and location of shunt Right-to-left shunt and location of shunt Anatomic definition
Peripheral pulmonary artery stenoses	Intrapulmonary arterial pressure Pulmonary angiogram	Intrapulmonary arterial pressure gradients Pulmonary arterial branch stenoses
Major pulmonary arterial occlusion by clot, or tumor*	Continuous pressure recording from distal pulmonary artery to main pulmonary artery Selective or main pulmonary angiography	Focal pressure gradient in a lobar or larger pulmonary artery, intravascular filling defect or narrowing
Mitral stenosis Cor triatriatum Supravalvular mitral ring	Simultaneous wedge and left ventricular pressure recording	An elevated wedge pressure and mean mitral valve diastolic pressure gradient >3 mm Hg at rest, both of which increase with exercise
Mitral regurgitation	Simultaneous wedge and left ventricular pressure recording Left ventriculogram	Large systolic pressure wave in wedge tracing. Regurgitation of contrast from left ventricular angiogram into the left atrium.
Left ventricular diastolic dysfunction	Left ventricular pressure	Left ventricular end-diastolic pressure >15 mm Hg LVEDP response to intravenous fluid challenge; normalization of LVEDP with marked reduction in pulmonary artery pressure with intravenous nitroprusside.

* Ventilation and perfusion lung scans precede catheterization.
LVEDP = left ventricular end-diastolic pressure
Modified from Reeves, J. T., and Groves, B. M.: Approach to the patient with pulmonary hypertension. *In* Weir, E. K., and Reeves, J. T.: Pulmonary Hypertension. Mt. Kisco, NY, Futura Publishing Co., 1984, p. 20.

can Edwards Laboratories, Irvine, California) which has an extra port for the placement of a 0.32-inch guidewire to provide better stiffness to the catheter.[135] The risk associated with cardiac catheterization in patients with PPH is extremely low in experienced hands, but deaths have been reported.[65]

DIAGNOSIS

(Table 25–3)

It is essential that diagnostic efforts be pursued vigorously in patients with severe pulmonary hypertension in order to ensure that no patient with secondary pulmonary hypertension is erroneously classified as having PPH. Secondary pulmonary hypertension is often treatable in that the cause can be attacked directly. Patients with PPH may tolerate diagnostic procedures poorly. These individuals can experience sudden cardiovascular collapse and even death during or shortly after the induction of general anesthesia for surgical procedures, during cardiac catheterization and angiography.

The *differential diagnosis* of PPH includes a number of well-defined causes of secondary pulmonary hypertension. Exclusion of mitral stenosis, congenital cardiac defects (including cor triatriatum), pulmonary thromboembolism, and pulmonary venous obstruction by means of catheterization and angiography is imperative. "Silent" mitral stenosis, i.e., without the characteristic diastolic murmur, can be excluded by means of echocardiographic visualization of the motion of the mitral valve and the absence of a transvalvular pressure gradient (Chap. 32). *Congenital cardiac defects* with Eisenmenger syndrome can usually be ruled out if significant left-to-right or right-to-left shunts are absent, although occasional patients with equal pulmonary and systemic vascular resistances may have no detectable shunt at rest. Transesophageal echocardiography can reliably detect congenital cardiac defects and distinguish an atrial septal defect from a patent foramen ovale.[136] *Cor triatriatum* (see p. 923) is recognized by appropriate hemodynamic studies and angiographic visualization of the left atrial membrane. This entity presents a characteristic left atrial echocardiogram with normal mitral valve motion. Cardiac catheterization reveals a hemodynamic pattern similar in some ways to mitral stenosis, i.e., a diastolic pressure gradient between the left ventricle and the pulmonary capillary bed. *Pulmonary embolism* (Chap. 46) can be excluded by pulmonary angiography,[137] and *sickle cell disease with in situ pulmonary vascular thrombosis* (Chap. 57) can be evaluated by hemoglobin electrophoresis. The presence of severe *pulmonary parenchymal disease* can be recognized by the characteristic physical findings, chest roentgenogram, pulmonary function tests, and high-resolution chest computed tomography. *Collagen vascular disease* is suggested by the involvement of other organ systems or the presence of abnormal immunological phenomena, such as antinuclear antibodies and LE cells (Chap. 56).

TREATMENT

LIFE STYLE CHANGES. The diagnosis of PPH does not necessarily imply total disability for the patient. However, physical activity can be associated with elevated pulmonary artery pressures, as marked hemodynamic changes have been documented to occur early in the onset of increased physical activity.[138] For that reason, graded exercise activities, such as bike riding or swimming, in which patients can gradually increase their workload and easily limit the extent of their work, are thought to be safer than isometric activities. Isometric activities such as lifting weights or stair climbing can be associated with syncopal events and should be limited or avoided.

The subject of pregnancy should also be discussed with women of childbearing age. The physiological changes that occur in pregnancy can potentially activate the disease and result in the death of the mother and/or the child.[139] Besides the increased circulating blood volume and oxygen consumption that will increase right ventricular work, circulating procoagulant factors and the risk of pulmonary embolism from deep vein thrombosis and amniotic fluid are serious concerns. Syncope and cardiac arrest have also been reported to occur during active labor and delivery, and a syndrome of postpartum circulatory collapse has also been described.[140] For these reasons surgical sterilization should be given strong consideration by women with PPH or their husbands.

TABLE 25–3   DIAGNOSTIC STUDIES USEFUL FOR ELUCIDATING CAUSES OF PULMONARY HYPERTENSION

POTENTIAL CAUSE OF PULMONARY HYPERTENSION	POSSIBLE DIAGNOSTIC STUDIES
Pulmonary thromboembolic disease	Ventilation/perfusion scans and/or pulmonary angiography
Pulmonary venous thrombosis or obstruction	Chest x-ray, angiography, computed tomography, magnetic resonance imaging
Congenital intra-cardiac shunts causing increased pulmonary blood flow	Transesophageal echocardiography
Increased left atrial pressure; secondary to mitral or aortic valve disease, left ventricular dysfunction, or systemic hypertension	Pulmonary artery wedge pressure or left atrial pressure (via patent foramen ovale) (>15 mm Hg)
Pulmonary airways disease (e.g., chronic bronchitis and emphysema)	Respiratory function tests (FVC/FEV$_1$)
Hypoxic pulmonary hypertension associated with (i) impaired ventilation; either central (CNS) or peripheral (chest wall problems or upper airway obstruction); (ii) residence at high altitude	Sleep apnea studies and respiratory tests
Interstitial lung disease, pneumoconioses and fibrosis (e.g., silicosis, rheumatoid disease, and sarcoidosis)	Chest x-ray, spirometry and carbon monoxide diffusion, high-resolution chest computed tomography
Collagen disease (e.g., SLE, polyarteritis nodosa, scleroderma)	Serology, immunogenetic studies, skin, muscle, or other tissue biopsy, esophageal motility studies
Parasitic disease (schistosomiasis or filariasis)	Rectal biopsy, complement fixation, skin tests, blood smears
Cirrhosis or portal hypertension	Liver function tests
Peripheral pulmonary artery stenosis (including Takayasu's disease and fibrosing mediastinitis)	Selective pulmonary angiography, or pressure gradient at catheterization
Sickle cell disease	Erythrocyte morphology, hemoglobin electrophoresis
Choriocarcinoma and hydatidiform mole	Serum or urinary beta subunit of chorionic gonadotrophin
Intravenous injection of pulverized pills	Lung biopsy

Modified from Weir, E. K.: Diagnosis and management of primary pulmonary hypertension. *In* Weir, E. K., and Reeves, J. T.: Pulmonary Hypertension. Mt. Kisco, NY, Futura Publishing Co., 1984, p. 141.

DIGOXIN. The value of digoxin in patients with PPH has never been studied specifically. Animal studies performed on the utility of digoxin in right ventricular systolic overload show that prior administration helped prevent the reduction in contractility of the right ventricle.[141] More recently, digoxin has been shown to have sympatholytic properties and to restore baroreceptor tone toward normal in patients with congestive heart failure (see p. 499). Given that patients with advanced PPH have low cardiac outputs with resting tachycardia and systemic venous congestion, it makes intuitive sense to believe that digoxin may be as helpful in these patients as it is in patients with left ventricular failure.

DIURETIC THERAPY. Diuretics appear to be of marked benefit in symptom relief in patients with PPH. Their traditional role has been limited to patients manifesting right ventricular failure and systemic venous congestion. However, patients with advanced PPH can have increased left ventricular filling pressures that contribute to the symptoms of dyspnea and orthopnea which can be relieved with diuretics.[142] Diuretics may also serve to reduce right ventricular wall stress in patients with concomitant tricuspid regurgitation and volume overload. The fear that diuretics will induce systemic hypotension is unfounded, as the main factor limiting the cardiac output is pulmonary vascular resistance and not pulmonary blood volume. Patients with severe venous congestion may require high doses of loop diuretics or the use of combined diuretics. In these instances electrolytes need to be carefully watched for hyponatremia and hypokalemia.

SUPPLEMENTAL OXYGEN THERAPY. Hypoxic pulmonary vasoconstriction can contribute to pulmonary vascular disease in patients with alveolar hypoxia from parenchymal lung disease.[143,144] Supplemental low-flow oxygen alleviates arterial hypoxemia and attenuates the pulmonary hypertension in these disorders[143]; in contrast, most patients with PPH do not exhibit resting hypoxemia and derive little benefit from supplemental oxygen therapy.[145] Patients who experience arterial oxygen desaturation with activity, however, may benefit from ambulatory supplemental oxygen as they develop increased oxygen extraction in the face of a fixed oxygen delivery. Patients with severe right-sided heart failure and resting hypoxemia resulting from a markedly increased oxygen extraction at rest should be treated with continuous oxygen therapy to maintain their arterial oxygen saturation above 90 per cent. Patients with hypoxemia due to a right-to-left shunt via a patent foramen ovale do not improve their level of oxygenation to an appreciable degree with supplemental oxygen.

VASODILATOR TREATMENT

Because of early reports showing a reduction in pulmonary artery pressure following the acute administration of vasodilators,[50–52] it has been presumed that vasodilators are the mainstay of treatment in patients with PPH. This, however, is not supported by the published literature over the past two decades. Vasodilators appear to be effective in a subset of patients with PPH, but many complexities regarding vasodilator administration make their use in these patients very difficult.

The first principle in utilizing vasodilators in patients with PPH is to establish accurate baseline hemodynamics. Because substantial hemodynamic variability has been reported to exist in the pulmonary vascular bed which will produce changes in cardiac output and pulmonary artery pressure from moment to moment, serial baseline recordings are required in order to evaluate the magnitude of change in hemodynamics that may be attributed to variability rather than to drug effect.[146] The practice of attributing "peak" effect of the drug to an administered agent introduces bias into the assessment. Thus, by choosing the highest level of pulmonary artery pressure as the baseline and the subsequent lowest one as drug effect, one may be misled to attribute a favorable influence from a medication when, in fact, no effect, or even an adverse one, is occurring.

It must also be emphasized that the hemodynamic assessment of the entire circulatory system is essential when determining the influence of drugs in these patients. Small changes in pulmonary artery pressure are likely due to variability and are not related to direct drug influence. Changes in pulmonary vascular resistance cannot be directly measured but are computed by the change in pulmonary pressure and cardiac output simultaneously. Because thermodilution cardiac output, the method that is most commonly used in these patients, can have large errors in reproducibility, particular care should be taken in the methodology of thermodilution used in these patients. In addition, when an underlying right-to-left shunt exists or there is concern about severe tricuspid regurgitation, the Fick determination of cardiac output is preferred.

Changes in pulmonary capillary wedge pressure can have important influences on the determination of pulmonary vascular resistance. A

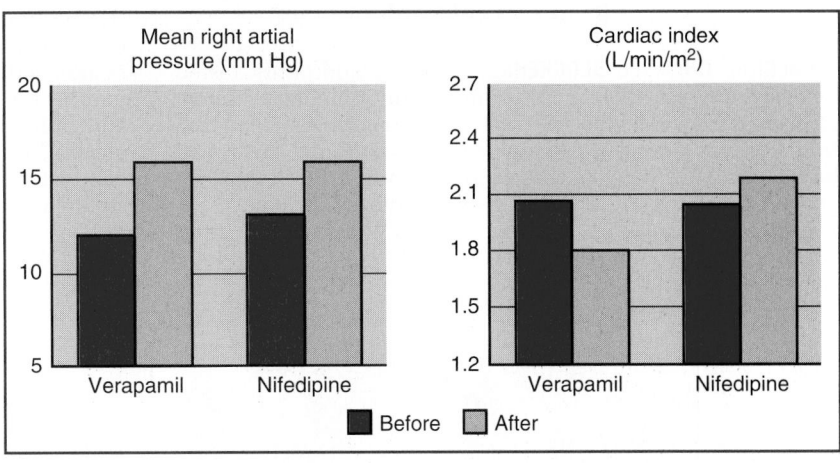

FIGURE 25–11. Adverse effects of calcium blockers in pulmonary hypertension. The hemodynamic effects of verapamil and nifedipine in patients with pulmonary hypertension are shown. An increase in right atrial pressure in association with no significant change in cardiac index as produced by nifedipine suggests that right ventricular dysfunction is occurring. The increased right atrial pressure associated with a fall in cardiac index, as produced by verapamil, suggests that negative inotropic effects are producing overt right ventricular failure. (Adapted from Packer, M., Medina, N., and Yushak, M.: Adverse hemodynamic and clinical effects of calcium channel blockade in pulmonary hypertension secondary to obliterative pulmonary vascular disease. Reprinted with permission from the American College of Cardiology. J. Am. Coll. Cardiol. 4:890, 1994.)

rising capillary wedge pressure due to an increased cardiac output may be the first sign of impending left ventricular failure and an adverse effect of a drug, whereas the calculated pulmonary vascular resistance may become lower and suggest a beneficial effect. The right atrial pressure also reflects the filling characteristics of the right ventricle. Right atrial pressure increase in the face of a rising cardiac output suggests right ventricular diastolic dysfunction[147] (Fig. 25–11). Resting heart rate is a physiological parameter of marked importance in patients with congestive heart failure, and treatments that cause an increased heart rate are likely to yield deleterious long-term results. Finally, systemic arterial oxygen content should be evaluated in patients with PPH. Effective vasodilator drugs can result in vasodilatation of blood vessels supplying poorly ventilated areas of the lung and worsen hypoxemia.[148] This is particularly noticeable in patients with underlying chronic lung disease. For all of these reasons it has been advocated that vasodilators be initiated only in the hospital setting with central catheter placement for direct hemodynamic recordings and never initiated in the outpatient setting.[149]

ACUTE TESTING WITH INTRAVENOUS VASODILATORS

Intravenous vasodilators may be of value in the short-term assessment of pulmonary vasodilator reserve in patients with PPH. Historically, tolazoline received attention as an agent to acutely test the responsiveness of the pulmonary vascular bed in patients with pulmonary hypertension from several causes.[150,151] However, it is poorly tolerated acutely owing to its side effects and has largely been replaced by other agents. Acetylcholine was one of the first medications used to evaluate patients with PPH.[152,153] It is rapidly inactivated by the lung, which explains why the intravenous administration seems to produce selective pulmonary vasodilator effects. Although it has been reported to produce substantial acute reductions in pulmonary artery pressure in some patients, chronic therapy with this drug is not feasible. Isoproterenol is a potent beta-adrenergic agent that affects both the systemic and pulmonary vascular beds and increases cardiac output by chronotropic and inotropic mechanisms. It is considered a pulmonary vasodilator because it results in a lowering of the calculated pulmonary vascular resistance.[154] However, it rarely results in a substantial lowering of the pulmonary artery pressure in patients with pulmonary hypertension because of its more direct effect in increasing cardiac output.[155] Phentolamine is a potent alpha-adrenergic blocker that has been shown to cause pulmonary vasodilatation in animals and humans.[156,157] Its widespread use is limited by the profound systemic hypotension that occurs upon administration, and it is generally not used in the evaluation of PPH.[158] Sodium nitroprusside is a potent vasodilator that acts on arterial and venous beds. Its short half-life is also an advantage because the effects rapidly dissipate when infusion of the drug is stopped. Like phentolamine, its use as a test of vasodilator reserve is limited by the marked lowering in systemic blood pressure that occurs.

ADENOSINE. This substance is an intermediate product in the metabolism of adenosine triphosphate that has potent vasodilator properties through its action on specific vascular receptors.[159] In addition to pulmonary vasodilatation, it can also produce systemic and coronary vasodilatation.[160,161] It is believed to stimulate the endothelial cell and vascular smooth muscle receptors of the A2 type, which induce vascular smooth muscle relaxation by increasing cyclic AMP.[162] In patients with PPH, adenosine has been shown to be an extremely potent vasodilator and predictive of the subsequent effects of intravenous prostacyclin and oral calcium channel blockers[163,164] (Fig. 25–12). Adenosine has an extremely short half-life (less than 5 seconds), which provides a safety net by its rapid dissolution should any adverse side effects occur. It is administered intravenously in doses of 50 ng/kg/min and titrated upward every 2 minutes until the patient develops uncomfortable symptoms (such as chest tightness or dyspnea). It should be noted that adenosine is given as an infusion, and not as an intravenous bolus as is used to treat supraventricular tachyarrhythmias.

PROSTACYCLIN. This substance (epoprostenol sodium, or PGI$_2$) is a metabolite of arachidonic acid that is synthesized and released from vascular endothelium and smooth muscle.[35] The vasodilatory effects are thought to be mediated by activation of specific membrane PGI$_2$ receptors that are also coupled to the adenylate cyclase system.[35,165] Other effects include the inhibition of platelet activation and aggregation as well as leukocyte adhesion to the endothelium.[166] Prostacyclin has been used as an acute test of vasodilator reserve in patients with PPH.[167] Like adenosine, its short half-life allows the drug to be discontinued if any acute adverse effects result. Also similar to adenosine, it is administered incrementally, at 2 ng/kg/min and increased every 15 to 30 minutes until systemic effects such as headache, flushing, or nausea occur which limit the acute dose titration. Favorable acute effects from prostacyclin appears to be predictive of a favorable response to oral calcium channel blockers[168] and determination of this effect.

NITRIC OXIDE (NO). This substance, whose activity is identical to that of EDRF, is produced from L-arginine by NO synthase.[38a,169] NO diffuses to the vascular smooth muscle and mediates vasodilatation by stimulating soluble guanylate cyclase to produce cyclic GMP. Because it binds very rapidly to hemoglobin with a high affinity and is thereby inactivated, inhalation of NO gas results in selective pulmonary vascular effects without influencing the systemic circulation.[38a,169] The inhalation of NO by patients with PPH has been shown to produce a reduction in pulmonary vascular resistance acutely, similar to that achieved with intravenous adenosine.[170] NO has also been shown to be effective in patients with pulmonary hypertension secondary to congenital heart disease and the adult respiratory distress syndrome.[171] Although as yet untested, NO should produce vasodilatory effects similar to those of adenosine and prostacyclin in the initial assessment of pulmonary vasodilator reserve in these patients.

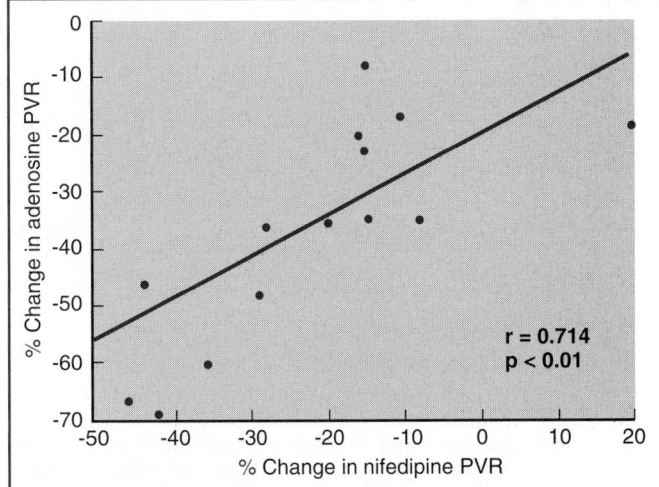

FIGURE 25–12. Testing of pulmonary vasodilator reserve with an infusion of intravenous adenosine. The per cent reduction in pulmonary vascular resistance (PVR) from intravenous adenosine challenge and the subsequent effect of nifedipine in patients with primary pulmonary hypertension are shown. The relative vasodilatory effect on PVR was greater for adenosine than for nifedipine. However, failure to respond to adenosine predicted failure to respond to nifedipine. (From Schrader, B., Inbar, S., Kaufmann, E., et al.: Comparison of the effects of adenosine and nifedipine in pulmonary hypertension. Reprinted with permission from the American College of Cardiology. J. Am. Coll. Cardiol. 19:1060, 1992.)

CALCIUM CHANNEL BLOCKERS. Of the vasodilators tested in patients with PPH, the calcium channel blockers appear to have the widest usage. Early reports utilizing conventional doses failed to demonstrate a chronic sustained benefit.[172-175] Moreover, the calcium channel blockers have properties that could worsen the underlying pulmonary hypertension, including negative inotropic effects on right ventricular function (Fig. 25–11) and reflex sympathetic stimulation, which may increase resting heart rate.[147,176] Recently it has been reported that patients with PPH who are challenged with very high doses of calcium blockers may manifest a dramatic reduction in pulmonary artery pressure and pulmonary vascular resistance which, upon serial catheterization, has been maintained for over 5 years[117,177] (Fig. 25–13A). Importantly, the patient's quality of life is restored with improved functional class, and survival (94 per cent at 5 years) is improved compared with nonresponders and historical control subjects (36 per cent) (Fig. 25–13B).

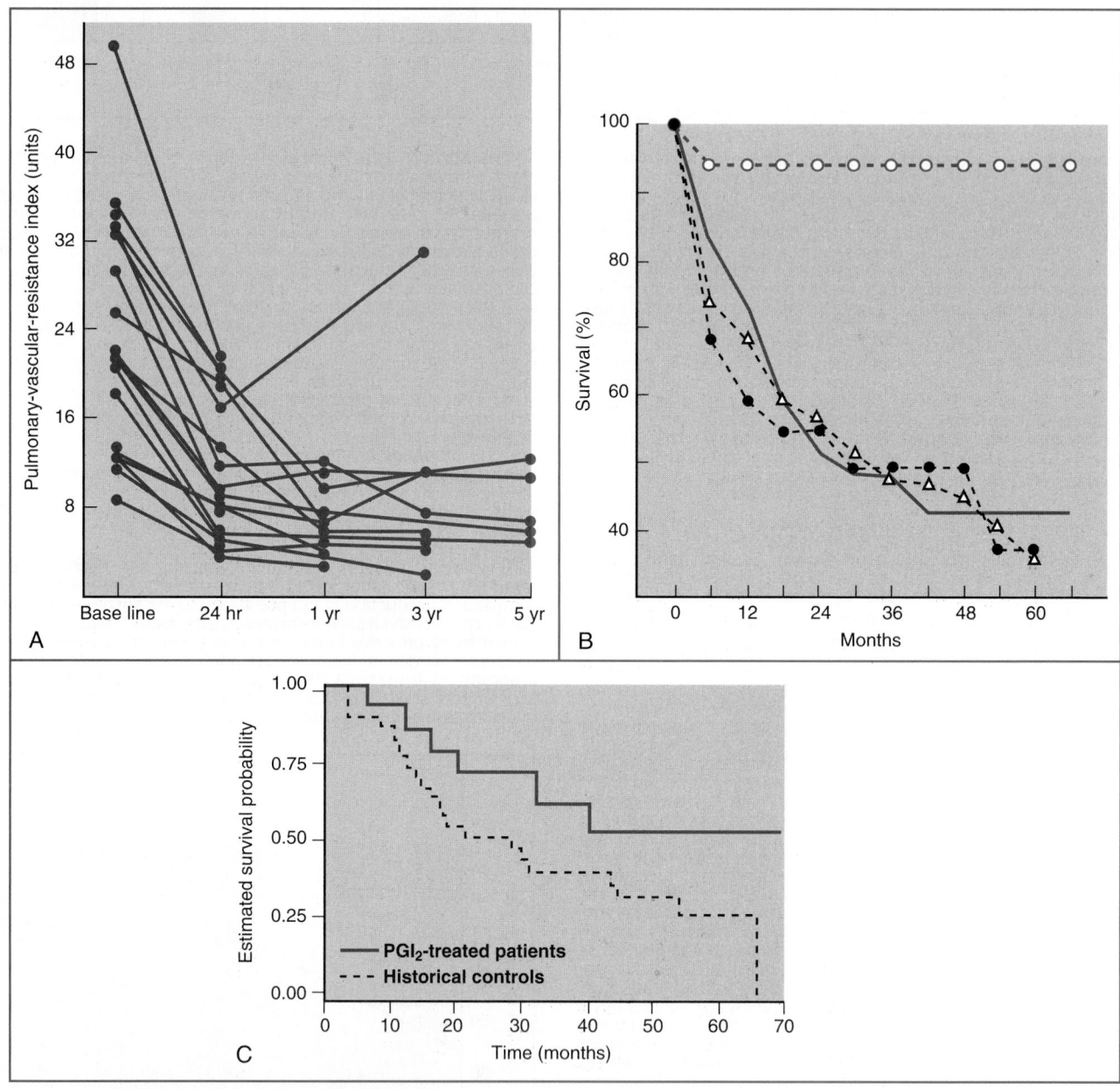

FIGURE 25–13. *A,* Hemodynamic effects of high doses of calcium channel blockers on patients with primary pulmonary hypertension followed over 5 years. The acute reduction in pulmonary vascular resistance that was achieved after 24 hours was maintained over 5 years, as documented by serial catheterizations. The patient who appeared not to have the sustained reduction in pulmonary vascular resistance was studied only after 3 years and was found not to be taking the high dose of calcium channel blockers as prescribed. *B,* The effect of high doses of calcium channel blockers on survival over 5 years in patients with primary pulmonary hypertension. Patients who responded to the high-dose regimen *(open circles)* had a 95 per cent 5-year survival compared with the nonresponders *(solid line),* who had a 36 per cent 5-year survival. This was similar to patients studied in the National Institutes of Health Registry on PPH *(triangles),* as well as patients from the University of Illinois only *(solid circles). C,* The effect of intravenous prostacyclin on survival in patients with primary pulmonary hypertension. The survival of patients given a chronic infusion of prostacyclin and followed out to 5.5 years is compared to functional class III and IV patients from the NIH Registry (historical controls). (*A* and *B* from Rich, S., Kaufmann, E., and Levy, P. S.: The effects of high doses of calcium channel blockers on survival of primary pulmonary hypertension. N. Engl. J. Med. *327:*76, 1992. *C,* from Barst, R. J., Rubin, L. J., McGoon, M. D., et al.: Survival of primary pulmonary hypertension with longterm continuous intravenous prostacyclin. Ann. Intern. Med. *121:*409, 1994.)

This experience suggests that some patients with PPH have the ability to have their pulmonary hypertension reversed and their quality of life and survival enhanced. It is unknown if the response to calcium channel blockers identifies two subsets of patients with PPH, or different stages of PPH, or a combination of both. However, it is essential to point out that patients who do not exhibit a dramatic hemodynamic response to calcium channel blockers do not appear to benefit from their long-term administration. Unfortunately, it is becoming common practice for physicians to prescribe calcium channel blockers at conventional doses to all patients with pulmonary hypertension, often without hemodynamic guidance. This unfortunate practice may result in a quicker deterioration of these patients and should be strongly discouraged.

CHRONIC PROSTACYCLIN INFUSION THERAPY. Continuous infusion prostacyclin therapy has now been shown in prospective randomized trials to improve quality of life and symptoms related to PPH, exercise tolerance, hemodynamics, and survival.[178-180,180a] The initial enthusiasm for prostacyclin was based on the demonstration of pulmonary vasodilator effects when administered to experimental animals with acute pulmonary vasoconstriction, and subsequently to patients with primary pulmonary hypertension.[181-185] More recently, however, a prospective treatment trial was undertaken in which patients were randomized to receive chronic intravenous prostacyclin therapy independent of any acute response to the drug, with substantial benefits noted as well[180] (Fig. 25-13C). The long-term effects of prostacyclin in PPH may be related to its ability to restore the integrity of the pulmonary vascular endothelium and to produce antithrombotic effects, as well as to its vasodilator properties.

Prostacyclin is generally administered through a central venous catheter that is surgically implanted and delivered by an ambulatory infusion system. The delivery system is complex and requires patients to learn the techniques of sterile drug preparation, operation of the pump, and care of the intravenous catheter. Most of the serious complications that have occurred with prostacyclin therapy have been attributable to the delivery system and include catheter-related infections and thrombosis and temporary interruption of the infusion due to pump malfunction. Anecdotal reports of rebound pulmonary hypertension occurring in patients in whom the infusion was interrupted suggest that great care must be taken to ensure that the infusion is never stopped.

Side effects related to the prostacyclin therapy include flushing, headache, nausea, diarrhea, and a unique type of jaw discomfort that occurs with eating. In most patients these symptoms are minimal and well tolerated. Tachyphylaxis to the drug also develops, requiring a constant periodic dose increase to maintain its efficacy. To date chronic prostacyclin has been given in patients with PPH for over 5 years with continued favorable effectiveness. In some patients (Class IV) who are critically ill, it serves as a bridge to lung transplantation, stabilizing the patient to a more favorable preoperative state. Patients who are less critically ill may do so well on prostacyclin that they may delay the need to consider transplantation, perhaps indefinitely. Currently prostacyclin has been used only in Class III and IV patients, and it is not known how effective it may be in patients with less advanced disease.

ANTICOAGULANTS. Oral anticoagulant therapy is widely recommended for patients with PPH, although its clinical efficacy as a therapy is difficult to prove. A retrospective review of patients with PPH followed over a 15-year period at the Mayo Clinic suggested that patients who received warfarin had improved survival over those who did not.[65] Recently, the influence of warfarin therapy was investigated in patients with PPH who failed to respond to high doses of calcium channel blockers.[117] A significant improvement in survival was observed in those who

received anticoagulation, with a 1-year survival of 91 per cent and 3-year survival of 47 per cent, compared with 1 and 3 years of 62 per cent and 31 per cent, respectively, in patients who were not anticoagulated. The current recommendation is to use warfarin in relatively low doses, as has been recommended for prophylaxis of venous thromboembolism, controlling the INR to 1.5 to 2.5 times control.[47] Heparin, given its inhibitory effects on smooth muscle cell proliferation, might be a more suitable anticoagulant in PPH, although its use is more difficult. Adjusting to a partial thromboplastin time of 1.3 to 1.5 times control would make it a viable alternative treatment in patients considered to have a greater risk of hemorrhagic events (such as prior episodes of hemoptysis), or patients who for some reason cannot safely take warfarin.

ATRIAL SEPTOSTOMY

It has been presumed that intracardiac shunting, allowing blood flow from right to left, provides some type of protection to the right ventricle in the presence of pulmonary hypertension. It has also been noted that sudden cardiac death may be a more common occurrence in patients with PPH than in patients with Eisenmenger's physiology.[186]

Since 1983 there have been several reports of atrial septostomies performed in patients with PPH.[187-190] It has been suggested that it provides palliation to select patients, manifested primarily by improvement in the symptoms of syncope and right-sided heart failure, and possibly improving survival until more definitive therapy can be instituted. However, because it does not affect the underlying pulmonary vascular disease, it should be considered an adjunct palliative therapy only. Because it creates hypoxemia, only patients with fairly normal resting systemic arterial oxygen saturations can be considered candidates. At the present time this technique should be considered investigational. It is not an appropriate measure in the setting of acute right ventricular failure and impending cardiogenic shock.

HEART-LUNG AND LUNG TRANSPLANTATION
(See also p. 529)

Heart-lung transplantation has been performed successfully in patients with PPH for more than a decade.[191-194] Because these patients have pulmonary vascular disease and severe right ventricular dysfunction, it was originally believed that heart-lung transplant was the only transplantation option. The widespread application of heart-lung transplant, however, has been limited by the number of centers with expertise to perform the procedure, the scarcity of suitable donor organs, and the very long waiting times required for patients with end-stage right-heart failure. More recently, bilateral or double lung transplantation and single lung transplantation have been performed successfully in patients with PPH.[195,196] Hemodynamic studies have shown an immediate reduction in pulmonary artery pressure and

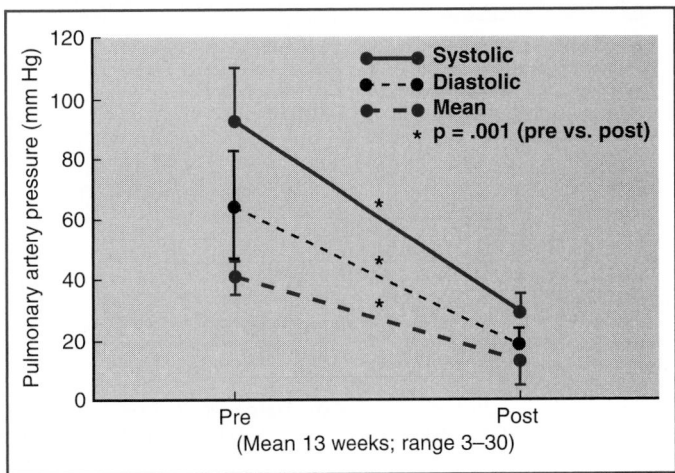

FIGURE 25-14. The hemodynamic effects of single lung transplantation in patients with pulmonary hypertension. The reduction in mean pulmonary artery pressure after a mean of 13 weeks following single lung transplantation in patients with pulmonary hypertension is shown. A significant reduction, approaching normal values, was achieved in almost all patients. (Reproduced with permission from Pasque, M. Q., Trulock, E. P., Kaiser, L. R., and Cooper, J. D.: Single lung transplantation for pulmonary hypertension. Circulation 84:2275, 1991. Copyright 1991 American Heart Association.)

pulmonary vascular resistance associated with improvement in right ventricular function[196] (Fig. 25–14).

The advantage of bilateral lung transplantation is that pulmonary blood flow is relatively evenly distributed between both lungs postoperatively and thus there is greater reserve for the patient should the patient sustain rejection or infection. The advantage of single lung transplantation is that it is a simpler operation, and there would be more potential suitable donors and shorter waiting times. However, studies have shown that more than 90 per cent of the pulmonary blood flow postoperatively goes to the transplanted lung, thus leaving the potential for marked ventilation-perfusion mismatch and little reserve should the transplanted lung sustain perioperative problems.[197]

The concern regarding restoration of right ventricular function has lessened by the finding that, as in patients undergoing pulmonary thromboendarterectomy for pulmonary hypertension, marked re-gression of right ventricular hypertrophy occurs in the postoperative recovery period following lung transplantation, with a dramatic improvement in right ventricular performance.[196] The major long-term problem in patients who survive the operation is the high incidence of bronchiolitis obliterans in the transplanted lungs, acute organ rejection, and opportunistic infection. In most series 4-year survival remains below 60 per cent for lung transplantation, with patients being transplanted for pulmonary hypertension having the worst long-term outcome. This reason, as well as the expense of the operation and the early mortality rate, render lung transplantation a treatment of last resort for PPH. Many advocate that patients with PPH not undergo lung transplantation until they manifest clinical right ventricular failure. Early data suggest that prostacyclin may prove to be the ideal bridge to keep these patients alive and stable until organs become available.

SECONDARY PULMONARY HYPERTENSION

Several secondary causes of pulmonary hypertension have been well established, although the mechanisms for the pulmonary hypertension often remain in doubt (Table 25–4). In many instances, increased resistance to pulmonary blood flow downstream leads to what has been referred to as "passive" pulmonary hypertension, because in many cases there is elevation of the pulmonary artery pressure but no significant elevation in pulmonary vascular resistance. Reactive pulmonary hypertension often coexists in these states, elevating the pulmonary artery pressure and pulmonary vascular resistance to levels higher than can be accounted for purely by increased downstream resistance to blood flow. In some instances, relieving the downstream obstruction results in normalization of pulmonary artery pressure and pulmonary vascular resistance, whereas in other instances it may not. This has been believed to be related to the chronicity of the reactive pulmonary hypertension leading to irreversible vascular changes, although this hypothesis has never been proven. When reactive pulmonary hypertension occurs, it often results in right ventricular failure, which can predominate in the patient's clinical symptomology and lead to a marked deterioration in functional class and death.

INCREASED RESISTANCE TO PULMONARY VENOUS DRAINAGE

PATHOPHYSIOLOGY. Increased resistance to pulmonary venous drainage is a mechanism common to several conditions of diverse causes in which pulmonary arterial hypertension occurs. Altered resistance to pulmonary venous drainage may be the result of diseases affecting the left ventricle or pericardium, mitral or aortic valvular disease, or rare entities such as cor triatriatum, left atrial myxoma, or pulmonary veno-occlusive disease (see below).

The magnitude of pulmonary hypertension depends, in part, on the performance of the right ventricle. In response to an acute stress, such as pulmonary embolism, the normal right ventricle of an adult living at sea level can develop systolic pulmonary pressures of 45 to 50 mm Hg, above which right ventricular failure supervenes. Systolic pressures of 80 to 100 mm Hg can be generated only by a hypertrophied right ventricle that is normally perfused. If right ventricular infarction or ischemia has occurred,[198–200] or if the right and left ventricles are both affected by a myopathic process, right ventricular failure occurs at lower pulmonary vascular pressures, and significant pulmonary hypertension may not develop despite an increase in pulmonary vascular resistance.

In the presence of a healthy, nonischemic right ventricle, an increase in left atrial pressure from subnormal levels up to 7 mm Hg results in a fall in both pulmonary vascular resistance and the pressure gradient across the lungs. These reductions may reflect distention of a population of compliant small vessels or recruitment of additional vascular channels or both. With further increases in left atrial pressure, pulmonary arterial pressure rises along with pulmonary venous pressure; i.e., at a constant pulmonary blood flow, the pressure gradient between the pulmonary artery and veins and the pulmonary vascular resistance remains constant. Finally, when pulmonary venous pressure approaches or exceeds 25 mm Hg on a chronic basis, a disproportionate elevation of pulmonary artery pressure occurs; i.e., the pressure gradient between the pulmonary artery

TABLE 25–4 CLASSIFICATION OF PULMONARY HYPERTENSION BASED ON ESTABLISHED CAUSES

LEFT VENTRICULAR DIASTOLIC FAILURE
  Hypertension
  Aortic stenosis
  Coronary artery disease
  Constrictive pericarditis
  Cardiomyopathy
    Hypertrophic
    Restrictive
    Dilated

LEFT ATRIAL HYPERTENSION
  Mitral stenosis
  Mitral regurgitation
  Cor triatriatum
  Left atrial myxoma or thrombus

LUNG DISEASE
  Parenchymal
    Chronic obstructive pulmonary disease
    Restrictive lung disease
    Interstitial lung disease
  Disorders of ventilation
    Obesity-hypoventilation syndromes
    Neuromuscular disorders
    Chest wall deformities
  Congenital anomalies
  Induced hypoxia

PULMONARY VASCULAR OBSTRUCTION
  Chronic thromboembolic pulmonary hypertension
  Mediastinal fibrosis
  Peripheral artery stenosis
  Foreign body embolization
  Tumor embolization

PULMONARY VASCULAR DISEASE
  Collagen vascular disease
  Congenital heart disease with post-tricuspid left-to-right shunting
  Increased pulmonary blood flow
    Atrial septal defect
    Anomalous pulmonary venous drainage
    High-output cardiac failure
      Beriberi
      Arteriovenous fistula
  Persistent fetal circulation of the newborn
  Primary pulmonary hypertension

OTHER RARE VASCULAR DISEASES
  Takayasu's arteritis
  Sarcoidosis
  Hemoglobinopathies
  Alveolar proteinosis

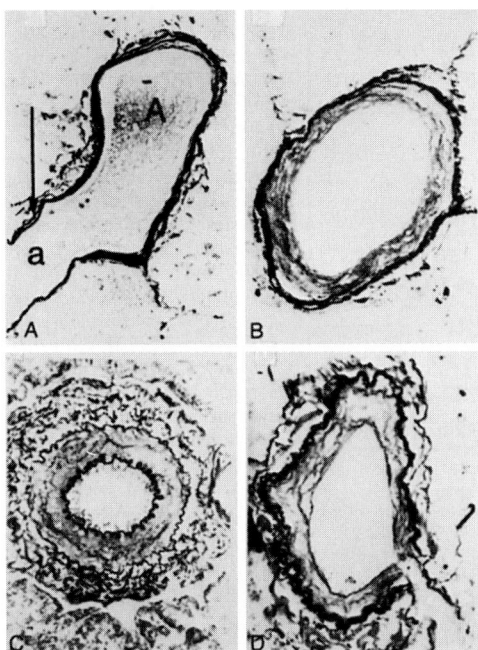

FIGURE 25–15. *A,* Oblique section through a muscular pulmonary artery, *A,* showing the characteristic thin media bounded by inner and outer elastic laminae. An arteriolar branch, *a,* arises from the parent vessel and passes downward and to the left. Its wall consists of a single elastic lamina except near its origin from its parent artery where the remains of a thin media bounded by two elastic laminae can still be seen *(arrow)* (Elastic–van Gieson × 284). *B,* Transverse section of a normal pulmonary venule. The wall consists of a single elastic lamina. There is considerable intimal fibrosis due to age change. (Elastic–van Gieson × 375). Muscular pulmonary artery *(C)* and venule *(D)* in a young woman with severe mitral stenosis. Note the marked hypertrophy in the artery and the crenated internal elastic lamina, suggesting constriction. The venule shows severe intimal fibrosis. (Modified from Harris, P., and Heath, D.: The Human Pulmonary Circulation. 3rd ed. New York, Churchill Livingstone, 1986, pp. 338 and 341.)

and veins rises while pulmonary blood flow remains constant or falls, indicating an elevation in pulmonary vascular resistance that is due, in part, to pulmonary vasoconstriction. The latter occurs to a variable extent in response to passive elevations of pulmonary venous pressure and probably reflects the reactivity of the pulmonary vasculature, which may be variable between and within species.

There is considerable variability in pulmonary arterial vasoconstriction in response to pulmonary venous hypertension. Marked reactive pulmonary hypertension, with pulmonary artery systolic pressures in excess of 80 mm Hg, occurs in somewhat less than one-third of patients with pulmonary venous pressures elevated chronically in excess of 25 mm Hg. The fact that less than one-third of patients with severe mitral stenosis develop severe reactive pulmonary hypertension also argues in favor of a spectrum of pulmonary vascular reactivity to chronic increases in pulmonary venous pressure.

The mechanism involved in elevating pulmonary vascular resistance is unclear. There may be a neural component; also, an elevation of pulmonary venous pressure may narrow or close airways, which may diminish ventilation and lead to hypoxia and, in turn, elevate pulmonary artery pressure. Finally, interstitial pulmonary edema secondary to pulmonary venous hypertension may encroach on the vascular lumen and contribute to the pulmonary arterial hypertension.

PATHOLOGY. Structural changes in the pulmonary vascular bed develop in association with chronic pulmonary venous hypertension, irrespective of its etiology. At the ultrastructural level, these changes include swelling of the pulmonary capillary endothelial cells, thickening of their basal lamina, and wide separation of groups of connective tissue fibrils, indicative of interstitial edema. With persistence of the edema, there is proliferation of reticular and elastic fibrils, so that the alveolar capillaries become embedded in dense connective tissue.[5] The permeability of interendothelial junctions depends on pulmonary capillary pressure, with leakage of large molecules (40,000 to 60,000

daltons) occurring at capillary pressures in excess of approximately 30 mm Hg.[201,202]

Light microscopic examination of the lungs of patients with pulmonary venous hypertension shows distention of pulmonary capillaries, thickening and rupture of the basement membranes of endothelial cells, and transudation of erythrocytes through these ruptured membranes into the alveolar spaces, which contain fragments of disintegrating erythrocytes. Pulmonary hemosiderosis is commonly observed and may progress to extensive fibrosis. In the late stages of pulmonary venous hypertension, areas of hemorrhage may be scattered throughout the lungs, edema fluid and coagulum may collect in the alveolar spaces, and there may be widespread organization and fibrosis of pulmonary alveoli. Occasionally, particularly in patients with chronic pulmonary venous hypertension due to mitral valve disease, ossification of alveolar spaces occurs.[203,204] Pulmonary lymphatics may become markedly distended, giving the appearance of lymphangiectasis, particularly when the pulmonary venous pressure chronically exceeds 30 mm Hg. Structural alterations in the small pulmonary arteries, arterioles, and venules include medial hypertrophy and intimal fibrosis and, rarely, necrotizing arteritis (Fig. 25–15). However, vasodilatation and plexiform lesions are not seen. The latter characterize the "irreversible" forms of pulmonary arterial hypertension, and their absence in that form of pulmonary hypertension associated with chronic pulmonary venous pressure elevation correlates with the reversibility of the pulmonary hypertension.

PULMONARY HYPERTENSION SECONDARY TO ELEVATION OF LEFT VENTRICULAR DIASTOLIC PRESSURE

LEFT VENTRICULAR DIASTOLIC FAILURE. This may result from hypertension; aortic stenosis; ischemic heart disease; hypertrophic, restrictive, and congestive cardiomyopathies; and constrictive pericarditis. Because chronic increases in mean left ventricular filling pressure exceeding 25 mm Hg are uncommon, the resulting pulmonary arterial hypertension is only moderate unless reactive pulmonary hypertension also occurs. In the absence of the latter, a normal pulmonary artery mean pressure of 15 mm Hg may rise to approximately 30 mm Hg as a result of left ventricular diastolic dysfunction. Because cardiac output is usually reduced in such patients, the mean pulmonary artery pressure would be considerably less than 30 mm Hg if pulmonary vascular resistance remains unchanged. However, many patients with left ventricular diastolic dysfunction exhibit increased pulmonary vascular resistance and moderately severe pulmonary hypertension.

PULMONARY HYPERTENSION SECONDARY TO LEFT ATRIAL HYPERTENSION

Mitral Valve Disease (see also Chap. 32)

MITRAL STENOSIS. This valvular lesion represents an important cause of pulmonary hypertension. Although the pulmonary hypertension associated with mitral stenosis is initially a result of an increase in resistance to pulmonary venous drainage and backward transmission of the elevated left atrial pressure, many patients subsequently exhibit marked pulmonary vasoconstriction and anatomical changes in vessels, so that the pulmonary hypertension is "reactive" as well as "passive." The elevation of pulmonary vascular resistance and the associated pulmonary hypertension may come to dominate the clinical picture in mitral stenosis (Fig. 25–16).[206,207] Thus, patients with mitral stenosis often develop what might be considered to be a more proximal obstruction at the level of the pulmonary arterioles and small muscular arteries, with resultant pulmonary hypertension equal to or exceeding systemic arterial pressure during exertion and sometimes even at rest. The clinical picture in such patients is characterized by right ventricular failure with distended neck veins, hepatomegaly, and ascites. These patients exhibit marked fatigue, occasionally a more serious complaint than dyspnea. The murmur of mitral stenosis may be soft or even inaudible, and the opening snap of the stenotic mitral valve may be indistinguishable from a loud pulmonic component of S_2, owing to narrowing of the S_2-opening snap interval. Pulmonary congestion and edema may not be prominent clinically. Cardiac output is usually markedly reduced. This constellation of findings may obscure the underlying diagnosis of mitral stenosis and suggest instead either PPH or pulmonary hypertension secondary to some other disorder.

Diagnostic Studies. The echocardiogram shows left atrial enlargement and thickened mitral valve leaflets whose mobility is markedly reduced (see p. 1012). At cardiac catheterization, the pulmonary arterial hypertension is associated with substantial elevations of the pulmonary wedge pressure, and there is generally a sizable (>10 mm

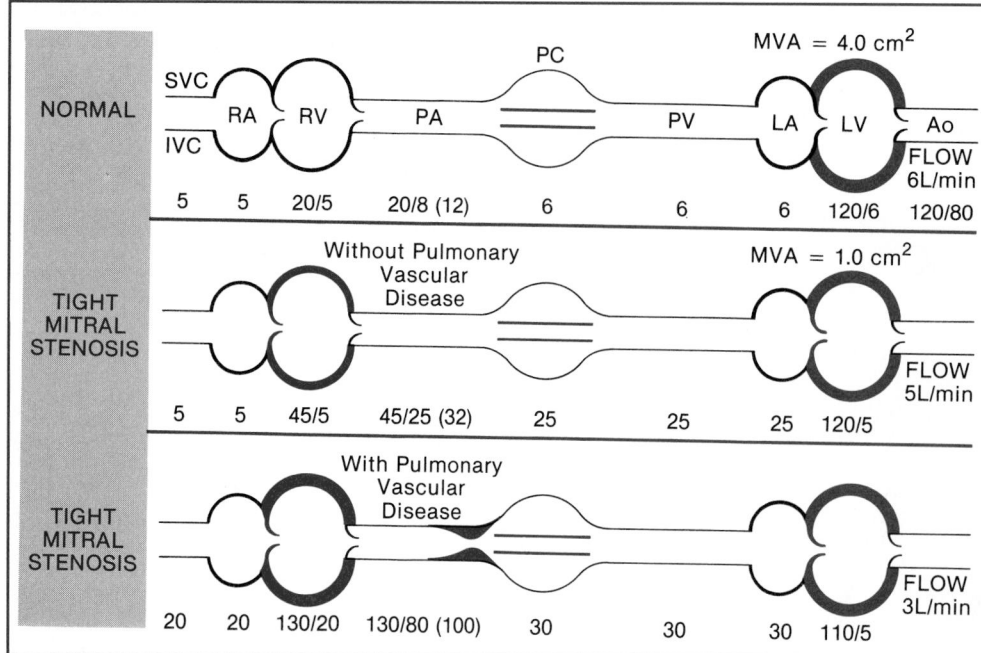

FIGURE 25–16. Schematic diagram of cardiopulmonary circulation in patients with tight mitral stenosis with and without pulmonary vascular disease. Pressures (in mm Hg) are listed for the superior and inferior venae cavae (SVC and IVC), right atrium (RA), right ventricle (RV), pulmonary arteries (PA), capillaries (PC), veins (PV), left atrium (LA), left ventricle (LV), and aorta (Ao) for the normal circulation *(upper panel)* and for the two types of mitral stenosis *(middle and lower panels).* Note that with pulmonary vascular disease (the "second stenosis") severe pulmonary hypertension occurs, and right ventricular failure develops. (Modified from Dexter, L.: Physiologic changes in mitral stenosis. N. Engl. J. Med. 254:829, 1956. Schlant, R. C.: Altered cardiovascular function of rheumatic heart disease and other acquired valvular disease. *In* Hurst, J. L., and Logue, R. B. (eds.): The Heart. 4th ed. New York, McGraw-Hill Book Co., 1978, p. 971.)

Hg) pressure gradient between pulmonary capillary wedge and left ventricular diastolic pressures. These findings are of key importance in distinguishing mitral stenosis from primary pulmonary hypertension, a condition in which left atrial size and the wedge pressure are normal and in which there is no diastolic pressure gradient between the wedge and left ventricular pressures.

Protection Against Pulmonary Edema. At least three mechanisms that tend to protect against pulmonary edema formation are operative in patients with mitral stenosis and chronic elevations of pulmonary venous pressure in excess of 25 mm Hg (Chap. 15). First, lymphatic drainage of the pulmonary interstitium increases abruptly when pulmonary venous pressure is increased to 25 mm Hg.[208,209] Acute increases in pulmonary lymph flow of up to eight times the resting level occur when pulmonary venous pressure is raised to 30 mm Hg for a 10-minute interval, and the increased lymphatic flow persists at high levels for 30 to 60 minutes after pulmonary venous pressure has returned to normal.[208] In models of *chronic* pulmonary venous pressure elevation, increases in pulmonary lymph flow of up to 28 times normal have been observed.[209]

Diminished permeability of the capillary alveolar barrier is a second protective mechanism that might be operative in patients with *chronic* pulmonary venous hypertension in excess of 25 mm Hg. There is morphological evidence of thickening of the layer between the capillary lumen and the alveolar space.[210–213] A third mechanism operating in patients with chronic increased resistance to pulmonary venous drainage is the reactive constriction of small muscular pulmonary arteries and arterioles (Fig. 25–15). This constriction, which results in considerable elevation of pulmonary artery pressure, is usually associated with a significant decline in right ventricular output (and therefore pulmonary blood flow). The lower pulmonary blood flow tends to diminish the formation of pulmonary edema because it results in substantially lower left atrial and pulmonary venous pressures at any given size of the mitral valve orifice[214] or for any given impairment of left ventricular function.

Effects of Surgery. After corrective surgery on the mitral valve or mitral balloon valvuloplasty (see p. 1014), both pulmonary vascular resistance and pulmonary hypertension decline,[215,216] the major extent of which is noted within the first postoperative week. The extent of reversal of pulmonary vascular obstruction has varied depending on the adequacy of the procedure in producing an increase in mitral orifice area and whether the patient develops mitral valve restenosis.[217]

MITRAL REGURGITATION. Although pulmonary hypertension is widely recognized as developing in patients with left atrial hypertension due to mitral stenosis, it can also occur in patients with pure mitral regurgitation.[218] In one series, nearly half of a cohort of 41 patients with severe mitral regurgitation had pulmonary artery systolic pressures in excess of 50 mm Hg. In this subgroup of patients, pulmonary vascular resistance was three times normal and cardiac output was substantially depressed, compared with that in patients in whom severe mitral regurgitation was associated with only minimal pulmonary artery pressure elevation.[218] Presumably, the pulmonary hypertension in these patients is reversible, just as it is in mitral stenosis, although data on this point have not been reported.

COR TRIATRIATUM (see also p. 923). This is a malformation in which partitioning of the left atrium creates two left atrial subchambers. The posterior subchamber receives the pulmonary venous inflow, which then drains through an opening in the partition into the anterior subchamber and then through the mitral orifice into the left ventricle. When the opening in the partition separating the two left atrial subchambers is small, severe pulmonary venous and pulmonary arterial hypertension result.[219]

INCREASED RESISTANCE TO FLOW THROUGH THE PULMONARY VASCULAR BED

Pulmonary Parenchymal Disease

Pulmonary hypertension is a common sequela to chronic bronchitis and emphysema (Chap. 47).[220] It had long been believed that the elevated pulmonary artery pressures in patients with emphysema resulted from destruction of the pulmonary vascular bed. Current views minimize this pathogenic pathway; because no direct correlation exists between the severity of the emphysema and the degree of right ventricular hypertrophy.[220,221]

PATHOPHYSIOLOGY. Hypoxia-induced vasoconstriction (see p. 781) probably plays a major role in producing pulmonary hypertension in patients with chronic bronchitis and emphysema.[222–224] There is also evidence for a pulmonary vasoconstrictive action by hydrogen ions, particularly in the presence of hypoxia. In this regard, in patients with chronic obstructive lung disease pulmonary artery pressure correlates inversely with arterial oxygen saturation and directly with arterial P_{CO_2},[225–228] providing indirect evidence for a role for hypoxia and hypercapnia in the production of pulmonary hypertension. When patients with chronic bronchitis and emphysema inspire high concentrations of oxygen acutely, there is only a modest decrease in pulmonary artery pressure and vascular resistance,[226,229–231] both of which remain considerably elevated. This suggests that muscular hypertrophy of pulmonary arterioles may in itself be of importance in maintaining the hypoxic pulmonary hypertension.

TRIALS WITH OXYGEN THERAPY. The results of two large trials designed to assess the role of long-term oxygen therapy in cor pulmonale due to chronic bronchitis and emphysema have been disappointing insofar as pulmonary vascular dynamics are concerned (see p. 1617).[232,233] Long-term domiciliary oxygen therapy in one study was associated with no change in mean pulmonary artery pressure after 500 days of oxygen treatment, compared with a 3-mm Hg increase in the control group.[232] In another study, nocturnal oxygen administration was associated with a 7 per cent increase in pulmonary vascular resistance after 6 months, compared with an 11 per cent decrease in patients receiving continuous oxygen.[233]

Blood volume and red cell mass, in particular, increase during acute respiratory failure and may contribute to the development of elevated pulmonary arterial pressures. By increasing blood viscosity, increases in hematocrit to within the range commonly seen in chronic bronchitis and emphysema (i.e., 50 to 55 per cent) result in 30 to 50 per cent increases in the transpulmonary arteriovenous pressure gradient at constant blood flow.

SPECIFIC DISORDERS

Progressive interstitial pulmonary fibrosis may be associated with pulmonary hypertension. The latter may occur in patients with *progressive systemic sclerosis* (see p. 1781), in whom the fibrotic process leads to major reduction in the cross-sectional area of the pulmonary vascular bed due to obliteration of alveolar capillaries and narrowing and obliteration of many small arteries and arterioles.[2,5] Moreover, a marked elevation of pulmonary artery pressure ($\geq$ 100 mm Hg systolic) and resistance ($\geq$ 2000 dynes-sec-cm^{-5}) in patients with a variant of scleroderma, the *CREST syndrome* (*c*alcinosis, *R*aynaud's phenomenon, *e*sophageal dysmotility, *s*clerodactyly, and *t*elangiectasia), has been reported[235] (see p. 1781). In patients with the CREST form of *scleroderma,* marked right ventricular dysfunction may be present with right ventricular ejection fractions less than 30 per cent, presumably reflecting systolic overload of the right ventricle due to severe pulmonary vascular disease,[154,236] in the absence of interstitial lung disease.

Fibrous obliteration of the pulmonary vascular bed and pulmonary hypertension have also been described in patients with various forms of pulmonary vasculitis (Table 25-5). These include isolated Raynaud's phenomenon,[237,238] dermatomyositis,[239] rheumatoid arthritis,[240] and systemic lupus erythematosus.[241,242] In the latter a *lupus anticoagulant* may be present in the IgG or IgM fractions of the serum; this may cause a paradoxical hypercoagulable state, intrapulmonary microthrombi, and pulmonary hypertension.[242] Pulmonary hypertension is an uncommon accompaniment of the Hamman-Rich syndrome,[243] desquamative

TABLE 25-5 PULMONARY VASCULITIDES

VASCULITIDES IN WHICH LUNG IS THE MAJOR ORGAN INVOLVED
Wegener's granulomatosis
Lymphomatoid granulomatosis
Lymphocytic angiitis and granulomatosis
Churg-Strauss syndrome
Overlap vasculitis
Necrotizing sarcoid granulomatosis

VASCULITIDES IN WHICH LUNG MAY BE INVOLVED
Henoch-Schönlein syndrome
Disseminated leukocytoclastic vasculitis
Cryoglobulinemia
Disseminated giant cell arteritis
Behçet's disease
Takayasu's disease
Polyarteritis nodosa

DISEASES IN WHICH PULMONARY VASCULITIS MAY BE PART OF THE SPECTRUM OF PATHOLOGY
Collagen-vascular disorders
  Rheumatoid arthritis
  Systemic lupus erythematosus
  Progressive systemic sclerosis
Eosinophilic pneumonias
Sarcoidosis
Immunoblastic lymphadenopathy
Organic dust diseseases (hypersensitivity pneumonitides)
Bronchocentric granulomatosis
Ulcerative colitis
Ankylosing spondylitis
Hughes-Stovin syndrome

From Fulmer, J. D., and Kaltreider, H. B.: The pulmonary vasculitides. Chest 82:615, 1982.

interstitial pneumonia, idiopathic pulmonary hemosiderosis,[244] and sarcoidosis.[245] It is not clear whether significant pulmonary hypertension may result from pulmonary fibrosis due to radiation therapy.

Diffuse lymphatic spread of carcinoma may also cause pulmonary hypertension and right heart failure.[246] In many cases tumor microemboli and the attendant thrombotic and fibrotic reaction lead to vascular obstruction. Obstruction of the major pulmonary arteries by tumor (usually sarcoma) may be a cause of right ventricular and main pulmonary artery hypertension.[247] Congenital pulmonary aplasia or hypoplasia, the latter often observed in Down syndrome,[248] may be responsible for an elevation of pulmonary vascular resistance and pulmonary hypertension.

Eisenmenger Syndrome
(See also pp. 750 and 967)

Decreased cross-sectional area of the pulmonary arteriolar bed with irreversible pulmonary hypertension characterizes the so-called Eisenmenger syndrome. This term was used by Wood[249] to refer to patients with congenital cardiac lesions and severe pulmonary hypertension in whom reversal of a left-to-right shunt has occurred. Left-to-right shunts are due usually to congenital cardiovascular malformations[250-254] (e.g., atrial and ventricular septal defects, patent ductus arteriosus).

PATHOPHYSIOLOGY (see p. 967). Pulmonary hypertension in congenital heart disease may occur simply because of increased pulmonary blood flow. When chronic, the increased pulmonary flow is often associated with a passive reduction in pulmonary resistance and little elevation of pulmonary vascular pressures. In a normal adult with a pulmonary blood flow (PBF) of 5 liters/min, a pulmonary vascular resistance (PVR) of 60 dynes-sec-cm^{-5}, and a mean left atrial pressure (LA) of 6 mm Hg, the pulmonary artery mean pressure (PA) may be calculated from the expression

$$PVR = \frac{(PA - LA)80}{PBF} = \frac{(PA - 6)80}{5} = 60 \text{ dynes-sec-cm}^{-5}$$

$$PA = \frac{60 \times 5}{80} + 6 = 10 \text{ mm Hg}$$

If PBF is doubled, a reduction in PVR to 30 dynes-sec-cm^{-5} maintains PA mean pressure at a normal level of 10 mm Hg. However, if PBF is increased four- to sixfold, the reserve capacity of the pulmonary vascular bed is exceeded, and pulmonary artery pressure rises. Thus, if the PVR is 30 dynes-sec-cm^{-5}, a PBF of 30 liters/min is associated with a mean PA pressure that is only minimally elevated at 17 mm Hg, although the high right ventricular stroke volumes associated with the augmentation in pulmonary blood flow result in considerably higher values (40 to 45 mm Hg) for pulmonary artery and right ventricular systolic pressures. If no underlying arteriolar vascular disease exists, abolition of the shunt by corrective operation restores pulmonary blood flow and PA pressure to normal.

If a congenital cardiovascular defect causes pulmonary hypertension from the time of birth, the small, muscular arteries of the fetal lung may undergo delayed or only partial involution, resulting in persistently high levels of pulmonary vascular resistance (see p. 781). This is true especially in those lesions in which a left-to-right shunt enters the right ventricle or pulmonary artery directly (i.e., a post-tricuspid valve shunt, such as ventricular septal defect or patent ductus arteriosus); these patients experience a higher incidence of severe and irreversible pulmonary vascular damage than those in whom the shunt is proximal to the tricuspid valve (pre-tricuspid shunts, as in atrial septal defect and partial anomalous pulmonary venous drainage). In the latter category, pulmonary hypertension may result from a large pre-tricuspid left-to-right shunt, which enhances the risk of pulmonary vascular damage.

PATHOLOGY. The extent of reversibility of pulmonary vascular obstructive disease in the presence of congenital heart disease varies. From an anatomical point of view, reversible conditions are those in which the decreased pulmonary arteriolar cross-sectional area is the result of medial hypertrophy and vasoconstriction; irreversibility is associated with the presence of necrotizing arteritis and plexiform lesions in these small vessels.[250-253] The classification by Heath and Edwards[109] of six grades of structural change is widely employed to assess the potential reversibility of pulmonary vascular disease and is summarized as follows: *Grade I* is characterized by hypertrophy of the media of small muscular pulmonary arteries and arterioles.

In *Grade II*, intimal cellular proliferation is added to the medial hypertrophy. *Grade IIII* is characterized by advanced medial thickening with hypertrophy and hyperplasia, together with progressive intimal proliferation and concentric fibrosis that results in obliteration of many arterioles and small arteries. In *Grade IV*, dilatation and so-called "plexiform lesions" of the muscular pulmonary arteries and arterioles are observed (Fig. 25–17). The latter consist of a plexiform network of capillary-like channels within a dilated segment of a muscular pulmonary artery. The channels are separated by proliferating endothelial cells, which often contain thrombi; indeed, the network of capillary channels may constitute recanalization of a thrombus. *Grade V* changes include complex plexiform, angiomatous, and cavernous lesions and hyalinization of intimal fibrosis. Finally, *Grade VI* is characterized by the presence of necrotizing arteritis.

The Heath and Edwards classification implies that the morphological alterations are sequential, with Grade I being the earliest stage and Grade VI being the "end stage" of pulmonary vascular obliterative disease. That such an orderly progression may not in fact occur is suggested by the findings of Wagenvoort, which indicate that plexiform lesions develop gradually in areas affected by necrotizing arteritis. They have suggested that fibrinoid necrosis of a

small segment of a pulmonary arterial branch leads to medial destruction and subsequent aneurysmal dilatation of the vessel as well as the formation of a fibrin clot in the lumen, often with admixture of platelets.[250] Organization of the fibrin clot by strands of intimal cells leads to formation of the plexus; the small capillary-like channels within the plexus (Fig. 25–17) provide continuity to the distal portion of the artery, which undergoes poststenotic dilatation. With time, the inflammatory component of the process subsides, fibrin disappears, and the strands of intimal cells become fibrotic. Wagenvoort's view is supported by animal experiments in which end-to-end systemic-pulmonary anastomoses resulted in arteritis and fibrinoid necrosis before the appearance of plexiform lesions.[255,256] Thus, although Heath-Edwards Grades I, II, and III may represent chronological progression, evidence exists that Grade VI (necrotizing arteritis) changes appear next, followed by Grades IV and V as end-stage alterations.

CLINICAL CONSIDERATIONS. As already mentioned, *Eisenmenger syndrome* is the term used by Wood to refer to patients with congenital central communications with severe pulmonary hypertension, in whom reversal of a left-to-right shunt has occurred across the pulmonary-systemic communication.[249] The patients described originally by Eisenmenger had ventricular septal defects, and the term *Eisenmenger complex* is applied to patients with severe pulmonary hypertension and right-to-left shunt through such a defect. The broader term *Eisenmenger syndrome* is applied to any anomalous circulatory communication that leads to obliterative pulmonary vascular disease, including pre- and post-tricuspid shunts. Health-Edwards Grades IV to VI changes are usual in these patients; occasionally, lesser anatomical changes predominate and may be reversible after successful corrective operation.

When the pulmonary vascular resistance has increased so that it equals or exceeds systemic resistance, and the anatomical changes of the pulmonary vessels are predominantly those of Grades IV to VI, surgical closure of the anomalous circulatory communication will be associated with a prohibitive immediate risk and if the patient survives will usually fail to relieve pulmonary hypertension. Operation may, in fact, hasten death in most survivors who had either balanced shunts or predominant right-to-left shunts because closure of the right-to-left communication merely increases the load on an already overburdened right ventricle. Structural changes in the pulmonary vascular bed are evident in pulmonary arteriograms, which reveal dilated central pulmonary arteries and narrowing of the peripheral branches. These changes can be evaluated by means of quantitative analysis of the pulmonary wedge angiogram.[257] This technique has been employed successfully by Rabinovitch, Reid, and coworkers, who have demonstrated progressively more abrupt tapering of the pulmonary arteries in patients with increasingly abnormal hemodynamics and increasingly severe structural changes in lung biopsy tissue.[257]

OTHER CONDITIONS ASSOCIATED WITH DECREASED CROSS-SECTIONAL AREA OF THE PULMONARY VASCULAR BED

PERSISTENT FETAL CIRCULATION IN THE NEWBORN (see also p. 883). This condition has been reported as a cause of severe pulmonary hypertension.[260–262] Affected infants exhibit cyanosis, tachypnea, acidemia, normal pulmonary parenchymal markings on chest radiography, and anatomically normal hearts. Cyanosis is the result of right-to-left shunting across the foramen ovale and through a patent ductus arteriosus.[260] The condition may be due to persistence of extremely muscular small pulmonary arteries, a diminution in the absolute number of these resistance vessels, or a combination of the two.[262]

INCREASED RESISTANCE TO FLOW THROUGH LARGE PULMONARY ARTERIES

PULMONARY THROMBOEMBOLISM (Chap. 46). Pulmonary thromboembolism, as a single event or as repeated events, rarely leads to the development of chronic pulmonary hypertension.[263] However, in a

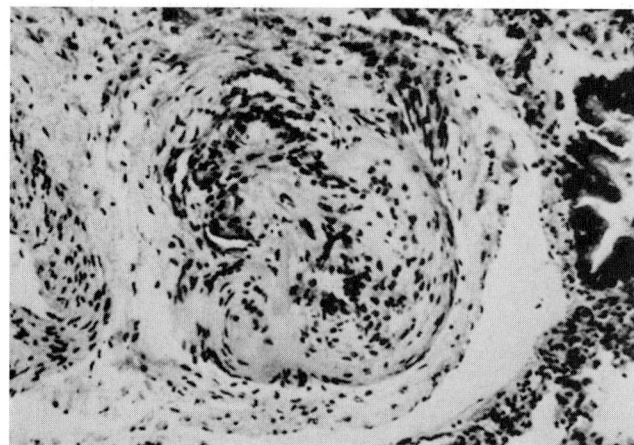

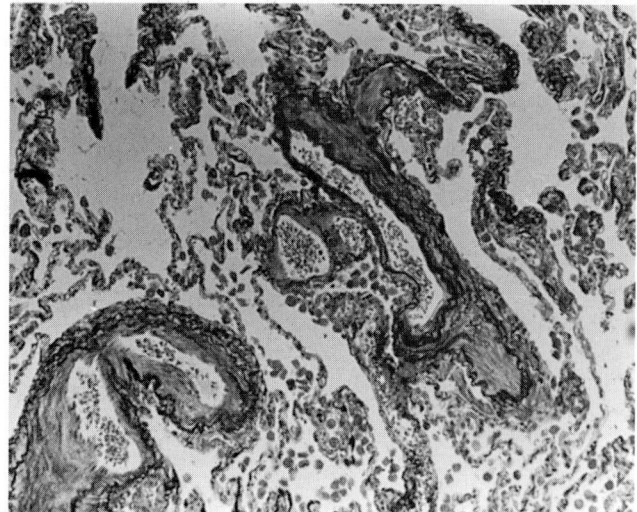

FIGURE 25–17. *Top,* Histological section from the lung of a 3-year-old boy with a common atrioventricular canal and severe pulmonary hypertension. A muscular pulmonary artery with an early plexiform lesion is seen as well as fibrinoid necrosis of the media and active proliferation of intimal cells. (From Wagenvoort, C. A., and Wagenvoort, N.: Pathology of Pulmonary Hypertension. 2nd ed. New York, John Wiley and Sons, 1977.) *Bottom,* Photomicrograph of a lung biopsy specimen from a 35-year-old man with a patent ductus arteriosus and systemic pulmonary hypertension. A predominance of advanced changes is seen, including plexiform and dilatation lesions.

subset of patients (believed to be less than 0.1 per cent of all patients suffering from pulmonary embolism), the outcome is unusual.[264] Rather than having inherent fibrinolytic resolution of the thromboembolism with restoration of vascular patency, the thromboemboli in these patients fail to resolve adequately (see p. 1598). They undergo organization and incomplete recanalization and become incorporated into the vascular wall. Commonly they are at the subsegmental and segmental and lobar vessels, although it is believed that the chronic thromboembolism tends to propagate retrogradely, leading to slowly progressive vascular obstruction.[263] It appears that the vast majority of these patients have suffered one major thromboembolic event rather than multiple recurrences.

The slowly progressive nature of the course of the disease allows right ventricular hypertrophy to ensue and compensate for the increased pulmonary vascular resistance. However, owing to either progressive thrombosis or vascular changes in the "uninvolved" vascular bed,[264,265] the pulmonary hypertension becomes progressive and the patients manifest the clinical symptoms of dyspnea, fatigue, hypoxemia, and right heart failure. It is particularly critical that these patients be identified and distinguished from patients with primary pulmonary hypertension or other causes, as a large proportion of patients are amenable to surgical thromboendarterectomy with an extraordinarily good outcome[264] (Fig. 46–16, p. 1599). The perfusion lung scan should adequately select out patients with this entity and is another reason why lung perfusion scanning is recommended for all patients who present with pulmonary hypertension (Fig.25–9).

Because the lung scan typically underestimates the severity of the central pulmonary arterial obstruction, any patient who presents with one or more mismatched segmental or larger defects should be considered to have this entity and should undergo pulmonary angiography.[262,263] Pulmonary angiography can be performed safely in these patients if particular attention is given to the hemodynamic state, and immediate treatment with atropine for any vagally induced response to contrast injection is considered.[263]

Patients suitable to undergo pulmonary thromboendarterectomy must have thrombi that are accessible to surgical removal and demonstrate a significant increase in pulmonary vascular resistance.[264] Although the published operative mortality is fairly high, survivors have immediate hemodynamic improvement with a good long-term prognosis. Right ventricular dysfunction of any magnitude is not a contraindication to surgery, as right ventricular function has been noted to improve once the obstruction of pulmonary blood flow is removed.

PERIPHERAL PULMONIC STENOSIS. This is a congenital lesion that occurs particularly in association with supravalvular aortic stenosis or as a sequela of the rubella syndrome (see p. 924). Hypertension in the proximal pulmonary arteries depends on the extent, location, and severity of the stenotic lesions.[266,267]

TAKAYASU'S (GIANT CELL) ARTERITIS (see also p. 1572). This frequently involves the pulmonary vessels; the pathological changes resemble those seen in systemic arteries. In the vast majority of these patients, the aorta and major arch vessels are involved as well. This condition can also be distinguished from PPH by the fact that the occlusive changes occur in the large and intermediate vessels rather than in the more distal vessels characteristic of PPH.[258,259]

HYPOVENTILATION

As discussed earlier (see p. 781), conditions associated with hypoxia may cause pulmonary hypertension, particularly if there is associated acidemia.[31] A number of disorders that affect the upper airways, neuromuscular control, or pulmonary parenchyma lead to hypoventilation and (in the setting of a reactive pulmonary vascular bed) pulmonary hypertension.

THE OBESITY-HYPOVENTILATION SYNDROME[270,271] (see also p. 1614). Also called the Pickwickian syndrome, this condition may lead to substantial pulmonary hypertension (mean pulmonary artery pressure $\geq$ 50 mm Hg), which correlates with the presence of hypoxemia and acidosis (Fig. 47–5, p. 1608). *Pharyngeal-tracheal obstruction* occurs in the presence of hypertrophied tonsils and adenoids[272,273] and may cause reversible pulmonary hypertension.

NEUROMUSCULAR DISORDERS. These include myasthenia gravis, poliomyelitis, and damage to the central respiratory center.[274] They may cause hypoventilation of sufficient severity to result in pulmonary hypertension (see p. 1877). *Disorders of the chest wall* (kyphoscoliosis, pectus excavatum) may also cause hypoventilation and pulmonary hypertension (see p. 1865).

The pulmonary hypertension in all of these conditions subsides with restoration of normal respiration and correction of the hypoxia. It should also be recognized that hypoxia may intensify pulmonary hypertension of other causes. For example, severe pulmonary hypertension occurring in children with a left-to-right shunt who reside at high altitude is often due to the combination of high pulmonary blood flow and superimposed hypoxic pulmonary vasoconstriction; pulmonary pressures may fall rapidly toward normal when residence is established at sea level.

OTHER CAUSES OF PULMONARY HYPERTENSION

HIGH-ALTITUDE PULMONARY EDEMA (see also p. 465). This entity is associated with reversible pulmonary hypertension. It is observed particularly in individuals acclimatized to high altitudes who, after a stay of some days or weeks at sea level, return to high altitude.[275] The

finding of high-altitude pulmonary edema in four persons without a right pulmonary artery has been reported,[276] giving support to speculation concerning the combined role of hypoxia and hyperfusion in patients with this condition.[277]

HIGH-OUTPUT CARDIAC FAILURE. A chronic high-output cardiac state can lead to elevation in left ventricular end-diastolic filling pressure.[278] This, along with the chronically increased pulmonary blood flow, may lead to reactive pulmonary hypertension in some individuals.[97] Because these states are uncommon, pulmonary hypertension presenting in this way is rare. Two cases of high-output failure associated with pulmonary hypertension due to hyperthyroidism and cardiac beriberi have been reported.[98] In each instance the pulmonary hypertension subsided when the underlying high-output state was treated. We have recently seen a patient with a chronic arteriovenous fistula resulting in high-output cardiac failure with a similar profile of increased left ventricular end-diastolic pressure and severe reactive pulmonary hypertension. In this individual surgically correcting the arteriovenous fistula improved the high cardiac output state and pulmonary hypertension as well.

OTHER CONDITIONS. Severe pulmonary hypertension is an occasional but unusual finding in patients with *isolated partial anomalous pulmonary venous drainage.*[279] Speculation exists that the cause may be the increase in pulmonary blood flow associated perhaps with a reflex pulmonary arterial vasoconstriction secondary to distention of the right atrium.

The cause of the pulmonary hypertension that occasionally develops following surgical correction of *tetralogy of Fallot* is unclear. In these patients, pulmonary vascular thrombotic lesions are common and, if extensive, may predispose to pulmonary hypertension when operation—either complete correction or creation of a left-to-right shunt—causes a sudden increase in pulmonary blood flow.[280]

Sickle cell anemia may be complicated by in situ pulmonary thrombosis and infarction (see p. 1787), although this does not usually lead to pulmonary hypertension. There are two case reports of cor pulmonale associated with hemoglobin SC disease,[281,282] but the prevalence of pulmonary hypertension in patients with this condition is unknown.

Intravenous drug abuse may lead to diffuse pulmonary vascular occlusion and pulmonary hypertension. Moderately severe pulmonary hypertension developed in association with *alveolar proteinosis* has been reported.[284] Hypoxemia appears to be the mediating factor.

REFERENCES

NORMAL PULMONARY CIRCULATION

1. Comroe, J. H., Jr.: The main functions of the pulmonary circulation. Circulation 33:146, 1966.
2. Wagenvoort, C. A., and Wagenvoort, N.: Pathology of Pulmonary Hypertension. 2nd ed. New York, John Wiley and Sons, 1977.
3. Fritts, H. W., Harris, P., Chidsey, C. A., et al.: Estimation of flow rate through bronchial–pulmonary vascular anastomoses with use of T-1824 dye. Circulation 23:390, 1961.
4. Barratt-Boyes, B. G., and Wood, E. H.: Cardiac output and related measurements and pressure values in the right heart and associated vessels, together with an analysis of the hemodynamic response to the inhalation of high oxygen mixtures in healthy subjects. J. Lab. Clin. Med. 51:72, 1958.
5. Harris, P., and Heath, D.: The Human Pulmonary Circulation. 3rd ed. New York, Churchill Livingstone, 1986, 702 pp.
6. Harris, P., Segel, N., and Bishop, J. M.: The relation between pressure and flow in the pulmonary circulation in normal subjects and in patients with chronic bronchitis and mitral stenosis. Cardiovasc. Res. 1:73, 1968.
7. Rudolph, A. M.: The changes in the circulation after birth. Their importance in congenital heart disease. Circulation 41:343, 1970.
8. Friedman, W. F., Molony, D. A., and Kirkpatrick, S. E.: Prostaglandins: Physiological and clinical correlations. Adv. Pediatr. 25:151, 1978.
9. Naeye, R. L.: Arterial changes during the perinatal period. Arch. Pathol. 71:121, 1961.
10. Davidson, W. R., Jr., and Fee, E. C.: Influence of aging on pulmonary hemodynamics in a population free of coronary artery disease. Am. J. Cardiol. 65:1454, 1990.
11. Ghali, J. K., Liao, Y., Cooper, R. S., and Cao, G.: Changes in pulmonary hemodynamics with aging in a predominantly hypertensive population. Am. J. Cardiol. 70:367, 1992.
12. Cacciapuoti, F., D'Avino, M., Lama, D., et al.: Hemodynamic change in pulmonary circulation induced by effort in the elderly. Am. J. Cardiol. 7:1481, 1993.
13. Heath, D.: Structural changes in the pulmonary vasculature associated with aging. In Carder, L., and Moyer, J. H. (eds.): Aging of the Lung. New York, Grune & Stratton, 1964, pp. 70–76.
14. Spirito, P., and Maron, B. J.: Influence of aging on Doppler echocardiographic indices of left ventricular diastolic function. Br. Heart J. 59:672, 1988.
15. Rich, S., Chomka, E., Hasara, L., et al.: The prevalence of pulmonary hypertension in the United States. Chest 96:236, 1989.
16. Fishman, A. P.: Hypoxia on the pulmonary circulation: How and where it acts. Circ. Res. 38:221, 1976.
17. Haneda, T., Nakajima, T., Shirato, K., et al.: Effects of oxygen breathing on pulmonary vascular input impedance in patients with pulmonary hypertension. Chest 83:520, 1983.

18. Weir, E. K., Tucker, A., Reeves, J. T., and Will, D. H.: Pulmonary hypertension in cattle at high altitude. Cardiovasc. Res. 8:745, 1975.
19. Fishman, A. P.: The enigma of hypoxic pulmonary vasoconstriction. In Fishman, A. P. (ed.): The Pulmonary Circulation: Normal and Abnormal. Philadelphia, University of Pennsylvania Press, 1990, pp. 109–129.
20. Griffith, T. M., Edwards, D. H., Davies, R. L., et al.: EDRF coordinates the behaviour of vascular resistance vessels. Nature 329:442, 1987.
21. Hickey, K. A., Rubanyi, G., Paul, R. J., and Highsmith, R. F.: Characterization of a coronary vasoconstrictor produced by cultured endothelial cells. Am. J. Physiol. 248:C550, 1985.
22. Stewart, D. J., Levy, R. D., Cernacek, P., and Langleben, D.: Increased plasma endothelin-1 in pulmonary hypertension: Marker or mediator of disease? Ann. Intern. Med. 114:464, 1991.
23. Kotlikoff, M. I., and Fishman, A. P.: Endothelin: Mediator of hypoxic vasoconstriction? In Fishman, A. P. (ed.): The Pulmonary Circulation: Normal and Abnormal. Phildelphia, University of Pennsylvania Press, 1990, pp. 85–89.
24. McMurtry, I. F.: Bay K 8644, a Ca^{++} channel facilitator, potentiates hypoxic vasoconstriction in isolated rat lungs. Fed. Proc. 44:2389, 1985.
25. McMurtry, I. F.: Humeral control. In Bergofsky, E. (ed.): Abnormal Pulmonary Circulation. New York, Churchill Livingstone, 1986, pp. 83–126.
26. Rabinovitch, M., Gamble, W., Nadas, A. S., et al.: Rat pulmonary circulation after chronic hypoxia: Hemodynamic and structural features. Am. J. Physiol. 236:H818, 1979.
27. Rabinovitch, M., Gamble W. J., Miettinen, O. S., and Reid, L.: Age and sex influence on pulmonary hypertension of chronic hypoxia and on recovery. Am. J. Physiol. 240:H62, 1981.
28. Glazier, J. B., and Murray, J. F.: Sites of pulmonary vasomotor reactivity in the dog during alveolar hypoxia and serotonin and histamine infusion. J. Clin. Invest. 50:2550, 1971.
29. Bergofsky, E. H.: Mechanisms underlying vasomotor regulation of regional pulmonary blood flow in normal and disease states. Am. J. Med. 57:378, 1974.
30. Hauge, A.: Hypoxia and pulmonary vascular resistance: The relative effects of pulmonary arterial and alveolar pO$_2$. Acta Physiol. Scand. 76:121, 1969.
31. Enson, Y., Giuntini, C., Lewis, M. L., et al.: The influence of hydrogen ion concentration and hypoxia on the pulmonary circulation. J. Clin. Invest. 43:1146, 1964.
32. Kadowitz, P. J., Joiner, P. D., and Hyman, A. L.: Effect of sympathetic nerve stimulation on pulmonary vascular resistance in the intact spontaneously breathing dog. Proc. Soc. Exp. Biol. Med. 147:68, 1974.
33. Fritts, H. W., Harris, P., Clauss, R. H., et al.: The effect of acetylcholine on the human pulmonary circulation under normal and hypoxic conditions. J. Clin. Invest. 37:99, 1958.
34. Kadowitz, P. J., and Hyman, A. L.: Differential effects of prostaglandins A$_1$ and A$_2$ on pulmonary vascular resistance in the dog. Proc. Soc. Exp. Biol. Med. 149:282, 1975.
35. Moncada, S.: Prostacyclin, from discovery to clinical application. J. Pharmacol. 16(Suppl):71, 1985.
36. Vane, J. R., Anggard, E. E., and Botting, R. M.: Regulatory functions of the vascular endothelium. N. Engl. J. Med. 323:27, 1990.
37. Radomski, M. W., Palmer, R. M., and Moncada, S.: The anti-aggregating properties of vascular endothelium: Interactions between prostacyclin and nitric oxide. Br. J. Pharmacol. 92:639, 1987.
37a. Cooper, C. J., Landzberg, M. J., Anderson, T. J., et al.: Role of nitric oxide in the local regulation of pulmonary vascular resistance in humans. Circulation 93:266, 1996.
38. DeNucci, G., Gryglewski, R. J., Warner, T. D., and Vane, J. R.: Receptor-mediated release of endothelium-derived relaxing factor and prostacyclin from bovine aortic endothelial cells is coupled. Proc. Natl. Acad. Sci. U.S.A. 85:2334, 1988.
38a. Mehta, S., Stewart, D. J., Langleben, D., and Levy, R. D.: Short-term pulmonary vasodilation with L-arginine in pulmonary hypertension. Circulation 92:1539, 1995.
39. Kay, J. M., Waymire, J. C., and Grover, R. F.: Lung mast cell hyperplasia and pulmonary histamine forming capacity in hypoxic rats. Am. J. Physiol. 226:178, 1974.
40. Haas, F., and Bergofsky, E. H.: Role of the mast cell in the pulmonary pressor response to hypoxia. J. Clin. Invest. 51:3154, 1972.
41. Goldring, R. M., Turino, G. M., Cohen, G., et al.: The catecholamines in the pulmonary arterial pressor response to acute hypoxia. J. Clin. Invest. 41:1211, 1962.
42. Long, W. A., and Brown, D. L.: Central neural regulation of the pulmonary circulation. In Fishman, A. P. (ed.): The Pulmonary Circulation: Normal and Abnormal. University of Pennsylvania Press, Philadelphia, 1990, pp. 131–149.
43. Tucker, A., Hoffman, E. A., and Weir, E. K.: Histamine receptor antagonism does not inhibit hypoxic pulmonary vasoconstriction in dogs. Chest 71(Suppl):261, 1977.
44. Moret, P., Covarrubias, E., Coudert, J., and Duchosall, F.: Cardiocirculatory adaptation to chronic hypoxia. Acta Cardiol. (Brux.) 27:596, 1972.
45. Vogel, J. H. K., Weaver, W. F., Rose, R. L., et al.: Pulmonary hypertension on exertion in normal men living at 10,150 feet (Leadville, Colorado). Med. Thorac. 19:461, 1962.

46. Hatano, S., and Strasser, T. (eds.): Primary Pulmonary Hypertension. Geneva, World Health Organization, 1975, pp. 7–45.
47. Rubin, L. J.: ACCP concensus statement. Primary pulmonary hypertension. Chest 104:236, 1993.
48. Abenhaim, L., Moride, Y., Rich, S., et al.: The International Primary Pulmonary Hypertension Study. Chest 105(2):37S, 1994.
49. Wood, P.: Pulmonary hypertension with special reference to the vasoconstrictive factor. Br. Heart J. 20:557, 1958.
50. Daoud, F. S., Reeves, J. T., and Kelly, D. B.: Isoproterenol as a potential pulmonary vasodilator in primary pulmonary hypertension. Am. J. Cardiol. 42:817, 1978.
51. Shepherd, J. T., Edwards, J. E., Burchell, H. B., et al.: Clinical, physiological and pathological considerations in patients with idiopathic pulmonary hypertension. Br. Heart J. 19:70, 1957.
52. Marshall, R. J., Helmholz, H. F., and Shepherd, J. T.: Effect of acetylcholine on pulmonary vascular resistance in a patient with idiopathic pulmonary hypertension. Circulation 20:391, 1959.
53. Uren, N. G., Ludman, P. E., Crake, T., and Oakley, C. M.: Response of the pulmonary circulation to acetylcholine, calcitonin, gene-related peptide, substance P, and oral nicardipine in patients with primary pulmonary hypertension. J. Am. Coll. Cardiol. 19:835, 1992.
54. Celermajer, D. S., Cullen, S., and Deanfield, J. E.: Impairment of endothelium-dependent pulmonary artery relaxation in children with congenital heart disease and abnormal pulmonary hemodynamics. Circulation 87:440, 1993.
55. Luscher, T. F.: Endothelin: Systemic arterial and pulmonary effects of a new peptide with potent biologic properties. Am. Rev. Respir. Dis. 146:S56, 1992.
56. Okada, M., Yamashita, C., Okada, M., and Okada, K.: Endothelin receptor antagonists in a beagle model of pulmonary hypertension: Contribution of possible potential therapy. J. Am. Coll. Cardiol. 25:1213, 1995.
57. Pietra, G. G., Edwards, W. D., Kay, J. M., et al.: Histopathology of primary pulmonary hypertension. A qualitative and quantitative study of pulmonary blood vessels from 58 patients in the National Heart, Lung, and Blood Institute, Primary Pulmonary Hypertension Registry. Circulation 80:1198, 1989.
58. Edwards, W. D., and Edwards, J. E.: Clinical primary pulmonary hypertension—three pathological types. Circulation 56:884, 1977.
59. Lindner, V., et al.: Role of basic fibroblast growth factor in vascular lesion formation. Circ. Res. 63:106, 1991.
60. Pierce, G. F., et al.: Platelet-derived growth factor β and transforming growth factors induce in vivo and in vitro tissue repair structures by unique mechanisms. J. Cell Biol. 109:429, 1989.
61. Botney, M. D., et al.: Vascular remodeling in primary pulmonary hypertension. Potential role for transforming growth factor β. Am. J. Pathol. 144:286, 1994.
62. Bodreau, N., and Rabinovich, M.: Developmentally regulated changes in extracellular matrix in endothelial and smooth muscle cells in the ductus arteriosus may be related to intimal proliferation. Lab. Invest. 64:187, 1991.
63. Botney, M. D., et al.: Active collagen synthesis by pulmonary arteries in human primary pulmonary hypertension. Am. J. Pathol. 143:121, 1993.
64. Rich, S., and Brundage, B. H.: Pulmonary hypertension: A cellular basis for understanding the pathophysiology and treatment. J. Am. Coll. Cardiol. 14:545, 1989.
65. Fuster, V., Steele, P. M., Edwards, W. D., et al.: Primary pulmonary hypertension: Natural history and the importance of thrombosis. Circulation 70:580, 1984.
66. Inglesby, T. V., Singer, J. W., and Gordon, D. S.: Abnormal fibrinolysis in familial pulmonary hypertension. Am. J. Med. 55:5, 1973.
67. Anderson, E. G., Simon, G., and Reid, L.: Primary and thromboembolic pulmonary hypertension: A quantitative pathological study. J. Pathol. 110:273, 1973.
68. Stuard, I. D., Heusinkveld, R. S., and Moss, A. J.: Microangiopathic hemolytic anemia and thrombocytopenia in primary pulmonary hypertension. N. Engl. J. Med. 287:869, 1972.
69. Franz, R. C., Ziady, F., Coetzee, W. J. C., and Hugo, N.: A possible causal relationship between defective fibrinolysis and pulmonary hypertension. S. Afr. Med. J. 55:170, 1979.
70. Tubbs, R. R., Levin, R. D., Shirey, E. K., and Hoffman, G. C.: Fibrinolysis in familial pulmonary hypertension. Am. J. Clin. Pathol. 71:384, 1979.
71. Geggel, R. L., Carvalho, A. C., Hoyer, L. N., et al.: Von Willebrand factor abnormalities in primary pulmonary hypertension. Am. Rev. Respir. Dis. 135:294, 1987.
72. Ware, J. A., and Helstad, D. D.: Platelet-endothelium interactions. N. Engl. J. Med. 328:628, 1993.
73. Hopkins, W. E., Waggoner, A. D., and Barzilai, B.: Frequency and significance of intrapulmonary right-to-left shunting in end-stage hepatic disease. Am. J. Cardiol. 70:516, 1992.
74. McDonnell, P. J., Toye, P. A., and Hutchins, G. M.: Primary pulmonary hypertension and cirrhosis: Are they related? Am. Rev. Respir. Dis. 127:437, 1983.
75. Lopez-Talavera, J. C., Merrill, W. M., and Groszmann, R. J.: Tumor necrosis factor α: A major contributor to the hyperdynamic circulation in prehepatic portal-hypertensive rats. Gastroenterology 108:761, 1995.
76. Stephens, K. E., Ishizaka, A., Larryk, J. W., and Raffin, T. A.: Tumor

necrosis factor causes increased pulmonary permeability and edema. Comparison to septic lung injury. Am. Rev. Respir. Dis. *137:*1364, 1988.

77. Goto, M., Takei, Y., Kuwano, S., et al.: Tumor necrosis factor and endotoxin in the pathogenesis of liver and pulmonary injuries after orthotopic liver transplantation in the rat. Hepatology *16:*487, 1992.

78. Groves, B. M., Brundage, B. H., Elliott, C. G., et al.: Pulmonary hypertension associated with hepatic cirrhosis. In Fishman, A. P. (ed.): The Pulmonary Circulation: Normal and Abnormal. Philadelphia, University of Pennsylvania Press, 1990, pp. 359–369.

79. Naeye, R. L.: "Primary" pulmonary hypertension with coexisting portal hypertension. A retrospective study of six cases. Circulation *22:*376, 1960.

80. Segel, N., Kay, J. M., Bayley, T. J., and Paton, A.: Pulmonary hypertension with hepatic cirrhosis. Br. Heart J. *30:*575, 1968.

81. Senior, R. M., Britton, R. C., Turino, G. M., et al.: Pulmonary hypertension associated with cirrhosis of the liver and with portacaval shunts. Circulation *37:*88, 1968.

82. Robalino, B. D., and Moodie, D. S.: Association between primary pulmonary hypertension and portal hypertension: Analysis of its pathophysiology and clinical, laboratory and hemodynamic manifestations. J. Am. Coll. Cardiol. *17:*492, 1991.

83. Gurtner, H. P.: Pulmonary hypertension, "plexogenic pulmonary arteriopathy" and the appetite depressant drug aminorex: Post or propter? Bull. Eur. Physiopathol. Resp. *15:*897, 1979.

84. Douglas, J. G., Monro, J. F., Kitchin, A. H., et al.: Pulmonary hypertension and fenfluramine. Br. Med. J. *283:*881, 1981.

85. McMurray, J., Bloomfield, P., and Miller, H. C.: Irreversible pulmonary hypertension after therapy with fenfluramine. Br. Med. J. *292:*239, 1986.

86. Brenot, F., Herve, P., Pettipretz, P., et al.: Primary pulmonary hypertension and fenfluramine use. Br. Heart J. *70:*537, 1993.

87. Roche, N., Labrune, S., Braune, J. M., and Huchon, G. J.: Pulmonary hypertension and dexfenfluramine. Lancet *339:*437, 1992.

88. Polos, P. G., Wolfe, D., Harley, R. A., et al.: Pulmonary hypertension and human immunodeficiency virus infection. Chest *101:*474, 1992.

89. Jacques, C., Richmond, G., Tierney, L., et al.: Primary pulmonary hypertension and human immunodeficiency virus infection in a non-hemophiliac man. Hum. Pathol. *23:*191, 1992.

90. Maliakkal, R., Freedman, S. A., and Sridhar, S.: Progressive pulmonary thromboembolism in association with HIV disease. N.Y. State J. Med. *92:*403, 1992.

91. Petitpretz, P., Brenot, F., Azarian, R., et al.: Pulmonary hypertension in patients with human immunodeficiency virus infection. Circulation *89:*2772, 1994.

92. Mette, S. A., Palevsky, H. I., Pietra, G. G., et al.: Primary pulmonary hypertension in association with human immunodeficiency virus infection. Am. Rev. Respir. Dis. *145:*1196, 1992.

93. Alpert, M. A., Bauer, J. H., Parker, B. M., et al.: Pulmonary hypertension in systemic hypertension. South Med. J. *78:*784, 1995.

94. Guazzi, M. D., Polese, A., Bartonelli, A., et al.: Evidence of a shared mechanism of vasoconstriction in pulmonary and systemic circulation in hypertension: A possible role of intracellular calcium. Circulation *66:*881, 1982.

95. Guazzi, M. D., DeCasare, N., Fiorentini, C., et al.: Pulmonary vascular supersensitivity to catecholamines in systemic high blood pressure. J. Am. Coll. Cardiol. *8:*1137, 1986.

96. Moruzzi, P., Sganzerla, P., and Guazzi, M. D.: Pulmonary vasoconstriction overreactivity in borderline systemic hypertension. Cardiovasc. Res. *23:*666, 1989.

97. Yamaki, S., Horiuchi, T., Miura, M., et al.: Pulmonary vascular disease in secundum atrial septal defect with pulmonary hypertension. Chest *89:*694, 1986.

98. Okura, H., and Takatsu, Y.: High-output heart failure as a cause of pulmonary hypertension. Intern. Med. *33:*363, 1994.

99. Robertson, B., Rosenhamer, G., and Lindberg, J.: Idiopathic pulmonary hypertension in two siblings. Acta Med. Scand. *186:*569, 1969.

100. Melmon, K. L., and Braunwald, E.: Familial pulmonary hypertension. N. Engl. J. Med. *269:*770, 1963.

101. Rogge, J. D., Mishkin, M. E., and Genovese, P. D.: The familial occurrence of primary pulmonary hypertension. Ann. Intern. Med. *65:*672, 1966.

102. Kingdon, H. S., Cohen, L. S., Roberts, W. C., and Braunwald, E.: Familial occurrence of primary pulmonary hypertension. Arch. Intern. Med. *118:*422, 1966.

103. Lloyd, J. E., Butler, M. G., Foroud, T. M., et al.: Fewer males at birth and genetic anticipation are features of familial primary pulmonary hypertension. Am. Rev. Respir. Dis. *147:*A928, 1993.

104. Lloyd, J. E., Primm, R. K., and Newman, J. H.: Transmission of familial primary pulmonary hypertension. Am. Rev. Respir. Dis. *129:*194, 1984.

105. Rich, S., Kieras, K., Hart, K., et al.: Antinuclear antibodies in primary pulmonary hypertension. J. Am. Coll. Cardiol. *8:*1307, 1986.

106. Barst, R. J., Flaster, E. R., Menom, A., et al.: Evidence for the association of unexplained pulmonary hypertension in children with the major histocompatibility complex. Circulation *85:*249, 1992.

107. Wagenvoort, C. A., and Wagenvoort, N.: Primary pulmonary hypertension: A pathologic study of the lung vessels in 156 clinically diagnosed cases. Circulation *42:*1163, 1970.

108. Bjornsson, J., and Edwards, W. D.: Primary pulmonary hypertension: A histopathologic study of 80 cases. Mayo Clin. Proc. *60:*16, 1969.

109. Clausen, K. P., and Geer, J. C.: Hypertensive pulmonary arteritis. Am. J. Dis. Child. *118:*718, 1969.

110. Wagenvoort, C. A.: Pulmonary veno-occlusive disease: Entity or syndrome. Chest *69:*82, 1976.

111. Rich, S.: Primary pulmonary hypertension. Prog. Cardiovasc. Dis. *31:*205, 1988.

112. Wagenvoort, C. A.: Capillary hemangiomatosis of the lung. Histopathology *2:*401, 1978.

113. Magee, F., Wright, J. L., Kay, M. J., et al.: Pulmonary capillary hemangiomatosis. Am. Rev. Resp. Dis. *132:*922, 1985.

114. Whittaker, J. S., Pickering, C. A. C., Heath, D., et al.: Pulmonary capillary hemangiomatosis. Diag. Histopathol. *6:*77, 1983.

115. Nootens, M., Wolfkiel, C. J., Chomka, E. V., and Rich, S.: Understanding right and left ventricular systolic function and interactions at rest and with exercise in primary pulmonary hypertension. Am. J. Cardiol. *75:*379, 1995.

116. D'Alonzo, G. E., Barst, R. J., Ayres, S. M., et al.: Survival in patients with primary pulmonary hypertension: Results from a national prospective registry. Ann. Intern. Med. *115:*343, 1991.

117. Rich, S., Kaufmann, E., and Levy, P. S.: The effect of high doses of calcium-channel blockers on survival in primary pulmonary hypertension. N. Engl. J. Med. *327:*76, 1992.

118. Sandoval, J., Bauerle, O., Palomar, A., et al.: Survival in primary pulmonary hypertension. Validation of a prognostic equation. Circulation *89:*1733, 1994.

119. Brooks, H., Kirk, E. S., Vokanas, P. S., et al.: Performance of the right ventricle under stress: Relation to right coronary flow. J. Clin. Invest. *50:*2176, 1971.

120. Murray, P. A., and Vatner, S. F.: Reduction of maximal coronary vasodilator capacity in conscious dogs with severe right ventricular hypertrophy. Circ. Res. *48:*27, 1981.

121. Doty, D. B., Wright, C. B., Hirratzka, L. F., et al.: Coronary reserve in volume-induced right ventricular hypertrophy from septal defect. Am. J. Cardiol. *54:*1059, 1984.

122. Vlhakes, G. J., Turley, K., and Hoffman, J. I. E.: The pathophysiology of failure in acute right ventricular hypertension: Hemodynamic and biochemical correlations. Circulation *63:*87, 1981.

123. Murray, P. A., and Vatner, S. F.: Carotid sinus baroreceptor control of right coronary circulation in normal, hypertrophied, and failing right ventricles of conscious dogs. Circ. Res. *49:*1339, 1981.

124. Wilmhurst, P. T., Webb-Peploe, M. M., and Corker, R. J.: Left recurrent laryngeal nerve palsy associated with primary pulmonary hypertension and recurrent pulmonary embolism. Br. Heart J. *49:*141, 1983.

124a. Chobanian, A. V., and Dzau, V. J.: Renin antiotensin system and atherosclerotic vascular disease. In Fuster, V., Ross, R., and Topol, E. J. (eds.): Atherosclerosis and coronary artery disease. Philadelphia, Lippincott-Raven Publishers, 1996, pp.237–242.

125. Kanemoto, N.: Electrocardiographic and hemodynamic correlations in primary pulmonary hypertension. Angiology *39:*781, 1988.

126. Kanemoto, N., Furuya, H., Etoh, T., Sasamoto, H., and Matsuyama, S.: Chest roentgenograms in primary pulmonary hypertension. Chest *76:*45, 1979.

127. Anderson, G., Reid, L., and Simon, G.: The radiographic appearances in primary and in thromboembolic pulmonary hypertension. Clin. Radiol. *24:*113, 1973.

128. Kuriyama, K., Gamsu, G., Stern, R. G., et al.: CT-determined pulmony artery diameters in predicting pulmonary hypertension. Invest. Radiol. *19:*16, 1984.

129. Goodman, D. J., Harrison, D. C., and Popp, R. L.: Echocardiographic features of primary pulmonary hypertension. Am. J. Cardiol. *33:*438, 1974.

130. Louie, E. K., Rich, S., and Brundage, B. H.: Doppler echocardiographic assessment of impaired left ventricular filling with right ventricular pressure overload due to primary pulmonary hypertension. J. Am. Coll. Cardiol. *8:*1298, 1986.

131. Rich, S., Pietra, G. G., Kieras, K., et al.: Primary pulmonary hypertension: Radiographic and scintigraphic patterns of histologic subtypes. Ann. Intern. Med. *105:*499, 1986.

132. Fishman, A. J., Moser, K. M., and Fedullo, P. F.: Perfusion lung scans vs pulmonary angiography in the evaluation of suspected primary pulmonary hypertension. Chest *84:*679, 1983.

133. Levin, R. I., and Glassman, E.: Left atrial-pulmonary artery wedge pressure relation: Effect of elevated pulmonary vascular resistance. Am. J. Cardiol. *55:*856, 1985.

134. Rozkovic, A., Montanes, D., and Oakley, C. M.: Factors that influence the outcome of primary pulmonary hypertension. Br. Heart J. *55:*449, 1986.

135. Groves, B. M., Ditchey, R. V., Reeves, J. T., et al.: Multicenter trial of a new guide wire thermodilution catheter. J. Am. Coll. Cardiol. *3:*599, 1984.

136. Nootens, M. T., Berarducci, L. A., Kaufmann, E., et al.: The prevalence and significance of a patent foramen ovale in pulmonary hypertension. Chest *104:*1673, 1993.

137. Benotti, J. R., and Grossman, W.: Pulmonary angiography. In Grossman, W., and Baim, D. S. (eds.): Cardiac Catheterization, Angiography and Intervention. 4th ed. Philadelphia, Lea and Febiger, 1991.

138. Janiki, J. S., Weber, K. T., Likoff, M. J., et al.: The pressure-flow response of the pulmonary circulation in patients with heart failure and pulmonary vascular disease. Circulation *72:*1270, 1985.

139. McCaffrey, R. M., and Dunn, L. J.: Primary pulmonary hypertension in pregnancy. Obstet. Gynecol. Surg. *19*:567, 1964.

140. Nelson, D. M., Main, E., Crafford, W., et al.: Peripartum heart failure due to primary pulmonary hypertension. Obstet. Gynecol. *62*:58S, 1983.

141. Spann, J. F., Buccino, R. A., Sonnenblick, E. H., et al.: Contractile state of cardiac muscle obtained from cats with experimentally produced ventricular hypertrophy. Circ. Res. *21*:431, 1967.

142. Fishman, A. P.: Chronic cor pulmonale. Am. Rev. Respir. Dis. *114*:775, 1976.

143. Abraham, A. S., Cole, R. B., and Bishop, J. B.: Reversal of pulmonary hypertension by prolonged oxygen administration to patients with chronic bronchitis. Circ. Res. *23*:147, 1968.

144. Swan, H. J. C., Burchell, H. B., and Wood, E. H.: Effect of oxygen on pulmonary vascular resistance in patients with pulmonary hypertension associated with atrial septal defect. Circulation *20*:66, 1959.

145. Morgan, J. M., Griffiths, M., du Bois, R. M., and Evans, T. W.: Hypoxic pulmonary vasoconstriction in systemic sclerosis and primary pulmonary hypertension. Chest *99*:551, 1991.

146. Rich, S., D'Alonzo, G. E., Dantzker, D. R., et al.: Magnitude and implications of spontaneous hemodynamic variability in primary pulmonary hypertension. Am. J. Cardiol. *55*:159, 1985.

147. Packer, M., Medine, N., and Yushak, M.: Adverse hemodynamic and clinical effects of calcium channel blockade in pulmonary hypertension secondary to obliterative pulmonary vascular disease. J. Am. Coll. Cardiol. *4*:890, 1984.

148. Melot, C., Hallemans, R., Naeije, R., et al.: Deleterious effect of nifedipine on pulmonary gas exchange in chronic obstructive pulmonary disease. Am. Rev. Respir. Dis. *130*:612, 1984.

149. Rich, S., and Kaufmann, L: High dose titration of calcium channel blocking agents for primary pulmonary hypertension: Guidelines for short-term drug testing. J. Am. Coll. Cardiol. *18*:1323, 1991.

150. Grover, R. F., Reeves, J. T., and Blount, S. F., Jr.: Tolazoline hydrochloride (Priscoline): An effective pulmonary vasodilator. Am. Heart J. *61*:5, 1961.

151. Rudolph, A. M., Paul, M. H., Sommer, L. S., et al.: Effects of tolazoline hydrochloride (Priscoline) on circulatory dynamics in patients with pulmonary hypertension. Am. Heart J. *56*:424, 1958.

152. Samet, P., Bernstein, W. H., and Widrich, J.: Intracardiac infusion of acetylcholine in primary pulmonary hypertension. Am. Heart J. *60*:433, 1960.

153. Charms, B. L.: Primary pulmonary hypertension: Effect of unilateral pulmonary artery occlusion and infusion of acetylcholine. Am. J. Cardiol. *99*:94, 1961.

154. Shettigar, U. R., Hultgren, H. N., Specter, M., et al.: Primary pulmonary hypertension: Favorable effect of isoproterenol. N. Engl. J. Med. *295*:1414, 1976.

154a. Morgan, J. M., Griffiths, M., du Bois, R. M., and Evans, T. W.: Hypoxic pulmonary vasoconstriction in systemic sclerosis and primary pulmonary hypertension. Chest *99*:551, 1991.

154b. Heath, D., and Edwards, J. E.: The pathology of hypertensive pulmonary vascular disease. A description of six grades of structural changes in the pulmonary arteries with special references to congenital cardiac septal defects. Circulation *18*:533, 1958.

155. Person, B., and Proctor, R. G.: Primary pulmonary hypertension: Responses to indomethacin, terbutaline and isoproterenol. Chest *76*:601, 1979.

156. Bergofsky, E. H.: Mechanisms underlying vasomotor regulation of regional pulmonary blood flow in normal and disease states. Am. J. Med. *57*:378, 1974.

157. Fishman, A. P.: Autonomic vasomotor tone in the pulmonary circulation. J. Anesthesiol. *45*:1, 1976.

158. Ruskin, J. N., and Hutter, A. M.: Primary pulmonary hypertension treated with oral phentolamine. Ann. Intern. Med. *90*:772, 1979.

159. Beladinelli, L., Linden, J., and Berne, M. R.: The cardiac effects of adenosine. Prog. Cardiovasc. Dis. *32*:73, 1989.

160. Watt, A. H., Penny, W. J., Singh, H., et al.: Adenosine causes transient dilatation of coronary arteries in man. Br. J. Clin. Pharmacol. *24*:665, 1987.

161. Bush, A., Busst, C. M., Clarke, B., and Barnes, P. J.: Effect of infused adenosine on cardiac output and systemic resistance in normal subjects. Br. J. Clin. Pharmacol. *27*:165, 1989.

162. McCormack, D. G., Clarke, B., and Barnes, P. J.: Characterization of adenosine receptors in human pulmonary arteries. Am. J. Physiol. *256*:H41, 1989.

163. Schrader, B., Inbar, S., Kaufmann, L., et al.: Comparison of the effects of adenosine and nifedipine in pulmonary hypertension. J. Am. Coll. Cardiol. *19*:1060, 1992.

164. Nootens, M., Schrader, B., Kaufmann, E., et al.: Comparative acute effects of adenosine and prostacyclin in primary pulmonary hypertension. Chest *107*:54, 1995.

165. Muller, B.: Pharmacology of thromboxane A_2, prostacyclin and other ecosanoids in the cardiovascular system. Therapie *46*:217, 1991.

166. Dusting, G. J., and MacDonald, P. S.: Prostacyclin and vascular function: Implications for hypertension and atherosclerosis. Pharmacol. Ther. *48*:323, 1990.

167. Rubin, L. J., Groves, B. M., Reeves, J. T., et al.: Prostacyclin-induced pulmonary vasodilation in primary pulmonary hypertension. Circulation *66*:334, 1982.

168. Barst, R. J.: Pharmacologically induced pulmonary vasodilatation in

169. Frostell, C., Fratacci, M. D., Wain, J. C., et al.: Inhaled nitric oxide:`A selective pulmonary vasodilator reversing hypoxic pulmonary vasoconstriction. Circulation *83*:2038, 1991.

170. Pepke-Zaba, J., Higgenbottam, W., Tuan Ding-Xuan, A., et al.: Inhaled nitric oxide as a cause of selective pulmonary vasodilation in pulmonary hypertension. Lancet *338*:1173, 1991.

171. Roberts, J. D., Lang, P., Bigatello, L. M., et al.: Inhaled nitric oxide in congenital heart disease. Circulation *87*:447, 1993.

172. Rubin, L. J., Nicod, P., Hillis, L. D., and Firth, B. G.: Treatment of primary pulmonary hypertension with nifedipine. A hemodynamic and scintigraphic evaluation. Ann. Intern. Med. *99*:433, 1983.

173. Fisher, J., Borer, J. S., Moses, J. W., et al.: Hemodynamic effects of nifedipine versus hydralazine in primary pulmonary hypertension. Am. J. Cardiol. *54*:646, 1984.

174. Melot, C., Naejie, R., Mols, P., et al.: Effects of nifedipine on ventilation/perfusion matching in primary pulmonary hypertension. Chest *83*:203, 1983.

175. Olivari, M. T., Cohn, J. N., Carlyle, P., and Levine, T. B.: Beneficial hemodynamic and exercise response to nifedipine in primary pulmonary hypertension. J. Am. Coll. Cardiol. *1*:735, 1983.

176. Packer, M., Medina, N., Yushak, M., and Wiener, I.: Detrimental effects of verapamil in patients with primary hypertension. Br. Heart J. *52*:106, 1984.

177. Rich, S., and Brundage, B. H.: High-dose calcium channel-blocking therapy for primary pulmonary hypertension: Evidence of long-term reduction in pulmonary arterial pressure and regression of right ventricular hypertrophy. Circulation *76*:135, 1987.

178. Jones, D. K., Whigenbottam, T. W., and Wallwork, J.: Treatment of primary pulmonary hypertension with intravenous epoprostenol (prostacyclin). Br. Heart J. *57*:270, 1987.

179. Rubin, L. J., Mendoza, J., Hood, M., et al.: Treatment of primary pulmonary hypertension with continuous intravenous prostacyclin (epoprostenol). Ann. Intern. Med. *112*:485, 1990.

180. Barst, R. J., Rubin, L. J., McGoon, M. D., et al.: Survival in primary pulmonary hypertension with long-term continuous intravenous prostacyclin. Ann. Intern. Med. *121*:409, 1994.

180a. Raffy, O., Azarian, R., Brenot, F., et al.: Clinical significance of the pulmonary vasodilator response during short-term infusion of prostacyclin in primary pulmonary hypertension. Circulation *93*:484, 1996.

181. Guadagni, D. N., Ikram, H., and Maslowski, A. H.: Haemodynamic effects of prostacyclin (PGI_2) in pulmonary hypertension. Br. Heart J. *45*:385, 1981.

182. Rubin, L. J., Groves, B. M., Reeves, J. T., et al.: Prostacyclin-induced acute pulmonary vasodilation in primary pulmonary hypertension. Circulation *66*:334, 1982.

183. Groves, B. M., Rubin, L. J., Frosolono, M. F., et al.: A comparison of the acute hemodynamic effects of prostacyclin and hydralazine in primary pulmonary hypertension. Am. Heart J. *110*:1200, 1985.

184. Rozkovec, A., Stradling, J. R., Shepherd, G., et al.: Prediction of favourable responses to long term vasodilator treatment of pulmonary hypertension by short-term administration of epoprostenol (prostacyclin) or nifedipine. Br. Heart J. *59*:696, 1988.

185. Lock, J. E., Olley, P. M., Coceani, P. M., et al.: Use of prostacyclin in persistent fetal circulation. Lancet *1*:1343, 1979.

186. Young, D., and Mark, H.: Fate of the patient with Eisenmenger's syndrome. Am. J. Cardiol. *65*:655, 1971.

187. Rich, S., and Lam, W.: Atrial septostomy as palliative therapy for refractory primary pulmonary hypertension. Am. J. Cardiol. *51*:1560, 1983.

188. Nihill, M. R., O'Laughlin, M. P., and Mullins, C. E.: Effects of atrial septostomy in patients with terminal cor pulmonale due to pulmonary vascular disease. Cathet. Cardiovasc. Diagn. *24*:166, 1991.

189. Hausknecht, M. J., Sims, R. E., Nihill, M. R., and Cashion, W. R.: Successful palliation of primary pulmonary hypertension by atrial septostomy. Am. J. Cardiol. *65*:1045, 1990.

190. Kirstein, D., Levy, P. S., Hsui, D. T., et al.: Blade balloon atrial septostomy in patients with severe primary pulmonary hypertension. Circulation *91*:2028, 1995.

191. Jamieson, S. W., Stinson, E. B., Oyer, P. E., et al.: Heart and lung transplantation for pulmonary hypertension. Am. J. Surg. *147*:740, 1984.

192. Dawkins, K. D., Jamieson, S. W., Hunt, S. A., et al.: Long-term results, hemodynamics, and complications after combined heart and lung transplantation. Circulation *71*:919, 1985.

193. Dawkins, K. D., Haverich, A., Derby, G. C., et al.: Long-term hemodynamics following combined heart and lung transplantation in primates. J. Thorac. Cardiovasc. Surg. *89*:55, 1985.

194. Reitz, B. A., Wallwork, J. L., Hunt, S. A., et al.: Heart-lung transplantation: Successful therapy for patients with pulmonary vascular disease. N. Engl. J. Med. *306*:557, 1982.

195. Kaiser, L. R., and Cooper, J. D.: The current status of lung transplantation. Adv. Surg. *25*:259, 1992.

196. Pasque, M. K., Trulock, E. P., Kaiser, L. R., and Cooper, J. D.: Single-lung transplantation for pulmonary hypertension: Three-month hemodynamic follow-up. Circulation *84*:2275, 1991.

197. Levine, S. M., Jenkinson, S. G., Bryan, C. L., et al.: Ventilation-perfusion inequalities during graft rejection in patients undergoing single lung transplantation for primary pulmonary hypertension. Chest *101*:401, 1992.

children and young adults with primary hypertension. Chest *89*:497, 1986.

198. Brooks, H. L., Kirk, E. S., Vokonas, P. S., et al.: Performance of the right ventricle under stress. J. Clin. Invest. 50:2176, 1971.

199. Berman, J. L., Green, L. G., and Grossman, W.: Right ventricular diastolic pressure in coronary artery disease. Am. J. Cardiol. 44:1263, 1979.

200. Lorell, B. H., Leinbach, R. C., Pohost, G. M., et al.: Right ventricular infarction. Am. J. Cardiol. 43:463, 1979.

201. Kay, J. M., and Edwards, F. R.: Ultrastructure of the alveolar-capillary wall in mitral stenosis. J. Pathol. 111:239, 1973.

202. Szidon, J. P., Pietra, G. G., and Fishman, A. P.: The alveolar-capillary membrane and pulmonary edema. N. Engl. J. Med. 286:1200, 1972.

203. Hicks, J. D.: Acute arterial necrosis in the lungs. J. Pathol. Bacteriol. 65:333, 1953.

204. Whitaker, W., Black, A., and Warrack, A. J. N.: Pulmonary ossification in patients with mitral stenosis. J. Fac. Radiol. (Lond.) 7:29, 1955.

205. Jordan, S. C., Hicken, P., Watson, D. A., et al.: Pathology of the lungs in mitral stenosis in relation to respiratory function and pulmonary haemodynamics. Br. Heart J. 28:101, 1966.

206. Grossman, W.: Profiles in valvular heart disease. In Grossman, W., and Baim, D. S. (eds.): Cardiac Catheterization, Angiography and Intervention. 4th ed. Philadelphia, Lea and Febiger, 1991.

207. Dexter, L.: Physiologic changes in mitral stenosis. N. Engl. J. Med. 254:829, 1956.

208. Robin, E. R., and Meyer, E. C.: Cardiopulmonary effects of pulmonary venous hypertension with special reference to pulmonary lymphatic flow. Circ. Res. 8:324, 1960.

209. Uhley, H. N., Leeds, S. E., Sampson, J. J., and Friedman, M.: Role of pulmonary lymphatics in chronic pulmonary edema. Circ. Res. 11:966, 1962.

210. Parker, F., and Weiss, S.: The nature and significance of the structural changes in the lungs in mitral stenosis. Am. J. Pathol. 12:573, 1936.

211. Coalson, J. J., Jacques, W. E., Campbell, G. S., and Thompson, W. M.: Ultrastructure of the alveolar capillary membrane in congenital and acquired heart disease. Arch. Pathol. 83:377, 1967.

212. Kay, J. M., and Edwards, F. R.: Ultrastructure of the alveolar capillary wall in mitral stenosis. J. Pathol. 111:239, 1973.

213. Heath, D., and Edwards, J. E.: Histological changes in the lung in diseases associated with pulmonary venous hypertension. Br. J. Dis. Chest 53:8, 1959.

214. Carabello, B. A., and Grossman, W.: Calculation of stenotic valve orifice area. In Grossman, W., and Gaim, D. S. (eds.): Cardiac Catheterization, Angiography, and Intervention. 4th ed. Philadelphia, Lea and Febiger, 1991.

215. Braunwald, E., Braunwald, N. S., Ross, J., Jr., and Morrow, A. G.: Effects of mitral valve replacement on pulmonary vascular dynamics of patients with pulmonary hypertension. N. Engl. J. Med. 273:509, 1965.

216. Dalen, J. E., Matloff, J. M., Evans, G. L., et al.: Early reduction of pulmonary vascular resistance after mitral valve replacement. N. Engl. J. Med. 277:387, 1967.

217. Levine, M. J., Weinstein, J. S., Diver, D. J., et al.: Progressive improvement in pulmonary vascular resistance following percutaneous mitral valvuloplasty. Circulation 79:1061, 1989.

218. Alexopoulos, D., Lazzam, C., Borrica, S., et al.: Isolated chronic mitral regurgitation with preserved systolic left ventricular function and severe pulmonary hypertension. J. Am. Coll. Cardiol. 14:319, 1989.

219. Magidson, A.: Cor triatriatum. Severe pulmonary arterial hypertension and pulmonary venous hypertension in a child. Am. J. Cardiol. 9:603, 1962.

220. Cromie, J. B.: Correlation of anatomic pulmonary emphysema and right ventricular hypertrophy. Am. Rev. Respir. Dis. 84:657, 1961.

221. Hicken, P., Heath, D., and Brewer, D.: The relation between the weight of the right ventricle and the percentage of abnormal air space in the lung in emphysema. J. Pathol. Bacteriol. 92:519, 1966.

221a. Burrow, B., Kettel, L. J., Niden, A. H., et al.: Patterns of cardiovascular dysfunction in chronic obstructive lung disease. N. Engl. J. Med. 286:912, 1972.

222. Harvey, R. M., Ferrer, M. I., Richards, D. W., and Cournand, A.: Influence of chronic pulmonary disease on the heart and circulation. Am. J. Med. 10:719, 1951.

223. Abraham, A. S., Cole, R. B., Green, I. D., et al.: Factors contributing to the reversible pulmonary hypertension in patients with acute respiratory failure studied by serial observation during recovery. Circ. Res. 24:51, 1969.

224. Abraham, A. S., Cole, R. B., and Bishop, J.: Effects of prolonged oxygen administration on the pulmonary hypertension of patients with chronic bronchitis. Circ. Res. 23:147, 1968.

225. Segel, N., and Bishop, J. M.: The circulation in patients with chronic bronchitis and emphysema at rest and during exercise with special reference to the influence of changes in blood viscosity and blood volumes on the pulmonary circulation. J. Clin. Invest. 45:1555, 1966.

226. Horsfield, K., Segel, N., and Bishop, J. M.: The pulmonary circulation in chronic bronchitis at rest and during exercise breathing air and 80% oxygen. Clin. Sci. 34:473, 1968.

227. Harvey, R. M., Ferrer, M. I., Richards, D. W., Jr., and Cournand, A.: Influence of chronic pulmonary disease on the heart and circulation. Am. J. Med. 10:719, 1951.

228. Yu, P. N., Lovejoy, F. W., Joos, H. A., et al.: Studies of pulmonary hypertension. I. Pulmonary circulatory dynamics in patients with pulmonary emphysema at rest. J. Clin. Invest. 32:130, 1953.

229. Kitchin, A. H., Lowther, C. P., and Matthews, M. B.: The effect of exercise and of breathing oxygen-enriched air on the pulmonary circulation in emphysema. Clin. Sci. 21:93, 1961.

230. Wilson, R. H., Hoseth, W., and Dempsey, M. E.: The effects of breathing 99.6% oxygen on pulmonary vascular resistance and cardiac output in patients with pulmonary emphysema and chronic hypoxia. Ann. Intern. Med. 42:629, 1955.

231. Aber, G. M., Harris, A. M., and Bishop, J. M.: The effect of acute changes in inspired oxygen concentration of cardiac, respiratory and renal function in patients with chronic obstructive airways disease. Clin. Sci. 26:133, 1964.

232. Stuart-Harris, C., Bishop, J. M., Clark, T. J. H., et al.: Long-term domiciliary oxygen therapy in chronic hypoxic cor pulmonale complicating chronic bronchitis and emphysema. Lancet 1:681, 1981.

233. Nocturnal Oxygen Therapy Trial Group: Continuous or nocturnal oxygen therapy in hypoxic chronic obstructive airways disease? Ann. Intern. Med. 93:391, 1980.

234. Foreman, S., Weill, H., Duke, R., et al.: Bullous disease of the lung: Physiologic improvement after surgery. Ann. Intern. Med. 69:757, 1968.

235. Salerni, R., Rodnan, G. P., Leon, D. F., and Shaver, J. A.: Pulmonary hypertension in the CREST syndrome variant of progressive systemic sclerosis (scleroderma). Ann. Intern. Med. 86:394, 1977.

236. Follansbee, W. P., Curtiss, E. I., Medsger, T. A., et al.: Myocardial function and perfusion in the CREST syndrome variant of progressive systemic sclerosis. Am. J. Med. 77:489, 1984.

237. Seldin, D. W., Ziff, M., and DeGraff, A. V., Jr.: Raynaud's phenomenon associated with pulmonary hypertension. Tex. State J. Med. 58:654, 1962.

238. Winters, W. L., Jr., Joseph, R. R., and Lerner, N.: "Primary" pulmonary hypertension and Raynaud's phenomenon. Arch. Intern. Med. 114:821, 1964.

239. Caldwell, I. W., and Aitchison, J. D.: Pulmonary hypertension in dermatomyositis. Br. Heart J. 18:273, 1956.

240. Walker, W. C., and Wright, V.: Pulmonary lesions and rheumatoid arthritis. Medicine 47:501, 1968.

241. Santini, D., Fox, D., Kloner, R. A., et al.: Pulmonary hypertension in systemic lupus erythematosus: Hemodynamics and effects of vasodilator therapy. Clin. Cardiol. 3:406, 1980.

242. Asherson, R. A., Mackworth-Young, C. G., Boey, M. L., et al.: Pulmonary hypertension in systemic lupus erythematosus. Br. Med. J. 287:1024, 1983.

243. Muschenheim, C.: Some observations on the Hamman-Rich disease. Am. J. Med. Sci. 241:279, 1961.

244. Soergel, K. H., and Sommers, S. C.: Idiopathic pulmonary hemosiderosis and related syndromes. Am. J. Med. 32:499, 1962.

245. Manglo, A., Fisher, J., Libby, D. M., and Saddekni, S.: Sarcoidosis, pulmonary hypertension, and acquired peripheral pulmonary artery stenosis. Cathet. Cardiovasc. Diagn. 11:69, 1985.

246. Kane, R. D., Hawkins, H. K., Miller, J. A., and Noce, P. S.: Microscopic pulmonary tumor emboli associated with dyspnea. Cancer 36:1473, 1975.

247. Jacques, J. E., and Barclay, R.: The solid sarcomatous pulmonary artery. Br. J. Dis. Chest 11:123, 1974.

248. Cooney, T. P., and Thurlbeck, W. M.: Pulmonary hypoplasia in Down's syndrome. N. Engl. J. Med. 307:1170, 1982.

249. Wood, P.: The Eisenmenger syndrome, or pulmonary hypertension with reversed central shunt. Br. Med. J. 2:755, 1958.

250. Yamaki, S., and Wagenvoort, C. A.: Comparison of primary plexogenic arteriopathy in adults and children. A morphometric study in 40 patients. Br. Heart J. 54:428, 1985.

251. Haworth, S. G.: Pulmonary vascular disease in different types of congenital heart disease. Implications for interpretation of lung biopsy findings in early childhood. Br. Heart J. 52:557, 1984.

252. Rabinovitch, M., Keane, J. F., Norwood, W. I., et al.: Vascular structure in lung tissue obtained at biopsy correlated with pulmonary hemodynamic findings after repair of congenital heart defects. Circulation 69:655, 1984.

253. Davies, N. J. H., Shinebourne, E. A., Scallan, M. J., et al.: Pulmonary vascular resistance in children with congenital heart disease. Thorax 39:895, 1984.

254. Takahashi, T., and Wagenvoort, C. A.: Density of muscularized arteries in the lung. Arch. Pathol. Lab. Med. 107:23, 1983.

255. Harley, R. A., Friedman, P. J., Saldana, M., et al.: Sequential development of lesions in experimental extreme pulmonary hypertension. Am. J. Pathol. 52:52A, 1968.

256. Saldana, M. E., Harley, R. A., Liebow, A. A., and Carrington, C. B.: Extreme experimental pulmonary hypertension in relation to polycythemia. Am. J. Pathol. 52:935, 1968.

257. Rabinovitch, M., Keane, J. F., Fellows, K. E., et al.: Quantitative analysis of the pulmonary wedge angiogram in congenital heart defects. Circulation 63:152, 1981.

258. Kawai, C., Ishikawa, K., Kato, M., et al.: Pulmonary pulseless disease: Pulmonary involvement in so-called Takayasu's disease. Chest 73:651, 1978.

259. Lande, A., and Bard, R.: Takayasu's arteritis: An unrecognized cause of pulmonary hypertension. Angiography 27:114, 1976.

260. Levin, D. E., Heymann, M. A., Kitterman, J. A., et al.: Persistent pulmonary hypertension of the newborn infant. J. Pediatr. 89:626, 1976.

261. Finn, M. C., Williams, L. C., and King, T. D.: Persistent fetal circulation in the newborn. J. La. State Med. Soc. *129*:169, 1977.

262. Haworth, S. G., and Reid, L.: Persistent fetal circulation: Newly recognized structural features. J. Pediatr. *88*:614, 1976.

263. Rich, S., Levitsky, S., and Brundage, B. H.: Pulmonary hypertension from chronic pulmonary thromboembolism. Ann. Intern. Med. *108*:425, 1988.

264. Moser, K. M., Daily, P. O., Peterson, K., et al.: Thromboembolic pulmonary hypertension. Ann. Intern. Med. *107*:560, 1987.

265. Shure, D., Gregoratos, G., and Moser, K. M.: Fiberoptic angioscopy: Role in diagnosis of chronic pulmonary arterial obstruction. Ann. Intern. Med. *103*:844, 1985.

266. Delaney, T. B., and Nadas, A. S.: Peripheral pulmonic stenosis. Am. J. Cardiol. *13*:451, 1964.

267. McCue, C. M., Robertson, L. W., Lester, R. G., and Mauck, H. P.: Pulmonary artery coarctations. J. Pediatr. *67*:222, 1965.

268. Pool, P. E., Vogel, J. H. K., and Blount, S. G., Jr.: Congenital unilateral absence of a pulmonary artery. Am. J. Cardiol. *10*:706, 1962.

269. Cohn, L. H., Sanders, J. H., Jr., and Collins, J. J., Jr.: Surgical treatment of congenital unilateral pulmonary arterial stenosis with contralateral pulmonary hypertension. Am. J. Cardiol. *38*:257, 1976.

270. Burwell, C. S., Robin, E. D., Whaley, R. D., and Bickelmann, A. G.: Extreme obesity associated with alveolar hypoventilation. Am. J. Med. *21*:811, 1956.

271. James, T. N., Frame, B., and Coates, E. D.: De subitaneis mortibus. III. Pickwickian syndrome. Circulation *48*:1311, 1973.

272. Noonan, A. J.: Reversible cor pulmonale due to hypertrophied tonsils and adenoids: Studies in two cases. Circulation *32*(Suppl. II):164, 1965.

273. Menashe, V. D., Farrchi, C., and Miller, M.: Hypoventilation and cor pulmonale due to chronic upper airway obstruction. J. Pediatr. *57*:198, 1965.

274. Naeye, R. L.: Alveolar hypoventilation and cor pulmonale secondary to damage to the respiratory center. Am. J. Cardiol. *8*:416, 1961.

275. Hultgren, H. N., Lopez, C. E., Lundberg, E., and Miller, H.: Physiologic studies of pulmonary edema at high altitude. Circulation *29*:393, 1964.

276. Hackett, P. H., Creagh, C. E., Grover, R. F., et al.: High altitude pulmonary edema in persons without the right pulmonary artery. N. Engl. J. Med. *302*:1070, 1980.

277. Staub, N. C.: Pulmonary edema—Hypoxia and overperfusion. N. Engl. J. Med. *302*:1085, 1980.

278. Ingram, C., Satler, L. F., and Rackley, C. E.: Progressive heart failure secondary to a high output state. Chest *92*:1117, 1987.

279. Saaluke, M. G., Shapiro, S. R., Perry, L. W., and Scott, L. P.: Isolated partial anomalous pulmonary venous drainage associated with pulmonary vascular obstructive disease. Am. J. Cardiol. *39*:439, 1977.

280. Heath, D., DuShane, J. W., Wood, E. H., and Edwards, J. E.: The etiology of pulmonary thrombosis in cyanotic congenital heart disease with pulmonary stenosis. Thorax *13*:213, 1958.

281. Durant, J. R., and Cortes, F. M.: Occlusive pulmonary vascular disease associated with hemoglobin SC disease. Am. Heart J. *71*:100, 1966.

282. Rowley, P. T., and Enlander, D.: Hemoglobin SC disease presenting as acute cor pulmonale. Am. Rev. Respir. Dis. *98*:494, 1968.

283. Houck, R. J., Bailey, G. L., Doaroca, P. J., et al.: Pentazocine abuse: Report of a case with pulmonary arterial cellulose granulomas and pulmonary hypertension. Chest *77*:2, 1980.

284. Oliva, P. B., and Vogel, J. H. K.: Reactive pulmonary hypertension in alveolar proteinosis. Chest *58*:167, 1970.

285. Rose, A. G., Halper, J., and Factor, S. M.: Primary arteriopathy in Takayasu's disease. Arch. Pathol. Lab. Med. *108*:644, 1984.

Chapter 26
Systemic Hypertension: Mechanisms and Diagnosis

NORMAN M. KAPLAN

DEFINITIONS, PREVALENCE, AND CONSEQUENCES OF HYPERTENSION

Hypertension, despite its widely recognized high prevalence and associated danger, remains inadequately treated in the majority of patients. In the representative sample of the U.S. population examined in the 1988–1991 National Health and Nutrition Examination Survey (NHANES III), only 21 per cent of hypertensives had their blood pressure well controlled, as defined by a reading below 140/90 mm Hg[1] (Fig. 26–1). Although most hypertension had been identified previously, only about half of hypertensives were currently being treated. Even in a group of hypertensive health care workers with an insurance plan that covered all costs, only 12 per cent of those surveyed in 1992 had their blood pressure adequately managed.[2]

Despite these disturbing figures, the management of hypertension is now the leading indication for both visits to physicians and the use of prescription drugs in the United States. According to the National Ambulatory Care Survey, over 85 million office visits related to hypertension were made in 1991.[3] Clearly, more attention is being directed toward hypertension, but its adequate control remains elusive. This reflects, in large part, the asymptomatic nature of the disease for the first 15 to 20 years, even as it progressively damages the cardiovascular system.[4] Asymptomatic patients often are unwilling to alter life style or take medication to forestall some far-off, poorly perceived danger, particularly when they are made uncomfortable in the process.

In view of these built-in barriers to effective control of the individual patient, the population-wide application of preventive measures becomes inherently more attractive. Although the specific mechanisms for most hypertension remain unknown, it is highly likely that the process could be slowed, if not prevented, by the prevention of obesity, moderate reduction in sodium intake, higher levels of physical activity, and avoidance of excessive alcohol consumption.[5] Since most people will eventually develop hypertension during their lifetime, the need for more widespread adoption of potentially effective and totally safe preventive measures is obvious. In the meantime, better management of those already afflicted must be practiced, starting with careful documentation of the diagnosis.

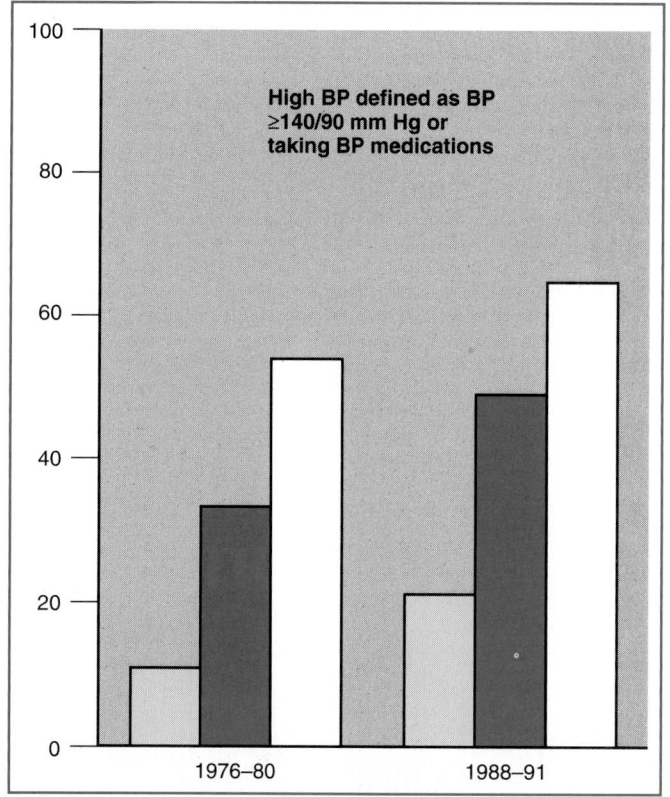

High BP defined as BP ≥140/90 mm Hg or taking BP medications

FIGURE 26–1. Percentage of U.S. adults aged 18 to 74 years surveyed in 1976–1980 and 1988–1991 with hypertension controlled *(left-hand bars)*, treated *(middle)*, and diagnosed *(right)*. Hypertension was defined as use of antihypertensive drug therapy or raised systolic (≥140) or diastolic (≥90) blood pressure on a single occasion. (Adapted from Joint National Committee on Detection, Evaluation, and Treatment of High Blood Pressure: The fifth report of the Joint National Committee on Detection, Evaluation, and Treatment of High Blood Pressure [JNC V]. *Arch. Intern. Med.* *153*:154, 1993. Copyright 1993 American Medical Association.)

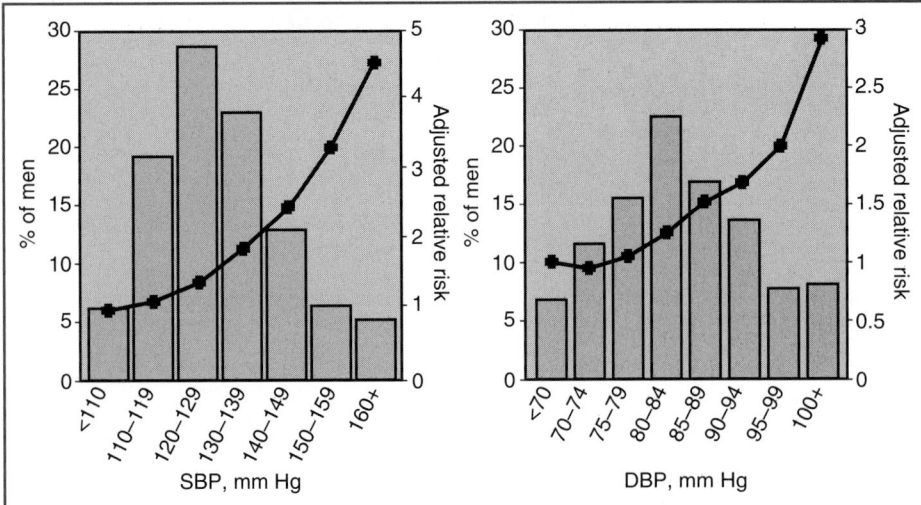

FIGURE 26–2. *Left,* **Percentage distribution of systolic blood pressure (SBP) for men screened for the Multiple Risk Factor Intervention Trial who were aged 35 to 57 years and had no history of myocardial infarction (*n* = 347978) *(shaded bars)* and corresponding 12-year rates of cardiovascular mortality by SBP level adjusted for age, race, total serum cholesterol level, cigarettes smoked per day, reported use of medication for diabetes mellitus, and imputed household income (using census tract of residence). *Right,* Same as at left but for diastolic blood pressure (DBP) (*n* = 356222).** (From National High Blood Pressure Education Program Working Group: National High Blood Pressure Education Program Working Group report on primary prevention of hypertension. Arch. Intern. Med. *153:*186, 1993. Copyright 1993 American Medical Association.)

DEFINITION OF HYPERTENSION

Blood pressure is distributed in a typical bell-shaped curve within the overall population (Fig. 26–2). As seen in the 12-year experience of the 350,000 men screened for the Multiple Risk Factor Intervention Trial (MRFIT) study, the long-term risks for cardiovascular mortality associated with various levels of pressure rise progressively over the entire range of blood pressure, with no threshold that clearly identifies potential danger. Therefore, the definition of hypertension is somewhat arbitrary, usually taken as that level of pressure associated with a doubling of long-term risk.[4] Perhaps the best operational definition is "the level at which the benefits (minus the risks and costs) of action exceed the risks and costs (minus the benefits) of inaction."[6]

The issue as to what blood pressure level should be taken to signify hypertension is further complicated by its typically marked variability. Such variability is seldom recognized by the relatively few office readings taken by most practitioners[7] but can easily be identified by automatically recorded measurements taken throughout the day and night (Fig. 26–3). This variability often can be attributed to physical activity or emotional stress but is frequently without obvious cause.

In a few patients, markedly elevated levels clearly indicate serious disease requiring immediate treatment. However, in most cases, initial readings are not high enough to indicate immediate danger, and the diagnosis of hypertension should be substantiated by repeated readings. The reason for such caution is obvious: The diagnosis of hypertension imposes psychological[8] and socioeconomic burdens on an individual and usually implies the need for a commitment to lifelong therapy.

Both transient and persistent elevations of pressure are common when it is taken in the physician's office or hospital.[7] To obviate "white coat" hypertension, more widespread use of out-of-the-office readings, either with semiautomatic inexpensive devices or automatic ambulatory recorders, is encouraged both to establish the diagnosis and to monitor the patient's response to therapy.[9] A large body of data provides normal ranges for both home self-recorded[10] and automatic ambulatory measurements.[11] Both average about 10/5 mm Hg lower than the average of multiple office readings. A closer correlation between the presence of various types of target organ damage, specifically left ventricular hypertrophy,[12] proteinuria, and retinopathy,[13] has been noted with ambulatory levels than with office levels. However, in the absence of adequate long-term follow-up evidence of the risks associated with either home or ambulatory monitoring, office readings should

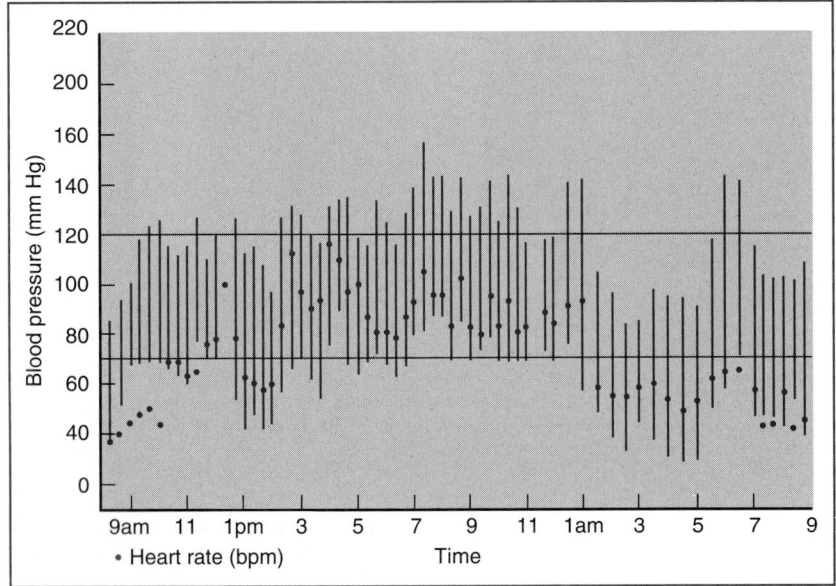

FIGURE 26–3. **Computer printout of blood pressures obtained by ambulatory blood pressure monitoring over 24 hours beginning at 9 A.M. in a 50-year-old man with hypertension receiving no therapy. The patient slept from midnight until 6 A.M.** *Solid circles,* Heart rate. (From Zachariah, P. K., Sheps, S. G., and Smith, R. L.: Defining the roles of home and ambulatory monitoring. Diagnosis *10:*39, 1988.)

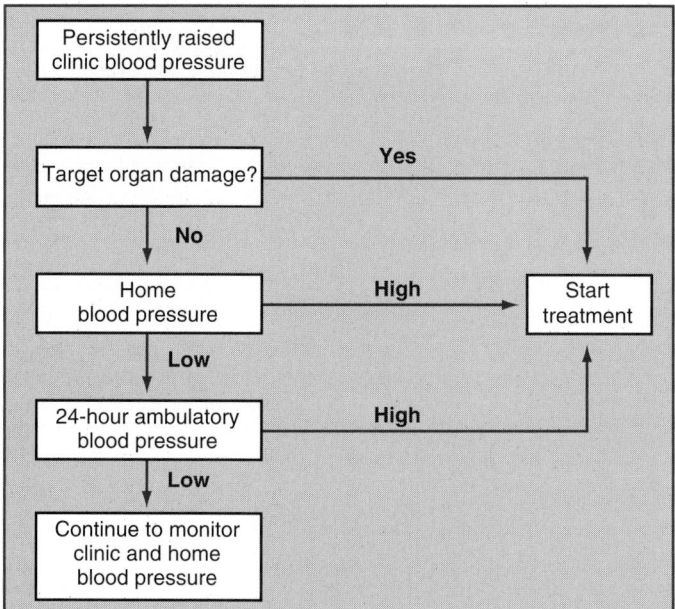

FIGURE 26–4. Schema for evaluation of hypertensive patients by use of clinic, home, and ambulatory monitoring of blood pressure. (From Pickering, T. G.: Blood pressure measurement and detection of hypertension. Lancet *344:*31, 1994.)

continue to be the basis for the diagnosis and management of hypertension.

Whenever possible, office readings should be supplemented by out-of-the-office measurements, particularly when there is an apparent discrepancy between the level of blood pressure and the degree of target organ damage, wherein white coat hypertension should be suspected. Pickering has provided a scheme for the use of home and ambulatory monitoring in such a circumstance[7] (Fig. 26–4). In as many as half of patients with office readings that remain elevated despite the use of three or more drugs, hypertension in as many as half is found to be well controlled by out-of-the-office readings.[14] Purely white coat hypertension, that is, persistently elevated office readings but persistently normal out-of-the-office readings, is found in 20 to 30 per cent of patients.[7] Most are found to be free of the target organ damage[15] and metabolic abnormalities (dyslipidemia, hyperinsulinemia)[16] that are often found in patients with sustained hypertension, so close observation and life style modifications but not antihypertensive drug therapy seem appropriate management for such patients.

In addition to their role in the recognition of white coat hypertension, out-of-the-office readings are essential for the recognition of persistently elevated pressures soon after awakening, when the largest proportion of sudden deaths, myocardial infarctions, and strokes occur.[17] Increased awareness of the role of the abrupt and marked rise of pressure after awakening in the etiology of these early morning cardiovascular catastrophes has prompted therapeutic strategies to ensure control of hypertension at that time, including late evening dosing with currently available medications[18] and the development of tablets that are delayed in releasing active drug so that they can be taken at bedtime but not become active until the hours before awakening.[19]

In view of the usual nocturnal fall in pressure (Fig. 26–3), the addition of the maximal antihypertensive effect of medication taken before bedtime could incite myocardial and cerebral ischemia during sleep. Therefore, the best way to blunt the early morning surge in pressure is to use formulations that provide full 24-hour coverage and to take them as early in the morning as possible.

Although a nocturnal fall in pressure is usual, various groups of hypertensives who have a more serious degree of target organ damage or subsequent major cardiovascular

events[20] have been noted to have little or no nocturnal fall. These include patients with left ventricular hypertrophy,[21] diabetes,[22] or renal damage[23] and blacks.[24] The recognition of abnormal nocturnal patterns of blood pressure, presumably adding an additional stress to the cardiovascular system, is a potential indication for more widespread use of automatic recordings.

Another source of potentially useful prognostic information is the blood pressure response to exercise, usually ascertained in treadmill testing. An exaggerated response in normotensive adults, defined as a systolic pressure above 210 mm Hg in men or 190 mm Hg in women, has been found to be followed 5 years later by a 1.7 times increased incidence of hypertension over that seen in those with a normal response.[25] Over a 16-year follow-up, those middle-aged men with resting systolic pressures of 140 mm Hg or higher who increased their pressure to 200 mm Hg or higher within the first 6 minutes of a bicycle exercise test at a workload of 600 kpm/min had a cardiovascular death rate of 16.1 per cent compared with a rate of 6.0 per cent in those with a lesser pressure response.[26]

DOCUMENTATION OF HYPERTENSION. For most patients who are in no immediate danger from markedly elevated pressure, i.e., below approximately 170/110 mm Hg, the following guidelines are offered:

1. Multiple readings should be obtained using appropriate techniques (pp. 20 to 21, Table 26–1). If possible, the readings should be taken under varying conditions and at various times for at least 4 to 6 weeks with a semiautomatic home device. If there is a need to establish the diagnosis more rapidly, a set of readings obtained by an automatic monitor over a single 24-hour period will be adequate.

2. Although the logical approach would be to calculate the average values from multiple readings when deciding whether or not hypertension is present, even a single high measurement should not be disregarded. In large populations, a single set of casual measurements has been found to predict a greater likelihood of subsequent cardiovascular disease.[27] However, such elevated measurements do not necessarily predict either fixed hypertension or increased risk for each individual. For example, in one study, only 10.8 per cent of 719 men aged 18 to 30 with initial systolic values of 140 to 170 began to exhibit systolic pressures persistently above 140 over the next 12 to 15 years.[28] Nonetheless, persistently elevated pressures were found 2.3 times more often among those with initially high readings, obviously placing them at higher risk.

3. Systolic elevations pose a risk that is equal to or greater than that posed by diastolic elevations.[27] Isolated systolic hypertension, as is commonly seen among the elderly, presents a risk both for stroke and myocardial infarction.[29]

4. The elderly often have sclerotic brachial arteries that may not become occluded until very high pressures are exerted by the balloon; therefore, cuff diastolic levels may be considerably higher than those measured intraarterially. In patients with high cuff readings but little or no hypertensive retinopathy, cardiac hypertrophy, or other evidence of longstanding hypertension, "pseudohypertension" should be suspected and ruled out before treatment is begun.[30]

5. Elderly persons with elevated systolic pressure should be monitored carefully for significant falls in pressure either with sudden upright posture or after meals.[31] These changes probably reflect a progressive loss of baroreceptor responsiveness with age. This condition makes the elderly particularly susceptible to marked orthostatic hypotension after even small decreases in vascular volume.

For the individual patient, hypertension can be definitively diagnosed when most readings are at a level known to be associated with a significantly higher cardiovascular risk without treatment. The recommendations of the Fifth Joint National Committee are shown in Table 26–2.[32] Note that systolic levels of 130 to 139 mm Hg and diastolic levels of 85 to 89 mm Hg are classified as *high normal blood pressure,* a recommendation stemming from a prospective 8.6-year observation of over 7000 white American men aged 40 to 59. A 52 per cent increase in *relative risk* for coronary disease was noted among those in the middle quintile, whose diastolic pressures were between 80 and 87 mm Hg, compared with patients with diastolic pressures below 80 mm Hg.[33] Therefore, persons with relatively high systolic or diastolic pressures should be advised that they may be at increased risk and counseled to follow better health habits in the hope of slowing the progression toward definite hypertension.

The criteria shown in Table 26–2 are based on at least three sets of measurements taken over at least a 3-month interval. Even more readings may be needed to establish a patient's usual level.

Even though they are diagnosed as hypertensive, not all persons with usual levels above 140/90 mm Hg need be treated with drugs, although all should be advised to use the various life style modifications described in Chapter 27. The threshold level recommended by various expert committees for institution of drug therapy varies between diastolic levels of 90 to 100 mm Hg and systolic levels between

TABLE 26–1   GUIDELINES IN MEASURING BLOOD PRESSURE

I. CONDITIONS FOR THE PATIENT
  A. Posture
    1. For patients who are over age 65, diabetic, or receiving antihypertensive therapy, check for postural changes by taking readings immediately and 2 minutes after patient stands.
    2. Sitting pressures usually are adequate for routine follow-up. Patient should sit quietly with back supported for 5 minutes and arm supported at level of heart.
  B. Circumstances
    1. No caffeine for preceding hour.
    2. No smoking for preceding 15 minutes.
    3. No exogenous adrenergic stimulants, e.g., phenylephrine in nasal decongestants or eye drops for pupillary dilation.
    4. A quiet, warm setting.
    5. Home readings taken under varying circumstances and 24-hour ambulatory recordings may be preferable and more accurate in predicting subsequent cardiovascular disease.

II. EQUIPMENT
  A. Cuff size: The bladder should encircle and cover two-thirds of the length of the arm; if not, place the bladder over the brachial artery; if bladder is too small, spuriously high readings may result.
  B. Manometer: Aneroid gauges should be calibrated every 6 months against a mercury manometer.
  C. For infants, use ultrasound equipment, e.g., the Doppler method.

III. TECHNIQUE
  A. Number of readings
    1. On each occasion, take at least two readings, separated by as much time as is practical. If readings vary by more than 5 mm Hg, take additional readings until two are close.
    2. For diagnosis, obtain at least 3 sets of readings at least a week apart.
    3. Initially, take pressure in both arms; if pressure differs, use arm with higher pressure.
    4. If arm pressure is elevated, take pressure in one leg, particularly in patients below age 30.
  B. Performance
    1. Inflate the bladder quickly to a pressure 20 mm Hg above the systolic, as recognized by disappearance of the radial pulse.
    2. Deflate the bladder 3 mm Hg every second.
    3. Record the Korotkoff phase V (disappearance) except in little children, in whom use of phase IV (muffling) may be preferable.
    4. If Korotkoff sounds are weak, have the patient raise the arm, and open and close the hand 5 to 10 times, after which the bladder should be inflated quickly.
  C. Recordings
    1. Note the pressure, patient position, the arm, cuff size (e.g., 140/90, seated, right arm, large adult cuff).

140 and 170 mm Hg.[34] As will be noted on p. 813, the most rational approach is to incorporate age, gender, and the presence of other major cardiovascular risk factors in the decision process along with the level of blood pressure. The threshold for therapy is important, since over 60 per cent of all hypertensives have diastolic blood pressures between 90 and 100 mm Hg (Fig. 26–2).

BORDERLINE HYPERTENSION. In view of the usual variability in blood pressure levels, the term *labile* is inappropriate for describing diastolic pressures that only occasionally exceed 90 mm Hg. Instead, the term *borderline* should be used. In 30 to 40 per cent of patients whose initial diastolic measurement exceeds 90 mm Hg, repeat readings taken soon after will be well below this value.[35] Such patients should be advised that their blood pressure level is *borderline elevated* and should be checked at least annually while they follow general health measures. Tracking of patients with borderline hypertension has not been conducted for a sufficiently long period to provide firm data

TABLE 26–2   CLASSIFICATION OF BLOOD PRESSURE FOR ADULTS AGED 18 YEARS AND OLDER*

CATEGORY	SYSTOLIC	DIASTOLIC
Normal†	<130	<85
High normal	130–139	85–89
Hypertension‡		
Stage 1 (mild)	140–159	90–99
Stage 2 (moderate)	160–179	100–109
Stage 3 (severe)	180–209	110–119
Stage 4 (very severe)	>210	>120

From Joint National Committee: The fifth report of the Joint National Committee on Detection, Evaluation, and Treatment of High Blood Pressure (JNC V). Arch. Intern. Med. *153*:154, 1993.
* These definitions apply to adults who are not taking antihypertensive drugs and who are not acutely ill. When systolic and diastolic blood pressures fall into different categories, the higher category should be selected to classify the individual's blood pressure status. Isolated systolic hypertension is defined as a systolic blood pressure of 140 mm Hg or more and a diastolic blood pressure of less than 90 mm Hg and staged appropriately.
† Optimal blood pressure with respect to cardiovascular risk is less than 120 mm Hg systolic and less than 80 mm Hg diastolic. However, unusually low readings should be evaluated for clinical significance.
‡ Based on the average of two or more readings taken at each of two or more visits after an initial screening.

regarding the likelihood that persistent hypertension will develop.

HYPERTENSION IN CHILDREN AND ADOLESCENTS (see also p. 822).   Upper limits of normal in children of various ages were proposed in the Fifth Joint National Committee report[32] (Table 26–3). Premature labeling of children whose readings are above these limits as hypertensive should be avoided, since long-time tracking is only now being carried out.[36] Appropriate management for asymptomatic children with sustained elevations in blood pressure has not been established. Although many maintain similarly high readings over 3- to 4-year periods, most become normotensive. Such patients should be followed carefully, with particular emphasis placed on regular exercise and weight reduction for those who are overweight in the hope of preventing progression of the disease. If life style modifications are not successful, antihypertensive agents probably should be prescribed for those with sustained hypertension.

TABLE 26–3   CLASSIFICATION OF HYPERTENSION IN THE YOUNG*

AGE GROUP	≥95TH PERCENTILE	≥99TH PERCENTILE
Infants (≤2 y)		
SBP	≥112	≥118
DBP	≥74	≥82
Children, y		
3–5		
SBP	≥116	≥124
DBP	≥76	≥84
6–9		
SBP	≥122	≥130
DBP	≥78	≥86
10–12		
SBP	≥126	≥134
DBP	≥82	≥90
13–15		
SBP	≥136	≥144
DBP	≥86	≥92
Adolescents (16–18 y)		
SBP	≥142	≥150
DBP	≥92	≥98

From 1993 Joint National Committee: The 1993 report of the Joint National Committee on Detection, Evaluation, and Treatment of High Blood Pressure. Arch. Intern. Med. *153*:154, 1993. Copyright 1993, American Medical Association.
* SBP indicates systolic blood pressure; DBP, diastolic blood pressure. Classification based on report of Second Task Force on Blood Pressure Control in Children—1987. All values expressed as millimeters of mercury.

PREVALENCE OF HYPERTENSION

As noted previously, the criteria used for the diagnosis greatly affect the number of people considered hypertensive: The prevalence almost doubles when the level of 140/90 instead of 160/95 mm Hg is used. Most surveys prior to 1980 using single measurements assigned a level of 160/95 mm Hg as the minimum blood pressure denoting hypertension for adults. The levels used to define hypertension shown in Table 26–2 are lower; however, if the diagnosis is based on multiple measurements taken under reasonably controlled circumstances, as it should be, these lower levels seem appropriate. With the lower numbers, hypertension is common, and its frequency increases with the age of the population[5] (Fig. 26–5). The apparent decreases from the 1976–1980 survey may reflect more careful measurements or a true decrease in prevalence by adoption of preventive measures. The incidence of hypertension among blacks is greater at every age beyond adolescence, and they have a higher proportion of more severe disease[37] with a higher mortality rate than whites at every level of income.[38]

SECONDARY HYPERTENSION. Among the large number of people with hypertension, it is helpful to know whether some secondary process—perhaps curable by operation or more easily controlled by a specific drug—may be present (Table 26–4) so that the clinician can determine whether more definitive diagnostic testing is in order.[38a] Most surveys to determine the relative proportion of various secondary diseases are biased as a result of the selection process, with only the increasingly suspect population "funneled" to an investigator interested in a particular disease. Thus estimates as high as 20 per cent for certain secondary forms of hypertension have been reported; however, these do not reflect the incidence in the population at large. Estimates more likely to be indicative of the situation in usual clinical practice are shown in Table 26–5.[39–41] The closest approximation of usual medical practice is the survey by Rudnick et al. with middle-class white patients seen in a family practice in Hamilton, Canada, from 1965 to 1974.[39] In this as in the other surveys, many of the patients underwent intravenous pyelography in addition to providing a history and undergoing a physical examination and routine urine and blood tests. Although a few

patients with secondary diseases may have been missed, the similarity of data strongly supports the view that in more than 90 per cent of all hypertensive persons there will be no recognizable cause; i.e., they have essential hypertension.

811

Ch 26

TABLE 26–4   TYPES OF HYPERTENSION

I. SYSTOLIC AND DIASTOLIC HYPERTENSION

A. Primary, essential, or idiopathic
B. Secondary
  1. Renal
    a. Renal parenchymal disease
      (1) Acute glomerulonephritis
      (2) Chronic nephritis
      (3) Polycystic disease
      (4) Diabetic nephropathy
      (5) Hydronephrosis
    b. Renovascular
      (1) Renal artery stenosis
      (2) Intrarenal vasculitis
    c. Renin-producing tumors
    d. Renoprival
    e. Primary sodium retention (Liddle's syndrome, Gordon's syndrome)
  2. Endocrine
    a. Acromegaly
    b. Hypothyroidism
    c. Hyperthyroidism
    d. Hypercalcemia (hyperparathyroidism)
    e. Adrenal
      (1) Cortical
        (a) Cushing's syndrome
        (b) Primary aldosteronism
        (c) Congenital adrenal hyperplasia
        (d) Apparent mineralocorticoid excess (licorice)
      (2) Medullary: Pheochromocytoma
    f. Extraadrenal chromaffin tumors
    g. Carcinoid
    h. Exogenous hormones
      (1) Estrogen
      (2) Glucocorticoids
      (3) Mineralocorticoids
      (4) Sympathomimetics
      (5) Tyramine-containing foods and monoamine oxidase inhibitors
  3. Coarctation of the aorta
  4. Pregnancy-induced hypertension
  5. Neurological disorders
    a. Increased intracranial pressure
      (1) Brain tumor
      (2) Encephalitis
      (3) Respiratory acidosis
    b. Sleep apnea
    c. Quadriplegia
    d. Acute porphyria
    e. Familial dysautonomia
    f. Lead poisoning
    g. Guillain-Barré syndrome
  6. Acute stress, including surgery
    a. Psychogenic hyperventilation
    b. Hypoglycemia
    c. Burns
    d. Pancreatitis
    e. Alcohol withdrawal
    f. Sickle cell crisis
    g. Postresuscitation
    h. Postoperative
  7. Increased intravascular volume
  8. Alcohol and drug use

II. SYSTOLIC HYPERTENSION

A. Increased cardiac output
  1. Aortic valvular insufficiency
  2. A-V fistula, patent ductus
  3. Thyrotoxicosis
  4. Paget's disease of bone
  5. Beriberi
  6. Hyperkinetic circulation
B. Rigidity of aorta

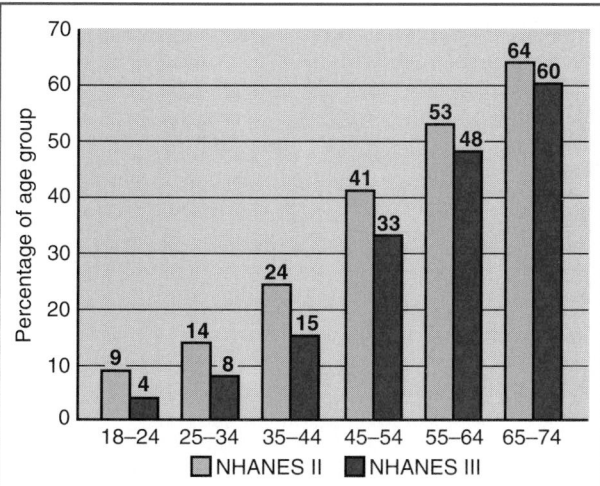

FIGURE 26–5. Incidence of hypertension in U.S. adults according to data from the National Health and Nutrition Examination Surveys conducted during 1976–1980 (NHANES II) and 1988–1991 (NHANES III). Hypertension is defined as mean blood pressure of 140/90 mm Hg or higher based on three readings taken on a single occasion or the use of antihypertensive mediations. (From Centers for Disease Control and Prevention, National Center for Health Statistics [Composed from National High Blood Pressure Education Program Working Group]): Report on primary prevention of hypertension. Arch. Intern. Med. *153*:186, 1993.)

TABLE 26–5   FREQUENCY OF VARIOUS DIAGNOSES IN HYPERTENSIVE SUBJECTS

DIAGNOSIS	RUDNICK et al.[39]	SINCLAIR et al.[40]	ANDERSON et al.[41] *
Essential hypertension	94%	92.1%	89.5%
Chronic renal disease	5%	5.6%	1.8%
Renovascular disease	0.2%	0.7%	3.3%
Coarctation of aorta	0.2%		
Primary aldosteronism		0.3%	1.5%
Cushing's syndrome	0.2%	0.1%	0.6%
Pheochromocytoma		0.1%	0.3%
Oral contraceptive–induced	0.2%	1.0%	
No. of patients	665	3783	4429

Data from Rudnick, K. V., et al.: Hypertension in family practice. Can. Med. Assoc. J. *117*,492, 1977; Sinclair, A. M., et al.: Secondary hypertension in a blood pressure clinic. Arch. Intern. Med. *147*:1289, 1987; Anderson, G. H., Jr., et al.: The effect of age on prevalence of secondary forms of hypertension in 4429 consecutively referred patients. J. Hypertens. *12*:609, 1994.

* The patients screened by Anderson et al. were referred for evaluation of secondary causes; those screened by Rudnick and Sinclair were all those seen in a primary setting.

THE CHANGING NATURE OF CHILDHOOD HYPERTENSION (see also p. 822).

Even among children, secondary hypertension is less common than indicated by previous surveys of hospital-based populations. As more apparently normal children are being screened and more are found to be hypertensive, the clinical presentation of childhood hypertension is changing from that of a rare and serious disease, usually related to renal damage, to a more common and usually asymptomatic process, in most cases without recognizable cause.[36] Some prepubertal hypertensive children do not have recognizable secondary diseases, whereas most identified after puberty have primary hypertension.

SCREENING FOR SECONDARY HYPERTENSION

Because of the relatively low frequency of the various secondary diseases, the clinician should be selective in carrying out various screening and diagnostic tests. The presence of features *inappropri-*

TABLE 26–6   FEATURES OF "INAPPROPRIATE" HYPERTENSION

1. Onset before age 20 or after age 50
2. Level of blood pressure >180/110 mm Hg
3. Organ damage
   a. Funduscopic findings of Grade 2 or higher
   b. Serum creatinine >1.5 mg/100 ml
   c. Cardiomegaly (on x-ray) or left ventricular hypertrophy (on electrocardiogram)
4. Features indicative of secondary causes
   a. Unprovoked hypokalemia
   b. Abdominal bruit
   c. Variable pressures with tachycardia, sweating, tremor
   d. Family history of renal disease
5. Poor response to therapy that is usually effective

ate for usual uncomplicated primary hypertension indicates the need for additional tests (Table 26–6). However, for the 9 out of 10 hypertensive patients without these features, a hematocrit, urine analysis, automated blood biochemical profile (including plasma glucose, potassium, creatinine, and total and high-density lipoprotein cholesterol), and an electrocardiogram are all that is required. Although some would include other tests, an inordinate number of screening tests for relatively rare diseases will increase the likelihood of a false-positive result. For example, according to Bayes' theorem (see p. 162), using a prevalence rate of 2 per cent for renovascular hypertension, which is probably higher than seen in the overall hypertensive population, the predictive value of an intravenous pyelogram (IVP) or isotopic renogram suggestive of this diagnosis is only 10 per cent, and an abnormal IVP or renogram is more likely to be a false-positive result than true-positive indicating a specific diagnosis.[42]

NATURAL HISTORY OF UNTREATED HYPERTENSION

A meta-analysis of nine major prospective observational studies involving 420,000 individuals free of known coronary or cerebral vascular disease at baseline who were followed for 6 to 25 years (mean of 10 years) shows a "direct, continuous and apparently independent association" of diastolic blood pressure (DBP) with both stroke and coronary heart disease (CHD)[43] (Fig. 26–6). The data indicate that prolonged increases in usual DBP of 5 and 10 mm Hg were associated with at least 34 and 56 per cent increases in stroke risk and with at least 21 and 37 per cent increases in CHD risk, respectively.

SYMPTOMS AND SIGNS. Because uncomplicated hypertension is almost always asymptomatic, a person may be unaware of the consequent progressive cardiovascular damage for as long as 10 to 20 years. Only if blood pressure is measured frequently and people are made aware that hypertension may be harmful even if asymptomatic will the majority of people with unrecognized or inadequately

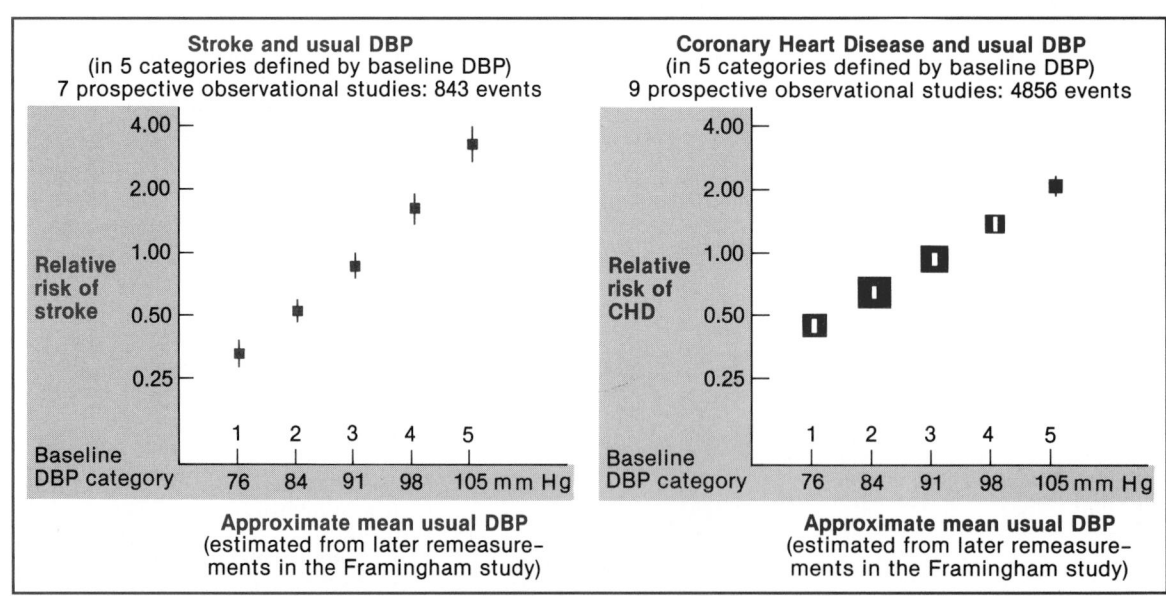

FIGURE 26–6.   The relative risks of stroke and of coronary heart disease, estimated from the combined results of the prospective observational studies, for each of five categories of diastolic blood pressure. (Estimates of the usual DBP in each baseline DBP category are taken from mean DBP values 4 years post-baseline in the Framingham study.) The solid squares represent disease risks in each category relative to risk in the whole study population; the sizes of the squares are proportional to the number of events in each DBP category, and 95 per cent confidence intervals for the estimates of relative risk are denoted by vertical lines. (From MacMahon, S., Peto, R., Cutler, J., et al.: Blood pressure and coronary heart disease: Part I, prolonged differences in blood pressure: Prospective observational studies corrected for the regression dilution bias. Lancet *335*:765, 1990. © by the Lancet Ltd.)

treated hypertension be managed effectively. Symptoms often attributed to hypertension—headache, tinnitus, dizziness, and fainting—may be observed just as commonly in the normotensive population.[44] Moreover, many symptoms attributed to the elevated blood pressure are psychogenic in origin,[8] often reflecting hyperventilation induced by anxiety over the diagnosis of a lifelong, insidious disease which threatens well-being and survival. Even headache, long considered a frequent symptom of hypertension, is poorly related to the level of blood pressure,[45] as noted in 10 to 20 per cent of those with DBP levels from below 90 to above 120 mm Hg.

COURSE OF UNTREATED HYPERTENSION. As noted in Figure 26-6, even minimal hypertension is accompanied by significant increases in coronary disease and stroke. However, these figures may be misleading, since they seem to imply that most hypertensives, including those with minimally elevated pressures, will experience adverse consequences of hypertension, and rather quickly. The issue is well identified in the data from the Pooling Project,[33] which includes multiple prospective follow-up studies including the Framingham cohort. As noted previously, these data indicate that those white men with diastolic pressures of 80 to 87 mm Hg had a 52 per cent greater *relative* risk of having a major coronary event over an 8.6-year period than did those with diastolic pressures below 80. However, this large increased *relative* risk translates to an *absolute* excess risk of only 3.5 men per 100 over the 8.6-year interval. Obviously, the majority of those with even higher diastolic pressures did not suffer a major coronary event.

Nonetheless, because there are so many persons with hypertension, the fact that even a minority of them will suffer a premature cardiovascular event in the course of their disease makes hypertension a major societal problem. In fact, when the death rates for various levels of diastolic blood pressure are multiplied by the proportion of people in the population who have these various levels, the majority of excess deaths attributable to hypertension are found to occur among those with minimally elevated pressures[5] (Fig. 26-2).

As the public and the medical profession have become aware of the overall societal consequences of even mild hypertension, enthusiasm for its early recognition and aggressive treatment has continued to mount. A closer look at the issue of deciding on the need for therapy is provided in Chapter 27. However, further consideration of the natural course of hypertension, as it applies to the individual patient, is needed in order to answer a basic question: Are the blood pressure and the consequent risk high enough to justify medical intervention? Unless the risk is high enough to mandate some form of intervention, there seems to be no need to identify and label the person as hypertensive, since psychological and socioeconomic burdens accompany this label; unless risks clearly outweigh these burdens, caution is obviously advised. A cogent view of this issue has been offered by Rose[46]:

> In reality the care of the symptomless hypertensive person is preventive medicine, not therapeutics. If a preventive measure exposes many people to a small risk, the harm it does may readily . . . outweigh the benefits, since these are received by relatively few. . . . We may thus be unable to identify that small level of harm to individuals from long-term intervention that would be sufficient to make that line of prevention unprofitable or even harmful. Consequently we cannot accept long-term mass preventive medication.

We are thus left with a dilemma: For hypertensive individuals as a group, even those with the least elevated pressures, risk is increased; for the individual hypertensive, the risk may not justify the labeling or treatment of the condition.

Guidelines are available to help practitioners resolve this dilemma in dealing with the individual patient. These guidelines are based on the overall assessment of cardiovascular risk and the biological aggressiveness of the hypertension. They are intended to apply only to those with stage 1 (formerly referred to as mild) hypertension, that is, diastolic pressure between 90 and 99 mm Hg; those with diastolic levels persistently at or above 100 mm Hg have been shown to be at high enough risk from the hypertension per se to justify immediate intervention. Recall, however, that most hypertensives are in the range between 90 and 99 mm Hg (Fig. 26-2).

OVERALL CARDIOVASCULAR RISK. The Framingham Study and other epidemiological surveys have clearly defined certain risk factors for premature cardiovascular disease in addition to hypertension (see Chap. 35). For varying levels of blood pressure, the Framingham data (available in the *Coronary and Stroke Risk Handbooks* published by the American Heart Association) show the increasing likelihood of a vascular event over the next 10 years for both men and women at various ages as more and more risk factors are added[29] (Fig. 26-2). For example, a 55-year-old man with a systolic blood pressure of 160 mm Hg who is otherwise at low risk would have a 13.7 per cent chance of a vascular event in the next 10 years (Fig. 26-7). A man of the same age with the same pressure but with all the additional risk factors (elevated serum total cholesterol, low HDL-cholesterol, cigarette smoking, glucose intolerance, and left ventricular hypertrophy on the electrocardiogram) has a 59.5 per cent chance. Obviously, the higher the overall risk, the more intensive the interventions should be.

An interesting—and disturbing—connection between untreated hypertension and *hypercholesterolemia* has been noted in multiple populations.[47] This connection may be mediated through insulin resistance and hyperinsulinemia, anticipated in those with upper body obesity[48] but also found in nonobese hypertensives[49] (see p. 820). Clearly, through this association, hypertensives are often burdened with an even greater risk than that imposed by their blood pressure alone.

Complications of Hypertension

The higher the level of blood pressure, the more likely that various cardiovascular diseases will develop prematurely through acceleration of atherosclerosis, the pathological hallmark of uncontrolled hypertension. If untreated, about 50 per cent of hypertensive patients die of coronary heart disease or congestive failure, about 33 per cent of stroke, and 10 to 15 per cent of renal failure. Those with

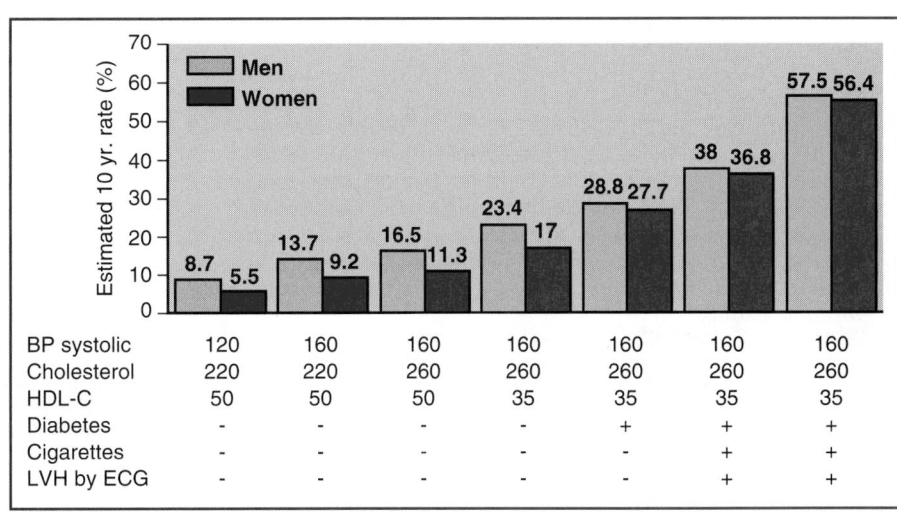

FIGURE 26-7. Estimated 10-year risk of coronary artery disease in hypothetical 55-year-old men and women according to levels of various risk factors. Lipid units are milligrams per deciliter. (From Wilson, P. W. F.: Established risk factors and coronary artery disease: The Framingham Study. Am. J. Hypertens. *7*:7S, 1994.)

BP systolic	120	160	160	160	160	160	160
Cholesterol	220	220	260	260	260	260	260
HDL-C	50	50	50	35	35	35	35
Diabetes	-	-	-	-	+	+	+
Cigarettes	-	-	-	-	-	+	+
LVH by ECG	-	-	-	-	-	+	+

TABLE 26–7 VASCULAR COMPLICATIONS OF HYPERTENSION

HYPERTENSIVE	ATHEROSCLEROTIC
Accelerated-malignant phase	Coronary heart disease
Hemorrhagic stroke	Sudden death
Congestive heart failure	Other arrhythmias
Nephrosclerosis	Atherothrombotic stroke
Aortic dissection	Peripheral vascular disease

Adapted from Smith, W. M.: Treatment of mild hypertension. Results of a ten-year intervention trial. Circ. Res. *25* (Suppl. I):98, 1977. Copyright 1977 by the American Heart Association.

rapidly accelerating hypertension die more frequently of renal failure, as do those who are diabetic, once proteinuria or other evidence of nephropathy develops. It is easy to underestimate the role of hypertension in producing the underlying vascular damage that leads to these cardiovascular catastrophes. Death is usually attributed to stroke or myocardial infarction instead of to the hypertension that was largely responsible. Moreover, hypertension may not persist after a myocardial infarction or stroke.

In general, the vascular complications of hypertension can be considered as either "hypertensive" or "atherosclerotic" (Table 26–7). The former are more directly caused by the increased blood pressure per se and can be prevented by lowering this level; the latter have more multiple causations (Chap. 35). Although hypertension may represent the most significant of the known risk factors of atherosclerosis in quantitative terms, lowering blood pressure may not by itself halt the atherosclerotic process.

The path from hypertension to vascular disease likely involves three interrelated processes: *pulsatile flow, endothelial cell dysfunction,* and *smooth muscle cell hypertrophy.* Higher systolic pressures are probably more responsible for these changes than are lower diastolic levels, providing an explanation for the closer approximation of cardiovascular risk to systolic pressure.

These three interrelated processes are probably responsible for the arteriolar and arterial sclerosis that is the usual consequence of longstanding hypertension leading to the target organ damage to be described as the features included in overall assessment of hypertension risks. Beyond the damage to eyes, heart, brain, and kidney, the large vessels such as the aorta may be directly affected, leading to aneurysms and dissection.

Target Organ Damage

The biological aggressiveness of a given level of hypertension varies among individuals. This inherent propensity to induce vascular damage can be ascertained best by examination of the eyes, heart, and kidney.

FUNDUSCOPIC EXAMINATION. As described by Keith et al. in 1939, vascular changes in the fundus reflect both hypertensive retinopathy and arteriosclerotic retinopathy (Fig. 2–1, p. 16).[50] The two processes induce first narrowing of the arteriolar lumen (Grade 1) and then sclerosis of the adventitia and/or thickening of the arteriolar wall, visible as arteriovenous nicking (Grade 2). Progressive hypertension induces rupture of small vessels, seen as hemorrhages and exudates (Grade 3) and eventually papilledema (Grade 4). The Grade 3 and 4 changes are clearly indicative of an accelerated-malignant form of hypertension, whereas the lesser changes have been correlated with other evidence of target organ damage.[51]

CARDIAC INVOLVEMENT. Hypertension places increased tension on the left ventricular myocardium, causing it to stiffen and hypertrophy, and accelerates the development of atherosclerosis within the coronary vessels.[51a] The combination of increased demand and lessened supply increases the likelihood of myocardial ischemia, leading to higher incidences of myocardial infarction, sudden death,

arrhythmias, and congestive failure in hypertensives (Figs. 26–2 and 26–6).

Abnormalities of Left Ventricular Function. Even before left ventricular hypertrophy (LVH) develops, changes in both systolic and diastolic function may be seen. Those with minimally increased left ventricular muscle mass may have supernormal contractility reflecting an increased inotropic state with a high percentage of fractional shortening and increased wall stress.[52] The earliest functional cardiac changes in hypertension are in left ventricular diastolic function with prolongation and incoordination of isovolumic relaxation, reduced rate of rapid filling, and an increase in the relative amplitude of the *a* wave, probably caused by increased passive stiffness.[53]

With increasing hemodynamic load, either systolic or diastolic dysfunction may evolve, progressing to different forms of congestive heart failure[54] (Fig. 26–8) (see also p. 394). The syndrome of severe concentric hypertrophy with a small ventricular cavity leading to dyspnea and pulmonary congestion has been most frequently reported in black hypertensive women.[55] In addition, impaired coronary flow reserve and thallium perfusion defects may be observed in hypertensives without obstructive coronary disease.[56]

Left Ventricular Hypertrophy (LVH). Hypertrophy as a response to the increased afterload of an elevated systemic vascular resistance can be viewed as necessary and protective up to a certain point. Beyond that point, a variety of dysfunctions accompany LVH.

In the past, LVH was recognized by electrocardiography (Fig. 4–11, p. 116), based on increased voltage of QRS complexes, intrinsicoid deflection over lead V_5 or V_6 greater than 0.06 sec, and ST-segment depression greater than 0.5 mm (see p. 139). Increasingly, echocardiography is being used (see p. 66) because it is much more sensitive in recognizing early cardiac involvement. By echocardiography, left ventricular mass is shown to progressively increase with increases in blood pressure[57,58] (Fig. 26–9). LVH may be noted by echocardiography even before blood pressures become overtly abnormal in young offspring of hypertensive parents,[59] and larger left ventricular mass by echocardiography may identify subjects at risk of developing hypertension.[60] Left ventricular mass is greater in those whose pressure does not fall during sleep, reflecting a more persistent pressure load.[61]

The pathogenesis of LVH involves a number of variables other than the pressure load. One of these is hemodynamic volume load; Devereux et al.[62] found a closer correlation between left ventricular (LV) stroke volume and LV mass with diastolic than with systolic blood pressure. Other determinants are obesity,[63] levels of sympathetic nervous system and renin-angiotensin activity, and whole blood viscosity, presumably by way of its influence on peripheral resistance.[62] The

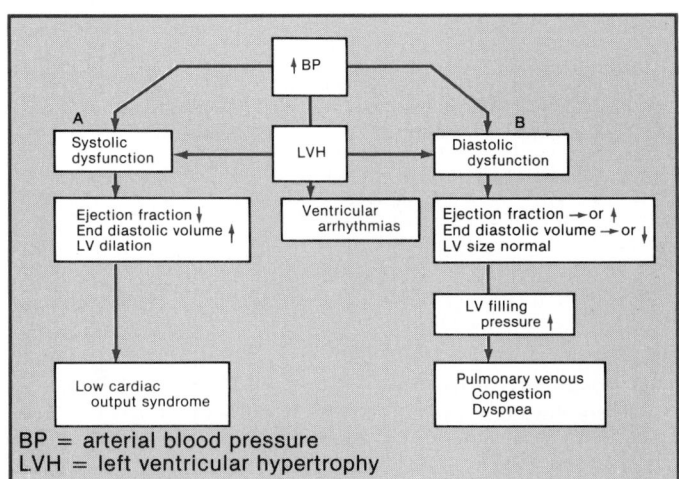

FIGURE 26–8. Consequences of systolic and diastolic dysfunction related to hypertension. *A,* Systolic dysfunction and congestive heart failure may occur late in the evolution of hypertensive heart disease, because of impaired ventricular contraction. *B,* Diastolic dysfunction is the most common manifestation of the effect of hypertension on cardiac function and also can lead to congestive heart failure due to increased filling pressures. LV = left ventricular. (From Shepherd, R. F. J., Zachariah, P. K., Shub, C.: Hypertension and left ventricular diastolic function. Mayo Clin. Proc. *64*:1521, 1989. By permission)

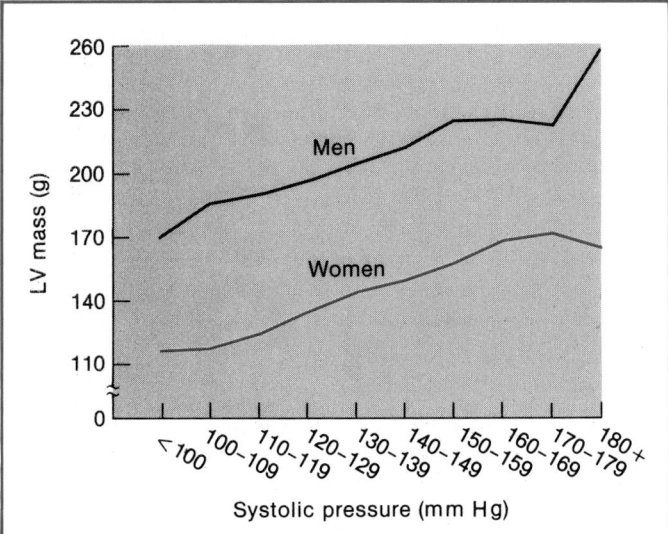

FIGURE 26–9. Mean left ventricular mass by sex and by systolic pressure, including participants taking antihypertensive medications, aged 17 to 90 years. These data were obtained by M-mode echocardiograms taken on 2226 men and 2746 women in the Framingham Study, cohort examination 16 and offspring cycle 2, 1979 to 1983. (From Savage, D. D., Levy, D., Danneberg, A. L., et al.: Association of echocardiographic left ventricular mass with body size, blood pressure and physical activity [the Framingham Study]. Am. J. Cardiol. 65:371, 1990.)

correlation is much closer between LVH and pressures taken during the stresses of work by ambulatory monitoring than between LVH and casual pressures.[63] Blacks have more extensive LVH and more impairment of LV diastolic function than do whites with equal levels of blood pressure.[64]

The basic signals that initiate and maintain myocardial hypertrophy probably include a number of growth factors whose effects may be transmitted via the alpha$_1$-adrenergic receptor to activate intracellular transducing proteins and ribonucleic acid (RNA) transcription factors.[65] The renin-angiotensin-aldosterone mechanism may be involved in both functional[66] and structural[67] changes in the myocardium.

Different patterns of hypertrophy may evolve, often starting with asymmetrical LV remodeling due to isolated septal thickening, noted in 22 per cent of untreated hypertensives with normal LV mass.[68] The pattern of LVH may have important prognostic implications. In a 10-year follow-up of 253 hypertensives, all-cause mortality was higher and cardiovascular events were most frequent in those with concentric LVH.[69] The degree of increased muscle mass is a strong and independent risk factor for cardiac mortality over and above the extent of coronary artery disease.[70] In addition, the risk of ventricular arrhythmias is increased at least twofold in the presence of LVH.[71]

Since the presence of LVH may connote a number of deleterious effects of hypertension on cardiac function, a great deal of effort has been expended in showing that treatment of hypertension will cause LVH to regress. Treatment with all antihypertensive drugs except those which further activate sympathetic nervous system activity, e.g., diuretics and direct vasodilators such as hydralazine when used alone, has been shown to cause LVH regression.[72] With regression, left ventricular function usually improves.[73]

Features of Coronary Artery Disease. As detailed elsewhere (see p. 1168), hypertension is a major risk factor for myocardial ischemia and infarction.[27,29] Moreover, in the Framingham cohort, the prevalence of silent myocardial infarction was significantly increased in hypertensive subjects.[74] They are also more susceptible to silent ischemia[75] and sudden death.[74] Beyond these multiple additional risks associated with hypertension, a higher incidence of coronary events has been recognized when elevated diastolic blood pressures are reduced with either diuretic or beta-blocker–based therapies to levels below 85 to 90 mm Hg.[76] This J-shaped curve in the incidence of coronary disease probably reflects a reduction in perfusion pressure through coronary vessels either narrowed or having impaired vasodilatory reserve in the presence of a hypertrophied myocardium.

RENAL FUNCTION. Renal dysfunction, too subtle to be recognized, may be responsible for the development of

most cases of essential hypertension. As discussed on p. 817, increased renal retention of salt and water may be a mechanism initiating primary hypertension, but the retention is so small that it escapes detection. With detailed study, both structural damage and functional derangements reflecting intraglomerular hypertension often reflected by microalbuminuria[77] can be found in almost all hypertensive persons. Microalbuminuria has been correlated with both high blood pressure and evidence of endothelial cell dysfunction.[78] In patients with longstanding hypertension, a loss of concentrating ability may be manifested by nocturia, creatinine clearance falls, and the development of more significant proteinuria. As hypertension-induced nephrosclerosis proceeds, the plasma creatinine level begins to rise, and eventually renal insufficiency with uremia may develop, making hypertension a leading cause for end-stage renal disease, particularly in blacks.[79]

CEREBRAL INVOLVEMENT. Hypertension, particularly systolic, is a major risk factor for initial and recurrent stroke and for transient ischemic attacks caused by extracranial atherosclerosis.[80] Usually with, but sometimes without, hypertension, increasing LV mass on echocardiography was associated with progressively higher risk for stroke in an elderly cohort.[81] The blood pressure usually rises further during the acute phases of a stroke, and caution is advised in lowering the blood pressure during this crucial period.[82]

PLASMA RENIN ACTIVITY AS A PROGNOSTIC GUIDE. In 1972, Bruner et al. published data showing that a group of hypertensives with low levels of plasma renin activity (PRA) had a benign course, with no heart attacks or strokes uncovered on retrospective analysis.[83] Subsequently, many investigators have examined the relationship between renin levels and cardiovascular complications and found that, with few exceptions,[84] patients with low PRA do not have a more benign course than do those with normal PRA.

On the basis of the aforementioned assessments of overall cardiovascular risk and severity of hypertension, it should be possible to determine the approximate risk status and prognosis for individual patients. This can most easily be accomplished with the Framingham data, as described on page 813.

SHORT-TERM COURSE OF LOW-RISK HYPERTENSION. Data on the 4-year experiences of over 1600 "low-risk" hypertensives who served as controls in the Australian Therapeutic Trial document the validity of this assessment.[85] To enter this placebo versus drug trial, the patients had to be free of all identifiable cardiovascular disease, with the second set of diastolic pressures between 95 and 109 mm Hg. Thus they could be considered "low-risk" hypertensives. Over the next 4 years, in the majority of these patients, who were given placebo tablets but neither nondrug nor drug therapy, blood pressures dropped progressively, from an average of 157/102 to 144/91 mm Hg. Diastolic pressure was below 95 mm Hg in 47.5 per cent at the end of the trial. The fall in blood pressure was not related to any recognizable change in the patients' status; similar decreases occurred independent of changes in or stability of body weight. Of great interest was the lack of excess morbidity or mortality among those whose diastolic pressures remained below 100 mm Hg.

These results support strongly the view that certain patients can be characterized as being at relatively low risk and can therefore safely do without drug therapy long enough for the clinician to monitor both their blood pressure levels over time and the effectiveness of nondrug measures, if indicated. The large number of patients whose pressures fell and the high average degree of fall may seem surprising, but none of these patients started with any identifiable cardiovascular disease or complications due to hypertension. Moreover, placebo may be more effective than no therapy.

Similar results were observed in the even larger Medical Research Council (MRC) trial in England, in which over 18,000 patients with pretreatment diastolic pressures between 95 and 109 mm Hg were randomly assigned to antihypertensive drugs or placebo.[86] At the end of 5 years, these pressures had dropped to below 90 mm Hg in 43 per cent of the men and 50 per cent of the women on placebo.

THE POTENTIAL FOR PROGRESSION. Although these data reflect the benign nature of "low-risk" hypertension over the short term, it should be noted that the diastolic blood pressure rose above 110 mm Hg in 12 per cent of the nondrug-treated patients in both the Australian and English trials. Therefore, continued monitoring of the blood pressure levels is obviously needed for all patients with even the mildest "low-risk" hypertension.

A SYNTHESIS OF RISK. In the MRC trial, older age, male sex, hypercholesterolemia, and cigarette smoking, along with an increased level of systolic blood pressure at entry, were related significantly to the subsequent development of cardiovascular complications.[86] Although the ability to discriminate between those who did and did not suffer a coronary or cerebrovascular event in this 5-year trial was not precise, the degree of risk from hypertension can be categorized with reasonable accuracy, taking into account (1) the level of blood pressure, (2) the biological nature of the hypertension, based on the degree of target organ damage, and (3) the coexistence of other risks. Although risk is increased for the hypertensive population as a whole, problems are more likely in those with higher levels of pressure (diastolic above 100 mm Hg), considerable target organ damage (retinopathy, cardiomegaly, renal damage), and other risk factors (hypercholesterolemia, cigarette smoking, diabetes). For them, immediate and effective reduction of pressure appears to be indicated. But for the majority, who are at relatively low risk, the more reasonable approach would be to continue to monitor the blood pressure while encouraging healthful habits, such as weight control, moderate sodium restriction, isotonic exercise, and relaxation, in hopes of slowing progression of the disease (Chap. 27).

A group of physicians from New Zealand has formalized this approach into a nomogram based on the concept that "decisions to treat raised blood pressure should be based primarily on the estimated absolute risk of cardiovascular disease rather than on blood pressure alone."[87] They separate patients by levels of blood pressure, gender, and age and take various risk factors and evidences of target organ damage into account. After consideration of the available data both on the ability of therapy to reduce cardiovascular risk and on the financial and other costs of therapy, they propose active drug therapy for those patients whose overall risk status of a major cardiovascular event in 10 years (based on the Framingham data) is more than about 20 per cent. They believe that at that level of absolute risk, "150 people would require treatment to reduce the annual number of cardiovascular events by about one."

Although one could argue that their limit for active therapy is too high, excluding some patients who would benefit from therapy, I believe that their concept is absolutely correct and should be followed in making the crucial decision for the institution of therapy, as will be detailed in the next chapter.

It is obvious that since there is no certain way to predict the course of the blood pressure, even hypertensives who are not treated should be followed, and recognition of their hypertension should motivate them to follow good health habits. In this way, no harm should be done, and the potential benefit may be considerable if progression of the disease can be slowed by life style modifications.

MECHANISMS OF PRIMARY (ESSENTIAL) HYPERTENSION

No single or specific cause is known for most hypertension, referred to as *primary* in preference to *essential*. Since persistent hypertension can develop only in response to an increase in cardiac output or a rise in peripheral resistance, defects may be present in one or more of the multiple factors that affect these two forces (Fig. 26–10). The interplay of various derangements in factors affecting cardiac output and peripheral resistance may precipitate the disease, and these may differ in both type and degree in different patients.

Hemodynamic Patterns

Before describing specific abnormalities in the various factors shown in Figure 26–10 to affect the basic equation BP = CO × PR, the hemodynamic patterns that have been measured in patients with hypertension will be considered. One cautionary factor should be kept in mind: The development of the disease is slow and gradual. By the time blood pressure becomes elevated, the initiating factors may no longer be apparent, because they may have been "normalized" by multiple compensatory interactions. Nonetheless, when a group of untreated young hypertensive patients was studied initially, cardiac output was normal or slightly increased and peripheral resistance was normal.[88] Over the next 20 years, cardiac output fell progressively, while peripheral resistance rose. In a much larger study involving over 2600 subjects in Framingham followed for 4 years by echocardiography, an increased cardiac index and

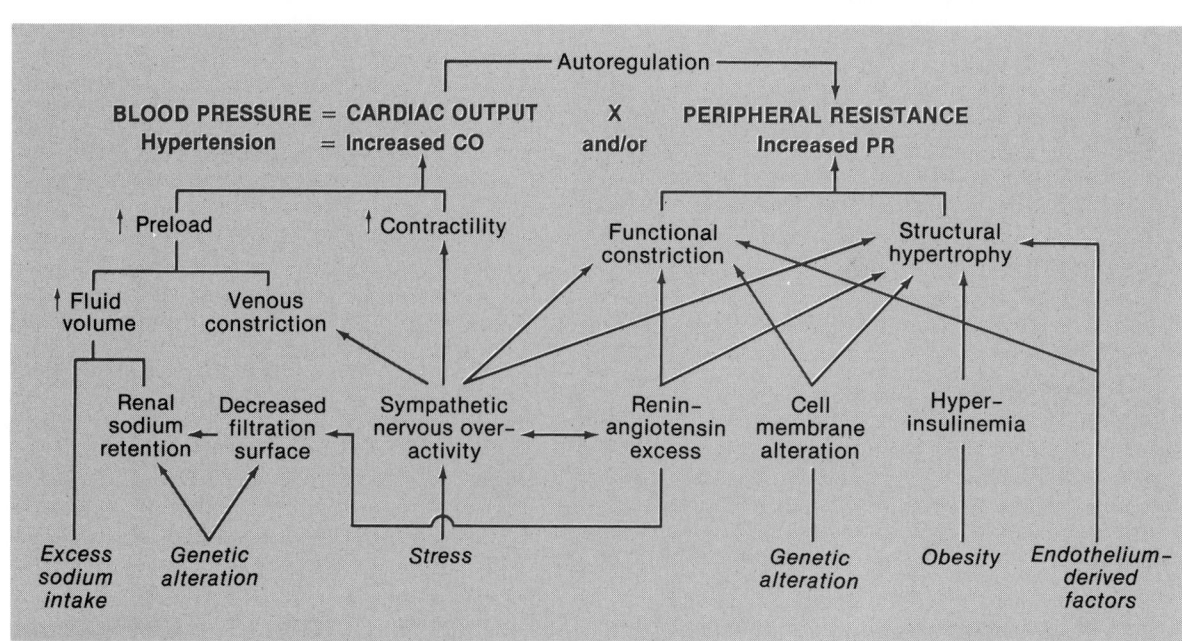

FIGURE 26–10. Some of the factors involved in the control of blood pressure that affect the basic equation: Blood pressure = cardiac output (CO) × peripheral resistance (PR). Cellular hyperplasia may be seen along with hypertrophy. (From Kaplan, N. M.: Clinical Hypertension. 6th ed. Baltimore, © by Williams and Wilkins, 1994, p. 57.)

end-systolic wall stress were related to the development of hypertension, but these hemodynamic measures were no longer significant predictors when adjustments for age and baseline blood pressure were made.[89]

Regardless of how hypertension begins, the eventual primacy of increased resistance can be shown even in models of hypertension that feature an initial increase in fluid volume and cardiac output.[90]

Genetic Predisposition

As discussed on p. 1677 and shown in Figure 26–10, genetic alterations may initiate the cascade to permanent hypertension. Clearly, heredity plays a role, although only one linkage has been described, involving regions within or close to the angiotensinogen gene.[91,91a] In studies of twins and family members in which the degree of familial aggregation of blood pressure levels is compared with the closeness of genetic sharing, the genetic contributions have been estimated to range from 30 to 60 per cent.[92] Unquestionably, environment plays some role, and Harrap[92] offers as a working model an interaction between genes and environment "in which the average population pressure is determined by environment, but blood pressure rank within the distribution is decided largely by genes."

If genetic markers of a predisposition to develop hypertension are found, specific environmental manipulations could then be directed toward those susceptible subjects. For now, children and siblings of hypertensives should be more carefully screened. They should be vigorously advised to avoid environmental factors known to aggravate hypertension and increase cardiovascular risk (e.g., smoking, inactivity, and excess sodium).

The Fetal Environment

Environmental factors may come into play very early. Low birth weight as a consequence of fetal undernutrition is followed by an increased incidence of high blood pressure later in life.[93] Increased postnatal feeding of low-birth-weight infants does not alter their blood pressure levels at 8 years of age,[94] suggesting that permanent imprinting has already occurred. Brenner and Chertow[95] hypothesize that a decreased number of nephrons could very well serve as this permanent, irreparable defect that eventuates in hypertension (Fig. 26–11). In their words: "This hypothesis

draws on observations suggesting (1) a direct relationship between birth weight and nephron number, (2) an inverse relationship between birth weight and childhood, adolescent, and adult blood pressures, and (3) an inverse relationship between nephron number and blood pressure, irrespective of whether nephron number is reduced congenitally or in postnatal life (as from partial renal ablation or acquired renal disease)."

This hypothesis fits nicely with Brenner's explanation for the inexorable progression of renal damage once it begins and the concept that hypertension may begin by renal sodium retention induced by the decreased filtration surface area.[96]

Renal Retention of Excess Sodium

A considerable amount of circumstantial evidence supports a role for sodium in the genesis of hypertension (Table 26–8). To induce hypertension, some of that excess sodium must be retained by the kidneys. Such retention could arise in a number of ways, including

- A decrease in filtration surface by a congenital or acquired deficiency in nephron number or function.[96]
- A resetting of the normal pressure-natriuresis relationship, wherein a rise in pressure invokes an immediate increase in renal sodium excretion, shrinking fluid volume and returning the pressure to normal. Guyton[97] has long argued for a resetting of this relationship as a fundamental defect that must be present to explain the persistence of an elevated pressure.
- Nephron heterogeneity, as hypothesized by Sealey et al.,[98] as the presence of "a subpopulation of nephrons that is ischemic either from afferent arteriolar vasoconstriction or from an intrinsic narrowing of the lumen. Renin secretion from this subgroup of nephrons is tonically elevated. This increased renin secretion then interferes with the compensatory capacity of intermingled normal nephrons to adaptively excrete sodium and, consequently, perturbs overall blood pressure homeostasis."
- An acquired inhibitor of the sodium pump that "affects sodium transport across cell membranes. In the kidney, it adjusts urinary sodium excretion so that sodium balance is near that of normal subjects on the same intake of sodium, thus making it difficult to demonstrate an increase in extracellular fluid volume. In the arteriole, it causes a rise in intracellular sodium concentration, which in turn raises the intracellular calcium concentration and thus increases vascular reactivity."[99] A great deal of work has gone into identification of a circulating sodium pump inhibitor. Some believe it to be ouabain,[100,101] but others do not.[102]

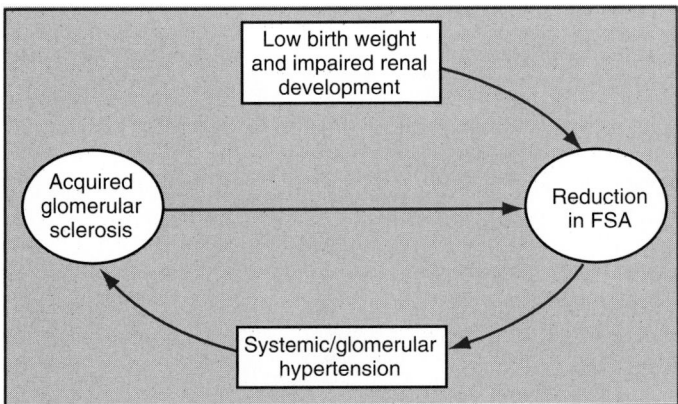

FIGURE 26–11. Hypothesis. The risks of developing essential hypertension and progressive renal injury in adult life are increased as a result of congenital oligonephropathy, an inborn deficit of filtration surface area (FSA) due to impaired renal development. Low birth weight, due to intrauterine growth retardation or prematurity, contributes to this oligonephropathy. Systemic and glomerular hypertension in later life results in progressive glomerular sclerosis, further reducing FSA and thereby perpetuating a vicious cycle, leading, in the extreme, to end-stage renal failure. (From Brenner, B. M., and Chertow, G. M.: Congenital oligonephropathy: An inborn cause of adult hypertension and progressive renal injury? Curr. Opin. Nephrol. Hypertens. 2:691, 1993.)

TABLE 26–8 EVIDENCE FOR A ROLE OF SODIUM IN PRIMARY (ESSENTIAL) HYPERTENSION

1. In multiple populations, the rise in blood pressure with age is directly correlated with increasing levels of sodium intake.
2. Multiple, scattered groups who consume little sodium (less than 50 mmol/day) have little or no hypertension. When they consume more sodium, hypertension appears.
3. Animals given sodium loads, if genetically predisposed, develop hypertension.
4. Some people, when given large sodium loads over short periods, develop an increase in vascular resistance and blood pressure.
5. An increased concentration of sodium is present in the vascular tissue and blood cells of most hypertensives.
6. Sodium restriction, to a level of 60 to 90 mmol per day, will lower blood pressure in most people. The antihypertensive action of diuretics requires an initial natriuresis.

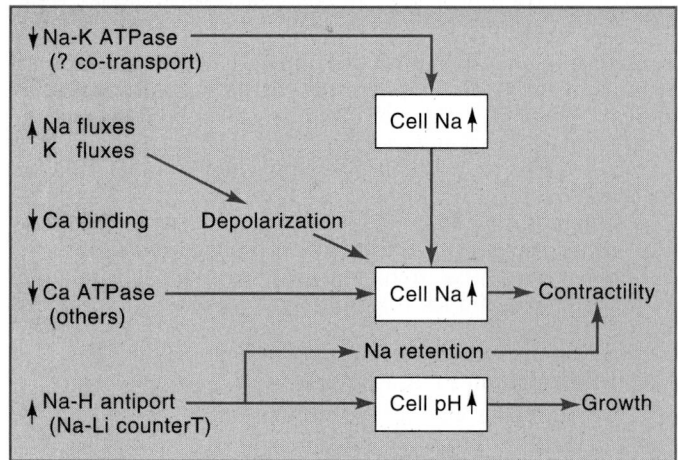

FIGURE 26–12. Hypotheses linking abnormal ionic fluxes to increased peripheral resistance through increases in cell sodium, calcium, or pH. *CounterT* = countertransport. (From Swales, J. D.: Functional disturbance of the cell membrane in hypertension. J. Hypertens. *8* [Suppl. 7]:S203, 1990.)

- A deficient responsiveness of the atrial natriuretic hormone.[103] Although the atrial and brain natriuretic peptides likely play an important role in maintenance of sodium balance and blood pressure regulation,[104] the evidence for their involvement in the genesis of hypertension is weak at best.

There are, then, more than enough possible ways to incite renal retention of even a very small bit of the excess sodium typically ingested that could eventually expand body fluid volume. Variations in sensitivity to sodium also have been noted and may explain why only some people respond to excess sodium and others do not.[105]

Defects in Cell Transport or Binding

A host of defects in various cell membrane functions has been shown mostly in red blood cells. Most involve increased movement of sodium into the cell, thereby increasing intracellular calcium, which, in turn, would increase vascular tone and contractility[106] (Fig. 26–12). John Swales questions their pathogenetic role, concluding that "the best unifying hypothesis is that all the reported abnormalities are markers for a disturbance of physicochemical properties of the cell membrane lipids of hypertensive patients."[107]

Vascular Hypertrophy

Both excess sodium intake and renal sodium retention would presumably work primarily on increasing fluid volume and cardiac output. A number of other factors may work primarily on the second part of the equation, BP = CO × PR (Fig. 26–10). Most of these can cause both functional contraction and structural remodeling and hypertrophy.

Multiple vasoactive substances act as growth factors for vascular hypertrophy.[108] As seen in Figure 26–13, these pressor-growth promoters may result in both vascular contraction and hypertrophy simultaneously, but the perpetuation of hypertension involves hypertrophy. The various hormonal mediators shown at the top of Figure 26–13 may serve as the initiator of what eventuates as increased peripheral resistance. From the study of certain "pure" forms of hormonally induced hypertension, Lever and Harrap[109] have postulated that "most forms of secondary hypertension have two pressor mechanisms: a primary cause, e.g., renal clip, and a second process, which is slow to develop, capable of maintaining hypertension after removal of the primary cause, and probably self-perpetuating in nature. We suggest that essential hypertension also has two mechanisms, both based upon cardiovascular hypertrophy: (1) a growth-promoting process in children (equivalent to the

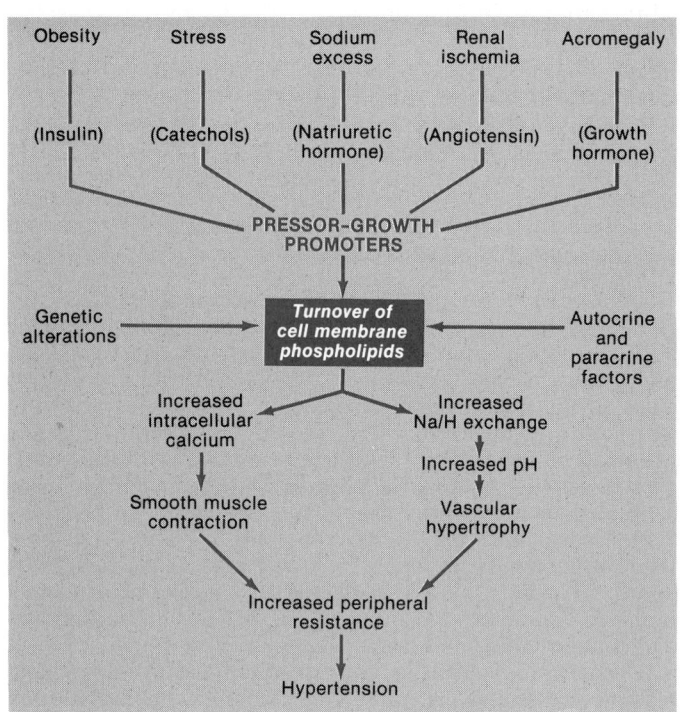

FIGURE 26–13. Scheme for the induction of hypertension by numerous pressor hormones that act as vascular growth promoters. (From Kaplan, N. M.: Clinical Hypertension. 6th ed. Baltimore, © by Williams and Wilkins, 1994, p. 84.)

primary cause in secondary hypertension) and (2) a self-perpetuating mechanism in adults."

These investigators have built on the original proposal of Folkow[110] of a "positive feedback interaction" wherein even mild functional pressor influences, if repeatedly exerted, may lead to structural hypertrophy, which, in turn, reinforces and perpetuates the elevated pressure (Fig. 26–14). Lever and Harrap[109] have added two hypotheses to Folkow's first: a reinforcement of the hypertrophic response to stimuli that initially raise the pressure, e.g., defects in the vascular cell membrane, and the action of various trophic mechanisms that may cause vascular hypertrophy directly, as the "slow pressor mechanism." Whereas the immediate pressor effect is mediated by increased free intracellular calcium, the slowly developing vascular hypertrophy is postulated to involve phosphati-

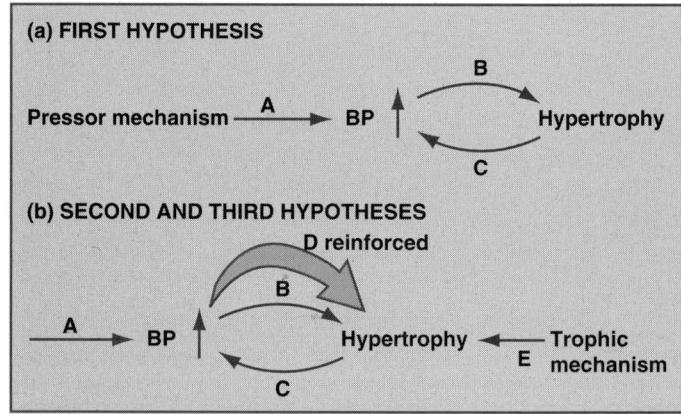

FIGURE 26–14. Hypotheses for the initiation and maintenance of hypertension: A, Folkow's first proposal that a minor overactivity of a pressor mechanism (A) raises blood pressure slightly, initiating positive feedback (BCB) and a progressive rise of blood pressure. B, As in A with two additional signals: D, an abnormal or "reinforced" hypertrophic response to pressure, and E, increase of a humoral agent causing hypertrophy directly. (From Lever, A. F., and Harrap, S. B.: Essential hypertension: A disorder of growth with origins in childhood? J. Hypertens. *10*:101, 1992.)

dyl-inositol metabolism and activation of tyrosine kinase[111] in the cell membrane.

This scheme to explain an immediate pressor action and a slow hypertrophic effect is thought to be common to the action of pressor-growth promoters. When present in high concentrations over long periods, as with angiotensin II in renal artery stenosis, each of these pressor-growth promoters causes hypertension. Moreover, when the source of the excess pressor-growth promoter is removed, hypertension may recede slowly, presumably reflecting the time needed to reverse vascular ·hypertrophy.

No marked excess of any known pressor hormone is identifiable in the majority of hypertensive patients. Nonetheless, a lesser excess of one or more may have been responsible for intiation of a process sustained by the positive feedback postulated by Folkow[110] and the trophic effects emphasized by Lever and Harrap.[109] This sequence encompasses a variety of specific initiating mechanisms that accentuate and maintain the hypertension by a nonspecific feedback-trophic mechanism (Fig. 26–14). If this double process is fundamental to the pathogenesis of primary hypertension, the difficulty in recognizing the initiating causal factor is easily explained. As formulated by Lever[112]:

> The primary cause of hypertension will be most apparent in the early stages; in the later stages, the cause will be concealed by an increasing contribution from hypertrophy. . . . A particular form of hypertension may wrongly be judged to have "no known cause" because each mechanism considered is insufficiently abnormal by itself to have produced the hypertension. The cause of essential hypertension may have been considered already but rejected for this reason.

A large number of circulating hormones and locally acting substances may be involved. Support exists for each of those shown as potential instigators in Figure 26–10. They will be considered in the order shown without attempting to prioritize their role.

Sympathetic Nervous Hyperactivity

Young hypertensives tend to have increased levels of circulating catecholamines,[113] augmented sympathetic nerve traffic in muscles,[114] faster heart rate,[115] and heightened vascular reactivity to norepinephrine.[116] These could raise blood pressure in a number of ways—either alone or in concert with stimulation of renin release by catecholamines—by causing arteriolar and venous constriction, by increasing cardiac output, or by altering the normal renal pressure-volume relationship. In addition to cardiac stimulation by sympathetic activity, vagal inhibitory responses to baroreceptors and other stimuli also may be important. In humans with denervated transplanted hearts, both pulse and blood pressure fail to display the usual nocturnal fall, and hypertension is frequent.[117] The transient increase in epinephrine during stress reactions may invoke a more prolonged pressor response by facilitating the release of norepinephrine from sympathetic neurons.[118]

Repetitive stress or an accentuated, exaggerated response to stress is the logical means by which sympathetic activation would arise. Young hypertensives tend to be hyperresponsive,[119] and at least among middle-aged men in Framingham, the development of hypertension over 18 to 20 years was associated with heightened anxiety and anger intensity and suppressed expression of anger at baseline.[120] Moreover, in the 29-year-old normotensives in the Tecumseh Blood Pressure Study, increased sympathetic activity was closely correlated with higher hematocrit levels (presumably reflecting a decrease in plasma volume from vasoconstriction), and higher hematocrits have been found repeatedly to be associated with higher blood pressures.[115]

The Tecumseh subjects with higher plasma catecholamines also tended to have higher plasma renin activity (PRA) levels. Other investigators have noted that hypertensives with high PRA had more anxiety, suppressed anger, and susceptibility to emotional distress.[121] Obviously, the sympathetic and renin mechanisms may be connected in various ways.

Sympathetic nervous activity could be activated from the brain without the mediation of stress or emotional distress. Hypertension has been induced in animals by various neurogenic defects. An intriguing association has been reported between essential hypertension and compression of the ventrolateral medulla by loops of the posterior inferior cerebellar artery or an ectatic vertebral artery seen by magnetic resonance tomography.[122]

Whatever the specific role of sympathetic activity in the pathogenesis of hypertension, it appears to be involved in the increased cardiovascular morbidity and mortality that affect hypertensive patients during the early morning hours. Increased alpha-sympathetic activity occurs in the early morning, associated with the preawakening increase in REM sleep[123] and the assumption of upright posture after overnight recumbency.[124] As a consequence of the increased sympathetic activity, blood pressure rises abruptly and markedly. This rise must be at least partly responsible for the increase in cardiovascular catastrophes in the early morning hours.[17]

The Renin-Angiotensin System

Both as a direct pressor and as a growth promoter, the renin-angiotensin mechanism also may be involved in the pathogenesis of hypertension.[124a] All functions of renin are mediated through the synthesis of angiotensin II. This system is the primary stimulus for the secretion of aldosterone and hence mediates the mineralocorticoid responses to varying sodium intakes and volume loads. When sodium intake is reduced or effective plasma volume shrinks, the increase in renin–angiotensin II stimulates aldosterone secretion, and this, in turn, is responsible for a portion of the enhanced renal retention of sodium and water (Fig. 26–15).

According to the feedback shown in Figure 26–15, any rise in blood pressure inhibits release of renin from the renal juxtaglomerular (JG) cells. Therefore, primary (essential) hypertension would be expected to be accompanied by low, suppressed levels of PRA. When large populations of hypertensives are surveyed, only about 30 per cent have low PRA, whereas 50 per cent have normal levels and the remaining 20 per cent high levels.[125]

NORMAL AND HIGH RENIN HYPERTENSION

A number of explanations have been offered for these "inappropriately normal" or high levels, beyond the proportion expected in a normal gaussian distribution curve. One of the more attractive is the concept of "nephron heterogeneity" described by Sealey et al.,[98] which assumes a mixture of normal and ischemic nephrons caused by afferent arteriolar narrowing. Excess renin from the ischemic nephrons could raise the total blood renin level to varying degrees and cause some persons to have normal or high renin hypertension.

This hypothesis is similar to that proposed by Goldblatt, who believed that "the primary cause of essential hypertension in man is intrarenal obliterative vascular disease, from any cause, usually arterial and arteriolar sclerosis, or any other condition which brings about the same disturbance of intrarenal hemodynamics."[126] When Goldblatt placed the clamp on the main renal arteries in canine studies, he was trying to explain the pathogenesis of primary (essential) hypertension rather than what he ended up explaining: the pathogenesis of renovascular hypertension.[126a] Nonetheless, his experimental concept is the basis for the more modern model of Sealey et al. The elevated renin from the ischemic population of nephrons, although diluted in the systemic circulation, provides the "normal" renin levels that are usual in patients with primary hypertension who would otherwise be expected to shut down renin secretion and in whom levels would be low. These diluted levels are still high enough to impair sodium excretion in the nonischemic hyperfiltering nephrons

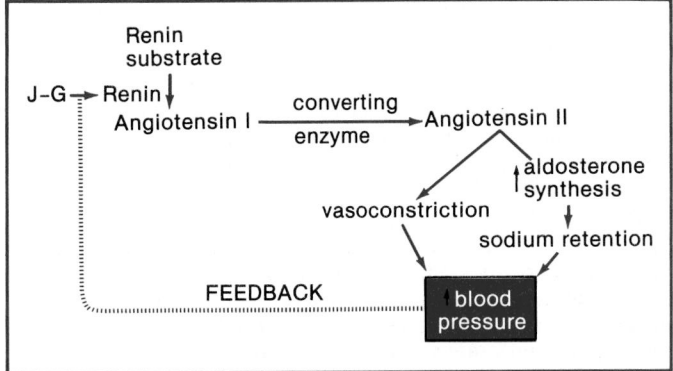

FIGURE 26–15. Overall scheme of the renin-angiotensin mechanism.

but are too low to support efferent tone in the ischemic nephrons, thereby reducing sodium excretion in them as well.

Sealey and associates' concept of nephron heterogeneity differs from Brenner and associates' concept of nephron scarcity previously noted. Nevertheless, Sealey et al. agree that "a reduction in nephron number related to either age or ischemia could amplify the impaired sodium excretion and promote hypertension."[98]

The renin-angiotensin system is active in multiple organs, either from in situ synthesis of various components or by transport from renal JG cells through the circulation. The presence of the complete system in endothelial cells, the brain, the heart, and the adrenal cortex[127] broadens the potential roles of this mechanism far beyond its previously accepted boundaries. Angiotensin may have a direct role in vascular hypertrophy: When local expression of vascular angiotensin-converting enzyme (ACE) was increased by in vivo gene transfer, local hypertrophy of the vessel way occurred, independent of systemic factors or hemodynamic effects.[128]

Hyperinsulinemia/Insulin Resistance

An association between hypertension and hyperinsulinemia has been recognized for many years, particularly with accompanying obesity,[49] but also in nonobese hypertensives.[129] The association does not apply to some ethnic groups such as Pima Indians but has been found in blacks and Asians as well as whites.[130]

All obese people are hyperinsulinemic secondary to insulin resistance and even more so if the obesity is predominantly visceral, i.e., abdominal or upper body, wherein decreased hepatic uptake of insulin contributes to the hyperinsulinemia.[131] The hyperinsulinemia of hypertension also arises as a consequence of resistance to the effects of insulin on peripheral glucose utilization.[132] The cause for the insulin resistance is unknown. It could reflect a simple inability of insulin to reach the skeletal muscle cells, wherein its major peripheral actions on glucose metabolism occur. This, in turn, may result from a defect in the usual vasodilatory effect of insulin, mediated through increased synthesis of nitric oxide,[133] which normally counters the multiple pressor effects of insulin[134] (Fig. 26–16). These pressor effects, in addition to activation of sympathetic activity, include a trophic action on vascular hypertrophy and increased renal sodium reabsorption.

The failure of vasodilation to antagonize the multiple pressor effects of insulin presumably eventuates in a rise in blood pressure that may be either a primary cause of hy-

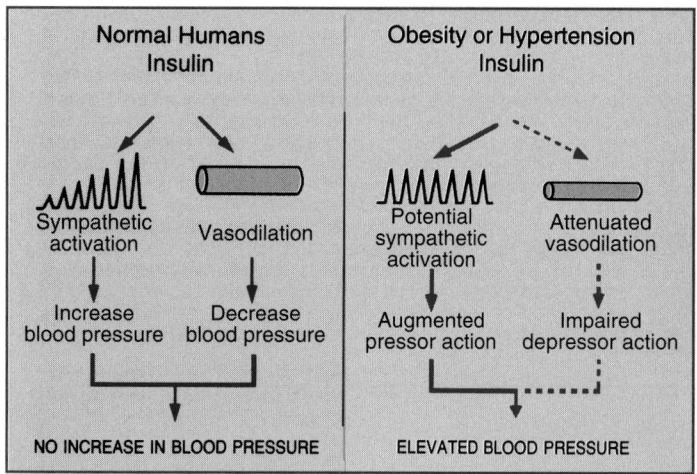

FIGURE 26–16. *Left panel,* Insulin's actions in normal humans. Although insulin causes a marked increase in sympathetic neural outflow which would be expected to increase blood pressure, it also causes vasodilation which would decrease blood pressure. The net effect of these two opposing influences is no change or a slight decrease in blood pressure. There may be an imbalance between the sympathetic and vascular actions of insulin in conditions such as obesity or hypertension. *Right panel,* Insulin may cause potentiated sympathetic activation or attenuated vasodilation. An imbalance between these pressor and depressor actions of insulin may result in elevated blood pressure. (From Anderson, E. A., and Mark, A. L.: Cardiovascular and sympathetic actions of insulin: The insulin hypothesis of hypertension revisited. Cardiovasc. Risk Factors 3:159, 1993.)

pertension or, at least, a secondary potentiator. In addition, the underlying insulin resistance is often associated with a full syndrome, including dyslipidemia and diabetes along with hypertension, which combine to be a major risk factor for premature coronary disease.[132]

Endothelial Cell Dysfunction

The impairment of normal vasodilation seen in the insulin resistance syndrome has been shown to involve a failure to synthesize the normal endothelium-derived relaxing factor nitric oxide (NO).[133] This is one of the rapidly increasing evidences for an active role for the endothelial cells, now known to be the source of multiple relaxing and constricting substances, most having a local, paracrine influence on the underlying smooth muscle cells[135] (Fig. 26–17).

NITRIC OXIDE (see also p. 1164). Hypertensive patients have been shown by some[136] but not all[137] to have a reduced vasodilatory response to various stimuli of NO release. In addition, hypertensives display a less pronounced decrease in forearm blood flow when an inhibitor of NO synthesis is infused, indicating a decreased basal release of NO by the endothelial cells of hypertensive endothelial cells. The forearm responsiveness has been restored by normalization of blood pressure by antihypertensive drugs with different modes of action.[138]

The previously noted frequent association of dyslipidemia with hypertension may be based on an inhibition of endothelium-dependent vasodilation by oxidized lipoproteins.[139]

ENDOTHELIN. A number of endothelium-derived constricting factors are shown in the middle portion of Figure 26–17. Of these, endothelin-1 appears to be of particular importance because it causes pronounced and prolonged vasoconstriction[140] and because inhibitors of its synthesis or binding cause significant vasodilation.[141] Its role in human hypertension, however, remains uncertain.

OTHER POSSIBLE MECHANISMS

The preceding description of the possible roles of the various mechanisms portrayed in Figure 26–10 does not exhaust the list of putative contributors to the pathogenesis of primary hypertension.

Other pressor hormones are known, including vasopressin,[142] but their possible role in human hypertension remains unknown. Similarly, a number of vasodepressor hormones are known, but their function, too, remains uncertain. These include kallikrein[143] and medullipin, a renomedullary lipid.[144]

Contributions from excesses of various minerals, particularly lead,[145] and changing ratios among dietary sodium, potassium, calcium, and magnesium also have been postulated.[146] Support for these and other postulated mechanisms is meager, and the overall schemes involving intracellular sodium and calcium and the pressor-growth promotor mechanisms for vascular hypertrophy seem more than adequate to explain the pathogenesis of primary hypertension. However, a number of associations between hypertension and other conditions have been noted and may offer additional insights into the potential causes and possible prevention of the disease.

ASSOCIATION OF HYPERTENSION WITH OTHER CONDITIONS

OBESITY. Even though obese hypertensives may have lower rates of coronary mortality than lean hypertensives,[147] hypertension is more common among obese individuals and probably adds to their increased risk of developing ischemic heart disease. In the Framingham offspring study, adiposity, as measured by subscapular skinfold thickness, was the major controllable contributor to hypertension.[148] This finding corroborates the crucial importance of the *distribution* of body fat, since blood pressure as well as blood lipids, glucose levels, and insulin levels tends to

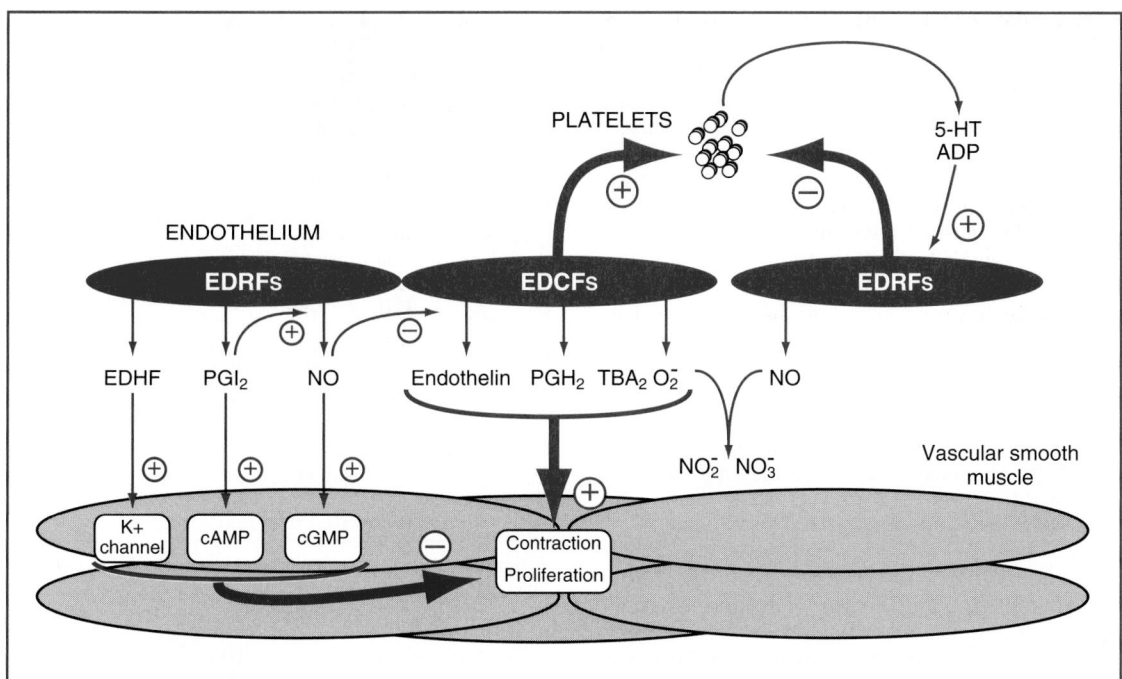

FIGURE 26–17. Schematic diagram of proposed interactions between endothelial mediators. *PGI₂*, prostacyclin; *NO*, nitric oxide; *EDHF*, endothelium-derived hyperpolarizing factor; *PGH₂*, prostaglandin H₂; *TBA₂*, thromboxane A₂; *O₂⁻*, superoxide anion; *5-HT*, serotonin; *ADP*, adenosine diphosphate; *EDRFs*, endothelium-derived relaxing factors; *EDCFs*, endothelium-derived contracting factors. (From Flavahan, N. A.: Atherosclerosis or lipoprotein-induced endothelial dysfunction: Potential mechanism underlying reduction in EDRF/nitric oxide activity. Circulation 85:1927, 1992.)

be highest in those with visceral or upper body obesity.[131] As noted previously, these may all be interconnected via insulin resistance and hyperinsulinemia. Children seem particularly vulnerable to the hypertensive effects of weight gain.[36] Therefore, avoidance of childhood obesity with the hope of avoiding subsequent hypertension seems important. The evidence that weight reduction will lower established hypertension is discussed on p. 844.

SLEEP APNEA. One of the contributors to the hypertension in obese people is sleep apnea. Snoring and sleep apnea are clearly associated with hypertension, and this, in turn, may be induced by increased sympathetic activity in response to hypoxemia during apnea.[149]

PHYSICAL INACTIVITY. Physical fitness may help prevent hypertension, and persons who are already hypertensive may lower their blood pressure by means of regular isotonic exercise. The relationship may involve insulin resistance, because increased resistance was coupled with low physical fitness in normotensive men with a family history of hypertension.[150] Regular exercise may prevent hypertension and thereby protect against the development of cardiovascular disease.[151] Among 16,936 Harvard male alumni followed for 16 to 50 years, those who did not engage in vigorous sports play were at 35 per cent greater risk for developing hypertension, whether or not they had higher blood pressures while at Harvard, a family history of hypertension, or obesity—factors that also increased the risk of hypertension.[152]

ALCOHOL INTAKE. Alcohol in small amounts (less than two usual portions a day) provides protection from coronary mortality[153] and atherosclerosis[154] but in larger amounts (more than two portions a day) increases blood pressure[155] and overall mortality.[153] The reduction in coronary disease in persons who ingest small amounts of alcohol may reflect an improvement in the lipid profile,[156] a reduction in factors that encourage thrombosis,[157] and an improvement in insulin sensitivity.[158]

The pressor effect of larger amounts of alcohol primarily reflects an increase in cardiac output and heart rate, possibly a consequence of increased sympathetic nerve activ-

ity.[159] Alcohol also alters cell membranes, allowing more calcium to enter, perhaps by inhibition of sodium transport.[160]

SMOKING (see also p. 844). Cigarette smoking raises blood pressure, probably through the nicotine-induced release of norepinephrine from adrenergic nerve endings. In addition, smoking causes an acute and marked reduction in radial artery compliance, independent of the increase in blood pressure.[161] When smokers quit, a trivial rise in blood pressure may occur, probably reflecting a gain in weight.[162]

HEMATOLOGIC FINDINGS. Polycythemia vera is frequently associated with hypertension (see p. 1792). More common is a "pseudo-" or "stress" polycythemia with a high hematocrit[115] and increased blood viscosity[163] but contracted plasma volume as well as normal red cell mass and serum erythropoietin levels. High white blood cell counts are predictive of the development of hypertension.[164]

HYPERURICEMIA. Hyperuricemia is present in 25 to 50 per cent of individuals with untreated primary hypertension, about five times the frequency found in normotensive persons. Hyperuricemia likely reflects decreased renal blood flow, presumably a reflection of nephrosclerosis.[165] In addition to these conditions which are often associated with hypertension, distinctive features of hypertension may be important in various special groups of people.

HYPERTENSION IN SPECIAL GROUPS

Blacks

Although, on average, blood pressure in blacks is not higher than that in whites during adolescence,[36] adult blacks have hypertension more frequently, producing higher rates of morbidity and mortality. These higher rates may reflect a lesser tendency for the pressure to fall during sleep[24] and greater degrees of left ventricular hypertrophy,[64] but the lower socioeconomic status and lesser access to adequate health care of blacks as a group are likely more important. In particular, blacks suffer more renal damage, even with effective blood pressure control, leading to a significantly greater prevalence of end-stage disease.[166] When given a high-sodium diet, blacks but not whites tend to have increases in glomerular filtration rates, providing a possible mechanism for increased glomerular sclerosis.[167] Hypertension in blacks has been characterized as having a relatively greater component of fluid volume excess, including a higher prevalence of low plasma renin activity and a greater responsiveness to diuretic therapy.[168]

Perhaps blacks evolved the physiological machinery that would offer protection in their ancestral habitat, i.e., hot, arid climates in which avid sodium conservation was necessary for survival because the diet was relatively low in sodium.[169] When they migrate to areas where sodium intake is excessive, they are then more susceptible to "sodium overload." In addition, blacks also may be more susceptible to hypertension because as a group they tend to ingest less potassium.[170]

Women

In general, women suffer less cardiovascular morbidity and mortality than men for any degree of hypertension.[171] Moreover, before menopause, hypertension is less common in women than in men. Perhaps the lower frequency and severity of hypertension reflect the lower blood volume afforded women by menses. Eventually, however, more women than men suffer a hypertension-related cardiovascular complication because there are more elderly women than elderly men and hypertension is both more common and dangerous in the elderly.[172]

Children and Adolescents
(See also Chap. 31)

As in adults, care is needed in establishing the presence of persistently elevated blood pressures in children using the upper limits of normal shown in Table 26–3. Recall that these are the averages of the first blood pressure value obtained; since the pressure usually falls on repeated measurements, levels below those shown in Table 26–3 may be abnormally high for a given child. In addition, the recent inclusion of height along with age and weight to the nomograms for children and adolescents likely improves their diagnostic accuracy.[173] Uncertainty remains as to the meaning of readings above the 95th percentile in an asymptomatic child, since the tracking of blood pressure as children grow older does not tend to be persistent; the positive predictive value of a blood pressure above the 95th percentile in a 10-year-old boy being at a hypertensive level at age 20 is only 0.44.[174] Moreover, the sensitivity of this high blood pressure in a 10-year-old to detect hypertension 10 years later is only 0.17.

Nonetheless, most authorities[36,175,176] agree that those with "significant" hypertension (levels above the 95th percentile) should be given a limited work-up for target organ damage and secondary causes (perhaps including an echocardiogram and likely including a renal isotopic scan); if these are negative, they should be carefully monitored and given nonpharmacological therapy. Those with "severe" hypertension (levels above the 99th percentile) should be more rapidly and completely evaluated and given appropriate pharmacological therapy.

EPIDEMIOLOGY. The older the child, the more likely the hypertension is of unknown cause, i.e., primary or essential. In prepubertal children, chronic hypertension is more likely caused by congenital or acquired renal parenchymal or vascular disease[176] (Table 26–9).

In adolescents, primary hypertension is the most likely diagnosis. Factors that increase the likelihood for early onset of hypertension include a positive family history of hypertension, obesity, poor physical fitness, and an increase in thickness of the interventricular septum during systole on echocardiography.[177,178] Among black children, a

TABLE 26-9 MOST COMMON CAUSES OF CHRONIC HYPERTENSION IN CHILDHOOD

- **NEWBORN**
  Renal artery stenosis or thrombosis
  Congenital renal structural abnormalities
  Coarctation of the aorta
  Bronchopulmonary dysplasia
- **INFANCY TO 6 YEARS**
  Renal structural and inflammatory diseases
  Coarctation of the aorta
  Renal artery stenosis
  Wilms' tumor
- **6–10 YEARS**
  Renal structural and inflammatory diseases
  Renal artery stenosis
  Essential (primary) hypertension
  Renal parenchymal diseases
- **ADOLESCENCE**
  Primary hypertension
  Renal parenchymal diseases

From Loggie, J. M. H.: Hypertension in children. Heart Dis Stroke May/June:147, 1994.

greater blood pressure reactivity to stress also may be predictive.[179]

MANAGEMENT. Once persistently elevated blood pressures are identified and an appropriate work-up has been performed, weight reduction if the patient is overweight and moderate restriction of dietary sodium should be encouraged. In particular, regular dynamic exercise should be encouraged with few restrictions except for those with severe hypertension.[180] Those deemed to be in need of drug therapy are usually treated in the way adults are managed, as described in the next chapter. Unfortunately, there are very few controlled trials of various therapies in children, so most have adopted newer drugs, i.e., ACE inhibitors and calcium channel blockers, as appropriate therapies.[181] The pharmacological management of life-threatening hypertension follows the guidelines given later in this chapter with appropriate reductions in doses.[36,182]

Elderly

As more people live longer, more hypertension, particularly systolic, will be seen. By the usual criteria of the average of three blood pressure measurements on one occasion at or above 140 mm Hg systolic and/or 90 mm Hg diastolic or the taking of antihypertensive medication, 54 per cent of men and women aged 65 to 74 have hypertension; among blacks, the prevalence is 72 per cent.[183] In elderly patients with significant hypertension of recent onset, chronic renal disease or atherosclerotic renovascular disease is more likely to be found.

The risks of both pure systolic and combined systolic and diastolic hypertension at every level are greater in the elderly than in younger patients, reflecting the adverse effects of age-related atherosclerosis and concomitant conditions. It comes as no surprise that the elderly achieved even greater reductions in coronary disease and heart failure by effective therapy than the younger hypertensives in multiple clinical trials.[183,184]

The elderly may display two features that reflect age-related cardiovascular changes. The first is pseudohypertension from markedly sclerotic arteries that do not collapse under the cuff, presenting much higher cuff pressures than are present within the vessels. If arteries feel rigid but there are few retinal or cardiac findings to go along with marked hypertension, direct intraarterial measurements may be needed before therapy is begun to avoid inordinate lowering of blood pressures that are not, in fact, elevated. The second feature, seen in about 20 per cent of the elderly, is postural and postprandial hypotension, usually reflecting a progressive loss of baroreceptor responsiveness with age.[31,184] A standing blood pressure should always be taken in patients over age 65, particularly if seated or supine hypertension is noted; if postural hypotension is present, maneuvers to overcome the precipitous falls in pressure should be utilized before the seated and supine hypertension is cautiously treated. More about the special therapeutic challenges often found in the elderly is provided in the next chapter.

Diabetes Mellitus
(See also p. 1900)

Hypertension and diabetes coexist more commonly than predicted by chance. They feed on each other to markedly accelerate cardiovascular damages that are, in turn, responsible for the premature disabilities and higher rates of mortality that afflict diabetics. Among some 1500 diabetics followed by Danish investigators, 51 per cent of the insulin-dependent diabetics and 80 per cent of the non-insulin-dependent diabetics had blood pressures above 140/90 mm Hg.[185] In more than half these hypertensive diabetics, isolated systolic hypertension was noted.

Not only is hypertension more common in diabetics, but it also tends to be more persistent, with less of the usual nocturnal fall in pressure.[22] The absence of a nocturnal fall in pressure may reflect autonomic neuropathy or incipient diabetic nephropathy.[186]

The presence of hypertension increases all the microvascular and macrovascular complications seen in diabetes. Even at the initial presentation of diabetes, the presence of hypertension is associated with about a doubling of the prevalence of microalbuminuria, left ventricular hyper-

trophy, and electrocardiographic signs of myocardial ischemia.[187] As these newly diagnosed diabetics were followed for about 5 years, those with hypertension suffered almost a twofold greater incidence of cardiovascular morbidity and mortality than did the nonhypertensive diabetics.

When hypertensive, patients with diabetes mellitus may confront some interesting problems. With progressive renal insufficiency, they may have few functional juxtaglomerular cells, and as a result, the syndrome of hyporeninemic hypoaldosteronism may appear, usually manifested by hyperkalemia. If hypoglycemia develops because of too much insulin or other drugs, severe hypertension may occur as a result of stimulated sympathetic nervous activity.

Diabetics are also susceptible to special problems associated with antihypertensive therapy. High doses of both diuretics and beta blockers may worsen diabetic control, probably by inducing further insulin resistance. Those who are prone to hypoglycemia may have difficulties with beta-blocking agents, since these drugs blunt their protective catecholamine response, and severe hypoglycemia may develop with sweating as the only warning. Diabetic neuropathy may add to the postural hypotension and impotence that frequently complicate antihypertensive therapy. Diabetic nephropathy will impair sodium excretion and diminish the effectiveness of diuretics. On the other hand, successful control of hyperglycemia and reduction of blood pressure will protect such patients from the otherwise inexorable progress of diabetic nephropathy. Angiotensin-converting enzyme inhibitors may be especially effective in reducing the high intraglomerular pressures that are probably responsible for the progressive glomerulosclerosis of diabetes.[188]

SECONDARY FORMS OF HYPERTENSION
(See Tables 26–4 and 26–5, pp. 811 and 812)

Oral Contraceptive and Postmenopausal Estrogen Use

The use of estrogen-containing oral contraceptive pills is probably the most common cause of secondary hypertension in young women. Most women who take them experience a slight rise in blood pressure, and about 5 per cent develop hypertension (i.e., blood pressure above 140/90 mm Hg) within 5 years of oral contraceptive use. This is more than twice the incidence seen among women of the same age who do not use these agents.[172] Although the hypertension is usually mild, it may persist after the oral contraceptive is discontinued, it may be severe, and it is almost certainly a factor in the increased cardiovascular mortality seen among young women who take these agents.[189] Despite these facts, these drugs have provided effective and safe birth control for millions of women, and the need for oral contraceptives remains.

The dangers of oral contraceptives should be kept in proper perspective. While it is true that use of these drugs is associated with increased morbidity and mortality, the absolute numbers are quite small, and overall mortality from cardiovascular disease has been declining progressively among women in the United States at a rate equal to that noted among American men. Moreover, the risks appear to have been lessened by more careful selection of users and lower doses of hormones.[190] Most adverse effects occur in women who smoke and have other cardiovascular risk factors and who take formulations with more than 50 μg of estrogen. Thus, the currently used low-estrogen and progesterone forms seem quite safe for the purposes of temporary birth control.

INCIDENCE. The best data on the incidence of oral contraceptive–induced hypertension came from a large study of the Royal College of General Practitioners. The incidence of hypertension was 2.6 times greater among 23,000 pill users compared with 23,000 nonusers, resulting in a 5 per cent incidence over 5 years of oral contraceptive use.[191] In addition, this incidence increased with long duration of pill use, being only slightly higher than that among controls during the first year but rising to almost three times higher by the fifth year. In a much smaller but more carefully performed prospective study of 186 Scottish women, systolic pressure rose in 164 (by more than 25 mm Hg in 8) and diastolic pressure rose in 150 (by more than 20 mm Hg in 2) during the first 2 years of oral contraceptive use.[192] After 3 years, the mean rise in 83 of these women was 9.2 mm Hg. The current use of smaller amounts of estrogen (20 to 35 μg) than the 50 μg taken by most of these women may induce less hypertension.

CLINICAL FEATURES. The likelihood of developing hypertension among women using oral contraceptives is much greater among those who are over age 35 or obese or who drink large quantities of alcohol.[193] The presence of hypertension during a prior pregnancy increases this likelihood but not enough to preclude pill use in such women who require contraception. In most women the hypertension is mild; however, in some it may accelerate rapidly and cause severe renal damage.[194] When the pill is discontinued, blood pressure falls to normal within 3 to 6 months in about half the patients. Whether the pill caused permanent hypertension in the other half or just uncovered primary hypertension at an earlier time is not clear.

MECHANISMS OF HYPERTENSION. Oral contraceptive use probably causes hypertension by renin-aldosterone–mediated volume expansion. Estrogens and the synthetic progestogens used in oral contraceptive pills both cause sodium retention.[195] In keeping with the probable role of hyperinsulinemia in other hypertensive states (see p. 820), this may be involved in oral contraceptive–induced hypertension as well because plasma insulin levels are increased after start of oral contraceptive use, reflecting peripheral insulin resistance.[196]

MANAGEMENT. The use of estrogen-containing oral contraceptives should be restricted in women over age 35, particularly if they also smoke or are hypertensive or obese. Women given the pill should be properly monitored as follows: (1) the supply should be limited initially to 3 months and thereafter to 6 months; (2) they should be required to return for a blood pressure check before an additional supply is provided; and (3) if blood pressure has risen, an alternative contraceptive should be offered. If the pill remains the only acceptable contraceptive, the elevated blood pressure can be reduced with appropriate therapy. In view of the probable role of aldosterone, use of a diuretic-spironolactone combination seems appropriate. In those who stop taking oral contraceptives, evaluation for secondary hypertensive diseases should be postponed for at least 3 months to allow the changes in the renin-angiotensin-aldosterone system to remit. If the hypertension does not recede, additional work-up and therapy may be needed.

POSTMENOPAUSAL ESTROGEN USE. Millions of women use estrogen for its potential benefits after menopause. It does not appear to induce hypertension, even though it does induce various changes in the renin-angiotensin-aldosterone system seen with oral contraceptive use.[197] Moreover, the majority of case-control studies have shown a significantly *lower* mortality rate from coronary artery disease among postmenopausal estrogen users than nonusers.[198] Such cardioprotection likely reflects improvement in endothelium-dependent, flow-mediated vasodilation, either from a direct effect on endothelial function or through changes in blood lipids.[199]

Renal Parenchymal Disease

In the overall population, renal parenchymal disease is the most common cause of secondary hypertension, responsible for 2 to 5 per cent of cases (Table 26–5). As chronic glomerulonephritis becomes less common, hypertensive nephrosclerosis and diabetic nephropathy have become the most common causes of end-stage renal disease (ESRD).[200] The higher prevalence of hypertension among U.S. blacks is probably responsible for their significantly higher rate of ESRD, with hypertension as the underlying cause in as many as one-half of these patients.[201]

Not only does hypertension cause renal failure and renal failure cause hypertension, but also more subtle renal dysfunction may be involved in patients with primary hypertension. As discussed earlier (see p. 817), the kidneys may initiate the hemodynamic cascade eventuating in primary hypertension. As that disease progresses, some renal dysfunction is demonstrable in most patients; progressive renal damage is the end result and is the cause of death in perhaps 10 per cent of hypertensives. Since early treatment of hypertension will likely protect against nephrosclerosis, there is hope that improved control of hypertension will slow the progression and reduce the frequency of ESRD.

In hypertension with renal parenchymal disease the sequence of progressively worsening renal damage is (1) acute renal diseases that are often reversible, (2) unilateral and bilateral diseases without renal insufficiency, (3) chronic renal disease with renal insufficiency, and (4) hypertension in the anephric state and after renal transplantation.

ACUTE RENAL DISEASES. Hypertension may appear with any sudden, severe insult to the kidneys that either markedly impairs the excretion of salt and water, which leads to volume expansion, or reduces renal blood flow, which sets off the renin-angiotensin-aldosterone mechanism. Bilateral ureteral obstruction is an example of the former; sudden bilateral renal artery occlusion, as by emboli, is an example of the latter. Relief of either may dramatically reverse severe hypertension. This has been particularly striking in men with high-pressure chronic retention of urine, who may manifest both renal failure and severe hypertension, both of which may be relieved by relief of the obstruction.[202] Some of the collagen diseases also may produce rapidly progressive renal damage. The more common acute processes are glomerulonephritis and oliguric renal failure.

ACUTE GLOMERULONEPHRITIS. Although the classic syndrome of type-specific poststreptococcal nephritis has become much less common, glomerular lesions of various types may be associated with hypertension. Moreover, although the epidemic poststreptococcal disease is usually self-limited, the disease in some patients follows a progressive, smoldering course that may lead to renal insufficiency.[203] Typically, hypertension accompanies the fluid retention of acute renal injury and is best relieved by sodium and fluid restriction and potent diuretics. Dialysis and parenteral antihypertensive drugs may be needed if encephalopathy supervenes. In milder cases, the hypertension recedes as the edema is relieved.

ACUTE OLIGURIC RENAL FAILURE. Acute renal failure may occur after hypotension, particularly in patients in whom renin levels are already high, such as those with cirrhosis and ascites or at the end of pregnancy. The release of even more renin by decreased blood pressure and effective circulating blood volume may flood the renal vasculature and cause such intense renal vasoconstriction that renal function shuts down. Hypertension in this setting is usually not an important problem and can be controlled by preventing volume overload. High doses of furosemide may be helpful, but dialysis is often needed. When acute renal failure occurs in the setting of accelerated or malignant hypertension, aggressive therapy (including dialysis) may be followed by sustained recovery of renal function.[203] The use of nonsteroidal antiinflammatory agents (NSAIDs) may cause acute renal failure usually in the setting of chronic renal damage.[204]

VASCULITIS. Rapidly progressive renal deterioration with severe hypertension occurs not infrequently during the course of scleroderma and other forms of vasculitis (p. 799). Therapy with antihypertensives, particularly angiotensin-converting enzyme inhibitors, may reverse the process.[205]

EXTRACORPOREAL SHOCK WAVE LITHOTRIPSY. As this procedure has been utilized increasingly to treat nephrolithiasis, at least transient rises in blood pressure have been observed in from 20 to 30 per cent of patients,[206] but persistent hypertension is unusual.[207]

RENAL DISEASE WITHOUT RENAL INSUFFICIENCY

Although an entire kidney may be removed without obvious effect and no rise in blood pressure,[208] hypertension may be associated with unilateral and bilateral renal parenchymal diseases in the absence of significant renal insufficiency. Although such hypertension may reflect other unrecognized processes, most likely it is caused by activation of the renin-angiotensin-aldosterone mechanism. However, in some patients whose hypertension has been relieved by correction of a renal defect, the levels of renin have not been high.

UNILATERAL PARENCHYMAL RENAL DISEASE. A number of unilateral kidney diseases may be associated with hypertension, and in some of these the affected kidney may appear shrunken. Nonetheless, most small kidneys do not cause hypertension, and when they are indiscriminately removed from patients with hypertension, the condition is relieved in only about 25 per cent.[209] Of that 25 per cent, most have arterial occlusive disease, either as the primary cause of the renal atrophy or secondary to irregular scarring of the parenchyma.[210]

POLYCYSTIC KIDNEY DISEASE. Although patients with adult polycystic kidney disease usually progress to renal insufficiency, some retain reasonably normal glomerular filtration rates (GFR) and display no azotemia. Hypertension, although more common in those with renal failure, is present in perhaps half of those with a normal GFR and probably reflects variable degrees of both renin excess and fluid retention.[211]

CHRONIC PYELONEPHRITIS. The relationship between pyelonephritis and hypertension is multifaceted: Pyelonephritis, either unilateral or bilateral, may cause hypertension; hypertensive individuals may be more susceptible to renal infection. In pyelonephritic patients with hypertension but fairly normal renal function, renin levels are high,[212] probably from interstitial scarring with obstruction of intrarenal vessels.

CHRONIC RENAL DISEASES WITH RENAL INSUFFICIENCY. As dialysis and transplantation prolong the lives of more patients with renal insufficiency, their hypertension must be dealt with over much longer periods. Hypertension in most patients with renal insufficiency is predominantly caused by volume overload resulting from the inability of the reduced functioning renal mass to handle the usual sodium and water intake. With proper attention to sodium and water intake and, if needed, adequate dialysis, control of blood pressure may not be particularly difficult. Unfortunately, some patients are much more fragile, alternating between low and high pressures, and some are much more resistant, presumably because of a greater contribution of high renin levels to the hypertension. Moreover, their pressures may not fall much during sleep, posing an additional burden on the heart and vasculature.[23] Nonetheless, with judicious use of available therapy, hypertension should not be a major problem for most patients with renal insufficiency.

In view of increasing evidence that glomerular capillary hypertension is responsible for the progressive loss of renal function once renal damage begins (Fig. 26–11), aggressive reduction of intraglomerular hypertension in order to prevent further renal loss is being actively pursued. Angiotensin-converting enzyme (ACE) inhibitors may be particularly effective in this regard.[188]

Three aspects of hypertension with end-stage renal disease (ESRD) should be recognized: (1) hypertension contributes to the cardiovascular diseases that are the cause of death in about half of patients with ESRD;[213] (2) renal damage may progress despite apparent control of hypertension, particularly among blacks;[201] and (3) a significant proportion of ESRD may reflect bilateral renovascular disease that may be made worse by antihypertensive drug therapy but markedly improved by revascularization.[214]

Diabetic Nephropathy (see also p. 1900). Hypertension often accompanies diabetic nephropathy, reflecting inability to handle volume loads because of loss of nephrons as a result of progressive intercapillary glomerulosclerosis. As shown in Figure 26–18, intrarenal hypertension accelerates the progress of the glomerulosclerosis, and antihypertensive therapy has been shown to slow the progression of renal failure.[188] Although more effective relief of glomerular capillary hypertension may be possible with ACE inhibitors, long-term protection has been obtained with traditional antihypertensive drugs, not including ACE inhibitors.[215] As common as it is, hypertension may not be as severe or as likely to progress to an accelerated-malignant phase in diabetics with nephropathy for two reasons: first, these patients often have a diminished intravascular volume because of the hypoalbuminemia of the nephrotic syndrome; second, they have low renin levels, presumably owing to hyalinization of juxtaglomerular cells, which may present as hyporeninemic hypoaldosteronism.

Analgesic Nephropathy. In addition to acute renal insufficiency that may accompany the inhibition of renal prostaglandins by nonsteroidal antiinflammatory agents,[204] permanent interstitial renal damage may supervene after prolonged exposure to analgesics, particularly phenacetin and, to a lesser degree, acetaminophen.[216] Until late in their course, these patients have a greater propensity for salt wasting and therefore may have less severe hypertension.

HYPERTENSION DURING CHRONIC DIALYSIS AND AFTER RENAL TRANSPLANTATION. In patients with end-stage renal disease, blood pressure depends mainly upon body fluid volume. Hypertension may be accentuated by the accumulation of endogenous inhibitors of nitric oxide synthase, withdrawing the vasodilation provided by nitric oxide.[217] With neither the vasoconstrictor effects of renal renin nor the vasodepressor actions of various renal hormones, blood pressure may be particularly labile and sensitive to changes in adrenergic activity. Among patients receiving maintenance hemodialysis every 48 hours, elevated blood pressures tend to fall progressively after dialysis is completed, remain depressed during the remainder of the first 24 hours, and rise again during the second day.[218] Thus antihypertension therapy may be needed only on the days between dialyses.

Whereas successful renal transplantation may cure primary hypertension,[219] various problems may result, with about half the recipients becoming hypertensive within 1 year.[220] These problems include stenosis of the renal artery at the site of anastomosis, rejection reactions, high doses of adrenal steroids and cyclosporine, and excess renin derived from the retained diseased kidneys. ACE inhibitor therapy may obviate the need to remove the native diseased kidneys in order to relieve hypertension caused by their persistent secretion of renin.[221] The source of the donor kidney also may play a role in the subsequent development of hypertension in the recipient: More hypertension has been observed when donors had a family history of hypertension or when the donors had died of subarachnoid hemorrhage and had probably been hypertensive.[222]

Renovascular Hypertension

Renovascular hypertension is the most common secondary form of hypertension and is not easily recognizable. Although no more than 1 per cent of all adults with hypertension have renovascular hypertension (Table 26–5), the prevalence is much higher in those with sudden onset of severe hypertension and other suggestive features[223] (Table 26–10). Mann and Pickering classify patients into low, moderate, and high "clinical index of suspicion" as a guide to the selection of additional work-up for renovascular hypertension. Those with characteristics listed under moderate are considered to have a 5 to 15 per cent likelihood of the diagnosis and therefore are in need of a noninvasive screening test. Those with characteristics listed under high

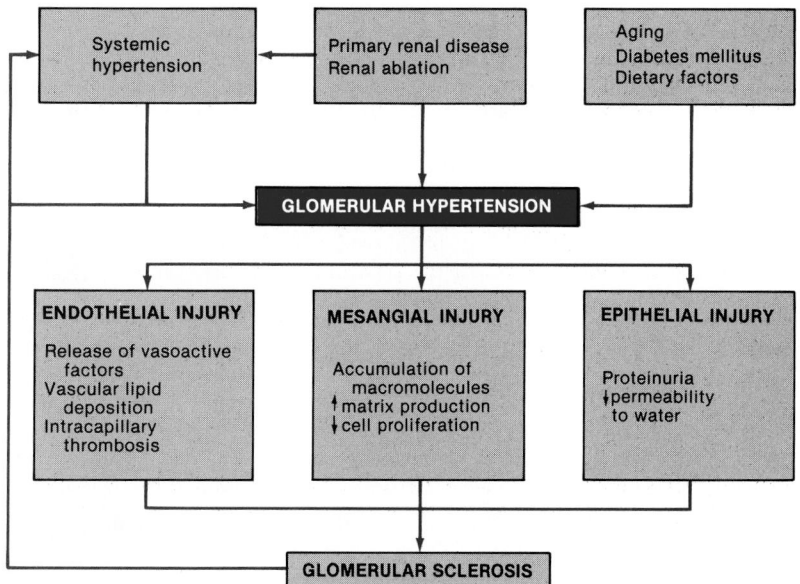

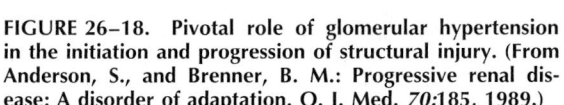

FIGURE 26–18. Pivotal role of glomerular hypertension in the initiation and progression of structural injury. (From Anderson, S., and Brenner, B. M.: Progressive renal disease: A disorder of adaptation. Q. J. Med. 70:185, 1989.)

TABLE 26–10   TESTING FOR RENOVASCULAR HYPERTENSION: CLINICAL INDEX OF SUSPICION AS A GUIDE TO SELECTING PATIENTS FOR WORK-UP

LOW (SHOULD NOT BE TESTED): Borderline, mild, or moderate hypertension, in the absence of clinical clues

MODERATE (NONINVASIVE TESTS RECOMMENDED):

Severe hypertension (diastolic blood pressure greater than 120 mm Hg)

Hypertension refractory to standard therapy

Abrupt onset of sustained, moderate to severe hypertension at age < 20 or age > 50

Hypertension with a suggestive abdominal bruit (long, high-pitched, and localized to the region of the renal artery)

Moderate hypertension (diastolic blood pressure exceeding 105 mm Hg) in a smoker, in a patient with evidence of occlusive vascular disease (cerebrovascular, coronary, peripheral vascular), or in a patient with unexplained but stable elevation of serum creatinine

Normalization of blood pressure by an angiotensin-converting enzyme inhibitor in a patient with moderate or severe hypertension (particularly a smoker or a patient with recent onset of hypertension)

HIGH (MAY CONSIDER PROCEEDING DIRECTLY TO ARTERIOGRAPHY):

Severe hypertension (diastolic blood pressure greater than 120 mm Hg with either progressive renal insufficiency or refractoriness to aggressive treatment, particularly in a patient who has been a smoker or has other evidence of occlusive arterial disease)

Accelerated or malignant hypertension (grade III or IV retinopathy)

Hypertension with recent elevation of serum creatinine, either unexplained or reversibly induced by an angiotensin-converting enzyme inhibitor

Moderate to severe hypertension with incidentally detected asymmetry of renal size

From Mann, S. J., Pickering, T. G.: Detection of renovascular hypertension. State of the art: 1992. Ann. Intern. Med. *117*:845, 1992.

are considered to have a greater than 25 per cent likelihood of the diagnosis so that renal arteriography should be the initial test.

In multiple series, renovascular disease has been found less commonly in black hypertensives than in whites.[224,225] In the large series described by Novick et al.,[225] the blacks had more severe hypertension and extensive atherosclerosis in other vascular beds.

CLASSIFICATION. In adults, the two major types of renovascular disease tend to appear at different times and affect the sexes differently (Table 26–11). Atherosclerotic disease affecting mainly the proximal third of the main renal artery is seen mostly in older men. Fibroplastic disease involving mainly the distal two-thirds and branches of the renal arteries appears most commonly in younger women. Overall, about two-thirds of cases are caused by atherosclerotic dis-

ease and one-third by fibroplastic disease. While the non-atherosclerotic stenoses involve all layers of the renal artery, the most common is medial fibroplasia.

There are a number of other intrinsic and extrinsic causes of renovascular hypertension, including emboli within the renal artery or compression of this vessel by nearby tumors. Most renovascular hypertension develops from partial obstruction of one main renal artery, but only a branch need be involved; segmental disease was found in 11 per cent of cases in one large series.[226] On the other hand, if apparent complete occlusion of the renal artery is slow in developing, enough collateral flow will become available to preserve the viability of the kidney. In this way, the seemingly nonfunctioning kidney may be responsible for continued renin secretion and hypertension. If recognized, such totally occluded vessels can sometimes be repaired, with return of renal function and relief of hypertension.[227]

Renovascular stenosis is often bilateral, although usually one side is clearly predominant. In the Cooperative Study on Renovascular Hypertension, 25 per cent of the subjects had bilateral atherosclerotic or fibroplastic disease.[228] The possibility of bilateral disease should be suspected in those with renal insufficiency, particularly if rapidly progressive oliguric renal failure develops without evidence of obstructive uropathy and even more so if it develops after start of ACE inhibitor therapy.[228]

MECHANISMS. Since Goldblatt produced renovascular hypertension in the dog in 1934, the pathophysiology of this disease has been studied extensively. Confusion has arisen because of the use of one-kidney models, which are more appropriate to the study of renal parenchymal hypertension. The sequence of changes in the two-kidney (one-clip) model and in patients with renovascular hypertension almost certainly starts with the release of increased amounts of renin when sufficient ischemia is induced to diminish pulse pressure against the juxtaglomerular cells in the renal afferent arterioles. A reduction of renal perfusion pressure by 50 per cent leads to an immediate and persistent increase in renin secretion from the ischemic kidney, with suppression of secretion from the contralateral one. With time, renin levels fall (but not to the low levels expected based on the elevated blood pressure), accompanied by an expanded body fluid volume and increased cardiac output.[229]

DIAGNOSIS. The presence of the clinical features listed under moderate in Table 26–10 indicates the need for a screening test for renovascular hypertension in perhaps 5 to 10 per cent of all hypertensives. A positive screening test, or very strong clinical features, calls for more definitive confirmatory tests.

Some patients have renovascular hypertension but none of the clinical features listed in Table 26–10, clinically resembling patients with mild primary hypertension. Nonetheless, these features should be used to exclude the major-

TABLE 26–11   FEATURES OF THE TWO MAJOR FORMS OF RENAL ARTERY DISEASE

CAUSE	INCIDENCE (%)	AGE (yr)	LOCATION OF LESION IN RENAL ARTERY	NATURAL HISTORY
Atherosclerosis	65	> 50	Proximal 2 cm; branch disease rare	Progression in 50 per cent, often to total occlusion
Fibromuscular dysplasias				
Intimal	1–2	Birth–25	Mid-main renal artery and/or branches	Progression in most cases; dissection and/or thrombosis common
Medial	30	25–50	Distal main renal artery and/or branches	Progression in 33 per cent; dissection and/or thrombosis rare
Periarterial	1–2	15–30	Middle to distal main renal artery or branches	Progression in most cases; dissection and/or thrombosis common

From Kaplan, N. M.: Clinical Hypertension. 6th ed. Baltimore, Williams and Wilkins, 1994, p. 326.

ity of hypertensives from additional work-up and to identify the 10 per cent or so who should undergo a work-up.

Functional Diagnostic Tests. Isotopic renography and plasma renin measurements after an oral captopril challenge are currently the best initial tests in patients with those suggestive clinical features listed under moderate in Table 26–10, to be followed by renal arteriography and then renal vein renin assays.[230,231] The latter procedure may not be needed if isotopic renography after captopril indicates significant renal ischemia in the kidney with renal artery disease by arteriography. In some centers with facilities dedicated to the performance of renal artery duplex sonography, that procedure is being utilized for initial screening.[230] In the future, magnetic resonance arteriography may be utilized.

The captopril challenge test depends on the abrupt inhibition of circulating angiotensin II by the ACE inhibitor removing the major support for perfusion through a stenotic renal artery to a kidney. The acutely ischemic kidney immediately releases more renin and undergoes a marked decrease in glomerular filtration and renal blood flow. Therefore, both plasma renin levels and the isotopic flow through the kidneys 1 hour after a single 50-mg dose of the ACE inhibitor should be measured. To measure the plasma renin response, the patient should be on normal sodium dietary intake and off diuretics and ACE inhibitors; if possible, other antihypertensive medications should be withdrawn for at least a week, although the test was originally found to be almost equally valid among those examined while on therapy.[232] After the patient sits for 30 minutes, venous blood is obtained for basal PRA, and 50 mg of captopril is given orally. At 60 minutes, another blood sample for stimulated PRA is obtained. The original criteria for a positive test for renovascular hypertension were (1) a stimulated PRA of 12 ng/ml/hr or more, (2) an absolute increase in PRA of 10 ng/ml/hr or more, and (3) a 150 per cent or greater increase in PRA or, if baseline PRA is below 3 ng/ml/hr, a 400 per cent increase. The authors have subsequently reported a high prevalence of false-positive responses in patients with high baseline renin levels.[233] Others report sensitivity ranging from 0.73 to 1.0 and specificity ranging from 0.73 to 0.95.[231]

The performance of isotopic renography 1 hour after the oral captopril dose provides additional diagnostic information that appears to be more accurate than the renin response.[234] The renogram may use labeled hippurate, a measure of renal blood flow, or diethylenetriaminepentaacetic acid (DTPA) or mercaptoacetyltriglycine (MAG3), measures of glomerular filtration rate. If the postcaptopril test shows a significant difference between the two kidneys, the procedure should be repeated without captopril to document the ischemic origin of the differences in blood flow or GFR. With captopril renography, renal vein renin measurements are needed less often to localize the affected side when renovascular disease is bilateral.

MANAGEMENT

Medical. The availability of ACE inhibitors (see p. 494) may be considered a two-edged sword; one edge provides better control of renovascular hypertension than may be possible with other antihypertensive medications, while the other edge exposes the already ischemic kidney to a further loss of blood flow by removing the high levels of angiotensin II that were supporting its circulation.[231] Calcium entry blockers and other antihypertensive drugs may be almost as effective as ACE inhibitors and considerably safer.[235]

Angioplasty. Angioplasty has been shown to improve 60 to 70 per cent of patients, more with fibromuscular disease than with atherosclerosis, as is also the case for surgery.[236] It is being performed more and more frequently as the initial procedure, particularly in patients who are poor candidates for major surgery, even in the presence of severe stenoses.[237]

Surgery. Surgical repair has been shown to relieve renovascular hypertension in an increasing number of patients, including the elderly[238] and those with renal insufficiency.[239] Most agree that surgery is indicated in patients whose hypertension is not well controlled or whose renal function deteriorates on medical therapy and in those with only a transient response to angioplasty or when lesions are not amenable to that procedure.

RENIN-SECRETING TUMORS

Made up of juxtaglomerular cells or hemangiopericytomas, these tumors have been found mostly in young patients with severe hypertension, very high renin levels in both peripheral blood and the kidney harboring the tumor, and secondary aldosteronism manifested by hypokalemia.[240] The tumor usually can be recognized by selective renal angiography, usually performed for suspected renovascular hypertension, although a few are extrarenal.[241] More commonly, children with Wilms' tumors (nephroblastoma) may have hypertension and high plasma renin and prorenin levels that revert to normal after nephrectomy.[242]

Adrenal Causes of Hypertension
(See Chap. 61)

Adrenal causes of hypertension include primary excesses of aldosterone, cortisol, and catecholamines; more rarely, excess deoxycorticosterone (DOC) is present along with congenital adrenal hyperplasia. Together these cause less than 1 per cent of all hypertensive diseases. Each can usually be recognized with relative ease, and patients suspected of having these disorders can be screened by means of readily available tests. More of a problem than the diagnosis of these adrenal disorders is the need to exclude their presence because of the increasing identification of incidental adrenal masses when abdominal computed tomography (CT) is done to diagnose intraabdominal pathology. Unsuspected adrenal tumors have been found in from 1 to 2 per cent of abdominal CT scans obtained for reasons unrelated to the adrenal gland. Most of these "incidentalomas" appear to be nonfunctional on the basis of normal basal adrenal hormone levels. However, when more detailed studies are done, a significant number show incomplete suppression of cortisol by dexamethasone, i.e., subclinical Cushing's disease which does not appear to progress to overt hypercortisolism, and a few have unsuspected catecholamine hypersecretion.[243] Nonfunctioning adenomas have significantly less lipid content than do functioning adenomas by chemical-shift magnetic resonance imaging,[244] so this procedure may have clinical usefulness. The threat of malignancy probably can be best excluded by adrenal scintigraphy with the radioiodinated derivative of cholesterol, NP-59.[245] Benign lesions almost always take up the isotope, while malignant ones almost always do not. Osella et al.[243] found lower plasma dehydroepiandrosterone sulfate (DHEA-S) levels in most with nonfunctioning benign adenomas and high levels in those with adrenal malignancies. Most tumors larger than 4 cm are resected, since a significant number of them are malignant.

Primary Aldosteronism
(See also p. 1895)

This disease is relatively rare in unselected populations (Table 26–5), although it has been recognized in considerably more patients screened by a plasma aldosterone/renin activity ratio.[246]

PATHOPHYSIOLOGY. Primary aldosterone excess usually arises from solitary benign adenomas. As diagnostic tests have improved and become more readily available, larger numbers of patients with minimal features have been recognized.[246] Many of these patients have been found to have bilateral adrenal hyperplasia, the number averaging about one-third of all cases of aldosteronism.

MINERALOCORTICAL HYPERTENSION. The pathogenesis of the familial glucocorticoid-suppressible aldosteronism has now been elucidated, and it is not as rare as once thought.[247] The syndrome is caused by a mutation in the genes involved in the coding for the aldosterone synthase enzyme normally found only in the outer zona glomerulosa and the 11-beta-hydroxylase enzyme in the zona fasciculata.[248] The chimeric gene induces an enzyme that catalyzes the synthesis of 18-hydroxylated cortisol in the zona fasciculata. Since this zone is under the control of ACTH, the glucocorticoid suppressibility of the syndrome is explained.

Another unusual form of mineralocorticoid hypertension also has been explained by the recognition of deficiency of the enzyme 11-beta-hydroxysteroid dehydrogenase (11-β-OHSD) in the renal tubule, where it normally converts cortisol (which has the ability to act on the mineralocorticoid receptor) to cortisone (which does not). The persistence of high levels of cortisol induces all the features of mineralocorticoid excess. The 11-β-OHSD enzyme may be congenitally absent (the syndrome of apparent mineralocorticoid excess)[249] or inhibited by the glycyrrhetenic acid contained in licorice.[250] More subtle deficiencies of 11-β-OHSD have been recognized in some patients with chronic renal disease[251] and low-renin essential hypertension.[252]

Whatever the source, excess mineralocorticoid usually causes hypertension and hypokalemia, defined as a plasma potassium level below 3.2 mEq/liter. Very rarely, mineralocorticoid excess has been recognized in normotensive persons.[246] Not so rarely, hypokalemia may be absent or only intermittent, but in most patients with adenomas, persistent hypokalemia is observed.[253]

The hypertension begins as a volume overload but soon converts, as do apparently all forms of hypertension, to increased peripheral resistance. Hypertension may be severe, with a mean pressure in one group of 136 patients of 205/123 mm Hg and 4 of the patients showing histological evidence of malignant hypertension on renal biopsy.[254] Furthermore, 23 per cent of these patients had a serious vascular complication such as stroke or myocardial infarction. In association with the increased pressure and expanded blood volume, renin secretion is suppressed. Although this finding has been almost invariable with hyperaldosteronism, the overwhelming majority of hypertensive patients with suppressed renin do not have mineralocorticoid excess.

DIAGNOSIS. Serious consideration should be given to the diagnosis of primary aldosteronism when hypertension and hypokalemia coexist. If normokalemic patients with the disease are thereby missed, little will be lost as long as the patients are protected by appropriate treatment of the hypertension. Since this is likely to include a diuretic, significant hypokalemia will likely soon become manifested,

making the diagnosis obvious. If hypokalemia is present, excessive urinary potassium excretion (above 30 mmol/day) is strongly suggestive of mineralocorticoid excess.

A high plasma aldosterone/renin ratio in plasma is a useful screening test that can be performed immediately upon recognition of hypokalemia in a hypertensive patient, without special conditions or preparation.[246] Not only should plasma renin levels be low, but plasma aldosterone levels should be elevated, giving a ratio of well above 30.[255] Although this ratio is being used increasingly to screen for primary aldosteronism, it has not always been found to be abnormal in patients with the syndrome.[256] Therefore, the finding of increased urinary aldosterone levels or the failure to suppress plasma aldosterone levels by volume expansion also may be useful.

ESTABLISHING THE PATHOLOGY. Once the diagnosis of primary aldosteronism is made, the type of adrenal pathology should be determined, and only those patients with a tumor should be subjected to operation and those with bilateral hyperplasia kept on medical therapy. The best initial study is an adrenal CT or MRI scan (Fig. 26–19). However, the ability of these scans to identify hitherto hidden degrees of adrenal pathology may engender confusion; the usual modularity seen in the remainder of a gland that harbors a solitary adrenal adenoma may give the appearance of bilateral hyperplasia, and some larger hyperplastic modules may look like adenomas.[257] Therefore, unless the scan is unequivocal, additional tests to discriminate between adenoma and hyperplasia should be done (Fig. 26–19).

Various maneuvers are available.[253] Basal levels of serum 18-hydroxycorticosterone (18-OHB) and changes in plasma aldosterone levels after 2 hours of upright posture from 8 A.M. to 10 A.M. usually distinguish patients with adenomas (who usually have basal 18-OHB levels above 65 ng/dl and falls in upright plasma aldosterone) from those with bilateral hyperplasia (who usually have basal 18-OHB levels below 50 ng/dl and postural rises in plasma aldosterone presumably invoked by their supersensitivity to posture-mediated rises in renin-angiotensin). In addition, most adenomas but few hyperplastic glands secrete increased amounts of 18-hydroxylated cortisol, suggesting that they harbor similar mutant genes as found in the glucocorticoid-suppressible syndrome. If there is still uncertainty, bilateral adrenal vein catheterization with analysis of venous aldosterone and cortisol levels should be performed.

THERAPY. Once the diagnosis of primary aldosteronism is made and the type of adrenal disorder has been established, the choice of therapy is fairly easy: Patients with a solitary adenoma should have the tumor resected, now

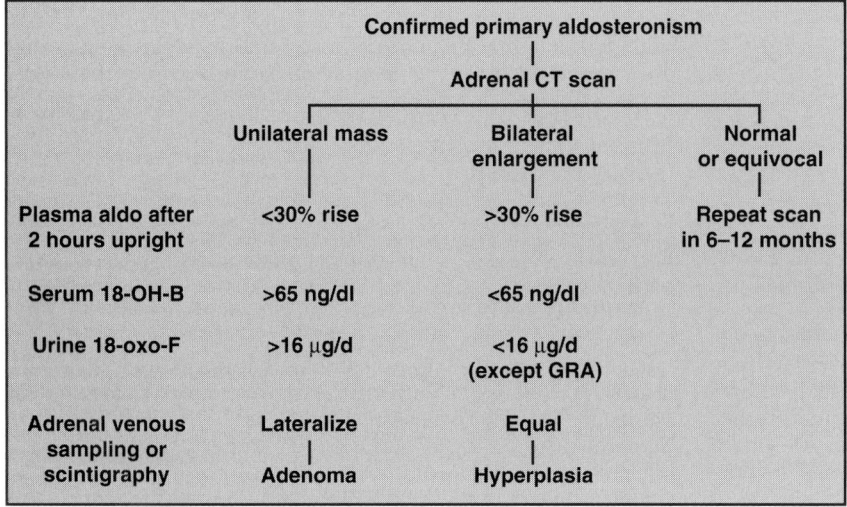

	Unilateral mass	Bilateral enlargement	Normal or equivocal
Confirmed primary aldosteronism			
Adrenal CT scan			
Plasma aldo after 2 hours upright	<30% rise	>30% rise	Repeat scan in 6–12 months
Serum 18-OH-B	>65 ng/dl	<65 ng/dl	
Urine 18-oxo-F	>16 μg/d	<16 μg/d (except GRA)	
Adrenal venous sampling or scintigraphy	Lateralize / Adenoma	Equal / Hyperplasia	

FIGURE 26–19. A flow diagram for the progressive work-up of confirmed primary aldosteronism, with additional steps for when initial studies are aberrant. Rare, angiotensin II–responsive adenomas may demonstrate features of hyperplasia but lateralize by venous sampling or scintigraphy. On the other hand, primary adrenal hyperplasia may demonstrate features of an adenoma except for equally high steroid levels by venous sampling. *18-OH-B*, 18-hydroxycorticosterone; *18-oxo-F*, 18-hydrocortisol; *GRA*, glucocorticoid-remediable aldosteronism. (From Kaplan, N. M.: Primary aldosteronism. *In* Kaplan, N. M. [ed.]: Clinical Hypertension. 6th ed. Baltimore, Williams and Wilkins, 1994, p. 404.)

more and more frequently done by laparoscopic surgery.[258] Those with bilateral hyperplasia should be treated with spironolactone (see p. 1897) and if necessary a thiazide diuretic or other antihypertensive drugs.[259] Fortunately, the doses of spironolactone required for chronic therapy are usually low enough to avoid bothersome side effects. When an adenoma is resected, about half of patients will become normotensive, while the others, though improved, remain hypertensive, either from preexisting primary hypertension or from renal damage due to prolonged secondary hypertension.[253]

CUSHING'S SYNDROME (see also p. 1896)

Hypertension occurs in about 80 per cent of patients with Cushing's syndrome. If left untreated, it can cause marked left ventricular hypertrophy and congestive heart failure.[260] As with hypertension of other endocrine causes, the longer it is present, the less likely it is to disappear when the underlying cause is relieved.

MECHANISM OF HYPERTENSION. Blood pressure may increase for a number of reasons. The secretion of mineralocorticoids also may be increased along with cortisol. The excess cortisol may overwhelm the renal 11-β-OHSD enzyme's ability to convert it to the inactive cortisone so that it activates renal mineralocorticoid receptors to retain sodium and expand fluid volume.[261] Cortisol stimulates the synthesis of renin substrate and the expression of angiotensin II receptors, which may be responsible for enhanced pressor effects.[262]

DIAGNOSIS. The syndrome should be suspected in patients with truncal obesity, thin skin, muscle weakness, and osteoporosis. If clinical features are suggestive, the diagnosis can be either ruled out or virtually ensured by the measurement of free cortisol in a 24-hour urine or the simple overnight *dexamethasone suppression test*.[263] In normal subjects, the level of plasma cortisol in a sample drawn at 8 A.M. after a bedtime dose of 1 mg of dexamethasone should be below 7 μg/100 mg. If the level is higher, additional work-up is in order to establish both the diagnosis of cortisol excess and the pathological type. Measurement of urine free cortisol levels is almost as good a screening test: Most patients who do not have Cushing's syndrome excrete less than 100 μg/24 hours.

When an abnormal screening test is found, some would immediately perform pituitary and adrenal CT or MRI scans to elucidate the type of pathology. However, most authorities continue to recommend longer dexamethasone suppression tests using 0.5 mg every 6 hours and then 2.0 mg every 6 hours, each for 2 days, measuring urinary free cortisol excretion and plasma cortisol levels on the second day of each dose. Patients with Cushing's syndrome fail to suppress urine free cortisol to below 25 μg/day on the 0.5-mg dose; if Cushing's syndrome is caused by excess pituitary ACTH drive with bilateral adrenal hyperplasia, urinary free cortisol will be suppressed to below 40 per cent of the control value on the 2.0-mg dose. Plasma ACTH assays provide an additional means of differentiating pituitary and ectopic ACTH excess from adrenal tumors with ACTH suppression.[264] The response to corticotropin-releasing hormone (CRH) and inferior petrosal sinus sampling may help identify the pituitary cause for the syndrome.[265]

THERAPY. In about two-thirds of patients with Cushing's syndrome, the process begins with overproduction of ACTH by the pituitary, which leads to bilateral adrenal hyperplasia. Although pituitary hyperfunction may reflect a hypothalamic disorder, the majority of patients have discrete pituitary adenomas that usually can be resected by selective transsphenoidal microsurgery.[266]

If an adrenal tumor is present, it should be removed surgically. With earlier diagnosis and more selective surgical therapy, it is hoped that more patients with Cushing's syndrome will be cured without the need for lifelong glucocorticoid replacement therapy and with permanent relief of their hypertension. Temporarily, and rarely permanently, therapy may require one of a number of medical approaches.[267]

CONGENITAL ADRENAL HYPERPLASIA (see also p. 1678).

Two other enzymatic defects may induce hypertension by interfering with cortisol biosynthesis. The low levels of cortisol lead to increased ACTH, which increases the accumulation of precursors proximal to the enzymatic block, specifically deoxycorticosterone (DOC), which induces mineralocorticoid hypertension. The more common of these is *11-hydroxylase deficiency*, which leads to virilization (from excessive androgens) and hypertension with hypokalemia (from excessive DOC).[268] A partial deficiency has been recognized in 15 patients with what appeared to be ordinary primary hypertension.[269] The other is *17-hydroxylase deficiency*, which also causes hypertension from excess DOC but, in addition, causes failure of secondary sexual development because sex hormones are also defi-

cient.[270] Affected children are hypertensive, but the defect in sex hormone synthesis may not become obvious until after puberty. Thereafter, affected males display ambiguity of sexual development and fail to mature.

PHEOCHROMOCYTOMA (see also p. 1897)

The wild fluctuations in blood pressure and dramatic symptoms of pheochromocytoma usually alert both the patient and the physician to the possibility of this diagnosis. However, such fluctuations may be missed or, as occurs in half the patients, the hypertension may be persistent. The symptoms may be incorrectly ascribed to psychoneurosis by practitioners not sensitized to "spells," which usually represent menopausal hot flushes or anxiety-induced hyperventilation. Unfortunately, if the diagnosis is missed, severe complications may arise from exceedingly high blood pressure and damage to the heart by catecholamines (see p. 1447). Stroke and hypertensive crises with encephalopathy and retinal hemorrhages may occur, probably because blood pressure levels soar in vessels unprepared by a chronic hypertensive condition. Fortunately, a simple and inexpensive test will detect the disease with virtual certainty, so that diagnostic indecision should be minimized.

PATHOPHYSIOLOGY. The cells of the sympathetic nervous system arise from the primitive neural crest as primitive stem cells, called *sympathogonia*. These cells differentiate into ganglion cells, neuroblasts, and chromaffin cells. Tumors develop from each of these cell types; ganglioneuromas and neuroblastomas usually occur in children, whereas tumors arising from chromaffin cells, i.e., pheochromocytomas, occur at all ages anywhere along the sympathetic chain and rarely in aberrant sites.[271] About 15 per cent of pheochromocytomas are extraadrenal; nonsecreting ones are called *paragangliomas* or *chemodectomas*.

Of the 85 per cent of pheochromocytomas that arise in the adrenal medulla, 10 per cent are bilateral and another 10 per cent are malignant. Multiple adrenal tumors are particularly common in patients with simple familial pheochromocytoma and multiple endocrine neoplasia (MEN) Type 2A in association with medullary carcinoma of the thyroid (Sipple's syndrome) or with mucosal ganglioneuromas in addition (Type 2B). The MEN2 syndromes are inherited as autosomal dominants with mutations at the same locus on chromosome 10.[272] Diffuse medullary hyperplasia may precede the development of tumors, and the tumors may, in fact, reflect extreme degrees of nodular hyperplasia.[273] Adrenal pheochromocytomas have been found to produce a number of other hormones in addition to catecholamines, which in turn are co-secreted with the soluble protein chromogranin A.[274]

Secretion from nonfamilial pheochromocytomas varies considerably, with small tumors tending to secrete larger proportions of active catecholamines. If the predominant secretion is epinephrine, which is formed primarily in the adrenal medulla, the symptoms reflect its effects—mainly systolic hypertension due to increased cardiac output, tachycardia, sweating, flushing, and apprehension. If norepinephrine is predominantly secreted, as from some of the adrenal tumors and from almost all the extraadrenal tumors, the symptoms include both systolic and diastolic hypertension from peripheral vasoconstriction but less tachycardia, palpitations, and anxiety. The hemodynamic features of 24 untreated patients with surgically proven pheochromocytomas were quite similar to those found in 24 untreated patients of similar sex, age, weight, and blood pressure with primary hypertension, with increased total peripheral resistance as the primary in both groups.[274]

The episodic hypertension often seen in patients with a pheochromocytoma may arise from catecholamines released from the tumor, stored in the sympathetic nerves, and released when the sympathetic nerves are activated by various stresses rather than directly from the tumor.[275]

DIAGNOSIS. Many more hypertensive patients have variable blood pressures and "spells" than the 0.1 per cent or so who harbor a pheochromocytoma. Spells with paroxysmal hypertension may occur with a number of stresses, and a large number of conditions may involve transient catecholamine release. A pheochromocytoma should be suspected in patients with hypertension that is either paroxysmal or persistent and accompanied by the symptoms and signs listed in Table 26-12. In addition, children and patients with rapidly accelerating hypertension should be screened. Those whose tumors secrete predominantly epinephrine are prone to postural hypotension from a contracted blood volume and blunted sympathetic reflex tone. Suspicion should be heightened if activities such as bending over, exercise, palpation of the abdomen, smoking, or dipping snuff cause repetitive spells that begin abruptly, advance rapidly, and subside within minutes.

High levels of catecholamines may induce myocarditis (Chap. 41), which may progress to cardiomyopathy and left ventricular failure.[276] Electrocardiographic changes of ischemia also may be seen.[277] Beta blockers given to such patients may raise the pressure and induce coronary spasm through blockade of beta-mediated vasodilation.[278]

LABORATORY CONFIRMATION. The easiest and best procedure is either a 24-hour or spot urine assay for total metanephrine. This catecholamine metabolite is least affected by various interfering sub-

TABLE 26–12 FEATURES SUGGESTIVE OF PHEOCHROMOCYTOMA

HYPERTENSION: PERSISTENT OR PAROXYSMAL
 Markedly variable blood pressures (± orthostatic hypotension)
 Sudden paroxysms (± subsequent hypertension) in relation to:
  Stress: anesthesia, angiography, parturition
  Pharmacological provocation: histamine, nicotine, caffeine,
   beta blockers, glucocorticoids, tricyclic antidepressants
  Manipulation of tumors: abdominal palpation, urination
 Rare patients persistently normotensive
 Unusual settings
  Childhood, pregnancy, familial
  Multiple endocrine adenomas: medullary carcinoma of thy-
   roid (MEN2), mucosal neuromas (MEN2B)
  Neurocutaneous lesions: Neurofibromatosis

ASSOCIATED SYMPTOMS:
 Sudden spells with headache, sweating, palpitations, nervous-
  ness, nausea, and vomiting
 Pain in chest or abdomen

ASSOCIATED SIGNS:
 Sweating, tachycardia, arrhythmia, pallor, weight loss

stances including antihypertensive drugs, with the exception of labetalol, which may cause markedly elevated levels of all catecholamines.[279] In addition to the effects of labetalol, urinary metanephrine excretion will be increased if patients are taking sympathomimetic or dopaminergic drugs or are under acute, severe stress such as an acute myocardial infarction or severe congestive heart failure. Interference with the measurement of metanephrine may occur for the next few days after use of radiograph contrast media containing methylglucamine, leading to a falsely low value. Therefore, the urine should be collected before coronary angiography or other such procedures are done.

If urine assays are equivocal, measurement of a plasma norepinephrine level 3 hours after a single 0.3-mg oral dose of the adrenergic inhibitor clonidine has been shown to separate the nonpheochromocytoma patients, whose levels are suppressed, from those with disease whose levels are not suppressed.[274]

LOCALIZATION OF THE TUMOR. Once the diagnosis has been made, medical therapy should be started and the tumor localized by CT or MRI scans, which usually demonstrate these typically large tumors with ease. Radioisotopes that localize in chromaffin tissue are available and are of additional help in the few patients in whom localization is not possible by CT or MRI.[274]

THERAPY. Once diagnosed and localized, pheochromocytomas should be resected. Great care should be taken in preparing patients for operation and managing them through the procedure.[274] The most important part of their preoperative management is alpha-adrenergic receptor blockade sufficient to overcome vasoconstriction and allow the reduced blood volume to reexpand. If the tumor is unresectable, chronic medical therapy with the alpha blocker phenoxybenzamine (Dibenzyline) or the inhibitor of catechol synthesis, α-methyl-tyrosine (Demser), can be used.

Other Causes of Hypertension

A host of other causes of hypertension are known (Table 26–4). One that is likely becoming more common is ingestion of various drugs—prescribed (e.g., cyclosporine[280] and erythropoietin[281]), over the counter (e.g., phenylpropanolamine[282]), and illicit (e.g., cocaine).

COARCTATION OF THE AORTA (see pp. 911 and 965). Congenital narrowing of the aorta may occur at any level of the thoracic or abdominal aorta. It is usually found just beyond the origin of the left subclavian artery or distal to the insertion of the ligamentum arteriosum. The coarctation may be localized or more diffuse. Other cardiac anomalies usually accompany the latter, giving rise to considerable mortality during the first year of life, although operative treatment of both the coarctation and associated anomalies may reduce this mortality rate. With less severe postductal lesions, damage is more insidious, and symptoms may not appear until the teenage years or later.

Hypertension in the arms and weak or absent femoral pulses are the classic features of coarctation. The pathogenesis of the hypertension may be more complicated than simple mechanical obstruction; a generalized vasoconstrictor mechanism is likely to be involved, which may be ei-

ther renin-angiotensin or sympathetic nervous activity.[283] The lesion may be detected by two-dimensional echocardiography (Fig. 29–28, p. 912), and aortography proves the diagnosis. To diminish the development of congestive heart failure, endocarditis, and stroke, the obstruction should be corrected in early childhood either by surgery[284] or by angioplasty.[285] Immediately after either, the blood pressure may transiently rise even further, and mesenteric arteritis may develop. These changes may reflect very high levels of renin-angiotensin and catecholamines and can be prevented by the prophylactic use of beta blockers.[286]

HORMONAL DISTURBANCES

Hypertension is seen in as many as half of patients with a variety of hormonal disturbances, including acromegaly,[287] hypothyroidism,[41] and hyperparathyroidism.[288] The diagnosis of the latter two conditions has been made easier by readily available blood tests, and affected hypertensives may be relieved of their high blood pressure by correction of the hormonal disturbance. This happens more frequently with hypothyroidism than with hyperparathyroidism.[289]

Hypertension After Heart Surgery
(See also p. 1723)

Transient hypertension may develop postoperatively for various reasons: pain, physical and emotional excitement, hypoxia, hypercapnia, and excessive volume loads.[290] More severe hypertension has been noted to follow a number of cardiovascular surgical procedures:

1. *Coronary bypass surgery.* The incidence, exceeding 33 per cent, is far higher than after other major cardiac or noncardiac surgery.[291] The problem appears more commonly on the background of preexisting hypertension, greater than 50 per cent obstruction of the left main coronary artery, or the preoperative use of beta blockers. The hemodynamic pattern of increased peripheral resistance can be explained by the markedly elevated plasma catecholamine levels measured in such patients in the presence of normal renin-angiotensin levels.[292] In those patients who had previously received beta-blocker therapy, the postoperative hypertension also may reflect a rebound phenomenon. Therefore, continuation of beta-blocker therapy through the perioperative period is likely to reduce the frequency of the problem. If it occurs, parenteral therapy is often required, and intravenous nicardipine has been found to be very effective.[293]

2. *Aortic valve replacement.* Transient hypertension may give way to more permanent hypertension. In one series, 53 per cent of 116 patients were hypertensive 5 years after surgery, and hypertension was a major determinant of late failure of the homograft valve.[294]

3. *Closure of an atrial septal defect.*[295]

4. *Cardiac transplantation.* With current immunosuppression using cyclosporine and high doses of adrenal steroids, hypertension is almost invariable and can be resistant to intensive therapy.[296] Fortunately, with effective antihypertensive therapy, left ventricular hypertrophy may be prevented.[297]

HYPERTENSION DURING PREGNANCY
(See also p. 1852)

In as many as 10 per cent of first pregnancies in previously normotensive women, hypertension appears during the last trimester or immediately after delivery, in the syndrome called *preeclampsia, pregnancy-induced hypertension,* or *gestational hypertension.*[298] This disorder should be distinguished from chronic hypertension, although both may progress into eclampsia, defined as the occurrence of convulsions. Gestational hypertension is of unknown cause but occurs more frequently in primigravid women or in subsequent pregnancies with a different father,[299] suggesting an immunological mechanism. Additional predisposing factors include increased age, black race, multiple gestations, concomitant heart or renal disease, and chronic hypertension.[300]

The diagnosis is usually based on a rise in pressure of 30/15 mm Hg or more to a level above 140/90.[301] Though some measure the Korotkoff fourth sound (muffling), the fifth sound (disappearance) is closer to the true diastolic and should be used.[301]

CLINICAL FEATURES. The features shown in Table 26–13 should help distinguish gestational hypertension from chronic, primary hypertension. The distinction should be made because management and prognosis are different: Gestational hypertension is self-limited and rarely recurs in subsequent pregnancies, whereas chronic hypertension progresses and usually complicates subsequent pregnancies. The separation may be difficult because of a lack of knowledge of prepregnancy blood pressure and because of the usual tendency for high pressure to fall considerably during the middle trimester so that hypertension present before pregnancy may not be recognized.

In gestational hypertension, the blood pressure usually rises only late in pregnancy. Among 84 patients with the onset of hypertension before 37 weeks' gestation, 55 had renal disease documented by kidney biopsy 6 months post partum when morphological changes due solely to gestational hypertension should have subsided.[302] Gestational hypertension was the diagnosis in only 10 per cent of primiparous women with onset of hypertension before 37 weeks, whereas it was the diagnosis in three-fourths of primigravid women with onset of hypertension after 37 weeks.

The hemodynamic features of gestational hypertension are a further rise in cardiac output than that usually seen in normal pregnancy accompanied by profound vasoconstriction that reduces the intravascular capacity even more than blood volume.[298] The mother may be particularly vulnerable to encephalopathy because of her previously normal blood pressure. As is described in more detail on p. 832, cerebral blood flow is normally maintained constant over a fairly narrow range of mean arterial pressure, roughly between 60 to 100 mm Hg in normotensive individuals. In a previously normotensive young woman, an acute rise in blood pressure to 150/100 mm Hg may exceed the upper limit of autoregulation, resulting in a "breakthrough" of cerebral blood flow (acute dilation) that leads to cerebral edema, convulsions, and all the clinical manifestations of eclampsia.

Beyond the common associations with proteinuria and edema, no other tests have been found to accurately predict the development of preeclampsia.[303]

PATHOGENESIS. The common factor that predisposes to development of gestational hypertension is *reduced uteroplacental perfusion*. Increasing evidence supports a failure of normal invasion of the uterus by trophoblasts as the mechanism.[304] As explained by D. A. Clark[305]:

> The key lesion in preeclampsia is failure of extravillous cytotrophoblast cells to invade the maternal uterine spiral arteries to a sufficient depth during the first and second trimester. Consequently, the arterial wall does not distend enough to allow sufficient blood flow to the placenta in late pregnancy. The placenta is thereby subjected to ischaemia, and compensatory mechanisms are activated which lead to increased vascular volume and blood pressure. Some of these mechanisms may involve release of prostacyclins, since administration of aspirin can reduce the incidence of preeclampsia. Endothelins, which are potent vasoconstrictors, may also be implicated in the systemic effects, and vascular spasm (leading to encephalopathy and seizures) may result from endothelial damage by shed trophoblast membrane vesicles in the bloodstream.

The defect in trophoblastic invasion may be prevented by suppression of maternal immune responses that produce antibodies against trophoblast antigens.[306] Support for this hypothesis comes from the observation that the incidence of preeclampsia is reduced by repeated exposure to semen,[299] presumably allowing the mother to develop immunological tolerance to the fetal antigenic load. The lesser degree of immunological reaction within the maternal decidua would thereby allow more extensive trophoblastic invasion.[306]

The failure of trophoblastic invasion may, as noted by Clark,[305] lead to a number of secondary phenomena that are responsible for the rise in blood pressure, renal damage, and edema. A decreased synthesis of nitric oxide may be involved,[307] along with increased levels of vasoconstricting prostaglandins.

PREVENTION. Along with more prolonged exposure to semen, as suggested by the data from Robillard et al.,[299] small doses of aspirin[308] and calcium supplements[309] have been found to reduce the incidence of preeclampsia in high-risk women.

Treatment

GESTATIONAL HYPERTENSION. Women with gestational hypertension and their fetuses can be protected from excessive morbidity and mortality by maneuvers that lower the blood pressure without impairing uteroplacental perfusion. These maneuvers include modified bed rest, a nutritious diet with normal amounts of sodium, and antihypertensive agents when diastolic blood pressure above 100 mm Hg indicates impairment of renal function and predisposition to overt eclampsia.

However, as noted by Redman and Roberts,[310] "The cure is achieved by delivery, which removes the diseased tissue—the placenta. In short, the need is to deliver before it is too late. To achieve this apparently simple end, the clinician must detect the symptomless prodromal condition by screening all pregnant women, admit to hospital those with advanced preeclampsia so as to keep track of an unpredictable situation, and time preemptive delivery to maximize the safety of mother and baby."

Caution is advised in the use of drugs for mild gestational hypertension, traditionally limited to methyldopa. In one of the few controlled studies comparing modified bed rest versus antihypertensive drug therapy, half of 200 primigravid women with relatively mild hypertension at 26 to 35 weeks' gestation were given labetalol and the other half were monitored while in the hospital.[311] Those given labetalol had a significant fall in blood pressure, whereas the controls did not, but those in both groups had some worsening of renal function. However, the number of small-for-gestational age infants was higher in the labetalol group (19 versus 9 per cent). Thus, drug treatment of maternal blood pressure did not improve perinatal outcome and was associated with fetal growth retardation. Most authorities recommend antihypertensive drugs if diastolic pressures re-

TABLE 26–13 DIFFERENCES BETWEEN PREECLAMPSIA AND CHRONIC HYPERTENSION

	PREECLAMPSIA	CHRONIC HYPERTENSION
Age	Young (< 20)	Older (> 30)
Parity	Primigravida	Multigravida
Onset	After 20 weeks of pregnancy	Before 20 weeks of pregnancy
Weight gain and edema	Sudden	Gradual
Systolic blood pressure	< 160	> 160
Funduscopic findings	Spasm, edema	Arteriovenous nicking, exudates
Proteinuria	Present	Absent
Plasma uric acid	Increased	Normal
Blood pressure after delivery	Normal	Elevated

main above 100 mm Hg.[312] The only drugs that are contraindicated are ACE inhibitors because of their propensity to induce neonatal renal failure and hypotension.[313]

If the syndrome advances and eclampsia threatens before the 32nd week of gestation, expectant management (bed rest, oral antihypertensives, and intensive fetal monitoring) provides better eventual outcomes than more aggressive therapy (glucocorticoids for 48 hours followed by delivery either by induction or cesarean).[314] If parenteral antihypertensives are needed, hydralazine works well.[315]

CHRONIC HYPERTENSION. If pregnancy begins while a woman is on antihypertensive drug therapy, the medications, including diuretics, are usually continued, on the basis of the belief that the mother should be protected and that the fetus will not suffer from any sudden hemodynamic shifts such as occur when therapy is first begun. Among women with chronic hypertension who were not undergoing treatment, therapy with either hydralazine or methyldopa significantly reduced the incidence of gestational hypertension when compared with that in a placebo-treated group.[316] However, despite modern treatment, the incidence of perinatal mortality and fetal growth retardation remains higher in patients with chronic hypertension.[317]

MANAGEMENT OF ECLAMPSIA. With appropriate care of gestational hypertension, eclampsia hardly ever supervenes; when it does, however, maternal and fetal mortality remain very high.[318] Excellent results have been reported with the use of magnesium sulfate to prevent convulsions.[319] Patients with severe eclampsia who have persistent oliguria after a fluid challenge should undergo hemodynamic monitoring, since management may require additional volume or a reduction in preload or afterload.[320]

CONSEQUENCES OF PREGNANCY-RELATED HYPERTENSION. The long-term prognosis of women with gestational hypertension is excellent. When 200 women with the most severe form, eclampsia, were followed for up to 44 years, the distribution of blood pressure was identical to that in the general population.[321] Chesley concludes that "eclampsia neither is a sign of latent essential hypertension nor causes hypertension." The long-term mortality rate in black women having eclampsia and of white women having eclampsia as multiparas is increased, probably because they had underlying but previously unrecognized chronic hypertension or renal disease.

After delivery, women may develop transient or persistent hypertension. In many, early primary hypertension may have been masked by the hemodynamic changes of pregnancy. Some women develop postpartum heart failure that may be an idiopathic cardiomyopathy but is usually related to hypertension, preexisting heart disease, or complications of pregnancy.[322]

HYPERTENSIVE CRISES

DEFINITIONS. A number of clinical circumstances may require rapid reduction of the blood pressure (Table 26–14). These may be separated into *emergencies*, which require immediate reduction of blood pressure (within 1 hour), and *urgencies*, which can be treated more slowly. A persistent diastolic pressure exceeding 130 mm Hg is often associated with acute vascular damage; some patients may suffer vascular damage from lower levels of pressure, while others manage to withstand even higher levels without apparent harm. As discussed below, the rapidity of the rise may be more important than the absolute level in producing acute vascular damage. Therefore, in practice, all patients with diastolic blood pressures above 130 mm Hg should be treated, some more rapidly with parenteral drugs, others more slowly with oral agents, as described on p. 858.

TABLE 26–14 CIRCUMSTANCES REQUIRING RAPID TREATMENT OF HYPERTENSION

ACCELERATED-MALIGNANT HYPERTENSION WITH PAPILLEDEMA

CEREBROVASCULAR
Hypertensive encephalopathy
Atherothrombotic brain infarction with severe hypertension
Intracerebral hemorrhage
Subarachnoid hemorrhage

CARDIAC
Acute aortic dissection
Acute left ventricular failure
Acute or impending myocardial infarction
After coronary bypass surgery

RENAL
Acute glomerulonephritis
Renal crises from collagen-vascular diseases
Severe hypertension after kidney transplantation

EXCESSIVE CIRCULATING CATECHOLAMINES
Pheochromocytoma crisis
Food or drug interactions with monoamine-oxidase inhibitors
Sympathomimetic drug use (cocaine)
Rebound hypertension after sudden cessation of antihypertensive drugs

ECLAMPSIA

SURGICAL
Severe hypertension in patients requiring immediate surgery
Postoperative hypertension
Postoperative bleeding from vascular suture lines

SEVERE BODY BURNS

SEVERE EPISTAXIS

From Kaplan, N. M.: Management of hypertensive emergencies. Lancet *344*:1335, 1994. © by the Lancet Ltd.

When the rise in pressure causes acute damage to retinal vessels, the term *accelerated-malignant hypertension* is used. The separation has been based on the presence of retinal hemorrhages or exudates (accelerated) and papilledema (malignant). The clinical features and survival rates of those with or without papilledema are so similar that there is no reason to separate the two.[323]

Hypertensive encephalopathy is characterized by headache, irritability, alterations in consciousness, and other manifestations of central nervous dysfunction with sudden and marked elevations in blood pressure. Symptoms can be reversed by a reduction in the pressure.

INCIDENCE. In fewer than 1 per cent of patients with primary hypertension, the disease progresses to an accelerated-malignant phase. Although the incidence likely is falling as a consequence of more widespread treatment of hypertension, no difference was found in the numbers of patients seen in Birmingham, England, from 1970 to 1993.[324]

Any hypertensive disease can initiate a crisis. Some, including pheochromocytoma and renovascular hypertension, do so at a higher rate than does primary hypertension. However, since hypertension is of unknown cause in over 90 per cent of all patients, most hypertensive crises appear in the setting of preexisting primary hypertension.[324]

PATHOPHYSIOLOGY. Whenever blood pressure rises and remains above a critical level, various processes set off a series of local and systemic effects that cause further rises in pressure and vascular damage that eventuate in accelerated-malignant hypertension (Fig. 26–20).

Studies in animals and humans by Strandgaard and Paulson have elucidated the mechanism of hypertensive encephalopathy.[325] First, they directly measured the caliber of pial arterioles over the cerebral cortex in cats whose blood pressure was varied over a wide range of infusion by vasodilators or angiotensin II. As the pressure fell, the arterioles

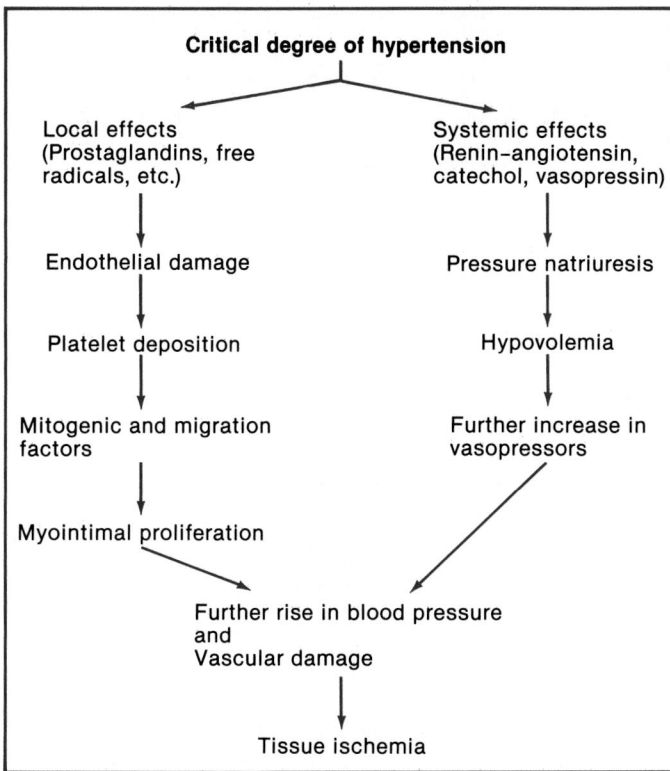

Critical degree of hypertension

Local effects
(Prostaglandins, free
radicals, etc.)

Systemic effects
(Renin-angiotensin,
catechol, vasopressin)

Endothelial damage

Pressure natriuresis

Platelet deposition

Hypovolemia

Mitogenic and migration
factors

Further increase in
vasopressors

Myointimal proliferation

Further rise in blood pressure
and
Vascular damage

Tissue ischemia

FIGURE 26–20. A scheme for the initiation and progression of malignant hypertension. (From Kaplan, N. M.: Clinical Hypertension. 6th ed. Baltimore, © by Williams and Wilkins, 1994, p. 283.)

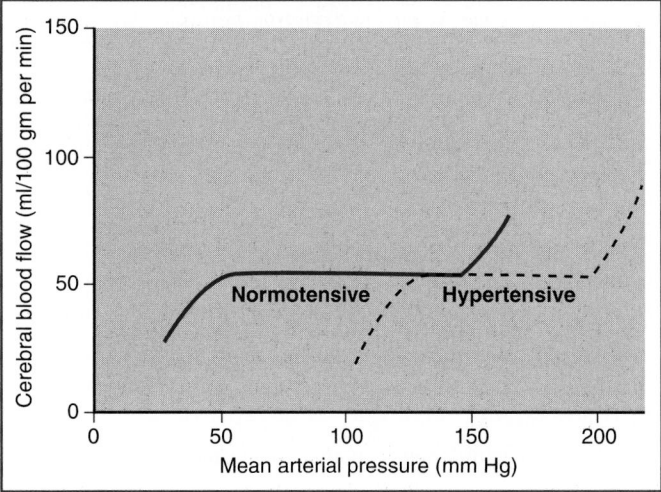

FIGURE 26–21. Idealized curves of cerebral blood flow at varying levels of systemic blood pressure in normotensive and hypertensive subjects. Rightward shift is shown in autoregulation with chronic hypertension. (Adapted from Strandgaard, S., Olesen, J., Skinhøj, and Lassen, N. A.: Autoregulation of brain circulation in severe arterial hypertension. Br. Med. J. 1:507, 1973.)

became dilated; as the pressure rose, they become constricted. Thus a constant cerebral blood flow was maintained by means of autoregulation, which is dependent on the cerebral sympathetic nerves. However, when mean arterial pressure rose above 180 mm Hg, the tightly constricted vessels could no longer withstand the pressure and suddenly dilated. This began in an irregular manner, first in areas with less muscle tone and then diffusely, producing generalized vasodilatation. This "breakthrough" of cerebral blood flow hyperperfuses the brain under high pressure, causing leakage of fluid into the perivascular tissue and resulting in cerebral edema and the syndrome of hypertensive encephalopathy.

In human subjects, cerebral blood flow was measured repetitively by an isotopic technique while blood pressure was lowered or raised with vasodilators or vasoconstrictors in a manner similar to that employed in the animal studies.[325] Curves depicting cerebral blood flow as a function of arterial pressure demonstrated autoregulation with a constancy of flow over mean pressures in normotensive persons from about 60 to 120 mm Hg and in hypertensive patients from about 110 to 180 mm Hg (Fig. 26–21). This "shift to the right" in hypertensive patients is the result of structural thickening of the arterioles as an adaptation to the chronically elevated pressures. When pressures were raised beyond the upper limit of autoregulation, the same "breakthrough" with hyperperfusion occurred as was seen in the animal studies. In previously normotensive persons whose vessels have not been altered by prior exposure to high pressure, breakthrough occurred at a mean arterial pressure of about 120 mm Hg; in hypertensive patients, the breakthrough occurred at about 180 mm Hg.

These studies confirm clinical observations. In previously normotensive persons, severe encephalopathy occurs with relatively little hypertension. In children with acute glomerulonephritis and in women with eclampsia, convulsions may occur owing to hypertensive encephalopathy with blood pressures as low as 150/100 mm Hg. Obviously, chronically hypertensive patients withstand such pressures

without difficulty; however, when pressures increase significantly, they too may develop encephalopathy.

MANIFESTATIONS AND COURSE. The symptoms and signs of hypertensive crises are usually dramatic (Table 26–15). However, some patients may be relatively asymptomatic, despite markedly elevated pressures and extensive organ damage. Young black men are particularly prone to hypertensive crisis with severe renal insufficiency but little obvious prior distress. When the blood pressure is so high as to induce encephalopathy or accelerated-malignant hypertension, the following clinical features are frequently present:

1. Renal insufficiency with protein and red cells in the urine and azotemia; acute oliguric renal failure also may develop.

2. Elevated levels of plasma renin from the diffuse intrarenal ischemia, resulting in secondary aldosteronism, often manifested by hypokalemia. Although not causal, the secondarily elevated renin and aldosterone levels most likely exacerbate the hypertensive process.

3. Microangiopathic hemolytic anemia with red cell fragmentation and intravascular coagulation.

4. Cardiac size and function may *not* be abnormal in those who suddenly develop malignant hypertension.[326]

If left untreated, patients die quickly from brain damage or more gradually from renal damage. Before effective therapy was available, fewer than 25 per cent of patients with malignant hypertension survived 1 year and only 1 per cent survived 5 years.[327] With therapy including renal dialysis, over 90 per cent survive 1 year and about 80 per cent survive 5 years. Death in patients with severe hypertension is usually from stroke or renal failure if it occurs in the

**TABLE 26–15   CLINICAL CHARACTERISTICS OF
HYPERTENSIVE CRISIS**

Blood pressure: Usually > 140 mm Hg diastolic
Funduscopic findings: Hemorrhages, exudates, papilledema
Neurological status: Headache, confusion, somnolence, stupor, visual loss, focal deficits, seizures, coma
Cardiac findings: Prominent apical impulse, cardiac enlargement, congestive failure
Renal: Oliguria, azotemia
Gastrointestinal: Nausea, vomiting

From Kaplan, N. M.: Clinical Hypertension. 6th ed. Baltimore, © by Williams and Wilkins, 1994, p. 283.

TABLE 26–16 CONDITIONS TO BE DIFFERENTIATED FROM A HYPERTENSIVE CRISIS

Acute left ventricular failure
Uremia from any cause, particularly with volume overload
Cerebrovascular accident
Subarachnoid hemorrhage
Brain tumor
Head injury
Epilepsy (postictal)
Collagen diseases, particularly lupus, with cerebral vasculitis
Encephalitis
Overdose and withdrawal from narcotics, amphetamines, etc.
Hypercalcemia
Acute anxiety with hyperventilation syndrome

first few years after onset. If therapy keeps patients alive for longer than 5 years, death will usually be due to coronary artery disease, in which factors other than the high pressure per se are probably also involved.[323]

DIFFERENTIAL DIAGNOSIS. The presence of hypertensive encephalopathy or accelerated-malignant hypertension demands immediate, aggressive therapy to lower blood pressure effectively, often before the specific cause is known. However, certain serious diseases as well as psychogenic problems, i.e., acute anxiety with hyperventilation or panic attacks,[328] can mimic a hypertensive crisis (Table 26–16), and management of these conditions obviously requires different diagnostic and therapeutic approaches. In particular, blood pressure should not be lowered too abruptly in a patient with a stroke.[82,329] Specific therapy of hypertensive crises is described in the next chapter (p. 858).

REFERENCES

1. Whelton, P. K.: Epidemiology of hypertension. Lancet 344:101, 1994.
2. Stockwell, D. H., Madhavan, S., Cohen, H., et al.: The determinants of hypertension awareness, treatment, and control in an insured population. Am. J. Public Health 84:1768, 1994.
3. Schappert, S. M.: National ambulatory medical survey: 1991 summary. NCHS Advance Data, no. 230, Vital and Health Statistics of the National Center for Health Statistics, Hyattsville, MD, U.S. Department of Health and Human Services Publication (PHS) 93-1250. March 29, 1993.
4. Kaplan, N. M.: Clinical Hypertension. 6th ed. Baltimore, Williams and Wilkins, 1994.
5. National High Blood Pressure Education Program Working Group: National High Blood Pressure Education Program Working Group Report on Primary Prevention of Hypertension. Arch. Intern. Med. 153:186, 1993.
6. Rose, G.: Epidemiology. In Marshall, A. J., and Barritt, D. W. (eds.): The Hypertensive Patient. Kent, England, Pitman Medical, 1980, p. 1.
7. Pickering, T. G.: Blood pressure measurement and detection of hypertension. Lancet 344:31, 1994.
8. Alderman, M. H., and Lamport, B.: Labelling of hypertensives: A review of the data. J. Clin. Epidemiol. 43:195, 1990.
9. Sheps, S. G., and Canzanello, V. J.: Current role of automated ambulatory blood pressure and self-measured blood pressure determinations in clinical practice. Mayo Clin. Proc. 69:1000, 1994.
10. de Gaudemaris, R., Chau, N. P., and Mallion, J.-M.: Home blood pressure: Variability, comparison with office readings and proposal for reference values. J. Hypertens. 12:831, 1994.
11. Staessen, J. A., O'Brien, E. T., Amery, A. K., et al.: Ambulatory blood pressure in normotensive and hypertensive subjects: Results from an international database. J. Hypertens. 12 (Suppl. 7):S1, 1994.
12. Clement, D. L., De Buyzere, M., and Duprez, D.: Prognostic value of ambulatory blood pressure monitoring. J. Hypertens. 12:857, 1994.
13. Tseng, Y.-Z., Tseng, C.-D., Lo, H.-M., et al.: Characteristic abnormal findings of ambulatory blood pressure indicative of hypertensive target organ complications. Eur. Heart J. 15:1037, 1994.
14. Mejia, A. D., Egan, B. M., Schork, N. J., and Zweifler, A. J.: Artifacts in measurement of blood pressure and lack of target organ involvement in the assessment of patients with treatment-resistant hypertension. Ann. Intern. Med. 112:270, 1990.
15. Høegholm, A., Bank, L. E., Kristensen, K. S., et al.: Microalbuminuria in 411 untreated individuals with established hypertension, white coat hypertension, and normotension. Hypertension 24:101, 1994.
16. Marchesi, E., Perani, G., Falaschi, F., et al.: Metabolic risk factors in white coat hypertensives. J. Hum. Hypertens. 8:475, 1994.
17. Muller, J. E., Abela, G. S., Nesto, R. W., and Tofler, G. H.: Triggers, acute risk factors and vulnerable plaques: The lexicon of a new frontier. J. Am. Coll. Cardiol. 23:809, 1994.
18. Pickering, T. G., Levenstein, M., and Walmsley, P.: Nighttime dosing of doxazosin has peak effect on morning ambulatory blood pressure: Results of the HALT study. Am. J. Hypertens. 7:844, 1994.
19. Anders, R. J., White, W. B., Grimm, R. H., et al.: Pharmacodynamic profile of delayed release verapamil gastrointestinal therapeutic system (GITS) following nocturnal dosing. J. Hypertens. 12 (Suppl. 3):S25, 1994.
20. Verdecchia, P., Porcellati, C., Schillaci, G., et al.: Ambulatory blood pressure: An independent predictor of prognosis in essential hypertension. Hypertension 34:793, 1994.
21. Palatini, P., Penzo, M., Racioppa, A., et al.: Clinical relevance of nighttime blood pressure and of daytime blood pressure variability. Arch. Intern. Med. 152:1855, 1992.
22. Lurbe, A., Redón, J., Pascual, J. M., et al.: Altered blood pressure during sleep in normotensive subjects with type I diabetes. Hypertension 21:227, 1993.
23. Rosansky, S. J., Johnson, K. L., Hutchinson, C., and Erdel, S.: Blood pressure changes during daytime sleep and comparison of daytime and nighttime sleep-related blood pressure changes in patients with chronic renal failure. J. Am. Soc. Nephrol. 4:1172, 1993.
24. Gretler, D. D., Fumo, M. T., Nelson, K. S., and Murphy, M. B.: Ethnic differences in circadian hemodynamic profile. Am. J. Hypertens. 7:7, 1994.
25. Manolio, T. A., Burke, G. L., Savage, P. J., et al.: Exercise blood pressure response and 5-year risk of elevated blood pressure in a cohort of young adults: The CARDIA Study. Am. J. Hypertens. 7:234, 1994.
26. Mundal, R., Kjeldsen, S. E., Sandvik, L., et al.: Exercise blood pressure predicts cardiovascular mortality in middle-aged men. Hypertension 24:56, 1994.
27. Neaton, J. D., and Wentworth, D.: Serum cholesterol, blood pressure, cigarette smoking, and death from coronary heart disease. Arch. Intern. Med. 152:56, 1992.
28. Froom, P., Bar-David, M., Ribak, J., et al.: Predictive value of systolic blood pressure in young men for elevated systolic blood pressure 12 to 15 years later. Circulation 68:467, 1983.
29. Wilson, P. W. F.: Established risk factors and coronary artery disease: The Framingham Study. Am. J. Hypertens. 7:7S, 1994.
30. Zweifler, A. J., and Shahab, S. T.: Pseudohypertension: A new assessment. J. Hypertens. 11:1, 1993.
31. Schutzman, J., Jaeger, F., Maloney, J., and Fouad-Tarazi, F.: Head-up tilt and hemodynamic changes during orthostatic hypotension in patients with supine hypertension. J. Am. Coll. Cardiol. 24:454, 1994.
32. Joint National Committee on Detection, Evaluation, and Treatment of HIgh Blood Pressure: The fifth report of the Joint National Committee on Detection, Evaluation, and Treatment of High Blood Pressure (JNC V). Arch. Intern. Med. 153:154, 1993.
33. The Pooling Project Research Group: Relationship of blood pressure, serum cholesterol, smoking habit, relative weight and ECG abnormalities to incidence of major coronary events: Final report of the pooling project. J. Chron. Dis. 31:201, 1978.
34. Swales, J. D.: Guidelines on guidelines. J. Hypertens. 11:899, 1993.
35. Hypertension Detection and Follow-up Program Cooperative Group: Blood pressure studies in 14 communities: A two-stage screen for hypertension. JAMA 237:2385, 1977.
36. Lieberman, E.: Hypertension in childhood and adolescence. In Kaplan, N. M. (ed.): Clinical Hypertension. 6th ed. Baltimore, Williams and Wilkins, 1994, p. 437.
37. Cooper, R. S., and Liao, Y.: Is hypertension among blacks more severe or simply more common? Circulation 85(Abs.):12, 1992.
38. Sorlie, P., Rogot, E., Anderson, R., et al.: Black-white mortality differences by family income. Lancet 340:346, 1992.
38a. Frohlich, E. D.: Hypertension: Clinical classifications. In Fuster, V., Ross, R., and Topol, E. J. (eds.): Atherosclerosis and Coronary Artery Disease. Philadelphia, Lippincott-Raven Publishers, 1996, pp. 243–258.
39. Rudnick, J. V., Sackett, D. L., Hirst, S., and Holmes, C.: Hypertension in family practice. Can. Med. Assoc. J. 3:492, 1977.
40. Sinclair, A. M., Isles, C. G., Brown, I., et al.: Secondary hypertension in a blood pressure clinic. Arch. Intern. Med. 147:1289, 1987.
41. Anderson, G. H., Jr., Blakeman, N., and Streeten, D. H. P.: The effect of age on prevalence of secondary forms of hypertension in 4429 consecutively referred patients. J. Hypertens. 12:609, 1994.
42. Coughlin, S. S., Trock, B., Criqui, M. H., et al.: The logistic modeling of sensitivity, specificity, and predictive value of a diagnostic test. J. Clin. Epidemiol. 45:1, 1992.
43. MacMahon, S., Peto, R., Cutler, J., et al.: Blood pressure, stroke, and coronary heart disease: I. Prolonged differences in blood pressure: Prospective observational studies corrected for the regression dilution bias. Lancet 335:765, 1990.
44. Weiss, N. S.: Relation of high blood pressure to headache, epistaxis, and selected other symptoms. N. Engl. J. Med. 287:631, 1972.
45. Cooper, W. D., Glover, D. R., Hormbrey, J. M., and Kimber, G. R.: Head-

ache and blood pressure: Evidence of a close relationship. J. Hum. Hypertens. 3:41, 1989.

46. Rose, G.: Strategy of prevention: Lessons from cardiovascular disease. Br. Med. J. 282:1847, 1981.

47. Lemne, C., Hamsten, A., Karpe, F., et al.: Dyslipoproteinemic changes in borderline hypertension. Hypertension 24:605, 1994.

48. Kaplan, N. M.: The deadly quartet: Upper-body obesity, glucose intolerance, hypertriglyceridemia, and hypertension. Arch. Intern. Med. 149:1514, 1989.

49. Maheux, P., Jeppesen, J., Sheu, W. H.-H., et al.: Additive effects of obesity, hypertension, and type 2 diabetes on insulin resistance. Hypertension 24:695, 1994.

50. Keith, N. M., Wagener, H. P., and Barker, N. W.: Some different types of essential hypertension: Their course and prognosis. Am. J. Med. Sci. 197:332, 1939.

51. Dahlöf, B., Stenkula, S., and Hansson, L.: Hypertensive retinal vascular changes: Relationship to LV hypertrophy and arteriolar changes before and after treatment. Blood Press. 1:35, 1992.

51a. Phillips, R. A., and Diamond, J. A.: Hypertensive Heart Disease. In Fuster, V., Ross, R., and Topol, E. J. (eds.): Atherosclerosis and Coronary Artery Disease. Philadelphia, Lippincott-Raven Publishers, 1996, pp. 275–302.

52. de Simone, G., Devereux, R. B., Roman, M. J., et al.: Assessment of left ventricular function by the midwall fractional shortening/end-systolic stress relation in human hypertension. J. Am. Coll. Cardiol. 23:1444, 1994.

53. Ren, J.-F., Pancholy, S. B., Iskandrian, A. S., et al.: Doppler echocardiographic evaluation of the spectrum of left ventricular diastolic dysfunction in essential hypertension. Am. Heart J. 127:906, 1994.

54. Shepherd, R. F. J., Zachariah, P. K., and Shub, C.: Hypertension and left ventricular diastolic function. Mayo Clin. Proc. 64:1521, 1989.

55. Karam, R., Lever, H. M., and Healy, B. P.: Hypertensive hypertrophic cardiomyopathy or hypertrophic cardiomyopathy with hypertension? A study of 78 patients. J. Am. Coll. Cardiol. 13:580, 1989.

56. Houghton, J. L., Frank, M. J., Carr, A. A., et al.: Relations among impaired coronary flow reserve, left ventricular hypertrophy and thallium perfusion defects in hypertensive patients without obstructive coronary artery disease. J. Am. Coll. Cardiol. 15:43, 1990.

57. Savage, D. D., Levy, D., Dannenberg, A. L., et al.: Association of echocardiographic left ventricular mass with body size, blood pressure and physical activity (the Framingham Study). Am. J. Cardiol. 65:371, 1990.

58. Devereux, R. B., Roman, M. J., Ganau, A., et al.: Cardiac and arterial hypertrophy and atherosclerosis in hypertension. Hypertension 23 (part 1):802, 1994.

59. Nielsen, J. R., Oxhøj, H., and Fabricius, J.: Left ventricular structural changes in young men at increased risk of developing essential hypertension: Assessment by echocardiography. Am. J. Hypertens. 2:885, 1989.

60. Post, W. S., Larson, M. G., and Levy, D.: Impact of left ventricular structure on the incidence of hypertension. Circulation 90:179, 1994.

61. Verdecchia, P., Schillaci, G., Guerrieri, M., et al.: Circadian blood pressure changes and left ventricular hypertrophy in essential hypertension. Circulation 81:528, 1990.

62. Devereux, R. B., Koren, M. J., de Simone, G., et al.: LV mass as a measure of preclinical hypertensive disease. Am. J. Hypertens. 5:175S, 1992.

63. Gottdiener, J. S., Reda, D. J., Materson, B. J., et al.: Importance of obesity, race and age to the cardiac structural and functional effects of hypertension. J. Am. Coll. Cardiol. 24:1492, 1994.

64. Mayet, J., Shahi, M., Foale, R. A., et al.: Racial differences in cardiac structure and function in essential hypertension. Br. Med. J. 308:1011, 1994.

65. Frohlich, E. D., Apstein, C., Chobanian, A. V., et al.: The heart in hypertension. N. Engl. J. Med. 327:998, 1992.

66. Clarkson, P. B. M., Wheeldon, N. M., MacLeod, C., et al.: Effects of angiotensin II and aldosterone on diastolic function in vivo in normal man. Clin. Sci. 87:397, 1994.

67. Weber, K. T., Sun, Y., and Guarda, E.: Structural remodeling in hypertensive heart disease and the role of hormones. Hypertension 23 (Part 2):869, 1994.

68. Verdecchia, P., Porcellati, C., Zampi, I., et al.: Asymmetric left ventricular remodeling due to isolated septal thickening in patients with systemic hypertension and normal left ventricular masses. Am. J. Cardiol. 73:247, 1994.

69. Koren, M. J., Devereux, R. B., Casale, P. N., et al.: Relation of left ventricular mass and geometry to morbidity and mortality in uncomplicated essential hypertension. Ann. Intern. Med. 114:345, 1991.

70. Ghali, J. K., Liao, Y., Simmons, B., et al.: The prognostic role of LV hypertrophy in patients with or without coronary artery disease. Ann. Intern. Med. 117:831, 1992.

71. Schmieder, R. E., and Messerli, F. H.: Determinants of ventricular ectopy in hypertensive cardiac hypertrophy. Am. Heart J. 123:89, 1992.

72. Dahlöf, B., Pennert, K., and Hansson, L.: Reversal of left ventricular hypertensive patients: A metaanalysis of 109 treatment studies. Am. J. Hypertens. 5:95, 1992.

73. Habib, G. B., Mann, D. L., and Zoghbi, W. A.: Normalization of cardiac structure and function after regression of cardiac hypertrophy. Am. Heart J. 128:333, 1994.

74. Kannel, W. B.: Contribution of the Framingham Study to preventive cardiology. J. Am. Coll. Cardiol. 15:206, 1990.

75. Hedblad, B., and Janzon, L.: Hypertension and ST segment depression during ambulatory electrocardiographic recording: Results from the prospective population study "men born in 1914" in Malm, Sweden. Hypertension 20:32, 1992.

76. Lindblad, U., Råstam, L., and Rydén, L.: The J-curve phenomenon: Inverse relation between achieved diastolic blood pressure and risk of acute myocardial infarction. In Kendall, M. J., Kaplan, N. M., and Horton, R. C. (eds.): Difficult Hypertension, Practical Management and Decision Making. London, Martin Dunitz, 1995, pp. 79–96.

77. Harvey, J. M., Howie, A. J., Lee, S. J., et al.: Renal biopsy findings in hypertensive patients with proteinuria. Lancet 340:1435, 1992.

78. Pedrinelli, R., Giampietro, O., Carmassi, F., et al.: Microalbuminuria and endothelial dysfunction in essential hypertension. Lancet 344:14, 1994.

79. Perneger, T. V., Klag, M. J., Feldman, H. I., and Whelton, P. K.: Projections of hypertension-related renal disease in middle-aged residents of the United States. JAMA 269:1272, 1993.

80. Alter, M., Friday, G., Lai, S. M., et al.: Hypertension and risk of stroke recurrence. Stroke 25:1605, 1994.

81. Bikkina, M., Levy, D., Evans, J. C., et al.: Left ventricular mass and risk of stroke in an elderly cohort. JAMA 272:33, 1994.

82. O'Connell, J. E., and Gray, C. S.: Treating hypertension after stroke. Br. Med. J. 308:1523, 1994.

83. Bruner, H. R., Laragh, J. H., Baer, L., et al.: Essential hypertension: Renin and aldosterone, heart attack and stroke. N. Engl. J. Med. 286:441, 1972.

84. Alderman, M. H., Madhavan, S., Ooi, W. L., et al.: Association of the renin-sodium profile with the risk of myocardial infarction in patients with hypertension. N. Engl. J. Med. 324:1098, 1991.

85. Management Committee: Untreated mild hypertension. Lancet 1:185, 1982.

86. Medical Research Council Working Party: MRC trial of treatment of mild hypertension: Principal results. Br. Med. J. 291:97, 1985.

87. Jackson, R., Barham, P., Bills, J., et al.: Management of raised blood pressure in New Zealand: A discussion document. Br. Med. J. 307:107, 1993.

MECHANISMS OF ESSENTIAL HYPERTENSION

88. Lund-Johansen, P.: Central haemodynamics in essential hypertension at rest and during exercise: A 20-year follow-up study. J. Hypertens. 7 (Suppl. 6):S52, 1989.

89. Post, W. S., Larson, M. G., and Levy, D.: Hemodynamic predictors of incident hypertension. Hypertension 24:585, 1994.

90. Julius, S., Mejia, A. D., Schork, N. J., and Krause, L. C.: Neurogenic hyperkinetic borderline hypertension (BHT) in Tecumseh, Michigan. Circulation 81:16, 1990.

91. Jeunemaitre, X., Soubrier, F., Kotelevtsev, Y. V., et al.: Molecular basis of human hypertension: Role of angiotensinogen. Cell 71:169, 1992.

91a. Hunt, S. C., Hopkins, P. N., and Williams, R. R.: Hypertension: Genetics and mechanisms. In Fuster, V., Ross, R., and Topol, E. J. (eds.): Atherosclerosis and Coronary Artery Disease. Philadelphia, Lippincott-Raven Publishers, 1996, pp. 209–236.

92. Harrap, S. B.: Hypertension: genes versus environment. Lancet 344:169, 1994.

93. Law, C. M., de Sweit, M., Osmond, C., et al.: Initiation of hypertension in utero and its amplification throughout life. Br. Med. J. 306:24, 1993.

94. Lucas, A., and Morley, R.: Does early nutrition in infants born before term programme later blood pressure? Br. Med. J. 309:304, 1994.

95. Brenner, B. M., and Chertow, G. M.: Congenital oligonephropathy: An inborn cause of adult hypertension and progressive renal injury? Curr. Opin. Nephrol. Hypertens. 2:691, 1994.

96. Brenner, B. M., and Anderson, S.: The interrelationships among filtration surface area, blood pressure, and chronic renal disease. J. Cardiovasc. Pharmacol. 19 (Suppl. 6):S1, 1992.

97. Guyton, A. C.: Kidneys and fluids in pressure regulation: Small volume but large pressure changes. Hypertension 19 (Suppl. I):I-2, 1992.

98. Sealey, J. E., Blumenfeld, J. D., Bell, G. M., et al.: On the renal basis for essential hypertension: Nephron heterogeneity with discordant renin secretion and sodium excretion causing a hypertensive vasoconstriction-volume relationship. J. Hypertens. 6:763, 1988.

99. de Wardener, H. E., and MacGregor, G. A.: Dahl's hypothesis that a saluretic substance may be responsible for a sustained rise in arterial pressure: Its possible role in essential hypertension. Kidney Int. 18:1, 1980.

100. Woolfson, R. G., Poston, L., and de Wardener, H. E.: Digoxin-like inhibitors of active sodium transport and blood pressure: The current status. Kidney Int. 46:297, 1994.

101. Hamlyn, J. M., Laredo, J., Lu, Z., et al.: Do putative endogenous digitalis-like factors have a physiological role? Hypertension 24:641, 1994.

102. Lewis, L. K., Yandle, T. G., Lewis, J. G., et al.: Ouabain is not detectable in human plasma. Hypertension 24:549, 1994.

103. Richards, A. M.: The natriuretic peptides and hypertension. J. Intern. Med. 235:543, 1994.

104. Buckley, M. G., Markandu, N. D., Sagnella, G. A., and MacGregor, G. A.: Brain and atrial natriuretic peptides: A dual peptide system of potential importance in sodium balance and blood pressure regulation in patients with essential hypertension. J. Hypertens. 12:809, 1994.

105. Kimura, G., and Brenner, B. M.: A method for distinguishing salt-sensitive from non–salt-sensitive forms of human and experimental hypertension. Curr. Opin. Nephrol. Hypertens. 2:341, 1993.

106. Resnick, L. M., Gupta, R. K., DiFabio, B., et al.: Intracellular ionic consequences of dietary salt loading in essential hypertension. J. Clin. Invest. 94:1269, 1994.

107. Swales, J. D.: Membrane transport of ions in hypertension. Cardiovasc. Drug Ther. 4:367, 1990.

108. Dzau, V. J., Gibbons, G. H., Cooke, J. P., and Omoigui, N.: Vascular biology and medicine in the 1990s: Scope, concepts, potentials, and perspectives. Circulation 87:705, 1993.

109. Lever, A. F., and Harrap, S. B.: Essential hypertension: A disorder of growth with origins in childhood? J. Hypertens. 10:101, 1992.

110. Folkow, B.: "Structural factor" in primary and secondary hypertension. Hypertension 16:89, 1990.

111. Davis, M. G., Ali, S., Leikauf, G. D., and Dorn, G. W., II: Tyrosine kinase inhibition prevents deformation-stimulated vascular smooth muscle growth. Hypertension 24:706, 1994.

112. Lever, A. F.: Slow pressor mechanisms in hypertension: A role for hypertrophy of resistance vessels? J. Hypertens. 4:515, 1986.

113. Müller, R., Steffen, H. M., Weller, P., and Krone, W.: Plasma catecholamines and adrenoceptors in young hypertensive patients. J. Hum. Hypertens. 8:351, 1994.

114. Floras, J. S., and Hara, K.: Sympathoneural and haemodynamic characteristics of young subjects with mild essential hypertension. J. Hypertens. 11:647, 1993.

115. Smith, S., Julius, S., Jamerson, K., et al.: Hematocrit levels and physiologic factors in relationship to cardiovascular risk in Tecumseh, Michigan. J. Hypertens. 12:455, 1994.

116. Ziegler, M. G., Mill, P., and Dimsdale, J. E.: Hypertensives' pressor response to norepinephrine: Analysis by infusion rate and plasma levels. Am. J. Hypertens. 4:586, 1991.

117. Reeves, R. A., Shapiro, A. P., Thompson, M. E., and Johnsen, A.-M.: Loss of nocturnal decline in blood pressure after cardiac transplantation. Circulation 73:401, 1986.

118. Vincent, H. H., Boomsma, F., Man in'T Veld, A. J., and Schalekamp, M. A. D. H.: Stress levels of adrenaline amplify the blood pressure response to sympathetic stimulation. J. Hypertens. 4:255, 1986.

119. al'Absi, M., Lovallo, W. R., McKey, B. S., and Pincomb, G. A.: Borderline hypertensives produce exaggerated adrenocortical responses to mental stress. Psychosom. Med. 56:245, 1994.

120. Markovitz, J. H., Matthews, K. A., Kannel, W. B., et al.: Psychological predictors of hypertension in the Framingham Study: Is there tension in hypertension? JAMA 270:2439, 1993.

121. Perini, C., Smith, D. H. G., Neutel, J. M., et al.: A repressive coping style protecting from emotional distress in low-renin essential hypertensives. J. Hypertens. 12:601, 1994.

122. Naraghi, R., Geiger, H., Crnac, J., et al.: Posterior fossa neurovascular anomalies in essential hypertension. Lancet 344:1466, 1994.

123. Somers, V. K., Dyken, M. E., Mark, A. L., and Abboud, F. M.: Sympathetic-nerve activity during sleep in normal subjects. N. Engl. J. Med. 328:303, 1993.

124. Cohen, M. C., and Muller, J. E.: Onset of acute myocardial infarction: Circadian variation and triggers. Cardiovasc. Res. 26:831, 1992.

125. Brunner, H. R., Sealey, J. E., and Laragh, J. H.: Renin subgroups in essential hypertension. Circ. Res. 32/33 (Suppl. I):I-99, 1973.

126. Goldblatt, H.: Reflections. Urol. Clin. North Am. 2:219, 1975.

126a. Jackson, E. K., and Garrison, J. C.: Renin and angiotensin. In Hardman, J. G., et al. (eds.): Goodman and Gilman's The pharmacological basis of therapeutics. 9th ed. New York, McGraw-Hill, 1996, pp. 733–758.

127. Johnston, C. J.: Renin-angiotensin system: A dual tissue and hormonal system for cardiovascular control. J. Hypertens. 10 (Suppl. 7):S13, 1992.

128. Morishita, R., Gibbons, G. H., Ellison, K. E., et al.: Evidence for direct local effect of angiotensin in vascular hypertrophy. J. Clin. Invest. 94:978, 1994.

129. Nilsson, P. M., Lind, L., Andersson, P.-E., et al.: On the use of ambulatory blood pressure recordings and insulin sensitivity measurements in support of the insulin-hypertension hypothesis. J. Hypertens. 12:965, 1994.

130. Wing, J. R., Van Der Merwe, M. T., Joffe, B. I., et al.: Insulin-mediated glucose disposal in black South Africans with essential hypertension. Q. J. Med. 87:431, 1994.

131. Lemieux, S., Després, J. P., Moorjani, S., et al.: Are gender differences in cardiovascular disease risk factors explained by the level of visceral adipose tissue? Diabetologia 37:757, 1994.

132. Reaven, G. M., and Laws, A.: Insulin resistance, compensatory hyperinsulinaemia, and coronary heart disease. Diabetologia 37:948, 1994.

133. Steinberg, H. O., Brechtel, G., Johnson, A., et al.: Insulin-mediated skeletal muscle vasodilation is nitric oxide dependent. J. Clin. Invest. 94:1172, 1994.

134. Anderson, E. A., and Mark, A. L.: Cardiovascular and sympathetic actions of insulin: The insulin hypothesis of hypertension revisited. Cardiovasc. Risk Factors 3:159, 1994.

135. Flavahan, N. A.: Atherosclerosis or lipoprotein-induced endothelial dysfunction: Potential mechanisms underlying reduction in EDRF/nitric oxide activity. Circulation 85:1927, 1992.

136. Panza, J. A., Casino, P. R., Kilcoyne, C. M., and Quyyumi, A. A.: Role of endothelium-derived nitric oxide in the abnormal endothelium-dependent vascular relaxation of patients with essential hypertension. Circulation 87:1468, 1993.

137. Cockroft, J. R., Chowienczyk, P. J., Benjamin, N., and Ritter, J. M.: Preserved endothelium-dependent vasodilatation in patients with essential hypertension. N. Engl. J. Med. 330:1036, 1994.

138. Lyons, D., Webster, J., and Benjamin, N.: The effect of antihypertensive therapy on responsiveness to local intra-arterial N^G-monomethyl-L-arginine in patients with essential hypertension. J. Hypertens. 12:1047, 1994.

139. Galle, J., Öchslen, M., Schollmeyer, P., and Wanner, C.: Oxidized lipoproteins inhibit endothelium-dependent vasodilation. Hypertension 23:556, 1994.

140. Kiowski, W., Linder, L., and Erne, P.: Vascular effects of endothelin-1 in humans and influence of calcium channel blockade. J. Hypertens. 12 (Suppl. 1):S21, 1994.

141. Haynes, W. G., and Webb, D. J.: Contribution of endogenous generation of endothelin-1 to basal vascular tone. Lancet 344:852, 1994.

142. Henneberry, H. P., Slater, J. D. H., Eisen, V., and Führ, S.: Arginine vasopressin response to hypertonicity in hypertension studied by arginine vasopressin assay in unextracted plasma. J. Hypertens. 10:221, 1992.

143. Fitzgibbon, W. R., Ploth, D. W., and Margolius, H. S.: Kinins and vasoactive peptides. Curr. Opin. Nephrol. Hypertens. 2:283, 1993.

144. Muirhead, E. E., Brooks, B., and Byers, L. W.: Biologic differences between vasodilator prostaglandins and medullipin I. Am. J. Med. Sci. 303:86, 1992.

145. Maheswaran, R., and Beevers, D. G.: Lead and blood pressure. J. Hypertens. 7 (Suppl. 6):S381, 1989.

146. Witteman, J. C. M., Willett, W. C., Stampfer, M. J., et al.: A prospective study of nutritional factors and hypertension among U.S. women. Circulation 80:1320, 1989.

147. Carman, W. J., Barrett-Connor, E., Sowers, M., and Khaw, K.: Higher risk of cardiovascular mortality among lean hypertensive individuals in Tecumseh, Michigan. Circulation 89:703, 1994.

148. Sonne-Holm, S., Sørensen, T. I. A., Jensen, G., and Schnohr, P.: Independent effects of weight change and attained body weight on prevalence of arterial hypertension in obese and non-obese men. Br. Med. J. 299:767, 1989.

149. Hla, K. M., Young, T. B., Bidwell, T., et al.: Sleep apnea and hypertension. Ann. Intern. Med. 120:382, 1994.

150. Endre, T., Mattiasson, I., Hulthén, U. L., et al.: Insulin resistance is coupled to low physical fitness in normotensive men with a family history of hypertension. J. Hypertens. 12:81, 1994.

151. Blair, S. N., Kohl, H. W., III, Paffenbarger, R. S., Jr., et al.: Physical fitness and all-cause mortality: A prospective study of healthy men and women. JAMA 262:2395, 1989.

152. Paffenbarger, R. S., Jr.: Contributions of epidemiology to exercise science and cardiovascular health. Med. Sci. Sports Exerc. 20:426, 1988.

153. Grøbæk, M., Deis, A., Sørensen, T. I. A., et al.: Influence of sex, age, body mass index, and smoking on alcohol intake and mortality. Br. Med. J. 308:302, 1994.

154. Kiechl, S., Willeit, J., Egger, G., et al.: Alcohol consumption and carotid atherosclerosis: Evidence of dose-dependent atherogenic and antiatherogenic effects. Stroke 25:1593, 1994.

155. Marmot, M. G., Elliott, P., Shipley, M. J., et al.: Alcohol and blood pressure: The INTERSALT study. Br. Med. J. 308:1263, 1994.

156. Gaziano, J. M., Buring, J. E., Breslow, J. L., et al.: Moderate alcohol intake, increased levels of high-density lipoprotein and its subfractions, and decreased risk of myocardial infarction. N. Engl. J. Med. 329:1829, 1993.

157. Ridker, P. M., Vaughan, D. E., Stampfer, M. J., et al.: Association of moderate alcohol consumption and plasma concentration of endogenous tissue-type plasminogen activator. JAMA 272:929, 1994.

158. Facchini, F., Chen, Y.-D. I., and Reaven, G. M.: Light-to-moderate alcohol intake is associated with enhanced insulin sensitivity. Diabetes Care 17:115, 1994.

159. Grassi, G. M., Somers, V. K., Renk, W. S., et al.: Effects of oral alcohol intake on blood pressure and sympathetic nerve activity in normotensive humans: A preliminary report. J. Hypertens. 7 (Suppl. 6):S20, 1989.

160. Kojima, S., Kawano, Y., Abe, H., et al.: Acute effects of alcohol ingestion on blood pressure and erythrocyte sodium concentration. J. Hypertens. 11:185, 1993.

161. Giannattasio, C., Mangoni, A. A., Stella, M. L., et al.: Acute effects of smoking on radial artery compliance in humans. J. Hypertens. 12:691, 1994.

162. Terres, W., Becker, P., and Rosenberg, A.: Changes in cardiovascular risk profile during the cessation of smoking. Am. J. Med. 97:242, 1994.

163. Smith, W. C. S., Lowe, G. D. O., Lee, A. J., and Tunstall-Pedoe, H.: Rheological determinants of blood pressure in a Scottish adult population. J. Hypertens. 10:467, 1992.

164. Friedman, G. D., Selby, J. V., and Quesenberry, C. P., Jr.: The leukocyte count: A predictor of hypertension. J. Clin. Epidemiol. 43:907, 1990.

165. Messerli, F. H., Frohlich, E. D., Dreslinski, G. R., et al.: Serum uric acid in essential hypertension: An indicator of renal vascular involvement. Ann. Intern. Med. 93:817, 1980.

HYPERTENSION IN SPECIAL GROUPS

166. Walker, W. G., Neaton, J. D., Cutler, J. A., et al.: Renal function change in hypertensive members of the Multiple Risk Factor Intervention Trial. JAMA 268:3085, 1992.

167. Parmer, R. J., Stone, R. A., and Cervenka, J. H.: Renal hemodynamics in essential hypertension: Racial differences in response to changes in dietary sodium. Hypertension 24:752, 1994.

168. Luft, F. C., Miller, J. Z., Grim, C. E., et al.: Salt sensitivity and resistance of blood pressure. Hypertension 17 (Suppl. 1):102, 1991.

169. Wilson, T. W., and Grim, C. E.: Biohistory of slavery and blood pressure differences in blacks today. Hypertension 17 (Suppl. 1):122, 1991.

170. Barlow, R. J., Connel, M. A., and Milne, F. J.: A study of 48-hour faecal and urinary electrolyte excretion in normotensive black and white South African males. J. Hypertens. 401:197, 1986.

171. Isles, C. G., Hole, D. J., Hawthorn, V. M., and Lever, A. F.: Relation between coronary risk and coronary mortality in women of the Renfrew and Paisley survey: Comparison of men. Lancet 339:702, 1992.

172. Kaplan, N. M.: The treatment of hypertension in women. Arch. Intern. Med. 155:563, 1995.

173. Rosner, B., Prineas, R. J., Loggie, J. M. H., and Daniels, S. R.: Blood pressure nomograms for children and adolescents, by height, sex, and age, in the United States. J. Pediatr. 123:871, 1993.

174. Gillman, M. W., Cook, N. R., Rosner, B., et al.: Identifying children at high risk for the development of essential hypertension. J. Pediatr. 122:837, 1993.

175. Morgenstern, B. Z.: Hypertension in pediatric patients: Current issues. Mayo Clin. Proc. 69:1089, 1994.

176. Loggie, J. M. H.: Hypertension in children. Heart Dis. Stroke May/June:147, 1994.

177. Lauer, R. M., Burns, T. L., Clarke, W. R., and Mahoney, L. T.: Childhood predictors of future blood pressure. Hypertension 18 (Suppl. I):I-74, 1991.

178. Hansen, H. S., Nielsen, J. R., Nyldebrandt, N., and Froberg, K.: Blood pressure and cardiac structure in children with a parental history of hypertension: The Odense Schoolchild Study. J. Hypertens. 10:677, 1992.

179. Murphy, J. K., Alpert, B. S., and Walker, S. S.: Ethnicity, pressor reactivity, and children's blood pressure. Hypertension 20:327, 1992.

180. Kaplan, N. M., Deveraux, R. B., and Miller, H. S., Jr.: Task Force 4: Systemic hypertension. J. Am. Coll. Cardiol. 24:885, 1994.

181. Gruskin, A. B., Dabbagh, S., Fleischmann, L. E., and Atiyeh, B. A.: Application since 1980 of antihypertensive agents to treat pediatric disease. J. Hum. Hypertens. 8:381, 1994.

182. Deal, J. E.: Treatment of children with hypertension. In Kendall, M., Kaplan, N. M., and Horton, R. (eds.): Difficult Hypertension, Practical Management and Decision Making. London, Martin Dunitz, 1995, pp. 7–20.

183. National High Blood Pressure Education Program Working Group: National High Blood Pressure Education Program Working Group report on hypertension in the elderly. Hypertension 23:275, 1994.

184. Kaplan, N. M.: The promises and perils of treating the elderly hypertensive. Am. J. Med. Sci. 305:183, 1993.

185. Tarnow, L., Rossing, P., Gall, M.-A., et al.: Prevalence of arterial hypertension in diabetic patients before and after the JNC-V. Diabetes Care 17:1247, 1994.

186. Berrut, G., Hallab, M., Bouhanick, B., et al.: Value of ambulatory blood pressure monitoring in type I (insulin-dependent) diabetic patients with incipient diabetic nephropathy. Am. J. Hypertens. 7:222, 1994.

187. The Hypertension in Diabetes Study Group: Hypertension in diabetes study (HDS): I. Prevalence of hypertension in newly presenting type 2 diabetic patients and the association with risk factors for cardiovascular and diabetic complications. J. Hypertens. 11:309, 1993.

188. Lewis, E. J., Hunsicker, L. G., Bain, R. P., and Rohde, R. D.: The effect of angiotensin-converting enzyme inhibition on diabetic nephropathy. N. Engl. J. Med. 329:1456, 1993.

SECONDARY HYPERTENSION

189. Hannaford, P. C., Croft, P. R., and Kay, C. R.: Oral contraception and stroke. Evidence from the Royal College of General Practitioners' Oral Contraception Study. Stroke 25:935, 1994.

190. Rosenberg, L., Palmer, J. R., and Shapiro, S.: Use of lower dose oral contraceptives and risk of myocardial infarction. Circulation 83(Abs.):8, 1991.

191. Royal College of General Practitioners: Hypertension. In Oral Contraceptives and Health. From the Oral Contraceptive Study of the Royal College of General Practice. New York, Pitman Publishing, 1974, p. 37.

192. Weir, R. J.: Effect on blood pressure of changing from high to low dose steroid preparation in women with oral contraceptive induced hypertension. Scott. Med. J. 27:212, 1982.

193. Wallace, R. B., Barrett-Connor, E., Criqui, M., et al.: Alteration in blood pressures associated with combined alcohol and oral contraceptive use: The Lipid Research Clinics Prevalence Study. J. Chron. Dis. 35:251, 1982.

194. Lim, K. G., Isles, C. G., Hodsman, G. P., et al.: Malignant hypertension in women of childbearing age and its relation to the contraceptive pill. Br. Med. J. 294:1057, 1987.

195. McAreavey, D., Cumming, A. M. M., Boddy, K., et al.: The renin-angiotensin system and total body sodium and potassium in hypertensive women taking estrogen-progestogen oral contraceptives. Clin. Endocrinol. 18:111, 1983.

196. Gosland, I. F., Walton, C., Felton, C., et al.: Insulin resistance, secretion, and metabolism in users of oral contraceptives. J. Clin. Endocrinol. Metab. 74:64, 1992.

197. Nabulsi, A. A., Folsom, A. R., White, A., et al.: Association of hormone-replacement therapy with various cardiovascular risk factors in postmenopausal women. N. Engl. J. Med. 328:1069, 1993.

198. Rosenberg, L., Palmer, J. R., and Shapiro, S.: A case-control study of myocardial infarction in relation to use of estrogen supplements. Am. J. Epidemiol. 137:54, 1993.

199. Lieberman, E. H., Gerhard, M. D., Uehata, A., et al.: Estrogen improves endothelium-dependent, flow-mediated vasodilation in postmenopausal women. Ann. Intern. Med. 121:936, 1994.

200. Perneger, T. V., Brancati, F. L., Whelton, P. K., and Klag, M. J.: End-stage renal disease attributable to diabetes mellitus. Ann. Intern. Med. 121:912, 1994.

201. Smith, S. R., Svetkey, K. P., and Dennis, V. W.: Racial differences in the incidence and progression of renal diseases. Kidney Int. 40:815, 1991.

202. Ghose, R. R., and Harindra, V.: Unrecognized high pressure chronic retention of urine presenting with systemic arterial hypertension. Br. Med. J. 298:1626, 1989.

203. Bakir, A. A., Bazilinski, N., and Dunea, G.: Transient and sustained recovery from renal shutdown in accelerated hypertension. Am. J. Med. 80:173, 1986.

204. Shankel, S. W., Johnson, D. C., Clark, P. S., et al.: Acute renal failure and glomerulopathy caused by nonsteroidal anti-inflammatory drugs. Arch. Intern. Med. 152:986, 1992.

205. Coruzzi, P., and Novarini, A.: Which antihypertensive treatment in renal vasculitis? Nephron 62:372, 1992.

206. Hammond, J. J., Raffaele, J., Liddel, N., et al.: A prospective study to evaluate the effects of extracorporeal shock wave lithotripsy (ESWL) on blood pressure (BP), renal function (RF) and glomerular filtration (GFR). J. Am. Coll. Cardiol. 21(Abs.):257, 1993.

207. Smith, L. H., Drach, G., Hall, P., et al.: National High Blood Pressure Education Program (NHBPEP) review paper on complications of shock wave lithotripsy for urinary calculi. Am. J. Med. 91:635, 1991.

208. Najarian, J. S., Chavers, B. M., McHugh, L. E., and Matas, A. J.: 20 years or more of follow-up on living kidney donors. Lancet 340:807, 1992.

209. Smith, H. W.: Unilateral nephrectomy in hypertensive disease. J. Urol. 76:685, 1956.

210. Lüscher, T. F., Wanner, C., Hauri, D., et al.: Curable renal parenchymatous hypertension: Current diagnosis and management. Cardiology 72 (Suppl. 1):33, 1985.

211. Torres, V. E., Donovan, K. A., Scicli, G., et al.: Synthesis of renin by tubulocystic epithelium in autosomal-dominant polycystic kidney disease. Kidney Int. 42:364, 1992.

212. Siamopoulos, K., Sellars, L., Mishra, S. C., et al.: Experience in the management of hypertension with unilateral chronic pyelonephritis: Results of nephrectomy in selected patients. Q. J. Med. 207:34, 1983.

213. Rostand, S. G., Brunzell, J. D., Cannon, R. O., III, and Victor, R. G.: Cardiovascular complications in renal failure. J. Am. Soc. Nephrol. 2:1053, 1991.

214. Breyer, J. A., and Jacobson, H. R.: Ischemic nephropathy. Curr. Opin. Nephrol. Hypertens. 2:216, 1993.

215. Parving, H.-H., Smidt, U. M., Mathiesen, E. R., et al.: Effective antihypertensive treatment postpones renal insufficiency in diabetic nephropathy. Am. J. Kidney Dis. 22:188, 1993.

216. Dubach, U. C., Rosner, B., and Stürmer, T.: An epidemiologic study of abuse of analgesic drugs: Effects of phenacetin and salicylate on mortality and cardiovascular morbidity (1968 to 1987). N. Engl. J. Med. 324:155, 1991.

217. Brenner, B. M., and Yu, A. S. L.: Uremic syndrome revisited: A pathogenetic role for retained endogenous inhibitors of nitric oxide synthesis. Curr. Opin. Nephrol. Hypertens. 1:3, 1992.

218. Henrich, W. L.: Hemodynamic instability during hemodialysis. Kidney Int. 30:605, 1986.

219. Curtis, J. J., Luke, R. G., Dustan, H. P., et al.: Remission of essential hypertension after renal transplantation. N. Engl. J. Med. 309:1009, 1983.

220. Raman, G. V.: Posttransplant hypertension. J. Hum. Hypertens. 5:1, 1991.

221. Bresticker, M., Nelson, J., Wolf, J., and Anderson, B.: Plasma renin activity in renal transplant patients with hypertension. Am. J. Hypertens. 4:623, 1991.

222. Strandgaard, S., and Hansen, U.: Hypertension in renal allograft recipients may be conveyed by cadaveric kidneys from donors with subarachnoid hemorrhage. Br. Med. J. 292:1041, 1986.

223. Mann, S. J., and Pickering, T. G.: Detection of renovascular hypertension: State of the art: 1992. Ann. Intern. Med. 227:845, 1992.

224. Svetkey, L. P., Kadir, S., Dunnick, N. R., et al.: Similar prevalence of renovascular hypertension in selected blacks and whites. Hypertension 17:678, 1991.

225. Novick, A. C., Zaki, S., Goldfarb, D., and Hodge, E. E.: Epidemiologic and clinical comparison of renal artery stenosis in black patients and white patients. J. Vasc. Surg. 20:1, 1994.

226. Bookstein, J. J.: Segmental renal artery stenosis in renovascular hypertension. Radiology 90:1073, 1968.

227. Geyskes, G. G., Klinge, O. J., Kooiker, C. J., et al.: Renovascular hypertension: The small kidney updated. Q. J. Med. 66:203, 1988.

228. Rimmer, J. M., and Gennari, F. J.: Atherosclerotic renovascular disease and progressive renal failure. Ann. Intern. Med. 228:712, 1993.

229. Pickering, T. G.: Renovascular hypertension: Etiology and pathophysiology. Semin. Nucl. Med. 19:79, 1989.

230. Canzanello, V. J., and Textor, S. C.: Noninvasive diagnosis of renovascular disease. Mayo Clin. Proc. 69:1172, 1994.

231. Derkx, F. H. M., and Schalekamp, M. A. D. H.: Renal artery stenosis and hypertension. Lancet 344:237, 1994.

232. Muller, F. B., Sealey, J. E., Case, D. B., et al.: The captopril test for identifying renovascular disease in hypertensive patients. Am. J. Med. 80:6433, 1986.

233. Gerber, L. M., Mann, S. J., Müller, F. B., et al.: Response to the captopril test is dependent on baseline renin profile. J. Hypertens. 12:173, 1994.

234. Elliott, W. J., Martin, W. B., and Murphy, M. B.: Comparison of two noninvasive screening tests for renovascular hypertension. Arch. Intern. Med. 153:755, 1993.

235. Mimran, A.: Renal effects of antihypertensive agents in parenchymal renal disease and renovascular hypertension. J. Cardiovasc. Pharmacol. 19 (Suppl. 6):45, 1992.

236. Losinno, F., Zuccalà, A., Busato, F., and Zucchelli, P.: Renal artery angioplasty for renovascular hypertension and preservation of renal function: Long-term angiographic and clinical follow-up. A.J.R. 162:853, 1994.

237. Tykarski, A., Edward, R., Dominiczak, A. F., and Reid, J. L.: Percutaneous transluminal renal angioplasty in the management of hypertension and renal failure in patients with renal artery stenosis. J. Hum. Hypertens. 7:491, 1993.

238. Bedoya, L., Ziegelbaum, M., Vidt, D. G., et al.: Baseline renal function and surgical revascularization in atherosclerotic renal arterial disease in the elderly. Cleveland Clin. J. Med. 56:415, 1989.

239. Libertino, J. A., Bosco, P. J., Ying, C. Y., et al.: Renal revascularization to preserve and restore renal function. J. Urol. 147:1485, 1992.

240. McVicar, M., Carman, C., Chandra, M., et al.: Hypertension secondary to renin-secreting juxtaglomerular cell tumor: Case report and review of 38 cases. Pediatr. Nephrol. 7:404, 1993.

241. Geddy, P. M., and Main, J.: Renin-secreting retroperitoneal leiomyosarcoma: An unusual cause of hypertension. J. Hum. Hypertens. 4:57, 1990.

242. Leckie, B. J., Birnie, G., and Carachi, R.: Renin in Wilms' tumor: Prorenin as an indicator. J. Clin. Endocrinol. Metab. 79:1742, 1994.

243. Osella, G., Terzolo, M., Borretta, G., et al.: Endocrine evaluation of incidentally discovered adrenal masses (incidentalomas). J. Clin. Endocrinol. Metab. 79:1532, 1994.

244. Tsushima, Y.: Different lipid contents between aldosterone-producing and nonhyperfunctioning adrenocortical adenomas: In vivo measurement using chemical-shift magnetic resonance imaging. J. Clin. Endocrinol. Metab. 79:1759, 1994.

245. Gross, M. D., Shapiro, B., Gouffard, J. A., et al.: Distinguishing benign from malignant euadrenal masses. Ann. Intern. Med. 109:613, 1988.

246. Gordon, R. D.: Mineralocorticoid hypertension. Lancet 344:240, 1994.

247. Rich, G. M., Ulick, S., Cook, S., et al.: Glucocorticoid-remediable aldosteronism in a large kindred: Clinical spectrum and diagnosis using a characteristic biochemical phenotype. Ann. Intern. Med. 116:813, 1992.

248. Lifton, R. P., Dluhy, R. G., Powers, M., et al.: A chimaeric 11β-hydroxylase/aldosterone synthase gene causes glucocorticoid-remediable aldosteronism and human hypertension. Nature 355:262, 1992.

249. Stewart, P. M., Corrie, J. E. T., Shackleton, C. H. L., and Edwards, C. R. W.: Syndrome of apparent mineralocorticoid excess: A defect in the cortisol-cortisone shuttle. J. Clin. Invest. 82:340, 1988.

250. Stewart, P. M., Wallace, A. M., Valentino, R., et al.: Mineralocorticoid activity of liquorice: 11-Beta-hydroxysteroid dehydrogenase deficiency comes of age. Lancet 2:821, 1987.

251. Vierhapper, H., Derfler, K., Nowotny, P., et al.: Impaired conversion of cortisol to cortisone in chronic renal insufficiency: A cause of hypertension or an epiphenomenon? Acta Endocrinol. 125:160, 1991.

252. Walker, B. R., Stewart, P. M., Shackleton, C. H. L., et al.: Deficient inactivation of cortisol by 11β-hydroxysteroid dehydrogenase in essential hypertension. Clin. Endocrinol. 39:221, 1993.

253. Blumenfeld, J. D., Sealey, J. E., Schlussel, Y., et al.: Diagnosis and treatment of primary hyperaldosteronism. Ann. Intern. Med. 121:877, 1994.

254. Ferriss, J. B., Beevers, D. G., Brown, J. J., et al.: Clinical, biochemical and pathological features of low renin ("primary") hyperaldosteronism. Am. Heart J. 95:375, 1978.

255. Weinberger, M. H., and Fineberg, N. S.: The diagnosis of primary aldosteronism and separation of two major subtypes. Arch. Intern. Med. 153:2125, 1993.

256. Bravo, E. L., and Canale, M. P.: Clinical utility of some screening tests in the evaluation of suspected primary aldosteronism. Hypertension 24(Abs.):58, 1994.

257. Radin, D. R., Manoogian, C., and Nadler, J. L.: Diagnosis of primary hyperaldosteronism: Importance of correlating CT findings with endocrinologic studies. A.J.R. 158:553, 1992.

258. Guazzoni, G., Montorsi, F., Bergamaschi, F., et al.: Effectiveness and safety of laparoscopic adrenalectomy. J. Urol. 152:1375, 1994.

259. Young, W. F., Jr.: Primary aldosteronism. In Rakel, R. E. (ed.): Conn's Current Therapy. Philadelphia, W. B. Saunders Company, 1993, p. 610.

260. Sugihara, N., Shimizu, M., Kita, Y., et al.: Cardiac characteristics and postoperative courses in Cushing's syndrome. Am. J. Cardiol. 69:1475, 1992.

261. Ulick, S., Tedde, R., and Wang, J. Z.: Defective ring A reduction of cortisol as the major metabolic error in the syndrome of apparent mineralocorticoid excess. J. Clin. Endocrinol. Metab. 74:593, 1992.

262. Sato, A., Suzuki, H., Murakami, M., et al.: Glucocorticoid increases angiotensin II type 1 receptor and its gene expression. Hypertension 23:25, 1994.

263. Montwill, J., Igoe, D., and McKenna, T. J.: The overnight dexamethasone test is the procedure of choice in screening for Cushing's syndrome. Steroids 59:296, 1994.

264. Orth, D. N.: Differential diagnosis of Cushing's syndrome. N. Engl. J. Med. 325:957, 1991.

265. Trainer, P. J., and Grossman, A.: The diagnosis and differential diagnosis of Cushing's syndrome. Clin. Endocrinol. 34:317, 1991.

266. Klibanski, A., and Zervas, N. T.: Diagnosis and management of hormone-secreting pituitary adenomas. N. Engl. J. Med. 324:822, 1991.

267. Trainer, P. J., and Besser, M.: Cushing's syndrome: Therapy directed at the adrenal glands. Endocrinol. Metab. Clin. North Am. 23:571, 1994.

268. Helmberg, A., Ausserer, B., and Kofler, R.: Frame shift by insertion of 2 basepairs in codon 394 of CYP11B1 causes congenital adrenal hyperplasia due to steroid 11β-hydroxylase deficiency. J. Clin. Endocrinol. Metab. 75:1278, 1992.

269. de Simone, G., Tommaselli, A. P., Rossi, R., et al.: Partial deficiency of adrenal 11-hydroxylase: A possible cause of primary hypertension. Hypertension 7:204, 1985.

270. Cottrell, D. A., Bello, F. A., and Falko, J. M.: Case report: 17-Alpha-hydroxylase deficiency masquerading as primary hyperaldosteronism. Am. J. Med. Sci. 300:380, 1990.

271. Whalen, R. K., Althausen, A. F., and Daniels, G. H.: Extra-adrenal pheochromocytoma. J. Urol. 147:1, 1992.

272. Nanes, M. S., and Catherwood, B. D.: The genetics of multiple endocrine neoplasia syndromes. Annu. Rev. Med. 43:253, 1992.

273. Gagel, R. F., Tashjian, A. H., Jr., Cummings, T., et al.: The clinical outcome of prospective screening for multiple endocrine neoplasia type 2a: An 18-year experience. N. Engl. J. Med. 318:478, 1988.

274. Bravo, E. L.: Evolving concepts in the pathophysiology, diagnosis, and treatment of pheochromocytoma. Endocrinol. Rev. 15:356, 1994.

275. Atuk, N. O., Hanks, J. B., Weltman, J., et al.: Circulating dihydroxyphenylglycol and norpinephrine concentrations during sympathetic nervous system activation in patients with pheochromocytoma. J. Clin. Endocrinol. Metab. 79:1609, 1994.

276. Scott, I., Parkes, R., and Cameron, D. P.: Phaeochromocytoma and cardiomyopathy. Med. J. Aust. 148:94, 1988.

277. Haas, G. J., Tzagournis, M., and Boudoulas, H.: Pheochromocytoma: Catecholamine-mediated electrocardiographic changes mimicking ischemia. Am. Heart J. 116:1363, 1988.

278. Goldbaum, T. S., Henochowicz, S., Mustafa, M., et al.: Pheochromocytoma presenting with Prinzmetal's angina. Am. J. Med. 81:921, 1986.

279. Feldman, J. M.: Falsely elevated urinary excretion of catecholamines and metanephrines in patients receiving labetalol therapy. J. Clin. Pharmacol. 27:288, 1987.

280. Textor, S. C., Canzanello, V. J., Taler, S. J., et al.: Cyclosporine-induced hypertension after transplantation. Mayo Clin. Proc. 69:1182, 1994.

281. Fahal, I. H., Yaqoob, M., and Ahmad, R.: Phlebotomy for erythropoietin-induced malignant hypertension. Nephron 61:214, 1992.

282. Lake, C. R., Gallant, S., Masson, E., and Miller, P.: Adverse drug effects attributed to phenylpropanolamine: A review of 142 case reports. Am. J. Med. 89:195, 1990.

283. Ross, R. D., Clapp, S. K., Gunther, S., et al.: Augmented norepinephrine and renin output in response to maximal exercise in hypertensive coarctation patients. Am. Heart J. 123:1293, 1992.

284. Stewart, A. B., Ahmed, R., Travill, C. M., and Newman, C. G. H.: Coarctation of the aorta—life and health 20–44 years after surgical repair. Br. Heart J. 69:65–70, 1993.

285. Shaddy, R. E., Boucek, M. M., Sturtevant, J. E., et al.: Comparison of angioplasty and surgery for unoperated coarctation of the aorta. Circulation 87:793, 1993.

286. Gidding, S. S., Rocchini, A. P., Beekman, R., et al.: Therapeutic effect of propranolol on paradoxical hypertension after repair of coarctation of the aorta. N. Engl. J. Med. 312:1224, 1985.

287. Ritchie, C. M., Sheridan, B., Fraser, R., et al.: Studies on the pathogenesis of hypertension in Cushing's disease and acromegaly. Q. J. Med. 76:855, 1990.

288. Lind, I., Hvarfner, A., Palmer, M., et al.: Hypertension in primary hyperparathyroidism in relation to histopathology. Eur. J. Surg. 157:457, 1991.

289. Jespersen, B., Brock, A., Charles, P., et al.: Unchanged noradrenaline reactivity and blood pressure after corrective surgery in primary hyperparathyroidism. Scand. J. Clin. Lab. Invest. 53:470, 1993.

290. Heuser, D., Guggenberger, H., and Fretschner, R.: Acute blood pressure increase during the perioperative period. Am. J. Cardiol. 63:26C, 1989.

291. Colvin, J. R., and Kenny, G. N. C.: Automatic control of arterial pressure after cardiac surgery. Anaesthesia 44:37, 1989.

292. Weinstein, G. S., Zabetakis, P. M., Clavel, A., et al.: The renin-angiotensin system is not responsible for hypertension following coronary artery bypass grafting. Ann. Thorac. Surg. 43:74, 1987.

293. Kaplan, J. A.: Clinical considerations for the use of intravenous nicardipine in the treatment of postoperative hypertension. Am. Heart J. 119:443, 1990.

294. Estafanous, F. G., Tarazi, R. C., Buckley, S., and Taylor, P. C.: Arterial hypertension in immediate postoperative period after valve replacement. Br. Heart J. 40:718, 1978.

295. Cockburn, J. S., Benjamin, I. S., Thomson, R. M., and Bain, W. H.: Early systemic hypertension after surgical closure of atrial septal defect. J. Cardiovasc. Surg. 16:1, 1975.

296. Brozena, S. C., Johnson, M. R., Ventura, J. O., and Naftel, D. C.: Effectiveness of diltiazem or lisinopril for treatment of hypertension in car-

diac transplant patients: A prospective, randomized multi-center trial. Circulation *88* (Part 2):480, 1993.

297. Leenen, F. H. H., Holliwell, D. L., and Cardella, C. J.: Blood pressure and left ventricular anatomy and function after heart transplantation. Am. Heart J. *122*:1087, 1991.

298. Roberts, J. M., and Redman, C. W. G.: Pre-eclampsia: More than pregnancy-induced hypertension. Lancet *341*:1447, 1993.

299. Robillard, P.-Y., Hulsey, T.C., Périanin, J., et al.: Association of pregnancy-induced hypertension with duration of sexual cohabitation before conception. Lancet *344*:973, 1994.

300. Eskenazi, B., Fenster, L., and Sidney, S.: A multivariate analysis of risk factors for preeclampsia. JAMA *266*:231, 1991.

301. Brown, M. A., Reiter, L., Smith, B., et al.: Measuring blood pressure in pregnant women: A comparison of direct and indirect methods. Am. J. Obstet, Gynecol. *171*:661, 1994.

302. Ihle, B. U., Long, P., and Oats, J.: Early onset pre-eclampsia: Recognition of underlying renal disease. Br. Med. J. *294*:79, 1987.

303. Dekker, G. A., and Sibai, B. M.: Early detection of preeclampsia. Am. J. Obstet. Gynecol. *165*:160, 1991.

304. Zhou, Y., Damsky, C. H., Chiu, K., et al.: Preeclampsia is associated with abnormal expression of adhesion molecules by invasive cytotrophoblasts. J. Clin. Invest. *91*:950, 1993.

305. Clark, D. A.: Does immunological intercourse prevent pre-eclampsia? Lancet *344*:969, 1994.

306. Chen, G., Wilson, R., Cumming, G., et al.: Immunological changes in pregnancy-induced hypertension. Eur. J. Obstet, Gynecol. *53*:21, 1994.

307. Seligman, S. P., Buyon, J. P., Clancy, R. M., et al.: The role of nitric oxide in the pathogenesis of preeclampsia. Am. J. Obstet. Gynecol. *171*:944, 1994.

308. Sibai, B. M., Caritis, S. N., Thom, E., et al.: Prevention of preeclampsia with low-dose aspirin in healthy, nulliparous pregnant women. N. Engl. J. Med. *329*:1213, 1993.

309. Carroli, G., Duley, L., Belizán, J. M., and Villar, J.: Calcium supplementation during pregnancy: A systematic review of randomised controlled trials. Br. J. Obstet. Gynaecol. *202*:753, 1994.

310. Redman, C. W. G., and Roberts, J. M.: Management of pre-eclampsia. Lancet *341*:1451, 1993.

311. Sibai, B. M., Gonzalez, A. R., Mabie, W. C., and Moretti, M.: A comparison of labetalol plus hospitalization versus hospitalization alone in the management of preeclampsia remote from term. Obstet. Gynecol. *70*:323, 1987.

312. National High Blood Pressure Education Program Working Group: Report on high blood pressure in pregnancy. Am. J. Obstet. Gynecol. *163*:1689, 1990.

313. Rosa, F. W., Bosco, L. A., Graham, C. F., et al.: Neonatal anuria with maternal angiotensin-converting enzyme inhibition. Obstet. Gynecol. *74*:371, 1989.

314. Sibai, B. M., Mercer, B. M., Schiff, E., and Friedman, S. A.: Aggressive versus expectant management of severe preeclampsia at 28 to 32 weeks' gestation: A randomized controlled trial. Am. J. Obstet. Gynecol. *171*:818, 1994.

315. Paterson-Brown, S., Robson, S. C., Redfern, N., et al.: Hydralazine boluses for the treatment of severe hypertension in pre-eclampsia. Br. J. Obstet. Gynaecol. *101*:409, 1994.

316. Welt, S. I., Dorminy, J. H., Jelovsek, F. R., et al.: The effect of prophylactic management and therapeutics on hypertension disease in pregnancy: Preliminary studies. Obstet. Gynecol. *57*:557, 1981.

317. Rey, E., and Couturier, A.: The prognosis of pregnancy in women with chronic hypertension. Am. J. Obstet. Gynecol. *171*:410, 1994.

318. Moodley, J.: Treatment of eclampsia. Br. J. Obstet. Gynaecol. *97*:99, 1990.

319. Pritchard, J. A., Cunningham, F. G., and Pritchard, S. A.: The Parkland Memorial Hospital protocol for treatment of eclampsia: Evaluation of 245 cases. Am. J. Obstet. Gynecol. *148*:951, 1984.

320. Clark, S. L., Greenspoon, J. S., Aldahl, D., and Phelan, J. P.: Severe preeclampsia with persistent oliguria: Management of hemodynamic subsets. Am. J. Obstet. Gynecol. *154*:490, 1986.

321. Chesley, L. C.: Hypertension in pregnancy: Definitions, familial factor, and remote prognosis. Kidney Int. *18*:234, 1980.

322. Marin-Neto, J. A., Maciel, B. C., Urbanetz, L. L. T., et al.: High output failure in patients with peripartum cardiomyopathy: A comparative study with dilated cardiomyopathy. Am. Heart J. *121*:134, 1991.

HYPERTENSIVE CRISES

323. Webster, J., Petrie, J. C., Jeffers, T. A., and Lovell, H. G.: Accelerated hypertension: Patterns of mortality and clinical factors affecting outcome in treated patients. Q. J. Med. *86*:485, 1993.

324. Lip, G. Y. H., Beevers, M., and Beevers, G.: The failure of malignant hypertension to decline: A survey of 24 years' experience in a multiracial population in England. J. Hypertens. *12*:1297, 1994.

325. Strandgaard, S., and Paulson, O. B.: Cerebral blood flow and its pathophysiology in hypertension. Am. J. Hypertens. *2*:486, 1989.

326. Shapiro, L. M., and Beevers, D. G.: Malignant hypertension: Cardiac structure and function at presentation and during therapy. Br. Heart J. *49*:477, 1983.

327. Kaplan, N. M.: Management of hypertensive emergencies. Lancet *344*:1335, 1994.

328. White, W. B., and Baker, L. H.: Episodic hypertension secondary to panic disorder. Arch. Intern. Med. *146*:1129, 1986.

329. Carlberg, B.: Blood pressure in acute stroke: Causes and consequences. Hypertens. Res. *17* (Suppl. I):S77, 1994.

Chapter 27
Systemic Hypertension: Therapy

NORMAN M. KAPLAN

As noted at the beginning of Chapter 26, the number of patients being treated for hypertension has expanded markedly over the last 25 years so that it is now the leading reason for office visits to physicians. Nonetheless, a recent survey of well-informed hypertensive patients whose costs were completely covered by insurance found that only 12 per cent had their disease under good control.[1] This apparent paradox of expanded coverage but continued poor control is not the consequence of either the ineffectiveness of available therapy or an unwillingness of physicians to provide it. In controlled trials, most patients with the most prevalent form of hypertension, previously called "mild" but now referred to as grade 1, i.e., diastolic blood pressure (DBP) between 90 and 100 mm Hg, achieve excellent control with one of multiple drugs.[2] Relatively few patients are truly resistant to therapy.[3] Moreover, physicians in the United States begin treatment of virtually all patients with blood pressure levels above 140/90 mm Hg.

The problem derives from the inherent nature of hypertension: induced by common but unhealthy life styles, asymptomatic and persistent, with overt consequences delayed by 10 to 30 years so that the costs of therapy, both in money and in adverse effects, seem to outweigh benefits to be derived from adherence to the regimen. Furthermore, behind the inherent nature of the disease that often interferes with patient adherence to their physician's requests, there lurks yet another disquieting feature to the therapy of most hypertension: it may not benefit the majority of patients who adhere faithfully to their treatment. Among "mild" hypertensives, only about one in 500 are saved from a serious adverse effect per year of therapy.[4] Moreover, in some population settings, those who take antihypertensive therapy have higher rates of coronary mortality than those who do not, particularly if they start with relatively mild hypertension.[5] Presumably, the minimum protection they could receive from lower blood pressure is negated by the adverse effects of therapy. Those with higher initial risk have more to gain even if these putative adverse effects persist. Such potential harm from misdirected therapy underscores the need for caution, as called for by Geoffrey Rose[6] and formalized by Jackson et al.,[7] in the use of medication as a preventive measure. Their advice, detailed in the next section, needs to be kept in mind as we consider the general principles and specific details of the treatment of hypertension.

Yet another element, the issue of cost-effectiveness, has been introduced into the debate about the value of treating all patients with any degree of hypertension.[8] As the escalating costs of health care consume a greater share of society's resources, two opposing forces have risen: one, the need for less expensive illness care and the other, the relatively large cost of prevention when indiscriminately applied to low-risk subjects. Therefore, it is likely that the calls for more selective and targeted antihypertensive therapy[7] will be more widely listened to in the future.

We will examine the evidence for benefits of therapy and then apply this evidence to the criteria for the initiation of therapy to individual patients.

BENEFITS OF THERAPY

The treatment of hypertension is aimed not at the simple reduction of blood pressure but at the prevention of the cardiovascular complications that are known to accompany the high pressure.[8a] Over the past 25 years, multiple randomized controlled trials have tested the ability of a limited number of antihypertensive drugs—primarily diuretics and adrenergic inhibitors—to prevent strokes and heart attacks.

A series of meta-analyses from 1986 on have portrayed the effects of therapy in a progressively enlarging number of completed trials.[9–11] They have shown a uniform and persistent reduction in morbidity and mortality from stroke averaging 40 per cent, a reduction that fits exactly to what was predicted from epidemiological evidence if the attributable risk had been completely reversed.[12] On the other hand, the impact on coronary heart disease reported in 1986 on the basis of data from nine trials was not significant, averaging only 8 per cent.[9] By 1990, with analysis of five more sets of data, the reduction was 14 per cent, still below the 20 to 25 per cent predicted if the risk attributed to blood pressure had been completely reversed.[12] By 1993, however, data from three recently reported trials in elderly patients[13–15,15a] brought the overall impact on coronary events to a 16 per cent reduction, with confidence limits of 8 to 23 per cent, which overlap the excess 20 to 25 per cent risk predicted from epidemiological evidence (Figure 27–1).

Some have assumed that these data now prove that treatment of hypertension completely reverses the risk of both stroke and coronary disease, providing "the maximum attainable reduction over a short interval."[16] Caution is advised in assuming that the diuretic and adrenergic blocking drugs used in all of the trials now completed have, in fact, provided all of the protection against coronary disease that could be obtained. Recall that the evidence for the impact on stroke is uniform and equal to that expected, but the evidence on coronary disease is spotty and less impressive. Moreover, only one of the trials involving patients under age 60 showed a significant reduction in coronary events. This trial, the Hypertension Detection and Follow-up Program (HDFP), has been faulted both for its design, by which the control group received less medical care beyond antihypertensive therapy, and for its loose criteria for the diagnosis of coronary events.[4] The large number of coro-

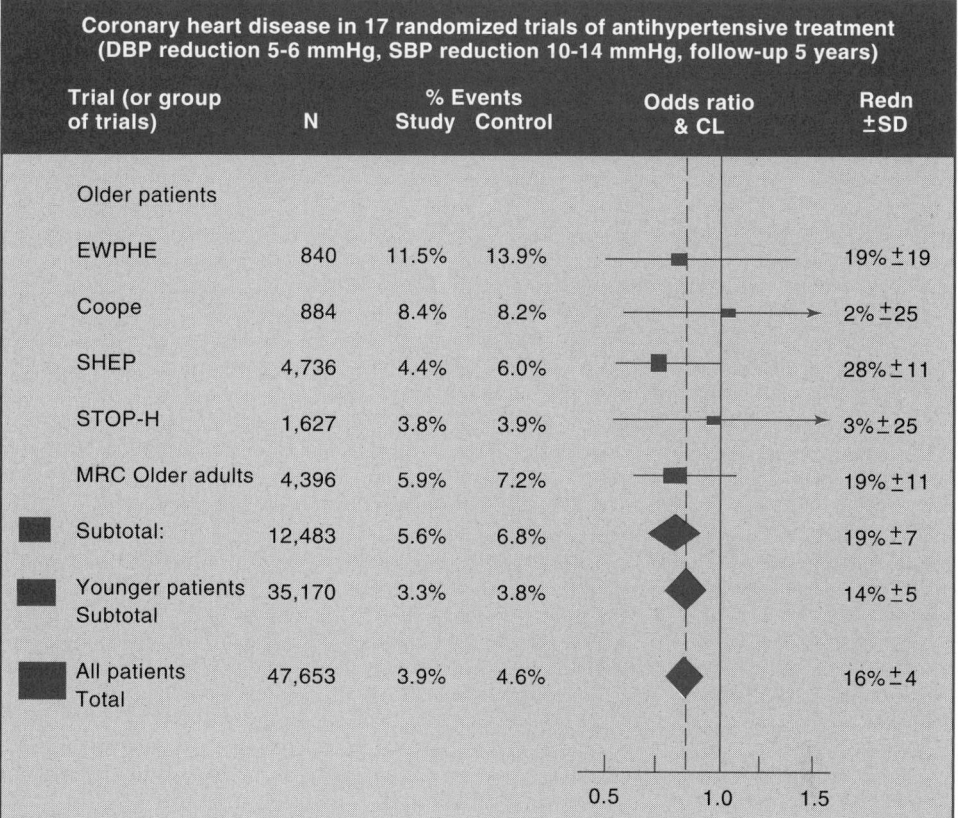

Coronary heart disease in 17 randomized trials of antihypertensive treatment (DBP reduction 5–6 mmHg, SBP reduction 10–14 mmHg, follow-up 5 years)					
Trial (or group of trials)	N	% Events Study	Control	Odds ratio & CL	Redn ±SD
Older patients					
EWPHE	840	11.5%	13.9%		19% ±19
Coope	884	8.4%	8.2%		2% ±25
SHEP	4,736	4.4%	6.0%		28% ±11
STOP-H	1,627	3.8%	3.9%		3% ±25
MRC Older adults	4,396	5.9%	7.2%		19% ±11
Subtotal:	12,483	5.6%	6.8%		19% ±7
Younger patients Subtotal	35,170	3.3%	3.8%		14% ±5
All patients Total	47,653	3.9%	4.6%		16% ±4

FIGURE 27–1. Effects of blood pressure reduction on coronary heart disease incidence in 12 randomized controlled trials of young patients (most under age 60) and 5 trials in older patients (all over age 60). Box size is proportional to number of events recorded. Horizontal lines denote 99 per cent confidence intervals of odds ratios from individual trial results and diamonds denote 95 per cent confidence intervals for odds ratios for combined trial results. (From MacMahon, S., and Rodgers, A.: The effects of blood pressure reduction in older patients: An overview of five randomized controlled trials in elderly hypertensives. Clin. Exper. Hypertens. *15:* 967, 1993.)

nary events in HDFP provided 31 per cent of the total included in the 1993 meta-analysis, suggesting that "there may have been a systematic bias as a result of flawed design."[4]

Swales concludes, "Despite such misgivings, the consistent trend in all the major trials for a reduction in coronary events, and the impressive significant impact in some trials, particularly in the elderly, allow us to conclude that treatment reduces the frequency of ischaemic heart disease. Nevertheless, the extent of that impact is uncertain and is likely to remain so for some years, and the observed effect may well be heterogeneous, depending on patient groups studied (particularly in relation to age) and classes of drugs used. Meta-analyses that pool disparate studies cannot help us to make such fine distinctions, but where findings are reasonably consistent, as for stroke, they provide robust overall conclusions."[4]

Just as the risks of untreated hypertension rise progressively with every increment in pressure (Fig. 27–2), so do the benefits of treatment increase progressively the higher the level.

BENEFITS FOR SEVERE HYPERTENSION. The evidence for protection from overall and cause-specific mortality by therapy of patients with more severe hypertension (DBP above 110 mm Hg, Table 26–2) is incontrovertible.[17] Whereas most patients with accelerated or malignant hypertension died within a year if left untreated, survival rates of well beyond 50 per cent after 10 years have been reported since effective therapy has been provided.[18] For those with nonmalignant but severe hypertension, the evidence is almost as impressive.[10]

BENEFITS FOR MODERATE HYPERTENSION. Those patients with initial DBP between 100 and 110 mm Hg (grade 2 or moderate) enrolled in the multiple clinical trials have generally been found to benefit from therapy.[10] Nonetheless, there is a need to ensure that their pressure is *persistently* elevated: Even among the patients enrolled in the Australian trial whose DBP was between 105 and 109 after two sets of readings 4 weeks apart, 11 per cent of those given only placebo pills had DBP persistently below 90 mm Hg for the next 4 years.[19] Their blood pressure fell mostly during the first 4 months. Therefore, unless there is an obvious need for the more immediate institution of drug therapy, such as progressive target organ damage or blood pressures so high as to threaten immediate danger, all patients should be given the opportunity to achieve a spontaneous reduction of their initially high pressures over a 4- to 6-month interval. During that time they should have their pressures carefully moni-

tored, since if it goes up—as it did in 10 to 15 per cent of the placebo-treated patients in the multiple trials shown in Figure 27–1—immediate institution of drug therapy may be indicated.

As noted in the preceding chapter, the monitoring logically can be done at home and, for some, with ambulatory 24-hour monitoring, which may provide, in a condensed manner, better prognostic evidence than multiple blood pressure measurements taken in the office. While the blood pressure is being monitored, the use of appropriate nondrug therapies may help lower the pressure even more, without risk and with relatively little inconvenience. Such nondrug therapies may not only lower the blood pressure but also reduce overall cardiovascular risk by amelioration of such conditions as hyperlipidemia, glucose intolerance, and alcohol abuse.

BENEFITS FOR MILD HYPERTENSION. The majority of people with elevated blood pressure, defined as above 140/90 mm Hg, have "mild" hypertension (grade 1) with DBP between 90 and 100 mm Hg (see Chap. 26, Fig. 26–2). As shown in Figure 26–2, even though the risk rises progressively, the sheer number of patients with minimally elevated pressure causes them to make a major contribution to the overall population risk from hypertension. Therefore, the call for population-wide preventive measures makes sense and should be heeded.[20]

However, when individual patients are involved, the issues are not so simple and the answer not so obvious. The rate of cardiovascular complications falls progressively with lower levels of pressure, whether they are naturally lower or lowered by therapy. However, the fall in risk observed in the clinical trials is not a straight-line, linear one, shown as line A in Figure 27–2. Rather, in some studies it follows a curvilinear pattern, with a sharp downward trend at higher levels and a much lower rate of decrease in risk at lower levels, shown as line B in Figure 27–2. As we shall note subsequently, the data from most trials follow a J curve, with an upward trend below some crucial level, shown as line C in Figure 27–2. Disregarding the presence of this J curve for now, it is obvious that less benefit is provided when diastolic pressures are lowered below 100 mm Hg and much less when lowered below 95 mm Hg than when lowered from higher levels (Fig. 27–3). These data are from a trial comparing two forms of therapy[21] and are not included in the meta-analyses of placebo-controlled trials, although the data in them are similar. Thus, in the MRC trial,[22] to prevent one stroke, therapy had to be given for 1 year to 333 patients with entry blood pressure in the 105 to 109 range, but to 666 patients with blood pressure of 100 to 104 and to 2000 patients with blood pressure of 95 to 99 mm Hg.

Thus, lowering, the threshold of treatment from a DBP of 100 down to 95 means that an additional 1334 patients will be treated for 1 year without apparent benefit. The number will be far greater if the threshold is lowered to a DBP of 90. Not only will more patients be treated without apparent benefit, but a far greater number of patients will be treated if a lower threshold is used. In the large population screened for the HDFP, 25.3 per cent had a DBP of 90 or higher,

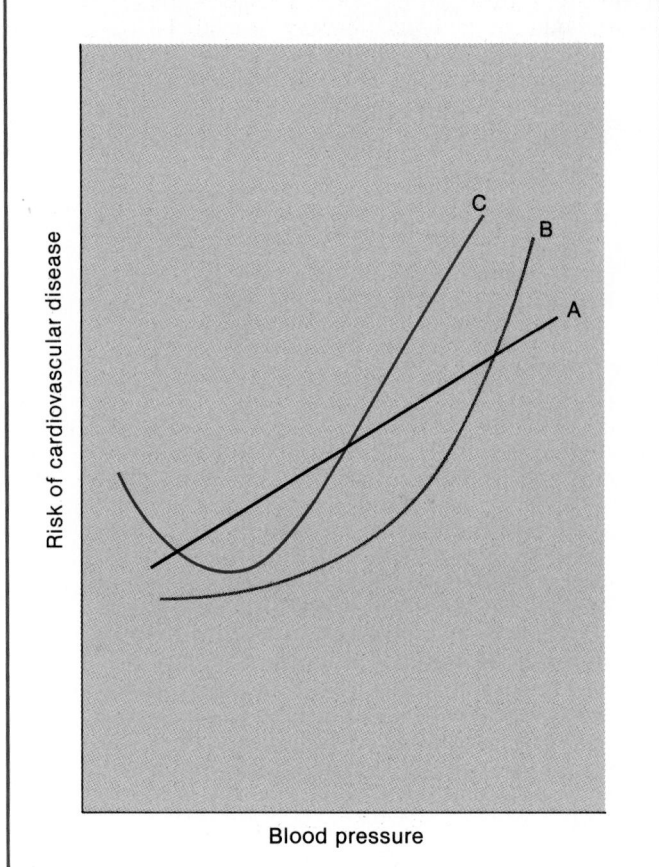

FIGURE 27–2. Three models representing hypothetical relationships between levels of blood pressure and risk of cardiovascular disease. (From Epstein, F. H.: Proceedings of the XVth International Congress of Therapeutics, September 5–9, 1979. Brussels, Excerpta Medica, 1980.)

but 40 per cent of these readings were between 90 and 94 and two-thirds were below 100 mm Hg.

RESULTS OF CLINICAL TRIALS

Whereas the evidence for overall protection of patients with DBP between 95 and 100 is reasonably strong, the evidence for those between 90 and 95 is weak at best and nonexistent in most trials that have included such patients.[23] Part of this failure may reflect the finding that many of the patients in these trials were not, in fact, hypertensive: None of the trials required more than a 2-month run-in period before randomization to active or placebo therapy, and it has been shown that readings in as many as one-third to one-half of patients with DBP above 95 mm Hg will be persistently below 90 mm Hg after 4 to 6 months without therapy.[19]

In addition, as noted, the risks are relatively small at such low levels of elevated blood pressure, and the trials, despite their size and duration, may not have been adequate to show protection with so little preexisting risk. Moreover, the trials mainly involved low-risk, otherwise healthy patients, unlike many seen in clinical practice. In the HDFP trial, those patients with initial DBP between 90 and 95 mm Hg whose pressures were lowered more aggressively (the stepped-care group) had fewer cardiovascular events than did those whose pressures were lowered less.[24] However, the more intensively treated (Special Intervention) half of the patients in the Multiple Risk Factor Intervention Trial (MRFIT) whose initial DBP was between 90 and 94 mm Hg had a *higher* total and coronary death rate than did those given less therapy (Usual Care),[25] so that the evidence from the two large nonplacebo-controlled trials done in the U.S. remains contradictory.

THRESHOLD FOR THERAPY

There is legitimate cause for the disagreement as to the level at which to institute drug therapy, some expert groups such as the U.S. Joint National Committee[26] believing that drug therapy should be given to most with DBP above 90 mm Hg, and others such as the British[27] and Ca-

nadian[28] expert committees believing that it should be given only to those with DBP above 100 mm Hg in the absence of coexisting risk factors or target organ damage. The disagreement is not only of academic interest. As many as 40 million persons in the United States alone are in that 90 to 100 mm Hg range, and so obviously the issue has great clinical and economic relevance.

A compromise position was adopted by a conference sponsored by the World Health Organization and the International Society of Hypertension.[29] In substance, it states that after 3 to 6 months of observation, 95 mm Hg DBP should be used as the level for institution of active drug therapy. Patients with DBP between 90 and 95 who are at high overall risk of developing coronary artery disease should be "considered" for treatment.

The recommendations of all these expert committees call for therapy at lower levels of blood pressure when other major risk factors or target organ damage is present. Although it is not possible to predict with certainty which patients will develop complications, the larger the number of other cardiovascular risk factors present, the larger the number of complications observed and the greater the potential for protection by the amelioration of these other risks as well.[30] Because of their relatively lower degree of risk at every level of pressure, women are relatively less in need of therapy than are men.[31]

A Rational Approach

A group of experts from New Zealand have taken into account all of these considerations—level of blood pressure, age, gender, other risk factors, and target organ damage (Table 27–1)—and have constructed a rational approach based on their assessment of the evidence of benefit that has been shown.[7]

Their recommendation is that "people with an estimated absolute risk of cardiovascular disease of about 20 per cent or more in 10 years and a sustained blood pressure greater than 150 mm Hg systolic or 90 mm Hg diastolic (phase 5) should be considered for treatment to lower blood pressure

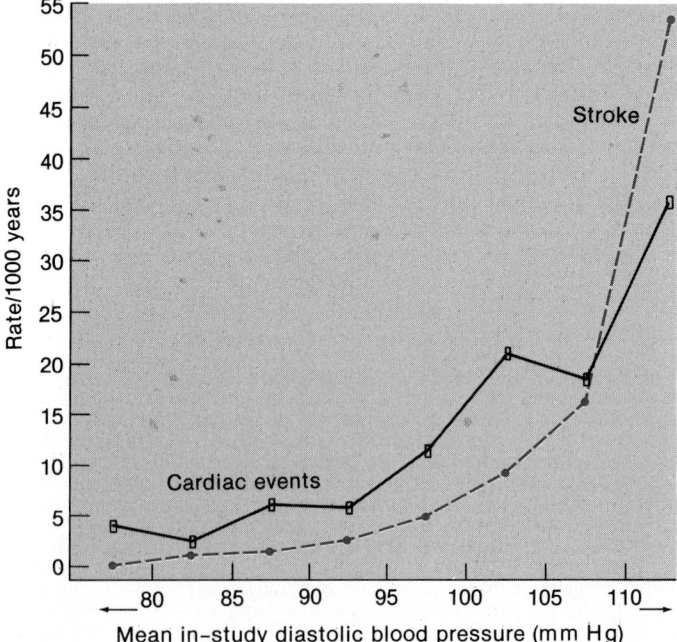

FIGURE 27–3. Absolute rate of cardiac events and stroke related to diastolic blood pressure during antihypertensive treatment. The extremes of the diastolic pressure scale include all values at or below 80 and above 110 mm Hg. Square = cardiac events; Circle = stroke. (From IPPPSH Collaborative Group: Cardiovascular risk and risk factors in a randomized trial of treatment based on the beta-blocker oxprenolol: The International Prospective Primary Prevention Study in Hypertension [IPPPSH]. J. Hypertens. *3:*388, 1985.)

TABLE 27–1 FEATURES CONSIDERED IN THE DECISION TO TREAT

OTHER RISK FACTORS
  Cigarette smoking
  Total cholesterol/HDL cholesterol ratio >6
  Diabetes
  Obesity (body mass index >30)
  Family history of premature cardiovascular disease (in parent
    or sibling before age 55)
SYMPTOMATIC CARDIOVASCULAR DISEASE
  Angina or silent ischemia
  Myocardial infarction
  Coronary angioplasty or bypass surgery
  Heart failure
  Left ventricular hypertrophy demonstrated by ECG or echo-
    cardiography
  Transient ischemic attacks
  Stroke
  Peripheral vascular disease
  Familial hyperlipidemia
  Other target organ damage such as renal disease

From Jackson, R., et al.: Management of raised blood pressure in New Zealand: A discussion document. Br. Med. J. *307*:107, 1993.

(see Figure 27–4 to estimate risk). Lowering the blood pressure of these patients by an average of 5 to 6 mm Hg diastolic (and 10 mm Hg systolic) would reduce their risk of cardiovascular disease by about one-third. In those with an absolute risk of 20 per cent in 10 years, the risk would be reduced to about 13 per cent in 10 years, meaning that one event would be prevented for every 150 patients treated each year. Any adverse effects of treatment are unlikely to outweigh the benefits of treatment at this level of risk, and treatment is likely to be relatively cost-effective. The absolute benefits and cost-effectiveness of treatment would be greater if larger reductions of blood pressure could be achieved.

Notice from Figure 27–4 that the threshold for therapy decreases progressively with degree of hypertension, age, and numbers of other risk factors. Therapy is advised in all patients with sustained average blood pressures above 170/100 regardless of degree of absolute risk. They also recommend that patients under age 40 with levels above 150/90 be referred to a specialist for work-up of secondary causes. These recommendations, as rational as they are, may be too conservative for many practitioners who have accepted the need for "more aggressive" therapy at much lower levels of blood pressure and overall risk. Perhaps the absolute level of risk should be placed at 10 per cent or 15 per cent, but that would obviously expose many more patients to the potential adverse effects and financial costs of therapy without the expectation of benefit. Regardless of whether this really quite simple and rational approach gains widespread acceptance, there is little reason for patients or physicians to be concerned about "watchful waiting." Recall the experience of the placebo-treated half of the patients in the Australian trial[32]: Over 4 years, the average DBP fell below 95 in 47.5 per cent of patients with baseline DBP of 95 to 109, and increased morbidity and mortality were seen only in those whose average DBP remained above 100.

If drug therapy is not given, close surveillance of all patients must be provided, because from 10 to 17 per cent of the placebo-treated patients in various trials had progression of their blood pressure to a level above that considered an indication for active treatment. Moreover, all patients should be strongly advised to use the appropriate life style modifications described on p. 844.

Systolic Pressure in the Elderly

The New Zealand recommendations rationally recommend that therapy be given to the elderly at lower levels of pressure because they "generally have a higher absolute risk of cardiovascular disease and therefore derive greater

benefit from treatment."[7] They recognize that little evidence about the value of therapy is available for people aged 80 or over. Since survival seems to be better at higher pressures in those over 80,[33] caution is obviously needed for the older elderly. As seen in Figure 27–1, the elderly achieved even greater protection from coronary disease in the three recently published trials. Furthermore, protection from congestive heart failure was even more impressive, therapy reducing the incidence by over 50 per cent.[13,14]

The New Zealand data include systolic levels in the decision to treat. This is based on the epidemiological evidence reviewed in Chapter 26 that systolic levels are more predictive of long-term prognosis than are diastolic levels and the evidence from the Systolic Hypertension in the Elderly Program (SHEP) trial,[13] wherein excellent protection was shown in a large group of elderly patients with isolated systolic hypertension, the average pretreatment blood pressure being 170/77. A consensus has been reached that systolic blood pressure over 160 mm Hg should be treated, at least to age 80. However, as seen in Figure 27–4, some older women with no other risk factors likely do not need therapy until systolic levels are above 170 mm Hg.

USE OF SURROGATE INDICATIONS. All of the preceding coverage of the benefits of therapy and the threshold for treatment has involved "hard" endpoints: morbidity and mortality. Some argue that softer endpoints should also be taken into account, using as surrogates one or another evidence of cardiovascular damage that may be easier to assess and quicker to appear. These include regression of left ventricular hypertrophy or carotid artery stenosis and reduction of proteinuria. Most, however, hold to the need for the hard endpoints.

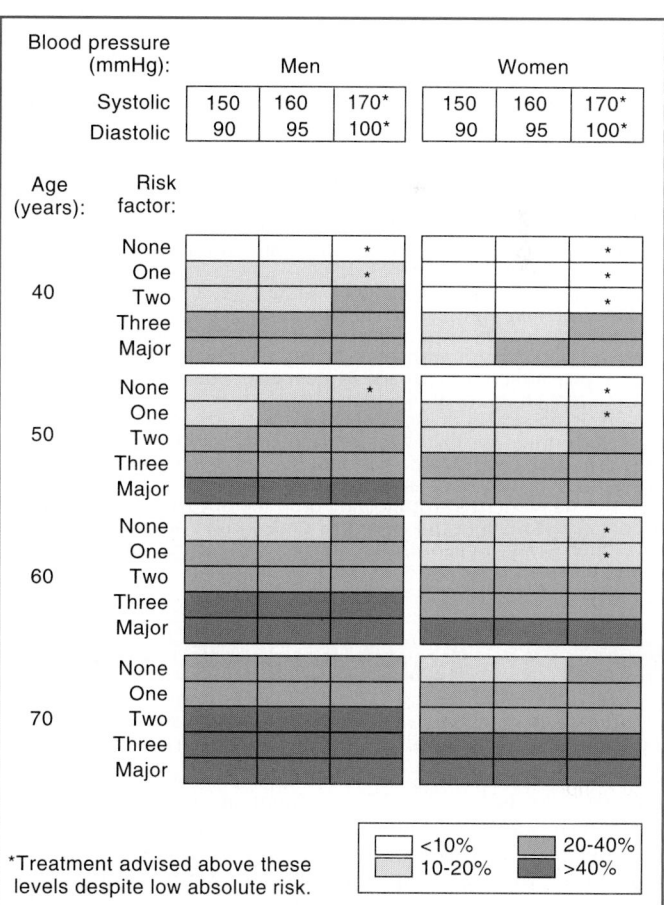

FIGURE 27–4. Absolute risk (percentage) of having a cardiovascular event in 10 years according to age, blood pressure, and other risk factors shown in Table 27–1. (From Jackson, R., et al.: Management of raised blood pressure in New Zealand: A discussion document. Br. Med. J. *307*:107, 1993.)

GOAL OF THERAPY

Once having decided to treat, the clinician must consider the goal of therapy. In the past, most physicians assumed that the effects of reduction of blood pressure on cardiovascular risk would fit a straight line downward (line A in Fig. 27–2),[34] justifying the opinion "the lower, the better." However, as noted, data from large trials indicated a more gradual decline in risk when pressures were reduced to moderate levels (line B in Fig. 27–2), around 95 mm Hg in the IPPPSH trial (Fig. 27–3).[21] Subsequently, Cruickshank[35] called attention to a J curve (line C in Fig. 27–2), reflecting a progressive fall in risk as pressure is lowered, but only to a certain level; below that level, the risk for coronary ischemic events goes back up.

Additional evidence for the J curve has been added to the six retrospective studies analyzed by Cruickshank, including two prospective studies of sizeable numbers of patients.[36,37] Recall, too, the data from HDFP and MRFIT showing higher coronary mortality rates among mild hypertensives with baseline ECG abnormalities if they were given more intensive therapy.[38,39] The apparent propensity to induce myocardial ischemia when pressures are lowered below a certain crucial threshold may not apply to other vital organs. Therefore, maximal protection against stroke or renal damage may require greater falls in pressure than the coronary circulation can safely handle.

The presence of a J curve has been stoutly defended[40] and almost as aggressively denied.[41] Some deny that it occurs except as an "irregularity" of small sets of data in a particularly vulnerable group of patients.[12] On the other hand, the denial of a J-curve on the basis of the absence of a lower threshold of risk in long-term observations on normotensive and mildly hypertensive people free of coronary artery disease and given no antihypertensive therapy[12] should be given no credence as evidence against the presence of such a threshold in more significantly hypertensive patients, often with preexisting coronary artery disease, who are given antihypertensive therapy and whose pressures are thereby "artificially" lowered. This is particularly important in the elderly, who may experience an increase in coronary events with even small decrements in blood pressure, whether induced by antihypertensive therapy or not.[42] The Hypertension Optimal Treatment (HOT) Trial should provide more conclusive evidence about the J curve in patients who were randomized to different target blood pressures.[43] For now, the prudent course is to accept the considerable evidence that a J curve does exist and hope to avoid it by careful, gradual reduction in pressure with agents that do not simultaneously incite other risks.

Once good control of blood pressure in a patient has been achieved, it may be possible to reduce or withdraw drug therapy. Perhaps one-fourth of patients with initially mild hypertension who achieve good control with therapy will remain normotensive for at least 1 year after their therapy is stopped.[44] However, such patients need to remain under observation.

There is no simple or single answer to the questions of whom to treat with drugs for mild hypertension and how much the pressure should be reduced. Each patient must be considered separately, taking various factors into account. The foregoing discussion should indicate the wisdom of withholding drug therapy from many of these patients, at least until the effects of time and life style modifications have been given a chance, thereby avoiding too fast and too great falls in pressure.

LIFE STYLE MODIFICATIONS

Interest in the use of various nondrug therapies, better called life style modifications, for the treatment of hypertension has risen markedly in the past few years. Yet many practitioners either do not use them or use them in a casual, perfunctory manner. This hesitant attitude can be attributed both to the sparseness of firm evidence indicating that these therapies succeed and to the difficulty many have faced in convincing patients to adhere to them. This situation is likely to change: Evidence for the effectiveness of these approaches in lowering blood pressure is growing,[2,45,46] techniques for improving adherence are being popularized, and patients seem increasingly willing to adopt changes in life style. These changes come at a pro-

pitious time, when many more people are being identified as hypertensive and are considered in need of lowering of blood pressure. Although most have turned first to drugs, the evidence presented in the previous section suggests that these can be safely withheld from many hypertensives to allow life style modifications a chance to be effective. The need for strong and immediately effective therapy was clear when the majority of patients had fairly severe hypertension; however, as a larger number of patients with mild hypertension have entered the picture, a more gradual approach to their management seems more appropriate. In addition, increasing awareness of the need to address other risk factors, such as dyslipidemia and glucose intolerance, along with hypertension has given additional emphasis to the value of life style modifications that can impact favorably on them as well.

Just as the increased awareness of the problem of patients' frequent poor adherence to drug therapy has led to attempts to improve the situation, similar attention toward adherence to life style modifications is likely to improve their effectiveness. These measures should be introduced gradually and gently. Too many and too drastic changes in life style may discourage patients from accepting them. Eventually, however, all hypertensive patients should benefit from moderate restriction of dietary salt, reduction of excess body weight, regular exercise, and moderation of alcohol intake.[26] As will be noted, when used together these can postpone the onset of hypertension and reduce the severity of existing disease. We will first examine the effect of each modification used alone. The data shown in Figure 27–5 are from the largest and best-controlled study comparing the effects of most of the individual modifications on blood pressure, not in hypertensives but in subjects with high-normal levels, DBP 80 to 89 mm Hg.[45] Altogether, 2182 men and women, aged 30 to 54, were randomly assigned to one of three life style changes (weight reduction, sodium restriction, or stress management) for 18 months or to one of four nutritional supplements (calcium, magnesium, potassium, or fish oil) for 6 months with placebo controls for each group. The results demonstrate a significant effect of weight loss, averaging 3.9 kg, and sodium restriction, averaging 44 mmol/day, but no effect of the other modalities. Obviously, different effects could be seen in various hypertensive patients.

AVOIDANCE OF TOBACCO. Until recently, the major pressor effect of tobacco was missed because patients have not been allowed to smoke in places where blood pressures are recorded. With automatic monitoring, the effect is easy to demonstrate[47] (Fig. 27–6). Patients who smoke or dip snuff should be strongly and repeatedly told to stop. Failing that, they should be advised to monitor their blood pressure while they smoke because such pressures are at least partially responsible for increased risks for cardiovascular disease and should be the target of antihypertensive therapy.

WEIGHT REDUCTION. In most published studies, weight loss has been shown to reduce blood pressure. In a review of adequately controlled intervention studies, a 1.0-kilogram decrease in body weight was accompanied by an average reduction of 1.6/1.3 mm Hg in blood pressure.[48] There may be a threshold, around 4 kg, to observe an effect,[49] but significant falls in pressure have been noted with only modest weight loss.[50] Use of a very low calorie supplement may achieve faster weight loss and marked falls in blood pressure.[51] Moreover, weight loss may reduce the sensitivity of blood pressure to sodium.[52] Although the rate of recidivism among obese people is high, an attempt at weight reduction in all obese hypertensive patients should be made, using whatever level of caloric restriction the patient is able to maintain.

DIETARY SODIUM RESTRICTION. On page 817 evidence was presented incriminating the typically high sodium content of the diet of people living in developed, industri-

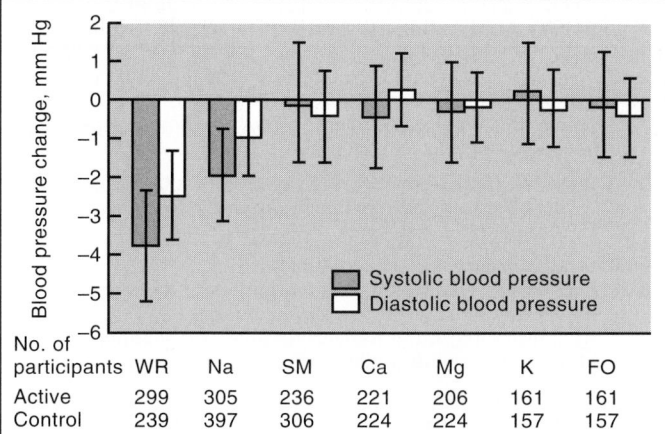

No. of participants	WR	Na	SM	Ca	Mg	K	FO
Active	299	305	236	221	206	161	161
Control	239	397	306	224	224	157	157

FIGURE 27–5. Net mean changes in systolic and diastolic blood pressure (baseline minus follow-up), with 95 per cent confidence intervals. WR = weight reduction; Na = sodium reduction; SM = stress management; Ca = calcium supplementation; Mg = magnesium supplementation; K = potassium supplementation; FO = fish oil supplementation. (From The Trials of Hypertension Prevention Collaborative Research Group: The effects of nonpharmacologic interventions on blood pressure of persons with high normal levels. Results of the Trials of Hypertension Prevention, Phase I. JAMA 267:1213, 1992. Copyright 1992 American Medical Association.)

alized societies as a cause of hypertension. Once hypertension is present, modest salt restriction may help lower the blood pressure. In a review by Cutler et al. of 20 well-controlled intervention studies in which daily intake (based on urinary sodium excretion) was reduced by as little as 16 to as much as 171 mmol/day, blood pressure reductions (beyond those seen in controls) averaged 4.9/2.6 mm Hg.[53] There is probably a dose-response relation—the more sodium reduction, the greater the blood pressure fall. In a small but well-controlled study, the fall in blood pressure was shown to be 8/5 mm Hg on a daily sodium intake of 100 mmol and 16/9 mm Hg on a 50 mmol per day intake.[54]

However, rigid degrees of sodium restriction are not only difficult for patients to achieve but may also be counterproductive.[55] The marked stimulation of renin-aldosterone that accompanies rigid sodium restriction may prevent the blood pressure from falling and increase the amount of potassium wastage if diuretics are concomitantly used. Not all hypertensives will respond to a moderate degree of sodium restriction to a level of 70 to 100 mmol sodium, or approximately 2 gm per day. Blacks and elderly patients may be more responsive to sodium restriction, perhaps because of their usually lower renin responsiveness.[56]

Even if the blood pressure does not fall with moderate degrees of sodium restriction, the patient may still benefit: Improved beta-adrenergic responsiveness,[57] increased antihypertensive effectiveness of other drugs,[58] less diuretic-induced potassium wastage,[55] and reduction in left ventricular hypertrophy[59] have all been reported among patients on moderate sodium restriction. Although there is no certainty that moderate sodium restriction will help, there is little evidence that it will hurt.[55] For example, neither the intake of other vital nutrients[60] nor exercise tolerance in a hot environment[61] is reduced by a lower sodium intake.

Therefore, I consider it to be useful for all persons, as a preventive measure in those who are normotensive, and, more certainly, as partial therapy in those who are hypertensive. Population-wide reductions may be possible[62] with a considerable potential thereby to reduce cardiovascular mortality.[63] Although some believe that a "wholesale recommendation to add sodium restriction to antihypertensive therapy is not warranted,"[64] I believe that the potential benefits far outweigh the costs.

The easiest way to accomplish moderate sodium restriction is to substitute natural foods for processed foods, since natural foods are low in sodium and high in potassium, whereas most processed foods have had sodium added and potassium removed. Additional guidelines include the following:

1. Add no sodium chloride to food during cooking or at the table.
2. If a salty taste is desired, use a half sodium and half potassium chloride preparation (such as Lite Salt) or a pure potassium chloride substitute.
3. Avoid or minimize the use of "fast" foods, many of which have high sodium content.
4. Recognize the sodium content of some antacids and proprie-

tary medications. (For example, Alka-Seltzer contains more than 500 mg of sodium; Rolaids are virtually sodium free.)

POTASSIUM SUPPLEMENTATION. Some of the advantages of a lower sodium intake may relate to its tendency to increase body potassium content, both by a coincidental increase in dietary potassium intake and by a decrease in potassium wastage if diuretics are being used. Potassium deficiency exerts multiple effects that may increase blood pressure,[65] and potassium infusions increase the vasodilating effect of acetylcholine, apparently through the nitric oxide pathway.[66] Potassium supplements have been shown to reduce the blood pressure an average of 8.2/4.5 mm Hg in 19 trials published up to 1990.[67] Nonetheless, potassium supplements are too costly and potentially hazardous for routine use in normokalemic hypertensives. Patients should be protected from potassium depletion and encouraged to increase dietary potassium intake, which may be enough to lower blood pressure.[68]

MAGNESIUM SUPPLEMENTATION. In controlled trials little effect on blood pressure is seen with magnesium supplements.[69] However, those who are magnesium depleted may not be able to replete concomitant potassium deficiency.[70]

CALCIUM SUPPLEMENTATION. As noted on page 818, an increase in free calcium concentration in vascular smooth muscle cells may be a final step in the pathogenesis of primary hypertension. Nonetheless, some hypertensive patients have a lower calcium intake and higher urinary calcium excretion than do normotensives.[71] In 22 mostly short-term studies, about one-third of hypertensives given 1 to 2 gm of supplemental calcium per day exhibited a fall in blood pressure.[72] Elderly hypertensives appeared to be even less responsive.[73] Because some given calcium supplements have a rise in blood pressure, the best course is to ensure that calcium intake is not inadvertently reduced by reduction of milk and cheese consumption in an attempt to reduce saturated fat and sodium intake when supplemental calcium is not taken.

OTHER DIETARY CHANGES. Some lowering of the blood pressure has been noted in studies of a lacto-ovo-vegetarian diet,[74] high fiber intake,[75] and high doses of omega-3 fatty acids from fish oil.[76] No additional effect of 6-gm daily supplements of fish oil was found in those who regularly ate fish three or more times a week.[77] Decreases in total dietary fat do not seem to alter blood pressure.[78] In the attempt to reduce calories and overall coronary risk, substitution of carbohydrate for fat may aggravate further the hyperinsulinemia often present in primary hypertension and therefore may be counterproductive.[79] Consumption of dried garlic powder lowered diastolic pressure in four of seven trials compared with placebo.[80]

When consumed by noncoffee drinkers, caffeine equivalent to the amount in two to three cups of coffee raises the blood pressure, probably by activation of the sympathetic nervous system.[81] However, chronic caffeine ingestion is not associated with significant rises in blood pressure because of tolerance to the hemodynamic effects.

MODERATION OF ALCOHOL. Moderate alcohol consumption, less than 1 oz of ethanol per day, does not increase the prevalence of hypertension. Heavier drinking clearly exerts a pressor effect that makes alcohol abuse the most common cause of reversible hypertension.[64] One to two portions of alcohol-containing beverages a day, containing 0.5 to 1.0 oz of ethanol, need not be prohibited, particu-

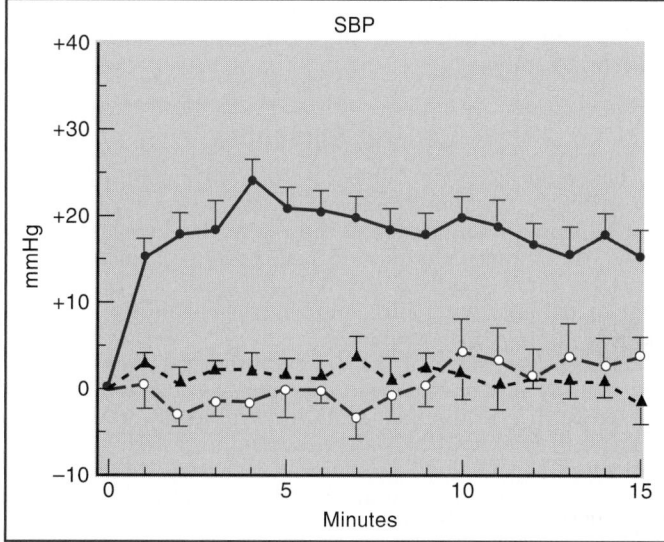

FIGURE 27–6. Changes in systolic blood pressure (SBP) over 15 minutes after smoking the first cigarette of the day within the first 5 minutes (solid circles), during no activity (open circles), and during sham-smoking (triangles) in normotensive smokers. (From Groppelli, A., et al.: Blood pressure and heart rate response to repeated smoking before and after beta blockade and selective α_1 inhibition. J. Hypertens. 10:495, 1992.)

larly because fewer coronary events and lower mortality have been noted in those who consume that amount.[82]

PHYSICAL EXERCISE. Although the systolic pressure rises considerably during dynamic (aerobic) exercise, vascular compliance increases[83] and resting blood pressure usually falls[84] in hypertensives after regular exercise programs. Unfit patients are at increased risk for coronary ischemia if they engage in heavy exercise,[85] and so a gradual buildup is advisable. Although pure static exercise acutely raises both systolic and diastolic pressures, repetitive circuit weight training also lowers blood pressure.[86]

RELAXATION TECHNIQUES. A review of 26 reports of various forms of relaxation—transcendental meditation, yoga, biofeedback, psychotherapy—reports that they were no more effective in lowering blood pressure than were sham controls.[87]

COMBINED THERAPIES

When multiple life style modifications are combined, additional antihypertensive effects may be seen. The best study is the placebo arm of the Treatment of Mild Hypertension Study (TOMHS),[2] in which 234 mild hypertensives followed a 48-month regimen of moderate sodium restriction, weight loss, regular exercise, and moderation of alcohol. Despite relatively small changes in weight (average loss of 6.6 lbs), sodium intake (reduction of 10 per cent), exercise level, and alcohol consumption, these patients had an 8.6/8.6 mm Hg fall in blood pressure at the end of the 4-year program. Moreover, they experienced improvements in lipid profile and reduction in left ventricular mass.

THE POTENTIAL OF LIFE STYLE MODIFICATIONS

Part of the antihypertensive effect reported in this and other trials of life style modification may be attributable to the nonspecific fall in blood pressure so often seen when repeated readings are taken. Such decreases may reflect a statistical regression toward the mean, a placebo effect, or a relief of anxiety and stress with time. The same phenomenon is probably also responsible for much of the initial response to drug therapy, so that success may be attributed to both drugs and nondrugs when it is deserved by neither.

Nonetheless, increasingly long and strong evidence from controlled studies attests to the efficacy of multifaceted nondrug programs to reduce the blood pressure. Whether such success can be achieved by individual practitioners is uncertain. However, because help is available, including various educational materials for patients, professional assistants such as dietitians and psychologists, and groups organized for weight reduction, exercise, and relaxation therapies, the effort seems both increasingly easy and likely to be successful in lowering blood pressure.

ANTIHYPERTENSIVE DRUG THERAPY

If the life style modifications just described are not followed or prove to be ineffective, or if the level of hypertension at the onset is so high that immediate drug therapy is deemed necessary, the general guidelines listed in Table 27–2 should be helpful in improving patient adherence to lifelong treatment.

General Guidelines

The points listed in Table 27–2 are all aimed at providing effective, 24-hour control of hypertension in a manner that encourages adherence to the regimen. The approach is based on known pharmacological principles and proven ways to improve adherence. It is designed for the 90 per cent of patients with fairly mild hypertension, in whom a gradual approach is feasible.

Once the selection of the most appropriate agent for initial therapy has been made (by a process that will be discussed further in the next section), a relatively low dose of a single drug should be started, aiming for a reduction of 5 to 10 mm Hg in blood pressure at each step. Many physicians, by nature and training, desire to control a patient's hypertension rapidly and completely. Regardless of which drugs are used, this approach often leads to easy fatigability, weakness, and postural dizziness, which many patients find intolerable, particularly when they felt well before therapy was begun. Although hypokalemia and other electrolyte abnormalities may be responsible for some of these symptoms, a more likely explanation has been provided by the studies of Strandgaard and Haunsø.[88] As shown in Fig-

TABLE 27–2   GENERAL GUIDELINES TO IMPROVE PATIENT ADHERENCE TO ANTIHYPERTENSIVE THERAPY

1. Be aware of the problem of nonadherence and be alert to signs of patient nonadherence.

2. Establish the goal of therapy: to reduce blood pressure to normotensive levels with minimal or no side effects.

3. Educate the patient about the disease and its treatment.
   a. Involve the patient in decision-making.
   b. Encourage family support.

4. Maintain contact with the patient.
   a. Encourage visits and calls to allied health personnel.
   b. Allow the pharmacist to monitor therapy.
   c. Give feedback to the patient via home BP readings.
   d. Make contact with patients who do not return.

5. Keep care inexpensive and simple.
   a. Do the least work-up needed to rule out secondary causes.
   b. Obtain follow-up laboratory data only yearly unless indicated more often.
   c. Use home blood pressure readings.
   d. Use nondrug, no-cost therapies.
   e. Use the fewest daily doses of drugs needed.
   f. If appropriate, use combination tablets.
   g. Tailor medication to daily routines.

6. Prescribe according to pharmacological principles.
   a. Add one drug at a time.
   b. Start with small doses, aiming for 5 to 10 mm Hg reductions at each step.
   c. Prevent volume overload with adequate diuretic and sodium restriction.
   d. Take medication immediately upon awakening or after 4 A.M. if patient awakens to void.
   e. Ensure 24-hour effectiveness by home or ambulatory monitoring.
   f. Continue to add effective and tolerated drugs, stepwise, in sufficient doses to achieve the goal of therapy.
   g. Be willing to stop unsuccessful therapy and try a different approach.
   h. Adjust therapy to ameliorate side effects that do not spontaneously disappear.

From Kaplan, N. M.: Clinical Hypertension. 6th ed. Baltimore, © Williams & Wilkins, 1994, p. 197.

ure 27–7, they demonstrated the constancy of cerebral blood flow by autoregulation over a range of mean arterial pressures from about 60 to 120 mm Hg in normal subjects and from 110 to 180 mm Hg in patients with hypertension. This shift to the right protects the hypertensive patient from a surge of blood flow, which could cause cerebral edema. However, the shift also predisposes the hypertensive patient to cerebral ischemia when blood pressure is lowered.

The lower limit of autoregulation necessary to preserve a constant cerebral blood flow in hypertensive patients is a mean of about 110 mm Hg. Thus acutely lowering the pressure from 160/110 (mean = 127) to 140/85 (mean = 102) may induce cerebral hypoperfusion, although hypotension in the accepted sense has not been produced. This provides an explanation for what many patients experience at the start of antihypertensive therapy, i.e., manifestations of cerebral hypoperfusion, even though blood pressure levels do not seem inordinately low.

Thus, there should be a gradual approach to antihypertensive therapy in order to avoid symptoms related to overly aggressive blood pressure reduction. Fortunately, as shown in the middle of Figure 27–7, if therapy is continued for a period of time, the curve of cerebral autoregulation shifts back toward normal, allowing patients to tolerate greater reductions in blood pressure without experiencing symptoms.

STARTING DOSAGES. The need to start with a fairly small dosage also reflects a greater responsiveness of some patients to doses of medication that may be appropriate for the majority. All drugs exert increasing effect with increasing dosages, portrayed by a log-linear dose-response curve[89] (Fig. 27–8). However, different patients re-

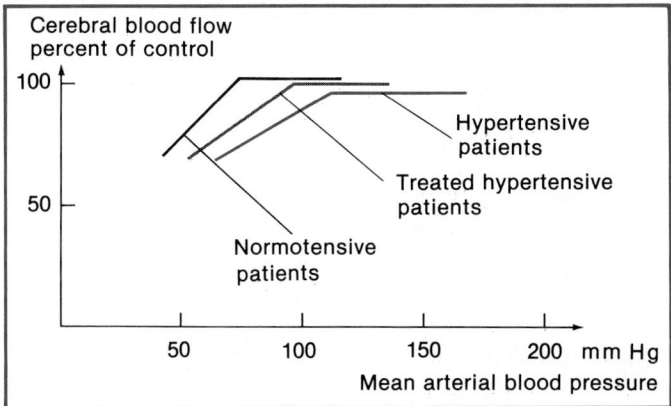

FIGURE 27–7. Mean cerebral blood flow autoregulation curves from normotensive, severely hypertensive, and effectively treated hypertensive patients are shown. (Modified from Strandgaard [Circulation 53:720, 1976.] From Strandgaaard, S., Haunsø, S.: Why does antihypertensive treatment prevent stroke but not myocardial infarction? Lancet 2:658, 1987. © by the Lancet Ltd.)

---

quire different absolute amounts of drug for their own dose response.

As a hypothetical example, for the majority of patients, 50 mg of the beta blocker atenolol would provide a moderate response, shown as point A on the Therapeutic Effect curve, whereas a dose of 25 mg would provide only a minimal response. At the dose A, providing the significant albeit partial response, the side effects would be minimal, as shown by point A' on the curve of Toxic Effect. If a starting dose of 100 mg were used, the therapeutic effect would be near maximal (point B) but the side effects would be much greater as well (point B'). Therefore, a lower starting dose is preferable for most patients.

However, the response to a given dose is not the same for all patients but rather assumes a bell-shaped curve; some patients are very sensitive to that dose and some very resistant, the majority having a moderate response. Therefore, a significant minority of patients—the very sensitive ones—would obtain a near-maximal response to the 25-mg dose and would better be started on 12.5 mg in order to achieve a moderate therapeutic effect (point A) with minimal side effects (point A'). Without knowing how individual patients will respond, the safest and easiest approach is to start at a dose that probably is not enough for most patients.

The situation was well described by Herxheimer.[90] "For a new drug to penetrate the market quickly, it should be rapidly effective in a high proportion of patients and simple to use. To achieve this, the dosage of the first prescription is therefore commonly set at about the ED_{90} level, i.e., the dose which the early clinical (phase 2) studies have shown to be effective in 90 per cent of the target population, provided that the unwanted effects at this dose are considered acceptable. In 25 per cent of patients a smaller—perhaps much smaller—

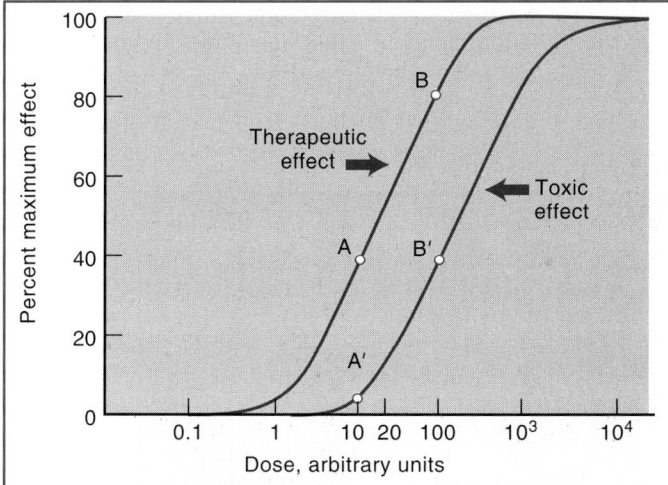

FIGURE 27–8. Theoretical therapeutic and toxic logarithmic-linear dose-response curves. The horizontal axis is a logarithmic scale with arbitrary dose units. The vertical axis is a linear scale showing percentage of maximum possible response. See text for discussion. (From Fagan, T. C.: Remembering the lessons of basic pharmacology. Arch. Intern. Med. 154:1430, 1994. Copyright 1994 American Medical Association.)

---

dose (the ED_{25}) will be effective. The patients in this quartile are the most sensitive to the drug and are liable to receive far more than they need if they are given the ED_{90}. They are also likely to be more sensitive to the dose-related side effects of the drug."

As I have written,[91] Herxheimer goes on to recommend a logical solution: starting doses should be less than the usual maximal effective dose. For this to be effective, however, physicians must be willing to start most patients with a dose of medication that will not be fully effective. As he states, "The disadvantage from the marketing standpoint is that for the majority of patients the dose must be titrated. That is time-consuming for doctors and patients and more difficult to explain to them. A drug requiring dose titration cannot be presented as the 'quick fix', the instant good news that marketing departments love."[90] The quick fix is inappropriate for most hypertensive patients. To allow for autoregulation of blood flow to maintain perfusion to vital organs when perfusion pressure is lowered, the fall in pressure should be relatively small and gradual.[88] More precipitous falls in pressure as frequently seen with larger starting doses may induce considerable hypoperfusion that results in symptoms that are at least bothersome (fatigue, impotence) and that may be potentially hazardous (postural hypotension, coronary ischemia). It is far better to start low and go slow.[91]

DRUG COMBINATIONS. Combinations of smaller doses of two drugs from different classes have been marketed to take advantage of the differences in the dose-response curves for therapeutic and toxic (side) effects shown in Figure 27–8.[91a] By combining two drugs, each at a dose near point A, a greater antihypertensive effect will be provided (up to point B), but because the side effects are not additive for different classes of drugs, they remain at point A'. A combination of low doses of a beta blocker (bisoprolol) and a diuretic (hydrochlorothiazide) has been approved for initial therapy for hypertension, after it was shown to provide antihypertensive efficacy far beyond that of each component but with no more side effects than seen with each separately.[92] More and more low-dose combinations are likely to become available.

COMPLETE COVERAGE WITH ONCE DAILY DOSING. A number of choices within each of the six major classes of antihypertensive drugs now available provide full 24-hour efficacy. Therefore, single daily dosing should be feasible for virtually all patients, thereby improving adherence to therapy.[93] Moreover, the use of longer-acting agents avoids the potential of inducing too great a peak effect in order to provide an adequate effect at the end of the dosing interval (the trough). As seen in Figure 27–9, when the angiotensin-converting enzyme (ACE) inhibitor enalapril was given in a once-daily dose large enough to achieve a trough effect, the peak effect was greater than desired.[94] When the same total dosage of the drug was given in two doses, a much smoother effect with excellent peak and trough effects was obtained.

Rather than adding to the patient's burden (and expense) of taking two doses a day, the better way to accomplish the desired sustained effect is to use inherently longer-acting drugs (or sustained-release formulations of shorter-acting ones). As noted, such choices are available within each class.[95] However, because patients differ not only as to degree of response but also as to the duration of effect, the prudent course is to document the patient's response at the end of the dosing interval by home or ambulatory monitoring. With this approach the abrupt surge in blood pressure that occurs on awakening will be blunted, and, it is hoped, patients can be better protected from the increased incidence of cardiovascular catastrophes at this crucial time.

If medications are taken at bedtime in order to ensure coverage in the early morning, ischemia to vital organs might be induced by the combination of the maximal effect of the drug within the first 3 to 6 hours after intake and the usual nocturnal fall in pressure. Therefore, the safest course is to take medications with 24-hour duration of action as early in the morning as possible, as early as 4 or 5 A.M. if the patient awakens to urinate.

THE INITIAL CHOICE. The initial choice of antihypertensive therapy is perhaps the most important decision made in the treatment process. That drug is likely to be effective in about half the patients and, if no significant overt side

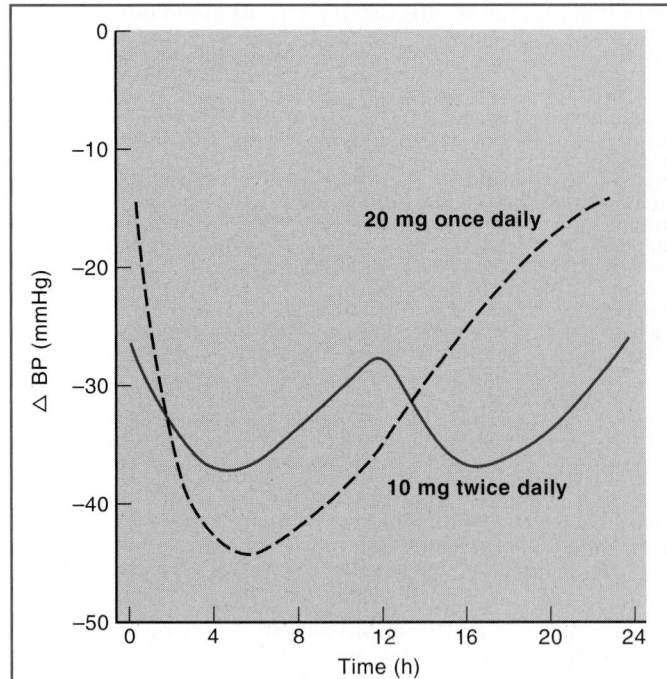

FIGURE 27–9. Comparison of blood pressure (BP) response profiles (placebo-controlled) in a representative patient following 20 mg enalapril once a day and 10 mg twice a day. (From Elliott, H.L.: Trough: Peak ratio and twenty-four-hour blood pressure control. J. Hypertens. *12*[Suppl. 5]:S29, 1994.)

effects occur, may be taken for many years. If the choice is ineffective or bothersome, the patient's confidence may be shaken, postponing or preventing adequate control. A number of guidelines by expert committees have been recently published. About half of them, including the U.S. Joint National Committee (JNC),[26] recommend diuretics or beta blockers for initial therapy.[96] The rationale is simple, as stated in the JNC-5 report: "Because diuretics and beta blockers are the only classes of drugs that have been used in long-term controlled clinical trials and have been shown to reduce morbidity and mortality, they are recommended as first-choice agents." The preference given to diuretics and beta blockers has been roundly criticized as a backward step, going against the rapidly rising use of newer agents.[97,98] However, the critics have failed to read the remainder of the JNC-5 statement: ". . . unless they are contraindicated or unacceptable, or unless there are special indications for other agents."[26]

There are multiple considerations listed in JNC-5 that may be taken into account when choosing initial therapy. These include demography, the presence of concomitant conditions, quality of life, physiological measurements, and cost. The importance of demography is nicely portrayed in the results of a large Veterans Administration cooperative trial in which younger and older and black and white hypertensive men were randomly assigned to a drug representing each of the six major classes or a placebo.[99] When the percentage of responders to each drug was determined for each demographic group, the same drug (the ACE inhibitor captopril) was found to be the most effective drug for the younger whites but the least effective drug for the older blacks.

INDIVIDUALIZED THERAPY. Perhaps the most crucial factor in the selection process is the presence of one or more concomitant conditions, some that could be worsened by the drug chosen, others that could be improved. Table 27–3 is my formulation of the relative appropriateness of members of the five major classes, not including centrally acting alpha-agonists, which are not included in the JNC-5 choices for initial therapy. Most of these preferences or contraindications are obvious; others will be defended later in this chapter. Regardless of the correctness of this formulation, the concept is absolutely valid: The choice of therapy should be individualized.

SUBSTITUTION. Even after a careful attempt to select the most appropriate drug for an individual patient, the choice may be either ineffectual in perhaps a third or unacceptable because of side effects in another 10 to 20 per cent of all patients. Although the overall effectiveness of all approved drugs is about equal in the general population,[2] individual patients show considerable variability in their response to different drugs.[100] Therefore, the physician must be willing to discontinue the initial choice and try a drug from another category. A more structured trial and error approach has been described in which each patient is put through multiple double-blind, randomized crossover trials against placebos to determine the best drug.[101] However, this approach probably is too much trouble for most physicians and patients. Other approaches have been recommended, including one based on the renin profile[102] and another on multiple hemodynamic features.[103] The general principles shown in Tables 27–2 and 27–3 should serve well to ensure that each patient receives a drug likely to provide good control and few side effects.

For patients with more severe hypertension, in whom the first choice can be expected to be only partially effective, the stepped-care approach is logical. A diuretic will enhance the effectiveness of most other drugs used, preventing the "pseudotolerance" that develops because of the fluid retention that frequently follows the use of some adrenergic blocking drugs and vasodilators. Increasingly, an

TABLE 27–3   INDIVIDUALIZED CHOICES OF THERAPY

COEXISTING CONDITION	DIURETIC	BETA BLOCKER	ALPHA BLOCKER	CALCIUM BLOCKER	ACEI
Older age (> 65)	++	+/−	+	+	+
Black race	++	+/−	+	+	+/−
Angina	+/−	++	+	++	+
Post-myocardial infarction	+	++	+	+/−*	++
Congestive failure	++	+/−	+	−	++
Cerebrovascular disease	+	+	+/−	++	+
Renal insufficiency	++	+/−	+	++	++
Diabetes	+/−	−	++	+	++
Dyslipidemia	−	−	++	+	+
Asthma or COPD	+	−	+	+	+
Benign prostatic hypertrophy			++		

++ = preferred; + = suitable; +/− = usually not preferred; − = usually contraindicated; * = dihydropyridines may be contraindicated; ACEI = angiotensin-converting enzyme inhibitors.

ACE inhibitor or calcium antagonist is being chosen as the second or third drug when triple therapy is needed.

THE GOAL OF THERAPY. As discussed earlier in the chapter, caution is advised in lowering diastolic pressure below 85 mm Hg, the apparent nadir of the J curve, particularly in patients prone to coronary disease. On the other hand, lower levels may prove to be maximally effective in other groups such as diabetics with nephropathy.

THE PLACE OF GUIDELINES. As noted, a number of guidelines on the treatment of hypertension by expert committees have recently been published (see p. 1991). Although considerable differences exist between them and a number of valid objections have been raised to the entire process of establishing such guidelines,[96] these structured recommendations are finding increased use in the rapidly expanding world of managed care.[104] Like them or not they have a place, and I believe they should be used, not as rigid legal documents but as gentle persuasions coming from the best-thinking of independent, informed experts who wish to ease the way for the harried practitioner.

DIURETICS

(See also pp. 498 to 499)

Diuretics useful in the treatment of hypertension may be divided into four major groups by their primary site of action within the tubule, starting in the proximal portion and moving to the collecting duct: (1) agents acting on the proximal tubule, such as carbonic anhydrase inhibitors, which have limited antihypertensive efficacy; (2) loop diuretics; (3) thiazides and related sulfonamide compounds; and (4) potassium-sparing agents (Fig. 16–3, p. 476). A thiazide is the usual choice, often in combination with a potassium-sparing agent. Loop diuretics should be reserved for those patients with renal insufficiency or resistant hypertension.

MECHANISM OF ACTION. All diuretics initally lower the blood pressure by increasing urinary sodium excretion and by reducing plasma volume, extracellular fluid volume, and cardiac output.[91a] Within 6 to 8 weeks the lowered plasma, extracellular fluid volume, and cardiac output return toward normal. At this point and beyond, the lower blood pressure is related to a fall in peripheral resistance, thereby improving the underlying hemodynamic defect of hypertension. The mechanism responsible for the lowered peripheral resistance is unknown, but there is a need for an initial diuresis, because diuretics fail to lower the blood pressure when the excreted sodium is returned or when given to chronic dialysis patients with nonfunctioning kidneys. With the shrinkage in blood volume and lower blood pressure, increased secretion of renin and aldosterone retards the continued sodium diuresis. Both renin-induced vasoconstriction and aldosterone-induced sodium retention prevent continued diminution of body fluids and progressive fall in blood pressure while diuretic therapy is continued.

CLINICAL EFFECTS. With continuous diuretic therapy, blood pressure usually falls about 10 mm Hg, although the degree depends on various factors, including the initial height of the pressure, the quantity of sodium ingested, the adequacy of renal function, and the intensity of the counterregulatory renin-aldosterone response. The antihypertensive effect of the diuretic persists indefinitely, although it may be overwhelmed by dietary sodium intake above 8 gm per day.

If other antihypertensive drugs are used, a diuretic may also be needed. Without a concomitant diuretic, antihypertensive drugs that do not block the renin-aldosterone mechanism may cause sodium retention. This mechanism probably reflects the success of the drugs in lowering the blood pressure and may involve the abnormal renal pres-

sure–natriuresis relationship that is presumably present in primary hypertension. Just as it takes more pressure to excrete a given load of sodium in the hypertensive individual, so does a lowering of pressure toward normal incite sodium retention.

The crucial need for adequate diuretic therapy to keep intravascular volume diminished has been repeatedly documented.[105] Therefore, diuretics are likely to continue to be widely used in antihypertensive therapy. Drugs that inhibit the renin-aldosterone mechanism, such as ACE inhibitors, or drugs that induce some natriuresis themselves, such as calcium antagonists, may continue to work without the need for concomitant diuretics. However, a diuretic will enhance the effectiveness of all other types of drugs, including calcium antagonists.[106]

DOSAGE AND CHOICE OF AGENT. Most patients with mild to moderate hypertension and serum creatinine concentrations below 2.0 mg/dl will respond to the lower doses of the various diuretics listed in Table 27–4. An amount equivalent to 12.5 mg of hydrochlorothiazide is usually adequate; larger doses will have some additional antihypertensive effect but at the price of additional potassium wastage and insulin resistance.[107] For uncomplicated hypertension, a moderately long-acting thiazide is a logical choice, and a single morning dose of hydrochlorothiazide will provide a 24-hour antihypertensive effect. The nonthiazide agent indapamide has special properties that make it an attractive choice; it seldom disturbs lipid or glucose levels.[108] With renal failure, manifested by a serum creatinine level above 2.0 mg/dl or creatinine clearance below 25 ml/min, thiazides are usually not effective, and multiple doses of furosemide, one or two doses of torsemide,[109] or a single dose of metolazone will be needed.

SIDE EFFECTS. A number of biochemical changes often accompany successful diuresis, including a decrease in plasma potassium and increases in glucose, insulin, and cholesterol (Fig. 27–10).

Hypokalemia. Serum potassium falls an average of 0.67 mmol/liter after institution of continuous, daily diuretic

TABLE 27–4 DIURETICS AND POTASSIUM-SPARING AGENTS

AGENT	DAILY DOSAGE (mg)	DURATION OF ACTION (hr)
THIAZIDES		
Bendroflumethiazide (Naturetin)	2.5–5.0	More than 18
Benzthiazide (Aquatag, Exna)	12.5–50	12–18
Chlorothiazide (Diuril)	125–500	6–12
Cyclothiazide (Anhydron)	0.5–2	18–24
Hydrochlorothiazide (Esidrix, HydroDIURIL, Oretic)	6.25–50	12–18
Hydroflumethiazide (Saluron)	12.5–50	18–24
Methyclothiazide (Enduron)	2.5–5.0	More than 24
Polythiazide (Renese)	1–4	24–48
Trichlormethiazide (Metahydrin, Naqua)	1–4	More than 24
RELATED SULFONAMIDE COMPOUNDS		
Chlorthalidone (Hygroton)	12.5–50	24–72
Indapamide (Lozol)	2.5	24
Metolazone (Zaroxolyn, Diulo)	0.5–10	24
Quinethazone (Hydromox)	25–100	18–24
LOOP DIURETICS		
Bumetanide (Bumex)	0.5–5	4–6
Ethacrynic acid (Edecrin)	25–100	12
Furosemide (Lasix)	40–480	4–6
Torsemide (Demadex)	5–40	12
POTASSIUM-SPARING AGENTS		
Amiloride (Midamor)	5–10	24
Spironolactone (Aldactone)	25–100	8–12
Triamterene (Dyrenium)	50–100	12

From Kaplan, N. M.: Clinical Hypertension. 6th ed. Baltimore, © by Williams and Wilkins, 1994, p. 200.

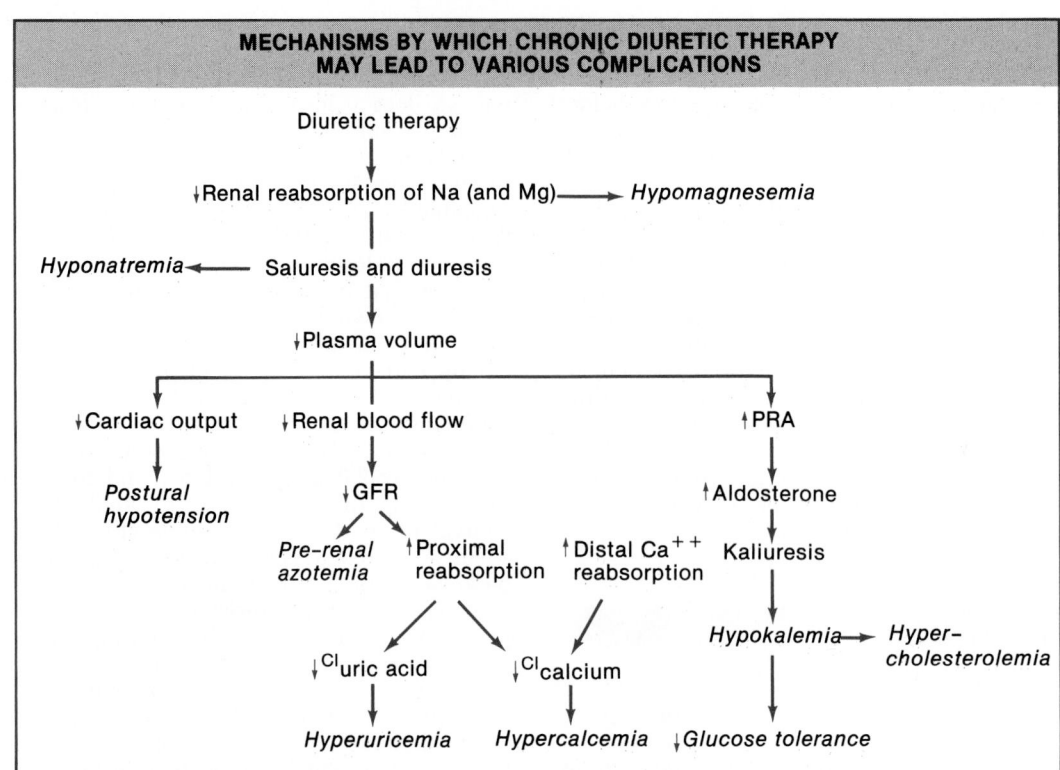

FIGURE 27–10. The mechanisms by which chronic diuretic therapy may lead to various complications. The mechanism for hypercholesterolemia remains in question, although it is shown as arising via hypokalemia. Cl = clearance; PRA = plasma renin activity; GFR = Glomerular filtration rate. (From Kaplan, N. M.: Clinical Hypertension. 6th ed. Baltimore, © by Williams & Wilkins, 1994, p. 203.)

therapy for hypertension.[110] Among 158 hypertensives given diuretics for 2 years, plasma potassium levels fell to between 3.0 and 3.3 mmol/liter in 29 per cent and to between 2.6 and 2.9 mmol/liter in 7 per cent.[111] This fall in serum concentration may not reflect a significant decrease in total body potassium nor may it progress after the initial decline. Nevertheless, it may precipitate potentially hazardous ventricular ectopic activity and increase the risk of primary cardiac arrest,[112] even in patients not known to be susceptible because of concomitant digitalis therapy or myocardial irritability. The arrhythmogenic effect of diuretic-induced hypokalemia may become manifested only at times of stress, when catecholamines may lower the plasma potassium level another 0.5 to 1.0 mmol/liter or when beta-adrenergic agonists are used as bronchodilators.[113]

Most patients are unaware of mild diuretic-induced hypokalemia, although it may contribute to leg cramps, polyuria, and muscle weakness, but subtle interference with antihypertensive therapy may accompany even mild hypokalemia, and correction of hypokalemia may result in a fall in blood pressure.[114] In addition to increasing the propensity to ventricular ectopic activity, hypokalemia may be responsible for the worsening of insulin resistance, the loss of carbohydrate tolerance, and the rise in plasma lipids seen with diuretic use.[115]

Prevention of hypokalemia is preferable to correction of potassium deficiency. The following maneuvers should help prevent diuretic-induced hypokalemia:

- Use the smallest dose of diuretic needed.
- Use a moderately long-acting (12- to 18-hour) diuretic, such as hydrocholorothiazide, because longer-acting drugs (e.g., chlorthalidone) may increase potassium loss.
- Restrict sodium intake to less than 100 mmol per day (i.e., 2 gm sodium).
- Increase dietary potassium intake.
- Restrict concomitant use of laxatives.

- Use a combination of a thiazide with a potassium-sparing agent except in patients with renal insufficiency or in association with an ACE inhibitor.
- The concomitant use of a beta blocker or an ACE inhibitor will diminish potassium loss by blunting the diuretic-induced rise in renin-aldosterone.

If hypokalemia is to be treated, these principles should be followed, along with some form of supplemental potassium. Potassium chloride is preferred for correction of the associated alkalosis. If tolerated, granular potassium chloride can be given as a salt substitute; thereby, extra potassium will be provided while sodium intake is reduced. Caution is necessary when supplemental potassium chloride is given to older patients with borderline renal function in whom hyperkalemia may be induced.

HYPOMAGNESEMIA. In some patients concomitant diuretic-induced magnesium deficiency will prevent the restoration of intracellular deficits of potassium[116] so that hypomagnesemia should be corrected. Magnesium deficiency may also be responsible for some of the arrhythmias ascribed to hypokalemia.[117]

HYPERURICEMIA. The serum uric acid level is elevated in as many as one-third of untreated hypertensive patients. With chronic diuretic therapy, hyperuricemia appears in another third of patients, probably as a consequence of increased proximal tubular reabsorption accompanying volume contraction. Diuretic-induced hyperuricemia precipitates acute gout, most frequently in those who are obese and consume large amounts of alcohol.[118] Since asymptomatic hyperuricemia does not cause urate deposition, most investigators agree that it need not be treated. If therapy is used, a uricosuric drug such as probenecid should be given. Although allopurinol is often used, it is more likely to cause side effects and is a less rational choice, since the problem is a failure to excrete uric acid and not its overproduction.

HYPERLIPIDEMIA. Serum cholesterol levels often rise after diuretic therapy.[119] Although the rise in lipids can be prevented by a diet low in saturated fat, the propensity toward worsening of the lipid profile may inhibit the potential for diuretic therapy to reduce the incidence of coronary disease while it lowers blood pressure.

HYPERGLYCEMIA AND INSULIN RESISTANCE. Diuretics may impair glucose tolerance and precipitate diabetes mellitus,[115] probably because they increase insulin resistance and hyperinsulinemia.[120] The manner by which diuretics increase insulin resistance is uncertain, but in view of the multiple potential pressor actions of hyperinsulinemia (see p. 820), this could be a significant problem.

HYPERCALCEMIA. A slight rise in serum calcium, less than 0.5 mg/dl, is frequently seen with thiazide diuretic therapy, at least in part because increased calcium reabsorption accompanies the increased sodium reabsorption in the proximal tubule induced by contraction of extracellular fluid volume.[121] The rise is of little concern except in patients with previously unrecognized hyperparathyroidism, who may experience a much more marked rise. On the other hand, the diuretic-induced positive calcium balance is associated with a reduction in the incidence of osteoporosis in the elderly.[122]

IMPOTENCE. A high incidence of impotence (22.6 per cent) was found among men taking 10 mg of bendroflumethiazide per day, compared with a rate of 10.1 per cent among those on placebo and 13.2 per cent among those on propranolol in the large MRC trial.[123]

LOOP DIURETICS. Loop diuretics are usually needed in the treatment of hypertensive patients with renal failure defined here as a serum creatinine exceeding approximately 2.0 mg/dl. Furosemide has been most widely used, although either torsemide[109] or metolazone may be as effective, and each requires only a single daily dose. Many physicians use furosemide in the management of uncomplicated hypertension, but this drug provides less antihypertensive action when given once or twice a day than do longer-acting diuretics, which maintain a slight volume contraction.

POTASSIUM-SPARING AGENTS. These drugs are normally used in combination with a thiazide diuretic. Of the three currently available, one (spironolactone) is an aldosterone antagonist, while the other two (triamterene and amiloride) are direct inhibitors of potassium secretion. In combination with a thiazide diuretic, they will diminish the amount of potassium wasting. Although they are more expensive than thiazides alone, they may decrease the total cost of therapy by reducing the need to monitor and treat potassium depletion.

An Overview of Diuretics in Hypertension

Diuretics have been effective for the treatment of millions of hypertensive patients during the past 30 years. They reduce DBP and maintain it below 90 mm Hg in about half of all hypertensive patients, providing the same degree of effectiveness as most other antihypertensive drugs.[2] In two groups that constitute a rather large portion of the hypertensive population, the elderly[124] and blacks,[99] diuretics may be particularly effective. One-half of a diuretic tablet per day is usually all that is needed, minimizing cost and maximizing adherence to therapy. Even lower doses, i.e., 6.25 mg of hydrochlorothiazide, may be adequate when combined with other drugs.[92]

The side effects of high-dose diuretic therapy are usually not overtly bothersome, but the hypokalemia, hypercholesterolemia, hyperinsulinemia, and worsening of glucose tolerance that often accompany prolonged diuretic therapy gave rise to concerns about their long-term benignity. However, lower doses are usually just as potent as higher doses in lowering the blood pressure and less likely to induce metabolic mischief.[107] Therefore, the advocacy of low-dose diuretic therapy in the 1993 JNC-5 report[26] and by most expert committees[96] and reviewers[4] is appropriate.

ADRENERGIC INHIBITORS

A number of drugs that inhibit the adrenergic nervous system are available, including some that act centrally on vasomotor center activity, peripherally on neuronal catecholamine discharge, or by blocking alpha- and/or beta-adrenergic receptors (Table 27–5); some act at multiple sites. Figure 27–11, a schematic view of the ending of an adrenergic nerve and the effector cell with its receptors, depicts how some of these drugs act. When the nerve is stimulated, norepinephrine, which is synthesized intraneuronally and stored in granules, is released into the synaptic cleft. It binds to postsynaptic alpha- and beta-adrenergic receptors and thereby initiates various intracellular processes. In vascular smooth muscle, alpha stimulation causes constriction and beta stimulation causes relaxation. In the central vasomotor centers, sympathetic outflow is inhibited by alpha stimulation; the effect of central beta stimulation is unknown.

An important aspect of sympathetic activity involves the feedback of norepinephrine to alpha- and beta-adrenergic receptors located on the neuronal surface, i.e., presynaptic

1. PERIPHERAL NEURONAL INHIBITORS
  a. Reserpine
  b. Guanethidine (Ismelin)
  c. Guanadrel (Hylorel)
  d. Bethanidine (Tenathan)

2. CENTRAL ADRENERGIC INHIBITORS
  a. Methyldopa (Aldomet)
  b. Clonidine (Catapres)
  c. Guanabenz (Wytensin)
  d. Guanfacine (Tenex)

3. α-RECEPTOR BLOCKERS
  a. α_1- and α_2-receptor
    (1) Phenoxybenzamine (Dibenzyline)
    (2) Phentolamine (Regitine)
  b. α_1-receptor
    (1) Doxazosin (Cardura)
    (2) Prazosin (Minipress)
    (3) Terazosin (Hytrin)

4. β-RECEPTOR BLOCKERS
  a. Acebutolol (Sectral)
  b. Atenolol (Tenormin)
  c. Betaxolol (Kerlone)
  d. Bisoprolol (Zebeta)
  e. Carteolol (Cartrol)
  f. Metoprolol (Lopressor, Toprol)
  g. Nadolol (Corgard)
  h. Penbutolol (Levatol)
  i. Pindolol (Visken)
  j. Propranolol (Inderal)
  k. Timolol (Blocadren)

5. α- AND β-RECEPTOR BLOCKER
Labetalol (Normodyne, Trandate)

receptors. Presynaptic alpha-adrenergic receptor activation inhibits release, whereas presynaptic beta activation stimulates further norepinephrine release. The presynaptic receptors probably play a role in the action of some of the drugs to be discussed.

Elucidation and quantitation of the various actions of these drugs remain incomplete. The listing in Table 27–5 is based on the predominant site of action according to currently available data. The action of beta-adrenergic receptor blockers involves a peripheral effect, but they almost certainly also act on central vasomotor mechanisms.

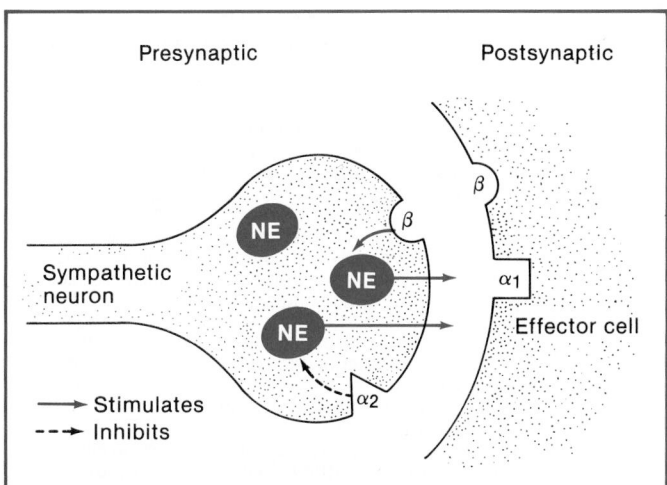

FIGURE 27–11. Simplified schematic view of the adrenergic nerve ending showing that norepinephrine (NE) is released from its storage granules when the nerve is stimulated and enters the synaptic cleft to bind to alpha$_1$ and beta receptors on the effector cell (postsynaptic). In addition, a short feedback loop exists, in which NE binds to alpha$_2$ and beta receptors on the neuron (presynaptic), to inhibit or to stimulate further release, respectively.

Reserpine, guanethidine, and related compounds act differently to inhibit the release of norepinephrine from peripheral adrenergic neurons.

RESERPINE. Reserpine, the most active and widely used of the derivatives of the rauwolfia alkaloids, depletes the postganglionic adrenergic neurons of norepinephrine by inhibiting its uptake into storage vesicles, exposing it to degradation by cytoplasmic monoamine oxidase. The peripheral effect is predominant, although the drug enters the brain and depletes central catecholamine stores as well. This probably accounts for the sedation and depression seen with reserpine use. The drug has certain advantages. Only one dose a day is needed; in combination with a diuretic, the antihypertensive effect is significant, greater than that noted with propranolol in one comparative study[125]; little postural hypotension is noted; and many patients experience no side effects. The drug has a relatively flat dose-response curve, so that a dose of only 0.05 mg per day will give almost as much antihypertensive effect as 0.125 or 0.25 mg per day but fewer side effects.[126] However, the psychological depression that occurs in perhaps 2 per cent of patients may be severe but difficult to recognize and treat. Although it remains popular in some places, the use of reserpine has declined progressively because it has no commercial sponsor.[127]

GUANETHIDINE. This agent and a series of related guanidine compounds, including guanadrel, bethanidine, and debrisoquine, act by inhibiting the release of norepinephrine from the adrenergic neurons, perhaps by a local anesthetic-like effect on the neuronal membrane. In order to act, the drug must be transported actively into the nerve through an amine pump. Various drugs, in particular tricyclic antidepressants, amphetamines, and ephedrine, competitively block the uptake of guanethidine into the nerves and thereby antagonize its effects.

Their low lipid solubility prevents guidance compounds from entering the brain, so that sedation, depression, and other side effects involving the central nervous system are not seen. Initially, the predominant hemodynamic effect is to decrease cardiac output; after continued use, peripheral resistance declines. Blood pressure is reduced further when the patient is upright, owing to gravitational pooling of blood in the legs, since compensatory sympathetic nervous system–mediated vasoconstriction is blocked. This results in the most common side effect, postural hypotension. Patients should be advised to arise slowly, sleep with the head of the bed elevated, and wear elastic hose to minimize this potential problem. Unlike reserpine, guanethidine has a steep dose-response curve, so that it can be successfully used in treating hypertension of any degree in daily doses of 10 to 300 mg. Like reserpine, it has a long biological half-life and may be given once daily. As other drugs have become available, guanethidine and related compounds have been relegated mainly to the treatment of severe hypertension unresponsive to all other agents.

Drugs That Act on Receptors

Predominantly Central Alpha Agonists

Until the mid-1980's, methyldopa was the most widely used of the adrenergic receptor blockers, but its use has fallen off as beta blockers and other drugs have become more popular. In addition, three other drugs—clonidine, guanabenz, and guanfacine, which act similarly to methyldopa but have fewer serious side effects—have become available.

METHYLDOPA. The primary site of action of methyldopa is within the central nervous system, where alpha-methylnorepinephrine, derived from methyldopa, is released from adrenergic neurons and stimulates central alpha-adrenergic receptors, reducing the sympathetic outflow from the central nervous system.[128] The blood pressure mainly falls as a result of a decrease in peripheral resistance with little effect on cardiac output. However, methyldopa, in concert with other antihypertensive agents that decrease sympathetic activity, may reduce the degree of left ventricular hypertrophy as noted by echocardiography.[129] Renal blood flow is well maintained, and significant postural hypotension is unusual. Therefore, the drug has been widely used in hypertensive patients with renal failure or cerebrovascular disease.

Methyldopa need be given no more than twice daily, in doses ranging from 250 to 3000 mg per day.

Side effects include some that are common to centrally acting drugs that reduce sympathetic outflow: sedation, dry mouth, impotence, and galactorrhea. However, methyldopa causes some unique side effects that are probably of an autoimmune nature, since a positive antinuclear antibody test is seen in about 10 per cent of patients who take the drug, and red cell autoantibodies occur in about 20 per cent. Clinically apparent hemolytic anemia is rare, probably because methyldopa also impairs reticuloendothelial function so that antibody-sensitized cells are not removed from the circulation and hemolyzed.[130] Inflammatory disorders in various organs have been re-

ported, most commonly involving the liver (with diffuse parenchymal injury similar to viral hepatitis).[131]

CLONIDINE. Although of different structure, clonidine shares many features with methyldopa. It probably acts at the same central sites, has similar antihypertensive efficacy, and causes many of the same bothersome but less serious side effects (e.g., sedation, dry mouth). It does not, however, induce the autoimmune and inflammatory side effects.

As an alpha-adrenergic receptor agonist, the drug also acts on presynaptic alpha receptors and inhibits norepinephrine release (Fig. 27–11), and plasma catecholamine levels fall.[132] The drug has a fairly short biological half-life, so that when it is discontinued, the inhibition of norepinephrine release disappears within about 12 to 18 hours, and plasma catecholamine levels rise. This is probably responsible for the rapid rebound of the blood pressure to pretreatment levels and the occasional appearance of withdrawal symptoms, including tachycardia, restlessness, and sweating. Rarely, the blood pressure increases beyond the pretreatment level. If the rebound requires treatment, clonidine may be reintroduced or alpha-adrenergic receptor antagonists given. Similar "overshoots" have been reported less commonly after the discontinuation of a variety of other antihypertensives.[133]

Clonidine is available in a *transdermal* preparation, which may provide smoother blood pressure control for as long as 7 days with fewer side effects. However, bothersome skin rashes preclude its use in perhaps one-fourth of patients.[134]

GUANABENZ. This drug differs in structure but shares many characteristics with both methyldopa and clonidine, acting primarily as a central alpha agonist. It may differ, however, in not causing fluid retention,[135] so that it may turn out to be effective without the need for a concomitant diuretic. Moreover, unlike diuretics, guanabenz has been found to reduce serum cholesterol.[136]

GUANFACINE. This drug is also similar to clonidine but is longer acting, which enables once-a-day dosing and minimizes rebound hypertension.[137]

Alpha-Adrenergic Receptor Antagonists

Before 1977 the only alpha blockers used to treat hypertension were phenoxybenzamine (Dibenzyline) and phentolamine (Regitine). These drugs are effective in acutely lowering blood pressure, but their effects are offset by an accompanying increase in cardiac output, and side effects are frequent and bothersome. Their limited efficacy may reflect their blockade of presynaptic alpha-adrenergic receptors, which interferes with the feedback inhibition of norepinephrine release (Fig. 27–11). Increased catecholamine release would then blunt the action of postsynaptic alpha-adrenergic receptor blockade. Their use has largely been limited to the treatment of patients with pheochromocytomas.

PRAZOSIN. This was the first of a group of selective antagonists of the postsynaptic alpha$_1$ receptors. By blocking alpha-mediated vasoconstriction, prazosin induces a fall in peripheral resistance with both venous and arteriolar dilation. Because the presynaptic alpha-adrenergic receptor is left unblocked, the feedback loop for the inhibition of norepinephrine release is intact, an action that is also certainly responsible for the greater antihypertensive effect of the drug and the absence of concomitant tachycardia, tolerance, and renin release. The inhibition of norepinephrine release may also account for the propensity toward greater first-dose falls in blood pressure.

OTHER ALPHA BLOCKERS. Two other alpha blockers, terazosin[138] and doxazosin,[139] are available. Beyond longer duration of action and less propensity for first-dose hypotension, they appear to differ little from prazosin.

Selective alpha blockers are as effective as other first-line antihypertensives.[2] When given to patients whose condition is poorly controlled on standard triple therapy (diuretic, beta blocker, and vasodilator), they may reduce blood pressure even more than anticipated.[140] They can be safely and effectively used in patients with renal failure. The favorable hemodynamic changes—a fall in peripheral resistance with maintenance of cardiac output—make them an attractive choice for patients who wish to remain physically active. In addition, blood lipids are not adversely altered and may actually improve with alpha blockers, unlike the adverse effects observed with diuretics and beta blockers.[141] Moreover, improved insulin sensitivity with lesser rises in plasma glucose and insulin levels after a glucose load has been observed with alpha blockers.[142] Alpha blockers decrease the smooth muscle tone of the bladder neck and prostate, relieving the obstructive symptoms of prostatism.[143] They are then an excellent choice for older men with benign prostatic hypertrophy.

Side effects, beyond first-dose postural hypotension, include the nonspecific effects of lower blood pressure, such as dizziness, weakness, fatigue, and headaches. Most patients, however, find the drugs easy to take, with little sedation, dry mouth, or impotence.

Beta-Adrenergic Receptor Antagonists
(See also p. 610)

In the 1980's, beta-adrenergic receptor blockers became the most popular form of antihypertensive therapy after diuretics, reflecting their relative effectiveness and freedom from many bothersome side effects. For the majority of patients, beta blockers are usually easy to take, because somnolence, dry mouth, and impotence are seldom encountered. Because beta blockers have been found to reduce mortality if taken either before or after acute myocardial infarction,[144] i.e., secondary prevention, it was assumed that they might offer special protection against initial coronary events, i.e., primary prevention. However, in four large clinical trials, a beta blocker provided no more protection than did a diuretic.[15,123,145,146] In the continuation of the HAPPHY trial, the group who remained on metoprolol experienced a lower eventual coronary mortality and morbidity rate than did the one who continued on a diuretic.[147,148]

THE VARIETY OF BETA BLOCKERS. Beta blockers now available in the United States are listed in Table 27–5, and others are available in other countries. A number of agents with additional vasodilatory effects will probably soon be approved for use in the United States, and they may be free of many of the unfavorable hemodynamic and adverse effects of currently available agents.[149] Pharmacologically, those now available differ considerably from one another with respect to degree of absorption, protein binding, and bioavailability. However, the three most important differences affecting their clinical use are cardioselectivity, intrinsic sympathomimetic activity, and lipid solubility. Despite these differences, they all seem to be about equally as effective as antihypertensives.

Cardioselectivity. As seen in Figure 27–12, beta blockers can be classified by their degree of cardioselectivity relative to their blocking effect on the beta$_1$-adrenergic receptors in the heart compared with that on the beta$_2$ receptors in the bronchi, peripheral blood vessels, and elsewhere. Such cardioselectivity can be easily shown using small doses in acute studies; with the rather high

doses used to treat hypertension, much of this selectivity is lost.

Intrinsic Sympathomimetic Activity (ISA). Some of these drugs have ISA, interacting with beta receptors to cause a measurable agonist response but at the same time blocking the greater agonist effects of endogenous catecholamines. As a result, while in usual doses they lower the blood pressure about the same degree as do other beta blockers, they cause a smaller decline in heart rate, cardiac output, and renin levels. As noted under Side Effects, ISA may blunt the adverse effects on lipid metabolism seen with non-ISA beta blockers.[150]

Lipid Solubility. Atenolol and nadolol are among the least lipid-soluble of the beta blockers. This could translate into two clinically important advantages. First, because they escape hepatic inactivation and are excreted virtually unchanged through the kidneys (Fig. 27–13), they remain as active drugs in the plasma much longer, allowing once-a-day dosage. Second, because they do not enter the brain as readily, they may cause fewer central nervous system side effects.[151]

Mechanism of Action. Despite these and other differences, the various beta blockers now available are approximately equipotent as antihypertensive agents. How they lower the blood pressure remains uncertain, although a number of possible mechanisms are likely to be involved. In those without ISA, cardiac output falls 15 to 20 per cent and renin release is reduced about 60 per cent. Central nervous system beta-adrenergic receptor blockade may reduce sympathetic discharge, but similar antihypertensive effects are seen with those drugs that are more lipid-soluble, and therefore in high concentration within the central nervous system, and those that are less lipid-soluble.

At the same time that beta blockers lower blood pressure through various means, their blockade of peripheral beta-adrenergic receptors inhibits vasodilation, leaving alpha receptors open to catecholamine-mediated vasoconstriction. However, over time, vascular resistance tends to return to normal, which presumably preserves the antihypertensive effect of a reduced cardiac output.[152]

Clinical Effects. Even in small doses, beta blockers begin to lower the blood pressure within a few hours, although their maximal effect may not be noted for some weeks. Even though progressively higher doses have usually been given, careful study has shown a near-maximal effect from smaller doses. For example, in a double-blind crossover study involving 24 patients, 40 mg of propranolol twice a day provided the same antihypertensive effects as 80, 160, or 240 mg twice a day.[153] The degree of blood pressure reduction is at least comparable to that noted with other antihypertensive drugs. Because beta blockers, along with diuretics, are the only class of antihypertensive drugs tested in large clinical trials and thereby shown to reduce mortality, they have been given preference in JNC-5 and elsewhere.[4] They may be particularly well suited for younger and middle-aged hypertensives, especially non-blacks, and in patients with myocardial ischemia and high levels of stress.[154] However, since the hemodynamic responses to stress are reduced, they may interfere with athletic performance.[155]

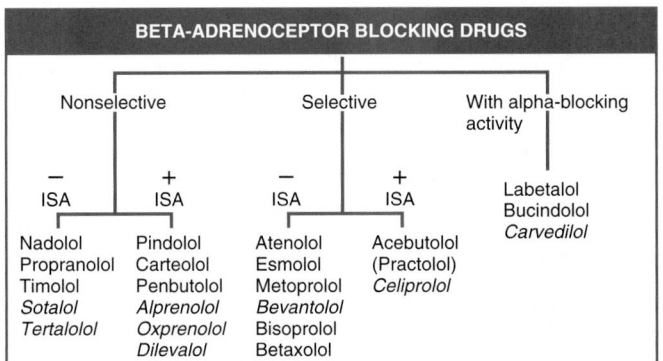

FIGURE 27–12. Classification of beta-adrenergic receptor blockers based on cardioselectivity and intrinsic sympathomimetic activity (ISA). Those not approved for use in the United States are in italics. (From Kaplan, N. M.: Clinical Hypertension. 6th ed. Baltimore, © by Williams & Wilkins, 1994, p. 221.)

SPECIAL USES FOR BETA BLOCKERS

COEXISTING ISCHEMIC HEART DISEASE. Even without evidence that beta blockers protect patients from initial coronary events, the antiarrhythmic and antianginal effects of these drugs make them especially valuable in hypertensive patients with coexisting coronary disease.

PATIENTS NEEDING ANTIHYPERTENSIVE VASODILATOR THERAPY. If a diuretic and an adrenergic receptor blocker are inadequate to control blood pressure, the addition of a vasodilator is a logical third step. When used alone, direct vasodilators induce reflex sympathetic stimulation of the heart. The simultaneous use of beta blockers prevents this undesirable increase in cardiac output, which not only

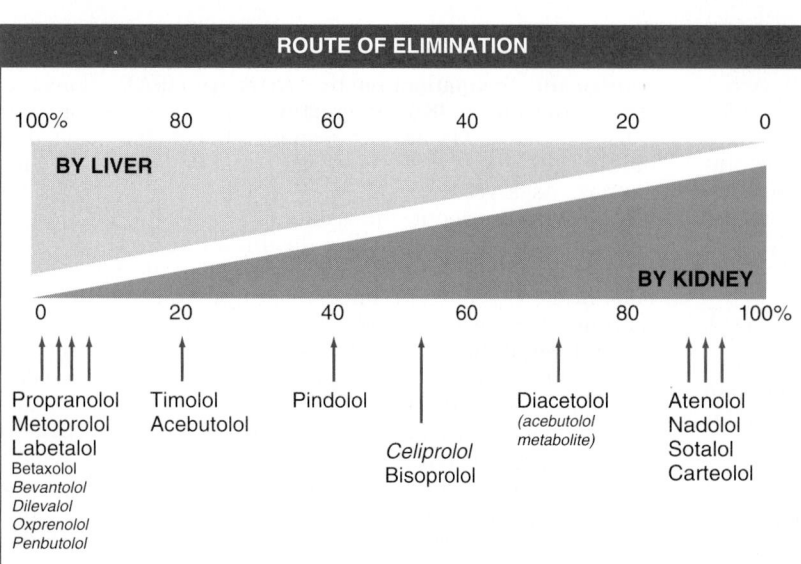

FIGURE 27–13. The relative degree of clearance by hepatic uptake and metabolism (liver) and renal excretion (kidney) of 10 beta-adrenoceptor blocking agents. The differences largely reflect differences in lipid solubility, which progressively diminishes from left to right. (Modified from Meier, J.: Beta-adrenoceptor-blocking agents: Pharmacokinetic differences and their clinical implications illustrated on pindolol. Cardiology 64[Suppl. 1]:1, 1979.)

bothers the patient but also dampens the antihypertensive effect of the vasodilator.

PATIENTS WITH HYPERKINETIC HYPERTENSION. Some hypertensive patients have increased cardiac output that may persist for many years. Beta blockers are particularly effective in such patients, but a reduction in exercise capacity may necessitate restriction of their use in young athletes.

PATIENTS WITH MARKED ANXIETY. The somatic manifestations of anxiety—tremor, sweating, and tachycardia—can be helped, without the undesirable effects of methods commonly used to control anxiety, such as alcohol and tranquilizers.

PERIOPERATIVE STRESS. The ultra–short-acting cardioselective agent esmolol has been successfully used to prevent postintubation tachycardia and hypertension.[156]

SIDE EFFECTS. Most of the side effects of beta blockers relate to their major pharmacological action, the blockade of beta-adrenergic receptors. Certain concomitant problems may worsen when beta-adrenergic receptors are blocked. These include peripheral vascular disease, bronchospasm, and congestive heart failure. However, cautious use of beta blockers in patients with systolic dysfunction may prove to be valuable.[157]

Diabetics may have additional problems with beta blockers, more so with nonselective ones. The responses to hypoglycemia, both the symptoms and the counterregulatory hormonal changes that raise blood sugar levels, are partially dependent on sympathetic nervous activity. Diabetics who are susceptible to hypoglycemia may not be aware of the usual warning signals and may not rebound as quickly. The majority of noninsulin-dependent diabetics can take these drugs without difficulty, although their diabetes may be exacerbated, probably from beta blocker interference with insulin sensitivity.[142]

The most common side effect is fatigue, which is probably a consequence of decreased cardiac output and also of the decrease in cerebral blood flow that may accompany successful lowering of the blood pressure by any drug (Fig. 27–7). More direct effects on the central nervous system—insomnia, nightmares, and hallucinations—occur in some patients.[158] An association with depression appears to be accounted for by various confounding variables.[159]

When a beta blocker is discontinued, angina pectoris and myocardial infarction may occur.[160] Since patients with hypertension are more susceptible to coronary disease, they should be weaned gradually and given appropriate coronary vasodilator therapy. Perturbations of lipoprotein metabolism accompany the use of beta blockers.[141] Nonselective agents cause greater rises in triglycerides and falls in cardioprotective high-density lipoprotein-cholesterol levels, whereas ISA agents cause less or no effect and some agents such as celiprolol may raise HDL-cholesterol levels.[161] Patients with renal failure may take beta blockers without additional hazard, although modest falls in renal blood flow and glomerular filtration rate have been measured, presumably from renal vasoconstriction.

Caution is advised in the use of beta blockers in patients suspected of harboring a pheochromocytoma (see p. 828), because unopposed alpha-adrenergic agonist action may precipitate a serious hypertensive crisis if this disease is present. The use of beta blockers during pregnancy has been clouded by scattered case reports of various fetal problems. Moreover, prospective studies have found that the use of beta blockers during pregnancy may lead to fetal growth retardation.[162]

AN OVERVIEW OF BETA BLOCKERS IN HYPERTENSION. Beta blockers are likely to continue to be popular in the treatment of hypertension. If a beta blocker is chosen, those agents that have ISA and are more cardioselective and lipid-insoluble offer the likelihood of fewer perturbations of lipid and carbohydrate metabolism and greater patient adherence to therapy; only one dose a day is needed and side effects probably are minimized.

Alpha- and Beta-Adrenergic Receptor Antagonists

The combination of an alpha and a beta blocker in a single molecule is available in the form of labetalol, which combines both alpha- and beta-blocking actions in a ratio between 1:3 and 1:7. The fall in pressure mainly results from a decrease in peripheral resistance, with little or no fall in cardiac output.[163] The most bothersome side effects are related to postural hypotension; the most serious side effect is hepatotoxicity.[164] Intravenous labetalol is used to treat hypertensive emergencies.

VASODILATORS

Until recently, direct-acting arteriolar vasodilators were used mainly as third drugs, when combinations of a diuretic and adrenergic blocker failed to control blood pressure. However, with the availability of vasodilators of different types that can be easily tolerated when used as first or second drugs, a wider and earlier application of vasodilators in therapy of hypertension has begun (Table 27–6).

TABLE 27–6 VASODILATOR DRUGS USED TO TREAT HYPERTENSION

DRUG	RELATIVE ACTION ON ARTERIES (A) OR VEINS (V)
Direct	
Hydralazine	A >> V
Minoxidil	A >> V
Nitroprusside	A = V
Diazoxide	A > V
Nitroglycerin	V > A
Calcium entry blockers	A >> V
Converting enzyme inhibitors	A > V
Alpha blockers	A = V

Direct Vasodilators

Hydralazine is the most widely used agent of this type. Minoxidil is more potent but is usually reserved for patients with severe, refractory hypertension associated with renal failure.[91a] Diazoxide and nitroprusside are given intravenously for hypertensive crises and are discussed on page 858.

HYDRALAZINE. Since the early 1970's, hydralazine, in combination with a diuretic and a beta blocker, has been used increasingly to treat severe hypertension. The drug acts directly to relax the smooth muscle in precapillary resistance vessels with little or no effect on postcapillary venous capacitance vessels. As a result, blood pressure falls by a reduction in peripheral resistance, but in the process a number of compensatory processes, which are activated by the arterial baroreceptor arc, blunt the decrease in pressure and cause side effects.[165] When a diuretic is used to overcome the tendency for fluid retention and an adrenergic inhibitor is used to prevent the reflex increase in sympathetic activity and rise in renin, the vasodilator is more effective and causes few, if any, side effects. Without the protection conferred by concomitant use of an adrenergic blocker, numerous side effects (tachycardia, flushing, headache, and precipitation of angina) may be seen.

The drug need be given only twice a day. Its daily dosage should be kept below 400 mg to prevent the lupus-like syndrome that appears in 10 to 20 per cent of patients who receive more. This reaction, although uncomfortable to the patient, is almost always reversible. In fact, the reaction is uncommon with daily doses of 200 mg or less and is more common in slow acetylators of the drug.

MINOXIDIL. This drug vasodilates by opening potassium channels in vascular smooth muscle. Its hemodynamic effects are similar to those of hydralazine, but minoxidil is even more effective and may be used once a day. It is particularly useful in managing patients with severe hypertension and renal failure.[166] Even more than with hydralazine, diuretics and adrenergic receptor blockers must be used with minoxidil to prevent the reflex increase in cardiac output and fluid retention. Pericardial effusions have appeared in about 3 per cent of those given minoxidil, in some without renal or cardiac failure.[167] The drug also causes hair to grow profusely, and the facial hirsutism precludes use of the drug in most women.

Calcium Antagonists
(See also p. 475)

These drugs have become the most popular class of agents used in the treatment of hypertension. They differ in both their sites and modes of action (Table 27–7), with major pharmacological differences between the various dihydropyridines.[168] Dihydropyridines have the greatest peripheral vasodilatory action with little effect on cardiac automaticity, conduction, or contractility. However, comparative trials have shown that verapamil and diltiazem, which do affect these properties, are also effective antihypertensives, and they may cause fewer side effects related to vasodilation, such as flushing and ankle edema. Calcium antagonists are effective in hypertensive patients of all ages and races.[99]

Calcium antagonists may cause at least an initial natriuresis, probably by producing renal vasodilation,[169] which may obviate the need for concurrent diuretic therapy. In fact, unlike all other antihypertensive agents, they may have their effectiveness reduced rather than enhanced by concomitant dietary sodium restriction,[170] whereas most careful studies show an enhancement of their effect by concomitant diuretic therapy.[106] Their renal vasodilatory effect allows glomerular filtration rate and renal blood flow to be well maintained as they reduce systemic blood pressure.[171] Because they act primarily to dilate afferent arterioles,

TABLE 27–7 PHARMACOLOGICAL EFFECTS OF CALCIUM ANTAGONISTS*

	DILTIAZEM	VERAPAMIL	DIHYDRO-PYRIDINES
Heart rate	↓	↓	↑–
Myocardial contractility	↓	↓↓	↓–
Nodal conduction	↓	↓↓	–
Peripheral vasodilation	↑	↑	↑↑

* The ↓ indicates decrease; ↑, increase; and –, no change.

these agents could accelerate a decline in renal function by increasing flow within the glomeruli. Although they do not decrease proteinuria as well as ACE inhibitors,[172] they seem to preserve renal function as well[171] and, in some studies, better than the latter drugs.[173] They have been used successfully for treatment of hypertension associated with diabetes without altering glucose tolerance or lipid levels.[174]

A potentially serious adverse effect from the use of calcium antagonists to treat hypertension was described in a case-control study wherein more hypertensives who had a myocardial infarction were taking short-acting calcium antagonists than were hypertensives who had not had an infarct.[174a] The most likely explanation for the finding is exclusion bias, which is an inherent problem with case-control studies wherein the cases are at greater risk for the complication than the controls; i.e., higher-risk patients are excluded from the control group but not from the case group. Specifically, short-acting calcium antagonists, which were not approved for the treatment of hypertension and which were more expensive and more difficult to use because they require three doses a day compared with the other approved antihypertensive agents, were probably given to patients considered at higher risk for coronary events. Similar case-control studies claiming that the use of reserpine was associated with a threefold increase in breast cancer were subsequently shown to be erroneous because of exclusion bias.[174b] No data incriminating the long-acting calcium antagonists approved for the treatment of hypertension have been presented.

Along with freedom from most of the side effects seen with other classes, calcium antagonists may be unique in not having their antihypertensive efficacy blunted by nonsteroidal antiinflammatory agents.[175]

Liquid nifedipine has been used effectively to reduce high levels of blood pressure quickly. Doses of 5 to 10 mg provide almost uniform reduction of blood pressure by 25 per cent within 30 minutes.[176] Intravenous nicardipine is available for hypertensive emergencies.[177]

Renin-Angiotensin Inhibitors
(See also p. 473)

Activity of the renin-angiotensin system may be inhibited in four ways (Fig. 27–14), three of which can be applied clinically.[177a] The first, use of adrenergic receptor blockers to inhibit the release of renin, was discussed earlier (p. 851). The second, direct inhibition of renin activity by specific renin inhibitors, is being actively investigated.[178] The third, inhibition of the enzyme that converts the inactive decapeptide angiotensin I to the active octapeptide angiotensin II (AII), is being widely utilized with orally effective ACE inhibitors. The fourth approach to inhibiting the renin-angiotensin system, blockade of angiotensin's actions by a

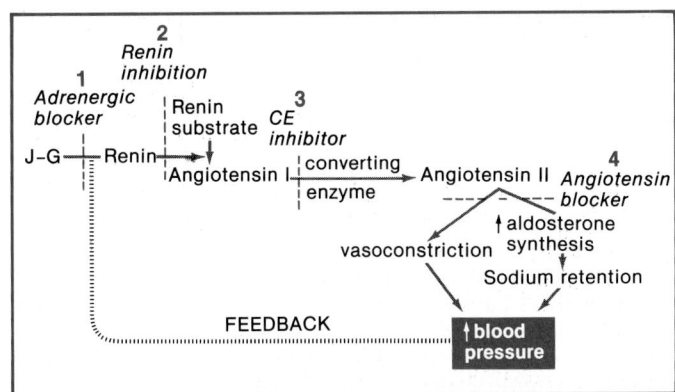

FIGURE 27–14. The four sites of action of inhibitors of the renin-angiotensin system. J-G = juxtaglomerular apparatus. (From Kaplan, N. M.: Clinical Hypertension. 6th ed. Baltimore, © by Williams & Wilkins, 1994, p. 241.)

competitive blocker, is now feasible, and orally effective AII receptor blockers are now approved for clinical use.[179] The AII receptor blockers may offer additional benefits, but their immediate advantage is the absence of cough and angioedema that often accompany ACE inhibitors. Because they are so widely used, the remainder of this section will examine ACE inhibitors.

MECHANISM OF ACTION. The first of these ACE inhibitors, captopril, was synthesized as a specific inhibitor of the converting enzyme that breaks the peptidyldipeptide bond in angiotensin I, preventing the enzyme from attaching to and splitting the angiotensin I structure. Because angiotensin II cannot be formed and angiotensin I is inactive, the ACE inhibitor paralyzes the renin-angiotensin system, thereby removing the effects of endogenous angiotensin II as both a vasoconstrictor and a stimulant to aldosterone synthesis. Subsequently, a number of other ACE inhibitors, differing primarily by the presence of a carboxyl or phosphoryl group rather than a sulfhydryl group, act in a similar manner but with a slower onset and a longer duration of action.

Interestingly, the plasma angiotensin II levels actually return to previous readings with chronic use of ACE inhibitors while the blood pressure remains lowered[180]; this suggests that the antihypertensive effect may involve other mechanisms. Since the same enzyme that converts angiotensin I to angiotensin II is also responsible for inactivation of the vasodepressor hormone bradykinin, by inhibiting the breakdown of bradykinin, ACE inhibitors increase the concentration of a vasodepressor hormone while they decrease the concentration of a vasoconstrictor hormone.[181] The increased plasma kinin levels may contribute to the improvement in insulin sensitivity observed with ACE inhibitors,[182] but they are also responsible for the most common and bothersome side effect of their use, a dry, hacking cough.[183] ACE inhibitors may also vasodilate by increasing levels of vasodilatory prostaglandins and decreasing levels of vasoconstricting endothelins.[184] Their effects may also involve inhibition of the renin-angiotensin system within the heart and other tissues,

Regardless of the manner in which they work, ACE inhibitors lower blood pressure mainly by reducing peripheral resistance with little, if any, effect on heart rate, cardiac output, or body fluid volumes. After a year of treatment with an ACE inhibitor, the structure and function of subcutaneous resistance vessels were improved whereas no changes were observed with a beta blocker.[185] The lack of a rise in heart rate despite a significant fall in blood pressure has been explained by a blunting of the adrenergic nervous system.[186]

CLINICAL USE. In patients with uncomplicated primary hypertension, ACE inhibitors provide antihypertensive effects that are equal to those seen with other classes, but they are less effective in blacks,[99] perhaps because blacks tend to have lower renin levels. They are equally effective in elderly and younger hypertensive patients.

The initial dose of ACE inhibitor may precipitate a rather dramatic but transient fall in blood pressure,[187] but the full effect may not be seen for 7 to 10 days. The initial dosage may be as little as 12.5 mg of captopril twice a day or 5 mg once a day of most of the other members of this class. The response to an ACE inhibitor is usually well maintained, perhaps because its suppression of aldosterone mitigates the tendency toward volume expansion that often antagonizes the effects of other antihypertensives.

These drugs have been a mixed blessing for patients with renovascular hypertension. On the one hand, the response of plasma renin to a single dose of captopril may provide a simple diagnostic test for the disease (see p. 827). More importantly, they usually control the blood pressure effectively.[188] On the other hand, the removal of the high levels of angiotensin II that they produce may deprive the stenotic kidney of the hormonal drive to its blood flow, thereby causing a marked fall of renal perfusion so that patients with solitary kidneys or bilateral disease may develop acute and sometimes persistent renal failure.[189]

Patients with intraglomerular hypertension, specifically those with diabetic nephropathy or reduced renal functional mass, may benefit especially from the reduction in efferent arteriolar resistance that follows reduction in angiotensin II. The clinical evidence for modulation of the progressive loss of renal function in diabetic nephropathy is now unequivocal.[190] Whether this effect is quantitatively better with ACE inhibitors than that provided by other drugs is less certain as is the ability of ACE inhibitors to also slow the progress of other forms of renal disease.[191] Because of their ability to improve insulin sensitivity, ACE inhibitors are particularly attractive for diabetics, with or without nephropathy,[192] and for hypertensives with visceral obesity.[193]

SIDE EFFECTS. Most patients who take an ACE inhibitor experience no side effects nor the biochemical changes often seen with other drugs that may be of even more concern even though they are not so obvious; neither rises in lipids, glucose, or uric acid nor falls in potassium levels are seen, and insulin sensitivity may improve.

To be sure, ACE inhibitors may cause both specific and nonspecific adverse effects. Among the specific ones are rash, loss of taste, glomerulopathy manifested by proteinuria, and leukopenia. In addition, these drugs may cause a hypersensitivity reaction with angioneurotic edema[194] or a cough, although often persistent, is infrequently associated with pulmonary dysfunction.[194a] The cough, seen in over 10 per cent of women and about half as many men,[195] may not disappear for 3 weeks after the ACE inhibitor is discontinued.[196] The recently approved angiotensin II receptor blockers do not induce the cough, which presumably arises from the increased levels of kinins that occur when the ACE enzyme is inhibited.

There is at least a potential problem for those patients taking an ACE inhibitor who coincidentally develop volume depletion, as from gastroenteritis, since they may be unable to marshal the compensatory homeostatic responses that involve increased angiotensin II and aldosterone. Lastly, patients on potassium supplements or sparing agents may not be able to excrete potassium loads and therefore may develop hyperkalemia.

AN OVERVIEW OF ACE INHIBITOR THERAPY. These drugs are widely used for all degrees and forms of hypertension. Their use is likely to increase further because of their particular ability to decrease intrarenal hypertension, to unload the hemodynamic burden of congestive heart failure, and to protect against ventricular dysfunction after myocardial infarction. Angiotensin II receptor blockers may offer all of the advantages of ACE inhibitors and fewer side effects.

Other Vasodilators

A variety of other forms of antihypertensive therapy are under investigation. These include endothelin receptor antagonists,[197] agents that serve as exogenous atrial natriuretic factor[198] or prolong its endogenous effectiveness,[199] and a host of renin inhibitors and angiotensin antagonists.[200,200a]

SPECIAL CONSIDERATIONS IN THERAPY

RESISTANT HYPERTENSION. There are multiple causes for resistance to therapy, usually defined as the failure of diastolic blood pressure to fall below 90 mm Hg despite the use of three or more drugs,[105] although some believe the definition should extend to the use of only two drugs in maximal doses.[201] Often patients do not respond well because they do not take their medications. On the other hand, what appears to be a poor response based on office readings of blood pressure may turn out to be an adequate response when home readings are obtained.[202] However, a number of factors may be responsible for a poor response even if the appropriate medication is taken regularly (Table 27–8). Most common is volume overload owing either to inadequate diuretic or excessive dietary sodium intake. Larger doses or more potent diuretics often bring resistant hypertension under control. On the other hand, blood pressure of a few patients is resistant to therapy because of overly vigorous diuresis, which contracts vascular volume and activates both renin and catecholamines.

Resistance is particularly common in patients with visceral obesity and associated insulin resistance.[203] A frequently overlooked cause is the interference with virtually all antihypertensive drugs (with the possible exception of calcium antagonists) by NSAIDs.[204]

Resistance can usually be overcome by adequate doses of a diuretic, a calcium antagonist, and an ACE inhibitor.

ANESTHESIA IN HYPERTENSIVE PATIENTS. In the absence of significant cardiac dysfunction, hypertension does not add

to the cardiovascular risks of surgery.[205] However, if possible, hypertension should be well controlled by means of medications before anesthesia and surgery to reduce the risk of myocardial ischemia.[206] Therefore, patients taking antihypertensive medications should continue these drugs, as long as the anesthesiologist is aware of their use and takes reasonable precautions to prevent wide swings in pressure. The very short-acting beta blocker esmolol has been successful in preventing surges in blood pressure during intubation.[156] Patients receiving calcium antagonists may occasionally manifest adverse effects when inhalation agents such as halothane, enflurane, and isoflurane are used, either because the cardiovascular effects of these agents are similar to those of calcium antagonists or because these agents may increase the plasma levels of the calcium antagonists.[207]

Hypertension is often observed during and immediately after coronary bypass surgery (see p. 830); various intravenous agents have been successfully used to lower the pressure. Nitroprusside has been the usual choice during the postoperative period, but toxicity, often in the form of loss of consciousness and cyanide or thiocyanate toxicity, may develop in those who are critically ill and given the drug for prolonged periods.[208] Esmolol, labetalol, or nicardipine may be a better choice.[209]

HYPERTENSIVE CHILDREN (see also p. 822). Almost nothing is known about the effects of various antihypertensive medications given to children over long periods. In the absence of adequate data, an approach similar to that advocated for adults is advised.[210] The dosages of drugs are shown in Table 31–5, p. 998. Emphasis should be placed on weight reduction in hypertensive children who are obese, in the hope of attempting to control hypertension without the need for drug therapy.

HYPERTENSION DURING PREGNANCY. This topic is discussed in Chapter 59.

HYPERTENSION IN THE ELDERLY. As noted on page 822, a few elderly persons may have high blood pressure as measured by the sphygmomanometer but may have less or no hypertension when direct intraarterial readings are made. Presumably their pseudohypertension is related to the failure of the sphygmomanometer cuff to collapse the rigid artery beneath the cuff. The cuff systolic pressure may more frequently underestimate the intraarterial level, whereas the cuff diastolic level tends to be higher than the direct measurement.[211] If both systolic and diastolic pressures are elevated, elderly patients should be treated in a manner similar to that for younger persons; they seem to respond as well[11] but may have a number of problems with the medications[212] (Table 27–9). In view of the reduced effectiveness of the baroceptor reflex and the failure of peripheral resistance to rise appropriately with standing,[213] drugs with a propensity to cause postural hypotension

TABLE 27–8 CAUSES FOR INADEQUATE RESPONSIVENESS TO THERAPY

PSEUDORESISTANCE
  "White coat" or office elevations
  Pseudohypertension in elderly

NONADHERENCE TO THERAPY
  Side effects of medication
  Cost of medication
  Lack of consistent and continuous primary care
  Inconvenient and chaotic dosing schedules
  Instructions not understood
  Inadequate patient education
  Organic brain syndrome (e.g., memory deficit)

DRUG-RELATED CAUSES
  Doses too low
  Inappropriate combinations (e.g., two centrally acting adrenergic inhibitors)
  Rapid inactivation (e.g., hydralazine)
  Drug interactions
    Nonsteroidal antiinflammatory drugs   Oral contraceptives
    Sympathomimetics   Adrenal steroids
      Nasal decongestants   Licorice (chewing tobacco)
      Appetite suppressants   Cyclosporine
      Cocaine   Erythropoietin
      Caffeine   Cholestyramine
    Antidepressants (MAO inhibitors, tricyclics)
  Excessive volume contraction with stimulation of renin-aldosterone
  Hypokalemia (usually diuretic-induced)
  Rebound after clonidine withdrawal

ASSOCIATED CONDITIONS
  Smoking
  Increasing obesity
  Sleep apnea
  Insulin resistance/hyperinsulinemia
  Ethanol intake more than 1 ounce a day (>3 portions)
  Anxiety-induced hyperventilation or panic attacks
  Chronic pain
  Intense vasoconstriction (Raynaud's, arteritis)

SECONDARY HYPERTENSION
  Renal insufficiency
  Renovascular hypertension
  Pheochromocytoma
  Primary aldosteronism

VOLUME OVERLOAD
  Excess sodium intake
  Progressive renal damage (nephrosclerosis)
  Fluid retention from reduction of blood pressure
  Inadequate diuretic therapy

Modified from Joint National Committee. Fifth report of the Joint National Committee on detection, evaluation, and treatment of high blood pressure (JNC V). Arch. Intern. Med. *153*:154, 1993. Copyright 1993 American Medical Association.

TABLE 27–9 FACTORS THAT MIGHT CONTRIBUTE TO INCREASED RISK OF PHARMACOLOGICAL TREATMENT OF HYPERTENSION IN THE ELDERLY

FACTORS	POTENTIAL COMPLICATIONS
Diminished baroreceptor activity	Orthostatic hypotension
Decreased intravascular volume	Orthostatic hypotension, dehydration
Sensitivity to hypokalemia	Arrhythmia, muscular weakness
Decreased renal and hepatic function	Drug accumulation
Polypharmacy	Drug interaction
CNS changes	Depression, confusion

should be avoided, and all drugs should be given in slowly increasing doses to prevent extensive lowering of the pressure.

Including the data shown in Figure 27–1, the results of all 13 randomized trials lasting at least 1 year involving over 16,000 elderly hypertensives demonstrate that treating healthy old patients is highly efficacious.[214] By design, the patients enrolled in these trials were healthier than most elderly hypertensives so that caution is advised in extrapolating these excellent results to the patients usually seen in clinical practice.

Isolated systolic hypertension is common in the elderly and presents a serious risk, particularly for strokes. The results of the SHEP indicated that these risks could be significantly reduced by small doses of diuretic and, if needed, a beta blocker.[13] Calcium antagonists also work well in the elderly.[215] The average level of systolic pressure reached by the SHEP participants, 145 mm Hg, seems a reasonable goal for most elderly patients.

HYPERTENSION WITH CONGESTIVE HEART FAILURE. Cardiac output may fall so markedly in hypertensive patients who are in heart failure with systolic dysfunction that their blood pressure is reduced, obscuring the degree of hypertension; often, however, the diastolic pressure is raised by intense vasoconstriction while the systolic pressure falls as a result of the reduced stroke volume. Lowering the blood pressure may, by itself, relieve the heart failure. Chronic unloading has been most efficiently accomplished with ACE inhibitors[216] (see p. 856). Caution is needed for those elderly hypertensives with diastolic dysfunction related to marked left ventricular hypertrophy, because unloaders may worsen their status, whereas beta blockers or calcium antagonists may be beneficial.

As noted in Chapter 26, left ventricular hypertrophy (LVH) is frequently found by echocardiography, even in patients with mild hypertension. All antihypertensive drugs except direct vasodilators have been shown to regress LVH, and regression may continue for as long as 5 years of treatment.[217]

HYPERTENSION WITH ISCHEMIC HEART DISEASE. The coexistence of ischemic heart disease makes antihypertensive therapy even more essential, since relief of the hypertension may ameliorate the coronary disease. Beta blockers and calcium antagonists are particularly useful if angina or arrhythmias are present. Caution is needed to avoid decreased coronary perfusion that is likely to be responsible for the J curve seen in multiple trials[35–37] (see p. 841).

The often markedly high levels of blood pressure during the early phase of an acute myocardial infarction may reflect sympathetic nervous hyperreactivity to pain. Cautious use of antihypertensive drugs that do not decrease cardiac output may be useful in the immediate postinfarction period, whereas beta blockers and ACE inhibitors have been shown to provide long-term benefit.

THERAPY FOR HYPERTENSIVE CRISES

When diastolic blood pressure exceeds 140 mm Hg, rapidly progressive damage to the arterial vasculature is demonstrable experimentally, and a surge of cerebral blood flow may rapidly lead to encephalopathy (p. 832). If such high pressures persist or if there are any signs of encephalopathy, the pressures should be lowered using parenteral agents in those patients considered to be in immediate danger or with oral agents in those who are alert and in no other acute distress.

A number of drugs for this purpose currently are available (Table 27–10). If diastolic pressure exceeds 140 mm Hg and the patient has any complications, such as an aortic dissection, a constant infusion of nitroprusside is most effective and will almost always lower the pressure to the desired level. Constant monitoring with an intraarterial line is mandatory because a slightly excessive dose may lower the pressure abruptly to levels that will induce shock. The potency and rapidity of action of nitroprusside have made it the treatment of choice for life-threatening hypertension. However, nitroprusside acts as a venous and arteriolar dilator, so that venous return and cardiac output are lowered[218] and intracranial pressures may increase.[219] Therefore, other parenteral agents are being more widely used. These include labetalol[163] and the calcium antagonist nicardipine.[177]

With any of these agents, intravenous furosemide is often needed to lower the blood pressure further and prevent retention of salt and water. Diuretics should not be given if volume depletion is initially present.

For patients in less immediate danger, oral therapy may be used. Almost every drug has been used and most will, with repeated doses, reduce high pressures. The current

TABLE 27–10 PARENTERAL DRUGS FOR TREATMENT OF HYPERTENSIVE EMERGENCY (IN ORDER OF RAPIDITY OF ACTION)

DRUG	DOSAGE	ONSET OF ACTION	ADVERSE EFFECTS
VASODILATORS			
Nitroprusside (Nipride, Nitropress)	0.25–10 μg/kg/min as I.V. infusion	Instantaneous	Nausea, vomiting, muscle twitching, sweating, thiocyanate intoxication
Nitroglycerin	5–100 μg/min as I.V. infusion	2–5 min	Tachycardia, flushing, headache, vomiting, methemoglobinemia
Diazoxide (Hyperstat)	50–100 mg/I.V. bolus, repeated or 15–30 mg/min by I.V. infusion	2–4 min	Nausea, hypotension, flushing, tachycardia, chest pain
Nicardipine (Cardene)	2–10 mg/hr I.V.	5–10 min	Tachycardia, headache, flushing, local phlebitis
Hydralazine (Apresoline)	10–20 mg I.V. / 10–50 mg I.M.	10–20 min / 20–30 min	Tachycardia, flushing, headache, vomiting, aggravation of angina
Enalapril (Vasotec IV)	1.25–5 mg q 6 hr	15 min	Precipitous fall in BP in high renin states; response variable
ADRENERGIC INHIBITORS			
Phentolamine (Regitine)	5–15 mg I.V.	1–2 min	Tachycardia, flushing
Trimethaphan (Arfonad)	0.5–5 mg/min as I.V. infusion	1–5 min	Paresis of bowel and bladder, orthostatic hypotension, blurred vision, dry mouth
Esmolol (Brevibloc)	500 μg/kg/min for 4 min, then 150–300 μg/kg/min I.V.	1–2 min	Hypotension
Labetalol (Normodyne, Trandate)	20–80 mg I.V. bolus every 10 min / 2 mg/min I.V. infusion	5–10 min	Vomiting, scalp tingling, burning in throat, postural hypotension, dizziness, nausea

preference of many is nifedipine, 10 mg by mouth or sublingually, repeated in 30 minutes if needed.[176] The sublingual route provides a slower route and probably, therefore, a safer one. The pressure almost always falls about 25 per cent within the first 30 minutes. Rarely, and not unexpectedly, a few patients may suffer tissue ischemia with such rapid and marked falls in pressure. A safer course for many patients, particularly if their current high pressures are simply a reflection of stopping previously effective oral medication, is simply to restart that medication and monitor their response closely. If their nonadherence to therapy was caused by side effects, appropriate changes should be made.

With some exceptions,[220] most centers are seeing fewer patients in hypertensive crisis, presumably because more patients are diagnosed and treated before the disease enters this malignant course. The continued successful treatment of many more hypertensive persons will prevent the more frequent long-range cardiovascular complications of hypertension.

REFERENCES

BENEFITS OF THERAPY

1. Stockwell, D. H., Madhavan, S., Cohen, H., et al.: The determinants of hypertension awareness, treatment, and control in an insured population. Am. J. Public Health 84:1768, 1994.
2. Neaton, J. D., Grimm R. H., Jr., Prineas, R. J., et al.: Treatment of mild hypertension study. JAMA 270:713, 1993.
3. Kaplan, N. M.: Treatment of hypertension: Drug therapy. In Kaplan, N. M. (ed.): Clinical Hypertension. 6th ed. Baltimore, Williams and Wilkins, 1994, p. 191.
4. Swales, J. D.: Pharmacological treatment of hypertension. Lancet 344:380, 1994.
5. Thürmer, H. H., Lund-Larsen, P. G., and Tverdal, A.: Is blood pressure treatment as effective in a population setting as in controlled trials? Results from a prospective study. J. Hypertens. 12:481, 1994.
6. Rose, G.: The Strategy of Preventive Medicine. Oxford, Oxford University Press, 1992.
7. Jackson, R., Barham, P., Bills, J., et al.: Management of raised blood pressure in New Zealand: A discussion document. Br. Med. J. 307:107, 1993.
8. Johannesson, M.: Economic evaluation of hypertension treatment—methods and empirical results. In Swales, J. D. (ed.): Textbook of Hypertension. Oxford, Blackwell Scientific Publications, 1994, p. 1292.
8a. Kaplan, N. M.: Management of hypertension. In Fuster, V., Ross, R., and Topol, E. J. (eds.): Atherosclerosis and Coronary Artery Disease. Philadelphia, Lippincott-Raven Publishers, 1996, pp. 259–274.
9. MacMahon, S. W., Cutler, J. A., Furberg, C. D., and Payne, G. H.: The effects of drug treatment for hypertension on morbidity and mortality from cardiovascular disease: A review of randomized controlled trials. Prog. Cardiovasc. Dis. 29:99, 1986.
10. Collins, R., Peto, R., MacMahon, S., et al.: Blood pressure, stroke, and coronary heart disease. Part II: Short-term reductions in blood pressure: Overview of randomized drug trials in their epidemiological context. Lancet 335:827, 1990.
11. MacMahon, S., and Rodgers, A.: The effects of blood pressure reduction in older patients: An overview of five randomized controlled trials in elderly hypertensives. Clin. Exper. Hypertens. 15:967, 1993.
12. MacMahon, S., Peto, R., Cutler, J., et al.: Blood pressure, stroke and coronary heart disease: Part I. Prolonged differences in blood pressure: Prospective observational studies corrected for the regression dilution bias. Lancet 335:765, 1990.
13. SHEP Cooperative Research Group: Prevention of stroke by antihypertensive drug treatment in older persons with isolated systolic hypertension. JAMA 265:3255, 1991.
14. Dahlöf, B., Lindholm, L. H., and Hansson, L.: Morbidity and mortality in the Swedish Trial in Old Patients with Hypertension (STOP-Hypertension). Lancet 338:1281, 1991.
15. Medical Research Council Working Party: Medical Research Council trial of treatment of hypertension in older adults: Principal results. Br. Med. J. 304:405, 1992.
15a. Chobanian, A. V.: Have long-term benefits of antihypertensive therapy been underestimated? Provocative findings from the Framingham Heart Study. Circulation 93:638, 1996.
16. Hebert, P. R., Moser, M., Mayer, J., et al.: Recent evidence on drug therapy of mild to moderate hypertension and decreased risk of coronary heart disease. Arch. Intern. Med. 153:578, 1993.
17. Kaplan, N. M.: Management of hypertensive emergencies. Lancet 344:1335, 1994.
18. Bing, R. F., Heagerty, A. M., Russell, G. I., et al.: Prognosis in malignant hypertension. J. Hypertens. 4(Suppl. 6):S42, 1986.
19. Management of Committee of the Australian Therapeutic Trial in Mild Hypertension: Untreated mild hypertension. Lancet 1:185, 1982.

20. National High Blood Pressure Education Program Working Group: National High Blood Pressure Education Program Working Group Report on primary prevention of hypertension. Arch. Intern. Med. 153:186, 1993.
21. IPPPSH Collaborative Group: Cardiovascular risk and risk factors in a randomized trial of treatment based on the beta-blocker oxprenolol: The International Prospective Primary Prevention Study in Hypertension (IPPPSH). J. Hypertens. 3:379, 1985.
22. Medical Research Council Working Party: MRC trial of treatment of mild hypertension: principal results. Br. Med. J. 291:97, 1985.
23. Kaplan, N. M. (ed.): Treatment of Hypertension: Rationale and Goals. Baltimore, Williams and Wilkins, 1994, p. 145.
24. Hypertension Detection and Follow-Up Program Cooperative Group: The effect of treatment on mortality in "mild" hypertension. N. Engl. J. Med. 307:976, 1982.
25. Multiple Risk Factor Intervention Trial Research Group: Multiple risk factor intervention trial. Risk factor changes and mortality results. JAMA 248:1465, 1982.

THRESHOLD FOR THERAPY

26. Joint National Committee on Detection, Evaluation, and Treatment of High Blood Pressure: The fifth report of the Joint National Committee on Detection, Evaluation and Treatment of High Blood Pressure (JNC V). Arch. Intern. Med. 153:154, 1993.
27. Sever, P., Beevers, G., Bulpitt, C., et al.: Management guidelines in essential hypertension: Report of the second working party of the British Hypertension Society. Br. Med. J. 306:983, 1993.
28. Haynes, R. B., Lacourcière, Y., Rabkin, S. W., et al.: Report of the Canadian Hypertension Society Consensus Conference: 2. Diagnosis of hypertension in adults, Can. Med. Assoc. J. 149:409, 1993.
29. The Guidelines Subcommittee of the WHO/ISH Mild Hypertension Liaison Committee: 1993 Guidelines for the management of mild hypertension. Hypertension 22:392, 1993.
30. Samuelsson, O.: Experiences from hypertension trials. Impact of other risk factors. Drugs 36(Suppl. 3):9, 1988.
31. Kaplan, N. M.: The treatment of hypertension in women. Arch. Intern. Med. 155:563, 1995.
32. Management Committee: The Australian therapeutic trial in mild hypertension. Lancet 1:1261, 1980.
33. Bulpitt, C. J., and Fletcher, A. E.: Aging, blood pressure and mortality. J. Hypertens. 10(Suppl. 7):45, 1992.
34. Epstein, F. H.: Proceedings of the XVth International Congress of Therapeutics, Sept. 5–9, 1979. Brussels, Excerpta Medica, 1980.
35. Cruickshank, J. M.: Coronary flow reserve and the J curve relation between diastolic blood pressure and myocardial infarction. Br. Med. J. 297:1227, 1988.
36. Lindblad, U., Råstam, L., Rydén, L., et al.: Control of blood pressure and risk of first acute myocardial infarction: Skaraborg hypertension project. Br. Med. J. 308:681, 1994.
37. Madhavan, S., Ooi, W. L., Cohen, H., and Alderman, M. H.: Relation of pulse pressure and blood pressure reduction to the incidence of myocardial infarction. Hypertension 23:395, 1994.
38. Kuller, L. H., Hulley, S. B., Cohen, J. D., and Neaton, J.: Unexpected effects of treating hypertension in men with electrocardiographic abnormalities. A critical analysis. Circulation 73:114, 1986.
39. Cooper, S. P., Hardy, R. J., Labarthe, D. R., et al.: The relation between degree of blood pressure reduction and mortality among hypertensives in the hypertension detection and follow-up program. Am. J. Epidemiol. 127:387, 1988.
40. Cruickshank, J. M.: J curve in antihypertensive therapy: Does it exist? A personal point of view. Cardiovasc. Drug Ther. 8:757, 1994.
41. Amery, A., Berglund, G., Cruickshank, J. M., et al.: How much should blood pressure be lowered? The problem of the J-shaped curve. J. Hypertens. 7(Suppl. 6):S338, 1989.
42. Tervahauta, M., Pekkanen, J., Enlund, H., and Nissinen, A.: Change in blood pressure and 5-year risk of coronary heart disease among elderly men: The Finnish cohorts of the Seven Countries Study. J. Hypertens. 12:1183, 1994.
43. The HOT Study Group: The Hypertension Optimal Treatment (HOT) Study: a prospective study of the optimal therapeutic goal and of the value of a low dose aspirin in anti-hypertensive treatment. Blood Press 2:62, 1993.
44. Schmieder, R. E., Rockstroh, J. K., and Messerli, F. H.: Antihypertensive therapy. To stop or not to stop? JAMA 256:1566, 1991.

LIFE STYLE MODIFICATIONS

45. The Trials of Hypertension Prevention Collaborative Research Group: The effects of nonpharmacologic interventions on blood pressure of persons with high normal levels. Results of the Trials of Hypertension Prevention, Phase I. JAMA 267:1213, 1992.
46. Geleijnse, J. M., Witteman, J. C. M., Bak, A. A. A., et al.: Reduction in blood pressure with a low sodium, high potassium, high magnesium salt in older subjects with mild to moderate hypertension. Br. Med. J. 309:436, 1994.
47. Groppelli, A., Giorgi, D. M. A., Omboni, S., et al.: Persistent blood pressure increase induced by heavy smoking. J. Hypertens. 10:495, 1992.
48. Staessen, J., Fagard, R., Lijnen, P., and Amery, A.: Body weight, sodium intake and blood pressure. J. Hypertens. 7(Suppl. 1):S19, 1989.

49. Smoller, S. W., Blaufox, M. D., Oberman, A., et al.: TAIM Study: Adequate weight loss as effective as drug therapy for mild hypertension. Circulation *81*:4, 1990.
50. Schotte, D. E., and Stunkard, A. J.: The effects of weight reduction on blood pressure in 301 obese patients. Arch. Intern. Med. *150*:1701, 1990.
51. Wadden, T. A., Foster, G. D., Letizia, K. A., and Stunkard, A. J.: A multicenter evaluation of a proprietary weight reduction program for the treatment of marked obesity. Arch. Intern. Med. *152*:961, 1992.
52. Rocchini, A. P., Key, J., Bondie, D., et al.: The effect of weight loss on the sensitivity of blood pressure to sodium in obese adolescents. N. Engl. J. Med. *321*:580, 1989.
53. Cutler, J. A., Follmann, D., Elliott, P., and Suh, I.: An overview of randomized trials of sodium reduction and blood pressure. Hypertension *17*(Suppl. I):I-27, 1991.
54. MacGregor, G. A., Markandu, N. D., Sagnella, G. A., et al.: Double-blind study of three sodium intakes and long-term effects of sodium restriction in essential hypertension. Lancet *2*:1244, 1989.
55. Alderman, M. H., Madhaven, S., Cohen, H., et al.: Low urinary sodium is associated with greater risk of myocardial infarction among treated hypertensive men. Hypertension *25*:1144, 1995.
56. Weinberger, M. H., and Fineberg, N. S.: Sodium and volume sensitivity of blood pressure. Age and pressure change over time. Hypertension *18*:67, 1991.
57. Feldman, R. D.: A low-sodium diet corrects the defect in β-adrenergic response in older subjects. Circulation *85*:612, 1992.
58. Singer, D. R. J., Markandu, N. D., Sugden, A. L., et al.: Sodium restriction in hypertensive patients treated with a converting enzyme inhibitor and a thiazide. Hypertension *17*:798, 1991.
59. Jula, A., Karanko, H., and Rönnemaa, T.: Effects of long-term sodium restriction on left ventricular hypertrophy in mild to moderate essential hypertension. (Abstract) J. Hypertens. *10*(Suppl. 4):104, 1992.
60. Nowson, C. A., and Morgan, T. O.: Change in blood pressure in relation to change in nutrients effected by manipulation of dietary sodium and potassium. Clin. Exp. Pharmacol. Physiol. *15*:225, 1988.
61. Hargreaves, M., Morgan, T. O., Snow, R., and Guerin, M.: Exercise tolerance in the heat on low and normal salt intakes. Clin. Sci. *76*:553, 1989.
62. Kumanyika, S. K., Hebert, P. R., Cutler, J. A., et al.: Feasibility and efficacy of sodium reduction in the Trials of Hypertension Prevention, Phase I. Hypertension *22*:502, 1993.
63. Joossens, J. V., and Kesteloot, H.: Trends in systolic blood pressure, 24-hour sodium excretion, and stroke mortality in the elderly in Belgium. Am. J. Med. *90*(Suppl. 3A):5, 1991.
64. Alderman, M. H.: Non-pharmacological treatment of hypertension. Lancet *344*:307, 1994.
65. Krishna, G. G., and Kapoor, S. C.: Potassium depletion exacerbates essential hypertension. Ann. Intern. Med. *115*:77, 1991.
66. Taddei, S., Mattei, P., Virdis, A., et al.: Effect of potassium on vasodilation to acetylcholine in essential hypertension. Hypertension *23*:485, 1994.
67. Cappuccio, F. P., and MacGregor, G. A.: Does potassium supplementation lower blood pressure? A meta-analysis of published trials. J. Hypertens. *9*:465, 1991.
68. Siani, A., Strazzullo, P., Giacco, A., et al.: Increasing the dietary potassium intake reduces the need for antihypertensive medication. Ann. Intern. Med. *115*:753, 1991.
69. Wirell, M. P., Wester, P. O., and Stegmayr, B. G.: Nutritional dose of magnesium in hypertensive patients on beta blockers lowers systolic blood pressure: A double-blind, cross-over study. J. Intern. Med. *236*:189, 1994.
70. Whang, R., Whang, D. D., and Ryan, M. P.: Refractory potassium repletion. A consequence of magnesium deficiency. Arch. Intern. Med. *152*:40, 1992.
71. Lind, L., Lithell, H., Gustafsson, I. B., et al.: Calcium metabolism and sodium sensitivity in hypertensive subjects. J. Hum. Hypertens. *7*:53, 1993.
72. Grobbee, D. E., and Waal-Manning, H. J.: The role of calcium supplementation in the treatment of hypertension. Current evidence. Drugs *39*:7, 1990.
73. Morris, C. D., and McCarron, D. A.: Effect of calcium supplementation in an older population with mildly increased blood pressure. Am. J. Hypertens. *5*:230, 1992.
74. Sciarrone, S. E. G., Strahan, M. T., Beilin, L. J., et al.: Ambulatory blood pressure and heart rate responses to vegetarian meals. J. Hypertens. *11*:277, 1993.
75. Eliasson, K., Ryttig, K. R., Hylander, B., and Rössner, S.: A dietary fibre supplement in the treatment of mild hypertension. A randomized, double-blind, placebo-controlled trial. J. Hypertens. *10*:195, 1992.
76. Morris, M. C., Sacks, F., and Rosner, B.: Does fish oil lower blood pressure? A meta-analysis of controlled trials. Circulation *88*:523, 1993.
77. Bønaa, K. H., Bjerve, K. S., Straume, B., et al.: Effect of eicosapentaenoic and docosahexaenoic acids on blood pressure in hypertension. A population-based intervention trial from the Tromsø study. N. Engl. J. Med. *322*:795, 1990.
78. Sacks, F. M.: Dietary fats and blood pressure: A critical review of the evidence. Nutr. Rev. *47*:291, 1989.
79. Parillo, M., Coulston, A., Hollenbeck, C., and Reaven, G.: Effect of a low fat diet on carbohydrate metabolism in patients with hypertension. Hypertension *11*:244, 1988.

80. Silagy, C. A., and Neil, H. A. W.: A meta-analysis of the effect of garlic on blood pressure. J. Hypertens. *12*:463, 1994.
81. Sung, B. H., Whitsett, T. L., Lovallo, W. R., et al.: Prolonged increase in blood pressure by a single oral dose of caffeine in mildly hypertensive men. Am. J. Hypertens. *7*:755, 1994.
82. Grønbæk, M., Deis, A., Sørensen, T. I. A., et al.: Influence of sex, age, body mass index, and smoking on alcohol intake and mortality. Br. Med. J. *308*:302, 1994.
83. Cameron, J. D., and Dart, A. M.: Exercise training increases total systemic arterial compliance in humans. Am. J. Physiol. *266*:H693, 1994.
84. Dubbert, P. M., Martin, M. E., Cushman, W. C., et al.: Endurance exercise in mild hypertension: Effects on blood pressure and associated metabolic and quality of life variables. J. Hum. Hypertens. *8*:265, 1994.
85. Shaper, A. G., Wannamethee, G., and Walker, M.: Physical activity, hypertension and risk of heart attack in men without evidence of ischaemic heart disease. J. Hum. Hypertens. *8*:3, 1994.
86. Steward K. J.: Weight training in coronary artery disease and hypertension. Prog. Cardiovasc. Dis. *35*:159, 1992.
87. Eisenberg, D. M., Delbanco, T. L., Berkey, C. S., et al.: Cognitive behavioral techniques for hypertension: Are they effective? Am. J. Hypertens. *4*:416, 1993.

ANTIHYPERTENSIVE DRUG THERAPY

88. Strandgaard, S., and Haunsø, S.: Why does antihypertensive treatment prevent stroke but not myocardial infarction? Lancet *2*:658, 1987.
89. Fagan, T. C.: Remembering the lessons of basic pharmacology. Arch. Intern. Med. *154*:1430, 1994.
90. Herxheimer, A.: How much drug in the tablet? Lancet *337*:346, 1991.
91. Kaplan, N. M.: The appropriate goals of antihypertensive therapy: Neither too much nor too little. Ann. Intern. Med. *116*:686, 1992.
91a. Oates, J. A.: Antihypertensive agents and the drug therapy of hypertension. *In* Hardman, J. G., et al. (eds.): Goodman and Gilman's The Pharmacological Basis of Therapeutics. 9th ed. New York, McGraw-Hill, 1996, pp. 781–808.
92. Frishman, W. H., Bryzinski, B. S., Coulson, L. R., et al.: A multifactorial trial design to assess combination therapy in hypertension. Arch. Intern. Med. *154*:1461, 1994.
93. Eisen, S. A., Miller, D. K., Woodward, R. S., et al.: The effect of prescribed daily dose frequency on patient medication compliance. Arch. Intern. Med. *150*:1881, 1990.
94. Elliott, H. L.: Trough: Peak ratio and 24-hour blood pressure control. J. Hypertens. *12*(Suppl. 5):S29, 1994.
95. Anderson, A., Morgan, O., and Morgan, T.: Effectiveness of blood pressure control with once daily administration of enalapril and perindopril. Am. J. Hypertens. *7*:371, 1994.
96. Swales, J. D.: Guidelines on guidelines. J. Hypertens. *11*:899, 1993.
97. Weber, M. A., and Laragh, J. H.: Hypertension: Steps forward and steps backward. Arch. Intern. Med. *153*:149, 1993.
98. Tobian, L., Brunner, H. R., Cohn, J. N., et al.: Modern strategies to prevent coronary sequelae and stroke in hypertensive patients differ from the JNC V consensus guidelines. J. Hypertens. *7*:859, 1994.
99. Materson, B. J., Reda, D. J., and Cushman, W. C.: Department of Veterans Affairs Single-Drug Therapy of Hypertension Study. Revised figures and new data. Am. J. Hypertens. *8*:189, 1995.
100. Attwood, S., Bird, R., Burch, K., et al.: Within-patient correlation between the antihypertensive effects of atenolol, lisinopril and nifedipine. J. Hypertens. *12*:1053, 1994.
101. Guyatt, G. H., Keller, J. L., Jaeschke, R., et al.: The n-of-1 randomized controlled trial: Clinical usefulness. Our three-year experience. Ann. Intern. Med. *112*:293, 1990.
102. Laragh, J. H.: Perspectives in choosing therapy for hypertension. *In* Kaplan, N. M., Brenner, B. M., and Laragh, J. H. (eds.): New Therapeutic Strategies in Hypertension. New York, Raven Press, 1989, p. 141.
103. Bravo, E. L.: Rational drug therapy based on understanding the pathophysiology of hypertension. Cleveland Clin. J. Med. *56*:362, 1989.
104. Woolf, S. H.: Practice guidelines: A new reality in medicine. III. Impact on patient care. Arch. Intern. Med. *153*:2646, 1993.

Diuretics

105. Kaplan, N. M.: Difficult to treat hypertension. Am. J. Med. Sci. *309*:339, 1995.
106. Burris, J. F., Weir, M. R., Oparil, S., et al.: An assessment of diltiazem and hydrochlorothiazide in hypertension. Application of factorial trial design to a multicenter clinical trial of combination therapy. JAMA *263*:1507, 1990.
107. Harper, R., Ennis, C. N., Sheridan, B., et al.: Effects of low dose versus conventional dose thiazide diuretic on insulin action in essential hypertension. Br. Med. J. *309*:226, 1994.
108. Hall, W. D., Weber, M. A., Ferdinand, K., et al.: Lower dose diuretic therapy in the treatment of patients with mild to moderate hypertension. J. Hum. Hypertens. *8*:571, 1994.
109. Baumgart, P.: Torsemide in comparison with thiazides in the treatment of hypertension. Cardiovasc. Drug Ther. *7*:63, 1993.
110. Morgan, D. G., and Davidson, C.: Hypokalemia and diuretics: An analysis of publications. Br. Med. J. *280*:905, 1980.
111. Sandor, F. F., Pickens, P. T., and Crallan, J.: Variations of plasma potassium concentrations during long-term treatment of hypertension with diuretics without potassium supplements. Br. Med. J. *284*:711, 1982.

112. Siscovick, D. S., Raghunathan, T. E., Psaty, B. M., et al.: Diuretic therapy for hypertension and the risk of primary cardiac arrest. N. Engl. J. Med. 330:1852, 1994.

113. Lipworth, B. J., McDevitt, D. G., and Struthers, A. D.: Electrocardiographic changes induced by inhaled salbutamol after treatment with bendrofluazide: Effects of replacement therapy with potassium, magnesium and triamterene. Clin. Sci. 78:225, 1990.

114. Kaplan, N. M., Carnegie, A., Raskin, P., et al.: Potassium supplementation in hypertensive patients with diuretic-induced hypokalemia. N. Engl. J. Med. 312:746, 1985.

115. Samuelsson, O., Hedner, T., Berglund, G., et al.: Diabetes mellitus in treated hypertension: Incidence, predictive factors and the impact of non-selective beta-blockers and thiazide diuretics during 15 years treatment of middle-aged hypertensive men in the Primary Prevention Trial Göteborg, Sweden. J. Hum. Hypertens. 8:257, 1994.

116. Dørup, I., Skajaa, K., and Thybo, N. K.: Oral magnesium supplementation restores the concentrations of magnesium, potassium and sodium-potassium pumps in skeletal muscle of patients receiving diuretic treatment. J. Intern. Med. 233:117, 1993.

117. Horner, S. M.: Efficacy of intravenous magnesium in acute myocardial infarction in reducing arrhythmias and mortality. Meta-analysis of magnesium in acute myocardial infarction. Circulation 86:774, 1992.

118. Waller, P. C., and Ramsay, L. E.: Predicting acute gout in diuretic-treated hypertensive patients. J. Hum. Hypertens. 3:457, 1989.

119. Kasiske, B. L., Ma, J. Z., Kalil, R. S. N., and Louis, T. A.: Effects of antihypertensive therapy on serum lipids. Ann. Intern. Med. 122:133, 1995.

120. Pollare, T., Lithell, H., and Berne, C.: A comparison of the effects of hydrochlorothiazide and captopril on glucose and lipid metabolism in patients with hypertension. N. Engl. J. Med. 321:868, 1989.

121. Gesek, F. A., and Friedman, P. A.: Mechanism of calcium transport stimulated by chlorothiazide in mouse distal convoluted tubule cells. J. Clin. Invest. 90:429, 1992.

122. Morton, D. J., Barrett-Connor, E. L., and Edelstein, S. L.: Thiazides and bone mineral density in elderly men and women. Am. J. Epidemiol. 139:1107, 1994.

123. Medical Research Council Working Party on Mild to Moderate Hypertension: Adverse reactions to bendrofluazide and propranolol for the treatment of mild hypertension. Lancet 2:539, 1981.

124. Beard, K., Bulpitt, C., Mascie-Taylor, H., et al.: Management of elderly patients with sustained hypertension. Br. Med. J. 304:412, 1992.

Adrenergic Inhibitors

125. Veterans Administration Cooperative Study Group on Antihypertensive Agents: Propranolol in the treatment of essential hypertension. JAMA 237:2303, 1977.

126. Participating Veterans Administration Medical Centers: Low dose vs. standard dose of reserpine. JAMA 248:2471, 1982.

127. Lederle, F. A., Applegate, W. B., and Grimm, R. H., Jr.: Reserpine and the medical marketplace. Arch. Intern. Med. 153:705, 1993.

128. Struthers, A. D., Brown, M. J., Adams, E. F., and Dollery, C. T.: The plasma noradrenaline and growth hormone response to α-methyldopa and clonidine in hypertensive subjects. Br. J. Clin. Pharmacol. 19:311, 1985.

129. Fouad, F. M., Nakashima, Y., Tarazi, R. C., and Salcedo, E. E.: Reversal of left ventricular hypertrophy in hypertensive patients treated with methyldopa. Am. J. Cardiol. 49:795, 1982.

130. Kelton, J. G.: Impaired reticuloendothelial function in patients treated with methyldopa. Am. J. Cardiol. 49:795, 1982.

131. Kaplowitz, N., Aw, T. Y., Simon, F. R., and Stolz, A.: Drug-induced hepatotoxicity. Ann. Intern. Med. 104:826, 1986.

132. van Zwieten, P. A.: Different types of centrally acting antihypertensive drugs. Eur. Heart J. 13:18, 1992.

133. Houston, M. C.: Abrupt cessation of treatment in hypertension: Consideration of clinical features, mechanisms, prevention and management of the discontinuation syndrome. Am. Heart J. 102:415, 1981.

134. Schmidt, G. R., Schuna, A. A., and Goodfriend, T. L.: Transdermal clonidine compared with hydrochlorothiazide as monotherapy in elderly hypertensive males. J. Clin. Pharmacol. 29:133, 1989.

135. Gehr, M., MacCarthy, E. P., and Goldberg, M.: Guanabenz: A centrally acting, natriuretic antihypertensive drug. Kidney Int. 29:1203, 1986.

136. Kaplan, N. M., and Grundy, S.: Comparison of the effects of guanabenz and hydrochlorothiazide on plasma lipids. Clin. Pharmacol. Ther. 44:297, 1988.

137. Lewin, A., Alderman, M. H., and Mathur, P.: Antihypertensive efficacy of guanfacine and prazosin in patients with mild to moderate essential hypertension. J. Clin. Pharmacol. 30:1081, 1990.

138. Lenz, M. L., Pool, J. L., Laddu, A. R., et al.: Combined terazosin and verapamil therapy in essential hypertension: Hemodynamic and pharmacokinetic interactions. Am. J. Hypertens. 8:133, 1995.

139. Pickering, T. G., Levenstein, M., and Walmsley, P.: Nighttime dosing of doxazosin has peak effect on morning ambulatory blood pressure. Results of the HALT study. Am. J. Hypertens. 7:844, 1994.

140. Heagerty, A. M., Russell, G. I., Bing, R. F., et al.: The addition of prazosin to standard triple therapy in the treatment of severe hypertension. Br. J. Clin. Pharmacol. 13:539, 1982.

141. Rabkin, S. W., Huff, M. W., Newman, C., et al.: Lipids and lipoproteins during antihypertensive drug therapy. Comparison of doxazosin and atenolol in a randomized, double-blind trial: The Alpha Beta Canada study. Hypertension 24:241, 1994.

142. Andersson, P.-E., Johansson, J., Berne, C., and Lithell, H.: Effects of selective alpha₁ and beta₁-adrenoreceptor blockade on lipoprotein and carbohydrate metabolism in hypertensive subjects, with special emphasis on insulin sensitivity. J. Hum. Hypertens. 8:219, 1994.

143. Monda, J. M., and Oesterling, J. E.: Medical treatment of benign prostatic hyperplasia: 5α-reductase inhibitors and α-adrenergic antagonists. Mayo Clin. Proc. 68:670, 1993.

144. Viscoli, C. M., Horwitz, R. I., and Singer, B. H.: Beta-blockers after myocardial infarction: influence of first-year clinical course on long-term effectiveness. Ann. Intern. Med. 118:99, 1993.

145. IPPPSH Collaborative Group: Cardiovascular risk and risk factors in a randomized trial of treatment based on the beta-blocker oxprenolol: The International Prospective Primary Prevention Study in Hypertension (IPPPSH). J. Hypertens. 3:379, 1985.

146. Wilhelmsen, L., Berglund, G., Elmfeldt, D., et al.: Beta-blockers versus diuretics in hypertensive men: Main results from the HAPPHY Trial. J. Hypertens. 5:561, 1987.

147. Wikstrand, J., Warnold, I., Olsson, G., et al.: Primary prevention with metoprolol in patients with hypertension. Mortality results from the MAPHY study. JAMA 259:1976, 1988.

148. Wikstrand, J., Warnold, I., Tuomilehto, J., et al.: Metoprolol versus thiazide diuretics in hypertension. Hypertension 17:579, 1991.

149. Fitzgerald, J. D.: The applied pharmacology of beta-adrenoceptor antagonists (beta blockers) in relation to clinical outcomes. Cardiovasc. Drug Ther. 5:561, 1991.

150. Lithell, H., Pollare, T., and Vessby, B.: Metabolic effects of pindolol and propranolol in a double-blind cross-over study in hypertensive patients. Blood Pressure 1:92, 1992.

151. Yudofsky, S. C.: β-blockers and depression. The clinician's dilemma. JAMA 267:1295, 1991.

152. Man in't Veld, A. J., Van Den Meiracker, A. H., and Schalekamp, M. A.: Do beta-blockers really increase peripheral vascular resistance? Review of the literature and new observations under basal conditions. Am. J. Hypertens. 1:91, 1988.

153. Serlin, M. M., Orme, M. L'E., Baber, N. A., et al.: Propranolol in the control of blood pressure: A dose-response study. Clin. Pharmacol. Ther. 27:586, 1980.

154. Cruickshank, J. M.: The case for beta-blockers as first-line antihypertensive therapy. J. Hypertens. 10:S21, 1992.

155. Gullestad, L., Birkeland, K., Nordby, G., et al.: Effects of selective β₂-adrenoceptor blockade on serum potassium and exercise performance in normal men. Br. J. Clin. Pharmacol. 32:201, 1991.

156. Oxorn, D., Knox, J. W. D., and Hill, J.: Bolus doses of esmolol for the prevention of perioperative hypertension and tachycardia. Can. J. Anaesth. 37:206, 1990.

157. Eichhorn, E. J., and Hjalmarson, A.: β-Blocker treatment for chronic heart failure. The frog prince. Circulation 90:2153, 1994.

158. Dahlöf, C., and Dimenäs, E.: Side effects of β-blocker treatments as related to the central nervous system. Am. J. Med. Sci. 299:236, 1990.

159. Bright, R. A., and Everitt, D. E.: β-blockers and depression. Evidence against an association. JAMA 267:1783, 1992.

160. Psaty, B. M., Koepsell, T. D., Wagner, E. H., et al.: The relative risk of incident coronary heart disease associated with recently stopping the use of β-blockers. JAMA 263:1653, 1990.

161. Dujovne, C. A., Ferraro, L., Goldstein, R. J., et al.: Comparative effects of atenolol versus celiprolol on serum lipids and blood pressure in hyperlipidemic and hypertensive subjects. Am. J. Cardiol. 72:1131, 1993.

162. Butters, L., Kennedy, S., and Rubin, P. C.: Atenolol in essential hypertension during pregnancy. Br. Med. J. 301:587, 1990.

163. Goa, K. L., Benfield, P., and Sorkin, E. M.: Labetalol. A reappraisal of its pharmacology, pharmacokinetics and therapeutic use in hypertension and ischaemic heart disease. Drugs 37:583, 1989.

164. Clark, J. A., Zimmerman, H. J., and Tanner, L. A.: Labetalol hepatotoxicity. Ann. Intern. Med. 113:210, 1990.

Vasodilators

165. Shepherd, A. M. M., and Irving, N. A.: Differential hemodynamic and sympathoadrenal effects of sodium nitroprusside and hydralazine in hypertensive subjects. J. Cardiovasc. Pharmacol. 8:527, 1986.

166. Halstenson, C. E., Opsahl, J.A., Wright, E., et al.: Disposition of minoxidil in patients with various degrees of renal function. J. Clin. Pharmacol. 29:798, 1989.

167. Houston, M. C., McChesney, J. A., and Chatterjee, K.: Pericardial effusion associated with minoxidil therapy. Arch. Intern. Med. 131:69, 1981.

168. Kelly, J. G., and O'Malley, K.: Clinical pharmacokinetics of calcium antagonists. Clin. Pharmacokinet. 22:416, 1992.

169. Cappuccio, F. P., Antonios, T. F. T., Markandu, N. D., et al.: Acute natriuretic effect of nifedipine on different sodium intakes in essential hypertension: Evidence for distal tubular effect? J. Hum. Hypertens. 8:627, 1994.

170. Luft, F. C., Fineberg, N. S., and Weinberger, M. H.: Long-term effect of nifedipine and hydrochlorothiazide on blood pressure and sodium homeostasis at varying levels of salt intake in mildly hypertensive patients. Am. J. Hypertens. 4:752, 1991.

171. ter Wee, P. M., De Micheli, A. G., and Epstein, M.: Effects of calcium antagonists on renal hemodynamics and progression of nondiabetic chronic renal disease. Arch. Intern. Med. 154:1185, 1994.

172. Ranieri, G., Andriani, A., Lamontanara, G., and De Cesaris, R.: Effects

of lisinopril and amlodipine on microalbuminuria and renal function in patients with hypertension. Clin. Pharmacol. Ther. 56:323, 1994.

173. Siewert-Delle, A., Ljungman, S., Hartford, M., and Wikstrand, J.: Effects of intensified blood-pressure reduction on renal function and albumin excretion in primary hypertension. Addition of felodipine or ramipril to long-term treatment with β-blockade. Am. J. Hypertens. 8:113, 1995.

174. Zanetti-Elshater, F., Pingitore, R., Beretta-Piccoli, C., et al.: Calcium antagonists for treatment of diabetes-associated hypertension. Am. J. Hypertens. 7:36, 1994.

174a. Psaty, B. M., Heckbert, S. R., Koepsell, T. D., et al.: The risk of myocardial infarction associated with antihypertensive drug therapies. JAMA 274:620, 1995.

174b. Horwitz, R. I., Feinstein, A. R.: Exclusion bias and the false relationship of reserpine use and breast cancer. Arch. Intern. Med. 145:1873, 1995.

175. Klassen, D. K., Jane, L. H., Young, D. Y., and Peterson, C. A.: Assessment of blood pressure during naproxen therapy in hypertensive patients treated with nicardipine. Am. J. Hypertens. 8:146, 1995.

176. Jaker, M., Atkin, S., Soto, M., et al.: Oral nifedipine vs oral clonidine in the treatment of urgent hypertension. Arch. Intern. Med. 149:260, 1989.

177. Neutel, J. M., Smith, D. H. G., Cook, W. E., et al.: A comparison of intravenous nicardipine and sodium nitroprusside in the immediate treatment of severe hypertension. Am. J. Hypertens. 7:623, 1994.

177a. Jackson, E. K., and Garrison, J. C.: Renin and angiotensin. In Hardman, J. G., et al. (eds.): Goodman and Gilman's The Pharmacological Basis of Therapeutics. 9th ed. New York; McGraw-Hill, 1996, pp. 733–758.

178. Kobrin, I., Viskoper, R. J., Laszt, A., et al.: Effects of an orally active renin inhibitor, RO 42-5892, in patients with essential hypertension. Am. J. Hypertens. 6:349, 1993.

179. Grossman, E., Peleg, E., Carroll, J., et al.: Hemodynamic and humoral effects of the angiotensin II antagonist losartan in essential hypertension. Am. J. Hypertens. 7:1041, 1994.

180. van den Meiracker, A. H., Man in't Veld, A. J., Admiraal, P. J. J., et al.: Partial escape of angiotensin converting enzyme (ACE) inhibition during prolonged ACE inhibitor treatment: Does it exist and does it affect the antihypertensive response? J. Hypertens. 10:803, 1992.

181. Pellacani, A., Brunner, H. R., and Nussberger, J.: Plasma kinins increase after angiotensin-converting enzyme inhibition in human subjects. Clin. Sci. 87:567, 1994.

182. Tomiyama, H., Kushiro, T., Abeta, H., et al.: Kinins contribute to the improvement of insulin sensitivity during treatment with angiotensin converting enzyme inhibitor. Hypertension 23:450, 1994.

183. Fletcher, A. E., Palmer, A. J., and Bulpitt, C. J.: Cough with angiotensin converting enzyme inhibitors: how much of a problem? J. Hypertens. 12(Suppl. 2):S43, 1994.

184. Ferri, C., Laurenti, O., Bellini, C., et al.: Circulating endothelin-1 levels in lean noninsulin-dependent diabetic patients: Influence of ACE-inhibition. Am. J. Hypertens. 8:40, 1995.

185. Schiffrin, E. L., Deng, L. Y., and Larochelle, P.: Effects of a β-blocker or a converting enzyme inhibitor on resistance arteries in essential hypertension. Hypertension 23:83, 1994.

186. Giannattasio, C., Cattaneo, B. M., Omboni, S., et al.: Sympathomoderating influence of benazepril in essential hypertension. J. Hypertens. 10:373, 1992.

187. Postma, C. T., Dennesen, P. J. W., de Boo, T., and Thien, T.: First dose hypotension after captopril; Can it be predicted? A study of 240 patients. J. Hum. Hypertens. 6:205, 1992.

188. Kaplan, N. M.: Renal vascular hypertension. In Kaplan, N. M. (ed.): Clinical Hypertension. 6th ed. Baltimore, Williams & Wilkins, 1994, p. 319.

189. Devoy, M. A. B., Tomson, C. R. V., Edmunds, M. E., et al.: Deterioration in renal function associated with angiotensin converting enzyme inhibitor therapy is not always reversible. J. Intern. Med. 232:493, 1992.

190. Lewis, E. J., Hunsicker, L. G., Bain, R. P., and Rohde, R. D.: The effect of angiotensin-converting-enzyme inhibition on diabetic nephropathy. N. Engl. J. Med. 329:1456, 1993.

191. Buzio, C., Regolisti, G., Perazzoli, F., et al.: Renal effects of nifedipine and captopril in patients with essential hypertension and reduced renal reserve. Hypertension 24:763, 1994.

192. Hypertension in Diabetes Study Group: Hypertension in Diabetes Study III. Prospective study of therapy of hypertension in type 2 diabetic patients: Efficacy of ACE inhibition and β-blockade. Diabetic Med. 11:773, 1994.

193. Raccah, D., Pettenuzzo-Mollo, M., Provendier, O., et al.: Comparison of the effects of captopril and nicardipine on insulin sensitivity and thrombotic profile in patients with hypertension and android obesity. Am. J. Hypertens. 7:731, 1994.

194. Chu, T. J., and Chow, N.: Adverse effects of ACE inhibitors. Ann. Intern. Med. 118:313, 1993.

194a. Wood, R.: Bronchospasm and cough as adverse reactions to the ACE inhibitors captopril, enalapril and lisinopril. Br. J. Clin. Pharmacol. 39:265, 1995.

195. Os, I., Bratland, B., Dahlöf, B., et al.: Female preponderance for lisinopril-induced cough in hypertension. Am. J. Hypertens. 7:1012, 1994.

196. Lip, G. Y. H., Zarifis, J., Beevers, M., and Beevers, D. G.: Duration of cough following cessation of ACE inhibitor therapy. Am. J. Hypertens. 8:98, 1995.

197. Warner, T. D., Battistini, B., Doherty, A. M., and Corder, R.: Endothelin receptor antagonists: Actions and rationale for their development. Biochem. Pharmacol. 48:625, 1994.

198. Vesely, D. L., Douglass, M. D., Dietz, J. R., et al.: Three peptides from the atrial natriuretic factor prohormone amino terminus lower blood pressure and produce diuresis, natriuresis, and/or kaliuresis in humans. Circulation 90:1129, 1994.

199. Ogihara, T., Rakugi, H., Masuo, K., et al.: Antihypertensive effects of the neutral endopeptidase inhibitor SCH 42495 in essential hypertension. Am. J. Hypertens. 7:943, 1994.

200. Cody, R. J.: The clinical potential of renin inhibitors and angiotensin antagonists. Drugs 47:586, 1994.

200a. Awan, N. A., and Mason, D. T.: Direct selective blockade of the vascular angiotensin II receptors in therapy for hypertension and severe congestive heart failure. Am. Heart J. 131:177, 1996.

SPECIAL CONSIDERATIONS IN THERAPY

201. Setaro, J. F., and Black, H. R.: Refractory hypertension. N. Engl. J. Med. 8:543, 1992.

202. Mejia, A. D., Egan, B. M., Schork, N. J., and Zwiefler, A. J.: Artefacts in measurement of blood pressure and lack of target organ involvement in the assessment of patients with treatment-resistant hypertension. Ann. Intern. Med. 117:270, 1990.

203. Isaksson, H., Cederholm, T., Jansson, E., et al.: Therapy-resistant hypertension associated with central obesity, insulin resistance, and large muscle fibre area. Blood Pressure 2:46, 1993.

204. Johnson, A. G., Nguyen, T. V., and Day, R. O.: Do nonsteroidal anti-inflammatory drugs affect blood pressure? Ann. Intern. Med. 121:289, 1994.

205. Estafanous, F. G.: Hypertension in the surgical patient: Management of blood pressure and anesthesia. Cleveland Clin. J. Med. 56:385, 1989.

206. Wolfsthal, S. D.: Is blood pressure control necessary before surgery? Med. Clin. North Am. 77:349, 1993.

207. Haworth, R. A., Goknur, A. B., and Berkoff, H. A.: Inhibition of Na-Ca exchange by general anesthetics. Circ. Res. 65:1021, 1989.

208. Patel, C. G., Laboy, V., Venus, B., et al.: Use of sodium nitroprusside in post-coronary bypass surgery. A plea for conservatism. Chest 80:663, 1986.

209. Halpern, N. A., Goldberg, M., Neely, C., et al.: Postoperative hypertension: A multicenter, prospective, randomized comparison between intravenous nicardipine and sodium nitroprusside. Crit. Care Med. 20:1637, 1992.

210. Lieberman, E.: Hypertension in childhood and adolescence. In Kaplan, N. M. (ed.): Clinical Hypertension. 6th ed. Baltimore, Williams and Wilkins, 1994, p. 437.

211. Lewis, R. R., Evans, P. J., McNabb, W. R., and Padayachee, T. S.: Comparison of indirect and direct blood pressure measurements with Osler's manoeuvre in elderly hypertensive patients. J. Hum. Hypertens. 8:879, 1994.

212. Kaplan, N. M.: The promises and perils of treating the elderly hypertensive. Am. J. Med. Sci. 305:183, 1993.

213. Lye, M., Vargas, E., Faragher, E. B., et al.: Haemodynamic and neurohumoral responses in elderly patients with postural hypotension. Eur. J. Clin. Invest. 20:90, 1990.

214. Mulrow, C. D., Cornell, J. A., Herrera, C. R., et al.: Hypertension in the elderly. Implications and generalizability of randomized trials. JAMA 272:1932, 1994.

215. Stein, G. H., Hamilton, B. P., Hamilton, J. H., et al.: One year experience of elderly hypertensive patients with isradipine therapy. J. Hum. Hypertens. 8:911, 1994.

216. Groden, D. L.: Vasodilator therapy for congestive heart failure. Arch. Intern. Med. 153:445, 1993.

217. Franz, I.-W., Ketelhut, R., Behr, U., and Tönnesmann, U.: Time course of reduction in left ventricular mass during long-term antihypertensive therapy. J. Hum. Hypertens. 8:191, 1994.

218. Brush, J. E., Jr., Udelson, J. E., Bacharach, S. L., et al.: Comparative effects of verapamil and nitroprusside on left ventricular function in patients with hypertension. J. Am. Coll. Cardiol. 14:515, 1989.

219. Cottrell, J. E., Patel, K., Turndorf, H., and Ransohoff, J.: Intracranial pressure changes induced by sodium nitroprusside in patients with intracranial mass lesions. J. Neurosurg. 48:329, 1978.

220. Lip, G. Y. H., Beevers, M., and Beevers, G.: The failure of malignant hypertension to decline: A survey of 24 years' experience in a multiracial population in England. J. Hypertens. 12:1297, 1994.

Chapter 28
Syncope and Hypotension

WISHWA N. KAPOOR

Syncope is defined as a sudden temporary loss of consciousness associated with a loss of postural tone with spontaneous recovery not requiring electrical or chemical cardioversion. Syncope is a common symptom accounting for 1 to 6 per cent of hospital admissions and up to 3 per cent of emergency department visits. Loss of consciousness is also common in healthy young adults (12 to 48 per cent), although most do not seek medical attention. Syncope is a frequent symptom in the elderly; a 6 per cent incidence and 23 per cent previous lifetime episodes were reported in one long-term care institution.

CLINICAL AND PATHOPHYSIOLOGICAL CLASSIFICATION

Although syncope has a large differential diagnosis, the causes can be classified into four major categories (Table 28–1).

Reflex-Mediated Vasomotor Instability Syndromes

Neurally mediated, neurocardiogenic, reflex, and neuro-regulatory syncope are broad terms, used synonymously, referring to syncope resulting from reflex mechanisms associated with inappropriate vasodilatation and/or brady-

TABLE 28–1 ETIOLOGIES OF SYNCOPE

REFLEX-MEDIATED VASOMOTOR INSTABILITY	DECREASED CARDIAC OUTPUT
Vasovagal	**Obstruction to Flow**
Situational	Obstruction to LV outflow
Micturition	Aortic stenosis, HCM
Cough	Mitral stenosis, myxoma
Swallowing	Obstruction to RV outflow
Defecation	Pulmonic stenosis
Carotid sinus syncope	PE, pulmonary hypertension
Neuralgias	Myxoma
High altitude	
Psychiatric disorders	**Other Heart Disease**
Others (exercise, selected drugs)	Pump failure
	MI, CAD, coronary spasm
ORTHOSTATIC HYPOTENSION	Tamponade, aortic dissection
	Arrhythmias
NEUROLOGICAL DISEASES	Bradyarrhythmias
Migraines	Sinus node disease
TIAs	Second and third degree atrio-ventricular block
Seizures	Pacemaker malfunction
	Drug-induced bradyarrhythmias
	Tachyarrhythmias
	Ventricular tachycardia
	Torsades de pointes (e.g., associated with congenital long Q-T syndromes or acquired Q-T prolongation)
	Supraventricular tachycardia

LV = left ventricle; HCM = hypertrophic cardiomyopathy; MI = myocardial infarction; TIA = transient ischemic attack; CAD = coronary artery disease.

cardia.[1] These terms incorporate more specific syndromes such as vasovagal, vasodepressor, situational, or carotid sinus syncope. Currently, various neurally mediated syndromes are believed to have common pathophysiological elements as well as differences in triggering factors, afferent and efferent neural arcs, and central nervous system (CNS) processing that ultimately result in hypotension and loss of consciousness[1] (Fig. 28–1). For all of these syndromes, there are facilitating factors, such as emotional state, volume status, and posture, predisposing to syncope.

Receptors that respond to pain, mechanical stimuli, and temperature appear to serve as the origins of the afferent signals triggering the various neurally mediated syncopal syndromes.[1–3] For example, in carotid sinus hypersensitivity, carotid artery baroreceptors and in vasovagal syncope, left ventricular baroreceptors (mechanoreceptors) serve as triggers. Similar receptors in the aortic arch, carotid arteries, atrial and ventricular myocardium, respiratory tree, bladder, and gastrointestinal tract may trigger various other neurally mediated syndromes.[1] The afferent pathway consists of neural fibers (e.g., vagal C fibers in vasovagal syncope) that transmit signals to the CNS sites (in the medulla, particularly the nucleus tractus solitarius). The efferent outflow results in vasodilation and bradycardia. Ventricular mechanoreceptors are sensitized by catecholamines and arginine vasopressin, high levels of which are often found before vasovagal syncope. Provocation of syncope with upright tilt testing after heart transplantation has raised questions about this mechanism, because evidence for reinnervation is not found in some patients.[4–6] Central inhibition of sympathetic excitatory neurons has been considered to be an alternative mechanism with vasopressin release and opiate receptor activation playing possible roles.[7,8] Additionally, the role of serotonin[2,9] and endogenous nitric oxide as mediators of central inhibitory activity has been postulated.[2] More complete understanding of the mechanism of neurally mediated syncope has to await further studies. Current understanding of the clinical and pathophysiological mechanism of specific entities is described below.

VASOVAGAL SYNCOPE. Vasodepressor or vasovagal syncope is characterized by a sudden fall in blood pressure with or without bradycardia in association with autonomic and humoral activity such as pallor, nausea, sweating, mydriasis, bradycardia, hyperventilation, and antidiuresis. Vasodepressor syncope often occurs in young people and generally in response to fear or injury. Predisposing factors include fatigue, prolonged standing, venipuncture, blood donation, heat, dental surgery, and eye surgery. Vasovagal syncope may also occur without any identifiable predisposing factors and may be provoked by standing still in an upright posture in susceptible individuals.

Vasovagal syncope has three phases. During the first phase, blood pressure and heart rate increase largely owing to a baroreceptor-mediated rise in sympathetic tone. This is followed by abrupt hypotension and bradycardia (occasionally asystole of 10 to 20 sec or greater) with premonitory symptoms culminating in syncope. The third phase consists of rapid recovery upon recumbency.

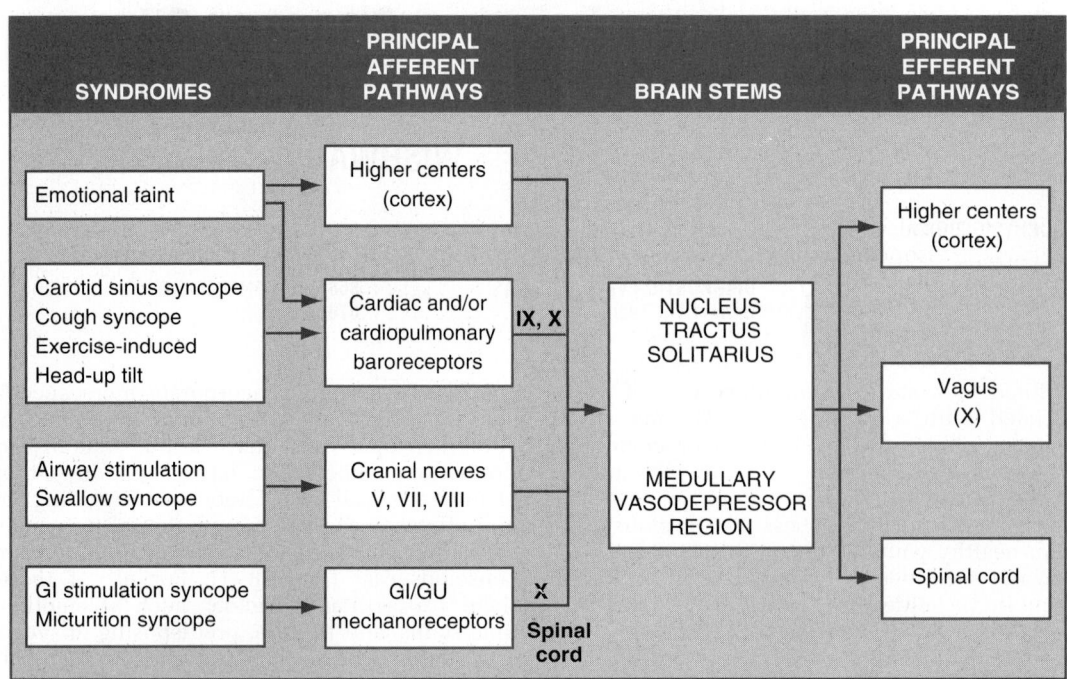

SYNDROMES	PRINCIPAL AFFERENT PATHWAYS	BRAIN STEMS	PRINCIPAL EFFERENT PATHWAYS

FIGURE 28–1. The mechanisms for various reflex-mediated vasomotor syndromes showing similarities and differences in the mechanisms of these entities IX and X refer to the ninth and tenth cranial nerves. (Adapted from Benditt, D.G., et al.: Tilt table testing for evaluation of neurally mediated (cardioneurogenic) syncope: Rationale and proposed protocols. PACE *14*:1528, 1991.)

Generally, vasovagal syncope occurs in an upright posture. During upright standing, there is decreased venous return, stroke volume, and arterial pressure leading to compensatory responses mediated by arterial and cardiopulmonary baroreceptors. Normally, afferent neural input from baroreceptors is relayed to the medullary centers; this results in increased sympathetic and decreased parasympathetic activity. However, occasionally abrupt decrease in venous return (e.g., with hemorrhage) may result in a relatively "empty ventricle" that contracts vigorously, leading to excessive stimulation of ventricular mechanoreceptors and paradoxical vasodilatation and bradycardia.[2,3] Increased circulating epinephrine level and higher CNS centers may augment this response.

SITUATIONAL SYNCOPE. Syncope in association with various daily activities (e.g., micturition, defecation, cough, and swallowing) is termed *situational syncope.*

Micturition syncope was originally described in healthy young men who, after rising from bed in the early morning hours, experienced sudden loss of consciousness during or immediately after urination. Predisposing factors having a facilatatory role include reduced food intake, recent upper respiratory tract infection, fatigue, and ingestion of alcohol. Older patients (mean age 60 years) with multiple acute and chronic medical problems may experience micturition syncope[10] often associated with orthostatic hypotension. Isolated case reports have associated micturition syncope and presyncope with bladder neck obstruction, psychomotor epilepsy, complete AV block, and pheochromocytoma of the bladder.

The mechanism of micturition syncope is probably similar to that of vasovagal syncope except for the site or nature of the trigger factors. Mechanoreceptors in the bladder have been implicated in micturition syncope. A combination of physiological changes during sleep and urination may predispose to micturition syncope. These changes include sudden decompression of the bladder, a decline of blood pressure and heart rate mediated by decreased peripheral resistance during sleep, possible Valsalva maneuver during micturition, and orthostatic hypotension (in the elderly).

In *defecation syncope,* vagal afferents transmit neural impulses from gut wall tension receptors. These signals are then presumably transmitted to the CNS, resulting in hypotension and bradycardia. A variety of gastrointestinal tract conditions (Meckel's diverticulum, ruptured appendix) and cardiovascular diseases (ventricular arrhythmias), as well as orthostatic hypotension and transient ischemic attacks, have been reported to contribute to syncope.[11] Cases of association with pulmonary embolism and foreign body (toothpick) in the rectum have been reported. Syncope in association with rectal and pelvic examination and during sigmoidoscopy probably has a similar mechanism.

Syncope in association with *swallowing* probably results from afferent neural impulses in the upper gastrointestinal tract served by the glossopharyngeal or vagus nerves with transmission to the CNS. Most patients with syncope during or immediately following swallowing have had structural abnormalities of the esophagus or the heart (diverticula, diffuse esophageal spasm, achalasia, and stricture). Cardiac conditions have included acute rheumatic carditis treated with digitalis, acute myocardial infarction, and a calcified mass over the aortic valve and septum. Bradyarrhythmias (sinus arrest or asystole, complete AV block, nodal or sinus bradycardia, and sinoatrial block) have been demonstrated during swallow syncope.

Airway stimulation (e.g., during endotracheal intubation or bronchoscopy) may also result in marked bradycardia resulting from similar mechanisms involving vagal afferent neural transmission to the CNS with subsequent vagal efferents leading to bradycardia and hypotension. A similar mechanism is probably operative in *cough syncope,* which consists of the very brief loss of consciousness after paroxysms of severe cough, described almost exclusively (> 90 per cent) in middle-aged men who drink ethanol, smoke, and have chronic lung disease. Coughing may produce very high intrathoracic pressure, with a sudden decrease in venous return and cardiac output and transmission of high intrathoracic pressure during cough to the subarachnoid space, which may reduce cerebral blood and lead to syncope. Alternatively, reflex syncope may be the predominant mechanism.

Rare case reports have associated cough syncope with Mobitz II or complete AV block, obstructive cardiomyopathy, hypersensitive carotid sinus syndrome, herniated-cerebellar tonsils, and severe bilateral cerebrovascular disease. A related syndrome, *sneeze syncope,* is probably due to similar mechanisms and has been associated with the Arnold-Chiari malformation. In the treatment of cough syncope due to underlying lung disease, smoking cessation is the most important factor, in addition to bronchodilators and cough suppressants.

CAROTID SINUS SYNCOPE. The carotid sinus baroreceptors consist of sensory nerve endings located in the internal carotid artery just above the bifurcation of the common carotid artery. Afferent impulses travel via the sinus nerve of Hering and join the glossopharyngeal nerve and perhaps cervical sympathetic and vagus nerves to enter the sensory nucleus of the vagus (solitary tract) and the vasomotor center. Efferent pathways include sympathetic adrenergic nerves to the heart, resistance and capacitance vessels, and cardiac vagus nerve.[12,13]

Three types of carotid sinus hypersensitivity are generally recognized.[12,13] *Cardioinhibitory carotid sinus hypersensitivity* is widely defined as cardiac asystole of 3 sec or more. The pure *vasodepressor type* is defined as a systolic blood pressure decline of 50 mm Hg or more (in the absence of significant bradycardia). A *mixed type* consists of a combination of cardioinhibitory and vasodepressor response. The prevalence of carotid sinus hypersensitivity in an asymptomatic population is reported to be 5 to 25 per cent, occurring primarily in older individuals ($\geq$ 60 years); the condition is found more commonly in men. The cardioinhibitory variety accounts for 34 to 78 per cent and vasodepressor 5 to 10 per cent of cases of carotid sinus hypersensitivity.

Five to 20 per cent of individuals with abnormal carotid sensitivity suffer spontaneous fainting, termed *carotid sinus syncope.* Attacks may be precipitated by factors that exert pressure on the carotid sinus (e.g., tight collar, shaving, sudden turning), a history of which is obtained in only a quarter of patients with this syndrome. Syncope occurs predominantly in men, 70 per cent of whom are 50 years of age or older. The majority have coronary artery disease and hypertension. Other predisposing factors include neck pathology such as enlarged lymph nodes, tissue scars, carotid body tumors, parotid, thyroid, and head and neck tumors. Possible associations with digitalis, alpha-methyldopa, and propranolol have been reported. Abnormalities of sinus node function and atrioventricular conduction are often found in patients with carotid sinus hypersensitivity.

Survival in patients with carotid sinus hypersensitivity is similar to that in the general population and is largely related to underlying diseases. Survival appears to be unrelated to pacemaker therapy.[14] Prior studies had reported symptom recurrence in 20 to 25 per cent of untreated or medically treated patients with carotid sinus syndrome. However, syncope recurred in 57 per cent of those without pacemakers vs. 9 per cent of a paced group in a prospective study of patients with severe carotid sinus syndrome (i.e., patients with recurrent syncope, trauma, and reproduction of symptoms upon massage).[15]

GLOSSOPHARYNGEAL NEURALGIA. This is a severe unilateral paroxysmal pain in the oropharynx, tonsillar fossa, base of tongue, or ear precipitated by swallowing, chewing, or coughing. Occasionally, syncope and seizures occur during the attack, which in most instances is caused by asystole or bradycardia and rarely by a vasodepressor reaction. Seizures are consistent with hypoxemic convulsions. Neoplasms have been reported in one-sixth of the patients with syncope and consist of neck tumors or lymphoma with meningeal involvement. Trigeminal neuralgia has also been associated with syncope and seizures due to bradycardia and asystole or a vasodepressor reaction. Syncope is probably due to spread of afferent impulses from the trigger zone in the pharynx (conducted in the glossopharyngeal nerve) to the dorsal motor nucleus of the vagus, causing intense vagal stimulation. In the vasodepressor variety, inhibition of peripheral sympathetic activity is implicated.

HIGH-ALTITUDE SYNCOPE. A young healthy individual's recent arrival at moderate or very high altitudes can result in syncope without long-term adverse sequelae.[16] Possible mechanisms include reflex bradycardia, hyperventilation, and subsequent hypocapnia resulting in reflex cerebral vasoconstriction, which may decrease cerebral oxygen delivery. Mild volume depletion due to diuresis at high altitude or due to physical activity may lead to vasovagal syncope.

PSYCHIATRIC ILLNESSES. Stress and psychiatric illnesses probably cause syncope by precipitating vasovagal reactions. Patients with psychiatric syncope are generally young, are more often female, and have recurrent syncope but no organic heart disease.[17-19] Generalized anxiety disorder, panic disorder, and major depression account for the majority of psychiatric causes. Several epidemics of fainting described in young individuals have been attributed to transitory anxiety attacks in response to environmental stresses. Syncope constitutes a somatic complaint in up to 9 per cent of the patients with panic disorder. Major depression may lead to syncope through the common association with anxiety disorder, or syncope may be a somatic manifestation of depression, because medical patients with depression often present with nonspecific cardiopulmonary and other physical complaints indicating masked or atypical depression.

OTHER ENTITIES. Neurally mediated reflex mechanism is also implicated for syncope in association with exercise, especially syncope occurring immediately after exercise in individuals without structural heart disease.[20-22] An increase in catecholamines and force of ventricular contraction may stimulate the cardiac mechanoreceptors in the setting of mild volume depletion and shifts of blood flow to dissipate heat.

NEURALLY MEDIATED SYNCOPE. This may also occur with drugs that decrease venous return to the heart in an upright position. For example, nitrates lead to marked venous dilatation, decreased venous return, and diminished cardiac output, which normally results in tachycardia and increased cardiac inotropic state. However, in susceptible individuals, this may lead to stimulation of cardiac mechanoreceptors and syncope.[23] Syncope with aortic stenosis,[24] hypertrophic cardiomyopathy,[25] supraventricular tachycardias,[26] paroxysmal atrial fibrillation,[27] and that related to pacemakers[28] (i.e., pacemaker syndrome), appears to be neurally mediated.

Orthostatic Hypotension

When a person assumes upright posture, 500 to 700 ml of blood is pooled in the lower extremities and the splanchnic circulation. The consequent reduction in venous return to the heart results in decreased cardiac output and stimulation of aortic, carotid, and cardiopulmonary baroreceptors. This stimulation reflexly increases sympathetic outflow and inhibits parasympathetic activity. These adjustments lead to an increase in heart rate and vascular resistance to maintain systemic blood pressure upon standing upright.[29] Orthostatic hypotension results when a defect exists in regulation of systemic blood pressure in any element of this system, from the circulating volume to neural input to the vascular system.

Symptoms due to orthostatic hypotension include dizziness or light-headedness, blurring or loss of vision, a sense of profound weakness, and syncope. Loss of consciousness is generally brief, and there are no associated symptoms of autonomic hyperactivity. These symptoms are often worse on arising in the morning and may be especially prominent after meals or exercise.

Decreased intravascular volume and adverse effects of drugs are the most common causes of symptomatic orthostatic hypotension (Table 28-2).[29] Drugs cause syncope by leading to alterations of vascular volume or tone (e.g., antihypertensive agents, nitrates) or by causing an allergic or anaphylactic reaction. Drugs are responsible for 2 to 9 per cent of symptoms in patients presenting with syncope. Elderly patients are especially vulnerable to symptoms resulting from drugs and volume depletion because of reduced baroreceptor sensitivity, decreased cerebral blood flow, excessive renal sodium wasting, and an impaired thirst mechanism that develops with aging.[30]

Orthostatic hypotension is an important manifestation of diseases affecting the autonomic nervous system (Table 28-2).[31] *Idiopathic orthostatic hypotension* is a rare illness that affects men five times more frequently than women, and is often associated with other autonomic disturbances such as sphincter malfunction, impotence, impaired erection and ejaculation, and impaired sweating. Plasma norepinephrine levels are markedly reduced at rest and remain unchanged on standing, suggesting peripheral dysfunction. Shy-Drager syndrome is associated with autonomic failure and involvement of the corticospinal, extrapyramidal, and cerebellar tracts including a parkinson-like syndrome. This disease may also be associated with cholinergic dysfunction

TABLE 28–2   CAUSES OF ORTHOSTATIC HYPOTENSION

1. PRIMARY

Pure autonomic failure (idiopathic orthostatic hypotension)
Autonomic failure with multiple system atrophy (Shy-Drager syndrome)
Autonomic failure with Parkinson's disease

2. SECONDARY

General medical disorders: diabetes; amyloid; alcoholism
Autoimmune disease: Guillain-Barré syndrome; mixed connective tissue disease; rheumatoid arthritis; Eaton-Lambert syndrome; systemic lupus erythematosus
Carcinomatous autonomic neuropathy
Metabolic disease: Vitamin B12-deficiency; porphyria; Fabry's disease; Tangier disease
Hereditary sensory neuropathies, dominant or recessive
Infections of the nervous system: syphilis; Chagas' disease; HIV infection; botulism; herpes zoster
Central brain lesions: vascular lesion or tumors involving the hypothalamus and midbrain, for example craniopharyngioma; multiple sclerosis; Wernicke's encephalopathy
Spinal cord lesions
Familial dysautonomia
Familial hyperbradykininism
Renal failure
Dopamine beta-hydroxylase deficiency
Ageing

3. DRUGS

Selective neurotoxic drugs; alcoholism
Tranquilizers: phenothiazines; barbiturates
Antidepressants: tricyclics; monoamine oxidase inhibitors
Vasodilators: prazosin; hydralazine; calcium channel blockers
Centrally acting hypotensive drugs: methyldopa; clonidine
Adrenergic neuron blocking drugs: guanethidine
Alpha-adrenergic blocking drugs: phenoxybenzamine; labetalol
Ganglion-blocking drugs: hexamethonium; mecamylamine
Angiotensin-converting enzyme inhibitors: captopril; enalapril; lisinopril

Adapted from Bannister, S. R. (ed.): Autonomic Failure. 2nd ed. Oxford, Oxford University Press, 1988, p. 8.

affecting the vagal, ocular, bladder, and sweat glands. Norepinephrine levels are normal at rest but remain unchanged on standing, suggesting an inability to stimulate normally functioning peripheral neurons.

Postprandial syncope can be a rare problem in the elderly due to hypotension after meals. Possible mechanism includes failure to maintain compensatory norepinephrine levels and cardioacceleratory responses. A systolic blood pressure decline of about 20 mm Hg after a meal has been reported in up to 36 per cent of elderly nursing home residents, occurring at 45 to 60 minutes in most patients.[32] This decline is often asymptomatic but rarely may lead to syncope and presyncope.

Neurological Disorders

These are infrequent causes of syncope.

CEREBROVASCULAR DISEASE. Approximately 6 per cent of ischemic strokes or transient ischemic attacks (TIAs) are associated with syncope. In 483 syncope patients seen in an emergency department, 7.7 per cent had TIAs.[33] All patients had concurrent neurological symptoms, most frequently vertigo, ataxia, and paresthesia. Almost all patients had vertebrobasilar TIAs.[33] Syncope is a rare manifestation of bilateral severe carotid artery disease. TIAs may result from atherosclerotic disease, inflammatory disorders (e.g., giant cell arteritis, systemic lupus erythematosus), aortic arch syndrome, dissection of extracranial arteries, cardiac diseases leading to emboli (e.g., rheumatic heart disease, myxoma), sickle cell disease, and anomalies of the cervical spine or cervical spondylosis. Syncope is also a manifestation of subclavian steal syndrome in which there is a stenosis of the subclavian artery and reversal of blood flow in the ipsilateral vertebral artery leading to vertebrobasilar ischemia.

MIGRAINES. A "faint sensation" is reported in 12 to 18 per cent of patients with migraine. Basilar artery migraine is a rare disorder affecting adolescents when syncope is associated with symptoms of brainstem ischemia. Localized brain stem ischemia due to spasm is the postulated mechanism. Migraine may result in syncope and orthostatic hypotension possibly because of hyper-responsiveness of

dopamine receptors with inhibition of the vasomotor center. Migraines may also lead to a vasovagal reaction secondary to pain.

SEIZURE. Fewer than 2 per cent of patients presenting with syncope are diagnosed as having a seizure disorder as a cause of their loss of consciousness.[34,35] Atonic seizures or epileptic "drop attacks" are nonconvulsive seizures found most commonly with secondary generalized epilepsy or partial epilepsy affecting mesial frontal or central cortical regions. Sudden falls also occur with temporal lobe epilepsy.[36] *Temporal lobe syncope* is the term used for complex partial seizure when patients also have drop attacks resembling syncope.[37] Patients may have a brief loss of consciousness followed by partial responsiveness or confusion and may exhibit formed speech or reactive automatisms. Characteristically, an interictal electroencephalogram (EEG) shows temporal lobe epileptic abnormalities. Temporal lobe epilepsy has been rarely associated with bradyarrhythmias.[38]

Cardiac Syncope

Severe obstruction to cardiac output or rhythm disturbance can lead to syncope. Occasionally, obstructive lesions and arrhythmias coexist, and one disorder may accentuate the other.

OBSTRUCTION TO FLOW. This may be due to structural lesions of either the left or right side of the heart (Table 28–1). Exertional syncope is a common manifestation of all types of heart disease in which cardiac output is fixed and does not rise (or even falls) with exercise. Syncope occurs in up to 42 per cent of patients with severe aortic stenosis (see p. 1039), commonly with exercise.[24] The most likely mechanisms of exertional syncope in aortic stenosis, as in other entities that cause left ventricular outflow obstruction, are ventricular baroceptor-mediated hypotension and bradycardia. Exercise leads to a marked increase in left ventricular systolic pressure without a corresponding increase in aortic pressure. This results in excessive stimulation of left ventricular mechanoreceptors leading to inhibition of sympathetic and activation of parasympathetic tone through cardiac vagal afferent fibers.[24,39] Myocardial ischemia may be present during syncope (even in patients without coexistent coronary artery disease), suggesting ischemia as contributing to vasodepressor syncope or reduction in coronary artery perfusion due to hypotension and bradycardia.[39] Other rare potential causes of syncope include ventricular tachyarrhythmias, paroxysmal AV block, and atrial fibrillation with loss of "atrial kick." Syncope is prognostically important in aortic stenosis, with an average survival of 2 to 3 years after its onset in the absence of valve replacement.

Similar pathophysiological processes may be responsible for syncope in hypertrophic cardiomyopathy (see p. 1419).[25] Syncope is reported in as many as 30 per cent of patients with hypertrophic cardiomyopathy. Left ventricular outflow obstruction is dynamic and worsened by an increase in contractility, a decrease in chamber size, or a decrease in afterload and distending pressure. Thus, Valsalva maneuver, severe coughing paroxysm, or specific drugs (e.g., digitalis) may precipitate hypotension and syncope. Myocardial ischemia is frequently found with syncope.[40] Ventricular tachycardia is reported in approximately 25 per cent of adult patients with hypertrophic cardiomyopathy and is an important cause of syncope.[41] Predictors of syncope include age less than 30 years, left ventricular end-diastolic volume index less than 60 ml/m^2, and nonsustained ventricular tachycardia.[42] Extensive hypertrophy and ventricular tachycardia are associated with poorer prognosis.[43]

Effort syncope commonly occurs in pulmonary hypertension (up to 30 per cent in primary pulmonary hypertension [see p. 788]). The limitations to right ventricular outflow may lead to diminished capacity to increase cardiac output, which, in association with lowered peripheral resistance with exercise, may lead to hypotension and syncope. Exertional syncope may also occur with severe pulmonic stenosis on the basis of a similar mechanism (see p. 1059). Patients with congenital heart disease (e.g., tetralogy of Fallot, patent ductus arteriosus, and interventricular or interatrial septal defects) can experience syncope with effort or crying as a result of sudden reversal of a left-to-right shunt and a fall in arterial oxygen saturation.

Syncope, which may occasionally occur with exertion, is reported in 10 to 15 per cent of patients with pulmonary embolism and is more likely to occur with massive embolism (> 50 per cent obstruction of the pulmonary vascular bed) (Chap. 46). Massive pulmonary embolism results in acute right ventricular failure, which leads to increased right ventricular filling pressure and reduced stroke volume. Subsequent decreased cardiac output and hypotension may lead to loss of consciousness. Consciousness may be regained if the embolus migrates to a distal location in the pulmonary artery. Alternatively, activation of cardiopulmonary mechanoreceptors in the setting of increased force of ventricular contraction may be the cause of syncope.

Atrial myxomas may result in obstruction of the mitral or tricuspid valve leading to symptoms of cardiac failure and rarely syncope (see p. 1466). Syncope, dyspnea, and cardiac murmurs that change with body position are particularly indicative of myxoma. Mitral stenosis rarely leads to syncope; it may be due to severe obstruction to outflow, atrial fibrillation with rapid ventricular response, pulmonary hypertension, or a cerebral embolic event.

OTHER ORGANIC HEART DISEASE. Syncope may be the presenting symptom in 5 to 12 per cent of elderly patients with acute myocardial infarction (see p. 1199). Mechanisms responsible for syncope include (1) sudden pump failure producing hypotension and a decrease in perfusion of the brain, and (2) rhythm disturbance that may include ventricular tachycardia or bradyarrhythmias. Vasovagal reactions resulting from stimulation of left ventricular baroreceptors may occur during acute inferior infarction or ischemia involving the right coronary artery. Unstable angina and coronary artery spasm also have been rarely associated with syncope.

Syncope occurs in 5 per cent of patients with aortic dissection. Loss of consciousness may be due to stroke or related to rupture into the pericardial space, resulting in sudden cardiac tamponade.

ARRHYTHMIAS. Bradycardia leads to a prolonged ventricular filling period resulting in increased stroke volume to maintain cardiac output (see p. 449). Severe bradycardia may result in an inadequate compensatory increase in stroke volume and lead to syncope. Mild to moderate tachycardias increase cardiac output, whereas markedly fast rates lead to a decrease in diastolic filling and cardiac output resulting in hypotension and syncope. Supraventricular tachycardias and paroxysmal atrial fibrillation may activate cardiac mechanoreceptors because of diminished cardiac volume and vigorous ventricular contraction, leading to neurally mediated syncope.[26,27]

Sinus bradycardia may be from excessive vagal tone, decreased sympathetic tone, or sinus node disease. Sinus bradycardia in healthy young athletes is generally attributed to increased vagal tone and decreased sympathetic activity but rarely results in syncope. Sinus bradycardia also occurs with eye surgery, myxedema, intracranial and mediastinal tumors, and with use of many parasympathomimetic, sympatholytic, beta blocker, and other drugs. Conjunctival instillation of beta blockers may also cause symptomatic bradycardia.

Syncope is reported in 25 to 70 per cent of patients with sick sinus syndrome (see p. 648). This syndrome is characterized by disturbance of sinoatrial impulse formation or conduction. Electrocardiographic manifestations include sinus bradycardia, pauses, arrest, or exit block. Supraventricular tachycardia or atrial fibrillation may also occur in association with bradycardia or atrial fibrillation with slow ventricular response (bradycardia-tachycardia syndrome). Sick sinus syndrome may overlap with neurally mediated syndromes leading to recurrent syncope despite pacemaker therapy.[44]

Ventricular tachycardias generally occur in the setting of known organic heart disease. Severity of symptoms is related to the rate, duration, and myocardial pump function (see p. 679). Torsades de pointes and syncope occur in the setting of syndromes of congenital prolongation of Q-T interval (with or without deafness) as well as acquired long Q-T syndromes, which occur with drugs, electrolyte abnormalities, and CNS disorders (see p. 685). Antiarrhythmic drugs are the most common cause of torsades de pointes, occurring with quinidine (quinidine syncope), procainamide, disopyramide, flecainide, encainide, amiodarone, and satolol.

Other tachyarrhythmias that may cause syncope include atrial fibrillation or flutter with rapid ventricular response and AV nodal reentrant tachycardia (see p. 663). Syncope in Wolff-Parkinson-White syndrome may be related to rapid rate of reciprocating supraventricular tachycardia or to a rapid ventricular response over the accessory pathway during atrial fibrillation.[45] Syncope alone in Wolff-Parkinson-White syndrome may not predict risk of sudden death.[46,47]

Distribution of Causes of Syncope

There has been a wide variation in the proportion of patients diagnosed with various causes of syncope.[34,35,48–50] This is largely due to patient selection (differences ranging from emergency department to ICU patients) and lack of uniform criteria for assigning causes of syncope. The most common etiologies are vasovagal syncope (1 to 29 per cent), situational syncope (1 to 8 per cent), orthostatic hypotension (4 to 12 per cent), and drug-induced syncope (2 to 9 per cent). Organic cardiac diseases constitute 3 to 11 per cent and arrhythmias 5 to 30 per cent of causes of syncope. Each of the other causes is found in less than 5 per cent of patients. In studies in the 1980's, a cause of syncope was not diagnosed in 38 to 42 per cent. However, the proportion undiagnosed is probably substantially lower with wider use of event monitoring, tilt testing, electrophysiological studies, attention to psychiatric illnesses, and recognition that syncope in the elderly may be multifactorial. In a cardiology tertiary care referral center where patients underwent electrophysiological studies and tilt testing, a cause was not established in 26 per cent.[51]

Outcome in Syncope of Various Etiologies

The one-year mortality of patients with cardiac causes of syncope has been consistently high, ranging between 18 and 33 per cent.[34,35,49,50] These rates have been found to be higher than those in patients with a noncardiac cause (0 to 12 per cent) or in patients with unknown cause (6 per cent). The incidence of sudden death in patients with cardiac causes was also markedly higher as compared with the other two groups.[34,35] Even when adjustments for differences in comorbidity were made, cardiac syncope was still an independent predictor of mortality and sudden death. It is not known whether syncope predisposes to increased risk of mortality independent of underlying diseases. In the Framingham study, patients younger than age 60 experiencing syncope who did not have cardiovascular or neurological diseases had rates of mortality, sudden death, stroke, and myocardial infarction similar to patients without syncope.[52] In a study of patients with advanced heart failure, poor left ventricular function was associated with a high risk of sudden death regardless of the cause of syncope.[53,54] A comparative outcome study of unselected patients with and without syncope showed that underlying heart disease was associated with higher mortality.

There is an important difference in prognosis between cardiac syncope and neurally mediated or neurocardiogenic syncope. Neurocardiogenic syncope has excellent long-term prognosis, although recurrences are common and a major reason for seeking medical care. Similarly, syncope associated with psychiatric disease has no increased mortality but has one-year recurrence rates of 26 to 50 per cent.[17]

In patients presenting with syncope, the recurrence rate is 34 per cent over 3-year follow-up and it is lower in patients with cardiac causes as compared with the other groups, but not significantly so.[55] Although recurrences are associated with fractures and soft tissue injury in 12 per cent of patients, they do not predict an increased risk of mortality or sudden death.[55]

DIAGNOSTIC EVALUATION

The most important elements in the evaluation of syncope are (1) determining whether the patient has actually experienced syncope, (2) risk stratification, and (3) selective use of diagnostic tests to define the cause.

DETERMINING WHETHER THE PATIENT HAD SYNCOPE. A history from the patient and a witness, if present, is needed to separate syncope from other entities such as dizziness, vertigo, drop attacks, coma, and seizure. A particularly important issue is the distinction between syncope and seizure. Videometric analysis of patients with syncope has shown myoclonic activity in 90 per cent, predominantly consisting of multifocal arrhythmic jerks both in proximal and distal muscles.[56] Other findings include head turns, oral automatism, and visual and auditory hallucinations. Eyes remained open throughout syncope and upward deviation was common. Despite these findings, historical features are often sufficient to distinguish syncope from seizures. A comparison of seizures and syncope shows that seizures are associated with a blue face (or not pale), frothing at the mouth, tongue biting, disorientation, aching muscles, sleepiness after the event, and a duration of unconsciousness of more than 5 minutes. On the other hand, patients with syncope often report sweating or nausea before the event. The best discriminatory symptom is disorientation after the episode, which often signifies a seizure.[57] Tilt testing (see p. 870) may be useful to distinguish vasovagal syncope from seizure by provoking symptoms and hemodynamic changes with syncope that can be observed.[58]

RISK STRATIFICATION. This is important for initial management decisions such as admission to the hospital and the use of invasive testing such as electrophysiological studies. The issues include prediction of risk of sudden death and likelihood of cardiac syncope. In the assessment of risk, cause of syncope, presence of underlying cardiac disease, and abnormalities on electrocardiogram (ECG) are important.

Previous studies have consistently shown increased mortality and sudden death rates in patients with cardiac causes of syncope, thus identifying these patients as a high-risk subset. Examples include those with aortic stenosis, pulmonary hypertension, and arrhythmic syncope. Arrhythmias are primarily of concern in patients with heart disease or abnormal ECG. Thus, the presence of heart disease and certain abnormalities on ECG helps stratify patients into low- and high-risk groups. Patients with congestive heart failure, valvular heart disease, hypertrophic cardiomyopathy, and other types of organic heart disease constitute a high-risk group. Bundle branch block, old myocardial infarction, Wolff-Parkinson-White syndrome, and other evidence of AV block are also considered high-risk findings on ECG. If the presence or absence of heart disease cannot be determined clinically, specific tests such as echocardiogram, stress test, and ventricular function studies may be needed for risk stratification.

SELECTIVE USE OF DIAGNOSTIC TESTS. The evaluation of syncope is best approached by using the history and physical examination, ECG, and risk stratification to guide further diagnostic tests.

History, Physical Examination, and Baseline Laboratory Tests

A detailed account of syncope, the events leading to loss of consciousness, and symptoms following the episode is crucial to diagnosing specific entities. In diagnosing vasovagal syncope, precipitating factors, in conjunction with autonomic symptoms, can lead to diagnosis. Syncope during or immediately after micturition, cough, defecation, and swallowing is well described and easily diagnosed by history. Syncope associated with neurological symptoms of brain stem ischemia suggests transient ischemic attacks, basilar artery migraines, and subclavian steal syndrome. A detailed drug history may provide clues to possible drug-induced syncope. Table 28–3 shows other clinical presentations that may suggest specific entities.

Physical examination is used to diagnose specific entities and exclude others. Orthostatic hypotension, cardiovascular findings, and neurological examination are crucial in this regard. Orthostatic hypotension is generally defined as a decline of 20 mm Hg or more in systolic pressure upon assuming the upright position. However, this finding is reported in up to 24 per cent of the elderly and is frequently not associated with symptoms.[29] Thus, the clinical diagnosis of orthostatic hypotension should incorporate the presence of symptoms (e.g., dizziness and syncope) in association with a decrease in systolic blood pressure.

In the detection of orthostatic hypotension, supine blood pressure and heart rate should be measured after the patient has been recumbent for at least 5 minutes. Standing measurements should be obtained immediately and for at least 2 minutes. These measurements should be carried out to 10 minutes if there is a high suspicion of orthostatic hypotension without a drop in blood pressure having been

TABLE 28–3 CLINICAL FEATURES SUGGESTIVE OF SPECIFIC CAUSES

SYMPTOM OR FINDING	DIAGNOSTIC CONSIDERATION
After sudden unexpected pain, unpleasant sight, sound, or smell	Vasovagal syncope
During or immediately after micturition, cough, swallow, or defecation	Situational syncope
With neuralgia (glossopharyngeal or trigeminal)	Bradycardia or vasodepressor reaction
Upon standing	Orthostatic hypotension
Prolonged standing at attention	Vasovagal syncope
Well-trained athlete after exertion	Neurally mediated
Changing position (from sitting to lying, bending, turning over in bed)	Atrial myxoma, thrombus
Syncope with exertion	Aortic stenosis, pulmonary hypertension, pulmonary embolus, mitral stenosis, idiopathic hypertrophic subaortic stenosis, coronary artery disease, neurally-mediated
With head rotation, pressure on carotid sinus (as in tumors, shaving, tight collars)	Carotid sinus syncope
Associated with vertigo, dysarthria, diplopia, and other motor and sensory symptoms of brain stem ischemia	TIA, subclavian steal, basilar artery migraine
With arm exercise	Subclavian steal
Confusion after episode	Seizure

found earlier.[59] Sitting blood pressures are not reliable for detection of orthostatic hypotension.

Several cardiovascular findings are crucial diagnostically. Differences in the pulse intensity and blood pressure (generally over 20 mm Hg) in the two arms are suggestive of aortic dissection or subclavian steal syndrome. Special focus on cardiovascular examination for aortic stenosis, idiopathic hypertrophic subaortic stenosis, pulmonary hypertension, myxomas, and aortic dissection may uncover clues to these entities.

In those patients in whom the cause can be defined, the history and physical examination identify a potential cause in 49 to 85 per cent.[34,35,48–50] Furthermore, organic cardiac diseases causing syncope (e.g., aortic stenosis, idiopathic hypertrophic subaortic stenosis, pulmonary embolism), and neurological diseases (e.g., subclavian steal syndrome) can be strongly suspected by the history and physical examination. Testing for these diseases should be selective and based on findings of a careful history and physical examination. In one study, suggestive findings on history and physical examination were helpful in assigning the ultimate cause of syncope by directed testing in 8 per cent of additional patients.[34]

Initial laboratory blood tests rarely yield diagnostically helpful information. Hypoglycemia, hyponatremia, hypocalcemia, or renal failure is found in 2 to 3 per cent of patients, but most of these appear to result in seizures rather than syncope. These tests are often confirmatory of clinical suspicion of these laboratory abnormalities. Bleeding as a cause of syncope is generally diagnosed clinically and confirmed by a complete blood count or hemoccult tests.

Carotid Massage

The technique of carotid massage is not standardized. Commonly, massage is done in the supine position, and occasionally repeated in the sitting and standing positions if the vasodepressor variety is suspected and the test in the supine position is negative. Electrocardiographic and blood pressure monitoring is necessary. Mixed cardioinhibitory and vasodepressor response is diagnosed when carotid sinus massage is performed after cardioinhibitory response is abolished with atropine or atrioventricular sequential pacing. The duration of massage has varied from 5 sec to 40 sec,[12] but recent studies have used 6 to 10 sec.[14,15,60] Simultaneous bilateral massage should never be done. At least 15 seconds should be allowed to elapse between massage from one side to the other. Complications of carotid sinus massage include prolonged asystole, ventricular fibrillation, transient or permanent neurological deficit, and sudden death. Complication rates are not available but are considered extremely low; however, in patients with cerebrovascular disease the test should be done only if all other diagnostic modalities are exhausted and the pretest probability of carotid sinus syncope remains high.

Carotid sinus syncope is diagnosed in patients who are found to have carotid sinus hypersensitivity and have reproduction of spontaneous symptoms during carotid sinus massage. In the absence of symptom reproduction, carotid sinus syncope is likely when carotid sinus hypersensitivity is found and spontaneous episodes are related to activities that press or stretch the carotid sinus, or the patient has recurrent syncope with a negative workup.

Diagnostic Tests for Arrhythmias

Ascribing syncope to arrhythmias is often difficult because, in most patients, symptoms have already resolved by the time of testing; thus, a causal inference is often made on the basis of tests performed during asymptomatic periods. In diagnosing arrhythmias, every attempt should be made to attain symptomatic correlation. When this is not possible, uncertainty may remain regarding the cause of syncope because currently there are no validated criteria

for attributing syncope to most arrhythmias by the use of electrocardiographic or electrophysiological abnormalities during asymptomatic periods.

ELECTROCARDIOGRAM. An abnormal ECG may be found in 50 per cent of patients presenting with syncope.[34] The most common abnormalities include bundle branch or bifascicular block, old myocardial infarction, and left ventricular hypertrophy. Arrhythmias as cause of syncope are assigned by ECG in 2 to 11 per cent of patients.[34,35,49,50] Exercise ECG (Chap. 5) can be used to evaluate syncope with exercise for the diagnosis of ischemia, exercise-induced tachyarrhythmias, or bradyarrhythmias after abrupt termination of exercise. However, the yield of this test for arrhythmias is very low.

Signal-averaged ECG, used for detection of low amplitude signals (late potentials) (see p. 583), has a sensitivity of 73 to 89 per cent and specificity of 89 to 100 per cent for prediction of inducible sustained ventricular tachycardia in patients with syncope.[61–63] Signal-averaged ECG has been used as a screening test in selecting patients for electrophysiological studies when ventricular tachycardia is the only concern. However, complete electrophysiological studies are generally needed to evaluate syncope when the decision is made to perform this test because abnormalities other than ventricular tachycardia (e.g., sinus node dysfunction, other conduction system disease, induced supraventricular tachycardia) as well as multiple abnormalities are often of concern.

PROLONGED ELECTROCARDIOGRAPHIC MONITORING. The central problem in attributing syncope to arrhythmias is that the vast majority of detected arrhythmias in syncope patients are brief and result in no symptoms.[64–67] On the other hand, arrhythmias are commonly reported in normal or ambulatory asymptomatic individuals, including sinus bradycardia, brief episodes of supraventricular tachycardia, and PACs or PVCs. Sinus pauses of more than 2 sec and brief runs of unsustained ventricular tachycardia (mostly less than 5 beat runs) are reported in up to 4 per cent of asymptomatic subjects. Mobitz II or complete AV block are very rare.

One method of assessing the impact of ambulatory monitoring in syncope is to determine the presence or absence of arrhythmias in patients who develop symptoms during monitoring. In studies that evaluated syncope or presyncope with approximately 12 hours of monitoring and reported on symptoms, only 4 per cent of patients had symptomatic correlation with arrhythmias.[67] In approximately 17 per cent of patients, symptoms were not associated with arrhythmias, thus potentially excluding rhythm disturbance as an etiology for syncope. In approximately 80 per cent of patients, no symptoms occurred but arrhythmias were often found. The causal relation between these arrhythmias and syncope therefore is uncertain. Furthermore, the finding of brief or no arrhythmias (without symptoms) on monitoring does not exclude arrhythmic syncope because of the episodic nature of arrhythmias. In patients with high pretest likelihood of arrhythmias, further evaluation for arrhythmias should be pursued by event monitoring or electrophysiological studies. Extending the duration of monitoring to 72 hours may increase the yield of brief arrhythmias detected (14.7 per cent during the first day, an additional 11.1 per cent the second day, and an additional 4.2 per cent the third day[65]), but not the yield for arrhythmias associated with symptoms.

Long-term monitoring (weeks to months) is possible with patient-activated intermittent loop recorders that can capture the rhythm during syncope after the patient has regained consciousness, because several minutes of retrograde electrocardiographic recording can be obtained. In one study of patients with multiple recurrences of syncope (median of 10 episodes), 7 of the 57 patients had an arrhythmia found with recurrent symptoms of which three were due to neurally mediated syncope.[68] Seven others had negative findings, therefore excluding arrhythmias as a cause of syncope. However, in 18 patients there were technical problems with use of the recorder that precluded a diagnosis. Thus, loop monitoring is most useful in patients with history of recurrent unexplained syncope because the probability of recurrence in these patients is higher, making it more likely that arrhythmias can be captured during an event.

ELECTROPHYSIOLOGICAL STUDIES (see p. 577). The indications for electrophysiological studies in patients with syncope have not been systematically defined, but they are more likely to be "positive" in patients with known heart disease, abnormal ventricular function, or abnormalities on the ECG or on ambulatory monitoring.[69–74] These tests are also more likely to be positive in patients with bundle branch block, identifying isolated conduction disease or ventricular tachyarrhythmias. Predictors of ventricular tachycardia by electrophysiological studies include organic heart disease, PVCs by ECG, and nonsustained ventricular tachycardia by Holter monitoring.[75] Sinus bradycardia, first-degree AV block, and bundle branch block by ECG predict bradyarrhythmic outcome.[75]

Predictors of a negative electrophysiological study in patients with syncope include the absence of heart disease, an ejection fraction over 40 per cent; normal ECG and Holter monitoring, absence of injury during syncope, and multiple or prolonged (> 5 minutes) episodes of syncope.[71] In studies of patients with syncope who have electrophysiological testing, the proportion of patients with positive findings has ranged between 18 and 75 per cent (mean of 60 per cent).[69] Approximately 35 per cent (range 0 to 80) had inducible ventricular tachycardia, 20 per cent (range 0 to 60) supraventricular tachycardia, 35 per cent (range 11 to 60) conduction disturbance (abnormal sinus node, atrioventricular node, or His-Purkinje function), and 10 per cent (range 0 to 24) other abnormalities (including hypervagotonia and carotid hypersensitivity).

Several issues need to be considered in using electrophysiological studies in the evaluation of syncope: First, induced arrhythmias presumed to be diagnostic should be associated with or capable of producing symptomatic hypotension. Second, the clinical significance of some of the electrophysiological abnormalities may be difficult to determine because of problems with sensitivity and specificity of several electrophysiological findings. For example, prolonged sinus node recovery time has a low sensitivity for diagnosis of sinus node dysfunction (18 to 69 per cent), but high specificity (88 to 100 per cent) when electrophysiological results are compared with ambulatory monitoring.[72,73] Tests for atrioventricular nodal conduction and refractoriness are also difficult to interpret and vary considerably with autonomic tone. A prolonged H-V interval and block between H and V with atrial pacing is a marker of significant conduction disease that may have resulted in bradyarrhythmias and syncope; however, cutpoints for the length of H-V interval have varied widely when syncope is attributed to conduction system disease (criteria have ranged from over 55 msec to over 100 msec).

Supraventricular tachycardia and atrial fibrillation or flutter may be occasionally initiated during electrophysiological studies, especially if aggressive induction procedures are used. The significance of these induced arrhythmias is uncertain unless they reproduce the patient's spontaneous symptoms.

Patients with structural heart disease have higher rates of inducible ventricular tachycardia as compared with those without cardiac disease (approximately 55 to 70 per cent vs. less than 20 per cent). The finding of *sustained monomorphic ventricular tachycardia* (see p. 679) has a high sensitivity and specificity for the presence of spontaneous ventricular tachycardia. However, induction of *polymorphic* or *nonsustained ventricular tachycardia* may frequently represent a nonspecific response to an aggressive ventricular stimulation protocol.

Third, the variations in the proportion of patients with positive findings on electrophysiological testing in syncope may be due to patient selection, testing methodology, and criteria for abnormal results. Patients have included those with single as well as multiple episodes and with many types of organic heart diseases as well as without heart disease. Testing variations include performance of left ventricular stimulation, use of isoproterenol, use of procainamide infusion during testing, and the number of extrastimuli for induction procedures.

In evaluation of outcomes, recurrence in follow-up is used as a measure of the effectiveness of testing with the assumption that treatment based on abnormal results leads to resolution of symptoms. In those who have normal studies, recurrence rates are 8 to 80 per cent with a mean of 35 per cent, while recurrence rates in those with abnormal testing are 0 to 32 per cent with a mean of 15 per cent over a mean length of follow-up of 11 to 36 months.[69] These data suggest potential outcome benefit for patients with an abnormal study. The interpretation of the rate of recurrence is, however, complicated because it may be caused by the side effects of drugs, noncompliance, inadequate treatment, or an incorrect initial diagnosis. Furthermore, recurrences are sporadic; thus, analysis of their rate over time may be difficult.

Mortality and incidence of sudden death in patients with positive findings are higher than in those with negative findings. For example, a 3-year sudden death rate of 48 per cent in patients with positive studies as compared with 9 per cent in those with negative studies has been found.[70] These differences are probably largely due to higher prevalence of cardiac comorbidity in patients with positive findings. These differences suggest that aggressive treatment of underlying heart disease should be pursued, in addition to the treatment of arrhythmia. A low rate of mortality and sudden death in patients with negative studies can also be reassuring because this defines a low-risk group of syncope patients.[76]

Upright Tilt Testing

Upright tilt testing refers to maintaining the patient in an upright position for a brief period to provoke vasovagal syncope. Upright tilt leads to pooling of blood in the lower limbs, resulting in decreased venous return (Fig. 28–2). Normal compensatory response to upright posture is reflex tachycardia, more forceful contraction of the ventricles, and vasoconstriction. However, in individuals susceptible to vasovagal syncope, this forceful ventricular contraction[76a] in the setting of a relatively empty ventricle, may activate the cardiac mechanoreceptors, triggering reflex hypotension and/or bradycardia. Catecholamine release (as may occur with anxiety, fear, and panic), by increasing ventricular contraction, may also activate the nerve endings responsible for triggering this reflex. Thus, catecholamines have been used to facilitate positive responses during upright tilt testing.[1,2]

Almost all tilt testing protocols employ tilt tables with footboard support. Saddle support is not used clinically because of poor specificity.[77] Testing is often performed in a fasting state and vasoactive drugs (e.g., calcium channel blockers, vasodilators, diuretics) are withheld before testing (approximately for 5 half-lives). The test should generally be performed in a quiet room, minimizing surrounding noise such as beepers and traffic. There should be ample lighting, and the temperature should be kept comfortably cool.

Monitoring of blood pressure during upright tilt testing has been done either noninvasively (e.g., with blood pressure cuff or digital plethysmography) or by invasive intra-arterial blood pressure monitoring. Although concern has been voiced that invasive procedures may provoke vasova-

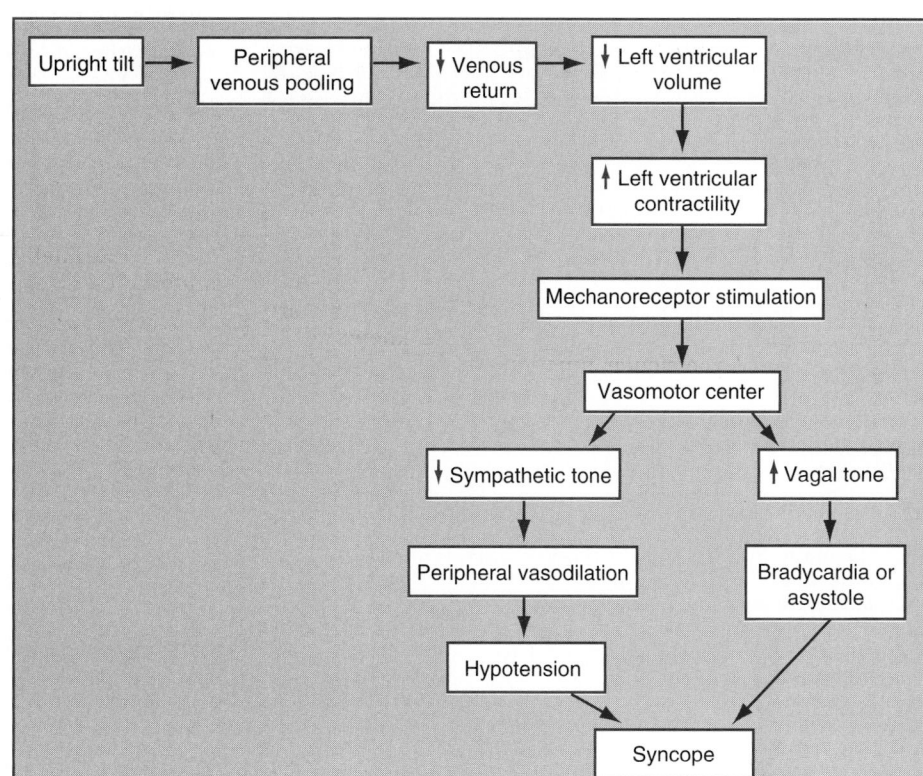

FIGURE 28–2. A pathophysiological mechanism for induction of vasovagal syncope during upright tilt testing.

gal reactions, the effect of monitoring has not been clearly established. Whenever possible, invasive monitoring should be avoided because of the provocation of vasovagal responses and increase in cost and complexity of testing.

The two general types of testing procedures are upright tilt testing alone (passive testing) and tilt testing in conjunction with a chemical agent. The vast majority of the reported studies employ passive testing[77–83] or use isoproterenol after a brief period of passive tilt testing.[51,84–93] Limited experiences with epinephrine,[94] edrophonium,[95] intravenous or sublingual nitroglycerin,[23] and esmolol tilt testing with esmolol withdrawal[96] are reported. These protocols cannot be recommended for general use because of limited data on their performance characteristics.

During passive tilt testing protocols, after baseline supine measurements of blood pressure and continuous monitoring of heart rate, patients are suddenly brought to an upright position. As shown in Table 28–4, most studies using passive testing protocols have employed a tilt angle of 60 degrees. Although protocols consisting of 60 minutes of testing have been studied, a total duration of 45 minutes is recommended because that time is two standard deviations away from mean time to positive responses (approximately 24 minutes).[77]

All testing protocols incorporating *isoproterenol* employ a passive phase of testing. The most common duration of this phase has been 10 to 15 minutes. If an endpoint of the study is not reached, the patient is generally brought to a supine position. Isoproterenol infusion is started while the patient is supine. The most common starting infusion rate is 1 μg/min; the most common duration of tilt testing with isoproterenol at each dose is 10 to 15 minutes. If patients do not develop an endpoint during this phase of testing, they are again brought to a supine position, isoproterenol infusion rate is increased, and patients are retilted for a similar duration of testing as during the initial dose of isoproterenol. This procedure is continued with increasing doses of isoproterenol until a positive response or another endpoint (e.g., maximum dosage, adverse effects, or development of severe tachycardia) is reached. The maximum dosage of isoproterenol used in reported studies is 3 to 5 μg/min. The endpoints of a positive response are syncope or presyncope in association with hypotension and/or bradycardia, although no standard definitions of hypotension or bradycardia are used across the studies.

POSITIVE RESPONSES IN PATIENTS WITH UNEXPLAINED SYNCOPE. In studies using passive upright tilt testing, 49 per cent (range 26 to 90 per cent) have had a positive response to tilt testing (Table 28–5), while in studies using isoproterenol, overall positive responses are approximately 64 per cent (range 39 to 87 per cent).[97] Approximately two-thirds of the positive responses occur during the isoproterenol phase. With either type of testing, about two-thirds of the responses appear to be cardioinhibitory (defined as bradycardia with or without associated hypotension), and the rest are pure vasodepressor reactions (defined as hypotension without significant bradycardia).

Higher angles and longer duration of testing are associated with higher positive responses to tilt testing.[97] The angle of testing during passive protocols has been 60 degrees, while with isoproterenol it predominantly has been 80 degrees, although studies have reported testing at 60, 70, and 90 degrees (Table 28–4). The duration of the passive phase of testing has also been variable, ranging from 5 to 60 minutes.[97] Additionally, the dosing of isoproterenol has also been variable, including bolus infusions starting at 2 μg as well as infusions based on body weight and heart rate increase (Table 28–4).[97] The maximum dosage of isoproterenol has also varied. The differences between positive responses on passive protocols and testing with isoproterenol appear to be due to differences in the angle and duration of testing. When studies of tilt testing with isoproterenol using 60 degree angles are compared with passive tilt testing at 60 degrees for 60 minutes, the positive responses are similar at 52 versus 54 per cent, respectively.[97]

SENSITIVITY AND SPECIFICITY. Sensitivity is determined by calculating the ratio of number of patients with positive tests over the number of patients who have the disease. The disease has to be diagnosed independently of the test by using a separate gold standard. In small studies of patients who have clinical vasovagal syncope, 67 to 83 per cent have had positive response, thus equalling the sensitivity of this test.[93,94] Specificity is defined as the propor-

TABLE 28-4   TILT TESTING PROTOCOLS

	PASSIVE (NO. OF STUDIES)	ISOPROTERENOL (NO. OF STUDIES)
Tilt Angle		
40°	1	—
60°	9	3
70°	—	1
80°	—	11
90°	—	1
Other*	1	—
Duration of Passive Tilt (in minutes)		
10	—	5
15	1	4
20	1	1
30	—	5
60	8	1
Other†	1	
Dose of Isoproterenol		
Starting dose		
1 μg/min		12
2 μg/min		1
0.02-0.04 μg/kg/min		1
2 μg‡		1
Other§		1
Increment in dose		
1 μg/min		10
2 μg/min		2
3 μg/min		1
0.05-0.1 μg/kg/min		1
2 μg‡		1
Other§		1
Highest		
3 μg/min		6
4 μg/min		1
5 μg/min		7
8 μg		1
0.05-0.1 μg/kg/min		1
Endpoints**		
Syncope	3	5
Syncope/Presyncope	2	3
Syncope or Presyncope in association with hypotension and/or bradycardia	4	8
Other	2††	6

* Endpoints were not specifically stated.

† 26 minutes.

‡ One study used bolus infusion starting only at 2 μg and increasing dose by 2 mg.

§ One study gave isoproterenol to elicit a 20 per cent increase in heart rate.

** 15°, 30°, 45° for 2 minutes, then 60° for 20 minutes.

†† Studies with isoproterenol report multiple other endpoints that are not mutually exclusive.

Adapted from Kapoor, W. N., et al.: Upright tilt testing in evaluating syncope: A comprehensive literature review. Am. J. Med. 97:78, 1994.

tion of subjects without the disease or disorder who have a negative test. Specificity has generally been evaluated by performing upright tilt testing in subjects who have not had syncope previously. With passive tilt testing, specificity

TABLE 28-5   POSITIVE RESPONSES

	TOTAL SUBJECTS	NO. POSITIVE	% POSITIVE	POSITIVE RANGE
Passive tilt only	425	210	49	26-90
Isoproterenol tilt				
Passive phase	592	133	23	0-57
Isoproterenol phase	459	220	48	12-81
Overall	592	378*	64	39-87

* These 378 patients include 25 positive patients from one study that did not specify whether those patients were positive during the isoproterenol phase or the passive phase.

Adapted from Kapoor, W. N., et al.: Upright tilt testing in evaluating syncope: A comprehensive literature review. Am. J. Med. 97:78, 1994.

has been variable and has ranged between 0 and 100 per cent, although an overall rate is approximately 90 per cent.[97] The overall specificity of upright tilt testing with isoproterenol is approximately 75 per cent and range of 35 to 100 per cent.[97-99] Subjects of studies reporting poor specificity of tilt testing with isoproterenol were generally younger as compared with those reporting higher specificity.[97,98]

REPRODUCIBILITY. Reproducibility of upright tilt testing of 67 to 85 per cent has been adequate,[86,97,100-103] except for a recent study that showed remarkable lack of reproducibility.[104] In a study of 109 patients undergoing 2 consecutive days of passive testing, there was a 63 per cent rate of discordance between day 1 and day 2 of testing.[104] Of patients who had vasovagal syncope on day one, only 31 per cent had it on the second day.

Neurological Testing

Skull films, lumbar puncture, radionuclide brain scan, and cerebral angiography do not generally yield diagnostic information for a cause of syncope in the absence of clinical findings suggestive of a specific neurological process.[48] Studies of the EEG in patients with syncope have shown that an epileptiform abnormality was found in 1 per cent of patients; almost all of these were suspected clinically.[34,105] Treatment based on the EEG was initiated in 1 to 2 per cent of patients.[105] Head computed tomography (CT) scans are rarely useful to assign an etiology but are needed if a subdural hemorrhage due to head injury is suspected or in patients suspected to have a seizure as a cause of loss of consciousness.[34]

Specific tests of autonomic function are on occasion useful in defining further the nature of disease responsible for postural hypotension or when no clear reason for orthostasis is apparent.[31] These tests include cardiovascular responses to deep breathing, hyperventilation, stress (handgrip, noise, mental arithmetic, and cold pressor test), breath holding, and Valsalva maneuver. Protocols are also available for sweating and pupillary responses and pharmacological and biochemical testing of sympathetic and parasympathetic systems.[31] These tests are not recommended routinely because clinical data with a focus on autonomic symptoms, diseases causing orthostatic hypotension, and drugs frequently provide clues to the etiology of orthostatic hypotension, and there is often little need for additional diagnostic testing or for therapy selection.

Psychiatric Assessment

Psychiatric illnesses need to be considered as a cause of syncope, especially in young patients and those with multiple syncopal episodes who also have other nonspecific complaints. A high clinical suspicion for these disorders is needed because they are often not diagnosed in medical patients. Screening instruments for generalized anxiety disorder, panic attack and disorder, depression, and somatization disorder are recommended. A high rate of recurrence of syncope in these patients makes detection of these illnesses especially important.

Approach to Diagnostic Evaluation

As shown in Figure 28-3, history and physical examination are the starting points in the evaluation of the patient with syncope. Furthermore, the history and physical examination may reveal findings suggestive of specific entities as possible causes (e.g., findings of aortic stenosis or neurological signs and symptoms suggestive of a seizure disorder) that may require further noninvasive or invasive directed tests for establishing a diagnosis and initiating treatment.

An ECG is generally needed for the evaluation of patients with syncope, the cause of which is not evident from the history and physical examination. Although the diagnostic

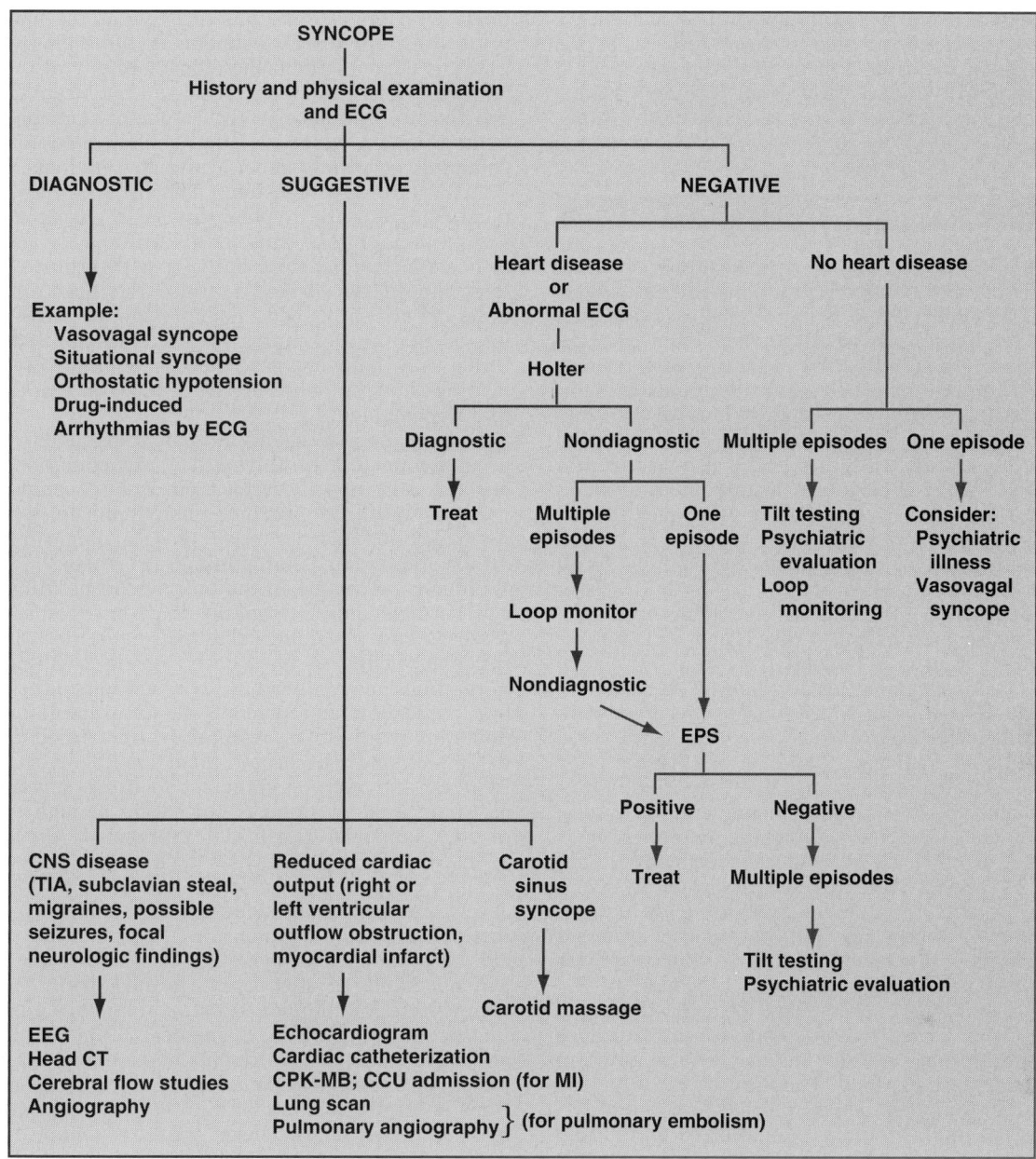

FIGURE 28–3. A flow diagram showing the approach to the evaluation of syncope.

yield of an ECG is low (e.g., for arrhythmias or suspicion of myocardial infarction), abnormalities can be treated quickly if found. Furthermore, patients with a normal ECG have a low likelihood of arrhythmias as a cause of syncope and are at low risk of sudden death. Thus, the ECG can offer both diagnostic and prognostic information which may have an important role in further evaluation and management.

In patients in whom a cause of syncope is not determined by the history, physical examination, and ECG, further testing can be approached by stratifying patients into those with and without heart disease and/or ECG abnormalities. If the presence or absence of heart disease cannot be determined clinically, specific tests such as echocardiogram, stress test, and ventricular function studies may be needed.

In patients with coronary artery disease, congestive heart failure, valvular heart disease, hypertrophic cardiomyopathy, or ECG abnormalities (e.g., bundle branch block or bifascicular block), prolonged ECG monitoring is the first step in evaluation. If prolonged monitoring is nondiagnostic, electrophysiological studies should be considered if symptoms are consistent with arrhythmic syncope. The findings of electrophysiological studies can form the basis

for therapy. Patients with negative electrophysiological studies have a favorable prognosis, and thus empiric therapy with a pacemaker or antiarrhythmics is not justified. In patients with negative electrophysiological studies and recurrent unexplained syncope, upright tilt testing may help define neurally mediated syncope as a potential cause.

Younger patients (less than 60 years of age) with syncope and without heart disease have an excellent prognosis.[106] Furthermore, in patients with a normal ECG, the likelihood of arrhythmias is low, and prolonged electrocardiographic monitoring rarely leads to a specific diagnosis. The yield of electrophysiological studies in patients without heart disease is low. Thus, these studies are not justified in most patients. Many patients (especially those with recurrent syncope) probably have vasovagal syncope or psychiatric disorders that should be investigated. Although similar conclusions probably apply to older patients without heart disease, further studies are needed to better define the role of tests for detection of arrhythmias, especially for diagnosis of bradyarrhythmias.

Patients with recurrent syncope constitute a group in which management is difficult. Patients with multiple episodes (more than 5 in the last year) are less likely to have arrhythmias[71] and are more likely to have psychiatric illnesses.[17] The extent of initial evaluation of these patients is guided by the presence or absence of heart disease. In patients with frequent recurrent syncope in whom there is a high suspicion of arrhythmias, loop event recorders are especially valuable if a cause is not established by other means.

MANAGEMENT

Management issues include hospitalization decision, treatment selection, and patient instructions and education.

HOSPITAL ADMISSION. There are no studies evaluating the need for hospital admission in patients with syncope. Generally, patients are admitted if a rapid diagnostic evaluation is needed because of concerns about serious arrhythmias, sudden death, newly diagnosed serious cardiac disease (e.g., aortic stenosis, myocardial infarction), and new onset of seizure or stroke. Admission is also needed for treatment when etiology is clear (e.g., management of dehydration). In the large group of patients with unexplained syncope after initial history, physical examination, and ECG, risk stratification for arrhythmias and sudden death should guide the admission decision.

TREATMENT SELECTION. Because the treatment largely depends on the cause of syncope, a discussion of the treatment of all of the causes is beyond the scope of this review. General management issues and treatments of neurally mediated syncope that have recently received considerable attention will be reviewed.

Neurally Mediated Syncope. Patients may have a cluster of syncopal episodes at one time that may diminish or resolve spontaneously. Thus, the frequency and severity of events need to be considered when long-term therapy is started. Because of potential side effects, treatment should be reserved for patients with frequent or disabling symptoms. Because psychiatric illnesses probably lead to vasovagal reactions, screening for the psychiatric illnesses should be performed. Treatment of the psychiatric illness often will result in resolution of recurrent syncope.

Various drugs and pacemakers have been tried for patients with vasovagal syncope, and a decrease in recurrence of syncope or resolution of symptoms has been reported in almost every uncontrolled study. The most commonly used drugs are beta blockers (e.g., metoprolol 50 to 200 mg/day, atenolol 25 to 200 mg/day, and propranolol 40 to 160 mg/day),[97] which may inhibit the activation of cardiac mechanoreceptors by decreasing cardiac contractility. Anticholinergic drugs, such as transdermal scopolamine 1 patch every 2 to 3 days, have been tried,[97] particularly in patients with profound bradycardia during upright tilt testing. Disopyramide (200 to 600 mg/day) (see p. 609) has anticholinergic and negative inotropic effects that may inhibit activation of cardiac mechanoreceptors.[107,108] Measures to expand volume, such as increased salt intake, custom-fitted counterpressure support garments from ankle to waist, and fludrocortisone acetate (0.1 to 1 mg per day) are frequently used.[89,90,97] Potential side effects may include recumbent hypertension, hypokalemia, fluid retention, and congestive heart failure.

Theophylline (6 to 12 mg/kg/day) has been tried on occasion.[109] The mechanism of action of theophylline in the treatment of vasovagal syncope is not known; a blockade of effects of adenosine, which has vasodilatory effects, is postulated. Limited uncontrolled but favorable experiences are reported with serotonin reuptake inhibitors fluoxetine[110] and sertraline,[111] ephedrine,[112] etilephrine,[113] dihydroergotamine,[113] dextroamphetamine,[114] and pseudoephedrine.[115]

Finally, atrioventricular pacing has been utilized in patients with significant bradycardia in response to upright tilt testing.[116–118] Pacemakers may ameliorate symptoms but vasodepressor reactions still continue to occur. Even in patients with bradycardia and asystole as the major response to tilt testing, drug treatment is the therapy of choice. There is concern about the efficacy of any of the treatments for vasovagal syncope because one randomized trial showed no difference in recurrence of syncope between 15 treated (with a variety of drugs such as atenolol, dihydroergotamine, cafedrine) and 15 untreated patients.[113]

Orthostatic Hypotension. The initial approach to treatment of orthostatic hypotension is to ensure adequate salt and volume intake and to discontinue drugs that cause orthostatic hypotension. Patients with orthostatic hypotension should be advised to raise the head of the bed at night, to rise from bed or chair slowly, and to avoid prolonged standing. Compressive stockings applied up to thigh levels may help decrease venous pooling. Frequent small feedings may be helpful in patients with marked postprandial hypotension.

Pharmacological agents of potential benefit include fludrocortisone (0.1 to 1.0 mg/day), in conjunction with increased salt intake. Various adrenergic agents have been used, including ephedrine, phenylephrine, and others. A more detailed discussion of pharmacological treatment of orthostatic hypotension is found elsewhere.[31]

Elderly. Syncope in the elderly can be difficult to manage because elderly patients may have multiple chronic diseases and physiological impairments that predispose to syncope.[30] Thus, in the elderly, several seemingly mild abnormalities may contribute to a sudden reduction of cerebral blood flow and syncope. As an example, mild volume depletion with upper respiratory tract infection in an elderly patient with chronic renal insufficiency and systolic hypertension may be sufficient to cause syncope, whereas any one problem alone is not severe enough to cause loss of consciousness. The initial approach to the management of the elderly should be to search for a single condition as a cause of syncope. If a single condition is found (such as severe aortic stenosis, symptomatic bradycardia, or symptomatic orthostatic hypotension), treatment of that disease can be planned. However, a single disease as the cause of syncope is often not apparent. In these patients, inability to compensate for common situational stresses may be a factor in the setting of multiple medical problems, medications, and physiological impairments. A careful assessment of the effect of underlying pathological conditions and medications is important to determine whether multiple pathological processes could have led to syncope. Once these potential processes are identified, treatment should be directed to correcting these factors. As an example, consider an elderly patient presenting with syncope, who has taken enalapril 10 mg/day, has anemia (hemoglobin 9.0), mild orthostatic hypotension, and a recent upper respiratory tract infection. In this patient, if no other etiology of syncope is apparent on the basis of clinical findings and selective use of laboratory tests, volume repletion, treatment of anemia and adjustment or change of antihypertensive medication may help prevent further episodes of syncope.

PATIENT INSTRUCTIONS AND EDUCATION. Issues in patient education include instructions in prevention of syncope, non-pharmacologic treatment, and restriction of activities. Many patients with vasovagal syncope have precipitating factors or situations that should be identified and the patient instructed to avoid these situations. Common triggers include prolonged standing, venipuncture, large meals, and heat (such as hot baths or sunbathing). Additionally, fasting, lack of sleep, and alcohol intake may predispose to vasovagal syncope and should be avoided. Postexercise vasovagal syncope may occasionally be related to chronic inadequate salt and fluid replacement. Syncope may be prevented with the use of electrolyte-containing solutions and water in such instances. In other patients, exercise may have to be curtailed.

Patients with syncope should also be instructed to assume a supine position as soon as they develop premonitory symptoms. They should remain supine for 15 to 30 minutes. Patients with potential recurrences need to be instructed to avoid activities that may lead to serious injury to the patient or others. Activities such as swimming, mountain climbing, operating milling machines and saws, and other similar work should be curtailed or performed in the presence of a companion.

Although 84 per cent of states in the United States have specific regulations for driving restriction for seizures, only 26 states (52 per cent) have regulations that limit driving after an episode of loss of consciousness other than seizure (e.g., vasovagal syncope, arrhythmias, diabetic coma).[119] In nonseizure loss of consciousness, the average mandated duration of driving restriction is 4.3 months. In addition to adhering to state regulations on driving, the likelihood of recurrent episodes and the probability of treatment efficacy should be considered in restricting driving.[119,120]

REFERENCES

1. Benditt, D. G., Remole, S., Bailin, S., et al.: Tilt table testing for evaluation of neurally-mediated (cardioneurogenic) syncope: Rationale and proposed protocols. PACE 14:1528, 1991.
2. Abboud, F. M.: Neurocardiogenic syncope. N. Engl. J. Med. 15:1117, 1993.
3. Waxman, M. B., Cameron, D. A., and Wald, R. W.: Role of ventricular vagal afferents in the vasovagal reaction. J. Am. Coll. Cardiol. 21:1138, 1993.
4. Scherrer, U., Vissing, S., Morgan, B. J., et al.: Vasovagal syncope after infusion of a vasodilator in a heart transplant recipient. N. Engl. J. Med. 32:602, 1990.
5. Fitzpatrick, A. P., Banner, N., Cheng, A., et al.: Vasovagal reactions may occur after orthotopic heart transplantation. J. Am. Coll. Cardiol. 21:1132, 1993.
6. Lightfoot, J. T., Rowe, S. A., and Fortney, S. M.: Occurrence of presyncope in subjects without ventricular innervation. Clin. Sci. 85:695, 1993.
7. Moorita, H., Nishida, Y., Motochigawa, H., et al.: Opiate receptor-mediated decrease in renal nerve activity during hypotensive hemorrhage in conscious rabbits. Circ. Res. 63:165, 1988.
8. Smite, M. L., Carlson, M. D., and Thames, M. D.: Naloxone does not prevent vasovagal syncope during simulated orthostatis in humans. J. Am. Nerv. 45:1, 1993.
9. Schadt, J. C., and Ludbrook, J.: Hemodynamic and neurohumoral responses to acute hypovolemia in conscious mammals. Am. J. Physiol. (Heart Circ. Physiol. 29) 260:H305, 1991.
10. Kapoor, W. N., Peterson, J., and Karpf, M.: Micturition syncope. JAMA 253:796, 1985.
11. Kapoor, W. N., Peterson, J., and Karpf, M.: Defecation syncope. A symptom with multiple etiologies. Arch. Intern. Med. 146:2377, 1986.
12. Strasberg, B., Sagie, A., Erdman, S., et al.: Carotid sinus hypersensivity and the carotid sinus syndrome. Prog. Cardiovasc. Dis. 5:379, 1989.
13. Katritsis, D., Ward, D. E., and Camm, A. J.: Can we treat carotid sinus syndrome? PACE 14:1367, 1991.
14. Brignole, M., Oddone, D., Cogorno, S., et al.: Long-term outcome in symptomatic carotid sinus hypersensitivity. Am. Heart J. 123:687, 1992.
15. Brignole, M., Menozzi, C., Lolli, G., et al.: Long-term outcome of paced and nonpaced patients with severe carotid sinus syndrome. Am. J. Cardiol. 69:1039, 1992.
16. Nicholas, R., O'Meara, P. D., and Calonge, N.: Is syncope related to moderate altitude exposure? JAMA 268:904, 1992.
17. Kapoor, W. N., Fortunato, M., Hanusa, B. H., and Schulberg, H. C.: Psychiatric illnesses in patients with syncope. Am. J. Med. 99:505, 1995.
18. Koenig, D., Linzer, M., Pontinenn, M., and Divine, G. W.: Syncope in young adults: evidence for a combined medical and psychiatric approach. J. Intern. Med. 232:169, 1992.
19. Linzer, M., Felder, A., Hackel, A., et al.: Psychiatric syncope. Psychosom. Med. 31:181, 1990.
20. Grubb, B. P., Temesy-Armos, P. N., Samoil, D., et al.: Tilt table testing in the evaluation and management of athletes with recurrent exercise-induced syncope. Med. Sci. Sports Exerc. 28:24, 1993.
21. Osswald, S., Brooks, R., O'Nunain, S. S., et al.: Asystole after exercise in healthy persons. Ann. Intern. Med. 120:1008, 1994.
22. Sneddon, J. F., Scalia, G., Ward, D. E., et al.: Exercise-induced vasodepressor syncope. Br. Heart J. 71:554, 1994.
23. Raviele, A. N., Gasparini, G., DiPede, F., et al.: Nitroglycerine infusion during upright tilt: A new test for the diagnosis of vasovagal syncope. Am. Heart J. 127:103, 1994.
24. Grech, E. D., and Ramsdale, D. R.: Exertional syncope in aortic stenosis. Am. Heart J. 121:603, 1991.
25. Gilligan, D. M., Nihoyannopoulos, P., Chan, W. L., and Oakley, C. M.: Investigation of a hemodynamic basis for syncope in hypertrophic cardiomyopathy. Use of head-up tilt testing. Circulation 85:2140, 1992.
26. Leitch, J. W., Klein, G. J., Yee, R., et al.: Syncope associated with supraventricular tachycardia: An expression of tachycardia rate or vasomotor response? Circulation 85:1064, 1992.
27. Brignole, M., Gianfranchi, L., Menozzi, C., et al.: Role of autonomic reflexes in syncope associated with paroxysmal atrial fibrillation. J. Am. Coll. Cardiol. 22:1123, 1993.
28. Pavlovic, S. U., Kocovic, D., Djordjevic, M., et al.: The etiology of syncope in pacemaker patients. PACE 14:2086, 1991.
29. Lipsitz, L.: Orthostatic hypotension in the elderly. N. Engl. J. Med. 321:952, 1989.
30. Kapoor, W. N.: Syncope in the older person. J. Am. Geriatr. Soc. 42:426, 1994.
31. Bannister, S. R. (ed.): Autonomic Failure: A Textbook of Clinical Disorders of the Autonomic Nervous System. 2nd ed. Oxford, Oxford Medical Publishers, 1988, pp. 1–20.
32. Vaitkevicius, P. V., Esserwein, D. M., Maynard, A. K., et al.: Frequency and importance of postprandial blood pressure reduction in elderly nursing-home patients. Ann. Intern. Med. 115:865, 1991.
33. Davidson, E., Rotenbeg, Z., Fuchs, J., et al.: Transient ischemic attack–related syncope. Clin. Cardiol. 14:141, 1991.
34. Kapoor, W.: Evaluation and outcome of patients with syncope. Medicine 69:160, 1990.
35. Kapoor, W., Karpf, M., Wieand, S., et al.: A prospective evaluation and follow-up of patients with syncope. N. Engl. J. Med. 309:197, 1983.
36. Gambardella, A., Reutens, D. C., Andermann, F., et al.: Late-onset drop attacks in temporal lobe epilepsy: A reevaluation of the concept of temporal lobe syncope. Neurology 44:1074, 1994.
37. Jacome, D. E.: Temporal lobe syncope: Clinical variants. Clin. Electroencephal. 20:58, 1989.
38. Constantin, L., Martins, J. B., Fincham, R. W., and Dagli, R. D.: Bradycardia and syncope as manifestations of partial epilepsy. J. Am. Coll. Cardiol. 15:900, 1990.
39. Baltazar, R. F., Go, E. H., Benesh, S., and Mower, M. M.: Case report: Myocardial ischemia: an overlooked substrate in syncope of aortic stenosis. Am. J. Med. Sci. 303:105, 1992.
40. Dilsizian, V., Bonow, R. O., Epstein, S. E., and Fananapazir, L.: Myocardial ischemia detected by thallium scintigraphy is frequently related to cardiac arrest and syncope in young patients with hypertrophic cardiomyopathy. J. Am. Coll. Cardiol. 22:796, 1993.
41. Fananapazir, L., Tracy, C. M., Leon, M. B., et al.: Electrophysiologic abnormalities in patients with hypertrophic cardiomyopathy. Circulation 80:1259, 1989.
42. Nienaber, C. A., Hiller, S., Spielmann, R. P., et al.: Syncope in hypertrophic cardiomyopathy: Multivariate analysis of prognostic determinants. J. Am. Coll. Cardiol. 15:948, 1990.
43. Bradenburg, R. O.: Syncope and sudden death in hypertrophic cardiomyopathy. J. Am. Coll. Cardiol. 15:962, 1990.
44. Sgarbossa, E. B., Pinski, S. L., Jaeger, F. J., et al.: Incidence and predictors of syncope in paced patients with sick sinus syndrome. PACE 15:2055, 1992.
45. Paul, T., Guccione, P., and Garson, A.: Relationship of syncope in young patients with Wolff-Parkinson-White syndrome to rapid ventricular response during atrial fibrillation. Am. J. Cardiol. 65:318, 1990.
46. Auricchio, A., Klein, H., Trappe, H., and Wenzlaff, P.: Lack of prognostic value of syncope in patients with Wolff-Parkinson-White syndrome. J. Am. Coll. Cardiol. 17:152, 1991.
47. James, T. N.: Syncope and sudden death in the Wolff-Parkinson-White syndrome. J. Am. Coll. Cardiol. 17:159, 1991.
48. Kapoor, W., Karpf, M., Maher, Y., et al.: Syncope of unknown origin: The need for a more cost-effective approach to its diagnostic evaluation. JAMA 247:2687, 1982.
49. Silverstein, M. D., Singer, D. E., Mulley, A., et al.: Patients with syncope admitted to medical intensive care units. JAMA 248:1185, 1982.
50. Martin, G. J., Adams, S. L., Martin, H. G., et al.: Prospective evaluation of syncope. Ann. Emerg. Med. 13:499, 1984.
51. Sra, J. S., Anderson, A. J., Sheikh, S. H., et al.: Unexplained syncope evaluated by electrophysiologic studies and head-up tilt testing. Ann. Intern. Med. 114:1013, 1991.
52. Savage, D. D., Corwin, L., McGee, D. L., et al.: Epidemiologic features of isolated syncope. The Framingham Study. Stroke 16:626, 1985.
53. Middlekauff, H. R., Stevenson, W. G., and Sacon, L. A.: Prognosis after syncope: Impact of left ventricular function. Am. Heart J. 125:121, 1993.
54. Middlekauff, H. R., Stevenson, W. G., Stevenson, L. W., and Saxon, L. A.: Syncope in advanced heart failure: High risk of sudden death regardless of origin of syncope. J. Am. Coll. Cardiol. 21:110, 1993.
55. Kapoor, W., Peterson, J., Wieand, H. S., and Karpf, M.: Diagnostic and prognostic implications of recurrences in patients with syncope. Am. J. Med. 83:700, 1987.
56. Lempert, T., Bauer, M., and Schmidt, D.: Syncope: A video metric analysis of 56 episodes of transient cerebral hypoxia. Ann. Neurol. 36:233, 1994.
57. Hoefnagels, W. A. J., Padberg, G. W., Overweg, J., et al.: Syncope or seizure? The diagnostic value of the EEG and hyperventilation test in transient loss of consciousness. J. Neurol. 54:953, 1991.
58. Grubb, B. P., Gerard, G., Roush, K., et al.: Differentiation of convulsive syncope and epilepsy with head-up tilt testing. Ann. Intern. Med. 115:871, 1991.
59. Atkins, D., Hanusa, B., Sefcik, T., and Kapoor, W.: Syncope and orthostatic hypotension. Am. J. Med. 91:179, 1991.
60. Kenny, R. A., and Traynor, G.: Carotid sinus syndrome: Clinical characteristics in elderly patients. Age Ageing 20:449, 1991.
61. Winters, S. L., Stewart, D., and Gomes, J. A.: Signal averaging of the surface QRS complex predicts inducibility of ventricular tachycardia in

patients with syncope of unknown origin: A prospective study. J. Am. Coll. Cardiol. *10*(4):775, 1987.

62. Gang, E. S., Peter, T., Rosenthal, M. E., et al.: Detection of late potentials on the surface electrocardiogram in unexplained syncope. Am. J. Cardiol. *58*(10):14, 1986.

63. Steinberg, J. S., Prytowsky, E., Freedman, R. A., et al.: Use of the signal-averaged electrocardiogram for predicting inducible ventricular tachycardia in patients with unexplained syncope: Relation to clinical variables in a multivariate analysis. J. Am. Coll. Cardiol. *23*:99, 1994.

64. Gibson, T. C., and Heitzman, M. R.: Diagnostic efficacy of 24-hour electrocardiographic monitoring for syncope. Am. J. Cardiol. *53*:1013, 1984.

65. Bass, E. B., Curtiss, E. L., Arena, V. C., et al.: The duration of Holter monitoring in patients with syncope: Is 24 hours enough? Arch. Intern. Med. *150*:1073, 1990.

66. Kapoor, W., Cha, R., Peterson, J., et al.: Prolonged electrocardiographic monitoring in patients with syncope: The importance of frequent or repetitive ventricular ectopy. Am. J. Med. *82*:20, 1987.

67. DiMarco, J. P., and Philbrick, J. T.: Use of ambulatory electrocardiographic (Holter) monitoring. Ann. Intern. Med. *113*:53, 1990.

68. Linzer, M., Pritchett, E. L. C., Pontinenn, M., et al.: Incremental diagnostic yield of loop electrocardiographic recorders in unexplained syncope. Am. J. Cardiol. *66*:214, 1990.

69. Kapoor, W. N., Hammill, S. C., and Gersh, B. J.: Diagnosis and natural history of syncope and the role of invasive electrophysiologic testing. Am. J. Cardiol. *63*:730, 1989.

70. Bass, E. B., Elson, J. J., Fogoros, R. N., et al.: Long-term prognosis of patients undergoing electrophysiologic studies for syncope of unknown origin. Am. J. Cardiol. *62*:1186, 1988.

71. Klein, G. J., Gersh, B. J., and Yee, R.: Electrophysiological testing: The final court of appeal for the diagnosis of syncope? Circulation *92*:1332, 1995.

72. DiMarco, J. P.: Electrophysiologic studies in patients with unexplained syncope. Circulation *75*(Suppl III):140, 1987.

73. McAnulty, J. H.: Syncope of unknown origin: The role of electrophysiologic studies. Circulation *75*(Suppl III):144, 1987.

74. Moazes, F., Peter, T., Simonson, J., et al.: Syncope of unknown origin: clinical, noninvasive, and electrophysiologic determinants of arrhythmia induction and symptom recurrence during long-term follow-up. Am. Heart J. *121*:81, 1991.

75. Bachinsky, W. B., Linzer, M., Weld, L., and Estes, N. A. M.: Usefulness of clinical characteristics in predicting the outcome of electrophysiologic studies in unexplained syncope. Am. J. Cardiol. *69*:1044, 1992.

76. Kushner, J. A., Kou, W. H., Kadish, A. H., and Morady, F.: Natural history of patients with unexplained syncope and a nondiagnostic electrophysiologic study. J. Am. Coll. Cardiol. *14*:391, 1989.

76a. Yamanouchi, Y., Jaalouk, S., Shehadeh, A. A., et al.: Changes in left ventricular volume during head-up tilt in patients with vasovagal syncope. An echocardiographic study. Am. Heart J. *131*:73, 1996.

77. Fitzpatrick, A. P., Theodorakis, G., Vardas, P., and Sutton, R.: Methodology of head-up tilt testing in patients with unexplained syncope. J. Am. Coll. Cardiol. *17*:125, 1991.

78. Hackel, A., Linzer, M., Anderson, N., and Williams, R.: Cardiovascular and catecholamine responses to head-up tilt in the diagnosis of recurrent unexplained syncope in elderly patients. J. Am. Geriatr. Soc. *39*:663, 1991.

79. Kenny, R. A., Ingram, A., Bayliss, J., and Sutton, R.: Head-up tilt: A useful test for investigating unexplained syncope. Lancet *1*:1352, 1986.

80. Lerman-Sagie, T., Rechavia, E., Strasberg, B., et al.: Head-up tilt for the evaluation of syncope of unknown origin in children. J. Pediatr. *118*:676, 1991.

81. Raviele, A., Gasparini, G., DiPede, F., et al.: Usefulness of head-up tilt test in evaluating patients with syncope of unknown origin and negative electrophysiologic study. Am. J. Cardiol. *65*:1322, 1990.

82. Strasberg, B., Rechavia, E., Sagie, A., et al.: The head-up tilt table test in patients with syncope of unknown origin. Am. Heart J. *118*:923, 1989.

83. Abi-Samra, F., Maloney, J. D., Fouad-Tarazi, F. R., and Castle, L. W.: The usefulness of head-up tilt testing and hemodynamic investigations in the workup of syncope of unknown origin. PACE *11*:1202, 1988.

84. Almquist, A., Goldenberg, I. F., Milstein, S., et al.: Provocation of bradycardia and hypotension by isoproterenol and upright posture in patients with unexplained syncope. N. Engl. J. Med. *320*:346, 1989.

85. Chen, M. Y., Goldenberg, I. F., Milstein, S., et al.: Cardiac electrophysiologic and hemodynamic correlates of neurally mediated syncope. Am. J. Cardiol. *63*:66, 1989.

86. Chen, X. C., Chen, M. Y., Remole, S., et al.: Reproducibility of head-up tilt-table testing for eliciting susceptibility to neurally mediated syncope in patients without structural heart disease. Am. J. Cardiol. *69*:755, 1992.

87. Grubb, B. P., Temesy-Armos, P., Hahn, H., and Elliott, L.: Utility of upright tilt-table testing in the evaluation and management of syncope of unknown origin. Am. J. Med. *90*:6, 1991.

88. Grubb, B. P., Gerard, G., Roush, K., et al.: Cerebral vasoconstriction during head-upright tilt-induced vasovagal syncope. Circulation *84*:1157, 1991.

89. Grubb, B. P., Temesy-Armos, P., Moore, J., et al.: Head-upright tilt-table testing in evaluation and management of the malignant vasovagal syndrome. Am. J. Cardiol. *69*:904, 1992.

90. Grubb, B. P., Temesy-Armos, P., Moore, J., et al.: The use of head-upright tilt table testing in the evaluation and management of syncope in children and adolescents. PACE *15*:742, 1992.

91. Pongiglione, G., Fish, F. A., Strasburger, J. F., and Benson, D. W.: Heart rate and blood pressure response to upright tilt in young patients with unexplained syncope. J. Am. Coll. Cardiol. *16*:165, 1990.

92. Sheldon, R., and Killam, S.: Methodology of isoproterenol-tilt table testing in patients with syncope. J. Am. Coll. Cardiol. *19*:773, 1992.

93. Waxman, M. B., Yao, L., Cameron, D. A., et al.: Isoproterenol induction of vasodepressor-type reaction in vasodepressor-prone persons. Am. J. Cardiol. *63*:58, 1989.

94. Calkins, H., Kadish, A., Sousa, J., et al.: Comparison of responses to isoproterenol and epinephrine during head-up tilt in suspected vasodepressor syncope. Am. J. Cardiol. *67*:207, 1991.

95. Lurie, K. G., Dutton, J., Mangat, R., et al.: Evaluation of edrophonium as a provocative agent for vasovagal syncope during head-up tilt-table testing. Am. J. Cardiol. *72*:1286, 1993.

96. Ovadia, M., and Thoele, D.: Esmolol tilt testing with esmolol withdrawal for the evaluation of syncope in the young. Circulation *89*:228, 1994.

97. Kapoor, W. N., Smith, M., and Miller, N. L.: Upright tilt testing in evaluating syncope: a comprehensive literature review. Am. J. Med. *97*:78, 1994.

98. Kapoor, W. N., and Brant, N.: Evaluation of syncope by upright tilt testing with isoproterenol. Ann. Intern. Med. *116*:358, 1992.

99. Nwosu, E. A., Rahkoo, P. S., Hanson, P., and Grogan, E. W.: Hemodynamic and volumetric response of the normal left ventricle to upright tilt test. Am. Heart J. *128*:106, 1994.

100. Sheldon, R., Splawinski, J., and Killam, S.: Reproducibility of isoproterenol tilt table tests in patients with syncope. Am. J. Cardiol. *69*:1300, 1992.

101. Blanc, J. J., Mansourati, J., Maheu, B., et al.: Reproducibility of a positive passive upright tilt test at a seven-day interval in patients with syncope. Am. J. Cardiol. *72*:469, 1993.

102. Fish, F. A., Strasburger, J. F., and Benson, D. W.: Reproducibility of a symptomatic response to upright tilt in young patients with unexplained syncope. Am. J. Cardiol. *70*:605, 1992.

103. de Buitleir, M., Grogan, E. W., Picone, M., and Casteen, J. A.: Immediate reproducibility of the tilt-table test in adults with unexplained syncope. Am. J. Cardiol. *71*:304, 1993.

104. Brooks, R., Ruskin, J. N., Powell, A. C., et al.: Prospective evaluation of day-to-day reproducibility of upright tilt-table testing in unexplained syncope. Am. J. Cardiol. *71*:1289, 1993.

105. Davis, T. L., and Freemoon, F. R.: Electroencephalography should not be routine in the evaluation of syncope in adults. Arch. Intern. Med. *150*:2027, 1990.

106. Kapoor, W., Snustad, D., Peterson, J., et al.: Syncope in the elderly. Am. J. Med. *80*:419, 1986.

107. Kelly, P. A., Mann, D. E., Adler, S. W., et al.: Low-dose disopyramide often fails to prevent neurogenic syncope during head-up tilt testing. PACE *17*:573, 1994.

108. Morilo, C. A., Leith, J. W., Yee, R., and Klein, G. J.: A placebo-controlled trial of intravenous and oral disopyramide for prevention of neurally mediated syncope induced by head-up tilt. J. Am. Coll. Cardiol. *22*:1843, 1993.

109. Nelson, S. D., Stanley, M., Love, C. J., et al.: The autonomic and hemodynamic effects of oral theophylline in patients with vasodepressor syncope. Arch. Intern. Med. *151*(12):2425, 1991.

110. Grubb, B. P., Wolfe, D. A., Samoil, D., et al.: Usefulness of fluoxetine hydrochloride for prevention of resistant upright tilt induced syncope. PACE *16*:458, 1993.

111. Grubb, B. P., Samoil, D., Kosinski, D., et al.: Use of sertraline hydrochloride in the treatment of refractory neurocardiogenic syncope in children and adolescents. J. Am. Coll. Cardiol. *24*:490, 1994.

112. Janoski, D., Holt, D., Fredman, C., and Bjerregaard, P.: Efficacy of oral ephedrine sulfate in preventing neurocardiogenic syncope (abst). Circulation *84*:929, 1991.

113. Brignole, M., Menozzi, C., Gianfranchi, L., et al.: A controlled trial of acute and long-term medical therapy in tilt-induced neurally mediated syncope. Am. J. Cardiol. *70*:339, 1992.

114. Susmano, A., Volgman, A. S., and Buckingham, T. A.: Beneficial effects of dextro-amphetamine in the treatment of vasodepressor syncope. PACE *16*:1235, 1993.

115. Strieper, M. J., and Campbell, R. M.: Efficacy of alpha-adrenergic agonist therapy for prevention of pediatric neurocardiogenic syncope. J. Am. Coll. Cardiol. *22*:594, 1994.

116. Benditt, D. G., Petersen, M., Lurie, K. G., et al.: Cardiac pacing for prevention of recurrent vasovagal syncope. Ann. Intern. Med. *122*:204, 1995.

117. Petersen, M. E. V., Price, D., Williams, T., et al.: Short AV interval VDD Pacing does not prevent tilt induced vasovagal syncope in patients with cardioinhibitory vasovagal syndrome. PACE *17*:882, 1994.

118. Sra, J. S., Jazayeri, M. R., Avitall, B., et al.: Comparison of cardiac pacing with drug therapy in the treatment of neurocardiogenic (vasovagal) syncope with bradycardia or asystole. N. Engl. J. Med. *328*:1085, 1993.

119. Strickberger, S. A., Cantillon, C. O., and Friedman, P. L.: When should patients with lethal ventricular arrhythmia resume driving? An analysis of state regulations and physician practices. Ann. Intern. Med. *115*:560, 1991.

120. Decter, B. M., Goldner, B., and Cohen, T. J.: Vasovagal syncope as a cause of motor vehicle accidents. Am. Heart J. *127*:1619, 1994.

Part III
Diseases of the Heart, Pericardium, Aorta, and Pulmonary Vascular Bed

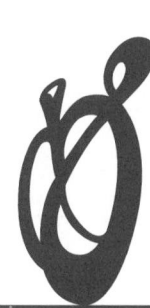

Chapter 29

Congenital Heart Disease in Infancy and Childhood

WILLIAM F. FRIEDMAN

GENERAL CONSIDERATIONS

DEFINITION

Congenital cardiovascular disease is defined as an *abnormality in cardiocirculatory structure or function that is present at birth, even if it is discovered much later.* Congenital cardiovascular malformations usually result from altered embryonic development of a normal structure or failure of such a structure to progress beyond an early stage of embryonic or fetal development. The aberrant patterns of flow created by an anatomical defect may, in turn, significantly influence the structural and functional development of the remainder of the circulation. For instance, the presence in utero of mitral atresia may prohibit normal development of the left ventricle, aortic valve, and ascending aorta. Similarly, constriction of the fetal ductus arteriosus may result directly in right ventricular dilatation and tricuspid regurgitation in the fetus and newborn, contribute importantly to the development of pulmonary arterial aneurysms in the presence of ventricular septal defect and absent pulmonic valve, or, further, result in an alteration in the number and caliber of fetal and newborn pulmonary vascular resistance vessels.

POSTNATAL EVENTS. These may markedly influence the clinical presentation of a specific "isolated" malformation. The infant with Ebstein's malformation of the tricuspid valve may improve dramatically as the magnitude of tricuspid regurgitation diminishes with normal fall in pulmonary vascular resistance after birth; the infant with hypoplastic left heart syndrome or interrupted aortic arch may not exhibit circulatory collapse; and the baby with pulmonic atresia or severe stenosis may not become cyanotic until normal spontaneous closure of a patent ductus arteriosus occurs. Ductal constriction many days after birth also may be a central factor in some infants in the development of coarctation of the aorta. Still later in life the patient with a ventricular septal defect may experience spontaneous closure of the abnormal communication, or develop right ventricular outflow tract obstruction and/or aortic regurgitation or pulmonary vascular obstructive disease. These selected examples serve to emphasize that anatomical and physiological changes in the heart and circulation may continue indefinitely from prenatal life in association with any specific congenital cardiocirculatory lesion.

Certain congenital defects are not apparent on gross inspection of the heart or circulation. Examples include the electrophysiological pathways for ventricular preexcitation or interruptions in the cardiac conduction system giving rise to paroxysmal supraventricular tachycardia or congenital complete heart block, respectively. Similarly, abnormalities in the development of myocardial autonomic innervation or in the ultrastructure of myocardial cells may ultimately prove to contribute to asymmetrical septal hypertrophy and left ventricular outflow tract obstruction. These examples make clear that occasional difficulties arise in distinguishing between congenital anomalies that are readily apparent at or shortly after birth and lesions that may have as their basis a subtle or undetectable abnormality that is present at birth.

INCIDENCE. The true incidence of congenital cardiovascular malformations is difficult to determine accurately, partly because of the difficulties in definition discussed above. About 0.8 per cent of live births are complicated by a cardiovascular malformation.[1] This figure does not take into account what may be the two most common cardiac anomalies: the congenital, nonstenotic bicuspid aortic valve[2] and the leaflet abnormality associated with mitral valve prolapse.[3] Moreover, the widely quoted 0.8 per cent incidence figure fails to include small preterm infants, almost all of whom have persistent patent ductus arteriosus. Further, if the calculations were to include stillbirths and abortuses, the incidence would be greatly increased. Cardiac malformations occur 10 times more often in stillborn than in liveborn babies, and many early spontaneous abortions are associated with chromosomal defects (see Chapter 49).[1] Thus, it is clear that past statistical analyses have seriously *underestimated* the incidence of congenital heart disease.

Precise data concerning the frequency of individual congenital lesions also are lacking, and the results of many analyses differ, depending on the source (living or dead) and the selection of the study population. Table 29–1 is a compilation from both clinical and pathological studies that approximates the frequency of occurrence of specific cardiovascular malformations.[4,5,5a]

Taken in toto, children with congenital heart disease are predominantly male. Moreover, specific defects may show a definite gender preponderance; patent ductus arteriosus, Ebstein's anomaly of the tricuspid valve, and atrial septal defect are more common in *females,* whereas valvular aor-

TABLE 29–1   RELATIVE FREQUENCY OF OCCURRENCE OF CARDIAC MALFORMATIONS AT BIRTH

DISEASE	PERCENTAGE
Ventricular septal defect	30.5
Atrial septal defect	9.8
Patent ductus arteriosus	9.7
Pulmonic stenosis	6.9
Coarctation of the aorta	6.8
Aortic stenosis	6.1
Tetralogy of Fallot	5.8
Complete transposition of the great arteries	4.2
Persistent truncus arteriosus	2.2
Tricuspid atresia	1.3
All others	16.5

Data based on 2310 cases.

tic stenosis, coarctation of the aorta, hypoplastic left heart, pulmonary and tricuspid atresia, and transposition of the great arteries are more common in *males.*[6]

Extracardiac anomalies occur in about 25 per cent of infants with significant cardiac disease,[7] and their presence may significantly increase mortality. The extracardiac anomalies often are multiple, in part involving the musculoskeletal system; one third of infants with both cardiac and extracardiac anomalies have some established syndrome.

ETIOLOGY

Malformations appear to result from an interaction between multifactorial genetic and environmental systems too complex to allow a single specification of cause[8]; in most instances, a causal factor cannot be identified. Maternal rubella, ingestion of thalidomide and isoretinoin early during gestation, and chronic maternal alcohol abuse are environmental insults known to interfere with normal cardiogenesis in humans.[9-11] *Rubella syndrome* consists of cataracts, deafness, microcephaly, and, either singly or in combination, patent ductus arteriosus, pulmonic valvular and/or arterial stenosis, and atrial septal defect. *Thalidomide* exposure is associated with major limb deformities and, occasionally, with cardiac malformations without predilection for a specific lesion. Tricuspid valve anomalies are associated with the ingestion of *lithium* during pregnancy. The *fetal alcohol syndrome* consists of microcephaly, micrognathia, microphthalmia, prenatal growth retardation, developmental delay, and cardiac defects. The latter—often defects of the ventricular septum—occur in about 45 per cent of affected infants. *Maternal lupus erythematosus* during pregnancy has been linked to congenital complete heart block (see p. 949). Animal experiments have incriminated hypoxia, deficiency or excess of several vitamins, intake of several categories of drugs, and ionizing irradiation as teratogens capable of causing cardiac malformations. The precise relation of these animal teratogens to human malformations is not clear.

The genetic aspects of congenital heart disease are discussed extensively in Chap. 49. A single gene mutation may be causative in the familial forms of atrial septal defect with prolonged AV conduction, mitral valve prolapse, ventricular septal defect, congenital heart block, situs inversus, pulmonary hypertension, and the syndromes of Noonan, LEOPARD, Ellis–van Creveld, and Kartagener. In recent years, the genes responsible for several defects have either been mapped (e.g., long QT syndrome, Holt-Oram syndrome) or identified (e.g., Marfan syndrome, hypertrophic cardiomyopathy, supravalvular aortic stenosis). Contiguous gene defects on the long arm of chromosome 22 likely underlie the conotruncal malformations of the DiGeorge and velocardiofacial syndromes.[12,13] Table 29–2 provides a partial list of syndromes in which cardiovascular anomalies may be manifestations of the pleiotropic effects of single genes or examples of gross chromosomal defects. Less than 10 per cent of all cardiac malformations can be accounted for by chromosomal aberrations or genetic mutations or transmission.

The finding that, with some exceptions, only one of a pair of monozygotic twins is affected by congenital heart disease indicates that the vast majority of cardiovascular malformations are not inherited in a simple manner.[14] However, this observation may have led, in the past, to an underestimation of genetic contribution, because most recent twin studies reveal more than double the incidence of heart defects in monozygotic twins but usually only one of the pair.[15] Family studies indicate a twofold to tenfold increase in the incidence of congenital heart disease in siblings of affected patients or in the offspring of an affected parent. Malformations often are concordant or partially concordant within families.[16,17] Because the incidence of congenital heart disease in the offspring or siblings of an index patient is only 2 to 10 per cent, it is seldom wise to discourage the parents of one affected child from having additional children if either parent is free of a cardiovascular anomaly.[1] Moreover, the low recurrence rate and the increasing possibilities for effective treatment for nearly all cardiac lesions usually justify a positive approach to family counseling. When two or more members of the family are affected, the recurrence risk may be quite high, and a pedigree should be obtained before further counseling. If a dominant or recessive mendelian pattern is established, the mendelian laws apply, and the risk of recurrence in each pregnancy is equal.

PREVENTION

The feasibility of preventive programs depends on what is learned in the future about the 90 per cent or more of cardiovascular anomalies for which no cause currently is known. Strict testing in animals of new drugs that may be teratogenic when taken during pregnancy may be expected to reduce the chances of another thalidomide tragedy. In this regard, the dictum cannot be emphasized too strongly that no medication should be taken during pregnancy without prior consultation with a physician. Physicians who deal with pregnant women should be aware of known teratogens as well as drugs that may have a functional rather than structural damaging influence on the fetal and newborn heart and circulation, and should recognize that drugs abound for which there is inadequate information concerning their teratogenic potential. Similarly, appropriate radiological equipment and techniques for reducing gonadal and fetal radiation exposure should always be used to reduce the potential hazards of this likely cause of birth defects.

Detection of abnormal chromosomes in fetal cells obtained from amniotic fluid or chronic villus biopsy (Chap. 49) may predict cardiac malformation as one component of the multisystem involvement that may exist in such syndromes as Down, Turner, or trisomy 13–15 (D1) or 16–18 (E). Similarly, identification in such cells of the enzyme disorders observed in the mucopolysaccharidoses, homocystinuria, or type II glycogen storage disease may allow one to predict the ultimate presence of cardiac disease. Finally, immunization of children with rubella vaccine will avoid the effects of maternal rubella and its cardiac consequences.

EMBRYOLOGY

NORMAL CARDIAC DEVELOPMENT. Correlation of anatomical features of malformed hearts and embryonic cardiac morphology allows a developmental analysis of various anomalies. Detailed accounts of the normal development of the cardiovascular system are provided elsewhere.[18–20] In brief, during the first month of gestation the primitive, straight cardiac tube is formed, comprising the sinuatrium, the primitive ventricle, the bulbus cordis, and the truncus arteriosus in series, from cephalad to caudad. In the second month of gestation this tube doubles over on itself to form two parallel pumping systems, each with two chambers and a great artery. The two atria develop from the sinuatrium; the atrioventricular canal is divided by the endocardial cushions into tricuspid and mitral orifices; and the right and left ventricles develop from the primitive ventricle and bulbus cordis. Differential growth of myocardial cells causes the straight cardiac tube to bear to the right, and the bulboventricular portion of the tube doubles over on itself, bringing the ventricles side by side. Migration of the atrioventricular canal to the right and of the ventricular septum to the left serves to align each ventricle with its appropriate atrioventricular valve. At the distal end of the cardiac tube the bulbus cordis divides into a subaortic muscular conus and a subpulmonic muscular conus; the subpulmonic conus elongates and the subaortic conus resorbs, allowing the aorta to move posteriorly and connect with the left ventricle.

ABNORMAL DEVELOPMENT. A host of anomalies may result from defects in this basic developmental pattern. Thus, double-inlet left ventricle (see p. 944) is observed if the tricuspid orifice does not align over the right ventricle. The various types of persistent truncus arteriosus (p. 907) result from failure of the truncus to divide into main pulmonary artery and aorta. Double-outlet anomalies of the right ventricle (p. 941) are produced by failure of either the subpulmonic or subaortic conus to resorb, whereas resorption of the subpulmonic instead of the subaortic conus may be central to transposition of the great arteries (p. 935).

THE ATRIA. The primitive sinuatrium is separated into right and left atria by the downgrowth from its roof of the septum primum toward the atrioventricular canal, thereby creating an inferior intraatrial ostium primum opening (Fig. 29–1). Multiple perforations form in the anterosuperior portion of the septum primum as the septum secundum begins to develop to the right of the former. The coalescence of these perforations forms the ostium secundum. The septum secundum completely separates the atrial chambers except for a central opening—the fossa ovalis—which is covered by tissue of the septum primum, forming the valve of the foramen ovale.

Fusion of the endocardial cushions anteriorly and posteriorly divides the atrioventricular canal into tricuspid and mitral inlets (Fig. 29–2). The inferior portion of the atrial septum, the superior portion of the ventricular septum, and portions of the septal leaflets of both the tricuspid and mitral valves are formed from the endocardial cushions. The integrity of the atrial septum depends on growth of the septum primum and septum secundum and proper fusion of the endocardial cushions. Atrial septal defects (see p. 896) and varying degrees of endocardial cushion defect (see p. 898) are the result of developmental deficiencies of this process.

THE VENTRICLES. Partitioning of the ventricles occurs as cephalic growth of the main ventricular septum results in its fusion with the endocardial cushions and the infundibular or conus septum. Defects in the ventricular septum may occur owing to a deficiency of septal substance; malalignment of septal components in different planes, preventing their fusion; or an overly long conus, keeping the septal components apart. Isolated defects probably result from the first mechanism, whereas the latter two appear to generate the ventricular defects seen in tetralogy of Fallot (p. 929) and transposition complexes (p. 935).

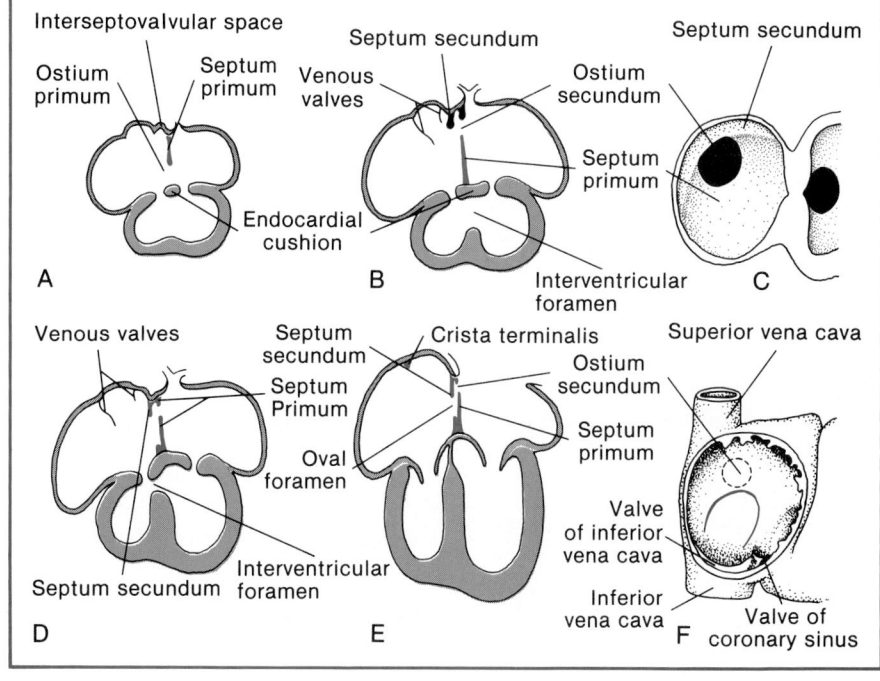

FIGURE 29–1. Diagrammatic representation of the atrial septa at 30 days *(A)*, at 33 days *(B)*, at 33 days (seen from the right side) *(C)*, at 37 days *(D)*, and in the newborn *(E)*; the newborn atrial septum viewed from the right *(F)*. (From Clark, E. B., and Van Mierop, L. H. S.: Development of the cardiovascular system. *In* Moss' Heart Disease in Infants, Children, and Adolescents. Baltimore, © Williams and Wilkins, 1989.)

SYNDROME	MAJOR CARDIOVASCULAR MANIFESTATIONS	MAJOR NONCARDIAC ABNORMALITIES
Heritable and Possibly Heritable		
Ellis–van Creveld	Single atrium or atrial septal defect	Chondrodystrophic dwarfism, nail dysplasia, polydactyly
TAR (thrombocytopenia–absent radius)	Atrial septal defect, tetralogy of Fallot	Radial aplasia or hypoplasia, thrombocytopenia
Holt-Oram	Atrial septal defect (other defects common)	Skeletal upper limb defect, hypoplasia of clavicles
Kartagener	Dextrocardia	Situs inversus, sinusitis, bronchiectasis
Laurence-Moon-Biedl-Bardet	Variable defects	Retinal pigmentation, obesity, polydactyly
Noonan	Pulmonic valve dysplasia, cardiomyopathy (usually hypertrophic)	Webbed neck, pectus excavatum, cryptorchidism
Tuberous sclerosis	Rhabdomyoma, cardiomyopathy	Phakomatosis, bone lesions, hamartomatous skin lesions
Multiple lentigines (LEOPARD)	Pulmonic stenosis	Basal cell nevi, broad facies, rib anomalies, deafness
Rubinstein-Taybi	Patent ductus arteriosus (others)	Broad thumbs and toes, hypoplastic maxilla, slanted palpebral fissures
Familial deafness	Arrhythmias, sudden death	Sensorineural deafness
Weber-Osler-Rendu	Arteriovenous fistulas (lung, liver, mucous membranes)	Multiple telangiectasias
Apert	Ventricular septal defect	Craniosynostosis, midfacial hypoplasia, syndactyly
Crouzon's	Patent ductus arteriosus, aortic coarctation	Ptosis with shallow orbits, craniosynostosis, maxillary hypoplasia
Hypertrophic cardiomyopathy	Asymmetric septal hypertrophy	Family history of sudden death
Incontinentia pigmenti	Patent ductus arteriosus	Irregular pigmented skin lesions, patchy alopecia, hypodontia
Alagille (arteriohepatic dysplasia)	Peripheral pulmonic stenosis, pulmonic stenosis	Biliary hypoplasia, vertebral anomalies, prominent forehead, deep-set eyes
DiGeorge	Interrupted aortic arch, tetralogy of Fallot, truncus arteriosus	Thymic hypoplasia or aplasia, parathyroid aplasia or hypoplasia, ear anomalies
Friedreich's ataxia	Cardiomyopathy and conduction defects	Ataxia, speech defect, degeneration of spinal cord dorsal columns
Muscular dystrophy	Cardiomyopathy	Pseudohypertrophy of calf muscles, weakness of trunk and proximal limb muscles
Cystic fibrosis	Cor pulmonale	Pancreatic insufficiency, malabsorption, chronic lung disease
Sickle cell anemia	Cardiomyopathy, mitral regurgitation	Hemoglobin SS
Conradi-Hünermann	Ventricular septal defect, patent ductus arteriosus	Asymmetrical limb shortness, early punctate mineralization, large skin pores
Cockayne	Accelerated atherosclerosis	Cachectic dwarfism, retinal pigment abnormalities, photosensitivity dermatitis
Progeria	Accelerated atherosclerosis	Premature aging, alopecia, atrophy of subcutaneous fat, skeletal hypoplasia
Connective Tissue Disorders		
Cutis laxa	Peripheral pulmonic stenosis	Generalized disruption of elastic fibers, diminished skin resilience, hernias
Ehlers-Danlos	Arterial dilatation and rupture, mitral regurgitation	Hyperextensible joints, hyperelastic and friable
Marfan	Aortic dilatation, aortic and mitral incompetence	Gracile habitus, arachnodactyly with hyperextensibility, lens subluxation
Osteogenesis imperfecta	Aortic incompetence	Fragile bones, blue sclerae
Pseudoxanthoma elasticum	Peripheral and coronary arterial disease	Degeneration of elastic fibers in skin, retinal angioid streaks
Inborn Errors of Metabolism		
Pompe disease	Glycogen storage disease of heart	Acid maltase deficiency, muscular weakness
Homocystinuria	Aortic and pulmonary artery dilatation, intravascular thrombosis	Cystathionine synthetase deficiency, lens subluxation, osteoporosis

TABLE 29–2   SYNDROMES WITH ASSOCIATED CARDIOVASCULAR INVOLVEMENT—*Continued*

SYNDROME	MAJOR CARDIOVASCULAR MANIFESTATIONS	MAJOR NONCARDIAC ABNORMALITIES
Inborn Errors of Metabolism, *continued*		
Mucopolysaccharidoses: Hurler; Hunter	Multivalvular and coronary and great artery disease; cardiomyopathy	Hurler: Deficiency of α-L-iduronidase, corneal clouding, coarse features, growth and mental retardation Hunter: Deficiency of L-idurano-sulfate sulfatase, coarse facies, clear cornea, growth and mental retardation
Morquio; Scheie; Maroteaux-Lamy	Aortic regurgitation	Morquio: Deficiency of *N*-acetylhexosamine sulfate sulfatase, cloudy cornea, severe bone changes involving vertebrae and epiphyses Scheie: Deficiency of α-L-iduronidase, cloudy cornea, normal intelligence, peculiar facies Maroteaux-Lamy: Deficiency of arylsulfatase B, cloudy cornea, osseous changes
Chromosomal Abnormalities		
Trisomy 21 (Down syndrome)	Endocardial cushion defect, atrial or ventricular septal defect, tetralogy of Fallot	Hypotonia, hyperextensible joints, mongoloid facies, mental retardation
Trisomy 13(D)	Ventricular septal defect, right ventricle patent ductus arteriosus, double-outlet right ventricle	Single midline intracerebral ventricle with midfacial defects, polydactyly, nail changes, mental retardation
Trisomy 18(E)	Congenital polyvalvular dysplasia, ventricular septal defect, patent ductus	Clenched hand, short sternum, low arch dermal ridge pattern on fingertips, mental retardation
Cri du chat (short-arm deletion-5)	Ventricular septal defect	Cat cry, microcephaly, antimongoloid slant of palpebral fissures, mental retardation
XO (Turner)	Coarctation of aorta, bicuspid aortic valve, aortic dilatation	Short female, broad chest, lymphedema, webbed neck
XXXY and XXXXX	Patent ductus arteriosus	XXXY: Hypogenitalism, mental retardation, radial-ulnar synostosis XXXXX: Small hands, incurving of fifth fingers, mental retardation
Sporadic Disorders		
VATER association	Ventricular septal defect	Vertebral anomalies, anal atresia, tracheoesophageal fistula, radial and renal anomalies
CHARGE association	Tetralogy of Fallot (other defects common)	Colobomas, choanal atresia, mental and growth deficiency, genital and ear anomalies
Williams	Supravalvular aortic stenosis, peripheral pulmonic stenosis	Mental deficiency, elfin facies, loquacious personality, hoarse voice
Cornelia de Lange	Ventricular septal defect	Micromelia, synophrys, mental and growth deficiency
Shprintzen (velocardiofacial)	Ventricular septal defect, tetralogy of Fallot, right aortic arch	Cleft palate, prominent nose, slender hands, learning disability
Long Q-T (Jervell and Lange-Nielsen, Romano-Ward)	Long Q-T interval, ventricular arrhythmias	Family history of sudden death, congenital deafness (not in Romano-Ward)
Teratogenic Disorders		
Rubella	Patent ductus arteriosus, pulmonic valvular and/or arterial stenosis, atrial septal defect	Cataracts, deafness, microcephaly
Alcohol	Ventricular septal defect (other defects)	Microcephaly, growth and mental deficiency, short palpebral fissures, smooth philtrum, thin upper lip
Dilantin	Pulmonic stenosis, aortic stenosis, coarctation, patent ductus arteriosus	Hypertelorism, growth and mental deficiency, short phalanges, bowed upper lip
Thalidomide	Variable	Phocomelia
Lithium	Ebstein's anomaly, tricuspid atresia	None

Modified from Friedman, W. F.: Congenital heart disease. *In* Isselbacher, K. I., Braunwald, E. et al. (eds.): Harrison's Principles of Internal Medicine. 13th ed. New York, McGraw-Hill Book Co., 1994, p. 1038. © 1994 The McGraw-Hill Companies, Inc.

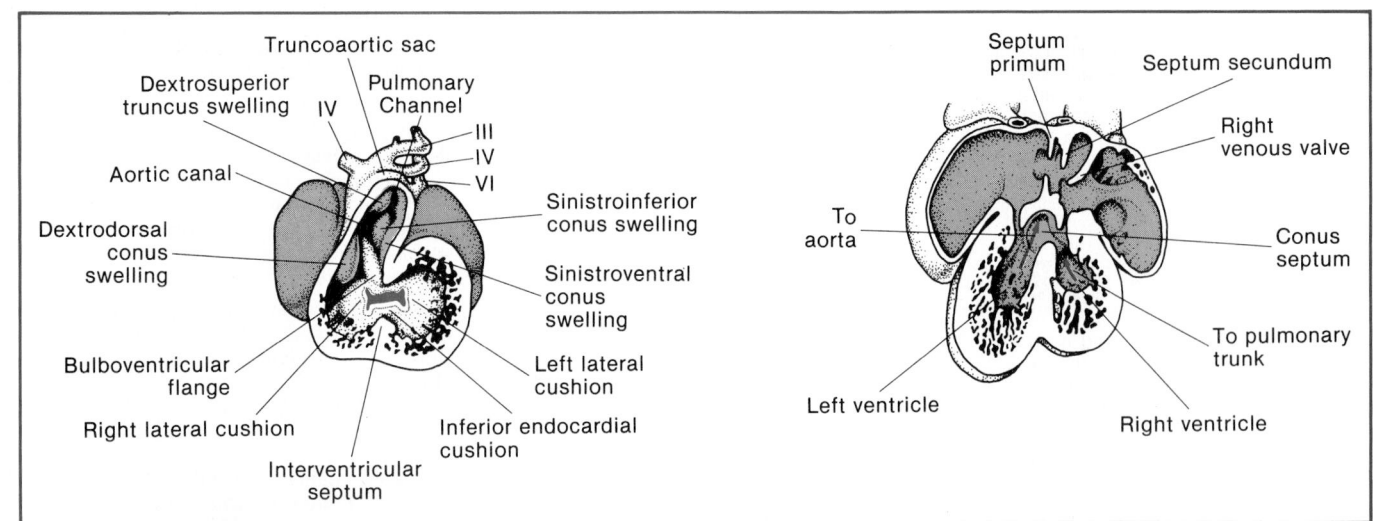

FIGURE 29-2. Frontal section through the heart of a 9-mm embryo (left panel) and 15-mm embryo (right panel). At 9 mm, development is noted of the cushions in the atrioventricular canal, and the truncus and conus swellings are visible. At 15 mm, the conus septum is completed; note the septation in the atrial region. (From Clark, E. B., and Van Mierop, L. H. S.: Development of the cardiovascular system. *In* Moss' Heart Disease in Infants, Children, and Adolescents. Baltimore, © Williams and Wilkins, 1989.)

THE LUNGS. These structures arise from the primitive foregut and are drained early in embryogenesis by channels from the splanchnic plexus to the cardinal and umbilicovitelline veins. An outpouching from the posterior left atrium forms the common pulmonary vein, which communicates with the splanchnic plexus, establishing pulmonary venous drainage to the left atrium. The umbilicovitelline and anterior cardinal vein communications atrophy as the common pulmonary vein is incorporated into the left atrium. Anomalous pulmonary venous connections (see p. 946) to the umbilicovitelline (portal) venous system or to the cardinal system (superior vena cava) result from failure of the common pulmonary vein to develop or establish communications to the splanchnic plexus. Cor triatriatum (see p. 923) results from a narrowing of the common pulmonary vein–left atrial junction.

THE GREAT ARTERIES. The truncus arteriosus is connected to the dorsal aorta in the embryo by six pairs of aortic arches. Partition of the truncus arteriosus into two great arteries is a result of the fusion of tissue arising from the back wall of the vessel and the truncus septum. Rotation of the truncus coils the aorticopulmonary septum and creates the normal spiral relation between aorta and pulmonary artery. Semilunar valves and their related sinuses are created by absorption and hollowing out of tissue at the distal side of the truncus ridges. Aorticopulmonary septal defect (see p. 906) and persistent truncus arteriosus (see p. 907) represent varying degrees of partitioning failure.

Although the six aortic arches appear sequentially, portions of the arch system and dorsal aorta disappear at different times during embryogenesis (Fig. 29-3). The first, second, and fifth sets of paired

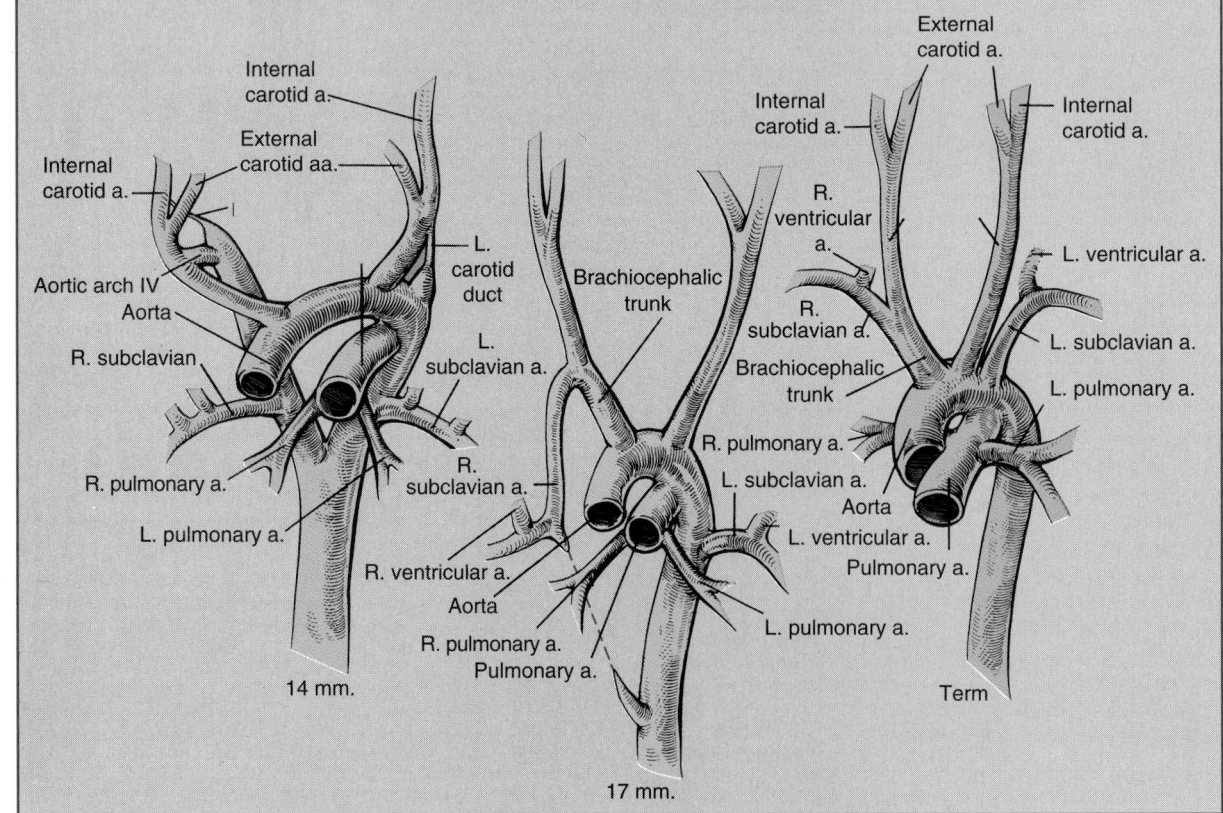

FIGURE 29-3. Transformation of the aortic arches and dorsal aortae into the definitive vascular pattern is a process of fusion and segmental resorption of the paired first to sixth branchial arches with the paired dorsal aortae. (From Castaneda, A., et al.: Cardiac Surgery of the Neonate and Infant. Philadelphia, W.B. Saunders Company, 1994, p. 398.)

arches regress completely. The proximal portions of the sixth arches become the right and left pulmonary arteries and the distal left sixth arch becomes the ductus arteriosus. The third aortic arch forms the connection between internal and external carotid arteries, while the left fourth arch becomes the arterial segment between left carotid and subclavian arteries; the proximal portion of the right subclavian artery forms from the right fourth arch. An abnormality in regression of the arch system in a number of sites can produce a wide variety of arch anomalies, whereas a failure of regression usually results in a double aortic arch malformation.

FETAL AND TRANSITIONAL CIRCULATIONS

Although the illness created by the presence of a cardiac malformation is almost always recognized only after an affected baby is born, important effects on the circulation have existed from early in pregnancy until the time of delivery. Thus knowledge of the changes in cardiocirculatory structure, function, and metabolism that accompany development is central to a systematic comprehension of congenital heart disease.

FETAL CIRCULATORY PATHWAYS. Dynamic alterations occur in the circulation during the transition from fetal to neonatal life when the lungs take over the function of gas exchange from the placenta. The single fetal circulation consists of parallel pulmonary and systemic pathways (Fig. 29-4) in contrast to the two-circuit system in the newborn and adult, in whom the pulmonary vasculature exists in series with the systemic circulation. Prenatal survival is not endangered by major cardiac anomalies as long as one side of the heart can drive blood from the great veins to the aorta; in the fetus, blood can bypass the nonfunctioning lungs both proximal and distal to the heart.

Oxygenated blood returns from the placenta through the umbilical vein and enters the portal venous system. A variable amount of this stream bypasses the hepatic microcirculation and enters the inferior vena cava by way of the ductus venosus. Inferior vena caval blood is composed to flow from the ductus venosus, hepatic vein, and lower body venous drainage, which is summarily deflected to a significant extent across the foramen ovale into the left atrium. Almost all superior vena caval blood passes directly through the tricuspid valve entering the right ventricle. Most of the blood that reaches the right ventricle bypasses the high-resistance, unexpanded lungs and passes through the ductus arteriosus into the descending aorta. The right ventricle contributes about 55 per cent and the left 45 per cent to the total fetal cardiac output. The major portion of blood ejected from the left ventricle supplies the brain and upper body, with lesser flow to the coronary arteries; the balance passes across the aortic isthmus to the descending aorta, where it joins with the large stream from the ductus arteriosus before flowing to the lower body and placenta.

FETAL PULMONARY CIRCULATION. In fetal life, pulmonary arteries and arterioles are surrounded by a fluid medium, have relatively thick walls and small lumina, and resemble comparable arteries in the systemic circulation. The low pulmonary blood flow in the fetus (7 to 10 per cent of the total cardiac output) is the result of high pulmonary vascular resistance. Fetal pulmonary vessels are highly reactive to changes in oxygen tension or in the pH of blood perfusing them as well as to a number of other physiological and pharmacological influences.

EFFECTS OF CARDIAC MALFORMATIONS ON THE FETUS. Although fetal somatic growth may be unimpaired, the hemodynamic effects in utero of many cardiac malformations may alter the development and structure of the fetal heart and circulation.[21] Thus, total anomalous pulmonary venous connection in utero may result in underdevelopment of the left atrium and left ventricle (see p. 944), and premature closure of the foramen ovale may result in hypoplasia of the left ventricle. Moreover, postnatally, the caliber of the aortic isthmus may be reduced (see p. 913) in the presence of lesions in utero that create left ventricular hypertrophy and impede filling because of reduced compliance of that chamber. It may also be reduced in the presence of a lesion that interferes with left ventricular filling directly (e.g., mitral stenosis) or indirectly by diverting a proportion of left ventricular output away from the ascending aorta while increasing right ventricular output and ductus arteriosus flow (e.g., atrioventricular septal defect with left ventricular-right atrial shunt or aortic or subaortic stenosis with ventricular septal defect). Similarly, obstruction in utero to right ventricular outflow is associated with an increase in proximal aortic flow and diameter and almost never with aortic coarctation (see p. 965). In these and other examples it is important to recognize that malformations compatible with fetal survival may nonetheless result in abnormal development of the circulation in utero and also affect circulatory adjustments after birth.

FUNCTION OF THE FETAL HEART. Compared with the adult heart, the fetal and newborn heart is unique with respect to its ultrastructural appearance,[22] its mechanical and biochemical properties,[23-27] and its autonomic innervation.[24,27] During late fetal and early neonatal development there is maturation of the excitation-contraction coupling process[25,26,30,31] and the biochemical composition of the heart's energy-utilizing myofibrillar proteins and of adenosine triphosphate and creatine phosphate energy-producing proteins.[27] Moreover, fetal and neonatal myocardial cells are small in diameter and reduced in density, so that the young heart contains relatively more noncontractile mass (primarily mitochondria, nuclei, and surface membranes) than later in postnatal life. As a result, force generation and the extent and velocity of shortening are decreased, and stiffness and water content of ventricular myocardium are increased in the fetal and early newborn periods.

The diminished function of the young heart is reflected in its limited ability to increase cardiac output in the presence of either a volume load or a lesion that increases resistance to emptying.[32] Although functional integrity exists of efferent and afferent cardiac autonomic pathways early in life, fetal and newborn myocardium lacks the complete development of sympathetic but not cholinergic innervation. Thus, adaptation to cardiocirculatory stress in fetal or early newborn life may be less effective than in adulthood.

CHANGES AT BIRTH. The fundamental change that normally occurs at birth is a division of the single parallel fetal circulation into separate, independent circulations. Inflation of the lungs at the first inspiration produces a marked reduction in pulmonary vascular resistance owing partly to the sudden suspension in air of fetal pulmonary vessels previously supported by fluid media. The reduced extravascular pressure assists new vessels to open and already patent vessels to enlarge. The rapid decrease in pulmonary vascular resistance is related more importantly to vasodilatation owing to the increase in oxygen tension to which pulmonary vessels are exposed rather than to physical expansion of alveoli with gas. Great interest exists currently in defining the role of nitric oxide in the mediation of changes in pulmonary vascular tone in these events.[22,33] Pulmonary arterial pressure falls, and pulmonary blood flow increases greatly. Systemic vascular resistance rises when clamping of the umbilical cord removes the low-resistance placental circulation. Increased pulmonary blood flow increases the return of blood to the left atrium and raises left atrial pressure, which in turn closes the foramen ovale.

The shift in oxygen dependence from the placenta to the lungs produces a sudden increase in arterial blood oxygen tension, which, in concert with alterations in the local prostaglandin milieu, initiates constriction of the ductus arteriosus.[35] Pulmonary pressure falls further as the ductus constricts. In healthy mature infants the ductus

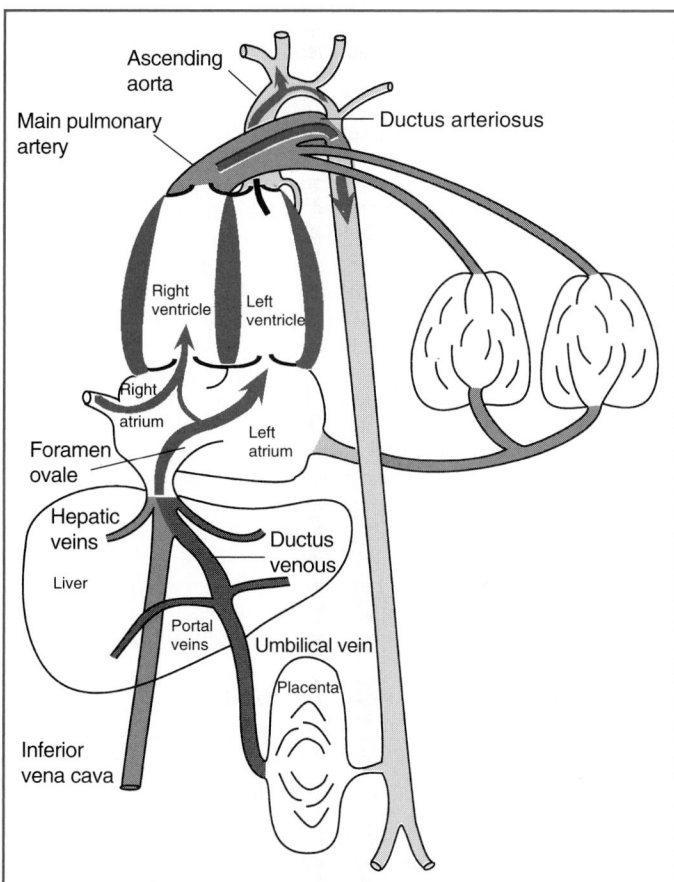

FIGURE 29-4. The fetal circulation with arrows indicating the directions of flow. A fraction of umbilical venous blood enters the ductus venosus and bypasses the liver. This relatively low-oxygenated blood flows across the foramen ovale to the left heart, preferentially perfusing the coronary arteries, head, and upper trunk. The output of the right ventricle flows preferentially across the ductus arteriosus and circulates to the placenta as well as to the abdominal viscera and lower trunk. (Courtesy of David Teitel, M.D.)

Labels in figure: Ascending aorta; Main pulmonary artery; Ductus arteriosus; Right ventricle; Left ventricle; Right atrium; Left atrium; Foramen ovale; Hepatic veins; Liver; Ductus venosus; Portal veins; Umbilical vein; Placenta; Inferior vena cava arteriosus is profoundly constricted at 10 to 15 hours and is closed functionally by 72 hours, with total anatomical closure following within a few weeks by a process of thrombosis, intimal proliferation, and fibrosis. A high incidence exists in preterm infants of persistent patency of the ductus arteriosus because of an immaturity of those mechanisms responsible for constriction (see p. 905). In surviving preterm infants the ductus arteriosus spontaneously closes within 4 to 12 months of birth.

The ductus venosus, ductus arteriosus, and foramen ovale remain potential channels for blood flow after birth. Thus persistent patency of the ductus venosus may mask the most marked signs of pulmonary venous obstruction in infants with total anomalous pulmonary venous connection below the diaphragm (see p. 944). Similarly, lesions producing right or left atrial volume or pressure overload may stretch the foramen ovale and render incompetent the flap valve mechanism for its closure. Anomalies that depend on patency of the ductus arteriosus for preserving pulmonary or systemic blood flow remain latent until the ductus arteriosus constricts. A common example is the rapid intensification of cyanosis observed in the infant with tetralogy of Fallot when the magnitude of pulmonary hypoperfusion is unmasked by spontaneous closure of the ductus arteriosus. Moreover, there is increasing evidence that ductal constriction is a key factor in the postnatal development of coarctation of the aorta (see p. 965). Lastly, it should be recognized that because the ductus arteriosus is potentially patent after birth and the pulmonary resistance vessels are hyperreactive, hypoxic pulmonary vasoconstriction of diverse causes may result in a right-to-left shunt through the ductus.

PATHOLOGICAL CONSEQUENCES OF CONGENITAL CARDIAC LESIONS

CONGESTIVE HEART FAILURE

Although the basic mechanisms of cardiac failure, as outlined in Chapter 13, are similar for all ages, the pediatric cardiologist should clearly recognize that the common causes, time of onset, and often the approach to treatment vary with age.[36-38] The development of fetal echocardiography has allowed the diagnosis of intrauterine cardiac failure.[39-41] The cardinal findings of fetal heart failure are scalp edema, ascites, pericardial effusion, and decreased fetal movements. Although abnormalities in several organ systems may result in nonimmunological fetal hydrops, cardiac causes include a host of structural, functional, rhythm, and metabolic disturbances of the heart. Infants under 1 year of age with cardiac malformations account for 80 to 90 per cent of pediatric patients who develop congestive failure. Moreover, cardiac decompensation in the infant is a medical emergency necessitating immediate treatment if the patient is to be saved.

CAUSES OF HEART FAILURE. In the preterm infant, especially under 1500 gm birthweight, persistent patency of the ductus arteriosus is the most common cause of cardiac decompensation, and other forms of structural heart disease are rare.[42] In the full-term newborn the earliest important causes of heart failure are the hypoplastic left heart and coarctation of the aorta syndromes, sustained tachyarrythmia, cerebral or hepatic arteriovenous fistula, and myocarditis. Among the lesions commonly producing heart failure beyond age 1 to 2 weeks, when diminished pulmonary vascular resistance allows substantial left-to-right shunting, are ventricular septal and atrioventricular septal defects, transposition of the great arteries, truncus arteriosus, and total anomalous pulmonary venous connection, often with pulmonary venous obstruction. Although heart failure usually is the result of a structural defect or of myocardial disease, it should be recognized that the newborn myocardium may be severely depressed by such abnormalities as hypoxemia and acidemia, anemia, septicemia, marked hypoglycemia, hypocalcemia, and polycythemia. In the older child, heart failure often is due to acquired disease (Chap. 31) or is a complication of open-heart surgical procedures. In the acquired category are rheumatic and endomyocardial diseases, infective endocarditis, hematological and nutritional disorders, and severe cardiac arrhythmias.

CLINICAL MANIFESTATIONS IN THE INFANT. The clinical expression of cardiac decompensation in the infant consists of distinctive signs of pulmonary and systemic venous congestion and altered cardiocirculatory performance that resemble, but often are not identical to, those of the older child or adult (Table 29-3).[36,43] These reflect the interplay between the hemodynamic burden and adaptive responses. Common symptoms and signs are feeding difficulties and failure to gain weight and grow, tachypnea, tachycardia, pulmonary rales and rhonchi, liver enlargement, and cardio-megaly. Less frequent manifestations include peripheral edema, ascites, pulsus alternans, gallop rhythm, and inappropriate sweating. Pleural and pericardial effusions are exceedingly rare. The distinction between left and right heart failure is less obvious in the infant than in the older child or adult because most lesions that create a left ventricular pressure or volume overload also result in left-to-right shunting of blood through the foramen ovale and/or patent ductus arteriosus as well as pulmonary hypertension owing to elevated pulmonary venous pressures. Conversely, augmented filling or elevated pressure of the right ventricle in the infant reduces left ventricular compliance disproportionately when compared with the older child or adult and gives rise to signs of both systemic and pulmonary venous congestion.[37]

Fatigue and dyspnea on exertion express themselves as a feeding problem in the infant. Characteristically, the respiratory rate in heart failure is rapid (50 to 100 breaths/min). In the presence of left ventricular failure, interstitial pulmonary edema reduces pulmonary compliance and results in tachypnea and retractions. Excessive pulmonary blood flow by way of significant left-to-right shunts may further decrease lung compliance. Moreover, upper airway obstruction may be produced by selective enlargement of cardiovascular structures. In patients with large left-to-right shunts and left atrial and main pulmonary artery enlargement, the left main stem bronchus may be compressed, resulting in emphysematous expansion of the left upper or lower lobe or left lower lobe collapse.[44] Respiratory distress with grunting, flaring of the alae nasi, and intercostal retractions is observed when failure is severe and especially when pulmonary infection precipitates cardiac decompensation, which often is the case. Under these circumstances pulmonary rales may be due to the infection or failure, or both. A resting heart rate with little variability is also characteristic of heart failure. Hepatomegaly is regularly seen in infants in failure, although liver tenderness is uncommon. Cardiomegaly may be assessed roentgenographically, but it

TABLE 29-3 FEATURES OF HEART FAILURE IN INFANTS

Poor feeding and failure to thrive
Respiratory distress—mainly tachypnea
Rapid heart rate (160 to 180 beats/min)
Pulmonary rales or wheezing
Cardiomegaly and pulmonary edema on radiogram
Hepatomegaly (peripheral edema unusual)
Gallop sounds
Color—ashen pale or faintly cyanotic
Excessive perspiration
Diminished urine output

must be recognized that in the normal newborn infant, the cardiac diameter may be as much as 60 per cent of the thoracic diameter, and the large thymus gland in infants occasionally interferes with evaluation of heart size. Two-dimensional and Doppler echocardiography provide a good estimate of cardiac performance and chamber dimensions, and values may be compared with data derived from normal infants.[45-49]

Cardiac decompensation may progress with extreme rapidity in the first hours and days of life, producing a clinical picture of advanced cardiogenic shock and a profoundly obtunded infant. The presence of marked hepatomegaly and gross cardiomegaly usually allows distinction from noncardiac causes of diminished systemic perfusion.

The management of the infant with congenital heart disease and heart failure is described on p. 889.

CYANOSIS

Cyanosis is produced by reduced hemoglobin in cutaneous vessels in excess of approximately 3 gm/dl (see p. 891). Peripheral cyanosis usually reflects an abnormally great extraction of oxygen from normally saturated arterial blood, commonly the result of peripheral cutaneous vasoconstriction. Central cyanosis is a result of arterial blood oxygen unsaturation, most often in patients with congenital heart disease caused by shunting of systemic venous blood into the arterial circuit. Infants especially (as compared with adults) may appear cyanotic when in heart failure because of both peripheral and central factors[50]; the latter may include severe impairment of pulmonary function that commonly exists with alveolar hypoventilation, ventilation-perfusion inequality, or impaired oxygen diffusion.

In patients with central cyanosis owing to arterial oxygen unsaturation, the degree of cutaneous discoloration depends on the absolute amount of reduced hemoglobin, the magnitude of the right-to-left shunt relative to systemic flow, and the oxyhemoglobin saturation of venous blood. The last of these depends in turn on the tissue extraction of oxygen. Commonly, cyanosis appears or intensifies with physical activity or exercise as the saturation of systemic venous blood declines concurrent with an increase in right-to-left shunting across a defect as peripheral vascular resistance decreases. Oxygen transfer to the tissues is affected by shifts in the oxygen hemoglobin dissociation relation, which may be altered by blood pH and levels of red blood cell 2,3-diphosphoglycerate concentration.

The clinical approach to the infant with cyanosis is discussed on pp. 890 to 894.

CLUBBING AND POLYCYTHEMIA/ERYTHROCYTOSIS. Prominent accompaniments of arterial hypoxemia are polycythemia and clubbing of the digits. The latter is associated with an increased number of capillaries with increased blood flow through extensive arteriovenous aneurysms and an increase of connective tissue in the terminal phalanges of the fingers and toes. Polycythemia is a physiological response to chronic hypoxemia that stimulates erythrocytosis. The extremely high hematocrits observed in patients with arterial oxygen unsaturation cause a progressive increase in blood viscosity. Because the relationship is nonlinear between hematocrit and blood viscosity, relatively small increases beyond packed blood cell volumes of 60 per cent result in large increases in viscosity. Also, the apparent viscosity of blood increases in the microcirculation where lower shear rates exist, an increasingly important factor as the hematocrit exceeds 70 per cent.

Both the hematocrit and the circulating whole blood volume are increased in polycythemia accompanying cyanotic congenital heart disease; the hypervolemia is the result of an increase in red cell volume. The augmented red blood cell volume provoked by hypoxemia provides an increased oxygen-carrying capacity and enhanced oxygen supply to the tissues. The compensatory polycythemia often is of such severity that it becomes a liability and produces such adverse physiological effects as hyperviscosity, cellular aggregation, and thrombotic lesions in diverse organs and a hemorrhagic diathesis.[51] In this regard, oral steroid contraceptives are contraindicated in the adolescent cyanotic female because of the enhanced risk of cerebral thrombosis.

Management. Red cell volume reduction and replacement with plasma or albumin (erythrophoresis) lower blood viscosity and increase systemic blood flow and systemic oxygen transport, and thus may be helpful in the management of patients with severe hypoxic polycythemia (hematocrit $\geq$ 65 per cent). A final hematocrit of 55 to 63 per cent should be achieved; the higher level is necessary in patients with low initial oxygen saturation to avoid a severe reduction in arterial oxygen content. Acute phlebotomy without fluid replacement is contraindicated.

CEREBRAL AND PULMONARY COMPLICATIONS. Cerebrovascular accidents and brain abscesses occur particularly in cyanotic patients with substantial arterial desaturation.[52,53] *Cerebral thrombosis* is most common under age 2 years in severely cyanotic children, even in the presence of relatively low hematocrits, and occurs especially in a clinical setting in which oxygen requirements are raised by fever or, if blood viscosity is increased, dehydration.

Brain Abscess. This is an important complication of cyanotic heart disease.[53] Such abscesses are rare under 18 months of age and commonly are of insidious onset marked by headache, low-grade fever, vomiting, and a change in personality. Seizures or paralysis less frequently herald the onset of a brain abscess. Abscess must be suspected in any cyanotic child with focal neurological signs. Morbidity and mortality are related inversely to oxygen saturation levels. Brain abscess is thought to occur in about 2 per cent of the population with cyanotic congenital heart disease; a mortality rate of 30 to 40 per cent often is related to delay in diagnosis and treatment.

Paradoxical Embolus. This is a rare complication of cyanotic heart disease, usually observed only at necropsy.[54] Emboli arising in systemic veins may pass directly to the systemic circulation, because right-to-left intracardiac shunts allow venous blood to bypass the normal filtering action of the lungs.

Retinopathy. Dilated tortuous vessels progressing to papilledema, and retinal edema occasionally are observed in cyanotic patients, and appear to be related to decreased arterial oxygen saturation and/or to erythrocytosis but not to hypercapnia.

Hemoptysis. This is an uncommon but major complication in cyanotic patients with congenital heart disease, and occurs most often in the presence of pulmonary vascular obstructive disease or in patients with an extensive bronchial collateral circulation or pulmonary venous congestion.[55] Massive hemoptysis almost always represents rupture of a dilated bronchial artery.

SQUATTING. After exertion, patients with cyanotic heart disease, especially tetralogy of Fallot, typical assume a squatting posture to obtain relief from breathlessness.[56] Squatting appears to improve arterial oxygen saturation by increasing systemic vascular resistance, thereby diminishing the right-to-left shunt, and also by the pooling of markedly desaturated blood in the lower extremities. In addition, systemic venous return, and therefore pulmonary blood flow, may increase.

HYPOXIC SPELLS. Hypercyanotic or hypoxemic spells commonly complicate the clinical course in younger children with certain types of cyanotic heart disease, especially tetralogy of Fallot (see p. 929).[56] The spells are characterized by anxiety, hyperpnea, and a sudden marked increase in cyanosis; they are the result of an abrupt reduction in pulmonary blood flow. Unless terminated, the hypercyanotic episodes may lead to convulsions and may even be fatal. The sudden reduction in pulmonary blood flow may be precipitated by fluctuations in arterial pCO_2 and pH, a sudden fall in systemic or increase in pulmonary vascular resistance, or an acute increase in the severity of right ventricular outflow tract obstruction either by augmented contraction of the hypertrophied muscle in the right ventricular outflow tract or by a decrease in right ventricular cavity volume owing to tachycardia.

Treatment. This consists of oxygen administration, placing the child in the knee-chest position, and administration of morphine sulfate. Additional medications that may prove of value include the intravenous administration of sodium bicarbonate to correct the accompanying acidemia, alpha-adrenoceptor stimulants such as phenylephrine hydrochloride (Neo-Synephrine) or methoxamine to raise peripheral resistance and diminish right-to-left shunting, and beta-adrenoceptor blocking agents, which reduce cardiac sympathetic tone and depress cardiac contractility directly and increase ventricular volume by reducing heart rate.

ACID-BASE IMBALANCE

Disturbances in blood gas and acid-base equilibrium are noted particularly in infants with either congestive heart failure or cyanosis.[57] Large-volume left-to-right shunts, especially with pulmonary edema, may be associated with moderate respiratory acidemia and a lowering of arterial oxygen tensions, reflecting an increase in the alveolar-arterial oxygen tension gradient and ventilation-perfusion imbalance. Interference with carbon dioxide transport implies moderate to severe failure in these infants. Lesions associated with a reduced systemic cardiac output, such as severe coarctation of the aorta or critical aortic stenosis in infancy, often present as cardiac failure complicated by a severe metabolic acidemia and relatively high values of arterial oxygen tension. The latter finding, even in the presence of right-to-left shunting across a patent ductus arteriosus, is a result of diminished systemic perfusion and an elevated pulmonary-systemic blood flow ratio.

Respiratory acidemia and depressed levels of oxygen tension are observed in infants with obstruction to pulmonary venous return and right-to-left atrial shunting. Many infants with severe hypoxemia caused by lesions such as transposition of the great arteries or pulmonic atresia show metabolic acidemia and marked reductions in carbon dioxide tension secondary to hyperventilation, resulting from hypoxic stimulation of peripheral chemoreceptors.

IMPAIRED GROWTH

Impaired growth and physical development and delayed onset of adolescence are common features of many cyanotic and, to a lesser extent, acyanotic forms of congenital heart disease.[58-60] Mental development seldom is affected. The severity of growth disturbance depends on the anatomical lesion and its functional effect. Most children with mild defects grow normally. Weight gain is commonly slower than linear growth in acyanotic patients with large left-to-right shunts, whereas in cyanotic congenital heart disease, height and weight usually parallel each other. Boys appear to be more retarded in growth than girls, especially in the second decade. Skeletal maturity (i.e., bone age) is delayed in cyanotic children in relation to the severity of hypoxemia.

In some children, prenatal factors such as intrauterine infection and chromosomal and other hereditary and nonhereditary syndromes are responsible for growth retardation. In other patients, extracardiac malformations may contribute to poor weight gain and linear growth. Additional explanations for the mechanisms of growth interference have implicated malnutrition as a result of anorexia and inadequate nutrient and caloric intake, hypermetabolic state, acidemia and cation imbalance, tissue hypoxia, diminished peripheral blood flow, chronic cardiac decompensation, malabsorption or protein loss, recurrent respiratory infections, and endocrine or genetic factors. In some instances, the underdevelopment is influenced little by operative correction of the underlying cardiac anomaly.

Among factors that may be responsible for persistent growth retardation postoperatively are age at operation, hemodynamically significant residual lesions, and sequelae or complications of operation. As a general rule, it is unwise preoperatively to guarantee to the parents of a child with heart disease that surgery will result in accelerated growth and development.

PULMONARY HYPERTENSION

(See also Chap. 25)

Pulmonary hypertension is a common accompaniment of many congenital cardiac lesions, and the status of the pulmonary vascular bed often is the principal determinant of the clinical manifestations, the course, and whether surgical treatment is feasible.[61] Increases in pulmonary arterial pressure result from elevations of pulmonary blood flow and/or resistance, the latter sometimes caused by an increase in vascular tone, but usually the result of underdevelopment and/or obstructive, obliterative structural changes within the pulmonary vascular bed.[62-64]

Pulmonary vascular resistance normally falls rapidly immediately after birth, owing to onset of ventilation and subsequent release of hypoxic pulmonary vasoconstriction. Subsequently the medial smooth muscle of pulmonary arterial resistance vessels thins gradually.[65] This latter process often is delayed by several months in infants with large aorticopulmonary or ventricular communications, at which time levels of pulmonary vascular resistance are still somewhat elevated. In patients with high pulmonary arterial pressure from birth, failure of normal growth of the pulmonary circulation may occur, and anatomical changes in the pulmonary vessels in the form of proliferation of intimal cells and intimal and medial thickening often progress, so that in the older child or adult vascular resistance ultimately may become fixed by obliterative changes in the pulmonary vascular bed. The causes of pulmonary vascular obstructive disease remain unknown, although increased pulmonary arterial blood pressure, elevated pulmonary venous pressure, polycythemia, systemic hypoxia, acidemia, and the nature of the bronchial circulation have all been implicated. Quite likely, injury to pulmonary vascular endothelial cells initiates a cascade of events that involve the release or activation of factors that alter the extracellular matrix, induce hypertrophy, cause proliferation of vascular smooth muscle cells, and promote connective tissue protein synthesis. Taken together these may permanently alter vessel structure and function.[66,67]

There are many patients with pulmonary vascular obstruction whose cardiac anomaly places them at particular risk quite early in life, precluding survival to adulthood. Patients at particularly high risk for the development of significant pulmonary vascular obstruction are those with certain forms of cyanotic congenital heart disease, such as complete transposition of the great arteries with or without ventricular septal defect or patent ductus arteriosus, single ventricle without pulmonary stenosis, double-outlet right ventricle, and truncus arteriosus. Other conditions in which pulmonary vascular obstruction appears to progress rapidly include large ventricular septal defect, as well as the less common conditions of unilateral pulmonary artery absence, congenital left-to-right shunts in an environment of high altitude or in association with the Down syndrome of trisomy 21, and complete atrioventricular canal defects, even those unassociated with a chromosomal anomaly.

MECHANISMS OF DEVELOPMENT. Intimal damage appears to be related to shear stresses because endothelial cell damage occurs at high-flow shear rates. A reduction in pulmonary arteriolar lumen size due to either thickened medial muscle or vasoconstriction increases the velocity of flow. Shear stress also increases as blood viscosity rises; therefore, infants with hypoxemia and high hematocrits as well as increased pulmonary blood flow are at increased risk of developing pulmonary vascular disease. In patients with left-to-right shunts, pulmonary arterial hypertension, if not present in infancy or childhood, may never occur or may not develop until the third or fourth decade or later. Once developed, intimal proliferative changes with hyalinization and fibrosis are not reversible by repair of the underlying cardiac defect. In severe pulmonary vascular obstructive disease, arteriovenous malformations may develop and predispose to massive hemoptysis.

Most vexing is the variability among patients with the same or similar cardiac lesions in both the time of appearance and rate of progression of their pulmonary vascular obstructive process. Although genetic influences may be operative (an example is the apparent acceleration of pulmonary vascular disease in patients with congenital heart disease and trisomy 21), evidence is now accumulating for important prenatal and postnatal modifiers of the pulmonary vascular bed that appear, at least in part, to be lesion-dependent. Thus a quantitative variability exists in the pulmonary vascular bed related to the *number*, not just the size and wall structure, of arterial vessels within the pulmonary circulation.[68,69]

Modeling of the blood vessels occurs proximal to and within terminal bronchioles (preacinar and intraacinar vessels, respectively) continuously from before birth. The intraacinar vessels, in particular, increase in size and number from late fetal life throughout childhood with minimal muscularization of their walls. The ensuing increase in the cross-sectional area of the pulmonary arterial circulation allows the cardiac output to rise substantially without an increase in pulmonary arterial pressure. If, however, the presence of a cardiac lesion interferes with the normal growth and multiplication of these most peripheral arteries, the resulting elevation of pulmonary vascular resistance may first be related to failure of the intraacinar pulmonary circulation to develop fully, and then secondarily to the morphological changes of obliterative vascular disease—medial thickening, intimal proliferation, hyalinization and fibrosis, angiomatoid and plexiform lesions, and ultimately, arterial necrosis.[64,70]

In essence, the morphometric framework adds an important dimension, that of growth and development of the pulmonary circulation, to the traditional view of pulmonary vascular obstructive disease occurring primarily as a result of anatomical changes in the individual pulmonary arterioles. Research attention currently focuses on the cellular and molecular biology of the vessel wall and abnormalities in endothelial cell–smooth muscle interactions in pulmonary hypertension.[62,66,67,69,70]

ASSESSMENT OF THE PATIENT WITH PULMONARY HYPERTENSION. It is important to understand the difficulties that exist with standard methods of assessing the severity of pulmonary vascular obstructive disease. Clinical and electrocardiographic observations do not distinguish between reversible and irreversible elevations in pulmonary vascular resistance. Echocardiography and Doppler interrogation of the heart may enable one to diagnose the presence of pulmonary hypertension but do not provide an accurate estimate of pressure or a reliable calculation of pulmonary vascular resistance.[71] Thus, hemodynamic measurements at cardiac catheterization are the mainstay in assessing the pulmonary vascular bed, especially its reactivity. The premium on accuracy is high because the presence, degree, and reactivity of pulmonary vascular obstruction determine the feasibility and long-term outcome of operation. Surgery must not be offered to patients with severe, fixed pulmonary vascular obstruction, even when the cardiac defect is anatomically correctable. Such patients either do not survive operation or, if they do, are not benefited and more often than not are harmed.

The aims of hemodynamic study are to quantify and compare the pulmonary and systemic flows and resistances and to determine the reactivity of the pulmonary vascular bed in patients with pulmonary hypertension. Because resistance to pulmonary blood flow cannot be measured directly, it is calculated from the ratio of pressure gradient to flow across the pulmonary bed according to Poiseuille's equation, which refers to steady flow of a newtonian fluid through straight, rigid tubes. There are potential errors in applying the equation and errors inherent in the methods of measurement. Furthermore, it is not possible in every patient to catheterize the pulmonary artery; when this is the case pulmonary venous wedge pressures may be used, but they are not always reliable indicators of pulmonary artery pressure, and the moment of hemodynamic evaluation may not be representative of potentially variable states of the pulmonary circulation. Nonetheless, a practical index of pulmonary vascular resistance can be established from measurements of pulmonary and systemic arterial pressures and calculated flows. One can then determine whether administration of drugs or oxygen or nitric oxide reduces the pulmonary vascular resistance, implying that the resistance is not fixed and therefore may decrease or at least not progress after successful operation.[72] A reduction in calculated pulmonary vascular resistance in response to oxygen or nitric oxide inhalation or pharmacological invention does not exclude coexisting anatomical pulmonary vascular disease but does imply a component of potentially reversible vasoconstriction contributing to the high resistance.

Other Diagnostic Methods. Because of the aforementioned shortcomings, additional methods have been developed to study the morphology of the small pulmonary arteries in patients with pulmonary hypertension. An example is the use of high-resolution magnification for *pulmonary wedge angiography* to determine the presence and extent of obstructive pulmonary vascular changes.[73] Pulmonary wedge angiograms, assessed quantitatively, appear to correlate well with both hemodynamic findings and histological observations of the structural state of the pulmonary vascular bed. Of additional interest is the current practical application of morphometric structural analyses that attempt to identify for operation patients whose postoperative pulmonary hemodynamics might be expected to improve, if not normalize.[74] Thus, *lung biopsy* at surgery has been proposed in patients with equivocal hemodynamic data to aid in determining whether to proceed with operation in reasonable anticipation of postoperative regression of elevated pulmonary vascular resistance.

THE MORPHOMETRIC APPROACH. Decisions on optimal timing of operations often are difficult because of the varying rates of development of pulmonary vascular disease in different patients with the same anomaly and because the evaluation of pulmonary vascular resistance and reactivity in the catheterization laboratory is a less than perfect science. Preoperative lung biopsy using the Heath-Edwards criteria has enjoyed little popularity, especially because sampling errors may result from the scatter of different grades of lesion in different parts of the lung. Accordingly, it is attractive to seek an alternative method that would obviate these problems. In this regard, application of a morphometric approach holds promise because the described changes in pulmonary vessel morphological characteristics are more uniformly distributed throughout the lung and, importantly, lend themselves to quantification.

Three abnormalities have been identified as anatomical markers of elevated pulmonary vascular resistance: (1) an excessive and premature extension of vascular smooth muscle into intraacinar pulmonary arteries, (2) failure of preacinar arterial wall thickness to regress normally, and (3) failure of pulmonary arteries to grow and proliferate normally during postnatal development. Frozen-section lung biopsy provides a firmer basis for judgment of whether reparative or palliative operation should proceed. The technique has proved useful in patients with univentricular hearts or tricuspid atresia in determining the feasibility of a Fontan procedure (see p. 933) and in patients with lesions known to

exhibit early and rapidly progressive pulmonary vascular disease, such as complete transposition of the great arteries, complete atrioventricular canal defect, and nonrestrictive ventricular septal defect.[75]

CLINICAL MANIFESTATIONS OF PULMONARY HYPERTENSION. When this condition is associated with a large left-to-right shunt, the clinical manifestations reflect the specific malformation responsible. When pulmonary vascular resistance is elevated and a significant right-to-left shunt exists, the patient is cyanotic, and polycythemia and clubbing are noted. A dominant *a* wave in the jugular venous pulse may be seen, reflecting vigorous right atrial contraction caused by diminished compliance of the right ventricle. In some instances there are large systolic *c-v* waves, which suggest tricuspid regurgitation. A prominent right ventricular parasternal lift and palpable systolic expansion of the pulmonary artery are present. A soft pulmonary systolic ejection murmur preceded by an ejection sound and followed by a markedly accentuated pulmonic component of the second heart sound often is audible on auscultation; an early diastolic decrescendo blowing murmur of pulmonary regurgitation may be heard. If right ventricular failure and dilatation supervene, the systolic murmur of tricuspid regurgitation may be audible at the lower left sternal border. Right ventricular enlargement may be evident on the chest roentgenogram and electrocardiogram. The former examination also reveals a conspicuously enlarged pulmonary artery, prominent hilar pulmonary vascular markings, and attenuated peripheral vessels. The presence of pulmonary hypertension is suggested by analysis of Doppler waveforms of right and left ventricular ejection.[76,77] The site of the underlying defect may be localized by means of two-dimensional and Doppler echocardiography and/or cardiac catheterization and angiocardiography. Pressures in the right side of the heart are essentially identical to systemic pressures in cyanotic patients if the shunt is at the ventricular or aorticopulmonary levels, but they usually are lower than systemic pressures in patients with an intraatrial shunt. No specific treatment has proved beneficial for obstructive pulmonary vascular disease.

This fact underscores the importance of efforts to define the optimal age at operation to provide the highest probability of postoperative normalization of the pulmonary vascular bed. It is important to emphasize that almost all congenital cardiovascular defects are amenable to surgical repair in infancy, and it is likely that the surgical art will progress to the point that virtually all patients with lesions associated with pulmonary hypertension will be operated on within the first 3 to 18 months of life. When this goal is reached without increased operative mortality, the incidence of postoperative pulmonary vascular obstruction may well achieve the status of a bygone concern.

OTHER CONSEQUENCES OF CONGENITAL HEART DISEASE

INFECTIVE ENDOCARDITIS (see also Chap. 33). Infective endocarditis is uncommon under age 2 years and thereafter most often affects children with tetralogy of Fallot (especially after systemic-pulmonary anastomosis), ventricular septal defect, aortic stenosis, and patent ductus arteriosus. Postsurgical patients with prosthetic heterograft or homograft valves or conduits are at particular risk. Infants and children with normal cardiac anatomy are at increased risk now that the use of central venous catheters is routine, and drug addiction in adolescents is an emerging risk factor.[78,79]

A causative organism can be isolated in about 90 per cent of children, usually either alpha-streptococci (usually *Streptococcus viridans*) or *Staphylococcus aureus*, although uncommon organisms may also be identified.[78,80,81] Fungal endocarditis is quite rare in the pediatric age group. Mortality appears to be highest when coagulase-positive *Staphylococcus* is the offending organism and when the endocarditis involves the left, rather than the right, side of the heart. Most recent data suggest 75 to 80 per cent overall survival.[80] Factors predisposing to endocarditis may be identified in about one-third of cases. These include cardiovascular surgery with infection during the perioperative period, respiratory tract infections, and ear, nose, throat, and dental procedures. Less often, contamination during a surgical procedure or cardiac catheterization or an infection involving the skin, genitourinary tract, or other organ system has been the cause.

Although routine antimicrobial prophylaxis is recommended for all children with congenital heart disease and for the majority of patients after operative repair of the lesion,[82] it should be recognized that many different microbes are responsible for the disease and that an effective preventive approach ultimately may center on active immunization rather than antibiotics. Antibiotic prophylaxis currently is recommended for all dental procedures known to induce gingival or mucosal bleeding, including cleaning, oral trauma, and other procedures such as tonsillectomy, gastrointestinal surgery, genitourinary surgery, and incision and drainage of infected tissue (Table 29–4). The risk of endocarditis is undoubtedly related both to the magnitude of bacteremia and to the type of underlying heart disease. Because infection on a prosthetic heart valve or conduit may be devastating, combinations of antibiotics given parenterally are advisable in these patients.

CHEST PAIN (see also pages 3 and 1291). *Angina pectoris* is an uncommon symptom of cardiac disease in infants and children, occurring in association with anomalous pulmonary origin of a coronary artery or, occasionally, in association with severe aortic stenosis, pulmonic stenosis, or pulmonary hypertension owing to pulmonary vascular obstruction. Cardiac pain in the infant with anomalous coronary artery (see p. 909) usually takes the form of irritability and crying during feeding or straining at bowel movement. In children with severe or right ventricular outflow tract obstruction, chest pain commonly follows effort and is identical to angina observed in adults. Cardiac pain associated with *pulmonary vascular obstruction* may be anginal in nature but often is evanescent and pleuritic in type. Atypical forms of chest pain associated with the syndrome of *mitral valve prolapse* are much less usual in children than in adults. A sensation of chest discomfort or cardiac awareness frequently is interpreted as pain by the parents of children with cardiac arrhythmias. Careful questioning serves to identify palpitations rather than pain as the symptom and often elicits an additional history of anxiety, pallor, and sweating. Pain caused by *pericarditis* is commonly of acute onset and associated with fever, and can be identified by specific physical, roentgenographic, and echocardiographic findings.

Most commonly, chest pain in children is *musculoskeletal* in origin and may be reproduced on upper-extremity movement or by palpation; chest wall pain often is the result of *costochondritis*.[83] Finally, children, like adults, may suffer chest pain of nonspecific form owing to *anxiety*, with or without hyperventilation; a history often is elicited of a family member or friend who had recently died from or suffered myocardial infarction.

SYNCOPE (see also Chap. 28). Syncope is an unusual feature of heart disease in children; its presence suggests specific diagnoses, the most common being an arrhythmia. The symptom is observed in patients with long QT syndrome and in children with complete atrioventricular block that is less often of congenital origin than a sequela of cardiac operation. Syncope caused by abrupt episodes of either bradycardia or tachycardia occurs in association with the sick sinus syndrome. The latter is most commonly produced in children after surgical procedures that involve the region of the sinoatrial node, e.g., atrial septal defect closure or Mustard's venous switch procedure for transposition of the great arteries (see p. 835). Syncope is an occasional but ominous symptom if associated with severe aortic stenosis, pulmonary vascular obstruction, or a left atrial myxoma that transiently occludes left ventricular inflow.[84]

In children with an anatomically normal heart, transient episodes of vasovagally mediated hypotension and bradycardia (neurocardiogenic syncope) may be diagnosed by autonomic function testing and head-upright tilt table testing (see p. 584). The latter is especially helpful in assessing the adequacy of prophylactic therapy, usually by volume expansion (e.g., salt and fludrocortisone), or by beta-adrenergic blockade or alpha-adrenergic agonist or serotonin reuptake inhibitor therapy.[85–87]

SUDDEN DEATH (see also Chap. 24). The sudden infant death syndrome is not likely due to a cardiac cause but rather to pulmonary and/or central nervous system causes. In contrast to adults, children seldom die suddenly and unexpectedly from cardiovascular disease. Arrhythmias, hypoxemia, and coronary insufficiency secondary to left ventricular outflow tract obstruction are the most frequent causes of death.[88–91] Sudden death most often is reported in patients with postoperative heart disease or dilated cardiomyopathy. It is also observed in patients with aortic stenosis or hypertrophic obstructive cardiomyopathy, primary pulmonary hypertension, the Eisenmenger syndrome of pulmonary vascular obstruction, myocarditis, congenital complete heart block, primary endocardial fibroelastosis, anomalies of the coronary arteries, and cyanotic congenital heart disease with pulmonic stenosis or atresia. A relation exists between strenuous exercise and sudden death in patients with aortic stenosis or obstructive cardiomyopathy, thus providing justification for restricting patients with these lesions from gymnastic activities and strenuous competitive sports.

TABLE 29–4 PROPHYLACTIC ANTIBIOTICS FOR PROTECTION FROM BACTERIAL ENDOCARDITIS

I. STANDARD PROPHYLACTIC REGIMEN FOR DENTAL/ORAL/UPPER RESPIRATORY TRACT PROCEDURES
Amoxicillin 3.0 gm orally 1 hour before procedure, then 1.5 gm 6 hours after initial dose.
For amoxicillin/penicillin-allergic individuals:
  Erythromycin ethylsuccinate 800 mg or erythromycin stearate 1 gm orally 2 hours before a procedure, then one-half the dose 6 hours after the initial administration.

-OR-

  Clindamycin 300 mg 1 hour before a procedure, and 150 mg 6 hours after initial dose.

II. ALTERNATIVE PROPHYLACTIC REGIMENS FOR DENTAL/ORAL/UPPER RESPIRATORY TRACT PROCEDURES
For patients unable to take oral medications:
  Ampicillin 2.0 gm IV (or IM) 30 minutes before procedure, then 1.0 gm ampicillin IV (or IM) or 1.5 gm amoxicillin orally 6 hours after initial dose.
For ampicillin/amoxicillin/penicillin-allergic patients unable to take oral medications:
  Clindamycin 300 mg IV 1 hour before a procedure and 150 mg IV (or orally) 6 hours after initial dose.
Optional regimen for individuals considered to be at very high risk who are not candidates for the standard regimen:
  Ampicillin 2.0 gm IV (or IM) plus gentamicin 1.5 mg/kg IV (or IM) (not to exceed 80 mg) one-half hour before procedure, followed by 1.5 gm oral amoxicillin 6 hours after the initial dose. Alternatively, the parenteral regimen may be repeated 8 hours after the initial dose.
Optional regimen for amoxicillin/ampicillin/penicillin-allergic patients:
  Vancomycin 1.0 gm IV administered over 1 hour, starting 1 hour before the procedure. No repeat dose is necessary.

III. REGIMENS FOR GENITOURINARY/GASTROINTESTINAL PROCEDURES
Standard regimen:
  Ampicillin 2.0 gm IV (or IM) plus gentamicin 1.5 mg/kg IV (or IM) (not to exceed 80 mg) one-half hour before procedure, followed by 1.5 gm oral amoxicillin 6 hours after the initial dose. Alternatively, the parenteral regimen may be repeated once 8 hours after the initial dose.
For amoxicillin/ampicillin/penicillin-allergic patients:
  Vancomycin 1.0 gm IV administered over 1 hour plus gentamicin 1.5 mg/kg IV (or IM) (not to exceed 80 mg) 1 hour before the procedure. May be repeated once 8 hours after initial dose.
Alternative oral regimen in low-risk patients:
  Amoxicillin 3.0 gm orally 1 hour before the procedure, then 1.5 gm 6 hours after the initial dose.
Note: Initial pediatric dosages are listed below. Follow-up doses should be one-half the initial dose. Total pediatric dose should not exceed total adult dose.

Amoxicillin: 50 mg/kg
Ampicillin: 50 mg/kg
Clindamycin: 10 mg/kg
Gentamicin: 2.0 mg/kg
Vancomycin: 20 mg/kg
Erythromycin
ethylsuccinate or stearate: 20 mg/kg

Adapted from Dajani, A. S., et al.: Prevention of bacterial endocarditis. Recommendations by the American Heart Association. JAMA *264*:2919, 1990. Copyright 1990 American Medical Association.

Without prompt recognition, accurate diagnosis, and treatment, about one-third of all infants born with congenital heart disease die in the first months of life. Heart failure and cyanosis are the two cardinal signs in the high-risk infant with heart disease, and this section provides an approach for the management of each.

HEART FAILURE

The causes and clinical manifestations of heart failure in the infant with congenital heart disease are discussed on p. 884. Care of the infant with heart failure must include careful consideration of the underlying structural or functional disturbance. The general aims of treatment are to achieve an increase in cardiac performance, augment peripheral perfusion, and decrease pulmonary and systemic venous congestion.[36,37] It must be emphasized, however, that under many conditions medical management cannot control the effects of the abnormal loads imposed by a host of congenital cardiac lesions. Under these circumstances cardiac diagnosis and interventional catheter or operative intervention may be urgently required.[28,68] Thus initial therapy is aimed at stabilizing the infant's condition for diagnostic ultrasonography or hemodynamic or angiocardiographic study as soon as possible. In almost all situations the decision to intervene surgically or to continue medical management requires a definitive anatomical diagnosis.

RESERVE MECHANISMS IN THE NEONATAL HEART

Pediatricians in particular should be aware of the important concept of cardiac reserve because it is in this regard that important differences exist between the young heart (of the preterm or newborn infant) and the fully developed heart of the older child, adolescent, and adult (Fig. 29-5).

Clinicians have long recognized the unique fragility and lability of the neonatal circulation in response to disease states and various physiological stimuli. Moreover, it often is apparent that newborns may exhibit suboptimal therapeutic responses to drugs such as digitalis, which directly stimulate cardiac contractility. The age dependency of these observations have their basis in the reduced ability of the hearts of premature and full-term newborns, when compared with the hearts and circulation of older children or adults, to call on a functional reserve capacity to adapt to stress.[36,92,93]

Studies from the author's and other laboratories have shown that structural, functional, biochemical, and pharmacological properties of the young heart differ considerably from those of its older counterpart.[22-32] The young heart contains fewer myofilaments to generate force with and to shorten during contraction. In addition, the chamber stiffness of the young heart's ventricles is greater than that seen later in life.

PRELOAD RESERVE. Any increase in ventricular filling or volume in the small, young heart results in a disproportionately greater rise in ventricular wall tension or stress. Similarly, it takes a smaller increase in ventricular filling to reach the limits of assistance given to cardiac pump and muscle function by stretching the myofilaments; that is, *preload or diastolic reserve is limited.*

The young heart generates relatively less force; it cannot generate the same ventricular systolic pressure or wall tensions, or obtain the same stroke volume augmentation from any initial stretch, as can the older heart. With these facts in mind, it must be remembered that the oxygen consumption of the normal newborn is considerably higher than later in life; accordingly, the newborn at rest has a much higher cardiac output/m² than the child or adult. Thus, even in the absence of stress, the young heart must function near peak performance just to satisfy the normal demands of the peripheral tissues. Because newborn cardiac performance at rest is so close to its ceiling, or limits of function, little *systolic reserve* is available to adapt to an acute or chronic stress such as pressure or volume load from an obstructive lesion or left-to-right circulatory shunt, respectively, or asphyxia.

HEART RATE RESERVE. This consists of the ability of the heart to change its rate of pumping to raise the level of cardiac output. In this regard the newborn also is limited because in this age group the intrinsic heart rate normally is quite high. In addition, heart failure per se raises the frequency of contraction even further, primarily as a result of high circulating levels of catecholamines. In this sense, the

newborn's heart rate also is closer than the child's or adult's to its ceiling, or upper limits of effectiveness. Furthermore, increases in heart rate occur largely at the expense of diastolic filling time. Thus, at very rapid heart rates, there is a disproportionately diminished diastolic time and therefore diminished time for perfusion of the myocardium by its own coronary arterial system. In addition, rapid heart rates result in elevated myocardial energy expenditure and increased myocardial demand for oxygen. The sum of these considerations indicates that newborn *heart rate reserve* is reduced.

TREATMENT (see also Chap. 17). Table 29-5 lists supportive and pharmacological measures in the treatment of the newborn with heart failure. The supportive measures are designed to increase tissue oxygen supply, decrease tissue oxygen consumption, and correct metabolic abnormalities. Digitalis glycosides and certain diuretic agents provide the most important elements of medical therapy, but it is important to recognize that the dosage regimen of drugs administered to young patients must be adjusted to take into account the age and size of the patient and the maturity-dependent pharmacological properties of cardioactive drugs.[92,94] Because this is especially true in early in-

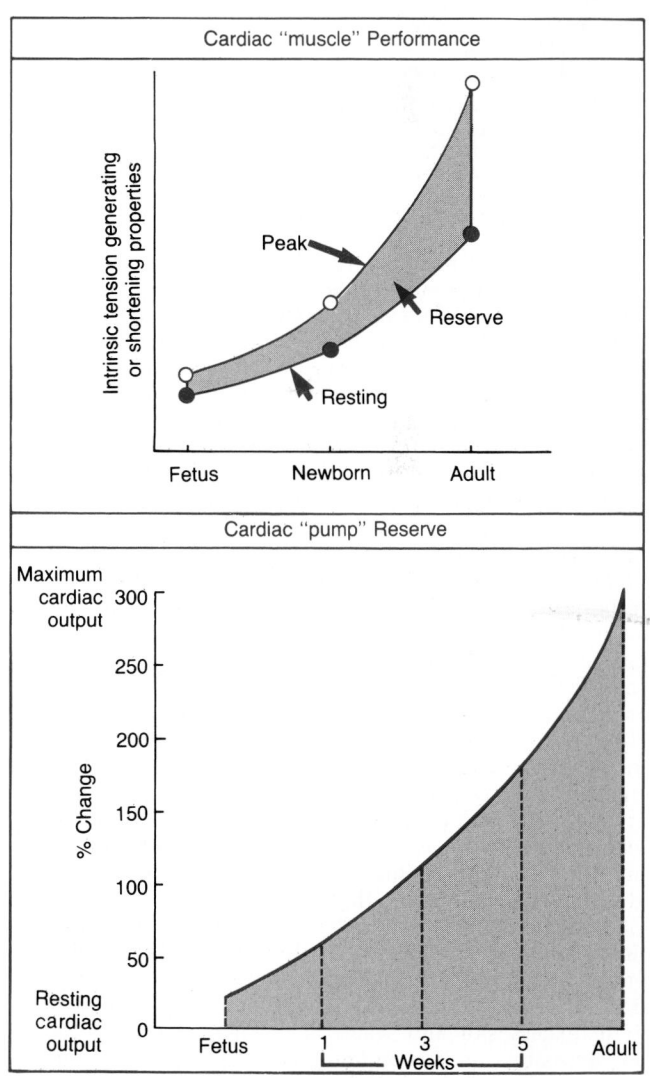

FIGURE 29-5. Schema of reduced cardiac reserve in fetal and newborn hearts compared with the adult's. In the newborn infant, resting cardiac muscle performance *(top panel)* is close to the peak of ventricular function because of limitations in diastolic, systolic, and heart rate reserve. Similarly, pump reserve *(bottom panel)* early in life is limited by these factors, as well as by a much higher resting cardiac output relative to body weight, compared with the adult.

TABLE 29–5 TREATMENT OF CONGESTIVE HEART FAILURE

I. GENERAL INTERVENTIONS
Rest (occasional sedation)
Semi-Fowler position
Temperature and humidity control
Oxygen
Decrease sodium load
Avoid aspiration
Treat infection, if present

II. SPECIFIC INTERVENTIONS
Preload manipulation
Move ventricular function curve up by volume infusion to increase venous return
Move ventricular function curve down with diuretics, venodilators
Afterload reduction
Facilitate ventricular emptying by reducing wall tension
Reduce blood viscosity
Drugs, arteriolar dilators, mechanical counterpulsation
Inotropic stimulation
Improve physical and metabolic milieu: pH, PaO_2, glucose, calcium, hemoglobin
Inotropic drugs: digitalis, catecholamines, dobutamine, dopamine
Heart rate
Control rhythm disturbances with pacing, drugs
Other
Mechanical ventilation
Prostaglandin manipulation
Peritoneal dialysis

III. INTERVENTIONAL CATHETER-DIRECTED THERAPY or SURGERY (may include transplantation)

fancy, Table 29–6 provides the dosages of digoxin and diuretics commonly used for infants.

Digitalis and Diuretics. Digoxin is the glycoside used exclusively to treat pediatric patients in most cardiac centers because it is readily absorbed, available in convenient dosage form, and excreted rapidly from the body. Premature infants are more sensitive to digitalis than are full-term newborns, who, in turn, are more sensitive than older infants. Infants absorb and excrete digoxin as well as adults do, and their relative distribution of the glycoside to different body tissues is also similar. The prevailing dose schedules for digoxin produce higher serum concentrations in infants than would be considered optimal for adults.[95] The basis for the higher digitalis requirement in infancy is unclear, although it may relate to an age-dependent alteration in the sensitivity of the myocardium per se to the glycosides. In this regard, infants tolerate higher serum digoxin concentrations than adults without developing signs of toxicity. In the adult, the usual therapeutic concentrations of digoxin are less than 2 ng/ml blood, and toxicity commonly occurs above that level. In contrast, in infants, therapeutic levels of digoxin range from 1 to 5 ng/ml (mean = 3.5), while toxicity is associated with concentrations in excess of 3 ng/ml. Older children have therapeutic and toxic levels similar to those of adults.

A restricted fluid intake (65 ml/kg/day) and a low-sodium diet (1 to 2 mEq/kg/day) should accompany diuretic therapy in the most seriously ill infants with heart failure. Furosemide is the agent of choice when the rapid elimination of excess salt and water is needed. Hydrochlorothiazide, occasionally in conjunction with spironolactone or triamterene to reduce potassium loss and sodium retention, is convenient for long-term therapy.

Other Pharmacological Approaches. These may prove to be of significant benefit in selected instances in which digitalis and diuretics are relatively ineffective. In situations in which cardiac decompensation is not the result of an obstructive lesion, catecholamines may be used tempo-

rarily to alleviate cardiac failure while the patient is awaiting more definitive operative treatment (Table 29–7).[92] In infants with the coarctation of the aorta syndrome, in whom ductal constriction unmasks the aortic branch point producing aortic narrowing (see p. 911), or with aortic arch interruption, heart failure may be reversed dramatically by the intravenous infusion of prostaglandin E_1 (0.03–0.1 mg/kg/min), which results in dilatation of the ductus arteriosus and relief of the obstruction.[96,97] Conversely, in preterm infants in whom patent ductus arteriosus is responsible for profound cardiopulmonary deterioration, constriction of the ductus arteriosus may be accomplished by inhibition of prostaglandin synthesis with the nonsteroidal anti-inflammatory agent indomethacin (0.2 mg/kg IV).[98,99]

Vasodilator therapy also is used in infants or children with heart disease in whom preload or afterload alterations may be expected to improve cardiac performance (Table 29–8).[36,37,92,100] Moreover, treatment of severe cardiac failure often requires combining inotropic and afterload-reducing agents (see p. 495). Combinations of dopamine, dobutamine, and nitroprusside have been used extensively and effectively in the pediatric population, primarily in the setting of low cardiac output after open-heart surgery.[92] Use of oral afterload-reducing agents, e.g., hydralazine or captopril, in association with digoxin is worthwhile in the long-term therapy of outpatients with congestive cardiomyopathy and/or significant mitral or aortic regurgitation.

Rapid developments in molecular biology have begun to revolutionize our understanding of cardiovascular regulation, both before and after birth and at all ages. As knowledge is gained about the mechanisms responsible for the variability of gene expression in the heart, it is apparent that the future holds the opportunity for clinicians to modify gene expression in ways that will importantly enhance the heart's ability to respond to both the heart failure state

TABLE 29–6 DIURETIC AND DIGITALIS DOSAGES FOR INFANTS

PREPARATION	DOSAGE AND ROUTE OF ADMINISTRATION
Furosemide	IV, 1 mg/kg/dose; oral, 2 to 6 mg/kg/day
Ethacrynic acid	IV, 1 mg/kg/dose; oral, 2 to 3 mg/kg/day
Hydrochlorothiazide	Oral, 2 to 5 mg/kg/day
Spironolactone	Oral, 1 to 3 mg/kg/day
Triamterene	Oral, 2 to 4 mg/kg/day
Digoxin	
Elixir	0.05 mg/ml
Parenteral	0.10 mg/ml

AGE AND WEIGHT	DOSE AND ROUTE*	
	Acute Digitalization	Maintenance
Prematures < 1.5 kg	10–20 μg/kg IV TDD: ½, ¼, ¼ of dose q 8h	4 μg/kg/day IV (may increase to 4 μg/kg q 12h at age 1 month)
1.5–2.5 kg	Same as above	4 μg/kg q 12h IV
Full-term newborns	30 μg/kg IV, TDD	4–5 μg/kg q 12h IV
Infants (1–12 months)	35 μg/kg IV, TDD	5–10 μg/kg q 12h IV
> 12 months	40 μg/kg IV, TDD (maximum 1.0 mg)	5–10 μg/kg q 12h IV
Older children (over 20 kg)	1.0–2.0 mg IV, TDD over 48 hours	0.125–0.250 mg IV q day

* po = Oral dose approximately 20 per cent greater than IV dose except in "older children." In older children, IV = oral dose.
TDD = Total digitalizing dose.

TABLE 29-7 DOSAGE REGIMENS: INOTROPIC AGENTS

891

Ch 29

DRUG	DOSE	COMMENTS
Epinephrine (Adrenalin)	0.05–1.0 μg/kg/min IV	May cause hypertension and cardiac arrhythmias; inactivated in alkaline solution
Isoproterenol (Isuprel)	0.05–0.5 μg/kg/min IV	May decrease coronary blood flow; results in peripheral and pulmonary vasodilation
Norepinephrine (Levophed)	0.05–0.5 μg/kg/min IV	Causes significant vasoconstriction
Dobutamine (Dobutrex)	2–10 μg/kg/min IV (Max 40 μg/kg/min)	No direct effect on renal perfusion, little or no peripheral vaso-dilatation or tachycardia
Dopamine (Intropin)	2–20 μg/kg/min IV (Max 50 μg/kg/min) 2–5 μg/kg/min 5–8 μg/kg/min >8 μg/kg/min >10 μg/kg/min 15–20 μg/kg/min	Significant renal vasodilatation Inotropic ± heart rate acceleration Significant heart rate acceleration ± Vasoconstriction Significant vasoconstriction
	(Above dose/effect relations speculative in neonates)	
Amrinone	Dose schedule not established for infants and children Adults: 40 μg/kg/min IV for 1 hr, then 6–10 μg/kg/min; 50–450 mg/day po divided TID	May cause thrombocytopenia, hepatic and GI disturbance, fever, and arrhythmias

From Friedman, W. F., and George, B. L.: New concepts and drugs in the treatment of congestive heart failure. Pediatr. Clin. North Am. *31*:1197, 1984.

and those diseases that are responsible for the abnormalities leading to cardiac disease.[101,102]

CYANOSIS

Cyanosis in the infant (see p. 885) often presents as a diagnostic emergency, necessitating prompt detection of the underlying cause. The schema in Figure 29–6 outlines a general approach to diagnosis. The cardiologist must distinguish between three types of cyanosis—peripheral, differential, and central—while recognizing that cyanosis may accompany diseases of the central nervous, hematological, respiratory, and cardiac systems.

PERIPHERAL CYANOSIS. Peripheral cyanosis (normal arterial oxygen saturation and widened arteriovenous oxygen differences) usually indicates stasis of blood flow in the periphery. The level of reduced hemoglobin in the capillaries of the skin usually exceeds 3 gm/100 dl. The most prominent causes of peripheral cyanosis in the newborn are autonomically controlled alterations in the cutaneous distribution of capillary blood flow (acrocyanosis) and septicemia associated with evidence of a low cardiac output, i.e., hypotension, weak pulse, and cold extremities. In many instances, peripheral cyanosis is clearly the result of a cold environment or high hemoglobin content. When cyanosis is caused by the former, vasodilatation produced by immersing the extremity in warm water for several minutes reverses the cyanosis.

CENTRAL CYANOSIS. Oxygen unsaturation in central cyanosis may result from inadequately oxygenated pulmonary venous blood, in which case inhalation of 100 per cent oxygen may diminish or clear the discoloration (see below). Conversely, in instances in which cyanosis is due to an intracardiac or extracardiac right-to-left shunt, pulmonary venous blood is fully saturated, and inhalation of 100 per cent oxygen usually does not improve the infant's color. It is necessary to qualify the latter statement because oxygen may act directly in infants with elevated pulmonary vascular resistance to dilate the pulmonary blood vessels and thus reduce the magnitude of the veno-arterial shunt. Central cyanosis also may be due to the replacement of normal by abnormal hemoglobin, as in methemoglobinemia.

Several factors influence the oxygen saturation produced at any given arterial pO_2. These include temperature, pH, ratio of fetal to adult hemoglobin, and erythrocyte concentration of 2,3-diphosphoglycerate. For example, fetal hemoglobin has a higher affinity for oxygen than does adult hemoglobin and therefore would be more highly saturated at any given pO_2. Thus, determination of the systemic arterial oxygen tension may provide a more accurate picture of the underlying pathophysiology than simply measuring the oxygen saturation.[50,103]

DIFFERENTIAL CYANOSIS. Differential cyanosis virtually always indicates the presence of congenital heart disease, often with patency of the ductus arteriosus and coarctation of the aorta as components of the abnormal anatomical complex. If the upper part of the body is pink and the lower part of the body blue, coarctation of the aorta or interruption of the aortic arch is probable, with oxygenated blood supplying the upper body and desaturated blood supplying the lower body by way of right-to-left flow through the ductus arteriosus. The latter also occurs in patients with patent ductus arteriosus and markedly elevated pulmonary vascular resistance. A patient with transposition of the great arteries and coarctation of the aorta with retrograde flow through a patent ductus arteriosus demonstrates the reverse situation, i.e., the lower part of the body is pink and the upper part blue. Simultaneous determinations of oxygen saturation in the temporal or right brachial artery and the femoral artery are helpful in confirming the presence of differential cyanosis.

TABLE 29-8 DOSAGE REGIMENS: VASODILATORS IN INFANTS AND CHILDREN

DRUG	DOSE AND ROUTE OF ADMINISTRATION	COMMENTS
Nitroglycerin	0.5–20 μg/kg/min IV (Max 60 μg/kg/min IV)	Dosage schedule for IV and other routes of administration not well established for children
Hydralazine (Apresoline)	0.5 mg/kg/day po q 6–8h (Max 200 mg/day or 7 mg/kg/day) 1.5 μg/kg/min IV or 0.1–0.5 mg/kg/dose IV q 6h (Max 2 mg/kg q 6h)	May cause tachycardia, GI symptoms, neutropenia, lupus-like syndrome
Captopril (Capoten)	0.1–0.4 mg/kg/dose po given q 6–24h as needed	May cause neutropenia/proteinuria
Nitroprusside (Nipride)	0.5–8 μg/kg/min IV	May result in thiocyanate or cyanide toxicity if used in high doses or for prolonged periods of time; light-sensitive
Prazosin (Minipress)	1st dose: 5 μg/kg/po (Max 25 μg/kg/dose q 6h)	Initial dose used to elevate hypotensive effects; orthostatic hypotension, attenuation of hemodynamic effects may occur.

From Friedman, W. F., and George, B. L.: New concepts and drugs in the treatment of congestive heart failure. Pediatr. Clin. North Am. *31*:1197, 1984.

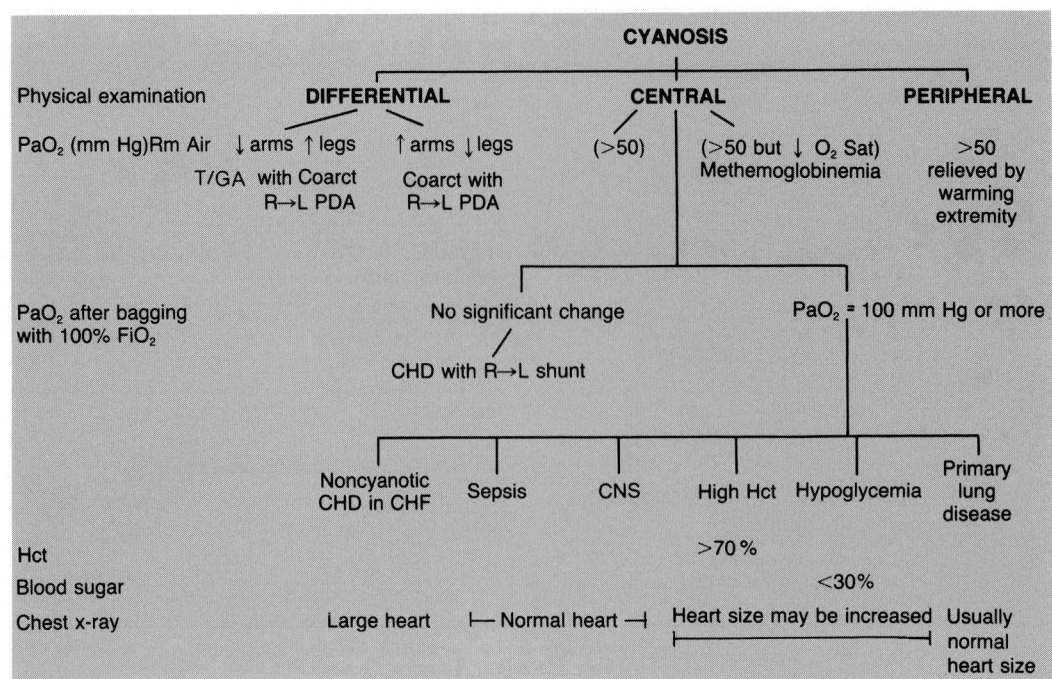

FIGURE 29–6. Flow chart for the evaluation of cyanotic infants. Tests to be done are listed at the left. The response to each of these tests leads along the line to the proper diagnostic category. CHD = congenital heart disease, CHF = congestive heart failure, CNS = central nervous system, Hct = hematocrit, PDA = patent ductus arteriosus, T/GA = transposition of great arteries. (From Kirkpatrick, S. E., et al.: Differential diagnosis of congenital heart disease in the newborn—University of California, San Diego, School of Medicine, and University Hospital, San Diego [Specialty Conference]. West. J. Med. *128*:127, 1978.)

Differentiating Between Pulmonary and Cardiac Causes of Cyanosis

The distinction between respiratory signs and symptoms arising from cyanotic cardiac disease and those associated with a primary pulmonary disorder is an important challenge to the cardiologist.[43] Upper airway obstruction precipitates cyanosis by producing alveolar hypoventilation owing to reduced pulmonary ventilation. Mechanical obstruction may occur from the nares to the carina, and the important diagnostic possibilities among congenital abnormalities are choanal atresia, vascular ring, laryngeal web, and tracheomalacia. Acquired causes include vocal cord paresis, obstetrical injury to the cricothyroid cartilage, and foreign body. Structural abnormalities in the lungs resulting from intrapulmonary disease are more frequently a basis for cyanosis among newborns than is upper airway obstruction. Hyaline membrane disease, atelectasis, or pneumonitis causing inflammation, collapse, and fluid accumulation in the alveoli results in reduction of the oxygenation of blood reaching the systemic circulation.

Successfully distinguishing between these various causes of cyanosis depends on interpretation of the respiratory pattern, the cardiac physical examination, evaluation of arterial blood gases (Table 29–9), and interpretation of the electrocardiogram, chest x-ray, and echocardiogram.

RESPIRATORY PATTERNS. The key to differential diagnosis at the bedside commonly is the proper evaluation of the pattern of respiration. Term infants normally exhibit a progressive reduction in respiratory rate during the first day of life from 60 to 70 per minute to 35 to 55 per minute. Moreover, mild intercostal retractions and minimal expiratory grunting disappear within several hours of birth. An increased depth of respiration in the presence of cyanosis, but without other signs of respiratory distress, often is associated with congenital cardiac disease in which inadequate pulmonary blood flow is the most important functional component.

Apnea. The most important variations from normal respiratory patterns are apnea and bradypnea, and tachypnea. Intermittent apneic episodes are common in premature infants with central nervous system immaturity or disease. In addition, higher centers may be depressed as a result of severe hypoxemia, acidemia, or the administration of pharmacological agents to mother or baby. The association of apneic episodes, lethargy, hypotonicity, and a reduction of spontaneous movement most often points to intracranial disease as an underlying cause.

Tachypnea. Diverse conditions result in tachypnea in the newborn period. Tachypnea in the presence of intrinsic pulmonary disease with upper or lower airway obstruction usually is accompanied by flaring of the alae nasi, chest-

TABLE 29–9   ARTERIAL BLOOD GAS PATTERNS IN VARIOUS DISORDERS CAUSING CYANOSIS IN INFANTS

PATTERN	pH	pO₂	pCO₂	RESPONSE TO O₂	VENOUS pH	SUGGESTED CONDITION
1	↓	↓↓	↑	↑↑	↓	Hyaline membrane or other pulmonary parenchymal disease
2	↓	↓	↑↑↑	↑	↓	Hypoventilation
3	—	↓	—	↑	—	Venous admixture
4	↓	↓↓	—	—	↓	Decreased or ineffective pulmonary blood flow
5	↓↓↓	↓	—↑	—↑	↓↓↓	Systemic hypoperfusion

— = no effect. For description of patterns, see p. 893.

wall retractions, and grunting. In contrast, tachypnea associated with intense cyanosis in the absence of obvious respiratory distress suggests the presence of cyanotic congenital heart disease. In general, highest respiratory rates (80 to 110/min) are seen in association with primary lung, and not heart, disease. Initial chest radiography frequently is diagnostic, especially if the problem is aspiration, mucous plug, adenomatoid malformation, lobar emphysema, diaphragmatic hernia, pneumothorax, lung agenesis, pulmonary hemorrhage, or an abnormal thoracic cage configuration. Choanal atresia may be excluded by passing a feeding tube through the nares, and the more common types of esophageal atresia and tracheoesophageal fistula may be excluded by passing the tube farther into the stomach.

CARDIAC EXAMINATION. Specific findings on cardiovascular examination may direct attention to a cardiac cause for cyanosis. Peripheral perfusion is poor in the presence of severe primary myocardial disease or the hypoplastic left heart syndrome. In contrast, peripheral pulses are bounding and the dorsalis pedis and palmar pulses are easily palpable in infants with patent ductus arteriosus, truncus arteriosus, or aorticopulmonary window. A marked discrepancy between upper- and lower-extremity blood pressures helps to identify the infant with coarctation of the aorta. Inspection and palpation of the precordium allow an overall estimate of cardiac activity. A thrill in the suprasternal notch and/or over the precordium occasionally may be felt in the infant with patent ductus arteriosus, critical aortic stenosis, or coarctation of the aorta. Characterization of the second heart sound may be of help because it often is single in infants with a hypoplastic left heart complex, pulmonary atresia with or without an intact ventricular septum, or truncus arteriosus. Wide splitting of the second heart sound may occur in infants with total anomalous pulmonary venous return. Ejection sounds often are detectable in infants with persistent truncus arteriosus and occasionally with critical aortic or pulmonic stenosis. The presence of a third heart sound is normal, but a gallop rhythm may provide a clue to myocardial failure. Wide splitting of the first and second heart sounds may produce the characteristically rhythmic auscultatory cadence of Ebstein's anomaly of the tricuspid valve (see p. 934). The presence of a cardiac murmur may point clearly to underlying cardiac disease, but the absence of a murmur does not exclude the presence of a cardiac malformation. Moreover, cardiac murmurs of specific anomalies often are atypical in the newborn period. However, certain cardiac murmurs such as the decrescendo holosystolic murmur of tricuspid regurgitation in Ebstein's anomaly or the transient tricuspid regurgitation of infancy may point clearly to an accurate diagnosis. Auscultation of the head and abdomen may detect the murmur of an arteriovenous malformation at those sites in infants who present with findings of severe heart failure.

BLOOD GAS AND pH PATTERNS. Arterial blood gas analysis may be a reliable method of evaluating cyanosis, suggesting the type of altered physiology, and assessing responses to therapeutic maneuvers.[57] Specimens for blood gas analysis should be obtained in room air and in 100 per cent oxygen. Stick capillary samples from the patient's warmed heel may be used, although determinations obtained by arterial puncture are preferable for evaluation of oxygenation because they are less susceptible to alterations in regional blood flow in the critically ill infant. Sampling of right radial or temporal arterial blood is preferable because these sites are proximal to flow through a ductus arteriosus and do not reflect right-to-left ductal shunting, as would a sample from the descending aorta obtained by means of an umbilical artery catheter. A trial of continuous positive airway pressure may improve oxygenation in infants with either hyaline membrane disease or pulmonary edema.

Arterial blood gas patterns in various pathophysiological conditions are listed in Table 29–9. Pattern 1 typically is observed in infants with ventilation-perfusion abnormali-

ties resulting from primary respiratory disease, often associated with elevated pulmonary vascular resistance and venoarterial shunting across a patent foramen ovale or patent ductus arteriosus. Pulmonary hypoventilation with CO_2 retention produces pattern 2. In the presence of a lesion causing obligatory venous admixture, such as total anomalous pulmonary venous connection (pattern 3), the response to oxygen may reflect an increase in pulmonary venous return secondary to a fall in pulmonary vascular resistance. Pattern 4 typically is seen in infants with a cardiac malformation that results in reduced pulmonary blood flow. Oxygen administration in these infants does not alter the arterial pO_2. The alterations of pattern 5 are observed when systemic hypoperfusion is the principal hemodynamic problem. In these babies the arteriovenous oxygen difference is high, and the acidemia may be progressive and unrelenting.

ELECTROCARDIOGRAM (see also Chap. 4). This is less helpful in suggesting a diagnosis of heart disease in the premature and newborn infant than in the older child. Right ventricular hypertrophy is a normal finding in the neonate, and the range of normal voltages is wide. However, specific observations may offer major clues to the presence of a cardiovascular anomaly. A counterclockwise, superiorly oriented frontal QRS loop with absent or reduced right ventricular forces suggests the diagnosis of tricuspid atresia (see p. 932). In contrast, when the QRS axis is normal but left ventricular forces predominate, the diagnosis of pulmonic atresia must be considered (see p. 926). The counterclockwise, superior QRS orientation also is observed in infants with an endocardiac cushion defect (see p. 898) and in some with double-outlet right ventricle (see p. 941); right ventricular forces in these babies are increased.

The initial septal vector should be assessed from the electrocardiogram. Often Q waves are not clearly seen in the lateral precordial leads in the first 72 hours of life. A leftward, posteriorly directed septal vector giving rise to Q waves in the right precordial leads is abnormal and suggests the presence of marked right ventricular hypertrophy, single ventricle (see p. 947), or inversion of the ventricles. T-wave alterations may be seen in a normal neonatal electrocardiogram and may be of no particular consequence. However, by 72 hours of age the T waves should be inverted in V_3 and V_1 and upright in the lateral precordium; persistently upright T waves in the right precordial leads are a sign of right ventricular hypertrophy. Depressed or flattened T waves in the lateral precordium may suggest subendocardial ischemia and a left heart outflow tract obstructive lesion, electrolyte disturbance, acidosis, or hypoxemia. An electrocardiographic pattern of myocardial infarction suggests a diagnosis of anomalous pulmonary origin of the coronary artery (see p. 909). Finally, rhythm disturbances such as complete heart block or supraventricular tachycardia can be detected readily by electrocardiography.

RADIOGRAPHIC EXAMINATION (see also Chap. 7). Chest radiography often is useful in differentiating between respiratory and cardiac causes of cyanosis in the newborn period. Determination of a normal cardiac and abdominal situs aids in ruling out several kinds of complex cyanotic cardiac malformations associated with asplenia or polysplenia with abdominal heterotaxy and dextrocardia (see p. 966). The distinct appearance of pulmonary parenchymal disease, such as the classic reticulogranular pattern of hyaline membrane disease, may allow a specific radiological diagnosis. In those premature infants with a large ductus arteriosus the radiographic appearance often evolves from the typical findings of hyaline membrane disease to increased pulmonary vascular markings and finally to perihilar and generalized pulmonary edema.

Most important, the pediatric cardiologist depends heavily on the evaluation of pulmonary vascular markings to categorize congenital cardiac malformations in the newborn infant according to function. In the presence of cyanosis, diminished pulmonary vascular markings call attention to the group of anomalies that includes tetralogy of Fallot, pulmonic stenosis with intact ventricular septum, pulmonic atresia, tricuspid atresia, and Ebstein's malformation of the tricuspid valve. Reduced pulmonary blood flow is responsible for the systemic arterial desaturation in these babies. Increased pulmonary vascular markings in the cyanotic infant are associated with lesions in which an obligatory admixture of systemic venous and pulmonary venous blood occurs. The more common anomalies in this category include transposition of the great arteries, hypoplastic left heart syndrome, truncus arteriosus, and total anomalous pulmonary venous drainage.

As mentioned earlier, overall heart size in the normal newborn infant is greater than in the older child, and cardiothoracic ratios up to 0.60 are within normal limits. The thymus shadow occasionally obscures the cardiac silhouette and prohibits accurate estimation of heart size. An enlarged heart on x-ray examination suggests a cardiac disorder. However, in the presence of severe respiratory difficulties with an increase in carbon dioxide tension and a decrease in both pH and arterial oxygen tension, cardiomegaly may be only moderate. A right aortic arch suggests the presence of either tetralogy of Fallot or persistent truncus arteriosus. An ovoid heart with a narrow base associated with increased pulmonary vascular marking is typical of transposition of the great arteries. A boot-shaped heart with concavity of the pulmonary outflow tract suggests tetralogy of Fallot, pulmonic atresia, or tricuspid atresia.

LABORATORY STUDIES IN CONGENITAL HEART DISEASE

FETAL ECHOCARDIOGRAPHY (see also p. 54). Ultrasound technology now allows examination of human fetal cardiac development and function in utero.[39-41,104-106] Diagnostic-quality images of the fetal heart in utero can be obtained as early as 16 weeks of gestation. Cardiac structures are imaged primarily by cross-sectional echocardiography and augmented by a combination of range-gated pulse Doppler ultrasonography and M-mode echocardiography. The analysis of the structure and function of the fetal heart during the second and third trimesters of pregnancy has allowed cardiologists to counsel prospective parents, and in a number of instances to formulate management plans for pregnancy, delivery, and the immediate postnatal period. Using fetal echocardiography, major forms of congenital heart disease have been diagnosed in utero, and cardiac rhythm abnormalities have been detected, permitting direct efforts at transplacental therapy. In particular, it has been established that a high incidence exists of cardiac pathology in the presence of nonimmune fetal hydrops. It appears clear that hydrops fetalis often represents end-stage fetal cardiac decompensation (Fig. 29–7). Atrioventricular valve insufficiency often causes fetal right ventricular volume overload and systemic venous hypertension leading to hydrops fetalis.

Pulsed Doppler ultrasound examination of the fetus importantly supplements the echocardiographic findings in identifying the responsible defects, such as Ebstein's malformation of the tricuspid valve, atrial isomerism with atrioventricular septal defects, and the absent pulmonary valve and hypoplastic left heart syndromes.

Fetal cardiac ultrasonography is of special importance in analyzing disturbances of fetal cardiac rhythm, which usually are first suspected on the basis of auscultatory findings. Transabdominal electrocardiography cannot identify atrial depolarization and is of limited value in the analysis of cardiac arrhythmias in utero. However, M-mode recordings of cardiac motion versus time allow conclusions regarding electrical events in the fetal heart, as they are reflected by the mechanical responses that are recorded

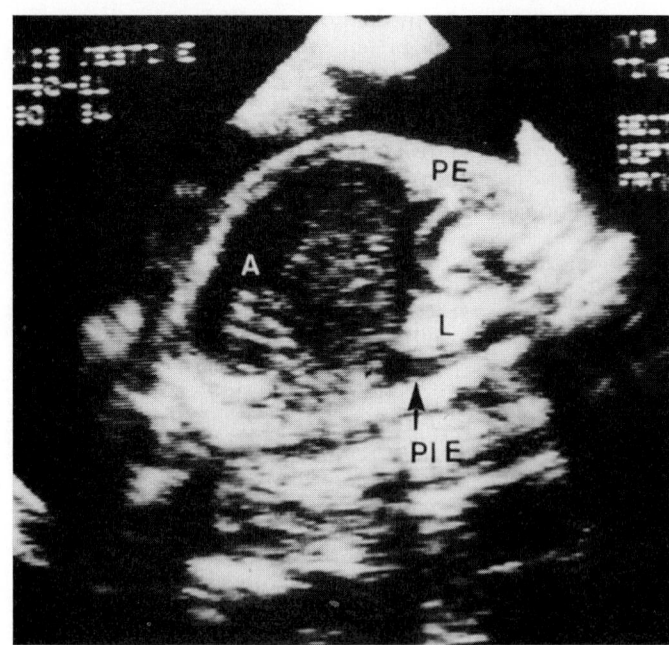

FIGURE 29–7. Abdominal ultrasound examination of a 28-week fetus with nonimmunological hydrops fetalis. A = ascites, PE = pericardial effusion, L = lung, PlE = pleural effusion. The fetal heart is to the right and inferior of the arrow showing the pericardial effusion.

echocardiographically. Supraventricular tachyarrhythmias are a common cause of nonimmune fetal hydrops (Fig. 29–8). Detection is of practical use in the management of these patients because the arrhythmia is treatable with use of various antiarrhythmic drugs, such as digoxin, procainamide, propranolol, and flecainide, administered to the mother and reaching the fetus transplacentally or, rarely, under sonographic guidance, by means of injection of drugs, such as amiodarone, into the umbilical vein.[107]

ECHOCARDIOGRAPHY IN THE NEONATE. Echocardiography is of immense value in differentiating between heart dis-

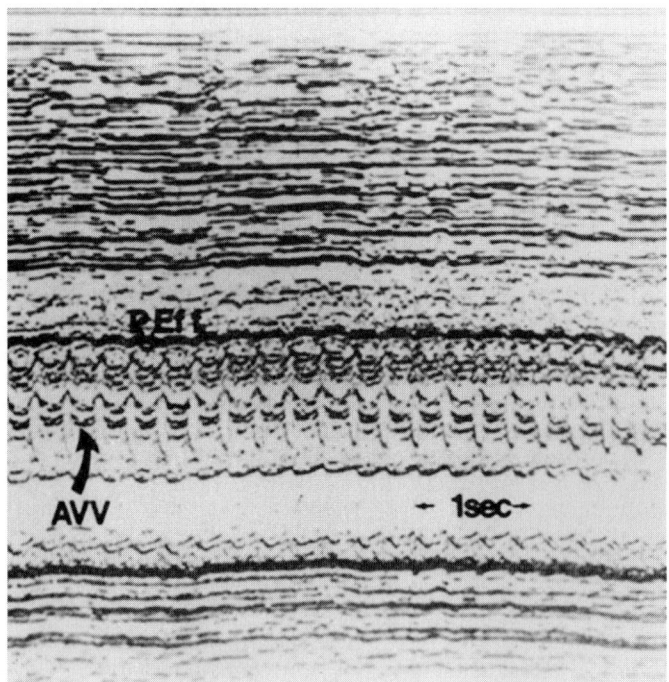

FIGURE 29–8. M-mode echocardiogram at 35 weeks' gestation, showing fetal supraventricular tachycardia and pericardial effusion (PEff). The tracing, taken at the midventricular level, allows the heart rate to be calculated from atrioventricular valve (AVV) motion (250 beats/min). (Courtesy of Charles Kleinman, M.D.)

ease and lung disease in the newborn.[108] Echocardiographic diagnoses that often can be made with certainty include hypoplastic left heart syndrome, aortic valve stenosis, membranous and fibromuscular subvalvular aortic stenosis, aortic coarctation, hypertrophic cardiomyopathy, cor triatriatum, atrial septal defect, tricuspid atresia, Ebstein's anomaly of the tricuspid valve, valvular pulmonic stenosis, atrioventricular septal defect, single ventricle, double-outlet right ventricle, transposition of the great arteries, and patent ductus arteriosus. The echocardiogram provides suggestive and often conclusive evidence for tetralogy of Fallot, truncus arteriosus, total anomalous pulmonary venous connection, and pulmonary atresia with an intact ventricular septum.

Doppler ultrasonography (see p. 56) supplements the two-dimensional echocardiographic examination by its ability to quantify valve gradients, cardiac output, blood flow patterns in the cardiac chambers and great arteries, and often shunt size.[108–111] For example, the pulmonary-systemic blood flow ratio can be calculated by multiplying the square of the ratio of the great vessel diameters by the ratio of the peak systolic flow velocities, the pulmonary variable being the numerator in each ratio.[109] The coupling of Doppler ultrasonographic techniques with the two-dimensional echocardiogram, and the representation in color of abnormalities in flow, volume, and direction (see p. 63), greatly improve diagnostic accuracy.

CARDIAC CATHETERIZATION (see also Chap. 6). If certain cardiac anomalies are identified by noninvasive studies or if a clear-cut differentiation cannot be made between cardiac and pulmonary disease, heart catheterization and angiocardiography may be necessary to define the underlying state precisely. However, fewer cardiac catheterizations have been performed in infants and children of all ages since the beginning of aggressive pursuit of preoperative diagnoses by noninvasive imaging modalities, particularly two-dimensional Doppler flow echocardiography.[111,112] Hemodynamic study of the newborn infant carries a small but distinct risk.[113] As a general rule, cardiac catheterization is not performed unless the information sought is central to the management of the infant. Most infants with serious heart disease require therapeutic intervention, and thus catheterization should be performed only when surgical support is readily available. Cardiac catheterization usually is indicated in most newborns who experience congestive heart failure in the first days after birth if the cause is an anatomical abnormality rather than an arrhythmia or a metabolic disturbance. Preferably, medical measures will have been instituted to stabilize the clinical state before a hemodynamic study is performed.

It is generally agreed that some newborns with cyanotic congenital heart disease require prompt cardiac catheterization because of the considerable risk of rapid deterioration.[21] Under these circumstances hemodynamic and angiographic study may not only provide the anatomical diagnosis required before emergency operation but also allow the opportunity for therapeutic maneuvers such as balloon atrial septostomy to facilitate intercirculatory mixing in patients with complete transposition of the great arteries or to augment interatrial shunting in patients with a restrictive patent foramen ovale and either tricuspid, pulmonic, or mitral atresia, or total anomalous pulmonary

venous connection. The selective infusion of low doses of prostaglandin E_1 (0.05–0.1 $\mu g/kg/min$) intravenously has been used before and at cardiac catheterization for the emergency palliation of ductus-dependent cardiac lesions such as pulmonary atresia, aortic coarctation, and interruption of the aortic arch.[96] Because a patent ductus arteriosus maintains pulmonary and systemic blood flow, respectively, in these infants, dilatation of the ductus with vasodilatory prostaglandins may retard their clinical deterioration. Thus, prostaglandin E_1 infusion has been shown to be an effective short-term measure to correct hypoxemia and acidemia and to improve the preoperative and intraoperative status of infants who require surgical relief of the congenital cardiac lesion that is causing pulmonary or systemic hypoperfusion.

Therapeutic Catheterization (see also Chap. 39). Balloon atrial septostomy was the first catheter intervention that proved useful to treat congenital heart disease, and it remains the standard initial palliation in infants with complete transposition of the great arteries unless the arterial switch operation is performed imminently.[114] Many additional transcatheter techniques are now used successfully to treat congenital heart disease. These include knife blade atrial septostomy, umbrella or coil closure of patent ductus arteriosus, umbrella closure of atrial septal defect,[112,115] balloon-expandable intravascular stents for peripheral pulmonary artery and selected postoperative stenoses, and balloon and coil embolization of large systemic pulmonary artery collateral vessels and arteriovenous fistulas. Other procedures that have expanded the role of the cardiac catheter from a diagnostic tool to a therapeutic instrument include transvenous or transarterial pacemaker insertion and retrieval of foreign bodies from the cardiovascular system. Transluminal balloon angioplasty currently is used principally in pediatrics for dilation of pulmonic and aortic valve stenosis, native and recoarctation of the aorta, and peripheral pulmonary artery stenosis. Unresolved questions continue to exist about transluminal angioplasty in native neonatal coarctation and congenital subaortic and mitral stenosis. Lastly, electrode catheter radiofrequency ablative techniques for the treatment of tachycardias are now performed routinely in centers with pediatric electrophysiology programs.[116,117]

Electrophysiological Studies (see also Chap. 21). The cardiac catheterization laboratory also is being used with increasing frequency to define the anatomical and physiological diagnoses of arrhythmias, thus facilitating an accurate prognosis and providing a rational basis for pharmacological, catheter ablative, or surgical treatment.[118–121] The invasive electrophysiological approach provides unique information that cannot be obtained noninvasively. These include determination of conduction times of individual components of the conducting system and measurement of refractory periods for structures such as the atrioventricular node, His bundle, and bundle branches. In addition, one can determine the origin or anatomical circuit, sustaining mechanisms, and possible perturbations that terminate the arrhythmia. This last maneuver is particularly important because it may enable the planning of effective drug treatment. It also may determine the advisability of catheter ablation, pacemaker control, or surgical treatment of the rhythm disturbance.

SPECIFIC CARDIAC DEFECTS

Many classifications of congenital cardiovascular lesions have been proposed on the basis of hemodynamic, anatomical, and radiographic factors. Although there is overlapping between groups, the following arrangement of cardiac anomalies is used in this chapter: (1) communications between the systemic and pulmonary circulations without cyanosis (left-to-right shunts), (2) obstructing valvular and vascular lesions with or without associated right-to-left shunt, (3) abnormalities in the origins of the great arteries and veins (the transposition complexes), (4) malpositions of the heart and cardiac apex, and (5) miscellaneous anomalies.

Atrial Septal Defect
(See also p. 1660)

MORPHOLOGY. Atrial septal defect is one of the most commonly recognized congenital cardiac anomalies in adults but is very rarely diagnosed and even less commonly results in disability in infants.[122] The anatomical sites of interatrial defects are shown in Figure 29–9. Defects of the sinus venosus type are high in the atrial septum near the entry of the superior vena cava and may be created by a deficiency in the wall that normally separates the pulmonary veins from the right lung and the superior vena cava and right atrium, thereby also resulting in partial anomalous pulmonary venous drainage.[99,123] Most often the atrial septal defect involves the fossa ovalis, is midseptal in location, and is of the ostium secundum type. This type of defect is a true deficiency of the atrial septum and should not be confused with a patent foramen ovale. Embryologically the left side of the atrial septum is derived from the septum primum, which possesses an opening—the interatrial ostium secundum (Fig. 29–1). The ostium secundum lies forward and superior to the position of the foramen ovale. The latter is formed by the septum secundum and occupies the right side of the atrial septum. Tissue of the septum primum lying to the left of the foramen ovale serves as a flap valve that usually becomes fused postnatally with the side of the foramen ovale, yielding an anatomically closed or sealed foramen. "Probe patency," or an incomplete seal of the foramen ovale, occurs in about 25 per cent of adults. A widely patent foramen ovale may be considered an acquired form of atrial septal defect that occurs especially when a disproportion exists between the size of the foramen ovale and the effective length of its valve. Enlargement of the foramen ovale per se is commonly associated with obstructive lesions on the right side of the heart, whereas a short valve relative to the size of the foramen often is seen in large-volume left-to-right shunts in which left atrial dilatation is prominent.

Ostium primum atrial septal anomalies are a form of atrioventricular septal defect and are dealt with in the next section. Lutembacher's syndrome is a designation applied to the rare combination of atrial septal defect and mitral stenosis, which is almost invariably the result of acquired rheumatic valvulitis.[124] Ten to 20 per cent of patients with ostium secundum atrial septal defect also have prolapse of the mitral valve as an associated anomaly.[125]

HEMODYNAMICS. The magnitude of the left-to-right shunt through an atrial septal defect depends on the size of the defect and the relative compliance of the ventricles, and the relative resistance in both the pulmonary and the systemic circulation.[126] In patients with a small atrial septal defect or patent foramen ovale, the left atrial pressure may exceed the right by several millimeters of mercury, whereas the mean pressures in both atria are nearly identical when the defect is large. Left-to-right shunting occurs predominantly in late ventricular systole and early diastole with some augmentation during atrial contraction. The shunt results in diastolic overloading of the right ventricle and increased pulmonary blood flow. During the first few days and weeks of life, pulmonary resistance falls and systemic resistance rises, facilitating right ventricular emptying and impeding left ventricular emptying; the left-to-right shunt rises. Early in infancy left-to-right flow through even a large interatrial communication commonly is limited by both the reduced chamber compliance of the thick neonatal right ventricle and the elevated pulmonary and reduced systemic vascular resistance of the neonate. The pulmonary vascular resistance commonly is normal or low in the older infant or child with atrial septal defect, and the volume load usually is well tolerated, even though pulmonary blood flow may be two to five times greater than systemic. A transient and small right-to-left shunt occurring with the onset of left ventricular contraction and especially during respiratory periods of decreasing intrathoracic pressure is common in patients with ostium secundum defect, even in the absence of pulmonary hypertension.

CLINICAL FINDINGS. Patients with atrial septal defect usually are asymptomatic early in life, although occasional reports exist of congestive heart failure and recurrent pneumonia in infancy.[122] Children with atrial septal defect may experience easy fatigability and exertional dyspnea. They tend to be somewhat underdeveloped physically and prone to respiratory infection. Atrial arrhythmias, pulmonary arterial hypertension, development of pulmonary vascular obstruction, and heart failure are exceedingly uncommon in the pediatric age range, in contrast to their common appearance in adults with atrial septal defect. In the former group, diagnosis often is entertained after detection of a heart murmur on routine physical examination prompts a more extensive cardiac evaluation.

Physical Examination. Common findings include a prominent right ventricular cardiac impulse and palpable pulmonary artery pulsation. The first heart sound is normal or split, with accentuation of the tricuspid valve closure sound. Increased flow across the pulmonic valve is responsible for a midsystolic pulmonary ejection murmur. After the normal postnatal drop in pulmonary vascular resistance, the second heart sound is split widely and is relatively fixed in relation to respiration in patients with normal pulmonary pressures and low pulmonary vascular impedance because of a delay in pulmonic valve closure. With pulmonary hypertension the splitting interval is a function of the electromechanical intervals of each ventricle; wide splitting occurs with shortening of the left and/or lengthening of the right ventricular electromechanical interval.[127] If the shunt is large, increased blood flow across the tricuspid valve is responsible for a mid-diastolic rumbling murmur at the lower left sternal border. In patients with associated prolapse of the mitral valve, an apical holosystolic or late systolic murmur radiating to the axilla often is heard, but a midsystolic click may be difficult to discern. Moreover, left ventricular precordial overactivity usually is absent because mitral regurgitation is mild in most patients.

In the teenage patient, the physical findings may be altered when an increase in pulmonary vascular resistance results in diminution of the left-to-right shunt. Both the pulmonary and the tricuspid murmurs decrease in intensity, whereas the pulmonic component of the second heart sound becomes accentuated and the two components of the second heart sound may fuse; a diastolic murmur of pul-

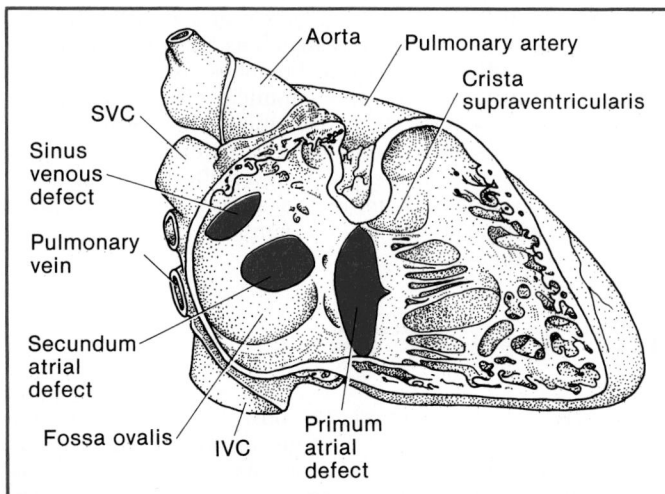

FIGURE 29–9. Composite locations of atrial defects. SVC = superior vena cava, IVC = inferior vena cava.

monic incompetence appears. Cyanosis and clubbing accompany development of a right-to-left shunt.

Electrocardiogam. In patients with an ostium secundum defect, the electrocardiogram usually shows right-axis deviation, right ventricular hypertrophy, and rSR′ or rsR′ pattern in the right precordial leads with a normal QRS duration (Fig. 29–10). It is not clear whether the delay in right ventricular activation is a manifestation of right ventricular volume overload or a true conduction delay in the right bundle branch and peripheral Purkinje system.[128] Left-axis deviation of the P wave in the frontal plane (manifested by a negative P wave in lead III) suggests the presence of a sinus venosus rather than an ostium secundum type of atrial septal defect. Left-axis deviation and superior orientation and counterclockwise rotation of the QRS loop in the frontal plane suggests the presence of either an ostium primum defect or a secundum atrial septal defect in association with mitral valve prolapse. Prolongation of the P-R interval may be seen with all types of atrial septal defects; the prolonged internodal conduction time may be related to both the increased size of the atrium and the increased distance for internodal conduction produced by the defect itself.[128]

Chest Roentgenogram (Figs. 7–43, p. 232). This usually reveals enlargement of the right atrium and ventricle, dilatation of the pulmonary artery and its branches, and increased pulmonary vascular markings. Dilatation of the proximal portion of the superior vena cava occasionally is noted in patients with a sinus venosus defect. Left atrial dilatation is extremely rare but may be observed when significant mitral regurgitation exists.

Echocardiographic Features. These include pulmonary arterial and right ventricular dilatation and anterior systolic (paradoxical) or "flat" interventricular septal motion if significant right ventricular volume overload is present.[108] The defect may be visualized directly by two-dimensional echo imaging, particularly from a subcostal view of the interatrial septum[46] (Fig. 29–11; also see Fig. 3–77, p. 82). Transesophageal color-coded Doppler echocardiography

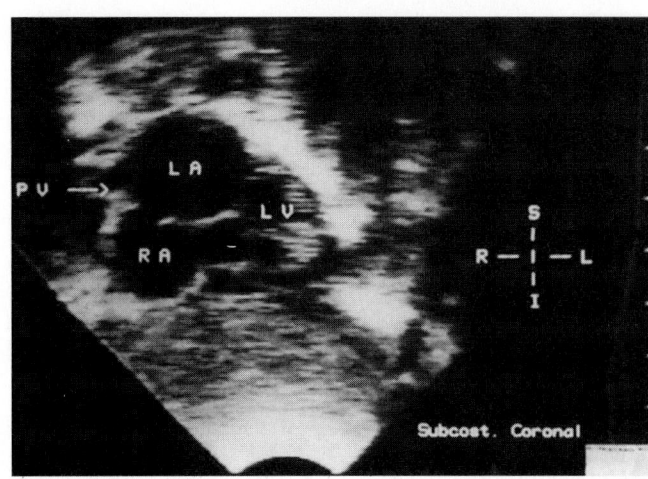

FIGURE 29–11. Subcostal coronal view showing a secundum atrial septal defect between the left atrium (LA) and the right atrium (RA). The right upper pulmonary vein (PV) is seen entering the left atrium. This view is posterior to the major portion of the ventricles; the left ventricle (LV) is seen, but only a small portion of the right ventricle (unlabeled) is apparent. I = inferior, L = left, R = right, S = superior. (Courtesy of Norman Silverman, M.D.)

provides excellent visualization of defects of the atrial septum.[129,130] Associated mitral valve prolapse also may be identified by echocardiographic examination (Figs. 3–51, p. 73 and 3–52, p. 74). Findings on ultrafast computed tomographic scanning are discussed on page 342.

Two-dimensional echocardiography, supplemented by conventional or color-coded Doppler flow and/or contrast echocardiography, has supplanted cardiac catheterization as the confirmatory test for atrial septal defect.[131,132] Cardiac catheterization is then used if inconsistencies exist in the clinical data or if significant pulmonary hypertension is suspected.

Cardiac Catheterization. Diagnosis may be readily confirmed by passage of the catheter across the atrial defect. The site at which the catheter crosses, if high in the cardiac silhouette, may suggest a sinus venosus defect; if midseptal, a patent foramen ovale or ostium secundum defect; or, if low, a primum defect.[133] Serial determinations of the oxygen saturation or indicator dilution curve techniques may be used to estimate the magnitude of the shunt. In the absence of pulmonary hypertension, pressures on the right side of the heart often are normal, despite a large shunt. When a high oxygen saturation is found in the superior vena cava or when the catheter enters pulmonary veins directly from the right atrium, a sinus venosus defect is likely, and indicator dilution curves and selective angiography aid in identifying the number and location of the anomalous veins. *Partial anomalous pulmonary venous connection,* although usually associated with sinus venosus defect, may accompany secundum defects. Selective left ventricular angiography identifies prolapse of the mitral valve and allows assessment of the magnitude of mitral regurgitation that may be present in such patients.

MANAGEMENT. In contrast to adults, children with sinus venosus or secundum types of atrial septal defect seldom require treatment for heart failure or antiarrhythmic medications for atrial fibrillation or supraventricular tachycardia. Respiratory tract infections should be treated promptly. Although the risk of infective endocarditis is low, antibiotics should be administered prophylactically before dental procedures.

Operative Repair. This should be advised for all patients with uncomplicated atrial septal defects in whom there is evidence of significant left-to-right shunting, i.e., with pulmonary-systemic flow ratios exceeding about 1.5 : 1.0. Ideally, this should be carried out in those 2 to 4

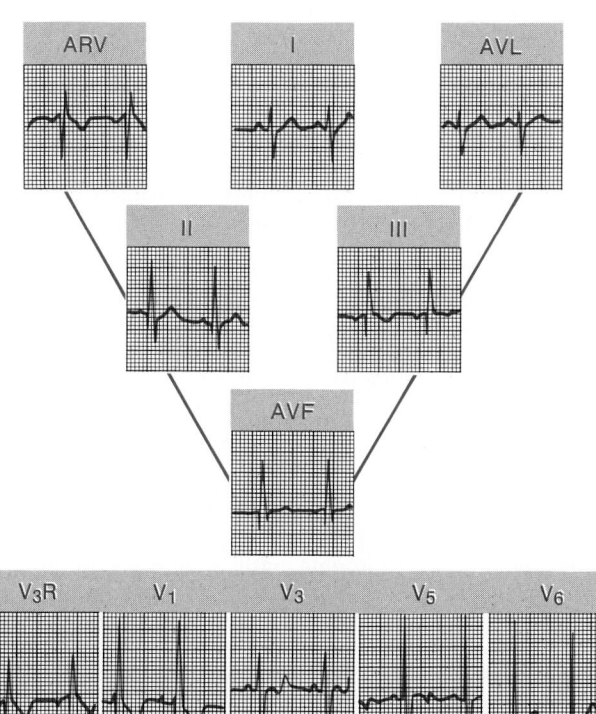

FIGURE 29–10. Typical electrocardiographic tracing in secundum atrial septal defect showing right axis deviation, rSR′ in the right pericordial leads, and right ventricular hypertrophy. (Courtesy of Delores A. Danilowicz, M.D.)

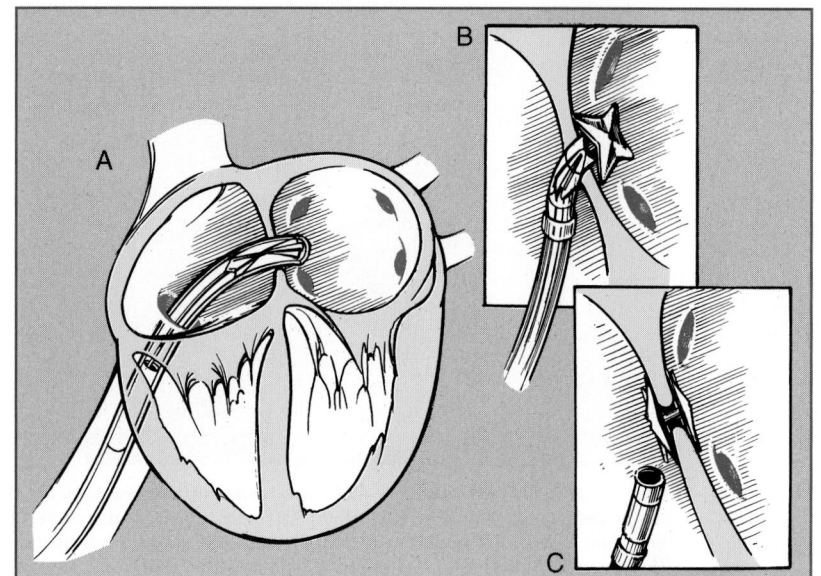

FIGURE 29–12. Clam-shell umbrella occlusion of an ostium secundum atrial septal defect. A long sheath is positioned in the left atrium (*A*). *B*, The distal umbrella arms are opened in the left atrium and the umbrella and sheath are pulled back together to the atrial septum. *C*, The proximal set of arms is then delivered on the right atrial side of the atrial septum. The correct position of the device is confirmed by fluoroscopy, angiography, and echocardiography before it is released. (From Castaneda, A., et al.: Cardiac Surgery of the Neonate and Infant. Philadelphia, W.B. Saunders Company, 1994, p. 136.)

years of age. Rarely, an atrial septal aneurysm is seen in association with a secundum-type atrial septal defect.[134] Such patients may experience spontaneous closure and may be followed more conservatively until an older age before advising operation. The defect is closed by suture or with a patch of prosthetic material with the patient on cardiopulmonary bypass. Earlier surgical repair is definitive treatment for the small number of infants and young children with significant symptoms or congestive failure. The surgical mortality rate is less than 1 per cent, and results usually are excellent. Although the mitral valve may be examined directly at operation, it seldom is necessary in childhood to attempt plication or replacement of a ballooning or prolapsing mitral valve.

Operation should *not* be carried out in patients with small defects and trivial left-to-right shunts (pulmonary-systemic flow ratio $\leq 1.5:1.0$) or in those with severe pulmonary vascular disease (pulmonary-systemic resistance ratio $\geq 0.7:1.0$) without a significant left-to-right shunt.[135] Still investigational is the use of transcatheter closure by way of a clam-shell-configuration double umbrella or a buttoned device using fluoroscopic or transesophageal echocardiographic imaging guidance[114,136–138a] (Fig. 29–12). Limitations include difficulties in centering the device, the need to use a large sheath delivery system, the need to have more than a 4-mm separation between the edges of the defect and other important cardiac structures, and the inability to close defects whose stretched diameter exceeds 22 mm.[114,136–138a]

Subtle evidence of left ventricular dysfunction may be observed preoperatively at cardiac catheterization in children with isolated large atrial septal defects but without overt left or right ventricular failure.[139] Thus decreased left ventricular stroke volume and cardiac output have been observed in children with both low and normal left ventricular end-diastolic volumes. In routine catheterization studies carried out on patients whose atrial septal defects were closed during preadolescence or later, a residual reduced cardiac output response to intense upright exercise in the absence of residual shunts, arrhythmias, or pulmonary arterial hypertension has been observed.[140] Normal myocardial function is preserved in patients in whom the defects were closed in early childhood.[141]

Electrophysiological Abnormalities. Intracardiac electrophysiological studies reveal a high incidence of intrinsic dysfunction of the sinoatrial and atrioventricular nodes, which persists after surgical repair. These intrinsic nodal abnormalities are more common in sinus venosus than in ostium secundum defects[142,143] but occur in both varieties.

There also is evidence that the type of venous cannulation at the time of operative repair may contribute to the incidence and severity of arrhythmias observed at long-term follow-up.[144]

Atrioventricular (AV) Septal Defect

AV septal defects account for 4 to 5 per cent of congenital heart defects and comprise a range of malformations characterized by varying degrees of incomplete development of the inferior portion of the atrial septum, the inflow portion of the ventricular septum, and the AV valves (Fig. 29–1). These anomalies also have been called endocardial cushion defects and AV canal defects. The basic defect is a deficiency of the AV septum which separates the left ventricular inlet from the right atrium; it causes anomalies that range in severity from a small ostium primum atrial defect to a complete AV septal malformation that also involves defects in the interventricular septum and the mitral and tricuspid valves. The latter often are abnormal to varying degrees, with five or six leaflets present of variable size, and variability also in the completeness of their commissures. Often AV septal defects are encountered in association with other congenital abnormalities, such as asplenia or polysplenia syndromes, trisomy 21 (Down syndrome), and Ellis–van Creveld syndrome of ectodermal dysplasia and polydactyly.

OSTIUM PRIMUM DEFECT (PARTIAL AV CANAL). Ostium primum atrial septal defects lie immediately adjacent to the AV valves, either of which may be deformed and incompetent. Most often only the anterior or septal leaflet of the mitral valve is displaced, and it commonly is cleft; the tricuspid valve usually is not involved. A cleft often is considered to be present in the mitral valve, although it is likely that the valve is in fact a trileaflet structure, with the cleft representing an abnormal commissure. The interatrial defect often is large, and the size of the left-to-right interatrial shunt in these patients is controlled by the same factors that exist in patients with ostium secundum atrial septal defect. Moreover, the clinical features are quite similar and principally consist of right ventricular precordial hyperactivity, a wide and persistently split second heart sound, a right ventricular outflow tract systolic ejection murmur, and a mid-diastolic tricuspid flow rumble. The murmurs of AV valve regurgitation may be audible if either valve is significantly abnormal; however, serious AV valve regurgitation usually is absent. In the occasional patient, mitral regurgitation is substantial and creates prominent signs of left ventricular overload.

Chest roentgenography usually reveals right atrial and ventricular cardiomegaly, prominence of the right ventricular outflow tract, and increased pulmonary vascular markings. The *electrocardiogram* is characteristic, and shows a right ventricular conduction defect accompanied by left anterior division block, left-axis deviation, and superior orientation and counterclockwise rotation of the QRS loop in the frontal plane (Fig. 4–21, p. 123).[145] Hemodynamic factors do not appear to be important in producing the characteristic electrocardiogram. Rather, the superior QRS vector in patients with a shortened H-V interval appears to be related to early activation of the posterobasal left ventricular wall; in other patients with a normal conduction time between the bundle of His and the ventricles, the counterclockwise superior inscription of the frontal plane vector appears to be related to late activation of the anterolateral left ventricular wall.[146] A prolonged P-R interval is observed in many patients with an ostium primum atrial septal defect; prolonged internodal conduction may be related to displacement of the AV node in a posteroinferior direction in some patients or to the enlarged right atrium, or both.[147]

Echocardiography. Two-dimensional echocardiography is considered the standard for the diagnosis of all forms of AV septal defect (Fig. 3–77, p. 82). Important features include enlargement of both the right ventricle and the pulmonary artery, systolic anterior ventricular septal motion, prolonged mitral-septal apposition in diastole, and various abnormalities in mitral valve motion.[148,149] The defect is easily visualized from the precordial apical and subxiphoid positions, with the latter views best demonstrating the relation between the atrial defect, AV valves, and the interventricular septum (Figs. 29–13 and 3–81, p. 83, color plate No. 4). Interatrial septal tissue is absent in the region of the crest of the interventricular septum; the trileaflet configuration of the mitral valve also may be identified. The subxiphoid long-axis view of the left ventricular outflow tract exhibits the "gooseneck" deformity in a manner similar to that with a right anterior oblique left ventricular angiogram. Echocardiography is particularly useful for detecting and characterizing double-orifice mitral valve, an association in about 3 per cent of patients with ostium primum atrial defect. It also allows detection of single left ventricular papillary muscle, hypoplasia of the left ventricle, and coarctation of the aorta, seen especially in symptomatic infants with an ostium primum atrial defect but without trisomy 21.[150] The *angiographic features* resemble those in the complete form of AV septal defect and are discussed below.

Morphology. The complete form of the AV septal defect includes, in addition to the ostium primum atrial septal defect, a ventricular septal defect in the posterior basal inlet portion of the ventricular septum and a common AV orifice. The common AV valve usually has six leaflets: left superior and inferior, left and right lateral, and right superior and inferior. The left and right superior leaflets together often are referred to as the "anterior" bridging leaflet. No attachment exists between the left superior and inferior leaflets and the right superior and inferior leaflets. The left superior leaflet may cross the crest of the ventricular septum to reside partially on the right ventricular side. A classification of complete AV canal defect into types A, B, and C reflects the variability and the degree of anterior leaflet bridging of the ventricular septum (Fig. 29–14). Thus in type A the anterior leaflet is almost entirely committed to the left ventricle and is attached by chordae tendineae to the crest of the ventricular septum. In type C there is marked rightward displacement of the anterior bridging leaflet, which floats freely over the crest of the ventricular septum and is not attached to it by chordae tendineae. In type B chordal attachments extend medially to an anomalous papillary muscle adjacent to the septum in the right ventricle.

A high incidence (about 35 per cent) of additional cardiovascular lesions exists in patients with common AV canal. Principal among those associated with type C are tetralogy of Fallot, double-outlet right ventricle, transposition of the great arteries, and asplenia and polysplenia syndromes. Moreover, the type A complete AV septal anomaly commonly is seen in patients with Down syndrome.

The designation *unbalanced atrioventricular canal* is applied to the condition in which one ventricle is hypoplastic and the other receives most of the common AV valve. Subaortic obstruction may be due to abnormal features of the left side of the common AV valve or to hypoplasia of the left ventricle. The left-sided (mitral) component may also be the site of a potential form of double orifice mitral stenosis postoperatively.

Diagnosis. Patients with common AV septal defects present clinically under age 1 year with a history of frequent respiratory infections and poor weight gain. Heart failure in infancy is extremely common. The *physical findings* are similar to those observed in patients with ostium primum atrial septal defect but may include as well the holosystolic, lower left sternal border murmur of an interventricular communication and/or the decrescendo, holosystolic apical murmur of mitral regurgitation. The *electro-*

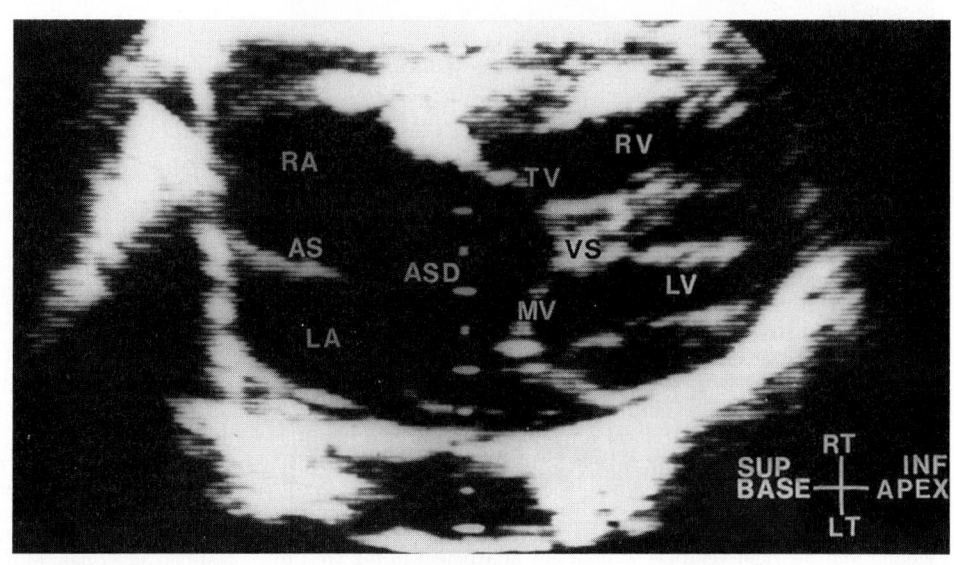

FIGURE 29–13. Subcostal four-chamber view showing an ostium primum atrial septal defect (ASD). There is echo dropout in the inferior portion of the atrial septum (AS). RA = right atrium, LA = left atrium, TV = tricuspid valve, MV = mitral valve, VS = ventricular septum, RV = right ventricle, LV = left ventricle. (Courtesy of Thomas DiSessa, M.D.)

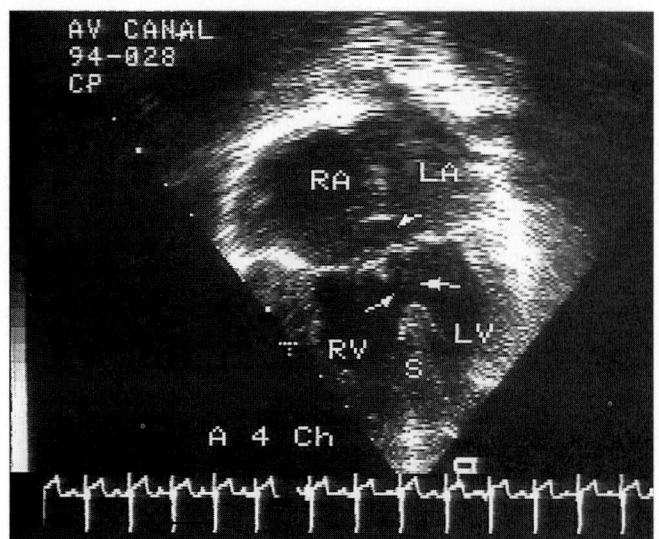

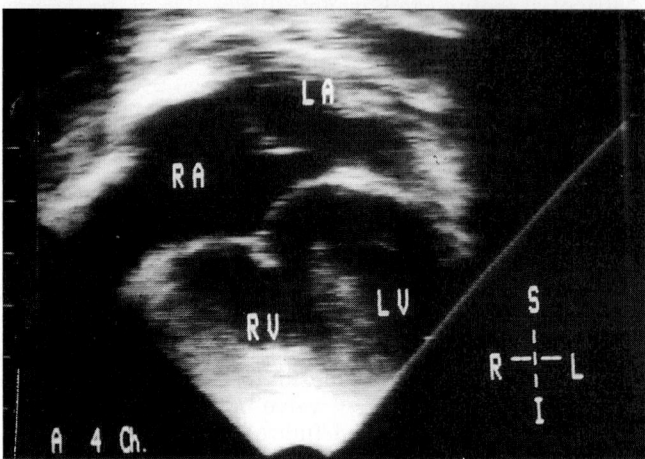

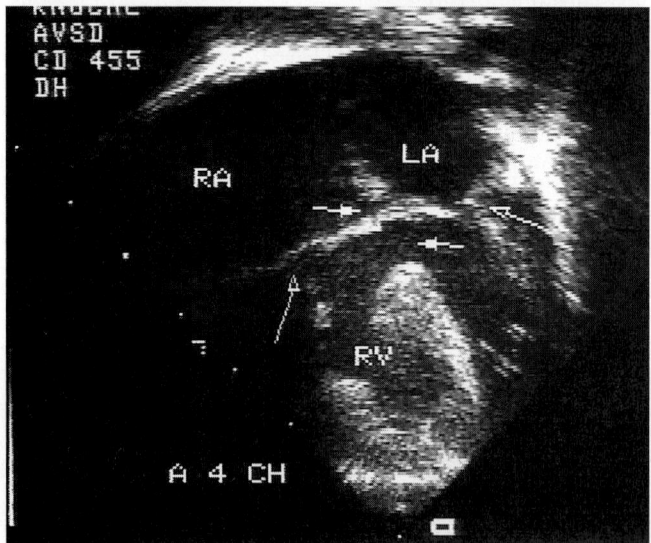

FIGURE 29–14. Composite of atrioventricular septal defects in apical four chamber views. *Top,* Atrioventricular septal defect of Rastelli type A variety. The arrows indicate the positions of the interatrial and interventricular communications. A common atrioventricular valve leaflet can be seen to straddle the defects, and the arrows in the ventricle identify the position of the chordae tendineae attached to the crest of the septum from the anterior superior bridging leaflet. *Middle,* Atrioventricular septal defect, Rastelli type B, in which the anterior superior bridging leaflet is not attached to the crest of the septum, but rather attaches to a papillary muscle within the right ventricle. *Bottom,* Rastelli type C, the so-called free-floating anterior superior bridging leaflet, indicated by the arrows. The leaflet arises from a papillary muscle within the left ventricle and straddles the septum into the right ventricle without any attachment to the crest of

cardiographic features of complete AV canal defects resemble those in the partial ostium primum variety of AV septal anomalies (Fig. 29–11). *Radiographically,* the usual findings are generalized cardiomegaly and engorged pulmonary vessels.

Two-dimensional echocardiography is diagnostic (Figs. 29–14 and 3–79, p. 83).[148,149] Apical and subcostal views are used to determine the size of the septal defects, the commitment of valve tissue and chordal attachments to the ventricles, ventricular size, the magnitude of AV valve insufficiency, and the anatomy of the left ventricular outflow tract. The subcostal oblique coronal view is often best to evaluate the commitment of AV valve tissue to each ventricle. Patterns of shunting and the number and magnitude of regurgitant jets are best evaluated by using pulsed, continuous-wave, and color flow Doppler imaging. On *hemodynamic study,* patients with persistent common AV canal invariably have elevated pulmonary arterial pressures; beyond age 2 years a significant number of these patients have progressively severe pulmonary vascular obstructive disease.

Diagnosis also is reliably established by selective left ventricular *angiocardiography* using rapid injection of relatively large quantities of contrast material.[151] The findings include an absence of the AV septum and a deficiency of the inlet portion of the ventricular septum, with elongation of the left ventricular outflow tract in relation to the inflow tract. The aortic valve is elevated and displaced anteriorly relative to the AV valves, changing the relation between the anterior components of the left AV valve and the aorta, which produces a pathognomonic "gooseneck" deformity seen angiographically in diastole.

Management. In patients with complete AV canal, cardiac decompensation should be controlled initially. Even if there is an adequate response to medical therapy early in life, operation should be considered before age 6 months because infants with a complete form of the AV septal defect are at high risk of obstructive pulmonary vascular disease. The level of major shunting should be determined by echocardiographic–Doppler data, or less often during initial hemodynamic and angiographic study because if it is mainly at the ventricular level, pulmonary artery banding occasionally may be advised for intractable heart failure and failure to thrive. Often, however, there is a significant left ventricular–right atrial shunt either directly or indirectly by way of mitral regurgitation and left-to-right interatrial shunting, which will be unaffected by pulmonary artery banding and requires complete surgical correction.

SURGICAL REPAIR. In most centers primary repair in patients who have intractable heart failure, growth failure, or severe pulmonary hypertension is the preferred approach at any age.[152] Mild to moderate regurgitation often persists after surgical repair, particularly if significant AV valve incompetence existed preoperatively.[153] Rarely, if left AV leaflet tissue is remarkably deficient or deformed, mitral valve replacement may be required. Recent advances in the surgical approach to complex forms of AV septal defects have greatly improved the outlook for patients born with this malformation.[154,155] These include better reconstruction of the mitral valve (Fig. 29–15) and a more precise preoperative detection of such anatomical features as additional muscular ventricular septal defects, malalignment of the complete AV septum, and left ventricular hypoplasia. Operative improvement is primarily related to a clearer understanding of the anatomy of this complex lesion and to the ability to reconstruct the left AV valve, often by splitting of

the ventricular septum and attaches to the anterior papillary muscle lying within the right ventricle. Orientation: S = superior, I = inferior, R = right, L = left. LA = left atrium, LV = left ventricle, RA = right atrium, RV = right ventricle, S = ventricular septum. (Courtesy of Norman Silverman, M.D.)

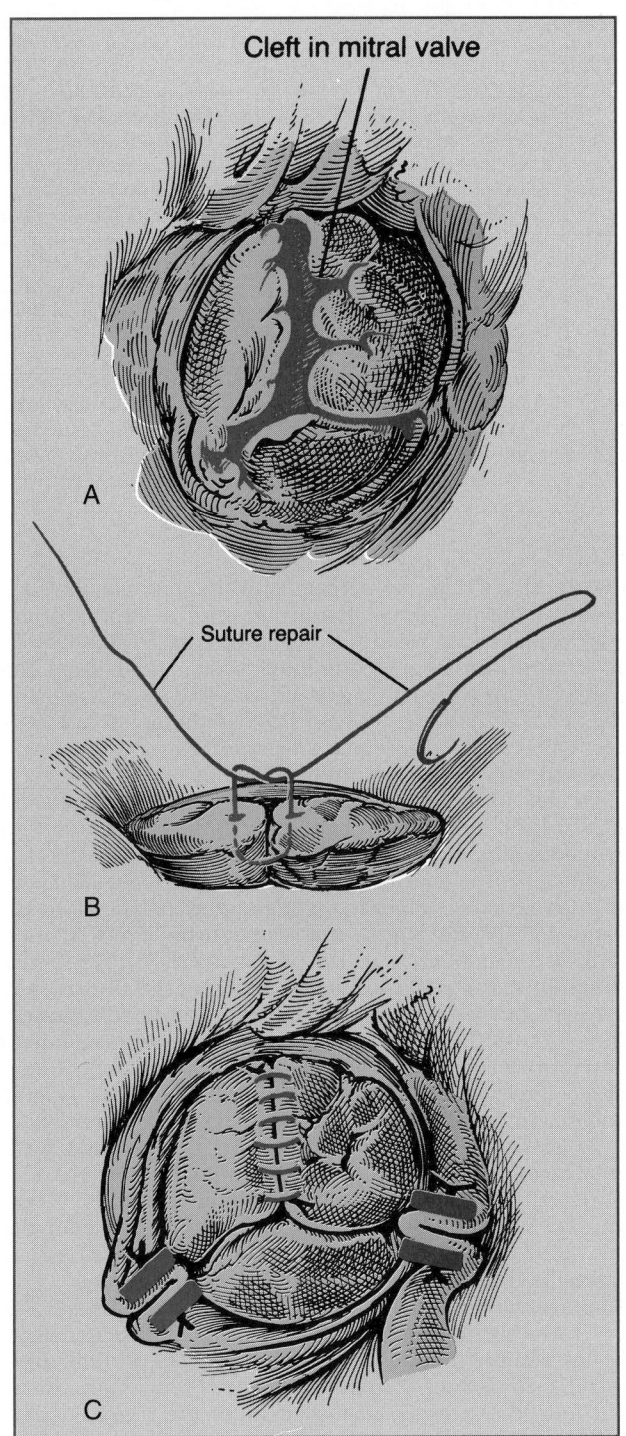

Cleft in mitral valve

A

Suture repair

B

C

FIGURE 29–15. A suture technique is illustrated for repair of a cleft mitral valve *(A)*. Absolute alignment of the cleft in all its dimensions is of critical importance with placement of the sutures where the edges naturally coapt *(B)*. *C,* The cleft repair is accompanied by annuloplasty. (From Castaneda, A., et al.: Cardiac Surgery of the Neonate and Infant. Philadelphia, W.B. Saunders Company, 1994, p. 174.)

papillary muscles and shortening of cordae tendineae, with or without annuloplasty. Many surgeons prefer to close the septal defects with a single patch rather than separating ventricular and atrial patches. Suture placement is avoided in the region of the AV node and the bundle of His.

Ventricular Septal Defect
(See also p. 967)

MORPHOLOGY. Among the most prevalent of cardiac malformations, defects of the ventricular septum occur commonly, both as isolated anomalies and in combination with other anomalies. The ventricular septum is made up of four compartments: the membranous septum, the inlet septum, the trabecular septum, and the outlet, or infundibular, septum. Defects result from a deficiency of growth or a failure of alignment or fusion of component parts. Defects most commonly are classified as occurring in or adjacent to one or more of the septal components (Fig. 29–16).[156–159]

The most common defects occur in the region of the membranous septum, and are referred to as *paramembranous* or *perimembranous defects* because they are larger than the membranous septum itself and are associated with a muscular defect at a portion of their perimeter. They also are known as infracrital, subaortic, or conoventricular defects. These perimembranous defects also can be defined by their adjacent areas as inlet, trabecular, or outlet. A second type of defect is one with an entirely muscular rim. Such muscular defects also can be defined as inlet, trabecular, central, apical, marginal or "Swiss cheese," or outlet and vary greatly in size, shape, and number. A third type of defect occurs when the outlet septum is deficient and commonly is referred to as supracristal, subpulmonary, outlet, infundibular, or conoseptal. Because the aortic and pulmonary valves are in fibrous continuity, this type of defect also may be referred to as doubly committed subarterial. A septal deficiency of the site of the atrioventricular septum characterizes defects called atrioventricular septal, atrioventricular canal, or inlet septal defects.

The other feature of any defect may be a malalignment of the septal components. Either the inlet or the outlet septum can be malaligned. Malalignment of the inlet septum produces either mitral or tricuspid valve override and/or straddle. Malalignment of the outlet septum can be to the right or the left of the trabecular septum; when to the left of the trabecular septum, the ventricular septal defect is characteristic of tetralogy of Fallot, double-outlet ventricle, truncus arteriosus, and, in some cases, transposition of the great arteries.

ECHOCARDIOGRAPHY. Two-dimensional and Doppler echocardiography identify the type of defect in the ventricular septum.[160–163] Perimembranous ventricular septal defects are identified by septal dropout in the area behind the septal leaflet of the tricuspid valve and below the right border of the aortic annulus. The subaortic or anterior malalignment type of ventricular septal defect appears just below the posterior semilunar valve cusps, entirely superior to the tricuspid valve. The subpulmonary ventricular septal defect appears as echo dropout within the outflow septum, which extends to the pulmonary annulus. One or two of the aortic cusps may be visualized protruding through the defect into the right ventricular outflow tract. The inlet atrioventricular septal–type of ventricular septal defect extends from the fibrous annulus of the tricuspid valve into the muscular septum and often is entirely beneath the septal tricuspid leaflet. Muscular defects may appear anywhere throughout the ventricular septum and may be either large and single or small and multiple. Anatomical localization of all ventricular septal defects is facilitated by coupling two-dimensional ultrasound images (Fig. 3–75, p. 82) with a Doppler system and also by superimposing a color-coded direction and velocity of blood flow on the real-time images.[163–167]

Pulmonary and systemic blood flow can be calculated from arterial velocity profiles and cross-sectional areas of the great vessels. The calculation of pulmonary/systemic flow ratios is reasonably accurate. The detection of jets within the right ventricle allows determination of right ventricular pressure by subtracting the product using the Bernoulli equation, which gives the pressure difference, from the systemic systolic blood pressure. Continuous-wave Doppler has been helpful in determining the right ventricular pressure from tricuspid insufficiency which is found fairly often with ventricular septal defects. Many other techniques of Doppler measurement have been used with

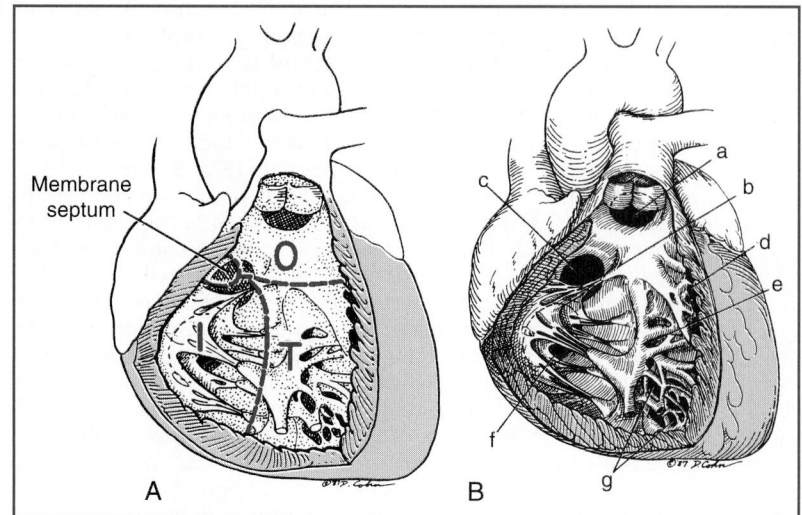

Membrane
septum

FIGURE 29–16. *A,* The four components of the ventricular septum viewed from the right ventricular side. I = inlet component extends from tricuspid annulus to attachments of the tricuspid valve, T = trabecular septum extends from inlet out to the apex and up to the smooth-walled outlet, O = outlet septum or infundibular septum extends up to the pulmonary valve and membranous septum. *B,* The anatomical position of ventricular septal defects. a = outlet defect, b = papillary muscle of the conus, c = perimembranous defect, d = marginal muscular defects, e = central muscular defects, f = inlet defect, g = apical muscular defects. (From Graham, T. P., Jr., and Gutgesell, H. P.: Ventricular septal defects. *In* Emmanouilides, G. C., Allen, H. D., et al. (eds.): Moss and Adams' Heart Disease in Infants, Children and Adolescents. 5th ed. Baltimore, © Williams and Wilkins, 1994, p. 724.)

varying success in efforts to accurately determine pulmonary arterial pressure.

PATHOPHYSIOLOGY. The functional disturbance caused by a ventricular septal defect depends primarily on its size and the status of the pulmonary vascular bed rather than on the location of the defect. A small ventricular septal defect with high resistance to flow permits only a small left-to-right shunt. A large interventricular communication allows a large left-to-right shunt only if there is no pulmonic stenosis or high pulmonary vascular resistance because these factors also determine shunt flow. Resistance to left ventricular emptying also affects shunt flow because it is an important factor in determining left ventricular pressure. Large defects allow both ventricles to function hemodynamically as a single pumping chamber with two outlets, equalizing the pressure in the systemic and pulmonary circulations. In such patients the magnitude of the left-to-right shunt varies inversely with pulmonary vascular resistance.

A wide spectrum exists in the natural history of ventricular septal defects, ranging from spontaneous closure to congestive cardiac failure and death in early infancy. Within this spectrum are possible development of pulmonary vascular obstruction, right ventricular outflow tract obstruction, aortic regurgitation, and infective endocarditis.[167–176]

INFANTS. It is unusual for a ventricular septal defect to cause difficulties in the immediate postnatal period, although congestive heart failure during the first 6 months of life is a frequent occurrence. Early diagnosis is helpful to ensure more careful observation of the affected infant.[172] The examining physician usually suspects the diagnosis because of a harsh systolic murmur at the lower left sternal border. The electrocardiogram and chest roentgenogram are within normal limits in the immediate neonatal period because appreciable left-to-right shunting occurs only after the pulmonary vascular resistance decreases as the pulmonary vessels lose their fetal characteristics. It is desirable to follow these infants closely.

A ventricular septal defect that either decreases in size or closes completely during the first year of life presents no problems to the practicing physician. Spontaneous closure occurs by age 3 years in about 45 per cent of patients born with ventricular septal defect; occasional patients, however, do not experience spontaneous closure until age 8 to 10 years or even later.[170] Closure is more common in patients born with a small ventricular septal defect; nonetheless, about 7 per cent of infants with a large defect and congestive heart failure early in life also may experience spontaneous closure. Partial rather than complete closure is common in patients with both large and small ventricular septal defects. Anatomically, reduction of the ventricular septal defect often is based on adherence of the tricuspid valve to the defect, hypertrophy of septal muscle, or ingrowth of fibrous tissue. Rarely, closure of the ventricular septal defect is the result of prolapse of an aortic cusp[173] or infective endocarditis.[176] Some defects close when an aneurysm forms in the ventricular septum.[171] On auscultation a click may be heard in early systole as the aneurysm tenses toward the right; the septal aneurysm may be detected by echocardiography as an anterior systolic bulge in the right ventricular outflow tract. A persistent minute ventricular septal defect is not life-threatening unless infective endocarditis develops. With proper precautions (see p. 974), the incidence of this complication is less than 1 per cent.

If a moderate or large defect maintains its size after birth, the net left-to-right shunt increases during the first month of life as pulmonary vascular resistance falls. *Physical examination* during this time usually reveals a thrill along the lower left sternal border, and the holosystolic murmur of flow across the interventricular defect is accompanied by a low-pitched diastolic rumble at the apex, reflecting increased flow across the mitral valve. *Chest roentgenograms* reveal increased pulmonary vascular markings; evidence of left or biventricular hypertrophy may be observed on the electrocardiogram. Infants with a large left-to-right shunt tend to do poorly, with recurrent upper and lower respiratory tract infections, failure to gain weight, and congestive heart failure. Congestive heart failure may be severe and intractable despite intensive medical management.

Management. This author currently recommends primary intracardiac repair of the ventricular septal defect at any age rather than surgical banding of the pulmonary artery[177,178] to reduce pulmonary blood flow and alleviate heart failure. An exception is made for the rare infant with multiple ventricular septal defects and a sievelike septum, who is at higher risk for complications following operative repair. Operation usually is deferred, along with debanding of the pulmonary artery, until the child reaches 3 to 5 years. Primary closure of the ventricular septal defect, preferably through the right atrium, may be performed in infancy using cardiopulmonary bypass, profound hypothermia and cardiocirculatory arrest, or a combination of the two techniques. Mortality approaches zero in major centers if the defect is isolated and uncomplicated but approaches 10 per cent if multiple anomalies are present.[179]

Fortunately, medical treatment often is successful in controlling congestive heart failure. Nevertheless, these infants should be referred for cardiac catheterization to evaluate pulmonary vascular resistance and to detect associated defects that may require operation, such as patent ductus arteriosus and coarctation of the aorta.

CHILDREN. Beyond the first year of life a variable clinical picture emerges in children with ventricular septal defect.[170–172,176] If a small defect is present, the child usually is asymptomatic, the electrocardiogram usually is normal, and the chest roentgenogram shows normal or only a mild increase in pulmonary vascular markings. Effort intolerance and fatigue are associated with moderate left-to-right shunts. These children exhibit cardiomegaly with a forceful left ventricular impulse and a prominent systolic thrill along the lower left sternal border. The second heart sound normally is split, with moderate accentuation of the pulmonic component; a third heart sound and rumbling diastolic murmur that reflects increased flow across the mitral valve are audible at the cardiac apex. The characteristic murmur resulting from flow across the defect is harsh and holosystolic, is best heard along the third and fourth interspaces to the left of the sternum, and is widely transmitted over the precordium. A basal midsystolic ejection murmur due to increased flow across the pulmonic valve also may be heard. The electrocardiogram reveals left or combined ventricular hypertrophy, and the chest roentgenogram and CT scan (Fig. 7–43, p. 232) show cardiomegaly, left atrial enlargement, and vascular engorgement.

PULMONARY HYPERTENSION. It is of utmost importance to identify patients who may develop irreversible pulmonary vascular obstructive disease (the Eisenmenger reaction).[180–182] Retrospective analyses of children who develop this complication indicate that infants with systemic or near systemic pressures in the pulmonary artery at the time of initial hemodynamic study are most at risk. If early primary closure is not recommended, recatheterization before age 18 months and a second determination of pulmonary vascular resistance should be performed in these patients to decide whether surgical intervention is obligatory to prevent development of fixed obliterative changes in the pulmonary vessels.

Mechanisms. It is likely that multiple factors are involved in the development of pulmonary vascular disease (Chap. 25, p. 781).[61–69] The anatomically large ventricular septal defect allows some or all of the systemic pressure to be transmitted to the pulmonary arteries, thereby retarding regression of their muscular media. Medial hypertrophy in the first months of life is responsible for higher pulmonary vascular resistance than would be anticipated for the amount of pulmonary blood flow. The shearing forces created by the high velocity of flow through narrowed pulmonary arterioles cause endothelial damage that is progressive.

Although an elevation in left atrial pressure may contribute to the rise in pulmonary vascular resistance, it is not an essential factor because pulmonary venous pressures can be low in patients who later develop pulmonary vascular disease. Nonetheless, pulmonary venous hypertension also may contribute to pulmonary arterial vasoconstriction and thus to increased shear forces. In this same regard, pulmonary vasoconstriction enhancing the risk of pulmonary vascular obstruction also may be caused by hypoxia due to either high altitude or lung disease. At high altitudes, large ventricular septal defects have higher pulmonary vascular resistances and smaller shunts than at low altitudes.

Clinical Features. If a child who previously had a loud murmur and thrill associated with poor growth suddenly has a growth spurt, fewer respiratory infections, and a diminution of the intensity of the cardiac murmur and disappearance of the thrill, he or she may be developing severe obliterative changes in the pulmonary vascular bed. An increase in intensity of the pulmonic component of the second heart sound, a reduction in heart size on the chest roentgenogram, and more pronounced right ventricular hypertrophy on the electrocardiogram also are noted. These changes occur because the increased pulmonary vascular resistance causes a decrease in the left-to-right shunt. If these changes are suspected, cardiac catheterization should be repeated; if they are confirmed, prompt surgical repair is indicated before an inoperable predominant right-to-left shunt ensues. If operation is performed under age 2 years, pulmonary vascular resistance may be expected to fall to normal levels.[182]

In older patients the degree to which pulmonary vascular resistance is elevated before operation is a critical factor determining prognosis. If the pulmonary vascular resistance is one-third or less of the systemic value, progressive pulmonary vascular disease after operation is unusual. However, if a moderate-to-severe increase in pulmonary vascular resistance exists preoperatively, either no change or progression of pulmonary vascular disease is common postoperatively. Moreover, the presence of increased pulmonary vascular resistance results in a higher immediate postoperative mortality rate for surgical closure of ventricular septal defect. These observations make it clear that a large ventricular septal defect should be approached surgically very early in life when pulmonary vascular disease is still reversible or has not yet developed (Fig. 29–17).

RIGHT VENTRICULAR OUTFLOW TRACT OBSTRUCTION. With time, the clinical picture changes in 5 to 10 per cent of patients with ventricular septal defect and a moderate to large left-to-right shunt early in

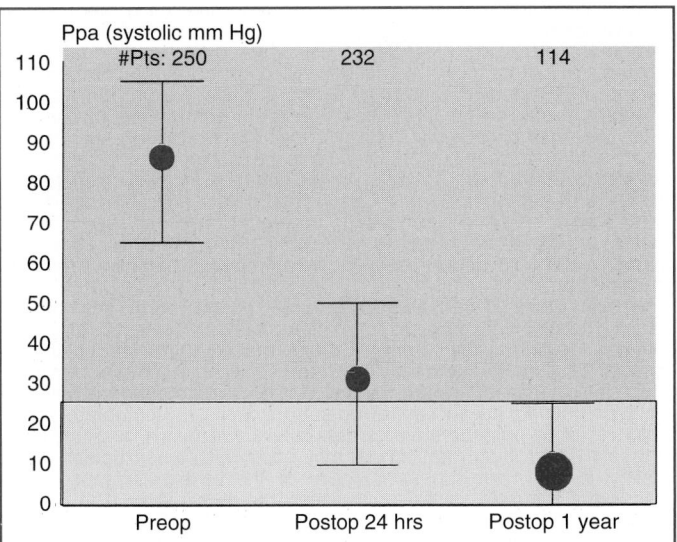

FIGURE 29–17. Early and late postoperative changes of pulmonary artery pressure after closure of ventricular septal defects in infants. (From Castaneda, A., et al.: Cardiac Surgery of the Neonate and Infant. Philadelphia, W.B. Saunders Company, 1994, p. 200.)

life. It begins to resemble more closely the tetralogy of Fallot (see p. 929); i.e., subvalvular right ventricular outflow tract obstruction develops owing to progressive hypertrophy of the crista supraventricularis. Depending on the severity of the latter process, it ultimately may result in reduced blood flow and a right-to-left shunt across the ventricular septal defect. As right ventricular outflow tract obstruction develops, the holosystolic murmur is replaced by the crescendo-decrescendo ejection systolic murmur of pulmonic stenosis, and the pulmonary closure sound becomes softer. Right ventricular hypertrophy is evident on the electrocardiogram, and the chest roentgenogram shows a reduction in pulmonary vascular markings and a smaller heart size with a right ventricular configuration. Infundibular hypertrophy may progress quite rapidly within the first year of life, but the typical evolution to a clinical picture of cyanotic tetralogy of Fallot often takes 1 to 4 years. In those infants who develop right ventricular outflow obstruction the incidence of spontaneous closure or reduction in size of a ventricular septal defect is low.

VENTRICULAR SEPTAL DEFECT WITH AORTIC REGURGITATION. This well-described complication of ventricular septal defect occurs in about 5 per cent of patients.[183,184] It usually is noted after age 5 years when a physician detects the early diastolic blowing murmur and wide pulse pressure of aortic regurgitation while following a patient with a ventricular septal defect. The diagnosis is readily confirmed by Doppler echocardiography. In such patients aortic regurgitation may become the predominant hemodynamic abnormality. It is of interest that ventricular septal defect with aortic regurgitation is rare in Europe and the United States, with an incidence of about 4 per cent of all cases of isolated ventricular septal defect, whereas in Japan the incidence is substantially higher (about 10 per cent). In the Japanese, in particular, aortic regurgitation is the result of herniation of an aortic leaflet (usually the right coronary) through a subpulmonic supracristal ventricular septal defect. In these patients, closure of the ventricular septal defect may be all that is required to relieve aortic regurgitation. In many patients, however, especially in the Western world, the ventricular septal defect is below the infundibular septum (crista supraventricularis). Although aortic leaflet herniation, especially of the right or noncoronary cusp, may occur in some of these patients, quite often aortic regurgitation results from a primary abnormality of the valve, usually one defective commissure. In the latter situation, plication of the elongated leaflet may lessen, but not abolish, the aortic regurgitation; in some patients prosthetic aortic valve replacement may be necessary to provide hemodynamic relief.

In most patients with ventricular septal defect and aortic regurgitation, the ventricular septal defect is small to moderate in size, and mild right ventricular outflow tract obstruction exists. The latter is caused by either subpulmonic infundibular stenosis or projection of the herniated aortic cusp into the right ventricular outflow tract. The distinction between types of ventricular septal defect with aortic regurgitation usually can be made by two-dimensional and Doppler echocardiography and by selective left ventricular angiocardiography to define the site of the interventricular communication in combination with retrograde aortography to assess the anatomy and competence of the aortic valve.[184,185]

Management. Treatment of the patient with ventricular septal defect and aortic regurgitation is controversial. In patients with a large, hemodynamically significant left-to-right shunt, repair of the ventricular septal defect is indicated, but aortic regurgitation is repaired only if at least moderate aortic regurgitation exists. If a supracristal ventricular septal defect without aortic regurgitation is identified at cardiac catheterization in early childhood, a sensible argument for prophylactic closure of the ventricular septal defect can be put forth to prevent the potential complication of aortic valve incompetence. In the presence of moderate or severe aortic regurgitation, valvuloplasty is preferred to valve replacement, in recognition of the fact that the severity of aortic regurgitation may increase in subsequent years and that reoperation with valve replacement may be necessary.[186] Operation should probably be deferred in asymptomatic patients with a subcristal ventricular septal defect and an insignificant left-to-right shunt in whom aortic regurgitation is not severe. If the defect is supracristal in the same clinical setting, its closure may not alleviate the mild degree of aortic incompetence but may retard its progression.

OTHER FORMS OF VENTRICULAR DEFECT. Unusual forms of ventricular septal defect include multiple muscular defects and left ventricular–right atrial communications. Defects in the muscular ventricular septum frequently are multiple small fenestrations that produce a large net left-to-right shunt.[168,187] Their recognition is a necessary preliminary to successful operation because incomplete repair may result in postoperative cardiac failure and death. A shunt from the left ventricle to right atrium may occur with a ventricular septal defect in the most superior portion of the ventricular septum because the tricuspid valve is lower than the mitral valve. The clinical, electrocardiographic, and radiological findings in these patients do not differ appreciably from those in patients with a simple ventricular septal defect, although right atrial enlargement may provide a clue to correct diagnosis of left ventricular–right atrial communication.[188]

The pathophysiology of a single or common ventricle (p. 947) may resemble that of a large ventricular septal defect, although these defects are dissimilar embryologically. The single chamber frequently is the morphological left ventricle; malposition of the great arteries is quite common. There may be no detectable cyanosis if selective streaming and increased pulmonary blood flow rather than complete mixing occurs. Pulmonary hypertension invariably is present unless pulmonic stenosis exists. It is imperative to differentiate a single ventricle from a large ventricular septal defect by echocardiography[162] and angiography[151] because the operative approaches to the former malformation require the atriopulmonary Fontan connection.

MANAGEMENT OF VENTRICULAR SEPTAL DEFECT. It is rarely necessary to restrict the activities of a child with an isolated ventricular septal defect. Infective bacterial endocarditis is always a threat, and antibiotic prophylaxis for dental procedures and minor surgery is indicated (Table 29–4).[189] Respiratory infections require prompt evaluation and treatment. These children should be seen at least once or twice yearly to detect changes in the clinical picture that suggest the development of pulmonary vascular obliterative changes.

Surgical Treatment. When clinical findings suggest a moderate shunt but no pulmonary hypertension, elective hemodynamic evaluation should be advised between ages 3 and 6 years. Of prime importance in the hemodynamic evaluation is a determination of pressure and blood flow in the pulmonary artery.[190] Surgical treatment is not recommended for children who have normal pulmonary arterial pressures with small shunts (pulmonary-systemic flow ratios of less than 1.5 to 2.0:1).[191] In such patients the remaining risk of infective endocarditis does not exceed the risk of operation. Moreover, although the inherent risk of operation is small, the possibility of postoperative heart block, infection, or other complications of operation and cardiopulmonary bypass dictates a conservative approach when the cardiac defect may be well tolerated for life.

In some centers, the use of intraoperative transesophageal echocardiography has provided an accurate assessment of patch integrity and the presence of additional muscular defects after termination of cardiopulmonary bypass.[192,193]

With larger shunts, elective operation may be advised before the child enters school, thus minimizing any subsequent distinction of these patients from their normal classmates. A total assessment of the psychosocial dynamics of the family and child is helpful in determining the proper age for elective operation in each patient.

Under investigation is transcatheter closure by umbrella or clamshell occluder devices (see p. 898) inserted by crossing the ventricular defect by way of the left ventricle to guide a venous catheter through a long sheath, and, ultimately, placing the device across the ventricular septum from the right ventricular side.[194]

Complete heart block is the most significant surgically induced conduction system abnormality, occurring immediately after surgery in fewer than 1 per cent of patients. Late-onset complete heart block occasionally is a problem, especially in the 10 to 25 per cent of patients whose postoperative electrocardiographic findings show complete right bundle branch block with left anterior hemiblock.[195] When the latter electrocardiographic pattern is observed in patients with transient complete heart block in the early postoperative period, electrophysiological studies should be conducted at postoperative cardiac catheterization. Patients presenting postoperatively with right bundle block and left anterior hemiblock appear to fall into two populations, defined by either peripheral damage to the conduction system or damage to the bundle of His or its proximal branches.[195] The former has not been associated with transient postoperative complete heart block, and these patients usually have a benign course. Trifascicular damage may be demonstrated in the latter population by a prolonged H-V interval, which implies a higher risk of complete heart block later in life. Although the prophylactic use of permanent pacemakers in asymptomatic patients with evidence of trifascicular damage is not currently recommended, this group certainly requires careful follow-up and continued study.

Treadmill exercise studies in patients who preoperatively had normal or only moderately elevated pulmonary vascular resistance and essentially normal postoperative cardiac catheterization data may uncover late abnormalities in circulatory function.[196,197] Despite normal cardiac output at rest, an impaired cardiac output response to exercise is noted in some. Moreover, despite a normal pulmonary arterial pressure at rest, markedly abnormal increases in pulmonary arterial pressure may be noted during exercise. These findings may be related to abnormal left ventricular function after closure of the ventricular septal defect and/or to persistent pathological changes in the pulmonary arterioles or to abnormal pulmonary vascular reactivity.[198] A direct relation exists between age at operation and the magnitude of the pulmonary arterial pressure response to intense exercise, suggesting that early operation may prevent permanent impairment of the functional capacity of the myocardium and pulmonary vascular bed.

Occasionally a child may come to medical attention who has already developed pulmonary vascular obstruction and a net right-to-left shunt across the ventricular septal defect. Symptoms may consist of exertional dyspnea, chest pain, syncope, and hemoptysis; the right-to-left shunt leads to cyanosis, clubbing, and polycythemia. There currently is little to offer this group of patients other than continuing support to the patient and family.

Patent Ductus Arteriosus
(See also p. 966)

The ductus arteriosus normally exists in the fetus as a widely patent vessel connecting the pulmonary trunk and the descending aorta just distal to the left subclavian artery (Fig. 29–4). In the fetus most of the output of the right ventricle bypasses the unexpanded lungs by way of the ductus arteriosus and enters the descending aorta, where it travels to the placenta, the fetal organ of oxygenation.

It was earlier assumed that during fetal life the ductus arteriosus was a passively open channel that constricted postnatally by means of undefined molecular mechanisms in response to the abrupt rise in arterial pO_2 accompanying the first breath of life.[199] Even in utero the lumen of the ductus arteriosus may be influenced by vasoactive substances, particularly prostaglandins.[98,99,200–202] Thus inhibition of prostaglandin synthesis causes profound constriction of the ductus arteriosus in the mammalian fetus that may be reversed by administration of vasodilatory E-type prostaglandins. Initial contraction and functional closure of the ductus arteriosus shortly after birth is related both to the sudden increase in the partial pressure of oxygen that accompanies ventilation and to changes in the synthesis and metabolism of vasoactive eicosanoids. Intimal proliferation and fibrosis proceed more gradually, so that anatomical closure may take as long as several weeks for completion.[203]

The ductus arteriosus is a unique structure after birth because its patency may, on the one hand, result in cardiac decompensation but may, on the other hand, provide the only life-sustaining conduit to preserve systemic or pulmonary arterial blood flow in the presence of certain cardiac malformations.[96] Appreciable left-to-right shunting across the patent ductus arteriosus frequently complicates the clinical course of infants born prematurely.[204] The ductal shunt has been implicated specifically in the deterioration of pulmonary function in infants with the respiratory distress syndrome in whom severe congestive heart failure often is unresponsive to digitalis and diuretics.[99]

A distinction should be made between patency of the ductus arteriosus in the *preterm* infant, who lacks the normal mechanisms for postnatal ductal closure because of immaturity, and the full-term newborn, in whom patency of the ductus is a true congenital malformation, probably related to a primary anatomical defect of the elastic tissue within the wall of the ductus.[203] In the former circumstance, delayed spontaneous closure of the ductus may be anticipated if the infant does not succumb to the cardiopulmonary difficulties caused by the ductus itself or to some lethal complication of prematurity, such as hyaline membrane disease, intraventricular hemorrhage, or necrotizing enterocolitis. In a similar manner, some full-term newborns have persistent patency of the ductus arteriosus for weeks or months because their relative hypoxemia contributes to vasodilatation of the channel. In the latter category are infants born at high altitude; those born with congenital malformations causing hypoxemia, such as pulmonary atresia with or without ventricular septal defect; or malformations in which ductal flow supplies the systemic circulation, such as hypoplastic left heart syndrome, interruption of the aortic arch, or some examples of coarctation of the aorta syndrome.

In the clinical settings in which the ductus preserves pulmonary blood flow, the essentially inevitable spontaneous closure of the vessel is associated with profound clinical deterioration. The latter may be reversed medically within the first 4 to 5 days of life by infusion of prostaglandin E₁ intravenously. By dilating the constricted ductus arteriosus, a temporary increase occurs in arterial blood oxygen tension and oxygen saturation and correction of acidemia.[96] These infants can then undergo operative repair or a palliative systemic-pulmonary anastomosis, under more optimal circumstances. Pharmacological dilation of the ductus arteriosus also is effective in the preoperative restoration of systemic blood flow and the alleviation of heart failure, especially in infants with aortic coarctation or hypoplastic left heart syndrome, and in infants with complete transposition of the great arteries in whom intercirculatory mixing is augmented.[96]

PREMATURE INFANTS. In most, if not all, preterm infants under 1500 gm birthweight, persistence of a patent ductus arteriosus is prolonged, and in about one-third of these infants a large aortico-pulmonary shunt is responsible for significant cardiopulmonary deterioration.[204–206] Radiographic, echocardiographic, and Doppler ultrasound signs of significant left-to-right shunting usually precede the appearance of physical findings suggesting ductal patency.[42,203,207,208] A significant increase in the cardiothoracic ratio is seen on sequential roentgenograms as well as increased pulmonary arterial markings progressing to perihilar and generalized pulmonary edema. Serial echocardiographic evaluations that demonstrate increases in left ventricular end-diastolic and left atrial dimensions, especially when correlated with the aforementioned radiographic signs, are highly suggestive of a large shunt.[207] Two-dimensional and Doppler echocardiography directly visualize and define the flow characteristics of the ductus arteriosus with great accuracy (Fig. 3–82, p. 84).[42,208,209]

Clinical Findings. These include bounding peripheral pulses, an infraclavicular and interscapular systolic murmur (occasionally a continuous murmur), precordial hyperactivity, hepatomegaly, and either multiple episodes of apnea and bradycardia or respiratory dependency. Cardiac catheterization carries a high risk in the preterm infant and seldom is indicated unless the diagnosis is obscure.

Treatment. Management of the preterm infant with a patent ductus arteriosus varies with the magnitude of shunting and the severity of hyaline membrane disease because the ductus may contribute importantly to mortality in the respiratory distress syndrome. Intervention in an asymptomatic infant with a small left-to-right shunt is unnecessary because the patent ductus arteriosus almost invariably undergoes spontaneous closure and does not require late surgical ligation and division. Those infants who demonstrate unmistakable signs of a significant ductal left-to-right shunt during the course of the respiratory distress syndrome often are unresponsive to medical measures to control congestive heart failure and require closure of the patent ductus arteriosus to survive. These infants are best managed within the first 2 to 7 days of life by pharmacological inhibition of prostaglandin synthesis with indomethacin to constrict and close the ductus[204,210–214]; surgical ligation is required in the estimated 10 per cent of infants who are unresponsive to indomethacin.[210,215] Early intervention is advised to reduce the likelihood of necrotizing enterocolitis and of bronchopulmonary dysplasia related to prolonged respirator and oxygen dependency.[214] Less often, indications for pharmacological or surgical closure of the ductus consist of life-threatening episodes of apnea and bradycardia or a prolonged failure to gain weight and grow.

FULL-TERM INFANTS AND CHILDREN. In full-term newborns and older infants and children, patency of the ductus arteriosus occurs particularly in females and in the offspring of pregnancies complicated by first-trimester rubella. Although most frequent in isolated form, the anomaly may coexist with other malformations, particularly coarctation of the aorta, ventricular septal defect, pulmonic stenosis, and aortic stenosis. Flow across the ductus is determined by the pressure relation between the aorta and the pulmonary artery and by the cross-sectional area and length of the ductus itself.[216] Pulmonary pressures most commonly are normal, and a persistent gradient and shunt from aorta to pulmonary artery exist throughout the cardiac cycle.

Physical examination reveals a characteristic thrill and a continuous "machinery" murmur with a late systolic accentuation at the upper left sternal border. The left atrium and left ventricle enlarge to accommodate the increased pulmonary venous return, and flow murmurs across the mitral and aortic valves may be detected. With significant left-to-right shunting, the runoff of blood through the ductus causes a widened systemic pulse pressure and bounding peripheral pulses. The hemodynamic abnormality is reflected in the electrocardiogram by left ventricular and occasionally left atrial hypertrophy, and in the chest roentgenogram by left atrial and ventricular enlargement, prominent ascending aorta and pulmonary artery, and pulmonary vascular engorgement (Fig. 7–43, p. 232 and Fig. 30–6, p. 967).

The clinical diagnosis may be difficult when the findings do not conform to the classic presentation.[217] As mentioned above, disappearance of the diastolic component of the murmur is common in premature infants because higher pulmonary arterial diastolic pressures exist at that age. In older patients both heart failure and pulmonary hypertension are associated with a reduction in the pressure gradient across the ductus arteriosus and result in atypical systolic murmurs. When severe pulmonary vascular obstructive disease results in reversal of flow through the ductus and preferential shunting of unoxygenated blood to

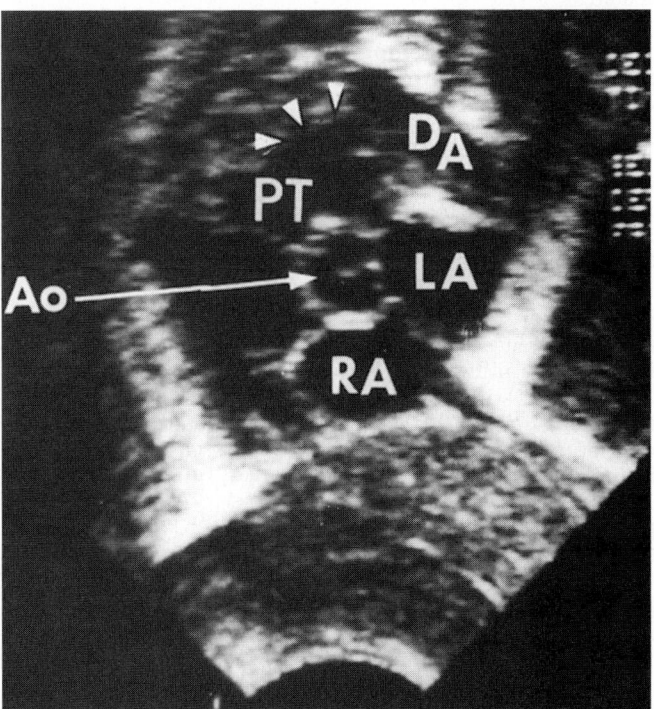

FIGURE 29–18. Parasternal short-axis view of a patent ductus arteriosus (arrowheads) in an infant. The pulmonic valve is the linear echo just beneath the pulmonary trunk (PT). AO = aortic valve, DA = descending aorta, RA = right atrium, LA = left atrium. (From Perloff, J.: The Clinical Recognition of Congenital Heart Disease. 3rd ed. Philadelphia, W.B. Saunders Company, 1986.)

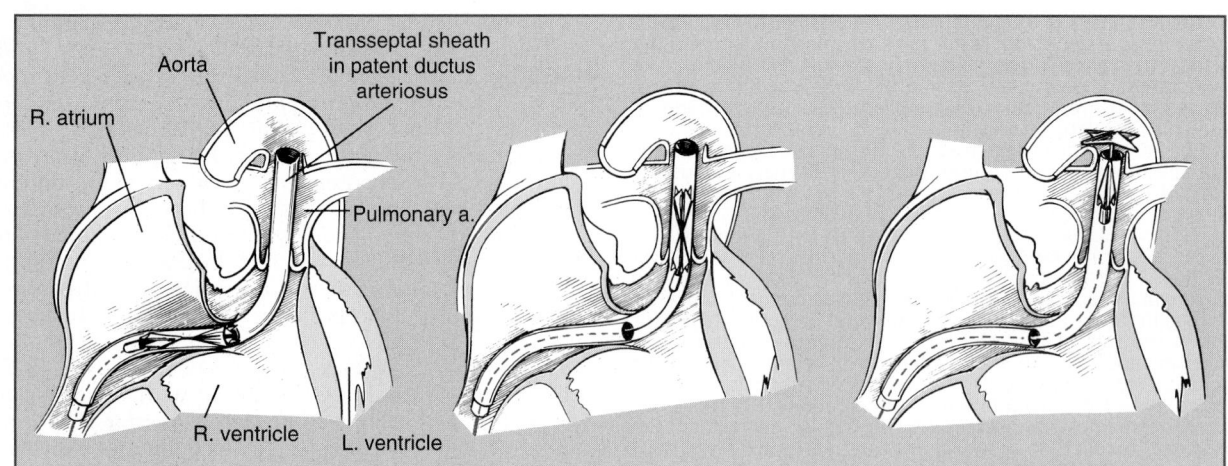

FIGURE 29–19. Transcatheter closure of a patent ductus arteriosus is illustrated using the Rashkind double-umbrella technique. The catheter approaches the ductus via a long sheath advanced from the femoral vein. The right panel shows expansion of the distal umbrella. (From Castaneda, A., et al.: Cardiac Surgery of the Neonate and Infant. Philadelphia, W.B. Saunders Company, 1994, p. 136.)

the descending aorta, the toes, rather than the fingers, may show cyanosis and clubbing.

The full-term infant with patent ductus arteriosus may survive for a number of years, although occasionally a large defect results in heart failure and pulmonary edema early in life. The leading causes of death in older children are infective endocarditis and heart failure. Beyond the third decade severe pulmonary vascular obstruction has been known to cause aneurysmal dilatation, calcification, and rupture of the ductus.[217]

The patent ductus usually can be directly visualized by two-dimensional echocardiography (Fig. 29–18); range-gated pulse Doppler echocardiography shows the characteristic flow abnormalities across the ductus, as well as a continuous flow disturbance in the pulmonary artery. Cardiac catheterization may be indicated when additional lesions or pulmonary vascular obstruction is suspected.

Management. In the absence of severe pulmonary vascular disease with predominant right-to-left shunting, the anatomical presence of a patent ductus usually is considered sufficient indication for operation. Ligation or division of the ductus carries a low risk, whether performed electively in the asymptomatic child or at any age if symptoms are present. The operative risk is reduced if heart failure can be compensated by medical measures before surgery. Operation should be deferred for several months in patients treated successfully for infective endarteritis because the ductus may remain somewhat edematous and friable. Rarely, when the infection does not subside with intensive antibiotic treatment, surgical ligation may be necessary to eradicate the infection.

Although still investigational, substantial experience exists with transcatheter closure of the patent ductus using a variety of approaches, including coils, buttons, plugs, and umbrellas, with each occluder device introduced through a relatively large-diameter sheath from the femoral vein (Fig. 29–19).[218–224a] The approach is especially feasible in patients who weigh more than 10 kg, and with neither a long tubular ductus nor a ductus with a long, narrow aortic end. In experienced hands, initial occlusion is successful in 85 to 90 per cent of patients; reocclusion adds 5 to 7 per cent to the overall success rate. Potential complications in 5 to 10 per cent of patients include embolization of the device, endocarditis, and hemolysis.[114,224] Ductal closure by thoracoscopy will undoubtedly undergo future evaluation.

Aorticopulmonary Septal Defect

Aorticopulmonary window or fenestration, partial truncus arteriosus, and aortic septal defect are other designations applied to this

relatively uncommon anomaly. Septation of the aortopulmonary trunk occurs by fusion of the conotruncal ridges (Fig. 29–2). The right and left sixth aortic arches, destined to become the pulmonary arteries, join the pulmonary artery to complete great artery development (Fig. 29–5). Congenital defects between the ascending aorta and the pulmonary artery result from faulty development of this area during embryonic life. The typical aortopulmonary septal defect results because of incomplete fusion of the distal aortopulmonary septum.[225] Malalignment of the conotruncal ridges results in unequal partitioning of the aortopulmonary trunk, which may result in partial or complete fusion of the right pulmonary artery to the aorta.

The usual defect consists of a communication between the aorta and pulmonary artery just above the semilunar valves. Persistent patency of the ductus arteriosus is an associated lesion in 10 to 15 per cent of cases. Less common accompanying cardiovascular lesions include ventricular septal defect, aortic origin of the right pulmonary artery, aortic arch interruption, coarctation of the aorta, and right aortic arch. Aorticopulmonary septal defects usually are large and are accompanied by severe pulmonary arterial hypertension and early-onset pulmonary vascular obstruction.

PHYSICAL EXAMINATION. The pulses typically are bounding, like those of a large patent ductus arteriosus. The murmur, however, seldom is continuous, and a basal systolic murmur is most common. Cardiomegaly is present, and pulmonary hypertension is reflected in a loud and palpable sound of pulmonary valve closure. Aorticopulmonary septal defect should be suspected whenever a large shunt into the pulmonary artery is demonstrated at catheterization. Diagnosis of the anomaly and its distinction from patent ductus and persistent truncus arteriosus usually can be done by two-dimensional echocardiography, but definitive identification of the aortopulmonary window and associated malformations requires hemodynamic study and selective angiocardiography with the injection of contrast mate-

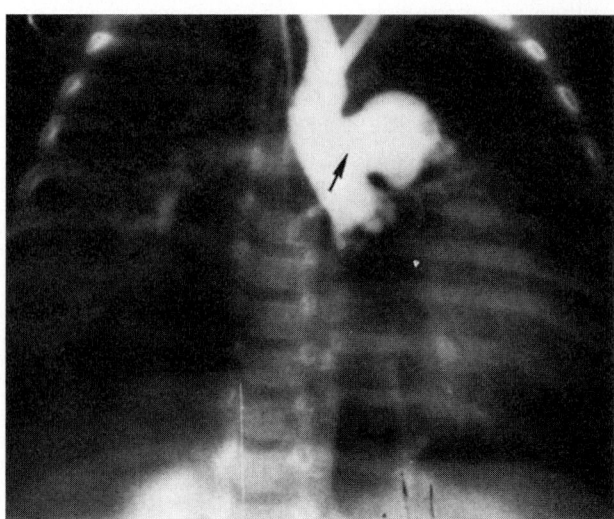

FIGURE 29–20. Aortic root injection of contrast material in the frontal view produces simultaneous opacification of aorta and pulmonary artery through a large aorticopulmonary septal defect (arrow). (Courtesy of Robert White, M.D.)

rial into the left ventricle and/or the root of the aorta (Fig. 29–20). Although some patients may survive to adulthood with uncorrected aorticopulmonary septal defect, most die early in life unless surgical treatment is undertaken. Operative correction is indicated in all symptomatic infants when the diagnosis is made. Elective repair is advised at 3 to 6 months. Profound hypothermic total circulatory arrest or total cardiopulmonary bypass is required, and the defect is closed by way of a transaortic approach, usually with a prosthetic or xenograft pericardial patch.[226,227]

Persistent Truncus Arteriosus

MORPHOLOGY. Persistent truncus arteriosus is a rare but serious anomaly in which a single vessel forms the outlet of both ventricles and gives rise to the systemic, pulmonary, and coronary arteries.[228] The defect results from failure of septation of the embryonic truncus by the infundibular truncal ridges (Fig. 29–4). It is always accompanied by a ventricular septal defect, frequently with a right-sided aortic arch. The ventricular septal defect is due to the absence or underdevelopment of the distal portion of the pulmonary infundibulum. The truncal valve usually is tricuspid but is quadricuspid in about one-third of patients and rarely can be bicuspid. Truncal valve regurgitation and truncal valve stenosis are each seen in 10 to 15 per cent of patients. There may be a single coronary artery, displacement of the coronary ostia (usually the left ostium posteriorly), or a single posterior descending coronary artery arising from the right coronary or, less often, from the left circumflex artery, especially in patients with a single coronary artery.[229,230]

Truncus malformations may be classified either anatomically according to the mode of origin of pulmonary vessels from the common trunk or from a functional point of view, based on the magnitude of blood flow to the lungs.[231] In the common type (type I) of truncus arteriosus malformation a partially separate pulmonary trunk of variable length exists because of the presence of an incompletely formed aorticopulmonary septum. The pulmonary trunk usually is very short and gives rise to left and right pulmonary arteries. When the aorticopulmonary septum is absent, there is no discrete main pulmonary artery component, and both pulmonary artery branches arise directly from the truncus.

In type II, each pulmonary artery arises separately but close to the other from the posterior aspect of the truncus (Fig. 29–21). In type III, each pulmonary artery arises from the lateral aspect of the truncus. Less commonly, one pulmonary artery branch may be absent, with collateral arteries supplying the lung that does not receive a pulmonary artery branch from the truncus. Truncus arteriosus malformation should not be confused with "pseudotruncus arteriosus," which is the severe form of tetralogy of Fallot with pulmonary atresia in which the single aorta arises from the heart accompanied by a remnant of atretic pulmonary artery.

HEMODYNAMICS. Pulmonary blood flow is governed by the size of the pulmonary arteries and the pulmonary vascular resistance. In infancy, pulmonary blood flow is usually excessive because pulmonary vascular resistance is not greatly increased. Thus, despite an obligatory admixture of systemic and pulmonary venous blood in the common trunk, only minimal cyanosis is present. Rarely, pulmonary blood flow is restricted by hypoplastic or stenotic pulmonary arteries arising from the truncus. Pulmonary vascular obstruction usually does not restrict pulmonary blood flow before 1 year of age.[232]

CLINICAL FEATURES. The infant with truncus arteriosus usually presents with mild cyanosis coexisting with the cardiac findings of a large left-to-right shunt. Symptoms of heart failure and poor physical development usually appear in the first weeks or months of life. The most frequent physical findings include cardiomegaly, a systolic ejection sound accompanied by a thrill, a loud single second heart sound, a harsh systolic murmur, and a low-pitched mid-diastolic rumbling murmur and bounding pulses. Truncus arteriosus often is a measure of the *DiGeorge syndrome* (Table 29–2); thus facial dysmorphism, a high incidence of extracardiac malformations (particularly of the limbs, kidneys, and intestines), atrophy or absence of the thymus gland, T-lymphocyte deficiency, and predilection to infection also may be features of the clinical presentation.[233] Recent evidence suggests that embryonic abnormalities in the cardiac neural crest play a major role in the creation of the cardiovascular malformation as well as the other components of the syndrome.[234]

Truncal valve incompetence is suggested by the presence of a diastolic decrescendo murmur at the base of the heart.[235] The physical findings are quite different if pulmonary blood flow is restricted by either high pulmonary vascular resistance or pulmonary arterial stenosis: Cyanosis is prominent, congestive failure is rare, and only a short systolic ejection may be audible occasionally accompanied by continuous murmurs posteriorly of bronchial collateral flow.

ECG AND RADIOGRAPHY. Left ventricular hypertrophy alone or in

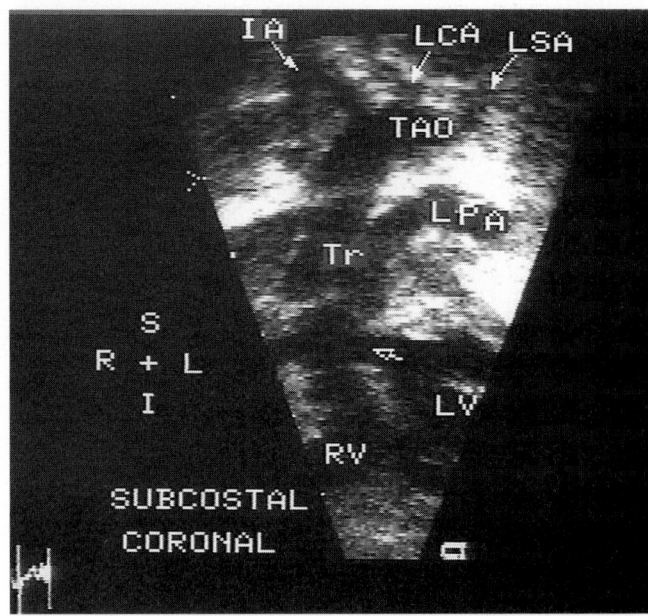

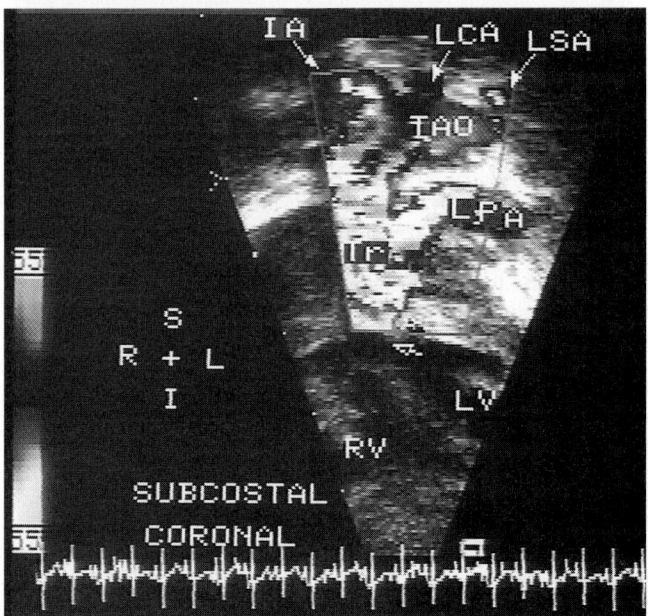

FIGURE 29–21. *Top,* Subcostal coronal view of truncus arteriosus (Tr). The truncal valve lies above the ventricular septal defect (open arrow), which appears above the left ventricle (LV) and right ventricle (RV). The truncus arteriosus (Tr) is seen dividing into the transverse aortic arch (TAO), which gives rise to the vessels supplying the head and neck: the innominate artery (IA), the left carotid artery (LCA), and the left subclavian artery (LSA). *Bottom,* Doppler color flow image showing the superimposition of color flow into the truncus arteriosus, left pulmonary artery, transverse aorta, and branches to the head and neck. Orientation: S = superior, I = inferior, R = right, L = left. (Courtesy of Norman Silverman, M.D.)

combination with right ventricular hypertrophy is present electrocardiographically when a prominent left-to-right shunt exists; right ventricular hypertrophy is observed in patients with restricted pulmonary blood flow. The radiographic findings depend on the hemodynamic circumstances. Gross cardiomegaly with left or combined ventricular enlargement, left atrial enlargement, and a small or absent main pulmonary artery segment with pulmonary vascular engorgement are the usual radiographic features. A right aortic arch is common (25 to 30 per cent of patients). When pulmonary blood flow is reduced, both heart size and pulmonary vascular markings are less prominent.

The *echocardiographic* features of truncus arteriosus (Fig. 29–21) include the detection of a large truncal root overriding the ventricular septum, truncal valve abnormalities, an increase in the right ventricular dimension, and mitral valve–truncal root continuity. Differentiation be-

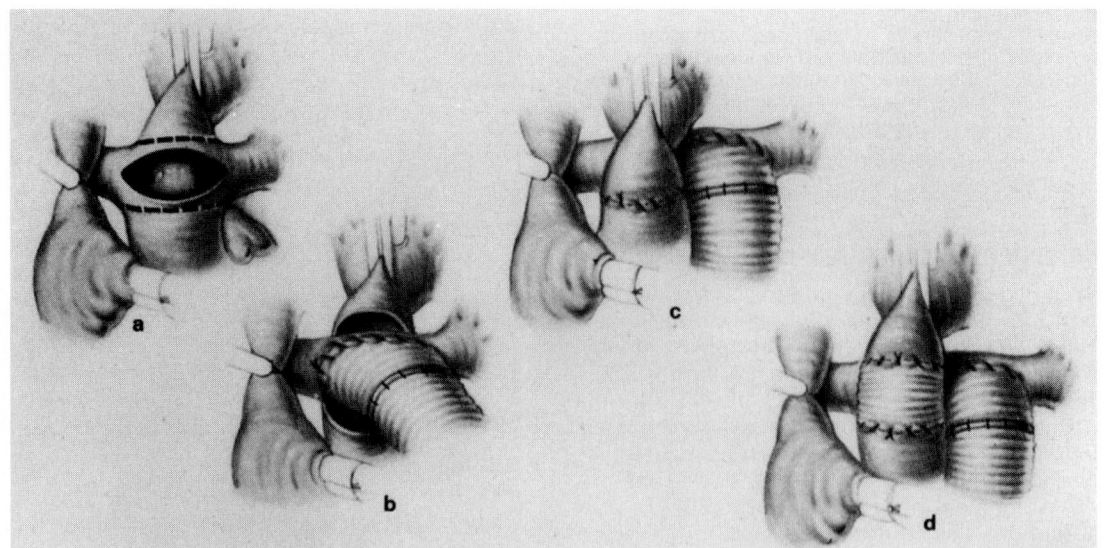

FIGURE 29–22. Operative correction of truncus arteriosus, type III. The pulmonary arteries arise separately from the truncus. An anterior incision is made and a segment of aorta containing the orifices of both pulmonary arteries is excised from the truncus (a). The cuff of tissue containing the two pulmonary arteries is anastomosed to an extracardiac valved conduit (b). Aortic continuity is restored by direct suture (c) or by interposing a preclotted graft (d). The diagram does not show closure of the ventricular septal defect. (From Stark, J., and DeLaval, M.: Surgery for Congenital Heart Defects. New York, Grune and Stratton, 1983, p. 420.)

tween truncus arteriosus and tetralogy of Fallot by ultrasonography may be difficult unless either the separate origin of the pulmonary arteries or a single trunk from the ascending portion of a single arterial root can be identified. The origin of the pulmonary arteries is detected best from high short-axis views, scanning superiorly from the semilunar valve. Diagnosis should be suspected at cardiac catheterization if the catheter fails to enter the central pulmonary arteries from the right ventricle. Selective angiocardiography and retrograde aortography are necessary to establish a precise diagnosis and to reveal the common trunk arising from the heart and the origin of the pulmonary arteries from the truncus.[236]

The early fatal course as well as early development of pulmonary vascular obstructive disease in patients surviving infancy is responsible for the poor prognosis associated with truncus arteriosus. In infants and young children with large left-to-right shunts, surgical banding of one or both pulmonary arteries to reduce pulmonary flow has been used with little success. Corrective operation is indicated before age 3 months to avoid the development of severe pulmonary vascular obstructive disease.[237]

SURGICAL TREATMENT. Operation consists of closure of the ventricular septal defect, leaving the aorta arising from the left ventricle; the pulmonary arteries are excised from their truncus origin and a valve-containing prosthetic conduit or aortic homograft valve conduit is used to establish continuity between the right ventricle and the pulmonary arteries (Fig. 29–22). Important risk factors for perioperative death are severe truncal valve regurgitation, interrupted aortic arch, coronary artery anomalies, and age at operation greater than 100 days.[238] Patients with only one pulmonary artery are especially prone to early development of severe pulmonary vascular disease but otherwise are not at increased risk from surgery.

With truncus arteriosus defects, the possible inequalities of pressure and flow between the two pulmonary arteries often make precise calculation of pulmonary resistance difficult. Corrective operation may be performed in patients with at least one adequate pulmonary artery having low distal pressure or arteriolar resistance. Conversely, significant systemic arterial desaturation in a patient with two pulmonary arteries and with neither pulmonary artery stenosis nor a previous pulmonary artery band signifies that high pulmonary vascular resistance exists and that the condition is probably inoperable. It is not yet clear how often and at what age the conduit between the right ventricle and pulmonary artery must be replaced with a larger prosthesis because of either growth of the patient, in

whom a small conduit causes eventual obstruction, heterograft valve degeneration, or obstruction created by neointimal proliferation within a prosthetic conduit.[239] When operation is carried out within a conduit in the first year of life, conduit replacement often is required within 3 to 5 years.

Coronary Arteriovenous Fistula

Coronary arteriovenous fistula (see also p. 967) is an unusual anomaly that consists of a communication between one of the coronary arteries and a cardiac chamber or vein. The right coronary artery, or its branches, is the site of the fistula in about 55 per cent of cases; the left coronary artery is involved in about 35 per cent, and both coronary arteries in 5 per cent. Connections between the coronary system and a cardiac chamber appear to represent persistence of embryonic intertrabecular spaces and sinusoids. Most of these fistulas drain into the right ventricle, right atrium, or coronary sinus; fistulous communication to the pulmonary artery, left atrium, or left ventricle is much less frequent. Most often the shunt through the fistula is of small magnitude, and myocardial blood flow is not compromised.[240] Rarely, spontaneous closure may occur. Potential complications include pulmonary hypertension and congestive heart failure if a large left-to-right shunt exists, bacterial endocarditis, rupture or thrombosis of the fistula or an associated arterial aneurysm, and myocardial ischemia distal to the fistula due to decreased coronary blood flow.

Most pediatric patients are asymptomatic and are referred because of a cardiac murmur that is loud, superficial, and continuous at the lower or midsternal border. The site of maximal intensity of the murmur is related to the site of drainage and usually is different from the second left intercostal space—the classic site of the continuous murmur of persistent ductus arteriosus—except when the fistula drains into the pulmonary artery or right ventricle. In the latter situation the murmur is louder in diastole than in systole because of compression of the fistula by contracting myocardium. The electrocardiogram and chest roentgenogram quite often are normal and seldom show selective chamber enlargement or myocardial ischemia. Significantly enlarged coronary arteries may be detected by two-dimensional echocardiography, and the actual diagnosis of an arteriovenous fistula occasionally can be made by combining two-dimensional echocardiography and Doppler techniques to detect the entrance site of the shunt, which is characterized by a continuous turbulent systolic and diastolic flow pattern (Fig. 30–8, p. 968).[241,242]

Standard retrograde thoracic aortography, balloon occlusion angiography of the aortic root with a 45-degree caudal tilt of the frontal camera ("laid back" aortogram),[243] or coronary arteriography can be used reliably to identify the size and anatomical features of the fistulous tract, which can be closed by transcatheter coil embolization or suture obliteration in most cases.[243,244] In the presence of a large left-to-right shunt and symptoms of heart failure, the decision to operate is clearly justified. Most often the fistula is closed in asymptomatic patients to prevent future symptoms or complications, such as infective endocarditis. The prognosis after successful closure of a coronary artery–cardiac chamber fistula is excellent.

Anomalous Pulmonary Origin of the Coronary Artery

This rare malformation occurs in about 0.4 per cent of patients with congenital cardiac anomalies. In almost all patients the left coronary artery originates from the posterior sinus of the pulmonary artery.[246]

Unusual cases have been reported in which the right coronary artery, or the entire coronary artery system, originates from the main pulmonary trunk. Embryologically the distal coronary artery system is formed by 9 weeks from solid angioblastic buds that extend throughout the epicardium to form the major coronary artery branches. Proximally the coronary network forms a ring around the truncus arteriosus, joining with coronary buds from the primitive aortic sinuses as the truncus partitions to form the great arteries. The varieties of anomalous pulmonary origin of the coronary artery are the result of displacement in this proximal process.

PATHOPHYSIOLOGY. During fetal life pulmonary artery pressure is slightly greater than aortic pressure, and perfusion of the left coronary artery is antegrade (Fig. 29–23A). After birth, when pulmonary artery pressure falls below aortic pressure, perfusion of the left coronary artery from the pulmonary artery ceases, and the direction of flow in the anomalous vessel reverses. Blood flows from the aorta to the right coronary artery, then through collateral channels to the left coronary artery, and finally to the pulmonary artery (Fig. 29–23B). In effect, the left coronary artery behaves as a fistulous communication between the aorta and pulmonary artery.[245] If adequate collateral channels exist or develop between the two coronary artery circulations, total myocardial perfusion through the right coronary artery increases (Fig. 29–23C). In 10 to 15 per cent of patients myocardial ischemia never develops because extensive intercoronary collaterals

allow survival to adolescence or adulthood.[245] In fact, if collateral blood flow is considerable, the patient may develop the clinical manifestations of a large arteriovenous shunt and a continuous or diastolic murmur.

By far the most common clinical presentation is that of the infant who suffers a myocardial infarction and develops congestive heart failure.[247–249] The infant syndrome usually becomes manifested at age 2 to 4 months with angina-like symptoms that may be misinterpreted as colic. Feeding and defecation often are accompanied by dyspnea, irritability and crying, pallor, diaphoresis, and occasional loss of consciousness. Older children or adults usually present with a continuous murmur or with mitral regurgitation resulting from dysfunction of ischemic or infarcted papillary muscles. In some instances the coronary anomaly is unsuspected until a previously well adolescent or adult experiences angina, heart failure, or sudden death.

DIAGNOSIS. The diagnosis of anomalous origin of the coronary artery is supported by the electrocardiographic demonstration of deep Q waves in association with ST-segment alterations and T-wave inversions in leads I, aV_L, V_5, and V_6 (Fig. 29–24). These findings greatly assist the distinction of this anomaly from myocarditis and dilated cardiomyopathy.[250] Chest roentgenograms show moderate to severe enlargement of the left atrium and ventricle. Echocardiography with Doppler color-flow mapping is replacing cardiac catheterization as the standard method of diagnosis. The color flow mapping demonstrates retrograde flow in the left coronary system and an abnormal flow jet from the left coronary artery into the pulmonary trunk. Moreover, detection of antegrade flow in the left coronary system helps to exclude the diagnosis.[251] The origin of the anomalous left coronary artery occasionally may be visualized echocardiographically from long- or short-axis views of the pulmonary artery.[252] Absence of the left coronary artery from its usual origin in the left sinus of Valsalva does not distinguish this lesion from single coronary artery. Color-flow Doppler examination may also reveal associated mitral regurgitation. Ischemia or infarction is suggested by the echocardiographic findings of segmental wall motion abnormalities, particularly involving the anterolateral free wall of the left ventricle. Stress thallium scintigraphy shows a characteristic defect of the anterolateral wall of the left ventricle. Positron emission tomography reveals both

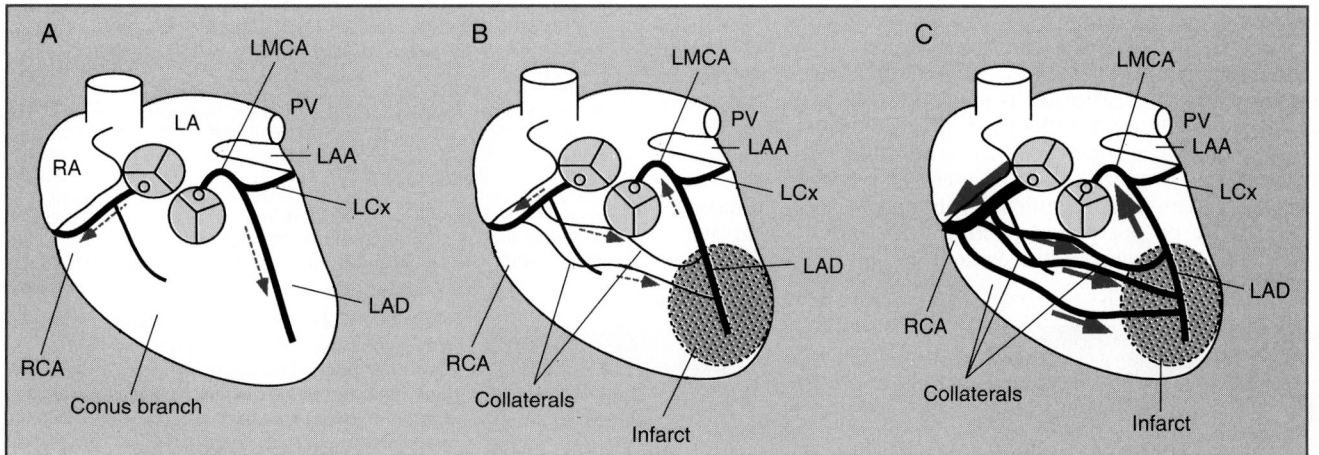

FIGURE 29–23. Anomalous origin of left main coronary artery from pulmonary artery. A, In fetus, both right and left coronary arteries receive forward flow from their respective great arteries. B, Early after birth, before collaterals are well developed, there may be an anterolateral infarct and slight retrograde flow from the left coronary artery to the pulmonary artery. C, After collaterals have enlarged, there is high flow in the enlarged right coronary artery and the collaterals and significant retrograde flow into the pulmonary artery. Dotted arrows indicate direction and approximate magnitude of flow in the right and left coronary arteries and the collaterals between them. SVC = superior vena cava, PV = pulmonary vein, LA = left atrium, LAA = left atrial appendage, RA = right atrium, LMCA = left main coronary artery, LCx = left circumflex coronary artery, LAD = left anterior descending coronary artery, RCA = right coronary artery, RVI = right ventricular infundibulum (outflow tract). (From Hoffman, J. I. E.: In Moss and Adams' Heart Disease in Infants, Children, and Adolescents. 5th ed. Baltimore, © Williams and Wilkins, 1994, p. 776.)

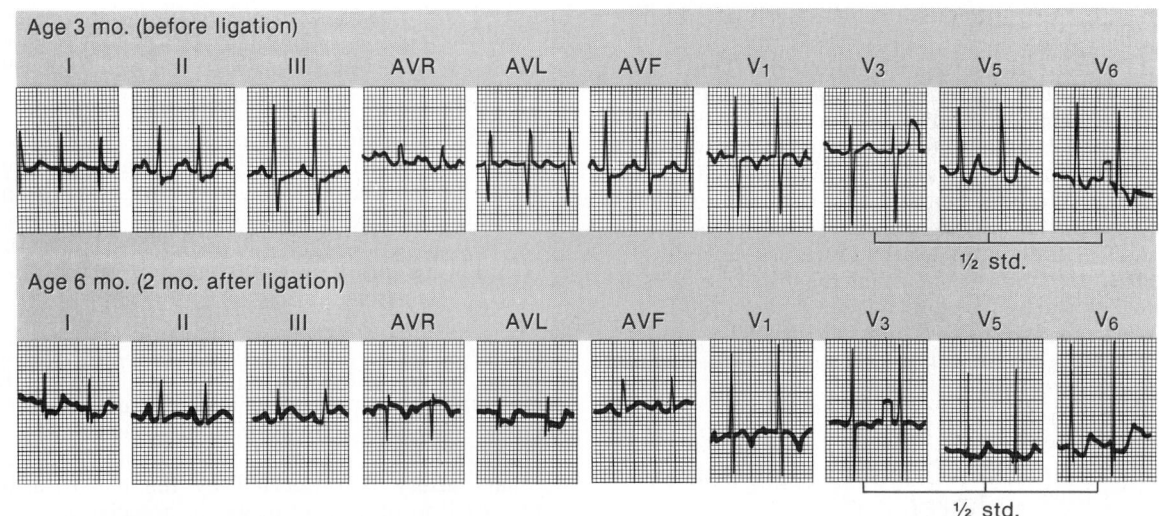

Age 3 mo. (before ligation)

| I | II | III | AVR | AVL | AVF | V₁ | V₃ | V₅ | V₆ |

½ std.

Age 6 mo. (2 mo. after ligation)

| I | II | III | AVR | AVL | AVF | V₁ | V₃ | V₅ | V₆ |

½ std.

FIGURE 29–24. Typical electrocardiogram of an infant with anomalous left coronary artery before *(above)* and after *(below)* ligation of the anomalous left coronary artery. Note the abnormal Q waves in I, AV$_L$, and V$_6$. (Courtesy of Delores A. Danilowicz, M.D.)

the perfusion defect and its metabolic consequences (Fig. 29–25).

Aortography or coronary angiography demonstrates the retrograde drainage of the coronary vessel into the pulmonary artery. It should be recognized that ventricular arrhythmias may complicate the course of hemodynamic study. The magnitude of shunting into the pulmonary artery may be determined by oximetry, indicator dilution curves, or angiography.

MANAGEMENT. *Medical treatment* is indicated in infants with myocardial infarction for congestive heart failure, arrhythmias, and cardiogenic shock. In patients with a small left-to-right shunt or no shunt at all, the prognosis is exceedingly poor with conservative management, justifying an attempt to reestablish a two–coronary artery system. The *operations* that have been used include reimplanting the left coronary artery into the aortic root, surgically creating an aortopulmonary window and a tunnel to convey blood from the window across the back of the pulmonary trunk to the origin of the anomalous left coronary artery, with reconstruction of the anterior wall of the pulmonary trunk, and anastomosis of the left coronary artery with the subclavian artery or with the aorta by means of a graft.[253-255] If clinical deterioration occurs in infants in whom a sizable left-to-right shunt into the pulmonary artery exists, simple ligation of the left coronary artery at its origin prevents retrograde flow and allows perfusion of the left ventricle with blood supplied through anastomoses with the right coronary artery. If medical management stabilizes the infant with significant intercoronary collaterals, operation may be postponed to allow the patient to grow, because increased size of the vessels enhances the likeli-

hood of successful reimplantation or coronary arterial bypass surgery. The outcome of surgery and ultimate prognosis are significantly influenced by the degree of myocardial damage suffered preoperatively.[256] Uncommonly, it is necessary to consider aneurysmectomy or mitral valve replacement.

Aortic Sinus Aneurysm and Fistula

Congenital aneurysm of an aortic sinus of Valsalva (see also p. 967), particularly the right coronary sinus, is an uncommon anomaly that occurs three times more often in males than in females. The malformation consists of a separation, or lack of fusion, between the media of the aorta and the annulus fibrosis of the aortic valve.[257] The receiving chamber of the aorticocardiac fistula usually is the right ventricle, but occasionally, when the noncoronary cusp is involved, the fistula drains into the right atrium.

Five to 15 per cent of aneurysms originate in the posterior or noncoronary sinus; seldom is the left aortic sinus involved. Associated anomalies are common and include bicuspid aortic valve, ventricular septal defect, and coarctation of the aorta.

The deficiency in the aortic media appears to be congenital. Reports in infants are exceedingly rare[258] and are infrequent in children, because progressive aneurysmal dilatation of the weakened area develops but may not be recognized until the third or fourth decade of life, when rupture into a cardiac chamber occurs.

The *unruptured aneurysm* usually does not produce a hemodynamic abnormality, although pressure on the intracardiac conduction system by an unruptured aneurysm may be a rare cause of complete atrioventricular block; rarely, myocardial ischemia may be caused by coronary arterial compression. Rupture is often of abrupt onset, causes chest pain, and creates continuous arteriovenous shunting and volume loading of both right and left heart chambers, which results in heart failure. An additional complication is infective endo-

NH₃–Perfusion

FDG–Metabolism

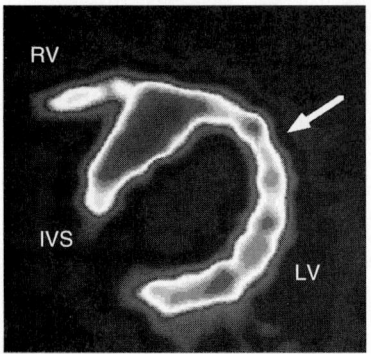

RV

IVS

LV

A
R ─┼─ L
P

FIGURE 29–25. Positron emission tomography (PET) transaxial images depict myocardial perfusion and glucose metabolism in a 7-month-old infant with anomalous origin of left coronary artery from the pulmonary artery. The ammonia (NH₃) scan demonstrates hypoperfusion *(left panel)*, whereas the fluorodeoxyglucose scan shows increased glucose metabolism *(right panel)* in the anterior lateral left ventricular wall (arrows) in the region perfused by left coronary artery (LCA). Under fasting conditions, normal myocardium has minimal glucose (FDG) uptake, whereas, in this figure, hypoperfused myocardium preferentially metabolizes glucose. The "mismatch" pattern in this figure indicates ischemic but viable myocardium. This patient underwent reimplantation of the LCA with subsequent complete recovery of cardiac function and normalization of PET perfusion and metabolism. RV = right ventricle, LV = left ventricle, IVS = interventricular septum, A = anterior, L = lateral, P = posterior, R = right.

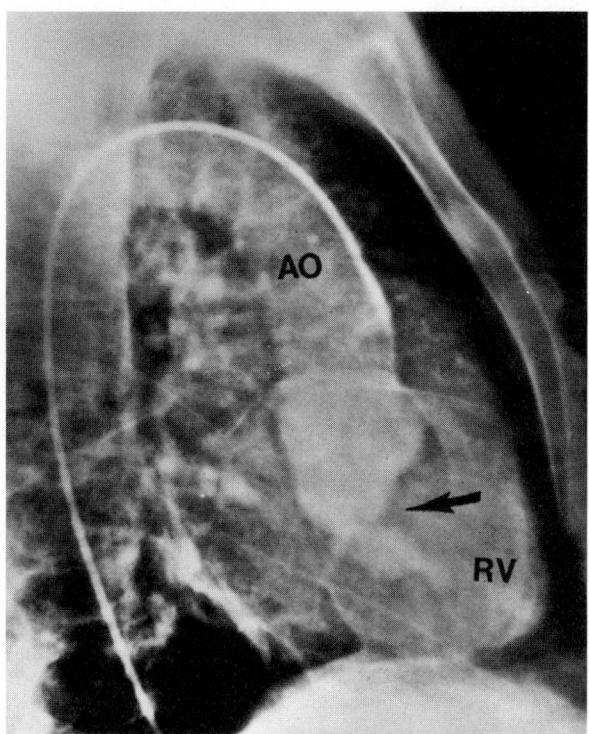

FIGURE 29–26. A retrograde aortogram shows the fistulous connection between the noncoronary sinus of Valsalva and the right ventricle (RV) (arrow). AO = aorta. (Courtesy of Robert White, M.D.)

carditis, which may originate either on the edges of the aneurysm or on those areas in the right side of the heart that are traumatized by the jet-like stream of blood flowing through the fistula.

DIAGNOSIS. The presence of this anomaly should be suspected in a patient with a history of chest pain of recent onset, symptoms of diminished cardiac reserve, bounding pulses, and a loud superficial continuous murmur accentuated in diastole when the fistula opens into the right ventricle, as well as a thrill along the right or left lower parasternal border. The *physical findings* may be difficult to distinguish from those produced by a coronary arteriovenous fistula. *Electrocardiography* shows biventricular hypertrophy, and chest roentgenography demonstrates generalized cardiomegaly. Two-dimensional and pulsed Doppler *echocardiographic* studies may detect the walls of the aneurysm and disturbed flow within the aneurysm or at the site of perforation, respectively.[259] *Transesophageal echocardiography* may provide more precise information than the transthoracic approach. *Cardiac catheterization* reveals a left-to-right shunt at the ventricular or, less commonly, the atrial level; the diagnosis may be established definitively by retrograde thoracic aortography (Fig. 29–26).

MANAGEMENT. Preoperative medical management consists of measures to relieve cardiac failure and to treat coexistent arrhythmias or endocarditis, if present. At operation the aneurysm is closed and amputated, and the aortic wall is reunited with the heart, either by direct suture or with a prosthesis.[260] Every effort should be made to preserve the aortic valve in children because patch closure of the defect combined with prosthetic valve replacement greatly enhances the risk of operation in small patients.

VALVULAR AND VASCULAR LESIONS WITH OR WITHOUT RIGHT-TO-LEFT SHUNT

Aortic Arch Obstruction

The conventional anatomical and clinical divisions into preductal and postductal coarctation or infantile and adult types, respectively, are misleading because the anatomical

localization is inaccurate and the age-dependency of the clinical presentation does not hold true (i.e., the adult type often is seen in the first weeks of life). A spectrum of anatomical lesions exists, causing obstruction of the aortic arch or proximal portion of the descending aorta. These range from a localized coarctation or constriction of the lumen, most commonly located just distal to the origin of the left subclavian artery and closely related to the attachment of the ductus arteriosus with the aorta, to diffuse narrowing or interruption of a portion of the aortic arch. In this chapter, aortic arch obstruction is divided into three types: (1) localized juxtaductal coarctation, (2) hypoplasia of the aortic isthmus, and (3) aortic arch interruption. *Pseudocoarctation* is used synonymously with "kinking" or "buckling" of the aorta, which is a subclinical form of localized juxtaductal coarctation of the aorta.[261]

Localized Juxtaductal Coarctation
(See also p. 965)

MORPHOLOGY. This lesion consists of a localized shelf-like thickening and infolding of the media of the posterolateral aortic wall opposite the ductus arteriosus; the wall of the aorta into which the ductus or ligamentum arteriosum inserts is not involved.[262] Juxtaductal coarctation occurs two to five times more commonly in males than in females, and there is a high degree of association with gonadal dysgenesis (Turner syndrome) and bicuspid aortic valve. Other common associated anomalies include ventricular septal defect and mitral stenosis or regurgitation. The most important extracardiac anomaly is aneurysm of the circle of Willis.

PATHOGENESIS. Juxtaductal coarctation is probably related to an abnormality in the pattern of ductus arteriosus blood flow in utero, which, in turn, may be the result of associated intracardiac anomalies.[262,263] Thus, in fetal life, blood flow through the aortic isthmus constitutes only 12 to 17 per cent of the total cardiac output, while blood flow through the ductus arteriosus exceeds that across the aortic valve. The dorsal aortic wall directly opposite the ductus arteriosus resembles morphologically the apex of a normal branch point of the aorta if ductal flow pathways in utero diverge, with some flow directed cephalad into the aortic isthmus and the remainder proceeding into the descending aorta. The aortic branch point is identical histologically to the posterior shelf of juxtaductal aortic coarctation. A divergence of ductal flow is fostered by the presence of lesions in the fetus that create an imbalance between left and right ventricular outputs, with right-sided flow predominating (e.g., bicuspid aortic valve, mitral valve anomaly). In the absence of an anomaly fostering augmented ductal flow, a branch point may be created by an alteration in the angle at which the ductus arteriosus meets the aorta, pointing the ductal stream directly against the posterior aortic wall rather than obliquely down into the descending aorta. Cardiac anomalies that cause augmented ascending aortic blood flow (e.g., pulmonic atresia or stenosis, tetralogy of Fallot) prevent development of a branch point and indeed are almost never seen in association with juxtaductal coarctation of the aorta.

During fetal life the posterior aortic shelf is not obstructive because blood may pass readily from the ascending aorta to the descending aorta by traversing the anterior aortic segment and the aortic end of the ductus arteriosus. Postnatally, however, when the ductus undergoes obliteration at its aortic end, the shelf-like projection of the posterior aortic wall unmasks the obstruction to aortic flow (Fig. 29–27). After pharmacological interventions that dilate the ductus arteriosus (prostaglandin E₁ infusion) the pressure difference may be obliterated across the site of coarctation because the fetal flow pattern is reestablished.[96,264]

The pathogenesis of juxtaductal coarctation already described explains the prevalence of associated intracardiac anomalies that foster reduced ascending aortic flow and augmented ductus arteriosus flow in utero, and the absence of associated intracardiac anomalies in which the converse flow conditions exist in utero. The dependence of aortic obstruction on constriction of the ductus arteriosus postnatally explains the variable onset after birth of the clinical manifestations of coarctation, as well as the dramatic alleviation of the obstruction produced pharmacologically by dilatation of the ductus arteriosus.

CLINICAL FINDINGS. The manifestations of juxtaductal coarctation of the aorta depend on the prominence of the posterolateral aortic shelf, which determines the intensity of obstruction and on the rapidity with which obstruction develops.

911

Ch 29

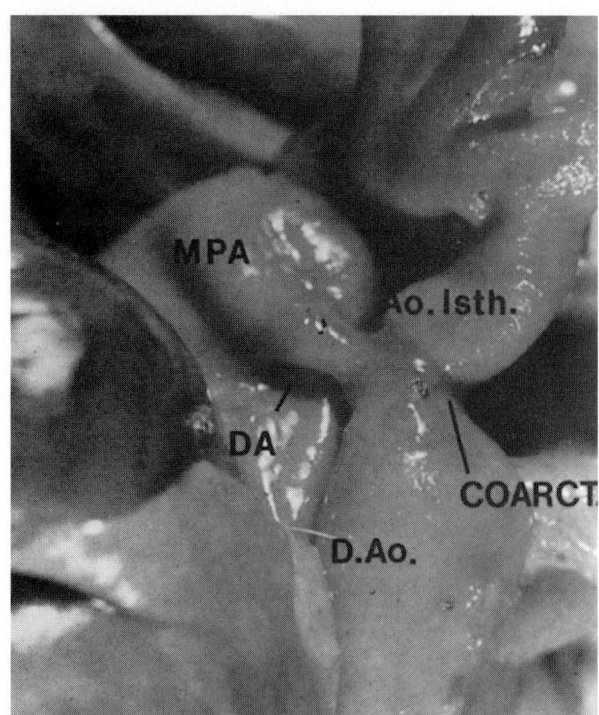

FIGURE 29–27. Juxtaductal coarctation (COARCT) unmasked by constriction of the ductus arteriosus (DA). MPA = main pulmonary artery, D.Ao. = descending aorta, Ao.Isth. = aortic isthmus. (Courtesy of Norman Talner, M.D.)

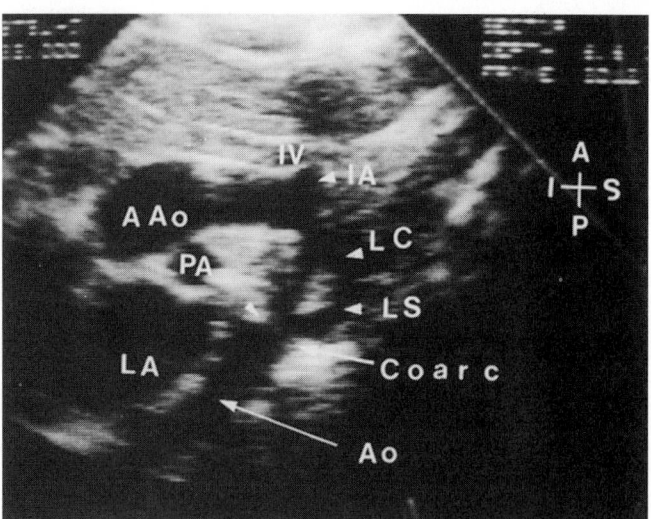

FIGURE 29–28. Aortic coarctation (Coarc) is visualized from the suprasternal notch. The aorta (Ao) can be traced from the ascending aorta (AAo). The aortic arch is somewhat narrowed, and the relationship of the left subclavian artery (LS) to the coarctation is identified clearly. LA = left atrium, PA = pulmonary artery, IA = innominate artery, LC = left carotid artery. (Courtesy of Norman Silverman, M.D.)

NEONATES AND INFANTS. Rapid, severe obstruction in infancy is a prominent cause of left ventricular failure and systemic hypoperfusion. Substantial left-to-right shunting across a patent foramen ovale and pulmonary venous hypertension secondary to heart failure cause pulmonary arterial hypertension. Because little or no aortic obstruction existed during fetal life, the collateral circulation in the newborn period is often poorly developed. Characteristically in these infants, peripheral pulses are weak throughout the body until left ventricular function is improved with medical management; a significant pressure difference then develops between the arms and the legs, allowing detection of a pulse discrepancy. Cardiac murmurs are nonspecific in infancy and commonly are derived from associated lesions.

The *electrocardiogram* shows the right-axis deviation and right ventricular hypertrophy; the *chest radiograph* shows generalized cardiomegaly and pulmonary arterial and venous engorgement. Two-dimensional and Doppler echocardiography provide an accurate noninvasive assessment of the anatomy and physiology in most patients. Hemodynamic study also allows delineation of the site and extent of aortic obstruction and the detection of associated cardiac malformations. Most infants with early-onset severe heart failure respond poorly to medical management, and balloon angioplasty, surgical excision of the coarctation, or a subclavian flap angioplasty often is required.

Aortic obstruction may develop slowly in infants in whom the posterolateral aortic shelf is not prominent at birth and in whom ductus arteriosus constriction is gradual. In these babies compensatory myocardial hypertrophy and an extensive collateral circulation have time to develop. If the obstruction does not intensify and cardiac failure does not occur by age 6 or 9 months, circulatory compensation is likely until adult life.

CHILDREN. Most children with isolated juxtaductal coarctation are asymptomatic. Complaints of headache, cold extremities, and claudication with exercise may be noted, although attention usually is directed to the cardiovascular system by detection of a heart murmur of upper-extremity hypertension on routine physical examination. Mechanical factors rather than those of renal origin play the primary role in the production of hypertension. Absent, markedly diminished, or delayed pulsations in the femoral arteries and a low or unobtainable arterial pressure in the lower extremities with hypertension in the arms are the basic clues to the diagnosis. A midsystolic murmur over the anterior chest, back, and spinous processes is most frequent, becoming continuous if the lumen is sufficiently narrowed to result in a high-velocity jet across the lesion throughout the cardiac cycle. Additional systolic and continuous murmurs over the lateral thoracic wall may reflect increased flow through dilated and tortuous collateral vessels.

Electrocardiography reveals left ventricular hypertrophy of varying degrees, depending on the height of arterial pressure above the obstruction and the patient's age. Combined with right ventricular hypertrophy, this usually implies a complicated lesion. *Chest roentgenograms* (Fig. 7–42, p. 232) may show a dilated left subclavian artery high on the left mediastinal border and a dilated ascending aorta. Indentation of the aorta at the site of coarctation and prestenotic and poststenotic dilatation (the "3" sign) along the left premediastinal shadow is almost pathognomonic. Poststenotic dilation also may be detected by indentation of the barium-filled esophagus. Notching of the ribs, an important radiographic sign, is due to erosion by dilated collateral vessels, increases with age, and usually becomes apparent between the 4th and 12th years of life. The aortic coarctation may be visualized directly by two-dimensional

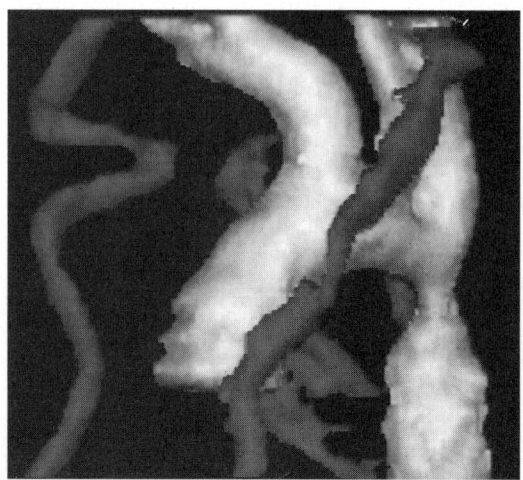

FIGURE 29–29. Three-dimensional computer reconstruction of magnetic resonance images in a child with discrete coarctation and numerous large collateral vessels, displayed in a lateral projection. Dilated brachiocephalic and internal mammary arteries are evident. (Courtesy of W. James Parks, M.D., The Children's Heart Center, Emory University, Atlanta, Georgia.)

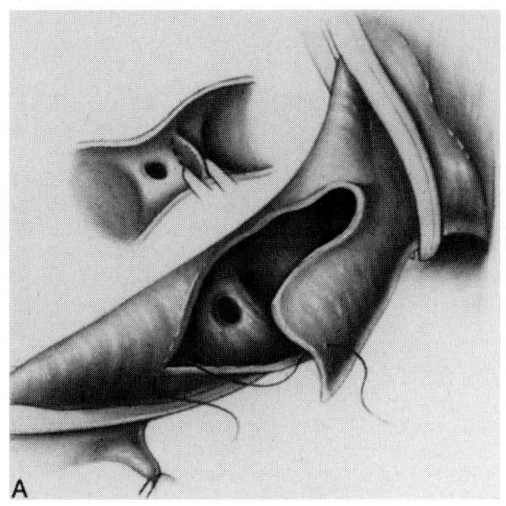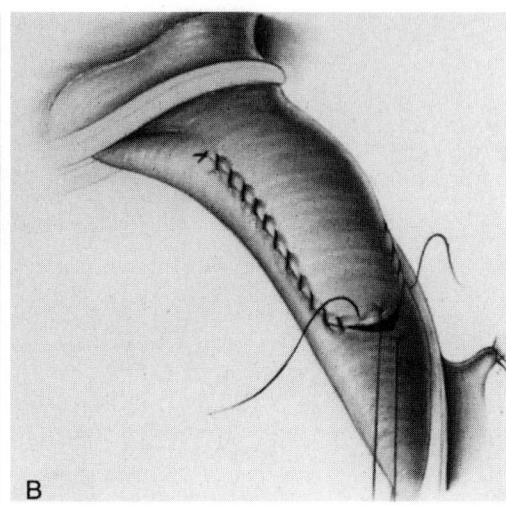

FIGURE 29–30. Subclavian flap aortoplasty repair of aortic coarctation. A, The left subclavian artery has been ligated and divided; the aorta is incised from below the coarctation ridge of tissue, which is carefully excised. B, The distal end of the subclavian artery forms a flap, which is sutured to the aortotomy. (From Stark, J., and DeLaval, M.: Surgery for Congenital Heart Defects. New York, Grune and Stratton, 1983, p. 216.)

echocardiography from high parasternal or suprasternal notch views with short focused transducers and from the subxiphoid window with extended focal range transducers (Fig. 29–28). Doppler examination reveals a flow disturbance and high-velocity jet at the site of obstruction and provides a reasonable estimate of the transcoarctation pressure gradient.[265,266] Computed tomography,[267] magnetic resonance imaging[268] (Fig. 29–29 and Fig. 10–22, p. 328), or cardiac catheterization and aortography also accurately localizes the site of obstruction, determines the length of coarctation, and, particularly, identifies associated malformations. Preoperative catheterization is avoided for selected patients with typical clinical and two-dimensional and Doppler echocardiographic findings.[269] Intravascular ultrasonography provides interesting morphological images suitable especially for comparison to postoperative status.[270,271]

MANAGEMENT. Controversy exists concerning the role of balloon angioplasty (see p. 1366) in the treatment of native coarctation, especially in neonates.[271–274] There is concern about residual pressure gradients, aneurysm formation, aortic dissection and rupture, and femoral arterial complications, especially late after angioplasty. It is clear that angioplasty can effectively reduce obstruction in many patients, albeit with an unpredictable late outcome.

Subclavian flap aortoplasty (Fig. 29–30), particularly in neonates and infants, or surgical resection and end-to-end anastomosis of uncomplicated juxtaductal coarctation of the aorta can be accomplished with excellent results in most patients[275,276]; some surgeons prefer an on-lay patch across the site of obstruction. In children who are asymptomatic it is preferable to delay surgery until age 4 to 6 years, at which time coarctation seldom recurs.[277] Paradoxical hypertension of short duration often is noted in the immediate postoperative period, a phenomenon much less common after balloon angioplasty.[278] A resetting of carotid baroreceptors and increased catecholamine secretion appears to be responsible for the initial phase of postoperative systemic hypertension with a later, second phase of prolonged elevation of systolic and particularly diastolic blood pressure related to activation of the renin-angiotensin system.[279] A necrotizing panarteritis of the small vessels of the gastrointestinal tract of uncertain cause occasionally complicates the course of recovery.

A 5 to 10 per cent risk of recurrent narrowing exists after repair of coarctation in infancy. Such narrowing is best detected by magnetic resonance imaging or Doppler ultrasonography.[280] This problem is treated most effectively by transcutaneous balloon angioplasty,[281,281a] which may be expected to markedly reduce, but not abolish entirely, the pressure differences across the site of recoarctation.

In those patients who survive the first 2 years of life, complications of juxtaductal coarctation are uncommon be-

fore the second or third decade. The chief hazards to patients with coarctation result from severe hypertension and include the development of cerebral aneurysms and hemorrhage, hypertensive encephalopathy, rupture of the aorta, left ventricular failure, and infective endocarditis. Systemic hypertension in the absence of residual coarctation has been observed in resting or exercise-stressed patients postoperatively and appears to be related to the duration of preoperative hypertension.[282–284] Lifelong observation is desirable because of the late onset of hypertension in some postoperative patients.[285–288]

Hypoplasia of the Aortic Arch

MORPHOLOGY. The aortic isthmus, the portion of the aorta between the left subclavian artery and the ductus arteriosus, normally is narrowed in the fetus and newborn. The lumen of the aortic isthmus is about two-thirds that of the ascending and descending portions of the aorta until age 6 to 9 months, when the physiological narrowing disappears.[289] Pathological tubular hypoplasia of the aortic arch usually is noted in the aortic isthmus and often is referred to as preductal or infantile coarctation of the aorta.[290] Associated major cardiac malformations occur in virtually all such infants and include large ventricular septal defect, atrioventricular septal defect, transposition of the great arteries, the Taussig-Bing type of anomaly, and double-outlet right ventricle. The ventricular septal defect most often is subpulmonary, lying within the substance of the infundibular septum. Thus, muscle persists between the aortic and pulmonary valve leaflets, which, when displaced leftward, produces subaortic stenosis. Persistent patency of the ductus arteriosus commonly coexists, and right-to-left flow across the ductus arteriosus usually provides filling of the descending aorta. The adequacy of blood flow to the lower body depends on the degree of aortic hypoplasia, the caliber of the ductus arteriosus, and the relationship between pulmonary and systemic vascular resistance. Substantial right-to-left shunting through a wide-open ductus arteriosus minimizes the arterial blood pressure difference between the upper and lower body.

CLINICAL FINDINGS. Differential cyanosis of the toes and feet with normal color of the fingers and hands may be difficult to discern because intracardiac left-to-right shunting and pulmonary edema attenuate the differences in oxygen saturation in the ascending and descending aorta. Clinical deterioration is associated with ductal constriction or a fall in pulmonary vascular resistance. Moreover, the clinical presentation often is dictated by the hemodynamic effects of complex associated intracardiac malformations. Infants most often present with findings of a large left-to-right intracardiac shunt, pulmonary hypertension, and marked cardiac decompensation. Although tubular hypoplasia is detectable by two-dimensional echocardiography, cardiac catheterization may be required to evaluate the full extent of intracardiac and extracardiac lesions.[291] Surgical repair of aortic arch hypoplasia usually must be accompanied by operative palliation or correction of associated intracardiac lesions. An extended end-to-end anastomosis (Fig. 29–31), classic or reversed subclavian flap angioplasty, patch aortography, and bypass grafting are among the operative approaches to correct long segment narrowing.[292–294] Recoarctation is common and often necessitates transcatheter balloon aortoplasty and/or a second operation later in life to relieve anastomotic stenosis.

AORTIC ARCH INTERRUPTION

Aortic arch interruption is a rare and usually lethal anomaly; unless treated surgically almost all infants die within the first

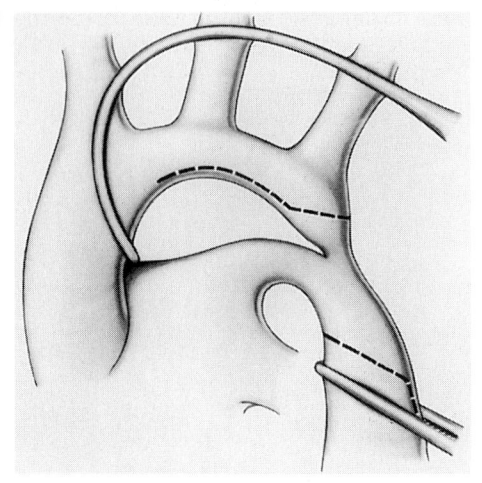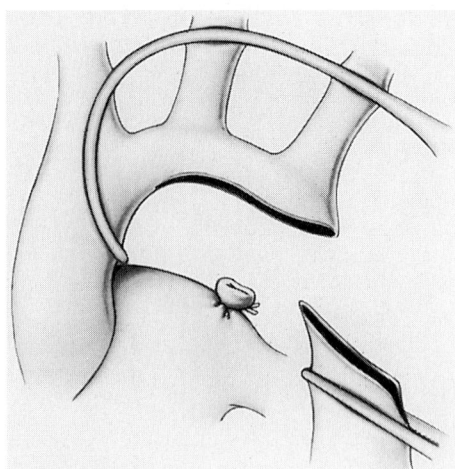

FIGURE 29–31. An extended repair of aortic coarctation is employed in the presence of a hypoplastic aortic arch. The dashed lines in the left panel delineate resection sites of the coarcted segment. In the right panel, the ductus arteriosus has been ligated and the incisions are extended to the undersurface of the aortic arch and onto the distal aorta. When the suture line is completed, the reconstruction of the arch is generally excellent. (From Stark, J., and DeLaval, M.: Surgery for Congenital Heart Defects. 2nd ed. Philadelphia, W.B. Saunders Company, 1994, p. 292.)

month of life.[295] Interruptions distal to the left subclavian artery (Type A) occur with almost equal frequency to interruptions distal to the left common carotid artery (Type B); interruptions distal to the innominate artery (Type C) are extremely uncommon. The right subclavian artery often is of variable origin, frequently arising from the descending aortic segment distal to the interruption. The clinical presentation resembles that seen in tubular hypoplasia or severe juxtaductal coarctation of the aorta with a patent ductus arteriosus.

Virtually all patients have associated intracardiac anomalies. A patent ductus arteriosus almost always connects the main pulmonary artery with the descending aorta. With rare exceptions, patients with interrupted aortic arch have either a ventricular septal defect (80 to 90 per cent of cases) or an aorticopulmonary window (10 to 20 per cent). Because the ductus arteriosus provides lower-body blood flow, its spontaneous constriction results in profound clinical deterioration. The latter may be temporarily ameliorated by prostaglandin E$_1$ infusion.[96,264] The ventricular septal defect most often is subpulmonary, lying within the substance of the infundibular septum. Thus, muscle persists between the aortic and pulmonary valve leaflets, which, when displaced leftward, produces subaortic stenosis. Other complex intracardiac malformations, such as transposition of the great arteries, aortopulmonary window, and truncus arteriosus, are common.[296]

CLINICAL FEATURES. An association is frequent with DiGeorge syndrome, a constellation of cardiac, parathyroid, thymic, and facial anomalies attributed to disruption of the interaction of premigratory neural crest cells with endodermal pharyngeal pouch cells. In this syndrome thymic hypoplasia or aplasia is accompanied by immunological and hypocalcemia problems.[297,298] The major clinical problem is severe congestive heart failure as a consequence of volume overload of the left ventricle resulting from an associated intracardiac left-to-right shunt and of pressure overload imposed by systemic hypertension.

Management. The perioperative clinical condition of most patients can be improved by intensive medical management with mechanical ventilation, inotropic support, and prostaglandin infusion. Various forms of palliative operative techniques have fair to poor results. There has been increasing success with complete primary repair in infancy as the procedure of choice.[299–301] In some circumstances, a two-stage approach with initial arch repair and pulmonary artery banding is followed by later repair of the intracardiac lesion. Recurrent narrowing at the aortic suture line can be treated by balloon angioplasty or reoperation.

Congenital Valvular Aortic Stenosis
(See also p. 1035)

MORPHOLOGY. Congenital valvular aortic stenosis is a relatively common anomaly, estimated to occur in 3 to 6 per cent of patients with congenital cardiovascular defects. However, it must be appreciated that the true incidence of the malformation is probably grossly underestimated because the congenital bicuspid aortic valve may be undetected in early life and becomes stenotic and of clinical significance only in adult life, at a time when it may be indistinguishable from the acquired forms of aortic stenosis (Fig. 30–1, p. 964). Congenital valvular aortic stenosis occurs much more frequently in males than in females, with the gender ratio approximating 4:1. Associated cardiovascular anomalies have been noted in as many as 20 per cent of patients.[302] Patent ductus arteriosus and coarc-

tation of the aorta occur most frequently with valvular aortic stenosis; all three of these lesions may coexist.

The basic malformation consists of thickening of valve tissue with varying degrees of commissural fusion. The valve most commonly is bicuspid with a single fused commissure and an eccentrically place orifice. Sometimes a third commissure, incomplete or rudimentary, is apparent. Less commonly, the valve has three fused cusps with a stenotic central orifice. In some patients the stenotic aortic valve is unicuspid and dome-shaped with no or one lateral attachment to the aorta at the level of the orifice. In infants and young children with severe aortic stenosis the aortic valve ring may be relatively underdeveloped. This lesion forms a continuum with the hypoplastic left heart syndrome and the aortic atresia and hypoplasia complexes. Secondary calcification of the valve is extremely rare in childhood, but the dynamics of blood flow associated with the congenitally deformed aortic valve ultimately lead to thickening of the cusps and calcification in adult life. When the obstruction is hemodynamically significant, concentric hypertrophy of the left ventricular wall and dilatation of the ascending aorta occur.

HEMODYNAMICS (see also Figs. 6–12, p. 194, and 32–27, p. 1036). The hemodynamic abnormalities produced by obstruction to left ventricular outflow are discussed on p. 1036. A peak systolic gradient exceeding 75 mm Hg in association with a normal cardiac output or an effective aortic orifice less than 0.5 cm^2/m^2 body surface area is considered to reflect critical or severe obstruction to left ventricular outflow.[302,303] The normal outflow orifice approximates 2.0 cm^2/m^2 body surface area; areas of 0.5 to 0.8 cm^2/m^2 signify moderate obstruction; when the area is larger than 0.8 cm^2/m^2, the obstruction is considered to be mild.

The resting cardiac output and stroke volume usually are within normal limits. During exercise, most children with critical stenosis show an elevation of the cardiac output and an associated elevation in the transvalvular pressure gradient.[304,305] When left ventricular failure occurs, the cardiac output decreases, and the left atrial, left ventricular end-diastolic, and pulmonary vascular pressures increase.

Studies of left ventricular performance in children with aortic stenosis often indicate that supernormal pump function exists, as indicated by increases in ejection fraction and circumferential fiber shortening.[306] Despite high left ventricular systolic pressures, left ventricular wall stress appears to be lower than normal throughout systole, presumably because increases in wall thickness provide overcompensation for the pressure overload. Undoubtedly, a spectrum exists, from well-compensated patients at one end, who have supernormal pump function and normal contractile function, to patients with heart failure at the opposite end, who have both impaired pump function and a reduced contractile state.

Whereas pressure overload hypertrophy may preserve systolic function, it may also result in abnormal left ventricular early diastolic filling.[307,308] Thus, clinical studies seeking to analyze the determinants of left ventricular filling by a separate assessment of dynamic (elastic recoil, ventricular relaxation rate, and atrial driving pressure) and static (chamber stiffness and left ventricular hypertrophy) determinants suggest that diastolic function most importantly varies according to the severity of left ventricular hypertrophy and systolic function. Studies in children suggest that hypertrophy is a more important factor than excessive wall stress and depressed ejection performance in accounting for abnormal diastolic filling.

The blood supply to the myocardium may be significantly compromised in infants and children with aortic stenosis, despite normal patency of the coronary arteries.[309] Coronary blood flow and arterial oxygen content are critical determinants of oxygen supply to the myocardium. Because intramyocardial compressive forces are greatest in the subendocardium, blood flow to that region of the left ventricle is entirely diastolic in the presence of elevated left ventricular systolic pressure. In patients with left ventricular outflow tract obstruction, coronary vasodilatation may give an inadequate response to an increase in the demands of the myocardium for oxygen at rest or with exercise. When subendocardial vessels are maximally dilated, the coronary artery driving pressure and the duration of diastole determine the magnitude of subendocardial flow. When the duration of systolic ejection lengthens across the stenotic orifice, diastole is shortened, especially at high heart rates. Moreover, a reduction occurs in coronary driving pressure if left ventricular end-diastolic pressure is high or if aortic diastolic pressure is low, e.g., with aortic regurgitation or heart failure. In patients with severe aortic stenosis the redistribution of flow away from the subendocardium and the ischemia that results in that portion of ventricular muscle may be estimated by relating the diastolic pressure–time index (DPTI) (i.e., the area between the aortic and left ventricular pressures in diastole) to the systolic pressure–time index (SPTI) (a measure of myocardial oxygen demands). Inadequate subendocardial oxygen delivery has been shown to exist when the ratio [DPTI × arterial oxygen content/SPTI] falls below 10.[309]

NEONATES AND INFANTS. Reports exist of cardiac dysfunction and even nonimmunological fetal hydrops fetalis in association with severe aortic stenosis.[310] The hydrops may be the result of in utero left ventricular myocardial infarction or profound left ventricular systolic and diastolic dysfunction. Balloon dilation using coronary balloon catheters has been attempted via transabdominal echo-guided needle puncture of the fetal left ventricle. This approach is not established and it remains conjectural whether it will become a management option.[311]

Fortunately, isolated aortic valvular stenosis seldom causes symptoms in infancy.[312–314] This lesion, however, occasionally may be responsible for profound and intractable heart failure. Despite normal coronary arterial anatomy, infarction of left ventricular papillary muscles may occur, resulting in an acquired form of mitral valvular regurgitation that intensifies the heart failure state. In addition, endocardial fibroelastosis may result from limited subendocardial oxygen delivery, and myocardial degeneration may be significant.[314] The symptomatic infant with isolated valvular aortic stenosis is irritable, pale, and hypotensive and presents with tachycardia, cardiomegaly, and pulmonary congestion manifested by dyspnea, tachypnea, subcostal retractions, and diffuse rales. Cyanosis may be observed secondary to pulmonary venous desaturation. The systolic murmur in infants often is atypical; it is best heard at the apex or along the lower left sternal border and may be confused with that caused by a ventricular septal defect. In infants with heart failure the murmur occasionally may be absent or extremely soft, becoming louder when myocardial contractility is improved with digitalis and other medical

measures. The response to medical management of the infant with heart failure is frequently poor.

The *electrocardiographic findings* may not be characteristic; left ventricular hypertrophy and/or strain as well as right atrial enlargement and right ventricular hypertrophy may be detected shortly after birth.[312] The latter signs of right heart involvement result from both pulmonary hypertension secondary to elevated left ventricular diastolic and left atrial pressures and from volume loading of the right ventricle caused by left-to-right shunting across the foramen ovale. Survival past the early neonatal period does not preclude subsequent difficulties, and clinical deterioration may recur with the onset of physiological anemia.

MANAGEMENT. Congenital aortic stenosis must be considered a medical emergency in the seriously ill newborn, and echocardiography, and sometimes cardiac catheterization and angiocardiography, may be indicated in the first 24 hours of life. Two-dimensional echocardiographic studies show a severe immobility of the aortic valve, with little or no systolic opening, poststenotic dilation of the aorta, left ventricular hypertrophy, right ventricular enlargement, and a severely disturbed Doppler-determined pattern of ascending aortic flow velocity. The echo-Doppler examination must also identify associated intracardiac and extracardiac anomalies, one of the most important of which is severe aortic arch obstruction.

In many centers, expeditious balloon aortic valvuloplasty follows the echo-Doppler examination in infants who are unstable and markedly symptomatic.[315–316b] A number of approaches have been reported for performing this procedure, including the use of a carotid artery cutdown, which thus far does not appear to result in any abnormalities of the carotid pulse or any neurological sequelae.[317] A transumbilical technique of balloon valvuloplasty can be performed quickly, safely, and effectively with preservation of the femoral artery.[314] Because of a high risk of iliofemoral artery complications in infants with the transfemoral route to valvuloplasty, when this route is employed it is advisable to use double-balloon techniques to allow insertion of small valvuloplasty catheters. The complications of balloon valvuloplasty are related to the small size and young age of the patient. Accordingly, if arterial access is a problem, and in infants less than 1 month of age, surgical valvotomy remains a satisfactory option. Open repair under direct vision is the preferred type of operation.

Hemodynamic findings in neonates and infants frequently include left-to-right shunting at the atrial level, an elevated left atrial and left ventricular end-diastolic pressure, and a small pressure drop across the aortic valve as a result of markedly reduced cardiac output. Right-to-left shunting across a patent ductus arteriosus is encountered occasionally. The lesion may be distinguished from the hypoplastic left heart syndrome echocardiographically and angiographically by the presence of normal or enlarged left ventricular cavity and normal or dilated ascending aorta. Establishment of the diagnosis and prompt catheter valvuloplasty or surgical valvotomy are justified because prolonged periods of stabilization are uncommon with medical therapy. Poor myocardial performance resulting from endocardial fibroelastosis, subendocardial ischemia, reduced left ventricular compliance, and inadequate relief of obstruction with or without aortic insufficiency are some of the factors accounting for high mortality and morbidity following catheter-directed treatment or operation.

At the extreme end of the spectrum of critical valvar aortic stenosis in the newborn are patients with multiple small left-sided structures in whom the adverse effects of small inflow, outflow, and/or cavity size of the left ventricle appear to be cumulative.[318–320] It is in this group that traditional treatment by aortic valvuloplasty or valvotomy, which is a two-sided ventricle repair, may be less effective than a multistaged Norwood approach.[321] The latter consists of an initial single-ventricle repair in which the main pulmonary artery is anastomosed to the aorta with creation of a systemic-to-pulmonary arterial shunt, followed later by a Fontan-type operation that creates an atriopulmonary connection, with or without a prior superior cavapulmonary connection. The single-ventricle repair results in the functional sacrifice of the left ventricle and the right ventricle supporting the systemic circulation without a pulmonary ventricle.

CHILDREN. Congenital aortic stenosis may be responsible for severe obstruction to left ventricular outflow in the absence of clinical symptoms of diminished cardiac reserve that are so frequent in other forms of congenital heart disease.[322] Most children with congenital aortic stenosis grow and develop normally and are asymptomatic. Attention usually is called to these children when a murmur is detected on routine examination. When symptoms occur, those noted most commonly are fatigability, exertional dyspnea, angina pectoris, and syncope. Less often described are abdominal pain, profuse sweating, and epistaxis. The symptomatic child usually has critical stenosis. There is a distinct threat of sudden death in patients with severe obstruction[303] (p. 885). Although the precise cause is poorly understood, ventricular arrhythmias, perhaps initiated by acute myocardial ischemia, are probably the most common inciting event. It has been speculated that an abrupt rise in intracavity left ventricular systolic pressure elicits a reflex hypotensive syncope that promotes acute ischemia and ventricular fibrillation.[323] Bacterial endocarditis occurs in about 4 per cent of patients with congenital valvular aortic stenosis.[324]

DIAGNOSIS. Physical Findings. When the magnitude of obstruction is significant, a left ventricular lift usually is palpable, and a precordial systolic thrill often is palpated over the base of the heart with transmission to the jugular notch and along the carotid arteries; presystolic expansion often is palpable. The obstruction usually is mild if neither a left ventricular lift nor a thrill is present.

Opening of the aortic valve produces a systolic aortic ejection sound that typically is present at the cardiac apex when the valve is mobile, particularly in patients with mild to moderate stenosis. A delay in closure of the stenotic aortic valve leads to a single or a closely split second heart sound, and paradoxical splitting may be present. A fourth heart sound normally is associated with severe obstruction. A loud, harsh, rhomboid-shaped systolic murmur starts after completion of left ventricular isometric contraction and is best heard at the base of the heart. The murmur, like the thrill, radiates to the suprasternal notch and carotid vessel as well as to the apex. An early diastolic blowing murmur of aortic regurgitation is present in some patients, but unless the valve leaflets have been eroded by bacterial endocarditis, the regurgitation usually is not hemodynamically significant; uncommonly, in patients with a congenitally bicuspid valve, aortic regurgitation may be severe and may predominate.

Electrocardiography. There is a tendency for electrocardiographic signs of left ventricular hypertrophy to vary with the severity of obstruction, although a normal or near-normal electrocardiogram does not exclude severe aortic stenosis, and excessive left ventricular voltages may be observed in children with mild obstruction.[322] The lack of a good correlation between the ECG and the transvalvular pressure gradient emphasizes the potential hazard of relying on the ECG in patient management. The most reliable index of the severity of obstruction is the presence of a left ventricular "strain pattern," consisting of left ventricular hypertrophy combined with ST-segment depressions and T-wave inversion in the left precordial leads (Fig. 29–32).

Roentgenography. Overall heart size is normal or the degree of enlargement is slight in most children with congenital valvular aortic stenosis. Concentric left ventricular hypertrophy accompanies moderate or severe obstruction and is manifested by rounding of the cardiac apex in the frontal projection and posterior displacement in the lateral view.

Echocardiography. Two-dimensional and Doppler echocardiography are the current methods of choice for defining the anatomy and the hemodynamic severity of valvular aortic stenosis.[325–328] Real-time cross-sectional echocardiography reveals impaired mobility of cusp tissue, an alteration in the phasic movement of the aortic valve with reduced lateral and increased superior excursions of valve echoes, and an increase in the internal aortic root dimension beyond the level of the valve annulus.[302] Imaging of the valve must be performed many times in order to display the valve through the long axis of the left ventricular outflow tract and then through a plane parallel to the valve annulus. The long-axis view of the left ventricular outflow tract allows evaluation of the valve mobility and cusp separation; it is the best view for demonstrating doming of the aortic valve. The parasternal short-axis view bisects the face of the valve, demonstrating the anatomy of the commissures (Fig. 29–33).

The echocardiogram also reveals associated left ventricular hypertrophy and the presence of endocardial fibroelastosis (seen as bright endocardial echoes). Further, the measurement of mitral valve diameter, left ventricular end-diastolic dimension, and left ventricular cross-sectional area serve to distinguish those infants with critical aortic stenosis from those with a hypoplastic left ventricle.[326] Among these calculations suggesting the latter are an end-

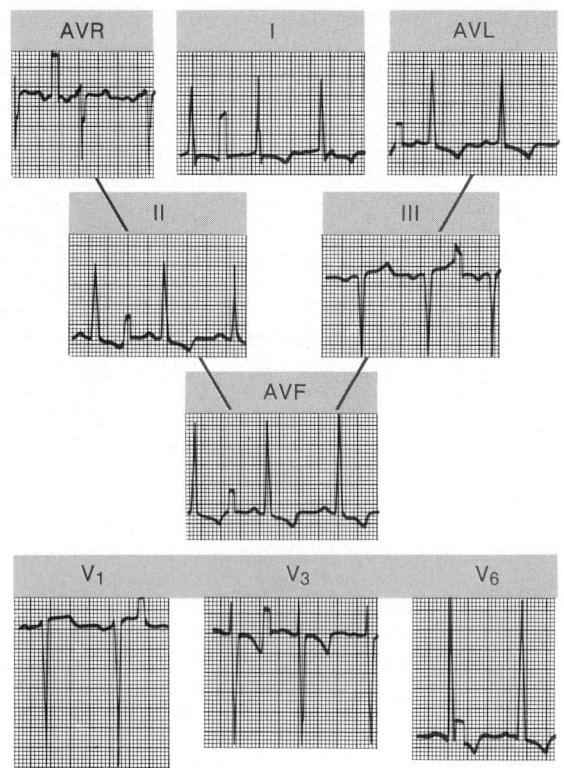

FIGURE 29–32. Electrocardiogram in congenital aortic stenosis. This tracing shows left ventricular hypertrophy and the typical left ventricular "strain" pattern (V_6, *arrow*). (Courtesy of Delores A. Danilowicz, M.D.)

diastolic volume less than 20 ml/m², an inflow dimension of 25 mm, a narrow ventricular aortic junction less than 5 mm, or a small mitral orifice less than 9 mm. Pulse-Doppler echocardiography allows inspection of the pattern of flow velocity within the circulation.[325,327] This technique detects the altered and disturbed turbulence of flow in patients with aortic stenosis. A highly accurate noninvasive approach to quantifying the severity of obstruction combines continuous-wave Doppler flow analysis with the cross-sectional echocardiographic determination of the area of the orifice.[329] A simplified Bernoulli equation uses the measurement of the maximum velocity of the aortic jet and time-averaged pressure drop obtained from planimetry of the maximal velocity spectral reading. A simpler estimate of the transvalvular gradient (in mm Hg) may be calculated as four times the square of the peak Doppler velocity (m/sec).

The Doppler method records a peak instantaneous pressure difference, which may differ importantly from the gradient recorded by a cardiac catheter, which is a peak-to-peak pressure difference.[330] Doppler mean gradient is more accurate than the instantaneous gradient when compared with the pressures found at cardiac catheterization. Management decisions often depend on the estimation of the severity of obstruction, and all pressure gradient estimations depend on flow velocity across the valve, which may be confounded by low cardiac output or concomitant valvar regurgitation. Thus, an important argument can be made that the determination of the stenotic valve systolic area is often more important than calculation of a systolic gradient.[327–329]

The most widely accepted technique for correcting the gradient for flow is to use the continuity equation, which measures the flow velocity ratio across the aortic valve and, therefore, corrects for high and low flow rates. The continuity equation presumes that for flow in a series, the product of mean velocity and cross-sectional area is constant at all points in the flow circuit. In patients with aortic stenosis, the area of the left ventricular outflow tract is deter-

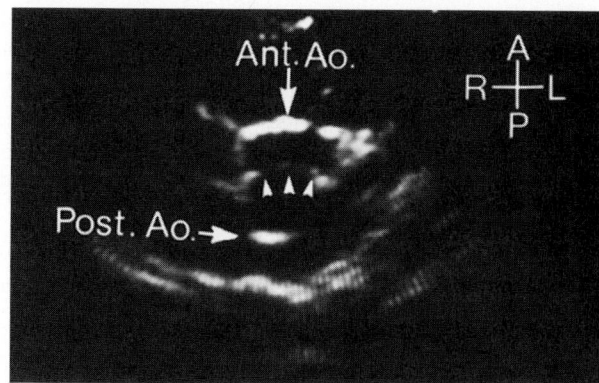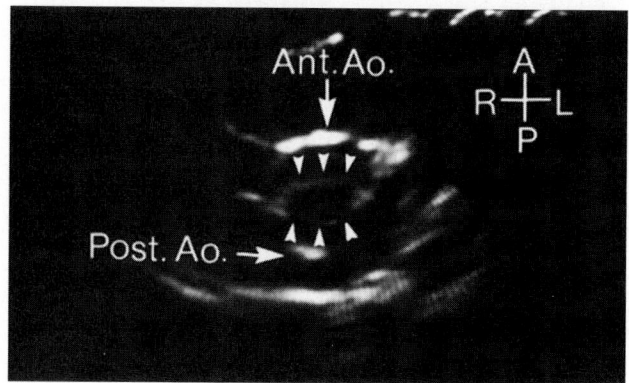

FIGURE 29–33. Short-axis view at the base of the heart of a bicuspid aortic valve. In the left panel the valve is imaged as a single diastolic echo (arrows) in the aortic root. In systole *(right panel)*, the valve opens (arrows) with a typical fish-mouth appearance. Ant.Ao. = anterior aorta, Post.Ao. = posterior aorta. (From DiSessa, T. G., and Friedman, W. F.: Cardiovascular Clinics. Fowler, N. [ed.], Philadelphia, F. A. Davis Co., 1983.)

mined by two-dimensional echocardiography, the flow velocity of the outflow tract by pulse-Doppler, and the flow velocity immediately above the valve by continuous-wave Doppler, all of which, taken together, allow the determination of the valve area by the continuity equation: Aortic valve area (area) LVOT × (V)LVOT/(V)AV (obtained by converting the diameter to area and assuming that it is circular); (V)LVOT = peak outflow tract velocity, and (V)AV = peak velocity across the aortic valve.

Transesophageal two-dimensional echocardiographic determination of aortic valve area has been applied in adults with aortic stenosis.[331,332] The approach offers considerably better resolution of cardiac anatomy than does conventional transthoracic two-dimensional echocardiography and may also prove to be more accurate in estimating pressure gradients and aortic valve areas. The approach has not yet been reported in children in sufficient detail to make specific recommendations.

Diagnostic Cardiac Catheterization. Cardiac catheterization is now rarely used to establish the site and severity of obstruction to left ventricular outflow because the malformation is readily diagnosed and the evaluation of the intensity of stenosis is accurate by echo-Doppler examination.[333] Instead, catheterization is undertaken when

therapeutic interventional transcatheter balloon aortic valvuloplasty is indicated.

During the catheterization procedure, cardiac output is measured by the indicator-dilution, thermodilution, or Fick technique. Retrograde left heart catheterization allows withdrawal pressure recordings across the site of stenosis, and left ventricular angiocardiography can be carried out, permitting an evaluation of the size of the left ventricular cavity, the thickness of the wall, the competency of the mitral valve, the patency of the coronary arteries, and the diameter of the aortic root and ascending aorta. If aortic insufficiency is thought to be present, cineaortography is performed with injection of contrast material into the aortic root. The severity of aortic insufficiency can be assessed qualitatively by cineaortography and quantitatively by ventriculography with calculation of regurgitant volume by subtraction of net forward flow (calculated by the Fick method) from angiographically determined total forward flow.[336] The typical angiocardiographic features of valvar stenosis are thickening of the aortic cusps, poststenotic dilation of the ascending aorta, and, occasionally, a jet of contrast material entering the ascending aorta through a central or eccentric narrowed valve orifice (Fig. 29–34). The leaflets of the bicuspid valve are domed in systole, and

FIGURE 29–34. *A,* Left ventricular angiocardiogram obtained by the transseptal method in a patient with congenital valvular aortic stenosis. Ao = poststenotic dilatation of the aorta; LV = left ventricle. Arrow denotes the thickened valve cusp. *B,* Selective angiocardiogram in a patient with discrete subvalvular stenosis (bottom arrow). Associated mitral regurgitation is evident from the reflux of contrast into an enlarged left atrium (LA). The aortic valve (top arrow) is normal, and the right coronary artery is visualized. (From Friedman, W. F., Kirkpatrick, S. E.: Congenital aortic stenosis. *In* Moss, A. J., Adams, F. H., and Emmanouilides, G. C. [eds.]: Heart Disease in Infants, Children and Adolescents. 2nd ed. Baltimore, © Williams and Wilkins, 1977.)

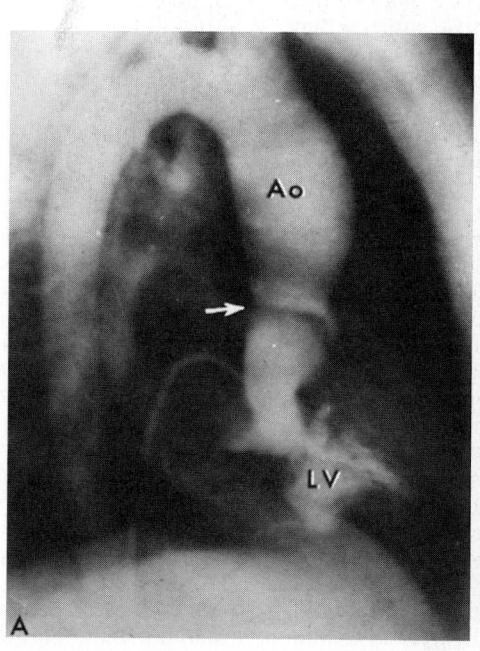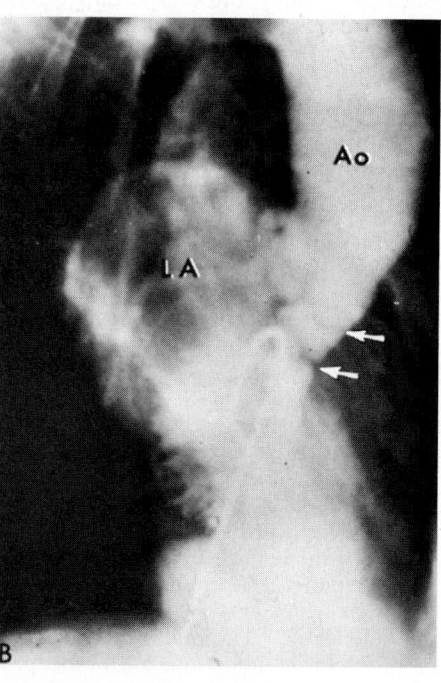

a central jet corresponds to the orifice of the stenotic valve. In contrast, the stenotic orifice of the unicommissural valve can be visualized by the systolic jet in contact with the posterior wall of the aorta, with leaflet tissue and valve motion seen only anteriorly.[302]

Balloon Valvuloplasty. Balloon dilatation may be indicated in any child with a clinical diagnosis of aortic stenosis in whom the clinical examination, roentgenogram, resting or exercise ECG, or Doppler echocardiogram suggests the possibility of severe obstruction.[334,335] Even in the absence of such findings, balloon valvuloplasty may be performed if symptoms that might be related to AS exist, such as dizziness, fainting, or angina.

This author prefers to catheterize the left side of the heart via a retrograde approach by femoral percutaneous puncture. The goals of the study are to analyze the severity of obstruction and assess the function of the left ventricle. In most centers, balloon valvuloplasty is recommended if the severity of the AS would otherwise require surgical treatment, that is, a peak systolic pressure gradient exceeding 70 mm Hg measured in the basal state or a calculated effective orifice less than 0.5 cm^2/m^2 of body surface area. In the presence of symptoms or left ventricular strain pattern on the ECG or an abnormal exercise ECG, there is less rigid regard to the hemodynamic assessment of the severity of stenosis. Further, some centers go forward with balloon valvuloplasty with peak systolic gradients greater than or equal to 50 mm Hg. There is general agreement that there be no significant aortic regurgitation (less than grade 2 of 4) and that other associated cardiac anomalies be absent, except aortic coarctation.

Balloon dilatation of the aortic valve began in the mid-1980s; truly long-term follow-up studies are not yet available. Early studies and the experience of the author suggest that the diameter of the balloon should not exceed that of the aortic valve ring. Most centers prefer a balloon with a diameter 80 to 100 per cent that of, or at least 1 mm smaller than, the aortic annulus. The expected hemodynamic result is a reduction in the catheterization-measured peak-to-peak ejection gradient of about 60 to 70 per cent. The appearance of aortic regurgitation or its progression is the major complication of valvuloplasty, although the aortic regurgitation is mild in the great majority of patients.[316b,334] Significant aortic regurgitation appears to accompany the development of aortic valve prolapse, which is likely due to tearing of the valve cusp or its raphe or partial detachment of the valve from the valve ring, all of which undermine the support mechanism of the valve.[335] In those patients whose balloon valvuloplasty has resulted in very significant aortic regurgitation, valve surgery may be required to either replace the valve or repair a tear in the valve. Other complications from balloon aortic valvuloplasty include bleeding, arrhythmias, cerebral vascular accidents, iliofemoral arterial complications, injury to the mitral valve, and, rarely beyond infancy, death.[334]

Natural History. Congenital aortic stenosis frequently is a progressive disorder, even early in life, in a significant fraction of patients presenting initially with mild obstruction.[337-340] Thus, clinical deterioration may be anticipated because of an intensification in the severity of stenosis rather than the development of significant aortic regurgitation. Progression of obstruction usually is the result of the increase in cardiac output that occurs concurrent with increased body growth. Less often, a decrease in the area of the orifice is an added factor in the intensification of obstruction. The onset of symptoms or changes in the phonocardiogram or graphic pulse tracings, chest roentgenograms, electrocardiograms, or vectorcardiograms cannot be depended on to indicate progressive obstruction in the individual patient; Doppler echocardiography is most reliable.

MANAGEMENT. The malformed aortic valve is a potential site of bacterial infection; antibiotic prophylaxis is recommended for all patients, regardless of the severity of obstruction. Strict avoidance of strenuous physical activity is advised if severe aortic stenosis is present. Participation in competitive sports also should probably be restricted in patients with milder degrees of obstruction. Digitalis should be administered to patients who have symptoms of diminished cardiac reserve and also should be considered in patients with left ventricular hypertrophy, even if they are not in heart failure.

Surgery. Percutaneous balloon aortic valvuloplasty is a useful palliation to delay open valvulotomy or valve replacement. For those patients in whom balloon valvuloplasty is unsuccessful, operation is carried out under direct vision after institution of cardiopulmonary bypass, and the fused commissures are opened. When this is done precisely and judiciously, the commissural incision enlarges the valve orifice and does not result in significant aortic insufficiency.[341] When operation is performed in childhood, a mortality rate of less than 2 per cent can be expected.[341,342] Among the factors influencing the indications, techniques, and results of operation are the patient's age, the nature of the valvar deformity, and the experience of the surgical team.

Long-term follow-up studies indicate that aortic valvotomy is a safe and effective means of palliative treatment with excellent relief of symptoms.[341-343] Occasionally, aortic insufficiency may be progressive and require valve replacement. Moreover, following commissurotomy, the valve leaflets remain somewhat deformed; and it is likely that further degenerative changes, including calcification, will lead to significant stenosis in later years.[302] Thus, prosthetic valve replacement is required in approximately 35 per cent of patients within 15 to 20 years of the original operation.[342,343] Because the valve is not rendered normal, antibiotic prophylaxis is indicated in the postoperative patient, even if the systolic pressure gradient has been abolished.[342] For those patients eventually requiring aortic valve replacement, the surgical options include replacement with a prosthetic aortic valve, an aortic homograft, or a pulmonary autograft in the aortic position.[344-347a] Evidence is beginning to accumulate that the pulmonary autograft may ultimately be preferable to the aortic homograft for aortic reconstruction. Neither homografts nor autografts require anticoagulation. There is a finite incidence of valve degeneration of approximately 2 per cent per patient per year with the former, whereas primary tissue failure has not been observed among pulmonary autografts.

Discrete Subaortic Stenosis

This malformation accounts for 8 to 10 per cent of all cases of congenital aortic stenosis and occurs twice as frequently in males as in females. The lesion consists of a membranous diaphragm or fibrous ring encircling the left ventricular outflow tract or a long fibromuscular narrowing just beneath the base of the aortic valve. Subaortic stenosis is rarely diagnosed in infancy, when it is usually the result of a malalignment ventricular septal defect with deviation posteriorly of the outlet septum into the left ventricular outflow tract, often associated with coarctation of the aorta or interruption of the aortic arch.

Distinction of subvalvular from valvular aortic stenosis is extremely difficult by means of clinical findings alone.[302] Rarely, a systolic ejection sound is heard, and the diastolic murmur of aortic regurgitation is more common than it is in valvular aortic stenosis. Dilatation of the ascending aorta is common, but valvular calcification is not observed.

Echocardiography is useful in the differentiation between valvular and subvalvular stenosis (Figs. 3–71, p. 80, and 3–72, p. 81).[348,349] The criterion for diagnosis of the latter is the demonstration of a localized subvalvar discrete ridge or long segment narrowing in the left ventricular outflow tract. Further, because of the possibility of recurrence of subvalvular aortic stenosis, careful postoperative follow-up echocardiography is required. Two-dimensional echocardiographic studies from the apical two-chamber and left parasternal and subxiphoid long-axis views demonstrate persistent, prominent echoes in the subaortic left ventricle in both systole and diastole (Fig. 29–35). Doppler sampling proximal to the aortic valve shows increased flow velocity.[348] Most important, echocardiography also can identify hypertrophic subaortic stenosis when it coexists with fixed subaortic stenosis and can differentiate between the two forms of obstruction.

Definitive distinction between valvular and subvalvular obstruction is also provided by transesophageal Doppler echocardiography[350] and by recording pressure tracings as a catheter is withdrawn across the outflow tract and valve, or by localizing the site of obstruction with selective left ventricular angiocardiography (Fig. 29–34).

Mild degrees of aortic valvular regurgitation commonly are observed in patients with discrete subaortic stenosis and appear to be caused by thickening of the valve and impaired mobility of the cusps secondary to the trauma created by the high-velocity jet passing through the subaortic diaphragm. Further deformation of these abnormal valve cusps by the vegetations of bacterial endocarditis often results in severe aortic regurgitation.

MANAGEMENT. Because of the likelihood of both progressive obstruction and aortic regurgitation, the presence of even mild or moderate subaortic stenosis warrants consideration of elective operation.[351,352] Reports exist of transluminal balloon dilation for discrete subaortic stenosis. This palliative approach may be an acceptable alternative in selected patients,[353] but the relief of obstruction is not likely to be as complete or as long as in those patients undergoing surgical resection. It is clear that further study is required to delineate which forms of subaortic stenosis are most favorable for balloon dilation in comparing the long-term results of this approach with those of surgical treatment.

The risks of operation in patients with discrete subaortic stenosis and valvular aortic stenosis are essentially the same. The surgical treatment of discrete subaortic stenosis has evolved from simply excising the membrane or fibrous ridge to adding a generous ventricular myotomy and myectomy to the membranectomy.[354] Operation may be expected to improve the hemodynamic state substantially; it frequently is totally curative.[361]

Recent evidence indicates that muscle resection combined with membrane excision lowers the risk of reoperation for recurrent subaortic stenosis.[355] A tendency appears

to exist for discrete membranous subaortic stenosis to recur after operation, although this author and others consider these recurrences to be often related, at least in part, to incomplete removal of the lesion at initial operation. Intraoperative echocardiography has been used as an adjunct to operation to enable immediate assessment of the adequacy of relieving obstruction.[356] Studies have suggested that abnormal flow patterns may predispose to pathological proliferation of subvalvar aortic tissue, which reinforces the requirement that careful echocardiographic and surgical exploration of the outflow tract, even well below the subvalvar stenosis, be undertaken to detect and resect structures that cause turbulence.[357]

UNCOMMON FORMS OF SUBAORTIC STENOSIS

Combined Valvular and Subvalvular Stenosis

In some patients, valvular and subvalvular aortic stenosis coexist with hypoplasia of the aortic valve ring and thickened valve leaflets, producing a tunnel-like narrowing of the left ventricular outflow tract. Additional findings often include a small ascending aorta. The subvalvular fibrous process usually extends onto the aortic valve cusps and almost always makes contact with the ventricular aspect of the anterior mitral leaflet at its base. The presence of "tunnel stenosis" may be suspected echocardiographically or angiographically from the appearance of the outflow tract and the aortic root. Operative treatment often is complicated by the need for an aortoventriculoplasty, consisting of prosthetic or homograft replacement of the aortic valve as well as enlarging the aortic annulus, proximal aorta, and left ventricular outlet tract (the Konno-Rastan operation). The *modified* Konno-Rastan operation preserves the native aortic valve if the annulus is normal or near normal. Alternatively, a conal enlargement technique may be used.[358–360]

Various anatomical lesions other than a discrete membrane or ridge may produce subaortic stenosis.[362–364] Among these are abnormal adherence of the anterior leaflet of the mitral valve to the left septal surface, and the presence in the left ventricular outflow tract of accessory endocardial cushion tissue. In some patients with atrioventricular canal, the part of the ventricular septum that contributes to the wall of the left ventricular outflow tract is deficient, and the ventricular aspect of the anterior leaflet of the common atrioventricular valve is adherent to the posterior edge of the deficient septum, resulting in a narrow left ventricular outflow tract. Malalignment of the conoventricular septum, resulting in an inferior ventricular septal defect, produces a leftward superior deviation and insertion of the conal septum, obstructing left ventricular outflow.[364] In patients with a single ventricle and an outflow chamber, the bulboventricular foramen serves as a potential site of aortic outflow obstruction. Additionally, rarer causes of subaortic stenosis include redundant dysplastic left atrioventricular valve tissue in patients with congenitally corrected transposition of the great arteries and anomalous muscle bundles of the left ventricular outflow tract.

MUSCULAR SUBAORTIC STENOSIS. A muscular type of subaortic stenosis may result from a convergence of all the mitral chordae into one or two fused papillary muscles; a "parachute" deformity of the mitral valve is produced that often is seen in association with supravalvular stenosis of the left atrium and coarctation of the aorta. In some of these patients, discrete membranous subvalvular aortic obstruction also has been noted.

In patients with ventricular septal defect, muscular subaortic stenosis has been shown to develop after surgical banding of the pulmonary artery, possibly as a result of hypertrophy of the conal septum or crista supraventricularis encroaching on the left ventricular outflow tract above the septal defect.

Subaortic muscular hypertrophy secondary to diffuse involvement of the myocardium by glycogen storage disease (Pompe's disease) is an extremely rare cause of obstruction to left ventricular outflow. A positive family history, symptoms of muscle weakness, heart failure in infancy, and the characteristic electrocardiographic findings of a short PR interval, high-voltage QRS and T waves, and left ventricular hypertrophy warrant skeletal muscle biopsy or fibroblast culture, permitting an antemortem diagnosis.

The last, relatively uncommon form of subaortic stenosis to be mentioned occurs infrequently in patients with congenitally corrected transposition of the great arteries in whom an anomalous muscle bundle in the subaortic area of the arterial ventricle obstructs outflow.

Supravalvular Aortic Stenosis

Supravalvular aortic stenosis is a congenital narrowing of the ascending aorta that may be localized or diffuse, originating at the superior margin of the sinuses of Valsalva just above the levels of the coronary arteries.

The clinical picture of supravalvular obstruction usually differs in major respects from that observed in the other

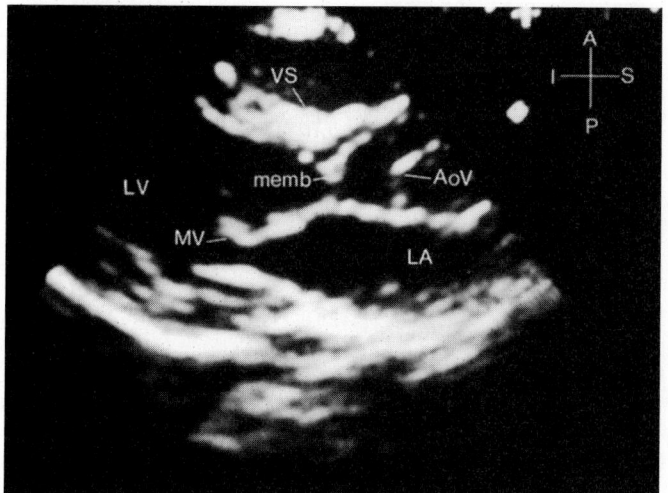

FIGURE 29–35. Long-axis view of discrete membranous subaortic stenosis. A discrete membrane (memb) is imaged in the left ventricular (LV) outflow tract beneath and parallel to the aortic valve (AoV), extending from the ventricular septum (VS) to the anterior leaflet of the mitral valve (MV). LA = left atrium.

forms of aortic stenosis. Chief among these differences is the association of supravalvular aortic stenosis with idiopathic infantile hypercalcemia, a disease that occurs in the first years of life and may be related to deranged vitamin D metabolism.[365-368]

It is helpful to classify patients according to their clinical presentation into nonfamilial, sporadic cases with normal facies and intelligence; autosomal dominant familial cases with normal facies and intelligence; and the Williams syndrome with abnormal facial appearance and mental retardation (Fig. 29–36). In contrast to the other forms of aortic stenosis, there appears to be no gender predilection in any of these three categories.

WILLIAMS SYNDROME. The designations supravalvular aortic stenosis syndrome or Williams syndrome or Williams-Beuren syndrome[369,370] have been applied to the distinctive picture produced by coexistence of the cardiac and multiple-system disorder. Beyond infancy in these patients, a challenge with vitamin D or calcium loading tests unmask abnormalities in the regulation of circulating 25-hydroxyvitamin D.[371,372] Unanimity of opinion does not exist of the exact relation between Williams syndrome and calcium metabolism. Some have suggested that the abnormalities of calcium metabolism might be explained by a defect in synthesis or release of calcitonin, whereas others have concluded recently that calcitonin deficiency is not present in patients with Williams syndrome.

Infants with Williams syndrome often exhibit feeding difficulties, failure to thrive, and gastrointestinal problems in the form of vomiting, constipation, and colic. The entire spectrum of clinical manifestations includes auditory hyperacusis, inguinal hernia, a hoarse voice, and a typical personality that is outgoing and engaging. Other manifestations of this syndrome include mental retardation, "elfin facies" (Fig. 29–33), narrowing of peripheral systemic and pulmonary arteries, strabismus, and abnormalities of dental development consisting of microdontia, enamel hypoplasia, and malocclusion.

Many medical conditions can complicate the course of Williams syndrome,[372] including systemic hypertension, gastrointestinal problems, and urinary tract abnormalities. Particularly in the older child or adult, progressive joint limitation and hypertonia may become a problem. Adult patients are usually handicapped by their developmental disabilities.

Hypervitaminosis D in the pregnant rabbit has resulted in craniofacial and dental abnormalities and malformations resembling supravalvular aortic stenosis in the offspring.[365-367] Skin fibroblast cultures from patients with Williams syndrome show enhanced metachromasia upon addition of vitamin D and calcium.[371] In humans, chromosome studies have revealed normal karyotypes, with the exception of one patient who demonstrated a 46/47 mosaic pattern with an extra chromosome resembling the 19 to 20 group.

Until recently, Williams syndrome was considered to be nonfamilial. Interestingly, three families have been identified in which parent-to-child transmission of Williams syndrome has occurred. These are not families with autosomal dominant supravalvular aortic stenosis whose members are normal in appearance and intelligence. All of these families show a parent and child to be affected with Williams syndrome, including one instance of male-to-male transmission. This supports autosomal dominant inheritance as the likely pattern, with most cases of Williams syndrome probably occurring as the result of a new mutation.

FAMILIAL AUTOSOMAL DOMINANT PRESENTATION. Most commonly, supravalvular aortic stenosis is a feature of the distinctive Williams syndrome described above.[374] However, the aortic anomaly and peripheral pulmonary arterial stenosis are also seen in familial and sporadic forms *unassociated* with the other features of the syndrome.[375] Thus, affected patients have normal intelligence and are normal in facial appearance. Genetic studies suggest that when the anomaly is familial, it is transmitted as autosomal dominant with variable expression. Some family members may have peripheral pulmonary stenosis either as an isolated lesion or in combination with the supravalvular aortic anomaly.

Recently, linkage analyses in two unrelated families with autosomal dominant supravalvular aortic stenosis were performed. Linkage was identified between the supravalvular aortic stenosis phenotype and polymorphic markers on the long arm of chromosome 7.[376] These findings indicate that a gene for supravalvular aortic stenosis may be located in the same chromosomal subunit as elastin. Further, a family has been identified with autosomal dominant supravalvular aortic stenosis in which a balanced translocation was identified, which disrupts the elastin gene and cosegregates with the disease in this family, supporting the hypothesis that mutations in the elastin gene may cause supravalvular aortic stenosis.[377] Hemizygosity at the elastin locus is likely responsible for the vascular pathology in Williams syndrome, although it is unlikely that elastin deletions account for all features of the syndrome. Because the deletions responsible for Williams syndrome extend well beyond the elastin locus, it is probable that the syndrome is a contiguous gene disorder.[377a]

MORPHOLOGY. Three anatomical types of supravalvular aortic stenosis are recognized, although some patients may have findings of more than one type. Most common is the hourglass type, in which marked thickening and disorganization of the aortic media produce a constricting annular ridge at the superior margin of the sinuses of Valsalva. The membranous type is the result of fibrous or fibromuscular semicircular diaphragm with a small central opening stretched across the lumen of the aorta. Uniform hypoplasia of the ascending aorta characterizes the hypoplastic type.[378]

Because the coronary arteries arise proximal to the site of outflow obstruction in supravalvular aortic stenosis, they are subjected to the elevated pressure that exists within the left ventricle. These vessels often are dilated and tortuous, and premature coronary arteriosclerosis has been observed. Moreover, if the free edges of some or all of the aortic cusps adhere to the site of supravalvular stenosis, coronary artery inflow may be reduced. The formation of thoracic aortic aneurysms has been described in several patients.

CLINICAL FEATURES. Patients with Williams syndrome are mentally retarded and resemble one another in their facial features. The typical appearance is similar to that of the elfin facies observed in the severe form of idiopathic infantile hypercalcemia and is characterized by a high prominent forehead, stellate or lacy iris patterns, epicanthal folds, underdeveloped bridge of the nose and mandible, overhanging upper lip, strabismus, and anomalies of dentition (Fig. 29–36). Recognition of this distinctive appearance, even in infancy, should alert the physician to the

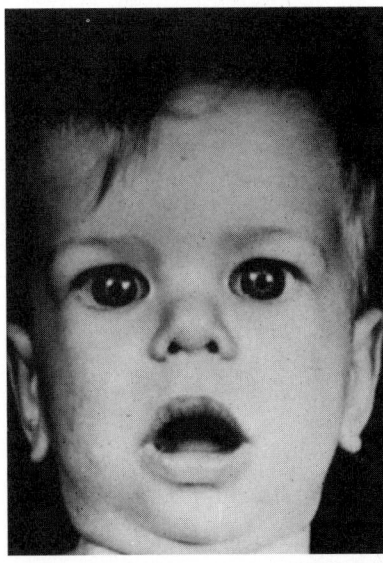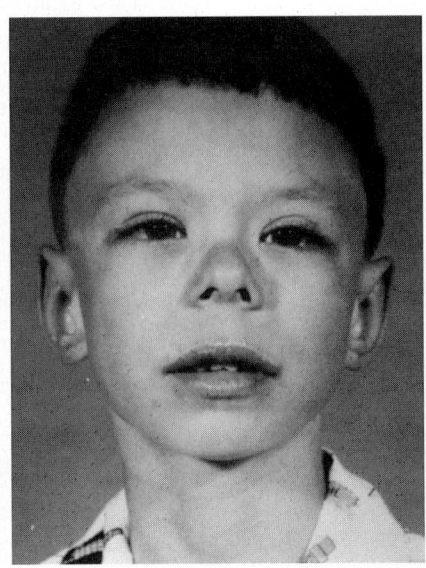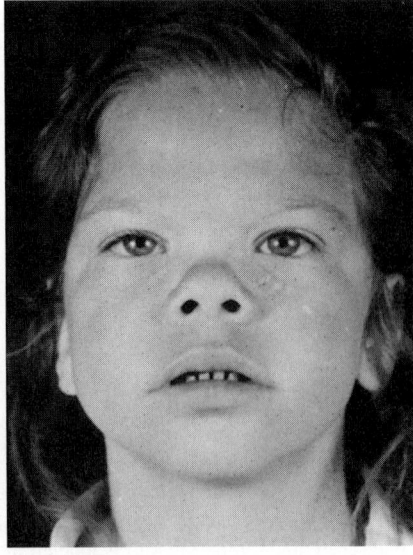

FIGURE 29–36. Typical elfin facies in three patients with supravalvular aortic stenosis. (Friedman, W. F., Kirkpatrick, S. E.: Congenital aortic stenosis. *In* Moss, A. J., Adams, F. H., and Emmanouilides, G. C. [eds.]: Heart Disease in Infants, Children and Adolescents. 2nd ed. Baltimore, © Williams and Wilkins, 1977.)

possibility of underlying multisystem disease. In addition, a positive family history in a patient with a normal appearance and clinical signs suggesting left ventricular outflow obstruction should lead to the suspicion of either supravalvular aortic stenosis or hypertrophic obstructive cardiomyopathy.[291]

Patients with supravalvular aortic obstruction appear to be subject to the same risks of unexpected sudden death [in some of whom myocardial infarction has been found at autopsy[379]] and endocarditis as those with valvular aortic stenosis. Studies of the natural history of the principal vascular lesions in these patients[380,381]—supravalvular aortic stenosis and peripheral pulmonary artery stenosis—indicate that the aortic lesion is usually progressive, with an increase in the intensity of obstruction related often to poor growth of the ascending aorta. In contrast, the patients with pulmonary branch stenosis, whether or not associated with the aortic lesion, tend to show no change or a reduction in right ventricular pressure with time.

With few exceptions, the major *physical findings* resemble those observed in patients with valvular aortic stenosis. Among these exceptions are accentuation of aortic valve closure due to elevated pressure in the aorta proximal to the stenosis, an infrequent systolic ejection sound, and the especially prominent transmission of a thrill and murmur into the jugular notch and along the carotid vessels. Uncommonly, there is an early diastolic, decrescendo, blowing murmur of aortic regurgitation caused by the fusion of one or more cusps to the area of stenosis. The narrowing of the peripheral pulmonary arteries that often coexists in these patients frequently produces a late systolic or continuous murmur that may help to distinguish this anomaly from valvular aortic stenosis. This differentiation is reinforced by the frequent finding of a significant disparity between the arterial pressures in the upper extremities in supravalvular aortic stenosis; the systolic pressure in the right arm tends to be the higher of the two and occasionally exceeds that in the femoral arteries. The disparity in pulses may relate to the tendency of a jet stream to adhere to a vessel wall (Coanda effect) and selective streaming of blood into the innominate artery.[382,383]

Electrocardiography usually reveals left ventricular hypertrophy when obstruction is severe. Biventricular, or even right ventricular, hypertrophy may be found if significant narrowing of peripheral pulmonary arteries coexists. Radiographically, in contrast to valvular and discrete subvalvular aortic stenosis, poststenotic dilation of the ascending aorta seldom is seen. The sinuses of Valsalva usually are dilated, and the ascending aorta and aortic arch are of normal size or appear small.

Echocardiography is the most valuable technique for localizing the site of obstruction to the supravalvular area (Fig. 29–37). Most often the sinuses of Valsalva are dilated and the ascending aorta and arch are of normal size or appear small. A useful ratio can be constructed of the measurements of the aortic annulus and the sinotubular junction, in which the latter is always less than the former in patients with supravalvular stenosis, a finding not present in normals.[384] Recently, intraluminal ultrasound imaging has been used to visualize the vascular pathology in Williams syndrome.[385] Doppler examination and retrograde aortic catheterization can determine the degree of hemodynamic abnormality.[386]

Because of the nature of the anatomical defect, this author does not think that transcatheter balloon angioplasty will be an effective treatment option. For several reasons, depending primarily on the anatomical variant of the lesion, supravalvular aortic stenosis may be less amenable to operative treatment than either valvular or discrete subvalvular stenosis. The lumen of the aorta at the supravalvular level may be widened by the insertion of an oval- or diamond-shaped fabric prosthesis in those patients with a normal or near normal ascending aorta.[387] However, if the

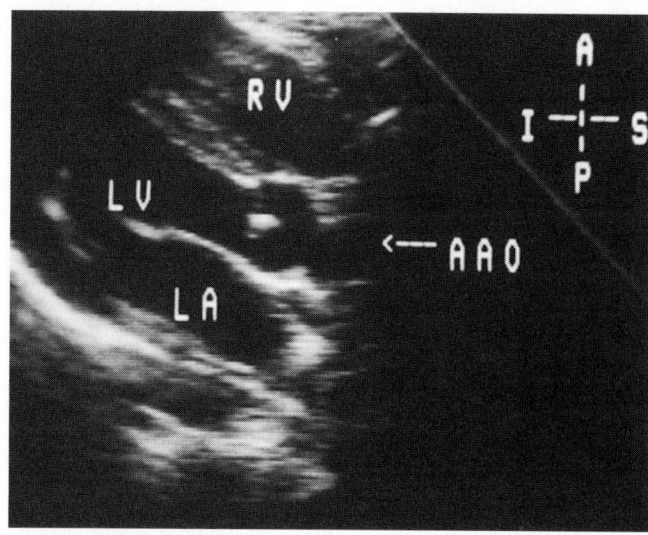

FIGURE 29–37. Supravalvar aortic stenosis is seen in a parasternal long-axis view. The constriction is distal to the sinuses of Valsalva in the ascending aorta (AAO). RV = right ventricle, LV = left ventricle, LA = left atrium. (Courtesy of Norman Silverman, M.D.)

aorta is markedly hypoplastic, this operation merely displaces the pressure gradient distally without abolishing the obstruction. Under these circumstances, repair may require replacement or widening of the entire hypoplastic aorta with an appropriate prosthesis.[387]

Hypoplastic Left Heart Syndrome

This designation is used to describe a group of closely related cardiac anomalies characterized by underdevelopment of the left cardiac chambers, atresia or stenosis of the aortic and/or the mitral orifices, and hypoplasia of the aorta.[388] These anomalies are an especially common cause of heart failure in the first week of life. The left atrium and ventricle often exhibit *endocardial fibroelastosis*. Pulmonary venous blood traverses a patent foramen ovale, and a dilated and hypertrophied right ventricle acts as the systemic, as well as pulmonary, ventricle; the systemic circulation receives blood by way of a patent ductus arteriosus (Fig. 29–38).

The diagnosis should be considered in infants, particularly males, with the sudden onset of heart failure, systemic hypoperfusion, and nonspecific murmur. *Electrocardiography* frequently reveals right axis deviation, right atrial and ventricular enlargement, and ST and T-wave abnormalities in the left precordial leads. Chest roentgenography may show only slight enlargement shortly after birth, but with clinical deterioration there are marked cardiomegaly and increased pulmonary venous and arterial vascular markings. The *echocardiographic* findings usually are diagnostic (Fig. 29–39), and include a diminutive aortic root and left ventricular cavity and absence or poor visualization of aortic and mitral valve echoes, which, when seen, are of diminished amplitude and mobility.[389] *Retrograde aortography* shows hypoplasia of the ascending aorta.

MANAGEMENT. Medical therapy directed at cardiac decompensation, hypoxemia, and metabolic acidemia seldom prolongs survival beyond the first days of life. Constriction of the patent ductus arteriosus and limited flow through a restrictive patent foramen ovale are the principal factors responsible for early death. Prostaglandin E_1 infusion is effective in maintaining ductal patency.

SURGICAL TREATMENT. Some centers are attempting staged surgical management in an effort to provide long-term palliation.[388,390–392] The first stage, often referred to as the *Norwood procedure,* consists of creating an unobstructed communication between the right ventricle and aorta, and enlargement of the ascending aorta. The right ventricular–aortic connection has been accomplished with homograft or prosthetic conduits from the right ventricle or pulmonary trunk to

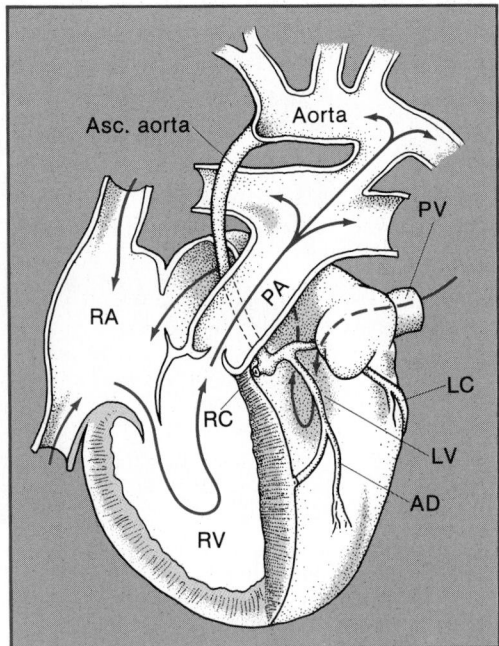

FIGURE 29–38. Hypoplastic left heart with aortic hypoplasia, aortic valve atresia, and a hypoplastic mitral valve and left ventricle. RA = right atrium, RV = right ventricle, RC = right coronary artery, PA = pulmonary artery, PV = pulmonary vein, LC = left coronary artery, LV = left ventricle, AD = anterior descending coronary artery. (From Neufeld, H. N., et al.: Diagnosis of aortic atresia by retrograde aortography. Circulation 25:278, 1962. Copyright American Heart Association.)

the descending aorta, or by direct connection between the proximal pulmonary trunk and ascending aorta, which also enlarges the ascending aorta. Pulmonary blood flow and pressure are controlled by a tubed interposition systemic-pulmonary shunt to the distal pulmonary artery. The patent ductus arteriosus is ligated. A large interatrial communication also must be assured in stage 1 to allow free access of pulmonary venous blood to the tricuspid valve.

In stage 2 an interatrial baffle is created to provide continuity between left atrium and tricuspid valve; the pulmonary arterial circulation is provided by direct anastomosis of the right atrium to the pulmonary arteries (the Fontan connection).[393] Many surgeons prefer

to perform a modified superior vena cava–pulmonary artery shunt (bidirectional Glenn operation) as an intermediate step before the Fontan procedure. In some centers, the preferred operation is cardiac transplantation.[394,395,395a] Stenting of the ductus arteriosus may be used as an ambulatory bridge to transplantation.[396]

Congenital Aortic Regurgitation

Congenital aortic valve regurgitation is a rare isolated congenital cardiac lesion.[397,398] Aortic regurgitation most often occurs in association with congenital valvular aortic stenosis in which the valve commissures are fused, inhibiting cusp mobility; subvalvular aortic stenosis in which the aortic ring is dilated and the valve cusps are deformed; coarctation of the aorta when the aortic ring is dilated and the aortic valve is bicuspid; ventricular septal defect (see p. 901); and endocardial fibroelastosis. Aortic valve regurgitation also may accompany aortic sinus aneurysm or be secondary to dilatation of the ascending aorta in patients with Marfan syndrome, Turner syndrome, cystic medial necrosis, or osteogenesis imperfecta, in which the aortic lesions are manifestations of the underlying connective tissue disorder.

Severe aortic regurgitation also may occur through channels other than the aortic valve.[399,400] Thus aortico–left ventricular tunnel is a rare anomaly that must be distinguished from congenital aortic valve regurgitation, because the approach to management of the former usually does not include consideration for prosthetic valve replacement. The aortico–left ventricular tunnel is an abnormal channel beginning in the ascending aorta above the right coronary orifice and ending in the left ventricle below the right aortic cusp. The channel usually passes behind the right ventricular infundibulum and through the ventricular septum.

Echocardiography, Doppler studies, and aortography combine to establish a precise diagnosis. Exercise testing[401] and magnetic resonance velocity mapping[402] are useful to assess the severity of the lesion. In infants and children with congenital aortic regurgitation the severity of regurgitation increases with time, and valve replacement, rather than plication, is almost always necessary to correct the lesion. Operation should be deferred until symptoms, signs, and noninvasive assessment dictate its necessity. Conversely, closure of an aortic–left ventricular communication is advisable before progressive dilation of the aortic annulus creates secondary changes in the aortic valve itself which may necessitate aortic valve replacement.

Pulmonary Vein Atresia and Stenosis

Pulmonary vein atresia is a rare anomaly in which the pulmonary veins do not connect with the heart or with a major systemic vein.[403] The lesion is incompatible with life, but infants may survive for days, probably because communications exist between the pulmonary veins and the bronchial or esophageal veins that allow limited egress for pulmonary venous blood. Pulmonary vein stenosis may occur as a focal stenosis at the atrial junction or generalized hypoplasia of one

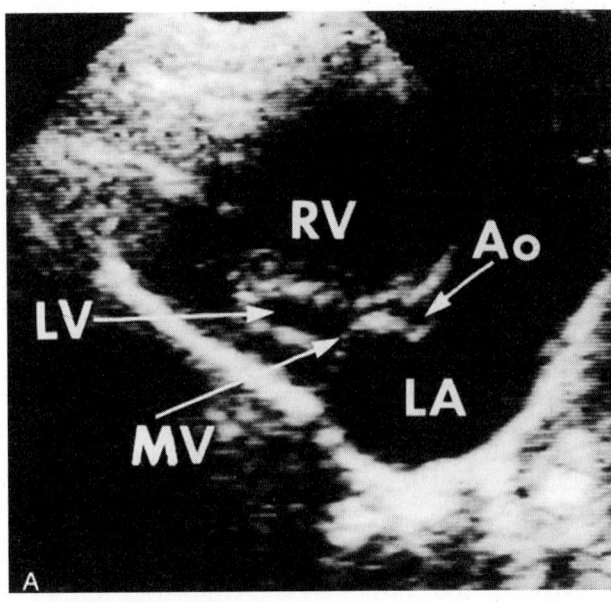

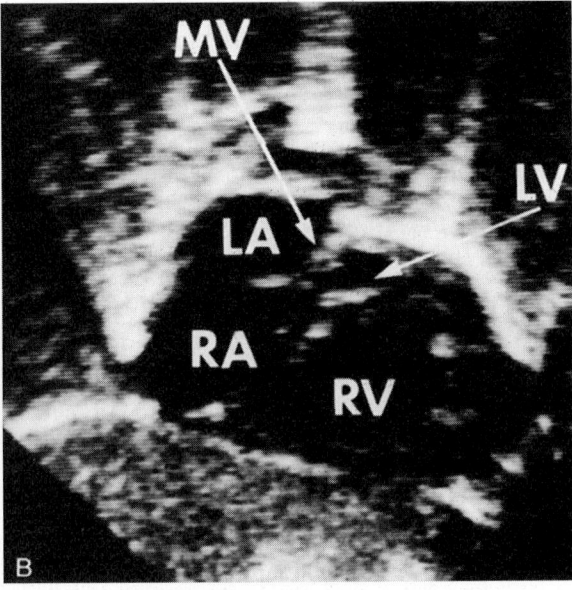

FIGURE 29–39. A, Hypoplastic left heart in a parasternal long-axis view in a newborn with aortic atresia, intact ventricular septum, and patent but hypoplastic mitral valve (MV). The left ventricular (LV) cavity is diminutive and the ascending aorta (Ao) is hypoplastic. Right ventricular (RV) dilation is noted. B, In the subcostal four-chamber view dilatation of the right atrium (RA) and right ventricle (RV) is noted. The endocardial echoes are very bright owing to fibroelastosis. (From Perloff, J.: The Clinical Recognition of Congenital Heart Disease. 3rd ed. Philadelphia, W.B. Saunders Company, 1986.)

or more pulmonary veins. There is an extremely high incidence of associated cardiac malformations, including atrial septal defect, tetralogy of Fallot, tricuspid and mitral atresia, and endocardial cushion defect. The severe pulmonary vein obstruction imposed by pulmonary vein abnormalities causes severe cyanosis, congestive cardiac failure, and early death. Focal stenosis of one or more pulmonary veins at the atrial junction, recognized by two-dimensional echocardiography or angiography, may be relieved surgically.[404] Results of transcutaneous balloon angioplasty have been disappointing.

Cor Triatriatum

In this malformation failure of resorption of the common pulmonary vein results in a left atrium divided by an abnormal fibromuscular diaphragm into a posterosuperior chamber receiving the pulmonary veins and an anteroinferior chamber giving rise to the left atrial appendage and leading to the mitral orifice.[405] The communication between the divided atrial chambers may be large, small, or absent, depending on the size of the opening in the subdividing diaphragm, which determines the degree of obstruc-

tion to pulmonary venous return. Elevations of both pulmonary venous pressure and pulmonary vascular resistance result in severe pulmonary artery hypertension.

The diagnosis is established by two-dimensional or transesophageal echocardiography; cardiac catheterization and angiography are necessary only if major associated cardiac anomalies are suspected.[406–406b] The obstructive membrane is visualized in the parasternal long- and short-axis and four-chamber (Fig. 29–40) views and can be distinguished from a supravalvular mitral ring[406a] by its position superior to the left atrial appendage, which forms part of the distal chamber. Also present are diastolic fluttering of the mitral leaflets and high-velocity flow detected by Doppler examination in the distal atrial chamber and at the mitral orifice.

The diagnosis should be suspected at cardiac catheterization if the pulmonary arterial wedge pressure is higher than a simultaneous left atrial pressure. The diagnosis also may be established by visualizing the obstructing lesion angiographically. Although rare, it is important to recognize the malformation because it may be easily correctable at operation.[407]

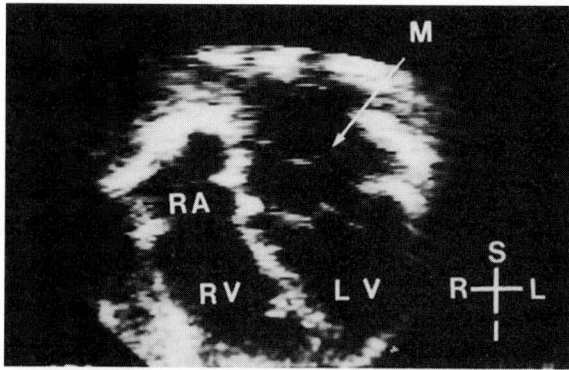
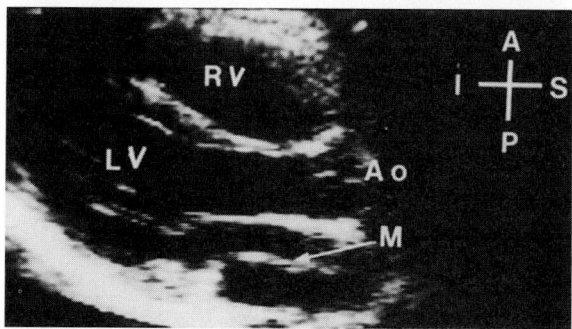
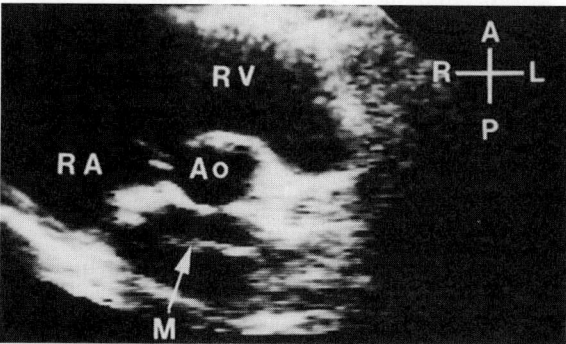

FIGURE 29–40. Echocardiograms demonstrating the membrane (M) of cor triatriatum. The apical four-chamber view *(top panel)* shows the membrane lying within the left atrial chamber. The atrial appendage is distal to the membrane and the pulmonary veins drain into the proximal portion. The parasternal long-axis view *(center panel)* shows the membrane posterior to the aortic root (AO) and mitral valve, dividing the left atrium into two chambers. In the parasternal short-axis view *(bottom panel)*, the membrane is within the left atrium close to the posterior aortic root. RA = right atrium, RV = right ventricle, LV = left ventricle. (Courtesy of Norman Silverman, M.D.)

Congenital Mitral Stenosis

Anatomical types of mitral stenosis include the parachute deformity of the valve, in which shortened chordae tendineae converge and insert into a single large papillary muscle; thickened leaflets with shortening and fusion of the chordae tendineae; an anomalous arcade of obstructing papillary muscles; accessory mitral valve tissue; and a supravalvular circumferential ridge of connective tissue arising at the base of the atrial aspect of the mitral leaflets.[408,409] Associated cardiac defects are common, including endocardial fibroelastosis, coarctation of the aorta, patent ductus arteriosus, and left ventricular outflow tract obstruction. Two-dimensional echocardiography, combined with Doppler studies, often provides a complete analysis of the anatomy and function of congenital left ventricular inflow lesions.[410,411] The clinical and hemodynamic consequences of isolated congenital mitral stenosis are similar to those of acquired mitral obstruction with modifications imposed by coexisting anomalies.

The prognosis is poor; symptoms attributable to pulmonary vein obstruction begin usually in infancy and the majority of patients expire before age 1 year unless catheter balloon dilation or operation is successful.[411–412a] Conduit bypass of the mitral valve and prosthetic valve replacement are required if a reparative operation is not possible.[413,414] The use of a porcine bioprosthesis is contraindicated because of its rapid degeneration in the infant or young child.

Congenital Mitral Regurgitation

The syndrome of *mitral valve prolapse* is discussed on p. 1029. This condition usually is quite benign in children. However, occasional difficulties exist with infective endocarditis, arrhythmias, atypical chest pain, and sudden death.[415] *Isolated congenital mitral regurgitation* of hemodynamic significance is an unusual lesion in infants and children.

MORPHOLOGY. Congenital malformations of the mitral valve producing insufficiency most often are encountered in association with endocardial cushion defect, congenitally corrected transposition of the great arteries, endocardial fibroelastosis, anomalous pulmonary origin of the coronary artery, congenital subaortic stenosis, hypertrophic obstructive cardiomyopathy, and coarctation of the aorta. Mitral valve dysfunction also commonly is seen in various metabolic disorders (e.g., the mucopolysaccharidoses), primary and secondary cardiomyopathies, connective tissue disease (e.g., rheumatoid arthritis, Marfan syndrome, Ehlers-Danlos syndrome, pseudoxanthoma elasticum), and rheumatic and nonrheumatic inflammatory diseases of the myocardium.[416]

The various anatomical lesions that result in isolated congenital mitral regurgitation include prolapse of one or both mitral leaflets, cleft or perforated mitral leaflet, inadequate leaflet tissue, double orifice of the mitral valve, anomalous insertion of chordae tendineae (anomalous mitral arcade), redundant leaflet tissue, displacement inferiorly of the ring of the inferior leaflet into the left ventricle, and abnormal length of the chordae tendineae.[416]

CLINICAL FINDINGS. The clinical, echocardiographic, and hemodynamic findings in patients with isolated congenital mitral incompetence resemble those observed in acquired mitral regurgitation.[417] Mitral annuloplasty (which is preferred) and prosthetic valve replacement are procedures reserved for infants and children who are at least moderately symptomatic despite comprehensive medical management, often with repeated episodes of pulmonary infection, or cardiac failure with anorexia and retarded growth and development.[416] Operative condidates are shown by echocardiographic, Doppler, hemodynamic, and angiographic studies to have pulmonary hypertension, a regurgitant fraction in excess of 50 per cent, and a marked increase in left ventricular end-diastolic volume.[418]

Pulmonary Arteriovenous Fistula

Abnormal development of the pulmonary arteries and veins in a common vascular complex is responsible for this rare congenital anomaly (see also p. 967). A variable number of pulmonary arteries communicate directly with branches of the pulmonary veins; in some cases the fistula receives systemic arterial branches.[419] Most patients have an associated Weber-Osler-Rendu syndrome; additional associated problems include bronchiectasis and other malformations of the bronchial tree, and absence of the right lower lobe. Venoarterial shunting depends on the extent of the fistulous communications and may result in cyanosis and secondary polycythemia. Paradoxical emboli and brain abscess may cause major neurological deficits.

Patients with hereditary hemorrhagic telangiectasis often are anemic owing to repeated blood loss and may have less obvious cyanosis. Systolic and continuous murmurs are audible over areas of the fistula. Rounded opacities of variable size in one or both lungs on chest roentgenogram may suggest the presence of the lesion. Pulmonary angiography reveals the site and extent of the abnormal communication (Fig. 30–8, p. 968). Unless the lesions are widespread throughout both lungs, surgical treatment aimed at removing the lesions with preservation of healthy lung tissue commonly is indicated to avoid the complications of massive hemorrhage, bacterial endocarditis, and rupture of arteriovenous aneurysms.

Transcatheter balloon or plug or coil occlusion embolotherapy may prove to be the therapeutic procedure of choice.[420,421]

Peripheral Pulmonary Artery Stenosis

Stenosis of the pulmonary artery may occur as single or multiple lesions located anywhere from the main pulmonary trunk to the smaller peripheral arterial branches.[422] Associated defects are observed in most patients and include pulmonic valvular stenosis, ventricular septal defect, tetralogy of Fallot, and supravalvular aortic stenosis.

ETIOLOGY. The most important cause of significant pulmonary artery stenoses producing symptoms in the newborn is intrauterine rubella infection.[423] Diagnosis is facilitated in these infants by finding elevations of the IgM fraction and rubella antibody titer. Other cardiovascular malformations commonly seen in association with congenital rubella include patent ductus arteriosus, pulmonic valve stenosis, and atrial septal defect. Generalized systemic arterial stenotic lesions also may be a feature of the rubella embryopathy, often involving large and medium-sized vessels such as the aorta and coronary, cerebral, mesenteric, and renal arteries. Cardiovascular lesions are but one manifestation of intrauterine rubella infection because cataracts, microphthalmia, deafness, thrombocytopenia, hepatitis, and blood dyscrasias also are common. Thus, the clinical picture in infants with rubella syndrome depends on the severity of the cardiovascular lesions and the associated abnormalities of other organs and systems. Peripheral pulmonary stenosis also often is associated with supravalvular aortic stenosis in patients with the familial form of the latter anomaly or in patients with the Williams syndrome (see also p. 920).

MORPHOLOGY. Obstruction within the pulmonary arterial tree may be classified into four types: (1) stenosis of the main pulmonary trunk or the main left or right branch; (2) narrowing at the bifurcation of the pulmonary artery, extending into both right and left branches; (3) multiple sites of peripheral branch stenosis; and (4) a combination of main and peripheral stenosis. Pulmonary artery obstruction may be produced by localized narrowing, diffuse constrictions, or, rarely, a membrane or diaphragm. Poststenotic dilatation is usual when the stenosis is localized but may be absent or minimal with elongated constriction. It should be recognized that a physiological branch pulmonary artery stenosis often is present in the normal newborn in whom both right and left main pulmonary arteries are small and arise almost perpendicular from a large main pulmonary artery.[424] The branch vessels increase in size with growth and become less angulated in their take-off from the main pulmonary artery.

CLINICAL FINDINGS. The degree of obstruction is the principal determinant of clinical severity; the type of obstruction determines the feasibility of direct surgical relief. The clinical features vary; most infants and children are asymptomatic.[425] An ejection systolic murmur at the upper left sternal border that is well transmitted to the axillae and back is most common. The presence of an ejection sound suggests that pulmonic valve stenosis coexists. The pulmonic component of the second heart sound may be slightly accentuated, but occasionally is extremely loud if multiple peripheral stenoses exist. A continuous murmur is audible, especially in patients with main or branch steno-

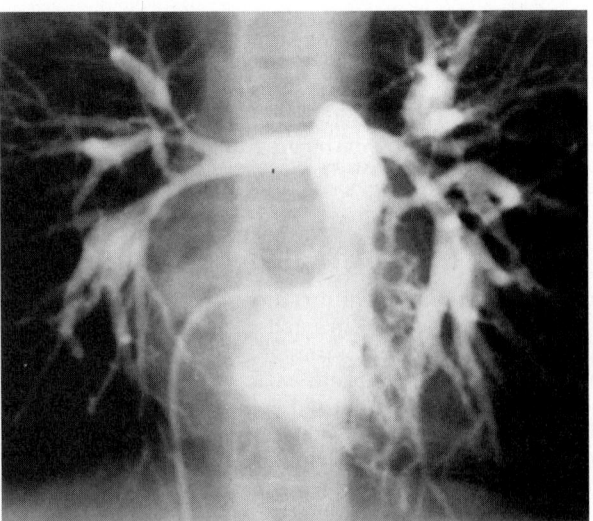

FIGURE 29–41. Right ventricular angiocardiogram showing multiple sites of peripheral pulmonic stenosis and poststenotic dilatation of the peripheral pulmonic arteries.

sis, and particularly if an associated cardiovascular anomaly produces increased pulmonary blood flow. Electrocardiography shows right ventricular hypertrophy when obstruction is severe; left-axis deviation with counterclockwise orientation of the frontal QRS vector is common in the rubella syndrome and when the lesion coexists with supravalvular aortic stenosis. Mild or moderate stenosis usually produces a normal chest roentgenogram; detectable differences in vascularity between regions of the lungs or dilated pulmonary artery segments are uncommon. When obstruction is bilateral and severe, right atrial and ventricular enlargement may be observed.

Diagnosis. This is confirmed by observing pressure gradients within the pulmonary arterial system at cardiac catheterization; digital subtraction and/or selective pulmonary angiography defines the exact location, extent, and distribution of the lesion (Fig. 29–41). Mild to moderate unilateral or bilateral stenosis does not require surgical relief; numerous stenotic areas are not amenable to correction, even with intraoperative balloon angioplasty. Well-localized obstruction of severe degree in the main pulmonary artery or its major branches may be alleviated by percutaneous transcatheter balloon angioplasty (see p. 1313),[426] often accompanied by endovascular stent implantation,[427] or with a patch graft or bypassed with a tubular conduit. The natural history of peripheral pulmonary stenosis is not clear. Obstruction may increase by discrepant growth between a stenotic area and normal portions of the pulmonary artery tree, or as a result of an increase in cardiac output, especially during adolescence. Rarely, hypertrophy of right ventricular infundibular muscle is progressive and results in hypercyanotic spells.

Pulmonic Stenosis with Intact Ventricular Septum

Valvular pulmonic stenosis, resulting from fusion of the valve cusps during mid to late intrauterine development, is the most common form of isolated right ventricular obstruction and occurs in about 7 per cent of patients with congenital heart disease. Hypertrophy of the septal and parietal bands narrowing the right ventricular infundibulum often accompanies the pulmonic valve lesion, especially if it is severe. Fused cusps of varying thickness and rigidity form a fibrous dome in the severest forms. Pulmonic valve dysplasia, especially common in patients with Noonan syndrome (see p. 1663), produces obstruction in the absence of adherent leaflets because leaflets are thickened, rigid, and myxomatous and are limited in their lateral movement because of the presence of tissue pads within the pulmonic valve sinuses.[428]

NEONATES AND INFANTS. The clinical presentation and course of circulation in the newborn with pulmonic stenosis depends on the severity of obstruction and the degree of development of the right ventricle and its outflow tract, the tricuspid valve, and the pulmonary arterial tree. The greater the degree of pulmonic valve stenosis, the more closely the manifestations resemble those observed with pulmonary atresia and intact ventricular septum (see p. 922). Severe pulmonic stenosis is characterized by cyanosis caused by right-to-left shunting through the foramen ovale, cardiomegaly, and diminished pulmonary blood flow in the absence of persistent patency of the ductus arteriosus. Hypoxemia and metabolic acidemia, rather than right ventricular failure, are the main clinical disturbances in the symptomatic neonate and can be alleviated temporarily by infusion of prostaglandin E₁ to dilate the ductus arteriosus and increase pulmonary blood flow. Distinction of these babies from those with tetralogy of Fallot or tricuspid or pulmonary atresia usually is possible because infants with tetralogy usually do not have roentgenographic evidence of cardiomegaly; infants with tricuspid and pulmonary atresia show a preponderance of left ventricular forces by electrocardiography in contrast to the right ventricular hypertrophy usually observed with critical pulmonic stenosis in the absence of right ventricular hypoplasia.

Combined two-dimensional echocardiographic and continuous-wave Doppler examination (Fig. 3–68, p. 79) characterizes the anatomical valve abnormality and its severity, and has essentially eliminated the requirement for cardiac catheterization and angiographic studies to establish a precise diagnosis (Fig. 29–42).[429,430]

Balloon Valvuloplasty. Balloon dilatation of the pulmonary valve (see p. 968) is the therapeutic procedure of choice,[430a,430b] but a pulmonary valvotomy and systemic-to-pulmonary arterial shunt may be necessary in infants with underdevelopment of the right ventricular cavity.[431] In this group, recent success has been achieved by modification of balloon valvuloplasty with predilation initially using a coronary dilatation catheter to facilitate introduction of a definitive balloon catheter.[432] Transcatheter balloon valvuloplasty may be expected to reduce, but not abolish, the pressure difference in neonates with mobile doming valves. This approach is of lesser efficacy in those patients with dysplastic valves, and is contraindicated if valve dysplasia is associated with annular hypoplasia.[433,434]

CHILDREN. The clinical profile of patients with valvular pulmonic stenosis beyond infancy usually is distinctive.[435] The severity of obstruction is the most important determinant of the clinical course. In the presence of a normal cardiac output a peak systolic transvalvular pressure gradient between 50 and 80 mm Hg or a peak systolic right ventricular pressure between 75 and 100 mm Hg is considered to be indicative of moderate stenosis; levels below and above that range are classified as mild and severe, respectively. Most patients with mild pulmonic stenosis are asymptomatic, and the condition is discovered during routine examination. In patients with more significant obstruction the severity of stenosis may increase with time. Progression may be relative and reflect disproportional physical growth of the patient, infundibular narrowing due to progressive hypertrophy of the right ventricular outflow tract, or fibrosis of the valve cusps.

Symptoms, when present, vary from mild exertional dyspnea and mild cyanosis to signs and symptoms of heart failure, depending on the degree of obstruction and the level of myocardial compensation. Exertional fatigue, syncope, and chest pain are related to an inability to augment pulmonary blood flow during exercise in some patients with moderate or severe obstruction.

Physical Examination. The severity of obstruction often is suggested by the physical findings. Right ventricular hypertrophy reduces compliance of that chamber, and a forceful right atrial contraction is necessary to augment right ventricular filling. Prominent a waves in the jugular venous pulse, a fourth heart sound, and, occasionally, presystolic pulsations of the liver reflect a vigorous atrial contraction and suggest the presence of severe stenosis. Cardiomegaly and a right ventricular parasternal lift accompany moderate or severe obstruction. A systolic thrill is palpable along the upper left sternal border in all but the mildest forms of stenosis. The first heart sound is normal and is followed by a systolic ejection sound at the upper left sternal edge produced by sudden opening of the stenotic valve; an ejection sound is not heard in patients with pulmonic valve dysplasia. The ejection sound typically is louder during expiration; when it is inaudible or occurs less than 0.08 second from the onset of the Q wave on electrocardiogram, severe obstruction is suggested. Right ventricular ejection is prolonged in patients with moderate or severe stenosis, and the sound of pulmonic valve closure is delayed and soft. The characteristic feature of valvular pulmonic stenosis on auscultation is a harsh, diamond-shaped systolic ejection murmur heard best at the upper left sternal border. The systolic murmur becomes louder and its crescendo occurs later in systole, obscuring the aortic component of the second sound with more severe degrees of valvular obstruction because these patients have a greater prolongation of right ventricular systole. The holosystolic decrescendo murmur of tricuspid regurgitation may accompany severe pulmonic stenosis, especially in the presence of congestive heart failure. Cyanosis, reflecting venoarterial shunting through a patent foramen ovale, is absent with mild stenosis and infrequent with moderate obstruction. Cyanosis may not be apparent in patients with severe obstruction if the atrial septum is intact.

Electrocardiography (Fig. 30–9, p. 969). This technique may be helpful in assessing the degree of obstruction to right ventricular output.[436] In mild cases the electrocardiogram often is normal, whereas moderate and severe steno-

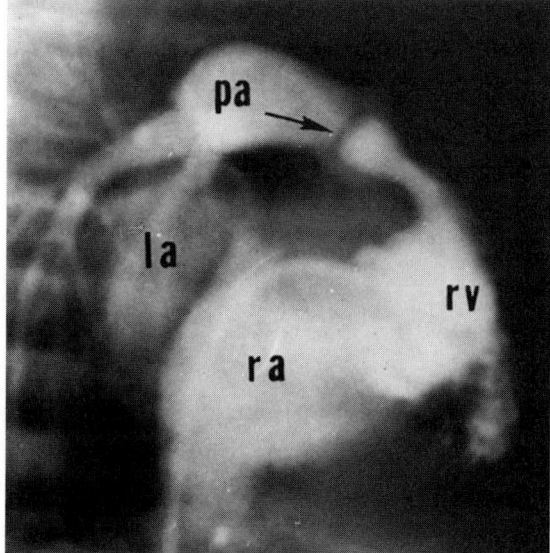
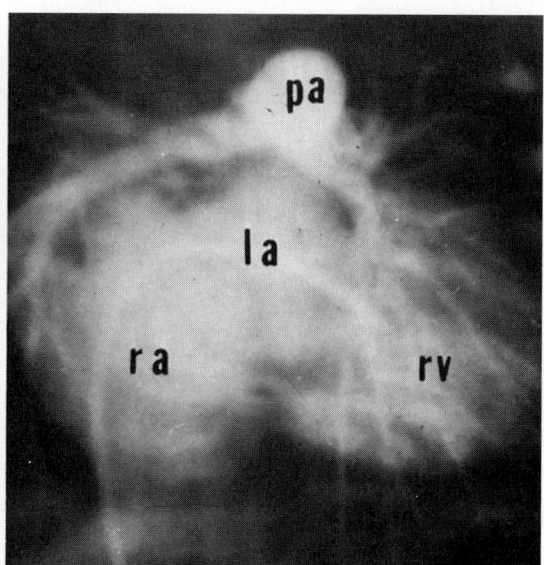

FIGURE 29–42. Right ventriculogram in an infant with critical pulmonic stenosis shows the thickened, nonmobile pulmonic valve (arrow) in the lateral projection *(left)*. Both the lateral and frontal *(right)* projections show regurgitation of contrast material across the tricuspid valve into the right atrium (ra), with subsequent shunting across the foramen ovale to the left atrium (la). rv = right ventricle; pa = pulmonary artery. (Courtesy of Norman Talner, M.D.)

ses are associated with right axis deviation and right ventricular hypertrophy. In the latter patients between ages 2 and 20 years, an estimate of right ventricular pressure can be made by multiplying the height of the R wave in lead V_{4R} or V_1 by 5.[436] A tall QR wave in the right precordial leads with T-wave inversion and ST-segment suppression (right ventricular "strain") reflects severe stenosis. When an rSR' pattern is observed in lead V_1 (20 per cent of patients) lower right ventricular pressures are found than in patients with a pure R wave of equal amplitude. High-amplitude P waves in leads II and V_1 indicating right atrial enlargement are associated with severe stenosis.

Chest Roentgenography. In patients with mild or moderate pulmonic stenosis chest roentgenography often shows a heart of normal size and normal pulmonary vascularity (Fig. 7–20, p. 218). Poststenotic dilatation of the main and left pulmonary arteries often is evident. Right atrial and right ventricular enlargement are observed in patients with severe obstruction and resultant right ventricular failure. The pulmonary vascularity may be reduced in patients with severe stenosis, right ventricular failure, and/or a venoarterial shunt at the atrial level (see p. 983).

Echocardiography. Reliable localization of the site of obstruction and assessment of its severity are obtained by combined continuous-wave or pulsed Doppler and two-dimensional echocardiography[429–431,437] (Figs. 3–68, p. 79, 30–4, p. 965, and Fig. 29–43). The latter usually shows quite prominent pulmonary valve echoes with restricted systolic motion as well as poststenotic dilation of the main pulmonary artery and its branches. In contrast to these findings in classical valvular pulmonic stenosis, patients with a dysplastic valve show thickened and immobile leaflets with hypoplasia of the pulmonary valve annulus and absent poststenotic dilatation of the pulmonary artery. Parasternal and subcostal views are required to detect most accurately maximal pulmonary artery blood flow velocity, which is converted to a pressure difference across the valve utilizing a modified Bernoulli equation (pressure difference [mm Hg] = 4 × the squared peak Doppler velocity [m/s]). A semiquantitative estimation of pulmonary and tricuspid regurgitation can be obtained. The peak systolic velocity of the tricuspid regurgitant jet provides a reliable indirect measurement of the severity of obstruction because the reverse gradient between the right ventricle and right atrium allows derivation of the ventricular peak systolic pressure. The constant value of 14 is used for right atrial pressure in the calculation.

Cardiac Catheterization and Angiocardiography. These techniques are now used only rarely to establish or exclude other diagnostic possibilities. The usual indication for cardiac catheterization is to provide definitive therapy for the lesion. Cardiac catheterization, however, may also localize the site of obstruction, evaluate its severity, and document the coexistence of additional cardiac malformations. The resting cardiac output usually is normal, even in cases of severe stenosis, and most children show the ability to increase cardiac output with exercise.[438] Right ventricular dysfunction occurs especially when venoarterial shunting is significant and produces systemic arterial desaturation. In patients with critical stenosis, care must be taken during hemodynamic study that the cardiac catheter does not dangerously occlude the stenotic valve opening. The angiographic appearance of a typical valvular pulmonic stenosis differs from that of a dysplastic valve. The former is thickened and domes during systole, returning to normal configuration in diastole. Poststenotic dilatation of the main pulmonary trunk and sometimes of the left pulmonary artery is usual. The leaflets of the dysplastic valve are not fused anatomically but are thickened and immobile, creating little change in the angiographic picture during the cardiac cycle. Moreover, a small annulus and narrow sinuses of Valsalva are common accompaniments of valve dysplasia. With either type of valve, systolic narrowing of the right ventricular infundibulum usually is associated with moderate or severe obstruction.

Natural History. Mild and moderate pulmonic valve stenoses have a generally favorable course; uncommonly, progression occurs in the severity of obstruction.[439,440] Serial hemodynamic studies reveal unchanged pressure gradients over 4- to 8-year intervals in three-fourths of patients. Equal percentages of the remainder have an increase or a decrease in the severity of obstruction; significant increases in the pressure gradient occur especially in children with a gradient in excess of 50 mm Hg at initial examination.[435]

Management. Percutaneous transluminal balloon valvuloplasty (see p. 1313) is the initial procedure of choice in patients with typical pulmonary valve stenosis and moderate to severe degrees of obstruction (Fig. 29–44).[114,434] This approach provides palliative improvement with the great likelihood that the improvement is permanent. In these same patients *surgical relief* also can be accomplished at extremely low risk.[441] The valve is approached through an incision in the pulmonary arterial trunk, and resection of infundibular muscle, if necessary, may be accomplished through the pulmonic valve. Reoperation or subsequent balloon valvuloplasty is seldom required. In patients with a dysplastic valve, in whom transcatheter valvuloplasty is ineffective, the thickened valve tissue is removed and a patch often is required to widen the annulus and proximal main pulmonary artery. In children with mild pulmonic valve stenosis, prophylaxis against infective endocarditis is recommended; these patients need not restrict their physical activities.

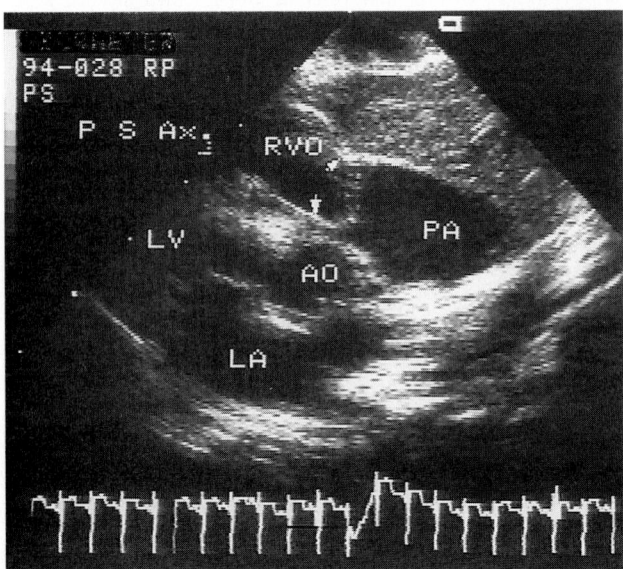

FIGURE 29–43. Severe valvular pulmonic stenosis seen from a parasternal short-axis view. The thickened pulmonary valve can be seen lying between the right ventricular outflow tract (RVO) and a dilated pulmonary artery (PA). The arrows are at the annulus of the pulmonary valve; the thickened, domed valve can be identified clearly. LV = left ventricle, AO = aorta, LA = left atrium. (Courtesy of Norman Silverman, M.D.)

Pulmonic Atresia with Intact Ventricular Septum

MORPHOLOGY. This anomaly is an uncommon and highly lethal cause of cyanosis in the neonatal period that may respond well to aggressive medical and surgical treatment.[442–444] In almost all infants the pulmonic valve is atretic; in the majority both the valve ring and the main pulmonary artery are hypoplastic. The right ventricular infundibulum occasionally may be atretic or extremely narrowed. A spectrum exists in right ventricular cavity size and configuration, from a diminutive right ventricular chamber, often with tricuspid stenosis, to a large right ventricle, frequently with tricuspid regurgitation (Fig. 29–45). In most infants the right ventricle is hypoplastic, and

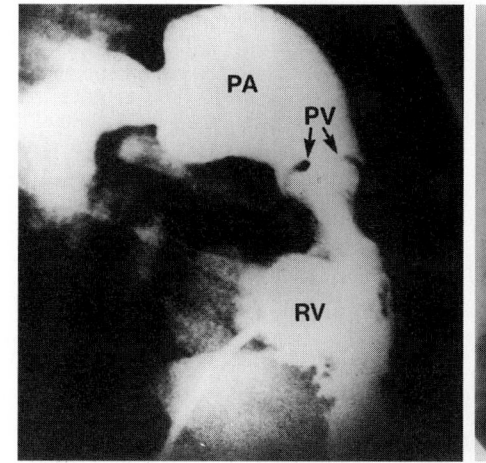

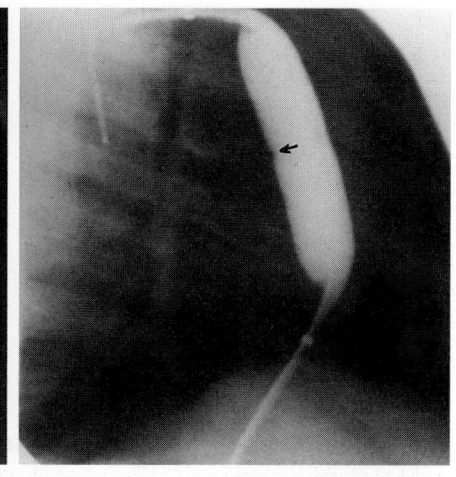

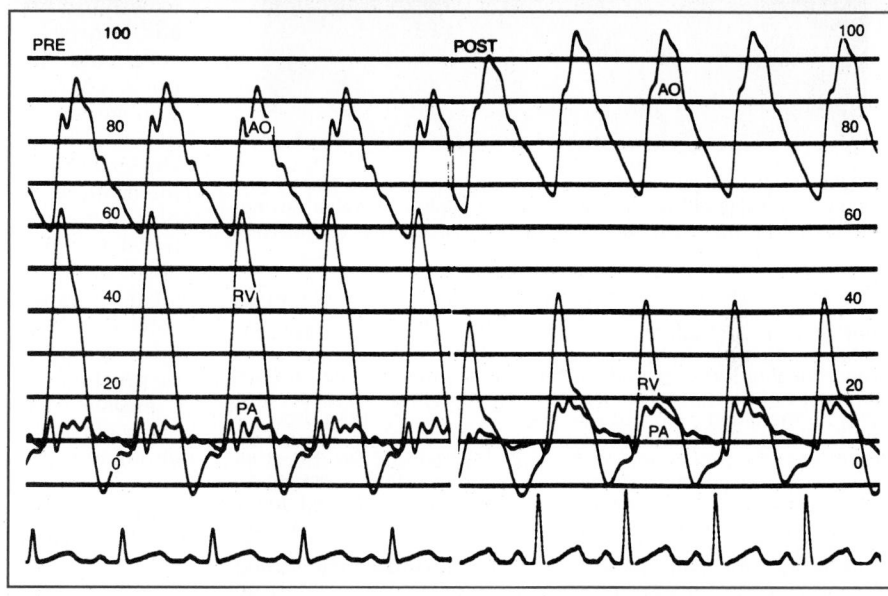

FIGURE 29–44. Right ventriculogram (RV) in the lateral projection *(top left)* from a patient with valvular pulmonic stenosis. The pulmonic valve (PV) is thickened and domes in systole. There is poststenotic dilatation of the pulmonary artery (PA). At the top right, successful balloon valvuloplasty shows almost complete disappearance of the stenotic waist (arrow). The bottom panel shows the pre *(left)* and post *(right)* valvuloplasty hemodynamics, showing a reduction from moderately severe to mild pulmonic stenosis. Ao = aorta. (Courtesy of Dr. Thomas G. DiSessa.)

sinusoidal communications exist in half the patients between the right ventricular cavity and the coronary circulation.[444,445]

The intramyocardial sinusoids may end blindly or communicate with coronary arteries. Further, these communications may be multiple and feed both the left and right coronary systems, or they may be fed via a single, dilated vessel. The proximal coronary arteries in some patients may be atrophic, proximal to a communication between the sinusoids and the distal coronary artery, particularly in

hearts with severe hypoplasia of the right ventricle. In these circumstances, the distal coronary vessels are supplied by communications with the right ventricle, and the coronary circulation is, therefore, right ventricle–dependent. In this group, decompression of the right ventricle by a surgical procedure would be associated with a high risk of myocardial ischemia and death.[448]

Because the pulmonic valve is imperforate and completely obstructed, systemic venous blood returning to the heart bypasses the

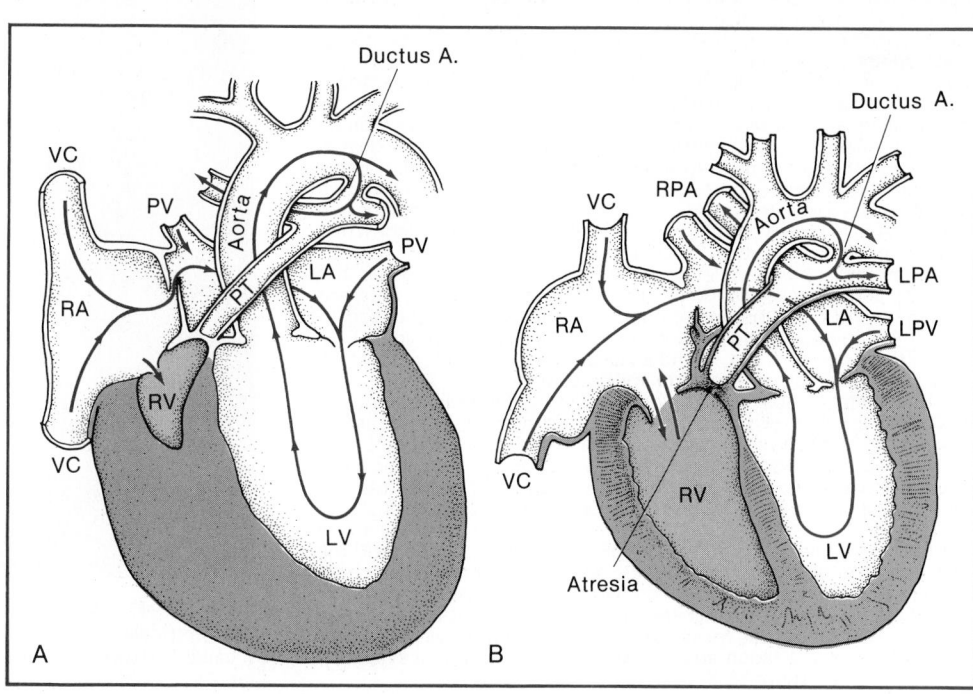

FIGURE 29–45. Pulmonic atresia with intact ventricular septum. With a competent tricuspid valve the right ventricular chamber is diminutive (*A*); Significant tricuspid regurgitation is associated with a normal or large right ventricular cavity (*B*). VC = vena cava, RA = right atrium, RV = right ventricle, PT = pulmonary trunk, PV = pulmonary vein, LA = left atrium, LV = left ventricle, Ductus A. = ductus arteriosus, LPA = left pulmonary artery, RPA = right pulmonary artery, LPV = left pulmonary vein. (From Edwards J. E.: Congenital malformations of the heart and great vessels. *In* Gould, S. E. [ed.]: Pathology of the Heart. 2nd ed. Springfield, Ill., Charles C Thomas, 1960.)

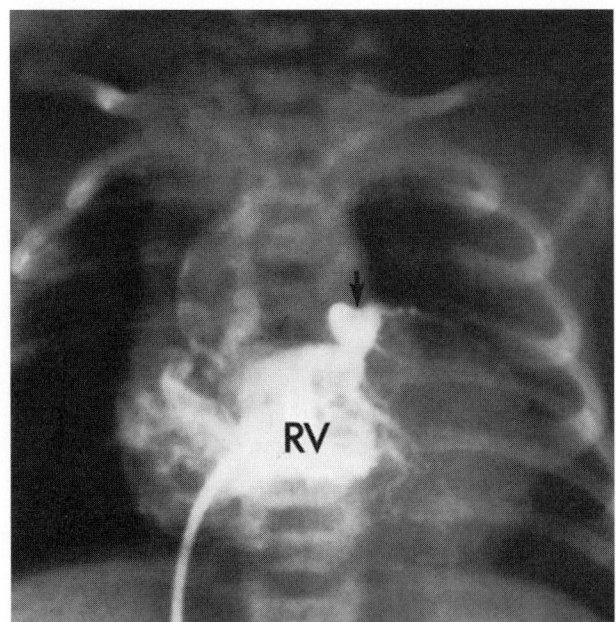

FIGURE 29–46. Right ventricular angiocardiogram in the frontal projection in a 1-day-old infant with an atretic pulmonic valve (arrow). The cavity of the right ventricle (RV) is small and eccentrically shaped. (Courtesy of Robert Freedom, M.D.)

right ventricle through an interatrial communication. Right ventricular output does not contribute to the effective cardiac output and is proportional to the magnitude of tricuspid regurgitation and the size and extent of the sinusoidal communications with the coronary arterial tree. The blood supply to the lungs is derived from the bronchial circulation and from flow through a persistently patent ductus arteriosus. The size and patency of the ductus arteriosus are critical determinants in postnatal survival; ductus closure results in death. Reduced pulmonary blood flow by way of a partially constricted ductus arteriosus results in profound hypoxemia, tissue hypoxia, and metabolic acidemia.

DIAGNOSIS. The diagnosis is suggested by roentgenographic findings of pulmonary hypoperfusion and the electrocardiographic observation of a normal QRS axis, absent or diminished right ventricular forces, and/or dominant left ventricular forces. In the minority of infants with marked tricuspid regurgitation, the right ventricle and right atrium are massively enlarged. The echocardiogram in the usual infant shows a small right ventricular cavity and diminutive or absent pulmonic valve echoes.[446,447] Doppler examination shows continuous retrograde flow to the pulmonary artery and/or its branches through a patent ductus arteriosus, which usually is narrow and tortuous. Only if tricuspid valve echoes are imaged by ultrasound examination can tricuspid atresia be distinguished from pulmonic atresia.

Although the diagnosis of this entity can be made by echocardiography, angiocardiography is required to assess treatment options because key determinants are the identification and nature of ventriculocoronary connections, which are not well characterized by echocardiography. Cardiac catheterization usually is performed on an emergency basis. Because survival depends on patency of the ductus arteriosus, infusion of prostaglandin E₁ (0.05 – 0.1 μg/kg/min) intravenously may dramatically reverse clinical deterioration and improve arterial blood gases and pH.[96] The usual hemodynamic findings are right atrial and right ventricular hypertension, with right ventricular pressure often greater than systemic pressure, and a massive right-to-left interatrial shunt. Selective angiocardiography establishes the diagnosis and allows evaluation of the degree of separation between the right ventricular infundibular and pulmonary trunk, the size of the right ventricular cavity and of the pulmonary arteries (Fig. 29–46), the anatomy and function of the tricuspid valve, and the anatomical and functional details of the coronary circulation.

MANAGEMENT. Initial stabilization is usually required in infants, necessitating infusion of prostaglandin E₁ to dilate the ductus arteriosus and measures to correct metabolic acidosis. The rare infant with membranous pulmonary atresia may be a candidate for balloon valvotomy.[447a] Initial surgical considerations focus on whether the patient is a candidate for a biventricular or univentricular (Fontan) repair (Fig. 29–46).[448–456] The angiographic delineation of coronary artery anatomy determines the feasibility of early decompression of the right ventricle, because this approach is contraindicated when there are ventriculocoronary connections with part or all of the coronary circulation right ventricle–dependent. Patients in this latter group are ultimately candidates for a lateral tunnel Fontan procedure, after initial palliation by balloon atrial septostomy followed by a systemic-pulmonary artery shunt.[457,458]

At the other end of the spectrum, babies with only mild hypoplasia of the right ventricle and tricuspid valve are candidates for a transventricular closed pulmonary valvotomy, followed later by balloon angioplasty or repeat surgical valvotomy. In infants with moderate right ventricular hypoplasia, a biventricular repair is preferred, often using a homograft valve in the outflow tract. In this group, the smaller the size of the right ventricle and tricuspid valve, the more likely a partial biventricular repair will be necessary, relieving the outflow tract obstruction with insertion of a valve, coupled with a bidirectional cavopulmonary (Glenn) shunt to ensure obligatory pulmonary blood flow.

Intraventricular Right Ventricular Obstruction

Infundibular pulmonic stenosis with an intact ventricular septum and the presence of anomalous muscle bundles are the two principal causes of intraventricular right ventricular obstruction (Fig. 29–47).[459]

SUBPULMONIC INFUNDIBULAR STENOSIS. This anomaly usually occurs at the proximal portion of the infundibulum and consists of a fibrous band at the junction of the right ventricular cavity and outflow tract. The clinical manifestations, course, and prognosis of patients with infundibular stenosis are similar to those of patients with valvular stenosis, although the former diagnosis is suggested by the absence of a systolic ejection sound and a systolic murmur lower along the left sternal border. Doppler echocardiography, withdrawal pressure tracings, and selective right ventricular angiocardiography permit localization of the site of obstruction and assessment of its extent and severity. Surgical treatment consists of resection of the fibrotic narrowed area and hypertrophied muscle. Occasionally it may be necessary to widen the outflow tract with a pericardial or prosthetic patch.

ANOMALOUS MUSCLE BUNDLES. A two-chambered right ventricle is formed by right ventricular obstruction due to anomalous muscle bundles; most of the patients have an associated malalignment or perimembranous ventricular septal defect, and about 5 per cent have subaortic stenosis.[459,460] Aberrant hypertrophied muscle bands traverse the

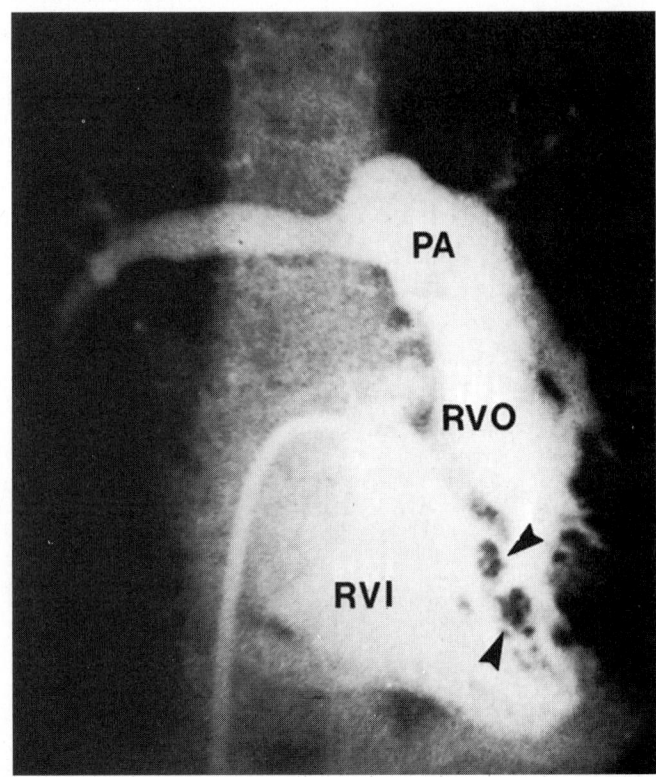

FIGURE 29–47. Intraventricular right ventricular obstruction. The right ventricular inflow (RVI) and outflow (RVO) tracts are separated by bands (arrows), creating intraventricular right ventricular obstruction. PA = pulmonary artery.

right ventricular cavity, extending from its anterior wall to the crista supraventricularis and/or the portion of the adjacent interventricular septum. The anomalous pyramid-shaped muscle mass obstructs blood flow through the body of the right ventricle and produces a proximal high-pressure inflow chamber and a distal low-pressure chamber. Thus this type of obstruction is distinguishable from that in tetralogy of Fallot, in which hypertrophied infundibular muscle protrudes into but does not cross the cavity of the right ventricle.

The clinical, electrocardiographic, and chest roentgenographic findings resemble those observed in pulmonic valvular or subvalvular infundibular obstruction, although the systolic thrill and murmur may be displaced lower along the left sternal border. Progressive obstruction occurs in some patients. The diagnosis may be established by two-dimensional echocardiography.[460] Selective right ventricular angiocardiography provides the most accurate diagnosis and reveals a filling defect in the midportion of the right ventricle which often does not change significantly with systole and diastole.

Management. The treatment for anomalous muscle bundles consists of surgical removal.[461] In the absence of preoperative recognition of the anomaly, the surgeon should be alerted to the correct diagnosis by the presence of a dimple during contraction on the ordinarily smooth anterior surface of the right ventricle and/or the inability to view the tricuspid valve through a longitudinal ventriculotomy because of the presence of the abnormal muscle mass.

Tetralogy of Fallot

DEFINITION. The overall incidence of this anomaly approaches 10 per cent of all forms of congenital heart disease, and it is the most common cardiac malformation responsible for cyanosis after 1 year of age.[462] The four components of this malformation are (1) ventricular septal defect, (2) obstruction to right ventricular outflow, (3) overriding of the aorta, and (4) right ventricular hypertrophy. The basic anomaly is the result of an anterior deviation of the septal insertion of the infundibular ventricular septum from its usual location in the normal heart between the limbs of the trabecular septum. The interventricular malalignment defect usually is large, approximating the aortic orifice in size, and is located high in the septum just below the right cusp of the aortic valve, separated from the pulmonic valve by the crista supraventricularis. The aortic root may be displaced anteriorly and straddle or override the septal defect, but, as in the normal heart, it lies to the right of the origin of the pulmonary artery. In most cases no dextroposition of the aorta exists; overriding of the aorta is a phenomenon secondary to the subaortic location of the ventricular septal defect.

HEMODYNAMICS. The degree of obstruction to pulmonary blood flow is the principal determinant of the clinical presentation. The site of obstruction is variable[463–465]; infundibular stenosis is the only major obstruction in about 50 per cent of patients and coexists with valvular obstruction in another 20 to 25 per cent (Fig. 29–48). Supravalvular and peripheral pulmonary arterial narrowing may be observed, and unilateral absence of a pulmonary artery (usually the left) is found in a small number of patients. Circulation to the abnormal lung is accomplished by bronchial and other collateral arteries.[465–467] Atresia of the pulmonic valve, infundibulum, or main pulmonary artery occasionally is referred to as "pseudotruncus arteriosus." True truncus arteriosus with absent pulmonary arteries (Type 4) differs from Fallot's tetralogy, in which pulmonary artery branches are present but are fed by a patent ductus arteriosus and/or bronchial arteries (see Fig. 29–51).[462] A right-sided aortic knob, aortic arch, and descending aorta occur in about 25 per cent of patients with tetralogy of Fallot. The coronary arteries may have surgically important variations[468]: the an-

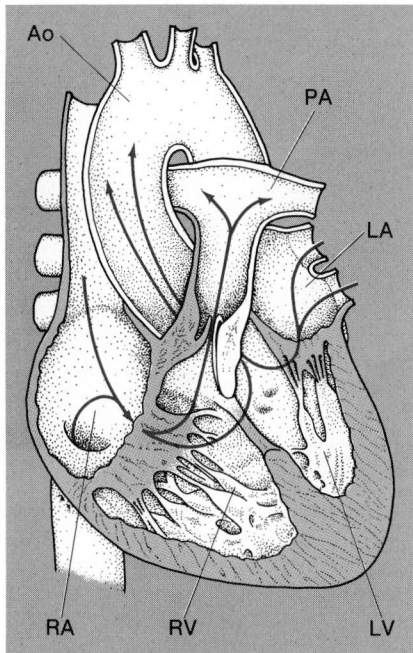

FIGURE 29–48. Tetralogy of Fallot with infundibular and valvular pulmonic stenosis. The arrows indicate direction of blood flow. A substantial right-to-left shunt exists across the ventricular septal defect. RA = right atrium, LA = left atrium, RV = right ventricle, LV = left ventricle, Ao = aorta, PA = pulmonary artery.

terior descending artery may originate from the right coronary artery; a single right coronary artery may give off a left branch that courses anterior to the pulmonary trunk; a single left coronary artery may give off a right branch that crosses the infundibulum of the right ventricle. Enlargement of the infundibulum branch of the right coronary artery often presents a problem with respect to a right ventriculotomy.

Associated cardiac anomalies exist in about 40 per cent of patients. Major associated cardiac anomalies include patent ductus arteriosus, multiple (usually muscular) ventricular septal defects, and complete atrioventricular septal defects. Localized single or multiple peripheral pulmonary arterial stenotic lesions are common; rarely, the right or left pulmonary artery may arise anomalously from the ascending aorta. Infrequently, aortic valve regurgitation results from aortic cusp prolapse. Associated extracardiac anomalies are present in 20 to 30 per cent of patients.

The relation between the resistance of blood flow from the ventricles into the aorta and into the pulmonary vessels plays a major role in determining the hemodynamic and clinical picture.[469] Thus, the severity of obstruction to right ventricular outflow is of fundamental significance. When right ventricular outflow tract obstruction is severe, the pulmonary blood flow is markedly reduced, and a large volume of unsaturated systemic venous blood is shunted from right to left across the ventricular septal defect. Severe cyanosis and polycythemia occur, and symptoms and sequelae of systemic hypoxemia are prominent. At the opposite end of the spectrum, the term "acyanotic" or "pink" tetralogy of Fallot often is used to describe an interventricular communication and a milder degree of obstruction to right ventricular outflow with little or no venoarterial shunting. In many infants and children the obstruction to right ventricular outflow is mild but progressive, so that early in life pulmonary exceeds systemic blood flow, and the symptoms resemble those produced by a simple ventricular septal defect.

CLINICAL MANIFESTATIONS. Few children with tetralogy of Fallot remain asymptomatic or acyanotic. Most are cyanotic from birth or develop cyanosis before age 1 year. In general, the earlier the onset of systemic hypoxemia, the

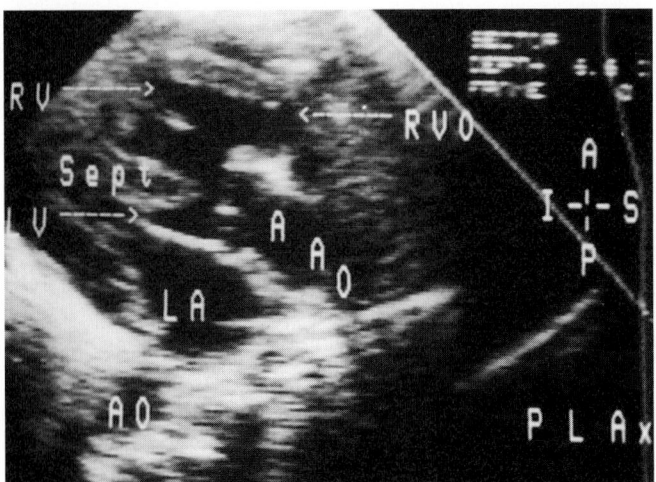

FIGURE 29–49. Tetralogy of Fallot in a parasternal long-axis (PLAx) view, which demonstrates the aorta overriding the ventricular septum (Sept). RV = right ventricle, RVO = right ventricular outflow tract, LV = left ventricle, LA = left atrium, AO = ascending aorta. (Courtesy of Norman Silverman, M.D.)

more likely the possibility that severe pulmonary outflow tract stenosis or atresia exists. Dyspnea with exertion, clubbing, and polycythemia is common. When resting after exertion, children with tetralogy characteristically assume a squatting posture (see p. 885). The latter may be obvious even in infancy; many cyanotic infants prefer to lie in a knee-chest position. Spells of intense cyanosis related to a sudden increase in venoarterial shunting and a reduction in pulmonary blood flow most often have their onset between 2 and 9 months of age and constitute an important threat to survival.[470–472] The attacks are not restricted to patients with severe cyanosis; they are most common in the morning after awakening and are characterized by hyperpnea and increasing cyanosis that progresses to limpness and syncope and occasionally terminates in convulsions, a cerebrovascular accident, and death.

Physical Examination. This reveals variable degrees of underdevelopment and cyanosis. Clubbing of the terminal digits may be prominent after the first year of life. The heart is not hyperactive or enlarged; a right ventricular impulse and systolic thrill often are palpable along the left sternal border. An early systolic ejection sound that is aortic in origin may be heard at the lower left sternal border and apex; the second heart sound is single, the pulmonic component rarely being audible. A systolic ejection murmur is produced by flow across the narrowed right ventricular infundibulum or pulmonic valve. The intensity and duration of the murmur vary inversely with the severity of obstruction—the opposite of the relation that exists in patients with pulmonic stenosis and an intact ventricular sep-

tum. Polycythemia, decreased systemic vascular resistance, and increased obstruction to right ventricular outflow may all be responsible for a decrease in intensity of the murmur; with extreme outflow tract stenosis or pulmonic atresia and during an attack of paroxysmal hypoxemia, there may be no or only a very short, faint murmur. A continuous murmur faintly audible over the anterior or posterior chest reflects flow through enlarged bronchial collateral vessels. A loud continuous murmur of flow through a patent ductus arteriosus occasionally may be heard at the upper left sternal border.

LABORATORY EXAMINATIONS. The *electrocardiogram* ordinarily shows right ventricular and, less frequently, right atrial hypertrophy. In a patient with acyanotic tetralogy, combined ventricular hypertrophy may be noted initially, progressing to right ventricular hypertrophy as cyanosis develops. *Roentgenographic* examination characteristically reveals a normal-sized, boot-shaped heart (coeur en sabot) with prominence of the right ventricle and a concavity in the region of the underdeveloped right ventricular outflow tract and main pulmonary artery. The pulmonary vascular markings typically are diminished, and the aortic arch and knob may be on the right side; the ascending aorta usually is large. A uniform, diffuse, fine reticular pattern of vascular markings is noted in the presence of prominent collateral vessels.

Echocardiography. Findings include aortic enlargement, aortic–septal discontinuity, and aortic overriding of the ventricular septum.[473] Two-dimensional echocardiography (Fig. 3–84, p. 84) shows the right ventricular outflow tract to be narrowed and in a more horizontal orientation than normal. The main pulmonary artery and its branches are mildly to severely hypoplastic. The usual ventricular septal malalignment defect lies superior to the tricuspid valve and immediately below the aortic valve cusps. These findings are best displayed in views of the long axis of the right ventricular outflow tract, which are the subxiphoid short axis and the high transverse parasternal echo windows. Echo views that show the anteroposterior coordinates best indicate the overriding of the aorta; these are the parasternal long-axis, apical two-chamber, and subxiphoid views (Fig. 29–49). The echocardiographic examination also reveals the origin of the main pulmonary artery from the right ventricle, and continuity of the main pulmonary artery with its right and left branches, and is accurate for diagnosing coronary abnormalities, although the latter are identified best by angiography.[467,471] The demonstration of mitral–semilunar valve continuity helps to distinguish tetralogy from double-outlet right ventricle with pulmonic stenosis, in which discontinuity of the mitral valve echo and the aortic cusp echo is a critical feature.

Cardiac Catheterization and Angiocardiography (Fig. 29–50). Despite the accuracy of noninvasive approaches, many centers still consider invasive study necessary to

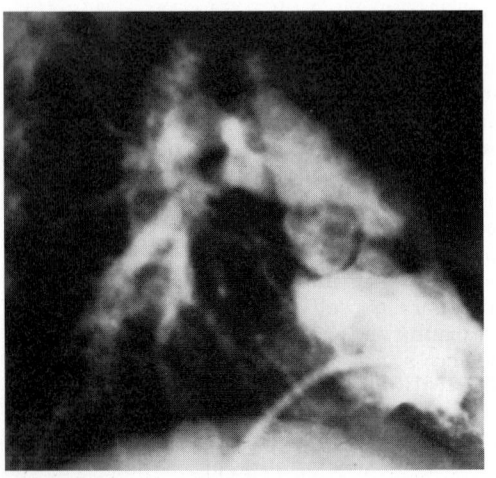

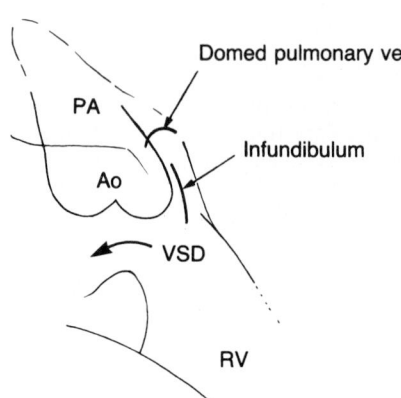

FIGURE 29–50. Lateral view of a right ventriculogram in a child with tetralogy of Fallot showing simultaneous opacification of the pulmonary artery (PA) and aorta (Ao). PV = pulmonic valve, VSD = ventricular septal defect, RV = right ventricle.

confirm the diagnosis; assess the magnitude of right-to-left shunting; provide details of additional muscular ventricular septal defects, if present; evaluate the architecture of the right ventricular outflow tract, pulmonic valve, and annulus and the morphology and caliber of the main branches of the pulmonary arteries; and analyze the anatomy of the coronary arteries. *Axial cineangiography*, utilizing the sitting-up projection, greatly facilitates evaluation of the pulmonary outflow tract and arteries.[151] The preoperative assessment of tetralogy with pulmonic atresia must include delineation of the arterial supply to both lungs by selective catheterization and visualization of bronchial collateral arteries with late serial filming; pulmonary arteries may be opacified only after the bronchial collateral arteries have cleared of contrast material (Fig. 29–51).[463] A patient with pulmonic atresia should not be ruled out as a candidate for surgical correction unless an inadequate pulmonary arterial supply to the lungs is clearly demonstrated.[466] Rarely, injection of contrast through a catheter in the pulmonary venous capillary wedge position is required to assess the possibility that anatomical pulmonary arteries are present. Computer-assisted axial tomography may visualize central pulmonary arteries when conventional angiography cannot.

MANAGEMENT. Among the factors that may complicate the management of patients with tetralogy are iron deficiency anemia, infective endocarditis, paradoxical embolism, polycythemia, coagulation disorders, and cerebral infarction or abscess. Paroxysmal hypercyanotic spells may respond quickly to oxygen, placing the child in the knee-chest position, and morphine. If the spell persists, metabolic acidosis will develop from prolonged anaerobic metabolism, and infusion of sodium bicarbonate may be necessary to interrupt the attack. Vasopressors, beta-adrenoceptor receptor blockade, or general anesthesia occasionally may be necessary.[472]

Total Surgical Correction. This operation is advisable ultimately for almost all patients with tetralogy of Fallot.[474–479] Early definitive repair, even in infancy, currently is advocated in most centers that are experienced in intracardiac surgery in infants. Successful early correction appears to prevent the consequences of progressive infundibular obstruction and acquired pulmonic atresia, delayed growth and development, and complications secondary to hypoxemia and polycythemia with bleeding tendencies. The anatomy of the right ventricular outflow tract and the size of the pulmonary arteries, rather than the age or size of the infant or child, are the most important determinants in assessing candidacy for primary repair; a transannular patch may be used in infants with severe outflow narrowing.[479] Marked hypoplasia of the pulmonary arteries is a relative contraindication for early corrective operation.

Palliative Surgery. When marked hypoplasia of the pulmonary arteries exists, a palliative operation designed to increased pulmonary blood flow is recommended and usually consists in the smallest infants of a systemic-pulmonary arterial anastomosis.[480] A transventricular infundibulectomy or valvulotomy is an alternative palliative procedure that may be considered. Balloon dilatation of the pulmonary valve may afford palliation in selected infants.[481,481a] Total correction can then be carried out at a lower risk later in childhood. The palliative procedures relieve hypoxemia caused by diminished pulmonary blood flow and reduce the stimulus to polycythemia. Because pulmonary venous return is augmented, the left atrium and ventricle are stimulated to enlarge their capacity in anticipation of total correction. In the most severe forms of tetralogy of Fallot with pulmonic atresia, the goals of operation include establishment of nonstenotic continuity between the right ventricle and pulmonary arteries, closure of the intracardiac shunt, and interruption of surgically created shunts or major collateral arteries to the lungs. When atresia is confined to the infundibulum or pulmonic valve, repair may be accomplished by infundibular resection and reconstruction of the outflow tract with a pericardial patch. If a long segment of pulmonary arterial atresia exists, a valve-containing conduit is inserted from the right ventricle to the distal pulmonary artery.[482] The presence of a single pulmonary artery in the hilus of either lung is a prerequisite for repair of pulmonic atresia. Prior unifocalization to incorporate multiple systemic to pulmonary artery collaterals into a neo–pulmonary artery may be required in selected patients. A conduit also may be necessary in less severe forms of right ventricular outflow tract obstruction when an anomalous coronary artery crosses the right ventricular outflow tract.

Postoperative Complications. A variety of complications are common in the postoperative period after palliative or corrective operation. Mild-to-moderate left ventricular decompensation may be secondary to the sudden increase in pulmonary venous return; varying degrees of pulmonic valvular regurgitation increase right ventricular cavity size further.[483] Patients with progressive pulmonary insufficiency and severe right ventricular dilatation are candidates for prosthetic pulmonary valve insertion.[484,485]

Bleeding problems frequently are seen, especially in older polycythemic patients. Complete right bundle branch block or the pattern of left anterior hemiblock often is seen, but disabling dysrhythmias are infrequent.[486] Restricted pulmonary arterial flow is the greatest cause for early and late mortality and poor late results.[462] After convalescence from intracardiac repair, symptoms of hypoxemia and severe exercise intolerance are relieved even in the presence of some residual right ventricular outflow tract obstruction, pulmonic valve incompetence, and/or cardiomegaly.[479,487] However, cardiovascular performance at rest or during exercise may remain below normal,[488,489] and major complications, such as trifascicular block, complete heart block, ventricular arrhythmias, and sudden death, may rarely occur many years after surgical treatment.

Late ventricular arrhythmias are rare in patients with successful early correction of the malformation unless complex or multiple operations were performed. Because widespread use of ambulatory electrocardiographic monitoring has resulted in greater detection of ventricular arrhythmias, usually isolated ventricular extrasystoles or nonsustained tachycardia, some have suggested that the asymptomatic patients in this category should have pharmacological suppression of their arrhythmias. Most recent studies, how-

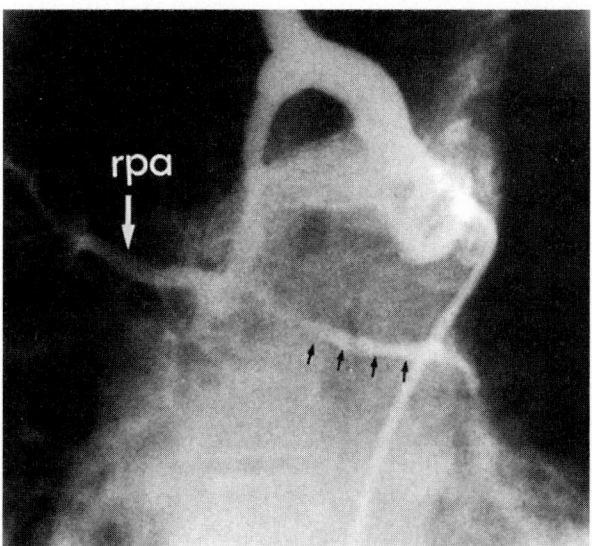

FIGURE 29–51. Selective systemic collateral bronchial arteriogram demonstrates "gull-wing" configuration of the hypoplastic right pulmonary artery (rpa) and left pulmonary artery (arrows) in a patient with tetralogy of Fallot and pulmonic atresia. (Courtesy of Robert Freedom, M.D.)

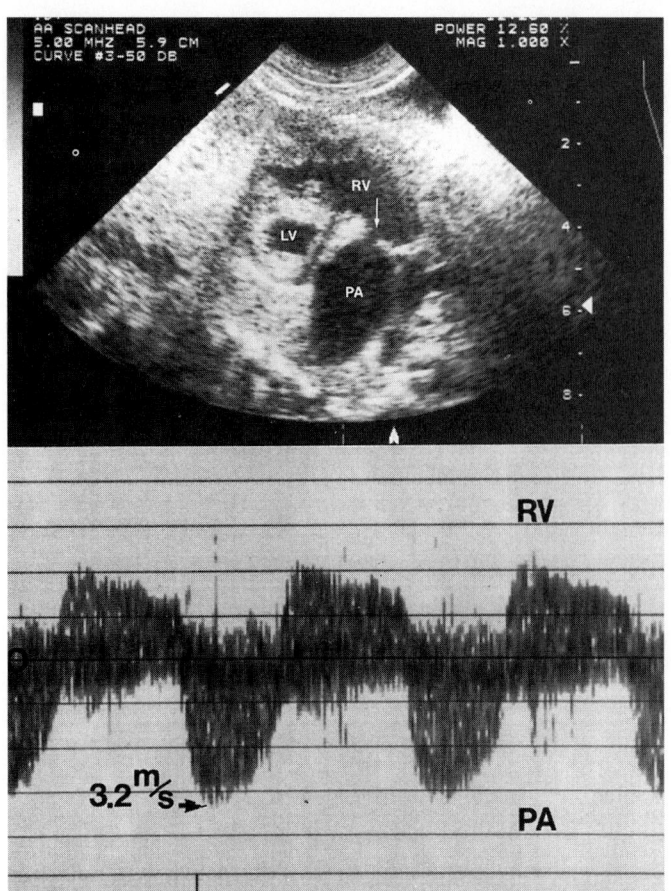

FIGURE 29–52. Two-dimensional *(top panel)* and Doppler *(lower panel)* echocardiogram of a 30-week gestation fetus with tetralogy of Fallot and absent pulmonary valve. The pulmonary artery (PA) is aneurysmally dilated and the right ventricle (RV) is also dilated. The arrow points to the stenotic pulmonary valve annulus. Pulmonary valve leaflets are not detectable. The Doppler study at the level of the pulmonary valve annulus demonstrates to-and-fro flow with increased forward velocity in systole. LV = left ventricle. (Courtesy of James C. Huhta, M.D.)

marked aneurysmal dilatation of the pulmonary arteries. The combination of anomalies often is referred to as tetralogy of Fallot with absent pulmonic valve. The obstructing lesion principally consists of underdeveloped, primitive valve tissue within a hypoplastic annulus; infundibular obstruction and the ventricular septal defect do not differ from classic tetralogy of Fallot. Recent reports indicate that deletion within chromosome 22 is common in patients with this anomaly.[494b]

The massively dilated pulmonary arteries often are the major determinant of the clinical course because they frequently result in upper airway obstruction and severe respiratory distress in infancy.[495] Smaller intrapulmonary bronchi may also be compressed by abnormally branching distal pulmonary arteries, and in some cases a reduction exists in the number of bronchial generations or alveolar multiplications.[496,497] Poststenotic pulmonary artery aneurysms develop in utero, and their size and location appear to be related to the magnitude of pulmonic regurgitation in fetal life, the orientation of the right ventricular infundibulum to the right or left, and the size of the ductus arteriosus.[498]

CLINICAL AND LABORATORY FINDINGS. The *clinical* features often are distinctive, with an early onset of severe respiratory distress caused by tracheobronchial compression accompanied by a systolic ejection and a widely transmitted low-pitched, decrescendo diastolic murmur at the upper left sternal border. In the absence of pulmonary complications cyanosis is commonly mild. *Roentgenographically* the heart is moderately enlarged; hyperinflated lung fields are observed with large hilar densities representing the aneurysmally dilated pulmonary arteries. The *echocardiographic* features are similar to those seen in classic tetralogy of Fallot, in addition to massive dilatation of the main pulmonary artery and branch pulmonary arteries. Remnants of pulmonary cusps may be visible. Right ventricular dilatation is produced by significant pulmonary regurgitation; the latter is identified by retrograde diastolic flow in the pulmonary arteries and right ventricle at Doppler examination. These findings may be detected before birth (Fig. 29–52). Definitive diagnosis is established by cardiac catheterization and selective angiocardiography.

NATURAL HISTORY AND MANAGEMENT. Prognosis is related to the intensity of upper airway obstruction; pulmonary complications are the usual cause of death in infancy. If survival beyond infancy is accomplished, the respiratory symptoms usually diminish, probably because of maturational changes in the structure of the tracheobronchial tree. The surgical approach in infancy often is unsatisfactory; a variety of procedures have been attempted, ranging from aneurysmorrhaphy to pulmonary artery suspension to transection and reanastomosis of pulmonary artery segments to homograft insertion.[499,500] Also suggested are ligation of the main pulmonary artery and creation of a systemic-pulmonary shunt, and primary repair of the ventricular septal defect with pulmonary arterial plication. In older patients the stenotic annulus may be widened with a patch and the ventricular septal defect closed. It seldom is necessary to replace the pulmonic valve.

ever, do not support the use of potentially dangerous long-term antiarrhythmic treatment for asymptomatic postoperative patients.[490–494a]

Congenital Absence of the Pulmonic Valve

PATHOLOGY AND PATHOGENESIS. In the majority of cases of this rare malformation the lesion is associated with a ventricular septal defect, a narrowed obstructive annulus of the pulmonic valve, and

Tricuspid Atresia

MORPHOLOGY. This anomaly is characterized by absence of the tricuspid orifice, an interatrial communication, hypoplasia of the right ventricle, and the presence of a communication between the systemic and pulmonary circulations, usually a ventricular septal defect.[501] Thus there is a univentricular atrioventricular connection, consisting of a left-sided mitral valve between the morphological left

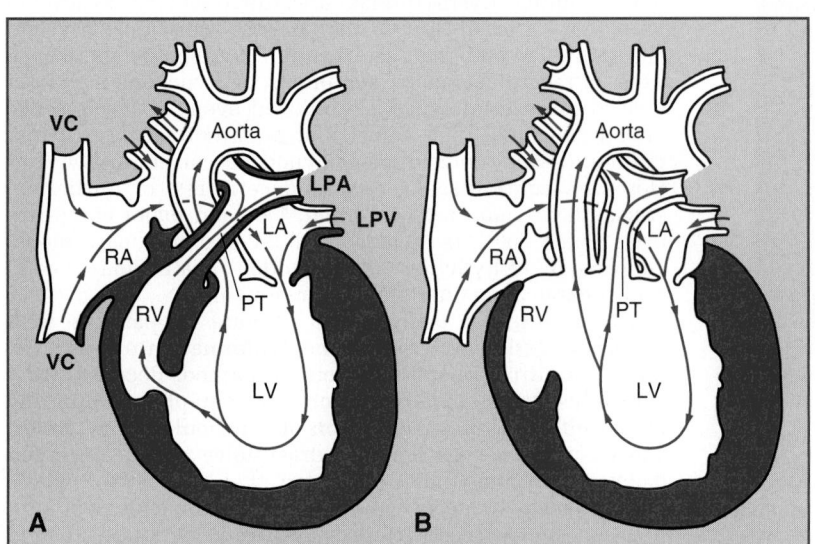

FIGURE 29–53. *A,* Tricuspid atresia with normally related great arteries, a small ventricular septal defect, diminutive right ventricular chamber, and narrowed outflow tract. *B,* An example of tricuspid atresia and complete transposition of the great arteries in which the left ventricular chamber is essentially a common ventricle, with the aorta arising from an infundibular component (RV) of the common ventricle. VC = vena cava, RA = right atrium, LA = left atrium, RV = right ventricle, LV = left ventricle, LPV = left pulmonary vein, LPA = left pulmonary artery. (Modified from Edwards, J. E., and Burchell, H. B.: Congenital tricuspid atresia: Classification. Med. Clin. North Am. *33*:1177, 1949.)

atrium and left ventricle. Unequal division of the atrioventricular canal by fusion of the right-sided endocardial cushions has been proposed as the embryological fault. Patients may be subdivided into those with normally related great arteries (70 to 80 per cent of cases) and those with D-transposition of the great arteries; further classification depends on the presence of pulmonic stenosis or atresia and the absence or size of the ventricular septal defect (Fig. 29–53). Additional cardiovascular malformations often are present, especially in patients with D-transposition of the great arteries, and include persistent left superior vena cava, patent ductus arteriosus, coarctation of the aorta, and juxtaposition of the atrial appendages.

PATHOPHYSIOLOGY. The association with other cardiac malformations determines whether or not pulmonary blood flow is decreased, normal, or increased and therefore the degree of systemic hypoxemia.[502] The clinical picture usually is dominated by symptoms resulting from greatly diminished pulmonary blood flow with severe cyanosis. Cyanosis results from an obligatory admixture of systemic and pulmonary venous blood in the left atrium, and its intensity primarily depends on the magnitude of pulmonary blood flow. Heart failure, rather than cyanosis, is the predominant problem in infants with torrential pulmonary blood flow, which results when D-transposition of the great arteries, a ventricular septal defect, and an unobstructed pulmonary outflow tract coexist. If these patients survive infancy, they are candidates for pulmonary vascular obstructive disease; a favorable response to pulmonary arterial banding is common early in life.

CLINICAL FEATURES. The diagnosis is easily established in the vast majority of infants with tricuspid atresia and pulmonary hypoperfusion. The *electrocardiographic* findings of left-axis deviation, right atrial enlargement, and left ventricular hypertrophy in a cyanotic infant strongly suggest tricuspid atresia.[502] *Echocardiography* reveals a small or absent right ventricle, large left ventricle, and absent tricuspid valve echoes (Figs. 29–54 and 3–19, p. 60); further, it may demonstrate the relation of the great arteries unless pulmonic atresia is present. Color flow and pulsed Doppler echocardiography reveals the abnormal flow patterns; apical and subxiphoid cross-sectional views best reveal the atretic tricuspid orifice. *Roentgenographically,* there are diminished pulmonary vascular markings and a concavity in the region of the cardiac silhouette usually occupied by the main pulmonary artery. The right atrial shadow may be prominent unless left-sided juxtaposition of the atrial appendages exists, which produces a straight and flattened right heart border.

CARDIAC CATHETERIZATION AND ANGIOGRAPHY. The right ventricle cannot be entered directly from the right atrium. When the great arteries are related normally, pulmonary blood flow is found to be derived from shunting through a ventricular septal defect or by way of a patent ductus arteriosus; the latter and the bronchial collaterals are the source of pulmonary flow if the ventricular septum is intact. In complete transposition the pulmonary artery fills directly from the left ventricle and the aorta indirectly through a ventricular septal defect and the hypoplastic right ventricle. Because complete admixture exists in the left atrium of pulmonary and systemic venous return, the degree of systemic arterial hypoxemia depends on the pulmonary-systemic flow ratio. Right atrial angiography does not opacify the right ventricle unless by way of a ventricular septal defect. Selective left ventricular *angiography* permits identification of the hypoplastic right ventricle, the size and location of the ventricular septal defect, the type of pulmonary obstruction, the relation between the great arteries, and the size of the distal pulmonary arterial tree.

MANAGEMENT. *Balloon atrial septostomy* in those infants with a restrictive interatrial communication and palliative operations designed to increase pulmonary blood flow (systemic arterial—or venous—pulmonary artery anastomosis)

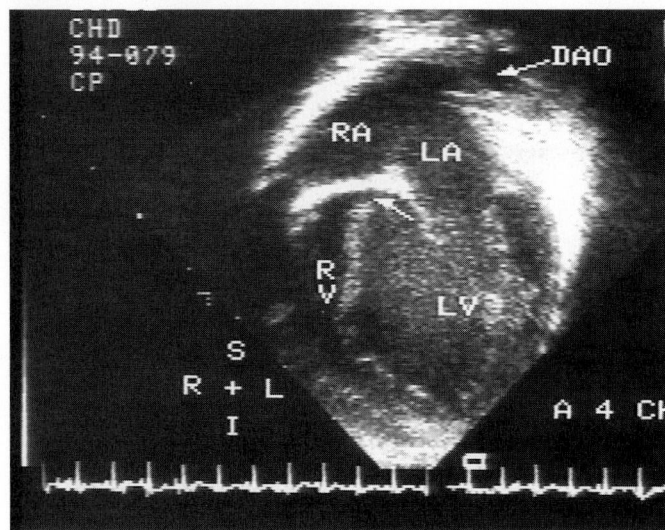

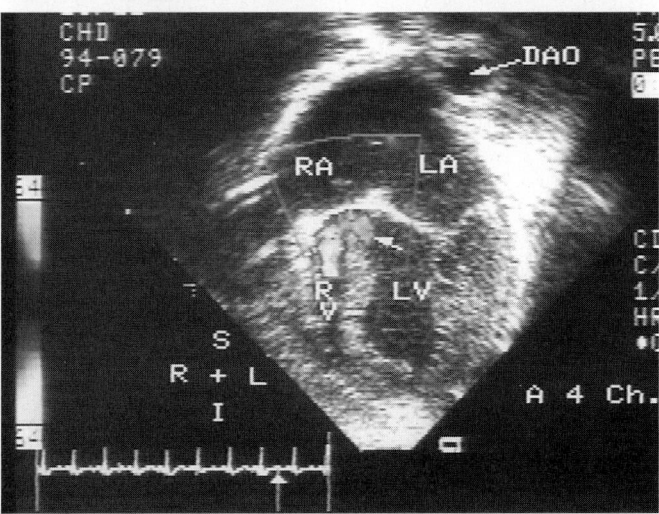

FIGURE 29–54. Apical four-chamber views of a patient with tricuspid atresia. In these views the right atrium (RA) and left atrium (LA) can be seen above, and the small right ventricle (RV) and large left ventricle (LV) can be seen below. *Top,* Diastole with the mitral valve in the open position. Note the intense tissue echoes from the right atrioventricular groove between the right atrium (RA) and right ventricle (RV), indicating the absence of the tricuspid valve. The descending aorta (DAO) can be identified posterior to the left atrium (LA). *Bottom,* Doppler color flow map of the same patient taken toward end-systole, showing the passage of blood across the ventricular septal defect (arrow). Orientation: S = superior, I = inferior, R = right, L = left. (Courtesy of Norman Silverman, M.D.)

are capable of producing clinical improvement of significant duration in patients with diminished blood flow.[502]

Functional correction of the anomaly has been accomplished in children beyond age 12 months by an intraatrial cavopulmonary baffle (lateral tunnel Fontan) (Fig. 29–55) or connection of the left pulmonary artery to the superior vena cava and inferior vena cava to the right pulmonary artery.[502a] An adjustable snare around the atrial septal defect or a fenestrated cavocaval baffle with later transcatheter closure appears to prevent acute increases in systemic venous pressure, improve cardiac output, and enhance surgical survival.[503–504a] In patients with tricuspid atresia and complete transposition of the great arteries, subaortic obstruction can be anticipated when the ventricular septal defect becomes restrictive, also referred to as an obstructive bulboventricular foramen. In most patients, the subaortic tissue must be resected, or preferably, a main pulmonary artery to ascending aorta anastomosis (Damus-Stansel-Kaye procedure) is performed at the time of the Fontan operation.[505] Candidates for these corrective procedures must

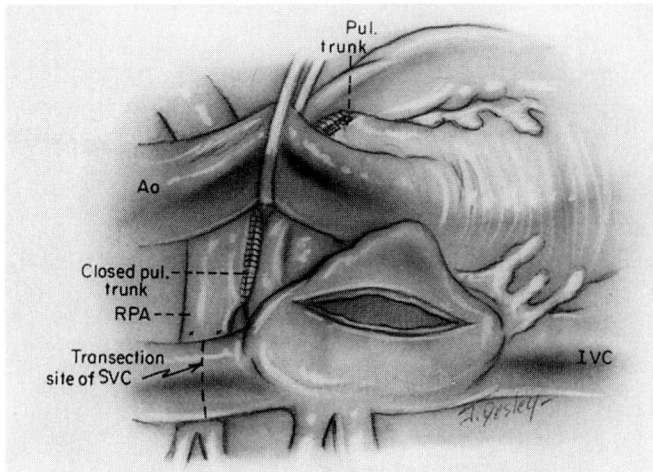

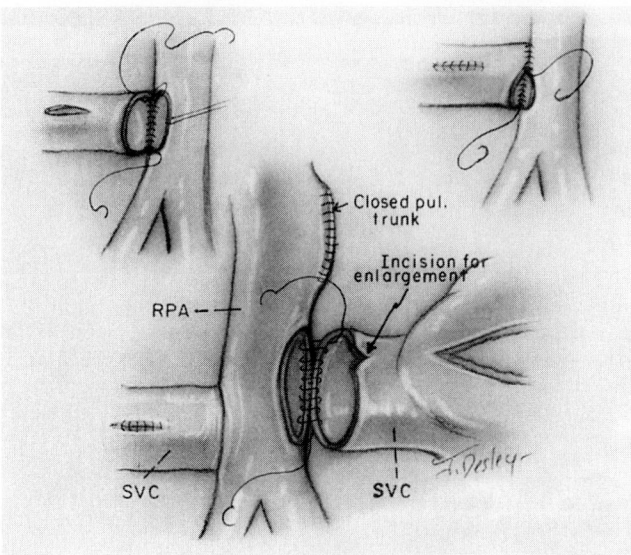

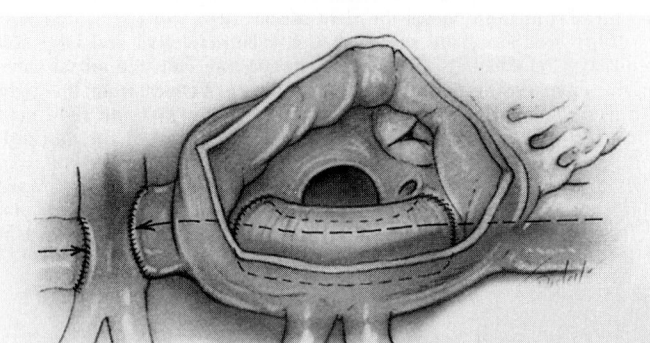

have normal pulmonary vascular resistance and a mean pulmonary artery pressure less than 20 mm Hg, pulmonary arteries of adequate size, and good left ventricular function.[506–508] The postoperative period usually is characterized transiently by a superior vena cava syndrome with right heart failure, edema, ascites, and hepatomegaly. Long-term results have been good.[509–511a] Late atrial arrhythmias may be a consequence of adverse preoperative hemodynamic function.[512]

Ebstein's Anomaly of the Tricuspid Valve
(See also p. 966)

This malformation is characterized by a downward displacement of the tricuspid valve into the right ventricle due to anomalous attachment of the tricuspid leaflets (Fig. 29–56).[513] Case-control studies suggest that maternal exposure in the first trimester to lithium carbonate, used in the management of manic-depressive psychosis, is associated with a greatly increased risk of this anomaly in exposed offspring.[514] Tricuspid valve tissue is dysplastic, and a variable portion of the septal and inferior cusps adhere to the right ventricular wall some distance away from the atrioventricular junction. Because of the abnormally situated tricuspid orifice, a portion of the right ventricle lies between the atrioventricular ring and the origin of the valve, which is continuous with the right atrial chamber. This proximal segment is "atrialized," and a distal, functionally small ventricular chamber exists. The degree of impairment of right ventricular function depends primarily on the extent to which the right ventricular inflow portion is atrialized and on the magnitude of tricuspid valve regurgitation.

CLINICAL MANIFESTATIONS. These are variable because the spectrum of pathology varies widely and because of the presence of associated malformations.[515,516] If the tricuspid valve is deformed severely, neonatal heart failure or even

FIGURE 29–55. The Fontan operation by total cavopulmonary connection. *Top,* The pulmonary trunk has been divided close to the pulmonary valve and both ends closed. The right atrium is opened and a pump sump sucker is placed across the foramen ovale and into the left atrium (not shown). Marking stitches are placed at the proposed site of transection of the superior vena cava and at the proposed sites of the two longitudinal incisions on the superior and inferior aspects of the right pulmonary artery. *Middle,* The anastomosis made between the distal end of the divided superior vena cava and the incision in the superior aspect of the right pulmonary artery. The cardiac end of the superior vena cava is rarely enlarged; anastomosis is made to an incision in the inferior aspect of the right pulmonary artery. *Bottom,* A tunnel is created from a cylinder of either Dacron, Gore-Tex, or pericardium connecting the inferior vena cava to the atrial orifice of the superior vena cava. The right pulmonary veins drain behind the tunnel. (From Kirklin, J. W., and Barratt-Boyes, B. G.: Cardiac Surgery. 2nd ed. New York, Churchill Livingstone, 1993, p. 1068.)

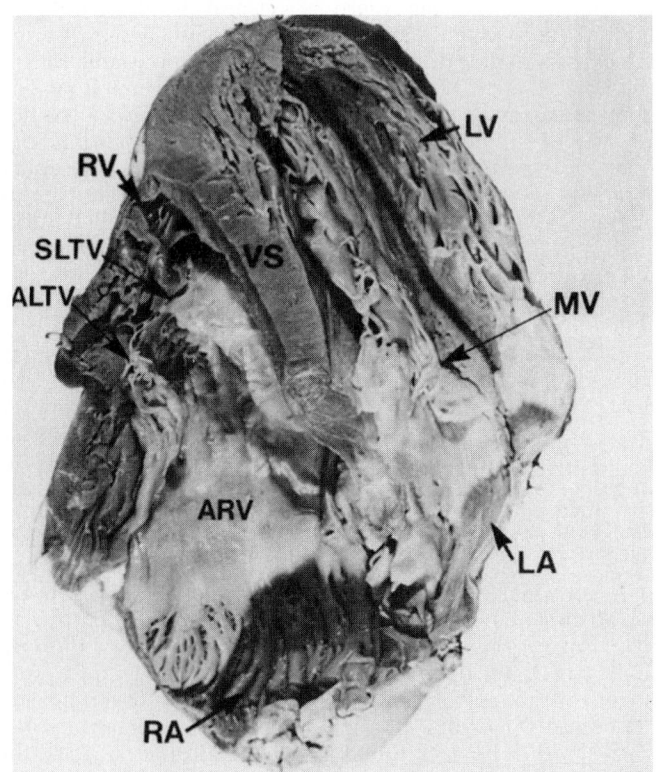

FIGURE 29–56. Anatomical specimen of Ebstein's anomaly of the tricuspid valve, cut in the same place as an apical four-chamber echocardiographic view (Fig. 29–57). The septal and anterior leaflets of the tricuspid valve (SLTV, ALTV) are displaced into the right ventricle (RV), producing a large atrialized right ventricle (ARV). VS = ventricular septum, RA = right atrium, LA = left atrium, MV = mitral valve, LV = left ventricle. (Courtesy of Thomas DiSessa, M.D.)

fetal hydrops and intrauterine death may occur.[517] At the other end of the spectrum, patients with a mildly deformed tricuspid valve may remain symptom free well into adulthood. The severity of symptoms also depends upon the presence or absence of associated malformations. An interatrial communication consisting of a patent foramen ovale or an ostium secundum atrial septal defect is present in more than half the cases. The most common important associated defect is pulmonic stenosis or atresia. Other coexistent anomalies may include an ostium primum type of atrial septal defect and ventricular septal defect alone or in combination with other lesions. The Ebstein's lesion commonly is observed in association with congenitally corrected transposition of the great arteries, in which the tricuspid valve is in the left atrioventricular orifice (see p. 940). The usual manifestations in infancy are cyanosis, a cardiac murmur, and severe congestive heart failure. The magnitude of tricuspid regurgitation in the neonate is enhanced because the pulmonary vascular resistance is normally high early in life.[518] In this regard, newborn infants with Ebstein's anomaly and massive tricuspid regurgitation must be distinguished by two-dimensional and Doppler echocardiography from those with organic pulmonary atresia and the presence of elevated perinatal pulmonary vascular resistance.[519]

The tricuspid regurgitation in infants with Ebstein's anomaly may lessen substantially, and cyanosis may disappear early in life as pulmonary vascular resistance falls, only to occur at a later age when right ventricular dysfunction and/or paroxysmal arrhythmias develop. In some infants with Ebstein's malformation, cyanosis is suddenly intensified as the degree of pulmonary hypoperfusion is unmasked by spontaneous closure of a patent ductus arteriosus.

Beyond infancy the onset of symptoms is insidious; the most common complaints are exertional dyspnea, fatigue, and cyanosis. About 25 per cent of patients suffer episodes of paroxysmal atrial tachycardia. A prominent systolic pulsation of the liver and a large *v* wave in the jugular venous pulse accompany the systolic thrill and murmur of tricuspid regurgitation. Wide splitting of the first and second heart sounds and prominent third and fourth heart sounds may produce a characteristically rhythmic auscultatory cadence with a triple, quadruple, and quintuple combination of sounds.

LABORATORY FINDINGS. The electrocardiographic abnormalities commonly fall into two categories—those with a right bundle branch block pattern and those with a Wolff-Parkinson-White syndrome (Fig. 4-28, p. 126). The pattern in the latter is always Type B, resembling left bundle branch block with predominant S waves in the right pericardial leads. The presence of a preexcitation (Fig. 30-7, p. 968) pattern increases the risk of supraventricular paroxysmal tachycardia.[520] The electrocardiogram most often shows giant P waves, a prolonged P-R interval, and prolonged terminal QRS depolarization, producing variable degrees of right bundle branch block. These distinctive findings help to distinguish Ebstein's anomaly from other forms of right ventricular dysplasia whose presenting problem often is an arrhythmia. Roentgenographic studies (Fig. 7-46, p. 234) usually demonstrate an enlarged right atrium, a small right ventricle, and a pulmonary artery with reduced pulsations; the pulmonary vascularity may be reduced if a large right-to-left shunt is present.

Echocardiographic Findings. The principal echocardiographic findings observed in patients with this anomaly, as well as in those with other forms of right ventricular volume overload, are an increase in right ventricular dimension, paradoxical ventricular septal motion, an increase in tricuspid valve excursion, and an abnormal closing velocity of the tricuspid valve. More specific findings for Ebstein's anomaly include a delay in tricuspid valve closure relative to mitral closure and a decrease in the E-F slope of the tricuspid valve, an abnormal anterior position of the tricuspid valve during diastole, and the detection of tricuspid valve echoes with more lateral placement of the transducer than usual.[521] Two-dimensional echocardiographic techniques are superior for observation of the inferior and leftward displacement of the tricuspid valve and simultaneously demonstrate the abnormal positional relation between the tricuspid and mitral valves (Figs. 29-57 and 3-69, p. 80). Moreover, the boundaries of the atrialized right ventricle may be defined.

Specific diagnosis requires identification, usually from an apical four-chamber view, of displacement of the septal tricuspid leaflet.[522]

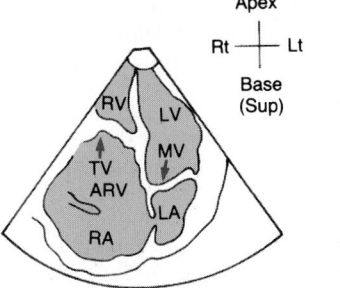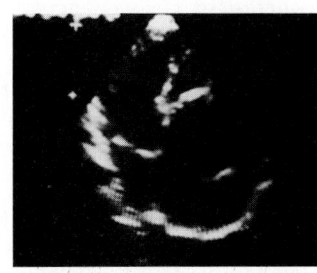

FIGURE 29–57. Apical four-chamber view of Ebstein's anomaly, corresponding to the anatomical specimen in Figure 29–56. RA = right atrium, LA = left atrium, MV = mitral valve, LV = left ventricle, TV = tricuspid valve, ARV = atrialized right ventricle, RV = right ventricle. (Courtesy of Thomas DiSessa, M.D.)

Tricuspid regurgitation, if present, is detected by Doppler examination.

Invasive Study. These are rarely necessary. When *cardiac catheterization* is performed, the intracavitary electrocardiogram recorded just proximal to the tricuspid valve shows a right ventricular type of complex, while the pressure recorded is that of the right atrium. A right-to-left atrial shunt normally is present. The hemodynamic findings depend on the degree of tricuspid regurgitation. The cardiac muscle is unusually irritable, and a high incidence of significant arrhythmias during catheterization has been noted. Selective right ventricular *angiocardiography* shows the position of the displaced tricuspid valve, the size of the right ventricle, and the configuration of the outflow portion of the right ventricle.

MANAGEMENT. Ebstein's anomaly may be compatible with a relatively long and active life, with most patients surviving into the the third decade.[515,523,524] In symptomatic infants with severe cardiomegaly, the initial surgical approach is similar to that in patients with tricuspid atresia, creating a systemic pulmonary shunt, and at a later age the Fontan approach. Consideration may be given in some of these patients to the creation of a bidirectional Glenn shunt from the superior vena cava to the pulmonary arteries, to divert systemic venous return from the right atrium and to increase pulmonary blood flow. In older patients, significant benefit has resulted from reconstruction of the tricuspid valve, closure of the atrial septal defect, plication of the free wall of the right ventricle, posterior tricuspid annuloplasty, and a reduction in right atrial size.[515] Because late results of this latter approach are encouraging, we now recommend operation for all symptomatic patients and even asymptomatic patients if their heart size is increasing significantly. In patients with a preexcitation syndrome (see p. 673) that is producing life-threatening rhythm disturbances, the accessory conduction pathways are either catheter ablated or surgically divided.

TRANSPOSITION COMPLEXES

The term *transposition* identifies a group of malformations that have in common an abnormal relation between the cardiac chambers and great arteries. In this chapter the term is used to include both anomalous insertion of the pulmonary veins and cardiac malpositions.

Complete Transposition of the Great Arteries

MORPHOLOGY. This is a common and potentially lethal form of heart disease in newborns and infants.[525] The malformation consists of the origin of the aorta arising from the morphological right ventricle and that of the pulmonary artery from the morphological left ventricle. With rare exceptions there is no fibrous continuity between the aortic and mitral valves. The origin of the aorta usually is to the right and anterior to, but may be lateral to, the main pulmonary artery. Thus, dextro- or D-transposition is a term often used interchangeably with complete transposition. In other classifications the anomaly is described as concordant atrioventricular and discordant ventriculoarterial connections. The embryogenesis of complete transposition of the great arteries is controversial. There is consensus that the ventricular origins of the great arteries are reversed after development of a straight rather than a spiral infundibulotruncal septum. Transposition appears to result from a transfer of the pulmonary artery, instead of the aorta, from the heart tube's outlet zone to the left ventricle.[526] The latter may result from maldevelopment of the infundibulum, or a combination of both infundibulum maldevelopment and truncal malseptation; the former results if the subpulmonary, rather than the subaortic, infundibulum is absorbed.

The anatomical arrangement results in two separate and parallel circulations. Some communication between the two circulations must exist after birth to sustain life; otherwise, unoxygenated systemic venous blood is directed inappropriately to the systemic circulation and oxygenated pulmonary venous blood is directed to the pulmonary circulation. Almost all patients have an interatrial communication (Fig. 29–58). Two-thirds have a patent ductus arteriosus, and about one-third have an associated ventricular septal defect. Complete transposition occurs more frequently in the offspring of diabetic mothers and more often in males than in females. Without treatment, about 30 per cent of these infants die within the first week of life, 50 per cent within the first month, 70 per cent within 6 months, and 90 per cent within the first year.[525] Those who live beyond infancy have, as a general rule, either an isolated large atrial septal defect or a single ventricle, or ventricular septal defect and pulmonic stenosis. Current aggressive medical and surgical approaches to this group of patients have transformed the prognosis for an infant with this malformation from hopeless to very good.

HEMODYNAMICS. The *clinical course* is determined by the degree of tissue hypoxia, the ability of each ventricle to sustain an increased workload in the presence of reduced coronary arterial oxygenation, the nature of the associated cardiovascular anomalies, and the anatomical and functional status of the pulmonary vascular bed.[525] A bidirec-

tional shunt is always present because continuous unidirectional shunting would result in a progressive depletion of the circulating volume in either the pulmonary or the systemic vascular bed.

A major determinant of the systemic arterial oxygen saturation is the amount of blood exchanged between the two circulations by intercirculatory shunts. The net volume of blood passing left to right from the pulmonary to the systemic circulation represents the anatomical left-to-right shunt and is in fact the effective systemic blood flow (i.e., the amount of oxygenated pulmonary venous return reaching the systemic capillary bed). Conversely, the volume of blood passing right to left from the systemic to the pulmonary circulation constitutes the anatomical right-to-left shunt and is in fact the effective pulmonary blood flow (i.e., the net volume of unsaturated systemic venous return perfusing the pulmonary capillary bed).

The net volume exchange between the two circulations per unit time is equal. The magnitude of the intercirculatory mixing volume is modified by the number of intercirculatory communications that exist, the presence of associated obstructive intracardiac and extracardiac anomalies, the extent of the bronchopulmonary circulation, and the relation between pulmonary and systemic vascular resistance. For example, in the newborn with an intact ventricular septum and a constricted or closed patent ductus arteriosus, inadequate mixing through a small patent foramen ovale often is the cause of severe hypoxemia. If a large interatrial communication or a ventricular septal defect exists, systemic arterial oxygen saturation is influenced more importantly by the pulmonary–systemic blood flow relation than by the adequacy of mixing; augmented pulmonary blood flow produces a higher systemic arterial saturation if the left ventricle can sustain a high-output state without the intervention of congestive heart failure and pulmonary edema. The systemic arterial oxygen saturation is quite low, despite adequate intercirculatory mixing sites, if pulmonary blood flow is reduced by left ventricular outflow tract obstruction or increased pulmonary vascular resistance.

Pulmonary Vascular Changes. Infants with complete transposition of the great arteries are particularly susceptible to the early development of *pulmonary vascular obstructive disease*.[63,527] Moderately severe morphological alterations develop in the pulmonary vascular bed by the age of 6 to 12 months in many infants and by 2 years in almost all patients with an associated large ventricular septal defect or large patent ductus arteriosus in the absence of obstruction to left ventricular outflow. Advanced pulmonary vascular disease also is seen within this same time frame in 15 to 30 per cent of patients without a patent ductus arteriosus and with an intact ventricular septum. Systemic arterial hypoxemia, increased pulmonary blood flow, and pulmonary hypertension contribute to the development of pulmonary vascular obstruction in these patients as they do in other forms of congenital heart disease. Among the additional factors implicated in the accelerated and more widespread pulmonary vascular obstruction found in patients with complete transposition is the presence of extensive bronchopulmonary anastomotic channels, which enter the pulmonary vascular bed proximal to the pulmonary capillary bed; thus, oxygen tension is reduced at the precapillary level, causing pulmonary vasoconstriction.[528]

Beyond the early neonatal period many patients have an abnormal distribution pattern of pulmonary blood flow, with preferential flow to the right lung.[529] The asymmetrical distribution of pulmonary blood flow in these individuals results from an abnormal rightward inclination of the main pulmonary artery in the transposition malformation that favors flow from the main to the right pulmonary artery. Persistently increased pulmonary blood flow to the right lung would be expected to contribute to pulmonary

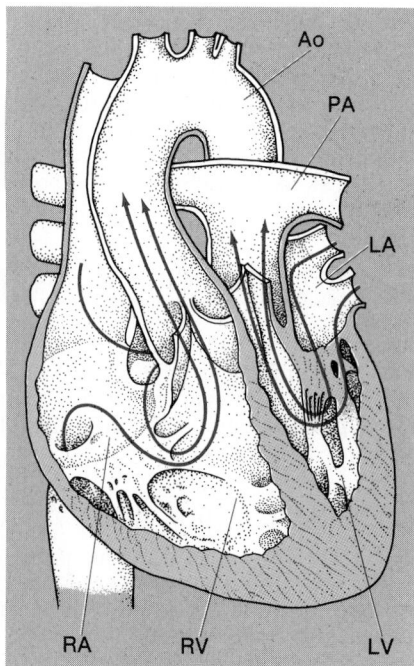

FIGURE 29–58. Complete transposition of the great arteries. Intercirculatory mixing occurs only at the atrial level. RA = right atrium, LA = left atrium, RV = right ventricle, LV = left ventricle, Ao = aorta, PA = pulmonary artery.

vascular obstructive changes within the lung; in the left pulmonary vascular bed, thrombotic changes may occur because of the combination of reduced flow and polycythemia. Finally, it should be recognized that a prenatal alteration in pulmonary vascular smooth muscle may exist because blood perfusing the fetal lungs in complete transposition of great arteries has a higher than normal pO_2 and may serve to dilate pulmonary vessels in utero. Postnatally such vessels may have an enhanced capacity to constrict in response to vasoactive stimuli and suffer anatomical, obliterative changes.

CLINICAL FINDINGS. Average birthweight and size of infants born with complete transposition of the great arteries are greater than normal. The usual clinical manifestations are dyspnea and cyanosis from birth, progessive hypoxemia, and congestive heart failure. Early in postnatal life the clinical manifestations and course are influenced principally by the magnitude of intercirculatory mixing. The most severe cyanosis and hypoxemia are observed in infants with only a small patent foramen ovale or ductus arteriosus and an intact ventricular septum in whom mixing is inadequate, or in those infants with relatively reduced pulmonary blood flow because of left ventricular outflow tract obstruction.[530] With a large persistent patent ductus arteriosus or a large ventricular septal defect, cyanosis may be minimal and heart failure is the usual dominant problem after the first few weeks of life.[525] It should be recognized that a patent ductus arteriosus is present in about half of newborn infants with transposition, although it closes functionally and anatomically soon after birth in almost all cases. If the ductus arteriosus remains open, better mixing of the venous and arterial circulations usually is at the expense of pulmonary artery hypertension.[531]

Cardiac murmurs are of little diagnostic significance and are absent or insignificant in about 30 to 50 per cent of infants with complete transposition of the great arteries and an intact ventricular septum. In infants with a large persistent patent ductus arteriosus, fewer than half exhibit physical signs typical of ductus arteriosus, such as continuous murmur, bounding pulses, or a prominent mid-diastolic rumble. Moreover, *differential cyanosis* caused by reversed pulmonary-to-systemic shunting across the ductus arteriosus is difficult to detect because of generalized arterial desaturation. In those infants with a large ventricular septal defect, a pansystolic murmur usually emerges within the first 7 to 10 days of life. In newborns with transposition and severe pulmonic stenosis or atresia, the clinical findings are similar to those in the infant with tetralogy of Fallot.

ELECTROCARDIOGRAPHY AND ROENTGENOGRAPHY. The most usual *electrocardiographic findings* include right-axis deviation, right atrial enlargement, and right ventricular hypertrophy, reflecting that the right ventricle is the systemic pumping chamber. Combined ventricular hypertrophy may be present in those patients with a large ventricular septal defect and elevated pulmonary blood flow. Isolated left ventricular hypertrophy is encountered rarely in patients with a ventricular septal defect and a hypoplastic right ventricle, in many of whom the tricuspid valve is displaced abnormally and straddles a ventricular septal defect. In the first days of life the chest radiogram may appear normal, particularly in infants with an intact ventricular septum. Thereafter, roentgenographic findings often are highly suggestive of the diagnosis,[532] and consist of (1) progressive cardiac enlargement in early infancy; (2) a characteristic oval or egg-shaped cardiac configuration in the anteroposterior view, and a narrow vascular pedicle created by superimposition of the aortic and pulmonary artery segments; and (3) increased pulmonary vascular markings (Fig. 29–59). A right aortic arch is seen in about 4 per cent of infants with an intact ventricular septum and 11 per cent of infants with a ventricular septal defect.

CT scanning (see p. 342) and MR imaging (Fig.

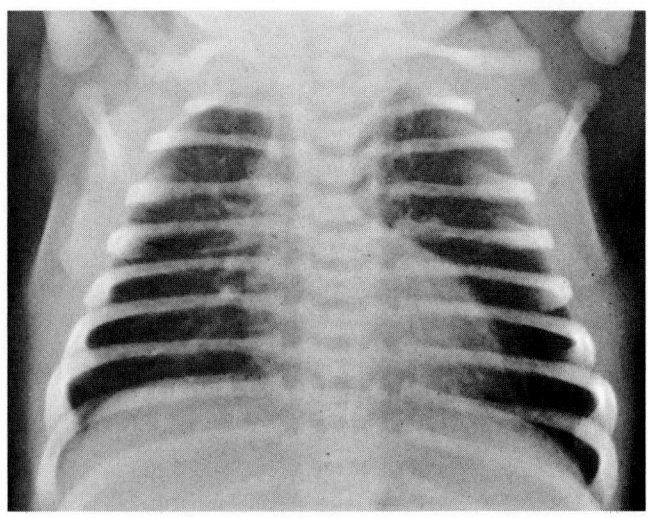

FIGURE 29–59. Chest roentgenogram in a 4-day-old infant with complete transposition of the great arteries showing an oval-shaped heart with a narrow base and increased pulmonary vascular markings.

10–20, p. 327) are also capable of establishing the diagnosis.

ECHOCARDIOGRAPHY. Two-dimensional echocardiography is the procedure of choice in the diagnosis of complete transposition of the great arteries and the detection of significant associated cardiac anomalies[533–535] (Figs. 29–60 and 29–61). In sagittal cross sections the aorta is observed to ascend retrosternally, in contrast to the normal posterior sweep of the pulmonary artery. With transverse short-axis cross-sectional imaging, the diagnosis is confirmed by demonstrating that the anterior great artery (the aorta) is to the right of the posterior great artery (pulmonary) or that the two arteries are visualized side by side (Fig. 29–60). Moreover, from subcostal views (Fig. 29–61) the course of the two great arteries may be traced to delineate their ventricle of origin, demonstrating that the anterior rightward vessel (aorta) originates from the right ventricle and the posterior leftward vessel (pulmonary artery) originates from the left ventricle (Fig. 29–61). Echocardiography also may assist in identifying associated defects. Ventricular septal defects may be localized to the membranous, atrioventricular, and trabecular muscular septa, and malalignment types of ventricular septal defects may be identified if the infundibular septum is shifted either anteriorly or posteriorly.[536] A subaortic obstruction may be created by anterior shifting of the infundibular septum, whereas a posterior shift may narrow the subpulmonary area. The nature of left ventricular outflow tract obstruction may be further identified as a fixed obstruction caused by a fibromuscular ridge or as a dynamic obstruction caused by deviation of the interventricular septum toward the left ventricular cavity and the apposition between a thickened interventricular septum and systolic anterior motion of the mitral valve.

Ultrasound imaging may also be used to guide catheter placement and manipulation during balloon atrial septostomy and to assess the anatomical adequacy of the septostomy.

CARDIAC CATHETERIZATION AND ANGIOCARDIOGRAPHY. The major abnormal hemodynamic findings include right ventricular pressure at systemic levels and either a high or low left ventricular pressure, depending on pulmonary blood flow, pulmonary vascular resistance, and the presence or absence of left ventricular outflow tract obstructive lesions. Oxygen saturation in the aorta is lower than that in the pulmonary artery. Application of the Fick principle to the calculation of pulmonary and systemic blood flow rates in these patients is an important source of error. Assumed values of oxygen consumption are unreliable in the severely hypoxemic infant. Moreover, because systemic and

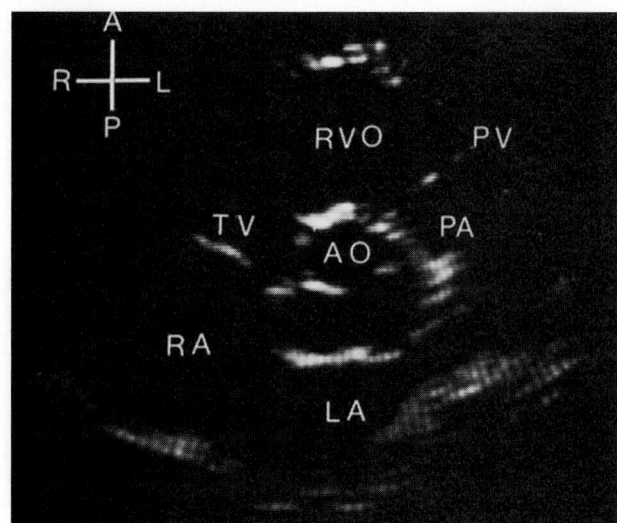

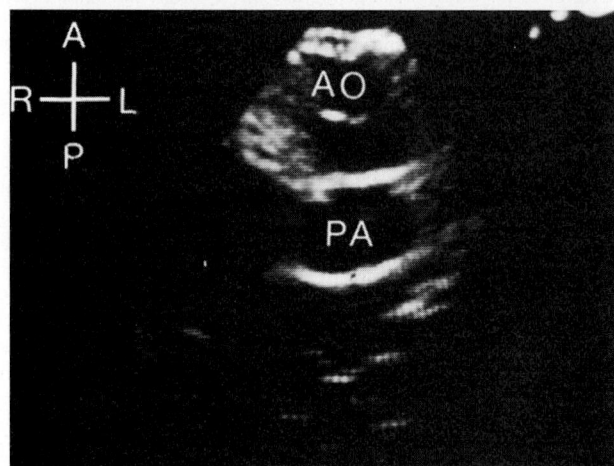

FIGURE 29–60. *Top,* A two-dimensional echocardiographic short-axis scan demonstrates normal great artery relations. The right ventricular outflow tract (RVO) wraps around the aorta (AO) in a clockwise manner. The pulmonic valve (PV) is to the left of the aortic valve. *Bottom,* Short-axis scan shows the abnormal great artery relations in an infant with transposition of the great arteries. The aorta (AO) is directly anterior and slightly to the right of the pulmonary artery (PA). The clockwise partial encirclement of the aorta by the right ventricular outflow tract is no longer observed. A = anterior, L = left, P = posterior, R = right, LA = left atrium, RA = right atrium, TV = tricuspid valve.

particularly pulmonary arteriovenous oxygen differences may be quite reduced, small errors in oxygen saturation values result in large errors in flow calculations. Furthermore, because bronchial collaterals enter the pulmonary circuit at the precapillary level, a true mixed pulmonary artery saturation cannot be sampled; pulmonary blood flow is therefore overestimated when one uses a sample from the central pulmonary artery, and pulmonary vascular resistance values often are underestimated.

Infants with simple, complete transposition of the great arteries who present in the first few weeks of life to a center prepared to correct the anomaly by the arterial switch operation (see below) often are taken to the operating room shortly after two-dimensional echocardiography and Doppler examination are performed.[535] In these cases, transcatheter balloon atrial septostomy is not performed unless a delay is expected in taking the patient to the operating room. In essentially all other patients, cardiac catheterization and balloon septostomy are components of the initial approach to the patient.

The diagnostic portion of the cardiac catheterization allows confirmation of the anatomical derangement of the great arteries and establishes the presence of associated le-sions; in the newborn, unless prompt arterial switch repair is planned, it should always be accompanied by a palliative balloon atrial septostomy, which serves to enlarge the interatrial communication and improve oxygenation. In the older neonate, usually beyond age 3 weeks, thickening of the atrial septum may preclude satisfactory balloon septostomy. In those instances, transcatheter blade septostomy is the preferred approach to palliation. Two-dimensional echocardiography, with or without fluoroscopy, may be used as the imaging mode for both balloon and blade creation of an atrial septal defect.[536] Subcostal four-chamber and sagittal views image cardiac anatomy and catheter position during the procedure, substantially reducing radiation dosage.[537]

Both the diagnostic and the palliative procedures can be performed by percutaneous entry into the femoral vein, umbilical vein catheterization, or direct cutdown into the femoral or saphenous vein. The catheter passes easily across the foramen ovale into the left atrium and left ventricle and may be manipulated into the pulmonary artery by means of a flow-directed balloon-guided catheter or by manipulation of a standard catheter bent in the form of a J loop within the left ventricle, with the tip pointed posteriorly to the pulmonary artery. When a large ventricular septal defect is present, the catheter often can be manipulated directly across it from the right ventricle into the pulmonary artery.[538]

Selective Ventricular Angiography. This is diagnostic and demonstrates that the anteriorly placed aorta arises from the right ventricle and that the posteriorly placed pulmonary artery in continuity with the mitral valve arises from the left ventricle. The status of the ductus arteriosus and the site and size of a ventricular septal defect can be well visualized by angiography. Interventricular defects posterior and inferior to the crista supraventricularis occur in about half of these patients; less often the defects are anterior and superior to the crista supraventricularis or are of the atrioventricular septal type.[539] A variety of lesions may be identified as the cause of left ventricular outflow tract obstruction, including ventricular septal hypertrophy with systolic anterior movement of the mitral valve, discrete or tunnel fibromuscular subpulmonic stenosis, valvular and supravalvular stenosis, and, rarely, an aneurysm of the membranous ventricular septum or redundant tricuspid valve tissue protruding through a ventricular septal defect.

Both angiographic and echocardiographic imaging may be required to detect the coronary arterial patterns that are seen in patients with complete transposition of the great arteries.[540–542a] In the majority, the left coronary artery originates in the left sinus and the right coronary artery originates in the posterior sinus, with a single ostium above both the left and the posterior sinus. In almost 20 per cent of patients the left circumflex artery arises as a branch of the right coronary artery; a single coronary artery is present in about 6 per cent; in 3 to 4 per cent of patients either the right coronary and anterior descending arteries originate in the left sinus, with the left circumflex originating in the posterior sinus, or two ostia are present above one sinus, one giving rise to the right and the other to the left coronary artery. To avoid the danger of excision during transfer of the coronary arteries as part of the arterial switch corrective operation, the intramural course of the left coronary artery or the left anterior descending coronary artery should be identified, a finding in up to 5 per cent of patients. An intramural course should be assumed when the vessel has an aberrant origin from the right sinus or when it is in intimate relationship with the commissure between the right and left sinuses and courses between the great arteries.[542]

MANAGEMENT. Medical treatment often is of limited help but should be vigorous because both functional and anatomical corrections of the malformation achieve good results. Conservative measures include the use of oxygen,

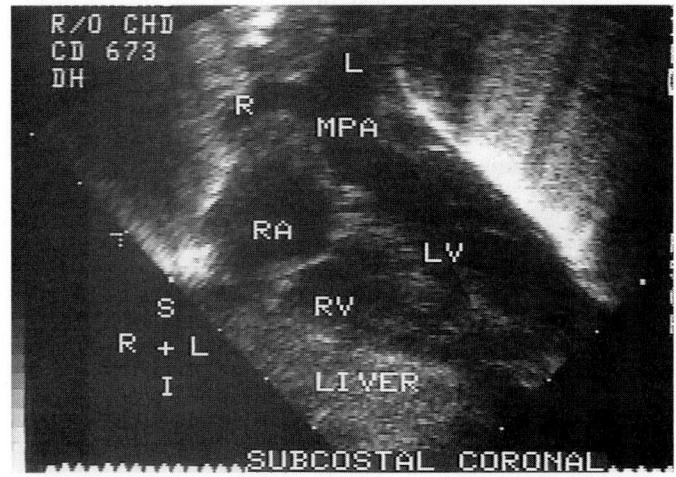

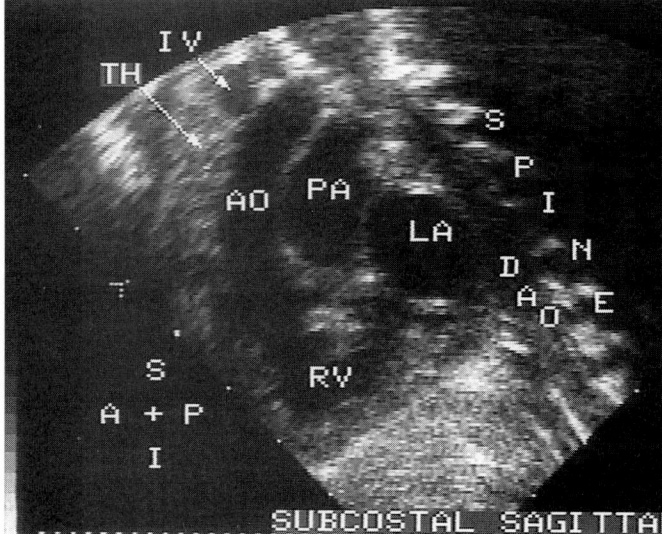

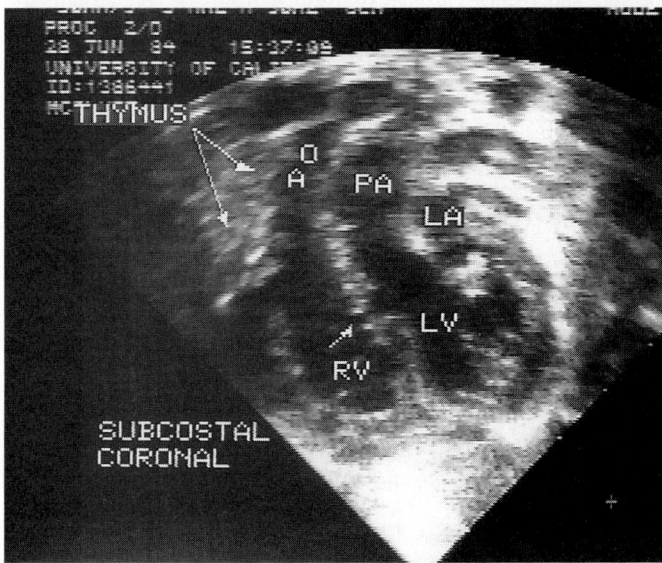

digitalis, diuretics, iron (if an associated iron-deficiency anemia is present), and intravenous sodium bicarbonate for severe hypoxemic metabolic acidosis. Dilatation of the ductus arteriosus by prostaglandin E_1 in the early neonatal period both augments pulmonary blood flow and enhances intercirculatory mixing.

Atrial Septostomy. The creation or enlargement of an interatrial communication is the simplest procedure for providing increased intracardiac mixing of systemic and pulmonary venous blood; preferably this is achieved by rupturing the valve of the foramen ovale by balloon catheter during transseptal catheterization of the left side of the heart (Rashkind's procedure), or by blade septostomy. Surgical atrial septectomy seldom is required. The balloon should be inflated to a diameter of about 15 mm before pullback to the right atrium. Salutary results consist of a fall in left atrial pressure, equalization of mean left and right atrial pressures, and an increase in the systemic arterial oxygen saturation. When the foramen ovale is stretched by the balloon without accomplishing rupture of the septum primum valve of the fossa ovalis, the improvement in oxygenation is short-lived. Infusion or reinfusion intravenously of prostaglandin E_1 (0.05 to 0.1 mg/kg/min) has been shown to improve systemic oxygenation temporarily in the latter situation, by dilating the ductus arteriosus and thereby facilitating intercirculatory mixing.[96] Although balloon atrial septostomy usually is successful in stabilizing the infant's condition and allowing survival in the neonatal period, the initial rise in systemic arterial oxen saturation to 65 to 75 per cent often is not sustained beyond 6 to 9 months of age.

SURGICAL TREATMENT

The development of *corrective operations* for infants born with transposition of the great arteries has greatly improved prognosis.[543,544]

ATRIAL (VENOUS) SWITCH OPERATION. This correction, by the *Mustard* technique, is accomplished by excision of the interatrial septum and creation of a new interatrial septum with a pericardial baffle diverting the systemic venous return into the left ventricle through the mitral valve and thence to the left ventricle and pulmonary artery, while the pulmonary venous blood is diverted through the tricuspid valve and right ventricle to the aorta.[545,545a] The *Senning* procedure is based on a similar principle and consists of diversion of left pulmonary venous blood by a coronary sinus flap and rerouting of caval flow by the use of an atrial wall flap.[546]

After physiological correction by atrial switch, postoperative complications are observed that are directly related to the intraatrial repair (shunts across the intraatrial patch and obstruction to either systemic or pulmonary venous return or both).[547–550] There is a high incidence of early and late postoperative dysrhythmias that are more likely to have their basis in injury to the sinoatrial node and/or its arterial supply than in disruption of internodal tracts or damage to the atrioventricular node.[551] Tricuspid regurgitation is a less common complication of operation and may be related in some patients to a preexisting abnormality of the tricuspid valve, whereas in most it is related to right ventricular dysfunction. Although the assessment of right ventricular contractility is difficult, the right ventricular pump function appears to be impaired before Mustard operation and does not return to normal after successful surgery.[552–554] It seems likely that the right ventricle can perform as a systemic pumping chamber for the duration of a normal life span.

ARTERIAL SWITCH OPERATION. A one-stage anatomical correction is now the approach of choice in major centers that care for infants with congenital heart disease.[555–557] In this operation both coronary arteries are transposed to the posterior artery; the aorta and pulmonary arteries are transsected, contraposed, and anastomosed (Jatene operation) (Fig. 29–62). The arterial switch anatomical correction may be complicated by coronary ostial stenosis, acquired supravalvular aortic and/or pulmonary stenosis, and pulmonic and/or aortic incompetence. The major advantages of the arterial switch procedure,

---

FIGURE 29–61. Composite subcostal views of transposition of the great arteries. *Top,* Subcostal coronal view showing the main pulmonary artery (MPA) arising directly from the left ventricle (LV) and dividing into the right (R) and left (L) pulmonary arteries. The right atrium (RA) and right ventricle (RV) lie adjacent in this view to the liver. *Middle,* The scan plane has been rotated 90 degrees clockwise (note the change in spatial orientation and the position of the spine). The thymus (TH) is seen anteriorly, and the innominate vein (IV) lies anterior to the aortic arch. The right ventricle (RV) lies anteriorly above the diaphragm and behind the thymus and gives rise to the aorta (AO), its arch, and the descending aorta (DAO). The main pulmonary artery (PA) lies in the crux of the aortic arch. *Bottom,* An intermediate subcostal view, lying oblique in a plane between the top two panels. The entire ventriculoarterial connection is imaged in this plane, showing the right ventricle connecting to the aortic arch, a small ventricular septal defect (VSD) indicated by the small arrow, and the pulmonary artery (PA) arising from the left ventricle (LV). The left atrium (LA) can be seen below the pulmonary artery. (Courtesy of Norman Silverman, M.D.)

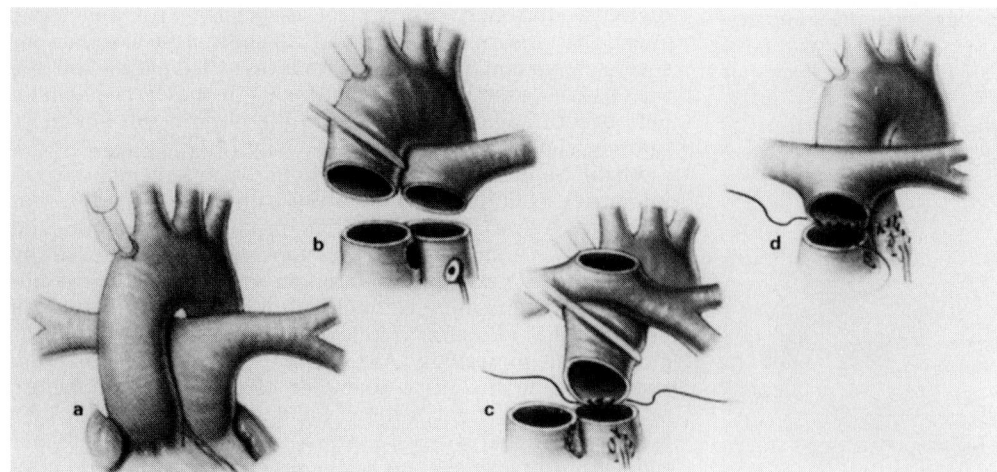

FIGURE 29–62. Complete transposition of the great arteries, corrected by a modified arterial switch operation. The aorta and pulmonary artery are transected and the orifices of the coronary arteries are excised with a rim of adjacent aortic wall (b). The aorta is brought under the bifurcation of the pulmonary artery, and the proximal pulmonary artery and the aorta are anastomosed without necessitating graft interposition. The coronary arteries are transferred to the pulmonary artery (c). The mobilized pulmonary artery is directly anastomosed to the proximal aortic stump (d). (From Stark, J., and DeLaval, M.: Surgery for Congenital Heart Defects. New York, Grune and Stratton, 1983, p. 379.)

when compared with the atrial switch procedure, are the restoration of the left ventricle as the systemic pump and the potential for long-term maintenance of sinus rhythm.[558–561]

Within the first month of life the arterial switch operation may be performed as a single-stage repair. In such patients, the origin and branching patterns of the coronary arteries are defined reliably preoperatively by two-dimensional echocardiography.[525] In older infants it appears necessary to prepare the left ventricle to withstand the systemic pressure that is produced after switching the great arteries because, if the ventricular septum is intact, left ventricular pressure and left ventricular wall thickness diminish normally in relation to the postnatal reduction in pulmonary artery pressure. In these infants a two-stage approach is used, the first of which consists of banding the pulmonary artery; the arterial switch is performed soon thereafter, in some centers as early as 1 to 2 weeks later.[562,563]

In the unusual infant with an intact ventricular septum and a significant patent ductus arteriosus, an early neonatal arterial switch corrective operation with closure of the ductus is indicated. The optimal management of patients with a large ventricular septal defect is a one-stage intraarterial switch anatomical correction as early in life as possible.

In some patients after early arterial repair of transposition of the great arteries, abnormally enlarged bronchial arteries are identified at postoperative catheterization and they explain continuous murmurs or persistent cardiomegaly. When these vessels are large enough to produce a volume load to the systemic ventricle, catheter-directed coil embolization is indicated.[564] Follow-up studies after the arterial switch operation have demonstrated good left ventricular function and normal exercise capacity. Potential sequelae of the operation include supravalvular pulmonary stenosis, which may be treated either by reoperation or balloon angioplasty, supravalvular aortic stenosis, and neo–aortic regurgitation, usually mild.[565,566] Long-term patency and growth of the coronary arteries appear satisfactory.[557–570] Infants with transposition of the great arteries plus a ventricular septal defect and left ventricular outflow tract obstruction may require a systemic–pulmonary artery anastomosis when a pronounced diminution in pulmonary blood flow exists. A later corrective procedure for these patients bypasses the left ventricular outflow obstruction and uses an intracardiac ventricular baffle connecting the left ventricle to the aorta and an extracardiac prosthetic conduit between the right ventricle and the distal end of a divided pulmonary artery (Rastelli procedure).[571] An alternative approach (the Lecompte procedure) couples an intraventricular tunnel and the arterial switch operation, avoiding the use of an extracardiac conduit.[572]

In patients with significant pulmonary vascular obstructive disease the risk associated with definitive repair (anatomical correction or intraatrial baffle and closure of the ventricular septal defect) is great. In this group of patients a "palliative" Mustard or Senning procedure leaving the ventricular septal defect open often provides good, short-term, symptomatic improvement by increasing arterial oxygen tension and reducing the stimulus to progressive polycythemia.[573]

Congenitally Corrected Transposition of the Great Arteries

This term is applied to two distinctly different anomalies: anatomically corrected transposition or malposition of the great arteries and physiologically corrected levo- or L-transposition of the great arteries.

MORPHOLOGY. Anatomically corrected malposition of the great arteries is a rare form of congenital heart disease in which the great arteries are abnormally related to each other and to the ventricles but arise, nonetheless, above the anatomically correct ventricles.[574,575]

Because of this, the term *malposition*, rather than *transposition*, is preferable. The anomaly results from either leftward looping of the ventricular segment of the embryonic heart tube in the situs solitus heart, or rightward looping in the situs inversus heart. In this unusual malformation the aorta is anterior and to the left (levo- or L-malposition) and the pulmonary artery is posteromedial and to the right, presumably because of a subaortic conus which causes mitral-aortic discontinuity.

When no other defect exists, the circulation proceeds normally. When an associated lesion prompts echocardiographic examination, the diagnosis is indicated by the finding of atrioventricular concordance in association with wide mitral-aortic discontinuity with an anteriorly placed aorta. At cardiac catheterization, the diagnosis of the abnormal relation between the great arteries may be made by biplane angiocardiography. Anomalies commonly associated with anatomically corrected malposition of the great arteries include ventricular septal defect, left juxtaposition of the atrial appendages, tricuspid atresia or stenosis, and valvular and subvalvular pulmonic stenosis.

DEFINITION. Invariably, the term *congenitally corrected transposition* is applied to the heart in which a functional correction of the circulation exists by virtue of the relation between the ventricles and great arteries.[576,577] Corrected or L-transposition occurs when the primitive cardiac tube loops to the left, instead of to the right, during embryogenesis. The anatomical right ventricle comes to lie on the left and receives oxygenated blood from the left atrium; this blood is ejected into an anteriorly placed, left-sided aorta. The anatomical left ventricle lies to the right and connects the right atrium to a posteriorly placed pulmonary artery. Thus, there are both ventriculoarterial and atrioventricular discordant connections, with ventricular inversion. This arrangement of the great arteries and ventricles (in contrast to the uncorrected, complete, or D-transposition) permits functional correction, so that systemic venous blood passes into the pulmonary trunk while arterialized pulmonary venous blood flows into the aorta. In the heart with congenitally corrected transposition, the venae cavae and coronary sinus drain into a right atrium that is normal in position and structure.

PHYSIOLOGY. Venous blood flows from the right atrium, designated as the "venous atrium," across an atrioventricular valve that has the structure of a normal mitral valve and into the right-sided "venous ventricle." The venous ventricle, however, has the morphological characteristics of a normal left ventricle; i.e., its interior lining is trabeculated, it has no crista supraventricularis, and the atrioventricular valve is in continuity with the posteriorly placed semilunar valve. It ejects blood into the pulmonary trunk, which arises posterior to the ascending aorta. Oxygenated blood returns from the lungs to the left atrium, which is normal in position and structure; from there it flows into the left-sided "arterial ventricle" across an atrioventricular valve that has the structure of a normal tricuspid valve. The interior lining of the arterial ventricle has the morphological characteristics of a normal right ventricle (i.e., it has coarse trabeculations and a crista supraventricularis), and the tricuspid atrioventricular valve is not in continuity with the anteriorly placed semilunar valve. The arterial ventricle ejects blood into the aorta, which arises anterior to the pulmonary trunk. In addition to inversion of the cardiac ventricles, there is inversion of the conduction system and coronary arteries. Commonly associated anatomical lesions include atrial and ventricular septal defects, often accompanied by valvular or subvalvular pulmonary stenosis; single ventricle with an outlet chamber with or without pulmonic stenosis; left atrioventricular valve regurgitation, usually because of an Ebstein's malformation of the left-sided tricuspid valve; and abnormalities of visceral and atrial situs.[578]

CLINICAL MANIFESTATIONS. The clinical presentation, course, and prognosis of patients with congenital functionally corrected transposition vary, depending on the nature and severity of the complicating intracardiac anomalies.[579,579a] Patients in whom corrected transposition exists as an isolated anomaly present no functional alterations and have no symptoms. Asymptomatic children with an increase in the size of the systemic ventricle, due to significant left-to-right shunting or tricuspid regurgitation, usually develop symptoms of systemic ventricular dysfunction by the third or fourth decade.[580]

The *physical findings* in congenitally corrected transposition are those of the associated lesions with two exceptions: (1) a single accentuated second heart sound usually is present in the second left intercostal space, representing closure of the aortic valve lying lateral and anterior to the pulmonic valve; and (2) there is a high incidence of cardiac dysrhythmias.

LABORATORY EXAMINATION. Because of the inversion of the heart's conduction system, the *electrocardiogram* may provide important clues in the diagnosis. An abnormal direction of initial (septal) depolarization from right to left causes leftward, anterior, and superior orientation of the initial QRS forces and reversal of the precordial Q-wave pattern (Q waves are present in the right precordial leads and absent in the left). In addition to inversion of the conduction system, the His bundle is elongated because of the greater distance between the atrioventricular node and the base of the ventricular septum.[581] The His bundle is located beneath the pulmonic valve in the position of mitral pulmonary continuity; thus, it is subject to significant excursions during mitral valve closure. This arrangement may be a causal factor in the arrhythmias and atrioventricular conduction disturbances commonly observed in these patients. First-degree atrioventricular (AV) block occurs in about 50 per cent, and complete AV block occurs in 10 to 15 per cent of patients. Other degrees of AV dissociation may be observed as well as paroxysmal supraventricular tachycardia and ventricular extrasystoles. In some patients, Kent bundle connections provide the anatomical substrate for preexcitation.[582]

Roentgenographic examination characteristically reveals absence of the normal pulmonary artery segment and a smooth convexity of the left supracardiac border produced by the displaced ascending aorta (Fig. 7–45, p. 233). The latter may be visualized by radionuclide scintillation scans of the central circulation. The main pulmonary trunk is medially displaced and absent from the cardiac silhouette; the right pulmonary hilus often is prominent and elevated compared with the left, producing a right-sided "waterfall" appearance.

Two-dimensional echocardiography seeks to identify the morphology of each ventricle by defining the characteristics of the inflow and outflow tracts and papillary and trabecular muscle morphology, ventricular shape, and great artery position.[583] By tracing the great arteries back to their ventricles of origin in subxiphoid and parasternal short-axis planes, one would find that the anterior leftward great artery (the aorta) arises from the left-sided ventricle and is not in continuity with the left-sided atrioventricular valve. The great arteries exit the heart in parallel fashion; the position, origin, and branching pattern of the great arteries are observed in subxiphoid and suprasternal views, while the anteroposterior and right-left positions of the great arteries can be seen from the parasternal short-axis view. Because the ventricular septum lies in the anteroposterior

plane parallel to the echo beam, it may not be visualized from a left parasternal view. In apical-basal or subxiphoid, four-chamber echocardiographic views, the right and left ventricular morphology and the inverted position of the atrioventricular valves may be ascertained correctly. The latter views also demonstrate the level of attachment of the atrioventricular valves and allow detection of inferior displacement of the left-sided tricuspid valve when Ebstein's anomaly coexists.

At *cardiac catheterization* the diagnosis should be suspected when the venous catheter enters a posterior and midline main pulmonary trunk. Retrograde arterial catheter passage establishes the typical position of the ascending aorta at the upper left cardiac border. Hemodynamic abnormalities depend on the lesions associated with corrected transposition. Selective *angiocardiography* allows visualization of the transposed great arteries and morphological differentiation of the two ventricles (Fig. 29–63). The ventricles usually lie side by side, with the ventricular septum oriented in an anteroposterior direction. Selective aortography demonstrates the inverted coronary arterial pattern that is invariably present in corrected transposition. The competence of the left atrioventricular valve may be determined by injection of contrast material into the arterial ventricle.[584] When a left-sided Ebstein's malformation exists, the leaflets are displaced distal to the true valve annulus. The level of the annulus may be determined by visualization of the circumflex branch of the left coronary artery, which courses posteriorly in the AV groove.

Specific problems have attended operative repair of the lesions associated with congenitally corrected transposition, owing primarily to the course of the atrioventricular conduction system and the coronary arterial pattern.[585-587] Intraoperative electrophysiological mapping of the course of the conduction system has been proposed to reduce, but not abolish, the risk of surgically induced heart block. The AV bundle is located anteriorly and in relation to the anterolateral quadrant of the pulmonary outflow tract. Thus, when a ventricular septal defect is present, the bundle usually is related to the anterior and superior margins of the defect and lies beneath the pulmonic valve. In corrected transposition, the coronary arteries have a course appropriate to their ventricles; i.e., the anterior descending and circumflex arteries supply the morphological left ventricle, and the right coronary artery supplies the morphological right ventricle. However, because the great arteries are transposed, the noncoronary sinus is the anterior sinus of the aortic valve.

The inversion of the coronary arterial system occasionally may limit and preclude an incision into the venous ventricle, thereby interfering with exposure of intracardiac defects in the usual manner. The disadvantage in approaching intracardiac anomalies using an incision in the morphological right ventricle is that this is the systemic ventricle. When significant pulmonary stenosis exists within a ventricular septal defect, a valved extracardiac conduit often is a required part of the surgical repair. Surgical risks are especially high in patients in whom significant regurgitation exists from the arterial ventricle to the arterial atrium. In these patients, annuloplasty, or more usually valve replacement, is required. In all operative approaches, if complete heart block has been present intermittently or permanently preoperatively or intraoperatively, permanent epicardial atrial and ventricular pacemaker leads are implanted.

Double-Outlet Right Ventricle

MORPHOLOGY. Other designations applied to this lesion include origin of both great arteries from the right ventricle, partial transposition, complete transposition of the aorta and levo-position of the pulmonary artery, complete dextroposition of the aorta, and the Taussig-Bing complex. This is an extremely heterogeneous category of malformations in which an abnormal relation exists between the aorta and the pulmonary trunk, which arise wholly or in large part from the right ventricle.[588]

DEFINITIONS. A uniform definition or classification of double-outlet right ventricle does not exist. To some, double-outlet right ventricle means origin of one great artery and at least 50 per cent of the other over the right ventricle; others require the presence of bilateral conus muscle between both great arteries and the atrioventricular annulus. One or both great arteries may arise from an infundibular chamber; there may be considerable variability in the amount of subarterial conus muscle. Thus, the semilunar valves may lie side by side, or with the pulmonary valve more anterior and superior, or with a more anterior and superior aortic valve. Commonly, neither semilunar valve is in fibrous continuity with either atrioventricular valve, and usually a ventricular septal defect is present and represents the

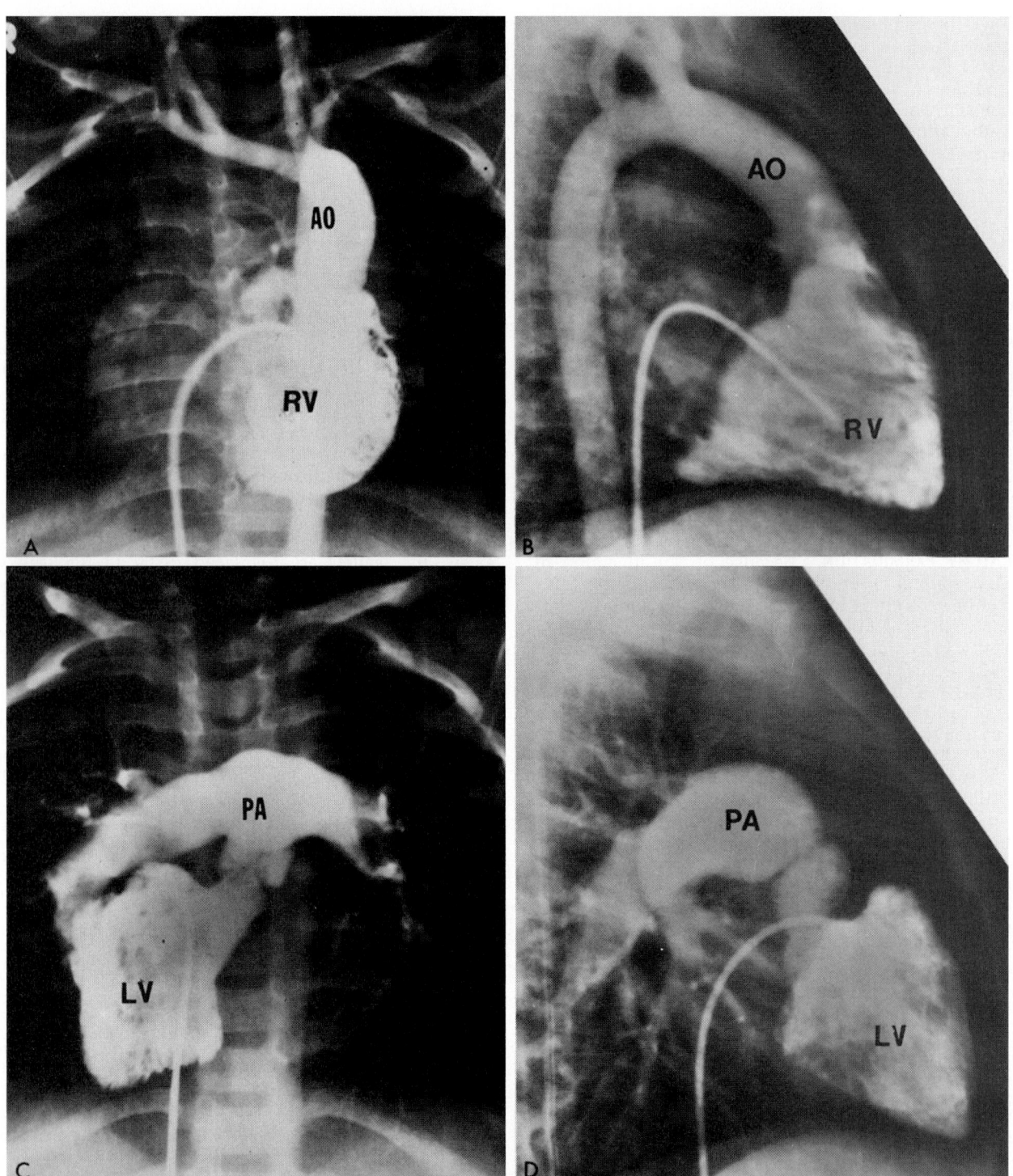

FIGURE 29–63. Congenitally corrected (levo-)transposition of the great arteries in a 4-year-old boy. *A,* Antero-posterior ventriculogram in left-sided ventricle with mesocardia. The morphological right ventricle (RV) is left-sided, indicating an L-ventricular loop (inverted ventricles in *situs solitus*). The aorta (AO) originates above the morphological right ventricle and is thus transposed and in classic levo-transposition. *B,* Lateral ventriculo-gram in left-sided ventricle (same frame as *A*). The aorta originates anteriorly above the morphological right ventricle (RV). *C,* Anteroposterior ventriculogram in right-sided morphological left ventricle (LV). The trans-posed pulmonary artery (PA) arises from this ventricle, and the ventricular septum appears intact. Pulmonic valve thickening is also evident. The aorta (A) is to the left of the pulmonary artery. Note that the ventricular septum in the L-ventricular loop is visualized best in the anteroposterior views. *D,* Lateral ventriculogram in right-sided ventricle (same frame as *C*). The pulmonary artery is posterior to the aorta, and supravalvular pulmonic narrowing is seen. (Reproduced with permission from Freedom, R. M., et al.: The differential diagnosis of levo-transposed or malposed aorta. An angiocardiographic study. *Circulation 50*:1040, 1974. Copyright 1974 the American Heart Association.)

only outlet from the left ventricle. The ventricular septal defect is of the malalignment type because the infundibular septum is positioned abnormally.

When the amount of conus muscle beneath the two great arteries varies, the ventricular septal defect commonly is positioned beneath the more posterior semilunar valve, which in fact usually overrides

the interventricular septum through this ventricular septal defect. The amount of conus muscle underneath the valve determines the position of the semilunar root in relation to the ventricles below. Thus double-outlet right ventricle resides within the spectrum of conotruncal abnormalities ranging from tetralogy of Fallot to trans-position of the great arteries. The ventricular septal defect occasion-

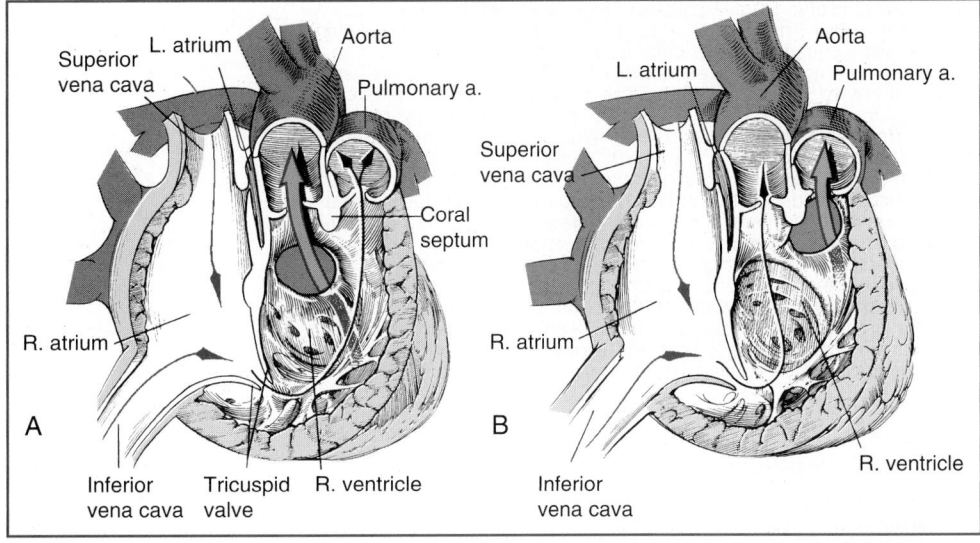

FIGURE 29–64. Double-outlet right ventricle (RV) with side-by-side relation of great arteries is illustrated in both panels. A subaortic ventricular septal defect (VSD) below the crista supraventricularis *(left)* favors delivery of left ventricular blood to the aorta *(A)*. Subpulmonary location of the VSD above the crista *(right)* favors streaming to the pulmonary trunk *(B)*. (From Castaneda, A., et al.: Cardiac Surgery of the Neonate and Infant. Philadelphia, W.B. Saunders Company, 1994, p. 446.)

ally extends beneath both great arteries and is referred to as doubly committed. In some instances, the ventricular septal defect is remote to both great arteries, or is considered uncommitted, in which case the defect often lies in the inlet or muscular portion of the interventricular septum.

ASSOCIATED LESIONS. More than half of patients with double-outlet right ventricle have associated anomalies of the right atrioventricular valves.[588] Mitral atresia associated with a hypoplastic left ventricle is common; less often observed are tricuspid stenosis, Ebstein's anomaly of the tricuspid valve, complete atrioventricular septal defect, and overriding or straddling of either atrioventricular valve. Aortic coarctation may be associated with double-outlet right ventricle, particularly when the subaortic area is narrowed by malalignment of the infundibular septum. Double-outlet right ventricle also may be a component of the multiple cardiovascular anomalies of the splenic dysgenesis or heterotaxy syndromes. An increased incidence of the anomaly occurs in infants with the trisomy 18 syndrome.

The pathological features in most patients include side-by-side pulmonic and aortic valves and discontinuity between the mitral and aortic valves. The latter exists because muscular infundibulum is usual beneath both semilunar valves. The ventricular septal defect may be remote from or closely related to one or both semilunar valves (Fig. 29–64).[588] When the interventricular defect is subpulmonic, with or without a straddling pulmonary trunk, the complex is designated "Taussig-Bing." In most patients the interventricular septal defect is below the crista supraventricularis and is subaortic in location. Least often the defect either is remote from both semilunar valves ("uncommitted") or underlies both ("doubly committed").

CLINICAL MANIFESTATIONS. The clinical and physiological picture is determined by the size and location of the ventricular septal defect and the presence or absence of pulmonic stenosis. In the Taussig-Bing form of double-outlet right ventricle, the malformation resembles physiologically and clinically complete transposition with ventricular septal defect and pulmonary hypertension. When the ventricular septal defect is subaortic, the stream of blood from the left ventricle is directed preferentially to the aorta. Thus, there may be little or no detectable cyanosis, and these patients usually clinically resemble those with an isolated, large ventricular septal defect and pulmonary hypertension.

The most important determinant of the natural history in both these types of double-outlet right ventricle is the progression of pulmonary vascular obstruction. In contrast, when there is pulmonary outflow tract obstruction, which often is severe and found commonly in these patients in whom the ventricular septal defect is subaortic, clinical findings are similar to those of cyanotic tetralogy of Fallot. In some patients, especially without pulmonic stenosis, the electrocardiogram shows a superiorly oriented counterclockwise frontal plane QRS loop in addition to right ventricular hypertrophy.[589] The pattern appears to result from relative hypoplasia of the antero-superior left bundle and preferential activation of the posteroinferior left ventricular wall. The presence of the latter electrocardiographic pattern in patients with double-outlet right ventricle should raise the possibility of a coexistent atrioventricular septal defect or abnormality of the mitral valve.

DIAGNOSIS. Two-dimensional *echocardiography* may reliably distinguish double-outlet right ventricle from other lesions causing cyanosis, such as tetralogy of Fallot and transposition of the great arteries.[590] The three key imaging features are origin of both great arteries from the anterior right ventricle, mitral-semilunar valve discontinuity, and absence of left ventricular outflow other than the ventricular septal defect. The relative anteroposterior positions of the great arteries can be determined from the parasternal short-axis view. The parasternal long-axis view shows the position of the more posterior semilunar root relative to the interventricular septum and

anterior mitral leaflet and is the best view for demonstrating the presence of subarterial conus muscle. Subxiphoid views best demonstrate the position of both great arteries over the ventricles. Each great artery is displayed on long- and short-axis subxiphoid sweeps.

In reporting echocardiographic results, it is imperative to state each component's anatomical feature, i.e., the position of both great arteries, the presence and amount of infundibulum under each semilunar valve, the anatomy of both subpulmonary and subaortic outflow tracts, the position and size of the associated ventricular septal defect, and the presence of all other associated lesions, particularly atrioventricular valve anomalies and coarctation of the aorta.

In each of the different types of double-outlet right ventricle, precise delineation of the malformation also depends on careful angiocardiographic analysis. The diagnosis can be established with confidence when the angiographic findings include simultaneous opacification of both great vessels from the right ventricle, aortic and pulmonic valves at the same transverse level, and separation of the aortic valve from the aortic leaflet of the mitral valve by the crista supraventricularis (Fig. 29–65).[591] The position of the ventricular septal defect and the relation between the great arteries must be defined to plan surgical procedures appropriately.

Experience is growing with the application of transesophageal echocardiography in analyzing the complex anatomical and spatial relationships encountered in double-outlet right ventricle, requiring a biplane or multiplane format for adequate assessment.

SURGICAL TREATMENT. The goals of operative treatment are to establish left ventricle-to-aorta continuity, create adequate right ventricle–to-pulmonary continuity and repair associated lesions.[592] Because of the complexity of intracardiac repair of these anomalies,

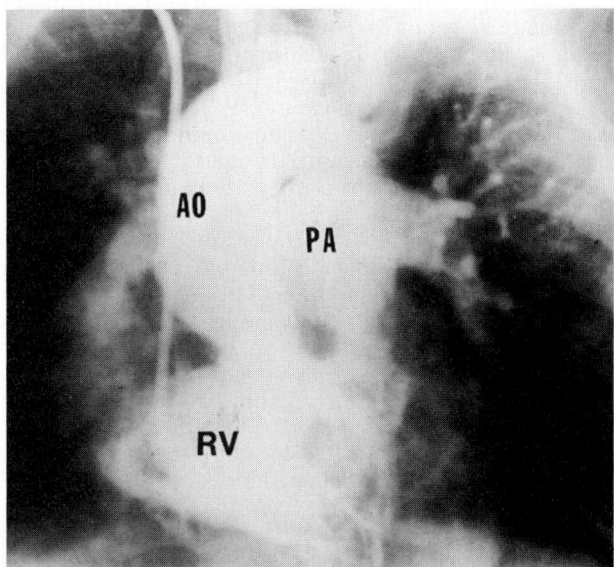

FIGURE 29–65. Simultaneous opacification of both great arteries from a right ventricular injection of contrast material in a patient with double-outlet right ventricle (RV). The aortic and pulmonic valves are at the same transverse level. AO = aorta, PA = pulmonary artery. (Courtesy of Robert White, M.D.)

many centers prefer to give palliation to infants, attempting reparative surgery after the age of 1 to 2 years. In double-outlet right ventricle with subaortic ventricular septal defect, repair is accomplished by creating an intraventricular baffle that conducts left ventricular blood to the aorta. When the ventricular septal defect is subpulmonic, repair is accomplished by closure of the ventricular septal defect and arterial switch.[592,593] When the ventricular septal defect is doubly committed, i.e., both subaortic and subpulmonic, operation consists of creating an intraventricular baffle that conducts left ventricular blood to the aorta. The type of double-outlet right ventricle in which the ventricular septal defect is remote and uncommitted to either semilunar orifice may be approached by a venous switch operation, permitting the right ventricle to eject into the aorta, followed by placement of a conduit between the left ventricle and the pulmonary trunk. Alternatively, some patients may be candidates for a modified Fontan procedure (see p. 933), particularly if additional findings include a common atrioventricular orifice, hypoplastic ventricles, a straddling tricuspid valve, or a straddling mitral valve.[594]

Double-Outlet Left Ventricle

One of the rarest cardiac anomalies consists of the origin of both great arteries from the morphological left ventricle. Conal musculature or an infundibulum usually is absent or deficient beneath the orifices of both semilunar valves.[595] A broad spectrum of associated malformations exists. A ventricular septal defect and valvular or subvalvular pulmonic stenosis have been present in most patients. Supportive diagnostic information is provided by magnetic resonance imaging.[596] Echocardiographic[597] and angiocardiographic assessment of the spatial relations of the origins of the great arteries is essential to an accurate diagnosis and to evaluating the possibility of operative repair. In most patients, the latter consists of closure of the ventricular septal defect and placement of a right ventricle–pulmonary artery conduit.

Total Anomalous Pulmonary Venous Connection

This anomaly has been estimated to account for 1 to 3 per cent of all cases of congenital heart disease and 2 per cent of deaths therefrom in the first year of life.[403,598] The anomaly is the result of persistence during embryogenesis of communications between the pulmonary portion of the foregut plexus and the cardinal or umbilicovitelline system of veins, resulting in the connection of all the pulmonary veins either to the right atrium directly or to the systemic veins and their tributaries. Because all venous blood returns to the right atrium, an interatrial communication is an integral part of this malformation. Additional major cardiac malformations occur in about 30 per cent of patients.[598] Among these are common atrium, single ventricle, truncus arteriosus, and anomalies of the systemic veins. Extracardiac malformations, particularly of the alimentary, endocrine, and genitourinary systems, are present in 25 to 30 per cent of cases.

MORPHOLOGY. The anatomical varieties of total anomalous pulmonary venous connection may be subdivided, depending on the level of the abnormal drainage (Fig. 29–66). Table 29–10 provides average figures of the distribution of the sites of anomalous connection.[403] The anomalous connection usually is supradiaphragmatic and to the left brachiocephalic vein, right atrium, coronary sinus, or superior vena cava. In about 13 per cent, particularly in males, the distal site of connection is below the diaphragm. In this situation a common trunk originates from the confluence of pulmonary veins and descends in front of the esophagus, penetrating the diaphragm through the esophageal hiatus. The anomalous trunk then connects into the portal vein or one of its tributaries, the ductus venosus, or, rarely, to one of the hepatic veins. In rare cases various combinations of anomalous connection occur in which drainage is to multiple levels.

HEMODYNAMICS. The physiological consequences and, accordingly, the clinical picture depend on the size of the interatrial communication and on the magnitude of the pulmonary vascular resistance. When the interatrial communication is small, systemic blood flow is markedly limited.[599] Right atrial and systemic venous pressures are elevated, and hepatic enlargement and peripheral edema are present. The size of the interatrial communication also is an important determinant in the development in utero and postnatally of the left atrium and left ventricle. Left atrial

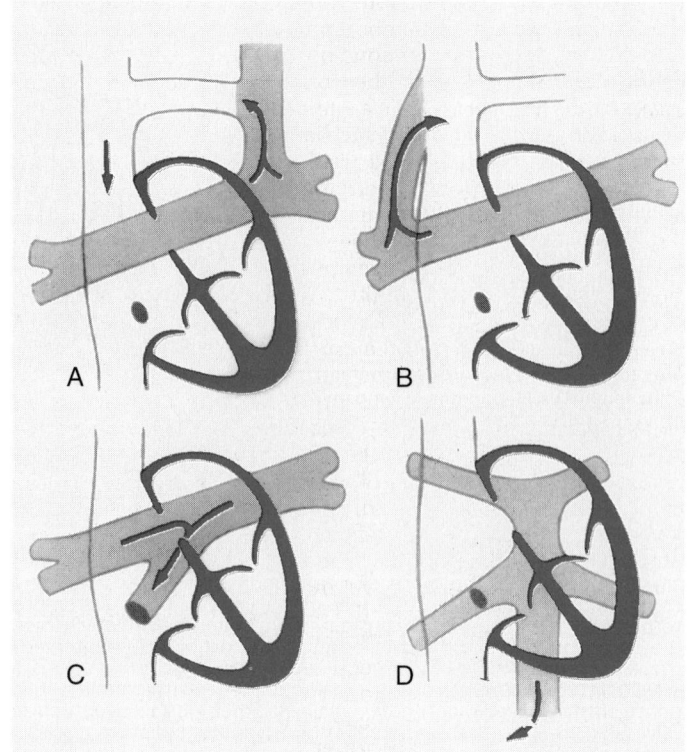

FIGURE 29–66. Anatomical types of total anomalous pulmonary venous return. Supracardiac, in which the pulmonary veins drain either via the vertical vein to the anomalous vein *(A)* or directly to the superior vena cava with the orifice close to the orifice of the azygos vein *(B)*. *C* shows drainage directly into the right atrium or into the coronary sinus. *D* shows infracardiac drainage via a vertical vein into the portal vein or the inferior vena cava. (From Stark, J., and DeLeval, M.: Surgery for Congenital Heart Defects. 2nd ed. Philadelphia, W.B. Saunders Company, 1994, p. 330.)

cavity size usually is somewhat reduced, whereas left ventricular volumes may be reduced or normal. The magnitude of pulmonary blood flow and therefore the ratio of oxygenated to unoxygenated blood that returns to the right atrium are a function of pulmonary vascular resistance. The arterial oxygen saturation, which ranges from markedly reduced to normal values, is inversely related to the pulmonary vascular resistance. In this regard, in most patients the principal determinant of pulmonary pressures and resistance is related less to augmented pulmonary blood flow and pulmonary arteriolar vascular obstruction than to the presence and intensity of pulmonary venous obstruction.[600–602]

Obstruction to pulmonary venous return and pulmonary venous hypertension are invariably present in patients with

TABLE 29–10   SITE OF CONNECTION IN TOTAL ANOMALOUS PULMONARY VENOUS CONNECTION

1. **Connection to right atrium**	15%
2. **Connection to common cardinal system**	
a. (Right) superior vena cava	11%
b. Azygos vein	1%
3. **Connection to left common cardinal system**	
a. Left innominate vein	36%
b. Coronary sinus	16%
4. **Connection to umbilicovitelline system**	
a. Portal vein	6%
b. Ductus venosus	4%
c. Inferior vena cava	2%
d. Hepatic vein	1%
5. **Multiple sites**	7%
6. **Unknown**	1%

infradiaphragmatic anomalous pulmonary venous connection and in many with a subdiaphragmatic pathway. In the former type, pulmonary venous obstruction results from the length and narrowness of the common pulmonary venous trunk, compression at the esophageal hiatus of the diaphragm, constriction at the subdiaphragmatic site of insertion, or pulmonary venous return that must pass first through the portal-hepatic circulation before returning to the right atrium. When venous obstruction occurs in supradiaphragmatic types of drainage, constriction may exist at the entrance site of the anomalous veins into the systemic venous circulation, and/or the anomalous venous channel may be kinked or situated abnormally and compressed between the left pulmonary artery and left bronchus.[602,603] The presence of a small, restrictive patent foramen ovale occasionally results in pulmonary venous obstruction. Pulmonary vascular obstructive disease is rare during infancy, although exceptions have been reported.[604] In patients without pulmonary venous obstruction the risk of developing the Eisenmenger reaction is comparable to that in patients with an atrial septal defect.

CLINICAL MANIFESTATIONS. The majority of patients with total anomalous pulmonary venous connection have symptoms during the first year of life, and 80 per cent die before age 1 year if left untreated.[598] The few who remain asymptomatic have a relatively good prognosis; once the condition is detected, operation may be elected later in childhood. Symptomatic infants with total anomalous pulmonary venous connection present with signs of heart failure and/or cyanosis. Infants with pulmonary venous obstruction present with the early onset of severe dyspnea, pulmonary edema, cyanosis, and right heart failure. Cardiac murmurs often are not prominent. In the unobstructed forms of total anomalous pulmonary venous connection the characteristic physical findings include right ventricular precordial overactivity and minimal cyanosis unless congestive heart failure intervenes. Multiple heart sounds often are audible, consisting of a first heart sound followed by an ejection sound; a fixed, widely split second heart sound with an accentuated pulmonic component; and a third and often a fourth heart sound. A soft systolic ejection murmur is usual along the left sternal border, and a mid-diastolic murmur of flow across the tricuspid valve commonly is audible at the lower left sternal border.

LABORATORY FINDINGS. The *electrocardiogram* shows right-axis deviation and right atrial and right ventricular hypertrophy. *Roentgenograms* of the chest reveal increased pulmonary blood flow; the right atrium and ventricle are dilated and hypertrophied, and the pulmonary artery segment is enlarged (Fig. 29-67). In addition, the specific site of anomalous connection may cause a characteristic appearance of the cardiac silhouette. Thus, in patients with total anomalous pulmonary venous connection to the left brachiocephalic vein, the superior vena cava on the right, left brachiocephalic vein superiorly, and vertical vein on the left produce a cardiac shadow that resembles a snowman or figure of eight. The upper right cardiac border may be prominent when the anomalous connection is to the right superior vena cava.

Echocardiography demonstrates marked enlargement of the right ventricle and a small left atrium.[605] The objective of ultrasound imaging in these patients is to confirm the clinical diagnosis and to locate the site of connection of the common pulmonary vein. Doppler studies are required to assess the presence of obstruction within individual pulmonary veins and along the vertical vein. An echo-free space representing the common pulmonary venous chamber occasionally may be seen to lie behind the left atrium on ultrasound examination. Diagnostic echocardiographic findings include an absence of pulmonary vein connections and a small left atrium in the presence of right to left bulging of the septum primum at the foramen ovale. Positive diagnosis is made by identifying pulmonary

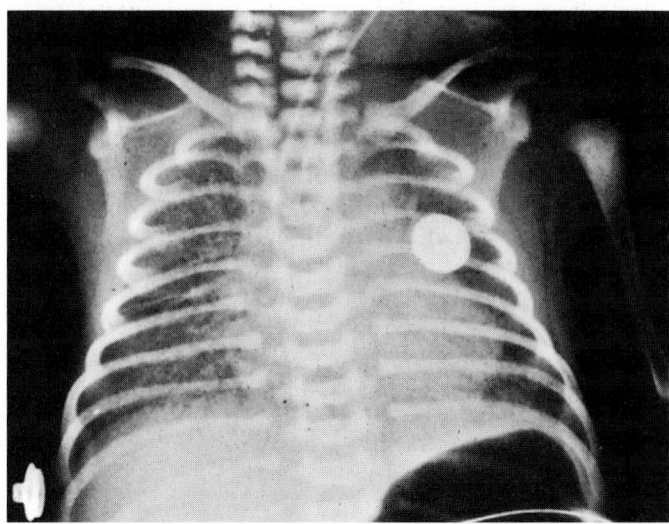

FIGURE 29-67. Chest roentgenogram in an infant with total anomalous pulmonary venous connection below the diaphragm shows normal overall heart size but diffuse pattern of pulmonary venous hypertension in both lung fields.

venous connection to the systemic veins, coronary sinus, or right atrium, rather than to the left atrium. All four pulmonary veins and their connections must be identified to diagnose mixed types accurately.[605] There is no standard echocardiographic method for tracing pulmonary venous pathways because of their diverse anatomical positions.

Infradiaphragmatic total anomalous pulmonary venous connection usually connects to the portal venous system but can connect to the hepatic veins. Doppler is utilized to distinguish between the abdominal vessels. Thus, the flow pattern in the inferior vena cava is phasic, nearly continuous, and toward the heart, in contrast to flow in the descending aorta, which has a laminar profile in systole in a direction away from the heart. Flow in the common pulmonary vein resembles that of the inferior vena cava except that its direction is away from the heart. Although not often employed, especially in infants, magnetic resonance imaging may also delineate the site of connections of the various types of total anomalous pulmonary venous return.

At *cardiac catheterization* those patients found to have systemic arterial saturations below 70 per cent and with pulmonary artery pressure at or above systemic levels are likely to have pulmonary venous obstruction. Variations in oxygen saturation in the systemic venous circulation may be helpful. In the subdiaphragmatic type, a step-up may not be apparent in inferior vena caval oxygen saturations obtained by way of femoral vein cannulation because of the contribution of highly oxygenated renal venous blood to the caval stream. In contrast, sampling of the hepatic or portal vein by way of a catheter inserted through the umbilical vein yields diagnostically higher oxygen saturations, indicating anomalous return to those vessels. If the cardiac catheter can be manipulated directly into the anomalous trunk through its site of connection, selective injection of contrast material into the common channel provides anatomical definition of the pulmonary venous tree. If the pulmonary veins cannot be entered directly, selective right and left main pulmonary artery injection of contrast material often is more helpful than is injection into a main pulmonary artery because many infants have a persistent patent ductus arteriosus through which the contrast agent flows right to left. Moreover, the drainage from both lungs must be outlined clearly to exclude a mixed type of anomalous venous drainage. Pulmonary venous obstruction may be detected by noting a pressure difference between the pulmonary artery wedge pressure and the right atrium.

MANAGEMENT. Corrective surgery for the sick infant should be performed as soon as possible, usually on the basis of two-dimensional and Doppler echocardiography, avoiding the additional stress of invasive diagnostic study. Before age 1 month, survival greater than 75 per cent is anticipated. Infants with the worst prognosis are those in whom individual pulmonary vein sizes are smallest, measurements that can be made preoperatively by echocardiogram.[606] Unless pulmonary vascular disease is present, results of operation for total anomalous pulmonary venous connection in patients beyond infancy are generally good.[607] The procedure consists of creating an anastomosis between the common pulmonary venous channel and left atrium and closing the atrial defect and the anomalous venous pathway. Improved results of operation in infancy require that postoperative pulmonary venous hypertension be averted by construction of a generally large anastomosis with or without enlargement of the left atrium. Normal hemodynamics and cardiac function have been demonstrated after surgical correction.

Partial Anomalous Pulmonary Venous Connection

In this condition one or more of the pulmonary veins, but not all, are connected to the right atrium or to one or more of its venous tributaries (see p. 944). An atrial septal defect, particularly one of the sinus venosus type, commonly accompanies this anomaly; the usual connection involves the veins of the right upper and middle lobes and the superior vena cava.[598] Exclusive of atrial septal defects, major additional cardiac malformations occur in about 20 per cent of patients; these include ventricular septal defect, tetralogy of Fallot, and a variety of complex anomalies.

In the absence of associated anomalies the physiological disturbance is determined by the number of anomalous veins and their site of connection, the presence and size of an atrial septal defect, and the state of the pulmonary vascular bed.[608] In the usual patient with isolated partial pulmonary venous connection the hemodynamic state and physical findings are similar to those in atrial septal defect. Rarely, venous drainage of the right lung is into the inferior vena cava. This condition often is associated with hypoplasia of the right lung, dextroposition of the heart, pulmonary parenchymal abnormalities, and anomalous system supply to the lower lobe of the right lung from the abdominal aorta or its main branches. This complex has been designated the "scimitar syndrome" because of the characteristic roentgenographic finding of a crescent-like shadow in the right lower lung field that is produced by the anomalous venous channel.[609,610]

At *cardiac catheterization*, partial anomalous pulmonary venous connection to the coronary sinus, azygos vein, or superior vena cava may be identified by careful and frequent oximetry sampling. Oximetry is of limited value when the anomalous connection is to the inferior vena cava because of both reduced flow through the right lung and the contribution to the vena caval stream of highly oxygenated blood from the renal veins. Selective angiography is most helpful in cases in which the anomalous veins connect far away from the right atrium. Surgical repair offers definitive therapy at low risk if pulmonary vascular obliterative disease has not yet developed.

Malpositions of the Heart and Cardiac Apex

Positional anomalies of the heart are conditions in which the cardiac apex is located in the right side of the chest (dextrocardia) or is centrally located (mesocardia) or in which there is a normal location of the heart in the left side of the chest but abnormal position of the viscera (isolated levocardia). Such hearts commonly are abnormal with respect to chamber localization and great artery attachments; associated complex intracardiac and extracardiac lesions are common.

Problems of terminology abound in the literature describing these complex cardiac anomalies, although sensible and uniform systems of classification are available.[611, 612]

ANATOMICAL FEATURES. Defining the cardiac anatomy in instances of cardiac malposition requires a description of three cardiac segments—the visceroatrial situs, the ventricular loop, and the conotruncus (the atria, ventricles, and great arteries, respectively). In addition to defining positional interrelation, the description of the malposed heart also must include the connections of the ventricles to the atria and great arteries as well as chamber identification, both morphologically and functionally.

DIAGNOSIS. To accomplish accurate diagnosis may require a synthesis of findings from noninvasive tests such as two-dimensional echocardiography, computed tomography, and magnetic resonance imaging, as well as hemodynamic and cineangiographic findings obtained at cardiac catheterization. Expert echocardiographers analyze, separately and independent of adjacent segments, each cardiac seg-

ment (atria, atrioventricular canal, ventricles, infundibulum, and great arteries) in terms of both situs and alignments.[613-616]

In general, the determination of the body situs indicates the position of the atria. The visceral situs usually can be determined by the location of the stomach bubble and liver on a routine roentgenogram and of the inferior vena cava by means of echocardiography or the position of a cardiac catheter, or by means of a computed axial tomogram or venous or radioisotope angiocardiogram. Atrial anatomy is best investigated noninvasively by using subxiphoid long- and short-axis and apical four-chamber echocardiographic views. Venous contrast injections may be useful to define systemic venous connections.

Situs solitus is the normal arrangement of viscera and atria, with the right atrium right-sided and the left atrium left-sided. Situs solitus is further characterized by a trilobed right lung and eparterial bronchus (i.e., the right upper lobe bronchus passes above the right pulmonary artery), a bilobed left lung and hyparterial bronchus (i.e., the left bronchus passes below the left pulmonary artery), the major lobe of the liver on the right, a left-sided stomach and spleen, and right-sided venae cavae. *Situs inversus* is a mirror image of normal. *Situs ambiguus* or visceral heterotaxy refers to an anatomically uncertain or indeterminate body configuration. The latter often is seen in association with congenital asplenia, which resembles bilateral right-sidedness, and congenital polysplenia, which resembles bilateral left-sidedness.[617-620]

ASPLENIA. Cardiac anomalies associated commonly with asplenia include anomalous systemic venous connection, atrial septal or complete endocardial cushion defect, common ventricle, transposition of the great arteries, severe pulmonic stenosis or atresia, and anomalous pulmonary venous connection. Polysplenia commonly is associated with absence of the hepatic portion of the inferior vena cava with azygos continuation, bilateral superior venae cavae, anomalous pulmonary venous connection, and atrial septal defect (either ostium secundum or endocardial cushion). Pulmonic stenosis and double-outlet right ventricle are each observed in about 25 per cent of cases. It is important to recognize these complex syndromes to distinguish them from forms of cyanotic heart disease that may be more amenable to corrective surgical therapy. In many of these patients, improvement results from palliation by modifications of the Fontan procedure, despite anomalies of systemic and pulmonary venous return in association with single ventricle anatomy.[621,622] Diagnosis is suggested by a symmetrical liver shadow roentgenographically and, in asplenia, by the presence of Howell-Jolly and Heinz bodies in red blood cells demonstrated on blood smear, and it is confirmed by a negative or abnormal radioactive spleen scan.

Once the visceral situs is defined, it is necessary to describe the bulboventricular loop. The primitive cardiac tune normally bends to the right (D-loop), which brings the anatomical right ventricle to the right of the anatomical left ventricle. An L-loop brings the morphological right ventricle left-sided relative to the morphological left ventricle. The L-loop is normal in the presence of situs inversus, but in situs solitus it is synonymous with inverted ventricles.

VENTRICULAR MORPHOLOGY. The number, morphology, and size of the ventricles can be ascertained by using a variety of echocardiographic views. The morphological features of each ventricle also can be identified angiographically. The anatomical right ventricle is equipped with a tricuspid valve, is highly trabeculated, and contains the septal band of the single papillary muscle; its infundibulum lies anterior to and superiorly beyond the outlet of the left ventricle. The anatomical right ventricle usually connects with whichever of the two great arteries is the more anterior. The anatomical left ventricle is smooth-walled and contains an outlet that lies posterior to the right ventricular infundibulum; its entrance is guarded by a bicuspid mitral valve, the anterior leaflet of which is normally in continuity with elements of the semilunar valve at its outlet.

GREAT ARTERIES. The great arteries are described in terms of their positional interrelations and their ventricular connections. Each outflow tract and semilunar valve should be examined in both long- and short-axis echocardiographic views.[613,615] The ventriculoarterial alignments may be determined by direct visualization from the subxiphoid window. The relation between the great arteries can best be demonstrated noninvasively using parasternal short-axis echocardiographic views, which display the semilunar roots. The aortic arch and brachiocephalic arteries are seen well using suprasternal notch views. The pulmonary artery is seen from high parasternal or suprasternal notch short-axis sections. The ventricular attachments may be normal or may form the anomalies of double-outlet right or left ventricle or transposition. The arterial interrelations are described as D (dextro), in which the ascending aorta sweeps toward the right and lies to the right of the main pulmonary artery; L (levo), in which the ascending aorta sweeps toward the left and lies to the left of the main pulmonary artery; or A (antero), which is the rare situation in which the aorta lies directly in front of the pulmonary artery. The D, L, and A descriptions of the aorticopulmonary artery interrelations should not be confused with the D- or L-loop designation of the ventricular interrelations.[612]

Using segmental sets composed of descriptive units of visceroatrial situs/ventricular loop/great artery relations greatly simplifies expression of the type of cardiac anatomy present in cardiac malposition. For example, the normal heart in a patient with situs inversus and dextrocardia is referred to as inversus/L loop/L normal; complete transposition of the great arteries in a patient with situs inversus is referred to as inversus/L loop/L transposition; functionally corrected transposition in a patient with situs solitus is referred to as solitus/L loop/L transposition; dextrocardia and functionally corrected transposition is designated solitus/D loop/D transposition with dextrocardia.

After the cardiac chambers are diagnosed functionally (arterial and venous), the positional and morphological relations are understood, and the presence of associated anomalies is established, the principles of medical and surgical treatment apply to these cardiac malpositions as they do to normally located hearts.

OTHER CONDITIONS

Congenital Pericardial Defects

Isolated pericardial defects (see p. 1522) are rare. They most commonly occur in males and usually are left-sided, although they may be right-sided, diaphragmatic, or total.[623] The anomaly is produced by deficient formation of the pleuropericardial membrane, or, if diaphragmatic, defective formations of the septum transversum. Associated congenital anomalies of the heart and lungs occur in about 30 per cent of cases. Most patients with the isolated defect are asymptomatic. Nonspecific anterior chest pain may be the result of torsion of the great arteries due to absence of the stabilizing forces of the left pericardium.

With complete absence of the left pericardium a conspicuous apical impulse may be noted shifted leftward to the anterior or midaxillary line. Electrocardiographic changes may be related to levo-position of the heart; a leftward displacement of the QRS transition in the precordial leads and vertical or right-axis deviation are usual. The diagnosis may be suggested by chest roentgenograms.[624] With complete left pericardial absence, the heart is levo-posed, and the aortic knob, pulmonary artery, and ventricles form three prominent left heart border convexities.

A partial left pericardial defect may be suspected on the basis of varying degrees of prominence of the pulmonary artery and/or the left atrial appendage. Echocardiographic findings often mimic those observed in patients with right ventricular volume overload (enlarged right ventricle and abnormal ventricular septal motion), probably owing to the altered cardiac position and motion with the thorax.[625] Other echocardiographic clues include lateral extension of the left atrial appendage as it herniates through the pericardial defect; this is best seen in short-axis views. The anomaly can be definitively diagnosed by computed tomography or magnetic resonance imaging. Cardiac catheterization is of little diagnostic value.

Complete absence of the left pericardium requires no treatment. However, partial defects may impose serious risks, including herniation and strangulation of the ventricles or left atrial appendage with left-sided defects, or the possibility of a superior vena cava obstructive syndrome with right-sided defects.[626] In the diaphragmatic type, cardiac compression by abdominal contents requires surgical repair.[627] Partial left or right defects may be closed with a patch of mediastinal pleura.

Single Atrium

Single or common atrium is a rare, isolated defect. The anomaly consists of an absent atrial septum, usually with a cleft in the anteromedial leaflet of the mitral valve and, occasionally, with a cleft tricuspid valve as well. The lesion may be seen as one component of the Ellis–van Creveld syndrome (Table 29–2) or of the complex cardiac anomalies seen in patients with asplenia or polysplenia.

Single atrium may be suspected clinically by the presence of cardiac murmurs of an atrial septal defect and mitral regurgitation associated with mild cyanosis, roentgenographic evidence of cardiac enlargement and increased pulmonary blood flow, and electrocardiographic features of

atrioventricular septal defect. An absence of echoes from any part of the atrial septum is the essential feature of two-dimensional echocardiographic examination, which also may show a cleft anterior mitral leaflet, increased right ventricular end-diastolic dimension, paradoxical ventricular septal motion, and dilated, pulsatile pulmonary trunk. Angiographically, the absence of the atrial septum produces a large, globe-shaped single atrial structure. Selective left ventricular angiocardiography shows the characteristic gooseneck appearance seen in the various forms of atrioventricular septal defect. In the absence of pulmonary vascular obstructive disease surgical correction is indicated by means of a prosthetic patch.

Single Ventricle
(Univentricular Atrioventricular Connection)

Hearts with univentricular atrioventricular connection constitute a family of complex lesions in which both atrioventricular valves, or a common atrioventricular valve, open into a single ventricular chamber.[628] Terminology is varied, and the anomaly often is referred to as single or common ventricle, which is imprecise but useful shorthand for the entity. The definition excludes examples of tricuspid or mitral atresia. Single ventricle is almost always accompanied by abnormal great artery positional relations; the incidence of L-malposition of the great arteries is about equal to that of D-malposition. Associated anomalies are common, and include, in particular, pulmonic valvular or subvalvular stenosis, subaortic stenosis, total or partial anomalous pulmonary venous connection, and coarctation of the aorta.

MORPHOLOGY. In about 80 per cent of patients the single ventricle morphologically resembles a left ventricular chamber that is separated from an infundibular outlet chamber by a bulboventricular septum.[629] The opening is variously called the bulboventricular foramen and ventricular septal defect. The infundibular chamber is considered to represent developmentally the outflow tract of the right ventricle. When the great arteries are malposed the infundibulum lying anterior at the basal position of the single ventricle communicates with the aorta and may be in one of two positions: noninverted (D-malposition), when it is situated at the right basal aspect of the heart, or inverted (L-malposition), when it is located at the left base of the heart. In the unusual situation in which the great arteries are normally related, the infundibulum communicates with the pulmonary trunk.[629] Double-inlet left ventricle is a term used synonymously to describe the most frequently encountered single ventricular chamber that has the anatomical characteristics of the left ventricle. Less commonly the single ventricular chamber resembles a right ventricle (double-inlet right ventricle) or contains features suggestive of both ventricles or neither one; the latter two situations occasionally have been designated common ventricle and single ventricle of the primitive type, respectively.

CLINICAL FINDINGS. Depending on the associated anomalies, the clinical presentation of single ventricle mimics other conditions in which cyanosis and decreased or increased pulmonary blood flow coexist, e.g., tetralogy of Fallot or tricuspid atresia in the former instance or complete transposition of the great arteries and double-outlet right ventricle in the latter. The electrocardiogram in double-inlet left ventricle without inversion of the infundibulum (D-malposition) usually shows features of left ventricular hypertrophy. With infundibular inversion (L-malposition) the electrical forces are directed anteriorly and rightward, as they are in ventricular inversion without associated defects. In patients with the more primitive types of common or single ventricle there is a repetitious rS pattern in all the precordial electrocardiographic leads. Chest roentgenographic findings resemble those observed in patients with complete (dextro-) transposition of the great arteries or functionally corrected (levo-) transposition of the great arteries without features distinctive for single ventricle.

ECHOCARDIOGRAPHY. Two-dimensional and Doppler echocardiography are extremely important to demonstrate ventricular anatomy and to recognize associated intra- and extracardiac anomalies (Fig. 29–68). A segmental approach should be employed for accurate and complete echocardiographic evaluation. Thus, precise details are required of the basic anatomy of atrial and visceral situs, location of the cardiac apex, the extracardiac course of the great arteries, and systemic and pulmonary venous connections.

In those patients in whom two separate atrioventricular valves communicate with the single ventricular chamber, echocardiography (Fig. 3–85, p. 85) suggests the correct diagnosis when echoes are visualized from the two valves without an intervening interventricu-

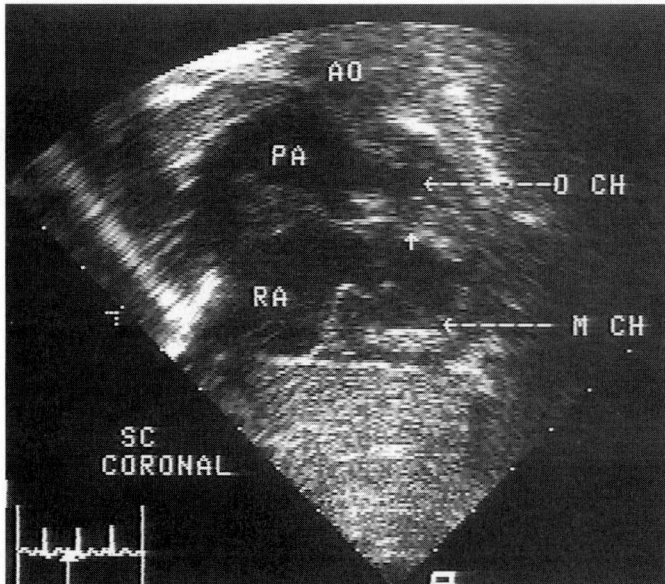

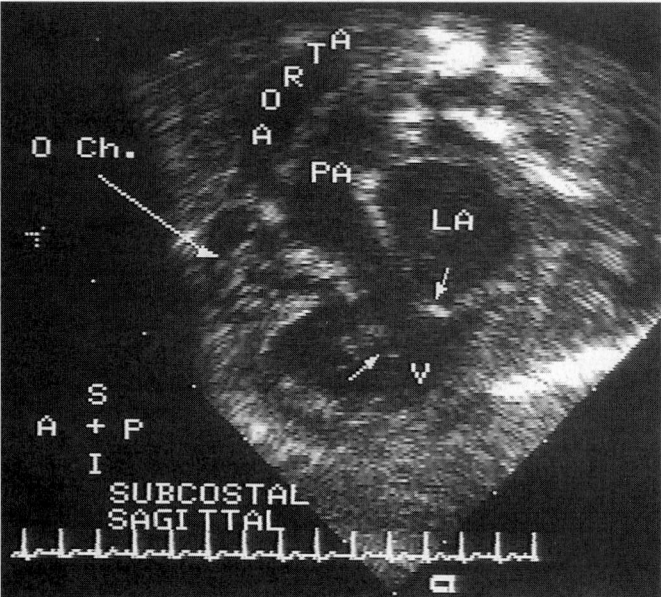

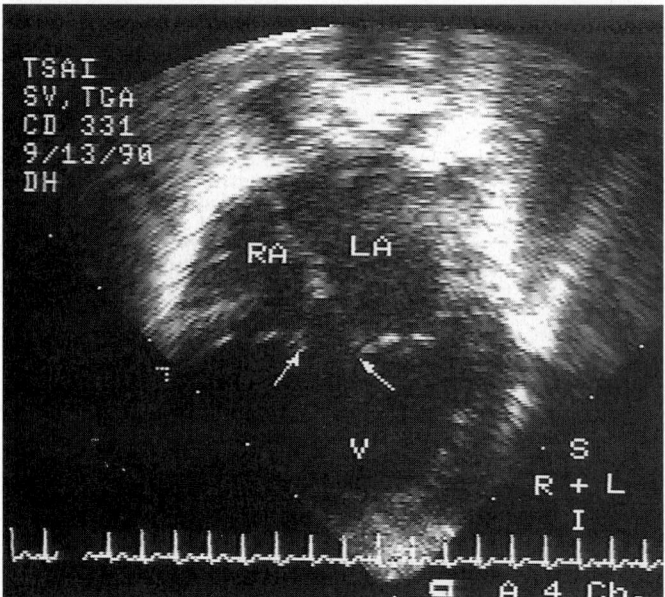

FIGURE 29–68. Echo images of a double-inlet left ventricle type of univentricular heart. *Top,* Subcostal coronal view shows the right atrium (RA) giving rise to a tricuspid valve guarding entry into a main

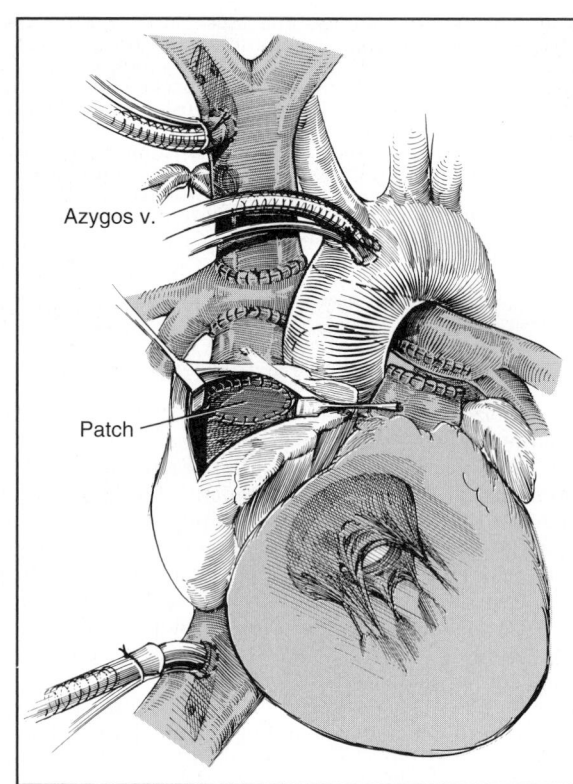

FIGURE 29–69. A bidirectional cavopulmonary artery shunt with patch occlusion of the superior vena cava right atrial junction (hemi-Fontan procedure) using direct cannulation of the superior and inferior venae cavae and a single arterial cannula. The main pulmonary artery is shown divided and oversewn, but in some cases it may be allowed to remain patent. Connections are made between both ends of the divided superior vena cava and the pulmonary artery. A subsequent Fontan operation involves only removal of the patch at the junction of the superior vena cava and the right atrium and placement of the intraatrial baffle to divert the inferior vena caval blood up to the superior vena cava orifice. (From Castaneda, A., et al.: Cardiac Surgery of the Neonate and Infant. Philadelphia, W.B. Saunders Company, 1994, p. 263.)

lar septum.[630,631] In the absence of ventricular septal echoes when the two valves are not visualized simultaneously, they may be identified separately with a careful long-axis sweep of the ventricle. It is possible to detect the presence of a small outflow chamber anterior to the atrioventricular valves by using subcostal or parasternal short-axis views, and a plane orthogonal to the long-axis plane (Fig. 29–64).

The single ventricle with a single atrioventricular valve is suspected when the excursion of echoes from the single valve located posteriorly in the ventricular chamber is of large amplitude. Enhanced assessment of the atrioventricular valve in patients with single ventricle is provided by Doppler echocardiography.[632] Magnetic resonance imaging provides valuable complementary information to echocardiographic study.[630,631] Selective ventriculography is necessary to delineate with certainty the anatomical type of single ventricle and to diagnose the associated great artery interrelations and the presence or absence of additional lesions.[633]

chamber (M CH) of left ventricular morphology from which the pulmonary artery (PA) arises. The arrow indicates the small ventricular septal defect (bulboventricular foramen) entering into an outflow chamber (O CH) which gives rise to the aorta (AO). *Middle,* Orthogonal subcostal sagittal equivalent to the top frame. The left atrium (LA) is seen above the main chamber of left ventricular morphology (V). The arrows indicate the origin of the left and right atrioventricular valves within the same ventricular chamber. The pulmonary artery (PA) arises from the main chamber and the long narrow bulboventricular foramen is shown to enter the outlet chamber (O CH) with its connection to the aorta. *Bottom,* Apical four-chamber view shows the right atrium (RA) and the left atrium (LA) with their corresponding valves (arrows) entering into the common large ventricle (V). (Courtesy of Norman Silverman, M.D.)

SURGICAL TREATMENT. Attempts to partition the single ventricle with a Dacron or Teflon prosthetic patch have met with limited success as well as a high incidence of postoperative complete heart block. Modifications of the Fontan approach are generally applied to patients with all types of anatomical and functional single ventricle.[634-636] Surgical outcome is related to the creation of an unobstructed pathway from the systemic veins to the pulmonary arteries, low pulmonary vascular resistance, and a compliant, well-functioning ventricle. In most centers, the Fontan procedure is divided into two stages, an initial superior vena cava–pulmonary artery anastomosis (bidirectional Glenn shunt or hemi-Fontan procedure; Fig. 29-69, p. 948), followed later by completion of the Fontan procedure directing flow from the inferior vena cava to the amalgamation of the superior vena cava and the branch pulmonary arteries. At first-stage operation, prior systemic–pulmonary shunts are eliminated and any areas of distortion or narrowing of the pulmonary arteries are repaired, particularly if a prior pulmonary artery banding was performed to limit pulmonary blood flow.

At the author's center, the complete Fontan procedure is accompanied by placement of a snare around the atrial septal defect to control its size postoperatively, whereas in other centers, fenestrations in the atrial baffle may be used. These procedures appear to reduce significantly postoperative morbidity from pericardial effusions and significantly improve survival. Results of early bidirectional cavopulmonary shunting in young infants are encouraging. The objective of this approach early in life is to yield a more suitable Fontan candidate while reducing ventricular volume overload and repeated palliative procedures. Subaortic stenosis, a common occurrence in patients with univentricular heart and malposed great arteries, occurs as a result of a restrictive bulboventricular foramen (ventricular septal defect) or as a consequence of ventricular hypertrophy from a previous pulmonary banding operation.

The *Damus-Kaye-Stansel operation*, consisting of anastomosis of the pulmonary artery to the ascending aorta, is a generally successful approach to this problem.[637-641] After operation, all patients need continued close surveillance.[642-646] Complications include thromboembolic phenomena and atrial arrhythmias. Survivors generally lead active lives with exercise levels less than normal, but relevant to ordinary daily life.

VASCULAR RINGS

MORPHOLOGY. The normal development of the aortic arch system is described on page 882 (Fig. 29-3). The term *vascular ring* is used for those aortic arch or pulmonary artery malformations that exhibit an abnormal relation with the esophagus and trachea, causing compression, dysphagia, and/or respiratory symptoms.[647] The most common and serious vascular ring is produced by a double aortic arch in which both the right and left fourth embryonic aortic arches persist. In the most common type of double aortic arch there is a left ligamentum arteriosum or ductus arteriosus, and both arches are patent, the right being larger than the left. A right aortic arch with a left ductus or ligamentum arteriosum connecting the left pulmonary artery and the upper part of the descending aorta, and with an anomalous right subclavian artery arising from the left descending aorta, are additional important vascular ring arrangements.[648] The latter anomaly frequently exists in cases of tetralogy of Fallot and otherwise uncomplicated coarctation of the aorta. An unusual cause of tracheal compression is the "vascular sling" created by an anomalous left pulmonary artery that arises from a rightward, elongated pulmonary trunk and courses between the trachea and esophagus before it branches normally within the left lung.[649] This arrangement commonly is associated with other cardiac and extracardiac anomalies.

CLINICAL FINDINGS. The symptoms produced by vascular rings depend on the tightness of anatomical constriction of the trachea and esophagus and consist principally of respiratory difficulties, cyanosis (associated especially with feeding), stridor, and dysphagia. The electrocardiogram is normal unless associated cardiovascular anomalies are present. The barium esophagogram is a useful screening procedure. Prominent posterior indentation of the esophagus is observed in the common vascular ring arrangements, although the pulmonary artery "vascular sling" produces an anterior indentation. Unusual and rare aortic arch anomalies may create rings that impinge on the trachea but

do not compress the esophagus and are detected not by this simple radiographic procedure but rather by bronchoscopy. Selective contrast angiography delineates the anatomy of the aorta and its branches or the course of the main pulmonary arteries. Computed axial tomography and magnetic resonance imaging offer excellent imaging alternatives.[650,651]

MANAGEMENT. The severity of symptoms and the anatomy of the malformation are the most important factors in determining treatment. Patients, particularly infants, with respiratory obstruction require prompt surgical intervention. Operative repair of the double aortic arch requires division of the minor arch (usually the left).[652] A reported 20 to 30 per cent operative mortality is related, in part, to problems in postoperative respiratory care, especially when there is coexistent residual anatomical tracheal narrowing. Patients with a right aortic arch and a left ductus or ligamentum arteriosum require division of the ductus or ligamentum and/or ligation and division of the left subclavian artery, which is the posterior component of the ring. Operation seldom is indicated for patients with an aberrant right subclavian artery derived from a left aortic arch and left descending aorta. In patients with a pulmonary artery vascular sling, operation consists of detachment of the left pulmonary artery at its origin and anastomosis to the main pulmonary artery directly or by way of a conduit of its proximal end brought anterior to the trachea.[652] Some patients with persistent respiratory symptoms require postoperative evaluation of residual anatomical obstruction, tests of pulmonary function, and bronchodilator therapy.[653]

CONGENITAL ARRHYTHMIAS

This classification refers to arrhythmias that are present in infancy, whose causes, when known, relate to a structural malformation or defect of the conduction system or to an acquired prenatal condition such as myocarditis, hypoxia acidosis, or transplacental passage of a drug or substance from mother to fetus. In these latter examples, the substrate for the postnatal expression of the rhythm disturbance existed before birth and the arrhythmia is therefore designated "congenital." Complete heart block and supraventricular and ventricular tachycardias are the most common important congenital arrhythmias.[654] The electrophysiological and electrocardiographic features of these arrhythmias are discussed elsewhere in the text (Chaps. 22 and 23).

Congenital Complete Heart Block
(See also p. 966)

The atrioventricular node and the His bundle originate during fetal development as separate structures and later join together. Anatomical studies have shown the basic lesion in congenital complete heart block to consist of discontinuity between the atrial musculature and the AV node or the His bundle, if the AV node is absent. The anatomical interruption occasionally may be situated between the AV node and the main His bundle, or within the bundle itself.[655] No cause is known for the vast majority of cases of congenital heart block in infants, who usually have otherwise anatomically normal hearts. However, fetal myocarditis, idiopathic hemorrhage and necrosis involving conduction tissue, and degeneration and fibrosis related in some instances to the transplacental passage of anti-Ro/ss-A antibody and other immune complexes from mothers with systemic lupus erythematosus are all entities capable of causing congenital heart block.[656,657] Less often, congenital heart block may be associated with various forms of congenital heart disease, the most common malformation being congenitally corrected transposition of the great arteries.[655a]

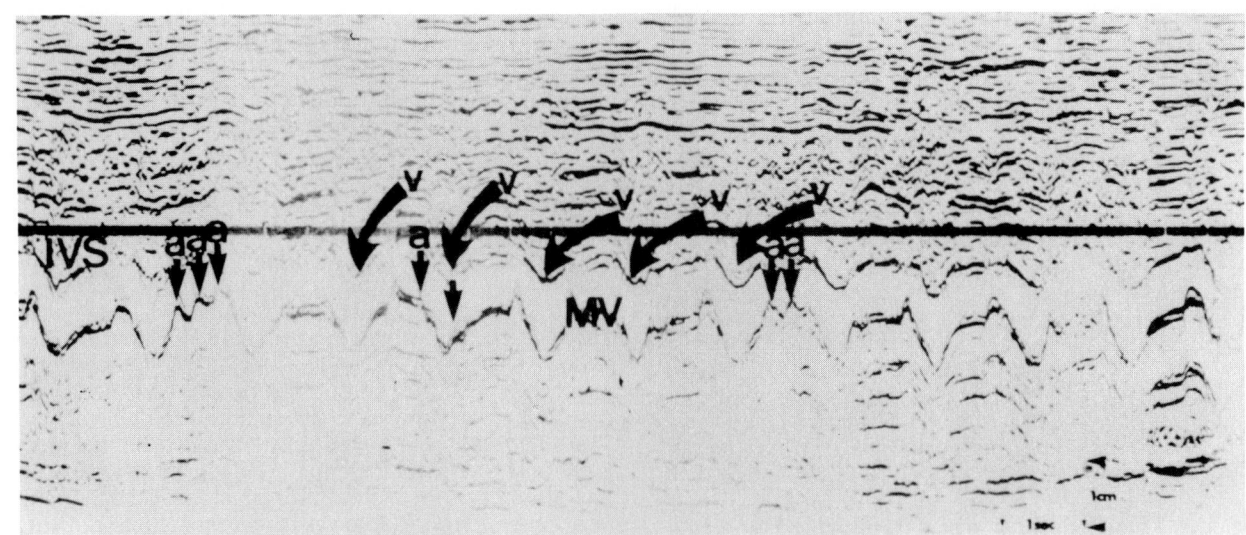

FIGURE 29-70. Fetal M-mode echocardiogram of complete heart block at 28 weeks' gestation. A slow ventricular rate of 45 to 50 beats/min is seen by the undulations (v, *curved arrows*) of the interventricular septum (IVS). Atrial contractions (a, *straight vertical arrows*) cause regular undulations of the mitral valve (MV) at a rate of 120 to 130 beats/min. The atrial activity has no fixed relationship to the idioventricular rhythm. (Courtesy of Charles Kleinman, M.D.)

Detection of consistent fetal bradycardia (heart rate 40 to 80 beats/min) by auscultation, fetal echocardiography (Fig. 29–70), or electronic monitoring allows anticipation of the correct diagnosis. The newborn, especially with a ventricular rate less than 50 beats/min and atrial rate in excess of 150 beats/min, is at highest risk; the presence of an associated cardiovascular anomaly greatly lessens the chances of survival. Treatment is not required for the asymptomatic infant. Digitalization is recommended for the baby in congestive heart failure, irrespective of complete heart block. Isoproterenol and other sympathomimetic drugs and atropine do not have permanent or beneficial effect. Congestive heart failure and Stokes-Adams attacks require pacemaker treatment at any age. This requires transvenous or transatrial placement of endocardial leads in the older child or permanent epicardial pacemaker insertion in infants and small children. A variety of problems may be anticipated after pacemaker implantation related to growth of the patient, which stresses the electrical lead system; the fragility of the lead system in a physically active young patient; and the limited life span of the pulse generator. Patients with congenital complete heart block who survive infancy usually remain asymptomatic until late in childhood or adolescence.[662]

Supraventricular Tachycardia

Paroxysmal tachycardia of supraventricular origin may have its origin in utero or in the immediate postnatal period. The most frequent arrhythmias producing symptoms are paroxysmal atrial tachycardia with or without ventricular preexcitation, atrial flutter, and junctional tachycardia. The arrhythmia may cause intrauterine cardiac failure; its detection and persistence prenatally should prompt consideration of administration of digitalis, or if that fails, of propranolol, quinidine, flecainide, or amiodarone to the mother if amniocentesis indicates surfactant deficiency and fetal lung immaturity because early delivery is not indicated if the baby will have hyaline membrane disease. Experience is limited with antiarrhythmic drugs, delivered by umbilical venous infusion.[107] Cesarean delivery or induced labor may be indicated if the fetus is close to term. No cause is recognized for the disorder in the majority of infants. The transplacental passage of long-acting thyroid-stimulators (LATS) and immune gamma 2 globulin from hyperthyroid mothers, hypoglycemia, and Ebstein's anomaly of the tricuspid valve occasionally are causative.[665] Wolff-Parkinson-White syndrome (see p. 667) is present in 10 to 50 per cent of infants with supraventricular tachycardia.[666] Symptoms produced by the tachyarrhythmia after birth are subtle and often go undetected until signs of heart failure have been present for 24 to 36 hours. Conversion to normal sinus rhythm usually is accomplished by administration of digitalis or adenosine, direct-current cardioversion, transesophageal atrial pacing, or a diving reflex elicited by covering the face with an ice-cold wet washcloth for 4 to 5 seconds.[667] Conversion should be followed by digitalization on a prophylactic basis. Common practice consists of digitalis treatment for 9 to 12 recurrence-free months followed by its abrupt cessation. Recurrence of tachycardia, particularly in those infants with ventricular preexcitation, is not uncommon; maintenance of normal rhythm may require the administration, alone or in combination, of digitalis, phenytoin sodium, flecainide, and propranolol.[667] The rate of recurrence falls substantially between ages 2 and 10 years, with a slight rise during adolescence. In general, the prognosis is excellent.[668]

ELECTROPHYSIOLOGICAL STUDIES. Beyond infancy, patients whose condition is refractory to medical treatment are candidates for electrophysiological catheter evaluation, which facilitates differentiation of a causative ectopic anatomical focus within the atria from accessory conduction pathways.[654,669] Endocardial mapping is performed to specifically localize the site of earliest activation in the atrium, or to identify multiple foci of ectopic impulses. Electrophysiological studies should include measurement of resting intervals and sinus and atrioventricular node function, including recovery times, effective refractory period, and Wenckebach conduction. Premature atrial stimulation may be used to interrupt tachycardia. Premature ventricular stimulation is used to measure retrograde conduction and localize the site of earliest atrial activation, and to assess the effective refractory period of the accessory pathway. Coronary sinus and right atrial catheters provide localization of the site of earliest atrial activation during tachycardia, and allow measurement of the antegrade effective refractory period of the accessory pathway.

If the tachyarrhythmia is refractory to pharmacological therapy, it may be treated definitively by radiofrequency catheter ablation of accessory pathways (see p. 621). This procedure has become the primary treatment modality for most symptomatic rhythm disturbances in children.[670-674]

Among the advantages of this approach is that successful ablation represents a cure; the heart is left structurally normal, and the cause of the arrhythmia is eliminated. Further, the need for antiarrhythmic agents with the concomitant risk of side effects or proarrhythmia is eliminated. This author has used transesophageal biplanar cross-sectional imaging during ablation procedures to precisely localize the ablation catheter tip and its stability.

ATRIAL FLUTTER. Uncommonly, atrial flutter is the cause of supraventricular tachycardia,[675–677] especially in the setting of newborn infants with hydrops fetalis, whose intrauterine tachyarrhythmia is an alternation between supraventricular tachycardia with Wolff-Parkinson-White syndrome and atrial flutter. Another common clinical setting for atrial flutter is in the infant under age 6 months with an otherwise normal heart, who shows frequent premature atrial contractions. In infants, classic flutter waves may not be present on a surface electrocardiogram or rhythm strip; detection may require recordings of transesophageal atrial electrograms. Acute treatment with electrical conversion or transesophageal overdrive pacing effectively terminates the rhythm disturbance.[677,678] If synchronized direct-current electrocardioversion is used, standby pacing should be available; if overdrive pacing is used, the same pacing catheter can be used to pace the heart in the event of asystole. Uncommonly, chronic drug treatment with digitalis, digitalis plus quinidine, or amiodarone may be required.

Junctional automatic tachycardia is characterized by a narrow QRS complex and AV dissociation, with the ventricular rate faster than the normal atrial rate. Ventricular dysfunction and congestive heart failure occur early, and the rhythm disturbance usually is not convertible to sinus rhythm by any medical treatment. When the latter fails and because sudden death is a risk, pacemaker implantation is recommended with subsequent catheter ablation.

VENTRICULAR TACHYCARDIA. Ventricular tachycardia is defined as three or more consecutive premature ventricular contractions. The definition, however, fails to identify a high-risk group. Infants or children who meet this criterion but seldom require treatment and seem to be at little risk have no symptoms and no evidence of anatomical heart disease. Potentially serious ventricular tachycardia in the newborn is associated with Q-T prolongation, mitral valve prolapse, and Marfan syndrome. In these settings the tachycardia is potentially life-threatening and always merits treatment.[654]

The genes have been mapped for the long Q-T syndrome (see p. 685). The two most effective treatments are beta blockade and high thoracic left sympathectomy, which reduce the incidence of syncope and sudden death without affecting the Q-T interval.

The treatment of ventricular tachycardia (see p. 619) consists of intravenous administration of lidocaine, followed by direct-current electrical cardioversion. In the absence of Q-T prolongation but in the presence of mitral prolapse or other cardiac abnormalities, chronic treatment should be undertaken of multiform premature ventricular contractions, couplets, or ventricular tachycardia. In infants and children unresponsive to conventional or investigational antiarrhythmic drugs, consideration should be given to pacemaker implantation, cardiac sympathetic denervation, and perhaps implantation of a defibrillator.[680]

REFERENCES

1. Hoffman, J. I. E.: Congenital heart disease. Ped. Clin. North Am. 37:45, 1990.
2. Roberts, W. C.: Anatomically isolated aortic valvular disease: The case against its being of rheumatic etiology. Am. J. Cardiol. 49:151, 1970.
3. Warth, D. C., King, M. E., Cohen, J. M., et al.: Prevalence of mitral valve prolapse in normal children. J. Am. Coll. Cardiol. 5:1173, 1985.
4. Fontana, R. S., and Edwards, J. E.: Congenital Cardiac Disease: A Review of 357 Cases Studied Pathologically. Philadelphia, W.B. Saunders Company, 1962.
5. Bankl, H.: Congenital Malformations of the Heart and Great Vessels: Synopsis of Pathology, Embryology and Natural History. Baltimore-Munich, Urban and Schwarzenberg, 1977.
5a. Gerlis, L. M.: Covert congenital cardiovascular malformations discovered in an autopsy series of nearly 5000 cases. Cardiovasc. Pathol. 5:11, 1996.
6. Samanek, M.: Boy:girl ratio in children born with different forms of cardiac malformation: A population-based study. Pediatr. Cardiol. 15:53, 1994.
7. Greenwood, R. D.: Cardiovascular malformations associated with extracardiac anomalies and malformation syndromes. Clin. Pediatr. 23:145, 1984.
8. Ferencz, C., and Villasenor, A. C.: Epidemiology of cardiovascular malformations: The state of the art. Cardiol. Young. 1:264, 1991.
9. de la Cruz, M. V., Munoz-Castellanos, L., and Nadal-Ginard, S.: Extrinsic factors in the genesis of congenital heart disease. Br. Heart J. 33:203, 1971.
10. Ruttenberg, H. D.: Concerning the etiology of congenital cardiac disease. Am. Heart J. 84:437, 1972.
11. Ouelette, E. M., Rossett, H. L., Rossman, M. P., and Wiener, L.: Adverse effects on offspring of maternal alcohol abuse during pregnancy. N. Engl. J. Med. 297:528, 1977.
12. Stevens, C. A., Carey, J. C., and Shigeoka, A. O.: DiGeorge anomaly and velocardiofacial syndrome. Pediatrics 85:526, 1990.
13. Dietz, H. C., and Pyeritz, R. E.: Molecular genetic approaches to the study of human cardiovascular disease. Annu. Rev. Physiol. 56:763, 1994.
14. Noonan, J.: Twins, conjoined twins, and cardiac defects. Am. J. Dis. Child. 132:17, 1978.
15. Burn, J.: Consequences of chromosome 22q11.2 deletions. Circulation 90:II–ID, 1994.
16. Corone, P., Bonaiti, C., Feingold, J., et al.: Familial congenital heart disease: How are the various types related? Am. J. Cardiol. 51:942, 1983.
17. Whittemore, R., Wells, J. A., and Castellsague, X.: A second-generation study of 427 probands with congenital heart defects and their 837 children. J. Am. Coll. Cardiol. 23:1459, 1994.
18. Anderson, R. H., and Ashley, G. T.: Anatomic development of the cardiovascular system. In Davies, J., and Dobbing, J. (eds.): Scientific Foundations of Paediatrics. London, Heinemann, 1974, p. 165.
19. Langman, J., and van Mierop, L. H. S.: Development of the cardiovascular system. In Moss, A. J., and Adams, F. H. (eds.): Heart Disease in Infants, Children, and Adolescents. Baltimore, Williams and Wilkins, 1968, p. 3.
20. Los, J. A.: Embryology. In Watson, H. (ed.): Pediatric Cardiology. London, Lloyd Luke Ltd., 1968, p. 1.
21. Rudolph, A. M.: Congenital Diseases of the Heart. Chicago Year Book Medical Publishers, 1974.
22. Sheldon, C. A., Friedman, W. F., and Sybers, H. D.: Scanning electron microscopy of fetal and neonatal lamb cardiac cells. J. Mol. Cell. Cardiol. 8:853, 1976.
23. McPherson, R. A., Kramer, M. F., Covell, J. W., and Friedman, W. F.: A comparison of the active stiffness of fetal and adult cardiac muscle. Pediatr. Res. 10:660, 1976.
24. Friedman, W. F.: The intrinsic physiologic properties of the developing heart. Prog. Cardiovasc. Dis. 15:87, 1972.
25. Huynh, T. V., Wetzel, G. T., Friedman, W. F., and Klitzner, T. S.: Developmental changes in membrane Ca^{2+} and K^+ currents in fatal, neonatal, and adult heart cells. Circ. Res. 70:508, 1992.
26. Chen, F., Wetzel, G. T., Friedman, W. F., and Klitzner, T. S.: ATP sensitive potassium channels in isolated neonatal and adult rabbit ventricular myocytes. Pediatr. Res. 32:230, 1992.
27. Ingwall, J. S., Kramer, M. F., Woodman, D., and Friedman, W. F.: Maturation of energy metabolism in the lamb: Changes in myosin ATPase and creatine kinase activities. Pediatr. Res. 15:1128, 1981.
28. Friedman, W. F.: Physiological properties of the developing heart. Paediatric Cardiology. Vol. 6. New York, Churchill Livingstone, 1987, p. 3.
29. Geis, W. P., Tatooles, C. J., Priola, D. V., and Friedman, W. F.: Factors influencing neurohumoral control of the heart and newborn. Am. J. Physiol. 228:1685, 1975.
30. Klitzner, T. S., and Friedman, W. F.: Excitation contraction coupling in developing mammalian myocardium. Pediatr. Res. 23:428, 1988.
31. Klitzner, T. S., and Friedman, W. F.: A diminished role for the sarcoplasmic reticulum in newborn myocardial contraction. Pediatr. Res. 26:98, 1989.
32. Romero, T. E., and Friedman, W. F.: Limited left ventricular response to volume overload in the neonatal period. Pediatr. Res. 13:910, 1979.
33. Finer, N. N., Etches, P. C., Kamstra, B., et al.: Inhaled nitric oxide in infants referred for extracorporeal membrane oxygenation: Dose response. J. Pediatr. 124:302, 1994.
34. Geggel, R. L.: Inhalational nitric oxide: A selective pulmonary vasodilator for treatment of persistent pulmonary hypertension of the newborn. J. Pediatr. 123:76, 1993.
35. Friedman, W. F., Printz, M. P., Kirkpatrick, S. E., and Hoskins, E. J.: The vasoactivity of the fetal lamb ductus arteriosus studied in utero. Pediatr. Res. 17:331, 1983.

PATHOLOGICAL CONSEQUENCES

36. Friedman, W. F., and George, B. L.: Medical progress—Treatment of congestive heart failure by altering loading conditions of the heart. J. Pediatr. 106:697, 1985.
37. Friedman, W. F., and George, B. L.: Treatment of cardiac failure in infants. Compr. Ther. 12:8, 1986.
38. Artman, M., Parrish, M. D., and Graham, T. P., Jr.: Congestive heart failure in childhood and adolescence: Recognition and management. Am. Heart J. 105:471, 1983.
39. Schmidt, K. G., Araujo, L., and Silverman, N. H.: Evaluation of structural and functional abnormalities of the fetal heart by echocardiography. Am. J. Cardiol. Imag. 2:57, 1988.
40. Wyllie, J., Wren, C., and Stewart, H.: Screening for fetal cardiac malformations. Br. Heart J. 71:20, 1994.
41. Meijboom, E. J., Van Engelen, A. D., Van de Beek, E. W., et al.: Fetal arrhythmias. Curr. Opin. Cardiol. 9:97, 1994.
42. Milne, M. J., Sung, R. Y. T., Fok, T. F., and Crozier, I. G.: Doppler echocardiographic assessment of shunting via the ductus arteriosus in newborn infants. Am. J. Cardiol. 64:102, 1989.
43. Sahn, D. J., and Friedman, W. F.: Difficulties in distinguishing cardiac from pulmonary disease in the neonate. Pediatr. Clin. North Am. 20:293, 1973.
44. Stanger, P., Lucas, R. V., Jr., and Edwards, J. E.: Anatomic factors causing respiratory distress in acyanotic congenital cardiac disease: Special reference to bronchial obstruction. Pediatrics 43:760, 1969.

45. DiSessa, T. G., and Friedman, W. F.: Echocardiographic evaluation of cardiac performance. Cardiol. Clin. 1:487, 1983.

46. DiSessa, T. G., and Friedman, W. F.: Echocardiographic evaluation of cardiac performance. In Friedman, W. F., and Higgins, C. B. (eds.): Pediatric Cardiac Imaging. Philadelphia, W. B. Saunders Company, 1984, p. 219.

47. Mercier, J. C., DiSessa, T. G., Jarmakani, J., and Friedman, W. F.: Two dimensional echocardiographic assessment of left ventricular volumes and ejection fraction. Circulation 65:962, 1982.

48. Huwez, F. U., Houston, A. B., Watson, J., et al.: Age and body surface area related normal upper and lower limits of M mode echocardiographic measurements and left ventricular volume and mass from infancy to early adulthood. Br. Heart J. 72:276, 1994.

49. Wessel, A., Schüller, W. C., Yelbuz, T. M., and Bürsch, J. H.: Effect of increased wall thickness on indices of left ventricular pump function in children. Br. Heart J. 72:182, 1994.

50. Teitel, D., and Rudolph, A. M.: Perinatal oxygen delivery and cardiac function. Adv. Pediatr. 32:321, 1985.

51. Rosenthal, A., Nathan, D. G., Marty, A. T., et al.: Acute hemodynamic effects of red cell volume reduction, polycythemia of cyanotic congenital heart disease. Circulation 42:297, 1970.

52. Voigt, G. C., and Wright, J. R.: Cyanotic congenital heart disease and sudden death. Am. Heart J. 87:773, 1974.

53. Fischbein, C. A., Rosenthal, A., Fischer, E. G., et al.: Risk factors for brain abscess in patients with congenital heart disease. Am. J. Cardiol. 34:97, 1974.

54. Corrin, C.: Paradoxical embolism. Br. Heart J. 26:549, 1964.

55. Haroutunian, L. M., and Neill, C. A.: Pulmonary complications of congenital heart disease: Hemoptysis. Am. Heart J. 84:540, 1972.

56. Guntheroth, W. G., Morgan, B. C., and Mullens, G. L.: Physiologic studies of paroxysmal hyperpnea in cyanotic congenital heart disease. Circulation 31:70, 1965.

57. Talmer, N. S.: Congestive heart failure in the infant. Pediatr. Clin. North Am. 18:1011, 1971.

58. Rosenthal, A., and Castaneda, A. R.: Growth and development after cardiovascular surgery in infants and children. In Rosenthal, A., Sonnenblick, E. H., and Lesch, M. (eds.): Postoperative Congestive Heart Disease. New York, Grune and Stratton, 1975, p. 110.

59. Gingell, R. I., and Hornung, M. G.: Growth problems associated with congenital heart disease in infancy. In Lebenthal, E. (ed.): Textbook of Gastroenterology and Nutrition in Infancy. New York, Raven Press, 1989, p. 639.

60. Salzer, H. R., Haschke, F., Wimmer, M., et al.: Growth and nutritional intake of infants with congenital heart disease. Pediatr. Cardiol. 10:17, 1989.

61. Friedman, W. F., Heiferman, M. F., and Perloff, J. K.: Late postoperative pulmonary vascular disease—Clinical concerns. In Engle, M. A., and Perloff, J. K. (eds.): Congenital Heart Disease After Surgery. New York, York Medical Publishers, 1983, p. 151.

62. Rabinovitch, M.: Structure and function of the pulmonary vascular bed: An update. Cardiol. Clin. 7:227, 1989.

63. Rabinovitch, M., Keane, J. F., and Norwood, W. I.: Vascular structure and lung biopsy tissue correlated with pulmonary hemodynamic findings after repair of congenital heart defects. Circulation 69:655, 1984.

64. Heath, D., and Edwards, J. E.: The pathology of hypertensive pulmonary vascular disease. Circulation 18:533, 1958.

65. Levin, D. L., Rudolph, A. M., Heymann, M. A., and Phibbs, R. H.: Morphological development of the pulmonary vascular bed in the fetal lamb. Circulation 53:144, 1976.

66. Burchenal, J. E. B., and Loscalzo, J.: Endothelial dysfunction and pulmonary hypertension. Primary Cardiol. 20:28, 1994.

67. Celermajer, D. S., Dollery, C., Burch, M., and Deanfield, J. E.: Role of endothelium in the maintenance of low pulmonary vascular tone in normal children. Circulation 89:2041, 1994.

68. Rabinovitch, M., and Reid, L. M.: Quantitative structural analysis of the pulmonary vascular bed in congenital heart defects. In Engle, M. A. (ed.): Pediatric Cardiovascular Disease. Philadelphia, F. A. Davis, 1981, p. 149.

69. Friedman, W. F.: Proceedings of the National Heart, Lung and Blood Institute Pediatric Cardiology Workshop: Pulmonary Hypertension. Pediatr. Res. 20:8, 1986.

70. Aiello, V. D., Higuchi, M., Lopes, E. A., et al.: An immunohistochemical study of arterial lesions due to pulmonary hypertension in patients with congenital heart defects. Cardiol Young 4:37, 1994.

71. Hopkins, W., and Waggoner, A. D.: Right and left ventricular area and function determined by two-dimensional echocardiography in adults with the Eisenmenger syndrome from a variety of congenital anomalies. Am. J. Cardiol. 72:90, 1993.

72. Roberts, J. D., Lang, P., Bigatello, L. M., et al.: Inhaled nitric oxide in congenital heart disease. Circulation 87:447, 1992.

73. Rabinovitch, M., Keane, J. F., Fellows, K. E., et al.: Quantitative analysis of the pulmonary wedge angiogram in congenital heart defects. Circulation 63:152, 1981.

74. Rabinovitch, M., Castaneda, A. R., and Reid, L.: Lung biopsy with frozen section as a diagnostic aid in patients with congenital heart defects. Am. J. Cardiol. 47:77, 1981.

75. Rabinovitch, M.: Pathophysiology of pulmonary hypertension. In Emmanouilides, G. C., et al. (eds.): Moss and Adams' Heart Disease in Infants, Children, and Adolescents. 5th ed. Baltimore, Williams and Wilkins, 1994, p. 1659.

76. Zeller, S. T., and Gutgesell, H. P.: Noninvasive estimation of pulmonary artery pressure. J. Pediatr. 114:735, 1989.

77. Morera, J., Hoadley, S. D., Roland, J. M., et al.: Estimation of the ratio of pulmonary to systemic pressures by pulsewave Doppler echocardiography for assessment of pulmonary artery pressures. Am. J. Cardiol. 63:862, 1989.

78. Awadallah, S. M., Kavey, R. E., Byrum, C. J., et al.: The changing pattern of infective endocarditis in childhood. Am. J. Cardiol. 68:90, 1991.

79. Saiman, L., Prince, A., and Gersony, W. M.: Pediatric infective endocarditis in the modern era. J. Pediatr. 122:847, 1993.

80. Van Hare, G. F., Ben-Shachar, G., Liebman, J., et al.: Infective endocarditis in infants and children during the past 10 years: A decade of change. Am. Heart J. 107:1235, 1984.

81. Dajani, A. S.: Prevention of bacterial endocarditis. Pediatr. Infect. Dis. 4:349, 1985.

82. Dajani, A. S., Bisno, A. L., Chung, K. J., et al.: Prevention of bacterial endocarditis: Recommendations by the American Heart Association. JAMA 264:2919, 1990.

83. Selbst, S. M., Ruddy, R. M., Clark, B. J., et al.: Pediatric chest pain: A prospective study. Pediatrics 82:319, 1988.

84. Graham, T. P., Gessner, I. H., Friedman, W. F., et al.: Recommendations for use of laboratory studies for pediatric patients with suspected or proven heart disease: A statement of the Committee on Congenital Cardiac Defects of the Council on Cardiovascular Disease in the Young of the AHA. Circulation 74:443a, 1986.

85. Strieper, M. J., and Campbell, R. M.: Efficacy of alpha-adrenergic agonist therapy for prevention of pediatric neurocardiogenic syncope. J. Am. Coll. Cardiol. 22:594, 1993.

86. Grubb, B. P., Samoil, D., Kosinski, D., et al.: Use of sertraline hydrochloride in the treatment of refractory neurocardiogenic syncope in children and adolescents. J. Am. Coll. Cardiol. 24:490, 1994.

87. Perry, J., and Garson, A.: The child with recurrent syncope: Autonomic function testing and beta-adrenergic hypersensitivity. J. Am. Coll. Cardiol. 17:1168, 1991.

88. Driscoll, D. J., and Edwards, W. D.: Sudden unexpected death in children and adolescents. J. Am. Coll. Cardiol. 5:118B, 1985.

89. Denfield, S. W., and Garson, A., Jr.: Sudden death in children and young adults. Ped. Clin. North Am. 37:215, 1990.

90. Klitzner, T. S.: Sudden cardiac death in children. Circulation 82:629, 1990.

91. Gillette, P. C., and Garson, A.: Sudden cardiac death in the pediatric population. Circulation 85:I, 1992.

APPROACH TO THE HIGH-RISK INFANT

92. Friedman, W. F., and George, B. L.: New concepts and drugs in the treatment of congestive heart failure. Pediatr. Clin. North Am. 31:1197, 1984.

93. Anderson, P. A. W.: Maturation in cardiac contractility. Cardiol. Clin. 7:209, 1989.

94. Talner, N. S., and Lister, G.: Perioperative care of the infant with congenital heart disease. Cardiol. Clin. 7:419, 1989.

95. Park, M. K.: Use of digoxin in infants and children, with specific emphasis on dosage. J. Pediatr. 108:871, 1986.

96. Freed, M. D., Hegmann, M. A., Lewis, A. B., et al.: Prostaglandin E_1 in infants with ductus arteriosus dependent congenital heart disease. Circulation 64:899, 1981.

97. Lewis, A. B., Freed, M. D., Hegmann, M. A., et al.: Side effects of therapy with prostaglandin E_1 in infants with critical congenital heart disease. Circulation 64:893, 1981.

98. Friedman, W. F., Kurlinski, J., Jacob, J., et al.: Inhibition of prostaglandin and prostacyclin synthesis in clinical management of PDA. Semin. Perinatol. 4:125, 1980.

99. Friedman, W. F.: Patent ductus arteriosus in respiratory distress syndrome. Pediatr. Cardiol. 4(Suppl. 2):3, 1983.

100. Montigny, M., Davignon, A., Fouron, J. C., et al.: Captopril in infants for congestive heart failure secondary to a large ventricular to right shunt. Am. J. Cardiol. 63:631, 1989.

101. Schwartz, K., Chassagne, C., and Boheler, K. R.: The molecular biology of heart failure. J. Am. Coll. Cardiol. 22:30A, 1993.

102. Carter, L. F., and Rubin, S. A.: The molecular and cellular biology of heart failure. Curr. Opin. Cardiol. 8:361, 1993.

103. Snyder, J. V.: Assessment of systemic oxygen transport. In Snyder, J. V. (ed.): Oxygen Transport in the Clinically Ill. Chicago, Year Book Medical Publishing Co., 1987, p. 179.

104. Kleinman, C. S., and Donnerstein, R. L.: Ultrasonic assessment of cardiac function in the intact human fetus. J. Am. Coll. Cardiol. 5:84S, 1985.

105. Silverman, N. H., Kleinman, C. S., Rudolph, A. M., et al.: Fetal atrioventricular valve insufficiency associated with nonimmune hydrops: A two-dimensional echocardiographic and pulsed Doppler ultrasound study. Circulation 72:825, 1985.

106. Reed, K. L., Appelton, C. P., Anderson, C. F., et al.: Doppler studies of venacaval flows in human fetuses. Circulation 81:498, 1990.

107. Gembruch, U., Manz, M., Bald, R., et al.: Repeated intravascular treatment with amiodarone in a fetus with refractory supraventricular tachycardia and hydrops fetalis. Am. Heart J. 118:1335, 1989.

108. Silverman, N. H., and Schmidt, K. G.: The current role of Doppler echocardiography in the diagnosis of heart disease in children. Cardiol. Clin. 7:265, 1989.

109. Cloez, J. L., Schmidt, K. G., Birk, E., and Silverman, N. H.: Determina-

tion of pulmonary systemic blood flow ratio in children by simplified Doppler echocardiographic method. J. Am. Coll. Cardiol. *11*:825, 1988.

110. Sahn, D. J.: Applications of color flow mapping in pediatric cardiology. Cardiol. Clin. *7*:255, 1989.

111. Krabill, K. A., Ring, W. S., Foker, J. E., et al.: Echocardiographic versus cardiac catheterization diagnosis of infants with congenital heart disease requiring cardiac surgery. Am. J. Cardiol. *60*:351, 1987.

112. Beekman, R. P., Filippini, L. H. P. M., and Meijboom, E. J.: Evolving usage of pediatric cardiac catheterization. Curr. Opin. Cardiol. *9*:721, 1994.

113. Stanger, P., Heymann, M. A., Tarnoff, H., et al.: Complications of cardiac catheterization of neonates, infants and children. Circulation *50*:595, 1974.

114. Allen, H. D., Driscoll, D. J., Fricker, F. J., et al.: Guidelines for pediatric therapeutic cardiac catheterization. Circulation *84*:2248, 1991.

115. Tynan, M., and Qureshi, S.: Interventional catheterization in congenital heart disease. Curr. Opin. Cardiol. *8*:114, 1993.

116. Hebe, J., Schluter, M., and Kuck, K. H.: Catheter ablation in children with supraventricular tachycardia mediated by accessory pathways— use of radiofrequency current as a first line of therapy. Cardiol. Young *4*:28, 1994.

117. Kugler, J. D., Danford, D. A., and Deal, B. J.: Radiofrequency catheter ablation for tachyarrhythmias in children and adolescents. N. Engl. J. Med. *330*:1481, 1994.

118. Zipes, D. P., Akthar, M., Denes, P., et al.: Guidelines for clinical intracardiac electrophysiologic studies: A report of the American College of Cardiology/AHA Task Force on assessment of diagnostic and therapeutic cardiovascular procedures. J. Am. Coll. Cardiol. *14*:1827, 1989.

119. Klitzner, T. S., Wetzel, G. T., Saxon, L. A., and Stevenson, W. G.: Radiofrequency ablation: A new era in the management of pediatric arrhythmias. Am. J. Dis. Child. *147*:769, 1993.

120. Van Hare, G. F., Lesh, M. D., and Stanger, P.: Radiofrequency catheter ablation of supraventricular arrhythmias in patients with congenital heart disease: Results and technical considerations. J. Am. Coll. Cardiol. *22*:883, 1993.

121. Dhala, A., Bremner, S., Deshpande, S., et al.: Efficacy and safety of atrioventricular nodal modification for atrioventricular nodal reentrant tachycardia in the pediatric population. Am. Heart J. *128*:903, 1994.

SPECIFIC CARDIAC DEFECTS

122. Hunt, C. E., and Lucas, R. V., Jr.: Symptomatic atrial septal defect in infancy. Circulation *42*:1042, 1973.

123. Van Praagh, S., Carrera, M. E., Sanders, S. P., et al.: Sinus venosus defects: Unroofing of the right pulmonary veins—anatomic and echocardiographic findings and surgical treatment. Am. Heart J. *128*:365, 1994.

124. Bashi, V. V., Ravikumar, E., Jairaj, P. S., et al.: Coexistent mitral valve disease with left-to-right shunt at the atrial level: Clinical profile, hemodynamics, and surgical considerations in 67 consecutive patients. Am. Heart J. *114*:1406, 1987.

125. Leachman, R. D., Cokkinos, D. V., and Cooley, D. A.: Association of ostium secundum atrial septal defects with mitral valve prolapse. Am. J. Cardiol. *38*:167, 1976.

126. Levin, A. R., Spach, M. S., Boineau, J. P., et al.: Atrial pressure flow dynamics and atrial septal defects (secundum type). Circulation *37*:476, 1968.

127. O'Toole, J. D., Reddy, I., Curtiss., E. I., and Shaver, J. A.: The mechanism of splitting the second heart sound in atrial septal defect. Circulation *41*:1047, 1977.

128. Clark, E. B., and Kugler, J. D.: Preoperative secundum atrial septal defect with coexisting sinus node and atrioventricular node dysfunction. Circulation *65*:976, 1982.

129. Konstantinides, S., Kasper, W., Geibel, A., et al.: Detection of left-to-right shunt in atrial septal defect by negative contrast echocardiography: A comparison of transthoracic and transesophageal approach. Am. Heart J. *126*:909, 1993.

130. Ishii, M., Kato, H., Inoue, O., et al.: Biplane transesophageal echo-Doppler studies of atrial septal defects: Quantitative evaluation and monitoring for transcatheter closure. Am. Heart J. *125*:1363, 1993.

131. Shub, C., Tajik., A. J., Seward, J. B., et al.: Surgical repair of uncomplicated atrial septal defect without "routine" preoperative cardiac catheterization. J. Am. Coll. Cardiol. *6*:49, 1985.

132. Freed, M. D., Nadas, A. S., Norwood, W. I., and Castaneda, A. R.: Is routine preoperative cardiac catheterization necessary before repair of secundum and sinus venosus atrial septal defects? J. Am. Coll. Cardiol. *4*:333, 1984.

133. Taketa, R. M., Sahn, D. J., Simon, A. L., et al.: Catheter positions in congenital cardiac malformations. Circulation *51*:749, 1975.

134. Brand, A., Keren, A., Branski, D., et al.: Natural course of atrial septal aneurysm in children and the potential for spontaneous closure of associated septal defect. Am. J. Cardiol. *64*:996, 1989.

135. Steele, P. M., Fuster, V., Cohen, M., et al.: Isolated atrial septal defect with pulmonary vascular obstructive disease—long term follow up and prediction of outcome after surgical correction. Circulation *76*:1037, 1987.

136. Lloyd, T. R., Rao, P. S., Beekman, R. H., et al.: Atrial septal defect occlusion with the buttoned device (a multi-institutional U.S. trial). Am. J. Cardiol. *73*:286, 1994.

137. Hausdorf, G., Schneider, M., Franzbach, B., et al.: Transcatheter closure of secundum atrial septal defects with the atrial septal defect occlusion system (ASDOS): Initial experience in children. Heart *75*:83, 1996.

138. Reddy, S. C. B., Rao, P. S., Ewenko, J., et al.: Echocardiographic predictors of success of catheter closure of atrial septal defect with the buttoned device. Am. Heart J. *129*:76, 1995.

138a. Auslender, M., Beekman, R. H., and Lloyd, T. R.: Transcatheter closure of atrial septal defects. J. Interven. Cardiol. *8*:533, 1995.

139. Levin, A. R., Liebson, P. R., Ehlers, K. H., and Daimant, B.: Assessment of left ventricular function in atrial septal defect. Pediatr. Res. *9*:894, 1975.

140. Epstein, S. E., Beiser, G. D., Goldstein, R. E., et al.: Hemodynamic abnormalities in response to mild and intense upright exercise following operative correction of an atrial septal defect or tetralogy of Fallot. Circulation *42*:1065, 1973.

141. Murphy, J. G., Gersh, B. J., McGoon, M. D., et al.: Long term outcome after surgical repair of isolated atrial septal defect. N. Engl. J. Med. *323*:1645, 1990.

142. Karpawich, P. P., Antillon, J. R., Cappola, P. R., and Agarwal, K. C.: Pre- and postoperative electrophysiologic assessment of children with secundum atrial septal defect. Am. J. Cardiol. *55*:519, 1985.

143. Bink-Boelkens, M. T. E., Bergstra, A., and Landsman, M. L. J.: Functional abnormalities of the conduction system in children with an atrial septal defect. Int. J. Cardiol. *20*:263, 1988.

144. Bink-Boelkens, M. T. E., Meuzelaar, K. J., and Eygelaar, A.: Arrhythmias after repair of secundum atrial septal defect: The influence of surgical modification. Am. Heart J. *115*:629, 1988.

145. Borkon, A. M., Pieroni, D. R., Varghese, P. J., et al.: The superior QRS axis in ostium primum ASD. Am. Heart J. *92*:15, 1975.

146. Jacobsen, J. R., Gillette, P. C., Corbett, B. N., et al.: Intracardiac electrography in endocardial cushion defects. Circulation *54*:599, 1976.

147. Waldo, A. L., Kaiser, G. A., Bowman, F. O., Jr., and Malm, J. R.: Etiology of prolongation of the PR interval in patients with an endocardial cushion defect. Circulation *43*:19, 1973.

148. Zellers, T. M., Zehr, R., Weinstein, E., et al.: Two-dimensional and Doppler echocardiography alone can adequately define preoperative anatomy and hemodynamic status before repair of complete atrioventricular septal defect in infants <1 year old. J. Am. Coll. Cardiol. *24*:1565, 1994.

149. Minich, L. A., Snider, A. R., Bove, E. L., et al.: Echocardiographic evaluation of atrioventricular orifice anatomy in children with atrioventricular septal defect. J. Am. Coll. Cardiol. *19*:149, 1992.

150. DeBia, S. E. L., DiCommo, V., Ballerini, L., et al.: Prevalence of left-sided obstructive lesions in patients with atrial ventricular canal without Down's syndrome. J. Thorac. Cardiovasc. Surg. *91*:467, 1986.

151. Elliott, L. P., Bargeron, L. M., Jr., and Green, C. E.: Angled angiography: General approach and findings. *In* Friedman, W. F., and Higgins, C. B. (eds.): Pediatric Cardiac Imaging. Philadelphia, W. B. Saunders Company, 1984, p. 1.

152. Merrill, W. H., Hammon, J. W., Jr., and Bender, H. W., Jr.: Technique of repair of atrioventricular septal defect with a common atrioventricular orifice. Cardiol. Young *1*:379, 1991.

153. Kadoba, K., and Jonas, R. A.: Replacement of the left atrioventricular valve after repair of atrioventricular septal defect. Cardiol. Young *1*:383, 1991.

154. DeLeon, S. Y., Ilbawi, M. N., Wilson, W. R., et al.: Surgical options in subaortic stenosis associated with endocardial cushion defects. Ann. Thorac. Surg. *52*:1076, 1991.

155. Gatzoulis, M. A., Yacoub, M., and Shinebourne, E. A.: Complete atrioventricular septal defect with tetralogy of Fallot: Diagnosis and management. Br. Heart J. *71*:579, 1994.

156. Soto, B., Ceballos, R., and Kirklin, J. W.: Ventricular septal defects: A surgical viewpoint. J. Am. Coll. Cardiol. *14*:1291, 1989.

157. Van Praagh, R., Geva, T., and Kreutzer, J.: Ventricular septal defects: How shall we describe, name and classify them? J. Am. Coll. Cardiol. *14*:1298, 1989.

158. Hagler, D. J., Edwards, W. D., Seward, J. B., and Tajik, A. J.: Standardized nomenclature of the ventricular septum and ventricular septal defects, with applications for two-dimensional echocardiography. Mayo Clin. Proc. *60*:741, 1985.

159. Baker, E. J., Leung, M. P., Anderson, R. H., et al.: The cross-sectional anatomy of ventricular septal defects: A reappraisal. Br. Heart J. *69*:339, 1988.

160. Helmcke, F., Souza, A., Nanda, N. C., et al.: Two-dimensional and color Doppler assessment of ventricular septal defect of congenital origin. Am. J. Cardiol. *63*:1112, 1989.

161. Sharif, D. S., Huhta, J. C., Marantz, P., et al.: Two-dimensional echocardiographic determination of ventricular septal defect size: Correlation of autopsy. Am. Heart J. *117*:1333, 1989.

162. Ortiz, E., Robinson, P. J., Deanfield, J. E., et al.: Localisation of ventricular septal defects by simultaneous display of superimposed colour Doppler and cross sectional echocardiographic images. Br. Heart J. *54*:53, 1985.

163. Pieroni, D. R., Nishimura, R. A., Bierman, F. Z., et al.: Second natural history study of congenital heart defects: Ventricular septal defect: Echocardiography. Circulation *87*:I, 1993.

164. Murphy, D. J., Ludomirsky, A., and Huhta, J. C.: Continuous-wave Doppler in children with ventricular septal defect: Noninvasive estimation of interventricular pressure gradient. Am. J. Cardiol. *57*:428, 1986.

165. Kurokawa, S., Takahashi, M., Katoh, Y., et al.: Noninvasive evaluation of the ratio of pulmonary to systemic flow in ventricular septal defect

by means of Doppler two-dimensional echocardiography. Am. Heart J. *116*:1033, 1988.

166. Williams, R. G.: Doppler color-flow mapping and prediction of ventricular defect outcome. J. Am. Coll. Cardiol. *13*:1119, 1989.

167. Hornberger, L. K., Sahn, D. J., Krabill, K. A., et al.: Elucidation of the natural history of ventricular septal defects by serial Doppler color-flow mapping studies. J. Am. Coll. Cardiol. *13*:1111, 1989.

168. Friedman, W. F., Mehrizi, A., and Pusch, A. L.: Multiple muscular ventricular septal defects. Circulation *32*:35, 1964.

169. Dickinson, D. F., Arnold, R., and Wilkinson, J. L.: Ventricular septal defects in children born in Liverpool: Evaluation of natural course and surgical implications in an unselected population. Br. Heart J. *46*:47, 1981.

170. Weidman, W. H., Blount, S. G., Jr., DuShane, J. W., et al.: Clinical course in ventricular septal defect: Natural history study. Circulation *56*(Suppl.):I, 1977.

171. Ramaciotti, C., Keren, A., and Silverman, N. H.: Importance of (perimembranous) ventricular septal aneurysm in the natural history of isolated perimembranous ventricular septal defect. Am. J. Cardiol. *57*:268, 1986.

172. Friedman, W. F., and Pitlick, P. T.: Ventricular septal defect in infancy —University of California, San Diego (Specialty Conference). West. J. Med. *120*:295, 1974.

173. Moe, D. J., and Guntheroth, W. G.: Spontaneous closure of uncomplicated ventricular septal defect. Am. J. Cardiol. *60*:674, 1987.

174. Neutze, J. M., Ishikawa, T., Clarkson, P. M., et al.: Assessment and follow up of patients with ventricular septal defect and elevated pulmonary vascular resistance. Am. J. Cardiol. *63*:327, 1989.

175. Van Den Heuvel, F., Timmers, T., and Hess, J.: Morphological, haemodynamic, and clinical variables as predictors for management of isolated ventricular septal defect. Br. Heart J. *73*:49, 1995.

176. Kidd, L., Driscoll, D. J., Gersony, W. M., et al.: Second natural history study of congenital heart defects: Results of treatment of patients with ventricular septal defects. Circulation *87*:I, 1993.

177. Yeager, S. B., Freed, M. D., Keane, J. F., et al.: Primary surgical closure of ventricular septal defect in the first year of life: Results in 128 infants. J. Am. Coll. Cardiol. *3*:1269, 1984.

178. Kirkllin, J. W., and Barrett-Boyes, B. J. (eds.): Cardiac Surgery. 2nd ed. New York, Churchill Livingstone, 1993, p. 798.

179. McDaniel, N., Gutgesell, H. P., Nolan, S. P., and Kron, I. L.: Repair of large muscular ventricular septal defects in infants employing left ventriculotomy. Ann. Thorac. Surg. *47*:593, 1989.

180. Gheen, K. M., and Reeves, J. T.: Effects of size of ventricular septal defect and age on pulmonary hemodynamics at sea level. Am. J. Cardiol. *75*:66, 1995.

181. Hislop, A., Haworth, S. G., Shinebourne, E. A., and Reid, L.: Quantitative structural analysis of pulmonary vessels in isolated ventricular septal defect in infancy. Br. Heart J. *37*:1014, 1975.

182. DuShane, J. W., and Kirklin, J. W.: Late results of the repair of ventricular septal defect on pulmonary vascular disease. *In* Kirklin, J. W. (ed.): Advances in Cardiovascular Surgery. New York, Grune and Stratton, 1973, p. 9.

183. Rhodes, L. A., Keane, J. F., Keane, J. P., et al.: Long-term follow up (up to 43 years) of ventricular septal defect with audible aortic regurgitation. Am. J. Cardiol. *66*:340, 1990.

184. Schmidt, K. G., Cassidy, S. C., Silverman, N. H., and Stanger, P.: Doubly committed subarterial ventricular septal defects: Echocardiographic features and surgical implications. J. Am. Coll. Cardiol. *12*:1538, 1988.

185. Wang, J. K., Lue, H. C., Wu, M. H., et al.: Assessment of ventricular septal defect with aortic valve prolapse by means of echocardiography and angiography. Cardiol. Young *4*:44, 1994.

186. Bonhoeffer, P., Fabbrocini, M., Lecompte, Y., et al.: Infundibular septal defect with severe aortic regurgitation: A new surgical approach. Ann. Thorac. Surg. *53*:851, 1992.

187. Ramaciotti, C., Vetter, J. M., Bornemeier, R. A., and Chin, A. J.: Prevalence, relation to spontaneous closure, and association of muscular ventricular septal defects with other cardiac defects. Am. J. Cardiol. *75*:61, 1995.

188. Leung, M. P., Mok, C. K., Lo, R. N. S., and Lau, K. C.: An echocardiographic study of perimembranous ventricular septal defect with left ventricular to right atrial shunting. Br. Heart J. *55*:45, 1986.

189. Gersony, W. M., and Hayes, C. J.: Bacterial endocarditis in patients with pulmonary stenosis, aortic stenosis, or ventricular septal defect: Natural history study. Circulation *56*(Suppl.):I, 1977.

190. deLeval, M.: Ventricular septal defects. *In* Stark, J., and deLeval, M. (eds.): Surgery for Congenital Heart Defects. New York, Grune and Stratton, Inc., 1983, p. 271.

191. Waldman, J. D.: Why not close a small ventricular septal defect? Ann. Thorac. Surg. *56*:1011, 1993.

192. Van Der Velde, M. E., Sanders, S. P., Keane, J. F., et al.: Transesophageal echocardiographic guidance of transcatheter ventricular septal defect closure. J. Am. Coll. Cardiol. *23*:1660, 1994.

193. Tee, S. D. C., Shiota, T., Weintraub, R., et al.: Evaluation of ventricular septal defect by transesophageal echocardiography: Intraoperative assessment. Am. Heart J. *127*:585, 1994.

194. Rigby, M., and Redington, A. N.: Primary transcatheter umbrella closure of perimembranous ventricular septal defect. Br. Heart J. *72*:368, 1994.

195. Okarama, E. O., Guller, B., Molony, J. D., and Weidman, W. H.: Etiology of right bundle-branch block pattern after surgical closure of ventricular-septal defects. Am. Heart J. *90*:14, 1975.

196. Otterstad, J. E., Simonsen, S., and Erikssen, J.: Hemodynamic findings at rest and during mild supine exercise in adults with isolated uncomplicated ventricular septal defects. Circulation *71*:650, 1985.

197. Maron, B. J., Redwood, D. R., Hirschfield, J. W., Jr., et al.: Postoperative assessment of patients with ventricular septal defect and pulmonary hypertension: Response to intense upright exercise. Circulation *48*:864, 1973.

198. Graham, T. P., Jr., Atwood, G. F., Boucek, R. J., Jr., et al.: Right ventricular volume characteristics in ventricular septal defect. Circulation *54*:800, 1976.

199. Heymann, M. A., and Rudolph, A. M.: Control of the ductus arteriosus. Physiol. Rev. *55*:62, 1975.

200. Friedman, W. F., Printz, M. P., Kirkpatrick, S. E., and Hoskins, E. J.: The vasoactivity of the fetal lamb ductus arteriosus studied in utero. Pediatr. Res. *17*:331, 1983.

201. Skidgel, R. A., Friedman, W. F., and Printz, M. P.: Prostaglandin biosynthetic activities of the fetal lamb ductus arteriosus, other blood vessels and fetal lung. Pediatr. Res. *18*:12, 1984.

202. Printz, M. P., Skidgel, R. A., and Friedman, W. F.: Studies of pulmonary prostaglandin biosynthetic and catabolic enzymes as factors in ductus arteriosus patency and closure: Evidence for a shift in products with gestational age. Pediatr. Res. *18*:19, 1984.

203. Gittenberger-DeGroot, A. C.: Persistent ductus arteriosus: Most probably a primary congenital malformation. Br. Heart J. *39*:610, 1977.

204. Friedman, W. F., Hirschklau, M. J., Printz, M. P., et al.: Pharmacologic closure of patent ductus arteriosus in the premature infant. N. Engl. J. Med. *295*:526, 1976.

205. Douidar, S. M., Richardson, J., and Snodgrass, W. R.: Use of indomethacin in ductus closure: An update evaluation. Dev. Pharmacol. Ther. *11*:196, 1988.

206. Shimada, S., Kasai, T., Konishi, M., et al.: Effects of patent ductus arteriosus on left ventricular output and organ blood flows in preterm infants with respiratory distress syndrome treated with surfactant. J. Pediatr. *125*:270, 1994.

207. Sahn, D. J., Vaucher, Y., Williams, D. E., et al.: Echocardiographic detection of large left to right shunts and cardiomyopathies in infants and children. Am. J. Cardiol. *38*:73, 1976.

208. Liao, P. K., Su, W. J., and Hung, J. S.: Doppler echocardiographic flow characteristics of isolated patent ductus arteriosus: Better delineation by Doppler color-flow mapping. J. Am. Coll. Cardiol. *12*:1285, 1988.

209. Hiraishi, S., Horiguchi, Y., Misawa, H., et al.: Noninvasive Doppler echocardiographic evaluation of shunt flow dynamics of the ductus arteriosus. Circulation *75*:1146, 1987.

210. Yeh, T. F., Achanti, B., Patel, H., and Pildes, R. S.: Indomethacin therapy in premature infants with patent ductus arteriosus—determination of therapeutic plasma levels. Dev. Pharmacol. Ther. *12*:169, 1989.

211. Jacob, J., Gluck, L., DiSessa, T. G., et al.: The contribution of PDA in the neonate with severe RDS. J. Pediatr. *96*:79, 1980.

212. Merritt, T. A., Harris, J. P., and Roghmann, K.: Early closure of the patent ductus arteriosus in very low birth weight infants: A controlled trial. J. Pediatr. *99*:281, 1981.

213. Gersony, W. M., Peckham, G. J., Ellison, R. C., et al.: Effects of indomethacin in premature infants with patent ductus arteriosus: Results of a national collaborative study. J. Pediatr. *102*:895, 1983.

214. Cassady, G., Crouse, D. T., Kirklin, J. W., et al.: A randomized control trial of very early prophylactic ligation of the ductus arteriosus in babies who weighed 1000 g or less at birth. N. Engl. J. Med. *320*:1511, 1989.

215. Wagner, H. R., Ellison, R. C., Zierler, S., et al.: Surgical closure of patent ductus arteriosus in 268 preterm infants. J. Thorac. Cardiovasc. Surg. *87*:870, 1984.

216. Jarmakini, M. M., Graham, T. P., Jr., Canent, R. V., Jr., et al.: Effect of site of shunt on left heart volume characteristics in children with ventricular septal defect and patent ductus arteriosus. Circulation *40*:411, 1969.

217. Bessenger, F. B., Jr., Blieden, L. C., and Edwards, J. E.: Hypertensive pulmonary vascular disease associated with patent ductus arteriosus. Circulation *52*:157, 1975.

218. Moore, J. W., George, L., Kirkpatrick, S. E., et al.: Percutaneous closure of the small patent ductus arteriosus using occluding spring coils. J. Am. Coll. Cardiol. *23*:759, 1994.

219. Magee, A. G., Stumper, O., Burns, J. E., et al.: Medium-term follow up of residual shunting and potential complications after transcatheter occlusion of the ductus arteriosus. Br. Heart J. *71*:63, 1994.

220. Verin, V. E., Saveliev, S. V., Kolody, S. M., et al.: Results of transcatheter closure of the patent ductus arteriosus with the Botallooccluder. J. Am. Coll. Cardiol. *22*:1509, 1993.

221. Schräder, R., Kneissl, G. D., Sievert, H., et al.: Nonoperative closure of the patent ductus arteriosus: The Frankfurt experience. J. Interven. Cardiol. *5*:89, 1992.

222. Galal, O., de Moor, M., Al-Fadley, F., and Hijazi, Z. M.: Transcatheter closure of the patent ductus arteriosus: Comparison between the Rashkind occluder device and the anterograde Gianturco coils technique. Am. Heart J. *131*:368, 1996.

223. Gray, D. T., Fyler, D. C., Walker, A. M., et al.: Clinical outcomes and costs of transcatheter as compared with surgical closure of patent ductus arteriosus. N. Engl. J. Med. *329*:1517, 1993.

224. Gray, D. T., Walker, A. M., Fyler, D. C., et al.: Examination of the early "learning curve" for transcatheter closure of patent ductus arteriosus using the Rashkind occluder. Circulation *90*:36, 1994.

224a. Moore, J. W., and Cambier, P. A.: Transcatheter occlusion of patent ductus arteriosus. J. Interven. Cardiol. 8:517, 1995.

225. Kutsche, L. M., and Van Mierop, L. H. S.: Anatomy and pathogenesis of aorticopulmonary septal defect. Am. J. Cardiol. 59:443, 1987.

226. Matsuki, O., Yagihara, T., Yamamoto, F., et al.: New surgical technique for total-defect aortopulmonary window. Ann. Thorac. Surg. 54:991, 1992.

227. Prasad, T. R., Valiathan, M. S., Chyamakrishnan, K. G., et al.: Surgical management of aortopulmonary septal defect. Ann. Thorac. Surg. 47:877, 1989.

228. Crupi, G., Macartney, F. J., and Anderson, R. H.: Persistent truncus arteriosus: A study of 66 autopsy cases with special reference to definition and morphogenesis. Am. J. Cardiol. 40:569, 1977.

229. Shrivastava, F., and Edwards, J. E.: Coronary arterial origin and persistent truncus arteriosus. Circulation 55:551, 1977.

230. Suzuki, A., Ho, S. Y., Anderson, R. H., and Deanfield, J. E.: Coronary arterial and sinusal anatomy in hearts with a common arterial trunk. Ann. Thorac. Surg. 48:792, 1989.

231. Calder, L., Van Praagh, R., Sears, W. P., et al.: Truncus arteriosus communis. Am. Heart J. 92:23, 1976.

232. Juaneda, E., and Haworth, S. G.: Pulmonary vascular disease in children with truncus arteriosus. Am. J. Cardiol. 54:1314, 1984.

233. Radford, D. J., Perkins, L., Lachman, R., and Thong, Y. H.: Spectrum of DiGeorge syndrome in patients with truncus arteriosus: Expanded DiGeorge syndrome. Pediatr. Cardiol. 9:95, 1988.

234. Kirby, M. L., and Waldo, K. L.: Role of neural crest in congenital heart disease. Circulation 82:332, 1990.

235. Gelband, H., Van Meter, S., and Gersony, W. M.: Truncal valve abnormalities in infants with persistent truncus arteriosus. Circulation 45:397, 1972.

236. Yoshizato, T., and Julsrud, P. R.: Truncus arteriosus revisited: An angiographic demonstration. Pediatr. Cardiol. 11:36, 1990.

237. Bove, E. L., Beekman, R. H., Snider, A. R., et al.: Repair of truncus arteriosus in the neonate and young infant. Ann. Thorac. Surg. 47:499, 1989.

238. Hanley, F. L., Heinemann, M. K., Jonas, R. A., et al.: Repair of truncus arteriosus in the neonate. J. Thorac. Cardiovasc. Surg. 105:1047, 1993.

239. Heinemann, M. K., Hanley, F. L., Fenton, K. N., et al.: Fate of small homograft conduits after early repair of truncus arteriosus. Ann. Thorac. Surg. 55:1409, 1993.

240. Davis, J. T., Allen, H. D., Wheler, J. J., et al.: Coronary artery fistula in the pediatric age group: A 19-year institutional experience. Ann. Thorac. Surg. 58:760, 1994.

241. Yoshikawa, J., Katao, H., Yanagihara, K., et al.: Noninvasive visualization of the dilated main coronary arteries in coronary artery fistulas by cross-sectional echocardiography. Circulation 65:600, 1993.

242. Miyatake, K., Okamoto, M., Kinoshita, N., et al.: Doppler echocardiographic features of coronary arteriovenous fistula: Complementary roles of cross sectional echocardiography and the Doppler technique. Br. Heart J. 51:508, 1984.

243. Hofbeck, M., Wild, F., and Singer, H.: Improved visualisation of a coronary artery fist by the "laid-back" aortogram. Br. Heart J. 70:272, 1993.

244. Perry, S. B., Rome, J., Keane, J. F., et al.: Transcatheter closure of coronary artery fistulas. J. Am. Coll. Cardiol. 20:205, 1992.

245. Ruttenhouse, E. A., Doty, D. B., and Ehrenhaft, J. L.: Congenital coronary artery-cardiac chamber fistula: Review of operative management. Ann. Thorac. Surg. 20:468, 1975.

246. Angelini, P.: Normal and anomalous coronary arteries: Definitions and classification. Am. Heart J. 117:418, 1989.

247. Celermajer, D. S., Sholler, G. F., Howman-Giles, R., and Celermajer, J. M.: Myocardial infarction in childhood: Clinical analysis of 17 cases and medium term follow up of survivors. Br. Heart J. 65:332, 1991.

248. Hurwitz, R. A., Caldwell, R. L., Girod, D. A., et al.: Clinical and hemodynamic course of infants and children with anomalous left coronary artery. Am. Heart J. 118:1176, 1989.

249. Menahem, S., and Venables, A. W.: Anomalous left coronary artery from the pulmonary artery: A 15-year sample. Br. Heart J. 58:378, 1987.

250. Johnsrude, C. L., Perry, J. C., Cecchin, F., et al.: Differentiating anomalous left main coronary artery originating from the pulmonary artery in infants from myocarditis and dilated cardiomyopathy by electrocardiogram. Am. J. Cardiol. 75:71, 1995.

251. Karr, S. S., Parness, I. A., Spevak, P. J., et al.: Diagnosis of anomalous left coronary artery by Doppler color flow mapping: Distinction from other causes of dilated cardiomyopathy. J. Am. Coll. Cardiol. 19:1271, 1992.

252. Schmidt, K. G., Cooper, M. J., Silverman, N. H., and Stanger, P.: Pulmonary artery origin of the left coronary artery: Diagnosis by two-dimensional echocardiography, pulsed Doppler ultrasound and color-flow mapping. J. Am. Coll. Cardiol. 11:396, 1988.

253. Vouhe, P. R., Tamisier, D., Sidi, D., et al.: Anomalous left coronary artery from the pulmonary artery: Results of isolated aortic reimplantation. Ann. Thorac. Surg. 54:621, 1992.

254. Fernandes, E. D., Kadivar, H., Hallman, G. L., et al.: Congenital malformations of the coronary arteries: The Texas Heart Institute experience. Ann. Thorac. Surg. 54:732, 1992.

255. Francois, K., Provenier, F., Jordaens, L., and Van Nooten, G. J.: Anomalous origin of the left coronary artery from the pulmonary artery. Ann. Thorac. Surg. 56:1168, 1993.

256. Dua, R., Smith, J. A., Wilkinson, J. L., et al.: Long-term follow-up after two coronary repair of anomalous left coronary artery from the pulmonary artery. J. Cardiovasc. Surg. 8:384, 1993.

257. Boutefeu, J. M., Morat, P. R., Hahn, C., and Hauf, E.: Aneurysms of the sinus of Valsalva: Report of seven cases in review of the literature. Am. J. Med. 65:18, 1978.

258. Perry, L. W., Martin, G. R., Galioto, F. M., Midgley, F. M.: Rupture of congenital sinus of valsalva aneurysm in a newborn. Am. J. Cardiol. 68:1255, 1991.

259. Holdright, D. R., Brecker, S., and Sheppard, M.: Ruptured aneurysm of the sinus of Valsalva—difficulties in establishing the diagnosis. Cardiol. Young 5:75, 1995.

260. Barragry, T. P., Ring, W. S., Moller, J. H., and Lillehei, C. W.: 15 to 30 year follow up of patients undergoing repair of ruptured congenital aneurysms of the sinus of Valsalva. Ann. Thorac. Surg. 46:515, 1988.

261. Smyth, P. T., and Edwards, J. E.: Pseudocoarctation, kinking or buckling of the aorta. Circulation 46:1027, 1972.

262. Hutchins, G. M.: Coarctation of the aorta explained as a branch point of the ductus arteriosus. Am. J. Pathol. 63:203, 1971.

263. Talner, N. S., and Berman, M. A.: Postnatal development of obstruction in coarctation of the aorta: Role of the ductus arteriosus. Pediatrics 56:562, 1975.

264. Heymann, M. A., Berman, W., Jr., Rudolph, A. M., and Whitman, V.: Dilatation of the ductus arteriosus by prostaglandin E₁ in aortic arch abnormalities. Circulation 59:169, 1979.

265. Van Son, J. A. M., Skotnicki, S. H., Van Asten, W. N., et al.: Quantitative assessment of coarctation in infancy by Doppler spectral analysis. Am. J. Cardiol. 63:1282, 1989.

266. Rao, P. S., and Carey, P.: Doppler ultrasound in the prediction of pressure gradients across aortic coarctation. Am. Heart J. 118:299, 1989.

267. Godwin, G. D., Herfkens, R. L., Brundage, D. H., and Lipton, N. J.: Evaluation of coarctation of the aorta by computed tomography. J. Comput. Assist. Tomogr. 5:153, 1981.

268. Mohiaddin, R. H., Kilner, P. J., Rees, S., et al.: Magnetic resonance volume flow and jet velocity mapping in aortic coarctation. J. Am. Coll. Cardiol. 22:1515, 1993.

269. George, B., DiSessa, T. G., Williams, R. G., et al.: Coarctation repair without cardiac catheterization in infants. Am. Heart J. 114:1421, 1987.

270. DeGroff, C. G., Rice, M. J., Reller, M. D., et al.: Intravascular ultrasound can assist angiographic assessment of coarctation of the aorta. Am. Heart J. 128:836, 1994.

271. Rao, P. S., Galal, O., Smith, P. A., and Wilson, A. D.: Five- to nine-year follow-up results of balloon angioplasty of native aortic coarctation in infants and children. J. Am. Coll. Cardiol. 27:462, 1996.

271a. Ino, T., Nishimoto, K., Akimoto, K., et al.: Prospective study on a new therapeutic strategy for infants and children with aortic coarctation. Cardiol. Young 5:36, 1995.

271b. Fletcher, S., Nihill, M. R., Grifka, R. G., et al.: Balloon angioplasty of native coarctation of the aorta: Midterm follow-up and prognostic factors. J. Am. Coll. Cardiol. 25:730, 1995.

271c. Mendelsohn, A. M.: Balloon angioplasty for native coarctation of the aorta. J. Interven. Cardiol. 8:487, 1995.

272. Johnson, M. C., Canter, C. E., Strauss, A. W., et al.: Repair of coarctation of the aorta in infancy: Comparison of surgical and balloon angioplasty. Am. Heart J. 125:464, 1993.

273. Rao, P. S., Chopra, P. S., Koscik, R., et al.: Surgical versus balloon therapy for aortic coarctation in infants ≤3 months old. J. Am. Coll. Cardiol. 23:1479, 1994.

274. Shaddy, R. E., Boucek, M. M., Sturtevant, J. E., et al.: Comparison of angioplasty and surgery for unoperated coarctation of the aorta. Circulation 87:793, 1993.

275. Merrill, W. H., Hoff, S. J., Stewart, J. R., et al.: Operative risk factors and durability of repair of coarctation of the aorta in the neonate. Ann. Thorac. Surg. 58:399, 1994.

276. Kopf, G. S., Hellenbrand, W., Kleinman, C., et al.: Repair of aortic coarctation in the first three months of life: Immediate and long-term results. Ann. Thorac. Surg. 41:425, 1986.

277. Beekman, R. H., Rocchini, A. P., Behrendt, D. M., and Rosenthal, A.: Reoperation for coarctation of the aorta. Am. J. Cardiol. 48:1108, 1981.

278. Choy, M., Rocchini, A. P., Beekman, R. H., et al.: Paradoxical hypertension after repair of coarctation of the aorta in children: Balloon angioplasty versus surgical repair. Circulation 75:1186, 1987.

279. Gidding, S. S., Rocchini, A. P., Beekman, R., et al.: Therapeutic effect of propranolol on paradoxical hypertension after repair of coarctation of the aorta. N. Engl. J. Med. 312:1224, 1985.

280. Mühler, E. G., Neuerburg, J. M., Rüben, A., et al.: Evaluation of aortic coarctation after surgical repair: Role of magnetic resonance imaging and Doppler ultrasound. Br. Heart J. 70:285, 1993.

281. Fawzy, M. E., Dunn, B., Galal, O., et al.: Balloon coarctation angioplasty in adolescents and adults: Early and intermediate results. Am. Heart J. 124:167, 1992.

281a. Hijazi, A. M., Geggel, R. L.: Balloon angioplasty for postoperative recurrent coarctation of the aorta. J. Interven. Cardiol. 8:509, 1995.

282. Kimball, T. R., Reynolds, J. M., Mays, W. A., et al.: Persistent hyperdynamic cardiovascular state at rest and during exercise in children after successful repair of coarctation of the aorta. J. Am. Coll. Cardiol. 24:194, 1994.

283. Balderston, S. M., Daberkow, E., Clarke, D. R., et al.: Maximal voluntary exercise variables in children with postoperative coarctation of the aorta. J. Am. Coll. Cardiol. 19:154, 1992.

284. Murphy, A. M., Blades, M., Daniels, S., and James, F. W.: Blood pres-

285. Krogmann, O. N., Rammos, S., Jakob, M., et al.: Left ventricular diastolic dysfunction late after coarctation repair in childhood: Influence of left ventricular hypertrophy. J. Am. Coll. Cardiol. *21*:1454, 1993.

286. Johnson, M. C., Gutierrez, F. R., Sekarski, D. R., et al.: Comparison of ventricular mass and function in early versus late repair of coarctation of the aorta. Am. J. Cardiol. *73*:698, 1994.

287. Mathew, P., Moodie, D., Blechman, G., et al.: Long-term follow-up of aortic coarctation in infants, children and adults. Cardiol. Young *3*:20, 1993.

288. Gardiner, H. M., Celermajer, D. S., Sorensen, K. E., et al.: Arterial reactivity is significantly impaired in normotensive young adults after successful repair of aortic coarctation in childhood. Circulation *89*:1745, 1994.

289. Van Woezik, E. V. M., Kline, H. W., and Krediet, P.: Normal internal calibers of ostia, great arteries and aortic isthmus in children. Br. Heart J. *39*:860, 1977.

290. Bharati, S., and Lev, M.: The surgical anatomy of the heart in tubular hypoplasia of the transverse aorta (preductal coarctation). J. Thorac. Cardiovasc. Surg. *91*:79, 1986.

291. Graham, T. P., Jr., Atwood, G. F., Boerth, R. C., et al.: Right and left heart size and function in infants with symptomatic coarctation. Circulation *56*:641, 1977.

292. Zannini, L., Gargiulo, G., Albanese, S. B., et al.: Aortic coarctation with hypoplastic arch in neonates: A spectrum of anatomic lesions requiring different surgical options. Ann. Thorac. Surg. *56*:288, 1993.

293. Hoff, S. J., Stewart, J. R., and Bender, H. W., Jr.: Aortic obstructions in infants and children: Surgery for complex aortic coarctation. Prog. Pediatr. Cardiol. *3*:62, 1994.

294. Ino, T., Nishimoto, K., Akimoto, K., et al.: Prospective study on a new therapeutic strategy for infants and children with aortic coarctation. Cardiol. Young *5*:36, 1995.

295. Johns, J. A., and Graham, T. P., Jr.: Aortic obstructions in infants and children: Pathophysiology and clinical presentation of interrupted aortic arch. Prog. Pediatr. Cardiol. *3*:87, 1994.

296. Dekker, A. O., Gittenberger-DeGroot, A. C., and Roozendaal, H.: The ductus arteriosus and associated cardiac anomalies in interruption of the aortic arch. Pediatr. Cardiol. *2*:185, 1982.

297. Stevens, C. A., Carey, J. C., and Shigeoka, A. O.: DiGeorge anomaly and velocardiofacial syndrome. Pediatrics *85*:526, 1990.

298. Buck, S. H., Graham, T. P., Jr., and Lawton, A. R.: DiGeorge syndrome: Implications for aortic arch obstruction. Prog. Pediatr. Cardiol. *3*:94, 1994.

299. Hoff, S. J., Merrill, W. H., and Bender, H. W., Jr.: Aortic obstructions in infants and children: Surgery for interrupted aortic arch. Prog. Pediatr. Cardiol. *3*:100, 1994.

300. Matsuki, O., Yagihara, T., Yamamoto, F., et al.: One-stage repair for intracardiac malformations associated with interrupted aortic arch or aortic coarctation in the first year of life. Cardiol. Young *5*:15, 1995.

301. Foker, J. E.: Surgical repair of aortic arch interruption. Ann. Thorac. Surg. *53*:369, 1992.

302. Friedman, W. F.: Congenital aortic stenosis. *In* Emmanoulides, G., et al. (eds.): Moss and Adams' Heart Disease in Infants, Children, and Adolescents. 5th ed. Baltimore, Williams and Wilkins, 1994, p. 1087.

303. Friedman, W. F., and Pappelbaum, S. J.: Indications for hemodynamic evaluation and surgery in congenital aortic stenosis. Pediatr. Clin. North Am. *18*:1207, 1971.

304. Kveselis, D. A., Rocchini, A. P., Rosenthal, A., et al.: Hemodynamic determinants of exercise-induced ST-segment depression in children with valvar aortic stenosis. Am. J. Cardiol. *55*:1133, 1985.

305. Driscoll, D. J., Wolfe, R. R., Gersony, W. M., et al.: Cardiorespiratory responses to exercise of patients with aortic stenosis, pulmonary stenosis, and ventricular septal defect. Circulation *87*(Suppl. I):I, 1993.

306. Graham, T. P., Louis, B. J., Jarmakani, J. M., et al.: Left heart volume and mass quantification in children with left ventricular pressure overload. Circulation *41*:203, 1970.

307. Fifer, M. A., Borow, K. M., Colan, S. D., et al.: Early diastolic left ventricular function in children and adults with aortic stenosis. J. Am. Coll. Cardiol. *5*:1147, 1985.

308. Villari, B., Hess, O. M., Kaufmann, P., et al.: Effect of aortic valve stenosis (pressure overload) and regurgitation (volume overload) on left ventricular systolic and diastolic function. Am. J. Cardiol. *69*:927, 1992.

309. Lewis, A. L., Heymann, M. A., Stanger, P., et al.: Evaluation of subendocardial ischemia in valvar aortic stenosis in children. Circulation *49*:978, 1974.

310. Strasburger, J. F., Kugler, J. D., Cheatham, J. P., and McManus, B. M.: Nonimmunologic hydrops fetalis associated with congenital aortic valvular stenosis. Am. Heart J. *108*:1380, 1984.

311. Maxwell, D., Allan, L., and Tynan, M. J.: Balloon dilation of the aortic valve in the fetus: A report of two cases. Br. Heart J. *55*:53, 1991.

312. Lakier, J. B., Lewis, A. B., Heymann, M. A., et al.: Isolated aortic stenosis of the neonate: Natural history and hemodynamic considerations. Circulation *50*:801, 1974.

313. Karl, T. R., Sano, S., Brawn, W. J., and Mee, R. B. B.: Critical aortic stenosis in the first month of life: Surgical results in 26 infants. Ann. Thorac. Surg. *50*:105, 1990.

314. Broderick, T. W., Higgins, C. B., and Friedman, W. F.: Critical aortic stenosis in neonates. Radiology *129*:393, 1978.

315. Donti, A., Bonvicini, M., Gargiulo, G., et al.: Criteria for selection of

316. Beekman, R. H., Rocchini, A. P., and Andes, A.: Balloon valvuloplasty for critical aortic stenosis in the newborn: Influence of new catheter technology. J. Am. Coll. Cardiol. *17*:1172, 1991.

316a. Donti, A., Bonvicini, M., Gargiulo, G., et al.: Criteria for selection of balloon valvuloplasty for treatment of aortic stenosis in neonates. Cardiol. Young *5*:31, 1995.

316b. Sandhu, S. K., Silka, M. J., and Reller, M. D.: Balloon aortic valvuloplasty for aortic stenosis in neonates, children, and young adults. J. Interven. Cardiol. *8*:477, 1995.

317. Fischer, D. R., Ettedgui, J. A., Park, S. C., et al.: Carotid artery approach for balloon dilation of aortic valve stenosis in the neonate: A preliminary report. J. Am. Coll. Cardiol. *14*:1633, 1990.

318. Rhodes, L. A., Colan, S. D., Perry, S. B., et al.: Predictors of survival in neonates with critical aortic stenosis. Circulation *84*:2325, 1991.

319. Leung, M. P., McKay, R., Smith, A., et al.: Critical aortic stenosis in early infancy. J. Thorac. Cardiovasc. Surg. *101*:526, 1991.

320. Vogel, M., Sebening, F., Sauer, U., and Buhlmeyer, K.: Left ventricular function and myocardial mass after aortic valvotomy in infancy. Pediatr. Cardiol. *13*:5, 1992.

321. Rychik, K., Murdison, K. A., Chin, A. J., and Norwood, W. I.: Surgical management of severe aortic outflow obstruction in lesions other than the hypoplastic left heart syndrome: Use of the pulmonary artery to aorta anastomosis. J. Am. Coll. Cardiol. *18*:809, 1991.

322. Braunwald, E., Goldblatt, A., Aygen, M. M., et al.: Congenital aortic stenosis. I. Clinical and hemodynamic findings in 100 patients. Circulation *27*:426, 1963.

323. Johnson, A. M.: Aortic stenosis, sudden death, and the left ventricular baroreceptors. Br. Heart J. *33*:1, 1971.

324. Gersony, W. M., Hayes, C. J., Driscoll, D. J., et al.: Bacterial endocarditis in patients with aortic stenosis, pulmonary stenosis, or ventricular septal defect. Circulation *87*(Suppl. I):I, 1993.

325. Bengur, A. R., Snider, A. R., Serwer, G. A., et al.: Usefulness of the Doppler mean gradient in evaluation of children with aortic valve stenosis in comparison to gradient at catheterization. Am. J. Cardiol. *64*:756, 1989.

326. Parsons, N. K., Moreau, G. A., Graham, T. P., Jr., et al.: Echocardiographic estimation of critical left ventricular size in infants with isolated aortic valve stenosis. J. Am. Coll. Cardiol. *18*:1049, 1991.

327. Bengur, A. R., Snider, A. R., Meliones, J. M., and Vermilion, R. P.: Doppler evaluation of aortic valve area in children with aortic stenosis. J. Am. Coll. Cardiol. *18*:1499, 1991.

328. Nishimura, R. A., Pieroni, D. R., Bierman, F. Z., et al.: Second natural history study of congenital heart defects: Aortic stenosis: Echocardiography. Circulation *87*:I, 1993.

329. Gutgesell, H. P., and French, M.: Echocardiographic determination of aortic and pulmonary valve areas in subjects with normal hearts. Am. J. Cardiol. *68*:773, 1991.

330. Beekman, R. H., Rocchini, A. P., Gillon, J. H., et al.: Hemodynamic determinants of the peak systolic left ventricular–aortic pressure gradient in children with valvar aortic stenosis. Am. J. Cardiol. *69*:813, 1992.

331. Stoddard, M. F., Arce, J., and Liddell, N. E.: Kupersmith two-dimensional transesophageal echocardiographic determination of aortic valve area in adults with aortic stenosis. Am. Heart J. *122*:1415, 1991.

332. Tribouilloy, C., Shen, W. F., Pelrier, M., et al.: Quantitation of aortic valve area in aortic stenosis with multiplane transesophageal echocardiography: Comparison with monoplane transesophageal approach. Am. Heart J. *128*:526, 1994.

333. Shah, P. M., and Graham, B. M.: Management of aortic stenosis: Is cardiac catheterization necessary? Am. J. Cardiol. *67*:1031, 1991.

334. McCrindle, B. W., for the Valvuloplasty and Angioplasty of Congenital Anomalies (VACA) Registry Investigators: Independent predictors of immediate results of percutaneous balloon aortic valvotomy in childhood. Am. J. Cardiol. *77*:286, 1996.

335. Witsenburg, M., Cromme-Dijkhuis, A., Frohn-Mulder, I. M. E., and Hess, J.: Short and midterm results of balloon valvuloplasty for valvular aortic stenosis in children. Am. J. Cardiol. *69*:945, 1992.

336. Kennedy, J. W., Twiss, R. D., Blackmon, J. R., et al.: Quantitative angiography. III. Relationships of left ventricular pressure, volume and mass in aortic valve disease. Circulation *38*:838, 1968.

337. El-Said, G., Gallioto, F. J., Mullens, C. E., and McNamara, D. G.: Natural hemodynamic history of congenital aortic stenosis in childhood. Am. J. Cardiol. *30*:6, 1972.

338. Hurwitz, R. A.: Aortic valve stenosis in childhood: Clinical and hemodynamic history. J. Pediatr. *82*:228, 1973.

339. Friedman, W. F., Modlinger, J., and Morgan, J.: Serial hemodynamic observations in asymptomatic children with valvar aortic stenosis. Circulation *43*:91, 1971.

340. Cohen, L. S., Friedman, W. F., and Braunwald, E.: Natural history of mild congenital aortic stenosis elucidated by serial hemodynamic studies. Am. J. Cardiol. *30*:1, 1972.

341. DeBoer, B. A., Robbins, R. C., Maron, B. J., et al.: Late results of aortic valvotomy for congenital valvular aortic stenosis. Ann. Thorac. Surg. *50*:69, 1990.

342. Keane, J. F., Driscoll, D. J., Gersony, W. M., et al.: Second natural history study of congenital heart defects. Circulation *87*(Suppl. I):I, 1993.

343. Kitchiner, D., Sreeram, N., Malaiya, N., et al.: Long-term follow-up of treated clinical aortic stenosis. Cardiol. Young *5*:9, 1995.

344. Gerosa, G., McKay, R., Davies, J., and Ross, O. N.: Comparison of the

aortic homograft and the pulmonary autograft for aortic valve or root replacement in children. J. Thorac. Cardiovasc. Surg. *102*:51, 1991.

345. Gerosa, G., McKay, R., and Ross, D. N.: Replacement of the aortic valve or root with a pulmonary autograft in children. Ann. Thorac. Surg. *51*:424, 1991.

346. Ross, D. B., Trusler, G. A., Coles, J. G., et al.: Small aortic root in childhood: Surgical options. Ann. Thorac. Surg. *58*:1617, 1994.

347. Elkins, R. C., Knott-Craig, C. J., Ward, K. E., et al.: Pulmonary autograft in children: Realized growth potential. Ann. Thorac. Surg. *57*:1387, 1994.

347a. Westaby, S.: Pulmonary autograft replacement of the aortic valve. Br. Heart J. *74*:1, 1995.

348. Kinney, E. L., Machado, H., Cortada, X., and Galbut, D. L.: Diagnosis of discrete subaortic stenosis by pulsed and continuous wave echocardiography. Am. Heart J. *110*:1069, 1985.

349. Frommelt, M. A., Snider, A. R., Bove, E. L., and Lupinetti, F. M.: Echocardiographic assessment of subvalvular aortic stenosis before and after operation. J. Am. Coll. Cardiol. *19*:1018, 1992.

350. Mugge, A., Daniel, W. G., Wolpers, H. G., et al.: Improved visualization of discrete subvalvular aortic stenosis by transesophageal color-coded Doppler echocardiography. Am. Heart J. *117*:474, 1989.

351. Choi, J. Y., and Sullivan, I. D.: Fixed subaortic stenosis: Anatomical spectrum and nature of progression. Br. Heart J. *65*:280, 1991.

352. DeVries, A. G., Hess, J., Witsenburg, M., et al.: Management of fixed subaortic stenosis: A retrospective study of 57 cases. J. Am. Coll. Cardiol. *19*:1013, 1992.

353. Ritter, S. B.: Discrete subaortic stenosis and balloon dilation: The four questions revisited. J. Am. Coll. Cardiol. *18*:1316, 1991.

354. Drinkwater, D. C., and Laks, H.: Surgery for subvalvular aortic stenosis. Prog. Pediatr. Cardiol. *3*:189, 1994.

355. Lupinetti, F. M., Pridjian, A. K., Callow, L. B., et al.: Optimum treatment of discrete subaortic stenosis. Ann. Thorac. Surg. *54*:467, 1992.

356. Sreeram, N., Sutherland, G. R., Bogers, A. J. J. C., et al.: Subaortic obstruction: Intraoperative echocardiography as an adjunct to operation. Ann. Thorac. Surg. *50*:579, 1990.

357. Gewillig., M., Daenen, W., Dumoulin, M., and Van Der Hauwaert, L.: Rheologic genesis of discrete subvalvular aortic stenosis: A Doppler echocardiographic study. J. Am. Coll. Cardiol. *19*:818, 1992.

358. Frommelt, P. C., Lupinetti, F. M., and Bove, E. L.: Aortoventriculoplasty in infants and children. Circulation *86*:II, 1992.

359. DeLeon, S. Y., Iobawi, M. N., Robertson, D. A., et al.: Conal enlargement for diffuse subaortic stenosis. J. Thorac. Cardiovasc. Surg. *102*:814, 1991.

360. Van Son, J. A. M., Schaff, H. V., Danielson, G. K., et al.: Surgical treatment of discrete and tunnel subaortic stenosis. Circulation *88*:159, 1993.

361. Coleman, D. M., Smallhorn, J. F., McCrindle, B. W., et al.: Postoperative follow-up of fibromuscular subaortic stenosis. J. Am. Coll. Cardiol. *24*:1558, 1994.

362. Waldman, J. D., Schneeweiss, A., Edwards, W. D., et al.: The obstructive subaortic conus. Circulation *70*:339, 1984.

363. Ow, E. P., DeLeon, S. Y., Freeman, J. E., et al.: Recognition and management of accessory mitral tissue causing severe subaortic stenosis. Ann. Thorac. Surg. *57*:952, 1994.

364. Reeder, G. S., Danielson, G. K., Seward, J. B., et al.: Fixed subaortic stenosis in atrioventricular canal defect: A Doppler echocardiographic study. J. Am. Coll. Cardiol. *20*:386, 1992.

365. Friedman, W. G., and Roberts, W. C.: Vitamin D and the subvalvular aortic stenosis syndrome: The transplacental effects of vitamin D on the aorta of the rabbit. Circulation *34*:77, 1966.

366. Friedman, W. F.: Vitamin D embryopathy. Adv. Teratol. *3*:85, 1968.

367. Friedman, W. F., and Mills, L. F.: The relationship between vitamin D and the craniofacial and dental anomalies of the supravalvular aortic stenosis syndrome. Pediatrics *43*:12, 1969.

368. Garcia, R. C., Friedman, W. F., Kaback, M. M., and Rowe, R. D.: Idiopathic hypercalcemia and supravalvular aortic stenosis: Documentation of a new syndrome. N. Engl. J. Med. *271*:117, 1964.

369. Williams, J. C. P., Barrett-Boyes, B. G., and Low, J. B.: Supravalvular aortic stenosis. Circulation *24*:1311, 1961.

370. Zalzstein, E., Moes, C. A. F., Musewe, N. N., and Freedom, R. M.: Spectrum of cardiovascular anomalies in Williams-Beuren syndrome. Pediatr. Cardiol. *12*:219, 1991.

371. Becroft, D. M., and Chamber, D.: Supravalvular aortic stenosis—infantile hypercalcemia syndrome: In vitro hypersensitivity to vitamin D and calcium. J. Med. Genet. *13*:223, 1976.

372. Taylor, A. B., Stern, P. H., and Bell, N. H.: Abnormal regulation of circulating 25-hydroxy vitamin D in the Williams syndrome. N. Engl. J. Med. *306*:972, 1982.

373. Kruse, K., Pankau, R., Gosch, A., and Wohlfahrt, K.: Calcium metabolism in Williams-Beuren syndrome. J. Pediat. *121*:902, 1992.

374. Morris, C. A., Demsey, S. A., Leonard, C. O., et al.: Natural history of Williams syndrome: Physical characteristics. J. Pediatr. *113*:318, 1988.

375. Kahler, R. L., Braunwald, E., Plauth, W. H., Jr., and Morrow, A. G.: Familial congenital heart disease. Am. J. Med. *40*:384, 1966.

376. Ewart, A. K., Morris, C. A., Ensing, G. J., et al.: A human vascular disorder, supravalvular aortic stenosis, maps to chromosome 7. Proc. Natl. Acad. Sci. *90*:3226, 1993.

377. Curran, M., Atkinson, D. L., Ewart, A. K., et al.: The elastin gene is disrupted by a translocation associated with supravalvular aortic stenosis. Cell *73*:159, 1993.

377a. Keating, M. T.: Genetic approaches to cardiovascular disease, supra-

378. Zalzstein, E., Moes, C. A. F., Musewe, N. N., and Freedom, R. M.: Spectrum of cardiovascular anomalies in Williams-Beuren syndrome. Pediatr. Cardiol. *12*:219, 1991.

379. Conway, E. E., Noonan, J., Marion, R. W., and Steeg, C. N.: Myocardial infarction leading to sudden death in the Williams syndrome: Report of three cases. J. Pediatr. *117*:593, 1990.

380. Ino, T., Nishimoto, K., Iwahara, M., et al.: Progressive vascular lesions in Williams-Beuren syndrome. Pediatr. Cardiol. *9*:55, 1988.

381. Wren, C., Oslizlok, P., and Bull, C.: Natural history of supravalvular aortic stenosis and pulmonary artery stenosis. J. Am. Coll. Cardiol. *15*:1625, 1990.

382. French, J. W., and Guntheroth, W. G.: An explanation of asymmetric upper extremity blood pressure in supravalvular aortic stenosis: The Coanda effect. Circulation *42*:31, 1970.

383. Goldstein, R. E., and Epstein, S. E.: Mechanism of elevated innominate artery pressures in supravalvular aortic stenosis. Circulation *42*:23, 1970.

384. Masura, J., Bzduch, J., Lolan, M., et al.: Diagnosis of supravalvular aortic stenosis by means of two-dimensional echocardiography (in Slovak). Bratisl. Lek. Listy. *90*:895, 1989.

385. Rein, A. J. J. T., Preminger, T. J., Perry, S. B., et al.: Generalized anteriopathy in Williams syndrome: An intravascular ultrasound study. J. Am. Coll. Cardiol. *21*:1727, 1993.

386. Brand, A., Keren, A., Reifen, R. M., et al.: Echocardiographic and Doppler findings in the Williams syndrome. Am. J. Cardiol. *63*:633, 1989.

387. Permut, L. C., and Laks, H.: Surgery for valvar and supravalvar aortic stenosis. Prog. Pediatr. Cardiol. *3*:177, 1994.

388. Sade, R. M., Crawford, F. A., Jr., and Fyfe, D. A.: Symposium on hypoplastic left heart syndrome. J. Thorac. Cardiovasc. Surg. *91*:937,1986.

389. Bash, S. E., Huhta, J. C., Vick, G. W., III, et al.: Hypoplastic left heart syndrome: Is echocardiography accurate enough to guide surgical palliation? J. Am. Coll. Cardiol. *7*:610, 1986.

390. Rossi, A. F., Sommer, R. J., Lotvin, A., et al.: Usefulness of intermittent monitoring of mixed venous oxygen saturation after stage I palliation for hypoplastic left heart syndrome. Am. J. Cardiol. *73*:1118, 1994.

391. Norwood, W. I., Jacobs, M. L., and Murphy, J. D.: Fontan procedure for hypoplastic left heart syndrome. Ann. Thorac. Surg. *54*:1025, 1992.

392. Guntheroth, W. G.: Fontan procedure for hypoplastic left heart syndrome. Circulation *86*:1662, 1992.

393. Rossi, A. F., Sommer, R. J., Steinberg, L. G., et al.: Effect of older age on outcome for stage one palliation of hypoplastic left heart syndrome. Am. J. Cardiol. *77*:319, 1996.

394. Bailey, L. L., and Gundry, S. R.: Hypoplastic left heart syndrome. Pediatr. Clin. North Am. *37*:137, 1990.

395. Canter, C. E., Moorhead, S., Huddleston, C. B., and Spray, T. L.: Restrictive atrial septal communication as a determinant of outcome of cardiac transplantation for hypoplastic left heart syndrome. Circulation *88*:456, 1993.

395a. Gutgesell, H. P., and Massaro, T. A.: Management of hypoplastic left heart syndrome in a consortium of university hospitals. Am. J. Cardiol. *76*:809, 1995.

396. Slack, M. C., Kirby, W. C., Towbin, J. A., et al.: Stenting of the ductus arteriosus in the hypoplastic left heart syndrome as an ambulatory bridge to cardiac transplantation. Am. J. Cardiol. *74*:636, 1994.

397. Frahm, C. J., Braunwald, E., and Morrow, A. G.: Congenital aortic regurgitation. Am. J. Med. *31*:63, 1961.

398. Donofrio, M. T., Engle, M. A., O'Loughlin, J. E., et al.: Congenital aortic regurgitation: Natural history and management. J. Am. Coll. Cardiol. *20*:336, 1992.

399. Tuna, I. C., and Edwards, J. E.: Aortico-left ventricular tunnel and aortic insufficiency. Ann. Thorac. Surg. *45*:5, 1988.

400. Hovaguimian, H., Cobanoglu, A., and Starr, A.: Aortico-left ventricular tunnel: A clinical review and new surgical classification. Ann. Thorac. Surg. *45*:106, 1988.

401. Goforth, D., James, F. W., Kaplan, S., and Donner, R.: Maximal exercise in children with aortic regurgitation: An adjunct to noninvasive assessment of disease severity. Am. Heart J. *108*:1306, 1984.

402. Sondergaard, L., Lindvig, K., Hildebrandt, P., et al.: Quantification of aortic regurgitation by magnetic resonance velocity mapping. Am. Heart J. *125*:1081, 1993.

403. Lucas, R. V., Jr.: Anomalous venous connection, pulmonary and systemic. In Adams, F. H., and Emmanouilides, G. C. (eds.): Moss' Heart Disease in Infants, Children and Adolescents. 4th ed. Baltimore, Williams and Wilkins, 1989, p. 580.

404. Pacifico, A. D., Mandke, N. V., McGrath, L. B., et al.: Repair of congenital pulmonary venous thrombosis with living autologous atrial tissue. J. Thorac. Cardiovasc. Surg. *89*:604, 1985.

405. Marin-Garcia, J., Tandon, R., Lucas, R. V., Jr., and Edwards, J. E.: Cor triatriatum: Study of 20 cases. Am. J. Cardiol. *35*:59, 1975.

406. Burton, D. A., Chin, A., Weinberg, P. M., and Pigott, J. D.: Identification of cor triatriatum dexter by two-dimensional echocardiography. Am. J. Cardiol. *59*:409, 1987.

406a. Tulloh, R. M. R., Bull, C., Elliott, M. J., and Sullivan, I. D.: Supravalvar mitral stenosis: Risk factors for recurrence or death after resection. Br. Heart J. *73*:164, 1995.

406b. Shuler, C. O., Fyfe, D. A., Sade, R., and Crawford, F. A.: Transesophageal echocardiographic evaluation of cor triatriatum in children. Am. Heart J. *129*:507, 1995.

407. Oglietti, J., Cooley, D. A., Izquierdo, J. P., et al.: Cor triatriatum: Operative results in 25 patients. Ann. Thorac. Surg. 35:415, 1983.

408. Ruckman, R. N., and Van Praagh, R.: Anatomic types of congenital mitral stenosis: Report of 49 autopsy cases with consideration of diagnosis and surgical implications. Am. J. Cardiol. 42:592, 1978.

409. Parr, G. V. S., Fripp, R. A., Whitman, V., et al.: Anomalous mitral arcade: Echocardiographic and angiographic reception. Pediatr. Cardiol. 4:163, 1983.

410. Ortiz, E., and Somerville, J.: Assessment by cross-sectional echocardiography of surgical mitral valve disease in children and adolescents. Br. Heart J. 56:267, 1986.

411. Moore, P., Adatia, I., Spevak, P. J., et al.: Severe congenital mitral stenosis in infants. Circulation 89:2099, 1994.

412. Fawzy, M. E., Mimish, L., Awad, M., et al.: Mitral balloon valvotomy in children with Inoue balloon technique: Immediate and intermediate-term result. Am. Heart J. 127:1559, 1994.

412a. Tulloh, R. M. R., Bull, C., Elliott, M. J., and Sullivan, I. D.: Supravalvular mitral stenosis: Risk factors for recurrence or death after resection. Br. Heart J. 73:164, 1995.

413. Mazzera, E., Corno, A., Di Donato, R., et al.: Surgical bypass of the systemic atrioventricular valve in children by means of a valve conduit. J. Thorac. Cardiovasc. Surg. 96:321, 1988.

414. Zweng, T. N., Bluett, M. K., Mosca, R., et al.: Mitral valve replacement in the first 5 years of life. Ann. Thorac. Surg. 47:720, 1989.

415. Perloff, J. K.: Evolving concepts of mitral valve prolapse. N. Engl. J. Med. 307:369, 1982.

416. Carpentier, A.: Congenital malformations of the mitral valve. In Stark, J., and deLeval, M. (eds.): Surgery for Congenital Heart Defects. New York, Grune and Stratton, 1983, p. 467.

417. Wu, Y. T., Chang, A. C., and Chin, A. J.: Semiquantitative assessment of mitral regurgitation by Doppler color flow imaging in patients aged <20 years. Am. J. Cardiol. 71:727, 1993.

418. Lamberti, J. J., Gensen, T. S., Grehl, T. M., et al.: Late reoperation for systemic atrioventricular valve regurgitation after repair of congenital heart defects. Ann. Thorac. Surg. 47:517, 1989.

419. Gonzalez, V. R., Pieper, W. M., and Kap-herr, S. H.: Pulmonary arteriovenous fistula in childhood. Z. Kinderchir. 40:101, 1985.

420. Grady, R. M., Sharkey, A. M., and Bridges, N. D.: Transcatheter coil embolisation of a pulmonary arteriovenous malformation in a neonate. Br. Heart J. 71:370, 1994.

421. Puskas, J. D., Allen, M. S., Moncure, A. C., et al.: Pulmonary arteriovenous malformations: Therapeutic options. Ann. Thorac. Surg. 56:253, 1993.

422. D'Cruz, I. A., Agustssou, M. M., Bicoff, J. P., et al.: Stenotic lesions of the pulmonary arteries: Clinical hemodynamic findings in 84 cases. Am. J. Cardiol. 13:441, 1964.

423. Venables, A. W.: The syndrome of pulmonary stenosis complicating maternal rubella. Br. Heart J. 27:49, 1965.

424. Friedman, D. M., Fernandes, J., Rutkowski, M., and Danilowicz, D.: Doppler evaluation of physiologic peripheral pulmonic stenosis in newborns. Cardiol. Young 2:179, 1992.

425. Eldredge, W. J., Tingelstad, J. B., Robertson, L. W., et al.: Observations on the natural history of pulmonary artery coarctation. Circulation 45:404, 1972.

426. Kan, J. S., Marvin, W. J., Jr., Bass, J. L., et al.: Balloon angioplasty-branch pulmonary artery stenosis: Results from the valvuloplasty and angioplasty of congenital anomalies registry. Am. J. Cardiol. 65:798, 1990.

427. O'Laughlin, M. P., Slack, M. C., Grifka, R. G.: Implantation and intermediate-term follow-up of stents in congenital heart disease. Circulation 88:605, 1993.

428. Burch, M., Sharland, M., Shinebourne, E., et al.: Cardiologic abnormalities in Noonan syndrome: Phenotypic diagnosis and echocardiographic assessment of 118 patients. J. Am. Coll. Cardiol. 22:1189, 1993.

429. Aldousany, A. W., DiSessa, T. G., Dubois, R., et al.: Doppler estimation of pressure gradient in pulmonary stenosis: Maximal instantaneous vs peak-to-peak, vs mean catheter gradient. Pediatr. Cardiol. 10:145, 1989.

430. Frantz, E. G., and Silverman, N. H.: Doppler ultrasound evaluation of valvular pulmonary stenosis from multiple transducer positions in children requiring pulmonary valvuloplasty. Am. J. Cardiol. 61:844, 1988.

430a. Fedderly, R. T., and Beekman, R. H.: Balloon valvuloplasty for pulmonary valve stenosis. J. Interven. Cardiol. 8:451, 1995.

430b. Tabatabaei, H., Boutin, C., Nykanen, D. G., et al.: Morphologic and hemodynamic consequences after percutaneous balloon valvotomy for neonatal pulmonary stenosis: Medium-term follow-up. J. Am. Coll. Cardiol. 27:473, 1996.

431. Srinivasan, V., Konyer, A., Broda, J. J., and Subramanian, S.: Critical pulmonary stenosis in infants less than three months of age: A reappraisal of closed transventricular pulmonary valvotomy. Ann. Thorac. Surg. 34:46, 1982.

432. Burzynski, J. B., Kveselis, D. A., Byrum, C. J., et al.: Modified technique for balloon valvuloplasty of critical pulmonary stenosis in the newborn. J. Am. Coll. Cardiol. 22:1944, 1993.

433. Radtke, W., and Lock, J.: Balloon dilation. Pediatr. Clin. North Am. 37:193, 1990.

434. Fedderly, R. T., Lloyd, T. R., Mendelsohn, A. M., et al.: Determinants of successful balloon valvotomy in infants with critical pulmonary stenosis or membranous pulmonary atresia with intact ventricular septum. J. Am. Coll. Cardiol. 25:460, 1995.

435. Lange, P. E., Onnasch, G. W., and Heintzen, P. H.: Valvular pulmonary stenosis: Natural history and right ventricular function in infants and children. Eur. Heart J. 6:706, 1985.

436. Mahra-Pour, M., Whitney, A., Liebman, J., et al.: Quantification of the Frank and MacFee-Parungao orthogonal electrocardiogram in valvular pulmonic stenosis: Correlation with hemodynamic measurements. J. Electrocardiol. 12:69, 1979.

437. Nishimura, R. A., Pieroni, D. R., Bierman, F. Z., et al.: Second natural history of congenital heart defects: Pulmonary stenosis: Echocardiography. Circulation 87:I, 1993.

438. Krabill, K. A., Wang, Y., Einzig, S., and Moller, J. H.: Rest and exercise hemodynamics in pulmonary stenosis: Comparison of children and adults. Am. J. Cardiol. 56:360, 1985.

439. Danilowicz, D., Hoffman, J. I. E., and Rudolph, A. M.: Serial studies of pulmonary stenosis in infancy and childhood. Br. Heart J. 37:808, 1975.

440. Wennevold, A., and Jacobsen, J. R.: Natural history of valvular pulmonary stenosis in children below the age of two years: Long-term follow-up with serial heart catheterizations. Eur. J. Cardiol. 8:371, 1978.

441. Hayes, C. J., Gersony, W. M., Driscoll, D. J., et al.: Second natural history study of congenital heart defects: Results of treatment of patients with pulmonary valvar stenosis. Circulation 87:I, 1993.

442. Laks, H., and Billingsley, A. M.: Advances in the treatment of pulmonary atresia with intact ventricular septum: Palliative and definitive repair. Cardiol Clin. 7:387, 1989.

443. Coles, J. G., Freedman, R. M., Lightfoot, N. E., et al.: Long-term results in neonates with pulmonary atresia and intact ventricular septum. Ann. Thorac. Surg. 47:213, 1989.

444. Vosa, C., Arciprete, P., Caianiello, G., and Palma, G.: Pulmonary atresia with intact ventricular septum: Is it possible to improve survival? Cardiol. Young 2:391, 1992.

445. Daliento, L., Scognamiglio, R., Thiene, G., et al.: Morphologic and functional analysis of myocardial status in pulmonary atresia with intact ventricular septum—an angiographic, histologic and morphometric study. Cardiol. Young 2:361, 1992.

446. Hanseus, K., Bjorkhem, G., Lundstrom, N. R., and Laurin, S.: Cross-sectional echocardiographic measurements of right ventricular size and growth in patients with pulmonary atresia and intact ventricular septum. Pediatr. Cardiol. 12:135, 1991.

447. Leung, M. P., Mok, C. K., and Hui, P. W.: Echocardiographic assessment of neonates with pulmonary atresia and intact ventricular septum. J. Am. Coll. Cardiol. 12:719, 1988.

447a. Fedderly, R. T., Lloyd, T. R., Mendelsohn, A. M., et al.: Determinants of successful balloon valvulotomy in infants with critical pulmonary stenosis or membranous pulmonary atresia with intact ventricular septum. J. Am. Coll. Cardiol. 25:460, 1995.

448. Freedom, R. M., Wilson, G., Trusler, G., et al.: Pulmonary atresia and intact ventricular septum: A review of the anatomy, myocardium and factors influencing right ventricular growth and guidelines for surgical intervention. Scand. J. Thorac. Cardiovasc. Surg. 17:1, 1983.

449. Leung, M. P., Mok, C. K., Lee, J., et al.: Management evolution of pulmonary atresia and intact ventricular septum. Am. J. Cardiol. 71:1331, 1993.

450. Giglia, T. M., Jenkins, K. J., Matitiau, A., et al.: Influence of right heart size on outcome in pulmonary atresia with intact ventricular septum. Circulation 88:22, 1993.

451. Laks, H., Pearl, J. M., Drinkwater, D. C., et al.: Partial biventricular repair of pulmonary atresia with intact ventricular septum: Use of an adjustable atrial septal defect. Circulation 86:II, 1992.

452. Hanley, F. L., Sade, R. M., Blackstone, E. H., et al.: Outcomes in neonatal pulmonary atresia with intact ventricular septum: A multi-institutional study. J. Thorac. Cardiovasc. Surg. 105:406, 1993.

453. Pawade, A., Capuani, A., Penny, D. J., et al.: Pulmonary atresia with intact ventricular septum: Surgical management based on right ventricular infundibulum. J. Cardiovasc. Surg. 8:371, 1993.

454. Steinberger, J., Berry, J. M., Bass, J. L., et al.: Results of a right ventricular outflow patch for pulmonary atresia with intact ventricular septum. Circulation 86:II, 1992.

455. Gentles, T. L., Colan, S. D., Giglia, T. M., et al.: Right ventricular decompression and left ventricular function in pulmonary atresia with intact ventricular septum. Circulation 88:II, 1992.

456. Schmidt, K. G., Cloe, J-L., and Silverman, N. H.: Changes of right ventricular size and function after valvotomy for pulmonary atresia or critical pulmonary stenosis and intact ventricular septum. J. Am. Coll. Cardiol. 19:1032, 1992.

457. Latson, L. A.: Nonsurgical treatment of a neonate with pulmonary atresia and intact ventricular septum by transcatheter puncture and balloon dilation of the atretic valve. Am. J. Cardiol. 68:277, 1991.

458. Leung, M. P., Lo, R. N. S., Cheung, H., et al.: Balloon valvuloplasty after pulmonary valvotomy for babies with pulmonary atresia and intact ventricular septum. Ann. Thorac. Surg. 53:864, 1992.

459. Danilowicz, D., and Ishmael, R.: Anomalous right ventricular muscle bundle: Clinical pitfalls and extracardiac anomalies. Clin. Cardiol. 4:146, 1981.

460. Wong, P. C., Sanders, S. P., Jonas, R. A., et al.: Pulmonary valve–moderator band distance and association with development of double-chambered right ventricle. Am. J. Cardiol. 68:1681, 1991.

461. Ford, D. K., Bollaboy, C. A., Derkac, W. M., et al.: Transatrial repair of double-chambered right ventricle. Ann. Thorac. Surg. 46:412, 1988.

462. Pinsky, W. W., and Arciniegas, E.: Tetralogy of Fallot. Pediatr. Clin. North Am. 37:179, 1990.

463. Soto, B., and McConnell, M. E.: Tetralogy of Fallot: Angiographic and pathological correlation. Semin. Thorac. Cardiovasc. Surg. 2:12, 1990.

464. Rabinovitch, M.: Pathology and anatomy of pulmonary atresia and ventricular septal defect. Prog. Pediatr. Cardiol. 1:9, 1992.

465. Castaneda, A. R., Mayer, J. E., Jr., and Lock, J. E.: Tetralogy of Fallot pulmonary atresia and diminutive pulmonary arteries. Prog. Pediatr. Cardiol. 1:50, 1992.

466. Barbero-Marcial, M., and Jatene, A. D.: Surgical management of the anomalies of the pulmonary arteries in the tetralogy of Fallot with pulmonary atresia. Semin. Thorac. Cardiovasc. Surg. 2:93, 1990.

467. Hiraishi, S., Misawa, H., Hirota, H., et al.: Noninvasive quantitative evaluation of the morphology of the major pulmonary artery branches in cyanotic congenital heart disease. Angiocardiographic and echocardiographic correlative study. Circulation 89:1306, 1994.

468. Carvalho, J. S., Silva, C. M. C., Rigby, M. L., et al.: Angiographic diagnosis of anomalous coronary artery in tetralogy of Fallot. Br. Heart J. 70:75, 1993.

469. Feldt, R. H., Liao, P., and Puga, F. J.: Clinical profile and natural history of pulmonary atresia and ventricular septal defect. Prog. Pediatr. Cardiol. 1:18, 1992.

470. Santoro, G., Marino, B., Di Carlo, D., et al.: Echocardiographically guided repair of tetralogy of Fallot. Am. J. Cardiol. 73:808, 1994.

471. Morgan, B. C., Guntheroth, W. G., Blume, R. S., and Fyler, D. C.: A clinical profile of paroxysmal hyperpnea in cyanotic congenital heart disease. Circulation 31:66, 1965.

472. Shaddy, R. E., Viney, J., Judd, V. E., and McGough, E. C.: Continuous intravenous phenylephrine infusion for treatment of hypoxemic spells in tetralogy of Fallot. J. Pediatr. 114:468, 1989.

473. McConnell, M. E.: Echocardiography in classical tetralogy of Fallot. Semin. Thorac. Cardiovasc. Surg. 2:2, 1990.

474. Castaneda, A. R.: Classical repair of tetralogy of Fallot: Timing, technique, and results. Semin. Thorac. Cardiovasc. Surg. 2:70, 1990.

475. Pacifico, A. D., Kirklin, J. K., Colvin, E. V., et al.: Transatrial-transpulmonary repair of tetralogy of Fallot. Semin. Thorac. Cardiovasc. Surg. 2:76, 1990.

476. Puga, F. J.: Surgical treatment of pulmonary atresia and ventricular septal defect. Prog. Pediatr. Cardiol. 1:37, 1992.

477. Groh, M. A., Meliones, J. N., Bove, E., et al.: Repair of tetralogy of Fallot in infancy: Effect of pulmonary artery size on outcome. Circulation 84(Suppl. III):206, 1991.

478. Permut, L. C., Laks, H., Haas, G. S., et al.: Surgical management of pulmonary atresia and ventricular septal defect with major systemic-pulmonary collaterals. J. Am. Coll. Cardiol. 15:79A, 1990.

479. Kirklin, J. W., Blackstone, E. H., Jonas, R. A., et al.: Morphologic and surgical determinants of outcome events after repair of tetralogy of Fallot and pulmonary stenosis. J. Thorac. Cardiovasc. Surg. 103:706, 1992.

480. Rosankranz, E. R.: Modified Blalock-Taussig shunts in the treatment of tetralogy of Fallot. Semin. Thorac. Cardiovasc. Surg. 2:27, 1990.

481. Sreeram, N., Saleem, M., Jackson, M., et al.: Results of balloon pulmonary valvuloplasty as a palliative procedure in tetralogy of Fallot. J. Am. Coll. Cardiol. 18:59, 1991.

481a. Sluysmans, T., Neven, B., Rubay, J., et al.: Early balloon dilatation of the pulmonary valve in infants with tetralogy of Fallot. Circulation 91:1506, 1995.

482. Chan, K. C., Fyfe, D. A., McKay, C. A., et al.: Right ventricular outflow reconstruction with cryopreserved homografts in pediatric patients: Intermediate-term follow-up with serial echocardiographic assessment. J. Am. Coll. Cardiol. 24:483, 1994.

483. Naito, Y., Fujita, T., Yagihara, T., et al.: Usefulness of left ventricular volume in assessing tetralogy of Fallot for total correction. Am. J. Cardiol. 56:356, 1985.

484. Rebergen, S. A., Chin, J. G. J., Ottenkamp, J., et al.: Pulmonary regurgitation in the late postoperative follow-up of tetralogy of Fallot: Volumetric quantitation by nuclear magnetic resonance velocity mapping. Circulation 88:2257, 1993.

485. Warner, K. G., Anderson, J. E., Fulton, D. R., et al.: Restoration of the pulmonary valve reduces right ventricular volume overload after previous repair of tetralogy of Fallot. Circulation 88:189, 1993.

486. Garson, A., Jr., Randall, D. C., Gillette, P. C., et al.: Prevention of sudden death after repair of tetralogy of Fallot: Treatment of ventricular arrhythmias. J. Am. Coll. Cardiol. 6:221, 1985.

487. Oku, H., Shirotani, H., Sunakawa, A., and Yokoyama, T.: Postoperative long-term results in total correction of tetralogy of Fallot: Hemodynamics and cardiac function. Ann. Thorac. Surg. 41:413, 1986.

488. Rosenthal, A., Behrendt, D., Sloan, H., et al.: Long-term prognosis (15 to 26 years) after repair of tetralogy of Fallot: I. Survival and symptomatic status. Ann. Thorac. Surg. 38:151, 1984.

489. Sandor, G. G. S., Patterson, M. W. H., Tipple, M., et al.: Left ventricular systolic and diastolic function after total correction of tetralogy of Fallot. Am. J. Cardiol. 60:1148, 1987.

490. Cullen, S., Celermajer, D. S., Franklin, R. C. G., et al.: Prognostic significance of ventricular arrhythmia after repair of tetralogy of Fallot: A 12-year prospective study. J. Am. Coll. Cardiol. 23:1151, 1994.

491. Joffe, H., Georgakopoulos, D., Celermajer, D. S., et al.: Late ventricular arrhythmia is rare after early repair of tetralogy of Fallot. J. Am. Coll. Cardiol. 23:1146, 1994.

492. Ross, B. A.: From the bedside to the basic science laboratory: Arrhythmias in Fallot's tetralogy. J. Am. Coll. Cardiol. 21:1738, 1993.

493. Vaksmann, G., Kohen, M. E., Lacroix, D., et al.: Influence of clinical

and hemodynamic characteristics on signal-averaged electrocardiogram in postoperative tetralogy of Fallot. Am. J. Cardiol. 71:317, 1993.

494. Misaki, T., Tsubota, M., Watanabe, G., et al.: Surgical treatment of ventricular tachycardia after surgical repair of tetralogy of Fallot: Relation between intraoperative mapping and histological findings. Circulation 90:264, 1994.

494a. Bricker, J. T.: Sudden death and tetralogy of Fallot. Risks, markers, and causes. Circulation 92:162, 1995.

494b. Johnson, M. C., Strauss, A. W., Dowton, S. B., et al.: Deletion within chromosome 22 is common in patients with absent pulmonary valve syndrome. Am. J. Cardiol. 76:66, 1995.

495. Fouron, J. C.: Tetralogy of Fallot with absent pulmonary valve: Clarification of a complex malformation and of its therapeutic challenge. Circulation 82:1531, 1990.

496. Rabinovich, M., Grady, S., David, J., et al.: Compression of intrapulmonary bronchi by abnormally branching pulmonary valves. Am. J. Cardiol. 50:804, 1982.

497. Milanesi, O., Talenti, E., Pallegrino, P. A., and Thiene, G.: Abnormal pulmonary artery branching in tetralogy of Fallot with absent pulmonary valve. Int. J. Cardiol. 6:375, 1984.

498. Fischer, D. R., Neches, W. H., Beerman, L. B., et al.: Tetralogy of Fallot with absent pulmonic valve: Analysis of 17 patients. Am. J. Cardiol. 53:1433, 1984.

499. Dunnigan, A., Oldham, H. N., and Benson, D. W.: Absent pulmonary valve syndrome in infancy: Surgery reconsidered. Am. J. Cardiol. 48:117, 1981.

500. Kron, I. L., Johnson, A. M., Carpenter, M. A., et al.: Treatment of absent pulmonary valve syndrome with homograft. Ann. Thorac. Surg. 46:579, 1988.

501. Rigby, M. L., Carvalho, J. S., Anderson, R. H., and Redington, A.: The investigation and diagnosis of tricuspid atresia. Int. J. Cardiol. 27:1, 1990.

502. Sade, R. M., and Fyfe, D. A.: Tricuspid atresia: Current concepts in diagnosis and treatment. Pediatr. Clin. North Am. 7:151, 1990.

502a. Laks, H., Ardehali, A., Grant, P. W., et al.: Modification of the Fontan procedure. Superior vena cava to left pulmonary artery connection and inferior vena cava to right pulmonary artery connection with adjustable atrial septal defect. Circulation 91:2943, 1995.

503. Pearl, J. M., Laks, H., Drinkwater, D. C., et al.: Modified Fontan procedure in patients less than 4 years of age. Circulation 86:II, 1992.

504. Bridges, N. D., Mayer, J. E., Lock, J. E., et al.: Effect of baffle fenestration on outcome of the modified Fontan operation. Circulation 86:1762, 1992.

504a. Kuhn, M. A., Jarmakani, J. M., Laks, H., et al.: Effect of late postoperative atrial septal defect closure on hemodynamic function in patients with a lateral tunnel Fontan procedure. J. Am. Coll. Cardiol. 26:259, 1995.

505. Carter, T., Mainwaring, R. D., and Lamberti, J. J.: Damus-Kaye-Stansel procedure: Midterm follow-up and technical considerations. Ann. Thorac. Surg. 58:1603, 1994.

506. Gross, G. J., Jonas, R. A., Castaneda, A. R., et al.: Maturational and hemodynamic factors predictive of increased cyanosis after bidirectional cavopulmonary anastomosis. Am. J. Cardiol. 74:705, 1994.

507. Senzaki, H., Isoda, T., Ishizawa, A., and Hishi, T.: Reconsideration of criteria for the Fontan operation: Influence of pulmonary artery size on postoperative hemodynamics of the Fontan operation. Circulation 89:1196, 1994.

508. Sandor, G. G. S., Patterson, M. W. H., and LeBlanc, J. G.: Systolic and diastolic function in tricuspid valve atresia before the Fontan operation. Am. J. Cardiol. 73:292, 1994.

509. Frommelt, P. C., Snider, R., Meliones, J. N., and Vermilion, R. P.: Doppler assessment of pulmonary artery flow patterns and ventricular function after the Fontan operation. Am. J. Cardiol. 68:1211, 1991.

510. Mair, D. D., Puga, F. J., and Danielson, G. K.: Late functional status of survivors of the Fontan procedure performed during the 1970s. Circulation 86:II, 1992.

511. Driscoll, D. J., Offord, K. P., Feldt, R. H., et al.: Five- to fifteen-year follow-up after Fontan operation. Circulation 85:469, 1992.

511a. Rosenthal, M., Bush, A., Deanfield, J., et al.: Comparison of cardiopulmonary adaptation during exercise in children after the atriopulmonary and total cavopulmonary connection Fontan procedures. Circulation 91:372, 1995.

512. Gewillig, M., Wyse, R. K., de Leval, M. R., and Deanfield, J. E.: Early and late arrhythmias after the Fontan operation: Predisposing factors and clinical consequences. Br. Heart J. 67:72, 1992.

513. Gussenhoven, E. J., Stewart, P. A., Becker, A. E., et al.: "Offsetting" of the septal tricuspid leaflet in normal hearts and in hearts with Ebstein's anomaly. Am. J. Cardiol. 53:172, 1984.

514. Zalzstein, E., Koran, G., Einarson, T., and Freedom, R. M.: A case control study on the association between first trimester exposure to lithium and Ebstein's anomaly. Am. J. Cardiol. 65:817, 1990.

515. Mair, D. D.: Ebstein's anomaly: Natural history and management. J. Am. Coll. Cardiol. 19:1047, 1992.

516. Celermajer, D. S., Bull, C., Till, J. A., et al.: Ebstein's anomaly: Presentation and outcome from fetus to adult. J. Am. Coll. Cardiol. 23:170, 1994.

517. Oberhoffer, R., Cook, A. C., Lang, D., et al.: Correlation between echocardiographic and morphological investigations of lesions of the tricuspid valve diagnosed during fetal life. Br. Heart J. 68:580, 1992.

518. Boucek, R. J., Jr., Graham, T. P., Jr., Morgan J. P., et al.: Spontaneous

resolution of massive congenital tricuspid insufficiency. Circulation 54:795, 1976.

519. Freedom, R. M., Culham, J. A. G., Olley, P. M., et al.: The differentiation of functional from organic pulmonary atresia: The role of aortography. Am. J. Cardiol. 41:914, 1978.

520. Kastor, J. A., Goldreier, B. N., Josephson, M. E., et al.: Electrophysiologic characteristics of Ebstein's anomaly of the tricuspid valve. Circulation 52:987, 1975.

521. Gussenhoven, W. J., Spitaels, S. E. C., Bom, N., and Becker, A. E.: Echocardiographic criteria for Ebstein's anomaly of tricuspid valve. Br. Heart J. 43:31, 1980.

522. Hirschklau, M. J., Sahn, D. J., Hagan, A. D., et al.: Cross-sectional echocardiographic features of Ebstein's anomaly of the tricuspid valve. Am. J. Cardiol. 40:400, 1977.

523. Hong, Y. M., and Moller, J. H.: Ebstein's anomaly: A long-term study of survival. Am. Heart J. 125:1419, 1993.

524. Hurwitz, R. A.: Left ventricular function in infants and children with symptomatic Ebstein's anomaly. Am. J. Cardiol. 73:716, 1994.

525. Paul, N. H., and Wernodsky, G.: Transposition of the great arteries. In Emmanoulides, G. C., Allen, H. D., et al. (eds.): Moss and Adams' Heart Disease in Infants, Children and Adolescents. 5th ed. Baltimore, Williams and Wilkins, 1994, p. 1154.

526. Anderson, R. H., Henry, G. W., and Becker, A. E.: Morphologic aspects of complete transposition. Cardiol. Young 1:41, 1991.

527. Lakier, J. B., Stanger, P., Heymann, M. A., et al.: Early onset of pulmonary vascular obstruction in patients with aortopulmonary transposition and intact ventricular septum. Circulation 51:875, 1975.

528. Aziz, K. U., Paul, M. H., and Rowe, R. D.: Bronchopulmonary circulation in D-transposition of the great arteries: Possible role and genesis of accelerated pulmonary vascular disease. Am. J. Cardiol. 39:432, 1977.

529. Muster, A. J., Paul, M. H., Van Grondell, E. A., and Conway, J. J.: Asymmetric distribution of the pulmonary blood flow between the right and left lungs in D-transposition of the great arteries. Am. J. Cardiol. 38:352, 1976

530. Chiu, I., Anderson, R. H., Macartney, F. J., et al.: Morphologic features of an intact ventricular septum susceptible to subpulmonary obstruction in complete transposition. Am. J. Cardiol. 53:1633, 1984.

531. Waldman, J. D., Paul, M. H., Newfeld, E. A., et al.: Transposition of the great arteries with intact ventricular septum and patent ductus arteriosus. Am. J. Cardiol. 39:232, 1977.

532. Tonkin, I. L., Kelley, M. J., Bream, P. R., and Elliott, L. P.: The frontal chest film as a method of suspecting transposition complexes. Circulation 53:1016, 1976.

533. Deal, B. J., Chin, A. J., Sanders, S. P., et al.: Subxiphoid two-dimensional echocardiographic identification of tricuspid valve abnormalities in transposition of the great arteries with ventricular septal defect. Am. J. Cardiol. 55:1146, 1985.

534. Chin, A. J., Yeager, S. B., Sanders, S. P., et al.: Accuracy of prospective two-dimensional echocardiographic evaluation of left ventricular outflow tract in complete transposition of the great arteries. Am. J. Cardiol. 55:759, 1985.

535. Rigby, M. L., and Chan, K-Y.: The diagnostic evaluation of patients with complete transposition. Cardiol. Young 1:26, 1991.

536. Pasquini, L., Sanders, S. P., Parness, I. A., et al.: Conal anatomy in 119 patients with D-loop transposition of the great arteries and ventricular septal defect: An echocardiographic and pathologic study. J. Am. Coll. Cardiol. 21:1712, 1993.

537. DiSessa, T. G., Childs, W., Ti, C. C., and Friedman, W. F.: Systolic anterior motion of the mitral valve in a one day old infant with transposition of the great vessels. J. Clin. Ultrasound 6:186, 1978.

538. Lin, A. E., DiSessa, T. G., Williams, R. G., et al.: Balloon and blade atrial septostomy facilitated by two-dimensional echocardiography. Am. J. Cardiol. 57:273, 1986.

539. Moene, R. J., Oppenheimer-Dekker, A., Wenink, A. C. G., et al.: Morphology of ventricular septal defect in complete transposition of the great arteries. Am. J. Cardiol. 55:1566, 1985.

540. Amato, J. J., Zelen, J., and Bushong, J.: Coronary arterial patterns in complete transposition—classification in relation to the arterial switch procedure. Cardiol. Young 4:329, 1994.

541. Sim, E. K. W., van Son, J. A. M., Edwards, W. D., et al.: Coronary artery anatomy in complete transposition of the great arteries. Ann. Thorac. Surg. 57:890, 1994.

542. Pasquini, L., Parness, I. A., Colan, S. D., et al.: Diagnosis of intramural coronary artery in transposition of the great arteries using two-dimensional echocardiography. Circulation 88:1136, 1993.

542a. Chiu, I. S., Chu, S. H., Wang, J. K., et al.: Evolution of coronary artery pattern according to short-axis aortopulmonary rotation: A new categorization for complete transposition of the great arteries. J. Am. Coll. Cardiol. 26:250, 1995.

543. Kirklin, J. W., Colvin, E. V., McConnell, M. E., and Bargeron, L. M.: Complete transposition of the great arteries: Treatment in the current era. Pediatr. Clin. North Am. 37:171, 1990.

544. Kirklin, J. W.: The surgical repair for complete transposition. Cardiol. Young 1:13, 1991.

545. Oelert, H.: Modification of the Mustard operation for surgical treatment of complete transposition by creating a confluence of the caval veins. Cardiol. Young 1:71, 1991.

545a. Sagin-Saylam, G., and Somerville, J.: Palliative Mustard operation for transposition of the great arteries: Late results after 15–20 years. Heart 75:72, 1996.

546. Merrill, W. H., Stewart, J. R., Hammon, J. W., Jr., et al: The Senning

547. Wong, K. Y., Venables, A. W., Kelly, M. J., and Kalff, V.: Longitudinal study of ventricular function after the Mustard operation for transposition of the great arteries: A long-term follow up. Br. Heart J. 60:316, 1988.

548. Dihmis, W. C., Hutter, J. A., Joffe, H. S., et al.: Medium-term clinical results after the Senning procedure with haemodynamic and angiographic evaluation of the venous pathways. Br. Heart J. 69:436, 1993.

549. Hochreiter, C., Snyder, M. S., Borer, J. S., et al.: Right and left ventricular performance 10 years after Mustard repair of transposition of the great arteries. Am. J. Cardiol. 74:478, 1994.

550. Reybrouck, T., Gewillig, M., Dumoulin, M., et al.: Cardiorespiratory exercise performance after Senning operation for transposition of the great arteries. Br. Heart J. 70:175, 1993.

551. Deanfield, J. E., Cullen, S., and Gewillig, M.: Arrhythmias after surgery for complete transposition: Do they matter? Cardiol. Young 1:91, 1991.

552. Hurwitz, R. A., Caldwell, R. L., Girod, D. A., and Brown, J.: Right ventricular systolic function in adolescents and young adults after Mustard operation for transposition of the great arteries. Am. J. Cardiol. 77:294, 1996.

553. Ensing, G. J., Heise, C. T., and Driscoll, D. J.: Cardiovascular response to exercise after the Mustard operation for simple and complex transposition of great arteries. Am. J. Cardiol. 62:617, 1988.

554. Turina, M. I., Siebenmann, R., Von Segesser, L., et al.: Late functional deterioration after atrial correction for transposition of the great arteries. Circulation 80(Suppl. I):162, 1989.

555. Gutgesell, H. P., Massaro, T. A., and Kron, I. L.: The arterial switch operation for transposition of the great arteries in a consortium of university hospitals. Am. J. Cardiol. 74:959, 1994.

556. Castaneda, A. R., Mayer, J. E., Jonas, R. A., et al.: Transposition of the great arteries: The arterial switch operation. Cardiol. Clin. 7:369, 1989.

557. Planche, C., Serraf, A., Lacour-Gayet, F., et al.: Anatomic correction of complete transposition with ventricular septal defect in neonates: Experience with 42 consecutive cases. Cardiol. Young 1:101, 1991.

558. Colan, S. D., Trowitz, S. C. H. E., Wernvosky, et al.: Myocardial performance after arterial switch operation for transposition of the great arteries with intact ventricular septum. Circulation 78:132, 1988.

559. Gleason, M. M., Chin, A., Andrews, B. A., et al.: Two-dimensional and Doppler echocardiographic assessment of neonatal arterial repair for transposition of the great arteries. J. Am. Coll. Cardiol. 13:1320, 1989.

560. Martin, M. M., Snider, R., Bove, E. L., et al.: Two-dimensional and Doppler echocardiographic evaluation after arterial switch repair in infancy for complete transposition of the great arteries. Am. J. Cardiol. 63:332, 1989.

561. Villafane, J., White, S., Elbl, F., et al.: An electrocardiographic midterm follow up study after anatomic repair of transposition of the great arteries. Am. J. Cardiol. 66:350, 1990.

562. Boutin, C., Wernovsky, G., Sanders, S. P., et al.: Rapid two-stage arterial switch operation: Evaluation of left ventricular systolic mechanics late after an acute pressure overload stimulus in infancy. Circulation 90:1294, 1994.

563. Boutin, C., Jonas, R. A., Sanders, S. P., et al.: Rapid two-stage arterial switch operation: Acquisition of left ventricular mass after pulmonary artery banding in infants with transposition of the great arteries. Circulation 90:1304, 1994.

564. Wernovsky, G., Bridges, N. D., and Mandell, V. S.: Enlarged bronchial arteries after early repair of transposition of the great arteries. J. Am. Coll. Cardiol. 21:465, 1993.

565. Nakanishi, T., Matsumoto, Y., Seguchi, M., et al.: Balloon angioplasty for postoperative pulmonary artery stenosis in transposition of the great arteries. J. Am. Coll. Cardiol. 22:859, 1993.

566. Martin, R. P., Ettedgui, J. A., Qureshi, S. A., et al.: A quantitative evaluation of aortic regurgitation after anatomic correction of transposition of the great arteries. J. Am. Coll. Cardiol. 12:1281, 1988.

566a. Redington, A. N.: Functional assessment of the heart after corrective surgery for complete transposition. Cardiol. Young 1:84, 1991.

567. Hourihan, M., Colan, S. D., Wernovsky, G., et al.: Growth of the aortic anastomosis, annulus, and root after the arterial switch procedure performed in infancy. Circulation 88:615, 1993.

568. Weindling, S. N., Wernovsky, G., Colan, S. D., et al.: Myocardial perfusion, function and exercise tolerance after the arterial switch operation. J. Am. Coll. Cardiol. 23:424, 1994.

569. Lupinetti, F. M., Bove, E. L., Minich, L. L., et al.: Intermediate-term survival and functional results after arterial repair for transposition of the great arteries. J. Thorac. Cardiovasc. Surg. 103:421, 1992.

570. Elkins, R. C., Knott-Craig, C. J., Ahn, J. H., et al.: Ventricular function after the arterial switch operation for transposition of the great arteries. Ann. Thorac. Surg. 57:826, 1994.

571. Corno, A., George, B., Pearl, J., and Laks, H.: Surgical options for complex transposition of the great arteries. J. Am. Coll. Cardiol 14:742, 1989.

572. Lecompte, Y., Neveux, J. Y., Leca, F., et al.: Reconstruction of the pulmonary outflow tract without prosthetic conduit. J. Thorac. Cardiovasc. Surg. 87:727, 1982.

573. Corno, A. F., Parisi, F., Marino, B., et al.: Palliative Mustard operation: An expanded horizon. Eur. J. Cardiothorac. Surg. 1:144, 1987.

574. Colli, A. M., De Leval, M., and Somerville, J.: Anatomically corrected malposition of the great arteries. Am. J. Cardiol. 55:1367, 1985.

575. Kirklin, J. W., Pacifico, A. D., Bargeron, L. M., Jr., and Soto, B.: Cardiac

repair and anatomically corrected malposition of the great arteries. Circulation 48:153, 1973.

576. Berry, W. B., Roberts, W. C., Morrow, A. G., and Braunwald, E.: Corrected transposition of the aorta and pulmonary trunk: Clinical, hemodynamic, and pathologic findings. Am. J. Med. 36:35, 1964.

577. Freedberg, D. Z., and Nadas, A. S.: Clinical profile of patients with congenital corrected transposition of the great arteries. N. Engl. J. Med. 282:1053, 1970.

578. Bjarke, B. B., and Kidd, B. S. L.: Congenitally corrected transposition of the great arteries: A clinical study of 101 cases. Acta Paediatr. Scand. 65:153, 1976.

579. Lundstrom, U., Bull, C., Wyse, R. K. H., et al.: The natural and "unnatural" history of congenitally corrected transposition. Am. J. Cardiol. 65:1222, 1990.

579a. Presbitero, P., Somerville, J., Rabajoli, F., et al.: Corrected transposition of the great arteries without associated defects in adult patients: Clinical profile and follow up. Br. Heart J. 74:57, 1995.

580. Dimas, A. P., Moodie, D. S., Strba, R., and Gill, C. C.: Long-term function of the morphologic right ventricle in adult patients with corrected transposition of the great arteries. Am. Heart J. 118:526, 1989.

581. Waldo, A. L., Pacifico, A. D., Bargeron, L. M., Jr., et al.: Electrophysiological delineation of specialized AV conduction system in patients with corrected transposition of the great vessels and ventricular septal defect. Circulation 52:435, 1975.

582. Bharati, B., Rosen, K., Steinfeld, L., et al.: The anatomic substrate for pre-excitation in corrected transposition. Circulation 62:831, 1980.

583. Meissner, M. D., Panidis, I. P., Eshaghpour, E., et al.: Corrected transposition of the great arteries: Evaluation by two-dimensional and Doppler echocardiography. Am. Heart J. 111:599, 1986.

584. Freedom, R. M., Harrington, D. P., and White, R. I., Jr.: The differential diagnosis of levotransposed or malposed aorta: An angiocardiographic study. Circulation 50:1040, 1974.

585. Russo, P., Danielson, G. K., and Driscoll, D. J.: Transaortic closure of ventricular septal defect in patients with corrected transposition with pulmonary stenosis or atresia. Circulation 76(Suppl. III):88, 1987.

586. McGrath, L. B., Kirklin, J. W., Blackstone, E. H., et al.: Death and other events after cardiac repair in discordant atrioventricular connection. J. Thorac. Cardiovasc. Surg. 90:711, 1985.

587. Yoshimura, N., Yamaguchi, M., Oshima, Y., et al.: Systemic atrioventricular valve replacement in an infant with corrected transposition of the great arteries. Ann. Thorac. Surg. 54:573, 1992.

588. Hagler, D. J.: Double-outlet right ventricle. In Emmanoulides, G. C., Allen, H. D., et al. (eds.): Moss and Adams' Heart Disease in Infants, Children and Adolescents. 5th ed. Baltimore, Williams and Wilkins, 1994, p. 1246.

589. Goitein, K. J., Neches, W. H., Park, S. C., et al.: Electrocardiogram in double chamber right ventricle. Am. J. Cardiol. 45:604, 1980.

590. Roberson, D. A., and Silverman, N. H.: Malaligned outlet septum with subpulmonary ventricular septal defect and abnormal ventriculoarterial connection: A morphologic spectrum defined echocardiographically. J. Am. Coll. Cardiol. 16:459, 1990.

591. Sridaromont, S., Ritter, D. G., Feldt, R. H., et al.: Double outlet right ventricle: Anatomic and angiocardiographic correlations. Mayo Clin. Proc. 53:555, 1978.

592. Kirklin, J. W., Pacifico, A. D., Blackstone, E. H., et al.: Current risks and protocols for operations for double-outlet right ventricle. J. Thorac. Cardiovasc. Surg. 92:913, 1986.

593. Russo, P., Danielson, G. K., Puga, F. J., et al.: Modified Fontan procedure for biventricular hearts with complex forms of double-outlet right ventricle. Circulation 78(Suppl. III):20, 1988.

594. Day, R., Laks, H., Milgalter, E., et al.: Partial biventricular repair for double-outlet right ventricle with left ventricular hypoplasia. Ann. Thorac. Surg. 49:1003, 1990.

595. Van Praagh, R., Weinberg, P. M., and Srebro, J. P.: Double-outlet left ventricle. In Emmanouilides, G. C., et al. (eds.): Moss and Adams' Heart Disease in Infants, Children, and Adolescents. 4th ed. Baltimore, Williams and Wilkins, 1989, p. 461.

596. Rebergen, S. A., Guit, G. L., and de Roos, A.: Double outlet left ventricle: Diagnosis with magnetic resonance imaging. Br. Heart J. 66:381, 1991.

597. Marino, B., and Bevilacqua, M.: Double-outlet left ventricle: Two-dimensional echocardiographic diagnosis. Am. Heart J. 123:1075, 1992.

598. Krabill, K. A., and Lucas, R. V., Jr.: Abnormal pulmonary venous connections. In Emmanouilides, G. C., Allen, H. D., et al. (eds.): Moss and Adams' Heart Disease in Infants, Children, and Adolescents. 5th ed. Baltimore, Williams and Wilkins, 1994, p. 838.

599. Ward, K. E., Mullins, C. E., Huhta, J. C., et al.: Restrictive interatrial communication in total anomalous pulmonary venous connection. Am. J. Cardiol. 57:1131, 1986.

600. Lucas, R. V., Jr., Lock, J. E., Tandon, R., and Edwards, J. E.: Gross and histologic anatomy of total anomalous pulmonary venous connections. Am. J. Cardiol. 62:292, 1988.

601. Lincoln, C. R., Rigby, M. L., Marcanti, C., et al.: Surgical risk factors in total anomalous pulmonary venous connection. Am. J. Cardiol. 61:608, 1988.

602. Wang, J. K., Lue, H. C., Wu, M. H., et al.: Obstructed total anomalous pulmonary venous connection. Pediatr. Cardiol. 14:28, 1993.

603. Elliott, L. P., and Edwards, J. E.: The problem of pulmonary venous obstruction in total anomalous pulmonary venous connection to the left innominate vein. Circulation 25:913, 1962.

604. Newfeld, E. A., Wilson, A., Paul, M. H., and Reisch, J. S.: Pulmonary

vascular disease in total anomalous pulmonary venous drainage. Circulation 61:103, 1980.

605. Chin, A. J., Sanders, S. P., Sherman, F., et al.: Accuracy of subcostal two-dimensional echocardiography in prospective diagnosis of total anomalous pulmonary venous connection. Am. Heart J. 113:1153, 1987.

606. Jenkins, K. J., Sanders, S. P., Orav, E. J., et al.: Individual pulmonary vein size and survival in infants with totally anomalous pulmonary venous connection. J. Am. Coll. Cardiol. 22:201, 1993.

607. Lamb, R. K., Qureshi, S. A., Wilkinson, J. L., et al.: Total anomalous pulmonary venous drainage: 17-year surgical experience. J. Thorac. Cardiovasc. Surg. 96:368, 1988.

608. Van Meter, C., Jr., LeBlanc, J. G., Culpepper, W. S., III, and Ochsner, J. L.: Partial anomalous pulmonary venous return. Circulation 82(Suppl. IV):195, 1990.

609. Gao, Y. A., Burrows, P. E., Benson, L. N., et al.: Scimitar syndrome in infancy. J. Am. Coll. Cardiol. 22:873, 1993.

610. Dupuis, C., Charaf, L. A. C., Breviere, G. M., and Abou, P.: "Infantile" form of the scimitar syndrome with pulmonary hypertension. Am. J. Cardiol. 71:1326, 1993.

611. Stanger, P., Rudolph, A. M., and Edwards, J. E.: Cardiac malpositions: An overview based on a study of 65 necropsy specimens. Circulation 56:159, 1977.

612. Van Praagh, R.: Diagnosis of complex congenital heart disease: Morphologic-anatomic method and terminology. Cardiovasc. Intervent. Radiol. 7:115, 1984.

613. Silverman, N. H.: An ultrasonic approach to the diagnosis of cardiac situs, connections, and malposition. In Friedman, W. F., and Higgins, C. B. (eds.): Pediatric Cardiac Imaging. Philadelphia, W. B. Saunders Company, 1984, p. 188.

614. Geva, T., Vick, W., Wendt, R., and Rokey, R.: Role of spin echo and cine magnetic resonance imaging in presurgical planning of heterotaxy syndrome: Comparison with echocardiography and catheterization. Circulation 90:348, 1994.

615. Geva, T., Sanders, S. P., Ayres, N. A., et al.: Two-dimensional echocardiographic anatomy of atrioventricular alignment discordance with situs concordance. Am. Heart J. 125:459, 1993.

616. Wang, J. K., Li, Y. W., Chiu, I. S., et al.: Usefulness of magnetic resonance imaging in the assessment of venoatrial connections, atrial morphology, bronchial situs, and other anomalies in right isomerism. Am. J. Cardiol. 74:701, 1994.

617. Anderson, C., Devine, W. A., Anderson, R. H., et al.: Abnormalities of the spleen in relation to congenital malformations of the heart: Survey of necropsy findings in children. Br. Heart J. 63:122, 1990.

618. Peoples, W. M., Moller, J. H., and Edwards, J. E.: Polysplenia: A review of 146 cases. Pediatr. Cardiol. 4:129, 1983.

619. Phoon, C. K., and Neill, C. A.: Asplenia syndrome—risk factors for early unfavorable outcome. Am. J. Cardiol. 73:1235, 1994.

620. Phoon, C. K., and Neill, C. A.: Asplenia syndrome: Insight into embryology through an analysis of cardiac and extracardiac anomalies. Am. J. Cardiol. 73:581, 1994.

621. Culbertson, C. B., George, B. L., Day, R. W., et al.: Factors influencing survival of patients with heterotaxy syndrome undergoing the Fontan procedure. J. Am. Coll. Cardiol. 20:678, 1992.

622. Oku, H., Iemura, J., Kitayama, H., et al.: Bivalvation with bridging for common atrioventricular valve regurgitation in right isomerism. Ann. Thorac. Surg. 57:1324, 1994.

623. Gehlman, H. R., and Van Ingen, G. J.: Symptomatic congenital complete absence of the left pericardium: Case report and review of the literature. Eur. Heart J. 10:670, 1989.

624. Pernot, C., Hoeffel, J. C., and Henry, M.: Radiologic patterns of congenital malformation of the pericardium. Radiol. Clin. (Basel) 44:505, 1975.

625. Rowland, T. W., Twible, E. A., Norwood, W. I., Jr., and Keane, J. F.: Partial absence of the left pericardium: Diagnosis by two-dimensional echocardiography. Am. J. Dis. Child. 136:628, 1982.

626. Jones, J. W., and McManus, B. M.: Fatal cardiac strangulation by congenital partial pericardial defect. Am. Heart J. 107:183, 1984.

627. Rowland, T. W., Twible, E. A., Norwood, W. J., Jr., and Keane, J. F.: Partial absence of the left pericardium. Am. J. Dis. Child. 136:628, 1982.

628. Anderson, R. H., Macartney, F. J., Tynan, M., et al.: Univentricular atrioventricular connection: The single ventricle trap unsprung. Pediatr. Cardiol. 4:273, 1983.

629. Thies, W. R., Soto, B., Diethelm, E., et al.: Angiographic anatomy of hearts with one ventricular chamber: The true single ventricle. Am. J. Cardiol. 55:1363, 1985.

630. Change, A. C., Hanley, F. L., Wernovsky, G., et al.: Early bidirectional cavopulmonary shunt in young infants. Circulation 88:149, 1993.

631. Calderon-Colmenero, J., Ramirez, S., Rijlaarsdam, M., et al.: Use of bidirectional cavopulmonary shunt in patients under one year of age. Cardiol. Young 5:28, 1995.

632. Moak, J. P., and Gersony, W. M.: Progressive atrioventricular valvular regurgitation in single ventricle. Am. J. Cardiol. 59:656, 1987.

633. Mair, D. D., Hagler, D. J., Julsrud, P. R., et al.: Early and late results of the modified Fontan procedure for double-inlet left ventricle: The Mayo Clinic experience. J. Am. Coll. Cardiol. 18:1727, 1991.

634. DiSessa, T. G., Isabel-Jones, J. G., Heins, H., et al.: Two dimensional echocardiographic features of the univentricular heart. Cardiovasc. Ultrason. 3:89, 1984.

635. Jacobs, M. I., and Norwood, W. I.: Fontan operation: Influence of modifications on morbidity and mortality. Ann. Thorac. Surg. 58:945, 1994.

636. Bevilacqua, M., Sanders, S. P., and van Praagh, S.: Double-inlet single

left ventricle: Echocardiographic anatomy with emphasis on the morphology of the atrioventricular valves and ventricular septal defect. J. Am. Coll. Cardiol. 18:559, 1991.

637. Fogel, M. A., Weinberg, P. M., Fellows, K. E., and Hoffman, E. A.: Magnetic resonance imaging of constant total heart volume and center of mass in patients with functional single ventricle before and after staged Fontan procedure. Am. J. Cardiol. 72:1435, 1993.

638. Matitiau, A., Geva, T., Colan, S. D., et al.: Bulboventricular foramen size in infants with double-inlet left ventricle or tricuspid atresia with transposed great arteries: Influence on initial palliative operation and rate of growth. J. Am. Coll. Cardiol. 19:142, 1992.

639. Huggon, I. C., Baker, E. J., Maisey, M. N., et al.: Magnetic resonance imaging of hearts with atrioventricular valve atresia or double inlet ventricle. Br. Heart J. 68:313, 1992.

640. Mayer, J. E.: Surgical aortico-pulmonary anastomosis for a complex aortic obstruction with single ventricle. Prog. Pediatr. Cardiol. 3:106, 1994.

641. Lui, R. C., Williams, W. G., Trusler, G. A., et al.: Experience with the Damus-Kaye-Stansel procedure for children with Taussig-Bing hearts or univentricular hearts with subaortic stenosis. Circulation 88:170, 1993.

642. Gewillig, M., Wyse, R. K., De Leval, M. R., et al.: Early and late arrhythmias after the Fontan operation: Predisposing factors and clinical consequences. Br. Heart J. 67:72, 1992.

643. Parikh, S. R., Hurwitz, R. A., Caldwell, R. L., and Girod, D. A.: Ventricular function in the single ventricle before and after Fontan surgery. Am. J. Cardiol. 67:1390, 1991.

644. Kurer, C. C., Tanner, C. S., and Vetter, V. L.: Electrophysiologic findings after Fontan repair of functional single ventricle. J. Am. Coll. Cardiol. 17:174, 1991.

645. Sluysmans, T., Sanders, S. P., van der Velde, M., et al.: Natural history and patterns of recovery of contractile function in single left ventricle after Fontan operation. Circulation 86:1753, 1992.

646. Rosenthal, M., Bush, A., Deanfield, J., and Redington, A.: Comparison of cardiopulmonary adaptation during exercise in children after the atriopulmonary and total cavopulmonary connection Fontan procedures. Circulation 91:372, 1995.

647. Stevenson, O., Soderlund, S., Thoren, C., and Wallgren, G.: Arterial anomalies causing compression of the trachea and/or the esophagus. Acta Paediatr. Scand. 60:81, 1971.

648. Park, C. D., Waldhausen, J. A., Friedman, S., et al.: Tracheal compression by the great arteries in the mediastinum: Report of 39 cases. Arch. Surg. 103:626, 1971.

649. Ashwinikumar, P., de Leval, M. R., Elliott, M. J., et al.: Pulmonary artery sling. Ann. Thorac. Surg. 54:967, 1992.

650. Baron, R. L., Gutierrez, F. R., and McKnight, R. C.: Computed tomographic evaluation of the great arteries and aortic arch malformations. In Friedman, W. F., and Higgins, C. B. (eds.): Pediatric Cardiac Imaging. Philadelphia, W. B. Saunders Company, 1983, p. 135.

651. Azarow, K. S., Pearl, R. H., Hoffman, M. A., et al.: Vascular ring: Does magnetic resonance imaging replace angiography? Ann. Thorac. Surg. 53:882, 1992.

652. deLeval, M.: Vascular rings. In Stark, J., and deLeval, M. (eds.): Surgery for Congenital Heart Defects. New York, Grune and Stratton, 1983, p. 227.

653. Anand, R., Dooley, K. J., Williams, W. H., et al.: Follow-up of surgical correction of vascular anomalies causing tracheobronchial compression. Pediatr. Cardiol. 15:58, 1994.

654. Perry, J. C., and Garson, A., Jr.: Diagnosis and treatment of arrhythmias. Adv. Pediatr. 36:177, 1989.

655. Anderson, R. H., Wenick, A. C. G., Losekoot, T. G., and Becker, A. E.: Congenitally complete heart block. Circulation 56:90, 1977.

655a. Michaelsson, M.: Congenital complete atrioventricular block. Progr. Pediatr. Cardiol. 4:1, 1995.

656. Derksen, R. H., and Meilof, J. F.: Anti-Ro/SS-A and anti-La/SS-B autoantibody levels in relation to systemic lupus erythematosus disease activity and congenital heart block. Arthritis Rheum. 35:953, 1992.

657. Horsfall, A. C., and Rose, L. M.: Cross-reactive maternal autoantibodies and congenital heart block. J. Autoimmun. 5:479, 1992.

658. Ross, B. A.: Congenital complete atrioventricular block. Pediatr. Clin. North Am. 37:69, 1990.

659. Kugler, J. D., and Danford, D. A.: Pacemakers in children: An update. Am. Heart J. 117:665, 1989.

660. Hoyer, M. H., Beerman, L. B., Ettedgui, J. A., et al.: Transatrial lead placement for endocardial pacing in children. Ann. Thorac. Surg. 58:97, 1994.

661. Dreifus, L. S., Fisch, C., Griffin, J. C., et al.: Guidelines for implantation of cardiac pacemakers and antiarrhythmia devices: A report of the American College of Cardiology/American Heart Association Task Force on assessment of diagnostic and therapeutic cardiovascular procedures (Committee on Pacemaker Implantation). J. Am. Coll. Cardiol. 18:1, 1991.

662. Michaelsson, M., and Engle, M. A.: Congenital complete heart block: An international study of the natural history. Cardiovasc. Clin. 4:85, 1982.

663. Ko, J. K., Deal, B. J., Strasburger, J. F., et al.: Supraventricular tachycardia mechanisms and their age distribution in pediatric patients. Am. J. Cardiol. 69:1028, 1992.

664. Kleinman, C. S., Donnerstein, R. L., DeVore, G. R., et al.: Fetal echocardiography for evaluation of in utero congestive heart failure. N. Engl. J. Med. 306:568, 1982.

665. Radford, D. J., Izukawa, T., and Rowe, R. D.: Congenital paroxysmal atrial tachycardia. Arch. Dis. Child. 51:613, 1976.

666. Deal, B. J., Keane, J. F., Gillette, P. C., and Gardon, A., Jr.: Wolff-Parkinson-White syndrome and supraventricular tachycardia during infancy: Management and follow-up. J. Am. Coll. Cardiol. 5:130, 1985.

667. Klitzner, T. S., and Friedman, W. F.: Cardiac arrhythmias: The role of pharmacologic intervention. Cardiol. Clin. 7:299, 1989.

668. Benson, D. W., Jr., Dunnigan, A., and Benditt, D. G.: Follow-up evaluation of infant paroxysmal atrial tachycardia: Transesophageal study. Circulation 75:542, 1987.

669. Zipes, D. P., et al.: Guidelines for clinical intracardiac electrophysiologic studies: A report of the American College of Cardiology/American Heart Association Task Force on Assessment of Diagnostic and Therapeutic Cardiovascular Procedures. J. Am. Coll. Cardiol. 14:1827, 1989.

670. Klitzner, T. S., Wetzel, G. T., Saxon, L. A., et al.: Radiofrequency ablation: A new era in the treatment of pediatric arrhythmias. Am. J. Dis. Child. 147:769, 1993.

671. Lai, W. W., Al-Khatib, Y., Klitzner, T. S., et al.: Biplanar transesophageal echocardiographic direction of radiofrequency catheter ablation in children and adolescents with the Wolff-Parkinson-White syndrome. Am. J. Cardiol. 71:872, 1993.

672. Dhala, A., Bremner, S., Deshpande, S., et al.: Efficacy and safety of atrioventricular nodal modification for atrioventricular nodal reentrant tachycardia in the pediatric population. Am. Heart J. 128:903, 1994.

673. Hebe, J., Schlüter, M., and Kuck, K. H.: Catheter ablation in children with supraventricular tachycardia mediated by accessory pathways — use of radiofrequency current as a first line of therapy. Cardiol. Young 4:28, 1994.

674. Kugler, J. D., Danford, D. A., Deal, B. J., et al.: Radiofrequency catheter ablation for tachyarrhythmias in children and adolescents. N. Engl. J. Med. 330:1481, 1994.

675. Garson, A., Jr., Bink-Boelkens, M., Hesslein, P. S., et al.: Atrial flutter in the young: A collaborative study of 380 cases. J. Am. Coll. Cardiol. 6:871, 1985.

676. Mendelsohn, A., Dick, M., and Serwer, G. A.: Natural history of isolated atrial flutter in infancy. J. Pediatr. 119:386, 1991.

677. Dunnigan, A., Benson, W., Jr., and Benditt, D. G.: Atrial flutter in infancy: Diagnosis, clinical features and treatment. Pediatrics 75:725, 1985.

678. Dick, M., Scott, W. A., Serwer, G. S., et al.: Acute termination of supraventricular tachyarrhythmias in children by transesophageal atrial pacing. Am. J. Cardiol. 61:925, 1988.

679. Jiang, C., Atkinson, D., Towbin, J. A., et al.: Two long QT syndrome loci map to chromosomes 3 and 7 with evidence for further heterogeneity. Nature Genetics 8:141, 1994.

680. Garson, A., Jr., Dick, M., II, Fournier, A., et al.: The long QT syndrome in children: An international study of 287 patients. Circulation 87:1866, 1993.

Chapter 30
Congenital Heart Disease in Adults

JOSEPH K. PERLOFF

Advances in diagnostic techniques and in the surgical and medical management of infants and children with congenital malformations of the heart and circulation have had a major impact upon longevity.[1-3] The number of older patients with congenital heart disease is steadily increasing, and the trend promises to continue. Congenital heart disease in adults has emerged as a special area of cardiovascular interest[4] that includes patients who have never undergone cardiac surgery, those who have undergone cardiac surgery and require no further operation, those who have had palliation with or without anticipation of reparative surgery, and those whose condition is inoperable apart from organ transplantation. This chapter begins with a brief historical perspective and then focuses upon the multidisciplinary facilities for comprehensive care, survival patterns (without operation and postoperative), medical considerations, surgical considerations, and postoperative residua and sequelae.[2]

HISTORICAL PERSPECTIVES

Congenital heart disease is, by definition, present at birth (con, together; genitus, born), but survival patterns vary widely.[2,5] In 1888, Etienne-Louis Arthur Fallot wrote, "We have seen from our observations that cyanosis, especially in the adult, is the result of a small number of cardiac malformations well determined."[6] Fallot referred to the tetralogy that still bears his name as one of the most familiar eponyms in cardiovascular medicine.

In the first half of the twentieth century, the untiring work of Maude Abbott culminated in her remarkable Atlas of Congenital Heart Disease, which was based upon 1000 pathology specimens personally studied.[7] The atlas was not only a landmark in the classification of congenital malformations of the heart but also provided invaluable information on survival patterns before the advent of cardiac surgery. The seminal contributions of Gross, Blalock, and Crafoord appreciably modified those survival patterns, and the sense of despair that had surrounded congenital cardiac anomalies—those "hopeless futilities"—began to dissipate.

In 1939, Robert Gross, a pediatric surgeon in Boston, ligated a patent ductus arteriosus in a 7½-year-old girl.[8] A few years later, Helen Brooke Taussig, a pediatric cardiologist in Baltimore, conceived the idea of "creating" a patent ductus in cyanotic children suffering from deficient pulmonary blood flow, and in 1945, Alfred Blalock, a vascular surgeon at Johns Hopkins Hospital, implemented Taussig's idea by suturing the end of a subclavian artery to the side of a pulmonary artery in a patient with Fallot's tetralogy, thus establishing the Blalock-Taussig anastomosis.[9] Before this operation, ". . . a blue baby with a malformed heart was considered beyond the reach of surgical aid." In the early 1940's, Clarence Crafoord, at the Karolinska Institute in Sweden, while operating on patients with patent ductus arteriosus, "began to wonder whether it might not also be possible to treat coarctation of the aortic isthmus by surgical means."[10] The introduction of cardiac catheterization after World War II, a technique for which Andre F. Cournand and Dickenson W. Richards in the United States and Werner Forssman in Germany received the Nobel Prize in 1956, was a major step forward both diagnostically and in the study of circulatory physiology.[2] The development of extracorporeal circulation in the early to mid-1950's was destined to make virtually all congenital malformations of the heart accessible to the skills of cardiac surgeons. The stage was set for "accurate visualization of structures within the heart for a period sufficient to permit precise corrective measures."[11]

The culmination of these historical landmarks was one of the most successful diagnostic and therapeutic achievements that medicine has witnessed. Formidable technical resources became accessible, permitting remarkably accurate anatomical and physiological diagnoses and astonishing feats of reparative surgery. Survival patterns were affected, often profoundly. Congenital heart disease should therefore be considered not only in terms of age of onset but also in terms of the age range that survival now permits—an uninterrupted continuum from fetal life to senescence.[2,4] Although long-term management remains concerned with unoperated patients, medical management increasingly focuses on the growing numbers of postoperative patients who need surveillance. The quality of care provided by pediatric cardiologists from birth to maturity must be matched with care of equal quality for adults.

Unoperated adults experience improved longevity because of refinements in the management of arrhythmias and conduction disturbances, ventricular failure, pulmonary vascular disease, hematological disorders, renal function, urate metabolism, infective endocarditis, pregnancy, and noncardiac surgery. The management of patients after cardiac surgery or interventional catheterization requires knowledge of the intrinsic congenital cardiac or vascular malformation, the nature and effects of the therapeutic intervention, and the presence, type, and extent of postinterventional residua and sequelae. The ideal of cure in the literal sense is rarely achieved, however, so that a broad range of residua and sequelae are left behind and require prolonged, if not indefinite, medical attention that is essential if the concerns inherent in this new and increasing patient population are to be addressed properly.[2,4]

MULTIDISCIPLINARY CARE OF ADULTS WITH CONGENITAL HEART DISEASE

In the United States and abroad, increasing numbers of specialized facilities are emerging for the care of adults with congenital heart disease.[2,4] Relevant to these facilities are staffing, diagnostic laboratories, criteria for patient entry, referral patterns, outpatient and inpatient management, multidisciplinary consultants, and educational, training, and research commitments.[2]

Patients are best managed, at least for the foreseeable future, by collaboration between medical and pediatric cardiologists and cardiac surgeons with the assistance of cardiovascular nurse specialists or physician assistants. Cardiac surgeons who have the knowledge and skills needed to deal with congenital heart disease can, as a rule, adapt those skills to coexisting acquired cardiac diseases and obviate the need for two cardiac surgeons to perform one operation. An adult congenital heart disease facility should be a collaborative effort, especially in the setting of a university hospital in which intellectual interchange, teaching, and research are as paramount as optimal patient care. Cardiologists with special expertise in this area are now recognized as part of the profile of cardiovascular specialists.[12]

Consultative needs should be anticipated rather than solicited as ad hoc opinions. Noncardiac consultants are best incorporated into the adult congenital heart disease facility and include electrophysiologists, hematologists, nephrologists, rheumatologists, transplant cardiologists, pulmonologists, high-risk pregnancy obstetricians, gynecologists, psychiatrists, cardiac anesthesiologists, cardiac pathologists, and social service personnel for insurance and vocational counseling.

Criteria for patient entry into the specialized facilities are based on age and psychological and physical maturity. Adolescents are neither children nor adults, and adolescent medicine, at least at present, is best dealt with by the more knowledgeable pediatricians or by medical cardiologists with pediatric experience. In some centers, adolescent patients remain the province of pediatric cardiologists, whereas in others, adolescents are included within the adult congenital heart disease facility, provided that facility has a pediatric cardiologist on its staff.[4]

Tertiary centers for congenital heart disease in adults do not compete with practicing physicians or community hospitals but instead offer services that are difficult if not impossible to duplicate. Broadly speaking, the base of the referral pyramid is the primary care physician in the community (general pediatrician, general physician). The next level (stratum) is the cardiologist in the community (pediatric, medical) who provides both consultative and primary care. Tertiary care depends upon regional specialized facilities that have experience even with rare and complex malformations.

There is a mounting consensus that adults with congenital heart disease are best managed in an adult setting, both outpatient and inpatient. Pediatric cardiology clinics tend to reinforce a sense of dependency that patients must overcome if they are to function as mature adults. Inpatient policy depends in part on whether medicine and pediatrics share the same hospital. When that is the case, adults with congenital heart disease are admitted to adult inpatient facilities under the care of the cardiologist with inpatient privileges. Hospitalized adults are an important part of the educational experience of house staff and fellows. Admissions are for cardiac or noncardiac surgery, for labor and delivery, for cardiac intensive care (generally arrhythmias), for heart failure, or for coexisting general medical disorders.

Noninvasive, exercise, catheterization, angiographic, and magnetic resonance imaging (MRI) laboratories must provide the same high quality of care for adults with congenital heart disease as that provided by pediatric laboratories for infants and children. Quality cannot be compromised for expediency.

Medical records serve multiple purposes. The goal should be a quality standard appropriate for the use of records for research purposes. Reports to referring physicians should be both practical and educational. It is useful to have a dual record system, with one set for hospital files and a second for the congenital heart disease facility. When patients move to another area, copies of their records should be carried for delivery to their new cardiologist. Patients have proved to be responsible emissaries.

The educational and training commitments of an adult congenital heart disease facility extend to community physicians, house staff, fellows, medical students, visiting physicians, nurses (especially nurse specialists), and the patients themselves. Tertiary care centers should assume responsibility for informing community physicians that adults with congenital heart disease require special expertise seldom available in local hospitals. That level of awareness is important in channeling patients to tertiary facilities.

Adult congenital heart disease centers, especially in university hospitals, should be committed to research prompted by a desire to address unresolved questions posed by this patient population. A rich harvest is in store if advantage is taken of collaboration with colleagues in other disciplines. A research base must be provided for fellows with career interests in adult congenital heart disease.

SURVIVAL PATTERNS

Unoperated Patients

The term *natural history* is a misnomer, because mortality and morbidity for patients who have not undergone cardiac surgery have been materially influenced by advances in *medical* management. Accordingly, "natural history" should be replaced by "unoperated survival."

Unoperated patients include those with malformations that do not require surgery, malformations that are amenable to operation in adulthood, and malformations that are inoperable except for heart, lung, or heart-lung transplantation. Management of unoperated adults must take into account not only the congenital disorder per se but also the medical disorders that are inherent components of certain types of congenital heart disease, as well as acquired disorders of the heart and circulation that coexist with and modify the physiological expressions of the congenital malformation. This section deals chiefly with common or uncommon defects in which unoperated adult survival is expected and with certain defects that are common and therefore familiar but for which adult survival is exceptional.

Common Defects in Which Unoperated Adult Survival is Expected

BICUSPID AORTIC VALVE (see also p. 914, and Fig. 3–67, p. 79, and Fig. 29–33, p. 917). This malformation is the most

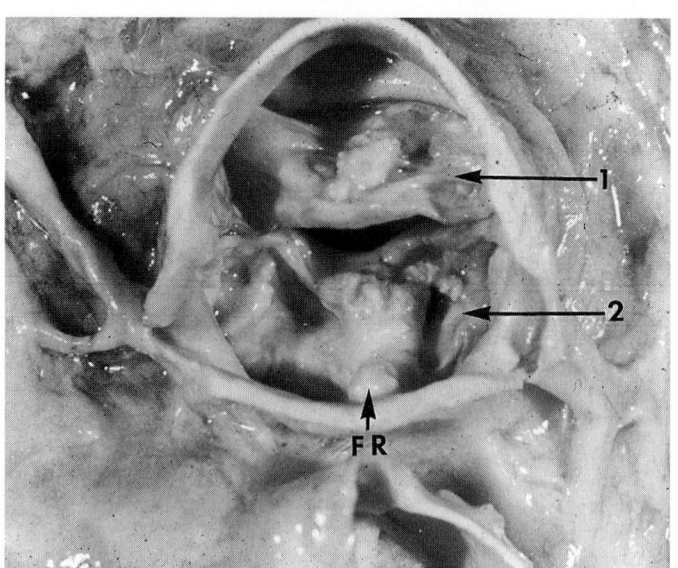

FIGURE 30–1. Necropsy specimen from an adult with bicuspid aortic stenosis. The first arrow points to one calcified leaflet, the second arrow points to a second calcified leaflet, and the vertical arrow points to calcium in the false raphe (FR). (Courtesy of Dr. William C. Roberts.

frequent congenital anomaly to which that structure is subject and is one of the most common gross morphological congenital anomalies of the heart or great arteries.[13] Bicuspid aortic valves that are functionally normal at birth can remain so throughout a normal life span. Progressive stenosis results from fibrocalcific thickening, a substrate that accounts for about one-half of surgical cases of isolated calcific aortic valve stenosis in adults (Fig. 30–1).[14] Conversely, a functionally normal bicuspid aortic valve may develop progressive incompetence and is an important cause of anatomically isolated aortic regurgitation in adults.[5] A bicuspid aortic valve may be modified, sometimes suddenly and appreciably, by infective endocarditis, to which the malformation is highly susceptible.[15] An inherent relationship exists between a congenital bicuspid aortic valve and an abnormality of the aortic root that takes the form of cystic medial necrosis related to the bicuspid

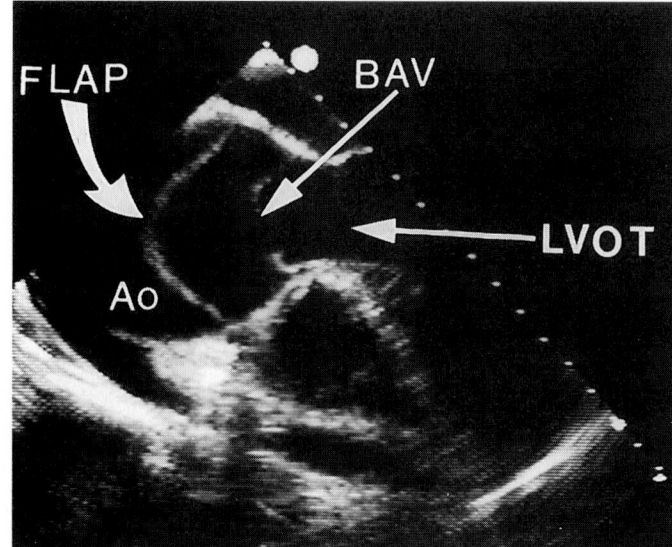

FIGURE 30–2. Transesophageal echocardiogram from a 37-year-old man with a biscuspid aortic valve, aortic regurgitation, and a dissecting aneurysm of the ascending aorta. The flap of the aortic dissection (FLAP) moved freely within the dilated aortic root (Ao). The dissection began just distal to the bicuspid aortic valve (BAV). LVOT = left ventricular outflow tract.

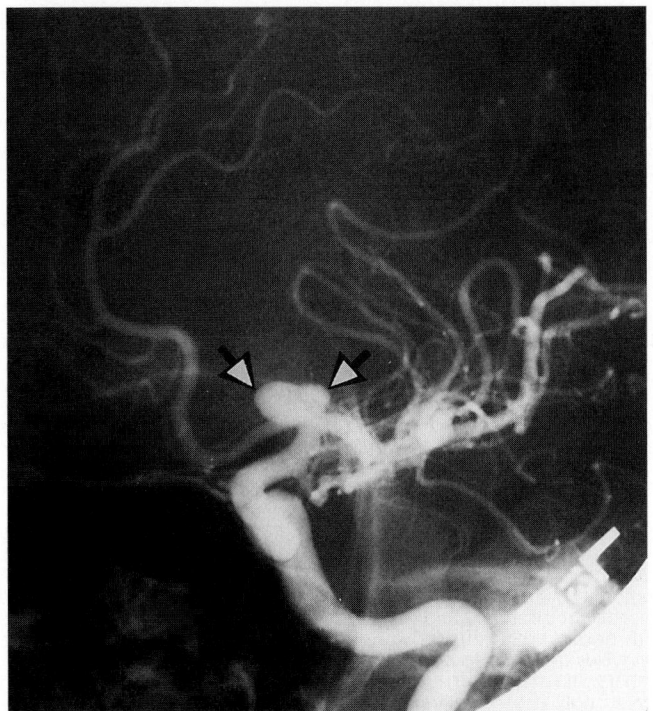

FIGURE 30–3. Congenital berry aneurysm of the circle of Willis in a 28-year-old woman with Fallot's tetralogy and pulmonary atresia. This type of congenital cerebral aneurysm is usually found in conjunction with coarctation of the aorta.

quarters by age 50.[17] The oldest recorded survivor was a 92-year-old man reported by Reynaud in 1828.[18]

Survival and morbidity in adults with aortic coarctation are influenced by coexisting congenital and acquired cardiac and vascular diseases. The most common associated congenital malformation is the bicuspid aortic valve[5] (see above). Infective endocarditis is more likely to involve the bicuspid aortic valve than the site of coarctation.[5] A less common but potentially lethal coexisting malformation is a congenital aneurysm of the circle of Willis (Fig. 30–3), which typically becomes manifested by sudden rupture.[19] Dissection or rupture of the aorta itself is a dramatic complication with peak incidence in the third and fourth decades.[5] The proximal ascending aorta is the most common site, susceptibility influenced in part by a coexisting bicuspid aortic valve or by XO Turner's syndrome.[5] The second site of rupture or dissection is in the postcoarctation aorta, which, like the aortic root, histologically resembles cystic medial necrosis.[20] Left ventricular failure in unoperated patients with coarctation of the aorta occurs either before the first year of life or after age 40 but seldom in between.[5] Systemic hypertension predisposes to premature coronary artery disease.[21]

PULMONARY VALVE STENOSIS (see also p. 968, and Fig. 29–42, p. 925). Represented by a pliant conical or dome-shaped valve with a narrow outlet at its apex, this malformation typically occurs as an isolated anomaly and is the most common variety of congenital obstruction to right ventricular outflow.[5] Survival into adolescence and adulthood is the rule, except for pinpoint pulmonary stenosis in neonates. Longevity depends chiefly on three variables: (1) the initial severity of obstruction, (2) whether a given degree of obstruction remains constant or progresses, and (3) the functional adequacy of the pressure-overloaded right ventricle.[22–24] The orifice size of isolated pulmonary valve stenosis usually increases appropriately with body growth. However, the development of secondary hypertrophic subpulmonary stenosis (Fig. 30–4) or fibrocalcific thickening in older patients may augment the degree of obstruction. Although subjective complaints become more prevalent as years go by, equivalent degrees of stenosis may limit one patient in childhood yet leave another relatively unencumbered as an adult.[5] Right ventricular failure is the most common cause of death. Infective endocarditis is a risk, except perhaps in mild pulmonary valve stenosis.

valve, whether functionally normal, stenotic, or incompetent.[5,16,16a] This aortic root disease can express itself in older adults as an aneurysm with aortic regurgitation or can announce itself dramatically in younger adults as aortic dissection (Fig. 30–2).

COARCTATION OF THE AORTA (see also p. 911). This malformation is likely to produce significant symptoms either in early infancy or after age 20 to 30 years.[5,17] The majority of patients who survive early life live to reach adulthood, but sporadic examples of exceptional longevity should not obscure the inherent risks that shorten life span.[5] Half of unoperated patients die by age 30, and more than three-

FIGURE 30–4. A, Continuous-wave Doppler across the right ventricular outflow tract of a 33-year-old man with severe pulmonary valve stenosis (PS) and secondary hypertrophic subpulmonary stenosis. The peak instantaneous gradient across the valve was 120 mm Hg. Within the major symmetrical flow disturbance envelope, there is an asymmetrical, lower-velocity pattern (unmarked arrow) caused by the hypertrophic subpulmonary stenosis. a = presystolic flow in response to an increased force of right atrial contractions; PR = pulmonary regurgitation. B, After balloon dilatation, the gradient at valve level was virtually abolished, leaving only the subpulmonary (PS) gradient, which subsequently resolved.

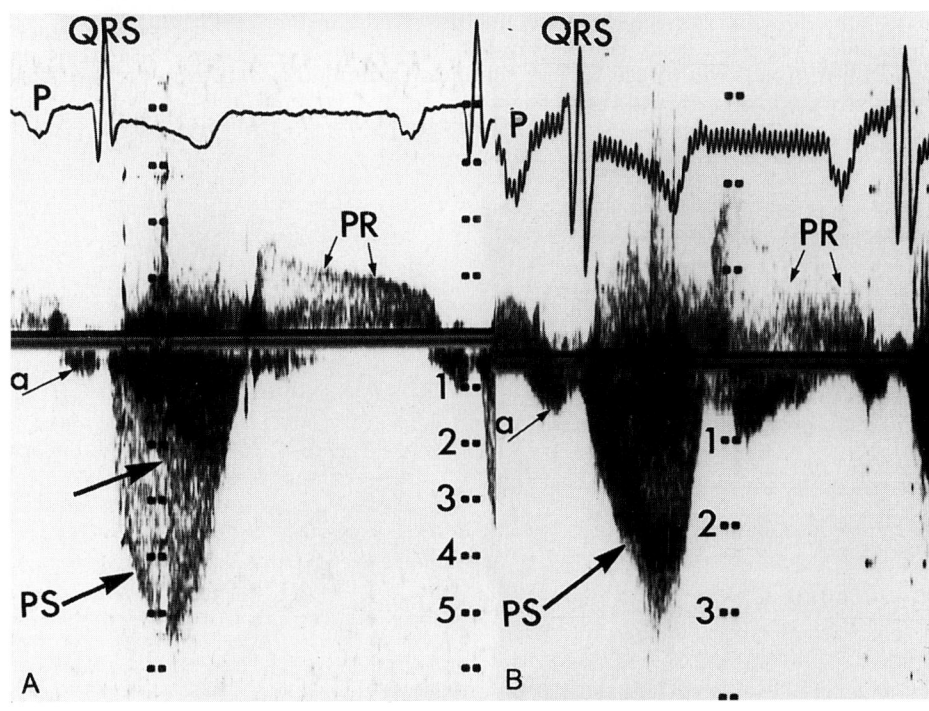

OSTIUM SECUNDUM ATRIAL SEPTAL DEFECT (see also p. 896 and Figs. 3–80, p. 83, and 29–11, p. 897). This anomaly is among the most common congenital cardiac malformations in unoperated adults and is by far the most common shunt lesion.[25–27] Although life expectancy is not normal, survival into adulthood is the rule.[5] Ostium secundum atrial septal defects are sporadically found in patients beyond age 70 years and occasionally in patients in their 80's or 90's.[26–28] One of the author's patients died at age 87 (Fig. 30–5), and another lived relatively comfortably until 3 months before his 95th birthday.[29]

Almost all patients who survive beyond the sixth decade are symptomatic. Death may be unrelated to the malformation, but when a relationship exists, cardiac failure is the most common cause of death. Older patients deteriorate chiefly on three counts[5]: (1) A decrease in left ventricular distensibility (acquired coronary artery disease, systemic hypertension) augments the left-to-right shunt; (2) atrial tachyarrhythmias, especially fibrillation, less commonly flutter or atrial tachycardia, increase in frequency after the fourth decade and serve to precipitate right ventricular failure; (3) the majority of symptomatic adults beyond age 40 have mild to moderate pulmonary hypertension despite the presence of a persistent, large left-to-right shunt, so the aging right ventricle is doubly beset by both pressure and volume overload.

The incidence, extent, and degree of associated mitral valve disease increase with age and the disease is characterized morphologically by thick, fibrotic leaflets and short, fibrotic chordae tendineae.[30,31] These mitral valve abnormalities have been attributed to abnormal cusp movement (trauma) caused by the effects of left ventricular cavity deformity (abnormal position and motion of the ventricular septum in response to volume overload of the right ventricle).[32,33] The abnormalities are believed to be the basis for the mitral regurgitation that tends to develop with age in about 15 per cent of patients.[29–31]

PATENT DUCTUS ARTERIOSUS (see also p. 971 and Fig. 29–19, p. 906). A large ductus is a relatively common cause of congestive heart failure in term infants, but after the first year of life, most patients with patent ductus arteriosus are asymptomatic.[34] In the second decade, the risk of infective endarteritis exceeds the risk of heart failure.[34] Beginning with the third decade (occasionally earlier), more patients with significant left-to-right shunts develop heart failure,[35] whereas those with small shunts remain asymptomatic. One of the author's patients was an 84-year-old woman with a moderately restrictive patent ductus, atrial fibrillation, and congestive heart failure (Fig. 30–6), and there is one report of survival to age 90.[36] A significant cumulative risk of infective endarteritis exists, especially if the ductus is restrictive. Patients with nonrestrictive patent ductus arteriosus seldom reach adulthood unless a rise in pulmonary vascular resistance relieves the left ventricle of excessive volume overload.[37] Survival to adulthood is then the rule, with differential cyanosis a distinctive feature of the reversed shunt.[5]

Uncommon Defects in Which Unoperated Adult Survival is Expected

SITUS INVERSUS WITH DEXTROCARDIA (see also p. 946). This cardiac malposition usually occurs with an otherwise structurally and functionally normal heart.[5] Symptoms related to *acquired* cardiac or noncardiac disease may lead to the discovery of the hitherto unsuspected malposition. If angina pectoris or myocardial infarction occurs with complete situs inversus, the pain is located in the *right* anterior chest with radiation to the right shoulder and right arm.[38] The pain of appendicitis is referred to the *left* lower quadrant, and the pain of biliary colic presents in the *left* upper quadrant, owing to the mirror image positions of abdominal viscera. The cardiac malposition is occasionally associated with sinusitis and bronchiectasis—Kartagener's triad.[5] Symptoms of bronchiectasis usually develop in early adulthood and may prompt investigations that lead to the discovery of the malposition. Situs inversus is common in men with infertility secondary to sperm immotility,[39] an observation that led to identification of a generalized disorder of ciliary motility in Kartagener's triad.[40] When situs inversus with dextrocardia coexists with congenital malformations of the heart, survival is determined by the associated anomalies.[5]

SITUS SOLITUS WITH DEXTROCARDIA. This cardiac malposition occurs only occasionally with a structurally normal heart, which permits adult survival but delays clinical recognition.[5] A routine chest radiograph may provide the first evidence of the malposition. Coexisting congenital cardiac anomalies, which are usually present, determine survival.

CONGENITAL COMPLETE HEART BLOCK (see also pp. 691 and 904). Adult survival is the rule, although the ultimate fate of large numbers of older patients with congenital complete heart block dampens optimism, and mortality even in infancy and childhood is not negligible.[41–43] A substantial majority of young patients are asymptomatic, but mild, serious, or even fatal sequelae sometimes occur.[5] Key determinants of clinical stability in uncomplicated congenital complete heart block are the ventricular rate, the hemodynamic adjustments at rest and with exercise, and the presence of intrinsically normal myocardium.[5]

CONGENITALLY CORRECTED TRANSPOSITION OF THE GREAT ARTERIES (see also p. 940 and Fig 29–62, p. 940). When this malformation is isolated (uncomplicated), survival is good but not normal because of the vulnerability of a morphological right ventricle in the systemic location.[44–47] A major variable that decreases long-term survival is the presence and degree of incompetence of the inverted left atrioventricular valve (Ebstein-like anomaly) that may be mistaken for acquired mitral regurgitation.[5] Survival into the sixth or seventh decade is uncommon, but not unknown, with an occasional patient reaching the eighth decade.[48] Complete atrioventricular block accrues at a rate of about 2 per cent per year and may become manifested with a Stokes-Adams attack or sudden death.[49]

EBSTEIN'S ANOMALY OF THE TRICUSPID VALVE (see also p. 969 and Figs. 29–56, p. 934, and 29–57, p. 935). Longevity ranges from intrauterine or neonatal death to asymptomatic survival into late

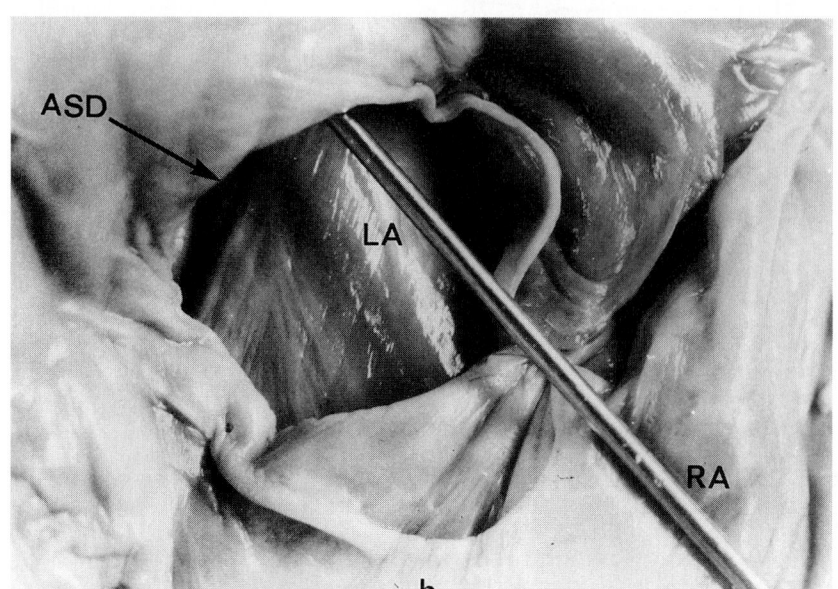

FIGURE 30–5. Necropsy specimen from an 87-year-old woman with a nonrestrictive ostium secundum atrial septal defect (ASD). The left atrium (LA) is seen through the defect. RA = right atrium.

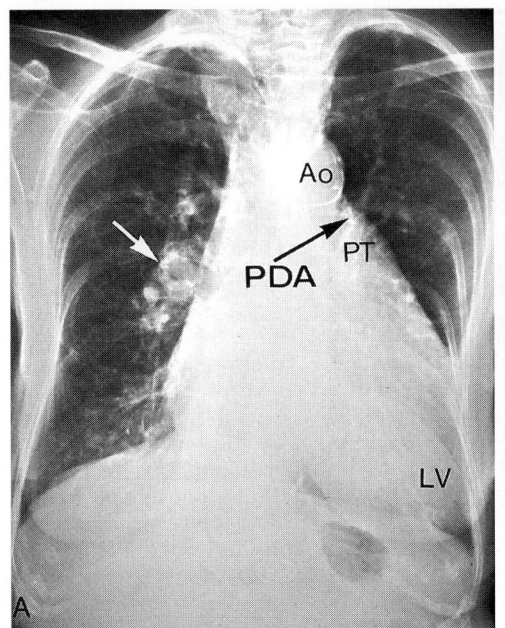
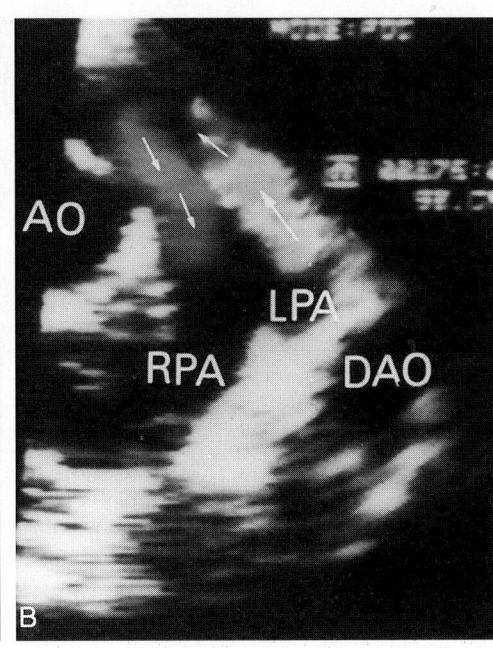

FIGURE 30–6. *A*, Radiograph from an 84-year-old woman with a moderately restrictive calcified patent ductus arteriosus (PDA). The pulmonary trunk (PT) and its right branch (unmarked white arrow) are dilated. Pulmonary arterial pressure was 90/40 mm Hg. The enlarged left ventricle (LV) occupies the apex. The aortic knuckle (Ao) is calcified. *B*, Black and white print of a color flow image (parasternal short axis). Arrows trace the direction of ductal flow, moving first down the left lateral wall of the pulmonary trunk, then up the opposite wall. LPA = left pulmonary artery; RPA = right pulmonary artery; DAo = descending aorta.

adulthood.[50–52] The majority of patients fall between these extremes. Factors chiefly limiting survival in adults are functional class, marked increase in cardiac size, cyanosis, and recurrent paroxysmal rapid heart action, especially when accompanied by accelerated conduction through accessory pathways (Fig. 30–7).[53,54] Left ventricular function is an additional matter of concern.[55,56] Syncope heightens suspicion of accelerated bypass conduction (rapid atrial fibrillation or one-to-one atrial flutter). The rapid ventricular response has been responsible for sudden death. For patients who survive the first year of life, there is a cumulative mortality of approximately 12 per cent, which is distributed about evenly throughout childhood and adolescence.[53,54] Nevertheless, there are accounts of patients with Ebstein's anomaly who have survived into their eighth decade.[57,58] The oldest patient recorded with the anomaly lived to age 85 and had no cardiac symptoms until age 79.[59]

CONGENITAL PULMONARY VALVE REGURGITATION (see also p. 1059). Because the degree of regurgitation is seldom more than moderate, and because the right ventricle readily adapts to low pressure volume overload, most patients tolerate this anomaly into adulthood, through middle age, and occasionally into their sixth, seventh, or even eighth decade.[60–62] However, right heart failure may occur in older adults after decades of stability, because acquired cardiopulmonary disorders serve to increase the amount of regurgitation across the congenitally incompetent pulmonary valve.[5]

LUTEMBACHER'S SYNDROME. The disorder consists of a congenital atrial septal defect upon which *acquired* mitral stenosis is imposed.[5] Mitral stenosis augments the left-to-right interatrial shunt, while the atrial septal defect decompresses the left atrium and reduces the mean left atrial pressure and the gradient across the stenotic mitral valve. Lutembacher's patient was a 61-year-old woman who had seven pregnancies,[63] and Firkett's patient was a 74-year-old woman who had 11 pregnancies.[64] The oldest recorded patient was an 81-year-old woman who experienced no cardiac symptoms until her 75th year.[65] These favorable reports should not obscure the fact that survival in patients with ostium secundum atrial septal defects is unfavorably influenced by mitral stenosis that augments the left-to-right shunt and predisposes to atrial fibrillation and right ventricular failure.[5]

SINUS OF VALSALVA ANEURYSM (see also p. 910). The malformation begins as a blind pouch or diverticulum that takes origin from a localized site in one aortic sinus.[66] A substantial majority of ruptures occur before age 30 (rarely in infancy or early childhood), generally in men, at an average age of 34 years with a range of 11 to 67 years.[66,67] The physiological consequences and clinical course depend upon the rapidity with which the rupture develops, the amount of blood flowing through the abnormal communication, and the chamber (site) that receives the shunt.[68] Complete heart block is an occasional cause of syncope or sudden death when a ruptured or unruptured aneurysm penetrates the base of the ventricular septum.[69] Small perforations may come to light because of an asymptomatic continuous murmur, because of a right ventricular outflow tract systolic murmur (subpulmonary obstruction by the aneurysm), or because of aortic regurgitation.[5] Small chronic perforations are susceptible to infective endocarditis. About 20 per cent of congenital sinus of Valsalva aneurysms are unperforated and are discovered at necropsy, cardiac surgery, or operation for ventricular septal defect, which sometimes coexists with an aortic sinus aneurysm.[68] In one of our patients, an 85-year-old man, an unsuspected unperforated aortic sinus aneurysm was diagnosed by echocardiography.

CORONARY ARTERIAL FISTULAS. These anomalies represent one of the most common major congenital malformations of the coronary circulation that permit adult survival.[70] Both coronary arteries arise from the aorta at their normal sites, but a fistulous branch of one or more arteries communicates directly with a cardiac chamber or with the pulmonary trunk, coronary sinus, vena cava, or a pulmonary vein. Clinically occult coronary arterial fistulas, generally to the pulmonary artery, have been found in a small but consistent percentage of adults undergoing diagnostic coronary angiography for other reasons.[71] Survival into adulthood is the rule, although life span is not normal.[70] Longevity depends upon the amount of blood traversing the communication, the chamber or vessel into which the fistula drains, and the presence and degree of myocardial ischemia that might result when the fistula causes a coronary steal.[72] Occasional survivals have been recorded in the seventh and eighth decades, with one report of a patient living to age 84.[73] Death, when it comes, may be due to noncardiac causes or to acquired coronary artery disease.

CONGENITAL PULMONARY ARTERIOVENOUS FISTULA. These fistulas can be solitary or multiple, unilateral or bilateral, or minute and diffuse throughout both lungs, and are usually associated with hereditary hemorrhagic telangiectasia (Rendu-Osler-Weber syndrome).[74] A substantial majority go unrecognized until adulthood.[5] Dyspnea and fatigue are often related to anemia caused by bleeding telangiectases rather than to the pulmonary arteriovenous fistulas per se. Two of the author's patients without telangiectasia were siblings aged 71 and 73 years (Fig. 30–8).[75]

Common Defects in Which Unoperated Adult Survival is Exceptional

VENTRICULAR SEPTAL DEFECT (see also p. 901, Fig. 29–16, p. 902). These defects are among the most common congenital cardiac malformations at birth but are seldom found in adulthood.[76,77] Adult survivors comprise two widely disparate groups[78–80]: (1) those with defects that have either closed spontaneously or decreased to a small or moderately restrictive size, and (2) those with nonrestrictive defects with elevated pulmonary vascular resistance that relieves the left ventricle of volume overload while imposing no additional afterload upon the systemic right ventricle (Eisenmenger's complex).

The chief reason for adult survival in patients with ventricular septal defects is spontaneous closure.[81] Paul Wood asked, "Where's the *maladie de Roger*? Assuming it does not provide immortality, it must either close spontaneously in middle life or have long since run its mortal course."[82] Early spontaneous closure by formation of septal aneurysm leaves the patient with a functionally normal heart that still harbors a morphological abnormality.[83] The occasional adult survivor with persistent patency of a small perimembranous ventricular septal defect confronts a cumulative risk of infective endocarditis.[84]

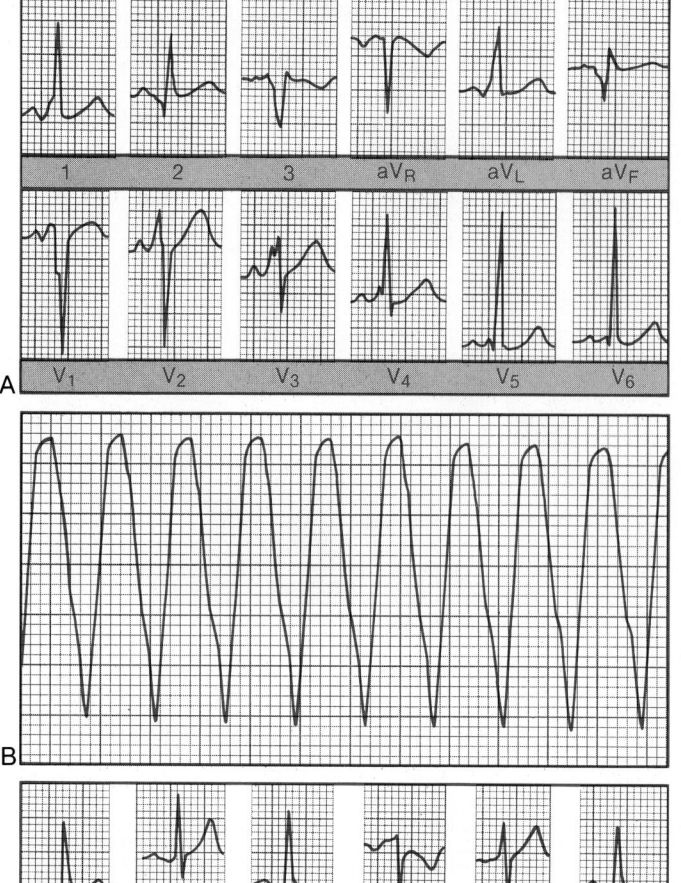

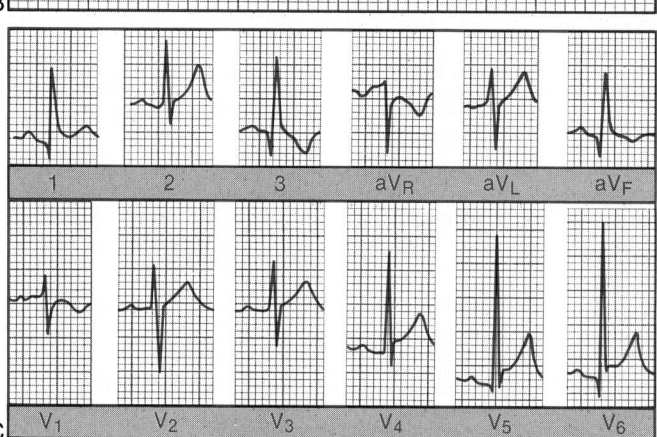

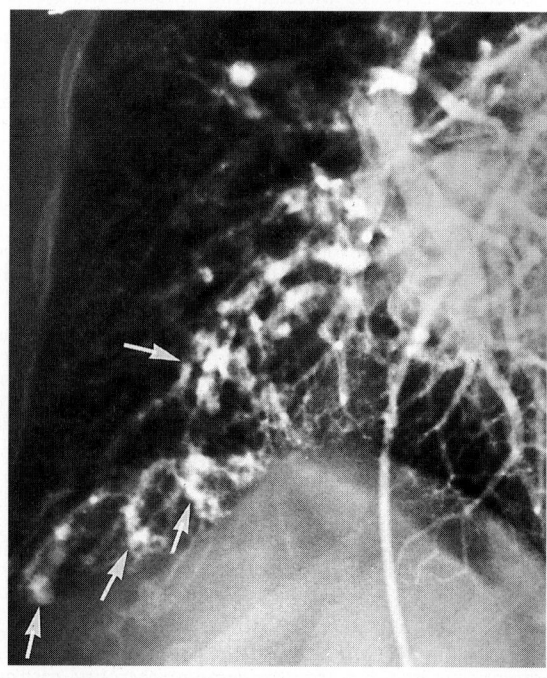

FIGURE 30–7. *A,* Twelve-lead electrocardiogram from a patient with Ebstein's anomaly of the tricuspid valve. There are typical fusion beats due to a right atrioventricular bypass tract. The delta wave is directed to the left, superior and posterior. *B,* Lead V₁ showing antegrade wide QRS tachycardia via the right bypass tract. *C,* Twelve-lead electrocardiogram after tricuspid valve reconstruction with interruption of the bypass tract by surgical dissociation between right atrium and right ventricle. The delta wave is absent.

It is the rule rather than the exception for patients with Eisenmenger's complex to reach adulthood. The author's oldest patient died from noncardiac causes at age 69 years.

FALLOT'S TETRALOGY (see also p. 929). Arthur Fallot recognized that ". . . cyanosis, especially in the adult, is the result of a small number of cardiac malformations. . . . One of these cardiac malformations is much more frequent than others . . ."[6] namely, the tetralogy to which he referred. Fallot's tetralogy represents the largest proportion of adults with cyanotic congenital heart disease, but only 6 per cent of unoperated patients are alive at age 30 and 3 per cent at age 40.[85,86] There are individual reports of survival into the seventh decade.[85] Fallot's tetralogy with pulmonary atresia and adequate but not excessive aortic-to-pulmonary collateral circulation occasionally permits survival not only to adolescence but to adulthood.[87] One of the author's patients lived to age 55, despite acquired calcific aortic stenosis.

Systemic hypertension is a special problem in adult sur-

vivors, because the increase in afterload is imposed on both the left and right ventricles (biventricular aorta).[5] The rise in right ventricular systolic pressure may augment pulmonary blood flow and reduce cyanosis but at the price of right ventricular (or biventricular) failure. Infective endocarditis on an incompetent biventricular aortic valve may incur catastrophic acute severe aortic regurgitation into both right and left ventricles.

Late Survival After Cardiac Surgery or Interventional Catheterization

An understanding of long-term outcomes requires knowledge of the preoperative or preinterventional congenital malformation, the nature and effects of the therapeutic intervention, and the subsequent residua and sequelae.[2] Success is measured not only by the length of survival but also by the quality of life and the need for reoperation. Surgical refinements affect long-term outcome, often significantly. Techniques have evolved and will continue to do so. Patients who underwent cardiac surgery decades ago benefited from the anatomical repairs but often suffered from deleterious effects of inadequate intraoperative myocardial protection.[2] Prosthetic materials—valves, patches, conduits—that were previously state of the art have been superseded by many generations of improved devices and materials.

Congenitally Malformed Cardiac Valves

ISOLATED PULMONARY VALVE STENOSIS (see also pp. 965 and 924). Balloon dilatation has largely replaced surgery for typical isolated congenital pulmonary valve stenosis, provided that the stenotic valve is thin, pliant, and mobile (Fig. 30–9).[88,89] Secondary hypertrophic subpulmonary stenosis tends to regress after successful dilatation of the stenotic valve (Fig. 30–4). Long-term results of balloon valvuloplasty have thus far been as good as those of surgical valvotomy.[87] If pulmonary stenosis is relieved during childhood, long-term survival patterns are similar to those in age- and sex-matched controls.[87] Exemplary results are qualified by age at intervention and by the severity of the stenosis before relief. The more severe and protracted the obstruction, the less optimal the long-term outcome, including late death from right ventricular failure. These con-

FIGURE 30–8. Selective right pulmonary arteriogram from a 71-year-old man with congenital bilateral pulmonary arteriovenous fistulas (arrows). His 73-year-old sister was similarly afflicted. Neither had telangiectasia.

tis is not affected by either balloon dilatation or surgical reconstruction. The enhanced ejection performance of the left ventricle in young patients with congenital aortic stenosis[92] tends to be maintained after relief of the obstruction, provided relief is achieved before contractility begins to decline.[92,93] If the aortic valve is replaced, the fate of the prosthesis and the need for anticoagulants are important determinants of late postoperative outcome. The inherent risk of aortic root dissection (Fig. 30–2) persists after either balloon dilatation, direct reconstruction, or aortic valve replacement.

A functionally normal bicuspid aortic valve may develop gradually progressive *aortic regurgitation* that requires surgical relief using a prosthetic valve. Prime objectives of valve replacement are removal of left ventricular volume overload and preservation or restoration of satisfactory left ventricular systolic function. Even if these objectives are achieved, a minority of patients die late after operation, not because of heart failure but because of what is presumed to be a disturbance in ventricular rhythm (sudden death). Infective endocarditis can convert a bicuspid aortic valve that is functionally normal into the catastrophic hemodynamic fault of acute severe aortic regurgitation that, with few exceptions, requires emergency valve replacement.[15]

EBSTEIN'S ANOMALY (see also pp. 934 and 966). This malformation is the most common cause of surgically important congenital tricuspid regurgitation.[94] The timing and success of operation in large part depend on whether or not the malformed valve can be reconstructed rather than replaced. Transesophageal echocardiography provides a se-

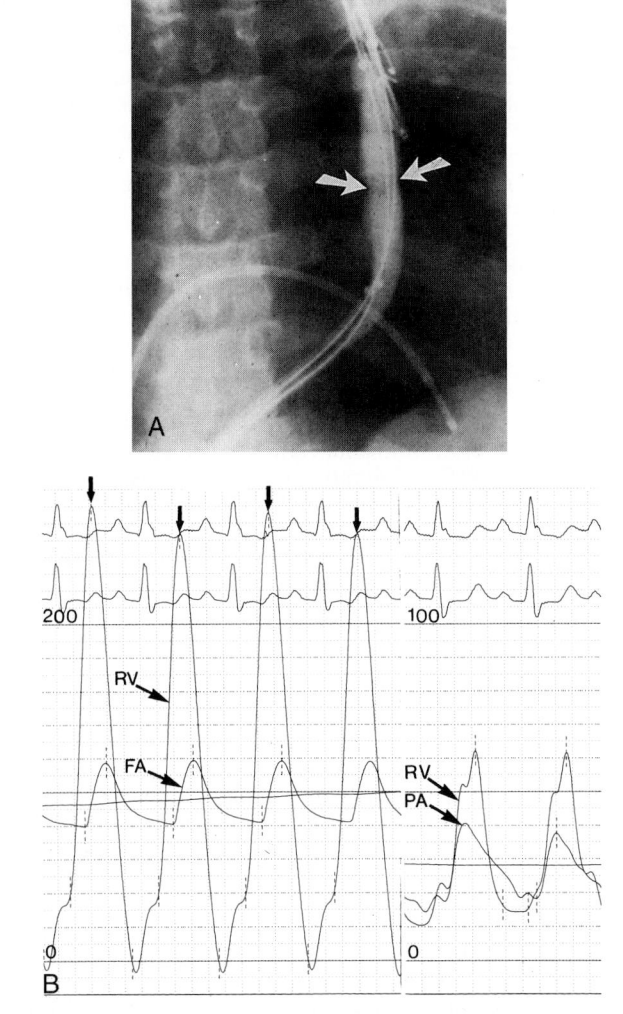

FIGURE 30–9. *A*, Single balloon across a severely stenotic mobile pulmonary valve of an 18-year-old pregnant woman near term. *B*, Pressure pulses before *(left)* and after *(right)* balloon dilatation. The right ventricular (RV) pressure fell from 280 to 60 mm Hg. The right ventricular to pulmonary arterial gradient fell to 40 mm Hg. Right ventricular pulsus alternans was present before dilatation, indicating depressed right ventricular systolic function. Three days after balloon dilatation, the patient went into spontaneous uncomplicated labor. FA = femoral arteries; PA = pulmonary artery.

clusions support the practice of relieving hemodynamically significant pulmonary valve stenosis during childhood but underscore the desirability of surveillance through adolescence and adulthood. With few exceptions, postinterventional or postoperative pulmonary regurgitation is no more than mild to moderate. Residual dilatation of the pulmonary trunk is of no clinical significance even when marked. Susceptibility to infective endocarditis is believed to be low if not absent if the postinterventional gradient is small and if pulmonary regurgitation is absent or mild.

CONGENITAL AORTIC VALVE STENOSIS (see also pp. 964 and 914). Balloon dilatation in young patients with congenital bicuspid aortic stenosis is feasible provided the valve is thin and mobile, with no calcific deposits (Fig. 30–10*A*). The best that can be achieved, however, is separation of the fused commissures that results in a functionally normal bicuspid aortic valve (Fig. 30–10*B*) with an outlook analogous to that of surgical reconstruction.[90,91] The repaired valve has at least the same tendency as an unoperated, functionally normal bicuspid aortic valve to develop regurgitation or to thicken, calcify, and become stenotic with the passage of time (Fig. 30–1). The risk of infective endocardi-

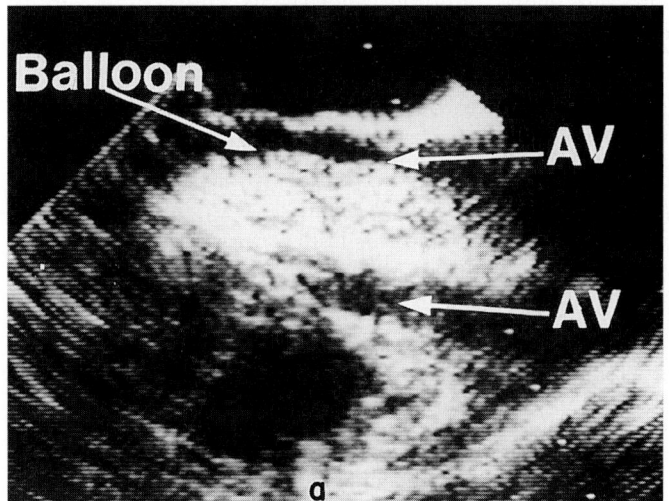

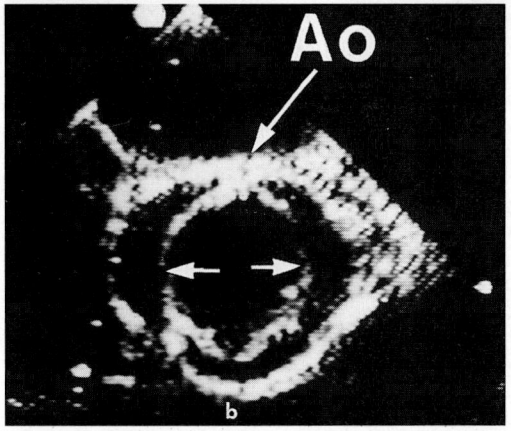

FIGURE 30–10. *A*, Balloon dilatation of bicuspid aortic stenosis using transesophageal echocardiographic monitoring in a 32-year-old man. The inflated balloon is across the stenotic bicuspid aortic valve (AV). *B*, A short-axis image after balloon dilatation showing a mobile functionally normal bicuspid aortic valve (Ao) with no commissural fusion. There was mild residual aortic regurgitation.

cure basis for judging whether a large mobile anterior tricuspid leaflet can be used to create a competent unicuspid valve. Successful operation relieves right ventricular volume overload, improves right ventricular function, removes the risk of paradoxical emboli through an interatrial communication, and interrupts right atrioventricular bypass tracts, eliminating the hazard of rapid ventricular response to atrial flutter or fibrillation (Fig. 30–7). Supraventricular arrhythmias may recur postoperatively, but if the accessory pathways have been divided, the ventricular response is not accelerated, and the arrhythmias are more likely to respond to pharmacological management. Tissue valves are used for tricuspid replacement because mechanical prostheses function poorly in the tricuspid location in addition to posing the risk of pulmonary embolization even with anticoagulation.

ISOLATED INCOMPETENCE OF THE LEFT-SIDED ATRIOVENTRICULAR VALVE IN CONGENITALLY CORRECTED TRANSPOSITION OF THE GREAT ARTERIES. The Ebstein-like anomaly that causes incompetence of the tricuspid valve in the systemic (inverted) position is analogous to, but not identical to, Ebstein's anomaly as just described.[5] The anterior leaflet is smaller in size than in right-sided Ebstein's anomaly and is usually malformed. Accordingly, when surgical relief of regurgitation is indicated, the left-sided tricuspid valve almost always requires replacement. Long-term outcome is then determined by the duration of preoperative regurgitation, the functional adequacy (or inadequacy) of a morphological right ventricle in the systemic location, and an accrued incidence of high-degree atrioventricular heart block.

ATRIAL SEPTAL DEFECT (OSTIUM SECUNDUM) (see also pp. 896 and 966). Children, adolescents, and young adults with this malformation usually have few or no symptoms.[5] An assessment of asymptomatic or minimally symptomatic patients with ostium secundum or sinus venosus atrial septal defects who were over 25 at the time of presentation disclosed no difference in survival or symptoms and no difference in the incidence of new arrhythmias, stroke, embolic phenomena, or cardiac failure between medically and surgically managed patients after a mean follow-up of 25 years.[95] The study confirmed that progressive pulmonary vascular disease does not develop in this patient population, so its anticipation is not a rationale for operation.[95,96] Long-term observations after closure of atrial septal defects found that actuarial 27-year rates of survival in patients 12 to 24 years of age at operation were the same as for normal patients; operation at 25 to 41 years of age was followed by long-term survival that was good but not normal, whereas closure after age 41 years was associated with a significant increase in late mortality and in the frequency of late cardiac failure, stroke, and atrial fibrillation.[97] The age beyond which surgery should not be offered has been questioned.[95,98] However, in patients older than age 40 years, a recent multivariate analysis of 84 postoperative patients with atrial septal defects was compared with results in 95 patients who had been treated medically; there was a significant reduction in overall mortality and considerable improvement in long-term functional status of the surgically treated patients.[99] Long-term functional improvement was sustained in 69 per cent of patients who had suffered from severe heart failure before surgery.[99] In contrast to the clear benefit of surgery with respect to long-term survival and symptomatic improvement, repair later in life did not significantly reduce the prevalence of atrial fibrillation or flutter or morbidity associated with thromboembolic complications.[99]

COMPLETE TRANSPOSITION OF THE GREAT ARTERIES (see also p. 935). A relatively large number of patients with this malformation have reached adulthood because of a Rashkind balloon atrial septostomy as neonates followed by intraatrial redirection of venous return (Mustard or Senning atrial switch operations).[2] Twenty-year survival after atrial switch has been reported at 80 to 90 per cent, but major

late postoperative sequelae are the rule.[100,101] Intraatrial repair involves excision of the atrial septum and insertion of a pericardial or Dacron baffle that directs systemic venous return across the mitral valve into the left ventricle and pulmonary artery and that directs pulmonary venous return across the tricuspid valve into the right ventricle and aorta.[102] Electrophysiological sequelae of this extensive reconstruction are damage to the sinus node, atrial arrhythmias (atrial fibrillation or flutter), and damage to the atrioventricular node (Fig. 30–11).[103,104] During long-term follow-up, 2 to 8 per cent of patients die suddenly due to bradyarrhythmias, atrial tachyarrhythmias, or high-degree atrioventricular block. A second major postoperative concern is the long-term performance of a morphological right ventricle in the systemic location.[105,106] Progressive systolic dysfunction is not uncommon, and there is a relatively high incidence of coexisting left ventricular dysfunction.[106,107] Aortic regurgitation, still another late postoperative concern, exerts a negative impact on already depressed function of the morphological right ventricle.

FALLOT'S TETRALOGY (see also p. 929). Assessment of the postoperative course must take into account the morphological variations of the basic malformation, previous shunt procedures, age at intracardiac repair, and the presence and degree of postoperative residua and sequelae.[108,110] Patients who had undergone palliative shunts, followed by intracardiac repair in early childhood, experienced 87 per cent survival 10 to 20 years after operation.[109] All but a minority were free from significant cardiac or vascular symptoms and were leading normal lives. Some patients who reach adulthood after successful shunt operations in infancy or early childhood maintain improvement for decades and ultimately benefit from intracardiac repair as adults. The outlook for patients who had a Waterston or Potts shunt before intracardiac repair is more guarded, because these shunts lend themselves to the risk of excessive pulmonary blood flow, pulmonary vascular disease, or kinking of a pulmonary artery.[109] A technically good intracardiac repair in infancy substantially improves cumulative survival, reduces incidence of complications, and improves quality of life.[109,110] Older age at the time of intraventricular repair was a powerful predictor of poor late survival.[109,111,112]

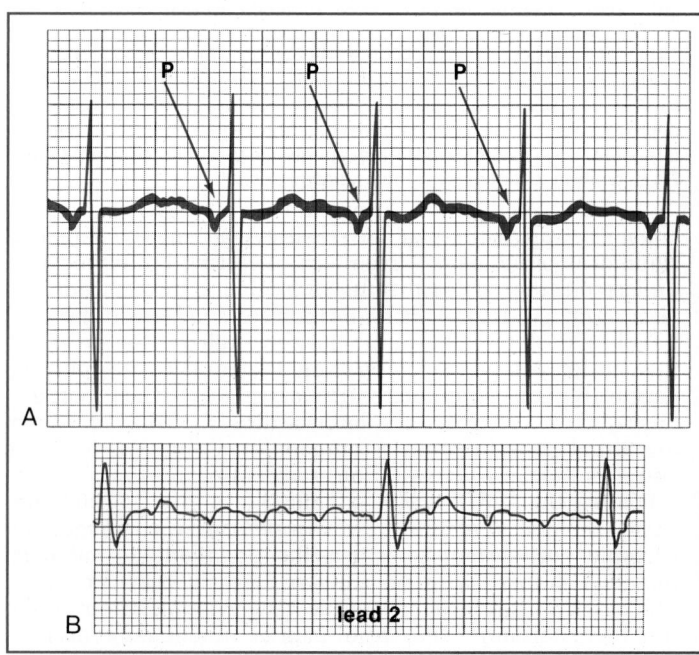

FIGURE 30–11. *A,* Junctional ectopic rhythm early after a Mustard repair for complete transposition of the great arteries. *B,* Late-onset atrial flutter with a slow ventricular response (impaired atrioventricular conduction) in a 25-year-old man who had a Mustard repair in infancy. The patient developed sinus node dysfunction in addition to atrial tachyarrhythmias.

The effectiveness of surgery must take into account not only survival but symptomatic status, postoperative residua and sequelae, and the need for reoperation.[113] Late postoperative sudden death has been a legitimate concern. Ventricular electrical instability, rather than high-degree heart block, is now considered the major risk factor.[108,109,109a] Ventricular ectopic rhythms correlate with older age at intracardiac repair, with postoperative right ventricular pressure or volume overload, and with depressed right ventricular function.[108,109] Postoperative *left* ventricular dysfunction is related to age at the time of intracardiac repair and to previous shunt procedures. A decrease in *left* ventricular volume and ejection fraction is a feature of severe cyanotic Fallot's tetralogy because of reduced pulmonary arterial blood flow (underloading).[114] A shunt operation increases left ventricular volume, sometimes excessively, setting the stage for late postoperative electrical instability. If primary intracardiac repair is undertaken after 2 years of age, left heart volumes approach normal, but left ventricular function may remain subnormal.[114,115]

The emphasis on disturbances in ventricular rhythm after intracardiac repair of Fallot's tetralogy should not obscure the importance of disturbances in atrial rhythm.[116] Atrial fibrillation, atrial flutter, and supraventricular tachycardia were important determinants of morbidity in approximately one-third of patients. Attention was also called to the incidence of sinus node dysfunction, with pacemakers needed twice as often for sinus bradycardia as for atrioventricular block.[116]

PATENT DUCTUS ARTERIOSUS (see also p. 905). Division of an isolated restrictive patent ductus arteriosus in childhood represents one of the few literal cures of congenital malformations of the heart and circulation. Transcatheter ductal occlusion must compete with this record, which is ideal except for the thoracotomy.[117] The risk of infective endocarditis is eliminated. When a ductus is moderately restrictive or nonrestrictive, division in early childhood usually results in regression of left atrial and left ventricular enlargement and normalization of pulmonary arterial and right ventricular systolic pressures. Adult survival of patients with a nonrestrictive patent ductus depends on a rise in pulmonary vascular resistance that relieves the left ventricle of volume overload but incurs inoperability when the shunt is reversed.

COARCTATION OF THE AORTA (see also p. 911). Repair in early childhood results in 89 per cent survival at 15 years and 83 per cent at 25 years.[118] Postoperative residua and sequelae are common, however, and require long-term follow-up.[119,120] Three principal postoperative concerns include residual systolic hypertension despite absence of a coarctation gradient, bicuspid aortic valve, and recoarctation. A major risk factor for persistent postoperative hypertension is older age at repair: i.e., the duration of preoperative hypertension that results in baroreceptor abnormalities and compliance changes in the walls of the major arteries.[121,122]

The fate of a coexisting functionally normal bicuspid aortic valve is the same as that of an isolated congenitally bicuspid aortic valve as described earlier. Recurrence of coarctation after reparative surgery is related chiefly to the technique used for the initial repair.[123] Resection with end-to-end anastomosis, when technically feasible, is associated with the lowest incidence of recoarctation. Balloon dilatation has been a step forward in the management of recoarctation, but *not* of the native obstruction.[124] The histology of the aorta immediately distal to the coarctation resembles that of the Marfan syndrome. Balloon dilatation further injures this inherently vulnerable segment.[20] Conversely, resection with end-to-end anastomosis removes the vulnerable segment, an advantage to women during subsequent pregnancy. Premature coronary artery atherosclerosis, myocardial infarction, and congestive heart failure were causes of death in 12 per cent of patients 11 to 25 years after coarctectomy.[119] Early successful repair promises to minimize these late complications. Congenital aneurysms of the circle of Willis (Fig. 30-3) are uncommon but well-established coexisting malformations in patients with coarctation of the aorta and set the stage for catastrophic cerebral hemorrhage. Rupture of an aneurysm has been reported in normotensive patients long after successful coarctation repair.[125] Abnormalities of the mitral apparatus occur in 26 to 58 per cent of patients with coarctation and vary from clinically occult and functionally benign to overt stenosis or incompetence of the mitral orifice.[126]

CONGENITAL SINUS OF VALSALVA ANEURYSMS (see also p. 910). An acute large rupture announces itself dramatically, whereas as a small perforation that develops gradually or an unruptured aneurysm may go unnoticed, at least initially.[5] In any event, surgical mortality is low, and late results of repair are excellent, especially when aortic valve regurgitation is absent.

THE FONTAN PROCEDURE (see Figs. 29-55, p. 934, and 29-69, p. 948). In 1971, Fontan and Baudet reported a new operation for tricuspid atresia (caval-to-pulmonary artery anastomosis)[127] that bears the first author's name as an eponym. The Fontan operation has emerged as a landmark in the surgical treatment of congenital heart disease.[128] Complete bypass of the right ventricle was a logical extension of its predecessor, the partial right heart bypass procedure introduced by Glenn.[129] The original Glenn shunt consisted of an anastomosis of the superior vena cava to the right pulmonary artery that was divided from the pulmonary trunk.[129] Acquired right lower-lobe pulmonary arteriovenous fistulas were late postoperative complications.[130] The procedure has now been modified as the "bidirectional Glenn shunt," represented by anastomosis of the superior vena cava to an undivided right pulmonary artery.[130] The bidirectional Glenn shunt is used as palliation in patients for whom a Fontan operation is not considered feasible or as the first stage in anticipation of total caval-to-pulmonary arterial connection, which is the most recent modification of the Fontan repair.[130-132,132a] Among 352 patients who had a Fontan operation prior to 1995, the 10-year survival was 60 per cent.[132] Survival was adversely affected by depressed ventricular function, increased pulmonary arterial pressure, and atrioventricular valve dysfunction.[132] Meticulous selection of patients increases late survival and reduces morbidity. As experience has accumulated, operative risk has declined, survival has improved, morbidity has decreased, and the quality of life has improved, sometimes appreciably.[132-134]

The Fontan operation for patients 18 years or older has also been successful, occasionally achieving remarkable degrees of rehabilitation.[133] There are, however, a number of caveats. Because of the importance of ventricular function, postoperative afterload reduction using angiotensin-converting enzyme inhibitors is common practice, and the importance of maintaining sinus rhythm has been emphasized.[133,134] Atrial arrhythmias, especially atrial flutter or fibrillation, adversely affect ventricular function and may precipitate congestive heart failure. Thrombotic and thromboembolic events are additional concerns and do not appear to be related to ventricular function or disturbances in atrial rhythm.[132] Thrombi have been identified in the superior vena cava, inferior vena cava, lateral tunnel, right atrium, and the ventricular chamber, setting the stage for pulmonary and systemic emboli. Anticoagulation is an important consideration.

MEDICAL MANAGEMENT OF ADULT CONGENITAL HEART DISEASE

Cyanotic

Cyanotic congenital heart disease can be viewed as a multisystem, systemic disorder that affects red blood cells and hemostasis, the kidneys, urate metabolism, the digits and long bones, bilirubin kinetics, respiration and ventilation, the coronary and systemic vascular beds, and the central nervous system.[135]

REGULATION OF RED CELL MASS

Erythrocytosis is a physiologically appropriate response to a decrease in tissue oxygenation (arterial hypoxemia) that stimulates elaboration of erythropoietin from specialized sensor cells in the kidney, resulting in an increase in the number of circulating red blood cells and in an expanded blood volume.[136,137] The increase in erythrocyte mass offsets the deficit in tissue oxygenation. When erythrocytosis is sufficient to raise the tissue oxygen concentration above the threshold for release of erythropoietin by the renal oxygen sensors, a new equilibrium is established at a higher hematocrit level.[138] Should tissue oxygen concentration fail to reach that threshold, or should the renal oxygen sensors fail to respond appropriately, a stable equilibrium at a higher hematocrit level is not achieved.[138] Erythropoietin secretion and red blood cell mass continue to rise (negative feedback inhibition does not seem to occur) despite potentially harmful effects that accompany a further increase in hematocrit level.[138]

The adaptive increase in red blood cell mass of cyanotic congenital heart disease is fundamentally different from polycythemia rubra vera (primary polycythemia), which is an idiopathic clonal disorder of the bone marrow characterized by autonomous overproduction of red blood cells, thrombocytosis, leukocytosis, an increase in leukocyte alkaline phosphatase, and basophilia (see Chap. 57). To make that distinction clear, the increase in red blood cell mass prompted by the hypoxemia of cyanotic congenital heart disease is properly called "erythrocytosis" rather than "polycythemia."[135]

The erythrocytosis of cyanotic congenital heart disease falls into two categories: compensated and decompensated, defined in terms of erythrocyte indices and hyperviscosity symptoms.[138,139] *Compensated* erythrocytosis refers to patients who establish equilibrium hematocrit levels in iron-replete states and who have absent, mild, or moderate hyperviscosity symptoms, even at high hematocrit levels, even in excess of 70 per cent. *Decompensated* erythrocytosis refers to patients who fail to establish equilibrium conditions, who manifest unstable, rising hematocrit levels that are uncontrolled by negative feedback inhibition and who experience marked-to-severe hyperviscosity symptoms. Hematocrit levels should be determined by automated techniques, because microhematocrit centrifugation results in plasma trapping and falsely elevated levels.[135]

IRON AND IRON DEFICIENCY. The role of iron and the effects of iron deficiency are important clinical aspects of the erythrocytosis of cyanotic congenital heart disease. Iron is an integral part of myoglobin and of certain mitochondrial enzymes and plays a pivotal role in oxidative metabolism. Iron deficiency decreases work capacity in both experimental animals and in human subjects.[140,141] The consequences of iron deficiency are related not only to anemia per se but also to a decrease in the activity or concentration of iron-containing enzymes in muscle mitochondria and to impaired red cell deformability.[135,140] During iron repletion, muscle oxidases approach control values, reflecting a shift to greater dependence upon oxidative metabolism. An important effect of iron deficiency is on red blood cell shape.[140]

Whole-blood viscosity is a function of hematocrit level and of a number of other variables including deformability of erythrocytes, aggregation and dispersion of cellular elements, flow velocity (shear rate), temperature, vessel bore, endothelial integrity, and plasma viscosity. The normal biconcave disc-shaped erythrocyte is a flexible membrane partially filled with a viscous, noncompressible hemoglobin solution that allows deformation into an infinite variety of shapes with little or no change in cell volume or surface area. Conversely, iron-deficient red blood cells are relatively rigid microspherocytes that resist deformation in the microcirculation, thus increasing whole-blood viscosity. Accordingly, for an equivalent red blood cell mass, whole-blood viscosity is higher in an iron-deficient state.[140]

PHLEBOTOMIES. Adults with cyanotic congenital heart disease and erythrocytosis are frequently phlebotomized and occasionally anticoagulated. The rationale for phlebotomy assumes an inherent increase in the risk of cerebral arterial thrombotic stroke, a risk that has not withstood scrutiny in a study of 112 adults with cyanotic congenital heart disease observed for a total of 748 patient years.[142]

In cyanotic adults, cerebrovascular accidents are often associated with excessive, injudicious phlebotomies or with the use of antiplatelet agents (aspirin) or anticoagulants that reinforce intrinsic hemostatic defects and risk intracranial bleeding.[134,142] As the risk of stroke due to cerebral arterial thrombosis has not materialized, because the circulatory effects of phlebotomy are transient and because the result of phlebotomy-induced iron deficiency is an increase in whole-blood viscosity, phlebotomy is not recommended on the basis of hematocrit level per se.[134,142] For patients with *compensated* erythrocytosis, phlebotomy is not advised, even when the hematocrit level exceeds 70 per cent, as long as symptoms attributed to hyperviscosity are absent, mild, or moderate. Hyperviscosity symptoms at hematocrit levels less than 65 per cent are almost always due to iron deficiency. Phlebotomy further depletes iron stores and aggravates rather than alleviates the symptoms that respond instead to iron repletion. Iron therapy must be monitored closely, because hematocrit levels tend to rise rapidly.[134]

The firmest indication for phlebotomy is marked-to-severe symptomatic hyperviscosity in patients with hematocrit levels exceeding 65 per cent, provided that dehydration is not the cause. The objective of phlebotomy is temporary alleviation of intrusive hyperviscosity symptoms while minimizing the degree of phlebotomy-induced iron deficiency. A comparatively simple and safe outpatient method of phlebotomy for adults involves removal of 500 ml of blood over 30 to 45 minutes followed by quantitative replacement of the volume with isotonic saline. Saline is as efficacious as albumin for volume replacement, but if saline is clinically undesirable, isovolumetric repletion can be achieved with dextran 40 (5 per cent dextrose in water), which is salt free.

HEMOSTASIS. Bleeding tendencies tend to be mild to moderate in cyanotic adults, and are principally mucocutaneous.[143] However, epistaxis and hemoptysis vary from occasional and mild to copious and recurrent. In addition, serious and sometimes fatal bleeding can occur with accidental trauma or with surgical procedures. A decrease or absence of high molecular weight forms of the von Willebrand factor in plasma has recently been established and correlated with cyanosis, pulmonary vascular disease, and turbulent blood flow.[143] The von Willebrand abnormality in congenital heart disease is believed to be acquired, and the types and prevalence of bleeding are similar to the patterns in other forms of acquired von Willebrand disease.[143] Platelet counts are generally in the low range of normal in cyanotic adults but occasionally are moderately to markedly reduced.[134]

The hemostatic defect(s), especially in cyanotic patients, tend to be reinforced by an increase in tissue vascularity.[143] Aspirin, oral anticoagulants, and nonsteroidal antiinflammatory agents increase these intrinsic bleeding tendencies. Bronchoscopy should not be used to investigate hemoptysis, because the procedure is accompanied by risks while providing no additional basis for therapeutic judgment.

Hematocrit levels above 65 per cent incur an increased likelihood of perioperative hemorrhage. Preoperative phlebotomy designed to reduce the hematocrit level to just below 65 per cent serves to improve hemostasis and decrease the perioperative risk.[134] Phlebotomized units should be stored for potential postoperative autologous transfusion.

Another therapeutic issue in cyanotic adults is the use of nasal oxygen. From both the hematological and respiratory points of view, there is little evidence that oxygen is beneficial,[144] and the drying effect on nasal mucous membranes increases the risk of epistaxis.

RENAL INVOLVEMENT. Involvement of the kidneys in cyanotic congenital heart disease has been known for over four decades, but the pathogenesis of the lesion has only recently been clarified.[145] Renal histopathology resides chiefly in the glomerulus.[146] The abnormality takes the form of a vascular response including dilatation of hilar arterioles, dilatation and engorgement of capillaries and enlargement of the glomerular tuft, and also a nonvascular response characterized by an increase in mesangial matrix and cellularity, and an increase in endothelial cell proliferation.[145] The *vascular* response has been ascribed to release of L-arginine–derived nitric oxide that acts as an autocrine hormone, modulating the increased glomerular vascular resistance incurred by erythrocytosis.[145] The *nonvascular* response has been assigned to local release of platelet-derived growth factor from the cytoplasm of circulating systemic venous megakaryocytes that are delivered into the systemic arterial circulation through the right-to-left shunt.[145]

URATE METABOLISM. Hyperuricemia and proteinuria are common features of cyanotic congenital heart disease.[147] The mechanism of proteinuria is unclear, but a relationship appears to exist between proteinuria and hyperviscosity.[147] High plasma uric acid levels are secondary to inappropriately low renal fractional uric acid excretion rather than to urate overproduction.[147] Hyperuricemia therefore serves as a marker of abnormal intrarenal hemodynamics but appears to exert little or no deleterious effect on renal function and is not routinely treated.[134] Acute gouty arthritis is relatively uncommon, despite elevated uric acid levels, an observation similar to that in other forms of secondary hyperuricemia.[147,148]

Intravenous colchicine, the preferred treatment for acute gouty arthritis in cyanotic adults, is followed by a rapid clinical response and minimizes the undesirable dehydrating gastrointestinal side effects of oral colchicine. Prophylaxis after resolution of acute gouty arthritis is best achieved with low-dose oral colchicine (0.6 mg once or twice daily), a dose schedule that prevents recurrences in 75 to 90 per cent of patients and is usually tolerated without gastrointestinal side effects. Recurrent gouty arthritis is treated with allopurinol, probenicid, sulfinpyrazone, or combined therapy.

CLUBBING OF THE DIGITS AND HYPERTROPHIC OSTEOARTHROPATHY (Fig. 2–4, p. 17). These abnormalities are also believed to be responses to local release of platelet-derived growth factor from the cytoplasm of megakaryotes that are shunted from right to left and that impact in the capillary beds of the fingers, toes, and periosteum.[149] Clubbing is asymptomatic, but hypertrophic osteoarthropathy not uncommonly causes arthralgias over long bones. If therapy is indicated, salsalate is sometimes helpful. The drug is a nonacetylated analog of aspirin but does not interfere with normal platelet function.

GALLSTONES. Cyanotic adults with erythrocytosis are at risk for cholelithiasis caused by calcium bilirubinate gallstones[134] (Fig. 30–12A). An expanded red blood cell mass provides the substrate for an in-

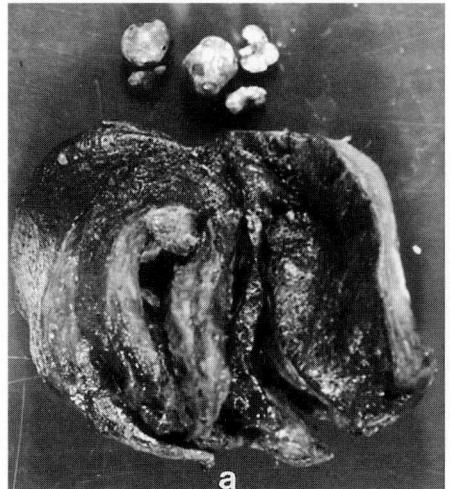
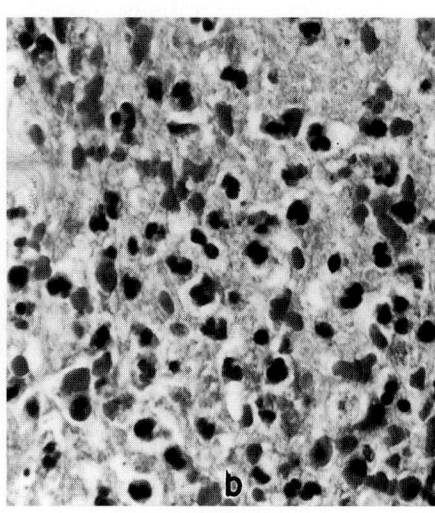

FIGURE 30–12. *A*, Thick-walled gallbladder with calcium bilirubinate gallstones shown above the specimen which was removed from a 47-year-old cyanotic man with Eisenmenger's complex and acute cholecystitis. *B*, Microscopic section of the gallbladder showing acute inflammatory cells.

crease in unconjugated bilirubin, which is believed to cause pigment stones because the compound is largely insoluble in water. Biliary colic may become clinically overt years after surgical relief of the cyanosis. An additional hazard of acute cholecystitis is infective endocarditis caused by bacteremia associated with septic inflammation of the gallbladder (Fig. 30–12*B*).

OXYGEN UPTAKE AND CONTROL OF VENTILATION. Diversion of venous blood into the systemic arterial circulation is a basic pathological fault in cyanotic congenital heart disease. Exercise serves to increase significantly the degree of venoarterial shunting and materially influences the dynamics of oxygen uptake ($\dot{V}O_2$) and ventilation.[150,151] Patients with cyanotic congenital heart disease experience markedly abnormal responses in achieving a steady state for $\dot{V}O_2$ after the onset of dynamic (isotonic) exercise. The prolonged onset and recovery of $\dot{V}O_2$ kinetics result in large O_2 deficits and hypoxemia, even with low levels of isotonic exercise; this suggests that patients with significant right-to-left shunts rely to an unusual degree on anaerobic metabolism. Unlike in the prolonged $\dot{V}O_2$ kinetics, cyanotic patients exhibit large increases in ventilation in phase I of exercise, and, in contrast to normal subjects, ventilation increases much more rapidly than $\dot{V}O_2$ in phase II (Fig. 30–13).[150,151] Ventilatory stimuli that are augmented by exercise in patients with right-to-left shunts include hypoxemia, metabolic acidosis, and shunting of CO_2 into the systemic arterial circulation. Because these patients have a substantially greater increase in ventilation during isotonic exercise than do normal subjects, "dyspnea" may be a prominent subjective complaint.[134] The New York Heart Association functional class is inappropriate because "dyspnea" is, in fact, hyperventilation unrelated to heart failure. The functional classification shown in Table 30–1 is recommended for patients with congenital heart disease.

THE CORONARY VASCULAR BED. It has long been known that the extramural coronary arteries in older patients with cyanotic congenital heart disease tend to become enlarged and tortuous, sometimes dramatically so.[152] The reason may lie in the dilating effects of nitric oxide and perhaps of prostaglandins that are elaborated by endothelium in response to the viscosity-induced increase in shear stress.[143] Of potentially greater functional importance is the effect of cyanotic congenital heart disease on myocardial perfusion. Recent studies using positron emission tomography (PET) disclosed that myocardial perfusion at rest is normal, but perfusion reserve is reduced after pharmacological stress, implying a perfusion deficit during physical exercise.[153]

DISORDERS OF THE CENTRAL NERVOUS SYSTEM. Prominent among these in adults with congenital heart disease are brain abscess, cerebral emboli, subclavian steal, syncope, intracerebral and subarachnoid hemorrhage, and seizures.[154]

The pathogenesis of a brain abscess is not always clear. Right-to-left shunts in patients with cyanotic congenital heart disease bypass the pulmonary filter, permitting bacteria to enter the systemic and therefore cerebral circulations. However, a focal zone of cerebral vulnerability appears to be necessary for formation of abscess.[154] Brain abscess should be suspected when adults with cyanosis experience headache, focal neurological signs, seizures, and fever. The diagnosis of a recent brain abscess can be established by computed tomography (CT), which identifies the lesion and the distinctive ring enhancement. Seizures may accompany the fresh abscess and may persist or recur years later because of focal brain injury at the site of the healed abscess.

Paradoxical Emboli. Cerebral emboli (see p. 885) can be bland or infected. Relatively unique to congenital heart

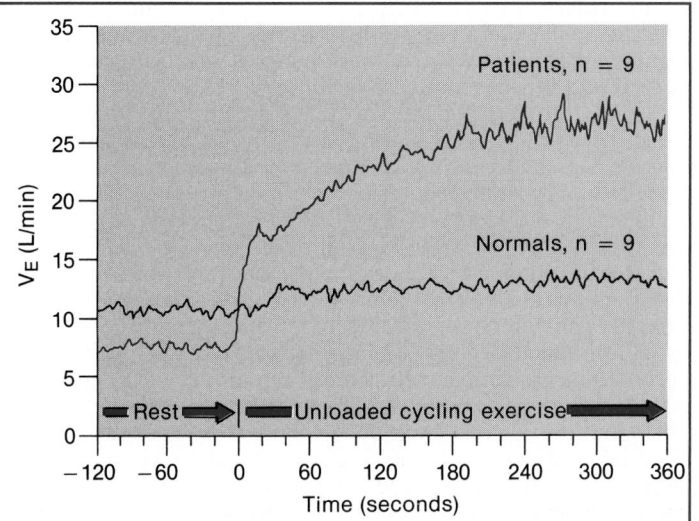

FIGURE 30–13. The increase in ventilation in response to unloaded cycle ergometric exercise in nine adults with right-to-left shunts and in nine normal subjects. The patients had higher minute ventilation both at rest and in response to exercise. (From Sietsema, K. E., et al.: Control of ventilation during exercise in patients with central venous to systemic arterial shunts. J. Appl. Physiol. *64*:234, 1988.)

TABLE 30–1 CONGENITAL HEART DISEASE FUNCTIONAL CLASSIFICATION (PRESENCE AND DEGREE OF SYMPTOMS)

Class 1	Asymptomatic at all levels of activity
Class 2	Symptoms are present but do not curtail average everyday activity
Class 3	Symptoms significantly curtail most but not all average everyday activity
Class 4	Symptoms significantly curtail virtually all average everyday activity and may be present at rest

disease—usually, but not necessarily, cyanotic—are paradoxical emboli.[154] In cyanotic patients, paradoxical emboli originate in lower-extremity or pelvic veins and reach the brain by peripheral venous blood that has direct access to the systemic arterial circulation due to the right-to-left shunt. Anticoagulants may reduce the risk of paradoxical embolization, but reinforce the intrinsic hemostatic defects in cyanotic patients and increase the risk of cerebral hemorrhage.

A potential source of paradoxical embolization in hospitalized cyanotic patients is an intravenous line inserted for infusions or drugs.[155] Particles or air accidentally introduced into peripheral veins may be delivered into the systemic circulation through the right-to-left shunt.

Paradoxical emboli in acyanotic patients occur when an interatrial communication—ostium secundum atrial septal defect or patent foramen ovale—permits inferior caval blood to stream across the atrial septum into the left atrium and systemic circulation. Recent interest has focused upon young adults with stroke ascribed to paradoxical emboli through a patent foramen ovale,[156] a pathway analogous to that of an ostium secundum atrial septal defect. Platelet/fibrin particles that circulate in the systemic nervous bed are removed by the efficient lytic system in the lungs. Isometric exercise, the Valsalva maneuver, or vigorous coughing may provoke transient venoarterial mixing that delivers clusters of these particles through a patent foramen ovale into the systemic circulation and into a cerebrovascular bed that lacks a lytic system. The Valsalva maneuver is used diagnostically to initiate a transient right-to-left shunt through a foramen ovale during contrast echocardiography or transcranial contrast ultrasound.[156]

An atrial septal aneurysm may be the source of fibrin/platelet thrombi and embolic strokes, generally manifested by transient ischemic attacks in acyanotic patients.[157] The aneurysm can be suspected in a transthoracic echocardiogram but is best established by transesophageal echocardiography (see Fig. 3–16, p. 59).

Cerebral Hemorrhage. This complication tends to occur in adults with congenital heart disease under a limited number of circumstances. One cause is the injudicious use of anticoagulants or antiplatelet agents in cyanotic patients. An uncommon but potentially catastrophic cause of a hemorrhagic cerebrovascular accident is rupture of a congenital aneurysm of the circle of Willis, especially but not exclusively in patients with coarctation of the aorta (Fig. 30–3).

Mycotic aneurysms (better termed *septic aneurysms*) (Fig. 30–14) result from inflammatory weakening of the wall of a cerebral artery caused by septic microemboli to vasa vasora or by impaction of an infected embolus in the lumen of the artery.[154] Cerebral mycotic aneurysms may enlarge and rupture despite antibiotic eradication of the offending organism. Headaches or seizures announce an enlarging or perforating aneurysm, which can be diagnosed by CT scan and cerebral angiography. Aneurysms approaching 1 cm in diameter are treated by surgical excision to prevent catastrophic rupture.

Other Neurological Complications. The subclavian steal is an occasional neurological complication of a Blalock-Taussig anastomosis.[158] The classic shunt operation may create an anatomical and physiological substrate analogous to that of an atherosclerotic subclavian steal. Symptoms of the steal may appear decades after the shunt is established, depending on the development of cervical and intrathoracic collaterals. The steal is not necessarily corrected by intracardiac repair, even though the anastomosis is ligated. Congenital subclavian steal is rare.

In patients with congenital aortic stenosis, cerebral symptoms may consist of mere giddiness, faintness, or lightheadedness with effort. Conversely, syncopal episodes are sometimes recurrent and potentially dangerous.

Infective Endocarditis: Risks and Prophylaxis
(See also Chap. 33)

The clinical and bacteriological profiles of infective endocarditis changed significantly after the advent of cardiac surgery and prosthetic devices. Certain operations (division of a patent ductus arteriosus) eliminate the risk, whereas other operations (shunts, prosthetic valves or conduits) materially increase the risk.[2] However, certain general principles still prevail: namely, that the two major predisposing factors that increase the risk of infective endocarditis are a susceptible cardiac or vascular substrate and the presence of bacteremia. Susceptible lesions are those associated with high-velocity turbulent flow, jet impact, and focal increases in the rate of shear. An exception is the peculiar lack of susceptibility associated with the high-velocity diastolic flow accompanying pulmonary hypertensive pulmonary regurgitation. Portals of entry include the oral cavity, the genitourinary tract in men, the upper and lower gastrointestinal tracts, the airways and respiratory tract, and treatments such as obstetrical and gynecological procedures, and certain types of noncardiac surgery.

Susceptibility to infective endocarditis in congenital heart disease has been classified according to low-risk unoperated anomalies, low- or no-risk postoperative, intermediate-risk unoperated, intermediate-risk postoperative, and high-risk postoperative.[2] Low-risk unoperated anomalies are represented by ostium secundum atrial septal defect and mild pulmonary valve stenosis. A no-risk postoperative lesion is typified by a patent ductus arteriosus after ligation. Intermediate-risk unoperated lesions are represented by a functionally normal bicuspid aortic valve, aortic regurgitation, restrictive ventricular septal defect, or patent ductus arteriosus, especially restrictive. Intermediate-risk postoperative lesions include bicuspid aortic stenosis and residual aortic or left atrioventricular valve regurgitation. High-risk postoperative substrates include rigid prosthetic valves (especially left-sided), external-valved conduits, and aortopulmonary shunts.

Prophylaxis for infective endocarditis consists of both nonchemotherapeutic and chemotherapeutic (antimicrobial) measures. Nonchemotherapeutic prophylaxis involves day-to-day oral hygiene, skin care, nail care, and female contraception. The spongy, fragile gums of patients with cyanotic

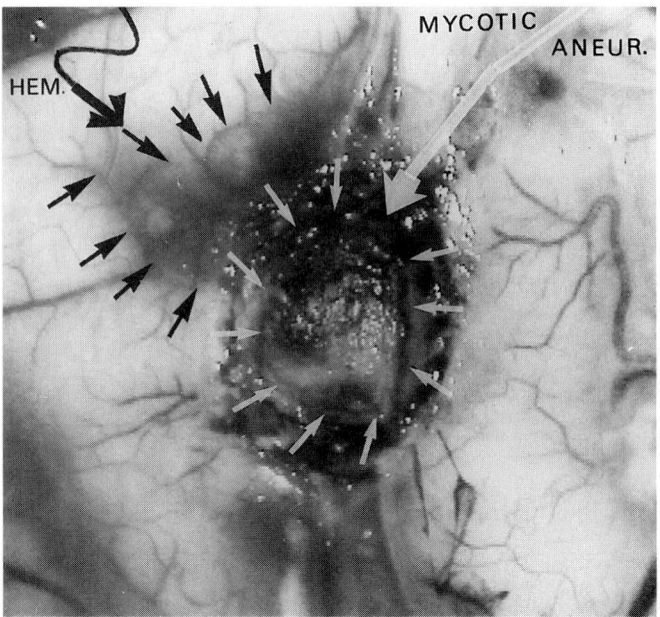

FIGURE 30–14. Mycotic aneurysm photographed at craniotomy in a 27-year-old man with *Streptococcus viridans* infective endocarditis, status postintracardiac repair of congenitally corrected transposition of the great arteries, ventricular septal defect, and pulmonary stenosis. Hemorrhage (HEM) adjacent to the aneurysm indicated impending rupture had surgery not intervened.

congenital heart disease are of special concern. A soft-bristled toothbrush should be used. Dental appointments for prophylaxis should be at least twice yearly. Meticulous skin care is important, especially in adolescents and young adults with acne that may be distributed beyond the face. Biting or picking of fingernails risks injury to contiguous skin and predisposes to paronychial infection with staphylococci. Intrauterine devices are best avoided because of the risk of bacteremia.

Pregnancy and Congenital Heart Disease: The Mother and the Fetus
(See also pp. 1846–1848)

Central to this topic is the intricate interplay between maternal circulatory and respiratory physiology and maternal congenital heart disease and the effects of this interplay upon the fetus. The fetus is exposed to risks that threaten its intrauterine viability and to risks that subsequently express themselves as developmental defects or transmitted congenital malformations of the heart or circulation.[159]

An important aspect of congenital heart disease and pregnancy is contraception.[159] Barrier methods include the condom (male) and the diaphragm with spermicide for the female. Tubal ligation can be accomplished safely, even in relatively high-risk women. The levonorgestrel implant (controlled release of progestin) is a safe and efficacious contraceptive for cyanotic women with pulmonary vascular disease. Retention of fluid is modest and does not preclude use of the implant for patients with controlled heart failure. Progestin injections are not recommended for patients with heart failure because of the associated retention of fluid. Low estrin is the lowest estrogen-containing oral contraceptive, and is considered safe and nonthrombogenic with a low rate of failure if no dose is missed. Use of the intrauterine device within a monogamous relationship probably does not increase the risk of infection or of infective endocarditis, but endometrial irritation may induce excessive bleeding, especially in patients with cyanotic congenital heart disease and hemostatic defect(s).

THE UNOPERATED PATIENT

There are a number of common congenital malformations that are found in unoperated adult women (Table 30–2).

OSTIUM SECUNDUM ATRIAL SEPTAL DEFECT. This malformation is of special relevance because the history without operation spans the reproductive years and because the majority of affected patients are female.[5] Young women with uncomplicated ostium secundum atrial septal defects generally tolerate pregnancy with no ill effects. An important risk, however, is a paradoxical embolus that originates in pelvic and leg veins and is carried by inferior vena caval blood across the atrial septal defect into the systemic circulation.[160] Accordingly, meticulous leg care and early ambulation after delivery are mandatory. Acute blood loss poses a potential risk because hemorrhage provokes a rise in systemic vascular resistance and a fall in systemic venous return, augmenting the left-to-right shunt, sometimes appreciably.[159]

PATENT DUCTUS ARTERIOSUS. This anomaly predominates in women but is of limited practical importance as a complication of pregnancy, because the clinical diagnosis is simple, and division of the ductus in childhood is curative. A small or moderate-sized patent ductus with normal pulmonary arterial pressure poses no risk apart from susceptibility to infective endocarditis during delivery. In the presence of a moderately restrictive patent ductus (Fig. 30–15), the gestational fall in systemic vascular resistance serves to decrease

TABLE 30–2 COMMON MALFORMATIONS WITH EXPECTED ADULT SURVIVAL (ORDER OF FEMALE PREVALENCE)

Acyanotic
Atrial septal defect (secundum)
Patent ductus arteriosus
Pulmonary valve stenosis
Coarctation of the aorta
Aortic valve disease
Cyanotic
Fallot's tetralogy

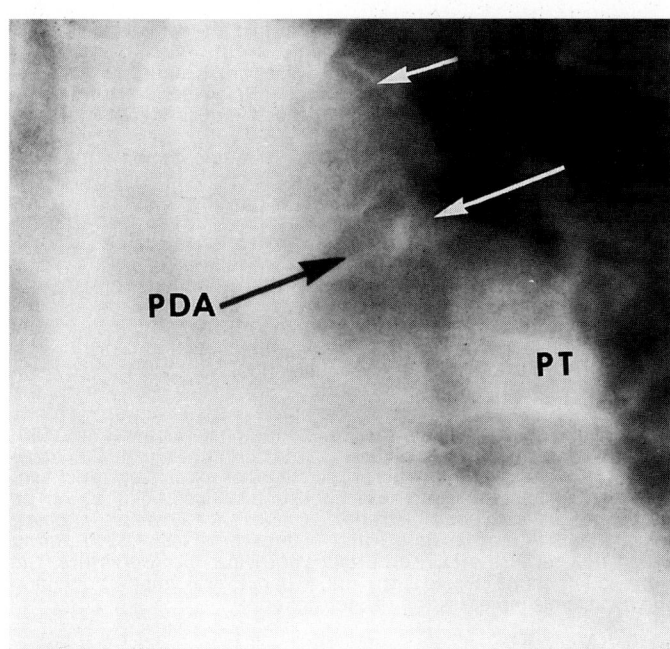

FIGURE 30–15. Chest radiograph (closeup) from a 57-year-old woman with a calcified patent ductus arteriosus (PDA, dark arrow) that was moderately restrictive. She had 20 pregnancies with 12 live births. The pulmonary trunk (PT) is dilated. The aorta also contains calcium (top white arrow).

ductal flow, but if the shunt is large, that benefit is unlikely to compensate for the hemodynamic burden of pregnancy. At highest risk is the patient with a nonrestrictive patent ductus, pulmonary vascular disease, and reversed shunt.[159] The gestational decline in systemic vascular resistance augments the right-to-left shunt through the ductus, further lowering uterine arterial oxygen saturation, which poses potential harm to the fetus.

ISOLATED PULMONARY VALVE STENOSIS. Fifty per cent of patients with this malformation are women and adult survival is the rule, even in the presence of significant obstruction to right ventricular outflow.[5] Severe pulmonary stenosis is occasionally tolerated despite gestational volume overload imposed upon an already pressure-loaded right ventricle. Infective endocarditis prophylaxis is advisable during delivery, although the probability of infection in patients with mild obstruction to right ventricular outflow is believed to be negligible.

COARCTATION OF THE AORTA. The malformation occurs chiefly in men but is dealt with here because maternal morbidity—cardiovascular complications without death—is relatively high.[159,161] The hypertension of coarctation is accompanied by a comparatively low incidence of toxemia compared to other forms of systemic hypertension.[5] Connective tissue changes in the walls of systemic arteries during normal pregnancy[162] increase the risk of aortic rupture or dissection, especially in the vulnerable postcoarctation segment and in the aortic root,[20] and increase the risk of cerebral hemorrhage from rupture of an aneurysm of the circle of Willis (Fig 30–3). Left ventricular failure is exceptional, despite augmented volume imposed upon the pressure-loaded left ventricle. Susceptibility to infective endocarditis is determined chiefly by coexistence of a bicuspid aortic valve.

BICUSPID AORTIC STENOSIS. Because of the low incidence of this malformation among women, bicuspid aortic stenosis is only an occasional complication of pregnancy. The increased cardiac output tends to be tolerated in women with mild-to-moderate bicuspid aortic stenosis, but severe obstruction encroaches on limited circulatory reserve. Dyspnea, angina pectoris, or cerebral symptoms that precede conception or appear early in gestation are matters of grave concern.

BICUSPID AORTIC REGURGITATION. Moderate-to-severe chronic bicuspid aortic regurgitation is generally well tolerated during pregnancy, provided that the adaptive response of the left ventricle preserves normal function. The gestational fall in systemic vascular resistance, together with a more rapid heart rate (shorter diastole), results in a decrease in regurgitant flow.[159] The risk of infective endocarditis is high; therefore, antibiotic prophylaxis is obligatory during labor and delivery.

FALLOT'S TETRALOGY. About half of patients with this anomaly are women, and Fallot's tetralogy is the most common cyanotic malformation that might permit unoperated survival into reproductive age. A gestational fall in systemic vascular resistance and augmented venous return to an obstructed right ventricle result in an increase in the right-to-left shunt and a fall in systemic arterial oxygen saturation, changes that are especially harmful to the fetus. During labor and delivery, a sudden fall in systemic vascular resistance may precipitate intense cyanosis, syncope, and death. Conversely, bearing down during labor may abruptly and dangerously reduce systemic arterial blood flow.

CONGENITAL COMPLETE HEART BLOCK. This uncommon congenital conduction defect permits survival into childbearing age, and about one-half of the patients are female.[5] Asymptomatic young women usually experience an uneventful pregnancy, provided that the QRS duration is not prolonged and the rate response to exercise is satisfactory.[159,163,164] Stokes-Adams attacks occasionally occur during gestation, and the heart and circulation may not respond appropriately to the volatile demands of labor and delivery.

EBSTEIN'S ANOMALY OF THE TRICUSPID VALVE. About half of the patients with this malformation are women, and the majority reach adulthood.[5] The functionally inadequate right ventricle, already volume-overloaded by tricuspid regurgitation, copes poorly with the gestational increase in cardiac output.[165] Atrial tachyarrhythmias occur in approximately one-third of nonpregnant patients with Ebstein's anomaly and are potential hazards during pregnancy.[166] Wolff-Parkinson-White bypass tracts set the stage for excessively rapid ventricular rates in response to atrial fibrillation or flutter (Fig. 30–7). The consequences can be catastrophic. Cyanosis in Ebstein's anomaly (right-to-left interatrial shunt) may first become manifested during pregnancy because of a rise in right ventricular filling pressure. The right-to-left shunt increases the risk of paradoxical embolization, and the hypoxemia increases the risk to the fetus.

THE POSTOPERATIVE PATIENT

There is a consensus that successful surgery before gestation can be pivotal in reducing maternal risks of congenital heart disease. Surgery should therefore be anticipatory. The objectives of reparative surgery are to increase the safety and success of pregnancy, to preserve the health of the mother, and to reduce the risk to the fetus. Closure of an *ostium secundum atrial septal defect* in children or young adults permits pregnancy without maternal risk. The complication of paradoxical embolization from the inferior vena cava is eliminated. However, an increase in incidence of atrial tachyarrhythmias should be considered when the defect is closed after young adulthood.

Division of a small nonpulmonary hypertensive *patent ductus* early in life is curative. Division of a nonrestrictive or moderately restrictive ductus is sometimes followed by incomplete resolution of elevated pulmonary vascular resistance or by less than adequate functional recovery of the volume-overloaded left ventricle, important residua that might confront the pregnant woman. In any event, division of a patent ductus eliminates the risk of infective endocarditis.

Successful response of congenital *pulmonary valve stenosis* to balloon dilatation or to direct repair permits the pregnant woman to anticipate a normal pregnancy except for a low, if not altogether absent, risk of infective endocarditis. Mild-to-moderate low-pressure postinterventional pulmonary regurgitation is not a concern, with few exceptions. Balloon dilatation has proven efficacious during pregnancy (Fig. 30–9).

After repair of *coarctation of the aorta*, the risk of pregnancy depends on relief of the isthmic obstruction (and reduction of systemic blood pressure), the surgical technique, and whether or not a bicuspid aortic valve coexists. To what extent correction of coarctation reduces the hazard of gestational rupture of an aneurysm of the circle of Willis is open to question. The histology of the aorta immediately distal to the coarctation resembles that of cystic medionecrosis, and balloon dilatation injures this already vulnerable aortic segment.[20] Relief of the isthmic obstruction by partial resection and roofing with a graft leaves the vulnerable postcoarctation aortic segment largely in place. The procedure of choice in women is resection that includes the segment of aorta distal to the coarctation, with end-to-end anastomosis. Should a bicuspid aortic valve coexist, two additional postoperative concerns persist: susceptibility to infective endocarditis and the risk inherent in the histological abnormalities of the aortic root.

Surgical relief or balloon dilatation of congenital bicuspid *aortic stenosis* (Fig. 30–10) significantly lowers the risk of pregnancy (see earlier), but not the risk of infective endocarditis. In the presence of hemodynamically significant bicuspid aortic regurgitation, it is usually better to advise pregnancy before aortic valve replacement, provided that left ventricular function is normal or nearly normal. If a stenotic or incompetent aortic valve requires replacement in a woman of childbearing age, a tissue valve has the advantage of good hemodynamics without the need for anticoagulants (but with the caveats commented upon later).

Pregnancy after repair of *Fallot's tetralogy* is accompanied by a gratifyingly small risk, especially when outflow obstruction is relieved without inducing significant low-pressure pulmonary regurgitation. Elimination of cyanosis increases the probability of successful conception,[167] improves the stability of pregnancy, and results in normal fetal growth and development. Postoperative electrophysiological sequelae cannot be ignored but are comparatively infrequent when successful repair is accomplished at a young age (see p. 982).

Closure of a nonrestrictive or moderately restrictive perimembranous *ventricular septal defect* in infancy or early childhood serves to preclude the development of pulmonary vascular disease and to relieve the left ventricle of volume overload. Pregnancy can be anticipated with optimism. Postoperative electrophysiological sequelae are exceptional.

A pacemaker is occasionally required in young women with *congenital complete heart block*, but with relative confidence that pregnancy can then safely proceed if ventricular function is normal, which is usually the case. Although a dual-chamber pacemaker is preferable, a fixed-rate system provides satisfactory physiological support.

Surgical repair of *Ebstein's anomaly of the tricuspid valve* ideally takes the form of reconstruction using the large mobile anterior tricuspid leaflet to create a competent unicuspid atrioventricular valve. Active or potential bypass tracts are eliminated by surgical dissociation of right atrium from right ventricle (Fig. 30–7). The maternal risk of pregnancy, including susceptibility to infective endocarditis, is reduced but not eliminated.

Pregnancy after repair of certain forms of *complex cyanotic congenital heart disease* is now a practical objective. However, menstrual patterns of women who were cyanotic before operation differ significantly from normal women, implying abnormalities of gynecological endocrinology that may influence fertility.[167] After a *Fontan procedure*, a twofold increment in cardiac index can usually be achieved in response to isotonic exercise.[168] The corollary is that women who have undergone successful Fontan repairs and have good if not normal ventricular function confront the physiological burden of pregnancy with circulations that potentially possess adequate hemodynamic reserve. However, other variables may influence outcome.[133]

Medical Management of the Pregnant Woman with Congenital Heart Disease

PRENATAL CARE. A major objective of medical management is to minimize the factors that encroach upon the limited circulatory reserve of pregnant women with heart disease. Cardiac reserve is encroached upon by the hemodynamic burden of pregnancy and by the heart disease itself. Anxiety is a special concern in the primigravida as she anticipates her first gestational experience. The expectant mother should be prepared for what awaits her during pregnancy, labor, delivery, and puerperium in order to decrease if not eliminate fear of the unknown. Diuretics can be used judiciously for the edema of cardiac failure but should not be used for the edema of normal pregnancy.[159] The pregnant woman with heart disease should limit herself to moderate isotonic exercise. Heat and humidity add to the hemodynamic burden; a dry cool atmosphere is therapeutic. The physiological anemia of pregnancy must be distinguished from pathological anemia, and the latter assiduously addressed. Meticulous leg care reduces the gestational tendency for lower-extremity venous stasis and the attendant risk of thromboembolism. Passive standing should be avoided, the supine position minimized (compression of the inferior vena cava by the enlarged uterus), and the pregnant woman should minimize or avoid sitting with knees flexed and legs dependent. As term approaches, an important element in reducing anxiety is assurance that the pain of labor and delivery will be minimized.

The efficacy of oxygen administration during gestation in cyanotic women is open to question, with little or no convincing evidence of benefit to the mother. There is less-than-convincing evidence that oxygen administration exerts a favorable effect on growth retardation of the fetus in cyanotic women.

Maternal mortality in pregnant women with heart disease has been coupled with functional class. Symptoms associated with congenital heart disease, especially cyanotic, have prompted the use of the functional classification shown in Table 30–1. In addition to and apart from symptoms and functional limitations, certain congenital cardiac malformations impose such a formidable threat to maternal survival that pregnancy is proscribed or should be interrupted. Of the two major maternal cardiac risks—pulmonary vascular disease and pulmonary edema—the former is more relevant to congenital heart disease. Primary pulmonary hypertension epitomizes this risk (see Chap.

25), but pulmonary vascular disease in any context is a major hazard, limiting if not precluding rapid adaptive responses to the circulatory changes of pregnancy and to the volatile changes during labor, delivery, and the puerperium.

LABOR AND DELIVERY. In women with functionally mild unoperated lesions and in patients after successful cardiac surgery, management of labor and delivery is the same as for normal pregnant women. The need for infective endocarditis prophylaxis during routine delivery in pregnant cardiac patients has been questioned because of the low incidence of bacteremia that accompanies a normal uncomplicated vaginal delivery.[169] It should not be assumed, however, that a given delivery will be uncomplicated. An episiotomy and vacuum extraction are, strictly speaking, not "normal." Accordingly, pregnant women with cardiac lesions susceptible to infective endocarditis should receive appropriate antibiotic prophylaxis from the onset of labor through the third or fourth postpartal day.[170]

For pregnant women with functionally important congenital cardiac disease—unoperated or operated—the management of labor, delivery, and the puerperium is crucial if risk is to be minimized. The first necessity is to underscore the beneficial effects of induced vaginal delivery. Cesarean section should be reserved for cephalopelvic disproportion, for breech presentation, or for preterm labor in a woman receiving coumadin anticoagulation. Cesarean section results in about twice the blood loss as vaginal delivery, in addition to the risks of wound and uterine infection, thrombophlebitis (delayed ambulation), and potential postoperative complications.

Amniocentesis around the 37th week determines whether or not fetal lung maturity has been achieved and whether induced delivery can safely proceed. The pregnant woman is then admitted for induction, with delivery planned as far as possible during the working day so that a high-risk obstetrician, neonatologist, and cardiologist can more readily be available. On admission, prostaglandin vaginal gel is applied to soften and dilate the cervix.[159] *Laminaria*, derived from the stems of a special seaweed, can be used for the same purpose because of its hydrophilic properties. Oxytocin may be required for augmentation of uterine contractions that are usually initiated by absorbed prostaglandin. The sequence of cervical softening and dilatation precedes the onset of uterine contractions, as in normal spontaneous vaginal delivery.

After contractions are under way, artificial rupture of the membranes is performed. The woman should labor in a lateral decubitus position in order to attenuate the hemodynamic fluctuations provoked by major uterine contractions in the supine position. Meperidine is used selectively for relief of pain and apprehension. The anesthetic of choice is a lumbar epidural preparation, such as fentanyl, that exquisitely controls pain without reducing the strength of uterine contractions, which are monitored together with fetal rate (Fig. 30–9A). The fetus is allowed to pass through the pelvis in response to the force of uterine contractions unsupplemented by straining in order to avoid the undesirable circulatory effects of the Valsalva maneuver. Delivery is assisted by vacuum extraction and low forceps.

Systemic arterial pressure should be monitored during labor, because lumbar epidural anesthetics may cause hypotension. In patients with Fallot's tetralogy or Eisenmenger's complex, a sudden fall in systemic vascular resistance poses a special threat. Use of a flotation catheter for hemodynamic monitoring is an individual cardiological decision, rather than routine policy. In Eisenmenger's complex, for example, the risks of a flotation catheter far outweigh the benefits.[171] Oxygen is often intuitively administered during labor, especially in cyanotic women, although without proven efficacy.

After expulsion of the placenta, bleeding is reduced by uterine massage. If intravenous oxytocin is used, the drug should be administered slowly because of its potential hypotensive effect. In the postpartum period, meticulous leg care, use of elastic support stockings, and early ambulation are important preventive measures that reduce the risk of thromboembolism.

BREAST FEEDING. This practice may encroach upon cardiac reserve and increase the risk of mastitis and bacteremia. Nursing should therefore be advised with caution in patients with congenital cardiac disease, and its duration should be minimized. Engorgement of the breasts and suppression of lactation are managed with binding, cold packs, and analgesics rather than with bromocriptine, which can cause hypotension.

Maternal congenital heart disease exposes the fetus to risks that threaten its intrauterine viability and to risks of potential congenital and developmental malformations.[172] Intrauterine viability is influenced by the functional class of the mother (with the qualifications noted above), by maternal cyanosis, and by oral anticoagulants. Maternal cyanosis threatens the growth, development, and viability of the fetus and materially increases fetal wastage, dysmaturity, and prematurity. The risk to the fetus of oral anticoagulants has not been satisfactorily resolved, so the need for anticoagulation should be minimized (see p. 1066). Valve reconstruction is recommended in women of childbearing age. A bioprosthetic valve obviates the need for anticoagulants but subjects the patient to subsequent reoperation. In addition, there is concern that pregnancy itself might accelerate degeneration of a bioprosthetic valve because of the inherent gestational changes in connective tissue. Aspirin is not a viable alternative to anticoagulants because of its potential for closing the fetal ductus and because of low efficacy.

There is no consensus on how best to administer anticoagulants. It is currently believed that the risk of fetal wastage from heparin is not of the same order as from coumadin,[173] previous reports notwithstanding. Whichever regimen of heparin and/or coumadin is chosen, the patient and her partner should be so advised before conception. There is a mounting consensus that warfarin should be replaced with heparin before conception in order to avoid the teratogenic risk of coumadin in early gestation.

The change from coumadin to heparin is best accomplished in the hospital. A nurse specialist instructs the patient and her partner on the technique of subcutaneous administration of heparin using a short 25-gauge needle and an abdominal site for injection at right angles to the elevated skin surface. The needle should be withdrawn slowly, and the site should not be massaged.

Heparin can either be continued throughout gestation (provided that the anticoagulant response is carefully monitored) or replaced with warfarin in the second trimester, returning to heparin in the 36th week. Because of harmful effects that coumadin might exert on the fetal central nervous system—which continues to develop throughout gestation—it has been argued that heparin is the preferred drug because it does not cross the placental barrier and is therefore not teratogenic either during initial organogenesis or during subsequent maturation of the higher centers of the brain. That is, the risk of coumadin lies not only in warfarin embryopathy but potentially in the effect of the oral anticoagulant on central nervous system development.[174] In light of concern that the risk of embryopathy varies directly with blood level, warfarin dosage should be monitored using the International Normalized Ratio (INR) in order to achieve a therapeutic range at the lowest possible dose.[175]

Preterm labor in a pregnant woman taking warfarin threatens the fetus with fatal hemorrhage because fetal anticoagulation cannot be promptly reversed. Emergency cesarean section is required if the fetus is to be saved. Maternal administration of vitamin K and infusion of fresh frozen plasma do not reverse fetal anticoagulation quickly enough to obviate fatal hemorrhage, but fresh frozen plasma should be administered to the newborn. There are, however, four concerns regarding the administration of heparin throughout pregnancy[173]: (1) greater difficulty in achieving a stable therapeutic response; (2) the inconvenience of parenteral administration, an inconvenience that the woman may not be prepared to sustain; (3) the risk of heparin-induced thrombocytopenia; and (4) the risk of bone demineralization.

Extracorporeal circulation is associated with a high incidence of fetal wastage, but cardiac surgery is rarely employed during gestation, especially in the pregnant woman with congenital heart disease. Should cardiac surgery be necessary, it is best to await the 25th to 26th week of gestation.

In addition to threats to its intrauterine viability, the fetus is exposed to risks that take the form of genetic parental transmission, teratogenic effects of certain cardiac drugs, and the harmful effects of certain environmental toxins. A substantial majority of congenital heart diseases cannot be attributed to either a syndrome or a single-gene defect that exhibits mendelian inheritance.[172] A number of studies have concluded that the risk of recurrence of congenital cardiac defects in offspring is greater if the mother rather than the father is the affected parent.[172] A hypothesis that might account for this pattern is cytoplasmic or maternal inheritance based on the observation that mitochondrial DNA is inherited only from the mother.[172] A second hypothesis, "parental imprinting" or "genomic imprinting," refers to gene expression that varies according to its maternal or paternal origin.[176] The imprinting factor is believed to be DNA methylation.

Exercise Before and After Surgery or Interventional Catheterization

Certain types of congenital disorders of the heart or circulation expose patients to the risk of complications or sudden death during strenuous exercise or competitive sports.[177] Consideration must be given to (1) the type, intensity, and duration of exercise; (2) the risk of body collision inherent in a given type of athletic activity; (3) the training program (conditioning) required for a given sport; (4) the emotional stress that the participant experiences in anticipation of or during a particular sport event; (5) the risk of injury to either the participant or spectators if the athletic activity induces loss of consciousness; and (6) the sometimes arbitrary distinction between competitive and recreational athletics.[178]

Two general types of exercise are recognized: isotonic (dynamic) and isometric (static).[2] *Isotonic exercise* is associated with changes in muscle length and with rhythmic muscular contractions that develop comparatively little force. A steady state can be achieved. *Isometric exercise* results in sudden development of a comparatively large force with little or no change in muscle length; a steady state cannot be achieved, even temporarily. There is usually a continuum between the two types, with most physical activity incorporating isotonic and isometric components. The risk incurred by conditioning (training) may equal or exceed the risk of the competitive event itself. The heightened emotional response of an athlete before or during a sporting event may trigger a disturbance in cardiac rhythm and a loss of consciousness, putting the athlete, as well as bystanders, at risk of injury. Central to the following discussion are the type and severity of a given congenital malformation, whether or not the patient had undergone cardiac surgery, and, if so, the type and success of the operation.

CONGENITAL HEART BLOCK. Patients with congenital complete heart block occasionally perform optimally,[5] but prolonged, high-intensity isotonic exercise is ill advised, and strenuous isometric exercise is unwise, even if tolerated. If a pacemaker is required, patients are allowed isotonic or isometric exercise within the limits of sensible moderation and according to the type of pacemaker used. Contact sports risk damage to the pacemaker.

ABERRANT CORONARY ARTERY BETWEEN THE AORTA AND RIGHT VENTRICULAR OUTFLOW TRACT (see Fig. 8–28, p. 262). This uncommon anomaly can cause angina pectoris, myocardial infarction, and sudden death.[179] The risk is greatest, especially in men, when the *left* coronary artery arises from the right aortic sinus and passes between the aorta and right ventricular outflow tract (Fig. 30–16). Sudden death typically accompanies or immediately follows relatively strenuous physical effort. Expansion of the aortic root and pulmonary trunk during exercise is believed to increase preexisting acute angulation of the proximal course of the aberrant coronary artery and to reduce its lumen, especially if the lumen is slit-like.[180,181] If the coronary anomaly is identified and surgically corrected, subsequent athletic activity is not restricted, provided that flow is unobstructed and myocardial ischemia is absent.

COARCTATION OF THE AORTA. In this condition the proximal aorta is less distensible than is the postcoarctation aorta, accounting, in part, for the disproportionate rise in systolic blood pressure in the proximal compartment.[5] The excessive rise in systolic blood pressure during isotonic exercise represents an exaggeration of the disproportionate systolic hypertension in the resting state. A disproportionate exercise-induced postoperative rise in systolic pressure

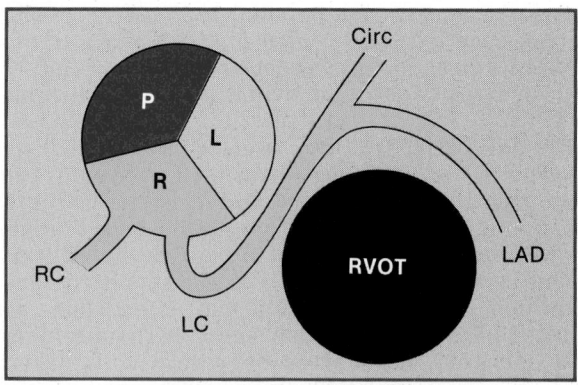

FIGURE 30–16. Illustration of the left coronary artery (LC) arising from a right aortic sinus (R) and coursing between the aorta and the right ventricular outflow tract (RVOT). P = posterior aortic sinus; L = left aortic sinus; RC = right coronary artery; Circ = circumflex coronary artery; and LAD = left anterior descending artery.

is in large part related to age at the time of repair and the adequacy of repair.

CONGENITAL AORTIC STENOSIS. Unoperated patients with *mild* congenital aortic valve stenosis (resting gradient 20 mm Hg or less) are not restricted, provided that the electrocardiogram (ECG) is normal, the response to exercise stress testing is normal, left ventricular function is normal or supernormal, and no significant disturbances in rhythm are recorded during 24-hour ambulatory electrocardiography. Patients with *moderate* congenital aortic stenosis (resting gradients higher than 20 but less than 50 mm Hg), especially those at the upper range, should confine athletics to low-intensity isotonic exercise. Isometric exercise, by increasing aortic root systolic pressure, reduces the gradient, but increases an already elevated left ventricular afterload. Peak systolic gradients in excess of 50 mm Hg warn against high-intensity isotonic or isometric exercise or competitive sports.

The potential risk of sudden death is a legitimate concern when advising exercise limitations in patients with aortic stenosis. Syncope that precedes sudden death is believed to be initiated by left ventricular baroreceptors activated by an exercise-induced increase in left ventricular pressure or stretch, which causes vasodilatation in skeletal muscle followed by systemic hypotension.[182] Malignant ventricular arrhythmias seldom *initiate* syncope but are thought to be the chief cause of death *after* a faint. Syncope-induced hypotension is more likely to provoke disturbances in ventricular rhythm in adults with coexisting coronary artery disease than in younger patients with normal coronary arteries and no myocardial ischemia.

After valvotomy or valvuloplasty for congenital aortic stenosis, recommendations based on the above criteria do not necessarily apply, because risk is not determined by the gradient, even when it is relatively small. Athletic activity should be limited to low or moderate intensity when left ventricular internal dimensions at end diastole are increased, when aortic regurgitation is more than mild, when the scalar ECG shows residual abnormalities of repolarization at rest or with exercise, or when important disturbances in ventricular rhythm are present at rest, with exercise, or on 24-hour ambulatory ECG. These recommendations are appropriate even if left ventricular systolic function is within normal range.

PULMONARY STENOSIS. Patients with mild pulmonary valve stenosis (peak systolic gradient < 25 mm Hg) are allowed unrestricted athletic activity. When obstruction is moderate (gradient between 25 and 50 mm Hg), high-intensity competitive sports are unwise even if tolerated, because right ventricular systolic pressure can rise appreciably. When the resting peak systolic gradient exceeds 50 mm Hg—especially if there is impaired right ventricular function—isotonic exercise should be limited to mild intensity and short duration. After successful balloon dilatation or valvotomy, patients generally need few restrictions, and, as a rule, may safely participate in high-intensity competitive athletics, provided that right ventricular size, wall thickness, and function are normal. If postinterventional obstruction to right ventricular outflow is moderate or greater, athletic activity should be limited to noncompetitive low-to-moderate—intensity exercise, especially if right ventricular internal dimensions are increased and systolic function is less than normal.

ATRIAL SEPTAL DEFECT. The majority of young adults with uncomplicated ostium secundum atrial septal defect are asymptomatic and often have relatively normal tolerance to exercise. High-intensity competitive sports may be tolerated but are probably unwise. When surgery abolishes the shunt in childhood or young adulthood, long-term outlook is excellent, and athletic activity is unrestricted, provided that pulmonary vascular resistance is normal, sinus node function and atrioventricular conduction are normal, and the right atrial and right ventricular volumes are normal or nearly so.

VENTRICULAR SEPTAL DEFECT. A restrictive ventricular septal defect with a functionally normal heart imposes no exercise limitations. Although patients can safely participate in competitive sports without restriction, adults in this category are uncommon. An important variation on the theme is the adult who had a moderately restrictive perimembranous ventricular septal defect that decreased in size or closed spontaneously in infancy. There is consensus that such patients are physiologically normal and should be permitted unrestricted physical activity. However, two-dimensional echocardiography with Doppler interrogation and color flow imaging should be performed to determine whether the defect closed by formation of a "septal aneurysm."[5] Although there is no evidence that strenuous athletic exercise, especially isotonic, risks rupturing a septal aneurysm, it is prudent to be aware of the morphological substrate.

After surgical closure of a moderate-to-large ventricular septal defect, recommendations regarding physical activity and competitive sports depend on the postoperative pulmonary arterial pressure; the absence of significant disturbances in ventricular rhythm during maximal exercise stress testing and during 24-hour ambulatory electrocardiography; and two-dimensional echocardiographic evidence of an intact ventricular septum together with normalization of left ventricular and left atrial size and left ventricular function. It is also desirable that the 12-lead scalar ECG exhibit little or no evidence of left ventricular volume overload or right ventricular pressure overload. If these criteria are met, patients are permitted unrestricted exercise. Persistent postoperative elevation of pulmonary arterial pressure, especially if accompanied by exercise-induced right ventricular ectopic rhythms, requires limitation to isotonic physical activity of low intensity and short duration.

PATENT DUCTUS ARTERIOSUS. A small patent ductus arteriosus is of little or no physiological significance, and there are no postoperative limitations after division of an isolated restrictive patent ductus. Recommendations after division of a moderately restrictive or nonrestrictive patent ductus with large left-to-right shunt and variable elevations of pulmonary arterial pressure depend upon the guidelines just set forth for postoperative moderately restrictive to nonrestrictive ventricular septal defect.

Pulmonary vascular disease in these cyanotic patients is a contraindication to strenuous exercise. In patients with suprasystemic pulmonary vascular resistance and right-to-left shunts, even low levels of isotonic exercise tend to be accompanied by decrements in systemic arterial oxygen content and the development of tissue lactic acidosis. The exercise-induced increase in right-to-left shunt poses a special problem regarding the elimination of metabolically produced carbon dioxide, resulting in high ventilatory requirements, subjective dyspnea (Fig. 30–13), and occasionally, respiratory acidosis.[150,151] In nonrestrictive patent ductus arteriosus with suprasystemic pulmonary vascular resistance and reversed shunt, exercise may cause leg fatigue but comparatively little dyspnea, because the ventilatory stimuli of hypoxemia, hypercapnia, and acidemia circumvent the respiratory center. (Venous blood is delivered to the lower body but not to the vital centers of the head and neck.[5])

FALLOT'S TETRALOGY. In patients with this anomaly isotonic exercise provokes a fall in systemic vascular resistance and an augmentation of venous return to a right ventricle with fixed obstruction to outflow, so the right-to-left shunt increases. The subjective sensation of breathlessness is caused chiefly by the response of the respiratory center to the sudden change and blood gas composition and pH as just described. The relief of effort-induced dyspnea by squatting (see p. 885), a time-honored hallmark of Fallot's tetralogy in children, is seldom seen in adults.[5] Squatting exerts its salutary effect by countering the exercise-induced fall in systemic vascular resistance and by decreasing the amount of low oxygen content inferior vena caval blood that is received by the right ventricle and shunted into the aorta during exercise. High-intensity *isometric* exercise in Fallot's tetralogy abruptly reduces flow from the right ventricle into the aorta in the face of fixed obstruction to right ventricular outflow, so systemic flow suddenly falls, risking syncope and occasionally sudden death. All but low-intensity isometric exercise is proscribed.

After repair of Fallot's tetralogy, recommendations regarding physical activity and participation in athletics depend upon patient age at operation and the presence and degree of postoperative residua and sequelae.[183] After repair of Fallot's tetralogy, patients should undergo two-dimensional echocardiography with Doppler interrogation and color flow imaging, exercise stress testing, and 24-hour ambulatory electrocardiography. If obstruction to right ventricular outflow is mild or absent, if the shunt is absent or trivial, if low-pressure pulmonary regurgitation is no more than mild to moderate, if there are no significant disturbances in ventricular rhythm, and if right ventricular size and function are normal or nearly so, limitations are not imposed upon athletic activity, either isotonic or isometric.[183] Of particular concern are residual right ventricular outflow gradients that increase significantly during exercise and are accompanied by right ventricular ectopic rhythms believed to originate at the site of the ventriculotomy scar. Postoperative bifascicular block (Fig. 30–17) is uncommon with current surgical techniques. Bifascicular block without the aforementioned residua or sequelae does not in itself preclude unrestricted physical activity, provided that the 24-hour ambulatory ECG records no additional evidence of impaired atrioventricular conduction.

COMPLETE TRANSPOSITION OF THE GREAT ARTERIES. Data regarding this anomaly are derived chiefly from patients who have undergone atrial switch operations in early life. With few exceptions, important postoperative residua and sequelae require that isotonic physical activity be restricted to mild or moderate intensity and limited duration. Recommendations regarding athletic activity after the *arterial* switch operation cannot currently be made. However, there is an air of cautious optimism that uncomplicated arterial switch repairs may circumvent the electrophysiological sequelae so common after atrial switch operations (Fig. 30–11), while allowing the morphological left ventricle to serve as the systemic pump.

The *Fontan operation* permits study of the human circulation in which total right atrial or total caval flow is channeled directly into the pulmonary artery or into a small right ventricle that serves only as a conduit. Exercise per-

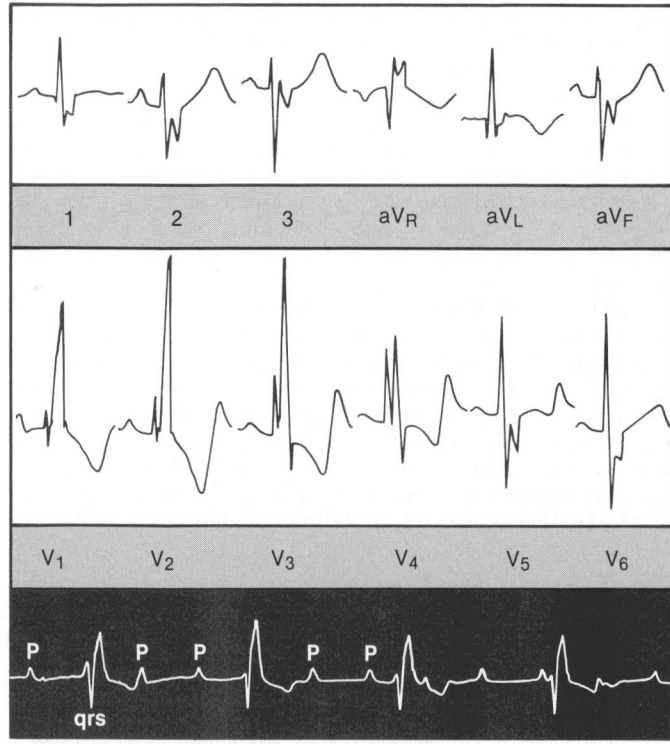

FIGURE 30–17. Twelve-lead electrocardiogram *(top and center panels)* and single-channel electrocardiogram from a patient with Fallot's tetralogy after intracardiac repair. Bifascicular block (right bundle branch block with left anterior fascicular block) *(top)* progressed to complete atrioventricular block *(bottom)*.

formance improves but remains subnormal and the cardiac index increases, but seldom more than twofold.[132a,168,184] Patients with optimal repairs are permitted moderate-intensity isotonic exercise if the following criteria are met: (1) a satisfactory working capacity as judged by exercise stress testing, (2) stable sinus rhythm with no significant disturbances in atrial or ventricular rhythm in response to exercise or on 24-hour ambulatory electrocardiography, (3) normal ventricular function as determined by two-dimensional echocardiography or radionuclide imaging, and (4) normal systemic arterial oxygen saturation.

Employability and Psychosocial Considerations

EMPLOYABILITY. Opportunities for employment of adults with congenital heart defects are influenced by the type of cardiac lesion, cardiac surgery, job discrimination, and educational level.[185] Legislation has been enacted to protect the rights of patients and to provide assistance in seeking employment. Overprotective attitudes of parents and teachers combined with absence of self-discipline may seriously reduce competitive spirit and curtail educational achievement. Job discrimination is one of the most important factors affecting employment opportunities for patients with congenital heart disease. The smaller the company, the greater the reluctance to hire an employee with a thoracotomy scar or with preexisting cardiac disease.

In selected occupations (bus drivers and airline pilots, for example), the safety of others is in the hands of a single individual. To make sensible recommendations regarding fitness for these occupations, the patient's risk of incapacity or sudden death must be defined. The National Rehabilitation Act of 1973 and the Vocational Rehabilitation Act of 1920 offer a wide range of services that are significantly underutilized, especially by cardiac patients.

PSYCHOSOCIAL CONSIDERATIONS. Special if not unique psychological problems confront patients who have experienced dramatic and sometimes traumatic diagnostic and therapeutic interventions during key developmental phases of their lives.[186] The trend toward early diagnosis and reparative surgery in congenital heart disease has made it difficult to generalize from results of studies done 10 to 20 years ago. Despite methodological difficulties and a number of constraints, a reasonable understanding has been achieved by critical assessment of available data combined with clinical experience.

Most patients with congenital heart disease function within normal psychological range, although low self-esteem, insecurity, and feeling of vulnerability are matters of concern.[186] Parental knowledge, understanding, and attitude significantly affect psychosocial adjustments. Difficulty in accepting illness may be manifested by denial and by potentially self-destructive behavior, especially in adolescents. Adults with congenital heart disease face problems in the workplace, in dating, in marriage, and in parenthood. Cyanosis impairs intellectual function, although the degree of impairment is generally mild and often overestimated by IQ tests that depend upon gross motor function at a young age. Early surgery in cyanotic patients appears to improve intellectual and psychological development.[187] Circulatory arrest with deep hypothermia may have subtle adverse effects upon intellectual function, especially if the circulatory arrest and hypothermia are prolonged.[188]

Surgical Considerations

Operation or reoperation for adults with congenital heart disease involves special surgical considerations peculiar to an older patient population.[2] When preoperative phlebotomy is required to improve hemostasis in cyanotic patients, the blood should be stored for potential autologous transfusion. Reoperation after palliative procedures involves revision of Blalock-Taussig shunts, Glenn shunts, Potts or Waterston shunts, and pulmonary arterial bands. Important considerations at reoperation after reparative surgery are reconstruction of cardiac valves and replacement of conduits or prosthetic valves. Operative planning requires knowledge of the basic congenital malformation, of the initial surgical procedure, and of postoperative residua, sequelae, and complications. Perhaps the most important variable that precludes reparative or palliative surgery or reoperation is pulmonary vascular disease. Depressed ventricular function, which is the second major impediment to operability or reoperability, is a consequence of volume or pressure overload, myocardial ischemia, and inherent ventricular morphology.

Certain important principles apply intraoperatively, including myocardial protection, cardioplegia, and hypothermia. Intraoperative salvage of red blood cells and platelet-rich plasma before cardiopulmonary bypass has diminished the need for nonautologous blood and blood products. Minimizing the need for donor blood and blood products is more important at reoperation because of the greater risk of bleeding. The sternotomy incision at reoperation is a technical problem, posing a significant risk when an enlarged right ventricle is apposed to the sternum and when right ventricular outflow conduits adhere. The risk can be reduced materially if reoperation is anticipated at the time of initial repair with placement of an anterior patch of synthetic pericardium.

There are three categories of prostheses: patches, valves, and conduits. The devices and materials selected must achieve an immediately successful technical result, while taking into account the long-term postoperative effects on morbidity and mortality. The choice of materials is based on the patient's age and size, the nature of the congenital malformation, the type of repair, whether or not subsequent repairs are anticipated, the availability of various synthetic and biological materials and devices, complications of long-term anticoagulation, and the risk of infection.

Cardiac Catheterization as a Therapeutic Intervention
(See also Chap. 39)

Therapeutic cardiac catheterization, like cardiac surgery, has three principal objectives: (1) preservation or improvement of cardiac function, (2) an increase in longevity, and (3) maintenance or improvement of the quality of life. When the catheterization technique achieves these ends, surgical morbidity and mortality are circumvented. *Corrective* or *reparative* interventional catheterization procedures currently apply to pulmonary valve stenosis (Fig. 30–9), recoarctation of the aorta, patent ductus arteriosus, and selected patients with atrial septal defect. *Palliative* interventions can be either in lieu of surgery or as adjuncts to surgery. Procedures performed in lieu of surgery apply to lesions such as aortic valve stenosis (Fig. 30–10), postoperative systemic or pulmonary venous obstruction, native coarctation of the aorta, obstructed bioprosthetic valves, and pulmonary arteriovenous fistulas (Fig. 30–8). Palliative procedures that are adjuncts to surgery deal with systemic-to-pulmonary arterial collaterals, systemic-to-pulmonary arterial surgical shunts, pulmonary or systemic venous obstruction, certain intraatrial communications, and selected patients with pulmonary artery stenosis.

Noncardiac Surgery in Adults with Congenital Heart Disease

(See also Chap. 54)

When adults with congenital heart disease require noncardiac surgery, perioperative risks can be reduced, often appreciably, if problems inherent in that patient population are anticipated.[2,155] The following discussion includes patients with cyanotic or acyanotic congenital heart disease who have *not* undergone cardiac surgery, and patients who have undergone reparative cardiac surgery.

SITUS INVERSUS WITH DEXTROCARDIA (see p. 946). This cardiac malposition may go unrecognized until an illness that requires noncardiac surgery brings the adult to medical attention.[5] Accompanying symptoms are likely to be misconstrued and diagnostic conclusions incorrect unless the mirror-image visceral positions are known. In acute appendicitis, the abdominal pain is in the *left* lower quadrant, whereas biliary colic is in the *left* upper quadrant. The risk of noncardiac surgery is the same in the presence of situs inversus as in patients with normal situs, provided no congenital malformations coexist in the mirror-image heart.

CONGENITAL COMPLETE HEART BLOCK (see p. 949). This conduction defect requires electrocardiographic monitoring during and immediately after noncardiac surgery. Intraoperative vagotonic stimuli during ophthalmic or gastrointestinal surgery should be minimized and treated with intravenous atropine expectantly or if there is a sudden decrease in heart rate.[155] If the preoperative scalar ECG shows wide QRS complexes and a relatively slow ventricular rate, especially if there is a history of syncope or near syncope, a temporary right ventricular pacemaker should be inserted.

BICUSPID AORTIC VALVE (see p. 914). If the valve is functionally normal, or nearly normal, noncardiac surgery incurs nothing more than the risk of infective endocarditis. When emergency noncardiac surgery is required in an adult with severe calcific bicuspid aortic stenosis and marginal left ventricular function, hemodynamic monitoring with a flotation catheter should be used. If surgery is elective, consideration should be given to preemptive aortic valve replacement. Balloon valvuloplasty is problematic, even more so if stenosis is due to calcification of a congenitally *bicuspid* aortic valve rather than to calcification of a *trileaflet* aortic valve. Coronary angiography may shed light on whether or not angina pectoris is caused by coexisting coronary artery disease or by augmented oxygen demands of the afterloaded left ventricle. The margin of safety during noncardiac surgery is sometimes improved by preoperative coronary angioplasty. Intraoperative monitoring of systemic blood pressure is important because a sudden fall in systemic vascular resistance may not be associated with an adequate increase in stroke volume, owing to fixed obstruction to left ventricular outflow. An attempt to correct hypotension with rapid infusion of intravenous fluids may cause pulmonary edema.[155] Pharmacological support of systemic resistance is safer than an intravenous infusion and just as efficacious.

Patients with hemodynamically significant *bicuspid aortic regurgitation* confront noncardiac surgery with risks determined by left ventricular function and susceptibility to infective endocarditis. If ventricular function is normal, the risk of noncardiac surgery is small. Moderate intraoperative anesthetic hypotension is not a hazard, serving instead to decrease regurgitant flow and reduce the volume overload of the left ventricle. If left ventricular function is depressed, elective noncardiac surgery raises the question of preemptive replacement of the aortic valve. A tissue valve is preferred to avoid anticoagulants if subsequent noncardiac surgery is anticipated. Emergency noncardiac operation in the presence of depressed left ventricular function calls for hemodynamic monitoring and reduction of postoperative pharmacological afterload.

EBSTEIN'S ANOMALY OF THE TRICUSPID VALVE (see p. 934). Patients with the acyanotic form of the anomaly confront noncardiac surgery with four risks: (1) the functionally inadequate right ventricle, (2) atrial tachyarrhythmias with or without accessory pathways, (3) paradoxical embolism through an intraatrial communication, and (4) infective endocarditis on the malformed tricuspid valve. Right ventricular failure is less a perioperative risk than sudden atrial flutter or fibrillation, especially with rapid antegrade conduction through bypass tracts. Patients with histories of rapid heart action or fusion beats (type B Wolff-Parkinson-White) on scalar ECG require electrocardiographic monitoring. Postoperative thrombophlebitis and the attendant risk of paradoxical embolization are reduced by the use of support hose and early ambulation.

OSTIUM SECUNDUM ATRIAL SEPTAL DEFECT (see p. 896). Young adults with uncomplicated defects experience comparatively little risk during noncardiac surgery, with two exceptions. In response to hemorrhage, systemic resistance rises and venous return diminishes, a combination that augments the left-to-right interatrial shunt, sometimes considerably. An additional concern is the risk of paradoxical emboli from leg veins because thrombi carried by the inferior vena cava tend to stream across the atrial septal defect into the systemic circulation. Meticulous leg care and early ambulation minimize venous stasis.

CYANOTIC CONGENITAL HEART DISEASE. Cyanotic adults have an increased incidence of acute cholecystitis caused by *calcium bilirubinate gallstones* (Fig. 30–12). Perioperative improvement in *hemostasis* in cyanotic patients can be addressed if surgery is elective, with guidelines set forth earlier. Inhalation of oxygen may raise arterial oxygen saturation even in the presence of a right-to-left shunt, but there is little evidence that its routine perioperative use is beneficial. *Intravenous lines, infusions,* and *drugs* must be managed with special care in cyanotic patients. Introduction of air or particles into peripheral veins risks delivery into the systemic circulation because of the right-to-left shunt. Use of an air/particle filter obviates the risk.

Older patients with *Fallot's tetralogy* may come to noncardiac surgery without intracardiac repair or with only a shunt inserted in infancy or childhood. Meticulous perioperative monitoring of oxygen saturation (pulse oximeter) and blood pressure is important, because a sudden fall in systemic resistance may precipitate intense cyanosis and occasionally death, or a sudden rise in systemic resistance may abruptly and dangerously depress systemic blood flow.[155] The risk of postoperative postural hypotension is mentioned below. Susceptibility to infective endocarditis requires prophylaxis.

Cyanotic patients with *elevated pulmonary vascular resistance* face noncardiac surgery with risks inherent in the cyanosis itself in addition to the formidable risks of pulmonary vascular disease. Fixed pulmonary resistance precludes rapid adaptive responses to labile intraoperative or postoperative hemodynamic changes. In Eisenmenger's complex or physiologically analogous lesions, a sudden fall or a sudden rise in systemic vascular resistance precipitates responses similar to those already described in Fallot's tetralogy. Every effort should be made to minimize the postural hypotension that tends to occur during early conva-lescence in patients having general anesthesia.[155] Because the attendant drop in systemic vascular resistance suddenly augments the right-to-left shunt, convalescent cyanotic patients with pulmonary vascular disease should change positions slowly until the risk of postoperative postural hypotension has abated.

Noncardiac Surgery in Adults with Repaired Congenital Heart Disease

Adults who have undergone reparative surgery for congenital heart disease comprise an increasing percentage of patients who require subsequent noncardiac operations. If cardiac surgery is curative (division of a small patent ductus arteriosus), there is no added risk of a noncardiac surgical procedure. Early correction of simple pulmonary valve stenosis is also close to a cure. Subsequent noncardiac surgery imposes little or no risk, including, in all probability, susceptibility to infective endocarditis. Closure of an ostium secundum atrial septal defect in childhood is close to a cure.

Valvular residua and *sequelae* after cardiac surgery or therapeutic catheterization are relevant in the medical management of patients who undergo noncardiac surgery in adulthood.[189] Successful repair of coarctation of the aorta may leave behind a functionally normal bicuspid aortic valve that is susceptible to infective endocarditis. After complete relief of congenital pulmonary valve stenosis by direct repair or balloon dilatation, the risk of infective endocarditis is low if not absent, but the functional adequacy of the right ventricle is an important perioperative variable. In Fallot's tetralogy, reconstruction of the right ventricular outflow tract may largely or entirely abolish the gradient. If the function of the right ventricle is satisfactory, and if postoperative pulmonary regurgitation is no more than moderate, the risk of noncardiac surgery is small. Infective endocarditis prophylaxis is advisable even though susceptibility is relatively low.

After surgical repair of *Ebstein's anomaly of the tricuspid valve* (tricuspid reconstruction and division of bypass tracts), atrial arrhythmias remain a concern during noncardiac surgery, but without fear of accelerated conduction (Fig. 30–7). Closure of the intraatrial communication eliminates cyanosis, so the hematological derangements are no longer issues, and the potential for paradoxical embolization is eliminated. The postoperative right ventricle is not functionally normal, but the hemodynamic risk during subsequent noncardiac surgery is small. If residual tricuspid regurgitation is more than mild, prophylaxis for infective endocarditis is advisable.

PROSTHETIC MECHANICAL VALVES. These devices (see p. 1066) complicate the management of noncardiac surgery. The immediate issue is anticoagulation in addition to and apart from the risk of infective endocarditis. If noncardiac surgery is elective, and if the prosthesis carries a high thromboembolic risk (mitral location with atrial fibrillation), warfarin should be replaced with an in-hospital continuous infusion of heparin that is discontinued 4 to 6 hours before the elective surgery, restarted within 48 hours after surgery, and then replaced by warfarin. For a lower-risk prosthetic valve in the aortic location, it is relatively safe to discontinue warfarin 2 to 3 days before noncardiac surgery and resume the drug 2 to 3 days after surgery.

Emergency noncardiac surgery in an anticoagulated patient with a mechanical prosthesis is managed differently. Prompt restitution of hemostasis requires infusion of fresh frozen plasma. Cessation of warfarin and administration of vitamin K do not achieve immediate reversal of the anticoagulant effects, which persist for 24 hours or more. If vitamin K is used, the preoperative response to readministration of warfarin is blunted.

ELECTROPHYSIOLOGICAL SEQUELAE. Electrophysiological sequelae after reparative surgery are important concerns during management of subsequent noncardiac surgery. The most diverse and complex sequelae are incurred by intraatrial repairs (Mustard or Senning operations) for complete transposition of the great arteries, and require monitoring during noncardiac surgery. Intraventricular surgery may result in electrophysiological sequelae that are potentially important. Awareness of the presence or potential presence of these sequelae decreases perioperative risk.

After repair of coarctation of the aorta, *systemic hypertension* may persist or recur even if the obstruction has been completely relieved, but the incidence is declining owing to the success of early operation. Nevertheless, pharmacological control of perioperative hypertension is sometimes necessary during noncardiac surgery. The greater the duration of systemic hypertension before repair, the greater the likelihood of premature coronary artery disease—a point to be considered in subsequent perioperative management.

VENTRICULAR FUNCTION. The adequacy of ventricular function (left, right, or single ventricle) is a major determinant of risk during noncardiac surgery in adults. Excessive intravenous fluids should be avoided, and hemodynamic monitoring used when the morphological substrate permits insertion of a flotation catheter.[155]

Medical management during noncardiac surgery must also take into account acquired diseases of the heart and circulation, especially coronary artery disease and systemic hypertension, as well as noncardiac acquired medical disorders such as renal, respiratory, gastrointestinal, or endocrinological.

Postoperative Residua and Sequelae

Residua are defined as cardiac, vascular, or noncardiovascular disorders that are unavoidably left behind at the time of reparative heart surgery[189] (Table 30-3). With few exceptions, residua do not result from surgery having fallen short of its goal, at least in a technical sense.[190] By contrast, *sequelae* are defined as alterations or disorders that are intentionally incurred—occasionally or invariably—at the time of reparative surgery and are looked upon as necessary and acceptable consequences of surgery[189] (Table 30–4). *Complications* are unintentional aftermaths of reparative surgery that range in degree from inconsequential to fatal. Complications and sequelae imperceptibly merge. Surgery is *curative* if there are no cardiac or vascular residua, sequelae, or complications after surgery. "Curative" means that normal cardiovascular structure and function are achieved and maintained, life expectancy is normal, and further medical or surgical treatment for the congenital heart disease is unnecessary. This ideal seldom is realized, and even curative cardiac surgery does not preclude noncardiac residua.[189]

Residua

ELECTROPHYSIOLOGICAL RESIDUA. With some exceptions, these residua are inherent components of certain congenital cardiac malformations.[189] The abnormalities are often evident in standard preoperative 12-lead ECG's, and persist—sometimes harmlessly, sometimes not so harmlessly—after reparative surgery. Electrophysiological residua include (1) axis deviation, especially left; (2) conduction defects, especially atrioventricular; (3) disorders of impulse formation, especially of the sinus node; and (4) arrhythmias, especially atrial.

RESIDUAL ABNORMALITIES OF CARDIAC VALVES. These residua fall into three general categories: (1) congenitally malformed cardiac valves that are functionally normal and

---

TABLE 30–3   RESIDUA AFTER REPARATIVE SURGERY FOR CONGENITAL HEART DISEASE

1. Electrophysiological
2. Valvular
3. Ventricular
   a. Chamber morphology
   b. Chamber mass
   c. Chamber function
   d. Myocardial connective tissue
4. Vascular
   a. Anatomical (morphological) vascular anomalies or defects
   b. Elevated resistance and/or pressure: systemic, pulmonary
5. Noncardiovascular
   a. Developmental abnormalities
   b. Somatic defects
   c. Medical disorders

TABLE 30–4 SEQUELAE OF REPARATIVE SURGERY FOR CONGENITAL HEART DISEASE

A. **Electrophysiological**
   1. **Atriotomy**
      a. Intraatrial repair
      b. Intraventricular repair
   2. **Ventriculotomy**
      a. Incision site
      b. Intracardiac repair
B. **Native valves**
   1. Left ventricular or right ventricular *outflow* repair
   2. Left ventricular or right ventricular *inflow* repair
C. **Prosthetic materials**
   1. Patches
   2. Valves
   3. Conduits
D. **Myocardial and endocardial sequelae**

do not require attention during reparative surgery; (2) intrinsically normal cardiac valves that are rendered incompetent because of the physiological stress imposed by the congenital malformation that prompted surgical repair; and (3) residually incompetent or stenotic congenitally malformed cardiac valves that do not lend themselves to complete repair. Aortic valve abnormalities that represent unimportant residua include functionally normal bicuspid aortic valve with coarctation of the aorta and mild aortic regurgitation that may accompany Fallot's tetralogy. Residual congenital mitral valve abnormalities that are functionally unimportant include the "cleft" but competent anterior mitral leaflet of an atrioventricular septal defect and the reduction in interpapillary muscle distance associated with coarctation of the aorta. Postoperative residual incompetence of an intrinsically normal pulmonary or tricuspid valve is usually the result of pulmonary hypertension or obstruction to right ventricular outflow.

RESIDUAL VENTRICULAR ABNORMALITIES. Certain ventricular abnormalities are obligatory and permanent after reparative surgery, such as the morphology of a chamber, or may change with the passage of time, such as alterations in chamber mass and function. In patients undergoing either an atrial switch operation for complete transposition of the great arteries, or operation for congenitally corrected transposition of the great arteries, a postoperative residuum of fundamental importance is the presence of a morphological right ventricle in the systemic location. A pivotal question is whether that right ventricle, perfused by a right coronary artery, can, in the long term, perform as a systemic chamber as well as a morphological left ventricle perfused by a left coronary artery.

The development of increased ventricular mass and its regression after reparative surgery are important properties of ventricular myocardium.[190–192] An increase in ventricular mass in excess of the normal process of growth is determined by the nature of the inciting stimulus (hemodynamic or hypoxic), the duration and type of the hemodynamic stimulus (pressure or volume overload), myocardial age (maturity) at the time the stimulus is imposed, and the cell type that is involved.[191–193] The response of a given cell type to a hemodynamic or hypoxic stimulus depends chiefly upon myocyte maturity. If overload or hypoxia is imposed on the immature heart, the cellular response is characterized by replication (hyperplasia) of myocytes and fibroblasts.[194] If the stimulus continues beyond immaturity, myocytes respond by hypertrophy (enlargement) and fibroblasts by hyperplasia (replication).[192] An unresolved concern is the cellular basis for the regression in mass after surgical relief from ventricular overload or hypoxia (Fig. 30–18). The fate of myocytes that replicate in excess of their genetically regulated numbers has not been established.[195] A postoperative reduction in ventricular mass in the setting of hyperplasia implies, at least in part, that the numerically excessive myocytes become smaller in size, but

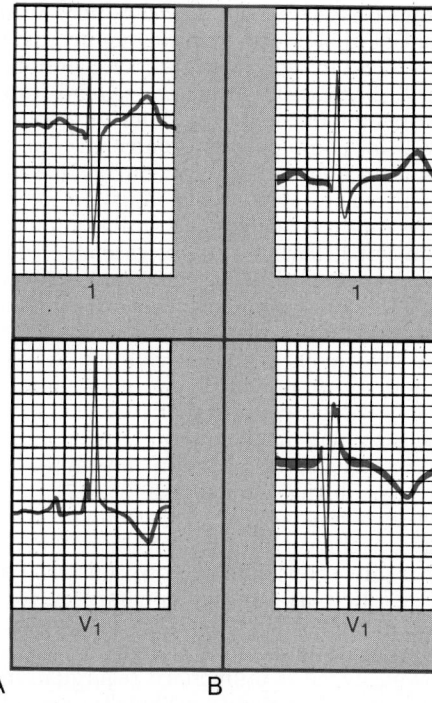

FIGURE 30–18. *A,* Leads 1 and V$_1$ from a 2-year-old boy with severe pulmonary valve stenosis. *B,* Leads 1 and V$_1$, 7 years after surgical pulmonary valvotomy. Right axis deviation has resolved and the rR′ in lead V$_1$ has been replaced with an rSr′. These are electrocardiographic features of regression of right ventricular hypertrophy.

not fewer in number. If this contention is valid, its long-term functional significance is unknown. The response of connective tissue cell hyperplasia to operative removal of the overload or hypoxic stimulus is also unknown, although there is evidence that connective tissue cells do not regress as readily as myocytes.[196]

VASCULAR RESIDUA. Vascular residua consist of anatomical anomalies or defects or elevated resistance and/or pressure in the systemic or pulmonary circulation. Examples include the relationship between aortic root disease and bicuspid aortic valve and rupture of an aneurysm of the circle of Willis associated with coarctation of the aorta.

Congenital anomalies of the coronary arteries coexist with a number of congenital malformations of the heart.[5] Examples include Fallot's tetralogy and the residual coronary artery disease (intimal proliferation, medial thickening, premature atherosclerosis) initiated by the hypertension of coarctation of the aorta. The preoperative status of the pulmonary vascular bed, especially the resistance vessels, is a major determinant of the presence and degree of residual postoperative pulmonary vascular disease. Refinements and improved safety that currently permit surgical repairs within the first 6 to 12 months of life make it likely that postoperative pulmonary vascular disease will become less and less a postoperative residuum.

NONCARDIOVASCULAR RESIDUA. These can be important long-term concerns after reparative surgery.[189] Developmental abnormalities such as the mental retardation of Down syndrome or the physical abnormalities of Turner's or the Ellis-van Creveld syndrome are examples. Residual somatic defects include dysmorphism and limb abnormalities. Psychosocial disorders may exist as important postoperative residua, and a healed brain abscess can serve as a focus of a seizure disorder. Cataracts and deafness persist as residua after division of the patent ductus in children with the rubella syndrome.

Sequelae

Sequelae relate to electrophysiological disturbances, native cardiac valves, prosthetic materials, myocardium, and endocardium (Table 30–4). *Electrophysiological sequelae* after intraatrial repair are represented by disturbances in rhythm and conduction, sinoatrial dysfunction, junctional rhythm, atrial fibrillation, atrial flutter, and impaired atrioventricular conduction varying from prolongation of the P-R interval to complete atrioventricular block. Electrophysiological sequelae after intraventricular repair through a right atrial incision result from injury to internodal pathways and to the proximal right bundle branch alone or in combination with the left anterior fascicle.[197] A right ventriculotomy is responsible for two electrophysiological sequelae: an alteration in the sequence of ventricular activation and electrical instability of the incised right ventricle. The surface ECG is useful in determining the proximal origin of abnormal right ventricular activation when right bundle branch block coexists with left anterior fascicular block.[197] Bifascicular block sets the stage for postoperative complete heart block, which is an uncommon but hazardous electrophysiological sequel (Fig. 30–17).

Sequelae involving native cardiac valves occur after left ventricular or right ventricular *outflow* repairs, or left ventricular or right ventricular *inflow* repairs. Postoperative aortic regurgitation as a sequel of surgery for congenital bicuspid aortic stenosis is an example. Surgical repair or balloon dilatation of congenital pulmonary valve stenosis is often followed by mild pulmonary regurgitation, a physiologically minor and therefore acceptable sequel. Repair of complex obstruction to right ventricular outflow, as in Fallot's tetralogy, usually induces pulmonary regurgitation, the importance of which depends on the degree of regurgitant flow and the functional state of the right ventricle.

Sequelae associated with left ventricular *inflow* repairs accompany operations for congenital mitral regurgitation or congenital obstruction to left ventricular inflow. Assuming complete relief of the mitral regurgitation associated with an atrioventricular septal defect, morphological abnormalities intrinsic to the congenitally malformed valve leave the left ventricular inflow guarded by an abnormal mitral apparatus. Reconstruction of the tricuspid valve in Ebstein's anomaly is somewhat analogous. Repair is necessarily followed by sequelae intrinsic to the basic tricuspid valve malformation, even if competence is established.

PROSTHETIC MATERIALS. Insertion of these materials represents a special category of sequelae after reparative surgery for congenital heart disease. Certain materials are exceptions, such as an endogenous pericardial patch for closure of an ostium secundum atrial septal defect or a synthetic patch that is entirely covered by a neointimal layer. Valve replacement results in sequelae that vary in significance according to the physical and hemodynamic characteristics of the prosthetic device (bioprosthetic or rigid), the site of insertion, and patient age at the time of operation. Reoperation is required when an infant or child outgrows the original valve prosthesis. Bioprosthetic valves degenerate at rates determined chiefly by patient age at the time of insertion, and by the tissue characteristics of the device (endogenous or exogenous materials, homografts or xenografts). Susceptibility to infective endocarditis varies from negligible with aortic homografts to high with mechanical prostheses. The incidence of thromboembolic complications is low with an aortic homograft and high with a rigid mitral prosthesis. Anticoagulants reduce but do not eliminate thromboembolic complications and carry the inherent risk of anticoagulant-induced bleeding and the risk of teratogenicity during pregnancy.

Conduits can be nonvalved (usually synthetic) or valved (bioprosthetic or mechanical) and pose the risks of degeneration, thrombogenicity, anticoagulation, and infective endocarditis. In addition, conduits—especially valved—are subject to pseudointimal proliferation (peel).[2] Conduit obstruction can therefore result from both nongrowth of the device and pseudointimal proliferation.

MYOCARDIAL SEQUELAE. Morphological or mechanical se-

quelae at the site of the ventriculotomy or atriotomy are usually negligible unless there is formation of an aneurysm, which is more properly considered a complication. Electrophysiological sequelae were discussed earlier. Certain *endocardial sequelae* after intraventricular repair have been called "surgical fibroelastosis."[198,199] The cause and functional significance of these endocardial lesions, which are not necessarily confined to the chamber in which the intracardiac repair was done, have not been established.

REFERENCES

1. Perloff, J. K.: Pediatric congenital cardiac becomes a postoperative adult. The changing population of congenital heart disease. Circulation *47*:606, 1973.
2. Perloff, J. K., and Child, J. S.: Congenital Heart Disease in Adults. Philadelphia, W. B. Saunders Company, 1991.
3. Perloff, J. K.: Congenital heart disease in adults: A new cardiovascular subspecialty. Circulation *84*:1881, 1991.
4. Perloff, J. K. (Chairman): 22nd Bethesda Conference: Congenital heart disease after childhood: An expanding patient population. J. Am. Coll. Cardiol. *18*:311, 1991.
5. Perloff, J. K.: The Clinical Recognition of Congenital Heart Disease. 4th ed. Philadelphia, W. B. Saunders Company, 1994.
6. Fallot, A.: Contribution a l'anatomie pathologique de la maladie bleue (cyanose cardiaque). Marseilleméd. *25*:418, 1888.
7. Abbott, M. E.: Atlas of Congenital Heart Disease. New York, The American Heart Association, 1936.
8. Gross, R. E., and Hubbard, J. P.: Surgical ligation of a patent ductus arteriosus: report of first successful case. JAMA *112*:729, 1939.
9. Blalock, A., and Taussig, H. B.: Surgical treatment of malformations of the heart in which there is pulmonary stenosis or pulmonary atresia. JAMA *128*:189, 1945.
10. Crafoord, C., and Nylin, G.: Congenital coarctation of the aorta and its surgical treatment. J. Thorac. Surg. *14*:347, 1945.
11. Kirklin, J. W., DuShane, J. W., Patrick, R. T., et al.: Intracardiac surgery with the aid of a mechanical pump-oxygenator system (Gibbon type): Report of eight cases. Proc. Staff Meet. Mayo Clin. *30*:201, 1955.
12. Ritchie, J. L., Cheitlin, M. D., Hlatky, M. A., et al.: Task Force 5: Profile of the cardiovascular specialist: Trends in needs and supply and implications for the future. J. Am. Coll. Cardiol. *24*:313, 1994.
13. Roberts, W. C.: The congenitally bicuspid aortic valve: a study of 85 autopsy cases. Am. J. Cardiol. *26*:72, 1970.

SURVIVAL PATTERNS

14. Subramanian, R., Olson, L. J., and Edwards, W. D.: Surgical pathology of pure aortic stenosis: A study of 374 cases. Mayo Clin. Proc. *59*:683, 1984.
15. Morganroth, J., Perloff, J. K., Zeldes, S. M., and Dunkman, W. B.: Acute severe aortic regurgitation. Ann. Intern. Med. *87*:223, 1977.
16. Larson, E. W., and Edwards, W. D.: Risk factors for aortic dissection: A necropsy study of 161 cases. Am. J. Cardiol. *53*:849, 1984.
16a. Hahn, R. T., Roman, M. J., Maftader, A. H., and Devereux, R. B.: Association of aortic dilatation with regurgitant, stenotic and functionally normal bicuspid aortic values. J. Am. Coll. Cardiol. *19*:283, 1992.
17. Campbell, M.: Natural history of coarctation of the aorta. Br. Heart J. *32*:633, 1970.
18. Jarcho, S.: Coarctation of the aorta (Reynaud, 1828). Am. J. Cardiol. *9*:591, 1962.
19. Hodes, H. L., Steinfeld, L., and Blumenthal, S.: Congenital cerebral aneurysms and coarctation of the aorta. Arch. Pediatr. *76*:28, 1959.
20. Isner, J. M., Donaldson, R. F., Fulton, D., et al.: Cystic medial necrosis in coarctation of the aorta. Circulation *75*:689, 1987.
21. Vladover, Z., and Neufeld, H. N.: Coronary arteries in coarctation of the aorta. Circulation *37*:449, 1968.
22. Campbell, M.: The natural history of congenital pulmonic stenosis. Br. Heart J. *31*:394, 1969.
23. Nugent, E. W., Freedom, R. M., Nora, J. J., et al.: Clinical course in pulmonary stenosis. Circulation *56*(Suppl. 1):38, 1977.
24. Moller, J. H., and Adams, P. Jr.: Natural history of pulmonary valvular stenosis: Serial cardiac catheterization in 21 children. Am. J. Cardiol. *16*:654, 1965.
25. Campbell, M.: Natural history of atrial septal defect. Br. Heart J. *32*:820, 1970.
26. Craig, R. J., and Selzer, A.: Natural history and prognosis of atrial septal defect. Circulation *37*:805, 1968.
27. Markman, P. G., Horvitt, E. G., and Wade, E. G.: Atrial septal defect in the middle-aged and elderly. Q. J. Med. *34*:409, 1965.
28. Colmers, R. E.: Atrial septal defects in elderly patients: Report of three patients aged 68, 72, and 78. Am. J. Cardiol. *1*:768, 1958.
29. Perloff, J. K.: Ostium secundum atrial septal defect—survival for 87 and 94 years. Am. J. Cardiol. *53*:388, 1984.
30. Nagata, S., Yasuharu, N., Sakakibara, H., et al: Mitral valve lesion associated with secundum atrial septal defect. Br. Heart J. *49*:51, 1983.
31. Boucher, C. A., Liberthson, R. R, and Buckley, M. J.: Secundum atrial

septal defect and significant mitral regurgitation: Incidence, management and morphologic basis. Chest 75:697, 1979.

32. Popio, K. A., Gorlin, R., Teichholz, L., et al.: Abnormalities of left ventricular function and geometry in adults with an atrial septal defect. Am. J. Cardiol. 36:302, 1975.

33. Wanderman, K. L., Ovsyheer, I., and Gueron, M.: Left ventricular performance in patients with atrial septal defect: Evaluation with noninvasive methods. Am. J. Cardiol. 41:487, 1978.

34. Campbell, M.: Natural history of persistent ductus arteriosus. Br. Heart J. 30:4, 1968.

35. Marquis, R. M., Miller, H. C., McCormack, R. J. M., et al: Persistence of ductus arteriosus with left to right shunt in the older patient. Br. Heart J. 48:469, 1982.

36. White, P. D., Maxurkie, S. J., and Boschetti, A. E.: Patency of the ductus arteriosus at 90. N. Engl. J. Med. 280:146, 1969.

37. Wood, P.: The Eisenmenger syndrome or pulmonary hypertension with reversed central shunt. Br. Med. J. 2:701 and 755, 1958.

38. Hynes, K. M., Gau, G. T., Titus, J. L.: Coronary heart disease in situs inversus totalis. Am. J. Cardiol. 31:666, 1973.

39. Afzlius, B. A.: Genetical and ultrastructural aspects of the immobile cilia syndrome. Am. J. Human Genet. 33:852, 1981.

40. Davey, R. D., Nadol, J. B., Holmes, L. B., et al.: Kartagener's syndrome: A blinded, controlled study of cilia ultrastructure. Arch. Otolaryngol. Head Neck Surg. 112:646, 1986.

41. McHenry, M. M.: Factors influencing longevity in adults with congenital complete heart block. Am. J. Cardiol. 29:416, 1972.

42. Reybrouck, T., Vanden Eynde, B. B., Dumoulin, M., and Van der Hauwaert, L. G.: Cardiorespiratory response to exercise in congenital complete atrioventricular block. Am. J. Cardiol. 64:896, 1989.

43. Dewey, R. C., Capeless, M. A., and Levy, A. M.: Use of ambulatory electrocardiographic monitoring to identify high-risk patients with congenital complete heart block. N. Engl. J. Med. 316:835, 1987.

44. Bjarke, B. B., and Kidd, B. S. L.: Congenitally corrected transposition of the great arteries: a clinical study of 101 cases. Acta Paediatr. Scand. 65:153, 1976.

45. Cumming, G. R.: Congenital corrected transposition of the great vessels without associated intracardiac anomalies. Am. J. Cardiol. 10:605, 1962.

46. Nagle, J. P., Cheitlin, M. D., and McCarty, R. J.: Corrected transposition of the great vessels without associated anomalies. Chest 60:363, 1971.

47. Schiebler, G. L., Edwards, J. E., Burchell, H. B., et al.: Congenital corrected transposition of the great vessels. Pediatrics 27:851, 1961.

48. Lieberson, A. D., Schumacker, R., and Childress, D.: Corrected transposition of the great vessels in a 73-year-old man. Circulation 39:96, 1969.

49. Huhta, J. C., Danielson, G. K., Ritter, D. G., and Ilstrup, D. M.: Survival in atrioventricular discordance. Pediatr. Cardiol. 6:57, 1985.

50. Anderson, K. R., Zuberbuhler, J. R., Anderson, R. H., et al.: Morphologic spectrum of Ebstein's anomaly of the heart. Mayo Clin. Proc. 54:174, 1979.

51. Watson, H.: Natural history of Ebstein's anomaly of tricuspid valve in childhood and adolescence: An international cooperative study of 505 cases. Br. Heart J. 36:417, 1974.

52. Radford, D. J., Graff, R. F., and Neilson, G. H.: Diagnosis and natural history of Ebstein's anomaly. Br. Heart J. 54:517, 1985.

53. Giuliani, E. R., Fuster, V., Brandenburg, R. O., and Mair, D. D.: Ebstein's anomaly: the clinical features and natural history of Ebstein's anomaly of the tricuspid valve. Mayo Clin. Proc. 54:163, 1979.

54. Leung, M. P., Baker, E. J., Anderson, R. H., and Zuberbuhler, J. R.: Cineangiographic spectrum of Ebstein's malformations: Its relevance to clinical presentation and outcome. J. Am. Coll. Cardiol. 11:154, 1988.

55. Benson, L. N., Child, J. S., Schwaiger, M., Perloff, J. K., et al.: Left ventricular geometry and function in adults with Ebstein's anomaly of the tricuspid valve. Circulation 75:353, 1987.

56. Saxena, A., Fona, L. V., Tristam, M., et al.: Left ventricular function in patients >20 years of age with Ebstein's anomaly of the tricuspid valve. Am. J. Cardiol. 67:217, 1991.

57. Makous, N., and Vander Veer, J. B.: Ebstein's anomaly and life expectancy: Report of a survival to over seventy-nine. Am. J. Cardiol. 18:100, 1966.

58. Adams, J. C. L., and Hudson, R.: Case of Ebstein's anomaly surviving to age 79. Br. Heart J. 18:129, 1956.

59. Seward, J. B., Tajik, A. J., Feist, D. J., and Smith, H. C.: Ebstein's anomaly in an 85 year old man. Mayo Clin. Proc. 54:193, 1979.

60. Collins, N. P., Braunwald, E., and Morrow, A. G.: Isolated congenital pulmonary valvular regurgitation. Am. J. Med. 28:159, 1960.

61. Cortes, F. M., and Jacoby, W. J.: Isolated congenital pulmonary valvular insufficiency. Am. J. Cardiol. 10:287, 1962.

62. Pouget, J. M., Kelly, C. E., and Pilz, C. G.: Congenital absence of the pulmonic valve: Report of a case in a 73 year old man. Am. J. Cardiol. 19:732, 1967.

63. Lutembacher, R.: De la stenose mitrale avec communication interauriculaire. Arch. Mal. Coeur 9:237, 1916.

64. Firkett, C. H.: Examen anatomique d'un cas de pesistence du trou ovale de botal, avec lesions valvulaires considerables du coueur gauche, chez une femme de 74 ans. Ann. Soc. Med. Chir. Liege 19:188, 1880.

65. Rosenthal, L.: Atrial septal defect with mitral stenosis (Lutembacher's syndrome) in a woman of 81. Br. Med. J. 2:1351, 1956.

66. Botefeu, J. M., Moret, P. R., Hahn, C., and Hauf, E.: Aneurysms of the sinus of Valsalva: Report of seven cases and review of the literature. Am. J. Med. 65:18, 1983.

67. Mayer, E. D., Ruffman, K., Saggau, W., et al.: Ruptured aneurysms of the sinus of Valsalva. Ann. Thorac. Surg. 42:81, 1986.

68. Sakakibara, S., and Konno, S.: Congenital aneurysm of the sinus of Valsalva: A clinical study. Am. Heart J. 63:708, 1962.

69. Onat, A., Ersanli, O., Kanuni, A., and Aykan, T. B.: Congenital aortic sinus aneurysms with particular reference to dissection of the interventricular septum. Am. Heart J. 72:158, 1966.

70. Liberthson, R. R., Sagar, K., Berkoben, J. P., et al.: Congenital coronary arteriovenous fistula: Report of 13 patients, review of the literature and delineation of management. Circulation 59:849, 1979.

71. Gillebert, C., Van Hoof, R., Van de Werf, F, et al.: Coronary artery fistulas in an adult population. Eur. Heart J. 7:437, 1986.

72. Cheng, T. O.: Left coronary artery-to-left ventricular fistula: Demonstration of coronary steal phenomenon. Am. Heart J. 104:870, 1982.

73. Paul, O., Sweet, R. H., and White, P. D.: Coronary arteriovenous fistula case report. Am. Heart J. 37:441, 1949.

74. Dines, D. E., Seward, J. B., and Bernatz, P. E.: Pulmonary arteriovenous fistula. Mayo Clin. Proc. 58:176, 1983.

75. Wong, L. B., and Perloff, J. K.: Familial occurrence of congenital pulmonary arteriovenous fistulae in octogenarian siblings. Am. J. Cardiol. 62:1149, 1988.

76. Corone, P., Doyon, F., Gaudeau, S., et al.: Natural history of ventricular septal defect: A study involving 790 cases. Circulation 55:908, 1977.

77. Campbell, M.: Natural history of ventricular septal defect. Br. Heart J. 33:246, 1971.

78. Weidman, W. H., DuShane, J. W., and Ellison, R. C.: Clinical course in adults with ventricular septal defect. Circulation 56(Suppl. I):78, 1977.

79. Ellis, J. H. IV, Moodie, D. S., Sterba, R., and Gill, C. C.: Ventricular septal defect in the adult: Natural and unnatural history. Am. Heart J. 114:115, 1987.

80. Otterstad, J. E., Nitter-Hauge, S., and Myhre, E.: Isolated ventricular septal defect in adults: Clinical and haemodynamic findings. Br. Heart J. 50:343, 1983.

81. Moe, D. G., and Guntheroth, W. G.: Spontaneous closure of uncomplicated ventricular septal defect. Am. J. Cardiol. 60:674, 1987.

82. Wood, P.: Foreword. Bedford, E. D., and Caird, F. L.: Valvular Diseases of the Heart in Old Age. Boston, Little, Brown, and Co., 1960.

83. Ramaciotti, C., Keren, A., and Silverman, N. H.: Importance of (perimembranous) ventricular septal aneurysm in the natural history of isolated perimembranous ventricular septal defect. Am. J. Cardiol. 57:268, 1986.

84. Shah, P., Singh, W. S. A., Rose, V., and Keith, J. D.: Incidence of bacterial endocarditis in ventricular septal defects. Circulation 34:127, 1966.

85. Abraham, K. A., Cherian, G., Rao, V. D., et al.: Tetralogy of Fallot in adults: A report on 147 patients. Am. J. Med. 66:811, 1979.

86. Bertranou, E. G., Blackstone, E. H., Hazelrig, J. B., et al.: Life expectancy without surgery in tetralogy of Fallot. Am. J. Cardiol. 42:458, 1978.

87. Marelli, A. J., Perloff, J. K., Child, J. S., and Laks, H.: Pulmonary atresia with ventricular septal defect in adults. Circulation 89:243, 1994.

88. Stanger, P., Cassidy, S. C., Girod, D. A., et al.: Balloon pulmonary angioplasty: Results of the Valvuloplasty and Angioplasty of Congenital Anomalies Registry. Am. J. Cardiol. 65:775, 1990.

89. Nishimura, R. A., Holmes, D. R., and Reeder, G. S.: Percutaneous balloon valvuloplasty. Mayo Clin. Proc. 65:198, 1990.

90. Sandor, G. G. S., Olley, P. M., Trusler, G. A., et al.: Long-term follow-up of patients after valvotomy for congenital valvular aortic stenosis in children. J. Thorac. Cardiovasc. Surg. 80:171, 1980.

91. Hsieh, K., Keane, J. F., Nadas, A. S., et al.: Long-term follow-up of valvulotomy before 1968 for congenital aortic stenosis. Am. J. Cardiol. 58:338, 1986.

92. Donner, R. M., Carabello, B. A., Black, I., and Spann, J. F.: Left ventricular wall stress in compensated aortic stenosis in children. Am. J. Cardiol. 51:946, 1983.

93. Assey, M. E., Wisenbaugh, T., Spann, J. F., et al.: Unexpected persistence into adulthood of low wall stress in patients with congenital aortic stenosis: Is there a fundamental difference in the hypertrophic response to a pressure overload present from birth? Circulation 75:973, 1987.

94. Danielson, G. K., and Fuster, V.: Surgical repair of Ebstein's anomaly. Ann. Surg. 196:499, 1982.

95. Shah, D., Azhar, M., Oakley, C. M., et al.: Natural history of secundum atrial septal defect in adults after medical or surgical treatment: A historical prospective study. Br. Heart J. 71:224, 1994.

96. Steele, P. M., Fuster, V., Cohen, M., et al.: Isolated atrial septal defect with pulmonary vascular obstructive disease: Long-term follow-up and prediction of outcome after surgical correction. Circulation 76:1037, 1987.

97. Murphy, J. G., Gersh, B. J., McGoon, D. C., et al.: Long-term outcome after surgical repair of isolated atrial septal defect. N. Engl. J. Med 323:1645, 1990.

98. Ward, C.: Secundum atrial septal defect: Routine surgical treatment is not of proven benefit. Br. Heart J. 71:219, 1994.

99. Konstantinides, S., Gerbel, A., Olschewski, M., et al.: Clinical course of atrial septal defect in patients older than 40 years: Benefits of surgical repair compared with medical treatment. N. Engl. J. Med. 333:469, 1995.

100. Williams, W. G., Trusler, G. A., Kirklin, J. W., et al.: Early and late

results of a protocol for simple transposition leading to an atrial switch (Mustard) repair. J. Thorac. Cardiovasc. Surg. 45:717, 1988.

101. Turina, M., Siebenmann, R., Nussbaumer, P., and Senning, A.: Long-term outlook after atrial correction of transposition of the great arteries. J. Thorac. Cardiovasc. Surg. 95:828, 1988.

102. Mustard, W. T.: Successful two-stage correction of transposition of the great vessels. Surgery 55:469, 1964.

103. Gillette, P. C., Kugler, J. D., Garson, A., et al.: Mechanism of the cardiac arrhythmias after the Mustard operation for transposition of the great arteries. Am. J. Cardiol. 45:1225, 1980.

104. Vetter, V. L., Tanner, C. S., Horowitz, L. N.: Inducible atrial flutter after the Mustard repair of complete transposition of the great arteries. Am. J. Cardiol. 61:428, 1988.

105. Musewe, N. N., Reisman, J., Benson, L. N., et al.: Cardiopulmonary adaptation at rest and during exercise 10 years after Mustard atrial repair for transposition of the great arteries. Circulation 77:1055, 1988.

106. Parrish, M. D., Graham, T. P., Bender, H. W., et al.: Radionuclide angiographic evaluation of right and left ventricular function during exercise after repair of transposition of the great arteries. Circulation 67:178, 1983.

107. Ramsay, J. M., Venables, A. W., Kelly, M. J., and Kalff, V.: Right and left ventricular function at rest and with exercise after the Mustard operation for transposition of the great arteries. Br. Heart J. 51:364, 1984.

108. Waien, S. A., Liu, P. P., Ross, B. L., et al.: Serial follow-up of adults with repaired tetralogy of Fallot. JAMA 20:295, 1992.

109. Murphy, J. G., Gersh, B. J., Mair, D. D., et al.: Long-term outcome in patients undergoing surgical repair of tetralogy of Fallot. N. Engl. J. Med. 329:593, 1993.

109a. Gatzoulis, M. A., Till, J. A., Somerville, J., and Redington, A. N.: Mechanoelectrical interaction in tetralogy of Fallot. Circulation 92:231, 1995.

110. Walsh, E. P., Rockenmacher, S., Keane, J. F., et al.: Late results in patients with tetralogy of Fallot repaired during infancy. Circulation 77:1062, 1988.

111. Hu, D. C. K., Seward, J. B., Puga, F. J., et al: Total correction of tetralogy of Fallot at age 40 years or older: Long-term follow-up. J. Am. Coll. Cardiol. 5:40, 1985.

112. Hughes, C. F., Lim, Y. C., Cartmill, T. B., et al.: Total intracardiac repair for tetralogy of Fallot in adults. Ann. Thorac. Surg. 43:634, 1987.

113. Zhao, H., Miller, D. C., Reitz, B. A., and Shumway, N. E.: Surgical repair of tetralogy of Fallot: Long-term follow-up with particular emphasis on late death and reoperation. J. Thorac. Cardiovasc. Surg. 89:204, 1985.

114. Jarmakani, J. M., Graham, T. P., and Canent, R. V.: Left heart function in children with tetralogy of Fallot before and after palliative or corrective surgery. Circulation 46:478, 1972.

115. Borow, K. M., Green, L. H., Castenada, A. R., and Keane, J. F.: Left ventricular function after repair of tetralogy of Fallot and its relationship to age of surgery. Circulation 61:1150, 1980.

116. Roos-Hesselink, J., Perlroth, M. G., McGhie, J., and Spitaels, S.: Atrial arrhythmias in adults after repair of tetralogy of Fallot: Correlations with clinical, exercise and echocardiographic findings. Circulation 91:2214, 1995.

117. Fisher, R. G., Moodie, D. S., Sterba, R., and Gill, C. G.: Patent ductus arteriosus in adults—long-term follow-up: Nonsurgical versus surgical treatment. J. Am. Coll. Cardiol. 8:280, 1986.

118. Kirklin, J. W., and Barratt-Boyes, B. G.: Cardiac Surgery. New York, John Wiley and Sons, 1986, p. 1059.

119. Koller, M., Rothlin, M., and Senning, A.: Coarctation of the aorta: Review of 362 operated patients. Long-term follow-up and assessment of prognostic variables. Eur. Heart J. 8:670, 1987.

120. Presbitero, P., Demarie, D., Villani, M., et al.: Long-term results (15 to 30 years) of surgical repair of aortic coarctation. Br. Heart J. 57:462, 1987.

121. Daniels, S. R., James, F. W., Loggie, J. M. H., and Kaplan, S.: Correlates of resting and maximal exercise systolic blood pressure after repair of coarctation of the aorta: a multivariate analysis. Am. Heart J. 113:349, 1987.

122. Clarkson, P. M., Nicholson, M. R., Barratt-Boyes, B. G., et al.: Results after repair of coarctation of the aorta beyond infancy: A 10 to 28 year follow-up with particular reference to late systemic hypertension. Am. J. Cardiol. 51:1481, 1983.

123. Hesslein, P. S., McNamara, D. G., Morriss, M. J. H., et al.: Comparison of resection versus patch aortoplasty for repair of coarctation in infants and children. Circulation 64:164, 1981.

124. Hellenbrand, W., Allen, H., Golinko, R., et al.: Balloon angioplasty for aortic recoarctation: Results of the valvuloplasty and angioplasty of congenital anomalies Registry. Am. J. Cardiol. 65:793, 1990.

125. Liberthson, R. L., Pennington, D. G., Jacobs, M. L., and Daggett, W. M.: Coarctation of the aorta: Review of 234 patients and clarification of management problems. Am. J. Cardiol. 43:835, 1979.

126. Celano, V., Pieroni, D. R., Morera, J. A., et al.: Two-dimensional echocardiographic examination of mitral valve abnormalities associated with coarctation of the aorta. Circulation 69:924, 1984.

127. Fontan, F., and Baudet, E.: Surgical repair of tricuspid atresia. Thorax 26:240, 1971.

128. Cowgill, L. D.: The Fontan procedure: A historical review. Ann. Thorac. Surg. 51:1026, 1991.

129. Glenn, W. W. L.: Circulatory bypass of the right side of the heart. IV Shunt between superior vena cava and distal right pulmonary artery: Report of clinical application. N. Engl. J. Med. 259:117, 1958.

130. Kopf, G. S., Laks, H., Stansel, H. C., et al.: Thirty-year follow-up of superior vena cava-pulmonary artery (Glenn) shunts. J. Thorac. Cardiovasc. Surg. 100:662, 1990.

131. de Leval, M. R., Kilner, P., Gewillig, M., and Bull, C.: Total cavopulmonary connection: A logical alternative to atriopulmonary connection for complex Fontan operations. Experimental studies and early clinical experience. J. Thorac. Cardiovasc. Surg. 96:682, 1988.

132. Stein, D. G., Laks, H., Drinkwater, D. C., et al.: Results of total cavopulmonary connection in the treatment of patients with a functional single ventricle. J. Thorac. Cardiovasc. Surg. 102:280, 1991.

132a. Rosenthal, M., Bush, A., Deanfield, J., and Redington, A.: Comparison of cardiopulmonary adaptation during exercise in children after the atriopulmonary and total cavopulmonary connection Fontan procedures. Circulation 91:372, 1995.

133. Driscoll, D. J., Offord, K. P., Feldt, R. H., et al.: Five-to-fifteen follow-up after Fontan operation. Circulation 85:469, 1992.

134. Humes, R. A., Mair, D. D., Porter, C. J., et al.: Results of the modified Fontan operation in adults. Am. J. Cardiol. 61:602, 1988.

MEDICAL MANAGEMENT OF ADULT CONGENITAL HEART DISEASE

135. Perloff, J. K.: Systemic complications of cyanosis in adults with congenital heart disease. Cardiol. Clin. 11:689, 1993.

136. Berman, W., Jr., Wood, S. C., Yabek, S. M., et al.: Systemic oxygen transport in patients with congenital heart disease. Circulation 75:360, 1987.

137. Tyndall, M. R., Teitel, D. F., Lutin, W. A., et al.: Serum erythropoietin levels in patients with congenital heart disease. J. Pediatr. 110:538, 1987.

138. Rosove, M. H., Perloff, J. K., Hocking, W. G., et al.: Chronic hypoxaemia and decompensated erythrocytosis in cyanotic congenital heart disease. Lancet 2:313, 1986.

139. Perloff, J. K., Rosove, M. H., Child, J. S., and Wright, G. B.: Adults with cyanotic congenital heart disease: Hematologic management. Ann. Intern. Med. 109:406, 1988.

140. Linderkamp, O., Klose, H. J., Betke, K., et al.: Increased blood viscosity in patients with cyanotic congenital heart disease and iron deficiency. J. Pediatr. 95:567, 1979.

141. Giddings, S. S., and Stockman, J. A.: Effect of iron deficiency on tissue oxygen delivery in cyanotic congenital heart disease. Am. J. Cardiol. 61:605, 1988.

142. Perloff, J. K., Marelli, A. J., and Miner, P. D.: Risk of stroke in adults with cyanotic congenital heart disease. Circulation 87:1954, 1993.

143. Territo, M. C., Perloff, J. K., Rosove, M. H., and Moake, J.: von Willebrand factor abnormalities in adults with congenital heart disease: A hematologic/pathophysiologic correlative study. (In preparation.)

144. Bowyer, J. J., Busst, C. M., Denison, D. M., and Shinebourne, E. A.: Effect of long-term oxygen treatment at home in children with pulmonary vascular disease. Br. Heart J. 55:385, 1986.

145. Perloff, J. K., Latta, H., and Barsotti, P.: Pathogenesis of the abnormal glomerulus in cyanotic congenital heart disease (in preparation).

146. Spear, G. S.: The glomerular lesion of cyanotic congenital heart disease. Bull. Johns Hopkins Hosp. 140:185, 1977.

147. Ross, E. A., Perloff, J. K., Danovitch, G. M., et al.: Renal function and urate metabolism in late survivors with cyanotic congenital heart disease. Circulation 73:396, 1986.

148. German, D. C., and Holmes, E. W.: Hyperuricemia and gout. Med. Clin. North Am. 70:419, 1986.

149. Martinez-Lavin, M.: Cardiogenic hypertrophic osteoarthropathy. Clin. Exp. Rheum. 10:19, 1992.

150. Sietsema, K. E., Cooper, D. M., Perloff, J. K., et al.: Dynamics of oxygen uptake during exercise in adults with cyanotic congenital heart disease. Circulation 73:1137, 1986.

151. Sietsema, K. E., Cooper, D. M., Perloff, J. K., et al.: Control of ventilation during exercise in patients with central venous-to-systemic arterial shunts. J. Appl. Physiol. 64:234, 1988.

152. Perloff, J. K., Urschell, C. W., Roberts, W. C., and Caulfield, W. H.: Aneurysmal dilatation of the coronary arteries in cyanotic congenital heart disease. Am. J. Med. 45:802, 1968.

153. Czernin, J., Brunken, R. C., Perloff, J. K., et al.: Myocardial perfusion and perfusion reserve in adults with cyanotic congenital heart disease. (In preparation.)

154. Perloff, J. K., and Marelli, A. J.: Neurological and psychosocial disorders in adults with congenital heart disease. Heart Dis. Stroke 1:218, 1992.

155. Baum, V. C., and Perloff, J. K.: Anesthetic implications of adults with congenital heart disease. Anesth. Analg. 76:1342, 1993.

156. Karnik, R., Stollberger, C., Valentin, A., et al.: Detection of patent foramen ovale by transcranial contrast Doppler ultrasound. Am. J. Cardiol. 69:560, 1992.

157. Pearson, A. C., Nagelhout, D., Castello, R., et al.: Atrial septal aneurysm and stoke: A transesophageal echocardiographic study. JAMA 18:1223, 1991.

158. Kurlan, R., Krall, R. L., and Deweese, J. A.: Vertebrobasilar ischemia after total repair of tetralogy of Fallot: Significance of subclavian steal created by Blalock-Taussig anastomosis. Stroke 15:359, 1984.

159. Perloff, J. K.: Congenital heart disease and pregnancy. Clin. Cardiol. *17*:579, 1994.

160. Loscalzo, J.: Paradoxical embolization: Clinical presentation, diagnostic strategies, and therapeutic options. Am. Heart J. *112*:141, 1986.

161. Pitkin, R. M., Perloff, J. K., Koos, B. J., and Beall, M. H.: Pregnancy and congenital heart disease. Ann. Intern. Med. *112*:445, 1990.

162. Manalo-Estrella, P., and Barker, A. E.: Histopathologic findings in human aortic media associated with pregnancy. Arch. Pathol. *83*:336, 1967.

163. Esscher, E. B.: Congenital complete heart block in adolescence and adult life: A follow-up study. Eur. Heart J. *2*:281, 1981.

164. Esscher, E. B.: Congenital complete heart block (Review). Acta Paediatr. Scand. *70*:131, 1981.

165. Waickman, L. A., Skorton, D. J., Varner, M. W., et al.: Ebstein's anomaly and pregnancy. Am. J. Cardiol. *53*:357, 1984.

166. Saxon, L. A., and Perloff, J. K.: Arrhythmias and conduction disturbances associated with pregnancy. *In* Podrid, P. J. and Kowey, P. R. (eds.): Cardiac Arrhythmia. Baltimore, Williams and Wilkins, 1995, p. 1161.

167. Canobbio, M. M., Rapkin, A. J., Perloff, J. K., et al.: Menstrual patterns in women with congenital heart disease. Pediatr. Cardiol. *16*:12, 1995.

168. Barber, G., DiSessa, T., Child, J. S., et al.: Hemodynamic responses to isolated increments in heart rate by atrial pacing after a Fontan procedure. Am. Heart J. *115*:837, 1988.

169. Baker, T. H., Machikawa, J. H., Stapleton, J. J.: Asymptomatic peripheral bacteremia. Am. J. Obstet. Gynecol. *94*:903, 1966.

170. Child, J. S., and Perloff, J. K.: Infective endocarditis: Risks and prophylaxis. *In* Perloff, J. K., and Child, J. S. (eds.): Congenital Heart Disease in Adults. Philadelphia, W. B. Saunders Company, 1991.

171. Devitt, J. H., Noble, W. H., and Byrick, R. J.: A Swan-Ganz catheter-related complication in a patient with Eisenmenger's syndrome. Anesthesiology *57*:335, 1982.

172. Clarke, C. F., Beall, M. H., Perloff, J. K.: Genetics, epidemiology, counseling, and prevention. *In* Perloff, J. K., and Child, J. S. (eds.): Congenital Heart Disease in Adults. Philadelphia, W. B. Saunders Company, 1991.

173. Ginsberg, J. S., Kowalchuk, G., Hirsh, J., et al.: Heparin therapy during pregnancy: Risks to mothers and fetus. Arch. Intern. Med. *149*:2233, 1989.

174. Zakzouk, M. S.: The congenital warfarin syndrome. J. Laryngol. Otol. *100*:215, 1986.

175. Hirsh, J., and Fuster, V.: AHA medical/scientific statement. Guide to anticoagulant therapy part 2: Oral anticoagulants. Circulation *89*:1469, 1994.

176. Barlow, D. P.: Methylation and imprinting: From host defense to gene regulation? Science *260*:309, 1993.

177. Maron, B. J., Epstein, S. E., and Mitchell, J. H.: Sixteenth Bethesda Conference: Cardiovascular abnormalities in the athlete: Recommendations regarding eligibility for competition. J. Am. Coll. Cardiol. *6*:1189, 1985.

178. Mitchell, J. H., Blomqvist, G., Haskell, W. L., et al.: Classification of sports. Am. J. Coll. Cardiol. *6*:1189, 1985.

179. Barth, C. W., and Roberts, W. C.: Left main coronary artery originating from the right sinus of Valsalva and coursing between the aorta and pulmonary trunk. J. Am. Coll. Cardiol. *7*:366, 1986.

180. Cheitlin, M. D., De Castro, C. M., and McAllister, H. A.: Sudden death as a complication of anomalous left coronary origin from the anterior sinus of Valsalva: A not so minor congenital anomaly. Circulation *50*:780, 1974.

181. Maron, B. J., Roberts, W. C., McAllister, H. A., et al.: Sudden death in young athletes. Circulation *62*:218, 1980.

182. Mark, A. L., Abboud, F. M., Schmidt, P. G., and Heistad, D. D.: Reflex vascular responses to left ventricular outflow obstruction and activation of ventricular baroreceptors in dogs. J. Clin. Invest. *52*:1147, 1982.

183. Garson, A., Gillette, P. C., Gutgesell, H. P., and McNamara, D. G.: Stress-induced ventricular arrhythmias after repair of tetralogy of Fallot. Am. J. Cardiol. *46*:1006, 1980.

184. Driscoll, D. J., Danielson, O. K., Puga, F. J., et al.: Exercise tolerance and cardiorespiratory response to exercise after the Fontan operation for tricuspid atresia or functional single ventricle. J. Am. Coll. Cardiol. *7*:1087, 1986.

185. Manning, J. A.: Insurability and employability of young cardiac patients. *In* Engle, M. A. (ed.): Pediatric Cardiovascular Disease. Philadelphia, F. A. Davis Co., 1981.

186. Sillanpaa, M.: Social adjustment and functioning of chronically ill and impaired children and adolescents. Acta. Paediatr. Scand. *340*[Suppl]:1, 1987.

187. Baer, P. E., Freedman, D. A., and Garson, A.: Long-term psychological follow-up of patients after corrective surgery for tetralogy of Fallot. J. Am. Acad. Child Psychiatry *5*:622, 1984.

188. Dickinson, D. F., and Sambrooks, J. E.: Intellectual performance in children after circulatory arrest with profound hypothermia in infancy. Arch. Dis. Child. *54*:1, 1979.

189. Perloff, J. K.: Residua and sequelae. *In* Perloff, J. K., and Child, J. S. (eds.): Congenital Heart Disease in Adults. Philadelphia, W. B. Saunders Company, 1991, p. 251.

190. Stark, J.: Do we really correct congenital heart defects? J. Thorac. Cardiovasc. Surg. *97*:1, 1989.

191. Grossman, W.: Cardiac hypertrophy: useful adaptation or pathologic process? Am. J. Med. *69*:576, 1980.

192. Zak, R., Kizu, A., and Bugaisay, L.: Cardiac hypertrophy: its characteristics as a growth process. Am. J. Cardiol. *44*:941, 1979.

193. Anversa, P., Ricci, R., and Olivetti, G.: Quantitative structural analysis of the myocardium during physiologic growth and induced cardiac hypertrophy: A review. J. Am. Coll. Cardiol. *7*:1140, 1986.

194. Ghani, Q. P., and Hollenberg, M.: Poly-adenosine biphosphate ribose metabolism and regulation of myocardial cell growth by oxygen. Biochem. J. *170*:378, 1978.

195. Hathaway, D. R., and March, K. L.: Molecular cardiology: New avenues for the diagnosis and treatment of cardiovascular disease. J. Am. Coll. Cardiol. *13*:265, 1989.

196. Cutilleta, A. F., Bowell, R. T., Rudnik, M., et al.: Regression of myocardial hypertrophy: I. Experimental model, changes in heart weight, nucleic acids and collagen. J. Molec. Cell. Cardiol. *7*:67, 1975.

197. Horowitz, L. N., Alexander, J. A., and Edmunds, L. H.: Postoperative right bundle branch block: Identification of three levels of block. Circulation *62*:319, 1980.

198. Bharati, S., and Lev, M.: Sequelae of atriotomy on the endocardium, conduction system and coronary arteries. *In* Engle, M. A. and Perloff, J. K. (eds.): Congenital Heart Disease after Surgery. New York, Yorke Medical Books, 1983.

199. Miller, A. J., Pick, R., and Katz, L. N.: Ventricular endomyocardial change after impairment of cardiac lymph flow in dogs. Br. Heart J. *25*:182, 1963.

Chapter 31
Acquired Heart Disease in Infancy and Childhood

WILLIAM F. FRIEDMAN

Because many of the topics discussed in this chapter are given more substantial coverage elsewhere in this text, the emphasis herein is placed on features of acquired heart disease that are relatively unique to or common in infancy and childhood, although the disease processes per se may not recognize age-related boundaries. Acute rheumatic fever and rheumatic heart disease are discussed in Chapter 55. The hyperlipidemias are discussed in Chapter 35.

NONRHEUMATIC INFLAMMATORY DISEASE

Infective Myocarditis
(See also Chapter 41)

Infectious processes that cause inflammatory disease of the heart may occur at any age, including fetal life. Causative agents include viruses, ricketsiae, bacteria, spirochetes, fungi, protozoa, and helminths. As a general rule, few of the generalized illnesses caused by these agents feature significant involvement of the heart. Myocardial involvement may be demonstrated histologically, but in most cases little or no expression of cardiac inflammation is detected clinically. Important exceptions are infections caused by certain viruses, diphtheria, and trypanosomes; these are discussed individually below.

VIRAL MYOCARDITIS. Coxsackie B and rubella viruses are the most common causative agents in infective myocarditis of the newborn. The rubella embryopathy and its associated cardiovascular malformations are discussed on page 878. Active *rubella myocarditis* occurs in utero, and may cause varying degrees of myocardial damage.[1] Invariably, however, other cardiovascular manifestations of the rubella syndrome dominate the clinical picture.

Coxsackie B typically causes outbreaks of epidemic myocarditis but may occur in the isolated infant in the newborn nursery, commonly with a fatal outcome.[2] The illness is of sudden onset and is characterized by fever, tachycardia, signs of systemic hypoperfusion, cyanosis, and, occasionally, cardiac failure. In some infants signs and symptoms of encephalomyelitis and hepatitis predominate. The diagnosis is suggested by electrocardiographic findings of atrial and/or ventricular arrhythmias, generalized ST-segment and T-wave changes, and low-voltage QRS complexes, accompanied by the appearance of marked generalized cardiomegaly and pulmonary vascular congestion on the chest roentgenogram. Echocardiography reveals dilatation of both ventricles and depressed indices of cardiac performance. Echocardiography is especially helpful in excluding congenital cardiac structural anomalies. The diagnosis is strongly suggested or confirmed when the virus can be isolated from pericardial fluid, pharyngeal secretions, or feces and when elevations occur in type-specific–neutralizing, hemagglutination-inhibiting, or complement-fixing antibody.[3] The immune system plays a role in the pathogenesis of myocarditis, and pathogenic autoantibodies to cardiac sarcolemma and myofibrils (known antigens in various anti-inflammatory heart diseases) have been identified.[4] These antibodies are up-regulated by viral stimulation, fix complement, and exert cytolytic and cytotoxic effects in vitro. Digitalis, diuretics, and general supportive measures are of limited benefit. Although increased sensitivity to the toxic effects of the glycosides is common, digitalis should be administered cautiously and continued until heart size is normal because cardiac failure may recur when the drug is discontinued.

Numerous viral agents have been identified as a cause of myocarditis in childhood beyond infancy.[5–7] The most common are Coxsackie A and B, influenza, adenovirus, and ECHO virus. Moreover, myocarditis, usually of mild degree, may be associated with the common viral infectious diseases of childhood, including mumps, measles, infectious mononucleosis, varicella, and variola. Although the diagnosis usually is one of exclusion, it may be suggested by the presence of sustained tachycardia out of proportion to fever, cardiomegaly without significant murmurs, poor-quality heart sounds, a gallop rhythm, an unexplained arrhythmia, and the electrocardiographic findings already mentioned.

Radionuclide gallium-67 scanning of the heart, showing a dense gallium uptake, provides suggestive evidence of active myocarditis.[8] Technetium-labeled leukocyte scanning may also prove useful in evaluation.[9] Magnetic resonance imaging holds promise for the noninvasive diagnosis of acute myocarditis, showing consistently greater than normal myocardial/skeletal muscle signal intensity ratios.[10] Although endomyocardial biopsy is a reasonably safe procedure in infants, children, and adolescents, a poor correlation exists between clinical and endomyocardial biopsy diagnoses of acute myocarditis in these age groups.[11–14] However, the recent development of in situ hybridization and polymerase chain reaction gene amplification technology may provide direct evidence by detecting enterovirus genome in the myocardium, greatly facilitating etiological diagnosis.[14a] Important differential diagnostic possibilities include endocardial fibroelastosis, glycogen storage disease with cardiac involvement, anomalous pulmonary origin of a coronary artery, critical aortic stenosis in infancy, and coarctation of the aorta or hypoplastic left heart syndromes.

The vast majority of these children recover from the acute episode of myocarditis with few or no sequelae. The results of treating patients with antiviral therapy or with immunosuppressants and antiinflammatory drugs have been inconclusive or disappointing.[13,15,16] Evidence that viral persistence in the myocardium may signify a poor prognosis raises the hope that antiviral therapy may prove beneficial in the future.[17] In some centers, high-dose intravenous gamma-globulin is administered to all children with presumed acute myocarditis. Results suggest that this approach results in better survival and improved recovery of left ventricular function.[18] Some patients may retain a permanent conduction defect or mild cardiac enlargement as a result of the acute illness. Moreover, a child may progress from the acute episode to a chronic dilated cardiomyopathy, characterized by signs of left ventricular dysfunction and mitral valve insufficiency. Unfortunately there are no predictive criteria to identify the latter situation.[19] Cardiac transplantation has been successful in some of these children with cardiomyopathy and a chronic, relentless, and refractory course of heart failure. However, cardiac transplantation in children, especially in infants or very young children, is complicated by growth suppression related to the required corticosteroid doses, and the complexity and severity of the immunosuppression in these infection-prone age groups.

DIPHTHERITIC CARDIOMYOPATHY

Diphtheria usually occurs in unimmunized children, especially in the western United States. Cardiac involvement is the result of the bacterial endotoxin rather than cardiac invasion by the bacillus.[20] Cardiac dysfunction appears to be related to abnormal fat metabolism because diphtheria toxin causes marked depletion of myocardial carnitine, a cofactor required for the beta-oxidation of fats.[21] Thus, what was formerly designated a form of myocarditis is now considered an acute metabolic cardiomyopathy. The pathology includes extensive intracellular fat vacuolization and glycogen depletion. Plasma carnitine deficiencies have also been found in children with other forms of dilated cardiomyopathy.[22]

Cardiac involvement occurs in about 10 per cent of affected patients and is the most common cause of death from this disease. Heart disease is most reliably indicated by electrocardiographic changes, which range from ST-segment and T-wave changes to arrhythmias and conduction disturbances, including complete heart block.[23] Occasionally, the electrocardiographic pattern of myocardial infarction may emerge. The electrocardiogram is a fair indicator of the extent of myocardial involvement and of prognosis. The latter usually is favorable if only ST-segment and T-wave changes are observed in the absence of conduction system disturbances. Right or left bundle branch block and complete atrioventricular block are associated with mortality rates of 50 to 80 per cent. The electrocardiographic findings may be accompanied by evidence of myocardial dysfunction and ventricular chamber dilatation on cardiac ultrasound.

MANAGEMENT. Treatment of diphtheritic cardiomyopathy usually is unsatisfactory. All patients should receive diphtheria anti-toxin and intravenous penicillin after appropriate skin testing. Corticosteroid therapy is of no value. Digitalis should be administered cautiously because it may increase atrioventricular block. Diuretics and antiarrhythmic medications usually are indicated; transvenous pacemaker therapy is instituted for complete AV block.[23a] Parenteral administration of carnitine (100 mg/kg/day) has been found to partially reverse diphtheritic cardiac dysfunction and reduce the risk of cardiac death.[24] This observation requires confirmation. If the child recovers from the acute episode of diphtheritic cardiomyopathy, the prognosis is quite good.

MYOCARDITIS CAUSED BY TRYPANOSOMAL INFECTION

Chagas' disease (p. 1442) is a chronic parasitosis caused by *Trypanosoma cruzi*, transmitted to humans by the bite of insects in the reduviid family. In the United States the disease is seen mostly in the southern states; endemic infection occurs in Latin America. Its most important clinical manifestation is a late-developing, chronic myocarditis and, much less frequently, an early acute myocarditis that is fatal in up to 10 per cent of cases.[25] In approximately 30 per cent of patients who survive the acute stage, cardiomyopathy may occur after an interval of 10 to 30 years.

DIAGNOSIS. The cardiac findings are often accompanied by digestive and autonomic disorders. It has been suggested that parasitic neuroaminodase may alter cell membrane gangliosides in target tissues.[26]

Diagnosis of the acute illness is supported by findings of edema and adenitis in the region of the insect bite, associated with low-grade intermittent fever, sweating, muscle pain, and, at times, diarrhea and vomiting; weeks or months later cardiomegaly, gallop rhythm, and conduction disturbances may be noted. Xenodiagnosis (examination of the excreta of laboratory-bred insects fed on the patient) or complement-fixation tests provide confirmation. Newer approaches are promising to improve direct detection of parasites by polymerase chain reaction amplification techniques.[27–29] Endomyocardial biopsy reveals mitochondrial, nuclear, and cell membrane abnormalities early in the myocardial degenerative pro-

cess. Late stages are characterized by severe myofibrillar lysis and variable amounts of fibrous tissue and cellular infiltrates.[30]

There is no satisfactory treatment.[30a] Administrtion of mixed gangliosides intramuscularly may be beneficial in reducing arrhythmias.[31] Treatment of ventricular tachycardia with drugs guided by electrophysiological study may improve survival in chronic chagasic patients with this complication.[32] Prophylaxis consists of control of the carrier of the parasites, reduviid bugs, by benzene hexachloride. Nitrofuran compounds, nifurtimox and benznidazole, appear effective in the acute stage of infection but not during the intracellular parasitic infection period.[33] Recently, binary and tertiary combinations of sterol biosynthesis inhibitors (ketoconazole, terbinafine, mevanolin) have shown strong antiproliferative, synergistic action in vitro on *T. cruzi* and in a murine model,[34,35] suggesting that this novel approach may achieve clinical significance.

Trypanosoma rhodesiense, which causes African sleeping sickness, may also produce myocardial hemorrhage, interstitial edema, mononuclear infiltration, and myocardial degeneration.[36] Cardiac involvement is usually relatively mild, and the clinical picture is dominated by evidence of encephalitis.

MYOCARDITIS CAUSED BY HUMAN IMMUNODEFICIENCY VIRUS

(see also p. 1438). In infants and children, the cardiac complications of the acquired immunodeficiency syndrome (AIDS) range from incidental microscopic inflammatory findings at necropsy to clinically significant, extensive, and chronic cardiac dysfunction.[37–39] In most children infected with the human immunodeficiency virus (HIV), the virus appears to have been transmitted from mother to child; other routes of transmission include contaminated blood products. Older children or adolescents also can be infected by routes more commonly associated with adults, such as sharing needles used for the injection of drugs, and sexual activity.

Cardiovascular abnormalities have been observed in as many as 65 per cent of infants or children with AIDS, whether induced by opportunistic infection or by the HIV infection itself.[40] As the prevalence of AIDS escalates, it is predictable that the cardiac involvement in infants and children with this disease will become better defined. Ventricular dysfunction, pericardial effusion, dilated cardiomyopathy, and rhythm disturbances (including high-grade atrial and ventricular ectopy and sudden death) provide evidence that HIV infection may have multiple direct or indirect effects on the heart. The latter may be due to infection with a variety of opportunistic organisms as well as to toxins, drugs, and autoimmunity.[40a] Other possible contributors to the cardiomyopathy include the myocardial depressant action of overwhelming noncardiac infection, the hypoxic and ischemic influence of severe lung disease, renal failure, autonomic dysfunction, chronic anemia, malnutrition, elevated endogenous catecholamines, vasoactive substances related to stress, and therapeutic interventions, including the use of steroids. Serial noninvasive assessment of this patient population, particularly by echocardiography, will, it is hoped, enable early or even anticipatory medical therapy, improving the cardiovascular status of children with HIV infection.

MYOCARDITIS IN LYME DISEASE (see also p. 1440). Transmitted to humans via the saliva of the deer tick *Ixodes dammini*, Lyme disease is caused by the spirochete, *Borrelia burgdorferi*. The disease is endemic in the northeastern United States, Wisconsin, and Minnesota and is associated with carditis in approximately 10 per cent of cases. Lyme disease occurs usually in stages, manifested initially by a characteristic skin lesion (erythema chronicum migrans) and flulike symptoms. If left untreated, it may progress to neurological, arthritic, and cardiac manifestations. Attempts to culture the organism are usually unsuccessful; an enzyme-linked immunosorbent assay is commonly employed to detect antibody to *B. burgdorferi*.[41] Cardiac involvement is usually a late manifestation expressed as various degrees of atrioventricular block, myopericarditis, and myocardial dysfunction. Nuclear isotope testing showing increased gallium-67 uptake, or by means of indium-111 antimyosin antibody scintigraphy, supports but is not specific for cardiac involvement. Early antibiotic treatment with penicillin, amoxicillin, doxycline, or ceftriaxone may prevent Lyme carditis.[42] Despite scattered reports of possible benefit from corticosteroids or salicylates, their therapeutic role has not been established. In children with high degrees of atrioventricular block, a finding that usually resolves with treatment, temporary transvenous pacing may be necessary.

Infective Pericarditis
(See also p. 1505)

Numerous infectious agents may be responsible for infective pericarditis. Viral and tuberculous inflammatory pericardial diseases are discussed in detail in Chapter 43. Of special concern in infancy and childhood is disease caused by pyogenic bacteria.[43,44] Purulent pericarditis occurs most often in the first two decades of life and is especially common in children under 6 years of age. Acute bacterial pericarditis usually is fatal if misdiagnosed or incorrectly treated. The most common pathogens are *Staphylococcus aureus, Streptococcus pneumoniae, Haemophilus influenzae,* and *Neisseria meningitides.* Unusual organisms that cause purulent pericarditis include *Escherichia coli, Pseudomonas, Salmonella, Klebsiella, Proteus,* and *Bacteroides. H. influenzae,* in particular, affects infants and young children, usually in association either with upper respiratory tract infection and croup, with lower respiratory tract pneumonia, bronchitis, or, occasionally, with meningitis.

Presenting clinical signs and symptoms vary, depending on the age of the patient, the responsible organism, and the site(s) of associated infection. The latter two require identification if therapy is to be effective. Fever, tachycardia, dyspnea, and chest pain are invariably present. Pericardial exudate resulting from the acute suppurative process commonly produces signs of life-threatening cardiac tamponade. Physical findings suggestive of purulent pericarditis include neck vein distention and hepatomegaly, pulsus paradoxus, and/or systemic hypotension with a narrow pulse pressure, muffled and distant heart sounds, marked cardiomegaly, and a point of maximal cardiac impulse well within the area of percussed dullness. Although the presence of a pericardial friction rub clearly points to pericardial involvement, this sign occurs infrequently.

An enlarged, globular cardiac configuration on chest radiography, electrocardiographic findings of diminished QRS amplitude, and abnormalities of the ST segment (usually elevated) and T waves (often inverted) usually focus attention on the pericardium. Echocardiographic evaluation (see p. 93) is reliable for establishing the diagnosis of significant pericardial effusion and for directing and guiding pericardiocentesis.[45] Culture and examination of pericardial fluid obtained by pericardiocentesis are essential for diagnosis and treatment.[46] Unless effective surgical drainage is combined with antibiotic treatment, the mortality rate is high. Operation should consist of creation of a subxiphoid pericardial window with placement of a drainage tube, or anterior pericardiectomy with tube drainage.[47] Early aggressive diagnosis and treatment reduce the risk of death substantially (10 to 20 per cent).[46] Pericardial constriction is uncommon, but all patients should be followed carefully for this complication.[48]

Postpericardiotomy Syndrome
(See also p. 1520)

In the first year after cardiac operation in which the pericardium is opened, and seldom in the second or third postoperative year, a febrile illness may occur, consisting of a pericardial and pleural inflammatory reaction with effusion and often with pulmonary parenchymal involvement. The illness occurs in 25 to 30 per cent of children undergoing pericardiotomy and usually is self-limiting; infants undergoing open-heart surgery are seldom affected. It is characterized by fever; chest, neck, or shoulder pain that becomes worse with inspiration; anorexia; and laboratory findings of leukocytosis and an elevated erythrocyte sedimentation rate.[49] Recurrences are uncommon and usually mild. Physical, electrocardiographic, and roentgenographic signs of pericardial involvement vary with the magnitude of the effusion. Echocardiographic detection of the effusion is common between 4 and 10 days postoperatively.[50] Cardiac tamponade, although not usual, occurs with sufficient frequency to warrant careful observation of the patient.

Viral infection and an autoimmune reaction have been implicated in the pathogenesis. Serum antibodies and a rise in titer frequently are found in reaction to adenovirus, Coxsackievirus, and cytomegalovirus. Elevations in levels of heart-reactive antibody are common.

An association recently has been shown between antinuclear antibodies, which are immunoglobulins directed toward antigenic nuclear material, and postpericardiotomy syndrome.[51]

The syndrome must be distinguished from infective endocarditis and the postperfusion syndrome of atypical lymphocytosis and hepatosplenomegaly, which occurs about 3 to 6 weeks after extracorporeal circulation and is caused by cytomegalovirus infection.[52]

Treatment of the postpericardiotomy syndrome depends on the degree of patient discomfort and the magnitude of pericardial and/or pleural effusion. In some patients signs of cardiac tamponade require pericardiocentesis. Bed rest and salicylates or indomethacin

lessen patient discomfort and diminish the production of pleural or pericardial fluid. Corticosteroids are employed by some in all cases; most consider them indicated for severe illness because steroids promptly relieve fever and symptoms.[53] Antibiotics are not useful in the treatment. Prolonged therapy is seldom necessary because of the self-limited nature of this postoperative complication. Late or recurrent tamponade, although rare, may require reinstitution of treatment.[54]

PRIMARY CARDIOMYOPATHIES
(See also Chap. 41)

The important *nonobstructive* cardiomyopathies, of special concern in infants and children, are idiopathic dilated (congestive) cardiomyopathy and the familial forms of endocardial fibroelastosis,[55,56] which afflict many of the patients also designated as having *dilated cardiomyopathy.*[57-61] By definition these diagnostic terms exclude patients whose myocardial dysfunction is caused by active infection, a congenital cardiac anomaly, or increased preload or afterload. Dilated (congestive) cardiomyopathy often is a disease of infants, with most cases becoming manifested before the age of 1 year, with a history of respiratory or diarrheal illness preceding the onset of cardiac symptoms. Severely ill patients may have endocardial fibroelastosis, although the latter can be confirmed definitely only after myocardial biopsy or autopsy.[62] Beyond age 2 years, dilated cardiomyopathy, like the condition in adults, is characterized by an unobstructed, dilated, and poorly contracting left ventricle.[63] For this group of children, debate exists as to whether endocardial fibroelastosis should be categorized as a separate entity under dilated or congestive cardiomyopathy, and whether it is an end stage of dilated cardiomyopathy of *any* cause.

Idiopathic Dilated Cardiomyopathy in Childhood

Approximately 90 per cent of all children presenting with dilated cardiomyopathy have no clearly identifiable cause, although it has long been speculated that a viral disease is a pivotal factor in the pathogenesis of the entity.[64-67] The application of molecular biology to clinical diagnosis, particularly techniques for gene amplification, have strengthened this hypothesis. Viral cytotoxicity, immunological responses, viral RNA persistence, and spasm of the coronary microvasculature have all been implicated in the development of the cardiomyopathy.

Dilated cardiomyopathy is characterized by a large dilated heart with poor biventricular systolic function. Signs and symptoms of congestive heart failure prevail. Symptoms consisting most often of fatigue and breathlessness are usually rapidly progressive. Examination reveals tachycardia, cardiomegaly, gallop rhythm, and hepatosplenomegaly. Cardiac murmurs are present in about half of patients, most of whom have the characteristic apical systolic murmur of mitral regurgitation.[68]

Chest roentgenography reveals marked generalized cardiomegaly with normal or congested pulmonary vascular markings. Most children have abnormal electrocardiograms showing hypertrophy, conduction disturbance, or ST-segment and T-wave abnormalities. Approximately 20 per cent of patients have arrhythmias, most of which are ventricular in origin. Two-dimensional echocardiography is virtually diagnostic of cardiomyopathy (Fig. 31–1). Dilated cardiac chambers are observed with generalized poor ventricular function. Mitral valve closure may be delayed, and aortic valve closure may occur earlier than normal. Valve regurgitation is detected readily by Doppler echocardiography. Calculations of left ventricular shortening fraction are helpful in both initial diagnosis and following the course of the disease, although measures of shortening fraction, left ven-

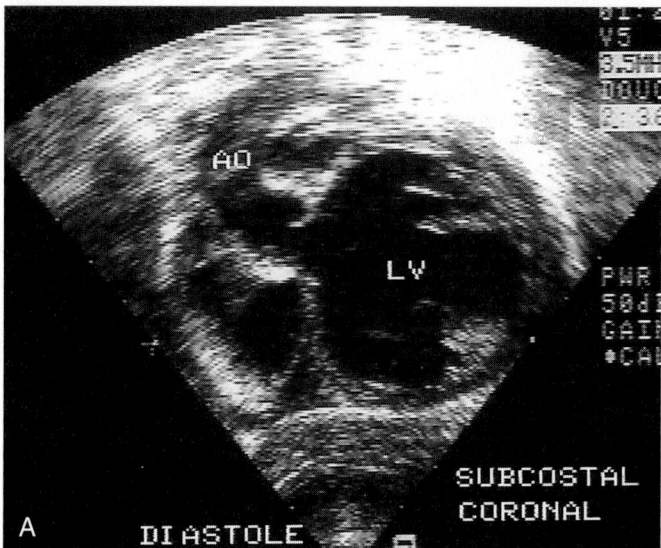

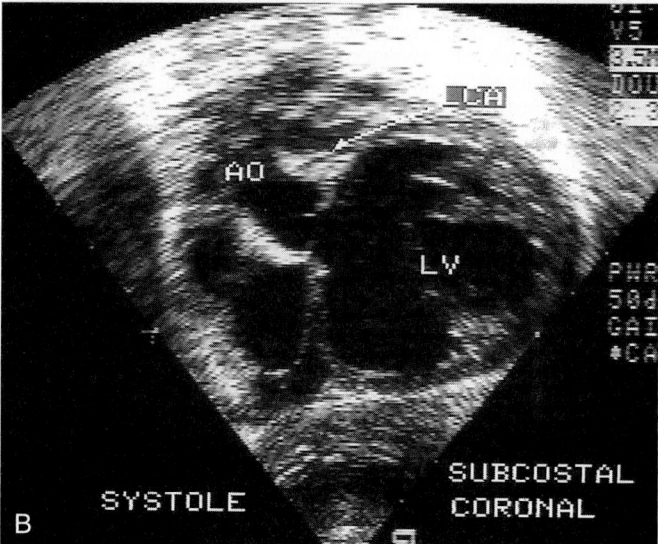

FIGURE 31–1. Subcostal coronal echocardiographic views at end-diastole *(top)* and end-systole *(bottom)* from a 4-year-old with idiopathic dilated cardiomyopathy, demonstrating minimal contraction of the left ventricle (LV). Identification at end-systole of the left coronary artery (LCA) from the aortic root (AO) indicates this is not an example of anomalous pulmonary origin of the left coronary artery. (Courtesy of Norman H. Silverman, M.D.)

tricular diastolic diameter, and wall mass have not been predictive of ultimate clinical outcome.[69–72,72a–c]

DIAGNOSIS. The diagnosis of dilated cardiomyopathy is generally one of exclusion. Differential diagnosis includes anomalous pulmonary origin of the left coronary artery, myocarditis, hypertrophic obstructive cardiomyopathy, anomalies that cause left ventricular outflow tract obstruction, and glycogen storage disease of the heart. The first four of these entities differ appreciably from dilated cardiomyopathy in their electrocardiographic or echocardiographic features; the skeletal muscle biopsy in glycogen storage disease is diagnostic.

Hemodynamic studies reveal evidence of left ventricular dysfunction. This includes elevations in left ventricular end-diastolic and left atrial pressures, moderate pulmonary hypertension, widened arteriovenous oxygen differences, and reduced left ventricular stroke volume and cardiac output. Angiography usually demonstrates a markedly dilated left ventricle, a reduced ejection fraction, and varying degrees of mitral regurgitation.

MANAGEMENT. This is directed at alleviating the signs and symptoms of congestive heart failure and includes the use of diuretics, inotropic support, afterload reduction, and

antiarrhythmic therapy when indicated.[73–76] Heart transplantation is an acceptable therapy for end-stage cardiomyopathy.[77,78] The overall 2-year survival for children between the ages of 1 and 18 years exceeds 72 per cent. Identifying the child who is most gravely ill is the biggest problem in determining the timing of transplantation. The overall mortality of dilated cardiomyopathy approaches 35 per cent, the vast majority of fatal cases occurring during the first episode of cardiac failure.

Endocardial Fibroelastosis (EFE)

Various designations have been applied to this condition, including endocardial sclerosis, fetal endocarditis, fetal endomyocardial fibrosis, and elastic tissue hyperplasia.[58] In recent years familial cases have been encountered more commonly than has the isolated form. The data provided by family studies fit neither an autosomal recessive nor a multifactorial mode of inheritance. Although the reasons are obscure, a marked reduction has been observed in the past decade of isolated, nonfamilial EFE. No definite cause for this condition has been established, although a host of theories have been proposed; inadequate subendocardial blood flow and/or prenatal or postnatal inflammation or infection currently are considered the most likely pathogenetic pathways.[62,79]

A distinction has been made between primary EFE, in which there is no cardiac malformation, and EFE secondary to congenital malformations of the heart.[55] In the *secondary* variety, focal areas of opaque fibroelastotic thickening of the mural endocardium or cardiac valves are observed in association with cardiac malformations. Underlying cardiovascular anomalies are almost always obstructive lesions, particularly of the left side of the heart, and these create cardiac hypertrophy and an imbalance in the myocardial oxygen supply-demand relation. Thus, secondary EFE quite commonly occurs in aortic stenosis, coarctation of the aorta, and hypoplastic left heart syndrome.

The *primary* form of EFE invariably involves the left ventricle and mitral and aortic valves without significant associated cardiac defects. Although the use of the term "primary" implies that this form of EFE is a specific disease entity, most would agree that it is the end result of many different diseases.[62] Further, as already discussed, clear separation may not exist clinically between primary EFE and dilated cardiomyopathy. Primary EFE commonly produces a marked dilatation of the left ventricle; rarely, a "contracted" type of primary EFE is observed, in which the left ventricle is relatively hypoplastic or normal in size. In the latter situation the right and left atria and the right ventricle are markedly enlarged and hypertrophied, with minimal or no endocardial sclerosis. In the common, dilated type of primary EFE, microthrombi may be found adherent to the endocardium. The diffuse endocardial hyperplasia may be several millimeters thick (Fig. 31–2). The aortic and mitral valve leaflets are thickened and distorted; mitral regurgitation is especially common. The papillary muscles and chordae tendineae are involved in the fibroelastic process and are shortened and distorted.

Primary EFE is a disease of infancy; symptoms usually develop between 2 and 12 months of age, although rarely they may be present shortly after birth. Clinical features reflect left ventricular dysfunction and congestive heart failure.[80]

Echocardiographic features include an increase in left atrial and left ventricular dimensions, reduced left ventricular septal and posterior wall motion, reduced ejection fraction, and abnormal mitral valve motion. Dense echoes along the endocardium of the left ventricle are a diagnostic clue. *Endomyocardial biopsy* shows a diagnostic invasion of the endocardium and subendocardium by fibroelastic tissue.[11,14,81] The *contracted form* of primary EFE produces a clinical picture of left-sided obstructive disease, particu-

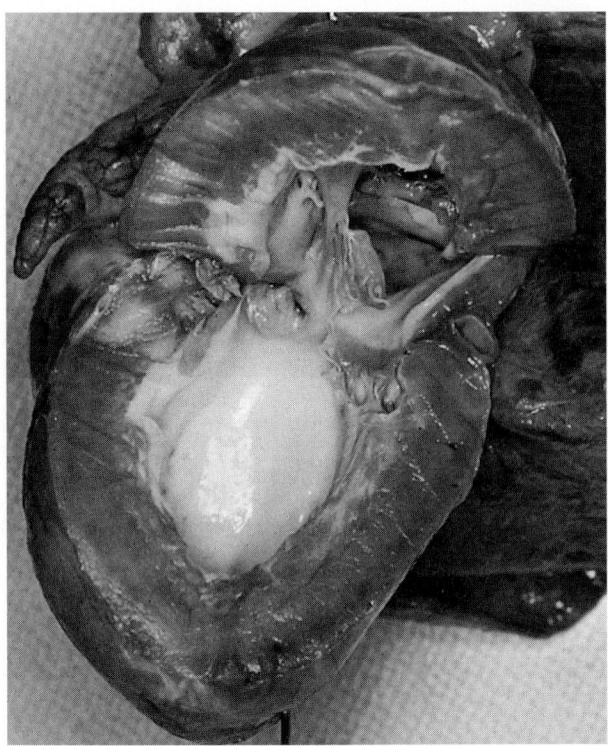

FIGURE 31–2. Diffuse left ventricular endocardial fibroelastosis. There is myocardial hypertrophy and obliteration of the papillary muscles as well as encroachment of the sclerotic subendocardial process onto the base of the aortic cusps. (From Tingelstaad, J. B., et al.: The electrocardiogram in the contracted type of primary endocardial fibroelastosis. Am. J. Cardiol. *27:*304, 1971.)

larly if the mitral valve is small. Left atrial pressure is elevated, with pulmonary artery pressures at or near systemic arterial levels.

The optimal management of patients with primary EFE consists of early and prolonged treatment with digitalis. Glycoside therapy should be continued for many years after the disappearance of symptoms, because cessation of the drug may result in acute cardiac failure, even when the heart size has returned to normal. The results of pericardial poudrage and mitral valve replacement in seriously afflicted infants have been disappointing. Cardiac transplantation may be recommended for those patients with end-stage disease.

SECONDARY CARDIOMYOPATHIES

The designation "secondary" cardiomyopathy refers to intrinsic myocardial disease that is secondary to or associated with systemic disease or diseases of other organs or in other systems. Myocardial disease coexisting with collagen vascular disorders (Chap. 56), neuromuscular disorders (Chap. 60), neoplasms (Chap. 57), acute glomerulonephritis (Chap. 62), and thalassemia and sickle cell disease (Chap. 57) are discussed elsewhere in this text. An abbreviated list of secondary cardiomyopathies in children is provided in Table 31–1. Of special interest to those caring for infants and children are the conditions seen in infants of diabetic mothers, and associated with glycogen storage disease, neonatal thyrotoxicosis, infantile beriberi, protein-calorie malnutrition, tropical endomyocardial fibrosis, anthracycline toxicity, and the mucocutaneous lymph node syndrome. Attention is directed to each of these latter disorders.

Cardiomyopathy in Infants of Diabetic Mothers

Infants born of gestational or established diabetic mothers are exposed to chronic hyperinsulinism in utero

and to reactive hypoglycemia after birth. They are large for gestational age, often weighing more than 4 kg at birth, have organomegaly, and are subject to hypocalcemia and polycythemia. Such infants occasionally display two basic forms of cardiomyopathy, both of which usually are transient.[82–85] Evidence exists that suboptimal metabolic control of maternal diabetes during pregnancy increases the incidence of these abnormalities.[85] In some of these infants, hypertrophy and hyperplasia of myocardial cells constitute a diffuse process, producing reversible signs and symptoms that resemble those of congestive cardiomyopathy. In other infants, the clinical findings are indistinguishable from those of hypertrophic obstructive cardiomyopathy.[86] The natural history in this latter group has been one of gradual spontaneous regression within 1 to 12 months of obstructive murmurs, cardiomegaly, and electrocardiographic and echocardiographic abnormalities typical of hypertrophic obstructive cardiomyopathy.

Glycogen Storage Disease

Glycogen storage disease is the result of a deficiency of one or more of the enzymes involved in the biosynthesis and degradation of glycogen. Cardiomyopathy is rare but may be observed in types III, IV, and VI of this disease, each representing an enzymatic defect on the glycolytic pathway.[87] The heart is importantly involved in type II (Pompe's disease), which results from a deficiency of alpha-1,4-glucosidase (acid maltase), a lysosomal enzyme that hydrolyzes glycogen into glucose.[88] This disease is a hereditary error of metabolism transmitted through a single recessive gene. Generalized glycogenesis takes place, occurring especially in the heart, the skeletal muscles, and the liver. The glycogen within cardiac muscle cells is biochemically normal but is present in excessive amounts, both within lysosomes and free in the cytoplasm. As a result, the heart enlarges, often to a marked degree, and congestive heart failure supervenes. Glycogen deposition within the myocardium usually is uniform, although occasionally the

TABLE 31–1 COMMON SECONDARY CARDIOMYOPATHIES IN CHILDREN

Inflammatory
  Postinfectious (viral, bacterial, fungal, protozoal, rickettsial, spirochetal)
  Hypersensitivity
  Giant cell

Neuromuscular
  Muscular dystrophy
  Myotonic dystrophy

Toxic
  Alcohol
  Anthracyclines (doxorubicin)
  Lead
  Cyclophosphamide
  Vincristine

Infiltrative/fibrotic
  Glycogen storage
  Mucopolysaccharidoses
  Hemochromatosis
  Endomyocardial fibrosis

Metabolic
  Infants of diabetic mothers
  Carnitine deficiency
  Nutritional deficiency (thiamine, kwashiorkor, selenium)
  Thyroid disease
  Catecholamine cardiomyopathy

Ischemic/anemic
  Kawasaki disease
  Familial hypercholesterolemia
  Congenital coronary artery malformation
  Sickle cell anemia

interventricular septum is especially involved, producing subpulmonic obstruction or a constellation of features indistinguishable from hypertrophic obstructive cardiomyopathy. Selective angiography has revealed a distinctive trabeculation of the left ventricle in some infants.[89]

Clinical signs of type II glycogen storage disease usually become prominent in the early neonatal period.[90,91] Characteristic symptoms include failure to thrive, progressive hypotonia, lethargy, and a weak cry. Prominent early features include nonspecific cardiac murmurs, cardiomegaly, signs of congestive heart failure, macroglossia, poor skeletal muscle tone, and weakness. The electrocardiogram shows extremely tall, broad QRS complexes with a short P-R interval (commonly less than 0.09 sec) (Fig. 31–3).

The short P-R interval may be the result of facilitated atrioventricular conduction owing to myocardial glycogen deposition. Less often, deep Q waves are observed over the mid or left precordium as are T-wave inversion and ST-segment elevation. Chest roentgenograms show an enlarged globular heart associated with pulmonary vascular congestion (Fig. 31–4). In rare patients with cardiac glycogenosis the cardiac murmur suggests left ventricular outflow tract obstruction and/or mitral regurgitation; the echocardiographic, hemodynamic, and angiographic features in this subgroup are indistinguishable from those in infants with hypertrophic obstructive cardiomyopathy. Diagnosis is confirmed by demonstrating the enzymatic deficiency in lymphocytes, skeletal muscle, or liver. Skeletal muscle biopsy reveals histological and histochemical evidence of glycogen deposition.

Cardiac glycogenosis may be confused with other entities that cause cardiac failure in the early months of life, including idiopathic dilated cardiomyopathy and endocardial fibroelastosis, anomalous pulmonary origin of the left coronary artery, fixed and dynamic forms of left ventricular outflow tract obstruction, coarctation of the aorta, and myocarditis. The short P-R interval and the skeletal muscle hypotonia in glycogen storage disease help to distinguish this disorder from dilated cardiomyopathy and *endocardial fibroelastosis.* Infants with an anomalous pulmonary origin of the *left coronary artery* usually have a distinctive elec-

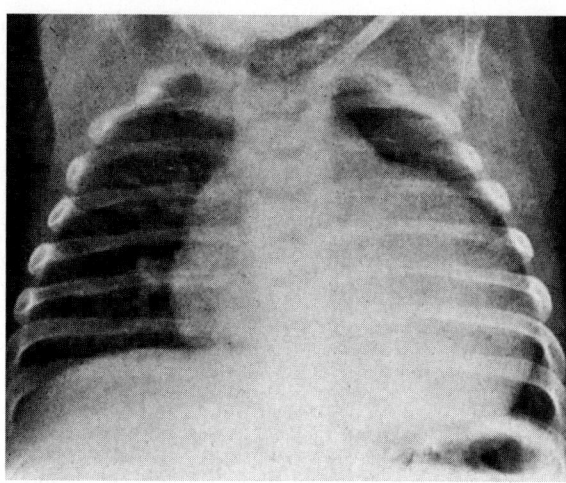

FIGURE 31–4. Chest roentgenogram of an infant with glycogen storage disease showing massive cardiomegaly and pulmonary edema. (From Taussig, H.: Congenital Malformations of the Heart. Vol. 2. 2nd ed. Boston, Harvard University Press, Copyright © 1947, 1960 by The Commonwealth Fund.)

trocardiographic pattern of anterolateral myocardial infarction. In infants with *coarctation of the aorta* the pulse and blood pressure discrepancies between the upper and lower extremities point to the proper diagnosis (see p. 965). *Myocarditis* usually is of abrupt onset in a previously healthy child and is not associated with marked hypotonia; the generally low-voltage electrocardiogram does not show the short P-R interval. The skeletal muscle hypotonia and the macroglossia in infants with glycogen storage disease occasionally raise the possibilities of amyotonia congenita and cretinism or mongolism, respectively.

Cardiac glycogenosis leads to progressive impairment of myocardial function; Pompe's disease is uniformly fatal, usually within the first year of life. Death quite often is the result of either cardiac failure or complications of respiratory management such as pneumonia or aspiration.

Neonatal Thyrotoxicosis

Thyroid-stimulating immunoglobulin traverses the placental barrier and stimulates the fetal thyroid gland when maternal hyperthyroidism exists. Many infants are born prematurely or are small for gestational age. Jitteriness and irritability are noted early. Thyroid hormone has both direct and indirect effects on the heart and circulation.[92] Cardiac findings include tachycardia, bounding pulses, systolic hypertension, and a precordial systolic murmur. Congestive heart failure frequently is present, and the presenting finding occasionally is an episode of paroxysmal atrial tachycardia. A neonatal goiter may be observed, especially if the mother received iodine therapy during pregnancy.

Diagnosis should be anticipated whenever a history of hyperthyroidism exists in the mother. Neonatal thyrotoxicosis occurs in the offspring of about 1 to 2 per cent of these women. A maternal level of thyroid-stimulating immunoglobulin should be obtained before delivery in anticipation of the problem arising in the newborn infant because high levels often are observed in both mother and offspring. The serum levels of thyroxine are increased in the newborn.

The infant who has heart failure may be treated with digitalis and propylthiouracil or carbimazole. The latter two drugs are not completely effective for many weeks; a beta blocker usually is helpful in addition to these agents. Supportive measures such as sedation and minimal stimulation may be helpful. Exchange transfusion or corticosteroid treatment is of no proven benefit.

Infants usually improve between the second and third month of life, although lack of attention to the problem or inadequate therapy may result in a fatal outcome.

Infantile Beriberi
(See also p. 461)

Thiamine (vitamin B₁) deficiency mainly occurs in regions of Southeast Asia, India, Brazil, and Africa, in which the dietary staple is polished rice or cassava. Thiamine functions as a coenzyme in decarboxylation of alpha-keto acids and in the utilization of pentose in the hexose monophosphate shunt. A reduction in myocardial energy production causes symptoms in the infant, usually between 1 and 4

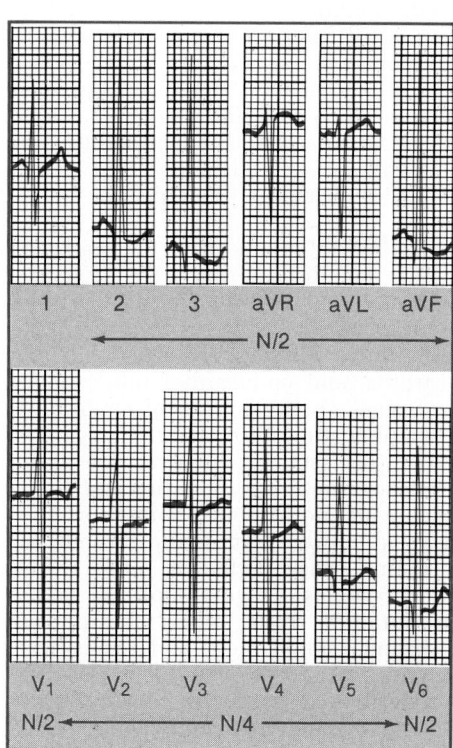

FIGURE 31–3. Electrocardiogram of an infant with glycogen storage disease showing a short PR interval and left ventricular hypertrophy.

months of age, who is breast fed by a thiamine-deficient mother.[93] Rarely, improper and ill-advised parental feeding practices lead to the vitamin deficiency.[93a] Such infants usually are edematous, irritable, pale, and anorectic. Hoarseness or aphonia is common, owing to involvement of the recurrent laryngeal nerve; blepharoptosis occurs in one-third of infants. Typically, cardiac involvement manifests as dilation of the right ventricle and prominent signs of systemic venous congestion. Electrocardiographic findings are nonspecific, and radiological findings principally consist of right ventricular dilatation. Infantile beriberi may be rapidly fatal but responds quickly and well to administration of thiamine (25 to 50 mg intravenously initially, with reduction of the dose to 10 mg/day for several days, and then orally for several weeks). Dramatic amelioration occurs within a few days of the cardiac findings. Cure is complete with no known sequelae.

Protein-Calorie Malnutrition
(See also p. 1907)

This is a major public health problem in underdeveloped areas of the tropics.[94] In infants inadequate diet results in a state of emaciation termed "marasmus"; "kwashiorkor" is a designation applied to this syndrome in children beyond 1 year of age. The disease results from a deficiency of protein relative to calories, although the latter and other essential nutrients often are lacking as well. General muscle wasting, loss of subcutaneous fat, and atrophy of most organs, including the heart, are typical in marasmic infants. In both marasmus and kwashiorkor, thinning and atrophy of cardiac muscle fibers and interstitial edema or vacuolization of the myocardial fibers are noted.[95] As the condition progresses, listlessness becomes prominent. Cardiovascular collapse is easily precipitated in these infants by the stress of infection.

In both infancy and childhood the principal physical findings reflect systemic hypoperfusion and principally consist of hypothermia, hypotension, tachycardia, and low-amplitude peripheral arterial pulsations. Peripheral usually nonpitting edema is prominent, as are wasting of the skeletal musculature, exfoliative dermatitis, and gray or red discoloration of the hair. Changes seen on electrocardiogram and on radiographic examination are nonspecific.

Treatment should be directed at correction of fluid and electrolyte imbalance, eradication of infection, and management of such associated problems as anemia and parasitic infestation. Care is required in the correction of dehydration or severe anemia because volume overload of the heart is easily produced. Supplements of potassium and magnesium often are required, and because of deficiencies in these elements, digitalis should probably be avoided or used with extreme caution. If the infant or child survives the initial phase, a well-balanced diet effects an impressive recovery over several months' duration.

Tropical Endomyocardial Fibrosis
(See also p. 1431)

Endomyocardial fibrosis (endomyocardial disease) is a rare, acquired, progressive disease, usually involving children and young adults from Africa, Southeast Asia, and South America. This cardiomyopathy of unknown cause is characterized by focal endocardial fibrosis of one or, rarely, both ventricles.[96] Controversy exists as to whether or not endomyocardial fibrosis, which is not associated with eosinophilia, and Löffler's endocarditis with eosinophilia (Chap. 41) are the same disorder described from temperate climates.[97] Endocardial fibrosis is located almost exclusively in the inflow tracts of the ventricles and commonly involves one or the other atrioventricular valve. Partial obliteration of either cardiac chamber results in reduced ventricular compliance with impairment of filling. The fibrotic process often involves the chordae tendineae, resulting in mitral and/or tricuspid regurgitation. Plaques of heaped-up fibrous tissue without elastic fibers are especially common within the left ventricle. Endomyocardial fibrosis involving the right ventricle may have to be differentiated from Ebstein's anomaly of the tricuspid valve (see p. 934), and endomyocardial fibrosis involving the left ventricle may have to be differentiated from rheumatic mitral regurgitation.

When left ventricular disease predominates, the clinical findings often resemble those of mitral stenosis or regurgitation. When endocardial involvement of the right ventricle is more severe than that of the left ventricle, the patient usually presents with findings of markedly elevated systemic venous pressure and tricuspid regurgitation.

Treatment is supportive. Survival usually depends on the extent of endocardial and valvular involvement and is better when right ventricular disease predominates.[98] Mean survival after the onset of symptoms is about 24 months. Specific treatment does not exist, and corticosteroid therapy has not proved efficacious. Surgical excision (decortication) of affected tissue with prosthetic valve replacement has been associated with clinical improvement.[99] However, children most severely affected by this disease commonly reside in regions of the tropics and subtropics where cardiac surgery is not readily available.

Kawasaki Disease
(Mucocutaneous Lymph Node Syndrome)

Kawasaki disease was first described in Japan in 1967. It is a generalized vasculitis of unknown etiology and a leading cause of acquired heart disease in the United States. Eighty per cent of cases occur in children less than 5 years of age, and most are under 2. Fewer than 2 per cent of patients have recurrences.

The syndrome presents with fever and ocular and oral manifestations followed in 5 days by a rash and indurative edema of the hands and feet, with palmar and plantar erythema. Finally, after about 2 weeks, cutaneous desquamation occurs. Diagnostic criteria include (1) a fever lasting for 5 or more days that is unresponsive to antibiotics; (2) bilateral congestion of the ocular conjunctiva; (3) peripheral limb changes that include an indurative peripheral edema and erythema of the palms and feet, followed later in the course of the illness by a membranous desquamation of the fingertips; (4) changes in the lips and mouth, including dry, erythematous, and fissured lips, injected oropharyngeal mucosa, and a strawberry tongue; (5) a polymorphous exanthema of the trunk without crusts or vesicles; and (6) cervical lymphadenopathy. Diagnosis is accepted when the first criterion and at least four of the remainder are present.[100]

In addition to the mucous membrane and cutaneous effects, multiple organ system involvement has been noted. Noncardiovascular complications of the illness include arthritis, cerebrospinal fluid pleocytosis, pulmonary infiltrates, hepatic dysfunction, and hydrops of the gallbladder. The illness often is accompanied by diarrhea, vomiting and abdominal pain, leukocytosis with a predominance of neutrophils, thrombocytosis, sterile pyuria and proteinuria, elevated liver transaminases, an elevation in the erythrocyte sedimentation rate, alpha$_1$-antitrypsin and serum immunoglobulin E, and a positive C-reactive protein.[100]

An extensive search for the cause of Kawasaki disease has been unproductive. The epidemiology and clinical presentation are highly suggestive of an infectious agent; person-to-person transmission is highly unlikely. Multiple immunoregulatory abnormalities have been suggested to be involved in the pathogenesis of the illness, with speculation that they result from profound superantigenic stimulation from microbial toxins. Abnormalities include marked polyclonal B-cell expansion; T-cell, monocyte, and macrophage activation; increased interleukins-1, -2, -6, and -8, tumor necrosis factor-alpha, and antibodies against endothelial cell antigens; and increased expression of heat shock protein.[101,102] Recent studies do not support a retroviral etiology.[103]

NATURAL HISTORY. On the basis of pathological data, progression of the disease may be divided into four stages.[104] In stage I, lasting for 1 to 9 days, acute perivasculitis of the small arteries is evident and involves the vasa vasorum of the major coronary arteries. Pericarditis, interstitial myocarditis, and endocardial inflammation also are seen; these changes chiefly consist of neutrophilic, eosinophilic, and lymphocytic infiltrations. In stage II, of 12 to 25 days' duration, panvasculitis involves the major coronary arteries. It affects the intima, media, and adventitia and results in aneurysm and thrombus formation. In stage III, of 28 to 31 days' duration, granulating thrombi and marked intimal thickening cause partial or total occlusion of the major coronary arteries. Stage IV follows and may be of many years' duration, during which healing occurs, consisting of scarring, calcification, and recanalization of occluded arteries.

The syndrome has an associated acute mortality of less than 1 per cent, secondary to complications from coronary artery involvement, myocarditis, or pericarditis, with a majority of deaths occurring in the third or fourth week of children aneurysms of the coronary arteries with narrowing, tortuosity, and obstruction are detected by two-dimensional echocardiography, aortography, and coronary angiography (Fig. 31–6).[107–112] The appearance more than 6 weeks after the onset of illness is uncommon.

Echocardiography is the primary tool for evaluation and follow-up of coronary abnormalities (Fig. 31–7). Detailed examination displays the left main, anterior descending, and left circumflex coronary arteries as well as the proximal, middle, and distal segments of the right and posterior coronary arteries. These vessels are seen in multiple planes using a combination of view windows. A conclusion that the coronary arteries are normal should not be reached until all major vessel segments have been visualized and determined to be normal.[107a] Intravascular imaging may

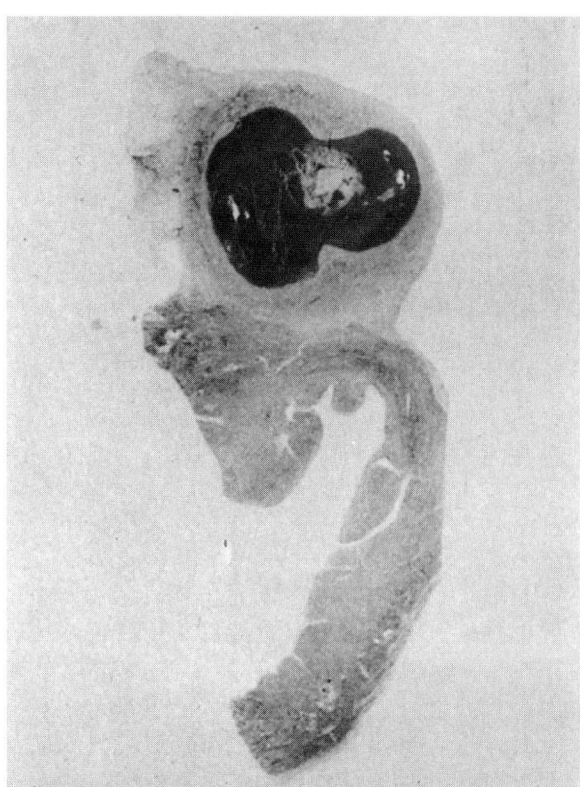

FIGURE 31–5. Low-power photomicrograph of a coronary artery aneurysm with recent occlusive thrombosis in a patient with mucocutaneous lymph node syndrome. (From Landing, B. H., and Larson, E. J.: Are infantile periarteritis nodosa with coronary artery involvement and fatal mucocutaneous lymph node syndrome the same? Comparison of 20 patients from North America with patients from Hawaii and Japan. Pediatrics 59:651, 1977. Copyright American Academy of Pediatrics, 1977.)

illness.[105] Other children may die later in life as a result of myocardial infarction.[106,107] Autopsy examination has almost uniformly demonstrated coronary arterial aneurysms, with occlusion caused by thromboendarteritis (Fig. 31–5). The clinical and laboratory features are shown in Table 31–2 and the spectrum of cardiovascular involvement is outlined in Table 31–3. The factors associated with increased risk of developing coronary aneurysms include male gender, age less than 1 year, signs of pancarditis including arrhythmias, prolonged period of inflammation including fever lasting for more than 10 days, and recurrence of fever after an afebrile period of at least 24 hours.

The disease often has been misdiagnosed in the United States as scarlet fever, drug reaction, measles or other febrile viral exanthems, Stevens-Johnson syndrome, Rocky Mountain spotted fever, staphylococcal scalded skin syndrome, leptospirosis, or mercury poisoning.[100]

CARDIAC MANIFESTATIONS. Infants and children with this syndrome should be closely watched for signs of cardiac involvement. A significant number of patients show evidence of myocarditis or pericarditis, or both, in the early phases of the disease.[104] Pericardial effusion is detected by echocardiography in approximately 30 per cent of patients. It rarely progresses to tamponade and usually resolves without specific therapy. Electrocardiographic evidence of myocarditis with low voltage and nonspecific ST-T wave changes is seen in 45 per cent of patients, echocardiographic evidence of poor left ventricular function in 25 per cent, cardiomegaly on chest radiographs in 25 per cent, and a gallop rhythm in 12 per cent. Coronary arterial abnormalities develop in approximately 20 per cent of untreated patients and are the most common case of both short- and long-term morbidity and mortality.[107a] In these

TABLE 31–2   CLINICAL AND LABORATORY FEATURES OF KAWASAKI DISEASE

Diagnostic criteria (principal clinical findings*)
Fever of at least 5 days' duration†
Presence of four of the following principal features:
Changes in extremities
Polymorphous exanthem
Bilateral conjunctival injection
Changes in the lips and oral cavity
Cervical lymphadenopathy
Exclusion of other diseases with similar findings
Other clinical and laboratory findings
Cardiac findings
Pancarditis, in early stages of disease
Coronary artery abnormalities, usually beyond 10 days of onset of illness
Noncardiac findings
Musculoskeletal system
Arthritis, arthralgia
Gastrointestinal tract
Diarrhea, vomiting, abdominal pain
Hepatic dysfunction
Hydrops of the gallbladder
Central nervous system
Extreme irritability
Aseptic meningitis
Respiratory tract
Post-respiratory illness
Otitis media
Pulmonary infiltrates
Other findings
Erythema and induration at Bacille Calmette-Guérin (BCG) inoculation site
Auditory abnormalities
Testicular swelling
Peripheral gangrene
Aneurysms of medium-sized noncoronary arteries
Laboratory findings
Neutrophilia with immature forms
Elevated erythrocyte sedimentation rate
Positive C-reactive protein
Elevated serum alpha$_1$-antitrypsin
Anemia
Hypoalbuminemia
Elevated serum immunoglobulin E
Thrombocytosis
Proteinuria
Sterile pyuria
Elevated serum transaminases

* Patients with fever and fewer than four principal clinical features can be diagnosed as having Kawasaki disease when coronary artery disease is detected by two-dimensional echocardiography or coronary angiography.

† Many experts believe that, in the presence of classic features, the diagnosis of Kawasaki disease can be made by experienced practitioners before the fifth day of fever.

From Dajani, A. S., Taubert, K. A., Gerber, M. A., et al.: Diagnosis and therapy of Kawasaki disease in children. Circulation 87:1776–1780, 1993. Copyright 1993 American Heart Association.

TABLE 31–3 SPECTRUM OF CARDIOCIRCULATORY FINDINGS IN KAWASAKI DISEASE

CARDITIS (myocarditis, pericarditis)
  Congestive heart failure
  Arrhythmias
CORONARY ANGIITIS
  Thromboendarteritis—aneurysms
    Regression
    Thrombosis—recanalization
    Obstruction—stenosis
    Collaterals
    Rupture
  Myocardial ischemia or infarction
    Ventricular aneurysm
    Papillary muscle dysfunction—mitral regurgitation
ARTERIAL INVOLVEMENT
  Pulmonary/renal angiitis—pulmonary/renal hypertension
  Arteritis, aneurysms: Femoral, iliac, brachial, cerebral, hepatic, etc.

allow more detailed visualization of coronary wall morphology and the healing process, as well as the analysis of coronary artery distensibility.[113]

About half of the children with coronary aneurysms diagnosed shortly after the acute phase of the disease subsides have normal-appearing vessels by angiography 1 or 2 years later.[114–116] Patients with giant aneurysms (internal diameter ≥ 8 mm) have the worst prognosis and greatest chance of developing coronary thrombosis, stenosis, or myocardial infarction. In those patients with residual cardiac abnormalities after recovery from the acute illness phase, a variety of findings have been described. These include impairment of left ventricular function secondary to the coronary arterial involvement, papillary muscle dys-

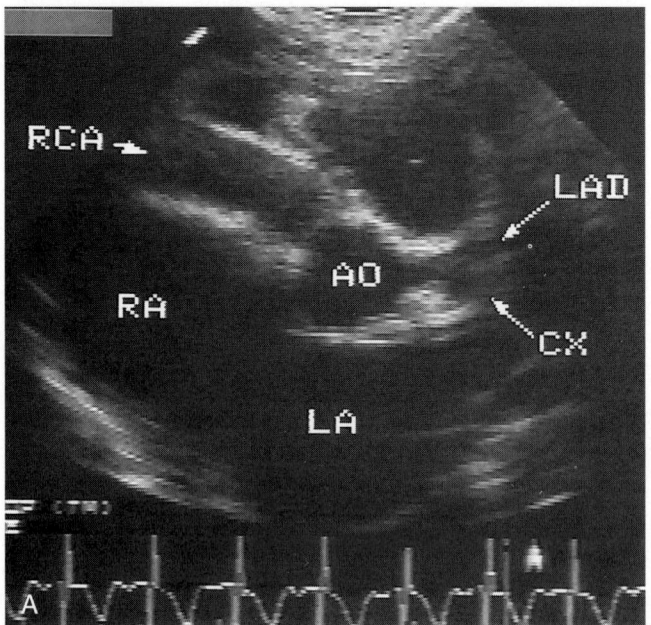

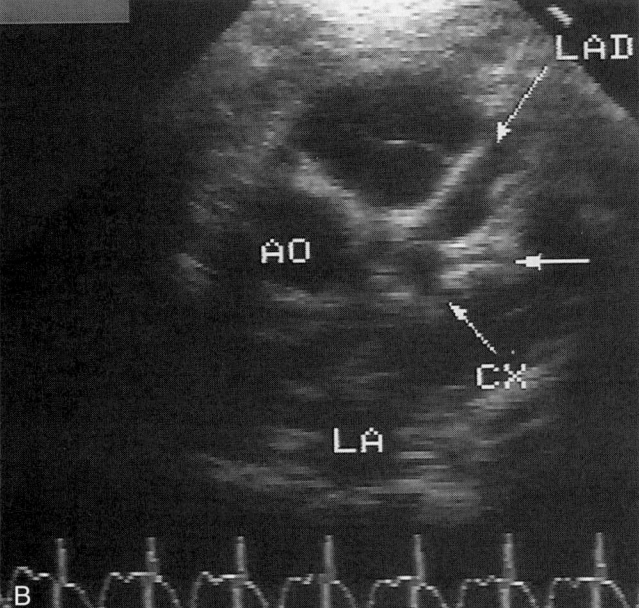

FIGURE 31–7. Parasternal short-axis echocardiographic views of the coronary arteries in a 2-year-old boy with Kawasaki disease. *A,* At the level of the aortic root (AO), a giant fusiform coronary aneurysm of the right coronary artery (RCA) and enlargement of the left anterior descending (LAD) and circumflex (Cx) coronary arteries. *B,* A close-up view of the left coronary artery system demonstrating a fusiform aneurysm of the left anterior descending coronary artery (LAD) and a proximal aneurysm of the circumflex coronary artery (Cx). The arrow between the LAD and Cx indicates a prominent obtuse marginal branch. RA = right atrium, LA = left atrium. (Courtesy of Norman H. Silverman, M.D.)

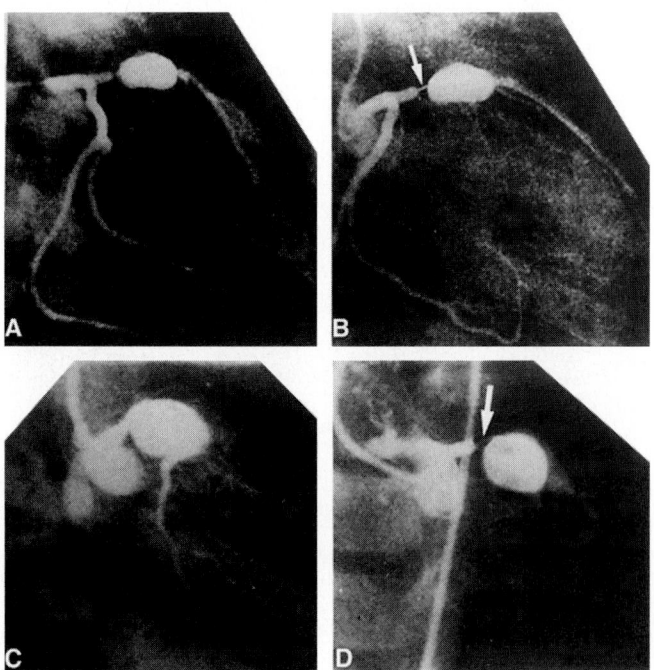

FIGURE 31–6. *A,* Left selective coronary angiogram at 30 degrees right anterior oblique projection, showing localized stenosis of about 75 per cent. *B,* Selective coronary angiogram, inclining to 60 degrees right anterior oblique, shows a 99 per cent stenosis (white arrow). *C,* Left selective coronary angiogram failed to demonstrate a localized stenosis because the catheter tip had been pushed into the aneurysm. *D,* In this selective coronary angiogram, the catheter tip at the ostium shows a localized 99 per cent stenosis at the inlet of the aneurysm *(arrow).* (From Tsubata, S., Suzuki, A., Ono, Y. et al.: Coronary arterial lesions due to Kawasaki disease: Selective coronary angiography in five cases with difficult-to-detect localized stenosis. Pediatr. Cardiol. *14:*169, 1993.)

function with mitral regurgitation,[117] impaired left ventricular function,[118] and abnormalities of the distensibility of the coronary arteries (even after aneurysms have disappeared and no morphological abnormalities are recognized by coronary arteriography).[119]

MANAGEMENT. Initial therapy during the acute stage for Kawasaki disease is directed at reducing inflammation, especially in the coronary arterial tree and myocardium. Later, treatment is directed toward preventing coronary thrombosis by inhibiting platelet aggregation. Specific treatment awaits discovery of the etiological agent.[100]

Current therapy is outlined in Table 31–4. It appears that corticosteroid therapy is detrimental during the acute ill-

TABLE 31–4 TREATMENT FOR ACUTE STAGE OF KAWASAKI DISEASE

Intravenous gamma-globulin (IVGG) 2 gm/kg as single infusion over 12 hours
PLUS
Aspirin 80–100 mg/kg/day orally in four equally divided doses until patient is afebrile
THEN
3–5 mg/kg orally once daily up to 6–8 weeks*

* Discontinue 6–8 weeks after onset of illness if no coronary artery abnormalities are present by echocardiography. Continue indefinitely if there are coronary artery abnormalities.

ness. Many children with Kawasaki disease fail to achieve therapeutic serum concentrations of salicylate despite high oral dosage because of impaired gastrointestinal absorption.[120,121] Therefore, monitoring of serum salicylate levels is advisable.

All children diagnosed with Kawasaki disease within 10 days of onset of fever should receive intravenous gamma-globulin and high-dose aspirin as early as possible.[100] Trials comparing single with multiple dose gamma-globulin schedules favor the former.[122,123] Intravenous gamma-globulin reduces the likelihood of development of giant coronary artery aneurysms and appears to have a direct beneficial effect on abnormalities in cardiac function associated with the acute phase of Kawasaki disease. Intravenous gamma-globulin should also be considered for patients in whom a diagnosis of Kawasaki disease is made after day 10 of the illness if they have signs of ongoing inflammation or evolving coronary artery disease. Also, some patients already have coronary arterial abnormalities within 10 days of onset of fever. These patients should receive aspirin and intravenous gamma-globulin. It should be recognized that the mechanism of action of intravenous gamma-globulin in Kawasaki disease is unknown. Although the costs of intravenous gamma-globulin are high, studies have shown that lower rates of coronary artery involvement result in lower overall medical costs.[124]

In some patients with acute coronary thrombosis, especially those with giant coronary aneurysms, intracoronary thrombolytic therapy may prevent total occlusion of the artery.[125] The prognosis of children with vascular involvement should be guarded[125a]; some are candidates for percutaneous transluminal coronary angioplasty, bypass grafting, and cardiac transplantation.[126–128] The patency rate of saphenous vein grafts is generally unsatisfactory; bypasses using the internal mammary artery and gastroepiploic artery grafts appear to offer better long-term patency and growth in caliber than saphenous vein grafts.[129]

The approach to follow-up of patients with coronary involvement employs the judicious use of exercise testing,[129a] echocardiography, and radionuclide and angiographic studies to detect and evaluate occlusive lesions.

Anthracycline Toxicity
(See also p. 1800)

Anthracycline drugs such as doxorubicin and daunorubicin and the newer derivatives, used as cancer chemotherapeutic agents, cause a dose-related cardiomyopathy.[130,131] The risk of cardiac involvement increases significantly with doses in excess of 400 mg/m². The onset of cardiac symptoms often is delayed, occurring 2 to 3 months after the anthracycline dose. Cardiac dysfunction usually presents first as unexplained tachycardia, progressing to dyspnea, congestive heart failure, hepatomegaly, and, often, death. The cardiomyopathy most often is reversible only in its early stages.[132] Later, it usually is poorly responsive to digitalis, diuretics, and afterload-reducing agents. Quite often patients are in remission from their neoplasm when the drug's cardiotoxicity proves lethal. Sequential monitoring of cardiac function of patients undergoing chemotherapy allows identification of subclinical cardiotoxicity.[131] Guidelines have been formulated for cardiac monitoring for both modifying therapy and long-term assessment (Fig. 31–8).[131] Long-term follow-up has disclosed ele-

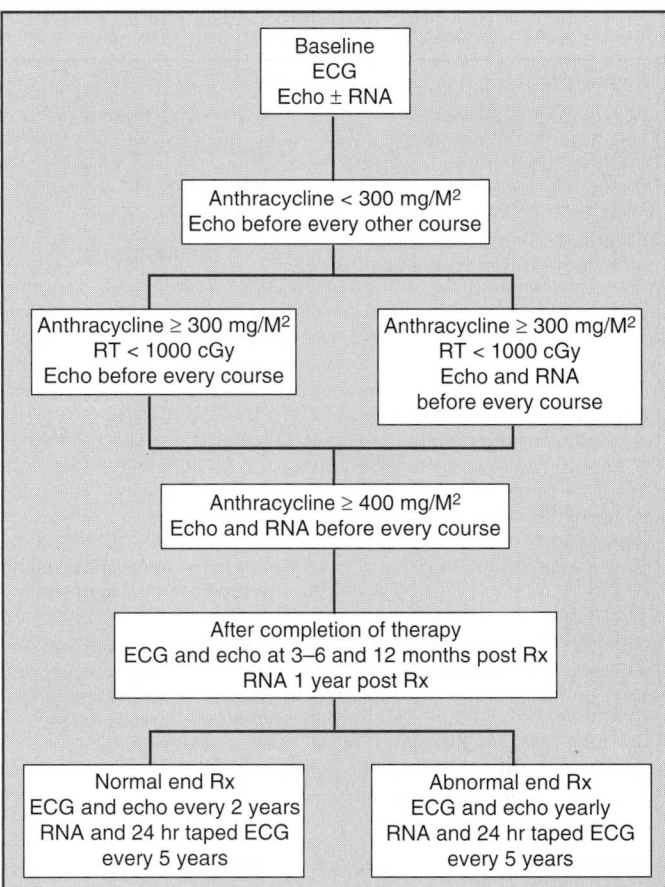

FIGURE 31–8. The monitoring of patients receiving anthracycline. ECG = electrocardiogram; Echo = echocardiogram; RNA = radionuclide angiocardiogram; RT = radiation therapy; Rx = therapy. (From Steinherz, L. J., Graham, T., Hurwitz, R., et al.: Guidelines for cardiac monitoring of children during and after anthracycline therapy: Report of the Cardiology Committee of the Children's Cancer Study Group. Pediatrics 89:942–949, 1992. Copyright American Academy of Pediatrics, 1992.)

vated levels of left ventricular wall stress and impairment of diastolic function in children without overt cardiomyopathy. Further, there are occasional reports of late-onset heart failure in previously asymptomatic children many years after their cancer chemotherapy.

SYSTEMIC HYPERTENSION
(See also p. 822)

Unfortunately, many physicians consider hypertension a disease of adults and not children. Thus, all too frequently, blood pressure is not recorded during the pediatric physical examination. It should be emphasized that elevations in systemic blood pressure may occur in as many as 2 per cent of children, and it has been well documented that undetected or untreated hypertension may lead to unfortunate consequences.[133] Three points in particular require recognition[134]:

1. Causes of hypertension in infants and children differ markedly from those in adults. Most children have secondary rather than essential forms of hypertension (Table 31–5); therefore, it is important to search for a remedial cause.

2. Offspring of hypertensive parents are known to have an increased susceptibility to blood pressure elevation.

3. Children with elevated blood pressure require the same surveillance and treatment as adults.

Accurate blood pressure measurements require cuffs of different sizes because of the variation in arm size from infancy through adolescence. To measure blood pressure

TABLE 31–5   CONDITIONS AND DRUGS ASSOCIATED WITH HYPERTENSION IN INFANTS AND CHILDREN

CONGENITAL	*ACQUIRED, RENAL*
Coarctation of the aorta	Unilateral hydronephrosis
Gonadal dysgenesis (Turner syndrome)	Unilateral pyelonephritis
Rubella syndrome	Renal trauma
Pseudoxanthoma elasticum (Ehlers-Danlos syndrome)	Renal tumors
Ask-Upmark syndrome (segmental renal artery dysplasia)	Unilateral multicystic kidney
	Unilateral ureteral occlusion
Renal arterial abnormalities	Renal artery stenosis
Multiple systemic and pulmonary artery stenoses	Renal arteritis
Solitary renal cyst	Fibromuscular dysplasia of the renal artery
Hydronephrosis	Renal fistula
GENETIC	Renal artery aneurysm
Diabetes mellitus	Chronic pyelonephritis superimposed on abnormal kidneys
Neurofibromatosis (von Recklinghausen's disease)	
Adrenogenital syndrome	Nephritis: shunt nephritis, acute poststreptococcal disease, anaphylactoid purpura, disseminated lupus erythematosus
Pheochromocytoma	
Polycystic kidney disease (infantile and adult forms)	
Familial nephritis (Alport syndrome)	Renal tuberculosis
Little syndrome	Renal cortical necrosis: hemolytic uremic syndrome; sepsis
Fabry's disease (angiokeratoma corporis diffusum)	
Familial dysautonomia (Riley-Day syndrome)	Renal vein thrombosis
Essential hypertension	Radiation nephritis
Tuberous sclerosis with angiolipomas	Postrenal transplantation
Primary hyperparathyroidism	*ACQUIRED, OTHER THAN RENAL*
Porphyria	Hyperthyroidism
PHARMACOLOGICAL	Retrosternal goiter
Sympathomimetics: ephedrine, epinephrine, isoproterenol	Guillain-Barré syndrome or poliomyelitis
	Cerebral edema
Adrenal steroids	Stevens-Johnson syndrome
Heavy metals: mercury, lead	Neuroblastoma
Licorice	Hypercalcemia or hypernatremia
	Adrenal adenoma or hyperplasia: primary aldosteronism or Cushing's syndrome
	Hyperuricemic nephropathy
	Burns

Modified from Lieberman, E.: Diagnostic evaluation of hypertensive children. Pediatr. Ann. *6*:390, 1977.

correctly, width of the inner rubber cuff bladder should be 40 per cent of the circumference of the upper arm or thigh while leaving the antecubital or popliteal fossa free. A cuff that is too small is likely to produce spuriously high readings. In infants under age 2 years the flush technique may be used, although a Doppler instrument is preferred.[135] Because disappearance of the Korotkoff sound may cause underestimation of the diastolic pressure, both muffling (the fourth phase of the Korotkoff sound) and disappearance (fifth phase) should be recorded. The fourth phase is the more accurate measure of diastolic pressure in most prepubertal children; beyond adolescence the fifth phase sound more closely reflects diastolic pressure.[136]

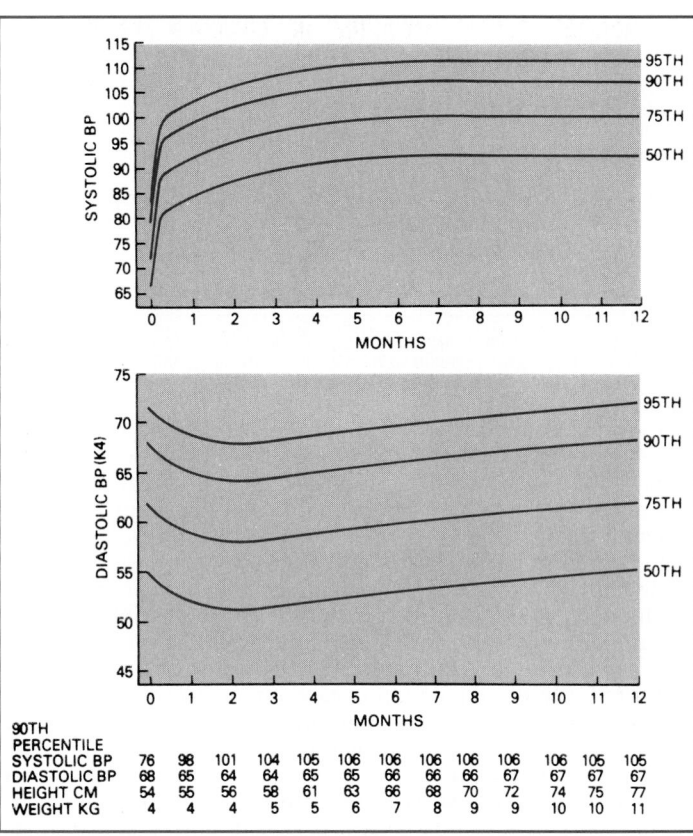

90TH PERCENTILE													
SYSTOLIC BP	76	98	101	104	105	106	106	106	106	106	106	105	105
DIASTOLIC BP	68	65	64	64	65	65	66	66	66	67	67	67	67
HEIGHT CM	54	55	56	58	61	63	66	68	70	72	74	75	77
WEIGHT KG	4	4	4	5	5	6	7	8	9	9	10	10	11

FIGURE 31–9. Age-specific percentiles of blood pressure measurements in girls—birth to 12 months of age. Korotkoff phase IV used for diastolic blood pressure. (From Horan, M. J., et al.: Report of the second task force on blood pressure control in children—1987. Pediatrics *79*:1, 1987. Copyright American Academy of Pediatrics, 1987.)

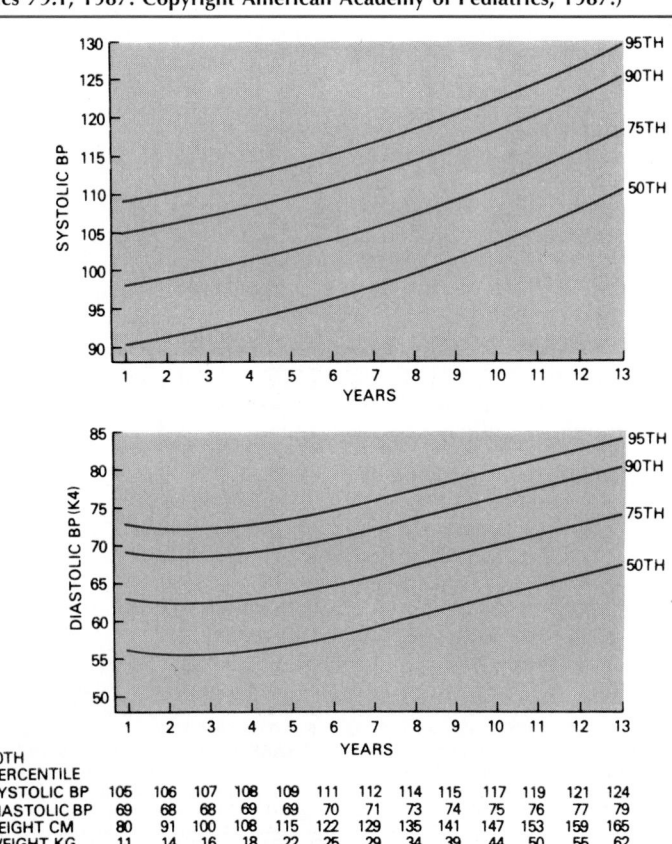

90TH PERCENTILE													
SYSTOLIC BP	105	106	107	108	109	111	112	114	115	117	119	121	124
DIASTOLIC BP	69	68	68	69	69	70	71	73	74	75	76	77	79
HEIGHT CM	80	91	100	108	115	122	129	135	141	147	153	159	165
WEIGHT KG	11	14	16	18	22	25	29	34	39	44	50	55	62

FIGURE 31–10. Age-specific percentiles of blood pressure measurements in boys—1 to 13 years of age. Korotkoff phase IV used for diastolic blood pressure. (From Horan, M. J., et al.: Report of the second task force on blood pressure control in children—1987. Pediatrics *79*:1, 1987. Copyright American Academy of Pediatrics, 1987.)

NORMAL BLOOD PRESSURE IN CHILDREN. The normal ranges of blood pressure relative to age are shown in Figures 31–9 through 31–13 and serve as a guide in judging unsafe levels. Because considerable variation exists in most children's pressures, it should be recognized that a single blood pressure recording at or higher than the 90th percentile at a single point in time may not be an abnormal finding. In an apparently healthy child measurements should be repeated serially; further investigation is warranted if the blood pressure persists at or above the 90th percentile.[137,138] In contrast, definite or severe hypertension (i.e., pressures repeatedly well beyond the broad limits of normal) requires prompt investigation and treatment.[139,140] Particularly urgent attention must be paid to those children whose systolic and diastolic pressures are remarkably high (i.e., equal to or greater than 180 and 110 mm Hg, respectively). Other findings identifying the patient at acute risk include localized neurological signs and/or generalized seizures; blurred vision or such eye ground changes as retinal hemorrhage, exudate, papilledema, or retinal arterial constriction; renal or abdominal pain; evidence of left ventricular hypertrophy or cardiac decompensation; renal dysfunction; palpation of an abdominal mass or enlargement of the kidneys; or auscultation of an abdominal bruit.

ASSESSMENT. Evaluation of the asymptomatic child or adolescent with a blood pressure level above the 90th percentile on three or more occasions includes a careful history focusing on conditions or drugs known to be associated with or to predispose to high blood pressure. These include oral contraceptives (see p. 823), use of glucocorticoids, renal disease, and symptoms that suggest aldosteronism (see p. 827) (i.e., spells, weakness, polyuria, muscle cramps) or pheochromocytoma (see p. 1897) (i.e., excessive sweating, palpitations). The family history should be re-

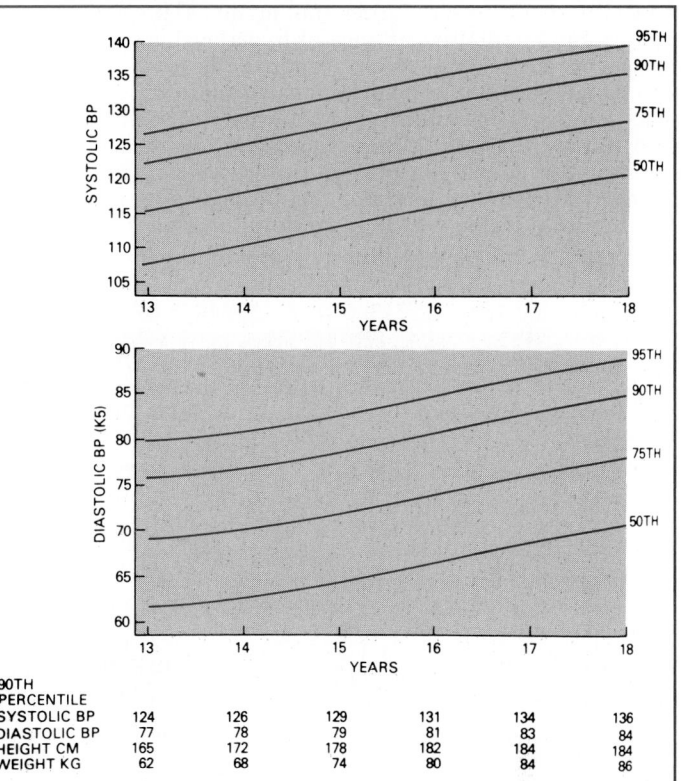

90TH PERCENTILE						
SYSTOLIC BP	124	126	129	131	134	136
DIASTOLIC BP	77	78	79	81	83	84
HEIGHT CM	165	172	178	182	184	184
WEIGHT KG	62	68	74	80	84	86

FIGURE 31–12. Age-specific percentiles of blood pressure measurements in boys—13 to 18 years of age. Korotkoff phase V used for diastolic blood pressure. (From Horan, M. J., et al.: Report of the second task force on blood pressure control in children—1987. Pediatrics 79:1, 1987. Copyright American Academy of Pediatrics, 1987.)

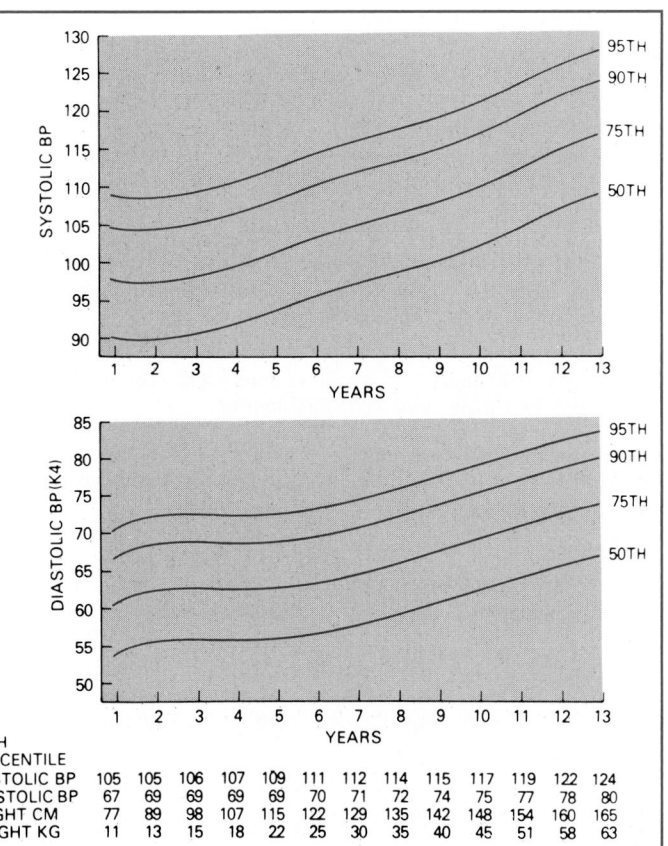

90TH PERCENTILE													
SYSTOLIC BP	105	105	106	107	109	111	112	114	115	117	119	122	124
DIASTOLIC BP	67	69	69	69	69	70	71	72	74	75	77	78	80
HEIGHT CM	77	89	98	107	115	122	129	135	142	148	154	160	165
WEIGHT KG	11	13	15	18	22	25	30	35	40	45	51	58	63

FIGURE 31–11. Age-specific percentiles of blood pressure measurements in girls—1 to 13 years of age. Korotkoff phase IV used for diastolic blood pressure. (From Horan, M. J., et al.: Report of the second task force on blood pressure control in children—1987. Pediatrics 79:1, 1987. Copyright American Academy of Pediatrics, 1987.)

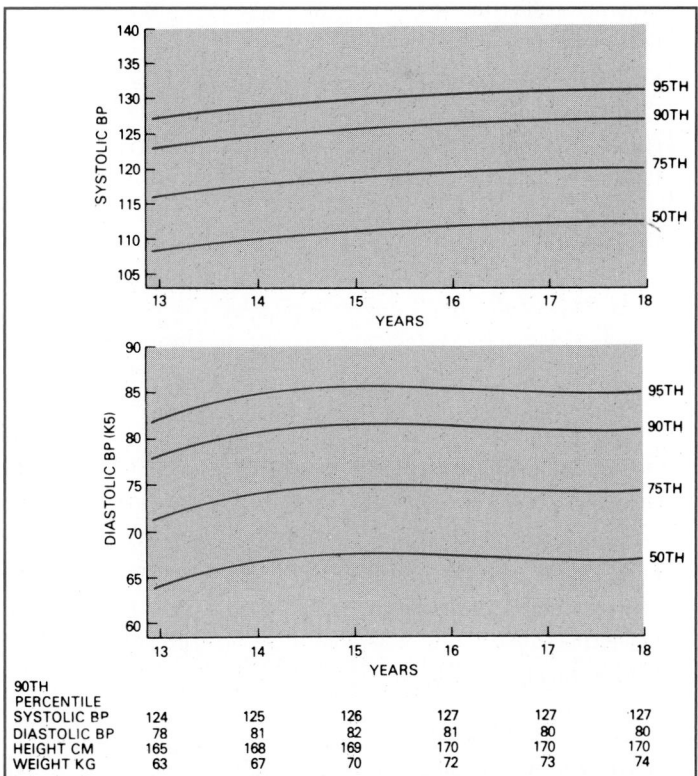

90TH PERCENTILE						
SYSTOLIC BP	124	125	126	127	127	127
DIASTOLIC BP	78	81	82	81	80	80
HEIGHT CM	165	168	169	170	170	170
WEIGHT KG	63	67	70	72	73	74

FIGURE 31–13. Age-specific percentiles of blood pressure measurements in girls—13 to 18 years of age. Korotkoff phase V used for diastolic blood pressure. (From Horan, M. J., et al.: Report of the second task force on blood pressure control in children—1987. Pediatrics 79:1, 1987. Copyright American Academy of Pediatrics, 1987.)

viewed for eclampsia during the mother's pregnancy as well as any familial occurrence of hypertension, premature coronary artery disease, stroke, or renal failure.

Common *symptoms* in hypertensive children are headache, nausea and vomiting, loss of appetite, epistaxis, and palpitation. A dietary history should be obtained with an emphasis on sodium intake. The *physical examination* is directed at detecting conditions associated with secondary hypertension (Table 31–5) and finding evidence of target organ damage on funduscopic and cardiac examination. Typically, the physical findings in hypertensive disorders in children reflect the underlying cause of the elevated pressure; distinctive physical findings accompany many of the conditions listed in Table 31–5 (see also Chap. 26).

LABORATORY STUDIES. These are aimed primarily at identifying secondary causes of hypertension.[139] The minimal laboratory tests required are a urinalysis, complete blood count, serum electrolytes, blood urea nitrogen, serum

TABLE 31–6 DOSAGES OF DRUGS COMMONLY USED IN PEDIATRIC CARDIOLOGY

DRUG	ROUTE OF ADMINISTRATION	DOSAGE
Acetaminophen (Tylenol)	PO or PR	<1 year 60 mg (q4h); 1 to 3 years 120 mg (q4h); >3 years 120 to 240 mg (q4h)
Acetylsalicylic acid (aspirin)	PO or PR	30 to 100 mg/kg/day (q4h)
ε-Aminocaproic acid (Amicar)	IV	Total 100 mg/kg/dose (q6h)
Aminophylline	PO, PR, or IV	12 mg/kg/day (q6h)
Amiodarone	PO	10 mg/kg/day for 10 to 14 days, then 5 mg/kg/day for 1 to 2 mo, then 2.5 mg/kg/day
Ammonium chloride	PO	75 mg/kg/day (q6h)
Atropine	IV, SC, or PO	0.01 to 0.03 mg/kg (q4–6h)
Bicarbonate sodium	IV	1 to 2 mEq/kg/5 min
Bishydroxycoumarin (Dicumarol)	PO	Loading dose: 50 to 100 mg Maintenance: 10 to 50 mg/day (regulate according to prothrombin times)
Bretylium	IV	5 mg/kg/dose over 10 minutes, then 50 to 100 μg/kg/min
Calcium chloride	IV	1 to 4 ml of 10% solution; for cardiac arrest, 10 mg/kg/dose
Calcium gluconate	IV PO	2 to 6 ml of 10% solution; for cardiac arrest, 10 mg/kg/dose 500 mg/kg/day (q6h)
Captopril	PO	0.1 to 0.4 mg/kg/day (infants) 0.5 to 1.0 mg/kg/day (q8h) (children)
Chlorothiazide (Diuril)	PO	20 to 40 mg/kg/day (q12h)
Chlorthalidone	PO	1 to 2 mg/kg/day (q12h)
Cholestyramine (Questran)	PO	250 to 1500 mg/kg/day (q6–12h)
Clonidine (Catapres)	PO	0.002 to 0.008 mg/kg/day in divided doses
Codeine	PO	0.5 to 1.5 mg/kg/dose (q3h)
Dexamethasone (Decadron)	IV	0.2 to 0.5 mg/kg/dose (q6h) for cerebral edema
Diazoxide	IV	1 to 3 mg/kg/dose over 30 sec (q2–6h) (careful of severe hypotension)

Digitalis (Digoxin)		Loading dose:
		  Premature infants 0.01–0.02 mg/kg IV or IM
		  Term infants
		    Parenteral:
		      Up to 4 wk: 0.03 mg/kg; 4 wk to 12 mo: 0.035 mg/kg; over 12 mo: 0.040 mg/kg; beyond 2 yr: 0.03 mg/kg
		
		  Oral: Approximately 20% greater than IV dose
		Maintenance: ⅓ to ¼ of loading dose, given in two divided doses/24 hr

Digoxin immune Fab fragments (Ovine)	IV	0.6 mg digoxin bound by 40 mg Fab fragments
Dobutamine	IV	2 to 15 μg/kg/min
Dopamine	IV	1 gm in 250 ml D₅W; 2 to 20 μg/kg/min
Edrophonium chloride (Tensilon)	IV	0.05 to 0.2 mg/kg/dose
Enalapril maleate (Vasotec)	PO	0.1 to 0.4 mg/kg/day
Ephedrine sulfate	IM or PO	0.8 to 1.6 mg/kg/day (q6h)
Epinephrine (Adrenalin)	IV	For cardiac arrest: single dose: 0.1 to 1.0 ml of 1:1000; 0.1 to 1.0 μg/min infusion
Ethacrynic acid (Edecrin)	IV	1.0 mg/kg/day
Ethylenediaminetetraacetic acid (EDTA) disodium salt	IV	20 mg/ml: 10 to 50 mg/kg (q12h)
Flecainide acetate (Tambocor)	PO	3 to 6 mg/kg/day (q8h)
Furosemide (Lasix)	IV or IM PO	1 to 2 mg/kg/dose 1 to 4 mg/kg/day
Glucagon	IV	0.05 to 0.10 mg/kg/hr

DRUG	ROUTE OF ADMINISTRATION	DOSAGE
Glucose 50%	IV	1 mg/kg/dose
Glucose 50% + Insulin	IV	1 gm glucose/kg (50% solution) with insulin, 1 unit/3 gm glucose
Heparin	IV	100 units/kg (q4h)
Hydralazine hydrochloride (Apresoline)	IV PO	0.8 to 3.0 mg/kg/day (q4–6h) 0.75 to 7.5 mg/kg/day (q6–8h)
Hydrochlorothiazide	PO	1 to 3 mg/kg/day (q12h)
Hydrocortisone sodium succinate (Solu-Cortef)	IV	For shock: 50 to 75 mg/kg (q6h)
Indomethacin	IV	0.1 to 0.25 mg/kg/dose (premature, for ductal closure)
Innovar (fentanyl citrate & droperidol)	IV	0.01 to 0.02 ml/kg
Isoproterenol hydrochloride (Isuprel hydrochloride)	IV	0.05 to 0.25 μg/kg/min
Lidocaine (Xylocaine hydrochloride)	IV	Single dose: 1 mg/kg; 10 to 50 μg/kg/min infusion
Magnesium sulfate, 3%	IV	For neonatal seizure: single dose: 2 to 6 ml
Mannitol	IV	For cerebral edema: 1 to 2 gm/kg Repeated doses: 250 mg/kg (q4h) For hemoglobinuria: single dose: 0.5 gm/kg; 5% solution infusion if necessary
Meperidine hydrochloride (Demerol)	IM or IV	1 mg/kg/dose (q3h)
Metaraminol (Aramine metaraminol bitartrate)	IV	Single dose: 0.1 mg/kg or 50 mg/500 ml; titrate to effect infusion
Methyldopa (Aldomet)	PO or IV	10 to 40 mg/kg/day (q6–8h)
Methylprednisolone (Solu-Medrol)	IV	For shock: 30 mg/kg/dose; for cerebral edema: 4 to 5 mg/kg/dose
Mexiletine	PO	4 to 20 mg/kg/day (q8h)
Minoxidil	PO	0.05 to 2.0 mg/kg/day
Morphine sulfate	SC	0.1 to 0.2 mg/kg/dose (q3h)
Naloxone hydrochloride (Narcan)	IM or IV	0.01 to 0.1 mg/kg/dose
Nifedipine (Procardia)	PO	0.25 to 0.5 mg/kg/dose (hypertension) 0.6 to 0.9 mg/kg/day (q6–8h) (hypertrophic cardiomyopathy)
Nitroglycerine	IV	1 to 3 μg/kg/min
Nitroprusside, sodium	IV	0.5 to 0.8 μg/kg/min initial rate; titrate to effect
Norepinephrine (Levophed bitartrate)	IV	0.1 to 1.0 μg/kg/min
Pentobarbital (Nembutal)	PO or IM	2 to 3 mg/kg/dose
Phenobarbital	PO or IM	3 to 5 mg/kg/day (q8h)
Phenoxybenzamine	IV	0.5 to 1.0 mg/kg
Phentolamine	IV	0.05 to 0.10 mg/kg
Phenylephrine (Neo-Synephrine hydrochloride)	IV	10 mg/100 ml D_5W; 0.1 to 0.5 μg/kg/min, titrate to effect
Phenytoin (Dilantin)	PO or IV	For seizures: 5 to 10 mg/kg/day (q8h); for arrhythmias: 1 to 5 mg/kg/5 min, not to exceed 15 mg/kg
Potassium chloride	PO IV	1 to 4 mEq/kg/day 0.5 mEq/kg/hr not to exceed 2 mEq/kg, as 40 to 80 mEq/liter solution
Potassium gluconate (Kaon) and potassium triplex	PO	1 to 2 mEq/kg/day
Prazosin HCl (Minipress)	PO	25 to 150 μg/kg/day (q6h)
Procainamide hydrochloride (Pronestyl)	PO IM IV	15 to 50 mg/kg/day (q4–6h), not to exceed 4 g/day 20 to 30 mg/kg (q6h) 2 to 6 mg/kg/dose over 5 min, maintenance 20 to 80 μg/kg/min
Promethazine	PO	0.5 to 2 mg/kg/day (q6–8h)

Table continues on following page

DRUG	ROUTE OF ADMINISTRATION	DOSAGE
Propranolol hydrochloride (Inderal)	PO	1.0 to 6.0 mg/kg/day (divided q6h)
	IV	0.01 to 0.15 mg/kg (q6–8h)
	IM	0.5 to 1.0 mg/kg (q4–6h)
Prostaglandin E$_1$	IV	0.1 μg/kg/min, reduce to 0.01 μg/kg/min to maintain effect
Protamine sulfate	IV	1 mg for every 100 units of heparin
Quinidine gluconate	IV	2 to 10 mg/kg/dose (q3–6h), not recommended
Quinidine sulfate	PO	15 to 60 mg/kg/dose (q6h)
Sodium polystyrene sulfonate (Kayexalate)	PO, PR	1 gm/kg mixed with sorbitol
Spironolactone (Aldactone)	PO	1 to 3 mg/kg/day (q6–12h)
Succinylcholine chloride (Anectine chloride)	IV	1 to 2 mg/kg dose
Tolazoline (Priscoline)	IV	1 mg/kg/dose, then 1 to 3 mg/kg/hr
Triamterene (Dyrenium)	PO	2–4 mg/kg/day
Trimethaphan camsylate (Arfonad)	IV	50 mg in 100 ml D$_5$W, titrate to effect
Tris buffer (THAM) (Tromethamine)	IV	(0.3M) weight (kg) × base deficit = dose in ml
Tubocurarine chloride (curare)	IM or IV	Initial dose: 0.3 to 0.5 mg/kg; subsequent dose: 0.1 mg/kg
Verapamil (Isopten)	IV	0.1 to 0.2 mg/kg/dose over 2 min
Vitamin K (AquaMEPHYTON)	IM or IV	Single dose (neonate): 1 mg
Warfarin sodium crystalline (Coumadin)	PO or IM	Initial dose: 0.5 mg/kg Maintenance: 1 to 5 mg/day (regulate according to prothrombin times)

creatinine, uric acid, echocardiogram, electrocardiogram, and chest roentgenogram. Because the most common cause of secondary hypertension in children is renal disease, evaluation often proceeds to include plasma renin activity with 24-hour urinary sodium excretion[141] or plasma renin in response to captopril (see p. 827), rapid-sequence intravenous pyelogram, ultrasonography of the kidneys, and isotopic or angiographic analysis of the kidneys and/or their blood supply. Fortunately, most identifiable causes of correctable hypertension in children and adolescents are associated with clinical findings that direct attention to a particular organ system (renal, endocrine, central nervous, and cardiovascular). Less often, hypertension may result from tumors (ganglioneuroma, pheochromocytoma, Wilms', and neuroblastoma) or collagen vascular disease. Laboratory studies should be as specific as possible to avoid an unselected analysis of every organ system theoretically associated with hypertension. In general, the younger the child and the higher the blood pressure elevation, the more vigorous should be the laboratory evaluation. It should be recognized that although essential hypertension often is a diagnosis by exclusion in prepubertal children, it is a viable diagnosis, particularly in adolescents.[137,142,143] In the author's opinion the need for extensive laboratory investigations has been overemphasized in children or adolescents with mild sustained elevations in blood pressure.

MANAGEMENT. Asymptomatic children and adolescents with borderline or only mildly elevated blood pressure (<5 to 10 mm Hg beyond the 90th percentile values for age) may not require antihypertensive pharmacological agents but should receive counseling regarding weight control, salt abuse, and avoidance of agents with pressor effects (e.g., caffeine, some bronchoconstrictors, nicotine). These patients should be encouraged to be physically active, especially in exercises improving cardiovascular fitness. Isometric or static exercise such as wrestling and weight lifting should be avoided, especially in children with evidence of left ventricular hypertrophy. If the latter exists or if these conservative measures do not result in normalization of

blood pressure, treatment with antihypertensive drugs is indicated.

Drug therapy (Table 31–6) is aimed at prescribing the least complex regimen with the fewest side effects (see also Chap. 27). Pharmacological management is usually undertaken if diastolic blood pressure is greater than 85 mm Hg in children less than age 12 years, and greater than 90 mm Hg in children older than 12 years. If left ventricular hypertrophy is evident by echocardiogram, drug treatment is advisable at lower diastolic pressures. An oral thiazide diuretic usually is the initial drug of choice and may be combined with a potassium-sparing drug or with a dietary regimen that provides adequate potassium. If blood pressure control is not achieved, an angiotensin-converting en-

TABLE 31–7 FASTING LIPID AND LIPOPROTEIN LEVELS (mg/dl) IN CHILDREN BY AGE

	MALES			FEMALES		
	5%	50%	95%	5%	50%	95%
Cholesterol						
0–4 yr	114	155	203	112	156	200
5–9 yr	121	160	203	126	164	205
10–14 yr	119	158	202	124	160	201
15–19 yr	113	150	197	120	158	203
Triglycerides						
0–4 yr	29	56	98	34	64	112
5–9 yr	30	56	101	32	60	105
10–14 yr	32	66	125	37	75	131
15–19 yr	37	78	148	39	75	132
HDL Cholesterol						
5–9 yr	38	56	74	36	53	73
10–14 yr	37	55	74	37	52	70
15–19 yr	30	46	63	35	52	74
LDL Cholesterol						
5–9 yr	63	93	129	68	100	140
10–14 yr	64	100	140	68	97	132
15–19 yr	62	94	130	59	96	137

Data from Lipid Research Clinics: Population Studies Data Book. Dept. of Health and Human Services (NIH) 80-1527, Vol. I: The Prevalence Study.

zyme inhibitor may be added to the regimen. Occasionally it is necessary to use a beta-adrenergic blocking agent such as atenolol, a calcium channel blocker such as nifedipine, or a central sympathetic inhibitor such as clonidine.

Acute, life-threatening episodes of hypertension occur rarely and in a variety of clinical situations.[144] Encephalopathy is the most severe complication of an acute hypertensive crisis; its presence demands immediate lowering of the systemic arterial blood pressure. Diazoxide is the agent of choice as a first drug for the patient with encephalopathy. If diazoxide is ineffective, catecholamine-producing tumors must be suspected and consideration given to using alpha-adrenergic blocking agents such as phentolamine or phenoxybenzamine. Sodium nitroprusside usually is considered the agent to be administered when all others have failed. If a cause for sustained hypertension has been detected, medical and/or surgical treatment should be directed at the underlying disease process.

The importance of prevention of arteriosclerosis in childhood is widely accepted.[145,146] Hyperlipidemic children are at high risk of becoming hyperlipidemic adults and are therefore at greater risk of future atherosclerotic disease.[147,148] Although opinions vary about the feasibility of maintaining low serum lipid levels in normal children by dietary modification, there is consensus that children whose serum cholesterol or triglyceride levels are beyond the 95th percentile for their age and gender should be treated. Guidelines for abnormal levels in the first two decades of life are provided in Table 31–7.

Controversy exists concerning the value of selective versus universal cholesterol and lipid screening strategies for children.[147–151] The National Cholesterol Education Pro-

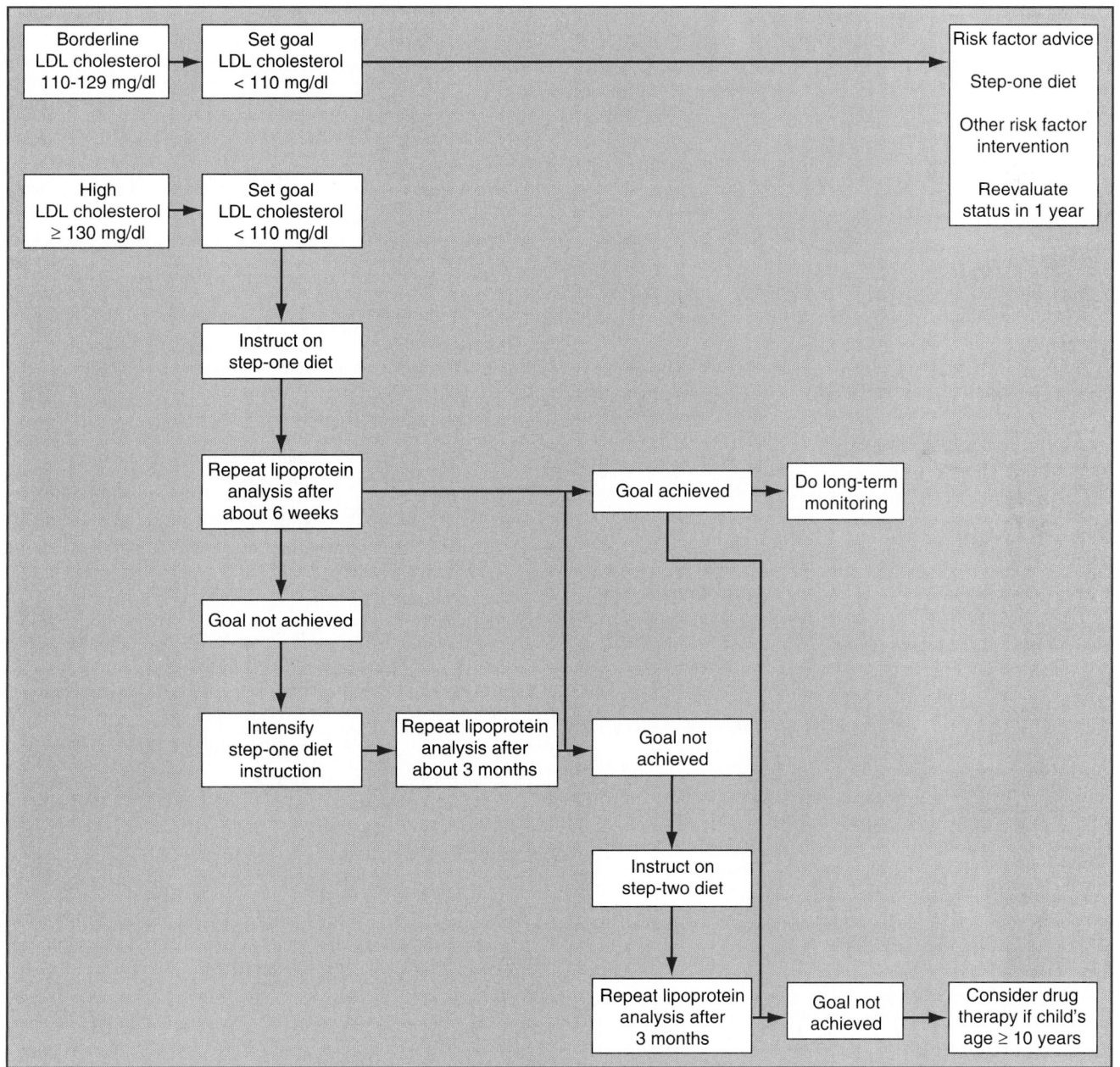

FIGURE 31–14. The National Cholesterol Education Program recommendation for dietary treatment of hypercholesterolemia in children. LDL = low density lipoprotein. (From The Report of the Expert Panel on Blood Cholesterol Levels in Children and Adolescents. Pediatrics 89:525–584, 1992. Copyright American Academy of Pediatrics, 1992.)

gram recommendations for management of hypercholesterolemia in children is shown in Fig. 31–14. In the author's opinion, as part of routine pediatric practice, a careful family history of cardiovascular disease should be obtained and all children should have a random nonfasting cholesterol test performed. If the cholesterol level exceeds 200 mg/dl, a lipid profile should be obtained and, if the LDL cholesterol exceeds 130 mg/dl, appropriate therapy should be instituted. Serum lipid levels should be analyzed at regular intervals in all children from families with hyperlipidemia or with histories that include hypertension, myocardial infarction, stroke, or peripheral vascular disease among parents or grandparents before age 50.[145,150] Differentiation is necessary between acquired hyperlipidemia and one of the familial, and presumably genetic, hyperlipidemias.[152]

Homozygous familial hypercholesterolemia causes severe atherosclerosis of the coronary arteries and myocardial infarction in childhood; rarely it causes atherosclerosis of the aortic valve, leading to critical aortic stenosis that requires surgical treatment.[153]

REFERENCES

NONRHEUMATIC INFLAMMATORY DISEASE

1. Ainger, L. E., Lawyer, N. G., and Fitch, C. W.: Neonatal rubella myocarditis. Br. Heart J. 28:691, 1966.
2. Ayuthya, T. S. N., Jayavasu, J., and Pongpanich, B.: Coxsackie group B virus in primary myocardial disease in infants and children. Am. Heart J. 88:311, 1974.
3. Lerner, A. M., and Wilson, F. M.: Virus myocardiopathy. Progr. Med. Virol. 15:63, 1973.
4. Maisch, B., Drude, L., Hengstenberg, C., et al.: Cytolytic anticardiac membrane antibodies in the pathogenesis of myopericarditis. Postgrad. Med. J. 68(Suppl. 1):S11, 1992.
5. Oda, T., Hamamoto, K., and Morinaga, H.: Clinical aspects of nonrheumatic myocarditis in children. Jpn. Circ. J. 43:443, 1979.
6. Wink, K., and Schmitz, H.: Cytomegalovirus myocarditis. Am. Heart J. 100:667, 1980.
7. Arita, M., Ueno, Y., and Masuyama, Y.: Complete heart block in mumps myocarditis. Br. Heart J. 46:342, 1981.
8. O'Connell, J. B.: Gallium-67 imaging in patients with dilated cardiomyopathy and biopsy proven myocarditis. Circulation 70:58, 1984.
9. Kao, C-H., Hsieh, K-S., Wang, Y-L., and Wang, S-J.: The use of technetium-99m hexamethylpropylene amine oxime labelled white blood cells to detect subclinical inflammation of the heart after cardiopulmonary bypass in children with congenital heart disease. Eur. J. Nucl. Med. 19:960, 1992.
10. Gagliardi, M. G., Bevilacqua, M., DiRenzi, P., et al.: Usefulness of magnetic resonance imaging for diagnosis of acute myocarditis in infants and children, and comparison with endomyocardial biopsy. Am. J. Cardiol. 68:1089, 1991.
11. Leatherbury, L., Chandra, R. S., Shapiro, S. R., and Perry, L. W.: Value of endomyocardial biopsy of infants, children and adolescents with dilated or hypertrophic cardiomyopathy and myocarditis. J. Am. Coll. Cardiol. 12:1547, 1988.
12. Schmaltz, A. A., Apitz, J., Hort, W., and Maisch, B.: Endomyocardial biopsy in infants and children: Experience in 60 patients. Pediatr. Cardiol. 11:15, 1990.
13. Fisher, L. L., and Fisher, B. A.: Recognition and treatment of viral myocarditis. Primary Cardiol. 16:46, 1990.
14. Yoshizato, T., Edwards, W. D., Alboliras, E. T., et al.: Safety and utility of endomyocardial biopsy in infants, children and adolescents: Our view of 66 procedures in 53 patients. J. Am. Coll. Cardiol. 15:436, 1990.
14a. Martin, A. B., Webber, S., Fricker, F. I., et al.: Acute myocarditis: Rapid diagnosis by PCR in children. Circulation 90:330, 1994.
15. Rezkalla, S. H., and Kolner, R. A.: Management strategies in viral myocarditis. Am. Heart J. 117:706, 1989.
16. Chan, K. Y., Iwahara, M., Benson, L. N., et al.: Immunosuppressive therapy in the management of acute myocarditis in children: A clinical trial. J. Am. Coll. Cardiol. 17:458, 1991.
17. Richardson, P. I., Why, H. J. F., and Archard, L. C.: Virus infection and dilated cardiomyopathy. Postgrad. Med. J. 68(Suppl. 1):S17, 1992.
18. Driucker, N. A., Colan, S. D., Willis, A. B., et al.: δ-globulin treatment of acute myocarditis in the pediatric population. Circulation 89:252, 1994.
19. Taliercio, C. P., Seward, J. B., Driscoll, D. J., et al.: Idiopathic dilated cardiomyopathy in the young: Clinical profile and natural history. J. Am. Coll. Cardiol. 6:1126, 1985.
20. Wittels, B., and Bressler, R. J.: Biochemical lesions of diphtheria toxin in the heart. J. Clin. Invest. 43:630, 1964.
21. Challoner, D. R., and Prols, H. G.: Free fatty acid oxidation and carnitine levels in diphtheritic guinea pig myocardium. J. Clin. Invest. 51:2071, 1972.

22. Ino, T., Sherwood, W. G., Benson, L. N. et al.: Cardiac manifestations and disorders of fat and carnitine metabolism in infancy. J. Am. Coll. Cardiol. 11:1301, 1988.
23. Srivastava, S. C., Puri, D. S., and Lumba, S. T.: An electrocardiographic study of myocarditis and diphtheria. J. Assoc. Phys. India 14:365, 1966.
23a. Stockins, B. A., Lanas, F. T., Saavedra, J. G., et al.: Prognosis in patients with diphtheric myocarditis and bradyarrhythmias: Assessment of results of ventricular pacing. Br. Heart J. 72:190, 1994.
24. Ramos, A., Elias, P., Barrucand, L., and DaSilva, J.: The protective effect of carnitine in human diphtheritic myocarditis. Pediatr. Res. 18:815, 1984.
25. Prata, A.: Chagas' heart disease. Cardiologia 52:79, 1968.
26. Libby, P., Alroy, J., and Pereiro, M. E. A.: A neuraminidase from Trypanosoma cruzi removes sialic acid from the surface of membrane myocardial and endothelial cells. J. Clin. Invest. 77:127, 1986.
27. Breniere, S. F., Bosseno, M. F., Revollo, S., et al.: Direct identification of Trypanosoma cruzi natural clones in vectors and mammalian hosts by polymerase chain reaction amplification. Am. J. Trop. Med. Hyg. 46:335, 1992.
28. Moncayo, A., and Luquetti, A. O.: Multicentre double blind study for the evaluation of Trypanosoma cruzi defined antigens as diagnostic reagents. Mem. Inst. Oswaldo Cruz 85:489, 1990.
29. Quiassi, A., Aguirre, T., Plumas-Marty, B., et al.: Cloning and sequencing of a 24 kDa Trypanosoma cruzi specific antigen released in association with membrane vesicles and defined by a monoclonal antibody. Biol. Cell. 75:11, 1992.
30. Guerra, H. A. C., Palacios-Prue, E., Scorza, C. D., et al.: Clinical, histochemical, and ultrastructural correlation in septal endomyocardial biopsies from chronic chagasic patients: Detection of early myocardial damage. Am. Heart J. 113:716, 1987.
30a. Mady, C., Cardoso, R. H. A., Barreto, A. C. P., et al.: Survival and predictors of survival in patients with congestive heart failure due to Chagas' cardiomyopathy. Circulation 90:3098, 1994.
31. Iosa, D., Massari, D. C., and Dorsey, F. C.: Chagas' cardioneuropathy: Effect of ganglioside treatment in chronic dysautonomic patients—A randomized, double-blind, parallel, placebo controlled study. Am. Heart J. 122:775, 1991.
32. Ginger, A. G., Retyk, E. O., Laino, R. A., et al.: Ventricular tachycardia in Chagas' disease. Am. J. Cardiol. 970:459, 1992.
33. Abramowicz, M. (ed.): Drugs for parasitic infections. In The Medical Letter of Drugs and Therapeutics, Vol. 28 (Issue 706). New Rochelle, The Medical Letter, Inc., January 1986.
34. Urbina, J. A., Maldonado, R. A., Pallares, G., et al.: In vitro and in vivo synergism of binary and ternary combinations of ergosterol biosynthesis inhibitors as antiproliferative agents against Trypanosoma cruzi: Therapeutic implications. Mem. Inst. Oswaldo Cruz 86:33, 1991.
35. Durand, J. B., O'Connell, J. B., and Costanzo-Nordin, M. R.: Specific heart muscle disease. Curr. Opin. Cardiol. 7:445, 1992.
36. Koten, J. W., and DeRaadt, P.: Myocarditis and Trypanosoma rhodesiense infections. Trans. R. Soc. Trop. Med. Hyg. 63:485, 1969.
37. Stewart, J. M., Kaul, A., Gromisch, D. S., et al.: Symptomatic cardiac dysfunction in children with immunodeficiency virus infection. Am. Heart J. 117:140, 1989.
38. Lipshultz, S. E., Chanock, S., Sanders, S. P., et al.: Cardiovascular manifestations of human immunodeficiency virus infection in infants and children. Am. J. Cardiol. 63:1489, 1989.
39. Lipshultz, S. E., Orav, E. J., Sanders, S. P., et al.: Cardiac structure and function in children with human immunodeficiency virus infection treated with zidovudine. N. Engl. J. Med. 327:1260, 1992.
40. Herskowitz, A., Vlahov, D., Willoughby, S., et al.: Prevalence and incidence of left ventricular dysfunction in patients with human immunodeficiency virus infection. Am. J. Cardiol. 71:955–958, 1993.
40a. Domanski, M. J., Sloas, M. M., Follmann, D. A., et al.: Effect of zidovudine and didanosine treatment on heart function in children infected with human immunodeficiency virus. J. Pediatr. 127:137, 1995.
41. Gerber, M. A., and Shapiro, E. D.: Diagnosis of Lyme disease in children. J. Pediatr. 121:157, 1992.
42. Salazar, J. C., Gerber, M. A., and Goff, C. W.: Long-term outcome of Lyme disease in children given early treatment. J. Pediatr. 122:591, 1993.
43. Okoroma, E. O., Terry, L. W., and Scott, L. T.: Acute bacterial pericarditis in children: Report of 25 cases. Am. Heart J. 90:709, 1975.
44. VanReken, D., Strauss, A., Hernandez, A., and Feigin, R. D.: Infectious pericarditis in children. J. Pediatr. 85:165, 1974.
45. Callahan, J. A., Seward, J. B., Nishimura, R. A., et al.: Two dimensional echocardiographically guided pericardiocentesis: Experience in 117 consecutive patients. Am. J. Cardiol. 55:476, 1985.
46. Sagrista-Sauleda, J., Barrabes, J. A., Permanyer-Miralda, G., and Solar-Soler, J.: Purulent pericarditis: Review of a twenty year experience in a general hospital. J. Am. Coll. Cardiol. 22:1661, 1993.
47. Lajos, T. Z., Black, H. E., Cooper, R. G., and Wanka, J.: Pericardial decompression. Ann. Thorac. Surg. 19:47, 1975.
48. Oh, J. K., Hatle, L. K., Seward, J. B., et al.: Diagnostic role of Doppler echocardiography in constrictive pericarditis. J. Am. Coll. Cardiol. 23:154, 1994.
49. Engle, M. A., Ehlers, K. H., O'Laughlin, J. E., et al.: The post-pericardiotomy syndrome: Iatrogenic illness with immunologic and virologic components. In Engle, M. A. (ed.): Pediatric Cardiovascular Disease. Philadelphia, F. A. Davis Co., 1981, p. 381.

50. Clapp, S. K., Garson, J., Jr., Gutgesell, H. P., et al.: Postoperative pericardial effusion and its relation to post-pericardiotomy syndrome. Pediatrics 66:585, 1980.
51. Mason, T. G., Neal, W. A., and DiBartolomeo, A. G.: Elevated antinuclear antibody titers and the postpericardiotomy syndrome. J. Pediatr. 116:403, 1990.
52. Paloheimo, J. A., Van Essen, R., Klemola, E., et al.: Sub-clinical cytomegalovirus infections and cytomegalovirus mononucleosis after open heart surgery. Am. J. Cardiol. 22:624, 1968.
53. Wilson, N. J., Webber, S. A., Patterson, M. W. H., et al.: Double-blind placebo-controlled trial of corticosteroids in children with post pericardiotomy syndrome. Pediatr. Cardiol. 15:62, 1994.
54. Kron, I. L., Rheuban, K., and Nolan, S. P.: Late cardiac tamponade in children. Ann. Surg. 199:173, 1984.
55. Moller, J. N., Lucas, R. V., Adams, P., et al.: Endocardial fibroelastosis: A clinical and anatomic study of 47 patients with emphasis on its relationship to mitral insufficiency. Circulation 30:759, 1964.
56. Haunkoglu, A., Fried, D., and Somekh, E.: Inheritance of familial primary endocardial fibroelastosis. Clin. Pediatr. 25:272, 1986.
57. Taliercio, C. P., Seward, J. B., Driscoll, D. J., et al.: Idiopathic dilated cardiomyopathy in the young: Clinical profile and natural history. J. Am. Coll. Cardiol. 6:1126, 1985.

PRIMARY CARDIOMYOPATHIES

58. Greenwood, R. D., Nadas, A. S., and Fyler, D. C.: The clinical course of primary myocardial disease in infants and children. Am. Heart J. 92:549, 1976.
59. Guntheroth, W. G.: Congestive cardiomyopathy in children. J. Am. Coll. Cardiol. 15:194, 1990.
60. Chen, S., Nouri, S., Balfour, I., et al.: Clinical profile of congestive cardiomyopathy in children. J. Am. Coll. Cardiol. 15:189, 1990.
61. Griffin, M. L., Hernandez, A., Martin, T. C., et al.: Dilated cardiomyopathy in infants and children. J. Am. Coll. Cardiol. 11:139, 1988.
62. Lurie, P. R.: Endocardial fibroelastosis is not a disease. Am. J. Cardiol. 62:468, 1988.
63. Friedman, R. A., Moak, J. P., and Garson, A., Jr.: Clinical course of idiopathic dilated cardiomyopathy in children. J. Am. Coll. Cardiol. 18:152, 1991.
64. Ferencz, C., and Neill, C. A.: Cardiomyopathy in infancy: Observations in an epidemiologic study. Pediatr. Cardiol. 13:65, 1992.
65. Sole, M. J., and Liu, P.: Viral myocarditis: A paradigm for understanding the pathogenesis and treatment of dilated cardiomyopathy. J. Am. Coll. Cardiol. 22(Suppl. A):99A, 1993.
66. Wiles, H. B.: Idiopathic dilated cardiomyopathy and myocarditis in children. Prim. Cardiol. 19:26, 1993.
67. Martino, T. A., Liu, P., and Sole, M. J.: Viral infection and the pathogenesis of dilated cardiomyopathy. Circ. Res. 74:182, 1994.
68. Akagi, T., Benson, L. N., Lightfoot, N. E., et al.: Natural history of dilated cardiomyopathy in children. Am. Heart J. 121:1502, 1991.
69. Lewis, A. B.: Prognostic value of echocardiography in children with idiopathic dilated cardiomyopathy. Am. Heart J. 128:133, 1994.
70. Kimball, T. R., Daniels, S. R., Meyer, R. A., et al.: Left ventricular mass in childhood dilated cardiomyopathy: A possible predictor for selection of patients for cardiac transplantation. Am. Heart J. 122:126,1991.
71. Wiles, H. B., McArthur, P. D., Taylor, A. B., et al.: Prognostic features of children with idiopathic dilated cardiomyopathy. Am. J. Cardiol. 68:1372, 1991.
72. Lewis, A. B., and Chabot, M.: Outcome of infants and children with dilated cardiomyopathy. Am. J. Cardiol. 68:365, 1991.
72a. Lewis, A. B.: Prognostic value of echocardiography in children with Idiopathic dilated cardiomyopathy. Am. Heart J. 128:133, 1994.
72b. Burch, M., Siddiqi, S. A., Celermajer, D. S., et al.: Dilated cardiomyopathy in children: determinants of outcome. Br. Heart J. 72:246, 1994.
72c. Matitiau, A., Perez-Atayde, A., Sanders, S. P., et al.: Infantile dilated cardiomyopathy: Relation of outcome to left ventricular mechanics, hemodynamics, and histology at the time of presentation. Circulation 90:1310, 1994.
73. Gersony, W. M.: The child with dilated cardiomyopathy: Prognostic considerations and management decisions. J. Am. Coll. Cardiol. 18:157, 1991.
74. Lewis, A. B., and Chabot, M.: The effect of treatment with angiotensin-converting enzyme inhibitors on survival of pediatric patients with dilated cardiomyopathy. Pediatr. Cardiol. 14:9, 1993.
75. Latson, L. A.: Captopril in children with cardiomyopathies. Circulation 83:707, 1991.
76. Bengur, A. R., Beekman, R. H., Rocchini, A. P., et al.: Acute hemodynamic effects of captopril in children with a congestive or restrictive cardiomyopathy. Circulation 83:523, 1991.
77. Radley-Smith, R. C., and Yacoub, M.: Long-term results of pediatric heart transplantation. J. Heart Lung Transplant. 11:S277, 1992.
78. Armitage, J. M., Fricker, F. I., Del Nido, P., et al.: A decade (1982–1992) of pediatric cardiac transplantation and the impact of FK-506 immunosuppression. J. Thorac. Cardiovasc. Surg. 105:464, 1993.
79. Carceller, A. M., Maroto, E., and Fouron, J. C.: Dilated and contracted forms of primary endocardial fibroelastosis: A single fetal disease with two stages of development. Br. Heart J. 63:311, 1990.
80. Ino, T., Benson, L. N., Freedom, R. M., and Rowe, R. D.: Endocardial fibroelastosis: Natural history and prognostic risk factors. Am. J. Cardiol. 62:431, 1988.

81. Billingham, M. E.: The safety and utility of endomyocardial biopsy in infants, children and adolescents. J. Am. Coll. Cardiol. 15:443, 1990.
82. Gutgesell, H. P., Speer, M. E., and Rosenberg, H. S.: Characterization of the cardiomyopathy in infants with diabetic mothers. Circulation 51:441, 1980.
83. Trowitzsch, E., Bigalke, U., Gisbertz, R., and Kallfelz, H. C.: Echocardiographic profile of infants of diabetic mothers. Eur. J. Pediatr. 140:441, 1983.
84. Walther, F. J., Siassi, B., King, J., and Wu, P. Y-K.: Cardiac output in infants of insulin-dependent diabetic mothers. J. Pediatr. 107:109, 1985.
85. Miller, E., Hare, J. W., Cloherty, J. P., et al.: Elevated maternal hemoglobin A_{1C} in early pregnancy and major congenital anomalies in infants of diabetic mothers. N. Engl. J. Med. 304:1331, 1981.
86. Deorari, A. K., Saxena, A., Singh, M., and Shrivastava, S.: Echocardiographic assessment of infants born to diabetic mothers. Arch. Dis. Child. 64:721, 1989.
87. Labrune, P. H., Huguet, P., and Odievre, M.: Cardiomyopathy in glycogen-storage disease type III: Clinical and echographic study of 18 patients. Pediatr. Cardiol. 12:161, 1991.
88. Bordiuk, J. N., Logato, M. J., Lovelace, R. E., and Blumenthal, S.: Pompe's disease: Electron myographic, electron microscopic and cardiovascular aspects. Arch. Neurol. 23:113, 1970.
89. Dickenson, E. F., Houlsby, W. T., and Wilkinson, J. L.: Unusual angiographic appearance of the left ventricle in two cases of Pompe's disease (glycogenosis type 2). Br. Heart J. 41:238, 1979.
90. Hwang, G., Meng, C. C., Lin, C. Y., and Hsu, H. C.: Clinical analysis of five infants with glycogen storage disease of the heart—Pompe's disease. Jpn. Heart J. 27:25, 1986.
91. DeDominicis, E., Finocchi, G., Vincenzi, M., et al.: Echocardiographic and pulsed Doppler features in glycogen storage disease type II of the heart (Pompe's disease). Acta Cardiologica 46:107, 1991.
92. Polikar, R., Burger, A. G., Scherrer, U., and Nicod, P.: The thyroid and the heart. Circulation 87:1435, 1993.
93. Sanstead, H. H.: Clinical manifestations of certain vitamin deficiencies. In Goodhart, M. S., and Shils, M. E. (eds.): Modern Nutrition in Health and Disease, 5th ed. Philadelphia, Lea and Febiger, 1973, p. 593.
93a. Fujita, I., Sata, T., Gondo, K., et al.: Cardiac beriberi (Shoshin beriberi) caused by excessive intake of isotonic drink. Acta Paediatr. Jpn. 34:466, 1992.
94. Sanstead, H. H.: Mineral metabolism and protein malnutrition. In Olson, R. E. (ed.): Protein Calorie Malnutrition. New York, Academic Press, 1975, p. 213.
95. Nutter, D. O., Murray, T. G., Heymsfield, S. B., and Fuller, E. O.: The effect of chronic protein-calorie undernutrition in the rate on myocardial function and cardiac function. Circ. Res. 45:144, 1979.
96. Roberts, W. C., and Ferrans, V. J.: Pathological aspects of certain cardiomyopathies. Circ. Res. 34(Suppl. II):II–128, 1974.
97. Roberts, W. C., Buja, L. M., and Ferrans, V. J.: Löffler's fibroplastic parietal endocarditis, eosinophilic leukemia, and Davies' endomyocardial fibrosis: The same disease at different stages? Pathol. Microbiol. 35:90, 1970.
98. Barretto, A. C. P., DaLuz, T. L., Oliveira, S. A., et al.: Determinants of survival in endomyocardial fibrosis. Circulation 80(Suppl. I):177, 1989.
99. Valithan, M. S., Balkrishnan, K. G., Sankarkumar, R., and Kartha, C. C.: Surgical treatment of endomyocardial fibrosis. Ann. Thorac. Surg. 43:68, 1987.
100. Dajani, A. S., Taubert, K. A., Gerber, M. A., et al.: Diagnosis and therapy of Kawasaki disease in children. Circulation 87:1776, 1993.
101. Lin, C. Y., Lin, C. C., Hwang, B., and Chiang, B.: Serial changes of serum interleukin-6, interleukin-8, and tumor necrosis factor alpha among patients with Kawasaki disease. J. Pediatr. 121:924, 1992.
102. Takeshita, S., Kawase, H., Yamamoto, M., et al.: Increased expression of human 63-kD heat shock protein gene in Kawasaki disease determined by quantitative reverse transcription-polymerase chain reaction. Pediatr. Res. 35:179, 1994.
103. Rowley, A., Castro, B., Levy, J., et al.: Failure to confirm the presence of a retrovirus in cultured lymphocytes with Kawasaki syndrome. Pediatr. Res. 29:417, 1991.
104. Hiraishi, S., Yashiro, K., Oguchi, K., and Nakazawa, K.: Clinical course of cardiovascular involvement in the mucocutaneous lymph node syndrome. Am. J. Cardiol. 47:323, 1981.
105. Nakamura, Y., Yanagawa, H., and Kawasaki, T.: Mortality among children with Kawasaki disease in Japan. N. Engl. J. Med. 323:1246, 1992.
106. Kato, H., Ichinose, E., and Kawasaki, T.: Myocardial infarction in Kawasaki disease: Clinical analyses in 195 cases. J. Pediatr. 108:923, 1986.
107. Ishwata, S., Fuse, K., Nishyama, S., et al.: Adult coronary artery disease secondary to Kawasaki disease in childhood. Am. J. Cardiol. 69:692, 1992.
107a. Dajani, A.S., Taubert, K. A., and Takahashi, M.: Guidelines for long-term management of patients with Kawasaki disease. Circulation 89:917, 1994.
108. Nakanishi, T., Takao, A., Nakazawa, M., et al.: Mucocutaneous lymph node syndrome: Clinical, hemodynamic, and angiographic features of coronary obstructive disease. Am. J. Cardiol. 55:6662, 1985.
109. Yoshida, H., Maeda, T., and Taniguchi, N.: Subcostal two-dimensional

echocardiographic imaging of peripheral right coronary artery in Kawasaki disease. Circulation 65:956, 1982.

110. Tsubata, S., Suzuki, A., Ono, Y., et al.: Coronary arterial lesions due to Kawasaki disease: Selective coronary angiography in five cases with difficult-to-detect localized stenosis. Pediatr. Cardiol. 14:169, 1993.

111. Ichida, F., Fatica, N. S., O'Loughlin, J. E., et al.: Correlation of electrocardiographic and echocardiographic changes in Kawasaki disease. Am. Heart. J. 116:812, 1988.

112. Fujiwara, T., Fujiwara, H., Ueda, T., et al.: Comparison of macroscopic, postmortem, angiographic and two-dimensional echocardiographic findings of coronary aneurysms in children with Kawasaki disease. Am. J. Cardiol. 6:199, 1986.

113. Sugimura, T., Kato, H., Inoue, O., et al.: Intravascular ultrasound of coronary arteries in children. Circulation 89:258, 1994.

114. Akagi, T., Rose, V., Benson, L. N., et al.: Outcome of coronary artery aneurysms after Kawasaki disease. J. Pediatr. 121: 689, 1992.

115. Kato, H., Ichinose, E., Matsunaga, S., et al.: Fate of coronary aneurysms in Kawasaki disease: Serial coronary angiography and long-term follow-up study. Am. J. Cardiol. 49:1758, 1982.

116. Suzuki, A., Kamiya, T., Yasuo, O., and Kuroe, K.: Extended long-term follow-up of study of coronary arterial lesions in Kawasaki disease. J. Am. Coll. Cardiol. 17:33A, 1991.

117. Akagi, T., Kato, H., Inoue, O., et al.: Valvular heart disease in Kawasaki syndrome: Incidence and natural history. Am. Heart J. 120:366, 1990.

118. Kosuda, T., and Sone K.: Assessment of left ventricular function in Kawasaki disease by dipyridamole-loading cineventriculography. Am. J. Cardiol. 70:863, 1992.

119. Sugimura, T., Kato, H., Inoue, O., et al.: Vasodilatory response of the coronary arteries after Kawasaki disease: Evaluation by intracoronary injection of isosorbide dinitrate. J. Pediatr. 121:684, 1992.

120. Koren, G., and MacLaod, S. M.: Difficulty in achieving therapeutic serum concentrations of salicylate in Kawasaki's disease. J. Pediatr. 105:991, 1984.

121. Umezawa, T., Matsuo, N., and Saji, T.: Treatment of Kawasaki disease using the intravenous aspirin anti-inflammatory effect of salicylate. Acta Paediatr. Jpn. 34:584, 1992.

122. Newburger, J. W., Takahashi, M., Burns, J. C., et al.: The treatment of Kawasaki syndrome with intravenous gamma globulin. N. Engl. J. Med. 315:341, 1986.

123. Newburger, J. W., Takahashi, M., Beiser, A. S., et al.: A single intravenous infusion of gamma globulin as compared with four infusions in the treatment of acute Kawasaki syndrome. N. Engl. J. Med. 324:1633, 1991.

124. Klassen, T. P., Rowe, P. C., and Gafni, A.: Economic evaluation of intravenous immune globulin therapy for Kawasaki syndrome. J. Pediatr. 122:538, 1993.

125. Kato, H., Inoue, O., Ichinose, E., et al.: Intracoronary urokinase in Kawasaki disease: Treatment and prevention of myocardial infarction. Acta Paediatr. Jpn. 33:27, 1991.

125a. Hijazi, Z. M., Udelson, J. E., Snapper, H., et al.: Physiologic significance of chronic coronary aneurysms in patients with Kawasaki disease. J. Am. Coll. Cardiol. 24:1633, 1994.

126. Ino, T., Nishimoto, K., Akimoto, K., et al.: Percutaneous transluminal coronary angioplasty for Kawasaki disease: A case report and literature review. Pediatr. Cardiol. 12:33, 1991.

127. Kitamura, S.: Surgical management for cardiovascular lesions in Kawasaki disease. Cardiol. Young 1:240, 1991.

128. Travaline, J. M., Hamilton, S. M., Ringle R. E., et al.: Cardiac transplantation for giant coronary artery aneurysms complicating Kawasaki disease. Am. J. Cardiol. 68:560, 1991.

129. Kawachi, K., Kitamura, S., Seki, T., et al.: Hemodynamics and coronary blood flow during exercise after coronary artery bypass grafting with internal mammary arteries in children with Kawasaki disease. Circulation 84:618, 1991.

129a. Pahl, E., Sehgal, R., Chrystof, D., et al.: Feasibility of exercise stress echocardiography for the follow-up of children with coronary involvement secondary to Kawasaki disease. Circulation 91:122, 1995.

130. Lipshultz, S. E., Colan, S. D., Gelber, R. D., et al.: Late cardiac effects of doxorubicin therapy for acute lymphoblastic leukemia in childhood. N. Engl. J. Med. 324:808, 1991.

131. Steinherz, L. J., Graham, T., Hurwitz, R., et al.: Guidelines for cardiac monitoring of children during and after anthracycline therapy: Report of the Cardiology Committee of the Children's Cancer Study Group. Pediatrics 89:942, 1992.

132. Sharkey, A. M., Carey, A. B., Heise, C. T., and Barber, G.: Cardiac rehabilitation after cancer therapy in children and young adults. Am. J. Cardiol. 71:1488, 1993.

SYSTEMIC HYPERTENSION

133. New, M. I., and Levine, L. S.: Hypertension in childhood and adolescence. Cardiovasc. Rev. 3:115, 1982.

134. Lieberman, E.: Diagnostic evaluation of hypertensive children. Pediatr. Ann. 6:390, 1977.

135. Horan, M. J., Falkner, B., Kimm, Y. S., et al.: Report of the second task force on blood pressure control in children—1987. Pediatrics 79:1, 1987.

136. Berenson, G. S., Webber, L. S., and Voors, A. W.: Diagnosing hypertension in children. J. Cardiovasc. Med. 6:273, 1982.

137. Gillman, M. W., Cook, N. R., Rosner, B., et al.: Identifying children at high risk for the development of essential hypertension. J. Pediatr. 122:837, 1993.

138. Gillman, M. W., Rosner, B., Evans, D. A., et al.: Use of multiple visits to increase blood pressure tracking correlations in childhood. Pediatrics 87:708, 1991.

139. Schieken, R. M.: Hypertension and atherosclerosis in children. Curr. Opin. Cardiol. 9:130, 1994.

140. The Fifth Report of the Joint National Committee on Detection. Evaluation, and Treatment of High Blood Pressure. Arch. Intern. Med. 153:154, 1993.

141. Harshfield, G. A., Pulliam, D. A., Albert, B. S., et al.: Ambulatory blood pressure patterns in children and adolescents: Influence of renin-sodium profiles. Pediatrics 87:94, 1991.

142. Daniels, S. R.: Left ventricular mass in childhood essential hypertension. Prim. Cardiol. 18:100, 1992.

143. Lauer, R. M., and Clarke, W. R.: Childhood risk factors for high adult blood pressure: The Muscatine study. Pediatrics 84:633, 1989.

144. Fleischmann, L. E.: Management of hypertensive crises in children. Pediatr. Ann. 6:410, 1977.

HYPERLIPIDEMIAS

145. Schieken, R. M.: The management of the family at high risk for coronary heart disease. In Friedman, W. F., and Talner, N. S. (eds.): Cardiology Clinics: Update in Pediatric Cardiology. Philadelphia, W. B. Saunders Company, Vol. 7, No. 2, 1989, pp. 467–477.

146. Ruttenberg, H. D.: Preventive cardiology in children. In Yanowitz, F. G. (ed.): Coronary Heart Disease Prevention. New York, Marcel Dekker Inc., 1992.

147. Lauer, R. M., Lee, J., and Clarke, W. R.: Factors affecting the relationship between childhood and adult cholesterol levels: The Muscatine study. Pediatrics 82:309, 1988.

148. Wilcken, D. E. L., Wang, X. L., Greenwood, J., and Lynch, J.: Lipioprotein (a) and apolipoproteins B and A-1 in children and coronary vascular events in their grandparents. J. Pediatr. 123:519, 1993.

149. Fuchs, G. J., Farris, R. P., DeWier, M., et al.: Effect of dietary fat on cardiovascular risk factors in infancy. Pediatrics 93:756, 1994.

150. National Cholesterol Education Program: Report of the expert panel on blood cholesterol levels in children and adolescents. National Institutes of Health publication 91-2732. Rockville, MD, U. S. Department of Health and Human Services, 1991.

151. Garcia, R. E., and Moodie, D. S.: Routine cholesterol surveillance in childhood. Pediatrics 84:751, 1989.

152. Breslow, J. L.: Genetic basis of lipoprotein disorders. J. Clin. Invest. 84:373, 1989.

153. Forman, M. B., Kinsley, R. M., DuPlessis, J. P., et al.: Surgical correction of combined supravalvular and valvular aortic stenosis in homozygous familial hypercholesterolemia. S. Afr. Med. J. 1:579, 1982.

Chapter 32
Valvular Heart Disease

EUGENE BRAUNWALD

MITRAL STENOSIS

ETIOLOGY AND PATHOLOGY

The predominant cause of mitral stenosis (MS) is rheumatic fever[1] (see p. 1776). Far less frequently, MS is congenital in etiology,[3] and this form is observed almost exclusively in infants and young children (see p. 923) Very rarely, mitral stenosis is a complication of malignant carcinoid, systemic lupus erythematosus, rheumatoid arthritis,[2] and the mucopolysaccharidoses of the Hunter-Hurley phenotype.[3] Amyloid deposits may occur on rheumatic valves and contribute to the obstruction to left atrial emptying. Methysergide therapy is an unusual but documented cause of MS.[4] MS, generally of rheumatic origin, may be associated with atrial septal defect in Lutembacher's syndrome (see p. 967). Left atrial tumor, particularly myxoma (see p. 1466); ball-valve thrombus in the left atrium (usually associated with MS)[5]; infective endocarditis with large vegetations; and a congenital membrane in the left atrium, i.e., cor triatriatum (see p. 923), may also obstruct left atrial outflow and therefore simulate MS. Although calcification of the mitral annulus usually causes mitral regurgitation (MR), when subvalvular or intravalvular extension is extensive, MS may result.[5] Approximately 25 per cent of all patients with rheumatic heart disease have pure MS, and an additional 40 per cent have combined MS and MR.[6,7] Two-thirds of all patients with rheumatic MS are female.

Rheumatic fever results in four forms of fusion of the mitral valve apparatus leading to stenosis: (1) commissural, (2) cuspal, (3) chordal, and (4) combined.[8] Thickening of the commissures alone occurs in 30 per cent, of the cusps alone in 15 per cent, and of the chordae alone in 10 per cent; in the remainder, thickening of more than one of these structures is involved. Characteristically, mitral valve cusps fuse at their edges, and fusion of the chordae results in thickening and shortening of these structures. The leaflets exhibit fibrous obliteration and revascularization. The stenotic mitral valve is typically funnel-shaped, and the orifice is frequently shaped like a "fish mouth" or buttonhole, with calcium deposits in the valve leaflets sometimes extending to involve the valve ring, which may become quite thick[8] (Fig. 32-1). The thickened leaflets may be so adherent and rigid that they cannot open or shut, reducing or rarely even abolishing the first heart sound (S_1) and leading to combined MS and MR. There is a rough correlation between the severity of calcification and the transvalvular gradient.[8] When rheumatic fever results exclusively or predominantly in contraction and fusion of the chordae tendineae, with little fusion of the valvular commissures, dominant MR results.[9]

It probably takes a minimum of 2 years after the onset of acute rheumatic fever for severe MS to develop, and most patients in temperate climates remain asymptomatic for at least a decade more.[10] Symptoms commence most commonly in the third or fourth decade, although mild MS in the aged is becoming a more frequent finding.[11] In the tropics, particularly in underdeveloped areas, the disease advances more rapidly, and severe MS may be present in early adolescence.[12] The debate continues about whether the anatomical changes in severe MS result from a smoldering rheumatic process or whether, once the valve has been deformed by the initial episode, the constant trauma produced by the turbulent blood flow leads to progressive fibrosis, thickening, and calcification of the valve apparatus.[13]

Enlargement of the left atrium and resultant elevation of the left main stem bronchus, calcification of the left atrial wall, the development of mural thrombi, and obliterative changes in the pulmonary vascular bed (see p. 797) may all result from chronic MS.

PATHOPHYSIOLOGY

In normal adults the cross-sectional area of the mitral valve orifice is 4 to 6 cm². When the orifice is reduced to approximately 2 cm², which is considered to represent mild MS, blood can flow from the left atrium to the left ventricle only if propelled by a small, although abnormal, pressure gradient. When the mitral valve opening is reduced to 1 cm², which is considered to represent critical MS,[12a] a left atrioventricular pressure gradient of approximately 20 mm Hg (and therefore, in the presence of a normal left ventricular diastolic pressure, a mean left atrial pressure of approximately 25 mm Hg) is required to maintain normal cardiac output at rest (Figs. 32-2, p. 1009 and 6-13, p. 194). The elevated left atrial pressure in turn raises pulmonary venous and capillary pressures, resulting in exertional dyspnea. The first bouts of dyspnea in patients with MS are usually precipitated by exercise, emotional stress, sexual intercourse, infection, or atrial fibrillation, all of which **1007**

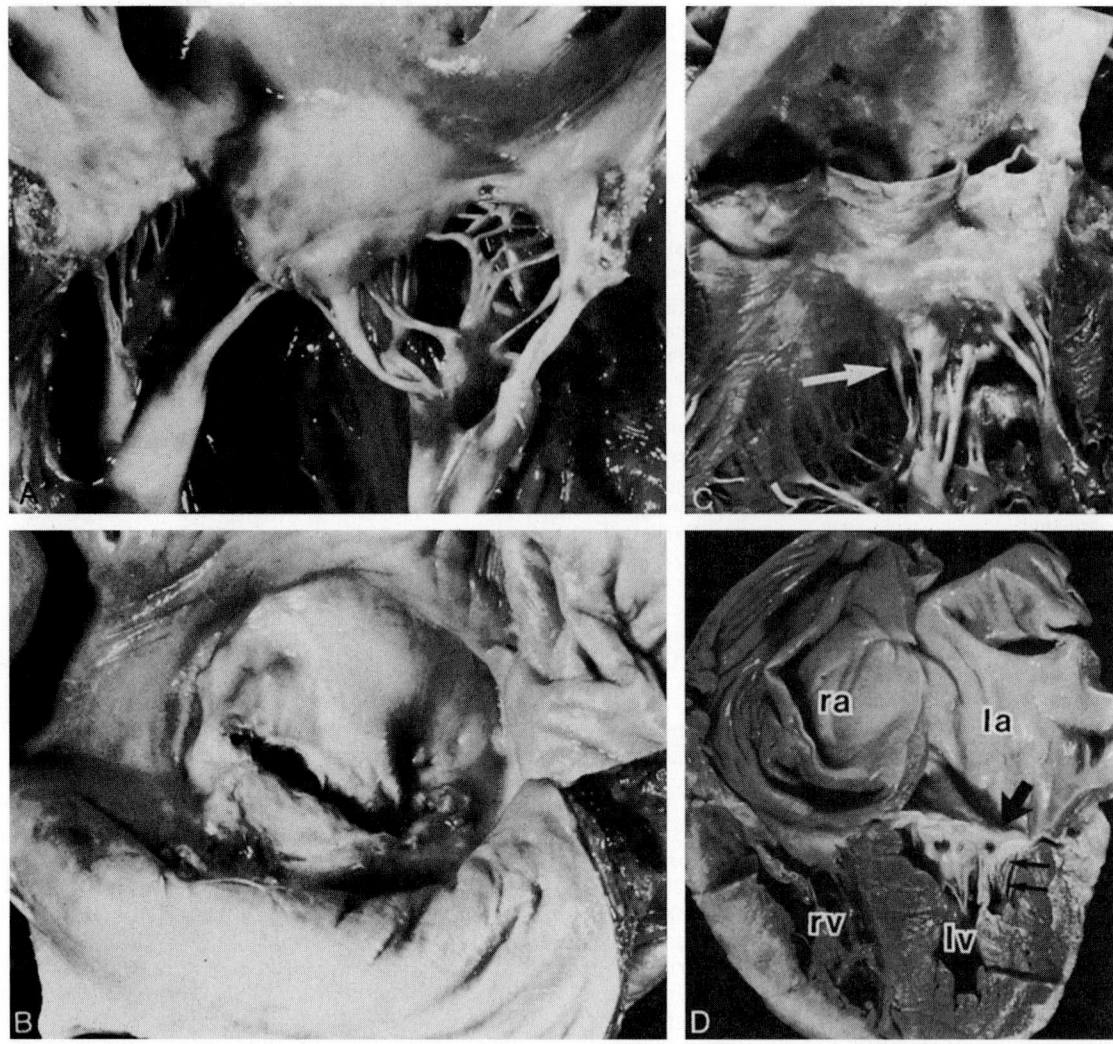

FIGURE 32–1. Rheumatic mitral stenosis. *A,* Moderate valvular changes including diffuse leaflet fibrosis, commissural fusion, and chordal thickening and fusion. In another case, atrial view *(B)* and subvalvular and aortic aspects *(C)* show prominent subvalvular involvement; severe subvalvular distortion is evident (arrow). *D,* Severe rheumatic mitral stenosis with specimen shown in apical four-chamber echocardiographic view, demonstrating small left ventricle (lv) and enlarged left atrium (la), right ventricle (rv), and right atrium (ra). Note the calcified stenotic valve (arrow) and prominent subvalvular changes (double arrows). *(A* and *D* from Schoen, F. J., and St. John Sutton, M.: Contemporary issues in the pathology of valvular heart disease. Hum. Pathol. *18:*568, 1987.)

increase the rate of blood flow across the mitral orifice and result in further elevation of the left atrial pressure.[14,15]

In order to assess the severity of obstruction of the mitral valve (and, for that matter, of any valve), it is essential to measure both the transvalvular pressure gradient and the flow rate.[15a] The latter depends not only on cardiac output but on heart rate as well. An increase in heart rate shortens diastole proportionately more than systole and diminishes the time available for flow across the mitral valve. Therefore, at any given level of cardiac output, tachycardia augments the transmitral valvular pressure gradient and elevates left atrial pressures further.[16] This explains the sudden occurrence of dyspnea and pulmonary edema in previously asymptomatic patients with MS who develop atrial fibrillation with a rapid ventricular rate[17]; it also accounts for the equally rapid improvement in these patients when the ventricular rate is slowed by means of cardiac glycosides and/or beta-adrenoceptor blocking agents, even when the cardiac output per minute remains constant. Hydraulic considerations dictate that at any given orifice size the transvalvular gradient is a function of the square of the transvalvular flow rate (see p. 194).[18] Thus, a doubling of flow rate will quadruple the pressure gradient, so that a stress such as exercise in patients with moderate or severe MS will cause marked elevation of left atrial pressure.[18a] Pregnancy, hypervolemia, and hyperthyroidism all increase

mitral valve flow and thereby the transvalvular pressure gradient. Although the Gorlin formula has been the benchmark for evaluating stenotic valvular orifices since 1951[18] (see p. 194), there is increasing evidence that valvular orifices are not rigid and that, in fact, as transvalvular flow increases, the orifice becomes distended. Accordingly, it has been proposed that stenosis be expressed as valvular resistance, the quotient of the mean transvalvular pressure gradient and the mean transvalvular flow.[19]

Atrial contraction augments the presystolic transmitral valvular gradient by approximately 30 per cent in patients with MS. Withdrawal of atrial transport when atrial fibrillation develops decreases cardiac output by about 20 per cent. The more rapid ventricular rate that occurs in atrial fibrillation until it is pharmacologically controlled raises the transvalvular pressure gradient. Thus, hemodynamic considerations indicate the desirability of maintaining sinus rhythm in patients with MS.

Intracardiac and Intravascular Pressures

Left ventricular diastolic pressure is normal in patients with pure MS; coexisting MR, aortic valve lesions, systemic hypertension, ischemic heart disease, and cardiomyopathy may all be responsible for elevations of left ventricular diastolic pressure. In approximately 85 per cent of patients

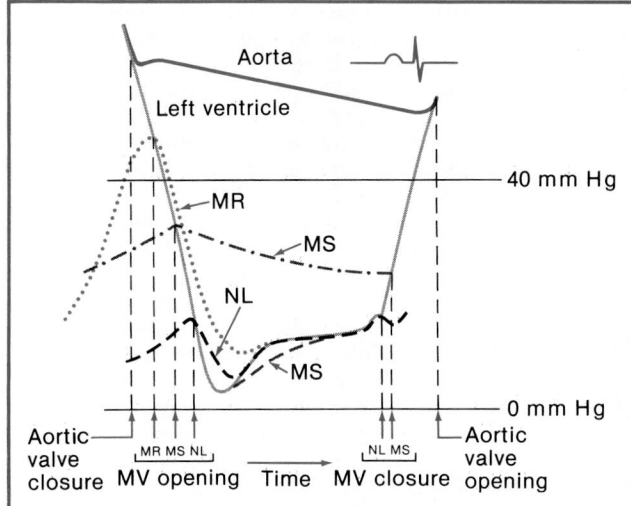

FIGURE 32–2. Schematic relationship of left ventricular (——), aortic (━━), and pulmonary atrial wedge (PAW) pressures. Note that the higher the left atrial *v* wave, the earlier the pressure crossover, and the earlier the mitral valve (MV) opening. The higher left atrial end-diastolic pressure with severe mitral stenosis (MS) also results in later closure of the mitral valve. PAW pressures in severe mitral regurgitation (MR) (· · · · ·), mitral stenosis (— · — · — ·), and normal (— — —). The LV diastolic pressure in mitral stenosis (━━━━━) rises slowly, denoting the absence of a rapid filling wave. (From Braunwald, E., and Turi, Z. G.: Pathophysiology of mitral valve disease. *In* Wells, F. C., and Schapiro, L. M. [eds.]: Mitral Valve Disease. London, Butterworths, 1996.)

with pure MS, the end-diastolic volume is within the normal range, whereas it is reduced in the remainder.[20] In approximately one-fourth of patients with pure MS the ejection fraction and other ejection indices of systolic performance (see p. 425) are below normal, most likely resulting from chronic reduction in preload and elevated afterload, the latter related to a chronically depressed cardiac output.[21] Regional hypokinesis is common,[22] perhaps caused by extension of the scarring process from the mitral valve into the adjacent posterior basal myocardium or by associated ischemic heart disease. Leftward displacement of the interventricular septum secondary to more rapid early filling of the right ventricle may be responsible for a reduction of left ventricular distensibility.[23] The left ventricular mass is normal or slightly reduced.[20] It has long been postulated that persistent myocardial dysfunction, perhaps caused by smoldering rheumatic myocarditis, may be responsible for the poor results following surgical treatment of some patients with pure MS.[24] The bulk of available evidence suggests that myocardial *contractility* is normal or slightly impaired in the majority of patients.[25] Associated ischemic heart disease may be responsible for myocardial dysfunction.[26] Most patients with MS show a normal elevation of ejection fraction and reduction of end-systolic volume during exercise.[27]

In MS and sinus rhythm, the *left atrial pressure pulse* generally exhibits a prominent atrial contraction (*a*) wave (Fig. 6–13, p. 194) and a gradual pressure decline after mitral valve opening (*y* descent); the mean left atrial pressure is elevated. In patients with mild to moderate MS without elevation of pulmonary vascular resistance, pulmonary arterial pressure may be normal or only slightly elevated at rest and may rise only during exercise. However, in patients with severe MS and/or those in whom the pulmonary vascular resistance is significantly increased, pulmonary arterial pressure is elevated when the patient is at rest, and in rare cases of extreme elevation of the pulmonary vascular resistance it may exceed the systemic arterial pressure. Further elevations of left atrial and pulmonary vascular pressures occur during exercise or tachycardia or

both. With moderate elevation of pulmonary artery pressure (systolic pressure 30 to 60 mm Hg), right ventricular performance is usually maintained.[28] However, an elevation of pulmonary arterial systolic pressure exceeding 60 mm Hg represents a serious impedance to emptying of the right ventricle and may cause right ventricular failure with elevations of the right ventricular end-diastolic and right atrial pressures. During exercise, patients with MS and pulmonary hypertension commonly fail to exhibit normal elevation of right ventricular ejection fraction.[24]

The *clinical and hemodynamic features* of MS of any given severity are dictated largely by the levels of cardiac output and pulmonary vascular resistance. The response to a given degree of mitral obstruction may be characterized at one end of the hemodynamic spectrum by a normal cardiac output and a high left atrioventricular pressure gradient or, at the opposite end of the spectrum, by a markedly reduced cardiac output and low transvalvular pressure gradient. Thus, in some patients with moderately severe stenosis (mitral valve area = 1.0 to 1.5 cm²) cardiac output at rest may be normal and it rises normally during exertion as well. In these patients, marked elevation of left atrial and pulmonary capillary pressures and the high transvalvular pressure gradient together lead to severe pulmonary congestion during exertion. In contrast, in the majority of patients with severe MS, cardiac output rises subnormally during exertion, thus reducing the pulmonary venous pressure and the severity of symptoms of pulmonary congestion more than would be the case if the output rose normally. In patients with severe stenosis (mitral valve area < 1.0 cm²), particularly when pulmonary vascular resistance is elevated, cardiac output is usually depressed at rest and may fail to rise at all during exertion. These patients frequently have prominent symptoms secondary to a low cardiac output, e.g., severe weakness and fatigue.

Pulmonary hypertension in patients with MS results from (1) passive backward transmission of the elevated left atrial pressure; (2) pulmonary arteriolar constriction, which presumably is triggered by left atrial and pulmonary venous hypertension (reactive pulmonary hypertension)[29]; and (3) organic obliterative changes in the pulmonary vascular bed, which may be considered to be a complication of longstanding and severe MS[30] (Chap. 25). In time, severe pulmonary hypertension results in right-sided failure, with dilatation of the right ventricle and its annulus, and secondary tricuspid and sometimes pulmonic regurgitation. It has been suggested that these changes in the pulmonary vascular bed may also exert a protective effect; the elevated precapillary resistance makes the development of symptoms of pulmonary congestion less likely by tending to prevent blood from surging into the pulmonary capillary bed and damming up behind the stenotic mitral valve, although this protection occurs at the expense of a reduced cardiac output. In patients with severe MS, pulmonary vein–bronchial vein shunts occur.[31] Patients with severe MS manifest a marked reduction in lung compliance, an increase in the work of breathing, and a redistribution of pulmonary blood flow from the bases to the apices.

The combination of mitral valve disease and atrial inflammation secondary to rheumatic carditis causes (1) left atrial dilatation, (2) fibrosis of the atrial wall, and (3) disorganization of the atrial muscle bundles. The third condition leads to disparate conduction velocities and inhomogeneous refractory periods. Premature atrial activation, due either to an automatic focus or to reentry, may stimulate the left atrium during the vulnerable period and may thus precipitate atrial fibrillation. Often this is episodic at first, but then it becomes more persistent. Atrial fibrillation per se causes diffuse atrophy of atrial muscle, further atrial enlargement,[32] and further inhomogeneity of refractoriness and conduction; these changes, in turn, lead to irreversible atrial fibrillation.

History

The principal symptom of MS is dyspnea, largely the result of reduced compliance of the lungs. Cough and wheezing may be accompanying symptoms. Vital capacity is reduced, presumably owing to the presence of engorged pulmonary vessels and interstitial edema. Patients with critical obstruction to left atrial emptying and dyspnea with ordinary activity (functional Class III) generally have orthopnea and are at risk of experiencing attacks of frank pulmonary edema. The latter may be precipitated by effort, emotional stress, respiratory infection, fever, sexual intercourse, pregnancy, atrial fibrillation with a rapid ventricular rate or other tachyarrhythmia, or, indeed, by any condition that increases blood flow across the stenotic mitral valve, either by increasing total cardiac output or by reducing the time available for this flow of blood to occur. In patients with a markedly elevated pulmonary vascular resistance, right ventricular function is often impaired.[32a]

HEMOPTYSIS. Wood has differentiated between several kinds of *hemoptysis* complicating MS.[14]

1. Sudden hemorrhage (sometimes called pulmonary apoplexy), while often profuse, is only rarely life-threatening.[33] It results from the rupture of thin-walled, dilated bronchial veins,[31,34] usually as a consequence of a sudden rise in left atrial pressure. With persistence of pulmonary venous hypertension, the walls of these veins thicken appreciably, and this form of hemoptysis tends to disappear.

2. Blood-stained sputum associated with attacks of paroxysmal nocturnal dyspnea.

3. Pink, frothy sputum characteristic of acute pulmonary edema with rupture of alveolar capillaries.

4. Pulmonary infarction, a late complication of MS associated with heart failure.

5. Blood-stained sputum complicating chronic bronchitis; the edematous bronchial mucosa in patients with chronic MS increases the likelihood of chronic bronchitis, a common complication of MS, particularly in Great Britain.

CHEST PAIN. A small fraction, perhaps 15 per cent, of patients with MS experience chest discomfort that is indistinguishable from angina pectoris.[14,15] This symptom may be caused by right ventricular hypertension or by coincidental coronary atherosclerosis,[26] or it may be secondary to coronary obstruction caused by coronary embolization.[35] In many such patients, however, a satisfactory explanation cannot be uncovered even after complete hemodynamic and angiographic studies.

THROMBOEMBOLISM. Prior to the advent of surgical treatment, this serious complication of MS developed in at least 20 per cent of patients at some time during the course of their disease, and as many as 10 to 15 per cent of this group died as a consequence.[36] Before the era of anticoagulant therapy and surgical treatment, approximately one-fourth of all fatalities in patients with mitral valve disease were secondary to embolism. The tendency for embolization correlates inversely with cardiac output and directly with the patient's age and the size of the left atrial appendage; 80 per cent of patients with MS in whom systemic emboli develop are in atrial fibrillation. When embolization occurs in patients in sinus rhythm, the possibility of transient atrial fibrillation and underlying infective endocarditis should be considered. There is no simple correlation between the incidence of embolism on one hand and the size of the mitral orifice on the other. Indeed, embolism may be the first symptom of MS and may occur in patients with mild MS even before the development of dyspnea. Patients older than 35 with atrial fibrillation, especially with a low cardiac output and dilation of the left atrial appendage, are at the highest risk for emboli and therefore should receive prophylactic anticoagulant treatment.

Because thrombi are found in the left atrium at operation in only a minority of patients with a history of recent embolism, it is likely that only fresh clots are discharged. Approximately half of all clinically apparent emboli are found in the cerebral vessels. Coronary embolism may lead to myocardial infarction, angina pectoris, or both, and renal emboli may be responsible for the development of systemic hypertension. Emboli are recurrent and multiple in approximately 25 per cent of patients subject to this complication. Rarely, massive thrombosis develops in the left atrium, resulting in a pedunculated ball-valve thrombus, which may suddenly aggravate obstruction to left atrial outflow when a specific body position is assumed, or it may cause sudden death.[5,37] Similar consequences occur in patients with free-floating thrombi in the left atrium. These two conditions are usually characterized by variability in the physical findings, often on a positional basis; they are very hazardous and require surgical treatment, often on an emergent basis.

INFECTIVE ENDOCARDITIS (see also Chap. 33). This complication tends to occur *less frequently* on rigid, thickened, calcified valves and is therefore more common in patients with mild than with severe MS.

OTHER SYMPTOMS. Compression of the left recurrent laryngeal nerve by a greatly dilated left atrium, enlarged tracheobronchial lymph nodes, and dilated pulmonary artery may cause hoarseness (Ortner's syndrome).[38] A history of repeated hemoptysis is common in patients with pulmonary hemosiderosis, and longstanding elevation of pulmonary venous pressure is present in patients with pulmonary ossification. Systemic venous hypertension, hepatomegaly, edema, ascites, and hydrothorax are all signs of severe MS with elevated pulmonary vascular resistance and right heart failure.

Physical Examination[39,40]

Patients with severe MS, a low cardiac output, and systemic vasoconstriction may exhibit the so-called mitral facies, characterized by pinkish-purple patches on the cheeks.[14] The *arterial pulse* is usually normal, but in patients in whom the stroke volume is reduced, it may be small in volume. The *jugular venous pulse* usually exhibits a prominent *a* wave in patients with sinus rhythm (Fig. 2–6A, p. 19) and elevated pulmonary vascular resistance. In atrial fibrillation, the *x* descent of the jugular pulse disappears, and there is only one crest, a prominent *v* or *c-v* wave, per cardiac cycle. *Palpation* of the cardiac apex usually reveals an inconspicuous left ventricle; the presence of either a palpable presystolic expansion wave or an early diastolic rapid filling wave speaks strongly against significant MS. A readily palpable, tapping first heart sound (S_1) suggests that the anterior mitral valve leaflet is pliable. When the patient is in the left lateral recumbent position, the low-pitched diastolic rumbling murmur of MS may be palpable as a thrill at the apex. Often a right ventricular lift is felt in the left parasternal region in patients with pulmonary hypertension. A markedly enlarged right ventricle may displace the left ventricle posteriorly and produce a prominent apex beat that can be confused with a left ventricular lift. A loud pulmonic closure sound (P_2) may be palpable in the second left intercostal space in patients with MS and pulmonary hypertension.

AUSCULTATION. The auscultatory (and phonocardiographic) features of MS (some of which are illustrated in Fig. 2–38, p. 42) include an accentuated S_1 with prolongation of the Q-S_1 interval, correlating with the level of the left atrial pressure. Accentuation of S_1 occurs when the mitral valve leaflets are flexible.[41] It is caused, in part, by the rapidity with which left ventricular pressure rises at the time of mitral valve closure as well as by the wide closing excursion of the valve leaflets.[42] Marked calcification or thickening of the mitral valve leaflets or both reduce the amplitude of S_1, probably because of diminished motion of the leaflets. As pulmonary artery pressure rises, P_2 at first becomes accentuated and widely transmitted and can often be readily heard and recorded at both the mitral and the aortic areas. With further elevation of pulmonary artery pressure, splitting of S_2 narrows because of reduced compliance of the pulmonary vascular bed, which shortens the "hangout interval." Finally, S_2 becomes single and accentuated. Other signs of pulmonary hypertension include a nonvalvular pulmonic ejection sound that diminishes during inspiration, owing to dilation of the pulmonary artery; the systolic murmur of tricuspid regurgitation; a Graham Steell murmur of pulmonic regurgitation; and an S_4 originating from the right ventricle.[43] An S_3 originating from the left ventricle is absent, unless significant mitral or aortic regurgitation coexists.

The *opening snap* (OS) of the mitral valve appears to be due to a sudden tensing of the valve leaflets after the valve cusps have completed their opening excursion. OS occurs when the movement of the mitral dome into the left ventricle suddenly stops.[42] It is most readily audible at the apex and with the diaphragm of the stethoscope and can usually be differentiated from P_2 because the OS occurs later, unless right bundle branch block is present. The mitral valve cannot be totally rigid if it produces an OS, which is usually accompanied by an accentuated S_1. The OS and the delayed S_1 are "reciprocal sounds," both caused by abrupt termination of movement of the fused mitral complex.[42] Calcification confined to the tip of the mitral valve leaflets does not preclude an OS, although calcification of the body and tip does. In patients with combined MS and regurgitation, the OS may be followed by an S_3. The mitral OS follows A_2 by 0.04 to 0.12 sec; this interval varies inversely with left atrial pressure.[41] Although a short A_2-OS interval is a reliable indicator of severe MS, the converse is not necessarily the case. $(Q-S_1)-(A_2-OS)$ correlates better with the height of the left atrial pressure than does either term alone.

The diastolic murmur of MS is a low-pitched, rumbling murmur, best heard at the apex and with the bell of the stethoscope (Fig. 2–38, p. 42). When this murmur is soft, it is limited to the apex, but when louder, it may radiate to the axilla or the lower left sternal area. Although the intensity of the diastolic murmur is not closely related to the severity of stenosis, the *duration* of the murmur is a guide to the severity of mitral narrowing. The murmur persists for as long as the left atrioventricular pressure gradient exceeds approximately 3 mm Hg. The murmur usually commences immediately after the mitral OS. In mild MS, the early diastolic murmur is brief but it resumes in presystole. In severe stenosis, the murmur is holodiastolic, with presystolic accentuation in patients with sinus rhythm.

Although a *presystolic murmur* is usually present in patients with sinus rhythm in whom transvalvular blood flow is accelerated by atrial contraction, a presystolic murmur may also occur in patients with atrial fibrillation, in whom it results from the increased velocity of blood flow across a mitral valve orifice that begins to narrow after the onset of left ventricular contraction. Because in patients with atrial fibrillation, this murmur results from motion of the mitral valve leaflets, a flexible mitral valve is required for its generation.

The *diastolic rumbling murmur* of MS may be masked by the presence of obesity, pulmonary emphysema, and a low cardiac output with a low flow rate across the mitral valve. This murmur may be sharply localized and thus missed unless palpation is used to detect the apex of the left ventricle and to pinpoint the area at which auscultation should be carried out. In so-called "silent" MS, there is usually marked right ventricular enlargement, so that the right ventricle occupies the cardiac apex, the left ventricle is rotated posteriorly, and cardiac output is reduced, so that the murmur either is not audible at all or can be heard only in the

mid- or posterior axillary line. Auscultation of the murmur is facilitated by placing the patient in the left lateral position and auscultating during expiration after a few sit-ups, walking up a flight of stairs, or other maneuvers described later.

Dynamic Auscultation. The diastolic murmur and OS of MS are often reduced during inspiration and augmented during expiration[39,40]—the opposite of what occurs when these findings are secondary to tricuspid stenosis (see p. 1054). During inspiration the A_2-OS interval widens, and three sequential sounds (A_2, P_2, and OS) are frequently audible. Sudden standing and the resultant reduction of venous return lower left atrial pressure and widen the A_2-OS interval; this maneuver is useful in distinguishing an A_2-OS combination from a split S_2, which narrows on standing. In contrast, A_2-OS is significantly narrowed during exercise as left atrial pressure rises. The diastolic rumbling murmur of MS is reduced during the strain of a Valsalva maneuver and in any condition in which transmitral valve flow rate declines. Amyl nitrite, coughing, isometric or isotonic exercise, and sudden squatting are all useful in accentuating a faint or equivocal murmur of MS. Progressive narrowing of A_2-OS on serial examinations suggests an increase in the severity of stenosis, whereas widening of A_2-OS after mitral commissurotomy indicates that the severity of stenosis has been reduced significantly.

DIFFERENTIAL DIAGNOSIS. A number of conditions other than MS may exhibit auscultatory findings that can be confused with MS. In addition to the findings listed in the table, the *Carey-Coombs murmur* of acute rheumatic fever is a sign of active mitral valvulitis and can be confused with the murmur of MS. The Carey-Coombs murmur is a soft, early diastolic murmur, usually varies from day to day, and is higher pitched than the diastolic rumbling murmur of established MS. In pure, severe MR—indeed, in any condition in which there is increased flow across a nonstenotic mitral valve—there may also be a short diastolic murmur following an S_3. *Left atrial myxoma* may produce auscultatory findings similar to those in rheumatic valvular MS (see p. 1466). A high-frequency early systolic murmur is audible along the lower left sternal border in one-third of patients with MS.[42] This should be distinguished from the apical (often holosystolic or late systolic) murmur of MR. In addition, a *pansystolic murmur of tricuspid regurgitation* and an S_3 originating from the right ventricle may be audible in the fourth intercostal space in the left parasternal region in patients with severe mitral stenosis. These signs, secondary to pulmonary hypertension, may be confused with the findings of MR. However, the inspiratory augmentation of the murmur and of the S_3 and the prominent v wave in the jugular venous pulse aid in establishing that the murmur originates from the tricuspid valve. A decrescendo diastolic murmur along the left sternal border in patients with MS and pulmonary hypertension is usually due to aortic regurgitation but occasionally represents a Graham Steell murmur of pulmonary regurgitation[43] (see p. 41); the latter, when present, characteristically increases during inspiration.

LABORATORY EXAMINATION

ELECTROCARDIOGRAPHY. The ECG and vectorcardiogram are relatively insensitive techniques for the detection of mild MS, but they do show characteristic changes in moderate or severe obstruction.[44,45] Left atrial enlargement (P-wave duration in lead II > 0.12 sec, terminal negative P force in lead V_1 > 0.003 mV/sec, P-wave axis between + 45 and − 30 degrees) is a principal electrocardiographic feature of MS and is found in 90 per cent of patients with significant MS and sinus rhythm.[46] The ECG signs of left atrial enlargement correlate more closely with left atrial volume than with left atrial pressure and often regress following successful valvulotomy.[14] When atrial fibrillation is present, the fibrillatory waves are usually coarse, i.e., greater than 0.1 mV in amplitude in V_1, also suggesting the presence of atrial enlargement.[47] Atrial fibrillation usually develops in the presence of preexistent ECG evidence of left atrial enlargement and is related to the size and the extent of fibrosis of the left atrial myocardium, the duration of atriomegaly, and the age of the patient.[48]

Whether or not there is ECG evidence of right ventricular hypertrophy depends largely on the height of right ventricular systolic pressure; an incomplete right bundle branch block pattern with an rSr pattern in V_1 is not usual. It is infrequent in patients with right ventricular systolic pressures less than 70 mm Hg.[46] Approximately half of all patients with right ventricular systolic pressures between 70 and 100 mm Hg manifest the electrocardiographic criteria for right ventricular hypertrophy, including both a mean QRS axis greater than 80 degrees in the frontal plane and an R:S ratio greater than 1.0 in V_1.[49] In other patients with this degree of pulmonary hypertension there is no frank evidence of right ventricular hypertrophy, but the R:S ratio fails to increase from right to midprecordial leads. When right ventricular systolic pressures exceed 100 mm Hg, electrocardiographic evidence of right ventricular hypertrophy is found quite consistently.

The *QRS axis in the frontal plane* often correlates with the severity of valve obstruction and with the level of pulmonary vascular resistance in pure MS; thus, a mean frontal axis between 0 and +60 degrees suggests that the mitral valve area exceeds 1.3 cm², whereas an axis greater than 60 degrees suggests that the valve area is less than 1.3 cm². In patients in whom pulmonary vascular resistance is greater than 650 dynes · sec · cm⁻⁵, the mean axis usually exceeds +110 degrees. In patients whose pulmonary artery systolic pressures approach systemic levels, the mean axis averages +150 degrees.[50]

VECTORCARDIOGRAPHY. The characteristic *vectorcardiographic finding* in MS is right ventricular hypertrophy Type C characterized by counterclockwise rotation in the horizontal plane and a terminal deflection directed to the right, posteriorly, and superiorly.[46,50,51]

RADIOLOGICAL FINDINGS (see also Figs. 7–8B, p. 209; 7–16, p. 215 and 7–35, p. 226). Although in patients with hemodynamically significant MS the cardiac silhouette may be normal in the frontal projection, with the exception of an enlarged atrial appendage, left atrial enlargement is almost invariably evident on the lateral and left anterior oblique views. The size of the left atrium does *not* correlate with the severity of obstruction. Extreme left atrial enlargement rarely occurs in pure MS; when it is present, MR is usually severe. Enlargement of the pulmonary artery, right ventricle, and right atrium (as well as the left atrium) is commonly seen in severe MS (Fig. 7–35, p. 226). Occasionally, calcification of the mitral valve is evident on the chest roentgenogram (Fig. 7–29, p. 222), but, more commonly, fluoroscopy is required to detect valvular calcification.

Radiological changes in the lung fields (Fig. 7–35, p. 226) are useful in estimating the height of pulmonary venous pressure and thereby the severity of MS. Interstitial edema, an indication of severe obstruction, is manifested as Kerley B lines (dense, short, horizontal lines most commonly seen in the costophrenic angles).[52] This finding is present in 30 per cent of patients with resting pulmonary artery wedge pressures below 20 mm Hg and in 70 per cent of patients with pressures exceeding 20 mm Hg. Severe, longstanding mitral obstruction often results in Kerley A lines (straight, dense lines up to 4 cm in length running toward the hilum) as well as the findings of pulmonary hemosiderosis (Fig. 7–35, p. 226) and rarely of parenchymal ossification. Pulmonary edema is rarely evident.

ANGIOGRAPHY. Angiograms exposed in the right and left anterior oblique projections afford the best views of the mitral valve. Although ideally contrast medium should be injected into the left atrium, it is often possible to achieve good visualization of the left side of the heart by injecting a large volume into the main pulmonary artery. Such angiograms provide an assessment of left atrial size, may demonstrate thickening and reduced motion of the valve leaflets, and may outline large intraluminal thrombi.[53] Left cine ventriculography is useful in the assessment of mitral valve motion. Although this technique allows visualization of only the ventricular aspect of the leaflet in patients with pure MS, it makes possible simultaneous assessment of left ventricular contractile function and of the subvalvular mitral apparatus. Angiography in the evaluation of patients with MS or suspected MS has been largely superseded by echocardiography.

ECHOCARDIOGRAPHY (see also p. 71). MS can ordinarily be readily diagnosed by M-mode echocardiography (Fig. 3–45, p. 71), but this technique does not allow a precise determination of its severity. Echocardiograms of a thickened, calcified stenotic rheumatic valve demonstrate increased acoustic impedence and fusion of the mitral valve leaflets and poor leaflet separation in diastole.[54] The leaflets fail to close normally in mid-diastole and may not reopen widely during atrial contraction. Normally, the posterior leaflet of the mitral valve moves posteriorly during early diastole, but in more than 90 per cent of patients with MS, both leaflets move anteriorly at this time. The left atrium is usually enlarged, and in isolated MS the left ventricular cavity is normal or reduced in size. Two-dimensional echocardiography may be helpful in the preop-

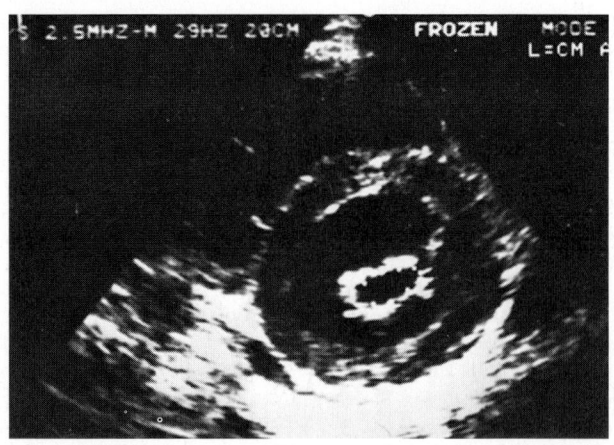

FIGURE 32–3. Two-dimensional parasternal short-axis view of the mitral valve orifice during diastole, demonstrating the echocardiographic method of mitral valve area calculation. The innermost border of the mitral orifice was planimetered with the use of a light-pen system to obtain the area (in cm²). (Reproduced with permission from Smith, M. D., et al.: Comparative accuracy of two-dimensional echocardiography and Doppler pressure half-time methods in assessing severity of mitral stenosis in patients with and without prior commissurotomy. Circulation 73:100, 1986. Copyright 1986 American Heart Association.)

erative recognition of left atrial thrombus and in assessing mitral valve calcification and left ventricular contractility.

Two-dimensional echocardiography (Fig. 32–3 and Fig. 3–46, p. 72) is more accurate than M-mode echocardiography in determining mitral orifice size.[55] It reveals restricted motion and doming of the valve leaflets. With progressive thickening and fibrosis of the leaflets, the orifice becomes fixed and can then often be imaged directly and measured. This technique also provides information on the pliability and extent of calcification of the valve, thickening of the subvalvular apparatus, and fusion and retraction of the chordae as well as calcification of the mitral annulus. The echocardiogram is helpful in determining whether the patient with MS is a suitable candidate for balloon mitral valvuloplasty (see p. 1385).

Doppler echocardiography is the most accurate noninvasive technique available for quantifying the severity of MS[55,56] (Fig. 3–47, p. 72). This technique is also useful for estimating pulmonary arterial pressure. Doppler color flow imaging can be used to enhance the accuracy of the Doppler data by guiding the position of the beam[56] and to determine whether mitral regurgitation and other valvular abnormalities coexist. Transesophageal two-dimensional echocardiography provides superior images of the mitral valve and may show thrombus in the left atrium. Pedunculated and free-floating thrombi are also usually readily detected by this technique.

A detailed echocardiographic examination including two-dimensional echocardiography, a Doppler study, and Doppler color flow imaging in a patient with MS can frequently provide sufficient information to allow development of a therapeutic plan without the need for cardiac catheterization. Of course, it provides no information on the state of the coronary arteries. If surgery is planned, it is important to ascertain whether or not bypass grafting is indicated in patients at risk of having coexisting coronary artery disease.

MANAGEMENT

Medical Treatment

Patients with rheumatic heart disease should receive penicillin prophylaxis for beta-hemolytic streptococcal infections and prophylaxis for infective endocarditis (see p.

1098). Anemia and infections should be treated promptly and aggressively in patients with valvular heart disease. Adolescents and young adults with serious valvular heart disease should be advised to avoid entering occupations requiring strenuous exertion.

In symptomatic patients with mitral valve disease, considerable improvement occurs with oral diuretics and the restriction of sodium intake. Digitalis glycosides do not alter the hemodynamics and usually do not benefit patients with MS and sinus rhythm[54,57] but are of great value in slowing the ventricular rate in patients with atrial fibrillation and in the treatment of right-sided heart failure. Measures designed to reduce pulmonary venous pressure, including sedation, assumption of the upright posture, and aggressive diuresis, are used to treat hemoptysis. Beta blockers may increase exercise capacity by reducing heart rate in patients with sinus rhythm[58] but especially in patients with atrial fibrillation.

In patients with rheumatic heart disease and heart failure, anticoagulant therapy is helpful in preventing venous thrombosis and pulmonary embolism in those who have experienced one or more previous embolic episodes, in those who are at high risk of embolization, i.e., with atrial fibrillation, and in those with mechanical prosthetic heart valves. However, no firm evidence exists that anticoagulant therapy reduces the incidence of pulmonary or systemic embolism in patients in sinus rhythm in whom such episodes have not previously occurred.

TREATMENT OF ARRHYTHMIAS. Frequent premature atrial contractions often presage atrial fibrillation, and the administration of antiarrhythmic drugs, as outlined on page 593, may be effective in preventing this complication. However, once atrial fibrillation has developed, these agents may be ineffective in restoring sinus rhythm or even in maintaining sinus rhythm following electrical cardioversion, because of the pathological changes that occur in the atrium secondary to the arrhythmia itself. After electrical cardioversion, sinus rhythm can often be maintained with antiarrhythmic drugs in young patients with mild MS without marked left atrial enlargement who have been in atrial fibrillation less than 6 months and who are maintained by adequate doses of quinidine. If elective cardioversion (pharmacological or electrical) is to be attempted in the patient with MS and atrial fibrillation, a preparatory 3-week course of anticoagulation should be given to minimize the risk of systemic embolism when sinus rhythm resumes (see Ch. 46). Immediate treatment of atrial fibrillation should be directed toward reducing the ventricular rate by means of digitalis and, if possible, toward reestablishing sinus rhythm by a combination of pharmacological treatment and cardioversion. Paroxysmal atrial fibrillation and repeated conversions, spontaneous or induced, carry the risk of embolization. In patients who cannot be converted or maintained in sinus rhythm, the ventricular rate at rest should be maintained at approximately 60 to 65 beats/min with digitalis. If this is not possible, small doses of a beta blocker, such as atenolol (25 mg daily), may be added. Multiple repeat cardioversions are *not* indicated if the patient has not sustained sinus rhythm while on adequate doses of quinidine. Patients with chronic atrial fibrillation who undergo open mitral repair or valve replacement may undergo the Cox maze procedure (atrial compartment operation). More than 80 per cent of such patients can be maintained in sinus rhythm postoperatively[59] and regain normal atrial function.[60,61]

Natural History

The development of effective surgical treatment has obscured our understanding of the natural history of MS (Fig. 32–4) and, for that matter, of all valvular lesions.[53] Although few meaningful data are available, it appears that in temperate zones such as the United States and Europe, after an attack of rheumatic fever there is an asymptomatic period of approximately 15 to 20 years before symptoms set in. It then takes approximately 3 years for most patients to progress from mild disability (i.e., early Class II) to severe disability (i.e., Class III or IV). The progression is much more rapid in patients in tropical and subtropical areas,[62] in Polynesians, as well as in Alaskan Eskimos. Economic as well as genetic conditions may play a role. In India, critical MS may be present in children as young as 6 to 12 years.

In the *presurgical era*, Olesen found 62 per cent 5-year and 38 per cent 10-year survival rates among patients in New York Heart Associ-

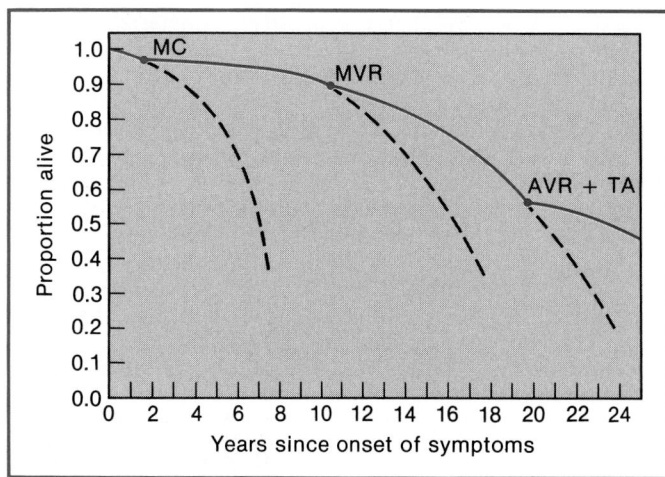

FIGURE 32–4. Schematic representation of the subsequent life history after the initial development of symptoms in a large group of patients with mitral stenosis. The colored solid circles and colored lines indicate a surgical procedure. The dashed lines represent estimated survival of patients not receiving the surgical procedure. MC = mitral commissurotomy, MVR = mitral valve replacement, TA = tricuspid annuloplasty, AVR = aortic valve replacement. (From Kirklin, J. W., and Barratt-Boyes, B. G. [eds.]: Cardiac Surgery. New York, John Wiley and Sons, 1986, p. 328.)

ation functional Class III but only 15 per cent 5-year survival rate in patients in Class IV.[63] Among asymptomatic patients (Class I) with MS treated medically, 40 per cent had a worsened course or had died within 10 years. Among mildly symptomatic patients (Class II), the comparable number was 80 per cent.[64] In medically treated patients with MS or with combined MS and MR, Munoz et al. found a 45 per cent 5-year survival rate.[65] In a comparable group of patients subjected to mitral commissurotomy, the 5-year survival rate was substantially better. In an unselected mix of patients with MS of varying severity, 80 per cent were alive after 5 years and 60 per cent after 10 years of medical treatment.[66]

Surgical Treatment

INDICATIONS FOR OPERATION. Patients with MS who are asymptomatic or minimally symptomatic frequently remain so for years. However, once moderate symptoms (Class II) develop, if the stenosis is not relieved mechanically, the disease may progress relatively rapidly, as already discussed. Operation (or balloon valvuloplasty) should therefore be carried out in symptomatic patients with moderate to severe MS (i.e., a mitral valve orifice size less than approximately 1.0 cm²/m² body surface area [BSA]—less than 1.5 to 1.7 cm² in normal-sized adults).

There has been considerable debate concerning the need for routine cardiac catheterization in determining whether operation is indicated.[67–69] A careful clinical evaluation and noninvasive assessment, particularly using two-dimensional and Doppler echocardiography, can provide sufficient information to permit an informed decision in the majority of patients. However, the consequences of valvular surgery, particularly valve replacement, are so profound that I recommend preoperative catheterization and angiography in the following groups of patients with MS: (1) patients with heart murmurs and other findings suggesting the presence of valve lesions in addition to MS, (2) patients with associated chronic obstructive pulmonary disease in which it is important to determine the contribution of MS to the symptoms, (3) patients in whom left atrial myxoma should be excluded, and (4) patients who have angina or angina-like chest pain or who have risk factors for coronary artery disease in whom associated coronary artery disease must be excluded. Critical narrowing of one or more coronary vessels occurs in approximately one-fourth of all adults with severe MS. It is more common in men over 45 years who have angina and risk factors for coronary artery disease.[26,70] I believe that preoperative catheterization can be omitted in the young (< 40 years) patient without angina and significant risk factors for coronary artery disease who has typical symptoms and classic findings of pure, severe MS on physical examination and by noninvasive tests, including two-dimensional and Doppler echocardiography.

Care of mildly symptomatic patients (Class II) must be individualized. It is necessary to consider and balance three important factors: (1) the size of the mitral orifice, (2) the degree to which the patient's life style is impaired by the mitral obstruction, (3) the history of complications, particularly systemic embolism, and (4) the risk of the procedure (operation or balloon valvuloplasty). If there are no obvious contraindications to one of these procedures, left heart catheterization should be performed to determine the size of the valve orifice. In general, mechanical relief of obstruction can be deferred in patients with mild symptoms and mild stenosis (i.e., mitral valve orifice size > approximately 1.0 cm²/m² BSA), whereas it should be recommended for those with mild symptoms and more severe stenosis (i.e., mitral valve orifice size < approximately 1.0 cm²/m² BSA). However, this plan is subject to qualification. For instance, mechanical relief of obstruction might well be deferred in a retired, sedentary septuagenarian with a mitral valve orifice of 0.8 cm²/m² BSA. On the other hand, a 30-year-old laborer whose family's economic well-being depends on his continued physical exertion might be an excellent candidate for mechanical relief of obstruction, although his mitral valve orifice size is 1.2 cm²/m² BSA.

Because of the high rate of recurrence, mechanical relief of obstruction is also indicated in patients with MS in whom systemic embolism has previously occurred, even if they are otherwise asymptomatic and even though there is no definitive evidence that the incidence of recurrent emboli will be significantly reduced. Anticoagulants should be administered up to the time of operation. Although the risk of operation is higher in patients with advanced disease characterized by severe pulmonary hypertension and right-sided heart failure, surviving patients nearly always show striking clinical and hemodynamic improvement, with a marked reduction in pulmonary vascular pressures. In the pregnant patient with MS, operative treatment should be carried out only if serious pulmonary congestion occurs despite intensive medical treatment including bed rest (p. 1849).

There is no evidence that surgical treatment improves the prognosis of patients with no or only slight functional impairment. Therefore, valvotomy is not indicated in patients who are entirely asymptomatic, except in unusual circumstances. For example, some years ago I saw a 33-year-old woman with MS who had had hemoptysis and pulmonary edema during the second trimester of a pregnancy 2 years previously. She then became asymptomatic but wished to have another child. Hemodynamic study showed a pulmonary wedge pressure of 17 mm Hg and a mitral orifice area of 1.7 cm²/m² BSA. Prophylactic mitral valvotomy was undertaken in this patient because it was virtually certain that another pregnancy would have resulted in serious heart failure. At present I would recommend balloon mitral valvuloplasty for such a patient (see p. 1016).

SURGICAL TECHNIQUES. Three basically different operative approaches are available for the treatment of rheumatic MS: (1) closed mitral valvotomy[71,72]; (2) open valvotomy, i.e., valvotomy carried out under direct vision with the aid of cardiopulmonary bypass; and (3) mitral valve replacement.[73] *Closed mitral valvotomy,* performed with the aid of a transventricular dilator,[72] is an effective operation, provided that MR, atrial thrombosis, or valvular calcification is not serious and that chordal fusion and shortening are not severe. Echocardiographic examination

is an important prerequisite. Unfortunately, few patients satisfy all these criteria, and they are difficult to identify preoperatively. In one large series,[72] hospital mortality was 1.5 per cent, and 0.3 per cent of patients developed severe MR. Marked symptomatic improvement occurred in 86 per cent of survivors. Actuarial survival rate was 89.5 per cent after 18 years. Closed valvotomy for restenosis was carried out with a 6.7 per cent mortality. Long-term follow-up has shown that the results are best if the operation is carried out before chronic atrial fibrillation and/or heart failure has occurred.[71] If possible, closed mitral valvotomy should be carried out with "pump standby"; if the surgeon is unable to achieve a satisfactory result, the patient can be placed on cardiopulmonary bypass, and the valvotomy carried out under direct vision or the valve replaced. Closed mitral valvotomy is rarely used in the United States today, having been replaced by balloon valvuloplasty, which is of similar effectiveness in patients who are candidates for closed mitral valvotomy (see p. 1016). Closed mitral valvotomy is more popular in developing nations, where the expense of open-heart surgery is a more important factor and where patients with mitral valve disease are younger. In any event, echocardiography is useful in selecting suitable candidates for closed mitral valvotomy by identifying patients without valvular calcification or dense fibrosis.

Most surgeons in North America and Western Europe now prefer to carry out *direct-vision* or *open valvotomy.*[73-75] Cardiopulmonary bypass is established, and in order to obtain a dry, quiet heart, body temperature is usually lowered, the heart is arrested, and the aorta is occluded intermittently. Thrombi are removed from the left atrium and its appendage, and the latter is often amputated in order to remove a potential source of postoperative emboli. The commissures are incised, and when necessary, fused chordae are separated, the underlying papillary muscle is split, and the valve leaflets are debrided of calcium; mild or even moderate mitral regurgitation may be corrected. Left atrial and ventricular pressures are measured after bypass has been discontinued to confirm that the valvotomy has in fact been effective. In patients with atrial fibrillation, conversion to sinus rhythm is carried out at the completion of the operation. In a series of open mitral valve reconstructive procedures for MS at Brigham and Women's Hospital, the actuarial probability of survival at 10 years was 95 per cent. The annual reoperation rate was 1.7 per cent.[76] A survival rate of 75 per cent over 20 years after surgical repair of MS has been reported.[7]

The mortality rate after mitral valvotomy, whether open or closed, ranges from 1 to 3 per cent, depending on the condition of the patient and the skill and experience of the surgical team.[74-76] Five-year survival rates are 90 to 96 per cent and event-free survival rates 72 to 94 per cent.[77-79] In general, open valvotomy provides better hemodynamic relief of mitral valve obstruction than does the closed procedure,[75,80,81] and the risk of dislodging thrombi from the atrium or calcium from the mitral valve is also less.[76] Left atrial size, the need for mitral or tricuspid annuloplasty, and the presence of left atrial thrombus are all "risk factors" for a less than optimal outcome.[81] However, it must be recognized that mitral valvotomy, whether open or closed, and valvuloplasty are *palliative* rather than curative procedures, and even when successful they merely "turn the clock back." (The generally more effective open valvulotomy turns the clock farther back than does the closed valvulotomy or balloon mitral valvuloplasty.) Thus, valvulotomy does not result in a normal mitral valve but, at best, results in one resembling the valve as it existed perhaps a decade earlier. Because the valve is not normal postoperatively, turbulent flow usually persists in the paravalvular region, and the resultant trauma may well play a role in restenosis. These changes are analogous to the gradual development of obstruction in a congenitally bicuspid aortic valve (see p. 964) and are not usually the result of recurrent rheumatic fever. When commissurotomy is attempted and the results are inadequate—most commonly due to severe distortion and calcification of the valve and subvalvular apparatus with the accompanying regurgitation that cannot be corrected—mitral valve replacement is carried out (see p. 1027).[82]

Although a contemporary control series of medically and surgically treated patients is not available (nor is it likely ever to be), appropriate surgical treatment appears to prolong survival substantially in patients with MS (Fig. 32–4).

Mitral Restenosis

This condition can be diagnosed with certainty only on the basis of three satisfactory hemodynamic or echocardiographic investigations: a preintervention study, a second study following a successful intervention in which an increase in the size of the valvular orifice has been demonstrated, and a third when a reduction in size relative to the earlier postintervention study is noted. On clinical grounds alone, i.e., based on the reappearance of symptoms, the incidence of "restenosis" has been estimated to range widely, from 2 to 60 per cent[83]; approximately 10 per cent

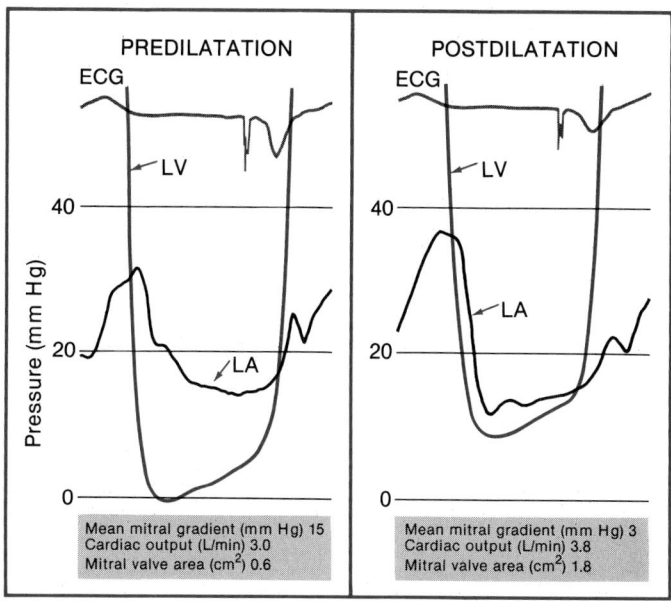

FIGURE 32–6. Simultaneous left atrial (LA) and left ventricular (LV) pressure before and after balloon valvuloplasty of the mitral valve in a patient with severe mitral stenosis. (Courtesy of Raymond G. McKay, M.D.)

of patients who have undergone mitral valvotomy require reoperation within 5 years, but that fraction increases to 60 per cent by 10 years.[84] The recurrence of symptoms is *not necessarily* due to restenosis. Recurrent symptoms may be due to one of four other conditions: (1) an inadequate first operation with residual stenosis; (2) the presence or development of MR, either at operation or as a consequence of infective endocarditis; (3) the progression of aortic valve disease; and (4) the development of symptoms due to an unrelated illness, such as ischemic heart disease or chronic obstructive lung disease. In a study in which the size of the mitral valve orifice was estimated using two-dimensional echocardiography in 18 patients who had undergone successful surgical valvotomy, no change in the mitral valve area occurred over a 10- to 14-year period in 13 patients, whereas in 5 (28 per cent) true restenosis developed.[84] The rate of restenosis is approximately 10 per cent within 6 years.[85]

Thus, in properly selected patients, mitral valvotomy results in a significant increase in the size of the mitral orifice and, at a low risk, favorably alters the clinical course of an otherwise progressive disease. Pulmonary artery pressure falls promptly and decisively when mitral obstruction is effectively relieved.[86,87] Some patients maintain clinical improvement for many (10 to 15) years of follow-up. When a second operation is required because of symptomatic deterioration, the valve is usually calcified and more seriously deformed than at the time of the first operation, and adequate reconstruction is not always possible. Accordingly, mitral valve replacement is often necessary at that time.

Also, in patients with combined MS and MR, and in those with extensive calcification involving the commissures of the valve, mitral replacement rather than valvotomy is often required. The operative mortality following mitral valve replacement ranges from 3 to 8 per cent in most hospitals. As described below (see p. 1027), the long-term fate of the prosthetic valves is not yet clear; also, the hazards of lifelong anticoagulant treatment in patients with mechanical prostheses cannot be neglected. Therefore, in patients in whom preoperative evaluation suggests that valve replacement may be required, the threshold for operation should be higher than in patients believed to require commissurotomy alone.

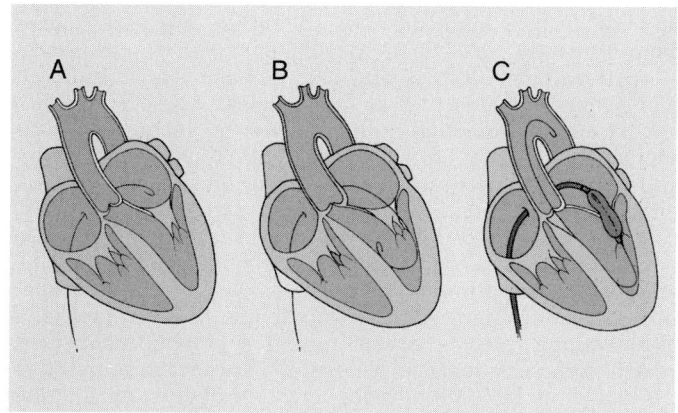

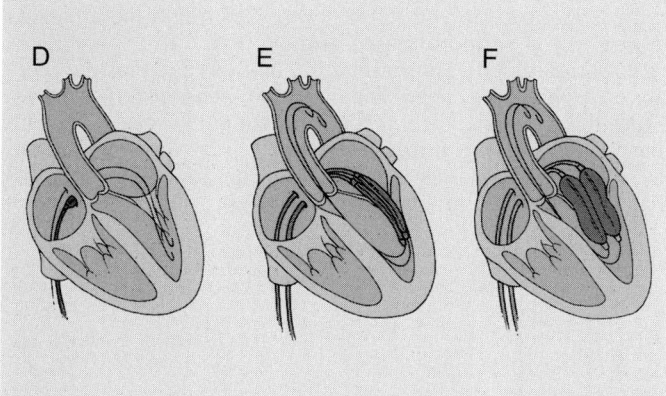

FIGURE 32–5. Technique of double-balloon mitral valvuloplasty. *A*, The position of the guidewire in the left atrium after left atrial puncture using the Brockenbrough needle. *B*, The position of the guidewire as it is advanced into the left ventricle across the stenotic mitral valve. *C*, Partial inflation of a single-balloon catheter across the stenotic mitral valve when a single-balloon valvuloplasty is to be performed. Notice that the guidewire may be advanced into the aorta in an antegrade fashion to provide greater stabilization. *D*, Dilatation of the atrial septum using an Olbert catheter in anticipation of performing a two-balloon mitral valvuloplasty. *E*, The two valvuloplasty catheters across the stenotic mitral valve. *F*, The appearance of the two simultaneously inflated balloons as the two-balloon valvuloplasty is being performed. (From Srebro, J. P., and Ports, T. A.: Catheter balloon valvuloplasty. *In* Chatterjee, K., et al. [eds.]: Cardiology: An Illustrated Text. Philadelphia, J.B. Lippincott, 1991, p. 9.54.)

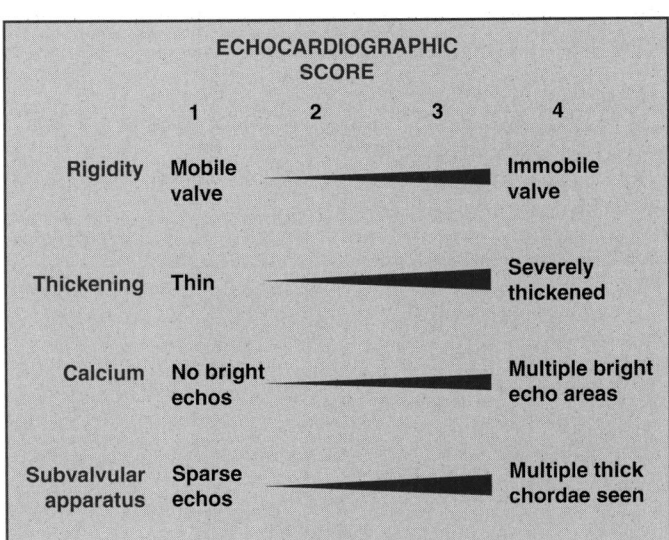

	1	2	3	4
Rigidity	Mobile valve			Immobile valve
Thickening	Thin			Severely thickened
Calcium	No bright echos			Multiple bright echo areas
Subvalvular apparatus	Sparse echos			Multiple thick chordae seen

FIGURE 32–7. Determination of echocardiographic score. Valve rigidity, thickening, calcification, and the amount of subvalvular disease are graded 1 to 4 depending on severity of abnormality. The sum of the four factors equals the echo score. (From Block, P. C.: Mitral balloon valvotomy: Why, when and how? Cardiol. Rev. 2:19, 1994.)

Balloon Mitral Valvuloplasty
(See also Chap. 39)

This procedure represents an alternative to surgical treatment of MS. The technique consists of advancing a small balloon flotation catheter across the interatrial septum (after transseptal puncture), enlarging the opening and advancing one large (23 to 25 mm) or two smaller (12 to 18 mm) balloons across the mitral orifice, and inflating them within the orifice[54,77,88–90a] (Fig. 32–5 and Fig. 39–14, p. 1385). Commissural separation and fracture of nodular calcium appear to be the mechanisms responsible for improvement in valvular function. In several series the hemodynamic results have been quite favorable (Fig. 32–6), with reduction of the transmitral pressure gradient from an average of approximately 18 to 6 mm Hg, a small (average 20 per cent) increase in cardiac output, and, on the average, a doubling of the calculated mitral valve area from 1.0 to 2.0 cm². The reported mortality averages 0.5 per cent. Complications include cerebral embolic events (despite absence of detectable thrombus on two-dimensional echocardiography) and cardiac perforation, each in approximately 1 per cent, and the development of mitral regurgitation severe enough to require operation in another 2 per cent (ap-

proximately 15 per cent develop lesser, but still undesirable, degrees of regurgitation). Results are especially impressive in younger patients without valvular thickening or calcification. Improvement in exercise tolerance has paralleled the favorable hemodynamic changes.

Approximately 10 per cent of patients are left with a small residual atrial septal defect, but this closes or decreases in size in the majority. Rarely, the defect is large enough to cause right heart failure.[91] Elevated pulmonary vascular resistance declines rapidly (but usually not completely) following mitral balloon valvuloplasty,[92] and pulmonary function improves as well. In follow-up studies over 3 years, hemodynamic benefit has been maintained in the majority of patients, and they have not required surgical treatment, i.e., with commissurotomy or mitral valve replacement. Approximately 10 per cent have developed restenosis.

The combination of significant symptoms and documented MS generally serves as an indication for balloon valvulotomy. The skill and experience of the operator (interventional cardiologist) must be considered. Detailed two-dimensional and Doppler echocardiographic studies are indicated before a decision is made. Left atrial thrombus must be excluded by echocardiography.

An echocardiographic scoring system developed by Wilkins et al.[93] has been found to be particularly valuable in patient selection. Leaflet rigidity, leaflet thickening, valvular calcification, and subvalvular disease are each scored from 0 to 4 (Fig. 32–7). Rigid, thickened valves with extensive subvalvular fibrosis and calcification lead to suboptimal results. A score of 8 or less is usually associated with an excellent immediate and long-term result, whereas scores exceeding 8 are associated with less impressive results (Fig. 32–8). Fluoroscopically visible calcium is another important predictor of outcome; patients with heavily calcified valves exhibit less increase in valve area and a poorer long-term survival than those with no or lesser degrees of calcification.[94,94a] The findings on echocardiography and fluoroscopy affect the outcome of both open and closed surgical commissurotomy in a similar manner. A trial in which patients with severe MS were randomized to percutaneous balloon valvuloplasty and open surgical commissurotomy resulted in similar clinical results from the two techniques. Indeed, after 3 years, mitral valve area was greater in the balloon-treated group[95] (Fig. 32–9).

In patients with symptomatic, hemodynamically severe stenosis, with an echocardiographic score of 8 or less, without left atrial thrombus, percutaneous balloon angioplasty is the procedure of choice.[89] The lower cost and morbidity are obvious advantages. The procedure is optimal for treating young patients with noncalcific MS in de-

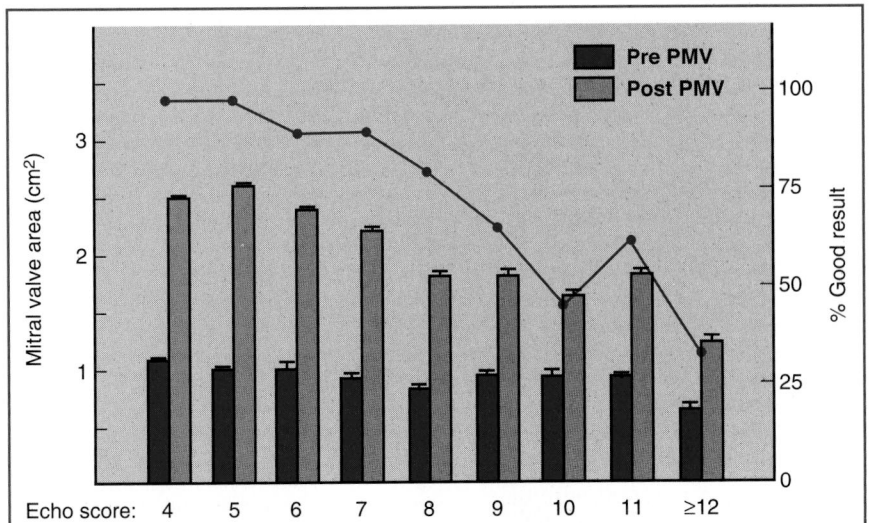

FIGURE 32–8. Relationship between echocardiographic score (X axis), the increase in mitral valve area produced by percutaneous mitral valvotomy (left Y axis), and the per cent of patients having a good result (mitral valve area > 1.5 cm²) (right Y axis). (From Block, P. C., and Palacios, I. F.: Aortic and mitral balloon valvuloplasty: The United States experience. In Topol, E. J. [ed.]: Textbook of Interventional Cardiology. Philadelphia, W.B. Saunders Company, 1990, p. 831.)

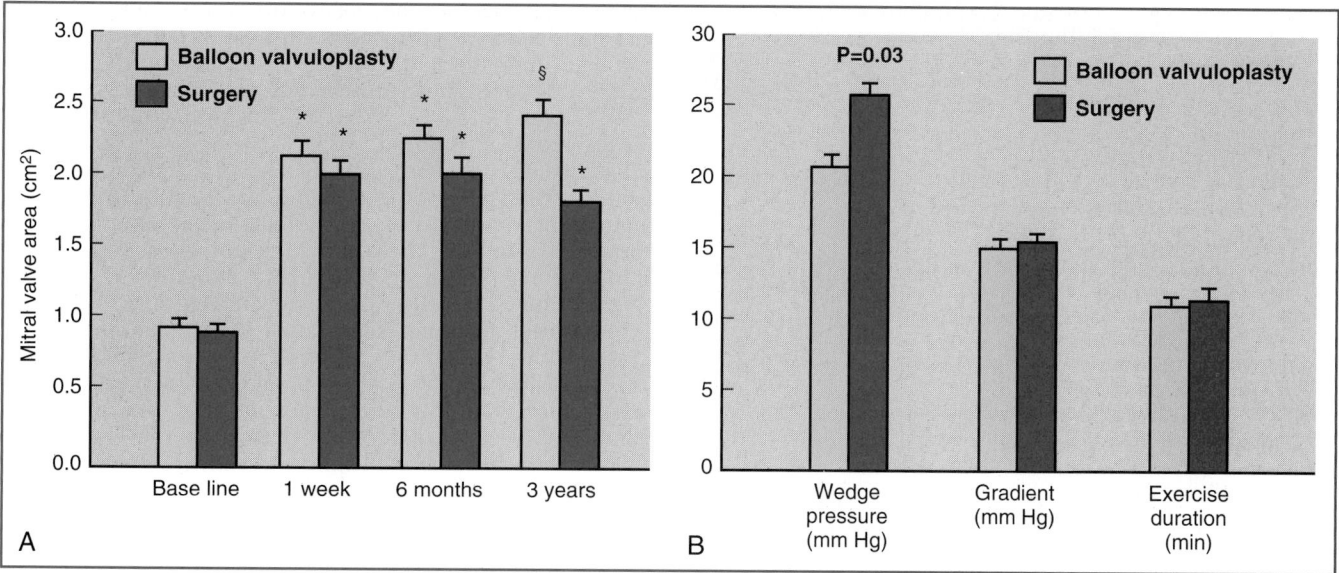

FIGURE 32–9. *A,* Hemodynamic variables at baseline and 1 week, 6 months, and 3 years after balloon mitral valvuloplasty or open surgical commissurotomy. The asterisk indicates P < 0.001 for the comparison with the baseline value. The section mark (§) indicates P < 0.001 for the comparison with the surgery group. The bars indicate the standard errors. *B,* Pulmonary artery wedge pressure and mitral valve gradient during exercise and duration of exercise at the 3-year follow-up examination. The bars indicate the standard errors. (From Reyes, V. P., Raju, B. S., Wynne, J., et al.: Percutaneous balloon valvuloplasty compared with open surgical commissurotomy for mitral stenosis. N. Engl. J. Med. *331*:961, 1994. Copyright Massachusetts Medical Society.)

veloping nations with limited facilities for open heart surgery.[90] It may also be used in patients with less favorable valves who are unsuitable for surgery because of high risk.[96,96a] These include very elderly patients and patients with associated severe ischemic heart disease, as well as patients in whom MS is complicated by pulmonary, renal, or neoplastic disease, women of childbearing age in whom valve replacement is undesirable, and pregnant women

with MS.[97] Balloon angioplasty can also be the initial procedure in patients with symptomatic, severe MS and unfavorable valves (echocardiographic score >8 and/or dense calcification on fluoroscopic examination)[94,98] without any of these characteristics but with the appreciation that the failure rate is considerable and that the patient may require follow-up surgical treatment, ordinarily mitral valve replacement.

MITRAL REGURGITATION

ETIOLOGY AND PATHOLOGY

The mitral valve apparatus involves the mitral leaflets per se, the chordae tendineae, the papillary muscles, and the mitral annulus. Abnormalities of any of these structures may cause mitral regurgitation (MR)[98a] (Table 32–1). The mitral valve prolapse syndrome, an important cause of MR, is discussed in a separate section (see p. 1029).

ABNORMALITIES OF VALVE LEAFLETS. MR due to predominant involvement of the valve leaflets occurs most commonly in chronic rheumatic heart disease and is more frequent in men than in women. It is a consequence of shortening, rigidity, deformity, and retraction of one or both cusps of the mitral valve, associated with shortening and fusion of the chordae tendineae and papillary muscles.[99,99a] Infective endocarditis can cause MR by perforating valve leaflets; vegetations can prevent leaflet coaptation, and valvular retraction during the healing phase of endocarditis can cause MR. Destruction of the mitral valve leaflets can also occur in penetrating and nonpenetrating trauma (see p. 1541). When severe MR accompanies acute rheumatic fever in children or in adolescents in developing countries, regurgitation is usually secondary to a combination of prolapse of the anterior leaflet, elongation of the chordae, and dilatation of the annulus.[100] Left ventricular submitral aneurysm has been reported as a cause of MR in sub-Saharan Africa. It appears to be caused by a congenital defect in the posterior portion of the annulus. Diagnosis by transesophageal echocardiography[101] and surgical repair have been reported.

ABNORMALITIES OF THE MITRAL ANNULUS. Dilatation. In a normal adult the mitral annulus measures approximately 10 cm in circumference; it is soft and flexible, and during systole contraction of the surrounding left ventricular muscle causes the annulus to constrict. This constriction contributes importantly to valve closure. MR secondary to dilatation of the mitral annulus can occur in any form of heart disease characterized by severe dilatation of the left ventricle,[102] especially dilated ischemic cardiomyopathy.[103] It is often difficult to differentiate this secondary from the primary form of MR, but it is notable that primary valvular regurgitation is often more severe than is regurgitation secondary to annular dilatation.

Calcification. Idiopathic (degenerative) calcification of the mitral annulus is one of the most common cardiac abnormalities found at autopsy; in most hearts it is of little functional consequence. However, when it is severe it may be an important cause of MR,[103a] and in contrast to MR secondary to rheumatic fever, this cause is more common in women than in men. The development of degenerative calcification of the mitral annulus is accelerated by systemic hypertension, aortic stenosis, and diabetes, as well as by an intrinsic defect in the fibrous skeleton of the heart, such as occurs in the Marfan and Hurler syndromes. In these two conditions, the mitral annulus is not only calcified but is also dilated, further contributing to MR. The incidence of mitral annular calcification is also increased in patients with chronic renal failure with secondary hyperparathyroidism.[104] The annulus may also become thick, rigid, and calcified secondary to rheumatic

TABLE 32–1 CAUSES OF ACUTE AND CHRONIC MITRAL REGURGITATION

ACUTE

Mitral Annulus Disorders
Infective endocarditis (abscess formation)
Trauma (valvular heart surgery)
Paravalvular leak due to suture interruption (surgical technical problems or infective endocarditis)

Mitral Leaflet Disorders
Infective endocarditis (perforation or interfering with valve closure by vegetation)
Trauma (tear during percutaneous mitral balloon valvotomy or penetrating chest injury)
Tumors (atrial myxoma)
Myxomatous degeneration
Systemic lupus erythematosus (Libman-Sacks lesion)

Rupture of Chordae Tendineae
Idiopathic, e.g., spontaneous
Myxomatous degeneration (mitral valve prolapse, Marfan syndrome, Ehlers-Danlos syndrome)
Infective endocarditis
Acute rheumatic fever
Trauma (percutaneous balloon valvotomy, blunt chest trauma)

Papillary Muscle Disorders
Coronary artery disease (causing dysfunction and rarely rupture)
Acute global left ventricular dysfunction
Infiltrative diseases (amyloidosis, sarcoidosis)
Trauma

Primary Mitral Valve Prosthetic Disorders
Porcine cusp perforation (endocarditis)
Porcine cusp degeneration
Mechanical failure (strut fracture)
Immobilized disc or ball of the mechanical prosthesis

CHRONIC

Inflammatory
Rheumatic heart disease
Systemic lupus erythematosus
Scleroderma

Degenerative
Myxomatous degeneration of mitral valve leaflets (Barlow's click-murmur syndrome, prolapsing leaflet, mitral valve prolapse)
Marfan syndrome
Ehlers-Danlos syndrome
Pseudoxanthoma elasticum
Calcification of mitral valve annulus

Infective
Infective endocarditis affecting normal, abnormal, or prosthetic mitral valves

Structural
Ruptured chordae tendineae (spontaneous or secondary to myocardial infarction, trauma, mitral valve prolapse, endocarditis)
Rupture or dysfunction of papillary muscle (ischemia or myocardial infarction)
Dilatation of mitral valve annulus and left ventricular cavity (congestive cardiomyopathies, aneurysmal dilatation of the left ventricle)
Hypertrophic cardiomyopathy
Paravalvular prosthetic leak

Congenital
Mitral valve clefts or fenestrations
Parachute mitral valve abnormality in association with:
Endocardial cushion defects
Endocardial fibroelastosis
Transposition of the great arteries
Anomalous origin of the left coronary artery

Data from Jutzy, K. R., and Al-Zaibag, M.: Acute mitral and aortic valve regurgitation. *In* Al-Zaibag, M., and Duran, C. M. G. (eds.): Valvular Heart Disease. New York, Marcel Dekker, 1994, pp. 345–382 (top portion) and Haffajee, C. I.: Chronic mitral regurgitation. *In* Dalen, J. E., and Alpert, J. S. (eds.): Valvular Heart Disease. 2nd ed. Boston, Little, Brown and Co., 1987, p. 112 (lower portion).

involvement; when this process is severe, it also can interfere with valve closure.

When annular calcification is severe, a rigid, curved bar or ring of calcium encircles the mitral orifice (Fig. 7–28, p. 222), and calcific spurs may project into the adjacent left ventricular myocardium.[105] The bulk of the calcium is located in the subvalvular region. The calcification may immobilize the basal portion of the mitral leaflets, preventing their normal excursion in diastole and coaptation in systole and aggravating the MR that results from loss of the normal sphincteric action of the mitral ring.[106] Rarely, when severe calcification encroaches on or protrudes into the mitral orifice, obstruction to left ventricular filling may occur. Calcification of the aortic valve cusps is an associated finding in approximately 50 per cent of patients with severe annular calcification, but this rarely causes aortic stenosis. In patients with severe calcification the conduction system may be invaded by calcium, leading to atrioventricular and/or intraventricular conduction defects.[105] Occasionally, calcific deposits extend into the coronary arteries.

ABNORMALITIES OF THE CHORDAE TENDINEAE. These are important causes of MR. The chordae may be congenitally abnormal; rupture may be spontaneous ("primary")[106] or may occur as a consequence of infective endocarditis, trauma, rheumatic fever, or rarely, osteogenesis imperfecta.[107,108] Lengthening and rupture of chordae tendineae are cardinal features of the mitral valve prolapse syndrome (see p. 1029). In most cases no cause for chordal rupture is apparent, other than increased mechanical strain. Chordae to the posterior leaflet rupture more frequently than those to the anterior leaflet. Patients with idiopathic rupture of mitral chordae tendineae frequently exhibit pathological fibrosis of the papillary muscles. It is possible that the dysfunction of the papillary muscles may have caused stretching and ultimately rupture of the chordae. Chordal rupture may also result from acute left ventricular dilatation, regardless of etiology. Depending on the number of chordae involved in rupture and rate at which rupture occurs, the resultant MR may be mild, moderate, or severe and acute, subacute, or chronic, respectively.

INVOLVEMENT OF THE PAPILLARY MUSCLES. Diseases of the left ventricular papillary muscles frequently cause MR.[109] Because these muscles are perfused by the terminal portion of the coronary vascular bed, they are particularly vulnerable to ischemia, and any disturbance in coronary perfusion may result in papillary muscle dysfunction (Fig. 32–10). When ischemia is transient, it results in temporary papillary muscle dysfunction and may cause transient episodes of MR sometimes associated with attacks of angina pectoris. When ischemia of papillary muscles is severe and prolonged, it causes papillary muscle dysfunction and scarring and chronic MR. The posterior papillary muscle, which is supplied by the posterior descending branch of the right coronary artery, becomes ischemic and infarcted more frequently than does the anterolateral papillary muscle, which is supplied by diagonal branches of the left anterior descending coronary artery and often by marginal branches from the left circumflex artery as well. Ischemia of the papillary muscle is caused most commonly by coronary artery disease, but it may also occur in severe anemia, shock, coronary arteritis of any etiology, and anomalous left coronary artery. MR occurs frequently in patients with healed myocardial infarcts, and is caused by dyskinesis of the left ventricular myocardium at the base of a papillary muscle.[110]

Left ventricular dilatation of any cause, including ischemia, can alter the spatial relationships between the papillary muscles and the chordae tendineae and thereby result in MR.[111] Although *necrosis of a papillary muscle* is a frequent complication of myocardial infarction,[112] frank rupture is far less common; the latter is usually fatal because of the extremely severe MR that it produces. However, rupture of one or two of the apical heads of a

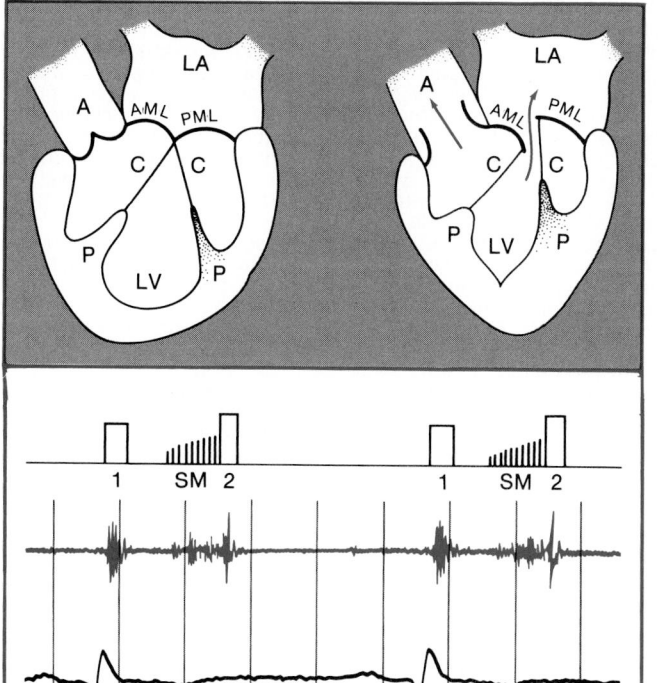

FIGURE 32–10. *Top,* Mitral regurgitation due to papillary muscle dysfunction. At the onset of systole (left), the anterior and posterior mitral valve leaflets (AML and PML) approximate. Later in systole (right), the anterior papillary muscle (P, nonhatched) contracts while the posterior papillary muscle (P, hatched) fails to contract because of ischemia or infarction. Part of the posterior leaflet is allowed to prolapse into the left atrium (LA) during systole, producing regurgitation. This process may involve either papillary muscle. C = chordae tendineae, LV = left ventricle, A = aorta. *Bottom,* Late systolic murmur (SM) that developed in a patient following an inferior myocardial infarction and is probably due to weakening of the posterior papillary muscle with prolapse of the mitral leaflet into the atrium during late systole. (From Ravin, A., et al.: Auscultation of the Heart. 3rd ed. Chicago, Year Book Medical Publishers, 1977, p. 99. Copyright © 1977 by Year Book Medical Publishers, Inc., Chicago.)

muscle, which results in a lesser degree of MR, makes survival possible, usually with surgical therapy (see p. 1243).

Some degree of MR is found in approximately 30 per cent of patients with coronary artery disease who are being considered for coronary bypass surgery,[110] and in them it is secondary to ischemic damage of the papillary muscles, dilatation of the mitral valve ring, or both. In most of these patients MR is mild, but in the small percentage in whom MR is severe (3 per cent in one large series of patients with coronary artery disease proved by coronary arteriography), it is associated with a poor prognosis.[113] The incidence and severity of regurgitation vary inversely with the left ventricular ejection fraction and directly with the left ventricular end-diastolic pressure.

A variety of other disorders of papillary muscles may also be responsible for the development of mitral regurgitation (Table 32–1). These include congenital malposition, absence of one papillary muscle, resulting in the so-called parachute mitral valve syndrome, and involvement or infiltration of papillary muscles by a variety of processes, including abscesses, granulomas, neoplasms, amyloidosis, and sarcoidosis.

Other causes of MR, discussed in greater detail elsewhere, include obstructive cardiomyopathy (see p. 1404), mitral valve prolapse (see p. 1029), the hypereosinophilic syndrome,[114] endomyocardial fibrosis,[115] trauma affecting the leaflets[116] and/or papillary muscles[117] (see p. 1541), Kawasaki disease[118] (see p. 994), left atrial myxoma, a variety

PATHOPHYSIOLOGY

Because the regurgitant mitral orifice is functionally in parallel with the aortic valve, the impedance to ventricular emptying is reduced in MR. Consequently, MR enhances left ventricular emptying. Almost half of the regurgitant volume is ejected into the left atrium before the aortic valve opens.[121] The volume of MR depends on the impedance to left ventricular emptying and is increased by hypertension and aortic stenosis and reduced in shock.

The volume of mitral regurgitation flow depends on a combination of the instantaneous size of the regurgitant orifice and the (reverse) pressure gradient between the left ventricle and left atrium[18a,122–124]; both of these factors—orifice size and pressure gradient—are labile. Left ventricular systolic pressure and therefore the left ventricular–left atrial gradient depends on systemic vascular resistance[122] and in patients in whom the mitral annulus is normally flexible, the cross-sectional area of the mitral annulus may be altered by many interventions. Thus, increases of both preload and afterload and depressions of contractility increase left ventricular size and enlarge the mitral annulus and thereby the regurgitant orifice.[124] When ventricular size is reduced by treatment with positive inotropic agents, diuretics, and particularly vasodilators, the volume of regurgitant flow declines, as reflected in the height of the *v* wave in the left atrial pressure pulse and in the intensity and duration of the systolic murmur. Conversely, left ventricular dilatation may increase MR.

In canine experiments in which the acute effects of equally severe MR and aortic regurgitation (AR) on the left ventricle were compared, left ventricular end-diastolic pressure, volume, and radius rose with both lesions, but far *less* so with MR.[125] Peak left ventricular wall tension rose markedly when AR was induced but either did not change greatly or actually declined with MR. According to Laplace's law, myocardial wall tension is related to the product of intraventricular pressure and ventricular radius. Because *acute* MR reduces both late systolic ventricular pressure and radius, left ventricular wall tension declines markedly (and proportionately to a greater extent than left ventricular pressure), permitting a reciprocal increase in both the extent and velocity of myocardial fiber shortening. Thus, the reduced left ventricular afterload allows a greater proportion of the contractile energy of the myocardium to be expended in shortening than in tension development and explains how the left ventricle can adapt to the load imposed by MR. The ratio of wall thickness (h) to ventricular radius (r) is lower and the fractional shortening of myocardium greater in patients with MR than AR.[126,127]

The left ventricle initially compensates for the development of acute MR in part by emptying more completely and in part by increasing preload, i.e., by use of the Frank-Starling principle. As regurgitation, particularly severe regurgitation, becomes chronic, the left ventricular end-diastolic volume increases. By the Laplace principle, this increases wall tension to normal or supranormal levels.[128] The resultant increase in left ventricular volume and mitral annular diameter may create a vicious circle in which "MR begets more MR."[129]

For many years it was thought that when heart failure occurred in patients with severe rheumatic MR and acute rheumatic fever, it was caused, at least in part, by the accompanying rheumatic myocarditis. However, the normalization of hemodynamics following valve replacement in such patients makes this unlikely and instead suggests that the heart failure is secondary to the valvular lesion itself.[130]

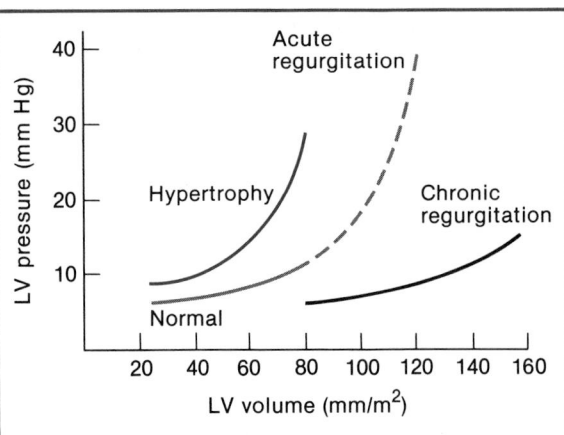

FIGURE 32–11. Diagrammatic representation of the changes in the diastolic pressure-volume relationship that occur in valve disease. Hypertrophy without significant ventricular dilatation (e.g., in aortic stenosis) produces a somewhat steeper curve than normal. Acute regurgitation produces a sudden volume load on the ventricle without time for other changes to occur and the ventricle operates at the upper (steep) end of the normal curve (broken line). Chronic aortic and mitral regurgitation with volume overload produces a flattened curve so that large volumes are accommodated without the large rise in end-diastolic pressure which occurs in acute regurgitation. (From Hall, R. J., and Julian, D. G.: Diseases of the Cardiac Valves. New York, Churchill Livingstone, 1989, p. 291.)

A large volume of MR induced experimentally produces only slightly increased myocardial oxygen consumption,[131] because myocardial fiber shortening, which is elevated in MR, is not one of the principal determinants of myocardial oxygen consumption.[132] One of these, mean left ventricular wall tension, may actually be reduced in MR whereas the other two, contractility and heart rate, may be little affected. These experimental observations correlate with the low incidence of clinical manifestations of myocardial ischemia in patients with severe MR compared with that occurring in aortic stenosis or aortic regurgitation, conditions in which myocardial oxygen demands are augmented.

In patients with chronic MR, both left ventricular end-diastolic volume and mass are increased; i.e., typical volume overload (eccentric) hypertrophy develops. The degree of hypertrophy is usually appropriate to the left ventricular dilatation, so that the ratio of left ventricular mass to end-diastolic volume is normal (Fig. 13–10, p. 401). A shift to the right occurs in the left ventricular diastolic pressure-volume curve with chronic MR (Fig. 32–11).[133]

ASSESSMENT OF MYOCARDIAL CONTRACTILITY IN MITRAL REGURGITATION

(See also p. 430)

Because the ejection phase indices of myocardial contractility are inversely correlated with afterload, patients with early MR (with reduced left ventricular afterload) often exhibit elevations in ejection phase indices of myocardial contractility, such as ejection fraction (EF), fractional fiber shortening (FS), and velocity of circumferential fiber shortening (VCF).[134] However, by the time patients become seriously symptomatic, EF, FS, and mean VCF have usually declined to *normal* levels or below. As MR persists, the reduction in afterload, which increases myocardial shortening and the above-mentioned ejection phase indices, is opposed by the impairment of myocardial function characteristic of severe chronic diastolic overload. However, even in patients with overt heart failure secondary to MR, the EF and FS may be only slightly reduced.[183,184,188] Therefore, *normal* values for the ejection phase indices of myocardial performance in patients with acute MR may actually reflect impaired myocardial function,[135,136] whereas moderately reduced values (e.g., an ejection fraction of 40 to 50 per cent) generally signify severe, often irreversible, impairment of contractility. An ejection fraction under 40 per cent in patients with severe MR usually represents advanced myocardial dysfunction; such patients are high operative risks and may not experience marked improvement following mitral valve replacement (see p. 1026). Indeed, long-term survival following replacement or repair of regurgitant mitral valves is reduced if the ejection fraction declines below 60 per cent.[136]

END-SYSTOLIC VOLUME. Preoperative myocardial contractility is an important determinant of the risk of operative death and of cardiac failure in the perioperative period and of the level of left ventricular function postoperatively. Therefore, it is not surprising that the end-systolic pressure (or stress/dimension) relation has emerged as a useful index for evaluating left ventricular function in patients with valvular regurgitation.[137] Indeed, the simple measurement of

end-systolic volume has been found to be more useful as a predictor of outcome than the ejection fraction, end-diastolic volume, or end-diastolic pressure.[138] Patients with severe MR with a normal preoperative end-systolic volume (<40 ml/m²) retained normal left ventricular function postoperatively, whereas marked enlargement of the end-systolic volume (>80 ml/m²) signified a high perioperative mortality and residual left ventricular dysfunction. An end-systolic volume of 55 ml/m² appears to discriminate between patients who do well after surgical correction and those who are at risk of irreversible dysfunction.[139] Patients with MR and modest enlargement of end-systolic volume (between 40 and 80 ml/m²) usually tolerate operation satisfactorily but may have reduced left ventricular function postoperatively. For any level of end-systolic volume, patients with MR have more severe left ventricular dysfunction than do patients with aortic regurgitation.[140] This finding reflects the lower afterload in MR and correlates with the clinical observation that patients with MR have a less favorable response to surgical intervention than do those with aortic regurgitation.[138]

A closely related variable, the end-systolic diameter, determined by echocardiography, is the most reliable noninvasive predictor of outcome (survival without severe heart failure) following mitral valve replacement. The outcome is excellent until the end-systolic diameter exceeds approximately 45 mm or 26 ml/m² (Fig. 32–12).[141]

HEMODYNAMICS. Effective (forward) *cardiac output* is usually depressed in seriously symptomatic patients, whereas *total* left ventricular output (the sum of forward and regurgitant flow, which can be measured by radionuclide ventriculography)[142] is usually elevated until quite late in the patient's course. The atrial contraction (a) wave in the left atrial pressure pulse is usually not as prominent in MR as in MS, but the v wave is often much taller[123] (Fig. 6–5, p. 184), because it is inscribed during ventricular systole, when the left atrium is being filled with blood from the pulmonary veins as well as from the left ventricle (Fig. 32–13). Occasionally, backward transmission of the tall v wave into the pulmonary arterial bed may result in an early diastolic "pulmonary arterial v wave."[143] In patients with pure MR, the y descent is particularly rapid as the distended left atrium empties rapidly during early systole. However, in patients with combined MS and MR, the y descent is gradual. Although a left atrioventricular pressure gradient persisting throughout diastole signifies the

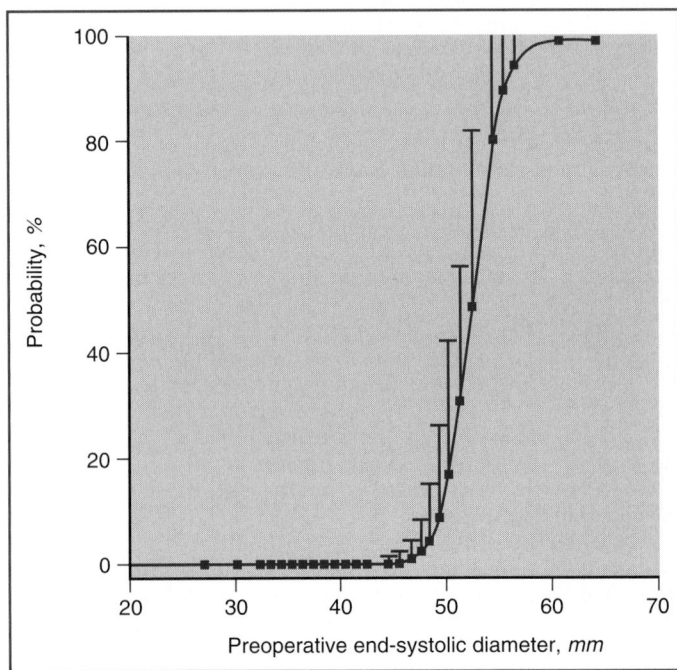

FIGURE 32–12. The probability of postoperative death or persistence of severe heart failure in patients with mitral regurgitation plotted against preoperative echocardiographic end-systolic diameter. As end-systolic diameter exceeded 45 mm, the incidence of a poor postoperative outcome increased abruptly. (Reproduced with permission from Wisenbaugh, T., et al.: Prediction of outcome after valve replacement for rheumatic mitral regurgitation in the era of chordal preservation. Circulation *89*:191, 1994. Copyright 1994 American Heart Association.)

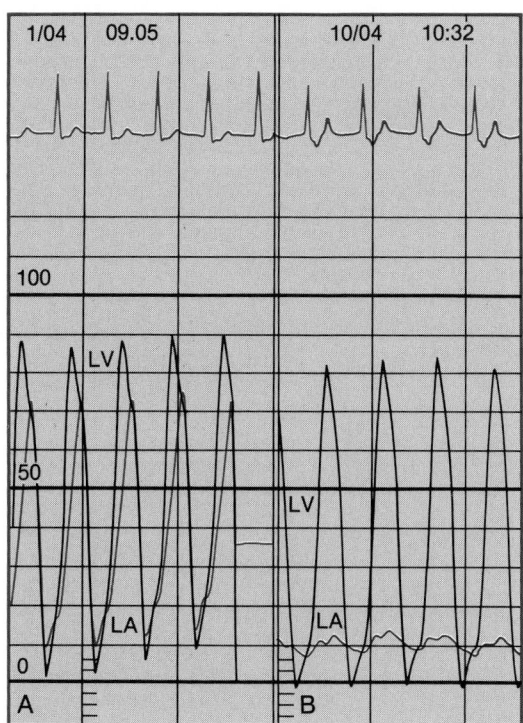

FIGURE 32–13. Intraoperative simultaneous left ventricular (LV) and left atrial (LA) pressures (mm Hg) before (*A*) and after (*B*) mitral valvuloplasty for correction of severe acute mitral regurgitation. Note the height of the *v* wave in the preoperative tracing. (From Barlow, J. B.: Perspectives on the Mitral Valve. Philadelphia, F. A. Davis Co., 1987, p. 257.)

presence of significant associated MS, a brief early diastolic gradient may occur in patients with isolated, severe regurgitation as a result of the torrential flow of blood across a normal-sized mitral orifice[143a] (Fig. 32–2).

LEFT ATRIAL COMPLIANCE

The compliance of the left atrium (and pulmonary venous bed) is an important determinant of the hemodynamic[144,145] and clinical picture in MR. Three major subgroups of patients with severe MR based on left atrial compliance have been identified[125,146,147] (Fig. 32–14) and are characterized as follows:

NORMAL OR REDUCED COMPLIANCE. There is little enlargement of the left atrium but marked elevation of the mean left atrial pressure, particularly of the *v* wave,[148,149] and pulmonary congestion is a prominent symptom. In most cases, severe MR has developed suddenly, as occurs with rupture of chordae tendineae, infarction of one of the heads of a papillary muscle, or perforation of a mitral leaflet as a consequence of trauma or endocarditis. Initially in acute MR the left atrium operates on the steep portion of its pressure-volume curve. Sinus rhythm is usually present; with the passage of weeks or a few months the left atrial wall frequently exhibits striking hypertrophy, is capable of contracting vigorously, and facilitates left ventricular filling.[144] The thicker atrium is less compliant than normal, increasing further the height of the *v* wave. Thickening of the walls of the pulmonary veins and proliferative changes in the pulmonary arteries as well as marked elevation of pulmonary vascular resistance usually develop over the course of 6 to 12 months.

MARKEDLY INCREASED COMPLIANCE. At the opposite end of the spectrum from patients in the first group are those with severe, longstanding MR with massive enlargement of the left atrium and normal or only slightly elevated left atrial pressure.[147] The atrial wall contains only a small remnant of muscle surrounded by a great deal of fibrous tissue. Longstanding MR in these patients has altered the physical properties of the left atrial wall and thereby displaced the atrial pressure-volume curve, allowing a normal or almost normal pressure to exist in a greatly enlarged left atrium. (This shift in the left atrial pressure-volume curve with persistent MR has been documented in animal experiments.[144]) Pulmonary artery pressure and pulmonary vascular resistance are normal or only slightly elevated at rest. Atrial fibrillation and a low cardiac output are almost invariably present.[147]

MODERATELY INCREASED COMPLIANCE. This, the most common subgroup, consists of patients between the ends of the spectrum represented by groups 1 and 2; these patients have severe chronic MR and exhibit variable degrees of enlargement of the left atrium, associated with significant elevation of the left atrial pressure.

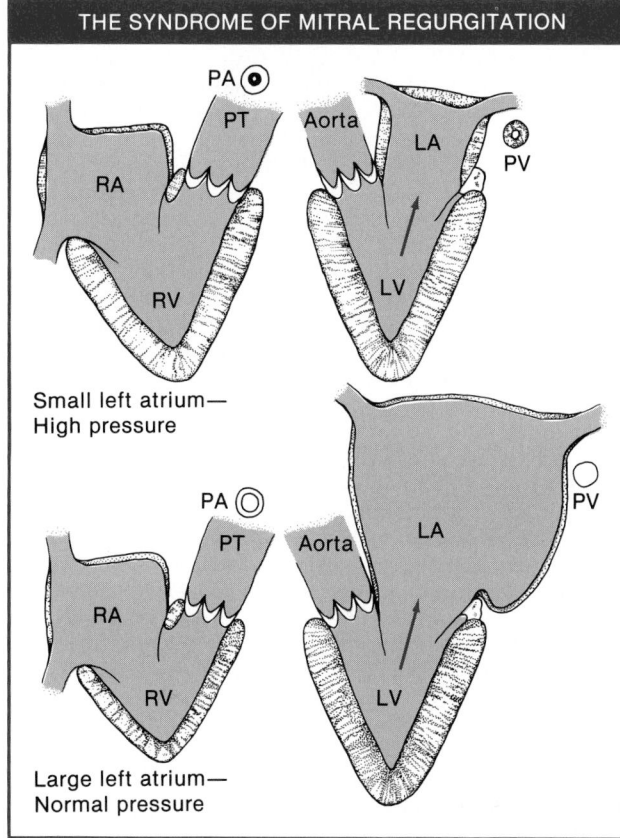

THE SYNDROME OF MITRAL REGURGITATION

Small left atrium—
High pressure

Large left atrium—
Normal pressure

FIGURE 32–14. Diagram depicting the two extremes of the spectrum in pure mitral regurgitation. When severe mitral regurgitation appears suddenly in individuals with previously normal or near-normal hearts (*top*), the left atrium (LA) is relatively small and the high pressure within it is reflected back into the pulmonary vessels and right ventricle (RV). The anatomical indicator of this latter physiological event is severe hypertrophy of the left atrial and right ventricular walls and marked intimal proliferation and medial hypertrophy of the pulmonary arteries (PA), arterioles, and veins (PV). At the other extreme with severe chronic mitral regurgitation (*bottom*), the left atrial cavity is of giant size and its wall is thin. It is thus able to "absorb" the left ventricular (LV) pressure without reflecting it back into the pulmonary vessels or right ventricle. As a consequence, pulmonary vessels remain normal, and the right ventricular wall does not thicken. PT = pulmonary trunk; RA = right atrium. (From Roberts, W. C., et al.: Nonrheumatic valvular cardiac disease. A clinicopathologic survey of 27 different conditions causing valvular dysfunction. *In* Likoff, W. [ed.]: Cardiovascular Clinics. Vol. 5, No. 2, Valvular Heart Disease. Philadelphia, F. A. Davis Co., 1973, p. 403.)

CLINICAL MANIFESTATIONS

History

The nature and severity of the symptoms of patients with chronic MR are functions of its severity, rate of progression, the level of pulmonary artery pressure, and the presence of associated valvular, myocardial, or coronary artery disease. Because symptoms usually do not develop in patients with chronic MR until the left ventricle fails, the time interval between the initial attack of rheumatic fever (when one has occurred) and the development of symptoms tends to be longer in MR than in MS and often exceeds two decades. The course in patients with chronic MR tends to be less dramatic and is punctuated with fewer acute complications than in patients with MS. Acute pulmonary edema occurs less frequently in chronic MR than in MS, presumably because sudden surges in left atrial pressure are less common.[15] Similarly, although hemoptysis and systemic embolization do occur in MR, they are less common than in MS. The development of atrial fibrillation affects the course adversely but perhaps not as dramatically as it does in MS. On the other hand, chronic weakness and fatigue secondary to a low cardiac output are more prominent features in MR.

Patients with mild MR may remain asymptomatic for their entire lives.[41] The majority of patients with MR of rheumatic origin have only mild disability, unless regurgitation progresses as a result of chronic rheumatic activity, infective endocarditis, or rupture of chordae tendineae.[147] However, the indolent course of MR may, in fact, be deceptive. By the time that symptoms secondary to a reduced cardiac output and/or pulmonary congestion become apparent, serious and sometimes even irreversible left ventricular dysfunction may have developed. In contrast, patients with MS have the benefit of an "early warning system," i.e., symptoms of pulmonary congestion with frequent, sudden elevations of left atrial pressure.

In patients with severe chronic MR with a greatly enlarged left atrium and with relatively mild left atrial hypertension (group 2 with increased left atrial compliance, described above), pulmonary vascular resistance does not usually rise appreciably. Instead, the major symptoms, fatigue and exhaustion, are related to a low cardiac output. Right heart failure, characterized by congestive hepatomegaly, edema, and ascites, is observed in patients with acute MR and elevated pulmonary vascular resistance. Angina pectoris is rare unless coronary artery disease coexists.

NATURAL HISTORY. This is variable and depends on a combination of the volume of regurgitation, the state of the myocardium, and the cause of the underlying disorder. The condition in asymptomatic patients with mild MR usually remains stable for many years[150]; severe regurgitation develops in only a small percentage of these, in some cases because of intervening infective endocarditis or rupture of chordae tendineae or both. Regurgitation tends to progress more rapidly in patients with connective tissue diseases, such as Marfan syndrome, than in those with chronic MR on a rheumatic basis. Isolated severe MR secondary to acute rheumatic fever occurs frequently in adolescents in developing nations. The course is often rapidly progressive. Because the natural history of severe MR has been altered greatly by surgical intervention, it is difficult now to predict the course of patients on medical therapy alone. However, in an unselected group of patients with MR who were treated medically before surgical treatment of severe MR became commonplace, approximately 80 per cent survived 5 years after the diagnosis and almost 60 per cent survived 10 years.[66] Patients with combined MS and MR had a poorer prognosis, with only 67 per cent surviving 5 years and 30 per cent surviving 10 years after diagnosis. Munoz et al., in studying a group of patients with greater disability, found that medically treated patients with severe MR had a 5-year survival rate of only 45 per cent.[65] Among medically treated patients with MR, the arteriovenous oxygen difference and ventricular end-diastolic volume were significant (inverse) predictors of survival.[148]

Physical Examination

Palpation of the arterial pulse is helpful in differentiating aortic stenosis from MR; both may produce a prominent systolic murmur at the base of the heart.[32a] The carotid arterial upstroke is sharp in severe MR[151] and delayed in aortic stenosis; the volume of the pulse may be normal or reduced in the presence of heart failure.

The cardiac impulse, like the arterial peel, is brisk and hyperdynamic, and it is displaced to the left[15] (Table 2–1, p. 24 and Fig. 32–15), and a prominent left ventricular filling wave is frequently palpable in early diastole. Systolic expansion of the enlarged left atrium may result in a late systolic thrust in the parasternal region, which may be confused with right ventricular enlargement.[152]

AUSCULTATION. With severe, chronic MR due to defective valve cusps, S_1, produced by valve closure, is usually

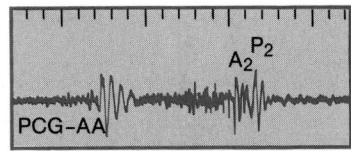
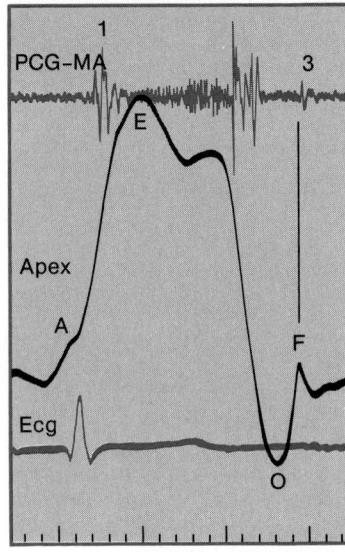

FIGURE 32–15. Hyperdynamic apexcardiogram in mitral regurgitation. The configuration of the tracing in systole is qualitatively similar to a normal curve, although the amplitude was clearly exaggerated by palpation. The rapid filling wave (F) is higher than normal and terminates in a sharp point coincident with its audible counterpart, the third heart sound (3). (From Craige, E., and Smith, D.: Heart sounds. *In* Braunwald, E. [ed.]: Heart Disease: A Textbook of Cardiovascular Medicine. 3rd ed, Philadelphia, W. B. Saunders Company, 1988, p. 58.)

diminished.[153,154] Wide splitting of S_2 is common and results from the shortening of left ventricular ejection and an earlier A_2 as a consequence of reduced resistance to left ventricular outflow. In the presence of MR with severe pulmonary hypertension, P_2 is louder than A_2. The abnormal increase in the flow rate across the mitral orifice during the rapid filling phase is usually associated with an S_3 (Fig. 32–15), the auscultatory counterpart of a palpable rapid filling wave. A left ventricular S_3, i.e., one that is not augmented by inspiration, excludes predominant MS (unless aortic regurgitation, ischemic heart disease, or another cause of an S_3 is present).

The *systolic murmur* is the most prominent physical finding in MR; it must be differentiated from the systolic murmur heard in aortic stenosis, tricuspid regurgitation, ventricular septal defect, and sometimes MS (Table 32–2). In most cases of severe MR the systolic murmur commences immediately after the soft S_1 and continues beyond and may obscure A_2 because of the persistence of the pressure difference between the left ventricle and left atrium (Figs. 2–31, p. 38, and 2–32, p. 39). The holosystolic murmur of chronic MR is usually constant in intensity, blowing, high-pitched, and loudest at the apex with radiation to the axilla and left infrascapular area; however, radiation toward the sternum or the aortic area may occur with abnormalities of the posterior leaflet. The murmur shows little change even in the presence of large beat-to-beat variations of left ventricular stroke volume, as occur in atrial fibrillation, in contrast to most midsystolic (ejection) murmurs, such as in aortic stenosis, which vary greatly in intensity with stroke volume and therefore with the duration of diastole.[155] There is little correlation between the intensity of the systolic murmur and the severity of MR. Indeed, in patients with severe MR due to left ventricular dilatation, acute myocardial infarction, or paraprosthetic valvular regurgitation, or in those who have marked emphysema, obesity,

TABLE 32-2 DIFFERENTIAL DIAGNOSIS OF MITRAL REGURGITATION, VENTRICULAR SEPTAL DEFECT, TRICUSPID REGURGITATION, AND AORTIC STENOSIS

PHYSICAL, ROENTGENOGRAPHIC, OR ELECTROCARDIOGRAPHIC FEATURE	MITRAL REGURGITATION	VENTRICULAR SEPTAL DEFECT	TRICUSPID REGURGITATION	AORTIC STENOSIS
Systolic murmur	Harsh and pansystolic	Harsh and pansystolic	Pansystolic	Ejection, crescendo-decrescendo
Primary location of murmur	Apex	Left sternal border	Left sternal border	Base of heart; occasionally apical
Radiation of murmur	Axilla; occasionally base and neck	Left precordium	Little	Carotids
Thrill	Occasionally present at apex	Usually present at left sternal border	Rare	Occasionally present at base
Murmur with inspiration	No change	No change	Increases	No change
Valsalva maneuver	May increase	Increases or no change	No change	Decreases
Venous pressure	Often normal	Slightly elevated with prominent A and V waves	Elevated, with very prominent V waves	Usually normal
Pulsatile liver	No	No	Yes	No
Pulmonary component of S_2	Normal; occasionally increased	Normal or loud; usually delayed	Usually increased	Normal
Apical impulse	Hyperkinetic; occasional heaving	Hyperkinetic	Weak or normal	Forceful and sustained
ECG	Left ventricular hypertrophy; left atrial hypertrophy	Biventricular hypertrophy (Katz-Wachtel phenomenon)	Right ventricular hypertrophy, occasional right atrial hypertrophy	Left ventricular hypertrophy with associated ST-T changes
Chest roentgenogram	Moderately enlarged heart, marked left atrial enlargement	Enlarged left and right ventricle	Enlarged right ventricle	Often normal heart size or left ventricular hypertrophy

From Haffajee, C. I.: Chronic mitral regurgitation. *In* Dalen, J. E., and Alpert, J. S. (eds.): Valvular Heart Disease. 2nd ed. Boston, Little, Brown and Company, 1987, p. 141.

chest deformity, or a prosthetic heart valve, the systolic murmur may be barely audible or even absent, a condition referred to as "silent MR."[156]

Pansystolic and late systolic murmurs (and pansystolic murmurs with late systolic accentuation) are characteristic of MR. When the murmur is confined to late systole, the regurgitation is usually mild and may be secondary to prolapse of the mitral valve or papillary muscle dysfunction. These causes of MR are frequently associated with a normal S_1 because initial closure of the mitral valve cusps may be unimpaired. The murmur of papillary muscle dysfunction is particularly variable; it may become accentuated or holosystolic during acute myocardial ischemia and often disappears when ischemia is relieved. The response of a mid- to late-systolic murmur to a number of maneuvers, as described on page 1032, helps to establish the diagnosis of prolapse of the mitral valve.

Dynamic Auscultation (Table 2-4, p. 46; Fig. 2-40, p. 42). The holosystolic murmur of rheumatic MR varies little during respiration. However, sudden standing and amyl nitrite inhalation usually diminish the murmur (Table 32-3), whereas squatting and methoxamine or phenylephrine augment it. The murmur is reduced during the strain of the Valsalva maneuver and shows a left-sided response, i.e., a transient overshoot, six to eight beats following release. The murmur of MR is usually intensified by isometric exercise, differentiating it from the systolic murmurs of valvular aortic stenosis and hypertrophic obstructive cardiomyopathy, both of which are reduced by this intervention. The murmur due to left ventricular dilatation *decreases* in intensity and duration with effective therapy with cardiac glycosides, diuretics, rest, and particularly vasodilators.

Differential Diagnosis. The holosystolic murmur of MR resembles that produced by a ventricular septal defect.

TABLE 32-3 EFFECT OF VARIOUS INTERVENTIONS ON SYSTOLIC MURMURS

INTERVENTION	HYPERTROPHIC OBSTRUCTIVE CARDIOMYOPATHY	AORTIC STENOSIS	MITRAL REGURGITATION	MITRAL PROLAPSE
Valsalva	↑	↓	↓	↑ or ↓
Standing	↑	↑ or unchanged	↓	↑
Handgrip or squatting	↓	↓ or unchanged	↑	↓
Supine position with legs elevated	↓	↑ or unchanged	Unchanged	↓
Exercise	↑	↑ or unchanged	↓	↑
Amyl nitrite	↑↑	↑	↓	↑
Isoproterenol	↑↑	↑	↓	↑

↑↑ = Markedly increased.

Modified from Paraskos, J. A.: Combined valvular disease. *In* Dalen, J. E., and Alpert, J. S. (eds.): Valvular Heart Disease. 2nd ed. Boston, Little, Brown and Company, 1987, p. 365.

However, the latter is usually loudest at the sternal border rather than the apex and is usually accompanied by a parasternal, rather than an apical, thrill. The murmur of MR may also be confused with that of tricuspid regurgitation, which is usually heard best along the left sternal border, is augmented during inspiration, and is accompanied by a prominent v wave and y descent in the jugular venous pulse.

When the chordae tendineae to the posterior leaflet of the mitral valve rupture, the regurgitant jet is often directed anteriorly, so that it impinges on the atrial septum adjacent to the aortic root and causes a systolic murmur most prominent at the base of the heart, which can be confused with that of aortic stenosis. The acoustic energy derived from the mitral regurgitant jet may be transmitted to the aorta by the impact of the jet on the portion of the left atrial wall adjacent to the aortic root.[157] On the other hand, when the chordae to the anterior leaflet rupture, the jet is usually directed to the posterior wall of the left atrium, and the murmur may be transmitted to the spine or even to the top of the head.[158]

Patients with rheumatic disease of the mitral valve exhibit a spectrum of abnormalities, ranging from pure MS to pure MR. The presence of an S_3, a rapid left ventricular filling wave and left ventricular impulse on palpation, and a soft S_1 all favor predominant MR. In contrast, an accentuated S_1, a prominent OS with a short A_2-OS interval, and a soft, short systolic murmur all point to predominant MS. Elucidation of the predominant valvular lesion may be complicated by the presence of a holosystolic murmur of tricuspid regurgitation in patients with pure MS and pulmonary hypertension; this murmur, as has already been noted, may sometimes be heard at the apex when the right ventricle is greatly enlarged and may therefore be mistaken for the murmur of MR. Many patients with severe tricuspid regurgitation have a low cardiac output and an inaudible or barely audible diastolic murmur of MS, further complicating the clinical diagnosis. An S_3 originating from the right ventricle in patients with MS and pulmonary hypertension may falsely suggest the presence of MR. On the other hand, systolic expansion of the left atrium, as occurs in severe MR, often produces a late systolic parasternal expansion that may be confused with right ventricular hypertrophy and falsely attributed to mitral stenosis.

LABORATORY EXAMINATION

ELECTROCARDIOGRAPHY. The principal *electrocardiographic* findings in patients with MR are left atrial enlargement and atrial fibrillation.[46,153,159] Electrocardiographic evidence of left ventricular enlargement occurs in about one-third of patients with severe MR. Approximately 15 per cent can exhibit electrocardiographic evidence of right ventricular hypertrophy, a change that reflects the presence of pulmonary hypertension of sufficient severity to counterbalance even the hypertrophied left ventricle of MR.

RADIOLOGICAL FINDINGS (Figs. 7-37, p. 227, and 7-38, p. 228). Cardiomegaly with left ventricular and particularly with left atrial enlargement is a common finding in patients with chronic severe MR.[160] However, there is little correlation between left atrial size and pressure. Changes in the lung fields are less prominent in MR than in MS, but interstitial edema with Kerley B lines is frequently seen with acute regurgitation or with progressive left ventricular failure.

In patients with combined MS and MR, overall cardiac enlargement and particularly left atrial dilatation are prominent findings. However, it is often difficult to determine which lesion is predominant from the plain chest roentgenogram because it may be difficult to distinguish between right and left ventricular enlargement. Predominant MS is suggested by relatively mild cardiomegaly, principally straightening of the left cardiac border with significant changes in the lung fields, whereas predominant MR is more likely when the heart is greatly enlarged and the changes in the lungs are relatively inconspicuous. When the left atrium is aneurysmally dilated, chronic MR is almost always the dominant lesion. Calcification of the mitral valve occurs in patients with stenosis, regurgitation, or mixed lesions.

Calcification of the mitral annulus, an important cause of MR in the elderly, is most prominent in the posterior third of the cardiac silhouette and is best visualized on films exposed in the lateral or right anterior oblique projection, in which it appears as a dense, coarse, C-shaped opacity (Fig. 7-28, p. 222).

LEFT VENTRICULAR ANGIOCARDIOGRAPHY. The diagnosis of MR can be established definitively by means of left ventricular angiocardiography.[161] The prompt appearance of contrast material in the left atrium following its injection into the left ventricle indicates the presence of MR (Fig. 32-16). The injection should be rapid enough to permit left ventricular opacification but slow enough to avoid the development of premature ventricular contractions, which can induce spurious regurgitation.

The regurgitant volume can be determined from the difference between the total left ventricular stroke volume, estimated angiocardiographically, and the simultaneous measurement of the effective forward stroke by Fick's method (see p. 192). The results of such studies suggest that in patients with severe regurgitation, the regurgitant volume may approach and in rare instances may even exceed the effective forward stroke volume.

Qualitative but clinically useful estimates of the severity of MR may be made by cineangiographic observation of the degree of opacification of the left atrium and pulmonary veins following the injection of contrast material into the left ventricle. MR secondary to rheumatic heart disease is characterized angiographically by a central regurgitant jet and by thickened leaflets that exhibit reduced motion, whereas in regurgitation due to other causes, particularly dilatation or calcification of the mitral annulus or ruptured chordae and papillary muscles, the systolic jet may be eccentric, and the valves consist of thin filaments that display excessive motion. The cause of the regurgitation, e.g., prolapse of the mitral valve, and a flail leaflet are often distinguishable angiographically.

MAGNETIC RESONANCE IMAGING. This technique, described on p. 319, is effective in measuring regurgitant flow and is the most accurate noninvasive technique that can provide these measurements[162,162a] (Fig. 10-28, p. 333).

ECHOCARDIOGRAPHY (see also p. 72). Two-dimensional transthoracic echocardiography is more useful in evaluating left ventricular function and in determining the etiology of MR than in estimating the severity of MR. Severe MR results in enlargement of the left atrium and left ventricle, with increased systolic motion of both of these chambers. The underlying cause of the regurgitation—e.g., rupture of chordae tendineae, mitral valve prolapse (Figs. 3–51, p. 73 and

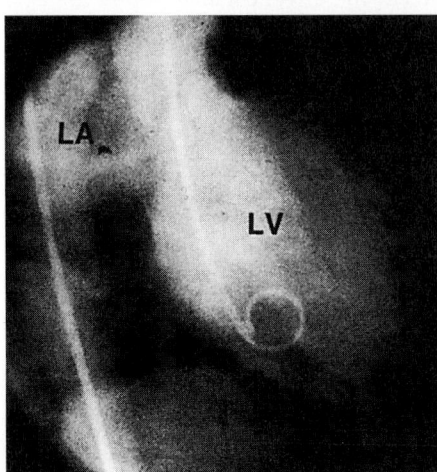
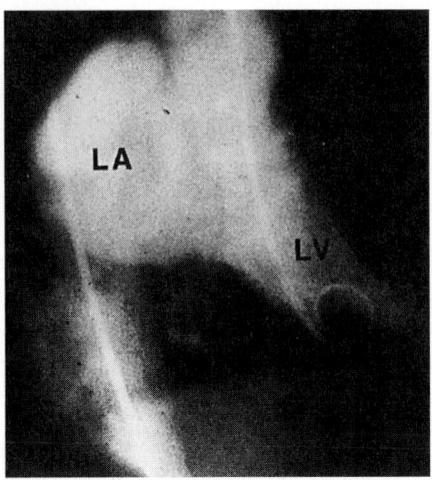

FIGURE 32–16. Diastolic *(left)* and systolic *(right)* frames of a left ventricular cineangiogram from a patient with severe mitral regurgitation. Dense opacification of the left atrium was seen in the first systolic frame. Left ventricular contraction is excellent. (From Hall, R. J., and Julian, D. G.: Diseases of the Cardiac Valves. New York, Churchill Livingstone, 1989, p. 66.)

3–52, p. 74), a flail leaflet[163] (Fig. 3–53, p. 74), and vegetation (Fig. 33–4, p. 1084)—can often be determined on the transthoracic echocardiogram, which may also show calcification of the mitral annulus as a band of dense echoes between the mitral apparatus and the posterior wall of the heart.[164] This technique is also useful for estimating the hemodynamic consequences of MR; with left ventricular dysfunction, end-diastolic and end-systolic volumes are increased. Doppler assessment of mitral regurgitant flow is provided by the difference between transmitral and transaortic flow.[165]

Doppler echocardiography in MR reveals a high-velocity jet in the left atrium during systole. The severity of the regurgitation is a function of the distance from the valve that the jet can be detected (Fig. 3–11, p. 57) and the size of the left atrium. Both color flow Doppler (Fig. 3–49, p. 73 color plate No. 2, and Fig. 3–50, p. 73, color plate No. 2) and pulsed techniques have been found to correlate well with angiographic methods in estimating the severity of MR. Other methods of assessing the severity of MR include measurement of the absolute mitral jet (>8 cm^2 specifies severe MR). However, color flow jet areas are influenced importantly by the cause of the regurgitation and jet eccentricity, limiting the accuracy of this approach.[166] However, the width of the proximal jet appears to correlate with established measures of MR.[167]

Transesophageal echocardiography is superior to transthoracic echocardiography in assessing the detailed anatomy of the regurgitant mitral valve, and therefore it is useful in the preoperative determination of whether valve replacement is necessary or repair is feasible.[168,169] Also, color flow mapping obtained by the transesophageal technique correlates better with angiographic grading of MR than does the transthoracic technique.[169a]

RADIONUCLIDE ANGIOGRAPHY. Gated pool imaging or first-pass angiography may reveal an increased end-diastolic volume; the regurgitant fraction can be estimated from the ratio of left ventricular to right ventricular stroke volume[142]; in patients with MR and impaired left ventricular function, ejection fraction fails to rise normally during exercise. Radionuclide angiograms are useful for interval follow-up of patients. Progressive increases in ventricular end-diastolic or end-systolic volume often suggest that surgical treatment is necessary (discussed later).

Acute Mitral Regurgitation

The causes of acute MR are shown in Table 32–1 (bottom). They are diverse and represent acute manifestations of disease processes that may, under other circumstances, cause chronic MR. Especially important causes of acute MR are infective endocarditis with disruption of valve leaflets or rupture of chordae tendineae, ischemic dysfunction or rupture of a papillary muscle, and malfunction of a prosthetic valve.

One major hemodynamic difference between acute and chronic MR derives from the differences in the compliance of the left atrium, as discussed on page 1020 and as illustrated in Figure 32–14. As shown in Table 32–4 (top), acute severe MR causes a marked reduction of forward stroke volume, a slight reduction of end-systolic volume, and an increase in end-diastolic volume. The differences in the clinical features between acute and chronic MR are summarized in Table 32–4 (bottom). Patients who develop acute MR usually have a normal-sized left atrium (group 1 with normal or reduced left atrial compliance, p. 1021). The left atrial pressure rises abruptly, possibly leading to pulmonary edema, marked elevation of pulmonary vascular resistance, and right-sided heart failure. Because the v wave is markedly elevated in acute MR, the pressure gradient between the left ventricle and atrium declines at the end of systole (Fig. 32–13), and the murmur may not be holosystolic but decrescendo, ending well before A$_2$. It is usually lower-pitched and softer than the murmur of chronic MR. A left-sided S$_4$ is common.[148] Pulmonary hypertension, common in acute MR, may increase the intensity of P$_2$ and the murmurs of pulmonary and tricuspid regurgitation, and a right-sided S$_4$ may also develop. Rarely in patients with severe acute MR, a v wave (late systolic pressure rise) in the pulmonary artery pressure pulse may cause premature

TABLE 32–4 DIFFERENTIAL DIAGNOSIS OF ACUTE VERSUS CHRONIC SEVERE MITRAL REGURGITATION

FINDING	CHRONIC SEVERE	ACUTE SEVERE
Clinical		
Onset	Chronic and gradual dyspnea	Acute
Appearance	Normal/mildly dyspneic	Severely ill
Blood pressure	Variable	Variable
Tachycardia	Variable/not striking	Almost always
Apical impulse	Displaced and forcible (large heart)	Not displaced
Apical systolic thrill	Common	No
S$_1$	Normal or soft	Usually normal or mildly increased
S$_2$	Wide splitting	Usually normal
S$_3$	Common	Common
S$_4$	Rare	Common
Apical mitral murmur	Harsh parasystolic	Soft or absent early systolic and decrescendo
X-radiation of murmur	Axilla	Axilla, spine, or base
Basal ejection systolic murmur	No	With posterior leaflet chordal rupture (not aortic in origin)
Apical rumbling diastolic murmur	Infrequent	Common and short
ECG/LVH	Almost always	No
Chest X-ray	Severe cardiomegaly	No cardiomegaly
Lung fields	Pulmonary venous congestion	Pulmonary edema
Echocardiography		
LV size	Dilated	Normal
LV function	Variable	Hyperactive
LA size	Dilated	Normal
Look for clues of underlying etiology		
Myocardial infarction	History, ECG, and echo	
Endocarditis	Peripheral signs, echo (vegetation)	
Leaking mitral prosthesis	Transesophageal echo and fluoroscopy (clots, vegetation)	

From Jutzy, K. R., and Al-Zaibag, M.: Acute mitral and aortic valve regurgitation. In Al-Zaibag, M., and Duran, C. M. G. (eds.): Valvular Heart Disease. New York, Marcel Dekker, 1994, pp. 345–382.

closure of the pulmonary valve, early P₂, and paradoxical splitting of S₂.[153] Acute MR, even if severe, often does not increase overall cardiac size of the chest roentgenogram and may produce only mild left atrial enlargement despite marked elevation of left atrial pressure. With acute MR, there may be little increase in the internal diameter of either of these chambers of the echocardiogram, but increased systolic motion of the ventricle is prominent.

Acute vs. Chronic Mitral Regurgitation

Both the clinical features and hemodynamic findings differ between acute and chronic MR. These differences are summarized in Table 32–4.

MANAGEMENT

Medical Treatment

This includes all the measures used in the treatment of heart failure, as outlined in Chapter 17. Afterload reduction is of particular benefit in the management of MR—both the acute and the chronic forms.[170,171] By reducing the impedance to ejection into the aorta, the volume of blood regurgitating into the left atrium is reduced. In addition, decreasing left ventricular volume reduces the diameter of the mitral annulus and thereby the regurgitant orifice.[170] Mean left atrial pressure and, in particular, the elevated *v* wave decline. Thus, in the management of MR, vasodilator therapy is actually directed at relieving the physiological abnormality rather than simply dealing with its consequences. Afterload reduction with intravenous nitroprusside may be lifesaving in acute MR due to rupture of the head of a papillary muscle occurring in the course of an acute myocardial infarction. It may permit stabilization of the patient's condition and thereby allow coronary arteriography and operation to be carried out with the patient in optimal condition. When surgical treatment is contraindicated, chronic afterload reduction with an angiotensin inhibitor[171] or oral hydralazine may improve the clinical state for months or even years in patients with severe, chronic MR. Digitalis glycosides play a more important role in the management of MR than of MS. Like diuretics, they are indicated in patients with severe MR and clinical evidence of heart failure. Cardiac glycosides are particularly helpful in patients with established atrial fibrillation. These patients should also receive anticoagulants.

Appropriate prophylaxis to prevent infective endocarditis (see p. 1097) is indicated in MR as in all valvular lesions. In patients with functional disability despite optimal medical management and/or in patients with only mild symptoms but progressively deteriorating left ventricular function on noninvasive examination, surgical treatment should be considered. Two-dimensional or transesophageal echocardiography with Doppler echocardiography and color flow Doppler imaging provide detailed assessment of mitral valve structure and function. However, left-sided cardiac catheterization, selective left ventricular angiocardiography, and coronary arteriography are indicated when surgery is considered. The objectives of these studies are to (1) confirm the presence of MR and estimate its severity; (2) aid in the identification of patients with primary myocardial disease and functional MR secondary to ventricular dilatation who are not likely to benefit from operation and in whom the operative risk is relatively high; (3) detect and assess the severity of any associated valve lesions; and (4) determine the presence and assess the extent of coronary artery disease. Because of the additional risks when surgical treatment is carried out in patients with severe left ventricular dysfunction, these left heart studies and consideration of surgical treatment should be carried out before the patient has developed severe heart failure.

Surgical Treatment

When operative treatment is under consideration, the chronic and often slowly but relentlessly progressive nature of MR must be weighed against the immediate risks and long-term uncertainties attendant upon surgery (Fig. 32–17). Surgical mortality depends on the patient's clinical and hemodynamic state (particularly the function of the left ventricle), on the presence of comorbid conditions such as renal, hepatic, or pulmonary disease, and on the skill and experience of the surgical team. The decision to replace (Fig. 32–18) or reconstruct (Figs. 32–19 and 32–20) the valve is of critical importance because replacement carries with it the risk of thromboembolism and anticoagulation in the case of mechanical prostheses and of valve deterioration in the case of bioprostheses (see p. 1061). Surgical mortality does not depend significantly on *which* of the currently used tissue or mechanical valve prostheses is used (see p. 1028).

The reconstructive procedure consists of annuloplasty, often with the use of a rigid (Carpentier) or a flexible prosthetic (Duran) ring (Fig. 32–19), or reconstruction of the valve[172–177] (Fig. 32–20). Prolapsed valves causing severe MR are usually treated with resection of the prolapsing

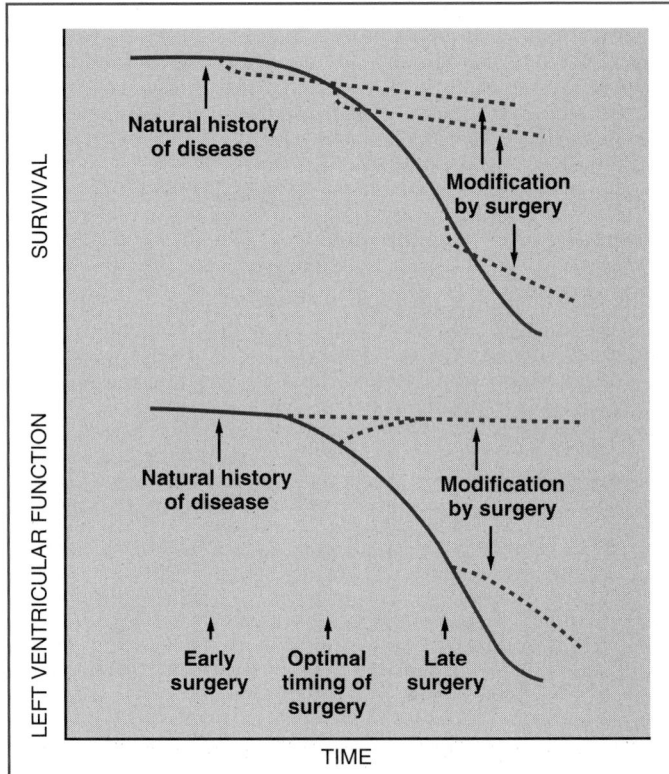

FIGURE 32–17. Schematic representation of the concept of optimal timing of valve replacement surgery. Early surgery yields low operative mortality and preservation of ventricular function. However, because of a finite postoperative risk of prosthesis-associated complications (the major determinant of the slope of the postoperative survival curve in either early or optimally timed surgery), postoperative risk exceeds that of pure medical treatment at this early phase of the disease. In contrast, if surgery is done too late, operative mortality is increased and ventricular function may progressively deteriorate after surgery. Thus, following late surgery, postoperative survival is primarily determined by both prosthesis-associated complications and congestive heart failure. Optimal timing of surgery balances the risks of maintained medical management with the new risks associated with postoperative complications. With optimally timed surgical intervention, operative mortality is relatively low, ventricular function is almost completely preserved, and postoperative risk is determined, as in early surgery, predominantly in the risk of prosthesis-associated complications. (From Schoen, F. J., and St. John Sutton, M.: Contemporary issues in the pathology of valvular disease. Hum. Pathol. *18*:568, 1987.)

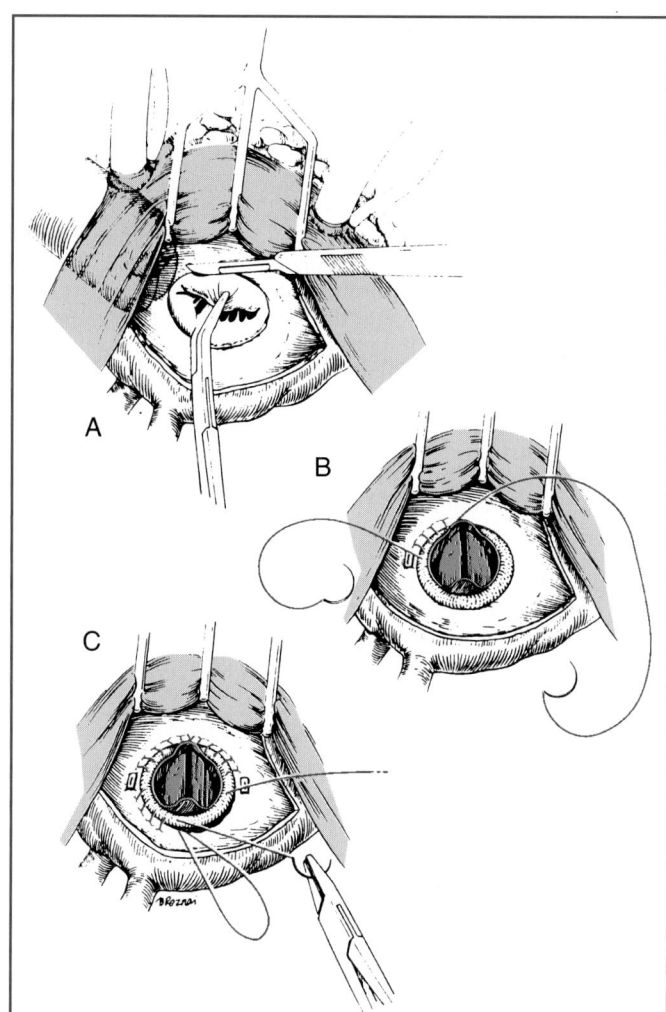

FIGURE 32–18. Continuous technique for mitral valve replacement. *A,* The excision of the valve is facilitated by applying traction to the anterior leaflet. A knife incision in the midportion of the leaflet allows precise initiation of the excision, which is usually completed by scissors. Position of the aorta, circumflex coronary artery, and conduction system should always be kept in mind. *B,* A 0-polypropylene double-armed pledgetted mattress suture is started in the anterolateral commissure. The valve without the holder is lowered in place at this point. *C,* The second 0-polypropylene pledgetted mattress suture is started at the posteromedial commissure. The two suture lines meet at one-half the distance in the anterior and posterior leaflet. The sutures are tied behind the pillar guard of the SJM prosthesis. (From Albertucci, M., and Karp, R. B.: Prosthetic valve replacement. *In* Al-Zaibag, M., and Duran, C. M. G. [eds.]: Valvular Heart Disease. New York, Marcel Dekker, 1994, pp. 601–634.)

segment and plication of the annulus (see p. 1029). Replacement,[178] reimplantation, elongation or shortening of chordae tendineae, splitting of the papillary muscle, and repair of the subvalvular apparatus have been successful in selected patients with pure or predominant MR.[173] Reconstruction of the mitral valve is often successful in patients with noncalcific MR who have pliable valves and a dilated mitral annulus and whose MR is secondary to ruptured chordae to the posterior leaflet or perforation of a mitral leaflet due to infective endocarditis but who do *not* have severe subvalvular chordal thickening and major loss of leaflet substance.[179] The results of these reconstructive operations have, in general, been more favorable in children and adolescents with pliable valves and in patients with MR secondary to mitral valve prolapse, annular dilatation, papillary muscle secondary to ischemia, dysfunction or rupture, or chordal rupture than they have been in older patients with the rigid, calcified, deformed valves of rheumatic heart disease. Many of the latter require mitral valve replacement, which is also usually the procedure of choice

in patients with badly scarred mitral valves who have previously undergone mitral commissurotomy. Young patients in developing countries with severe rheumatic MR in the absence of active carditis may undergo successful repair.[172]

Ischemic MR following acute myocardial infarction may be managed by reattaching the papillary muscle to adjacent myocardium[175] or by valve replacement. Ischemic MR secondary to severe annular dilatation may be treated with direct or ring annuloplasty. Episodic MR due to transient ischemia is often eliminated by coronary revascularization, whereas severe chronic MR secondary to fibrotic infarcted papillary muscle usually requires valve replacement.

Although mitral valve replacement[179a]—with mechanical or bioprostheses—has been used successfully in the treatment of MR for three and a half decades, there has been some dissatisfaction with the results of this operation. First, left ventricular function often deteriorates following this procedure, contributing to early and late mortality and late disability. The increase in afterload consequent to abolition of the low impedance leak was first believed to be responsible, but now it is clear that the loss of annular-chordal-papillary muscle continuity interferes with left ventricular function in patients who have undergone mitral valve replacement. This does not occur after mitral valve reconstruction.[178] Indeed, animal experiments have shown convincingly that the normal function of the mitral valve apparatus "primes" the left ventricle for normal contraction and that this is prevented when operation causes discontinuity of this apparatus. There is evidence, both from animal experiments[181] and patients,[182–185] that preservation of the papillary muscle and its chordal attachments to the mitral annulus is beneficial for postoperative left ventricular function, even when the mitral valve is replaced.

A second disadvantage of prosthetic mitral valve replacement results from the prosthesis itself: thromboembolism or hemorrhage in the case of mechanical prostheses, late mechanical dysfunction of bioprostheses, and the hazard of infective endocarditis with all prostheses. For these reasons, increasing efforts are being made to reconstruct the mitral valve whenever possible, especially in patients with pure and predominant regurgitation. Indeed, these procedures, widely employed in Europe since the early 1960's, are now frequently used by U.S. surgeons as well. In many centers in the United States, approximately half of all patients requiring operation for pure or predominant MR re

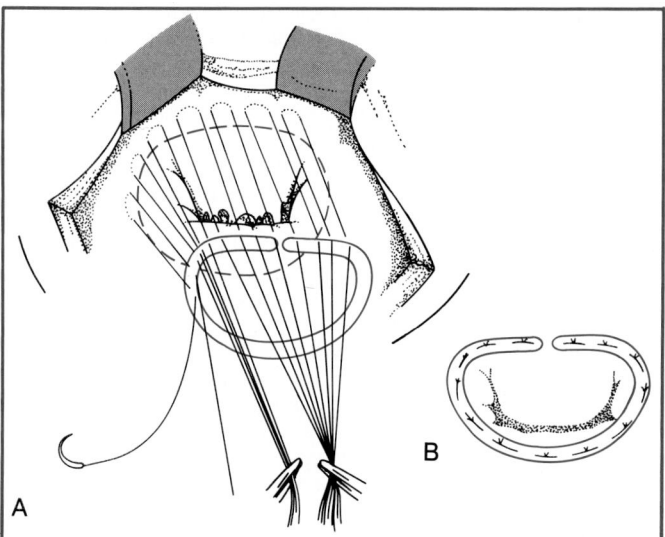

FIGURE 32–19. Illustration of insertion of annuloplasty ring. (Reproduced with permission from Galloway, A. C., Colvin, S. B., Baumann, F. G., et al.: Current concepts of mitral valve reconstruction for mitral insufficiency. Circulation *78*:1087, 1988. Copyright 1989 American Heart Association.)

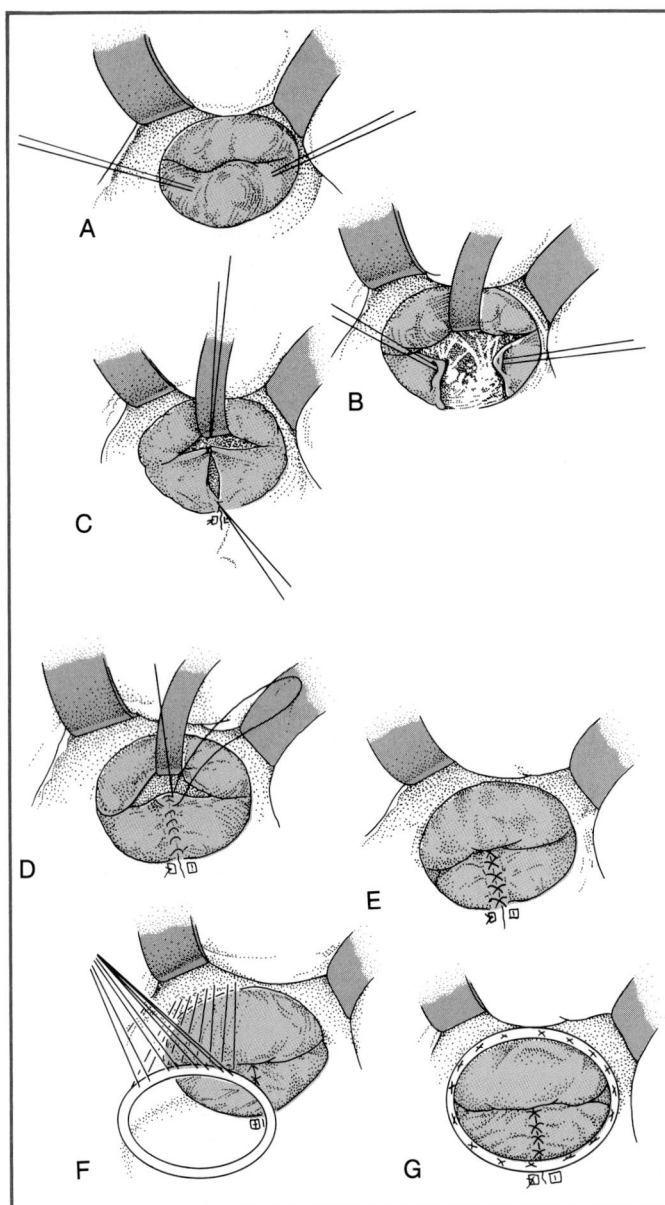

FIGURE 32–20. Valve repair techniques for quadrilateral resection of posterior leaflet of mitral valve. (From Cohn, L. H., DiSesa, V. J., Couper, G. S., et al.: Mitral valve repair for myxomatous degeneration and prolapse of the mitral valve. J. Thorac. Cardiovasc. Surg. 98:987, 1989.)

ceive reconstructive procedures and the other half valve replacement.

Intraoperative Doppler color flow mapping is extremely useful in assessing the adequacy of mitral valve repair. In the minority of patients with persistent severe MR in whom the results are unsatisfactory, the problem can usually be corrected before the chest is closed.[178] Left ventricular outflow tract obstruction due to systolic anterior motion of the mitral valve occurs in 5 to 10 per cent of patients following mitral valve repair. Its causes are not clear, but they may include excess valvular tissue with severe leaflet redundancy and/or an interventricular septum bulging into a small left ventricle.[176–186] This complication may be recognized intraoperatively by transesophageal echocardiography. Treatment with volume loading and beta-blockade is often helpful. The obstruction usually disappears with time, but if it does not, reoperation and re-repair or replacement may be necessary.

Progressive reduction in the prevalence of rheumatic heart disease—in which damaged valves often are not suitable for reconstructive surgery—with a simultaneous rise in degenerative causes of MR (including mitral valve pro-

lapse and rupture of chordae tendineae) as well as in ischemic causes is increasing the proportion of patients in whom reconstruction is carried out.

The potential advantages of repair of MR (as opposed to replacement with a prosthetic valve) are many; chronic anticoagulation and the hazards of bleeding and thromboembolism attendant upon implantation of a mechanical prosthesis are largely eliminated, as are the risks of late failure of a bioprosthesis. However, mitral repair is technically a more demanding procedure with a distinct learning curve for the surgeon.[187] Furthermore, many regurgitant valves, particularly those that are thickened, severely deformed, calcified, and partly stenotic, do not lend themselves to reconstruction: mitral valve replacement is necessary.

SURGICAL RESULTS. Mortality rates of 1 to 4 per cent in patients with predominant MS and of 2 to 7 per cent in patients with pure or predominant MR in functional Class II or III, who undergo elective isolated mitral valve replacement, are now common in many centers.[131,141,174,188,189] Operative mortality tends to be lower (1 to 4 per cent) in patients undergoing reconstructive surgery, but this may be related to the younger age and lower incidence of comorbid illnesses in these patients. Age per se is no barrier to successful surgery; mitral valve replacement can be carried out in patients older than 75 years if their general health status is adequate but with a higher risk than in younger patients.[183] Surgical treatment substantially improves survival in patients with symptomatic MR. Factors such as age less than 60 years, a preoperative New York Heart Association functional Class of II, a cardiac index exceeding 2.0 liters/min/m², a left ventricular end-diastolic pressure less than 12 mm Hg, and a normal ejection fraction and end-systolic volume all correlate with excellent immediate as well as long-term survival rates. Both preoperative and end-systolic diameter (Fig. 32–12) and ejection fraction (Fig. 32–21) are important predictors of short-term and long-term outcome. Excellent survival is observed in patients with end-systolic diameters less than 45 mm and ejection fractions of 60 per cent or more. Intermediate outcomes are seen in patients with diameters between 45 and 52 mm and ejection fractions between 50 and 60 per cent, with poor outcomes beyond these limits. In some series, only age and preoperative ejection fraction predicted long-term survival following mitral valve replacement.[190]

In a large proportion of survivors of operation, the clinical state and quality of life improve following valve replacement or repair. Severe pulmonary hypertension is re-

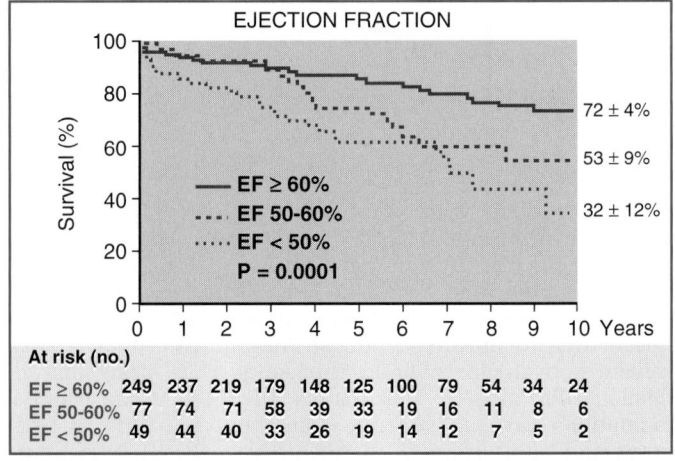

FIGURE 32–21. Graph of the late survival of operative survivors of surgical correction of MR according to preoperative echocardiographic ejection fraction (EF). Number at risk for each interval is indicated at bottom. (Reproduced with permission from Enriquez-Sarano, M., et al.: Echocardiographic prediction of survival after surgical correction of organic mitral regurgitation. Circulation 90:833, 1994. Copyright 1994 American Heart Association.)

lieved almost uniformly,[53] and left ventricular end-diastolic volume and mass are reduced. Depressed contractile function due to mitral regurgitation improves, especially after mitral valve reconstruction (or mitral valve repair if the chordae attachment to the annulus remains intact). However, patients with MR with marked left ventricular dysfunction preoperatively sometimes remain symptomatic with a depressed ejection fraction[192] after a technically satisfactory operation. Indeed, progressive left ventricular dysfunction and death from heart failure may occur. Long-term survival in patients with predominant MR who undergo mitral valve replacement may be poorer than in those with pure stenosis or mixed stenotic and regurgitant lesions, presumably because left ventricular dysfunction may be quite advanced and largely irreversible by the time patients with pure regurgitation become seriously symptomatic.[191,192] However, even though it is clearly desirable to operate on patients with MR before they develop marked left ventricular dysfunction, and despite the limitations of the results of surgical treatment in these patients, operation is still indicated in the majority of these patients because conservative therapy has little to offer.

The cause of MR also plays an important role in the outcome following surgical treatment. In patients in whom mitral dysfunction is secondary to ischemic heart disease, the 5-year survival rate is about 40 per cent, whereas in rheumatic mitral regurgitation it is much better, approximately 75 per cent. Occlusive coronary artery disease coexisting with, but not the primary cause of, mitral dysfunction requires simultaneous coronary artery bypass grafting and mitral valve replacement or repair. This is associated with decreased perioperative and long-term postoperative survival. Some improvement from mitral valve reconstruction or replacement can be expected even in patients with MR secondary to ischemic heart disease who are medically unresponsive and in congestive heart failure, as long as the cardiac index and ejection fraction exceed 1.8 liters/min/ m² and 40 per cent, respectively. When left ventricular dysfunction is more severe, however, the risk of perioperative death becomes prohibitive.[195]

Surgical Treatment of Acute Mitral Regurgitation. Emergency surgical treatment of acute left ventricular failure caused by acute MR due to myocardial infarction and rupture of the head of a papillary muscle, by trauma to the mitral valve, or by endocarditis is associated with higher mortality rate than is the elective surgical treatment of chronic MR. However, unless such patients with acute, severe MR and heart failure are treated aggressively, a fatal outcome is almost certain. If the condition of patients with MR secondary to acute infarction can be stabilized by medical treatment, it is preferable to defer operation until 4 to 6 weeks after infarction. Vasodilator treatment may be use-

ful during this period. However, medical management should not be prolonged if multisystem (renal or pulmonary or both) failure occurs. Surgical mortality is also higher in patients with refractory heart failure (functional Class IV), in those in whom a previously implanted prosthetic valve must be replaced because of thromboembolism or valve dysfunction, and in those with active infective endocarditis (of a natural or prosthetic valve). Despite the higher surgical risks, the efficacy of early operation has been established in patients with infective endocarditis complicated by medically uncontrollable congestive heart failure, recurrent emboli, or both (see p. 1096). Because fungal endocarditis responds poorly to medical management, it is now the practice to recommend valve replacement in these cases *before* the onset of heart failure or embolization.

INDICATIONS FOR OPERATION. In view of the reductions in operative mortality, and the improvements both in mitral reconstructive procedures and in artificial valves, as well as the poor long-term results in many patients whose MR is corrected after a long history of heart failure, a more aggressive stance concerning the desirability of operation is in order. Only a few years ago, I, along with many cardiologists, recommended operation for patients with chronic severe MR only if they were in functional Class III or IV, i.e., with symptoms at rest or on ordinary activity despite medical treatment. However, it is now my policy to recommend operation also for patients with severe MR who are in Class II, i.e., who become distinctly symptomatic only on heavy exertion, and if end-systolic volume and diameter are elevated (>50 ml/m² BSA and >45 mm, respectively).

The asymptomatic patient with severe MR presents a particularly challenging problem.[139,196,196a] Careful history and performance of an exercise test often reveal that these patients are not, in fact, truly asymptomatic, and if they are symptomatic they should be considered for operation, as indicated as above. However, patients with severe MR who are asymptomatic and perform well on an exercise test and have normal ventricular function (ejection fraction >70 per cent, end-systolic diameter <40 mm, end-systolic volume <40 ml/m²) are followed by echocardiography every 6 to 12 months. Operation should be considered even in asymptomatic patients if they are under age 70, if they are likely to be candidates for mitral valve repair, and if ventricular function as reflected in end-systolic volume and/or diameter shows *progressive* deterioration. If valve replacement is likely to be necessary, a somewhat higher threshold for clinical and hemodynamic impairment is employed than if valvular reconstruction is contemplated. Because of the higher operative mortality, older patients (>75 years) should, in general, be operated on only for symptoms.

MITRAL VALVE PROLAPSE

ETIOLOGY AND PATHOLOGY
(Fig. 32–22)

DEFINITION. The mitral valve prolapse (MVP) syndrome has been given many names, including the systolic click-murmur syndrome, Barlow syndrome, billowing mitral cusp syndrome, myxomatous mitral valve, floppy valve syndrome, and redundant cusp syndrome.[197–202,202a] It is a common but variable clinical syndrome that results from diverse pathogenic mechanisms of one or more portions of the mitral valve apparatus, the valve leaflets, chordae tendineae, papillary muscle, and valve annulus. The MVP syndrome has become recognized as one of the most prevalent cardiac valvular abnormalities, affecting as much as 3 to 5 per cent of the population.[203,204] It is twice as frequent

in females as in males. In 1963 Barlow et al. demonstrated that midsystolic clicks and late systolic murmurs, the auscultatory hallmarks of this syndrome, are frequently associated with prolapse of the mitral valve, often associated with regurgitation.[205]

Normally, the mitral valve billows slightly into the left atrium, and an exaggeration should be termed "billowing mitral valve." A "floppy valve" is regarded as an extreme form of billowing. MVP occurs when the leaflet edges of the valve do not coapt, causing MR. With chordal rupture, the prolapsed mitral valve is "flail." Obviously, these conditions blend into one another, and it is often difficult to distinguish them.

Perloff et al. have proposed specific clinical criteria for the diagnosis of MVP.[199] They have divided the findings into three groups (Table 32–5): (1) major criteria, the pres-

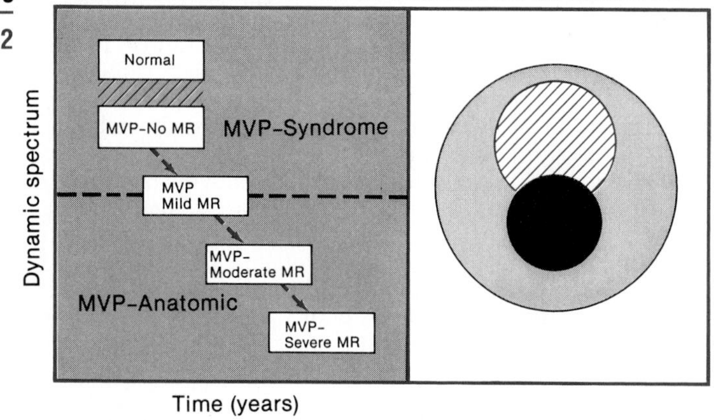

FIGURE 32–22. *Left panel,* The dynamic spectrum, time in years, and the progression of mitral valve prolapse (MVP) are shown. A subtle gradation (cross-hatched area) exists between the normal mitral valve and valves that produce mild MVP without mitral regurgitation (no MR). Progression from the level MVP–no MR to another level may or may not occur. Most of the MVP syndrome cases occupy the area above the dotted line, while progressive mitral valve dysfunction cases occupy the area below the dotted line. *Right panel,* The large circle represents the total number of patients with MVP. Patients with MVP may be symptomatic or asymptomatic. Symptoms may be directly related to mitral valve dysfunction (black circle), or to autonomic dysfunction (cross-hatched circle). Certain patients with symptoms directly related to mitral valve dysfunction may present with and continue to have symptoms secondary to autonomic dysfunction. (From Boudoulas, H., and Wooley, C. F.: Mitral Valve Prolapse and the Mitral Valve Prolapse Syndrome. Mount Kisco, NY, Futura Publishing Co., Inc., 1988.)

ence of one or more of which establishes the diagnosis of MVP; (2) minor criteria, which cannot be discounted and which raise the suspicion of MVP but which by themselves are not sufficient to establish the diagnosis; and (3) nonspecific findings which, although often present in patients with MVP, are quite nonspecific. Although they may alert the clinician, they do not aid in establishing the diagnosis. When rigorous two-dimensional echocardiography criteria (extension of leaflet tissue located cephalad to the plane of the mitral annulus) were employed, only 2 of 100 healthy young women displayed MVP.[200] In addition, Marks et al. have emphasized the importance of systolic displacement of one or both mitral leaflets into the left atrium in the *parasternal view* in the diagnosis of MVP. Such an approach avoids overdiagnosis, which may occur with posterior bowing of the mitral valve on the M-mode echocardiogram and even in the four-chamber view on two-dimensional echocardiography.

ETIOLOGY. Most frequently MVP occurs as a primary condition unassociated with other disease.[197,206] However, it has been reported to be associated with many conditions.[206–216] It is not clear how many of these are chance associations. MVP occurs quite commonly in heritable disorders of connective tissue that increase the size of the mitral leaflets and apparatus, including the Marfan syndrome (see p. 1669). Ehlers-Danlos syndrome[217,218] (see p. 1672), osteogenesis imperfecta, pseudoxanthoma elasticum,[219] and periarteritis nodosa, as well as with myotonic dystrophy,[210] von Willebrand's disease,[209] hyperthyroidism,[208] and congenital malformations such as Ebstein's anomaly of the tricuspid valve, atrial septal defect of the ostium secundum variety,[218] and the Holt-Oram syndrome (see p. 1661).[212] There appears to be a high incidence of MVP in patients with asthenic habitus[220] and a variety of congenital thoracic deformities, including a straight back, a pectus excavatum, and a shallow chest.[212,214] In these cases the association may be with a left ventricle that is small in relation to the mitral valve apparatus.

PATHOLOGY (Fig. 32–23). There is myxomatous proliferation of the mitral valve, in which the spongiosa com-

TABLE 32–5 DIAGNOSTIC CRITERIA AND NONSPECIFIC FINDINGS IN MITRAL VALVE PROLAPSE

MAJOR CRITERIA

Auscultation
  Mid- to late systolic clicks and late systolic murmur or "whoop" alone or in combination at the cardiac apex
Two-dimensional echocardiogram
  Marked superior systolic displacement of mitral leaflets with coaptation point at or superior to annular plane
  Mild to moderate superior systolic displacement of mitral leaflets with:
    Chordal rupture
    Doppler mitral regurgitation
    Annular dilatation
Echocardiogram plus auscultation
  Mild to moderate superior systolic displacement of mitral leaflets with:
    Prominent mid- to late systolic clicks at the cardiac apex
    Apical late systolic or holosystolic murmur in the young
    Late systolic "whoop"

MINOR CRITERIA

Auscultation
  Loud first heart sound with an apical holosystolic murmur
Two-dimensional echocardiogram
  Isolated mild to moderate superior systolic displacement of the posterior mitral leaflet
  Moderate superior systolic displacement of both mitral leaflets
Echocardiogram plus history of:
  Mild to moderate superior systolic displacement of mitral leaflets with:
    Focal neurologic attacks or amaurosis fugax in the young
    First-degree relatives with major criteria

NONSPECIFIC FINDINGS

Symptoms
  "Atypical" chest pain, dyspnea, fatigue, lassitude, giddiness, dizziness, syncope
  Psychological disturbances
Physical appearance
  Thoracic bony abnormalities
  Hypomastia
Electrocardiogram
  T-wave inversions in inferior limb leads or lateral precordial leads
  Premature ventricular beats at rest, during exercise, or on ambulatory ECG
  Supraventricular tachycardia
X-ray
  Scoliosis, pectus excavatum or carinatum, or loss of thoracic kyphosis
Two-dimensional echocardiogram
  Mild superior systolic displacement of anterior or anterior and posterior mitral leaflets

From Perloff, J. K., Child, J. S., and Edwards, J. E.: New guidelines for the clinical diagnosis of mitral valve prolapse. Am. J. Cardiol. *57*:1124, 1986.

ponent of the valve, i.e., the middle layer of the leaflet composed of loose, myxomatous material, is unusually prominent[221] and the quantity of acid mucopolysaccharide is increased secondary to a fundamental abnormality of collagen metabolism.[222,223] The concordance between inadequate production of type III collagen and echocardiographic findings of MVP in patients with type IV Ehlers-Danlos syndrome suggests that this abnormality of collagen is responsible for this subgroup.[222] Although the majority of patients with MVP exhibit myxomatous degeneration of the valve, postinflammatory changes also may be responsible for prolapse.[224]

Electron microscopy has shown haphazard arrangement, disruption, and fragmentation of collagen fibrils (Fig. 32–24). In mild cases, the valvular myxoid stroma is enlarged on histological examination but the leaflets are grossly normal. However, with increasing quantities of myxoid stroma, the leaflets become grossly abnormal and redundant and prolapse. Regions of endothelial disruption, possible sites of endocarditis or thrombus formation, are common.[225] The

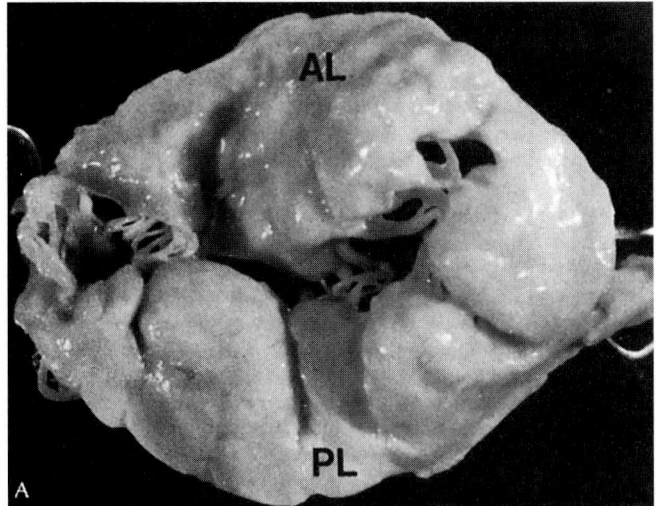

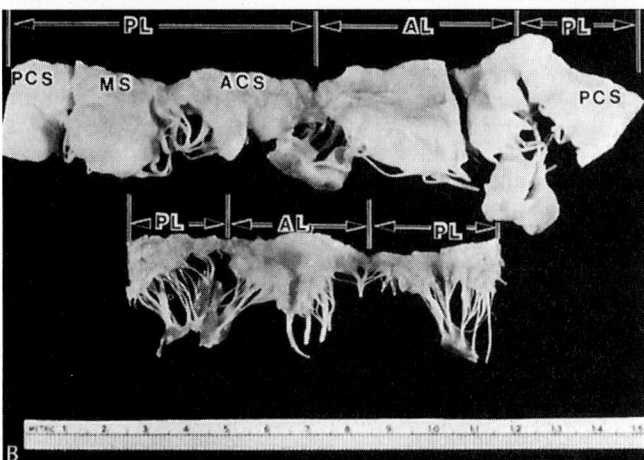

FIGURE 32–23. *A*, Myxomatous mitral valve, atrial view, from a patient with severe mitral regurgitation. The surface area of the valve is increased, with increased folding of the valve surface. The widths of the anterior leaflet (AL) and the posterior leaflet (PL) are almost equal. Individual scallops of the posterior leaflet are enlarged and redundant. *B*, Comparison of an excised myxomatous mitral valve from a patient with severe mitral regurgitation (top) with a normal mitral valve from a patient who died of noncardiac causes (bottom), showing the increased surface area of both anterior leaflets (AL) and posterior leaflets (PL) of the myxomatous valve with enlarged and redundant posterior leaflet scallops, enlarged mitral annulus, and elongated chordae tendineae. PCS = posteromedial commissural scallops; MS = middle scallop; ACS = anterolateral commissural scallop. (From Boudoulas, H., and Wooley, C. F.: Mitral valve prolapse and the mitral valve prolapse syndrome. *In* Yu, P., and Goodwin, J. [eds.]: Progress in Cardiology. Philadelphia, Lea and Febiger, 1986.)

severity of MR depends on the extent of the prolapse. The cusps of the mitral valve, the chordae tendineae, and the annulus may all be affected by myxomatous proliferation. Degeneration of collagen within the central core of the chordae tendineae is primarily responsible for chordal rupture, which occurs commonly in this syndrome and may intensify the severity of MR, although increased chordal tension resulting from the enlarged area of the valve cusps may play a contributory role.[226] Myxomatous changes in the annulus may result in annular dilatation and calcification—contributing to the severity of MR.

Myxomatous proliferation, although most commonly affecting the mitral valve, is not limited to this valve but has been described in the tricuspid,[215] aortic, and pulmonic valves, particularly in patients with Marfan syndrome, and may lead to regurgitation of these valves. The MVP syndrome appears to exhibit a strong hereditary component[197,221] and in some cases is transmitted as an autosomal dominant trait, with varying penetrance. Genetic segrega-

tion analyses of familial MVP have shown *no* linkage to fibrillar collagen genes.[227]

The MVP syndrome can coexist with rheumatic MS, and it may develop following mitral commissurotomy for this lesion. In hypertrophic obstructive cardiomyopathy, prolapse of the posterior leaflet of the mitral valve may accompany the usual anterior displacement of the anterior mitral valve leaflet.

Ischemic heart disease and MVP are both common disorders and coexist not infrequently; MVP may also occur secondary to papillary muscle dysfunction. In some patients, MVP has been documented to develop for the first time *following* myocardial infarction.[228] MVP may cause myocardial ischemia by increasing tension on the base of the involved muscle. During systole the tips of the papillary muscles move basally instead of apically. It has also been proposed that coronary artery spasm occurs as a reflex

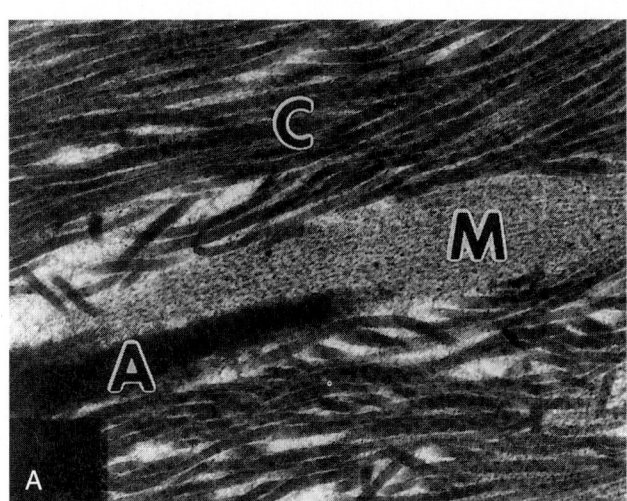

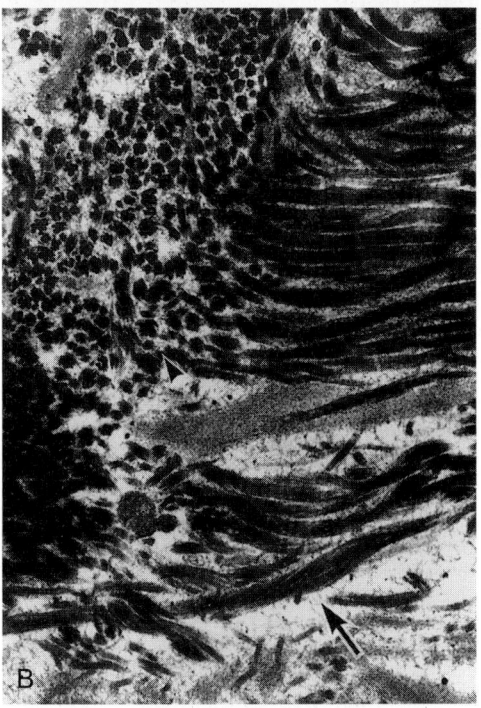

FIGURE 32–24. Electron micrographs of mitral valve. *A*, Normal valve: Elastic fiber is composed of amorphous component (A), associated with microfibrils (M) oriented in parallel. Collagen fibrils (C) are compactly arranged (Kajikawa stain; original magnification ×22,000). *B*, Prolapsed mitral valve. Collagen fibrils show spiraling appearance in longitudinal section (arrow) and flower-like appearance (arrowhead) in transverse section (Kajikawa stain; original magnification ×27,000). (From Tamura, K., Fukuda, Y., Ishizaki, M., et al.: Abnormalities in elastic fibers and other connective-tissue components of floppy mitral valve. Am. Heart J. *129*:1149, 1995.)

response to prolapse of the posterior mitral leaflet and that the resultant ischemia may be responsible for angina or angina-like pain, myocardial infarction, arrhythmias, and sudden death in this syndrome.

CLINICAL MANIFESTATIONS

The clinical presentations of the MVP syndrome are diverse.[197,229] The condition has been observed in patients of all ages and in both sexes. It is a common syndrome; indeed, prolapse of the mitral valve has been reported to occur in 6 per cent of healthy young women surveyed by echocardiography.[230] One series of 100 presumably healthy young women revealed that 17 had a midsystolic click or late systolic murmur or both and that 10 of these 17 had evidence of prolapse of the mitral valve on echocardiography.[231] However, as already noted, because billowing of the mitral valve is a normal variant and M-mode echocardiographic findings may be nonspecific, more rigorous criteria for diagnosis based on two-dimensional echocardiography will indicate a much lower prevalence.[199] Indeed, MVP is now the most common cause of isolated MR requiring surgical treatment.[202] Echocardiographic evidence of MVP has been found in more than 90 per cent of patients with Marfan syndrome[232] and in many of their first-degree relatives.

History

A large majority of patients with MVP are asymptomatic[233,234] (Fig. 32-22). In many cases, otherwise asymptomatic patients with MVP suffer from undue anxiety, perhaps precipitated by their having been informed of the presence of heart disease. Boudoulas et al. have called attention to an "MVP syndrome" with a characteristic systolic nonejection click and a variety of nonspecific symptoms, such as fatigability, palpitations, postural orthostasis, and neuropsychiatric symptoms, as well as symptoms of autonomic dysfunction.[234] How, and indeed whether, these symptoms relate to the presence of MVP is not clear. However, it has been suggested that many of the symptoms are related to dysfunction of the autonomic nervous system, which occurs frequently in the MVP syndrome.[235]

Patients may complain of syncope, presyncope, palpitations, chest discomfort, and, when MR is severe, symptoms of diminished cardiac reserve. Chest discomfort may be typical of angina but most often it is atypical in that it is prolonged, not clearly related to exertion, and punctuated by brief attacks or severe stabbing pain at the apex. The discomfort may be secondary to abnormal tension on papillary muscles.

Physical Examination

The body weight is often low. The blood pressure is usually normal or low; orthostatic hypotension may be present. As already mentioned, patients with MVP have a higher than expected prevalence of "straight back syndrome," scoliosis, and pectus excavatum.[195] MR ranges from nonexistent to severe and in the latter case palpation of the precordium and of the carotid pulses is characteristic (see p. 18).

The auscultatory findings are best elicited with the diaphragm of the stethoscope. The patient should be examined in the supine, left decubitus, and sitting positions. The physical findings unique to the MVP syndrome are detected by auscultation and can be corroborated by phonocardiography.[196] The most important is a systolic click at least 0.14 sec after S_1 (Fig. 2-34, p. 39). This can be differentiated from a systolic ejection click because it occurs distinctly after the beginning of the upstroke of the carotid pulse. Occasionally, multiple mid- and late-systolic clicks are audible most readily along the lower left sternal border

and are believed to be produced by sudden tensing of the elongated chordae tendineae and of the prolapsing leaflets. The click is often, although not invariably, followed by a mid- to late-crescendo systolic murmur that continues to A_2. This murmur is similar to that produced by papillary muscle dysfunction (Fig. 32-10, p. 1019), which is readily understandable because both result from mid- to late-systolic MR. In general, the duration of the murmur is a function of the severity of the MR, and when the murmur is confined to the latter portion of systole, MR usually is not severe. However, as MR becomes more severe, the murmur commences earlier and becomes holosystolic.

It is important to emphasize the variability of the physical findings in the MVP syndrome. Some patients exhibit both a midsystolic click and a mid- to late-systolic murmur; others present with one or the other of these two findings; still others have only a click on one occasion and only a murmur on another, both on a third examination, and no abnormality at all on a fourth. MVP may also cause an early diastolic sound or murmur, best heard at the apex or left sternal border 70 to 110 msec following A_2, at a time when the prolapsed posterior leaflet descends into the left ventricle. Conditions other than MVP cause midsystolic clicks; these include tricuspid valve clicks, atrial septal aneurysms,[236] and extracardiac causes.

DYNAMIC AUSCULTATION. The auscultatory and phonocardiographic findings are exquisitely sensitive to physiological and pharmacological interventions, and recognition of the changes induced by these interventions is of great value in the diagnosis of the MVP syndrome (Fig. 2-21, p. 31, and Fig. 2-29, p. 37; Table 32-3).[196] The mitral valve begins to prolapse when the reduction of left ventricular volume during systole reaches a critical point at which the valve leaflets no longer coapt; at that instant, the click occurs and the murmur commences. Any maneuver that decreases left ventricular volume, such as a reduction of impedance to left ventricular outflow, a reduction in venous return, or an augmentation of contractility, results in an earlier occurrence of prolapse during systole. As a consequence, the click and onset of the murmur move closer to S_1. When prolapse is severe or left ventricular size is markedly reduced or both, prolapse may begin with the onset of systole, and as a consequence, the click may not be audible and the murmur may be holosystolic. On the other hand, when left ventricular volume is augmented by an increase in venous return, a reduction of myocardial contractility, bradycardia, or an increase in the impedance to left ventricular emptying, both the click and the onset of the murmur will be delayed. Indeed, if the left ventricle becomes extremely large, prolapse may not occur at all, and the abnormal auscultatory features may disappear entirely.

During the straining phase of the Valsalva maneuver, upon sudden standing, and early during the inhalation of amyl nitrite, cardiac size decreases, and both the click and the onset of the murmur occur earlier in systole. In contrast, a sudden change from the standing to the supine position, leg-raising, squatting, maximal isometric exercise, and, to a lesser extent, expiration will delay the click and the onset of the murmur (Fig. 2-21, p. 31). During the overshoot phase of the Valsalva maneuver (i.e., six to eight cycles following release) and with prolongation of the R-R interval, either following a premature contraction or in atrial fibrillation, the click and onset of the murmur are usually delayed, and the intensity of the murmur is reduced. Maneuvers that elevate arterial pressure, such as isometric exercise, increase the intensity of the click and murmur.

In general, when the onset of the murmur is delayed, both its duration and intensity are diminished, reflecting a reduction in the severity of MR. With some maneuvers, however, there is a discrepancy between changes in the intensity and duration of the murmur. Following amyl nitrite inhalation, for example, the reduced left ventricular size results in an earlier click and longer murmur, but the lower left ventricular systolic pressure diminishes the severity of regurgitation and the intensity of the murmur. Conversely, phenylephrine and methoxamine delay the click and the onset of the murmur, but the larger volume of regurgitation consequent to the elevated left ventricular systolic pressure increases regurgitation and the intensity of the murmur.

There may be confusion between the systolic murmurs of hypertrophic cardiomyopathy (HCM) and of MVP, particularly because midsystolic clicks and a late systolic murmur have been reported in HCM and because the murmur may increase in intensity and duration with standing and decrease with squatting in both conditions (see p. 1420). However, the response to several interventions may be helpful in differentiating these two conditions. During the strain of the Valsalva maneuver, the murmur of HCM increases in intensity in contrast to that of MVP, which becomes longer but usually not louder. The murmur of HCM becomes louder after amyl nitrite inhalation, whereas that of MVP does not. Following a premature beat, the murmur of HCM increases in intensity and duration, whereas that due to MVP usually remains unchanged or decreases.

LABORATORY EXAMINATION

Electrocardiography

The electrocardiogram is usually normal in asymptomatic patients with typical auscultatory and echocardiographic findings. In a minority of asymptomatic patients and in many symptomatic patients, the electrocardiogram shows inverted or biphasic T waves and nonspecific ST-segment changes in leads II, III, and aV$_f$ and occasionally in the anterolateral leads as well.[196] The ST- and T-wave changes may become exaggerated during amyl nitrite inhalation and exercise. These electrocardiographic findings may be related to ischemia of the papillary muscles or of the left ventricle at their bases, resulting from increased tension on these structures produced by the prolapsing valve acting on the chordae. Alternatively, it is possible that the electrocardiographic abnormality reflects an underlying cardiomyopathy.

ARRHYTHMIAS. A spectrum of arrhythmias, including atrial and ventricular premature contractions and supraventricular and ventricular tachyarrhythmias[236–239] as well as bradyarrhythmias due to sinus node dysfunction or varying degrees of atrioventricular block,[239] have been observed. The mechanism of the arrhythmias is not clear. Diastolic depolarization of muscle fibers in the anterior mitral leaflet in response to stretch has been demonstrated experimentally, and the abnormal stretch of the prolapsed leaflet may be of pathogenetic significance. Wit et al. have shown that mitral valve leaflets contain atrium-like muscle fibers in continuity with left atrial myocardium. It is possible that mechanical stimulation of these fibers generates slow-response action potentials and sustained rhythmic action that penetrates the cardiac chambers.[240] Although most of these arrhythmias are of little clinical importance, recurrent ventricular tachycardia, refractory to the usual agents, and even ventricular fibrillation have been reported. These serious ventricular arrhythmias are significantly more frequent in patients with ST-segment and T-wave abnormalities on the resting electrocardiogram.

Paroxysmal supraventricular tachycardia is the most common sustained tachyarrhythmia in patients with MVP and may be related to what may be an increased incidence of left atrioventricular bypass tracts in this condition.[237] In the general population only 20 per cent of patients with paroxysmal supraventricular tachycardia have such bypass tracts, whereas the incidence in patients with MVP is three times as great. Conversely, there is evidence that the incidence of MVP among patients with the Wolff-Parkinson-White syndrome is increased.[241] Patients with MVP who develop paroxysmal supraventricular tachycardia should be subjected to electrophysiological investigation. The outcome of such studies may be important, because digitalis or propranolol, which may be useful in reentry tachycardias, may be hazardous in the presence of antegrade conduction over an atrioventricular bypass tract. There is also an increased association between MVP and prolongation of the Q-T interval, and this association may play a role in the genesis of ventricular arrhythmias.[237] Patients with MVP have an increased incidence of abnormal late potentials on signal-averaged electrocardiograms, as well as reduced heart rate variability[239]; the latter is a predictor of early mortality or of future need for valve surgery.

MVP AND SUDDEN DEATH. The relation between the MVP syndrome and sudden death is not clear.[238] However, the best evidence suggests that MVP increases the risk of sudden death slightly,[197] especially in patients with severe MR[240] or severe valvular deformity.[241]

The immediate cause of the sudden, unexpected death is probably ventricular fibrillation,[242] although complete heart block with prolonged asystole has also been reported in this syndrome.[237]

Kligfield et al. have identified the following as potential risks for sudden death in MVP: the presence of significant MR, complex ventricular arrhythmias, prolongation of Q-T interval, and a history of syncope and palpitations.[237]

Echocardiography
(See also p. 73)

Echocardiography plays a key role in the diagnosis of MVP and has been most useful in the delineation of this syndrome (Figs. 3–51, p. 73, and 3–52, p. 74). The most common electrocardiographic finding on M-mode echocardiography is abrupt posterior movement of the posterior leaflet or of both mitral leaflets in mid-systole with the leaflet interface greater than 2 mm posterior to the C-D line; this movement occurs simultaneously with the systolic click; a second finding is pansystolic posterior prolapse of one or both leaflets, giving rise to a U- or hammock-shaped configuration 3 mm or more posterior to the C-D segment. This is the opposite of what is seen in hypertrophic obstructive cardiomyopathy, in which the anterior leaflet of the mitral valve moves toward the ventricular septum in midsystole.

The two-dimensional echocardiogram shows one or both mitral valve leaflets billowing into the left atrium during systole (Fig. 32–25).[243,244] It is also helpful in the identification of patients at significant risk of developing severe MR or infective endocarditis; the leaflets are distinctly thickened or redundant[245] and the mitral annular diameter is abnormally increased in these patients.[243,246] Doppler echocardiography frequently reveals mild MR that is not always associated with an audible murmur. Color flow Doppler is useful in identifying the location and severity of the regurgitant jets. MR is moderate or severe in 10 per cent of patients, most commonly in men over the age of 50.[246,247] Transesophageal echocardiography provides additional details regarding the mitral valve apparatus and may demonstrate rupture of chordae tendineae.

The variability in physical findings in this syndrome, already commented upon, extends to the echocardiogram.[248] Thus, some patients have a systolic click with or without a murmur and show no evidence of MVP on the echocardiogram. Conversely, the echocardiographic findings of MVP may be observed in patients without the click or murmur. Others have both the typical echocardiographic and auscultatory features. The echocardiographic findings of MVP have been reported to occur in a large number of first-degree relatives of patients with established MVP.[249]

Two-dimensional echocardiography has also revealed prolapse of the tricuspid and aortic valves in approximately one-fifth of patients with MVP.[249,250] Conversely, however, prolapse of the tricuspid and aortic valves occurs *uncommonly* in patients without prolapse of the mitral valve.[250]

Stress Scintigraphy

The differential diagnosis between two common conditions—MVP associated with atypical chest pain and electrocardiographic abnormalities, and primary coronary artery disease associated with MVP—may be aided by exercise electrocardiography, but myocardial perfusion scintigraphy using thallium-201 or sestamibi during exercise pharmacological stress (see p. 290) is more specific. When findings are normal, i.e., when there is no evidence of stress-induced regional myocardial ischemia, the diagnosis of MVP unrelated to ischemic heart disease is favored.[251] Ejection fraction at rest determined by radionuclide angiography is usually normal in patients having MVP without associated MR.

Angiography

The configuration of the left ventriculogram during systole is helpful in the diagnosis of MVP. The right anterior oblique projection is most useful for defining the posterior leaflet of the mitral valve and

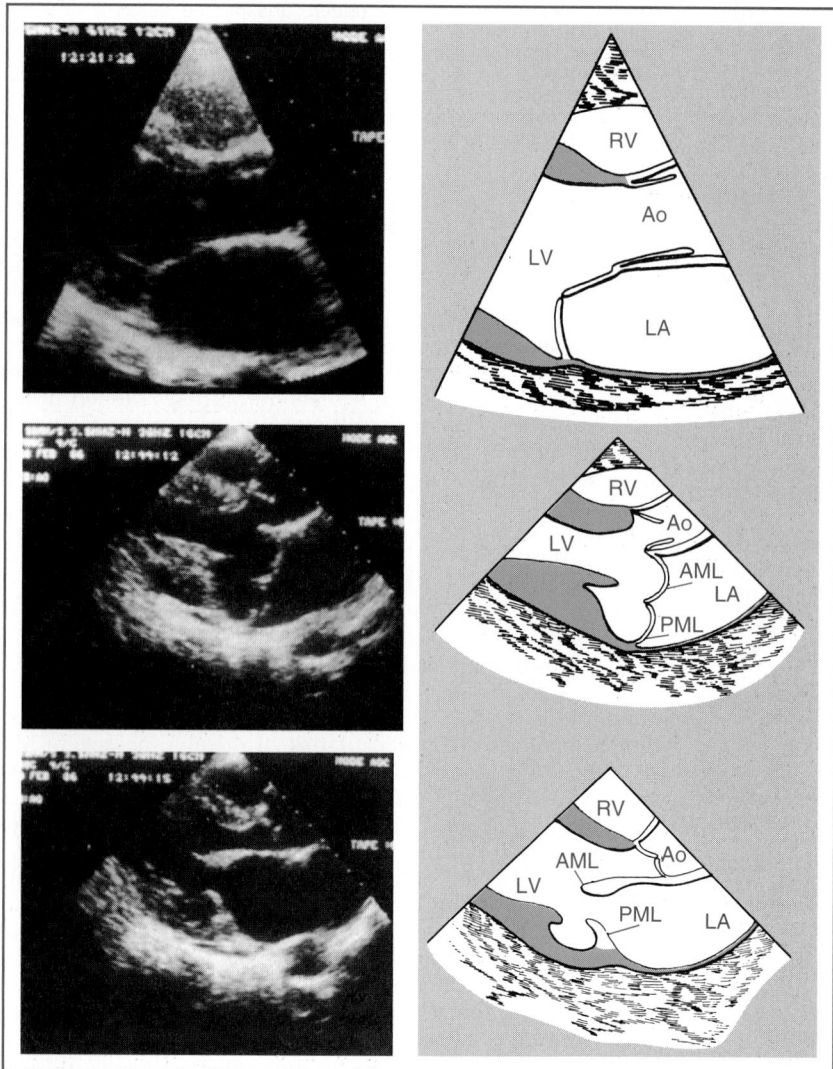

FIGURE 32–25. *Top,* Parasternal long-axis view of normal mitral valve leaflets during systole. RV = right ventricle, LV = left ventricle, Ao = aorta, and LA = left atrium. *Center,* Classic mitral valve prolapse. The parasternal long-axis view shows the mitral leaflets prolapsing into the left atrium during systole. Note the relation of the mitral leaflets to the mitral annulus. RV denotes right ventricle; LV = left ventricle, Ao = aorta, LA = left atrium, AML = anterior mitral leaflet, and PML = posterior mitral leaflet. *Bottom,* Classic mitral valve prolapse with leaflet thickening. The parasternal long-axis view of the same mitral valve as in center figure is shown during diastole. This view was used to measure the thickness of the leaflets. RV denotes right ventricle, LV = left ventricle, Ao = aorta, AML = anterior mitral leaflet, PML = posterior mitral leaflet, and LA = left atrium. (Reprinted by permission from Marks, A. R., Choong, C. Y., Sanfilippo, A. J., et al.: Identification of high-risk and low-risk subgroups of patients with mitral valve prolapse. N. Engl. J. Med. *320*:1031, 1989. Copyright 1989 Massachusetts Medical Society.)

the left anterior oblique projection for studying the anterior leaflet. The most helpful sign is extension of the mitral leaflet tissue inferiorly and posteriorly to the point of attachment of the mitral leaflets to the mitral annulus.[252] Angiography may also reveal scalloped edges of the leaflets, reflecting redundancy of tissue.

Other abnormalities noted on angiography of some patients with MVP include dilatation, decreased systolic contraction, and calcification of the mitral annulus and poor contraction of the basal portion of the left ventricle.[253] There may be an indentation at the base of the posteromedial papillary muscle associated with prolapse of the posterior leaflet and resulting from abnormal traction on this muscle. With involvement of both papillary muscles, there may be an indentation of the anterior as well as the inferior wall of the left ventricle, giving the cardiac silhouette an hourglass appearance. These left ventricular contraction abnormalities are secondary to redundancy of the mitral valve leaflets and transmission of the abnormal tension on these leaflets to the papillary muscles and underlying left ventricle.

NATURAL HISTORY

The outlook for MVP in children is excellent, a large majority remaining asymptomatic for many years without any change in clinical or laboratory manifestations.[197,233,254]

Progressive MR is the most frequent serious complication,[233,255,256] occurring in about 15 per cent of patients over a 10- to 15-year period; the incidence of this complication is significantly greater in patients with both murmurs and clicks than in those with an isolated click. In many patients, rupture of chordae tendineae is responsible for the intensification of the MR.[252] Severe MR occurs more frequently in men older than 50 years with MVP.[256] Patients with the MVP syndrome are also at risk of developing in-

fective endocarditis,[257,258] although the incidence appears to be extremely low in patients with a midsystolic click only; the incidence rises in patients with a systolic murmur.[258] It is higher in men than in women and in those more than 50 years of age. Endocarditis often aggravates the severity of MR and therefore the need for surgical treatment. Zuppiroli et al. followed 316 patients with MVP for an average of more than 8 years; 70 per cent were women and 29 per cent had familial MVP. Serious complications (cardiac death, need for cardiac surgery, acute infective endocarditis, or cerebral embolic events) occurred at a rate of 1 per 100 patient years.[233]

Acute hemiplegia, transient ischemic attacks, cerebellar infarcts, amaurosis fugax, and retinal arteriolar occlusions all appear to occur more frequently in patients with the MVP syndrome, suggesting that cerebral emboli are unusually common in this condition.[259,260] These neurological complications are often associated with shortened platelet survival. Loss of endothelial continuity and tearing of the endocardium overlying the myxomatous valve may initiate platelet aggregation and the formation of mural platelet-fibrin complexes.[259] The paroxysmal arrhythmias that occur in the MVP syndrome may contribute to the likelihood of embolization. Indeed, it is possible that cerebral embolization secondary to MVP may be a significant cause for unexplained strokes and other cerebral and retinal complications in young people without cerebrovascular disease. Similarly, myocardial infarction in patients with MVP and normal coronary arteries may be secondary to embolization.[261]

RISK LEVEL	PATIENTS	MANAGEMENT
Lowest	Subjects without mitral regurgitant murmurs or regurgitation revealed by Doppler echocardiography, especially women younger than age 45	Reassurance; peridental antibiotics not clearly necessary and if used should not include medication with risk of allergic reactions; reevaluation and echocardiography at moderate intervals (5 years)
Moderate	Subjects with intermittent or persistent mitral murmurs and mild regurgitation revealed by Doppler echocardiography	Antibiotic prophylaxis with erythromycin or amoxicillin; treatment of even mild established hypertension; reevaluation and echocardiography more frequently (2 to 3 years)
High	Subjects with moderate or severe mitral regurgitation	Antibiotic prophylaxis with amoxicillin (unless allergic); optimization of afterload (arterial pressure); reevaluation with Doppler echocardiography and other tests if needed annually; consider valve repair or replacement for exertional dyspnea or decline of left ventricular function into low-normal range

From Devereux, R. B.: Recent developments in the diagnosis and management of mitral valve prolapse. Curr. Opin. Cardiol. *10*:107, 1995. Modified from Devereux, R. B., and Kligfield, P.: Mitral valve prolapse. *In* Rakel, R.: Current Therapy. Philadelphia, W. B. Saunders Company, 1992, p. 237, 241.

MANAGEMENT

(Table 32–6)

Asymptomatic patients (or those whose principal complaint is anxiety) with no arrhythmias evident on a routine extended electrocardiographic tracing and on prolonged auscultation, with normal ST segments and without evidence of MR, have an excellent prognosis. They should be reassured about the favorable prognosis but should have follow-up examinations every 3 to 5 years. This should include a two-dimensional echocardiogram and a Doppler study. Patients with a long systolic murmur may show progression of MR and should be examined more frequently, at intervals of approximately 12 months. Mitral valve surgery, most commonly mitral valve repair,[202] should be carried out for patients with MVP and severe MR (see p. 1026). *Endocarditis prophylaxis* is advisable in patients with a typical systolic murmur and characteristic echocardiographic features of MVP and some evidence of MR. Prophylaxis does not appear to be necessary in patients, particularly women, with a midsystolic click without a systolic murmur.[257] Some, however, recommend prophylaxis when such patients are subjected to instrumentation of the upper respiratory or genitourinary tract (see p. 1097).

Patients with a history of palpitations, lightheadedness, dizziness, or syncope or those who have ventricular arrhythmias or Q-T prolongation on a routine electrocardiogram should undergo ambulatory (24-hour) electrocardiographic monitoring or exercise electrocardiography to detect arrhythmias. Because of the risk—albeit low—of sudden death,[237,238] electrophysiological studies should be carried out to characterize arrhythmias in symptomatic patients. Beta-adrenoceptor blockers are useful in the treatment of palpitations secondary to frequent ventricular premature contractions and for self-terminating episodes of supraventricular tachycardias. These drugs may also be useful in the treatment of chest discomfort, both in patients with associated coronary artery disease and in those with normal coronary vessels in whom the symptoms may be due to regional ischemia secondary to MVP. Radiofrequency ablation of atrioventricular bypass tracts is useful for frequent or prolonged episodes of supraventricular tachycardia.

In patients with MVP who have had any of the aforementioned cerebral events and in whom no other cause is apparent, anticoagulant therapy and/or aspirin should be given.

Patients with MVP and symptoms of left ventricular failure attributable to MR should be treated as are other patients with severe MR (see p. 1026), and those with severe regurgitation who are not responsive to medical management may require mitral valve surgery. Reconstructive surgery without valve replacement is often possible (Fig. 32–20).[202] Approximately half of all mitral valve reconstructions for MR are now carried out in patients with MVP. Among 252 such patients operated upon at the Brigham and Women's Hospital, resection of the most deformed leaflet segment and insertion of an annuloplasty ring to reduce the dilated annulus was the most commonly employed procedure. Rupture of the chords to the anterior leaflet could sometimes be treated by chordal transfer from the posterior leaflet. In other cases, shortening of the chordae and/or papillary muscle was necessary. The operative mortality was 2 per cent; structural valve degeneration occurred in 15 per cent at 5 years.

Coronary arteriography should be performed in patients with angina on effort and/or ischemic electrocardiographic changes or abnormalities on a thallium perfusion scan during exercise, and treatment should take into account both the responsiveness of symptoms to medical management and the coronary anatomy.

Although this discussion has focused attention on complications of the MVP syndrome, it should not be forgotten that, on the whole, this is a benign condition and that the *vast majority* of patients with this syndrome remain asymptomatic for their entire lives and require, at most, observation every few years and reassurance.[262]

AORTIC STENOSIS

ETIOLOGY AND PATHOLOGY

Obstruction to left ventricular outflow is localized most commonly at the aortic valve and is discussed in this section. However, obstruction may also occur above the valve (supravalvular stenosis [see p. 919]) or below the valve (discrete subvalvular aortic stenosis [see p. 918]) or may be caused by hypertrophic obstructive cardiomyopathy (see p. 1414). Valvular aortic stenosis (AS) *without accompanying mitral valve disease* is more common in men and very rarely occurs on a rheumatic basis but instead is usually either congenital or degenerative in origin[263–264a] (Figs. 32–26 and 32–27).

CONGENITAL AORTIC STENOSIS (see also pp. 914 and 969). Congenital malformations of the aortic valve may be

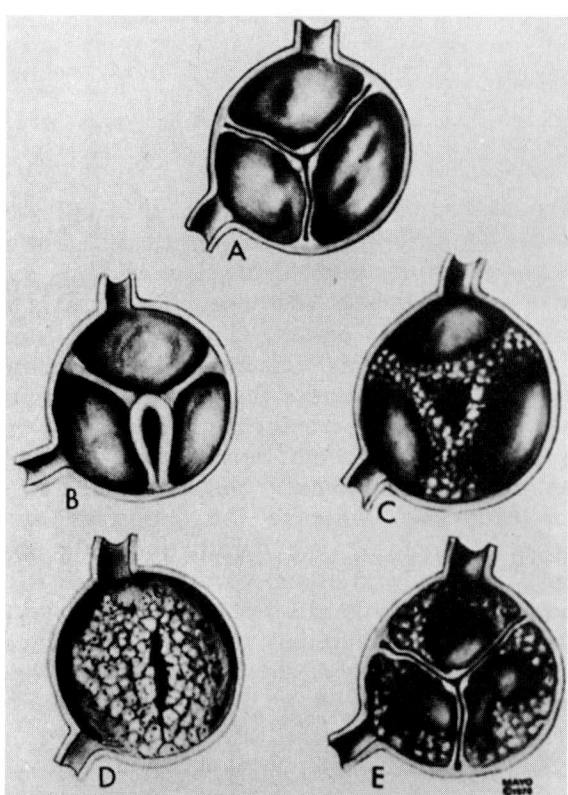

FIGURE 32–26. Types of aortic valve stenosis. *A*, Normal aortic valve. *B*, Congenital aortic stenosis. *C*, Rheumatic aortic stenosis. *D*, Calcific aortic stenosis. *E*, Calcific senile aortic stenosis. (From Brandenburg, R. O., et al.: Valvular heart disease—When should the patient be referred? Pract. Cardiol. *5:*50, 1979.)

unicuspid, bicuspid, or tricuspid, or there may be a dome-shaped diaphragm. *Unicuspid valves* produce severe obstruction in infancy and are the most frequent malformations found in fatal valvular aortic stenosis in children under the age of 1 year. Congenitally *bicuspid valves* may be stenotic with commissural fusion at birth, but more commonly they are not responsible for serious narrowing of the aortic orifice during childhood; their abnormal architecture induces turbulent flow, which traumatizes the leaflets and ultimately leads to fibrosis, increased rigidity, and calcification of the leaflets and narrowing of the aortic orifice[265,266] (Fig. 32–28). Infective endocarditis may develop on a congenitally bicuspid valve, which then becomes regurgitant. Rarely, a congenitally bicuspid valve is purely regurgitant in the absence of antecedent infection. It should be emphasized that in a majority of cases, a bicuspid valve is not stenotic at birth and the changes causing stenosis resemble those occurring in senile, degenerative calcific stenosis of a tricuspid aortic valve except that in the congenitally bicuspid valve these changes occur several decades earlier.

A third form of a congenitally malformed valve is *tricuspid,* with the cusps of unequal size and some commissural fusion. Although many of these valves retain normal function throughout life, it has been postulated that the turbulent flow produced by the mild congenital architectural abnormality may lead to fibrosis and ultimately to calcification and stenosis. Tricuspid stenotic aortic valves in adults may be congenital, rheumatic, or degenerative in origin.

ACQUIRED AORTIC STENOSIS. Rheumatic AS results from adhesions and fusions of the commissures and cusps and vascularization of the leaflets of the valve ring, leading to retraction and stiffening of the free borders of the cusps, with calcific nodules present on both surfaces and an orifice that is reduced to a small round or triangular opening. As a consequence, the rheumatic valve is often regurgitant

as well as stenotic.[263] The heart frequently exhibits other stigmata of rheumatic heart disease, especially mitral valve involvement. Rheumatic AS appears to be decreasing in frequency in industrialized nations with the decline in rheumatic fever.

In degenerative (senile) calcific AS, the cusps are immobilized by a deposit of calcium along their flexion lines at their bases. This most common cause of AS in adults (which is now the most frequent in patients with AS requiring aortic valve replacement)[267] appears to result from years of normal mechanical stress on the valve. Although degenerative calcification may extend in the direction of the cusps, no commissural fusion is present. Degenerative "wear and tear" appears to be the most likely cause of this form of AS, which is commonly accompanied by calcifications of the mitral annulus and coronary arteries but rarely by aortic regurgitation. Both diabetes mellitus and hypercholesterolemia are risk factors for the development of this lesion.[268] The stenosis is produced by the calcific deposits that prevent the cusps from opening normally during systole (Fig. 32–28).

In atherosclerotic aortic valvular stenosis, severe atherosclerosis involves the aorta and other major arteries; this form of AS occurs most frequently in patients with severe hypercholesterolemia and is observed in children with homozygous type II hyperlipoproteinemia, an extremely rare condition (see Ch. 35). Calcific aortic stenosis is observed in Paget's disease of bone[269] as well as in end-stage renal disease.[270] *Rheumatoid involvement* of the valve is a rare cause of AS and results in nodular thickening of the valve leaflets and involvement of the proximal part of the aorta (see p. 1776). *Ochronosis* is another rare cause of aortic stenosis.[271]

Roberts studied hearts with AS obtained at autopsy from patients between 15 and 65 years of age and found that almost 40 per cent were tricuspid. Because thickening of the mitral valve and a history of acute rheumatic fever were present in half of these cases, it is likely that the AS was rheumatic in etiology; in the remainder it was either congenital or degenerative in origin. In 90 per cent of hearts of patients with AS who were older than 65 years and who were examined at autopsy, the valves were tricuspid, with nodular calcific deposits on the aortic aspects of the cusps, but without commissural fusion,[264] indicative of degenerative disease.

Hemodynamically significant AS leads to severe concentric left ventricular hypertrophy,[272] with heart weights as great as 1000 gm. The interventricular septum often bulges into and encroaches on the right ventricular cavity. When

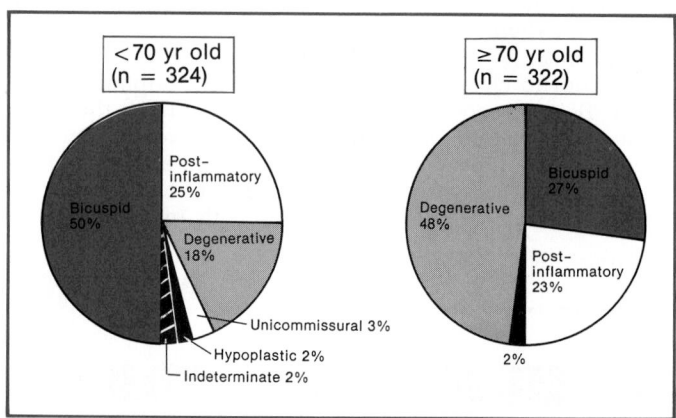

FIGURE 32–27. Causes of aortic stenosis, shown for two age groups. Among patients younger than 70 years *(left)*, calcification of congenitally bicuspid valves accounted for half of the surgical cases. In contrast, in those 70 years of age or older *(right)*, degenerative calcification accounted for almost half of the cases. (From Passik, C. S., et al.: Temporal changes in the causes of aortic stenosis: A surgical pathologic study of 646 cases. Mayo Clin. Proc. *62:*119, 1987.)

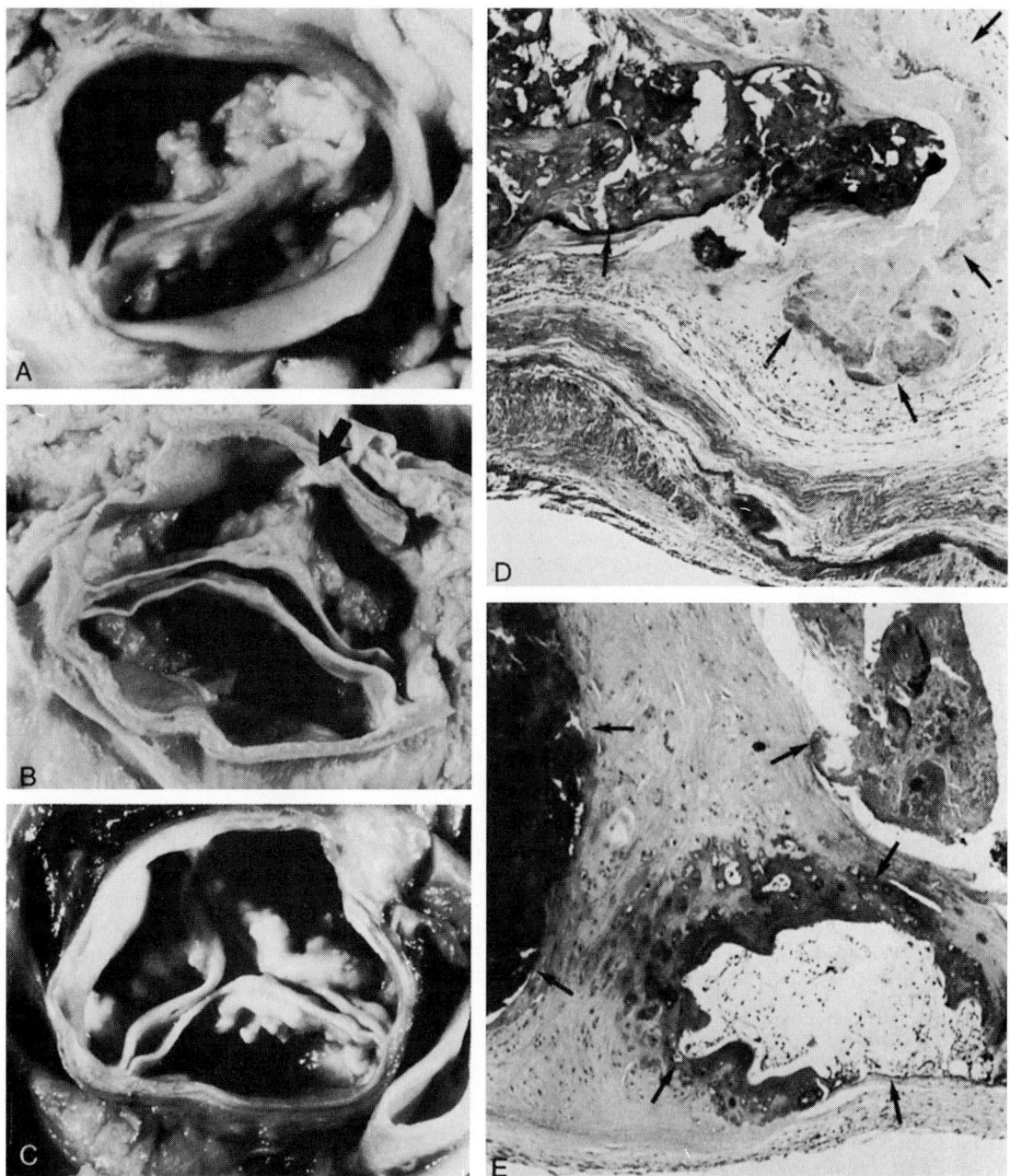

FIGURE 32–28. Calcific aortic stenosis. *A,* Congenitally bicuspid aortic valve, characterized by two equal cusps with basal mineralization. *B,* Congenitally bicuspid aortic valve having two unequal cusps, the larger with a central raphe (arrow). *C,* Otherwise anatomically normal tricuspid aortic valve in an elderly patient, characterized by isolated cusps with calcification localized to basilar aspect; cuspal free edges are not involved. *D* and *E,* Photomicrographs of calcific deposits in calcific aortic stenosis; deposits are rimmed by arrows (hematoxylin and eosin, ×15). *D,* Deposits with underlying cusp largely intact; transmural calcific deposits are shown in *E* (*A* and *C* from Schoen, F. J., and St. John Sutton, M.: Contemporary issues in the pathology of valvular heart disease. Hum. Pathol. *18*:568, 1987.)

left ventricular failure supervenes, the left ventricle dilates,[272] the left atrium enlarges, and changes secondary to backward failure occur in the pulmonary vascular bed, right side of the heart, and systemic venous bed.

PATHOPHYSIOLOGY

(Fig. 32–29)

The left ventricle responds to *sudden* severe obstruction to outflow by dilatation and reduction of stroke volume.[273] However, in adults with AS, the obstruction usually develops and increases gradually over a prolonged period. In infants and children with congenital AS, the valve orifice shows little change as the child grows, thereby intensifying the relative obstruction quite gradually. Left ventricular function can be well maintained in experimentally produced, chronic, gradually developing subcoronary AS.[274] Left ventricular output is maintained by the presence of left ventricular hypertrophy, which may sustain a large pressure gradient across the aortic valve for many years without a reduction in cardiac output, left ventricular dilatation, or the development of symptoms. A peak systolic pressure gradient exceeding 50 mm Hg in the presence of a normal cardiac output or an effective aortic orifice less than about 0.8 cm² in an average-sized adult, i.e., 0.5 cm²/m² of body surface area (less than approximately one-fourth of the normal orifice), is generally considered to represent critical obstruction to left ventricular outflow.[275]

As contraction of the left ventricle becomes progressively more isometric, the left ventricular pressure pulse exhibits

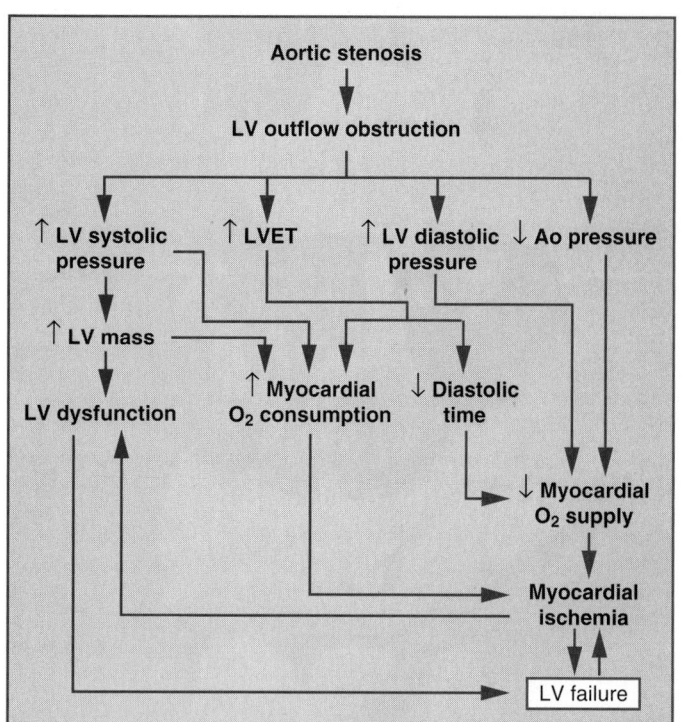

FIGURE 32–29. Pathophysiology of aortic stenosis. Left ventricular (LV) outflow obstruction results in an increased LV systolic pressure, increased left ventricular ejection time (LVET), increased left ventricular diastolic pressure, and decreased aortic (Ao) pressure. Increased LV systolic pressure with LV volume overload increases LV mass, which may lead to LV dysfunction and failure. Increased LV systolic pressure, LV mass, and LVET increase myocardial oxygen (O_2) consumption. Increased LVET results in a decrease of diastolic time (myocardial perfusion time). Increased LV diastolic pressure and decreased Ao diastolic pressure decrease coronary perfusion pressure. Decreased diastolic time and coronary perfusion pressure decrease myocardial O_2 supply. Increased myocardial O_2 consumption and decreased myocardial O_2 supply produce myocardial ischemia, which further deteriorates LV function ($\uparrow$ = increased, $\downarrow$ = decreased). (From Boudoulas, H., and Gravanis, M. B.: Valvular heart disease. In Gravanis, M. B.: Cardiovascular Disorders: Pathogenesis and Pathophysiology. St. Louis, C. V. Mosby, 1993, p. 64.)

a rounded, rather than flattened, summit. The elevated left ventricular end-diastolic pressure, which is characteristic of severe AS, does not necessarily signify the presence of left ventricular dilatation or failure but often reflects diminished compliance of the hypertrophied left ventricular wall; usually it results from a combination of both processes.[276,277]

In patients with severe AS, large a waves usually appear in the left atrial pressure pulse because of the combination of enhanced contraction of a hypertrophied left atrium and diminished left ventricular compliance. Atrial contraction plays a particularly important role in filling of the left ventricle in AS. It raises left ventricular end-diastolic pressure without producing a concomitant elevation of mean left atrial pressure.[278] This "booster pump" function of the left atrium prevents the pulmonary venous and capillary pressures from rising to levels that would produce pulmonary congestion, while at the same time maintaining left ventricular end-diastolic pressure at the elevated level necessary for effective left ventricular contraction. Loss of appropriately timed, vigorous atrial contraction, as occurs in atrial fibrillation or atrioventricular dissociation, may result in rapid clinical deterioration in patients with severe AS.

Although the *cardiac output* at rest is within normal limits in the majority of patients with severe AS,[275] it often fails to rise normally during exertion. Late in the course of the disease the cardiac output, stroke volume, and therefore the left ventricular–aortic pressure gradient all decline, whereas the mean left atrial, pulmonary capillary, pulmonary arterial, right ventricular systolic and diastolic, and right atrial pressures rise, often sequentially.[275a] AS intensifies the severity of any existing mitral regurgitation by increasing the pressure gradient responsible for driving blood from the left ventricle to the left atrium. In addition, the dilatation of the left ventricle, which occurs late in the course of aortic valve disease, may produce mitral regurgitation, superimposing the hemodynamic changes associated with this lesion on those produced by AS. Also, as a consequence of pulmonary hypertension or bulging of the hypertrophied septum into the right ventricular cavity or both, the a wave in the right atrial pressure pulse becomes prominent.

Left ventricular end-diastolic volume usually remains normal until quite late in the course of the disease, but left ventricular mass increases in response to the chronic pressure overload, resulting in an increase in the mass/volume ratio. However, the increase in mass may not be as great as that seen with aortic regurgitation (AR) or combined AS and AR.

Gender differences in the response of the left ventricle to AS have been reported.[279–280a] Women more frequently exhibit normal or even supernormal ventricular performance and smaller, thicker-walled concentrically hypertrophied left ventricles whereas men more frequently have eccentric hypertrophy and ventricular dilatation (Fig. 32–30).

MYOCARDIAL FUNCTION IN AORTIC STENOSIS

In experimental animals, when the aorta is suddenly constricted, left ventricular pressure rises, and there is a large increase in wall stress, whereas both extent and velocity of shortening decline. As pointed out in Chapter 13, the development of ventricular hypertrophy is one of the principal mechanisms by which the heart adapts

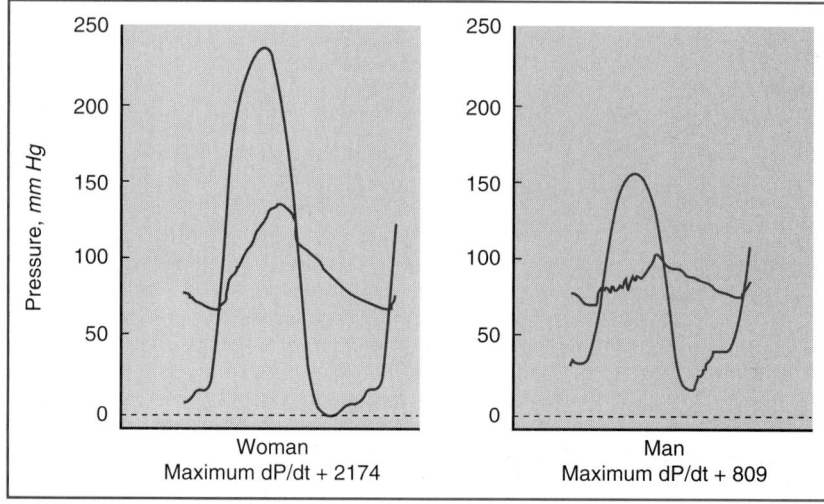

FIGURE 32–30. The difference in pressure-generating capabilities of the left ventricle in an 83-year-old woman and a 60-year-old man with a similar degree of aortic stenosis is shown. dP/dt—rate of pressure increase. (Reproduced with permission from Carroll, J. D., Carroll, E. P., Felman, T., et al.: Sex-associated differences in left ventricular function in aortic stenosis of the elderly. Circulation *86*:1099, 1992. Copyright 1992 American Heart Association.)

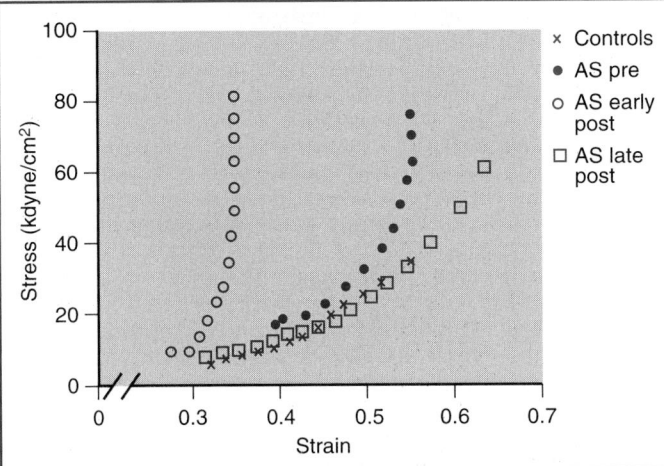

FIGURE 32–31. Representative plot of the diastolic stress-strain relation in a control subject and a patient with severe aortic stenosis (AS) before surgery (pre) as well as early and late after valve replacement (post). Early after surgery (early post), the curve is shifted to the left compared with the preoperative evaluation, and the constant of myocardial stiffness is increased. Late after valve replacement (late post) the curve is shifted to the right, and the constant of myocardial stiffness is normalized. (Reproduced with permission from Villari, B., et al.: Normalization of diastolic dysfunction in aortic stenosis late after valve replacement. Circulation *91*:2353, 1995. Copyright 1995 American Heart Association.)

to such an increased hemodynamic burden.[281] The increased systolic wall stress induced by AS apparently leads to parallel replication of sarcomeres and concentric hypertrophy (Fig. 13–10, p. 401), and the increase in left ventricular wall thickness is often sufficient to counterbalance the increased pressure so that peak systolic wall tension returns to normal or remains so if the obstruction develops slowly.[281–284] An inverse correlation between wall stress and ejection fraction exists in patients with AS.[284] This suggests that the depressed ejection fraction and velocity of fiber shortening that occur in *some* patients are a consequence of inadequate wall thickening,[285] resulting in "afterload mismatch."[286] Patients having AS with compensated pressure overload as well as some patients with depressed left ventricular ejection fraction and overt congestive failure may have normal values of intraventricular stress ($d\sigma/dt$)[287] and pressure (dP/dt) development, indicative of normal contractility.[279,280] In others, the lower ejection fraction is secondary to a depression of contractility; in the latter, surgical treatment is less effective.[288] Thus, both increased afterload and altered contractility are operative in depressing left ventricular performance.[279,280]

In order to evaluate myocardial function in patients with AS, the ejection phase indices, such as ejection fraction and myocardial fiber shortening, should be related to the existing wall tension. Wall thickness is a critical determinant of ventricular performance in patients with AS; inadequate hypertrophy, an intrinsic depression of myocardial contractility, or a combination of these two defects may lead to a depression of ventricular performance.[289] Impaired systolic function also occurs in prolonged, severe AS with massive hypertrophy (LV mass > 300 g/m²). It is associated with degenerative changes in the ultrastructure, including disruption of sarcomeres and increased interstitial fibrosis.

DIASTOLIC PROPERTIES (see p. 402). Although ventricular hypertrophy is a key adaptive mechanism to the pressure load imposed by AS, it has an adverse pathophysiological consequence; i.e., it increases diastolic stiffness (Figs. 32–11, and 32–31). As a result, greater intracavitary pressure is required for ventricular filling.[276,277,289a] Some patients with AS manifest an increase in stiffness of the left ventricle (chamber stiffness) due simply to an increase in muscle mass but with no alteration in the diastolic properties of each unit of myocardium (muscle stiffness); others exhibit increases in both chamber and muscle stiffness, which contribute to the elevation of ventricular diastolic filling pressure at any level of ventricular diastolic volume.[290,291] The diastolic dysfunction may be responsible for flash pulmonary edema in AS. Chamber stiffness may revert toward normal as hypertrophy regresses following relief of AS,[276,277] and at least in some patients muscle stiffness may also revert to normal. Whether this occurs in all patients is not clear. It is expected that this regression of stiffness would not occur in patients with extensive myocardial fibrosis. Indeed, in some patients stiffness increases postoperatively as ventricular hypertrophy regresses, while interstitial fibrosis remains unchanged.[292] The rate of ventricular thinning in diastole is slowed in AS.

STRUCTURE. A variety of changes in the myocardial ultrastructure have been documented in patients with severe AS. These include unusually large nuclei, loss of myofibrils, accumulation of mitochondria, large cytoplasmic areas devoid of contractile material, and proliferation of fibroblasts and collagen fibers in the interstitial space.[293] The depression of cardiac function that occurs late in the course of the disease may well be related to these morphological alterations. In adults with AS, both myocardial cellular hypertrophy and relative and absolute increases in connective tissue occur.[294] An inverse correlation between left ventricular ejection fraction and myocardial fiber diameter has been reported.[294]

ISCHEMIA. In AS, coronary blood flow at rest is elevated in absolute terms but is normal when corrected for myocardial mass.[295] There may be inadequate myocardial oxygenation in severe AS, even in the absence of coronary artery disease. The hypertrophied left ventricular muscle mass, the increased systolic pressure, and the prolongation of ejection all elevate myocardial oxygen consumption,[296] and the abnormally heightened pressure compressing the coronary arteries exceeds the coronary perfusion pressure, thereby interfering with coronary blood flow,[297,298] thus leading to a potential imbalance between myocardial oxygen supply and demand. Myocardial perfusion is also impaired by the relative decrease in myocardial capillary density and by the elevation of left ventricular end-diastolic pressure, which lowers the aortic–left ventricular pressure gradient in diastole, i.e., the coronary perfusion pressure gradient. The subendocardium in severe AS in particular is susceptible to ischemia, and this underperfusion may be responsible for the development of subendocardial ischemia.[297] Marcus et al. have demonstrated a reduction in the velocity of coronary blood flow during reactive hyperemia at the time of operation in patients with severe AS,[299] and this may correlate with the angina commonly observed in these patients. Metabolic evidence of myocardial ischemia, i.e., lactate production, can be demonstrated when myocardial oxygen needs are stimulated by exercise or isoproterenol in patients with AS, in both the presence and the absence of coronary arterial narrowing.

CLINICAL MANIFESTATIONS

History

In the natural history of adults with AS, a long latent period exists during which there is gradually increasing obstruction and an increase in the pressure load on the myocardium while the patient remains asymptomatic.[300] The cardinal manifestations of AS, which commence most commonly in the sixth decade of life, are angina pectoris, syncope, and heart failure.[301] In patients in whom the obstruction remains unrelieved, once these symptoms become manifested, the prognosis is poor; survival curves show that the interval from the onset of symptoms to the time of death is approximately 2 years in patients with heart failure, 3 years in those with syncope, and 5 years in those with angina.[302,303] *Angina* occurs in approximately two-thirds of patients with critical AS (about half of whom have associated significant coronary artery obstruction)[304] and usually resembles that observed in patients with coronary artery disease, in that it is commonly precipitated by exertion and relieved by rest. In patients without coronary artery disease it results from the combination of increased oxygen needs by the hypertrophied myocardium and reduction of oxygen delivery secondary to the excessive compression of coronary vessels[295,299] (see Ischemia, above). In patients with coronary artery disease, angina is caused by a combination of the epicardial coronary obstruction and the above-described oxygen imbalance characteristic of AS. Rarely, angina results from calcium emboli to the coronary vascular bed.[306]

Syncope is most commonly due to the reduced cerebral perfusion that occurs during exertion when arterial pressure declines consequent to systemic vasodilatation in the presence of a fixed cardiac output. Syncope has also been attributed to malfunction of the baroreceptor mechanism[266,308] and to vasodepressor response to a greatly elevated left ventricular systolic pressure during exercise.[309] Premonitory symptoms are common. Exertional hypotension may also be manifested as "graying out" spells or dizziness on effort. Syncope at rest may be due to transient ventricular fibrillation,[307] from which the patient recovers spontaneously; from transient atrial fibrillation with loss of the atrial contribution to left ventricular filling causing a precipitous decline in cardiac output; or transient atrioventricular block due to extension of the calcification of the valve into the conduction system. Exertional dyspnea with orthopnea, paroxysmal nocturnal dyspnea, and pulmonary edema reflect varying degrees of pulmonary venous hypertension. These are relatively late symptoms in AS, and their presence for more than 5 years should suggest the possibility of associated mitral valvular disease.

Gastrointestinal bleeding, idiopathic or due to angiodysplasia (most commonly of the right colon) or other vascular malformations, occurs more often in patients with calcific AS than in persons without this condition; it may cease after aortic valve replacement.[310] Infective endocarditis is a greater risk in younger patients with milder valvular deformity than in older patients with rocklike calcific aortic deformities. Cerebral emboli resulting in stroke or transient ischemic attacks may result from microthrombi on thickened bicuspid valves.[311] Calcific AS may cause embolization of calcium to a variety of organs, including the heart, kidney, and brain. Abrupt loss of vision has been reported when calcific emboli occluded the central retinal artery.[312]

Because cardiac output is usually well maintained for many years in patients with severe AS, marked fatigability, debilitation, peripheral cyanosis, and other manifestations of a low cardiac output are usually not prominent until quite late in the natural history of the disease. Atrial fibrillation, pulmonary hypertension, and systemic venous hypertension in patients with isolated AS are often preterminal findings. Although AS may be responsible for sudden death (see p. 749), this usually occurs in patients who had previously been symptomatic.

Physical Examination

The arterial pulse characteristically rises slowly and is small and sustained (pulsus parvus et tardus) (Fig. 2–8B, p. 21).[313,314] In the advanced stage, systolic and pulse pressures are both reduced. However, in patients with mild AS with associated AR and in older patients with an inelastic arterial bed, both systolic and pulse pressures may be normal or even increased. A systolic pressure exceeding 200 mm Hg is rare in patients with critical AS.[313] The anacrotic notch and coarse systolic vibrations are felt most readily in the carotid arterial pulse, producing the so-called carotid shudder. Simultaneous palpation of the apex and carotid arteries reveals a distinct lag in the latter in patients with severe AS.[315] Although left ventricular alternans occurs commonly in AS with left ventricular dysfunction[316] (Fig. 2–9, p. 23), obstruction of the aortic valve may prevent its recognition by examination of the peripheral arterial pulse. The jugular venous pulse usually shows prominent a waves, reflecting reduced right ventricular compliance consequent to hypertrophy of the ventricular septum.[317] With pulmonary hypertension and secondary right ventricular failure and tricuspid regurgitation, v or c-v waves may be prominent.

The cardiac impulse is sustained with left ventricular failure; it becomes displaced inferiorly and laterally (Fig. 2–11C). Presystolic distention of the left ventricle, i.e., a prominent precordial a wave, is often both visible and palpable. A hyperdynamic left ventricle suggests concomitant aortic and/or mitral regurgitation. A systolic thrill is usually best appreciated when the patient leans forward in full expiration. It is palpated most readily in the second left intercostal space on either side of the sternum or in the suprasternal notch and is frequently transmitted along the carotid arteries.

Rarely, right ventricular failure with systemic venous congestion, hepatomegaly, and edema precedes left ventricular failure. Probably this is caused by the so-called Bernheim effect, which results from the hypertrophied ventricular septum's bulging into and encroaching on the right ventricular cavity and leads to impairment of right ventricular filling. In such cases, the jugular venous pressure is elevated and the a wave is prominent.

AUSCULTATION (Tables 32–2 and 32–7). S_1 is normal or soft and S_4 is prominent, presumably because atrial contraction is vigorous and the mitral valve is partially closed during presystole.[318] S_2 may be single because calcification and immobility of the aortic valve make A_2 inaudible, be-

TABLE 32–7   DIFFERENTIAL DIAGNOSIS OF AORTIC STENOSIS: PHYSICAL FINDINGS

TYPE OF STENOSIS	MAXIMUM MURMUR AND THRILL	AORTIC EJECTION SOUND	AORTIC COMPONENT OF SECOND SOUND	REGURGITANT DIASTOLIC MURMUR	ARTERIAL PULSE
Acquired nonrheumatic or rheumatic	Second right sternal border to neck; may be at apex in the aged	Uncommon	Decreased or absent	Common	Delayed upstroke; anacrotic notch; ± small amplitude
Hypertrophic subaortic	Fourth left sternal border to apex (± regurgitant systolic murmur at apex)	Rare	Normal or decreased	Very rare	Brisk upstroke, sometimes bisferiens
Congenital valvular	Second right sternal border to neck (along left sternal border in some infants)	Very common in children, disappearing with decrease in valve mobility with age	Normal or increased in childhood; decreased with decrease in valve mobility with age	Uncommon in child; not uncommon in adult	Delayed upstroke; anacrotic notch; ± small amplitude
Congenital subvalvular	Discrete: like valvular; tunnel: left sternal border	Rare	Not helpful (normal, increased, decreased or absent)	Almost all	
Congenital supravalvular	First right sternal border to neck and sometimes to medial aspect of right arm; occasionally greater in neck than in chest	Rare	Normal or decreased	Uncommon	Rapid upstroke in right carotid, delayed in left carotid; right arm pulse pressure greater than left

From Levinson, G. E.: Aortic stenosis. *In* Dalen, J. E., and Alpert, J. S. (eds.): Valvular Heart Disease. 2nd ed. Boston, Little, Brown and Company, 1987, p. 202.

cause P_2 is buried in the prolonged aortic ejection murmur, or because prolongation of left ventricular systole makes A_2 coincide with P_2. Paradoxical splitting of S_2, which suggests associated left ventricular dysfunction, may also occur. With left ventricular failure and secondary pulmonary hypertension, P_2 may become accentuated. When the valve is rigid, A_2 may be inaudible, but when the valve is flexible, A_2 may be snapping and accentuated.

An aortic ejection sound (see p. 30) occurs simultaneously with the halting upward movement of the aortic valve (Fig. 2–17, p. 30). It is dependent on mobility of the valve cusps and disappears when they become severely calcified. Thus, it is common in children with congenital AS but is rare in elderly adults with acquired calcific AS and rigid valves. This sound occurs approximately 0.06 sec after the onset of S_1 and has a frequency similar to that of S_1. The ejection sound is heard most readily with the diaphragm of the stethoscope along the left sternal border, although it is often well transmitted to the apex, where it may be confused with S_1 (and the S_1 may be mistaken for an S_4). In contrast to a pulmonic ejection sound, aortic ejection sounds usually do not vary with respiration.

The *systolic murmur* of AS is usually late-peaking and heard best at the base of the heart but is often well transmitted along the carotid vessels and to the apex (Fig. 2–27, p. 36). Cessation of the murmur before A_2 is usually helpful in differentiating it from a pansystolic mitral murmur, but it may be falsely considered to be a pansystolic murmur because it may end with S_2, which represents pulmonic valve closure while A_2 is soft or even inaudible. In patients with calcified aortic valves, the murmur is harsh and rasping at the base, but high-frequency components selectively radiate to the apex (the so-called Gallavardin phenomenon [Fig. 2–28, p. 37]), where it may actually be more prominent and where it may be mistaken for the murmur of MR. Frequently, there is a "quiet area" between the base and apex where the murmur is diminished in intensity, supporting the erroneous impression that the apical and basal murmurs have different origins. In general, the more severe the stenosis, the longer the duration of the murmur[319] and the more likely that it peaks in mid-systole.[320]

In patients with degenerative AS, there may be heavy valvular calcification, but obstruction may not be severe because the commissural fusion characteristic of congenital and rheumatic AS is absent. The nonfused calcified cusps vibrate freely, resulting in a softer, more musical murmur, more prominent at the apex than the murmur of congenital or rheumatic AS.[319] High-pitched decrescendo diastolic murmurs secondary to AR are common in many patients with dominant AS.

In hypertrophic cardiomyopathy (HCM), the murmur is delayed in onset and may continue up to A_2 (see p. 1418); the carotid artery characteristically rises sharply and is bisferious. Palpation of the carotid pulse is also extremely helpful in differentiating between valvular AS on the one hand and HCM and MR on the other, because the arterial pulse generally rises slowly in AS but sharply in the other two conditions. However, confusion can arise in young patients with congenital AS, in whom sudden upward displacement ("doming") of the pliant aortic leaflet or leaflets with ventricular systole may result in a brisk initial upstroke in the carotid pulse, coincident with the systolic ejection click.

When the left ventricle fails and the cardiac output falls in AS, the murmur becomes softer or disappears altogether. The slow rise is more difficult to recognize. Stated simply, the clinical picture changes to that of severe left ventricular failure with a low cardiac output. Thus, occult AS may be a cause of intractable heart failure, and critical AS should be ruled out by echocardiography in patients with severe heart failure of unknown cause because operative treatment

may be life-saving and may result in substantial clinical improvement.[321]

Dynamic Auscultation (Table 32–3). The murmur of valvular AS is augmented by the inhalation of amyl nitrite and by squatting, which increase stroke volume. It is reduced in intensity during the Valsalva strain (which increases the murmur of HCM), with vasopressors, moderate isometric exercise, or standing, all of which reduce transvalvular flow.[322] The intensity of the systolic murmur varies from beat to beat when the duration of diastolic filling varies, as in atrial fibrillation or following a premature contraction. This characteristic is helpful in differentiating AS from MR, in which the murmur is usually unaffected.

LABORATORY EXAMINATION

ELECTROCARDIOGRAPHY

The principal electrocardiographic change is left ventricular hypertrophy, which is found in approximately 85 per cent of patients with severe AS. The absence of left ventricular hypertrophy does not exclude the presence of critical AS, and the correlation between the absolute voltages in precordial leads and the severity of obstruction, which is quite good in children with congenital AS, is not as good in adults. However, a good correlation has been reported between the sum of the QRS amplitudes in 12 leads and the height of the left ventricular systolic pressure.[323] T-wave inversion and ST-segment depression in leads with upright QRS complexes are common. ST-segment depressions greater than 0.2 mV in patients with AS (left ventricular "strain") suggest that severe ventricular hypertrophy is present. The progressive development of ST-segment and T-wave abnormalities suggests that hypertrophy has progressed. Occasionally, a "pseudoinfarction" pattern is present, characterized by a loss of r waves in the right precordial leads. There is evidence of left atrial enlargement in more than 80 per cent of patients with severe isolated AS[324]; the principal manifestation is prominent late negativity of the P wave in V_1 rather than an increased duration in lead II, suggesting hypertrophy rather than dilatation. Atrial fibrillation is an uncommon and late sign of pure AS, and its presence in a patient who does not appear to have end-stage aortic disease should suggest the coexistence of mitral valvular disease.

The extension of calcific infiltrates from the aortic valve into the conduction system may cause various forms and degrees of atrioventricular and intraventricular block in 5 per cent of patients with calcific AS.[325] Conduction defects are more common in patients who have associated mitral annular calcium.[325] Almost 10 per cent of all instances of left anterior hemiblock are secondary to aortic valvular disease.

Ambulatory electrocardiography frequently shows complex ventricular arrhythmias,[326] particularly in patients with myocardial dysfunction.

RADIOLOGICAL FINDINGS

Routine radiological examination may be entirely normal despite the presence of critical AS. The heart is usually of normal size or slightly enlarged, with a rounding of the left ventricular border and apex (Fig. 7–10A, p. 210), unless regurgitation or left ventricular failure is present and causes substantial cardiomegaly. Poststenotic dilatation of the ascending aorta is a common finding. Calcification of the aortic valve is found in almost all adults with hemodynamically significant AS;[327] it is more readily detected on fluoroscopy (or echocardiography) rather than on the roentgenogram. The *absence* of calcium in the region of the aortic valve on careful fluoroscopic examination in a patient older than 35 essentially rules out severe valvular AS. The converse is not true, however, and in patients over the age of 65 with degenerative AS, severe calcification of the valve may occur with only mild obstruction. The left atrium may be slightly enlarged, and there may be radiological signs of pulmonary venous hypertension. However, when left atrial enlargement is marked, particularly if the atrial appendage is prominent, the presence of associated mitral valvular disease should be suspected.

ANGIOGRAPHY. Angiographic studies of the aortic valve are best performed by injecting contrast medium into the left ventricle and filming in the 30-degree right anterior oblique and 60-degree left anterior oblique projections. These examinations often make it possible to ascertain the number of cusps of the stenotic valve and to demonstrate doming of a thickened valve and a systolic jet. There is some hazard associated with the rapid injection of a large volume of contrast material into a high-pressure left ventricle, and this is ordinarily not indicated in patients with AS, critical obstruction, and/or left ventricular failure.

ECHOCARDIOGRAPHY (see also p. 74). The normal range of opening of the aortic valve is 1.6 to 2.6 cm, and the normal aortic valve leaflets are barely visible in systole on the M-mode echogram. Two-dimensional transthoracic echocardiography may be helpful in the detection of valvular calcification, in outlining the valve leaflets, and sometimes in determining the severity of the stenosis, by imaging the orifice. The orifice may be more clearly defined by transesophageal echocardiography, which offers a precise short-axis view of the aortic valve[328] (Fig. 3–54, p. 74). Multiplanar transesophageal echocardiography is particularly useful.[329] Two-dimensional transthoracic echocardiography is invaluable in detecting associated mitral valve disease and in assessing left ventricular performance, dilatation, and hypertrophy. Doppler echocardiography allows calculation of the left ventricular-aortic pressure gradient[330,331] (Figs. 3–42, p. 70, and 3–55, p. 75) using a modified Bernoulli equation (Fig. 3–4, p. 69). The gradients noninvasively determined by this method correlate well with those determined by left heart catheterization.[332,333] Color flow Doppler imaging is helpful in the detection and determination of the severity of any accompanying aortic regurgitation.

NATURAL HISTORY

In contrast to MS, which leads to symptoms almost immediately after its development, patients with severe AS may be asymptomatic for many years despite the presence of severe obstruction.[300,305,334] The systolic pressure gradient can exceed 150 mm Hg, and the peak left ventricular systolic pressure can reach approximately 300 mm Hg with relatively little increase in overall heart size on radiographic examination and with normal left ventricular end-diastolic and end-systolic volumes.

Patients with severe chronic AS tend to be free of cardiovascular symptoms until relatively late in the course of the disease. In Rapaport's series, 40 per cent of patients treated medically survived for 5 years and 20 per cent for 10 years after diagnosis.[66] In another series of patients with hemodynamically significant valvular AS treated medically, the 5-year survival rate was 64 per cent. However, once patients with AS become symptomatic with angina or syncope, the average survival is 2 to 3 years, whereas with congestive heart failure it is 1.5 years[302,303] (Fig. 32–32). In an analysis of elderly patients with severe AS and symptoms of heart failure who declined surgery, 50 per cent had died by 18 months of follow-up; the ejection fraction correlated inversely with survival.[335]

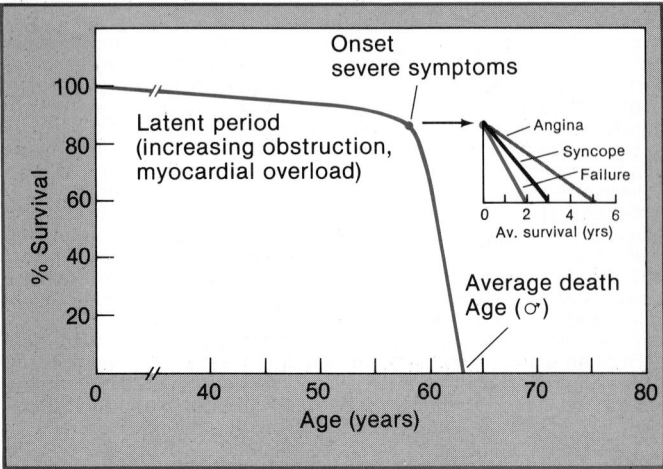

FIGURE 32–32. Natural history of aortic stenosis without operative treatment. (Reproduced with permission from Ross, J., Jr., and Braunwald, E.: Aortic stenosis. Circulation 38[Suppl. V]:61, 1968. Copyright 1968 American Heart Association.)

Asymptomatic patients have an excellent prognosis.[336,337] Sudden death, like syncope, in patients with severe AS may be due to cerebral hypoperfusion followed by arrhythmia. Although severe AS is a potentially lethal disease, death, even when sudden, usually occurs in *symptomatic* patients. A number of authors have followed asymptomatic patients with critical AS,[338] and sudden death is extremely rare. Of 229 asymptomatic patients with critical aortic stenosis, only 5 (2 per cent) died suddenly (certainly not higher than the mortality from operation).[339]

MANAGEMENT

Medical Treatment

Patients with known severe AS who are asymptomatic should be advised to report promptly the development of any symptoms possibly related to AS. Patients with critical obstruction should be cautioned to avoid vigorous athletic and physical activity. However, such restrictions do not apply to patients with mild obstruction. The necessity for endocarditis prophylaxis should be explained (see p. 1097). Because of the gradual increase in the severity of obstruction, noninvasive assessment of the severity of obstruction by Doppler echocardiography should be carried out at intervals. In patients with mild obstruction, this measurement should be repeated every 2 years. Doppler-derived gradients have been shown to increase by 4 to 8 mm Hg per year.[339–341] The rate of increase is greater in patients with coexisting coronary artery disease and lower in patients with rheumatic AS. In asymptomatic patients with severe obstruction, repeat echocardiography should be carried out every 6 to 12 months, with particular attention to possible changes in left ventricular function.

Digitalis glycosides are indicated if there is an increase in ventricular volume or reduced ejection fraction. Although diuretics are beneficial when there is abnormal accumulation of fluid, they must be used with caution, because hypovolemia may reduce the elevated left ventricular end-diastolic pressure, lower cardiac output, and produce orthostatic hypotension. Beta-adrenoceptor blockers can depress myocardial function and induce left ventricular failure and should be used only with great caution, if at all, in patients with AS.

Atrial flutter or fibrillation occurs in fewer than 10 per cent of patients with severe AS, perhaps because of the late occurrence of left atrial enlargement in this condition. When such an arrhythmia is observed in a patient with AS, the possibility of associated mitral valve disease should be considered. In light of the adverse hemodynamic effects of the loss of atrial booster pump function with atrial fibrillation in patients with AS,[278] an effort should be made to prevent the development of this arrhythmia by prophylaxis with an antiarrhythmic agent when premature atrial contractions are frequent. When atrial fibrillation does occur, the rapid ventricular rate may cause angina or electrocardiographic evidence of myocardial ischemia or both; the loss of the atrial contribution to ventricular filling and a sudden fall in cardiac output may cause serious hypotension. Therefore, this arrhythmia should be treated promptly (see p. 654), and a search for previously unrecognized mitral valve disease should be undertaken. If symptoms develop, adults considered to have severe AS should undergo left heart catheterization. In men over 35 years and women over 45 years, coronary arteriography is indicated. The purpose of catheterization is to confirm the site and document the severity of the obstruction, to determine the state of left ventricular function, and to ascertain the presence or absence of associated valvular disease and coronary artery disease.

Surgical Treatment

INDICATIONS FOR OPERATION. The most critical decision in the management of patients with AS—indeed, of all patients with valvular heart disease—concerns the advisability and timing of surgical treatment.[300,342] The indications for surgery as well as the techniques and results of operation depend on the patient's age and the nature of the valvular deformity. In children and adolescents with noncalcific congenital AS, who most commonly have bicuspid aortic valves, simple commissural incision under direct vision usually leads to substantial hemodynamic improvement at low risk, i.e., a mortality rate of less than 1 per cent (see p. 915).[343] Therefore, this procedure (or aortic balloon valvuloplasty) is indicated not only in symptomatic patients but also in asymptomatic children and adolescents with critical aortic stenosis, i.e., a calculated effective orifice less than 0.8 cm² or 0.5 cm²/m² BSA. Despite the salutary hemodynamic results following this procedure, the valve is not rendered entirely normal anatomically, and the turbulent blood flow through it may lead to further deformation, calcification, the development of regurgitation, and restenosis after 10 to 20 years, probably requiring reoperation and valve replacement later.

In most adults with calcific AS, satisfactory valvular function cannot be restored, even by careful sculpturing procedures carried out under direct vision, and valve replacement is the surgical treatment of choice.[344] Ultrasonic decalcification and other repairs may be effective immediately in a fraction of patients, but restenosis is a serious problem.[345] The aortic valve should, in general, be replaced (Fig. 32–33) in patients who have hemodynamic evidence of severe obstruction (aortic valve orifice < 0.8 cm² or < 0.5 cm²/m² BSA) and symptoms believed to result from AS. (Prosthetic valves are discussed on pp. 1061 to 1066). Surgical treatment should also be carried out in asymptomatic patients with progressive left ventricular dysfunction and/or significant ventricular ectopic activity at rest or an abnormal hemodynamic response (inadequate elevation of systolic arterial pressure) to exercise.[338] Although a prospective randomized controlled study has not been done, the long-term mortality in asymptomatic patients with critical AS and left ventricular dysfunction undergoing operation appears to be lower than that in medically treated patients without operation.[346] As artificial valves and surgical skills continue to improve, it is likely that patients with severe AS will become candidates for operation at progressively earlier stages in the natural history of their disease. At the present time, however, I do not recommend prophylactic replacement of a critically narrow calcific aortic valve in *asymptomatic* adults unless they exhibit progressive left ventricular dysfunction.

RESULTS. Successful replacement of the aortic valve results in substantial clinical and hemodynamic improvement in patients with AS, AR, or combined lesions.[347] In patients without frank left ventricular failure, the operative risk ranges from 2 to 8 per cent in most centers, and in patients under the age of 70 years it has been reported to be as low as 1 per cent.[280] Risk factors for higher mortality include high New York Heart Association (NYHA) class, impairment of left ventricular function, age, and the presence of associated AR.[343] The 5-year actuarial survival rate of hospital survivors is approximately 85 per cent. Risk factors for late death include higher preoperative NYHA class, advanced age, concomitant untreated coronary artery disease, preoperative impaired left ventricular function, preoperative ventricular arrhythmias, and associated significant AR. Symptoms secondary to elevations of left atrial pressure and myocardial ischemia are relieved in almost every patient. Hemodynamic results are equally impressive; elevated end-diastolic and end-systolic volumes show significant reduction. Impaired ventricular performance returns to normal more frequently in patients with AS than in those with aortic or mitral regurgitation. Diastolic function is normalized (Fig. 32–31).[276,277]

However, the finding that the strongest predictor of postoperative left ventricular dysfunction is preoperative dysfunction[346,348] suggests that patients should, if possible, be operated on before left ventricular function becomes seriously impaired. The increased left ventricular mass is reduced toward (but not to) normal within 18 months after aortic valve replacement in patients with AS.[349] When restudied 5 years postoperatively, left ventricular mass had returned to normal.[350] Myocyte hypertrophy regresses before fibrous tissue is resorbed.

When operation is carried out in patients with frank left

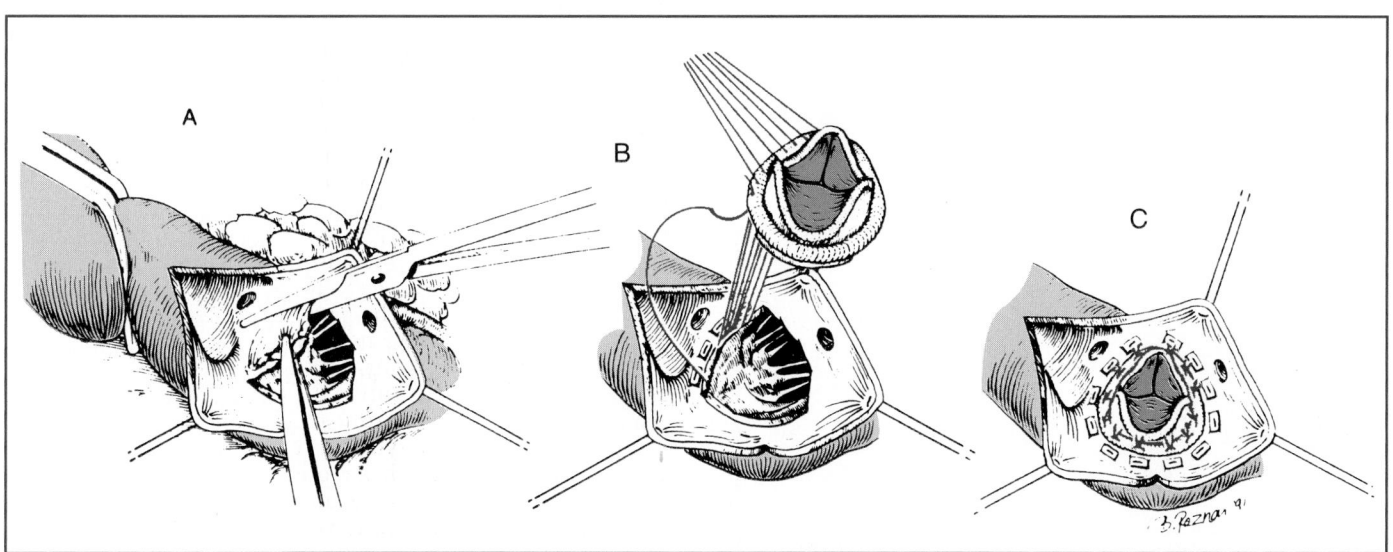

FIGURE 32–33. Interrupted suture technique for aortic valve replacement. *A,* The aortic valve is excised, leaving 1 or 2 mm of annular tissue as a sewing cuff. *B,* Pledgetted Tyeron mattress sutures (2-0) are placed with the pledget on the aortic side. Sutures are placed in the aortic ring and passed directly onto the prosthetic valve sewing ring held at a distance. *C,* After all sutures are placed, the valve is lowered in place and the sutures tied. The valve is then inspected for proper function and fit. (From Albertucci, M., and Karp, R. B.: Prosthetic valve replacement. *In* Al-Zaibag, M., and Duran, C. M. G. [eds.]: Valvular Heart Disease. New York, Marcel Dekker, 1994, pp. 601–634.)

ventricular failure or a depressed ejection fraction, the operative risk is higher, and the mortality ranges from 10 to 25 per cent, depending on the skill of the surgical team and the severity of depression of left ventricular function. A depressed relation between ejection fraction and wall stress is a poor prognostic index, as is a depressed level of dP/dt max at any given left ventricular end-diastolic pressure.[351] Obviously, it is desirable to perform surgery before the development of heart failure, but emergency operation is sometimes lifesaving even in the most desperate situations. In view of the extremely poor prognosis of such patients when they are treated medically, there is usually little choice but to advise immediate mechanical relief of obstruction, i.e., balloon angioplasty (see later discussion) or emergency surgery.[352] Many symptomatic patients with calcific AS are elderly, in whom particular attention must be directed to the adequacy of hepatic, renal, and pulmonary functions. However, the results of aortic valve replacement are satisfactory in patients older than 70[353] or even 80.[354] Age per se, while adding to the risk, should not be considered a contraindication to operation.

In patients with AS and obstructive coronary artery disease (a relatively common combination), aortic valve replacement and myocardial revascularization should be performed together.[354] Although the risk of aortic valve surgery is increased by the association of coronary artery disease, the operative mortality in patients undergoing the combined procedure is not necessarily higher than that of isolated aortic valve replacement in this group.[343] Indeed, the surgical risk rises if severe coronary artery disease is left untreated. The ability to avoid serious myocardial ischemia in the perioperative period is a major factor that has served to reduce operative mortality. After the patient has been placed on cardiopulmonary bypass, the heart is protected by means of hypothermic cardiac arrest alone or combined

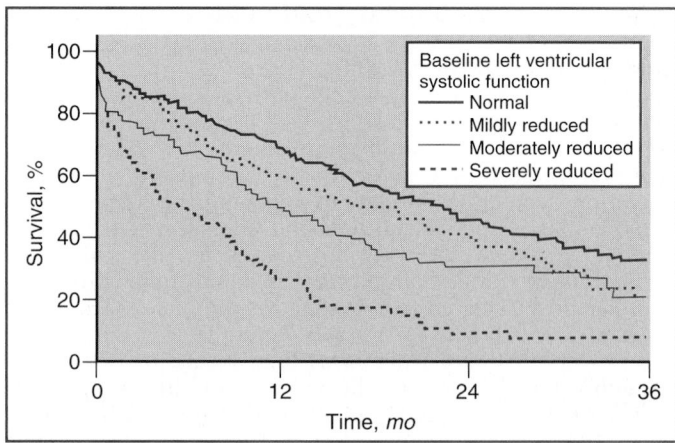

FIGURE 32–35. Kaplan-Meier survival curves following balloon aortic valvuloplasty for aortic stenosis, grouped according to left ventricular function. (Reproduced with permission from Otto, C. M., Mickel, M. C., Kennedy, J. W., et al.: Three-year outcome after balloon aortic valvuloplasty: Insights into prognosis of valvular aortic stenosis. Circulation *89*:642, 1994. Copyright 1994 American Heart Association.)

with cardioplegia. The calcified valve must be removed with great care to avoid embolization of calcified fragments into the systemic circulation.

Balloon Aortic Valvuloplasty
(See also Chap. 39)

This technique represents an increasingly attractive alternative to aortic valvotomy in children, adolescents, and young adults with congenital noncalcific AS (see p. 1385), but its value is limited in adults with calcific AS. A series of balloon dilatation catheters are advanced along a guidewire positioned at the left ventricular apex. In balloon dilatation of calcified stenotic aortic valves carried out on postmortem specimens and in the operating room, fracture of calcified nodules and/or separation of fused commissures were found to be responsible for the relief of obstruction[355]; stretching of the aortic valve ring is probably also involved.[356] There is considerable variation in patient response. However, balloon aortic valvuloplasty results initially in relief of obstruction in most patients[357–359] (Fig. 32–34). In a report of a multicenter registry involving 674 elderly (average age = 78 years) seriously ill patients treated at 24 centers, the procedural mortality was 3 per cent and the 30-day mortality 14 per cent. One-year mortality was 45 per cent. Valve area initially increased from 0.50 to 0.80 cm², and the mean gradient declined from approximately 55 to 29 mm Hg. Better survival was seen in patients with higher preoperative pressure gradients, in those with better preserved left ventricular systolic function (Fig. 32–35), and in women.[360] Left ventricular ejection fraction tends to rise in patients with depressed left ventricular function. In addition to the procedural mortality, another 6 per cent develop serious complications such as myocardial perforation, myocardial infarction, and severe aortic regurgitation.[362–364] The major disadvantage of balloon valvuloplasty in adults with critical, calcified AS is restenosis due to scarring, which occurs in about half of the patients within 6 months. Symptoms lessen in severity in the majority of patients but recur in approximately 30 per cent by 6 months. In most series, patients have been elderly, have had heart failure, and have been considered poor operative risks.

Although the overall intermediate-term (6 to 12 months) results of balloon aortic valvuloplasty have been disappointing, largely because of restenosis, the procedure does have a role in the management of severe calcific AS in patients who are not surgical candidates. This includes pa-

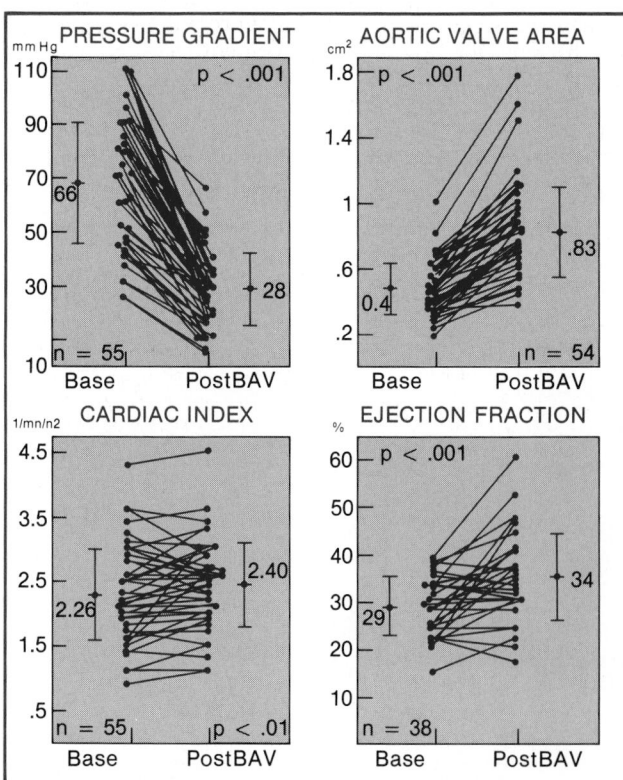

FIGURE 32–34. Plots of changes in pressure gradient, valve area, cardiac index, and ejection fraction at baseline (Base) after balloon aortic valvuloplasty (BAV). (Reproduced with permission from Berland, J., et al.: Percutaneous balloon valvuloplasty in patients with severe aortic stenosis and low ejection fraction. Circulation *79*:1189, 1989. Copyright 1989 American Heart Association.)

tients with cardiogenic shock due to critical AS,[365] patients with critical AS who require an urgent noncardiac operation, as a "bridge" to aortic valve replacement in patients with severe heart failure who are at extremely high operative risk, in pregnant women with critical AS,[366] and in patients with critical AS who refuse surgical treatment. However, in the adult with calcified AS, balloon aortic valvuloplasty is *not* a substitute for surgery (as balloon mitral valvuloplasty may be in the case of MS [see p. 1013]).

AORTIC REGURGITATION

ETIOLOGY AND PATHOLOGY

Aortic regurgitation (AR) may be caused by primary disease of either the aortic valve leaflets or the wall of the aortic root or both (Fig. 32–36).[367] Among patients with *pure* AR coming to valve replacement, the percentage with aortic root disease has been increasing steadily during the past few decades and now accounts for more than one-half of the patients.[263]

Valvular Disease

Rheumatic fever is a common cause of primary disease of the valve leading to regurgitation.[368,368a] The cusps become infiltrated with fibrous tissues and retract, a process that prevents cusp apposition during diastole and usually leads to regurgitation into the left ventricle through a defect in the center of the valve.[8] The associated fusion of the commissures may also restrict the opening of the valve, resulting in combined AS and AR; some associated mitral valve

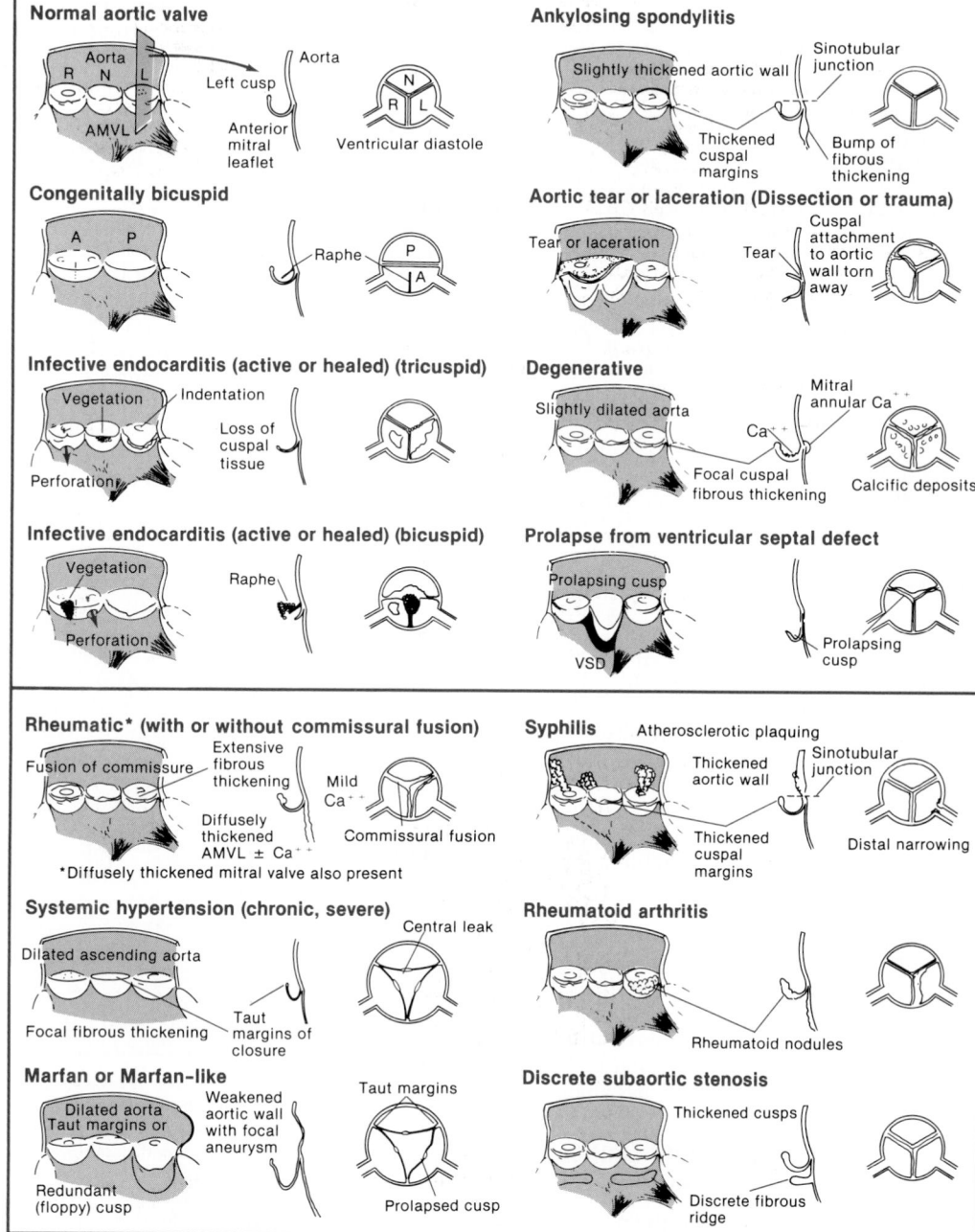

FIGURE 32–36. Diagram of various causes of pure aortic regurgitation. (From Waller, B. F.: Rheumatic and nonrheumatic conditions producing valvular heart disease. *In* Frankl, W. S., and Brest, A. N. [eds.]: Cardiovascular Clinics. Valvular Heart Disease: Comprehensive Evaluation and Management. Philadelphia, F. A. Davis Co., 1986, pp. 30–31.)

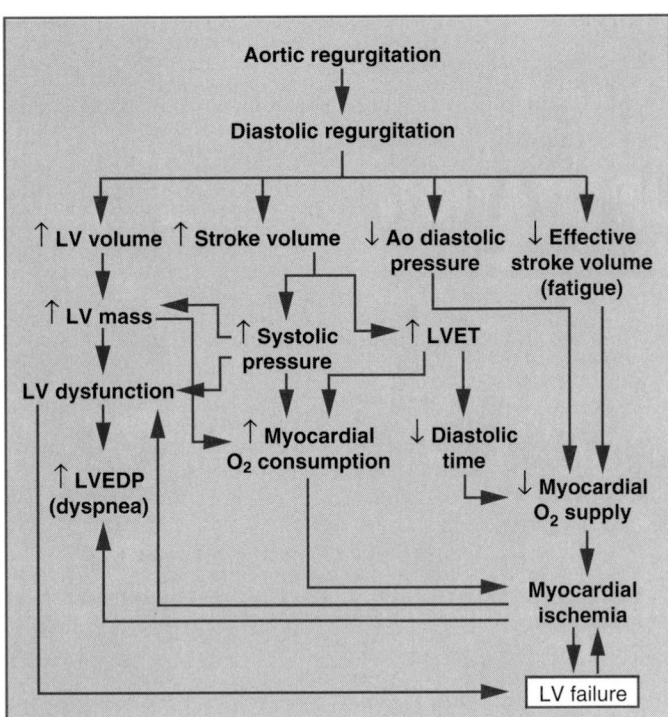

FIGURE 32-37. Pathophysiology of aortic regurgitation. Aortic regurgitation results in an increased left ventricular (LV) volume, increased stroke volume, increased aortic (Ao) systolic pressure, and decreased effective stroke volume. Increased LV volume results in an increased LV mass, which may lead to LV dysfunction and failure. Increased LV stroke volume increases systolic pressure and prolongation of left ventricular ejection time (LVET). Increased LV systolic pressure results in a decrease in diastolic time. Decreased diastolic time (myocardial perfusion time), diastolic aortic pressure, and effective stroke volume reduce myocardial O_2 supply. Increased myocardial O_2 consumption and decreased myocardial O_2 supply produce myocardial ischemia, which further deteriorates LV function (↑ = increased, ↓ = decreased). (From Boudoulas, H., and Gravanis, M. B.: Valvular heart disease. *In* Gravanis, M. B.: Cardiovascular Disorders: Pathogenesis and Pathophysiology. St. Louis, C. V. Mosby, 1993, p. 64.)

involvement is common. Other primary valvular causes of AR include *infective endocarditis* (Chap. 33), in which the infection may destroy or cause perforation of a leaflet, or the vegetations may interfere with proper coaptation of the cusps. *Trauma* (Fig. 44–9, p. 1542) resulting in a tear of the ascending aorta and loss of commissural support can cause prolapse of an aortic cusp. Although the most common complication of a congenitally *bicuspid valve* in adult life is stenosis, incomplete closure and/or prolapse of a bicuspid valve may cause isolated regurgitation or a combination of stenosis and regurgitation.[368-370] AR may develop in patients with large ventricular septal defects. Progressive regurgitation may also occur in patients with myxomatous proliferation of the aortic valve.[371] An increasingly common cause of valvular AR is structural deterioration of a bioprosthetic valve (see p. 1063). Less common causes of AR include a variety of forms of congenital AR: rupture of a congenitally fenestrated valve,[372] particularly in the presence of hypertension[373]; AR in association with systemic lupus erythematosus[374]; rheumatoid arthritis[375]; ankylosing spondylitis[376]; Jaccoud's arthropathy[377]; Takayasu's disease; Whipple's disease[378]; and Crohn's disease.[379] Isolated congenital AR is an uncommon lesion on necropsy studies, but when present, it is usually associated with a bicuspid valve.[380]

Aortic Root Disease
(See also Chap. 45)

A variety of diseases produce AR by causing marked dilatation of the ascending aorta (Fig. 32–36). AR secondary to root disease is now more common than primary valve disease in patients undergoing aortic root replacement.[263] These conditions include age-related (degenerative) aortic dilatation, cystic medial necrosis of the aorta (either isolated or associated with classic Marfan syndrome), aortic dissection, osteogenesis imperfecta, syphilitic aortitis, ankylosing spondylitis, Behçet's syndrome, psoriatic arthritis, arthritis associated with ulcerative colitis, relapsing polychondritis, Reiter's syndrome, giant cell arteritis, and systemic hypertension.[373,381-385]

When the aortic annulus becomes greatly dilated, the aortic leaflets separate, and AR may ensue. Dissection of the diseased aortic wall may occur and may aggravate the AR. Dilatation of the aortic root may also have secondary effects on the aortic valve, because it results in tension and bowing of the individual cusps, which may thicken, retract, and become too short to close the aortic orifice. This leads to intensification of the AR, which increases left ventricular stroke volume, further dilating the ascending aorta and thus leading to a vicious circle in which, just as is the case for MR, "regurgitation begets regurgitation."

AR, regardless of its cause, produces dilatation and hypertrophy of the left ventricle, dilatation of the mitral valve ring, and sometimes hypertrophy and dilatation of the left atrium. Endocardial pockets frequently develop in the left ventricular cavity at sites of impact of the regurgitant jet.

PATHOPHYSIOLOGY
(Fig. 32–37)

In contrast to MR, in which a fraction of the left ventricular stroke volume is ejected into the low-pressure left atrium, in AR the entire left ventricular stroke volume is ejected into a high-pressure chamber, i.e., the aorta (although the low aortic diastolic pressure does facilitate ventricular emptying during early systole). Whereas in MR the reduction of wall tension (i.e., reduced afterload) allows more complete systolic emptying, in AR the increase in left ventricular end-diastolic volume (i.e., increased preload) provides major hemodynamic compensation.[386,387]

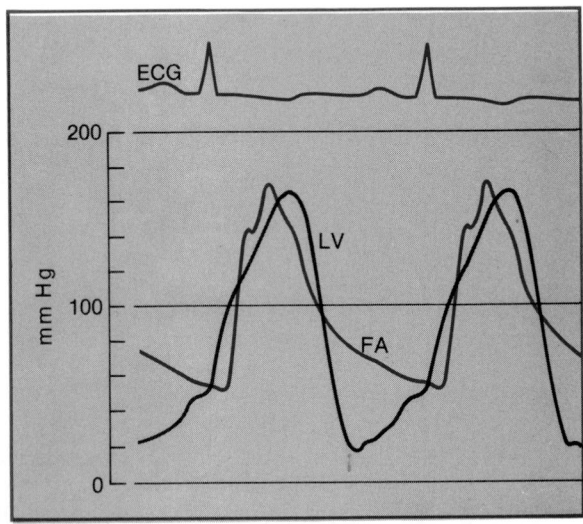

FIGURE 32-38. Pressure curves obtained from a 63-year-old man with symptoms of left ventricular failure and a loud decrescendo diastolic murmur. The femoral arterial (FA) pressure tracing demonstrates a widened pulse pressure of 115 mm Hg and equalization with left ventricular (LV) pressure late in diastole. The LV pressure curve exhibits a steady pressure increase throughout diastole, culminating in a markedly elevated end-diastolic pressure of 45 mm Hg. These findings are indicative of severe aortic regurgitation.

Severe AR may occur with a normal effective forward stroke volume and a normal ejection fraction (total [forward plus regurgitant] stroke volume/end-diastolic volume), together with an elevated left ventricular end-diastolic volume, pressure, and stress[388] (Figs. 32–38 and 32–39). In accord with Laplace's law (which indicates that wall tension is related to the product of intraventricular pressure and radius divided by wall thickness), left ventricular dilatation also increases the left ventricular systolic tension required to develop any level of systolic pressure. The increased end-diastolic wall stress leads to volume overload (eccentric) hypertrophy, with replication of sarcomeres largely in series, elongation of fibers, and sufficient wall thickening so that the ratio of ventricular wall thickness to cavity radius remains normal to maintain or return end-diastolic wall stress to normal levels.[389] This contrasts with the events in AS, in which there is pressure overload (concentric) hypertrophy with replication of sarcomeres largely in parallel and an increased ratio of wall thickness to radius. In AR, left ventricular mass is usually greatly elevated, often to levels even higher than in isolated AS[272] and sometimes exceeding 1000 gm.

Patients with severe chronic AR have the largest end-diastolic volumes of those with any form of heart disease (resulting in so-called *cor bovinium*). However, end-diastolic pressure is not uniformly elevated (i.e., left ventricular compliance often becomes increased [Fig. 32–11]).[392]

In the more severe cases of AR, the regurgitant flow may exceed 20 liters/min, so that the total left ventricular output at rest approaches 25 liters/min, a level that can be achieved acutely only by a trained endurance runner during maximal exercise. Thus, the adaptive response to gradually increasing, chronic AR permits the ventricle to function as an effective high-compliance pump, handling large end-diastolic and stroke volumes, often with little increase in filling pressure (Fig. 32–11). During exercise, peripheral vascular resistance declines, and with an increase in heart rate, diastole shortens and the regurgitation per beat decreases,[390,391] facilitating an increment in effective forward cardiac output without substantial increases in end-diastolic volume and pressure. The ejection fraction (total stroke volume/end-diastolic volume) and related ejection phase indices (see p. 425) are often within normal limits, both at rest and during exercise, even though myocardial function, as reflected in the slope of the end-systolic pressure-volume relation, is depressed. Thus, the latter appears to be a more sensitive index of contractility than the former (see p. 430).

LEFT VENTRICULAR FUNCTION. As left ventricular function deteriorates, the left ventricle dilates (Fig. 32–39D). Ventricular end-diastolic volume increases without further elevation of the aortic regurgitant volume; the ratio of left ventricular end-diastolic thickness to radius declines,[392] systolic wall tension rises, reducing ejection fraction, forward stroke volume, and ventricular emptying, while end-systolic volume rises. As the left ventricle decompensates, interstitial fibrosis increases and compliance may decline and left ventricular end-diastolic pressure rises. In advanced stages there may be considerable elevation of the left atrial, pulmonary artery wedge, pulmonary arterial, right ventricular, and right atrial pressures and lowering of the effective cardiac output, first during exercise[391] and then even at rest. There is failure of the normal decline in end-systolic volume or rise in ejection fraction during exercise.[393] Symptoms of heart failure, particularly those secondary to pulmonary congestion, develop.

As is the case in MR (see p. 1017), the end-systolic volume provides a useful overall index of myocardial function in patients with AR and

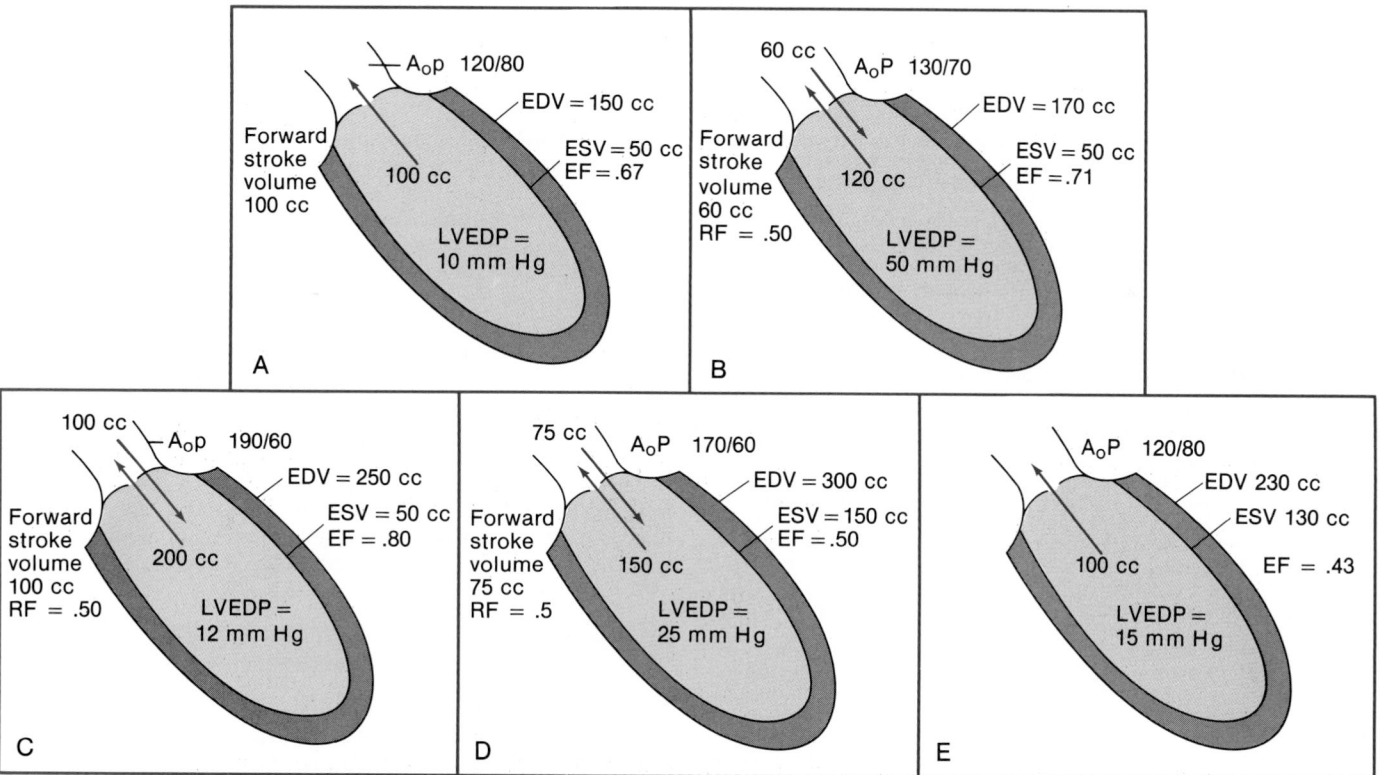

FIGURE 32–39. Hemodynamics of aortic regurgitation. *A,* Normal conditions. *B,* The hemodynamic changes that occur in severe acute aortic regurgitation. Although total stroke volume is increased, forward stroke volume is reduced. Left ventricular end-diastolic pressure rises dramatically. *C,* Hemodynamic changes occurring in chronic compensated aortic regurgitation are shown. Eccentric hypertrophy produces increased end-diastolic volume, which permits an increase in total as well as forward stroke volume. The volume overload is accommodated and left ventricular filling pressure is normalized. Ventricular emptying and end-systolic volume remain normal. *D,* In chronic decompensated aortic regurgitation, impaired left ventricular emptying produces an increase in end-systolic volume and a fall in ejection fraction, total stroke volume, and forward stroke volume. There is further cardiac dilatation and reelevation of left ventricular filling pressure. *E,* Immediately following valve replacement, preload estimated by end-diastolic volume decreases, as does filling pressure. End-systolic volume also is decreased but to a lesser extent. The result is an initial fall in ejection fraction. Despite these changes, elimination of regurgitation leads to an increase in forward stroke volume. AoP = aortic pressure; EDV = end-diastolic volume; ESV = end-systolic volume; EF = ejection fraction; LVEDP = left ventricular end-diastolic pressure; RF = regurgitant fraction. (From Carabello, B. A.: Aortic regurgitation: Hemodynamic determinants of prognosis. *In* Cohn, L. H., and DiSesa, V. J. [eds.]: Aortic Regurgitation: Medical and Surgical Management. New York, Marcel Dekker, Inc., 1986.)

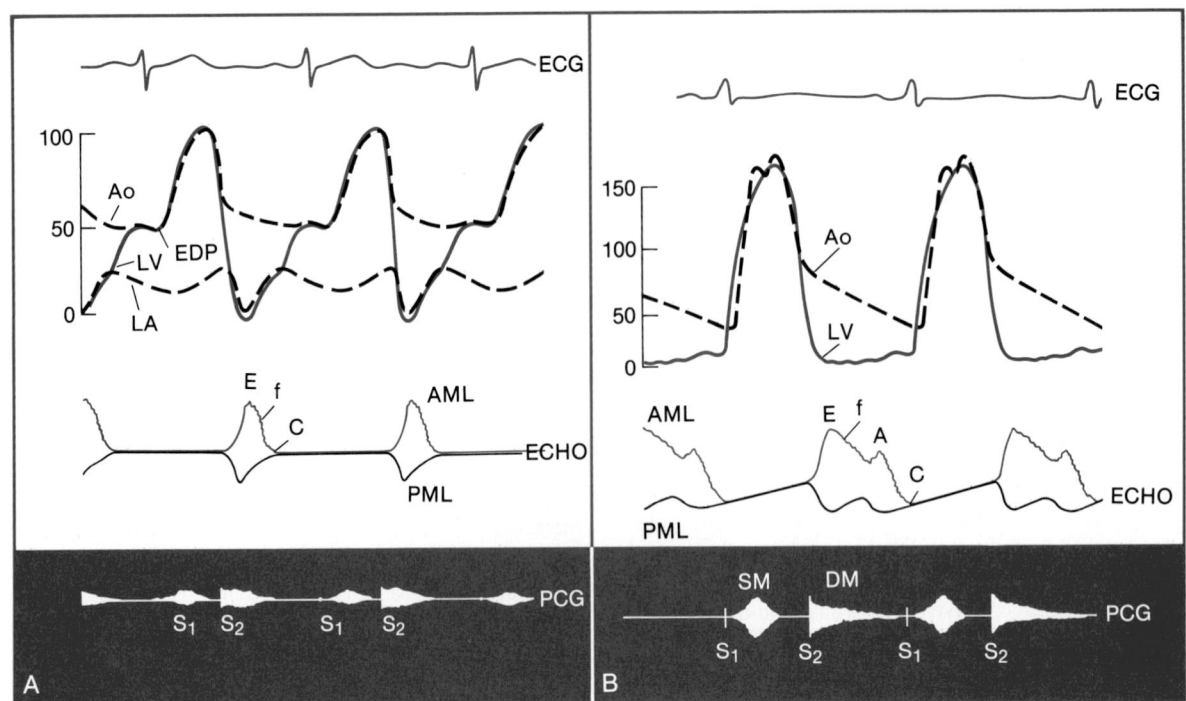

FIGURE 32–40. Schematic representations contrasting the hemodynamic, echocardiographic (ECHO), and phonocardiographic (PCG) manifestations of acute severe *(A)* and chronic severe *(B)* aortic regurgitation. Ao = aorta; LV = left ventricle; LA = left atrium; EDP = end-diastolic pressure; f = flutter of anterior mitral valve leaflet; AML = anterior mitral valve leaflet; PML = posterior mitral valve leaflet; SM = systolic murmur; DM = diastolic murmur; C = closure point of mitral valve. (From Morganroth, J., et al.: Acute severe aortic regurgitation. Ann. Intern. Med. *87:*225, 1977.)

correlates with operative mortality and postoperative left ventricular dysfunction.[138] Both the immediate and the long-term results are excellent in patients with normal left ventricular end-systolic volumes (<40 ml/m²), poor in patients in whom the index is elevated (>80 ml/m²), and variable in patients with intermediate values. In general, however, for any given preoperative level of impairment of left ventricular function, the outlook for left ventricular function in the postoperative period is somewhat better in patients with AR than with MR.

When *acute* AR is induced experimentally, preload, wall tension, and myocardial oxygen consumption all rise substantially,[131] secondary to an increase in wall tension. In patients with chronic, severe AR, total myocardial oxygen requirements are also augmented by the increase in left ventricular mass. Because the major portion of coronary blood flow occurs during diastole, when arterial pressure is lower than normal in AR, coronary perfusion pressure is reduced.[393] Studies in experimental AR have shown a reduction in coronary flow reserve with a change in forward coronary flow from diastole to systole.[394] The result—a combination of increased oxygen demand and reduced supply—sets the stage for the development of myocardial ischemia, especially during exercise.[395] Indeed, patients with severe AR exhibit a reduction of coronary reserve,[396] which may be responsible for myocardial ischemia, which in turn may play a role in the deterioration of left ventricular function.

The heightened activity of the adrenergic nervous system as a compensatory mechanism in patients with chronic AR is reflected in an abnormal increase in plasma catecholamine concentration during exercise, accompanied by a reduction in cardiac norepinephrine stores.[397]

Acute Aortic Regurgitation

In contrast to the pathophysiological events in chronic AR described above, in which the left ventricle has had the opportunity to adapt to the increased load, in acute AR (caused most commonly by infective endocarditis, aortic dissection, or trauma) the regurgitant volume fills a ventricle of normal size that cannot accommodate the combined large regurgitant volume and inflow from the left atrium.[398] Because the ability of total stroke volume to rise acutely is limited, forward stroke volume declines. The sudden increase in left ventricular filling causes the left ventricular diastolic pressure to rise rapidly to high levels, as the ventricle operates on a steep portion of its pressure-volume curve (Fig. 32–11).[386]

As left ventricular pressure rises rapidly above left atrial pressure during early diastole, the mitral valve closes prematurely in diastole (Fig. 32–40).[399] Preclosure of the mitral valve is accompanied by diastolic mitral regurgitation.[400] This protects the pulmonary venous bed from backward transmission of the greatly elevated end-diastolic pressure. Premature closure of the mitral valve, together with the tachycardia that shortens diastole, reduces the time interval during which the mitral valve is open. Left ventricular and aortic systolic pressures exhibit little change. Because aortic diastolic pressure cannot decline below the elevated left ventricular end-diastolic pressure, the systemic arterial pulse pressure widens relatively little. For a similar severe degree of AR, patients with acute AR have a lower effective forward stroke volume and pulse pressure, smaller end-diastolic and end-systolic volumes, and a more rapid heart rate than the patient with chronic AR.[409]

CLINICAL MANIFESTATIONS

History

CHRONIC AORTIC REGURGITATION. In patients with chronic, severe AR, the left ventricle gradually undergoes enlargement while the patient remains asymptomatic or almost so.[367] Symptoms of reduced cardiac reserve or myocardial ischemia develop, most often in the fourth or fifth decade and usually only *after* considerable cardiomegaly and myocardial dysfunction have occurred. Exertional dyspnea, orthopnea, and paroxysmal nocturnal dyspnea are the principal complaints. Syncope is rare, and although angina pectoris is less frequent than it is in patients with AS, nocturnal angina, often accompanied by diaphoresis that occurs when the heart rate slows and arterial diastolic pressure falls to extremely low levels, may be troublesome. These episodes are occasionally accompanied by abdominal discomfort, presumably caused by splanchnic ischemia. Patients with severe AR often complain of an uncomfortable awareness of the heartbeat, especially on lying down,

	CHRONIC SEVERE	ACUTE SEVERE
Clinical		
Onset	Chronic and gradual dyspnea	Acute
Appearance	Normal/mildly dyspneic	Severely ill
Blood pressure	Wide pulse pressure (very low diastolic and high systolic BP)	Not striking, normal, or even low
Tachycardia	Variable/not striking	Always
Peripheral arterial signs	Obvious	No
Apical impulse	Displaced and forcible (very large heart)	No
Basal diastolic thrill	Rare	More common (perforation)
Basal systolic thrill	Common	No
S_1	Usually normal	Soft
S_2	Usually normal (soft calcific valve)	Soft
S_3	Common with LV failure	Common
Basal ejection systolic murmur	Common and harsh	Common and soft
Basal early diastolic murmur	Long, blowing, and decrescendo	Short, soft, or loud and musical with perforation
Apical rumbling diastolic murmur	Common	Common but with no presystolic accentuation
ECG/LVH	Almost always	No
Chest X-ray		
Cardiomegaly	Severe	No
Lung fields	Usually normal	Pulmonary edema
Echocardiograph		
LV size	Severely dilated	Normal
LV function (EF)	Variable	Hyperactive
Premature closure of mitral valve	No	Common
Diastolic mitral regurgitation	No	Common
Late mitral valve opening	No	Common
Look for clues of underlying etiology		
Marfan's syndrome		
Aortic dissection		
Prosthetic aortic valve dysfunction		
Infective endocarditis		

From Jutzy, K. R., and Al-Zaibag, M.: Acute mitral and aortic valve regurgitation. *In* Al-Zaibag, M., and Duran, C. M. G. (eds.): Valvular Heart Disease. New York, Marcel Dekker, 1994, pp. 345–382.

and disagreeable thoracic pain due to pounding of the heart against the chest wall. Tachycardia, occurring with emotional stress or exertion, may produce palpitations and head pounding; premature ventricular contractions are particularly distressing because of the great heave of the volume-loaded left ventricle during the postpremature beat. These complaints may be present for many years before symptoms of overt left ventricular dysfunction develop.

ACUTE AORTIC REGURGITATION. In light of the limited ability of the left ventricle to tolerate severe, acute AR, patients with this valvular lesion often develop sudden clinical manifestations of cardiovascular collapse, with weakness, severe dyspnea, and hypotension secondary to the reduced stroke volume and elevated left atrial pressure, as discussed above (Table 32–8).

Physical Examination

In patients with chronic, severe AR, the head frequently bobs with each heartbeat *(de Musset's sign),*[401] and the pulses are of the water-hammer or collapsing type with abrupt distention and quick collapse (*Corrigan's pulse,* p. 22). The arterial pulse is often prominent in the carotid arteries and can be best appreciated by palpation of the radial artery with the patient's arm elevated. A *bisferious pulse* may be present (Fig. 2–8C, p. 21) and is more readily recognized in the brachial and femoral than in the carotid arteries. A variety of auscultatory findings provide confirmation of a wide pulse pressure. *Traube's sign* (also known as "pistol shot sounds"[402]) refers to booming systolic and diastolic sounds heard over the femoral artery, *Müller's*

sign consists of systolic pulsations of the uvula, and *Duroziez's sign* consists of a systolic murmur heard over the femoral artery when it is compressed proximally and a diastolic murmur when it is compressed distally. Capillary pulsations, i.e., *Quincke's sign,* can be detected by pressing a glass slide on the patient's lip or by transmitting a light through the patient's fingertips.

Systolic arterial pressure is elevated, and diastolic pressure is abnormally low. *Hill's sign* refers to popliteal cuff systolic pressure exceeding brachial cuff pressure by more than 60 mm Hg. Korotkoff sounds often persist to zero even though intraarterial pressure rarely falls below 30 mm Hg. The point of change in Korotkoff sounds, i.e., the muffling of these sounds in phase IV, correlates with the diastolic pressure. As heart failure develops, peripheral vasoconstriction may occur and arterial diastolic pressure may rise. This finding should not be interpreted as the presence of mild AR.

The apical impulse is diffuse and hyperdynamic and is displaced laterally and inferiorly; there may be systolic retraction over the parasternal region. A rapid ventricular filling wave is often palpable at the apex, as is a *systolic thrill* at the base of the heart or suprasternal notch and over the carotid arteries, resulting from the augmented stroke volume. In many patients, a carotid shudder is palpable or may be recorded.[403]

AUSCULTATION. In *chronic,* severe AR, there may be prolongation of the P-R interval, causing a soft S_1. A_2 is soft or absent, and P_2 may be obscured by the early diastolic murmur.[404] Thus, S_2 may be absent or single or exhibit narrow or paradoxical splitting. A systolic ejection sound, presumably related to abrupt distention of the aorta by the augmented stroke volume, is frequently audible. An S_3 gallop correlates with an increased left ventricular end-systolic volume and its development has been suggested as a sign of impaired left ventricular function, useful in identifying patients with severe regurgitation for surgical treatment.[405]

The aortic regurgitant murmur is one of high frequency that begins immediately after A_2 (Figs. 2–37, p. 41 and 2–41, p. 42). It may be distinguished from the murmur of pulmonic regurgitation (see p. 1059) by its earlier onset, i.e., immediately after A_2 rather than after P_2, and usually by the presence of a widened pulse pressure. The murmur is heard best with the diaphragm of the stethoscope while the patient is sitting up and leaning forward, with the breath held in deep expiration. In severe AR, the murmur reaches an early peak and then has a dominant decrescendo pattern throughout diastole.

The severity of the regurgitation correlates better with the *duration* than with the *intensity* of the murmur. In mild AR, the murmur may be limited to early diastole and is typically high-pitched and blowing; in severe regurgitation, the murmur is holodiastolic and may have a rough quality. When the murmur is musical ("cooing dove" murmur), it usually signifies eversion or perforation of an aortic cusp. In severe AR and left ventricular decompensation, equilibration of aortic and left ventricular pressures in late diastole (Fig. 32–38) abolishes this component of the regurgitant murmur. When regurgitation is due to primary valvular disease, the diastolic murmur is best heard along the left sternal border in the third and fourth intercostal spaces. However, when it is due mainly to dilatation of the ascending aorta,[406] the murmur is often more readily audible along the right sternal border.

A mid- and late-diastolic apical rumble, the *Austin Flint murmur,* is common in severe AR and may occur in the presence of a normal mitral valve (Fig. 2–41, p. 42). This murmur appears to be created by rapid antegrade flow across a mitral orifice that is narrowed by the rapidly rising left ventricular diastolic pressure caused by severe aortic reflux.[407] The Austin Flint murmur may be difficult to differentiate from that due to MS, but the presence of an opening snap and a loud S_1 in MS and the absence of these findings in AR are helpful clues. As the left ventricular end-diastolic pressure rises, the Austin Flint murmur commences and terminates earlier, and in acute AR with premature diastolic closure of the mitral valve, the presystolic portion of the Austin Flint murmur is eliminated. A short, midsystolic murmur, grades 1 to 4/6, related to the increased ejection rate and stroke volume, may be audible at the base of the heart and transmitted to the carotid vessels. It may be higher pitched and less rasping than the murmur of aortic stenosis but is often accompanied by a systolic thrill.

Dynamic Auscultation. The diastolic murmur of AR may be accentuated when the patient sits up and leans forward or by interventions that raise the arterial pressure, such as infusion of a vasopressor drug, squatting, or isometric exercise. The intensity of the murmur is reduced by interventions that lower the systolic pressure, such as amyl nitrite inhalation and the strain of the Valsalva maneuver.[408] The Austin Flint murmur, like that of AR, is augmented by isometric exercise and vasopressors and is reduced by amyl nitrite inhalation (Fig. 2–41, p. 42).[408]

ACUTE AORTIC REGURGITATION. When acute AR is severe, these patients appear gravely ill, with tachycardia, severe peripheral vasoconstriction and cyanosis, and sometimes pulmonary congestion and edema.[398,409,410] The peripheral signs of AR are often not impressive and certainly not as dramatic as in patients with chronic AR.[399] Duroziez's murmur, pistol shot sounds over the peripheral arteries (Traube's sign), and bisferious pulses are usually *absent* in

acute AR. The normal or only slightly widened pulse pressure may lead to serious underestimation of the severity of the valvular lesion. The left ventricular impulse is normal or nearly so, and the rocking motion of the chest characteristic of chronic AR is not apparent. S_1 may be soft or absent because of premature closure of the mitral valve.[411] Instead, the sound of mitral valve closure is occasionally audible. However, closure of the mitral valve may be incomplete, and diastolic mitral regurgitation may occur.[412] Evidence of pulmonary hypertension, with an accentuated P_2 and an S_3 and S_4, is frequently present. The early diastolic murmur of acute AR is lower pitched and shorter than that of chronic AR, because as left ventricular diastolic pressure rises, the pressure gradient between the aorta and the left ventricle is rapidly reduced. The Austin Flint murmur, if present, is brief and ceases when left ventricular pressure exceeds left atrial pressure in diastole.

LABORATORY EXAMINATION

ELECTROCARDIOGRAM. *Chronic* AR results in left axis deviation and a pattern of left ventricular diastolic volume overload, characterized by an increase in initial forces (prominent Q waves in leads I, aV_L, and V_3 to V_6) and a relatively small r wave in V_1 (Fig. 32–41). With the passage of time, these initial forces diminish, but the total QRS amplitude increases. The T waves may be tall and upright in left precordial leads early in the course, but more commonly they are inverted, with ST-segment depressions.[413] Left intraventricular conduction defects occur late in the course and are usually associated with left ventricular dysfunction. The electrocardiogram is not an accurate predictor of the severity of AR or cardiac weight.[414] When AR is caused by an inflammatory process, P-R prolongation may be present.[414]

In *acute* AR, the electrocardiogram may or may not show left ventricular hypertrophy, despite the presence of left ventricular failure, depending upon the severity and duration of the regurgitation. However, nonspecific ST-segment and T-wave changes are common.

RADIOLOGICAL FINDINGS (see also p. 225). Cardiac size is a function of the duration and severity of regurgitation and the state of left ventricular function. In acute AR, there may be little cardiac enlargement, but marked enlargement is a common finding in chronic AR. Typically, the left ventricle enlarges in an inferior and leftward direction, causing a significant increase in the long axis (Fig. 7–34, p. 226) but sometimes little or no increase in the transverse diameter of the heart. Calcification of the aortic valve is uncommon in patients with pure AR but is often present in patients with combined AS and AR. As in the case with AS, the presence of distinct left atrial enlargement in the absence of heart failure should suggest the possibility of associated mitral valve disease. Dilatation of the ascending aorta is usually more marked than in AS and may involve the entire aortic arch, including the aortic knob. Severe, aneurysmal dilatation of the aorta should suggest that aortic root disease (e.g., Marfan syndrome, cystic medionecrosis, or annuloaortic ectasia) is responsible for the AR. Linear calcifications in the wall of the ascending aorta are seen in syphilitic aortitis but are nonspecific and are observed in degenerative disease as well.

For angiographic assessment of AR, contrast material should be injected rapidly (i.e., 25 to 35 ml/sec) into the aortic root, and filming should be carried out in the right and left anterior oblique projections. Opacification may be improved by filming during a Valsalva maneuver. In acute AR, there is only a slight increase in ventricular end-diastolic volume, but with the passage of time both the end-diastolic volume and the thickness of the ventricular wall increase, usually in parallel.

ECHOCARDIOGRAPHY (Figs. 3–57 to 3–59, p. 76). Echocardiography is helpful in identifying the cause of AR. It may show thickening of the valve cusps, prolapse of the valve, a flail leaflet, vegetations, or dilatation of the aortic root.[415] Although transthoracic imaging is usually satisfactory, transesophageal echocardiography often provides more detail. Two-dimensional studies are useful for the measurement of left ventricular end-diastolic and end-systolic dimensions and volumes, shortening fractions, and ejection fractions. These measurements, when made serially, are of great value in selecting the optimal time for surgical intervention (see p. 1052).

In acute AR (Table 32–8; Fig. 3–59, p. 76), the echocardiogram reveals a reduction in amplitude of the opening

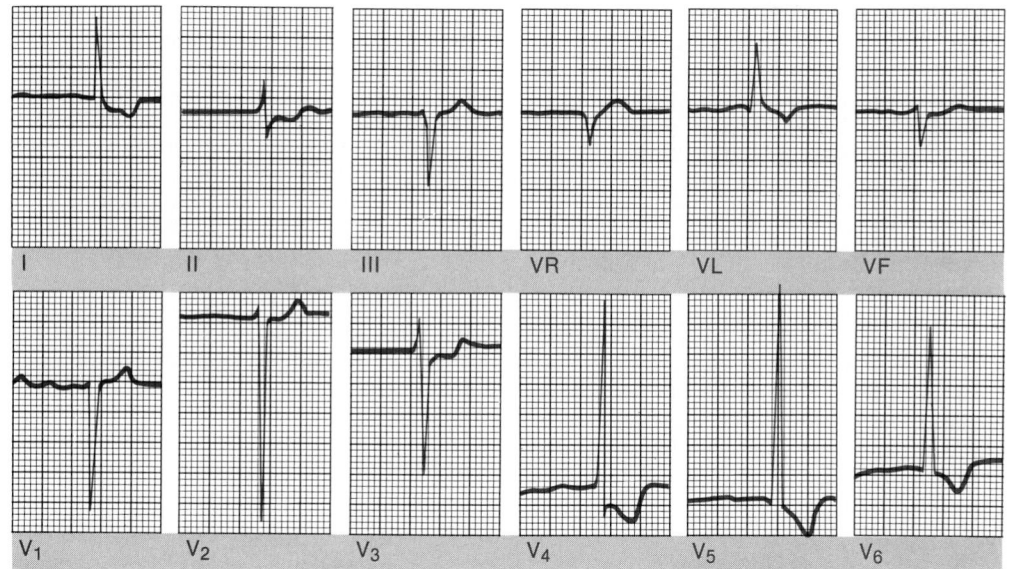

FIGURE 32-41. Atrial fibrillation and left ventricular hypertrophy. The most prominent features are the gross increase in precordial voltage (RV5 + SV2 = 70 mm) and the marked anterolateral ST/T wave changes (leads I, aVL, and V4-6). The patient had aortic regurgitation and normal coronary arteries and was not taking digitalis. (Normal standardization, i.e., 1 mV = 10 mm.) (From Hall, R. J., and Julian, D. G.: Diseases of the Cardiac Valves. New York, Churchill Livingstone, 1989, p. 39.)

movement of the mitral valve, premature closure and delayed opening of the mitral valve,[416] and, on the M-mode study, a reduction in the E-F slope, indicating that the left ventricle is operating on the steep portion of its pressure-volume curve. Left ventricular end-diastolic dimensions are not markedly increased, and fractional shortening is normal. This contrasts with the findings in chronic AR, in which end-diastolic dimensions and wall motion are increased. Occasionally, with equilibration of aortic and left ventricular pressures in diastole, premature opening of the aortic valve may be detected.[417]

High-frequency diastolic fluttering of the anterior leaflet of the mitral valve during diastole is an important echocardiographic finding in both acute and chronic AR; however, it does not occur when the mitral valve is rigid. This sign, which, unlike the Austin Flint rumble, occurs even in mild AR, results from the movement imparted to the anterior leaflet of the mitral valve by the jet of blood regurgitating from the aorta.

Doppler echocardiography and color flow Doppler imaging are the most sensitive and accurate noninvasive techniques in the detection of AR.[418,418a] They readily detect mild degrees of AR that may be inaudible by auscultation. In addition, by measuring the rate of decrease in velocity of the regurgitant jet in the left ventricle (see p. 332), they allow estimation of the severity. The aortic regurgitant orifice can be estimated, as can aortic regurgitant flow, from the difference between flow through the aortic and either the pulmonic or mitral valve orifice determined by continuous Doppler echocardiography.[419]

RADIONUCLIDE IMAGING. Radionuclide angiography, by allowing determination of the regurgitant fraction and of the left ventricular/right ventricular stroke volume ratio, provides an accurate noninvasive assessment of the severity of AR.[420] This technique is nonspecific because the ratio is increased by associated MR and reduced by tricuspid or pulmonary regurgitation. However, in the absence of these complicating lesions, a left ventricular/right ventricular stroke volume ratio of 2.0 or more denotes severe AR. Radionuclide angiography is of value in the assessment of left ventricular function in patients with AR.[393] Serial measurements are useful in the early detection of deterioration of left ventricular function.

NUCLEAR MAGNETIC RESONANCE IMAGING (Figs. 10-26 and

10-27, p. 332). This technique provides accurate measurements of regurgitant volumes, ventricular end-systolic and diastolic volumes, and the regurgitant orifice.[421] Although expensive, NMR imaging appears to be the most accurate noninvasive technique for assessing the patient with AR.[162,305]

MANAGEMENT

ACUTE AORTIC REGURGITATION. Since early demise due to left ventricular failure is frequent in patients with *severe acute* AR despite intensive medical management, prompt surgical intervention is indicated. Even a normal ventricle cannot sustain the burden of acute severe volume overload; therefore, the risk of *acute* AR is much greater than that of chronic AR.[398,409,410] While the patient is being prepared for surgery, intravenous treatment with a positive inotropic agent (dopamine or dobutamine) and/or vasodilator (nitroprusside) may be necessary. The agent and dosage should be selected on the basis of arterial pressure (Chap. 17). In hemodynamically stable patients with acute AR secondary to active infective endocarditis, operation may be deferred to allow 5 to 7 days of intensive antibiotic therapy.[410] However, aortic valve replacement should be undertaken at the earliest sign of hemodynamic instability, or if echocardiographic evidence of diastolic closure of the mitral valve develops.[422]

NATURAL HISTORY OF CHRONIC AORTIC REGURGITATION. Management must take into account the natural history of the lesion.[423] Moderately severe or even severe chronic AR may be associated with a generally favorable prognosis for many years. Approximately 75 per cent of patients survive for 5 years and 50 per cent for 10 years after diagnosis.[66] However, as is the case for AS, once the patient becomes symptomatic, the condition often deteriorates rapidly, and sudden death may occur, usually in previously symptomatic patients. Without surgical treatment, death usually occurs within 4 years after the development of angina and within 2 years after the onset of heart failure. Even during the asymptomatic period gradual deterioration of left ventricular function may occur; it is important, therefore, to intervene surgically before these changes have become irreversible.[423a]

Medical Treatment

Patients with mild or moderate AR who are asymptomatic with normal or only minimally increased cardiac size require no therapy but should be followed clinically and by echocardiography every 12 or 24 months if their clinical condition and echocardiogram remain stable, and with antibiotic prophylaxis for endocarditis. Patients with limitations of cardiac reserve and/or left ventricular dysfunction secondary to AR should not engage in vigorous sports or heavy exertion.[4] Cardiac glycosides may be employed in patients with severe AR and left ventricular dilatation, even in the absence of symptoms. Systemic arterial diastolic hypertension, if present, should be treated because it increases the regurgitant flow; however, drugs that impair left ventricular function, such as propranolol, should be avoided. Atrial fibrillation and bradyarrhythmias are poorly tolerated and should be prevented if possible. Because these and other cardiac arrhythmias and infections are poorly tolerated in patients with severe AR, such complications must be treated promptly and vigorously. Even though nitroglycerin and other nitrates are not as helpful in relieving anginal pain in patients with AR as they are in patients with coronary artery disease or AS, they are worth a trial. Although patients with left ventricular failure secondary to AR require surgical treatment, they respond, at least temporarily, to treatment with digitalis glycosides, salt restriction, and diuretics. The response to vasodilator therapy is often impressive. Hemodynamic studies have shown beneficial effects of intravenous hydralazine,[424] sublingual nifedipine,[425] and oral prazosin.[426] This form of therapy may be particularly helpful in stabilizing patients with acute lesions or those with decompensated chronic AR who are awaiting operation. However, because of the high incidence of side effects of hydralazine, attention has focused on nifedipine.[427] In a comparison of digoxin with nifedipine in asymptomatic patients with severe AR, the latter delayed the need for operation (the development of symptoms or of left ventricular dysfunction).[428]

Asymptomatic patients with severe chronic AR and normal left ventricular function should be examined at intervals of approximately 6 months. In addition to clinical examination, serial echocardiographic assessments of left ventricular size and ejection fraction should be made.

Surgical Treatment

INDICATIONS FOR OPERATION. Operative correction is usually deferred in patients with severe chronic AR who are asymptomatic, have good exercise tolerance, and have normal left ventricular function. Similarly, there is a consensus that in the absence of contraindications surgical treatment is advisable in patients with severe AR who are symptomatic as a result of this lesion and who have impaired left ventricular function. Between these two ends of the clinical-hemodynamic spectrum are many patients in whom it may be quite difficult to balance the immediate risks of operation and, in cases when it is required, the continuing risks of an implanted prosthetic valve on the one hand, against the hazards of allowing a severe volume overload to damage the left ventricle on the other.[429–432]

Postoperative left ventricular function is usually excellent in patients who have normal systolic function preoperatively.[433] However, changes in left ventricular function can develop in some patients with AR so that, even after successful correction of AR, they may have persistent cardiomegaly and depressed left ventricular function.[434,435] In such patients, symptoms of impaired left ventricular function present preoperatively may persist and occasionally even get worse despite successful valve replacement. Therefore, it is highly desirable to operate on patients *before* irreversible left ventricular changes have occurred. Patients whose ventricular function does not return to normal after aortic valve replacement often exhibit histological changes in the left ventricle, including massive fiber hypertrophy and increased interstitial fibrous tissue. However, even patients with irreversible left ventricular dysfunction may benefit from surgical treatment, whereas medical treatment has little to offer them.

In order to minimize the risk of postoperative left ventricular dysfunction, every effort should be made to operate on patients *before* serious left ventricular dysfunction occurs. Serial echocardiograms or radionuclide ventriculograms should be obtained to detect changes in left ventricular size and function. These examinations can provide valuable information concerning progressive deterioration in left ventricular function at rest. Both techniques allow repeated evaluation of ejection fraction and end-systolic volume (or dimensions) both at rest and during exercise. Impaired ventricular function at *rest* is the basis for selection of patients for operation; failure of a normal ejection fraction to respond normally to *exercise* portends impaired function at rest.

Because AR has complex effects on both preload and afterload, the selection of appropriate indices of ventricular contractility is a challenge.[436] Simple left ventricular end-diastolic volume and the ejection phase indices such as ejection fraction and ventricular fraction shortening are too strongly influenced by loading to be accurate indicators of ventricular contractility but may be useful empirical predictors of postoperative function.[348] On the other hand, preoperative left ventricular end-systolic volume and dimensions are largely preload dependent and are good predictors of postoperative left ventricular function.[437] The relationship between end-systolic wall stress and ejection fraction or per cent[438] fractional shortening may be even more useful. However, in the absence of such measurements, *serial* changes in ventricular end-diastolic and end-systolic volumes or dimensions can be employed to detect *relative* deterioration of ventricular function.

Patients with *severely* impaired left ventricular systolic function preoperatively are at high risk of developing irreversible left ventricular dysfunction and, indeed, of dying of congestive heart failure postoperatively. Other patients with impaired left ventricular function preoperatively, improve postoperatively—both symptomatically and insofar as left ventricular function is concerned. Bonow et al. have reported that, after valve replacement, survival was excellent in patients with normal resting ejection fractions preoperatively. However, patients with subnormal ejection fractions and only a relatively brief (< 1 year) duration of left ventricular dysfunction also did well postoperatively and maintained their preoperative levels of exercise tolerance. Asymptomatic patients with severe AR but normal left ventricular function have an excellent prognosis and do not warrant operation.[429] Less than 4 per cent per year require operation because of the development of symptoms of left ventricular dysfunction. On the other hand, patients with prolonged left ventricular dysfunction exhibited poor postoperative survival.[430] The end-systolic dimension determined by two-dimensional echocardiography is valuable in predicting outcome in asymptomatic patients. Patients with severe AR and an end-systolic diameter less than 40 mm almost invariably remain stable without cardiac failure or death, whereas those with an end-systolic diameter greater than 55 mm (Fig. 32–42), an end-systolic volume greater than 55 ml/m², an end-diastolic volume greater than 200 ml/m², or an ejection fraction less than 50 per cent have an increased risk of death secondary to left ventricular dysfunction.

Thus, the decision to recommend surgical treatment in some patients with severe AR remains difficult. Operation should be deferred in asymptomatic patients with normal and stable left ventricular function and should be recom-

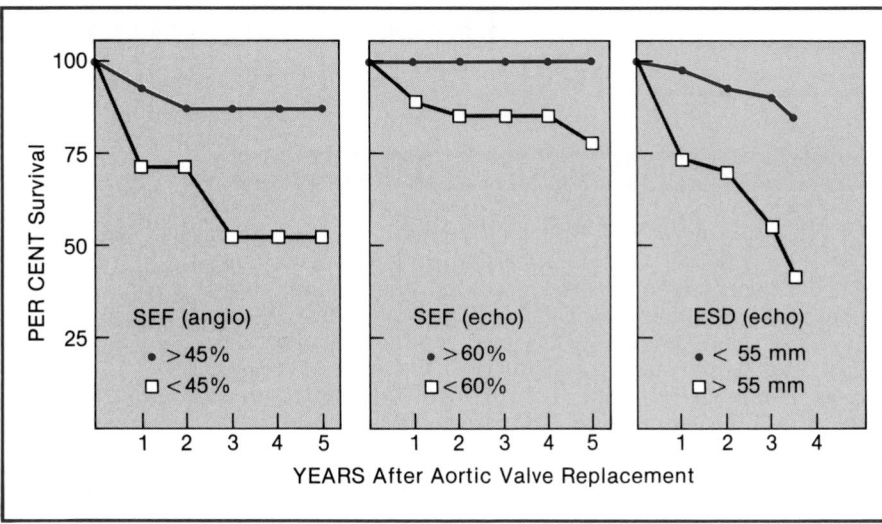

FIGURE 32–42. Relation of preoperative ventricular function to postoperative survival. Data of Greves et al. *(left)* and those of Bonow et al. *(right)* show remarkable agreement: Both groups incorporated limits clearly in abnormal range. Cunha et al. *(center)* selected a limit that was well within normal range. These and other published data indicate that preoperative ventricular function is an important determinant of postoperative survival. SEF = systolic ejection fraction; ESD = echocardiographically measured dimension at end-systole; angio = angiography; echo = echocardiography. (From Errichetti, A., et al.: Is valve replacement indicated in asymptomatic patients with aortic stenosis or aortic regurgitation? *In* Cheitlin, M. [ed.]: Dilemmas in Clinical Cardiology. Philadelphia, F. A. Davis Co., 1990, p. 204.)

mended in symptomatic patients regardless of the status of their left ventricular function. Asymptomatic patients with impaired left ventricular function must be treated individually, taking into account associated medical conditions and coronary artery disease that may add to the surgical risk, as well as the experience and results of the surgical team. A decision should be based not on a single abnormal measurement of impaired left ventricular function but rather on several observations of depressed performance and impaired exercise tolerance, carried out at intervals of 3 to 6 months. If abnormalities are progressive or consistent—i.e., if the left ventricular ejection fraction declines to 50 per cent, the left ventricular end-systolic diameter exceeds 45 to 50 mm, or the left ventricular end-systolic volume exceeds 55 ml/m²—operation should be carried out. If evidence of left ventricular dysfunction is borderline or is not consistent, continued close follow-up is indicated. The threshold for surgery may be lower when the surgeon believes that valve replacement will not be necessary (see below), but this prediction may be difficult.

OPERATIVE PROCEDURES. Because an increasing proportion of patients with severe, isolated AR coming to surgery now have primary aortic root rather than primary valve disease, an increasing proportion can be treated surgically by correcting the dilated aortic root.[439] One of two annuloplasty procedures may be employed—an encircling suture of the aorta or subcommissural annuloplasty. Aneurysmal dilatation of the ascending aorta requires excision, replacement with a graft, and reimplantation of the coronary arteries.[440] In patients with AR secondary to prolapse of an aortic leaflet, aortic cusp resuspension or cusp resection may be employed.[441,442] When AR is caused by leaflet perforation resulting from healed infective endocarditis, a pericardial patch can be used for repair.[443]

A large majority of patients with severe AR due to primary valve disease and almost all patients with combined AS and AR and calcific disease require placement with a prosthetic valve (see p. 1061). Because the aortic annulus in patients with severe AR is usually not as narrow as it is in patients with AS, a larger artificial valve can be inserted,

and mild postoperative obstruction to left ventricular outflow is less of a problem than it is in some patients with AS. Occasionally, when a leaflet has been torn from its attachments to the aortic annulus by trauma, surgical replacement without repair may be possible.

In general, the results of aortic valve replacement in patients with AR are similar to those in patients with AS, with a large percentage of patients exhibiting striking improvement in symptoms. Reductions in heart size and in left ventricular diastolic volume and mass occur in the majority of patients.[344,439] However, as already indicated, the extent of improvement in left ventricular function may not be as salutary in patients with AR as it is in patients with AS, perhaps because the ventricular dysfunction is more advanced and less reversible in patients with volume overload by the time they become symptomatic and are referred for surgical treatment[440] than it is in patients with pressure overload. As is the case of AS, the operative risk of aortic valve replacement in patients with AR depends on the general condition of the patient, the state of left ventricular function, and the skill and experience of the surgical team; the mortality rate ranges from 3 to 8 per cent in most medical centers. A late mortality of approximately 5 to 10 per cent per year is observed in survivors in whom cardiac enlargement was marked and prolonged left ventricular dysfunction was present preoperatively (Fig. 32–42). Follow-up studies have shown both early rapid and then slower long-term reductions of ventricular mass, ejection fraction, myocyte hypertrophy, and ventricular fibrous content.[294,350] By extending the indications for operation to symptomatic patients with normal left ventricular function as well as to asymptomatic patients with early left ventricular dysfunction, both early and late results are improving. It is likely that with the continued improvement of surgical techniques and results, it will become possible to extend the recommendation for operative treatment to asymptomatic patients with severe regurgitation and normal cardiac function. However, given the risks of operation and the long-term complications of artificial valves, I believe that the time for such a policy has not yet arrived.

TRICUSPID, PULMONIC, AND MULTIVALVULAR DISEASE

TRICUSPID STENOSIS

Etiology and Pathology

Tricuspid stenosis (TS) is almost always rheumatic in origin.[8] Other causes of obstruction to right atrial emptying are unusual and include congenital tricuspid atresia (see p. 932), right atrial tumors (which may produce a clinical picture suggesting rapidly progressive TS [see p. 1066]), and the carcinoid syndrome (which more frequently produces tricuspid regurgitation [TR] [see p. 1056] but which may occasionally produce TS). Rarely, obstruction to right ventricular inflow can be due to endomyocardial fibrosis, tricuspid valve vegetations, and extracardiac tumors.

The majority of cases of rheumatic tricuspid valve disease present with tricuspid regurgitation or a combination of stenosis and regurgitation. Rheumatic TS is uncommon and *almost* never occurs as an isolated lesion but generally accompanies mitral valve disease[442-444]; in many patients with TS, the aortic valve is also involved, i.e., trivalvular stenosis is present. TS is found at autopsy in about 15 per cent of patients with rheumatic heart disease but is of clinical significance in only about 5 per cent.[445]

Organic tricuspid valve disease is more common in India than in North America or Western Europe; it has been reported to occur in the hearts of more than one-third of patients with rheumatic heart disease studied at autopsy on the subcontinent.[446] The anatomical changes of rheumatic TS resemble those of MS, with fusion and shortening of the chordae tendineae and fusion of the leaflets at their edges producing a diaphragm with a fixed central aperture. However, valvular calcification is rare. As is the case with MS, TS is more common in women and, in the United States, TS is seen most commonly in persons between the ages of 20 and 60. Again, as in mitral valve disease, stenosis, regurgitation, or some combination of the two may exist.

The right atrium is often greatly dilated, and its walls are thickened. There may be evidence of severe passive congestion, with enlargement of the liver and spleen.

Pathophysiology

A diastolic pressure gradient between the right atrium and ventricle—the hemodynamic expression of TS—is augmented when the transvalvular blood flow increases during exercise or inspiration and is reduced when flow declines during expiration. A relatively modest diastolic pressure gradient, i.e., a mean gradient exceeding only 5 mm Hg, is usually sufficient to elevate mean right atrial pressure to levels that result in systemic venous congestion and, unless sodium intake has been restricted or diuretics have been given, is associated with jugular venous distention, ascites, and edema.

In patients with sinus rhythm, the right atrial *a* wave may be extremely tall (Fig. 32–43) and may even approach the level of the right ventricular systolic pressure. Resting cardiac output is usually markedly reduced and fails to rise during exercise, accounting for the normal or only slightly elevated left atrial, pulmonary arterial, and right ventricular systolic pressures, despite the presence of accompanying mitral valve disease.

A *mean* diastolic pressure gradient across the tricuspid valve as low as 2 mm Hg is sufficient to establish the diagnosis of TS. However, exercise, deep inspiration, and the rapid infusion of fluid or the administration of atropine may enhance greatly a borderline gradient in the presence of TS; expiration reduces or abolishes the gradient. There-fore, whenever this diagnosis is suspected, right atrial and ventricular pressures should be recorded simultaneously, using two catheters or a single catheter with a double lumen, with one lumen opening on either side of the tricuspid valve. The effects of respiration on any pressure difference should be examined.

Clinical Manifestations
(Table 32–9)

HISTORY. The low cardiac output characteristic of TS causes fatigue, and patients often complain of discomfort due to hepatomegaly, swelling of the abdomen, and anasarca.[447] The severity of these symptoms, which are secondary to an elevated systemic venous pressure, is out of proportion to the degree of dyspnea.[446] Some patients complain of a fluttering discomfort in the neck, caused by giant *a* waves in the jugular venous pulse. Despite the coexistance of MS, the symptoms characteristic of this valve lesion, i.e., hemoptysis, paroxysmal nocturnal dyspnea, and acute pulmonary edema, are usually absent in the presence of severe TS because the TS prevents surges of blood into the pulmonary circulation behind the stenotic mitral valve. Indeed, the *absence* of the symptoms of pulmonary congestion in a patient with obvious MS should suggest the possibility of TS.

PHYSICAL EXAMINATION. Because of the high frequency with which MS occurs in patients with TS and the similarity in the physical findings between the two valvular lesions, the diagnosis of TS is commonly missed. The physical findings are mistakenly attributed to MS, which is, of course, more common and may be more obvious. Therefore, a high index of suspicion is required to detect the tricuspid valve lesion. In the presence of sinus rhythm (which is surprisingly common in patients with TS), the *a* wave in the jugular venous pulse is tall, sharp, and flicking and on first impression may be confused with an arterial pulsation; a presystolic hepatic pulsation is often palpable. The *y* descent is slow and barely appreciable, indicating

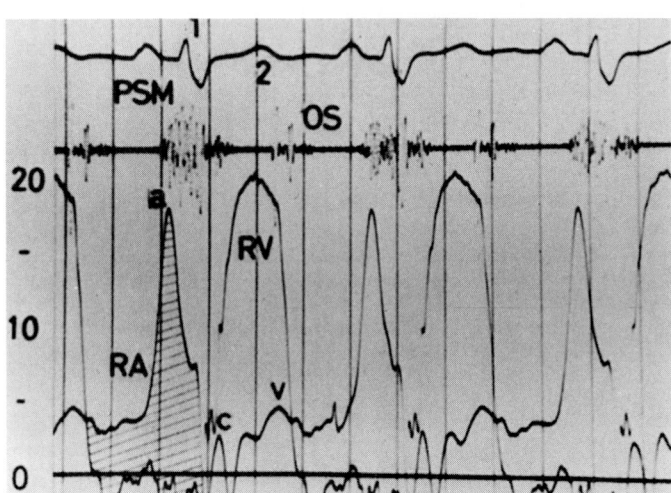

FIGURE 32–43. Phonocardiogram and right heart pressures in a patient with tricuspid stenosis. The giant right atrial *a* wave (a) nearly equals right ventricular (RV) systolic pressure and produces a large diastolic gradient (shaded area). A presystolic murmur (PSM), loud first heart sound (1), and early diastolic opening snap (OS) simulate the findings in mitral stenosis. (Time lines = 0.2 sec.) (From Criley, J. M., et al.: Departures from the expected auscultatory events in mitral stenosis. *In* Likoff, W. [ed.]: Valvular Heart Disease. Philadelphia, F. A. Davis Co., 1973, p. 214.)

TABLE 32–9 CLINICAL AND LABORATORY FEATURES OF RHEUMATIC TRICUSPID STENOSIS

HISTORY
Long history
Progressive fatigue, edema, anorexia
Minimal orthopnea, paroxysmal nocturnal dyspnea
Rheumatic fever in two-thirds of patients
Female preponderance
Orthopnea and paroxysmal nocturnal dyspnea are unusual
Pulmonary edema and hemoptysis are rare

PHYSICAL FINDINGS
Signs of multivalvular involvement
Wasting
Peripheral cyanosis
Neck vein distention, with prominent *v* waves
Right ventricular lift
Associated murmurs of mitral and aortic valve disease
Holosystolic murmur maximal at left lower sternal border, accentuating with inspiration
Hepatic pulsation
Ascites, peripheral edema

LABORATORY FINDINGS
Normal sinus rhythm is frequently present with large *a* waves in the neck veins
Absent right ventricular lift
Auscultation reveals a diastolic rumble at lower left sternal edge, increasing in intensity with inspiration
Electrocardiogram shows tall right atrial P waves and no right ventricular hypertrophy
Roentgenogram shows a dilated right atrium without an enlarged pulmonary artery segment

Modified from Ockene, I. S.: Tricuspid valve disease. *In* Dalen, J. E., and Alpert, J. S. (eds.): Valvular Heart Disease. 2nd ed. Boston, Little, Brown and Company, 1987, pp. 356, 390.

the absence of normal rapid early right ventricular filling. The lung fields are clear, and despite engorgement of the neck veins and the presence of ascites and anasarca, the patient may be comfortable while lying flat. A parasternal (right ventricular) lift is inconspicuous, and pulmonic valve closure is *not* palpable, but occasionally the pulsations of a greatly enlarged right atrium may be felt to the right of the sternum. Thus, the diagnosis of TS may be suspected from inspection and palpation from the combination of a prominent *a* wave in the jugular venous pulse in a patient with MS without evidence of pulmonary hypertension or right ventricular enlargement. This suspicion is strengthened when a diastolic thrill is felt at the lower left sternal edge, particularly if it appears or becomes more prominent during inspiration.[15]

The auscultatory findings of the accompanying MS are usually prominent and often overshadow the more subtle signs of TS. A tricuspid valvular opening snap (OS) may be audible but is often difficult to distinguish from a mitral OS. However, the tricuspid OS usually follows the mitral OS, and is localized to the lower left sternal border, whereas the mitral OS is usually most prominent at the apex and radiates more widely. The diastolic murmur of TS (Fig. 32–43) is commonly heard best along the lower left parasternal border in the fourth intercostal space and is usually softer, higher pitched, and shorter in duration than the murmur of MS. The presystolic component has a scratchy quality, commences earlier (0.06 sec after the P wave in TS compared with 0.12 in MS), and has a crescendo-decrescendo configuration, diminishing before S_1.[444] The diastolic murmur and OS of TS are both augmented by maneuvers that increase transtricuspid valve flow, including inspiration (Fig. 2–44, p. 44), the Mueller maneuver, assumption of the right lateral decubitus position, leg-raising, inhalation of amyl nitrite, squatting, and isotonic exercise. They are reduced during expiration or the strain of the Valsalva maneuver and return to control levels immediately (i.e., within two to three beats) after Valsalva release.

Laboratory Examination

ELECTROCARDIOGRAM. In a patient with valvular heart disease in the absence of atrial fibrillation, TS is suggested by the presence of ECG evidence of right atrial enlargement disproportionate to the degree of right ventricular hypertrophy. The P-wave amplitude in leads II and V exceeds 0.25 mV (see p. 115), and there may be depression of the P-R segment resulting from increased magnitude of the atrial T wave. Because most patients with TS have mitral valve disease, the ECG signs of biatrial enlargement (see p. 116) with abnormally tall, broad P waves in leads II, III, and aV_f and prominent positive and negative deflections in V_f are commonly found. Right atrial dilatation may rotate the ventricular septum and affect QRS morphology in a manner so that the large volume of the right atrium between the exploring electrode and the ventricles reduces the amplitude of the QRS complex in lead V_1 (which often has a Q wave), whereas the QRS complex is much taller in V_2.

RADIOLOGICAL FINDINGS. The key radiological findings in TS are marked cardiomegaly, with conspicuous enlargement of the right atrium (i.e., prominence of the right heart border), which extends into a dilated superior vena cava and azygos vein, but without dilatation of the pulmonary artery. The vascular changes in the lungs characteristic of mitral valve disease may be masked, with little or no interstitial edema or vascular redistribution, but left atrial enlargement may be present.

Angiography carried out following injection of contrast material into the right atrium and filming in the 30-degree right anterior oblique projection is useful for evaluating the appearance of the tricuspid valve. Thickening and decreased mobility of the leaflets, a jet through the constricted orifice, and thickening of the right atrial wall are characteristic findings.

ECHOCARDIOGRAM (see also p. 76). Although the motion of the normal tricuspid valve is similar to that of the normal mitral valve, it is more difficult to image. Not surprisingly, the changes in the echocardiogram of the tricuspid valve in TS resemble those observed in the mitral valve in MS (see p. 1012). Two-dimensional echocardiography characteristically shows diastolic doming of the leaflets, especially the anterior tricuspid valve leaflet, thickening and restriction of motion of the other leaflets, reduced separation of the tips of the leaflets,[448,449] and a reduction in diameter of the tricuspid orifice (Fig. 32–44). Transesophageal echocardiography allows added delineation of the details of valve structure.[450] Doppler echocardiography shows a prolonged slope of antegrade flow and compares well with cardiac catheterization in the quantification of TS and in the assessment of associated tricuspid regurgitation.[451]

Management

Although the fundamental approach to the management of severe TS is surgical treatment, intensive sodium restriction and diuretic therapy may diminish the symptoms secondary to the accumulation of excess salt and water. A prolonged preparatory period of diuresis may diminish hepatic congestion and thereby improve hepatic function sufficiently to diminish the risks of subsequent operation.

Most patients with TS have coexisting valvular disease that requires surgery. In patients with combined TS and MS, the former alone must not be corrected surgically because pulmonary congestion or edema may ensue.[452] Surgical treatment of TS should be carried out in patients with TS in whom the mean diastolic pressure gradients exceed 5 mm Hg and the tricuspid orifice is less than approximately 2.0 cm² at the time of mitral valve repair or replacement. The final decision concerning surgical treatment is often made at the operating table.[453] Because TS is almost always accompanied by some TR, simple finger fracture commissurotomy may not result in significant hemodynamic improvement but may merely substitute severe regurgitation for stenosis. However, open valvulotomy in which the stenotic tricuspid valve is converted into a functionally bicuspid one may result in substantial improvement. The commissures between the anterior and septal leaflets and between the posterior and septal leaflets are opened; it is not advisable to open the commissure between the anterior and posterior leaflets for fear of producing severe regurgitation. If open commissurotomy does not restore reasonable

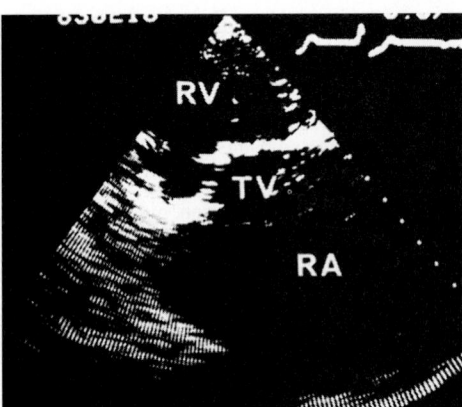

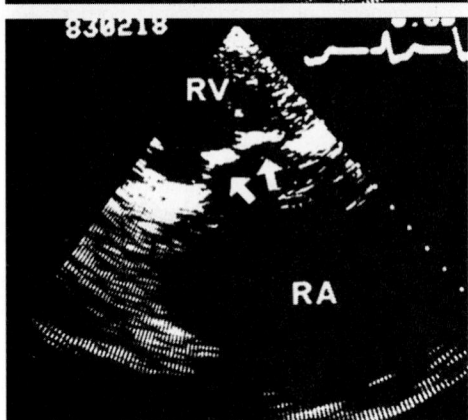

FIGURE 32–44. Two-dimensional echocardiograms in the long-axis view in a patient with tricuspid stenosis. *Top,* Systolic frame. *Bottom,* Diastolic frame that shows doming of both leaflets of the tricuspid valve (TV) (arrows). RA = right atrium; RV = right ventricle. (From Shimada, R., et al.: Diagnosis of tricuspid stenosis by M-mode and two-dimensional echocardiography. Am. J. Cardiol. *53:*164, 1984.)

TABLE 32–10 CAUSES AND MECHANISMS OF PURE TRICUSPID REGURGITATION

CAUSES

Anatomically ABNORMAL valve
  Rheumatic
  Nonrheumatic
    Infective endocarditis
    Ebstein's anomaly
    Floppy (prolapse)
    Congenital (non-Ebstein's)
    Carcinoid
    Papillary muscle dysfunction
    Trauma
    Connective tissue disorders (Marfan)
    Rheumatoid arthritis
    Radiation injury

Anatomically NORMAL valve (functional)
  Elevated right ventricular systolic pressure (dilated annulus)

MECHANISMS

Condition	Leaflet Area	Annular Circumference	Leaflet Insertion
Floppy	↑	↑	Normal
Ebstein's anomaly	↑	↑	Abnormal
Pulmonary/right ventricular systolic hypertension	Normal	↑	Normal
Papillary muscle dysfunction	Normal	Normal	Normal
Carcinoid	↓/Normal	Normal	Normal
Rheumatic	↓/Normal	Normal	Normal
Infective endocarditis	↓/Normal	Normal	Normal

Modified from Waller, B. F.: Rheumatic and nonrheumatic conditions producing valvular heart disease. *In* Frankl, W. S., and Brest, A. N. (eds.): Cardiovascular Clinics. Valvular Heart Disease: Comprehensive Evaluation and Management. Philadelphia, F. A. Davis Co., 1989, pp. 35, 95.

normal valve function, the tricuspid valve may have to be replaced.[454] A porcine bioprosthesis (see p. 1066) is preferred to a mechanical prosthesis in the tricuspid position because of the high risk of thrombosis of the latter[455] and the long-term durability of bioprostheses in the tricuspid position.[456–460] The feasibility of tricuspid balloon valvuloplasty has been demonstrated,[461] but it is not clear how this procedure will be used most effectively.

TRICUSPID REGURGITATION

Etiology and Pathology
(Table 32–10)

The most common cause of tricuspid regurgitation (TR) is not intrinsic involvement of the valve itself but *dilatation of the right ventricle* and of the tricuspid annulus, which may be complications of right ventricular failure of any cause and which cause secondary, functional TR. This is observed in patients with right ventricular hypertension secondary to any form of cardiac and pulmonary vascular disease, most commonly mitral valve disease,[454,461–464] right ventricular infarction[465] (see p. 1192), congenital heart disease (e.g., pulmonic stenosis and pulmonary hypertension secondary to Eisenmenger's syndrome), primary pulmonary hypertension, and rarely cor pulmonale. Severe TR has been reported to be the presenting manifestation in thyrotoxicosis.[466] In infants, TR may complicate right ventricular failure secondary to neonatal pulmonary diseases and pulmonary hypertension with persistence of the fetal pulmonary circulation.[467] In all of these cases, TR reflects the presence of, and in turn aggravates, severe right ventricular failure. Functional regurgitation may diminish or disappear as the right ventricle decreases in size with the treatment of

heart failure. TR can also occur as a consequence of dilatation of the annulus in Marfan syndrome, in which it is not associated with right ventricular dilatation secondary to pulmonary hypertension.

A variety of disease processes can affect the tricuspid valve apparatus *directly* and lead to regurgitation. Thus, organic TR may occur on a congenital basis, as part of *Ebstein's anomaly* (see p. 934), in atrioventricular canal, and when the tricuspid valve is involved in the formation of an aneurysm of the ventricular septum,[468] or it may occur as an isolated congenital lesion.[469] Rheumatic fever may involve the tricuspid valve directly,[460] and when it does so, it usually causes scarring of the valve leaflets and/or chordae, leading to limited leaflet mobility, pure TR, and/or a combination of TR and TS.

TR or the combination of TR and TS is an important feature of the *carcinoid syndrome* (Fig. 32–45), which leads to focal or diffuse deposits of fibrous tissue on the endocardium of the valvular cusps and cardiac chambers and on the intima of the great veins and coronary sinus.[470,471] The white, fibrous carcinoid plaques are most extensive on the right side of the heart, where they are usually deposited on the ventricular surfaces of the tricuspid valve and cause the cusps to adhere to the underlying right ventricular wall, thereby producing TR.

TR may result from prolapse of the tricuspid valve caused by myxomatous changes in the valve and chordae tendineae; this condition usually, but not always, accompanies prolapse of the mitral valve.[472,473] Prolapse of the tricuspid valve occurs in about one-third of all patients with mitral valve prolapse.[446] Tricuspid valve prolapse may also be associated with atrial septal defect. Other causes of TR include penetrating and nonpenetrating trauma,[474] dilated

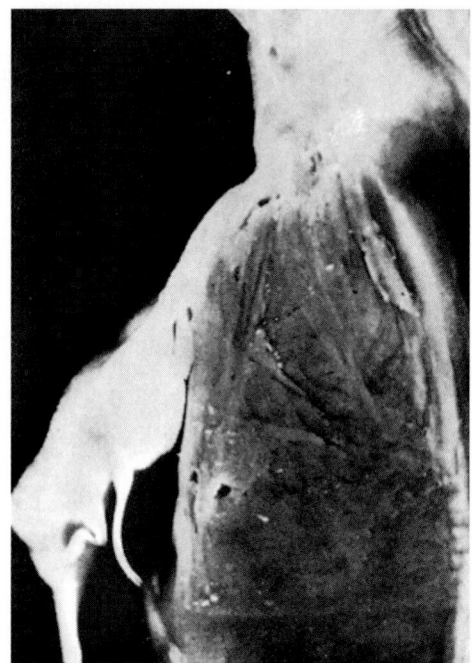

FIGURE 32–45. Septal tricuspid leaflet thickened by carcinoid plaques and fused to underlying ventricular septum. (From Callahan, J. A., et al.: Echocardiographic features of carcinoid heart disease. Am. J. Cardiol. *50:*766, 1982.)

cardiomyopathy,[475] infective endocarditis,[476] particularly staphylococcal endocarditis in narcotics addicts (see p. 1078), and surgical excision of the tricuspid valve that has been necessary in patients with infective endocarditis unresponsive to medical management.[477] Less common causes of TR include cardiac tumors, particularly right atrial myxoma; endomyocardial fibrosis; methysergide-induced valvular disease[478]; and systemic lupus erythematosus involving the tricuspid valve.[479]

Clinical Manifestations

HISTORY. In the absence of pulmonary hypertension, TR is generally well tolerated. However, when pulmonary hypertension and TR coexist, cardiac output declines, and the manifestations of right-sided heart failure become intensified.[480] Thus, the symptoms of TR result from a reduced cardiac output and from ascites, painful congestive hepatomegaly, and massive edema. Occasionally, patients complain of throbbing pulsations in the neck due to jugular venous distention, which intensify on effort,[15] and systolic pulsations of the eyeballs are sometimes noted.[481] In the many patients with TR who have mitral valve disease, the symptoms of the latter usually predominate. Symptoms of pulmonary congestion may abate as TR develops, but they are replaced by weakness, fatigue, and other manifestations of a depressed cardiac output.

PHYSICAL EXAMINATION (Fig. 2–7, p. 21). Evidence of weight loss and cachexia, cyanosis, and jaundice is often present on inspection. Atrial fibrillation is common. There is jugular venous distention,[482] the normal *x* and *x'* descents disappear, and a prominent systolic *("s")* wave, i.e., a *c-v* wave, is apparent. The descent of this wave, the *y* descent, is sharp and becomes the most prominent feature of the venous pulse (unless there is a coexisting TS, in which case it is slowed). The *s* waves and *y* descents become more prominent during inspiration.[483] A venous systolic thrill and murmur in the neck may be present in severe TR.[484] The right ventricular impulse is hyperdynamic and thrusting in quality. Rarely, a right atrial systolic impulse may be observed or palpated along the right lower sternal edge.[15] In patients with combined mitral

valve disease and TR, a relatively quiet zone may be present between the apex and the left sternal edge. Systolic pulsations of an enlarged tender liver are commonly present initially, but in chronic TR with congestive cirrhosis, the liver may be firm and nontender. Ascites and edema are frequent.

Auscultation (Table 32–2). This usually reveals an S_3 originating from the right ventricle, i.e., one accentuated by inspiration; when TR is associated with pulmonary hypertension, P_2 is accentuated as well. When TR occurs in the presence of pulmonary hypertension, the murmur is usually high-pitched, pansystolic, and loudest in the fourth intercostal space in the parasternal region but occasionally in the subxiphoid area. When TR is mild, the murmur may be short. When TR occurs in the absence of pulmonary hypertension, as for example in infective endocarditis or following trauma, the murmur is usually of low intensity and limited to the first half of systole. When the right ventricle is greatly dilated and occupies the anterior surface of the heart, the murmur may be the most prominent at the apex and difficult to distinguish from that produced by MR.

The response of the murmur to respiration and other maneuvers is of considerable aid in establishing the diagnosis of tricuspid regurgitation (Table 2–4, p. 46). It is usually augmented during inspiration (Carvallo's sign, p. 38). However, when the failing ventricle can no longer increase its stroke volume, the inspiratory augmentation may be elicited by standing and thereby reducing venous return. The murmur also increases during inspiration, the Mueller maneuver (forced inspiration against a closed glottis), exercise, leg-raising, hepatic compression, and amyl nitrite inhalation as well as after a prolonged diastole. It demonstrates an immediate overshoot after release of the Valsalva strain but is reduced in intensity and duration in the standing position and during the strain of the Valsalva maneuver. Rarely, TR is silent except for the selective appearance of a soft systolic murmur during inspiration.[485] Increased atrioventricular flow may cause a short early diastolic flow rumble in the left parasternal region following S_3. Tricuspid valve prolapse, like MVP, causes nonejection systolic clicks and late systolic murmurs. These findings are more prominent at the lower left sternal border. With inspiration the clicks occur later and the murmurs intensify and become shorter in duration.

Laboratory Examination

ELECTROCARDIOGRAM. This is usually nonspecific and characteristic of the lesion causing TR. Incomplete right bundle branch block, Q waves in lead V_1, and atrial fibrillation are commonly found.

RADIOLOGICAL FINDINGS. In patients with functional TR, marked cardiomegaly secondary to the condition responsible for the dilatation of the right ventricle is usually evident. The right atrium is prominent.[483] Evidence of elevated right atrial pressure may include distention of the azygos vein and the presence of pleural effusion. Ascites with upward displacement of the diaphragm may be present. Rarely, with prolonged elevation of right ventricular pressure, the tricuspid ring may calcify. The findings of pulmonary arterial and venous hypertension are common. Systolic pulsations of the right atrium may be present on fluoroscopy.

ECHOCARDIOGRAM (see also p. 76). The goal of echocardiography is to detect TR, estimate its severity, and assess pulmonary artery pressure and right ventricular function. In patients with TR secondary to dilation of the tricuspid annulus, usually associated with right ventricular systolic hypertension, the right atrium, right ventricle, and tricuspid annulus are all usually greatly dilated on echocardiography.[486,487] There is evidence of right ventricular diastolic overload with paradoxical motion of the ventricular septum similar to that observed in atrial septal defect. Exaggerated motion and delayed closure of the tricuspid valve are evident in patients with Ebstein's anomaly. In patients with TR secondary to right ventricular dilatation and pulmonary hypertension, the pulmonic valve echogram shows a diminished or absent *a* deflection. *Prolapse of the tricuspid valve* due to myxomatous degeneration may be evident on M-mode and two-dimensional echocardiography[472,473] (Fig. 3–60, p. 77). Simultaneous echocardiographic studies of the tricuspid valve and phonocardiography may reveal a nonejection systolic click originating from the right side of the heart that occurs at the onset of prolapse. Echocardiographic indications of tricuspid valve abnormalities, especially TR by Doppler examination, can be detected in the majority of patients with carcinoid heart disease.[470]

Contrast Echocardiography. This involves rapid ejection of saline or indocyanine green dye into an antecubital vein made while a two-dimensional echocardiogram is being recorded (see p. 58). It is both sensitive and specific for TR.[488] The injection produces microcavities that are readily visible on echocardiography and normally travel as a bolus through the circulation. In TR, these microcavities can be seen to travel back and forth across the tricuspid orifice and to pass into the inferior vena cava and hepatic veins during systole. TR secondary to carcinoid heart disease shows thickened, retracted valve leaflets, fixed in a semiopen position throughout the cardiac cycle,[489] whereas that due to endocarditis may reveal vegetations on the valve, or a flail valve. Transesophageal echocardiography enhances detection of TR.

Pulsed Doppler Echocardiography. This reveals systolic flow from right ventricle to right atrium and is an exquisitely sensitive technique for detecting TR.[490] Reverse flow can also be recorded in the inferior vena cava[491] and hepatic veins.[492] The peak velocity of TR flow is useful in the noninvasive estimation of right ventricular (and pulmonary artery) systolic pressure. Color Doppler imaging is an extremely accurate, sensitive, and specific method for assessing TR[493] and is helpful in selecting patients for surgical treatment and in assessing postoperative results.

HEMODYNAMIC AND ANGIOGRAPHIC FINDINGS. The right atrial and right ventricular end-diastolic pressures are characteristically elevated in TR, whether the condition is due to organic disease of the tricuspid valve or is secondary to right ventricular systolic overload (e.g., pulmonary hypertension and pulmonic stenosis). The right atrial pressure tracing reveals absence of the x descent and a prominent v or c-v wave ("ventricularization" of the atrial pressure). Therefore, as the severity of TR increases, the contour of the right atrial pressure pulse increasingly resembles that of the right ventricular pressure pulse (Fig. 32–46). A rise or no change in right atrial pressure on deep inspiration, rather than the usual fall, is characteristic.[483,494] Pulmonary artery (or right ventricular) systolic pressure may be helpful in determining whether the TR is primary (i.e., due to disease of the valve or its supporting structures) or functional (i.e., secondary to right ventricular dilatation). A pulmonary artery or right ventricular systolic pressure less than 40 mm Hg favors a primary etiology, whereas a pressure greater than 60 mm Hg suggests that TR is secondary.

Diagnosis and quantitative assessment of TR can be aided in many instances by right ventriculography, but the fact that the catheter must be positioned across the tricuspid valve cannot exclude the possibility of a false-positive diagnosis of TR. Modifications of previous angiographic techniques have been introduced in which a special, pre-formed catheter is positioned in the right ventricle, and angiography is carried out at low injection rates[495] or a special balloon catheter is employed to minimize the induction of extrasystoles, which can also cause spurious regurgitation.[496]

Management

TR in the absence of pulmonary hypertension usually does not require surgical treatment. Indeed, both patients and experimental animals with normal pulmonary artery pressure may tolerate total excision of the tricuspid valve, as long as right ventricular systolic pressure is normal for a period of time.[496] Dilatation of the right side of the heart usually occurs months or years after tricuspid valvectomy (usually carried out for acute infective endocarditis), and annuloplasty with insertion of a prosthetic valve can then be carried out after adequate sterilization of the valve ring. *Surgical treatment* of acquired regurgitation secondary to annular dilatation was greatly improved when Carpentier introduced the concept of suturing the annulus to a right prosthetic ring of appropriate dimensions.[497,498] Annuloplasty without insertion of a prosthetic ring (so-called De-Vega annuloplasty) has also been found to be effective in patients with annular dilatation. This technique is now widely employed.[453,480,499-501]

At the time of mitral valve surgery in patients with TR secondary to pulmonary hypertension, the severity of the regurgitation should be assessed by palpation of the valve and a determination made whether the TR is functional (secondary) or organic (primary). Patients with mild TR usually do not require surgical treatment[501]; pulmonary vascular pressures decline following successful mitral valve surgery, and the mild TR tends to disappear. Excellent results have been reported in patients with moderate TR with the use of suture annuloplasty of the posterior (unsupported) portion of the annulus.[453,502] Patients with severe TR and primary (organic) rheumatic valve disease with commissural fusion require commissurotomy and ring annuloplasty.[499,503] However, management of severe functional TR is more controversial. Although it is not clear whether severe TR should be treated by annuloplasty or valve replacement, most surgeons prefer the former approach and utilize a rigid (Carpentier) ring.[501] If it does not provide a good functional result at the operating table, as assessed by transesophageal echocardiography, they resort to valve replacement.

Organic disease of the tricuspid valve responsible for TR, as in Ebstein's anomaly[504] or carcinoid heart disease,[457] when severe enough to require surgery, usually requires valve replacement. The risk of thrombosis of mechanical prostheses is greater in the tricuspid than in the mitral or aortic positions, presumably because pressure and flow rates are lower in the right side of the heart. For this reason, the artificial valve of choice for the tricuspid position in adults at present is a large porcine heterograft.[458,459] Anticoagulants are not required, and a durability of more than 10 years has been established.

In treating the difficult problem of tricuspid endocarditis in heroin addicts, it has been noted that total excision of the tricuspid valve *without immediate replacement* can be tolerated by these patients, who usually do not have associated pulmonary hypertension. When antibiotic therapy is unsuccessful, valvular replacement frequently results in reinfection or continued infection. Therefore, diseased valvular tissue should be excised to eradicate the endocarditis, and antibiotic treatment can then be continued. Initially, most patients tolerate loss of the tricuspid valve without great difficulty, although a reduction in left ventricular ejection fraction may occur.[505] Later, right ventricular dysfunction usually occurs. Therefore, a bioprosthetic valve may be inserted 6 to 9 months after valve excision and control of the infection.

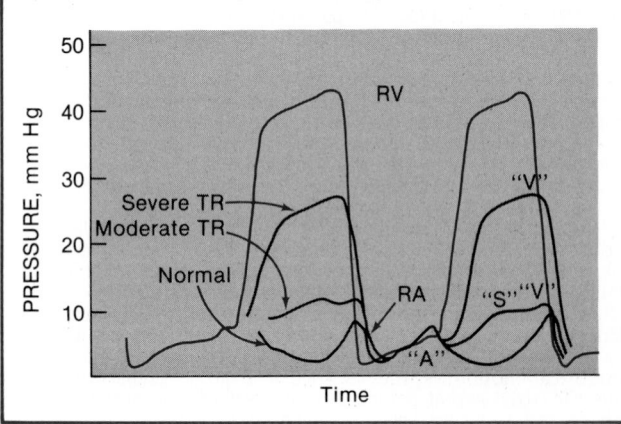

FIGURE 32–46. Appearance of right atrial (RA) pressure contour in patients with severe tricuspid regurgitation (TR), moderate TR, and no TR (normal). Note the regurgitant systolic ("S") wave that blends with the normal filling ("V") wave in severe TR. The resultant RA pressure waveform resembles a right ventricular (RV) pressure recording. (From Grossman, W. [ed.]: Cardiac Catheterization and Angiography. 3rd ed. Philadelphia, Lea and Febiger, 1986, p. 378.)

tricular septal defect, and pulmonic valvular stenosis. Less **1059**
common causes include trauma, carcinoid syndrome,[508] _____
rheumatic involvement,[515] injury produced by a pulmonary **Ch 32**

PULMONIC VALVE DISEASE

Etiology and Pathology

PULMONIC STENOSIS (PS). The *congenital* form is the most common cause of pulmonic stenosis.[506] Its manifestations in children are discussed on page 924 and in adults on page 965. *Rheumatic* inflammation of the pulmonic valve is very uncommon, is usually associated with involvement of other valves, and rarely leads to serious deformity. However, a high incidence of significant pulmonic valve involvement secondary to rheumatic fever has been reported in Mexico City, perhaps related to the pulmonary hypertension that occurs at high altitudes and the resultant greater stress on the pulmonic valve.[507] *Carcinoid* plaques, similar to those involving the tricuspid valve, are often present in the outflow tract of the right ventricle in patients with malignant carcinoid and result in constriction of the pulmonic valve ring, retraction and fusion of the valve cusps, and either PS or the combination of PS and pulmonic regurgitation (PR) (Fig. 32–47).[508,509] Obstruction in the region of the pulmonic valve may be extrinsic to the valve apparatus and may be produced by cardiac tumors or aneurysm of the sinus Valsalva.[510]

PULMONIC REGURGITATION (PR). By far the most common cause of PR is dilatation of the valve ring secondary to pulmonary hypertension (of any etiology) or to dilatation of the pulmonary artery, either idiopathic[511,512] or consequent to a connective tissue disorder such as Marfan syndrome. The second most common cause of PR is infective endocarditis.[508,513] Less frequently, it is iatrogenic and is induced at the time of surgical treatment of congenital PS or tetralogy of Fallot. PR may also result from a variety of lesions directly affecting the pulmonic valve. These include congenital malformations, such as absent, malformed, fenestrated, or supernumerary leaflets. These anomalies may occur as isolated lesions[514] but more often are associated with other congenital anomalies, particularly tetralogy of Fallot, ven-

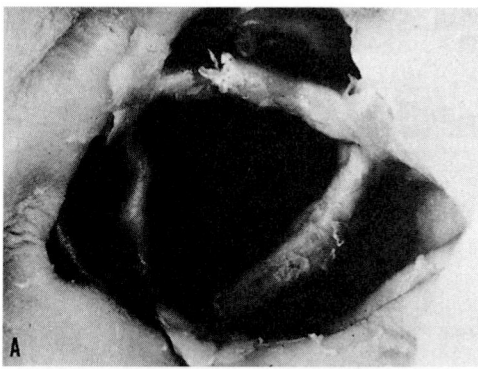

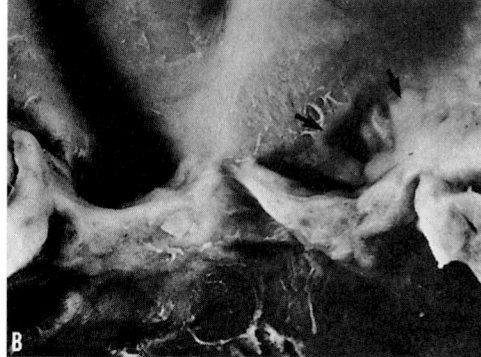

FIGURE 32–47. Carcinoid heart disease; pulmonary valve viewed from above *(A)* and opened *(B)*. The thickened and retracted cusps result in valvular incompetence. The constricted annulus results in valvular stenosis. Carcinoid plaques (arrows) extend onto the pulmonary trunk. (From Callahan, J. A., et al.: Echocardiographic features of carcinoid heart disease. Am. J. Cardiol. 50:767, 1982.)

artery flow-directed catheter,[516] syphilis,[517] and chest trauma.[518]

Clinical Manifestations

Like TR, isolated PR causes right ventricular volume overload and may be tolerated for many years without difficulty unless it complicates or is complicated by pulmonary hypertension, in which case it is usually accompanied by and aggravates right ventricular failure. Patients with PR caused by infective endocarditis who develop septic pulmonary emboli and pulmonary hypertension often exhibit severe right ventricular failure.[518] In most patients the clinical manifestations of the primary disease are severe and usually overshadow the PR, which often results only in incidental auscultatory findings. *Physical examination* reveals a hyperdynamic right ventricle, producing palpable systolic pulsations in the left parasternal area and an enlarged pulmonary artery that often results in palpable systolic pulsations in the second left intercostal space; sometimes systolic and diastolic thrills are felt in the same area. A tap reflecting pulmonic valve closure is usually easily palpable in the second intercostal space in patients with pulmonary hypertension and secondary PR.

AUSCULTATION. In patients with congenital absence of the pulmonic valve, P_2 is not audible, but this sound is accentuated in patients with PR secondary to pulmonary hypertension, particularly when the dilated pulmonary artery is near the chest wall. There may be wide splitting of S_2 due to prolongation of right ventricular ejection accompanying the augmented right ventricular stroke volume.[515] A nonvalvular systolic ejection click due to the sudden expansion of the pulmonary artery by the augmented right ventricular stroke volume frequently initiates a midsystolic ejection murmur, most prominent in the second left intercostal space. An S_3 and S_4 originating from the right ventricle are often audible, most readily in the fourth intercostal space at the left parasternal area, and are augmented by inspiration.

In the absence of pulmonary hypertension, the diastolic murmur of PR is low-pitched and is usually heard best at the third and fourth left intercostal spaces adjacent to the sternum (Fig. 2–42, p. 43). The murmur commences when pressures in the pulmonary artery and right ventricle diverge, approximately 0.04 sec after P_2. It is diamond-shaped in configuration and brief, reaching a peak intensity when the gradient between these pressures is maximal and ending with equilibration of the pressures.[517] The murmur becomes louder during inspiration and following inhalation of amyl nitrite.

Graham Steell Murmur. When pulmonary artery systolic pressure exceeds approximately 60 mm Hg, dilatation of the pulmonic annulus results in a regurgitant jet of high velocity that is responsible for the so-called Graham Steell murmur of PR. (Doppler ultrasound reveals pulmonary regurgitation at much lower pulmonary arterial pressures.)[518] The Graham Steell murmur is a high-pitched, blowing decrescendo murmur beginning immediately after P_2 and is most prominent in the left parasternal region in the second to fourth intercostal spaces. Thus, although it resembles the murmur of AR, it is usually accompanied by the findings of severe pulmonary hypertension, i.e., an accentuated P_2 or fused S_2, an ejection sound, and a systolic murmur of tricuspid regurgitation, and not by a widened arterial pulse pressure. Sometimes a low-frequency presystolic murmur is present, i.e., a right-sided Austin Flint murmur originating from the mitral valve.[519]

The Graham Steell murmur of PR secondary to pulmonary hypertension usually increases in intensity with inspiration, exhibits little change after amyl nitrite inhalation or vasopressors, is diminished during the Valsalva strain, and returns to baseline intensity almost immediately after release of the Valsalva strain. This murmur resembles and may be confused with the diastolic blowing murmur of AR. However, indicator dilution studies[520] and aortography have established that a diastolic blowing murmur along the left sternal border in patients with rheumatic heart disease and pulmonary hypertension—even in the absence of peripheral signs of AR—is usually due to AR and not PR.

Laboratory Examination

ELECTROCARDIOGRAM. In the absence of pulmonary hypertension, PR often results in an ECG that reflects right ventricular diastolic overload, i.e., an rSr' (or rSR') configuration in the right precordial leads. PR secondary to pulmonary hypertension is usually associated with ECG evidence of right ventricular hypertrophy.

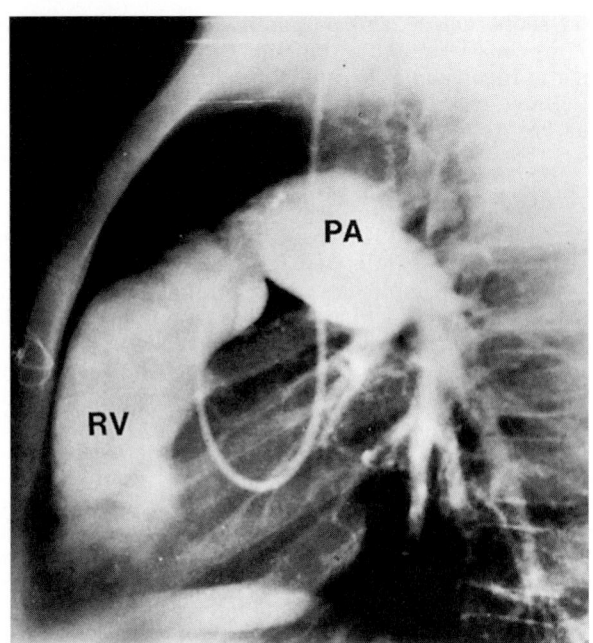

FIGURE 32–48. Pulmonic valvular regurgitation. Contrast medium has been injected into the main pulmonary artery (PA) and regurgitates back into an enlarged right ventricle (RV). (Reproduced with permission from Carlsson, E., et al.: The radiological diagnosis of cardiac valvular insufficiency. Circulation 55:921, 1977. Copyright 1977 American Heart Association.)

RADIOLOGICAL FINDINGS. Both the pulmonary artery and the right ventricle are usually enlarged, but these signs are nonspecific. Fluoroscopy may demonstrate pronounced pulsation of the main pulmonary artery. PR can be diagnosed by observing opacification of the right ventricle following injection of contrast material into the main pulmonary artery (Fig. 32–48). The diagnosis is supported by noting superimposition of the pulmonary artery and right ventricular pressure curves during mid and late diastole. Indicator dilution techniques with injections into the pulmonary artery and sampling from the right ventricle,[521] as well as intracardiac phonocardiography, can also be helpful in establishing the diagnosis in mild cases.

ECHOCARDIOGRAM. This shows right ventricular dilatation and, in patients with pulmonary hypertension, right ventricular hypertrophy as well. Abnormal motion of the septum characteristic of volume overload of the right ventricle in diastole and/or septal flutter[522] may be evident. The motion of the pulmonic valve may point to the cause of the pulmonic regurgitation.[523] Absence of *a* waves and systolic notching of the posterior leaflet suggest pulmonary hypertension; large *a* waves indicate pulmonic stenosis. PR can be detected by contrast echocardiography. The pulsed Doppler technique is extremely accurate in detecting PR. Abnormal Doppler signals in the right ventricular outflow tract whose velocity is sustained throughout diastole are generally observed in patients in whom dilatation of the valve ring (functional regurgitation) secondary to pulmonary hypertension is the cause. When the velocity falls during diastole, the pulmonary artery pressure is usually normal, and the regurgitation is caused by an abnormality of the valve itself.[523]

MANAGEMENT. PR per se is seldom severe enough to require specific treatment. Cardiac glycosides are useful in the management of right ventricular dilatation or failure. Treatment of the primary condition, such as infective endocarditis, or the lesion responsible for the pulmonary hypertension, such as surgical treatment of mitral valvular disease, often ameliorates the PR. Surgical treatment of *primary* PR directed specifically at the pulmonic valve is required only occasionally because of intractable right heart failure, and under such circumstances valve replacement may be carried out,[524] preferably with a porcine bioprosthesis.

MULTIVALVULAR DISEASE

Multivalvular involvement is caused most frequently by rheumatic fever, and a variety of clinical and hemodynamic syndromes can be produced by different combinations of valvular abnormalities. The Marfan syndrome and other connective tissue disorders may cause prolapse and dilatation of more than one valve annulus, causing multivalvular regurgitation. Degenerative calcification of the aortic valve may be associated with degenerative mitral annular calcification and cause AS and MR. Different pathological conditions may affect each valve, such as infective endocarditis on the aortic valve and ischemic

mitral regurgitation. Development of PR and TR secondary to dilatation of the pulmonic valve ring and tricuspid annulus, respectively, as a consequence of pulmonary hypertension secondary to disease involving the mitral or aortic valve or both, has already been discussed (see p. 1056), as has the combination of *organic* rheumatic tricuspid and mitral valvular disease (see p. 1011). In patients with multivalvular disease, the clinical manifestations depend on the relative severities of each of the lesions. When the valvular abnormalities are of approximately equal severity, as a general rule, clinical manifestations produced by the more proximal (upstream) of two valvular lesions, i.e., the mitral valve in patients with combined mitral and aortic valvular disease and the tricuspid valve in patients with combined tricuspid and mitral valvular disease, are more prominent than those produced by the distal lesion. Thus, the proximal lesion masks the distal lesion.

It is important to recognize multivalvular involvement preoperatively because failure to correct all significant valvular disease at the time of operation increases mortality considerably. In patients with multivalvular disease, the relative severity of each lesion may be difficult to estimate by clinical examination and noninvasive techniques, because one lesion may mask the manifestations of the other. For this reason, patients suspected of multivalvular involvement and in whom surgical treatment is under consideration should undergo (in addition to careful clinical examination and noninvasive workup, with emphasis on two-dimensional and Doppler echocardiography), right- and left-sided cardiac catheterization and angiography. If there is any question concerning the presence of significant AS in patients undergoing an operation on the mitral valve, the aortic valve should be inspected because overlooking this condition can lead to a high perioperative mortality. Similarly, it is useful to palpate the tricuspid valve at the time of operation on the mitral valve.

MITRAL STENOSIS AND AORTIC REGURGITATION

Approximately two-thirds of patients with severe MS have an early blowing diastolic murmur along the left sternal border with a normal pulse pressure; in 90 per cent of these the murmur is due to mild or moderate AR and is usually of little clinical importance. However, approximately 10 per cent of patients with MS have severe rheumatic AR,[525] which can usually be recognized by the peripheral signs of a widened pulse pressure, left ventricular dilatation and increased wall motion on echocardiography, and signs of left ventricular enlargement on radiological and electrocardiographic examinations.

In keeping with the general observation that a proximal lesion may mask a distal lesion, significant AR may be missed in patients with severe MS. The widened pulse pressure, in particular, may be absent. On the other hand, on clinical examination of patients with obvious AR, MS may be missed or, conversely, may be falsely diagnosed. An accentuated S₁ and an opening snap in a patient with AR should suggest the possibility of mitral valve disease. On the other hand, an Austin Flint murmur is often inappropriately considered to be the diastolic rumbling murmur of MS. These two murmurs may be distinguished at the bedside by means of amyl nitrite inhalation, which diminishes the Austin Flint murmur (Fig. 2–41, p. 42) but augments the murmur of MS; isometric handgrip and squatting augment both the diastolic murmur of AR and the Austin Flint murmur. Echocardiography, particularly pulsed Doppler echocardiography, is of decisive value in the detection of both lesions.

MITRAL STENOSIS AND AORTIC STENOSIS

The left ventricles of patients with these two lesions are usually small, stiff, and hypertrophied. When severe MS and AS coexist, the former masks many of the manifestations of the latter.[526] The cardiac output tends to be reduced further than in patients with isolated AS, and the atrial booster pump mechanism, so important in filling the ventricle in AS (see p. 1035), has little impact when MS is present. The reduction in cardiac output lowers both the transaortic valvular pressure gradient and the left ventricular systolic pressure, diminishes the incidence of angina, and retards the development of aortic valvular calcification and left ventricular hypertrophy.[527] On the other hand, clinical manifestations associated with MS, such as pulmonary congestion and hemoptysis, atrial fibrillation, and systemic embolization, occur more frequently than in patients with isolated AS.

On *physical examination*, presystolic distention of the left ventricle and an S₄, common in pure AS, are usually not present. The midsystolic murmur characteristic of AS may be reduced in intensity and duration because of stroke volume reduced by the MS. The *electrocardiogram* may fail to demonstrate left ventricular hypertrophy, but left atrial enlargement is common in patients in sinus rhythm. The *chest roentgenogram* is usually typical of MS except that calcium may be present in the region of the aortic valve. The two-dimensional and Doppler *echocardiograms* are of the greatest value because stenosis of both valves may be evident. However, the low cardiac output characteristic of the combination of lesions may reduce the transvalvular gradients estimated by Doppler echocardiography. The indirect *carotid pulse* tracing reveals a delayed upstroke.

It is vital to recognize the presence of hemodynamically significant aortic valvular disease (stenosis and/or regurgitation) preoperatively in patients who are to undergo surgical correction of MS because isolated mitral valvulotomy may be hazardous in such patients; this operation can impose a sudden hemodynamic load on the left ventricle that was previously protected by the MS and may lead to acute pulmonary edema.

AORTIC STENOSIS AND MITRAL REGURGITATION

The combination of severe AS and MR is a hazardous one, but fortunately it is relatively uncommon. Obstruction to left ventricular outflow augments the volume of MR flow,[122] whereas the presence of MR diminishes the ventricular preload necessary for maintenance of the left ventricular stroke volume in AS. The result is a reduced forward cardiac output and marked left atrial and pulmonary venous hypertension. The physical findings may be confusing because the delayed arterial pulse of AS may be counteracted by the sharp upstroke of MR, and it may be difficult to recognize two distinct systolic murmurs. Amyl nitrite tends to increase the intensity of the murmur of AS and to reduce that of MR. On echocardiography and roentgenography the left atrium and ventricle are usually larger than in isolated AS. Usually both valves must be treated surgically in patients with severe AS and MR.

AORTIC REGURGITATION AND MITRAL REGURGITATION

This relatively frequent combination of lesions[528] may be caused by rheumatic heart disease or by prolapse of both the aortic and mitral valves due to myxomatous degeneration,[529] or dilatation of both annuli in connective tissue disorders. The left ventricle is usually greatly dilated. The clinical features of AR usually predominate, and it sometimes is difficult to determine whether the MR is due to organic involvement of this valve or dilatation of the mitral valve ring secondary to left ventricular enlargement. When both valvular leaks are severe, this combination of lesions is poorly tolerated. The normal mitral valve ordinarily serves as a "backup" to the aortic valve, and premature (diastolic) closure of the mitral valve limits the volume of reflux that occurs in patients with acute AR.[386] With combined regurgitant lesions, regardless of the cause of the mitral lesion, blood may reflux from the aorta through both chambers of the left side of the heart into the pulmonary veins. Physical and laboratory examination will usually show evidence of both lesions. Both lesions are frequently associated with an S_3 and a brisk arterial pulse. The relative severity of each lesion can be assessed best by contrast angiography.

When MR occurs in patients with AR secondary to left ventricular dilatation, it often regresses following aortic valve replacement. If severe, it may be corrected by annuloplasty at the time of aortic valve replacement. An intrinsically normal mitral valve that is regurgitant due to a dilated annulus should not be replaced.

SURGICAL TREATMENT OF MULTIVALVULAR DISEASE

Combined aortic and mitral valve replacement is usually associated with a higher risk and poorer survival than is replacement of either of the two valves alone.[452] The operative risk of double-valve replacement is about 50 per cent higher than it is for single-valve replacement and, like the latter, has been slowly declining[530] and now ranges from 5 to 10 per cent. Kirklin reported a 5-year survival rate of 63 per cent after double-valve replacement compared with 80 per cent for single-valve replacement.[452] The long-term survival depends strongly on the preoperative functional status.[531] Patients operated on for the combination of AR and MR fare worse than patients receiving double-valve replacement for any of the other combinations, presumably because both of these valvular abnormalities may produce irreversible left ventricular damage. Mitral repair in combination with aortic valve replacement is preferable to double-valve replacement. Risk factors reducing long-term survival include advanced age, higher New York Heart Association class, greater left ventricular enlargement, and accompanying ischemic heart disease requiring coronary bypass surgery.[452]

Given the higher risks, a higher threshold is required for multivalve versus single-valve surgery. Thus, patients are generally not advised to undergo multivalve surgery until they reach late Class II or Class III (NY Heart Association). Despite detailed noninvasive and invasive workup, the decision to treat more than one valve is often made by palpation or direct inspection at the operating table.

THREE-VALVE DISEASE. Hemodynamically significant disease involving the mitral, aortic, and tricuspid valves is uncommon. Patients with trivalvular disease may present in advanced heart failure with marked cardiomegaly, and surgical correction of all three valvular lesions is imperative. However, triple-valve replacement is a long and complex operation. Early in the experience with this procedure, the mortality rate was 20 per cent in patients in functional Class III and 40 per cent in Class IV. More recently, it has declined to 5 per cent.[531,532] In some patients with trivalvular disease, it is possible to replace the mitral and aortic valves and carry out a tricuspid valvuloplasty.

Patients who survive three-valve surgery usually show substantial clinical improvement in the early postoperative period,[533,534] and postoperative catheterization studies show marked reductions in pulmonary arterial and capillary pressures. However, some patients succumb to arrhythmias[534] or congestive heart failure in the late postoperative period despite three normally functioning prostheses. The cause of cardiac failure in this situation is not known, but it may be related to intraoperative myocardial ischemia, microemboli from the multipole prosthesis, or continued subclinical episodes of rheumatic myocarditis.

When multiple prosthetic valves must be inserted, it is logical to select either two bioprostheses or mechanical prostheses for the left side of the heart. If the patient is to be exposed to the hazards of anticoagulants for one mechanical prosthesis, it seems unreasonable to add the potential risks of early failure of a bioprosthesis. However, if two mechanical prostheses on the left side of the heart are selected, the use of a bioprosthesis in the tricuspid position is suggested.[531]

PROSTHETIC CARDIAC VALVES

The first successful replacements of cardiac valves in the human were accomplished by Nina Braunwald,[535] Harken et al.,[536] and Starr[537] in 1960. Two major groups of artificial (prosthetic) valves are currently available in models designed for both the atrioventricular (mitral and tricuspid) and the aortic positions: mechanical prostheses and bioprostheses (tissue valves).[537a]

MECHANICAL PROSTHESES

Mechanical prosthetic valves are classified into two major groups: caged-ball and tilting-disc valves. The *Starr Edwards* caged-ball valve, the oldest prosthetic valve in continuous use (Figs. 32–49 and 32–50), has the longest record of predictable performance of any artificial valve.[538,539] The poppet is made of silicone rubber, the cage of stellite alloy, and the sewing ring of Teflon/polypropylene cloth. A disadvantage is its bulky cage design; it is not suitable in patients with a small left ventricular cavity or a small aortic annulus or in a valve–aortic arch composite graft. In a small number of patients it induces hemolysis, which may be greatly exaggerated and become of clinical importance if a perivalvular leak develops. In small sizes, this valve may cause mild obstruction, and the incidence of thromboembolism is slightly higher than with the tilting-disc valve.[540]

Several types of tilting-disc valves are widely employed; these are less bulky and have a lower profile than the caged-ball valve. The *St. Jude* valve (Fig. 32–49D), currently the most widely used prosthesis on a worldwide basis, is coated with pyrolytic carbon and has two semicircular discs that pivot between open and closed positions without the need for supporting struts (Fig. 32–50). It possesses favorable flow characteristics and causes a lower transvalvular gradient at any outer diameter and cardiac output than the caged-ball or tilting valves.[541,542] The St. Jude valve appears to have particularly favorable hemodynamic characteristics in the smaller sizes; therefore, it is especially useful in children. Thrombogenicity in the mitral position *may* be less than for other prosthetic valves. However, as with other mechanical prostheses, permanent anticoagulation is needed—antiplatelet agents alone are not sufficient.[541] A variation of the St. Jude valve, the *Carbomedics* prosthesis (Fig. 32–49E), is also a bileaflet valve composed of pyrolytic carbon with a titanium housing that can be rotated so as to avoid interference with disc excursion by subvalvular tissue.

The *Omniscience* valve (Fig. 32–49B), the successor to the *Lillehei-Kaster* pivoting-disc valve, consists of a titanium valve housing with a polyester knit sewing ring in which a pyrolytic disc is suspended. In the open position, the disc swings to an angle of 80 degrees, providing a large central flow orifice.[543,544] A closely related valve is the

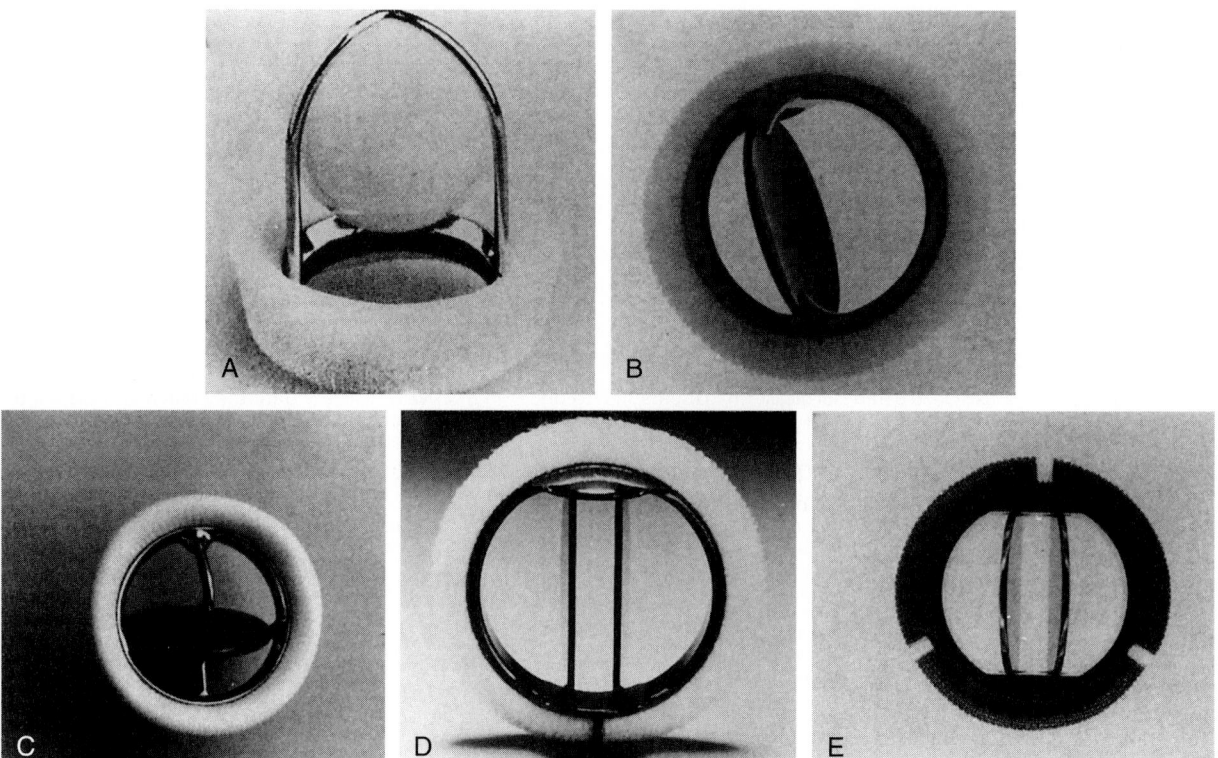

FIGURE 32–49. *A*, The Starr-Edwards ball and cage valve. *B*, The Omniscience valve. *C*, The Medtronic-Hall valve. *D*, The St. Jude valve. *E*, The Carbomedics bileaflet valve. (From Cohn, L. H.: Aortic valve prostheses. Cardiol. Rev. *2*:219, 1995.)

Medtronic-Hall valve (Fig. 32–49*C*), which has a Teflon sewing ring and titanium housing, and its thin, carbon-coated pivoting disc has a central perforation that allows improved hemodynamics. Thrombogenicity appears to be quite low—less than one episode per 100 patient-years in the mitral position[545]—and mechanical performance is excellent over the long term.

DURABILITY AND THROMBOGENICITY. Mechanical prosthetic valves all have an excellent record of durability—up to 35 years in the case of the Starr-Edwards valve. In the mitral position, perivalvular regurgitation appears to occur more frequently with mechanical than with tissue valves.[546] However, patients with any mechanical prosthesis—regardless of design or site of placement—require long-term anticoagulation because of the hazard of thromboembolism, which is greatest in the first postoperative year. Without anticoagulation, the incidence of thrombo-

embolism is three- to sixfold higher than with proper doses. Very rarely, thrombosis of the mechanical valve occurs. This may be a fatal event, but when non-fatal it interferes with prosthetic valve function and may sometimes be managed by thrombolytic therapy (see p. 1596).

Anticoagulation in patients with prosthetic valves is discussed on p. 1066. Sodium warfarin should begin about 2 days after operation, and the INR should be in the range of 2.5 to 3.5.[547] This relatively conservative approach reduces the risk of anticoagulant hemorrhage yet does not appear to be associated with a greater frequency of thromboembolism than an INR of 3.0 to 4.0, which was used in the past. Antiplatelet agents without anticoagulants do not provide adequate protection. However, the addition of 100 mg aspirin daily with coumadin may reduce the risk of embolism.[548]

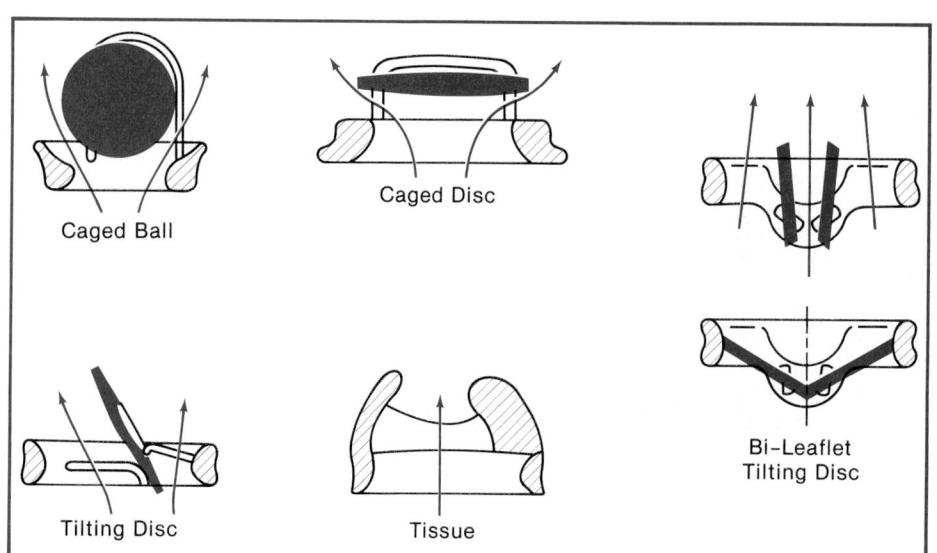

Caged Ball

Caged Disc

Tilting Disc

Tissue

Bi-Leaflet
Tilting Disc

FIGURE 32–50. Designs and flow patterns of major categories of prosthetic heart valves: caged-ball, caged-disc, tilting-disc, bileaflet tilting-disc, and bioprosthetic (tissue) valves. Whereas flow in mechanical valves must course along both sides of the occluder, bioprostheses have a central flow pattern. (Reproduced by permission from Schoen, F. J., et al.: Bioengineering aspects of heart valve replacement. Ann. Biomed. Eng. *10*:97, 1982. Copyright 1983, Pergamon Press Limited, 1983; and from Schoen, F. J.: Pathology of cardiac valve replacement. *In* Morse, D., Steiner, R. M., and Fernandez, J. [eds.]: Guide to Prosthetic Cardiac Valves. New York, Springer-Verlag, 1985, p. 209. Copyright 1985 Springer-Verlag, Inc.)

It must be recognized that (1) the administration of warfarin carries its own mortality and morbidity, estimated at 0.2 and 2.2 per 100 patient-years, respectively; and (2) despite treatment with anticoagulants, the incidence of thromboembolic complications with the best mechanical prosthesis is still about 0.2 (fatal) and 1 to 2 (nonfatal) per 100 patient-years for aortic valves and 2 to 3 for mitral valves.[549] Valve thrombosis, a particularly hazardous complication, occurs at an incidence of about 0.1 per cent per year in the aortic and 0.35 per cent per year in the mitral position. Thrombosis of mechanical prostheses in the tricuspid position is quite high, and for this reason bioprostheses are preferred at this site. The incidence of embolization in patients who have experienced repeated emboli from a prosthetic valve despite anticoagulants may be reduced by replacement with a tissue valve.

Mechanical prostheses regularly cause mild hemolysis,[550] but this is not severe enough to be of clinical importance unless the patient develops periprosthetic regurgitation.

TISSUE VALVES

Tissue valves (bioprostheses) have been developed largely to overcome the risk of thromboembolism that is inherent in all mechanical prosthetic valves and the attendant hazards and inconvenience of permanent anticoagulant therapy. The first of these to be widely used were chemically sterilized aortic homografts obtained from cadavers. However, these exhibited a high incidence of breakdown

within 3 years, and antibiotic-treated cryopreserved frozen-irradiated homografts were then developed. These are more durable[551-554] but, although they have many desirable properties, their use has been restricted by the problems inherent in their procurement (see below).

PORCINE HETEROGRAFTS. Porcine aortic heterografts were developed for both the mitral and the aortic positions and have been used clinically since 1965. Three porcine heterografts are widely used today.[544,551-554] (1) The *Hancock* valve (Fig. 32–51A) is fixed and preserved in glutaraldehyde and is mounted on a Dacron cloth–covered flexible polypropylene strut. In the smaller aortic models, the right coronary cusp is replaced by a posterior cusp from another valve to reduce obstruction resulting from the septal shelf of the valve. (2) The *Carpentier-Edwards* valve[551] (Fig. 32–51B) is pressure-fixed and then preserved in glutaraldehyde and is mounted on a Teflon-covered Eljiloy strut in a manner as to minimize the septal shelf. (3) The *Intact* valve is also glutaraldehyde-treated but at a fixation pressure of zero and with toluidine in an attempt to inhibit calcium deposition.

The hemodynamic profiles of the porcine heterografts are similar to those of comparably sized low-profile mechanical prostheses.[555,556] In contrast to the latter, however, the valve orifice is blood flow–dependent, with greater orifice size as transvalvular flow increases. The Hancock valve has been reported to have slightly better hemodynamics than the Carpentier-Edwards valve.[557]

During the first 3 postoperative months, while the sewing ring becomes endothelialized, the thromboembolic rate is high enough that anticoagulation is extremely desirable.

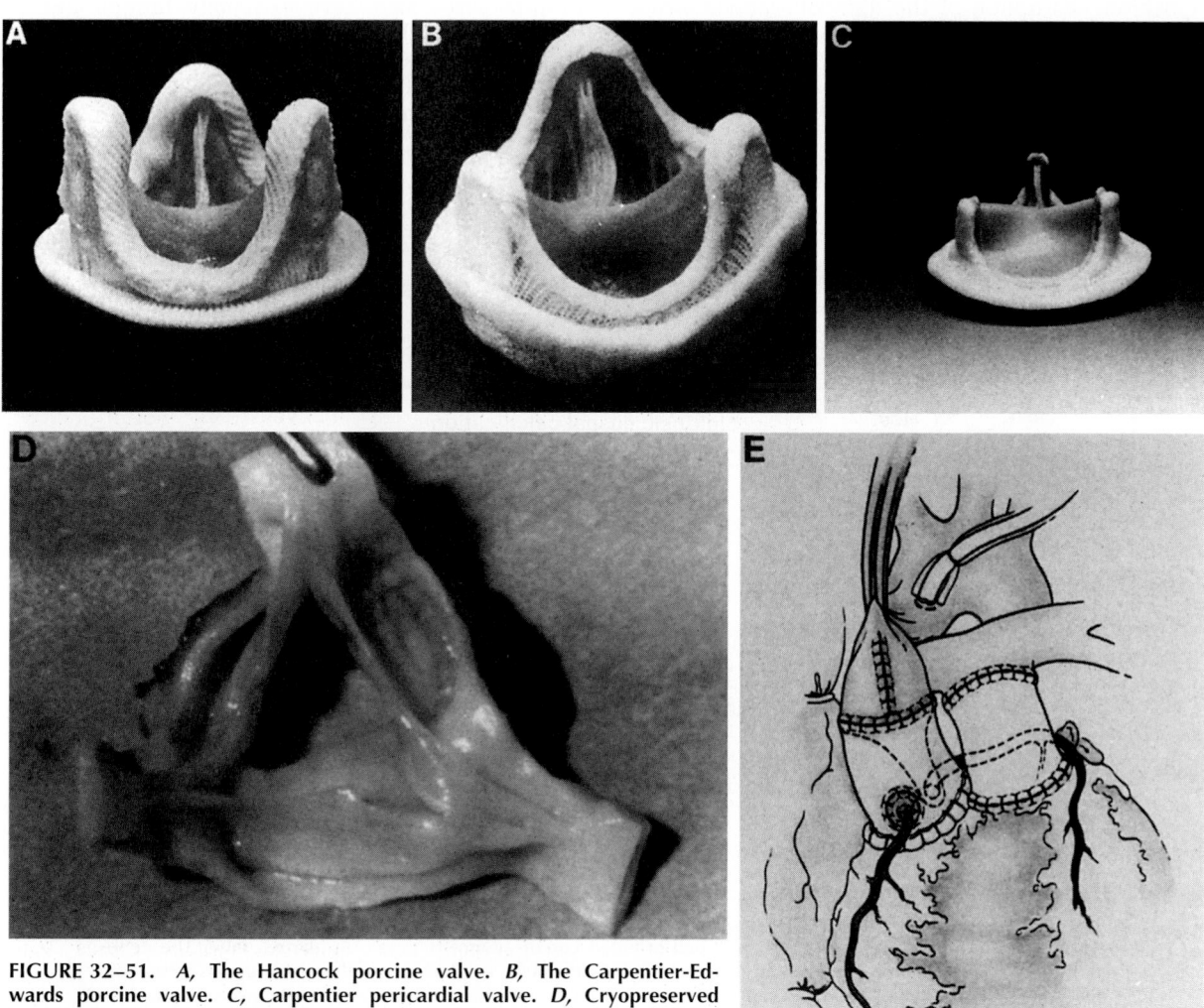

FIGURE 32–51. *A,* The Hancock porcine valve. *B,* The Carpentier-Edwards porcine valve. *C,* Carpentier pericardial valve. *D,* Cryopreserved homograft valve. *E,* Incisions for placement of pulmonary autograft valve into the aortic position. (From Oury, J. H.: Pulmonary autograft—past, present and future. J. Heart Valve Dis. 2:366, 1993.)

Thereafter, anticoagulants are not required for porcine valves in the aortic position, and the thromboembolic rate is approximately 1 to 2 episodes per 100 patient-years without these drugs.[558] When these valves have been placed in mitral position in patients who are in sinus rhythm, without heart failure, without thrombus in the left atrium or the left atrial appendage, and without a history of embolism preoperatively, anticoagulants are not needed (after the first 3 postoperative months), and the thromboembolic rate is also approximately 1 to 2 per 100 patient-years. This rate is comparable to that observed in patients with the St. Jude or other mechanical valves receiving anticoagulants and therefore subject to the risks of hemorrhage. It is unlikely that any replacement of the mitral valve can be associated with a thromboembolic rate much below 0.5 per 100 patient-years because some of the emboli in patients with longstanding mitral disease are derived from the left atrium rather than from the valve itself.[556] In patients undergoing mitral valve replacement who have experienced a previous embolus, in whom thrombus is found in the left atrium at operation, or who remain in atrial fibrillation postoperatively (approximately one-third of all patients receiving mitral valve replacements), the hazard of thromboembolism persists. Indeed, in patients with atrial fibrillation the incidence of postoperative emboli following implantation of a porcine bioprosthesis into the mitral position is three times as high as in patients in sinus rhythm. Therefore, anticoagulants are indicated in those patients with these three risk factors. The need for anticoagulants negates the principal advantage of the tissue valves.

The major problem with porcine bioprostheses is their limited durability (Fig. 32–52). Cuspal tears, degeneration, fibrin deposition, disruption of the fibrocollagenous structure, perforation, fibrosis, and calcification sufficiently severe to require reoperation begin to appear in some patients in the fourth or fifth postoperative year, and by 10 years the rate of primary tissue failure averages 30 per cent. It then accelerates, and by 15 years the actuarial freedom from bioprosthetic primary tissue failure has ranged from 30 to 60 per cent in several series.[552] Structural valve deterioration is more frequent in patients with bioprostheses in the mitral than in the aortic position, presumably because of the higher closing pressure. It is likely that with the passage of time even more of these valves will fail, and essentially all valves implanted into patients aged less than 60 years may have to be replaced.[559] Fortunately, however, these valves usually do not fail suddenly (as is often the case for structural failure or thrombosis of mechanical prostheses). Rereplacement of a bioprosthetic valve should be carried out when significant and/or progressive deterioration is evident before it becomes an emergency, and the second operation, when carried out on an elective basis, may be associated with a surgical mortality in the range of 10 to 15 per cent. Color Doppler echocardiography with two-dimensional imaging is extremely helpful in the early detection of bioprosthetic malfunction.[555] Transesophageal echocardiography is more sensitive than transthoracic imaging in detecting bioprosthetic valve deterioration. Even patients without new murmurs or other physical findings of valve dysfunction should have routine echocardiographic studies to look for early bioprosthetic valve dysfunction every year for 5 years after valve replacement and every 6 months beginning 8 years after surgery.

The time after implantation at which tissue valves fail varies inversely with age: It is prohibitively rapid in children and adults under 35 to 40 years of age. Therefore, bioprostheses are not advisable in these patient groups. On the other hand, degeneration is extremely rare when these valves are implanted into patients older than 70 years.[558] Bioprostheses also have extremely limited desirability in patients with chronic renal failure and hypercalcemia related to secondary hyperparathyroidism.

Prosthetic valve endocarditis, discussed on pp. 1079 to 1080, is a serious, often grave illness.

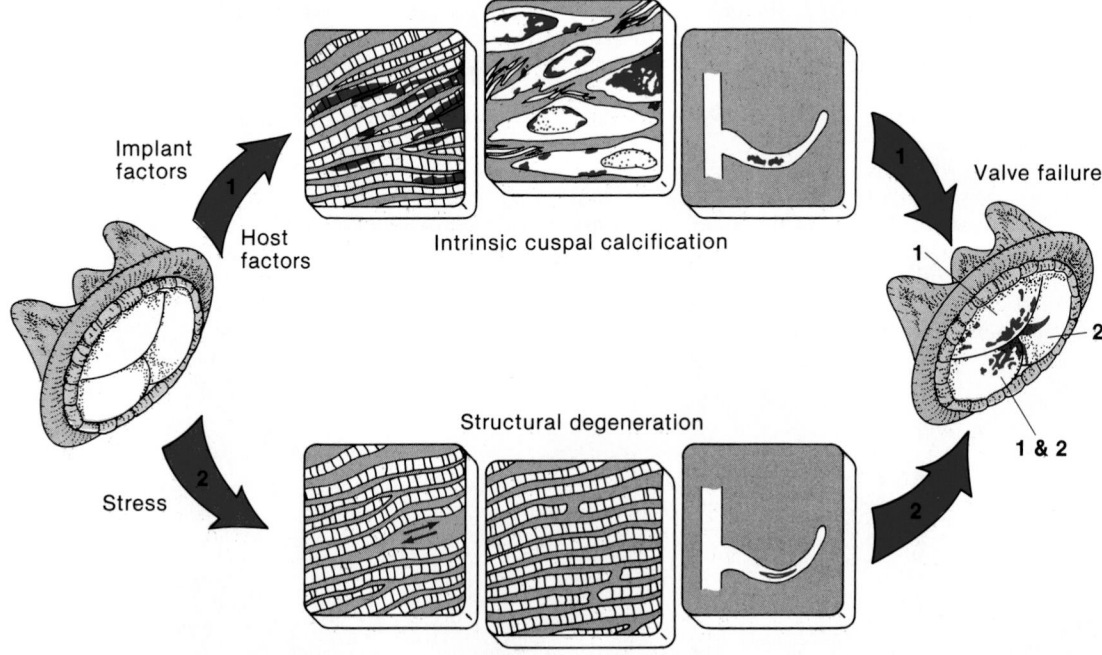

FIGURE 32–52. Unified model for bioprosthetic heart valve failure relating isolated tissue processes of mineralization and collagen degeneration to gross clinical failures. Such failures have calcification with cuspal stiffening (1), cuspal defects without calcific deposits (2), or cuspal tears associated with mineralization (1 and 2). These processes may occur independently or they may be synergistic. Specifically, implant and host factors interact to induce the collagen-oriented and cell-oriented calcific deposits noted ultrastructurally. The deposits predominate in the central portions of valve cusps, particularly at flexion points such as the commissures (Pathway 1). Stress causes shear between and fracture of collagen fibers, which may create gross cuspal defects (Pathway 2). Although dynamic mechanical activity is not a prerequisite for calcification, stress may promote (i.e., accelerate) this process through unknown mechanisms. (Amended from Schoen, F. I., and Levy, R. J.: Bioprosthetic heart valve failure: Pathology and pathogenesis. Cardiol. Clin. 2:717, 1984.)

HOMOGRAFT (ALLOGRAFT) AORTIC VALVES. These are harvested from cadavers, often along with kidneys, and are now usually preserved at $-196°C$ (Fig. 32-51D). They are inserted directly—usually in the aortic position—without being placed into a prosthetic stent. Their hemodynamics are superior to those of stented porcine valves. Like porcine xenografts, their thrombogenicity is low, but they appear to be subject to a similar rate of structural deterioration.[552] Homograft aortic valves are indicated in the presence of native or prosthetic valve endocarditis, but they are difficult to use when the aortic root and ascending aorta are greatly enlarged. Availability is often limited.[560,561]

PULMONARY AUTOGRAFTS. The patient's own pulmonary valve and adjacent main pulmonary artery are removed and used to replace the diseased aortic valve and often the neighboring aorta with reimplantation of the coronary arteries into the graft[562-564] (Fig. 32-51E). A human pulmonary or aortic homograft is then inserted into the pulmonary position. The autograft is nonthrombogenic and there is evidence in children and adolescents that it grows along with the patient; the risk of endocarditis is very low, anticoagulants are not required, and perhaps most important the long-term durability appears to be excellent.[565-567] While the pulmonary autograft is the replacement valve of choice in children, adolescents, and younger adults who have a long (>20 year) life expectancy, its use has been limited because the operation is technically much more complex than a simple aortic valve replacement. It should be carried out only by experienced surgeons.

HEMODYNAMICS OF VALVE REPLACEMENTS

The most commonly used prosthetic valves, mechanical prostheses and stented porcine xenografts, have an effective in vitro orifice size that is *smaller* than the normal valve at the same site.[568] (Unstented, i.e., free, homografts and pulmonary autografts have this problem.) After implantation, tissue ingrowth and endothelialization reduce the size of the in vivo effective orifice further. Therefore, the valves currently available must be considered to be mildly stenotic. However, postoperative hemodynamic measurements of the rigid prostheses show reasonably good function, with effective mitral valve orifice areas averaging 1.7 to 2.0 cm^2 and mitral valve gradients of 4 to 8 mm Hg at rest. The cloth-covered Starr-Edwards valve appears to be intrinsically slightly more stenotic than the Medtronic-Hall or Omniscience tilting-disc valves. The bileaflet St. Jude and Carbomedics valves, in turn, may be slightly superior to the latter. In hemodynamic studies, the porcine mitral valves behave in a manner similar to that of a mechanical prosthetic valve of the same diameter. Serious hemodynamic obstruction of an artificial valve (most commonly Starr-Ed-

wards) in the mitral position is quite uncommon, unless the valve is placed into a small left ventricular cavity or into an unusually small mitral annulus or unless the prosthesis chosen is inappropriate in size.

The problem of intrinsic stenosis may be more serious in patients who undergo aortic valve replacements for AS. The annulus into which the prosthesis is inserted in these patients is usually smaller than it is in patients with AR, and the surgeon may be forced to select an artificial valve of relatively small size. As a consequence, aortic valve replacement may not abolish obstruction in AS but may merely convert severe obstruction to a mild or moderate type. When the smaller models of the porcine xenograft or mechanical prosthesis are placed into the aortic position, effective orifice areas of about 1.1 to 1.3 cm^2 are common. In such patients, peak transvalvular gradients as high as 40 mm Hg during exercise have been recorded. It is possible that the poor late results observed in a minority of patients undergoing replacement of stenotic aortic valves may be the delayed effects of moderate stenosis of the prosthesis. In patients with AS who do not exhibit clinical improvement postoperatively, it is important to evaluate the function of both the prosthetic valve and the left ventricle. Rarely, reoperation to correct a malfunctioning prosthesis may be necessary.

SELECTION OF AN ARTIFICIAL VALVE

Most comparisons of mechanical and bioprostheses indicate similar overall results in terms of early and late mortality, prosthetic valve endocarditis and other complications, and the need for reoperation, at least for the first 5 years postoperatively. As indicated, there appear to be no significant differences insofar as hemodynamics are concerned, except that in patients with an unusually small left ventricular cavity or mitral or aortic annulus, the low-profile (tilting-disc) St. Jude or Carbomedics prosthesis or a tissue valve may perform better than other valves.[568,569] Patients with small aortic annuli may be better candidates for unstented homografts, heterografts, or pulmonary autografts.

The major task in selection of an artifical valve is to weigh the advantage of durability and the disadvantages of the risk of thromboembolism and of anticoagulant treatment inherent in mechanical prostheses on the one hand with the advantage of low thrombogenicity and the serious disadvantage of abbreviated durability of the bioprostheses on the other. Hammermeister et al.[570] has compared the outcome in 575 men who were randomized to replacement of the mitral or aortic valve with a mechanical versus a bioprosthetic valve. There was no difference in survival or in the probability of developing a valve-related complica-

TABLE 32-11 PROBABILITY OF DEATH DUE TO ANY CAUSE, ANY VALVE-RELATED COMPLICATION, AND INDIVIDUAL VALVE-RELATED COMPLICATIONS 11 YEARS AFTER RANDOMIZATION, ACCORDING TO TYPE AND LOCATION OF REPLACEMENT VALVE

EVENT	AORTIC VALVE		MITRAL VALVE	
	Mechanical Prosthesis (N = 198)	Bioprosthesis (N = 196)	Mechanical Prosthesis (N = 88)	Bioprosthesis (N = 93)
Death from any cause	0.53	0.59	0.64	0.67
Any valve-related complication	0.62	0.64	0.71	0.79
Systemic embolism	0.16	0.15	0.18	0.15
Bleeding	0.43	0.24*	0.41	0.28†
Endocarditis	0.07	0.08	0.11	0.17
Valve thrombosis	0.02	0.01	0.01	0.01
Perivalvular regurgitation	0.04	0.02	0.17	0.09†
Reoperation	0.07	0.16	0.21	0.47
Structural valve failure	0.00	0.15*	0.00	0.36*

P values are for the difference in the probability of event-free survival between patients with a mechanical prosthesis and those with a bioprosthesis at each site: *$P < 0.001$; †$P < 0.05$.

From Hammermeister, K. E., Sethi, G. K., Henderson, W. G., et al.: A comparison of outcomes in men 11 years after heart-valve replacement with a mechanical valve or bioprosthesis. N. Engl. J. Med. *328*:1289, 1993. Copyright 1993 Massachusetts Medical Society.

tion, including endocarditis, valve thrombosis, and systemic embolism. The rate of structurally-related valve failure requiring reoperation (which is associated with about twice the mortality of the initial procedure) was much higher in patients receiving tissue as opposed to mechanical valves. On the other hand, as anticipated, anticoagulant-related bleeding was higher in patients receiving mechanical valves. The latter also had a higher incidence of perivalvular regurgitation in the mitral position (Table 32–11). In the Edinburgh randomized trial, which also compared a mechanical with a porcine xenograft valve,[571] actuarial survival tended to be better and the freedom from all valve-related adverse events was significantly better with mechanical valves. Therefore, mechanical prostheses, usually of the bileaflet variety, are the valves of choice in the majority of patients. However, the following groups of patients should receive bioprostheses: (1) patients with coexisting disease who are prone to hemorrhage, such as those with bleeding disorders, intestinal polyposis, and angiodysplasia; (2) patients who are noncompliant with permanent anticoagulant treatment, who are unwilling to take anticoagulants on a regular basis, or who live in developing nations and cannot be monitored; (3) patients over the age of 65 to 70 years, in whom bioprosthetic valves deteriorate very slowly, who are unlikely to outlive their bioprostheses and who by reason of their age may also be at greater risk of hemorrhage while taking anticoagulants; (4) patients with a small aortic annulus in whom an unstented (free) autograft may provide superior hemodynamics; and (5) younger (<40 years) patients, especially women wishing to bear children, who require aortic valve replacement and in whom a pulmonary autograft may be preferable. However, the technical difficulties associated with the latter procedure must be taken into account.

Special Situations

PREGNANCY (see also p. 1856). Women with artificial valves can tolerate the hemodynamic burden of pregnancy well, but the hypercoagulable state of pregnancy increases the risk of thromboembolism in such patients with mechanical prostheses. Anticoagulation must not be interrupted, although an increased risk of fatal fetal hemorrhage is seen in those in whom it is continued. There is also a risk of fetal malformation caused by the probable teratogenic effect of warfarin. Although these problems represent arguments for the use of tissue valves in all women of childbearing age,[570,571] their limited durability in young adults makes their use unacceptable. Therefore, unless a pulmonary autograft can be employed (for patients who require aortic valve replacement), every effort should be made to defer valve replacement until after childbirth. In pregnant women with critical mitral or aortic stenosis, balloon valvuloplasty should be considered, and, if at all possible, mitral valve repair should be undertaken for patients with MR. Women of childbearing potential with a mechanical prosthesis should be counseled against pregnancy. When a woman in whom a mechanical prosthetic valve is already in place becomes pregnant, the risk to the fetus if the mother receives oral anticoagulants appears to be lower than the risk to the mother if anticoagulants are discontinued. Therefore, coumarin derivatives should be continued and the INR maintained between 2 and 3 until 2 weeks before expected delivery, when the patient should be switched to intravenous heparin.[570–572] Heparin should be discontinued at the onset of labor but may be restarted, along with coumarin, several hours after delivery.

NONCARDIAC SURGERY. When this is required in patients with prosthetic valves who are receiving anticoagulants, the risk is minimal when the drug regimen is stopped 1 to 3 days preoperatively and for a similar period postoperatively. It may be desirable, however, to protect the patient

with low molecular weight dextran during the perioperative period.

PATIENTS DESTINED TO RECEIVE ANTICOAGULANTS. Patients with earlier implantation of a mechanical prosthesis, chronic atrial fibrillation in the presence of an enlarged left atrium, a history of thromboembolism, or a thrombus in the left atrium at operation (and who therefore are destined to receive anticoagulants) should receive a mechanical prosthesis because the potential advantage of a tissue valve is negated.

CHILDREN AND PATIENTS RECEIVING CHRONIC HEMODIALYSIS. The high incidence of bioprosthetic valve failure in children and adolescents[573,574] and in patients on chronic hemodialysis virtually prohibits their use in these groups. In young adults between the ages of 25 and 35, the failure of bioprosthetic valves is somewhat higher than it is in older adults; this serves as a relative, but not an absolute, contraindication to their use in this age group.

In children, a mechanical prosthesis (generally the St. Jude valve) with its favorable hemodynamics is preferred despite the disadvantages inherent in anticoagulants in this age group.[575] Similarly, mechanical prostheses should be used in patients with chronic renal failure and/or hypercalcemia. Alternatively, if an experienced surgical team is available and the patient requires an aortic valve replacement, a pulmonary autograft may be employed.

TRICUSPID POSITION. The risk of thrombosis for all valves is highest in the tricuspid position because of the lower pressures and velocity of blood flow; this complication appears to be highest for tilting-disc valves, intermediate for caged-ball valves, and lowest for the bioprostheses, which are the valves of choice as tricuspid replacements. In the tricuspid position bioprostheses exhibit a much slower rate of mechanical deterioration than in the mitral or aortic position.

Detection of Prosthetic Valve Dysfunction

Artificial valves have distinctive auscultatory and phonocardiographic characteristics.[576] Transthoracic and transesophageal echocardiography, phonocardiography, and cineradiography are extremely useful in the identification of artificial valve dysfunction.[577,578] Two-dimensional and Doppler echocardiography are particularly useful in the follow-up of patients who demonstrate clinical deterioration in the postoperative period following porcine heterograft implantation. These techniques may prove capable of distinguishing between failure of a bioprosthesis (abnormal valve motion) and left ventricular dysfunction.

REFERENCES

MITRAL STENOSIS

1. Olson, L. J., Subramanian, R., and Ackermann, D. M.: Surgical pathology of the mitral valve: A study of 712 cases spanning 21 years. Mayo Clin. Proc. *62*:22, 1987.
2. Bortolotti, U., Valente, M., Agozzino, L., et al.: Rheumatoid mitral stenosis requiring valve replacement. Am. Heart J. *107*:1049, 1984.
3. Ladefoged, C., and Rohr, N.: Amyloid deposits in aortic and mitral valves. Virchows Arch. (A) *404*:301, 1984.
4. Misch, K. A.: Development of heart valve lesions during methylsergide therapy. Br. Med. J. *2*:365, 1974.
5. Wrisley, D., Giambartolomei, A., Lee, I., and Brownlee, W.: Left atrial ball thrombus: Review of clinical and echocardiographic manifestations with suggestions for management. Am. Heart. J. *121*:1784, 1991.
6. Kumar, A., Sinha, M., and Sinha, D. N. P.: Chronic rheumatic heart diseases in Ranchi. Angiology *33*:141, 1982.
7. Delahaye, F., Delahaye, J., Ecochard, R., et al.: Influence of associated valvular lesions on long-term prognosis of mitral stenosis: A 20-year follow-up of 202 patients. Eur. Heart J. *12*(Suppl B):77, 1991.
8. Schoen, F. J., and St. John Sutton, M.: Contemporary pathologic considerations in valvular disease. *In* Virmani, R., Atkinson, J. B., and Feuoglio, J. J. (eds.): Cardiovascular Pathology. Philadelphia, W. B. Saunders Co., 1991, p. 334.
9. Wells, F. C., and Shapiro, L. M. (eds.): Mitral Valve Disease. 2nd ed. London, Butterworths, 1996, 204 pp.
10. Bowe, J. C., Bland, F., Sprague, H. B., and White, P. D.: Course of mitral stenosis without surgery: 10 and 20 year perspectives. Ann. Intern. Med. *52*:741, 1960.

11. Bell, M. H., and Mintz, G. S.: Mitral valve disease in the elderly. *In* Frankl, W. S., and Brest, A. N. (eds.): Cardiovascular Clinics. Valvular Heart Disease: Comprehensive Evaluation and Management. Philadelphia, F. A. Davis, 1986, pp. 313–324.

12. Chopra, P., Tandon, H. D., Raizada, V., et al.: Comparative studies in mitral valves in rheumatic heart disease. Arch. Intern. Med. *143*:661, 1983.

12a. Kawanishi, D. T., and Rahimtoola, S. H.: Mitral stenosis. *In* Rahimtoola, S. H. (ed.): Valvular Heart Disease and Endocarditis. Atlas of Heart Diseases. Vol. 11. St. Louis, Mosby, 1996.

13. Dalen, J. E., and Alpert, J. S. (eds.): Valvular Heart Disease. 2nd ed. Boston, Little, Brown and Co., 1987, 600 pp.

14. Wood, P.: An appreciation of mitral stenosis. Br. Med. J. *1*:1051, and 1113, 1954.

15. Reichek, N., Shelburne, J. D., and Perloff, J. R.: Clinical aspects of rheumatic valvular disease. Prog. Cardiovasc. Dis. *15*:491, 1973.

15a. Grossman, W.: Profiles in valvular heart disease. *In* Baim, D. S., and Grossman, W. (eds.): Cardiac Catheterization, Angiography and Interventions. 5th ed. Baltimore, Williams and Wilkins, 1996, pp. 735–756.

16. Leavitt, J. L., Coats, M. H., and Falk, R. H.: Effects of exercise on transmitral gradient and pulmonary artery pressure in patients with mitral stenosis or a prosthetic mitral valve: A Doppler echocardiographic study. J. Am. Coll. Cardiol. *17*:1520, 1991.

17. Selzer, A.: Effects of atrial fibrillation upon the circulation in patients with mitral stenosis. Am. Heart J. *59*:518, 1960.

18. Gorlin, R., and Gorlin, S. G.: Hydraulic formula for calculation of the area of stenotic mitral valve, other cardiac valves and central circulatory shunts. Am. Heart J. *41*:1, 1951.

18a. Braunwald, E., and Turi, Z. G.: Pathophysiology of mitral valve disease. *In* Wells, F. C., and Shapiro, L. M. (eds.): Mitral Valve Disease. 2nd ed. London, Butterworths, 1996, pp. 28–36.

19. Ford, L. E., Feldman, T., and Carroll, J. D.: Valve resistance. Circulation *89*:893, 1994.

20. Kennedy, J. W.: The use of quantitative angiocardiography in mitral valve disease. *In* Duran, C., Angell, W. W., Johnson, A. D., and Oury, J. H. (eds.): Recent Progress in Mitral Valve Disease. London, Butterworths, 1984, pp. 149–159.

21. Gash, A. K., Carabello, B. A., Cepin, D., and Spann, J. F.: Left ventricular ejection performance and systolic muscle function in patients with mitral stenosis. Circulation *67*:148, 1983.

22. Colle, J. P., Rahal, S., Ohayon, J., et al.: Global left ventricular function and regional wall motion in pure mitral stenosis. Clin. Cardiol. *7*:573, 1984.

23. Gaasch, W. H., and Folland, E. D.: Left ventricular function in rheumatic mitral stenosis. Eur. Heart J. *12*(Suppl. B):66, 1991.

24. Harvey, R. M., Ferrer, M. I., Samet, P., et al.: Mechanical and myocardial factors in rheumatic heart disease in mitral stenosis. Circulation *11*:531, 1955.

25. Mohan, J. C., Khalilullah, M., and Arora, R.: Left ventricular intrinsic contractility in pure rheumatic mitral stenosis. Am. J. Cardiol. *64*:240, 1989.

26. Reis, R. N., and Roberts, W. C.: Amounts of coronary arterial narrowing by atherosclerotic plaques in clinically isolated mitral valve stenosis: Analysis of 76 necropsy patients older than 30 years. Am. J. Cardiol. *57*:1117, 1986.

27. Johnston, D. L., and Kotsuk, W. J.: Left and right ventricular function during symptom-limited exercise in patients with isolated mitral stenosis. Chest *89*:186, 1986.

28. Wroblewski, E., Spann, J. F., and Bove, A. A.: Right ventricular performance in mitral stenosis. Am. J. Cardiol. *47*:51, 1981.

29. Halperin, J. L., Brooks, K. M., Rothluf, E. B., et al.: Effect of nitroglycerin on the pulmonary venous gradient in patients after mitral valve replacement. J. Am. Coll. Cardiol. *5*:34, 1985.

30. Haworth, S. G., Hall, S. M., and Patel, M.: Peripheral pulmonary vascular and airway abnormalities in adolescents with rheumatic mitral stenosis. Int. J. Cardiol. *18*:405, 1988.

31. Babic, U. U., Popovic, Z., Grujicic, S., et al.: Systemic and pulmonary flow in mitral stenosis: Evidence for a bronchial vein shunt. Cardiology *78*:311, 1991.

32. Keren, G., Etzion, T., Sherez, J., et al.: Atrial fibrillation and atrial enlargement in patients with mitral stenosis. Am. Heart J. *114*:1146, 1987.

32a. Leatham, A.: Assessment of mitral valve function: clinical presentation, assessment and prognosis. *In* Wells, F. C., and Shapiro, L. M. (eds.): Mitral Valve Disease. 2nd ed. London, Butterworths, 1996, pp. 37–46.

33. Scarlat, A., Bodner, G., and Liron, M.: Massive haemoptysis as the presenting symptom in mitral stenosis. Thorax *41*:413, 1986.

34. Ohmichi, M., Tagaki, S., Nomura, N., et al.: Endobronchial changes in chronic pulmonary venous hypertension. Chest *94*:1127, 1988.

35. Baxter, R. H., Reid, J. M., McGuiness, J. B., and Stevenson, J. G.: Relation of angina to coronary artery disease in mitral and aortic valve disease. Br. Heart J. *40*:918, 1978.

36. Nielson, G. H., Galea, E. G., and Houssack, K. F.: Thromboembolic complications of mitral valve disease. Aust. N. Z. J. Med. *8*:372, 1978.

37. Lie, J. T., and Entmann, M. L.: "Hole-in-one" sudden death: Mitral stenosis and left atrial thrombus. Am. Heart J. *91*:798, 1976.

38. Sharma, N. G. K., Kapoor, C. P., Mahambre, L., and Borkar, M. P.: Ortner's syndrome. J. Indian Med. Assoc. *60*:427, 1973.

39. Horwitz, L. D., and Groves, B. M. (eds.): Signs and Symptoms in Cardiology. Philadelphia, J.B. Lippincott, 1985, 506 pp.

40. Abrams, J.: Mitral stenosis. *In* Essentials of Cardiac Physical Diagnosis. Philadelphia, Lea and Febiger, 1987, pp. 275–306.

41. Longhini, C., Baracca, E., Aggio, S., et al.: The first heart sound in mitral stenosis. Acta Cardiol. (Brux.) *46*:73, 1991.

42. Barrington, W. W., Boudoulas, J., Bashore, T., et al.: Mitral stenosis: Mitral dome excursion and M_1 and the mitral opening snap—the concept of reciprocal heart sounds. Am. Heart J. *115*:1280, 1988.

43. Perloff, J. K.: Auscultatory and phonocardiographic manifestations of pulmonary hypertension. Prog. Cardiovasc. Dis. *9*:303, 1967.

44. Saunders, J. L., Calatayud, J. B., Schultz, K. J., et al.: Evaluation of ECG criteria for P-wave abnormalities. Am. Heart J. *74*:757, 1967.

45. Walston, A., Harley, A., and Pipberger, H. V.: Computer analysis of the orthogonal electrocardiogram and vectorcardiogram in mitral stenosis. Circulation *50*:472, 1974.

46. Cooksey, J. D., Dunn, M., and Massie, E.: Clinical Vectorcardiography and Electrocardiography. 2nd ed. Chicago, Year Book Medical Publishers, 1977, p. 272.

47. Mounsey, P.: The atrial electrocardiogram as a guide to prognosis after mitral valvulotomy. Br. Heart J. *21*:617, 1961.

48. Probst, P., Goldschlager, N., and Selzer, A.: Left atrial size and atrial fibrillation in mitral stenosis: Factors influencing their relationship. Circulation *48*:1281, 1973.

49. Cueto, J., Toshima, J., Armyo, G., et al.: Vectorcardiographic studies in acquired valvular disease with reference to the diagnosis of right ventricular hypertrophy. Circulation *33*:588, 1967.

50. Taymor, R. C., Hoffman, I., and Henry, E.: The Frank vectorcardiogram in mitral stenosis. Circulation *30*:865, 1964.

51. Donoso, E., Jick, S., Braunwald, E., et al.: The spatial vectorcardiogram in mitral valve disease. Am. Heart J. *53*:760, 1957.

52. Melhem, R. E., Dunbar, J. D., and Booth, R. W.: "B" lines of Kerley and left atrial size in mitral valve disease: Their correlation with mean atrial pressure as measured by left atrial puncture. Radiology *76*:65, 1961.

53. Parker, B. M., Friedenberg, M. J., Templeton, A. W., and Burford, T. H.: Preoperative angiocardiographic diagnosis of left atrial thrombi in mitral stenosis. N. Engl. J. Med. *273*:136, 1965.

54. Rahimtoola, S. H.: Perspective on valvular heart disease: An update. J. Am. Coll. Cardiol. *14*:1, 1989.

55. Shapiro, L. M.: Echocardiography of the mitral valve. *In* Wells, F. C., and Shapiro, L. M. (eds.): Mitral Valve Disease. 2nd ed. London, Butterworths, 1996, pp. 47–50.

56. Shandheria, B. K., Tajik, A. J., Reeder, G. S., et al.: Doppler color flow imaging: A new technique for visualization and characterization of the blood flow jet in mitral stenosis. Mayo Clin. Proc. *61*:623, 1986.

57. Beiser, G. D., Epstein, S. E., Braunwald, E., et al.: Studies on digitalis. XVIII. Effects of ouabain on the hemodynamic response to exercise in patients with mitral stenosis in normal sinus rhythm. N. Engl. J. Med. *278*:131, 1968.

58. Klein, H. O., Sareli, P., Schamroth, C. L., et al.: Effects of atenolol on exercise capacity in patients with mitral stenosis with sinus rhythm. Am. J. Cardiol. *56*:598, 1985.

59. Kosakai, Y., Kawaguchi, A. T., Isobe, F., et al.: Cox maze procedure for chronic atrial fibrillation associated with mitral valve disease. J. Thorac. Cardiovasc. Surg. *108*:1049, 1994.

60. Shyu, K. G., Cheng, J. J., Chen, J. J., et al.: Recovery of atrial function after atrial compartment operation for chronic atrial fibrillation in mitral valve disease. J. Am. Coll. Cardiol. *24*:392, 1994.

61. Chua, Y. L., Schaff, H. V., Orszulak, T. A., and Morris, J. J.: Outcome of mitral valve repair in patients with preoperative atrial fibrillation: Should the maze procedure be combined with mitral valvuloplasty? J. Thorac. Cardiovasc. Surg. *107*:408, 1994.

62. Joswig, B. C., Glover, M. U., Handler, J. B., et al.: Contrasting progression of mitral stenosis in the Malayans versus American-born Caucasians. Am. Heart J. *104*:1400, 1982.

63. Olesen, K. H.: The natural history of 271 patients with mitral stenosis under medical treatment. Br. Heart J. *24*:349, 1962.

64. Rowe, J. C., Bland, E. F., Sprague, H. B., and White, P. D.: The course of mitral stenosis without surgery: Ten- and twenty-year perspectives. Ann. Intern. Med. *52*:741, 1960.

65. Munoz, S., Gallardo, J., Diaz-Gorrin, J. R., and Medina, O.: Influence of surgery on the natural history of rheumatic mitral and aortic valve disease. Am. J. Cardiol. *35*:234, 1975.

66. Rapaport, E.: Natural history of aortic and mitral valve disease. Am. J. Cardiol. *35*:221, 1975.

67. Sutton, M. J. St. J., Oldershaw, P., Sacchetti, R., et al.: Valve replacement without preoperative cardiac catheterization. N. Engl. J. Med. *305*:1233, 1981.

68. Slater, J., Gindea, A. J., Freedberg, R. S., et al.: Comparison of cardiac catheterization and Doppler echocardiography in the decision to operate in aortic and mitral valve disease. J. Am. Coll. Cardiol. *17*:1026, 1991.

69. O'Rourke, R. A.: Preoperative cardiac catheterization. Its need in most patients with valvular heart disease. JAMA *248*:745, 1982.

70. Ramsdale, D. R., Faragher, E. B., Bennett, D. H., et al.: Preoperative prediction of significant coronary artery disease in patients with valvular heart disease. Br. Med. J. *284*:223, 1982.

71. Gautam, P. C., Coulshed, N., Epstein, E. J., et al.: Preoperative clinical predictors of long-term survival in mitral stenosis: Analysis of 200 cases followed for up to 27 years after closed mitral valvotomy. Thorax *41*:401, 1986.

72. English, T.: Closed mitral valvotomy. *In* Wells, F. C., and Shapiro, L. M. (eds.): Mitral Valve Disease. 2nd ed. London, Butterworths, 1996, pp. 107–113.

73. de Vivie, E. R., and Hellberg, K.: Closed transventricular mitral commissurotomy. *In* Ionescu, M. I., and Cohn, L. H. (eds.): Mitral Valve Disease: Diagnosis and Treatment. London, Butterworths, 1985, pp. 139–152.

74. Duran, C.: Mitral reconstruction in predominant mitral stenosis. *In* Duran, C., Angell, W. W., Johnson, A. D., and Oury, J. H. (eds.): Recent Progress in Mitral Valve Disease. London, Butterworths, 1984, pp. 255–264.

75. Farhat, M. B., Boussadia, H., Gandjbakhch, I., et al.: Closed versus open mitral commissurotomy in pure noncalcific mitral stenosis: Hemodynamic studies before and after operation. J. Thorac. Cardiovasc. Surg. *99*:639, 1990.

76. Cohn, L. H., Allred, E. N., Cohn, L. A., et al.: Long-term results of open mitral valve reconstruction for mitral stenosis. Am. J. Cardiol. *55*:731, 1985.

77. John, S., Bashi, V. V., Jairaj, P. S., et al.: Closed mitral valvotomy: Early results and long-term follow-up of 3724 consecutive patients. Circulation *68*:891, 1983.

78. Cohen, D. J., Kuntz, R. E., Gordon, S. P. F., et al.: Predictors of long-term outcome after percutaneous balloon mitral valvuloplasty. N. Engl. J. Med. *327*:1329, 1992.

79. Hickey, M. S., Blackstone, E. H., Kirklin, J. W., and Dean, L. S.: Outcome probabilities and life history after surgical mitral commissurotomy: Implications for balloon commissurotomy. J. Am. Coll. Cardiol. *17*:29, 1991.

80. Eguaras, M. G., Luque, I., Montero, A., et al.: Conservative operation for mitral stenosis: Independent determinants of late results. J. Thorac. Cardiovasc. Surg. *95*:1031, 1988.

81. Gross, R. J., Cunningham, J. N., Jr., Snively, S. L., et al.: Long-term results of open radical mitral commissurotomy: Ten year follow-up study of 202 patients. Am. J. Cardiol. *47*:821, 1981.

82. Kirklin, J. W., and Barrat-Boyes, B. G.: Mitral commissurotomy. *In* Cardiac Surgery. 2nd ed. New York, Churchill-Livingstone, 1993, p. 444.

83. Aora, R., Khalilullah, M., Gupta, M. P., and Padmavati, S.: Mitral restenosis. Incidence and epidemiology. Indian Heart J. *30*:265, 1978.

84. Heger, J. J., Wann, L. S., Weyman, A. E., et al.: Long-term changes in mitral valve area after successful mitral commissurotomy. Circulation *59*:443, 1979.

85. Higgs, L. M., Glancy, D. L., O'Brien, K. P., et al.: Mitral restenosis: An uncommon cause of recurrent symptoms following mitral commissurotomy. Am. J. Cardiol. *26*:34, 1970.

86. Braunwald, E., Braunwald, N. S., Ross, J., Jr., and Morrow, A. G.: Effects of mitral valve replacement on the pulmonary vascular dynamics of patients with pulmonary hypertension. N. Engl. J. Med. *273*:509, 1965.

87. Foltz, B. D., Hessel, E. A., and Ivey, T. D.: The early course of pulmonary artery hypertension in patients undergoing mitral valve replacement with cardioplegic arrest. J. Thorac. Cardiovasc. Surg. *88*:238, 1984.

88. Shapiro, L. M.: Balloon dilatation of the stenotic mitral valve. *In* Wells, F. C., and Shapiro, L. M. (eds.): Mitral Valve Disease. London, Butterworths, 1996, pp. 181–186.

89. Palacios, I. F., Tuzeu, M. E., Weyman, A. E., et al.: Clinical follow-up of patients undergoing percutaneous mitral balloon valvotomy. Circulation *91*:671, 1995.

90. Chen, C-R., and Cheng, T. O.: Percutaneous balloon mitral valvuloplasty by the Inoue technique: A multicenter study of 4832 patients in China. Am. Heart J. *129*:1197, 1995.

90a. Berman, A. D., McKay, R. G., and Grossman, W.: Balloon valvuloplasty. *In* Baim, D. S., and Grossman, W. (eds.): Cardiac Catheterization, Angiography and Intervention. 2nd ed. Baltimore, Williams and Wilkins, 1996, pp. 659–688.

91. L'Epine, Y., Drobinski, G., Sotirov, Y., et al.: Right heart failure due to an inter-atrial shunt after percutaneous mitral balloon dilatation. Eur. Heart J. *10*:285, 1989.

92. Fawzy, M. E., Mimish, L., Sivanandam, V., et al.: Immediate and long-term effect of mitral balloon valvotomy on severe pulmonary hypertension in patients with mitral stenosis. Am. Heart J. *131*:89, 1996.

93. Wilkins, G. T., Weyman, A. E., Abascal, V. M., et al.: Percutaneous mitral valvotomy: An analysis of echocardiographic variables related to outcome and the mechanism of dilatation. Br. Heart. J. *60*:299, 1988.

94. Tuzcu, E. M., Block, P. C., Griffin, B., et al.: Percutaneous mitral balloon valvotomy in patients with calcific mitral stenosis: Immediate and long-term outcome. J. Am. Coll. Cardiol. *23*:1604, 1994.

95. Reyes, V. P., Raju, B. S., Wynne, J., et al.: Percutaneous balloon valvuloplasty compared with open surgical commissurotomy for mitral stenosis. N. Engl. J. Med. *331*:961, 1994.

96. Post, J. R., Feldman, T., Isner, J., and Herrmann, H. C.: Inoue balloon mitral valvotomy in patients with severe valvular and subvalvular deformity. J. Am. Coll. Cardiol. *25*:1129, 1995.

96a. Trevino, A. J., Ibarra, M., Garcia, A., et al.: Immediate and long-term results of balloon mitral commissurotomy for rheumatic mitral stenosis: Comparison between Inoue and double-balloon techniques. Am. Heart J. *131*:530, 1996.

97. Iung, B., Cormier, B., Elias, J., et al.: Usefulness of percutaneous balloon commissurotomy for mitral stenosis during pregnancy. Am. J. Cardiol. *73*:398, 1994.

98. Zhang, H. P., Allen, J. W., Lau, F. Y. K., and Ruiz, C. E.: Immediate and late outcome of percutaneous balloon mitral valvotomy in patients with significantly calcified valves. Am. Heart J. *129*:501, 1995.

98a. Carabello, B.: Mitral regurgitation. *In* Rahimtoola, S. H. (ed.): Valvular Heart Disease and Endocarditis. Atlas of Heart Diseases. Vol. 11. St. Louis, Mosby, 1996.

MITRAL REGURGITATION

99. Davies, M. J.: Aetiology and pathology of the diseased mitral valve. *In* Ionescu, M. I., and Cohn, L. H. (eds.): Mitral Valve Disease: Diagnosis and Treatment. London, Butterworths, 1985, pp. 27–42.

99a. Anderson, R. H., and Wilcox, B. R.: The anatomy of the mitral valve. *In* Wells, F. C., and Shapiro, L. M. (eds.): Mitral Valve Disease. 2nd ed. London, Butterworths, 1996, pp. 4–13.

100. Marcus, R. H., Sareli, P., Pocock, W. A., and Barlow, J. B.: The spectrum of severe rheumatic mitral valve disease in a developing country: Correlations among clinical presentation, surgical pathologic findings, and hemodynamic sequelae. Ann. Intern. Med. *120*:177, 1994.

101. Essop, M. R., Skoularigis, J., and Sareli, P.: Transesophageal echocardiography in congenital submitral aneurysm. Am. J. Cardiol. *71*:481, 1993.

102. Boltwood, C. M., Tei, C., Wong, M., and Shah, P. M.: Quantitative echocardiography of the mitral complex in dilated cardiomyopathy: The mechanism of functional mitral regurgitation. Circulation *68*:498, 1983.

103. Keren, G., Sonnenblick, E. H., and LeJemtel, T. H.: Mitral annulus motion: Relation to pulmonary venous and transmitral flows in normal subjects and in patients with dilated cardiomyopathy. Circulation *78*:621, 1988.

103a. Mann, J. M., and Davies, M. J.: The pathology of the mitral valve. *In* Wells, F. C., and Shapiro, L. M. (eds.): Mitral Valve Disease. 2nd ed. London, Butterworths, 1996, pp. 16–27.

104. Nestico, P. F., DePace, N. L., Kotler, M. N., et al.: Calcium phosphorus metabolism in dialysis patients with and without mitral anular calcium. Analysis of 30 patients. Am. J. Cardiol. *51*:497, 1983.

105. Mellino, M., Salcedo, E. E., Lever, H. M., et al.: Echographic-quantified severity of mitral annulus calcification: Prognostic correlation to related hemodynamic, valvular, rhythm, and conduction abnormalities. Am. Heart J. *103*:222, 1982.

106. Scott-Jupp, W., Barnett, N. L., Gallagher, P. J., et al.: Ultrastructural changes in spontaneous rupture of mitral chordae tendineae. J. Pathol. *133*:185, 1981.

107. Oliveira, D. B. G., Dawkins, K. D., Kay, P. H., and Paneth, M.: Chordal rupture I: Aetiology and natural history. Br. Heart J. *50*:312, 1983.

108. Hickey, A. J., Wilcken, D. E. L., Wright, J. S. and Warren, B. A.: Primary (spontaneous) chordal rupture: Relation to myxomatous valve disease and mitral valve prolapse. J. Am. Coll. Cardiol. *5*:1341, 1985.

109. Godley, R. W., Wann, L. S., Rogers, E. W., et al.: Incomplete mitral leaflet closure in patients with papillary muscle dysfunction. Circulation *63*:565, 1981.

110. Izumi, S., Miyatake, K., Beppu, S., et al.: Mechanism of mitral regurgitation in patients with myocardial infarction: A study using real-time two-dimensional Doppler flow imaging and echocardiography. Circulation *76*:777, 1987.

111. Ballester, M., Jajoo, J., Rees, S., et al.: The mechanism of mitral regurgitation in dilated left ventricle. Clin. Cardiol. *6*:333, 1983.

112. Tcheng, J. E., Jackman, J. D., Nelson, C. L., et al.: Outcome of patients sustaining acute ischemic mitral regurgitation during myocardial infarction. Ann. Intern. Med. *117*:18, 1992.

113. Hickey, M. St. J., Smith, L. R., Muhlbaier, L. H., et al.: Current prognosis of ischemic mitral regurgitation: Implications for future management. Circulation *78*(Suppl. I):I51, 1988.

114. Gottdiener, J. S., Maron, B. J., Schooley, R. T., et al.: Two-dimensional echocardiographic assessment of the idiopathic hypereosinophilic syndrome. Anatomic basis of mitral regurgitation and peripheral embolization. Circulation *67*:572, 1983.

115. Metras, D., Ouezzin-Coulibaly, A., Ouattara, K., et al.: Endomyocardial fibrosis masquerading as rheumatic mitral incompetence. A report of six surgical cases. J. Thorac. Cardiovasc. Surg. *86*:753, 1983.

116. Mazzucco, A., Rizzoli, G., Faggian, G., et al.: Acute mitral regurgitation after blunt chest trauma. Arch. Intern. Med. *143*:2326, 1983.

117. Jolly, D. T.: Traumatic rupture of a papillary muscle of the mitral valve due to blunt thoracic trauma. Can. Fam. Phys. *29*:1960, 1983.

118. Gidding, S. S., Shulman, S. T., Ibawi, M., et al.: Mucocutaneous lymph node syndrome (Kawasaki disease): Delayed aortic and mitral insufficiency secondary to active valvulitis. J. Am. Coll. Cardiol. *7*:894, 1986.

119. DiSegni, E., and Edwards, J. E.: Cleft anterior leaflet of the mitral valve with intact septa. A study of 20 cases. Am. J. Cardiol. *51*:919, 1983.

120. Nagata, S., Nimura, Y., Sakakibara, H., et al.: Mitral valve lesion associated with secundum atrial septal defect. Analysis of real-time two-dimensional echocardiography. Br. Heart J. *49*:151, 1983.

121. Eckberg, D. L., Gault, J. H., Bouchard, R. L., et al.: Mechanics of left ventricular contraction in chronic severe mitral regurgitation. Circulation *47*:1252, 1973.

122. Braunwald, E., Welch, G. H., Jr., and Sarnoff, S. J.: Hemodynamic effects of quantitatively varied experimental mitral regurgitation. Circ. Res. *5*:539, 1957.

123. Braunwald, E., and Turi, Z. G.: Pathophysiology of mitral valve disease. *In* Ionescu, M. I., and Cohn, L. H. (eds.): Mitral Valve Disease: Diagnosis and Treatment. London, Butterworths, 1985, pp. 3–10.

124. Yellin, E. L., Yoran, C., Frater, R. W. M., and Sonnenblick, E. H.: Dynamics of acute experimental mitral regurgitation. In Ionescu, M. I., and Cohn, L. H. (eds.): Mitral Valve Disease: Diagnosis and Treatment. London, Butterworths, 1985, pp. 11–26.

125. Braunwald, E.: Mitral regurgitation: Physiological, clinical and surgical considerations. N. Engl. J. Med. 281:425, 1969.

126. Corin, W. J., Monrad, E. S., Murakami, T., et al.: The relationship of afterload to ejection performance in chronic mitral regurgitation. Circulation 76:59, 1987.

127. Nwasokwa, O., Camesas, A., Weg, I., and Bodenheimer, M. M.: Differences in left ventricular adaptation to chronic mitral and aortic regurgitation. Chest 95:106, 1989.

128. Knotos, G. J., Jr., Schaff, H. V., Gersh, B. J., and Bove, A. A.: Left ventricular function in subacute and chronic mitral regurgitation: Effect on function early postoperatively. J. Thorac. Cardiovasc. Surg. 98:163, 1989.

129. Keren, G., Katz, S., Strom, J., et al.: Dynamic mitral regurgitation: An important determinant of the hemodynamic response to load alterations and inotropic therapy in severe heart failure. Circulation 80:306, 1989.

130. Essop, M. R., Wisenbaugh, T., and Sareli, P.: Evidence against a myocardial factor as the cause of left ventricular dilation in active rheumatic carditis. J. Am. Coll. Cardiol. 22:826, 1993.

131. Urschel, C. W., Covell, J. W., Graham, T. P., et al.: Effects of acute valvular regurgitation on the oxygen consumption of the canine heart. Circ. Res. 23:33, 1968.

132. Braunwald, E.: Control of myocardial oxygen consumption: Physiologic and clinical considerations. Am. J. Cardiol. 27:416, 1971.

133. Corin, W. J., Murakami, T., Monrad, E. S., et al.: Left ventricular passive diastolic properties in chronic mitral regurgitation. Circulation 83:797, 1991.

134. Ross, J., Jr.: Left ventricular function and the timing of surgical treatment in valvular heart disease. Ann. Intern. Med. 94:498, 1981.

135. Mirsky, I., Corin, W. J., Murakami, T., et al.: Correction for preload in assessment of myocardial contractility in aortic and mitral valve disease: Application of the concept of systolic myocardial stiffness. Circulation 78:68, 1988.

136. Enriquez-Sarano, M., Tajik, A. K., Schaff, H. V., et al.: Echocardiographic prediction of survival after surgical correction of organic mitral regurgitation. Circulation 90:830, 1994.

137. Ramanthan, K. B., Knowles, J., Connor, M. J., et al.: Natural history of chronic mitral insufficiency: Relation of peak systolic pressure/end-systolic volume ratio to morbidity and mortality. J. Am. Coll. Cardiol. 3:1412, 1984.

138. Borow, K., Green, L. H., Mann, T., et al.: End-systolic volume as a predictor of postoperative left ventricular performance in volume overload from valvular regurgitation. Am. J. Med. 68:655, 1980.

139. Mudge, G. H.: Asymptomatic mitral regurgitation. J. Cardiovasc. Surg. 9(Suppl.):248, 1994.

140. Wisenbaugh, T., Spann, J. F., and Carabello, B. A.: Differences in myocardial performance and load between patients with similar amounts of chronic aortic versus chronic mitral regurgitation. J. Am. Coll. Cardiol. 3:913, 1984.

141. Wisenbaugh, T., Skudicky, D., and Sareli, P.: Prediction of outcome after valve replacement for rheumatic mitral regurgitation in the era of chordal preservation. Circulation 89:191, 1994.

142. Boucher, C. A., Bingham, J. B., Osbakken, M. D., et al.: Early changes in left ventricular size and function after correction of left ventricular volume overload. Am. J. Cardiol. 47:991, 1981.

143. Grose, R., Strain, J., and Cohen, M. V.: Pulmonary arterial V waves in mitral regurgitation. Clinical and experimental observations. Circulation 69:214, 1984.

143a. Schofield, P. M.: Invasive investigation of the mitral valve. In Wells, F. C., and Shapiro, L. M. (eds.): Mitral Valve Disease. 2nd ed. London, Butterworths, 1996, pp. 84–91.

144. Kihara, Y., Sasayama, S., Miyazaki, S., et al.: Role of the left atrium in adaptation of the heart to chronic mitral regurgitation in conscious dogs. Circ. Res. 62:543, 1988.

145. Pape, L. A., Price, J. M., Alpert, J. S., et al.: Relation of left atrial size to pulmonary capillary wedge pressure in severe mitral regurgitation. Cardiology 78:297, 1991.

146. Braunwald, E., and Awe, W. C.: The syndrome of severe mitral regurgitation with normal left atrial pressure. Circulation 27:29, 1963.

147. Roberts, W. C., Braunwald, E., and Morrow, A. G.: Acute severe mitral regurgitation secondary to ruptured chordae tendineae. Clinical, hemodynamic and pathologic considerations. Circulation 33:58, 1966.

148. Cohen, L. S., Mason, D. T., and Braunwald, E.: Significance of an atrial gallop sound in mitral regurgitation: A clue to the diagnosis of ruptured chordae tendineae. Circulation 35:112, 1966.

149. Rippe, J. M., and Howe, J. P., III: Acute mitral regurgitation. In Dalen, J. E., and Alpert, J. S. (eds.): Valvular Heart Disease. 2nd ed. Boston, Little, Brown and Co., 1987, pp. 151–176.

150. Rosen, S. F., Borer, J. S., Hochreiter, C., et al.: Natural history of the asymptomatic patient with severe mitral regurgitation secondary to mitral valve prolapse and normal right and left ventricular performance. Am. J. Cardiol. 74:374, 1994.

151. Elkins, R. C., Morrow, A. G., Vasko, J. S., and Braunwald, E.: The effects of mitral regurgitation on the pattern of instantaneous aortic blood flow. Clinical and experimental observations. Circulation 36:45, 1967.

152. Basta, L. L., Wolfson, P., Eckberg, D. L., and Abboud, F. M.: The value of left parasternal impulse recordings in the assessment of mitral regurgitation. Circulation 48:1055, 1973.

153. Barlow, J. B.: Mitral regurgitation. In Perspectives on the Mitral Valve. Philadelphia, F. A. Davis Co., 1987, pp. 113–131.

154. Haffajee, C. I.: Chronic mitral regurgitation. In Dalen, J. E., and Alpert, J. S. (eds.): Valvular Heart Disease. 2nd ed. Boston, Little, Brown and Co., 1987, pp. 111–150.

155. Karliner, J. S., O'Rourke, R. A., Kearney, D. J., and Shabetai, R.: Haemodynamic explanation of why the murmur of mitral regurgitation is independent of cycle length. Br. Heart J. 35:397, 1973.

156. Schreiber, T. L., Fisher, J., Mangla, A., and Miller, D.: Severe "silent" mitral regurgitation: A potentially reversible cause of refractory heart failure. Chest 96:242, 1989.

157. Antman, E. M., Angoff, G. H., and Sloss, J. J.: Demonstration of the mechanism by which mitral regurgitation mimics aortic stenosis. Am. J. Cardiol. 42:1044, 1978.

158. Merendino, K. A., and Hessel, E. A.: The murmur on top of the head in acquired mitral insufficiency. JAMA. 199:392, 1967.

159. Morris, J. J., Estes, E. H., Whalen, R. E., et al.: P wave analysis in valvular heart disease. Circulation 29:242, 1964.

160. Priest, E. A., Finlayson, J. K., and Short, D. S.: The x-ray manifestations in the heart and lungs of mitral regurgitation. Prog. Cardiovasc. Dis. 5:219, 1962.

161. Wexler, L., Silverman, J. F., DeBusk, R. F., and Harrison, D. C.: Angiographic features of rheumatic and nonrheumatic mitral regurgitation. Circulation 44:1080, 1971.

162. Globits, S., and Higgins, C. B.: Assessment of valvular heart disease by magnetic resonance imaging. Am. Heart J. 129:369, 1995.

162a. Manzara, C. C., Pennell, D. J., and Underwood, S. R.: Assessment of the mitral valve by magnetic resonance imaging. In Wells, F. C., and Shapiro, L. M. (eds.): Mitral Valve Disease. 2nd ed. London, Butterworths, 1996, pp. 71–83.

163. Himelman, R. B., Kusumoto, F., Oken, K., et al.: The flail mitral valve: Echocardiographic findings by precordial and transesophageal imaging and Doppler color flow mapping. J. Am. Coll. Cardiol. 17:272, 1991.

164. Nair, C. K., Aronow, W. S., Sketch, M. H., et al.: Clinical and echocardiographic characteristics of patients with mitral annular calcification. Am. J. Cardiol. 51:992, 1983.

165. Jenni, R., Ritter, M., Eberli, F., et al.: Quantification of mitral regurgitation with amplitude-weighted mean velocity from continuous wave Doppler spectra. Circulation 79:1294, 1989.

166. Krivokapich, J.: Echocardiography in valvular heart disease. Curr. Opin. Cardiol. 9:158, 1994.

167. Mele, D., Vandervoort, P., Palacios, I., et al.: Proximal jet size by Doppler color flow mapping predicts severity of mitral regurgitation. Circulation 91:746, 1995.

168. Shyu, K., Lei, M., Hwang, J., et al.: Morphologic characterization and quantitative assessment of mitral regurgitation with ruptured chordae tendineae by transesophageal echocardiography. Am. J. Cardiol. 70:1152, 1992.

169. Smith, M. D., Cassidy, J. M., Gurley, J. C., et al.: Echo Doppler evaluation of patients with acute mitral regurgitation: Superiority of transesophageal echocardiography with color flow imaging. Am. Heart. J. 129:967, 1995.

169a. Bach, D.-S., Deeb, G. M., and Bolling, S. F.: Accuracy of intraoperative transesophageal echocardiography for estimating the severity of functional mitral regurgitation. Am. J. Cardiol. 76:508, 1995.

170. Yoran, C., Yellin, E. L., Becker, R. M., et al.: Mechanism of reduction of mitral regurgitation with vasodilator therapy. Am. J. Cardiol. 43:773, 1979.

171. Shimoyama, H., Sabbah, H. N., Roman, H., et al.: Effects of long-term therapy with enalapril on severity of functional mitral regurgitation in dogs with moderate heart failure. J. Am. Coll. Cardiol. 25:768, 1995.

172. Skoularigis, J., Sinovich, V., Joubert, G., and Sareli, P.: Evaluation of the long-term results of mitral valve repair in 254 young patients with rheumatic mitral regurgitation. Circulation 90:II–167, 1994.

173. Wells, F. C.: Conservation and surgical repair of the mitral valve. In Wells, F. C., and Shapiro, L. M. (eds.): Mitral Valve Disease. 2nd ed. London, Butterworths, 1996, pp. 114–134.

174. Straub, U., Feindt, P., Huwer, H., et al.: Mitral valve replacement with preservation of the subvalvular structures where possible: An echocardiographic and clinical comparison with cases where preservation was not possible. Thorac. Cardiovasc. Surg. 42:2, 1994.

175. David, T. E.: Techniques and results of mitral valve repair for ischemic mitral regurgitation. J. Cardiovasc. Surg. 9:274, 1994.

176. Odell, J. A., and Orszulak, T. A.: Surgical repair and reconstruction of valvular lesions. Curr. Opin. Cardiol. 10:135, 1995.

177. Oury, J. H., Cleveland, J. C., Duran, C. G., and Angell, W. W.: Ischemic mitral valve disease: Classification and systemic approach to management. J. Cardiovasc. Surg. 9(Suppl.):262, 1994.

178. Frater, R. W. M., Vetter, O., Zussa, C., and Dahm, M: Chordal replacement in mitral valve repair. Circulation 82(Suppl. IV):125, 1990.

179. Craver, J. M., Cohen, C., and Weintraub, W. S.: Case-matched comparison of mitral valve replacement and repair. Ann. Thorac. Surg. 49:964, 1990.

179a. Colon, R., and Frazier, O. H.: Mitral valve replacement techniques. In Wells, F. C., and Shapiro, L. M. (eds.): Mitral Valve Disease. 2nd ed. London, Butterworths, 1996, pp. 135–147.

180. Rozich, J. D., Carabello, B. A., and Usher, B. W.: Mitral valve replacement with and without chordal preservation in patients with chronic mitral regurgitation. Circulation 86:1718, 1992.

181. Nakano, K., Swindler, M. M., Spinale, F. B., et al.: Depressed contractile function due to canine mitral regurgitation improves after correction of the volume overload. J. Clin. Invest. 87:2077, 1991.

182. Duran, C. M., Gometza, B., and Saad, E.: Valve repair in rheumatic mitral disease: An unsolved problem. J. Cardiovasc. Surg. 9(Suppl.): 282, 1994.

183. Enriquez-Sarano, M., Schaff, H. V., Orszulak, T. A., et al.: Valve repair improves the outcome of surgery for mitral regurgitation. Circulation 91:1022, 1995.

184. Corin, W. J., Sutsch, G., Murakami, T., et al.: Left ventricular function in chronic mitral regurgitation. Preoperative and postoperative comparison. J. Am. Coll. Cardiol. 25:113, 1995.

185. Stewart, W. J., Currie, P. J., Salcedo, E. E., et al.: Intraoperative Doppler color flow mapping for decision-making in valve repair for mitral regurgitation. Circulation 81:556, 1990.

186. Lee, K. S., Stewart, W. J., Lever, H. M., et al.: Mechanism of outflow tract obstruction causing failed mitral valve repair: Anterior displacement of leaflet coaptation. Circulation 88:24, 1993.

187. Rankin, J. S., Feneley, M. P., Hickey, M. St. J., et al.: A clinical comparison of mitral valve repair versus valve replacement in ischemic mitral regurgitation. J. Thorac. Cardiovasc. Surg. 95:165, 1988.

188. Wisenbaugh, T., Skucicky, D., and Sarelli, P.: Prediction of outcome after valve replacement for rheumatic mitral regurgitation in the era of chordal preservation. Circulation 89:191, 1994.

189. Lee, S. J. K., and Bay, K. S.: Mortality risk factors associated with mitral valve replacement: A survival analysis of 10 year follow-up data. Can. J. Cardiol. 7:11, 1991.

190. Phillips, H. R., Levine, F. H., Carter, J. E., et al.: Mitral valve replacement for isolated mitral regurgitation: Analysis of clinical course and late postoperative left ventricular ejection fraction. Am. J. Cardiol. 48:647, 1981.

191. Peterson, K. L.: The timing of surgical intervention in chronic mitral regurgitation. Cathet. Cardiovasc. Diagn. 9:433, 1983.

192. Huikuri, H.: Effect of mitral valve replacement on left ventricular function in mitral regurgitation. Br. Heart J. 49:328, 1983.

193. Oury, J. H., Cleveland, J. C., Duran, C. G., and Angell, W. W.: Ischemic mitral valve disease: Classification and systemic approach to management. J. Cardiovasc. Surg. 9(Suppl.):262, 1994.

194. Akins, C. W., Hilgenberg, A. D., Buckley, M. J., et al.: Mitral valve reconstruction versus replacement for degenerative ischemic mitral regurgitation. Ann. Thorac. Surg. 58:668, 1994.

195. Connolly, M. W., Gelbfish, J. S., Jacobowitz, I. J., et al.: Surgical results for mitral regurgitation from coronary artery disease. J. Thorac. Cardiovasc. Surg. 91:379, 1986.

196. Gaasch, W. H., and Aurigemma, G. P.: Is corrective surgery ever indicated in the asymptomatic patient with mitral regurgitation? Cardiol. Rev. 2:138, 1994.

196a. Treasure, T.: Timing of surgery in chronic mitral regurgitation. In Wells, F. C., and Shapiro, L. M. (eds.): Mitral Valve Disease. 2nd ed. London, Butterworths, 1996, pp. 187–196.

THE MITRAL VALVE PROLAPSE SYNDROME

197. Devereux, R. B.: Recent developments in the diagnosis and management of mitral valve prolapse. Curr. Opin. Cardiol. 10:107, 1995.

198. Pocock, W. A.: Mitral leaflet billowing and prolapse. In Barlow, J. B. (ed.): Perspectives on the Mitral Valve. Philadelphia, F. A. Davis Co., 1987, pp. 45–112.

199. Perloff, J. K., Child, J. S., and Edwards, J. E.: New guidelines for the clinical diagnosis of mitral valve prolapse. Am. J. Cardiol. 57:1124, 1986.

200. Wann, L. S., Grove, J. R., Hess, T. R., et al.: Prevalence of mitral prolapse by two-dimensional echocardiography in healthy young women. Br. Heart J. 49:334, 1983.

201. Fontana, M. E., Sparks, E. A., Boudoulas, H., and Wooley, C. F.: Mitral valve prolapse and the mitral valve prolapse syndrome. Curr. Probl. Cardiol. 16:311, 1991.

202. Cohn, L. H., Couper, G. S., Aranki, S. F., et al.: Long-term results of mitral valve reconstruction for the regurgitating myxomatous mitral valve. J. Thorac. Cardiovasc. Surg. 107:143, 1994.

202a. Prabhu, S., and O'Rourke, R. A.: Mitral valve prolapse. In Rahimtoola, S. H. (ed.): Valvular Heart Disease and Endocarditis. Atlas of Heart Diseases. Vol. 11. St. Louis, Mosby, 1996.

203. Devereux, R. B., Hawkins, I., Kramer-Fox, R., et al.: Complications of mitral valve prolapse: Disproportionate occurrence in men and older patients. Am. J. Med. 81:751, 1986.

204. Levy, D., and Savage, D. D.: Prevalence and clinical features of mitral valve prolapse. Am. Heart J. 113:1281, 1987.

205. Barlow, J. B., Pocock, W. A., Marchand, P., and Denny, M.: The significance of the late systolic murmurs. Am. Heart J. 66:443, 1963.

206. Devereux, R. B., Kramer-Fox, R., and Kligfield, P.: Mitral valve prolapse: Etiology, clinical manifestations and management. Ann. Intern. Med. 111:305, 1989.

207. Goldhaber, S. Z., Brown, W. D., and St. John Sutton, M. G.: High frequency of mitral valve prolapse and aortic regurgitation among asymptomatic adults with Down's syndrome. J. A. M. A. 258:1793, 1987.

208. Noah, M. S., Sulimani, R. A., Famuyiwa, F. O., et al.: Prolapse of the mitral valve in hyperthyroid patients in Saudi Arabia. Int. J. Cardiol. 19:217, 1988.

209. Froom, P., Margulis, T., Grenadier, E., et al.: Von Willebrand factor and mitral valve prolapse. Thromb. Haemost. 60:230, 1988.

210. Streib, E. W., Meyers, D. G., and Sun, S. F.: Mitral valve prolapse in myotonic dystrophy. Muscle Nerve 8:650, 1985.

211. Johnson, G. L., Humphries, L. L., Shirley, P. B., et al.: Mitral valve prolapse in patients with anorexia nervosa and bulimia. Arch. Intern. Med. 146:1525, 1986.

212. Waite, P., and McCallum, C. A.: Mitral valve prolapse in craniofacial skeletal deformities. Oral Surg. Oral Med. Oral Pathol. 61:15, 1986.

213. Comens, S. M., Alpert, M. A., Sharp, G. C., et al.: Frequency of mitral valve prolapse in systemic lupus erythematosus, progressive systemic sclerosis and mixed connective tissue disease. Am. J. Cardiol. 63:59, 1989.

214. Chan, F. L., Chen, W. W., Wong, P. H. C., and Chow, J. S. F.: Skeletal abnormalities in mitral valve prolapse. Clin. Radiol. 34:207, 1983.

215. Zuppiroli, A., Roman, M. J., O'Gardy, M., and Devereux, R. B.: Lack of association between mitral valve prolapse and history of rheumatic fever. Am Heart J. 131:525, 1996.

216. Lu-Li, S., Guang-Gen, C., and Ru-Lian, L.: Valve prolapse in Behçet's disease. Br. Heart J. 54:100, 1985.

217. Levine, R. A., Handschumacher, M. D., Sanfilippo, A. J., et al.: Three-dimensional echocardiographic reconstruction of the mitral valve, with implications for the diagnosis of mitral valve prolapse. Circulation 80:589, 1989.

218. Cabeen, W. R., Jr., Reza, M. J., Kovick, R. B., and Stern, M. S.: Mitral valve prolapse and conduction defects in Ehlers-Danlos syndrome. Arch. Intern. Med. 137:1227, 1977.

219. Lebwohl, M. G., Distefano, D., Prioleau, P. G., et al.: Pseudoxanthoma elasticum and mitral valve prolapse. N. Engl. J. Med. 307:228, 1982.

220. Zema, M. J., Chiaramida, S., DeFilipp, G. J., et al.: Somatotype and idiopathic mitral valve prolapse. Cathet. Cardiovasc. Diagn. 8:105, 1982.

221. Malcolm, A. D.: Mitral valve prolapse associated with other disorders. Causal coincidence, common link, or fundamental genetic disturbance? Br. Heart J. 53:353, 1985.

222. Jaffe, A. S., Geltman, E. M., Rodey, G. E., and Uitto, J.: Mitral valve prolapse: A consistent manifestation of Type IV Ehlers-Danlos syndrome. The pathogenetic role of the abnormal production of Type III collagen. Circulation 64:121, 1981.

223. King, B. D., Clark, M. A., Baba, N., et al.: "Myxomatous" mitral valves: Collagen dissolution as the primary defect. Circulation 66:288, 1982.

224. Tomaru, T., Uchida, Y., Mohri, N., et al.: Postinflammatory mitral and aortic valve prolapse: A clinical and pathological study. Circulation 76:68, 1987.

225. Stein, P. D., Wang, C.-H., Riddle, J. M., et al.: Scanning electron microscopy of operatively excised severely regurgitant floppy mitral valves. Am. J. Cardiol. 64:392, 1989.

226. Baker, P. B., Bansal, G., Boudoulas, H., et al.: Floppy mitral valve chordae tendineae: Histopathologic alterations. Hum. Pathol. 19:507, 1988.

227. Wordsworth, P., Ogilvie, D., Akhras, F., et al.: Genetic segregation analysis of familial mitral valve prolapse shows no linkage to fibrillar collagen genes. Br. Heart J. 61:300, 1989.

228. Sanfilippo, A. J., Harrigan, P., Popovic, A. D., et al.: Papillary muscle traction in mitral valve prolapse: Quantitation by two-dimensional echocardiography. J. Am. Coll. Cardiol. 19:564, 1992.

229. Devereux, R. B., Kramer-Fox, R., and Kligfield, P.: Mitral valve prolapse: Causes, clinical manifestations, and management. Arch. Intern. Med. 111:305, 1989.

230. Procacci, P. M., Savran, S. V., Schreiter, S. L., and Bryson, A. L.: Prevalence of clinical mitral valve prolapse in 1,169 young women. N. Engl. J. Med. 294:1086, 1976.

231. Markiewicz, W., Stoner, J., London, E., et al.: Mitral valve prolapse in one hundred presumably healthy young females. Circulation 53:464, 1976.

232. Pan, C. W., Chen, C. C., Wang, S. P., et al.: Echocardiographic study of cardiac abnormalities in families of patients with Marfan's syndrome. J. Am. Coll. Cardiol. 6:1016, 1985.

233. Zuppiroli, A., Rinaldi, M., Kramer-Fox, R., et al.: Natural history of mitral valve prolapse. Am. J. Cardiol. 75:1028, 1995.

234. Boudoulas, H., Kolibash, A. J., Jr., Baker, P., et al.: Mitral valve prolapse and the mitral valve prolapse syndrome: A diagnostic classification and pathogenesis of symptoms. Am. Heart J. 118:796, 1989.

235. Davies, A. O., Mares, A., Pool, J. L., and Taylor, A. A.: Mitral valve prolapse with symptoms of beta-adrenergic hypersensitivity. Beta₂-adrenergic receptor supercoupling with desensitization on isoproterenol exposure. Am. J. Med. 82:193, 1987.

236. Alexander, M. D., Bloom, K. R., Hart, P., et al.: Atrial septal aneurysm: A cause of midsystolic click. Report of a case and review of the literature. Circulation 63:1186, 1981.

237. Kligfield, P., and Devereux, R. B.: Arrhythmia in mitral valve prolapse. In Podrid, P. R., and Kowey, P. R. (eds.): Cardiac Arrhythmia: Mechanisms, Diagnosis and Management. Baltimore, Williams and Wilkins Co., 1995, p. 1253.

238. Kligfield, P., Hochreiter, C., Niles, N., et al.: Relation of sudden death in pure mitral regurgitation with and without mitral valve prolapse, to repetitive ventricular arrhythmias and right and left ventricular ejection fraction. Am. J. Cardiol. 60:397, 1987.

239. Stein, K. M., Borer, J. S., Hochreiter, C., et al.: Prognostic value and physiological correlates of heart rate variability in chronic severe mitral regurgitation. Circulation 88:127, 1993.

240. Wit, A. L., Fenoglio, J. J., Hordof, A. J., and Reemtsma, K.: Ultrastructure and transmembrane potentials of cardiac muscle in the human anterior mitral valve leaflet. Circulation 59:1283, 1979.

241. Gallagher, J. J., Gilbert, M., and Svenson, R. H.: Wolff-Parkinson-White syndrome. The problem, evaluation and surgical correction. Circulation 57:767, 1975.

242. Pocock, W. A., Bosman, C. K., Chesler, E., et al.: Sudden death in primary mitral valve prolapse. Am. Heart J. 107:378, 1984.

243. Levine, R. A., Stathogiannis, E., Newell, J. B., et al.: Reconsideration of echocardiographic standards for mitral valve prolapse: Lack of association between leaflet displacement isolated to the apical four chamber view and independent echocardiographic evidence of abnormality. J. Am. Coll. Cardiol. 11:1010, 1988.

244. Alpert, M. A., Carney, R. J., Flaker, G. C., et al.: Sensitivity and specificity of two-dimensional echocardiographic signs of mitral valve prolapse. Am. J. Cardiol. 54:792, 1984.

245. Marks, A. R., Choong, C. Y., Sanfilippo, A. J., et al.: Identification of high-risk and low-risk subgroups of patients with mitral valve prolapse. N. Engl. J. Med. 320:1031, 1989.

246. Panidis, I. P., McAllister, M., Ross, J., and Mintz, G. S.: Prevalence and severity of mitral regurgitation in the mitral valve prolapse syndrome: A Doppler echocardiographic study of 80 patients. J. Am. Coll. Cardiol. 7:975, 1986.

247. Weissman, N. J., Pini, R., Roman, M. J., et al.: In vivo mitral valve morphology and function in mitral valve prolapse. Am. J. Cardiol. 73:1080, 1994.

248. Arvan, S., and Tunick, S.: Relationship between auscultatory events and structural abnormalities in mitral valve prolapse: A two-dimensional echocardiographic evaluation. Am. Heart J. 108:1298, 1984.

249. Sahn, D. J., Wood, J., Allen, H. D., et al.: Echocardiographic spectrum of mitral valve motion in children with and without mitral valve prolapse: The nature of false-positive diagnosis. Am. J. Cardiol. 39:422, 1977.

250. Rodger, J. C., and Morley, P.: Abnormal aortic valve echoes in mitral prolapse. Echocardiographic features of floppy aortic valve. Br. Heart J. 47:337, 1982.

251. Klein, G. J., Kostuk, W. J., Boughner, D. R., and Chamberlain, M. J.: Stress myocardial imaging in mitral leaflet prolapse syndrome. Am. J. Cardiol. 42:746, 1978.

252. Cohen, M. V., Shah, P. K., and Spindola-Franco, H.: Angiographic-echocardiographic correlation of mitral valve prolapse. Am. Heart J. 97:43, 1979.

253. Cipriano, P. R., Kline, S. A., and Baltaxe, H. A.: An angiographic assessment of left ventricular-function in isolated mitral valvular prolapse. Invest. Radiol. 15:293, 1980.

254. Mills, P., Rose, J., Hollingsworth, J., et al.: Long-term prognosis of mitral valve prolapse. N. Engl. J. Med 297:13, 1977.

255. Olson, L. J., Subramanian, R., Ackermann, D. M., et al.: Surgical pathology of the mitral valve: A study of 712 cases spanning 21 years. Mayo Clin. Proc. 62:22, 1987.

256. Wilcken, D. E., and Hickey, A. J.: Lifetime risk for patients with mitral prolapse of developing severe valve regurgitation requiring surgery. Circulation 78:10, 1988.

256a. Fakuda, N., Oki, T., Iuchi, A., et al.: Predisposing factors for severe mitral regurgitation in idiopathic mitral valve prolapse. Am. J. Cardiol. 76:503, 1995.

257. Hickey, A. J., MacMahon, S. W., and Wilcken, D. E. L.: Mitral valve prolapse and bacterial endocarditis: When is antibiotic prophylaxis necessary? Am. Heart J. 109:431, 1985.

258. Danchin, N., Briancon, S., Mathieu, P., et al.: Mitral valve prolapse as a risk factor for infective endocarditis. Lancet 1:743, 1989.

259. Schnee, M. A., and Bucal, A. A.: Fatal embolism in mitral valve prolapse. Chest 83:285, 1983.

260. Barletta, G. A., Gagliardi, R., Benvenuti, L., and Fantini, F.: Cerebral ischemic attacks as a complication of aortic and mitral valve prolapse. Stroke 16:219, 1985.

261. Makino, H., and Al-Sadir, J.: Myocardial infarction in patients with mitral valve prolapse and normal coronary arteries. J. Am. Coll. Cardiol. 1:661, 1983.

AORTIC STENOSIS

262. Levinson, G. E.: Aortic stenosis. In Dalen, J. E., and Alpert, J. S. (eds.): Valvular Heart Disease. 2nd ed. Boston, Little, Brown and Co., 1987, pp. 197–282.

263. Dare, A. J., Veinot, J. P., Edwards, W. D., et al.: New observations on the etiology of aortic valve disease. Hum. Pathol. 24:1330, 1993.

264. Roberts, W. C.: Valvular, subvalvular and supravalvular aortic stenosis. Morphologic features. Cardiovasc. Clin. 5:97, 1973.

264a. Rahimtoola, S. H.: Aortic stenosis. In Rahimtoola, S. H. (ed.): Valvular Heart Disease and Endocarditis. Atlas of Heart Diseases. Vol. 11. St. Louis, Mosby, 1996.

265. Braunwald, E., Goldblatt, A., Aygen, M. M., et al.: Congenital aortic stenosis: Clinical and hemodynamic findings in 100 patients. Circulation 27:426, 1963.

266. Selzer, A.: Changing aspects of the natural history of valvular aortic stenosis. N. Engl. J. Med. 317:91, 1987.

267. Passik, C. S., Ackermann, D. M., Pluth, J. R., and Edwards, W. D.: Temporal changes in the causes of aortic stenosis: A surgical pathologic study of 646 cases. Mayo Clin. Proc. 62:119, 1987.

268. Deutscher, S., Rockette, H. E., and Krishnaswami, V.: Diabetes and hypercholesterolemia among patients with calcific aortic stenosis. J. Chron. Dis. 37:407, 1984.

269. Strickberger, S. A., Schulman, S. P., and Hutchings, G. M.: Association

of Paget's disease of bone with calcific aortic valve disease. Am. J. Med. 82:953, 1987.

270. Maher, E. R., Young, G., Smyth-Walsh, B., et al.: Aortic and mitral valve calcification in patients with end stage renal diseases. Lancet 1:875, 1987.

271. Dereymacker, L., Van Parijs, G., Bayart, M., et al.: Ochronosis and alkaptonuria: Report of a new case with calcified aortic valve stenosis. Acta Cardiol. 45:98, 1990.

272. Kennedy, J. W., Twiss, R. D., and Blackmon, J. R.: Quantitative angiography. III. Relationships of left ventricular pressure volume and mass in aortic valve disease. Circulation 38:838, 1968.

273. Carabello, B. A.: Aortic stenosis. Cardiol. Rev. 1:59, 1993.

274. Carabello, B. A., Mee, R., Collins, J. J., Jr., et al.: Contractile function in chronic gradually developing subcoronary aortic stenosis. Am. J. Physiol. 240:H80, 1981.

275. Grossman, W.: Profiles in valvular heart disease. In Grossman, W., and Baim, D. (eds.): Cardiac Catheterization and Angiography. 4th ed. Philadelphia, Lea and Febiger, 1991.

275a. Laskey, W. K., Kussmaul, W. G., and Noordergraaf, A.: Valvular and systemic arterial hemodynamics in aortic valve stenosis. Circulation 9:1473, 1995.

276. Hess, O. L., Villari, B., and Krayenbuehl, H.: Diastolic dysfunction in aortic stenosis. Circulation 87(Suppl. 5):IV-73, 1993.

277. Villari, B., Vassalli, G., Monrad, E. S., et al.: Normalization of diastolic dysfunction in aortic stenosis late after valve replacement. Circulation 91:2353, 1995.

278. Braunwald, E., and Frahm, C. J.: Studies on Starling's law of the heart. IV. Observations on the hemodynamic functions of the left atrium in man. Circulation 24:633, 1961.

279. Carroll, J. D., Carroll, E. P., Feldman, T., et al.: Sex-associated differences in left ventricular function in aortic stenosis of the elderly. Circulation 86:1099, 1992.

280. Morris, J. J., Schaff, H. V., Mullany, C. J., et al.: Gender differences in left ventricular functional response to aortic valve replacement. Circulation 90:II-183, 1994.

280a. Legget, M. E., Kuusisto, J., Healy, N. L., et al.: Gender differences in left ventricular function at rest and with exercise in asymptomatic aortic stenosis. Am. Heart J. 131:94, 1996.

281. Donner, R., Carabello, B. A., Black, I., and Spann, J. F.: Left ventricular wall stress in compensated aortic stenosis in children. Am. J. Cardiol. 51:946, 1983.

282. Spann, J. F., Bove, A. A., Natarajan, G., and Kreulens, T.: Ventricular performance, pump function, and compensatory mechanisms in patients with aortic stenosis. Circulation 62:576, 1980.

283. Brouwer, C. B., Verwers, F. A., Alpert, J. S., and Goldberg, R. J.: Isolated aortic stenosis: Analysis of clinical and hemodynamic subsets. J. Appl. Cardiol. 4:565, 1989.

284. Krayenbuehl, H. P., Hess, O. M., Ritter, M., et al.: Left ventricular systolic function in aortic stenosis. Eur. Heart J. 9(Suppl. E):19, 1988.

285. Gunther, S., and Grossman, W.: Determinants of ventricular function in pressure overload hypertrophy in man. Circulation 59:679, 1979.

286. Ross, J., Jr.: Afterload mismatch and preload reserve: A conceptual framework for the analysis of ventricular function. Prog. Cardiovasc. Dis. 18:255, 1976.

287. Fifer, M. A., Gunther, S., Grossman, W., et al.: Myocardial contractile function in aortic stenosis as determined from the rate of stress development during isovolumic systole. Am. J. Cardiol. 44:1318, 1979.

288. Carabello, B. A., Green, L. H., Grossman, W., et al.: Hemodynamic determinants of prognosis of aortic valve replacement in critical aortic stenosis and advanced congestive heart failure. Circulation 62:42, 1980.

289. Huber, D., Grimm, J., Koch, R., and Krayenbuehl, H. P.: Determinants of ejection performance in aortic stenosis. Circulation 64:126, 1981.

289a. Movsowitz, C., Kussmaul, W. G., and Laskey, W. K.: Left ventricular diastolic response to exercise in valvular aortic stenosis. Am. J. Cardiol. 77:275, 1996.

290. Dineen, E., and Brent, B. N.: Aortic valve stenosis: Comparison of patients to those without chronic congestive heart failure. Am. J. Cardiol. 57:419, 1986.

291. Fifer, M. A., Borow, K. M., Colan, S. D., and Lorell, B. H.: Early diastolic left ventricular function in children and adults with aortic stenosis. J. Am. Coll. Cardiol. 5:1147, 1985.

292. Hess, O. M., Ritter, M., Schneider, J., et al.: Diastolic stiffness and myocardial structure in aortic valve disease before and after replacement. Circulation 69:855, 1984.

293. Schwarz, F., Flameng, W., Schaper, J., et al.: Myocardial structure and function in patients with aortic valve disease and their relation to postoperative results. Am. J. Cardiol. 41:661, 1978.

294. Krayenbuehl, H. P., Hess, O. M., Monrad, E. S., et al.: Left ventricular myocardial structure in aortic valve disease before, intermediate, and later after aortic valve replacement. Circulation 79:744, 1989.

295. Bertrand, M. E., LaBlanche, J. M., Tilmant, P. Y., et al.: Coronary sinus blood flow at rest and during isometric exercise in patients with aortic valve disease. Mechanism of angina pectoris in presence of normal coronary arteries. Am. J. Cardiol. 47:199, 1981.

296. Smucker, M. L., Tedesco, C. L., and Manning, S. B.: Demonstration of an imbalance between coronary perfusion and excessive load as a mechanism of ischemia during stress in patients with aortic stenosis. Circulation 78:573, 1988.

297. Vinten-Johansen, J., and Weiss, H. R.: Oxygen consumption in subepicardial and subendocardial regions of the canine left ventricle—The

effect of experimental acute valvular aortic stenosis. Circ. Res. 46:139, 1980.

298. Matsuo, S., Tsuruta, M., Hayano, M., et al.: Phasic coronary artery flow velocity determined by Doppler flowmeter catheter in aortic stenosis and aortic regurgitation. Am. J. Cardiol. 62:917, 1988.

299. Marcus, M. L., Dot, D. B., Hiratzka, L. F., et al.: Decreased coronary reserve. A mechanism for angina pectoris in patients with aortic stenosis and normal coronary arteries. N. Engl. J. Med. 307:1362, 1982.

300. Oakley, C. M.: Management of valvular stenosis. Curr. Opin. Cardiol. 10:117, 1995.

301. Kennedy, K. D., Nishimura, R. A., Holmes, D. R., et al.: Natural history of moderate aortic stenosis. J. Am. Coll. Cardiol. 17:313, 1991.

302. Ross, J., Jr., and Braunwald, E.: The influence of corrective operations on the natural history of aortic stenosis. Circulation 37(Suppl. V):61, 1968.

303. Frank, S., Johnson, A., and Ross, J., Jr.: Natural history of valvular aortic stenosis. Br. Heart J. 35:41, 1973.

304. Hakki, A.-H., Kimbiris, D., Iskandrian, A. S., et al.: Angina pectoris and coronary artery disease in patients with severe aortic valvular disease. Am. Heart. J. 100:441, 1980.

305. Baxley, W. A.: Aortic valve disease. Curr. Opin. Cardiol. 9:152, 1994.

306. Holley, K. E., Bahn, R. C., McGoon, D. C., and Mankin, H. T.: Spontaneous calcific embolization associated with calcific aortic stenosis. Circulation 27:197, 1963.

307. Grech, E. D., and Ramsdale, D. R.: Exertional syncope in aortic stenosis: Evidence to support inappropriate left ventricular baroreceptor response. Am. Heart J. 121:603, 1991.

308. Carabello, B. A.: Aortic stenosis. Cardiol. Rev. 1:59, 1993.

309. Schwartz, L. S., Goldfischer, J., Sprague, G. J., and Schwartz, S. P.: Syncope and sudden death in aortic stenosis. Am. J. Cardiol. 23:647, 1969.

310. Love, J. W.: The syndrome of calcific aortic stenosis and gastrointestinal bleeding: Resolution following aortic valve replacement. J. Thorac. Cardiovasc. Surg. 83:779, 1982.

311. Pleet, A. B., Massey, E. W., and Vengrow, M. E.: TIA, stroke, and the bicuspid aortic valve. Neurology 31:1540, 1981.

312. Brockmeier, L. B., Adolph, R. J., Gustin, B. W., et al.: Calcium emboli to the retinal artery in calcific aortic stenosis. Am. Heart J. 101:32, 1981.

313. Wood, P.: Aortic stenosis. Am. J. Cardiol. 1:553, 1958.

314. Aortic stenosis. In Fowler, N. O.: Diagnosis of Heart Disease. New York, Springer-Verlag, 1991, p. 134–145.

315. Abrams, J.: Aortic stenosis. In Essentials of Cardiac Physical Diagnosis. Philadelphia, Lea and Febiger, 1987, pp. 205–224.

316. Cooper, T., Braunwald, E., and Morrow, A. G.: Pulsus alternans in aortic stenosis: Hemodynamic observations in 50 patients studied by left heart catheterization. Circulation 18:64, 1958.

317. Perloff, J. K.: Clinical recognition of aortic stenosis. The physical signs and differential diagnosis of the various forms of obstruction to left ventricular outflow. Prog. Cardiovasc. Dis. 10:323, 1968.

318. Goldblatt, A., Aygen, M. M., and Braunwald, E.: Hemodynamic-phonocardiographic correlations of the fourth heart sound in aortic stenosis. Circulation 26:92, 1962.

319. Morton, B. C.: Natural history and management of chronic aortic valve disease. Can. Med. Assoc. J. 126:477, 1982.

320. Forssell, G., Jonasson, R., and Orinius, E.: Identifying severe aortic valvular stenosis by bedside examination. Acta Med. Scand. 218:397, 1985.

321. Dymond, D. S., Wolf, F. G., and Schmidt, D. H.: Severe left ventricular dysfunction in critical aortic stenosis—reversal following aortic valve replacement. Postgrad. Med. J. 59:781, 1983.

322. Delman, A. J., and Stein, E.: Valvular aortic stenosis. In Dynamic Cardiac Auscultation and Phonocardiography. Philadelphia, W. B. Saunders Co., 1979, p. 795.

323. Siegel, R. J., and Roberts, W. C.: Electrocardiographic observations in severe aortic valve stenosis: Correlative necropsy study of clinical, hemodynamic, and ECG variables demonstrating relation of 12-lead QRS amplitude to peak systolic transaortic pressure gradient. Am. Heart J. 103:210, 1982.

324. Gooch, A. S., Calatayud, J. B., Rogers, P. A., and Garman, P. A.: Analysis of the P wave in severe aortic stenosis. Dis. Chest 49:459, 1966.

325. Nair, C. K., Aronow, W. S., Stokke, K., et al.: Cardiac conduction defects in patients older than 60 years with aortic stenosis and without mitral annular calcium. Am. J. Cardiol. 53:169, 1984.

326. Klein, R. C.: Ventricular arrhythmias in aortic valve disease: Analysis of 102 patients. Am. J. Cardiol. 53:1079, 1984.

327. Szamosi, A., and Wassberg, B.: Radiologic detection of aortic stenosis. Acta Radiol. Diagn. 24:201, 1983.

328. Hoffmann, R., Flachskampf, F. A., and Hanrath, P.: Aortic stenosis using multiplane transesophageal echocardiography. J. Am. Coll. Cardiol. 22:529, 1993.

329. Tribouilloy, C., Shen, W. F., Peltier, M., et al.: Quantitation of aortic valve area in aortic stenosis with multiplane transesophageal echocardiography: Comparison with monoplane transesophageal approach. Am. Heart J. 128:526, 1994.

330. Galan, A., Zoghbi, W. A., and Quiñones, M. A.: Determination of severity of valvular aortic stenosis by Doppler echocardiography and relation of findings to clinical outcome and agreement with hemodynamic measurements determined at cardiac catheterization. Am. J. Cardiol. 67:1007, 1991.

331. Currie, P. J., Hagler, D. J., Seward, J. B., et al.: Instantaneous pressure

332. Agatston, A. S., Chengot, M., Rao, A., et al.: Doppler diagnosis of valvular aortic stenosis in patients over 60 years of age. Am. J. Cardiol. 56:106, 1985.

333. Yeager, M., Yock, P. G., and Popp, R. L.: Comparison of Doppler-derived pressure gradient to that determined at cardiac catheterization in adults with aortic valve stenosis: Implications for management. Am. J. Cardiol. 57:644, 1986.

334. Stone, P. H.: Management of the patient with asymptomatic aortic stenosis. J. Cardiovasc. Surg. 9(Suppl.):139, 1994.

335. Aronow, W. S., Ahn, C., Kronson, I., and Nanna, M.: Prognosis of congestive heart failure in patients aged ≥ 62 years with unoperated severe valvular aortic stenosis. Am. J. Cardiol. 72:846, 1993.

336. Cheitlin, M. D.: Should an asymptomatic patient with hemodynamically severe aortic stenosis ever have aortic valve surgery? Cardiol. Rev. 1:344, 1993.

337. Braunwald, E.: On the natural history of severe aortic stenosis (editorial). J. Am. Coll. Cardiol. 15:1018, 1990.

338. Pellikka, P. A., Nishimura, R. A., Bailey, K. R., and Tajik, A. J.: The natural history of adults with asymptomatic hemodynamically significant aortic stenosis. J. Am. Coll. Cardiol. 15:1012, 1990.

339. Davies, S. W., Gershlick, A. H., and Balcon, R.: The progression of valvular aortic stenosis: A long-term retrospective study. Eur. Heart J. 12:10, 1991.

340. Peter, M., Hoffman, A., Parker, C., et al.: Progression of aortic stenosis: Role of age and concomitant coronary artery disease. Chest 103:1715, 1993.

341. Brener, S. J., Duffy, C. I., Thomas, J. U. D., and Stewart, W. J.: Progression of aortic stenosis in 394 patients: Relation to changes in myocardial and mitral valve dysfunction. J. Am. Coll. Cardiol. 25:305, 1995.

342. Usher, B. W.: Valve surgery: Indications and long-term results. Curr. Opin. Cardiol. 6:219, 1991.

343. Kirklin, J. W., and Barratt-Boyes, B. G.: Congenital aortic stenosis. In Cardiac Surgery. 2nd ed. New York, Churchill-Livingstone, 1993, pp. 1195–1238.

344. Kirklin, J. W., and Barratt-Boyes, B. G.: Aortic valve disease. In Cardiac Surgery. 2nd ed. New York, Churchill-Livingstone, 1993, pp. 491–571.

345. McBride, L. R., Naunheim, K. S., Fiore, A. C., et al.: Aortic valve decalcification. J. Thorac. Cardiovasc. Surg. 100:36, 1990.

346. Lund, O.: Preoperative risk evaluation and stratification of long-term survival after valve replacement for aortic stenosis. Circulation 82:124, 1990.

347. Monrad, E. S., Hess, O. M., Murakami, T., et al.: Abnormal exercise hemodynamics in patients with normal systolic function late after aortic valve replacement. Circulation 77:613, 1988.

348. Hwang, M. H., Hammermeister, K. E., Oprian, C., et al.: Preoperative identification of patients likely to have left ventricular dysfunction after aortic valve replacement. Participants in the Veterans Administration Cooperative Study on Valvular Heart Disease. Circulation 80(Suppl. I):165, 1989.

349. Kennedy, J. W., Doces, J., and Stewart, D. K.: Left ventricular function before and following aortic valve replacement. Circulation 56:944, 1977.

350. Monrad, E. S., Hess, O. M., Murakami, T., et al.: Time course of regression of left ventricular hypertrophy after aortic valve replacement. Circulation 77:1345, 1988.

351. Mirsky, I., Henschke, C., Hess, O. M., and Krayenbuehl, H. P.: Prediction of postoperative performance in aortic valve disease. Am. J. Cardiol. 48:295, 1981.

352. Smith, N., McAnulty, J. H., and Rahimtoola, S. H.: Severe aortic stenosis with impaired left ventricular function and clinical heart failure: Results of valve replacement. Circulation 58:255, 1978.

353. Culliford, A. T., Galloway, A. C., Colvin, S. B., et al.: Aortic valve replacement for aortic stenosis in persons aged 80 years and over. Am. J. Cardiol. 67:1256, 1991.

354. Iung, B., Drissi, M. F., Michel, P.-L., et al.: Prognosis of valve replacement for aortic stenosis with or without coexisting coronary heart disease: A comparative study. J. Heart Valve Dis. 2:430, 1993.

355. Safian, R. D., Mandell, V. S., Thurer, R. E., et al.: Postmortem and intraoperative balloon valvuloplasty of calcific aortic stenosis in elderly patients: Mechanisms of successful dilation. J. Am. Coll. Cardiol. 9:655, 1987.

356. Beatt, K. J.: Balloon dilatation of the aortic valve in adults: A physician's view. Br. Heart J. 63:207, 1990.

357. Nishimura, R. A., Holmes, D. R., Jr., Michela, M. A., et al.: Follow-up of patients with low output, low gradient hemodynamics after percutaneous balloon aortic valvuloplasty: The Mansfield Scientific Aortic Valvuloplasty Registry. J. Am. Coll. Cardiol. 17:828, 1991.

358. Otto, C. M., Mickel, M. C., Kennedy, J. W., et al.: Three-year outcome after balloon aortic valvuloplasty: Insights into prognosis of valvular aortic stenosis. Circulation 89:642, 1994.

359. Elliott, J. M., and Tuzcu, E. M.: Recent developments in balloon valvuloplasty techniques. Curr. Opin. Cardiol. 10:128, 1995.

360. Otto, C. M., Mickel, M. C., Kennedy, J. W., et al.: Three-year outcome after balloon aortic valvuloplasty: Insights into prognosis of valvular aortic stenosis. Circulation 89:642, 1994.

361. Lieberman, E. B., Wilson, J. S., Harrison, J. K., et al.: Aortic valve replacement in adults after balloon aortic valvuloplasty. Circulation 90:II-205, 1994.

362. Berland, J., Cribier, A., Savin, T., et al.: Percutaneous balloon valvulo-

plasty in patients with severe aortic stenosis and low ejection fraction. Circulation 79:1189, 1989.

363. Isner, J. A., and the Mansfield Scientific Aortic Valvuloplasty Registry Investigators: Acute catastrophic complications of balloon aortic valvuloplasty. J. Am. Coll. Cardiol. 17:1436, 1991.

364. Holmes, D. R., Jr., Nishimura, R. A., and Reeder, G. S.: In-hospital mortality after balloon aortic valvuloplasty: Frequency and associated factors. J. Am. Coll. Cardiol. 17:189, 1991.

365. Moreno, P. R., Jang, I.-K., Newell, J. B., et al.: The role of percutaneous aortic balloon valvuloplasty in patients with cardiogenic shock and critical aortic stenosis. J. Am. Coll. Cardiol. 23:1071, 1994.

366. Angel, J. L., Chapman, C., and Knuppel, R. A.: Percutaneous balloon aortic valvuloplasty in pregnancy. Obstet. Gynecol. 72:438, 1988.

AORTIC REGURGITATION

367. Alpert, J. S.: Chronic aortic regurgitation. In Dalen, J. E., and Alpert, J. S. (eds.): Valvular Heart Disease. 2nd ed. Boston, Little, Brown and Co., 1987, pp. 283–318.

368. Stewart, W. J., King, M. E., Gillam, L. D., et al.: Prevalence of aortic valve prolapse with bicuspid aortic valve and its relation to aortic regurgitation: A cross-sectional echocardiographic study. Am. J. Cardiol. 54:1277, 1984.

368a. Rahimtoola, S. H.: Aortic regurgitation. In Rahimtoola, S. H. (ed.): Valvular Heart Disease and Endocarditis. Atlas of Heart Diseases. Vol. 11. St. Louis, Mosby, 1996.

369. Frahm, C. J., Braunwald, E., and Morrow, A. G.: Congenital aortic regurgitation. Clinical and hemodynamic findings in four patients. Am. J. Med. 31:63, 1961.

370. Roberts, W. C., Morrow, A. G., McIntosh, C. L., et al.: Congenitally bicuspid aortic valve causing severe, pure aortic regurgitation without superimposed infective endocarditis. Am. J. Cardiol. 47:206, 1981.

371. Tonnemacher, D., Reid, C., Kawanishi, D., et al.: Frequency of myxomatous degeneration of the aortic valve as a cause of isolated aortic regurgitation severe enough to warrant aortic valve replacement. Am. J. Cardiol. 60:1194, 1987.

372. Morain, S. V., Casanegra, P., Maturana, G., and Dubernet, J.: Spontaneous rupture of a fenestrated aortic valve. Surgical treatment. J. Thorac. Cardiovasc. Surg. 73:716, 1977.

373. Waller, B. F., Kishel, J. C., and Roberts, W. C.: Severe aortic regurgitation from systemic hypertension. Chest 82:365, 1982.

374. Chartash, E. K., Lans, D. M., Paget, S. A., et al.: Aortic insufficiency and mitral regurgitation in patients with severe systemic lupus erythematosus and the antiphospholipid syndrome. Am. J. Med. 86:407, 1989.

375. Kramer, P. H., Imboden, J. B., Jr., Waldman, F. M., et al.: Severe aortic insufficiency in juvenile chronic arthritis. Am. J. Med. 74:1088, 1983.

376. Demoulin, J. C., Lespagnard, J., Bertholet, M., and Soumagne, D.: Acute fulminant aortic regurgitation in ankylosing spondylitis. Am. Heart J. 105:859, 1983.

377. Tahakur, R., Gupta, L. C., Misra, M., et al.: Jaccoud's arthropathy— diagnostic and therapeutic implications. Postgrad. Med. J. 64:809, 1988.

378. Bostwick, D. G., Bensch, K. G., Burke, J. S., et al.: Whipple's disease presenting as aortic insufficiency. N. Engl. J. Med. 305:995, 1981.

379. Burdick, S., Tresch, D. D., and Komokowski, R. A.: Cardiac valvular dysfunction associated with Crohn's disease in the absence of ankylosing spondylitis. Am. Heart J. 118:174, 1989.

380. Darvill, F. R., Jr.: Aortic insufficiency of unusual etiology. J.A.M.A. 184:753, 1963.

381. Emanuel, R., Ng, R. A. L., Marcomichelakis, J., et al.: Formes frustes of Marfan's syndrome presenting with severe aortic regurgitation. Clinicogenetic study of 18 families. Br. Heart J. 39:190, 1977.

382. Reid, G. D., Patterson, M. W. H., Patterson, A. C., and Cooperberg, P. L.: Aortic insufficiency in association with juvenile ankylosing spondylitis. J. Pediatr. 95:78, 1979.

383. Paulus, H. E., Pearson, C. M., and Pitts, W., Jr.: Aortic insufficiency in five patients with Reiter's syndrome: A detailed clinical and pathologic study. Am. J. Med. 53:464, 1972.

384. Heppner, R. L., Babitt, H. I., Blanchine, J. W., and Warbasse, J. R.: Aortic regurgitation and aneurysm of sinus of Valsalva associated with osteogenesis imperfecta. Am. J. Cardiol. 31:654, 1973.

385. Esdah, J., Hawkins, D., Gold, P., et al.: Vascular involvement in relapsing polychondritis. Can. Med. Assoc. J. 116:1019, 1977.

386. Welch, G. H., Jr., Braunwald, E., and Sarnoff, S. J.: Hemodynamic effects of quantitatively varied experimental aortic regurgitation. Circ. Res. 5:546, 1957.

387. Iskandrian, A. S., Hakki, A-H., Manno, B., et al.: Left ventricular function in chronic aortic regurgitation. J. Am. Coll. Cardiol. 1:1374, 1983.

388. Borow, K. M., and Marcus, R. H.: Aortic regurgitation: The need for an integrated physiologic approach. J. Am. Coll. Cardiol. 17:898, 1991.

389. Grossman, W., Jones, D., and McLaurin, L. P.: Wall stress and patterns of hypertrophy in the human left ventricle. J. Clin. Invest. 56:56, 1975.

390. Kawanishi, D. T., McKay, C. R., Chandraratna, A. N., et al.: Cardiovascular response to dynamic exercise in patients with chronic symptomatic mild-to-moderate and severe aortic regurgitation. Circulation 73:62, 1986.

391. Massie, B. M., Kramer, B. L., Loge, D., et al.: Ejection fraction response to supine exercise in asymptomatic aortic regurgitation: Relation to simultaneous hemodynamic measurements. J. Am. Coll. Cardiol. 5:847, 1985.

392. Scognamiglio, R., Roelandt, J., Fasoli, G., et al.: Relation between myocardial contractility, hypertrophy and pump performance in patients with chronic aortic regurgitation: An echocardiographic study. Int. J. Cardiol. 6:473, 1984.

393. Dehmer, G. J., Firth, E. G., Hillis, L. D., et al.: Alterations in left ventricular volumes and ejection fraction at rest and during exercise in patients with aortic regurgitation. Am. J. Cardiol. 48:17, 1981.

394. Ardehall, A., Segal, J., and Cheitlin, M. D.: Coronary blood flow reserve in acute aortic regurgitation. J. Am. Coll. Cardiol. 25:1387, 1995.

395. Uhl, G. S., Boucher, C. A., Oliveros, R. A., and Murgo, J. P.: Exercise-induced myocardial oxygen supply-demand imbalance in asymptomatic or mildly symptomatic aortic regurgitation. Chest 80:686, 1981.

396. Nitenberg, A., Foult, J-M., Antony, I., et al.: Coronary flow and resistance reserve in patients with chronic aortic regurgitation, angina pectoris, and normal coronary arteries. J. Am. Coll. Cardiol. 11:478, 1988.

397. Maurer, W., Ablasser, A., Tschada, R., et al.: Myocardial catecholamine metabolism in patients with chronic aortic regurgitation. Circulation 66(Suppl. I):139, 1982.

398. Benotti, J. R.: Acute aortic insufficiency. In Dalen, J. E., and Alpert, J. S. (eds.): Valvular Heart Disease. 2nd ed. Boston, Little, Brown and Co., 1987, pp. 319–352.

399. Downes, T. R., Nomeir, A-M., Hackshaw, B. T., et al.: Diastolic mitral regurgitation in acute but not chronic aortic regurgitation: Implications regarding the mechanism of mitral closure. Am. Heart J.117:1106, 1989.

400. Eusebio, J., Louie, E. K., Edwards, D. C., et al.: Alterations in transmitral flow dynamics in patients with early mitral valve closure and aortic regurgitation. Am. Heart J. 128:941, 1994.

401. Sapira, J. D.: Quincke, DeMusset, Duroziez and Hill: Some aortic regurgitations. South. Med. J. 74:459, 1981.

402. Boudoulas, H., Triposkiadis, F., Dervenagas, J., et al.: Mechanisms of pistol shot sounds in aortic regurgitation. Acta Cardiol. 46:139, 1991.

403. Alpert, J. S., Veiweg, W. V. R., and Hagan, A. D.: Incidence and morphology of carotid shudders in aortic valve disease. Am. Heart J. 92:435, 1976.

404. Aortic insufficiency. In Fowler, N. O.: Diagnosis of Heart Disease. New York, Springer-Verlag, 1991, pp. 123–133.

405. Abdulla, A. M., Frank, M. J., Erdin, R. A., Jr., and Canedo, M. I.: Clinical significance and hemodynamic correlates of the third heart sound gallop in aortic regurgitation. A guide to optimal timing of cardiac catheterization. Circulation 64:464, 1981.

406. Harvey, W., Corrado, M. A., and Perloff, J. K.: "Right-sided" murmurs of aortic insufficiency. Am. J. Med. Sci. 245:53, 1963.

407. Fortuin, N. J., and Craige, E.: On the mechanism of the Austin Flint murmur. Circulation 45:558, 1972.

408. Delman, A. J., and Stein, E.: Aortic regurgitation. In Dynamic Cardiac Auscultation and Phonocardiography. Philadelphia, W. B. Saunders Co., 1979, pp. 811–1243.

409. Perloff, J. K.: Acute severe aortic regurgitation: Recognition and management. J. Cardiovasc. Med. 8:209, 1983.

410. Benotti, J. R., and Dalen, J. E.: Aortic valvular regurgitation: Natural history and medical treatment. In Cohn, L. H., and DiSesa, V. J. (eds.): Aortic Regurgitation: Medical and Surgical Management. New York, Marcel Dekker, 1986, pp. 1–54.

411. Spring, D. A., Folts, J. D., Young, W. P., and Rowe, G. G.: Premature closure of the mitral and tricuspid valves. Circulation 45:663, 1972.

412. Wong, M.: Diastolic mitral regurgitation. Hemodynamic and angiographic correlation. Br. Heart J. 31:468, 1969.

413. Estes, E. H.: Left ventricular hypertrophy in acquired heart disease: A comparison of the vectorcardiogram in aortic stenosis and aortic insufficiency. In Hoffman, I. (ed.): Vectorcardiography. Amsterdam, North Holland Publishing Co., 1976.

414. Roberts, W. C., and Day, P. J.: Electrocardiographic observations in clinically isolated, pure, and chronic, severe aortic regurgitation: Analysis of 30 necropsy patients aged 19 to 65 years. Am. J. Cardiol. 55:431, 1985.

415. DePace, N. L., Nestico, P. F., Kotler, M. N., et al.: Comparison of echocardiography and angiography in determining the cause of severe aortic regurgitation. Br. Heart J. 51:36, 1984.

416. Meyer, T., Sareli, P., Pocock, W. A., et al.: Echocardiographic and hemodynamic correlates of diastolic closure of mitral valve and diastolic opening of aortic valve in severe regurgitation. Am. J. Cardiol. 59:1144, 1987.

417. Weaver, W. F., Wilson, C. S., Rourke, T., and Caudill, C. C.: Mid-diastolic aortic valve opening in severe acute aortic regurgitation. Circulation 55:112, 1977.

418. Dolan, M. S., Castello, R., St. Vrain, J. A., et al.: Quantitation of aortic regurgitation by Doppler echocardiography: A practical approach. Am. Heart J. 129:1014, 1995.

418a. Shiota, T., Jones, M., Yamada, I., et al.: Effective regurgitant orifice area by the color Doppler flow convergence method for evaluating the severity of chronic aortic regurgitation: An animal study. Circulation 93:594, 1996.

419. Masuyama, T., Kodama, K., Kitabatake, A., et al.: Noninvasive evaluation of aortic regurgitation by continuous-wave Doppler echocardiography. Circulation 73:460, 1986.

420. Manyari, D. E., Nolewajka, A. J., and Kostuk, W. J.: Quantitative assessment of aortic valvular insufficiency by radionuclide angiography. Chest 81:170, 1982.

421. Reimold, S. C., Maier, S. E., Fleischmann, K. E., et al.: Dynamic nature of the aortic regurgitant orifice area during diastole in patients with chronic aortic regurgitation. Circulation 89:2085, 1994.

422. Sareli, P., Klein, H. O., Schamroth, C. L., et al.: Contribution of echocardiography and immediate surgery to the management of severe aortic regurgitation from active infective endocarditis. Am. J. Cardiol. 57:413, 1986.

423. Goldschlager, N., Pfeifer, J., Cohn, K., et al.: The natural history of aortic regurgitation. A clinical and hemodynamic study. Am. J. Med. 54:577, 1973.

423a. Klodas, E., Enriquez-Sarano, M., Tajik, A. J., et al.: Aortic regurgitation complicated by extreme left ventricular dilatation: Long-term outcome after surgical correction. J. Am. Coll. Cardiol. 27:670, 1996.

424. Elkayam, U., McKay, C. R., Weber, L., et al.: Favorable effects of hydralazine on the hemodynamic response to isometric exercise in chronic severe aortic regurgitation. Am. J. Cardiol. 54:1603, 1984.

425. Fioretti, P., Benussi, B., Scardi, S., et al.: Afterload reduction with nifedipine in aortic insufficiency. Am. J. Cardiol. 49:1728, 1982.

426. Jebavy, P., Koudelkova, E., and Henzlova, M.: Unloading effects of prazosin in patients with chronic aortic regurgitation. Am. Heart J. 105:567, 1983.

427. Rothlisberger, C., Sareli, P., and Wisenbaugh, T.: Comparison of single-dose nifedipine and captopril for chronic severe aortic regurgitation. Am. J. Cardiol. 71:799, 1993.

428. Scognamiglio, R., Rahimtoola, S. H., Fasoli, G., et al.: Nifedipine in asymptomatic patients with severe aortic regurgitation and normal left ventricular function. N. Engl. J. Med. 331:689, 1994.

429. Bonow, R. O.: Asymptomatic aortic regurgitation: Indications for operation. J. Cardiovasc. Surg. 9(Suppl):170, 1994.

430. Bonow, R. O., Lakatos, E., Maron, B. J., and Epstein S. E.: Serial long-term assessment of the natural history of asymptomatic patients with chronic aortic regurgitation and normal left ventricular systolic function. Circulation 84:1625, 1991.

431. Hancock, E. W.: When is the best time to operate for aortic regurgitation? Cardiol. Rev. 1:301, 1993.

432. Nishimura, R., McGoon, M. D., Schaff, H. V., and Giuliani, E. R.: Chronic aortic regurgitation: Indications for operation—1988. Mayo Clin. Proc. 63:270, 1988.

433. Bonow, R. O., Rosing, D. R., Kent, K. M., and Epstein, S. E.: Timing of operation for chronic aortic regurgitation. Am. J. Cardiol. 50:325, 1982.

434. Taniguchi, K., Nakano, S., Matsuda, H., et al.: Depressed myocardial contractility and normal ejection performance after aortic valve replacement in patients with aortic regurgitation. J. Thorac. Cardiovasc. Surg. 98:258, 1989.

435. Borow, K. M.: Surgical outcome in chronic aortic regurgitation: A physiologic framework for assessing preoperative predictors. J. Am. Coll. Cardiol. 10:1165, 1987.

436. Bonow, R. O., Dodd, J. T., Maron, B. J., et al.: Long-term serial changes in left ventricular function and reversal of ventricular dilatation after valve replacement for chronic aortic regurgitation. Circulation 78:1108, 1988.

437. Carabello, B. A., Usher, B. W., Hedrik, G. H., et al.: Predictors of outcome for aortic valve replacement in patients with aortic regurgitation and left ventricular dysfunction: A change in the measuring stick. J. Am. Coll. Cardiol. 10:991, 1987.

438. Wisenbaugh, T., Booth, D., DeMaria, A., et al.: Relationship of contractile state to ejection performance in patients with chronic aortic valve disease. Circulation 73:47, 1986.

439. Odell, J. A., and Orszulak, T. A.: Surgical repair and reconstruction of valvular lesions. Curr. Opin. Cardiol. 10:135, 1995.

440. David, T. E.: Aortic valve repair in patients with Marfan syndrome and ascending aorta aneurysms due to degenerative disease. J. Cardiovasc. Surg. 9(Suppl):182, 1994.

441. Cosgrove, M., Rosenkranz, E. R., Hendren, W. G., et al.: Valvuloplasty for aortic insufficiency. J. Thorac. Cardiovasc. Surg. 102:571, 1991.

442. Duran, C. M.: Present status of reconstructive surgery for aortic valve disease. J. Cardiovasc. Surg. 8:443, 1993.

443. Duran, C. M. G.: Conservative valve surgery. In Al-Zaibag, M., and Duran, C. M. G. (eds.): Valvular Heart Disease. New York, Marcel Dekker, 1994, p. 569.

TRICUSPID, PULMONIC, AND MULTIVALVULAR DISEASE

444. Wooley, C. F., Fontana, M. E., Kilman, J. W., and Ryan, J. M.: Tricuspid stenosis: Atrial systolic murmur, tricuspid opening snap and right atrial pressure pulse. Am. J. Med. 78:375, 1985.

445. Kitchin, A., and Turner, R.: Diagnosis and treatment of tricuspid stenosis. Br. Heart J. 26:354, 1964.

446. Ewy, G. A.: Tricuspid valve disease. In Chatterjee, K., Cheitlin, M. D., Karliner, J., et al. (eds.): Cardiology: An Illustrated Text Reference, Vol. 2. Philadelphia, J. B. Lippincott, 1991, p. 991.

447. Tricuspid valve disease. In Fowler, N. O.: Diagnosis of Heart Disease. New York, Springer-Verlag, 1991, pp. 181–186.

448. Pillai, M. G., Sharma, S., Munsi, S. C., et al.: Value of echocardiography in detecting rheumatic tricuspid stenosis. J. Cardiovasc. Ultrasonogr. 4:185, 1985.

449. Ribeiro, P. A., Al-Zaibag, M., and Sawyer, W.: A prospective study comparing the haemodynamic with the cross-sectional echocardiographic diagnosis of rheumatic tricuspid stenosis. Eur. Heart J. 10:120, 1989.

450. Lundin, L., Landelius, J., Adren, B., and Oberg, K.: Transesophageal echocardiography improves the diagnostic value of cardiac ultrasound in patients with carcinoid heart disease. Br. Heart J. 64:190, 1990.

451. Fawzy, M. E., Mercer, E. N., Dunn, B., et al.: Doppler echocardiography in the evaluation of tricuspid stenosis. Eur. Heart J. 10:985, 1989.

452. Kirklin, J. W., and Barratt-Boyes, B. G.: Combined aortic and mitral valve disease with or without tricuspid valve disease. In Cardiac Surgery. 2nd ed. New York, Churchill-Livingstone, 1993, pp. 573–588.

453. Kirklin, J. W., and Barratt-Boyes, B. G.: Tricuspid valve disease. In Cardiac Surgery. 2nd ed. New York, Churchill-Livingstone, 1993, pp. 589–608.

454. Thorburn, C. W., Morgan, J. J., Shanahan, M. X., and Chang, V. P.: Long-term results of tricuspid valve replacement and the problem of prosthetic valve thrombosis. Am. J. Cardiol. 51:1128, 1983.

455. Boskovic, D., Elezovic, I., Boskovic, D., et al.: Late thrombosis of the Björk-Shiley tilting disc valve in the tricuspid position. J. Thorac. Cardiovasc. Surg. 91:1, 1986.

456. Treasure, T.: Which prosthetic valve should we choose? Curr. Opin. Cardiol. 10:144, 1995.

457. Robiolio, P. A., Rigolin, V. H., Harrison, J. K., et al.: Predictors of outcome of tricuspid valve replacement in carcinoid heart disease. Am. J. Cardiol. 75:485, 1995.

458. Jegaden, O. L., Perinetti, M., Barthelet, M., et al.: Long-term results of porcine bioprostheses in the tricuspid position. Cardiothorac. Surg. 6:256, 1992.

459. McGrath, L. B., Chen, C., Bailey, B. M., et al.: Early and late phase events following bioprosthetic tricuspid valve replacement. J. Cardiovasc. Surg. 7:245, 1992.

460. Guerra, F., Bortolotti, U., Thiene, G., et al.: Long-term performance of the Hancock porcine bioprosthesis in the tricuspid position. A review of 45 patients with 14-year follow-up. J. Thorac. Cardiovasc. Surg. 99:838, 1990.

461. Goldenberg, I. F., Pedersen, W., Olson, J., et al.: Percutaneous double balloon valvuloplasty for severe tricuspid stenosis. Am. Heart J. 118:417, 1989.

462. Shafie, M. Z., Hayat, N., and Majid, O. A.: Fate of tricuspid regurgitation after closed valvotomy for mitral stenosis. Chest 88:870, 1985.

463. Cohen, S. R., Sell, J. E., McIntosh, C. L., and Clark, R. E.: Tricuspid regurgitation in patients with acquired, chronic, pure mitral regurgitation. 1. Prevalence, diagnosis, and comparison of preoperative clinical and hemodynamic features in patients with and without tricuspid regurgitation. J. Thorac. Cardiovasc. Surg. 94:481, 1987.

464. Morrison, D. A., Ovitt, T., and Hammermeister, K. E.: Functional tricuspid regurgitation and right ventricular dysfunction in pulmonary hypertension. Am. J. Cardiol. 62:108, 1988.

465. Vatterott, P. J., Nishimura, R. A., Gersh, B. J., and Smith, H. C.: Severe isolated tricuspid insufficiency in coronary artery disease. Int. J. Cardiol. 14:295, 1987.

466. Dougherty, M. J., and Craige, E.: Apathetic hyperthyroidism presenting as tricuspid regurgitation. Chest 63:767, 1973.

467. Scheck-Krejca, H., Zulstra, F., Roelandt, J., and Vletter-McGhie, J.: Diagnosis of tricuspid regurgitation: Comparison of jugular venous and liver pulse tracings with combined two-dimensional and Doppler echocardiography. Eur. Heart J. 7:973, 1986.

468. Esaghpour, E., Kawai, N., and Linhart, J. W.: Tricuspid insufficiency associated with aneurysm of the ventricular septum. Pediatrics 61:586, 1978.

469. Sakai, K., Inoue, Y., and Osawa, M.: Congenital isolated tricuspid regurgitation in an adult. Am. Heart J. 110:680, 1985.

470. Ohri, S. K., Schofield, J. B., Hodgson, H., et al.: Carcinoid heart disease: Early failure of an allograft valve replacement. Ann. Thorac. Surg. 58:1161, 1994.

471. Lundin, L., Norheim, I., Landelius, J., et al.: Carcinoid heart disease: Relationship of circulating vasoactive substances to ultrasound-detectable cardiac abnormalities. Circulation 77:264, 1988.

472. Jackson, D., Gibbs, H. R., and Zee-Cheng, C. S.: Isolated tricuspid valve prolapse diagnosed by echocardiography. Am. J. Med. 80:281, 1986.

473. Schlamowitz, R. A., Gross, S., Keating, E., et al.: Tricuspid valve prolapse: A common occurrence in the click-murmur syndrome. J. Clin. Ultrasound 10:435, 1982.

474. Gayet, C., Pierre, B., Delahaye, J-P., et al.: Traumatic tricuspid insufficiency: An underdiagnosed disease. Chest 92:429, 1987.

475. Dickerman, S. A., and Rubler, S.: Mitral and tricuspid valve regurgitation in dilated cardiomyopathy. Am. J. Cardiol. 63:629, 1989.

476. Ginzton, L. E., Siegel, R. J., and Criley, J. M.: Natural history of tricuspid valve endocarditis: A two-dimensional echocardiographic study. Am. J. Cardiol. 49:1853, 1982.

477. Arbulu, A., and Asfaw, I.: Tricuspid valvulectomy without prosthetic replacement. Ten years of clinical experience. J. Thorac. Cardiovasc. Surg. 82:684, 1981.

478. Mason, J. W., Billingham, M. E., and Friedman, J. P.: Methysergide induced heart disease: A case of multivalvular and myocardial fibrosis. Circulation 56:889, 1977.

479. Laufer, J., Frand, M., and Milo, S.: Valve replacement for severe tricuspid regurgitation caused by Libman-Sacks endocarditis. Br. Heart J. 48:294, 1982.

480. Pellegrini, A., Columbo, T., Donatelli, E., et al.: Evaluation and treatment of secondary tricuspid insufficiency. Eur. J. Cardiothorac. Surg. 6:288, 1992.

481. Allen, S. J., and Naylor, D.: Pulsation of the eyeballs in tricuspid regurgitation. Can. Med. Assoc. J. 133:119, 1985.

482. Abrams, J.: Tricuspid regurgitation. In Essentials of Cardiac Physical Diagnosis. Philadelphia, Lea and Febiger, 1987, pp. 375–400.

483. Cha, S. D., and Gooch, A. S.: Diagnosis of tricuspid regurgitation: Current status. Arch. Intern. Med. *143*:1763, 1983.

484. Amidi, M., Irwin, J. M., Salerni, R., et al.: Venous systolic thrill and murmur in the neck: A consequence of severe tricuspid insufficiency. J. Am. Coll. Cardiol. *7*:942, 1986.

485. Maisel, A. S., Atwood, J. E., and Goldberger, A. L.: Hepatojugular reflux: Useful in the bedside diagnosis of tricuspid regurgitation. Ann. Intern. Med. *101*:781, 1984.

486. Come, P. C., and Riley, M. F.: Tricuspid annular dilatation and failure of tricuspid leaflet coaptation in patients with tricuspid regurgitation. Am. J. Cardiol. *55*:599, 1985.

487. Popp, R. L.: When is tricuspid regurgitation important? Cardiol. Rev. *2*:183, 1994.

488. Meltzer, R. S., van Hoogenhuyze, D., Serruys, P. W., et al.: Diagnosis of tricuspid regurgitation by contrast echocardiography. Circulation *63*:1093, 1981.

489. Forman, M. B., Byrd, B. F., Oates, J. A., and Robertson, R. M.: Two-dimensional echocardiography in the diagnosis of carcinoid heart disease. Am. Heart J. *107*:492, 1984.

490. Curtius, J. M., Thyssen, M., Breuer, H. W. M., and Loogen, F.: Doppler versus contrast echocardiography for diagnosis of tricuspid regurgitation. Am. J. Cardiol. *56*:333, 1985.

491. Diebold, B., Touati, R., Blanchard, D., et al.: Quantitative assessment of tricuspid regurgitation using pulsed Doppler echocardiography. Br. Heart J. *50*:443, 1983.

492. Pennestri, F., Loperfido, F., Salvatori, M. F., et al.: Assessment of tricuspid regurgitation by pulsed Doppler ultrasonography of the hepatic veins. Am. J. Cardiol. *54*:363, 1984.

493. Suzuki, Y., Kambara, H., Kadota, K., et al.: Detection and evaluation of tricuspid regurgitation using a real-time, two-dimensional, color-coded, Doppler flow imaging system: Comparison with contrast two-dimensional echocardiography and right ventriculography. Am. J. Cardiol. *57*:811, 1986.

494. Lingameni, R., Cha, S. D., Maranhao, V., et al.: Tricuspid regurgitation: Clinical and angiographic assessment. Cathet. Cardiovasc. Diagn. *5*:7, 1979.

495. Cheitlin, M., and MacGregor, J. S.: Acquired tricuspid and pulmonary valve disease. *In* Rahimtoola, S. H. (ed.): Valvular Heart Disease and Endocarditis. Atlas of Heart Diseases. Vol. 11. St. Louis, Mosby, 1996.

496. Ubago, J. L., Figueroa, A., Colman, T., et al.: Right ventriculography as a valid method for the diagnosis of tricuspid insufficiency. Cathet. Cardiovasc. Diagn. *7*:433, 1981.

497. Carpentier, A., Deloche, A., and Dauptain, J.: A new reconstructive operation for correction of mitral and tricuspid insufficiency. J. Thorac. Cardiovasc. Surg. *61*:1, 1971.

498. Lambertz, H., Minale, C., Flachskampf, F. A., et al.: Long-term follow-up after Carpentier tricuspid valvuloplasty. Am. Heart J. *117*:615, 1989.

499. Duran, C. M., Kumar, N., Prabhakar, G., et al.: Vanishing De Vega annuloplasty for functional tricuspid regurgitation. J. Thorac. Cardiovasc. Surg. *106*:609, 1993.

500. Prabhakar, G., Kumar, N., Gometza, B., et al.: Surgery for organic rheumatic disease of the tricuspid valve. J. Heart Valve Dis. *2*:561, 1993.

501. Cohn, L. H.: Tricuspid regurgitation secondary to mitral valve disease: When and how to repair. J. Cardiovasc. Surg. *9*(Suppl.):237, 1994.

502. Chidambaram, M., Abdulali, S. A., Baliga, B. G., and Ionescu, M. I.: Long-term results of DeVega tricuspid annuloplasty. Ann. Thorac. Surg. *43*:185, 1987.

503. Duran, C. M.: Tricuspid valve surgery revisited. J. Cardiovasc. Surg. *9*(Suppl.):242, 1994.

504. Silver, M. A., Cohen, S. R., McIntosh, C. L., et al.: Late (5 to 132 months) clinical and hemodynamic results after either tricuspid valve replacement or annuloplasty for Ebstein's anomaly of the tricuspid valve. Am. J. Cardiol. *54*:627, 1984.

505. Lin, S. S., Reynerstonm, S. I., Louie, E. K., and Levitsky, S.: Right ventricular volume overload results in depression of left ventricular ejection fraction. Circulation *90*:II-209, 1994.

506. Kirshenbaum, H. D.: Pulmonary valve disease. *In* Dalen, J. E., and Alpert, J. S. (eds.): Valvular Heart Disease. 2nd ed. Boston, Little, Brown and Co., 1987, pp. 403–438.

507. Vela, J. E., Conteras, R., and Sosa, F. R.: Rheumatic pulmonary valve disease. Am. J. Cardiol. *23*:12, 1969.

508. Altrichter, P. M., Olson, L. J., Edwards, W. D., et al.: Surgical pathology of the pulmonary valve: A study of 116 cases spanning 15 years. Mayo Clin. Proc. *64*:1352, 1989.

509. Ohri, S. K., Schofield, J. B., Hodgson, H., et al.: Carcinoid heart disease: Early failure of an allograft valve. Ann. Thorac. Surg. *58*:1161, 1994.

510. Seymour, J., Emanuel, R., and Patterson, N.: Acquired pulmonary stenosis. Br. Heart J. *30*:776, 1968.

511. Brayshaw, J. R., and Perloff, J. K.: Congenital pulmonary insufficiency complicating idiopathic dilatation of the pulmonary artery. Am. J. Cardiol. *10*:282, 1962.

512. Runco, V., and Levin, H. S.: The spectrum of pulmonic regurgitation. *In* Physiologic Principles of Heart Sounds and Murmurs. American Heart Association Monograph No. 46, 1975, p. 175.

513. Cassling, R. S., Rogler, W. C., and McManus, B. M.: Isolated pulmonic valve infective endocarditis: A diagnostically elusive entity. Am. Heart J. *109*:558, 1985.

514. Collins, N. P., Braunwald, E., and Morrow, A. G.: Isolated congenital pulmonic valvular regurgitation. Am. J. Med. *28*:159, 1960.

515. Jacoby, W. J., Tucker, D. H., and Sumner, R. G.: The second heart sound in congenital pulmonary valvular insufficiency. Am. Heart J. *69*:603, 1965.

516. O'Toole, J. D., Wurtzbacher, J. J., Wearner, N. E., and Jain, A. C.: Pulmonary valve injury and insufficiency during pulmonary-artery catheterization. N. Engl. J. Med. *301*:1167, 1979.

517. Bousvaros, G. A., and Deuchar, D. C.: The murmur of pulmonary regurgitation which is not associated with pulmonary hypertension. Lancet *2*:962, 1961.

518. DePace, N. L., Nestico, P. F., Iskandrian, A. S., and Morganroth, J.: Acute severe pulmonic valve regurgitation: Pathophysiology, diagnosis and treatment. Am. Heart J. *108*:567, 1984.

519. Green, E. W., Agruss, N. S., and Adolph, R. J.: Right-sided Austin Flint murmur. Documentation by intracardiac phonocardiography, echocardiography and postmortem findings. Am. J. Cardiol. *32*:370, 1973.

520. Braunwald, E., and Morrow, A. G.: A method for detection and estimation of aortic regurgitant flow in man. Circulation *17*:505, 1958.

521. Collins, N. P., Braunwald, E., and Morrow, A. G.: Detection of pulmonic and tricuspid valvular regurgitation by means of indicator solutions. Circulation *20*:561, 1959.

522. Van Meurs-Van Woezik, H., McGhie, J., and Roelandt, J.: Septal flutter in pulmonary insufficiency. J. Cardiovasc. Ultrasonogr. *3*:159, 1984.

523. Miyatake, K., Okamoto, M., Kinoshita, N., et al.: Pulmonary regurgitation studied with the ultrasonic pulsed Doppler technique. Circulation *65*:969, 1982.

524. Emery, R. W., Landes, R. G., Moller, J. H., and Nicoloff, D. M.: Pulmonary valve replacement with a porcine aortic heterograft. Ann. Thorac. Surg. *27*:148, 1979.

525. Segal, J., Harvey, W. P., and Hufnagel, C. A.: Clinical study of one hundred cases of severe aortic insufficiency. Am. J. Med. *21*:200, 1956.

526. Zitnik, R. S.: The masking of aortic stenosis by mitral stenosis. Am. Heart J. *69*:22, 1965.

527. Schattenberg, T. T., Titus, J. L., and Parkin, T. W.: Clinical findings in acquired aortic valve stenosis. Effect of disease of other valves. Am. Heart J. *73*:322, 1967.

528. Melvin, D. B., Tecklenberg, P. L., Hollingsworth, J. F., et al.: Computer-based analysis of preoperative and postoperative prognostic factors in 100 patients with combined aortic and mitral valve replacement. Circulation *48*(Suppl. III):58, 1973.

529. Rippe, J. M.: Multiple floppy valves. An echocardiographic syndrome. Am. J. Med. *66*:817, 1979.

530. Nitter-Hauge, S., and Horstkotte, D.: Management of multivalvular heart disease. Eur. Heart J. *8*:643, 1987.

531. Coll-Mazzei, J. V., Jegaden, O., Janody, P., et al.: Results of triple valve replacement: Perioperative mortality and long-term results. J. Cardiovasc. Surg. *28*:369, 1987.

532. Michel, P. L., Houdart, E., Ghanem, G., et al.: Combined aortic mitral and tricuspid surgery: Results in 78 patients. Eur. Heart J. *8*:457, 1987.

533. MacManus, Q., Grunkemeier, G., and Starr, A.: Late results of triple valve replacement: A 14-year review. Ann. Thorac. Surg. *25*:402, 1978.

534. Vatterott, P. J., Gersh, B. J., Fuster, V., et al.: Long-term followup (2–20 years) of patients with triple valve replacement. J. Am. Coll. Cardiol. *1*(Abs.):586, 1983.

PROSTHETIC CARDIAC VALVES

535. Braunwald, N. S., Cooper, T. S., and Morrow, A. G.: Complete replacement of the mitral valve. J. Thorac. Cardiovasc. Surg. *40*:1, 1960.

536. Harken, D. E., Soroff, M. S., and Taylor, M. C.: Partial and complete prostheses in aortic insufficiency. J. Thorac. Cardiovasc. Surg. *40*:744, 1960.

537. Starr, A., and Edwards, M. L.: Mitral replacement: Clinical experience with a ball-valve prosthesis. Ann. Surg. *154*:726, 1961.

537a. Grunkemeier, G. L., Starr, A., and Rahimtoola, S. H.: Performance of prosthetic heart valves. *In* Rahimtoola, S. H. (ed.): Valvular Heart Disease and Endocarditis. Atlas of Heart Diseases. Vol. 11. St. Louis, Mosby, 1996.

538. Grunkemeier, G. L., and Starr, A.: Twenty-five year experience with Starr-Edwards heart valves: Follow-up methods and results. Can. J. Cardiol. *4*:381, 1988.

539. Pilegaard, H. K., Lund, O., Nielsen, T. T., et al.: Twenty-two-year experience with aortic valve replacement: Starr-Edwards ball valves versus disc valves. Texas Heart Inst. J. *18*:24, 1991.

540. Cohn, L. H.: Aortic valve prosthesis. Cardiol. Rev. *2*:219, 1994.

541. Nair, C. K., Mohiuddin, S. M., Hilleman, D. E., et al.: Ten-year results with the St. Jude medical prosthesis. Am. J. Cardiol. *65*:217, 1990.

542. Burckhardt, D., Streibel, D., Vogt, S., et al.: Heart valve replacement with St. Jude medical valve prosthesis: Long-term experience in 743 patients in Switzerland. Circulation *78*(Suppl. I):I18, 1988.

543. Stewart, S., Cianciotta, D., Hicks, G. L., and DeWeese, J. A.: The Lillehei-Kaster aortic valve prosthesis. J. Thorac. Cardiovasc. Surg. *95*:1023, 1988.

544. Starek, P. J. K., Beaudet, R. L., and Hall, K.-V.: The Medtronic-Hall valve: Development and clinical experience. *In* Crawford, F. A. (ed.): Cardiac Surgery: Current Heart Valve Prostheses. Vol. 1. Philadelphia, Hanley and Belfus, 1987, pp. 223–236.

545. Beaudet, R. L., Nakhle, G., Beaulieu, C. R., et al.: Medtronic-Hall prosthesis: Valve related deaths and complications. Can. J. Cardiol. *4*:376, 1988.

546. Hammermeister, K. E., Sethi, G. K., Henderson, W. G., et al.: A compar-

ison of outcomes in men 11 years after heart-valve replacement with a mechanical valve or bioprosthesis. N. Engl. J. Med. *328*:1289, 1993.

547. Horstkotte, D., Schulte, H., Bircks, W., et al.: Lower intensity anticoagulation therapy results in lower complication rates with the St. Jude medical prosthesis. J. Thorac. Cardiovasc. Surg. *107*:1136, 1994.

548. Turpie, A. G., Gent, M., Laupacis, A., et al.: A comparison of aspirin with placebo in patients treated with warfarin after heart-valve replacement. N. Engl. J. Med. *329*:524, 1993.

549. Turina, J., Hess, O. M., Turina, M., and Krayenbuehl, H. P.: Cardiac bioprosthesis in the 1990s. Circulation *88*:775, 1993.

550. Skoularigis, J., Essop, M. R., Skucicky, D., et al.: Frequency and severity of intravascular hemolysis after left-sided cardiac valve replacement with Medtronic-Hall, St. Jude Medical Protheses and influence of prosthetic type, position, size and number. Am. J. Cardiol. *71*:587, 1993.

551. Glower, D. D., White, W. D., Hatton, A. C., et al.: Determinants of reoperation after 960 valve replacements with Carpentier-Edwards prostheses. J. Thorac. Cardiovasc. Surg. *107*:381, 1994.

552. Grunkemeier, G. L., and Bodnar, E.: Comparison of structural valve failure among different "models" of homograft valves. J. Heart Valve Dis. *3*:556, 1994.

553. Barratt-Boyes, B. G., and Christie, G. W.: What is the best bioprosthetic operation for the small aortic root? Allograft, autograft, porcine, pericardial? Stented or unstented? J. Cardiovasc. Surg. *9*(Suppl.):158, 1994.

554. Bloomfield, P., Wheatley, D. J., Prescott, R. J., and Miller, H. C.: Twelve-year comparison of a Björk-Shiley mechanical heart valve with porcine bioprostheses. N. Engl. J. Med. *324*:573, 1991.

555. Khuri, S. F., Folland, E. D., Sethi, G. K., et al.: Six month postoperative hemodynamics of the Hancock heterograft and the Björk-Shiley prosthesis: Results of a Veteran's Administration cooperative prospective randomized trial. J. Am. Coll. Cardiol. *12*:8, 1988.

556. Janusz, M. T., Jamieson, W. R. E., Burr, L. H., et al.: Thromboembolism risks and role of anticoagulants in patients in chronic atrial fibrillation following mitral valve replacement with porcine bioprostheses. J. Am. Coll. Cardiol. *1*:587, 1983.

557. Khan, S. S., Mitchell, R. S., Derby, G. C., et al.: Differences in Hancock and Carpentier-Edwards porcine xenograft aortic valve hemodynamics: Effect of valve size. Circulation *82*(Suppl. IV):117, 1990.

558. Cohn, L. H., Collins, J. J., DiSesa, V. J., et al.: Fifteen-year experience with 1678 Hancock porcine bioprosthetic heart valve replacements. Ann. Surg. *210*:435, 1989.

559. Jamieson, W. R. E., Tyers, G. F. O., Janusz, M. T., et al.: Age as a determinant for selection of porcine bioprostheses for cardiac valve replacement: Experience with Carpentier-Edwards standard bioprosthesis. Can. J. Cardiol. *7*:181, 1991.

560. Kirklin, J. K., Smith, D., and Novick, W.: Long-term function of cryopreserved aortic homografts: A ten year study. J. Thorac. Cardiovasc. Surg. *106*:154, 1993.

561. Doty, D. B., Michielon, G., Wang, N-D., et al.: Replacement of the aortic valve with cryopreserved aortic allograft. Ann. Thorac. Surg. *56*:228, 1993.

562. Treasure, T.: The pulmonary autograft as aortic valve replacement. Lancet *343*:1308, 1994.

563. Kouchoukos, N. T., Davila-Roman, V. G., Spray, T. L., et al.: Replacement of the aortic root with a pulmonary autograft in children and young adults with aortic-valve disease. N. Engl. J. Med. *330*:1, 1994.

564. Elkins, R. C.: Pulmonary autograft—The optimal substitute for the aortic valve? N. Engl. J. Med. *330*:59, 1994.

565. Ross, D., Jackson, M., and Davies, J.: The pulmonary autograft: A permanent aortic valve. Eur. J. Cardiothorac. Surg. *6*:113, 1992.

566. Oury, J. H., Angell, W. W., Eddy, A. C., and Cleveland, J. C.: Pulmonary autograft—Past, present, and future. J. Heart Valve Dis. *2*:365, 1993.

567. Doty, D. B.: Replacement of the aortic valve with cryopreserved aortic allograft: The procedures of choice for young patients. J. Cardiac Surg. *9*(Suppl.):192, 1994.

568. Bloomfield, P., Wheatley, D. J., Prescott, R. J., and Miller, H. C.: Twelve-year comparison of a Björk-Shiley mechanical heart valve with porcine bioprostheses. N. Engl. J. Med. *324*:573, 1991.

569. Nashof, S. A. M., Sethia, B., Turner, M. A., et al.: Björk-Shiley and Carpentier-Edwards valves: A comparative analysis. J. Thorac. Cardiovasc. Surg. *93*:394, 1987.

570. Hammond, G. I., Geha, A. S., Klopf, G. S., and Hashim, S. W.: Biological versus mechanical valves: Analysis of 1116 valves inserted in 1012 adult patients with a 4818 patient-year and a 5327 valve-year followup. J. Thorac. Cardiovasc. Surg. *93*:182, 1987.

571. Sareli, P., England, M. J., Berk, M. R., et al.: Maternal and fetal sequelae of anticoagulation during pregnancy in patients with mechanical heart valve prostheses. Am. J. Cardiol. *63*:1462, 1989.

572. Iturbe-Alessio, I., Fonesca, M. D. C., Mutchinik, O., et al.: Risks of anticoagulant therapy in pregnant women with artificial heart valves. N. Engl. J. Med. *315*:1390, 1986.

573. John, S.: Valve replacement in the young patients with rheumatic heart disease: Review of a twenty year experience. J. Thorac. Cardiovasc. Surg. *99*:631, 1990.

574. Selwyn, L., Rao, S., Mardin, M. K., et al.: Prosthetic valves in children and adolescents. Am. Heart J. *121*:557, 1991.

575. Gardner, T. J.: Anticoagulants for children requiring heart valve replacement. *In* Dunn, J. M. (ed.): Cardiac Valve Disease in Children. New York, Elsevier, 1988, p. 359.

576. Smith, N. D., Raizada, V., and Abrams, J.: Auscultation of the normally functioning prosthetic valve. Ann. Intern. Med. *95*:594, 1981.

577. Klein, H. O., Schamroth, C. L., Marcus, B. D., et al.: Echo-phonocardiographic assessment of the Medtronic-Hall mitral valve prosthesis: Observations on normal and abnormal function. J. Cardiovasc. Ultrasonogr. *5*:115, 1986.

578. Alam, M., Serwin, J. B., Rosman, H. S., et al.: Transesophageal echocardiographic features of normal and dysfunctioning bioprosthetic valves. Am. Heart J. *121*:1149, 1991.

Chapter 33
Infective Endocarditis

ADOLF W. KARCHMER

DEFINITION

Infective endocarditis (IE) is the condition in which there is microbial infection of the endothelial surface of the heart. The characteristic lesion, the vegetation, is a variably sized amorphous mass of platelets and fibrin in which abundant microorganisms and scant inflammatory cells are enmeshed. Heart valves are most commonly involved; however, infection may occur at the site of a septal defect or on chordae tendineae or mural endocardium. Infection of arteriovenous shunts, arterioarterial shunts (patent ductus arteriosus), or coarctation of the aorta, although actually an endarteritis, is clinically and pathologically similar to IE. Many diverse species of bacteria, fungi, mycobacteria, rickettsiae, chlamydiae, and mycoplasma cause IE; nevertheless, streptococci, staphylococci, enterococci, and fastidious gram-negative coccobacilli that reside in the oral cavity and upper respiratory tract cause the majority of cases of IE.

IE has traditionally been classified as *acute* or *subacute.* Originally, these terms were applied to untreated patients and denoted a disease resulting in marked systemic toxicity and death in days to less than 6 weeks or an indolent, less toxic illness resulting in death in 6 weeks to 6 months or more, respectively. Today acute IE presents with marked toxicity and progresses over days to several weeks to valvular destruction and metastatic infection. In contrast, subacute IE evolves over weeks to months with only modest toxicity and rarely causes metastatic infection. Acute IE is caused typically, although not exclusively, by *Staphylococcus aureus*, whereas the subacute syndrome is more likely caused by viridans streptococci, enterococci, coagulase-negative staphylococci, or gram-negative coccobacilli. Classifications that indicate not only the temporal-toxicity aspects but also the etiology, the anatomical site of infection, and the relevant pathogenetic risk factors, if any, are preferred because they imply therapeutic and prognostic considerations.

EPIDEMIOLOGY

The incidence of IE is remarkably similar in developed countries. From 1950 through 1987, in Olmstead County, Minnesota, the incidence of IE remained relatively constant; it was 4.2 per 100,000 patient-years from 1970 to 1987.[1,2] During the 1980's, the yearly incidence of IE per 100,000 population was 2.0 in the United Kingdom and Wales, 1.9 in the Netherlands, and 1.7 in Louisiana.[3-5] Endocarditis occurred more frequently in men; gender derived ratios range from 1.6 to 2.5.[1,2,4] The age-specific incidence of endocarditis increased progressively after 30 years of age and exceeded 15 to 30 cases per 100,000 person-years in the sixth through eighth decades of life.[1,2,4] From 55 to 75 per cent of patients with native valve endocarditis (NVE) have predisposing conditions: rheumatic heart disease, congenital heart disease, mitral valve prolapse, degenerative heart disease, asymmetrical septal hypertrophy, or intravenous drug abuse.[2,6-8] From 7 to 25 per cent of cases involve prosthetic valves.[2,4,5,7,8] Predisposing conditions cannot be identified in 25 to 45 per cent of patients. The nature of predisposing conditions and, in part, the microbiology of IE correlate with the age of patients (Table 33–1).

CHANGE IN PATIENTS WITH IE. Infective endocarditis is an evolving disease. Changes in some aspects appear incontestable in spite of the

hazard of referral bias in available data. As a consequence of changes in the population at risk for IE, the median age of patients has gradually increased from 30 to 40 years of age in the preantibiotic and early antibiotic eras to 47 to 64 years in recent decades.[1,4,7-10] Rheumatic fever with subsequent rheumatic heart disease in children and young adults has been markedly reduced in developed countries. Patients with congenital and acquired valvular disease, who are vulnerable to IE, enjoy greater longevity. Additionally, during their later years many of these patients require valve replacement, which places them at greater risk for endocarditis. The increasing life span of the general population results in the emergence of degenerative heart disease as a major substrate for IE. Finally, nosocomial endocarditis presents with increased frequency among the elderly, who experience high rates of hospitalization for underlying illnesses.[9,11,12] In recent years, only the increasing role of intravenous drug abuse as predisposition for IE favors the occurrence of infection in younger patients.[10]

Changes have also occurred in the relative frequency of conditions that predispose to IE; the redistribution of predisposing conditions impacts on the age distribution of IE. Intravenous drug abuse, prosthetic heart valves, and nosocomial bacteremia have altered the epidemiological picture of IE over the past three decades. During this period mitral valve prolapse with a murmur of mitral regurgitation has been recognized as an important predisposition for endocarditis.[6,13-16]

CHANGES IN THE MICROBIOLOGY OF IE. The microbiology of IE is affected by the alterations in predisposing conditions and the age of patients with IE. Coagulase-negative staphylococci, previously a minor cause of NVE, are an important cause of prosthetic valve endocarditis (PVE) and nosocomial IE.[16-18] *S. aureus* is the predominant cause of IE among intravenous drug abusers, particularly of infection involving the tricuspid valve. In addition, *Pseudomonas aeruginosa*, other gram-negative bacilli, and *Candida* species, unusual causes of NVE in

TABLE 33–1 PREDISPOSING CONDITIONS AND MICROBIOLOGY OF NATIVE VALVE ENDOCARDITIS

	CHILDREN (%)		ADULTS (%)	
	Neonates	2 mo–15 yr	15–60 yr	> 60 yr
PREDISPOSING CONDITIONS				
RHD		2–10	25–30	8
CHD	28	75–90*	10–20	2
MVP		5–15	10–30	10
DHD			Rare	30
Parenteral drug abuse			15–35	10
Other			10–15	10
None	72†	2–5	25–45	25–40
MICROBIOLOGY				
Streptococci	15–20	40–50	45–65	30–45
Enterococci		4	5–8	15
S. aureus	40–50	25	30–40	25–30
Coagulase-negative staphylococci	10	5	3–5	5–8
GNB	10	5	4–8	5
Fungi	10	1	1	Rare
Polymicrobial	4		1	Rare
Other			1	2
Culture negative	4	0–15	3–10	5

RHD = Rheumatic heart disease; CHD = congenital heart disease; MVP = mitral valve prolapse; DHD = degenerative heart disease; GNB = gram-negative bacteria, frequently *Haemophilus* species, *Actinobacillus actinomycetemcomitans, Cardiobacterium hominis.*
* 50% of cases follow surgery and may involve implanted devices and foreign material.
† Often tricuspid valve IE.

other settings, are important causes of IE in drug abusers.[19] IE caused by enterococci, which are associated with genitourinary tract manipulations, and by *Streptococcus bovis*, which is associated with gastrointestinal malignancy and colonic polyps, occurs more frequently in the elderly, the population likely to experience these precipitating conditions.[1,3,9]

CLINICAL CLASSIFICATION

Cases of IE occurring in defined populations or settings often share clinical features and microbiology. Accordingly, it is useful to classify IE in terms of the population involved or a predisposing condition.

CHILDREN. The incidence of IE among hospitalized children ranges from 1 in 4500 to 1 in 1280.[20] In the Netherlands, IE was noted in 1.7 and 1.2 per 100,000 male and female children less than 10 years old, respectively.[4] Recently, IE has been noted in neonates with increasing frequency. Among neonates, IE typically involves the tricuspid valve of structurally normal hearts and is associated with very high mortality rates. It is likely that many of these episodes arise as a consequence of infected intravenous and right-heart catheters as well as cardiac surgery.[20-22]

The vast majority of children with IE occurring after the neonatal period have identifiable structural cardiac abnormalities (Table 33-1). In recent series, rheumatic heart disease was an infrequent predisposition for IE (≤4 per cent).[22-24] Congenital heart abnormalities, particularly those involving the aortic valve; ventricular septal defects; tetralogy of Fallot; and other complex structural anomalies associated with cyanosis are found in 75 to 90 per cent of cases. Of children with IE on congenital defects, 50 per cent develop infection after cardiac surgery; in these children, infection frequently involves prosthetic valves, valved conduits, or synthetic patches.[22-24] Secundum atrial septal defects are not associated with an increased risk for IE.[25] Since 1990 mitral valve prolapse has been recognized as a predisposition for IE in children; it, generally in association with a regurgitant murmur, was the predisposing cardiac abnormality in 15 per cent and 5 per cent of cases in two series.[23,24]

Endocarditis among neonates is caused primarily by *S. aureus*, coagulase-negative staphylococci, and group B streptococci.[20,21] Occasionally, infection is caused by gram-negative bacilli and *Candida* species.[20,22] Among older children, streptococci, the predominant cause, account for at least 40 per cent of cases, and *S. aureus* occurring as a nosocomial or community-acquired acute infection is the second most common cause of IE.[20,22-24] *Streptococcus pneumoniae*, a common cause of bacteremia in children, is nevertheless an uncommon cause of IE. Like *S. aureus*, *S. pneumoniae* may involve normal or abnormal valves, present as acute fulminant IE, cause rapid valve destruction and heart failure, and often result in death.[20] Although *Haemophilus influenzae* type B is also a frequent cause of bacteremia and meningitis in young children, it rarely causes IE.[20]

The clinical features and echocardiographic findings of IE in children are similar to those noted among adults with NVE or PVE, respectively.[20,23] In contrast, IE among neonates is more cryptic; the clinical picture is dominated by bacteremia, and classic signs of IE are rare.[20]

ADULTS. Some of the common features and evolving aspects of IE occurring in adults have been noted in considering the epidemiology of IE. Mitral valve prolapse has emerged as a predominant predisposing structural cardiac abnormality and accounts for 7 to 30 per cent of NVE in adults which is not related to drug abuse or nosocomial infection.[2,4,6-8,13] The frequency of mitral prolapse in IE is not a direct reflection of risk, however, because as many as 2 to 4 per cent of healthy persons have mitral valve prolapse, and rates increase to 20 per cent among young women.[26,27]

In case-control studies, the relative risk of endocarditis among patients with mitral valve prolapse ranges from 3.5 to 8.2.[13-17] This increased risk of endocarditis is almost entirely confined to patients with both prolapse and a mitral regurgitation murmur. Risk is also increased among men and patients over age 45.[14,16] Valve redundancy and thickened leaflets (>5 mm) by echocardiography also identify a population at increased risk for IE.[19,28] Among patients with mitral valve prolapse and a systolic murmur, the incidence of IE is 52 per 100,000 person-years, compared with a rate of 4.6 per 100,000 person-years among

those with prolapse and no murmur or among the general population.[16] Among 110 episodes of IE involving prolapsing mitral valves, infection was caused by streptococci in 53 per cent, *S. aureus* in 10 per cent, coagulase-negative staphylococci in 9 per cent, enterococci in 9 per cent, and *Haemophilus* species in 6 per cent.[29] The mortality rate was 14 per cent, similar to rates noted in NVE in general.[29]

Rheumatic heart disease was the predisposing cardiac lesion for IE in 20 to 25 per cent of cases in the 1970's and 1980's.[25] In reports from community hospitals in the United States in the 1980's, rheumatic heart disease predisposed to IE in only 7 and 10 per cent of cases.[7,8] In patients with rheumatic heart disease, endocarditis occurs most frequently on the mitral valve, a site at which women are more commonly infected. The aortic valve is the next most common site for IE; infection in this setting occurs more commonly in men.

Congenital heart disease is the substrate for IE in 10 to 20 per cent of younger adults and 8 per cent of older adults. Among adults, the common predisposing lesions are patent ductus arteriosus, ventricular septal defects, and bicuspid aortic valves, the latter seen particularly among older men (>60 years).

In settings where NVE among adults is not skewed dramatically by infection occurring among intravenous drug abusers and nosocomial disease, the microbiology is notably similar to that shown in Table 33-1.[2-4,30] *Coxiella burnetii*, an uncommon cause of IE in the United States, caused 3 per cent of all cases in the United Kingdom from 1976 to 1985 and is a prominent cause of IE in France.[3,31]

INTRAVENOUS DRUG ABUSERS. The risk for IE among intravenous drug abusers, 2 to 5 per cent per patient-year, is estimated to be severalfold greater than that of patients with rheumatic heart disease or prosthetic valves.[32] In one study IE was diagnosed in 74 (6.4 per cent) of 1150 intravenous drug abusers who were hospitalized during 12 months.[33] The ratio of men to women with IE in this study was 5.4:1, similar to that seen in other reports, and the average age of IE patients was 32.5 years. Intravenous cocaine use has been associated with an increased risk for endocarditis, and the intravenous use of pentazocine mixed with tripelennamine was associated with IE caused by *Pseudomonas aeruginosa* sero group 011 in both Detroit and Chicago.[34-36]

Endocarditis occurring in intravenous drug abusers has a unique propensity to infect right heart valves.[32,33] On postmortem examination of 80 addicts with active or healed IE involving 103 valves, evidence of infection was seen on the tricuspid valve in 44 per cent, the mitral valve in 43 per cent, the aortic valve in 40 per cent, and the pulmonic valve in 3 per cent.[37] Because mortality rates are higher in patients with left-sided versus right-sided IE, this distribution is undoubtedly skewed. In clinical series the typical distribution of valve involvement is tricuspid in 78 per cent, mitral in 24 per cent, and aortic in 8 per cent (8 patients had infection of multiple sites).[33] In intravenous drug abusers the valves were normal prior to infection in 75 to 93 per cent of patients.[32,33,37] The remaining patients have preexisting aortic or mitral valve abnormalities, resulting primarily from rheumatic heart disease, congenital heart disease, or prior episodes of IE. Intravenous drug abuse is a risk factor for recurrent NVE.[38]

The microbiology of IE occurring in intravenous drug abusers is unique in several respects (Table 33-2). In contrast to NVE among adults in general, *S. aureus* causes more than 50 per cent of these infections overall and more than 70 per cent of those involving the tricuspid valve. The well-established predilection for *S. aureus* to infect normal as well as abnormal left heart valves is seen in addicts. Although the phenomenon of *S. aureus* infection of normal tricuspid valves is not unique to addicts, the high frequency is characteristic.[32,39] Streptococcal and enterococcal infection of previously abnormal mitral or aortic valves in

TABLE 33–2 MICROBIOLOGY OF ENDOCARDITIS ASSOCIATED WITH INTRAVENOUS DRUG ABUSE

ORGANISM	PER CENT*		
	Right-sided (N = 346)	Left-sided (N = 204)	All Cases (N = 550)
Staphylococcus aureus	77	23	57
Streptococci	5	15	9
Enterococci	2	24	10
Gram-negative bacilli†	5	12	7
Fungi (predominantly *Candida* species)	0	12	5
Polymicrobial	6	7	6
Culture-negative	3	3	3
Miscellaneous	2	3	3

Data from references 32, 33, and 219.

* 10 cases with right- and left-sided IE are each counted twice.

† *P. aeruginosa, S. marcescens,* and Enterobacteriaceae.

addicts is comparable to that noted generally in NVE. In contrast, infection of right and left heart valves by *P. aeruginosa* and other gram-negative bacilli and left heart valves by fungi occurs with increased frequency among drug abusers. In addition, unusual organisms, some of which are likely related to injection of contaminated materials, cause endocarditis in these patients, e.g., *Corynebacterium* species, *Lactobacillus, Bacillus cereus,* and non-pathogenic *Neisseria* species. Polymicrobial endocarditis occurs with increased frequency in intravenous drug abusers. Among 85 cases of polymicrobial IE reported during the 1980's, intravenous drug abuse was a risk factor in 72 per cent.[40]

The clinical manifestations of IE in intravenous drug abusers depend on the valve(s) involved and, to a lesser degree, upon the infecting organism. Tricuspid valve endocarditis, particularly when caused by *S. aureus,* presents with pleuritic chest pain, shortness of breath, cough, and hemoptysis. In 75 per cent of patients, chest roentgenograms contain abnormalities due to septic pulmonary emboli. Murmurs of tricuspid regurgitation are noted in less than half of these patients. Infection of the aortic or mitral valve in addicts clinically resembles IE seen in other patients. That caused by *S. aureus* generally presents as acute endocarditis with marked systemic toxicity. Symptoms and signs of left heart failure, neurologic injury, systemic emboli, metastatic infections, and the classic peripheral stigmata of IE are strongly associated with left-sided endocarditis.[32]

Thirty-four human immunodeficiency virus (HIV)–infected and 12 HIV seronegative intravenous drug abusers were studied with 40 and 14 episodes of IE, respectively. Endocarditis in the two groups was similar in clinical presentation, microbiology, complications, and overall survival. Among HIV-infected patients, death attributed to IE was more frequent in CDC group IV patients (40 per cent) than in the non–group IV patients (10 per cent).[41]

PROSTHETIC VALVE ENDOCARDITIS (PVE). Epidemiologic studies suggest that PVE comprises 10 to 20 per cent of all cases of IE in developed countries.[2,4] In four studies with careful follow-up of valve recipients, the cumulative incidence of PVE estimated actuarially was 1.4 to 3.1 per cent at 12 months, 4.1 to 5.4 per cent at 4 years, and 3.2 to 5.7 per cent at 5 years.[42–45] The risk of PVE over time, however, is not uniform. The risk is greatest during the initial 6 months after valve surgery (particularly during the initial 5 to 6 weeks) and thereafter declines to a lower but persistent risk (0.2 to 0.35 per cent per year).[42–46]

PVE has been called "early" when symptoms begin within 60 days of valve surgery and "late" with onset thereafter. These terms were established to distinguish early PVE that arose as a complication of valve surgery from late infection that was more likely community ac-

quired. In fact, many cases with onset between 60 days and 1 year after surgery are likely to be nosocomial and in spite of their delayed presentation derive from events during the surgical admission.[47] Studies to identify risk factors for PVE have not resulted in a coherent picture. Data suggest that during the initial months after valve implantation mechanical prostheses are at greater risk of infection than bioprosthetic valves but that after 12 months the risk for infection of bioprostheses exceeds that of mechanical valves.[43–46] Patients with antecedent native valve endocarditis, particularly if active, are at increased risk for PVE.[43,44,46]

Microbiology of PVE. The microbiology of PVE is relatively predictable and reflects in part the presumed nosocomial or community acquisition of infection (Table 33–3). Coagulase-negative staphylococci, which when speciated are primarily *Staphylococcus epidermidis,* are the predominant causes of PVE diagnosed within 60 days after surgery. *S. aureus,* gram-negative bacilli, diphtheroids, and fungi (particularly *Candida* species) are also common causes of PVE during this period. Occasional cases of nosocomial PVE caused by *Legionella* species, atypical mycobacteria, mycoplasma, and fungi other than *Candida* have been reported. The spectrum and frequency of microorganisms causing PVE that occurs between 2 and 12 months after cardiac surgery and within the initial 60 postoperative days are similar. More than 80 per cent of the coagulase-negative staphylococci from either of these time periods are resistant to methicillin and all other beta-lactam antibiotics. In contrast, 30 per cent or fewer of the coagulase-negative staphylococci causing PVE with onset more than 1 year after valve surgery are methicillin-resistant.[45,48] PVE with onset 1 year or more postoperatively presumably results from transient bacteremia arising from dental, gastrointestinal, and genitourinary manipulations, breaks in the skin barrier, and intercurrent infections.[46,47] Consequently, the microbiology of these cases resembles that seen in community-acquired NVE in non-addicts: streptococci, *S. aureus,* enterococci, and fastidious gram-negative coccobacilli (*Haemophilus* species, *Actinobacillus actinomycetemcomitans, Cardiobacterium hominis, Eikenella,* and *Kingella*—the so-called HACEK group). Coagulase-negative staphylococci cause 15 per cent of these cases of PVE.

Pathology of PVE. The intracardiac pathology of PVE differs notably from the largely leaflet-confined pathology of NVE. Infection on mechanical prostheses commonly extends beyond the valve ring into the annulus and periannular tissue as well as the mitral-aortic intravalvular fibrosa, resulting in ring abscesses, septal abscesses, fistulous tracts, and dehiscence of the prosthesis with hemodynami-

TABLE 33–3 MICROBIOLOGY OF PROSTHETIC VALVE ENDOCARDITIS, 1975–1989

ORGANISM	TIME OF ONSET AFTER CARDIAC SURGERY (%)		
	< 2 Months (N = 73)	2–12 Months (N = 38)	> 12 Months (N = 94)
Coagulase-negative staphylococci	38	50	15
Staphylococcus aureus	14	11	13
Gram-negative bacilli	11	5	1
Streptococci	0	3	33
Enterococci	7	5	11
Diphtheroids	12	3	2
Fastidious gram-negative coccobacilli	0	3	12
Fungi	10	5	3
Miscellaneous	4	5	1
Culture-negative	4	11	10

Data from references 47 and 257–260.

cally significant paravalvular regurgitation (Fig. 33–1). In autopsy experience with 74 patients, which is clearly biased toward the most severe pathology, annular invasion was noted in 85 per cent, myocardial abscess in 32 per cent, and valve obstruction by vegetation overgrowth, a phenomenon of PVE at the mitral site, in 19 per cent.[47] Erosion through the aortic annulus to cause pericarditis occurred in 5 per cent.[47] In clinical series encompassing 85 patients, the rate of annulus invasion was 42 per cent, myocardial abscess 14 per cent, valve obstruction 4 per cent, and pericarditis 2 per cent.[47] The intracardiac pathology of bioprosthetic valve IE is more heterogeneous and includes invasive disease, comparable to that noted when PVE involves mechanical valves, as well as leaflet destruction (Figs. 33–1 and 33–2). Among 85 patients with bioprosthetic PVE, 29 (59 per cent) of 49 with infection within a year after surgery had invasive disease, in contrast to only 9 (25 per cent) of 36 patients with infection occurring more than 1 year postoperatively. Infection confined to the leaflets was proven in another 9 (25 per cent) with late onset and was assumed in the majority of the remaining 18 patients who survived without surgical intervention.[47] In a study of PVE involving either mechanical or bioprosthetic valves, aortic site and clinical onset within a year of valve surgery were significantly correlated with an increased risk for invasive infection.[49] Other studies have noted increased invasive disease with PVE at the aortic versus the mitral site.[50,51]

The clinical features of PVE resemble those found in non-drug abuse–associated NVE. Signs and symptoms in patients developing PVE within 60 days of cardiac surgery may be obscured by surgery or other postoperative complications. Peripheral signs of endocarditis (5 to 14 per cent) and central nervous system emboli (10 per cent) occur less frequently in these patients than in those with PVE occurring later after surgery. Among patients with later onset PVE, congestive heart failure occurs in 40 per cent, cerebrovascular complications in 26 to 28 per cent, and peripheral signs in 15 to 28 per cent.[47,52,53]

NOSOCOMIAL ENDOCARDITIS. Hospital-acquired endocarditis unrelated to concurrent cardiac surgery comprises 5 to 29 per cent of all cases of IE in various series.[7,8,11,12,54] Nosocomial IE has involved abnormal native cardiac valves, normal valves including the tricuspid, and prosthetic valves and occurs with similar frequency among patients with NVE and PVE (unrelated to valve surgery).[4,7,11] Infected intravascular devices and catheters give rise to 45 to 65 per cent of the

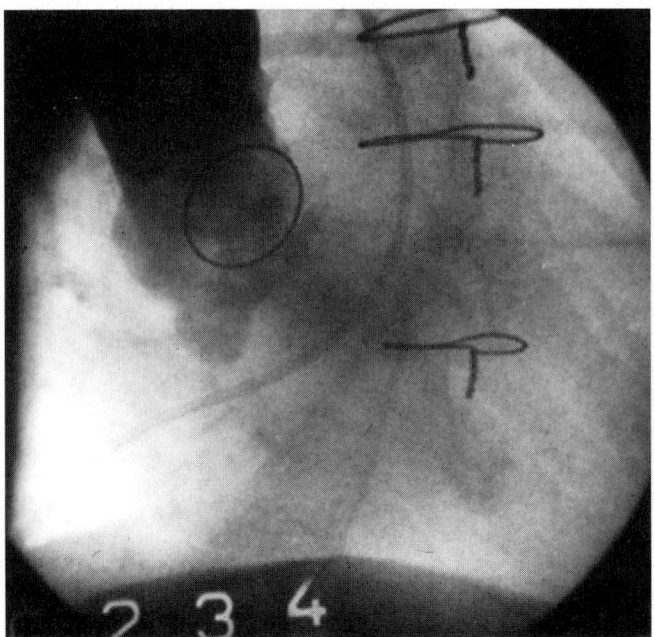

FIGURE 33–1. *S. epidermidis* infection of a bioprosthetic aortic valve 3 months after surgery. Contrast material injected supravalvularly fills a paravalvular abscess and regurgitates into the left ventricle.

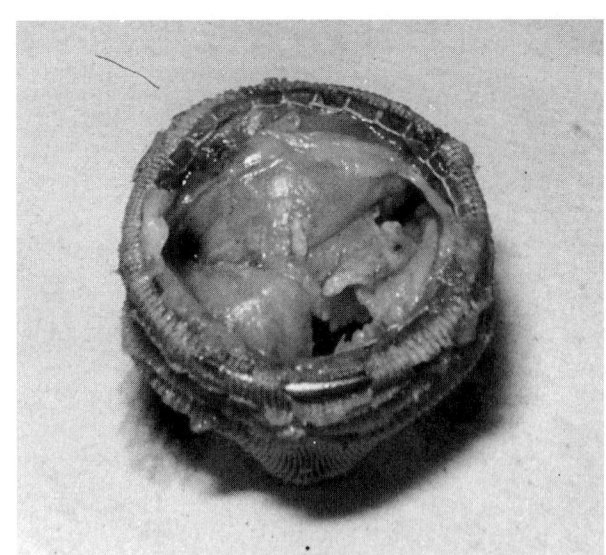

FIGURE 33–2. A bioprosthetic valve removed from the aortic position 18 months after insertion because of enterococcal PVE causing severe leaflet destruction and aortic regurgitation.

bacteremia that results in nosocomial IE.[11,12,54] Other sources of bacteremia include genitourinary and gastrointestinal tract instrumentation or surgery. In 141 bone marrow transplant recipients, prolonged placement (mean 98 days) of central venous catheters extending into or near the right atrium was associated with eight episodes of endocarditis, of which seven were right-sided.[55] In an autopsy study of 55 patients who had been managed using flow-directed pulmonary artery catheters, four were found to have right-sided endocarditis.[56]

Microbiology of Nosocomial IE. Gram-positive cocci are the predominant cause of nosocomial IE. Among 45 episodes from two series, *S. aureus* caused 44 per cent, coagulase-negative staphylococci 22 per cent, enterococci 18 per cent, streptococci and *Candida* species and gram-negative bacilli each 4 per cent. One patient (2 per cent) had negative cultures.[11,12] The frequency of endocarditis or other deep-seated *S. aureus* infections after catheter-related bacteremia ranges from 3 to 8 per cent; nevertheless, catheter-associated *S. aureus* bacteremia occurs with sufficient frequency to be the predominant predisposition for nosocomial IE.[11,12,57–60] IE complicates 0.85 to 3.1 per cent of nosocomial enterococcal bacteremia; although the risk of nosocomial enterococcal IE is increased in patients with abnormal valves, it remains small, relative to that for nosocomial *S. aureus* bacteremia.[11,12,61,62] Among 115 patients with prosthetic valves and a nosocomial bacteremia that was not the index test for PVE, 18 patients (15.6 per cent) subsequently developed PVE that was the apparent consequence of the bacteremia. *S. aureus* and *S. epidermidis* were that most common organisms in these cases of PVE, although gram-negative bacilli and fungi also caused episodes of PVE.[63] Bacteremia persisting for days prior to treatment or for 72 hours or more after removal of an infected catheter and initiation of treatment, especially in patients with abnormal heart valves or prosthetic valves, suggests the diagnosis of IE.[12,54,60]

The onset of nosocomial IE is usually acute and although a changing murmur may be heard, other classical signs of endocarditis are infrequent.[11,64] Mortality rates among these patients, many of whom are elderly and have serious underlying diseases, are high (40 to 56 per cent).[11,12,54]

Etiological Microorganisms

VIRIDANS STREPTOCOCCI. These streptococci, which cause 30 to 65 per cent of NVE unrelated to drug abuse, are normal inhabitants of the oropharynx, characteristically produce alpha-hemolysis when grown on sheep blood agar, and are usually nontypable using the Lancefield system. The viridans streptococci are not a species but rather a group of organisms composed of multiple species, many of which have recently undergone taxonomic redefinition. Using the previous classification, the species causing streptococcal NVE were distributed as follows: *Streptococcus mitior* (31 per cent of cases), *Streptococcus sanguis* (24 per cent), *Streptococcus bovis* (27 per cent), *Streptococcus mutans* (7 per cent), *Streptococcus milleri* (4 per cent), *Streptococcus faecalis* (now *Enterococcus faecalis*) (7 per cent), and *Streptococcus salivarius* and other species (2 per cent).[62] Another study, adjusted for the new taxonomy, has reported a similar distribution of streptococci causing IE.[65] Nutritionally variant streptococci, strains that require media supplemented with either pyridoxal hydrochloride or L-cysteine for growth and are now speciated as *Streptococcus adjacens* or *Streptococcus defectivus*, cause 5 per cent of streptococcal NVE.[62,66]

The viridans streptococci, other than the nutritionally variant organisms, are in general highly susceptible to penicillin (minimum inhibitory concentration [MIC] ≤ 0.1 μg/ml for 83 per cent) and are killed in an enhanced manner (synergistically) by penicillin plus gentamicin.[62,66,67] S. adjacens and S. defectivus appear more resistant to penicillin (MIC > 0.12 μg/ml in more than 30 per cent of strains).[66] Although penicillin-aminoglycoside synergy was not demonstrated in vitro with S. adjacens and S. defectivus, in therapy of experimental endocarditis caused by these organisms, penicillin-aminoglycoside combinations were more effective than penicillin alone; also, therapy with vancomycin alone was comparable to that with the penicillin-aminoglycoside combination.[66]

STREPTOCOCCUS BOVIS AND OTHER STREPTOCOCCI. S. bovis, part of the gastrointestinal tract normal flora, causes 27 per cent of the episodes of streptococcal NVE.[62] Although superficially resembling the enterococci, this species can be easily distinguished by its biochemical characteristics. The distinction is important because S. bovis is highly penicillin susceptible, in contrast to the relative penicillin resistance of enterococci. S. bovis NVE is frequently associated with coexistent colonic polyps or malignancy.[9,10,68]

Group A streptococci, which can infect normal valves, cause rare episodes of endocarditis. Among intravenous drug abusers, group A streptococci have caused tricuspid valve IE similar to that noted with S. aureus.[69] Group B organisms, Streptococcus agalactiae, are part of the normal flora of the mouth, genital tract, and gastrointestinal tract. Group B streptococci infect normal and abnormal valves and cause a very morbid NVE syndrome with a high incidence of systemic emboli.[70,71] The organisms' failure to produce fibrinolysin may result in large vegetations and a high rate of systemic emboli. Endocarditis caused by this organism may be associated with villous adenomas and colonic neoplasms.[72] Group G streptococci also produce a destructive, highly morbid left-sided NVE.[73] The Streptococcus milleri group, now divided into three species—Streptococcus intermedius, Streptococcus constellatus, and Streptococcus anginosus—are highly pyogenic organisms, some of which type as Lancefield group F.[74] These penicillin-susceptible organisms, which cause destructive infections similar to those caused by S. aureus, have accounted for 2 to 5 per cent of streptococcal NVE cases.[62,65]

STREPTOCOCCUS PNEUMONIAE. Although pneumococcal bacteremia occurs frequently, S. pneumoniae accounts for only 1 to 3 per cent of NVE cases. When causing IE, S. pneumoniae frequently involves a previously normal aortic valve and progresses rapidly with valve destruction, myocardial abscess formation, and acute congestive heart failure. Mortality rates range from 30 to 50 per cent.[75-77] Alcoholism is a risk factor for pneumococcal IE, and concurrent pneumonia or meningitis is common.[75,77] Although pneumococci causing endocarditis have been highly susceptible to penicillin, strains that are relatively penicillin-resistant (MIC ≥ 0.1 μg/ml to ≤ 1.0 μg/ml) and highly penicillin-resistant (MIC > 1.0 μg/ml) are increasingly common causes of pneumococcal infection, particularly in children.[78] Many of the highly resistant strains are also resistant to erythromycin, trimethoprim-sulfamethoxazole, and cephalosporins, including ceftriaxone. These strains remain susceptible to vancomycin. In the future these penicillin-resistant strains are likely to cause sporadic cases of IE.[79]

ENTEROCOCCI. These organisms, once considered Lancefield group D streptococci, have recently been accorded their own genus, Enterococcus. Although there are at present 12 species of enterococci, Enterococcus faecalis and Enterococcus faecium cause 85 per cent and 10 per cent of cases of enterococcal IE, respectively. Enterococci are part of the normal gastrointestinal flora and cause genitourinary tract infection. Enterococci account for 5 to 15 per cent of cases of NVE and a similar percentage of PVE cases (Tables 33–2 and 33–3).[47,80] Occasional cases occur in young women as a consequence of genitourinary tract manipulation or infection. The majority of cases occur, however, in older, predominantly male, patients and have the urinary tract as a likely portal of entry.[81] Enterococci infect either normal or previously abnormal valves and present as either acute or subacute IE.[80]

Enterococci are overtly resistant to cephalosporins, semisynthetic penicillinase-resistant penicillins (oxacillin and nafcillin), and therapeutic concentrations of aminoglycosides. Most enterococci are inhibited by modest concentrations of the cell wall–active antibiotics—penicillin, ampicillin, vancomycin, and teicoplanin (not licensed in the United States). Bactericidal anti-enterococcal activity can be achieved by combining an inhibitory cell wall–active agent and an appropriate aminoglycoside. This bactericidal activity, called synergy, is essential for optimal treatment of enterococcal IE.[80] Strains of enterococci that are highly resistant to penicillin and ampicillin, resistant to vancomycin, and highly resistant to all aminoglycosides have been identified as causes of nosocomial infections.[80,82] Although these resistant strains have caused only sporadic cases of IE, their wide distribution and frequency as nosocomial pathogens have increased the complexity of treating enterococcal IE (see Antimicrobial Therapy).[80-83]

STAPHYLOCOCCI. The coagulase-positive staphylococci are a single species, S. aureus. Of the 13 species of coagulase-negative staphylococci that colonize humans, one, S. epidermidis, has emerged as an important pathogen in the setting of implanted devices and hospitalized patients. S. aureus and S. epidermidis have surface receptors that bind to host proteins, including fibronectin and fibrinogen. These proteins, in turn, may be present at sites of endocardial injury and coat implanted foreign devices. Although the pathogenesis is un-

doubtedly far more complex, these receptors, by binding to host proteins, may facilitate the adherence of staphylococci to sites where they proliferate to generate endocarditis.[84,85] Coagulase-negative staphylococci are coated with a slime or glycocalyx layer that favors their survival on foreign devices. Embedded in this material, large populations of coagulase-negative staphylococci accumulate on the surface of foreign devices; these organisms in turn have altered phenotypes, including increased resistance to the bactericidal effects of many antibiotics.[86,87] A capsular polysaccharide/adhesin of S. epidermidis has increased the organism's resistance to eradication by host granulocytes and thus may allow an initial small inoculum to proliferate and ultimately cause IE.[88,89]

Antibiotic Resistance. In excess of 90 per cent of S. aureus, whether acquired in the hospital or community, produce beta-lactamase and thus are resistant to penicillin, ampicillin, and the ureidopenicillins. These organisms are, however, susceptible to the penicillinase-resistant beta-lactam antibiotics (oxacillin, nafcillin, cefazolin, and other first-generation cephalosporins). Resistance of S. aureus to methicillin and other beta-lactam antibiotics is based upon production of an altered penicillin-binding protein (called 2a or 2') with decreased affinity for beta-lactam antibiotics. Methicillin-resistant strains are increasingly prevalent in nosocomial settings and among selected, nonhospitalized populations (intravenous drug abusers, nursing home residents); methicillin-resistant strains must be considered when selecting initial empirical therapy for IE in patients from these groups.[33,90] Coagulase-negative staphylococci frequently produce beta-lactamase; furthermore, strains causing community-acquired infections are frequently methicillin-susceptible, while those causing nosocomial infections, including IE, are commonly methicillin-resistant.[48,91] Coagulase-negative staphylococci may not always phenotypically express methicillin resistance (a property called heteroresistance). Consequently, special testing may be required to detect this resistance.[48,90,91] Resistance to aminoglycosides and to fluoroquinolones is increasingly common among staphylococci, particularly those that are methicillin-resistant.[90,91] Most staphylococci are susceptible to rifampin; however, resistant strains are rapidly selected when rifampin is used alone to treat staphylococcal infections.[48,90] Staphylococci, including most strains that are resistant to methicillin, remain susceptible to vancomycin and teicoplanin.[48,90]

Clinical Features. S. aureus is a major cause of IE in all population groups (Tables 33–1 to 33–3). S. aureus IE is characterized by a highly toxic febrile illness, frequent focal metastatic infection, and a 30 to 50 per cent rate of central nervous system complications.[90] A cerebrospinal fluid polymorphonuclear pleocytosis, with or without S. aureus cultured from the cerebrospinal fluid, is common.[90] Heart murmurs are heard in 30 to 45 per cent of patients on initial evaluation and are ultimately heard in 75 to 85 per cent as a consequence of intracardiac damage. The mortality rate in nonaddicts with left-sided S. aureus endocarditis is 34 per cent overall and increases in those over 50 years of age, in those with significant underlying diseases, and when IE is complicated by a major neurologic event, valve dysfunction, or congestive heart failure.[90] Among addicts left-sided S. aureus IE resembles that seen in nonaddicts. In contrast, in patients with IE limited to the tricuspid valve, complications are rare, and mortality rates are only 2 to 4 per cent.[90,92] Occasionally tricuspid staphylococcal IE results in overwhelming septic pulmonary emboli, pyopneumothorax, and severe respiratory insufficiency.

Coagulase-Negative Staphylococci. These are a major cause of PVE, particularly during the initial year after valve surgery, an important cause of nosocomial IE, and the cause of 3 to 8 per cent of NVE, usually in the setting of prior valve abnormalities (Tables 33–1 and 33–3).[90,91] The vast majority of coagulase-negative staphylococci causing PVE, when speciated, are S. epidermidis.[48,90] In contrast, when infection involves native valves, only 50 per cent of isolates are S. epidermidis.[90,91] Staphylococcus lugdunensis, a coagulase-negative species, has caused highly destructive, often fatal NVE and PVE.[93,94] S. lugdunensis IE is usually community-acquired and the organism is often susceptible to many antistaphylococcal antibiotics, including penicillin.[94] Coagulase-negative staphylococcal NVE is generally subacute, and occasional patients have minimal or no fever throughout their illness. Nevertheless, destruction of intracardiac structures, metastatic infection including vertebral osteomyelitis, and central nervous system complications occur frequently in NVE caused by species other than S. lugdunensis.[90,91]

GRAM-NEGATIVE BACTERIA. Organisms of the so-called HACEK group, which are part of the upper respiratory tract and oropharyngeal flora, infect abnormal cardiac valves, causing subacute NVE, and cause PVE that occurs a year or more after valve surgery.[95-97] In NVE, the HACEK organisms have been associated with large vegetations and a high incidence of systemic emboli.[97] These organisms are fastidious and slow growing; when they are suspected, blood cultures should be incubated for 3 weeks. Haemophilus species, primarily H. aphrophilus followed by H. parainfluenzae and H. influenzae, account for 0.5 to 1.0 per cent of all IE. Among the other organisms in this group, A. actinomycetemcomitans and C. hominis are the next most common causes of IE, followed by E. corrodens, which is microaerophilic, and Kingella species. The HACEK group have been susceptible to penicillin, ampicillin, aminoglycosides, quinolones, and third-generation cephalosporins. Some recent isolates have produced a beta-lactamase; thus, penicillin and ampicillin must be used with caution when treating HACEK endocarditis.[29,95]

P. aeruginosa is the gram-negative bacillus that most commonly causes endocarditis. The proclivity of *P. aeruginosa,* as opposed to Enterobacteriaceae, to cause IE correlates with its resistance to the bactericidal activity of human sera and its adherence to cardiac valves and platelet-fibrin thrombi. Pseudomonal IE involves normal and abnormal valves on both sides of the heart and often causes valve destruction and heart failure (Fig. 33–3).[35,36,97]

The Enterobacteriaceae, in spite of causing frequent episodes of bacteremia, are implicated in only sporadic cases of IE. *Escherichia coli, Klebsiella-Enterobacter* species, and *Salmonella* species have infected normal as well as abnormal valves. *Salmonella* species also infect mural endocardial thrombi and atherosclerotic arterial aneurysms. Gram-negative bacillus IE is noted with increased frequency among intravenous drug abusers and during the initial year after prosthetic valve placement.[32,47] *Serratia marcescens* has caused regional epidemics of IE among addicts.[32,97]

Neisseria gonorrhoeae, a common cause of IE during the preantibiotic era, rarely causes endocarditis today.[98,99] Gonococci, similar to pneumococci, infect the aortic valve of young patients, resulting in valve destruction, abscess formation, and a probable need for valve replacement.[99] Penicillinase production and intrinsic resistance to penicillin are common among gonococci; however, all strains remain susceptible to ceftriaxone. Nonpathogenic *Neisseria* cause sporadic cases of IE.[99] *Brucella,* small aerobic slow-growing coccobacillary organisms, cause subacute IE in patients with valvular abnormalities, particularly among men exposed to infected foods and animals.[99,100] High antibody titers against *Brucella* can suggest the diagnosis when cultures are negative.

OTHER ORGANISMS. *Corynebacterium* species and other coryneform bacteria, often called diphtheroids, are commensals on the skin and mucous membranes. Prolonged incubation of blood cultures is often required to isolate these slow-growing, fastidious organisms from patients with IE. Although often contaminants in blood cultures, diphtheroids in multiple blood cultures cannot be ignored. They are an important cause of PVE occurring during the initial year after valve surgery and a surprisingly common cause of endocarditis involving abnormal valves.[47,101] Diphtheroids are often killed by the synergistic interaction of penicillin and an effective aminoglycoside as well as by vancomycin.[102] *Listeria monocytogenes,* a small gram-positive rod, causes occasional cases of IE involving abnormal left heart valves and prosthetic devices.[103] *Bartonella* species, formerly called *Rochalimaea,* can be isolated from patients with IE by prolonged incubation of blood cultures (2 weeks) followed by blind subculturing to fresh chocolate agar or sheep blood agar, which is in turn incubated for 2 to 3 weeks in 5 to 8 per cent CO_2.[104,105] *Bartonella quintana, Bartonella elizabethae,* and *Bartonella henselae* have caused subacute endocarditis with valvular damage. In the absence of special efforts in culturing, these cases would have been "culture negative."[104,105] Although *B. quintana* causes trench fever vectored by the body louse and cat-scratch disease, the role of ectoparasites and cats in the epidemiology of *Bartonella* endocarditis is not known.

The rickettsia *Coxiella burnetii,* a weakly gram-negative obligate intracellular organism, infects humans after inhalation of desiccated materials from infected animals or contact with infected parturient animals. At variable intervals after acute infection by *C. burnetii* (Q fever), persons with abnormal mitral or aortic valves who have not been able to eradicate the organism develop subacute IE with typical manifestations and often with valve dysfunction causing heart failure.[31,106] The diagnosis is typically based on high antibody titers to phase I and II *C. burnetii* antigens. However, the organism can be grown from blood (buffy coat) or valve tissue on human embryonic lung fibroblast cell culture and can be demonstrated in excised cardiac valves by immunohistological staining.[31,106] *Chlamydia psittaci,* the agent of psittacosis, has caused occasional episodes of subacute IE

and has resulted in hemodynamically significant valve damage. There may be concurrent pneumonia, and a history of contact with birds is often noted. The diagnosis can be suspected when routine blood cultures are negative and there is a strong serologic response. The organism can be cultured on cell monolayers from blood, the respiratory tract, or valve; it also can be demonstrated immunohistologically in excised valve tissue.[107] The many other organisms that have caused IE are beyond the scope of this chapter; some have been discussed in recent reviews.[99,108]

FUNGI. *Candida albicans,* non-albicans *Candida* species, *Torulopsis glabrata,* and *Aspergillus* species are the most common of the many fungal organisms identified as causing IE. Fungal endocarditis arises in specific settings. Valve replacement cardiac surgery and intravenous drug abuse are major predispositions. The most frequent fungi causing PVE are *C. albicans, Aspergillus* species, and non-albicans *Candida* species, while addict-associated fungal IE is most commonly caused by non-*albicans Candida* species, particularly *C. parapsilosis.*[109,110] Fungal IE resulting from prolonged intravenous antimicrobial therapy and parenteral alimentation is caused predominantly by *C. albicans* and *T. glabrata.* Patients who are severely immunodepressed occasionally experience IE caused by *Candida* species, *Aspergillus* species, or opportunistic mycelia fungi. Blood cultures frequently are positive when *Candida* species or *T. glabrata* cause IE but rarely yield organisms when IE is caused by mycelial organisms. Bulky vegetations, which embolize frequently, are common in fungal IE. Removal and careful microbiological evaluation of an embolic vegetation may provide an etiological diagnosis in fungal IE.[109,110]

PATHOGENESIS

The interactions between the human host and selected microorganisms that culminate in IE involve the vascular endothelium, hemostatic mechanisms, the host immune system, gross anatomic abnormalities in the heart, surface properties of microorganisms, and peripheral events that initiate bacteremia. Each component of these interactions is in itself complex, influenced by many factors and not fully elucidated. The rarity of endocarditis and endarteritis in the face of frequent transient asymptomatic and symptomatic bacteremia indicates that the intact endothelium is resistant to infection. The normal cardiac valve endothelium in rabbits is resistant to colonization by bacteria even with injection of 10^9 to 10^{10} organisms. If the endothelium on the valve surface is damaged, hemostasis is stimulated, leading to deposition of platelets and fibrin.[111] This resulting platelet-fibrin complex is more receptive to colonization by bacteria than is the intact endothelium.[112,113] It is hypothesized that platelet-fibrin deposition occurs spontaneously in persons vulnerable to endocarditis and that these deposits, called nonbacterial thrombotic endocarditis (NBTE), are the sites at which microorganisms adhere to initiate IE. Bacteremia allows organisms access to the NBTE. The relative uniformity of organisms causing IE, as contrasted with the variety of organisms causing overt and asymptomatic bacteremia, and the infectiousness of specific organisms in animal models of endocarditis, indicates that certain microorganisms are advantaged in their ability to colonize and infect NBTE. The events after colonization that lead to IE entail survival and multiplication of microorganisms and accrual of vegetation and are complex interactions as well. (Space limitations require that this summary of pathogenesis be abbreviated and incompletely referenced. For detailed reviews see references 114 to 119.)

DEVELOPMENT OF NONBACTERIAL THROMBOTIC ENDOCARDITIS. Two major mechanisms appear pivotal in the formation of NBTE: endothelial injury and a hypercoagulable state. NBTE has been found in 1.3 per cent of patients at autopsy and, while present at all ages, is more common with increasing age.[120] These lesions have also been noted frequently in patients with malignancy, disseminated intravascular coagulation, uremia, burns, systemic lupus erythematosus, valvular heart disease, and intracardiac catheters.[114,116,120] The platelet-thrombin deposits are found at the valve closure-contact line on the atrial surfaces of the mitral and tricuspid valves and the ventricular surfaces of the aortic and pulmonic valves. The sites of these NBTE

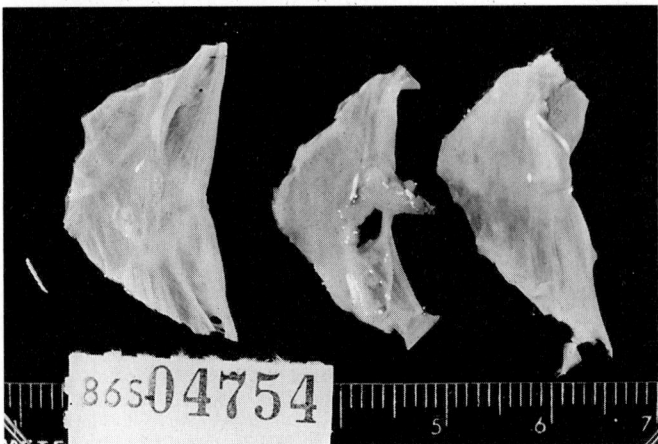

FIGURE 33–3. Aortic valve with multiple vegetations and valve destruction caused by *P. aeruginosa.* Surgery was required because of uncontrolled infection and congestive heart failure.

correspond closely with the location of infected vegetations in patients with IE.[120]

Three hemodynamic circumstances may injure the endothelium, initiating NBTE: (1) a high-velocity jet impacting endothelium; (2) flow from a high- to a low-pressure chamber; (3) flow across a narrow orifice at high velocity. Rodbard demonstrated that flow through a narrowed orifice, as a consequence of the Venturi effect, deposited bacteria maximally at the low-pressure sink immediately beyond an orifice or at the site where a jet stream impacts a surface. These are the same sites where NBTE forms as a result of hemodynamic circumstances. The superimposition of NBTE formation and preferential deposition of bacteria help explain the distribution of infected vegetations when IE complicates cardiac valvular abnormalities, septal defects, arteriovenous fistulas, coartation of the aorta, and a patent ductus arteriosus.[119,121,122] Additionally, the attenuation of these circumstances when intracardiac defects are associated with low flow and reduced turbulence (secundum atrial septal defect, atrial fibrillation, congestive heart failure) correlates with the observed reduction in frequency of IE in the respective circumstance.[119,121,122]

CONVERSION OF NBTE TO IE. The initiating event that ultimately converts NBTE to IE is the entry of microorganisms into the circulation as a consequence of localized infection or trauma to a body surface. The frequency and magnitude of bacteremia associated with daily activities and health care procedures appear related to specific mucosal surfaces and skin, the density of colonizing bacteria, the disease state of the surface, and the extent of the local trauma. Bacteremia rates are highest for events that traumatize the oral mucosa, particularly the gingiva, and progressively decrease with procedures involving the genitourinary tract and the gastrointestinal tract.[123,124] A diseased mucosal surface, particularly one that is infected, is associated with an increased risk of bacteremia. Thus, oral irrigation devices, prostate surgery, and urinary tract manipulation are associated with higher rates of bacteremia when there is severe gingivitis and poor dentition or infected urine, respectively, than when these states are absent.[123] In studies of rats with periodontitis and after teeth were extracted, the likelihood of endocarditis was not related to the magnitude of bacteremia by a specific organism; instead, the occurrence of endocarditis correlated with the capacity of bacterial organisms to adhere in vitro to platelet-fibrin aggregates.[125] The relationship between the magnitude of bacteremia with infection or after a procedure and the risk of endocarditis in humans is not known.

Although IE develops when circulating microorganisms are deposited at a site of NBTE, the coincidence of bacteremia and NBTE does not uniformly result in IE. To cause IE the organism must be able to persist and propagate on the endothelium. This requires resistance to host defenses. The impact of serum bactericidal activity is illustrated by the reduced frequency of IE caused by aerobic gram-negative bacilli. Only strains resistant to the complement-mediated bactericidal activity of serum, e.g., selected *E. coli*, *P. aeruginosa*, and *S. marcescens*, cause IE with significant frequency or are virulent in the rabbit model of endocarditis.[114,116] The precise role of granulocytes in eradicating early colonizing organisms is not clear. Platelet-released microbicidal material has been shown to eliminate recently adherent, susceptible viridans streptococci from valves in experimental endocarditis.[126]

The adherence of microorganisms to the NBTE is a pivotal early event in the development of IE. Those organisms that most frequently cause endocarditis adhere more vigorously in vitro to cardiac valves than do organisms that rarely cause IE. Multiple mechanisms promote this adherence, including the surface carbohydrates of bacteria.[116] Bacteremic streptococci that produce extracellular dextran cause endocarditis more frequently than do strains that do not produce dextran. Dextran on the surface of streptococci can be shown to mediate adherence to platelet fibrin lattices and injured valves. Dextran production, however, is not universal among the major microbial causes of IE; thus, other mechanisms of adherence are likely.

Fibronectin has been identified as an important factor in this process.[84] Fibronectin has been identified in lesions on heart valves and is produced by endothelial cells, platelets, and fibroblasts in response to vascular injury; a soluble form binds to exposed subendothelial collagen. Receptors for fibronectin are present on the surface of *S. aureus*, viridans streptococci, group A, C, and G streptococci, enterococci, *S. pneumoniae*, and *C. albicans*. Fibronectin has multiple binding domains and thus can bind simultaneously to fibrin, collagen, cells, and microorganisms and serve to facilitate adherence of bacteria to the valve at the site of injury or NBTE. Soluble fibronectin may coat circulating bacteria and subsequently bind to injured endothelium, or uncoated bacteria may adhere specifically to fibronectin bound to platelets, fibroblasts, and collagen at the endothelial surface. The glycocalyx or slime on the surface of *S. epidermidis* has been considered an adhesin in the pathogenesis of PVE. Other studies, however, have questioned the adhesin function, and recent observations suggest that the polysaccharide material may render organisms more virulent by virtue of enhancing their ability to avoid eradication by host defenses.[85,88,89]

The mechanism whereby virulent organisms colonize and infect intact valvular endothelium is less clearly understood. Endothelial cells in monolayers in vitro can phagocytize *S. aureus* and *Candida*. Multiplication of the organism intracellularly results in cell death, which in turn disrupts the endothelial surface and initiates formation of platelet-fibrin deposits.[127,128] Alternatively, fibronectin may facilitate the adherence of *S. aureus* to intact endothelium.[84]

After adherence to the NBTE or endothelium (in the case of virulent organisms), persistence and multiplication result in a complex dynamic process during which the infected vegetation increases in size by platelet-fibrin aggregation, microorganisms are shed into the blood, and vegetation fragments embolize. Staphylococci and streptococci promote platelet aggregation and growth of the vegetation. Surface antigens that promote platelet adhesion (Class I antigen) and aggregation (Class II antigen that functionally mimics a platelet interactive domain of collagen) are expressed by *S. aureus*. Strains of *S. sanguis* with the aggregation antigen cause more severe endocarditis in the rabbit model than do antigen-negative strains.[129] Fibrin deposition is enhanced by tissue factor (a tissue thromboplastin that binds to Factor VII) elaborated by endothelial cells, fibroblasts, or monocytes interacting with bacteria.[130,131] The vegetation has been considered a sheltered site wherein bacteria were protected from polymorphonuclear leukocytes. Recent studies indicate that platelet-fibrin deposits may do more than shield microorganisms from host defenses. Platelets elaborate a potent platelet microbicidal protein that kills some strains of streptococci and *S. aureus* and thus kills organisms in vegetations.[126,132,133]

PATHOPHYSIOLOGY

Aside from the constitutional symptoms of infection, which are likely mediated by cytokines, the clinical manifestations of IE result from (1) the local destructive effects of intracardiac infection; (2) the embolization of bland or septic fragments of vegetations to distant sites, resulting in infarction or infection; (3) the hematogenous seeding of remote sites during continuous bacteremia; and (4) an antibody response to the infecting organism with subsequent tissue injury due to deposition of preformed immune complexes or antibody-complement interaction with antigens deposited in tissues.

The intracardiac consequences of IE range from trivial, characterized by an infected vegetation with no attendant tissue damage, to catastrophic, when infection is locally destructive or extends beyond the valve leaflet. Distortion or perforation of valve leaflets, rupture of chordae tendineae, and perforations or fistulas between major vessels and cardiac chambers or between chambers themselves as a consequence of burrowing infection may result in congestive heart failure that is progressive (Figs. 33–3 and 33–4).[134–136] Infection, particularly that involving the aortic valve or prosthetic valves, may extend into paravalvular tissue and result in abscesses and persistent fever due to antibiotic unresponsive infection, disruption of the conduction system with electrocardiographic conduction abnor-

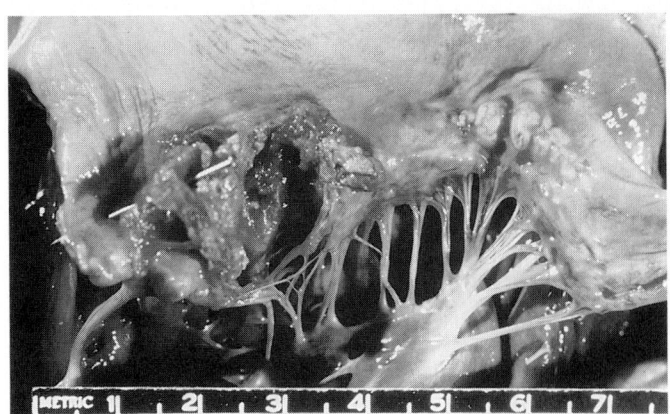

FIGURE 33–4. A large vegetation deforming and perforating the mitral valve. The nail probes an abscess that burrowed into the mitral valve annulus.

malities and clinically relevant arrhythmias, or purulent pericarditis.[30,137,138] Large vegetations, particularly at the mitral valve, can result in functional valvular stenosis and hemodynamic deterioration.[47,139] In general, intracardiac complications involving the aortic valve evolve more rapidly than those associated with the mitral valve; nevertheless, the progression is highly variable and unpredictable in individual patients.

Embolization of fragments from vegetations is clinically evident in 11 to 43 per cent of patients.[119,122,140,141] However, pathologic evidence of emboli at autopsy is found more frequently (45 to 65 per cent). Emboli from left-sided IE produce symptoms by infection or infarction at the site of lodgment, depending upon whether the vegetative material contains viable virulent organisms or is bland (sterile or contains avirulent organisms). Although not demonstrated in all studies, pooled data suggest that larger vegetations (>10 mm) are associated with a higher frequency of emboli, as are hypermobile vegetations.[142–144] Pulmonary emboli, which are often septic, occur in 75 per cent of intravenous drug abusers with tricuspid valve IE.[32]

The persistent bacteremia of IE, with or without septic emboli, may result in metastatic infection. In general, these infections originate before initiation of antimicrobial therapy; however, clinical manifestation may be delayed. These infections may present as local signs and symptoms or as persistent fever during therapy.[137,145] IE caused by virulent organisms, particularly S. aureus, is complicated more frequently by metastatic infection than is that due to avirulent bacteria, e.g., viridans streptococci. Virtually any organ or tissue may be hematogenously infected, including the spleen, kidney, brain, meninges, pericardium, bone (especially the vertebrae), synovium, and even vitreous humor. Metastatic abscesses are often small and miliary. Metastatic infection assumes particular importance when the required therapy is more than the antibiotics indicated for IE or when these infections constitute a focus that engenders relapse.[145]

The humoral and cell-mediated arms of the immune system are stimulated in patients with IE. Antibodies to the infecting organism in the three major classes—IgM, IgG, and IgA—with functional capacity including opsonization, agglutination, and complement fixation have been noted. Additionally, hypergammaglobulinemia and cryoglobulins have been noted. Cellular responses are suggested by activated circulating macrophages and splenomegaly.

Circulating immune complexes in high titer have been detected in most patients with bacteremic IE and PVE. The frequency and titer of the circulating immune complexes are highest in IE of long duration, in the presence of extravalvular manifestation, and in right-sided IE.[146] Although circulating immune complex titers fall with effective antibiotic therapy and rise or reappear with failure of therapy,

the finding of a fall in titers not widely used to monitor therapy. Immune complexes are clinically relevant when, with complement, they deposit subepithelially along the glomerular basement membrane to cause diffuse or focal glomerulonephritis.[122,147] Histological examination of affected glomeruli stained with fluorescent-labeled antibody to human globulin reveals a "lumpy-bumpy" pattern. The immunoglobulin eluted from the glomerular lesions reacts with bacterial antigens.[148] Rheumatological manifestations of IE and some peripheral manifestations of IE, such as Osler's nodes, have been attributed to local deposition of immune complexes.[122] Osler's nodes, however, have also been associated with septic embolization in S. aureus IE.

Rheumatoid factor (an IgM antibody directed against IgG) is present in half of the patients with IE of greater than 6 weeks' duration.[122,149] The titer of rheumatoid factor decreases slowly with effective antimicrobial therapy. Rheumatoid factor does not appear to play a role in the immune complex glomerulonephritis of IE.

CLINICAL FEATURES

The interval between the presumed initiating bacteremia and the onset of symptoms of IE is short. It is estimated that more than 80 per cent of patients with NVE develop symptoms within 2 weeks.[150] Interestingly, in some patients with intraoperative or perioperative infection of prosthetic valves, the incubation period may be prolonged (2 to 5 or more months).[47]

Fever is the most common symptom and sign in patients with IE (Table 33–4). In patients with subacute IE, fevers are low grade, rarely exceeding 39.4°C, remittent, and usually not associated with rigors. Fever may be absent or minimal in the elderly or in those with congestive heart failure, severe debility, or chronic renal failure and occasionally in patients with NVE caused by coagulase-negative staphylococci.[9,91]

Heart murmurs are noted in 80 to 85 per cent of patients with NVE and are emblematic of the lesion predisposing to IE. Murmurs are commonly not audible in patients with tricuspid valve IE. Similarly, in acute NVE due to S. aureus, murmurs are heard in only 30 to 45 per cent of patients on initial evaluation but are ultimately noted in 75 to 85 per cent. The new or changing murmurs (alterations

TABLE 33–4 CLINICAL FEATURES OF INFECTIVE ENDOCARDITIS

SYMPTOMS	PER CENT	SIGNS	PER CENT
Fever	80–85	Fever	80–90
Chills	42–75	Murmur	80–85
Sweats	25	Changing/new murmur	10–40
Anorexia	25–55		
Weight loss	25–35	Neurological abnormalities†	30–40
Malaise	25–40		
Dyspnea	20–40	Embolic event	20–40
Cough	25	Splenomegaly	15–50
Stroke	13–20	Clubbing	10–20
Headache	15–40	Peripheral manifestation	
Nausea/vomiting	15–20	Osler's nodes	7–10
Myalgia/arthralgia	15–30	Splinter hemorrhage	5–15
Chest pain*	8–35	Petechiae	10–40
		Janeway lesion	6–10
Abdominal pain	5–15	Retinal lesion/Roth spot	4–10
Back pain	7–10		
Confusion	10–20		

* More common in intravenous drug abusers.

† Central nervous system.

unrelated to heart rate or cardiac output) are relatively infrequent in subacute NVE and are more prevalent in acute IE and PVE.[47,151] They are frequently important harbingers of congestive heart failure.

Enlargement of the spleen is noted less commonly in recent reports than previously; in recent series splenomegaly has been noted in 15 to 50 per cent of patients and is more common in subacute IE of long duration.

Although 50 per cent of patients with IE were reported to have one or more of the classic peripheral manifestations of this illness, these findings are encountered less frequently today and are absent in IE restricted to the tricuspid valve.[1,7,9,32] *Petechiae* (Fig. 33–5), the most common of these manifestations, are found on the palpebral conjunctiva, the buccal and palatal mucosa, and the extremities. They are not specific for endocarditis even on the conjunctiva. *Splinter or subungual hemorrhages* (Fig. 33–6) are dark red, linear, or occasionally flame-shaped streaks in the nail bed of the fingers or toes. Distal lesions are likely due to trauma, whereas the more proximal ones are more likely related to IE. *Osler's nodes* are small, tender subcutaneous nodules that develop in the pulp of the digits or occasionally more proximally in the fingers and persist for hours to several days. These are not pathognomonic for this diagnosis. Osler's nodes have been described in patients with systemic lupus erythematosus, marantic endocarditis, and disseminated gonococcal disease and distal to infected arterial catheters.[151] Janeway lesions are small erythematous or hemorrhagic macular nontender lesions on the palms and soles and are the consequence of septic embolic events. Roth spots (Fig. 33–7), oval retinal hemorrhages with pale centers, are infrequent findings in patients with IE. They have been noted in patients with collagen vascular disease and hematologic disorders, including severe anemia.

Musculoskeletal symptoms, unrelated to focal infection, are relatively common in patients with IE.[152] These include arthralgias and myalgias, occasional true arthritis with nondiagnostic but inflammatory synovial fluid findings, and prominent back pain without evidence of vertebral body, disc space, or sacroiliac joint infection.[151,152] In patients with arthritis or back pain, focal infection must be excluded because additional therapy may be required.

Systemic emboli are among the most common clinical sequelae of IE, occurring in up to 40 per cent of patients, and are frequent subclinical events found only at autopsy.[119,122,140,141] Emboli often antedate diagnosis. Although

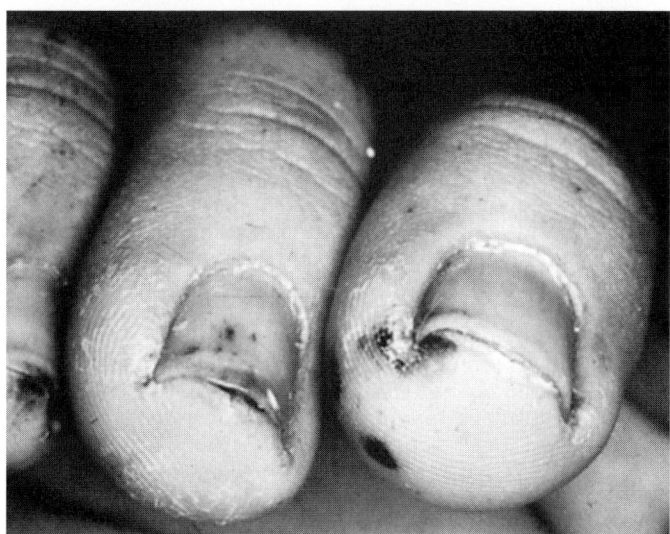

FIGURE 33–6. Subungual hemorrhages (splinter hemorrhages) and digital petechiae in a patient with IE. (From Korzeniowski, O. M., and Kaye, D.: Infective endocarditis. *In* Braunwald, E. (ed.): Heart Disease. 4th ed. Philadelphia, W. B. Saunders Company, 1992.)

embolic events may occur during or after antimicrobial therapy, the incidence decreases promptly during the administration of effective antibiotic therapy.[153,154] Embolic splenic infarction may cause left upper quadrant abdominal pain, left shoulder pain, and a small left pleural effusion and must be distinguished from the less common splenic abscess (see Treatment of Extracardiac Complications). Renal emboli may occur asymptomatically or with flank pain and may cause gross or microscopic hematuria but rarely result in clinically significant renal dysfunction. Embolic stroke syndromes, predominantly involving the middle cerebral artery territory, occur in 15 to 20 per cent of patients with NVE and PVE.[47,155–158] IE caused by *S. aureus* is associated with an increased risk of embolic complications.[153,158] Coronary artery emboli are common findings at autopsy but rarely result in transmural infarction. Emboli to the extremities may produce pain and overt ischemia, and those to mesenteric arteries may cause abdominal pain, ileus, and guaiac-positive stools. Embolic occlusion of a central retinal artery, which occurs in less than 3 per cent of IE cases, presents as sudden monocular blindness.[140,157]

Neurological symptoms and signs occur in 30 to 40 per cent of patients with IE, are more frequent when IE is

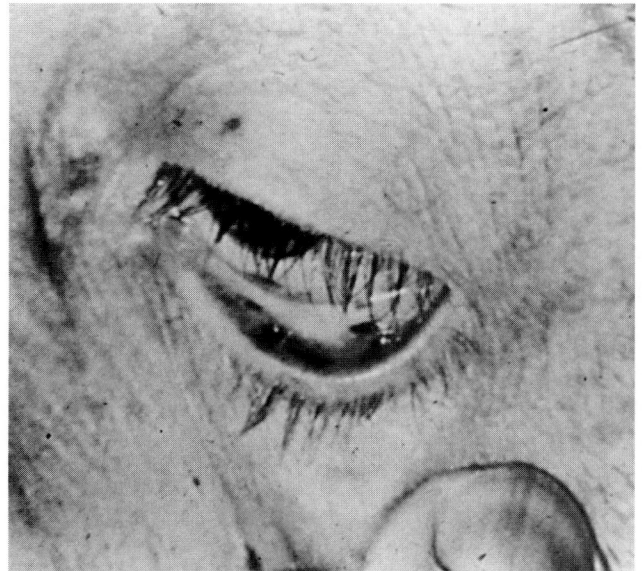

FIGURE 33–5. Conjunctival petechiae in a patient with IE. (From Kaye, D.: Infective Endocarditis. Baltimore, University Park Press, 1976.)

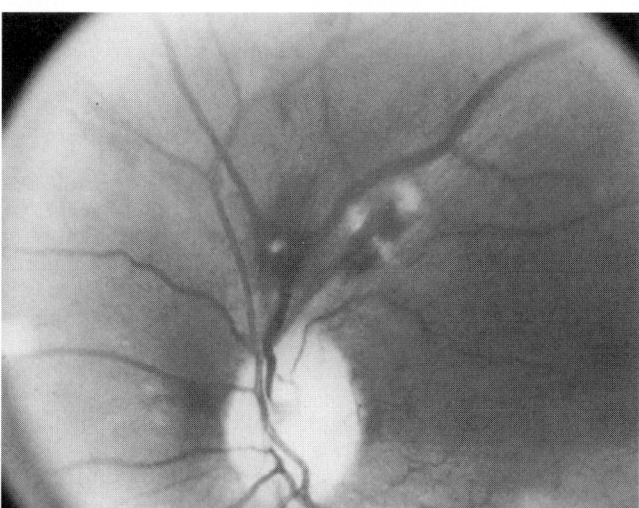

FIGURE 33–7. Roth spot (retinal hemorrhage with a clear center) in a patient with IE. (From Korzeniowski, O. M., and Kaye, D.: Infective endocarditis. *In* Braunwald, E. (ed.): Heart Disease. 4th ed. Philadelphia, W. B. Saunders Company, 1992.)

caused by *S. aureus,* and are associated with increased mortality rates.[140,151,155,157,158] Neurological manifestations, such as a stroke, intracerebral hemorrhage, or subarachnoid hemorrhage occurring at presentation, may be so dramatic that the diagnosis of IE is obscured. Embolic stroke is the most common and clinically important of the neurological manifestations. Intracranial hemorrhage occurs in 5 per cent of patients with IE. Bleeding results from rupture of a mycotic aneurysm, rupture of an artery due to septic arteritis at the site of embolic occlusion, or hemorrhage into an infarct.[159,160] Mycotic aneurysms, with or without rupture, occur in 2 to 10 per cent of patients with IE; approximately half of these involve intracranial arteries. Cerebritis with microabscesses complicates IE caused by invasive pathogens such as *S. aureus,* but large brain abscesses are rare.[155,158] Purulent meningitis complicates some episodes of IE caused by *S. aureus* or *S. pneumoniae,* but more typically the cerebrospinal fluid has an aseptic profile. Other neurological manifestations include severe headache (a potential clue to a mycotic aneurysm), seizure, and encephalopathy.

Congestive heart failure (CHF) complicating IE is primarily the result of valve destruction or distortion or rupture of chordae tendineae. Occasionally intracardiac fistulas, myocarditis, or coronary artery embolization may contribute to the genesis of CHF, as obviously can underlying cardiac disease. In the absence of surgery to correct valvular dysfunction, CHF, particularly that due to aortic insufficiency, was associated with very high mortality rates.[135,161] With appropriately-timed surgery, this increased mortality can be largely avoided.[135,140,161]

Renal insufficiency as a result of immune complex–mediated glomerulonephritis occurs in less than 15 per cent of patients with IE. Azotemia as a result of this process may develop or progress during initial therapy; it usually improves with continued administration of effective antibiotic therapy.[151] Focal glomerulonephritis and renal infarcts cause hematuria but rarely result in azotemia. Renal dysfunction in patients with IE is most commonly a manifestation of impaired hemodynamics or toxicities associated with antimicrobial therapy (interstitial nephritis or aminoglycoside-induced injury).

DIAGNOSIS

The symptoms and signs of endocarditis are often constitutional and, when localized, often result from a complication of IE rather than reflect the intracardiac infection itself (Table 33–4). Consequently, if physicians are to avoid overlooking the diagnosis of IE, a high index of suspicion must be maintained. The diagnosis must be investigated when patients with fever present with one or more of the cardinal elements of IE: a predisposing cardiac lesion or behavior pattern, bacteremia, embolic phenomenon, and evidence of an active endocardial process.

IE must be considered in a patient with significant valvular heart disease and a persistent unexplained fever, in the intravenous drug abuser with fever especially if there is cough and pleuritic chest pain, or in the young patient with an unexpected stroke or subarachnoid hemorrhage. The development of a new regurgitant murmur, which is indicative of an active endocardial process, must raise the possibility of IE. Because patients with prosthetic heart valves are always at risk for PVE, the presence of fever or new prosthesis dysfunction at any time warrants considering this diagnosis. In patients at risk for endocarditis, concurrent illnesses or iatrogenic events may create clusters of symptoms and signs that superficially mimic IE and require careful consideration to arrive at a correct diagnosis. For example, in an elderly patient with a murmur, low-grade fever, weight loss, myalgias and arthralgias, anemia, and elevated erythrocyte sedimentation rate, it may be difficult to distinguish IE from polymyalgia rheumatica. Even when the illness seems typical of endocarditis, the definitive diagnosis requires positive blood cultures or positive cultures (or histology) from the vegetation or embolus. There are many culture-negative mimics of IE: atrial myxoma, acute rheumatic fever, systemic lupus erythematosus or other collagen-vascular disease, marantic endocarditis, the antiphospholipid syndrome, carcinoid syndrome, renal cell carcinoma with increased cardiac output, and thrombotic thrombocytopenic purpura.

BACTEREMIA. Positive blood cultures may stimulate consideration of IE as a possible diagnosis. Sustained low-level (<100 organisms/ml) bacteremia is typical of IE. In evaluating positive blood cultures, sustained bacteremia (persisting over more than 1 hour) should be distinguished from transient bacteremia. When multiple blood cultures obtained over 24 hours or more are positive, the diagnosis of IE must be considered. The identity of the organism is also helpful in determining the intensity with which the diagnosis is entertained. Organisms can be divided into those that commonly cause IE, those that rarely cause IE, and the intermediate-behaving organisms, e.g., *S. aureus,* which, when in the blood, may or may not indicate IE. Lastly, the presence or absence of alternative sources for the bacteremia aids in the assessment of bacteremia. These considerations are embodied in the diagnostic criteria for IE (see Table 33–5).[162]

Among patients with *S. aureus* bacteremia, the risk of IE has been greatest in those with community-acquired infection, those who lack a peripheral site of infection, those who are intravenous drug abusers, those who have evidence of valvular disease, and those who are diabetic with chronic cutaneous infections. Screening of patients with community-acquired *S. aureus* bacteremia using transthoracic echocardiography demonstrated 20 per cent of the patients to have either occult IE or valve lesions predisposing to IE.[163,164] In contrast, among patients with catheter-associated nosocomial *S. aureus* bacteremia, the frequency of IE is 3 to 8 per cent.[57–60] Screening the latter group of patients with transthoracic echocardiography is not cost effective. Screening with transthoracic echocardiography is recommended for patients with *S. aureus* bacteremia acquired in a community setting or in a nosocomial setting, when patients have known underlying valvular heart disease, have a new significant heart murmur, or have persistent fever or bacteremia for 3 days or more after removal of the presumed primary focus of infection (intravascular catheter or drainage of an abscess) and initiation of therapy.[60,163,164]

When used judiciously over the entire evaluation sequence, i.e., not limited to initial findings, recently published criteria provide a sensitive and specific approach to the diagnosis of IE (Table 33–5).[162,165,166] Erroneous rejection of the diagnosis of endocarditis is unlikely. When using these diagnostic criteria to guide therapy, patients who are categorized with possible endocarditis should be treated as if they have IE. To use bacteremia due to coagulase-negative staphylococci or diphtheroids (organisms that may cause IE but more often contaminate blood cultures) to support the diagnosis of endocarditis, blood cultures must be persistently positive or the organisms recovered in multiple sporadically positive cultures must be proved to represent a single clone.[93,162]

Inclusion of echocardiographic evidence of endocardial infection in these criteria recognizes the high sensitivity of two-dimensional echocardiography with color Doppler, especially if the transesophageal approach is used, and the relative infrequency of false-positive studies when experienced operators use specific definitions for vegetations.[167–170] Although the sensitivity of transesophageal echocardiography to detect vegetations in patients with suspected infective endocarditis is 82 to 94 per cent (or higher if a follow-up study is performed), a negative study does not exclude the diagnosis or the need for therapy if

TABLE 33–5 DIAGNOSIS OF INFECTIVE ENDOCARDITIS

DEFINITIVE INFECTIVE ENDOCARDITIS
Pathological criteria
Microorganisms: demonstrated by culture or histology in a vegetation, *or* in a vegetation that has embolized, *or* in an intracardiac abscess, *or*
Pathological lesions: vegetation or intracardiac abscess present, confirmed by histology showing active endocarditis
Clinical criteria, using specific definitions listed below
Two major criteria, *or*
One major and three minor criteria, *or*
Five minor criteria

POSSIBLE INFECTIVE ENDOCARDITIS
Findings consistent with infective endocarditis that fall short of definite endocarditis but are not rejected

REJECTED
Firm alternative diagnosis for manifestations of endocarditis, *or*
Sustained resolution of manifestations of endocarditis, with antibiotic therapy for 4 days or less, *or*
No pathological evidence of infective endocarditis at surgery or autopsy, after antibiotic therapy for 4 days or less

CRITERIA FOR DIAGNOSIS OF INFECTIVE ENDOCARDITIS

MAJOR CRITERIA
Positive blood culture
Typical microorganism for infective endocarditis from two separate blood cultures
Viridans streptococci, *Streptococcus bovis*, HACEK group, *or*
Community-acquired *Staphylococcus aureus* or entero-cocci, in the absence of a primary focus, *or*
Persistently positive blood culture, defined as recovery of a microorganism consistent with infective endocarditis from:
Blood cultures drawn more than 12 hours apart, *or*
All of three or a majority of four or more separate blood cultures, with first and last drawn at least 1 hour apart
Evidence of endocardial involvement
Positive echocardiogram
Oscillating intracardiac mass, on valve or supporting structures, *or* in the path of regurgitant jets, *or* on implanted material, in the absence of an alternative anatomical explanation, *or*
Abscess, *or*
New partial dehiscence of prosthetic valve, *or*
New valvular regurgitation (increase or change in preexisting murmur not sufficient)

MINOR CRITERIA
Predisposition: predisposing heart condition *or* intravenous drug use
Fever ≥ 38.0°C (100.4°F)
Vascular phenomena: major arterial emboli, septic pulmonary infarcts, mycotic aneurysm, intracranial hemorrhage, conjunctival hemorrhages, Janeway lesions
Immunological phenomena: glomerulonephritis, Osler's nodes, Roth spots, rheumatoid factor
Microbiological evidence: positive blood culture but not meeting major criterion as noted previously* *or* serologic evidence of active infection with organism consistent with infective endocarditis
Echocardiogram: consistent with infective endocarditis but not meeting major criterion

* Excluding single positive cultures for coagulase-negative staphylococci and organisms that do not cause endocarditis.

Adapted from Durack, D. T., Lukes, A. S., and Bright, D. K.: New criteria for diagnosis of infective endocarditis: Utilization of specific echocardiographic findings. Am. J. Med. *96*:200, 1994.

the clinical suspicion is high.[169,170] In this population the false-negative rate for detection of vegetations on a single transesophageal echocardiogram ranges from 6 to 18 per cent; with repeat examinations, the likelihood of false-negative transesophageal studies is 4 to 13 per cent. Thus, these studies help to exclude the diagnosis when the clinical suspicion is low.[169,170] These guidelines are vulnerable

to misidentifying as culture-negative infective endocarditis the entity of NBTE that complicates marasmus, cryptic collagen-vascular disease, or the antiphospholipid antibody syndrome.

A microbial cause for infective endocarditis is established by recovering the infecting agent from the blood or from surgically removed endocardial vegetations or embolic material. Bacteremia in patients with endocarditis is continuous; hence, there is no advantage to obtaining blood cultures in relationship to fever. Furthermore, blood obtained from arterial and venous sources are culture positive at similar rates. In patients who have not received prior antibiotics and who will ultimately have blood culture–positive IE, it is likely that 95 to 100 per cent of all cultures obtained will be positive. In a study of 206 patients with IE who had not received prior antibiotics, among those with streptococcal IE, the first culture was positive in 96 per cent of patients and one of the first two cultures was positive in 98 per cent. Among patients with nonstreptococcal IE, the first culture was positive in 86 per cent of patients and the first or second culture was positive in all cases.[171] Prior antibiotic therapy is a major cause of blood culture–negative IE, particularly when the causative microorganism is highly antibiotic susceptible. In a recent study of 620 cases of IE, 88 (14 per cent) were culture-negative. In 31 (35 per cent) of the 88 culture-negative cases, the failure to isolate the causative agent from blood was attributed to prior antimicrobial therapy.[172] After subtherapeutic antibiotic exposure the time required for reversion to positive cultures is directly related to the duration of antimicrobial therapy and the susceptibility of the causative agent; days to a week or more may be required.

OBTAINING BLOOD CULTURES. Three separate sets of blood cultures, each from a separate venipuncture, obtained over 24 hours, are recommended to evaluate patients with suspected endocarditis.[173] Each set should include two flasks, one containing an aerobic medium and the other containing thioglycollate broth (anaerobic medium) into which at least 10 ml of blood should be placed. The laboratory should be advised that endocarditis is a possible diagnosis and which, if any, unusual bacteria are suspected (*Legionella* species, *Bartonella* species, HACEK organisms). If alerted, the laboratory can both hold the culture for a prolonged period and use special isolation techniques. If a clinically stable patient has received an antimicrobial agent during the past several weeks, it is prudent to delay therapy so that repeat cultures can be obtained on successive days. If fungal endocarditis is suspected, blood cultures should be obtained using the lysis-centrifugation method. The laboratory should be asked to save the organism causing endocarditis until successful therapy has been completed. Occasionally, serologic tests are used to make the presumptive etiological diagnosis of endocarditis caused by *Brucella* species, *Legionella* species, *Bartonella* species, *Coxiella burnetii,* or *Chlamydia* species. By special techniques these agents can be identified in or recovered from blood or vegetations.[31,104–107]

Laboratory Tests

Blood cultures are the crucial laboratory tests used in the diagnosis of IE (see Diagnosis). Other tests are inevitably obtained and merit mention.[174] Hematological parameters are commonly abnormal. Anemia, with normochromic normocytic red cell indices, a low serum iron, and low serum iron-binding capacity, is seen in 70 to 90 per cent of patients. Anemia worsens with increased duration of illness and thus in acute IE may be absent. In subacute IE the white blood cell count is usually normal; in contrast, a leukocytosis with increased segmented granulocytes is common in acute IE. Thrombocytopenia occurs only rarely.

The *erythrocyte sedimentation rate* (ESR) is elevated (average approximately 55 mm/hr) in almost all patients with IE; the exceptions are those with congestive heart failure, renal failure, or disseminated intravascular coagulation. Although a nonspecific test, the absence of an increased ESR, other than in selected circumstances, argues against the diagnosis of IE. Other tests often indicate immune stimulation or inflammation (see Pathophysiology): circulating immune complexes, rheumatoid factor, quantitative immune globulin determinations, cryoglobulins, and C-reactive protein. Although the results of these tests parallel disease activity, the tests are costly and not efficient ways to diagnose IE or monitor response to therapy. Very high serum concentrations of circulating immune complexes can help to distinguish transient bacteremia from endocarditis.[175] This test might, therefore, be useful when the results of blood cultures and echocardiography have not differentiated transient bacteremia from IE. Measurement of circulating immune complexes and complement may be useful in evaluating azotemia. Azotemia due to diffuse immune complex glomerulonephritis is associated with increased circulating immune complexes and hypocomplementemia.[146,147,174]

The *urine analysis* is often abnormal, even when renal function remains normal. Proteinuria and microscopic hematuria are noted in 50 per cent of patients. The urinalysis plays a standard role in the evaluation of azotemia.

Serological tests are used to evaluate blood culture–negative IE (see Diagnosis). Tests to detect antibodies to ribitol teichoic acids from staphylococci were developed in an attempt to distinguish uncomplicated *S. aureus* bacteremia from that associated with IE or other deep-seated infection. In clinical applications these tests have not been sufficiently specific or predictive.[164]

Echocardiography
(See also pp. 77 to 78)

Evaluation of patients with clinically suspected IE by this technique frequently allows the morphologic confirmation of infection and increasingly aids in decisions regarding management.[142,144,167–170] Echocardiography is not a useful screening test for the diagnosis of IE in unselected patients with positive blood cultures or in patients with fevers of unknown origin.[168,176] Nevertheless, echocardiographic evaluation should be performed in all patients with clinically suspected IE, including those with negative blood cultures. Although many patients with NVE involving the aortic or mitral valve can be imaged adequately by transthoracic echocardiography (TTE), transesophageal echocardiography (TEE) using biplane technology with incorporated color flow and continuous as well as pulsed Doppler is the state of the art.[168,177] TEE allows visualization of smaller vegetations and provides improved resolution compared with TTE. Not only is TEE the preferred approach in patients with clinically suspected IE in whom TTE is suboptimal, it is also the procedure of choice for imaging the pulmonic valve, patients with PVE (especially at the mitral site), and patients with signs of persistent or invasive infection in spite of adequate antimicrobial therapy.[167,168,177–179]

The sensitivity of echocardiographic detection of vegetations depends upon the technique and portal for the examination; M-mode is less sensitive than two-dimensional echocardiography and TTE is less sensitive than TEE. In two large studies of patients with proven IE examined by both approaches, the sensitivity of TEE was 100 and 90 per cent and that of TTE was 63 and 58 per cent, respectively.[142,180] In the setting of clinically suspected IE, the sensitivity of TEE ranges from 82 to 94 per cent (see Diagnosis).[169,170] In patients with PVE, TTE is limited by the shadowing effect of mitral valve prostheses. In two studies of PVE involving mechanical and bioprosthetic devices, the sensitivity of TEE to detect vegetations was 82 and 96 per cent, while that of TTE was 36 and 16 per cent.[178,181]

In spite of the sensitivity of TEE in detecting vegetations in patients with proven IE, echocardiography does not provide a specific diagnosis. Vegetations and valve dysfunction may be demonstrated, but determination of causality requires clinical or direct anatomical and microbiological confirmation. Infectious vegetations cannot be distinguished from marantic lesions on native valves, nor can vegetations be distinguished from thrombus or pannus on prostheses. Furthermore, it is usually not possible to distinguish active from healed vegetations in NVE.[168,182,183] Thickened valves, ruptured chordae or valves, valve calcification, and nodules may be mistaken for vegetations, indicating the specificity limitations of echocardiography.[142,168]

The natural history of vegetations during therapy is variable. On repeat echocardiogram 3 weeks to 3 months after initiation of ultimately effective antimicrobial therapy, 29 per cent of 41 initial vegetations were no longer detectable. Of the 29 vegetations that remained detectable, 58 per cent were unchanged, 24 per cent were smaller, and 17 per cent were larger. Mobility and extent (valves involved) of vegetations were unchanged in 86 and 65 per cent, respectively. The evolution of these vegetations was unrelated to the duration of therapy or initial vegetation size, nor did it predict late complications of IE.[183] In another study among patients, not all of whom were responding to therapy, persistence or increase in vegetation size during therapy was associated with an increased rate of complications.[184] Accordingly, changes in vegetations must be interpreted in a clinical context and do not in themselves reflect the efficacy of therapy. Vegetations persisting after effective therapy must not be misinterpreted as recurrence of IE unless there is supportive clinical and microbiological evidence.

Valve dysfunction due to tissue disruption or large obstructing vegetations can be visualized and quantitated by echocardiogram with Doppler.[143,168] Some degree of regurgitation by Doppler is almost universal early in the course of NVE and PVE and does not necessarily predict subsequent hemodynamic deterioration.[142,168,185,186] Extension of infection beyond the valve leaflet into surrounding tissue is an ominous step in the progression of IE. It can result in abscesses in various areas of the annulus or adjacent structures, mycotic aneurysms of the sinus of Valsalva or mitral valve, intracardiac fistulas, and purulent pericarditis. Using the knowledge of the anatomical relationships between the valve cusps and adjacent structures, the echocardiographer can define these perivalvular extensions of infection.[134,143] Myocardial abscesses are more readily detected by TEE than TTE in patients with NVE or PVE.[167,178] The sensitivity and specificity for abscess detection were 28 per cent and 98 per cent for TTE, compared with 87 per cent and 95 per cent for TEE.[167] Other studies have reported similar findings, especially in recognizing subaortic invasive disease.[187]

The stratification of patients into groups that are at high and low risk for congestive heart failure, systemic embolization, need for surgical intervention, and death based upon the presence or absence of vegetations remains controversial.[143,168] The heterogeneous nature of the patients examined, the technologies used, and the lack of correlation with other features of IE, as well as the increasing ability to visualize vegetations in most patients with IE using TEE, undermines this debate. Although not demonstrated in all individual studies, pooled data from two-dimensional echocardiographic studies suggest that patients with larger vegetations (>10 mm in diameter) are at increased risk for embolic complications (20 per cent versus 40 per cent).[143,168,186] This increased risk appears to be particularly associated with large vegetations involving the mitral valve and with the mobility of vegetations.[142,144,168] The correlation of aortic or mitral valve vegetation size, extent, mobility, and site with congestive heart failure, need for surgical intervention, and mortality (other than that associated with embolic events) has not been fully established.[142,144,168,186,188]

Among patients with right-sided IE, the visualization of vegetations by TTE has been correlated with prolonged fever during therapy and increased right ventricular end-diastolic dimensions. These findings were not related to vegetation size, nor did the presence of vegetations or their size predict the failure of medical therapy and a need for surgical intervention.[92]

MAGNETIC RESONANCE IMAGING. This technique has identified paravalvular extension of infection, aortic root aneurysms, and fistulas; however, its utility relative to echocardiography has not been established.[134,189]

SCINTIGRAPHY. Efforts to identify vegetations and intracardiac abscess in patients with IE and animal models have utilized scintigraphy with gallium-67 citrate, indium-111–labeled granulocytes, and indium-111–labeled platelets. These efforts have not been sufficiently sensitive nor anatomically localizing to be useful clinically.[134,190]

TREATMENT

Two major objectives must be addressed to effectively treat IE. The infecting microorganism must be eradicated. Failure to accomplish this results in relapse of infection. Also, the invasive, destructive intracardiac and focal extracardiac complications of infection must be addressed if morbidity and mortality are to be minimized. The second objective often exceeds the capacity of effective antimicrobial therapy and requires cardiac or other surgical intervention.

The principles that guide current treatment of endocarditis derive from observations made in vitro, in animal models of endocarditis, and in clinical studies. Bacteria in vegetations are able to multiply to population densities approaching 10^9 to 10^{10} organisms per gram of tissue.[116] Under the conditions in the vegetation, bacteria become metabolically dormant and less vulnerable to the killing action of antimicrobial agents, particularly the penicillins, cephalosporins, and vancomycin, which are the cornerstones of antibiotic therapy for IE. These observations, supplemented by clinical experience, suggest that optimal therapy should use bactericidal antibiotics or antibiotic combinations rather than bacteriostatic agents. Additionally, antibiotics reach the central areas of avascular vegetations by passive diffusion. To reach effective antibiotic concentrations in vegetations, high serum concentrations must be achieved, and even then penetration by some agents is limited.[191] Parenteral antimicrobial therapy is used whenever feasible in order to achieve suitable serum antibiotic concentrations and to avoid the potentially erratic absorption of orally administered therapy. Treatment is continued for prolonged periods to ensure the eradication of dormant microorganisms.

In selecting antimicrobial therapy for patients with IE, the ability of potential agents to kill the causative organism as well as the minimum inhibitory concentration (MIC) and minimum bactericidal concentration (MBC) of these antibiotics for the organism must be considered. The MIC is the lowest concentration that inhibits growth and the MBC is the lowest concentration that decreases a standard inoculum of organisms 99.9 per cent during 24 hours. For the vast majority of streptococci and staphylococci, the MIC and MBC of penicillins, cephalosporins, or vancomycin are the same or differ by only a factor of two to four. Occasionally, organisms are encountered for which the MBC for these antibiotics is 10-fold or greater than the MIC. This phenomenon has been termed tolerance.[108] Most of the tolerant strains are simply killed more slowly than nontolerant strains, and with prolonged incubation (48 hours) their MICs and MBCs are similar. Enterococci exhibit what superficially appears to be tolerance when tested against penicillins and vancomycin; however, these organisms are, in fact, not killed by these agents but are merely inhibited, even after longer incubation times. Enterococci can be killed by the combined activity of selected penicillins or vancomycin and an aminoglycoside. This enhanced antibiotic activity of the combination against enterococci, if of sufficient magnitude, is called synergy or a synergistic bactericidal effect.[80,108] A similar effect can be seen with these combinations against streptococci and staphylococci; this effect overcomes tolerance.[67,108]

A synergistic bactericidal effect is required for the optimal therapy of enterococcal endocarditis and has been employed to achieve more effective therapy or effective short-course therapy of IE caused by other organisms. The finding of tolerance in streptococci or staphylococci causing endocarditis has not been correlated with decreased cure rates or delayed responses to treatment with penicillins, cephalosporins, or vancomycin. Accordingly, the presence of tolerance in streptococci or staphylococci has not required combination therapy and, in fact, regimens are designed using the MICs of these organisms.[83]

The regimens recommended for the treatment of IE caused by specific organisms are designed to provide high concentrations of antibiotics (relative to the MIC of the target organism) in serum as well as concentrations deep in vegetations that exceed the organism's MIC throughout most, if not all, of the interval between doses. Although antibiotic concentrations in vegetations of patients with IE have been measured infrequently, the success of the recommended regimens suggests that this goal has been achieved. Accordingly, for optimal therapy, it is important that the recommended regimens be followed carefully.

Antimicrobial Therapy for Specific Organisms

The antimicrobial therapy for endocarditis should not only eradicate the causative agent but should do so while causing little or no toxicity. Therapy for a given patient requires modification to accommodate end-organ dysfunction, existing allergies, and other anticipated toxicities. With the exception of staphylococcal endocarditis, the antimicrobial regimens recommended for the treatment of patients with NVE and PVE are similar, although more prolonged treatment is often advised for patients with PVE.[47,83]

PENICILLIN-SUSCEPTIBLE VIRIDANS STREPTOCOCCI OR *STREPTOCOCCUS BOVIS*. Four regimens provide highly effective, comparable therapy for patients with endocarditis caused by penicillin-susceptible streptococci and *S. bovis* (Table 33–6).[83] The 4-week regimens yield bacteriologic cure rates of 98 per cent among patients who complete therapy. Treatment with the synergistic combination of penicillin plus gentamicin for 2 weeks is as effective in selected cases as treatment with the 4-week regimens. The combination regimen is recommended for patients with uncomplicated native valve endocarditis who are not at increased risk for aminoglycoside toxicity. Patients with endocarditis caused by nutritionally variant streptococci, endocarditis involving a prosthetic valve, or endocarditis complicated by a mycotic aneurysm, myocardial abscess, perivalvular infection, or an extracardiac focus of infection should not be treated with this short-course regimen. From 2 to 8 per cent of viridans streptococci and *S. bovis* causing endocarditis are highly resistant to streptomycin (MIC > 2000 µg/ml) and are not killed synergistically by penicillin plus streptomycin. These highly streptomycin-resistant strains are, however, killed synergistically by penicillin plus gentamicin.[67] Consequently, unless a causative streptococcus can be evaluated to exclude high-level resistance to streptomycin, gentamicin is recommended for use in the short-course combination regimen.[192] The nutritionally variant streptococci, *S. adjacens* and *S. defectivus,* are generally more resistant to penicillin than are other viridans streptococci.[62,66] Patients with endocarditis caused by these streptococci are treated with regimens recommended for enterococcal endocarditis (Table 33–8); however, outcome remains unsatisfactory.[193]

TABLE 33–6 TREATMENT FOR NATIVE VALVE ENDOCARDITIS DUE TO PENICILLIN-SUSCEPTIBLE VIRIDANS STREPTOCOCCI AND *STREPTOCOCCUS BOVIS* (MINIMUM INHIBITORY CONCENTRATION ≤ 0.1 µg/ml)*

ANTIBIOTIC	DOSAGE AND ROUTE†	DURATION (WEEKS)
Aqueous penicillin G	12–18 million U/24 hours IV either continuously or every 4 hours in six equally divided doses	4
Ceftriaxone	2 gm once daily IV or IM	4
Aqueous penicillin G *plus*	12–18 million U/24 hours IV either continuously or every 4 hours in six equally divided doses	2
Gentamicin	1 mg/kg IM or IV every 8 hours	2
Vancomycin	30 mg/kg per 24 hours IV in two equally divided doses, not to exceed 2 gm/24 hours unless serum levels are monitored	4

* For nutritionally variant streptococci (*Streptococcus adjacens, Streptococcus defectivus*), see Table 33–8.

† Dosages given are for patients with normal renal function. Vancomycin and gentamicin doses must be reduced for treatment of patients with renal dysfunction. Vancomycin and gentamicin doses are calculated using ideal body weight (men = 50 kg + 2.3 kg per inch over 5 feet; women = 45.5 kg + 2.3 kg per inch over 5 feet).

Modified from Wilson, W. R., Karchmer, A. W., Dajani, A. S., et al.: Antibiotic treatment of adults with infective endocarditis due to streptococci, enterococci, staphylococci, and HACEK microorganisms. JAMA *274*:1706, 1995. Copyright 1995 American Medical Association.

For the treatment of streptococcal endocarditis in patients with a history of immediate allergic reactions (urticarial or anaphylactic reactions) to a penicillin or cephalosporin antibiotic, vancomycin is recommended (Table 33–6). Patients with other forms of penicillin allergy (delayed maculopapular skin rash) may be treated cautiously with the ceftriaxone regimen (Table 33–6) or with cefazolin, 2 gm IV every 8 hours for 4 weeks.

For patients with PVE caused by penicillin-susceptible streptococci, treatment with 6 weeks of penicillin is recommended, with gentamicin given during the initial 2 weeks.[47]

RELATIVELY PENICILLIN-RESISTANT STREPTOCOCCI. Approximately 15 per cent of streptococci that cause endocarditis are relatively resistant to penicillin (MIC > 0.1 µg/ml).[62] Four weeks of high-dose parenteral penicillin plus an aminoglycoside (primarily gentamicin for the reasons noted previously) during the initial 2 weeks is recommended for treatment of patients with endocarditis caused by streptococci with MICs for penicillin between 0.2 and 0.5 µg/ml (Table 33–7). Patients who cannot tolerate penicillin because of immediate hypersensitivity reactions can be treated with vancomycin alone (Table 33–7). For those with nonimmediate penicillin hypersensitivity, effective treatment can be accomplished with either vancomycin alone or by adding gentamicin to the initial 2 weeks of the ceftriaxone regimen (Table 33–6). Patients with endocarditis caused by streptococci that are highly resistant to penicillin (MIC > 0.5 µg/ml) should be treated with one of the regimens recommended for enterococcal endocarditis (Table 33–8).

TABLE 33–7 TREATMENT FOR NATIVE VALVE ENDOCARDITIS DUE TO STRAINS OF VIRIDANS STREPTOCOCCI AND *STREPTOCOCCUS BOVIS* RELATIVELY RESISTANT TO PENICILLIN G (MINIMUM INHIBITORY CONCENTRATION > 0.1 µg/ml AND < 0.5 µg/ml)

ANTIBIOTIC	DOSAGE AND ROUTE*	DURATION (WEEKS)
Aqueous penicillin G *plus*	18 million U/24 h IV either continuously or every 4 hours in 6 equally divided doses	4
Gentamicin	1 mg/kg IM or IV every 8 hours	2
Vancomycin	30 mg/kg per 24 hours IV in 2 equally divided doses, not to exceed 2 gm/ 24 hours unless serum levels are monitored	4

* Dosages are for patients with normal renal function; see Table 33–6 footnote.

Modified from Wilson, W. R., Karchmer, A. W., Dajani, A. S., et al.: Antibiotic treatment of adults with infective endocarditis due to streptococci, enterococci, staphylococci, and HACEK microorganisms. JAMA *274*:1706, 1995. Copyright 1995 American Medical Association.

STREPTOCOCCUS PYOGENES, STREPTOCOCCUS PNEUMONIAE, AND GROUP B, C, AND G STREPTOCOCCI. Endocarditis caused by these streptococci has been either refractory to antibiotic therapy or associated with extensive valvular damage. Penicillin G in a dose of 3 million units intravenously every 4 hours for 4 weeks is recommended for the treatment of group A streptococcal and pneumococcal endocarditis. Pneumococci that are relatively resistant (MIC > 0.1 µg/ml to 1.0 µg/ml) and highly resistant (MIC > 1.0 µg/ml) to penicillin are widely distributed and likely to cause sporadic cases of endocarditis.[79] Although serum concentrations of penicillin G or ceftriaxone, using doses recommended for treatment of endocarditis, markedly exceed the MICs of these penicillin-resistant pneumococci, the efficacy of treatment with these antibiotics is not established. Treatment with vancomycin may be preferable. IE caused by group G, C, or B streptococci is more difficult to treat than that caused by penicillin-susceptible viridans streptococci. Consequently, the addition of gentamicin to the first 2 weeks of a 4-week regimen using high doses of penicillin is often advocated (Table 33–7).

ENTEROCOCCI. Optimal therapy for enterococcal endocarditis requires the synergistic bactericidal interaction of an antimicrobial targeted against the bacterial cell wall (penicillin, ampicillin, or vancomycin) and an aminoglycoside that is able to exert a lethal effect (primarily streptomycin or gentamicin). High-level resistance, defined as the inability of high concentrations of streptomycin (2000 µg/ml) or gentamicin (500 to 2000 µg/ml) to inhibit the growth of an enterococcus, is predictive of the agent's inability to exert this lethal effect and participate in the bactericidal synergistic interaction in vitro and in vivo.[80,82]

The standard regimens recommended for the treatment of enterococcal endocarditis (Table 33–8) are designed to achieve bactericidal synergy. Synergistic combination therapy has resulted in cure rates of approximately 85 per cent, compared with 40 per cent with single-agent, nonbactericidal treatment.[80,81] Some authorities prefer gentamicin doses of 1.5 mg/kg every 8 hours; however, because this dose may be associated with an increased frequency of nephrotoxicity, others advocate doses of 1 mg/kg every 8 hours. Peak serum gentamicin concentrations of approximately 5 µg/ml and 3.5 µg/ml are sought with these doses, respectively. In the absence of high-level resistance to streptomycin in a causative strain, streptomycin 9.5 mg/kg IM or IV, every 12 hours, to achieve a peak serum concentration of approximately 20 µg/ml, can be substituted for gentamicin in the standard regimens. For patients allergic to penicillin, the vancomycin-aminoglycoside regimen (Table 33–8) is recommended; alternatively, patients can be desensitized to penicillin. Desensitization may be desirable when pre-existing renal dysfunction favors avoiding the potentially more nephrotoxic vancomycin-aminoglycoside combination. Cephalosporins are not effective in the treatment of enterococcal endocarditis. Therapy is administered for 4 to 6 weeks, with the longer course used to treat patients with IE that was symptomatic for more than 3 months, with complicated disease, and when there is enterococcal PVE. During treatment, careful clinical follow-up of patients and aminoglycoside levels is required to prevent nephrotoxicity and ototoxicity.

Previously, 40 per cent of enterococci demonstrated high-level resistance to streptomycin, and none was highly resistant to gentamicin. Furthermore, penicillin, ampicillin, and vancomycin inhibited all

TABLE 33-8 STANDARD THERAPY FOR ENDOCARDITIS DUE TO ENTEROCOCCI*

ANTIBIOTIC	DOSAGE AND ROUTE†	DURATION (WEEKS)
Aqueous penicillin G *plus*	18–30 million U/24 hours IV given continuously or every 4 hours in six equally divided doses	4–6
Gentamicin	1 mg/kg IM or IV every 8 hours	4–6
Ampicillin *plus*	12 gm/24 hours IV given continuously or every 4 hours in six equally divided doses	4–6
Gentamicin	1 mg/kg IM or IV every 8 hours	4–6
Vancomycin‡ *plus*	30 mg/kg per 24 hours IV in two equally divided doses not to exceed 2 gm/24 hours unless serum levels are monitored	4–6
Gentamicin	1 mg/kg IM or IV every 8 hours	4–6

* All enterococci causing endocarditis must be tested for antimicrobial susceptibility in order to select optimal therapy. These regimens are for treatment of endocarditis caused by enterococci that are susceptible to vancomycin or ampicillin and not highly resistant to gentamicin. These may also be used for treatment of endocarditis caused by penicillin-resistant (MIC > 0.5) viridans streptococci and nutritionally variant streptococci (*S. defectivus, S. adjacens*), or enterococcal PVE.

† Dosages are for patients with normal renal function. See Table 33–6, footnote.

‡ Cephalosporins are not alternatives to penicillin/ampicillin in penicillin-allergic patients.

Modified from Wilson, W. R., Karchmer, A. W., Dajani, A. S., et al.: Antibiotic treatment of adults with infective endocarditis due to streptococci, enterococci, staphylococci, and HACEK microorganisms. JAMA *274*:1706, 1995. Copyright 1995 American Medical Association.

enterococci at concentrations achieved in the serum with standard intravenous doses. Accordingly, one of the standard regimens could be selected for treatment with confidence that bactericidal synergy would be achieved. Antimicrobial resistance among enterococci is now complex and cannot be predicted without in vitro testing. High-level resistance to gentamicin has been noted in 10 to 25 per cent of *E. faecalis* and 45 to 50 per cent of *E. faecium*, and resistance to penicillin, ampicillin, and vancomycin has become commonplace, especially in *E. faecium*. Resistance to these antibiotics is most commonly seen among enterococci isolated from hospitalized or previously hospitalized persons.[194]

Nevertheless, all enterococci causing endocarditis must be evaluated carefully in order to select effective therapy (Table 33–9). The strain causing endocarditis must be tested for high-level resistance to both streptomycin and gentamicin, as well as to determine its susceptibility to penicillin, ampicillin, and vancomycin. If the strain is either resistant to achievable serum concentrations of the cell wall–active agent or highly resistant to the aminoglycosides, synergy and optimal therapy cannot be obtained with a standard regimen that includes the inactive antimicrobial. Furthermore, high-level resistance to gentamicin predicts resistance to all other aminoglycosides except streptomycin. These susceptibility data allow the selection of a bactericidal synergistic regimen, if one is possible, or alternative treatment (Table 33–9).[82]

STAPHYLOCOCCI. More than 90 per cent of coagulase-positive and coagulase-negative staphylococci are penicillin resistant. Methicillin resistance is common among coagulase-negative staphylococci and is a less frequent but important characteristic among *S. aureus*. Methicillin-resistant strains are resistant to all beta-lactam antibiotics but remain susceptible to vancomycin. Although staphylococci are killed by cell wall–active antibiotics, the bactericidal effects of these agents can be enhanced by aminoglycosides. Combinations of semisynthetic penicillinase-resistant penicillins or vancomycin with rifampin do not result in predictable bactericidal synergism; nevertheless, rifampin has unique activity against staphylococcal infections that involve foreign material.[195,196] Staphylococcal infections involving prosthetic heart valves are treated differently from native valve endocarditis caused by the same species (Table 33–10).[47,83,91]

STAPHYLOCOCCAL NATIVE VALVE ENDOCARDITIS. The semisynthetic penicillinase-resistant penicillins are the cornerstones of the treatment of endocarditis caused by methicillin-susceptible staphylococci. When patients have a penicillin allergy that does not induce urticaria or anaphylaxis, a first-generation cephalosporin can be used. The synergistic interaction of beta-lactam antibiotics with an aminoglycoside has not increased the cure rates for staphylococcal endocarditis; however, treatment with these combinations has modestly accelerated the eradication of staphylococci in vegetations and from the blood. To achieve this potential benefit, gentamicin may be added to beta-lactam antibiotic therapy for *S. aureus* during the initial 3 to 5 days of treatment.[83] More prolonged administration of gentamicin has been associated with nephrotoxicity and should be avoided. The role for combination therapy is less well defined in NVE caused by coagulase-negative staphylococci; pooled data suggest improved cure rates with combination therapy.[91] Methicillin-susceptible *S. aureus* endocarditis in intravenous drug addicts that is apparently uncomplicated and limited to the right heart valves has been effectively treated with 2 weeks of semisynthetic penicillinase-resistant penicillin (but not vancomycin) plus an aminoglycoside (doses as noted in Table 33–10).[197,198] However, a significant proportion of patients with right-sided *S. aureus* endocarditis remain febrile and toxic after completing 2 weeks of combination therapy.[92] Hence, clinical judgment must be exercised when this abbreviated regimen is used. Therapy should be extended in those patients who remain febrile after 1 week of treatment or who develop signs suggesting left-sided infection. Endocarditis caused by methicillin-resistant staphylococci requires treatment with vancomycin (Table 33–10). Trimethoprim-sulfamethoxazole treatment of right-sided endocarditis caused by *S. aureus* susceptible to this antimicrobial has been only moderately successful.[199] Truly suitable alternatives to vancomycin are not available. Teicoplanin, a glycopeptide antibiotic similar to vancomycin but not available

TABLE 33-9 STRATEGY FOR SELECTING THERAPY FOR ENTEROCOCCAL ENDOCARDITIS CAUSED BY STRAINS RESISTANT TO COMPONENTS OF THE STANDARD REGIMEN

I. Ideal therapy includes a cell wall–active agent plus an effective aminoglycoside to achieve bactericidal synergy
II. Cell wall–active antimicrobial
   A. Determine MIC for ampicillin and vancomycin; test for beta-lactamase production (nitrocefin test)
   B. If ampicillin and vancomycin susceptible, use ampicillin
   C. If ampicillin resistant (MIC ≥ 16 μg/ml), use vancomycin
   D. If beta-lactamase produced, use vancomycin or consider ampicillin-sulbactam
   E. If ampicillin-resistant and vancomycin-resistant (MIC ≥ 16 μg/ml), consider teicoplanin*
   F. If ampicillin-resistant and highly resistant to vancomycin and teicoplanin (MIC ≥ 256 μg/ml), see alternatives in IV.
III. Aminoglycoside to be used with cell wall–active antimicrobial
   A. If no high-level resistance to streptomycin (MIC < 2000 μg/ml) or gentamicin (MIC < 500–2000 μg/ml), use gentamicin or streptomycin
   B. If high-level resistance to gentamicin (MIC > 500–2000 μg/ml), test streptomycin. If no high-level resistance to streptomycin, use streptomycin
   C. If high-level resistance to gentamicin and streptomycin, omit aminoglycoside therapy; use prolonged therapy with cell wall–active antimicrobial (8 to 12 weeks)
IV. Alternative regimens and approaches
   A. Consider ampicillin, vancomycin (or teicoplanin), and gentamicin (or streptomycin based on absence of high-level resistance)
   B. Treatment with fluoroquinolones, rifampin, or trimethoprim-sulfamethoxazole is of questionable efficacy
   C. Consider suppressive therapy with chloramphenicol or tetracycline and surgical intervention
   D. Consider quinupristin/dalfopristin* therapy for IE due to susceptible *E. faecium*
   E. Single drug therapy (III, C) and surgical intervention

* Not approved by the Food and Drug Administration for use in the United States; may be available through compassionate-use protocol.

TABLE 33–10 TREATMENT FOR STAPHYLOCOCCAL ENDOCARDITIS IN THE ABSENCE OF PROSTHETIC MATERIAL

ANTIBIOTIC	DOSAGE AND ROUTE*	DURATION (WEEKS)
METHICILLIN-SUSCEPTIBLE STAPHYLOCOCCI†		
Nafcillin or oxacillin	2 gm IV every 4 hours	4–6
With optional addition of gentamicin	1 mg/kg IM or IV every 8 hours	3–5 days
Cefazolin (or other first-generation cephalosporins in equivalent dosages)‡	2 gm IV every 8 hours	4–6
With optional addition of gentamicin	1 mg/kg IM or IV every 8 hours	3–5 days
Vancomycin‡	30 mg/kg per 24 hours IV in two equally divided doses, not to exceed 2 gm/24 hours unless serum levels are monitored	4–6
METHICILLIN-RESISTANT STAPHYLOCOCCI		
Vancomycin	30 mg/kg per 24 hours IV in two equally divided doses, not to exceed 2 gm/24 hours unless serum levels are monitored	4–6

* Dosages are for patients with normal renal function. See Table 33–6, footnote.

† For treatment of endocarditis due to penicillin-susceptible staphylococci (minimum inhibitory concentration ≤ 0.1 μg/ml), aqueous penicillin G (18 to 24 million U/24 hours) can be used for 4 to 6 weeks instead of nafcillin or oxacillin.

‡ Cefazolin, other first-generation cephalosporins, or vancomycin may be used in selected penicillin-allergic patients.

Modified from Wilson, W. R., Karchmer, A. W., Dajani, A. S., et al.: Antibiotic treatment of adults with infective endocarditis due to streptococci, enterococci, staphylococci, and HACEK microorganisms. JAMA 274:1706, 1995. Copyright 1995 American Medical Association.

in the United States, has been considered a possible alternative; however, some strains of S. aureus have become resistant to teicoplanin.[200] If the methicillin-resistant strain is susceptible to gentamicin, the aminoglycoside can be used in combination with vancomycin to enhance activity against these organisms. However, the frequency of renal toxicity may also be increased by this combination. The addition of rifampin to vancomycin for treatment of methicillin-resistant S. aureus endocarditis has not been beneficial.[201] Right-sided endocarditis caused by methicillin-resistant S. aureus is not treated with a 2-week regimen.

STAPHYLOCOCCAL PROSTHETIC VALVE ENDOCARDITIS. Evidence from in vitro studies, experimental animal models of infection, and clinical studies suggests that staphylococcal infections involving foreign bodies, such as prosthetic heart valves, should be treated with two or three antibiotics in combination. Rifampin provides unique antistaphylococcal activity when infection involves foreign bodies.[195,196] However, rifampin-resistant staphylococci emerge rapidly when rifampin is used alone or in combination with vancomycin to treat staphylococcal PVE.[47] Consequently, staphylococcal prosthetic valve endocarditis is treated with two antimicrobials plus rifampin.[47] This author prefers to delay rifampin therapy briefly until treatment with two effective antistaphylococcal agents is in place.

For PVE caused by methicillin-resistant staphylococci, treatment is initiated with vancomycin plus gentamicin, with rifampin added if the organism is susceptible to gentamicin. If the organism is resistant to gentamicin, an alternative aminoglycoside to which the organism is susceptible should be sought. Alternatively, for treatment of PVE caused by an organism resistant to all aminoglycosides, a quinolone to which it is susceptible may be used in lieu of an aminoglycoside.[47] For treatment of PVE caused by methicillin-susceptible staphylococci, a semisynthetic penicillinase-resistant penicillin should be substituted for vancomycin in the combination regimen (Table 33–11).

Patients with a nonimmediate penicillin allergy can be treated with a first-generation cephalosporin in lieu of the semisynthetic penicillin. PVE caused by coagulase-negative staphylococci that occurs within the initial year after valve placement is often complicated by perivalvular extension of infection, and valve replacement surgery is often required to eradicate infection and maintain suitable valve function.[47] Patients with S. aureus PVE have frequent intracardiac complications and exceptionally high mortality rates; they should be considered for early surgical intervention if antimicrobial therapy response is not prompt.[47,202]

HAEMOPHILUS PARAINFLUENZAE, HAEMOPHILUS APHROPHILUS, ACTINOBACILLUS ACTINOMYCETEMCOMITANS, CARDIOBACTERIUM HOMINIS,

***EIKENELLA CORRODENS, AND KINGELLA KINGII* (HACEK ORGANISMS).** Endocarditis caused by the HACEK group has in the past been treated with ampicillin administered alone or in combination with gentamicin. Occasional HACEK organisms that are ampicillin-resistant by virtue of beta-lactamase production have been isolated. Given the marked susceptibility of both beta-lactamase–producing and non-beta-lactamase–producing HACEK strains to third-generation cephalosporins, ceftriaxone or a comparable third-generation cephalosporin is recommended for treatment of NVE or PVE caused by these organisms (Table 33–12).[83] For endocarditis caused by strains that do not produce beta-lactamase, ampicillin combined with gentamicin can be used in lieu of ceftriaxone (Table 33–12).

OTHER PATHOGENS. The antimicrobial therapy for patients with IE caused by unusual organisms is based upon very limited clinical experience and data from animal models and in vitro studies. Therapeutic regimens for most of these infections are beyond the scope of this chapter; in fact, physicians are urged to review the published experience with a specific causative agent as well as to seek assistance from experienced infectious disease consultants when treating these patients. Among the more common of the unusual agents causing endocarditis are *P. aeruginosa, Candida* species, and *Corynebacterium* species. The preferred treatment for patients with endocarditis caused by *P. aeruginosa* is an antipseudomonal penicillin (ticarcillin or piperacillin) plus high doses of tobramycin (8 mg/kg/day

TABLE 33–11 TREATMENT OF STAPHYLOCOCCAL ENDOCARDITIS IN THE PRESENCE OF A PROSTHETIC VALVE OR OTHER PROSTHETIC MATERIAL

ANTIBIOTIC	DOSAGE AND ROUTE*	DURATION (WEEKS)
REGIMEN FOR METHICILLIN-RESISTANT STAPHYLOCOCCI		
Vancomycin	30 mg/kg per 24 hours IV in two equally divided doses, not to exceed 2 gm/24 hours unless serum levels are monitored	≥6
plus Rifampin *and*	300 mg p.o. every 8 hours	≥6
Gentamicin†	1.0 mg/kg IM or IV every 8 hours	2
REGIMEN FOR METHICILLIN-SUSCEPTIBLE STAPHYLOCOCCI		
Nafcillin or Oxacillin *plus*	2 gm IV every 4 hours	≥6
Rifampin *and* Gentamicin†	300 mg p.o. every 8 hours	≥6
	1.0 mg/kg IM or IV every 8 hours	2

* Dosages are for patients with normal renal function. See Table 33–6, footnote.

† Use during initial 2 weeks of treatment. If strain is gentamicin-resistant, see text for alternatives.

Modified from Wilson, W. R., Karchmer, A. W., Dajani, A. S., et al.: Antibiotic treatment of adults with infective endocarditis due to streptococci, enterococci, staphylococci, and HACEK microorganisms. JAMA 274:1706, 1995. Copyright 1995 American Medical Association.

TABLE 33-12 TREATMENT FOR ENDOCARDITIS DUE TO HACEK MICROORGANISMS*

ANTIBIOTIC	DOSAGE AND ROUTE†	DURATION (WEEKS)
Ceftriaxone‡	2 gm once daily IV or IM	4
Ampicillin	12 gm/24 hours IV given continuously or every 4 hours in six equally divided doses	4
plus		
Gentamicin	1 mg/kg IM or IV every 8 hours	4

* HACEK microorganisms are *Haemophilus parainfluenzae*, *Haemophilus aphrophilus*, *Actinobacillus actinomycetemcomitans*, *Cardiobacterium hominis*, *Eikenella corrodens*, and *Kingella kingii*.

† Dosages are for those with normal renal function. (Table 33–6, footnote.)

‡ Cefotaxime or ceftizoxime in comparable doses may be substituted for ceftriaxone.

Modified from Wilson, W. R., Karchmer, A. W., Dajani, A. S., et al.: Antibiotic treatment of adults with infective endocarditis due to streptococci, enterococci, staphylococci, and HACEK microorganisms. JAMA *274*:1706, 1995. Copyright 1995 American Medical Association.

IM or IV in divided doses every 8 hours to achieve peak serum concentrations of 15 μg/ml).[203] Endocarditis caused by *P. aeruginosa* is often both destructive and poorly responsive to antibiotic therapy (Fig. 33–2). As a result, many patients with *P. aeruginosa* endocarditis require cardiac surgery.

Amphotericin at full doses is recommended for treatment of *Candida* endocarditis. Several patients with *Candida* endocarditis are reported to have been cured by prolonged treatment with fluconazole.[204] Nevertheless, surgical intervention shortly after beginning amphotericin treatment remains the standard treatment for *Candida* endocarditis.

The antimicrobial susceptibility of corynebacteria causing endocarditis must be carefully evaluated. Many remain susceptible to penicillin, vancomycin, and aminoglycosides. Strains susceptible to aminoglycosides are killed synergistically by penicillin in combination with the aminoglycoside.[102] *Corynebacterium jeikeium*, while often resistant to penicillin and aminoglycosides, is killed by vancomycin.[102] NVE or PVE caused by *Corynebacterium* species can be treated with the combination of penicillin plus an aminoglycoside or vancomycin, contingent upon the susceptibilities of the causative strain.[101,102,205]

The Enterobacteriaceae (*E. coli* and *Klebsiella*, *Enterobacter*, *Serratia*, and *Proteus* species) are highly susceptible to third-generation cephalosporins, imipenem, and aztreonam. One of these antimicrobial agents in high doses is combined with an aminoglycoside to treat IE caused by an Enterobacteriaceae.

The optimal treatment of IE caused by *Coxiella burnetii* has not been established. Prolonged therapy (3 years) using doxycycline (100 mg twice daily) or another tetracycline is used but is not curative.[31,206] Adding a quinolone to doxycycline therapy is advocated.[206] Surgery is important in effective treatment.

CULTURE-NEGATIVE ENDOCARDITIS. Special studies to diagnose IE caused by fastidious bacteria and other organisms must be performed (see Diagnosis). Thereafter, unless clinical or epidemiologic clues suggest an etiologic diagnosis, the recommended treatment for culture-negative NVE is ampicillin plus gentamicin (see standard regimen for enterococcal endocarditis, Table 33–8); for patients with culture-negative PVE, vancomycin is added to this regimen.[47,207] Mortality rates are lower for patients with culture-negative endocarditis who received antibiotics prior to obtaining blood cultures and those who become afebrile during the initial week of antimicrobial treatment.[172,207] Surgical intervention should be considered for those who do not fully respond to empirical antimicrobial therapy. If surgical intervention is undertaken, a detailed microbiological and pathological examination of excised material must be performed in order to establish an etiologic diagnosis.

TIMING THE INITIATION OF ANTIMICROBIAL THERAPY. Current cost-containment pressures frequently result in initiation of antimicrobial therapy for suspected endocarditis immediately after blood cultures have been obtained. This practice is appropriate in the management of patients with acute IE in whom infection is highly destructive and rapidly progressive and of patients presenting with hemodynamic decompensation requiring urgent or emergent surgical intervention. Immediate therapy may have a favorable impact on outcome in these patients. In contrast, precipitous initiation of therapy in hemodynamically stable patients with suspected subacute endocarditis does not prevent early complications and may, by compromising subsequent blood cultures, obscure the etiological diagnosis of endocarditis. In these latter patients, it is prudent to briefly delay antibiotic therapy pending the results of the initial blood cultures. If these cultures are not positive promptly, this delay provides an important opportunity to obtain additional blood cultures without the confounding effect of empirical treatment. This opportunity is particularly important when patients have received antibiotics recently.

MONITORING THERAPY FOR ENDOCARDITIS. Patients must be monitored carefully during therapy and for several months thereafter to detect complications of endocarditis or therapy. Failure of antimicrobial therapy, myocardial or metastatic abscess, emboli, hypersensitivity to antimicrobial agents, and other complications of therapy (catheter-related infection, thrombophlebitis) or intercurrent illness may be manifested by persistent or recurrent fever. Clinical events may indicate a need for potentially life-saving revision of antimicrobial therapy or adjunctive surgical therapy.

The serum bactericidal titer (SBT), the highest dilution of the patient's serum during therapy that in vitro kills 99.9 per cent of a standard inoculum of the patient's infecting organism, has been used to assess the adequacy of antimicrobial therapy. The use of this test has, however, become controversial. The SBT has correlated poorly with outcome of therapy. These poor correlations can be attributed to performance of the test in a nonstandardized manner and the marked impact of complications on outcome. Several studies suggested, however, that peak and trough titers of at least 1:64 or 1:32 and 1:32, respectively, obtained with a standardized SBT method correlate with bacteriological cure.[208,209] When using regimens considered optimal on the basis of clinical experience, monitoring therapy with this test is not recommended.[83] The SBT may be useful when treating patients with endocarditis caused by organisms for which optimal therapy is not established or when using unconventional antimicrobial regimens.

The serum concentration of vancomycin or aminoglycosides should be measured periodically. This allows dose adjustment to ensure optimal therapy and avoid adverse events. Additionally, renal function should be monitored in patients receiving these two antimicrobials, and the complete blood count should be checked at least weekly in patients receiving high-dose beta-lactam antibiotics or vancomycin.

Repeat blood cultures should be obtained during the initial days of therapy or if fever persists to determine if the bacteremia has been controlled. It is common practice to confirm the eradication of infection by obtaining several blood cultures 2 to 8 weeks after completion of therapy. However, in patients with recrudescent fever after treatment, prompt cultures are essential to assess possible relapse of endocarditis.

OUTPATIENT ANTIMICROBIAL THERAPY. Technical advances allowing the safe administration of complex antimicrobial regimens, combined with well-developed home care systems that provide supplies and monitor outpatient treatment, make it feasible to treat patients with endocarditis on an outpatient basis. Doing so can reduce the cost of therapy significantly. However, only those patients who have responded to initial therapy and are free of fever, who are not experiencing threatening complications, who will be compliant with therapy, and who have a home situation that is physically suitable should be considered for outpatient treatment. Furthermore, patients being treated at home must be apprised of the potential complications of endocarditis, instructed to seek advice promptly when encountering unexpected or untoward clinical events, and have assiduous clinical and laboratory monitoring. Lastly, outpatient therapy must not result in compromises of antimicrobial therapy leading to suboptimal treatment.

Surgical Treatment of Intracardiac Complications

Cardiac surgical intervention plays an increasingly important role in the treatment of patients with intracardiac complications of endocarditis. Retrospective data suggest that mortality is unacceptably high when patients with these complications are treated with antibiotics alone, whereas mortality is reduced when treatment combines antibiotics and surgical intervention.[64,135,161,210–213] Accordingly, these complications have become indications for cardiac surgery (Table 33–13).

VALVULAR DYSFUNCTION. Medical therapy of patients with NVE that is complicated by moderate to severe (New York Heart Association Class III and IV) congestive heart failure due to new or worsening valvular dysfunction results in mortality rates of 50 to 90 per cent. Survival rates for a similar group of patients treated with antibiotics and cardiac surgery are 60 to 80 per cent.[64,135,210–213] Although survival rates among surgically treated patients with PVE complicated by valvular dysfunction and congestive heart failure are 45 to 64 per cent, few PVE patients with these complications are alive at 6 months when treated with antibiotics alone.[47] Worsening aortic valve incompetence is associated with more severe and more rapidly progressive congestive heart failure than is mitral valve incompetence. Hence, patients with aortic valve endocarditis not only account for the majority of surgically treated patients but also require surgery on a more urgent basis when heart failure supervenes. Severe mitral valve insufficiency, nevertheless, results in inexorable heart failure and ultimately requires surgical intervention. Doppler echocardiography and color flow mapping indicating significant valvular regurgitation during the initial week of endocarditis treatment does not reliably predict those patients who will require valve replacement during active endocarditis. Alternatively, despite the absence of significant valvular regurgitation on early echocardiography, marked congestive heart failure may still develop. Decisions regarding surgical intervention should not be made solely on the basis of echocardiographic findings but rather by integrating clinical data during careful serial monitoring.[185] On occasion, very large vegetations on the mitral valve, particularly a mitral valve prosthesis, result in significant obstruction and require surgery.[47]

UNSTABLE PROSTHESES. Dehiscence of an infected prosthetic valve is a manifestation of perivalvular infection and often results in hemodynamically significant valvular dysfunction. Surgical intervention is recommended for PVE patients with these complications.[47,210] The risk of invasive infection is increased among patients with onset of PVE within the year after valve implantation and those with infection of an aortic valve prosthesis.[49] Endocarditis in these patients is often caused by invasive antimicrobial-resistant organisms; consequently, the benefit of combined medical-surgical therapy is enhanced further. Patients who

appear clinically stable but who have overtly unstable and hypermobile prostheses, a finding indicative of dehiscence in excess of 40 per cent of the circumference, are likely to experience progressive valve instability and warrant surgical treatment. Occasional patients with PVE caused by noninvasive, highly antibiotic-susceptible organisms, e.g., streptococci, despite a favorable clinical course during antibiotic therapy, late in treatment experience minor valve dehiscence without prosthesis instability or hemodynamic deterioration. Surgical treatment of these patients can be deferred unless clear indications arise.

UNCONTROLLED INFECTION. Surgical intervention has improved the outcome of several forms of endocarditis when maximal antibiotic therapy fails to eradicate infection and, in some instances, even to suppress bacteremia. Amphotericin B is inadequate therapy for fungal endocarditis, including that caused by *Candida* species, and surgical intervention is recommended shortly after initiation of full doses of antifungal therapy. Endocarditis caused by some gram-negative bacilli, e.g., *P. aeruginosa, Achromobacter xylosoxidans,* may not be eradicated by maximum tolerable antibiotic therapy and may require surgical excision of the infected tissue to achieve cure. Similarly, standard therapy of endocarditis caused by *Brucella* species includes surgery because medical therapy is rarely successful.[100] Surgical intervention is recommended when patients with enterococcal endocarditis caused by a strain resistant to synergistic bactericidal therapy (see Antimicrobial Therapy for Specific Organisms—Enterococci) do not respond to initial therapy or relapse. Perivalvular invasive infection is in some instances a form of ineradicable infection. Relapse of PVE after optimal antimicrobial therapy reflects invasive disease. Patients with relapse of PVE are treated surgically.[47,49] In contrast, patients with NVE who relapse, unless it is associated with a highly resistant microorganism or demonstrable perivalvular infection, often are treated again with an intensified, prolonged course of antimicrobial therapy.[47,49,214]

PERIVALVULAR INVASIVE INFECTION. NVE at the aortic site and PVE are most commonly associated with perivalvular invasion with abscess or intracardiac fistula formation.[30,47,49,134,188] Invasive infection occurs in 10 to 14 per cent of patients with NVE and 45 to 60 per cent of those with PVE.[30,47,188] Persistent, otherwise unexplained fever in spite of appropriate antimicrobial therapy or pericarditis in patients with aortic valve endocarditis suggests infection extending beyond the valve leaflet.[137,167,215] New-onset and persistent electrocardiographic conduction abnormalities, although not a sensitive indicator of perivalvular infection (28 per cent), are relatively specific (85 to 90 per cent).[30,134] TEE is superior to TTE for detecting invasive infection in patients with NVE and PVE.[167] Doppler and color flow Doppler or contrast two-dimensional echocardiography optimally define fistulas.[134] Patients with IE in whom an abscess is suspected but not detected by TEE should undergo MRI, including MR angiography.[134] Cardiac catheterization may add little to these imaging studies and is not recommended unless coronary angiography is needed for patients undergoing valve surgery but also suspected of having significant coronary artery disease.[64,134]

In patients with endocarditis complicated by perivalvular extension of infection, cardiac surgery should be considered to debride invasive infection, ablate abscesses, and reconstruct anatomical damage. In patients with invasive disease that significantly disrupts cardiac structures, is associated with congestive heart failure, results in instability of a prosthetic valve, or renders infection uncontrolled (persistent fever), surgery is warranted. However, it is likely that increasingly sensitive imaging techniques will elucidate invasive infections that do not require immediate surgery. Patients with perivalvular infection detected by MRI have been effectively treated with antibiotics alone.[134] Also, conservative medical management has been effective

---

TABLE 33–13 CARDIAC SURGERY IN PATIENTS WITH INFECTIVE ENDOCARDITIS

ABSOLUTE INDICATIONS
  Moderate to severe congestive heart failure due to valve dysfunction
  Unstable prosthesis
  Uncontrolled infection: Persistent bacteremia, ineffective antimicrobial therapy, fungal endocarditis
  Relapse after optimal therapy (prosthetic valves)

RELATIVE INDICATIONS
  Perivalvular extension of infection
  Staphylococcus aureus endocarditis (aortic, mitral, prosthetic valve)
  Relapse after optimal antimicrobial therapy (native valves)
  Culture-negative endocarditis with persistent unexplained fever (≥ 10 days)
  Large (> 10 mm) vegetations

for selected patients with perivalvular infection detected by TEE.[216]

LEFT-SIDED *S. AUREUS* ENDOCARDITIS.
Because this infection is difficult to control, highly destructive, and associated with high mortality, some authors have suggested that these patients should be considered for surgical treatment when the response to antimicrobial therapy is not prompt and complete.[212,217,218] *S. aureus* PVE is associated with mortality rates exceeding 80 per cent and thus is an even stronger indication for surgical treatment.[47,202] In contrast, intravenous drug abusers with *S. aureus* endocarditis limited to the tricuspid or pulmonary valves often experience prolonged fever during antimicrobial therapy; nevertheless, the vast majority of these patients respond to antimicrobial therapy and do not require surgery.[92,219]

UNRESPONSIVE CULTURE-NEGATIVE ENDOCARDITIS.
Patients with culture-negative endocarditis who experience unexplained persistent fever during empirical antimicrobial therapy, particularly those with PVE, should be considered for surgical intervention. Persistent fever in these patients represents either unrecognized perivalvular infection or ineffective antimicrobial therapy.

LARGE VEGETATIONS (>10 MM) AND THE PREVENTION OF SYSTEMIC EMBOLI.
A meta-analysis suggested that the risk of systemic embolization was increased in patients with vegetations greater than 10 mm versus those with smaller or no detectable vegetations, 33 per cent versus 19 per cent.[143] The association of larger mitral valve vegetations (>10 mm) with systemic emboli was confirmed when sizing used transesophageal imaging; however, vegetation size was not related to development of congestive heart failure or increased mortality.[142] Although a relationship may exist between vegetation characteristics—including size, mobility, and extent (number of leaflets involved)—and complications, the implications for surgical intervention are not clear. Yet to be performed are multivariate analyses examining the relationship between outcome or the need for surgical intervention and variables including not only vegetation characteristics but also valve dysfunction, perivalvular invasion by infection, organism, and infection site. Nevertheless, some authors have concluded that vegetation characteristics alone might warrant surgery.[64,142] This recommendation can be questioned, even if it is focused on prevention of emboli as the complications that correlate best with vegetation size.

The rate of systemic or cerebral emboli in patients with NVE and PVE decreases during the course of effective antibiotic therapy.[153,154,156,157,220] Additionally, it is not clear that surgical intervention reduces the frequency of systemic emboli.[135,210] Finally, the morbidity and mortality of cerebral and coronary emboli are rarely compared to the immediate and long-term risks of valve replacement surgery. The latter include perioperative mortality, recrudescent endocarditis on the prosthesis, thromboembolic complications, early and late valve dysfunction requiring repeat valve replacement, the hazards of warfarin anticoagulation (including its contraindication during pregnancy), and the risk and morbidity of late-onset PVE.[210] In the author's opinion, vegetation size alone is rarely an indication for surgery. The clinical findings and echocardiographic evidence for other intracardiac complications must be weighed against the immediate and remote hazards of cardiac surgery when recommending therapy.[143,186] Thus, the risk for systemic embolization as related to vegetation size is only one of many factors to be considered when planning treatment. Prior systemic embolization should be considered in a manner analogous to vegetation size and not as an independent indication for surgical intervention.[153,154,156,157,220]

TECHNIQUES FOR REPAIR OF INTRACARDIAC DEFECTS.
New surgical techniques to address severe tissue destruction in NVE and PVE have been developed. Although these are beyond the scope of this discussion, examples include valve composite graft replacement of the aortic root, use of

sewing skirts attached to the prostheses, and homograft replacement of the aortic valve and root with coronary artery reimplantation.[221–225] Furthermore, repair of the mitral valve in patients with acute or healed endocarditis avoids insertion of prosthetic materials and the associated hazards.[226,227] Although tricuspid valvulectomy without valve replacement has been advocated for treatment of uncontrolled tricuspid valve infection in intravenous drug abusers at high risk of recidivism and recurrent endocarditis,[228] the likelihood of refractory right-heart failure with time after valvulectomy makes tricuspid valve repair preferable.[64] Cardiac transplantation has been used to salvage an occasional patient with refractory endocarditis.[229]

TIMING OF SURGICAL INTERVENTION.
When endocarditis is complicated by valvular regurgitation and significant impairment of cardiac function, surgical intervention before the development of severe intractable hemodynamic dysfunction is recommended, regardless of the duration of antimicrobial therapy.[210,211,230] Postoperative mortality correlates with the severity of preoperative hemodynamic dysfunction; consequently, this approach is justified. In patients with valvular dysfunction in whom infection is controlled and cardiac function is compensated, surgery may be delayed until antimicrobial therapy has been completed. However, if infection is not controlled, surgery should be performed promptly. Similarly, if a patient who requires valve replacement in the near future has a large vegetation, indicating a high risk for systemic embolization, early cardiac surgery is appropriate.

In order to avoid intracranial hemorrhagic complications in patients who have sustained recent neurological injury, the timing of surgical intervention may require modification. Where cardiac function permits, surgery should be delayed for patients who have had prior embolic infarcts until at least 4 and ideally 10 postinfarction days have elapsed[158,231–234] and for those who have sustained an intracranial hemorrhagic event until at least 21 days have elapsed.[232,234] It is prudent to evaluate the cerebral vasculature in patients who have sustained an embolic infarct or who have persistent headaches prior to cardiac surgery. If a mycotic aneurysm is found, the timing of cardiac surgery should be reconsidered and prostheses that require postoperative anticoagulant therapy should be avoided.

DURATION OF ANTIMICROBIAL THERAPY AFTER SURGICAL INTERVENTION.
Inflammatory changes and bacteria are commonly seen in culture-negative vegetations removed from patients who have received most or all of the standard antibiotic therapy recommended for endocarditis caused by the specific microorganism.[235] This does not indicate that antimicrobial therapy has failed nor a need for a full course of antibiotic therapy postoperatively. The duration of antimicrobial therapy after surgery depends upon the length of preoperative therapy, antibiotic susceptibility of the causative organism, the presence of paravalvular invasive infection, and the culture status of the vegetation. In general, for endocarditis caused by relatively antibiotic-resistant organisms with negative cultures of operative specimens, preoperative plus postoperative therapy should at least equal a full course of recommended therapy; for those patients with positive intraoperative cultures, a full course of therapy should be given postoperatively. Patients with PVE should be treated conservatively and receive a full course of antimicrobial therapy postoperatively when organisms are seen in resected material.[47]

Treatment of Extracardiac Complications

SPLENIC ABSCESS.
Three to 5 per cent of patients with IE develop a splenic abscess; these abscesses most commonly occur in patients with IE caused by *S. aureus*, streptococci, and gram-negative bacilli.[140,145] Although splenic defects can be identified by ultrasonography and CT, these tests usually cannot discriminate between abscess and infarct. Progressive enlargement of the lesion during antimicrobial therapy suggests that it is an abscess; this can be confirmed by

percutaneous needle aspiration. Successful therapy of splenic abscesses generally requires drainage, which can often be accomplished by percutaneous placement of a catheter.[145] In patients with endocarditis complicated by multiple splenic abscesses or in whom percutaneous drainage is unsuccessful, splenectomy is required.[145] Splenic abscesses should be effectively treated prior to valve replacement surgery in order to avoid recrudescent infection and seeding of the valve prosthesis.

MYCOTIC ANEURYSMS AND SEPTIC ARTERITIS. From 2 to 10 per cent of patients with endocarditis have mycotic aneurysms; in 1 to 5 per cent the aneurysms involve cerebral vessels.[157,158] Cerebral mycotic aneurysms occur at the branch points in cerebral vessels, are generally located distally over the cerebral cortex, and are found most commonly in branches of the middle cerebral artery. The aneurysms arise either from occlusion of vessels by septic emboli with secondary arteritis and vessel wall destruction or from bacteremic seeding of the vessel wall through the vasa vasorum. S. aureus is commonly implicated in the former and viridans streptococci in the latter.[159,160] Although many patients with mycotic aneurysms or septic arteritis present with devastating intracranial hemorrhage, focal deficits from embolic events and persistent focal headache may be premonitory symptoms. Cerebral angiography is required to evaluate patients with subarachnoid hemorrhage and has been recommended for patients experiencing premonitory symptoms or for those with neurologic symptoms in whom anticoagulant therapy is planned.[157,158] Mycotic aneurysms may resolve during antimicrobial therapy;[157] however, where anatomically feasible, aneurysms that have ruptured should be repaired surgically. Aneurysms that have not leaked should be followed angiographically during antimicrobial therapy. Surgery should be considered for a single lesion that enlarges during or following antimicrobial therapy. Anticoagulant therapy should be avoided in patients with a persisting mycotic aneurysm. Although persistent stable aneurysms may rupture after completion of standard antimicrobial therapy, there is no accurate estimation of risk for late rupture, and recommendations for surgical intervention are arbitrary. Nevertheless, prevaling opinion favors, whenever possible without serious neurological injury, the resection of single aneurysms that persist after therapy.[236] The potential existence of occult aneurysms in patients without neurological symptoms or those who have had a negative angiographic evaluation is not considered a contraindication to anticoagulant therapy after completion of antimicrobial therapy.[157]

Extracranial mycotic aneurysms should be followed during antibiotic therapy of IE in a manner analogous to that outlined for cerebral aneurysms. Those that leak, are expanding during therapy, or persist after therapy should be repaired. Particular attention should be given to aneurysms that involve intraabdominal arteries, rupture of which could result in life-threatening hemorrhage.

ANTICOAGULANT THERAPY. Patients with PVE involving devices that would usually warrant maintenance anticoagulation are continued on anticoagulant therapy.[47] Prothrombin times should be maintained at 1.5 times the control (INR = 3.0). Anticoagulation is not initiated as prophylaxis against thromboembolism in patients with PVE involving devices that do not usually require this therapy. Among patients with NVE there is no evidence that anticoagulant therapy prevents embolization, and in some instances it may contribute to intracranial hemorrhage, particularly in the presence of a recent cerebral infarct or a mycotic aneurysm.[157-159] Anticoagulant therapy in patients with NVE is limited to those patients for whom there is a clear indication for this therapy and for whom there is not a known increased risk for intracranial hemorrhage. If central nervous system complications occur in patients with IE who are receiving anticoagulant therapy, anticoagulation should be reversed immediately.[47]

Response to Therapy and Outcome

Temperature returns to normal in most patients with IE, including those with PVE, within a week after initiation of effective antimicrobial therapy.[47,137,237] Almost 75 per cent of patients are afebrile at the end of 1 week of therapy, and 90 per cent have defervesced by the end of the second week of treatment.[215,237] Prolonged fever during therapy is associated with IE due to S. aureus, P. aeruginosa, and culture-negative IE as well as IE characterized by microvascular phenomena and major embolic complications.[137,215,237] Persistence or recurrence of fever more than 7 to 10 days after initiation of antibiotic therapy identified patients with increased mortality rates and with complications of infection or therapy.[47,137,215,237] Those patients with prolonged or recurrent fever should be evaluated for intracardiac complications, focal extracardiac septic complications, intercurrent nosocomial infections, recurrent pulmonary emboli (patients with right-sided IE), drug-associated fever, additional underlying illnesses, and, if appropriate, in-hospital substance abuse.

Blood cultures should be repeated in search of persistent bacteremia or the presence of additional pathogens, e.g., previously unrecognized polymicrobial IE. The antimicrobial susceptibility of the causative organism should be reevaluated, as should the adequacy of antibiotic therapy. Drug reactions have accounted for fever in 17 to 19 per cent of these patients.[137,215] Drug fever attributed to the antimicrobial therapy itself may warrant revision of treatment if a suitable alternative is available. In the absence of effective alternative therapy, treatment can be continued with an antibiotic that is causing fever but is not causing significant end-organ toxicity. In 33 to 45 per cent of patients, persistent fever was associated with significant intracardiac complications, many of which required surgical intervention.[137,215]

Many clinical and laboratory features of IE are slow to resolve in spite of effective antimicrobial therapy. Peripheral manifestations of endocarditis and systemic emboli occur during the early weeks of treatment, although with decreasing frequency. Splenomegaly is slow to resolve, and murmurs may change throughout treatment. Normalization of the sedimentation rate and other inflammatory parameters, as well as correction of the anemia, may not occur until after therapy has been completed.

Mortality rates for large series of NVE treated between 1975 and 1990 range from 16 to 27 per cent.[4,7,8,30,238] Death due to IE has been associated with increased age (>65 to 70 years old), underlying diseases, infection involving the aortic valve, development of congestive heart failure, and central nervous system complications.[1,4,8,30] The treatment of heart failure due to valve dysfunction by early surgical intervention has decreased the mortality associated with congestive heart failure; but subsequently, neurological events and septic complications, e.g., uncontrolled infection and myocardial abscess, have accounted for a larger proportion of deaths and have been associated with high mortality rates.[140]

Mortality rates among patients with IE caused by viridans streptococci and S. bovis have ranged from 4 to 9 per cent.[1,4,7] Higher mortality rates are reported with left-sided NVE caused by other organisms: enterococci, 15 to 20 per cent[4,7,81]; S. aureus, 25 to 47 per cent[1,4,7,90]; nonviridans streptococci (groups B, C, and G), 50 per cent[239]; C. burnetti, 37 per cent[31]; P. aeruginosa, Enterobacteriaceae, and fungi, greater than 50 per cent.[35,97,109]

In a retrospective study of NVE patients with either Class III or IV heart failure (New York Heart Association), persistent hypotension, uncontrolled infection for over 21 days, aortic root abscess, or pericarditis, mortality rates for those treated with antibiotics plus surgery and those treated with antibiotics alone were 9 and 51 per cent, respectively.[135] Mortality rates among patients with NVE, particularly involving the aortic valve, who were treated surgically, have ranged from 5 to 26 per cent, with rates toward the high end of this range reported more frequently.[218,230,240-242] Severity of heart failure, abscess, S. aureus infection, and decreased renal function (possibly related to heart failure) have been associated with increased postoperative mortality.[218,242]

Outcome for patients with PVE, as contrasted with NVE, has been less desirable. Prior to 1980, mortality rates among patients with onset less than 60 days after surgery and later-onset PVE averaged 70 and 45 per cent, respectively.[47] With the recognition that PVE was frequently complicated by invasive infection and that patients would benefit from surgical intervention, mortality rates have decreased.[47,49] Long-term survival was adversely affected by the presence of moderate or severe heart failure at discharge.[49] Survival rates after aggressive surgery for PVE ranged from 75 to 80 per cent and were not related to time of onset after cardiac surgery.[49,243]

Among patients with NVE (nonaddicts) discharged after medical or medical-surgical therapy, long-term survival was

88 per cent at 5 years and 81 per cent at 10 years.[238] Among patients treated surgically for NVE, survival at 5 years ranged from 70 to 80 per cent.[64,240,241,243] Among patients with PVE treated surgically, survival rates at 4 to 6 years range from 50 to 80 per cent.[64,69,75,225]

RELAPSE AND RECURRENCE. Relapse of IE usually occurs within 2 months of discontinuing antibiotic treatment. Of patients with NVE caused by penicillin-susceptible viridans streptococci who receive a recommended course of therapy, less than 2 per cent relapse. From 8 to 20 per cent of patients with enterococcal IE relapse after standard therapy.[81,214] Patients with IE caused by S. aureus, Enterobacteriaceae, or fungi are more likely to experience overt failure of therapy rather than relapse; nevertheless, 4 per cent of patients with S. aureus IE relapse.[214] Relapse of fungal endocarditis at long intervals after treatment has been reported. At least 10 per cent of patients with PVE relapse.[49]

Among nonaddicts with an initial episode of NVE or PVE, 4.5 to 7 per cent experience one or more additional episodes.[49,214,238] Among these patients, recurrent IE shares the clinical, microbiological, and response to therapy noted in primary episodes of IE. Intravenous drug abuse is now the most common predisposition for recurrent IE (43 per cent of patients). This population is at increased risk for recurrence within the year after the initial episode.[38]

PREVENTION

A rationale for prophylaxis for endocarditis can be derived by considering the pathogenesis, epidemiology, and microbiology of the illness. This rationale, even in the absence of supporting clinical trials, has generated recommendations for prophylaxis against endocarditis that are routinely applied in developed countries.[244-246] During bacteremia provoked by daily activities, infections, or health care procedures, bacteria adhere to and colonize the platelet fibrin aggregates, NBTE, that have formed on the valve endothelium as a consequence of preexisting congenital or acquired cardiac disease. If the adherence and the subsequent multiplication of bacteria in the vegetation exceed the capacity of host defenses for bacterial eradication, IE results. Although many bacteria enter the bloodstream, those uniquely suited to adhere to NBTE cause the majority of cases of endocarditis. These organisms and the cardiac abnormalities resulting in vulnerable NBTE are evident from reported cases of IE. Events that predispose to bacteremia by organisms causing endocarditis have been identified.[123] By identifying the patients at risk, the causative bacteria and their respective antimicrobial susceptibility, and the events that induce bacteremia, strategies for prevention of some episodes of IE have been formulated. For practical consideration, these strategies have been focused on procedures inducing bacteremia by organisms frequently implicated as causes of IE.

Viridans streptococci, the most common cause of NVE and late-onset PVE, are the predominant aerobic flora of the oral cavity and the most frequent blood isolates after dental extractions and other procedures involving the oral cavity and upper respiratory tract.[123,247] Although gram-negative enteric bacilli are the organisms most commonly recovered from the blood after procedures involving the genitourinary tract, these organisms rarely cause IE.[123] In contrast, procedures involving the genitourinary and gastrointestinal tracts commonly precede the development of enterococcal endocarditis.[81,244] The prophylaxis for endocarditis used in conjunction with procedures involving these mucosal surfaces is targeted against the bacteremic isolates that are common causes of endocarditis. When incision and drainage of skin or soft tissue infections are undertaken, prophylaxis is focused on S. aureus. In identifying procedures for which IE prophylaxis is recommended, clinical evidence that a procedure is associated with IE is also considered.

Procedures for which IE prophylaxis is recommended or not recommended have been identified by the American Heart Association and others (Table 33–14).[124,244,245] Although prophylaxis is advised for all patients at risk who undergo dental procedures that cause gingival bleeding, extractions are the most strongly associated with subsequent IE.[150,248] Prophylaxis is recommended when patients at high or intermediate risk for endocarditis (Table 33–15) undergo esophageal dilatation, sclerotherapy for esophageal varices, and retrograde cholangiography when the bile ducts are obstructed. Because endocarditis has been reported only rarely in association with other gastrointestinal endoscopic procedures with or without biopsy, prophylaxis is not routinely recommended in this situation. However, some physicians may elect to give prophylaxis to high-risk patients who undergo these or other low-risk procedures.[244,245] Prophylaxis is not recommended with routine cardiac catheterization or TEE.[124,244,249]

The relative risk associated with specific cardiac lesions is reflected in the increased frequency of the lesion among

TABLE 33–14 PROCEDURES FOR WHICH PROPHYLAXIS AGAINST ENDOCARDITIS IS CONSIDERED

PROPHYLAXIS RECOMMENDED	PROPHYLAXIS NOT RECOMMENDED
Dental procedures known to induce gingival or mucosal bleeding, including professional cleaning and scaling	Dental procedures not likely to cause bleeding, such as adjustment of orthodontic appliances and simple fillings above the gum line
Tonsillectomy or adenoidectomy	Intraoral injection or local anesthetic
Surgery involving gastrointestinal or upper respiratory mucosa	Shedding of primary teeth
Bronchoscopy with rigid bronchoscope	Tympanostomy tube insertion
Sclerotherapy for esophageal varices	Endotracheal tube insertion
Esophageal dilation	Bronchoscopy with flexible bronchoscope, with or without biopsy†
Gallbladder surgery	Cardiac catheterization
Cytoscopy, urethral dilation	Gastrointestinal endoscopy, with or without biopsy†
Uretheral catheterization if urinary infection is present	Cesarean section
Urinary tract surgery, including prostate surgery	In the absence of infection: Urethral catheterization, dilatation and curettage, uncomplicated vaginal delivery, therapeutic abortion, insertion or removal of intrauterine device, sterilization procedures, laparoscopy†
Incision and drainage of infected tissue*	
Vaginal hysterectomy	
Vaginal delivery complicated by infection	

* Antibiotic prophylaxis should be directed against the most likely endocarditis-associated pathogen(s), often staphylococci.
† In patients at highest risk physicians may elect to use prophylaxis for these procedures.
Adapted from Dajani, A. S., Bisno, A. L., Chung, K. S., et al.: Prevention of bacterial endocarditis: Recommendations of the American Heart Association. JAMA 264:2919, 1990.

TABLE 33-15 RELATIVE RISK OF INFECTIVE ENDOCARDITIS ASSOCIATED WITH PREEXISTING CARDIAC DISORDERS

RELATIVELY HIGH RISK	INTERMEDIATE RISK	VERY LOW OR NEGLIGIBLE RISK*
Prosthetic heart valves†	Mitral valve prolapse with regurgitation (murmur)	Mitral valve prolapse without regurgitation (murmur)
Previous infective endocarditis†	Pure mitral stenosis	Trivial valvular regurgitation on echocardiography without structural abnormality
Cyanotic congenital heart disease†	Tricuspid valve disease	
Patent ductus arteriosus	Pulmonary stenosis	Isolated atrial septal defect (secundum)
Aortic regurgitation	Asymmetrical septal hypertrophy	Arteriosclerotic plaques
Aortic stenosis	Bicuspid aortic valve or calcific aortic sclerosis with minimal hemodynamic abnormality	Coronary artery disease
Mitral regurgitation		Cardiac pacemaker, implanted defibrillators
Mitral stenosis and regurgitation	Degenerative valvular disease in elderly patients	Surgically repaired intracardiac lesions, with minimal or no hemodynamic abnormality, more than 6 months after operation
Ventricular septal defect		
Coarctation of the aorta	Surgically repaired intracardiac lesions with minimal or no hemodynamic abnormality, less than 6 months after operation	
Surgically repaired intracardiac lesion with residual hemodynamic abnormality		Prior coronary bypass graft surgery
Surgically constructed systemic-pulmonary shunts†		Prior Kawasaki disease or rheumatic fever without valvular dysfunction

* Prophylaxis against endocarditis not recommended.
† Lesions considered at highest risk for endocarditis.
Adapted from Durack, D. T.: Prevention of infective endocarditis. N. Engl. J. Med. *332*:38, 1995; and Dajani, A. S., Bisno, A. L., Chung, K. J., et al.: Prevention of bacterial endocarditis: Recommendations of the American Heart Association. JAMA *264*:2919, 1990. Copyright 1990 American Medical Association.

patients with endocarditis compared with the general population. Accordingly, lesions have been assigned to high, intermediate, low, and negligible risk categories (Table 33–15).[25,124,250,251] The American Heart Association and the Expert Group of the International Society for Chemotherapy have identified patients with prosthetic valves, uncorrected cyanotic congenital heart disease, prior infective endocarditis, and surgically constructed systemic-pulmonary shunts or conduits as being at the highest risk for IE.[244,245] Currently, rheumatic heart disease is a less common predisposition for IE in most of the developed countries; however, the attack rate of IE among persons with rheumatic valvular disease approaches that seen with prosthetic valves and suggests that these lesions entail a high risk also.[251]

The risk of IE for patients with mitral valve prolapse and the resulting role of prophylaxis among these patients have been controversial. Mitral valve prolapse has been identified frequently among patients with IE. However, the risk of endocarditis among patients with mitral valve prolapse and a murmur of mitral regurgitation is still relatively low. It is 5- to 10-fold higher than that noted in the general population but 100-fold less than that among patients with rheumatic valvular heart disease.[251] As a result, mitral valve prolapse with a murmur of mitral regurgitation defines a patient with an intermediate risk for IE and one for whom prophylaxis against endocarditis is recommended when undergoing an endocarditis-prone procedure (Table 33–14). In the absence of a mitral regurgitation murmur, prophylaxis is not recommended.[244,245]

GENERAL METHODS. The incidence of IE can be significantly reduced by total surgical correction of some congenital lesions that otherwise predispose patients to IE, e.g., patent ductus arteriosus, atrial septal defect, ventricular septal defect, pulmonary stenosis, and tetralogy of Fallot.[250] Patients with persisting congenital lesions and those with acquired valvular heart disease who remain at risk for IE should be instructed regarding their risk for endocarditis and the potential benefits of antibiotic prophylaxis. Although the recommendations for chemoprophylaxis are

TABLE 33-16 REGIMENS FOR PROPHYLAXIS AGAINST ENDOCARDITIS FOR USE WITH DENTAL, ORAL, AND UPPER RESPIRATORY TRACT PROCEDURES

SETTING	REGIMEN*
Standard regimen†	Amoxicillin, 3.0 gm orally 1 hour before procedure; then 1.5 gm 6 hours after initial dose
Regimen for amoxicillin/penicillin–allergic patients	Erythromycin ethylsuccinate, 800 mg, or erythromycin stearate, 1.0 gm, orally 2 hours before procedure; then half the dose 6 hours after initial dose OR Clindamycin, 300 mg orally 1 hour before procedure and 150 mg 6 hours after initial dose
Regimen for patients unable to take oral medications	Ampicillin, 2.0 gm IM or IV 30 minutes before procedure; then either ampicillin, 1.0 g IM or IV, or amoxicillin, 1.5 gm orally, 6 hours after initial dose
Regimens for ampicillin/amoxicillin/penicillin–allergic patients unable to take oral medications	Clindamycin, 300 mg IV 30 minutes before procedure then 150 mg 6 hours after initial dose
Regimen for patients considered at highest risk and not candidates for standard regimen	Use standard regimen for genitourinary and gastrointestinal procedures
Regimen for ampicillin/amoxicillin/penicillin–allergic patients considered at highest risk	Use regimen for allergic patients undergoing genitourinary and gastrointestinal procedures

* Dosages for adults. Initial pediatric dosages are as follows: Ampicillin or amoxicillin, 50 mg/kg; clindamycin, 10 mg/kg; erythromycin ethylsuccinate or erythromycin stearate, 20 mg/kg; gentamicin, 2.0 mg/kg; and vancomycin, 20 mg/kg. Follow-up doses should be one-half the initial dose. **Total pediatric dose should not exceed total adult dose.**
† Generally recommended for patients at highest risk, including those with prosthetic heart valves; physician may elect more vigorous regimens.
Adapted from Dajani, A. S., Bisno, A. L., Chung, K. J., et al.: Prevention of bacterial endocarditis: Recommendations of the American Heart Association. JAMA *264*:2919, 1990. Copyright 1990 American Medical Association.

TABLE 33–17 PROPHYLAXIS AGAINST ENDOCARDITIS: REGIMENS FOR USE WITH GENITOURINARY/GASTROINTESTINAL PROCEDURES

SETTING	REGIMEN*
Standard regiment†	Ampicillin, 2.0 gm IV plus gentamicin, 1.5 mg/kg (not to exceed 80 mg) IV or IM 30 minutes before procedure; followed by amoxicillin, 1.5 gm orally 6 hours after initial dose Alternatively, the parenteral regimen may be repeated once 8 hours after initial dose
Regimen for ampicillin/amoxicillin/ penicillin–allergic patients†	Vancomycin, 1.0 gm IV infused over 1 hour plus gentamicin, 1.5 mg/kg (not to exceed 80 mg) IV or IM, 1 hour before procedure May be repeated once 8 hours after initial dose
Alternative regimen for low-risk patient/ low-risk procedure	Amoxicillin, 3.0 gm orally 1 hour before procedure; then 1.5 gm 6 hours after initial dose

* Dosages for adults. Repeat doses of vancomycin or gentamicin require adjustment for renal dysfunction. Initial pediatric dosages, see Table 33–16, footnote.

† Regimens identical to those of Expert Group of the International Society for Chemotherapy, reference 245.

Adapted from Dajani, A. S., Bisno, A. L., Chung, K. J., et al.: Prevention of bacterial endocarditis: Recommendations of the American Heart Association. JAMA 264:2919, 1990. Copyright 1990 American Medical Association.

often known to patients at risk, dentists, and physicians, compliance with these guidelines is poor.[18,248,252] Patients should be given written documentation of their predisposing cardiac lesion and the recommended prophylaxis.

Maintenance of good oral hygiene may be a more important preventive than procedure-focused chemoprophylaxis. Good oral hygiene decreases the frequency of bacteremias that accompany daily activities (chewing, tooth brushing), events that may entail more risks than the occasional defined endocarditis-prone procedure.[248,252] Oral hygiene should be addressed before prosthetic valves are placed electively.

Among patients at risk for IE, some activities or procedures likely to induce bacteremia should be avoided. Oral irrigating devices, which may produce bacteremia even in patients with normal gingiva, are not recommended. Similarly, the use of central intravascular catheters and urinary catheters should be minimized. Infections associated with bacteremia must be treated promptly and if possible eradicated before the involved tissues are incised or manipulated.[244,245]

CHEMOPROPHYLAXIS. The widely promulgated recommendations of antimicrobial prophylaxis for endocarditis are based upon circumstantial evidence supplemented by studies of prophylaxis using animal models.

Initial experiments in animal models demonstrated that bactericidal antibiotics could prevent endocarditis even in the face of a nonphysiological large inoculum of bacteria and with a foreign body at the target site. Recent studies, however, suggest that prophylactic antibiotics prevent endocarditis by inhibiting growth of the bacteria adherent to NBTE sufficiently to allow their subsequent complete elimination by host defenses.[124,125] With more numerous bacteria adherent to the valve, a longer period of antibiotic inhibitory activity is required to prevent endocarditis.[125] Although experimental studies that mimic single-dose amoxicillin prophylaxis in humans suggest adequate margins of efficacy, the more sustained inhibitory effect achieved through a postprocedure dose of antibiotics is likely to provide an even higher degree of efficacy.[125,253]

Clinical studies supporting the efficacy of antibiotic prophylaxis for endocarditis are limited. The frequency of viridans streptococcal bacteremia immediately after dental extractions is not reduced by prophylactic antibiotics.[247] This, however, is not inconsistent with effective prophylaxis as demonstrated in animal models.[125] A retrospective study of patients with prosthetic valves who underwent dental and surgical procedures suggested that antibiotic prophylaxis prevented PVE.[254] A small case-control study with several major design limitations suggested a 91 per cent protective effect for prophylaxis.[255] However, a second case-control study suggested only a 49 per cent protective effect for antibiotic prophylaxis.[256] Additionally, failures of

antibiotic prophylaxis unrelated to resistant bacteria have been noted.[124]

Risk-benefit and cost-benefit analyses have raised significant questions regarding antibiotic prophylaxis for patients with mitral valve prolapse. The conclusions of these studies depend highly upon initial assumptions. Nevertheless, it is clear that unless both the cost and risks of prophylaxis are very low, the cost per case of IE prevented is high and mortality or morbidity may not be reduced. From a population perspective, prophylaxis in low- to intermediate-risk settings may not be cost- or risk-beneficial, and prophylaxis might be reserved for patients with high-risk cardiac lesions who are undergoing high-risk procedures.[124]

Even if antibiotic prophylaxis is effective as well as safe and inexpensive, only a small percentage of the cases are preventable. For example, only 55 to 75 per cent of patients with NVE have preexisting endocarditis-prone valvular disease, and many are not aware of the lesion before the onset of NVE.[2,6–8,124,248] Additionally, among patients with IE, only a small fraction (5 per cent) had both a known valve lesion and a procedure within 30 days of onset of IE that would have warranted prophylaxis.[248] Nevertheless, the morbidity and mortality associated with IE justify the use of the recommended prophylaxis regimens (Tables 33–16 and 33–17) in patients with high- and intermediate-risk cardiac lesions (Table 33–15) who are to undergo bacteremia-inducing procedures (Table 33–14). Penicillin-resistant flora may emerge among patients who are receiving continuous penicillin for prevention of rheumatic fever. Consequently, a non–penicillin prophylaxis regimen is preferred for these patients. Similarly, when serial dental procedures are anticipated, resistance may emerge to a repetitively used antibiotic. Varying the regimens used or extending the intervals between dental procedures may reduce the emergence of resistant oral flora. Prophylactic antibiotics should be administered as recommended. Initiation of prophylaxis several days before a procedure encourages the emergence of antibiotic-resistant organisms at the mucosal site.

REFERENCES

EPIDEMIOLOGY

1. Steckelberg, J. M., Melton, L. J., III, Ilstrup, D. M., et al.: Influence of referral bias on the apparent clinical spectrum of infective endocarditis. Am. J. Med. 88:582, 1990.
2. Griffin, M. R., Wilson, W. R., Edwards, W. D., et al.: Infective endocarditis: Olmstead County, Minnesota, 1950 through 1981. JAMA 254:1199, 1985.
3. Young, S. E. J.: Aetiology and epidemiology of infective endocarditis in England and Wales. J. Antimicrob. Chemother. 20(Suppl. A):7, 1987.
4. van der Meer, J. T. M., Thompson, J., Valkenburg, H. A., and Michel, M. F.: Epidemiology of bacterial endocarditis in the Netherlands. I. Patient Characteristics. Arch. Intern. Med. 152:1863, 1992.
5. King, J. W., Nguyen, V. Q., and Conrad, S. A.: Results of a prospective statewide reporting system for infective endocarditis. Am. J. Med. Sci. 295:517, 1988.

6. McKinsey, D. S., Ratts, T. E., and Bisno, A. L.: Underlying cardiac lesions in adults with infective endocarditis: The changing spectrum. Am. J. Med. *82*:681, 1987.

7. Watanakunakorn, C., and Burkert, T.: Infective endocarditis at a large community teaching hospital, 1980–1990: A review of 210 episodes. Medicine *72*:90, 1993.

8. Kazanjian, P.: Infective endocarditis: Review of 60 cases treated in community hospitals. Infect. Dis. Clin. Pract. *2*:41, 1993.

9. Terpenning, M. S., Buggy, B. P., and Kauffman, C. A.: Infective endocarditis: Clinical features in young and elderly patients. Am. J. Med. *83*:626, 1987.

10. Kaye, D.: Changing pattern of infective endocarditis. Am. J. Med. *78*(Suppl. 6B):157, 1985.

11. Terpenning, M. S., Buggy, B. P., and Kauffman, C. A.: Hospital-acquired infective endocarditis. Arch. Intern. Med. *148*:1601, 1988.

12. Fernandez-Guerrero, M. L., Verdejo, C., Azofra, J., and de Gorgolas, M.: Hospital-acquired infectious endocarditis not associated with cardiac surgery: An emerging problem. Clin. Infect. Dis. *20*:16, 1995.

13. Clemens, J. D., Horwitz, R. I., Jaffe, C. C., et al.: A controlled evaluation of the risk of bacterial endocarditis in persons with mitral-valve prolapse. N. Engl. J. Med. *307*:776, 1982.

14. Hickey, A. J., MacMahon, S. W., and Wilcken, D. E. L.: Mitral valve prolapse and bacterial endocarditis: When is antibiotic prophylaxis necessary? Am. Heart J. *109*:431, 1985.

15. McMahon, S. W., Hickey, A. J., Wilcken, D. E. L., et al.: Risk of infective endocarditis in mitral valve prolapse with and without precordial systolic murmurs. Am. J. Cardiol. *58*:105, 1986.

16. MacMahon, S. W., Roberts, J. K., Kramer-Fox, R., et al.: Mitral valve prolapse and infective endocarditis. Am. Heart J. *113*:1291, 1987.

17. Danchin, N., Briancon, S., Mathieu, P., et al.: Mitral valve prolapse as a risk factor for infective endocarditis. Lancet *1*:743, 1989.

18. van der Meer, J. T. M., van Wijk, W., Thompson, J., et al.: Awareness of need and actual use of prophylaxis: Lack of patient compliance in the prevention of bacterial endocarditis. J. Antimicrob. Chemother. *29*:187, 1992.

19. Nishimara, R. A., McGoon, M. D., Shub, C., et al.: Echocardiographically documented mitral-valve prolapse: Long-term follow-up of 237 patients. N. Engl. J. Med. *313*:1305, 1985.

CLINICAL CLASSIFICATION

20. Stull, T. L., and LiPuma, J. J.: Endocarditis in children. *In* Kaye, D. (ed.): Infective Endocarditis. 2nd ed. New York, Raven Press, 1992, p. 313.

21. Millard, D. D., and Shulman, S. T.: The changing spectrum of neonatal endocarditis. Clin. Perinatol. *15*:587, 1988.

22. Baltimore, R. S.: Infective endocarditis in children. Pediatr. Infect. Dis. J. *11*:907, 1992.

23. Awadallah, S. M., Kavey, R. E. W., Byrum, C. J., et al.: The changing pattern of infective endocarditis in childhood. Am. J. Cardiol. *68*:90, 1991.

24. Normand, J., Bozio, A., Etienne, J., et al.: Changing patterns and prognosis of infective endocarditis in childhood. Eur. Heart J. *16*(Suppl. B):28, 1995.

25. Michel, P. L., and Acar, J.: Native cardiac disease predisposing to infective endocarditis. Eur. Heart J. *16*(Suppl. B):2, 1995.

26. Lavie, C. J., Khandheria, B. K., Seward, J. B., et al.: Factors associated with the recommendation for endocarditis prophylaxis in mitral valve prolapse. JAMA *262*:3308, 1989.

27. Savage, D. D., Garrison, R. J., Devereux, R. B., et al.: Mitral valve prolapse in the general population. I. Epidemiologic features: The Framingham study. Am. Heart J. *106*:571, 1983.

28. Marks, A. R., Choong, C. Y., Sanfilippo, A. J., et al.: Identification of high-risk and low-risk subgroups of patients with mitral-valve prolapse. N. Engl. J. Med. *320*:1031, 1989.

29. Baddour, L. M., and Bisno, A. L.: Infective endocarditis complicating mitral valve prolapse: Epidemiologic, clinical, and microbiologic aspects. Rev. Infect. Dis. *8*:117, 1986.

30. DiNubile, M. J., Calderwood, S. B., Steinhaus, D. M., and Karchmer, A. W.: Cardiac conduction abnormalities complicating native valve active infective endocarditis. Am. J. Cardiol. *58*:1213, 1986.

31. Stein, A., and Raoult, D.: Q fever endocarditis. Eur. Heart J. *16*(Suppl. B):19, 1995.

32. Sande, M. A., Lee, B. L., Mills, J., et al.: Endocarditis in intravenous drug users. *In* Kaye, D. (ed.): Infective Endocarditis. 2nd ed. New York, Raven Press, 1992, p. 345.

33. Levine, D. P., Crane, L. R., and Zervos, M. J.: Bacteremia in narcotic addicts at the Detroit Medical Center. II. Infectious endocarditis: A prospective comparative study. Rev. Infect. Dis. *8*:374, 1986.

34. Chambers, H. F., Morris, D. L., Tauber, M. G., and Modin, G.: Cocaine use and the risk for endocarditis in intravenous drug users. Ann. Intern. Med. *106*:833, 1987.

35. Komshain, S. V., Tablan, O. C., Palutke, W., and Reyes, M. P.: Characteristics of left-sided endocarditis due to *Pseudomonas aeruginosa* in the Detroit Medical Center. Rev. Infect. Dis. *12*:693, 1990.

36. Levin, M. H., Weinstein, R. A., Nathan, C., et al.: Association of infection caused by *Pseudomonas aeruginosa* serotype 011 with intravenous abuse of pentazocine mixed with tripelennamine. J. Clin. Microbiol. *20*:758, 1984.

37. Dressler, F. A., and Roberts, W. C.: Infective endocarditis in opiate addicts: Analysis of 80 cases studied at necropsy. Am. J. Cardiol. *63*:1240, 1989.

38. Baddour, L. M.: Twelve-year review of recurrent native-valve infective endocarditis: A disease of the modern antibiotic era. Rev. Infect. Dis. *10*:1163, 1988.

39. Clifford, C. P., Eykyn, S. J., and Oakley, C. M.: Staphylococcal tricuspid valve endocarditis in patients with structurally normal hearts and no evidence of narcotic abuse. Q. J. Med. *87*:755, 1994.

40. Baddour, L. M.: Polymicrobial infective endocarditis in the 1980's. Rev. Infect. Dis. *13*:963, 1991.

41. Nahass, R. G., Weinstein, M. P., Bartels, J., and Gocke, D. J.: Infective endocarditis in intravenous drug users: A comparison of human immunodeficiency virus type 1–negative and –positive patients. J. Infect. Dis. *162*:967, 1990.

42. Rutledge, R., Kim, J., and Applebaum, R. E.: Actuarial analysis of the risk of prosthetic valve endocarditis in 1,598 patients with mechanical and bioprosthetic valves. Arch. Surg. *120*:469, 1985.

43. Ivert, T. S. A., Dismukes, W. E., Cobbs, C. G., et al.: Prosthetic valve endocarditis. Circulation *69*:223, 1984.

44. Arvay, A., and Lengyel, M.: Incidence and risk factors of prosthetic valve endocarditis. Eur. J. Cardiothorac. Surg. *2*:340, 1988.

45. Calderwood, S. B., Swinski, L. A., Waternaux, C. M., et al.: Risk factors for the development of prosthetic valve endocarditis. Circulation *72*:31, 1985.

46. Horskotte, D., Piper, C., Niehues, R., et al.: Late prosthetic valve endocarditis. Eur. Heart J. *16*(Suppl. B):39, 1995.

47. Karchmer, A. W., and Gibbons, G. W.: Infections of prosthetic heart valves and vascular grafts. *In* Bisno, A. L., and Waldvogel, F. A. (eds): Infections Associated with Indwelling Devices. 2nd ed. Washington, D.C., American Society for Microbiology, 1994, p. 213.

48. Karchmer, A. W., Archer, G. L., and Dismukes, W. E.: *Staphylococcus epidermidis* causing prosthetic valve endocarditis: Microbiologic and clinical observations as guides to therapy. Ann. Intern. Med. *98*:447, 1983.

49. Calderwood, S. B., Swinski, L. A., Karchmer, A. W., et al.: Prosthetic valve endocarditis: Analysis of factors affecting outcome of therapy. J. Thorac. Cardiovasc. Surg. *92*:776, 1986.

50. Ismail, M. B., Hannachi, N., Abid, F., et al.: Prosthetic valve endocarditis: A survey. Br. Heart J. *58*:72, 1987.

51. Kuyvenhoven, J. P., van Rijk-Zwickker, G. L., Hermans, J., et al.: Prosthetic valve endocarditis: Analysis of risk factors for mortality. Eur. J. Cardiothorac. Surg. *8*:420, 1994.

52. Chastre, J., and Trouillet, J. L.: Early infective endocarditis on prosthetic valves. Eur. Heart J. *16*(Suppl. B):32, 1995.

53. Douglas, J. L., and Cobbs, C. G.: Prosthetic valve endocarditis. *In* Kaye, D. (ed.): Infective Endocarditis. 2nd ed. New York, Raven Press, 1992, p. 375.

54. Sobel, J. D.: Nosocomial infective endocarditis. *In* Kaye, D. (ed.): Infective Endocarditis. 2nd ed. New York, Raven Press, 1992, p. 361.

55. Martino, P., Micozzi, A., Venditti, M., et al.: Catheter-related right-sided endocarditis in bone marrow transplant recipients. Rev. Infect. Dis. *12*:250, 1990.

56. Rowley, K. M., Clubb, K. S., Smith, G. J. W., and Cabin, M. S.: Right-sided infective endocarditis as a consequence of flow-directed pulmonary artery catheterization: A clinicopathological study of 55 autopsies. N. Engl. J. Med. *311*:1152, 1984.

57. Jernigan, J. A., and Farr, B. M.: Short-course therapy of catheter-related *Staphylococcus aureus* bacteremia: A meta-analysis. Ann. Intern. Med. *119*:304, 1993.

58. Ehni, W. F., and Reller, L. B.: Short-course therapy for catheter-associated *Staphylococcus aureus* bacteremia. Arch. Intern. Med. *149*:533, 1989.

59. Mylotte, J. M., McDermott, C., and Spooner, J. A.: Prospective study of 114 consecutive episodes of *Staphylococcus aureus* bacteremia. Rev. Infect. Dis. *9*:891, 1987.

60. Raad, I. I., and Sabbagh, M. F.: Optimal duration of therapy for catheter-related *Staphylococcus aureus* bacteremia: A study of 55 cases and review. Clin. Infect. Dis. *14*:75, 1992.

61. Maki, D. G., and Agger, W. A.: Enterococcal bacteremia: Clinical features, the risk of endocarditis, and management. Medicine *67*:248, 1988.

62. Roberts, R. B., Krieger, A. G., Schiller, N. L., and Gross, K. C.: Viridans streptococcal endocarditis: The role of various species, including pyridoxal-dependent streptococci. Rev. Infect. Dis. *1*:955, 1979.

63. Fang, G., Keys, T. F., Gentry, L. O., et al.: Prosthetic valve endocarditis resulting from nosocomial bacteremia: A prospective, multicenter study. Ann. Intern. Med. *119*:560, 1993.

64. Larbalestier, R. I., Kinchla, N. M., Aranki, S. F., et al.: Acute bacterial endocarditis: Optimizing surgical results. Circulation *86*(Suppl. II):II68, 1992.

Etiologic Microorganisms

65. Douglas, C. W. I., Heath, J., Hampton, K. K., and Preston, F. E.: Identity of viridans streptococci isolated from cases of infective endocarditis. J. Med. Microbiol. *39*:179, 1993.

66. Bouvet, A.: Human endocarditis due to nutritionally variant streptococci: *Streptococcus adjacens* and *Streptococcus defectivus*. Eur. Heart J. *16*(Suppl. B):24, 1995.

67. Enzler, M. J., Rouse, M. S., Henry, N. K., et al.: In vitro and in vivo

studies of streptomycin-resistant, penicillin-susceptible streptococci from patients with infective endocarditis. J. Infect. Dis. *155*:954, 1987.

68. Ruoff, K. L., Miller, S. I., Garner, C. V., et al.: Bacteremia with *Streptococcus bovis* and *Streptococcus salivarius:* Clinical correlates of more accurate identification of isolates. J. Clin. Microbiol. *27*:305, 1989.

69. Burkert, T., and Watanakunakorn, C.: Group A streptococcus endocarditis: Report of five cases and review of the literature. J. Infect. *23*:307, 1991.

70. Gallagher, P. G., and Watanakunakorn, C.: Group B streptococcal endocarditis: Report of seven cases and review of the literature, 1962–1985. Rev. Infect. Dis. *8*:175, 1986.

71. Scully, B. E., Spriggs, D., and Neu, H. C.: *Streptococcus agalactiae* (group B) endocarditis—A description of twelve cases and review of the literature. Infection *15*:169, 1987.

72. Wiseman, A., Rene, P., and Crelinsten, G. L.: *Streptococcus agalactiae* endocarditis: An association with villous adenomas of the large intestine. Ann. Intern. Med. *103*:893, 1985.

73. Venezio, F. R., Gullberg, R. M., Westenfelder, G. O., et al.: Group G streptococcal endocarditis and bacteremia. Am. J. Med. *81*:29, 1986.

74. Shlaes, D. M., Lerner, P. I., Wolinsky, E., and Gopalakrishna, K. V.: Infections due to Lancefield group F and related streptococci *(S. milleri, S. anginosus).* Medicine *60*:197, 1981.

75. Ugolini, V., Pacifico, A., Stahlmann, T. C., and Mackowiak, P. A.: Pneumococcal endocarditis update: Analysis of 10 cases diagnosed between 1974 and 1984. Am. Heart J. *112*:813, 1986.

76. Powderly, W. G., Stanley, S. L., Jr., and Medoff, G.: Pneumococcal endocarditis: Report of a series and review of the literature. Rev. Infect. Dis. *8*:786, 1986.

77. Finley, J. C., Davidson, M., Parkinson, A. J., and Sullivan, R. W.: Pneumococcal endocarditis in Alaska natives: A population-based experience, 1978 through 1990. Arch. Intern. Med. *152*:1641, 1992.

78. Friedland, I. R., and McCracken, G. H., Jr.: Management of Infections caused by antibiotic-resistant *Streptococcus pneumoniae.* N. Engl. J. Med. *331*:377, 1994.

79. Okumura, A., Ito, K., Kondo, M., et al.: Infective endocarditis caused by highly penicillin-resistant *Streptococcus pneumoniae:* Successful treatment with cefuzonam, ampicillin and imipenem. Pediatr. Infect. Dis. J. *14*:327, 1995.

80. Eliopoulos, G. M.: Enterococcal endocarditis. *In* Kaye, D. (ed.): Infective Endocarditis. 2nd ed. New York, Raven Press, 1992, p. 209.

81. Rice, L. B., Calderwood, S. B., Eliopoulos, G. M., et al.: Enterococcal endocarditis: A comparison of prosthetic and native valve disease. Rev. Infect. Dis. *13*:1, 1991.

82. Eliopoulos, G. M.: Aminoglycoside resistant enterococcal endocarditis. Infect. Dis. Clin. North Am. *7*:117, 1993.

83. Wilson, W. R., Karchmer, A. W., Dajani, A. S., et al.: Antibiotic treatment of adults with infective endocarditis due to streptococci, enterococci, staphylococci, and HACEK microorganisms. JAMA *274*:1706, 1995.

84. Hamill, R. J.: Role of fibronectin in infective endocarditis. Rev. Infect. Dis. *9*(Suppl. 4):S360, 1987.

85. Vaudaux, P. E., Lew, D. P., and Waldvogel, F. A.: Host factors predisposing to and influencing therapy of foreign body infections. *In* Bisno, A. L., and Waldvogel, F. A. (eds.): Infections Associated with Indwelling Medical Devices. 2nd ed. Washington, D.C., American Society for Microbiology, 1994, p. 1.

86. Chuard, C., Vaudaux, P., Waldvogel, F. A., and Lew, D. P.: Susceptibility of *Staphylococcus aureus* growing on fibronectin-coated surfaces to bactericidal antibiotics. Antimicrob. Agents Chemother. *37*:625, 1993.

87. Anwar, H., Strap, J. L., and Costerton, J. W.: Establishment of aging biofilms: Possible mechanism of bacterial resistance to antimicrobial therapy. Antimicrob. Agents Chemother. *36*:1347, 1992.

88. Takeda, S., Pier, G. B., Kojima, Y., et al.: Protection against endocarditis due to *Staphylococcus epidermidis* by immunization with capsular polysaccharide/adhesin. Circulation *84*:2539, 1991.

89. Shiro, H., Muller, E., Gutierrez, N., et al.: Transposition mutants of *Staphylococcus epidermidis* deficient in elaboration of capsular polysaccharide/adhesin and slime are avirulent in a rabbit model of endocarditis. J. Infect. Dis. *169*:1042, 1994.

90. Karchmer, A. W.: Staphylococcal endocarditis. *In* Kaye, D. (eds.): Infective Endocarditis. 2nd ed. New York, Raven Press, 1992, p. 225.

91. Whitener, C., Caputo, G. M., Weitekamp, M. R., and Karchmer, A. W.: Endocarditis due to coagulase-negative staphylococci: Microbiologic, epidemiologic, and clinical considerations. Infect. Dis. Clin. North Am. *7*:81, 1993.

92. Bayer, A. S., Blomquist, I. K., Bello, E., et al.: Tricuspid valve endocarditis due to *Staphylococcus aureus:* Correlation of two-dimensional echocardiography with clinical outcome. Chest *93*:247, 1988.

93. Breen, J. D., and Karchmer, A. W.: Usefulness of pulsed-field gel electrophoresis in confirming endocarditis due to *Staphylococcus lugdunensis.* Clin. Infect. Dis. *19*:985, 1994.

94. Vandenesch, F., Etienne, J., Reverdy, M. E., and Eykyn, S. J.: Endocarditis due to *Staphylococcus lugdunensis:* Report of 11 cases and review. Clin. Infect. Dis. *17*:871, 1993.

95. Grace, C. J., Levitz, R. E., Katz-Pollak, H., and Brettman, L. R.: *Actinobacillus actinomycetemcomitans* prosthetic valve endocarditis. Rev. Infect. Dis. *10*:922, 1988.

96. Meyer, D. J., and Gerding, D. N.: Favorable prognosis of patients with prosthetic valve endocarditis caused by gram-negative bacilli of the HACEK group. Am. J. Med. *85*:104, 1988.

97. Hessen, M. T., and Abrutyn, E.: Gram-negative bacterial endocarditis. *In* Kaye, D. (ed.): Infective Endocarditis. 2nd ed. New York, Raven Press, 1992, p. 251.

98. Jackman, J. D., Jr., and Glamann, D. B.: Southwestern Internal Medicine Conference: Gonococcal endocarditis: Twenty-five year experience. Am. J. Med. Sci. *301*:221, 1991.

99. Siller, K. A., and Johnson, W. D., Jr.: Unusual bacterial causes of endocarditis. *In* Kaye, D. (ed.): Infective Endocarditis. 2nd ed. New York, Raven Press, 1992, p. 265.

100. Jacobs, F., Abramowicz, D., Vereerstraeten, P., et al.: Brucella endocarditis: The role of combined medical and surgical treatment. Rev. Infect. Dis. *12*:740, 1990.

101. Petit, A. I. C., Bok, J. W., Thompson, J., et al.: Native-valve endocarditis due to CDC coryneform group ANF-3: Report of a case and review of corynebacterial endocarditis. Clin. Infect. Dis. *19*:897, 1994.

102. Murray, B. E., Karchmer, A. W., and Moellering, R. C., Jr.: Diphtheroid prosthetic valve endocarditis: A study of clinical features and infecting organisms. Am. J. Med. *69*:838, 1980.

103. Lamothe, M., Simmons, B., Gelfand, M., and Schoettle, P.: *Listeria monocytogenes* causing endovascular infection. South. Med. J. *85*:193, 1992.

104. Drancourt, M., Mainardi, J. L., Brouqui, P., et al.: *Bartonella (Rochalimaea) quintana* endocarditis in three homeless men. N. Engl. J. Med. *332*:419, 1995.

105. Spach, D. H., Kanter, A. S., Daniels, N. A., et al.: *Bartonella (Rochalimaea)* species as a cause of apparent "culture-negative" endocarditis. Clin. Infect. Dis. *20*:1044, 1995.

106. Brouqui, P., Dumler, J. S., and Raoult, D.: Immunohistologic demonstration of *Coxiella burnetii* in the valves of patients with Q fever endocarditis. Am. J. Med. *97*:451, 1994.

107. Shapiro, D. S., Kenney, S. C., Johnson, M., et al.: Brief report: *Chlamydia psittaci* endocarditis diagnosed by blood culture. N. Engl. J. Med. *326*:1192, 1992.

108. Scheld, W. M., and Sande, M. A.: Endocarditis and intravascular infections. *In* Mandell, G. L., Bennett, J. E., and Dolin, R. (eds.): Mandel, Douglas and Bennett's Principles and Practice of Infectious Diseases. 4th ed. New York, Churchill Livingstone, 1995, p. 740.

109. Rubinstein, E., and Lang, R.: Fungal endocarditis. Eur. Heart J. *16*(Suppl. B):84, 1995.

110. Moyer, D. V., and Edwards, J. E., Jr.: Fungal endocarditis. *In* Kaye, D. (ed.): Infective Endocarditis. 2nd ed. New York, Raven Press, 1992, p. 299.

PATHOGENESIS

111. Richardson, M., Kinlough-Rathbone, R. L., and Groves, H. M.: Ultrastructural changes in re-endothelialized and non-endothelialized rabbit aorta neo-intima following reinjury with a balloon catheter. Br. J. Exp. Pathol. *65*:597, 1984.

112. Ferguson, D. J. P., McColm, A. A., and Savage, T. J.: A morphologic study of experimental rabbit staphylococcal endocarditis and aortitis. I. Formation and effect of infected and uninfected vegetations on the aorta. Br. J. Exp. Pathol. *67*:667, 1986.

113. Ferguson, D. J. P., McColm, A. A., and Savage, T. J.: A morphologic study of experimental rabbit staphylococcal endocarditis and aortitis. II. Interrelationship of bacteria, vegetation and cardiovasculature in established infections. Br. J. Exp. Pathol. *67*:679, 1986.

114. Livornese, L. L., Jr., and Korzeniowski, O. M.: Pathogenesis of infective endocarditis. *In* Kaye, D. (ed.): Infective Endocarditis. 2nd ed. New York, Raven Press, 1992, p. 19.

115. Baddour, L. M., Christensen, G. D., Lowrance, J. H., and Simpson, W. A.: Pathogenesis of experimental endocarditis. Rev. Infect. Dis. *11*:452, 1989.

116. Scheld, W. M.: Pathogenesis and pathophysiology of infective endocarditis. *In* Sande, M. A., Kaye, D., and Root, R. K. (eds.): Endocarditis. New York, Churchill Livingstone, 1984, p. 1.

117. Freedman, L. R.: The pathogenesis of infective endocarditis. J. Antimicrob. Chemother. *20*(Suppl. A):1, 1987.

118. Freedman, L. R.: Infective Endocarditis and Other Intravascular Infections. New York, Plenum Medical Book Company, 1982, p. 5.

119. Weinstein, L., and Schlesinger, J. J.: Pathoanatomic, pathophysiologic and clinical correlations in endocarditis (first of two parts). N. Engl. J. Med. *291*:832, 1974.

120. Lopez, J. A., Ross, R. S., Fishbein, M. C., and Siegel, R. J.: Nonbacterial thrombotic endocarditis: A review. Am. Heart J. *113*:773, 1987.

121. Rodbard, S.: Blood velocity and endocarditis. Circulation *27*:18, 1963.

122. Weinstein, L., and Schlesinger, J. J.: Pathoanatomic, pathophysiologic and clinical correlations in endocarditis (second of two parts). N. Engl. J. Med. *291*:1122, 1974.

123. Everett, E. D., and Hirschmann, J. V.: Transient bacteremia and endocarditis prophylaxis: A review. Medicine *56*:61, 1977.

124. Durack, D. T.: Prevention of infective endocarditis. N. Engl. J. Med. *332*:38, 1995.

125. Blatter, M., and Francioli, P.: Endocarditis prophylaxis: From experimental models to human recommendation. Eur. Heart J. *16*(Suppl. B):107, 1995.

126. Dankert, J., van der Werff, J., Zaat, S. A. J., et al.: Involvement of bactericidal factors from thrombin-stimulated platelets in clearance of adherent viridans streptococci in experimental infective endocarditis. Infect. Immun. *63*:663, 1995.

127. Hamill, R. J., Vann, J. M., and Proctor, R. A.: Phagocytosis of *Staphylococcus aureus* by cultured bovine aortic endothelial cells: Model for postadherence events in endovascular infections. Infect. Immun. *54*:833, 1986.

128. Rotrosen, D., Edwards, J. E., Jr., Gibson, T. R., et al.: Adherence of *Candida* to cultured vascular endothelial cells: Mechanisms of attachment and endothelial cell penetration. J. Infect. Dis. *152*:1264, 1985.

129. Herzberg, M. C., MacFarlane, G. D., Gong, K., et al.: The platelet interactivity phenotype of *Streptococcus sanguis* influences the course of experimental endocarditis. Infect. Immun. *60*:4809, 1992.

130. Drake, T. A., Rodgers, G. M., and Sande, M. A.: Tissue factor is a major stimulus for vegetation formation in enterococcal endocarditis in rabbits. J. Clin. Invest. *73*:1750, 1984.

131. Bancsi, M. J. L. M. F., Thompson, J., and Bertina, R. M.: Stimulation and monocyte tissue factor expression in an in vitro model of bacterial endocarditis. Infect. Immun. *62*:5669, 1994.

132. Sullam, P. M., Frank, U., Yeaman, M. R., et al.: Effect of thrombocytopenia on the early course of streptococcal endocarditis. J. Infect. Dis. *168*:910, 1993.

133. Yeaman, M. R., Puentes, S. M., Norman, D. C., and Bayer, A. S.: Partial characterization and staphylocidal activity of thrombin-induced platelet microbicidal protein. Infect. Immun. *60*:1202, 1992.

PATHOPHYSIOLOGY

134. Carpenter, J. L.: Perivalvular extension of infection in patients with infective endocarditis. Rev. Infect. Dis. *13*:127, 1991.

135. Croft, C. H., Woodward, W., Elliott, A., et al.: Analysis of surgical versus medical therapy in active complicated native valve infective endocarditis. Am. J. Cardiol. *51*:1650, 1983.

136. Watanabe, G., Haverich, A., Speier, R., et al.: Surgical treatment of active infective endocarditis with paravalvular involvement. J. Thorac. Cardiovasc. Surg. *107*:171, 1994.

137. Blumberg, E. A., Robbins, N., Adimora, A., and Lowy, F. D.: Persistent fever in association with infective endocarditis. Clin. Infect. Dis. *15*:983, 1992.

138. Arnett, E. N., and Roberts, W. C.: Valve ring abscess in active infective endocarditis: Frequency, location, and clues to clinical diagnosis from the study of 95 necropsy patients. Circulation *54*:140, 1976.

139. Douglas, J. L., and Dismukes, W. E.: Surgical therapy of infective endocarditis on natural valves. *In* Kaye, D. (ed.): Infective Endocarditis. 2nd ed. New York, Raven Press, 1992, p. 397.

140. Mansur, A. J., Grinberg, M., Lemos da Luz, P., and Bellotti, G.: The complications of infective endocarditis: A reappraisal in the 1980's. Arch. Intern. Med. *152*:2428, 1992.

141. Steckelberg, J. M., Murphy, J. G., and Wilson, W. R.: Management of complications of infective endocarditis. *In* Kaye, D. (ed.): Infective Endocarditis. 2nd ed. New York, Raven Press, 1992, p. 435.

142. Mugge, A., Daniel, W. C., Frank, G., and Lichtlen, P. R.: Echocardiography in infective endocarditis: Reassessment of prognostic implications of vegetation size determined by the transthoracic and transesophageal approach. J. Am. Coll. Cardiol. *14*:631, 1989.

143. Aragam, J. R., and Weyman, A. E.: Echocardiographic findings in infective endocarditis. *In* Weyman, A. E. (ed.): Principles and Practice of Echocardiography. 2nd ed. Philadelphia, Lea & Febiger, 1994, p. 1178.

144. Sanfilippo, A. J., Picard, M. H., Newell, J. B., et al.: Echocardiographic assessment of patients with infectious endocarditis: Prediction of risk for complications. J. Am. Coll. Cardiol. *18*:1191, 1991.

145. Allan, J. D., Jr.: Splenic abscess: Pathophysiology, diagnosis and management. *In* Remington, J. S., and Swartz, M. N. (eds.): Current Clinical Topics in Infectious Diseases. Boston, Blackwell Scientific Publications, 1994, p. 23.

146. Bayer, A. S., Theofilopoulos, A. N., Eisenberg, R., et al.: Circulating immune complexes in infective endocarditis. N. Engl. J. Med. *295*:1500, 1976.

147. Gutman, R. A., Striker, G. E., Gilliland, B. C., and Cutler, R. E.: The immune complex glomerulonephritis of bacterial endocarditis. Medicine *51*:1, 1972.

148. Levy, R. L., and Hong, R.: The immune nature of subacute bacterial endocarditis (SBE) nephritis. Am. J. Med. *54*:645, 1973.

149. Williams, R. C., Jr., and Kunkel, H. G.: Rheumatoid factor, complement, and conglutinin aberrations in patients with subacute bacterial endocarditis. J. Clin. Invest. *41*:666, 1962.

CLINICAL FEATURES

150. Starkebaum, M., Durack, D., and Beeson, P.: The "incubation period" of subacute bacterial endocarditis. Yale J. Biol. Med. *50*:49, 1977.

151. Bush, L. M., and Johnson, C. C.: Clinical syndrome and diagnosis. *In* Kaye, D. (ed.): Infective Endocarditis. 2nd ed. New York, Raven Press, 1992, p. 99.

152. Churchill, M. A., Jr., Geraci, J. E., and Hunder, G. G.: Musculoskeletal manifestations of bacterial endocarditis. Ann. Intern. Med. *87*:754, 1977.

153. Steckelberg, J. M., Murphy, J. G., Ballard, D., et al.: Emboli in infective endocarditis: The prognostic value of echocardiography. Ann. Intern. Med. *114*:635, 1991.

154. Paschalis, C., Pugsley, W., John, R., and Harrison, M. J. G.: Rate of cerebral embolic events in relation to antibiotic and anticoagulant therapy in patients with bacterial endocarditis. Eur. Neurol. *30*:87, 1990.

155. Pruitt, A. A., Rubin, R. H., Karchmer, A. W., and Duncan, G. W.: Neurologic complications of bacterial endocarditis. Medicine *57*:329, 1978.

156. Hart, R. G., Foster, J. W., Luther, M. F., and Kanter, M. C.: Stroke in infective endocarditis. Stroke *21*:695, 1990.

157. Salgado, A. V., Furlan, A. J., Keys, T. F., et al.: Neurologic complications of endocarditis: A 12-year experience. Neurology *39*:173, 1989.

158. Kanter, M. C., and Hart, R. G.: Neurologic complications of infective endocarditis. Neurology *41*:1015, 1991.

159. Hart, R. G., Kagan-Hallet, K., and Joerns, S. E.: Mechanisms of intracranial hemorrhage in infective endocarditis. Stroke *18*:1048, 1987.

160. Masuda, J., Yutani, C., Waki, R., et al.: Histopathological analysis of the mechanisms of intracranial hemorrhage complicating infective endocarditis. Stroke *23*:843, 1992.

161. Griffin, F. M., Jones, G., and Cobbs, C. G.: Aortic insufficiency in bacterial endocarditis. Ann. Intern. Med. *76*:23, 1972.

DIAGNOSIS

162. Durack, D. T., Lukes, A. S., and Bright, D. K.: New criteria for diagnosis of infective endocarditis: Utilization of specific echocardiographic findings. Am. J. Med. *96*:200, 1994.

163. Mortara, L. A., and Bayer, A. S.: *Staphylococcus aureus* bacteremia and endocarditis: New diagnostic and therapeutic concepts. Infect. Dis. Clin. North Am. *7*:53, 1993.

164. Bayer, A. S., Lam, K., Ginzton, L., et al.: *Staphylococcus aureus* bacteremia: Clinical, serologic, and echocardiographic findings in patients with and without endocarditis. Arch. Intern. Med. *147*:457, 1987.

165. Bayer, A. S., Ward, J. I., Ginzton, L. E., and Shapiro, S. M.: Evaluation of new clinical criteria for the diagnosis of infective endocarditis. Am. J. Med. *96*:211, 1994.

166. von Reyn, C. F., and Arbeit, R. D.: Case definitions for infective endocarditis. Am. J. Med. *96*:220, 1994.

167. Daniel, W. G., Mugge, A., Martin, R. P., et al.: Improvement in the diagnosis of abscesses associated with endocarditis by transesophageal echocardiography. N. Engl. J. Med. *324*:795, 1991.

168. Mugge, A.: Echocardiographic detection of cardiac valve vegetations and prognostic implications. Infect. Dis. Clin. North Am. *7*:877, 1993.

169. Shively, B. K., Gurule, F. T., Roldan, C. A., et al.: Diagnostic value of transesophageal compared with transthoracic echocardiography in infective endocarditis. J. Am. Coll. Cardiol. *18*:391, 1991.

170. Sochowski, R. A., and Chan, K. L.: Implication of negative results on a monoplane transesophageal echocardiographic study in patients with suspected infective endocarditis. J. Am. Coll. Cardiol. *21*:216, 1993.

171. Werner, A. S., Cobbs, C. G., Kaye, D., and Hook, E. W.: Studies on the bacteremia of bacterial endocarditis. JAMA *202*:127, 1967.

172. Hoen, B., Selton-Suty, C., Lacassin, F., et al.: Infective endocarditis in patients with negative blood cultures: Analysis of 88 cases from a one-year nationwide survey in France. Clin. Infect. Dis. *20*:501, 1995.

173. Washington, J. A.: The microbiologic diagnosis of infective endocarditis. J. Antimicrob. Chemother. *20*(Suppl. A):29, 1987.

174. Kaye, K. M., and Kaye, D.: Laboratory findings including blood cultures. *In* Kaye, D. (ed.): Infective Endocarditis. 2nd ed. New York, Raven Press, 1992, p. 117.

175. Kauffmann, R. H., Thompson, J., Valentijn, R. M., et al.: The clinical implications and the pathogenic significance of circulating immune complexes in infective endocarditis. Am. J. Med. *71*:17, 1981.

176. Stratton, J. R., Werner, J. A., Pearlman, A. S., et al.: Bacteremia and the heart: Serial echocardiographic findings in 80 patients with documented or suspected bacteremia. Am. J. Med. *73*:851, 1982.

177. Daniel, W. G., and Mugge, A.: Transesophageal echocardiography. N. Engl. J. Med. *332*:1268, 1995.

178. Vered, Z., Mossinson, D., Peleg, E., et al.: Echocardiographic assessment of prosthetic valve endocarditis. Eur. Heart J. *16*(Suppl. B):63, 1995.

179. Pedersen, W. R., Walker, M., Olson, J. D., et al.: Value of transesophageal echocardiography as an adjunct to transthoracic echocardiography in evaluation of native and prosthetic valve endocarditis. Chest *100*:351, 1991.

180. Lindner, J. R., Case, R. A., Dent, J. M., et al.: Diagnostic value of echocardiography in suspected endocarditis: An evaluation based on the pretest probability of disease. Circulation *93*:730, 1996.

181. Daniel, W. G., Mugge, A., Grote, J., et al.: Comparison of transthoracic and transesophageal echocardiography for detection of abnormalities of prosthetic and bioprosthetic valves in the mitral and aortic positions. Am. J. Cardiol. *71*:210, 1993.

182. Tak, T., Rahimtoola, S. H., and Kamar, A.: Value of digital image processing of two dimensional echocardiograms in differentiating active from chronic vegetations of infective endocarditis. Circulation *78*:116, 1988.

183. Vuille, C., Nidorf, M., Weyman, A. E., and Picard, M. H.: Natural history of vegetations during successful medical treatment of endocarditis. Am. Heart J. *128*:1200, 1994.

184. Rohmann, S., Erbel, R., and Darius, H.: Prediction of rapid versus prolonged healing of infective endocarditis in monitoring vegetation size. J. Am. Soc. Echocardiogr. *4*:465, 1991.

185. Karalis, D. G., Blumberg, E. A., Vilaro, J. F., et al.: Prognostic significance of valvular regurgitation in patients with infective endocarditis. Am. J. Med. *90*:193, 1991.

186. Jaffe, W. M., Morgan, D. E., Pearlman, A. S., and Otto, C. M.: Infective endocarditis, 1983–1988: Echocardiographic findings and factors in-

fluencing morbidity and mortality. J. Am. Coll. Cardiol. 15:1227, 1990.

187. Karalis, D. G., Bansal, R. C., Hauck, A. J., et al.: Transesophageal echocardiographic recognition of subaortic complications in aortic valve endocarditis: Clinical and surgical implications. Circulation 86:353, 1992.

188. Omari, B., Shapiro, S., Ginzton, L., et al.: Predictive risk factors for periannular extension of native valve endocarditis: Clinical and echocardiographic analyses. Chest 96:1273, 1989.

189. Akins, E. W., Slone, R. M., Wiechmann, B. N., et al.: Perivalvular pseudoaneurysm complicating bacterial endocarditis: MR detection in five cases. Am. J. Roentgenol. 156:1155, 1991.

190. Sokil, A. B.: Cardiac imaging in infective endocarditis. In Kaye, D. (ed.): Infective Endocarditis. 2nd ed. New York, Raven Press, 1992, p. 125.

TREATMENT

191. Cremieux, A. C., Maziere, B., Vallois, J. M., et al.: Evaluation of antibiotic diffusion into cardiac vegetations by quantitative autoradiography. J. Infect. Dis. 159:938, 1989.

Antimicrobial Therapy

192. Roberts, S. A., Lang, S. D. R., and Ellis-Pegler, R. B.: Short-course treatment of penicillin-susceptible viridans streptococcal infective endocarditis with penicillin and gentamicin. Infect. Dis. Clin. Pract. 2:191, 1993.

193. Stein, D. S., and Nelson, K. E.: Endocarditis due to nutritionally deficient streptococci: Therapeutic dilemma. Rev. Infect. Dis. 9:908, 1987.

194. Coque, T. M., Arduino, R. C., and Murray, B. E.: High-level resistance to aminoglycosides: Comparison of community and nosocomial fecal isolates of enterococci. Clin. Infect. Dis. 20:1048, 1995.

195. Chuard, C., Herrmann, M., Vaudaux, P., et al.: Successful therapy of experimental chronic foreign-body infection due to methicillin-resistant Staphylococcus aureus by antimicrobial combinations. Antimicrob. Agents Chemother. 35:2611, 1991.

196. Drancourt, M., Stein, A., Argenson, J. N., et al.: Oral rifampin plus ofloxacin for treatment of Staphylococcus-infected orthopedic implants. Antimicrob. Agents Chemother. 37:1214, 1993.

197. Chambers, H. F., Miller, T., and Newman, M. D.: Right-sided Staphylococcus aureus endocarditis in intravenous drug abusers: Two-week combination therapy. Ann. Intern. Med. 109:619, 1988.

198. Torres-Tortosa, M., de Cueto, M., Vergara, A., et al.: Prospective evaluation of a two-week course of intravenous antibiotics in intravenous drug addicts with infective endocarditis. Eur. J. Clin. Microbiol. Infect. Dis. 13:559, 1994.

199. Markowitz, N., Quinn, E. L., and Saravolatz, L. D.: Trimethoprim-sulfamethoxazole compared with vancomycin for the treatment of Staphylococcus aureus infection. Ann. Intern. Med. 117:390, 1992.

200. Mainardi, J. L., Shlaes, D. M., Goering, R. V., et al.: Decreased teicoplanin susceptibility of methicillin-resistant strains of Staphylococcus aureus. J. Infect. Dis. 171:1646, 1995.

201. Levine, D. P., Fromm, B. S., and Reddy, B. R.: Slow response to vancomycin or vancomycin plus rifampin in methicillin-resistant Staphylococcus aureus endocarditis. Ann. Intern. Med. 115:674, 1991.

202. Sett, S. S., Hudon, M. P. J., Jamieson, W. R. E., and Chow, A. W.: Prosthetic valve endocarditis: Experience with porcine bioprostheses. J. Thorac. Cardiovasc. Surg. 105:428, 1993.

203. Reyes, M. P., and Lerner, A. M.: Current problems in the treatment of infective endocarditis due to Pseudomonas aeruginosa. Rev. Infect. Dis. 5:314, 1983.

204. Venditti, M., DeBernardis, F., Micozzi, A., et al.: Fluconazole treatment of catheter-related right-sided endocarditis caused by Candida albicans and associated endophthalmitis and folliculitis. Clin. Infect. Dis. 14:422, 1992.

205. Morris, A., and Guild, I.: Endocarditis due to Corynebacterium pseudodiphtheriticum: Five case reports, review, and antibiotic susceptibility of nine strains. Rev. Infect. Dis. 13:887, 1991.

206. Levy, P. Y., Drancourt, M., Etienne, J., et al.: Comparison of different antibiotic regimens for therapy of 32 cases of Q fever endocarditis. Antimicrob. Agents Chemother. 35:533, 1991.

207. Tunkel, A. R., and Kaye, D.: Endocarditis with negative blood cultures. N. Engl. J. Med. 326:1215, 1992.

208. Stratton, C. W.: The role of the microbiology laboratory in the treatment of infective endocarditis. J. Antimicrob. Chemother. 20(Suppl. A):41, 1987.

209. Weinstein, M. P., Stratton, C. W., Ackley, A., et al.: Multicenter collaborative evaluation of a standardized serum bactericidal test as a prognostic indicator in infective endocarditis. Am. J. Med. 78:262, 1985.

Surgical Treatment of Intracardiac Complications

210. Alsip, S. G., Blackstone, E. H., Kirklin, J. W., and Cobbs, C. G.: Indications for cardiac surgery in patients with active infective endocarditis. Am. J. Med. 78(Suppl. 6B):138, 1985.

211. DiNubile, M. J.: Surgery in active endocarditis. Ann. Intern. Med. 96:650, 1982.

212. Mullany, C. J., McIsaacs, A. I., Rowe, M. H., and Hale, G. S.: The surgical treatment of infective endocarditis. World J. Surg. 13:132, 1989.

213. Al Jubair, K., Al Fagih, M., Ashmeg, A., et al.: Cardiac operations during active endocarditis. J. Thorac. Cardiovasc. Surg. 104:487, 1992.

214. Santoro, J., and Ingerman, M.: Response to therapy: Relapses and reinfections. In Kaye, D. (ed.): Infective Endocarditis. 2nd ed. New York, Raven Press, 1992, p. 423.

215. Douglas, A., Moore-Gillon, J., and Eykyn, S.: Fever during treatment of infective endocarditis. Lancet 1:1341, 1986.

216. Chan, K. L., and Sochowski, R. A.: Conservative medical treatment can be appropriate in the management of perivalvular abscess: Diagnosis and follow-up by transesophageal echocardiography. J. Am. Coll. Cardiol. 50(Abs.):322A, 1994.

217. Richardson, J. V., Karp, R. B., Kirklin, J. W., and Dismukes, W. E.: Treatment of infective endocarditis: A 10-year comparative analysis. Circulation 58:589, 1978.

218. D'Agostino, R. S., Miller, C., Stinson, E. B., et al.: Valve replacement in patients with native valve endocarditis: What really determines operative outcome? Ann. Thorac. Surg. 40:429, 1985.

219. Hecht, S. R., and Berger, M.: Right-sided endocarditis in intravenous drug users: Prognostic features in 102 episodes. Ann. Intern. Med. 117:560, 1992.

220. Davenport, J., and Hart, R. G.: Prosthetic valve endocarditis 1976–1987: Antibiotics, anticoagulation, and stroke. Stroke 21:993, 1990.

221. Ergin, M. A., Raissi, S., Follis, F., et al.: Annular destruction in acute bacterial endocarditis: Surgical techniques to meet the challenge. J. Thorac. Cardiovasc. Surg. 97:755, 1989.

222. Miller, D. C.: Predictors of outcome in patients with prosthetic valve endocarditis (PVE) and potential advantages of homograft aortic root replacement for prosthetic ascending aortic valve-graft infections. J. Cardiac Surg. 5:53, 1990.

223. Ross, D.: Allograft root replacement for prosthetic endocarditis. J. Cardiac Surg. 5:68, 1990.

224. McGiffin, D. C., Galbraith, A. J., McLachian, G. J., et al.: Aortic valve infection: Risk factors for death and recurrent endocarditis after aortic valve replacement. J. Thorac. Cardiovasc. Surg. 104:511, 1992.

225. Jault, F., Gandjbakheh, I., Chastre, J. C., et al.: Prosthetic valve endocarditis with ring abscesses: Surgical management and long-term results. J. Thorac. Cardiovasc. Surg. 105:1106, 1993.

226. Dreyfus, C., Serraf, A., Jebara, V. A., et al.: Valve repair in acute endocarditis. Ann. Thorac. Surg. 49:706, 1990.

227. Hendren, W. G., Morris, A. S., Rosenkranz, E. R., et al.: Mitral valve repair for bacterial endocarditis. J. Thorac. Cardiovasc. Surg. 103:124, 1992.

228. Arbulu, A., Holmes, R. J., and Asfaw, I.: Tricuspid valvulectomy without replacement: Twenty years' experience. J. Thorac. Cardiovasc. Surg. 102:917, 1991.

229. DiSesa, V. J., Sloss, L. J., and Cohn, L. H.: Heart transplantation for intractable prosthetic valve endocarditis. J. Heart Transplant. 9:142, 1990.

230. Middlemost, S., Wisenbaugh, T., Meyerowitz, C., et al.: A case for early surgery in native left-sided endocarditis complicated by heart failure: Results in 203 patients. J. Am. Coll. Cardiol. 18:663, 1991.

231. Maruyama, M., Kuriyama, Y., Sawada, T., et al.: Brain damage after open heart surgery in patients with acute cardioembolic stroke. Stroke 20:1305, 1989.

232. Ting, W., Silverman, N., and Levitsky, S.: Valve replacement in patients with endocarditis and cerebral septic emboli. Ann. Thorac. Surg. 51:18, 1991.

233. Zisbrod, Z., Rose, D. M., Jacobowitz, I. J., et al.: Results of open heart surgery in patients with recent cardiogenic embolic stroke and central nervous system dysfunction. Circulation 76(Suppl. V):V109, 1987.

234. Matsushita, K., Kuriyama, Y., Sawada, T., et al.: Hemorrhagic and ischemic cerebrovascular complications of active infective endocarditis of native valve. Eur. Neurol. 33:267, 1993.

235. Morris, A., Strickett, A., and MacCulloch, D.: Gram stain culture and histology results of heart valves removed during active bacterial endocarditis (Abs. 1174). Programs of the 31st Interscience Conference on Antimicrobial Agents and Chemotherapy, 1991.

236. Ojemann, R. G.: Surgical management of bacterial intracranial aneurysms. In Schmidek, H. H., and Sweet, W. H. (eds.): Operative Neurosurgical Techniques. 2nd ed. Orlando, Grune and Stratton, 1988, p. 997.

RESPONSE TO THERAPY AND OUTCOME

237. Lederman, M. M., Sprague, L., Wallis, R. S., and Ellner, J. J.: Duration of fever during treatment of infective endocarditis. Medicine 71:52, 1992.

238. Tornos, M. P., Permanyer-Miralda, G., Olona, M., et al.: Long-term complications of native valve infective endocarditis in non-addicts: A 15-year follow-up study. Ann. Intern. Med. 117:567, 1992.

239. Roberts, R. B.: Streptococcal endocarditis: The viridans and beta hemolytic streptococci. In Kaye, D. (ed.): Infective Endocarditis. 2nd ed. New York, Raven Press, 1992, p. 191.

240. Acar, J., Michel, P. L., Varenne, O., et al.: Surgical treatment of infective endocarditis. Eur. Heart J. 16(Suppl. B):94, 1995.

241. Amrani, M., Schoevaerdts, J. C., Eucher, P., et al.: Extension of native aortic valve endocarditis: Surgical considerations. Eur. Heart J. 16(Suppl. B):103, 1995.

242. Mullany, C. J., Chua, Y. L., Schaff, H. V., et al.: Early and late survival after surgical treatment of culture-positive active endocarditis. Mayo Clin. Proc. 70:517, 1995.

243. Lytle, B. W.: Surgical treatment of prosthetic valve endocarditis. Semin. Thorac. Cardiovasc. Surg. 7:13, 1995.

244. Dajani, A. S., Bisno, A. L., Chung, K. J., et al.: Prevention of bacterial endocarditis: Recommendations by the American Heart Association. J.A.M.A. 264:2919, 1990.

245. Leport, C., Horstkotte, D., Burckhardt, D., and Group of Experts of the International Society for Chemotherapy: Antibiotic prophylaxis for infective endocarditis from an international group of experts towards a European consensus. Eur. Heart J. 16(Suppl. B):126, 1995.

246. Hay, D. R., Chambers, S. T., Ellis-Pegler, R. B., et al.: Prevention of infective endocarditis associated with dental treatment and other medical interventions. N. Z. Med. J. 105:192, 1992.

247. Hall, G., Hedstrom, S. A., Heimdahl, A., and Nord, C. E.: Prophylactic administration of penicillins for endocarditis does not reduce the incidence of postextraction bacteremia. Clin. Infect. Dis. 17:188, 1993.

248. van der Meer, J. T. M., Thompson, J., Valkenburg, H. A., and Michel, M. F.: Epidemiology of bacterial endocarditis in the Netherlands. II. Antecedent procedures and use of prophylaxis. Arch. Intern. Med. 152:1869, 1992.

249. Melendez, L. J., Chan, K. L., Cheung, P. K., et al.: Incidence of bacteremia in transesophageal echocardiography: A prospective study of 140 consecutive patients. J. Am. Coll. Cardiol. 18:1650, 1991.

250. DeGevigney, G., Pop, C., and Delahaye, J. P.: The risk of infective endocarditis after cardiac surgical and interventional procedures. Eur. Heart J. 16(Suppl. B):7, 1995.

251. Steckelberg, J. M., and Wilson, W. R.: Risk factors for infective endocarditis. Infect. Dis. Clin. North Am. 7:9, 1993.

252. Wahl, M. J.: Myths of dental-induced endocarditis. Arch. Intern. Med. 154:137, 1994.

253. Fluckiger, U., Moreillon, P., Blaser, J., et al.: Simulation of amoxicillin pharmacokinetics in humans for the prevention of streptococcal endocarditis in rats. Antimicrob. Agents Chemother. 38:2846, 1994.

254. Horstkotte, D., Friedrichs, W., Pippert, H., et al.: Nutzen der endokarditisprophylaxe bei patienten mit prothetischen herzklappen. Kardiologie 75:8, 1986.

255. Imperiale, T. F., and Horwitz, R. I.: Does prophylaxis prevent postdental infective endocarditis? A controlled evaluation of protective efficacy. Am. J. Med. 88:131, 1990.

256. van der Meer, J. T., van Wuk, W., Thompson, J., et al.: Efficacy of antibiotic prophylaxis for prevention of native-valve endocarditis. Lancet 339:135, 1992.

257. Tornos, P., Sanz, E., Permanyer-Miralda, G., et al.: Late prosthetic valve endocarditis: Immediate and long-term prognosis. Chest 101:37, 1992.

258. Grover, F. L., Cohen, D. J., Oprian, C., et al.: Determinants of the occurrence of and survival from prosthetic valve endocarditis. J. Thorac. Cardiovasc. Surg. 108:207, 1994.

259. Keys, T. F.: Early-onset prosthetic valve endocarditis. Cleve. Clin. J. Med. 60:455, 1993.

260. Chen, S. C., Sorrell, T. C., Dwyer, D. E., et al.: Endocarditis associated with prosthetic cardiac valves. Med. J. Aust. 152:458, 1990.

Chapter 34
The Pathogenesis of Atherosclerosis

RUSSELL ROSS

Atherosclerosis, the principal cause of death in Western civilization,[1] is a progressive disease process that generally begins in childhood and has clinical manifestations in middle to late adulthood. Two decades ago, atherosclerosis was considered to be a degenerative process because of the accumulation of lipid and necrotic debris in the advanced lesions. We now recognize that it is a multifactorial process which, if it leads to clinical sequelae, requires extensive accumulation of smooth muscle cells within the intima of the affected artery. The form and content of the advanced lesions of atherosclerosis demonstrate the results of three fundamental biological processes. These are: (1) accumulation of intimal smooth muscle cells, together with variable numbers of accumulated macrophages and T-lymphocytes; (2) formation by the proliferated smooth muscle cells of large amounts of connective tissue matrix, including collagen, elastic fibers, and proteoglycans; and (3) accumulation of lipid, principally in the form of cholesteryl esters and free cholesterol within the cells as well as in the surrounding connective tissues.[2-5,5a] Despite the fact that the term "atherosclerosis" is derived from the Greek "athero" (gruel or porridge) and "sclerosis" (hardening), it is important to note that there may be great variability in the relative amounts of tissue formed by each of these processes in the lesions. Consequently, many lesions of atherosclerosis are dense and fibrous, whereas others may contain large amounts of lipid and necrotic debris, with most demonstrating combinations and variations of each of these characteristics. The distribution of lipid and connective tissue in these lesions determines whether they are stable or are at risk of rupture, thrombosis, and clinical sequelae.

RISK FACTORS

(See also Chap. 35)

The development of the concept of "risk factors" and their relationships to the incidence of coronary artery disease evolved from prospective epidemiological studies in the United States and Europe.[6-9] These studies demonstrated a consistent association among characteristics observed at one point in time in apparently healthy individuals with the subsequent incidence of coronary artery disease in those individuals. These associations include an increase in the concentration of plasma cholesterol, the incidence of cigarette smoking, hypertension, clinical diabetes, obesity, age, or male gender, and the occurrence of coronary artery disease.[10-12] As a result of these associations, each characteristic has been termed a risk factor for coronary artery disease, and this terminology has been generally accepted and has become part of the scientific literature associated with this problem.

It is important to remember, however, that the presence of a risk factor does not necessarily imply a direct causal relationship. In most instances, a risk factor is the trait that predicts the risk of development of clinically significant disease within a population. In some cases, it may be involved in the causation of the disease; however, to achieve the latter requires a proven epidemiological association that is statistically valid. The risk factor concept has been extremely useful because it permits one to assess the importance not only of the aforementioned risk factors but also of genetic traits in given individuals, such as a family history of premature coronary artery disease. Using such information, it has become possible to determine whether modification of a given risk factor will result in modification of the risk of a particular disease.

Thus, a risk factor may be defined broadly as "any habit or trait that can be used to predict an individual's probability of developing that disease."[9] A risk factor so defined may be a causative agent but is not necessarily one. A more limited and specific definition is that a risk factor is a causative agent or condition that can be used to predict an individual's probability of developing disease. Used in this fashion, there are at least three independent predictors of risk for individuals within a population of the incidence of atherosclerosis: plasma cholesterol concentration,[13-15] cigarette smoking,[16,17] and elevated blood pressure.[17-19]

THE NORMAL ARTERY

The normal artery (Fig. 34–1) consists of an intima lined by endothelium on the inner (luminal) aspect of the vessel and bounded by the internal elastic lamina on its outer aspect. The media is bounded by the internal elastic lamina and, in well-developed muscular and elastic arteries, by an external elastic lamina. The adventitia is bounded by the external elastic lamina and the exterior of the vessel itself.

The Intima

At birth, the intima consists of a relatively thin layer of connective tissue which contains occasional solitary smooth muscle cells. Most of the connective tissue at birth consists of basement membrane. With increasing age, the amount of connective tissue increases, principally as a result of thickening of the basement membrane and formation of collagen fibrils and new elastic fibers. With increasing age, there appears to be a concentric increase in the numbers of intimal smooth muscle cells.

The intima is the site at which the lesions of atherosclerosis form. The lesions of atherosclerosis appear to be able to form in two ways in different individuals. In those who develop clinical sequelae, the lesions form by a generally asymmetrical thickening of the intima which continually encroaches upon the lumen, resulting in a decrease in the flow of blood. The second form of intimal thickening is one in which the increase in the intima may be associated with

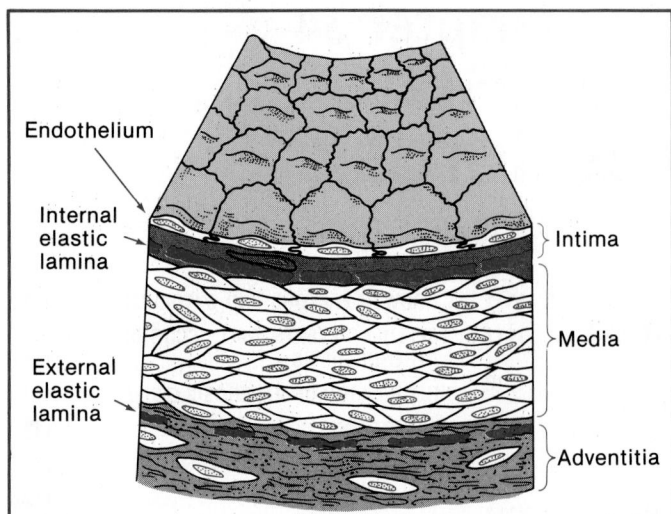

FIGURE 34–1. Structure of a normal muscular artery. (Reprinted by permission from Ross, R., and Glomset, J.: The pathogenesis of atherosclerosis. N. Engl. J. Med. 295:369, 1976. Copyright Massachusetts Medical Society.)

continued dilation of the artery so that the actual lumen changes little, if at all, in diameter. In the latter case, although lesions of atherosclerosis may form, they are generally more symmetrical and concentric; few if any clinical sequelae appear to result.

The Media

The media is the muscular wall of the artery, bounded by the internal and external elastic laminae (Fig. 34–1). These laminae consist of fenestrated sheets of elastic fibers with numerous openings large enough to permit both substances and cells to pass in either direction. The media of muscular arteries consists of spiraling layers of smooth muscle cells attached to one another, each cell surrounded by a discontinuous basement membrane and by interspersed collagen fibrils and proteoglycan. Elastic arteries contain multiple lamellae of smooth muscle cells, each equivalent to a single media in a small muscular artery, or arteriole. Each lamella is bounded by an elastic lamina on its inner and outer aspects. The number of lamellar units present in elastic arteries has been shown to be highly predictable in relation to the size of the animal and to other factors, such as the anatomical position of the artery. Twenty-nine lamellar units have been suggested to represent the thickest amount of artery wall capable of transporting oxygenated metabolites from the lumen of the aorta to the outermost lamella. When more than 29 lamellar units are present, vasa vasorum that are derived from the adventitia appear to be necessary. These can provide nutrients to the remaining outer lamellar units.[20,21]

The Adventitia

The adventitia consists of a dense collagenous structure containing numerous bundles of collagen fibrils, elastic fibers, and many fibroblasts, together with some smooth muscle cells (Fig. 34–1). It is a highly vascular tissue and contains many nerve fibers as well. As indicated earlier, the adventitia provides the outermost portion of the media of large elastic arteries with much of their nutrition via vasa vasorum, as well as with lymphatic channels and innervation. Wolinsky and Glagov[21] have observed that the abdominal aorta in humans lacks vasa vasorum in its outermost aspects and have suggested that this may be one of the reasons the abdominal aorta is particularly vulnerable to atherogenesis. Barger et al. have observed an increase in adventitial microvessels opposite fibrous plaques in the in-

tima of the coronary artery.[22,23] Using postmortem cinematography and silicon polymers injected into the lumen of the coronary artery, they noted not only an increase in adventitial vessels but in microvessels within the plaque itself. These may play an important role in hemorrhage and thrombosis should the plaques become unstable (see below).

CELLS OF THE ARTERY AND FROM THE BLOOD POTENTIALLY INVOLVED IN ATHEROGENESIS

Endothelium

The endothelial cells probably represent the largest and most extensive tissue in the body because they line the entire vascular tree. In the arterial system, the endothelial cells form a continuous, smooth, uninterrupted surface and represent the principal barrier between the elements of the blood and the artery wall (Fig. 34–2). In adulthood, the turnover of endothelial cells in those arteries that have been studied is relatively low; however, Schwartz and Benditt[24,25] have observed that there are "hot spots" where turnover of endothelium is high in the aorta, even in adults. These hot spots do not appear to be necessarily located at particular anatomical sites. The endothelium forms a highly selective permeability barrier,[26–30] is usually thought to be a nonthrombogenic surface,[31] is a highly active metabolic tissue,[32] and is capable of forming several

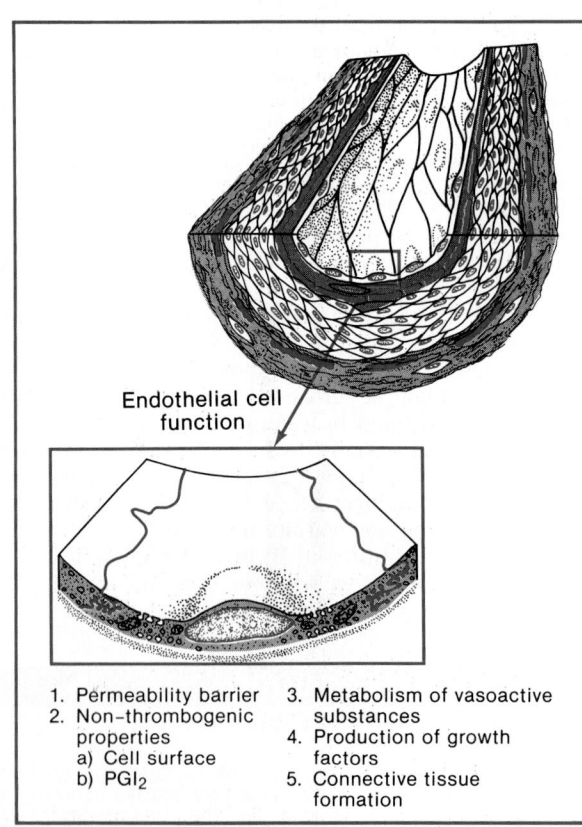

Endothelial cell function

1. Permeability barrier
2. Non-thrombogenic properties
   a) Cell surface
   b) PGI₂
3. Metabolism of vasoactive substances
4. Production of growth factors
5. Connective tissue formation

FIGURE 34–2. The endothelial barrier present in the normal artery wall. In the higher magnification inset, the borders between the endothelial cells are irregular, allowing the cells to interdigitate. Vesicles and infoldings at either cell surface permit the cells to transport materials from the lumen of the artery to the tissue by pinocytosis. Transport also occurs below the cell junctions, demonstrated by vesicles that fuse in these regions. In the artery, the cell rests on a connective tissue matrix that consists of a basement membrane intermixed with collagen fibrils. (Reprinted by permission from Ross, R., and Glomset, J.: The pathogenesis of atherosclerosis. N. Engl. J. Med. 295:371, 1976. Copyright Massachusetts Medical Society.)

vasoactive substances[31,33,34,36] and connective tissue macromolecules.[35] Endothelial cells examined in culture also have procoagulant properties[37]; however, it is probable that these procoagulant properties are manifested at times of "injury" to the endothelium and are probably not present in situ in the normal artery.

Although the endothelial cells, as seen *en face* by light and scanning electron microscopy (Fig. 34–3) and in cross section by light and transmission electron microscopy (Fig. 34–4), appear to be highly similar morphologically in different parts of the arterial tree, there may be functional differences in these lining cells in different anatomical sites. For example, capillary endothelial cells contain receptors on their surfaces for a potent growth-regulatory peptide, platelet-derived growth factor (PDGF), whereas these receptors are absent on arterial endothelium.[38] Other differences are likely to be found, not only between capillary and arterial endothelium, but among endothelial cells in different parts of the arterial tree itself. With these differences, one might anticipate that there might be differences in the way in which endothelial cells respond to injury after exposure to various injurious agents in different parts of the arterial tree. Endothelial cells are normally attached to each other by tight junctions and by gap junctions. They transport substances in both directions via the process of endocytosis, sometimes called *transcytosis*. Transendothelial channels have been observed in capillary endothelium; however, it is not clear whether they play a role in macromolecular transport in arterial tissue. It has also been suggested that the junctions between endothelial cells may serve as potential sites of increased endothelial transport, particularly when the endothelium has been injured.

Endothelial cells rest on a basement membrane that consists of a particular form of collagen (type IV collagen) intermixed with particular types of proteoglycan molecules. The endothelial cells are undoubtedly responsible for the synthesis of these connective tissue molecules.[35] The base-

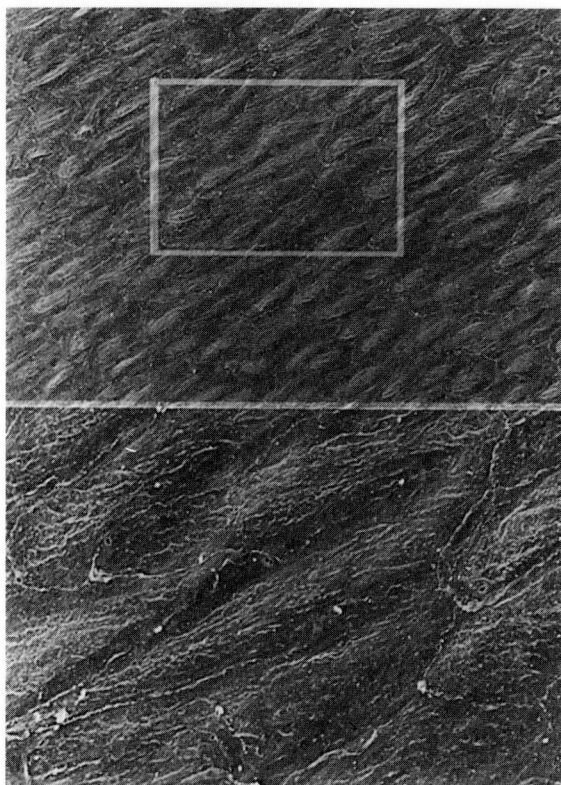

FIGURE 34–3. Scanning electron micrographs of the thoracic aorta endothelium from normal monkey *(Macaca nemestrina).* ×540. At somewhat higher magnification, the overlapping folds of the endothelial cells can be clearly visualized. The elongated and elliptical appearance of the endothelium can also be seen. The long axes of the cells appear to be diagonal and are oriented in the main direction of the flow of blood in the artery. ×2100. (Reproduced with permission from Ross, R.: Atherosclerosis: A problem of the biology of arterial wall cells and their interactions with blood components. Arteriosclerosis 1:297, 1981. Copyright 1981 American Heart Association.)

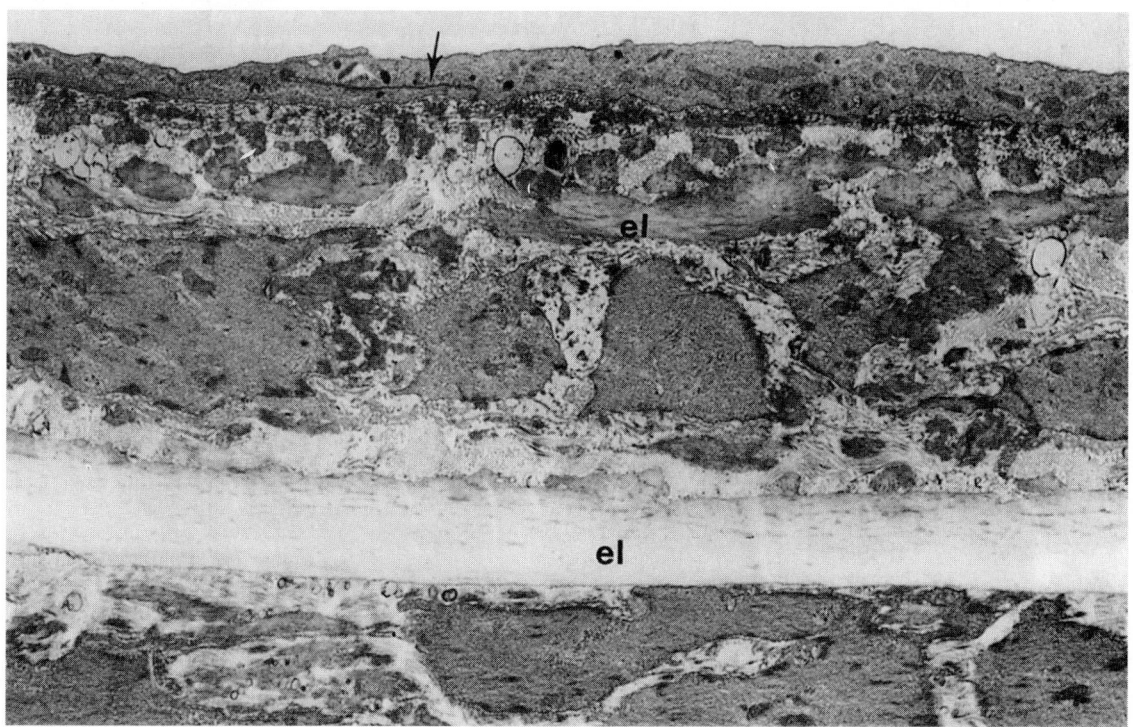

FIGURE 34–4. Transmission electron micrograph of a developing monkey aorta. Two endothelial cells can be seen at the lumen with a junction between them (arrow). Beneath the endothelial cells are newly forming elastic fibers (el) that are separated from the endothelium by basement membrane and collagen fibrils. Beneath the newly forming elastic fibers is a layer of smooth muscle cells separated from another layer by a well-formed elastica (el). No nuclei are apparent in the endothelial cells in this particular thin section.

ment membrane probably also serves as a crude form of filter.

Endothelial cells have receptors for many different molecules on their surface, including receptors for low-density lipoprotein (LDL),[39] for growth factors, and probably for a number of pharmacological agents. A special capacity of endothelium that may be particularly important in atherogenesis is its ability to modify lipoproteins. LDLs appear to be "modified" by a process of low-level oxidation when they are bound to LDL receptors, internalized, and transported through the endothelium. Such modified LDLs can bind to a specific type of receptor, termed a scavenger receptor, on the surface of macrophages, where they are ingested and contribute to the formation of foam cells. This activity is probably important in atherogenesis (see below). The endothelium normally provides a nonthrombogenic surface because of its capacity to form prostaglandin derivatives, particularly prostacyclin (PGI$_2$) (Chap. 59), a potent vasodilator that is an effective inhibitor of platelet aggregation,[31,34] and because of its surface coat of heparan sulfate. Endothelial cells also make the most potent vasodilator thus far discovered, endothelial-derived relaxing factor (EDRF), a thiolated form of nitric oxide (Chap. 36). EDRF formation by endothelium may be critical in maintaining a balance between vasoconstriction and vasodilation in the process of arterial homeostasis.[33,36] Endothelial cells can also secrete agents that are effective in lysing fibrin clots, including plasminogen, as well as procoagulant materials such as von Willebrand factor.[37] They also secrete a number of vasoactive agents, such as endothelin,[40] angiotensin-converting enzyme, and platelet-derived growth factor, which may be important in vasoconstriction.

A particular characteristic of the endothelium that may be of great importance is the fact that endothelial cells grow in an obligate monolayer. Such growth is representative of cells that line most body surfaces, including epithelial surfaces, and is characterized by the fact that the endothelial cells cannot crawl over one another at sites of injury to facilitate repair of a surface that has been deendothelialized. In other words, only the cells at the margin of an injury can participate in the regenerative response. Thus if a particular anatomical site is repeatedly injured over a prolonged period, and if the endothelial cells that regenerate lose their replication capacity, cells distal to the site, capable of replicating, may not be able to participate simply because they cannot reach the site to do so.

Arterial endothelial cells are capable of synthesizing and secreting several mitogens, one of which is a form of PDGF.[41–43] PDGF is a growth factor for mesenchymally derived, connective tissue–forming cells such as fibroblasts and smooth muscle, but not for arterial endothelial cells. The capacity of endothelium, when it has been appropriately "activated," to form such growth factors may be important in atherogenesis. This is discussed further in the section concerning the response-to-injury hypothesis of atherosclerosis (see p. 1114) (Fig. 34–5).

Thus, the endothelium forms an obligate monolayer that lines the entire arterial tree, is metabolically active, produces vasoactive substances, has a nonthrombogenic surface, and can form procoagulant materials.[44,45] It also serves as the permeability barrier that controls the passage of molecules into the artery. It can oxidize LDL and form nitric oxide (NO), the principal means by which vasodilation is maintained.[46] All of these activities demonstrate the dynamic nature of the endothelial lining and how potentially important this cell layer is in the maintenance of arterial homeostasis. If the endothelium forms oxLDL, the endothelium itself as well as the underlying cells in the artery wall may be injured. OxLDL may play an important initiating role in inducing increased adherence and migration of monocytes and T-lymphocytes from the lumen into the artery wall. OxLDL can induce the formation of at least two adhesive molecules on the surface of the endothelium, vas-

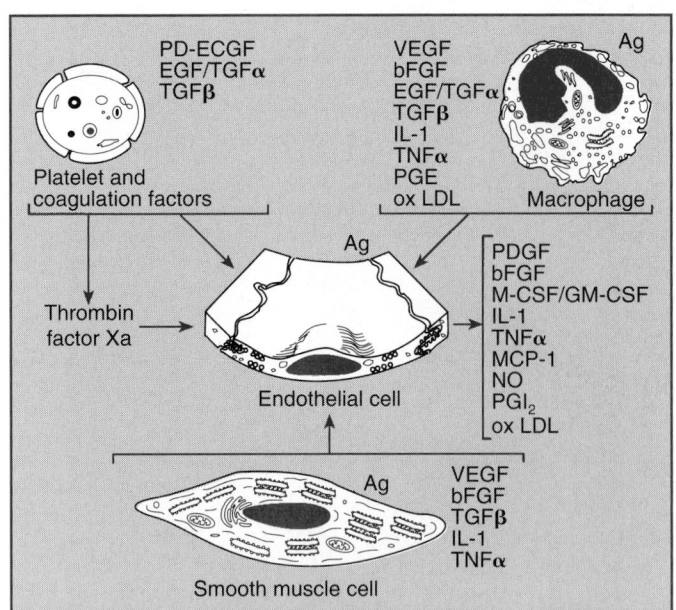

FIGURE 34–5. The endothelial cells normally present a barrier to the artery wall, have nonthrombogenic properties, and are capable of metabolizing numerous vasoactive substances, such as prostacyclin (PGI$_2$) and nitric oxide (NO). They are capable of producing growth factors and forming connective tissue matrix. The endothelial cells can also interact with platelets, monocytes, T-lymphocytes, and smooth muscle cells. The principal products of platelets, macrophages, and smooth muscle cells that may affect the endothelium are shown in this figure. Endothelial mitogens that can be produced by macrophages include vascular endothelial growth factor (VEGF), fibroblast growth factor (FGF), and transforming growth factor α (TGFα). Transforming growth factor β (TGFβ), as well as interleukin-1 (IL-1) and tumor necrosis factor α (TNFα), is capable of inhibiting endothelial proliferation and can also induce secondary gene expression of other growth-regulatory molecules by the endothelium. TGFβ is a potent inducer of connective tissue matrix synthesis.

Oxidized LDL (oxLDL), produced by endothelium, macrophages, or smooth muscle cells, can profoundly injure neighboring endothelial and smooth muscle cells. Platelets can provide a host of vasoactive substances, coagulation factors, and mitogens. Thrombin and Factor Xa from plasma may also stimulate the endothelium to a procoagulant state. Endothelial cells can also synthesize a number of growth-regulatory molecules, as noted to the right of the endothelial cell, that can induce proliferation of neighboring cells and their formation of connective tissue. Such cellular interactions are discussed in this chapter. Because oxLDL may be a principal cause of atherogenesis, it is important to note that the endothelial cells represent the first potential site of oxidation of LDL as it is transported into the artery wall. (From Ross, R.: The pathogenesis of atherosclerosis: A perspective for the 1990s. Nature 362:801, 1993. Copyright 1993 Macmillan Magazines Limited.)

cular cell adhesion molecule-1 (VCAM-1) and intercellular adhesion molecule-1 (ICAM-1). These two molecules can participate in the increased adhesion of monocytes and T cells to the endothelium through receptor-ligand–type interactions with appropriate molecules on the surface of the leukocytes. The roles of these molecules are discussed below.

Smooth Muscle

The cell that proliferates in the arterial intima to form the intermediate and advanced lesions of atherosclerosis, the smooth muscle cell, is originally derived from the media.[46a] In his early work, Wissler[47] described this cell as a "multifunctional medial mesenchymal cell." It is now widely accepted that accumulation of smooth muscle cells in the intima represents the sine qua non of the lesions of advanced atherosclerosis (Fig. 34–6).

Twenty-five years ago, the only functional capacity attributed to the smooth muscle cell was its ability to con-

PLATE 9

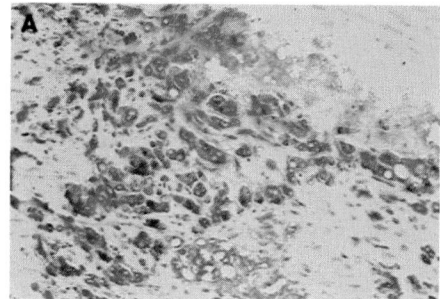
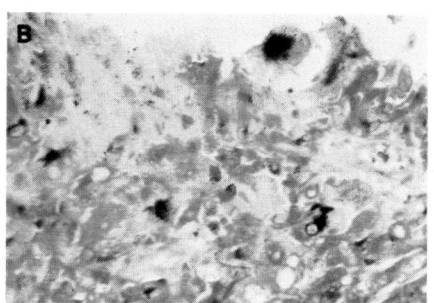
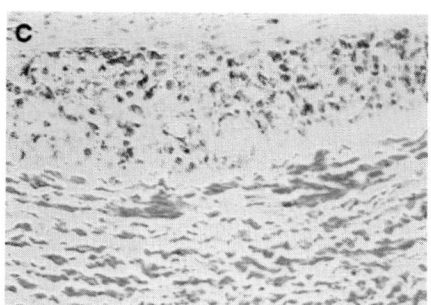

FIGURE 34–13. Double-immunostained preparations demonstrating the distribution of PDGF-B chain in methacarn-fixed, deparaffinized sections of advanced lesions of atherosclerosis from a high-level hypercholesterolemic nonhuman primate fed a hypercholesterolemic diet for 1 year. The sections were stained with a monoclonal antibody specific for PDGF-B-chain protein, and with cell-type-specific monoclonal antibodies for macrophages *(A, B)* or smooth muscle *(C)*, with IGSS and avidin-biotin immunoalkaline-phosphatase procedures. *A*, PDGF-B chain (black, granular reaction product) is localized to HAM56-positive macrophages (red reaction product). *B*, Positive cells at higher magnification. *C*, PDGF-B chain (black, granular reaction product) and HHF35–positive smooth muscle cells (red reaction product) are identified in nonoverlapping cell populations. All sections were counterstained with methyl green. *A* and *C* original magnifications, ×250; *B* original magnification, ×400. (From Ross, R., et al.: Localization of PDGF-B protein in macrophages in all phases of atherogenesis. Science *248:*1009, 1990. © Copyright 1990 by the American Association for the Advancement of Science.)

tract. In 1971, it became possible to maintain and propagate pure populations of smooth muscle cells in culture and to demonstrate that this cell, like the fibroblast, is one of the principal connective tissue—forming cells in the body.[48] It is capable of synthesizing and secreting several forms of collagen, both elastic fiber proteins and several different types of proteoglycans.[49] The principal role of the smooth muscle cell in the fully formed adult artery is presumably to maintain the tone of the arterial wall by its capacity to maintain the slow contractions peculiar to smooth muscle. The smooth muscle cell responds to numerous vasoactive agents, such as epinephrine and angiotensin, which induce contraction and vasoconstriction, and prostacyclin and NO, which can induce relaxation and vasodilation. Smooth muscle cells, like fibroblasts, contain specific high-affinity receptors for a number of ligands. These ligands include LDL[50] (see p. 1134) (which is the principal cholesterol-carrying plasma lipoprotein that participates in regulation of cholesterol metabolism), insulin (which is involved in glucose metabolism), and growth stimulators such as PDGF[51] and growth inhibitors such as transforming growth factor beta (TGF β) (which help to regulate cell multiplication). Arterial smooth muscle cells of the newborn rat, in contrast to adult rat smooth muscle, have been shown to be capable of synthesizing and secreting PDGF.[52] These observations suggest possible roles for smooth muscle in growth and development and possibly in atherosclerosis as well (to be discussed below).

Smooth muscle cells appear to be capable of presenting two different phenotypes in culture.[53,54] The first of these,

the *contractile phenotype,* is generally thought to be associated with cell contractility because the cells contain extensive myofibrils throughout their cytoplasm consisting of actin and myosin filaments. These contractile filaments bind to one another and to the subplasmalemmal surface of the cell by dense bodies. Such cells do *not* appear to be capable of responding to mitogens such as PDGF. When a smooth muscle cell becomes appropriately stimulated, it loses its contractile phenotype and changes to a cell that has decreased content of myofilaments and that contains an extensively developed rough endoplasmic reticulum and Golgi complex. Such a cell has been described as being in a *synthetic phenotype.* Smooth muscle cells in the synthetic phenotype appear to be involved in the formation of numerous secretory proteins, including connective tissue matrix macromolecules.

Smooth muscle cells rich in contractile elements can respond to agents that can induce vasoconstriction, such as endothelin (ET), catecholamines, or angiotensin II (AII). Agents that can induce vasodilation such as prostaglandin E, prostacyclin (PGI$_2$), neuropeptides, leukotrienes, or NO, can also have profound effects upon these cells. When the cells are rich in rough endoplasmic reticulum and Golgi complex (synthetic state), they can express genes for a number of the growth-regulatory molecules and cytokines (noted in Fig. 34–6). If smooth muscle cells are sufficiently injured, they can release growth factors such as FGF. In so doing they could stimulate neighboring smooth muscle or adjacent endothelium. The smooth muscle cell is the principal contributor to the reparative, fibroproliferative process in the development of the lesions of atherosclerosis.

It has been suggested that the phenotypic differentiation of the smooth muscle cell may be important in terms of its capacity to respond to mitogens such as PDGF and thus to form the proliferative lesions of atherosclerosis. Smooth muscle cells in the contractile phenotype have been described as nonresponsive to mitogens, whereas those in the synthetic phenotype have been described as responsive.[53,54] For the lesions of atherosclerosis to form, the smooth muscle cells must, in most cases, migrate from the media into the intima, where they can respond mitogenically. Consequently, control of the phenotypic state of smooth muscle cells could be important in understanding and preventing atherogenesis (Fig. 34–6).

Smooth muscle cells are derived locally from individual organ parenchyma during embryogenesis in contrast with the endothelium, which appears to be derived from the embryonic vasculature that invades the organ.[55] As a consequence, smooth muscle cells in different arteries may respond differently to agonists presented to them, which may explain in part why different arterial beds respond differently to local stimuli associated with the process of atherogenesis.[56]

One characteristic feature of the smooth muscle cells found in the lesions of atherosclerosis is the accumulation of lipid that results in formation of vacuolated cells, or foam cells.

Although smooth muscle cells were originally conceived of as only the receiver of signals such as those derived from mitogens, it has now been demonstrated not only that they can respond to mitogens such as PDGF but that they can synthesize and secrete substances such as PDGF and other growth-regulatory molecules so that they may stimulate themselves and their neighbors. Thus, smooth muscle cells may respond in autocrine fashion to molecules they themselves form. For example, it is well known that a marked intimal smooth muscle proliferative lesion can be induced by passing an intraarterial balloon embolectomy catheter through an artery. The pressure exerted by the balloon is sufficient to strip off the lining endothelium, expand the artery, and damage many of the smooth muscle cells in the wall of the artery. The exposed subendothelial connective tissue attracts platelets to adhere and degranulate, and many of the injured subendothelial smooth muscle cells undergo a change and migrate from the media into the intima, where they proliferate and form a myointimal hyperplastic fibrotic lesion. If the smooth muscle cells are cultured from such a lesion and are compared with those cultured from a contralateral uninjured artery, the cells from the proliferative lesion secrete a form of PDGF (see section on Growth Factors) and

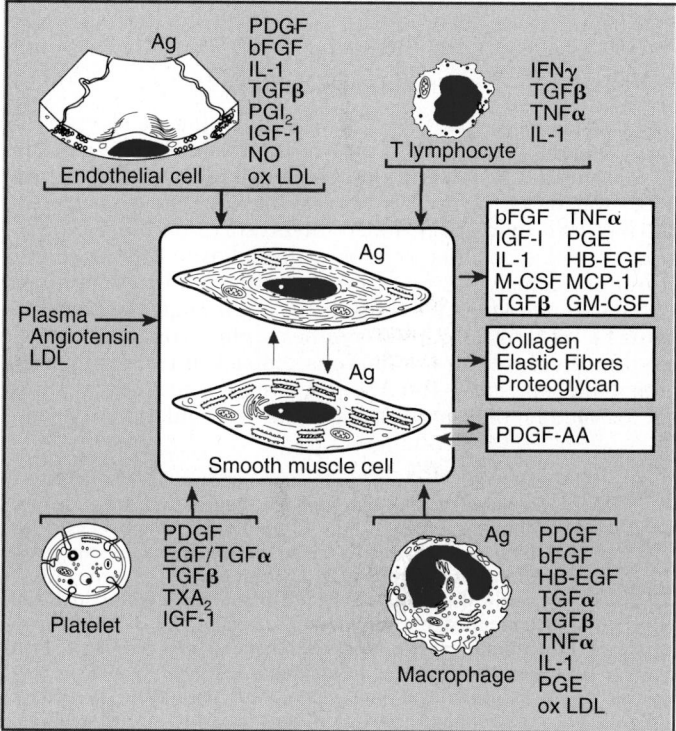

FIGURE 34–6. In the synthetic phenotype it is presumed that smooth muscle cells can form connective tissue molecules, as well as growth factors such as PDGF-AA and can stimulate themselves, as well as their neighbors. In their interactions with the overlying endothelium and neighboring cells T-lymphocytes, platelets, and macrophages, smooth muscle cells can respond to the different cytokines, growth-regulatory molecules, and vasodilator and vasoconstrictor substances that can be generated from these cells, as well as substances from the plasma, such as angiotensin. Thus, the genes that are expressed in the different phenotypic states by the smooth muscle (listed to the right), as well as those expressed by the neighboring cells (listed next to each cell) in the artery wall that result from these cellular interactions, determine whether a lesion progresses or regresses. (From Ross, R.: The pathogenesis of atherosclerosis: A perspective for the 1990s. *Nature* **362**:801, 1993. Copyright 1993 Macmillan Magazines Limited.)

thus may participate in further enlargement of the lesion by autocrine stimulation. Similarly, when smooth muscle cells derived from lesions of atherosclerosis are grown in culture, they secrete PDGF into the culture medium. Interestingly, data suggest that smooth muscle cells derived from human occlusive fibrous plaques of the superficial femoral arteries have a limited capacity to divide in culture. When placed in culture, these cells respond less well to mitogens and act like senescent cells that have already undergone numerous cell doublings.[57] Although the cells may secrete mitogens in culture, it remains to be determined whether they are capable of secreting mitogens and responding to them in vivo.

Some data relevant to these observations have come from studies in nonhuman primates where Northern blots of advanced lesions of atherosclerosis, using cDNA probes for different growth-regulatory peptides, have demonstrated increased messenger RNA for PDGF-B chain, and for both receptors of PDGF. Recent studies (see below), however, show that the principal source of the PDGF-B chain in these lesions is the macrophage. The smooth muscle cells appear to be the principal recipient of the growth regulatory peptides. Thus the regulation of smooth muscle cells via cellular interaction in the lesions of atherosclerosis needs to be further explored.

Macrophages

Macrophages in all tissues, whether they are resident macrophages or cells that have entered the tissue during an inflammatory response, are derived at some point in their life span from circulating monocytes.[58] When the monocyte enters a tissue, it appears to take on characteristics peculiar to the host tissue. In most inflammatory sites, the macrophage acts as a scavenger cell to remove foreign substances by phagocytosis and intracellular hydrolysis and as a second line of defense after the neutrophil against microbial organisms.[59] As a scavenger cell, the macrophage attempts to remove injurious materials such as oxLDL via scavenger receptors[60] and can oxidize LDL by such means as lipoxygenase enzymes (e.g., 15-lipoxygenase).[61] OxLDL can be taken up by the same macrophages or by neighboring macrophages. The importance of oxLDL in atherogenesis was first established in studies of the antioxidant drug probucol in hypercholesterolemic rabbits (discussed in greater detail below; see Lipids, Lipoproteins, and Modified LDL in Atherosclerosis). It has been recognized that not only do smooth muscle cells replicate in lesions of atherosclerosis, but macrophages may do so as well. Macrophage replication may represent as great, if not greater, source than smooth muscle cells in cell accumulation within the lesions. Thus, factors associated with their turnover, their replication, and programmed cell death (apoptosis) are all-important in determining whether macrophages accumulate in lesions (discussed in greater detail below; see The Response-to-Injury Hypothesis).

Macrophages are capable of secreting a large number of biologically important substances, including chemotactic agents such as leukotriene B4[62] and interleukin 1,[63] and oxygen metabolites such as superoxide anion,[64] which can be toxic to other cells. Macrophages have recently been shown to be capable of synthesizing and secreting at least six different growth factors.[65] These include (1) PDGF,[66] a growth factor for mesenchymal cells such as smooth muscle and fibroblasts; (2) interleukin 1, a cytokine that induces PDGF gene expression in fibroblasts[63,67]; (3) fibroblast growth factor (FGF),[68] a mitogen for endothelial cells and thus a potentially important angiogenic agent; (4) epidermal growth factor (EGF) and EGF-like molecules (e.g., transforming growth factor alpha [TGF α]), both of which bind to the same receptor and are capable of stimulating the growth of epithelial cells; (5) TGF β, a substance that participates in a synergistic way with some of the aforementioned growth factors in aiding the proliferation of many cells in different tissues and in many instances in inhibiting cell growth; and (6) M-CSF, a growth factor for monocyte macrophages[69] (Fig. 34–7).

As a result of its scavenging capacity and its ability to form and secrete growth factors, the macrophage is probably the key cell responsible for the promotion of connective tissue proliferation so commonly associated with chronic inflammatory responses. Macrophages, like smooth muscle, are a major source of foam cells in the lesions of atherosclerosis. In fact, they are the principal cells in the fatty streak, the initial lesion of atherosclerosis. They accumulate large amounts of lipid in the form of droplets that contain large amounts of cholesteryl ester. The role of the macrophage in atherogenesis is discussed below.

Platelets
(See also Chap. 58)

Although they may be uninvolved in the generation of many lesions, platelets are clearly implicated in the genesis of some of the lesions of atherosclerosis. (This is discussed in greater detail below.) However, platelets are also important because they are regularly involved in one of the principal sequelae of atherosclerosis, thrombosis. It is usually a mural or occlusive thrombus or both that lead to infarction.

Platelets are amazing cells in that, although they are capable of little to no protein synthesis, they contain, sequestered in their granules, numerous prepacked extraordinarily potent molecules[70,71] (Fig. 34–8). Among these are a number of factors that participate in the coagulation cascade

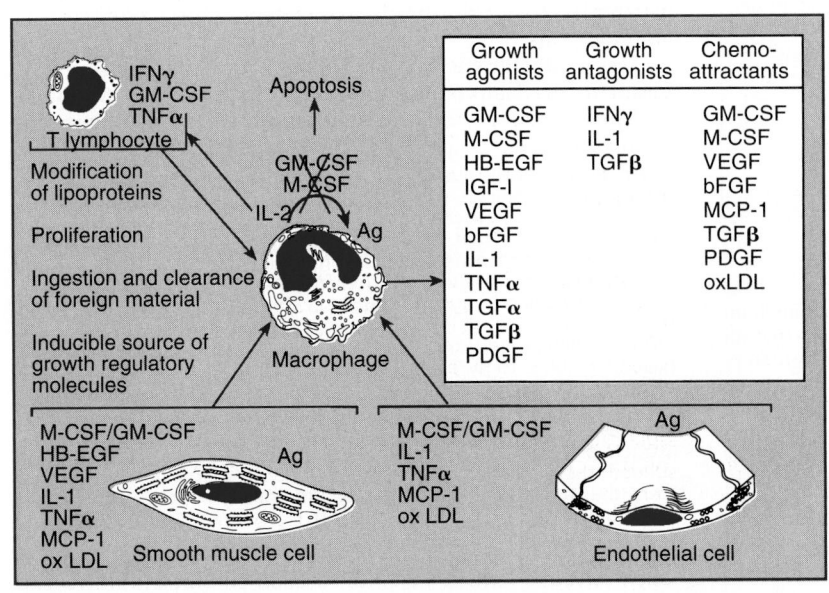

FIGURE 34–7. The reverse arrows between the T-lymphocyte and macrophage suggest that some form of immune response may occur during atherogenesis. Interactions between T cells and macrophages can result in proliferation of each of these cell types through IL-2 and CSFs, respectively. All of the cells with which the macrophage can interact, namely, the T-lymphocyte, smooth muscle, and endothelium, can present CSF to the macrophages to maintain cell viability and prevent apoptosis and cell death, and participate in further macrophage activation and replication. In addition, smooth muscle and endothelium can present antigens (Ag) at their surfaces and secrete chemoattractants for macrophages, including MCP-1 and oxLDL, as well as factors that can alter macrophage metabolism such as IL-1 or TNFα.

When macrophages are activated, they can produce an extraordinary number of biologically relevant molecules, some of which are listed in the box in relation to their capacity to induce or inhibit replication of endothelium, smooth muscle, or macrophages themselves, as well as their capacity to make chemoattractants for each of these cell types. (From Ross, R.: The pathogenesis of atherosclerosis: A perspective for the 1990s. *Nature* **362**:801, 1993. Copyright 1993 Macmillan Magazines Limited.)

and, in addition, at least four extremely potent growth factors or mitogens. These are the same growth factors that can be formed by the activated macrophage, namely, PDGF,[72] FGF, EGF[73] or TGF α, and TGF β.[74] It appears that each of these growth factors is present in a class of granules, the alpha granules, which were originally thought to represent a single class on the basis of cell fractionation studies. They may, however, represent several different granules that are similar in morphological and flotation characteristics. Thus, when they are separated by cell fractionation and density gradient centrifugation, they appear to sequester into a single population.

When the platelet is exposed to substrates that induce platelet adherence, aggregation, and degranulation, each of these growth factors is potentially released and thus is capable of eliciting a proliferative response by essentially all of the resident cells in a particular tissue. In other words, platelets contain growth factors potentially stimulatory for each of the cell types present in any tissue in which platelet aggregation and release may occur. Thus, at sites of injury in which collagen exposure, thrombin and fibrin formation, or adenosine diphosphate release occur, platelet aggregation and thrombosis can occur, leading to release of the numerous vasoactive, stimulatory, and proliferative agents carried by the platelets. Each of these agents may play an important role in stimulating an early vasoconstrictive and proliferative response.[75] This early reparative response to injury may be important in the initiation of the lesions of atherosclerosis as well.

Numerous factors may increase platelet activation in vitro, which could have profound effects on lesion formation or progression. High levels of circulating catecholamines, such as norepinephrine, may be associated with increased platelet activity and ability to aggregate.[76] Furthermore, chronic emotional stress, a history of cigarette smoking, or a strong family history of increased ability for platelets to aggregate have been shown to activate platelets in patients with coronary artery disease and thus decrease platelet survival.[77,78]

A lipid particle, lipoprotein (a) (Lp[a]), may also play an important role in atherogenesis and its progression. Lp(a) (see Chap. 35) consists of an LDL particle with a protein highly homologous to plasminogen covalently bound to the LDL moiety. It has been suggested that high levels of Lp(a) interfere with plasminogen by competing for plasminogen, and thus create a hyperthrombotic state. Potentially thrombogenic or high levels of Lp(a) have not yet been documented as a cause of an increase in the incidence of myocardial infarction. Nevertheless, children with high Lp(a) levels retrospectively show an increased incidence of myocardial infarction at a young age.[79-81] Thus, platelets may play an important role in atherogenesis but a potentially critical role in the progression of lesions and in the clinical sequelae of advanced lesions that may be susceptible to rupture and thrombosis (see below).

T-Lymphocytes

T-lymphocytes, both CD-8 + and CD-4 +, have been observed in all phases of atherogenesis in humans and in nonhuman primates.[82-85] Their involvement in the lesions of atherosclerosis supports the notion that these lesions may develop, at least in part, as a result of an immune or possibly autoimmune response. Experimentally induced autoimmunity has been shown to induce rampant proliferative lesions of atherosclerosis in rabbits.[86] In humans, rejected cardiac transplants characteristically have extensive occlusive lesions of atherosclerosis in the coronary arteries. However, in contrast to the lesions observed in common atherosclerosis, the majority of which are eccentric lesions, those observed in the rejected hearts are concentric in appearance. The nature of the antigen(s) that may play a role in common atherosclerosis is unknown. However, interac-

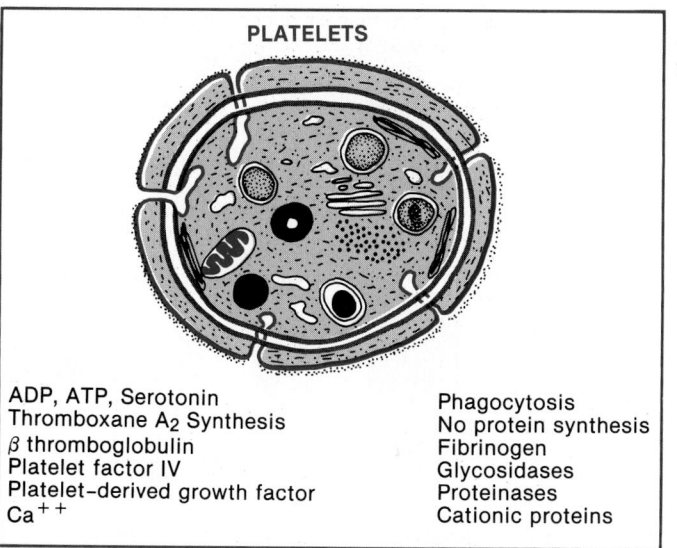

PLATELETS

ADP, ATP, Serotonin
Thromboxane A$_2$ Synthesis
β thromboglobulin
Platelet factor IV
Platelet-derived growth factor
Ca^{++}

Phagocytosis
No protein synthesis
Fibrinogen
Glycosidases
Proteinases
Cationic proteins

FIGURE 34–8. A platelet demonstrating its principal constituents which are listed beneath the figure. (Reproduced with permission from Ross, R.: Atherosclerosis: A problem of the biology of arterial wall cells and their interactions with blood components. Arteriosclerosis 1:301, 1981. Copyright 1981 American Heart Association.)

tions between T-lymphocytes and activated macrophages, both of which are prominent in the lesions, suggest that antigen presentation and the release of cytokines and growth factors between the activated macrophages and T cells may be important in this process.[87,88]

Libby and Hansson demonstrated that oxLDL may serve as one of the potential major antigens that stimulate macrophage–T-cell interactions. Many T cells and lesions are shown to be activated based upon their expression of the histocompatibility antigen HLA-DR. Nevertheless, clonal expansion of these lymphocytes does not appear to take place.[89] If oxLDL proves to be the antigen principally responsible for T-cell activation, this would provide a new approach to therapy and to the immune response in the process of atherogenesis.

THE LESIONS OF ATHEROSCLEROSIS

Although atherosclerosis has been known for centuries, its clinical effects are manifested principally in medium-sized muscular arteries, including the coronary, carotid, basilar, and vertebral arteries, as well as several arteries affecting the lower extremities, particularly the iliac and superficial femoral arteries. Larger arteries, such as the aorta and the iliac arteries, can also be involved, and the principal clinical sequelae in these large arteries is usually aneurysmal dilatation and its related effects.[90]

The earliest lesions of atherosclerosis can be found in young children and infants in the form of a lesion called the *fatty streak,* whereas the advanced lesion, the fibrous plaque, generally appears during early adulthood and progresses with age.[91-96] Until recently, most tissues that had been prepared for examination were derived from autopsy specimens and were sufficiently poorly preserved so that when the cells became laden with lipid and appeared as foam cells, it was virtually impossible to determine the origin of the cell. Advances in tissue fixation and embedding have permitted new modes of preservation. Furthermore, monoclonal antibodies have been developed that are specific for smooth muscle cells, for macrophages, and for lymphocytes. With the use of these antibodies and with improved preservation techniques, it has been possible to identify specifically the origin of the cells in the different lesions of atherosclerosis.

Studies of advanced complicated lesions of atherosclero-

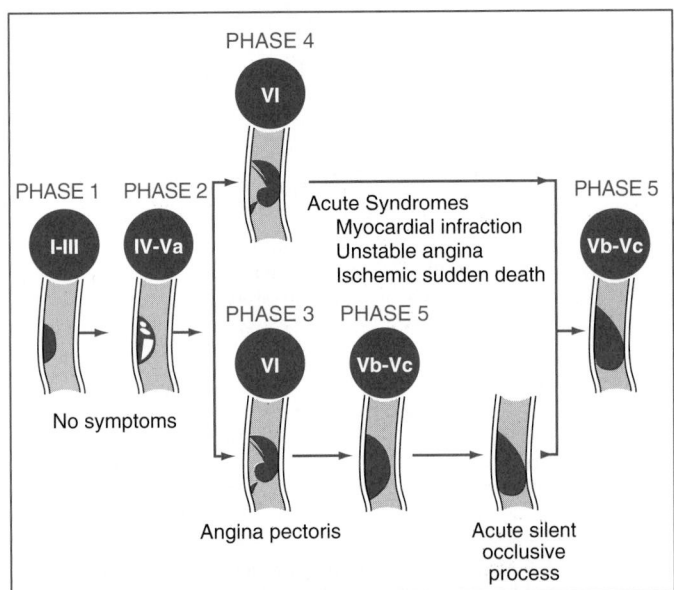

PHASE 4

VI

PHASE 1   PHASE 2

I-III   IV-Va

Acute Syndromes
Myocardial infraction
Unstable angina
Ischemic sudden death

PHASE 5

Vb-Vc

No symptoms

PHASE 3   PHASE 5

VI   Vb-Vc

Angina pectoris

Acute silent
occlusive
process

FIGURE 34–9. This figure shows the stages (phases) and lesion morphology of the progression of coronary atherosclerosis according to gross pathological and clinical findings. (Reproduced with permission from Fuster V.: Lewis A. Conner Memorial Lecture. Mechanisms leading to myocardial infarction: Insights from studies of vascular biology. Circulation *90*:2126, 1994. Copyright 1994 American Heart Association.)

sis have recently been aided by the use of the atherectomy catheter. Examination of atherectomy specimens has demonstrated virtually all of the cellular and structural features of atherosclerosis described in experimental animals and autopsy specimens. The use of freshly derived tissues and cells has demonstrated the nature and diversity of the connective tissue matrix and provided new data concerning proteoglycan constituents. Studies in progress use antibodies to PCNA, a nuclear marker of cells in cell cycle traverse, to determine cell replication in human lesions, which can be compared with lesions obtained from experimental studies.

A redefinition of lesion staging and phases of lesion pro-

gression has been completed by a committee of the American Heart Association. Fatty streaks have been included in Phase 1 lesions, which include types I to III (Fig. 34–9). The different types of fatty streaks (I and II) are based on the relative numbers of smooth muscle cells and macrophages and the amount of lipid contained within the lesions.[94] Lesions that progress to phase 2, which includes types IV and Va, can evolve into more stenotic, fibrotic lesions. Fibrotic lesions include types Vb and Vc, either of which can thrombose and lead to acute clinical sequelae. Type IV lesions can also rapidly progress to type VI, a complicated lesion, which can disrupt, thrombose, and lead to myocardial infarction or ischemic sudden death. Phase 3 lesions can also progress through phase 4 to phase 5 silently and gradually while developing collateral circulation (Fig. 34–9). This approach to categorizing lesions relates their progression with the clinical sequelae that may result.[95]

The Fatty Streak
(Lesion Types I to III)

Fatty streaks were observed by Stary[96] in his studies of a series of children and young adults. He demonstrated that by the age of 10 years, the fatty streaks consisted principally of lipid-laden macrophages, together with varying (but usually small) numbers of lipid-filled smooth muscle cells that accumulated beneath them as the lesions increased in size. Grossly, the fatty streak appears as an area of yellow discoloration due to the large amount of lipid deposited in the foam cells. The bulk of this lipid is in the form of cholesterol and cholesteryl ester, which probably enters the fatty streak by transport of lipoproteins from the plasma via the endothelial cells, after which it is taken up by macrophages and smooth muscle cells. The plasma lipids present in the intima are ingested by macrophages and are hydrolyzed and reesterified once they have been taken up by these cells.

Stary also studied fatty streaks in the coronary arteries of a series of children and young adults and observed that they were localized at anatomical sites that were the same as the sites in other older individuals that were occupied by advanced fibromuscular lesions or fibrous plaques. His data and that of others suggested that over a time, fatty

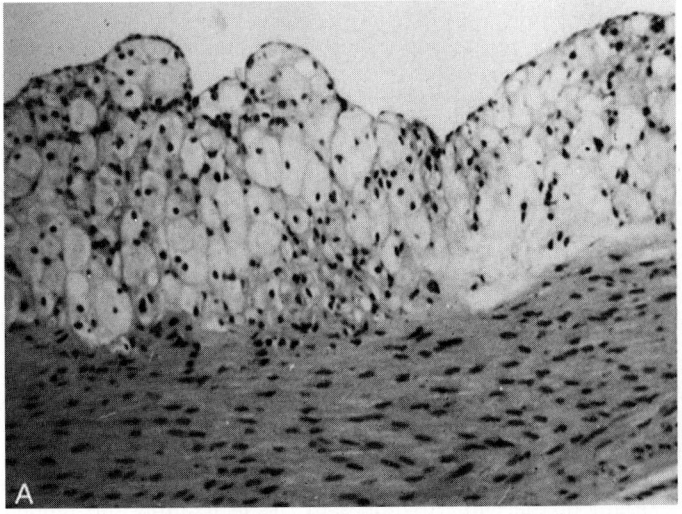
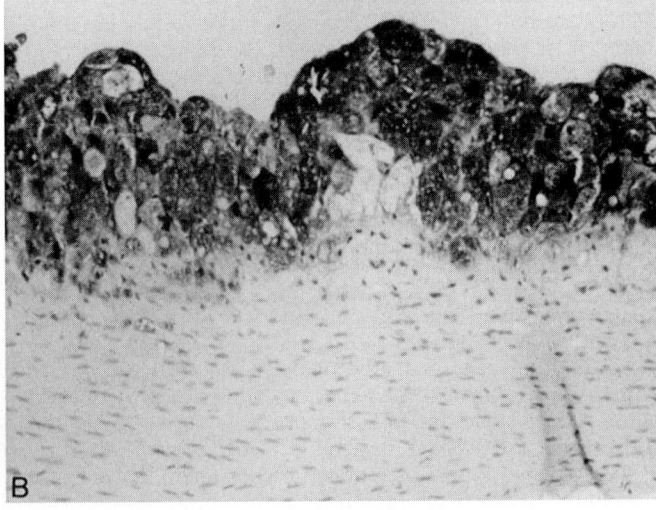

FIGURE 34–10. Light micrographs demonstrating portions of a fatty streak obtained from an aorta of a hypercholesterolemic monkey. This particular fatty streak contains several layers of macrophages. *A* is a routinely fixed and embedded paraffin section that has been stained with hematoxylin and eosin. The macrophage-rich areas are seen as clear because they are lipid-containing and the lipid has been extracted during the process of dehydration and embedding. *B* demonstrates an adjacent section that has been stained with immunoperoxidase coupled to an antibody specific for a cytoplasmic antigen present within the macrophage. The macrophages stain densely black in this micrograph, demonstrating that the large majority of the lipid-rich cells in the fatty streak are macrophages. Such antibodies make it possible to recognize cell type, even after the cells have become distorted by inclusions.

streaks at particular sites are converted by a series of changes into the more advanced fibroproliferative lesions of atherosclerosis, whereas fatty streaks at other anatomical sites either remain the same or regress and disappear. McGill[97] has gone on to review data to demonstrate that with time, fatty streaks occupy increasing surface areas of the coronary arteries and that these sites also precede the formation of advanced lesions. Thus, although it is difficult to derive firm conclusions from these types of data, such observations suggest that the fatty streak in many instances, if not the large majority, is the precursor lesion that becomes converted into the advanced occlusive form of atherosclerosis.

Once foam cells have formed in fatty streaks and in advanced lesions, it may become extremely difficult to define the cell of origin. The cells become filled with lipid droplets that appear as empty vacuoles in paraffin-embedded tissues which are often surrounded by a very thin rim of cytoplasm (Fig. 34–10). Electron microscopic examination may permit identification of some of these cells; however, large numbers remain difficult if not impossible to identify using standard techniques of tissue staining.

Several monoclonal antibodies have been developed, at least two of which appear to be specific for cell type. Tsudaka et al.[98] have developed monoclonal antibodies against smooth muscle–alpha actin and against a cytoplasmic antigen present in macrophages. Fortunately, these antigens resist some modes of fixation and embedding in paraffin. With these monoclonal antibodies, it has been possible to positively identify macrophages, T-lymphocytes, and smooth muscle cells in lesions of atherosclerosis. Thus it can be said definitively that the fatty streak consists principally of lipid-laden macrophages and T-lymphocytes, together with small and variable numbers of smooth muscle cells (Fig. 34–10).

Diffuse Intimal Thickening
(Lesion Type IV)

One form of lesion, described as a diffuse intimal thickening, consists of increased numbers of intimal smooth muscle cells surrounded by variable amounts of connective tissue. It is not entirely clear whether these sites of thickened intima represent developmental thickenings or whether such multilayered cushions of intimal smooth muscle cells are sites that formed because of increased stress on the artery wall but do not progress to advanced lesions of atherosclerosis. This is a somewhat poorly understood and controversial subject. These lesions may also have diffusely extracellular lipid intermixed with smooth muscle, macrophages, T cells, and connective tissue.

The Fibrous Plaque
(Lesion Types V and VI)

The advanced lesion of atherosclerosis is generally called a fibrous plaque. When the fibrous plaque becomes involved with thrombosis, hemorrhage, and/or calcification, it is often called a *complicated lesion*.

Fibrous plaques are grossly white in appearance and are usually elevated. In many cases they protrude into the lumen of the artery and, if sufficiently large, compromise the flow of blood. These lesions consist of large numbers of intimal smooth muscle cells, together with numerous macrophages and T-lymphocytes. When the macrophages and smooth muscle contain lipid, the lipid is primarily in the form of cholesterol and cholesteryl ester. The proliferated smooth muscle cells are surrounded by collagen and elastic fibers, by large amounts of proteoglycan, and, in individuals who are hypercholesterolemic, by varying amounts of lipid deposited in the cells and in the connective tissue. Fibrous plaques characteristically are covered by a fibrous cap.

In a study of a large series of male patients who had advanced occlusive lesions of the superficial femoral artery, we observed that the fibrous cap of each lesion consisted largely of a particular form of smooth muscle cell that is thin and pancake shaped and is surrounded by numerous lamellae of basement membrane, proteoglycan, and large numbers of collagen fibrils. The connective tissue in the fibrous cap is exceedingly dense. Beneath the fibrous cap lies a mixture of smooth muscle cells, macrophages, and numerous lymphocytes, principally CD-8 + and some CD-4 + T cells. Using the monoclonal antibodies already described, as well as antibodies to lymphocytes, it has been possible to identify definitively each of these cell types in the advanced lesions of atherosclerosis. In this highly cellular portion of the fibrous plaque, there are also large amounts of connective tissue. Beneath the cell-rich region, a zone of necrotic tissue and debris may contain cholesterol crystals and regions of calcification as well as numerous enlarged foam cells (Fig. 34–11).

Some plaques are densely fibrous and contain relatively little lipid, whereas others are rich in lipid deposits. Such differences can be found in different arteries within a given individual but are often associated with different risk factors. For example, it is common that the fibrous plaques observed in the superficial femoral arteries of those who are heavy cigarette smokers are extremely fibrous and contain relatively little lipid. On the other hand, individuals who are hypercholesterolemic and have advanced lesions in the coronary arteries often have large amounts of lipid within the lesions.[57]

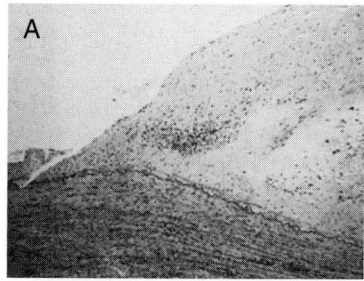 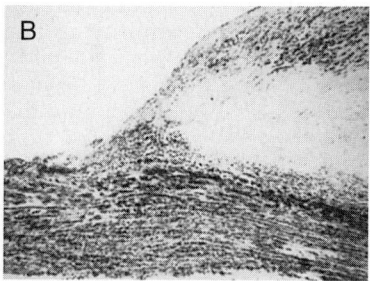 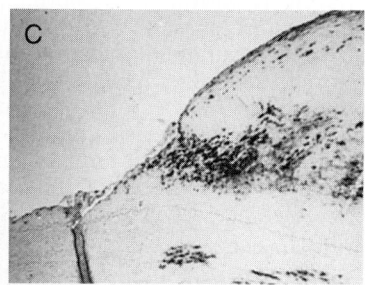

FIGURE 34–11. Three light micrographs demonstrating adjacent sections of a human fibrous plaque from a carotid endarterectomy specimen. *A* was stained with hematoxylin (H) and eosin (E). In the elevated portion of the lesion, the area adjacent to the lumen consists of a fibrous cap of parallel layers of smooth muscle cells covering a mixture of cells. With H & E it is impossible to determine cell type. *B* is an adjacent section that has been stained using immunoperoxidase coupled to an anti–smooth muscle actin antibody. The smooth muscle cells in the fibrous cap, in the media underlying the lesion, and in patches and individual cells located throughout the lesion are stained black. *C* is an adjacent section stained with immunoperoxidase coupled to an anti-macrophage antibody. Individual macrophages can be seen dispersed among the smooth muscle cells in the fibrous cap but are found principally in the area deep to the fibrous cap between the fibrous cap and the media, where most of the lipid-containing cells in this particular lesion can be found.

There appears to be a general pattern in the distribution of advanced lesions of atherosclerosis in humans. Generally, the abdominal aorta is more extensively involved than the thoracic aorta.[20] Lesions in the aorta are usually most prominent near the ostia of major branches that leave the aorta. Some arteries such as the renal arteries appear to be spared from atherosclerosis, except at their ostia.[99] The coronary arteries generally demonstrate the most intense involvement, with lesions of atherosclerosis located within the first 6 cm of the artery.[100] In hypertensive patients, lesions of the carotid, cerebral, and basilar arteries are more common. It has been suggested that the severity of lesion formation in a given artery may be related in part to the particular nature of the characteristics of the blood flow in the artery, and that rheological forces play a major role in determining the localization, extent, and severity of lesions in susceptible individuals.[101,102]

The principal clinical results of advanced lesions of atherosclerosis are derived either from the fact that they partially or totally occlude the lumen of the affected artery or because cracks and fissures develop in the lesions, leading to thrombosis and embolism or to aneurysmal dilatation (which usually occurs in large arteries such as the aorta). Many advanced lesions appear to be quite unstable, subject to rupture and thrombosis, and represent the principal cause of myocardial infarction and sudden ischemic death (discussed in detail below; see Thrombosis).

HYPOTHESES OF ATHEROGENESIS

Current theories of the pathogenesis of the lesions of atherosclerosis relate back to early proposals made by Virchow,[103] von Rokitansky,[104] and Duguid.[105] Virchow believed that a form of low-grade injury to the artery wall resulted in a type of inflammatory insudation, which in turn caused increased passage and accumulation of plasma constituents in the intima of the artery.[103] Rokitansky's belief, subsequently elaborated upon by Duguid, was that an encrustation of small mural thrombi existed at sites of arterial injury, that these thrombi went on to organize by the growth of smooth muscle cells into them, and that they would become incorporated into the lesions and thus serve as sites where the lesions would progress.[104,105]

In 1973, these two notions about atherogenesis were combined with new knowledge of the cellular and molecular biology of the artery wall in a hypothesis termed the *response-to-injury hypothesis of atherosclerosis.*[2] This hypothesis has been modified as new data have come forth. It now takes into account many aspects of the behavior of arterial and blood cells described above, as well as the numerous risk factors that have been associated with atherogenesis, including hyperlipidemia, hormone dysfunction, altered rheological forces as may occur in hypertension, and alteration of the endothelial barrier by factors associated with cigarette smoking, diabetes, and so on.[3,4,28,29,106]

A second hypothesis that was also formulated in 1973, the *monoclonal hypothesis,* suggests that the lesions of atherosclerosis may represent some form of neoplasia.[107] For further discussion of this hypothesis, the reader is referred to the review in reference number 3.

The Response-to-Injury Hypothesis

The response-to-injury hypothesis of atherosclerosis states that some form of "injury" may occur to the lining endothelial cells at particular anatomical sites in the artery wall. Injury to the endothelium is a key event in this hypothesis, and defining and understanding the subtleties of the nature of the various possible forms of injury are paramount in both testing the hypothesis and developing means of prevention and intervention. Sources of injury could include not only modified forms of lipoproteins but also viruses, such as herpesvirus,[108] and possibly other organisms, such as chlamydia, which have been observed in lesions.[109] However, the presence of organisms does not establish a causal relation. Thus, their role in the etiology and pathogenesis of the lesions remains to be determined.

Endothelial injury may be manifested as a number of forms of endothelial dysfunction.[108a] For example, interference with the permeability barrier role of the endothelium, alterations in the nonthrombogenic properties of the endothelial surface, promotion of the procoagulant properties of the endothelium, or increased release of vasoconstrictor or vasodilator molecules would all represent forms of dysfunction and injury that could result in some of the changes to be discussed below. Furthermore, maintenance of the continuity of the endothelial surface and maintenance of the normal low rates of turnover of the endothelial cells at most sites in the arterial tree are important in maintaining homeostasis. When turnover of the endothelium increases, it is possible that such turnover may be related to a series of changes in the endothelium, including the synthesis and secretion of vasoactive substances, of lipolytic enzymes, and of growth factors by the endothelial cells. Thus, endothelial injury could potentially lead to a host of changes in the functional activities of the lining endothelial cells, which could then lead to a critical sequence of cellular interactions, culminating in formation of lesions of atherosclerosis (Fig. 34–12).

In the case of chronic hyperlipidemia, the response-to-injury hypothesis proposes that an increase in plasma lipoproteins, principally oxidized LDL's and cholesterol, would result in toxic injury to the endothelium. It would also change the surface characteristics of both the endothelial cells and the circulating leukocytes, particularly circulating monocytes and possibly platelets as well. Hypercholesterolemia also somehow leads to increased adhesion of monocytes to endothelium at sites throughout the arterial tree.[110–113] When these monocytes adhere, they probe and are chemotactically attracted to migrate between endothelial cells and localize subendothelially, where they can become active as scavenger cells and are converted to macrophages. When they become macrophages, these cells take up lipid, principally modified, or oxidized LDL via receptors called scavenger receptors.[114–117] The lipid may enter the subendothelium in large quantities in the hypercholesterolemic state, resulting in the formation of foam cells and in the development of fatty streaks. The oxidized LDL may be toxic to the endothelium and to other cells in the microenvironment. The accumulation of macrophages in the intimal space would then establish conditions that could lead to further alterations in the endothelium.

Macrophages are well known to be capable of synthesizing and secreting numerous injurious agents that normally could play a role in killing ingested microorganisms or in nullifying toxic substances.[59] In this instance, the macrophages could potentially secrete oxidative metabolites such as oxidized LDL and superoxide anion, which could further injure the overlying endothelial cells. It has been demonstrated that lipid-laden macrophages are capable of oxidizing LDL and of forming peroxide and superoxide anion in vitro,[64] suggesting that this may occur in vivo as well.

An additional and potentially important reaction of the macrophage is related to its capacity to form growth regulatory molecules. Activated macrophages can, as already noted, synthesize and secrete at least four potent growth factors: PDGF, FGF, an EGF-like factor, and TGF β. PDGF is a potent mitogen for smooth muscle cells, as is FGF under some circumstances. The combination of these growth factors, together with TGF β, has been shown in vivo to be extremely potent in stimulating the migration and proliferation of fibroblasts and potentially of smooth muscle cells, and in stimulating formation of new connective tissue by these cells.[118]

stimulators of smooth muscle proliferation such as PDGF is probably critical in determining whether a net proliferative response of smooth muscle cells will occur, resulting in the formation of an atherosclerotic lesion. Thus, if the macrophage-derived foam cells are appropriately activated in the subendothelial space, they could potentially be involved in the secretion of growth factors that could chemotactically attract smooth muscle cells to migrate from the media into the intima, to proliferate within the intima, and to set up a series of conditions that could lead to the formation of an intimal, fibromuscular, proliferative lesion.

It has been demonstrated that PDGF-B-chain–containing protein is present in approximately 20 percent of the macrophages in both human and nonhuman atherosclerotic lesions in all phases of development. PDGF is present in the non–foam-cell macrophages that are distributed throughout the lesion, as well as in macrophages present among the smooth muscle cells in the fibrous cap portion of the fibrous plaque[120] (Fig. 34–13). The presence of PDGF-B protein in the macrophages in these lesions provides the first convincing basis for assigning the macrophage a key role in the induction and maintenance of the smooth muscle proliferative response during atherogenesis because PDGF-BB is one of the most potent growth factors, capable of stimulating smooth muscle migration, chemotaxis, and proliferation. Thus macrophage-derived PDGF-BB (Fig. 34–7) could be involved not only in the appearance of smooth muscle cells that migrate into macrophage-rich fatty streaks, but in the progression of these fatty streaks to intermediate or fibro-fatty lesions, which may ultimately become advanced occlusive lesions, or fibrous plaques. If the cycle of "endothelial injury" and macrophage accumulation and stimulation is repeated, at least two cells capable of releasing growth factors into the intima—the activated endothelial cell and the activated macrophage—may continue to contribute to progression of the lesions.

The response-to-injury hypothesis also provides an opportunity for the interaction of a third cell, the platelet. The hypothesis suggests that if the flow properties of the blood at particular anatomical sites are such that these properties participate in the endothelial injury, endothelial cell–cell attachment may be affected and cell disjunction may occur, leading to retraction of endothelial cells and exposure of the underlying foam cells or connective tissue or both. In either case, this would permit opportunities for platelets to interact, adhere, aggregate, and form mural thrombi.[121–125] Should this occur, the platelet could provide a third potent source of growth factors, including the same four factors that can be released by the activated macrophage. Thus, there are numerous opportunities for mitogens to be deposited in the artery wall, which, under proper circumstances, could play critical roles in the genesis of proliferative smooth muscle lesions of atherosclerosis (Fig. 34–13).

It is important to point out that injury to the endothelium need not result in denudation of the endothelial cells. Endothelial injury may simply be manifested by relatively rapid replacement of individual endothelial cells that are lost and is principally reflected in endothelial dysfunction such as alterations in endothelial permeability, increased adhesion of leukocytes to the endothelium, and release of vasoactive substances and growth factors.

Finally, it has been shown that human arterial smooth muscle cells removed from lesions of atherosclerosis have the capacity to express one of the PDGF genes and secrete a form of PDGF when they are grown in cell culture.[126] If this were to occur in vivo, then as the smooth muscle cells

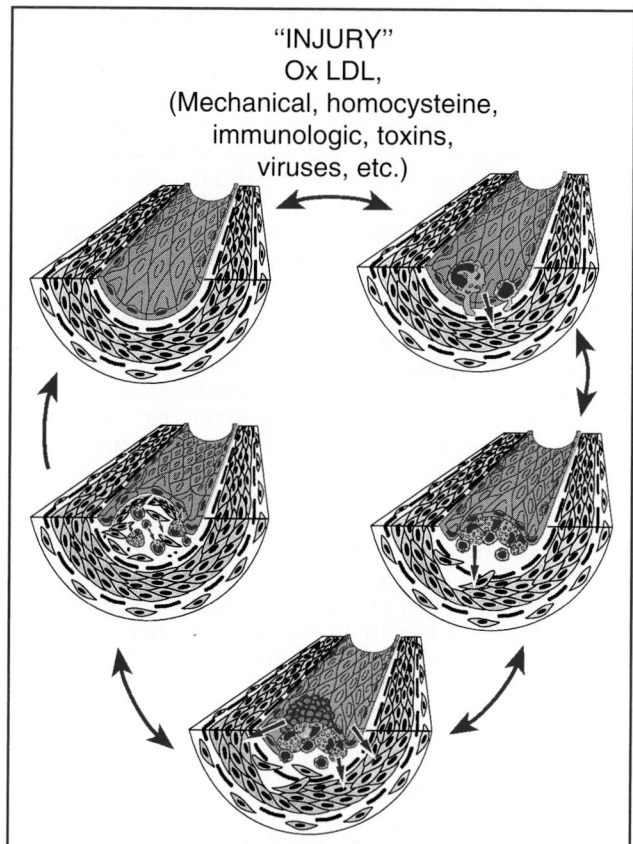

FIGURE 34–12. The response-to-injury hypothesis of atherosclerosis. Several different sources of injury to the endothelium can lead to endothelial cell dysfunction. One of the parameters associated with endothelial cell dysfunction that results from exposure to agents, such as oxLDL, is increased adherence of monocytes/macrophages and T-lymphocytes. These cells then migrate between the endothelium and localize subendothelially. The macrophages become large foam cells due to lipid accumulation and, with the T cells and smooth muscle, form a fatty streak. The fatty streak can then progress to an intermediate, fibrofatty lesion and ultimately to a fibrous plaque.

As the lesions accumulate increasing numbers of cells and the macrophages scavenge the lipid, some of the lipid-laden macrophages may emigrate back into the bloodstream by pushing apart the endothelial cells. Upon doing so, those at sites such as branches and bifurcations where blood flow is irregular with eddy currents and back currents may become thrombogenic sites that lead to formation of platelet mural thrombi. Such thrombi can release many potent growth-regulatory molecules from the platelets that can join with those released by the activated macrophages and possibly by lesion smooth muscle cells into the artery wall. Platelet thrombi can also form at sites where endothelial dysjunction may have occurred. Ultimately, the formation and release of numerous growth-regulatory molecules and cytokines from a network established between cells in the lesion, consisting of activated macrophages, smooth muscle, T cells, and endothelium, lead to progression of the lesions of atherosclerosis to a fibrous plaque or advanced, complicated lesion.

Each of the stages of lesion formation is potentially reversible. Thus, lesion regression can occur if the injurious agents are removed, or when protective factors intervene to reverse the inflammatory and fibroproliferative processes. (From Ross, R.: The pathogenesis of atherosclerosis: A perspective for the 1990s. Nature 362:801, 1993. Copyright 1993 Macmillan Magazines Limited.)

TGF β is not only a potent stimulator of connective tissue synthesis but is also the most potent inhibitor of smooth muscle proliferation thus far discovered.[119] It is ubiquitous in the sense that most cells have the capacity to form it, and rich sources of this molecule are the platelet and the activated macrophage. Much of the TGF β that is secreted by these cells is in a latent form that requires decreased pH or proteolytic cleavage for activity. Nevertheless, the balance between inhibitors such as TGF β and

FIGURE 34–13. See color plate 9.

proliferate in developing lesions, they could participate in inducing further progression of the lesions by release of PDGF. Thus a vicious circle might be established that would have to be stopped if one hoped to stop lesion progression and induce lesion regression.

LIPIDS, LIPOPROTEINS, AND MODIFIED LDL IN ATHEROSCLEROSIS

Because hypercholesterolemia is the major risk factor associated with the increased incidence of atherosclerosis in the United States and Western Europe, it is important to understand the role that lipids play in this process. Although many lesions of atherosclerosis are fibrous and contain relatively little lipid, the effects of lipid on endothelium, monocytes, and smooth muscle and the accumulation of lipid in the lesions of hypercholesterolemic individuals are critical components of the process of atherogenesis. Consequently, it is important to understand specifically how elevated levels of cholesterol-bearing lipoproteins are related to the process of atherogenesis. These subjects are discussed in detail on pp. 1127 to 1143.

The Lipid Research Clinic Trials have provided data suggesting that it would be beneficial to lower plasma LDL levels.[14,15] Those studies showed that the decrease in plasma cholesterol can be correlated with a reduction in the incidence of myocardial infarction and presumably atherosclerosis. The genetic basis for the increase in plasma LDL is not known for most individuals in the population who are hypercholesterolemic, although some may be heterozygous for the familial hypercholesterolemia (FH) trait. Nevertheless, our understanding of the LDL receptor control of HMG CoA reductase, and thus cholesterol synthesis, has been critical in permitting us to understand how cholesterol metabolism is regulated. As important as these studies are, however, they do not provide data that permit us to understand how the lesions of atherosclerosis form. In other words, although the LDL receptor pathway provides an understanding of the control of cholesterol metabolism, it yields no information concerning the basis of the cellular changes and interactions that occur when elevated plasma cholesterol leads to atherosclerosis.

To answer this question, it has been necessary to devise experiments using appropriate animal models and appropriate cell culture systems. These tests provide opportunities to determine how smooth muscle cells proliferate and under what circumstances, what cellular interactions occur during the pathogenesis of this disease process, and what factors are elaborated by the cells that control not only smooth muscle multiplication but also connective tissue formation and lipid accumulation.

The response-to-injury hypothesis of atherosclerosis already discussed can be taken one step further in terms of asking how chronic hypercholesterolemia may "injure" endothelium. Jackson and Gotto[127] have suggested that one form of endothelial injury which may occur upon exposure to chronically elevated levels of LDL may result from the effects of an increase in the number of cholesterol molecules in the plasma membranes of cells, including the endothelial cells. When the cholesterol/phospholipid ratio of endothelial plasma membranes is elevated, this could theoretically lead to an increase in the viscosity of the membranes. Changes such as these would decrease the malleability of the endothelial cell surface and, should this occur, could have critical effects at particular anatomical sites such as branches of bifurcations in the arterial tree, where the endothelial cells are exposed to changes in the flow of blood. Such rheological changes could cause an otherwise normally malleable endothelial surface, if it becomes more viscous and thus more rigid, to be incapable of dealing with the stresses caused by these changes in the flow

characteristics. This could lead to endothelial cell–cell separation and endothelial retraction, particularly at sites where the blood flow has already been modified owing to the formation of fatty streaks, as has been found to occur in hypercholesterolemic monkeys, swine, and humans. As already discussed, hypercholesterolemia also leads to changes in monocyte-endothelial adhesion properties and to the development of fatty streaks themselves.

It is also possible that hypercholesterolemia may alter the endothelial cells so that they are stimulated to produce increased amounts of growth factor. Recent studies with the Watanabe heritable hyperlipemic (WHHL) rabbit, an animal model of homozygous familial hypercholesterolemia, have demonstrated that probucol, a drug with mild lipid-lowering but powerful antioxidant properties, had a marked effect in significantly reducing the size and incidence of atherosclerotic lesions.[128,129] This led to studies suggesting that oxidized LDL might play a major role as an injurious agent responsible for many of the early events associated with atherogenesis, particularly because macrophages have scavenger receptors that can bind and permit phagocytosis of these oxidized lipid particles. The ingestion of oxidized LDL could lead to foam cell formation on the part of the macrophages, which can also engage in further oxidation of available molecules of LDL.

Recent studies in nonhuman primates with the antioxidant probucol[130] have further demonstrated that probucol decreases lesion formation and prevents the formation of fatty streaks. This antioxidant appears to have an early effect on the inflammatory processes that are required for lesion development. Unpublished data also suggest that there is a decreased turnover of both macrophages and smooth muscle cells in the lesions of the probucol-treated animals. Clinical trials are under way to determine the effectiveness of antioxidant therapy using oral antioxidants, including vitamins C, E, and beta-carotene. Results of these studies should provide further insight into the role of oxidation and other modifications of LDL, such as glycation, in the process of atherogenesis. Oxidized LDL is injurious to both endothelium and smooth muscle in vitro and has been found in both human and experimental lesions of atherosclerosis.[131] Thus the presence of this modified lipoprotein in the lesions suggests that it is the principal culprit in atherogenesis in hypercholesterolemic individuals and that interference with its formation could be an important step in lesion prevention.

GROWTH FACTORS AND CYTOKINES

As discussed earlier, growth factors and cytokines can be elaborated by all four cells potentially involved in the lesions of atherosclerosis: endothelium, monocyte/macrophages, platelets, and smooth muscle (Figs. 34–5 to 34–7). Although the first three of these cells can produce more than one growth factor, PDGF could play a critical role in the genesis of atherosclerosis because of its chemotactic and mitogenic effects on smooth muscle cells.

PDGF is a two-chain molecule of approximately 30,000 molecular weight that is highly cationic and highly disulfide bonded. It is an extraordinarily potent mitogen that binds with very high affinity to responsive cells[132] and is chemotactic for the same cells for which it is mitogenic.[133,134] When it binds to its high-affinity cell-surface receptor, it induces a series of biological events, some of which are probably related to induction of DNA synthesis and cell division. These cellular responses include phosphorylation of the PDGF receptor through the activation of a tyrosine kinase on the receptor, and the activation of C-kinase in the subplasmalemmal cytoplasm resulting from phospholipase activation at the cell surface. C-kinase activation could ultimately lead to calcium transfer from intracellular compartments, which in itself may possibly be important in induction of the mitogenic signal.[65]

PDGF also induces increased binding of LDL to cells by increasing the numbers of LDL receptors,[50,135] increased cholesterol synthesis, increased endocytosis, increased flux of ions into the cell, reorganization of actin cables within the cells, and change in cell shape. It also has recently been found to be a potent vasoactive agent, even more potent than angiotensin II.[65] Thus, if PDGF is released from platelets when they adhere to the artery wall at sites of injury, from activated macrophages where it is now known to present in these cells[120] after they enter the artery wall (particularly during fatty streak formation), from activated endothelial cells if they are appropriately stimulated, and perhaps in some special instances from appropriately activated smooth muscle cells, then such responses would enhance lesion formation.

PDGF has an extremely short half-life when it is injected into the circulation.[136] This short half-life suggests that PDGF that is not bound locally to tissue would be cleared rapidly and thus would be unavailable at sites distant from its release. Furthermore, PDGF binds to a number of proteins in the plasma, including alpha$_2$-macroglobulin. These binding proteins could serve to increase further the capacity of PDGF to act as a tissue mitogen at local sites where PDGF has been released and is bound to the tissue.[137]

There is a striking homology between the amino acid sequence of purified PDGF and that of a transforming protein derived from an oncogene of the simian sarcoma virus. This homology suggests that PDGF may be important in proliferation of cells transformed by the simian sarcoma virus.[138,139] Furthermore, numerous lines of transformed cells secrete a form of PDGF and have downregulated receptors for PDGF, suggesting that a form of PDGF may play a role in the proliferation of cells that are neoplastically transformed in other ways.[140] Both chains of PDGF and their receptors have been cloned. cDNA probes are available for each chain of PDGF and for both receptors. Investigations of these receptors have demonstrated a high degree of specificity of binding of the three different isomeric forms of PDGF (PDGF-AA, PDGF-AB, PDGF-BB) for the three different forms of the receptor (PDGF receptor $\alpha\alpha$, $\alpha\beta$, $\beta\beta$). For example, the A chain of PDGF can bind only to the alpha-receptor subunit; thus PDGF-AA can bind only to PDGF receptor $\alpha\alpha$. In contrast, PDGF-BB can bind to any one of the three forms of the PDGF receptor.[141] It therefore becomes important to understand the relative numbers of receptors on the different smooth muscle cells in different regions of the artery wall if one is to determine how effective the specific form of PDGF will be on these cells in a given site in the arterial tree. Our increased understanding of these degrees of specificity and responsivity will increase opportunities to make effective agents that can either induce smooth muscle proliferation or, potentially, prevent such a proliferative response.

Several animals form lesions of atherosclerosis similar to humans when they develop hypercholesterolemia from eating a fatty diet. This has made it possible to study the effects of hypercholesterolemia in terms of understanding the cellular interactions which occur that lead to the lesions of atherosclerosis. Such studies have been performed by Faggiotto et al.[142,143] and by Masuda and Ross[144,145] on nonhuman primates, by Gerrity[146–148] and his colleagues on swine, and by Rosenfeld et al.[149] on fat-fed rabbits and the WHHL rabbit. The latter studies have provided highly detailed observations concerning the sequence of cellular events that occur in endogenous hypercholesterolemia (the WHHL rabbit, a model of familial homozygous hypercholesterolemia) as compared with those that take place during diet-induced hypercholesterolemia.

Recently, genetically modified mice, in particular, the homozygous apoprotein E- (ApoE-) deficient transgenic mouse, have provided small murine models of atherosclerosis. The ApoE-deficient mouse, for example, develops lesions at anatomical sites similar to those found in humans. A sequence of cellular interactions and events similar to that in nonhuman primates and humans has been observed.[150,151] This model and other genetically modified mice provide opportunities to study which appropriate genetic combinations can be made by adding or removing specific molecules to determine their roles in the process of atherogenesis. An important new frontier of research has been opened in this area.

EARLY CHANGES. The data of Faggiotto et al.,[142,143] Masuda and Ross,[144,145] and Nakashima et al.[150] show that the first and most striking event occurs after 7 to 14 days of diet-induced hypercholesterolemia. This consists of the attachment of large numbers of leukocytes, principally monocytes, to the surface of the arterial endothelium (Fig. 34–14). The monocytes attach to the endothelial cells in clus-

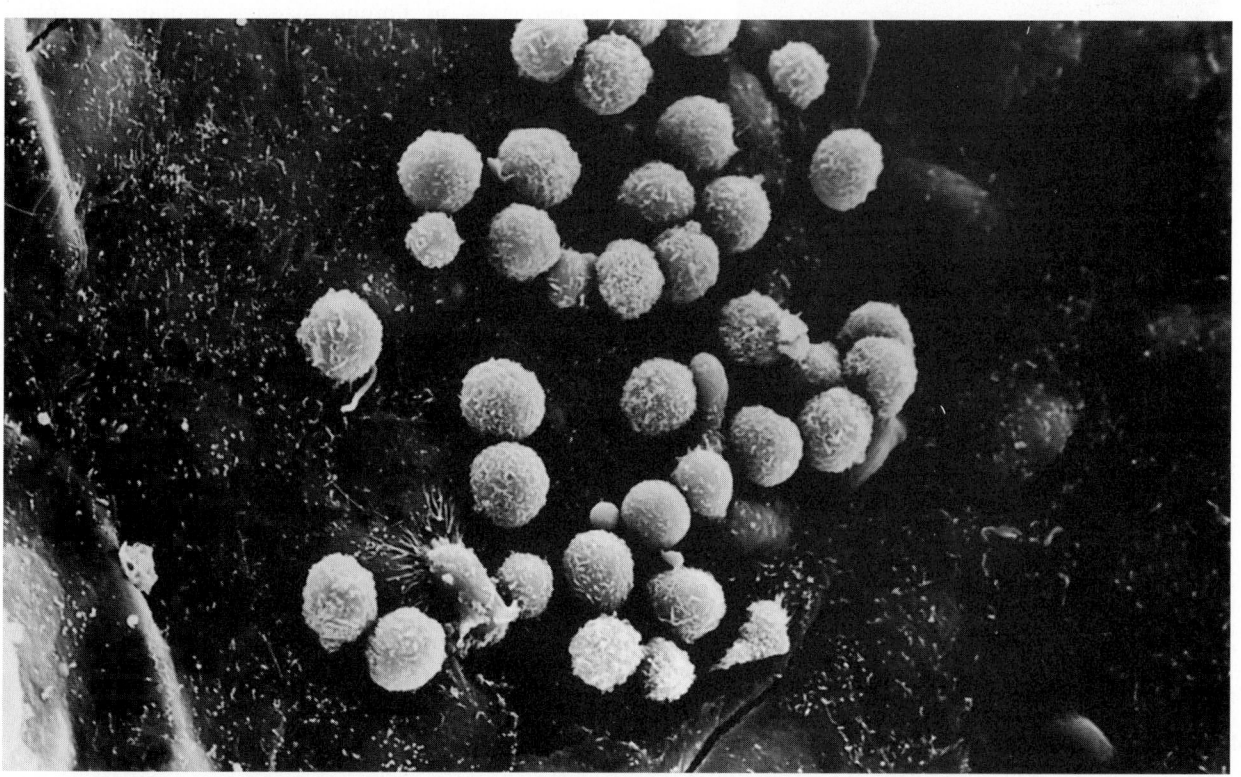

FIGURE 34–14. Electron micrograph demonstrating leukocytes adherent to the endothelium of the aorta of a hypercholesterolemic monkey after 14 days of an atherogenic diet. Adherent leukocytes (mostly monocytes) were found scattered in patches such as these randomly distributed at all levels of the aortic tree. Some of the cells appear spread on the surface, whereas others are rounded.

ters that appear to be located at branches and bifurcations throughout the arterial tree in all large and medium-sized arteries. The attached monocytes then migrate over the surface of the endothelium, where they probe, find a junction between the endothelial cells, and use this junctional site to slip between the cells and localize in the subendothelial space (Fig. 34–15). This process, as viewed in cell culture, appears to occur very rapidly and presumably does so in vivo as well. After finding their way into the subendothelial intimal space, the monocytes become converted into macrophages, so that within less than 1 month large numbers of foam cells, or lipid-filled macrophages, are found beneath an intact endothelium. These cells continue to enlarge as they fill with lipid. Such accumulations of foam cells represent the establishment of the first and ubiquitous lesion of atherosclerosis, the fatty streak (Fig. 34–16).

The fatty streaks continue to expand in hypercholesterolemic animals by continuing the process of monocyte adherence, subendothelial migration and localization, and lipid accumulation. As the fatty streaks expand, the surface of the artery becomes highly irregular and convoluted (Fig. 34–17). With increasing time, small numbers of smooth muscle cells begin to appear beneath the accumulated macrophages within the intima and also begin to accumulate deposits of lipid and take on the appearance of foam cells. As discussed earlier, monoclonal antibodies specific for

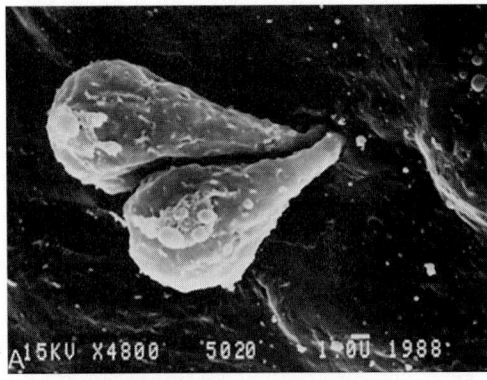

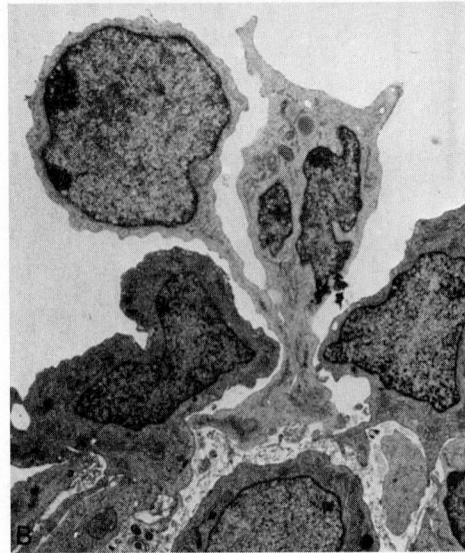

FIGURE 34–15. Scanning and transmission electron micrographs demonstrating leukocytes entering into the artery wall between endothelial junctions after 6 months and 1 year, respectively, of an atherogenic diet in nonhuman primates. *A*, Thoracic aorta, 6 months. ×4000. *B*, Thoracic aorta, 1 year. ×4700. (Reproduced with permission from Masuda, J., and Ross, R.: Atherogenesis during low level hypercholesterolemia in the nonhuman primate: I. Fatty streak formation. *Arteriosclerosis* 10:164, 1990. Copyright 1990 American Heart Association.)

smooth muscle and macrophages have made it possible to show that both types of cell become foam cells as the lesions expand. The cholesterol levels in the plasma of the fat-fed animals ranged between 500 and 1000 mg/dl, which are not dissimilar from the levels of plasma cholesterol found in humans with FH disease.

LATER CHANGES. After approximately 5 to 6 months at the very high cholesterol and LDL levels and after 1 year at levels closer to those observed in humans, a second series of changes occurred in the monkeys, initially at branches and bifurcations in the iliac arteries and subsequently at higher regions in the arterial tree. The changes that were found at branches and bifurcations suggest that they may be associated with the flow characteristics at these particular sites in the vessel. They consist of retraction of the endothelial cells covering some of the fatty streaks caused by endothelial cell-cell detachment. Endothelial retraction exposes the numerous lipid-filled macrophages to the circulation (Fig. 34–18) and permits them to remove the lipid they have ingested from the lesion by taking it with them into the circulation to the spleen and to lymph nodes. In this fashion, the macrophages play a role in the lesions of atherosclerosis similar to their role at sites of injury, where they are the principal scavenger cells. Thus, in a very real sense, the progressing lesions of atherosclerosis represent a special kind of inflammatory response in which macrophages (and perhaps T-lymphocytes) attempt initially to protect the tissues. With the continuing insult (hypercholesterolemia, diabetes, and so on), the response becomes excessive, and the resultant fibroproliferative events themselves become the disease process.

When the macrophages become exposed to the circulation they can serve as sites for platelet adherence and for microthrombi to form, demonstrating that the macrophages may represent a potent site for platelet interactions (Fig. 34–19). In these cases in which platelet interactions such as those just described occurred, similar anatomical sites were observed 1 to 2 months later to be occupied by space-filling lesions of advanced atherosclerosis, or fibrous plaques. These fibrous plaques had all of the characteristic appearances of fibrous plaques in humans, including a dense fibrous cap that overlay areas of extensive proliferation of smooth muscle cells intermixed with lipid-filled macrophages, beneath which were found areas of cell debris, lipid accumulation, and sometimes calcification (Fig. 34–20). The same changes occurred at the iliac bifurcation after approximately 7 months, in the abdominal aorta after 9 months, in the thoracic aorta by 11 months, and in the coronary arteries after 12 to 13 months. By analyzing the distribution of these changes and correlating this distribution with the levels of cholesterol in the animals with time, Faggiotto et al.[142,143] and Masuda and Ross[144,145] were able to demonstrate a correlation among three factors: the level of plasma cholesterol, the duration of the maintenance of this increased level of cholesterol, and the changes that occur at particular anatomical sites with time.

Another important observation was that many advanced lesions of atherosclerosis also occurred at sites where fatty streaks were present but where there was no clear evidence of endothelial cell-cell separation and exposure of the subendothelium.[143] Thus, one has to conclude that proliferative lesions of atherosclerosis can occur at sites where the endothelium remains intact over preexisting lesions such as fatty streaks. This can undoubtedly be explained by the fact that both activated macrophages and endothelium can serve as sources of growth factors so that platelet interactions are not required for smooth muscle proliferation to occur.

This leads to the need to determine what constitutes endothelial injury. It also suggests that nondenuding forms of injury or endothelial dysfunction are more important than the denuding forms described above. Reidy and

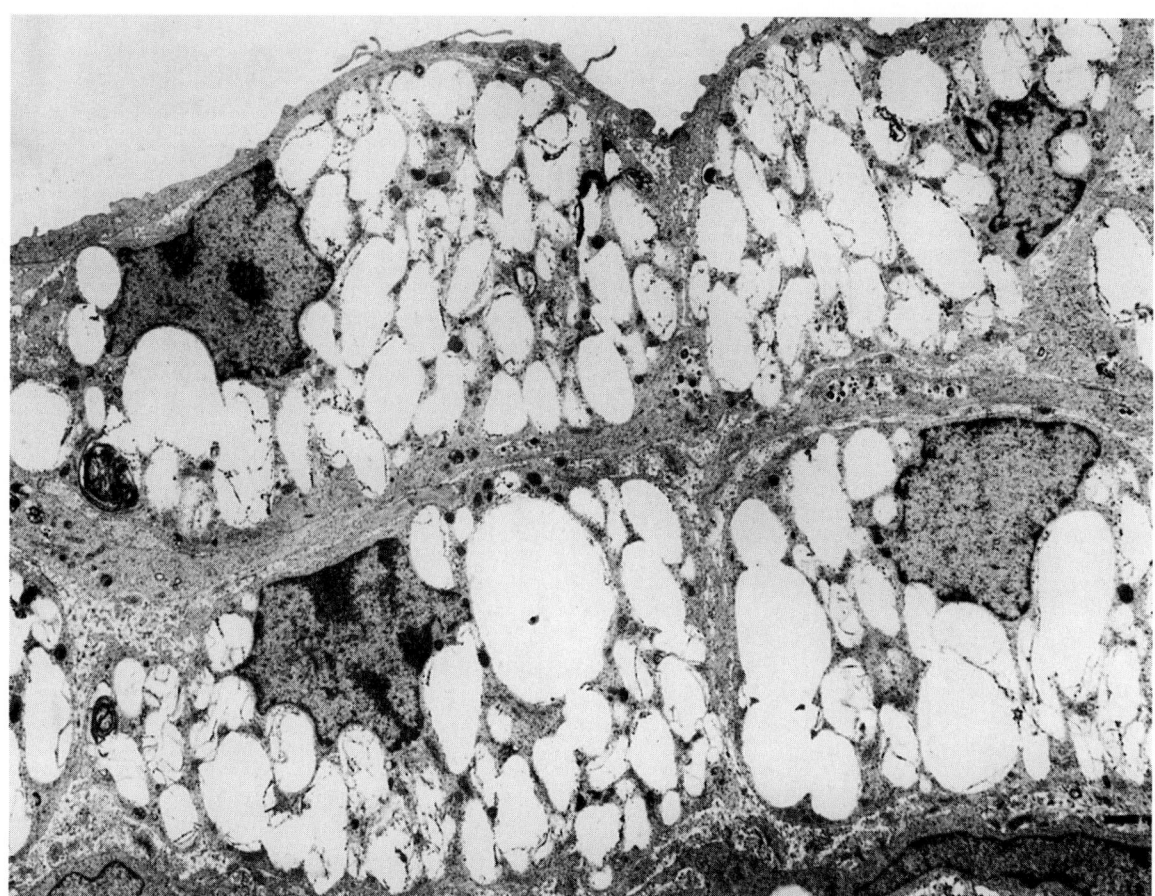

FIGURE 34–16. Transmission electron micrograph showing a fatty streak containing two layers of subendothelial foam cells after 2 months of hypercholesterolemia in a fat-fed nonhuman primate. The large lipid-filled macrophages are distributed focally in multilayers. The cells are four- to six-fold larger than lipid-laden macrophages observed in control animals. There is a small amount of intercellular matrix and some lipid debris. The macrophages maintain a close relationship to the intact endothelium. The endothelium is markedly stretched so that the endothelial cells have become very thin. (Reproduced with permission from Faggiotto, A., Ross, R., and Harker, L.: Studies of hypercholesterolemia in the nonhuman primate: I. Changes that lead to fatty streak formation. Arteriosclerosis 4:332, 1984. Copyright 1984 American Heart Association.)

Schwartz[152,153] have indicated that one of the most common results of endothelial injury may be detachment of individual endothelial cells, which are rapidly replaced by neighboring cells so that endothelial continuity is maintained. Several markers have been developed that can be used to

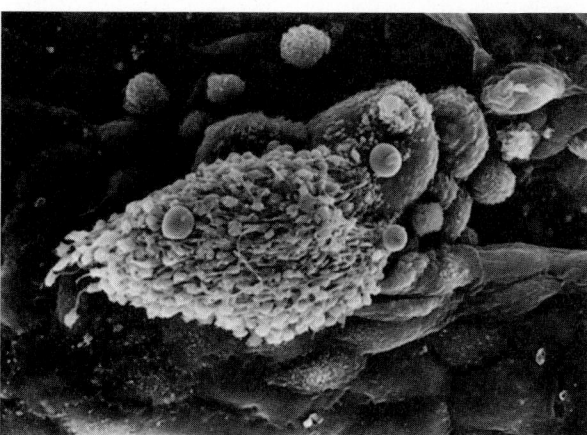

FIGURE 34–17. Scanning electron micrograph providing a surface view of a fatty streak from a fat-fed monkey after 2 months of hypercholesterolemia. The surface of the fatty streak has become highly irregular and has a striking nodular pattern with deep crevices between the nodules. Such a pattern forms by continuing adherence of monocytes to the endothelial cells that probe and migrate subendothelially between cells to continually expand the fatty streak.

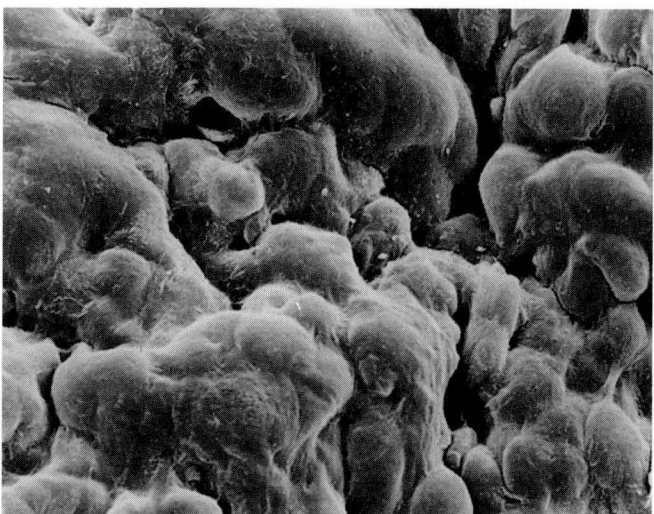

FIGURE 34–18. A scanning electron micrograph of the thoracic aorta of a nonhuman primate, showing the irregular surface of a fatty streak after 2 years of an atherogenic diet. Platelet microthrombi adherent to exposed macrophages are visible at a site of endothelial retraction. Many adherent leukocytes are also seen on the intact endothelial cells. ×720. (Reproduced with permission from Masuda, J., and Ross, R.: Atherogenesis during low level hypercholesterolemia in the nonhuman primate: II. Fatty streak conversion to fibrous plaque. Arteriosclerosis 10:178, 1990. Copyright 1990 American Heart Association.)

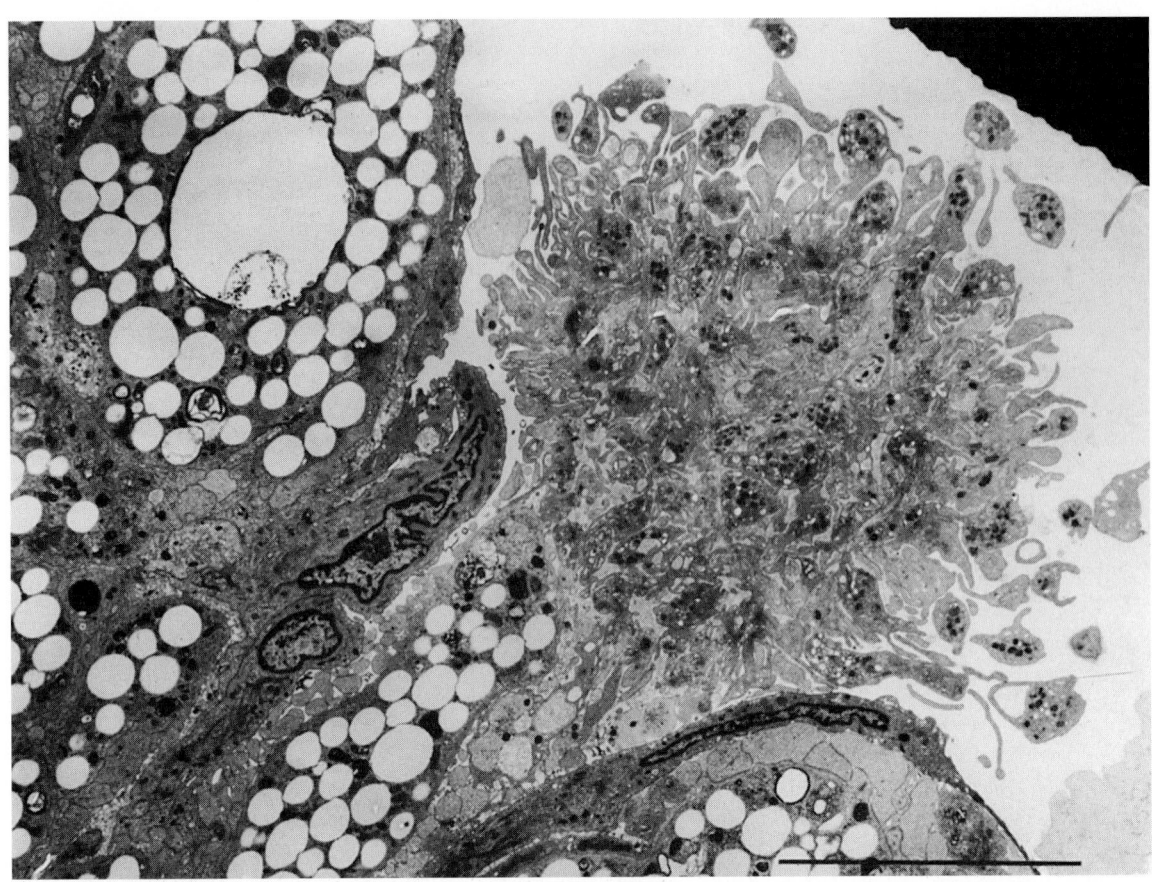

FIGURE 34-19. Transmission electron micrograph of platelets adherent to an exposed macrophage from a fatty streak in a fat-fed monkey that had been hypercholesterolemic for 6 months. The platelets in this thrombus are generally adherent to exposed foam cells and penetrate into the depth of a crevice in the fatty streak. Many of the platelets have undergone degranulation and have released their contents. Bar = 10 μ. (Reproduced with permission from Faggiotto, A., and Ross, R.: Studies of hypercholesterolemia in the nonhuman primate: II. Fatty streak conversion to fibrous plaque. Arteriosclerosis 4:349, 1984. Copyright 1984 American Heart Association.)

identify sites of endothelial injury. Hansson et al.[154] demonstrated that injured endothelial cells take up IgG whereas normal endothelium does not, and that such IgG uptake can be correlated with increased replication of the endothelium. Furthermore, Reidy and Schwartz[155] showed that a linear correlation exists between the extent of endothelial injury (the number of denuded cells) and the localization of indium-111–labeled platelets at these sites. Platelets

would adhere because injured endothelium appears to have lost its nonthrombogenic properties.

Thus, there may be several different forms of endothelial injury and more subtle techniques may be necessary to uncover them. This raises the interesting question, as suggested earlier, whether one subtle form of endothelial injury may be the stimulation of these cells to synthesize and secrete growth factors, including PDGF, that could then

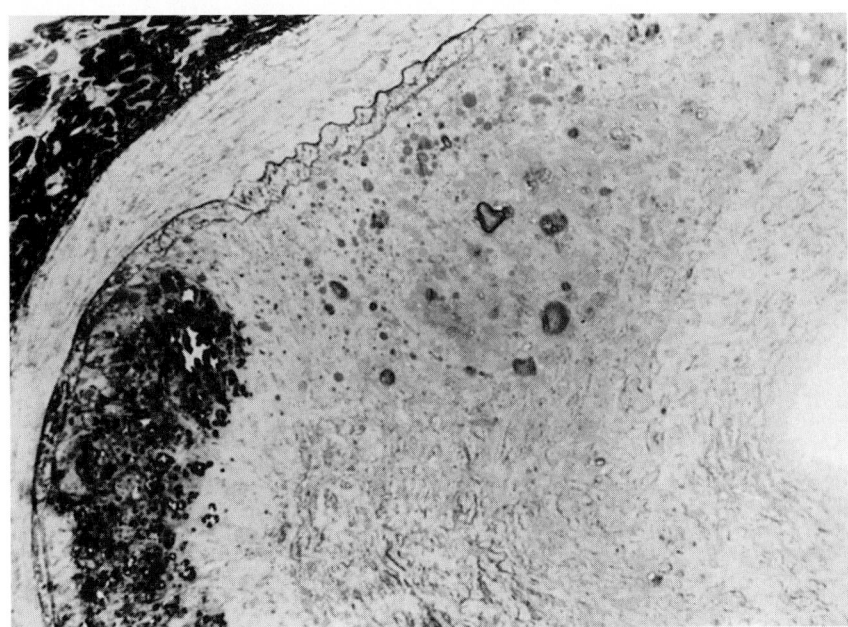

FIGURE 34-20. Light micrograph demonstrating an advanced fibrous plaque that formed in the internal iliac artery of a monkey that was hypercholesterolemic for 7 months. The lesion has occluded approximately 70 per cent of the arterial lumen and consists of numerous layers of smooth muscle cells surrounded by fibrous connective tissue. An area of lipid and necrotic tissue occupies the left side and upper portion of this lesion. (Reproduced with permission from Faggiotto, A., and Ross, R.: Studies of hypercholesterolemia in the nonhuman primate: II. Fatty streak conversion to fibrous plaque. Arteriosclerosis 4:345, 1984. Copyright 1984 American Heart Association.)

play a critical role in the genesis of the events previously described. If this were the case, then endothelial disjunction, retraction, and subendothelial exposure are clearly not necessary for lesions of atherosclerosis to develop because both activated endothelium and macrophages could be sufficient in themselves to provide a mitogenic stimulus for smooth muscle cells to form lesions of atherosclerosis.

REGRESSION OF ATHEROSCLEROSIS

ANIMAL STUDIES. A number of studies have demonstrated that lesions of experimentally induced atherosclerosis can in fact regress. When hypercholesterolemic swine and nonhuman primates that have developed severe lesions are fed a normocholesterolemic diet, these lesions can regress. Fatty streaks formed in the monkeys receiving the high-fat, high-cholesterol diet of Faggiotto et al.[142] were found to regress completely within 1 month after the animals resumed a normal diet. Most of the studies of regression of the advanced lesions of atherosclerosis have been performed in nonhuman primates, principally in different strains of macaques and in squirrel monkeys. The studies were performed by providing the monkeys with atherogenic diets that took them through stages of fatty streak development and on to fibrous plaque formation. When cholesterol was removed from the diet and plasma cholesterol concentrations returned to normal, Faggiotto et al.[142] observed that reasonably rapid regression of fatty streaks occurred. Of greater potential interest, significant reduction in the size of the smooth muscle proliferative lesions has been observed by several different investigators. Some of the earliest studies were performed by Armstrong et al.,[156] who demonstrated that coronary atherosclerosis could regress. These studies were subsequently confirmed by Wissler and Vesselinovitch.[157] Perhaps the largest number of studies have been performed by Clarkson and his colleagues.[158] They demonstrated the clear therapeutic benefit of lowering plasma cholesterol concentrations after having induced fibrous plaques in animals on hypercholesterolemic regimens for periods of 12 months and longer. Regression occurred principally in lesions in the abdominal aorta and in the coronary arteries, in contrast to those that formed at the carotid bifurcation, which appeared, on some occasions, to develop lesions relatively independently of plasma lipid concentrations. When regression occurs and plasma cholesterol levels return to baseline, the lesions of atherosclerosis become smaller, contain less lipid, and demonstrate marked decreases in their content of cholesterol and cholesteryl esters. Remodeling of connective tissue proteins also appears to take place, as shown by decreases in both collagen and elastic fiber proteins in these lesions. Thus it seems that, over a sufficiently long period, advanced lesions can in some cases also regress.

By decreasing lipid deposition or enhancing removal of lipids from the artery wall, for example, by reducing fat intake or increasing plasma HDL levels, it has been possible to show that lesion regression can be induced.[159] Similarly, as described above, antioxidants can induce lesion regression in the WHHL rabbit.[128,129]

HUMAN STUDIES. It has been demonstrated that advanced, semiocclusive lesions of human coronary atherosclerosis also can regress. In a quantitative image analysis study of coronary angiograms from a series of patients being aggressively treated with lipid-lowering regimens of either niacin and colestipol or lovastatin and colestipol, Brown and colleagues[160] have demonstrated statistically significant regression in association with decreases in plasma cholesterol and LDL. This provides clear evidence that the lesions of atherosclerosis are able to regress at apparently all stages of lesion development.

Various approaches have been used in clinical trials to induce lesion regression in humans. These trials have included lipid-lowering agents, including HMG–CoA reductase inhibitors, cholestyramine, colestipol/niacin therapy, as well as dietary and lifestyle changes, and even surgical approaches.[163–171] All of these trials have demonstrated decrease in incidence of acute cardiac events and, in some cases, extensive reduction with detectable, but minimal, lesion regression as determined angiographically. These approaches may increase the stability of advanced lesions of atherosclerosis without necessarily reducing their size as imaged angiographically. Because angiograms do not provide information on actual lesion size but only on lumen dimensions, it is not entirely clear what changes may have occurred in the lesions. Nevertheless, several trials have demonstrated substantial reduction in angina by reducing lipid levels.

A number of investigators have probed the capability of fish oils, which contain large amounts of omega-3 fatty acids, to decrease plasma cholesterol levels and potentially to induce lesion regression when added to the diet of hypercholesterolemic individuals.[172] Not only do these diets lead to decrease in plasma cholesterol levels, they also change the balance of prostaglandins that are formed by the cells. It is well known that platelets have the capacity to use arachidonic acid to form the prostaglandin derivative thromboxane A_2, a proaggregating factor for platelets. On the other hand, endothelial cells and smooth muscle use the same fatty acid to form, via cyclo-oxygenase, the prostaglandin metabolite prostacyclin (PGI_2), an extraordinarily potent antiaggregant and vasodilator. When the omega-3 fatty acids are fed to animals (and if they are particularly rich in eicosapentaenoic acid), they shift the balance because thromboxane A_3 derived from this fatty acid is inactive as a platelet aggregant, whereas PGI_3 is as active as PGI_2, thus favoring antiaggregant, vasodilator effects over effects that might lead to platelet aggregation and thrombosis.

Unstable Lesions and Sudden Death. The work of Davies and Thomas and Falk has provided evidence that many cases of sudden death result from lesion fissures or ruptures, which can induce hemorrhage or thrombosis and stenosis of the lumen.[161,162] Such lesions, discussed above, represent a new classification of lesions, which at present are extremely difficult to diagnose. Fibrous plaques susceptible to rupture are unstable in part due to the relative thinness of their fibrous cap, which may be partially explained by decreased formation of connective tissue by the smooth muscle cells of the lesion or by increased degradation of the matrix in the cap due to collections of macrophages often located at the shoulders of advanced lesions, which can provide connective tissue hydrolytic enzymes. If matrix removal exceeds that of deposition, then the fibrous cap that overlies the lipid-rich necrotic core of the fibrous plaque can become unstable. Stress increases on the fibrous cap of lesions located at branches and bifurcations where changes in blood flow may lead to induction of plaque rupture, hemorrhage, thrombosis, and either myocardial infarction or sudden death.

THROMBOSIS

(See also Chap. 58)

As described at the beginning of this chapter, thrombosis was originally considered to be an important component in the initiation and progression of the lesions of atherosclerosis. It now appears that thrombosis may play several roles. One prominent and potentially important clinical role is that of thrombi which become incorporated into existing advanced lesions of atherosclerosis, rapidly resulting in lumen narrowing and increase in lesion dimensions. Perhaps one of the most persistent and common complications of atherosclerosis is the formation of cracks and fissures in the advanced lesions of atherosclerosis that can act as sites for platelet attachment and formation of mural and potentially occlusive thrombi, which could lead to unstable angina or myocardial infarction.

As discussed earlier, there is good evidence in nonhuman primates and in rabbits that mural thrombi can contribute to the initiation and development of lesions of atherosclerosis.[121–125] This has also been demonstrated in humans at the perianastomotic site of coronary bypass surgery, where new lesions of atherosclerosis form in approximately 30 per cent of all bypass grafts.[173] In monkeys or rabbits receiving a hyperlipemic diet, intraarterial balloon catheter deendothelialization can lead to intimal smooth muscle proliferative lesions that appear very much like those found in hypercholesterolemic patients.

Thrombi have been observed in the coronary arteries of the vast majority of individuals who die of transmural myocardial infarction. However, thrombi are much less common in individuals who die of subendothelial infarction. Thrombosis is even less common in individuals who die of sudden cardiac death, although both thrombosis and embolism are well recognized as complications of cerebrovascular disease as well as peripheral vascular disease.

The role of the endothelium in the process of thrombosis is not entirely clear because, as discussed earlier, endothelial cells have both nonthrombogenic and procoagulant activities. Endothelial cells produce von Willebrand factor as well as plasminogen activator and prostacyclin. The development of agents that can alter thromboxane formation and thus prevent platelet interaction, or alter prostacyclin formation and thus promote platelet interactions, should make it possible to obtain a clearer idea of the role of these agents compared with others that can be produced by the endothelial cells in the process of thrombosis in general.

IMAGING ATHEROSCLEROSIS

Detection of occlusive lesions of atherosclerosis has until the present time required invasive methodology such as angiography and intravascular ultrasonography. For some peripheral arteries, it has been possible to use Doppler ultrasound techniques. However, the only current method that provides any information on the artery wall, the area occupied by the lesion, is intravascular ultrasonography (Fig. 3–95, p. 89), which is invasive and requires catheterization, possibly inducing some injury to the artery itself. Recently, Skinner et al. have taken advantage of magnetic resonance imaging (MRI) to visualize occlusive and aneurysmal lesions of atherosclerosis in rabbits[174] and more recently in nonhuman primates (unpublished observations).

With MRI not only is it possible to visualize the lumen using a procedure called "time of flight," but it also provides images similar to those seen on angiograms. This method also provides information on artery walls once they are thicker than 0.4 mm (the resolution of MRI), so that it is possible to see the lesion and fine structure of advanced lesions of atherosclerosis, such as a fibrous plaque containing a fibrous cap, necrotic core, and even fissuring. This method even allows serial imaging of experimental animals and, if used in patients, lesion progression and regression.

At present MRI can be used for peripheral arteries such as the iliac and superficial femoral arteries and for the abdominal aorta or the carotid artery. Because of motion due to breathing or heartbeat, it is not possible to use this method to visualize the thoracic aorta or the coronary arteries. However, new developments may make it feasible in the near future. Thus, on the immediate horizon is the advent of methodology to permit visualization of stenotic lesions that can be followed during therapy. Potentially dangerous lesions, which may have thin fibrous caps and may be subject to fissure, can be seen using this method, which could then permit intervention at a time prior to the disastrous consequences that can occur from rupture or fissuring of lesions.

CONCLUSIONS

Knowledge in the field of atherosclerosis has exploded and is changing rapidly. The opportunity to use the tools of cell and molecular biology, as well as new noninvasive methods for examining individuals at the clinical level, has broadened our understanding of the roles of the cells in atherogenesis. Cell and molecular biology has rapidly increased our understanding of the principal cells involved in atherosclerosis: endothelium, smooth muscle, platelets, and monocytes/macrophages and T-lymphocytes. How the risk factors that are commonly associated with an increased incidence of atherosclerosis are related to these cellular interactions is beginning to be understood, particularly in relation to hypercholesterolemia. Unfortunately, there are no good animal models that permit us to study the questions related to cigarette smoking, hypertension, diabetes, or some of the other risk factors that are epidemiologically associated with atherosclerosis. Without these, it is difficult to know the nature of the cellular interactions that occur during the genesis of the disease process as it is associated with each of these important risk factors.

Perhaps the most critical aspect of this problem is the need to understand the basis of the genetic susceptibility of individuals to these risk factors and thus to circumstances that can lead to these increased cellular interactions. Once the genetic loci for the various apoproteins are identified, and once it is possible to demonstrate altered genetic loci for these and other factors important in atherogenesis in individuals who are at increased risk for heart attack and/or stroke, it should be possible to begin to probe this question using these new tools.

Acknowledgments

This work was supported in part by US Public Health Service Grant HL-18645 and NIH grant RR-00166 to the Northwest Regional Primate Center. The author is particularly indebted to Elaine Raines, Agostino Faggiotto, Junichi Masuda, Michael Rosenfeld, Toyohiro Tsukada, Masakiyo Sasahara, Shogo Katsuda, Allen Gown, Daniel Bowen-Pope, Michael Skinner, and Yutaka Nakashima, with whom work reported from the author's laboratory was performed.

REFERENCES

RISK FACTORS

1. WHO-MONICA Project: Myocardial infarction and coronary deaths in the World Health Organization Monica Project: Registration procedures, event rates, and case-fatality rates in 38 populations from 21 countries in four continents. Circulation *90*:583, 1994.
2. Ross, R., and Glomset, J. A.: Atherosclerosis and the arterial smooth muscle cell. Science *180*:1332, 1973.
3. Ross, R., and Glomset, J. A.: The pathogenesis of atherosclerosis. N. Engl. J. Med. *295*:369, 420, 1976.
4. Ross, R., and Harker, L.: Hyperlipidemia and atherosclerosis. Science *193*:1094, 1976.
5. Fuster, V., Badimon, L., Badimon, J. J., and Chesebro, J. H.: The pathogenesis of coronary artery disease and the acute coronary syndromes. N. Engl. J. Med. *326*:242, 1992.
5a. Ross, R., and Fuster, V.: The pathogenesis of atherosclerosis. *In* Fuster, V., Ross, R., and Topol, E. J. (eds.): Atherosclerosis and Coronary Artery Disease. Philadelphia, Lippincott–Raven, 1996, pp. 441–462.
6. Dawber, T. R., Moore, F. E., and Mann, G. V.: Measuring the risk of coronary heart disease in adult population groups: II. Coronary heart disease in the Framingham study. Am. J. Public Health *47*:4, 1957.
7. American Heart Association: Heart and stroke facts. Dallas, American Heart Association National Center, 1992.
8. Cooper, E. S.: Prevention: The key to progress. Circulation *24*:629, 1993.
9. Report of the Working Group on Arteriosclerosis of the National Heart, Lung, and Blood Institute: DHEW Publication No. (NIH) 82–2035, Vol. 2. Washington, DC, US Government Printing Office, 1981.

10. Report of the Inter-Society Commission for Heart Disease Resources: Primary prevention of the atherosclerotic disease. Circulation 42:55, 1970.

11. Stamler, J., Berkson, D. M., and Lindberg, H. A.: Risk factors: Their role in the etiology and pathogenesis of the atherosclerotic diseases. In Wissler, R. W., Geer, J. C., and Kaufman, N. (eds.): The Pathogenesis of Atherosclerosis. Baltimore, Williams and Wilkins Co., 1972, p. 41.

12. Kuller, L. H.: Epidemiology of cardiovascular disease: Current perspectives. Am. J. Epidemiol. 104:425, 1976.

13. Inkeles, S., and Eisenberg, D.: Hyperlipidemia and coronary atherosclerosis: A review. Medicine 70:110, 1981.

14. Lipid Research Clinics Program: The Lipid Research Clinics Coronary Primary Prevention Trial Results: I. Reduction in incidence of coronary heart disease. JAMA 251:351, 1984.

15. Lipid Research Clinics Program: The Lipid Research Clinics Coronary Primary Prevention Trial Results: II. The relationship of reduction in incidence of coronary heart disease to cholesterol lowering. JAMA 251:365, 1984.

16. Smoking and Health, Ch. 3: Criteria for Judgment. DHEW Publication No. (NIH) 1103, Washington, DC, U.S. Government Printing Office, 1964.

17. The Pooling Project Research Group: Relationship of blood pressure, serum cholesterol, smoking habit, relative weight, and ECG abnormalities to incidence of major coronary events: Final report of the pooling project. J. Chronic Dis. 31:201, 1978.

18. Oberman, A., Harlan, W. R., Smith, M., and Graybiel, A.: The cardiovascular risk associated with different levels and types of elevated blood pressure. Minn. Med. 52:1283, 1969.

THE NORMAL ARTERY

19. 1988 Joint National Committee: The 1988 report of the Joint National Committee on detection, evaluation and treatment of high blood pressure. Arch. Intern. Med. 148:1023, 1988.

20. Glagov, S.: Hemodynamic risk factors: Mechanical stress, mural architecture, medial nutrition and the vulnerability of arteries to atherosclerosis. In Wissler, R. W., and Geer, J. C., (eds.): The Pathogenesis of Atherosclerosis. Baltimore, Williams and Wilkins, 1972, p. 164.

21. Wolinsky, H., and Glagov, S.: Comparison of abdominal and thoracic aortic medial structure in mammals: Deviation of man from the usual pattern. Circ. Res. 25:677, 1969.

22. Barger, A. C., Beeuwkes, R., Lainey, L. L., and Silverman, K. J.: Hypothesis: Vasa vasorum and neovascularization of human coronary arteries. N. Engl. J. Med. 310:175, 1984.

23. Barger, A. C., and Beeuwkes, R., III: Rupture of coronary vasa vasorum as a trigger of acute myocardial infarction. Am. J. Cardiol. 66:41G, 1990.

CELLS OF THE ARTERY AND FROM THE BLOOD POTENTIALLY INVOLVED IN ATHEROGENESIS

24. Schwartz, S. M., and Benditt, E. P.: Clustering of replicating cells in aortic endothelium. Proc. Natl. Acad. Sci. U.S.A. 73:651, 1976.

25. Schwartz, S. M., and Benditt, E. P.: Aortic endothelial cell replication. Effects of age and hypertension in the rat. Circ. Res. 41:248, 1977.

26. Simionescu, N., Simionescu, M., and Palade, G. E.: Permeability of muscle capillaries to small heme-peptides: Evidence for the existence of patent transendothelial channels. J. Cell. Biol. 64:586, 1975.

27. Gimbrone, M. A., Jr.: Culture of vascular endothelium. Prog. Hemost. Thromb. 3:1, 1976.

28. Ross, R.: The pathogenesis of atherosclerosis—an update. N. Engl. J. Med. 314:488, 1986.

29. Ross, R.: The pathogenesis of atherosclerosis: A perspective for the 1990s. Nature 362:801, 1993.

30. Renkin, E. M.: Multiple pathways of capillary permeability. Circ. Res. 41:735, 1977.

31. Moncada, S., Herman, A. G., Higgs, E. A., and Vane, J. R.: Differential formation of prostacyclin (PGX or PGI₂) by layers of the arterial wall: An explanation for the antithrombotic properties of vascular endothelium. Thromb. Res. 11:323, 1977.

32. Fielding, C. J.: Metabolism of cholesterol-rich chylomicrons: Mechanism of binding and uptake of cholesteryl esters by the vascular bed of the perfused rat heart. J. Clin. Invest. 62:141, 1978.

33. Furchgott, R. F.: Role of endothelium in responses of vascular smooth muscle. Circ. Res. 53:557, 1983.

34. Gimbrone, M. A., Jr., and Alexander, R. W.: Angiotensin II stimulation of prostaglandin production in cultured human vascular endothelium. Science 189:219, 1975.

35. Jaffe, E. A., Minick, C. R., Adelman, B., et al.: Synthesis of basement membrane by cultured human endothelial cells. J. Exp. Med. 144:209, 1976.

36. Lüscher, T. F.: Imbalance of endothelium-derived relaxing and contracting factors: A new concept in hypertension? Am. J. Hypertens. 3:317, 1990.

37. Jaffe, E. A., Hoyer, L. W., and Nachman, R. L.: Synthesis of antihemophilic factor antigen by cultured human endothelial cells. J. Clin. Invest. 52:2757, 1973.

38. Rubin, K., Tingström, A., Hansson, G. K., et al.: Induction of B-type receptors for platelet-derived growth factor in vascular inflammation: Possible implications for development of vascular proliferative lesions. Lancet 1:1353, 1988.

39. Steinberg, D.: Lipoproteins and atherosclerosis: A look back and a look ahead. Arteriosclerosis 3:283, 1983.

40. Yanagisawa, M., Kurihara, H., Kimura, S., et al.: A novel potent vasoconstrictor peptide produced by vascular endothelial cells. Nature 332:411, 1988.

41. Gajdusek, D. M., DiCorleto, P. E., Ross, R., and Schwartz, S. M.: An endothelial cell–derived growth factor. J. Cell Biol. 85:467, 1980.

42. DiCorleto, P. E., Gajdusek, C. M., Schwartz, S. M., and Ross, R.: Biochemical properties of the endothelium-derived growth factor: Comparison to other growth factors. J. Cell Physiol. 114:339, 1983.

43. DiCorleto, P. E., and Bowen-Pope, D. F.: Cultured endothelial cells produce a platelet-derived growth factor–like protein. Proc. Natl. Acad. Sci. U.S.A. 80:1919, 1983.

44. Loskutoff, D. J., and Curriden, S. A.: The fibrinolytic system of the vessel wall and its role in the control of thrombosis. Ann. N. Y. Acad. Sci. 598:238, 1990.

45. Sawdey, M. S., and Loskutoff, D. J.: Regulation of murine type 1 plasminogen activator inhibitor gene expression in vivo tissue specificity and induction by lipopolysaccharide tumor necrosis factor-alpha and transforming growth factor-beta. J. Clin. Invest. 88:1346, 1991.

46. Moncada, S., and Higgs, E. A.: Nitric oxide from L-arginine: A bioregulatory system. Amsterdam, Excerpta Medica, 1990.

46a. Owens, G. K.: Role of alterations in the differentiated state of smooth muscle cell in atherogenesis. In Fuster, V., Ross, R., and Topol, E. J. (eds.): Atherosclerosis and Coronary Artery Disease. Philadelphia, Lippincott–Raven, 1996, pp. 401–420.

47. Wissler, R. W.: The arterial medial cell, smooth muscle, or multifunctional mesenchyme? J. Atheroscler. Res. 8:201, 1968.

48. Ross, R.: The smooth muscle cells. II. Growth of smooth muscle in culture and formation of elastic fibers. J. Cell Biol. 50:172, 1971.

49. Burke, J. M., and Ross, R.: Synthesis of connective tissue macromolecules by smooth muscle. Int. Rev. Connect. Tissue Res. 8:119, 1979.

50. Chait, A., Ross, R., Albers, J. J., and Bierman, E. L.: Platelet-derived growth factor stimulates activity of low density lipoprotein receptors. Proc. Natl. Acad. Sci. U.S.A. 77:4084, 1980.

51. Bowen-Pope, D. F., Seifert, R. A., and Ross, R.: The platelet-derived growth factor receptor. In Boynton, A. L., and Leffert, H. L. (eds.): Control of Animal Cell Proliferation: Recent Advances, Vol. 1. New York, Academic Press, 1985, p. 281.

52. Seifert, R. A., Schwartz, S. M., and Bowen-Pope, D. F.: Developmentally regulated production of platelet-derived growth factor–like molecules. Nature 311:669, 1984.

53. Chamley-Campbell, J., Campbell, G., and Ross, R.: Phenotype-dependent response of cultured aortic smooth muscle to serum mitogens. J. Cell Biol. 89:379, 1981.

54. Thyberg, J., Palmberg, L., Nilsson, J., et al.: Phenotype modulation in primary cultures of arterial smooth muscle cells: On the role of platelet-derived growth factor. Differentiation 25:156, 1983.

55. Schwartz, S. M., Heimark, R. L., and Majesky, M. W.: Developmental mechanisms underlying pathology of arteries. Physiol. Rev. 70:1177, 1990.

56. Hultgardh-Nilsson, A., Krondahl, U., Querol-Ferrer, V., and Ringertz, N. R.: Differences in growth factor response in smooth muscle cells isolated from adult and neonatal rat arteries. Differentiation 47:99, 1991.

57. Ross, R., Wight, T. N., Strandness, E., and Thiele, B.: Human atherosclerosis. I. Cell constitution and characteristics of advanced lesions of the superficial femoral artery. Am. J. Pathol. 114:79, 1984.

58. Van Furth, R.: Current view on the mononuclear phagocyte system. Immunobiology 161:178, 1982.

59. Nathan, C. F., Murray, H. W., and Cohn, Z. A.: Current concepts: The macrophage as an effector cell. N. Engl. J. Med. 303:622, 1980.

60. Goldstein, J. L., Ho, Y. K., Basu, S. K., and Brown, M. S.: Binding site of macrophages that mediates uptake and degradation of acetylated low density lipoprotein, producing massive cholesterol deposition. Proc. Natl. Acad. Sci. U.S.A. 76:333, 1979.

61. Rosenfeld, M. E., Khoo, J. C., Miller, E., et al.: Macrophage-derived foam cells freshly isolated from rabbit atherosclerotic lesions degrade modified lipoproteins, promote oxidation of low-density lipoproteins, and contain oxidation-specific lipid-protein adducts. J. Clin. Invest. 87:90, 1990.

62. Martin, T. R., Altman, L. C., Albert, R. K., and Henderson, W. R.: Leukotriene B4 production by human alveolar macrophage: A potential mechanism for amplifying inflammation in the lung. Am. Rev. Respir. Dis. 129:106, 1984.

63. Bevilacqua, M. P., Pober, J. S., Cotran, R. S., and Gimbrone, M. A., Jr.: Interleukin 1 (IL 1) acts upon vascular endothelium to stimulate procoagulant activity and leukocyte adhesion. J. Cell. Biochem. 9A(Suppl. A):148, 1985.

64. Cathcart, M. K., Morel, D. W., and Chisolm, G. M.: Monocytes and neutrophils oxidize low-density lipoprotein making it cytotoxic. J. Leukoc. Biol. 38:341, 1985.

65. Ross, R., Raines, E. W., and Bowen-Pope, D. F.: The biology of platelet-derived growth factor. Cell 46:155, 1986.

66. Shimokado, K., Raines, E. W., Madtes, D. K., et al.: A significant part of macrophage-derived growth factor consists of at least two forms of PDGF. Cell 43:277, 1985.

67. Raines, E. W., Dower, S. K., and Ross, R.: Il-1 mitogenic activity for fibroblasts and smooth muscle cells is due to PDGF-AA. Science 243:393, 1989.

68. Baird, A., Mormede, P., and Bohlen, P.: Immunoreactive fibroblast-

growth factor in cells of peritoneal exudate suggests its identity with macrophage-derived growth factor. Biochem. Biophys. Res. Commun. *126*:358, 1985.

69. Ralph, P.: Colony stimulating factors. *In* Zembala, M., and Asherson, G. (eds.): Human Monocytes. New York, Academic Press, 1989, p. 228.

70. Holmsen, H., and Weiss, H. J.: Secretable storage pools in platelets. Annu. Rev. Med. *30*:119, 1979.

71. Pepper, D. S.: Macromolecules released from platelet storage organelles. Thromb. Haemost. *42*:1667, 1980.

72. Ross, R., Glomset, J., Kariya, B., and Harker, L.: A platelet-dependent serum factor that stimulates the proliferation of arterial smooth muscle cells in vitro. Proc. Natl. Acad. Sci. U.S.A. *71*:1207, 1974.

73. Oka, Y., and Orth, D. N.: Human plasma epidermal growth factor/beta-urogastrone is associated with blood platelets. J. Clin. Invest. *72*:249, 1983.

74. Assoian, R. K., Komoriya, A., Meyers, C. A., et al.: Transforming growth factor-β in human platelets: Identification of a major storage site, purification, and characterization. J. Biol. Chem. *258*:7155, 1983.

75. Baumgartner, H. R.: Platelet interaction with vascular structures. Thromb. Diath. Haemorrh. *51* (Suppl.):161, 1972.

76. Larsson, P. T., Wallen, N. H., and Hjemdahl, P.: Norepinephrine-induced human platelet activation in vivo is only partly counteracted by aspirin. Circulation *89*:1951, 1994.

77. Grignani, G., Soffiantino, F., Zucchella, M., et al.: Platelet activation by emotional stress in patients with coronary artery disease. Circulation *83* (Suppl. II):II128, 1991.

78. Fuster, V., Chesebro, J. H., Frye, R. L., and Elveback, L. R.: Platelet survival and the development of coronary artery disease in the young adult: Effects of cigarette smoking, strong family history, and medical therapy. Circulation *63*:546, 1981.

79. Ridker, P. M., Hennekens, C. H., and Stampfer, J. J.: A prospective study of lipoprotein(s) and the risk of myocardial infarction. JAMA *270*:2195, 1993.

80. Kostner, G. M., Czinner, A., Pfeiffer, K. H., and Bihari-Varga, M.: Lipoprotein(a) concentrations as indicators for atherosclerosis. Arch. Dis. Child. *66*:1054, 1991.

81. Bogalusa Heart Study: Racial (black/white) differences in serum lipoprotein(a) distribution and its relation to parental myocardial infarction in children: Bogalusa Heart Study. Circulation *84*:160, 1991.

82. Jonasson, L., Holm, J., Skalli, O., et al.: Regional accumulations of T cells, macrophages, and smooth muscle cells in the human atherosclerotic plaque. Arteriosclerosis *6*:131–138, 1986.

83. Gown, A. M., Tsukada, T., and Ross, R.: Human atherosclerosis. II. Immunocytochemical analysis of the cellular composition of human atherosclerotic lesions. Am. J. Pathol. *125*:191–207, 1986.

84. Munro, J. M., van der Walt, J. D., Munro, C. S., et al.: An immunohistochemical analysis of human aortic fatty streaks. Hum. Pathol. *18*:375, 1987.

85. Emeson, E. E., and Robertson, A. L., Jr.: T lymphocytes in aortic and coronary intimas: Their potential role in atherogenesis. Am. J. Pathol. *130*:369, 1988.

86. Minick, C. R., and Murphy, G. E.: Experimental induction of atheroarteriosclerosis by the synergy of allergic injury to arteries and lipid-rich diet. II. Effect of repeated injections of horse serum in rabbits fed a lipid-rich, cholesterol-poor diet. Am. J. Pathol. *73*:265, 1973.

87. Hansson, G. K., Holm, J., and Jonasson, L.: Detection of activated T lymphocytes in the human atherosclerotic plaque. Am. J. Pathol. *135*:169, 1989.

88. Hansson, G. K., Jonasson, L., Holm, J., and Clasesson-Welsh, L.: MHC antigen expression in the atherosclerotic plaque: Smooth muscle cells express HLA-DR, HLA-DQ, and the invariant gamma chain. Clin. Exp. Immunol. *64*:261, 1986.

89. Libby, P., and Hansson, G. K.: Involvement of the immune system in human atherogenesis: Current knowledge and unanswered questions. Lab. Invest. *64*:5, 1991.

THE LESIONS OF ATHEROSCLEROSIS

90. McGill, H. C., Jr. (ed.): The Geographic Pathology of Atherosclerosis. Baltimore, Williams and Wilkins Co., 1968.

91. Geer, J. C., McGill, H. C., Jr., and Strong, J. P.: The fine structure of human atherosclerotic lesions. Am. J. Pathol. *38*:263, 1961.

92. Geer, J. C.: Fine structure of human aortic intimal thickening and fatty streaks. Lab. Invest. *14*:1764, 1965.

93. Ghidoni, J. J., and O'Neal, R. M.: Recent advances in molecular pathology: A review: Ultrastructure of human atheroma. Exp. Mol. Pathol. *7*:378, 1967.

94. Stary, H. C., Chandler, A. B., Glagov, S., et al.: A definition of initial, fatty streak and intermediate lesions of atherosclerosis: A report from the Committee on Vascular Lesions of the Council on Arteriosclerosis, American Heart Association. Circulation *89*:2462, 1994.

95. A report from the Committee on Vascular Lesions of the Council on Arteriosclerosis, American Heart Association: Definitions of advanced types of atherosclerotic lesions and a historical classification of atherosclerosis. Circulation *15*:1512, 1995.

96. Stary, H. C.: Evolution of atherosclerotic plaques in the coronary arteries of young adults. Arteriosclerosis *3*:471a, 1983.

97. McGill, H. C., Jr.: Persistent problems in the pathogenesis of atherosclerosis. Arteriosclerosis *4*:443, 1984.

98. Tsudaka, T., Rosenfeld, M., Ross, R., and Gown, A. M.: Immunocytochemical analysis of cellular components in atherosclerotic lesions: Use of monoclonal antibodies with the Watanabe and fat-fed rabbit. Arteriosclerosis *6*:601, 1986.

99. Glagov, S., and Ozoa, A.: Significance of the relatively low incidence of atherosclerosis in the pulmonary, renal and mesenteric arteries. Ann. N. Y. Acad. Sci. *149*:940, 1968.

100. Strong, J. P., Eggen, D. A., and Oalmann, M. C.: The natural history, geographic pathology, and epidemiology of atherosclerosis. *In* Wissler, R. W., and Geer, J. C. (eds.): The Pathogenesis of Atherosclerosis. Baltimore, Williams and Wilkins Co., 1972, p. 20.

101. Glagov, S., Rowley, D. A., Cramer, D. B., and Page, R. G.: Heart rate during 24 hours of usual activity in 100 normal men. J. Appl. Physiol. *29*:799, 1970.

102. Wissler, R. W., and Vesselinovitch, D.: Atherosclerosis—relationship to coronary blood flow. Am. J. Cardiol. *52*:2A, 1983.

HYPOTHESES OF ATHEROGENESIS

103. Virchow, R.: Phlogose und thrombose in gefassystem. *In* Virchow, R. (ed.): Gesammelte Abhandlungen zur Wissenschaftlichen Medicin. Berlin, Meidinger Sohn and Co., 1856, p. 458.

104. von Rokitansky, C.: A Manual of Pathological Anatomy, translated by Day, G. E. Vol. 4. London, The Sydenham Society, 1852.

105. Duguid, J. B.: Thrombosis as a factor in the pathogenesis of coronary atherosclerosis. J. Pathol. Bacteriol. *58*:207, 1946.

106. Ross, R.: Atherosclerosis—a problem of the biology of arterial wall cells and their interaction with blood components. Arteriosclerosis *1*:293, 1981.

107. Benditt, E. P., and Benditt, J. M.: Evidence for a monoclonal origin of human atherosclerotic plaques. Proc. Natl. Acad. Sci. U.S.A. *70*:1753, 1973.

108. Hajjar, D. P., Fabricant, C. G., Minick, C. R., and Fabricant, J.: Virus-induced atherosclerosis: Herpes virus infection alters arterial cholesterol metabolism and accumulation. Am. J. Pathol. *122*:62, 1986.

108a. Glasser, S. P., Selwyn, A. F., and Ganz, P.: Atherosclerosis: Risk factors and the vascular endothelium. Am. Heart J. *131*:379, 1996.

109. Kuo, C. C., Gown, A. M., Benditt, E. P., and Grayston, J. T.: Detection of *Chlamydia pneumoniae* in aortic lesions of atherosclerosis by immunocytochemical stain. Arterioscler. Thromb. *13*:1501, 1993.

110. Leary, T.: The genesis of atherosclerosis. Arch. Pathol. *32*:507, 1941.

111. Springer, T. A.: Adhesion receptors of the immune system. Nature *346*:425, 1990.

112. Cybulsky, M. I., and Gimbrone, M. A., Jr.: Endothelial expression of a mononuclear leukocyte adhesion molecule during atherogenesis. Science *251*:788, 1991.

113. Navab, M., Hama, S. Y., Nguyen, T. B., and Fogelman, A. M.: Monocyte adhesion and transmigration in atherosclerosis. Cor. Art. Dis. *5*:198, 1994.

114. Parthasarathy, S., Quinn, M. T., Schwenke, D. C., et al.: Oxidative modification of beta-very low density lipoprotein: Potential role in monocyte recruitment and foam cell formation. Arteriosclerosis *9*:398, 1989.

115. Goldstein, J. L., Ho, Y. K., Basu, S. K., and Brown, M. S.: Binding site of macrophages that mediates uptake and degradation of acetylated low density lipoprotein, producing massive cholesterol deposition. Proc. Natl. Acad. Sci. U.S.A. *76*:333, 1979.

116. Steinberg, D.: Antioxidants and atherosclerosis: A current perspective. Circulation *86*:1420, 1991.

117. Kodama, T., Freeman, M., Rohrer, L., et al.: Type I macrophage scavenger receptor contains α-helical and collagen-like coiled coils. Nature *343*:531, 1990.

118. Assoian, R. K., Grotendorst, G. R., Miller, D. M., and Sporn, M. B.: Cellular transformation by coordinated action of three peptide growth factors from human platelets. Nature *309*:804, 1984.

119. Sporn, M. B., Roberts, A. B., Wakefield, L. M., and de Crombrugghe, B.: Some recent advances in the chemistry and biology of transforming growth factor-beta. J. Cell. Biol. *105*:1039, 1987.

120. Ross, R., Masuda, J., Raines, E. W., et al.: Localization of PDGF-B protein in macrophages in all phases of atherogenesis. Science *248*:1009, 1990.

121. Stemerman, M. B., and Ross, R.: Experimental arteriosclerosis. I. Fibrous plaque formation in primates, an electron microscope study. J. Exp. Med. *136*:769, 1972.

122. Shepard, B. L., and French, J. E.: Platelet adhesion in the rabbit abdominal aorta following the removal of the endothelium: A scanning and transmission electron microscopical study. Proc. R. Soc. Lond. (Biol.) *176*:427, 1971.

123. More, S.: Thromboatherosclerosis in normolipemic rabbits: A result of continued endothelial damage. Lab. Invest. *29*:478, 1973.

124. Friedman, R. J., Moore, S., and Singal, D. P.: Repeated endothelial injury and induction of atherosclerosis in normolipemic rabbits by human serum. Lab. Invest. *32*:404, 1975.

125. Harker, L. A., Ross, R., Slichter, S. J., and Scott, C. R.: Homocystine-induced arteriosclerosis: The role of endothelial cell injury and platelet response in its genesis. J. Clin. Invest. *58*:731, 1976.

126. Libby, P., Warner, S. J. C., Salomon, R. N., and Birinyi, L. K.: Production of platelet-derived growth factor–like mitogen by smooth-muscle cells from human atheroma. N. Engl. J. Med. *318*:1493, 1988.

LIPIDS AND LIPOPROTEINS AND MODIFIED LDL IN ATHEROSCLEROSIS

127. Jackson, R. L., and Gotto, A. M., Jr.: Hypothesis concerning membrane structure, cholesterol, and atherosclerosis. *In* Paoletti, R., and Gotto,

A. M., Jr. (eds.): Atherosclerosis Reviews. Vol. 1. New York, Raven Press, 1976, p. 1.

128. Carew, T. E., Schwenke, D. C., and Steinberg, D.: Antiatherogenic effect of probucol unrelated to its hypocholesterolemic effect: Evidence that antioxidants in vivo can selectively inhibit low density lipoprotein degradation in macrophage-rich fatty streaks and slow the progression of atherosclerosis in the Watanabe heritable hyperlipidemic (WHHL) rabbit. Proc. Natl. Acad. Sci. U.S.A. 84:7725, 1987.

129. Kita, T., Nagano, Y., Yokode, M., et al.: Probucol prevents the progression of atherosclerosis in Watanabe heritable hyperlipidemic rabbit, an animal model for familial hypercholesterolemia. Proc. Natl. Acad. Sci. U.S.A. 84:5928, 1987.

130. Sasahara, M., Raines, E. W., Chait, A., et al.: Inhibition of hypercholesterolemia-induced atherosclerosis in the nonhuman primate by probucol. I. Is the extent of atherosclerosis related to resistance of LDL to oxidation? J. Clin. Invest. 94:155, 1994.

131. Boyd, H. C., Gown, A. M., Wolfbauer, G., and Chait, A.: Direct evidence for a protein recognized by a monoclonal antibody against oxidatively modified LDL in atherosclerotic lesions from a Watanabe heritable hyperlipidemic rabbit. Am. J. Pathol. 135:815, 1989.

GROWTH FACTORS AND CYTOKINES

132. Bowen-Pope, D. F., and Ross, R.: Platelet-derived growth factor. II. Specific binding to cultured cells. J. Biol. Chem. 257:5161, 1982.

133. Grotendorst, G., Seppa, H. E. J., Kleinman, H. K., and Martin, G.: Attachment of smooth muscle cells to collagen and their migration toward platelet-derived growth factor. Proc. Natl. Acad. Sci. U.S.A. 78:3669, 1981.

134. Grotendorst, G. R., Chang, T., Seppa, H. E. J., et al.: Platelet-derived growth factor is a chemoattractant for vascular smooth muscle cells. J. Cell. Physiol. 113:261, 1982.

135. Witte, L. D., and Cornicelli, J. A.: Platelet-derived growth factor stimulates low density lipoprotein receptor activity in cultured human fibroblasts. Proc. Natl. Acad. Sci. U.S.A. 77:5962, 1986.

136. Bowen-Pope, D. F., Malpass, T. W., Foster, D. M., and Ross, R.: Platelet-derived growth factor in vivo: Levels, activity, and rate of clearance. Blood 64:458, 1984.

137. Raines, E. W., Bowen-Pope, D. F., and Ross, R.: Plasma binding proteins for platelet-derived growth factor that inhibit its binding to cell-surface receptors. Proc. Natl. Acad. Sci. U.S.A. 81:3424, 1984.

138. Doolittle, R. F., Hunkapiller, M. W., Hood, L. E., et al.: Simian sarcoma virus onc gene, v-sis, is derived from the gene (or genes) encoding a platelet-derived growth factor. Science 221:275, 1983.

139. Waterfield, M. D., Scrace, G. T., Whittle, N., et al.: Platelet-derived growth factor is structurally related to the putative transforming protein p28^sis of simian sarcoma virus. Nature 304:35, 1983.

140. Bowen-Pope, D. F., Vogel, A., and Ross, R.: Production of platelet-derived growth factor–like molecules and reduced expression of platelet-derived growth factor receptors accompany transformation by a wide spectrum of agents. Proc. Natl. Acad. Sci. U.S.A. 81:2396, 1984.

141. Seifert, R. A., Hart, C. E., Phillips, P. E., et al.: Two different subunits associate to create isoform-specific platelet-derived growth factor receptors. J. Biol. Chem. 264:8771, 1989.

CELLULAR EVENTS THAT OCCUR DURING ATHEROGENESIS

142. Faggiotto, A., Ross, R., and Harker, L.: Studies of hypercholesterolemia in the nonhuman primate. I. Changes that lead to fatty streak formation. Arteriosclerosis 4:323, 1984.

143. Faggiotto, A., and Ross, R.: Studies of hypercholesterolemia in the nonhuman primate. II. Fatty streak conversion to fibrous plaque. Arteriosclerosis 4:341, 1984.

144. Masuda, J., and Ross, R.: Atherogenesis during low-level hypercholesterolemia in the nonhuman primate. I. Fatty streak formation. Arteriosclerosis 10:164, 1990.

145. Masuda, J., and Ross, R.: Atherogenesis during low-level hypercholesterolemia in the nonhuman primate. II. Fatty streak conversion to fibrous plaque. Arteriosclerosis 10:178, 1990.

146. Gerrity, R. G., Naito, H. K., Richardson, M., and Schwartz, C. J.: Dietary induced atherogenesis in swine: Morphology of the intima in prelesion stages. Am. J. Pathol. 95:775, 1979.

147. Gerrity, R. G.: The role of the monocyte in atherogenesis. I. Transition of blood-borne monocytes into foam cells in fatty lesions. Am. J. Pathol. 103:181, 1981.

148. Gerrity, R. G., Goss, J. A., and Soby, L.: Control of monocyte recruitment by chemotactic factor(s) in lesion-prone areas of swine aorta. Arteriosclerosis 5:55, 1985.

149. Rosenfeld, M. E., Tsukada, T., Chait, A., et al.: Fatty streak expansion and maturation in Watanabe heritable hyperlipemic and comparably hypercholesterolemic fat-fed rabbits. Arteriosclerosis 7:24, 1987.

150. Nakashima, Y., Plump, A. S., Raines, E. W., et al.: ApoE-deficient mice develop lesions of all phases of atherosclerosis throughout the arterial tree. Arterioscler. Thromb. 14:133, 1994.

151. Reddick, R. L., Zhang, S. H., and Maeda, N.: Atherosclerosis in mice lacking apo E: Evaluation of lesional development and progression. Arterioscler. Thromb. 14:141, 1994.

152. Reidy, M. A., and Schwartz, S. M.: Endothelial regeneration. III. Time course of intimal changes after small defined injury to rat aortic endothelium. Lab. Invest. 44:301, 1981.

153. Reidy, M. A., and Schwartz, S. M.: Endothelial regeneration. IV. Endotoxin: A nondenuding injury to aortic endothelium. Lab. Invest. 48:25, 1983.

154. Hansson, G. K., Bondjers, G., Bylock, A., and Hjalmarsson, L.: Ultrastructural studies on nonatherosclerotic rabbits. Exp. Mol. Pathol. 33:301, 1980.

155. Reidy, M. A., and Schwartz, S. M.: Recent advances in molecular pathology: Arterial endothelium—assessment of in vivo injury. Exp. Mol. Pathol. 41:419, 1984.

REGRESSION OF ATHEROSCLEROSIS

156. Armstrong, M. L., Warner, E. D., and Conner, W. E.: Regression of coronary atheromatosis in rhesus monkeys. Circ. Res. 27:59, 1970.

157. Wissler, R. W., and Vesselinovitch, D.: Studies of regression of advanced atherosclerosis in experimental animals and man. Ann. N. Y. Acad. Sci. 275:363, 1976.

158. Clarkson, T. B., Bond, M. G., Bullock, B. C., et al.: A study of atherosclerosis regression in Macaca mulatta. V. Changes in abdominal aorta and carotid and coronary arteries from animals with atherosclerosis induced for 38 months and then regressed for 24 or 48 months at plasma cholesterol concentrations of 300 or 200 mg/dl. Exp. Mol. Pathol. 41:96, 1984.

159. Badimon, J. J., Badimon, L., and Fuster, V.: Regression of atherosclerotic lesions by high density lipoprotein plasma fraction in the cholesterol-fed rabbit. J. Clin. Invest. 85:1234, 1990.

160. Brown, B. G., Albers, J. J., Fisher, L. D., et al.: Treatment study: A randomized trial demonstrating coronary disease regression and clinical benefit from lipid altering therapy among men with high apolipoprotein B. N. Engl. J. Med. 323:1289, 1990.

161. Davies, M. J., and Thomas, A. C.: Plaque fissuring: The cause of acute myocardial infarction, sudden ischemic death and crescendo angina. Br. Heart J. 53:363, 1985.

162. Falk, E.: Unstable angina with fatal outcome: Dynamic coronary thrombosis leading to infarction and/or sudden death: Autopsy evidence of recurrent mural thrombosis with peripheral embolization culminating in total vascular occlusion. Circulation 71:699, 1985.

163. Blankenhorn, D. H., and Hodis, H. N.: Arterial imaging and atherosclerosis reversal. Arterioscler. Thromb. 14:177, 1994.

164. Brown, B. G., Zhao, X.-Q., Sacco, D. E., and Albers, J. J.: Lipid lowering and plaque regression: New insights into prevention of plaque disruption and clinical events in coronary disease. Circulation 87:1781, 1993.

165. Brensike, J. F., Levy, R. I., Kelsey, S. F., et al.: Effects of therapy with cholestyramine on progression of coronary arteriosclerosis: Results of the NHLBI Type II Coronary Intervention Study. Circulation 69:313, 1984.

166. Blankenhorn, D. H., Selzer, R. H., Mack, W. J., et al.: Evaluation of colestipol/niacin therapy with computer-derived coronary end point measures: A comparison of different measures of treatment effect. Circulation 86:1701, 1992.

167. Ornish, D., Brown, S. E., Scherwitz, L. W., et al.: Can lifestyle changes reverse coronary heart disease? The lifestyle heart trial. Lancet 336:129, 1990.

168. Buchwald, H., Matts, J. P., Fitch, L. L., et al., for the Program on the Surgical Control of the Hyperlipidemias (POSCH) Group: Changes in sequential coronary arteriograms and subsequent coronary events. JAMA 268:1429, 1992.

169. Kane, J. P., Malloy, M. J., Ports, T. A., et al.: Regression of coronary atherosclerosis during treatment of familial hypercholesterolemia with combined drug regimens. JAMA 264:3007, 1990.

170. Watts, G. F., Lewis, B., Brunt, J. N., et al.: Effects on coronary artery disease of lipid-lowering diet, or diet plus cholestyramine, in the St. Thomas' Atherosclerosis Regression Study (STARS). Lancet 339:563, 1992.

171. Haskell, W. L., Alderman, E. L., Fair, J. M., et al.: Effects of intensive multiple risk factor reduction on coronary atherosclerosis and clinical cardiac events in men and women with coronary artery disease: The Stanford Coronary Risk Intervention Project (SCRIP). Circulation 89:1994.

172. Cannon, P. J.: Eicosanoids and the blood vessel wall. Circulation 70:523, 1984.

THROMBOSIS

173. Chesebro, J. H., Clements, I. P., Fuster, V., et al.: A platelet-inhibitor–drug trial in coronary-artery bypass operations: Benefit of perioperative dipyridamole and aspirin therapy on early postoperative vein-graft patency. N. Engl. J. Med. 307:73, 1982.

174. Skinner, M. P., Yuan, C., Mitsumori, L., et al.: Serial magnetic resonance imaging of experimental atherosclerosis detects lesion fine structure, progression, and complications in vivo. Nature Med. 1:69, 1995.

Chapter 35
Dyslipidemia and Other Risk Factors for Coronary Artery Disease

JOHN A. FARMER, ANTONIO M. GOTTO, Jr.

DECLINING MORTALITY AND THE RISK FACTOR CONCEPT

Coronary artery disease (CAD) is the single most important disease entity in the United States and many other industrialized nations in terms of both mortality and morbidity. In the United States, CAD accounts for fully one-half of the nearly 1 million deaths each year from cardiovascular disease and is the leading cause of death in both genders.[1] Each year, about 1.5 million Americans suffer acute myocardial infarction, and almost all myocardial infarctions are due to atherosclerosis of the coronary arteries. Among the two-thirds who survive the myocardial infarction, about two-thirds do not make a full recovery; in 19 per cent of Americans aged 15 years or older who are categorized as disabled, the disability is from CAD or other cardiovascular disease.[1] CAD often strikes at the height of working careers. About 45 per cent of myocardial infarctions occur in people under age 65, and about 37 per cent of American males and 29 per cent of American females who die of CAD are younger than 55.[1] The economic burden of CAD to the nation is also enormous: An estimated $50 billion to $100 billion per year in medical interventions and lost wages.[2,3]

Nevertheless, an encouraging downward trend in CAD death rates in the United States began in the early 1960's and has continued. The CAD mortality rate fell 54 per cent between 1963 and 1990, accounting for 49 per cent of the decline in the total mortality rate.[4] In 1950, the annual age-adjusted death rate from myocardial infarction was 226.4 per 100,000; in 1991, it was 108.0.[1] The period of 1982 to 1992 alone saw a 31 per cent decline in myocardial infarction death rate.[1] These decreases have coincided with national risk reduction efforts—beginning in the 1960's, 1970's, and 1980's, respectively—against the major CAD risk factors of smoking, hypertension, and hypercholesterolemia, as well as with the improvement of therapies for myocardial infarction. The percentage of Americans who smoke has declined 37 per cent since 1965,[1] although there may now be a leveling off and even an increase in some groups, notably young women. The annual death rate from hypertension was 56.0 per 100,000 in 1950, compared with 6.5 in 1991.[1] Between 1960 and 1991, the average plasma cholesterol level decreased from 220 mg/dl to 205 mg/dl in Americans aged 20 to 74 years.[4] Nevertheless, these risk factors remain common: estimates are that 28 per cent of American men and 22 per cent of American women smoke,[5] 25 and 23 per cent have hypertension,[6] and 32 and 27 per cent have hypercholesterolemia[7] that requires di-

etary therapy by current National Cholesterol Education Program (NCEP) clinical guidelines.[2,3]

Risk factor reduction is the primary clinical approach to preventing CAD morbidity and mortality. Epidemiological studies have clearly demonstrated that risk factors such as dyslipidemia, hypertension, and the use of tobacco products act in a synergistic manner.[8] The concept of risk factor identification and modification is based on the premise that exposure to certain host and environmental factors increases the statistical risk for developing a disease and that alteration of these conditions decreases the risk. However, a given factor may not stand in a cause-and-effect relation to the disease but may be simply a nonspecific marker of the disease process. Criteria for determining whether an observed statistical association reflects causality include strength of the association, expressed by the relative risk of individuals exposed to a certain factor compared with individuals not exposed; whether the association represents a dose–response relation, so that relative risk is progressively increased at increasing levels of exposure to the factor; precedence of exposure to clinical onset of disease; consistency of results in different populations; independence of the association when controlling for other known risk factors; predictivity of disease incidence in different populations; and biological plausibility.[9]

Major CAD risk factors established by these criteria are dyslipidemia, hypertension, tobacco use, and diabetes mellitus. Other CAD risk factors include physical inactivity, obesity, family history of CAD, age, gender, hemostatic factors, homocysteinemia, alcohol consumption, and psychological factors. The identification of risk factors provides a means for decreasing CAD risk, through the reduction of modifiable risk factors, and for informing treatment decisions, through more accurate determination of overall risk status.

DYSLIPIDEMIA

Lipids are transported through the plasma compartment in lipoproteins, complex water-soluble molecules consisting of a core of cholesteryl ester and triglyceride covered by a surface monolayer of phospholipids, free cholesterol, and apolipoproteins. The major plasma lipoproteins—chylomicrons, very-low-density lipoprotein (VLDL), intermediate-density lipoprotein (IDL), low-density lipoprotein (LDL), and high-density lipoprotein (HDL)—are distinguished by lipid content, density on ultracentrifugation, size, mobility on electrophoresis, and the proteins on their

LIPOPROTEIN CLASS	MAJOR LIPIDS	APOLIPOPROTEINS	DENSITY (g/ml)	DIAMETER (Å)	ELECTROPHORETIC MOBILITY
Chylomicrons	Dietary triglyceride, cholesteryl ester	A-I, A-II, A-IV, B-48, C-I, C-II, C-III, E	<0.95	800–5000	Origin
Chylomicron remnants	Dietary cholesteryl ester	B-48, E	<1.006	>300	Origin
VLDL	Endogenous triglyceride	B-100, C-I, C-II, C-III, E	<1.006	300–800	Pre-beta
IDL	Cholesteryl ester, triglyceride	B-100, E	1.006–1.019	250–350	Broad-beta
LDL	Cholesteryl ester	B-100	1.019–1.063	180–280	Beta
HDL$_2$	Cholesteryl ester	A-I, A-II, C-I, C-II, C-III, E	1.063–1.125	90–120	Alpha
HDL$_3$	Cholesteryl ester	A-I, A-II, C-I, C-II, C-III, E	1.125–1.210	50–90	Alpha

Abbreviations: HDL = high-density lipoprotein; IDL = intermediate-density lipoprotein; LDL = low-density lipoprotein; VLDL = very-low-density lipoprotein.

surfaces (Table 35–1). The lipoproteins vary in their contribution to atherosclerotic risk: The triglyceride-rich lipoproteins—chylomicrons and VLDL—are not thought to be atherogenic, but the remnants of their lipolysis—chylomicron remnants and IDL, respectively—are believed to be atherogenic. The atherogenicity of LDL—the metabolic end product of VLDL—and lipoprotein(a) [Lp(a)] has been established, as has the cardioprotective effect of HDL (see below).

In dyslipidemia, circulating levels of lipid or lipoprotein fractions are abnormal because of genetic and/or environmental conditions that alter the production, catabolism, or clearance of plasma lipoproteins from the circulation. Dyslipidemias may be classified according to which lipoprotein levels are abnormal, as in the Fredrickson classification system (Table 35–2). The Fredrickson classification system is not diagnostic and does not consider HDL or Lp(a).

Hypercholesterolemia

The dyslipidemia most clearly associated with increased risk for CAD is hypercholesterolemia, particularly elevated plasma levels of cholesterol carried in LDL. LDL contains approximately 70 per cent of cholesterol in the blood and is the primary target of intervention in the guidelines of the second Adult Treatment Panel of the NCEP.[2,3]

The association between elevated blood cholesterol and CAD has been established in observational and interventional epidemiological studies, examples of which are presented here. These data support the lipid hypothesis: CAD risk is increased at increasing plasma cholesterol levels and can be decreased by decreasing plasma cholesterol.

Observational Studies

A continuous and graded positive relation was demonstrated between total cholesterol level and CAD mortality in the more than 350,000 men screened for the Multiple Risk Factor Intervention Trial (MRFIT).[10] The relation between total cholesterol level and coronary disease is not limited by nationality or ethnicity, as demonstrated in the Seven Countries Study, which determined that in areas such as Japan and countries surrounding the Mediterranean Sea, where the dietary intake of saturated fat is low and average plasma cholesterol level is relatively low, the mortality rate for CAD is also low, compared with countries such as Finland and the United States, where both the average plasma cholesterol level and the coronary mortality rate are higher.[11] Similarly, in the Ni-Hon-San Study, men of Japanese descent living in the United States consumed a diet higher in fat and cholesterol than Japanese men living in Japan[12] and had higher total cholesterol levels[13] and a higher age-adjusted incidence of myocardial infarction and CAD death.[14]

Interventional Studies in Primary Prevention

Although observational data lend credence to the lipid hypothesis, they do not demonstrate the effect of cholesterol lowering on coronary morbidity and mortality. Consequently, randomized, controlled clinical trials have employed a variety of interventions to determine the efficacy of cholesterol lowering in preventing CAD events in individuals free of known CAD, or primary prevention, and in preventing subsequent CAD events in subjects with known CAD, or secondary prevention.

Cholesterol-lowering interventions used to prevent CAD in subjects without known CAD have included pharmacological monotherapy and life style modification. Clinical events such as myocardial infarction and CAD death are typical endpoints in these studies.

LIPID RESEARCH CLINICS CORONARY PRIMARY PREVENTION TRIAL. The Lipid Research Clinics Coronary Primary Prevention Trial (LRC-CPPT) randomized 3806 hypercholesterolemic men (total cholesterol ≥265 mg/dl, LDL cholesterol ≥190 mg/dl, triglyceride ≤300 mg/dl), aged 35 to 59 years, to receive either the bile-acid sequestrant cholestyramine at a prescribed dosage of 24 gm/day or a placebo.[15] All subjects were to follow a moderate cholesterol-lowering diet (cholesterol 400 mg/day, polyunsaturated fat:saturated fat ratio 0.8). The study design predicted a 28 per cent decrease in total cholesterol in cholestyramine subjects ad-

TABLE 35–2   FREDRICKSON CLASSIFICATION OF THE HYPERLIPIDEMIAS*

PHENOTYPE	LIPOPROTEIN(S) ELEVATED	PLASMA CHOLESTEROL LEVEL	PLASMA TRIGLYCERIDE LEVEL	ATHEROGENICITY	RELATIVE FREQUENCY†
I	Chylomicrons	Normal to ↑	↑↑↑↑	None seen	<1%
IIa	LDL	↑↑	Normal	+++	10%
IIb	LDL and VLDL	↑↑	↑↑	+++	40%
III	IDL	↑↑	↑↑↑	+++	<1%
IV	VLDL	Normal to ↑	↑↑↑	+	45%
V	VLDL and chylomicrons	↑ to ↑↑	↑↑↑↑	+	5%

* The Fredrickson classification does not consider levels of high-density lipoprotein (HDL) cholesterol. It is not an etiological classification and does not differentiate primary and secondary hyperlipidemias.
† Approximate percentages of US patients with hyperlipidemia.
Abbreviations: IDL = intermediate-density lipoprotein; LDL = low-density lipoprotein; VLDL = very-low-density lipoprotein.
(From International Lipid Information Bureau: The ILIB Lipid Handbook for Clinical Practice: Blood Lipids and Coronary Heart Disease. Houston, International Lipid Information Bureau, 1995.)

hering to the prescribed dosage, but adherence was lower than expected because of gastrointestinal side effects and poor palatability of the drug. The actual cholestyramine dosage averaged 14 gm/day. The average time on trial was 7.4 years.

In the placebo group, diet alone decreased total cholesterol 5 per cent. Total cholesterol decreased 13 per cent from baseline in the group treated with diet and cholestyramine, and LDL cholesterol decreased 8 per cent and 20 per cent in the respective groups. In the cholestyramine group, the primary endpoint of nonfatal myocardial infarction and CAD death was significantly reduced 19 per cent. Development of new-onset angina pectoris was significantly reduced 20 per cent in the cholestyramine group, and incidence of new positive exercise stress test results was significantly reduced 25 per cent. Incidence of coronary bypass surgery was reduced 21 per cent, which was not statistically significant. CAD mortality was reduced 24 per cent, but total mortality was reduced only 7 per cent because of an increase in noncardiovascular deaths, particularly accidental and violent deaths; neither of these reductions in mortality was significant.

In the cholestyramine group, 32 per cent of subjects achieved a reduction in LDL cholesterol that was greater than 25 per cent. In this subgroup, the incidence of nonfatal myocardial infarction and CAD death was reduced 64 per cent.[16]

The LRC-CPPT provided the first major clinical substantiation of the lipid hypothesis. Its results were the first to give rise to the rule of thumb that a 1 per cent decrease in total cholesterol reduces the incidence of CAD events 2 to 3 per cent.

WORLD HEALTH ORGANIZATION COOPERATIVE TRIAL. The World Health Organization (WHO) Cooperative Trial randomized more than 10,000 men, aged 30 to 59 years, with total cholesterol level in the upper tertile of those screened for the trial, in which they received either the fibric-acid derivative clofibrate, 1600 mg/day, or a placebo.[17] Mean duration of treatment was 5.3 years. Results were not initially analyzed on an intent-to-treat basis, and data on subjects who dropped out of the trial because of morbid events, including nonfatal myocardial infarction, were not included in the original analysis.

In the group receiving clofibrate, total cholesterol decreased 9 per cent from baseline, and CAD incidence was significantly reduced 20 per cent. However, total mortality was increased in this group, largely due to an increase in noncardiovascular deaths. An analysis conducted almost 8 years after the trial ended indicated that the excess in mortality with clofibrate decreased from 47 per cent during the trial to 11 per cent during the entire 13 years of follow-up and was no longer statistically significant.[18]

HELSINKI HEART STUDY. The Helsinki Heart Study randomized 4081 men, aged 40 to 55 years, with non-HDL cholesterol greater than 200 mg/dl to receive the fibric-acid derivative gemfibrozil, 1200 mg/day, or placebo for 5 years.[19] Included in the trial were hypertriglyceridemic as well as hypercholesterolemic subjects. All subjects also received dietary counseling.

Compared with the placebo group, the gemfibrozil group had a 10 per cent decrease in total cholesterol, an 11 per cent decrease in LDL cholesterol, an 11 per cent increase in HDL cholesterol, and a 35 per cent decrease in triglyceride. The primary endpoint, incidence of cardiac events, defined as fatal and nonfatal myocardial infarction and cardiac death, was significantly reduced 34 per cent in the gemfibrozil group. CAD mortality was 26 per cent lower in the gemfibrozil group, but total mortality was slightly higher because of an increase in noncardiovascular deaths, particularly deaths due to accidents, violence, or intracranial hemorrhage; none of these differences was statistically significant.[20]

OSLO STUDY DIET AND ANTISMOKING TRIAL. The Oslo Study Diet and Antismoking Trial randomized 1232 men, aged 40 to 49 years, with total cholesterol of 290 to 380 mg/dl, systolic blood pressure below 150 mm Hg, and a coronary risk score, based on cholesterol, smoking, and blood pressure, in the highest quartile of the distribution.[21] Subjects in the intervention group were given dietary and antismoking advice. Approximately 80 per cent of each group were smokers.

During the 5-year trial, total cholesterol in the intervention group decreased approximately 13 per cent compared with the control group, and triglyceride decreased 20 per cent. Although the quantity of cigarettes smoked decreased 45 per cent more in the intervention group than in the control group, only 25 per cent of smokers in the intervention group stopped smoking, compared with 17 per cent of smokers in the control group. Incidence of fatal and nonfatal myocardial infarction and sudden coronary death was significantly reduced 47 per cent in the intervention group. The difference in CAD incidence between treatment groups was thought to be largely due to the reduction in total cholesterol, and 25 per cent was attributed to reduced cigarette consumption. Coronary mortality was reduced 55 per cent and total mortality was reduced 33 per cent in the intervention group, but these differences were not statistically significant.

At 102-month follow-up, 3 years after the trial was completed, the reduction in total cholesterol achieved by the intervention group during the trial was maintained.[22] Total cholesterol in the control group was reduced but remained higher than in the intervention group. Cigarette consumption in the intervention group was higher than at the end of the trial, although not as high as baseline; cigarette consumption in the control group remained about the same as at the end of the trial and only slightly higher than in the intervention group. Although the differences in risk factors between treatment groups were less than during the trial, between-group differences in incidence of fatal and nonfatal myocardial infarction and sudden coronary death remained the same as during the trial. Sudden death, coronary death, and total coronary events occurred significantly less frequently in the intervention group. Total mortality was reduced 40 per cent in the intervention group, which was a marginally significant difference.

WEST OF SCOTLAND CORONARY PREVENTION STUDY. The benefit of lipid-lowering with a 3-hydroxy-3-methylglutaryl coenzyme A (HMG-CoA) reductase inhibitor was extended to primary prevention in the West of Scotland Coronary Prevention Study (WOSCOPS), which randomized 6595 men, aged 45 to 64 years, with no history of myocardial infarction to receive pravastatin, 40 mg/day, or placebo.[22a] Eligible subjects had an LDL cholesterol level of at least 155 mg/dl on two assessments despite dietary therapy, at least 174 mg/dl on at least one assessment, and no more than 232 mg/dl on one assessment. Individuals with stable angina were not excluded if they had not been hospitalized within the previous year. The primary endpoint was either definite nonfatal myocardial infarction or CAD death as a first event. Mean follow-up was 4.9 years.

Lipid changes by intent-to-treat analysis are not available, but in subjects who actually received pravastatin, total plasma cholesterol was decreased 20 per cent, LDL cholesterol was decreased 26 per cent, triglyceride was decreased 12 per cent, and HDL cholesterol was increased 5 per cent.

For the primary endpoint, the relative risk in the group randomized to pravastatin was reduced 31 per cent compared with the group randomized to placebo, which was a significant difference. Noncardiovascular mortality was not significantly different between treatment groups. The group randomized to pravastatin had a 22 per cent reduction in death resulting from any cause compared with the group randomized to placebo, but this difference was of borderline statistical significance (P = .051).

TABLE 35–3   MAJOR ANGIOGRAPHICALLY MONITORED LIPID-LOWERING TRIALS IN PATIENTS WITH CORONARY ATHEROSCLEROSIS: LIPID AND ANGIOGRAPHIC RESULTS

| TRIAL* | SUBJECTS† | TRIAL PERIOD (YR) | INTERVENTION‡ | PER CENT LIPID RESPONSE (RX/CONTROL) | | ASSESSMENTS§ | PER CENT PATIENTS WITH CORONARY LESION | | EVENTS (RX/CONTROL)‖ |
				TC	LDL-C		Progression (Rx/Control)	Regression (Rx/Control)	
NHLBI	143 M + F	5	Ch	−17/−1	−26/−5	P	32/49	7/7	8/12
CLAS I	188 M	2	C + N	−26/−4	−43/−5	P	39/61	16/4	25/25
CLAS II	103 M	4	C + N	−25/−6	−40/−6	P	48/85	18/6	15/14
FATS	120 M	2.5	C + N	−23/−3	−32/−7	Q	25/46	39/11	2/10
			C + L	−34/−3	−46/−7	Q	21/46	32/11	3/10
UCSF-SCOR	72 M + F	2	C/N/L¶	−31/−9	−39/−12	Q	20/41	32/13	0/1
STARS	90 M	3	Ch	−25/−2	−36/−3	Q	12/46	33/4	1/10
			Diet alone	−14/−2	−16/−3	Q	15/46	38/4	3/10
POSCH	838 M + F	5**	PIB	−28/−5	−42/−7	P	37/65	13/5	
		10**		−22/−4	−39/−6	P	55/85	6/4	82/125
LHT	48 M + F	1	Life style	−24/−5	−37/−6	Q	18/53	82/42	Not available
MARS	270 M + F	2	L	−32/−2	−45/−3	Q	29/41	23/12	22/31
						P	47/65	23/11	
CCAIT	331 M + F	2	L	−21/−1	−29/−2	Q	33/50	10/7	15/20
REGRESS	885 M	2	P	−20/+2	−29/+2	Q	45/55	17/9	59/93
MAAS	381 M + F	4	S	−22/+3	−31/+7	Q	41/54	33/20	53/74

TC = total cholesterol; LDL-C = low-density lipoprotein cholesterol.

* NHLBI: National Heart, Lung, and Blood Institute Type II Coronary Intervention Study[30]; CLAS I: Cholesterol Lowering Atherosclerosis Study I[33]; CLAS II[35]; FATS: Familial Atherosclerosis Treatment Study[36]; UCSF-SCOR: University of California, San Francisco, Arteriosclerosis Specialized Center of Research Intervention Trial[37]; STARS: St. Thomas' Atherosclerosis Regression Study[38]; POSCH: Program on the Surgical Control of the Hyperlipidemias[39]; LHT: Lifestyle Heart Trial[41]; MARS: Monitored Atherosclerosis Regression Study[42]; CCAIT: Canadian Coronary Atherosclerosis Intervention Trial[44]; REGRESS: Regression Growth Evaluation Statin Study[46]; MAAS: Multicentre Anti-Atheroma Study.[47]

† M = male; F = female.

‡ All interventions included diet. C = colestipol; Ch = cholestyramine; L = lovastatin; N = nicotinic acid; P = pravastatin; PIB = partial ileal bypass; S = simvastatin.

§ P = panel assessment of lesion change (viewer estimation); Q = assessment by quantitative coronary angiography.

‖ Events variably defined among trials; generally, coronary death, myocardial infarction, unstable ischemia requiring revascularization.

¶ Various binary and ternary drug combinations.

** Follow-up rather than trial period (intervention was surgery).

Adapted from Jones, P. H., and Gotto, A. M., Jr.: Prevention of coronary heart disease in 1994: Evidence for intervention. Heart Dis. Stroke 3:290, 1994.

Interventional Studies in Secondary Prevention

Individuals with existing CAD or other clinical atherosclerotic disease are at the highest short-term risk for a CAD event. However, aggressive intervention has been shown to reduce that risk. Secondary-prevention trials using dietary, pharmacological, and/or surgical interventions have demonstrated a decrease in the progression of atherosclerotic lesions (Table 35–3) and a reduction in CAD morbidity and mortality with lipid-regulating therapy.[23] Recently published data also establish the beneficial effect of aggressive intervention on total mortality.

Early studies with angiographic endpoints were hampered by the limitation of visual interpretation as the only available means of assessing progression, regression, or stabilization of atherosclerotic lesions. The anatomical changes induced by therapeutic interventions are often quite modest and may be better assessed by computer-based quantitative techniques, which are more reproducible than visual assessment because they are not subject to the large interobserver and intraobserver variability that may occur in visual interpretation.[24] Quantitative coronary angiography can be used to evaluate a variety of parameters, including cross-sectional area and minimum lumen diameter. However, these measurements may not accurately reflect the clinical significance or overall severity of disease.[25] B-mode ultrasonography has been used in the carotid arteries to measure intima–media thickness, which has been suggested as a more accurate measurement of early atherosclerosis.[26] Positron emission tomography is now being used not only to quantify anatomic changes but also to determine the functional impact of these lesions on coronary flow reserve and myocardial viability.[27]

CORONARY DRUG PROJECT. The Coronary Drug Project tested the effects of pharmacological monotherapy with various agents in men, aged 30 to 64 years, with previous myocardial infarction.[28] Although 8341 men were randomized for the 5-year trial, three treatment arms were discontinued because of adverse effects. Conjugated estrogens,

5 mg/day, produced excess incidence of nonfatal myocardial infarction and insufficient efficacy; dextrothyroxine, 6 mg/day, produced excess mortality; and conjugated estrogens, 2.5 mg/day, produced excess incidence of thromboembolism, excess cancer mortality, and a small increase in total mortality.

Clofibrate, 1800 mg/day, was prescribed in 1103 subjects. In this treatment arm, total cholesterol decreased 6 per cent, and total triglyceride decreased 22 per cent. Combined incidence of CAD death and nonfatal myocardial infarction was reduced 9 per cent, but the difference was not statistically significant. Clofibrate treatment did not affect total mortality.

Nicotinic acid, 3 gm/day, was prescribed in 1119 subjects. In this treatment group, total cholesterol decreased 10 per cent, and total triglyceride decreased 26 per cent. During the trial period, there was a statistically significant 27 per cent decrease in incidence of nonfatal myocardial infarction compared with the placebo group but no difference in total mortality or CAD death. However, 15-year follow-up demonstrated an 11 per cent reduction in total mortality that was highly statistically significant and provided evidence that short-term reduction of coronary events translates into long-term mortality benefits.[29]

NATIONAL HEART, LUNG, AND BLOOD INSTITUTE TYPE II CORONARY INTERVENTION STUDY. The National Heart, Lung, and Blood Institute (NHLBI) Type II Coronary Intervention Study was the first major randomized trial to examine the effect of cholesterol lowering on angiographic parameters. This trial randomized 143 men and women, aged 21 to 55 years, to receive cholestyramine at a prescribed dosage of 24 gm/day or placebo for 5 years.[30] Entry criteria included angiographic evidence of CAD and an LDL cholesterol level above the 90th percentile for the general population despite dietary therapy (polyunsaturated fat:saturated fat ratio 2:1, cholesterol < 300 mg/day).[31] All subjects were to continue on the diet.

Total cholesterol decreased 17 per cent from baseline in

the cholestyramine group, and LDL cholesterol decreased 26 per cent, compared with respective decreases of 1 and 5 per cent in the placebo group. In the respective groups, HDL cholesterol increased 8 and 2 per cent, and triglyceride increased 28 and 26 per cent.

Angiograms taken at baseline and at 5-year follow-up were assessed visually to determine the primary endpoint of change in severity of CAD. Regression without progression was seen in approximately 7 per cent of both treatment groups. Progression without regression was seen in 32 per cent of subjects in the cholestyramine group and 49 per cent of subjects in the placebo group, which was a statistically significant difference. The benefit of cholestyramine treatment was most dramatic in lesions causing 50 per cent or greater stenosis at baseline: Progression in these lesions was seen in 12 per cent of subjects in the cholestyramine group compared with 33 per cent in the placebo group, which was a significant difference. The cholestyramine group had a 40 per cent reduced risk for progression, death, or nonfatal myocardial infarction, but this difference was not statistically significant.

Changes in HDL cholesterol:total cholesterol ratio and HDL cholesterol:LDL cholesterol ratio were the best predictors of angiographic change.[32] A significant inverse relation was found between lesion progression at 5 years and a combined increase in HDL cholesterol and decrease in LDL cholesterol.

CHOLESTEROL LOWERING ATHEROSCLEROSIS STUDY. The Cholesterol Lowering Atherosclerosis Study (CLAS) evaluated the effects of intensive combination-drug therapy on atherosclerosis in native coronary vessels and saphenous vein bypass grafts in a two-phase study. CLAS I randomized 188 nonsmoking men, aged 40 to 59 years, with previous coronary bypass surgery, progressive atherosclerosis, and total cholesterol of 185 to 350 mg/dl to receive either the bile-acid sequestrant colestipol, 30 gm/day, and nicotinic acid, 3 to 12 gm/day, or placebo for 2 years.[33] Both treatment groups were to follow a cholesterol-lowering diet, but that of the group randomized to combination-drug therapy was somewhat more restrictive (total fat 22 per cent, polyunsaturated fat 10 per cent, and saturated fat 4 per cent of total calories; cholesterol <125 mg/day) than that of the placebo group (total fat 26 per cent, polyunsaturated fat 10 per cent, and saturated fat 5 per cent of total calories; cholesterol <250 mg/day). All subjects received both study drugs for a 6-week pretrial period to ensure adequate compliance and a response of at least a 15 per cent decrease in total cholesterol.

In the group receiving combination-drug therapy, total cholesterol decreased 27 per cent, LDL cholesterol decreased 43 per cent, triglyceride decreased 22 per cent, and HDL cholesterol increased 37 per cent. The placebo group had decreases of 4 per cent, 5 per cent, and 5 per cent, and an increase of 2 per cent in the respective lipid levels.

A coronary global change score determined by visual assessment of angiograms obtained at baseline and 2-year follow-up was the primary endpoint. By this determination, progression was demonstrated in 39 per cent of subjects in the drug-treated group and 60 per cent of subjects in the placebo group. Regression was demonstrated in 16 per cent and 4 per cent of the respective groups, which was a statistically significant difference. Both native coronary arteries and saphenous vein bypass grafts showed improvement. Mean global change score in the drug-treated group was 0.3, compared with 0.8 in the placebo group, which represented a significant reduction in progression with combination-drug therapy. In each quartile of increased fat and polyunsaturated fat consumption, risk for new lesions was significantly increased.[34] Cardiovascular events occurred at similar rates in both treatment groups.

In CLAS II, 103 men completed an additional 2 years of treatment.[35] Lipid changes were maintained in the drug-treated group, and at 4-year follow-up, nonprogression or

regression was seen in significantly more subjects in the drug-treated group. Coronary global change score indicated progression in 48 per cent of subjects in the drug-treated group and 85 per cent of subjects in the placebo group. Regression was demonstrated in 18 per cent and 6 per cent of the respective groups, which was a significant difference.

FAMILIAL ATHEROSCLEROSIS TREATMENT STUDY. In the Familial Atherosclerosis Treatment Study (FATS), combination-drug therapy with the HMG-CoA reductase inhibitor lovastatin, 40 to 80 mg/day, and colestipol, 30 gm/day, or with nicotinic acid, 4 to 6 gm/day, and colestipol, 30 gm/day, was compared with placebo in 120 men, aged 62 years or less, with elevated plasma apolipoprotein (apo) B (>125 mg/dl), family history of CAD, and at least one coronary lesion causing 50 per cent or greater stenosis or three coronary lesions causing 30 per cent or greater stenosis.[36] All subjects received dietary therapy. Subjects randomized to placebo who had LDL cholesterol above the 90th percentile for age (43 per cent of the placebo group) also received colestipol, 30 gm/day. Average time on trial was 2.5 years.

Total cholesterol decreased 34 per cent in the group receiving lovastatin plus colestipol, 23 per cent in the group receiving nicotinic acid plus colestipol, and 3 per cent in the group receiving conventional therapy. In the respective groups, LDL cholesterol decreased 46, 32, and 7 per cent; HDL cholesterol increased 15, 43, and 5 per cent; and triglyceride decreased 9 and 30 per cent and increased 15 per cent. The large increase in HDL cholesterol reflects the use of nicotinic acid.

The primary endpoint, mean change in per cent stenosis of the worst lesion in each of nine proximal segments as assessed by quantitative coronary angiography, decreased 0.7 percentage point in the group receiving lovastatin plus colestipol and 0.9 percentage point in the group receiving nicotinic acid plus colestipol, indicative of lesion regression, and increased 2.1 percentage points in the group receiving conventional therapy, indicative of progression (Fig. 35–1). The change in the conventional-therapy group was significantly different from the changes in the combination-drug groups.

In the group receiving lovastatin plus colestipol, progression as the only angiographic change was seen in 21 per cent of subjects, and regression only was seen in 32 per cent of subjects. In the group receiving nicotinic acid plus colestipol, progression only was seen in 25 per cent of subjects, and regression only was seen in 39 per cent of subjects. In the group receiving conventional therapy, progression only was seen in 46 per cent of subjects, and regression only was seen in 11 per cent of subjects.

Cardiovascular events were defined as death, myocardial infarction, and need for peripheral or coronary bypass or angioplasty. These occurred in three subjects in the group receiving lovastatin plus colestipol, two subjects in the group receiving nicotinic acid plus colestipol, and ten subjects in the group receiving conventional therapy. Relative risk for a cardiovascular event was significantly greater in the conventional-therapy group than in the combination-drug groups.

UNIVERSITY OF CALIFORNIA, SAN FRANCISCO, ARTERIOSCLEROSIS SPECIALIZED CENTER OF RESEARCH INTERVENTION TRIAL. In the University of California, San Francisco, Arteriosclerosis Specialized Center of Research (UCSF-SCOR) Intervention Trial, 72 men and women aged 19 to 72 years with heterozygous familial hypercholesterolemia (FH) (described below) were randomized to receive combination-drug therapy consisting of colestipol, 15 to 30 gm/day; nicotinic acid, up to 7.5 gm/day; and lovastatin, 40 to 60 mg/day in various binary and ternary combinations or placebo.[37] During the 26-month trial, when the LRC-CPPT results were reported, UCSF-SCOR subjects randomized to placebo were given the option of receiving colestipol,

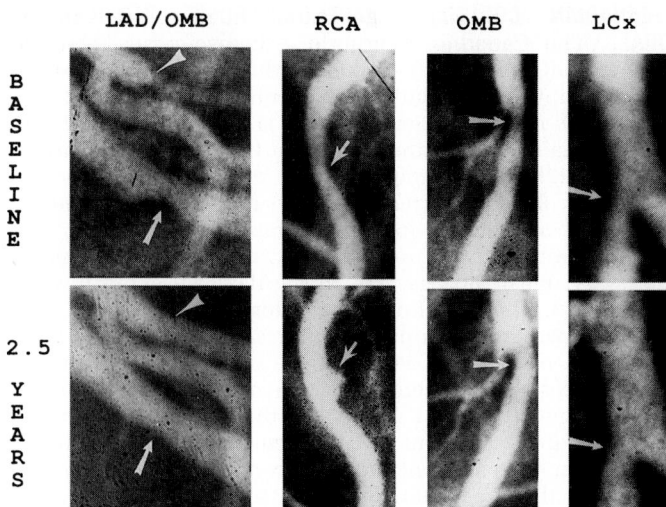

LAD/OMB   RCA   OMB   LCx

B
A
S
E
L
I
N
E

2.5

Y
E
A
R
S

FIGURE 35-1. Regression of coronary atherosclerotic lesions with lipid-regulating therapy: The Familial Atherosclerosis Treatment Study. LAD = left anterior descending artery; LCx = left circumflex artery; OMB = obtuse marginal branch; RCA = right coronary artery. Angiograms taken at baseline and after 2.5 years of treatment reflected improvement with aggressive lipid-regulating therapy. From left to right, stenosis decreased from 100 per cent to 28 per cent in the LAD and from 39 per cent to 18 per cent in the OMB, from 48 per cent to 30 per cent in the RCA, from 69 per cent to 37 per cent in the OMB, and from 44 per cent to 30 per cent in the LCx. (From Brown, G., Albers, J. J., Fisher, L. D., et al.: Regression of coronary artery disease as a result of intensive lipid-lowering therapy in men with high levels of apolipoprotein B. N. Engl. J. Med. 323:1289, 1990. Copyright Massachusetts Medical Society.)

15 gm/day; 44 per cent of UCSF-SCOR subjects in the placebo group took colestipol.

In the combination-drug group, total cholesterol decreased 31 percent, LDL cholesterol decreased 39 per cent, HDL cholesterol increased 25 per cent, and triglyceride decreased 21 per cent. Respective changes in the placebo group were decreases of 9 and 12 per cent and increases of 1 and 4 per cent.

The primary endpoint was mean within-patient change in per cent area stenosis as assessed by quantitative coronary angiography. This endpoint decreased 1.53 percentage points in the combination-drug group, indicative of lesion regression, and increased 0.80 percentage point in the placebo group, indicative of progression. The difference between groups was statistically significant. In subgroup analysis of women, the primary endpoint remained significantly different between treatment groups; the difference was not statistically significant in subgroup analysis of men.

In the combination-drug group, progression was reported in 20 per cent of subjects, and regression was reported in 32.5 per cent of subjects. In the placebo group, progression was reported in 41 per cent of subjects, and regression was reported in 12.5 per cent of subjects. Although the trend was toward more regression and less progression with combination-drug therapy, the difference was not significant.

ST THOMAS' ATHEROSCLEROSIS REGRESSION STUDY. The St Thomas' Atherosclerosis Regression Study (STARS) randomized 90 men with CAD, aged less than 66 years and with total cholesterol greater than 230 mg/dl, to receive a lipid-lowering diet plus cholestyramine, the same diet alone, or usual care.[38] The diet restricted total fat to 27 per cent and saturated fat to 8 to 10 per cent of total calories and increased omega-6 and omega-3 polyunsaturated fatty acids to 8 per cent of total calories; cholesterol was limited to 100 mg per 1000 kcal, and soluble fiber was increased to the equivalent of 3.6 gm polygalacturonate per 1000 kcal. Angiograms obtained at baseline and after an average of 39 months on trial were assessed quantitatively to determine the primary endpoint of change in the mean absolute width of coronary artery segments.

In the diet-plus-cholestyramine group, total cholesterol decreased 25 per cent, and LDL cholesterol decreased 36 per cent. Respective decreases in the diet-only group were 14 and 16 per cent, and respective decreases in the usual-care group were 2 and 3 per cent.

The primary endpoint was significantly improved in the active-treatment groups compared with the usual-care group. The mean absolute width of coronary artery segments increased 0.103 mm in the diet-plus-cholestyramine group and 0.003 mm in the diet-only group, indicative of lesion regression, but decreased 0.201 mm in the usual-care group, indicative of progression.

Significant improvement in clinical events was also demonstrated in the active-treatment groups. Cardiovascular events, defined as CAD death, myocardial infarction, coronary surgery, angioplasty, or stroke, were reported in one subject in the diet-plus-cholestyramine group, three subjects in the diet-only group, and ten subjects in the usual-care group.

PROGRAM ON THE SURGICAL CONTROL OF THE HYPERLIPID-EMIAS. The Program on the Surgical Control of the Hyperlipidemias (POSCH) randomized 838 men and women, aged 30 to 64 years, with one prior MI and hypercholesterolemia to receive partial ileal bypass surgery or usual care.[39] All subjects received dietary instruction (total fat < 25 per cent of calories; saturated, monounsaturated, and polyunsaturated fat each one-third of fat calories; cholesterol < 250 mg/day). Entry criteria included total cholesterol of at least 220 mg/dl or LDL cholesterol of at least 140 mg/dl after 6 weeks on diet. The primary endpoint was death of any cause. Angiograms were obtained at baseline and at 3-, 5-, and 7- or 10-year follow-up.

Compared with the control group, the surgery group had a 23 per cent decrease in total cholesterol, a 38 per cent decrease in LDL cholesterol, a 4 per cent increase in HDL cholesterol, and a 20 per cent increase in triglyceride at 5-year follow-up. Lesion progression as determined by a global change score was significantly reduced in the surgery group at each follow-up: 28 per cent compared with 41 per cent in the control group at 3 years, 37 per cent compared with 65 per cent of the control group at 5 years, 48 per cent compared with 77 per cent in the control group at 7 years, and 55 per cent compared with 85 per cent in the control group at 10 years. During the 10 years of the trial, total mortality was reduced 22 per cent and CAD mortality was reduced 28 per cent in the surgery group, but neither of these differences was significant. However, risk for CAD death or nonfatal myocardial infarction was significantly reduced 35 per cent in the surgery group. Changes between angiograms taken at baseline and at 3-year follow-up were significantly associated with total mortality and CAD mortality during the course of the study.[40]

POSCH demonstrated the effects of lipid lowering by a method that ensured compliance. Since the initiation of that trial, however, the availability of pharmacological agents with increased potency has reduced the need for such radical intervention.

LIFE STYLE HEART TRIAL. The Life style Heart Trial randomized 48 men and women aged 35 to 75 years and with angiographically documented CAD to a comprehensive life style-modification program, which included a low-fat vegetarian diet (as prescribed, total fat 10 per cent of calories, polyunsaturated fat:saturated fat ratio > 1, protein 15 to 20 per cent of calories, carbohydrate 70 to 75 per cent of calories and predominantly complex carbohydrates, cholesterol ≤ 5 mg/day), smoking cessation, stress management training, and moderate physical exercise, or to usual care.[41] Angiograms made at baseline and at 1-year follow-up were evaluated quantitatively.

In the life style-modification group, total cholesterol decreased 24 per cent and LDL cholesterol decreased 37 per cent. Respective decreases in the usual-care group were 5 and 6 per cent. The average per cent diameter stenosis in all detectable lesions decreased from 40 to 38 per cent in the life style-modification group and increased from 43 to 46 per cent in the usual-care group, which was a significant difference. In addition to the anatomical improvement, the life style-modification group had a significant 91 per cent decrease in frequency of angina, a nonsignificant 42 per cent decrease in duration of angina, and a significant 28 per cent reduction in severity of angina; respective increases in the control group were 165, 95, and 39 per cent. Although life style modifications of this magnitude require considerable dedication, this small trial demonstrated that substantial clinical benefit can be achieved by aggressive nonpharmacological intervention in highly motivated individuals.

MONITORED ATHEROSCLEROSIS REGRESSION STUDY. Monotherapy with an HMG-CoA reductase inhibitor has been evaluated in a number of angiographically monitored studies. The Monitored Atherosclerosis Regression Study (MARS) randomized 270 men and women, aged 37 to 67 years, to receive maximum-dosage lovastatin (80 mg/day) or placebo for 2 years.[42] Subjects were selected on the basis of angiographic evidence of CAD rather than dyslipidemia; total cholesterol could range from 190 to 295 mg/dl. All subjects were to follow a low-fat, low-cholesterol diet (total fat ≤27 per cent, saturated fat ≤7 per cent, monounsaturated fat ≤10 per cent, and polyunsaturated fat ≤10 per cent of total calories; cholesterol ≤250 mg/day).

Lovastatin therapy decreased total cholesterol 32 per cent, LDL cholesterol 45 per cent, and triglyceride 22 per cent and increased HDL cholesterol 8.5 per cent, compared with decreases of 2 and 3 per cent and increases of 3.5 and 2 per cent in the respective lipid levels in the placebo group.

Quantitative assessment of angiograms obtained at baseline and at 2-year follow-up did not demonstrate a significant improvement with lovastatin therapy in the primary endpoint of mean per-patient change in per cent diameter stenosis. Both groups showed lesion progression: Mean per cent diameter stenosis increased 1.6 per cent in the lovastatin group and 2.2 per cent in the placebo group. By this assessment, 29 per cent of lovastatin subjects and 41 per cent of placebo subjects demonstrated progression, and 23 and 12 per cent of the respective groups demonstrated regression; both of these differences were statistically significant. In lesions causing 50 per cent or greater stenosis at baseline, the lovastatin group showed a 4.1 per cent decrease in per cent diameter stenosis compared with a 0.9 per cent increase in the placebo group, which was a significant improvement. In the lovastatin group, the predominant predictor of progression in mild and moderate lesions was apo C-III, whereas the predominant predictor of progression in severe lesions was the LDL cholesterol:HDL cholesterol ratio; the predominant predictor of progression in both lesion categories in the placebo group was the total cholesterol:HDL cholesterol ratio.[43]

However, by a visually assessed global change score, there was significantly less progression in the lovastatin group, which had an average global change score of 0.41, than in the placebo group, which had an average score of 0.88. By this assessment, 47 per cent of lovastatin subjects and 65 per cent of placebo subjects demonstrated progression, and 23 per cent of lovastatin subjects and 11 per cent of placebo subjects demonstrated regression; both of these differences were statistically significant.

Between-group comparison of clinical coronary events—myocardial infarction, percutaneous transluminal coronary angioplasty, coronary artery bypass surgery, coronary death, and hospitalization for unstable angina—showed a slight reduction in events in the lovastatin group, which had 22 events compared with 31 in the placebo group, but this difference was not statistically significant.

CANADIAN CORONARY ATHEROSCLEROSIS INTERVENTION TRIAL. The Canadian Coronary Atherosclerosis Intervention Trial (CCAIT) also evaluated the benefit of lovastatin monotherapy in secondary prevention.[44] In this 2-year study, 331 men and women aged 21 to 70 years with angiographically demonstrated diffuse CAD and total cholesterol of 220 to 300 mg/dl were randomized to receive lovastatin dosed to reduce LDL cholesterol to 90 to 130 mg/dl or placebo. Initial lovastatin dosage was 20 mg/day and was titrated up to a maximum of 80 mg/day as necessary; mean dosage was 36 mg/day. All subjects were instructed in the Step I diet (see below).

In the lovastatin group, total cholesterol decreased 21 per cent, LDL cholesterol decreased 29 per cent, HDL cholesterol increased 7 per cent, and triglyceride decreased 8 per cent. Respective lipid levels in the placebo group decreased 1 and 2 per cent and increased 3 and 4 per cent.

The primary endpoint was a coronary change score defined as the quantitatively assessed mean per-patient change in minimum lumen diameter for all lesions measured. Although this assessment demonstrated lesion progression in both groups, the lovastatin group had significantly less progression than the placebo group: Mean lumen diameter decreased 0.05 mm and 0.09 mm in the respective groups. Progression as the only angiographic change was reported in 33 per cent of subjects in the lovastatin group and 50 per cent of subjects in the placebo group, which was a significant improvement. New lesion formation was significantly decreased in the lovastatin group, in which new lesions were seen in 16 per cent of subjects, compared with 32 per cent of subjects in the placebo group. Regression as the only angiographic change was not significantly different between treatment groups, occurring in 10 per cent of subjects in the lovastatin group and 7 per cent of subjects in the placebo group.

Fewer clinical coronary events, defined as cardiac death, myocardial infarction, and unstable angina, were reported in the lovastatin group, in which 14 subjects had 15 events, compared with the placebo group, in which 18 subjects had 20 events, but the difference was not statistically significant.

PRAVASTATIN LIMITATION OF ATHEROSCLEROSIS IN THE CORONARY ARTERIES. The Pravastatin Limitation of Atherosclerosis in the Coronary Arteries (PLAC I) study assessed the effect of pharmacological monotherapy with the HMG-CoA reductase inhibitor pravastatin on angiographic and clinical endpoints in 408 men and women with angiographic evidence of CAD (≥50 per cent stenosis in one or more coronary arteries) and LDL cholesterol of 130 to 190 mg/dl.[45] Subjects were randomized to receive pravastatin, 40 mg/day, or placebo for 3 years.

In the pravastatin group, the primary endpoint—mean change in diameter of 10 predetermined coronary artery segments as assessed by quantitative coronary angiography—decreased 0.02 mm/year, which was not significantly different from the 0.04 mm/year decrease in the placebo group. Pravastatin decreased total cholesterol 19 per cent, triglyceride 8 per cent, and LDL cholesterol 28 per cent and increased HDL cholesterol 7 per cent. Clinical cardiovascular events—fatal and nonfatal myocardial infarction, other cardiac death, stroke, bypass surgery, and coronary angioplasty—were significantly reduced in the pravastatin group.

REGRESSION GROWTH EVALUATION STATIN STUDY. In the Regression Growth Evaluation Statin Study (REGRESS), 885 men aged less than 70 years with total cholesterol between 155 mg/dl and 310 mg/dl and at least one coronary lesion causing at least 50 per cent stenosis in a major coronary artery were randomized to receive pravastatin, 40 mg/day, or placebo.[46] All subjects were to follow a diet that derived 10 to 15 per cent of total calories from protein, 30 to 35 per cent from lipid, and 50 to 55 per cent from carbohydrate. In subjects whose total cholesterol level was greater than

310 mg/dl on repeated assessments, cholestyramine was administered in addition to the study drug. Quantitative coronary angiography was performed at baseline and after 2 years of treatment.

In the pravastatin group, total cholesterol decreased 20 per cent, LDL cholesterol decreased 29 per cent, HDL cholesterol increased 10 per cent, and triglyceride decreased 7 per cent. All lipid values increased slightly in the placebo group.

Primary angiographic endpoints were the per-patient change in average mean segment diameter and the per-patient change in average minimum obstruction diameter. Both groups showed progression by both of these determinations. However, the pravastatin group showed significantly less decrease in the mean segment diameter (0.06 mm) than the placebo group (0.10 mm) and significantly less decrease in the minimum obstruction diameter (0.03 mm) than the placebo group (0.06 mm).

In the pravastatin group, 59 clinical events (fatal or non-fatal myocardial infarction, CAD death, unscheduled percutaneous transluminal coronary angioplasty or coronary artery bypass grafting, stroke or transient ischemic attack, and death of any other cause) were reported, compared with 93 in the placebo group.

MULTICENTRE ANTI-ATHEROMA STUDY. The effect of HMG-CoA reductase inhibitor monotherapy with simvastatin on known coronary atherosclerotic lesions was evaluated in the Multicentre Anti-Atheroma Study (MAAS).[47] In this study, 381 men and women, aged 30 to 67 years, were randomized to receive simvastatin, 20 mg/day, or placebo for 4 years. Entry criteria included angiographic evidence of atherosclerosis in at least two coronary artery segments, total cholesterol of 210 to 310 mg/dl, and triglyceride less than 350 mg/dl. Dietary instruction according to the usual practice of each center was given to all subjects.

Compared with placebo, simvastatin decreased total cholesterol 23 per cent, LDL cholesterol 31 per cent, and triglyceride 18 per cent and increased HDL cholesterol 9 per cent.

Angiograms obtained at baseline and at 2- and 4-year follow-up were assessed quantitatively. Change in diffuse coronary atherosclerosis was determined by the per-patient average of mean lumen diameter of all coronary artery segments, and change in focal coronary atherosclerosis was determined by the per-patient average of minimum lumen diameter of all segments that were atheromatous at baseline and/or follow-up. In both treatment groups, progression was seen in both measures of atherosclerotic disease, although there was significantly less progression by both determinations with simvastatin therapy. In the simvastatin group, mean lumen diameter decreased 0.02 mm and minimum lumen diameter decreased 0.04 mm; respective decreases in the placebo group were 0.08 mm and 0.13 mm. Progression as the only angiographic change was seen in 23 per cent of subjects in the simvastatin group and 32 per cent of subjects in the placebo group. Regression as the only angiographic change was seen in 19 per cent and 12 per cent of the respective groups.

Clinical event rates were similar between treatment groups. Myocardial infarction was reported in 11 subjects randomized to simvastatin and 7 subjects randomized to placebo. Cardiac death was reported in 4 subjects in each group.

SCANDINAVIAN SIMVASTATIN SURVIVAL STUDY. The Scandinavian Simvastatin Survival Study (4S) provided strong evidence that intensive lipid lowering improves survival in patients with coronary disease. This multicenter trial randomized 4444 men and women, aged 35 to 60 years, with a history of angina pectoris or myocardial infarction to receive placebo or simvastatin dosed to reduce total cholesterol to 115 to 200 mg/dl.[48] Other entry criteria were total cholesterol of 210 to 310 mg/dl and triglyceride of 220 mg/dl or less after dietary instruction. Simvastatin dosage was

increased from the initial 20 mg/day to 40 mg/day in 37 per cent of simvastatin subjects and decreased to 10 mg/day in 2 subjects. Median time on trial was 5.4 years. Analysis was intent to treat.

Simvastatin therapy decreased total cholesterol 25 per cent, LDL cholesterol 35 per cent, and triglyceride 10 per cent and increased HDL cholesterol 8 per cent. In the placebo group, respective lipid levels increased 1 per cent, 1 per cent, 7 per cent, and 1 per cent. Total mortality, the primary endpoint, was significantly decreased 30 per cent in the simvastatin group. Coronary mortality decreased 42 per cent, and there was no increase in noncardiovascular deaths, including deaths caused by violence or cancer, in the simvastatin group. Incidence of major coronary events, defined as coronary death, nonfatal myocardial infarction, and resuscitated cardiac arrest, was significantly decreased 34 per cent in the simvastatin group. Risk for major coronary events was similarly reduced in each quartile of baseline total cholesterol, LDL cholesterol, and HDL cholesterol distribution.[49]

Predetermined subgroup analyses compared clinical event rates by age and gender. In subjects aged 60 years or older, total mortality and incidence of major coronary events were significantly reduced with simvastatin treatment, although these reductions were less than in the overall study population. In women, total mortality was similar between treatment groups, but the incidence of major coronary events was significantly decreased 35 per cent in the simvastatin group.

Low Cholesterol and Mortality

Some epidemiological studies have found an increase in mortality at the lowest cholesterol levels,[50] and, as noted above, some early interventional trials of lipid lowering showed no improvement in total mortality, despite a reduction in coronary mortality, because of an increase in noncardiac mortality. These results have raised questions about a potential adverse effect of cholesterol lowering and about the causality of increased death rates at the lowest cholesterol levels reported in some studies.[51] The major controversy is whether the association between low cholesterol and increased mortality is causal or is attributable to confounding factors not adequately evaluated in epidemiological studies.[52]

The definition of low cholesterol has not been established, but many experts consider total cholesterol less than 160 mg/dl to be low. However, populations that consume low-fat, low-cholesterol diets have average total cholesterol levels in this general range. For example, in Shanghai, the mean total cholesterol level is 162 mg/dl, but no increase in cancer mortality or other causes of death has been demonstrated.[53]

In addition to diet, a variety of genetic and environmental conditions can decrease total cholesterol.[54] Genetic diseases characterized by low cholesterol include abetalipoproteinemia,[55] an autosomal recessive disorder characterized by a marked decrease or absence of apo B–containing lipoproteins and total cholesterol of 20 to 45 mg/dl, and hypobetalipoproteinemia,[56] an autosomal dominant disorder that in its homozygous form resembles abetalipoproteinemia and in its heterozygous form is characterized by total cholesterol of 90 to 140 mg/dl and LDL cholesterol of 30 to 50 mg/dl. Abnormalities associated with these conditions include peripheral neuropathies and fat malabsorption. However, patients with these disorders do not appear to have increased rates of death of malignancy or a shortened life span, despite lifelong exposure to cholesterol levels far below those obtained in clinical trials. Nongenetic factors associated with decreased plasma cholesterol include chronic disease states such as chronic obstructive pulmonary disease, bronchogenic carcinoma, and alcoholic cirrhosis. Preclinical malignancies may be the cause rather than the result of hypocholesterolemia.[57]

The Honolulu Heart Program demonstrated a definite U-shaped association between quintile of cholesterol and total mortality rate.[58] Subjects in quintile 3 (total cholesterol 210 to 239 mg/dl) had the lowest age-adjusted mortality rate (66.4 per 1000), subjects in quintiles 2 (total cholesterol 180 to 209 mg/dl) and 4 (total cholesterol 240 to 269 mg/dl) had slightly increased total mortality (69.5 per 1000 and 67.5 per 1000, respectively), and subjects in the lowest quintile (total cholesterol <180 mg/dl) and the highest quintile (total cholesterol 270 mg/dl or greater) had increased total mortality (97.3 per 1000 and 100.9 per 1000, respectively). However, in a reassessment of the Honolulu Heart Program data, excess mortality at low cholesterol levels was limited to subjects with confounding health problems, such as heavy alcohol consumption, heavy smoking, gastrectomy, cirrhosis, colectomy, or intestinal disease.[59] In additional analysis of traumatic deaths and suicides during 23 years of follow-up in the Honolulu Heart Program, total cholesterol at any level was found to be directly related to risk for suicide, and multivariate analysis did not find a relation between total cholesterol level and risk for traumatic death.[60]

Similarly, in the Whitehall Study, age-adjusted total mortality rate was slightly higher in the lowest quintile of total cholesterol (<129 mg/dl) than in the second-lowest quintile (129 to 174 mg/dl)—13.78 compared with 13.29 per 1000 person-years—but this difference was not statistically significant.[61] CAD mortality increased with each quintile of total cholesterol. The increase in noncardiovascular mortality was largely accounted for by confounding factors such as recent unexplained weight loss, respiratory symptoms, body mass index, marital status, and employment grade.

In a 30-year follow-up of subjects in the Framingham Heart Study who were without cancer or cardiovascular disease at initial assessment, total cholesterol level was directly related to total mortality and cardiovascular mortality in both men and women aged less than 50 years.[62] No association was found between cholesterol level and total mortality in subjects aged 50 years or older, presumably because of confounding by diseases that decrease cholesterol level.

When the increases in accidental and violent deaths reported in the LRC-CPPT and the Helsinki Heart Study were reanalyzed for potential confounding factors, it was noted that the two victims of homicide were both innocent victims and not offenders, and one had not been taking the study drug for more than 1 year.[63] The eight suicides include five subjects who had withdrawn from the trials and had not been taking the study drug for months or years. Of the ten accidental deaths, two were in subjects who had withdrawn from the study, three were in subjects with high blood alcohol concentrations at autopsy, and three were in subjects with a history of psychiatric disorders. Additionally, in both the LRC-CPPT and the Helsinki Heart Study, cholesterol lowering did not decrease cholesterol levels to what would be considered low.

Low cholesterol has been hypothesized to increase violent behavior because of a decrease in serotonin receptor activity in the brain.[64] However, lowering plasma cholesterol may not alter cholesterol level within the central nervous system, because essentially all the cholesterol in the central nervous system is produced locally, and the exchangeable pool of cholesterol is much lower in the central nervous system than in other organs.[65]

In 4S, cholesterol lowering decreased both coronary mortality and total mortality, demonstrating that noncoronary death rates did not offset improvement in cardiovascular mortality. Specifically, there was no increase in deaths due to violence or cancer.

In a prospectively planned pooled analysis of PLAC I, REGRESS, and two other regression studies using pravastatin 40 mg/day monotherapy for 2 or 3 years, combined incidence of nonfatal or fatal myocardial infarction was significantly reduced 62 per cent; this benefit was demonstrated in men and women and in patients older and younger than 65 years.[66] In this analysis, total mortality was decreased 46 per cent with pravastatin, but this difference was not significant.

Low-Density Lipoprotein Metabolism

LDL is the major carrier of cholesterol to the periphery and supplies the cholesterol essential for the integrity of nerve tissue, steroid synthesis, and cell membranes. Apo B-100 on the surface of LDL allows recognition, binding, and removal of the lipoprotein by the B/E (LDL) receptor, which removes approximately 75 per cent of LDL particles from the circulation and is downregulated as intracellular cholesterol increases. Scavenger receptors on macrophages and non–receptor-mediated pathways account for the clearance of the remaining LDL particles.

SMALL, DENSE LOW-DENSITY LIPOPROTEIN. In addition to LDL cholesterol level, LDL composition influences CAD risk. Triglyceride may be transferred from chylomicrons and VLDL to LDL, through the action of cholesteryl ester transfer protein (CETP), and subsequently hydrolyzed by hepatic lipase to produce LDL particles that are smaller and denser than normal. Large, buoyant LDL particles predominate in LDL subclass pattern A, and small, dense LDL particles predominate in LDL subclass pattern B.[67] LDL subclass pattern B is associated with a threefold-increased risk for myocardial infarction,[68] and LDL particles in individuals with angiographic evidence of CAD have been reported to be smaller and denser than LDL in individuals without angiographic evidence of CAD.[69] Although LDL subclass pattern B has been reported in approximately 37 per cent of males and 25 per cent of females, it is present in only 17 per cent of males aged 6 to 19 years and only 13 per cent of premenopausal females.[70] Genetic influences appear to account for 33 per cent to 50 per cent of the variation in LDL subclass,[71] indicating substantial environmental and thus potentially modifiable factors. Small, dense LDL frequently occurs in conjunction with elevated triglyceride level, low HDL cholesterol level, truncal obesity, and hypertension. Individuals with LDL subclass pattern B have been found to be more insulin resistant than individuals with LDL subclass pattern A,[72] suggesting that complex metabolic factors may also affect LDL subclass.

LDL subclass pattern can be altered to a potentially less atherogenic pattern. Pharmacological therapy, for example, with gemfibrozil[73] or bezafibrate,[74] has been shown to shift LDL particles toward a larger, more buoyant species.

The mechanism by which small, dense LDL confers increased atherosclerotic risk has not been totally determined and may be a combination of mechanisms. Compared with large, buoyant LDL, small, dense LDL has a lower sialic acid content, which may increase the binding capacity of LDL for proteoglycans localized to the arterial wall.[75] Hemostatic variables may be shifted to a more atherogenic pattern in the presence of small, dense LDL. A dose-dependent increase in thromboxane synthesis has been reported with increasing density of LDL particles.[76] Small, dense LDL appears to be more susceptible to in vitro oxidation than large, buoyant LDL.[77]

OXIDIZED LOW-DENSITY LIPOPROTEIN. LDL may be oxidized as a result of exposure to endothelial cells, smooth muscle cells, or macrophages.[78,78a] Oxidized LDL attracts circulating monocytes, which then adhere to the arterial wall, and precipitates their activation as macrophages, which are then prevented from leaving the arterial wall[79] (see Chap. 34). Scavenger receptors on macrophages recognize and bind oxidized LDL and, unlike the B/E receptor, are not downregulated as intracellular cholesterol accumulates. As uptake continues, the macrophages can become lipid-laden foam cells, the components of the fatty streak, which is the precursor atherosclerotic lesion.

Diagnosis and Treatment of Dyslipidemia

In the NCEP adult guidelines, the determination of lipid levels and estimation of the need for and intensity of lipid-regulating treatment are influenced by the individual's overall risk for CAD. Because, as noted above, individuals with existing CAD or other atherosclerotic disease, such as peripheral arterial disease or symptomatic carotid artery disease, are at the highest short-term risk for a CAD event, the initial risk stratification of the NCEP adult guidelines is according to the presence or absence of atherosclerotic disease. But it should be borne in mind that the distinction between primary and secondary prevention is at times semantic because many high-risk asymptomatic individuals have significant atherosclerosis.

Separate recommendations have been issued by the Expert Panel on Blood Cholesterol Levels in Children and Adolescents of the NCEP.[80] These guidelines, developed for individuals aged 2 to 19 years, recommend screening for dyslipidemia in children and adolescents who are from families with premature cardiovascular disease or dyslipidemia. LDL cholesterol of 170 mg/dl or greater should be treated by dietary therapy. If, after 6 months to 1 year of dietary therapy, LDL cholesterol remains 190 mg/dl or greater, or 160 mg/dl or greater in the presence of either a positive family history of cardiovascular disease before age 55 or two other risk factors that have not been successfully controlled, drug therapy should be considered in patients aged at least 10 years. Bile-acid sequestrant therapy is appropriate in this age group.

DETECTION OF DYSLIPIDEMIA. The NCEP adult guidelines recommend that all individuals aged 20 years or older without CAD or other atherosclerotic disease have their total cholesterol and, if accuracy can be assured, HDL cholesterol levels measured at least once every 5 years. These measurements can be obtained from nonfasting samples. At the discretion of the physician, a full fasting lipoprotein analysis may be performed instead. Lipoprotein analysis is the initial assessment in individuals with CAD or other atherosclerotic disease.

Primary Prevention. In individuals without atherosclerotic disease, estimation of risk status at a given cholesterol level is guided by the number of other risk factors present, although clinical judgment is required to evaluate the severity of each risk factor and the overall risk status of the individual. The following additional risk factors (besides LDL cholesterol elevation) are included in the NCEP's algorithm:

Positive risk factors
- Age (45 years or older in men; 55 years or older, or premature menopause without estrogen-replacement therapy, in women)
- Family history of premature CAD (myocardial infarction or sudden death before the age of 55 in father or other male first-degree relative, or before the age of 65 in mother or other female first-degree relative)
- Current cigarette smoking
  Hypertension (≥140/90 mm Hg, or on antihypertensive medication)
- Low HDL cholesterol (<35 mg/dl)
- Diabetes mellitus

Negative risk factor (subtract 1 of the additional risk factors if present)
- High HDL cholesterol (≥60 mg/dl)

Obesity is not included in the algorithm because it is usually found in conjunction with hypertension, hyperlipidemia, low HDL cholesterol, and diabetes mellitus, which are listed; nevertheless, it should be a target for intervention, as should physical inactivity. A concerted effort should be made to reduce all modifiable risk factors.

In primary prevention, total cholesterol less than 200 mg/dl is considered desirable, 200 to 239 mg/dl is

considered borderline high, and 240 mg/dl or greater is considered high (Fig. 35–2). At a total cholesterol level of 240 mg/dl, CAD risk is approximately twice that at a total cholesterol level of 200 mg/dl. However, because the relation between cholesterol level and CAD risk is continuous and graded, this categorization of cholesterol provides not absolute cutpoints but a guide for risk assessment.

In individuals without CAD whose total cholesterol is desirable and HDL cholesterol is 35 mg/dl or greater, no lipid-regulating intervention is required. These individuals should receive instruction in following dietary recommendations for the general population (Step I Diet) and in risk factor reduction. Retesting should be performed in 5 years. Individuals without CAD whose total cholesterol is borderline high and HDL cholesterol is 35 mg/dl or greater in the presence of fewer than two other risk factors should receive similar instruction and should be reevaluated in 1 to 2 years, at which time dietary instruction should be reinforced.

Individuals with low HDL cholesterol, borderline-high total cholesterol in the presence of two or more other risk factors, or high total cholesterol require full fasting lipoprotein analysis to help determine CAD risk. The analysis is performed on a sample obtained after a 12-hour fast to allow clearance of chylomicrons. Total cholesterol, HDL cholesterol, and total triglyceride levels are measured, and LDL cholesterol is calculated by the Friedewald formula:

LDL cholesterol (mg/dl)
= Total cholesterol − HDL cholesterol − (triglyceride/5)

The formula is not accurate if triglyceride is greater than 400 mg/dl or if the patient has type III hyperlipidemia or is homozygous for apo E_2; in these instances, LDL cholesterol needs to be determined by ultracentrifugation at a specialized laboratory.

The NCEP adult guidelines classify LDL cholesterol less than 130 mg/dl as desirable, 130 to 159 mg/dl as borderline high, and 160 mg/dl or greater as high in primary prevention (Fig. 35–3). Patients whose LDL cholesterol is desirable should receive instruction in dietary recommendations for the general population and in risk factor reduction. Low HDL cholesterol and hypertriglyceridemia require treatment as described below.

Patients who have borderline-high LDL cholesterol and fewer than two other risk factors should receive instruction in dietary modification and recommended physical activity. Retesting by lipoprotein analysis should be performed in 1 year. In patients who have borderline-high LDL cholesterol and two or more other risk factors, and in patients who have high LDL cholesterol, lipoprotein analysis should be repeated within 1 to 8 weeks. If the LDL cholesterol values vary by more than 30 mg/dl, the analysis should be repeated a third time. Treatment decisions should be based on the average of two, or, if necessary, three, LDL cholesterol values. Confirmation of borderline-high or high LDL cholesterol indicates the need for clinical evaluation and lipid-regulating intervention.

Secondary Prevention. Full fasting lipoprotein analysis should be performed at least once every year in individuals with CAD. Because LDL cholesterol may be decreased in patients recovering from an acute coronary event, analyses performed during the weeks immediately following the event may not accurately reflect the baseline LDL cholesterol level. However, elevated LDL cholesterol during this period suggests an even greater elevation upon recovery.

In patients with CAD, an LDL cholesterol level of 100 mg/dl or less is considered optimal (Fig. 35–4). Patients who have optimal LDL cholesterol should be given individualized instruction in dietary recommendations (Step II Diet) and physical activity. Retesting by lipoprotein analysis should be repeated annually. Low HDL cholesterol and hypertriglyceridemia require treatment as described below. Patients who have LDL cholesterol higher than opti-

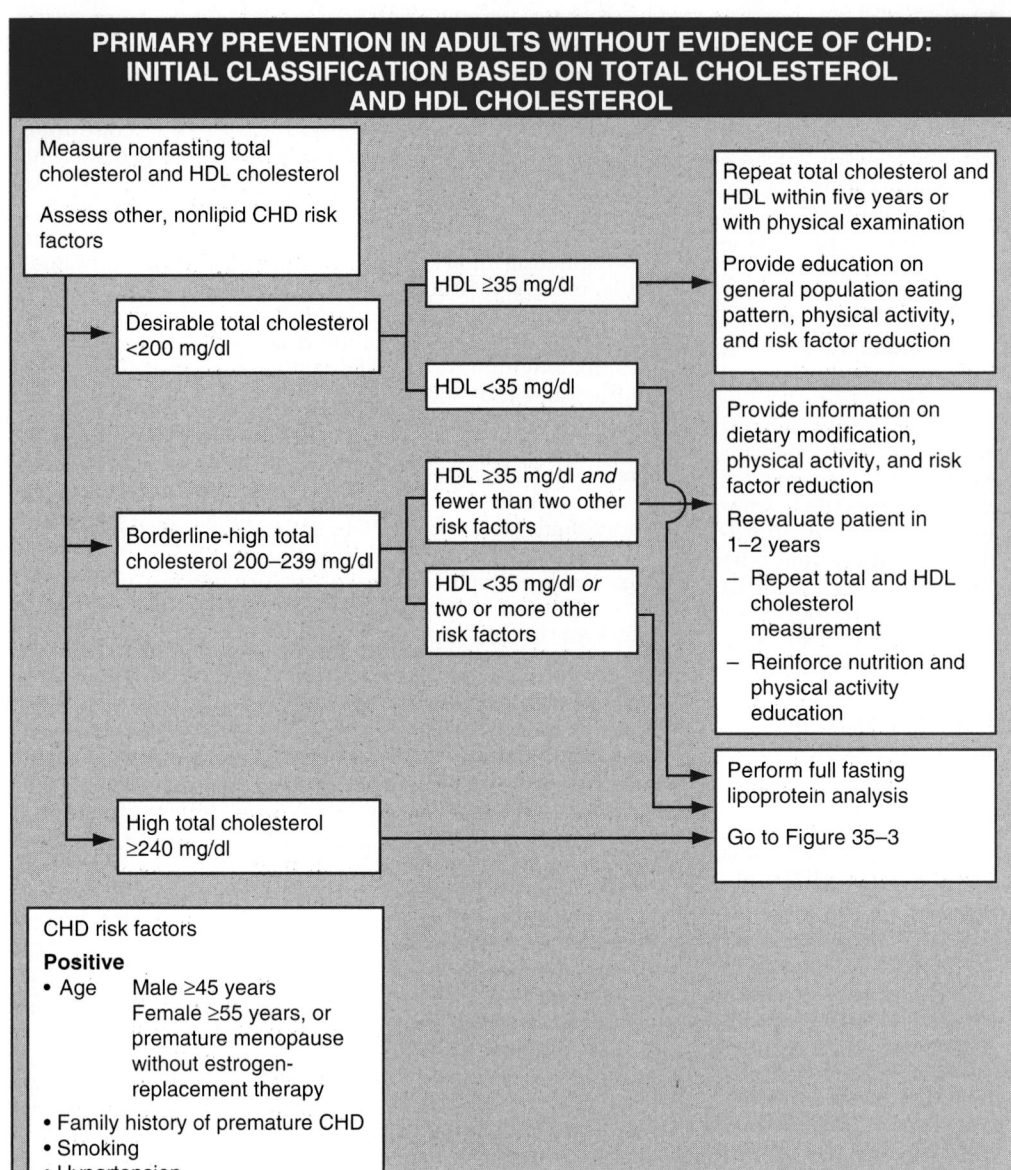

PRIMARY PREVENTION IN ADULTS WITHOUT EVIDENCE OF CHD: INITIAL CLASSIFICATION BASED ON TOTAL CHOLESTEROL AND HDL CHOLESTEROL

Measure nonfasting total cholesterol and HDL cholesterol

Assess other, nonlipid CHD risk factors

Desirable total cholesterol <200 mg/dl

HDL ≥35 mg/dl

HDL <35 mg/dl

Borderline-high total cholesterol 200–239 mg/dl

HDL ≥35 mg/dl *and* fewer than two other risk factors

HDL <35 mg/dl *or* two or more other risk factors

High total cholesterol ≥240 mg/dl

Repeat total cholesterol and HDL within five years or with physical examination

Provide education on general population eating pattern, physical activity, and risk factor reduction

Provide information on dietary modification, physical activity, and risk factor reduction

Reevaluate patient in 1–2 years

– Repeat total and HDL cholesterol measurement

– Reinforce nutrition and physical activity education

Perform full fasting lipoprotein analysis

Go to Figure 35–3

CHD risk factors
Positive
• Age   Male ≥45 years
            Female ≥55 years, or
            premature menopause
            without estrogen-
            replacement therapy
• Family history of premature CHD
• Smoking
• Hypertension
• HDL cholesterol <35 mg/dl
• Diabetes mellitus
Negative
• HDL cholesterol ≥60 mg/dl

FIGURE 35–2. Primary prevention classification by total cholesterol. In patients without coronary artery disease or other atherosclerotic disease, initial assessment for dyslipidemia is by total cholesterol and high-density lipoprotein cholesterol levels (minimum approach). The physician may choose the full fasting lipoprotein analysis as the first assessment. (From National Cholesterol Education Program.[2,3])

mal, as confirmed by multiple assessments as detailed above, should receive clinical evaluation and lipid-lowering intervention.

CLINICAL EVALUATION. The clinical evaluation estimates overall risk for CAD and attempts to determine whether the dyslipidemia is caused by a genetic disorder or is secondary to diet, to another condition such as diabetes mellitus, hypothyroidism, nephrotic syndrome, or obstructive liver disease, or to the use of drugs such as progestins, anabolic steroids, corticosteroids, beta blockers, or diuretics.

Essential components of the evaluation are personal and family history, physical examination, and basic laboratory tests. The physical examination should include careful assessment for manifestations of dyslipidemia, such as corneal arcus, xanthelasmas or xanthomas, and hepatosplenomegaly, and for manifestations of atherosclerosis, such as decreased peripheral pulses and vascular bruits. The clinical evaluation further refines estimation of the patient's CAD risk and provides additional targets for intervention through the identification of other risk factors. If genetic dyslipidemia is suspected, family members should be assessed. If dyslipidemia does not respond to treatment of

underlying conditions or removal or reduction of drugs that can cause dyslipidemia, it should be treated as a primary dyslipidemia.

Dietary Therapy

In the NCEP guidelines, the primary therapy for dyslipidemia is dietary. Reduction of saturated fat and cholesterol consumption is part of a triad of life style modifications that should also include weight loss if necessary and increased physical activity as appropriate. Dietary therapy judiciously employed is a risk-free intervention whose efficacy has been demonstrated in clinical trials.[81] The synergistic effects of dietary modification, regular exercise, and weight control are beneficial in reducing CAD risk by improving not only the lipid profile but also blood pressure and glucose tolerance.

In primary prevention in patients with fewer than two other risk factors, dietary therapy should be initiated if LDL cholesterol is 160 mg/dl or greater (Table 35–4). The goal of treatment in these patients is LDL cholesterol less than 160 mg/dl. In primary prevention in patients with two or more other risk factors, dietary therapy should be initiated

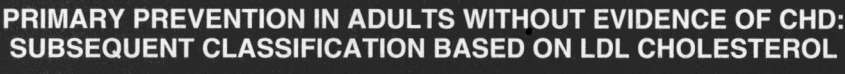

PRIMARY PREVENTION IN ADULTS WITHOUT EVIDENCE OF CHD: SUBSEQUENT CLASSIFICATION BASED ON LDL CHOLESTEROL

Full fasting lipoprotein analysis (fast 9–12 hours)

(may follow a total cholesterol determination or may be done at the outset)

Desirable LDL cholesterol <130 mg/dl

→ Repeat total cholesterol and HDL cholesterol measurement within five years

Provide education on general population eating pattern, physical activity, and risk factor reduction

Borderline-high LDL cholesterol 130–159 mg/dl and with fewer than two other risk factors

130–159 mg/dl* and with two or more other risk factors

Provide information on the Step I Diet and physical activity

Reevaluate patient status annually, including risk factor reduction

– Repeat lipoprotein analysis

– Reinforce nutrition and physical activity education

Clinical evaluation (history, physical examination, laboratory tests)

– Evaluate for causes of secondary dyslipidemia

– Evaluate for familial disorders

Consider influences of age, gender, other CHD risk factors

High-risk LDL cholesterol ≥160 mg/dl*

Initiate dietary therapy

*On the basis of the average of two determinations. If the first two LDL cholesterol determinations differ by more than 30 mg/dl, a third test should be obtained within 1–8 weeks and the average of the three tests used.

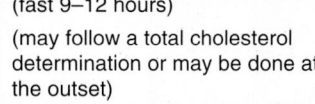

FIGURE 35–3. Primary prevention classification by low-density lipoprotein cholesterol. In patients without coronary artery disease or other atherosclerotic disease who have low high-density lipoprotein cholesterol, borderline-high total cholesterol in the presence of two or more other risk factors, or high total cholesterol, full fasting lipoprotein analysis is required to determine low-density lipoprotein cholesterol level. (From National Cholesterol Education Program.[2,3])

if LDL cholesterol is 130 mg/dl or greater. The goal of treatment in these patients is LDL cholesterol less than 130 mg/dl. The lower initiation level and goal reflect the additive impact of multiple risk factors on coronary disease, which justifies a more aggressive approach. In secondary prevention, dietary therapy should be initiated if LDL cholesterol is greater than 100 mg/dl. The goal of

TABLE 35–4 DIETARY THERAPY TREATMENT LEVELS IN ADULTS

RISK	LDL CHOLESTEROL LEVEL (mg/dl)	
	Initiation Level	Goal
Without CHD, fewer than two other risk factors	≥160	<160
Without CHD, two or more other risk factors	≥130	<130
With CHD or other atherosclerotic disease	>100	≤100

CHD = coronary heart disease; LDL = low-density lipoprotein.
From National Cholesterol Education Program: Second report of the Expert Panel on Detection, Evaluation, and Treatment of High Blood Cholesterol in Adults (Adult Treatment Panel II). Circulation 89:1329, 1994 Copyright American Heart Association.

treatment in these patients is LDL cholesterol of 100 mg/dl or less.

STEP I DIET. In primary prevention in patients following a typical Western diet, the initial diet is the Step I Diet (Table 35–5), which is recommended for the general population aged at least 2 years. The Step I Diet derives no more than 30 per cent of total calories from fat, 8 to 10 per cent of total calories from saturated fat, no more than 10 per cent of total calories from polyunsaturated fat, and no more than 15 per cent of total calories from monounsaturated fat.[81a] Cholesterol is limited to less than 300 mg/day, and total calories should be sufficient to achieve and maintain desirable weight.

STEP II DIET. In patients whose LDL cholesterol remains elevated despite adherence to the Step I Diet for 3 months, the Step II Diet should be instituted. The Step II Diet reduces saturated fat to less than 7 per cent of total calories and reduces cholesterol to less than 200 mg/day. In patients with CAD and in patients following the Step I Diet at the time of assessment, the Step II Diet is the initial therapy.

In patients previously consuming a typical Western diet, institution of the Step I Diet generally decreases total cholesterol 5 to 7 per cent, and institution of the Step II

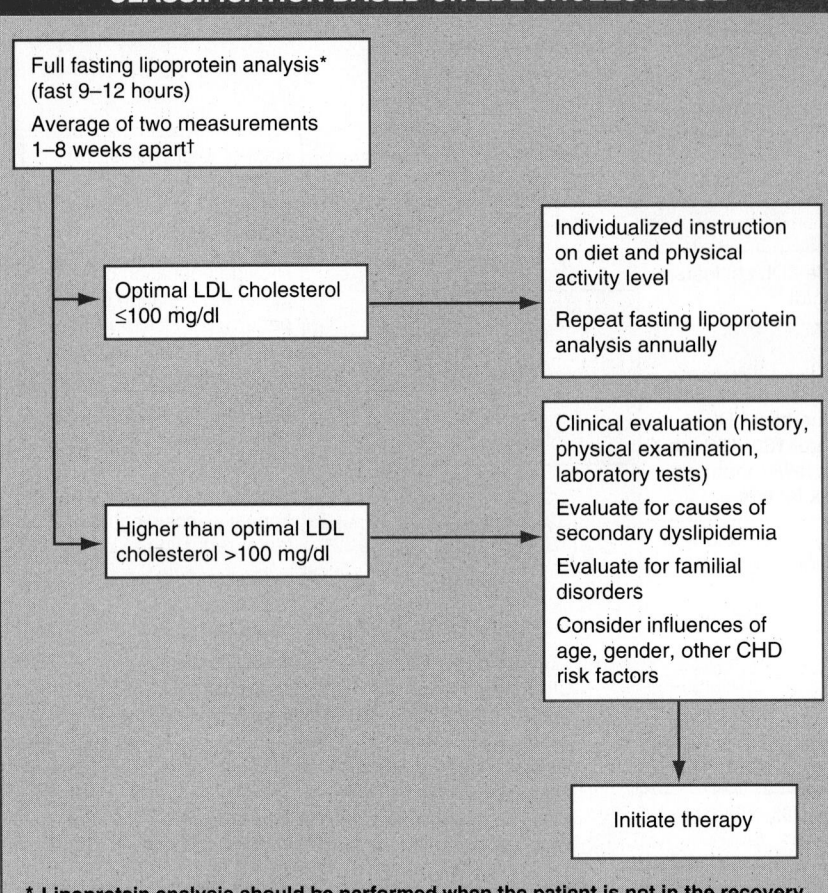

SECONDARY PREVENTION IN ADULTS WITH EVIDENCE OF CHD: CLASSIFICATION BASED ON LDL CHOLESTEROL

Full fasting lipoprotein analysis*
(fast 9–12 hours)

Average of two measurements
1–8 weeks apart†

Optimal LDL cholesterol
≤100 mg/dl

Individualized instruction
on diet and physical
activity level

Repeat fasting lipoprotein
analysis annually

Higher than optimal LDL
cholesterol >100 mg/dl

Clinical evaluation (history,
physical examination,
laboratory tests)

Evaluate for causes of
secondary dyslipidemia

Evaluate for familial
disorders

Consider influences of
age, gender, other CHD
risk factors

Initiate therapy

* Lipoprotein analysis should be performed when the patient is not in the recovery
phase from an acute coronary or other medical event that would lower his or her
usual LDL cholesterol level.

† If the first two LDL cholesterol determinations differ by more than 30 mg/dl, a third
test should be obtained within 1–8 weeks and the average of the three tests used.

FIGURE 35–4. Secondary prevention classification by low-density lipoprotein cholesterol. In patients with coronary artery disease or other atherosclerotic disease, initial assessment for dyslipidemia is by full fasting lipoprotein analysis to determine low-density lipoprotein cholesterol level. (From National Cholesterol Education Program.[2,3])

Diet decreases total cholesterol an additional 5 to 13 per cent.[82]

MONITORING DIETARY THERAPY. Total cholesterol may be used to monitor response to diet. In patients prescribed the Step I Diet, initial monitoring should occur 4 to 6 weeks and 3 months after the institution of therapy. Initial moni-

TABLE 35–5 DIETARY THERAPY OF HIGH BLOOD CHOLESTEROL

NUTRIENT	STEP I DIET*	STEP II DIET
Total fat	≤30% of total calories†	
Saturated fat	8–10% of total calories	<7% of total calories
Polyunsaturated fat	≤10% of total calories†	
Monounsaturated fat	≤15% of total calories†	
Carbohydrates	≥55% of total calories†	
Protein	~15% of total calories†	
Cholesterol	<300 mg/d	<200 mg/d
Total calories	Sufficient to achieve and maintain desirable weight	

* Recommended eating pattern for all healthy Americans aged 2 years or older.
† for both Step I and Step II Diet.
From National Cholesterol Education Program: Second report of the Expert Panel on Detection, Evaluation, and Treatment of High Blood Cholesterol in Adults (Adult Treatment Panel II). Circulation 89:1329, 1994. Copyright American Heart Association.

toring in patients prescribed the Step II Diet should occur 3 to 4 weeks and 3 months after the institution of therapy. Adherence to both diets should be assessed at 3 months. Some patients may require a longer trial before response to diet can be ascertained. More frequent follow-up may increase adherence. In most cases, an adequate trial of diet requires a minimum of 6 months' adherence. After LDL cholesterol goals have been achieved, long-term monitoring can be performed at 6-month intervals, providing an opportunity for continual reinforcement of dietary counseling.

Instituting and maintaining appropriate dietary therapy is a complex and frequently time-consuming process. Consultation with a dietitian provides an efficient means of assessing the patient's dietary habits. In addition, involvement of a dietitian is helpful in promoting adherence and ensuring adequate nutrition, particularly in patients prescribed the Step II Diet. A concerted effort should be made to maximize the effectiveness of dietary therapy, and the importance of this treatment should be stressed by the physician.

Drug Therapy

If, after an adequate trial of maximal dietary therapy, LDL cholesterol level remains above the initiation level for drug therapy (Table 35–6), pharmacological treatment of dyslipidemia should be considered in addition to dietary therapy (Table 35–7). Although an adequate trial of diet usually requires 6 months, a shorter time may be warranted in patients with CAD and in patients with severely ele-

TABLE 35-6 DRUG THERAPY TREATMENT LEVELS IN ADULTS

RISK	LDL CHOLESTEROL LEVEL (mg/dl)	
	Consideration Level	Goal
Without CHD, fewer than two other risk factors	≥ 190*	< 160
Without CHD, two or more other risk factors	≥ 160	< 130
With CHD or other atherosclerotic disease	≥ 130†	≤ 100

CHD = coronary heart disease; LDL = low-density lipoprotein.

* In younger patients (men aged < 35 years and premenopausal women) with LDL cholesterol 190–220 mg/dl, drug therapy may be delayed if other risk is absent.

† In patients with CHD and LDL cholesterol 100–130 mg/dl, the physician should exercise clinical judgment in deciding whether to initiate drug therapy.

From National Cholesterol Education Program: Second report of the Expert Panel on Detection, Evaluation, and Treatment of High Blood Cholesterol in Adults (Adult Treatment Panel II). Circulation 89:1329, 1994. Copyright American Heart Association.

vated cholesterol levels that would not be expected to be corrected by diet alone. The decision to initiate drug therapy requires careful weighing of the expected benefits and costs of potentially lifelong therapy, including possible adverse effects. Once drug therapy has been initiated, discontinuation quickly returns LDL cholesterol to pretreatment levels.

In primary prevention, drug therapy should be considered in patients with fewer than two other risk factors whose LDL cholesterol remains 190 mg/dl or greater on maximal dietary therapy. The goal of treatment in these patients is to reduce LDL cholesterol to less than 160 mg/dl. Because younger patients are at lower risk for CAD events, the NCEP guidelines recommend that drug therapy be delayed in men aged less than 35 years and in premenopausal women unless LDL cholesterol is 220 mg/dl or greater or unless additional risk is present. Clinical judgment is required to assess the patient's overall risk.

In patients without CAD who have two or more other risk factors, drug therapy should be considered if LDL cholesterol remains 160 mg/dl or greater on maximal dietary therapy. In these patients, the goal of treatment is to reduce LDL cholesterol to less than 130 mg/dl.

In secondary prevention, the high rate of recurrence of acute ischemic events warrants more intensive therapy. Drug therapy should be considered if maximal dietary therapy does not lower LDL cholesterol to 130 mg/dl or less. However, clinical judgment should be used in deciding whether drug therapy is needed in patients whose LDL cholesterol is 100 to 129 mg/dl. Clinical judgment is also required to recognize patients in whom lipid-regulating pharmacological therapy is not appropriate, such as patients with a very advanced age, poor cardiac prognosis, or severe concomitant medical conditions. In general, even

high-risk patients with limited life expectancy would not be expected to receive sufficient benefit from lipid-regulating drug therapy to justify its initiation.

Response to drug therapy should be monitored 6 to 8 weeks after initiation or, if nicotinic acid is used, 4 to 6 weeks after dosage stabilization; response should be reevaluated 6 weeks later. A minimum of two fasting lipoprotein analyses should be used to determine response, and adherence should be ascertained before adjusting dosage or considering another agent.

If 3 months' adherence to pharmacological monotherapy does not reduce LDL cholesterol to target levels, combination-drug therapy may be considered (Table 35–7). Although the addition of a second agent may increase the potential for side effects and drug interactions, combination therapy often decreases side effects and costs and increases adherence, because a lower dosage of each agent is required. In secondary prevention, clinical judgment is required to determine whether to add a second agent if LDL cholesterol is 100 to 129 mg/dl with pharmacological monotherapy.

Available lipid-regulating agents are bile-acid sequestrants, nicotinic acid, HMG-CoA reductase inhibitors, fibric-acid derivatives, and probucol (Table 35–8).[83a] In some postmenopausal women, estrogen-replacement therapy may provide an alternative to drug therapy.

BILE-ACID SEQUESTRANTS. The bile-acid sequestrants are quaternary ammonium salts, usually dispensed as a powdered preparation that requires mixing with liquids or foods prior to administration. However, a caplet and confectionery bar have been developed to increase ease of administration and palatability. The bile-acid sequestrants have a long history of clinical use, and their mechanisms of action, side effects, and clinical efficacy are well established. The use of bile-acid sequestrant monotherapy has declined in recent years because of the advent of more palatable and more potent drugs.

The mechanisms of action of the two available agents, cholestyramine and colestipol, are similar. These agents interrupt the enterohepatic circulation of bile acids by acting as polycationic exchange resins that bind the bile acids in the intestinal lumen and increase fecal loss.[83] Normally, approximately 97 per cent of the endogenously produced bile acids are reabsorbed and recycled in the enterohepatic circulation, and only 3 per cent are excreted. The increased excretion of bile acids with bile-acid sequestrant therapy causes an increase in the activity of 7-alpha-hydroxylase, the rate-limiting enzyme of bile acid synthesis, thereby increasing the conversion of cholesterol into bile acids. The resulting decrease in intrahepatic cholesterol causes increased activity of the B/E receptor and therefore the enhanced removal of apo B– and apo E–containing lipoproteins from the circulation. However, HMG-CoA reductase activity is also increased in response to the decrease in intrahepatic cholesterol, so that plasma cholesterol returns toward pretreatment levels.[84]

TABLE 35-7 DRUG SELECTION IN ADULTS: NATIONAL CHOLESTEROL EDUCATION PROGRAM RECOMMENDATIONS

HYPERLIPIDEMIA	SINGLE DRUG	COMBINATION DRUG
Elevated LDL cholesterol and triglyceride < 200 mg/dl	Bile-acid sequestrant	Bile-acid sequestrant + HMG-CoA reductase inhibitor
	HMG-CoA reductase inhibitor	Bile-acid sequestrant + nicotinic acid
	Nicotinic acid	HMG-CoA reductase inhibitor + nicotinic acid*
Elevated LDL cholesterol and triglyceride 200–400 mg/dl	Nicotinic acid	Nicotinic acid + HMG-CoA reductase inhibitor*
	HMG-CoA reductase inhibitor	HMG-CoA reductase inhibitor + gemfibrozil†
	Gemfibrozil	Nicotinic acid + bile-acid sequestrant
		Nicotinic acid + gemfibrozil

HMG-CoA = 3-hydroxy-3-methylglutaryl coenzyme A; LDL = low-density lipoprotein.

* Possible increased risk for myopathy or liver dysfunction.

† Increased risk for myopathy; must be used with caution.

From National Cholesterol Education Program: Second report of the Expert Panel on Detection, Evaluation, and Treatment of High Blood Cholesterol in Adults (Adult Treatment Panel II). Circulation 89:1329, 1994. Copyright American Heart Association.

TABLE 35–8 LIPID-LOWERING AGENTS: MECHANISMS, LIPID EFFECTS, AND SIDE EFFECTS

DRUG CLASS AND AGENTS	MECHANISM OF ACTION AND LIPID EFFECTS	SELECTED BIOCHEMICAL SIDE EFFECTS	SELECTED SYSTEMIC SIDE EFFECTS
Bile-acid sequestrants (resins) Cholestyramine (4–24 gm/day) Colestipol (5–30 gm/day)	Increase excretion of bile acids in the stool; increase LDL-receptor activity. Effectively decrease LDL cholesterol; HDL cholesterol increases slightly; may increase triglyceride	Binding and decreased absorption of certain other drugs; may prevent absorption of fat-soluble vitamins	No systemic toxicity; upper and lower gastrointestinal complaints common, such as constipation, bloating
Nicotinic acid (niacin) (1.5–6 gm/day)	Decreases plasma levels of free fatty acids; decreases hepatic VLDL synthesis; possibly inhibits cholesterol synthesis. Effectively decreases both LDL cholesterol and triglyceride; effectively increases HDL cholesterol	Altered liver function tests, increased uric acid, increased glucose intolerance	Cutaneous flushing, pruritus, gastrointestinal upset; side effects tend to limit compliance
HMG-CoA reductase inhibitors (statins) Fluvastatin (20–40 mg/day) Lovastatin (10–80 mg/day) Pravastatin (10–40 mg/day) Simvastatin (5–40 mg/day)	Inhibit HMG-CoA reductase, the rate-limiting step in cholesterol biosynthesis; increase LDL-receptor activity. Effectively decrease LDL cholesterol; moderate effect in decreasing triglyceride and in increasing HDL cholesterol	Elevated transaminase levels can occur (minor and usually transient); increased creatine kinase (uncommon)	Mild gastrointestinal symptoms; myositis syndrome (rare)
Fibric-acid derivatives (fibrates) Gemfibrozil (1.2 gm/day) Clofibrate (2 gm/day)	Decrease hepatic VLDL synthesis; increase lipoprotein lipase activity. Decrease triglyceride effectively; increase HDL cholesterol effectively; effect on LDL cholesterol variable, but may increase, especially in hypertriglyceridemia	Transient transaminase increases not infrequent; can potentiate effects of oral anticoagulants	Increased incidence of cholelithiasis; diarrhea, nausea, skin rash, myositis (rare)
Probucol (1 gm/day)	Enhances scavenger pathway removal of LDL. Slightly to moderately decreases LDL cholesterol; usually no effect on triglyceride; substantially decreases HDL cholesterol	Prolongation of QT interval and serious ventricular arrhythmias have occurred but are rare	Side effects usually infrequent and of short duration; chiefly, diarrhea, nausea, flatulence

HDL = high-density lipoprotein; HMG-CoA = 3-hydroxy-3-methylglutaryl coenzyme A; LDL = low-density lipoprotein; VLDL = very-low-density lipoprotein.

From Jones P. H., and Gotto, A. M., Jr.: Hyperlipidemia. *In* Hurst, J. W. (ed.): Medicine for the Practicing Physician, 4th ed. Norwalk, CT, Appleton & Lange 1996.

Cholestyramine dosed at 4 to 16 gm/day, up to a maximum of 24 gm/day, or colestipol dosed at 5 to 20 gm/day, up to a maximum of 30 gm/day, decreases LDL cholesterol 15 to 30 per cent on average. HDL cholesterol may increase 3 to 5 per cent, although it has not been determined if bile-acid sequestrants alter HDL synthesis or catabolic rates. Plasma triglyceride is not usually affected but may increase; this increase is more common in patients who are hypertriglyceridemic before therapy.

The major side effects of cholestyramine and colestipol are gastrointestinal disorders such as constipation, reflux esophagitis, and nausea. Because these drugs are not absorbed into the circulation, systemic side effects are uncommon. The same nonspecific binding by which the bile-acid sequestrants bind bile acids may cause decreased absorption of other drugs, including warfarin,[85] digitalis preparations,[86] thiazide diuretics,[87] and beta blockers.[88]

NICOTINIC ACID. Nicotinic acid is a B vitamin that was discovered to have lipid-regulating effects at high doses. Although nicotinic acid is a coenzyme in intermediary carbohydrate metabolism, this role is not related to its lipid-regulating action.

The mechanisms of action of nicotinic acid are complex and result in favorable changes in all lipoprotein fractions except chylomicrons. The primary action is a decrease in the hepatic synthesis and release of VLDL, thus also decreasing the circulating levels of IDL and LDL because of decreased production of precursor particles.[89] In addition, nicotinic acid causes a decrease in the release of free fatty acids from adipocytes, thereby decreasing hepatic production of triglyceride by decreasing the availability of the substrates for triglyceride synthesis. However, the long-term impact of this peripheral effect on the lipid profile has been questioned.[90]

Crystalline nicotinic acid dosed at 1.5 to 6 gm/day decreases LDL cholesterol 10 to 25 per cent. Triglyceride decreases 20 to 50 per cent, and HDL cholesterol increases 15 to 35 per cent. The increase in HDL cholesterol is caused by decreased catabolism of HDL and apo A-I.[91] Nicotinic acid has been shown to decrease Lp(a) levels,[92] which are not usually affected by lipid-regulating drugs. Nicotinic acid is also available in sustained-release preparations, which are administered at lower doses, but increased side effects and safety concerns have limited their use (see below).

Side effects of nicotinic acid include mild clinical irritations and potentially life-threatening complications. The rapid absorption of crystalline nicotinic acid from the gastrointestinal tract after oral administration may account for the agent's vasodilatory effects. Flushing is seen in virtually all patients and is secondary to the release of prostaglandin by the endothelium. Preadministration of prostaglandin inhibitors, such as aspirin, may decrease flushing. Hepatic toxicity, perhaps due to the high first-pass extraction of nicotinic acid by the liver, ranges from mild elevations of transaminase levels to fulminant hepatic failure,[93] although the latter is reported more often with sustained-release preparations.[94] Mild elevations of liver enzymes may be seen in as many as 5 per cent of patients receiving nicotinic acid[90] and are not in and of themselves indications for discontinuation of this drug. However, close clinical monitoring is warranted; an increase in liver enzymes to three times normal or greater requires discontinuation of nicotinic acid. On the other hand, a sudden decline in liver enzyme levels may indicate significant clinical deterioration and decreased synthetic ability and constitutes a medical emergency. Other gastrointestinal side effects include activation of peptic ulcer disease.[95] Nicotinic acid has also been reported to worsen glucose tolerance, precipitate gout, and cause ophthalmological complications that include worsening of glaucoma and cystic maculopathy secondary to increased fluid retention within the retina. Myositis is rare with nicotinic acid monotherapy[96] but may be somewhat more common when nicotinic acid is combined with an HMG-CoA reductase inhibitor.[97]

HMG-COA REDUCTASE INHIBITORS. The HMG-CoA reductase inhibitors represent a major therapeutic advance in lipid-regulating pharmacological therapy because of their increased efficacy, tolerability, and ease of administration. Fluvastatin, lovastatin, pravastatin, and simvastatin are the currently available agents.

Despite structural differences, the HMG-CoA reductase inhibitors appear to share a common mechanism of action, the partial inhibition of HMG-CoA reductase, the rate-limiting enzyme in cholesterol biosynthesis. The resultant reduction in intracellular cholesterol in the liver stimulates the upregulation of the B/E receptor and increases clearance of lipoproteins containing apo B or apo E from the plasma compartment. Although the predominant effect is to decrease circulating LDL cholesterol, VLDL and IDL particles are also removed. Inhibition of the synthesis of apo B–containing lipoproteins has also been postulated as a potential mechanism for these agents,[98] but this hypothesis remains controversial. Potential beneficial nonlipid effects include a reduction in plasminogen activator inhibitor 1 (PAI-1) in patients with hypercholesterolemia, reported with lovastatin[99] and pravastatin,[100] which provides a hemostatic mechanism for clinical improvement with HMG-CoA reductase inhibitor therapy.

Fluvastatin dosed at 20 to 40 mg/day, lovastatin dosed at 10 to 80 mg/day, pravastatin dosed at 10 to 40 mg/day, or simvastatin dosed at 5 to 40 mg/day may be expected to decrease LDL cholesterol 20 to 40 per cent. The dose-response effect of the HMG-CoA reductase inhibitors is log-linear: At higher doses, the cholesterol-lowering effect increases in smaller increments. HDL cholesterol increases 5 to 15 per cent, although the precise mechanism has not been elucidated, and triglyceride decreases 10 to 20 per cent, presumably because of increased clearance of VLDL by the B/E receptor.[101] Lp(a) level does not appear to be affected by HMG-CoA reductase inhibitor therapy.[102]

Because of their high patient acceptance rate and lipid-regulating efficacy, the HMG-CoA reductase inhibitors are frequently used as first-line pharmacological monotherapy. In addition, recently published clinical trial data have demonstrated improvements in clinical and anatomical endpoints. However, these agents are too new to have accumulated the long-term safety and efficacy data recorded for agents such as the bile-acid sequestrants; consequently, the NCEP does not recommend HMG-CoA reductase inhibitors as first-line drug therapy in primary prevention in young adults unless the underlying dyslipidemia is severe.

The side effects of the HMG-CoA reductase inhibitors are minimal. The major clinical problems that have been reported are hepatotoxicity and myopathy. Serum liver enzyme levels were greater than three times the upper limit of normal in less than 2 per cent of subjects who received maximum-dosage lovastatin in the 1-year Expanded Clinical Evaluation of Lovastatin (EXCEL) study, and at the usual dosage, the incidence was less than 1 per cent.[103] Most cases of transaminase elevation appear to occur within the first 3 months of therapy. Rhabdomyolysis has been documented in approximately 0.1 per cent of subjects

receiving lovastatin monotherapy[104] and appears to occur at about the same frequency for all the HMG-CoA reductase inhibitors. However, the exact incidence of myopathy, as defined by creatine kinase elevation, that is attributable to HMG-CoA reductase inhibitor use is difficult to establish: In subjects who continued in the EXCEL study a second year, creatine kinase elevations above the upper limit of normal were reported in 50 to 67 per cent of the groups receiving various dosages of lovastatin and 54 per cent of the placebo group.[105] Risk for myopathy may be increased when an HMG-CoA reductase inhibitor is combined with a fibric-acid derivative,[106] nicotinic acid,[107] cyclosporine,[108] or erythromycin.[109] Despite initial concern based on inhibitors of enzymes of cholesterol synthesis other than HMG-CoA, no evidence of increased lens opacity has been reported with the use of HMG-CoA reductase inhibitors.[110] Although it has been postulated that the lipophilic agents, lovastatin and simvastatin, may have a greater potential for sleep disturbances than the hydrophilic fluvastatin and pravastatin, because the former cross the blood–brain barrier, the incidence of sleep disturbances is uncommon with either lipophilic or hydrophilic agents.[111]

FIBRIC-ACID DERIVATIVES. The fibric-acid derivatives have been used clinically in a variety of lipoprotein disorders, and their efficacy and safety have been demonstrated. Clofibrate, which is little used, and gemfibrozil are currently available in the United States, and bezafibrate, ciprofibrate, and fenofibrate are available in other countries. Fenofibrate has been approved in the United States but is not yet available.

The mechanism of action of the fibric-acid derivatives is complex and has not been completely elucidated. The major effect is a decrease in VLDL secondary to increased lipoprotein lipase activity; lipoprotein lipase hydrolyzes triglyceride from VLDL to form IDL, which is either removed by the B/E receptor through apo E–mediated recognition and binding or further hydrolyzed by hepatic lipase to form LDL. The fibrates may also exert a peripheral effect by decreasing plasma levels of free fatty acids.[112]

Gemfibrozil dosed at 1200 mg/day or clofibrate dosed at 2000 mg/day decreases triglyceride 20 to 50 per cent and increases HDL cholesterol 10 to 15 per cent. LDL cholesterol is typically decreased 10 to 15 per cent but may increase in patients with hypertriglyceridemia, perhaps because of the inability of the B/E receptor to remove the increased number of LDL particles that result from enhanced VLDL catabolism. A decrease in Lp(a) has been reported with bezafibrate administration.[113]

In addition to their effects on lipoprotein levels, fibric-acid derivatives may alter the composition of lipoproteins. As noted above, gemfibrozil and bezafibrate have been shown to decrease the concentration of small, dense LDL. The fibrates may thus protect against coronary atherosclerosis not only by reducing LDL cholesterol level but also by shifting LDL particles to a less atherogenic phenotype.

Additionally, the fibric-acid derivatives provide nonlipid benefits, such as improvements in coagulation and fibrinolysis. A reduction in platelet aggregability and reactivity in response to epinephrine has been documented with gemfibrozil.[114] Gemfibrozil has also been shown to decrease the activity of PAI-1, thereby potentially improving fibrinolytic efficacy.[115] Bezafibrate has been reported to decrease circulating levels of fibrinogen[116]; fibrinogen has been directly associated with CAD risk in epidemiological studies (see below).

The side effects of the fibric-acid derivatives are generally mild and are encountered in approximately 5 to 10 per cent of patients treated with these agents. The majority of complaints are of nonspecific gastrointestinal symptoms such as nausea, flatulence, bloating, and dyspepsia. Increased lithogenicity of bile has been reported with clofibrate therapy[28] but has not been clearly demonstrated with the other fibrates. Fibrate monotherapy rarely results in muscle toxicity,[117] although mild elevations of creatine kinase may occasionally occur. However, the risk for myopathy is increased when a fibrate is used in combination with an HMG-CoA reductase inhibitor, as described above. Although recent studies have demonstrated that this combination may be used without severe muscle toxicity,[118] great caution is required, and careful patient education and surveillance are prerequisites.

PROBUCOL. Probucol is a complex agent that cannot be readily classified with the other lipid-regulating drugs in terms of structure or mechanism of action. It is a bisphenol derivative that is similar in structure to butylated hydroxytoluene, a compound with powerful antioxidant activity that has also been demonstrated to decrease the early microcirculatory changes induced by hypercholesterolemia in rabbits.[119]

The mechanism of action by which probucol lowers lipid levels has not been completely elucidated. Probucol does not appear to decrease the production of lipoproteins nor does it alter plasma clearance through the B/E receptor pathway. In the Watanabe heritable hyperlipidemic rabbit, which serves as an animal model for FH because it lacks functioning B/E receptors, the decreased rate of progression of atherosclerotic lesions with probucol administration appears to be predominantly attributable to the inhibitory effect of probucol on LDL oxidation.[120] In patients with FH, regression of tendinous xanthomas has been reported with probucol use.[121]

Probucol dosed at 1 gm/day decreases LDL cholesterol 5 to 15 per cent and decreases HDL cholesterol 20 to 30 per cent. Triglyceride is usually not affected. The effect on HDL cholesterol appears to be greater in patients with higher pretreatment levels of HDL cholesterol[122] and is of concern because of the inverse relation between HDL cholesterol level and CAD incidence established in epidemiological studies (see below). The composition of HDL particles is also altered by probucol therapy: The triglyceride content of HDL is increased, and the concentration of cholesteryl ester in HDL is decreased, apparently owing to increased CETP activity.[123] The clinical impact of the probucol-induced reduction in HDL cholesterol is controversial, but evidence suggests that probucol administration may enhance reverse cholesterol transport secondary to increased CETP activity and increased hepatic uptake of HDL.[124]

The side effects of probucol appear to be minimal. Probucol is highly lipophilic, so its absorption is enhanced after a fatty meal; therefore, administration should be separated from meals to prevent drug toxicity. Mild gastrointestinal symptoms are occasionally reported. The main clinical concern with probucol use is the possible potentiation of rhythm disorders associated with prolongation of repolarization. In experimental animals, increased incidence of sudden cardiac death with probucol administration was thought to be caused by induced ventricular arrhythmias.[125] Although no clear correlation between probucol use and sudden cardiac death has been established in humans, the Q-T interval should be monitored, especially in patients with baseline prolongation or receiving concomitant sotalol, quinidine, procainamide, tricyclic antidepressants, phenothiazines, or other agents known to increase the Q-T interval.

ESTROGEN. Women lose their relative protection against coronary atherosclerosis at menopause, when decreased estrogen production causes a gradual rise in LDL cholesterol levels. In a study in 542 healthy women, postmenopausal women had 14 per cent higher total cholesterol, 12 per cent higher triglyceride, and 27 per cent higher LDL cholesterol; HDL cholesterol was 7 per cent lower.[126] These potentially atherogenic alterations in the lipid profile have prompted an increased interest in estrogen-replacement therapy in postmenopausal women.

Estrogen-replacement therapy has been shown to de-

crease CAD morbidity and CAD mortality in observational epidemiological studies.[127] In a meta-analysis of case–control, cross-sectional, and prospective studies, the relative risk for CAD in postmenopausal subjects taking estrogen was 0.56 compared with postmenopausal subjects not taking estrogen.[128]

The precise mechanisms by which estrogen decreases CAD risk are not known. Increased HDL cholesterol and decreased LDL cholesterol have been demonstrated,[129] and other possible benefits include improved coronary tone and altered platelet aggregation. A decreased accumulation of LDL in the arterial wall has been reported in animal studies.[130] Circulating Lp(a) may also be decreased.[131]

Conjugated estrogen dosed at 0.625 mg/day or micronized estradiol dosed at 2 mg/day, administered orally, decreases LDL cholesterol 15 per cent and increases HDL cholesterol up to 15 per cent. Plasma triglyceride may increase, particularly if it is elevated before initiation of therapy. Transcutaneous or percutaneous administration of estrogen generally appears to have less effect on lipid levels than oral administration. Estrogen does not have a U.S. Food and Drug Administration indication for lipid regulation or CAD risk reduction.

Unopposed estrogen use increases risk for endometrial cancer and possibly increases risk for breast cancer. However, coadministration with progesterone moderates the risk for endometrial cancer without nullifying the lipid-regulating benefits of estrogen.[132]

Primary Dyslipidemias Characterized by Hypercholesterolemia

Fredrickson phenotypes in which hypercholesterolemia is the major dyslipidemia are types IIa and IIb. In type IIa, hypercholesterolemia is the only dyslipidemia, and in type IIb, triglyceride is also elevated. Both of these phenotypes are associated with increased risk for atherosclerotic disease. Among causes of secondary type II hyperlipidemia, which should be ruled out before a primary cause is considered, are diet, myxedema, obstructive liver disease, and nephrosis.

FAMILIAL HYPERCHOLESTEROLEMIA. The most clearly delineated familial disorder presenting as a type IIa and rarely as a type IIb phenotype is FH, an autosomal dominant disorder caused by a defect in the gene for the B/E receptor that results in decreased production or function of B/E receptors.[133,133a] Heterozygous FH occurs in approximately 1 in 500 individuals in the United States but has a higher frequency in Lebanon and in the Afrikaner population in South Africa, where the gene frequency is thought to be 1 per cent. Affected individuals have approximately half the number of functioning B/E receptors, and total cholesterol, which is elevated at birth, may reach 350 to 500 mg/dl. Symptomatic CAD typically develops by age 50 in men and age 60 in women. Clinical features include tendon xanthomas and corneal arcus. Heterozygous FH may be difficult to diagnose[134]; familial combined hyperlipidemia (FCH) and familial defective apo B-100 (see below) should be considered in the differential diagnosis. Treatment consists of dietary and drug therapy; combination-drug therapy is usually required.

Homozygous FH occurs in approximately 1 in 1 million individuals in the United States. Affected individuals have virtually no competent B/E receptors, and total cholesterol, which is elevated at birth, reaches 700 to 1200 mg/dl. Symptomatic CAD typically develops before age 20; premature atherosclerosis is the rule, and myocardial infarctions have been reported before the age of 2 years. Clinical features include cutaneous xanthomas, tendinous xanthomas, corneal arcus, and severe, diffuse atherosclerosis. The presence of xanthomas, which frequently occur in the buttocks, tongue, eyelid, and buccal mucosa, strongly suggests a diagnosis of FH, although tendinous xanthomas are not specific to FH but are also seen in other rare diseases such as cerebrotendinous xanthomatosis and sitosterolemia. Similarly, corneal arcus is a nonspecific finding for the diagnosis of FH; the presence of corneal arcus in a white patient aged less than 35 years suggests the presence of an underlying metabolic defect, but this sign loses its specificity in older patients and in black patients.

Low-Density Lipoprotein Apheresis. Because FH is usually resistant to dietary and pharmacological therapy, special techniques may be required to reduce circulating LDL cholesterol. LDL apheresis removes apo B–containing lipoproteins from blood by extracorporeal binding to dextran sulfate–cellulose columns, heparin precipitation, or immunoabsorption. In the LDL-Apheresis Regression Study, conducted in 37 subjects (7 patients with homozygous FH, 25 patients with heterozygous FH, and 5 hypercholesterolemic patients not diagnosed with FH), LDL cholesterol was reduced 78 per cent immediately after apheresis, and, after 1 year of apheresis treatments, regression was reported in 38 per cent of subjects.[135] The reduction in LDL cholesterol is only temporary, so the procedure must be repeated at 2- to 4-week intervals. In the Familial Hypercholesterolaemia Regression Study, 39 men and women with heterozygous FH were followed up by quantitative coronary angiography after a mean of 2.1 years of receiving either LDL apheresis every 2 weeks and simvastatin 40 mg/day or colestipol 20 gm/day and simvastatin 40 mg/day.[136] Entry criteria included total cholesterol of 310 mg/dl or greater plus either tendon xanthomas in the subject or a first-degree relative or total cholesterol of at least 310 mg/dl or myocardial infarction before age 60 in a first-degree relative or before age 50 in a second-degree relative, at least two abnormal coronary segments on angiographic assessment, and age of 20 to 64 years. Despite greater lowering of LDL cholesterol with apheresis plus simvastatin (53 per cent compared with 44 per cent with colestipol plus simvastatin), the primary angiographic endpoint of mean change in per cent diameter stenosis of the worst lesion in diseased segments was not significantly different between treatment groups, and the other primary endpoint—the number of patients demonstrating progression, regression, and no change or a mixed response—was also similar between groups. LDL apheresis is expensive and currently available only in selected centers.

Liver Transplantation. This procedure has been performed in patients with homozygous FH. In a 6-year-old patient, transplantation of a liver and heart from a normal donor decreased plasma LDL cholesterol 81 per cent and increased the fractional catabolic rate of radiolabeled LDL 2.5 times.[137]

Gene Therapy. This technique has recently been employed to introduce functioning B/E receptors in a patient with homozygous FH.[138] The ex vivo technique used requires partial hepatectomy, and the isolated hepatocytes are infected with retroviruses that express the normal B/E receptor. After the treated hepatocytes were infused into the patient, LDL cholesterol decreased 17 per cent. However, liver resection may cause a decrease in circulating LDL, because of decreased secretion of VLDL, and it has been suggested that gene therapy experiments demonstrate that LDL reductions are the result of increased B/E receptor activity, which should then be demonstrated to result from the exogenous gene.[139]

POLYGENIC HYPERCHOLESTEROLEMIA. The most common genetic cause of type IIa hyperlipidemia is polygenic hypercholesterolemia.[140] Although the prevalence of this disorder is unknown, it is thought to be between 1 in 20 and 1 in 100 in the United States. Total cholesterol level is usually less than in heterozygous FH, and xanthomas are absent. Severe cases may require treatment similar to that of heterozygous FH but may not require combination-drug therapy.

FAMILIAL COMBINED HYPERLIPIDEMIA. FCH[141] may present as type IIa, type IIb, or type IV hyperlipidemia. In type II

presentations, total cholesterol is usually 250 to 350 mg/dl. In type IIb and type IV presentations, triglyceride elevations are typically mild to moderate but may be severe. Presentation may vary within a family and within an individual. The disorder is relatively common in the United States, occurring in approximately 1 in 100 individuals. It is not known whether transmission is monogenic or polygenic; inheritance is autosomal dominant. The underlying mechanism is thought to be overproduction of apo B-100. Clinically, this disease may be distinguished from FH by a lack of tendinous xanthomas. Expression may or may not occur before adulthood. Premature coronary atherosclerosis is associated with FCH, and early recognition and treatment are required. The primary treatment is dietary; if diet proves inadequate, drug therapy should be added as appropriate for the dyslipidemia.

FAMILIAL DEFECTIVE APOLIPOPROTEIN B-100. Familial defective apo B-100 is an autosomal dominant disorder caused by a mutation in the gene for apo B-100 that results in apo B-100 with an abnormal structure and decreased binding by the B/E receptor.[142] Prevalence varies but is approximately 1 in 700 in whites. Cholesterol levels are similar to those in heterozygous FH but may be more moderate. In general, familial defective apo B-100 may be distinguished from heterozygous FH by the lack of tendinous xanthomas and by less severe hypercholesterolemia, but accurate diagnosis may require molecular analysis. Treatment is as for heterozygous FH and should begin with dietary therapy, to which may be added an HMG-CoA reductase inhibitor or a bile-acid sequestrant. Nicotinic acid is also useful in treating familial defective apo B-100.[143]

Low High-Density Lipoprotein Cholesterol

An inverse association has been established between HDL cholesterol level and CAD incidence in numerous epidemiological studies. For example, in the Framingham Heart Study, men and women with HDL cholesterol of 35 mg/dl or less had an eightfold increase in CAD incidence compared with men and women with HDL cholesterol of 65 mg/dl or greater.[144] Each 1 mg/dl increase in HDL cholesterol is estimated to decrease CAD risk 2 per cent in men and 3 per cent in women.[145]

Primary hypoalphalipoproteinemia may occur in up to 5 per cent of the general population. HDL cholesterol levels may also be lowered by cigarette smoking, the use of drugs such as anabolic steroids or beta blockers, and a diet very high in polyunsaturated fat.

High-Density Lipoprotein Metabolism

HDL is believed to be secreted by the liver and intestine as a discoidal precursor particle of phospholipid, cholesterol, and apolipoproteins. Through the activity of lecithin:cholesterol acyltransferase (LCAT), a core of cholesteryl ester is generated from the phospholipid and cholesterol, and the disk is transformed into mature, spherical HDL_3. HDL_3 acquires additional phospholipid and cholesterol from cell membranes and from the excess surface components of hydrolyzed triglyceride-rich lipoproteins. Through continued LCAT activity, HDL_3 is converted to HDL_2, which is larger and more cholesterol rich than HDL_3. Women have significantly higher plasma levels of HDL_2 than men[146]; increased levels of these larger, less dense particles may be partially responsible for the relative cardioprotection seen in premenopausal women.

The mechanism by which HDL confers decreased risk for CAD is complex and poorly understood. One proposed mechanism is as the possible vehicle of reverse cholesterol transport, the posited process by which cholesterol is returned from peripheral cells to the liver for excretion into the bile acid pool or for reconstitution into cell membranes or VLDL. Although the process by which cholesterol leaves the peripheral cell and is scavenged by HDL has not been clarified, a number of potential mechanisms have been proposed, including cholesterol efflux.[147]

Through the action of CETP, triglyceride from the triglyceride-rich lipoproteins is exchanged for cholesteryl ester in HDL. The transferred triglyceride then becomes a substrate for hepatic lipase, and the transferred cholesteryl ester continues with the triglyceride-rich lipoproteins in their respective lipolytic cascades and is removed with chylomicron remnants, IDL, and LDL. Because of the metabolic interrelation between HDL and the triglyceride-rich lipoproteins, high HDL cholesterol level may reflect rapid clearance of these triglyceride-rich particles, thereby decreasing the exposure of the vessel wall to potentially atherogenic remnant particles.[148] HDL levels would then serve as a marker of the efficiency of this metabolic process, rather than conferring direct protection against CAD.

Other potential mechanisms by which HDL may confer cardioprotection include enhancement of endothelial repair[149] and prostacyclin stabilization.[150] HDL has also demonstrated dose-dependent protection against peroxidation of LDL.[151]

Diagnosis and Treatment of Low High-Density Lipoprotein Cholesterol

As stated above, HDL cholesterol less than 35 mg/dl is considered low in the NCEP guidelines. The primary therapy for low HDL cholesterol is life style modification, emphasizing diet, regular exercise, smoking cessation, and weight reduction as appropriate. Intense efforts should also be made to control blood pressure and diabetes mellitus. If feasible, drugs that lower HDL cholesterol should be discontinued.

None of the available lipid-regulating agents acts exclusively to increase HDL cholesterol, and the NCEP does not recommend introducing a drug solely for this purpose in primary prevention in patients who are otherwise at low risk for CAD. However, if drug therapy is indicated to lower LDL cholesterol, a secondary goal of increasing HDL cholesterol should guide in selection of the agent. Lipid-regulating agents that are particularly effective in increasing HDL cholesterol are the fibric-acid derivatives, which have a greater effect in patients who also have increased plasma triglyceride, and nicotinic acid. In general, the same treatment plan should be used in secondary prevention, although the NCEP does recommend the consideration of nicotinic acid to increase HDL cholesterol even in patients whose LDL cholesterol is below the initiation level for drug therapy.

Primary Dyslipidemias Characterized by Low High-Density Lipoprotein Cholesterol

TANGIER DISEASE. Tangier disease, which was initially thought to be a lipid storage disorder, is a rare autosomal recessive disorder marked by low levels of both HDL cholesterol and apo A-I.[152] Cholesteryl ester is deposited in the tissues of the reticuloendothelial system, causing orange tonsils that in combination with low total cholesterol are diagnostic of this disease. Other symptoms include splenomegaly, peripheral neuropathy, and ocular abnormalities. Atherosclerotic risk does not appear to be increased.[153] This disorder results from markedly increased catabolism of HDL, apo A-I, and apo A-II[154] instead of from decreased synthesis.

LECITHIN:CHOLESTEROL ACYLTRANSFERASE DEFICIENCY. In familial LCAT deficiency disorder, LCAT activity is absent, resulting in increased plasma levels of cholesterol and lecithin and decreased plasma levels of cholesteryl ester and lysolecithin.[155] Composition, structure, and concentration of all lipoprotein fractions are altered.[156] HDL may remain as discoidal precursor particles or small, spherical particles. Clinical features include corneal opacities, anemia, renal failure, and proteinuria. Despite decreased HDL cholesterol, CAD risk is not usually increased, but atherosclerosis and tendon and planar xanthomas may result from hyperlipidemia and hypertension secondary to renal failure.

FISH-EYE DISEASE. Fish-eye disease resembles LCAT deficiency, but only LCAT activity toward HDL is decreased.[157] HDL particles are similar to those in LCAT deficiency, and triglyceride may be elevated. Corneal opacities are characteristic of this disease, and corneal transplantation is required in older patients. Atherosclerotic risk does not appear to be increased.

APO A-I$_{Milano}$. Individuals who have the apo A-I$_{Milano}$ mutation have low HDL cholesterol and hypertriglyceridemia. In a comparison of 29 affected individuals with age- and gender-matched controls, HDL cholesterol was decreased 67 per cent and triglyceride was increased 75 per cent.[158] Apo A-I$_{Milano}$ results from a mutation in the gene for apo A-I that has been shown to increase plasma clearance of apo A-I: Apo A-I$_{Milano}$ was catabolized more rapidly than normal apo A-I in normal subjects, and both apo A-I$_{Milano}$ and normal apo A-I were catabolized more rapidly in subjects with apo A-I$_{Milano}$ than in normal subjects.[159] Apo A-I$_{Milano}$ may also be more easily dissociated from HDL, thus potentially increasing the role of free apo A-I in cholesterol efflux. Despite low HDL cholesterol levels in these patients, CAD risk does not appear to be increased.[160]

APO A-I/APO C-III DEFICIENCY. A genetic disorder in which low HDL cholesterol is associated with increased atherosclerotic risk was reported in two sisters aged 29 and 31 years, who had HDL cholesterol levels of 4 mg/dl and 7 mg/dl and severe coronary atherosclerosis.[161] Apo A-I was not detectable on electrophoresis, and only traces were detectable on radioimmunoassay. Apo C-III was not detectable. The half-life of infused HDL was about half that in normal individuals. First-degree relatives also had low HDL cholesterol and low apo A-I. The underlying genetic abnormality is an inversion of the DNA i.e., DNA that contains parts of the genes for apo A-I and apo C-III.[162]

HIGH-DENSITY LIPOPROTEIN DEFICIENCY WITH XANTHOMAS. HDL deficiency with xanthomas has been described in a Turkish kindred with repetitive consanguinity.[163] The proband had HDL cholesterol of only 2 mg/dl and no apo A-I. Apo A-II level was approximately 15 per cent of normal, but apo A-IV and apo C-III levels were normal. Apo B and LDL cholesterol levels were increased, VLDL and IDL were decreased, and triglyceride level was normal. The underlying genetic defect, which has an autosomal dominant transmission, is a mutation in the apo A-I gene.

Hypertriglyceridemia

Although the relation between plasma triglyceride and CAD is not as well established as the relation between plasma cholesterol and CAD, epidemiological evidence suggests that triglyceride plays an important role in determining CAD risk. In prospective studies, univariate analyses have established a direct association between triglyceride level and CAD incidence, but the association often weakens in multivariate analyses and may disappear in analyses controlling for HDL cholesterol.[164]

In part, the weakening of association may be due to the metabolic interrelation between the triglyceride-rich lipoproteins and HDL. Variability of triglyceride measurements both within an individual and between individuals may also account for the uncertain relation between triglyceride and CAD.[165] Subjects may be misclassified in epidemiological and clinical trials, and controlling for more accurately measured lipids such as HDL cholesterol may cause the association of triglyceride and CAD to disappear.[166]

Triglyceride concentration is ordinarily determined from a fasting sample, but postprandial lipemia may also contribute to CAD risk. Recent studies have correlated the magnitude of elevation of remnants of triglyceride-rich lipoproteins with CAD, although fasting triglyceride level may be normal.[167] In one study, postprandial triglyceride level but not fasting triglyceride level was shown to be an independent predictor of CAD even in multivariate analysis controlling for HDL cholesterol.[168] These studies suggest that the inability to clear these lipid-rich and potentially cytotoxic remnant particles may play a role in atherogenesis. Gemfibrozil and lovastatin have been shown to decrease postprandial triglyceride levels.[169]

Epidemiological Evidence

A meta-analysis of 16 population-based, prospective studies, 12 that together enrolled 33,214 men and 4 that together enrolled 5836 women, with follow-up ranging from 3 to 14.5 years, triglyceride was established as a CAD risk factor even after adjusting for HDL cholesterol.[170] Although controlling for HDL cholesterol weakened the relation between triglyceride and CAD risk, the relation remained significant.

PROSPECTIVE CARDIOVASCULAR MÜNSTER STUDY. Among 4576 men in the observational Prospective Cardiovascular Münster (PROCAM) study, 39 per cent of subjects with myocardial infarction or CAD death, compared with 21 per cent of surviving subjects without myocardial infarction or stroke, had a triglyceride level of at least 200 mg/dl.[171] Triglyceride level was significantly related to CAD events in univariate analysis, but the association disappeared in multivariate analysis controlling for total cholesterol or HDL cholesterol. However, the combination of triglyceride level of at least 200 mg/dl and LDL cholesterol:HDL cholesterol ratio of at least 5 identified the subgroup at highest risk for a CAD event. Almost 25 per cent of CAD events occurred in this subgroup, which accounted for less than 4 per cent of subjects in this analysis.

CHOLESTEROL LOWERING ATHEROSCLEROSIS STUDY. Multivariate analysis of 2-year CLAS data (see p. 1130) found that the primary predictor of atherosclerotic lesion progression in subjects in the drug-treated group was the apo C-III content of HDL, and the primary predictor of atherosclerotic progression in subjects in the placebo group was non-HDL cholesterol.[172] In univariate analysis, apo C-III, which is thought to inhibit lipoprotein lipase activity, was a significant predictor of progression in both treatment groups. These findings indicate the importance of triglyceride-rich lipoprotein metabolism in atherosclerosis. Sequestration of apo C-III within HDL would presumably leave apo C-II unopposed, thereby increasing the catabolism of triglyceride-rich particles and decreasing the exposure of the vascular endothelium to their potentially atherogenic remnants.

HELSINKI HEART STUDY. Subsequent analysis of the Helsinki Heart Study (see p. 1128) determined that the relative risk for cardiac events was 3.8 in the subgroup with triglyceride higher than 200 mg/dl and LDL cholesterol:HDL cholesterol ratio greater than 5 compared with the subgroup with triglyceride of 200 mg/dl or less and LDL cholesterol:HDL cholesterol ratio of 5 or less.[173] In this high-risk subgroup, which accounted for approximately 10 per cent of study subjects, risk for cardiac events was reduced 71 per cent with gemfibrozil treatment.

Triglyceride-Rich Lipoprotein Metabolism

Chylomicrons are the largest lipoprotein particles and are produced in the endoplasmic reticulum of the gastrointestinal tract after a fatty meal. Apo B-48, which is produced by the insertion of a stop codon in the gene for apo B-100, is unique to chylomicrons and their metabolic remnants. VLDL particles are produced by the liver and contain apo B-100, which is characteristic of all particles in the endogenous lipolytic cascade. Chylomicrons and VLDL also contain C apolipoproteins, which modulate the metabolism of the triglyceride-rich lipoproteins, and apo E, which enables the metabolized remnant particle to be removed from the circulation.

As triglyceride from chylomicrons and VLDL is hydrolyzed through the action of lipoprotein lipase, which is activated by apo C-II on the lipoprotein surface, the surface components made redundant by the shrinking lipoprotein core are transferred to HDL. The C apolipoproteins transferred to HDL are subsequently transferred to newly secreted VLDL.

Unlike their precursor particles, chylomicron remnants and IDL are believed to increase CAD risk. Cholesterol from chylomicron remnants suppresses B/E receptor activity, thereby decreasing the removal of LDL from the circulation, and IDL was found to be predictive of atherosclerotic lesion progression in both the NHLBI Type II Coronary Intervention Study[174] and the nicardipine study of the Montreal Heart Institute.[175]

Hypertriglyceridemia

DETECTION. In the NCEP guidelines, triglyceride less than 200 mg/dl is normal, 200 to 400 mg/dl is borderline high, 400 to 1000 mg/dl is high, and greater than 1000 mg/dl is very high. As in hypercholesterolemia, treatment is influenced by the degree of CAD risk. Particularly in patients with CAD, FCH, diabetes, or a family history of premature CAD, elevated triglyceride should be reduced to decrease CAD risk. Causes of secondary hypertriglyceridemia include diabetes mellitus, obesity, hypothyroidism, dysglobulinemia, and use of beta blockers, diuretics, and estrogen. Underlying conditions should be treated and, as possible, offending drugs discontinued or decreased. High and very high triglyceride levels are usually caused by a combination of primary and secondary factors.

TREATMENT. The primary treatment for hypertriglyceridemia is life style modification, which should include weight control, a diet low in saturated fat and cholesterol, regular exercise, smoking cessation, and, in some patients, alcohol restriction. Frequent concomitants of elevated triglyceride are obesity, physical inactivity, and glucose intolerance.

The NCEP guidelines recommend the consideration of drug therapy in patients with borderline-high triglyceride in conjunction with CAD, family history of premature CAD, high total cholesterol combined with low HDL cholesterol, or a genetic hypertriglyceridemia known to increase CAD risk, such as dysbetalipoproteinemia (see below) or FCH. The agent should decrease LDL cholesterol, increase HDL cholesterol, and decrease VLDL and remnant particles. Suggested agents are nicotinic acid and fibric-acid derivatives.

High triglyceride may require drug therapy, especially in patients with a history of acute pancreatitis, to prevent an increase in triglyceride to a level that can cause pancreatitis. Treatment is as for borderline hypertriglyceridemia, but emphasis should be placed on controlling secondary causes, the most common of which is obesity.

Patients with very high triglyceride are at increased risk for pancreatitis and so require vigorous immediate intervention. Drugs that increase triglyceride should be discontinued, diabetes mellitus should be controlled, alcohol intake should be restricted, and dietary fat should be limited to 10 to 20 per cent of total calories. If triglyceride remains above 1000 mg/dl despite these measures, drug therapy should be initiated. Suggested agents are fibric-acid derivatives and, in patients who do not have diabetes mellitus, nicotinic acid. Triglyceride levels seldom return to normal in these patients; a reasonable treatment goal is triglyceride less than 500 mg/dl. There is no drug treatment for chylomicronemia (see below).

Fish Oil. In addition to the lipid-regulating drugs described above that affect triglyceride as well as cholesterol, omega-3 polyunsaturated fatty acids—predominantly eicosapentaenoic acid and docosahexaenoic acid—exert a triglyceride-lowering effect. In observational epidemiological studies, a diet rich in these compounds has been associated with decreased prevalence of atherosclerosis in populations such as Greenland Eskimos,[176] and in MRFIT, CAD mortality was found to be inversely related to the consumption of omega-3 polyunsaturated fatty acids.[177] However, the effect of long-term exposure to high doses of these compounds is not known, and the administration of fish oil supplements is not recommended by the NCEP.

Although the precise mechanism by which these compounds confer cardioprotection is not clear, high consumption of omega-3 fatty acids has been demonstrated to decrease the production of VLDL.[178] Fish oil also increases the proportion of HDL_2 to HDL_3,[179] thereby increasing the amount of cholesterol carried in HDL. Nonlipid benefits include a dose–response hypotensive effect, strongest in subjects with hypertension, hypercholesterolemia, or CAD, that was reported in a meta-analysis of placebo-controlled trials.[180] Prolonged bleeding has been reported with increased fish oil intake, but the alteration in hemostatic parameters may be less than previously suggested.[181] In some studies, fish oil supplementation has been shown to reduce restenosis after coronary angioplasty.[182]

Primary Dyslipidemias Characterized by Hypertriglyceridemia

FAMILIAL CHYLOMICRONEMIA. Familial chylomicronemia[183] is a rare disorder characterized by an elevation of circulating chylomicrons that persists in fasting plasma (Fredrickson phenotype I). The presence of chylomicrons is indicated by a creamy supernatant on plasma refrigerated for 12 hours. Blood cholesterol is normal to slightly elevated, and blood triglyceride is greatly increased. However, atherosclerotic risk does not appear to be increased.

Familial chylomicronemia results from decreased activity of lipoprotein lipase caused by genetic deficiency of lipoprotein lipase or of its activator apo C-II[184] or by the presence of an inhibitor to lipoprotein lipase.[185] Diagnosis is by determination of postheparin lipoprotein lipase activity. In patients with homozygous lipoprotein lipase deficiency or homozygous apo C-II deficiency, plasma triglyceride may exceed 1000 mg/dl. Inheritance of lipoprotein lipase and apo C-II deficiencies is autosomal recessive; the former genetic defect is more common than the latter.

Chylomicronemia usually causes diffuse abdominal pain and pancreatitis. Diagnosis is typically in childhood. Dermatological abnormalities include eruptive xanthomas that may be diffused over the entire body. These yellow, papular lesions consist of triglyceride-laden macrophages and may be controlled by lowering triglyceride levels. Lipemia retinalis may occur with more severe hypertriglyceridemia and is detected on funduscopic examination of the retina by diffuse pink discoloration caused by the dispersion of light by chylomicrons. Visual acuity is not affected, and there are no long-term ophthalmological sequelae.

The primary treatment for chylomicronemia is dietary and should include restriction of dietary fat to less than 10 per cent of total calories. Dietary fat should be in the form of short- and medium-chain triglycerides, which are absorbed directly into the portal vein instead of being formed into chylomicrons in the gastrointestinal tract. Agents that increase triglyceride production, such as estrogen and alcohol, should be avoided. Drug therapy is usually not effective in patients with this dyslipidemia.

DYSBETALIPOPROTEINEMIA (TYPE III HYPERLIPIDEMIA). Dysbetalipoproteinemia, or type III hyperlipidemia, is characterized by an elevation in IDL particles. Both cholesterol and triglyceride levels are elevated, and atherosclerotic risk is increased. Inheritance is most commonly autosomal recessive. This disorder, which occurs in approximately 1 in 5000 individuals in the United States, is most often found in individuals homozygous for apo E_2 but usually requires other metabolic or environmental factors for full clinical expression. Because the B/E receptor and possibly the putative chylomicron remnant receptor have decreased affinity for apo E_2, chylomicron and VLDL remnants accumulate instead of being cleared from the circulation by apo E–mediated removal. These remnant particles, which are known as beta-VLDL because they have beta electrophoretic mobility instead of the pre-beta mobility characteristic of normal VLDL, are enriched in cholesteryl ester.[186] Beta-VLDL particles can be taken up by macrophages, and because this uptake is not downregulated as intracellular cholesterol accumulates, the macrophages can become lipid-laden foam cells.[187]

Total cholesterol is typically 300 to 600 mg/dl, and total triglyceride is typically 400 to 800 mg/dl but may be much higher. Clinical signs of dysbetalipoproteinemia may include palmar xanthomas and tuberoeruptive xanthomas. Definitive diagnosis is by identification of apo E isoform, which requires special laboratory analysis. However, a VLDL cholesterol:plasma triglyceride ratio of 0.3 or greater supports the diagnosis of dysbetalipoproteinemia.[188] This disorder is not usually expressed in childhood and may be exacerbated by obesity, diabetes mellitus, hypothyroidism, myxedema, and excessive alcohol consumption.

Dysbetalipoproteinemia is extremely sensitive to dietary therapy, and reduction in saturated fat intake combined with weight reduction as necessary frequently corrects the dyslipidemia. If drug therapy is required, recommended agents are fibric-acid derivatives, HMG-CoA reductase inhibitors, and in patients who do not have diabetes or a prediabetic condition, nicotinic acid.

FAMILIAL ENDOGENOUS HYPERTRIGLYCERIDEMIA. Familial endogenous hypertriglyceridemia characterized by elevated VLDL (Fredrickson phenotype IV) occurs in approximately 1 in 300 individuals in the United States. In the type IV phenotype, blood triglyceride level is typically 200 to 500 mg/dl, and HDL cholesterol is usually decreased. Premature CAD is a feature in some kindreds but not in others. Treatment is as for hypertriglyceridemia, outlined above.

Rarely, this disease presents as type V hyperlipidemia, which may be recognized by a creamy supernatant of chylomicrons overlying a turbid layer of VLDL-rich fasting plasma. In this presentation, plasma triglyceride is typically greater than 1000 mg/dl, HDL cholesterol is usually decreased, and total cholesterol is normal to elevated. Atherosclerotic risk is increased. Triglyceride-lowering treatment, as outlined above, frequently alters the phenotype to type IV or IIb.

FAMILIAL COMBINED HYPERLIPIDEMIA. As noted above, FCH may present as type IV hyperlipidemia. Treatment should then be directed at triglyceride reduction.

Elevated Lipoprotein(a)

Lp(a) level has been shown in a number of clinical studies, primarily retrospective, to be an independent risk factor for CAD.[189] Structurally, Lp(a) is identical to LDL with the addition of a single apo(a) molecule attached by a disulfide bond to the apo B-100. The distribution of Lp(a) concentration is bell shaped in blacks but skewed in whites, who typically have levels below 20 mg/dl. A level above 30 mg/dl is generally considered elevated.

The primary determinant of Lp(a) level has been shown to be genetic. In one study in white families, more than 90 per cent of the variation in Lp(a) level was attributable to variation in the gene for apo(a).[190] Less than 10 per cent of the inherited variation in Lp(a) level may be attributable to variations in genes at other loci, such as the B/E receptor gene. Lp(a) concentration was reported to be three times higher in patients with heterozygous FH than in controls.[191] About 4 per cent of the variation in Lp(a) level may be attributable to variation in the gene for apo E: Compared with individuals with the gene for apo E_3, Lp(a) concentration was 25 per cent lower in individuals with the gene for apo E_2 and 25 per cent higher in individuals with the gene for apo E_4.[192]

The mechanism by which Lp(a) may increase risk for

CAD is complex. Lp(a) may interfere with the generation of plasmin because of structural similarity between apo(a) and plasminogen.[193] Lp(a) has been demonstrated to be deposited in the arterial wall, particularly in areas with atherosclerotic plaque, and apo(a) has been found co-localized with fibrinogen in the arterial wall.[194] Lp(a) that has been modified by malondialdehyde was reported to be removed by scavenger receptors on macrophages at a rate 20 times higher than that of native Lp(a).[195] Lp(a) appears to be more susceptible to oxidative modification than LDL[196] and thus may be preferentially taken up by scavenger receptors.

Treatment of elevated Lp(a) is problematic. Most lipid-regulating agents do not seem to lower Lp(a), except, as noted above, nicotinic acid, bezafibrate, and estrogen. Neomycin[197] and stanozolol[198] have also been reported to decrease Lp(a). Although lowering Lp(a) level is theoretically attractive, the clinical impact has not been determined. Because Lp(a) measurement is not a widely available laboratory determination and the clinical significance of alterations in Lp(a) level is not known, the NCEP does not recommend the routine measurement of this lipoprotein at this time.

TOBACCO USE

The use of tobacco products continues to be a major public health hazard in the United States[199,199a] and is one of the primary modifiable risk factors for CAD. In the United States, 46 million adults, or 25 per cent of the population aged 18 years or older, smoke.[5] Cigarette smoking is the leading preventable cause of premature death in the United States, and it is estimated that in 1990, approximately 417,000 Americans died of smoking-related causes.[1] Tobacco use is the largest single cause of premature death in the developed world among individuals aged 35 to 69 years, estimated to account for approximately 30 per cent of all deaths in this age group in the 1990s.[200] Cardiovascular diseases linked with tobacco use include CAD and cerebrovascular disease. Smoking multiplies the effect of other coronary risk factors and is estimated to be the cause of approximately 20 per cent of all deaths of cardiovascular disease in the United States in 1990.[201]

Epidemiological Evidence

In the Framingham Heart Study, cardiovascular mortality increased 18 per cent in men and 31 per cent in women for each 10 cigarettes smoked per day.[202] In addition, the use of tobacco products in individuals with other cardiac risk factors was found to have a synergistic effect on CAD morbidity and mortality: Smoking was found to increase the

risk for CAD, stroke, heart failure, and peripheral vascular disease at every level of blood pressure (Table 35–9). Smoking cessation in hypertensive patients who smoke 1 pack per day was estimated to reduce cardiovascular risk by 35 to 40 per cent.

Low-tar cigarettes and smokeless tobacco are *not* effective substitutes for discontinuing the use of tobacco products, despite claims to the contrary. In a multicenter case–control study, the relative risks for myocardial infarction in patients who smoked cigarettes with tar yield less than 10 mg, 10 to 15 mg, 15 to 20 mg, and greater than 20 mg were 3.8, 4.3, 3.2, and 3.7, respectively, compared with nonsmokers.[203] Compared with patients who smoked cigarettes with tar yield in the lowest category, the relative risks for myocardial infarction in patients who smoked cigarettes with tar yield in the subsequent categories were 1.2, 0.8, and 1.0. Smokeless tobacco is also associated with an increased risk for cardiovascular disease. In a 12-year observational epidemiological study conducted in 135,036 men, the age-adjusted relative risk for death of cardiovascular disease was 1.4 in users of smokeless tobacco, 1.8 in smokers of less than 15 cigarettes per day, and 1.9 in smokers of 15 or more cigarettes per day, compared with subjects who did not use any tobacco products.[204]

Passive exposure to smoke in individuals who have never smoked may also increase risk for CAD. In an analysis of nine epidemiological studies, the relative risk for heart disease death among individuals who had never smoked was as much as 3.0 in subjects who lived with current or former smokers compared with those who lived with nonsmokers.[205] In this analysis, among men who had never smoked, subjects who lived with a current or former smoker were estimated to have a 9.6 per cent chance of dying of ischemic heart disease by the age of 74, compared with a 7.4 per cent chance in subjects who lived with a nonsmoker; the respective risks in women were estimated to be 6.1 per cent and 4.9 per cent.

Mechanisms of Increased Risk

The use of tobacco products decreases HDL cholesterol. In an observational epidemiological study, HDL cholesterol was 12 per cent lower in male smokers and 7 per cent lower in female smokers than in nonsmokers.[206] Tobacco smoke may adversely affect HDL metabolism and structure by modifying the activity of LCAT. In an in vitro study, LCAT activity in human plasma exposed to the gas phase of cigarette smoke for only 15 minutes was reduced 7 per cent, and at 6 hours of exposure, LCAT activity was only 22 per cent of that in plasma exposed to filtered air.[207] Additionally, plasma exposure to cigarette smoke resulted in cross-linking between apo A-I and apo A-II, which may alter the function of HDL. Because of the cardioprotective

TABLE 35–9   RISK FOR CARDIOVASCULAR DISEASE BY SYSTOLIC BLOOD PRESSURE AND SMOKING STATUS: FRAMINGHAM 26-YEAR FOLLOW-UP OF MEN AGED 50 YEARS*

| | 8-YEAR RATES PER 1000 SUBJECTS | | | | | | | |
| | Any Cardiovascular Disease | | Intermittent Claudication | | Myocardial Infarction | | Stroke | |
SBP	Nonsmokers	Smokers	Nonsmokers	Smokers	Nonsmokers	Smokers	Nonsmokers	Smokers
105	37	64	3	10	17	26	7	11
120	47	81	4	12	21	32	8	13
135	60	102	5	15	26	39	9	15
150	76	128	6	19	31	47	11	18
165	96	160	7	23	39	58	13	21
180	121	198	9	29	47	70	15	25
195	151	242	11	36	58	86	18	29

Abbreviation: SBP = systolic blood pressure.
* Cholesterol 185 mg/dl; no glucose intolerance; no left ventricular hypertrophy.
From Kannel, W. B., and Higgins, M.: Smoking and hypertension as predictors of cardiovascular risk in population studies. J. Hypertens. Suppl. 8:S3, 1990.

effect of HDL, these alterations may provide a mechanism by which cigarette smoke increases risk for CAD.

Smoking may also have a detrimental effect on coronary flow. In a case–control study, smoking significantly increased the risk for vasospasm; the adjusted odds ratio for smoking as a risk factor for vasospasm was 2.41.[208] In addition, smoking adversely affects endothelial function,[209] fibrinogen level,[210] and platelet aggregation.[211]

Risk Factor Reduction

A computer model designed to measure the effect of risk factor modification on life expectancy in Americans who became 35 years old in 1990 predicted that the population-wide increase in life expectancy that would be gained with smoking cessation was 0.8 year in men and 0.7 year in women.[212] By comparison, reduction of cholesterol to 200 mg/dl, blood pressure control, and achievement of ideal body weight was predicted to increase life expectancy 0.7 year, 1.1 years, and 0.6 year, respectively, in men and 0.8 year, 0.4 year, and 0.4 year, respectively, in women. However, in individuals with a given risk factor, the effects of risk factor reduction are more impressive. Smoking cessation in smokers was estimated to increase life expectancy 2.3 years in men and 2.8 years in women. The elimination of CAD mortality in this age group was estimated to increase the average life expectancy 3.1 years in men and 3.3 years in women.

Smoking cessation improves other cardiovascular risk factors as well. In a recent study, LDL cholesterol decreased 5.6 per cent and HDL cholesterol increased 3.4 per cent in subjects who stopped smoking and stopped chewing nicotinic gum for at least 12 weeks.[213] Smoking cessation decreased platelet volume and increased the platelet cyclic adenosine monophosphate response to stimulation of adenylate cyclase by prostaglandin E_1. Elevation of platelet cyclic adenosine monophosphate levels has been associated with platelet reactivity, implying that the antiaggregating effect of vasoprotective prostaglandins may be increased after smoking cessation. Amounts of epinephrine and norepinephrine excreted in urine were decreased by smoking cessation, which may reflect improvement in vascular reactivity. Smoking cessation did not affect systolic blood pressure, but diastolic blood pressure was significantly increased.

Although smoking cessation has been reported to increase blood pressure in some studies, in the 3470 subjects in the interventional group in MRFIT who reported smoking at the initial screening and also attended the 72-month follow-up visit, the significantly increased incidence of hypertension, which occurred in 35 per cent of subjects who stopped smoking compared with 27 per cent of subjects who did not stop smoking, was found to be at least partially attributable to increased weight gain after smoking cessation.[214] At 72-month follow-up, weight gain of 2.7 kg (6 lb) occurred in 47 per cent of subjects who quit smoking, compared with 25 per cent of subjects who did not stop smoking. Stepped-care antihypertensive therapy was similarly effective in lowering diastolic blood pressure in hypertensive subjects who did or did not stop smoking.

Smoking cessation produces clinical benefits in a short period of time. In a population-based case–control study in which 1282 cases were compared with 2068 controls, the risk for myocardial infarction or coronary death in current smokers was 2.7 in men and 4.7 in women compared with the respective risks in nonsmokers.[215] After smoking cessation, the risk for CAD quickly declined and at approximately 3 years after smoking cessation became similar to that of subjects who had never smoked.

Smoking cessation, which is cost-free and has minimal adverse effects, should be encouraged in all patients. Approximately 70 per cent of current smokers report a desire to stop smoking completely.[5] However, data from the 1991 National Health Interview Survey of the Centers for Disease Control indicate that only slightly more than half of the smokers who had at least one outpatient visit with a physician or other health-care professional during a 1-year period were advised to quit.[216] It has been estimated that each year an additional 1 million individuals could be helped to stop smoking if all primary-care providers gave brief counseling to their smoking patients.[217] Brief counseling should include determining whether the patient smokes, advising any patient who smokes to quit, assisting the patient in quitting, for example, by setting a quit date and providing self-help material, and scheduling follow-up visits to reinforce adherence.[218]

HYPERTENSION

(See also Chaps. 25 and 26)

In the United States and other Western countries, the prevalence of hypertension is high and increases with age. The third and most recent National Health and Nutrition Examination Survey (NHANES III), conducted between 1988 and 1991, documented an overall prevalence of hypertension in adult Americans of 24 per cent, representing more than 43 million individuals[6] and ranging from 4 per cent of Americans aged 18 to 29 years to 65 per cent of Americans aged more than 80 years.[219]

Epidemiological Evidence

Numerous observational epidemiological studies in geographically and ethnically diverse populations have established a direct relation between blood pressure elevation and incidence of CAD and stroke. In a meta-analysis of nine prospective studies that together included almost 420,000 individuals without prior myocardial infarction or stroke who were followed up for an average of 10 years, baseline blood pressure level correlated with subsequent incidence rates of CAD death and nonfatal myocardial infarction.[220] The relative risk for CAD events in subjects in the highest quintile of diastolic blood pressure (mean, 105 mm Hg) was approximately 5 to 6 times that in subjects in the lowest quintile (mean, 76 mm Hg). Each 7.5 mm Hg difference in diastolic blood pressure was associated with an estimated 29 per cent difference in CAD risk. No threshold level of blood pressure was identified below which the association with CAD events changed.

In a meta-analysis of 14 randomized trials of hypotensive drug therapy, together enrolling almost 37,000 subjects, blood pressure was 6 mm Hg lower in treated subjects than in control subjects, and CAD event rate was 14 per cent lower,[221] which was a smaller improvement in CAD events than would have been expected on the basis of observational data. However, some of the hypotensive agents used in these interventional trials may adversely affect the lipid profile and may offset, at least partially, the reduction in risk obtained by lowering blood pressure. Thiazide diuretics and beta blockers without intrinsic sympathomimetic activity increase plasma triglyceride levels and may produce other metabolic adverse effects.[222]

Some studies have found a J-shaped relation between blood pressure and CAD events. In one study, in which this effect was limited to patients with evidence of CAD, the lowest incidence of fatal myocardial infarction was in patients whose diastolic blood pressure was 85 to 90 mm Hg; risk for fatal myocardial infarction was increased in patients whose blood pressure was either lower or higher than this range.[223] The precise clinical role of the J-shaped curve remains controversial but may be related to overzealous reduction of blood pressure in subjects with ostial coronary lesions, severe diastolic abnormalities that cause subendocardial ischemia, or potential adverse metabolic effects of hypotensive agents. In addition, left ventricular dysfunction may affect blood pressure and increase risk for coronary events immediately after a myocardial infarction.

TABLE 35–10 EFFECTS OF ANTIHYPERTENSIVE DRUGS ON OTHER CORONARY ARTERY DISEASE RISK FACTORS

RISK FACTORS	DIURETICS	INDAPAMIDE	BETA-BLOCKERS WITHOUT ISA	BETA-BLOCKERS WITH ISA	LABETALOL	GUANETHIDINE GUANADREL	CENTRAL ALPHA-AGONISTS	METHYLDOPA	DIRECT VASODILATORS	ALPHA-BLOCKERS	ACE INHIBITORS	CALCIUM BLOCKERS	RESERPINE
Hypertension	Reduced	Reduced	Reduced	Decreased	Decreased	Decreased	Decreased	Decreased	Decreased	Decreased	Decreased	Decreased	Decreased
Dyslipidemia	Increased	Neutral	Increased	No change	No change	No change	Decreased	Increased	No change	Decreased	No change	Decreased	Increased
Glucose intolerance	Increased	Neutral / Increased	Increased	Increased	Increased	No change	No change / No change	No change / No change	No change / No change	Decreased / Decreased	Decreased / Decreased	No change / No change	No change / Unknown
Insulin resistance	Increased	No change	Increased	Increased	Unknown	Unknown				Decreased	Decreased	Decreased	
LVH	No change / Increased	Reduced	No change	Increased	Decreased	Decreased	Decreased / No change	Decreased / No change	Increased / No change	Decreased / No change	Decreased / No change	Decreased / No change	Decreased / Decreased
Exercise	No change / Decreased	No change	Decreased	Decreased	No change / Decreased	Decreased	No change	No change	No change	No change	Increased	No change	No change
Potassium	Decreased	Decreased	No change / Increased	No change / Increased	No change	No change	No change	No change	No change	No change	No change / Increased	No change	No change
Magnesium	Decreased	Decreased	No change	No change	No change	No change	Decreased	No change	No change	No change	Decreased	No change	No change
Uric acid	Increased	Increased	Increased	Increased	Increased	No change	Decreased	Decreased	No change	Decreased	Increased	Decreased	
Blood viscosity	Increased	No change	No change	No change	No change	No change	No change	No change	Decreased	Decreased	No change	Unknown	Unknown
Blood velocity	No change / Increased	No change	Decreased	No change	No change	No change	Decreased	Increased	Increased	Decreased	Decreased	Decreased	Decreased
Catecholamines	Increased	Decreased	Increased	Increased	No change	Decreased	Decreased	Decreased	Increased	No change	Decreased	Decreased	Decreased
Angiotensin II	Increased	No change / Decreased	Decreased	No change	Decreased	Increased				Decreased			
Arrhythmia potential	Increased	No change	Decreased	No change / Increased	No change	Increased	Decreased	Decreased	Increased	No change / Decreased	Decreased	Decreased	Decreased
Fibrinogen	Increased	No change	Unknown	Unknown	Unknown	Unknown	Decreased	Decreased	Increased	No change	Decreased	Decreased	Increased
Platelet function	Increased	Decreased	No change / Decreased	Unknown	Unknown	Unknown	Unknown / Decreased	Unknown / No change	Unknown	Unknown	Unknown / Decreased	Unknown / Decreased	Unknown / Unknown
Thrombogenic potential	Increased	Decreased	Unknown	Unknown	Unknown	Unknown	Unknown	Unknown	Unknown	Unknown	Unknown	Decreased	Unknown
Antiatherogenic	No	Neutral	Yes (animal studies)	Unknown	Unknown	Yes	Unknown	Unknown	Unknown	Unknown	Decreased (animals)	Decreased (animals, humans)	Yes (animals)
CHD relative risk ratio Unfavorable/total	16/18	3–4/18	6/18	7/18	3/18	3/18	0/18	2/18	5/18	0/18	0/18	0/18	3/18

From Houston, M. C.: The management of hypertension and associated risk factors for the prevention of long-term cardiac complications. J. Cardiovasc. Pharmacol. *21*(Suppl. 2):S2, 1993.

Large-scale prospective interventional trials are under way to clarify this issue.[224]

Risk Factor Reduction

Elevated blood pressure frequently coexists with other risk factors.[225] The insulin-resistance syndrome (or metabolic syndrome X) described by Reaven[226] is characterized by resistance to insulin-mediated glucose intake, glucose intolerance, hyperinsulinemia, hypertension, increased triglyceride and decreased HDL cholesterol levels, and possibly microvascular angina, hyperuricemia, and increased PAI-1 level.[227] In addition, truncal obesity and coagulation abnormalities often coexist with hypertension. Evaluation of other risk factors that occur with hypertension is of special clinical importance because controlling blood pressure with certain antihypertensive medications may adversely affect other risk factors (Table 35–10).

DIABETES MELLITUS

(See also Chap. 61)

Almost 14 million individuals in the United States are estimated to have diabetes mellitus, although more than half have not been diagnosed.[228] Approximately 700,000 have insulin-dependent diabetes mellitus (IDDM), which occurs more often in whites and tends to cluster in families. More than 95 per cent of Americans with diabetes have non–insulin-dependent diabetes mellitus (NIDDM), which typically develops after age 30 but often is not recognized until serious complications occur. Risk for NIDDM increases with age, and among Americans aged 65 to 74 years, 17 per cent of whites, 25 per cent of blacks, and 33 per cent of Hispanics have NIDDM.[229]

Epidemiological Evidence

CAD is a major complication of both IDDM and NIDDM. In 14-year follow-up of the Rancho Bernardo Study, in which 334 men and women with NIDDM were compared with 2137 men and women without diabetes, the relative risk for CAD death was 1.9 in diabetic men and 3.3 in diabetic women compared with nondiabetic men and women after adjustment for other CAD risk factors.[230] CAD, cerebrovascular disease, or peripheral vascular disease is the cause of death in 75 to 80 per cent of adults with diabetes.[231] Atherosclerosis occurs earlier and more often in diabetic patients, and women with diabetes do not share the relative gender-mediated premenopausal protection against CAD of women without diabetes.

The relation between diabetes and cardiovascular disease is not uniform in all populations. In the WHO Multinational Study of Vascular Disease in Diabetics, the incidence of death in diabetic patients that was attributable to circulatory disease ranged from 32 per cent in men and 0 per cent in women in Tokyo to 67 per cent in men and 47 per cent in women in London.[232]

Mechanisms of Increased Risk

Diabetes frequently exists in the presence of other, often modifiable CAD risk factors. Hypertension and obesity are common in patients with diabetes, and the typical dyslipidemia in diabetes is increased plasma triglyceride and decreased HDL cholesterol, often in conjunction with small, dense LDL particles. Postprandial lipemia may also contribute to atherosclerotic risk in patients with diabetes. In a study in patients with NIDDM, VLDL level was increased but chylomicron level was similar compared with corresponding levels in subjects with normal glucose tolerance.[233] In the same study, significant correlations were found between postprandial insulin response and triglyceride response and between postprandial triglyceride response and fasting HDL cholesterol level. However, even

taken together, these other risk factors do not explain all of the increased risk associated with diabetes.[234]

Resistance to the action of circulating insulin may play a role in the dyslipidemia of diabetes.[235] Insulin normally suppresses plasma concentration of free fatty acids, and in insulin-resistance syndromes, the decreased suppression results in an increase in circulating levels of free fatty acids, which in turn stimulates triglyceride synthesis. Although elevated plasma triglyceride frequently occurs in conjunction with decreased HDL cholesterol, in part because of the metabolic interrelation of the triglyceride-rich lipoproteins and HDL, increased urinary loss of HDL has been demonstrated in patients with IDDM and albuminuria.[236]

In diabetic patients, lipoproteins may be altered by glycation, which affects their recognition and binding by receptors.[237] Glycation of LDL causes its accumulation in the circulation and may increase cholesteryl ester accumulation in macrophages.[238] Glycation of HDL may also promote cholesteryl ester accumulation in the arterial wall.[239] In addition to glycation, oxidation of LDL may be increased in diabetic individuals,[240] although extensive studies have not been performed.

The role of Lp(a) in diabetes is controversial and appears to be related at least in part to the type of diabetes. In a recent analysis of available data, patients with NIDDM generally did not have elevated Lp(a), nor was Lp(a) level a function of metabolic control; however, patients with IDDM tended to have increased Lp(a), especially patients with microalbuminuria or poor glycemic control.[241]

Atherosclerosis in diabetics is often complicated by a procoagulant state caused by increased platelet aggregability[242] and increased PAI-1.[243] Insulin may contribute to atherogenesis by promoting smooth muscle cell proliferation and cholesteryl ester accumulation in the arterial wall.[244]

Risk Factor Reduction

The relation between glycemic control and prevention of diabetic complications remains controversial. Epidemiological studies have estimated that approximately 25 per cent of patients with diabetes do not develop complications regardless of the degree of glycemic control; however, clinical trials have demonstrated decreased retinopathy and microalbuminuria with improved glycemic control, and blood lipoprotein levels show significant improvement when blood glucose is controlled near normal levels.[245] In addition, glycosylated hemoglobin, used as a marker of poor glycemic control, has been significantly correlated with death from diabetes and death from ischemic heart disease.[246]

The Diabetes Control and Complications Trial (DCCT) addressed the role of tight glycemic control in preventing complications of diabetes by analyzing 1441 patients with IDDM, aged 13 to 39 years, who were randomized to receive intensive insulin therapy or conventional treatment.[247] The intensive therapy consisted of administration of insulin by an external insulin pump three or more times daily as indicated by frequent blood glucose monitoring; conventional therapy consisted of one to two daily injections of insulin. After a mean of 6.5 years, intensive therapy significantly reduced risk for retinopathy, microalbuminuria, and clinical neuropathy. LDL cholesterol was lowered 34 per cent, and the combined occurrence of all major cardiovascular and peripheral vascular events was reduced 41 per cent, but this reduction in macrovascular events was not significant. However, the young cohort was not expected to produce enough macrovascular events to allow distinction of the treatment groups. The major adverse event was a significant threefold increase in incidence of severe hypoglycemia. Additional studies are needed to determine whether intensive glycemic control decreases risk for macrovascular complications without an offsetting increase in risk for hypoglycemia.

In risk factor reduction in patients with diabetes, great care must be taken not to exacerbate one condition while treating another. For example, as noted above, antihypertensive agents may adversely affect glucose tolerance, lipid levels, or both.[248,249] Thiazide diuretics have been implicated in worsening glucose control and in provoking dyslipidemia, and noncardioselective beta blockers that inhibit the adrenergic-mediated activation of lipoprotein lipase have been shown to worsen both glucose tolerance and triglyceride metabolism and, thus, should be used with caution in patients with brittle diabetes.

In treating dyslipidemia in patients with diabetes, the report of the American Diabetes Association (ADA) Consensus Development Conference on the Detection and Management of Lipid Disorders in Diabetes emphasizes the benefits of ideal body weight, appropriate diet, and a moderate exercise program.[231] Physical exercise may also decrease the risk for atherosclerotic disease in patients with diabetes by decreasing hyperinsulinemia, improving insulin resistance, and/or preventing increased intraabdominal adiposity.[250] If hygienic methods do not control the lipid abnormality, pharmacological therapy may be indicated. Many authorities, including the ADA consensus panel, recommend more stringent intervention levels and therapeutic goals in the diabetic patient. The ADA consensus panel recommends screening for dyslipidemia annually in all patients with diabetes by full fasting lipoprotein analysis and initiating treatment if LDL cholesterol is elevated (130 mg/dl or greater without evidence of macrovascular disease, greater than 100 mg/dl with evidence of macrovascular disease), if triglyceride is elevated (200 mg/dl or greater without macrovascular disease, greater than 150 mg/dl with macrovascular disease), or if HDL cholesterol is low (35 mg/dl or less).

PHYSICAL INACTIVITY

Almost 60 per cent of U.S. adults reported little or no leisure-time physical activity in the 1991 Behavioral Risk Factor Surveillance System of the Centers for Disease Control.[251] In this survey, prevalence of sedentary life style was similar in men and women and lower in whites (57 per cent) than in other races (64 per cent). Physical inactivity was directly related to age, ranging from 55 per cent in subjects aged 18 to 34 years to 62 per cent in subjects 55 years or older, and inversely related to income and education.

Epidemiological Evidence

Regular physical activity has been shown to reduce risk for CAD events in a number of observational epidemiological studies.[252] A meta-analysis of studies that compared CAD incidence in occupations with different activity levels determined that the relative risk for CAD death was 1.9 in sedentary occupations compared with active occupations.[253] In 10-year follow-up of MRFIT subjects, subjects in both treatment groups who engaged in moderate physical activity had a 27 per cent lower CAD mortality rate than less active subjects.[254]

Because of the methodological problems encountered in quantitating exercise and because of the potential for unreliability in self-reported estimates of physical activity, the level of physical fitness may provide a more accurate predictor of CAD risk. In the Lipid Research Clinics Mortality Follow-up Study, heart rate at stage 2 of a treadmill exercise test was used to determine physical fitness in 3106 healthy men and 649 men with symptoms suggestive of cardiovascular disease or taking antihypertensive medication.[255] Stage 2 heart rate ranged from 112 beats/min in subjects in the fittest quartile to 156 beats/min in subjects in the least fit quartile. Compared with the fittest quartile,

cardiovascular disease mortality was 8.5 times higher and CAD mortality was 6.5 times higher in the least fit quartile.

In a study in 1960 healthy men, physical fitness, measured as total work on a bicycle ergometer, and other coronary risk factors were assessed at baseline, and subjects were followed up for 16 years.[256] After adjustment for other cardiovascular risk factors, a graded, independent, inverse correlation was seen between physical fitness and cardiovascular mortality. Compared with subjects in the least fit quartile, relative risk for cardiovascular death in subjects in the fittest quartile was 0.41; relative risk in the second fittest quartile was 0.45, and relative risk in the third fittest quartile was 0.59. Compared with subjects in the least fit quartile, subjects in the fittest quartile had a 0.54 adjusted relative risk for death of any cause, but the relative risk for death of any cause was similar in the three fittest quartiles.

In addition to measurements of physical activity, maximum oxygen uptake during a monitored exercise test may be used as a marker for cardiorespiratory fitness. In 5-year follow-up of 1453 men, aged 42 to 60 years, with no history of cardiovascular disease, age-adjusted relative risk for myocardial infarction in subjects in the highest tertile of physical activity was 0.31 compared with subjects in the lowest tertile.[257] Similarly, the relative risk for myocardial infarction in subjects in the highest tertile of maximal oxygen uptake was 0.26 compared with subjects in the lowest tertile of maximal oxygen uptake, after adjustment for age, weight, height, and other variables. After controlling for 17 confounding variables, the relative risks for myocardial infarction in subjects in the highest tertile of physical activity and subjects in the highest tertile of maximal oxygen uptake were 0.34 and 0.35 compared with subjects in the lowest tertiles, which were statistically significant differences.

Risk Factor Reduction

The mechanisms by which increased exercise decreases risk for CAD events may include improvements in HDL cholesterol level,[258] insulin resistance,[259] body weight,[260] and blood pressure.[261] Exercise also increases maximal cardiac output and the amount of oxygen extracted from blood.[262] In addition to these direct benefits, exercise has been shown to increase the lipid-regulating effects of dietary therapy in moderately overweight, sedentary subjects.[263]

The optimal intensity and duration of exercise to produce cardiovascular benefit have not been firmly established and appear to relate to baseline activity level (Fig. 35-5). In 8-year follow-up of more than 10,000 Harvard University alumni, the self-reported initiation of moderately vigorous sports activity, defined as activity requiring 4.5 or more metabolic equivalents, was associated with a significant 41 per cent reduction in CAD mortality and a significant 23 per cent reduction in all-cause mortality.[264] Subjects who increased physical activity to 2000 kcal per week had a 17 per cent reduction in CAD mortality, but this reduction was not statistically significant.

Cardioprotective benefits may be obtained from a regular program of 30 minutes of moderate aerobic physical activity three times a week. Some experts recommend 30 minutes or more of moderately intensive physical activity daily for all adults.[265] Prudent exercise programs are cost-effective and have a low risk for adverse events in either primary or secondary prevention.[266] Exercise should be individualized to accommodate the patient's level of physical fitness, cardiac status, and preferred activities. In secondary prevention, a limited treadmill exercise test is required at discharge after an acute coronary event to determine prognostic stratification; a symptom-limited treadmill exercise test should be performed 6 weeks later to determine exercise recommendations.

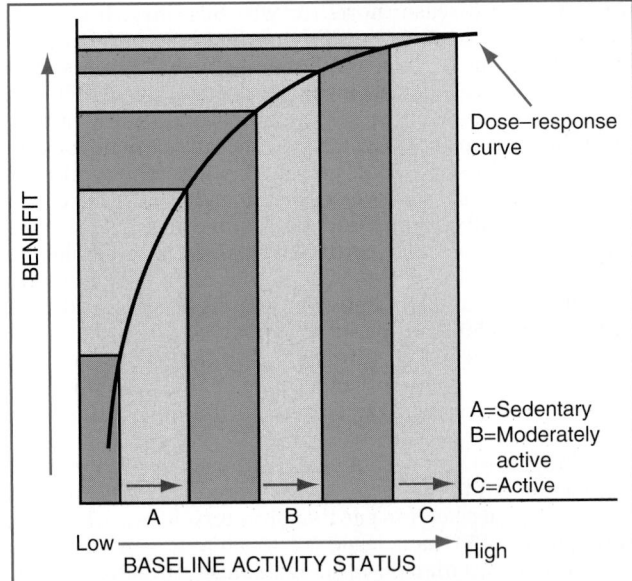

FIGURE 35-5. Dose–response relation between baseline physical activity and health benefit. The intensity and duration of physical activity required to produce a health benefit are related to the level of physical activity at baseline. In sedentary patients, even a modest increase in physical activity is beneficial. (From Pate, R. R., Pratt, M., Blair, S. N., et al.: Physical activity and public health: A recommendation from the Centers for Disease Control and Prevention and the American College of Sports Medicine. JAMA 273: 402–407, 1995. Copyright 1995 American Medical Association.)

OBESITY

In the third and most recent National Health and Nutrition Examination Survey (NHANES III), approximately 58 million U.S. adults—one-third of Americans aged 20 years or older—were estimated to be overweight, defined as a body mass index (weight in kg/height in m²) of 27.8 or greater in men and 27.3 or greater in women.[267] This increase in prevalence of 8 per cent since NHANES II was completed in 1988 reflects increases in all age groups and both genders. Prevalence ranges from a low of 31.2 per cent in black men to a high of 48.6 per cent in black women. The largest increase in prevalence occurred in white men and women, in whom prevalence of overweight increased 8 to 9 per cent.

The health risks of obesity not only increase with its severity but also may be affected by the distribution of body fat.[268] Visceral obesity, characterized by excessive adipose fat in the abdomen, appears to impart greater risk for CAD.[269] Recommended waist:hip ratios are less than 0.9 in men and less than 0.8 in middle-aged and elderly women.[270]

Epidemiological Evidence

In the Framingham Heart Study, obesity was found to be an independent risk factor for cardiovascular disease in both men and women. Among subjects aged less than 50 years, incidence of cardiovascular disease was two times higher in men and almost 2.5 times higher in women in the most obese tertile compared with the leanest tertile.[271]

Even individuals with a high-normal body mass index appear to be at increased risk for CAD. In a prospective cohort study conducted in 115,818 middle-aged women, the relative risk for a nonfatal myocardial infarction or fatal CAD was 1.46 in subjects with a body mass index of 23.0 to 24.9 and 2.06 in subjects with a body mass index of 25.0 to 28.9, compared with subjects with a body mass index less than 21.0, which were statistically significant increases.[272] Relative risk in subjects with a body mass index of 21 to 22.9 was 1.19, which was not significant, and

relative risk in subjects with a body mass index of 29 or more, which would be considered obese by the definition used in NHANES, was 3.56.

Risk Factor Reduction

Obesity frequently accompanies other cardiovascular risk factors such as hypercholesterolemia,[273] low HDL cholesterol,[274] hypertension,[275] and diabetes mellitus.[276] To improve lipid levels, blood pressure, and glucose tolerance, a concerted effort should be made to obtain ideal body weight by a combination of exercise and dietary interventions.

NONMODIFIABLE RISK FACTORS

Although risk factors such as a positive family history of CAD, age, and gender cannot be modified, their identification can help refine assessment of the patient's CAD risk profile.

Family History

Coronary atherosclerosis tends to aggregate in families. In studies that controlled for other risk factors, a family history of CAD has been shown to be a strong independent risk factor for CAD. For example, a study in relatives of 223 patients with angiographically demonstrated CAD and 57 control subjects found that, after stratification by age, gender, blood pressure, total cholesterol, smoking, diabetes, and left ventricular hypertrophy, relatives of patients had a significantly greater risk for CAD than relatives of controls, as reflected in odds ratios of 2.0 to 3.9 for various CAD endpoints.[277] In a 2-year study in 45,317 men, aged 40 to 75 years, without known CAD at baseline, relative risk for myocardial infarction was 2.2 in subjects whose parent had a myocardial infarction before the age of 70, compared with subjects without a family history of premature myocardial infarction.[278] In addition, risk for myocardial infarction was inversely related to the age at which myocardial infarction occurred in the parent.

Although symptomatic CAD typically does not occur until middle age, family history of CAD may influence atherosclerotic risk beginning in infancy. In an autopsy study of 136 infants aged less than 1 year, mean luminal narrowing in the left coronary artery was 1.4 times greater in infants with a family history of CAD than in infants with no family history of CAD, which was a statistically significant difference; there was no statistically significant difference in narrowing in the right coronary artery between groups.[279]

The increased CAD risk associated with a positive family history may be mediated by genetic effects on other risk factors such as obesity, hypertension, dyslipidemia, and diabetes.[280] Assessment of family history of these other risk factors may provide additional information about an individual's CAD risk and inform treatment decisions.

Age

Approximately four-fifths of fatal myocardial infarctions are in patients aged 65 years and older.[1] Because of the increased short-term risk for a CAD event in middle-aged and elderly patients, reduction of modifiable risk factors in this population is more likely to decrease CAD events in a shorter period of time than in younger patients with otherwise similar risk factors. For example, excess CAD mortality attributable to hypercholesterolemia increased more than five times with age in the observational Kaiser Permanente Coronary Heart Disease in the Elderly Study, conducted in 2746 men without CAD, aged 60 to 79 years.[281] Similarly, major cardiovascular events were reduced 32 per cent with antihypertensive drug therapy in men and women, aged 60 years or older, in the Systolic Hypertension in the Elderly Program (SHEP).[282]

Although older patients should not be excluded from aggressive risk factor reduction simply on the basis of age, overall health status and concomitant illnesses should be assessed in making treatment decisions. If pharmacological intervention is indicated, consideration must be given to the increased susceptibility to adverse drug effects in older patients. The patient's life expectancy should also guide treatment because risk factor reduction may not produce clinical benefit until after a few years of treatment. For example, in clinical trials, lipid-regulating therapy usually requires approximately 2 years before clinical benefit is demonstrated.

Gender

In the Framingham Heart Study, 26-year follow-up of men and women aged 35 to 84 years indicated that CAD morbidity was twice as high in men as in women, and 60 per cent of coronary events occurred in men.[283] The onset of symptomatic CAD is typically about 10 years earlier in men, but CAD incidence in women increases rapidly at menopause. Women have the same modifiable risk factors as men,[284] although diabetes appears to confer greater risk in women than in men,[285] as may low HDL cholesterol and elevated plasma triglyceride.[286]

OTHER RISK FACTORS

Hemostatic Factors

Thrombogenic factors have been demonstrated to predict CAD events. Although levels of coagulation factors, PAI-1, and fibrinolytic activity are not routinely measured to determine risk, their predictive power has been the subject of increasing research.

FIBRINOGEN. Fibrinogen levels vary among populations. Among blacks and whites in the United States, age-adjusted fibrinogen levels are 23 to 40 mg/dl higher in men and 25 to 67 mg/dl higher in women than in their counterparts in Japan, suggesting that low cholesterol levels in Japan may not fully explain the lower prevalence of CAD.[287]

Although elevated plasma fibrinogen occurs in conjunction with other CAD risk factors, such as age, cigarette smoking, hypertension, and obesity, fibrinogen has been demonstrated to be an independent CAD risk factor.[288] In 6-year follow-up of 2116 men in the PROCAM study, mean plasma fibrinogen level was significantly higher in men who had coronary events (2.88 gm/liter) than in men who did not have events (2.63 gm/liter), and the incidence of coronary events was 2.4 times higher in subjects in the highest tertile of plasma fibrinogen distribution (>2.77 gm/liter) than in subjects in the lowest tertile (<2.36 gm/liter).[289] In combined analysis of the Caerphilly and Speedwell prospective studies, which together evaluated almost 5000 men, age-adjusted relative risk for ischemic heart disease events was 4.1 for men in the highest quintile of fibrinogen distribution compared with men in the lowest quintile.[290]

COAGULATION FACTOR VII. Coagulation factor VII has been shown to increase CAD risk in a number of epidemiological studies.[291] factor VII levels are higher in individuals with a high intake of dietary fat,[292] and a direct association has been established between factor VII and total cholesterol level.[293] Elevated factor VII activity may increase thrombin production,[294] further leading to a hypercoagulant state.

FIBRINOLYTIC ACTIVITY. Decreased fibrinolytic activity has been reported in patients with coronary atherosclerosis. In the Northwick Park Heart Study, a difference of 1 stan-

dard deviation in fibrinolytic activity was significantly associated with a difference of 40 per cent in risk for ischemic heart disease events in men aged 40 to 54 years at entry into the study (mean follow-up, 16 years).[295] The association persisted after adjustment for plasma fibrinogen level, which was also directly associated with ischemic heart disease events. These results suggest that the decreased ability to lyse a clot and clear fibrin debris may play a role in atherosclerosis.

PLASMINOGEN ACTIVATOR INHIBITOR 1. Decreased fibrinolytic activity may result from elevated levels of PAI-1. In many case–control and cross-sectional studies, plasma PAI-1 has been reported to be increased in patients with CAD.[296] For example, in a study of men and women who had a myocardial infarction before age 45, PAI-1 level was higher than in healthy subjects.[297] This study also found PAI-1 level to be directly related to triglyceride level. In a study of almost 1500 men and women with angina pectoris, PAI-1 was found to be directly related to insulin level, confirming the role of PAI-1 in the insulin-resistance syndrome.[298] Increased PAI-1 has also been shown to be a risk factor for reinfarction in a prospective study of men whose first myocardial infarction occurred before age 45.[299] In addition to systemic increases in PAI-1, atherosclerotic lesions have been found to contain higher levels of PAI-1 than the normal arterial wall.[300]

Homocysteine

Plasma homocysteine is elevated in patients with homozygous homocystinuria, a rare autosomal recessive disorder, but levels are also increased in patients with CAD who do not have homocystinuria.[301,301a] Homocysteinemia has been established as an independent risk factor for coronary vascular disease, cerebrovascular disease, and peripheral vascular disease.[302]

In a study conducted in 482 hyperlipidemic men and women, 72 per cent of subjects with elevated serum homocysteine, defined as 16.2 nmol/ml or greater, had atherosclerotic vascular disease, compared with 44 per cent of those with normal serum homocysteine, which was a significant difference.[303] Compared with subjects in the lowest quintile of serum homocysteine (<6.9 nmol/ml), relative risk for atherosclerotic events was 2.8 in subjects in the highest quintile of serum homocysteine (≥11.4 nmol/ml).

In 271 men in the Physicians' Health Study who had a myocardial infarction during the 5-year study, plasma homocysteine level was significantly higher (mean, 11.1 nmol/ml) than in controls matched for age and smoking habits (mean, 10.5 nmol/ml).[304] Compared with subjects with plasma homocysteine no higher than the 90th percentile, relative risk for subjects with plasma homocysteine above the 95th percentile was 3.4 after adjustment for other cardiovascular risk factors.

Although the precise mechanism by which elevated plasma homocysteine increases risk for CAD has not been determined, possibilities include endothelial damage and altered anticoagulant activity.[305] Deficiency of vitamins B_6 and B_{12} and folic acid can cause elevated plasma homocysteine, and supplementation with these vitamins can decrease plasma homocysteine.

Alcohol

The role of alcohol in CAD risk is complicated by difficulties in obtaining accurate data on individual alcohol consumption. In a number of studies, moderate alcohol intake has been associated with decreased coronary risk,[306] and this protective effect may be mediated by an increase in HDL cholesterol.[307] In an analysis of subjects in the Honolulu Heart Program, approximately 50 per cent of the cardioprotection demonstrated with moderate alcohol consumption was attributable to increased HDL cholesterol, and 18 per cent was attributable to decreased LDL cholesterol, although the latter was offset by an increase in CAD risk of 17 per cent caused by increased systolic blood pressure.[308]

The mechanism responsible for the remaining cardioprotection is not known but may relate to decreased thrombogenicity. Alcohol may inhibit thrombosis[309] and may increase plasma levels of fibrinogen and decrease fibrinolytic activity.[310] Alcohol has been shown to increase tissue-type plasminogen activator (t-PA) secretion by endothelial cells.[311] In 631 men in the Physicians' Health Study, a direct relation was established between alcohol consumption and plasma level of t-PA antigen.[312] In subjects who drank alcohol daily, weekly, monthly, rarely, and never, mean t-PA antigen levels were 10.9, 9.7, 9.1, and 8.1 ng/ml, respectively. The relation persisted after controlling for other cardiovascular risk factors, including HDL cholesterol, supporting the hypothesis that alteration in fibrinolytic activity may contribute to alcohol-mediated protection against CAD.

In France, CAD incidence is relatively low despite mean plasma HDL cholesterol levels similar to those in other countries and fairly high intake of saturated fat. Suggested explanations for this so-called French paradox include alcohol-induced inhibition of platelet aggregation[313] and antioxidant effects of red wine.[314]

Type A Personality and Stress

The role of personality type[315] and emotional stress[316] in risk stratification for CAD remains controversial. Type A personalities are highly competitive, ambitious, and in constant struggle with their environment, whereas type B personalities are passive and less disturbed by environmental stress. Type A personality was reported to be an independent risk factor for CAD in 8.5-year follow-up of 3154 men, aged 39 to 59 years and without CAD at baseline, in the Western Collaborative Group Study: Type A subjects were twice as likely to have angina or myocardial infarction as type B subjects.[317] However, in 20 years of follow-up in 1289 men and women in the Framingham Heart Study, there was a significant twofold excess in risk for angina pectoris in both men and women with type A behavior but no association between personality type and risk for either myocardial infarction or fatal coronary events.[318] Similarly, in MRFIT subjects, type A behavior was not significantly associated with risk for first major coronary events, defined as coronary death and nonfatal myocardial infarction.[319] One possible explanation for the variable association between type A behavior and CAD risk is the use of different methods to determine behavior type.[320]

The mechanism by which personality types may predispose to increased coronary risk is not known but may include increased cardiovascular reactivity,[321] which may lead to increased endothelial injury and platelet aggregation, and increased sympathetic nervous system activity,[322] which increases blood pressure and heart rate.

Studies have been conducted to determine whether anger affects CAD risk. Findings indicate that the expression of anger may increase risk, because of increased cardiovascular reactivity, but that neither the experience nor the repression of anger has such an effect.[323] In a study in 12 patients undergoing cardiac catheterization for symptomatic myocardial ischemia, recalling a recent anger-provoking event significantly increased vasoconstriction, measured as decreases in mean and minimal diameters, in narrowed arteries but not in nonnarrowed arteries.[324]

Low Circulating Levels of Antioxidants

Blood concentrations of antioxidants may affect the susceptibility of LDL and Lp(a) to oxidation. Because lipoprotein oxidation is thought to be prerequisite to the recognition of these particles by the scavenger receptor on macrophages, decreased levels of substances that protect against oxidation may increase atherosclerotic risk.

Observational epidemiological studies have demonstrated an inverse relation between vitamin E intake and CAD events.[325] In the Health Professionals Follow-up Study, in which 39,910 American male health professionals aged 40 to 75 years were followed up for 4 years, risk for a CAD event (fatal coronary disease, nonfatal myocardial infarction, coronary artery bypass grafting, percutaneous transluminal coronary angioplasty) in subjects in the highest quintile of vitamin E intake (median, 419.0 IU/day) was significantly reduced 41 per cent, after adjustment for age, compared with subjects in the lowest quintile of vitamin E intake (median, 6.4 IU/day).[326] Similarly, in the Nurses' Health Study, in which 87,247 American female registered nurses aged 34 to 59 years were evaluated for 8 years, risk for major coronary disease (nonfatal myocardial infarction or CAD death) in subjects in the highest quintile of vitamin E intake (median, 208.0 IU/day) was significantly reduced 41 per cent, after adjustment for age, compared with subjects in the lowest quintile of vitamin E intake (median, 2.8 IU/day).[327] In both of these studies, vitamin E supplementation and not dietary sources alone appeared necessary to reduce risk for CAD events.

Additional observational data have come from information collected in interventional studies. During 13 years of follow-up of 1883 men in the placebo group of the LRC-CPPT, risk for a CAD event (nonfatal myocardial infarction or CAD death) in subjects in the highest quartile of serum carotenoid concentration ($>3.16 \mu mol/L$) was significantly reduced 36 per cent compared with subjects in the lowest quartile of serum carotenoid concentration ($<2.33 \mu mol/L$).[328] Among 156 CLAS subjects with 2-year angiograms evaluable by quantitative coronary angiography, evenly divided between drug and placebo groups, per cent stenosis in all coronary artery lesions decreased 0.8 percentage point, indicative of regression, in subjects with supplementary vitamin E intake of 100 IU/day or more, whereas per cent stenosis increased 2.0 percentage points, indicative of progression, in subjects with supplementary vitamin E intake less than 100 IU/day; this difference was statistically significant.[329] Lesion progression was not affected by supplementary intake of vitamin C or by dietary intake of vitamin E or vitamin C. In a case–control study of 270 subjects in the Helsinki Heart Study, the level of antibodies to oxidized LDL was significantly associated with an increased risk for a clinical event, defined as cardiac death or nonfatal myocardial infarction.[330] Compared with subjects in the lowest tertile of antibody level, subjects in the highest tertile had a 2.5-fold increased risk for a cardiac event after adjustment for age, smoking status, blood pressure, and HDL cholesterol level.

Few interventional data on the effect of antioxidants on CAD risk are available. In the Alpha-Tocopherol, Beta Carotene Cancer Prevention Study, 29,133 Finnish male smokers aged 50 to 69 years were randomized to receive alpha-tocopherol, 50 mg/day; beta-carotene, 20 mg/day; the combination; or placebo and followed up for a median of 6 years.[331] Although the study was designed to evaluate incidence of lung cancer, cardiovascular events were also recorded. Lung cancer incidence was reduced 2 per cent in subjects who received alpha-tocopherol, which was not a significant reduction, but was significantly increased 18 per cent in subjects who received beta-carotene. In subjects who received alpha-tocopherol, CAD mortality rate was 71.0 per 10,000 person-years, compared with 75.0 per 10,000 person-years in subjects who did not receive alpha-tocopherol, but total mortality increased 2 per cent, which was not a significant increase. In subjects who received beta-carotene, CAD mortality rate was 77.1 per 10,000 person-years, compared with 68.9 per 10,000 person-years in subjects who did not receive beta-carotene, and total mortality was significantly increased 8 per cent. These results, which appear to be in conflict with observational findings, may reflect the low dosages of the agents administered as well as the deleterious effects of tobacco use in the study population.

The NCEP does not recommend the use of antioxidant vitamin supplements to reduce CAD risk because of insufficient data supporting their cardiovascular benefits.[3] In addition, the effects of long-term use of antioxidants in large doses are not known.[332] Studies in progress, notably the Physicians' Health Study and the Women's Health Initiative, should help clarify this issue.

REFERENCES

DECLINING MORTALITY AND THE RISK FACTOR CONCEPT

1. American Heart Association: Heart and Stroke Facts: 1995 Statistical Supplement. Dallas, American Heart Association, 1994.
2. Expert Panel on Detection, Evaluation, and Treatment of High Blood Cholesterol in Adults: Summary of the second report of the National Cholesterol Education Program (NCEP) Expert Panel on Detection, Evaluation, and Treatment of High Blood Cholesterol in Adults (Adult Treatment Panel II). J. A. M. A. 269:3015, 1993.
3. National Cholesterol Education Program: Second report of the Expert Panel on Detection, Evaluation, and Treatment of High Blood Cholesterol in Adults (Adult Treatment Panel II). Circulation 89:1329, 1994.
4. Johnson, C. L., Rifkind, B. M., Sempos, C. T., et al.: Declining serum total cholesterol levels among US adults: The National Health and Nutrition Examination Surveys. J. A. M. A. 269:3002, 1993.
5. Cigarette smoking among adults—United States, 1993. M. M. W. R. 43:925, 1994.
6. Burt, V. L., Whelton, P., Roccella, E. J., et al.: Prevalence of hypertension in the US adult population: Results from the third National Health and Nutrition Examination Survey, 1988–1991. Hypertension 25:305, 1995.
7. Sempos, C. T., Cleeman, J. I., Carroll, M. D., et al.: Prevalence of high blood cholesterol among US adults: An update based on guidelines from the second report of the National Cholesterol Education Program Adult Treatment Panel. J. A. M. A. 269:3009, 1993.
8. Anderson, K. M., Wilson, P. W. F., Odell, P. M., and Kannel, W. B.: An updated coronary risk profile: A statement for health professionals. Circulation 83:356, 1991.
9. Stamler, J.: Epidemiology, established major risk factors, and the primary prevention of coronary heart disease. In Chatterjee, K., Cheitlin, M. P., Karlines, J., et al. (eds.): Cardiology: An Illustrated Text/Reference. Vol. 2, p. 1. Philadelphia, J. B. Lippincott, 1991.

DYSLIPIDEMIA

10. Stamler, J., Wentworth, D., and Neaton, J. D., for the MRFIT Research Group: Is relationship between serum cholesterol and risk of premature death from coronary heart disease continuous and graded? Findings in 356 222 primary screenees of the Multiple Risk Factor Intervention Trial (MRFIT). J. A. M. A. 256:2823, 1986.
11. Keys, A. (ed.): Coronary Heart Disease in Seven Countries. American Heart Association Monograph 29. Circulation 41(Suppl. 1):1, 1970.
12. Kagan A., Harris, B. R., Winkelstein, W., Jr., et al.: Epidemiologic studies of coronary heart disease and stroke in Japanese men living in Japan, Hawaii and California: Demographic, physical, dietary and biochemical characteristics. J. Chronic Dis. 27:345, 1974.
13. Marmot, M. G., Syme, S. L., Kagan, A., et al.: Epidemiologic studies of coronary heart disease and stroke in Japanese men living in Japan, Hawaii and California: Prevalence of coronary and hypertensive heart disease and associated risk factors. Am. J. Epidemiol. 102:514, 1975.
14. Robertson, T. L., Kato, H., Rhoads, G. G., et al.: Epidemiologic studies of coronary heart disease and stroke in Japanese men living in Japan, Hawaii and California: Incidence of myocardial infarction and death from coronary heart disease. Am. J. Cardiol. 39:239, 1977.
15. Lipid Research Clinics Program: The Lipid Research Clinics Coronary Primary Prevention Trial results. I. Reduction in incidence of coronary heart disease. J. A. M. A. 251:351, 1984.
16. Lipid Research Clinics Program: The Lipid Research Clinics Coronary Primary Prevention Trial results. II. The relationship of reduction in incidence of coronary heart disease to cholesterol lowering. J. A. M. A. 251:365, 1984.
17. Committee of Principal Investigators: A co-operative trial in the primary prevention of ischaemic heart disease using clofibrate. Br. Heart J. 40:1069, 1978.
18. Committee of Principal Investigators: WHO cooperative trial on primary prevention of ischaemic heart disease with clofibrate to lower serum cholesterol: Final mortality follow-up. Lancet 2:600, 1984.
19. Huttunen, J. K., Manninen, V., Mänttäri, M., et al.: The Helsinki Heart Study: Central findings and clinical implications. Ann. Med. 23:155, 1991.
20. Frick, M. H., Elo, O., Haapa, K., et al.: Helsinki Heart Study: Primary-prevention trial with gemfibrozil in middle-aged men with dyslipidemia: Safety of treatment, changes in risk factors, and incidence of coronary heart disease. N. Engl. J. Med. 317:1237, 1987.

21. Hjermann, I., Velve Byre, K., Holme, I., and Leren, P.: Effect of diet and smoking intervention on the incidence of coronary heart disease: Report from the Oslo Study Group of a randomised trial in healthy men. Lancet 2:1303, 1981.
22. Hjermann, I., Holme, I., and Leren, P.: Oslo Study Diet and Anti-smoking Trial: Results after 102 months. Am. J. Med. 80(Suppl. 2A):7, 1986.
22a. Shepherd, J., Cobbe, S. M., Ford, I., et al., for the West of Scotland Coronary Prevention Study Group: Prevention of coronary heart disease with provastatin in men with hypercholesterolemia. N. Engl. J. Med. 333:1301, 1995.
23. Brown, B. G., Zhao, X. -Q., Sacco, D. E., and Albers, J. J.: Lipid lowering and plaque regression: New insights into prevention of plaque disruption and clinical events in coronary disease. Circulation 87:1781, 1993.
24. Brown, B. G., Bolson, E. L., and Dodge, H. T.: Arteriographic assessment of coronary atherosclerosis: Review of current methods, their limitations, and clinical applications. Arteriosclerosis 2:2, 1982.
25. de Feyter, P. J., Serruys, P. W., Davies, M. J., et al.: Quantitative coronary angiography to measure progression and regression of coronary atherosclerosis: Value, limitations, and implications for clinical trials. Circulation 84:412, 1991.
26. Blankenhorn, D. H., and Hodis, H. N.: Arterial imaging and atherosclerosis reversal. Arterioscler. Thromb. 14:177, 1994.
27. Gould, K. L.: Reversal of coronary atherosclerosis: Clinical promise as the basis for noninvasive management of coronary artery disease. Circulation 90:1558, 1994.
28. Coronary Drug Project Research Group: Clofibrate and niacin in coronary heart disease. J. A. M. A. 231:360, 1975.
29. Canner, P. L., Berge, K. G., Wenger, N. K., et al., for the Coronary Drug Project Research Group: Fifteen year mortality in Coronary Drug Project patients: Long-term benefit with niacin. J. Am. Coll. Cardiol. 8:1245, 1986.
30. Brensike, J. F., Levy, R. I., Kelsey, S. F., et al.: Effects of therapy with cholestyramine on progression of coronary arteriosclerosis: Results of the NHLBI Type II Coronary Intervention Study. Circulation 69:313, 1984.
31. Brensike, J. F., Kelsey, S. F., Passamani, E. R., et al.: National Heart, Lung, and Blood Institute Type II Coronary Intervention Study: Design, methods, and baseline characteristics. Controlled Clin. Trials 3:91, 1982.
32. Levy, R. I., Brensike, J. F., Epstein, S. E., et al.: The influence of changes in lipid values induced by cholestyramine and diet on progression of coronary artery disease: Results of the NHLBI Type II Coronary Intervention Study. Circulation 69:325, 1984.
33. Blankenhorn, D. H., Nessim, S. A., Johnson, R. L., et al.: Beneficial effects of combined colestipol-niacin therapy on coronary atherosclerosis and coronary venous bypass grafts. J. A. M. A. 257:3233, 1987.
34. Blankenhorn, D. H., Johnson, R. L., Mack, W. J., et al.: The influence of diet on the appearance of new lesions in human coronary arteries. J. A. M. A. 263:1646, 1990.
35. Cashin-Hemphill, L., Mack, W. J., Pogoda, J. M., et al.: Beneficial effects of colestipol-niacin on coronary atherosclerosis: A 4-year follow-up. J. A. M. A. 264:3013, 1990.
36. Brown, G., Albers, J. J., Fisher, L. D., et al.: Regression of coronary artery disease as a result of intensive lipid-lowering therapy in men with high levels of apolipoprotein B. N. Engl. J. Med. 323:1289, 1990.
37. Kane, J. P., Malloy, M. J., Ports, T. A., et al.: Regression of coronary atherosclerosis during treatment of familial hypercholesterolemia with combined drug regimens. J. A. M. A. 264:3007, 1990.
38. Watts, G. F., Lewis, B., Brunt, J. N. H., et al.: Effects on coronary artery disease of lipid-lowering diet, or diet plus cholestyramine, in the St Thomas' Atherosclerosis Regression Study (STARS). Lancet 339:563, 1992.
39. Buchwald, H., Varco, R. L., Matts, J. P., et al.: Effect of partial ileal bypass surgery on mortality and morbidity from coronary heart disease in patients with hypercholesterolemia: Report of the Program on the Surgical Control of the Hyperlipidemias (POSCH). N. Engl. J. Med. 323:946, 1990.
40. Buchwald, H., Matts, J. P., Fitch, L. L., et al., for the Program on the Surgical Control of the Hyperlipidemias (POSCH) Group: Changes in sequential coronary arteriograms and subsequent coronary events. J. A. M. A. 268:1429, 1992.
41. Ornish, D., Brown, S. E., Scherwitz, L. W., et al.: Can lifestyle changes reverse coronary heart disease? The Lifestyle Heart Trial. Lancet 336:129, 1990.
42. Blankenhorn, D. H., Azen, S. P., Kramsch, D. M., et al.: Coronary angiographic changes with lovastatin therapy: The Monitored Atherosclerosis Regression Study (MARS). Ann. Intern. Med. 119:969, 1993.
43. Hodis, H. N., Mack, W. J., Azen, S. P., et al.: Triglyceride- and cholesterol-rich lipoproteins have a differential effect on mild/moderate and severe lesion progression as assessed by quantitative coronary angiography in a controlled trial of lovastatin. Circulation 90:42, 1994.
44. Waters, D., Higginson, L., Gladstone, P., et al.: Effects of monotherapy with an HMG-CoA reductase inhibitor on the progression of coronary atherosclerosis as assessed by serial quantitative arteriography: The Canadian Coronary Atherosclerosis Intervention Trial. Circulation 89:959, 1994.
45. Pitt, B., Mancini, G. B. J., Ellis, S. G., et al., for the PLAC I Investigators: Pravastatin Limitation of Atherosclerosis in the Coronary Arteries

(PLAC I): Reduction in atherosclerosis progression and clinical events. J. Am. Coll. Cardiol. 26:1133, 1995.

46. Jukema, J. W., Bruschke, A. V. G., van Boven, A. J., et al., on behalf of the REGRESS Study Group: Effects of lipid lowering by pravastatin on progression and regression of coronary artery disease in symptomatic men with normal to moderately elevated serum cholesterol levels: The Regression Growth Evaluation Statin Study (REGRESS). Circulation 91:2528, 1995.

47. MAAS Investigators: Effect of simvastatin on coronary atheroma: The Multicentre Anti-Atheroma Study (MAAS). Lancet 344:633, 1994.

48. Scandinavian Simvastatin Survival Study Group: Randomised trial of cholesterol lowering in 4444 patients with coronary heart disease: The Scandinavian Simvastatin Survival Study (4S). Lancet 344:1383, 1994.

49. Scandinavian Simvastatin Survival Study Group: Baseline serum cholesterol and treatment effect in the Scandinavian Simvastatin Survival Study (4S). Lancet 345:1274, 1995.

50. Neaton, J. D., Blackburn, H., Jacobs, D., et al.: Serum cholesterol level and mortality findings for men screened in the Multiple Risk Factor Intervention Trial. Arch. Intern. Med. 152:1490, 1992.

51. Lewis, B., Paoletti, R., Tikkanen, M. J. (eds.): Low Blood Cholesterol: Health Implications: Proceedings of a workshop held in Milan, July 1993, under the auspices of the International Task Force for the Prevention of Coronary Heart Disease, International Society and Federation of Cardiology, Giovanni Lorenzini Foundation. London, Current Medical Literature Ltd., 1993.

52. Rossouw, J. E., and Gotto, A. M., Jr.: Does low cholesterol cause death? (editorial) Cardiovasc. Drugs Ther. 7:789, 1993.

53. Chen, Z., Peto, R., Collins, R., et al.: Serum cholesterol concentration and coronary heart disease in population with low cholesterol concentrations. B. M. J. 303:276, 1991.

54. Ettinger, W. H., Jr., and Harris, T.: Causes of hypocholesterolemia. Coron. Artery Dis. 4:854, 1993.

55. Kane, J. P., and Havel, R. J.: Disorders of the biogenesis and secretion of lipoproteins containing the B apolipoproteins. In Scriver, C. R., Beaudet, A. L., Sly, W. S., and Valle, D. (eds.): The Metabolic and Molecular Bases of Inherited Disease, 7th ed. New York, McGraw-Hill, 1995, p. 1853.

56. Linton, M. F., Farese, R. V., and Young, S. G.: Familial hypobetalipoproteinemia. J. Lipid Res. 34:521, 1993.

57. Rose, G., and Shipley, M.: Plasma lipids and mortality: A source of error. Lancet 1:523, 1980.

58. Kagan, A., McGee, D. L., Yano, K., et al.: Serum cholesterol and mortality in a Japanese-American population: The Honolulu Heart Program. Am. J. Epidemiol. 114:11, 1981.

59. Iribarren, C., Dwyer, J. H., Burchfiel, C. M., and Reed, S. M.: Can the U-shaped relation between mortality and serum cholesterol be explained by confounding? (abstract) Circulation 87:684, 1993.

60. Iribarren, C., Reed, D. M., Wergowske, G., et al.: Serum cholesterol level and mortality due to suicide and trauma in the Honolulu Heart Program. Arch. Intern. Med. 155:695, 1995.

61. Davey Smith, G., Shipley, M. J., Marmot, M. G., and Rose, G.: Plasma cholesterol concentration and mortality: The Whitehall Study. J. A. M. A. 267:70, 1992.

62. Anderson, K. M., Castelli, W. P., and Levy, D.: Cholesterol and mortality: 30 years of follow-up from the Framingham Study. J. A. M. A. 257:2176, 1987.

63. Wysowski, D. K., and Gross, T. P.: Deaths due to accidents and violence in two recent trials of cholesterol-lowering drugs. Arch. Intern. Med. 150:2169, 1990.

64. Engelberg, H.: Low serum cholesterol and suicide. Lancet 339:727, 1992.

65. Hawton, K., Cowen, P., Owens, D., et al.: Low serum cholesterol and suicide. Br. J. Psychiatry 162:818, 1993.

66. Byington, R. P., Jukema, J. W., Salonen, J. T., et al.: Reduction in cardiovascular events during pravastatin therapy: Pooled analysis of clinical events of the pravastatin atherosclerosis intervention program. Circulation 92:2419, 1995.

67. Krauss, R. M.: The tangled web of coronary risk factors. Am. J. Med. 90(Suppl. 2A):2A–36S, 1991.

68. Austin, M. A., Breslow, J. L., Hennekens, C. H., et al.: Low-density lipoprotein subclass patterns and risk of myocardial infarction. J. A. M. A. 260:1917, 1988.

69. Coresh, J., Kwiterovich, P. O., Jr., Smith, H. H., and Bachorik, P. S.: Association of plasma triglyceride concentration and LDL particle diameter, density, and chemical composition with premature coronary artery disease in men and women. J. Lipid Res. 34:1687, 1993.

70. Austin, M. A., King, M-C., Vranizan, K. M., et al.: Inheritance of low-density lipoprotein subclass patterns: Results of complex segregation analysis. Am. J. Hum. Genet. 43:838, 1988.

71. Austin, M. A.: Genetic epidemiology of low-density lipoprotein subclass phenotypes. Ann. Med. 24:477, 1992.

72. Reaven, G. M., Chen, Y-D. I., Jeppesen, J., et al.: Insulin resistance and hyperinsulinemia in individuals with small, dense low density lipoprotein particles. J. Clin. Invest. 92:141, 1993.

73. Tilly-Kiesi, M., and Tikkanen, M. J.: Low density lipoprotein density and composition in hypercholesterolaemic men treated with HMG CoA reductase inhibitors and gemfibrozil. J. Intern. Med. 229:427, 1991.

74. Eisenberg, S., Gavish, D., Oschry, Y., et al.: Abnormalities in very low, low, and high density lipoproteins in hypertriglyceridemia: Reversal toward normal with bezafibrate treatment. J. Clin. Invest. 74:470, 1984.

75. La Belle, M., and Krauss, R. M.: Differences in carbohydrate content of low density lipoproteins associated with low density lipoprotein subclass patterns. J. Lipid Res. 31:1577, 1990.

76. Weisser, B., Locher, R., de Graaf, J., et al.: Low density lipoprotein subfractions increase thromboxane formation in endothelial cells. Biochem. Biophys. Res. Commun. 192:1245, 1993.

77. Dejager, S., Bruckert, E., and Chapman, M. J.: Dense low density lipoprotein subspecies with diminished oxidative resistance predominate in combined hyperlipidemia. J. Lipid Res. 349:295, 1993.

78. Steinberg, D., and Witztum, J. L.: Lipoproteins and atherogenesis: Current concepts. J. A. M. A. 264:3047, 1990.

78a. Thorne, S. A., Abbot, S. E., Winyard, P. G., et al.: Extent of oxidative modification of low density lipoprotein determines the degree of cytotoxicity to human coronary artery cells. Heart 75:11, 1996.

79. Schwartz, C. J., Valente, A. J., and Sprague, E. A.: A modern view of atherogenesis. Am. J. Cardiol. 71:9B, 1993.

80. National Cholesterol Education Program: Report of the Expert Panel on Blood Cholesterol Levels in Children and Adolescents. Pediatrics 39(3 pt 2):525, 1992.

81. Denke, M. A.: Cholesterol-lowering diets: A review of the evidence. Arch. Intern. Med. 155:17, 1995.

81a. Grundy, S. M.: Lipids, nutrition, and coronary heart disease. In Fuster, V., Ross, R., and Topol, E. J. (eds.): Atherosclerosis and Coronary Artery Disease. Philadelphia, Lippincott-Raven, 1996, pp. 45–68.

82. Kris-Etherton, P. M., Krummel, D., Russell, M. E., et al.: The effect of diet on plasma lipids, lipoproteins, and coronary heart disease. J. Am. Diet. Assoc. 88:1373, 1988.

83. Moore, R. B., Crane, C. A., and Frantz, I. D., Jr.: Effect of cholestyramine on the fecal excretion of intravenously administered cholesterol-4-¹⁴C and its degradation products in a hypercholesterolemic patient. J. Clin. Invest. 47:1664, 1968.

83a. Witztum, J. L.: Drugs used in the treatment of hyperlipoproteinemias. In Hardman, J. G., et al. (eds.): Goodman & Gilman's The pharmacological basis of therapeutics, 9th ed. New York, McGraw-Hill, 1996, pp. 875–898.

84. Grundy, S. M., Ahrens, E. H., Jr., and Salen, G.: Interruption of the enterohepatic circulation of bile acids in man: Comparative effects of cholestyramine and ileal exclusion on cholesterol metabolism. J. Lab. Clin. Med. 78:94, 1971.

85. Gallo, D. G., Bailey, K. R., and Sheffner, A. L.: The interaction between cholestyramine and drugs. Proc. Soc. Exp. Biol. Med. 120:60, 1965.

86. Bazzano, G., and Bazzano, G. S.: Digitalis intoxication: Treatment with a new steroid-binding resin. J. A. M. A. 220:828, 1972.

87. Hunninghake, D. B., King, S., and LaCroix, K.: The effect of cholestyramine and colestipol on the absorption of hydrochlorothiazide. Int. J. Clin. Pharmacol. Ther. Toxicol. 20:151, 1982.

88. Hibbard, D. M., Peters, J. R., and Hunninghake, D. B.: Effects of cholestyramine and colestipol on the plasma concentrations of propranolol. Br. J. Clin. Pharmacol. 18:337, 1984.

89. Grundy, S. M., Mok, H. Y. I., Zech, L., and Berman, M.: Influence of nicotinic acid on metabolism of cholesterol and triglycerides in man. J. Lipid Res. 22:24, 1981.

90. Brown, W. V., Howard, W. J., and Field, L.: Nicotinic acid and its derivatives. In Rifkind, B. M. (ed.): Drug Treatment of Hyperlipidemia. New York, Marcel Dekker, 1991, p. 189.

91. Shepherd, J., Packard, C. J., Patsch, J. R., et al.: Effects of nicotinic acid therapy on plasma high density lipoprotein subfraction distribution and composition and on apolipoprotein A metabolism. J. Clin. Invest. 63:858, 1979.

92. Carlson, L. A., Hamsten, A., and Asplund, A.: Pronounced lowering of serum levels of lipoprotein Lp(a) in hyperlipidaemic subjects treated with nicotinic acid. J. Intern. Med. 226:271, 1989.

93. Mullin, G. E., Greenson, J. K., and Mitchell, M. C.: Fulminant hepatic failure after ingestion of sustained-release nicotinic acid. Ann. Intern. Med. 111:253, 1989.

94. Rader, J. I., Calvert, R. J., and Hathcock, J. N.: Hepatic toxicity of unmodified and time-release preparations of niacin. Am. J. Med. 92:77, 1992.

95. Charman, R. C., Matthews, L. B., and Braeuler, C.: Nicotinic acid in the treatment of hypercholesterolemia: A long term study. Angiology 23:29, 1972.

96. Litin, S. C., and Anderson, C. F.: Nicotinic acid–associated myopathy: A report of three cases. Am. J. Med. 86:481, 1989.

97. Reaven, P., and Witztum, J. L.: Lovastatin, nicotinic acid, and rhabdomyolysis (letter). Ann. Intern. Med. 109:597, 1988.

98. Arad, Y., Ramakrishnan, R., and Ginsberg, H. N.: Lovastatin therapy reduces low density lipoprotein apoB levels in subjects with combined hyperlipidemia by reducing the production of apoB-containing lipoproteins: Implications for the pathophysiology of apoB production. J. Lipid Res. 31:567, 1990.

99. Isaacsohn, J. L., Setaro, J. F., Nicholas, C., et al.: Effects of lovastatin therapy on plasminogen activator inhibitor-1 antigen levels. Am. J. Cardiol. 74:735, 1994.

100. Wada, H., Mori, Y., Kaneko, T., et al.: Elevated plasma levels of vascular endothelial cell markers in patients with hypercholesterolemia. Am. J. Hematol. 44:112, 1993.

101. Gianturco, S. H., Bradley, W. A., Nozaki, S., et al.: Effects of lovastatin on the levels, structure, and atherogenicity of VLDL in patients with moderate hypertriglyceridemia. Arterioscler. Thromb. 13:472, 1993.

102. Kostner, G. M., Gavish, D., Leopold, B., et al.: HMG CoA reductase inhibitors lower LDL cholesterol without reducing Lp(a) levels. Circulation 80:1313, 1989.

103. Bradford, R. H., Shear, C. L., Chremos, A. N., et al.: Expanded Clinical Evaluation of Lovastatin (EXCEL) Study results. I. Efficacy in modifying plasma lipoproteins and adverse event profile in 8245 patients with moderate hypercholesterolemia. Arch. Intern. Med. 151:43, 1991.

104. Tobert, J. A., Shear, C. L., Chremos, A. N., and Mantell, G. E.: Clinical experience with lovastatin. Am. J. Cardiol. 65:23F, 1990.

105. Bradford, R. H., Shear, C. L., Chremos, A. N., et al.: Expanded Clinical Evaluation of Lovastatin (EXCEL) Study results: Two-year efficacy and safety follow-up. Am. J. Cardiol. 74:667, 1994.

106. Pierce, L. R., Wysowski, D. K., and Gross, T. P.: Myopathy and rhabdomyolysis associated with lovastatin-gemfibrozil combination therapy. J. A. M. A. 264:71, 1990.

107. Tobert, J. A.: Efficacy and long-term adverse effect pattern of lovastatin. Am. J. Cardiol. 62:28J, 1988.

108. Corpier, C. L., Jones, P. H., Suki, W. N., et al.: Rhabdomyolysis and renal injury with lovastatin use: Report of two cases in cardiac transplant recipients. J. A. M. A. 260:239, 1988.

109. Spach, D. H., Bauwens, J. E., Clark, C. D., and Burke, W. G.: Rhabdomyolysis associated with lovastatin and erythromycin use. West. J. Med. 154:213, 1991.

110. Laties, A. M., Shear, C. L., Lippa, E. A., et al.: Expanded Clinical Evaluation of Lovastatin (EXCEL) Study results. II. Assessment of the human lens after 48 weeks of treatment with lovastatin. Am. J. Cardiol. 67:447, 1991.

111. Illingworth, D. R., and Tobert, J. A.: A review of clinical trials comparing HMG-CoA reductase inhibitors. Clin. Ther. 16:366, 1994.

112. Levy, R. I., Morganroth, J., and Rifkind, B. M.: Treatment of hyperlipidemia. N. Engl. J. Med. 290:1295, 1976.

113. Bimmermann, A., Boerschmann, C., Schwartzkopff, W., et al.: Effective therapeutic measures for reducing lipoprotein (a) in patients with dyslipidemia: Lipoprotein (a) reduction with sustained-release bezafibrate. Current Therapeutic Research: Clinical and Experimental 49:635, 1991.

114. Todd, P. A., and Ward, A.: Gemfibrozil: A review of its pharmacodynamic and pharmacokinetic properties, and therapeutic use in dyslipidaemia. Drugs 36:314, 1988.

115. Andersen, P., Smith, P., Seljeflot, I., et al.: Effects of gemfibrozil on lipids and haemostasis after myocardial infarction. Thromb. Haemost. 63:174, 1990.

116. Bo, M., Bonino, F., Neirotti, M., et al.: Hemorheologic and coagulative pattern in hypercholesterolemic subjects treated with lipid-lowering drugs. Angiology 42:106, 1991.

117. Langer, T., and Levy, R. I.: Acute muscular syndrome associated with administration of clofibrate. N. Engl. J. Med. 279:856, 1968.

118. Wiklund, O., Angelin, B., Bergman, M., et al.: Pravastatin and gemfibrozil alone and in combination for the treatment of hypercholesterolemia. Am. J. Med. 94:13, 1993.

119. Xiu, R. J., Freyschuss, A., Ying, X., et al.: The antioxidant butylated hydroxytoluene prevents early cholesterol-induced microcirculatory changes in rabbits. J. Clin. Invest. 93:2732, 1994.

120. Carew, T. E., Schwenke, D. C., and Steinberg, D.: Antiatherogenic effect of probucol unrelated to its hypocholesterolemic effect: Evidence that antioxidants in vivo can selectively inhibit low density lipoprotein degradation in macrophage-rich fatty streaks and slow the progression of atherosclerosis in the Watanabe heritable hyperlipidemic rabbit. Proc. Natl. Acad. Sci. U. S. A. 84:7725, 1987.

121. Yamamoto, A., Matsuzawa, Y., Yokoyama, S., et al.: Effects of probucol on xanthomata regression in familial hypercholesterolemia. Am. J. Cardiol. 57:29H, 1986.

122. Mellies, M. J., Gartside, P. S., Glatfelder, L., et al.: Effects of probucol on plasma cholesterol, high and low density lipoprotein cholesterol, and apolipoproteins A1 and A2 in adults with primary familial hypercholesterolemia. Metabolism 29:956, 1980.

123. Franceschini, G., Sirtori, M., Vaccarino, V., et al.: Mechanisms of HDL reduction after probucol: Changes in HDL subfractions and increased reverse cholesteryl ester transfer. Arteriosclerosis 9:462, 1989.

124. McPherson, R., and Marcel, Y.: Role of cholesteryl ester transfer protein in reverse cholesterol transport. Clin. Cardiol. 14:131, 1991.

125. Buckley, M. M-T., Goa, K. L., Price, A. H., and Brogden, R. N.: Probucol: A reappraisal of its pharmacological properties and therapeutic use in hypercholesterolaemia. Drugs 37:761, 1989.

126. Stevenson, J. C., Crook, D., and Gosland, I. F.: Influence of age and menopause on serum lipids and lipoproteins in healthy women. Atherosclerosis 98:83, 1993.

127. Stampfer, M. J., Colditz, G. A., Willett, W. C., et al.: Postmenopausal estrogen therapy and cardiovascular disease: Ten-year follow-up from the Nurses' Health Study. N. Engl. J. Med. 325:756, 1991.

128. Stampfer, M. J., and Colditz, G. A.: Estrogen replacement therapy and coronary heart disease: A quantitative assessment of the epidemiologic evidence. Prev. Med. 20:47, 1991.

129. Granfone, A., Campos, H., McNamara, J. R., et al.: Effects of estrogen replacement on plasma lipoproteins and apolipoproteins in postmenopausal, dyslipidemic women. Metabolism 41:1193, 1992.

130. Wagner, J. D., St. Clair, R. W., Schwenke, D. C., et al.: Regional differences in arterial low density lipoprotein metabolism in surgically postmenopausal cynomolgus monkeys: Effects of estrogen and progesterone replacement therapy. Arterioscler. Thromb. 12:717, 1992.

131. Gotto, A. M., Jr.: Postmenopausal hormone-replacement therapy, plasma lipoprotein[a], and risk for coronary heart disease (editorial). J. Lab. Clin. Med. 123:800, 1994.

132. Writing Group for the PEPI Trial: Effects of estrogen or estrogen/progestin regimens on heart disease risk factors in postmenopausal women: The Postmenopausal Estrogen/Progestin Interventions (PEPI) trial. JAMA 273:199, 1995.

133. Goldstein, J. L., Hobbs, H. H., and Brown, M. S.: Familial hypercholesterolemia. In Scriver, C. R., Beaudet, A. L., Sly, W. S., and Valle, D. (eds.): The Metabolic and Molecular Bases of Inherited Disease, 7th ed. New York, McGraw-Hill, 1995, p. 1981.

133a. Brewer, H. B. Jr., Santamarina-Fojo, S., and Hoeg, J. M.: Genetic dyslipoproteinemias. In Fuster, V., Ross, R., and Topol, E. J. (eds.): Atherosclerosis and Coronary Artery Disease. Philadelphia, Lippincott-Raven, 1996, pp. 69–88.

134. Bild, D. E., Williams, R. R., Brewer, H. B., et al.: Identification and management of heterozygous familial hypercholesterolemia: Summary and recommendations from an NHLBI workshop. Am. J. Cardiol. 72:1D, 1993.

135. Tatami, R., Inoue, N., Itoh, H., et al., for the LARS Investigators: Regression of coronary atherosclerosis by combined LDL-apheresis and lipid-lowering drug therapy in patients with familial hypercholesterolemia: A multicenter study. Atherosclerosis 95:1, 1992.

136. Thompson, G. R., Maher, V. M. G., Matthews, S., et al.: Familial Hypercholesterolaemia Regression Study: A randomised trial of low-density-lipoprotein apheresis. Lancet 345:811, 1995.

137. Bilheimer, D. W., Goldstein, J. L., Grundy, S. M., et al.: Liver transplantation to provide low-density-lipoprotein receptors and lower plasma cholesterol in a child with homozygous familial hypercholesterolemia. N. Engl. J. Med. 311:1658, 1984.

138. Grossman, M., Raper, S. E., Kozarsky, K., et al.: Successful ex vivo gene therapy directed to liver in a patient with familial hypercholesterolaemia. Nat. Genet. 6:335, 1994.

139. Brown, M. S., Goldstein, J. L., Havel, R. J., and Steinberg, D.: Gene therapy for cholesterol (letter). Nat. Genet. 7:349, 1994.

140. Grundy, S. M.: Multifactorial etiology of hypercholesterolemia: Implications for prevention of coronary heart disease. Arterioscler. Thromb. 11:1619, 1991.

141. Kwiterovich, P. O., Jr.: Genetics and molecular biology of familial combined hyperlipidemia. Curr. Opin. Lipidol. 4:133, 1993.

142. Myant, N. B.: Familial defective apolipoprotein B-100: A review, including some comparisons with familial hypercholesterolaemia. Atherosclerosis 104:1, 1993.

143. Schmidt, E. B., Illingworth, D. R., Bacon, S., et al.: Hypolipidemic effects of nicotinic acid in patients with familial defective apolipoprotein B-100. Metabolism 42:137, 1993.

144. Gordon, T., Castelli, W. P., Hjortland, M. C., et al.: High density lipoprotein as a protective factor against coronary heart disease: The Framingham Study. Am. J. Med. 62:707, 1977.

145. Gordon, D. J., Probstfield, J. L., Garrison, R. J., et al.: High-density lipoprotein cholesterol and cardiovascular disease: Four prospective American studies. Circulation 79:8, 1989.

146. James, R. W., and Pometta, D.: Immunofractionation of high density lipoprotein subclasses 2 and 3: Similarities and differences of fractions isolated from male and female populations. Atherosclerosis 83:35, 1990.

147. Eisenberg, S.: High density lipoprotein metabolism. J. Lipid Res. 25:1017, 1984.

148. Patsch, J. R.: Triglyceride-rich lipoproteins and atherosclerosis. Atherosclerosis 110:S23, 1994.

149. Kuhn, F. E., Mohler, E. R., Satler, L. F., et al.: Effects of high-density lipoprotein on acetylcholine-induced coronary vasoreactivity. Am. J. Cardiol. 68:1425, 1991.

150. Aoyama, T., Yui, Y., Morishita, H., and Kawai, C.: Prostacyclin stabilization by high density lipoprotein is decreased in acute myocardial infarction and unstable angina pectoris. Circulation 81:1784, 1990.

151. Mackness, M. I., Abbott, C., Arrol, S., and Durrington, P. N.: The role of high-density lipoprotein and lipid-soluble antioxidant vitamins in inhibiting low-density lipoprotein oxidation. Biochem. J. 294:829, 1993.

152. Assmann, G., von Eckardstein, A., and Brewer, H. B., Jr.: Familial high density lipoprotein deficiency: Tangier disease. In Scriver, C. R., Beaudet, A. L., Sly, W. S., and Valle, D. (eds.): The Metabolic and Molecular Bases of Inherited Disease, 7th ed. New York, McGraw-Hill, 1995, p. 2053.

153. Schaefer, E. J., Zech, L. A., Schwartz, D. E., and Brewer, H. B., Jr.: Coronary heart disease prevalence and other clinical features in familial high-density lipoprotein deficiency (Tangier disease). Ann. Intern. Med. 93:261, 1980.

154. Schaefer, E. J., Blum, C. B., Levy, R. I., et al.: Metabolism of high density lipoprotein apoproteins in Tangier disease. N. Engl. J. Med. 299:905, 1978.

155. Glomset, J. A., and Norum, K. R.: The metabolic role of lecithin:cholesterol acyltransferase: Perspectives from pathology. Adv. Lipid Res. 11:1, 1973.

156. Glomset, J. A., Assmann, G., Gjone, E., and Norum, K. R.: Lecithin:cholesterol acyltransferase deficiency and fish eye disease. In Scriver, C. R., Beaudet, A. L., Sly, W. S., and Valle, D. (eds.): The Metabolic and Molecular Bases of Inherited Disease, 7th ed. New York, McGraw-Hill, 1995, p. 1933.

157. Carlson, L. A., and Holmquist, L.: Paradoxical esterification of plasma cholesterol in fish eye disease. Acta Med. Scand. 217:491, 1985.

158. Breslow, J. L.: Familial disorders of high density lipoprotein metabolism. In Scriver, C. R., Beaudet, A. L., Sly, W. S., and Valle, D. (eds.): The Metabolic and Molecular Bases of Inherited Disease, 7th ed. New York, McGraw-Hill, 1995, p. 2031.

159. Roma, P., Gregg, R. E., Meng, M. S., et al.: In vivo metabolism of a

mutant form of apolipoprotein A-I, apo A-I$_{Milano}$, associated with familial hypoalphalipoproteinemia. J. Clin. Invest. 91:1445, 1993.

160. Franceschini, G., Sirtori, C. R., Capurso, A., et al.: A-I$_{Milano}$ apoprotein: Decreased high density lipoprotein cholesterol levels with significant lipoprotein modifications and without clinical atherosclerosis in an Italian family. J. Clin. Invest. 66:892, 1980.

161. Norum, R. A., Lakier, J. B., Goldstein, S., et al.: Familial deficiency of apolipoproteins A-I and C-III and precocious coronary-artery disease. N. Engl. J. Med. 306:1513, 1982.

162. Karathanasis, S. K., Ferris, E., and Haddad, I. A.: DNA inversion within the apolipoproteins AI/CIII/AIV-encoding gene cluster of certain patients with premature atherosclerosis. Proc. Natl. Acad. Sci. U. S. A. 84:7198, 1987.

163. Lackner, K. J., Dieplinger, H., Nowicka, G., and Schmitz, G.: High density lipoprotein deficiency with xanthomas: A defect in reverse cholesterol transport caused by a point mutation in the apolipoprotein A-I gene. J. Clin. Invest. 92:2262, 1993.

164. Austin, M. A.: Plasma triglyceride and coronary heart disease. Arterioscler. Thromb. 11:2, 1991.

165. Austin, M. A.: Plasma triglyceride as a risk factor for coronary heart disease: The epidemiologic evidence and beyond. Am. J. Epidemiol. 129:249, 1989.

166. Criqui, M. H., Heiss, G., Cohn, R., et al.: Plasma triglyceride level and mortality from coronary heart disease. N. Engl. J. Med. 328:1220, 1993.

167. Groot, P. H. E., van Stiphout, W. A. H. J., Krauss, X. H., et al.: Postprandial lipoprotein metabolism in normolipemic men with and without coronary artery disease. Arterioscler. Thromb. 11:653, 1991.

168. Patsch, J. R., Miesenböck, G., Hopferwieser, T., et al.: Relation of triglyceride metabolism and coronary artery disease: Studies in the postprandial state. Arterioscler. Thromb. 12:1336, 1992.

169. Simo, I. E., Yakichuk, J. A., and Ooi, T. C.: Effect of gemfibrozil and lovastatin on postprandial lipoprotein clearance in the hypoalphalipoproteinemia and hypertriglyceridemia syndrome. Atherosclerosis 100:55, 1993.

170. Hokanson, J. E., and Austin, M. A.: Triglyceride is a risk factor for coronary disease in men and women: A meta-analysis of population-based prospective studies. Circulation 88(Abs.):I-510, 1993.

171. Assmann, G., and Schulte, H.: Role of triglycerides in coronary artery disease: Lessons from the Prospective Cardiovascular Münster study. Am. J. Cardiol. 70:10H, 1992.

172. Blankenhorn, D. H., Alaupovic, P., Wickham, E., et al.: Prediction of angiographic change in native human coronary arteries and aortocoronary bypass grafts: Lipid and nonlipid factors. Circulation 81:470, 1990.

173. Manninen, V., Tenkanen, L., Koskinen, P., et al.: Joint effects of serum triglyceride and LDL cholesterol and HDL cholesterol concentrations on coronary heart disease risk in the Helsinki Heart Study: Implications for treatment. Circulation 85:37, 1992.

174. Krauss, R. M., Lindgren, F. T., Williams, P. T., et al.: Intermediate-density lipoproteins and progression of coronary artery disease in hypercholesterolaemic men. Lancet 2:62, 1987.

175. Phillips, N. R., Waters, D., and Havel, R. J.: Plasma lipoproteins and progression of coronary artery disease evaluated by angiography and clinical events. Circulation 88:2762, 1993.

176. Bang, H. O., and Dyerberg, J.: Plasma lipids and lipoproteins in Greenlandic west coast Eskimos. Acta Med. Scand. 192:85, 1972.

177. Dolecek, T. A.: Epidemiological evidence of relationships between dietary polyunsaturated fatty acids and mortality in the Multiple Risk Factor Intervention Trial. Proc. Soc. Exp. Biol. Med. 200:177, 1992.

178. Nestel, P. J., Connor, W. E., Reardon, M. F., et al.: Suppression by diets rich in fish oil of very low density lipoprotein production in man. J. Clin. Invest. 74:82, 1984.

179. Abbey, M., Clifton, P., Kestin, M., et al.: Effect of fish oil on lipoproteins, lecithin:cholesterol acyltransferase, and lipid transfer protein activity in humans. Arteriosclerosis 10:85, 1990.

180. Morris, M. C., Sacks, F., and Rosner, B.: Does fish oil lower blood pressure? A meta-analysis of controlled trials. Circulation 88:523, 1993.

181. Braden, G. A., Knapp, H. R., and FitzGerald, G. A.: Suppression of eicosanoid biosynthesis during coronary angioplasty by fish oil and aspirin. Circulation 84:679, 1991.

182. Bairati, I., Roy, L., and Meyer, F.: Double-blind, randomized, controlled trial of fish oil supplements in prevention of recurrence of stenosis after coronary angioplasty. Circulation 85:950, 1992.

183. Chait, A., and Brunyell, J. D.: Chylomicronemia syndrome. Adv. Intern. Med. 37:249, 1991.

184. Santamarina-Fojo, S., and Brewer, H. B., Jr.: The familial hyperchylomicronemia syndrome: New insights into underlying genetic defects. JAMA 265:904, 1991.

185. Brunzell, J. D., Miller, N. E., Alaupovic, P., et al.: Familial chylomicronemia due to a circulating inhibitor of lipoprotein lipase activity. J. Lipid Res. 24:12, 1983.

186. Kane, J. P., Chen, G. C., Hamilton, R. L., et al.: Remnants of lipoproteins of intestinal and hepatic origin in familial dysbetalipoproteinemia. Arteriosclerosis 3:47, 1983.

187. Mahley, R. W., Innerarity, T. L., Weisgraber, K. H., and Rall, S. C., Jr.: Genetic defects in lipoprotein metabolism: Elevation of atherogenic lipoproteins caused by impaired catabolism. JAMA 265:78, 1991.

188. Mahley, R. W., and Rall, S. C., Jr.: Type III hyperlipoproteinemia (dysbetalipoproteinemia): The role of apolipoprotein E in normal and abnormal lipoprotein metabolism. In Scriver, C. R., Beaudet, A. L., Sly,

W. S., and Valle, D. (eds.): The Metabolic and Molecular Bases of Inherited Disease, 7th ed. New York, McGraw-Hill, 1995, p. 1953.

189. Loscalzo, J.: Lipoprotein(a): A unique risk factor for atherothrombotic disease. Arteriosclerosis 10:672, 1990.

190. Boerwinkle, E., Leffert, C. C., Lin, J., et al.: Apolipoprotein(a) accounts for greater than 90% of the variation in plasma lipoprotein(a) concentrations. J. Clin. Invest. 90:52, 1992.

191. Utermann, G., Hoppichler, F., Dieplinger, H., et al.: Defects in the low density lipoprotein receptor gene affect lipoprotein(a) levels: Multiplicative interaction of two gene loci associated with premature atherosclerosis. Proc. Natl. Acad. Sci. U. S. A. 86:4171, 1989.

192. De Knijff, P., Kaptein, A., Boomsma, D., et al.: Apolipoprotein E polymorphism affects plasma levels of lipoprotein(a). Atherosclerosis 90:169, 1991.

193. Loscalzo, J., Weinfeld, M., Fless, G. M., and Scanu, A. M.: Lipoprotein(a), fibrin binding, and plasminogen activation. Arteriosclerosis 10:240, 1990.

194. Beisiegel, U., Niendorf, A., Wolf, K., et al.: Lipoprotein(a) in the arterial wall. Eur. Heart J. 11(Suppl. E):174, 1990.

195. Haberland, M. E., Fless, G. M., Scanu, A. M., and Fogelman, A. M.: Malondialdehyde modification of lipoprotein(a) produces avid uptake by human monocyte–macrophages. J. Biol. Chem. 267:4143, 1992.

196. Naruszewicz, M., Selinger, E., and Davignon, J.: Oxidative modification of lipoprotein(a) and the effect of β-carotene. Metabolism 41:1215, 1992.

197. Gurakar, A., Hoeg, J. M., Kostner, G., et al.: Levels of lipoprotein Lp(a) decline with neomycin and niacin treatment. Atherosclerosis 57:293, 1985.

198. Albers, J. J., Taggart, H. M., Appelbaum-Bowden, D., et al.: Reduction of LCAT, apo D, and the Lp(a) lipoprotein with the anabolic steroid stanozolol. Biochim. Biophys. Acta 795:293, 1984.

TOBACCO USE

199. Bartecchi, C. E., MacKenzie, T. D., and Schrier, R. W.: The human costs of tobacco use (first of two parts). N. Engl. J. Med. 330:907, 1994.

199a. Stafford, R. S., and Becker, C. G.: Cigarette smoking and atherosclerosis. In Fuster, V., Ross, R., and Topol, E. J. (eds.): Atherosclerosis and Coronary Artery Disease. Philadelphia, Lippincott-Raven, 1996, pp. 303–326.

200. Peto, R., Lopez, A. D., Boreham, J., et al.: Mortality from tobacco in developed countries: Indirect estimation from national vital statistics. Lancet 339:1268, 1992.

201. Smoking-Related Deaths and Financial Costs: Estimates for 1990, rev. ed. Washington, D.C., Office of Technology Assessment, 1993.

202. Kannel, W. B., and Higgins, M.: Smoking and hypertension as predictors of cardiovascular risk in population studies. J. Hypertens. Suppl. 8:S3, 1990.

203. Negri, E., Franzosi, M. G., La Vecchia, C., et al.: Tar yield of cigarettes and risk of acute myocardial infarction. B. M. J. 306:1567, 1993.

204. Bolinder, G., Alfredsson, L., Englund, A., and de Faire, U.: Smokeless tobacco use and increased cardiovascular mortality among Swedish construction workers. Am. J. Public Health 84:399, 1994.

205. Steenland, K.: Passive smoking and the risk of heart disease. JAMA 267:94, 1992.

206. Sigurdsson, G., Jr., Gudnason, V., Sigurdsson, G., and Humphries, S. E.: Interaction between a polymorphism of the apo A-I promoter region and smoking determines plasma levels of HDL and apo A-I. Arterioscler. Thromb. 12:1017, 1992.

207. McCall, M. R., van den Berg, J. J., Kuypers, F. A., et al.: Modification of LCAT activity and HDL structure: New links between cigarette smoke and coronary heart disease risk. Arterioscler. Thromb. 14:248, 1994.

208. Sugiishi, M., and Takatsu, F.: Cigarette smoking is a major risk factor for coronary spasm. Circulation 87:76, 1993.

209. Pittilo, R. M., Mackie, I. J., Rowles, P. M., et al.: Effects of cigarette smoking on the ultrastructure of rat thoracic aorta and its ability to produce prostacyclin. Thromb. Haemost. 48:173, 1982.

210. Ogston, D., Bennett, N. B., and Ogston, C. M.: The influence of cigarette smoking on the plasma fibrinogen concentration. Atherosclerosis 11:349, 1970.

211. FitzGerald, G. A., Oates, J. A., and Nowak, J.: Cigarette smoking and hemostatic function. Am. Heart J. 115:267, 1988.

212. Tsevat, J., Weinstein, M. C., Williams, L. W., et al.: Expected gains in life expectancy from various coronary heart disease risk factor modifications. Circulation 83:1194, 1991.

213. Terres, W., Becker, P., and Rosenberg, A.: Changes in cardiovascular risk profile during the cessation of smoking. Am. J. Med. 97:242, 1994.

214. Gerace, T. A., Hollis, J., Ockene, J. K., and Svendsen, K.: Smoking cessation and change in diastolic blood pressure, body weight, and plasma lipids: MRFIT Research Group. Prev. Med. 20:602, 1991.

215. Dobson, A. J., Alexander, H. M., Heller, R. F., and Lloyd, D. M.: How soon after quitting smoking does risk of heart attack decline? J. Clin. Epidemiol. 44:1247, 1991.

216. Physician and other health-care professional counseling of smokers to quit—United States, 1991. M. M. W. R. 42:854, 1993.

217. Public Health Service: Healthy People 2000: National health promotion and disease prevention objectives—full report, with commentary. [DHHS publication no. (PHS)91-50212.] Washington, D.C., U.S. Department of Health and Human Services, Public Health Service, 1991.

218. Glynn, T. J., and Manley, M. W.: How to Help Your Patients Stop Smoking: A National Cancer Institute manual for physicians. [DHHS

publication no. (PHS)92-3064.] Bethesda, Md., U.S. Department of Health and Human Services, Public Health Service, National Institutes of Health, National Cancer Institute, 1992.

HYPERTENSION

219. National High Blood Pressure Education Program Working Group: Report on primary prevention of hypertension. Arch. Intern. Med. 153:186, 1993.
220. MacMahon, S., Peto, R., Cutler, J., et al.: Blood pressure, stroke, and coronary heart disease. Part 1. Prolonged differences in blood pressure: Prospective observational studies corrected for the regression dilution bias. Lancet 335:765, 1990.
221. Collins, R., Peto, R., MacMahon, S., et al.: Blood pressure, stroke, and coronary heart disease. Part 2. Short-term reductions in blood pressure: Overview of randomised drug trials in their epidemiological context. Lancet 335:827, 1990.
222. Black, H. R.: Metabolic considerations in the choice of therapy for the patient with hypertension. Am. Heart J. 121:707, 1991.
223. Samuelsson, O. G., Wilhelmsen, L. W., Pennert, K. M., et al.: The J-shaped relationship between coronary heart disease and achieved blood pressure level in treated hypertension: Further analyses of 12 years of follow-up of treated hypertensives in the Primary Prevention Trial in Gothenburg, Sweden. J. Hypertens. 8:547, 1990.
224. Hansson, L., and Zanchetti, A.: The Hypertension Optimal Treatment (HOT) Study—patient characteristics: Randomization, risk profiles, and early blood pressure results. Blood Press. 3:322, 1994.
225. Houston, M. C.: The management of hypertension and associated risk factors for the prevention of long-term cardiac complications. J. Cardiovasc. Pharmacol. 21(Suppl. 2):S2, 1993.
226. Reaven, G. M.: Role of insulin resistance in human disease (syndrome X): An expanded definition. Annu. Rev. Med. 44:121, 1993.
227. DeFronzo, R. A., and Ferrannini, E.: Insulin resistance: A multifaceted syndrome responsible for NIDDM, obesity, hypertension, dyslipidemia, and atherosclerotic cardiovascular disease. Diabetes Care 14:173, 1991.

DIABETES MELLITUS

228. American Diabetes Association: Diabetes Facts: The Dangerous Toll of Diabetes. Alexandria, Va., American Diabetes Association, 1994.
229. American Diabetes Association: Diabetes Facts: Profile of the Diagnosed. Alexandria, Va., American Diabetes Association, 1993.
230. Barrett-Connor, E. L., Cohn, B. A., Wingard, D. L., and Edelstein, S. L.: Why is diabetes mellitus a stronger risk factor for fatal ischemic heart disease in women than in men? The Rancho Bernardo Study. JAMA 265:627, 1991.
231. American Diabetes Association: Detection and management of lipid disorders in diabetes. Diabetes Care 16(Suppl. 2):106, 1993.
232. Head, J., and Fuller, J. H.: International variations in mortality among diabetic patients: The WHO Multinational Study of Vascular Disease in Diabetics. Diabetologia 33:477, 1990.
233. Chen, Y. D., Swami, S., Skowronski, R., et al.: Differences in postprandial lipemia between patients with normal glucose tolerance and non-insulin-dependent diabetes mellitus. J. Clin. Endocrinol. Metab. 76:172, 1993.
234. Pyörälä, K., Laakso, M., and Uusitupa, M.: Diabetes and atherosclerosis: An epidemiologic view. Diabetes Metab. Rev. 3:463, 1987.
235. Reaven, G. M., and Chen, Y-D. I.: Role of insulin in regulation of lipoprotein metabolism in diabetes. Diabetes Metab. Rev. 4:639, 1988.
236. Haaber, A. B., Deckert, M., Stender, S., and Jensen, T.: Increased urinary loss of high density lipoproteins in albuminuric insulin-dependent diabetic patients. Scand. J. Clin. Lab. Invest. 53:191, 1993.
237. Witztum, J. L., Mahoney, E. M., Branks, M. J., et al.: Nonenzymatic glycosylation of low-density lipoprotein alters its biologic activity. Diabetes 31:283, 1982.
238. Lopes-Virella, M. F., Klein, R. L., Lyons, T. J., et al.: Glycosylation of low-density lipoprotein enhances cholesteryl ester synthesis in human monocyte-derived macrophages. Diabetes 37:550, 1988.
239. Duell, P. B., Oram, J. F., and Bierman, E. L.: Nonenzymatic glycosylation of HDL and impaired HDL-receptor–mediated cholesterol efflux. Diabetes 40:377, 1991.
240. Morel, D. W., and Chisolm, G. M.: Antioxidant treatment of diabetic rats inhibits lipoprotein oxidation and cytotoxicity. J. Lipid Res. 30:1827, 1989.
241. Haffner, S. M.: Lipoprotein(a) and diabetes: An update. Diabetes Care 16:835, 1993.
242. Colwell, J. A., Winocour, P. D., Lopes-Virella, M., and Halushka, P. V.: New concepts about the pathogenesis of atherosclerosis in diabetes mellitus. Am. J. Med. 75:67, 1983.
243. Juhan-Vague, I., Roul, C., Alessi, M., et al.: Increased plasminogen activator inhibitor activity in non insulin dependent diabetic patients: Relationship with plasma insulin. Thromb. Haemost. 61:370, 1989.
244. Bierman, E. L.: Atherogenesis in diabetes. Arterioscler. Thromb. 12:647, 1992.
245. Strowig, S., and Raskin, P.: Glycemic control and diabetic complications. Diabetes Care 15:1126, 1992.
246. Moss, S. E., Klein, R., Klein, B. E., and Meuer, S. M.: The association of glycemia and cause-specific mortality in a diabetic population. Arch. Intern. Med. 154:2473, 1994.
247. Diabetes Control and Complications Trial Research Group: The effect of intensive treatment of diabetes on the development and progression of long-term complications in insulin-dependent diabetes mellitus. N. Engl. J. Med. 329:977, 1993.
248. Pandit, M. K., Burke, J., Gustafson, A. B., et al.: Drug-induced disorders of glucose tolerance. Ann. Intern. Med. 118:529, 1993.
249. Lardinois, C. K., and Neuman, S. L.: The effects of antihypertensive agents on serum lipids and lipoproteins. Arch. Intern. Med. 148:1280, 1988.
250. Ruderman, N. B., and Schneider, S. H.: Diabetes, exercise and atherosclerosis. Diabetes Care 15:1787, 1992.

PHYSICAL INACTIVITY

251. Prevalence of sedentary lifestyle—Behavioral Risk Factor Surveillance System, United States, 1991. M. M. W. R. 42:576, 1993.
252. Powell, K. E., Thompson, P. D., Caspersen, C. J., et al.: Physical activity and the incidence of coronary heart disease. Annu. Rev. Public Health 8:253, 1987.
253. Berlin, J. A., and Colditz, G. A.: A meta-analysis of physical activity in the prevention of coronary heart disease. Am. J. Epidemiol. 132:612, 1990.
254. Leon, A. S., Connett, J., for the MRFIT Research Group: Physical activity and 10.5 year mortality in the Multiple Risk Factor Intervention Trial (MRFIT). Int. J. Epidemiol. 20:690, 1991.
255. Ekelund, L-G., Haskell, W. L., Johnson, J. L., et al.: Physical fitness as a predictor of cardiovascular mortality in asymptomatic North American men: The Lipid Research Clinics Mortality Follow-up Study. N. Engl. J. Med. 319:1379, 1988.
256. Sandvik, L., Erikssen, J., Thaulow, E., et al.: Physical fitness as a predictor of mortality among healthy, middle-aged Norwegian men. N. Engl. J. Med. 328:533, 1993.
257. Lakka, T. A., Venalainen, J. M., Rauramaa, R., et al.: Relation of leisure-time physical activity and cardiorespiratory fitness to the risk of acute myocardial infarction. N. Engl. J. Med. 330:1549, 1994.
258. Blair, S. N., Cooper, K. H., Gibbons, L. W., et al.: Changes in coronary heart disease risk factors associated with increased treadmill time in 753 men. Am. J. Epidemiol. 118:352, 1983.
259. Helmrich, S. P., Ragland, D. R., Leung, R. W., and Paffenbarger, R. S., Jr.: Physical activity and reduced occurrence of non-insulin-dependent diabetes mellitus. N. Engl. J. Med. 325:147, 1991.
260. Després, J-P., Pouliot, M-C., Moorjani, S., et al.: Loss of abdominal fat and metabolic response to exercise training in obese women. Am. J. Physiol. 261:E159, 1991.
261. Arroll, B., and Beaglehole, R.: Does physical activity lower blood pressure: A critical review of the clinical trials. J. Clin. Epidemiol. 45:439, 1992.
262. Fletcher, G. F., Blair, S. N., Blumenthal, J., et al.: Statement on exercise: Benefits and recommendations for physical activity programs for all Americans: A statement for health professionals by the Committee on Exercise and Cardiac Rehabilitation of the Council on Clinical Cardiology, American Heart Association. Circulation 86:340, 1992.
263. Wood, P. D., Stefanick, M. L., Williams, P. T., and Haskell, W. L.: The effects on plasma lipoproteins of a prudent weight-reducing diet, with or without exercise, in overweight men and women. N. Engl. J. Med. 325:461, 1991.
264. Paffenbarger, R. S., Jr., Hyde, R. T., Wing, A. L., et al.: The association of changes in physical-activity level and other lifestyle characteristics with mortality among men. N. Engl. J. Med. 328:538, 1993.
265. Pate, R. R., Pratt, M., Blair, S. N., et al.: Physical activity and public health: A recommendation from the Centers for Disease Control and Prevention and the American College of Sports Medicine. J. A. M. A. 273:402, 1995.
266. Levine, G. N., and Balady, G. J.: The benefits and risks of exercise training: The exercise prescription. Adv. Intern. Med. 38:57, 1993.

OBESITY

267. Kuczmarski, R. J., Flegal, K. M., Campbell, S. M., and Johnson, C. L.: Increasing prevalence of overweight among US adults: The National Health and Nutrition Examination Surveys, 1960 to 1991. J. A. M. A. 272:205, 1994.
268. Bjorntorp, P.: Obesity and adipose tissue distribution as risk factors for the development of disease—a review. Infusiontherapie 17:24, 1990.
269. Larsson, B., Bengtsson, C., Bjorntorp, P., et al.: Is abdominal body fat distribution a major explanation for the sex difference in the incidence of myocardial infarction? The study of men born in 1913 and the study of women. Am. J. Epidemiol. 135:266, 1992.
270. Freedman, D. S., Jacobsen, S. J., Barboriak, J. J., et al.: Body fat distribution and male/female differences in lipids and lipoproteins. Circulation 81:1498, 1990.
271. Hubert, H. B., Feinleib, M., McNamara, P. M., and Castelli, W. P.: Obesity as an independent risk factor for cardiovascular disease: A 26-year follow-up of participants in the Framingham Heart Study. Circulation 67:968, 1983.
272. Willett, W. C., Manson, J. A. E., Stampfer, M. J., et al.: Weight, weight change, and coronary heart disease in women: Risk within the 'normal' weight range. J. A. M. A. 273:461, 1995.
273. Denke, M. A., Sempos, C. T., and Grundy, S. M.: Excess body weight: An underrecognized contributor to high blood cholesterol levels in white American men. Arch. Intern. Med. 153:1093, 1993.
274. Garrison, R. J., Wilson, P. W., Castelli, W. P., et al.: Obesity and lipoprotein cholesterol in the Framingham Offspring Study. Metabolism 29:1053, 1980.

275. Berchtold, P., Jorgens, V., Finke, C., and Berger, M.: Epidemiology of obesity and hypertension. Int. J. Obes. 5(Suppl. 1):1, 1981.
276. Hartz, A. J., Rupley, D. C., Kalkhoff, R. D., and Rimm, A. A.: Relationship of obesity to diabetes: Influence of obesity level and body fat distribution. Prev. Med. 12:351, 1983.

NONMODIFIABLE RISK FACTORS

277. Shea, S., Ottman, R., Gabrieli, C., et al.: Family history as an independent risk factor for coronary artery disease. J. Am. Coll. Cardiol. 4:793, 1984.
278. Colditz, G. A., Rimm, E. B., Giovannucci, E., et al.: A prospective study of parental history of myocardial infarction and coronary artery disease in men. Am. J. Cardiol. 67:933, 1991.
279. Kaprio, J., Norio, R., Pesonen, E., and Sarna, S.: Intimal thickening of the coronary arteries in infants in relation to family history of coronary artery disease. Circulation 87:1960, 1993.
280. Slyper, A., and Schectman, G.: Coronary artery disease risk factors from a genetic and developmental perspective. Arch. Intern. Med. 154:633, 1994.
281. Rubin, S. M., Sidney, S., Black, D. M., et al.: High blood cholesterol in elderly men and the excess risk for coronary heart disease. Ann. Intern. Med. 113:916, 1990.
282. SHEP Cooperative Research Group: Prevention of stroke by antihypertensive drug treatment in older persons with isolated systolic hypertension: Final results of the Systolic Hypertension in the Elderly Program (SHEP). J. A. M. A. 265:3255, 1991.
283. Lerner, D. J., and Kannel, W. B.: Patterns of coronary heart disease morbidity and mortality in the sexes: A 26-year follow-up of the Framingham population. Am. Heart J. 111:383, 1986.
284. Brezinka, V., and Padmos, I.: Coronary heart disease risk factors in women. Eur. Heart J. 15:1571, 1994.
285. Kannel, W. B., and McGee, D. L.: Diabetes and glucose tolerance as risk factors for cardiovascular disease: The Framingham Study. Diabetes Care 2:120, 1979.
286. Castelli, W. P.: Epidemiology of triglycerides: A view from Framingham. Am. J. Cardiol. 70:3H, 1992.

OTHER RISK FACTORS

287. Iso, H., Folsom, A. R., Sato, S., et al.: Plasma fibrinogen and its correlates in Japanese and US population samples. Arterioscler. Thromb. 13:783, 1993.
288. Ernst, E.: Plasma fibrinogen—an independent cardiovascular risk factor. J. Intern. Med. 227:365, 1990.
289. Heinrich, J., Balleisen, L., Schulte, H., et al.: Fibrinogen and factor VII in the prediction of coronary risk: Results from the PROCAM study in healthy men. Arterioscler. Thromb. 14:54, 1994.
290. Yarnell, J. W. G., Baker, I. A., Sweetnam, P. M., et al.: Fibrinogen, viscosity, and white blood cell count are major risk factors for ischemic heart disease: The Caerphilly and Speedwell collaborative heart disease studies. Circulation 83:836, 1991.
291. Miller, G. J.: Hemostasis and cardiovascular risk: The British and European experience. Arch. Pathol. Lab. Med. 116:1318, 1992.
292. Miller, G. J.: Environmental influences on hemostasis and thrombosis: Diet and smoking. Ann. Epidemiol. 2:387, 1992.
293. Kelleher, C. C.: Plasma fibrinogen and factor VII as risk factors for cardiovascular disease. Eur. J. Epidemiol. 8(Suppl. 1):79, 1992.
294. Meade, T. W.: Hypercoagulability and ischaemic heart disease. Blood Rev. 1:2, 1987.
295. Meade, T. W., Ruddock, V., Stirling, Y., et al.: Fibrinolytic activity, clotting factors, and long-term incidence of ischaemic heart disease in the Northwick Park Heart Study. Lancet 342:1076, 1993.
296. Juhan-Vague, I., and Alessi, M. C.: Plasminogen activator inhibitor 1 and atherothrombosis. Thromb. Haemost. 70:138, 1993.
297. Hamsten, A., Wiman, B., de Faire, U., and Blomback, M.: Increased plasma levels of a rapid inhibitor of tissue plasminogen activator in young survivors of myocardial infarction. N. Engl. J. Med. 313:1557, 1985.
298. Juhan-Vague, I., Thompson, S. G., Jespersen, J., on behalf of the ECAT Angina Pectoris Study Group: Involvement of the hemostatic system in the insulin resistance syndrome: A study of 1500 patients with angina pectoris. Arterioscler. Thromb. 13:1865, 1993.
299. Hamsten, A., de Faire, U., Walldius, G., et al.: Plasminogen activator inhibitor in plasma: Risk factor for recurrent myocardial infarction. Lancet 2:3, 1987.
300. Schneiderman, J., Sawdey, M. S., Keeton, M. R., et al.: Increased type 1 plasminogen activator inhibitor gene expression in atherosclerotic human arteries. Proc. Natl. Acad. Sci. U. S. A. 89:6998, 1992.
301. Robinson, K., Mayer, E., and Jacobsen, D. W.: Homocysteine and coronary artery disease. Cleve. Clin. J. Med. 61:438, 1994.
301a. Mayer, E. L., Jacobsen, D. W., and Robinson, K.: Homocysteine and coronary atherosclerosis. J. Am. Coll. Cardiol. 27:517, 1996.
302. Clarke, R., Daly, L., Robinson, K., et al.: Hyperhomocysteinemia: An independent risk factor for vascular disease. N. Engl. J. Med. 324:1149, 1991.
303. Glueck, C. J., Shaw, P., Lang, J. E., et al.: Evidence that homocysteine is an independent risk factor for atherosclerosis in hyperlipidemic patients. Am. J. Cardiol. 75:132, 1995.
304. Stampfer, M. J., Malinow, M. R., Willett, W. C., et al.: A prospective study of plasma homocyst(e)ine and risk of myocardial infarction in US physicians. J. A. M. A. 268:877, 1992.
305. Rodgers, G. M., and Conn, M. T.: Homocysteine, an atherogenic stimulus, reduces protein C activation by arterial and venous endothelial cells. Blood 75:895, 1990.
306. Pohorecky, L. A.: Interaction of alcohol and stress at the cardiovascular level. Alcohol 7:537, 1990.
307. Gaziano, J. M., Buring, J. E., Breslow, J. L., et al.: Moderate alcohol intake, increased levels of high-density lipoprotein and its subfractions, and decreased risk of myocardial infarction. N. Engl. J. Med. 329:1829, 1993.
308. Langer, R. D., Criqui, M. H., and Reed, D. M.: Lipoproteins and blood pressure as biological pathways for effect of moderate alcohol consumption on coronary heart disease. Circulation 85:910, 1992.
309. Criqui, M. H., Cowan, L. D., Heiss, G., et al.: Frequency and clustering of non-lipid coronary risk factors in dyslipoproteinemia. Circulation 73:I-40, 1986.
310. Meade, T. W., Vickers, M. V., Thompson, S. G., et al.: Epidemiological characteristics of platelet aggregability. B. M. J. 290:428, 1985.
311. Laug, W. E.: Ethyl alcohol enhances plasminogen activator secretion by endothelial cells. J. A. M. A. 250:772, 1983.
312. Ridker, P. M., Vaughan, D. E., Stampfer, M. J., et al.: Association of moderate alcohol consumption and plasma concentration of endogenous tissue-type plasminogen activator. J. A. M. A. 272:929, 1994.
313. Renaud, S., and de Lorgeril, M.: Wine, alcohol, platelets, and the French paradox for coronary heart disease. Lancet 339:1523, 1992.
314. Frankel, E. N., Kanner, J., German, J. B., et al.: Inhibition of oxidation of human low-density lipoprotein by phenolic substances in red wine. Lancet 341:454, 1993.
315. Lachar, B. L.: Coronary-prone behavior: Type A behavior revisited. Tex. Heart Inst. J. 20:143, 1993.
316. Littman, A. B.: Review of psychosomatic aspects of cardiovascular disease. Psychother. Psychosom. 60:148, 1993.
317. Rosenman, R. H., Brand, R. J., Jenkins, C. D., et al.: Coronary heart disease in the Western Collaborative Group Study: Final follow-up experience of 8½ years. J. A. M. A. 233:872, 1975.
318. Eaker, E. D., Abbott, R. D., and Kannel, W. B.: Frequency of uncomplicated angina pectoris in type A compared with type B persons (the Framingham Study). Am. J. Cardiol. 63:1042, 1989.
319. Shekelle, R. B., Hulley, S. B., Neaton, J. D., et al.: The MRFIT Behavior Pattern Study. II. Type A behavior and incidence of coronary heart disease. Am. J. Epidemiol. 122:559, 1985.
320. Matthews, K. A., and Haynes, S. G.: Type A behavior pattern and coronary disease risk: Update and critical evaluation. Am. J. Epidemiol. 123:923, 1986.
321. O'Rourke, D. F., Houston, B. K., Harris, J. K., and Snyder, C. R.: The type A behavior pattern: Summary, conclusions, and implications. In Houston, B. K., and Snyder, C. R. (eds.): Type A Behavior Pattern. Research, Theory, and Intervention. New York, John Wiley and Sons, 1988, p. 312.
322. Williams, R. B., Jr.: Biological mechanisms mediating the relationship between behavior and coronary heart disease. In Siegman, A. W., and Dembroski, T. M. (eds.): In Search of Coronary-Prone Behavior. Beyond Type A. Hillsdale, N. J., Lawrence Erlbaum Associates, 1989, p. 195.
323. Siegman, A. W.: Cardiovascular consequences of expressing, experiencing, and repressing anger. J. Behav. Med. 16:539, 1993.
324. Boltwood, M. D., Taylor, C. B., Burke, M. B., et al.: Anger report predicts coronary artery vasomotor response to mental stress in atherosclerotic segments. Am. J. Cardiol. 72:1361, 1993.
325. Hoffman, R. M., and Garewal, H. S.: Antioxidants and the prevention of coronary heart disease. Arch. Intern. Med. 155:241, 1995.
326. Rimm, E. B., Stampfer, M. J., Ascherio, A., et al.: Vitamin E consumption and the risk of coronary heart disease in men. N. Engl. J. Med. 328:1450, 1993.
327. Stampfer, M. J., Hennekens, C. H., Manson, J. E., et al.: Vitamin E consumption and the risk of coronary disease in women. N. Engl. J. Med. 328:1444, 1993.
328. Morris, D. L., Kritchevsky, S. B., and Davis, C. E.: Serum carotenoids and coronary heart disease: The Lipid Research Clinics Coronary Primary Prevention Trial and Follow-up Study. J. A. M. A. 272:1439, 1994.
329. Hodis, H. N., Mack, W. J., LaBree, L., et al.: Serial coronary angiographic evidence that antioxidant vitamin intake reduces progression of coronary artery atherosclerosis. J. A. M. A. 273:1849, 1995.
330. Puurunen, M., Mänttäri, M., Manninen, V., et al.: Antibody against oxidized low-density lipoprotein predicting myocardial infarction. Arch. Intern. Med. 154:2605, 1994.
331. Alpha-Tocopherol, Beta Carotene Cancer Prevention Study Group: The effect of vitamin E and beta carotene on the incidence of lung cancer and other cancers in male smokers. N. Engl. J. Med. 330:1029, 1994.
332. Steinberg, D.: Antioxidant vitamins and coronary heart disease (editorial). N. Engl. J. Med. 328:1487, 1993.

Chapter 36
Coronary Blood Flow and Myocardial Ischemia

Peter Ganz, Eugene Braunwald

HYPOXIA AND ISCHEMIA

Definitions

Hypoxia is the condition in which oxygen supply is reduced despite adequate perfusion; *anoxia* is the absence of oxygen supply despite adequate perfusion. These conditions should be distinguished from *ischemia,* in which oxygen deprivation is accompanied by inadequate removal of metabolites consequent to reduced perfusion. Although clinical manifestations of coronary insufficiency generally reflect the effects of ischemia, under selected experimental and clinical conditions, deprivation of oxygen can be separated from reduced washout of metabolites.[1] For example, cyanotic congenital heart disease, cor pulmonale, severe anemia, asphyxiation, and carbon monoxide poisoning are characterized by anoxia without ischemia because washout of metabolites is not hindered.

During ischemia an imbalance occurs between myocardial oxygen supply and demand (Fig. 36–1). Ischemia may be manifest as anginal discomfort, deviation of the ST segment on the electrocardiogram, reduced uptake of thallium-201 in myocardial perfusion images, or regional or global impairment of ventricular function. In the presence of coronary obstruction, an increase of myocardial oxygen requirements by exercise, tachycardia, or emotion leads to a transitory imbalance. This condition is frequently termed "demand ischemia" and is responsible for most episodes of chronic stable angina. In other situations the imbalance is caused by a reduction of oxygen supply secondary to increased coronary vascular tone or by platelet aggregates or thrombi; this condition, termed "supply ischemia," is responsible for myocardial infarction and most episodes of unstable angina. In many circumstances, ischemia results from both an increase in oxygen demand and a reduction in supply.

In this chapter we consider first the determinants of myocardial oxygen consumption, then the control of coronary blood flow, and finally, the hemodynamic and biochemical consequences of ischemia.

DETERMINANTS OF MYOCARDIAL OXYGEN CONSUMPTION

The heart is an aerobic organ; that is, it relies almost exclusively on the oxidation of substrates for the generation of energy, and it can develop only a small oxygen debt. Therefore, in a steady state, determination of the rate of myocardial oxygen consumption (MVO_2) provides an accurate measure of its total metabolism.[2] It has been known for many years that the total metabolism of the arrested, quiescent heart is only a small fraction of that of the working organ. The MVO_2 of the beating canine heart ranges from 8 to 15 ml/min/100 gm, whereas the MVO_2 of the noncontracting heart is approximately 1.5 ml/min/100 gm. The latter is required for those physiological processes not directly associated with contraction. Increases in the frequency of depolarization of the noncontracting heart are accompanied by only small increases of MVO_2[2-4] (Tables 36–1 and 36–2).

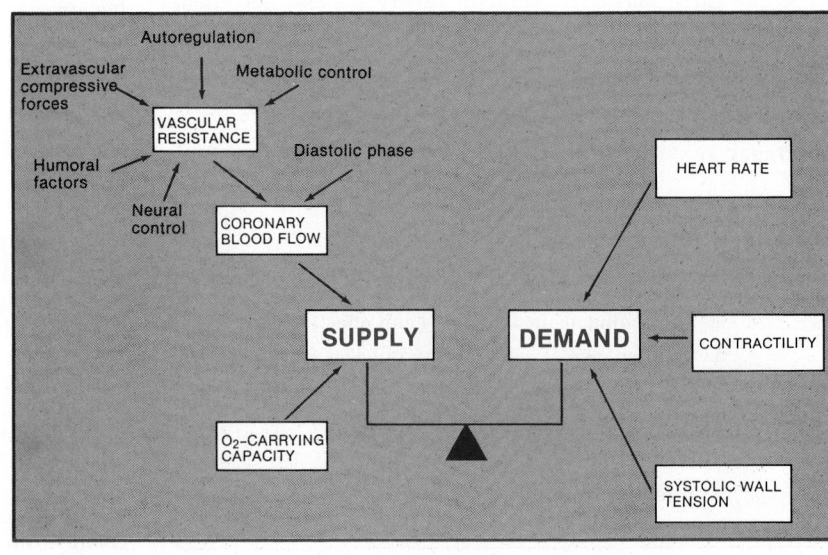

FIGURE 36–1. Factors influencing myocardial oxygen supply and demand. (From Ardehali, A., and Ports, T. A.: Myocardial oxygen supply and demand. Chest *98:*699, 1990.)

TABLE 36–1   MYOCARDIAL O₂ CONSUMPTION COMPONENTS

TOTAL: 6–8 cc/min/100 gm			
DISTRIBUTION			
Basal	20%	Volume work	15%
Electrical	1%	Pressure work	64%
EFFECTS ON MVO₂ of 50% INCREASES IN			
Wall stress	25%	Heart rate	50%
Contractility	45%	Volume work	4%
Pressure work	50%		

The table demonstrates the dominant contribution to MVO₂ made by pressure work and prominent effects of increasing pressure work and heart rate on MVO₂.

From Gould, K. L.: Coronary Artery Stenosis, New York, Elsevier, 1991, p. 8.

MYOCARDIAL TENSION. As early as 1915 Evans and Matsuoka concluded from studies of the Starling heart-lung preparation that "there is a relation between the tension set up on contraction and the metabolism of the contractile tissue."[5] In a systematic investigation of the relative effects of ventricular pressure, stroke volume, and heart rate on MVO₂, it was found that ventricular pressure development is a key determinant of MVO₂. These investigations suggested that MVO₂ per beat correlates well with the area under the left ventricular pressure curve, termed the "tension-time index." Subsequently, it was emphasized that the myocardial wall tension time integral is a more definitive determinant of MVO₂ than is the developed pressure.[6,7] Later studies demonstrated that frequency of contraction is an important determinant as well. An augmentation of heart rate elevates the MVO₂ by increasing the frequency of tension development per unit of time, as well as by increasing contractility.[6,8]

Rooke and Feigl have provided evidence that MVO₂ is influenced by stroke volume—that is, myocardial shortening—although less so than by tension development.[9] They have also provided an experimental basis for the use of the systolic pressure-rate product (plus an estimate of the oxygen requirements of the noncontracting heart) as a clinically useful index of MVO₂. Reexamination of the determinants of MVO₂ has emphasized that they correlate closely with the left ventricular systolic pressure volume area,[10,11] which consists of the sum of the area within the systolic pressure-volume loop (see Fig. 14-14, p. 431), that is, the external mechanical work and the end-systolic elastic potential energy in the ventricular wall, the area enclosed by the systolic pressure-volume trajectory and the E_{max} line (Fig. 36-2).[10a,11]

MYOCARDIAL CONTRACTILITY. In addition to the systolic pressure-volume area and heart rate, myocardial contractility is the third major determinant of MVO₂. The net effect of positive inotropic stimuli (such as Ca⁺⁺ and catecholamines) on MVO₂ is the end result of their influence on two of its major determinants that change in opposite di-

TABLE 36–2   DETERMINANTS OF MYOCARDIAL OXYGEN CONSUMPTION

1. Tension development
2. Contractile state
3. Heart rate
4. Shortening against a load (Fenn effect)
5. Maintenance of cell viability in basal state
6. Depolarization
7. Activation
8. Maintenance of active state
9. Direct metabolic effect of catecholamines
10. Fatty acid uptake

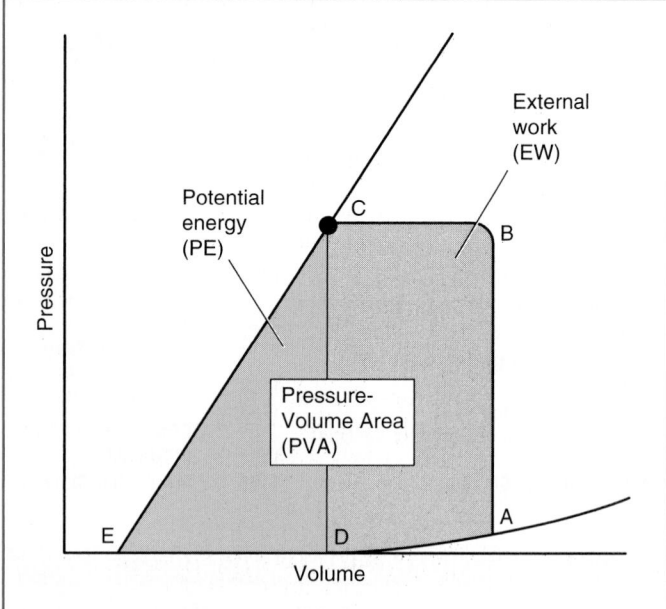

FIGURE 36–2. Myocardial oxygen consumption correlates with the left ventricular pressure–volume area (PVA). PVA is the area in the P-V diagram that is circumscribed by the end-systolic P-V line (E-C), the end-diastolic P-V relation curve (D-A), and the systolic segment of P-V trajectory (E-A-B-C-E). PVA consists of the external work (EW) performed during systole and the end-systolic elastic potential energy (PE) stored in the ventricular wall at end-systole. EW is the area within the P-V loop trajectory (A-B-C-D-A), and PE is the area between end-systolic P-V line and end-diastolic P-V relation curve to the left of EW (E-C-D-E). (Reproduced with permission from Kameyama, T., et al.: Energy conversion efficiency in human left ventricle. Circulation 85:988, 1992. Copyright American Heart Association.)

rections in the intact heart.[2] These are wall tension, which declines as a consequence of reduction in heart size, and myocardial contractility, which, by definition, is augmented by inotropic stimuli. In the failing, dilated ventricle, the increased contractility reduces the left ventricular end-diastolic pressure and volume. On the basis of the Laplace relation, the reduction in ventricular volume leads to a reduction in myocardial tension, which reduces MVO₂. However, the decrease in MVO₂ that might be expected to result from falling ventricular wall tension is opposed by the increase in contractility, which tends to augment MVO₂. Thus, the change in MVO₂ consequent to an inotropic stimulus depends on the extent to which intramyocardial tension is reduced in relation to the extent to which contractility is augmented. In the absence of heart failure, drugs that stimulate myocardial contractility elevate MVO₂ because heart size and therefore wall tension are not reduced substantially and do not offset the effect on metabolism of the simulation of contractility.

It has been suggested by Suga that almost the entire increase in MVO₂ produced by the administration of positive inotropic agents such as Ca⁺⁺ and epinephrine results from the energy costs of enhanced excitation-contraction coupling.[10] Specifically, the increased energy costs result from the greater and more rapid Ca⁺⁺ uptake by the sarcoplasmic reticulum as well as from the increased contractile activity, rather than from a direct stimulating effect of positive inotropic agents on basal myocardial metabolism. In experiments in which the relative effects of changes in tension development and in myocardial contractility on MVO₂ were assessed in the same heart, the quantitative effects of MVO₂ of changes in contractility and tension development were found to be both substantial and of the same order of magnitude.[12]

MVO₂ is also influenced by the substrate utilized. Specifically, it correlates directly with the fraction of energy derived from the metabolism of fatty acids, which in turn varies directly with the arterial concentration of fatty acids and inversely with that of glucose and insulin.[13]

REGULATION OF CORONARY BLOOD FLOW

During diastole, when the aortic valve is closed, aortic diastolic pressure is transmitted without impediment through the dilated sinuses of Valsalva to the coronary ostia. The aortic arch and sinuses then act as a miniature reservoir, facilitating maintenance of relatively uniform coronary inflow through diastole. The major coronary arteries and their principal branches course across the epicardial surface of the heart. They serve as conductance vessels and normally offer little resistance to coronary blood flow. The epicardial conductance vessels can constrict in response to alpha-adrenergic stimuli and dilate to nitroglycerin.[14] These vessels give rise to smaller penetrating vessels approximately at right angles (see Fig. 36–13, p. 1169). A large pressure drop occurs in these intramural vessels and in the coronary arterioles—hence their designation as "resistance vessels." The dense network of about 4000 capillaries per square millimeter is not uniformly patent because precapillary sphincters appear to serve a regulatory function[15] in accordance with the flow needs of the myocardium. This capillary density is reduced in the presence of ventricular hypertrophy.

As in any vascular bed, blood flow in the coronary bed depends on the driving pressure and the resistance offered by this bed. Coronary vascular resistance, in turn, is regulated by several control mechanisms that will be reviewed: myocardial metabolism (metabolic control), endothelial (and other humoral) control, autoregulation, myogenic control, extravascular compressive forces, and neural control. These individual control mechanisms may be impaired in a variety of conditions and contribute to the development of myocardial ischemia.

Metabolic Regulation

RELATIONSHIP BETWEEN CORONARY BLOOD FLOW AND MYOCARDIAL OXYGEN CONSUMPTION. Coronary blood flow is closely coupled to MVO_2 in normal hearts.[8,16] This linkage is necessary because the myocardium depends almost completely on aerobic metabolism. The oxygen content of coronary venous blood is low, permitting little additional oxygen extraction (baseline coronary venous oxygen saturation is 25 to 30 per cent), and oxygen stores in the heart are sparse.

Changes in myocardial oxygen balance lead to alterations in coronary vascular resistance with great rapidity, generally in less than 1 second. For example, occlusion of a coronary artery for less than 1 second produces an increase in coronary blood flow above baseline immediately following release of the occlusion.[17–19] This response is called coronary reactive hyperemia. In the dog, peak flow response follows coronary occlusion of 15 to 20 seconds.[20] The mechanisms that link metabolic activity and coronary vascular resistance have been extensively investigated. Investigations have focused on adenosine, other nucleotides, nitric oxide, prostaglandins, CO_2, and H^+ as the most likely potential mediators.

ADENOSINE. Degradation of adenine nucleotides under conditions in which ATP utilization exceeds the capacity of myocardial cells to resynthesize high-energy phosphate compounds (a process dependent on oxidative phosphorylation in mitochondria) results in the production of adenosine monophosphate (AMP). The enzyme 5'-nucleotidase is responsible for the formation of adenosine from AMP.[21] Accordingly, adenosine and its metabolites, inosine and hypoxanthine, appear in interstitial fluid and in the coronary sinus venous effluent. Adenosine is a powerful vasodilator that is considered to be an important, perhaps the

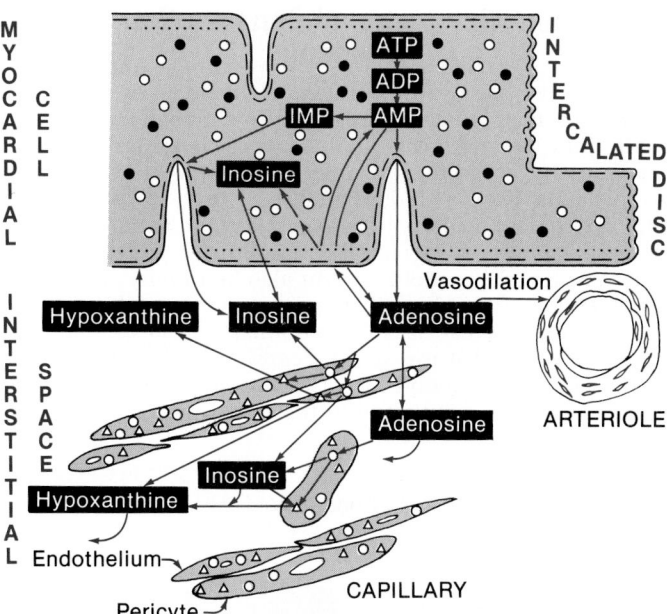

FIGURE 36–3. Schematic drawing depicting a myocardial interstitial space, an arteriole, and a capillary with the localization of enzymes involved in the formation and fate of adenosine. Adenosine formed by 5'-nucleotidase from AMP (which in turn arises from ATP) can enter the interstitial space. There it can induce arteriolar dilation and reenter the myocardial cell, where it is either phosphorylated to AMP by adenosine kinase or deaminated to inosine by adenosine deaminase, or it can enter the capillaries and leave the tissue. A large fraction of adenosine that crosses the capillary wall is deaminated to inosine, which in turn is split to hypoxanthine and ribose-1-PO_4 by nucleoside phosphorylase located in the endothelial cells, pericytes, and erythrocytes. Most of the adenosine is taken up by the myocardial cells, and that escaping into the circulation is largely in the form of inosine and hypoxanthine. Since adenylic acid deaminase (which deaminates AMP to IMP) is in low concentration in heart muscle, the major degradative pathway from AMP is via dephosphorylation to adenosine. ○, Adenosine deaminase; ●, adenylic acid deaminase; △, nucleoside phosphorylase; (---), 5'-nucleotidase; (···), adenosine kinase. (From Berne, R. M., and Rubio, R.: Coronary circulation. In Berne, R. M., Sperelakis, N., and Geiger, S. R. [eds.]: Handbook of Physiology, Section 2. The Cardiovascular System. Bethesda, Md., American Physiological Society, 1979, p. 924.)

critical, mediator linking metabolically induced vasodilation to diminished coronary perfusion[22] (Fig. 36–3). Its production increases at times of an imbalance in the supply-to-demand ratio for oxygen,[23] and the rise in the interstitial concentration of adenosine parallels the increase in coronary blood flow.[24]

Many investigators believe that adenosine fulfills most of the criteria for the metabolic regulation of blood flow.[22] Thus, it has been demonstrated that adenosine plays a significant role in the regulation of coronary blood flow during reactive hyperemia, hypoxia, inotropic stimulation with isoproterenol, dobutamine, and mental stress.[25–29] On the other hand, it has been reported that adenosine plays no significant role in the coronary vasodilation associated with inotropic stimulation with norepinephrine or the metabolic stress induced by rapid atrial pacing.[30,31] Thus, despite its acknowledged importance, adenosine is almost certainly not the *only* vasoactive factor involved in the metabolic regulation of coronary blood flow. Others include nitric oxide (see below) and prostanoids.

It is likely that vasoactive factors act in concert to regulate coronary flow in response to metabolic needs. Thus the reactive hyperemia following 10 to 20 seconds of occlusion can be reduced by approximately 30 per cent each by inhibitors of adenosine and nitric oxide. Simultaneous administration of these inhibitors attenuates reactive hyperemia by nearly 60 per cent.[32]

Endothelial Control of Coronary Vascular Tone

Vasoactive agents that influence the tone of large and small coronary vessels can arise from outside the vessel wall; they can circulate in the blood (e.g., epinephrine, vasopressin) or be derived from circulating elements such as platelets (e.g., serotonin, ADP) or from nerve endings (e.g., norepinephrine, vasoactive intestinal peptide). Vasoactive factors such as endothelium-derived relaxing factor, prostacyclin, and endothelin can also be formed in the vascular endothelium. Endothelium-derived vasoactive factors are of great interest because endothelium can be damaged by a variety of diseases and by cardiovascular risk factors. Endothelial dysfunction may lead to disturbances in coronary blood flow, contribute to the pathogenesis of myocar-

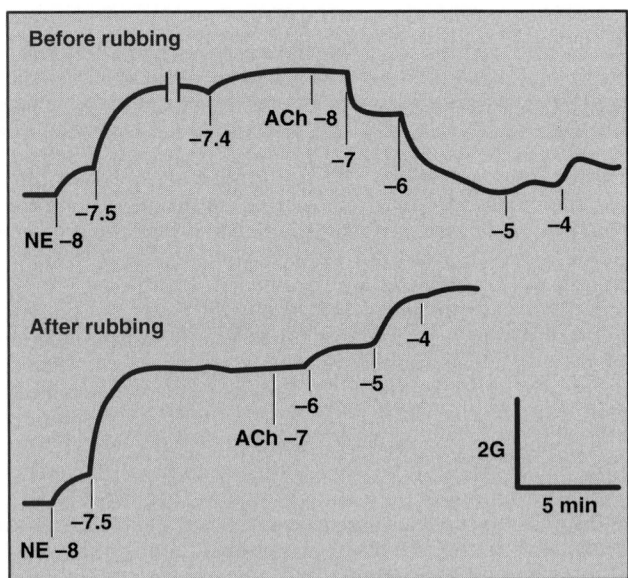

FIGURE 36-5. Relaxation by acetylcholine (ACh) of rings of rabbit thoracic aorta precontracted by norepinephrine (NE). Aortic rings were exposed to increasing concentrations of ACh with endothelium either intact or removed by rubbing with a wooden applicator stick. This representative tracing shows loss of relaxation in response to ACh with removal of endothelium and appearance of mild constriction. (Reproduced with permission from Furchgott, R. F.: Role of endothelium in responses of vascular smooth muscle. Circ. Res. 53:557, 1983. Copyright American Heart Association.)

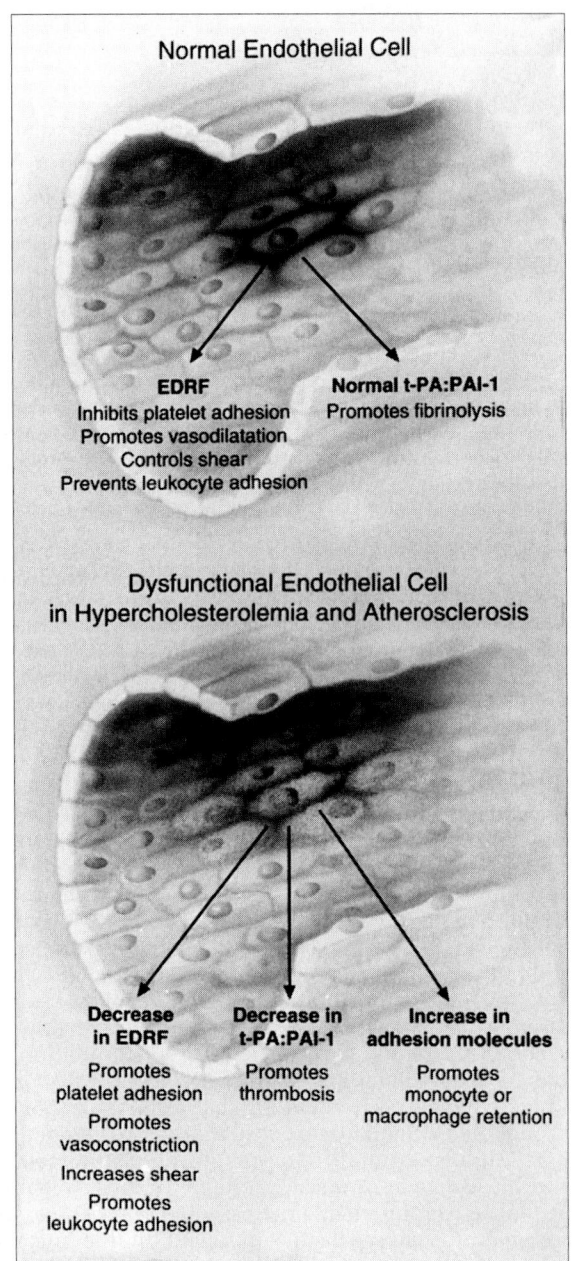

FIGURE 36-4. Normal and dysfunctional endothelial cells, with some of the functions adversely influenced by hypercholesterolemia and atherosclerosis that may contribute to acute coronary syndromes. The abbreviation t-PA:PAI-1 denotes the ratio of tissue plasminogen activator to plasminogen-activator inhibitor type 1. EDRF = endothelial derived relaxing factor. (From Levine, G. N., Keaney, J. F., and Vita, J. A.: Cholesterol reduction in cardiovascular disease. N. Engl. J. Med. 332:312, 1995. Copyright Massachusetts Medical Society.)

dial ischemia, and is a central feature in the evolution of atherosclerosis, thrombosis, inflammation, and atherogenesis[32a] (Fig. 36-4).

ENDOTHELIUM-DERIVED RELAXING FACTOR. The endothelium synthesizes several powerful vasodilators, including endothelium-derived relaxing factor (EDRF),[33] prostacyclin,[34] and endothelium-derived hyperpolarizing factor.[35] The discovery of these substances has changed the view that the vascular endothelium is simply an inert nonthrombogenic barrier separating the blood from the vascular smooth muscle.

The discovery of EDRF by Furchgott and Zawadzki[33] resulted from the observation that intact endothelium is a prerequisite for acetylcholine-induced vasodilation. In the presence of endothelium, acetylcholine produces dose-dependent vasodilation. When the endothelium is removed, only constriction is induced by acetylcholine (Fig. 36-5). It became apparent that acetylcholine has two distinct and opposite actions on blood vessels: a direct vasoconstrictor action and an indirect vasodilator action that is mediated by endothelium. In any blood vessel, the net response is related to the sum of these two actions. In most normal arteries, endothelium-dependent vasodilation predominates over direct vasoconstriction.

EDRF has been identified to be the nitric oxide (NO) radical[36,37] or a sulfhydryl complex containing it.[38] Nitric oxide is synthesized from the amino acid L-arginine[39] by the actions of the enzyme nitric oxide synthase.[40] Aside from acetylcholine, the release of nitric oxide is stimulated by aggregating platelets (serotonin, ADP), thrombin, the products of mast cells (histamine), and increased shear stress resulting from an increase in blood flow; the latter is responsible for so-called flow-mediated vasodilation[41] (Fig. 36-6). Vasoconstrictors such as alpha-adrenergic agonists may also stimulate the release of EDRF.[42] Although their net effect on the blood vessel may be vasoconstriction, the presence of an endothelium-dependent vasodilating influence attenuates this action. Only a few vasodilators can act independently of the endothelium and directly on vascular smooth muscle. These include the nitrovasodilators (e.g., nitroglycerin, nitroprusside), prostacyclin, and adenosine.

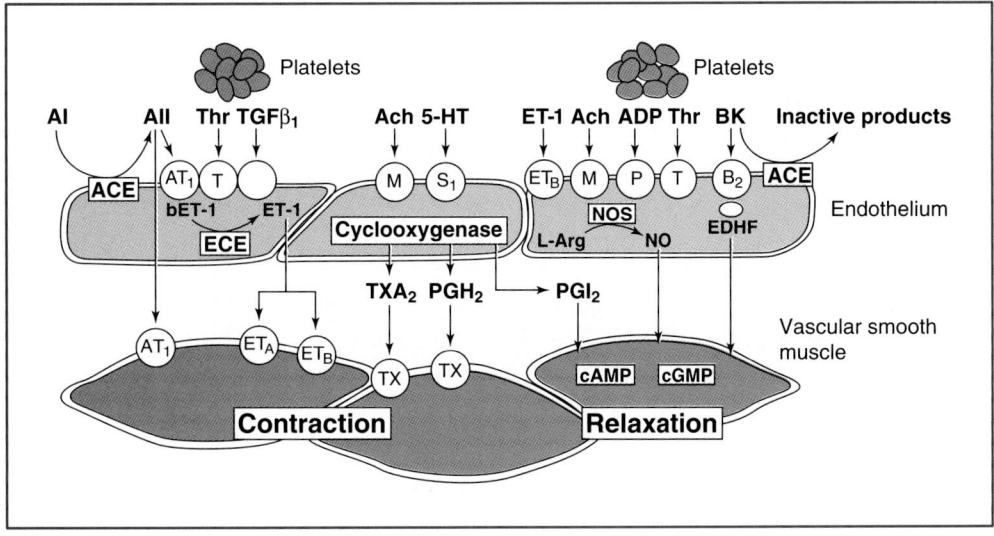

FIGURE 36–6. Endothelium-derived vasoactive substances. The endothelium is a source of relaxing (see bottom right) and contracting (see bottom left) factors. ACE = angiotensin converting enzyme; Ach = acetylcholine; ADP = adenosine diphosphate; BK = bradykinin; cAMP/cGMP = cyclic adenosine/guanosine monophosphate; ECE = endothelin converting enzymes; EDHF = endothelium-derived hyperpolarizing factor; ET-1 = endothelin-1; 5HT = 5-hydroxytryptamine (serotonin); L-arg = L-arginine; NO = nitric oxide; PGH$_2$ = prostaglandin H$_2$; PGI$_2$ = prostacyclin; TGFβ_1 = transforming growth factor β_1; Thr = thrombin; TXA$_2$ = thromboxane A$_2$; Circles represent receptors (AT = angiotensinergic; B = bradykinergic; M = muscarinic; P = purinergic; T = thrombin receptor). (From Lüscher, T. F., and Noll, G.: The endothelium in coronary vascular control. *In* Braunwald, E. (ed.): Heart Disease—Update 3. Philadelphia, W.B. Saunders Company, 1995, p. 2.)

ENDOTHELIUM-DEPENDENT VASODILATION IN EPICARDIAL ARTERIES.

The importance of endothelium-dependent vasodilation to vascular control has been established in many species and most vascular beds tested.[43–45] Intracoronary administration of acetylcholine, an endothelium-dependent agonist, has been shown to dilate normal coronary arteries in humans[46] (Fig. 36–7). Compelling evidence indicates that this is mediated by nitric oxide; inhibitors of nitric oxide such as N^G-monomethyl-L-arginine, hemoglobin and methylene blue abolish vasodilation and may even convert the vasodilator response to acetylcholine to vasoconstriction.[47,47a] Other substances that have been shown to dilate healthy human coronary arteries and increase blood flow by acting on the endothelium to release EDRF include serotonin, histamine, and substance P.[48–51]

One of the functions of the normal endothelium is to synthesize and release EDRF. It has been suggested that the tendency to vasoconstriction that characterizes atherosclerosis may be related to vasodilator dysfunction of the endothelium, resulting in the unopposed stimulation of vascular smooth muscle. Augmented vasoconstrictor responses resulting from an impairment of endothelium-dependent relaxation have been demonstrated in experimental models of atherosclerosis in several species.[52,53] Responses to endothelium-dependent stimuli that dilate healthy human coronary arteries have been found to be markedly impaired in patients with both early and advanced atherosclerosis. Acetylcholine constricts atherosclerotic coronary arteries,[46,54,55] presumably reflecting the loss of EDRF and acetylcholine's unopposed direct constrictor effects on vascular smooth muscle (Fig. 36–7). Although the role of acetylcholine in the physiological regulation of vascular tone has not been established, abnormal vasomotor responses to acetylcholine have served as convenient functional markers of endothelial dysfunction in atherosclerosis. This demonstration of endothelial vasodilator dysfunction has been confirmed using other stimuli that release EDRF, including serotonin,[48,56] ADP, and increased coronary blood flow (flow-mediated dilation).[50,57] For example, whereas serotonin, which is released by aggregating platelets, dilates normal human coronary arteries, it constricts atherosclerotic arteries.[48]

ENDOTHELIUM-DEPENDENT VASODILATION IN CORONARY RESISTANCE VESSELS.

Endothelium-dependent vasodilation operates not only in large (conductance) arteries, but it is also an important mechanism that controls resistance in small vessels.[58–62] Studies in the human forearm have suggested that *continuous* basal release of nitric oxide is an important determinant of resting vascular resistance.[60] When a specific inhibitor of nitric oxide synthesis was infused into the forearm, resting flow was reduced by half.

Atherosclerosis and hypercholesterolemia markedly im-

FIGURE 36–7. Responses of coronary arteries to intracoronary administration of an endothelium-dependent vasodilator (acetylcholine) and a direct smooth muscle vasodilator (nitroglycerin) in patients with atherosclerotic coronary arteries *(A)* and normal coronary arteries *(B)*. Atherosclerotic arteries exhibit a paradoxical constrictor response to acetylcholine with a preserved dilator response to nitroglycerin. C1 denotes control, C2 vehicle control, Ach$_{max}$ response to maximal dose of acetylcholine, C3 repeated control, and TNG nitroglycerin. Asterisks indicate that $P < 0.01$ for the comparison with C1. (Reprinted with permission from Ludmer, P. L., Selwyn, A. P., Shook, T. L., et al.: Paradoxical vasoconstriction induced by acetylcholine in atherosclerotic coronary arteries. N. Engl. J. Med. *315:*1046, 1986. Copyright Massachusetts Medical Society.)

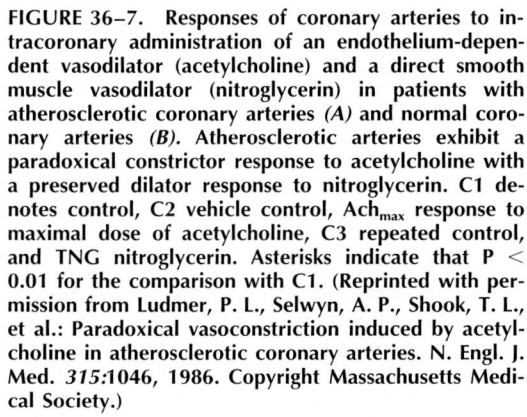

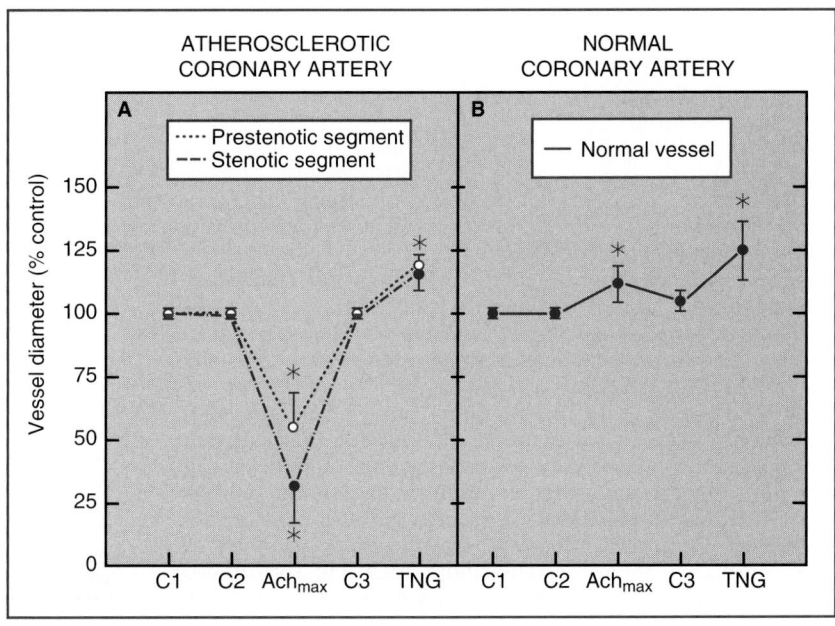

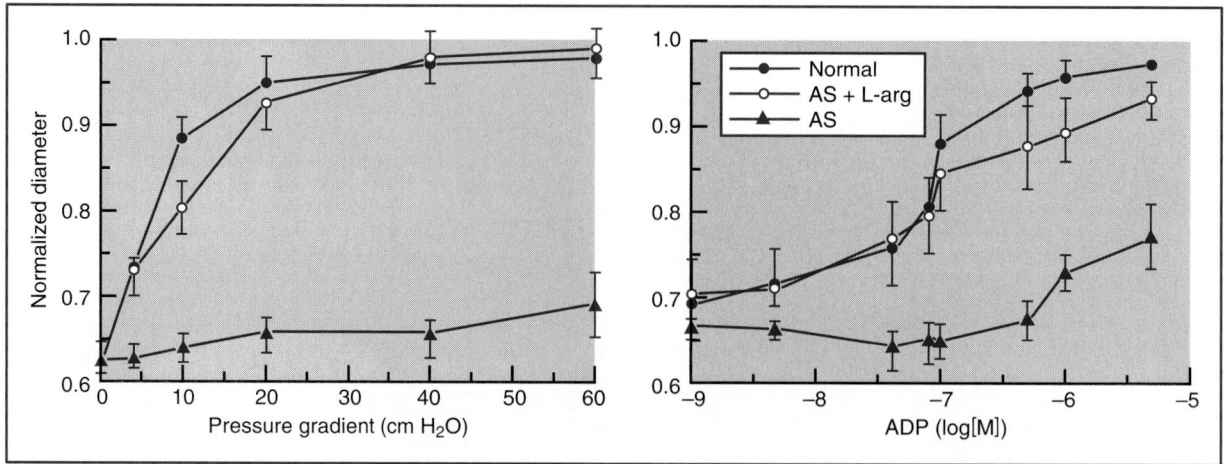

FIGURE 36–8. The effects of atherosclerosis on flow-dependent and pharmacological vasodilatation (adenosine diphosphate, ADP) in coronary arterioles. Pressure gradient (left) is proportional to blood flow. In vessels from normal control animals, both flow and ADP produced vasodilatation, whereas in atherosclerotic animals, this response was absent. Administration of L-arginine restored the responses in the atherosclerotic animals. (Reproduced with permission from Jones, C. J. H., Kuo, L., Davis, M. J., and Chilian, W. M.: Regulation of coronary blood flow: Coordination of heterogeneous control mechanisms in vascular microdomains. Cardiovasc. Res. 29:585, 1995. Adapted from Kuo, L., et al.: Pathophysiological consequences of atherosclerosis extend into the coronary microcirculation. Restoration of endothelium-dependent responses by L-arginine. Circ. Res. 70:465, 1992. Copyright American Heart Association.)

pair the responses of resistance vessels to endothelium-dependent vasodilators[61,63,64] (Fig. 36–8). The close correlation between the extent of endothelial dysfunction in resistance vessels and the failure of coronary blood flow to respond appropriately to metabolic stimuli suggests that endothelial dysfunction in resistance vessels may be an important factor in preventing coronary blood flow from rising appropriately during times of increased metabolic stress.[64a] An inappropriate increase in the tone of resistance vessels in the presence of an increase in metabolic demand may represent one of the mechanisms by which disturbances in endothelial function can lead to the development of myocardial ischemia in atherosclerosis.

ENDOTHELIAL DYSFUNCTION AND MYOCARDIAL ISCHEMIA. Several studies have demonstrated that reduced endothelium-dependent relaxation may play a role in the pathogenesis of myocardial ischemia in patients with stable angina. In such patients, mental stress caused dilation of the arteries with normal endothelium (evidenced by a normal response to acetylcholine) but constriction of vessels with evidence of endothelial dysfunction.[65] A similar pattern of dilation of normal coronary arteries and paradoxical constriction of atherosclerotic coronary arteries with dysfunctional endothelium has been observed with exercise,[66] the cold pressor test,[55] and an increase in heart rate.[67] These stimuli are normally accompanied by activation of the sympathetic nervous system, by an increase in circulating catecholamines, and by increases in coronary blood flow secondary to a rise in myocardial oxygen demand.[68] In patients with dysfunctional endothelium, the loss of flow-mediated[50,55,57] and catecholamine-stimulated EDRF release[69,70] allows the constrictor effects of catecholamines to act unopposed. Thus, the loss of EDRF may contribute to impaired dilator responses of epicardial and resistance vessel and thereby to myocardial ischemia.[68,71]

Plaque fissuring with superimposed platelet aggregation and occlusive thrombus formation is a hallmark of unstable angina,[72,72a] but coronary constriction also plays an important pathogenetic role in this condition[71,73] (see p. 1333). Endothelial vasodilator dysfunction has been implicated in the pathogenesis of coronary constriction, which is triggered by thrombosis and the products of platelet aggregation. As already mentioned, intracoronary administration of serotonin, a product released by aggregating platelets, dilates normal coronary arteries but constricts the atherosclerotic arteries of patients with coronary disease.[48] The

clinical significance of these findings is supported by the observations that patients with unstable coronary syndromes and complex plaques demonstrate augmented release of serotonin into the coronary circulation[74] and that aspirin is an effective agent in the treatment of this condition.

Patients with a recent history of myocardial infarction show evidence of endothelial vasodilator dysfunction in the infarct-related artery which is more pronounced than in patients with stable stenoses of similar severity. Available evidence suggests that endothelium damaged by the atherosclerotic process and by plaque fissuring contributes to coronary constriction in response to a variety of substances that would normally elicit vasodilation.

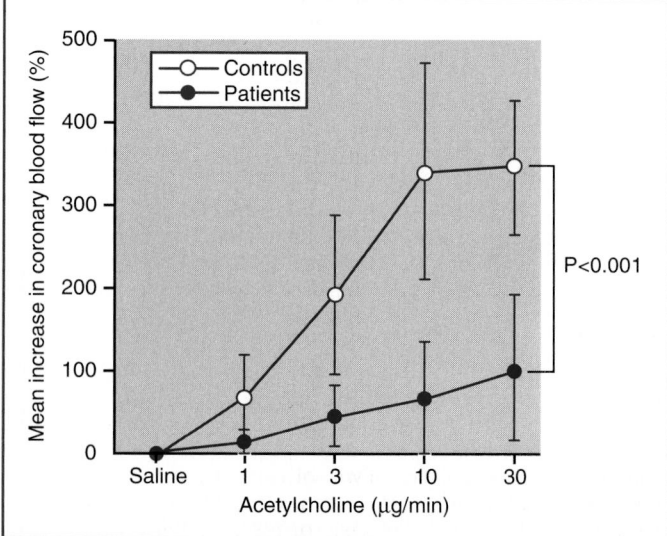

FIGURE 36–9. Increase in coronary blood flow evoked by graded doses of acetylcholine in control subjects and patients with microvascular angina. The dose-dependent increases in coronary blood flow produced by acetylcholine were significantly smaller in patients with microvascular angina than in control subjects ($P < 0.001$ by two-way analysis of variance). Bars indicate the standard deviation. (From Egashira, K., et al.: Evidence of impaired endothelium-dependent coronary vasodilatation in patients with angina pectoris and normal coronary angiograms. N. Engl. J. Med. 328:1659, 1993. Copyright Massachusetts Medical Society.)

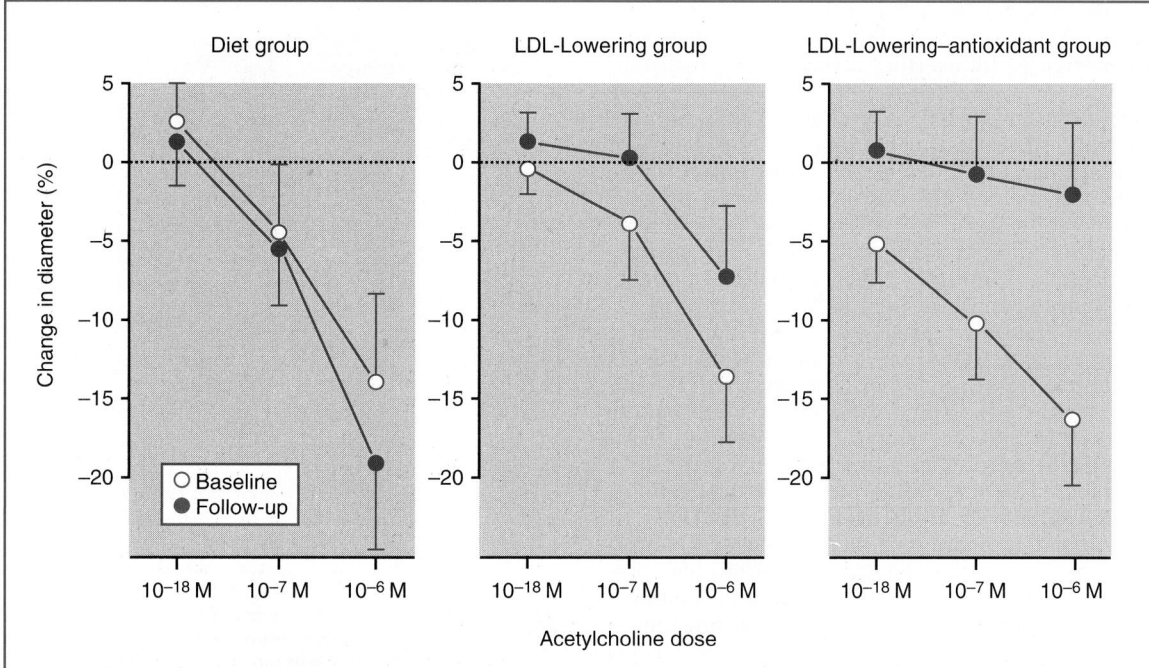

FIGURE 36–10. Mean (± SE) change in coronary artery diameter in response to serial infusions of acetylcholine at baseline and after 1 year of therapy in the three study groups. The improvement in the response from baseline to follow-up in the LDL-lowering–antioxidant group was significantly greater than that in the diet group (*P* > 0.05). Negative numbers indicate vasoconstriction. (From Anderson, T. J., et al.: The effect of cholesterol-lowering and antioxidant therapy on endothelium-dependent coronary vasomotion. N. Engl. J. Med. *332*:488, 1995. Copyright Massachusetts Medical Society.)

Endothelial dysfunction may involve the coronary resistance vessels in the *absence* of obstructive epicardial artery disease.[67,75] Impaired endothelium-dependent dilation of coronary resistance vessels has been demonstrated in patients with syndrome X, that is, anginal discomfort, evidence of myocardial ischemia on exercise testing, and angiographically normal coronary arteries (see p. 1343)[77–79] (Fig. 36–9). Impairment of endothelium-dependent vasodilation has also been observed in patients with coronary risk factors but without angiographic evidence of coronary artery disease. Lipid abnormalities, smoking, hypertension, and advanced age all may be associated with endothelial dysfunction.[68,80–81a]

Management. The use of cholesterol-lowering agents (lovastatin, pravastatin, or cholestyramine) for a period of 6 to 12 months has been associated with significantly improved responses to the endothelium-dependent vasodilator acetylcholine in both the epicardial arteries and resistance arterioles.[82–84a] The addition of the antioxidant probucol to lovastatin may yield an added benefit[82] (Figs. 36–10 and 36–11). These studies suggest that disturbances in vascular regulation associated with atherosclerosis may be reversible if coronary risk factors are aggressively treated.

ENDOTHELIUM-DERIVED CONSTRICTING FACTORS. The endothelium not only mediates vasodilation but is a source of vasoconstrictor factors as well (Fig. 36–6). The best characterized of these are the endothelins (see p. 415). Endothelin-1 (ET-1) is a 21-amino-acid peptide that has potent vasoconstrictor activity.[85] Two other forms of endothelin have been discovered (ET-2 and ET-3), but endothelium produces only ET-1.[86] Synthesis of ET-1 is complex, with a large precursor molecule, preproendothelin, which is first processed to "big endothelin" and finally converted by the action of endothelin-converting enzyme to the fully active ET-1.

Unlike nitric oxide, which is released rapidly in response to vasodilator stimuli and then inactivated in a few seconds, ET-1 has actions that last minutes to hours.[85] In addition, agents that stimulate ET-1, such as thrombin, angiotensin II, epinephrine, or vasopressin do so by *de novo*

Initial Study

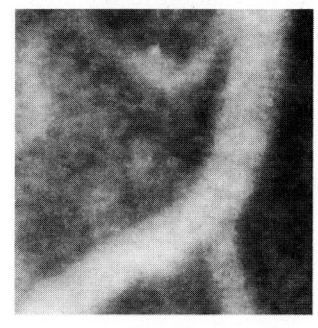 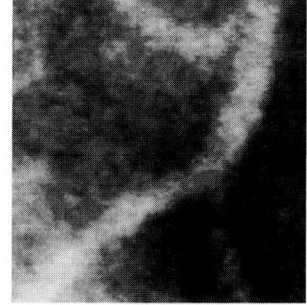

Follow-up Study

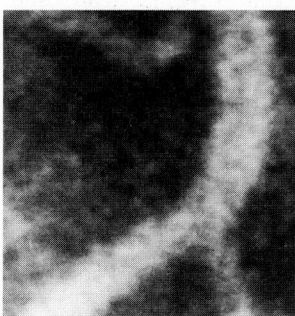 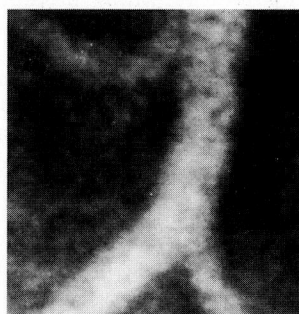

Control   Peak Acetylcholine

FIGURE 36–11. Segment of the circumflex coronary artery at the initial and follow-up (5.5 months) studies in a patient with coronary atherosclerosis assigned to lovastatin. Both left panels demonstrate baseline (control) arteriograms; both right panels demonstrate post-acetylcholine arteriograms. Substantial vasoconstriction occurs in response to the peak infusion of acetylcholine in the initial study, with marked improvement (a mild vasodilator response) in the follow-up study. (From Treasure, C. B., et al.: Beneficial effects of cholesterol-lowering therapy on the coronary endothelium in patients with coronary artery disease. N. Engl. J. Med. *332*:481, 1995. Copyright Massachusetts Medical Society.)

synthesis of m-RNA.[87] On the basis of these considerations, it is likely that ET-1 might contribute to the regulation of vascular tone primarily by exerting a tonic vasoconstrictor influence.

Plasma concentrations of ET-1 are elevated in a number of cardiovascular disorders, including atherosclerosis,[88] acute myocardial infarction,[89] congestive heart failure[90] (see p. 415), and hypertension.[91] ET-1 is also produced by activated human macrophages,[92] which are present in atherosclerotic lesions of patients with acute ischemic coronary syndromes and plaque rupture.[93,94] The plaques of patients with acute coronary syndromes (rest angina, crescendo angina, and post-infarction angina) expressed significantly greater ET-1 immunoreactivity than did plaques of patients with stable angina.[76] Two endothelin receptors, ET$_A$ and ET$_B$, have been characterized. Inhibitors of the ET receptors or of the endothelin-converting enzyme are becoming available[95] and should be helpful in assessing the role of ET-1 in diseases associated with abnormal vascular constrictions.

CLINICAL IMPLICATIONS OF ENDOTHELIAL DYSFUNCTION. It is now clear that the coronary anatomy as revealed by coronary angiography is a poor predictor of the clinical presentation and of the long-term course of individual patients with myocardial ischemia.[68] Many patients with only moderate stenoses but unstable plaques may develop serious complications, including unstable angina, myocardial infarction, or sudden death, whereas others with severe stenoses may have a stable pattern of symptoms.

Reductions of myocardial blood flow may be triggered by coronary vasoconstriction, by platelet aggregation and thrombosis, or by a combination of these factors. Normally functioning endothelium is important not only in the regulation of vascular tone but also in providing a nonthrombogenic surface and in preventing inflammation in the vessel wall that might lead to fissuring of a plaque. It is likely that endothelial dysfunction is a common link responsible for vasoconstrictor, inflammatory, and thrombotic manifestations of atherosclerosis. Reversal of endothelial dysfunction, as may be accomplished with the aggressive treatment of hypercholesterolemia (Fig. 36–10 and 36–11) may address the abnormal biology of atherosclerosis by improving coronary perfusion as well as other clinical sequelae of atherosclerosis.[96]

Autoregulation of Coronary Blood Flow

When sudden alterations in perfusion pressure are imposed in many arterial beds (including the coronary), the resulting abrupt changes in blood flow are only transitory, with flow returning promptly to the previous steady state level[97] (Fig. 36–12). This ability to maintain myocardial perfusion at constant levels in the face of changing driving pressure is termed *autoregulation*. Demonstration of autoregulation in the coronary bed is difficult in intact animals because modification of coronary perfusion pressure also changes myocardial oxygen demand and the extrinsic compression of the coronary vessels. However, under controlled experimental conditions in which perfusion pressure is altered but ventricular pressure, cardiac contractility, and heart rate—the principal determinants of myocardial oxygen demand—are maintained constant, autoregulation is clearly evident. Thus, in normal dogs, autoregulation is maintained at pressures as low as 60 mm Hg and as high as 130 mm Hg.[98] That is to say, when mean aortic pressure is within this range, coronary perfusion is relatively constant. When aortic pressure falls below 60 mm Hg, coronary blood flow declines. When aortic pressure exceeds 130 mm Hg, coronary flow rises sharply.

Although autoregulation cannot be studied in detail in humans, it does appear to play an important role in patients with coronary artery disease. Most patients with demand-induced angina have severe stenoses in epicardial

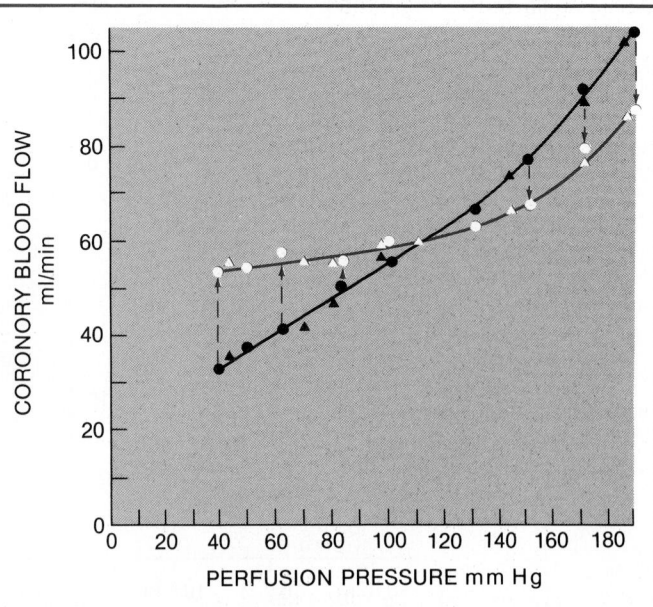

FIGURE 36–12. Autoregulation of coronary blood flow in the beating dog heart. The point where the curves cross represents the control steady-state pressure and flow. A sudden, sustained charge in perfusion pressure caused an abrupt change in flow represented by the filled symbols and black line (transient flow). The open symbols and red line represents the steady-state flows obtained at each perfusion pressure. The points represented by triangles were obtained after blockade of cardiac prostaglandin synthesis with indomethacin. (Reproduced by permission from Rubio, K., and Berne, K. M.: Regulation of coronary blood flow. Prog. Cardiovasc. Dis. 18:105, 1975.)

coronary arteries but no evidence of a resting perfusion deficit or myocardial ischemia. Reductions in perfusion pressure distal to stenoses are compensated for by autoregulatory dilation of the resistance vessels. However, in the presence of a critical stenosis, the ability of autoregulation to compensate for the effect of a proximal epicardial obstruction may be compromised by a reduction of aortic pressure. The latter can lower distal perfusion pressure below the critical levels at which autoregulation is no longer effective, thereby lowering myocardial perfusion, intensifying myocardial ischemia, and increasing left ventricular filling pressure, which decreases the perfusion pressure gradient further. These events may cause a vicious circle, especially in patients with extensive coronary artery disease. Insertion of an intraaortic balloon pump in this setting raises diastolic perfusion pressure and restores distal coronary pressure so that autoregulation is reestablished and myocardial ischemia is lessened.

Chronic hypertension and left ventricular hypertrophy narrow the range of autoregulation, especially in the subendocardium, in which autoregulation is ordinarily more limited than in the subepicardium.[99] This amplifies the detrimental effects of coronary stenoses on myocardial perfusion and in patients with severe hypertrophy may lead to subendocardial ischemia even in the absence of coronary stenosis.

Conditions that alter the function of vascular smooth muscle in coronary arteries can also attenuate autoregulation. Dilators of resistance vessels such as adenosine and dipyridamole reduce perfusion pressure distal to a stenosis by increasing subepicardial flow, abolish subendocardial autoregulation,[100,101] and reduce subendocardial perfusion, a phenomenon termed "transmural coronary steal." In the presence of coronary occlusion, perfusion of the ischemic myocardium is markedly pressure-dependent because coronary collaterals do not exhibit autoregulation.[102] This explains why patients with extensive collateral-dependent segments of myocardium tolerate hypotension poorly.

Mechanisms of Autoregulation

NITRIC OXIDE. Evidence strongly suggests a role for EDRF in coronary autoregulation. Inhibition of nitric oxide in conscious dogs raises the lower autoregulatory threshold by about 15 mm Hg.[103] Autoregulation is also impaired in guinea pig hearts when production of nitric oxide is inhibited but not with inhibition of the cyclooxygenase pathway.[104] These observations suggest that the endothelium modulates coronary autoregulation through the production of nitric oxide but not of prostanoids. The involvement of nitric oxide may be related to the ability of the endothelium to sense changes in perfusion pressure through specific pressure-sensitive channels.[105]

MYOGENIC CONTROL. Arteriolar smooth muscle reacts to increased intraluminal pressure by contracting.[106] The consequent augmentation of resistance tends to return blood flow toward normal despite the higher perfusion pressure. This regulatory mechanism, referred to as *myogenic control*,[106,107] is an important mechanism of autoregulation. Myogenic contraction can be demonstrated in organ chamber experiments; a stretch on a vascular ring or an increase in intravascular pressure in isolated perfused microvessels is followed by active contraction.[20]

Myogenic mechanisms are particularly prominent in arterioles smaller than 100 microns and less important in larger arterioles, in which other autoregulatory mechanisms play a greater role.[108] They are also more important in subepicardial than subendocardial arterioles.

Extravascular Compressive Forces

SYSTOLIC COMPRESSIVE FORCES. Because systolic ventricular wall tension compresses intramyocardial vessels, most of the coronary blood flow to the left ventricle occurs during diastole. Thus, the contracting heart obstructs its own blood supply. At peak systole, there is even backflow in the coronary arteries, particularly in the intramural and small epicardial vessels.[109] The extravascular systolic compressive force has two components. The first is left ventricular systolic intracavitary pressure, which is transmitted fully to the subendocardium but falls off to almost zero at the epicardial surface. The second, and perhaps even more important, is the vascular narrowing caused by compression and bending of small arterioles coursing through the ventricular wall as the heart contracts.[20,110]

The important resistance to coronary blood flow caused by left ventricular systolic compression can be demonstrated experimentally in a beating heart perfused at constant pressure in which transient asystole is induced by vagal stimulation. At that point, coronary blood flow suddenly increases by approximately 50 per cent because of the relief of the compressive effect.[111]

The "throttling" effect of systole on myocardial perfusion is particularly important when systolic intraventricular pressure is elevated to levels exceeding coronary perfusion pressure, as occurs with obstruction to left ventricular outflow by valvular or subvalvular aortic stenosis[111a] or with severe aortic regurgitation.[112] Because an increase in heart rate augments the total duration of systolic time per minute during which coronary vascular compression occurs, while augmenting myocardial oxygen demand, tachycardia may cause myocardial ischemia. The importance of extravascular compressive forces in limiting coronary blood flow is magnified when coronary vascular tone is diminished,[113] as may occur during the administration of arteriolar vasodilators or during metabolic vasodilation associated with physical activity.

Because compressive forces exerted by the right ventricle are ordinarily far smaller than those of the left ventricle, ventricular perfusion is reduced but not interrupted during systole. However, when right ventricular pressure is elevated, the phasic blood flow pattern of the arteries perfus-

ing the right ventricle resembles those of the left ventricle.[20]

DIASTOLIC COMPRESSIVE FORCES. The coronary perfusion or effective driving pressure has been assumed to be the pressure gradient between the coronary arteries and the pressure in either the right atrium or the left ventricle in diastole, because coronary flow drains primarily into these two chambers during this phase of the cardiac cycle. When coronary perfusion pressure is lowered, diastolic blood flow ceases when coronary driving pressure reaches approximately 50 mm Hg, the so-called pressure at zero flow (P_{zf}).[114,115] This pressure is determined largely by diastolic compressive forces.

Transmural Distribution of Myocardial Blood Flow

Extravascular compressive forces are greater in subendocardial than in subepicardial zones (Fig. 36–13). Subendocardial arterioles may be particularly susceptible to compression as they arborize from long, transmural vessels.[116] Therefore, *systolic* flow is more reduced in the subendocardium than the subepicardium. Nevertheless, in conscious dogs under resting physiological conditions, the ratio of endocardial to epicardial flow averaged throughout the cardiac cycle is approximately 1.25 : 1 as a consequence of preferential dilatation of the subendocardial vessels, causing a large increase in diastolic flow in the subendocardium.[117] The greater subendocardial blood flow appears to be secondary to the higher wall stress (and therefore oxygen consumption per unit weight), which is normally about 20 per cent greater than that of subepicardial muscle.[118]

SUBENDOCARDIAL ISCHEMIA. The subendocardium is more vulnerable to ischemic damage than the midmyocardium or subepicardium.[119] Epicardial coronary stenoses are associated with reductions in the subendocardial to subepicardial flow ratio.[120,122] When coronary arteries are constricted sufficiently to reduce total coronary flow to approximately 40 per cent of control, endocardial to epicardial flow ratio falls from 1.16 at baseline to 0.37.[121] This pattern of redistribution of flow away from the endocardium is further exaggerated during exercise and during pacing-induced tachycardia (Fig. 36–14).[120,122] Potent arteriolar vasodilators,

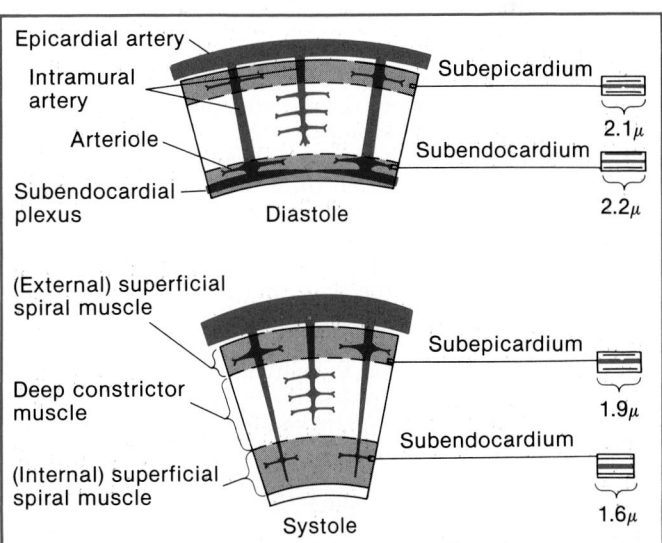

FIGURE 36–13. Cross-section of the left ventricular wall in diastole and systole. Factors involved in the susceptibility of the subendocardium to the development of ischemia include the greater dependence of this region on diastolic perfusion and the greater degree of shortening, and therefore of energy expenditure, of this region during systole. (From Bell, J. R., and Fox, A. C.: Pathogenesis of subendocardial ischemia. Am. J. Med. Sci. *268:*2, 1974.)

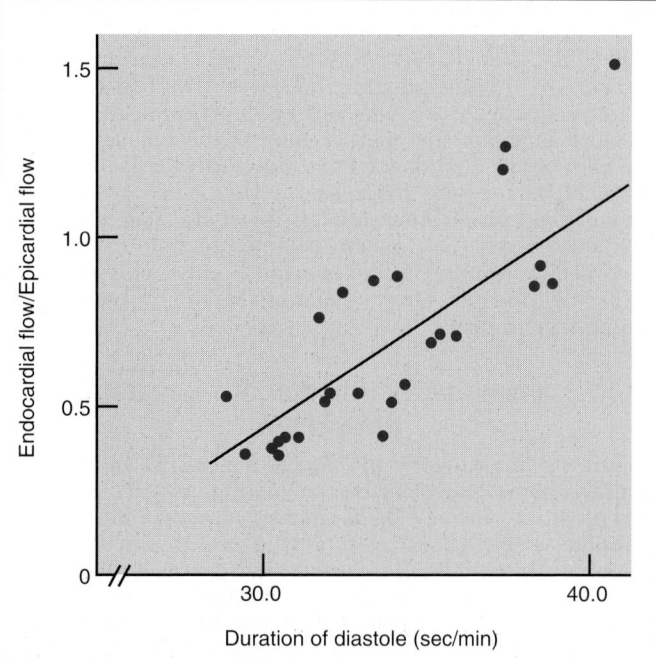

FIGURE 36–14. Relationship between subendocardial : subepicardial flow ratios and the duration of diastole during ventricular pacing at 100, 150, 200, and 250 beats per minute in seven dogs with maximal coronary vasodilation produced by intravenous infusion of adenosine, 4 μg/kg of body weight per minute. As heart rate is increased (shorter diastole), endocardial : epicardial flow falls. (Reproduced with permission from Bache, R. J., and Cobb, F. R.: Effect of maximal coronary vasodilation on transmural myocardial perfusion during tachycardia in the awake dog. Circ. Res. **41**:648, 1977. Copyright American Heart Association.)

such as adenosine, especially in the presence of an epicardial stenosis, can similarly affect transmural myocardial perfusion, causing an "intramural steal."[123,124] Severe pressure-induced left ventricular hypertrophy,[125] as well as heart failure with elevated left ventricular end-diastolic pressure, may also reduce the endocardial : epicardial flow ratio[126,127] (Fig. 36–15). When the markedly elevated left ventricular end-diastolic pressure in heart failure is corrected, subendocardial coronary flow reserve is restored and the endocardial : epicardial ratio is normalized.[127] Thus, impairment of endocardial perfusion in heart failure may be a direct consequence of the elevated left ventricular diastolic pressure and the diastolic compressive forces exerted on subendocardial perfusion (see p. 404).

A low subendocardial : subepicardial flow ratio can be increased by elevation of aortic pressure, which increases perfusion of the subendocardial region whose arterioles are maximally dilated and in which flow is pressure dependent. Overperfusion of the epicardial region is prevented by autoregulatory arteriolar constriction. Alpha-adrenergic constrictors[128] or inhibitors of adenosine-induced arteriolar dilation such as theophylline[129] cause constriction of subepicardial arterioles, resulting in a reduction of epicardial blood flow, thereby reducing the transstenotic pressure gradient and increasing pressure distal to the stenosis. This rise in distal pressure augments blood flow to the subendocardial region. Reduction of myocardial oxygen demand, for example by beta-blockers, also decreases epicardial blood flow and increases perfusion pressure and thereby flow to ischemic subendocardial region.[130,131]

Neural and Neurotransmitter Control

The coronary arteries are richly innervated by adrenergic and parasympathetic nerves,[14] and their activation can exert important influences on coronary vasomotor tone.

Both alpha₁ and alpha₂ adrenoceptors are present in coronary arteries,[132] and when activated by neuronally released or circulating norepinephrine both cause vasoconstriction,[133–135] which appears to be mediated by an increased concentration of calcium in coronary vascular smooth muscle.[134–136] When inotropic and chronotropic effects of norepinephrine are blocked[137] and the production of metabolic vasodilator stimuli inhibited, stimulation of sympathetic cardiac nerves causes coronary vasoconstriction. The activation of alpha₁ receptors induced by the infusion of methoxamine reduces the diameter of coronary arteries, despite increasing intraluminal pressure.[138] Activation of the carotid chemoreceptor reflex causes marked coronary constriction, which can be blocked by surgical denervation or by the alpha blocker phentolamine.[138] On the other hand, beta₂ adrenoceptors in the large and small coronary arteries mediate vasodilation.[139] Beta blockade induces coronary constriction, but this effect appears not to be a direct action on the coronary arteries. Instead, it results from blockade of beta-adrenoceptor mediated increase in myocardial oxygen demand.[140] Although parasympathetic stimulation appears to dilate small coronary arteries,[14] the extent of cholinergic regulation of large coronary arteries is also controversial.[141]

Intravenous use of norepinephrine induces a brief fall, followed by a sustained rise, in coronary vascular resistance, accompanied by a decline in coronary sinus pO₂.[142] The early vasodilatation can be eliminated by beta-adrenoceptor blockade and presumably results from the augmented myocardial oxygen consumption consequent to stimulation of myocardial beta receptors. The later increase in coronary vascular resistance can be prevented by alpha-adrenoceptor blockade and is caused by the stimulation of alpha receptors in the coronary vascular bed by norepinephrine. Blockade of alpha₁ receptors in patients with coronary artery disease attenuates the coronary vasoconstrictor response to the cold pressor test[143] and to cigarette smoking,[144] indicating that both responses are mediated by stimulation of these receptors.

REFLEX CONTROL. Baroreceptor activity affects coronary vascular resistance reflexly. With carotid occlusion, baroreceptor hypotension leads to reflex adrenergic stimulation, increased metabolic activity, and secondary coronary dilatation. When this augmentation of myocardial beta receptor–mediated activity is prevented by beta blockade, reflex coronary vasoconstriction secondary to carotid hypotension is unmasked.[145] Stimulation of the distal ends of the vagi produces coronary vasodilatation,[145,146] an effect

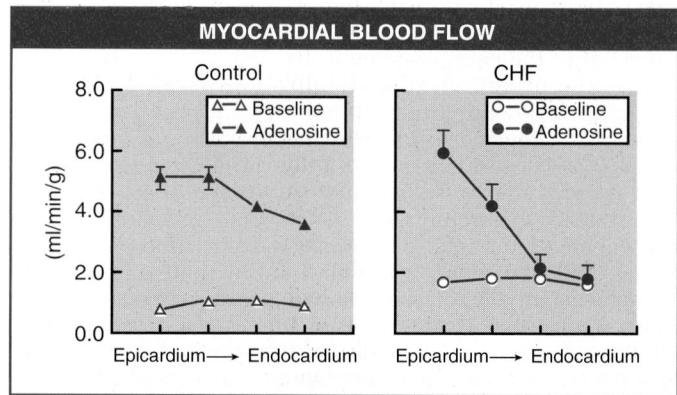

FIGURE 36–15. The reduction in subendocardial reserve as reflected by diminished responses of endocardial blood flow to near maximal vasodilation with adenosine. There was near exhaustion of subendocardial reserve in the dogs with left ventricular failure (CHF). (Reproduced with permission from Vatner, S. F., Shannon, R., and Hitinger, L.: Reduced subendocardial coronary reserve, a potential mechanism for impaired diastolic function in the hypertrophied and failing heart. Circulation **81**(Suppl. III):III-8, 1990. Copyright American Heart Association.)

mediated by the release of acetylcholine from vagal nerve endings that can be blocked by atropine.[111]

Stimulation of the carotid sinus nerves results in a substantial reduction in coronary vascular resistance,[147] an effect that can be prevented by alpha-receptor blockade. This finding indicates that adrenergic coronary constrictor tone is present in the resting conscious dog and the coronary vasodilation attendant upon stimulation of the carotid sinus nerves results from a reduction in this tone. Alpha receptor–mediated constrictor tone appears to persist in the coronary vascular bed during exercise, despite the coexisting metabolic vasodilation.[148] Alpha$_1$ adrenoceptor stimulation is capable of causing epicardial vasoconstriction in ischemic myocardium, thereby influencing favorably the transmural distribution of blood flow to the subendocardium[149,150] during exercise.

Efferent neural influences on the coronary vascular bed may also be activated reflexly by cardiopulmonary parasympathetic receptors. Stimulation of these receptors leads to reflex systemic and coronary vasodilation,[151] while stimulation of somatic afferent fibers increases coronary resistance through alpha-adrenergically mediated vasoconstriction.[152] Activation of chemoreceptors initially causes coronary dilation, a reflex that is mediated by the vagi and can be abolished by atropine.[111] Intracoronary injection of veratrum alkaloids, as well as other metabolically active substances, induces reflex bradycardia and hypotension (the Bezold-Jarisch reflex),[153] both the afferent and efferent limbs of which involve the vagus nerves.[151] Neurally controlled and alpha-adrenoceptor mediated constriction of stenotic lesions of the coronary vascular bed in humans has been observed on coronary arteriograms[150] during the handgrip test.[154]

TONIC CORONARY VASOCONSTRICTION. There is evidence for tonic coronary constriction mediated by adrenergic nerves.[147] Acute surgical denervation of the heart reduces coronary vascular resistance and lowers arteriovenous oxygen extraction and raises coronary venous O_2 content (primary vasodilation).[155] Coronary vascular resistance in dogs as well as patients with innervated hearts declines by almost 25 per cent in response to alpha-adrenoceptor blockade and the resultant release of basal coronary constrictor mediated by alpha receptors.[156] However, coronary vascular resistance does *not* diminish when patients with transplanted hearts are subjected to alpha-adrenoceptor blockade because in these patients, cardiac denervation, an element of transplantation, had already abolished the coronary constrictor tone.

An increase in adrenergic outflow does *not* appear to be responsible for the episodes of coronary spasm in most patients with Prinzmetal's (variant) angina[157] or in the genesis of ischemia in syndrome X (see p. 1343).[158] However, it has been reported that alpha-adrenoceptor stimulation can induce coronary spasm that can be prevented by phenoxybenzamine or prazosin in some patients with variant angina.[150] The finding in some patients with chronic stable angina that administration of alpha-receptor blockers can reduce exercise-induced ST-segment depression and angina[150,159,160] indicates that alpha receptor–mediated coronary vasoconstriction may play a contributory role in the development of myocardial ischemia resulting in these patients. It has also been reported that cocaine is a potent coronary vasoconstrictor both in dogs and humans,[161] and because this effect can be prevented by an alpha-receptor blocker, phentolamine, it appears to be mediated, at least in part, by alpha-adrenergic stimulation.[162]

Effects of Coronary Stenoses

Limitation of coronary blood flow by atherosclerotic plaques is related principally to their geometric features, including the severity and length of narrowings, their stiff-

ness or partial distensibility, and the presence of superimposed platelet aggregation and thrombosis.[163]

As blood traverses a stenosis, pressure (energy) is lost. To estimate this pressure loss, principles of fluid dynamics have been applied and tested in animal models as well as in patients.[164–166] Although the formulas are complex, they have been simplified as follows:[163]

$$\Delta P = \frac{1.8 \cdot Q}{d^4_{sten}} + \frac{6.1 \cdot Q^2}{d^4_{sten}}$$

where ΔP is the pressure drop across a stenosis in millimeters of mercury, Q is the flow across the stenosis in milliliters per second, and d_{sten} is the minimal stenosis lumen diameter in millimeters. The first term accounts for viscous friction between layers of fluid in the stenotic segment leading to frictional energy losses. The second term reflects energy losses occurring when the "pressure energy" of normal arterial flow is transferred first to the kinetic energy of high velocity flow and then, at the exit from the stenosis, to the turbulent energy of distal flow eddies (separation losses).

CORONARY BLOOD FLOW. At normal levels of arterial flow, both frictional and separation losses contribute to the stenosis resistance and to the presence of a pressure gradient. As flow increases, separation losses, which increase with the square of the flow, become increasingly prominent and viscous losses become negligible. Thus, increases in blood flow and pressure drops across the stenosis are related in an exponential manner (Fig. 36–16). Augmentation of coronary blood flow is associated with elevations in pressure gradients across the stenotic orifice and reductions in poststenotic perfusion pressure.

Brown et al.[163] have pointed out three common clinical situations in which the transstenotic pressure gradient elevations due to flow increases may be important in the pathogenesis of myocardial ischemia: (1) Pharmacological dilators of coronary resistance arterioles, such as dipyrida-

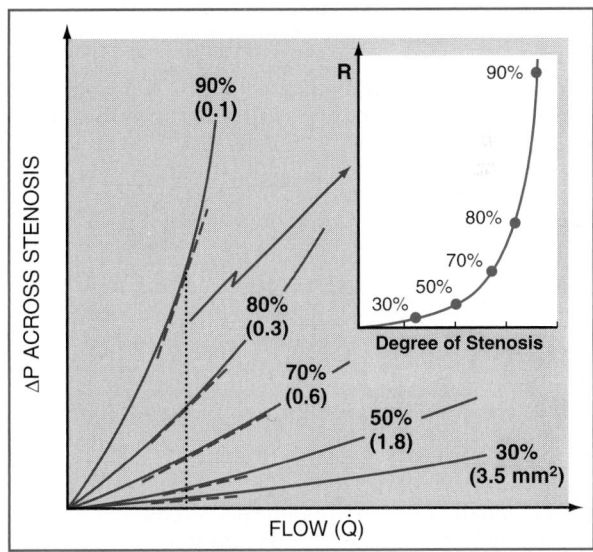

FIGURE 36–16. Relation between pressure reduction across a stenosis (ΔP) and flow through the stenosis (Q). Relations are shown for concentric stenoses of 30, 50, 70, 80, and 90 per cent internal diameter. The numbers in parentheses below each per cent diameter stenosis represent residual luminal cross-sectional area, calculated on the basis of a normal internal diameter of 3 mm and cross-sectional area of 7.1 mm². The level of flow corresponding to basal metabolic needs is represented by the vertical dotted line; stenosis resistances for this level of flow are shown as the dashed tangent lines to the individual pressure-flow relations. In the inset on the right, stenosis resistance (R) is plotted as a function of degree of stenosis. (From Klocke, F. J.: Measurements of coronary blood flow and degree of stenosis: Current clinical implications and continuing uncertainties. Newsletter of the Council on Clinical Cardiology of the American Heart Association. Vol 7, No. 3, July 1982.)

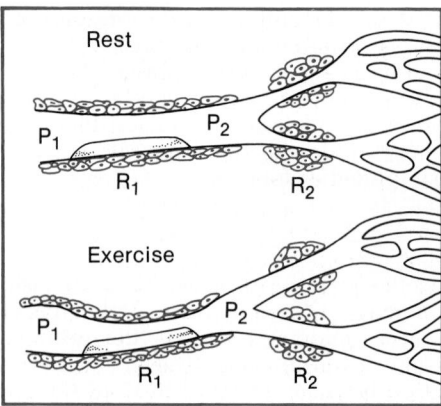

FIGURE 36–17. Diagrammatic representation of vessel collapse when myocardial flow increases. Under baseline conditions (Rest, *top*), flow across the stenosis (R₁) is modest and a large pressure gradient (P₁-P₂) does not develop. With a vasodilator intervention such as exercise *(bottom)*, the pressure gradient across the stenosis (P₁-P₂) increases. The resulting fall in intraluminal pressure may lead to collapse of the vessel at the level of the obstruction, thereby increasing the degree of stenosis. This leads to dilatation of the distal vessels (R₂). (From Epstein, S. E., Cannon, R. O., III, and Talbot, T. L.: Hemodynamic principles in the control of coronary blood flow. Am. J. Cardiol. *56*:9E, 1985.)

mole and adenosine, increase the transstenotic flow and pressure gradient. When subendocardial resistance vessels become fully dilated, their perfusion becomes perfusion pressure dependent. Redistribution of flow from the subendocardium to the subepicardium develops as the transstenotic pressure gradient increases and pressure distal to the stenosis falls. This is one mechanism of "coronary steal." A fall in aortic perfusion pressure reduces subendocardial flow further. (2) During physical activity, coronary blood flow rises to meet the increase in myocardial oxygen demand,[167,168] leading to an increase in transstenotic pressure gradient and a fall in the distal perfusion pressure, resulting in redistribution of blood flow from the subendocardium toward the subepicardium, an effect similar to that observed with the administration of pharmacological vasodilators (Fig. 36–17). Furthermore, the fall in intraluminal pressure may lead to collapse of the vessel at the level of the obstruction, thereby increasing the degree of stenosis. (3) The reduced oxygen-carrying capacity of anemia is compensated for by increases in coronary blood flow because the myocardium cannot sufficiently increase its oxygen extraction significantly. The augmentation of flow is associated with a marked increase in the transstenotic pressure gradient.[163,169] Not surprisingly, therefore, anemia is poorly tolerated in patients with coronary artery disease.

SEVERITY OF STENOSIS. At any level of blood flow, the single most important determinant of stenosis resistance is the minimum diameter of the stenosis. The transstenotic pressure drop is inversely proportional to the *fourth* power of the minimum luminal diameter. As a consequence, a relatively small change in luminal diameter (such as caused by active or passive vasomotion) is amplified to produce marked hemodynamic effects in the presence of severe stenoses.[163,170] For example, when the diameter stenosis is increased from 80 to 90 per cent, the resistance of a stenosis rises nearly threefold.[165]

ENTRANCE AND EXIT EFFECTS. Blood flow velocity (kinetic energy) increase and pressure (static energy) decreases in a narrowed arterial segment. The conversion of static to kinetic energy would occur with little loss of energy if the flow remained laminar, according to the Bernoulli principle.[163,166] Laminar flow can be preserved if the entrance and the exit of the stenotic segment are tapered gradually. However, most stenoses have abrupt transitions where energy losses associated with separation of laminar flow into eddy currents (vortices) occurs. The separation

energy losses are particularly pronounced at the exits of stenoses.

LENGTH OF STENOSES. For most stenoses, the length of the narrowed segment has only a modest effect on the physiological significance of the obstruction. However, in very long narrowed segments, significant turbulence occurs along the wall of the stenotic segment, and energy is dissipated as heat when eddies impact on the wall; stenosis length may become important under these conditions.[171]

DYNAMIC CHANGES IN STENOSIS SEVERITY. Examination of the morphology of pressure-fixed human coronary arteries has revealed eccentricity of atherosclerotic plaques which involve only a portion of the arterial wall while the remaining arc of the wall is relatively normal and often compliant.[172] This provides a mechanism by which changes in distending pressure or vascular tone may alter luminal caliber and stenosis resistance. For example, most atherosclerotic stenosis in patients can dilate actively in response to nitroglycerin or constrict in response to ergonovine or alpha-adrenergic stimuli.[173]

Dynamic changes in stenosis severity and resistance due to alterations in intraluminal distending pressure have been demonstrated in compliant stenoses, both in experimental models and in patients with coronary artery disease.[163,174,175] As blood flow velocity rises in the stenotic segment, distending pressure falls, leading to passive collapse of a pliable segment. Passive collapse of a stenosis associated with the use of vasodilators occurs with agents that selectively dilate distal resistance vessels. The administration of dipyridamole to patients with coronary artery disease causes narrowing of severely stenotic pliable segments as well as of the normal arterial segments distal to the stenoses.[176] Passive collapse of pliable stenosis may also occur when aortic pressure is lowered.

EFFECTS OF CORONARY STENOSIS IN THE INTACT CORONARY BED. The effect of a coronary stenosis depends on the degree to which the resistance to flow caused by the stenosis can be compensated for by dilation of arterioles distal to the stenosis.[177] Gould and Lipscomb[178] concluded that in normal dogs, resting coronary flow is not altered until the constriction reaches at least 85 per cent of the diameter. Therefore, resting coronary flow is little affected by mild or

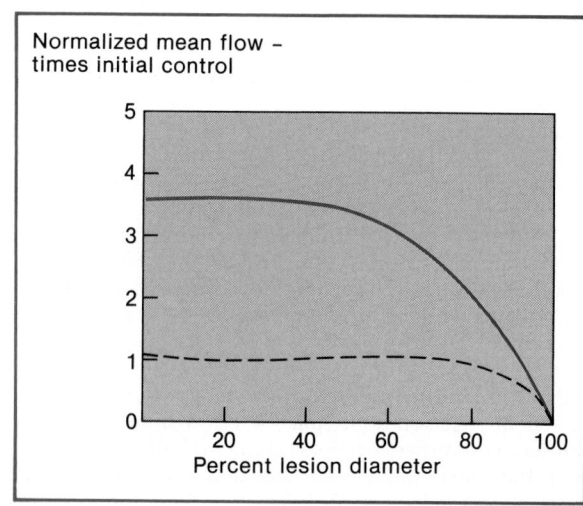

FIGURE 36–18. Relationship between resting *(dashed line)* and maximal coronary blood flow *(solid line)* and percentage of diameter stenosis in a dog. Progressive coronary stenosis was achieved by progressively narrowing a short segment of a proximal coronary artery. Resting coronary blood flow did not change until coronary diameter stenosis exceeded 80 per cent. Maximal coronary blood flow began to decrease when per cent diameter stenosis exceeded 50 per cent. (From Marcus, M. L.: The Coronary Circulation in Health and Disease. New York, McGraw-Hill, 1983, and modified from Gould, K. L., and Lipscomb, L.: Effects of coronary stenoses on coronary flow reserve and resistance. Am. J. Cardiol. *34*:50, 1974.)

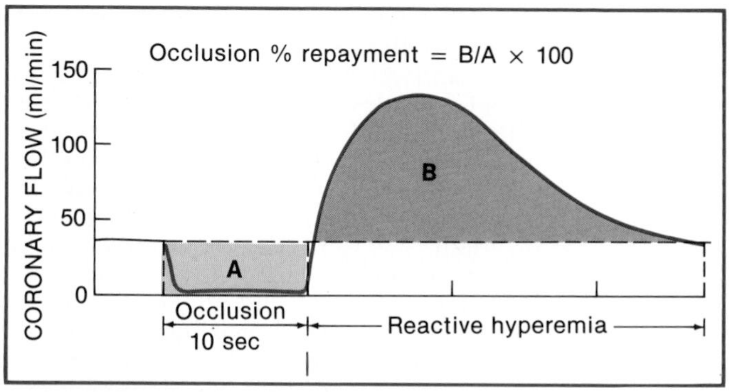

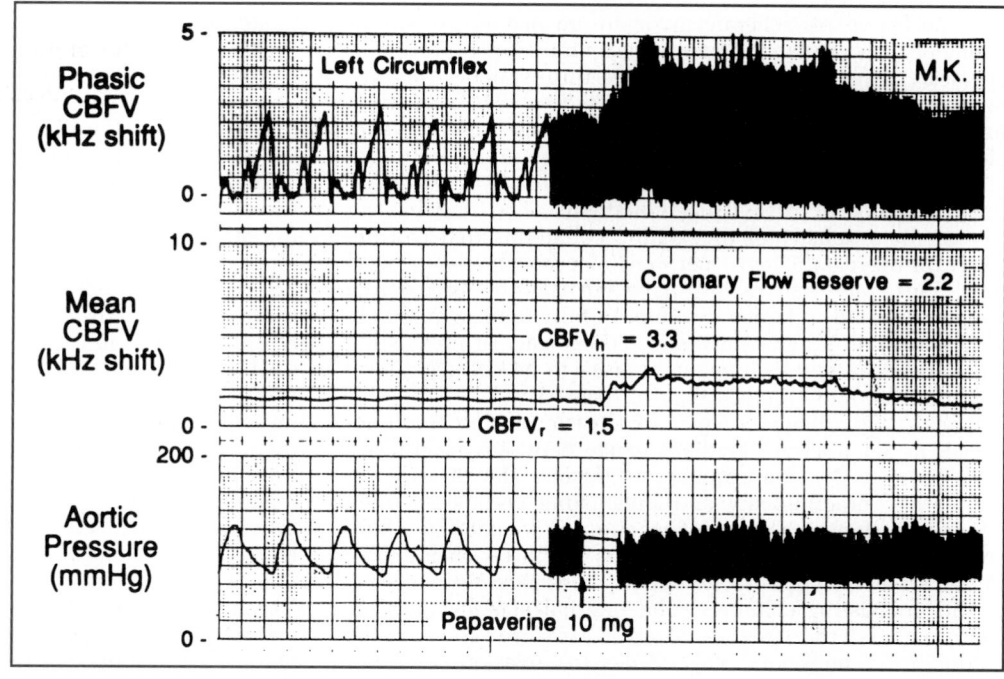

FIGURE 36–19. Mean coronary flow prior to, during, and following coronary occlusion. Arrow indicates the release of occlusion. Area A represents the flow debt, and area B its repayment. (From Gould, K. L.: Coronary Artery Stenosis. New York, Elsevier, 1991, p. 13.)

The marked vasodilation that characterizes reactive hyperemia is probably related to the accumulation of metabolites, especially adenosine (see p. 1163). The difference between basal coronary blood flow and peak flow during reactive hyperemia represents the *coronary flow reserve*.

Because of the limitations inherent in coronary angiography, attention has been directed to physiological approaches for assessing the severity of coronary stenoses. As noted earlier, maximal blood flow is a more sensitive index of stenosis severity than resting blood flow. Because methods for measuring maximal coronary flow in absolute terms are not readily available, the concept of *coronary flow reserve*, defined as the ratio of maximal flow to resting flow, has been developed and refined into an accepted functional measure of resistance to coronary blood flow. Abnormal resistance may be caused by stenosis and/or microcirculatory disorders.[170,179,181]

Three types of stimuli have been used to elicit maximal coronary blood flow: metabolic stress, pharmacological coronary dilation, and transient coronary occlusion. Intense treadmill or bicycle exercise yields near maximal four- to six-fold flow increases[182] and is thereby a widely accepted stimulus for assessing flow responses. Maximal increases in coronary blood flow can also be produced by pharmacological coronary vasodilators. Adenosine and papaverine (Fig. 36–20) have a rapid onset and brief duration of action, can be administered directly into the coronary artery, and are therefore particularly well-suited for studies in the catheterization laboratory.[183] Transient occlusion of a coronary artery by an angioplasty balloon with the measurement of reactive hyperemia is the third stimulus.

INVASIVE MEASUREMENT OF FLOW RESERVE. Several techniques for determining coronary flow reserve have been developed for use during cardiac catheterization. Catheter- or guidewire-based Doppler systems allow continuous measurement of phasic and mean coronary blood flow velocity.[184,185] Miniaturized Doppler crystals have been placed at the tip of angioplasty guidewires, permitting measurements of coronary blood flow velocity[186,187] (Fig. 36–20). The thermodilution method measures flow in the coronary venous system, either in the great cardiac vein (which drains the left anterior descending artery territory) or in the coronary sinus (which drains the left anterior descending and circumflex artery territories).[189] These approaches have demonstrated only a weak inverse correlation between angiographic estimates of per cent diameter stenosis and

moderate stenoses and is an insensitive measure for evaluating coronary artery disease. *Maximal* coronary blood flow, however, begins to decline when diameter stenosis exceeds 30 to 45 per cent (Fig. 36–18). The capacity to increase coronary blood flow in response to increased oxygen demand is abolished when diameter stenosis exceeds 90 per cent.

Insights derived from such animal studies need to be applied cautiously in clinical practice. The simple use of relative per cent diameter stenosis determined by coronary arteriography has important limitations, because it does not account for other geometric characteristics of the stenosis such as its absolute diameter, length, exit angle, or eccentricity. The determination of relative per cent diameter narrowing may be misleading in the setting of diffuse disease where segments adjacent to the stenosis are also reduced in caliber. The hemodynamic effects of serial stenoses are also difficult to assess from arteriograms.[170] It is not surprising, then, that the correlation between per cent diameter stenosis and the physiological significance of a given obstruction in patients is poor, especially for lesions of moderate severity.[179,180]

Coronary Flow Reserve and Hyperemia

Ischemia caused by transient coronary arterial occlusion is followed by an increase in blood flow above control levels, a response called reactive hyperemia (Fig. 36–19).

FIGURE 36–20. Assessment of coronary blood flow velocity (CBFV) in the normal circumflex artery of a patient with atherosclerotic disease of the left anterior descending coronary artery. Following intracoronary papaverine, an increase in coronary blood flow velocity 2.2 times the resting velocity was seen. (Normal coronary flow reserve > 3.5 : 1.) This reduction suggests the presence of microvascular disease. $CBFV_h$ = Coronary blood flow velocity hyperemia; $CBFV_r$ = coronary blood flow velocity at rest. (From White, C. W.: Clinical applications of Doppler coronary flow reserve measurements. Am. J. Cardiol. *71*:10D, 1993.)

coronary reserve, particularly for stenoses of moderate (intermediate) severity.[180]

NONINVASIVE MEASUREMENT OF FLOW RESERVE. Digital subtraction angiography can also be used to estimate regional coronary blood flow in a downstream area by measuring the time of arrival and/or the rapidity of clearance of injected x-ray contrast medium.[188] Radionuclide stress myocardial perfusion imaging (thallium-201, sestamibi) is used widely to quantify coronary flow reserve (see p. 288). Some laboratories are investigating the use of positron-emission tomography, ultrafast computed tomography, and nuclear magnetic resonance imaging for the same purpose.[190] Flow reserve is typically assessed by these techniques during exercise or with pharmacological vasodilators. In contrast to catheterization-based techniques that measure an *absolute* coronary flow reserve index (the quotient of maximal and basal flow), cardiac imaging techniques assess *relative* coronary flow reserve by comparing the perfusion of ischemic regions of the left ventricle with presumably normally perfused reference regions.[191]

Imaging techniques yield a less quantitative index of flow reserve than catheter-based techniques. In addition, results can be misleading in the setting of diffuse coronary disease when a normal reference region is not available. Together, absolute and relative coronary flow reserves provide a more complete description of physiological stenosis severity than does either alone.[191]

There is a poor correlation between the severity of stenoses and their propensity to cause myocardial infarction, sudden ischemic death, or unstable angina. Most atherosclerotic lesions responsible for these complications are either not appreciated on angiograms obtained shortly before the event or are mild stenoses of inconsequential hemodynamic significance.[192–194] Pathological studies have revealed that myocardial infarctions are usually caused by ruptures of plaques that are not necessarily severe, with formation of a superimposed occlusive thrombus.[195] These findings suggest that although measurements of coronary flow reserve may be useful in the assessment of the severity of stenoses and in the identification of severe lesions responsible for exertional angina, they are *not* likely to identify the more dangerous plaques responsible for unstable angina, acute myocardial infarction, and ischemic sudden death.

Coronary Collateral Circulation

Following total or near-total occlusion of a coronary artery, perfusion of ischemic myocardium occurs by way of collaterals—vascular channels that interconnect ordinary arteries.[190] Preexisting collaterals are thin-walled structures ranging in diameter from 20 to 200 μm.[196,197] The density of preexisting collaterals varies greatly among different species.[197] Acute coronary occlusion produces no infarction at all in guinea pigs because of an exceptionally well-developed network of preexisting collaterals. The dog has an intermediate density of preexisting collaterals that can deliver, on average, 5 to 10 per cent of preocclusional, basal flow. Pigs, rats, and rabbits have virtually no preexisting collaterals, and infarcts develop rapidly and completely with acute coronary occlusion.[197] The density of preexisting collateral channels in humans appears to be comparable to or somewhat more modest than in dogs.[198]

Preexisting collaterals are normally closed and nonfunctional, as no pressure gradient exists between the arteries they connect.[199] After coronary occlusion, the distal pressure drops precipitously and preexisting collaterals open virtually instantly. The transformation of preexisting collaterals into mature collaterals occurs in three stages. The initial stage (the first 24 hours) involves *passive widening* of the preexisting channels. The internal elastic lamina is ruptured and its fragments are displaced toward the media.[196,197] The second stage (1 day to 3 weeks) is characterized by *inflammation and cellular proliferation*.[196,197] Monocytes migrate into the vascular wall and secrete a variety of cytokines and growth factors.[201] This phase of vascular enlargement is marked by cellular proliferation involving endothelium, smooth muscle cells, and fibroblasts.[202] Over several weeks, these cells arrange themselves into circular and longitudinal layers.[198] During these first two phases, the luminal diameter of collateral channels increases nearly 10-fold. The third stage of collateral maturation (3 weeks to 6 months) involves thickening of the vessel wall due to *deposition of extracellular matrix* and further cellular proliferation.[203] In its final state, the mature collateral vessel may reach 1 mm in luminal diameter. Its three-layer structure is nearly indistinguishable from a normal coronary artery of the same size.[204]

Factors Promoting Collateral Growth

Mechanical forces determine the size of collateral channels in the early minutes and hours after coronary occlusion. Pressure gradients across preexisting collaterals augment blood flow and create shear stresses,[201] which in turn lead to activation of endothelial cells with expression of leukocyte adhesion molecules and secretion of growth factors.[205] Ischemia or hypoxia may initiate the process of vascular transformation by causing intense dilation of native coronary collateral channels, but these stimuli probably have only a limited role in further collateral angiogenesis.[201] Other chemical stimuli likely contribute to growth of collateral channels, including a variety of growth factors and proto-oncogenes. These are rapidly expressed following coronary occlusion, in part due to enhanced transcriptional activity.[206]

HEREDITARY FACTORS. These play an important role in determining the density of preexisting collaterals. For example, coronary occlusion in Black Russian rabbits results in a large infarct, as preexisting collaterals are virtually absent. New Zealand White rabbits, on the other hand, have a greater number of preexisting collaterals and are more resistant to the ischemic effects of a coronary occlusion.[197]

SEVERITY OF OBSTRUCTION. The severity of coronary obstruction is a critical determinant of the development of coronary collateral channels. In dogs, the growth of collaterals is not stimulated until a coronary stenosis reduces the luminal cross-sectional area by at least 80 per cent.[200] In patients, coronary collaterals do not develop until a stenosis of at least 70 per cent is present. Beyond this threshold value, the growth of collateral channels is directly related to stenosis severity.[207]

EXERCISE. This stimulus has no effect on the preexisting coronary collaterals in the absence of coronary occlusions or stenoses.[200] Even in the presence of severe coronary stenoses, the effects of exercise training have been inconsistent and overall quite small in animals.[208]

PHARMACOLOGICAL AGENTS. Coronary collaterals dilate in response to nitrates[200] and beta-adrenergic agonists.[204] On the other hand, calcium antagonists,[209] beta blockers,[210] and alpha-adrenergic agonists have no detectable direct effect on collateral function, whereas vasopressin[204] and serotonin[211] are potent constrictors of the collateral circulation. Such a constriction of collateral vessels may intensify myocardial ischemia during platelet aggregation or arterial thrombosis when serotonin is released locally into the coronary circulation, and it may contribute to episodes of myocardial ischemia and infarction during systemic vasopressin administration.[204]

Intracoronary and systemic administration of basic fibroblast growth factor (b-FGF) to dogs with coronary occlusion enhances endothelial cell proliferation, increases collateral density, and improves collateral blood flow.[212,213] Vascular endothelial growth factor (VEGF) is an endothelial cell–specific mitogen that markedly enhances collateral development following femoral artery occlusion in rabbits[214,215] and coronary occlusion in dogs.[216] Both b-FGF and VEGF are members of the family of heparin-binding growth factors, and some of their actions may be potentiated by the addition of heparin. Some[217,218] but not all[219] investigators have found that the administration of heparin can enhance or accelerate collateral development.

ENDOGENOUS VASODILATORS. The release of endogenous vasodilators such as prostacyclin and nitric oxide maintains collaterals in a dilated state.[219a] Inhibition of prostaglandin synthesis with indomethacin[220] or aspirin[221] results in marked reductions in collateral blood flow. Inhibition of nitric oxide synthesis with N^G-nitro-L-arginine methyl ester (L-NAME) also leads to marked reductions in collateral blood flow.[222] Thus, these two endothelium-derived factors play a central role in the maintenance of collateral flow.

FUNCTIONAL CAPACITY OF COLLATERALS. Mature collaterals can provide normal levels of perfusion to collateral-dependent regions at rest or during moderate exercise in dogs with chronic coronary occlusion.[200] However, during maximal exercise or maximal pharmacologically induced vasodilation, flow to regions perfused by collaterals may be less than normal, especially in subendocardial regions.[197] Relief of coronary occlusion leads to a rapid disappearance of functional and angiographic evidence of coronary collaterals. However, when a previously occluded vessel is reoccluded months later, the collateral circulation functions fully within 60 minutes.[200]

CORONARY COLLATERALS IN HUMANS. Controversy has existed in the past regarding the importance of coronary collaterals in humans.[197,200] However, it is now clear that coronary collaterals can mitigate the severity of myocardial ischemia and myocardial necrosis. Some patients with total occlusion of a major coronary artery may demonstrate no evidence of myocardial infarction and have normal ventricular function at rest.[200] Myocardium in the distribution of occluded coronary arteries with angiographically apparent collaterals has been shown to have better contractile function and less fibrosis than regions in the distribution of noncollateralized occluded vessels.[223]

Percutaneous transluminal coronary angioplasty (PTCA) has served as a model of controlled coronary artery occlusion in humans. During PTCA, collateral filling to the artery being dilated can be visualized by contrast injection into the contralateral coronary artery using a second angiographic catheter.[224] Filling through the collateral artery has been shown to increase significantly during balloon inflation,[225] with the opening of preformed collaterals. These recruitable collaterals afford protection from myocardial ischemia during balloon inflation as judged from the extent and severity of electrocardiographic ST-segment elevation, the appearance of wall-motion abnormalities,[225] and metabolic studies of transmyocardial lactate extraction.[226]

Coronary collaterals also limit the size of myocardial infarction and the clinical sequelae of coronary occlusion. Patients with acute myocardial infarction in whom thrombolytic therapy was unsuccessful may show subsequent improvement in regional and global wall motion if residual flow was improved by extensive collaterals.[218,227] Total occlusion of the left anterior descending coronary artery in association with poor collateral blood supply predisposes to left ventricular aneurysm formation after anterior myocardial infarction. However, coronary collaterals may prevent left ventricular aneurysm formation in such patients by limiting the progression of the wavefront of necrosis from the subendocardial to subepicardial layers and leaving a viable rim of myocardium or by improving the process of healing of the infarcted tissue.[218]

Recently, successful restoration of antegrade coronary blood flow several days or weeks after myocardial infarction has been shown to improve regional wall motion. The use of myocardial contrast echocardiography demonstrated an association between collateral blood flow and myocardial viability.[228] It may be presumed that low levels of

collateral blood flow, not detectable by angiography, maintained the myocardium in a viable although "hibernating" state (see p. 1176).

ENHANCING COLLATERAL FORMATION. There has been much interest in finding ways to enhance collateral function in patients with coronary stenoses. In experimental animals with coronary occlusion, exercise has no influence on collateral development.[197,208,229,230] In the few available clinical studies that utilized repeat coronary angiography, an increase in collaterals occurred only with progression in the severity of coronary artery stenoses, but not with long-term exercise programs.[231,232] The reduction of myocardial ischemia observed after an exercise program is most likely the result of exercise conditioning rather than collateral

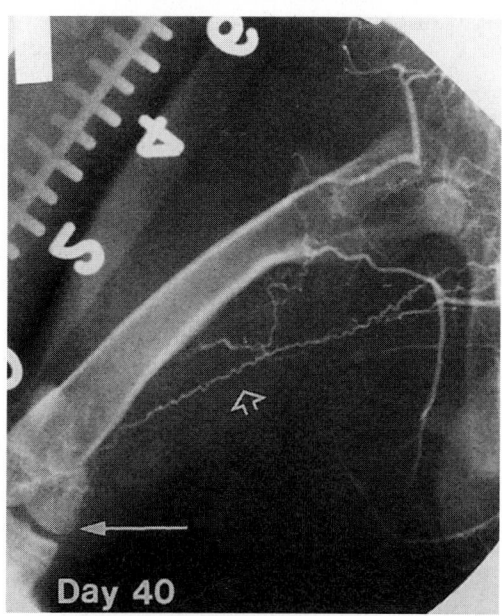

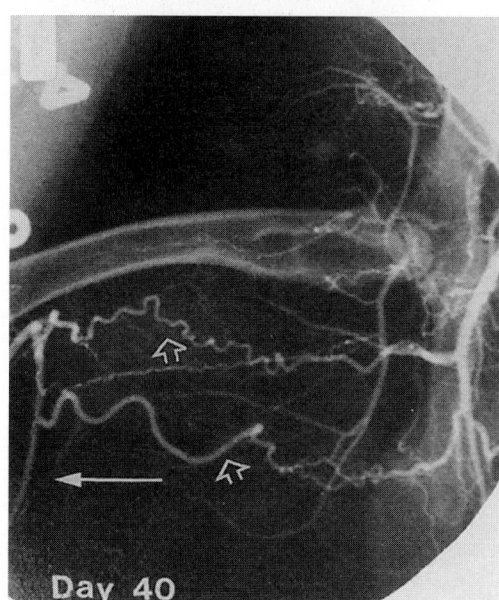

FIGURE 36–21. Selective internal iliac angiography of control rabbit performed at day 40 (control, untreated, *top*) and of VEGF-treated rabbit at day 40 (*bottom*). VEGF was administered as a single intraarterial bolus into the internal iliac artery of rabbits with severe ipsilateral ischemia. The angiogram shown here has yielded angiographic scores of 0.17 and 0.41. Distal reconstitution, barely apparent in the control group (arrows), was evident in the VEGF-treated group (arrows). Direct and linear extension of internal iliac artery to popliteal and/or saphenous arteries was also more evident in VEGF-treated group (open arrows). (From Takeshita, S., et al.: Therapeutic angiogenesis. J. Clin. Invest. *93*:662, 1994, by copyright permission of the American Society for Clinical Investigation.)

expansion. Preliminary studies have suggested that repeat exercise stress combined with injections of heparin may raise the ischemia threshold and improve collateral blood flow[218,233] and that heparin may improve collateral blood flow after myocardial infarction.[234]

Advances in molecular biology are bringing to clinical testing gene therapy for arterial disease.[235,236] After encouraging animal experiments (Fig. 36–21), a clinical trial has been initiated to evaluate whether local delivery of a gene encoding for vascular endothelial growth factor (VEGF) can enhance collateral development in patients with obstructive atherosclerosis involving the lower extremities. An improved understanding of the molecular and cellular mechanisms of angiogenesis should lead to other innovative approaches to augment collateral blood flow more effectively in patients with atherosclerotic stenoses in a variety of vascular beds.

CONSEQUENCES OF MYOCARDIAL ISCHEMIA

Myocardial Stunning and Hibernation
(See also pp. 89 and 388)

For four decades following Tennant and Wiggers' classic observation on the effects of coronary occlusion on myocardial contraction,[237] it was believed that transient severe ischemia caused either irreversible cardiac injury—that is, infarction, or prompt recovery. However, in the 1970's it became clear that after a brief episode of severe ischemia, prolonged myocardial dysfunction with gradual return of contractile activity occurred, a condition termed myocardial stunning[238–240] (Fig. 36–22). Stunning may occur following exercise-induced ischemia[241] and coronary spasm.[242] It affects both systolic and diastolic function[240,243] and can occur in the globally as well as the regionally ischemic heart. Clinically, myocardial stunning probably occurs most frequently in patients who have undergone ischemic cardiac arrest during cardiopulmonary bypass[244]; such hearts may not recover normal function for days. In patients with a myocardial infarction (both with and without the administration of reperfusion thrombolytic therapy), reversibly injured, functionally stunned myocardium lies adjacent to infarcted myocardium.[245,246] Myocardial stunning is an important feature of unstable angina (see p. 1332).

DETERMINANTS OF STUNNING. The severity of the ischemic stress is an important influence in the genesis of myocardial stunning. Bolli et al.[247] found a close relationship

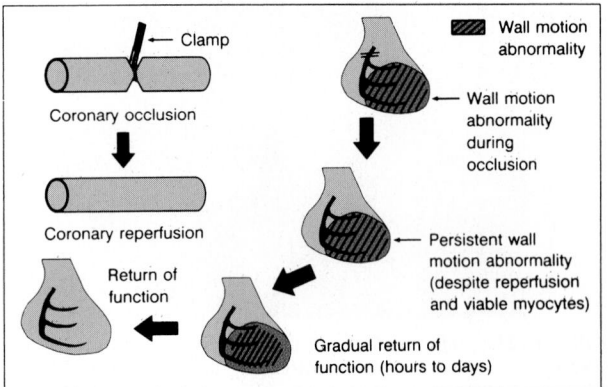

FIGURE 36–22. Schematic diagram of stunned myocardium. During coronary occlusion, a wall motion abnormality of the left ventricle is present in the region supplied by the occluded artery. With relief of ischemia and re-establishment of coronary blood flow, there is a persistent wall motion abnormality despite reperfusion and viable myocytes. There is then gradual improvement in function that requires hours to days for recovery. (From Kloner, R. A., Przyklenk, K., and Patel, B.: Altered myocardial states: The stunned and hibernating myocardium. Am. J. Med. *86*(Suppl. 1A):14, 1986.)

TABLE 36–3 THE PROPOSED MECHANISMS OF MYOCARDIAL STUNNING

1. **Insufficient energy production by mitochondria**
2. **Impaired energy use by myofibrils**
3. **Impaired sympathetic neuronal responsiveness**
4. **Impaired myocardial perfusion**
5. **Damage to the extracellular collagen matrix**
6. **Decreased sensitivity of myofilaments to calcium**
7. **Calcium overload**
8. **Excitation-contraction uncoupling due to dysfunction of sarcoplasmic reticulum**
9. **Generation of damaging oxygen free radicals**

Modified from Bolli, R.: Postischemic myocardial stunning. *In* Yellon, D. M., and Jennings, R. B. (eds.): Myocardial Protection: The Pathophysiology of Reperfusion and Reperfusion Injury. New York, Raven Press, Ltd., 1992.

between the magnitude of blood flow reduction during 15-minute periods of coronary artery occlusion and the degree of myocardial dysfunction after reperfusion. The severity of stunning is always greater in the subendocardial layers of the left ventricular wall which are more ischemic than the subepicardial layers.[247,248] The duration of ischemia is a second important factor.[248]

MECHANISMS OF STUNNING. The sequence of biochemical events whereby transient myocardial ischemia leads to protracted depression of myocardial contractility has not been elucidated definitively.[249] The proposed mechanisms are listed in Table 36-3. Insufficient energy production, impaired energy use by myofibrils, and impaired myocardial perfusion[250] are unlikely mechanisms because the contractility of the stunned myocardium can be transiently but rapidly restored by inotropic stimulation.[251–253] More likely mechanisms include a transient calcium overload of myocytes immediately after reperfusion,[254,255] excitation-contraction uncoupling due to ischemia-induced dysfunction of the sarcoplasmic reticulum,[256] and generation of oxygen free radicals.[257–260] Despite evidence that reperfusion-induced cellular changes are at least in part responsible for myocardial stunning, it is unlikely that reperfusion alone accounts for all of the postischemic damage. More likely, ischemia of the myocardium is associated with multiple and severe metabolic derangements, and recovery of function cannot be expected instantaneously even if no additional injury occurs upon reperfusion.[261,262]

MYOCARDIAL HIBERNATION. Chronic hypoperfusion of the myocardium ("hibernation") is a reversible cause of left ventricular dysfunction. Radionuclide imaging techniques, positron emission tomography, and stress (dobutamine) echocardiography are capable of assessing myocardial perfusion and viability and are helpful in determining whether myocardial dysfunction is due to necrosis or hibernation.

ISCHEMIC PRECONDITIONING. (See p. 1214)

Hemodynamic Consequences of Ischemia

Because the heart has virtually no stores of oxygen, within seconds of coronary occlusion its relatively high rate of energy expenditure results in a sudden, striking decline of myocardial oxygen tension and loss of contractility. If sufficiently widespread, regional impairment of myocardial contractile activity depresses global left ventricular function, causing reductions of stroke volume, stroke work, cardiac output, and ejection fraction while elevating ventricular end-diastolic volume and pressure. Clinical evidence of heart failure occurs when regional asynergy is so severe and extensive that the uninvolved myocardium cannot sustain the normal hemodynamic burden. Left ventricular failure usually develops when contraction ceases in 20 to 25 per cent of the left ventricle. With loss of 40 per cent

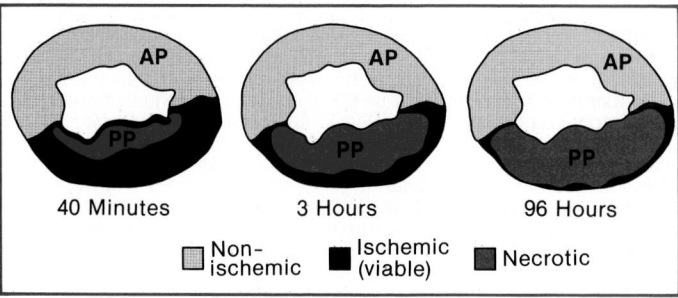

| Non-ischemic | Ischemic (viable) | Necrotic |

FIGURE 36–23. Progression of cell death versus time after circumflex coronary occlusion in dogs. Necrosis occurs first in the subendocardial myocardium. With longer occlusions, a wavefront of cell death moves from the subendocardial zone across the wall to involve progressively more of the transmural thickness of the ischemic zone. In contrast, the lateral margins in the subendocardial region of the infarct are established as early as 40 minutes after occlusion and are sharply defined by the anatomic boundaries of the ischemic bed. AP = anterior papillary muscle; PP = posterior papillary muscle. (From Reimer, K. A., Hill, M. L., and Jennings, R. B.: Prolonged depletion of ATP and of the adenine nucleotide pool due to delayed resynthesis of adenine nucleotides following reversible myocardial ischemic injury in dogs. J. Mol. Cell. Cardiol. *13*:229, 1981.)

or more of the left ventricular myocardium, severe pump failure ensues, and, if this loss is acute, cardiogenic shock develops.

Myocardial ischemia and infarction alter not only the contractile (systolic) properties of the heart but also its diastolic properties (see pp. 1194 and 1195). Ischemia causes both a leftward shift and an increase in the slope of the left ventricular end-diastolic pressure-volume relation so that ventricular pressure is higher at any volume[263] (Fig. 13–14, p. 403). Myocardial ischemia also impairs ventricular relaxation,[264] as evidenced by a decreased rate of the ventricular pressure decline (negative dP/dt) and ventricular wall thinning, and it prolongs the isovolumetric relaxation period.[264,265] With regional ischemia, the reduction of compliance is limited to the ischemic region, whereas the

nonischemic region operates on a higher and steeper portion of its (normal) pressure-volume curve. Thus, the ischemia-induced changes in diastolic properties increase the resistance to ventricular filling.

Thus, ischemia causes impairment of cardiac contraction and incomplete ventricular emptying (systolic failure). In addition, it impairs ventricular relaxation and shifts the diastolic pressure-volume curve leftward (diastolic failure). The combination of systolic and diastolic failure leads to elevated ventricular filling pressures, causing symptoms of pulmonary congestion.

The "Wavefront" of Ischemic Necrosis

As already noted (see p. 1174), within seconds of a coronary artery occlusion, blood begins to flow through preexisting collateral channels to the artery distal to the site of occlusion. Collateral flow is lowest and myocardial oxygen consumption highest in the subendocardium, and therefore ischemia is most severe in this region. In the normal myocardium, thickening and shortening are greater in the subendocardium, as is wall stress, accounting for the higher subendocardial energy requirements.[266,267] Consistent with these findings, higher rates of metabolic activity, lower tissue oxygen tension,[268] and greater oxygen extraction have been found in this region.[269] As a consequence, ischemia becomes most severe and myocardial cells undergo necrosis first in the subendocardium, commencing as early as 15 to 20 minutes after coronary artery occlusion. Necrosis progresses toward the epicardium, gradually involving the less severely ischemic outer layers (Fig. 36–23). The progression of the wavefront of necrosis[269a] is slowed by the presence of residual blood flow when the coronary occlusion is incomplete or when well-developed collaterals are present at the time of occlusion.[270] The progression of the wavefront is accelerated when myocardial ischemia is unusually severe, when collateral blood flow is low, in the presence of marked arterial hypotension (e.g., in patients in cardiogenic shock), and in the presence of elevated myocardial

FIGURE 36–24. Time course of metabolic changes during myocardial ischemia plotted by transmural layer (I = inner, subendocardial; M = middle; O = outer, subepicardial). Ischemia was induced by circumflex occlusion in anesthetized dogs. Data for different times are based on different groups of dogs; N = 4 to 6; brackets indicate plus or minus one standard error of the mean. *A*, More rapid depletion of ATP in the inner layer, highly significant after 5 min of ischemia (P < 0.01). *B*, Tissue lactate accumulation, with the most rapid accumulation in the subendocardium. For all layers there was a progressive increase in lactate content during the first 10 min of ischemia. Between 10 and 40 min there was continued lactate accumulation in the inner and middle layers, but not in the outer layer. *C*, Total adenine nucleotide content (ATP + ADP + AMP). Adenine nucleotide degradation was most rapid in the subendocardium. Note the time lag between ATP depletion (graph A) and adenine nucleotide breakdown. *D*, Total nucleosides and bases, which are the products of adenine nucleotide degradation. Accumulation was fastest in the subendocardium. As with lactate (graph B), nucleoside and

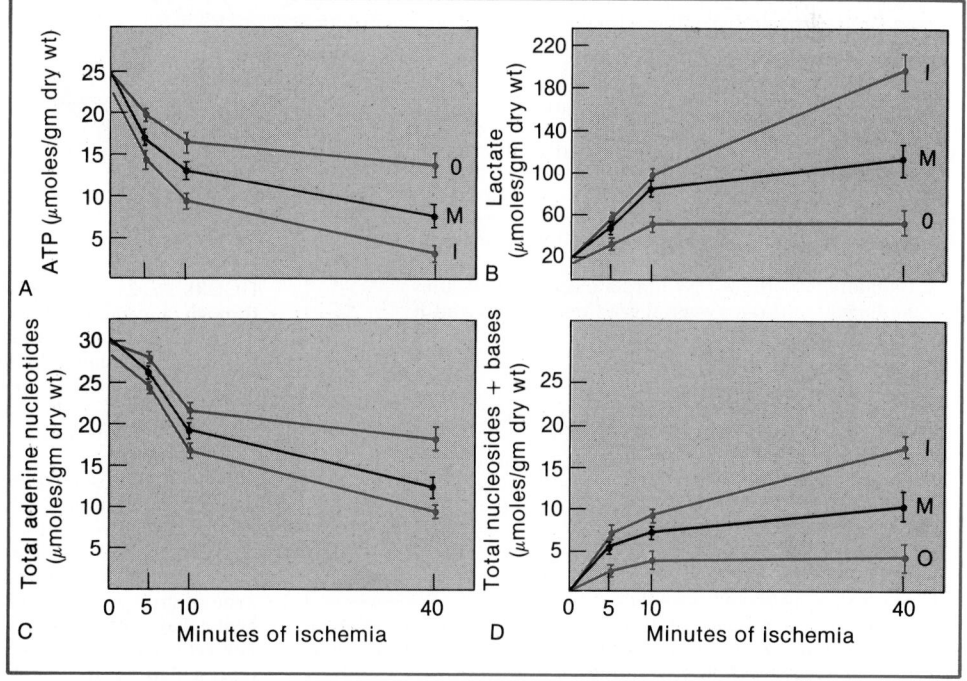

base content in the outer layer was maximal by 10 minutes and was not further increased at 40 minutes, even though adenine nucleotide breakdown in this layer continued (graph C). (From Reimer, K. A., and Jennings, R. B.: Myocardial ischemia, hypoxia, and infarction. *In* Fozzard, H. A., Jennings, R. B., Haber, E., Katz, A. M., and Morgan, H. E. [eds.]: The Heart and Cardiovascular System. 2nd ed. New York, Raven Press, 1991, p. 1888. From the studies of Murry, C. E., et al.: Collateral blood flow and transmural location: Independent determinants of ATP in ischemic canine myocardium. Fed. Proc. *44*:823, 1985.)

oxygen demand, as may be caused by inotropic stimulation (tachycardia or fever).

The transmural progression of necrosis has been demonstrated in dogs with a variable duration of coronary occlusion prior to reperfusion,[271] and in humans.[272] The recognition of the time-dependent progression of necrosis is the basis of interventions designed to arrest the progression of necrosis as rapidly as possible by reperfusion of occluded coronary arteries, using thrombolytic therapy or angioplasty.

Effects of Ischemia on Myocardial Metabolism

HIGH-ENERGY PHOSPHATE METABOLISM. During the first minutes of severe ischemia, the production of high-energy phosphates (the sum of ATP and creatine phosphate [CP]) declines and is greatly exceeded by their utilization. Therefore, tissue stores of high-energy phosphates decline progressively, with CP stores falling more rapidly than ATP stores. CP is depleted by transfer of high-energy phosphate to ADP as oxidative synthesis of ATP declines. In the absence of normal oxidative phosphorylation, ADP is converted to AMP (in the myokinase reaction), which in turn is broken down to adenosine and ultimately to inosine, hypoxanthine, and xanthine.[273] These changes are more striking in the subendocardium (Fig. 36–24). When tissue is only reversibly injured by ischemia (i.e., when its viability can still be maintained by reperfusion), ATP stores are usually greater than 60 per cent of control, and electron microscopy may reveal only glycogen loss, nuclear chromatin clumping, intermyofibrillar edema, and mitochondrial swelling but no sarcolemmal damage or accumulation of amorphous dense bodies in the mitochondria. When ATP content is reduced below 20 per cent of control values, cells become unable to regenerate high-energy phosphate or to maintain physiological ionic gradients and cell volume. The combination of reduced myocardial high-energy phosphate stores, cell swelling, and sarcolemmal damage (potentially attributable to oxygen-derived free radicals, causing lipid peroxidation) appears to play a key role in cell death with ischemia or reperfusion (Table 36–4).

OXIDATIVE PHOSPHORYLATION. The importance of oxidative phosphorylation—that is, the coupling of ATP synthesis to aerobic respiration—for the metabolic integrity of myocardium is underscored by some simple considerations. Complete oxidation of 1 mole of glucose gives rise to the net production of 36 moles of ATP. In contrast, only 2 moles of ATP are produced from anaerobic metabolism of 1 mole of glucose. Thus, even if the profound derangements in intermediary metabolism associated with increased production of reducing equivalents accompanying anaerobic glycolysis could be corrected, an 18-fold increase in glycolytic flux would be required for myocardium to synthesize comparable quantities of ATP via anaerobic compared with aerobic metabolism. The failure of energy production to keep pace with demand in ischemic cells is manifested by a prompt decline in the concentration of CP, a major constituent of myocardial high-energy phosphate stores.

ALTERATIONS IN CELLULAR ELECTROPHYSIOLOGY. The effects of ischemia on the electrophysiological properties of cardiac muscle are numerous and complex. Ischemia-induced ventricular tachyarrhyth-mias can be caused by increased automaticity, triggered activity, and reentry. The early electrophysiological hallmarks of ischemia include a marked diminution in the resting membrane potential, the action potential amplitude, the rate of upstroke of phase 0, and the action potential duration. Activation of ATP-sensitive K^+ channels appears to be responsible for the latter. Within 10 minutes of ischemia, action potential alterations in amplitude and duration become prominent, with subsequent diminution of excitability and conduction block. These alterations are discussed in Chap. 20.

ROLE OF CALCIUM IN ISCHEMIC INJURY. Myocardial injury induced by ischemia is associated with complexes of calcium in the tissue detectable by electron microscopy. As pointed out above, ischemia—whatever its cause—is characterized by a reduction of myocardial ATP stores, which interferes with the transsarcolemmal Na^+-K^+ exchange, which in turn elevates intracellular $[Na^+]$, raising intracellular $[Ca^{++}]$ through an enhanced Na^+-Ca^{++} exchange (see p. 386). Lowered ATP stores also reduce Ca^{++} uptake by the sarcoplasmic reticulum and reduce extrusion of Ca^{++} from cells. The resultant augmented intracellular $[Ca^{++}]$[274] causes mitochondrial Ca^{++} overload, which decreases ATP production further. Activation of intracellular Ca^{++} ATPases augments ATP usage and activates sarcolemmal phospholipases, which release membrane phospholipid degradation products whose detergent properties impair the integrity of the cell membrane.[275]

Calcium antagonists interfere with Ca^{++} influx through voltage-dependent channels. Beta-adrenoreceptor agonists recruit additional receptor-operated channels, and beta-adrenoreceptor blockers reduce Ca^{++} influx by interfering with this recruitment of receptor-operated channels. Thus, one would expect beta blockers and Ca^{++}

TABLE 36–4 POTENTIAL CAUSES OF IRREVERSIBILITY

High-energy phosphate depletion/cessation of anaerobic glycolysis
    Catabolism without resynthesis of macromolecules
    Reduced transsarcolemmal gradients of Na^+ and K^+
        Cell swelling
    Calcium overload
        Activation of phospholipases/proteases
        Impaired mitochondrial function
        Activation of ATPases

Catabolite accumulation (lactate, H^+ (acidosis), fatty acid derivatives, free radicals, ammonia, inorganic phosphate, etc.)
    Enzyme denaturation
    Membrane damage
    Increased intracellular osmolarity
    Cell swelling

Cell death may be related to the consequences of one or both general features of ischemic injury shown above. Some effects of ischemia may be related to both high-energy phosphate depletion and catabolite accumulation. For example, cell swelling may be due both to loss of ATP-dependent ion transport and to intracellular production of small-molecular-weight catabolites.

From Reimer, K. A., and Jennings, R. B.: Myocardial ischemia, hypoxia and infarction. *In* Fozzard, H. A., Haber, E., Jennings, R. B., et al. (eds.): The Heart and Cardiovascular System. 2nd ed. New York, Raven Press, 1991, pp. 1875–1974.

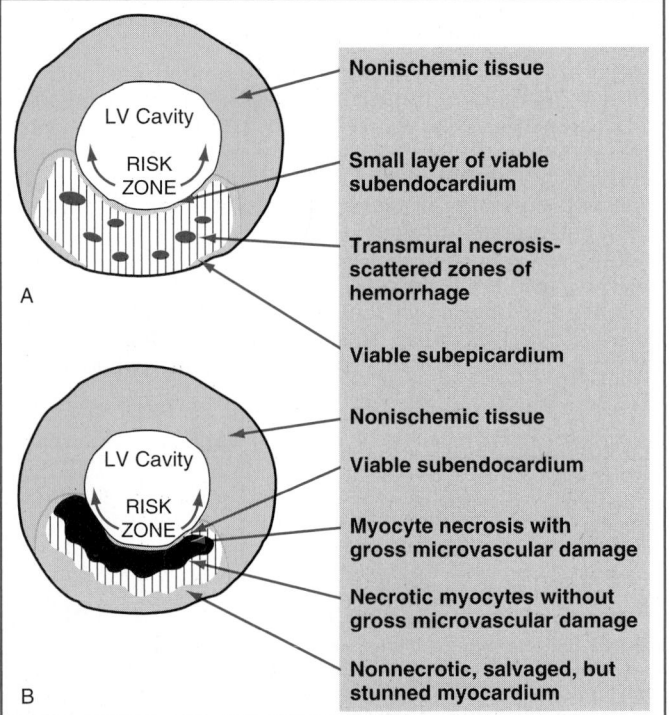

Nonischemic tissue

Small layer of viable subendocardium

Transmural necrosis-scattered zones of hemorrhage

Viable subepicardium

Nonischemic tissue

Viable subendocardium

Myocyte necrosis with gross microvascular damage

Necrotic myocytes without gross microvascular damage

Nonnecrotic, salvaged, but stunned myocardium

FIGURE 36–25. *A,* Schematic diagram showing a transverse section through a canine left ventricle subjected to a permanent coronary occlusion without reperfusion. The white area represents nonischemic myocardium supplied by the nonoccluded vessel. The infarct (hatched area) is transmural or near-transmural. There are scattered zones of hemorrhage (solid black). A small layer of viable subendocardium is present, which derives its oxygen directly from the ventricular cavity. Where collateral flow is high, there may be a small rim of surviving subepicardium (shaded areas). *B,* Schematic diagram showing a transverse section through a canine left ventricle subjected to coronary occlusion followed within 1 or 2 hours by coronary reperfusion. The hatched and solid black areas represent the infarct that is confined to the inner half of the myocardium. The solid black areas represent the zone of gross microvascular damage including zones of no-reflow and hemorrhage. It is smaller than and contained within the total infarct. The remainder of the infarct without severe microvascular damage is represented by the hatched area and is located in the midmyocardium. The epicardial portion of the ischemic zone (stippled area) has been salvaged by coronary reperfusion. It is nonnecrotic but stunned (postischemic ventricular dysfunction) for hours to days following coronary reperfusion. (From Braunwald, E., and Kloner, R. A.: Myocardial reperfusion: A double-edged sword? J. Clin. Invest. *76:*1715, 1985, by copyright permission of the American Society for Clinical Investigation.)

antagonists to have similar effects in the treatment of ischemia. Indeed, both groups of compounds delay ischemia-induced necrosis and, particularly when combined with reperfusion, reduce the extent of myocardial necrosis.[276-280]

REPERFUSION INJURY

Despite the unequivocal utility of reperfusion in limiting cell death in the presence of severe ischemia, reperfusion can elicit a number of adverse reactions that may limit its beneficial actions[281,282] (Fig. 36–25).

ACCELERATION OF MYOCYTE NECROSIS. After reperfusion, ischemic cells often suddenly develop ultrastructural changes indicative of cell death, including "explosive swelling"[283] and widespread architectural disruption. Nevertheless, it is likely that most—perhaps all—of the myocytes in which necrosis is accelerated by reperfusion were already irreversibly injured by the time reperfusion occurred and that reperfusion merely hastened the death of cells already destined not to recover. If reperfusion does cause necrosis of reversibly injured myocardium, the quantity of tissue so affected is likely small.

THE "NO-REFLOW" PHENOMENON. This refers to the failure to achieve sustained reperfusion after a prolonged period of ischemia. The areas of reduced or absent reflow often appear to result from ischemia-induced microvascular damage and myocardial contracture. However, the no-reflow phenomenon does not appear to augment myocyte death, because the zone of reflow is contained within areas in which myocytes were already necrotic at the time of the onset of reperfusion (Fig. 36–25).

REPERFUSION-INDUCED HEMORRHAGE. Reperfused infarcts frequently contain hemorrhagic areas.[284] Reperfusion-induced hemorrhage, like the "no-reflow" phenomenon, is caused largely by microvascular damage. It is generally contained within areas of myocardium already necrotic at the time of reperfusion.[285]

Thus, it appears that reperfusion can be detrimental by causing arrhythmias and can contribute to myocardial stunning, although it is not clear that this process causes necrosis of many *reversibly* injured ischemic cells.[286]

REFERENCES

DETERMINANTS OF MYOCARDIAL OXYGEN CONSUMPTION

1. Reimer, K. A., and Jennings, R. B.: Myocardial ischemia, hypoxia and infarction. In Fozzard, H. A., Haber, E., Jennings, R. B., et al. (eds.): The Heart and Cardiovascular System. 2nd ed. New York, Raven Press, 1991, pp. 1875–1974.
2. Braunwald, E.: Control of myocardial oxygen consumption: Physiologic and clinical considerations. Am. J. Cardiol. 27:416, 1971.
3. Klocke, F. J., Braunwald, E., and Ross, J., Jr.: Oxygen cost of electrical activation of the heart. Circ. Res. 18:357, 1966.
4. Loiselle, D. S.: Cardiac basal and activation metabolism. In Jacob, R., Just, H. J., and Holubarsch, D. H. (eds.): Cardiac Energetics: Basic Mechanisms and Clinical Implications. New York, Springer-Verlag, 1987, pp. 37–50.
5. Evans, C. L., and Matsuoka, Y.: The effect of various mechanical conditions on the gaseous metabolism and efficiency of the mammalian heart. J. Physiol. 49:378, 1915.
6. Sarnoff, S. J., Braunwald, E., Welch, G. H., Jr., et al.: Hemodynamic determinants of oxygen consumption of the heart with special reference to the tension-time index. Am. J. Physiol. 192:148, 1958.
7. Braunwald, E., Sarnoff, S. J., Case, R. B., et al.: Hemodynamic determinants of coronary flow: Effect of changes in aortic pressure and cardiac output on the relationship between myocardial oxygen consumption and coronary blood flow. Am. J. Physiol. 192:157, 1958.
8. Boerth, R. C., Covell, J. W., Pool, P. E., and Ross, J., Jr.: Increased myocardial oxygen consumption and contractile state associated with increased heart rate in dogs. Circ. Res. 24:725, 1969.
9. Rooke, G. A., and Feigl, E. O.: Work as a correlate of canine left ventricular oxygen consumption, and the problem of catecholamine oxygen wasting. Circ. Res. 50:273, 1982.
10. Suga, H.: Ventricular energetics. Physiol. Rev. 70:247, 1990.
10a. Kameyama, T., Asanoi, H., Ishizaka, S., et al.: Energy conversion efficiency in human left ventricle. Circulation 85:988, 1992.
11. Takaoka, H., Takeuchi, M., Odake, M., et al.: Comparison of hemodynamic determinants for myocardial oxygen consumption under different contractile states in human ventricle. Circulation 87:59, 1993.
12. Graham, T. P., Jr., Covell, J. W., Sonnenblick, E. H., et al.: Control of myocardial oxygen consumption: Relative influence of contractile state and tension development. J. Clin. Invest. 47:375, 1968.
13. Vik-Mo, H., and Mjos, O. D.: Influence of free fatty acids on myocardial oxygen consumption and ischemic injury. Am. J. Cardiol. 48:361, 1981.

REGULATION OF CORONARY BLOOD FLOW

14. Young, M. A., and Vatner, S. F.: Regulation of large coronary arteries. Circ. Res. 59:579, 1986.
15. Provenza, D. V., and Scherlis, S.: Coronary circulation in dog's heart: Demonstration of muscle sphincters in capillaries. Circ. Res. 7:318, 1959.
16. Olsson, R. A., and Bugni, W. J.: Coronary circulation. In Fozzard, H. A., Jennings, R. B., Haber, E., et al. (eds.): The Heart and Cardiovascular System. New York, Raven Press, 1986, pp. 987–1038.

17. Bache, R. J., and Hess, D. S.: Reactive hyperemia following one-beat coronary occlusions in the awake dog. Am. J. Physiol. 250:H474, 1986.
18. Sadick, N., Dube, G. P., McHale, P. A., and Greenfield, J. C., Jr.: Metabolic mediation of single brief diastolic occlusion reactive hyperemic responses. Am. J. Physiol. 253:H25, 1987.
19. Dube, G. P., Bemis, K. G., and Greenfield, J. C., Jr.: Distinction between metabolic and myogenic mechanisms of coronary hyperemic response to brief diastolic occlusion. Circ. Res. 68:1313, 1991.
20. Marcus, M. L.: The coronary circulation. In Marcus, M. L. (ed.): The Coronary Circulation in Health and Disease. New York, McGraw-Hill Book Co., 1983, pp. 65–92.
21. Sparks, H. V., Jr., and Bardenheuer, H.: Regulation of adenosine formation by the heart. Circ. Res. 58:193, 1986.
22. Berne, R. M.: The role of adenosine in the regulation of coronary blood flow. Circ. Res. 47:807, 1980.
23. Belardinelli, L., Linden, J., and Berne, R. M.: The cardiac effects of adenosine. Prog. Cardiovasc. Dis. 32:73, 1989.
24. Headrick, J. P., Ely, S. W., Matherne, G. P., and Berne, R. M.: Myocardial adenosine, flow, and metabolism during adenosine antagonism and adrenergic stimulation. Am. J. Physiol. 264:H61, 1993.
25. Radford, M. J., McHale, P. A., Sadick, N., et al.: Effect of aminophylline on coronary reactive and functional hyperaemic response in conscious dogs. Cardiovasc. Res. 18:377, 1984.
26. Sawmiller, D. R., Linden, J., and Berne, R. M.: Effects of xanthine amine congener on hypoxic coronary resistance and venous and epicardial adenosine concentrations. Cardiovasc. Res. 28:604, 1994.
27. Ely, S. W., Matherne, G. P., Coleman, S. D., and Berne, R. M.: Inhibition of adenosine metabolism increases myocardial interstitial adenosine concentrations and coronary flow. J. Mol. Cell. Cardiol. 24:1321, 1992.
28. Martin, S. E., Lenhard, S. D., Schmarkey, L. S., et al.: Adenosine regulates coronary blood flow during increased work and decreased supply. Am. J. Physiol. 264:H1438, 1993.
29. Billman, G. E.: Effects of aminophylline on behaviorally induced coronary blood flow increases. Am. J. Physiol. 253:H548, 1987.
30. Jones, C. E., Hurst, T. W., and Randall, J. R.: Effect of aminophylline on coronary functional hyperemia and myocardial adenosine. Am. J. Physiol. 243:H480, 1982.
31. Rossen, J. D., Oskarsson, H., Minor, R. L., et al.: Effect of adenosine antagonism on metabolically mediated coronary vasodilation in humans. J. Am. Coll. Cardiol. 23:1421, 1994.
32. Yamabe, H., Okumura, K., Ishizaka, H., et al.: Role of endothelium-derived nitric oxide in myocardial reactive hyperemia. Am. J. Physiol. 263:H8, 1992.
32a. DiCarleto, P. E., and Gimbrone, M. A. Jr.: Vascular endothelium. In Fuster, V., Ross, R., and Topol, E. J. (eds.): Atherosclerosis and Coronary Artery Disease. Philadelphia, Lippincott-Raven, 1996, pp. 387–400.
33. Furchgott, R. F., and Zawadzki, J. V.: The obligatory role of endothelial cells in the relaxation of arterial smooth muscle by acetylcholine. Nature 288:373, 1980.
34. Needleman, P., and Kaley, S.: Cardiac and coronary prostaglandin synthesis and function. N. Engl. J. Med. 298:1122, 1978.
35. Vanhoutte, P. M.: Endothelium-derived relaxing and contracting factors. Adv. Nephrol. 19:3, 1990.
36. Palmer, R. M., Ferrige, A. G., and Moncada, S.: Nitric oxide release accounts for the biological activity of endothelium-derived relaxing factor. Nature 327:524, 1987.
37. Ignarro, L. J., Byrns, R. E., Buga, G. M., and Wood, K. S.: Endothelium-derived relaxing factor from pulmonary artery and vein possesses pharmacological and chemical properties identical to those of nitric oxide radical. Circ. Res. 61:866, 1987.
38. Myers, P. R., Minor, R. L., Jr., Guerra, R., Bates, J. N., and Harrison, D. G.: The vasorelaxant properties of the endothelium-derived relaxing factor more closely resemble S-nitrosocysteine than nitric oxide. Nature 345:161, 1990.
39. Palmer, R. M., Ashton, D. S., and Moncada, S.: Vascular endothelial cells synthesize nitric oxide from L-arginine. Nature 333:664, 1988.
40. Lamas, S., Marsden, P. A., Li, G. K., et al.: Endothelial nitric oxide synthase: Molecular cloning and characterization of a distinct constitutive enzyme isoform. Proc. Natl. Acad. Sci. U.S.A. 89:6348, 1992.
41. Vanhoutte, P. M., and Shimokawa, H.: Endothelium-derived relaxing factor and coronary vasospasm. Circulation 80:1, 1989.
42. Martin, W., Furchgott, R. F., Villani, D., and Jothianandan, D.: Depression of contractile responses in rat aorta by spontaneously released endothelium-derived relaxing factor. J. Pharmacol. Exp. Ther. 237:529, 1986.
43. Vane, J. R., Anggard, E. E., and Botting, R. M.: Regulatory functions of the vascular endothelium. N. Engl. J. Med. 323:27, 1990.
44. Furchgott, R. F.: The 1989 Ulf von Euler lecture: Studies on endothelium-dependent vasodilation and the endothelium-derived relaxing factor. Acta. Physiol. Scand. 139:257, 1990.
45. Lüscher, T. F., and Tanner, F. C.: Endothelial regulation of vascular tone and growth. Am. J. Hypertens. 6:283S, 1993.
46. Ludmer, P. L., Selwyn, A. P., Shook, T. L., et al.: Paradoxical vasoconstriction induced by acetylcholine in atherosclerotic coronary arteries. N. Engl. J. Med. 315:1046, 1986.
47. Lefroy, D. C., Crake, T., Uren, N. G., et al.: Effect of inhibition of nitric oxide synthesis on epicardial coronary artery caliber and coronary blood flow in humans. Circulation 88:43, 1993.
47a. Quyyumi, A. A., Dakak, N., Andrews, N. P., et al.: Nitric oxide activity

in the human coronary circulation. Impact of risk factors for coronary atherosclerosis. J. Clin. Invest. 95:1747, 1995.

48. Golino, P., Piscione, F., Willerson, J. T., et al.: Divergent effects of serotonin on coronary artery dimensions and blood flow in patients with coronary atherosclerosis and control patients. N. Engl. J. Med. 324:641, 1991.

49. Matsuyama, K., Yasue, H., Okumura, K., et al.: Effects of H_1-receptor stimulation on coronary arterial diameter and coronary hemodynamics in humans. Circulation 81:65, 1990.

50. Nabel, E. G., Selwyn, A. P., and Ganz, P.: Large coronary arteries in humans are responsive to changes in blood flow: An endothelium-dependent mechanism that fails in patients with atherosclerosis. J. Am. Coll. Cardiol. 16:349, 1990.

51. Drexler, H., Zeiher, A. M., Wollschläger, H., et al.: Flow-dependent coronary artery dilatation in humans. Circulation 80:466, 1989.

52. Weidinger, F. F., McLenachan, J. M., Cybulsky, M. I., et al.: Hypercholesterolemia enhances macrophage recruitment and dysfunction of regenerated endothelium after balloon injury of the rabbit iliac artery. Circulation 84:755, 1991.

53. Shimokawa, H., Aarhus, L. L., and Vanhoutte, P. M.: Porcine coronary arteries with regenerated endothelium have a reduced endothelium-dependent responsiveness to aggregating platelets and serotonin. Circ. Res. 61:256, 1987.

54. Fish, R. D., Nabel, E. G., Selwyn, A. P., et al.: Responses of coronary arteries of cardiac transplant patients to acetylcholine. J. Clin. Invest. 81:21, 1988.

55. Zeiher, A. M., Drexler, H., Wollschläger, H., and Just, H.: Modulation of coronary vasomotor tone in humans: Progressive endothelial dysfunction with different early stages of coronary atherosclerosis. Circulation 83:391, 1991.

56. McFadden, E. P., Clarke, J. G., Davies, G. J., et al.: Effect of intracoronary serotonin on coronary vessels in patients with stable angina and patients with variant angina. N. Engl. J. Med. 324:648, 1991.

57. Cox, D. A., Vita, J. A., Treasure, C. B., et al.: Atherosclerosis impairs flow-mediated dilation of coronary arteries in humans. Circulation 80:458, 1989.

58. Furchgott, R. F., Carvalho, M. H., Khan, M. T., and Matsunaga, K.: Evidence for endothelium-dependent vasodilation of resistance vessels by acetylcholine. Blood Vessels 24:145, 1987.

59. Aalkjaer, C., Heagerty, A. M., Swales, J. D., and Thurston, H.: Endothelium-dependent relaxation in human subcutaneous resistance vessels. Blood Vessels 24:85, 1987.

60. Vallance, P., Collier, J., and Moncada, S.: Effects of endothelium-derived nitric oxide on peripheral arteriolar tone in man. Lancet 2:997, 1989.

61. Creager, M. A., Cooke, J. P., Mendelsohn, M. E., et al.: Impaired vasodilation of forearm resistance vessels in hypercholesterolemic humans. J. Clin. Invest. 86:228, 1990.

62. Treasure, C. B., Vita, J. A., Cox, D. A., et al.: Endothelium-dependent dilation of the coronary microvasculature is impaired in dilated cardiomyopathy. Circulation 81:772, 1990.

63. Sellke, F. W., Armstrong, M. L., and Harrison, D. G.: Endothelium-dependent vascular relaxation is abnormal in the coronary microcirculation of atherosclerotic primates. Circulation 81:1586, 1990.

64. Zeiher, A. M., Drexler, H., Wollschläger, H., and Just, H.: Endothelial dysfunction of the coronary microvasculature is associated with impaired coronary blood flow regulation in patients with early atherosclerosis. Circulation 84:1984, 1991.

64a. Quyyumi, A., Dakak, N., Andrews, N. P., et al.: Contribution of nitric oxide to metabolic coronary vasodilation in the human heart. Circulation 92:320, 1995.

65. Yeung, A. C., Vekshtein, V. I., Krantz, D. S., et al.: The effect of atherosclerosis on the vasomotor response of coronary arteries to mental stress. N. Engl. J. Med. 325:1551, 1989.

66. Gordon, J. B., Ganz, P., Nabel, E. G., et al.: Atherosclerosis influences the vasomotor response of epicardial coronary arteries to exercise. J. Clin. Invest. 83:1946, 1989.

67. Nabel, E. G., Selwyn, A. P., and Ganz, P.: Paradoxical narrowing of atherosclerotic coronary arteries induced by increases in heart rate. Circulation 81:850, 1990.

68. Meredith, I. T., Yeung, A. C., Weidinger, F. F., et al.: Role of impaired endothelium-dependent vasodilation in ischemic manifestations of coronary artery disease. Circulation 87:V–56, 1993.

69. Vita, J. A., Treasure, C. B., Yeung, A. C., et al.: Patients with evidence of coronary endothelial dysfunction as assessed by acetylcholine infusion demonstrate marked increase in sensitivity to constrictor effects of catecholamines. Circulation 85:1390, 1992.

70. Zeiher, A. M., Drexler, H., Wollschläger, H., et al.: Coronary vasomotion in response to sympathetic stimulation in humans: Importance of the functional integrity of the endothelium. J. Am. Coll. Cardiol. 14:1181, 1989.

71. Levine, G. N., Keaney, J. F., Jr., and Vita, J. A.: Cholesterol reduction in cardiovascular disease. N. Engl. J. Med. 332:512, 1995.

72. Fuster, V., Stein, B., Ambrose, J. A., et al.: Atherosclerotic plaque rupture and thrombosis: Evolving concepts. Circulation 82(Suppl. II):II–47, 1990.

72a. Stary, H. C., Chandler, A. B., Dinsmore, R. E., et al.: A definition of advanced types of atherosclerotic lesions and a histological classification of atherosclerosis. Circulation 92:1355, 1995.

73. Maseri, A., Severi, S., DeNes, D. M., et al.: "Variant" angina: One aspect of a continuous spectrum of vasospastic myocardial ischemia: Pathogenetic mechanisms, estimated incidence and clinical and coronary angiographic findings in 138 patients. Am. J. Cardiol. 42:1019, 1978.

74. Van den Berg, E. K., Schmitz, J. M., Benedict, C. R., et al.: Transcardiac serotonin concentration is increased in selected patients with limiting angina and complex coronary lesion morphology. Circulation 79:116, 1989.

75. Zeiher, A. M., Krause, T., Schächinger, V., et al.: Impaired endothelium-dependent vasodilatation of coronary resistance vessels is associated with exercise-induced myocardial ischemia. Circulation 91:2345, 1995.

76. Zeiher, A. M., Goebel, H., Schächinger, V., and Ihling, C.: Tissue endothelin-1 immunoreactivity in the active coronary atherosclerotic plaque. Circulation 91:941–947, 1995.

77. Motz, W., Vogt, M., Rabenau, O., et al.: Evidence of endothelial dysfunction in coronary resistance vessels in patients with angina pectoris and normal coronary angiograms. Am. J. Cardiol. 68:996, 1991.

78. Quyyumi, A. A., Cannon, R. O., III, Panza, J. A., et al.: Endothelial dysfunction in patients with chest pain and normal coronary arteries. Circulation 86:1864, 1992.

79. Egashira, K., Inour, T., Hirooka, Y., et al.: Evidence of impaired endothelium-dependent coronary vasodilatation in patients with angina pectoris and normal coronary angiograms. N. Engl. J. Med. 328:1659, 1993.

80. Vita, J. A., Treasure, C. B., Nabel, E. G., et al.: The coronary vasomotor response to acetylcholine relates to risk factors for coronary artery disease. Circulation 81:491, 1990.

81. Egashira, K., Inou, T., Hirooka, Y., et al.: Impaired coronary blood flow response to acetylcholine in patients with coronary risk factors and proximal atherosclerotic lesions. J. Clin. Invest. 91:29, 1993.

81a. Zeiher, A. M., Schächinger, V., and Minners, J.: Long-term cigarette smoking impairs endothelium-dependent coronary arterial vasodilator function. Circulation 92:1094, 1995.

82. Anderson, T. J., Meredith, I. T., Yeung, A. C., et al.: The effect of cholesterol-lowering and antioxidant therapy on endothelium-dependent coronary vasomotion. N. Engl. J. Med. 332:488, 1995.

83. Treasure, C. B., Klein, J. L., Weintraub, W. S., et al.: Beneficial effects of cholesterol-lowering therapy on the coronary endothelium in patients with coronary artery disease. N. Engl. J. Med. 332:481, 1995.

84. Egashira, K., Hirooka, Y., Kai, H., et al.: Reduction in serum cholesterol with pravastatin improves endothelium-dependent coronary vasomotion in patients with hypercholesterolemia. Circulation 89:2519, 1994.

84a. Leung, W. H., Lau, C. P., and Wong, C. K.: Beneficial effect of cholesterol-lowering therapy on coronary endothelium-dependent relaxation in hypercholesterolemic patients. Lancet 341:1496, 1993.

85. Yanagisawa, M., Kurihara, H., Kimura, S., et al.: A novel potent vasoconstrictor peptide produced by vascular endothelial cells. Nature 332:411, 1988.

86. Seo, B., Oemar, B. S., Siebenmann, R., et al.: Both ET_A and ET_B receptors mediate contraction to endothelin-1 in human blood vessels. Circulation 89:1203, 1994.

87. Lüscher, T. F.: Endothelin: Systemic arterial and pulmonary effects of a new peptide with potent biological properties. Am. Rev. Respir. Dis. 146:S56, 1992.

88. Lerman, A., Edwards, B. S., Hallett, J. W., et al.: Circulating and tissue endothelin immunoreactivity in advanced atherosclerosis. N. Engl. J. Med. 325:997, 1991.

89. Stewart, D. J., Kubac, G., Costello, K. B., and Cernacek, P.: Increased plasma endothelin-1 in the early hours of acute myocardial infarction. J. Am. Coll. Cardiol. 18:38, 1991.

90. Wei, C. M., Lerman, A., Rodeheffer, R. J., et al.: Endothelin in human congestive heart failure. Circulation 89:1580, 1994.

91. Lüscher, T. F., Boulanger, C. M., Dohi, Y., and Yang, Z.: Endothelium-derived contracting factors. Hypertension 19:117, 1992.

92. Ehrenreich, H., Anderson, R. W., Fox, C. H., et al.: Endothelins, peptides with potent vasoactive properties, are produced by human macrophages. J. Exp. Med. 172:1741, 1990.

93. Moreno, P. R., Falk, E., Palacios, I. F., et al.: Macrophage infiltration in acute coronary syndromes: Implications for plaque rupture. Circulation 90:775, 1994.

94. Van der Wal, A. C., Becker, A. E., Van der Loos, C. M., and Das, P. K.: Site of intimal rupture or erosion of thrombosed coronary atherosclerotic plaques is characterized by an inflammatory process irrespective of the dominant plaque morphology. Circulation 89:36, 1994.

95. Lüscher, T. F.: Endothelin, endothelin receptors, and endothelin antagonists. Curr. Opin. Nephrol. Hypertens. 3:92, 1994.

96. Scandinavian Simvastatin Survival Study Group: Randomised trial of cholesterol lowering in 4444 patients with coronary heart disease: The Scandinavian Simvastatin Survival Study (4S). Lancet 344:1383, 1994.

97. Johnson, P. C.: Autoregulation of blood flow. Circ. Res. 59:483, 1986.

98. Olsson, R. A., Bunger, R., and Spaan, J. A. E.: Coronary circulation. In Fozzard, H. A., Haber, E., Jennings, R. B., et al. (eds.): The Heart and Cardiovascular System. 2nd ed. New York, Raven Press, 1991, pp. 1392–1426.

99. Harrison, D. G., Florentine, M. S., Brooks, L. A., et al.: The effect of hypertension and left ventricular hypertrophy on the lower range of coronary autoregulation. Circulation 77:1108, 1988.

100. Rouleau, J., Boerboom, L. E., Surjadhana, A., and Hoffman, J. I. E.: The role of autoregulation and tissue diastolic pressures in the transmural distribution of left ventricular blood flow in anesthetized dogs. Circ. Res. 45:804, 1979.

101. Hoffman, J. I. E.: Maximal coronary flow and the concept of coronary vascular reserve. Circulation 70:153, 1984.

102. Marcus, M. L.: The coronary circulation. *In* Marcus, M. L. (ed.): The Coronary Circulation in Health and Disease. New York, McGraw-Hill Book Co., 1983, pp. 93–112.

103. Smith, T. P., Jr., and Canty, J. M., Jr.: Modulation of coronary autoregulatory responses by nitric oxide: Evidence for flow-dependent resistance adjustments in conscious dogs. Circ. Res. 73:232, 1993.

104. Ueeda, M., Silvia, S. K., and Olsson, R. A.: Nitric oxide modulates coronary autoregulation in the guinea pig. Circ. Res. 70:1296, 1992.

105. Lansman, J. B., Hallam, T. J., and Rink, T. J.: Single stretch-activated ion channels in vascular endothelial cells as mechanotransducers? Nature 325:811, 1987.

106. Oien, A. H., and Aukland, K.: A mathematical analysis of the myogenic hypothesis with special reference to autoregulation of renal blood flow. Circ. Res. 52:241, 1983.

107. Bayliss, W. M.: On the local reaction of the arterial wall to changes of internal pressure. J. Physiol. (Lond.) 28:220, 1902.

108. Rajagopalan, S., Dube, S., and Canty, J. M., Jr.: Regulation of coronary diameter by myogenic mechanisms in arterial microvessels greater than 100 microns in diameter. Am. J. Physiol. 268:H788, 1995.

109. Chilian, W. M., and Marcus, M. L.: Effects of coronary and extravascular pressure on intramyocardial and epicardial blood velocity. Am. J. Physiol. 248:H170, 1985.

110. Marcus, M. L., and Harrison, D. G.: Physiologic basis for myocardial perfusion imaging. *In* Schelbert, H. R., Skorton, D. J., and Wolf, G. L. (eds.): Cardiac Imaging, A Companion to Braunwald's Heart Disease. Philadelphia, W.B. Saunders Co., 1991, pp. 8–23.

111. Berne, R. M., and Rubio, R.: Coronary circulation. *In* Berne, R. M., Speralakis, N., and Geiger, S. R. (eds.): Handbook of Physiology: Section 2, The Cardiovascular System. Bethesda, American Physiologic Society, 1979, p. 897.

111a. Zhang, J., Duncker, D. J., Ya, X., et al.: Effect of left ventricular hypertrophy secondary to chronic pressure overload on transmural myocardial 2-deoxyglucose uptake. Circulation 92:1274, 1995.

112. Braunwald, E., Ross, J., Jr., and Sonnenblick, E. H.: Regulation of coronary blood flow. *In* Mechanisms of Contraction of the Normal and Failing Heart, 2nd ed. Boston, Little, Brown, and Co., 1976, p. 200.

113. Austin, R. E., Jr., Smedira, N. G., Squires, T. M., and Hoffman, J. I.: Influence of cardiac contraction and coronary vasomotor tone on regional myocardial blood flow. Am. J. Physiol. 266:H2542, 1994.

114. Farhi, E. R., Klocke, F. J., Mates, R. E., et al.: Tone-dependent waterfall behavior during venous pressure elevation in isolated canine hearts. Circ. Res. 68:392, 1991.

115. Hoffman, J. I., and Spaan, J. A.: Pressure-flow relations in coronary circulation. Physiol. Rev. 70:331, 1990.

116. Chilian, W. M.: Microvascular pressures and resistances in the left ventricular subepicardium and subendocardium. Circ. Res. 69:561, 1991.

117. Klocke, F. J.: Coronary blood flow in man. Prog. Cardiovasc. Dis. 19:117, 1976.

118. Weiss, H. R., Neubauer, J. A., Lipp, J. A., and Sinha, A. K.: Quantitative determination of regional oxygen consumption in the dog heart. Circ. Res. 42:394, 1978.

119. Hoffman, J. I.: Transmural myocardial perfusion. Prog. Cardiovasc. Dis. 29:429, 1987.

120. Gallagher, K. P., Osakada, G., Matsuzaki, M., et al.: Myocardial blood flow and function with critical coronary stenosis in exercising dogs. Am. J. Physiol. 243:H698, 1982.

121. Bache, R. J., McHale, P. A., and Greenfield, J. C., Jr.: Transmural myocardial perfusion during restricted coronary inflow in the awake dog. Am. J. Physiol. 232:H645, 1977.

122. Ball, R. M., and Bache, R. J.: Distribution of myocardial blood flow in the exercising dog with restricted coronary artery inflow. Circ. Res. 38:60, 1976.

123. Rembert, J. C., Boyd, L. M., Watkinson, W. P., and Greenfield, J. C., Jr.: Effect of adenosine on transmural myocardial blood flow distribution in the awake dog. Am. J. Physiol. 239:H7, 1980.

124. Gewirtz, H., Williams, D. O., Ohley, W. H., and Most, A. S.: Influence of coronary vasodilation on the transmural distribution of myocardial blood flow distal to a severe fixed coronary artery stenosis. Am. Heart J. 106:674, 1983.

125. O'Keefe, D. D., Hoffman, J. I., Cheitlin, R., et al.: Coronary blood flow in experimental canine left ventricular hypertrophy. Circ. Res. 43:43, 1978.

126. Hittinger, L., Shannon, R. P., Bishop, S. P., et al.: Subendocardial exhaustion of blood flow reserve and increased fibrosis in conscious dogs with heart failure. Circ. Res. 65:971, 1989.

127. Shannon, R. P., Komamura, K., Shen, Y. T., et al.: Impaired regional subendocardial coronary flow reserve in conscious dogs with pacing-induced heart failure. Am. J. Physiol. 265:H801, 1993.

128. Nathan, H. J., and Feigl, E. O.: Adrenergic vasoconstriction lessens transmural steal during coronary hypoperfusion. Am. J. Physiol. 250:H645, 1986.

129. Heller, G. V., Barbour, M. M., Dweik, R. B., et al.: Effects of intravenous theophylline on exercise-induced myocardial ischemia. I. Impact on the ischemic threshold. J. Am. Coll. Cardiol. 21:1075, 1993.

130. Kumada, T., Gallagher, K. P., Shirato, K., et al.: Reduction of exercise-induced regional myocardial dysfunction by propranolol. Circ. Res. 46:190, 1980.

131. Vatner, S. F., Baig, H., Manders, W. T., et al.: Effects of propranolol on regional myocardial function, electrograms, and blood flow in conscious dogs with myocardial ischemia. J. Clin. Invest. 60:353, 1977.

132. Vatner, S. F.: Alpha-adrenergic tone in the coronary circulation of the concious dog. Fed. Proc. 43:2867, 1984.

133. Woodman, O. L., and Vatner, S. F.: Coronary vasoconstriction mediated by alpha₁ and alpha₂ adrenoceptors in conscious dogs. Am. J. Physiol. 253:H388, 1987.

134. Young, M. A., Vatner, D. E., Knight, D. R., et al.: Alpha-adrenergic vasoconstriction and receptor subtypes in large coronary arteries of calves. Am. J. Physiol. 255:H1452, 1988.

135. Morgan, K. G., Papageorgiou, P., and Jiang, M. J.: Pathophysiologic role of calcium in the development of vascular smooth muscle tone. Am. J. Cardiol. 64:35F, 1989.

136. Johns, A., Leitjen, P., Yamamoto, H., et al.: Calcium regulation in vascular smooth muscle contractility. Am. J. Cardiol. 59:18A, 1987.

137. Rinkema, L. E., Thomas, J. X., Jr., and Randall, W. C.: Regional coronary vasoconstriction in response to stimulation of stellate ganglia. Am. J. Physiol. 243:H410, 1982.

138. Murray, P. A., Lavallee, M., and Vatner, S. F.: Alpha-adrenergic–mediated reduction in coronary blood flow secondary to carotid chemoreceptor reflex activation in conscious dogs. Circ. Res. 54:96, 1984.

139. Feldman, R. D., Christy, J. P., Paul, S. T., and Harrison, D. G.: Beta-adrenergic receptors on canine coronary collateral vessels: Characterization and function. Am. J. Physiol. 257:H1634, 1989.

140. Vatner, S. F., and Hintze, T. H.: Mechanism of constriction of large coronary arteries by beta-adrenergic receptor blockade. Circ. Res. 53:389, 1983.

141. Cox, D. A., Hintze, T. H., and Vatner, S. F.: Effects of acetylcholine on large and small coronary arteries in conscious dogs. J. Pharmacol. Exp. Ther. 225:764, 1983.

142. Vatner, S. F., Higgins, C. B., and Braunwald, E.: Effects of norepinephrine on coronary circulation and left ventricular dynamics in the conscious dog. Circ. Res. 34:812, 1974.

143. Kern, M. J., Horowitz, J. D., Ganz, P., et al.: Attenuation of coronary vascular resistance by selective alpha₁-adrenergic blockade in patients with coronary artery disease. J. Am. Coll. Cardiol. 5:840, 1985.

144. Winniford, M. D., Jansen, D. E., Reynolds, G. A., et al.: Cigarette smoking–induced coronary vasoconstriction in atherosclerotic coronary artery disease and its prevention by calcium antagonists and nitroglycerin. Am. J. Cardiol. 59:203, 1987.

145. Hackett, J. G., Abboud, F. M., Mark, A. L., et al.: Coronary vascular responses to stimulation of chemoreceptors and baroreceptors. Circ. Res. 31:8, 1972.

146. Higgins, C. B., Vatner, S. F., and Braunwald, E.: Parasympathetic control of the heart. Pharmacol. Rev. 25:119, 1973.

147. Vatner, S. F., Franklin, D., Van Citters, R. L., and Braunwald, E.: Effects of carotid sinus nerve stimulation on the coronary circulation of conscious dogs. Circ. Res. 27:11, 1970.

148. Heyndrickx, G. R., Muylaert, P., and Pannier, J. L.: Alpha-adrenergic control of oxygen delivery to myocardium during exercise in conscious dog. Am. J. Physiol. 242:H805, 1982.

149. Laxson, D. D., Dai, X. Z., Homans, D. C., and Bache, R. J.: The role of alpha₁- and alpha₂-adrenergic receptors in mediation of coronary vasoconstriction in hypoperfused ischemic myocardium during exercise. Circ. Res. 65:1688, 1989.

150. Heusch, G.: Alpha-adrenergic mechanisms in myocardial ischemia. Circulation 81:1, 1990.

151. Feigl, E. O.: Reflex parasympathetic coronary vasodilation elicited from cardiac receptors in the dog. Circ. Res. 37:175, 1975.

152. Pitetti, K. H., Iwamoto, G. A., Mitchell, J. H., and Ordway, G. A.: Stimulating somatic afferent fibers alters coronary arterial resistance. Am. J. Physiol. 256:R1331, 1989.

153. Jarisch, A., and Zotterman, Y.: Depressor reflexes from the heart. Acta Physiol. Scand. 16:31, 1948.

154. Brown, B. G., Lee, A. B., Bolson, E. L., and Dodge, H. T.: Reflex constriction of significant coronary stenosis as a mechanism contributing to ischemic left ventricular dysfunction during isometric exercise. Circulation 70:18, 1984.

155. Brachfeld, N., Monroe, R. G., and Gorlin, R.: Effects of pericoronary denervation on coronary hemodynamics. Am. J. Physiol. 199:174, 1960.

156. Macho, P., and Vatner, S. F.: Effects of prazosin on coronary and left ventricular dynamics in conscious dogs. Circulation 65:1186, 1982.

157. Chierchia, S., Davies, G., Berkenboom, G., et al.: Alpha-adrenergic receptors and coronary spasm: An elusive link. Circulation 69:8, 1984.

158. Galassi, A. R., Kaski, J. C., Pupita, G., et al.: Lack of evidence for alpha-adrenergic receptor mediated mechanisms in the genesis of ischemia in syndrome X. Am. J. Cardiol. 64:264, 1989.

159. Gould, L., Reddy, C. V., and Gombrecht, R. F.: Oral phentolamine in angina pectoris. Jpn. Heart J. 14:393, 1973.

160. Berkenboom, G. M., Abramowicz, M., Vandermoten, P., and Degre, S. G.: Role of alpha adrenergic coronary tone in exercise-induced angina pectoris. Am. J. Cardiol. 57:195, 1986.

161. Hayes, S. N., Moyer, T. P., Morley, D., and Bove, A. A.: Intravenous cocaine causes epicardial coronary vasoconstriction in the intact dog. Am. Heart J. 121:1639, 1991.

162. Lange, R. A., Cigarroa, R. G., Yancy, C. W., et al.: Cocaine-induced coronary-artery vasoconstriction. N. Engl. J. Med. 321:1557, 1989.

163. Brown, B. G., Bolson, E. L., and Dodge, H. T.: Dynamic mechanisms in human coronary stenosis. Circulation 70:917, 1984.

164. Young, D. F., Cholvin, N. R., and Roth, A. C.: Pressure drop across artificially induced stenoses in the femoral arteries of dogs. Circ. Res. 36:735, 1975.

165. Klocke, F. J.: Measurements of coronary blood flow and degree of ste-

nosis: Current clinical implications and continuing uncertainties. J. Am. Coll. Cardiol. *1*:31, 1983.

166. Gould, K. L.: Dynamic coronary stenosis. Am. J. Cardiol. *45*:286, 1980.

167. Ball, R. M., Bache, R. J., Cobb, F. R., and Greenfield, J. C., Jr.: Regional myocardial blood flow during graded treadmill exercise in the dog. J. Clin. Invest. *55*:43, 1975.

168. Bache, R. J., Vrobel, T. R., Ring, W. S., et al.: Regional myocardial blood flow during exercise in dogs with chronic left ventricular hypertrophy. Circ. Res. *48*:76, 1981.

169. Geha, A. S., and Baue, A. E.: Graded coronary stenosis and coronary flow during acute normovolemic anemia. World J. Surg. *2*:645, 1978.

170. Gould, K. L.: Pressure-flow characteristics of coronary stenoses in unsedated dogs at rest and during coronary vasodilation. Circ. Res. *43*:242–253, 1978.

171. Goldberg, S. J.: The principles of pressure drop in long segment stenosis. Herz *11*:291, 1986.

172. Freudenberg, H., and Lichtlen, P. R.: The normal wall segment in coronary stenosis—a postmortem study. Z. Kardiol. *70*:863, 1981.

173. Brown, B. G., Bolson, E. L., Petersen, R. B., et al.: The mechanisms of nitroglycerin action: Stenosis vasodilation as a major component of the drug response. Circulation *64*:1089, 1981.

174. Schwartz, J. S., Bache, R. J.: Effect of arteriolar dilation on coronary artery diameter distal to coronary stenoses. Am. J. Physiol. *249*:H981, 1985.

175. Santamore, W. P., and Walinsky, P.: Altered coronary flow response to vasoactive drugs in the presence of coronary arterial stenosis in the dog. Am. J. Cardiol. *45*:276, 1980.

176. Brown, B. G., Josephson, M. A., Petersen, R. B., et al.: Intravenous dipyridamole combined with isometric handgrip for near maximal acute increases in coronary flow in patients with coronary artery disease. Am. J. Cardiol. *48*:1077, 1981.

177. Klocke, F. J.: Measurements of coronary flow reserve: Defining pathophysiology versus making decisions about patient care. Circulation *76*:1183, 1987.

178. Gould, K. L., and Lipscomb, K.: Effects of coronary stenoses on coronary flow reserve and resistance. Am. J. Cardiol. *34*:48, 1974.

179. Wilson, R. F., Marcus, M. L., and White, C. W.: Prediction of the physiologic significance of coronary arterial lesions by quantitative lesion geometry in patients with limited coronary artery disease. Circulation *75*:723, 1987.

180. Donohue, T. J., Kern, M. J., Aguirre, F. V., et al.: Assessing the hemodynamic significance of coronary artery stenoses: Analysis of translesional pressure-flow velocity relationships in patients. J. Am. Coll. Cardiol. *22*:449, 1993.

181. Marcus, M., Wright, C., Doty, D., et al.: Measurements of coronary velocity and reactive hyperemia in the coronary circulation of humans. Circ. Res. *49*:877, 1981.

182. Vatner, S. F., Higgins, C. B., Franklin, D., and Braunwald, E.: Role of tachycardia in mediating the coronary hemodynamic response to severe exercise. J. Appl. Physiol. *32*:380, 1972.

183. Nahser, P. J., Brown, R. E., Oskarsson, H., et al.: Maximal coronary flow reserve and metabolic coronary vasodilation in patients with diabetes mellitus. Circulation *91*:635, 1995.

184. Doucette, J. W., Corl, P. D., Payne, H. M., et al.: Validation of a Doppler guide wire for intravascular measurement of coronary artery flow velocity. Circulation *85*:1899, 1992.

185. DiMario, C., Gil, R., and Serruys, P. W.: Long-term reproducibility of coronary flow velocity measurements in patients with coronary artery disease. Am. J. Cardiol. *75*:1177, 1995.

186. Kern, M. J., and Anderson, H. V. (eds.): A symposium: The clinical applications of the intracoronary Doppler guidewire flow velocity in patients: Understanding blood flow beyond the coronary stenosis. Am. J. Cardiol. *71*:1D–86D, 1993.

187. White, C. W., Wright, C. B., Doty, D. B., et al.: Does visual interpretation of the coronary arteriogram predict the physiological importance of a coronary stenosis? N. Engl. J. Med. *310*:819, 1984.

188. Reiber, J. H. C., Koning, G., Van der Zwet, P. M. J., et al.: Assessment of myocardial flow reserve with the DCI. Medica Mundi *38*:81, 1993.

189. Ganz, W., Tamura, K., Marcus, H. S., et al.: Measurement of coronary sinus blood flow by continuous thermodilution in man. Circulation *44*:181, 1971.

190. Marcus, M. L., Schelbert, H. R., Skorton, D. J., and Wolf, G. I. (eds.): Cardiac Imaging. Philadelphia, W. B. Saunders Co., 1991.

191. Gould, K. L., Kirkeeide, R. L., and Buchi, M.: Coronary flow reserve as a physiologic measure of stenosis severity. J. Am. Coll. Cardiol. *15*:459, 1990.

192. Little, W. C., Constantinescu, M., Applegate, R. J., et al.: Can coronary angiography predict the site of a subsequent myocardial infarction in patients with mild to moderate coronary artery disease? Circulation *78*:1157–1166, 1988.

193. Ambrose, J. A., Tannenbaum, M. A., Alexopoulos, D., et al.: Angiographic progression of coronary artery disease and the development of myocardial infarction. J. Am. Coll. Cardiol. *12*:56, 1988.

194. Giroud, D., Li, J. M., Urban, P., et al.: Relation of the site of acute myocardial infarction to the most severe coronary arterial stenosis at prior angiography. Am. J. Cardiol. *69*:729, 1992.

195. Davies, M. J., and Thomas, A. C.: Plaque fissuring: The cause of acute myocardial infarction, sudden ischaemic death and crescendo angina. Br. Heart J. *53*:363, 1985.

196. Kanazawa, T.: Coronary collateral circulation. Jpn. Circ. J. *58*:151, 1994.

197. Schaper, W., Gorge, G., Winkler, B., and Schaper, J.: The collateral circulation of the heart. Prog. Cardiovasc. Dis. *31*:57, 1988.

198. Goldstein, R. E., Michaelis, L. L., Morrow, A. G., and Epstein, S. E.: Coronary collateral function in patients without occlusive coronary artery disease. Circulation *51*:118, 1975.

199. Marcus, M. L., and Harrison, D. G.: Physiologic basis for myocardial perfusion imaging. *In* Schelbert, H. R., Skorton, D. J., and Wolf, G. L. (eds.): Cardiac Imaging, A Companion to Braunwald's Heart Disease. Philadelphia, W. B. Saunders Co., 1991, pp. 8–23.

200. Marcus, M. L.: The coronary circulation. *In* Marcus, M. L. (ed.): The Coronary Circulation in Health and Disease. New York, McGraw-Hill Book Co., 1983, pp. 221–241.

201. Schaper, W.: New paradigms for collateral vessel growth. Basic Res. Cardiol. *88*:193–198, 1993.

202. Pasyk, S., Schaper, W., Schaper, J., et al.: DNA synthesis in coronary collaterals after coronary artery occlusion in conscious dog. Am. J. Physiol. *242*:H1031, 1982.

203. Schaper, W., and Pasyk, S.: Influence of collateral flow on the ischemic tolerance of the heart following acute and subacute coronary occlusion. Circulation *53*(Suppl. 1):57, 1976.

204. Harrison, D. G., and Simonetti, I.: Neurohumoral regulation of collateral perfusion. Circulation *83*(Suppl. 3):62, 1991.

205. Nagel, T., Resnick, N., Atkinson, W. J., et al.: Shear stress selectively upregulates intercellular adhesion molecule-1 expression in cultured human vascular endothelial cells. J. Clin. Invest. *94*:885, 1994.

206. Knoll, R., Arras, M., Zimmermann, R., et al.: Changes in gene expression following short coronary occlusions studied in porcine hearts with run-on assays. Cardiovasc. Res. *28*:1062, 1994.

207. Rentrop, K. P., Thornton, J. C., Feit, F., and Van Buskirk, M.: Determinants and protective potential of coronary arterial collaterals as assessed by an angioplasty model. Am. J. Cardiol. *61*:677, 1988.

208. Schaper, W.: Influence of physical exercise on coronary collateral blood flow in chronic experimental two-vessel occlusion. Circulation *65*:905–912, 1982.

209. Pupita, G., Mazzara, D., Centanni, M., et al.: Ischemia in collateral-dependent myocardium: Effects of nifedipine and diltiazem in man. Am. Heart J. *126*:86, 1993.

210. Cohen, M. V.: Lack of effect of propranolol on canine coronary collateral development during progressive coronary stenosis and occlusion. Cardiovasc. Res. *27*:249–254, 1993.

211. Hollenberg, N.: Serotonin, atherosclerosis, and collateral vessel spasm. Am. J. Hypertens. *1*:312S–316S, 1988.

212. Unger, E. F., Banai, S., Shou, M., et al.: Basic fibroblast growth factor enhances myocardial collateral flow in a canine model. Am. J. Physiol. *266*:H1588, 1994.

213. Lazarous, D. F., Scheinowitz, M., Shou, M., et al.: Effects of chronic systemic administration of basic fibroblast growth factor on collateral development in the canine heart. Circulation *91*:145, 1995.

214. Bauters, C., Asahara, T., Zheng, L. P., et al.: Physiological assessment of augmented vascularity induced by VEGF in ischemic rabbit hindlimb. Am. J. Physiol. *267*:H1263, 1994.

215. Takeshita, S., Pu, L. Q., Stein, L. A., et al.: Intramuscular administration of vascular endothelial growth factor induces dose-dependent collateral augmentation in a rabbit model of chronic limb ischemia. Circulation *90*(Suppl. II):228, 1994.

216. Banai, S., Jaklitsch, M. T., Shou, M., et al.: Angiogenic-induced enhancement of collateral blood flow to ischemic myocardium by vascular endothelial growth factor in dogs. Circulation *89*:2183, 1994.

217. Carroll, S. M., White, F. C., Roth, D. M., and Bloor, C. M.: Heparin accelerates coronary collateral development in a porcine model of coronary artery occlusion. Circulation *88*:198, 1993.

218. Sasayama, S., and Fujita, M.: Recent insights into coronary collateral circulation. Circulation *85*:1197, 1992.

219. Cohen, M. V., Chukwuogo, N., and Yarlagadda, A.: Heparin does not stimulate coronary-collateral growth in a canine model of progressive coronary-artery narrowing and occlusion. Am. J. Med. Sci. *306*:75, 1993.

219a. Frank, M. W., Harris, K. R., Ahlin, K. A., and Klocke, F. J.: Endothelium-derived relaxing factor (nitric oxide) has a tonic vasodilating action on coronary collateral vessels. J. Am. Coll. Cardiol. *27*:658, 1996.

220. Altman, J. D., Dulas, D., Pavek, T., et al.: Endothelial function in well-developed canine coronary collateral vessels. Am. J. Physiol. *264*:H567, 1993.

221. Altman, J. D., Dulas, D., Pavek, T., and Bache, R. J.: Effect of aspirin on coronary collateral blood flow. Circulation *87*:583, 1993.

222. Randall, M. D., and Griffith, T. M.: EDRF plays central role in collateral flow after arterial occlusion in rabbit ear. Am. J. Physiol. *263*:H752, 1992.

223. Schwarz, F., Flameng, W., Ensslen, R., et al.: Effect of collaterals on left ventricular function at rest and during stress. Am. Heart J. *95*:570, 1978.

224. Rentrop, K. P., Cohen, M., Blanke, H., and Phillips, R. A.: Changes in collateral channel filling immediately after controlled coronary artery occlusion by an angioplasty balloon in human subjects. J. Am. Coll. Cardiol. *5*:587, 1985.

225. Cohen, M., and Rentrop, K. P.: Limitation of myocardial ischemia by collateral circulation during sudden controlled coronary artery occlusion in human subjects: A prospective study. Circulation *74*:469, 1986.

226. Mizuno, K., Horiuchi, K., Matui, M., et al.: Role of coronary collateral vessels during transient coronary occlusion during angioplasty assessed by hemodynamic, electrocardiographic and metabolic changes. J. Am. Coll. Cardiol. *12*:624, 1988.

227. Schwartz, H., Leiboff, R. L., Katz, R. J., et al.: Arteriographic predictors of spontaneous improvement in left ventricular function after myocardial infarction. Circulation *71*:466, 1985.

228. Sabia, P. J., Powers, E. R., Ragosta, M., et al.: An association between collateral blood flow and myocardial viability in patients with recent myocardial infarction. N. Engl. J. Med. 327:1825–1831, 1992.

229. Franklin, B. A.: Exercise training and coronary collateral circulation. Med. Sci. Sports Exerc. 23:648–653, 1991.

230. McKirnan, M. D., and Bloor, C. M.: Clinical significance of coronary vascular adaptations to exercise training. Med. Sci. Sports Exerc. 26:1262, 1994.

231. Hellerstein, H. K.: Acceleration of collaterals due to physical activity—dogma or fact. Bibl. Cardiol. 36:125, 1977.

232. Ferguson, R. J., Petitclerc, R., Choquette, G., et al.: Effect of physical training on treadmill exercise capacity, collateral circulation and progression of coronary disease. Am. J. Cardiol. 34:764, 1974.

233. Fujita, M., Sasayama, S., Asanoi, H., et al.: Improvement of treadmill capacity and collateral circulation as a result of exercise with heparin pretreatment in patients with effort angina. Circulation 77:1022, 1988.

234. Ejiri, M., Fujita, M., Miwa, K., et al.: Effects of heparin treatment on collateral development and regional myocardial function in acute myocardial infarction. Am. Heart J. 119:248, 1990.

235. Isner, J. M., and Feldman, L. J.: Gene therapy for arterial disease. Lancet 344:1653, 1994.

236. Isner, J. M., Walsh, K., Symes, J., et al.: Arterial gene therapy for therapeutic angiogenesis in patients with peripheral artery disease. Circulation 91:2687, 1995.

CONSEQUENCES OF MYOCARDIAL ISCHEMIA

237. Tennant, R., and Wiggers, C. J.: The effect of coronary occlusion on myocardial contractions. Am. J. Physiol. 112:351, 1935.

238. Heyndrickx, G. R., Millard, R. W., McRitchie, R. J., et al.: Regional myocardial functional and electrophysiological alterations after brief coronary occlusion in conscious dogs. J. Clin. Invest. 56:978, 1975.

239. Braunwald, E., and Kloner, R. A.: The stunned myocardium: Prolonged, postischemic ventricular dysfunction. Circulation 66:1146, 1982.

240. Ellis, S. G., Henschke, C. I., Sandor, T., et al.: Time course of functional and biochemical recovery of myocardium salvaged by reperfusion. J. Am. Coll. Cardiol. 1:1047, 1983.

241. Thaulow, E., Guth, B. D., Heusch, G., et al.: Characteristics of regional myocardial stunning after exercise in dogs with chronic coronary stenosis. Am. J. Physiol. 257:H113, 1989.

242. Fournier, C., Boujon, B., Hebert, J., et al.: Stunned myocardium following coronary spasm. Am. Heart J. 121:593, 1991.

243. Charlat, M. L., O'Neill, P. G., Hartley, C. J., et al.: Prolonged abnormalities of left ventricular diastolic wall thinning in the "stunned" myocardium in conscious dogs: Time course and relation to systolic function. J. Am. Coll. Cardiol. 13:185, 1989.

244. Braunwald, E.: The stunned myocardium: Newer insights into mechanisms and clinical implications. J. Thorac. Cardiovasc. Surg. 100:310, 1990.

245. Patel, B., Kloner, R. A., Przyklenk, K., and Braunwald, E.: Postischemic myocardial "stunning": A clinically relevant phenomenon. Ann. Intern. Med. 108:626, 1988.

246. Zimmermann, R., Mall, G., Rauch, B., et al.: Residual ^{201}Tl activity in irreversible defects as a marker of myocardial viability: Clinicopathological study. Circulation 91:1016, 1995.

247. Bolli, R., Patel, B. S., Hartley, C. J., et al.: Nonuniform transmural recovery of contractile function in the "stunned" myocardium. Am. J. Physiol. 257:H375, 1989.

248. Preuss, K. C., Gross, G. J., Brooks, H. L., and Warltier, D. C.: Time course of recovery of "stunned" myocardium following variable periods of ischemia in conscious and anesthetized dogs. Am. Heart J. 114:696, 1987.

249. Marban, E.: Myocardial stunning and hibernation: The physiology behind the colloquialisms. Circulation 83:681, 1991.

250. Bolli, R., Triana, J. F., and Jeroudi, M. O.: Prolonged impairment of coronary vasodilation after reversible ischemia: Evidence for microvascular "stunning." Circ. Res. 67:332, 1990.

251. Ellis, S. G., Wynne, J., Braunwald, E., et al.: Response of reperfusion-salvaged stunned myocardium to inotropic stimulation. Am. Heart J. 107:13, 1984.

252. Arnold, J. M. O., Braunwald, E., Sandor, T., and Kloner, R. A.: Inotropic stimulation of reperfused myocardium with dopamine: Effects on infarct size and myocardial function. J. Am. Coll. Cardiol. 6:1026, 1985.

253. Heusch, G., Schafer, S., and Kroger, K.: Recruitment of inotropic reserve in "stunned" myocardium by the cardiotonic agent AR-L 57. Basic Res. Cardiol. 83:602, 1988.

254. Lazdunski, M., Frelin, C., and Frelin, P.: The sodium/hydrogen exchange system in cardiac cells: Its biochemical and pharmacological properties and its role in regulating internal concentrations of sodium and internal pH. J. Mol. Cell. Cardiol. 17:1029, 1985.

255. Tani, M., and Neely, J. R.: Role of intracellular Na^+ in Ca^{2+} overload and depressed recovery of ventricular function of reperfused ischemic rat hearts: Possible involvement of H^+-Na^+ and Na^+-Ca^{2+} exchange. Circ. Res. 65:1045, 1989.

256. Krause, S. M., Jacobus, W. E., and Becker, L. C.: Alterations in cardiac sarcoplasmic reticulum calcium transport in the postischemic "stunned" myocardium. Circ. Res. 65:526, 1989.

257. Przyklenk, K., and Kloner, R. A.: Superoxide dismutase plus catalase improve contractile function in the canine model of the "stunned" myocardium. Circ. Res. 58:148, 1986.

258. Bolli, R., Patel, B. S., Jeroudi, M. O., et al.: Iron-mediated radical reactions upon reperfusion contribute to myocardial "stunning." Am. J. Physiol. 259:H1901, 1990.

259. Koerner, J. E., Anderson, B. A., and Dage, R. C.: Protection against postischemic myocardial dysfunction in anesthetized rabbits with scavengers of oxygen-derived free radicals: Superoxide dismutase plus catalase, N-2-mercaptopropionyl glycine and captopril. J. Cardiovasc. Pharmacol. 17:185, 1991.

260. Dage, R. C., Anderson, B. A., Mao, S. J. T., and Koerner, J. E.: Probucol reduces myocardial dysfunction during reperfusion after short-term ischemia in rabbit heart. J. Cardiovasc. Pharmacol. 17:158, 1991.

261. Bolli, R.: Postischemic myocardial stunning. In Yellon, D. M., and Jennings, R. B. (eds.): Myocardial Protection: The Pathophysiology of Reperfusion and Reperfusion Injury. New York, Raven Press, 1992.

262. Hearse, D. J.: Stunning: A radical re-view. Cardiovasc. Drugs Ther. 5:853, 1991.

263. Jennings, R. B., and Reimer, K. A.: Factors involved in salvaging ischemic myocardium: Effects of reperfusion of arterial blood. Circulation 68(Suppl. I):I-25, 1983.

264. Visner, M. S., Arentzen, C. E., Parrish, D. G., et al.: Effects of global ischemia on the diastolic properties of the left ventricle in the conscious dog. Circulation 71:610, 1985.

265. Momomura, S. I., Ferguson, J. J., Miller, M. J., et al.: Regional myocardial blood flow and left ventricular diastolic properties in pacing-induced ischemia. J. Am. Coll. Cardiol. 17:781, 1991.

266. Yin, F. C. P.: Ventricular wall stress. Circ. Res. 49:829, 1981.

267. Dunn, R. B., and Griggs, D. M.: Transmural gradients in ventricular tissue metabolites produced by stopping coronary blood flow in the dog. Circ. Res. 37:438, 1975.

268. Moss, A. J.: Intramyocardial oxygen tension. Cardiovasc. Res. 2:314, 1968.

269. Weiss, H. R., and Sinha, A. K.: Regional oxygen saturation of small arteries and veins in the canine myocardium. Circ. Res. 42:119, 1978.

269a. Reimer, K. A., and Jennings, R. B.: The "wavefront phenomenon" of myocardial ischemic cell death. II. Transmural progression of necrosis within the framework of ischemic bed size (myocardium at risk) and collateral flow. Lab. Invest. 40:633, 1979.

270. Naka, Y., Stern, D. M., and Pinsky, D. J.: The pathophysiology of myocardial ischemia, necrosis, and reperfusion. In Fuster, V., Ross, R., and Topol, E. J. (eds.): Atherosclerosis and Coronary Artery Disease. Philadelphia, Lippincott-Raven, 1996, pp. 807–818.

271. Ganz, W., Watanabe, I., Kanamasa, K., et al.: Does reperfusion extend necrosis? A study in a single territory of myocardial ischemia—half reperfused and half not reperfused. Circulation 82:1020, 1990.

272. Lee, J. T., Ideker, R. E., and Reimer, K. A.: Myocardial infarct size and location in relation to the coronary vascular bed at risk in man. Circulation 64:526, 1981.

EFFECTS OF ISCHEMIA ON MYOCARDIAL METABOLISM

273. Jennings, R. B., Reimer, K. A., Hill, M. L., and Mayer, S. E.: Total ischemia in dog hearts in vitro. I. Comparison of high energy phosphate production, utilization and depletion, and of adenine nucleotide catabolism in total ischemia in vitro vs. severe ischemia in vivo. Circ. Res. 49:892, 1981.

274. Marban, E., Koretsune, Y, Corretti, M., et al.: Calcium and its role in myocardial cell injury during ischemia and reperfusion. Circulation 80(Suppl. IV):80, 1989.

275. Sedlis, S. P., Corr, P. B., Sobel, B. E., and Ahumada, G. G.: Lysophosphatidyl choline potentiates Ca^{++} accumulation in rat cardiac myocytes. Am. J. Physiol. 244:H32, 1983.

276. Kloner, R. A., DeBoer, L. W. V., Carlson, N., and Braunwald, E.: The effect of verapamil on myocardial ultrastructure during and following release of coronary artery occlusion. Exp. Mol. Pathol. 36:277, 1982.

277. Braunwald, E., Muller, J. E., Kloner, R. A., and Maroko, P. R.: Role of beta-adrenergic blockade in the therapy of patients with myocardial infarction. Am. J. Med. 74:113, 1983.

278. Hammerman, H., Kloner, R. A., Briggs, L. L., and Braunwald, E.: Enhancement of salvage of reperfused myocardium by early beta-adrenergic blockade (timolol). J. Am. Coll. Cardiol. 3:1438, 1984.

279. Lo, H. M., Kloner, R. A., and Braunwald, E.: Effect of intracoronary verapamil on infarct size in the ischemic, reperfused canine heart: Critical importance of the timing of treatment. Am. J. Cardiol. 56:672, 1985.

280. Campbell, C. A., Kloner, R. A., Alker, K. J., and Braunwald, E.: Effect of verapamil on infarct size in dogs subjected to coronary artery occlusion with transient reperfusion. J. Am. Coll. Cardiol. 8:1169, 1986.

281. Forman, M. B., Virmani, R., and Puett, D. W.: Mechanisms and therapy of myocardial reperfusion injury. Circulation 81(Suppl. IV):69, 1990.

282. Lefer, A. M., Tsao, P. S., Lefer, D. J., and Ma, X.-L.: Role of endothelial dysfunction in the pathogenesis of reperfusion injury after myocardial ischemia. FASEB, J. 5:2029, 1991.

283. Jennings, R. B., Schaper, J., Hill, M. L., et al.: Effect of reperfusion late in the phase of reversible ischemic injury: Changes in cell volume, electrolytes, metabolites, and ultrastructure. Circ. Res. 56:262, 1985.

284. Kloner, R. A., Ellis, S. G., Lange, R., and Braunwald, E.: Studies of experimental coronary artery reperfusion: Effects on infarct size, myocardial function, biochemistry, ultrastructure, and microvascular damage. Circulation 68(Suppl. I):8, 1983.

285. Kloner, R. A., Ellis, S. G., Carlson, N. V., and Braunwald, E.: Coronary reperfusion for the treatment of acute myocardial infarction: Postischemic ventricular dysfunction. Cardiology 70:233, 1983.

286. Hearse, D. J., and Bolli, R.: Reperfusion-induced injury: Manifestations, mechanisms and clinical relevance. Cardiovasc. Res. 26:101, 1992.

Chapter 37
Acute Myocardial Infarction
ELLIOTT M. ANTMAN, EUGENE BRAUNWALD

CHANGING PATTERNS IN CLINICAL CARE OF PATIENTS WITH ACUTE MYOCARDIAL INFARCTION

Despite impressive strides in diagnosis and management over the last three decades, acute myocardial infarction (AMI) continues to be a major public health problem in the industrialized world. In the United States nearly 1.5 million patients annually suffer from AMI (about one patient every 20 seconds).[1] More than 1 million patients with suspected AMI are admitted yearly to coronary care units in the United States; in only 30 to 50 per cent of patients is the diagnosis confirmed.[2] Although the death rate from AMI has declined by about 30 per cent over the last decade, its development is still a fatal event in approximately one-third of patients.[1] About 50 per cent of the deaths associated with AMI occur within 1 hour of the event and are attributable to arrhythmias, most often ventricular fibrillation (Chap. 24). Because AMI may strike an individual during the most productive years, it can have profound deleterious psychosocial and economic ramifications. In the United States, the yearly economic burden of coronary artery disease is in excess of $60 billion.[1] Perhaps as much as half of this cost is related to AMI and its prevention and treatment. Utilizing national statistics and a previously validated Coronary Heart Disease Policy Model,[3] investigators at the Harvard School of Public Health estimate that the average annual cost of caring for a patient with AMI in 1996 is $12,000.

Driven in large part by the need for cost-saving measures,[4] contemporary care of patients with AMI is becoming increasingly influenced by managed care systems[5] and guidelines for clinical practice (Table 63–14, p. 1972).[2,5a] Coronary care practice is better equipped than other fields of cardiovascular medicine to face this transition from pathophysiologically based decision-making to evidence-based decision-making, given the rich data base of over 500,000 patients with suspected AMI studied in clinical trials and efforts at summarizing a vast amount of data using meta-analysis.[6–10] Valuable and often complementary insights are also available from observational registries and outcomes research projects using medical claims data bases.[11–13] New therapies for AMI are being evaluated not only for evidence of safety and efficacy but also for their cost-effectiveness in caring for patients and their impact on quality of life.[14–16] However, despite an abundance of cost-effectiveness information analyzed from a societal perspective using data from clinical trials, clinicians weighing the risk-benefit ratio at the bedside of an individual patient with AMI may have difficulty applying the findings for several reasons: uncertainty whether the benefits observed in a strictly defined trial population are applicable to a wider selection of patients,[17] limited data on specific subgroups, variations in the absolute level of baseline risk,[18,19] and variations in patient preferences.[20,21] The information in this chapter on various treatment strategies should therefore be used as a guide and not a substitute for carefully reasoned clinical decision-making on a case-by-case basis.

IMPROVEMENTS IN OUTCOME. A steady decline in the mortality rate from AMI has been observed across several population groups since 1960.[22–24a] This drop in mortality appears to be caused by a fall in the incidence of AMI (replaced in part by an increase in the rate of unstable angina[25,26]) and a fall in the case fatality rate once a myocardial infarction has occurred[27] (Fig. 37–1). In addition, clinicians are now more astute at identifying those patients who are at increased risk of AMI[28] and benefit from more aggressive prophylactic cardiovascular treatments to prevent it from occurring when they undergo noncardiac surgery (e.g., intravenous nitroglycerin perioperatively[29]).

Several landmarks in the management of patients have contributed to the decline in mortality from AMI.[30] In the mid-1960's the concept of coronary care units was introduced. The first decade of coronary care was notable for detailed analysis and vigorous management of cardiac arrhythmias. Subsequently, introduction of the pulmonary artery balloon flotation catheter set the stage for bedside hemodynamic monitoring and more precise management of heart failure and cardiogenic shock associated with AMI. The modern reperfusion era of coronary care was ushered in by intracoronary and then intravenous thrombolysis, increased use of aspirin, and development of primary percutaneous transluminal coronary angioplasty (PTCA) for AMI.[31] Drug therapy continues to be an integral aspect of the treatment of patients with AMI, with noteworthy advances in the use of beta-adrenoceptor blockers, antithrombotic regimens, nitrates, and angiotensin-converting enzyme (ACE) inhibitors.[7,32]

LIMITATIONS OF CURRENT THERAPY. Despite the gratifying success of medical therapy for AMI, several observations indicate that considerable room for improvement exists. The short-term mortality of patients with AMI who receive aggressive reperfusion therapy as part of a randomized trial is in the range of 6.5 per cent,[33] whereas observational data

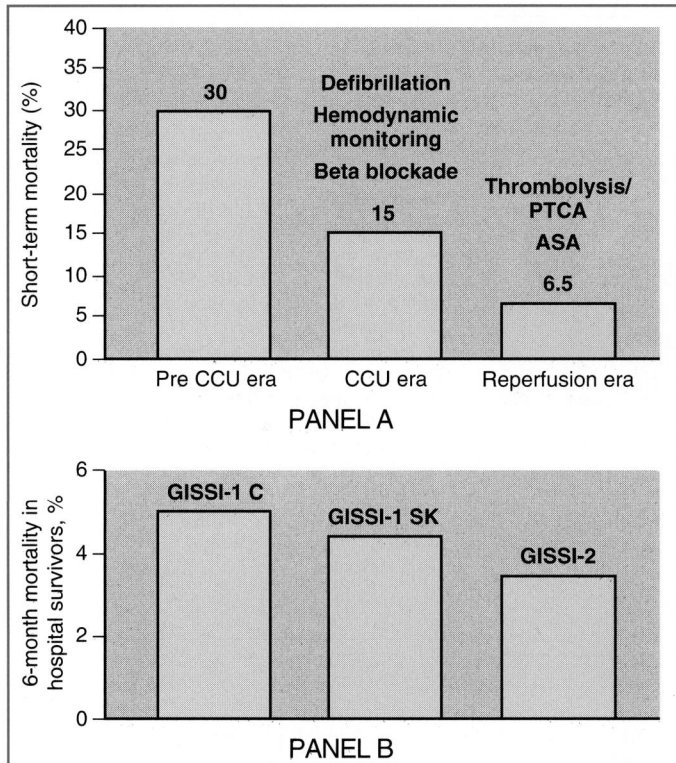

FIGURE 37–1. A, The impact of medical therapy for acute MI on short-term mortality. In the pre-CCU era acute MI short-term mortality (30-day) was estimated to be 30 per cent. Implementation of the CCU concept with defibrillation, sophisticated hemodynamic monitoring, and beta blockade reduced this to 15 per cent. A further mortality reduction was ushered in by the reperfusion era; combinations of thrombolysis, primary PTCA, and aspirin are now employed. (Modified from Antman, E. M.: General hospital management. *In* Julian, D., and Braunwald, E. (eds.): *Management of Acute Myocardial Infarction.* London, W. B. Saunders Company. Ltd., 1994, p. 31.) B, Six-month mortality for patients who survived the hospital phase of acute MI in the control (placebo) arm of the GISSI (GISSI-1 C) Study is compared with that in the GISSI-1 streptokinase arm (GISSI-1 SK). These results document the long-term benefits of thrombolytic therapy in reducing mortality. Further evidence that long-term use of aspirin and beta blockers contributes to a reduction in mortality can be seen in the third bar, which indicates 6-month mortality in GISSI-2. Compared with the GISSI-1 trial, at 6 months following infarction, greater proportions of patients in GISSI-2 were receiving aspirin (76 per cent versus 46 per cent, $P < 0.001$) and beta blockers (24 per cent versus 11 per cent, $P < 0.001$). (From Volpi, A., De Vita, C., Franzosi, M. G., et al.: Determinants of 6-month mortality in survivors of myocardial infarction after thrombolysis: Results of the GISSI-2 data base. Circulation **88**:416, 1993. Copyright 1993 American Heart Association.)

bases such as The National Registry of Myocardial Infarction suggest that the mortality rate in AMI patients not receiving reperfusion therapy is about 13 per cent.[12] In addition, the mortality rate from AMI in patients enrolled in randomized trials is considerably lower than that observed in patients who are excluded from such trials. For example, the 18-month mortality in the 2180 patients *excluded* from the Danish Verapamil Infarction Trial II (DAVIT II) was 25.6 per cent, whereas it was only 13.9 per cent in the placebo group enrolled in the trial.[34]

Although the survival of elderly patients (> age 65) following AMI has improved significantly,[35] advanced age consistently emerges as one of the principal determinants of mortality in AMI.[36–38] The 30-day and 1-year mortality rates for Medicare patients with AMI treated in 1990 were 23 per cent and 36 per cent, respectively.[35] Despite reluctance to use potentially life-saving drug therapies in the elderly, cardiac catheterization and other invasive procedures are being performed more commonly at some point during hospitalization in elderly AMI patients. Nevertheless, evidence suggests that the greatest reductions in mortality for elderly patients are derived from those strategies employed during the first 24 hours[39]—a time frame in which prompt and appropriate use of life-saving pharmacotherapy is of paramount importance, emphasizing the need to extend advances in drug therapy for AMI to the elderly.

Despite trends toward greater use of mortality-reducing therapies such as thrombolytics, aspirin, and beta-adrenoceptor blockers in patients with AMI,[40,41] these drugs still appear to be underutilized[42,43] (especially in the elderly[44,44a]), whereas calcium antagonists appear to be overutilized.[45,46] Considerable variation exists in practice patterns for management of patients with AMI.[47–50] This variation is seen not only on an international level[47,51] but also regionally within countries[49,50] and across medical specialties[52]; such variations in practice are correlated with differences in outcome after AMI.[52a]

Variation has also been observed in the treatment patterns of certain population subgroups with AMI—notably women and blacks. Although the unadjusted rates of thrombolytic use and referral for cardiac catheterization and angioplasty are lower[53,54] and mortality rates are higher in women with AMI,[10,55,56] gender differences are less apparent (but may not disappear entirely) once adjustment is made for baseline variables such as comorbidities and age[55–57] (Chap. 51). Although black patients with AMI in Veterans Administration Hospitals in the United States undergo fewer cardiac procedures such as cardiac catheterization than their white counterparts (even after adjustment for patient and hospital characteristics), they experience equivalent survival rates.[58]

PATHOLOGY

Almost all myocardial infarctions result from coronary atherosclerosis, generally with superimposed coronary thrombosis.[58a] Nonatherogenic forms of coronary artery disease are discussed on p. 1349 and causes of AMI without coronary atherosclerosis are shown in Table 37–1, p. 1193.

Prior to the thrombolytic era, clinicians typically divided AMI patients into those suffering a Q-wave or non-Q-wave infarct, based on the evolution of the pattern on the electrocardiogram (ECG) over several days following AMI. The term "Q-wave infarction" was frequently considered to be virtually synonymous with "transmural infarction," whereas "non-Q-wave infarctions" were often referred to as "subendocardial infarctions." Important advances have occurred in our understanding of the pathophysiology of AMI, leading to a reorganization of clinical presentations into what is now referred to as the *acute coronary syndromes,* the spectrum of which includes unstable angina, non-Q-wave infarction, and Q-wave infarction (Figs. 37–2 to 37–5).

ROLE OF ACUTE PLAQUE CHANGE

Slowly accruing high-grade stenoses of epicardial coronaries may progress to complete occlusion but do not usually precipitate AMI, probably because of the development of a rich collateral network (see p. 1174) over time. However, during the natural evolution of atherosclerotic plaques, especially those that are lipid-laden, an abrupt and catastrophic transition may occur, characterized by plaque rupture and exposure of substances that promote platelet activation and thrombin generation[59–65] (Figs. 37–2

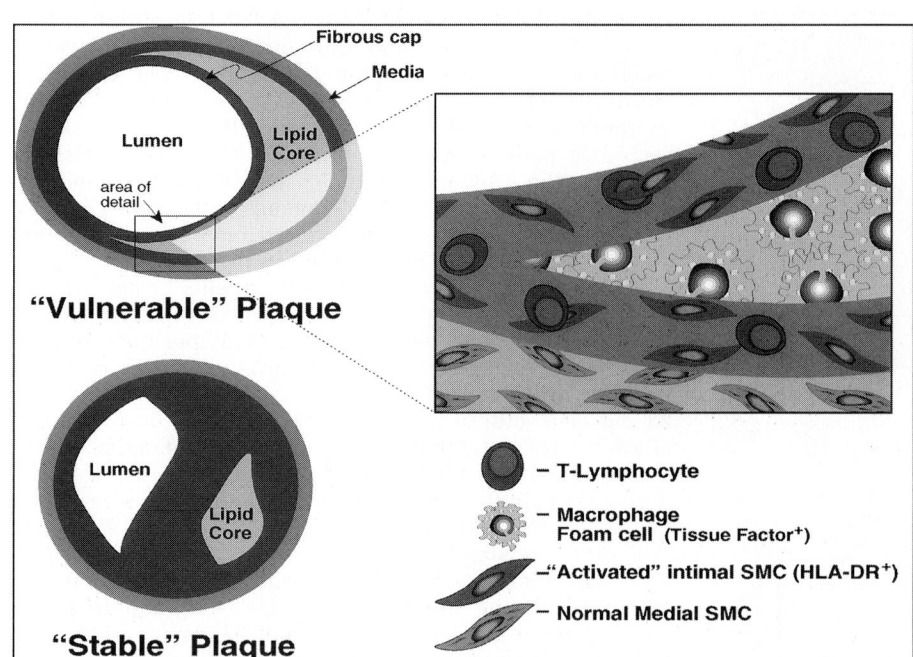

FIGURE 37–2. Comparison of the characteristics of "vulnerable" and "stable" plaques. Vulnerable plaques grow outward initially. The vulnerable plaque typically has a substantial lipid core and a thin fibrous cap separating the thrombogenic macrophages bearing tissue factor from the blood. At sites of lesion disruption, smooth muscle cells (SMCs) are often activated, as detected by their expression of the transplantation antigen HLA-DR. In contrast, the stable plaque has a relatively thick fibrous cap protecting the lipid core from contact with the blood. Clinical data suggest that stable plaques more often show luminal narrowing detectable by angiography than do vulnerable plaques. (Reproduced with permission from Libby, P.: Molecular bases of the acute coronary syndromes. Circulation *91*:2844, 1995. Copyright 1995 American Heart Association.)

to 37–4). The resultant thrombus interrupts blood flow and leads to an imbalance between oxygen supply and demand and, if this imbalance is severe and persistent, to myocardial necrosis (Fig. 36–23, p. 1177).

COMPOSITION OF PLAQUES. At autopsy, the atherosclerotic plaque of patients who died of MI is composed primarily of fibrous tissue of varying density and cellularity with superimposed thrombus.[66–67a] Calcium, lipid-laden foam cells, and extracellular lipid each constitute 5 to 10 per cent of the remaining area.[66] The atherosclerotic plaques that are associated with thrombosis and a total occlusion, located in infarct-related vessels, are generally more complex and irregular than those in vessels not associated with MI.[68] Histological studies of these lesions often

reveal plaque rupture or fissuring[60,68,69] (Fig. 37–6). Angiographic morphology suggestive of plaque rupture has been identified in the majority of stenoses associated with AMI or abrupt onset of unstable angina.[70] This finding is rare in the noninfarct-related vessels of AMI patients and in the vessels of patients with chronic stable angina.[70]

Platelet-rich thrombi are often associated with the surface of the most advanced atherosclerotic lesions, called complicated plaques, which are characterized by fibrocalcific degeneration, deposition of lipid, calcium, fibrous tissue, necrotic debris, extravasated blood, and a fibrous cap (Figs. 37–2 and 37–3). Impaired endothelial cell function may contribute to atherogenesis through release of growth factors.[68] Luminal narrowing may potentiate platelet activation

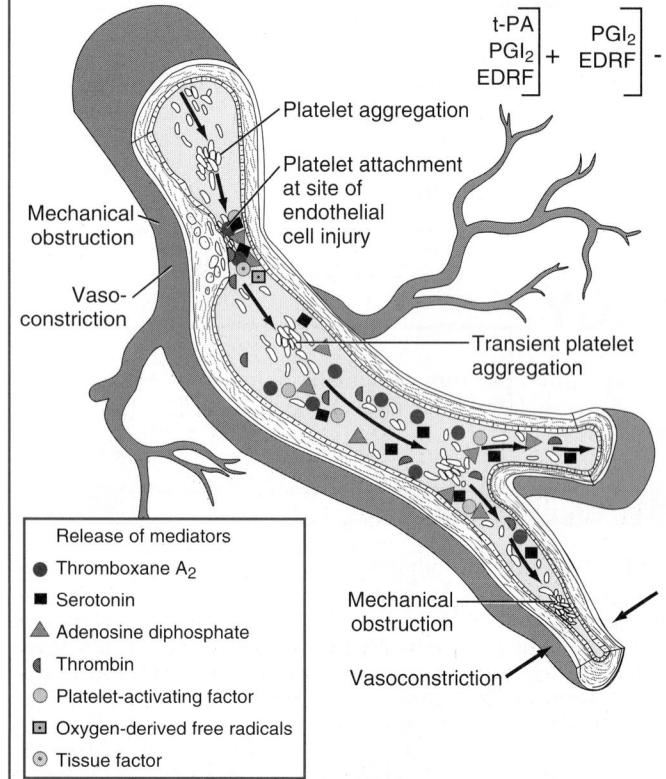

FIGURE 37–3. Schematic diagram suggesting probable mechanisms responsible for the conversion from chronic coronary heart disease to acute coronary artery disease syndromes. In this scheme, endothelial injury, usually at sites of atherosclerotic plaques and usually plaque ulceration or fissuring, is associated with platelet adhesion and aggregation and the release or activation of selected mediators, including thromboxane A_2, serotonin (5HT), adenosine diphosphate (ADP), platelet-activating factor (PAF), thrombin, tissue factor, and oxygen-derived free radicals. The accumulation of these mediators promotes platelet aggregation and mechanical obstruction of the narrowed artery. Thromboxane A_2, 5HT, thrombin, and PAF are vasoconstrictors at sites of endothelial injury. ADP, 5HT, and tissue factor have mitogenic influences and promote the development of neointimal proliferation. Therefore, the conversion from chronic stable to acute unstable coronary heart disease syndromes is most likely associated with endothelial injury, platelet aggregation, accumulation of platelet and other cell-derived mediators, further platelet aggregation, and vasoconstriction, with consequent dynamic narrowing of the coronary artery lumen. The relative absence of prostacyclin (PGI_2), t-PA (tissue plasminogen activator), and EDRF (nitrous oxide) at sites of endothelial injury contributes to the development of thrombosis, vasoconstriction, and neointimal proliferation. There are many different reasons for endothelial injury in addition to atherosclerotic plaque fissuring or ulceration, including flow shear stress, hypertension, immune complex deposition with complement activation, and mechanical injury to the endothelium as it occurs with coronary artery angioplasty, atherectomy, and stent placement and following heart transplantation. (From Willerson, J. T., Cohen, L. S., and Maseri, A.: Pathophysiology and clinical recognition. *In* Willerson, J. T., and Cohen, J. N. [eds.]: Cardiovascular Medicine. New York, Churchill Livingstone, 1995, p. 335.)

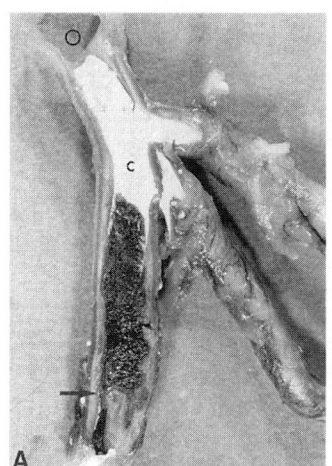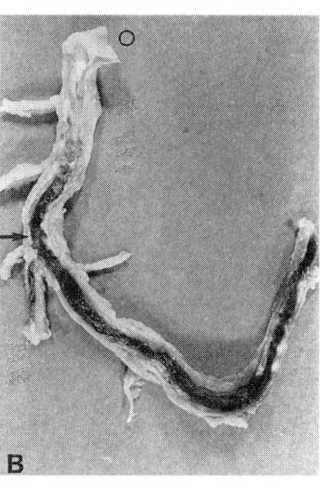

FIGURE 37–4. Thrombus propagation. *A*, Left anterior descending coronary artery cut open longitudinally, showing a dark (red) stagnation thrombosis propagating upstream from the initiating rupture/platelet-rich thrombus at the arrow. In this case, the thrombus has propagated proximally up to the nearest major side branch (the first diagonal branch). *B*, The right coronary artery cut open longitudinally, showing a huge stagnation thrombosis propagating downstream from the initiating rupture/platelet-rich thrombus at the arrow. Unlike upstream thrombus propagation, downstream propagation may, as in this case, occlude major side branches. O = coronary ostium; c = contrast medium injected postmortem. (From Falk, E.: Coronary thrombosis: Pathogenesis and clinical manifestations. Am. J. Cardiol. *68*:28B, 1991.)

through augmentation of shear forces. Young persons with coronary thrombotic events have been described as having a genetic polymorphism in glycoprotein IIb/IIIa, possibly altering platelet-fibrinogen interactions.[71] This observation raises the possibility of screening for patients at increased risk of coronary thrombosis in the event of plaque rupture.

In patients with MI, coronary thrombi are usually superimposed on or adjacent to atherosclerotic plaques (Figs. 37–3 and 37–4).[65] These coronary arterial thrombi, which are approximately 1 cm in length in most cases, adhere to the luminal surface of an artery and are composed of platelets, fibrin, erythrocytes, and leukocytes.[72] The composition of the thrombus may vary at different levels: A white thrombus is composed of platelets, fibrin, or both, and a red thrombus is composed of erythrocytes, fibrin, platelets, and leukocytes. Early thrombi are usually small and nonocclusive and are composed almost exclusively of platelets.

PLAQUE FISSURING AND RUPTURE. The process of plaque fissuring is an area of intense investigation and is likely to be multifactorial in nature[64] (Figs. 37–2 and 37–3). Libby has summarized the evidence suggesting that T lymphocytes in human atheroma elaborate the cytokine interferon-gamma (IFN-γ) that markedly inhibits the ability of vascular smooth muscle cells to form interstitial collagen in vulnerable regions of the fibrous cap over an atherosclerotic plaque.[68] Furthermore, in atherosclerotic plaques prone to rupture there is an increased rate of formation of metalloproteinase enzymes such as collagenase, gelatinase, and stromelysin that degrade components of the protective interstitial matrix.[65,68,73] These proteinases may be elaborated by activated macrophages and mast cells that have been shown to accumulate in high concentration at the site of atheromatous erosions and plaque rupture in patients who died of AMI.[63,74,75] Examination of specimens from directional atherectomy reveals a much higher content of macrophages in patients with unstable angina or AMI compared with patients with chronic stable angina.[64] In addition to these structural aspects of vulnerable plaques, stresses induced by intraluminal pressure, coronary vasomotor tone, tachycardia (cyclic stretching and compression),[65] and disruption of nutrient vessels[76] combine to produce plaque rupture at the margin of the fibrous cap near an adjacent plaque-free segment of the coronary artery wall (shoulder region of plaque).[65,77] A number of key physiological parameters such as systolic blood pressure, heart rate, blood viscosity, endogenous tissue plasminogen activator (t-PA) activity, plasminogen activator inhibitor-1 (PAI-1) levels, plasma cortisol levels, and plasma epinephrine levels that exhibit circadian variations act in concert to produce a heightened propensity to plaque rupture and coronary thrombosis between 6 and 11 A.M., yielding the circadian clustering of AMI and relative resistance to thrombolytic therapy in the early morning hours.[78,79]

ACUTE CORONARY SYNDROMES. If, when plaque rupture occurs, a sufficient quantity of thrombogenic substances is exposed, the coronary artery lumen may become obstructed

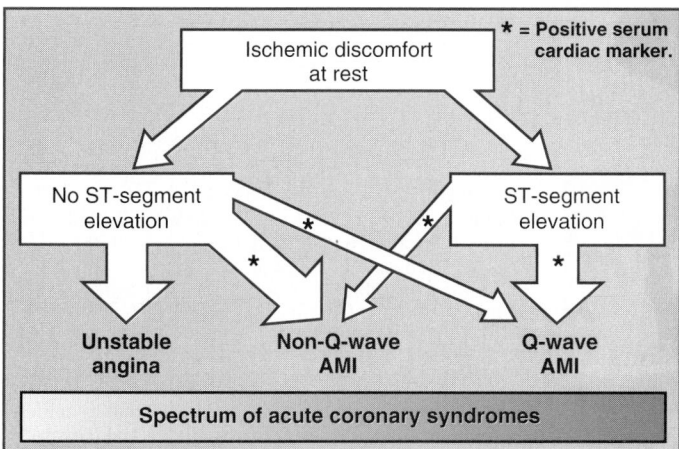

FIGURE 37–5. Acute coronary syndromes. Patients with ischemic discomfort may present with or without ST-segment elevation on the electrocardiogram. The majority (large arrow) of patients with ST-segment elevation ultimately develop a Q-wave acute myocardial infarction (AMI), whereas a minority (small arrow) develop a non-Q-wave AMI. Of the patients who present without ST-segment elevation, the majority (large arrows) are ultimately diagnosed with either unstable angina or non-Q-wave AMI based on the presence or absence of a cardiac marker such as CK-MB detected in the serum; a minority of such patients ultimately develop a Q-wave AMI. The spectrum of clinical conditions ranging from unstable angina to non-Q-wave AMI and Q-wave AMI is referred to as the acute coronary syndromes.

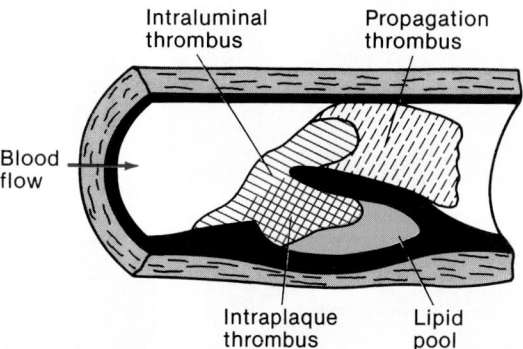

FIGURE 37–6. Representation of a longitudinal reconstruction of a coronary artery showing the histological components of an occluding thrombus. Much of the thrombus at the site of occlusion is contained within the plaque and compresses the lumen from outside. Intraluminal thrombus develops adjacent to a plaque fissure and then propagates downstream. A plug of lipid has extruded into the lumen. (Reproduced with permission from Davies, M. J.: A macro and micro view of coronary vascular insult in ischemic heart disease. Circulation *82*[Suppl. II]:38, 1990. Copyright 1990 American Heart Association.)

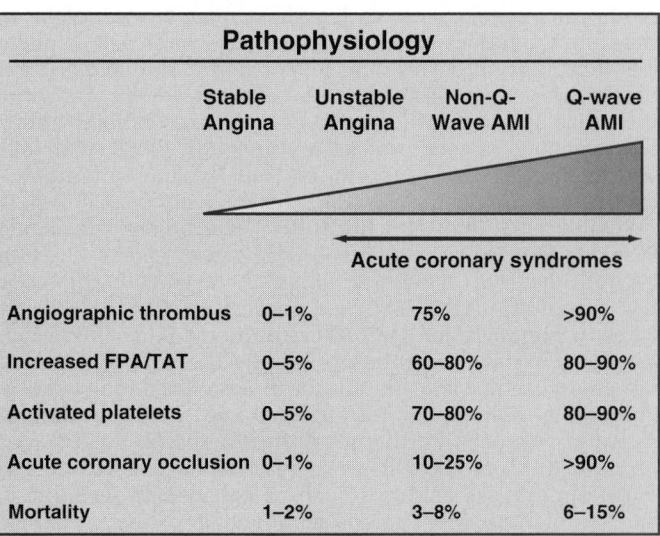

Pathophysiology	Stable Angina	Unstable Angina	Non-Q-Wave AMI	Q-wave AMI
		Acute coronary syndromes		
Angiographic thrombus	0–1%	75%		>90%
Increased FPA/TAT	0–5%	60–80%		80–90%
Activated platelets	0–5%	70–80%		80–90%
Acute coronary occlusion	0–1%	10–25%		>90%
Mortality	1–2%	3–8%		6–15%

FIGURE 37–7. Comparison of pathophysiological findings in patients with acute coronary syndromes. Progression from unstable angina to Q-wave AMI across the acute coronary syndrome spectrum is associated with a progressively increasing incidence of detection of thrombus at angiography, evidence of activation of the coagulation cascade (release of fibrinopeptide A [FPA] and generation of thrombin-antithrombin [TAT] complexes), activation and aggregation of platelets, and ultimately complete occlusion of the culprit coronary artery. The greater diminution in regional coronary blood flow and the larger amount of myocardium that progresses to necrosis with Q-wave AMI result in higher mortality rates than occurs in patients with unstable angina or non-Q-wave AMI. (From Cannon, C. P., and Rutherford, J. D.: The clinical spectrum of ischemic heart disease. *In* Antman, E. M., and Rutherford, J. D. [eds.]: Coronary Care Medicine: A Practical Approach. Boston, Marinus Nijhoff, 1996.)

by a combination of fibrin, platelet aggregates, and red blood cells[65] (Figs. 37–3, 37–4, and 37–6). An adequate collateral network that prevents necrosis from occurring can result in clinically silent episodes of coronary occlu-

sion.[80] The rupture of plaques is now considered to be the common pathophysiological substrate of the *acute coronary syndromes* that range from unstable angina through non-Q-wave AMI and Q-wave AMI (Figs. 37–5 and 37–7). The dynamic process of plaque rupture may evolve to a completely occlusive thrombus, typically producing ST elevation on the electrocardiogram and ultimately necrosis involving the full or nearly full thickness of the ventricular wall in a zone subtended by the affected coronary artery (i.e., transmural myocardial infarction, often with *Q wave* development on the ECG). Less obstructive thrombi and/or those that are constituted by less robust fibrin formation and a greater proportion of platelet aggregates produce the syndromes of *unstable angina* (see p. 1331) and *non-Q-wave AMI*, typically presenting as ST-segment depression and/or T-wave inversion on the ECG (Figs. 37–5 and 37–7). Relief of transient vasospasm (induced by thromboxane A_2 and serotonin released from activated platelets) or spontaneous lysis and restoration of antegrade flow in the culprit coronary vessel in less than 20 minutes usually does not result in histological evidence of necrosis, the release of biochemical markers of necrosis, or persistent changes on the electrocardiogram; the resulting condition is unstable angina (Figs. 37–5 and 37–7). Episodes of plaque rupture more prolonged and more severe than those producing unstable angina typically result in release of a biochemical marker of necrosis but a less extensive pattern of necrosis than is found in patients with ST-elevation MI. When clinical evidence of necrosis is detected (now possible in a greater number of patients with sensitive markers such as cardiac-specific troponin T or I) (see p. 1203) and no pathological Q waves evolve on the ECG, a diagnosis of non-Q-wave AMI is made, a condition midway between Q-wave infarction and unstable angina (Figs. 37–5 and 37–7). Often, patients with non-Q-wave MI have a pattern of myocardial necrosis that is less confluent in nature and more concentrated in the inner third of the ventricular wall because restoration of blood flow prevented the wavefront of necrosis from extending across the thickness of the ventricular wall.

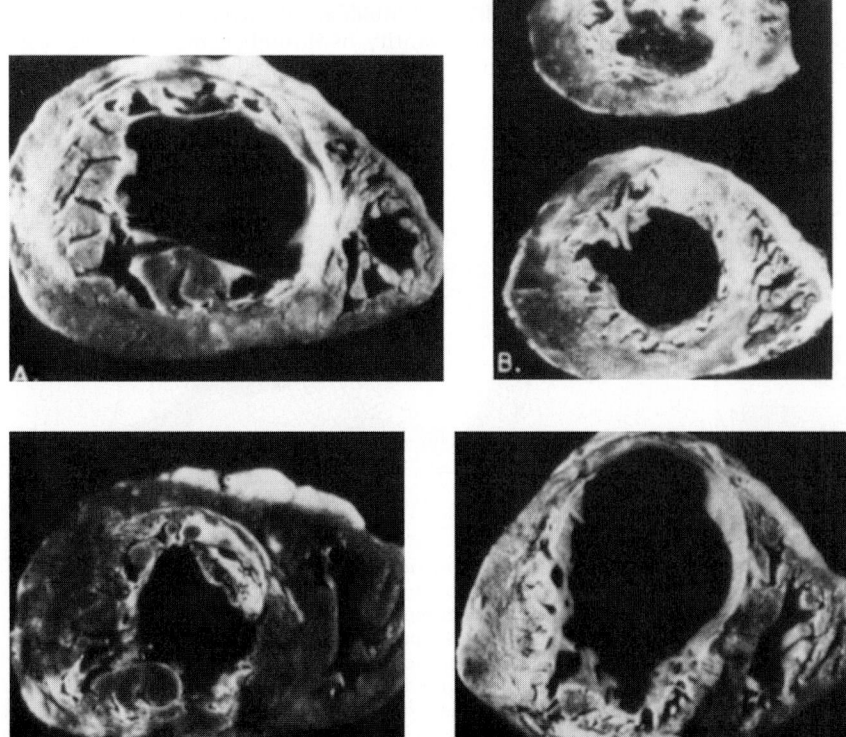

FIGURE 37–8. Examples of gross appearance of heart with healed MI. *A,* Healed extensive anteroseptal infarction. The involved part of the wall is thin. *B,* Two levels of section showing healed anterior infarction with mural thrombosis at the apex. *C,* Healed subendocardial anterior infarction with endocardial fibrosis. The inferolateral aspect shows scarring of healed infarction. *D,* Healed extensive anterior infarction and recent healing inferior infarction. The thin wall and endocardial fibrosis are characteristic of a healed extensive anterior infarct. The inferior wall contains an infarct that is undergoing healing. (From Edwards, B. S., and Edwards, J. E.: Pathology of acute myocardial infarction. *In* Francis, G. S., and Alpert, J. S. [eds.]: Modern Coronary Care. 2nd ed. Boston, Little, Brown and Co., 1995, p. 58.)

Some patients with stenotic atherosclerotic lesions experience AMI without evidence of plaque rupture or superimposed thrombosis. AMI occurs in clinical circumstances that produce a marked reduction in myocardial oxygen supply (e.g., prolonged severe vasospasm, as in Prinzmetal's variant angina (see p. 1340), or associated with a marked increase in myocardial oxygen demand (see below). These infarcts are located along the least well perfused inner one-third to one-half of the ventricular wall and often extend beyond the target territory perfused by a single coronary vessel. The ECG in such patients may show deep T-wave inversions or diffuse ST-segment depression.

Correlation with Evolutionary Changes on ECG

Autopsy data have shown that the ECG lacks sufficient sensitivity and specificity to permit reliable distinction of transmural from subendocardial infarcts because patients with transmural infarcts may not develop Q waves and Q waves may be seen in patients with autopsy evidence of a subendocardial (nontransmural) AMI.[81] These remarks not-

withstanding, a crude categorization of patients into Q-wave and non-Q-wave patterns based on the ECG is useful because Q-wave AMIs are usually associated with greater ventricular damage, a greater tendency to infarct expansion and remodeling, and a higher mortality rate.[82-84]

GROSS PATHOLOGICAL CHANGES

On gross inspection, AMI may be divided into two major types: transmural infarcts, in which myocardial necrosis involves the full thickness (or nearly full thickness) of the ventricular wall, and subendocardial (nontransmural) infarcts, in which the necrosis involves the subendocardium, the intramural myocardium, or both without extending all the way through the ventricular wall to the epicardium (Fig. 37–8).[58a]

An occlusive coronary thrombosis appears to be far more common when the infarction is transmural and localized to

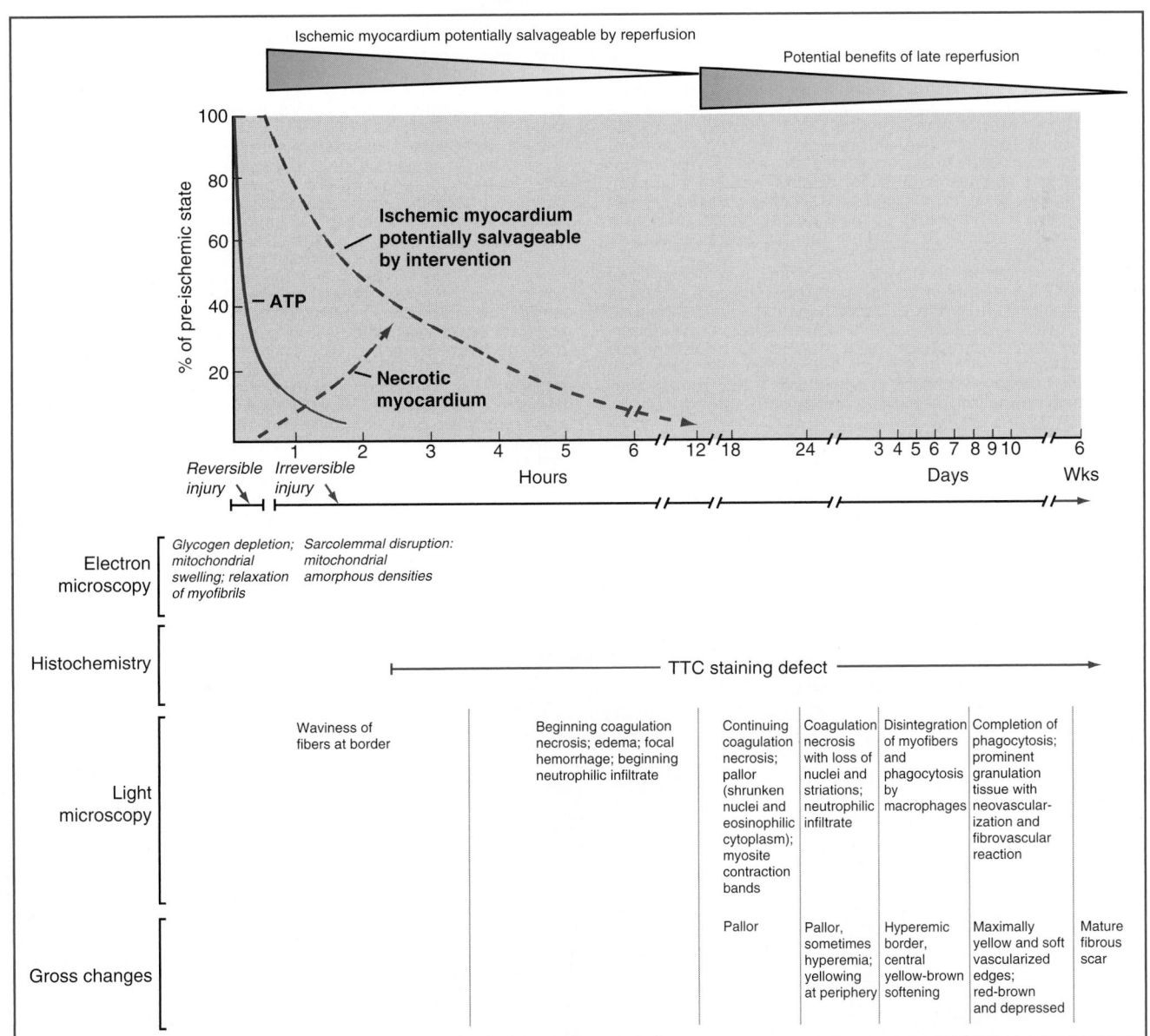

FIGURE 37–9. Temporal sequence of early biochemical, ultrastructural, histochemical, and histological findings after onset of MI. At the top of the figure are schematically shown the time frames for early and late reperfusion of the myocardium supplied by an occluded coronary artery. For approximately one-half hour following the onset of even the most severe ischemia, myocardial injury is potentially reversible; after that there is progressive loss of viability that is complete by 6 to 12 hours. The benefits of reperfusion (both early and late) are greatest when it is achieved early, with progressively smaller benefits occurring as reperfusion is delayed. (Figure developed in collaboration with Dr. Frederick J. Schoen.)

the distribution of a single coronary artery[85] (Figs. 37–4 and 37–7). Nontransmural infarctions, however, frequently occur in the presence of severely narrowed but still patent coronary arteries. Patchy nontransmural infarction may arise from thrombolysis or PTCA of an originally occlusive thrombus with restoration of blood flow *before* the wave-front of necrosis has extended from the subendocardium across the full thickness of the ventricular wall (Fig. 36–23, p. 1177). The histological pattern of necrosis may differ, with contraction band injury (see below) occurring almost twice as often in nontransmural as in transmural infarction.[85] Paradoxically, before their infarction, patients with nontransmural infarcts have, on average, a more severe stenosis in the infarct-related coronary artery than do patients suffering from transmural infarcts.[86] This finding suggests that a more severe obstruction occurring before infarction protects against the development of transmural infarction, perhaps by fostering the development of collateral circulation. It also accords with the concept that less severely stenotic but lipid-laden plaques with a fragile cap are responsible for the abrupt presentation of ST-segment elevation that may evolve to transmural infarctions.

Gross alterations of the myocardium are difficult to identify until at least 6 to 12 hours have elapsed following the onset of necrosis (Fig. 37–9). However, a variety of histochemical approaches have been used to identify zones of necrosis that can be discerned after only 2 to 3 hours. Tissue slices of suspected infarct sites are immersed in a solution of triphenyltetrazolium chloride (TTC), which stains viable myocardium brick red (because of preserved dehydrogenase enzymes that form a red formazen precipitate[87]) and leaves the infarcted region pale as a result of failure of uptake of the vital dye[88] (Fig. 37–9). The nitroblue tetrazolium (NBT) staining technique can similarly distinguish viable zones of myocardium, which stain dark blue, from necrotic areas of myocardium that therefore remain uncolored and identifiable.[89]

Initially, the myocardium in the affected region may appear pale and slightly swollen. Eighteen to 36 hours after the onset of the infarct, the myocardium is tan or reddish purple (due to trapped erythrocytes), with a serofibrinous exudate evident on the epicardium in transmural infarcts. These changes persist for approximately 48 hours; the infarct then turns gray, and fine yellow lines, secondary to neutrophilic infiltration, appear at its periphery. This zone gradually widens and during the next few days extends throughout the infarct.

Eight to 10 days following infarction, the thickness of the cardiac wall in the area of the infarct is reduced as necrotic muscle is removed by mononuclear cells. The cut surface of an infarct of this age is yellow, surrounded by a reddish purple band of granulation tissue that extends through the necrotic tissue by 3 to 4 weeks. Commencing at this time and extending over the next 2 to 3 months, the infarcted area gradually acquires a gelatinous, ground-glass, gray appearance, eventually converting into a shrunken, thin, firm scar,

which whitens and firms progressively with time[81] (Fig. 37–9). This process begins at the periphery of the infarct and gradually moves centrally. The endocardium below the infarct increases in thickness and becomes gray and opaque.

Histological and Ultrastructural Changes

ELECTRON MICROSCOPY. In experimental infarction, the earliest ultrastructural changes in cardiac muscle following ligation of a coronary artery, noted within 20 minutes, consist of reduction in the size and number of glycogen granules, intracellular edema, and swelling and distortion of the transverse tubular system, the sarcoplasmic reticulum, and the mitochondria (Figs. 37–9 and 37–10).[81,90] These early changes are reversible. Changes after 60 minutes of occlusion include myocardial cell swelling, mitochondrial abnormalities such as swelling and internal disruption, and development of amorphous, flocculent aggregation and margination of nuclear chromatin, and relaxation of myofibrils. After 20 minutes to 2 hours of ischemia, changes in some cells become irreversible, and there is progression of these alterations; additional changes include indistinct tight junctions at the intercalated discs, swollen sacs of the sarcoplasmic reticulum at the level of the A band, greatly enlarged mitochondria with few cristae, thinning and fractionation of myofilaments, disappearance of the heterochromatin, rarefaction of the euchromatin and peripheral aggregation of chromatin in the nucleus, disorientation of myofibrils, and clumping of mitochondria. Cells irreversibly damaged by ischemia are usually swollen, with an enlarged sarcoplasmic space; the sarcolemma may peel off the cells, defects in the plasma membrane may appear, and the mitochondria are fragmented. The swollen mitochondria obtained from ischemic myocardium contain deposits of calcium phosphate and amorphous matrix densities. Many of these changes become more intense when blood flow is restored.[81,90]

LIGHT MICROSCOPY. It was previously believed that no light microscopic changes could be seen in infarcted myocardium until 8 hours after interruption of blood flow. However, in some infarcts a pattern of wavy myocardial fibers may be seen 1 to 3 hours after onset, especially at the periphery of the infarct (Fig. 37–9). It is hypothesized that wavy fibers result from the stretching and buckling of noncontractile fibers as forces are transmitted to them from adjacent viable contractile fibers.[81,84] After 8 hours, edema of the interstitium becomes evident, as do increased fatty deposits in the muscle fibers, along with infiltration of neutrophilic polymorphonuclear leukocytes and red blood cells. Muscle cell nuclei become pyknotic and then undergo karyolysis, and small blood vessels undergo necrosis.

By 24 hours there is clumping of the cytoplasm and loss of cross striations, with appearance of focal hyalinization and irregular crossbands in the involved myocardial fibers. The nuclei become pyknotic and sometimes even disappear. The myocardial capillaries in the involved region dilate, and polymorphonuclear leukocytes accumulate, first at the periphery and then in the center of the infarct. During the first 3 days, the interstitial tissue becomes edematous and red blood cells may extravasate (Fig. 37–9). Generally, on about the fourth day after infarction, removal of necrotic fibers by macrophages begins, again commencing at the periphery (Fig. 37–9). Later, lymphocytes, macrophages, and fibroblasts infiltrate between myocytes, which become fragmented. At 8 days the necrotic muscle fibers have become

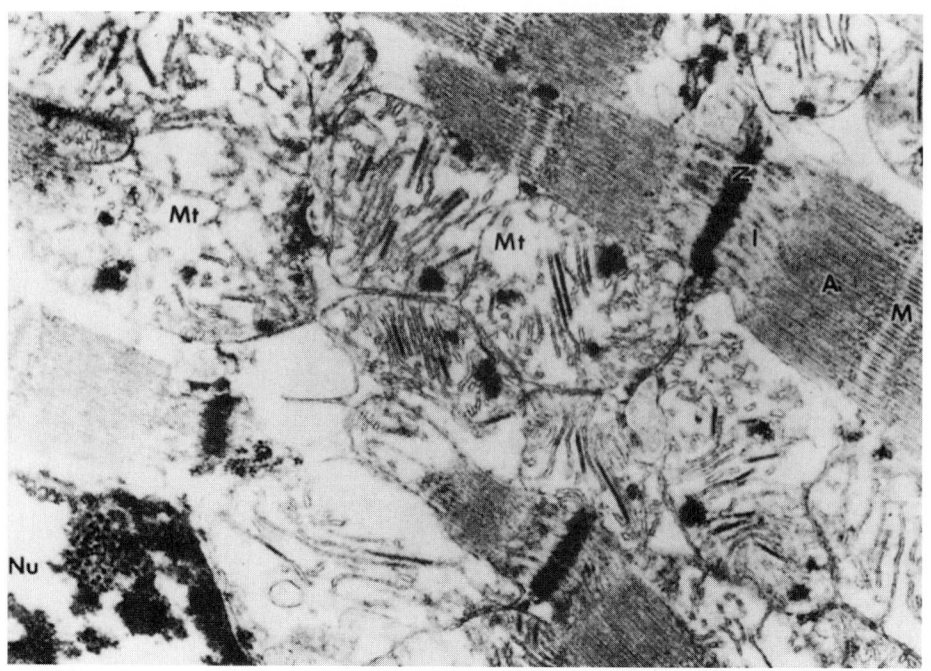

FIGURE 37–10. Electron micrograph of a muscle cell from the center of an infarct produced by permanent coronary occlusion in the dog. The myofibrils are fixed in a relaxed state and exhibit I, A, M, and Z bands. There is slight edema and no glycogen. (The clusters of granules resembling glycogen probably are ribosomes.) The mitochondria (Mt) are swollen and have linear densities and amorphous matrix (flocculent) densities. The nucleus (Nu) has clumped chromatin along the nuclear membrane and large lucent areas. (Tissue fixed with glutaraldehyde and osmium. Epoxy section stained with uranyl acetate and lead citrate, ×19,500.) (From Willerson, J. T., Hillis, L. D., and Buja, L. D. (eds.): Pathogenesis and pathology of ischemic heart disease. *In* Ischemic Heart Disease. Clinical and Pathophysiological Aspects. New York, Raven Press, 1982, p. 47.)

dissolved; by about 10 days the number of polymorphonuclear leukocytes is reduced, and granulation tissue first appears at the periphery. Ingrowth of blood vessels and fibroblasts continues, along with removal of necrotic muscle cells, until the fourth to sixth week following infarction, by which time much of the necrotic myocardium has been removed. This process continues along with increasing collagenization of the infarcted area. By the sixth week, the infarcted area has usually been converted into a firm connective tissue scar with interspersed intact muscle fibers (Fig. 37–9).

Patterns of Myocardial Necrosis

COAGULATION NECROSIS. This results from severe, persistent ischemia and is usually present in the central region of infarcts, which results in the arrest of muscle cells[91] in the relaxed state and the passive stretching of ischemic muscle cells. On light microscopy the myofibrils are stretched, many with nuclear pyknosis, vascular congestion, and healing by phagocytosis of necrotic muscle cells (Fig. 37–9). There is evidence of mitochondrial damage with prominent amorphous (flocculent) densities but no calcification.

NECROSIS WITH CONTRACTION BANDS. This form of myocardial necrosis, also termed *contraction band necrosis* or *coagulative myocytolysis*, results primarily from severe ischemia followed by reflow.[81] It is caused by increased Ca++ influx into dying cells, resulting in the arrest of cells in the contracted state. It is seen in the periphery of large infarcts and is present to a greater extent in nontransmural than in transmural infarcts.[85] The entire infarct may show this form of necrosis when reperfusion occurs experimentally or by surgery[91] (Fig.

37–11). Although patches of contraction band necrosis are found after successful reperfusion by thrombolytic therapy,[92] their presence in a large segment of the infarcts of patients who did not receive such therapy suggests that reperfusion through spontaneous thrombolysis or the release of spasm or both have occurred. It is characterized by hypercontracted myofibrils with contraction bands and mitochondrial damage, frequently with calcification, marked vascular congestion, and healing by lysis of muscle cells.

MYOCYTOLYSIS. Ischemia without necrosis generally causes no acute changes that are visible by light microscopy. However, severe prolonged ischemia can cause myocyte vacuolization, often termed myocytolysis. Prolonged severe ischemia, which is potentially reversible, causes cloudy swelling, as well as hydropic, vascular, and fatty degeneration.[93] Frequently seen at the borders of an infarct as well as in patchy areas of infarction in patients with chronic ischemic heart disease, myocytolysis is characterized by edema and cell swelling, lysis of myofibrils and nuclei, no neutrophilic response, and healing by lysis and phagocytosis of necrotic myocytes and ultimately scar formation.[94]

MODIFICATION OF PATHOLOGICAL CHANGES BY REPERFUSION

Early after the onset of ischemia, contractile dysfunction is observed that is believed to be due in part to shortening of the action potential duration, reduced cytosolic free calcium levels, and intracellular acidosis.[95] When reperfusion of myocardium undergoing the evolutionary changes from ischemia to infarction occurs sufficiently early (i.e., within 15 to 20 minutes), it may successfully prevent necro-

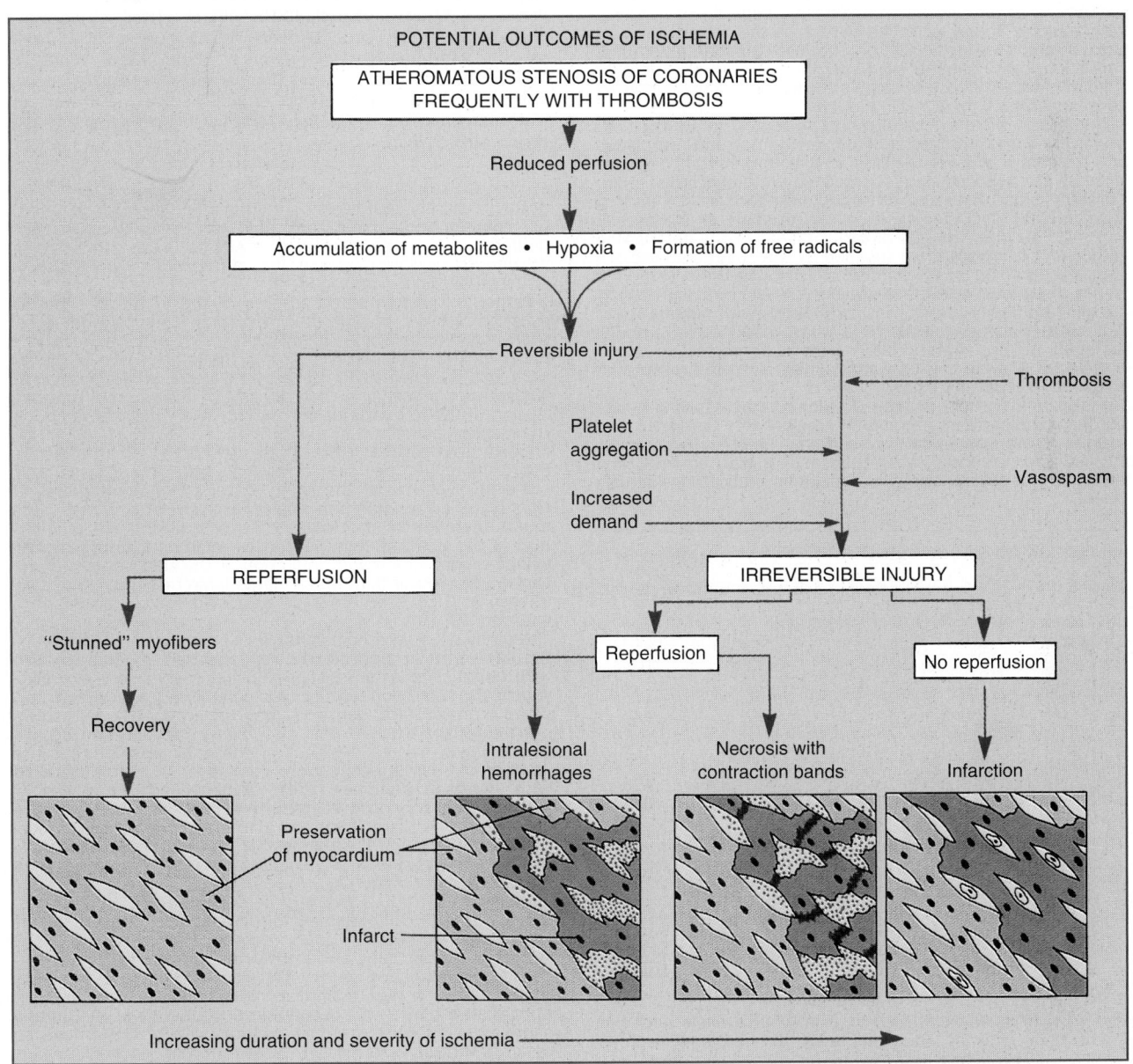

FIGURE 37–11. Several potential outcomes of reversible and irreversible ischemic injury to the myocardium. (From Schoen, F. J.: The heart. *In* Cotran, R. S., Kumar, V., and Robbins, S. L. (eds.): Pathologic Basis of Disease. 5th ed. Philadelphia, W. B. Saunders Company, 1994, p. 538.)

sis from developing. Beyond such a very early stage, the number of salvaged myocytes and therefore the amount of salvaged myocardial tissue (area of necrosis/area at risk) is directly related to the length of time the coronary artery has been totally occluded,[88] the level of myocardial oxygen consumption, and the collateral blood flow (Fig. 37–11). Typical pathological findings of reperfused infarcts include a histological mixture of necrosis, hemorrhage within zones of irreversibly injured myocytes,[96] coagulative myocytolysis with contraction bands, and distorted architecture of the cells in the reperfused zone[81] (Fig. 37–11). Following reperfusion, mitochondria in nonviable myocytes develop deposits of calcium phosphate and ultimately a large fraction of the cells may calcify. Reperfusion of infarcted myocardium also accelerates the washout of intracellular proteins ("serum cardiac markers"), producing an exaggerated and early peak value of substances such as CK-MB and cardiac-specific troponin T and I.[97]

CORONARY ANATOMY AND LOCATION OF INFARCTION

In over 75 per cent of patients with MI who come to autopsy, more than one coronary artery is severely narrowed.[94,98] One-third to two-thirds of patients with AMI have critical obstruction (to less than 25 per cent of luminal area) of all three coronary arteries, whereas the remainder are equally divided between those having one-vessel disease and those having two-vessel disease.[98,99] Coronary arteriographic studies in surviving patients show that a higher percentage have one-vessel disease. Angiographic studies performed in the earliest hours of AMI in patients presenting with ST-segment elevation have revealed approximately a 90 per cent incidence of total occlusion of the infarct-related vessel.[100,101] Recanalization from spontaneous thrombolysis[101,102] as well as attrition due to some mortality among those patients with total occlusion results in a diminishing incidence of angiographically totally occluded vessels in the period following myocardial infarction (Fig. 37–12).[99] In contrast to patients with a Q-wave infarction, those patients who sustain a non-Q-wave infarction have a much lower incidence of complete occlusion of the infarct-related coronary artery (Figs. 37–7 and 37–13).

Thus, transmural infarcts occur distal to an acutely totally occluded coronary artery with thrombus superimposed on a ruptured plaque. However, the converse is not the case, in that chronic total occlusion of a coronary artery is not always associated with myocardial infarction. Collateral blood flow and other factors—such as the level of myocardial metabolism, the presence and location of stenoses in other coronary arteries, the rate of development of the obstruction, and the quantity of myocardium supplied by the obstructed vessel—all influence the viability of myocardial cells distal to the occlusion. In many series of patients studied at necropsy or by coronary arteriography, a small number (<5 per cent) of patients with AMI are found to have normal coronary vessels.[94,99] In these patients, an embolus that has lysed, a transiently occlusive platelet aggregate, or a prolonged episode of severe coronary spasm may have been responsible for the reduction in coronary flow.

Studies of patients who ultimately develop AMI after having undergone coronary angiography at some time before its occurrence have been helpful in clarifying coronary anatomy before infarction. Although high-grade stenoses, when present,[103] more frequently lead to AMI than do less severe lesions, the majority of occlusions actually

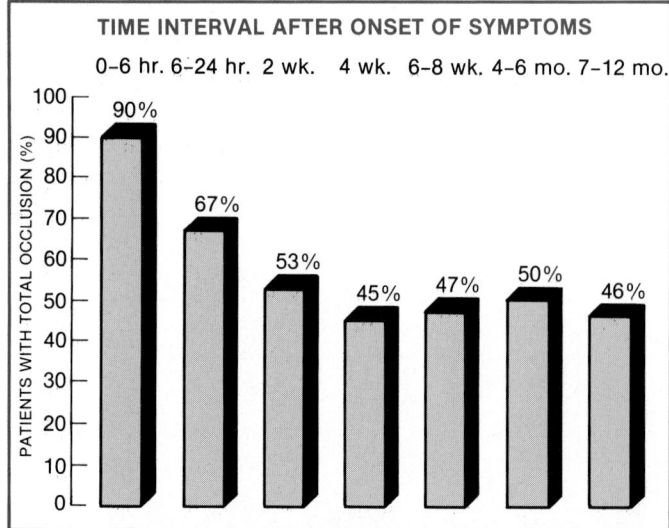

FIGURE 37–12. Percentage of patients with total coronary occlusion at different time intervals after the onset of symptoms of AMI. (Adapted from deFeyter, P. J., van den Brand, M., Serruys, P. W., and Wijns, W.: Early angiography after myocardial infarction: What have we learned? Am. Heart J. *109*:194, 1985.)

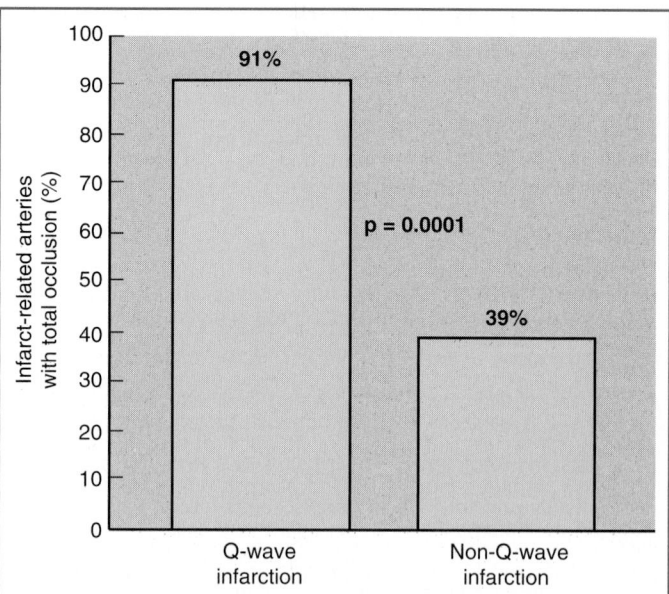

FIGURE 37–13. Prevalence of total occlusion of infarct-related artery in patients during the first 6 hours of acute Q-wave infarction versus non-Q-wave infarction. The infarct-related artery was totally occluded in 91 per cent of patients with Q-wave versus 39 per cent of patients with non-Q-wave infarction. (From Keen, W. D., Savage, M. P., Fischman, D. L., et al.: Comparison of coronary angiographic findings during the first 6 hours of non-Q-wave and Q-wave myocardial infarction. Am. J. Cardiol. *74*:324, 1994. Copyright 1994 by excerpta Medica Inc.)

occur in vessels with a previously identified stenosis of less than 50 per cent on angiograms performed months to years earlier.[104] This finding supports the concept that AMI occurs as a result of sudden thrombotic occlusion at the site of rupture of previously nonobstructive but lipid-rich plaques.[103]

Rather frequently, when an area of the ventricle is perfused by collateral vessels, an infarct occurs at a distance from a coronary occlusion. For example, following the gradual obliteration of the lumen of the right coronary artery, the inferior wall of the left ventricle may be maintained viable by collateral vessels arising from the left anterior descending coronary artery. In this circumstance, an occlusion of the left anterior descending artery may cause an infarct of the diaphragmatic wall.

RIGHT VENTRICULAR INFARCTION. Depending on the criteria used, approximately 50 per cent of patients with inferior infarction have some involvement of the right ventricle.[105] Among these patients, right ventricular infarction occurs exclusively in those with transmural infarction of the inferoposterior wall and the posterior portion of the septum. Right ventricular infarction almost invariably develops in association with infarction of the adjacent septum and left ventricular myocardium, but isolated infarction of the right ventricle is seen in 3 to 5 per cent of autopsy-proven cases of myocardial infarction.[106]

Regardless of whether or not it is combined with involvement of the left ventricle, right ventricular infarction is generally associated with obstructive lesions of the right coronary artery. However, right ventricular infarction occurs less commonly than would be anticipated from the frequency of atherosclerotic lesions involving the right coronary artery.[107] This discrepancy probably can be explained by the lower oxygen demands of the right ventricle, because right ventricular infarcts occur more commonly in conditions associated with increased right ventricular oxygen needs such as pulmonary hypertension and right ventricular hypertrophy.[105,108] Moreover, the intercoronary collateral system of the right ventricle is richer than that of the left, and the thinness of the right ventricular wall allows the chamber to derive some nutrition from the blood within the right ventricular cavity.

ATRIAL INFARCTION. This may be seen in up to 10 per cent of patients with AMI if PR segment displacement is used as the criterion for atrial infarction.[109] Although isolated atrial infarction may be observed in 3.5 per cent of autopsies of patients with AMI,[110] it often occurs in conjunction with ventricular infarction and can cause rupture of the atrial wall.[111] This type of infarct is more common on the right than the left side, occurs more frequently in the atrial appendages than in the lateral or posterior walls of the atrium, and can result in thrombus formation.[112] The difference in incidence between right and left atrial infarction might be explained by the considerably higher oxygen content of left atrial blood. Atrial infarction is frequently accompanied by atrial arrhythmias. It has also been reported to be associated with reduced secretion of atrial natriuretic peptide and a low cardiac output syndrome when right ventricular infarction coexists.[113]

CORONARY ARTERY SPASM (see also p. 1341). In addition to causing AMI in patients with Prinzmetal's angina (p. 1340), coronary artery spasm may also cause intimal damage that can initiate formation of an atherosclerotic plaque.[114] Epicardial coronary artery spasm has been identified in patients with fixed atherosclerotic coronary artery stenosis before, during, and after AMI. An association between coronary artery spasm and coronary artery thrombosis has also been documented clinically.[115]

COLLATERAL CIRCULATION IN ACUTE MYOCARDIAL INFARCTION (see also p. 1174)

The coronary collateral circulation is particularly well developed in patients with (1) coronary occlusive disease, especially when it is severe, with the reduction of the luminal cross-sectional area by more than 75 per cent in one or more major vessels; (2) chronic hypoxia, as occurs in severe anemia, chronic obstructive pulmonary disease, and cyanotic congenital heart disease; and (3) left ventricular hypertrophy, which intensifies coronary collaterals.

The magnitude of coronary collateral flow is one of the principal determinants of infarct size.[116] Indeed, it is rather common for patients with abundant collaterals to have totally occluded coronary arteries without evidence of infarction in the distribution of that artery; thus, the survival of the myocardium distal to such occlusions must depend on collateral blood flow. Even if collateral perfusion existing at the time of coronary occlusion is not successful in improving contractile function, it may still exert a beneficial effect by preventing the formation of a left ventricular aneurysm.[117] Some collaterals are seen in nearly 40 per cent of patients with an acute total occlusion,[118] and more begin to appear soon after the total occlusion occurs.[100] It is likely that the presence of a high-grade stenosis (>90 per cent), possibly with periods of intermittent total occlusion, permits the development of collaterals that remain only as potential conduits until a total occlusion occurs or recurs. The latter event then brings these channels into full operation.

The incidence of collaterals 1 to 2 weeks following AMI varies considerably and may be as high as 75 to 100 per cent in patients with persistent occlusion of the infarct vessel, or as low as 17 to 42 per cent in patients with subtotal occlusion.[119]

NONATHEROSCLEROTIC CAUSES OF ACUTE MYOCARDIAL INFARCTION

Numerous pathological processes other than atherosclerosis can involve the coronary arteries (see p. 1349) and result in myocardial infarction (Table 37-1).[90,119a] For example, coronary arterial occlusions can be the result of embolization of a coronary artery. Emboli most frequently lodge in the distribution of the left anterior descending coronary artery, commonly in the distal epicardial and intramural branches. The causes of coronary embolism are numerous: infective endocarditis and nonbacterial thrombotic endocarditis (see Chap. 33), mural thrombi, prosthetic valves,[120] neoplasms,[121] air that is introduced at the time of cardiac surgery,[122] and calcium deposits from manipulation of calcified valves at operation. In situ thrombosis of coronary arteries can occur secondary to chest wall trauma (see Chap. 44).

A variety of inflammatory processes can be responsible for coronary artery abnormalities, some of which mimic atherosclerotic disease and may predispose to true atherosclerosis.[123] Epidemiological evidence suggests that viral infections, particularly with coxsackie B, may be an uncommon cause of AMI.[124] Viral illnesses precede AMI occasionally in young persons who are later shown to have normal coronary arteries.[125]

Syphilitic aortitis may produce marked narrowing or occlusion of one or both coronary ostia,[126] whereas Takayasu's arteritis may result in obstruction of the coronary arteries (see Chap. 45).[127] Necrotizing arteritis, polyarteritis nodosa,[128] mucocutaneous lymph node syndrome (Kawasaki disease) (see p. 994),[129] systemic lupus erythematosus (see p. 1778) and giant cell arteritis[130] (see Chap. 56) can cause coronary occlusion. Therapeutic levels of mediastinal radiation can cause thickening and hyalinization of the walls of coronary arteries, with subsequent infarction.[131] AMI may also be the result of coronary arterial involvement in amyloidosis (see p. 1797), Hurler syndrome, pseudoxanthoma elasticum,[132] and homocystinuria (see Chap. 49).

As cocaine abuse has become more common, reports of AMI following the use of cocaine have appeared with increasing frequency. Cocaine may cause AMI in patients with normal coronary arteries, preexisting MI, documented coronary artery disease, or coronary artery spasm.[133–135] AMI associated with cocaine has also been reported following its topical use in nasal septoplasty[136] and in neonates whose mothers used the drug.[137] Recurrent MI after further cocaine abuse has been reported as well.

Cocaine may cause AMI by at least three mechanisms: (1) increasing myocardial oxygen demand through increases in heart rate and blood pressure, (2) diminishing coronary artery flow resulting from either coronary vasospasm and/or thrombosis, and (3) active myo-

carditis (either hypersensitivity or toxic).[134,135,138,139] In very high doses, cocaine appears to have a direct toxic effect on heart muscle which may produce cardiac failure and sudden death with extensive myocyte necrosis.[133,134]

TABLE 37-1 CAUSES OF MYOCARDIAL INFARCTION WITHOUT CORONARY ATHEROSCLEROSIS

CORONARY ARTERY DISEASE OTHER THAN ATHEROSCLEROSIS
Arteritis
  Luetic
  Granulomatous (Takayasu disease)
  Polyarteritis nodosa
  Mucocutaneous lymph node (Kawasaki) syndrome
  Disseminated lupus erythematosus
  Rheumatoid arthritis
  Ankylosing spondylitis
Trauma to coronary arteries
  Laceration
  Thrombosis
  Iatrogenic
  Radiation (radiotherapy for neoplasia)
Coronary mural thickening with metabolic disease or intimal proliferative disease
  Mucopolysaccharidoses (Hurler disease)
  Homocystinuria
  Fabry disease
  Amyloidosis
  Juvenile intimal sclerosis (idiopathic arterial calcification of infancy)
  Intimal hyperplasia associated with contraceptive steroids or with the postpartum period
  Pseudoxanthoma elasticum
  Coronary fibrosis caused by radiation therapy
Luminal narrowing by other mechanisms
  Spasm of coronary arteries (Prinzmetal's angina with normal coronary arteries)
  Spasm after nitroglycerin withdrawal
  Dissection of the aorta
  Dissection of the coronary artery

EMBOLI TO CORONARY ARTERIES
Infective endocarditis
Nonbacterial thrombotic endocarditis
Prolapse of mitral valve
Mural thrombus from left atrium, left ventricle, or pulmonary veins
Prosthetic valve emboli
Cardiac myxoma
Associated with cardiopulmonary bypass surgery and coronary arteriography
Paradoxical emboli
Papillary fibroelastoma of the aortic valve ("fixed embolus")
Thrombi from intracardiac catheters or guidewires

CONGENITAL CORONARY ARTERY ANOMALIES
Anomalous origin of left coronary from pulmonary artery
Left coronary artery from anterior sinus of Valsalva
Coronary arteriovenous and arteriocameral fistulas
Coronary artery aneurysms

MYOCARDIAL OXYGEN DEMAND-SUPPLY DISPROPORTION
Aortic stenosis, all forms
Incomplete differentiation of the aortic valve
Aortic insufficiency
Carbon monoxide poisoning
Thyrotoxicosis
Prolonged hypotension

HEMATOLOGICAL (IN SITU THROMBOSIS)
Polycythemia vera
Thrombocytosis
Disseminated intravascular coagulation
Hypercoagulability, thrombosis, thrombocytopenic purpura

MISCELLANEOUS
Cocaine abuse
Myocardial contusion
Myocardial infarction with normal coronary arteries
Complication of cardiac catheterization

Modified from Cheitlin, M., et al.: Myocardial infarction without atherosclerosis. JAMA 231:951, 1975. Copyright 1975, American Medical Association.

Approximately 6 per cent of all patients with AMI and perhaps four times that percentage of patients with this diagnosis under the age of 35 years do not have coronary atherosclerosis demonstrated by coronary arteriography or at autopsy.[99,100,140] Perhaps half of the patients of this group, in turn, have a variety of other lesions involving the coronary vessels or myocardium (Table 37–1), whereas the others have no detectable coronary obstructive lesions.[141,142] Patients with AMI and normal coronary arteries tend to be young and to have relatively few coronary risk factors, except that they often have a history of cigarette smoking.[140] Usually they have no history of angina pectoris prior to the infarction.[140] The infarction in these patients is usually not preceded by any prodrome, but the clinical, laboratory, and ECG features of AMI are otherwise indistinguishable from those present in the overwhelming majority of patients with AMI who have classic obstructive atherosclerotic coronary artery disease. In patients who recover, areas of localized dyskinesis and hypokinesis can often be demonstrated by left ventricular angiography. Many of these cases are caused by coronary artery spasm and/or thrombosis, perhaps with underlying endothelial dysfunction or small plaques that are not apparent on coronary angiography.[143] Additional suggested causes include (1) coronary emboli (perhaps from a small mural thrombus, a prolapsed mitral valve,[144] or a myxoma); (2) coronary artery disease in vessels too small to be visualized by coronary arteriography or coronary arterial thrombosis with subsequent recanalization (Table 37–1); (3) a variety of hematological disorders causing in situ thrombosis in the presence of normal coronary arteries (polycythemia vera, cyanotic heart disease with polycythemia,[145] sickle cell anemia,[146] disseminated intravascular coagulation, thrombocytosis, and thrombotic thrombocytopenic purpura); augmented oxygen demand (thyrotoxicosis,[147] amphetamine use[148]); (5) hypotension secondary to sepsis, blood loss, or pharmacological agents; and (6) anatomical variations such as anomalous origin of a coronary artery (see p. 909), coronary arteriovenous fistula (see p. 908), or a myocardial bridge (see p. 258).

PROGNOSIS. The long-term outlook for patients who have survived an AMI with angiographically normal coronary vessels on arteriography appears to be substantially better than for patients with MI and obstructive coronary artery disease.[149] Following recovery from the initial infarct, recurrent infarction, heart failure, and death are unusual in patients with normal coronary arteries.[150] Indeed, most of these patients have normal exercise electrocardiograms and only a minority develop angina pectoris.

PATHOPHYSIOLOGY

LEFT VENTRICULAR FUNCTION

Systolic Function

Upon interruption of antegrade flow in an epicardial coronary artery, the zone of myocardium supplied by that vessel immediately loses its ability to shorten and perform contractile work.[151,152] Four abnormal contraction patterns develop in sequence[153]: (1) dyssynchrony, i.e., dissociation in the time course of contraction of adjacent segments; (2) hypokinesis, reduction in the extent of shortening; (3) akinesis, cessation of shortening; and (4) dyskinesis, paradoxical expansion, systolic bulging.[154,155] Accompanying dysfunction of the infarcting segment initially is hyperkinesis of the remaining normal myocardium. The early hyperkinesis of the noninfarcted zones is thought to be the result of acute compensatory mechanisms, including increased activity of the sympathetic nervous system and the Frank-Starling mechanism.[84] A portion of this compensatory hyperkinesis is ineffective work because contraction of the noninfarcted segments of myocardium causes dyskinesis of the infarct zone.[156] Increased motion of the noninfarcted region subsides within 2 weeks of infarction, during which time some degree of recovery can be seen in the infarct region as well, particularly if reperfusion (see p. 1213) of the infarcted area occurs and myocardial stunning diminishes.[157]

Patients with AMI often also show reduced myocardial contractile function in noninfarcted zones. This may result from previous obstruction of the coronary artery supplying the noninfarcted region of the ventricle and loss of collaterals from the freshly occluded infarct related vessel, a condition that has been termed "ischemia at a distance."[158] Conversely, the presence of collaterals developing before MI may allow for greater preservation of regional systolic function in an area of distribution of the occluded artery and improvement in left ventricular ejection fraction early after infarction.[159]

If a sufficient quantity of myocardium undergoes ischemic injury, left ventricular pump function becomes depressed; cardiac output, stroke volume, blood pressure, and peak dP/dt are reduced[155]; and end-systolic volume is increased. In fact, the degree to which end-systolic volume increases is perhaps the most powerful predictor of mortality following AMI.[160] Paradoxical systolic expansion of an area of ventricular myocardium further decreases the left ventricular stroke volume. As necrotic myocytes slip past each other, the infarct zone thins and elongates, especially in patients with large anterior infarcts, leading to infarct expansion (see p. 1195). As the ventricle dilates during the first few hours to days following infarction, regional and global wall stress increases according to Laplace's law. In some patients a vicious circle of dilatation begetting further dilatation is initiated.[83,161] The degree of ventricular dilatation, which depends closely on infarct size, patency of the infarct-related artery,[162] and activation of the local renin-angiotensin system in the noninfarcted portion of the ventricle, can be favorably modified by ACE inhibition therapy even in the absence of symptomatic left ventricular dysfunction.[163–165]

With the passage of time, edema and cellular infiltration and ultimately fibrosis increase the stiffness of the infarcted myocardium back to and beyond control values. Increasing stiffness in the infarcted zone of myocardium improves left ventricular function because it prevents paradoxical systolic wall motion.

Rackley and collaborators have demonstrated a linear relationship between specific parameters of left ventricular function and the likelihood of developing clinical symptoms such as dyspnea and ultimately a shocklike state.[166] The earliest abnormality is a reduction in diastolic compliance (see below), which can be observed with infarcts that involve only 8 per cent of the total left ventricle on angiographic examination. When the abnormally contracting segment exceeds 15 per cent, the ejection fraction may be reduced and elevations of left ventricular end-diastolic pressure and volume occur. The risk of developing physical signs and symptoms of left ventricular failure also increase proportionally to increasing areas of abnormal left ventricular wall motion.[155] Clinical heart failure accompanies areas of abnormal contraction exceeding 25 per cent, and cardiogenic shock, often fatal, accompanies loss of more than 40 per cent of the left ventricular myocardium.[166]

Unless infarct extension occurs, some improvement in wall motion takes place during the healing phase, as recovery of function occurs in initially reversibly injured (stunned) myocardium (Fig. 37–11). Regardless of the age of the infarct, patients who continue to demonstrate abnormal wall motion of 20 to 25 per cent of the left ventricle are likely to manifest hemodynamic signs of left ventricular failure.

Diastolic Function

Left ventricular diastolic properties are altered in infarcted and ischemic myocardium, leading initially to an increase but later to a reduction in left ventricular compliance. These changes are associated with a decrease in the peak rate of decline in left ventricular pressure (peak (−) dP/dt), an increase in the time constant of left ventricular pressure fall (τ), and an initial rise in left ventricular end-diastolic pressure.[167] Over a period of several weeks, end-diastolic volume increases and diastolic pressure begins to fall toward normal.[84] As with impairment of systolic function, the magnitude of the diastolic abnormality appears to be related to the size of the infarct.

CIRCULATORY REGULATION

The abnormality in circulatory regulation that is present in AMI is diagrammed in Figure 37–14. The process begins with an anatomical or functional obstruction in the coronary vascular bed, which results in regional myocardial ischemia and, if the ischemia persists, in infarction. If the infarct is of sufficient size, it depresses overall left ventricular function so that left ventricular stroke volume falls and filling pressures rise. A marked depression of left ventricular stroke volume ultimately lowers aortic pressure and reduces coronary perfusion pressure; this condition may intensify myocardial ischemia and thereby initiate a vicious circle (Fig. 37–14). The inability of the left ventricle to empty also leads to an increased preload—that is, it dilates the well-perfused, normally functioning portion of the left ventricle. This compensatory mechanism tends to restore stroke volume to normal levels, but at the expense of a reduced ejection fraction. However, the dilatation of the left ventricle also elevates ventricular afterload, because Laplace's law (see p. 379) dictates that at any given arterial pressure the dilated ventricle must develop a higher wall tension. This increased afterload not only depresses left ventricular stroke volume but also elevates myocardial oxygen consumption, which in turn intensifies myocardial ischemia. When regional myocardial dysfunction is limited and the function of the remainder of the left ventricle is normal, compensatory mechanisms sustain overall left ventricular function. If a large portion of the left ventricle becomes necrotic, pump failure occurs; i.e., overall left

ventricular function becomes so depressed that the circulation cannot be sustained despite the dilatation of the remaining viable portion of the ventricle.

VENTRICULAR REMODELING

As a consequence of MI, the changes in left ventricular size, shape, and thickness involving both the infarcted and the noninfarcted segments of the ventricle described above occur and are collectively referred to as *ventricular remodeling.* This process, in turn, can influence ventricular function and prognosis.[83,84] A combination of changes in left ventricular dilation and hypertrophy of residual noninfarcted myocardium is responsible for remodeling. After the size of infarction, the two most important factors driving the process of left ventricular dilatation are ventricular loading conditions and infarct artery patency[83,162,168] (Fig. 37–15). Elevated ventricular pressure contributes to increased wall stress and the risk of infarct expansion, and a patent infarct artery accelerates myocardial scar formation and increases tissue turgor in the infarct zone, reducing the risk of infarct expansion and ventricular dilatation.

INFARCT EXPANSION. An increase in the size of the infarcted segment, known as infarct expansion, is defined as "acute dilatation and thinning of the area of infarction not explained by additional myocardial necrosis."[169] Infarct expansion appears to be caused by (1) a combination of slippage between muscle bundles, reducing the number of myocytes across the infarct wall; (2) disruption of the normal myocardial cells; and (3) tissue loss within the necrotic zone.[169] It is characterized by disproportionate thinning and dilation of the infarct zone prior to formation of a firm, fibrotic scar. The degree of infarct expansion appears to be related to the preinfarction wall thickness, with existing hypertrophy possibly protecting against infarct thinning.[170] The apex is the thinnest region of the ventricle and an area of the heart that is particularly vulnerable to infarct expansion.[171] Wall stress $(\sigma) = \dfrac{PR}{2h}$, where P = pressure, R = radius of curvature, and h = wall thickness.[171] Infarction of the apex secondary to occlusion of the left anterior descending coronary artery causes the radius of curvature at the apex to increase, exposing this normally thin region to a marked elevation in wall stress. This concept was reported by Picard et al., who observed greater infarct segment lengthening at the apex in dogs subjected to left anterior descending coronary artery occlusion than in the posterior zone of the left ventricle in dogs subjected to left circumflex coronary artery occlusion.[172]

When it is present, infarct expansion is associated with both a higher mortality and a higher incidence of nonfatal complications, such as heart failure and ventricular aneurysm.[84,173] Infarct expansion has been noted in more than three-fourths of the hearts of patients succumbing to AMI and one-third to one-half of all patients with anterior Q-wave infarctions.[173] Infarct expansion is best recognized echocardiographically as elongation of the noncontractile region of the ventricle.[174] When expansion is severe enough to cause symptoms, the most characteristic clinical finding is deterioration of systolic function associated with new or louder gallop sounds and new or worsening pulmonary congestion. Rupture of the ventricle may be considered to be a consequence of extreme infarct expansion.[175]

VENTRICULAR DILATATION. Although infarct expansion plays an important role in the ventricular remodeling that occurs early following myocardial infarction, remodeling is also caused by dilatation of the viable portion of the ventricle, commencing immediately following AMI, and progressing for months or years thereafter[176] (Fig. 37–15). As opposed to distention, dilatation may be accompanied by a shift of the pressure-volume curve of the left ventricle to

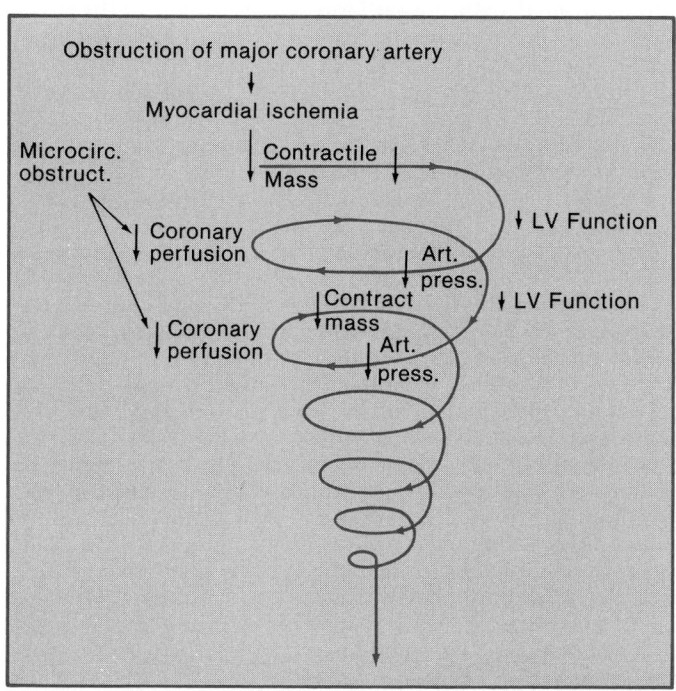

FIGURE 37–14. The sequence of events in the vicious circle in which coronary artery obstruction leads to cardiogenic shock and progressive circulatory deterioration. (From Pasternak, R. C., and Braunwald, E.: Acute myocardial infarction. *In* Isselbacher, K. J., et al. (eds.): Harrison's Principles of Internal Medicine. New York, McGraw-Hill Book Co., 1994.)

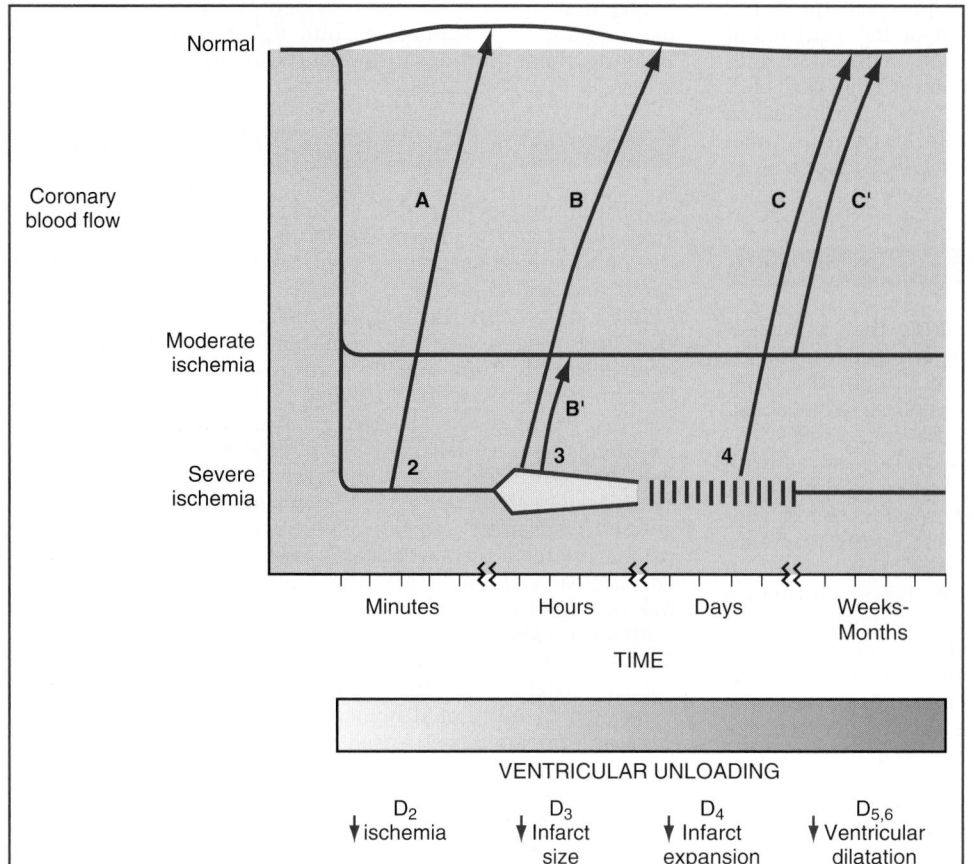

FIGURE 37–15. Therapeutic maneuvers in various stages of ischemia and infarction. Severely ischemic tissue (2) may be reperfused, thereby averting MI (A). Infarcting tissue (3) may be reperfused, leading to sparing of myocardial tissue (B). If blood flow is restored only in part (B'), the myocardium may remain noncontractile although viable, i.e., hibernating. After completion of the infarct (4), late reperfusion (C) may still be useful. Mechanical reperfusion of moderately ischemic myocardium (C') may restore contractility of hibernating myocardium to normal. Ventricular unloading may be useful throughout the pre- and post-infarct periods. Unloading may reduce ischemia (D_2), infarct size (D_3), infarct expansion (D_4), and ventricular dilation ($D_{5,6}$). (From Braunwald, E., and Pfeffer, M. A.: Ventricular enlargement and remodeling following acute myocardial infarction: Mechanisms and management. Am. J. Cardiol. **68**:4D, 1991.)

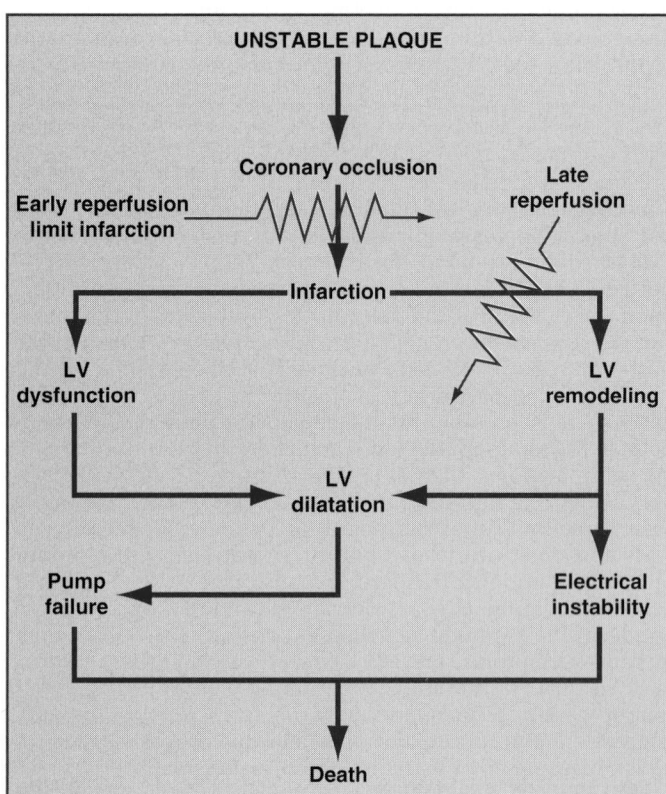

FIGURE 37–16. Flow chart showing postulated sequence of events from an unstable atherosclerotic plaque to death. The original paradigm emphasizing early reperfusion is shown at the left; the expanded paradigm illustrating the benefits of late reperfusion is shown at the right. (Reproduced with permission from Kim, C. B., and Braunwald, E.: Potential benefits of late reperfusion of infarcted myocardium: The open artery hypothesis. Circulation *88*:2426, 1993. Copyright 1993 American Heart Association.)

the right, resulting in a larger left ventricular volume at any given diastolic pressure (see p. 1194).[177] This global dilation of the noninfarct zone may be viewed as a compensatory mechanism that maintains stroke volume in the face of a large infarction. However, ventricular dilatation is also associated with nonuniform repolarization of the myocardium that predisposes the patient to life-threatening ventricular arrhythmias.[178]

Following AMI, an extra load is placed on the residual functioning myocardium,[84] a load that presumably is responsible for the compensatory hypertrophy of the uninfarcted myocardium. This hypertrophy could help to compensate for the functional impairment caused by the infarct and may be responsible for some of the hemodynamic improvement seen in the months after infarction in some patients.[179]

EFFECTS OF TREATMENT. Ventricular remodeling after AMI can be affected by several factors, the first of which is infarct size (Fig. 37–15). Acute reperfusion and other measures to restrict the extent of myocardial necrosis limit the increase in ventricular volume following AMI,[180] and evidence suggests that an open infarct artery per se achieved even late after coronary occlusion also attenuates ventricular enlargement[162,181] (Fig. 37–16). The second factor is scar formation in the infarct. Glucocorticosteroids and nonsteroidal anti-inflammatory agents given early after MI can cause scar thinning and greater infarct expansion,[182] whereas ACE inhibitors[83,84] attenuate ventricular enlargement (see p. 1229) (Figs. 37–15 and 37–16).

PATHOPHYSIOLOGY OF OTHER ORGAN SYSTEMS

PULMONARY

Changes in pulmonary gas exchange, ventilation, and distribution of perfusion all occur with AMI.[183] Hypoxemia is a frequent consequence, with a severity, in general, proportional to that of left ventricular failure. There is an inverse relation between pulmonary artery diastolic pressure and arterial oxygen tension in patients with AMI. This suggests that increased pulmonary capillary hydrostatic pressure leads to interstitial edema, which results in arteriolar and bronchiolar compression that ultimately causes perfusion of poorly ventilated alveoli with resultant hypoxemia.[184,185] In addition to hypoxemia, there is a fall in diffusing capacity.[185] Hyperventilation often occurs in patients with AMI and may cause hypocapnia and respiratory alkalosis, particularly in restless, anxious patients with pain. With reversal of heart failure, hypoxemia and intrapulmonary shunting diminish.

INCREASE IN INTERSTITIAL WATER. A positive correlation has been demonstrated between pulmonary extravascular (interstitial) water content, left ventricular filling pressure, and the clinical signs and symptoms of left ventricular failure.[185] The increase in pulmonary extravascular water may be responsible for the alterations in pulmonary mechanics observed in patients with AMI, i.e., reduction of airway conductance, pulmonary compliance, forced expiratory volume and midexpiratory flow rate, and an increase in closing volume—the last presumably related to the widespread closure of small, dependent airways during the first 3 days following AMI.[186] Ultimately, severe increases in extravascular water may lead to pulmonary edema. Recovery of left ventricular function or diuresis reduces abnormally elevated values for closing volumes—i.e., the lung volume at which airway closure commences—to normal.

The "closing volume" can encroach on and sometimes exceed functional residual volume. This can lead to arterial hypoxemia by the shunting of blood through alveoli that are not well ventilated.

REDUCTION OF VITAL CAPACITY. Virtually all lung volume indices—total lung capacity, functional residual capacity, and residual volume, as well as vital capacity—fall in the presence of AMI.[187] These reductions correlate with the elevations of left-sided filling pressures and are most probably due to increases in pulmonary extravascular water. Lung volumes, oxygenation, and airway resistance all return toward normal by the time of hospital discharge for most patients.[187] Increased pulmonary venous pressure also results in redistribution of pulmonary blood flow from the bases to the apices of the lung in patients with AMI,[188] altering the relationship between ventilation and perfusion. However, at follow-up examination 3 to 25 weeks after MI, the ventilation-perfusion relationship has usually returned to normal or almost so.

REDUCTION OF AFFINITY OF HEMOGLOBIN FOR OXYGEN. In patients with MI, particularly when complicated by left ventricular failure or cardiogenic shock, the affinity of hemoglobin for oxygen is reduced, i.e., the P_{50} is increased.[189] The increase in P_{50} results from increased levels of erythrocyte 2,3-diphosphoglycerate (2,3-DPG), which constitutes an important compensatory mechanism, responsible for an estimated 18 per cent increase in oxygen release from oxyhemoglobin in patients with cardiogenic shock.[189]

ENDOCRINE

PANCREAS. Hyperglycemia and impaired glucose tolerance are common in patients with AMI. Although the absolute levels of blood insulin are often in the normal range, they are usually inappropriately low for the level of blood sugar, and there may be relative insulin resistance as well. Patients with cardiogenic shock often demonstrate marked hyperglycemia and depressed levels of circulating insulin, often with complete suppression of insulin secretion in response to tolbutamide.[190] These abnormalities in insulin secretion and the resultant impaired glucose tolerance appear to be secondary to a reduction in pancreatic blood flow as a consequence of splanchnic vasoconstriction accompanying severe left ventricular failure. In addition, increased activity of the sympathetic nervous system with augmented circulating catecholamines inhibits insulin secretion and augments glycogenolysis, also contributing to the elevation of blood sugar.[191]

Glucose appears to be a more favorable energy source than free fatty acids for the ischemic myocardium by more efficiently replenishing Krebs cycle and stimulating contractile performance.[192,193] Because hypoxic heart muscle derives a considerable portion of its energy from the metabolism of glucose (see Chap. 36) and because insulin is essential for the uptake of glucose by the myocardium as well as for myocardial protein synthesis and inhibition of lysosomal activity, the deleterious effects of insulin deficiency are clear. These metabolic considerations, combined with epidemiological observations that diabetic patients have a markedly worse prognosis,[194] have served as the foundation for efforts to more aggressively administer insulin-glucose infusions to diabetics with AMI (see p. 1901).

ADRENAL MEDULLA. Excessive secretion of catecholamines produces many of the characteristic signs and symptoms of AMI. The plasma and urinary catecholamine levels are highest during the first 24 hours after the onset of chest pain,[191] with the greatest rise in plasma catecholamine secretion occurring during the first hour after the onset of MI.[195] These high levels of circulating catecholamines in patients with AMI correlate with the occurrence of serious arrhythmias and result in an increase in myocardial oxygen consumption, both directly and indirectly, as a consequence of catecholamine-induced elevation of circulating free fatty acids.[193] As might be anticipated, the concentration of circulating catecholamines correlates

with the extent of myocardial damage and incidence of cardiogenic shock, as well as both early and late mortality rates.[196]

Circulating catecholamines enhance platelet aggregation; when this occurs in the coronary microcirculation, the release of the potent vasoconstrictor thromboxane A_2 may further impair cardiac perfusion. The marked increase in sympathetic activity associated with AMI serves as the foundation for beta-adrenoceptor blocker regimens in the acute phase (see p. 1211).

LOCAL MYOCARDIAL AND SYSTEMIC RENIN-ANGIOTENSIN SYSTEM. Noninfarcted regions of the myocardium appear to exhibit activation of the tissue renin-angiotensin system with increased angiotensin II production.[84,165] Both locally and systemically generated angiotensin II may stimulate the production of various growth factors such as platelet-derived growth factor and transforming growth factor-β that promote compensatory hypertrophy in the noninfarcted myocardium as well as control the structure and tone of the infarct-related coronary and other myocardial vessels.[84,197,198] Additional potential actions of angiotensin II that have a more negative impact on the infarction process include release of endothelin, PAI-1, and aldosterone, which may cause vasoconstriction, impaired fibrinolysis, and increased sodium retention, respectively.[84,197,198] Inhibition of generation of circulating and tissue angiotensin II is one of the proposed mechanisms of benefit from ACE inhibitors in AMI.[84]

NATRIURETIC PEPTIDES. The peptides atrial natriuretic factor (ANF) and N-terminal pro-ANF are released from cardiac atria in response to elevation of atrial pressure. In a case-control study from the TIMI II trial, Hall and colleagues have shown that elevated N-terminal pro-ANF levels within the first 12 hours of AMI are highly predictive of an increased mortality risk in the year following infarction.[199] A novel protein, brain natriuretic peptide (BNP), originally isolated from porcine brain, has been shown to be secreted by human ventricular myocardium. It appears to be released early after AMI, peaking at about 16 hours.[200] Patients with anterior infarction, lower cardiac index, and more significant congestive heart failure after AMI have higher levels of BNP and also show a second peak of BNP release about 5 days after infarction.[200] These intriguing observations suggest that BNP levels may be a marker of the degree of left ventricular dysfunction in AMI and that markedly elevated levels of BNP correlate with a worse prognosis.

ADRENAL CORTEX. Plasma and urinary 17-hydroxycorticosteroids and ketosteroids, as well as aldosterone, are also markedly elevated in patients with AMI.[191] Their concentrations correlate directly with the peak level of serum creatine kinase,[196] implying that the stress imposed by larger infarcts is associated with greater secretion of adrenal steroids. The magnitude of the elevation of cortisol correlates with infarct size and mortality.[201] Glucocorticosteroids also contribute to the impairment of glucose tolerance.

THYROID GLAND. Although patients with AMI are generally euthyroid, evidence indicates a significant transient decrease in serum triiodothyronine (T_3), levels, a fall that is most marked on about the third day after the infarct.[202] This fall in T_3 is usually accompanied by a rise in reverse T_3, with variable changes or no change in thyroxine (T_4) and thyroid-stimulating hormone (TSH) levels. The alteration in peripheral T_4 metabolism appears to correlate with infarct size and may be mediated by the rise in endogenous levels of cortisol which accompanies AMI.[203]

RENAL FUNCTION

Both prerenal azotemia and acute renal failure can complicate the marked reduction of cardiac output that occurs in cardiogenic shock. On the other hand, an increase in circulating atrial natriuretic peptide (see p. 405) occurs following AMI, an increase that is correlated with the severity of left ventricular failure.[204] An increase in atrial natriuretic peptide is also found when right ventricular infarction accompanies inferior wall infarction, suggesting that this hormone may play a role in the hemodynamic disturbances that accompany right ventricular infarction (see p. 1240).[205]

HEMATOLOGICAL FUNCTION

PLATELETS. AMI generally occurs in the presence of extensive coronary and systemic atherosclerotic plaques, which may serve as the site for the formation of platelet aggregates, a sequence that has been suggested as the initial step in the process of coronary thrombosis, coronary occlusion, and subsequent MI. Circulating platelets are hyperaggregable in patients with AMI.[62,206] Findings suggestive of a hypercoagulable state as a risk factor for AMI are discussed on page 1153, and the role of platelets in AMI is discussed on page 1333. Platelets from AMI patients have an increased propensity for aggregation locally in the area of a disrupted plaque and also release vasoactive substances such as thromboxane A_2[62,207] (Figs. 37-2, 37-3, and 37-7).

COAGULATION TESTS. Elevated levels of serum fibrinogen degradation products, an end-product of thrombosis—as well as release of distinctive proteins when platelets are activated,[208] i.e., platelet factor 4 and beta-thromboglobulin—have been reported in some patients with AMI.[209,210] Fibrinopeptide A, a protein released from fibrin by thrombin, is a marker of ongoing thrombosis and is elevated during the early hours of AMI[211] (see Chap. 58 and Fig. 37-7, p. 1188). The interpretation of the coagulation tests in patients with AMI may be complicated by elevated blood levels of catecholamines, concomitant shock, and/or pulmonary embolism, conditions that are all capable of altering various tests of platelet and coagulation function. Thus, it is not yet clear whether the aforementioned changes are the causes or consequences of AMI.

LEUKOCYTES. AMI is usually accompanied by leukocytosis, which is related to the necrotic process and its magnitude and to elevated glucocorticoid levels. Activation of neutrophils may produce important intermediates, such as leukotriene B$_4$ and oxygen free radicals, that have important microcirculatory effects.[212]

BLOOD VISCOSITY. Clinical and epidemiological studies suggest that several hemostatic and hemorheological factors (e.g., fibrinogen, Factor VII, plasma viscosity, hematocrit, red blood cell aggregation,

total white cell count) are involved in the pathophysiology of atherosclerosis and also play an integral role in acute thrombotic events.[213] An increase in blood viscosity also occurs in patients with AMI. During the first few days after infarction, this is mainly attributable to hemoconcentration, but later the increases in plasma viscosity and red cell aggregation correlate with elevated serum concentrations of alpha$_2$ globulin and fibrinogen, which are nonspecific reactions to tissue necrosis and are also responsible for the elevated sedimentation rate characteristic of AMI.[214] The high values of blood viscosity indices are observed most frequently in patients with complications such as left ventricular failure, cardiogenic shock, and thromboembolism.

CLINICAL FEATURES

PREDISPOSING FACTORS

In as many one-half of patients with AMI, a precipitating factor or prodromal symptoms can be identified.[214a] Although adequate control studies have not been carried out, evidence suggests that unusually heavy exercise (particularly in fatigued or emotionally stressed patients) may play a role in precipitating AMI. Such infarctions could be the result of marked increases in myocardial oxygen consumption in the presence of severe coronary arterial narrowing. It has been suggested that unusually heavy exertion or mental stress such as that caused by anger[215,215a] may trigger plaque disruption, leading to AMI.[78] A number of reports have documented that upsetting life events occur commonly in patients who subsequently suffer an MI.[216,216a] Such events have been quantified and scored as "Life Change Units." Rahe and coworkers noted, on retrospective analysis, a significant buildup of Life Change Units in patients who subsequently suffered myocardial infarction or died suddenly.[216] Patients with known coronary disease who have been hospitalized for treatment of an acute coronary syndrome—related event and who subsequently report a high level of stress in their life have an increased risk of rehospitalization for cardiovascular reasons and also for "hard" events such as death and myocardial infarction.[217,218] Of interest, however, one study has provided evidence that in a multivariate analysis adjusting for other cardiac risk factors, job strain did not affect the outcome (including nonfatal AMI) in patients with angiographically proven coronary artery disease.[219]

Accelerating angina and rest angina, two patterns of unstable angina, may culminate as AMI (Fig. 37–7). Surgical procedures associated with acute blood loss have also been noted as precursors of AMI (see p. 1759). Reduced myocardial perfusion secondary to hypotension (e.g., hemorrhagic or septic shock) and increased myocardial oxygen demands secondary to aortic stenosis, fever, tachycardia, and agitation can also be responsible for myocardial necrosis. Other factors reported as predisposing to AMI include respiratory infections, hypoxemia of any cause, pulmonary embolism, hypoglycemia, administration of ergot preparations, use of cocaine, sympathomimetics, serum sickness, allergy, and on rare occasion wasp stings may all be triggers of AMI. In patients with Prinzmetal's angina (see p. 1340), AMI may develop in the territory of the coronary artery that repeatedly undergoes spasm.[220] Rarely, munition workers exposed to high concentrations of nitroglycerin may develop MI when they are withdrawn from this exposure, suggesting that it is caused by vasospasm.[221]

Trauma may precipitate an AMI in one of two ways. Myocardial contusion and hemorrhage into the myocardium may actually cause cell necrosis, or the injury may involve a coronary artery, causing occlusion of that vessel with resultant AMI (see Chap. 44). Neurological disturbances (transient ischemic attacks or strokes) may also precipitate AMI. Concern has been raised on the basis of a case-control study that patients with hypertension who are

receiving short-acting calcium antagonists, particularly in high doses, are at increased risk of developing AMI.[222] Because of possible selection bias in the patients who received calcium antagonists, these results must be viewed cautiously and clinicians should await the results of ongoing multicenter trials (e.g., ALLHAT) before withdrawing calcium antagonists from patients who might be benefiting from their antihypertensive effect (reduction of stroke).[223,224]

CIRCADIAN PERIODICITY. An analysis of a large number of patients hospitalized with MI, studied as a part of the Multicenter Investigation of Limitation of Infarct Size (MILIS), revealed a pronounced circadian periodicity for the time of onset of AMI, with peak incidence of events between 6 A.M. and 12 noon.[225] Circadian rhythms affect many physiological and biochemical parameters; the early morning hours are associated with rises in plasma catecholamines and cortisol and increases in platelet aggregability. Interestingly, the characteristic circadian peak was *absent* in patients receiving beta blocker or aspirin therapy before their presentation with AMI.[226,227]

HISTORY

PRODROMAL SYMPTOMS. Despite recent advances in the laboratory detection of AMI, the history remains of substantial value in establishing a diagnosis.[228,228a] The prodrome is usually characterized by chest discomfort, resembling classic angina pectoris (described on p. 1291), but it occurs at rest or with less activity than usual and can therefore be classified as unstable angina. However, the latter is often not disturbing enough to induce patients to seek medical attention, and if they do, they may not be hospitalized. Among patients who are hospitalized for unstable angina, fewer than 10 per cent develop AMI (see p. 1336). Of the patients with AMI presenting with prodromal symptoms of unstable angina, approximately one-third have had symptoms from 1 to 4 weeks before hospitalization; in the remaining two-thirds, symptoms predated admission by 1 week or less, with one-third of these patients (20 per cent of all with prodromes) having had symptoms for 24 hours or less.[229] A feeling of general malaise or frank exhaustion often accompanies other symptoms preceding AMI.

NATURE OF THE PAIN (see also p. 1291). The pain of AMI is variable in intensity; in most patients it is severe and in some instances intolerable. The pain is prolonged, usually lasting for more than 30 minutes and frequently for a number of hours. The discomfort is described as constricting, crushing, oppressing, or compressing; often the patient complains of a sensation of a heavy weight or a squeezing in the chest. Although the discomfort is typically described as a choking, viselike, or heavy pain, it may also be characterized as a stabbing, knifelike, boring, or burning discomfort. The pain is usually retrosternal in location, spreading frequently to both sides of the anterior chest, with predilection for the left side. Often the pain radiates down the ulnar aspect of the left arm, producing a tingling sensation in the left wrist, hand, and fingers. Some patients note only a dull ache or numbness of the wrists in association with severe substernal or precordial discomfort. In some instances, the pain of AMI may begin in the epigastrium and simulate a variety of abdominal disorders, a fact that often causes MI to be misdiagnosed as "indigestion." In other patients the discomfort of AMI radiates to the shoulders, upper extremities, neck, jaw, and interscapular region, again usually favoring the left side. In patients with preexisting angina pectoris, the pain of infarction usually resembles that of angina with respect to location. However, it is generally much more severe, lasts longer, and is not relieved by rest and nitroglycerin.

In some patients, particularly the elderly, AMI is manifested clinically not by chest pain but rather by symptoms of acute left ventricular failure and chest tightness or by marked weakness or frank syncope. These symptoms may be accompanied by diaphoresis, nausea, and vomiting.[230] The pain of AMI may have disappeared by the time the physician first encounters the patient (or the patient reaches the hospital), or it may persist for many hours. Opiates—in particular, morphine—usually relieve the pain. Both angina pectoris and the pain of AMI are thought to arise from nerve endings in ischemic or injured, but not necrotic, myocardium.[231] Thus, in MI, stimulation of nerve fibers in an ischemic zone of myocardium surrounding the necrotic central area of infarction probably gives rise to the pain.

Pain often disappears suddenly and completely when blood flow to the infarct territory is restored. In patients in whom reocclusion occurs after thrombolysis, pain recurs if the initial reperfusion has left viable myocardium. Thus, what has previously been thought of as the "pain of infarction," sometimes lasting for many hours, probably represents pain caused by ongoing ischemia. The recognition that pain implies ischemia and not infarction heightens the importance of seeking ways to relieve the ischemia, for which the pain is a marker. This finding suggests that the clinician should not be complacent about ongoing cardiac pain under any circumstances.

OTHER SYMPTOMS. Nausea and vomiting occur in more than 50 per cent of patients with transmural MI and severe chest pain,[232] presumably owing to activation of the vagal reflex or to stimulation of left ventricular receptors as part of the Bezold-Jarisch reflex (see p. 1171). These symptoms occur more commonly in patients with inferior MI than in those with anterior MI. Moreover, nausea and vomiting are common side effects of opiates. When the pain of AMI is epigastric in location and is associated with nausea and vomiting, the clinical picture may easily be confused with that of acute cholecystitis, gastritis, or peptic ulcer. Occasionally a patient complains of diarrhea or a violent urge to evacuate the bowels during the acute phase of MI. Other symptoms include feelings of profound weakness, dizziness, palpitations, cold perspiration, and a sense of impending doom. On occasion, symptoms arising from an episode of cerebral embolism or other systemic arterial embolism are the first signs of AMI. The aforementioned symptoms may or may not be accompanied by chest pain.

Differential Diagnosis

The pain of AMI may stimulate the pain of acute pericarditis (see p. 1481), which is usually associated with some pleuritic features; i.e., it is aggravated by respiratory movements and coughing and often involves the shoulder, ridge of the trapezius, and neck. An important feature that distinguishes pericardial pain from ischemic discomfort is that ischemic discomfort never radiates to the trapezius ridge, a characteristic site of radiation of pericardial pain.[233] Pleural pain is usually sharp, knife-like, and aggravated in a cyclical fashion by each breath, which distinguishes it from the deep, dull, steady pain of AMI. Pulmonary embolism (see Chap. 46) generally produces pain laterally in the chest, is

often pleuritic in nature, and may be associated with hemoptysis. The pain due to acute dissection of the aorta (see p. 1556) is usually localized in the center of the chest, is extremely severe and described by the patient as a "ripping" or "tearing" sensation, is at its maximal intensity shortly after onset, persists for many hours, and often radiates to the back or the lower extremities. Often one or more major arterial pulses are absent. Pain arising from the costochondral and chondrosternal articulations may be associated with localized swelling and redness; it is usually sharp and "darting" and is characterized by marked localized tenderness.

SILENT MI AND ATYPICAL PRESENTATION. Population studies suggest that between 20 and 60 per cent of nonfatal MIs are unrecognized by the patient and are discovered only on subsequent routine electrocardiographic[234,235] or postmortem examinations. Of these unrecognized infarctions, approximately half are truly silent, with the patients unable to recall any symptoms whatsoever. The other half of patients with so-called silent infarction can recall an event characterized by symptoms compatible with acute infarction when leading questions are posed after the electrocardiographic abnormalities are discovered. Unrecognized or silent infarction occurs more commonly in patients without antecedent angina pectoris[235] and in patients with diabetes and hypertension. Silent MI is often followed by silent ischemia (see p. 1344). The prognosis of patients with silent and symptomatic presentations of AMI appears similar.[235]

In an analysis of atypical presentations of AMI, Bean[236] lists the following: (1) congestive heart failure—beginning de novo or worsening of established failure; (2) classic angina pectoris without a particularly severe or prolonged attack; (3) atypical location of the pain; (4) central nervous system manifestations, resembling those of stroke, secondary to a sharp reduction in cardiac output in a patient with cerebral arteriosclerosis; (5) apprehension and nervousness; (6) sudden mania or psychosis; (7) syncope; (8) overwhelming weakness; (9) acute indigestion; and (10) peripheral embolization.

PHYSICAL EXAMINATION

GENERAL APPEARANCE. Patients suffering an AMI often appear anxious and in considerable distress.[228a] An anguished facial expression is common, and—in contrast to patients with severe angina pectoris, who often lie, sit, or stand still, recognizing that all forms of activity increase the discomfort—some patients suffering an AMI may be restless and move about in an effort to find a comfortable position. They often massage or clutch their chests and frequently describe their pain with a clenched fist held against the sternum (the "Levine" sign, named after Dr. Samuel A. Levine). In patients with left ventricular failure and sympathetic stimulation, cold perspiration and skin pallor may be evident; they typically sit or are propped up in bed, gasping for breath. Between breaths, they may complain of chest discomfort or a feeling of suffocation. Cough productive of frothy, pink, or blood-streaked sputum is common.

Patients in cardiogenic shock often lie listlessly, making few if any spontaneous movements. The skin is cool and clammy, with a bluish or mottled color over the extremities, and there is marked facial pallor with severe cyanosis of the lips and nailbeds. Depending on the degree of cerebral perfusion, the patient in shock may converse normally or may evidence confusion and disorientation.

HEART RATE. The heart rate may vary from a marked bradycardia to a rapid regular or irregular tachycardia, depending on the underlying rhythm and the degree of left ventricular failure. Most commonly, the pulse is rapid and regular initially (sinus tachycardia at 100 to 110 beats/

min), slowing as the patient's pain and anxiety are relieved; premature ventricular beats are common, occurring in more than 95 per cent of patients evaluated within the first 4 hours after the onset of symptoms.[237]

BLOOD PRESSURE. The majority of patients with uncomplicated AMI are normotensive, although the reduced stroke volume accompanying the tachycardia may cause declines in systolic and pulse pressures and elevation of diastolic pressure. Among previously normotensive patients, a hypertensive response occasionally is seen during the first few hours, with the arterial pressure exceeding 160/90 mm Hg, presumably as a consequence of adrenergic discharge secondary to pain and agitation. It is common for previously hypertensive patients to become normotensive without treatment following AMI, although many of these previously hypertensive patients eventually regain their elevated levels of blood pressure, generally 3 to 6 months after infarction. In patients with massive infarction, arterial pressure falls acutely, owing to left ventricular dysfunction and venous pooling secondary to administration of morphine or nitrates or both; as recovery occurs, the arterial pressure tends to return to preinfarction levels.

Patients in cardiogenic shock (see p. 1238), by definition, have systolic pressures below 90 mm Hg and evidence of end-organ hypoperfusion. However, hypotension alone does not necessarily signify cardiogenic shock because some patients with inferior infarction in whom the Bezold-Jarisch reflex is activated may also transiently have systolic blood pressure below 90 mm Hg.[238] Their hypotension eventually resolves spontaneously, although the process can be accelerated by intravenous atropine (0.5 to 1.0 mg) and assumption of the Trendelenburg position. Other patients who are initially only slightly hypotensive may demonstrate gradually falling blood pressures with progressive reduction in cardiac output over several hours or days as they develop cardiogenic shock as a consequence of increasing ischemia and extension of infarction (Fig. 37–14). Evidence of autonomic hyperactivity is common, varying in type with the location of the infarction. At some time in their initial presentation, more than half of patients with inferior MI have evidence of excess parasympathetic stimulation, with hypotension, bradycardia, or both, whereas about half of patients with anterior MI show signs of sympathetic excess, having hypertension, tachycardia, or both.[239]

TEMPERATURE AND RESPIRATION. Most patients with extensive AMI develop fever, a nonspecific response to tissue necrosis, within 24 to 48 hours of the onset of infarction. Body temperature often begins to rise within 4 to 8 hours after the onset of infarction, and rectal temperature may reach 101° to 102°F. Fever usually resolves by the fifth or sixth day following infarction.

The respiratory rate may be slightly elevated soon after the development of an AMI; in patients without heart failure, it results from anxiety and pain because it returns to normal with treatment of physical and psychological discomfort. In patients with left ventricular failure, the respiratory rate correlates with the severity of failure; patients with pulmonary edema may have respiratory rates exceeding 40 per minute. However, the respiratory rate is not necessarily elevated in patients with cardiogenic shock. Cheyne-Stokes (periodic) respiration (see p. 455) may occur in elderly individuals with cardiogenic shock and heart failure, particularly after opiate therapy and in the presence of cerebrovascular disease.

JUGULAR VENOUS PULSE. The height and contour of the jugular venous pulse reflect right atrial and right ventricular diastolic pressures (see p. 18). Because these pressures are usually normal or only slightly elevated in patients with AMI (even in the presence of mild to moderate left ventricular failure), it is not surprising that usually the jugular venous pulse fails to show any abnormalities. The *a* wave may be prominent in patients with pulmonary hypertension secondary to left ventricular failure or reduced compliance. In contrast, right ventricular infarction (whether or not it accompanies left ventricular infarction) often results in marked jugular venous distention and, when it is complicated by necrosis or ischemia of right ventricular papillary muscles, tall *c-v* waves of tricuspid regurgitation are evident. In patients with AMI and cardiogenic shock, the jugular venous pressure is usually elevated. In patients with AMI, hypotension, and hypoperfusion (findings that may resemble those of patients with cardiogenic shock) but who have flat neck veins, it is likely that the depression of left ventricular performance may be related, at least in part, to hypovolemia. The differentiation can be made only by assessing left ventricular performance using echocardiography or by measuring left ventricular filling pressure with a pulmonary artery flotation catheter.

CAROTID PULSE. Palpation of the carotid arterial pulse provides a clue to the left ventricular stroke volume; a small pulse suggests a reduced stroke volume, whereas a sharp, brief upstroke is often observed in patients with mitral regurgitation or ruptured ventricular septum with a left-to-right shunt. Pulsus alternans reflects severe left ventricular dysfunction.

THE CHEST. Moist rales are audible in patients who develop left ventricular failure and/or a reduction of left ventricular compliance with AMI. Diffuse wheezing may be present in patients with severe left ventricular failure. Cough with hemoptysis, suggesting pulmonary embolism with infarction, may also occur. In 1967 Killip proposed a prognostic classification scheme based on the presence and severity of rales detected in patients presenting with AMI.[240] Class I patients are free of rales and a third heart sound. Class II patients have rales but to only a mild-moderate degree (<50 per cent of lung fields) and may or may not have an S_3. Patients in Class III have rales in more than half of each lung field and frequently have pulmonary edema. Finally, Class IV patients are in cardiogenic shock. Despite overall improvement in mortality in each class, compared with data observed during the original development of the classification scheme, the latter remains useful today as evidenced by data from recent large MI trials.[10]

Cardiac Examination

PALPATION. Despite severe symptoms and extensive myocardial damage, the findings on examination of the heart may be quite unremarkable in patients with AMI.[241] Palpation of the precordium may yield normal findings, but in patients with transmural AMI it more commonly reveals a presystolic pulsation, synchronous with an audible fourth heart sound, reflecting a vigorous left atrial contraction filling a ventricle with reduced compliance. In the presence of left ventricular systolic dysfunction, an outward movement of the left ventricle may be palpated in early diastole, coincident with a third heart sound. When the anterior or lateral portion of the ventricle is dyskinetic, an abnormal systolic pulsation is present in the third, fourth, or fifth interspace to the left of the sternum. In some patients, this paradoxical precordial impulse is clearly separable from the point of maximal impulse, which is more lateral and to the left. In other patients, the abnormal impulse is a diffuse, rippling, precordial movement, approximately 5 to 10 cm in diameter, not clearly separable from the point of maximal impulse and can be appreciated near the left anterior axillary line. Patients with longstanding hypertension or previous infarction with left ventricular hypertrophy often demonstrate a laterally displaced, sustained apical impulse.

AUSCULTATION. The heart sounds, particularly the first sound, are frequently muffled and occasionally inaudible immediately after the infarct, and their intensity increases during convalescence. A soft first heart sound may also reflect prolongation of the P-R interval. Patients with marked ventricular dysfunction and/or left bundle branch block may have paradoxical splitting of the second heart sound (see p. 33). Patients with postinfarction angina may also develop a transient, paradoxically split second heart sound during anginal episodes.

A *fourth heart sound* is almost universally present in patients in sinus rhythm with AMI and is usually best heard between the left sternal border and the apex. This sound reflects the atrial contribution to ventricular filling and is particularly prominent in AMI patients due to a reduction in left ventricular compliance (see p. 1235) and elevation of left ventricular end-diastolic pressure, even in the absence of left ventricular systolic dysfunction. This finding is of limited diagnostic value because it is commonly audible in most patients with chronic ischemic heart disease and is recordable, although not often audible, in many normal subjects older than 45 years.

A *third heart sound* in AMI usually reflects severe left ventricular dysfunction with elevated ventricular filling pressure. It is caused by rapid deceleration of transmitral blood flow during protodiastolic filling of the left ventricle with resultant oscillations of the cardiohemic system (i.e., myocardium and stream of blood flowing from left atrium to left ventricle)[242] and is usually heard in patients with large infarctions. This sound is detected best at the apex, with the patient in the left lateral recumbent position, and is more common in patients with transmural anterior infarctions than in those with inferior or nontransmural infarctions. The mortality of patients who manifest a third heart sound during the acute phase of MI is higher than that of patients without such a sound.[243] A third heart sound may be caused not only by left ventricular failure but also by increased inflow into the left ventricle, as occurs when mitral regurgitation or ventricular septal defect complicates AMI. Third and fourth heart sounds emanating from the left ventricle are heard best at the apex; in patients with right ventricular infarcts, these sounds may be heard along the left sternal border and are intensified by inspiration.

Systolic murmurs, transient or persistent, are commonly audible in patients with AMI and generally result from mitral regurgitation secondary to dysfunction of the mitral valve apparatus (papillary muscle dysfunction, left ventricular dilatation). A new, prominent apical holosystolic murmur, accompanied by a thrill, may represent rupture of a head of a papillary muscle (see p. 1243). The findings in rupture of the interventricular septum are similar, although the murmur and thrill are usually most prominent along the left sternal border and may be audible at the right sternal border as well. The systolic murmur of tricuspid regurgitation (caused by right ventricular failure due to pulmonary hypertension and/or right ventricular infarction or by infarction of a right ventricular papillary muscle) is also heard along the left sternal border. It is characteristically intensified by inspiration and is accompanied by a prominent c-v wave in the jugular venous pulse and a right ventricular fourth sound.

Pericardial friction rubs are audible in 6 to 30 per cent of all patients with AMI and in a higher percentage of patients with transmural infarctions.[233] Rubs are notorious for their evanescence and, hence, are probably even more common than reported; frequent auscultation in patients with transmural infarction often results in the discovery of a rub that might otherwise have gone unnoticed. Although friction rubs may be heard within 24 hours or as late as 2 weeks after the onset of infarction, most commonly they are noted on the second or third day.[233] Occasionally, in patients with extensive infarction, a loud rub may be heard for many days. About 40 per cent of patients with AMI and a pericardial friction rub have a pericardial effusion on echocardiographic study,[244] but only rarely are the classic electrocardiographic changes of pericarditis (see p. 1483) seen.[233] Delayed onset of the rub and the associated discomfort of pericarditis (as late as 3 months postinfarction) are characteristic of the post–myocardial infarction (Dressler) syndrome (see p. 1256).

Pericardial rubs are most readily audible along the left sternal border or just inside the point of maximal impulse. Loud rubs may be audible over the entire precordium and even over the back. Occasionally, only the systolic portion of a rub is heard; it may be confused with a systolic murmur, and the diagnosis of rupture of the ventricular septum or mitral regurgitation may be incorrectly considered.

Other Findings

FUNDI. Hypertension, diabetes, and generalized atherosclerosis commonly accompany AMI, and because these conditions may produce characteristic changes in the fundus, a careful funduscopic examination may provide information concerning the underlying vascular status; this is particularly useful in patients unable to provide a detailed history.

ABDOMEN. As already noted, in patients with AMI, particularly in an inferior location with diaphragmatic irritation, the pain may be localized to the epigastrium or the right upper quadrant. Pain in the abdomen associated with nausea, vomiting, restlessness, and even abdominal distention is often interpreted by patients as a sign of "indigestion,"[236] resulting in self-medication with antacids, and it may suggest an acute abdominal process to the physician. Right heart failure, characterized by hepatomegaly and a positive abdominojugular reflux, is unusual in patients with acute left ventricular infarction but does occur in patients with severe and prolonged left ventricular failure or right ventricular infarction.

EXTREMITIES. Coronary atherosclerosis is often associated with systemic atherosclerosis, and it is therefore common for patients with AMI to have a history of intermittent claudication and to demonstrate physical findings of peripheral vascular disease. Thus, diminished peripheral arterial pulses, loss of hair, and atrophic skin in the lower extremities are noted frequently in patients with coronary artery disease. Peripheral edema is a manifestation of right ventricular failure and, like congestive hepatomegaly, is unusual in patients with acute left ventricular infarction. Cyanosis of the nailbeds is common in patients with severe left ventricular failure and is particularly striking in patients with cardiogenic shock.

NEUROPSYCHIATRIC FINDINGS (see also p. 1880). Except for the altered mental status that occurs in patients with AMI who have a markedly reduced cardiac output and cerebral hypoperfusion, the neurological examination is normal unless the patient has suffered cerebral embolism secondary to a mural thrombus. Indeed, an underlying MI is common in patients with cerebral embolic stroke.[245] In patients with cerebrovascular accidents, 13 per cent have an associated AMI (see p. 1879); in contrast, in a series of patients with AMI, only 2 per cent suffered a stroke. The relationship between stroke and AMI was confined to patients with large myocardial infarctions, as reflected in markedly elevated serum creatine kinase concentrations.[245] The coincidence between these two conditions may be explained by systemic hypotension due to MI precipitating a cerebral infarction and the converse, as well as by mural emboli from the left ventricle causing cerebral emboli.

Patients with AMI often exhibit alterations of the emotional state, including intense anxiety, denial, and depression. Medical staff caring for AMI patients must be sensitive to changes in the patient's emotional state—a calm, professional atmosphere, with thorough explanations of equipment and prognosis, can help alleviate the distress associated with AMI.[246]

LABORATORY EXAMINATIONS

Serum Markers of Cardiac Damage

The World Health Organization (WHO) criteria for the diagnosis of AMI require that at least two of the following three elements be present: a history of ischemic-type chest discomfort, evolutionary changes on serially obtained ECG tracings, and a rise and fall in serum cardiac markers.[247] There is considerable variability in the pattern of presentation of AMI with respect to these three elements, as exemplified by the following statistics. ST-segment elevation and Q waves on the ECG, two features that are highly indicative of AMI, are seen in only about half of AMI cases on presentation.[248] Approximately one-fourth of patients with AMI do not present with classic chest pain, and the event would go unrecognized unless an ECG were recorded fortuitously in temporal proximity to the infarction or permanent pathological Q waves are seen on later tracings.[249,250] Nondiagnostic ECGs are recorded in approximately half of patients presenting to emergency departments with chest pain suspicious for MI who ultimately are shown to have an AMI.[251] Among patients admitted to the hospital with a chest pain syndrome, fewer than 20 per cent are subsequently diagnosed as having had an AMI.[252,253] Therefore, in the majority of patients, clinicians must obtain serum cardiac marker measurements at periodic intervals to either establish or exclude the diagnosis of AMI[254]; such measurements may also be useful for a rough quantitation of the size of infarction.[255]

As myocytes become necrotic, the integrity of the sarcolemmal membrane is compromised and intracellular macromolecules (serum cardiac markers) begin to diffuse into the cardiac interstitium and ultimately into the microvasculature and lymphatics in the region of the infarct[97,256] (Fig. 37–17 and Table 37–2). The rate of appearance of these macromolecules in the peripheral circulation depends on several factors, including intracellular location, molecular weight, local blood and lymphatic flow, and the rate of elimination from the blood.[97,256,257]

Given the accelerated pace of decision-making in patients with acute coronary syndromes and emphasis on reduction of length of hospital stay,[258] there is considerable interest in evaluating new serum cardiac markers,[97] shortening assay time in the central chemistry laboratory,[259] and designing rapid whole blood bedside assays.[260] For optimal specificity, a serum marker of MI should be present in high concentration in the myocardium and be absent from nonmyo-

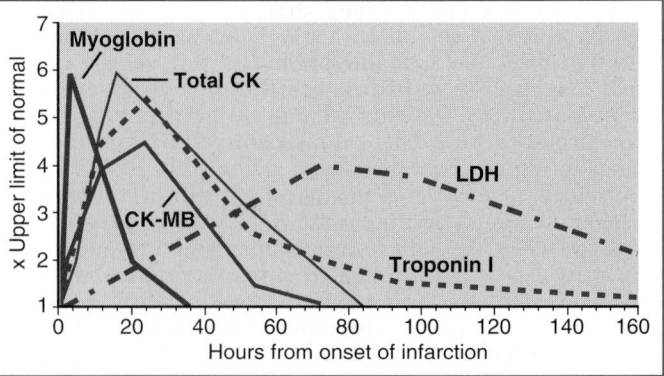

FIGURE 37–17. Time course of elevations of serum markers after AMI. This figure summarizes the relative timing, rate of rise, peak values, and duration of elevation above the upper limit of normal for multiple serum markers following AMI. Although traditionally total CK, CK-MB, and lactic dehydrogenase (LDH [with isoenzymes]) are measured, the relatively slow rate of rise above normal for CK and the potential confusion with noncardiac sources of enzyme release for both total CK and LDH have inspired the search for additional serum markers. The smaller molecule myoglobin is released quickly from infarcted myocardium but is not cardiac specific. Therefore, elevations of myoglobin that may be detected quite early after the onset of infarction require confirmation with a more cardiac-specific marker such as CK-MB or troponin I. Troponin I (and troponin T; not shown) rises more slowly than myoglobin and may be useful for diagnosis of infarction even up to 3 to 4 days after the event. Assays for cardiac-specific troponin I and troponin T using monoclonal antibodies are now available. (From Antman, E. M.: General hospital management. In Julian, D. G., and Braunwald, E. (eds.): Management of Acute Myocardial Infarction. London, W.B. Saunders Ltd., 1994, p. 63.)

cardial tissue and serum.[97,256] For optimal sensitivity it should be rapidly released into the blood after myocardial injury, and there should be a stoichiometric relationship between the plasma level of the marker and the extent of myocardial injury.[254] For ease of clinical use, the marker should persist in blood for an appropriate length of time to provide a convenient diagnostic time window (Table 37–2). Finally, the assay methodology should be inexpensive and easy to perform.

CREATINE KINASE (CK). Serum CK activity exceeds the normal range within 4 to 8 hours following the onset of AMI and declines to normal within 2 to 3 days (Fig. 37–7). Although the peak CK occurs on average at about 24 hours, peak levels occur earlier in patients who have had reperfu-

TABLE 37–2 MOLECULAR MARKERS USED OR PROPOSED FOR USE IN THE DIAGNOSIS OF ACUTE MYOCARDIAL INFARCTION

MARKER	MW (D)	RANGE OF TIMES TO INITIAL ELEVATION (h)	MEAN TIME TO PEAK ELEVATIONS (NONTHROMBOLYSIS)	TIME TO RETURN TO NORMAL RANGE	MOST COMMON SAMPLING SCHEDULE
hFABP	14,000–15,000	1.5	5–10 h	24 h	On presentation, then 4 h later
Myoglobin	17,800	1–4	6–7 h	24 h	Frequent; 1–2 h after CP
MLC	19,000–27,000	6–12	2–4 d	6–12 d	Once at least 12 h after CP
cTnI	23,500	3–12	24 h	5–10 d	Once at least 12 h after CP
cTnT	33,000	3–12	12 h–2 d	5–14 d	Once at least 12 h after CP
MB-CK	86,000	3–12	24 h	48–72 h	Every 12 h × 3*
MM-CK tissue isoform	86,000	1–6	12 h	38 h	60–90 min after CP
MB-CK tissue isoform	86,000	2–6	18 h	Unknown	60–90 min after CP
Enolase	90,000	6–10	24 h	48 h	Every 12 h × 3
LD	135,000	10	24–48 h	10–14 d	Once at least 24 h after CP
MHC	400,000	48	5–6 d	14 d	Once at least >2 d after CP

hFABP = heart fatty acid binding proteins; MLC = myosin light chain; cTnI = cardiac troponin I; cTnT = cardiac troponin T; MB-CK = MB isoenzyme of creatine kinase (CK); MM-CK = MM isoenzyme of CK; LD = lactate dehydrogenase; MHC = myosin heavy chain; CP = chest pain.

* Increased sensitivity can be achieved with sampling every 6 or 8 h.

Modified from Adams, J., III, Abendschein, D., and Jaffe, A.: Biochemical markers of myocardial injury. Is MB creatine kinase the choice for the 1990s? Circulation 88:750, 1993. Copyright 1993 American Heart Association.

sion as a result of the administration of thrombolytic therapy or mechanical recanalization (as well as in patients with early spontaneous thrombolysis). Because the time-activity curve of serum CK is influenced by reperfusion, and because reperfusion itself influences infarct size, reperfusion interferes with estimation of infarct size by enzyme analysis.[97,261]

Although elevation of the serum CK is a sensitive enzymatic detector of AMI that is routinely available in most hospitals,[97,262] important drawbacks include false-positive results in patients with muscle disease, alcohol intoxication, diabetes mellitus, skeletal muscle trauma, vigorous exercise, convulsions, intramuscular injections, thoracic outlet syndrome, and pulmonary embolism.[97,257,263]

CK ISOENZYMES. Three isoenzymes of CK (MM, BB, and MB) have been identified by electrophoresis. Extracts of brain and kidney contain predominantly the BB isoenzyme, skeletal muscle contains principally MM but does contain some MB (1 to 3 per cent),[264] and both MM and MB isoenzymes are present in cardiac muscle. The MB isoenzymes of CK may also be present in minor quantities in the small intestine, tongue, diaphragm, uterus, and prostate.[265] Strenuous exercise, particularly in trained long-distance runners or professional athletes, may cause elevation of both total CK and CK-MB.[97,266,267] Despite the fact that small quantities of CK-MB isoenzyme are found in tissues other than the heart, elevated serum activity of CK-MB may be considered, for practical purposes, to be the result of AMI (except in the case of trauma or surgery on the aforementioned organs, which contain small quantities of the enzyme). Earlier CK-MB assay methods that were in common use included radioimmunoassay and agarose gel electrophoresis techniques; these have now been largely supplanted by highly sensitive and specific enzyme immunoassays that utilize monoclonal antibodies directed against CK-MB.[268] Mass assays report results in nanograms per milliliter rather than units per milliliter and have been confirmed to be more accurate than CK-MB activity assays, especially in patients presenting within 4 hours of the onset of AMI.[269] It has been proposed that a ratio (relative index) of $\frac{\text{CK-MB mass}}{\text{CK activity}}$ of about 2.5 per cent is indicative of a myocardial rather than skeletal source of the CK-MB elevation.[270] Although this ratio may be satisfied by many patients with AMI, it is inaccurate in several circumstances: (1) When high levels of total CK are present because of skeletal muscle injury (a large quantity of CK-MB must be released from the myocardium to satisfy criteria); (2) Chronic skeletal muscle injury releases large amounts of CK-MB; (3) Total CK measurements are within the normal reference range for the laboratory and CK-MB is elevated (possibly indicating that a microinfarction has occurred).[97] Patients with minimally elevated CK-MB and normal CK have a prognosis that is generally worse than that for patients with suspected MI but no CK-MB elevation.[271] Thus, whether or not such elevations represent true "microinfarctions" may be less important than the prognostic connotations of this isolated elevation.

Clinicians should not rely on measurements of CK and CK-MB at a single point in time but instead should evaluate the temporal rise and fall of serially obtained values; skeletal muscle release of CK-MB generally remains elevated for a longer time than myocardial release of CK-MB and produces a "plateau" pattern of CK-MB values over several days, in contrast to the shorter time course of skeletal muscle CK-MB elevation, as depicted in Figure 37–17. Furthermore, the availability of new serum markers such as cardiac-specific troponin I and T (cTnI and cTnT) (Fig. 37–17 and Table 37–2) may help distinguish skeletal from cardiac muscle damage.

In addition to AMI secondary to coronary obstruction, other forms of injury to cardiac muscle—such as those resulting from myocarditis, trauma, cardiac catheterization,

shock, and cardiac surgery—may also produce elevated serum CK-MB levels.[97] These latter causes of elevation of serum CK-MB values can usually be readily distinguished from AMI by the clinical setting.

CK ISOFORMS. Isoforms of the MM and MB isoenzymes have been identified.[272] These are subtypes of the individual isoenzymes and are formed in the circulation when an enzyme known as carboxypeptidase cleaves lysine residues from the carboxy terminus of the myocardial form of the enzyme (CK-MM3 and CK-MB2), producing isoforms with a different electrophoretic mobility (CK-MM2, CK-MM1, and CK-MB1). Certain isoforms appear to be released into the blood quite rapidly—perhaps as soon as 1 hour—after the onset of infarction. In one study an absolute level of the CK-MB2 isoform > 1.0 U/L or ratio of $\frac{\text{CK-MB2}}{\text{CK-MB1}} > 1.5$ had a sensitivity for diagnosing AMI of 59 per cent at 2 to 4 hours and of 92 per cent at 4 to 6 hours.[273] A rapid high-voltage electrophoretic assay for these isoforms has been developed and preliminary results in experienced research laboratories suggest it may permit early identification of patients with AMI and early detection of successful reperfusion (peak $\frac{\text{CK-MB2}}{\text{CK-MB1}} > 3.8$ at 2 hours).[259,274]

MYOGLOBIN. This protein is released into the circulation from injured myocardial cells and can be demonstrated within a few hours after the onset of infarction[275,276] (Fig. 37–17 and Table 37–2). Peak levels of serum myoglobin are reached considerably earlier (1 to 4 hours) than peak values of serum CK.[97] In contrast to CK, myoglobin (which has a molecular weight of only 17,800) is readily excreted into the urine. A more rapid rise in serum myoglobin has been observed following reperfusion, and its measurement has been suggested as a useful index of successful reperfusion[97,277] and even infarct size.[278] However, the clinical value of serial determinations of myoglobin in AMI is limited by the brief duration of its elevation (< 24 hours) and by the lack of specificity. The latter results from the fact that myoglobin is a constituent of skeletal muscle. Because of its lack of cardiac specificity, an isolated measurement of myoglobin within the first 4 to 8 hours following onset of chest discomfort in patients with a nondiagnostic ECG should not be relied upon to make the diagnosis of AMI but should be supplemented by a more cardiac-specific marker such as CK-MB, cTnI, or cTnT (Table 37–2).

CARDIAC-SPECIFIC TROPONINS. The troponin complex consists of three subunits that regulate the calcium-mediated contractile process of striated muscle.[279] These are troponin C, which binds Ca^{++}; troponin I (TnI), which binds to actin and inhibits actin-myosin interactions; and troponin T (TnT), which binds to tropomyosin, thereby attaching the troponin complex to the thin filament (see Fig. 12–4, p. 364). Although the majority of TnT is incorporated in the troponin complex, approximately 6 per cent is dissolved in the cytosol[280]; about 2 to 3 per cent of TnI is found in a cytosolic pool.[281]

Although both TnT and TnI are present in cardiac and skeletal muscle, they are encoded by different genes and the amino acid sequence differs.[282] This permits the production of antibodies that are specific for the cardiac form (cTnT and cTnI) and has led to the development of quantitative assays for cTnT and cTnI that have been approved by the FDA for clinical use[281,283–286] (Fig. 37–17 and Table 37–2). Several studies have confirmed the reliability of these new quantitative assays for detecting myocardial injury, and measurement of cTnT or cTnI has been proposed as a new diagnostic criterion for MI.[97,257,263,281,286–288] A qualitative, rapid, bedside assay for cTnT has also been approved for diagnosing AMI.[288a]

Because CK-MB is found in skeletal muscle, the cut-off value for an elevated CK-MB is typically set a few units above the upper end of the reference range. However, because cTnT or cTnI is not detected in the peripheral circulation under normal circumstances, the cut-off value for these analytes may be set only slightly above the "noise" level of the assay.[257,285] Furthermore, whereas CK-MB usually increases 10- to 20-fold above the upper limit of the reference range, cTnT and cTnI typically increase more than 20 times above the reference range. These features of the cardiac-specific troponin assays provide an improved signal-to-noise ratio, enabling the detection of even minor degrees of myocardial necrosis.[260,289–291] In patients with AMI, cTnT and cTnI first begin to rise above the upper reference limit by 3 hours from the onset of chest pain.[287] Elevations of cTnI may persist for 7 to 10 days following AMI; elevations of cTnT may persist for up to 10 to 14 days.

The kinetics of release of cTnT are similar for patients with Q-wave and non-Q-wave AMI.[257,292] Patients with AMI who undergo successful recanalization of the infarct-related artery have a rapid release of cTnT that may be useful as an indicator of reperfusion.[97,293,294] In theory the same should hold true for cTnI, but criteria for reperfusion have not been established yet. Also, although CK-MB measurements return to the normal range by 72 hours following infarction, the degeneration of the contractile apparatus produces a continuous release of cTnI from the complex for 5 to 10 days and cTnT for 10 to 14 days after AMI, permitting late diagnosis of infarction.[97,257]

When comparing the diagnostic efficiency of cTnT versus CK-MB for AMI, it is important to bear in mind that the cTnT assay is probably capable of detecting episodes of myocardial necrosis that are below the detection limit of the current CK-MB assays. The somewhat vague term of "minor myocardial damage" has been used to describe the pathological process in patients who have a chest pain syndrome and elevated cTnT but in whom CK-MB is in the normal range.[282,289] At the present time it remains unclear whether such patients have release of cTnT from a cytosolic pool in response to reversible ischemia or they have actually sustained "microinfarctions." However, it has been established that patients with a chest pain syndrome suspicious for AMI who have a normal CK-MB and elevated cTnT have an increased risk for adverse clinical outcome, including death, recurrent nonfatal infarction, and need for revascularization with PTCA or CABG.[260,282,289,295]

The independent diagnostic and prognostic value of measurement of cTnT or cTnI versus CK-MB or other serum cardiac markers is currently under investigation.[296–299] Until sufficient information in a large enough sample of patients is available, no definitive recommendations regarding the prognostic implications of these markers can be made.

LACTIC DEHYDROGENASE (LDH). The activity of this enzyme exceeds the normal range by 24 to 48 hours after the onset of AMI, reaches a peak 3 to 6 days after the onset of pain, and returns to normal levels 8 to 14 days after the infarction[97] (Fig. 37–17). Total LDH, although sensitive, is not specific; false-positive elevations occur in patients with hemolysis, megaloblastic anemia, leukemia, liver disease, hepatic congestion, renal disease, a variety of neoplasms, pulmonary embolism, myocarditis, skeletal muscle disease, and shock.[300]

LDH comprises five isoenzymes, which are numbered in the order of the rapidity of their migration toward the anode of an electrophoretic field. LDH_1 moves most rapidly, whereas LDH_5 is the slowest. Fractionation of the serum LDH into its five isoenzymes increases diagnostic accuracy because the heart contains principally LDH_1. Most conditions causing elevated serum total LDH activity, such as liver or skeletal muscle disease or injury, are readily distinguished from AMI by analysis of LDH isoenzymes. Increased serum LDH_1 activity precedes elevation of serum total LDH and usually occurs within 8 to 24 hours after infarction.[97] Because hemolysis also raises serum LDH_1 activity, particular care must be taken in the withdrawal and handling of the blood specimens.

Many laboratories report a ratio of LDH_1/LDH_2 greater than 1.0 as a cut-off defining abnormality. However, even a ratio as low as 0.76 has been reported to be more than 90 per cent sensitive and specific for the diagnosis of AMI.[97] Although LDH isoenzyme testing may be useful, it is likely that LDH isoenzyme analysis for the diagnosis of AMI will be superseded by newer, more cardiac-specific late markers such as cTnT or cTnI (Table 37–2).

OTHER SERUM CARDIAC MARKERS. For many years the activity of serum glutamic oxaloacetic acid transferase (SGOT)—now generally referred to as aspartate aminotransferase (AST)—was monitored for diagnosis of AMI. However, because false-positive elevations occur frequently (with most hepatic or skeletal muscle diseases, following intramuscular injections or pulmonary embolism, with shock) and because the time course of elevation offers no advantage relative to other serum markers, its incremental benefit for the diagnosis of AMI is negligible, and it is no longer routinely used.

Other promising serum cardiac markers that are under development include heart fatty acid binding proteins (hFABP), myosin light chains (MLC), myosin heavy chains (MHC), and glycogen phosphorylase isoenzyme BB (GPBB).[97,301,302] These markers offer the potential for earlier diagnosis (hFABP, GPBB) and a longer diagnostic window (MLC, MHC), but their relative roles compared with traditional markers such as CK-MB and newer markers such as CK-MB isoforms, cTnT, or cTnI remain to be defined. Carbonic anhydrase III is a protein found only in skeletal muscle and not cardiac muscle.[303] With injury to skeletal muscle it is released in a fixed relationship to myoglobin, and therefore the ratio of myoglobin to carbonic anhydrase III may be a useful means of excluding a cardiac source of myoglobin elevation.[304]

RECOMMENDATIONS FOR MEASUREMENT OF SERUM MARKERS. Although most hospitals obtain CK and CK-MB measurements when evaluating patients with suspected AMI, this practice may change in the near future as assays for more rapidly released markers such as myoglobin and more cardiac-specific markers such as troponin T and troponin I become available clinically.[287]

It seems reasonable for clinicians to measure either cTnT or cTnI in patients with suspected AMI. From a cost-effectiveness perspective, it is unnecessary to measure both a cardiac-specific troponin and CK-MB at all time points. Routine diagnosis of AMI can be accomplished within 12 hours using CK-MB, cTnT, or cTnI by obtaining measurements approximately every 8 to 12 hours. Retrospective diagnosis or diagnosis of AMI in the presence of skeletal muscle injury is more readily accomplished with cTnT or cTnI. Future directions for research with the cardiac troponins involve evaluating their ability to aid in the diagnosis of AMI that occurs following cardiac[305] and noncardiac surgery[286] and interventional catheterization procedures and in identifying myocardial injury from conditions other than AMI, such as myocarditis.[306]

Other Laboratory Measurements

Numerous nonspecific manifestations may be recognized in patients with AMI. Although they are not generally employed in establishing the diagnosis, awareness of their coexistence with infarction is important in order to avoid misinterpretation or erroneous diagnosis of other disorders.

SERUM LIPIDS. These are often determined in patients with AMI. However, the results may be misleading because numerous factors that can alter the values are operating at the time of the patient's admission to the hospital. Serum triglycerides are affected by caloric intake, intravenous glucose, and recumbency.

During the first 24 to 48 hours after admission, total cholesterol and HDL cholesterol remain at or near baseline values but generally fall precipitously after that.[307,308] The fall in HDL cholesterol after AMI is greater than the fall in total cholesterol; thus, the ratio of total cholesterol to HDL cholesterol is no longer useful for risk assessment early after MI.[309] In review of the revised, more aggressive guidelines for management of hyperlipidemia in patients with clinical manifestations of coronary artery disease,[310] a lipid profile should be obtained on all AMI patients who are admitted within 24 to 48 hours of symptoms. For patients admitted beyond 24 to 48 hours, it is best to defer determinations of serum lipid levels until at least 8 weeks after the infarction has occurred.

HEMATOLOGICAL MANIFESTATIONS. The elevation of the white blood count usually develops within 2 hours after the onset of chest pain, reaches a peak 2 to 4 days following infarction, and returns to normal in 1 week; the peak white blood cell count usually ranges between 12 and 15×10^3 per cubic millimeter but occasionally rises to as high as 20×10^3 per cubic millimeter in patients with large transmural AMI. Often there is an increase in the percentage of polymorphonuclear leukocytes and a shift of the differential count to band forms. Using a combination of abnormal leukocyte differential count and CK-MB was found to be especially helpful in the recognition of AMI when the initial ECG tracing was nondiagnostic.[311]

The erythrocyte sedimentation rate (ESR) is usually normal during the first day or two after infarction, even though fever and leukocytosis may be present. It then rises to a peak on the fourth or fifth day and may remain elevated for several weeks. The increase in the ESR is secondary to elevated plasma alpha$_2$ globulin fibrinogen,[312] but the peak does not correlate well with the size of the infarction or with the prognosis. The hematocrit often increases during the first few days following infarction as a consequence of hemoconcentration.[214]

Electrocardiographic Findings
(See also p. 127)

In the majority of patients with AMI, some change can be documented when serial electrocardiograms (ECGs) are compared.[312a] However, many factors limit the ability of the ECG to diagnose and localize MI: the extent of myocardial injury, the age of the infarct, its location (e.g., the 12-lead ECG is relatively insensitive to infarction in the posterolateral region of the left ventricle), the presence of conduction defects, the presence of previous infarcts or acute pericarditis, changes in electrolyte concentrations, and the administration of cardioactive drugs. Nevertheless, serial standard 12-lead ECGs remain a clinically useful method for the detection and localization of MI.[255] Even when left bundle branch block is present on the ECG, MI can be diagnosed when striking ST-segment deviation is present beyond that which can be explained by the conduction defect.[312b]

Although general agreement exists on electrocardiographic and vectorcardiographic criteria for the recognition of infarction of the anterior and inferior myocardial walls (Table 4–3, p. 129), less agreement is found on criteria for lateral and posterior infarcts[313]; here even the terminology may be confusing. It has been reported that patients with an abnormal R wave in V$_1$ (0.04 sec in duration and/or R/S ratio ≥ 1 in the absence of preexcitation or right ventricular hypertrophy) with inferior or lateral Q waves have an increased incidence of isolated occlusion of a dominant left circumflex coronary artery without collateral circulation; such patients have a lower ejection fraction, increased end-systolic volume, and higher complication rate than patients with inferior infarction due to isolated occlusion of the right coronary artery.[314]

More sophisticated forms of ECG recordings including high-resolution electrocardiography, body surface potential mapping of ST segments, and continuous vectorcardiography have all been reported in small series of patients to augment the 12-lead ECG in diagnosing AMI, but the lack of ready availability of equipment and the special expertise required limits the use of these techniques.[315–317] Of potentially more widespread clinical applicability is a clinical and ECG algorithm for predicting the presence of AMI that provides a computerized reading of the tracing along with a statement of the patient's risk of adverse cardiovascular events with and without reperfusion therapy.[318]

Although most patients continue to demonstrate the ECG changes from an infarction for the rest of their lives, particularly if they evolve Q waves, in a substantial minority the typical changes disappear, Q waves can regress,[319] and the ECG can even return to normal after a number of years. Under many circumstances Q-wave patterns may simulate MI. Conditions that may mimic the electrocardiographic features of MI by producing a pattern of "pseudoinfarction" include ventricular hypertrophy, conduction disturbances, preexcitation, primary myocardial disease, pneumothorax,

pulmonary embolus, amyloid heart disease, primary and metastatic tumors of the heart, traumatic heart disease, intracranial hemorrhage, hyperkalemia, pericarditis, early repolarization, and cardiac involvement with sarcoidosis.[320]

Q-WAVE AND NON-Q-WAVE INFARCTION. As noted earlier (see p. 1189), the presence or absence of Q waves on the surface ECG does not reliably predict the distinction between transmural and nontransmural (subendocardial) AMI.[82,321] Q waves on the ECG signify abnormal electrical activity but are not synonymous with irreversible myocardial damage. Also, the absence of Q waves may simply reflect the insensitivity of the standard 12-lead ECG, especially in the posterior zones of the left ventricle.[82] True pathological subendocardial AMI, as recognized at autopsy, is seen with ST-segment depression and/or T-wave changes only about 50 per cent of the time.[322] Angiographic studies in AMI patients without ST-segment elevation show a higher incidence of subtotal occlusion of the culprit coronary vessel and greater collateral flow to the infarct zone[323,324] (Fig. 37–7). Observational data suggest that AMI without ST-segment elevation is seen more commonly in elderly patients and patients with a prior MI.[325,326]

Nevertheless, for the prognostic importance of identifying two different populations, a distinction should be made between AMI with and without Q waves, recognizing that the latter constitutes a heterogeneous group of abnormalities.[82,327,328] Changes in the ST segment and T wave are quite nonspecific and may occur in a variety of conditions, including stable and unstable angina pectoris, ventricular hypertrophy, acute and chronic pericarditis, myocarditis, early repolarization, electrolyte imbalance, shock, and metabolic disorders and following the administration of digitalis (see Chap. 4). Serial ECGs may be of considerable aid in differentiating these conditions from non-Q-wave infarction.[82,329] Transient changes favor angina or electrolyte disturbances, whereas persistent changes argue for infarction if other causes such as shock, administration of digitalis, and persistent metabolic disorders can be eliminated. In the final analysis, the diagnosis of nontransmural infarction rests more on the combination of clinical findings and the elevation of serum enzymes than on the ECG.

ISCHEMIA AT A DISTANCE. Patients with new Q waves and ST-segment elevation diagnostic for AMI in one territory often have ST-segment depression in other territories. These additional ST-segment changes may be caused by ischemia in a territory other than the area of infarction, termed "ischemia at a distance," or by reciprocal electrical phenomena.[330,331] A good deal of attention has been directed to associated ST-segment depression in the anterior leads, when it occurs in patients with acute inferior MI.[332,333] However, despite the clinical importance of differentiation among causes of anterior ST-segment depression in such patients—including anterior ischemia, posterior wall infarction, and true reciprocal changes—such a differentiation cannot be made reliably by electrocardiographic or even vectorcardiographic techniques. Although precordial ST-segment depression is more commonly associated with extensive infarction of the posterior, lateral, or inferior septal segments—rather than anterior wall subendocardial ischemia—imaging techniques such as two-dimensional echocardiography are necessary to ascertain whether an anterior wall motion abnormality is present. Regardless of whether the anterior ST-segment changes reflect anterior wall ischemia or are reciprocal to changes elsewhere, this finding, as with ischemia at a distance, implies a poorer prognosis than if such changes are not present.[330,331,333,334]

RIGHT VENTRICULAR INFARCTION. ST-segment elevation in right precordial leads (V$_1$, V$_3$R–V$_6$R) is a relatively sensitive and specific sign of right ventricular infarction.[335,336] Occasionally ST-segment elevation in leads V$_2$ and V$_3$ may be due to acute right ventricular infarction; this appears to occur only when the injury to the left inferior wall is minimal.[337] Usually, the concurrent inferior wall injury suppresses this anterior ST-segment elevation resulting from right ventricular injury. Likewise, right ventricular infarction appears to reduce the anterior ST-segment depression often observed with inferior wall myocardial infarction.[338] A QS or QR pattern in leads V_3R and/or V_4R also suggest right ventricular myocardial necrosis but has less predictive accuracy than ST-segment elevation in these leads.[339]

ATRIAL INFARCTION. The most common electrocardiographic patterns are depression or elevation of the PR segment, alterations in the contour of the P wave, and abnormal atrial rhythms, including atrial flutter, atrial fibrillation, wandering atrial pacemaker, and AV nodal rhythm.[340]

Imaging

ROENTGENOGRAPHY. The initial chest roentgenogram in patients with AMI is almost invariably a portable film obtained in the emergency room or the coronary care unit. Two findings are common: signs of left ventricular failure and cardiomegaly. Although the pulmonary vascular markings on the roentgenogram reflect left ventricular end-diastolic pressure, significant temporal discrepancies may occur because of what have been termed diagnostic lags and post-therapeutic lags. Up to 12 hours may elapse before pulmonary edema accumulates after ventricular filling pressure has become elevated. The post-therapeutic phase lag represents a longer time interval; up to 2 days are required for pulmonary edema to resorb and the radiographic signs of pulmonary congestion to clear after ventricular filling pressure has returned toward normal. The degree of congestion and the size of the left side of the heart on the chest film are useful for defining groups of patients with AMI who are at increased risk of dying after the acute event.[341]

Echocardiography

(See also pp. 87 to 90 and Fig. 3–87, p. 86)

TWO-DIMENSIONAL ECHOCARDIOGRAPHY. The relative portability of echocardiographic equipment makes this technique ideal for the assessment of patients with AMI hospitalized in the coronary care unit or even in the emergency department before admission.[342,342a] In patients with chest pain compatible with AMI but with a nondiagnostic ECG (Fig. 37–18), the finding on echocardiography of a distinct region of disordered contraction can be helpful diagnostically because it supports the diagnosis of myocardial ischemia.[343–345] Echocardiography is also useful in evaluating patients with chest pain and a nondiagnostic ECG who are suspected of having an aortic dissection. The identification of an intimal flap consistent with an aortic dissection is a crucial observation because it represents a major contraindication to thrombolytic therapy (see p. 1554).

Areas of abnormal regional wall motion are observed almost universally in patients with AMI, and the degree of wall motion abnormality can be categorized with a semi-quantitative wall motion score index.[346] Abnormal wall motion is less often noted echocardiographically when the infarction is nontransmural; however, abnormalities are still present in more than two-thirds of these patients. Left ventricular function estimated from two-dimensional echocardiograms correlates well with measurements from angiography and is useful in establishing prognosis following AMI.[347] Furthermore, the early use of echocardiography can aid in the early detection of potentially viable but stunned myocardium (contractile reserve),[348,349] residual provocable ischemia,[350] patients at risk for the development of congestive heart failure following AMI,[351] and mechanical complications of AMI.[352]

Whereas transthoracic imaging is adequate in most patients, occasional patients have poor echo windows, especially if they are undergoing mechanical ventilation. In such patients transesophageal echocardiography can be safely performed[353] and can be useful in evaluating ventricular septal defects and papillary muscle dysfunction.[352]

DOPPLER ECHOCARDIOGRAPHY. This technique (see p. 56) allows for assessment of blood flow in the cardiac chambers and across cardiac valves. Used in conjunction with two-dimensional echocardiography, it is helpful in detecting and assessing the severity of mitral or tricuspid regurgitation following AMI.[354] Identification of the site of acute ventricular septal rupture, as well as quantification of shunt flow across the resulting defect, is also possible.[355]

Other Imaging Modalities

COMPUTED TOMOGRAPHY (CT) (see p. 337). This technique can provide useful cross-sectional information in patients with MI. In addition to the assessment of cavity di-

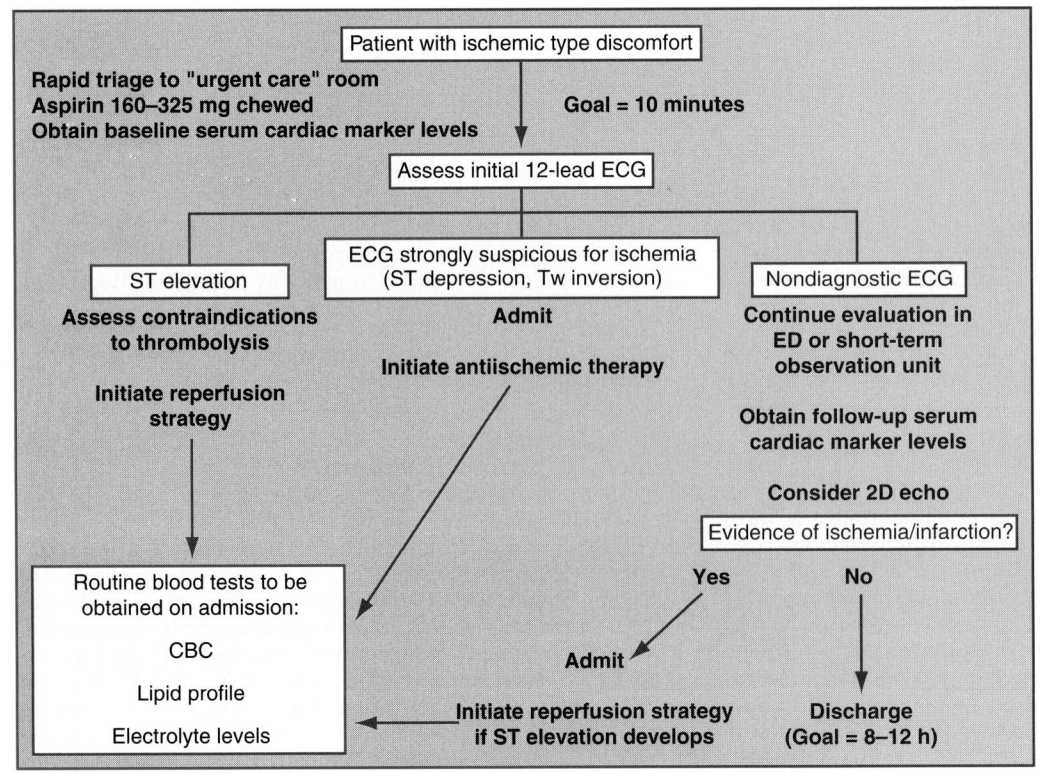

FIGURE 37–18. Algorithm for management of patients with suspected AMI in emergency department. All patients with ischemic-type discomfort should be rapidly evaluated and receive aspirin. The initial 12-lead electrocardiogram (ECG) is used to define the acute management strategy. Patients with ST-segment elevation should be considered candidates for reperfusion, whereas those without ST-segment elevation whose ECG and clinical history are strongly suspicious for ischemia should be admitted for initiation of antiischemic therapy. Patients with a nondiagnostic ECG should undergo further evaluation in the emergency department or short-term observation unit with ultimate disposition based on the results of serial serum cardiac marker levels and echocardiographic findings. Routine blood tests that should be obtained in all patients admitted include a complete blood count (CBC), lipid profile, and electrolyte levels.

mensions and wall thickness,[356] left ventricular aneurysms may be detected, and, of particular importance in AMI, intracardiac thrombi can be identified. Although cardiac CT is a less convenient technique, it probably is more sensitive for thrombus detection than is echocardiography.[357]

MAGNETIC RESONANCE IMAGING (MRI) (see Figs. 10–3, p. 320 and 10–4, p. 321). In addition to localizing and sizing the area of infarction, MRI techniques are capable of early recognition of MI and of providing an assessment of the severity of the ischemic insult.[358–360a] Although imaging with this technique presents practical problems for routine studies in coronary care unit patients because patients must be transported to the MRI facility, this modality holds much promise because of its ability to assess perfusion of infarcted and noninfarcted tissue as well as of reperfused myocardium; to identify areas of jeopardized but not infarcted myocardium; to identify myocardial edema, fibrosis, wall thinning, and hypertrophy; to assess ventricular chamber size and segmental wall motion; and to identify the temporal transition between ischemia and infarction.[358,361]

NUCLEAR IMAGING. Radionuclide angiography, perfusion imaging, infarct-avid scintigraphy, and positron-emission tomography have been used to evaluate patients with AMI. Nuclear cardiac imaging techniques (Fig. 9–21, p. 287, Figs. 9–30 and 9–31, p. 296) can be useful for detecting AMI[362]; assessing infarct size,[363] collateral flow,[116] and jeopardized myocardium; determining the effects of the infarct on ventricular function; and establishing prognosis of patients with AMI.[363,363a] However, the necessity of moving a critically ill patient from the coronary care unit (CCU) to the nuclear medicine department limits their practical application unless a portable gamma camera is available. The ACC/AHA Task Force Committee on Cardiac Radionuclide Imaging has *not* recommended the *routine* use of any radionuclide imaging technique for the purpose of diagnosing AMI, but considered rest radionuclide angiography for assessment of right and left ventricular function and stress myocardial perfusion imaging for detection of ischemia as usually appropriate and potentially useful (Class I).[362] The committee further emphasized that before ordering cardiac radionuclide imaging in individual patients, the quality of the laboratory, the expertise of the staff performing and evaluating the test results, and the potential impact of positive and negative results on subsequent clinical decision-making all be carefully considered.[362]

ELECTROCARDIOGRAPHY. Interest in limiting infarct size, in large part because of the recognition that the quantity of myocardium infarcted has important prognostic implications, has focused attention on the accurate determination of MI size. The sum of ST-segment elevations measured from multiple precordial leads correlates with the extent of myocardial injury in patients with anterior MI.[364] QRS scoring systems and planar or vectorcardiographic techniques to estimate infarct size have also been developed. Although they demonstrate good correlations with infarct size at autopsy and with enzymatic estimates, formal sizing of infarcts by ECG technique is not necessary in most patients. Of note, however, there is a relationship between the number of ECG leads showing ST elevation and mortality—patients with 8 or 9 of 12 leads with ST elevation have three to four times the mortality of those with only 2 or 3 leads with ST elevation.[365] The duration of ischemia time as estimated from continuous ST segment monitoring is correlated with infarct size, the ratio of infarct size to area at risk, and the extent of regional wall motion abnormality observed at 7 days and 30 days after AMI.[364]

SERUM CARDIAC MARKER METHODS. In order to estimate infarct size by analysis of serum cardiac marker levels, it is necessary to account for the quantity of the marker lost from the myocardium, its volume of distribution, and its release ratio.[97] Serial measurements of proteins released by necrotic myocardium, particularly CK and its MB isoenzyme, are helpful in determining AMI size. Clinically, the peak CK or CK-MB provides an approximate estimate of infarct size and is widely used prognostically. In the prethrombotic era, quantification of the cumulative release of CK or CK-MB correlated with other techniques for estimating infarct size in vivo as well as with the area of necrosis at autopsy. However, coronary artery reperfusion dramatically changes the wash-out kinetics of CK from myocardium, resulting in early and exaggerated peak enzyme levels and limiting the usefulness of CK curves as a measure of infarct size.[261] Whether structural proteins such as the troponins, whose release ratios are less affected by rapid changes in coronary flow, offer an advantage in this regard requires further investigation.[97]

NONINVASIVE IMAGING TECHNIQUES. Echocardiography (see Chap. 3), radionuclide scintigraphy[363] (see Chap. 9), CT scanning (see Chap. 10), and MRI[360] (see Chap. 10) have all been utilized for the clinical and experimental assessment of infarct size. Infarct-avid scintigraphy and myocardial perfusion imaging have been used to quantify infarct size. Estimation of infarct size by quantitative tomographic ^{99m}Tc-sestamibi imaging appears to be less limited by ventricular geometry and can distinguish small infarcts and ischemia from infarcted myocardium more readily than other noninvasive methods.[363] Tomography has improved on planar techniques employing technetium-99m pyrophosphate to image AMI (see p. 285).[366] Imaging of radiolabeled myosin-specific antibodies, which bind to myosin exposed by the loss of plasma membrane in early myocardial necrosis, holds promise for highly accurate quantification of infarct size.[87,367,368] Contrast-enhanced MRI imaging has been helpful in demonstrating the regional heterogeneity of infarction patterns in patients with persistently occluded infarct arteries versus those with successfully reperfused vessels.[369]

MANAGEMENT

Physician practices have changed dramatically as newer approaches to the care of the AMI patient have become available.[35,36,45] Almost all physicians in the United States have access to intensive care facilities for their patients with AMI. The current average hospital length of stay is 5 to 6 days, less than half of what it was in 1970. The National Registry of Myocardial Infarction, an observational data base of practice patterns reflecting treatment of 240,989 patients with AMI at 1073 hospitals between 1990 and 1993, reported that nearly 80 per cent of patients with AMI received aspirin.[12] Invasive and/or noninvasive procedures to evaluate prognosis and the need for further therapy are now used in most post-MI patients, whereas only a small percentage of patients had such procedures performed 25 years ago.[35,36,45] Finally, thrombolytic therapy and angioplasty are now the standard of care in appropriately selected patients.[370–374] The combination of these measures has led to a decline in the short-term mortality from AMI.[22]

PREHOSPITAL CARE

The prehospital care of patients with suspected acute myocardial infarction is a crucial element bearing directly on the likelihood of survival. Most deaths associated with AMI occur within the first hour of its onset and are usually due to ventricular fibrillation[375] (see also Chap. 24). Accordingly, the importance of the immediate implementation of definitive resuscitative efforts and of rapidly transporting the patient to a hospital cannot be overemphasized.[376] Major components of the delay from the onset of symptoms consistent with AMI to treatment include the following[375]: (1) the time for the patient to recognize the seriousness of the problem and seek medical attention; (2) prehospital evaluation, treatment, and transportation; (3) the time for diagnostic measures and initiation of treatment in the hospital.

Patients must be educated to seek immediate medical

attention should they develop manifestations of AMI. The GISSI investigators have analyzed the epidemiology of avoidable delays in the care of patients with AMI in Italy since 1990 and reported that the decision time by the patient played a more significant role than home-to-hospital time and in-hospital time in delay to treatment of AMI.[377] Patient-related factors that were correlated with longer decision to seek medical attention included advanced age, living alone, low intensity of initial symptoms, history of diabetes, occurrence of symptoms at night, and involvement of a general practitioner before arrival in the emergency department.[377]

Health care professionals should heighten the level of awareness of patients at risk for AMI (e.g., those with hypertension, diabetes, history of angina pectoris). They should review and reinforce with patients and their families the need for seeking urgent medical attention for a pattern of symptoms including chest discomfort, extreme fatigue, and dyspnea, especially if accompanied by diaphoresis, lightheadedness, palpitations, or a sense of impending doom.[378] Although many patients shun such discussions and tend to minimize the likelihood of ever needing emergency cardiac treatment, emphasis should be placed on the prevention and treatment of potentially fatal arrhythmias as well as salvage of the jeopardized myocardium by reperfusion, for which time is crucial.[379] Patients should also be instructed in the proper use of sublingual nitroglycerin that should be taken as one tablet at the onset of ischemic-type discomfort and repeated at 5-minute intervals for a total of three doses. If the symptoms have not dissipated within 15 minutes, the patient should be rapidly transported to a medical facility that has the capability of recording and interpreting an electrocardiogram, providing advanced cardiac life support and cardiac monitoring, and initiating reperfusion therapy with either thrombolysis or angioplasty if indicated.[2] Primary care physicians need to take a larger role in helping implement strategies to facilitate early treatment.[378]

Well-equipped ambulances and helicopters staffed by personnel trained in the acute care of the infarction victim (mobile CCUs) allow definitive therapy to commence while the patient is being transported to the hospital.[380] To be used effectively, they must be placed strategically within a community, and excellent radio communication systems must be available. These units should be equipped with battery-operated monitoring equipment, a DC defibrillator, oxygen, endotracheal tubes and suction apparatus, and commonly used cardiovascular drugs. A radiotelemetry system that allows transmission of the ECG signal to the hospital is desirable but not essential. The effectiveness of such a system depends upon the competency of paramedics, transmission distances, and the availability of expert consultation on the receiving end.[381] Observations of simple variables such as heart rate and blood pressure permit initial classification of patients into high- or low-risk subgroups[382] because those patients initially presenting with hypotension have a mortality in excess of 30 per cent, whereas young patients with isolated sinus bradycardia and a normal or elevated blood pressure appear to have a mortality that is under 5 per cent.[10]

In addition to prompt defibrillation, the efficacy of prehospital care appears to depend on several factors, including early relief of pain with its deleterious physiological sequelae, reduction of excessive activity of the autonomic nervous system, and abolition of prelethal arrhythmias, such as ventricular tachycardia. However, these efforts must not inhibit rapid transfer to the hospital, which might possibly diminish the benefit of the patient's early entry into the health care system.

PREHOSPITAL THROMBOLYSIS. The potential benefits of prehospital thrombolysis have been evaluated in five randomized trials that collectively randomized 6318 patients.[382-386] Although none of the individual trials showed a significant reduction in mortality with prehospital initiated thrombolytic therapy, there was a generally consistent observation of benefit from earlier treatment, and a meta-analysis of all the available trials demonstrated a 17 per cent reduction in mortality (95 per cent CI: 2 per cent to 29 per cent).[386]

Several factors must be weighed when communities consider whether their ambulances and emergency transport vehicles should have capabilities of initiating thrombolytic therapy. The greatest reduction in mortality is observed when reperfusion can be initiated within 60 to 90 minutes of the onset of symptoms.[10,375] It has been suggested that the streamlining of emergency department triage practices so that treatment can be started within 30 minutes, when coupled with the 15 to 30 minute transport time that is common in most urban centers, may be more cost effective than equipping all ambulances to administer prehospital thrombolytic therapy.[387] The latter would require extensive training of personnel, installation of computer-assisted electrocardiographs or systems for radio transmission of the ECG signal to a central station, and stocking of medicine kits with the necessary drug supplies.[381,388-390] However, in selected communities where transport delays may be 90 minutes or longer and experienced personnel or physicians are available on ambulances, prehospital thrombolytic therapy is probably beneficial.[390]

MANAGEMENT IN THE EMERGENCY DEPARTMENT

Physicians evaluating patients in the emergency department must confront the difficult task of rapidly identifying patients who require urgent reperfusion therapy, triaging lower risk patients to the appropriate facility within the hospital, and not discharging patients home inappropriately while avoiding unnecessary admissions.[375,391,392] As emphasized in Figure 37-18, a history of ischemic-type discomfort and the initial 12-lead electrocardiogram (Fig. 37-19) are the primary tools for screening patients with acute coronary syndromes in the emergency department.[376,393] ST-segment elevation on the electrocardiogram of a patient with a history compatible with AMI (see p. 1205) is highly suggestive of thrombotic occlusion of an epicardial coronary artery,[100,323,324] and its presence should serve as the trigger for a well-rehearsed sequence of rapid assessment of the patient for contraindications to thrombolysis and initiation of a reperfusion strategy[375,391] (Fig. 37-20).

Because lethal arrhythmias can occur suddenly in patients with an acute coronary syndrome, all patients should rapidly have a 12-lead ECG performed while a brief targeted history is taken[375,391] (Fig. 37-18). Patients should then be attached to a bedside ECG monitor and intravenous access obtained for infusion of 5 per cent dextrose in water. If the initial ECG shows ST-segment elevation of 1 mm or more in at least two contiguous leads (Fig. 37-19) or a new or presumably new left bundle branch block, the patient should be screened immediately for any contraindications to thrombolysis (Table 37-3) to help facilitate expeditious initiation of reperfusion therapy (see p. 1215). The National Heart Attack Alert Program recommends that emergency departments strive for a goal of treating eligible AMI patients with thrombolytic therapy within 30 minutes[375,391] (Fig. 37-21).

Patients with an initial ECG that reveals new or presumably new ST-segment depression and/or T-wave inversion, while not considered candidates for thrombolytic therapy, should be treated as though they are suffering from AMI without ST elevation or unstable angina (a distinction to be made subsequently after scrutiny of serial ECGs and serum cardiac marker measurements) (Fig. 37-5).

The available data fail to show a benefit of thrombolysis

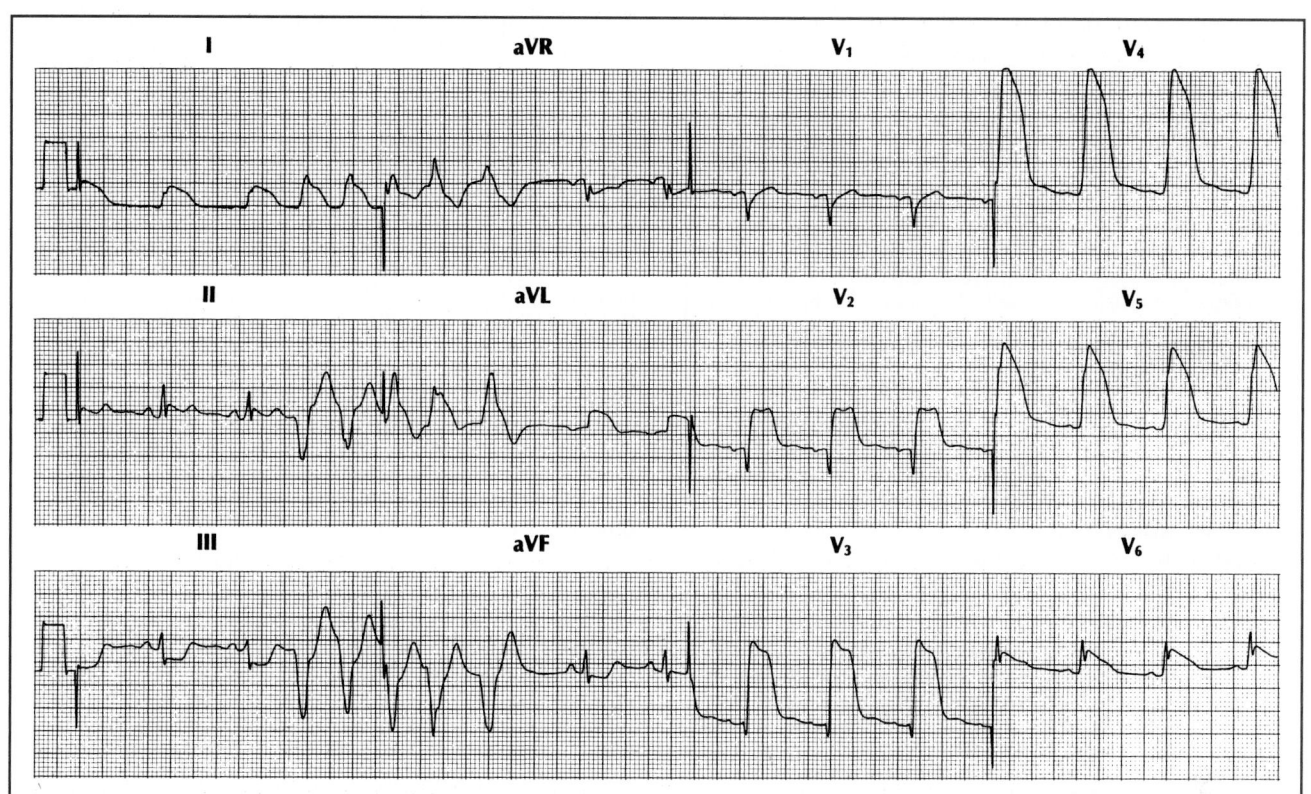

FIGURE 37–19. This 12-lead ECG was obtained from a middle-aged man admitted with an extensive anterior AMI. (Note pathological Q waves in the precordial leads and marked repolarization abnormalities in the anterior and lateral leads.) A five-beat salvo of nonsustained ventricular tachycardia is seen extending over the transition between leads III and aV$_f$. (From Antman, E. M., and Rutherford, J. D.: Coronary Care Medicine. Boston, Martinus Nijhoff Publishing, 1986, p. 81.)

in AMI patients who do not present with ST-segment elevation[10,394,395] (Fig. 37–18). Management of the AMI patient without ST-segment elevation is an important problem[396] because about 40 to 50 per cent of patients with AMI are not considered candidates for thrombolysis on the basis of an initial ECG that does not show ST-segment eleva-

tion.[397,398] Some patients without ST-segment elevation on the initial ECG may subsequently experience a worsening of ischemic discomfort, develop ST-segment elevation (presumably when a subtotal occlusion of the culprit coronary artery progresses to total occlusion), and become candidates for reperfusion therapy (Table 37–3). Therefore, pa-

FIGURE 37–20. Recommendations for management of patients with an acute Q-wave MI. All patients suspected of having a Q-wave MI (i.e., ST-segment elevation on electrocardiogram [ECG]) should receive aspirin (ASA), beta blockers (in the absence of contraindications), and an antithrombin (particularly if tissue-type plasminogen activator [t-PA] is used for thrombolytic therapy). Whether heparin is required in patients receiving streptokinase (SK) remains a matter of controversy; the small additional risk for intracranial hemorrhage may not be offset by the survival benefit afforded by adding heparin to SK therapy. Patients treated within 12 hours who are eligible for thrombolytics should expeditiously receive either front-loaded t-PA or SK or be considered for primary percutaneous transluminal coronary angioplasty (PTCA). Primary PTCA is also to be considered when lytic therapy is contraindicated. Individuals treated after 12 hours should receive the initial medical therapy noted above and, on an individual basis, may be candidates for angiotensin-converting enzyme (ACE) inhibitors (particularly if left ventricular function is impaired). Further information is required to place the role of magnesium in proper perspective. After discharge, all pa-

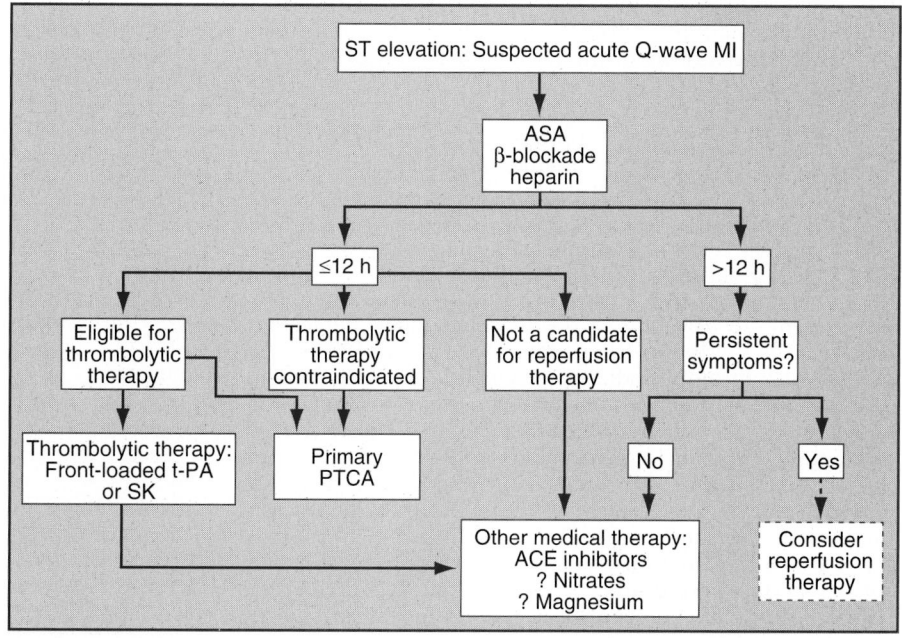

tients should receive aspirin and a beta blocker (in the absence of contraindications). Dietary modifications and, if needed, treatment to reduce LDL-cholesterol and elevate HDL-cholesterol are strongly encouraged, as is life style modification (including regular physical exercise and cessation of cigarette smoking). (Modified from Antman, E. M.: Medical therapy for acute coronary syndromes: An overview. *In* Califf, R. M. [ed.]: Acute Myocardial Infarction and Other Acute Ischemic Syndromes, vol. 8. Braunwald, E. (ed.): Atlas of Heart Diseases. Philadelphia, Current Science, 1996 [pp. 10–10.25].)

TABLE 37–3 CRITERIA FOR THROMBOLYSIS IN ACUTE MYOCARDIAL INFARCTION

Indications
1. Chest pain consistent with AMI
2. Electrocardiographic changes
   ST-segment elevation >0.1 mV in at least two contiguous leads
   New or presumably new left bundle branch block
3. Time from onset of symptoms
   < 6 hours: most beneficial
   6–12 hours: lesser but still important benefits
   >12 hours: diminishing benefits but may still be useful in selected patients

Absolute Contraindications
1. Active internal bleeding (excluding menses)
2. Suspected aortic dissection
3. Recent head trauma or known intracranial neoplasm
4. History of cerebrovascular accident known to be hemorrhagic
5. Major surgery or trauma < 2 wks

Relative Contraindications*
1. Blood pressure >180/110 mm Hg on at least two readings
2. History of chronic, severe hypertension with or without drug therapy
3. Active peptic ulcer
4. History of cerebrovascular accident
5. Known bleeding diathesis or current use of anticoagulants
6. Prolonged or traumatic cardiopulmonary resuscitation
7. Diabetic hemorrhagic retinopathy or other hemorrhagic ophthalmic condition
8. Pregnancy
9. Prior exposure to streptokinase or APSAC (This contraindication is particularly important in the initial 6- to 9-month period after streptokinase or APSAC administration and applies to reuse of any streptokinase-containing agent but does not apply to t-PA or urokinase.)

* These should be considered on a case-by-case analysis or risk versus benefit. In instances in which these contraindications (particularly 1 to 5) have paramount importance, such as more active peptic ulcer with history of bleeding, they become absolute contraindications when weighed against a less than life-threatening, evolving AMI.

Adapted from AHA Medical/Scientific Statement Special Report (1990): ACC/AHA guidelines for the early management of patients with acute myocardial infarction. Circulation 82:707; Anderson, H. V., and Willerson, J. T.: Thrombolyis in acute myocardial infarction. N. Engl. J. Med. 329:703, 1993. Copyright 1993 Massachusetts Medical Society.

tients whose ECG is highly suggestive of myocardial ischemia should be admitted to a hospital unit with facilities for continuous monitoring of the ECG (either the CCU or intermediate care unit) that will alert the staff if arrhythmias or ST elevation occurs. Arrangements should be made for 12-lead ECGs to be obtained approximately every 8 hours for the first 24 hours, or more frequently if ischemic discomfort recurs.

Patients with a history suggestive of AMI (see p. 1198) and an initial nondiagnostic ECG (i.e., no obvious ST-segment deviation or T-wave inversion) should have serial tracings obtained while being evaluated in the emergency department for AMI (Fig. 37–18). Emergency department staff may be alerted to the sudden development of ST segment elevation by periodic visual inspection of the bedside ECG monitor, by continuous ST-segment recording, or by auditory alarms when the ST-segment deviation exceeds programmed limits. Decision aids such as computer-based diagnostic algorithms,[399,399a] identification of high-risk clinical indicators,[400] rapid determination of cardiac serum markers,[260] two-dimensional echocardiographic screening for regional wall motion abnormalities,[343,344,401,402] and myocardial perfusion imaging[403] are of greatest clinical utility when the ECG is nondiagnostic. In an effort to improve the cost effectiveness of care of patients with a chest pain syndrome, nondiagnostic ECG, and low suspicion of AMI but in whom the diagnosis has not been entirely excluded, many medical centers have developed critical pathways[404,405] that involve a coronary observation unit with a goal of ruling out AMI in less than 12 hours[392,406,407] (Fig. 37–18).

General Treatment Measures

ASPIRIN. This agent is effective across the entire spectrum of acute coronary syndromes (Figs. 37–5 and 37–7) and now forms part of the initial management strategy of patients with suspected AMI (Fig. 37–18). The pharmacology of aspirin is presented on page 1819. The goal of aspirin treatment is to quickly block formation of thromboxane A_2 in platelets by cyclo-oxygenase inhibition.[408,409] Because low doses (40 to 80 mg) take several days to achieve full antiplatelet effect,[410] at least 160 to 325 mg should be administered acutely in the emergency department.[411] In order to achieve therapeutic blood levels rapidly, the patient should chew the tablet, thus promoting buccal absorption rather than absorption through the gastric mucosa.

Control of Cardiac Pain

Analgesia is an important element of management of AMI patients in the emergency department. Often there is a tendency to underdose the patient for fear of obscuring response to anti-ischemic or reperfusion therapy. This should be avoided because pain contributes to the heightened sympathetic activity that is particularly prominent during the early phase of AMI. Control of cardiac pain is typically accomplished with a combination of nitrates, analgesics (e.g., morphine), oxygen, and beta-adrenoceptor blockers. Similar pharmacological principles apply in the coronary care unit, where many of the therapies discussed below are continued after initial dosing in the emergency department.[412] Because the pain associated with MI is related to ongoing ischemia (see p. 1198), many interventions that act to improve the oxygen supply-demand relationship (by either increasing supply or decreasing demand) may lessen the pain associated with AMI.

ANALGESICS. Although a wide variety of analgesic agents has been used to treat the pain associated with AMI, including meperidine, pentazocine, and morphine, the latter remains the drug of choice, except in patients with well-documented morphine hypersensitivity. Four to 8 mg should be administered intravenously and doses of 2 to

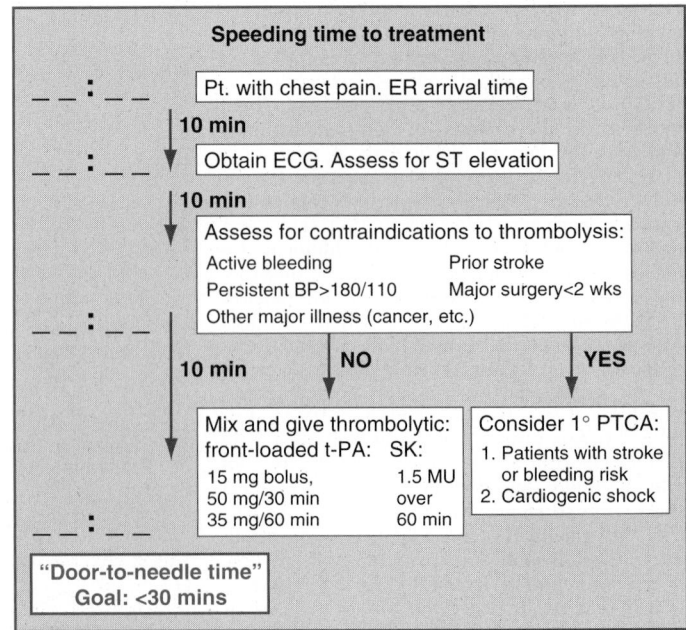

FIGURE 37–21. Algorithm for rapid triage of patients in the emergency room (ER) to provide thrombolysis with the shortest possible "door-to-needle" time. (From Cannon, C. P., Antman, E. M., Walls, R., and Braunwald, E.: Time as an adjunctive agent to thrombolytic therapy. J. Thromb. Thrombolysis 1:31, 1994.)

8 mg repeated at intervals of 5 to 15 minutes until the pain is relieved or evident toxicity—i.e., hypotension, depression of respiration, or severe vomiting—precludes further administration of the drug. In some patients, remarkably large cumulative doses of morphine (2 to 3 mg/kg) may be required and are usually tolerated.[30]

The reduction of anxiety resulting from morphine diminishes the patient's restlessness and the activity of the autonomic nervous system, with a consequent reduction of the heart's metabolic demands. The beneficial effect of morphine in patients with pulmonary edema is unequivocal and may relate to several factors, including peripheral arterial and venous dilatation (particularly among patients with excessive sympathoadrenal activity), reduction of the work of breathing, and slowing of heart rate secondary to combined withdrawal of sympathetic tone and augmentation of vagal tone.[30]

Hypotension following the administration of nitroglycerin (Fig. 37-22) and morphine can be minimized by maintaining the patient in a supine position and elevating the lower extremities if systolic arterial pressure declines below 100 mm Hg. Obviously, such positioning is undesirable in the presence of pulmonary edema, but morphine rarely produces hypotension under these circumstances. The concomitant administration of atropine in doses of 0.5 to 1.5 mg intravenously may be helpful in reducing the excessive vagomimetic effects of morphine, particularly when hypotension and bradycardia are present before it is administered. Respiratory depression is an unusual complication of morphine in the presence of severe pain or pulmonary edema, but as the patient's cardiovascular status improves, impairment of ventilation may supervene and should be watched for. It can be treated with naloxone, in doses of 0.1 to 0.2 mg intravenously initially, repeated after 15 minutes if necessary. Nausea and vomiting may be troublesome side effects of large doses of morphine and may be treated with a phenothiazine.

Other analgesics such as meperidine are less effective than is morphine but are equally likely to produce side effects and are prone to augment ventricular rate. Preliminary reports of treatment of AMI patients with the synthetic and semisynthetic narcotics fentanyl and sufentanil, patient controlled analgesia, and thoracic epidural anesthesia are encouraging, but the experience is too limited to recommend the use of these agents and modalities in routine practice.[413]

NITRATES. By virtue of their ability to enhance coronary blood flow by coronary vasodilation and to decrease ventricular preload by increasing venous capacitance, sublingual nitrates are indicated for most patients with an acute

coronary syndrome. At present, the only groups of patients with AMI in whom sublingual nitroglycerin should *not* be given are those with inferior MI and suspected right ventricular infarction[105] or marked hypotension (systolic pressure < 90 mm Hg), especially if accompanied by bradycardia.

Once it is ascertained that hypotension is not present, a sublingual nitroglycerin tablet should be administered and the patient observed carefully for improvement in symptoms or change in hemodynamics. If an initial dose is well tolerated and appears to be of benefit, further nitrates should be administered, with careful monitoring of the vital signs. Even small doses may produce sudden hypotension and bradycardia, a reaction that can be life-threatening but can usually be easily reversed with intravenous atropine if it is recognized quickly (Fig. 37-22). Long-acting oral nitrate preparations should be avoided in the very early course of AMI because of the frequently changing hemodynamic status of the patient. In patients with a prolonged period of waxing and waning chest pain, intravenous nitroglycerin may be of benefit in controlling symptoms and correcting ischemia, but frequent monitoring of blood pressure is required.[30]

BETA-ADRENOCEPTOR BLOCKERS. These drugs have been used in the early hours of AMI in attempts to limit the size of the infarct (see p. 1212). In the course of these studies, it has been recognized that beta blockers relieve pain and reduce the need for analgesics in many patients, presumably by reducing ischemia.[414] Patients most suited for the use of beta blockers early in the course of AMI are those who also have sinus tachycardia and hypertension because beta blockers lower both the heart rate and arterial blood pressure, thereby lowering myocardial oxygen demand. A popular and relatively safe protocol for the use of a beta blocker in this situation is as follows: (1) Patients with heart failure (rales > 10 cm up from diaphragm), hypotension (BP < 90 mm Hg), bradycardia (heart rate < 60 bpm), or heart block (PR > 0.24 sec) are first excluded.[415] (2) Metoprolol is given in three 5-mg boluses. (3) Patients are observed for 2 to 5 minutes after each bolus, and if heart rate falls below 60 beats/min or systolic blood pressure falls below 100 mm Hg, no further drug is given; a total of three intravenous doses (15 mg) is administered. (4) If hemodynamic stability continues, 15 minutes after the last intravenous dose, the patient is begun on oral metoprolol, 50 mg every 6 hours for 2 days, then switched to 100 mg twice daily. An infusion of an extremely short-acting beta blocker, esmolol (50 to 250 $\mu g/kg/min$), may be useful in patients with relative contraindications to beta blockade in whom heart rate slowing is considered highly desirable.[416]

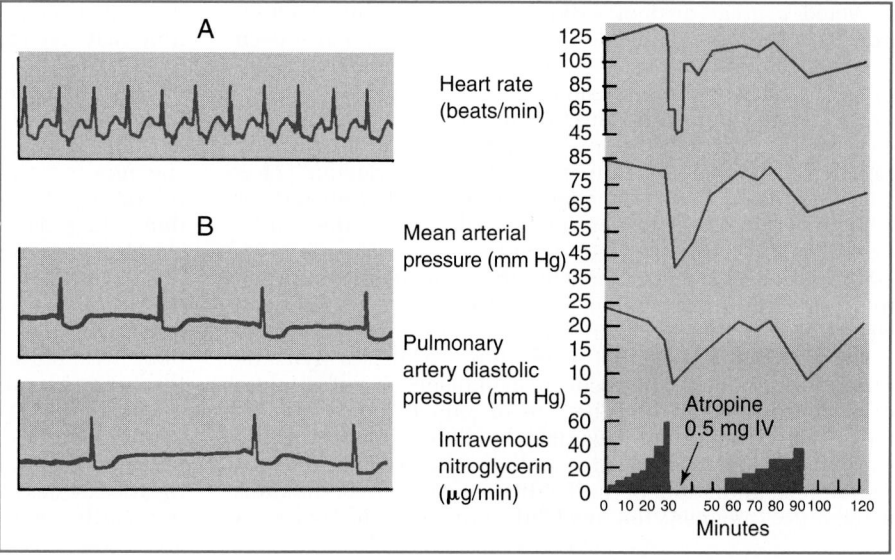

FIGURE 37-22. Sinus bradycardia and hypotension provoked by intravenous nitroglycerin in a patient with AMI. Intravenous nitroglycerin at a dose of 20 to 40 $\mu g/min$ in a patient with anteroseptal AMI and sinus tachycardia (A) provoked profound sinus bradycardia (B) and hypotension. This was quickly reversed with intravenous atropine, 0.5 mg, but recurred after reinstitution of intravenous nitroglycerin. (From Come, P. C., and Pitt, B.: Nitroglycerin-induced severe hypotension and bradycardia in patients with acute myocardial infarction. Circulation 54:624, 1976. Copyright 1976 American Heart Association.)

Unlike beta blockers, calcium antagonists are of little if any acute value in AMI and may, in fact, be hazardous.[414,417,418]

OXYGEN. Hypoxemia may occur in patients with AMI and is usually secondary to ventilation-perfusion abnormalities that are sequelae of left ventricular failure; pneumonia and intrinsic pulmonary disease are additional causes of hypoxemia. It is common practice to treat all patients hospitalized with AMI with oxygen for at least 24 to 48 hours, based on the empirical assumption of hypoxia and evidence that increased oxygen in the inspired air may protect ischemic myocardium.[419,420] However, this practice may not be cost effective. Augmentation of the fraction of oxygen in the inspired air does not elevate oxygen delivery significantly in patients who are not hypoxemic. Furthermore, it may increase systemic vascular resistance and arterial pressure and thereby lower cardiac output slightly.

In view of these considerations, arterial oxygen saturation may be estimated by pulse oximetry (an increasingly available technology), and oxygen therapy may be omitted if it is normal. On the other hand, oxygen should be administered to patients with AMI when arterial hypoxemia is clinically evident or can be documented by measurement. In these patients, serial arterial blood gas measurements may be employed to follow the efficacy of oxygen therapy. Although patients with AMI may exhibit a reduction in precordial ST-segment elevation during 100 per cent oxygen breathing, no long-term effect on survival or on the development of complications has been documented.[420]

In general, the delivery of 2 to 4 liters/min of 100 per cent oxygen by mask or nasal prongs for 6 to 12 hours is satisfactory for most patients with mild hypoxemia. If arterial oxygenation is still depressed on this regimen, the flow rate may have to be increased, and other causes for hypoxemia should be sought. In patients with pulmonary edema, endotracheal intubation and positive-pressure controlled ventilation may be necessary.

Limitation of Infarct Size

Infarct size is an important determinant of prognosis in patients with AMI.[421] Patients who succumb from cardiogenic shock generally exhibit either a single massive infarct or a small to moderate-sized infarct superimposed on multiple prior infarctions.[422,423] Survivors with large infarcts frequently exhibit late impairment of ventricular function,[356,424] and the long-term mortality rate is higher than for survivors with small infarcts, who tend not to develop cardiac decompensation.[84,171,425]

In view of the prognostic importance of infarct size, the concept that modification of infarct size is possible has attracted a great deal of experimental and clinical attention.[426] Efforts to limit the size of the infarct have been divided among three different (sometimes overlapping) approaches: (1) early reperfusion,[421,427] (2) reduction of myocardial energy demands, and (3) manipulation of sources of energy production in the myocardium.[193,428] Although early reperfusion ("time-dependent effect of reperfusion") has been the major focus of modern management strategies for AMI, it is important to note that in addition to the limitation of infarct size, even late reperfusion of ischemic myocardium conveys several benefits that contribute to mortality reduction ("time-independent effect of reperfusion,") (see p. 1213)[162,421,429] (Fig. 37-16).

THE DYNAMIC NATURE OF INFARCTION. AMI is a dynamic process that does not occur instantaneously but evolves over hours (Fig. 37-9). The fate of jeopardized, ischemic tissue may be affected favorably by interventions that restore perfusion, reduce myocardial oxygen requirements, inhibit accumulation of or facilitate wash-out of noxious metabolites, augment the availability of substrate for anaer-

obic metabolism,[192,193,421,430-433] or blunt the effects of mediators of injury (such as calcium overload or oxygen free radicals)[192,193,433-439] that compromise the structure and function of intracellular organelles and constituents of cell membranes. Strong evidence in experimental animals and suggestive evidence in patients indicate that ischemic preconditioning (see p. 1214) prior to sustained coronary occlusion decreases infarct size and is associated with a more favorable outcome, with decreased risk of extension of infarction and recurrent ischemic events.[440-444] Brief episodes of ischemia in one coronary vascular bed may precondition myocardium in a remote zone, attenuating the size of infarction in the latter when sustained coronary occlusion occurs.[441]

The perfusion of the myocardium in the infarct zone appears to be reduced maximally immediately following coronary occlusion. Up to one-third of patients may develop spontaneous recanalization of an occluded infarct-related artery beginning at 12 to 24 hours. This delayed spontaneous reperfusion has been associated with improvement of left ventricular function because it improves healing of infarcted tissue, prevents ventricular remodeling, and reperfuses hibernating myocardium. However, in order to *maximize* the amount of salvaged myocardium by *accelerating* the process of reperfusion and also implementing it in those patients who would otherwise have an occluded infarct-related artery, the strategies of pharmacologically induced thrombolysis and primary PTCA of the infarct vessel have been developed (see pp. 1215 and 1221).

Additional factors that may contribute to limitation of infarct size in association with reperfusion include relief of coronary spasm, improved systemic hemodynamics (augmentation of coronary perfusion pressure and reduced left ventricular end-diastolic pressure), and development of collateral circulation.[432] The prompt implementation of measures designed to protect ischemic myocardium and support myocardial perfusion may provide sufficient time for the development of anatomical and physiological compensatory mechanisms that limit the ultimate extent of infarction (Figs. 37-18 and 37-21).

AMI in hospitalized patients may be complicated by extension of infarction or early reinfarction (Fig. 37-23). Depending on the criteria utilized for detection, the incidence of these complications ranges from 8 to 30 per cent.[173] It is possible that interventions designed to protect ischemic myocardium during the initial event may also reduce the incidence of extension of infarction or early reinfarction.

ROUTINE MEASURES FOR INFARCT SIZE LIMITATION. Whereas reperfusion of ischemic myocardium is the most important technique for limiting infarct size, several routine measures to accomplish this goal are applicable to all patients with AMI, whether or not a reperfusion therapy is prescribed. The treatment strategies discussed in this section may be initiated in the emergency department (Fig. 37-18) and then continued in the coronary care unit.

It is important to maintain an optimal balance between myocardial oxygen supply and demand so that as much as possible of the jeopardized zone of the myocardium surrounding the most profoundly ischemic zones of the infarct can be salvaged. During the period before irreversible injury has occurred, myocardial oxygen consumption should be minimized by maintaining the patient at rest, physically and emotionally, and by utilizing mild sedation and a quiet atmosphere that may lower heart rate, a major determinant of myocardial oxygen consumption. If the patient was receiving a beta-adrenoceptor blocking agent at the time the clinical manifestations of the infarction commenced, the drug should be continued unless a specific contraindication develops, such as left ventricular systolic failure or bradyarrhythmia. Marked sinus bradycardia (heart rate less than approximately 50 beats/min) and the frequently coexisting hypotension should be treated with

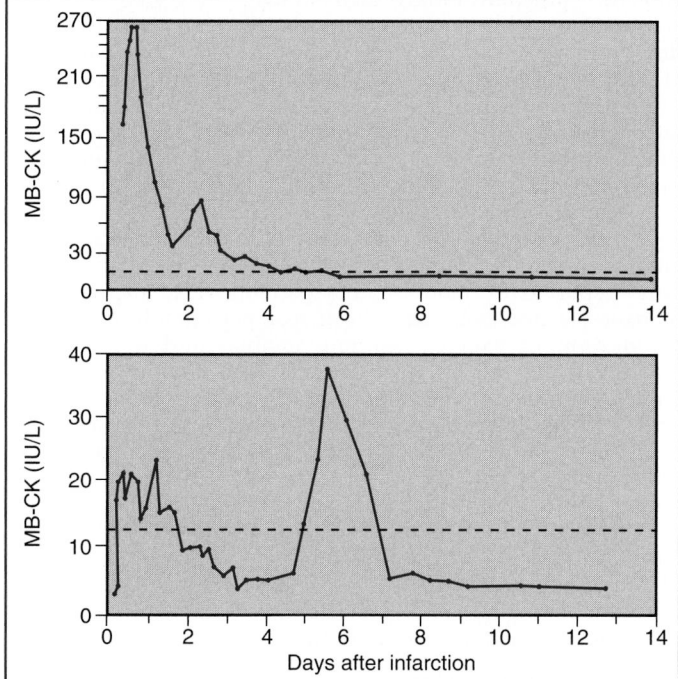

FIGURE 37-23. MB creatine kinase (MB-CK) time-activity curves for a patient in whom myocardial extension developed prior to return of plasma MB-CK to baseline (top) and a patient in whom extension occurred after return of MB-CK to baseline (bottom). (From Muller, J. E., Rude, R. E., Braunwald, E., et al.: Myocardial infarct extension: Occurrence, outcome, and risk factors in the MILIS. Ann. Intern. Med. **108**:1, 1988.)

postural maneuvers (the Trendelenburg position) to increase central blood volume and atropine and electrical pacing, but not with isoproterenol. On the other hand, the routine administration of atropine, with the resultant increase in heart rate, to patients without serious bradycardia is contraindicated. All forms of tachyarrhythmias require prompt treatment because they increase myocardial oxygen needs.

Congestive heart failure should be treated promptly. Given their multiple beneficial actions in AMI patients, ACE inhibitors are the first line of drugs indicated in the treatment of congestive heart failure associated with AMI unless the patient is hypotensive (see p. 495). Drugs such as isoproterenol that increase myocardial oxygen consumption should be avoided.

As discussed above, arterial oxygenation should be restored to normal in patients with hypoxemia, such as occurs in patients with chronic pulmonary disease, pneumonia, or left ventricular failure. Oxygen-enriched air should be administered to patients with hypoxemia, and bronchodilators and expectorants should be used when indicated. Severe anemia, which can also extend the area of ischemic injury, should be corrected by the cautious administration of packed red cells, accompanied by a diuretic if there is any evidence of left ventricular failure. Associated conditions, particularly infections and the accompanying tachycardia, fever, and elevated myocardial oxygen needs, require immediate attention.

Systolic arterial pressure should not be allowed to deviate by more than approximately 25 to 30 mm Hg from the patient's usual level unless marked hypertension had been present before the AMI. It is likely that each patient has an optimal range of arterial pressure; as coronary perfusion pressure deviates from this level, the unfavorable balance between oxygen supply (which is related to coronary perfusion pressure) and myocardial oxygen demand (which is related to ventricular wall tension) that ensues increases the extent of ischemic injury.

GENERAL CONCEPTS. Although reperfusion occurs spontaneously in some patients, persistent thrombotic occlusion is present in the majority of patients with AMI while the myocardium is undergoing necrosis.[100] Timely reperfusion of jeopardized myocardium represents the most effective way of restoring the balance between myocardial oxygen supply and demand. The extent of protection appears to be related directly to the rapidity with which reperfusion is implemented after the onset of coronary occlusion[382,427,445-449] (Fig. 37-9). Preliminary data exist suggesting that following thrombolytic therapy more rapid reperfusion (and smaller infarcts) occurs in patients with AMI preceded by unstable angina compared with those without preinfarction angina.[449a]

In some patients, particularly those with cardiogenic shock, tissue damage occurs in a "stuttering" manner rather than abruptly, a condition that might more properly be termed subacute infarction. This concept of the nature of the infarction process, as well as the observation that the incidence of complications of AMI in both the early and late postinfarction periods is a function of infarct size,[450] underscores the need for careful history-taking to ascertain whether the patient appears to have had repetitive cycles of spontaneous reperfusion and reocclusion. "Fixing" the time of onset of the infarction process in such patients can be difficult. In such patients with waxing and waning ischemic discomfort, a rigid time interval from the first episode of pain should not be used when determining whether a patient is "outside the window" for benefit from acute reperfusion therapy.

PATHOPHYSIOLOGY OF MYOCARDIAL REPERFUSION. Prevention of cell death by the restoration of blood flow depends on the severity and duration of pre-existing ischemia. Substantial experimental and clinical evidence exists indicating that recovery of left ventricular systolic function, improvement in diastolic function, and reduction in overall mortality are more favorably influenced, the earlier that blood flow is restored[10,421,427] (Fig. 37-16). Collateral coronary vessels also appear to play a role in the successful left ventricular function following reperfusion.[432,451] They provide sufficient perfusion of myocardium to retard cell death and are probably of greater importance in patients having reperfusion later rather than 1 to 2 hours after coronary occlusion.

Reperfusion Injury
(See p. 1179)

The process of reperfusion, although beneficial in terms of myocardial salvage, may come at a cost due to a process known as *reperfusion injury*[452,453] (Fig. 37-11) (see also Fig. 36-25, p. 1178). Kloner has summarized the data on the four types of reperfusion injury that have been observed in experimental animals.[454] These consist of (1) lethal reperfusion injury—a term referring to reperfusion-induced death of cells that were still viable at the time of restoration of coronary blood flow, (2) vascular reperfusion injury—progressive damage to the microvasculature such that there is an expanding area of no reflow and loss of coronary vasodilatory reserve,[455] (3) stunned myocardium—salvaged myocytes display a prolonged period of contractile dysfunction following restoration of blood flow owing to abnormalities of intracellular biochemistry leading to reduced energy production[88,436] (see pp. 388 and 1176) (Fig. 37-11), and (4) reperfusion arrhythmias—bursts of ventricular tachycardia and on occasion ventricular fibrillation that occur within seconds of reperfusion.[237] The available evidence suggests that vascular reperfusion injury, stunning, and reperfusion arrhythmias can all occur in patients with AMI. The concept of lethal reperfusion injury of potentially salvageable myocardium remains controversial, both in experimental animals and in patients.[81,454,456-459]

Reperfusion does increase the cell swelling that occurs with ischemia.[460,461] Reperfusion of the myocardium in which the microvasculature is damaged leads to the creation of a hemorrhagic infarct[462] (Fig. 37–11). Thrombolytic therapy appears more likely to produce hemorrhagic infarction than reperfusion by mechanical means. Although concern has been raised that this hemorrhage may lead to extension of the infarct, this does not appear to be the case.[463] Histological study of patients not surviving in spite of successful reperfusion has revealed hemorrhagic infarcts, but this hemorrhage usually does not extend beyond the area of necrosis.[96,464]

The loss of magnesium with ischemia, followed during reperfusion by the sudden exposure of severely ischemic cells to both calcium and oxygen upon restoration of flow, has been observed to affect the severity of ischemic damage in several animal species.[435-437,440,465,466] Toxicity from oxygen-derived free radicals mediated at least in part by stimulated leukocytes has attracted considerable attention for its possible role in extending myocardial injury and contributing to calcium overload and inability to regulate cell volume.[467,468] Observations in reperfused patients with AMI indicate that cardiac inflammatory responses are mediated by the cytokines IL-8 and IL-6, opening new options for reducing reperfusion injury by developing pharmacological interventions specifically targeted against specific cytokines.[469] Experimental models of AMI have revealed a consistent message—interventions that attenuate reperfusion injury exert their maximal beneficial effect if blood levels (and presumably myocardial tissue concentrations) are elevated at the time reperfusion occurs.[457-459,468,470,471] The effectiveness of agents such as superoxide dismutase and magnesium rapidly declines the later they are administered after reperfusion; eventually no beneficial effect is detectable in animal models after 45 to 60 minutes of reperfusion has elapsed.[459] This concept is strengthened further by investigations with novel agents such as liposomal PGE_1[472] and inhibitors of Na^+-H^+ exchange[473] that substantially reduce the amount of myocardial injury that occurs with reperfusion when they are administered prior to restoration of coronary blood flow. Drugs such as beta-adrenoceptor blockers, which delay the death of ischemic cells, may, if administered prophylactically to patients at high risk of occlusion (or reocclusion) or in the earliest phases of the development of an AMI, enhance the quantity of myocardium salvaged by early reperfusion.[474,475]

Ischemic Preconditioning

The intriguing observation that brief periods of experimental coronary occlusion and reperfusion prior to a more sustained period of occlusion lasting less than 1.5 to 3 hours result in marked reduction in the amount of necrosis that develops has led to the concept of *ischemic preconditioning*.[440,453,476] Recent data suggest that during the period of brief coronary occlusion adenosine receptors are activated which initiate a cascade of intracellular events culminating in phosphorylation of a membrane protein that is responsible for the protective effect. The leading candidate membrane protein is the ATP-dependent potassium channel that, when activated, causes a shortening of the action potential duration, a decrease in calcium influx, a reduction in contractile force generation, and thereby an energy-sparing effect.[477] The implications of ischemic preconditioning, including a possible modification of the severity of myocardial infarction, are profound and have stimulated interest in ATP-dependent potassium channel openers such as nicorandil, bimakalim, and other "preconditioning-mimetic" agents for potential use in patients with AMI.[440,478,479]

Another potential mechanism for the acute response to

ischemic preconditioning is a slowing of glycolysis with attenuation of intracellular acidosis.[480-480b] A "second window" of preconditioning has been described by Marber et al. that appears 24 hours or more after the initial preconditioning episodes and may be mediated by molecular adaptation leading to the production of heat shock protein.[481] Preconditioning appears to be associated with a more oxidized cellular redox state, which may contribute to protection against subsequent bouts of ischemia.[482]

Clinical observations consistent with the concept of ischemic preconditioning include the "warm-up phenomenon" reported by many angina patients (i.e., angina early in exercise necessitating a brief rest period followed by a resumption of exercise without angina) and a lower in-hospital death rate in AMI patients who have a history of angina within the 48-hour period that precedes infarction.[440,442] A history of preinfarction angina in patients with a first Q-wave MI has been reported to be associated with a lower peak CK activity, lower in-hospital incidence of sustained ventricular tachycardia and fibrillation, and a lower incidence of pump failure and cardiac mortality.[444] Of interest, in patients with a first anterior Q-wave MI, a history of preinfarction angina was associated with a higher ejection fraction, smaller end-diastolic volume, and a lower incidence of aneurysm formation.[444]

Reperfusion Arrhythmias

Transient sinus bradycardia occurs in many patients with inferior infarcts at the time of acute reperfusion; it is most often accompanied by some degree of hypotension. This combination of hypotension and bradycardia with a sudden increase in coronary flow has been ascribed to the activation of the Bezold-Jarisch reflex.[483] Premature ventricular contractions, accelerated idioventricular rhythm, and nonsustained ventricular tachycardia are also seen commonly following successful reperfusion. In experimental animals with AMI, ventricular fibrillation occurs shortly after reperfusion, but this arrhythmia is not as frequent in patients as in the experimental setting. Although some investigators have postulated that early afterdepolarizations participate in the genesis of reperfusion ventricular arrhythmias, Vera et al. have shown that early afterdepolarizations are present both during ischemia and during reperfusion and are therefore unlikely to be involved in the development of reperfusion ventricular tachycardia or fibrillation.[484]

When present, rhythm disturbances may actually be a marker of successful restoration of coronary flow.[485] However, although reperfusion arrhythmias have a high sensitivity for detecting successful reperfusion, the high incidence of identical rhythm disturbances in patients without successful coronary artery reperfusion limits their specificity for detection of restoration of coronary blood flow. In general, clinical features are poor markers of reperfusion, with no single clinical finding or constellation of findings being reliably predictive of angiographically demonstrated coronary artery patency.[486]

In an overview of randomized trials in which thrombolytic therapy was compared with placebo, Solomon et al. reported *no* increase in the risk of ventricular tachycardia or ventricular fibrillation in patients receiving thrombolytic therapy.[487] Thus, although reperfusion arrhythmias may show a temporal clustering at the time of restoration of coronary blood flow in patients with successful thrombolysis, the overall incidence of such arrhythmias appears to be similar in patients not receiving a thrombolytic agent who may develop these arrhythmias as a consequence of spontaneous coronary artery reperfusion or the evolution of the infarct process itself. These considerations, as well as the fact that the brief "electrical storm" occurring at the time of reperfusion is generally innocuous, indicate that no prophylactic antiarrhythmic therapy is necessary when thrombolytics are prescribed.[237]

Late Establishment of Patency of the Infarct Vessel

It has been suggested that improved survival and ventricular function after successful reperfusion are not due entirely to limitation of infarct size[162,421,488] (Fig. 37–16). Both experimental and clinical evidence indicate that the benefits of a patent artery include a favorable effect on ventricular remodeling (improved healing of infarcted tissue and prevention of infarct expansion),[83,171,425,489,489a] enhancement of collateral flow,[490] improvement in diastolic and systolic function,[491–495] increased electrical stability,[496–498] and reduced long-term mortality.[499,500] Late reperfusion of the artery perfusing an infarction provides a vascular scaffolding in the infarct zone[501] and increases the influx of inflammatory cells that participate in the formation of a mature fibrous scar.[502] The vascular scaffold and firmer myocardial scar prevent infarct segment lengthening and decrease the tendency to infarct expansion and aneurysm formation.[488] Poorly contracting or noncontracting myocardium in a zone that is supplied by a stenosed infarct-related artery with slow antegrade perfusion may still contain viable myocytes. This situation is referred to as *hibernating* myocardium[453] (see p. 1176), and its function can be improved by percutaneous transluminal coronary angioplasty (PTCA) to augment flow in the infarct-related artery.[503] Late reperfusion of the infarct-related artery by thrombolysis or late restoration of flow via PTCA[504] enhances the electrical stability of the infarcted zone and is probably related to the reduced incidence of ventricular fibrillation and automatic firing of implantable cardioverter-defibrillator devices.[505,506] The beneficial effect of late (within 16 days) reperfusion of the infarct-related artery is independent of left ventricular function and other mortality-reducing therapies such as ACE inhibitors[499] (see p. 1229).

Summary of Effects of Myocardial Reperfusion

As illustrated in Figure 37–16, rupture of an unstable plaque in the culprit vessel produces complete occlusion of the infarct-related coronary artery. AMI occurs with the ensuing development of left ventricular dilatation and ultimate death through a combination of pump failure and electrical instability. Early reperfusion (i.e., thrombolysis, primary PTCA) shortens the duration of coronary occlusion, minimizes the degree of ultimate left ventricular dysfunction and dilatation, and reduces the probability that the AMI patient will develop pump failure or malignant ventricular tachyarrhythmias. Late reperfusion (after approximately 4 to 6 hours have elapsed since the onset of coronary artery occlusion) appears to affect favorably the process of infarct healing and minimizes left ventricular remodeling and the ultimate development of pump dysfunction and electrical instability.

CORONARY THROMBOLYSIS

Many years elapsed between the first report of intracoronary clot lysis in an experimental animal and the widespread use of thrombolytic agents in AMI.[31,507] With publication of the first GISSI trial of over 11,000 patients in 1986,[508] in which intravenous streptokinase was shown to result in a significant reduction in mortality in patients treated within 6 hours of the onset of symptoms, the routine use of thrombolytic therapy in AMI was established. It is now clear that thrombolysis recanalizes thrombotic occlusion associated with AMI (Fig. 37–24), and restoration of coronary flow reduces infarct size and improves myocardial function and survival.[10,421]

INTRACORONARY THROMBOLYSIS. Clinical investigation in the area of pharmacological reperfusion of ischemic myocardium initially focused on the use of intracoronary thrombolysis in the early hours of AMI.[31,427,509,510] The fact that viability could be maintained in a portion of the suc-

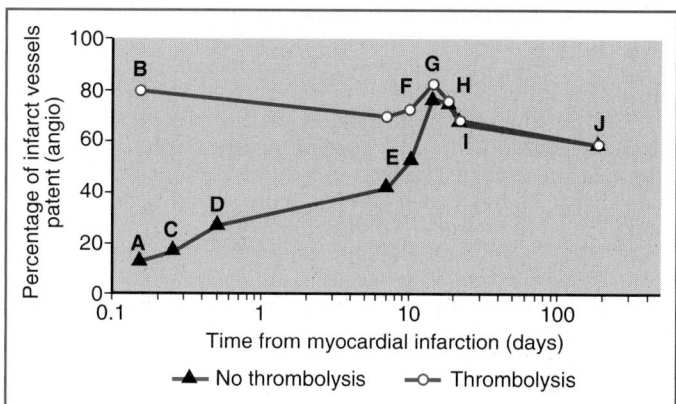

FIGURE 37–24. Comparison of angiographically documented infarct-related coronary artery patency rates in 10 separate clinical studies and time from MI as modulated by early administration of a thrombolytic agent versus nonthrombolytic (conventional) therapy. The x-axis is a semilogarithmic scale of time in days from myocardial infarction. Note that the difference in patency rates becomes diminishingly small within the first 2 to 3 weeks after infarction. (From Rumberg, J. A., and Gersh, B. J.: Coronary artery patency and left ventricular remodeling after myocardial infarction: mechanisms and mechanics. *In* Califf, R. M., Mark, D. B., and Wagner, G. S. [eds.]: Acute Coronary Care. St. Louis, Mosby-Year Book, 1995, p. 122.)

cessfully reperfused myocardium was reflected in studies showing the restoration of contractile activity.[511,512] Most reported experience with intracoronary thrombolysis has not been in randomized controlled trials, largely because it has been thought difficult to withhold thrombolytic therapy once a thrombotic coronary artery occlusion has been visualized angiographically, and it has not been considered ethical to catheterize patients if randomization to no thrombolytic therapy were possible for a portion of the patients. Because of the delay involved in catheterizing patients with AMI, current consensus is that intracoronary administration of thrombolytic therapy should be reserved for patients who develop coronary thrombosis during the course of an angiographic procedure and in whom either a coronary catheter is already in place or such placement is easily and rapidly achieved.

INTRAVENOUS THROMBOLYSIS. This form of thrombolytic therapy has several important advantages over intracoronary use. Because only the placement of a peripheral intravenous line is required, therapy may be initiated early, in a variety of locations (home, ambulance, helicopter, emergency department) and at relatively low cost. The subject of intravenous thrombolysis has perhaps been one of the most rapidly evolving areas in the management of patients with AMI, especially over the last decade.[512a]

PATENCY OF THE INFARCT-RELATED ARTERY. In the 1980's more than 20 trials were conducted that collectively enrolled over 8000 patients and established the patency rates of the infarct-related artery at 60 minutes, 90 minutes, 180 minutes, and 1 to 21 days following thrombolysis with a variety of regimens: conventional dose t-PA (alteplase), accelerated-dose t-PA, streptokinase, urokinase, anisoylated plasminogen streptokinase activator complex (APSAC) given alone or in combination (e.g., t-PA plus urokinase or streptokinase). The results of these trials have been summarized in several recent reviews.[427,513,514]

In order to provide a level of standardization for comparison of the various regimens, most investigators focus on the status of the infarct vessel at 90 minutes and describe the flow according to the TIMI grading system: Grade 0 = complete occlusion of the infarct related artery; Grade 1 = some penetration of the contrast material beyond the point of obstruction but without perfusion of the distal coronary bed; Grade 2 = perfusion of the entire infarct vessel into the distal bed but with delayed flow compared with a normal artery; Grade 3 = full perfusion of the infarct vessel with normal flow.[515,516] When evaluating reports of angiographic studies of thrombolytic agents, it must be kept in mind that only in studies in which a pretreatment coronary arteriogram documents occlusion of the culprit vessel can the term *recanalization* be applied if flow is restored. If the status of the culprit vessel is not known prior to treatment, the only fact that can be stated with certainty is the *patency rate* of the vessel at the moment contrast is injected.[513] This snapshot in time does not reflect the fluctuating status of flow in the infarct vessel that characteristically undergoes repeated cycles of patency and reocclusion, as has been documented angiographically[517] and by continuous ST-segment monitoring.[518]

Initially TIMI Grade 2 and Grade 3 flow were lumped into the favorable category of coronary patency that was compared with a combined TIMI Grade 0 and Grade 1 flow into an unfavorable category of persistent occlusion. However, TIMI Grade 2 flow should not be lumped with Grade 3 flow because it has been recognized that TIMI Grade 3 flow is far superior to Grade 2 in terms of infarct size reduction and both short-term[519] and long-term[520] mortality benefit. Therefore, TIMI Grade 3 flow should be considered to be the goal of reperfusion therapy.[521–523] However, Ito et al. have shown that even some patients with TIMI Grade 3 flow do not necessarily achieve adequate myocardial perfusion at the tissue level, as demonstrated on contrast echocardiography.[455] In an effort to provide a more quantitative statement of the briskness of coronary blood flow in the infarct artery and also to account for differences in the size and length of vessels (e.g., LAD versus RCA) and interobserver variability, Gibson and coworkers have developed the *TIMI frame count*—a simple count of the number of angiographic frames elapsed until the contrast arrives in the distal bed of the vessel of interest.[524] The TIMI frame count for patients with Grade 3 flow is in the range of 35 ± 13 frames, compared with 88 ± 31 frames for Grade 2 flow—this difference in frame counts correlates with CK release, left ventricular function, and clinical outcome.[524]

Despite the obvious mortality benefit afforded patients who rapidly achieve and maintain TIMI Grade 3 flow, the problems of "no reflow" at the myocardial level,[369] intermittent patency after successful clot lysis, and the risk of reocclusion has led Lincoff and Topol to pose the intriguing notion that there is an "illusion of reperfusion" because probably only one-quarter to one-third of patients treated with thrombolytics truly receive optimal reperfusion.[525] This has stimulated interest in development of alternative thrombolytic regimens (see p. 1220), evaluation of the benefits and risks of adjunctive therapies (see p. 1826), and evaluation of conjunctive therapies that help minimize myocardial damage (see p. 1221). Novel approaches to maintaining coronary artery patency after thrombolysis using tissue factor pathway inhibitor[526] and enhancing the concentration of nitric oxide in the coronary circulation[527] are being explored in experimental animals.

Effect on Mortality

There is no doubt that early intravenous therapy and thrombolytic drugs improve survival in patients with AMI[10,511] (Fig. 37–25). Mortality varies considerably depending on patients included for study and adjunctive therapies employed. The benefit of thrombolytic therapy appears to be greatest when agents are administered as early as possible, with the most dramatic results when the drug is given less than 1 to 2 hours after symptoms begin.[382,528] The impact of early treatment was first clearly shown in the initial GISSI trial[508] and confirmed in ISIS-2.[529] The GISSI-1 and ISIS-2 trials taken together with the ISAM[530] (streptokinase), AIMS[531] (APSAC), and ASSEST[532] (t-PA) trials are the critical elements of the port-

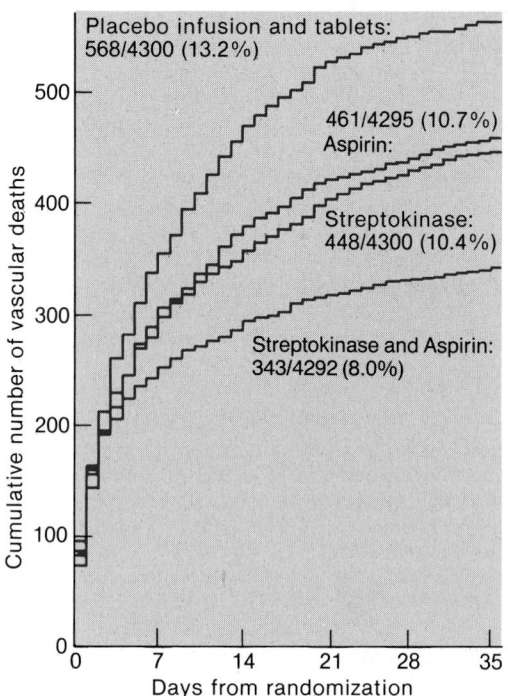

FIGURE 37–25. Cumulative vascular mortality (deaths from cardiac, cerebral, hemorrhagic, or other known vascular disease, or unknown causes) in days 0 to 35 of the Second International Study of Infarct Survival (ISIS-2). The four curves describe mortality for patients allocated (i) active streptokinase only, (ii) active aspirin only, (iii) both active treatments, and (iv) neither. Note that individually aspirin and streptokinase have a favorable effect of similar magnitudes and together the benefits appear additive. (From ISIS-2 [Second International Study of Infarct Survival] Collaborative Group: Randomized trial of intravenous streptokinase, oral aspirin, both, or neither among 17,187 cases of suspected acute myocardial infarction: ISIS-2. Lancet 2:349, 1988. © by The Lancet Ltd.)

folio of scientific evidence that thrombolytic therapy reduces mortality.[513]

The Fibrinolytic Therapy Trialists' (FTT) Collaborative Group has performed a comprehensive overview of nine trials of thrombolytic therapy, each of which enrolled more than 1000 patients[10] (Fig. 37–26). The data base for the FTT overview consisted of a total of 58,600 patients, including 6177 (10.5 per cent) who died, 564 (1.0 per cent) who sustained a stroke, and 436 (0.7 per cent) who sustained major noncerebral bleeds. A time-dependent effect[421] of thrombolytic therapy on mortality was evident in that the number of lives saved per 1000 patients treated in relation to the time from symptom onset to initiation of thrombolysis was as follows: 0 to 1 hour—35 per 1000; 2 to 3 hours—25 per 1000; 4 to 6 hours—19 per 1000; 7 to 12 hours—16 per 1000. The absolute mortality rates for the control and fibrinolytic groups stratified by presenting features are shown in Figure 37–26. The overall results indicated an 18 per cent reduction in short-term mortality, but as much as a 25 per cent reduction in mortality for the subset of 45,000 patients with ST-segment elevation or bundle branch block. There was a mortality reduction of 22 per cent in those patients with anterior ST-segment elevation and 11 per cent in those with inferior ST elevation. The patients presenting with ST-segment depression had an excess mortality of 11 per cent that serves as part of the foundaton for the observation that thrombolytic therapy does not benefit patients presenting with ST-segment depression. Two trials, LATE and EMERAS, viewed together provide evidence that a mortality reduction may still be observed in patients treated with thrombolytics between 6 and 12 hours from the onset of ischemic symptoms.[533,534] The data from LATE and EMERAS and the FTT overview form the basis for extending the "window" of treatment with thrombolytics up to 12 hours from the onset of symptoms.

The mortality effect of thrombolytic therapy in elderly patients is of considerable interest. Whereas patients greater than the age of 75 were initially excluded from randomized trials of thrombolytic therapy, they now constitute about 15 per cent of the patients studied in recent megatrials of thrombolysis.[33,535] Barriers to initiation of therapy in older patients with AMI include a protracted period of delay in seeking medical care, a lower incidence of ischemic discomfort and greater incidence of atypical symptoms and concomitant illnesses, and an increased incidence of nondiagnostic ECGs.[35,230,536,537] Younger patients with AMI achieve a slightly greater relative reduction in mortality compared with elderly patients, but the higher absolute mortality in the elderly results in similar absolute mortality reductions. Thus, as seen in Figure 37–26, there was a 26 per cent decrease in mortality in patients who were less than 55 years of age (11 lives saved per 1000 with thrombolytic therapy) and a 4 per cent reduction in

mortality in patients older than age 75 (10 lives saved per 1000 treated).

Other important baseline characteristics that impact on the mortality effect of thrombolytic therapy include the vital signs at presentation and the presence of diabetes mellitus (Fig. 37–26). For example, there was an 18 per cent decrease in mortality for patients presenting with a systolic pressure less than 100 mm Hg (62 lives saved per 1000 treated), compared with a 12 per cent reduction in mortality for patients with a systolic pressure of 175 mm Hg or more (10 lives saved per 1000 treated). Patients with a history of diabetes mellitus experienced a mortality reduction of 21 per cent (37 lives saved per 1000 treated), compared with a mortality reduction of 15 per cent (15 lives saved per 1000 treated) in patients without a history of diabetes.

A number of models have been developed to integrate the many clinical variables that affect a patient's mortality risk prior to administration of thrombolytic therapy. In the TIMI II trial, patients were classified as low risk if they *lacked* any of the following: age of 70 years or more,

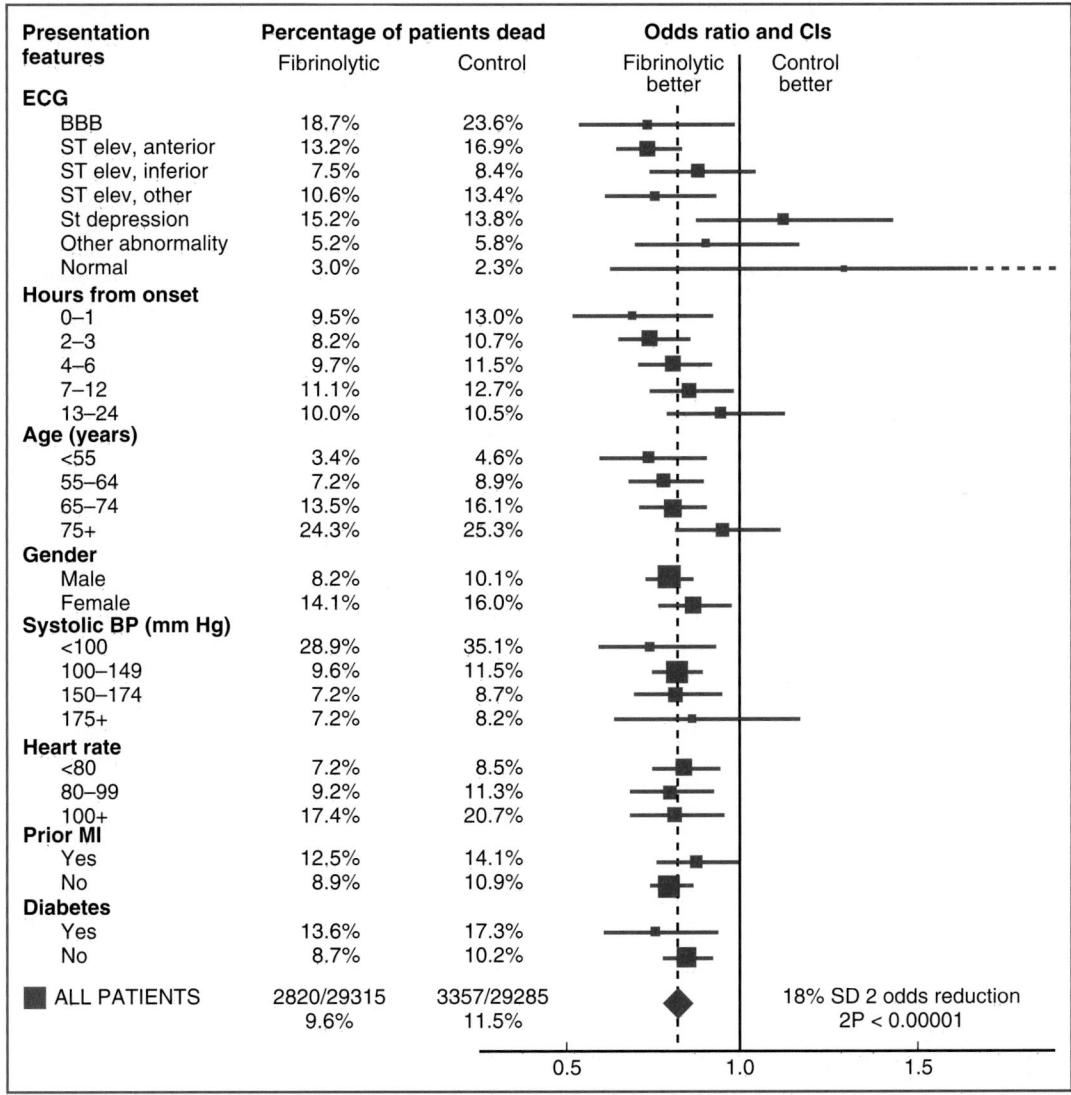

Presentation features	Percentage of patients dead		Odds ratio and CIs	
	Fibrinolytic	Control	Fibrinolytic better	Control better
ECG				
BBB	18.7%	23.6%		
ST elev, anterior	13.2%	16.9%		
ST elev, inferior	7.5%	8.4%		
ST elev, other	10.6%	13.4%		
St depression	15.2%	13.8%		
Other abnormality	5.2%	5.8%		
Normal	3.0%	2.3%		
Hours from onset				
0–1	9.5%	13.0%		
2–3	8.2%	10.7%		
4–6	9.7%	11.5%		
7–12	11.1%	12.7%		
13–24	10.0%	10.5%		
Age (years)				
<55	3.4%	4.6%		
55–64	7.2%	8.9%		
65–74	13.5%	16.1%		
75+	24.3%	25.3%		
Gender				
Male	8.2%	10.1%		
Female	14.1%	16.0%		
Systolic BP (mm Hg)				
<100	28.9%	35.1%		
100–149	9.6%	11.5%		
150–174	7.2%	8.7%		
175+	7.2%	8.2%		
Heart rate				
<80	7.2%	8.5%		
80–99	9.2%	11.3%		
100+	17.4%	20.7%		
Prior MI				
Yes	12.5%	14.1%		
No	8.9%	10.9%		
Diabetes				
Yes	13.6%	17.3%		
No	8.7%	10.2%		
■ ALL PATIENTS	2820/29315 9.6%	3357/29285 11.5%		18% SD 2 odds reduction 2P < 0.00001

0.5 1.0 1.5

FIGURE 37–26. **Mortality differences during days 0 to 35 subdivided by presentation features in a collaborative overview of results from nine trials of thrombolytic therapy. The absolute mortality rates are shown for fibrinolytic and control groups in the center portion of the figure for each of the clinical features at presentation listed on the left side of the figure. The ratio of the odds of death in the fibrinolytic group to that in the control group is shown for each subdivision (colored square), along with its 99 per cent confidence interval (horizontal line). The summary odds ratio at the bottom of the figure corresponds to an 18 per cent proportional reduction in 35-day mortality and is highly statistically significant. This translates to a reduction of 18 deaths per 1000 patients treated with thrombolytic agents.** (From Fibrinolytic Therapy Trialists' [FTT] Collaborative Group: Indications for fibrinolytic therapy in suspected acute myocardial infarction: Collaborative overview of mortality and major morbidity results from all randomized trials of more than 1000 patients. Lancet 343:311, 1994. © by The Lancet Ltd.)

TABLE 37–4 A) MORTALITY 6 WEEKS FOLLOWING THROMBOLYTIC THERAPY FOR EACH OF EIGHT RISK FACTORS IN 3261 PATIENTS*

RISK FACTOR	DEATHS BY 6 WEEKS (%)
None	1.5
Age ≥ 70 years	11.2
Previous infarction	7.9
Anterior infarction	5.6
Atrial fibrillation	10.6
Rales in more than one-third of lung fields	12.4
Hypotension and sinus tachycardia	10.1
Female gender	7.1
Diabetes mellitus	8.5

B) MORTALITY 6 WEEKS FOLLOWING THROMBOLYTIC THERAPY ACCORDING TO NUMBER OF RISK FACTORS† PRESENT INITIALLY

NO. OF RISK FACTORS	NO. OF PATIENTS	NO. OF DEATHS WITHIN 6 WEEKS	MORTALITY RATE (%)
0	864	13	1.5
1	1384	32	2.3
2	689	48	7.0
3	231	30	13.0
≥ 4	93	16	17.2

* Seventy-eight patients with cardiogenic shock or pulmonary edema were excluded.

† Possible risk factors listed in A.

Data from analysis of patients enrolled in Phase II of the Thrombolysis in Myocardial Infarction (TIMI) trial. Hillis, L. D., Foreman, S., and Braunwald, E.: Risk stratification before thrombolytic therapy in patients with acute myocardial infarction. Reprinted by permission of the American College of Cardiology. J. Am. Coll. Cardiol. 16:313, 1990.

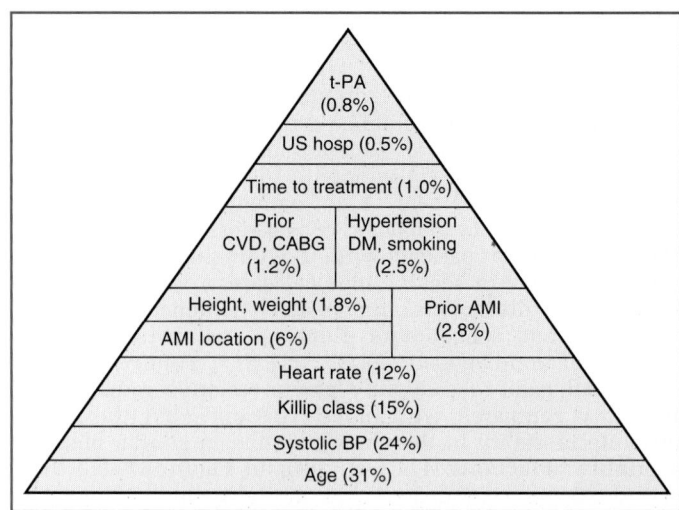

FIGURE 37–27. Influence of clinical characteristics on 30-day mortality after MI in patients treated with thrombolytic agents based on experience from the GUSTO Trial. Although considerable attention has been paid to optimizing thrombolytic regimens—indeed, the small absolute differences in mortality observed with different thrombolytic regimens are controversial—it should be emphasized that the choice of the agent is far less important than are certain clinical variables with respect to mortality. This pyramid depicts the importance of such clinical characteristics as calculated from a regression analysis in the GUSTO Trial. Numbers in parentheses represent the proportion of risk for 30-day mortality associated with the particular characteristics. AMI = acute myocardial infarction; BP = blood pressure; CABG = coronary artery bypass grating; CVD = cardiovascular disease; DM = diabetes mellitus; t-PA = tissue-type plasminogen activators; US Hosp = patients treated in a United States hospital. (Adapted from Lee, K. L., Woodlief, L. H., Topol, E. J., et al.: Predictors of 30-day mortality in the era of reperfusion for acute myocardial infarction: Results from an international trial of 41,021 patients. Circulation 91:1659, 1995. Copyright 1995 American Heart Association.)

previous infarction, atrial fibrillation, anterior infarction, rales in more than one-third of the lung fields, hypotension and sinus tachycardia, female gender, and diabetes mellitus[538] (Table 37–4). However, it should be noted that statistical modeling of mortality risk such as that cited above cannot cover all clinical scenarios and should not substitute for clinical judgment in individual cases. For example, patients with inferior MI who might otherwise be considered to have a low risk of mortality and for whom many physicians have questioned the benefits of thrombolytic therapy might be in a much higher mortality risk subgroup if their inferior infarction is associated with right ventricular infarction,[539] precordial ST-segment depression,[540] or ST-segment elevation in the lateral precordial leads.[541] The GUSTO I investigators developed a regression model to illustrate the relative importance of clinical characteristics on 30-day mortality in contemporary thrombolytic-treated patients.[542] The mortality "pyramid" shown in Figure 37–27 clearly demonstrates that much greater proportions of the risk of mortality are contributed by the systolic blood pressure and heart rate at presentation than precisely which thrombolytic agent was selected (e.g., the use of t-PA contributed less than 1 per cent to the proportional effect on mortality after adjusting for other clinical variables).

As a result of greater patency of the infarct vessel in patients treated with thrombolytic agents,[513] the clinical benefits that appear to accrue and contribute to the reduction in mortality include reductions in left ventricular failure,[543] malignant arrhythmias,[532,544] and serious complications of AMI such as septal rupture and cardiogenic shock.[530,532,544] The short-term survival benefit enjoyed by patients who receive thrombolytic therapy is maintained over the 1- to 5-year follow-up that has been reported in a number of studies.[545] However, room for improvement remains given reports of reocclusion rates of the infarct re-

lated artery as high as 10 per cent in hospital[513] and up to 30 per cent by 3 months,[546] and reinfarction rates as high as 5 per cent in hospital[513] and 7 per cent within the first year[547] in thrombolytic-treated patients.

Comparison of Thrombolytic Agents

There has been considerable controversy regarding the efficacy of various thrombolytic agents.[547a] Three megatrials comparing thrombolytic regimens have been reported. The first was GISSI-2,[548] which compared t-PA (alteplase, 100 mg over 3 hours) with streptokinase (1.5 MU over 30 to 60 minutes). All patients received oral aspirin; one-half received subcutaneous heparin. There was no difference in mortality in the group that received conventional dose t-PA (8.9 per cent) versus the group who received streptokinase (8.5 per cent). The ISIS-3 investigators reported no differences in mortality in a three-arm trial comparing streptokinase, 1.5 million units over 1 hour (10.6 per cent), t-PA (in the double-chain form as duteplase in contrast to the single-chain form as alteplase studied in GISSI-2) (10.3 per cent), and APSAC, 30 mg over 3 minutes (10.5 per cent).[535] A meta-analysis combining the GISSI-2 and ISIS-3 results summarized the information on a collective total of 48,294 patients.[535] Identical mortality rates of 10 per cent at 35 days were seen in the t-PA– and streptokinase-treated patients.

In the GUSTO I trial (Fig. 37–28), 41,021 patients were randomized into one of four treatment arms: streptokinase, 1.5 MU over 60 minutes with immediate intravenous heparin to a target APTT of 60 to 85 seconds; accelerated t-PA with immediate intravenous heparin; a combination arm of intravenous t-PA (1 mg/kg over 60 minutes) and streptokinase (1.0 MU over 60 minutes); and streptokinase, 1.5 MU over 60 minutes with subcutaneous heparin. The 30-day

FIGURE 37–28. *A* and *B*, Results of the Angiographic Substudy of the GUSTO Trial along with the 30-day mortality findings from the main study. The regimen that consisted of accelerated t-PA and intravenous (IV) heparin achieved the highest level of infarct-related artery patency (flow ≥ TIMI Grade II) by 90 minutes. Although the other regimens shown eventually "caught up" in terms of patency, it was apparently too late to provide the maximum reduction in mortality seen with the accelerated t-PA regimen. One drawback of regimens that achieve such early and sustained infarct-related patency is the associated small but definite increase in the risk for bleeding, the most serious complication being intracranial hemorrhage that results in a cerebrovascular accident (CVA). SC = subcutaneous; SK = streptokinase. (Adapted from The GUSTO Angiographic Investigators: The effects of tissue plasminogen activator, streptokinase, or both on coronary-artery patency, ventricular function, and survival after acute myocardial infarction. N. Engl. J. Med. *329:*1615, 1993; and The GUSTO Investigators: An international randomized trial comparing four thrombolytic strategies for acute myocardial infarction. N. Engl. J. Med. *329:*673, 1993. Copyright Massachusetts Medical Society.)

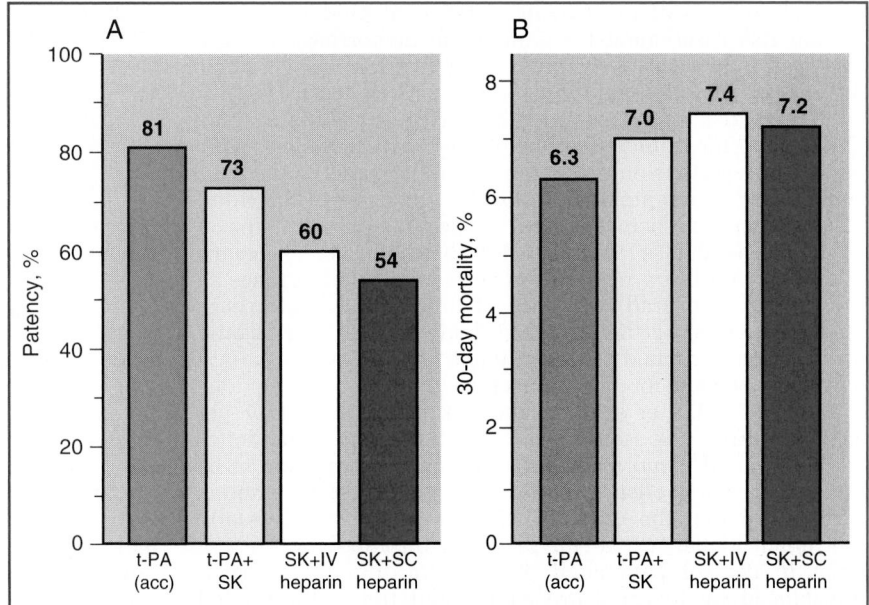

mortality for the accelerated t-PA group was 6.3 per cent, streptokinase plus subcutaneous heparin 7.2 per cent, streptokinase plus intravenous heparin 7.4 per cent, and streptokinase plus t-PA combination plus intravenous heparin 7.0 per cent (Fig. 37–28).

In the GUSTO Angiographic Substudy involving 2431 patients, those with TIMI Grade 0 or 1 flow had a 30-day mortality of 9.8 per cent that was reduced to 7.9 per cent in patients with TIMI Grade 2 flow and 4.3 per cent in those with TIMI Grade 3 flow.[519] The 90-minute patency rates for the infarct-related artery in the four treatment arms were as follows (Fig. 37–28): accelerated t-PA 81 per cent (54 per cent Grade 3 flow), combination t-PA plus streptokinase 73 per cent (38 per cent Grade 3 flow), streptokinase plus intravenous heparin 60 per cent (32 per cent Grade 3 flow), and streptokinase plus subcutaneous heparin 54 per cent (29 per cent Grade 3 flow). This early gradient in patency rates favoring t-PA was no longer apparent beyond 180 minutes, presumably because of a "catch-up" phenomenon whereby late patency rates with streptokinase approach those of front-loaded t-PA, albeit beyond a time when as much myocardial salvage is possible as with t-PA. A related observation on early arterial patency was made in the TIMI 4 trial that randomized patients with AMI presenting within 6 hours to receive either front-loaded t-PA, APSAC, or a combination of a reduced dose of both t-PA and APSAC.[549] The 90-minute patency rate for front-loaded t-PA was 84 per cent (60 per cent Grade 3), APSAC 73 per cent (43 per cent Grade 3), and the combination 68 per cent (45 per cent Grade 3). A mortality trend favoring t-PA compared with both of the other treatment regimens was seen at 1 year.[549]

EFFECT ON LEFT VENTRICULAR FUNCTION. Although precise measurements of infarct size would be an ideal endpoint for clinical reperfusion studies, such measures have been found to be impractical.[550] Attempts to use left ventricular ejection fraction as a surrogate for infarct size have not been productive because little difference is seen in ejection fraction between treatment groups that show a significant difference in mortality.[421,513] Alternative methods of assessing left ventricular function, such as end-systolic volume[551] or quantitative echocardiography,[552] are more revealing because patients with smaller volumes and better-preserved ventricular shape have an improved survival.

As with survival, improvement in global left ventricular function is related to the time of thrombolytic treatment, with greatest improvement occurring with earliest therapy.[513,553,554] Greater improvement in left ventricular func-

tion has been reported with anterior than with inferior infarcts.[421] Earlier trials failed to demonstrate any difference in global left ventricular function when streptokinase and t-PA were compared.[555,556] The angiographic substudy in GUSTO I reported detailed regional wall motion analyses stratified by thrombolytic regimen.[519] Patients who received the accelerated t-PA regimen had significantly less depression of regional wall motion in the ischemic zone, as evidenced by fewer abnormal chords when their ventricular silhouettes were subjected to segmental wall motion analysis. In addition, this patient group tended to have a slightly higher global ejection fraction and slightly reduced end-systolic volume index at 90 minutes following initiation of thrombolytic therapy. The totality of the data presented in the GUSTO angiographic substudy[519] is consistent with the hypothesis that more rapid and complete restoration of normal coronary blood flow in the infarct-related artery with t-PA was associated with an improvement in regional and global left ventricular function (presumably through greater myocardial salvage in the ischemic zone) and that this difference in function compared to that obtained with streptokinase may have contributed to the mortality differences observed at 30 days and beyond (Fig. 37–28).[372]

Complications of Thrombolytic Therapy

Recent (<1 year) exposure to streptococci or streptokinase produces some degree of antibody-mediated resistance to streptokinase (and APSAC) in most patients. Although this is of clinical consequence only rarely, it is recommended that patients not receive streptokinase for AMI if they have been treated with a streptokinase product within the last year. In the International t-PA/SK Mortality Trial, allergic reactions were seen in 1.7 per cent of patients given streptokinase. Hypotension can be expected in up to 10 per cent.[529] Bleeding complications are, of course, most common and potentially the most serious.[513,557] Most bleeding is relatively minor with all agents, with more serious episodes occurring in patients requiring invasive procedures.[558,559] Overall, 70 per cent of bleeding episodes occur at the site of vascular punctures.[558–560] Intracranial hemorrhage is the most serious complication of thrombolytic therapy[513,561–563]; its frequency varies with the clinical characteristics of the patient and the thrombolytic prescribed.[562,564]

Collaborators from the European Cooperative Society Group (ECSG) and GISSI, TAMI, TIMI, and ISAM groups pooled their respective data bases on thrombolytic-treated patients with AMI to develop a statistical model for individual risk assessment for intracranial hemorrhage using a case-control format.[564] The following four clinical variables known at hospital admission were shown to predict an increased risk of intracranial hemorrhage: age > 65 years (odds ratio for intracranial hemorrhage = 2.2), weight < 70 kg (2.1), hypertension on presentation (2.0), and use of t-PA as opposed to streptokinase (1.6). On the basis of the number of these risk factors present at the time of evaluation of a patient who is a candidate for thrombolysis, clinicians may estimate the probability of intracranial hemorrhage.[564] Assuming an overall incidence of intracranial hemorrhage of 0.75 per cent, the expected incidence of intracranial hemorrhage stratified by the number of risk factors would be 0.26 per cent for no risk factors, 0.96 per cent for one risk factor, 1.32 per cent for two risk factors, and 2.17 per cent for three risk factors.[544,565] The incremental incidence of intracranial hemorrhage with thrombolysis appears to be at least partially offset by a lower frequency of thrombotic strokes, so that the overall incidence of stroke is usually not much higher in patients receiving thrombolytic therapy than in control patients.[508,529,561] In addition to the risks introduced by invasive procedures and the features cited above, fibrinogen depletion and a prolonged activated partial thromboplastin time (aPTT) level (> 90 sec) during therapy confer an increased risk of bleeding in patients receiving thrombolytic therapy.[535,548,556,558,559]

There have been reports of an "early hazard" with thrombolytic therapy,[566,567] i.e., an excess of deaths in the first 24 hours in thrombolytic-treated patients compared with controls (especially in elderly patients treated > 12 hours).[10,568,569] However, this excess early mortality is more than offset by the deaths prevented beyond the first day, culminating in an 18 per cent (13 to 23 per cent) reduction in mortality by 35 days.[10] The mechanisms responsible for this early hazard are not clear but probably are multiple, including an increased risk of myocardial rupture[570] (particularly in the elderly),[567,571] fatal intracranial hemorrhage,[561] inadequate myocardial reperfusion resulting in pump failure and cardiogenic shock,[571,572] and possible reperfusion injury of reperfused myocardium.[454] Reports of more unusual complications such as splenic rupture,[573] aortic dissection,[574] and cholesterol embolization[575] have also appeared.

OTHER THROMBOLYTIC AGENTS

In addition to accelerated t-PA (alteplase) and streptokinase, two other thrombolytic agents—urokinase and anisoylated streptokinase plasminogen activator complex (APSAC, anistreplase)—have been approved by the United States Food and Drug Administration for the treatment of AMI. Urokinase (see p. 1821), a naturally occurring plasminogen activator, has been undergoing evaluation for treatment of AMI for at least three decades. Although it offers the potential advantage of less antigenicity than with streptokinase, infarct artery patency rates are about the same as those achieved with streptokinase.[513,514,576] Although it is prescribed in an intravenous regimen for AMI in some countries, given its high cost and lack of advantage over streptokinase, its use in the United States is almost exclusively for intracoronary infusion (6000 IU/minute to an average cumulative dose of 500,000 IU[577]) to lyse intracoronary thrombi that are believed to be responsible for an evolving AMI. APSAC, usually administered in a dose of 30 mg over 2 to 5 minutes intravenously, has a side-effect profile similar to that of streptokinase, a patency profile similar to that of conventional-dose t-PA, and a mortality benefit similar to that of streptokinase or t-PA (double-chain form, duteplase).[513,535,549,578,579] The lack of any compelling advantages (other than bolus administration) and costs higher than streptokinase have relegated APSAC to an extremely infrequently prescribed drug for AMI in the United States.

Recombinant human single-chain urokinase-type plasminogen activator (see p. 1821) (scuPA or pro-urokinase) has been produced both in nonglycosylated (e.g., saruplase) and glycosylated (e.g., Abbott-74187) forms. Pro-urokinase preparations have been studied alone[580] and in combination with urokinase[581] and t-PA.[582] Synergism has been suggested for these combinations, allowing for lower drug doses with higher clot specificity without an increase in bleeding complications. Combinations of urokinase and t-PA,[583,584] streptokinase and t-PA,[33,585] and APSAC and t-PA[579] have also been tested to take advantage of synergistic effects of multiple plasminogen activators. As yet, none of these combinations has proved clearly to be of additional benefit and none is recommended for routine use in AMI patients.

Site-directed mutagenesis has been used to produce t-PA molecules with altered pharmacokinetic and functional properties.[586] Reteplase (r-PA), a t-PA mutant that retains only the kringle-2 and protease domains and lacks glycosylated side chains, has a longer half-life than alteplase, permitting bolus administration.[587] Following encouraging results from phase 2 angiographic trials,[588,589] r-PA (two boluses of 10 MU separated by 30 minutes) was compared with streptokinase in a large phase 3 trial (INJECT).[590] The INJECT trial reported 35-day mortality rates of 9.02 per cent for r-PA and 9.53 per cent for streptokinase; at 6 months these rates were 11.0 per cent and 12.1 per cent, respectively (P = NS). Bleeding rates were similar in the two treatment arms. Given its demonstrated equivalence to streptokinase and advantage of ease of administration, r-PA may be a useful addition to the list of available thrombolytic agents; it is now being tested against accelerated t-PA in a large phase 3 mortality trial (GUSTO-3).

Another promising mutant of t-PA is TNK-tPA, which contains a new glycosylation site on kringle 1 (decreases rate of clearance), lacks another glycosylation on kringle 1 (decreases rate of clearance and increases fibrin specificity), and contains a 4-amino acid substitution in the protease domain (increases fibrin specificity and resistance to PAI-1).[591] Initial experience in patients (TIMI 10 Pilot) suggests that TNK-tPA has sufficiently slowed plasma clearance to permit single-bolus administration and greater fibrin specificity than alteplase t-PA and achieves a 90-minute patency rate that is at least comparable to that of alteplase t-PA.[592] Additional trials are under way.

Other approaches to development of new thrombolytic agents have included using recombinant DNA technology to produce staphylokinase[593] and vampire bat t-PA,[594] potent thrombolytics with fibrin specificity. It remains to be determined how immunogenic these molecules are and whether they will be useful clinically.

Recommendations for Thrombolytic Therapy

NET CLINICAL BENEFIT OF THROMBOLYSIS. Perhaps one of the most important messages from all of the available evidence is that thrombolytic therapy is underutilized in patients with AMI. Fendrick and colleagues have calculated that if every patient with AMI for whom thrombolytic therapy is recommended under current guidelines were treated with aspirin and a thrombolytic agent, more than 4000 additional lives would be saved annually in the United States.[595] Of all the currently approved regimens, accelerated t-PA is the most effective at recanalization of the infarct-related artery and restoration of normal coronary blood flow in the ischemic zone.[596] It is also the most expensive of the available treatment regimens, and this has engendered considerable discussion of the relative benefits of t-PA versus streptokinase, the intracranial hemorrhage risk difference in patients treated with t-PA versus streptokinase, and the cost effectiveness of substitution of t-PA for streptokinase in the treatment of AMI.[597-603]

Against the mortality benefits associated with administration of t-PA versus streptokinase must be weighed the excess risk of stroke that is estimated to be 2 to 3 per 1000 patients treated. When the entire cohort of patients enrolled in the GUSTO I trial was analyzed for the net clinical benefit of the various thrombolytic regimens (e.g., composite endpoint of 30 days' mortality or nonfatal stroke), a small but statistically significant benefit was still seen for the accelerated t-PA regimen (7.2 per cent) versus the streptokinase plus subcutaneous heparin regimen (7.9 per cent) and streptokinase plus intravenous heparin regimen (8.2 per cent).[33] However, this net clinical advantage of accelerated-dose t-PA regimen does not apply equally to all patients with AMI.[15,427] Patients with a higher baseline risk of mortality experience a greater mortality benefit with the accelerated t-PA regimen compared with streptokinase.[15,387] On average, the use of t-PA in place of streptokinase costs an additional $33,000 per year of life saved; t-PA is less cost effective in younger patients and more cost effective in older patients who are at higher risk of mortality.[15]

CHOICE OF AGENT. Analysis of the net clinical benefit and cost effectiveness of t-PA versus streptokinase does not easily yield recommendations for treatment because clinicians must weigh the risk of mortality and risk of intracranial hemorrhage when confronting a thrombolytic-eligible patient with AMI; additional considerations may be the constraints placed on physicians' therapeutic decision-making by the health care system in which they are practicing.[603] We are in agreement with the general recommendations by Martin and Kennedy[427] and Simoons and Arnold[604] that categorize patients into those that are at high risk of death (advanced age, female gender, depressed left ventricular function, anterior MI, bundle branch block, total magnitude of ST-segment elevation, diabetes, heart rate greater than 100 beats/min, systolic pressure less than 100 mm Hg, long delay since onset of ischemic discomfort),[427,604] and high risk of intracranial hemorrhage (age greater than 65 years). In the subgroup of patients presenting within 4 hours of symptom onset, the speed of reperfusion of the infarct vessel is of paramount importance and a high-intensity thrombolytic regimen such as accelerated t-PA is the preferred treatment, except in those individuals in whom the risk of death is low (e.g., a young patient with a small inferior MI) and the risk of intracranial hemorrhage is increased (e.g., acute hypertension), in whom streptokinase and accelerated t-PA are approximately equivalent choices. For those patients presenting between 4 and 12 hours after the onset of chest discomfort, the speed of reperfusion of the infarct vessel is of lesser importance, and therefore streptokinase and accelerated t-PA are generally equivalent options, given the difference in costs. Of note, for those patients presenting between 4 and 12 hours from symptom onset with a low mortality risk but an increased risk of intracranial hemorrhage (e.g., elderly patients with inferior MI, blood pressure greater than 100 mm Hg, and heart rate less than 100 beats/min), streptokinase is probably preferable to t-PA because of cost considerations if thrombolytic therapy is prescribed at all in such a patient.

LATE THERAPY. No mortality benefit was demonstrated in the LATE and EMERAS trials when thrombolytics were routinely administered to patients between 12 and 24 hours,[533,534] although we believe it is still reasonable to consider thrombolytic therapy in appropriately selected patients with persistent symptoms and ST elevation on ECG beyond 12 hours (Fig. 37–20). Persistent chest pain late after the onset of symptoms correlates with a higher incidence of collateral or antegrade flow in the infarct zone and is therefore a marker for patients with viable myocardium that might be salvaged.[605] Because elderly patients treated with thrombolytics more than 12 hours after the onset of symptoms are at increased risk of cardiac rupture,[567] it is our practice to restrict late thrombolytic administration to younger patients (<65 years) with ongoing ischemia, especially those with large anterior infarctions. The elderly patient with ongoing ischemic symptoms but presenting late (>12 hours) is probably better managed with direct (primary) PTCA (see below) than with thrombolytic therapy.

Before the institution of thrombolytic therapy, consideration should be given to the patient's need for intravascular catheterization, as would be required for the placement of an arterial pressure monitoring line, a pulmonary artery catheter for hemodynamic monitoring, or a temporary transvenous pacemaker. If any of these are required, ideally they should be placed as expeditiously as possible *before* infusion of the thrombolytic agent. If such procedures require an additional delay of more than 30 minutes, they should be deferred as long as possible after thrombolytic therapy is begun. In the early hours after institution of thrombolytic therapy, such catheterization should be performed only if crucial to survival, and then sites where excessive bleeding can be controlled should be chosen (e.g., subclavian vein catheterization should be avoided).

As noted above, all patients with suspected AMI should receive aspirin (160 to 325 mg) regardless of the thrombolytic agent prescribed. Aspirin should be continued indefinitely (see p.1264). The issues surrounding antithrombin therapy as an adjunct to thrombolysis are complex and are discussed in detail in a subsequent section (see p. 1224).

CORONARY ANGIOPLASTY

(See also p. 1313)

It is now established that reperfusion can be achieved by emergency PTCA.[606–610] Using a guidewire and balloon catheter, it is technically easier to cross a total occlusion consisting of a fresh thrombus than to cross a longstanding occlusion of a coronary artery. Thus, wire-guided balloon angioplasty can be useful to achieve reperfusion in two quite different circumstances[611]: (1) in lieu of thrombolytic therapy where it is referred to as *direct* or *primary angioplasty*,[612] and (2) as adjunctive therapy with thrombolysis or as a management strategy in the subacute phase of AMI (days 2 to 7) in patients who do not receive thrombolysis. Several clinical scenarios have been described that represent different categories of use of PTCA when it is not selected as the primary reperfusion strategy (see Chap. 39).[370,611,613] When thrombolysis has failed to reperfuse the infarct vessel or a severe stenosis is present in the infarct vessel, a *rescue PTCA* may be performed as soon as possible. Alternatively, strategies of empirical *immediate* (i.e., performed urgently within a few hours) or *deferred* (i.e., performed within the first week) PTCA have been proposed for all patients with residual critical stenosis (>70 per cent of lumen diameter) who receive thrombolysis. Finally, a more conservative approach of *elective* PTCA may be used to manage AMI patients only when spontaneous or exercise-provoked ischemia occurs whether or not they have received a previous course of thrombolytic therapy.

Primary Angioplasty

An important advantage of primary PTCA in AMI is the ability to achieve reperfusion of the infarct vessel without the risk of bleeding associated with thrombolytic therapy.[370,610,613–615a] In addition, primary PTCA (performed predominantly in experienced centers) as compared with thrombolytic therapy has been shown in several randomized trials and registries to yield higher patency rates of the infarct vessel both at 90 minutes (about 90 per cent for PTCA versus 65 per cent for thrombolysis).[519,546,606,610,616,617] In a randomized trial of primary PTCA versus intravenous streptokinase for AMI in patients presenting an average of 3 hours after symptom onset, de Boer et al.[617] found that infarct size measured by enzyme release was reduced by 23 per cent and global and regional left ventricular function was improved in the group undergoing PTCA. Systematic overviews[618,619] of seven trials of primary PTCA versus thrombolysis[606–608,620–623] collectively enrolling just under 1200 patients revealed a 40 per cent reduction in short-term mortality in patients treated with primary PTCA versus thrombolysis (Fig. 37–29); a similar reduction in the composite endpoint of death or nonfatal AMI by 6 weeks was also observed. When primary PTCA is performed in experienced centers with a well-staffed invasive angiography team, hospital length of stay and follow-up costs are less than for the patients with AMI who are treated by thrombolytic therapy.[16,608,609,624]

Why have these dramatic differences favoring primary PTCA over thrombolytic therapy been observed? In addition to the high level of technical expertise in the dedicated centers that have reported promising results with primary PTCA, differences in the adequacy of reperfusion and responses of ischemic myocardium to restoration of flow by thrombolysis and mechanical means should be considered.[617] Early patency of the infarct-related artery is higher

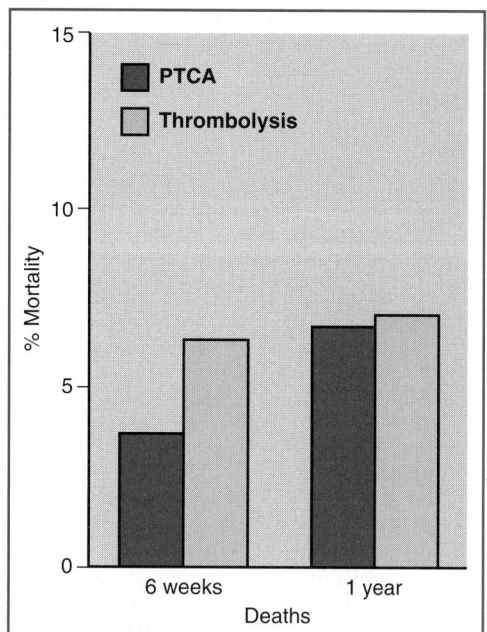

FIGURE 37–29. Comparison of mortality in AMI patients treated with primary PTCA versus thrombolysis. Pooled data from seven randomized trials reveal a significantly lower mortality at 6 weeks in the patients treated with PTCA. A nonsignificant trend favoring PTCA was present at 1 year. (Adapted from Michels, K. B., and Yusuf, S.: Does PTCA in acute myocardial infarction affect mortality and reinfarction rates?: A quantitative overview (meta-analysis) of the randomized clinical trials. Circulation 91:476, 1995; Copyright 1995 American Heart Association.)

with direct PTCA, full reperfusion (TIMI Grade 3 flow) is higher, the degree of residual stenosis is less,[617] reocclusion rates are lower,[546,616,625-627] and collateral flow to noninfarct-related myocardial zones is probably increased[607]—all features that promote better healing in the infarct zone, less left ventricular dilatation,[628] and reduced morbidity and mortality. Ohnishi and coworkers have reported in a canine model of AMI that pharmacological lysis of coronary thrombi associated with production of a systemic lytic state is associated with nonspecific protease activity, activation of neutrophils, complement activation, and platelet activation with release of vasoactive substances that appear to cause delayed recovery of contractile function due to reperfusion injury.[463] In contrast, mechanical recanalization of the infarct vessel does not produce the interstitial edema, contraction band necrosis, and microvascular hemorrhage seen with thrombolytic therapy[462] (Fig. 37–11).

The clinical trial results and intriguing experimental observations cited above must be placed in perspective when one considers implementing primary PTCA as a treatment strategy for the majority of patients with AMI. Fewer than 20 per cent of hospitals in the United States[609,629] and less than 10 per cent of hospitals in Europe[630] can perform primary PTCA, and an even smaller proportion are capable of performing it on an emergency basis 24 hours a day, 7 days a week. It remains to be determined whether lower-volume PTCA centers with less experienced investigators can replicate the encouraging results reported to date.[630,631] In addition, it is unclear whether on-site cardiac surgical backup is a necessary component of a primary PTCA strategy for AMI.[632] The potential cost implications of offering primary PTCA to all eligible patients with AMI are staggering and have been the subject of considerable ongoing debate in several countries.[614,633]

Angioplasty as an Adjunct to Thrombolysis

Ellis et al. have summarized the heterogeneous outcomes reported in observational series of *rescue* PTCA after failed thrombolysis.[634] Although procedural success was obtained

in about 80 per cent of patients, the average rate of reocclusion was 18 per cent, and the average mortality was 10.6 per cent. Two randomized trials subsequently compared rescue PTCA versus conservative therapy in patients with an occluded infarct vessel despite thrombolysis.[635,636] The RESCUE trial focused on the subset of AMI patients with an anterior infarction and reported a reduction in the composite endpoint of death or congestive heart failure by 30 days in the PTCA group.[636] When combined with the trial by Belenkie et al.,[635] a mortality rate of 5.4 per cent was seen in the rescue PTCA group versus 12.9 per cent in the conservative group, which was not statistically significant.[618]

Following thrombolytic therapy in patients who clinically appear to have reperfused, PTCA, whether applied immediately or deferred, has the theoretical benefit of further opening of a stenosed coronary artery to increase flow, perhaps enhancing myocardial recovery and diminishing the possibility of reocclusion. Several trials have compared immediate, early (within several hours to a few days), or deferred (delayed for 4 days) PTCA versus no PTCA, whereas others have compared immediate versus deferred PTCA or immediate versus deferred versus no PTCA; a summary of the design features and main findings of 16 trials that collectively enrolled about 6200 patients in these categories has been published along with meta-analysis of the mortality results.[618] Although none of the individual comparisons of strategies achieved conventional statistical significance, a consistent theme was observed—the *routine empirical* use of PTCA (either immediate or delayed) following thrombolysis was associated with a trend toward *increased* mortality.[370,613,618] In addition, there were higher rates of abrupt reclosure of the infarct-related coronary artery and complications, including reinfarction and the need for urgent coronary artery bypass surgery, while providing no benefit in terms of recovery of ventricular function.[565,637-639] Possible explanations for the increased hazard associated with PTCA soon after thrombolysis include exacerbation of platelet activation and thrombosis at the site of plaque rupture and increased bleeding, including hemorrhagic dissections of the target vessel.[637,640-643] There is also no evidence to support empirical deferred PTCA in patients without evidence of recurrent or provocable ischemia. The TOPS trial randomized patients with a negative exercise test several days following thrombolysis to either medical therapy or medical therapy plus PTCA.[644] There was no benefit in terms of rest or exercise ejection fraction, but there were disturbing trends toward a higher rate of abrupt vessel closure and non-Q-wave MI acutely and a lower rate of infarct-free survival at 1 year follow-up in the PTCA-treated patients.[644]

Recommendations for Use of PTCA in AMI

Although this field is evolving rapidly, at the time of this writing it appears that primary PTCA, when carried out by experienced interventional cardiologists in high-volume angiography laboratories, is at least as effective as and may actually be superior to thrombolytic therapy.[610a] It is our practice to refer thrombolytic-ineligible patients to primary PTCA and also to select primary PTCA as the reperfusion method of choice if the patient is at relatively high risk of intracerebral hemorrhage consequent to thrombolytic therapy (see p. 1220), or if the anticipated time to placement of angioplasty catheters is less than 1 hour from the patient's presentation to the emergency department. In the special circumstances of cardiogenic shock, a serious problem that affects about 5 to 7 per cent of patients with AMI,[422,645] the observational data to date appear to be more favorable with primary PTCA than thrombolysis[646-648] (see p. 1239) and in the absence of other life-threatening comorbidities (e.g., advanced cancer), we therefore refer cardiogenic shock patients for primary PTCA. Nonrandomized observational data from the GUSTO trial support the use of PTCA for management of shock both in patients who arrive in shock and in those who develop it during hospitalization (30-day mortality was 33 to 40 per cent in PTCA-treated patients, compared with 75 per cent in medically treated patients). An ongoing randomized study of PTCA versus medical therapy (SHOCK trial) will provide important, definitive data on the relative benefit of PTCA for cardiogenic shock.[646]

Patients in whom thrombolytic therapy fails to achieve reperfusion represent candidates for PTCA (rescue angioplasty), and in such patients PTCA can usually be safe and effective (greater than 80 per cent success rates).[649] Until there are better ways to recognize patients who might benefit from "rescue angioplasty," the question of optimal treatment of thrombolytic failure remains unresolved.[650] However, patients with evolving chest pain and ST-segment elevations that persist for 90 minutes following the onset of administration of a thrombolytic agent are candidates for emergency catheterization and, if the infarct-related vessel is occluded, for rescue angioplasty. Elective PTCA can be considered for most patients receiving thrombolytic therapy in whom ischemia develops at rest, during ambulation in the hospital, or during a prehospital discharge exercise test.[613,639,641,651] We do not consider it necessary to carry out routine coronary arteriography on asymptomatic patients with negative prehospital discharge exercise tests to identify patients who have severe obstruction in whom PTCA can be performed.

Evidence exists from observational studies, retrospective reviews of multicenter trials, as well as a recent randomized trial that routine prophylactic use of intra-aortic balloon counterpulsation following PTCA for AMI reduces the risk of reocclusion.[652–654] Whether or not thrombolysis was used, prophylactic intra-aortic balloon counterpulsation may be useful for 24 to 48 hours as an adjunct to maintain vessel patency following PTCA of the infarct vessel in those patients in whom it is judged that a sudden reocclusion of the target vessel would be associated with severe hemodynamic compromise.

SURGICAL REPERFUSION

There have been extensive improvements in intraoperative myocardial preservation with cardioplegia and hypothermia and in surgical techniques. These have allowed surgical reperfusion in patients with AMI to be carried out at quite low short- and long-term mortality rates—approximately 2 per cent in-hospital and 25 per cent 10-year mortality rates in selected centers. This has kept alive the concept of emergency coronary revascularization as a possible measure to protect jeopardized myocardium in patients suffering AMI.[655–657] As appears to be the case for all methods designed to limit infarct size, salvage of myocardium is most successful if surgery is performed within the first 4 to 6 hours of the onset of the acute event.[658] In the usual patient who develops an AMI outside of the hospital, it is logistically almost impossible to bring the patient to the hospital, carry out a clinical evaluation, outline the coronary anatomy by arteriography, assemble the surgical team, commence operation, and place the patient on cardiopulmonary bypass in less than 4 to 6 hours after the onset of the event. It is therefore unlikely that surgical reperfusion can or will be applied in the routine treatment of AMI. Indeed, the operation is contraindicated in patients with uncomplicated transmural infarcts more than 6 hours after the onset of the event. When carried out at this time, surgical reperfusion appears to produce marked hemorrhage into the area of infarction.[659] In some patients with AMI, including some with cardiogenic shock, infarction appears to occur in a stuttering manner over an interval of several days.[660] Revascularization carried out more than 6 hours after the onset of the

event might be of benefit in this group, but this has yet to be rigorously established.

About 10 to 20 per cent of AMI patients are currently referred for coronary bypass grafting for one of the following indications: persistent or recurrent chest pain despite thrombolysis or PTCA,[661] high-risk coronary anatomy (e.g., left main stenosis) discovered at catheterization, or a complication of AMI such as ventricular septal rupture or severe mitral regurgitation due to papillary muscle dysfunction. Patients with AMI with continued severe ischemic and hemodynamic instability are likely to benefit from emergency revascularization. PTCA is the preferable technique when revascularization is needed in the first 48 to 72 hours following AMI; surgery should be reserved for those in whom PTCA has been unsuccessful or whose anatomy dictates the need for coronary artery bypass grafting, such as patients with left main or extensive multivessel coronary artery disease.

Patients undergoing successful thrombolysis but with important residual stenoses, who on anatomical grounds are more suitable for surgical revascularization than for PTCA, have undergone coronary artery bypass surgery with quite low mortality (about 4 per cent) and morbidity *provided* that they are operated on more than 24 hours from AMI; those patients requiring urgent or emergency CABG within 24 to 48 hours of AMI have mortality rates between 15 and 20 per cent.[657,661,662] When surgery is performed under urgent conditions with active and ongoing ischemia or cardiogenic shock, operative mortality rises steeply.[663,664] At autopsy, such patients have extensive myocardial necrosis that is often hemorrhagic.[665] Patients who are referred urgently for CABG within 6 to 12 hours of receiving a thrombolytic should receive aprotinin and fresh-frozen plasma to correct their coagulation system deficit and minimize the requirements for blood transfusion. Although postoperative chest tube drainage with relatively minor bleeding occurs more commonly than after elective bypass surgery, this problem is not of major concern.[666]

ANTITHROMBOTIC AND ANTIPLATELET THERAPY

Antithrombotic Therapy

Despite 30 years of active clinical investigation, the use of antithrombotic agents after AMI remains controversial. The rationale for administering heparin (see p. 1978) acutely in AMI includes prevention of deep venous thrombosis, pulmonary embolism, ventricular thrombus formation, and cerebral embolization. In addition, establishing and maintaining patency of the infarct-related artery, whether or not a patient receives thrombolytic therapy, is another common rationale for heparin therapy in AMI.

Randomized trials in AMI conducted in the prethrombolytic era (between 1969 and 1973) showed that the risks of pulmonary embolism, stroke, and reinfarction were reduced in patients who received intravenous heparin.[667–669] Relative mortality was reduced by approximately 10 to 30 per cent, but hemorrhagic complications increased by a factor of 2- to 4-fold. A meta-analysis reported in 1977 indicated a significant reduction of mortality favoring the use of anticoagulation in the hospital phase of AMI[670]; some of the mortality reduction effects in this meta-analysis may have been due to long-term oral anticoagulant therapy superimposed on acute intravenous heparin initiated during the hospital phase.[671,672] With the introduction of the thrombolytic era and importantly after the publication of ISIS-2,[529] the situation became more complicated because of strong evidence of a substantial mortality reduction with aspirin alone and confusing and conflicting data regarding the risk-benefit ratio of heparin used as an adjunct to aspirin or in combination with aspirin and a thrombolytic agent. Several reviews have summarized the available information.[672–674]

EFFECT ON MORTALITY. In the SCATI trial of streptokinase for AMI, in which patients were randomized to receive either delayed subcutaneous heparin or placebo as the *sole* adjunctive therapy (i.e., no aspirin), there was a trend toward lower mortality in the heparin group.[675] No randomized trial data are available comparing aspirin alone versus aspirin plus heparin in patients not receiving thrombolytic therapy. In the combined data set of GISSI-2 and ISIS-3 (totaling over 62,000 patients), the 35-day mortality was 10.0 per cent in the patients receiving subcutaneous heparin versus 10.2 per cent in the patients not receiving any subcutaneous heparin.[672,674] In addition, in the GUSTO study, no difference was seen in the 35-day mortality rate in patients receiving streptokinase plus subcutaneous heparin (7.2 per cent) or intravenous heparin (7.4 per cent).[33] Nonrandomized subgroup analyses from the LATE trial of 2821 patients who received t-PA showed a 35-day mortality of 7.6 per cent when intravenous heparin was administered, compared with 10.4 per cent when no heparin was given.[533,672] Thus, the available information suggests that intravenous heparin is probably of no benefit in patients receiving streptokinase but may be helpful in patients receiving t-PA.

EFFECT ON PATENCY OF INFARCT ARTERY

A number of angiographic studies have examined the role of heparin therapy in establishing and maintaining patency of the infarct-related artery in patients with AMI. Comparison of these trials is difficult because of potentially important differences in study design, including whether aspirin was administered along with heparin, the thrombolytic agent that was administered, and variations in the time of diagnostic coronary arteriography. The Bleich[676] and HART[677] studies showed a higher infarct-related artery patency rate in AMI patients treated with t-PA plus heparin than t-PA plus placebo (71 to 82 per cent versus 43 to 52 per cent infarct-related artery patency at 7 to 72 hours). The European Cooperative Study Group performed angiograms relatively late, i.e., 48 to 120 hours following t-PA, and still showed a somewhat greater patency rate of the infarct-related artery in the heparin-treated patients.[678] The LIMITS (Liquemin in Myocardial Infarction During Thrombolysis with Saruplase) study investigators reported that AMI patients who are treated with unglycosylated single-chain urokinase-type plasminogen activator (saruplase) and are also treated with intravenous heparin (but no aspirin) achieve a higher patency rate of the infarct-related artery at 6 to 12 hours (79 per cent) than those in the control group (57 per cent).[580] The TAMI-3 study suggested that in patients receiving aspirin plus t-PA, no patency benefit was achieved by the immediate intravenous administration of heparin and that it could therefore be delayed for at least 60 to 90 minutes after thrombolysis.[679]

Although a slightly better 90-minute infarct-related artery patency rate was observed in the OSIRIS (streptokinase plus aspirin) study[680] in patients who received heparin versus placebo (82 per cent patency versus 72 per cent), the GUSTO angiographic substudy[519] showed no benefit of intravenous heparin versus subcutaneous heparin in patients who received streptokinase plus aspirin with respect to 90-minute infarct-related artery patency (60 per cent versus 54 per cent). Heparin afforded no benefit in terms of late patency (5-day) of the infarct-related artery in the DUCCS-1 study of patients receiving APSAC plus aspirin.[681]

In a randomized double-blind trial (APSIM) of APSAC versus conventional-dose heparin (500 IU/kg/24 hours), the patency rate of the infarct-related artery was 77 per cent in the thrombolytic group versus only 37 per cent in the heparin group.[682] However, the HEAP (Heparin in Early Patency) investigators have presented intriguing data that a large single intravenous bolus of 300 units per kilogram of heparin to AMI patients presenting in less than 6 hours with ST-segment elevation results in a 90-minute patency rate of the infarct-related artery of 60 per cent with 36 per cent TIMI Grade 3 flow.[683]

EFFECT ON LEFT VENTRICULAR THROMBUS. Anticoagulant therapy significantly reduces the incidence of echocardiographically documented left ventricular thrombi.[671] These benefits are observed most prominently in patients with anterior myocardial infarction, particularly those with a large area of wall motion abnormality. In the thrombolytic era, the incidence of left ventricular thrombi is reduced.[684,685] Although co-administration of heparin does not appear to affect the incidence of left ventricular thrombus formation in patients who receive thrombolytic therapy, the thrombi protrude less into the ventricular cavity when heparin is administered.[686]

COMPLICATIONS OF ANTITHROMBOTIC THERAPY

Although heparin may induce thrombocytopenia through an immunological mechanism, this is seen only rarely, probably occurring in only 2 to 3 per cent of patients.[687,687a] The most serious complication of antithrombotic therapy is bleeding—especially intracranial hemorrhage—when thrombolytic agents are prescribed (see p. 1219). Major hemorrhagic events occur more frequently in patients of low body weight, advanced age, and marked prolongation of the aPTT (greater than 90 to 100 seconds).[558,559] Frequent monitoring of the aPTT (facilitated by use of a bedside testing device) reduces the risk of major hemorrhagic complications in patients treated with heparin.[688] A standardized nomogram, adopted from treatment regimens for patients with pulmonary embolism, is commonly used to adjust heparin infusions in patients with AMI.[689] It should be noted, however, that during the first 12 hours following thrombolytic therapy, the aPTT may be elevated from the thrombolytic agent alone (particularly if streptokinase is administered), making it difficult to accurately interpret the effects of a heparin infusion on the patient's coagulation status.

NEW ANTITHROMBOTIC AGENTS
(See also p. 1821)

Potential disadvantages of infusions of unfractionated heparin include dependency on antithrombin III for inhibition of thrombin activity, sensitivity to platelet factor 4, inability to inhibit clot-bound thrombin, marked interpatient variability in therapeutic response, and the need for frequent aPTT monitoring. In an effort to circumvent these disadvantages of unfractionated heparin, there has been interest in the development of novel antithrombotic compounds.[690] The prototypical direct antithrombin is hirudin, which has been made available for clinical investigation using recombinant technology (see p. 1820). The TIMI-9 trial compared intravenous unfractionated heparin with intravenous hirudin in AMI patients receiving thrombolytic therapy (accelerated-dose t-PA or streptokinase). Hirudin was equal to heparin in effectiveness but was not superior when analyzed using a composite primary endpoint of the sum of death, nonfatal AMI, or congestive heart failure/cardiogenic shock, or the harder composite endpoint of the sum of death or nonfatal MI.[691] The GUSTO IIB study showed no statistically significant reduction in the incidence of death or nonfatal recurrent infarction by 30 days with hirudin versus heparin in MI patients with ST-segment elevation as well as those without.[691a]

The potential beneficial effects of low molecular weight heparin preparations, particularly those that have a high anti-X_a:anti-II_a ratio, are now being examined in AMI patients in both the presence and the absence of thrombolytic therapy.

Recommendations for Antithrombotic Therapy

Given the pivotal role thrombin plays in the pathogenesis of AMI, antithrombotic therapy remains an important therapeutic intervention. As reviewed on page 1225, all patients with an acute coronary syndrome should receive antiplatelet therapy (aspirin remains the recommended agent at this time). Until the results of ongoing studies are available, we believe that the recommendations below are a reasonable approach.

For patients who do *not* receive thrombolytic therapy, overviews of the available data indicate that heparin reduces mortality and morbidity from serious complications such as reinfarction and thromboembolism.[692,693] Therefore, in the absence of contraindications to anticoagulation we routinely use heparin in *all* AMI patients presenting with ST elevation who are not candidates for thrombolysis and also prescribe it for AMI patients presenting without ST elevation. Minimum therapy should consist of 7500 IU subcutaneously every 12 hours; however, it is the practice of many clinicians to administer intravenous heparin at full therapeutic dosage to such patients.[671] Dosing regimens that are based on weight (bolus 70 U/kg and infusion of 15 U/kg/hr) may more rapidly and safely establish a therapeutic level of heparin (target aPTT about 1.5 to 2 times control)[694,695]; in the average-sized patient this corresponds to an intravenous bolus of 5000 U and infusion of 1000 U/hr. The heparin infusion is continued for at least 48 hours, and then a decision is made about the patient's ongoing need for intravenous antithrombotic therapy based on factors such as the presence or absence of recurrent ischemia and plans for catheterization. Patients with a large anterior infarction with or without an echocardiographically demonstrated thrombus are at increased risk of cerebral embolism and should receive oral anticoagulant therapy (target INR 2.0 to 3.0) for at least 3 months following AMI.[684,685] Additional recommendations on long-term oral anticoagulant therapy after AMI are given on page 1265.

For patients receiving thrombolytic therapy with either streptokinase or APSAC, there is no apparent mortality benefit of immediate intravenous heparin, and we do not recommend its use if those thrombolytics are prescribed. The only exception to this are patients who have another compelling indication for anticoagulation such as a large anterior infarction with a significant wall motion abnormality[671] or atrial fibrillation (see p. 1253)—in this case we generally use intravenous heparin administered to a target aPTT of 60 to 70 seconds. The relative benefits of routine use of delayed (4 to 12 hours), high-dose (12,500 IU twice daily) subcutaneous heparin in patients receiving streptokinase remain unresolved.[695a]

On the basis of the principle that t-PA is a more fibrin-specific lytic agent and the evidence that infarct-related artery patency rates are higher in patients receiving intravenous heparin adjunctively with t-PA, it is commonly recommended that with t-PA, intravenous heparin should be administered.[671] A bolus of 5000 IU followed by an initial infusion of 1000 IU/hr or a bolus of 70 IU/kg followed by an initial infusion of 15 IU/kg/hr is appropriate.[696] In current practice the target aPTT range is 50 to 70 seconds.[2] Patients should be monitored for any signs of bleeding and frequent measurements of the aPTT (at least once every 12 to 24 hours) are recommended, because the incidence of hemorrhage increases with marked prolongation of the aPTT.[558,559] The infusion should be maintained for at least 24 to 48 hours following administration of t-PA.

Because of concern about the possibility of a rebound increase in thrombin generation and recurrent ischemia following cessation of heparin therapy[697,698] (see p. 1823), some clinicians have suggested a tapering of heparin infusions rather than abrupt discontinuation.

Antiplatelet Therapy

As discussed earlier (see p. 1110), platelets play a major role in the thrombotic response to rupture of a coronary artery plaque.[65,699] Aggregates of platelets are integrally involved in the development of AMI, both with and without ST-segment elevation.[207,699a] Platelet-rich thrombi are also more resistant to thrombolysis than are fibrin and erythrocyte-rich thrombi.[700,701] Thus, there is a sound scientific basis for inhibiting platelet aggregation in *all* AMI patients, regardless of whether a thrombolytic is prescribed. Comprehensive overviews of randomized trials of antiplatelet therapy have summarized the overwhelming evidence of benefit of antiplatelet therapy for a wide range of vascular disorders[9,702,703] (Fig. 37–30). In patients at risk for AMI, patients with a documented prior AMI, and patients in the acute phase of an AMI, dramatic reductions (between 25 to 50 per cent) in mortality, nonfatal reduction of recurrent infarction, and nonfatal stroke are achieved by antiplatelet therapy.[9] Not unexpectedly, the absolute benefits are greatest in those patients at highest baseline risk.[9] Although several antiplatelet regimens have been evaluated, the agent most extensively tested has been aspirin and this also is

the drug for which the most compelling evidence of benefit exists.[411,704]

The ISIS-2 study was the largest trial of aspirin in AMI and provides the single strongest piece of evidence that aspirin reduces mortality in AMI[529] (Fig. 37–25). Of interest, in contrast to the observations of a time-dependent mortality effect of thrombolytic therapy (see p. 1220), the mortality reduction with aspirin was similar in patients treated within 4 hours (25 per cent reduction in mortality), between 5 and 12 hours (21 per cent reduction), and between 13 and 24 hours (21 per cent reduction). There was an overall 23 per cent reduction in mortality from aspirin in ISIS-2 that was largely additive to the 25 per cent reduction in mortality from streptokinase, so that patients receiving both therapies experienced a 42 per cent reduction in mortality.[529] The mortality reduction was as high as 53 per cent in those patients who received both aspirin and streptokinase within 6 hours of symptoms. Of particular interest was the fact that the combination of streptokinase and aspirin reduced mortality from 23.8 per cent to 15.8 per cent (34 per cent reduction) *without* increasing the risk of stroke or hemorrhage.[671]

Recommendations for Antiplatelet Therapy

Some uncertainty about the optimal dose of aspirin for acute treatment of AMI remains.[705] In general, high doses of aspirin are not more effective than lower doses but are more likely to provoke gastrointestinal side effects.[411] However, adequate cyclo-oxygenase inhibition (and reduction in thromboxane A$_2$ production) takes several days to accomplish with less than 75 mg of aspirin, and loading doses of 160 to 325 mg (preferably chewed) are therefore recommended for all AMI patients without a history of aspirin allergy whether they present with ST elevation or not and whether they undergo reperfusion with thrombolytics or PTCA or are treated with a more conservative medical regimen (Fig. 37–18). Active peptic ulcer disease is a relative contraindication to antiplatelet therapy.[2] For patients with severe nausea and vomiting, aspirin suppositories (325 mg) can be used. Aspirin should be continued indefinitely in patients with AMI.

NEW ANTIPLATELET REGIMENS. Alternative regimens for inhibiting platelet function are under active development (see Chap. 58). Although thromboxane synthase inhibitors,[706] thromboxane and serotonin receptor antagonists,[707] and agents with combined actions on thromboxane synthesis and the thromboxane receptor have been explored,[708,709] the most promising class of agents are the glycoprotein IIb/IIIa receptor antagonists, which interfere with the final common pathway for platelet aggregation.[207,710] When combined with accelerated-dose t-PA and aspirin in patients with ST-elevation AMI, integrelin, a cyclic peptide antagonist of the IIb/IIIa receptor, achieves patency rates of the infarct-related artery between 70 and 80 per cent[711] and reduces the amount of ST-segment deviation observed over time with a continuous ECG monitor.[712]

FIGURE 37–30. Results of aspirin therapy after MI. Meta-analysis of several placebo-controlled trials of antiplatelet therapy after MI (predominantly aspirin), indicating a 25 per cent reduction in the odds for mortality in patients receiving the active therapy. (Adapted from Antiplatelet Trialists' Collaboration: Secondary prevention of vascular disease by prolonged antiplatelet treatment. BMJ 296:320, 1988.)

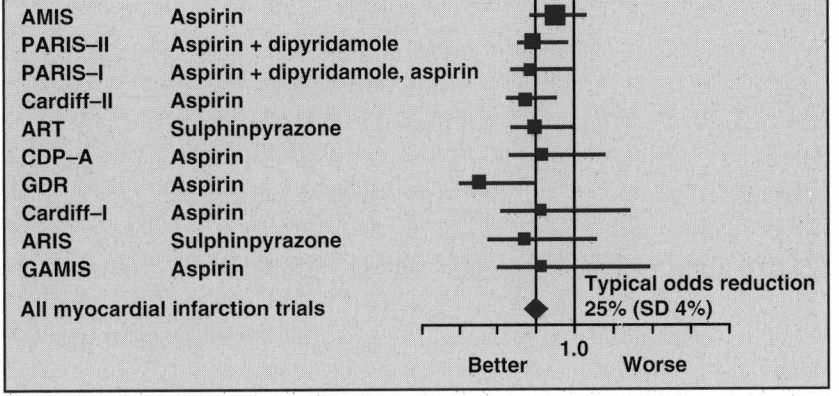

Coronary Care Units

Deaths from primary ventricular fibrillation in AMI have been prevented because the coronary care unit (CCU) allows continuous monitoring of cardiac rhythm by highly trained nurses with the authority to initiate immediate treatment of arrhythmias in the absence of physicians, and because of the specialized equipment (defibrillators, pacemakers) and drugs available. Although all of these benefits can be achieved for patients scattered throughout the hospital, the clustering of patients with AMI in the CCU has greatly improved the efficient use of the trained personnel, facilities, and equipment. In recent years, with increasing emphasis on hemodynamic monitoring and treatment of the serious complications of AMI with such modalities as thrombolytic therapy, afterload reduction, and intraaortic balloon counterpulsation, the CCU has assumed even greater importance.[30,713] As interventional strategies including thrombolytic therapy and acute coronary angioplasty are used more routinely in AMI patients, facilities in which patients may undergo diagnostic and therapeutic angiographic procedures are being integrated into the CCU structure.

At the same time, the value of CCUs for patients with uncomplicated AMI has been questioned and restudied.[30,714] With increasing attention directed to the limitation of resources and to the economic impact of intensive care, there have been efforts to select patients for whom hospitalization in a CCU would likely be of benefit (see p. 1749).[713] The ECG, on presentation, particularly in conjunction with previous tracings[715] and an immediate general clinical assessment, can be useful both for predicting which patients will have the diagnosis of AMI confirmed and identifying low-risk patients who may require less intensive care.[393,716,717] Of patients with a history of typical chest pain but with a normal ECG in the emergency department, less than 20 per cent ultimately have an AMI on that admission, and less than 1 per cent develop any significant complication.[718] Thus, a patient with a normal ECG may not require admission to a full-fledged CCU. Careful analysis of the quality of pain may help identify such low-risk patients as well. Patients without a history of angina pectoris or MI presenting with pain that is sharp or stabbing and pleuritic, positional, or reproduced by palpation of the chest wall are extremely unlikely to have an AMI.[719] Computer-guided decision protocols are being developed to aid clinicians in identifying those AMI patients who require admission to the CCU as opposed to a less intensive hospital ward.[720]

Contemporary CCUs typically have equipment available for noninvasive monitoring of single or multiple ECG leads, cardiac rhythm, ST-segment deviation, arterial pressure, and arterial oxygen saturation.[721] Computer algorithms for detection and analysis of arrhythmias are superior to visual surveillance by skilled CCU staff.[722] However, even the most sophisticated ECG monitoring systems are susceptible to artifacts due to patient movement or noise on the signal from poor skin preparation when monitoring electrodes are applied.[30] Noninvasive monitoring of arterial blood pressure using a sphygmomanometric cuff that undergoes cycles of inflation and deflation at programmed intervals is suitable for the majority of patients admitted to a CCU. Invasive arterial monitoring is preferred in patients with a low output syndrome under circumstances in which inotropic therapy is initiated for severe left ventricular failure (see p. 1194).[30]

The CCU remains the appropriate hospital unit for patients with complicated infarctions (e.g., hemodynamic instability, recurrent arrhythmias) and those patients requiring intensive nursing care for devices such as an intra-aortic balloon pump (see p. 1221). For patients with a low risk of mortality from AMI (see p. 1235), the clinician should consider admission to an intermediate care facility (see below) equipped with simple ECG monitoring and resuscitation equipment. This strategy has been shown to be cost effective[723] and may reduce CCU utilization by one-third, shorten hospital stays, and have no deleterious effect on patients' recovery. Intermediate care units for low-risk AMI patients may also be appealing to patients who stand to gain little benefit from the high staffing, intense activity, and elaborate technology available in current CCUs (with their attendant high costs) and who may be disturbed by that activity and equipment.

RECOMMENDATIONS FOR ADMISSION TO THE CCU. (1) Patients with clear-cut AMI, presenting within 12 to 24 hours of symptoms, should, in most instances, be admitted to an intensive CCU. (2) Most patients with severe unstable angina should also be admitted to the CCU, particularly if episodes of chest pain occur at rest, high doses of intravenous nitroglycerin (e.g., ≥ 300 $\mu g/min$) are required to relieve chest pain, or frequent adjustments of intravenous nitroglycerin infusions are required because of fluctuating symptoms and hemodynamic status. (3) Once an AMI is ruled out (ideally by 12 hours) and symptoms are controlled with oral or topical pharmacological agents, discharge from the CCU should be considered. (4) AMI patients with an uncomplicated status, such as those without a history of previous infarction, persistent ischemic-type discomfort, congestive heart failure, hypotension, heart block, or hemodynamically compromising ventricular arrhythmias, may be safely transferred out of the CCU within 24 to 36 hours. (5) In patients with a complicated AMI, the duration of the CCU stay should be dictated by the need for "intensive" care—that is, hemodynamic monitoring, close nursing supervision, intravenous vasoactive drugs, and frequent changes in the medical regimen.

General Measures for Management of AMI

The CCU staff must be sensitive to patient concerns about mortality, prognosis, and future productivity. A calm, quiet atmosphere and the "laying on of hands" with a gentle but confident touch helps allay anxiety and reduce sympathetic tone, ultimately leading to a reduction in hypertension, tachycardia, and arrhythmias.[30] To reduce the risk of nausea and vomiting early after infarction and to reduce the risk of aspiration, during the first 4 to 12 hours after admission patients should receive either nothing by mouth or a clear liquid diet. Subsequently a diet with 50 to 55 per cent of calories from complex carbohydrates and up to 30 per cent from mono- and unsaturated fats should be given. The diet should be enriched in foods that are high in potassium, magnesium, and fiber but low in sodium (Table 37–5).

The results of laboratory tests obtained in the CCU should be scrutinized for any derangements potentially contributing to arrhythmias, such as hypoxemia, hypovolemia, disturbances of acid-based balance or of electrolytes, and drug toxicity. Oxazepam, 15 to 30 mg orally four times a day, is useful to allay the anxiety that is common in the first 24 to 48 hours.[724] Delirium may be provoked by medications frequently used in the CCU, including antiarrhythmic drugs, H_2 blockers, narcotics, and beta blockers. Potentially offending agents should be discontinued in patients with an abnormal mental status. Haloperidol, a butyrophenone, may be used safely in patients with AMI beginning with a dose of 2 mg intravenously for mildly agitated patients and 5 to 10 mg for progressively more agitated patients.[724] Hypnotics, such as temazepam, 15 to 30 mg or an equivalent, should be provided as needed for sleep. Dioctyl sodium sulfosuccinate, 200 mg daily, or another stool softener should be used to prevent constipation and straining.

"Coronary precautions" that do *not* appear to be supported by evidence from clinical research[2] include the

TABLE 37–5 GUIDELINES FOR DIET THERAPY IN THE CARDIAC CARE UNIT

1. NPO prior to evaluation by physician

2. *Kilocalories and protein:* the diet should initially be planned to provide adequate kilocalories and protein to maintain the patient's initial weight. Caloric restrictions may subsequently be initiated for weight loss if needed

3. *Fats:* the diet should be limited to ≤30% of total calories from fat. Foods high in cholesterol and saturated fats should be avoided. One or two eggs per week may be given if requested and/or to ensure adequate protein intake; egg substitutes should also be available and encouraged

4. *Carbohydrates:* complex carbohydrates should constitute 50–55% of total calories

5. *Fiber:* the diet should contain fiber consistent with a balanced mixed diet, including fresh fruit and vegetables, whole-grain bread, and cereals. Foods that may cause gastrointestinal intolerance should be eliminated on an individual basis.

6. *Sodium:* a "no added salt" (NAS) diet (3–4 g Na+) is recommended, with adjustment as indicated by clinical status. The NAS diet order excludes a salt shaker as well as foods high in sodium (greater than 300 mg per serving)

7. *Potassium:* foods high in potassium should be encouraged except for patients with renal insufficiency

8. *Quantity:* small, frequent feedings may be recommended on an individual basis

9. *Fluids:* use of regular coffee should not be restricted. Decaffeinated beverages and weak tea may be offered as substitutes if desired by the patient

10. *Education:* the principal goal of patient education and long-term planning is to achieve and maintain ideal body weight and to adhere to dietary adjustments as ordered by the physician

Modified from Antman, E. M.: General hospital management. *In* Julian, D., and Braunwald, E. (eds.): Management of Acute Myocardial Infarction. London, W. B. Saunders Ltd., 1994, p. 35.

avoidance of iced fluids,[725,726] hot beverages,[727] caffeinated beverages,[728] rectal examinations,[729] back rubs,[730] and assistance with eating.[30]

PHYSICAL ACTIVITY. In the absence of complications, patients with AMI need not be confined to bed for more than 12 hours and, unless they are hemodynamically compromised, they may use a bedside commode shortly after admission.[731] Progression of activity should be individualized depending upon the patient's clinical status, age, and physical capacity; a suggested schedule for activity progression is shown in Table 37–6.

In patients without hemodynamic compromise, early ambulation—including dangling feet on the side of the bed, sitting in a chair, standing, and walking around the bed—does not cause important changes in heart rate, blood pressure, or pulmonary wedge pressure.[731] Although heart rate increases slightly (usually by less than 10 per cent), pulmonary wedge pressures fall slightly as the patient assumes the upright posture for activities. Early ambulatory activities are rarely associated with any symptoms, and when symptoms do occur, they generally are related to hypotension. Thus, when Levine and Lown proposed the "armchair" treatment of AMI in the 1950's, they were undoubtedly correct that stress to the myocardium is less in the upright position.[732] As long as blood pressure and heart rate are monitored carefully, early ambulation offers considerable psychological and physical benefit without any clear medical risk.

The Intermediate Coronary Care Unit

AMI patients are at risk for late in-hospital mortality from recurrent ischemia or infarction, hemodynamically significant ventricular arrhythmias, and severe congestive heart failure after discharge from the CCU. Therefore, continued surveillance in intermediate CCUs (also called step-down units) is justifiable. Risk factors for mortality in the hospital after discharge from the coronary care unit include significant congestive heart failure evidenced by persistent sinus tachycardia for more than 2 days and rales greater than one-third of the lung fields; recurrent ventricular tachycardia and ventricular fibrillation; atrial fibrillation or flutter while in the CCU; intraventricular conduction delays or heart block; anterior location of infarction; and recurrent episodes of angina with marked electrocardiographic ST-segment abnormalities at low activity levels.[538,733] Although it has not been shown rigorously,[734] it is likely that a reduction in late hospital mortality can be achieved with the use of intermediate CCUs, which permit prolonged continuous monitoring of the electrocardiogram and prompt, effective treatment of ventricular fibrillation and other serious arrhythmias.

The availability of intermediate care units may also be helpful in identifying those patients who remain free of complications and are suitable candidates for early discharge from the hospital. Several reports suggest that aggressive reperfusion protocols with angioplasty or thrombolytics can reduce length of hospital stay.[735,736] In patients who are believed to have undergone successful reperfusion, the *absence* of early sustained ventricular tachyarrhythmias, hypotension, or heart failure, coupled with a well-preserved left ventricular ejection fraction, predicts a low risk of late complications in-hospital. Such patients are suitable candidates for discharge from the hospital in less than 5 days from the onset of symptoms.

Following AMI, patients are often eager for information, in need of reassurance, confused by misinformation and prior impressions, capable of counterproductive denial, and

TABLE 37–6 ACTIVITY PROGRESSION FOLLOWING MYOCARDIAL INFARCTION

GENERAL GUIDELINES

When progressing through the stages noted below, specific activities should be stopped for increasing shortness of breath or the patient's perception of fatigue or detection of an increase in the heart rate of >20–30 beats/min⁻¹. Vital signs should be monitored before and following progression from one stage to the next and also from one level to the next within each stage. Energy-conserving techniques should be emphasized and the use of prophylactic nitroglycerin should be reviewed with the patient

STAGE I (DAY 1–2)

Use a bedpan/commode. Feed self-prepared tray with arm and back support. Complete assistance with bathing. Passive range of motion (ROM) to all extremities. Active ankle motion (with footboard if available). Emphasis on relaxation and deep breathing

Partially bathe upper body with back support. Bed to chair transfers for 1–2 hours per day. Active ROM to all extremities 5–10 times (sitting or supine)

STAGE II (DAY 3–4)

Bathe, groom, self-dress sitting on bed or chair. Bed to chair transfers ad lib. Ambulate in room with gradual increase in duration and frequency

May shower or stand at sink to bathe. May dress in own clothes. Supervised ambulation outside of room (100–600 feet several times per day) (33–200 meters)

Partially bathe upper body with back support. Bed to chair 20–30 min daily. Active assisted to active ROM all extremities: 5–10 times (sitting or supine)

STAGE III (DAY 5–7)

Ambulate 600 feet (200 meters) three times per day. May shampoo hair (e.g., activity with arms over head)

Supervised stair walking

Predischarge exercise tolerance test

From Antman, E. M.: General hospital management. *In* Julian, D., and Braunwald, E. (eds.): Management of Acute Myocardial Infarction. London, W. B. Saunders Ltd., 1994, p. 34.

simply frightened. Intermediate care facilities provide ideal settings and ample opportunities to begin the rehabilitation process. The capacity for the early detection of problems following AMI and the social and educational benefits of grouping such patients together strongly argue for continued utilization of intermediate CCUs. Furthermore, the economic advantage of grouping such patients together for sharing of skilled personnel and resources outweighs any questions raised by the lack of a clear consensus regarding reduced mortality. An additional potential advantage is the facilitation of patient education in a group setting with lectures and audiovisual programs.

PHARMACOLOGICAL THERAPY

The rationale and recommendations for initiation of several pharmacological measures to treat AMI in the emergency department have been reviewed previously (see p. 1210) (Fig. 37–18). The early use of beta blockers, ACE inhibitors, calcium antagonists, and magnesium and nitrates is discussed in this section. Secondary prevention with some of these agents is discussed subsequently (see p. 1263).

Beta Blockers
(See also p. 1978)

The effects of beta blockers on AMI can be divided into those that are immediate (when the drug is given very early in the course of infarction) and long-term (secondary prevention), when the drug is initiated sometime after infarction (see p. 1211).[736a] The immediate intravenous administration of beta-adrenoceptor blockers reduces cardiac index, heart rate, and blood pressure.[414] The net effect is a reduction in myocardial oxygen consumption per minute and per beat. Favorable effects of acute intravenous administration of beta-adrenoceptor blockers on the balance of myocardial oxygen supply and demand are reflected in reductions in chest pain,[737] in the proportion of patients with threatened infarction who actually evolve AMI,[738] and in the development of ventricular arrhythmias.[739,740] Because beta-adrenoceptor blockade diminishes circulating levels of free fatty acids by antagonizing the lipolytic effects of catecholamines and because elevated levels of fatty acids augment myocardial oxygen consumption and probably increase the incidence of arrhythmias, these metabolic actions of beta-blocking agents may also be beneficial to the ischemic heart.[739]

Objective evidence of beneficial effects of beta blockers in acute myocardial ischemia has been reported using the precordial ST-segment mapping technique.[741] Acute beta blockade probably reduces infarct size in AMI. Reduction in release of cardiac enzymes with beta blockade[742] is suggestive of a smaller infarct, as is the preservation of R waves and reduction in the development of Q waves.[743]

RESULTS OF MULTICENTER TRIALS. At least 27 randomized beta blocker trials involving more than 27,000 patients have been undertaken.[32,744] Several trials have been performed to test the effects of early beta blockade in myocardial infarction. The largest of these, ISIS-1, involving more than 16,000 patients, reported a significant reduction in mortality among the patients randomized to intravenous atenolol compared with placebo-treated patients.[745] The findings of a meta-analysis of data from the 27 early beta blocker trials (in the prethrombolytic era) are summarized in Figure 37–31. Intravenous followed by oral beta blocker therapy is associated with about a 15 per cent relative reduction in mortality, nonfatal reinfarction, and nonfatal cardiac arrest.[746] Although antagonism of sympathetic stimulation to the heart might be expected to exacerbate pulmonary edema in patients with occult heart failure, usually only small changes in pulmonary capillary wedge pressure

occur when the drug is used in patients with AMI.[739] Thus, in appropriately selected patients the benefits noted above occur at a cost of about a 3 per cent incidence of provocation of congestive heart failure or complete heart block and a 2 per cent incidence of the development of cardiogenic shock[746] (Fig. 37–31).

Because reduction of infarct size in AMI patients treated with beta blockers is likely to occur only with early treatment (≤ 4 hours from the onset of pain), investigators have sought other explanations for the reduction in the mortality in the acute phase which has been observed.[745] Intriguing observations from the ISIS-1 trial raise the possibility that a reduction in the development of cardiac rupture or electromechanical dissociation during the first day is achieved with early beta blockade.[747]

In the TIMI-II trial the addition of a beta blocker (metoprolol) to thrombolytic therapy was studied.[641] Although recurrent ischemia and reinfarction were reduced by immediate intravenous versus delayed use of metoprolol, mortality was not reduced nor was ventricular function improved. Thus, immediate intravenous beta blockade, although clinically beneficial, may not enhance salvage of myocardium in the setting of early reperfusion but may confer clinical benefit by means of its antiischemic effect.[475]

RECOMMENDATIONS. Given the overall favorable effects of beta blockade in the aforementioned clinical trials, patients in a hyperdynamic state (sinus tachycardia, hypertension, no evidence of heart failure or bronchospasm) as well as patients seen in the first 4 hours appear to be good candidates for this therapy, regardless of whether or not thrombolytic therapy is employed. Unless there are contraindications (see p. 1978), beta blockade probably should be continued in patients who develop AMI. In addition, beta blockers are indicated in patients in whom infarction is complicated by persistent or recurrent ischemic pain, progressive or repetitive serum enzyme elevations suggestive of infarct extension, or tachyarrhythmias early after the onset of infarction. If adverse effects of beta blockers develop or if patients present with complications of infarction that are contraindications to beta blockade such as heart failure or heart block, the beta blocker should be withheld.

SELECTION OF BETA BLOCKER. Favorable effects have been reported with atenolol, timolol, and alprenolol; these benefits probably occur with propranolol and with esmolol, an

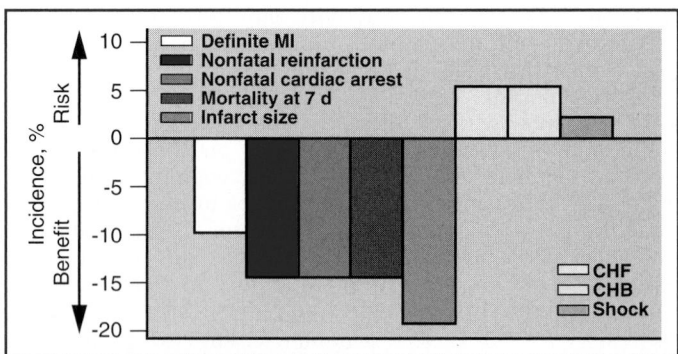

FIGURE 37–31. Results of intravenous beta blockade in acute MI: Acute phase of treatment. The benefits of beta blockers given intravenously followed by oral administration for 1 week in patients with suspected AMI include reductions in the rate of development of definite MI, in the incidence of nonfatal reinfarction and cardiac arrest, mortality at 7 days, and infarct size. In appropriately selected patients — i.e., those with a heart rate 60 beats/min or higher, systolic blood pressure 100 mm Hg or more, P-R interval less than 0.24 sec, rales in less than one-third of the lung field, and no history of bronchospastic lung disease—the risks for congestive heart failure (CHF), complete heart block (CHB), and cardiogenic shock are acceptably low. (Adapted from data in Yusuf, S.: The use of beta-blockers in the acute phase of myocardial infarction. *In* Califf, R. M., and Wagner, C. S. [eds.]: Acute Coronary Care 1986. Boston, Martinus Nijhoff, 1985, pp. 73–88.)

ultrashort-acting agent, as well. In the absence of any favorable evidence supporting the benefit of agents with intrinsic sympathomimetic activity (ISA), such as pindolol and oxprenolol, and with some unfavorable evidence for these agents in secondary prevention,[748] beta blockers with ISA probably should not be chosen for treatment of AMI. Occasionally the clinician may wish to proceed with beta blocker therapy even in the presence of relative contraindications, such as a history of mild asthma, mild bradycardia, mild heart failure, or first-degree heart block. In this situation, a trial of esmolol may help determine whether the patient can tolerate beta blockade.[416,748] Because the hemodynamic effects of this drug, with a half-life of 9 minutes, disappear in less than 30 minutes, it offers considerable advantage over longer-acting agents when the risk of a beta blocker complication is relatively high.

ACE Inhibitors

In 1992, with the publication of the SAVE trial,[749] ACE inhibitors were established as an important addition to the list of treatments for AMI. The rationale for their use includes experimental and clinical evidence of a favorable impact on ventricular remodeling, improvement in hemodynamics, and reductions in congestive heart failure.[84,171,425,750] There is now unequivocal evidence from eight randomized, placebo-controlled mortality trials collectively enrolling over 100,000 patients, that ACE inhibitors reduce death from AMI.[751] These eight trials may be grouped into two categories. The first *selected* AMI patients for randomization, based on features indicative of increased mortality such as left ventricular ejection fraction less than 40 per cent,[749] clinical signs and symptoms of congestive heart failure,[752] anterior location of infarction,[753] and abnormal wall motion score index[754] (Fig. 37–32). The second group were *unselective* trials that randomized all patients with AMI provided they had a minimum systolic pressure of approximately 100 mm Hg (ISIS-4 and GISSI-3 as shown in Figure 37–33; CONSENSUS II[755] and Chinese Captopril Study[756]). With the exception of the SMILE trial,[753] all of the selective trials initiated ACE inhibitor therapy between 3 and 16 days after AMI and maintained it for 1 to 4 years, whereas the unselective trials all initiated treatment within the first 24 to 36 hours and maintained it for only 4 to 6 weeks.

A consistent survival benefit was observed in all of the trials already noted, except for CONSENSUS II, the one study that utilized an intravenous preparation early in the course of AMI.[755] Estimates of the mortality benefit of ACE inhibitors in the unselective, short duration of therapy trials was 5 per 1000 patients treated. Recent analysis of these unselective short-term trials indicates that approximately one-third of the lives saved occurred within the first 1 to 2 days.[751] Not unexpectedly, greater survival benefits of 42 to 76 lives saved per 1000 patients treated were obtained in the selective, long duration of therapy trials. Of note, there was generally a 20 per cent reduction in the risk of death attributable to ACE inhibitor treatment in the selective trials. The mortality reduction with ACE inhibitors is accompanied by significant reductions in the development of congestive heart failure, supporting the underlying pathophysiological rationale for administering this class of drugs in AMI.[749,752,754,757] In addition, some data suggest that ischemic events, including recurrent infarction and the need for coronary revascularization, can also be reduced by chronic administration of ACE inhibitors after an AMI.[758]

The mortality benefits of ACE inhibitors are additive to those achieved with aspirin and beta blockers.[749,757] Thus, ACE inhibitors should not be considered a substitute for these other therapies with proven benefit in AMI patients. The benefits of ACE inhibition appear to be a class effect because mortality and morbidity have been reduced by several agents. However, to replicate these benefits in clinical

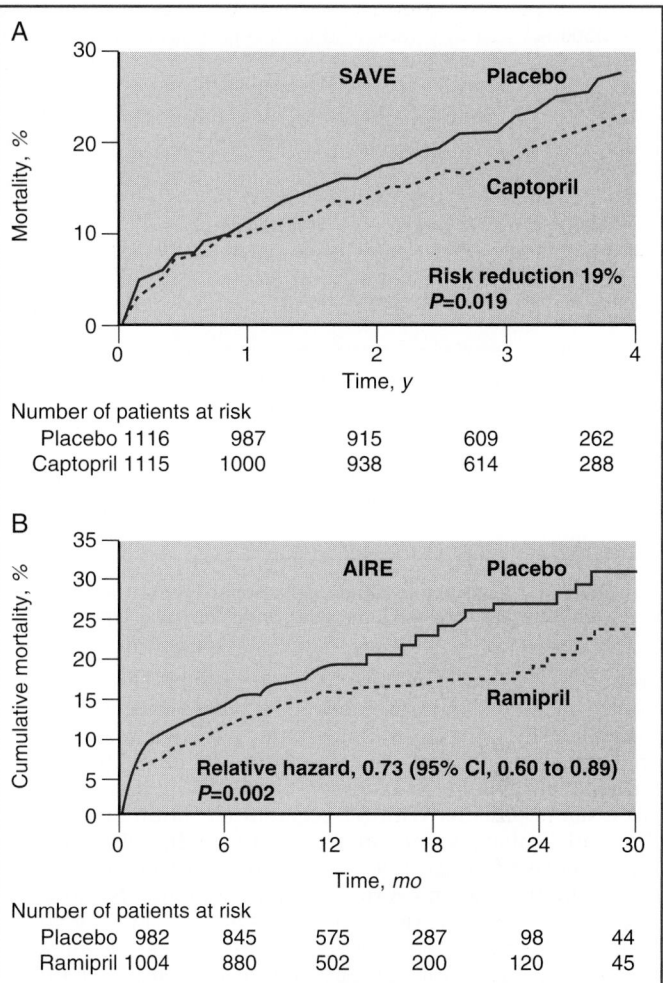

FIGURE 37–32. Benefits of long-term administration of angiotensin-converting enzyme (ACE) inhibitors to patients with AMI who have clinical evidence of left ventricular dysfunction. Among patients given active therapy (either captopril or ramipril) in the SAVE (Survival and Ventricular Enlargement) Trial (*A*) and the AIRE (Acute Infarction Ramipril Efficacy) Study (*B*), long-term mortality was reduced approximately 25 per cent. Additional benefits of ACE inhibitor therapy included reductions in recurrent hospitalizations for congestive heart failure and recurrent MI (not shown). (*A* adapted from Pfeffer, M. A., Braunwald, E., Moye, L. A., et al., on behalf of the SAVE Investigators: Effect of captopril on mortality and morbidity in patients with left ventricular dysfunction after myocardial infarction: Results of the Survival and Ventricular Enlargement Trial. N. Engl. J. Med. 327:669, 1992; *B* adapted from The Acute Ramipril Efficacy [AIRE] Study Investigators: Effect of ramipril on mortality and morbidity of survivors of acute myocardial infarction with clinical evidence of heart failure. Lancet 342:821, 1993. © by The Lancet Ltd.)

practice, physicians should select a specific agent and prescribe the drug according to the protocols utilized in the successful clinical trials reported to date.

The major *contraindications* to the use of ACE inhibitors in AMI include hypotension in the setting of adequate preload, known hypersensitivity, and pregnancy. Adverse reactions include hypotension, especially after the first dose, and intolerable cough with chronic dosing; much less commonly angioedema can occur (see p. 474).

RECOMMENDATIONS FOR USE OF ACE INHIBITORS. After administration of aspirin, initiating reperfusion strategies and where appropriate beta blockade (see p. 1228), *all* AMI patients should be considered for ACE inhibition therapy. Although there is little disagreement that high-risk AMI patients (elderly, anterior infarction, prior infarction, Killip class II or greater, and asymptomatic patients with evidence of depressed global ventricular function on an imaging study) should receive life-long treatment with ACE inhibitors,[425,759] short term (4 to 6 weeks) therapy to a broader

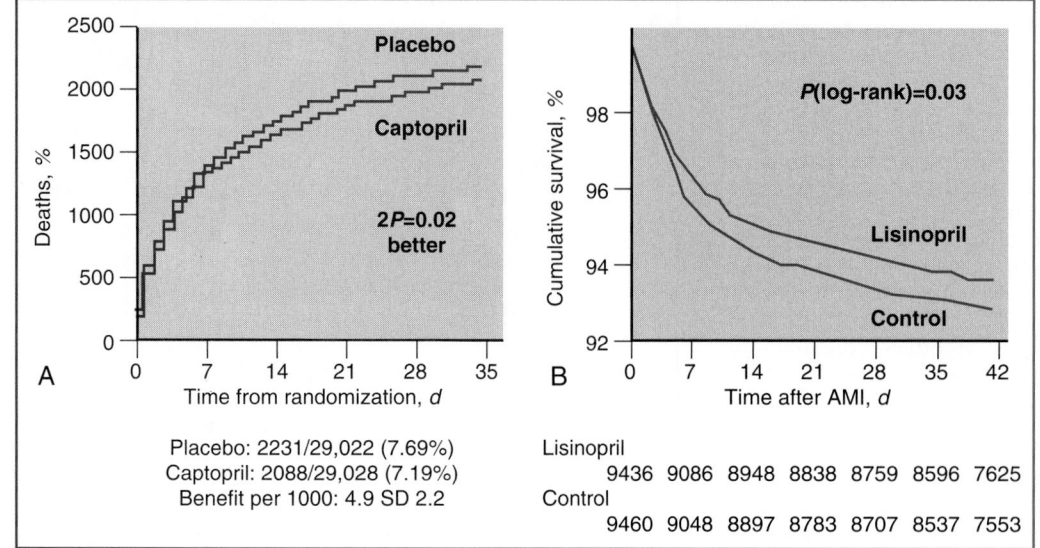

FIGURE 37-33. Results of treatment with angiotensin-converting enzyme (ACE) inhibitors after MI. Two trials of acute therapy in unselected patients (i.e., both with and without evidence of left ventricular dysfunction) have shown that ACE inhibitors reduce mortality at 4 to 6 weeks. This effect was seen in two different patient populations and with two different ACE inhibitors, captopril (*A*) and lisinopril (*B*), attesting to the consistency and general applicability of the observations. (Adapted from ISIS-4 [Fourth International Study of Infarct Survival] Collaborative Group: A randomized factorial trial assessing early oral captopril, oral mononitrate, and intravenous magnesium sulphate in 5850 patients with suspected acute myocardial infarction. Lancet *345:*669, 1995; and Gruppo Italiano per lo Studio della Sopravvivenza nell'Infarto Miocardico: GISSI-3: Effects of lisinopril and transdermal glyceryl trinitrate singly and together on 6-week mortality and ventricular function after acute myocardial infarction. Lancet *343:*1115, 1994. © by The Lancet Ltd.)

group of patients has also been proposed based on the pooled results of the unselective mortality trials.[18,760,761]

Considering all the available data, we favor a strategy of an initial trial of oral ACE inhibitors in all AMI patients with congestive heart failure as well as in hemodynamically stable patients with ST-segment elevation or left bundle branch block, commencing within the first 24 hours. In the absence of congestive heart failure, we do *not* recommend their use in AMI patients without ST-segment changes or only ST segment depression on ECG. Prior to hospital discharge, left ventricular function should be evaluated. ACE inhibition therapy should be continued indefinitely in patients with congestive heart failure, evidence of a reduction in global function, or a large regional wall motion abnormality. In patients without these findings at discharge, ACE inhibitors may be discontinued.

Nitrates
(See also p. 1211)

Sublingual nitroglycerin very rarely opens occluded coronary arteries. However, in patients with AMI the potential for reductions in ventricular filling pressures, wall tension, and cardiac work coupled with improvement in coronary blood flow, especially in ischemic zones,[762] and antiplatelet effects[763] make nitrates a logical and attractive pharmacological intervention in AMI.[764-766]

In patients with AMI, the administration of nitroglycerin and other nitrates such as isosorbide dinitrate reduces pulmonary capillary wedge pressure and systemic arterial pressure, left ventricular chamber volume, infarct size,[767,768] and the incidence of mechanical complications.[768] As with other interventions to spare ischemic myocardium in AMI, intravenous nitroglycerin appears to be of greatest benefit in patients treated earliest.[768]

CLINICAL TRIAL RESULTS. In the prethrombolytic era, 10 randomized trials of acute administration of intravenous nitroglycerin (or nitroprusside, another nitric oxide donor) collectively enrolled 2042 patients. A meta-analysis of these trial results showed a reduction in mortality of 35 per cent associated with nitrate therapy.[769]

In the thrombolytic era two megatrials of nitrate therapy have been conducted—GISSI-3[757] and ISIS-4.[761] In GISSI-3, there was no independent effect of nitrates on short-term mortality.[757] Similarly, in ISIS-4, no effect of a mononitrate on 35-day mortality was observed. A pooled analysis of over 80,000 patients treated with nitrate-like preparations intravenously or orally in 22 trials revealed a mortality rate

of 7.7 per cent in the control group, which was reduced to 7.4 per cent in the nitrate group. These data are consistent with a small treatment effect of nitrates on mortality such that 3 to 4 fewer deaths would occur for every 1000 patients treated.[761]

NITRATE PREPARATIONS AND MODE OF ADMINISTRATION. Intravenous nitroglycerin can be administered safely to patients with evolving MI as long as the dose is titrated carefully to avoid induction of reflex tachycardia or systemic arterial hypotension.[770] Patients with inferior wall infarction are particularly sensitive to an excessive fall in preload, particularly if concurrent right ventricular infarction is present.[771] In such cases nitrate-induced venodilatation could impair cardiac output and reduce coronary block flow, thus worsening myocardial oxygenation rather than improving it.[772]

A useful regimen employs an initial infusion rate of 5 to 10 μg/min with increases of 5 to 20 μg/min until the mean arterial blood pressure is reduced by 10 per cent of its baseline level in normotensive patients and by 30 per cent for hypertensive patients, but in no case below a systolic pressure of 90 mm Hg.[764,768] Alternatively, nitroglycerin may be administered as a sustained-release oral preparation (30 to 60 mg/day) or as an ointment (1 to 3 inches every 6 to 8 hours for patients with a systolic pressure greater than 120 mm Hg). Nitroglycerin can also be given sublingually at doses of 0.3 to 0.6 mg. This route may be more hazardous because the rate of absorption is difficult to control and arterial pressure may decline precipitously.

ADVERSE EFFECTS. Clinically significant methemoglobinemia has been reported to occur during administration of intravenous nitroglycerin.[773] Although uncommon, this problem is seen when unusually large doses of nitrates are administered. It is important not only for its potential to cause symptoms of lethargy and headache but also because elevated methemoglobin levels can impair the oxygen-carrying capacity of blood, potentially exacerbating ischemia. Dilatation of the pulmonary vasculature supplying poorly ventilated lung segments may produce a ventilation-perfusion mismatch.

Tolerance to intravenous nitroglycerin (as manifested by increasing nitrate requirements) develops in many patients, often as soon as 12 hours after the infusion is started.[774] Despite the theoretical and demonstrated benefit of sulfhydryl agents in diminishing tolerance, their use has not become widespread.[775]

RECOMMENDATIONS FOR NITRATES IN AMI. Nitroglycerin is indicated for the relief of persistent pain and as a vasodilator in patients with infarction associated with left ventricular failure. In the absence of recurrent angina or congestive heart failure, we do not routinely prescribe them in AMI patients. Higher-risk patients such as those with large transmural infarctions, especially of the anterior wall, have the most to gain from nitrates in terms of reduction of ventricular remodeling, and we therefore routinely use intravenous nitrates for 24 to 48 hours in such patients. There is no clear benefit to empirical long-term cutaneous or oral nitrates in the asymptomatic patient, and we therefore do not prescribe nitrates beyond the first 48 hours unless angina or ventricular failure is present.

Calcium Antagonists
(See also p. 1978)

Despite sound experimental and clinical evidence of an antiischemic effect,[776] calcium antagonists have *not* been found to be helpful in the acute phase of AMI, and concern has been raised in several systematic overviews about an increased risk of mortality when they are prescribed on a routine basis to AMI patients.[414,417,418] Perhaps in response to the lack of compelling data showing a beneficial effect and concerns about the risk of excess mortality coupled with more convincing evidence of benefit from aspirin and beta blockers, many clinicians have decreased their use of calcium antagonists in the setting of AMI.[12,40,41,45] A distinction should be made between the dihydropyridine type of calcium antagonists (e.g., nifedipine) and the nondihydropyridine calcium antagonists (e.g., verapamil and diltiazem).[417,777,777a]

NIFEDIPINE. In multiple trials involving a total of over 5000 patients, the immediate-release preparation of nifedipine has not shown any reduction in infarct size,[778–781] prevention of progression to infarction,[778,780] control of recurrent ischemia,[780] or lowering of mortality.[782] When trials of the immediate-release form of nifedipine are pooled in a meta-analysis, evidence suggests a dose-related increased risk of in-hospital mortality (especially above 80 mg of nifedipine),[418,783] although posthospital mortality does not appear to be increased in nifedipine-treated patients.[784,785] Nifedipine does not appear to be helpful in conjunction with either thrombolytic therapy[786] or beta blockade.[779,787] A potential mechanism by which the immediate release form of nifedipine may be harmful in AMI is coronary hypoperfusion due to an abrupt fall in systolic pressure from peripheral vasodilatation. The abrupt fall in arterial pressure may also provoke a reflex action of the renin-angiotensin system and sympathetic discharge that produces tachycardia.[776] Thus, we do not recommend use of immediate-release nifedipine early in the treatment of AMI. No trials of the sustained-release preparations of nifedipine in AMI have been reported to date.

VERAPAMIL AND DILTIAZEM. When administered during the acute phase of AMI, these drugs have not had any demonstrated favorable effect on infarct size or other important endpoints in patients with AMI, with the exception of control of supraventricular arrhythmias.[782,788] Although the possibility has been raised that verapamil and diltiazem in the first few days following AMI may be helpful in preventing reinfarction in patients with non-Q-wave infarction,[788–791] the data supporting this contention are not statistically robust and require further evaluation in future studies. Subgroup analyses of MDPIT and DAVIT-II trials with both diltiazem and verapamil have suggested that mortality is reduced in patients free of heart failure in the CCU.[792,793] These subgroup analyses must be interpreted with caution because in the MDPIT study about 50 per cent of patients in the placebo and diltiazem groups were also receiving beta blockers that may have contributed to the observed mortality reduction[792]; and in the DAVIT-II study patients with an indication for beta blockers were excluded from the trial.[793] Furthermore, both the MDPIT and DAVIT-

II studies were conducted in an era when aspirin, ACE inhibitors, and early use of coronary angiography for recurrent ischemia were not as common as they are now. Thus, based on the available data, we do *not* recommend the routine use of either verapamil or diltiazem in AMI regardless of whether it is believed that the patient is suffering from a Q-wave or non-Q-wave infarction. Their use should be avoided in patients with Killip class II or greater hemodynamic findings.

Magnesium

Patients with AMI may have a total body deficit of magnesium because of a low dietary intake, advanced age, or prior diuretic use. They may also acquire a functional deficit of available magnesium due to trapping of free magnesium in adipocytes, as soaps are formed when free fatty acids are released by catecholamine-induced lipolysis with the onset of infarction.[794–796] Myocardial and urinary losses of magnesium that occur during AMI may increase a patient's magnesium requirement. The magnesium cation serves as a critical cofactor in over 300 intracellular enzymatic processes, including several that are integrally involved in mitochondrial function, energy production, maintenance of trans-sarcolemmal ionic gradients, cell volume control, and resting membrane potential.[794,797,798] Experimental models of AMI in at least four different animal species have shown that supplemental administration of magnesium before coronary occlusion, during occlusion, coincident with reperfusion, or for a short time interval (15 to 45 minutes) after reperfusion reduces infarct size and prevents myocardial stunning due to reperfusion injury.[459] However, delayed administration of magnesium beyond a very short interval (15 to 60 minutes) following reperfusion is no longer effective in reducing myocardial damage.[459]

Since 1984, several trials of routine supplemental administration of intravenous magnesium in patients with suspected AMI have been conducted. By 1992 about 1300 patients had been randomized, and meta-analyses of the seven trials conducted to that point suggested that patients who received magnesium had a 45 per cent lower risk of mortality.[7,799] In 1992, the LIMIT-2 trial reported a 24 per cent reduction in mortality at 28 days in patients treated with magnesium compared with placebo (Fig. 37–34). This mortality reduction appeared to be mediated through a re-

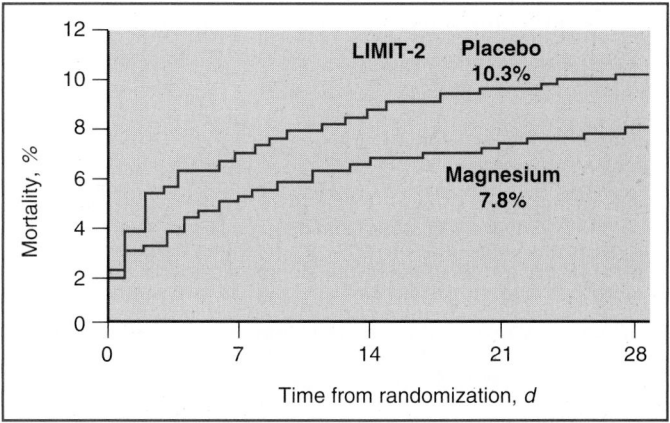

FIGURE 37–34. Results of intravenous (IV) magnesium therapy in acute MI. Two trials of magnesium conducted in the thrombolytic era. In LIMIT-2 (Second Leicester Intravenous Magnesium Intervention Trial), magnesium was administered relatively early and concurrently with thrombolytic agents in the 36 per cent of patients who received thrombolytic therapy. A 24 per cent reduction in mortality was seen at 28 days in patients treated with magnesium. (Adapted from Woods, K. L., Fletcher, S., Roffe, C., et al.: Intravenous magnesium sulphate in suspected acute myocardial infarction: results of the Second Leicester Intravenous Magnesium Intervention Trial [LIMIT 2]. Lancet *339*:1553, 1992. © by The Lancet Ltd.)

duction in congestive heart failure. Long-term follow-up of LIMIT-2 revealed a 20 per cent reduction in ischemic heart disease–related mortality over an average of 4.5 years.[800,801]

Unexpectedly, the ISIS-4 trial reported no effect of magnesium on 35-day mortality.[761] However, concern about interpretation has been raised over the low overall mortality of the control group in ISIS-4 (due to widespread use of aspirin and administration of thrombolytics to 75 per cent of patients) and the late administration of magnesium after pharmacological reperfusion and markedly delayed treatment (median of 12 hours) in patients who did not receive thrombolytic therapy.[459,800–802] Thus, despite the 58,050 patients randomized in ISIS-4, it is not clear that serum magnesium levels were elevated at the time of reperfusion in the cohort of patients randomized to magnesium or in any subgroup of them. Because of the trivial cost of magnesium, its ease of administration, its widespread availability, and the fact that it has the potential to reduce mortality in high-risk AMI patients (e.g., elderly patients who are not candidates for thrombolysis), another large-scale, randomized, multicenter trial (MAGIC)[459] is planned to define more explicitly the role of magnesium in AMI.

RECOMMENDATIONS. Because of the risk of cardiac arrhythmias when electrolyte deficits are present in the early phase of infarction, all patients with AMI should have a serum magnesium measurement on admission. We advocate repleting magnesium deficits to maintain a serum magnesium level of 2.0 mEq/liter or more. In the presence of hypokalemia (<4.0 mEq/liter) during the course of treatment of AMI, the serum magnesium should be rechecked and repleted if necessary because it is often difficult to correct a potassium deficit in the presence of a concurrent magnesium deficit. Episodes of torsades de pointes (see p. 684) should be treated with 1 to 2 gm of magnesium delivered as a bolus over about 5 minutes. Although routine early (ideally <6 hours from the onset of chest pain) supplemental magnesium administration may be helpful in certain high-risk patients such as the elderly or those for whom reperfusion therapy is contraindicated,[803] additional data are needed before definite recommendations regarding patient selection and dosing can be made. There does not appear to be any benefit to routine late (>6 hours) administration of magnesium to patients with uncomplicated AMI who do not have electrolyte deficits.

Because it may cause vasodilation and hypotension, magnesium infusions should not be administered in patients with a systolic pressure less than 80 to 90 mm Hg. Patients with renal failure may not excrete magnesium normally and should not be considered candidates for supplemental magnesium infusions.

Other Approaches

GLUCOSE-INSULIN-POTASSIUM. Administration of a solution of glucose-insulin-potassium (300 gm of glucose, 50 units of insulin, and 80 mEq of KCl in 1000 ml of water administered at a rate of 1.5 ml/kg/hr) lowers the concentration of plasma free fatty acids and improves ventricular performance, as reflected in systolic arterial pressure, cardiac output, and stroke work at any level of left ventricular filling pressure[804]; also the frequency of ventricular premature beats decreases.[805] In a nonrandomized study, mortality appeared to be reduced,[806] hemodynamics improved, global ejection fraction increased, and both asynergy in the ischemic zone and pulmonary artery diastolic pressure reduced.[805] However, no definitive effect on enzymatically estimated infarct size or long-term mortality has been described in a prospective, controlled, randomized trial.[805]

The DIGAMI (Diabetes Mellitus Insulin-Glucose Infusion in Acute Myocardial Infarction) Study reported a significant 30 per cent relative

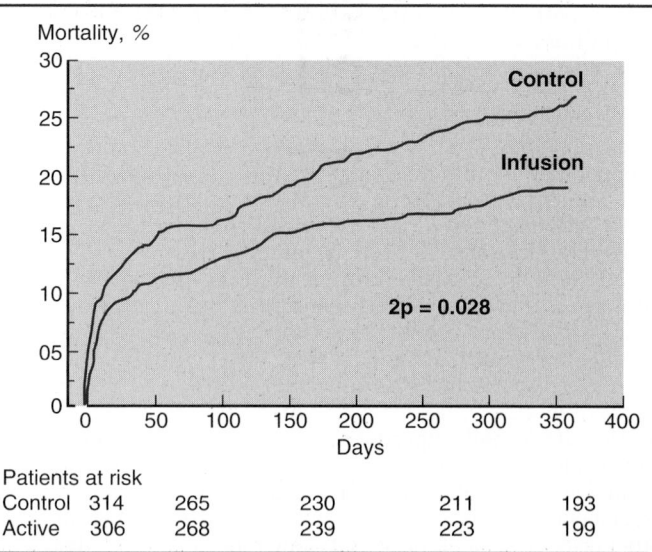

FIGURE 37–35. Actuarial mortality curves in patients receiving insulin-glucose infusion and in controls of the Diabetes Mellitus Insulin-Glucose Infusion in Acute Myocardial Infarction (DIGAMI) study during 1 year of follow-up. Numbers below graph indicate the number of patients at different times of observation. Active = patients receiving infusion. (From Malmberg, K., Ryden, L., Efendic, S., et al.: Randomized trial of insulin-glucose infusion followed by subcutaneous insulin treatment in diabetic patients with acute myocardial infarction (DIGAMI Study): Effects on mortality at 1 year. Reprinted with permission from the American College of Cardiology. J. Am. Coll. Cardiol. 26:57, 1995.)

decrease in mortality at 1 year in diabetics with AMI who received a strict regimen of an insulin-glucose infusion for 24 hours, followed by 3 months of subcutaneous injections of insulin four times daily as compared with standard therapy[807] (Fig. 37–35). Thus, "infusions of glucose-insulin-potassium (GIK) may provide necessary metabolic support for the ischemic myocardium; this may be particularly important in patients with large anterior infarcts and cardiogenic shock."[192,193]

INTRAAORTIC BALLOON COUNTERPULSATION (see also p. 1239). From a theoretical standpoint, intraaortic balloon counterpulsation might be expected to limit infarct size for several reasons. In experimental animals, intraaortic balloon counterpulsation decreases preload, increases coronary blood flow, and improves cardiac performance. No definitive information is available indicating that intraaortic balloon counterpulsation alters the prognosis in patients with relatively uncomplicated infarction. Leinbach et al., however, have reported an immediate, persistent fall in ST-segment elevation. This occurred in patients with anterior MI who had preservation of precordial R waves and good ventricular function,[808] in whom the left anterior descending coronary artery was not totally occluded and who underwent intraaortic balloon pumping within 6 hours.

Given the relatively frequent rate of complications[809] after intraaortic balloon insertion and the absence of convincing data for infarct size reduction, intraaortic balloon pumping should be reserved for hemodynamically compromised patients and for those with refractory ischemia. Although noninvasive external forms of counterpulsation have been developed, these approaches have not been rigorously studied in patients with AMI.

OTHER AGENTS. Oxygen-derived free radicals are abundant in ischemic tissue and may contribute to myocardial injury, particularly following reperfusion (see p. 1214). Although evidence from studies in animals suggested that the extent of myocardial necrosis and postischemic dysfunction can be affected favorably by treatment with oxygen free radical scavengers such as superoxide dismutase,[435,467] initial results in patients have not been encouraging.[468] Alternative forms of antioxidant therapy including vitamins E and C are being studied in experimental animals, but there is uncertainty about their potential role in patients.[810–812] Given the important role that nitric oxide (NO) plays in regulating platelet activation, interest has arisen in developing techniques for increasing NO production or providing exogenous NO donors in the setting of AMI other than the nitrates discussed above.[527,813]

HEMODYNAMIC ASSESSMENT

In patients with clinically uncomplicated AMI, invasive hemodynamic monitoring is not necessary because the status of the circulation can be assessed by careful clinical evaluation. This ordinarily consists of monitoring of heart rate and rhythm, repeated measurement of systemic arterial pressure by cuff, obtaining chest roentgenograms to detect heart failure, careful and repeated auscultation of the lung fields for pulmonary congestion, measurement of urine flow, examination of the skin and mucous membranes for evidence of the adequacy of perfusion, and arterial sampling for pO_2, PCO_2, and pH when hypoxemia or metabolic acidosis is suspected.

In contrast, in patients with AMI whose ventricular contractile performance is not normal, it is important to assess the degree of hemodynamic compromise in order to initiate therapy with drugs such as vasodilators and diuretics. In the past, central venous or right atrial pressure was used to gauge the degree of left ventricular failure in patients with AMI. However, this technique is fraught with error because central venous pressure actually reflects right rather than left ventricular function. Right ventricular function and therefore systemic venous pressure may be normal or nearly so in patients with significant left ventricular failure.[814] Conversely, patients with right ventricular failure due to right ventricular infarction or pulmonary embolism may exhibit elevated right atrial and central venous pressures despite normal left ventricular function.[813] Low values for right atrial and central venous pressures imply hypovolemia, whereas elevated right atrial pressures usually result from right ventricular failure secondary to left ventricular failure, pulmonary hypertension, or right ventricular infarction, or less commonly from tricuspid regurgitation or pericardial tamponade.

Major advances in the management of AMI have resulted from the hemodynamic monitoring that has become widespread in CCUs[816–818a] (Table 37–7). This often consists of both an intraarterial catheter and a pulmonary artery catheter for measurement of pulmonary artery, pulmonary artery occlusive (equivalent to pulmonary wedge), and right atrial pressures, and cardiac output by thermodilution. In patients with hypotension, a Foley catheter provides accurate and continuous measurement of urine output.

TABLE 37–7 INDICATIONS FOR HEMODYNAMIC MONITORING OF ACUTE MYOCARDIAL INFARCTION

Management of complicated AMI
  Hypovolemia vs. cardiogenic shock
  Ventricular septal rupture vs. acute mitral regurgitation
  Severe left ventricular failure
  Right ventricular failure
Refractory ventricular tachycardia
Differentiating severe pulmonary disease from left ventricular failure
Assessment of cardiac tamponade
Assessment of therapy in *selected* individuals
  Afterload reduction in patients with severe left ventricular failure
  Inotropic agent therapy
  Beta blocker therapy
  Temporary pacing (ventricular vs. atrioventricular)
  Intraaortic balloon counterpulsation
  Mechanical ventilation

From Gore, J. M., and Zwernet, P. L.: Hemodynamic monitoring of acute myocardial infarction. *In* Francis, G. S., and Alpert, J. S. (eds.): Modern Coronary Care. Boston, Little, Brown & Co., 1990, p. 138.

NEED FOR INVASIVE MONITORING. The use of invasive hemodynamic monitoring[814] is based on the following principal factors:

1. Difficulty of interpreting clinical and radiographic findings of pulmonary congestion because of phase lags, such as those occurring after diuretic therapy. Severe depression of cardiac index and/or elevation of left ventricular filling pressure may be unsuspected in as many as 15 per cent of patients when estimates are based exclusively on clinical criteria.[814]

2. Need for identifying noncardiac causes of arterial hypotension, particularly hypovolemia.

3. Possible contribution of reduced ventricular compliance to impaired hemodynamics, requiring judicious adjustment of intravascular volume to optimize left ventricular filling pressure.

4. Difficulty in assessing the severity and sometimes even determining the presence of lesions such as mitral regurgitation and ventricular septal defect when the cardiac output or the systemic pressures are depressed.

5. Establishing a baseline of hemodynamic measurements and guiding therapy in patients with clinically apparent pulmonary edema or cardiogenic shock.

6. Underestimation of systemic arterial pressure by the cuff method in patients with intense vasoconstriction.

The prognosis and the clinical status are related to both the cardiac output and the pulmonary artery wedge pressure. Patients with normal cardiac output after AMI have an extremely low expected mortality; prognosis worsens as cardiac output declines. Patients with intraventricular conduction defects, atrioventricular (AV) block, or both after anterior infarction have lower cardiac indices and higher pulmonary capillary wedge pressures than do patients without these conduction disturbances. On the other hand, patients with these conduction defects and inferior MI usually do not demonstrate such hemodynamic abnormalities.

PULMONARY ARTERY PRESSURE MONITORING. Patients most likely to benefit from pulmonary artery catheter monitoring include those whose AMI is complicated by (1) hypotension that is not easily corrected by fluid administration; (2) hypotension in the presence of congestive heart failure; (3) hemodynamic compromise severe enough to require intravenous vasopressors or vasodilators or intraaortic balloon counterpulsation; (4) mechanical lesions (or suspected ones) such as cardiac tamponade, severe mitral regurgitation, and a ruptured ventricular septum[819]; and (5) right ventricular infarction.[105] Other indications for hemodynamic monitoring include assessment of the effects of mechanical ventilation, differentiating pulmonary disease from left ventricular failure as the cause of hypoxemia, and management of septic shock[30] (Table 37–7).

Before inserting a pulmonary artery catheter into a patient with an AMI, the physician must decide that the potential benefit of the information to be obtained outweighs any potential risks. Major complications from pulmonary artery catheters are relatively rare (about 3 to 5 per cent of cases),[818] but severe problems can occur, including sepsis, pulmonary infarction, and pulmonary artery rupture. By minimizing the duration of catheterization and by strict adherence to aseptic techniques, risk can be diminished.[819]

Accurate determination of hemodynamics by clinical assessment is difficult in critically ill patients. The use of a pulmonary artery catheter often leads to important changes in therapy which would not have occurred if the hemodynamic information had not been available.[820] Some believe, however, that the pulmonary artery catheter is often overused. It has been suggested that until clinical trials assess-

TABLE 37-8   HEMODYNAMIC CLASSIFICATIONS OF PATIENTS WITH ACUTE MYOCARDIAL INFARCTION

A. BASED ON CLINICAL EXAMINATION[a]		B. BASED ON INVASIVE MONITORING[b]	
Class	Definition	Subset	Definition
I	Rales and S3 absent	I	Normal hemodynamics PCWP <18, CI >2.2
II	Rales over <50% of lung	II	Pulmonary congestion PCWP >18, CI <2.2
III	Rales over >50% of lung fields (pulmonary edema)	III	Peripheral hypoperfusion PCWP <18, CI >2.2
IV	Shock	IV	Pulmonary congestion and peripheral hypoperfusion PCWP >18, CI <2.2

Modified from (a) Killip, T. and Kimball, J.: Treatment of myocardial infarction in a coronary care unit. A two year experience with 250 patients. Am. J. Cardiol. *20*:457, 1967; and (b) Forrester, J., Diamond, G., Chatterjee, K., et al.: Medical therapy of acute myocardial infarction by the application of hemodynamic subsets. N. Engl. J. Med. *295*:1356, 1976.
PCWP = pulmonary capillary wedge pressure; CI = cardiac index.

ing its benefit are performed, the use of this technique should be curbed.[821,822] (At least one such trial has suggested that complications and mortality are actually higher in patients who received pulmonary artery catheterization,[823] although such patients might have been at higher risk initially.) These observations emphasize the importance of patient selection, meticulous technique, and correct interpretation of the data obtained.

Hemodynamic Abnormalities

In 1976, Swan, Forrester, and their associates measured the cardiac output and wedge pressure simultaneously in a large series of patients with AMI and identified four major hemodynamic subsets of patients (Table 37-8): (1) patients with normal perfusion and without pulmonary congestion (normal cardiac output and normal wedge pressure); (2) patients with normal perfusion and pulmonary congestion (normal cardiac output and elevated wedge pressure); (3) patients with decreased perfusion but without pulmonary congestion (reduced cardiac output and normal wedge pressure); and (4) patients with decreased perfusion and pulmonary congestion (reduced cardiac output and elevated wedge pressure).[817] This classification, which overlaps with a crude clinical classification proposed earlier by Killip and Kimball (Table 37-8), has proved to be quite useful, but it should be noted that patients frequently pass from one category to another with therapy and sometimes apparently even spontaneously.

HEMODYNAMIC SUBSETS. These are usually reflected in the patient's clinical status. Hypoperfusion usually becomes evident clinically when the cardiac index falls below approximately 2.2 liters/min/m², whereas pulmonary congestion is noted when the wedge pressure exceeds approximately 20 mm Hg. However, approximately 25 per cent of patients with cardiac indices less than 2.2 liters/min/m² and 15 per cent of patients with elevated

pulmonary capillary wedge pressures are not recognized clinically. Discrepancies in hemodynamic and clinical classification of patients with AMI arise for a variety of reasons. Patients may exhibit "phase lags" as clinical pulmonary congestion develops or resolves, symptoms secondary to chronic obstructive pulmonary disease may be confused with those resulting from pulmonary congestion, or long-standing left ventricular dysfunction may mask signs of hypoperfusion secondary to compensatory vasoconstriction.[817]

The hemodynamic findings shown in Tables 37-8 and 37-9 allow for rational approaches to therapy. The goals of hemodynamic therapy are to maintain ventricular performance, support blood pressure, and protect jeopardized myocardium. Because these goals occasionally may be at cross purposes, recognition of the hemodynamic profile, as assessed clinically or as available from hemodynamic monitoring, is required before optimal therapeutic interventions can be designed along the lines discussed below.

Hypotension in the Prehospital Phase

During the prehospital phase of AMI, invasive hemodynamic monitoring is not feasible, and during this period, therapy should be guided by frequent clinical assessment and measurement of arterial pressure by cuff, with the recognition that intense vasoconstriction can provide a falsely low pressure measured by this method. Hypotension associated with bradycardia often reflects excessive vagotonia. Relative or absolute hypovolemia is often present when hypotension occurs with a normal or rapid heart rate, particularly among patients receiving diuretics just prior to the occurrence of infarction. Marked diaphoresis, reduction of fluid intake, or vomiting during the period preceding and accompanying the onset of AMI may all contribute to the development of hypovolemia. Even if the effective vascular volume is normal, relative hypovolemia may be present because ventricular compliance is reduced in AMI and a

TABLE 37-9   HEMODYNAMIC PATTERNS FOR COMMON CLINICAL CONDITIONS

CARDIAC CONDITION	CHAMBER PRESSURES (mmHg)				
	RA	RV	PA	PCW	CI
Normal	0–6	25/0–6	25/0–12	6–12	≥2.5
AMI without LVF	0–6	25/0–6	30/12–18	≤18	≥2.5
AMI with LVF	0–6	30–40/0–6	30–40/18–25	>18	>2.0
Biventricular failure	>6	50–60/>6	50–60/25	18–25	>2.0
RVMI	12–20	30/12–20	30/12	≤12	<2.0
Cardiac tamponade	12–16	25/12–16	25/12–16	12–16	<2.0
Pulmonary embolism	12–20	50–60/12–20	50–60/12	<12	<2.0

From Gore, J. M. and Zwerner, P. L. Hemodynamic monitoring of acute myocardial infarction. In: Francis, G. S. and Alpert, J. S. (eds.) Modern Coronary Care, pp. 139–164, 1990. Boston, Little, Brown and Co.
AMI = acute myocardial infarction; CI = cardiac index; LVF = left ventricular failure; PA = pulmonary artery; PCW = pulmonary capillary wedge; RA = right atrium; RV = right ventricle; RVMI = right ventricular myocardial infarction.

left ventricular filling pressure as high as 20 mm Hg may be needed to provide an optimal preload.

MANAGEMENT. In the absence of rales involving more than one-third of the lung fields, the patient should be put in the reverse Trendelenburg position, and in those with sinus bradycardia and hypotension, atropine should be administered (0.3 to 0.6 mg intravenously repeated at 3- to 10-minute intervals up to 2.0 mg). If these measures do not correct the hypotension, normal saline should be administered intravenously, beginning with a bolus of 100 ml followed by 50-ml increments every 5 minutes. The patient should be carefully observed and the infusion stopped when the systolic pressure returns to approximately 100 mm Hg, if the patient becomes dyspneic, or if pulmonary rales develop or increase. Because of the poor correlation between left ventricular filling pressure and mean right atrial pressure, assessment of systemic (even central) venous pressure is of limited value as a guide to fluid therapy.

Administration of cardiotonic agents is indicated during the prehospital phase if systemic hypotension persists despite correction of hypovolemia and excessive vagotonia. In the absence of invasive hemodynamic monitoring, assessment of peripheral vascular resistance must be based on clinical observations. If cutaneous vasoconstriction is present, therapy with dobutamine, which stimulates cardiac contractility without unduly accelerating heart rate and which does not increase the impedance to ventricular outflow, may be helpful (see p. 1237). In hypotensive patients with AMI with clinical evidence of vasodilatation, an uncommon circumstance, phenylephrine hydrochloride is preferable, although this agent, which increases coronary as well as peripheral vascular tone, should be used with caution.

Hypovolemic Hypotension

Recognition of hypovolemia is of particular importance in hypotensive patients with AMI because of the hazard it poses and because of the improvement in circulatory dynamics that can be achieved so readily and safely by augmentation of vascular volume. Because hypovolemia is often occult, it is frequently overlooked in the absence of invasive hemodynamic monitoring. Hypovolemia may be absolute, with low left ventricular filling pressure (< 8 mm Hg), or relative, with normal (8 to 12 mm Hg) or even modestly increased (13 to 18 mm Hg) left ventricular filling pressures. Because of the reduction of left ventricular compliance that occurs with acute ischemia and infarction (see p. 1194), left ventricular filling pressures between 13 and 18 mm Hg, although above the upper limits of normal, may actually be suboptimal.

Exclusion of hypovolemia as the cause of hypotension requires the documentation of a reduced cardiac output despite left ventricular filling pressure exceeding 18 mm Hg. If, in a hypotensive patient, the pulmonary capillary wedge pressure (ordinarily measured as the pulmonary artery occlusive pressure) is below this level, fluid challenge should be carried out as described above. If hypovolemia is documented or suspected, the fluid replaced should resemble the fluid lost. Thus, when a low hematocrit complicates AMI, infusion of packed red blood cells or whole blood is the treatment of choice. On the other hand, crystalloid or colloid solutions should be administered when the hematocrit is normal or elevated.

Hypotension caused by right ventricular infarction may be confused with that caused by hypovolemia because both are associated with a low, normal, or minimally elevated left ventricular filling pressure. The findings and management of right ventricular infarction are discussed on page 1240.

The Hyperdynamic State

When infarction is not complicated by hemodynamic impairment, no therapy other than general supportive mea-

sures and treatment of arrhythmias is necessary. However, if the hemodynamic profile is of the hyperdynamic state, i.e., elevation of sinus rate, arterial pressure, and cardiac index, occurring singly or together in the presence of a normal or low left ventricular filling pressure, and if other causes of tachycardia such as fever, infection, and pericarditis can be excluded, treatment with beta-adrenoceptor blockers is indicated (see p. 1211). Presumably, the increased heart rate and blood pressure are the result of inappropriate activation of the sympathetic nervous system, possibly secondary to augmented release of catecholamines, pain and anxiety, or some combination of these.

LEFT VENTRICULAR FAILURE

Even in the thrombolytic era, left ventricular dysfunction remains the single most important predictor of mortality following AMI (Fig. 37–36). In patients with AMI, heart failure is characterized either by systolic dysfunction alone or by both systolic and diastolic dysfunction.[824] Left ventricular diastolic dysfunction leads to pulmonary venous hypertension and pulmonary congestion, whereas systolic dysfunction is principally responsible for a depression of cardiac output and of the ejection fraction. Clinical manifestations of left ventricular failure become more common

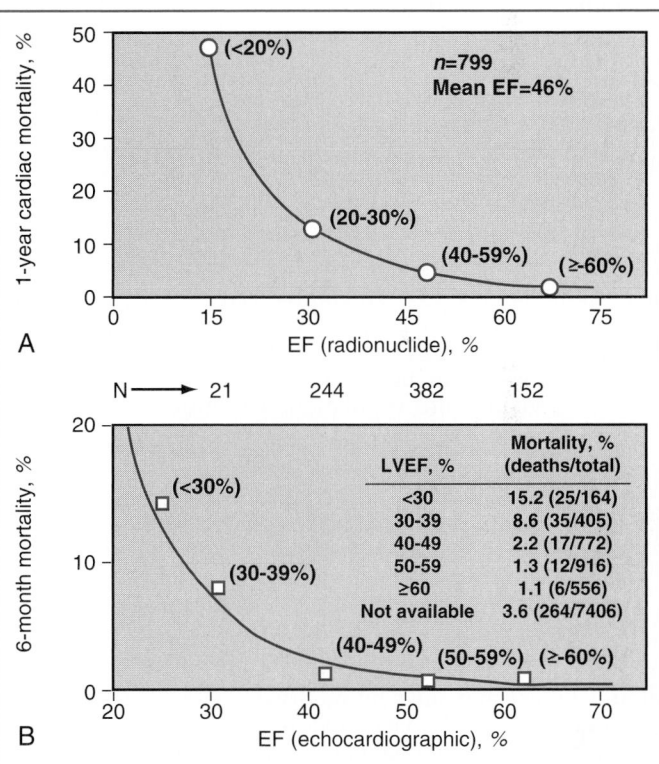

FIGURE 37–36. Impact of left ventricular (LV) function on survival following MI. The curvilinear relationship between LV ejection fraction (LVEF) is quite reproducible, whether EF is determined by the radionuclide method (*A*), as in the prethrombolytic era, or by the echocardiographic method (*B*), as in the thrombolytic era. Among patients with an LVEF below 40 per cent, mortality is markedly increased at 6 months and 1 year. Thus, interventions such as thrombolysis, aspirin, and angiotensin-converting enzyme (ACE) inhibitors should be of considerable benefit in patients with AMI to minimize the amount of LV damage and interrupt the neurohumoral activation seen with congestive heart failure. (*A* adapted from Multicenter Postinfarction Research Group: Risk stratification and survival after myocardial infarction. N. Engl. J. Med. *309*:331, 1983; *B* adapted from Volpi, A., De Vita, C., Franzosi, M. G., et al.: Determinants of 6-month mortality in survivors of myocardial infarction after thrombolysis: Results of the GISSI-2 data base. Circulation *88*:416, 1993. Copyright 1993 American Heart Association.)

as the extent of the injury to the left ventricle increases. Mortality increases in association with the severity of the hemodynamic deficit.[817]

THERAPEUTIC IMPLICATIONS. Classification of patients with AMI by hemodynamic subsets has therapeutic relevance. As already noted, patients with normal wedge pressures and hypoperfusion often benefit from infusion of fluids, because the peak value of stroke volume is usually not attained until left ventricular filling pressure reaches 18 to 24 mm Hg.[814] However, a low level of left ventricular filling pressure does not imply that left ventricular damage is necessarily slight. Such patients may be relatively hypovolemic and/or may have suffered a right ventricular infarct with or without severe left ventricular damage.[825]

The relation between ventricular filling pressure and cardiac index when preload is increased by an infusion of saline or dextran can provide valuable hemodynamic information, in addition to that obtained from baseline measurements. For example, the ventricular function curve rises steeply (marked increase in cardiac index, small increase in filling pressure) in patients with normal left ventricular function and hypovolemia, whereas the curve rises gradually or remains flat in those patients with a combination of hypovolemia and depressed cardiac function.

Invasive hemodynamic monitoring is essential to guide therapy of patients with severe left ventricular failure (pulmonary capillary wedge pressure > 18 mm Hg *and* cardiac index < 2.5 liters/min/m²).

AVOIDANCE OF HYPOXEMIA. Patients whose AMI is complicated by congestive heart failure characteristically develop hypoxemia due to a combination of pulmonary vascular engorgement (and in some cases pulmonary interstitial edema), diminished vital capacity, and respiratory depression from narcotic analgesics. Hypoxemia can impair the function of ischemic tissue at the margin of the infarct and thereby contribute to establishing or perpetuating the vicious circle (Fig. 37–14). The ventilation-perfusion mismatch that results in hypoxemia requires careful attention to ventilatory support. Increasing fractions of inspired oxygen (FiO₂) via face mask should be used initially, but if the oxygen saturation of the patient's blood cannot be maintained above 85 to 90 per cent on 100 per cent FiO₂, strong consideration should be given to endotracheal intubation with positive-pressure ventilation. The improvement of arterial oxygenation and hence myocardial oxygen supply may help to restore ventricular performance. Positive end-expiratory pressure (PEEP) may diminish systemic venous return and reduce effective left ventricular filling pressure. This may require reduction in the amount of PEEP, normal saline infusions to maintain left ventricular filling pressure, adjustment of the rate of infusion of vasodilators such as nitroglycerin, or some combination of the above. Because myocardial ischemia frequently occurs during the return to unsupported spontaneous breathing,[826] the weaning process should be accompanied by observation for signs of ischemia and is potentially facilitated by a period of intermittent mandatory ventilation before extubation. Continuous ST-segment monitoring has been recommended for these patients.[826]

When wheezing complicates pulmonary congestion, bronchodilators that act primarily on beta₂-adrenoceptors, such as isoetharine or metaproterenol, given as aerosols, or terbutaline, are more desirable than conventional bronchodilators, such as isoproterenol or epinephrine. The latter act primarily on beta₁-receptors, which, by increasing myocardial oxygen consumption, can increase ischemia.

Although positive inotropic agents may be useful, they do not represent the initial therapy of choice in patients with AMI. Instead, heart failure is managed most effectively first by reduction of ventricular preload, and then, if possible, by lowering afterload. Arrhythmias may contribute to hemodynamic compromise as discussed on page 1246 and should be treated promptly in patients with left ventricular failure.

DIURETICS (see also p. 498). Mild heart failure in patients with AMI frequently responds well to diuretics such as furosemide, administered intravenously in doses of 10 to 40 mg, repeated at 3- to 4-hour intervals if necessary. The resultant reduction of pulmonary capillary pressure reduces dyspnea, and the lowering of left ventricular wall tension that accompanies the reduction of left ventricular diastolic volume diminishes myocardial oxygen requirements and may lead to improvement of contractility and augmentation of the ejection fraction, stroke volume, and cardiac output. The reduction of elevated left ventricular filling pressure may also enhance myocardial oxygen delivery by diminishing the impedance to coronary perfusion attributable to elevated ventricular wall tension. It may also improve arterial oxygenation by reducing pulmonary vascular congestion.

The intravenous administration of furosemide reduces pulmonary vascular congestion and pulmonary venous pressure within 15 minutes, before renal excretion of sodium and water has occurred; presumably this action results from a direct dilating effect of this drug on the systemic arterial bed. It is important not to reduce left ventricular filling pressure much below 18 mm Hg, the lower range associated with optimal left ventricular performance in AMI, because this may reduce cardiac output further and cause arterial hypotension. Excessive diuresis may also result in hypokalemia, with its attendant risk of digitalis intoxication.

AFTERLOAD REDUCTION (see also p. 494). Myocardial oxygen requirements depend on left ventricular wall stress, which in turn is proportional to the product of peak developed left ventricular pressure, volume, and wall thickness. Vasodilator therapy is recommended in patients with AMI complicated by (1) heart failure unresponsive to treatment with diuretics, (2) hypertension, (3) mitral regurgitation, or (4) ventricular septal defect. In these patients, treatment with vasodilator agents increases stroke volume and may reduce myocardial oxygen requirements and thereby lessen ischemia. Hemodynamic monitoring of systemic arterial and, in many cases, pulmonary capillary wedge (or at least pulmonary artery) pressure and cardiac output in patients treated with these agents is important. Improvement of cardiac performance and energetics requires three simultaneous effects: (1) reduction of left ventricular afterload, (2) avoidance of excessive systemic arterial hypotension in order to maintain effective coronary perfusion pressure, and (3) avoidance of excessive reduction of ventricular filling pressure with consequent diminution of cardiac output. In general, pulmonary capillary wedge pressure should be maintained at approximately 20 mm Hg and arterial pressure above 90/60 mm Hg in patients who were normotensive before developing the AMI.

Vasodilator therapy is particularly useful when AMI is complicated by mitral regurgitation or rupture of the ventricular septum. In such patients, vasodilators alone or in combination with intraaortic balloon counterpulsation can sometimes serve as a "holding maneuver" and provide hemodynamic stabilization to permit definitive catheterization and angiographic studies to be carried out and to prepare the patient for early surgical intervention. Because of the precarious state of patients with complicated infarction and the need for meticulous adjustment of dosage, therapy is best initiated with agents that can be administered intravenously and that have a short duration of action, such as nitroprusside,[827,828] nitroglycerin,[829,830] or isosorbide dinitrate.[831] After initial stabilization, the medication of choice is generally an ACE inhibitor,[832] but long-acting nitrates given by mouth, sublingually, or by ointment[833] may also be useful.

Nitroglycerin. This drug has been shown in animal experiments to be less likely than nitroprusside to produce a "coronary steal," i.e., to divert blood flow from the ischemic to the nonischemic zone.[834] Therefore, apart from consideration of its routine use in AMI patients discussed earlier (see p. 1230), it may be a particularly useful vasodilator in patients with AMI complicated by left ventricular failure.[767,768,835] Ten to 15 μg/min is infused and the dose is increased by 10 μg/min every 5 minutes until (1) the desired effect (improvement of hemodynamics or relief of ischemic chest pain) is achieved or (2) a decline in systolic arterial pressure to 90 mm Hg, or by more than 15 mm Hg, has occurred. Although both nitroglycerin and nitroprusside lower systemic arterial pressure, systemic vascular resistance, and the heart rate–systolic blood pressure product, the reduction of left ventricular filling pressure is more prominent with nitroglycerin because of its relatively greater effect than nitroprusside on venous capacitance vessels. Nevertheless, in patients with severe left ventricular failure, cardiac output often increases despite the reduction in left ventricular filling pressure produced by nitroglycerin.

Oral Vasodilators. The use of oral vasodilators in the treatment of chronic congestive heart failure is discussed on page 474. In patients with AMI and persistent heart failure, long-term treatment with a converting enzyme inhibitor should be carried out. As noted on page 1229, this reduced ventricular load decreases the remodeling of the left ventricle that occurs commonly in the period after MI and thereby reduces the development of heart failure and risk of death.[83,84]

DIGITALIS (see also p. 480). Although digitalis increases the contractility and the oxygen consumption of normal hearts, when heart failure is present the diminution of heart size and wall tension frequently results in a net reduction of myocardial oxygen requirements.[836] In animal experiments it fails to improve ventricular performance immediately following experimental coronary occlusion, but salutary effects are elicited when it is administered several days later.[837] The absence of early beneficial effects may be due to the inability of ischemic tissue to respond to digitalis or the already maximal stimulation of contractility of the normal heart by circulating and neuronally released catecholamines.

Although the issue is still controversial, arrhythmias may be increased by digitalis glycosides when they are given to patients in the first few hours after the onset of MI, particularly in the absence of hypokalemia. Also, undesirable peripheral systemic and coronary vasoconstriction may result from the rapid intravenous administration of rapidly acting glycosides such as ouabain.[837]

Administration of digitalis to patients with AMI in the hospital phase should generally be reserved for the management of supraventricular tachyarrhythmias such as atrial flutter and fibrillation and of heart failure that persists despite treatment with diuretics, vasodilators, and beta-adrenoceptor agonists. There is no indication for its use as an inotropic agent in patients without clinical evidence of left ventricular dysfunction, and it is too weak an inotropic agent to be relied upon as the principal cardiac stimulant in patients with overt pulmonary edema or cardiogenic shock. It may, however, be useful as a supplement to vasodilator agents and in the treatment of persistent or recurrent left ventricular failure.[838]

Cardiac glycosides appear to become progressively more effective in the treatment of heart failure as the interval from onset of infarction lengthens; i.e., they are more effective in the treatment of chronic than of acute heart failure secondary to ischemic heart disease. Of note, in a direct comparison of captopril versus digoxin for prevention of left ventricular remodeling and dysfunction following AMI, Bonaduce and colleagues found that patients in whom captopril therapy was initiated 7 to 10 days after onset of infarction had less left ventricular remodeling and better-

preserved global left ventricular function than patients receiving digitalis.[839] In addition, the possibility that continued administration of digitalis might contribute to late mortality in the 2 years following AMI has been raised[840–844] and debated.[845,846] Although it is clear that mortality is greater in patients treated with digoxin after AMI, it is not clear that this increase in mortality is due to digoxin itself or to confounding variables that correlate with use of digoxin.[846,847] At this time, digoxin appears to be indicated in AMI patients only if they exhibit supraventricular tachyarrhythmias or overt heart failure that is not adequately controlled by ACE inhibitors and diuretics.

BETA-ADRENOCEPTOR AGONISTS. When left ventricular failure is severe, as manifested by marked reduction of cardiac index (<2 liters/min/m²), and pulmonary capillary wedge pressure is at optimal (18 to 24 mm Hg) or excessive (>24 mm Hg) levels despite therapy with diuretics, beta-adrenoceptor agonists are indicated. Although isoproterenol is a potent cardiac stimulant and improves ventricular performance, it should be avoided in AMI patients. It also causes tachycardia and augments myocardial oxygen consumption and lactate production[848]; in addition, it reduces coronary perfusion pressure by causing systemic vasodilation and in animal experiments it increases the extent of experimentally induced infarction.[849] Norepinephrine also increases myocardial oxygen consumption because of its peripheral vasoconstrictor as well as positive inotropic actions.

Dopamine and dobutamine (see p. 502) may be particularly useful in patients with AMI and reduced cardiac output, increased left ventricular filling pressure, pulmonary vascular congestion, and hypotension.[850] Fortunately, the potentially deleterious alpha-adrenergic vasoconstrictor effects exerted by dopamine occur only at higher doses than those required to increase contractility. Its vasodilating actions on renal and splanchnic vessels and its positive inotropic effects generally improve hemodynamics and renal function.[851] In patients with AMI and severe left ventricular failure, this drug should be administered at a dose of 3 μg/kg/min while monitoring pulmonary capillary wedge and systemic arterial pressures as well as cardiac output. The dose may be increased stepwise to 20 μg/kg/min, in order to reduce pulmonary capillary wedge pressure to approximately 20 mm Hg and elevate cardiac index to exceed 2 liters/min/m². However, it must be recognized that doses exceeding 5 μg/kg/min activate peripheral alpha receptors and cause vasoconstriction.

Dobutamine has a positive inotropic action comparable to that of dopamine but a slightly less positive chronotropic effect[852] and less vasoconstrictor activity. In patients with AMI, dobutamine improves left ventricular performance without augmenting enzymatically estimated infarct size.[853] It may be administered in a starting dose of 2.5 μg/kg/min and increased stepwise to a maximum of 30 μg/kg/min. Both dopamine and dobutamine must be given carefully and with constant monitoring of the ECG, systemic arterial pressure, and pulmonary artery or pulmonary artery occlusive pressure and, if possible, with frequent measurements of cardiac output. The dose must be reduced if the heart rate exceeds 100 to 110 beats/min, if supraventricular or ventricular tachyarrhythmias are precipitated, or if ST-segment changes increase.

OTHER POSITIVE INOTROPIC AGENTS. Amrinone and milrinone are noncatecholamine, nonglycoside, phosphodiesterase inhibitors with inotropic and vasodilating action[854] (see p. 502). Although these drugs have been used in patients undergoing cardiac surgery,[855,856] reported experience with them in the setting of AMI is limited.[857] In patients with left ventricular failure following AMI, amrinone increases cardiac output while reducing pulmonary wedge pressure and systemic vascular resistance[858,859]; heart rate increases only at relatively high doses.[859] In AMI patients studied, no exacerbation of angina or increased incidence of arrhythmias has been reported.[858] Thus, these phosphodiesterase inhibitors appear to be useful in selected patients whose heart failure persists despite treatment with diuretics, who are not hypotensive, and who are likely to benefit from both an enhancement in contractility and afterload reduction. The initial intravenous dosage of amrinone is 0.75 mg/kg infused slowly over several minutes. This is then followed by a maintenance infusion started at 5 to 10 μg/kg/min and titrated to the patient's hemodynamic response. The total daily dose should not exceed 10 mg/kg.[860] Milrinone should be given as a loading dose of 50 μg/kg over 10 minutes, followed by a maintenance infusion of 0.375 to 0.75 μg/kg/min.

CARDIOGENIC SHOCK

This severest clinical expression of left ventricular failure is associated with extensive damage to the left ventricular myocardium in more than 80 per cent of AMI patients in whom it occurs[860a]; the remainder have a mechanical defect such as ventricular septal or papillary muscle rupture or predominant right ventricular infarction.[646] In the past cardiogenic shock has been reported to occur in up to 20 per cent of patients with AMI,[861] but estimates from recent large randomized trials of thrombolytic therapy and observational data bases report an incidence rate in the range of 7 per cent.[422,423,645,862] About 10 per cent of patients with cardiogenic shock present with this condition at the time of admission, whereas 90 per cent develop it during hospitalization.[645] This low-output state is characterized by elevated ventricular filling pressures, low cardiac output, systemic hypotension, and evidence of vital organ hypoperfusion (e.g., clouded sensorium, cool extremities, oliguria, acidosis).[422,423,863] Patients with cardiogenic shock due to AMI are more likely to be older, to have a history of a prior MI or congestive heart failure, and to have sustained an anterior infarction at the time of development of shock.[422] When shock develops in the course of AMI, it usually is due to infarct extension[864] (Fig. 37–23). The prognosis of patients with cardiogenic shock is poor, with fatality rates of about 70 per cent.[422,646,862]

PATHOLOGICAL FINDINGS. At autopsy, more than two-thirds of patients with cardiogenic shock demonstrate stenosis of 75 per cent or more of the luminal diameter of all three major coronary vessels, usually including the left anterior descending coronary artery.[865] Almost all patients with cardiogenic shock are found to have thrombotic occlusion of the artery supplying the major region of recent infarction.[866,867] Page et al., who studied 20 cardiogenic shock patients at autopsy, found that all exhibited necrosis of at least 40 per cent of the left ventricle.[866] In contrast, 35 per cent or less of the left ventricle had been destroyed in all but 1 of 14 patients who succumbed without having been in cardiogenic shock.[866] Similar findings were reported by Alonso et al.[867] Patients with cardiogenic shock had lost an average of 51 per cent of the left ventricular myocardium (range: 35 to 68 per cent), whereas in a group of patients with AMI who died suddenly of arrhythmias and who had never been in cardiogenic shock, necrosis averaged 23 per cent (range: 14 to 31 per cent) of the left ventricle.[867]

Patients who die as a consequence of cardiogenic shock often have "piecemeal" necrosis, i.e., progressive myocardial necrosis from marginal extension of their infarct into an ischemic zone bordering on the infarction. This is generally associated with persistent elevation of CK-MB. Early deterioration in left ventricular function secondary to apparent extension of infarction may, in some cases, result from expansion of the necrotic zone of myocardium without actual extension of the necrotic process (Fig. 37–37).

Shear forces that develop during ventricular systole can disrupt necrotic myocardial muscle bundles, with resultant expansion and thinning of the akinetic zone of myocardium, which in turn results in deterioration of overall left ventricular function.

At autopsy, patients with cardiogenic shock consistently demonstrate marginal extension of recent areas of infarction (see p. 1194).[866,867] Additionally, focal areas of necrosis are frequently found in regions of the left and right ventricles that are not adjacent to the major area of recent infarction.[866] Such extensions and focal lesions are probably in part the result of the shock state itself because they can also be found in the hearts of patients dying of noncardiogenic shock. Infarction of the ischemic periinfarction zone can be precipitated by a number of factors that adversely affect the supply of oxygen or the metabolic demand in this zone of myocardium. These include a reduction of coronary perfusion pressure causing impaired myocardial perfusion in the presence of atherosclerotic obstructions of the nonculprit artery. An augmentation of myocardial oxygen demand resulting from the local release of catecholamines from ischemic adrenergic nerve endings in the heart as well as from circulating endogenous or infused catecholamines may also play a role. Patients with rupture of the ventricular septum or of a papillary muscle can also exhibit cardiogenic shock. These patients often have smaller infarcts than do those with cardiogenic shock secondary to ventricular failure without a mechanical lesion. The prognosis is better in such patients because the smaller infarct

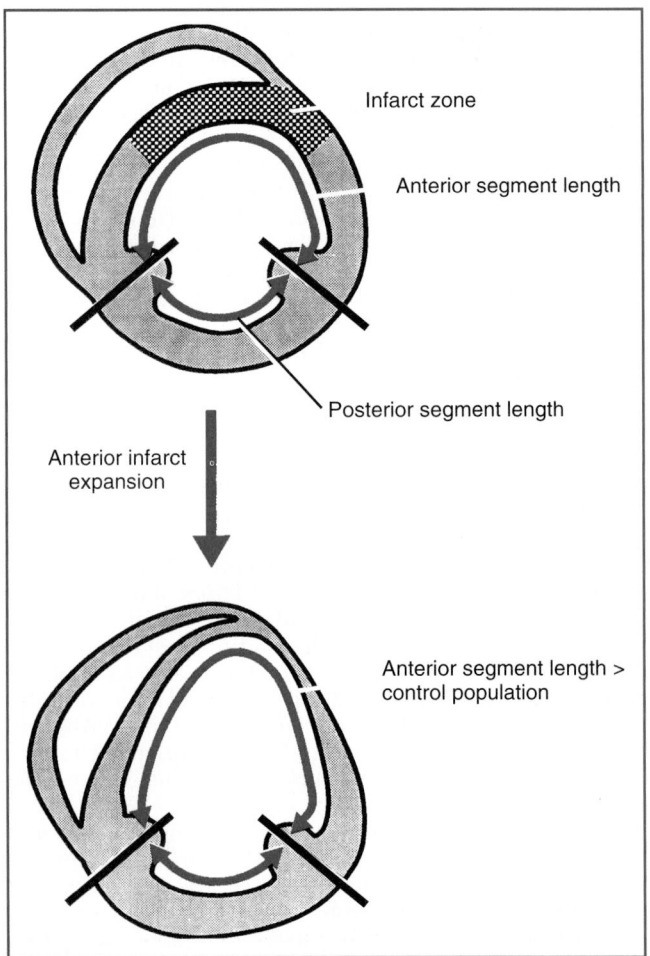

Infarct zone

Anterior segment length

Posterior segment length

Anterior infarct expansion

Anterior segment length > control population

FIGURE 37–37. Infarct expansion after transmural anterior myocardial infarction. (From Tice, F. D., and Kisslo, J.: Echocardiographic assessment and monitoring of the patient with AMI: Prospects for the thrombolytic era. *In* Califf, R. M., Mark, D. B., and Wagner, G. S. (eds.): Acute Coronary Care. St. Louis, Mosby-Year Book, 1995, p. 496.)

allows their left ventricle to support the circulation if the mechanical defect has been corrected surgically.

PATHOPHYSIOLOGY. The shock state in patients with AMI appears to be the result of a vicious circle, demonstrated in Figure 37–14 (see p. 1195).[422,423,863] According to this formulation, coronary obstruction leads to myocardial ischemia, which impairs myocardial contractility and ventricular performance. This, in turn, reduces arterial pressure and therefore coronary perfusion pressure, leading to further ischemia and extension of necrosis until the left ventricle has insufficient contracting myocardium to sustain life. The progressive nature of the myocardial insult in this syndrome is reflected in the stuttering and progressive evolution of elevations in the plasma enzyme–time activity curves of markers specific for myocardial injury. Consideration of the vicious circle also points to the hazard of hypovolemic hypotension in patients with AMI but without cardiogenic shock. Hypotension, whatever its cause, reduces coronary perfusion, especially of myocardium in the territory of obstructive arteries, and thereby may enhance necrosis.

DIAGNOSIS. Cardiogenic shock is characterized by marked and persistent (> 30 min) hypotension with systolic arterial pressure less than 80 mm Hg and a marked reduction of cardiac index (generally < 1.8 liters/mm/m²) in the face of elevated left ventricular filling pressure (pulmonary capillary wedge pressure > 18 mm Hg). Spurious estimates of left ventricular filling pressure based on measurements of the pulmonary artery wedge pressure can occur in the presence of marked mitral regurgitation, in which the tall v wave in the left atrial (and pulmonary artery wedge) pressure tracing elevates the mean pressure above left ventricular end-diastolic pressure. Accordingly, mitral regurgitation and other mechanical lesions such as ventricular septal defect, ventricular aneurysm, and pseudoaneurysm must be excluded before the diagnosis of cardiogenic shock due to impairment of left ventricular function can be established. Mechanical complications should be suspected in any patient with AMI in whom circulatory collapse occurs.[422,423,863] Immediate hemodynamic, angiographic, and echocardiographic evaluations are necessary in patients with cardiogenic shock. It is important to exclude mechanical complications because primary therapy of such lesions usually requires immediate operative treatment with intervening support of the circulation by intraaortic balloon counterpulsation.

Medical Management

When the aforementioned mechanical complications are not present, cardiogenic shock is due to impairment of left ventricular function. Although dopamine or dobutamine usually improves the hemodynamics in these patients, unfortunately neither appears to improve hospital survival significantly. Similarly, vasodilators have been utilized in an effort to elevate cardiac output and to reduce left ventricular filling pressure. However, by lowering the already markedly reduced coronary perfusion pressure, myocardial perfusion can be compromised further, accelerating the vicious circle illustrated in Figure 37–14 (see p. 1195). Vasodilators may nonetheless be used in conjunction with intraaortic balloon counterpulsation and inotropic agents in an effort to increase cardiac output while sustaining or elevating coronary perfusion pressure.[422,423,863]

The systemic vascular resistance is usually elevated in patients with cardiogenic shock, but occasionally resistance is normal and in a few cases vasodilation actually predominates. When systemic vascular resistance is not elevated (i.e., <1800 dynes/sec/cm⁵) in patients with cardiogenic shock, norepinephrine, which has both alpha- and beta-adrenoceptor agonist properties (in doses ranging from 2 to 10 μg/min), may be employed to increase diastolic arterial pressure, maintain coronary perfusion, and improve con-

tractility. However, there is no definitive evidence that ultimate outcome is affected by this drug.[868] Norepinephrine should be used only when other means, including balloon counterpulsation, fail to maintain arterial diastolic pressure above 50 to 60 mm Hg in a previously normotensive patient. The use of alpha-adrenoceptor agents such as phenylephrine and methoxamine is contraindicated in patients with cardiogenic shock (unless systemic vascular resistance is inordinately low).

Intraaortic Balloon Counterpulsation
(See also p. 535)

Intraaortic balloon counterpulsation may be useful in patients with cardiogenic shock due to mechanical defects following AMI (see pp. 1241 to 1245) or to severe left ventricular dysfunction when other medical measures fail.[869–872] The balloon is inserted percutaneously[873] or, rarely, via an arterial cutdown in the femoral artery and advanced into the thoracic aorta via the femoral artery. Phased pulsations, electrocardiographically synchronized, allow for inflation at the time of closure of the aortic valve and deflation just before the onset of systole. The augmented coronary perfusion pressure during diastole enhances coronary blood flow because coronary vascular resistance is minimal during this portion of the cardiac cycle. Because the balloon is deflated throughout systole, the left ventricle ejects against a lower impedance. Hemodynamic changes generally include a 10 to 20 per cent increase in cardiac output, a reduction in systolic and increase in diastolic arterial pressure with little change in mean pressure, a diminution of heart rate, and an increase in urine output.[869,872] The reduction in left ventricular afterload reduces myocardial oxygen consumption, and, as a consequence, anaerobic metabolism and myocardial ischemia are diminished.[869] Favorable effects are sometimes reflected in prompt resolution of electrocardiographic signs of ischemia.

INDICATIONS. Intraaortic balloon counterpulsation is utilized in the treatment of AMI in three groups of patients: (1) those whose conditions are hemodynamically unstable and in whom support of the circulation is required for the performance of cardiac catheterization and angiography carried out to assess lesions that are potentially correctable surgically or by angioplasty; (2) those with cardiogenic shock that is unresponsive to medical management; and (3) rarely, those with persistent ischemic pain that is unresponsive to treatment with inhalation of 100 per cent oxygen, beta-adrenoceptor blockade, and nitrates. Unfortunately, among patients with cardiogenic shock, improvement is often only temporary, and "balloon dependence" commonly develops.[870,872] Patients with cardiogenic shock treated with this modality can be successfully weaned from the supporting system only occasionally. Counterpulsation alone does not improve overall survival in patients either with or without a surgically remediable mechanical lesion.[870,871]

COMPLICATIONS. These occur infrequently but include damage to or perforation of the aortic wall, ischemia distal to the site of insertion of the balloon in the femoral artery, thrombocytopenia, hemolysis, renal emboli, and mechanical failure such as rupture of the balloon.[809,874] Those at highest risk include patients with peripheral vascular disease, the elderly, and women, particularly if they are small. These factors should be taken into consideration before an attempt is made to institute intraaortic balloon counterpulsation. Because of the potential for vascular bleeding complications, there has been reluctance to use intraaortic pumps in patients who have undergone thrombolytic therapy. However, despite the increased bleeding risk, because of the poor outcome among patients with shock following thrombolysis (usually ineffective thrombolysis), this modality should be considered in selected patients who are candidates for an aggressive approach to revascularization.

Reperfusion

Reversal of cardiogenic shock by acute reperfusion has been reported, usually with thrombolytic therapy, emergency PTCA, or a combination of these measures.[422,423,863] In several uncontrolled series of patients, the mortality of cardiogenic shock appears to have been reduced to about 35 per cent by early angioplasty or coronary artery bypass surgery.[875] Encouraging evidence favoring early angiography and revascularization has been reported in a cardiogenic shock registry.[646] Another small retrospective series reported that patients with cardiogenic shock who underwent a successful angioplasty had a better 1-year survival than either those who did not undergo a successful angioplasty or those who received only medical therapy.[876] These promising results must be interpreted cautiously because selection bias due to exclusion of elderly and moribund patients may have inflated the estimate of the beneficial effect of angioplasty.

Of the five therapies frequently used to treat patients with cardiogenic shock (vasopressors, intraaortic balloon counterpulsation, thrombolysis, angioplasty, and coronary artery bypass surgery), the first two are useful temporizing maneuvers, but only early revascularization appears to reduce mortality.[646] Because this conclusion is based on uncontrolled data, an international randomized trial (SHOCK) is underway to define whether revascularization with either angioplasty or bypass surgery is superior to conventional medical therapy. The results of randomized trials will also provide information on the overall costs to the health care system of implementing an aggressive treatment program.

We recommend assessment of patients on an individualized basis to determine their desire for aggressive care[877] and overall candidacy for further treatment (e.g., age, mental status, comorbidities). Patients who are potential candidates for revascularization should then rapidly receive intraaortic balloon counterpulsation and be referred for coronary arteriography. Those with suitable anatomy should be revascularized with angioplasty or coronary artery bypass surgery. In appropriately selected patients, emergency cardiac transplantation has also been used successfully to manage cardiogenic shock.[878]

SURGERY. Surgical treatment in cardiogenic shock (aside from correcting mechanical abnormalities) may involve bypassing occluded as well as severely obstructed nonoccluded vessels. Occlusion of one major vessel may cause left ventricular dysfunction and hypotension, which can then lead to hypoperfusion and ischemia of myocardium subserved by the other diseased vessels. Left ventricular function may be improved by relief of this ischemia with revascularization. It is possible that left ventricular bypass, a technique that reduces left ventricular oxygen demands more drastically, may ultimately prove to be more effective in improving survival in patients with cardiogenic shock than intraaortic balloon counterpulsation[879]; however, it is still experimental. Emergency percutaneous cardiopulmonary bypass has been used in a small series of patients before catheterization.[880] Although relatively successful in pilot studies, this complex strategy cannot be widely recommended until tested further.

RIGHT VENTRICULAR INFARCTION

A characteristic hemodynamic pattern (Table 37–10) has been observed in patients with right ventricular infarction,[881,882] which frequently accompanies inferior left ventricular infarction[541] or rarely occurs in isolated form.[883,884] Right-heart filling pressures (central venous, right atrial, and right ventricular end-diastolic pressures) are elevated whereas left ventricular filling pressure is normal or only slightly raised[825]; right ventricular systolic and pulse pres-

TABLE 37–10   FEATURES OF RIGHT VENTRICULAR INFARCTION

Inferior-posterior myocardial infarction
Clinical findings may include:
Normal or depressed right ventricular function
Shock
Tricuspid regurgitation
Ruptured ventricular septum
Hemodynamic measurements
Abnormally elevated right atrial pressure
Normal right ventricular and pulmonary artery systolic pressures
Increased ratio of right ventricular to left ventricular filling pressure
Depressed right ventricular function curve
Scintigraphy
Uptake in right ventricular free wall
Increased right ventricular dimensions and decreased wall motion
Echocardiography
Increased right ventricular dimension
Absence of pericardial effusion
Cardiac enzymes
Increased magnitude of enzyme values relative to degree of left ventricular dysfunction
Cardiac catheterization
Involvement of right (usually) or left (rarely) circumflex coronary arteries
Right ventricular akinesis
Differential diagnosis
Hypotension with acute myocardial infarction
Pericardial tamponade
Constrictive pericarditis
Pulmonary embolus

Modified from Rackley, C. E., Russell, R. O., Jr., Mantle, J. A., et al.: Right ventricular infarction and function. Am. Heart J. *101*:215, 1981.

sures are decreased, and cardiac output is often markedly depressed. Rarely, this disproportionate elevation of right-sided filling pressure causes right-to-left shunting through a patent foramen ovale.[885] This possibility should be considered in patients with right ventricular infarction who have unexplained systemic hypoxemia. The finding of an elevation in atrial natriuretic factor in this condition has led to the suggestion that abnormally high levels of this peptide might be in part responsible for the hypotension seen in right ventricular infarction.[205]

Diagnosis

Many patients with the combination of normal left ventricular filling pressure and depressed cardiac index have right ventricular infarcts (with accompanying inferior left ventricular infarcts). The hemodynamic picture may superficially resemble that seen in patients with pericardial disease (see Chap. 45).[825] It includes elevated right ventricular filling pressure; steep, right atrial *y* descent; and an early diastolic drop and plateau (square root sign) in the right ventricular pressure tracing. Moreover, Kussmaul's sign (an increase in jugular venous pressure with inspiration, p. 453) and pulsus paradoxus (a fall in systolic pressure of greater than 10 mm Hg with inspiration, p. 1488) may be present in patients with right ventricular infarction. In fact, Kussmaul's sign in the setting of inferior wall AMI is highly predictive of right ventricular involvement.

The ECG may provide the first clue that right ventricular involvement is present in the patient with inferior wall MI. Most patients with right ventricular infarction have ST-segment elevation in lead V_4R (right precordial lead in V_4 position)[339,886] (Fig. 4–39, p. 134). Transient elevation of the ST segment in any of the right precordial leads may occur with right ventricular MI, and the presence of ST-segment elevation of 0.1 mV or more in any one or combination of leads V_4R, V_5R, and V_6R in patients with the clinical picture of acute MI is highly sensitive and specific for the diagnosis of right ventricular MI.[339,887]

ECHOCARDIOGRAPHY AND RADIONUCLIDE ANGIOGRAPHY.
Echocardiography is helpful in the differential diagnosis[888] because in right ventricular infarction, in contrast to pericardial tamponade, no significant quantities of pericardial fluid are seen. On two-dimensional echocardiography, abnormal wall motion of the right ventricle as well as right ventricular dilatation and depression of right ventricular ejection fraction are noted.[888,889] Gated equilibrium radionuclide angiography is also useful for recognizing right ventricular MI.[881,890] Serial studies have shown that some degree of recovery of an initially depressed right ventricular ejection fraction is the rule with right ventricular MI,[754,881,891] whereas this is less apparent in left ventricular ejection fraction.

HEMODYNAMICS.
Loss of atrial transport in patients with right ventricular infarction can result in marked reductions in stroke volume and arterial blood pressure.[891] As already noted, disproportionate elevation of the right-sided filling pressure is the hemodynamic hallmark of right ventricular infarction. Therefore, ventricular pacing may fail to increase cardiac output, and atrioventricular sequential pacing may be required.[129,892] In general, the hemodynamic importance of right ventricular infarction in patients with inferior infarction is reflected in the observations of Marmor et al. They noted that although infarct sizes (reflected in CK release curves) were similar in patients with anterior and inferior infarcts, the former had severe depression of the left ventricular ejection fraction and the latter had more severe depression of the right ventricular ejection fraction.[893]

Treatment

In patients with hypotension due to right ventricular MI, hemodynamics may be improved by a combination of expanding plasma volume to augment right ventricular preload and cardiac output and, when left ventricular failure is present, arterial vasodilators. The initial therapy for hypotension in patients with right ventricular infarction should almost always be volume expansion. However, if hypotension has not been corrected after one or more liters of fluid have been administered briskly, consideration should be given to hemodynamic monitoring with a pulmonary artery catheter, because further volume infusion may be of little use and may produce pulmonary congestion.[815] Vasodilators reduce the impedance to left ventricular outflow and in turn left ventricular diastolic, left atrial, and pulmonary (arterial) pressures, thereby lowering the impedance to right ventricular outflow and enhancing right ventricular output. A remarkably high survival rate of 60 per cent, albeit in a small series of patients with right ventricular infarction and serious and prolonged hypotension, emphasizes the importance of recognition and vigorous medical therapy of this cause of serious hypotension in MI.[894]

Right ventricular infarction is common among patients with inferior left ventricular infarction. Therefore, otherwise unexplained systemic arterial hypotension or diminished cardiac output, or marked hypotension in response to small doses of nitroglycerin[771] in patients with inferior infarction, should lead to the prompt consideration of this diagnosis. In view of the importance of atrial transport, patients requiring pacing should have atrial or atrioventricular sequential pacing.[892] Replacement of the tricuspid valve and repair of the valve with annuloplasty rings have been carried out in the treatment of severe tricuspid regurgitation secondary to right ventricular infarction.

MECHANICAL CAUSES OF HEART FAILURE

Free Wall Rupture

The most dramatic complications of AMI are those that involve tearing or rupture of acutely infarcted tissue.[895,895a] The clinical characteristics of these lesions vary considerably and depend on the site of rupture, which may involve the papillary muscles, the interventricular septum, or the free wall of either ventricle. The overall incidence of these complications is hard to assess because clinical and autopsy series differ considerably.[896,897] However, as a group they are probably responsible for about 15 per cent of all deaths from AMI.[895,898] The comparative clinical profile of these complications, as gathered from different studies, is shown in Table 37–11. A large autopsy study in 1989 suggests that the incidence of myocardial rupture has increased since the late 1960's, with a rate of 31 per cent among necropsied cases.[897] The prior use of corticosteroids or nonsteroidal antiinflammatory agents has been implicated as predisposing to rupture as a result of impaired healing. Controversy remains about the actual relationship between the use of such agents and the frequency of rupture, with several series suggesting a correlation of rupture with their use[899,900] and others not.[896,901] Conversely, the early use of thrombolytic therapy appears to reduce the incidence of cardiac rupture,[464,567] an effect that is responsible in part for improved survival with effective thromboly-

TABLE 37–11   CLINICAL PROFILE OF MECHANICAL COMPLICATIONS OF MYOCARDIAL INFARCTION

VARIABLE	VENTRICULAR SEPTAL DEFECT	FREE WALL RUPTURE	PAPILLARY MUSCLE RUPTURE
Age (mean, years)	63	69	65
Days post-MI	3–5	3–6	3–5
Anterior MI	66%	50%	25%
New murmur	90%	25%	50%
Palpable thrill	Yes	No	Rare
Previous MI	25%	25%	30%
Echocardiographic findings			
Two-dimensional	Visualize defect	May have pericardial effusion	Flail or prolapsing leaflet
Doppler	Detect shunt	—	Regurgitant jet in LA
PA catheterization	Oxygen step-up in RV	Equalization of diastolic pressure	Prominent V wave in PCW tracing
Mortality			
Medical	90%	90%	90%
Surgical	50%	Case reports	40–90%

MI = myocardial infarction; LA = left atrium; PA = pulmonary artery; RV = right ventricle; PCW = pulmonary capillary wedge.
Modified from Labovitz, A. J., et al.: Mechanical complications of acute myocardial infarction. Cardiovasc. Rev. Rep. 5:948, 1984.

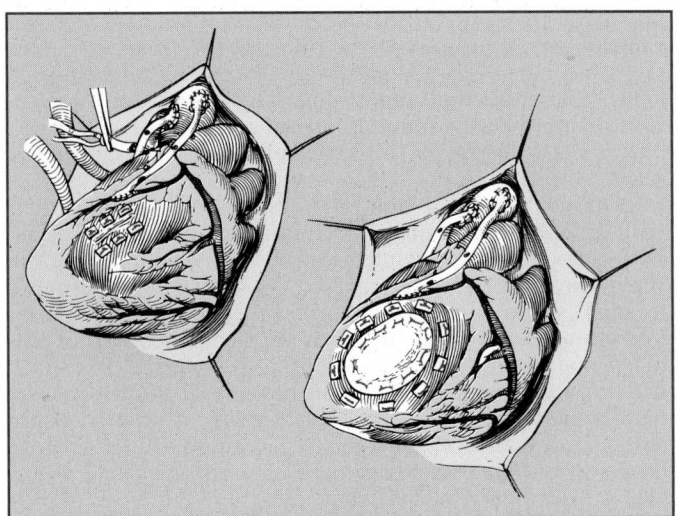

FIGURE 37–38. Free-wall perforation of the left ventricle. On the left is a direct suture repair of a small rupture. On the right is a Dacron patch closure of a larger rupture. Note the coronary artery bypass grafting which was also done at the time of surgery. (From Canacho, M. T., Muehrcke, D. D., and Loop. F. D.: Mechanical complications. In Julian, D. G., and Braunwald, E. [eds.]: Management of Acute Myocardial Infarction. London, W. B. Saunders Ltd., 1994, p. 310.)

sis. Late thrombolytic therapy may actually *increase* the risk of cardiac rupture despite improving overall survival.[567,902]

Rupture of the free wall of the infarcted ventricle (Fig. 37–38) occurs in up to 10 per cent of patients dying in the hospital of AMI.[895] Thinness of the apical wall, marked intensity of necrosis at the terminal end of the blood supply, poor collateral flow, the shearing effect of muscular contraction against an inert and stiffened necrotic area, and aging of the myocardium with laceration of the myocardial microstructure have all been proposed as the local factors that lead to rupture.[903–905]

CLINICAL CHARACTERISTICS. The following are some features that characterize this serious complication of AMI:

1. Occurs more frequently in the elderly and possibly more frequently in women than in men with infarction.[901]

2. Appears to be more common in hypertensive than in normotensive patients.[901,903]

3. Occurs approximately seven times more frequently in the left than the right ventricle and seldom occurs in the atria.

4. Usually involves the anterior or lateral walls[895,896] of the ventricle in the area of the terminal distribution of the left anterior descending coronary artery.

5. Is usually associated with a relatively large trans-

mural infarction involving at least 20 per cent of the left ventricle.[896]

6. Occurs between 1 day and 3 weeks, but most commonly 1 to 4 days, following infarction.

7. Is usually preceded by infarct expansion, i.e., thinning and a disproportionate dilatation within the softened necrotic zone.[907]

8. Most commonly results from a distinct tear in the myocardial wall or a dissecting hematoma that perforates a necrotic area of myocardium (Fig. 37–38).

9. Usually occurs near the junction of the infarct and the normal muscle.

10. Occurs less frequently in the center of the infarct, but when rupture occurs here, it is usually during the second rather than the first week following the infarct.

11. Rarely occurs in a greatly thickened ventricle or in an area of extensive collateral vessels.[904]

12. Most often occurs in patients *without* previous infarction.[896,906]

Rupture of the free wall of the left ventricle usually leads to hemopericardium and death from cardiac tamponade. Occasionally, rupture of the free wall of the ventricle occurs as the first clinical manifestation in patients with undetected or silent myocardial infarction, and then it may be considered a form of "sudden cardiac death" (see Chap. 24).

The course of rupture varies from catastrophic, with an acute tear leading to immediate death, to subacute with nausea, hypotension, and pericardial type of discomfort being the major clinical clues to its presence.[895,908] Survival depends on the recognition of this complication, hemodynamic stabilization of the patient—usually with inotropic agents and/or intraaortic balloon pump—and most importantly on prompt surgical repair.[908]

PSEUDOANEURYSM. Incomplete rupture of the heart may occur when organizing thrombus and hematoma, together with pericardium, seal a rupture of the left ventricle and thus prevent the development of hemopericardium (Fig. 37–39). With time, this area of organized thrombus and pericardium can become a pseudoaneurysm (false aneurysm) that maintains communication with the cavity of the left ventricle.[909] In contrast to true aneurysms, which always contain some myocardial elements in their walls, the walls of pseudoaneurysms are composed of organized hematoma and pericardium and lack any elements of the original myocardial wall. Pseudoaneurysms can become quite large, even equaling the true ventricular cavity in size, and they communicate with the left ventricular cavity through a narrow neck. Frequently, pseudoaneurysms contain significant quantities of old and recent thrombus, superficial portions of which can cause arterial emboli. Pseudoaneurysms can drain off a portion of each ventricular stroke volume exactly as do true aneurysms. The diagnosis

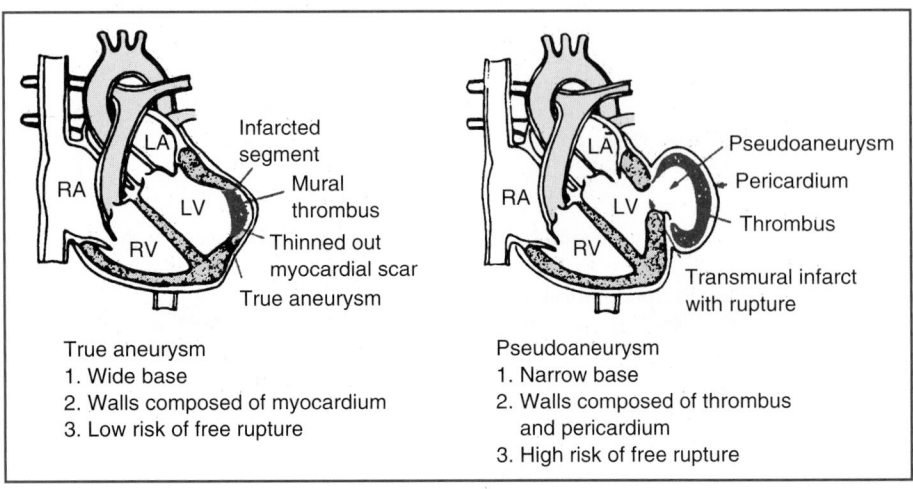

True aneurysm
1. Wide base
2. Walls composed of myocardium
3. Low risk of free rupture

Pseudoaneurysm
1. Narrow base
2. Walls composed of thrombus and pericardium
3. High risk of free rupture

FIGURE 37–39. Differences between a pseudoaneurysm and a true aneurysm. (From Shah, P. K.: Complications of acute myocardial infarction. In Parmley, W., and Chatterjee, K. [eds.]: Cardiology. Philadelphia, J. B. Lippincott, 1987.)

of pseudoaneurysm can usually be made by two-dimensional echocardiography (Fig. 3–91, p. 87) and contrast angiography, although at times differentiation between true aneurysm and pseudoaneurysm may be difficult by any imaging technique.[910]

DIAGNOSIS. The rupture usually is first suggested by the development of sudden profound shock, often rapidly leading to electromechanical dissociation due to pericardial tamponade. Immediate pericardiocentesis confirms the diagnosis and relieves the pericardial tamponade, at least momentarily. If the patient's condition is relatively stable, echocardiography may help in establishing the diagnosis of tamponade. Under the most favorable conditions, cardiac catheterization can be carried out, not necessarily to confirm the diagnosis of rupture but to delineate the coronary anatomy. This is helpful so that, in addition to ventricular repair, coronary artery bypass surgery can be performed in patients in whom high-grade obstructive lesions are present. In patients in whom hemodynamics are critically compromised, establishment of the diagnosis should be followed immediately by surgical resection of the necrotic and ruptured myocardium with primary reconstruction (Fig. 37–38). When rupture is subacute and a pseudoaneurysm is suspected or present, prompt elective surgery is indicated because rupture of the pseudoaneurysm occurs relatively frequently.[908]

Rupture of the Interventricular Septum

Although rupture of the interventricular septum previously was reported in up to 11 per cent of autopsied cases,[911] clinical experience suggests that its incidence is probably in the range of 2 per cent of AMI patients,[895,912,913] perhaps because death usually is not immediate, and patients frequently can reach a referral center where this complication is treated. Clinical features associated with an increased risk of rupture of the interventricular septum include lack of development of a collateral network, advanced age, hypertension, and possibly thrombolysis.[894,912–914]

The perforation may range in length from one to several centimeters. It may be a direct through-and-through opening, or it may be more irregular and serpiginous.[915,916] The size of the defect determines the magnitude of the left-to-right shunt and the extent of hemodynamic deterioration, which in turn affects the likelihood of survival.[895,917] As in

rupture of the free wall of the ventricle, transmural infarction underlies rupture of the ventricular septum. Rupture of the septum with an anterior infarction tends to be apical in location, whereas inferior infarctions are associated with perforation of the basal septum and with a worse prognosis than those in an anterior location.[918] Virtually all patients have multivessel coronary artery disease, with the majority exhibiting lesions in all of the major vessels. The likelihood of survival depends on the degree of impairment of ventricular function and the size of the defect.[918–920]

A ruptured interventricular septum is characterized by the appearance of a new harsh, loud holosystolic murmur that is heard best at the lower left sternal border and that is usually accompanied by a thrill. Biventricular failure generally ensues within hours to days. The defect can also be recognized by two-dimensional echocardiography with color flow Doppler imaging[921–923] or insertion of a pulmonary artery balloon catheter to document the left-to-right shunt.

Catheter placement of an umbrella-shaped device within the ruptured septum has been reported to stabilize the conditions of critically ill patients with acute septal rupture following AMI.[924]

Rupture of a Papillary Muscle

Partial or total rupture of a papillary muscle is a rare but often fatal complication of transmural MI[895,913,925] (Fig. 37–40). Inferior wall infarction can lead to rupture of the posteromedial papillary muscle,[926] which occurs more commonly than rupture of the anterolateral muscle, a consequence of anterolateral MI.[927,928] Rupture of a right ventricular papillary muscle is rare but can cause massive tricuspid regurgitation and right ventricular failure. Complete transection of a left ventricular papillary muscle is incompatible with life because the sudden massive mitral regurgitation that develops cannot be tolerated. Rupture of a portion of a papillary muscle, usually the tip or head of the muscle, resulting in severe, although not necessarily overwhelming, mitral regurgitation is much more frequent and is not immediately fatal. Unlike rupture of the ventricular septum, which occurs with large infarcts, papillary muscle rupture occurs with a relatively small infarction in approximately one-half of the cases seen.[929] The extent of coronary artery disease in these patients sometimes is modest as well.

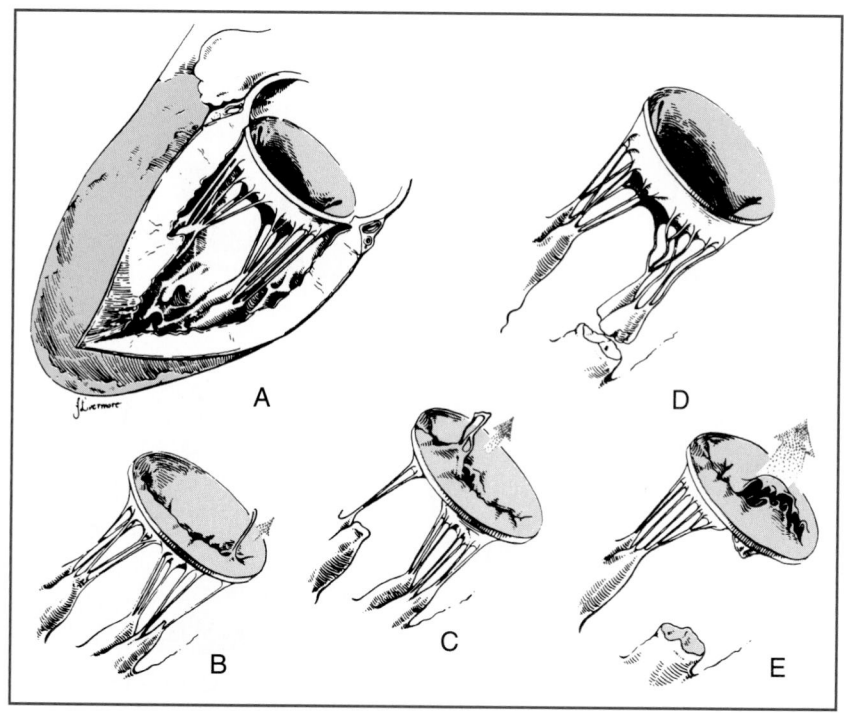

FIGURE 37–40. Mitral regurgitation after MI due to papillary head rupture. *A,* Normal annulus, chordae leaflets, and papillary structures. *B,* Ruptured posterolateral chordae with mild posterolateral regurgitant jet at the commissure. *C,* Partial papillary head rupture of the anterolateral papillary muscle with moderate mitral regurgitation of the anterolateral commissure. *D,* Complete rupture of the posteromedial papillary muscle. *E,* Severe regurgitation with anterior and posterior mitral leaflet flail segments due to the loss of the posterolateral papillary muscle. (From Camacho, M. T., Muehrcke, D. D., and Loop, F. D.: Mechanical complications. *In* Julian, D. G., and Braunwald, E. [eds.]: Management of Acute Myocardial Infarction. London, W. B. Saunders, Ltd., 1994, p. 305.)

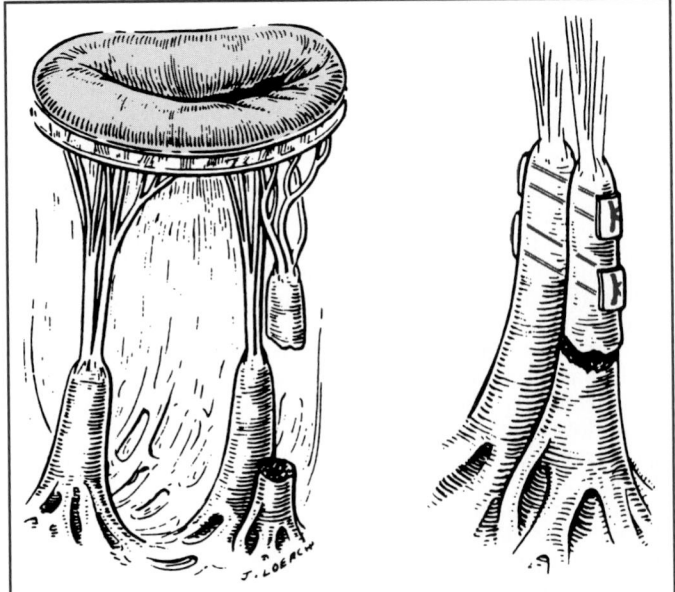

FIGURE 37–41. Repair of a totally ruptured papillary muscle head. On the left are the findings at surgery of a ruptured papillary head. On the right is a repair technique in which the ruptured papillary head is sutured to an adjacent papillary head for competence of the posterior medial papillary support structure. (From Camacho, M. T., Muehrcke, D. D., and Loop, F. D.: Mechanical complications. In Julian, D. G., and Braunwald, E. [eds.]: Management of Acute Myocardial Infarction. London, W. B. Saunders Ltd., 1994, p. 307.)

In a small number of patients, rupture of more than one cardiac structure is noted clinically[930] or at postmortem examination; all possible combinations of rupture of the free left ventricular wall, the interventricular septum, and papillary muscles have been described.[915]

As with patients who have a ruptured ventricular septal defect, those with papillary muscle rupture manifest a new holosystolic murmur and develop increasingly severe heart failure. In both conditions the murmur may become softer or disappear as arterial pressure falls. Mitral regurgitation due to partial or complete rupture of a papillary muscle may be promptly recognized echocardiographically.[931]

Color flow Doppler imaging is particularly helpful in distinguishing acute mitral regurgitation from a ventricular septal defect in the setting of AMI[932] (Table 37–11). Therefore, an echocardiogram should be obtained immediately on any patient in whom the diagnosis is suspected, because hemodynamic deterioration can ensue rapidly. Echocardiography also often permits differentiation of papillary muscle rupture from other, generally less severe forms of mitral regurgitation that occur with AMI.[933]

Differentiation Between Ventricular Septal Rupture and Mitral Regurgitation

It may be difficult, on clinical grounds, to distinguish between acute mitral regurgitation and rupture of the ventricular septum in patients with AMI who suddenly develop a loud systolic murmur.[934] This differentiation can be made most readily by color flow Doppler echocardiography.[932,935] In addition, a right-heart catheterization with a balloon-tipped catheter can readily distinguish between these two complications.[933] As already noted, patients with ventricular septal rupture demonstrate a "step-up" in oxygen saturation in blood samples from the right ventricle and pulmonary artery compared with those from the right atrium. Patients with acute mitral regurgitation lack this step-up; they may demonstrate tall c-v waves in both the pulmonary capillary and pulmonary arterial pressure tracings.

Invasive monitoring, which is essential in these patients, also allows for the critically important assessment of ventricular function. Right and left ventricular filling pressures (right atrial pressure and pulmonary capillary wedge pressure) dictate fluid administration or the use of diuretics, whereas measurements of cardiac output and mean arterial pressure are obtained for calculation of systemic vascular resistance as a guide for vasodilator therapy. Unless systolic pressure is below 90 mm Hg, this therapy, generally using nitroglycerin or nitroprusside, should be instituted as soon as possible once hemodynamic monitoring is available. This may be critically important for stabilizing the patient's condition in preparation for further diagnostic studies and surgical repair. If vasodilator therapy is not tolerated or if it fails to achieve hemodynamic stability, intraaortic balloon counterpulsation should be rapidly instituted.

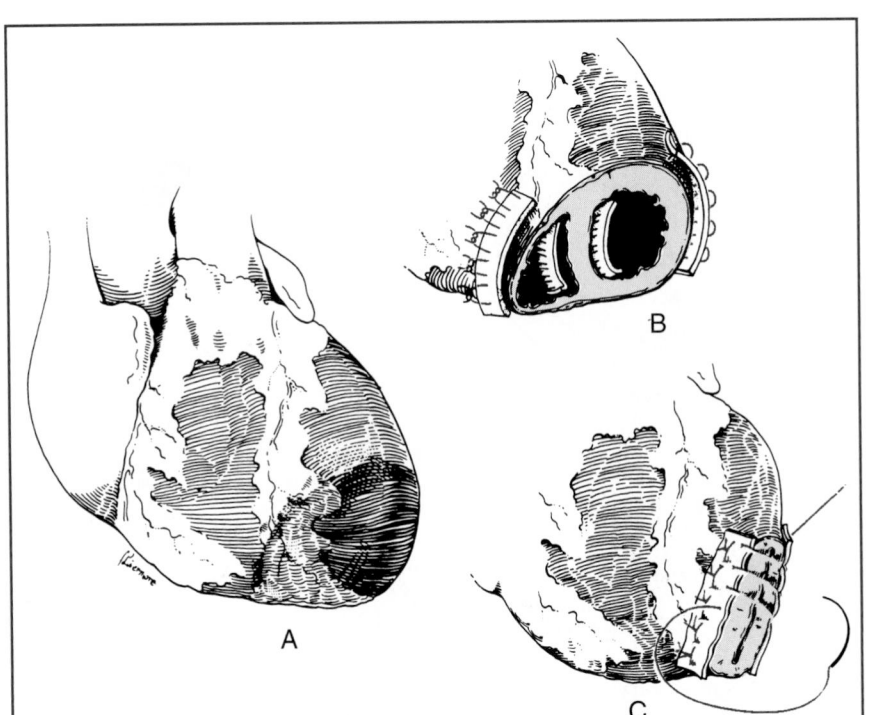

FIGURE 37–42. Repair of an apical ventricular septal defect. A, Large apical aneurysm with underlying ventricular septal defect. B, Interrupted suture repair is performed by excising the apex of the right and left ventricles, including the ventricular septal defect, with reapproximation of the left and right ventricular free walls along with the septum using Teflon felt strips for hemostasis. C, Over-and-over suture reinforcement of the repair for further hemostasis. (From Camacho, M. T., Muehrcke, D. D., and Loop, F. D.: Mechanical complications. In Julian, D. G., and Braunwald, E. [eds.]: Management of Acute Myocardial Infarction. London, W. B. Saunders Ltd., 1994, p. 296.)

Surgical Treatment

Operative intervention is most successful in patients with AMI and circulatory collapse when a surgically correctable mechanical lesion such as ventricular septal defect or mitral regurgitation can be identified and repaired.[913,936] In such patients the circulation should at first be supported by intraaortic balloon pulsation and a positive inotropic agent such as dopamine or dobutamine in combination with a vasodilator, unless the patient is hypotensive. Operation should not be delayed in patients with a correctable lesion who agree to an aggressive management strategy and require pharmacological and/or mechanical (counterpulsation) support.[912,936,937] Such patients frequently develop a serious complication—infection, adult respiratory distress syndrome, extension of the infarct, or renal failure—if operation is delayed. Surgical survival is predicted by early operation, short duration of shock, and mild degrees of right and left ventricular impairment.[912,934,936] When the hemodynamic status of a patient with one of these mechanical lesions complicating an AMI remains stable after the patient has been weaned from pharmacological and/or mechanical support, it may be possible to postpone operation for 2 to 4 weeks to allow some healing of the infarct to occur. Surgical repair may involve either correction of mitral regurgitation, insertion of a prosthetic mitral valve repair, or closure of a ventricular septal defect, usually accompanied by coronary revascularization[913] (Figs. 37–40 to 37–42).

ARRHYTHMIAS IN ACUTE MYOCARDIAL INFARCTION

The genesis and diagnosis of arrhythmias are presented in Chapters 20 and 22 and their treatment in Chapters 21 and 23. The role of arrhythmias in complicating the course of patients with AMI and the prevention and treatment of these arrhythmias in this setting are discussed here and summarized in Table 37–12.

The incidence of arrhythmias is higher in those patients seen earlier after the onset of symptoms. Many serious arrhythmias develop before hospitalization, even before the patient is monitored.[938] Some abnormality of cardiac rhythm also occurs in the majority of patients with AMI treated in CCUs.[939,940] When patients are seen very early during the course of MI, they almost invariably exhibit evidence of increased activity of the autonomic nervous system. Thus, sinus bradycardia, sometimes associated with AV block, and hypotension reflect augmented vagal activity.

TABLE 37–12   CARDIAC ARRHYTHMIAS AND THEIR MANAGEMENT DURING ACUTE MYOCARDIAL INFARCTION

CATEGORY	ARRHYTHMIA	OBJECTIVE OF TREATMENT	THERAPEUTIC OPTIONS
1. Electrical instability	Ventricular premature beats	Correction of electrolyte deficits and increased sympathetic tone	Potassium and magnesium solutions, beta blocker
	Ventricular tachycardia	Prophylaxis against ventricular fibrillation, restoration of hemodynamic stability	Antiarrhythmic agents; cardioversion/defibrillation
	Ventricular fibrillation	Urgent reversion to sinus rhythm	Defibrillation; bretylium tosylate
	Accelerated idioventricular rhythm	Observation unless hemodynamic function is compromised	Increase sinus rate (atropine, atrial pacing); antiarrhythmic agents
	Nonparoxysmal AV junctional tachycardia	Search for precipitating causes (e.g., digitalis intoxication); suppress arrhythmia only if hemodynamic function is compromised	Atrial overdrive pacing; antiarrhythmic agents; cardioversion relatively contraindicated if digitalis intoxication present
2. Pump failure/ Excessive sympathetic stimulation	Sinus tachycardia	Reduce heart rate to diminish myocardial oxygen demands	Antipyretics; analgesics; consider beta blocker unless CHF present; treat latter if present with anticongestive measures (diuretics, afterload reduction)
	Atrial fibrillation and/or atrial flutter	Reduce ventricular rate; restore sinus rhythm	Verapamil, digitalis glycosides; anticongestive measures (diuretics, afterload reduction); cardioversion; rapid atrial pacing (for atrial flutter)
	Paroxysmal supraventricular tachycardia	Reduce ventricular rate; restore sinus rhythm	Vagal maneuvers; verapamil, cardiac glycosides, beta-adrenergic blockers; cardioversion; rapid atrial pacing
3. Bradyarrhythmias and conduction disturbances	Sinus bradycardia	Acceleration of heart rate only if hemodynamic function is compromised	Atropine; atrial pacing
	Junctional escape rhythm	Acceleration of sinus rate only if loss of atrial "kick" causes hemodynamic compromise	Atropine; atrial pacing
	Atrioventricular block and intraventricular block		Insertion of pacemaker

Modified from Antman, E. M., and Rutherford, J. D. (eds): Coronary Care Medicine: A Practical Approach. Boston, Martinus Nijhoff Publishing, 1986, p. 78.

MECHANISM OF ARRHYTHMIAS. Activation of receptors within atrial and ventricular myocardium by ischemic or necrotic tissue may cause enhanced efferent sympathetic activity, increased concentrations of circulating catecholamines, and local release of catecholamines from nerve endings within the heart. The last phenomenon may also result from direct ischemic damage of adrenergic neurons.[940a] In addition, ischemic myocardium may be hyperreactive to the arrhythmogenic effects of norepinephrine,[941] which may vary strikingly in concentration in different portions of the ischemic heart.[942] Sympathetic stimulation of the heart may also enhance the automaticity of ischemic Purkinje fibers. Furthermore, catecholamines facilitate propagation of slow current responses mediated by calcium, and stimulation of ischemic myocardium by catecholamines may exacerbate arrhythmias dependent on such currents.[941] Finally, it has been demonstrated that transmural infarction can interrupt both afferent and efferent limbs of the sympathetic nervous system innervating myocardium distal to the area of infarction (but still viable)[942] (see p. 1192). In addition to the potential for modifying a variety of cardiovascular reflexes, this creation of autonomic imbalance may promote the development of arrhythmias.[942] This explains why beta-adrenoceptor blocking agents may also be helpful in the treatment of ventricular arrhythmias, particularly when the latter are associated with other signs of heightened adrenergic activity.

Experimental and clinical studies have suggested that electrolyte disturbances (e.g., hypokalemia, hypomagnesemia, acidosis), elevated free fatty acid levels, and oxygen-derived free radicals also contribute to the development of arrhythmias. The severity of these abnormalities, with the size of infarction and the perfusion status of the infarct-related coronary artery, appears to determine a patient's risk for developing the most serious rhythm disturbance—primary ventricular fibrillation (i.e., ventricular fibrillation occurring in the absence of congestive heart failure or cardiogenic shock).

The treatment of tachyarrhythmias involves not only the use of antiarrhythmic drugs but also correction of abnormalities of plasma electrolyte concentrations, acid-base balance disturbances, hypoxemia, anemia, and digitalis intoxication. In addition, it is essential to treat pericarditis, pulmonary emboli, and pneumonia or other infections, which may give rise to sinus tachycardia or other supraventricular tachyarrhythmias.

Arrhythmias occurring in patients with AMI require aggressive treatment when they (1) impair hemodynamics; (2) compromise myocardial viability by augmenting myocardial oxygen requirements; or (3) predispose to malignant ventricular arrhythmias, i.e., ventricular tachycardia, ventricular fibrillation, or asystole. Evidence indicates that both the diminished threshold to ventricular fibrillation[943] and the incidence of malignant ventricular arrhythmias associated with infarction[944] are affected by the extent of the underlying infarction.[945]

HEMODYNAMIC CONSEQUENCES. Patients with significant left ventricular dysfunction have a relatively fixed stroke volume and depend on changes in heart rate to alter cardiac output. However, there is a narrow range of heart rate over which the cardiac output is maximal, with significant reductions occurring at both faster and slower rates. Thus, all forms of bradycardia and tachycardia may depress the cardiac output in patients with AMI. Although the optimal rate insofar as cardiac output is concerned may exceed 100 per minute, it is important to consider that heart rate is one of the major determinants of myocardial oxygen consumption and that at more rapid heart rates myocardial energy needs can be elevated to levels that adversely affect ischemic myocardium. Therefore, in patients with AMI, the optimal rate is usually lower, in the range of 60 to 80 beats/min.

A second factor to consider in assessing the hemodynamic consequences of a particular arrhythmia is the loss of the atrial contribution to ventricular preload.[946] Studies in patients without AMI have demonstrated that loss of atrial transport decreases left ventricular output by 15 to 20 per cent.[947] However, in patients with reduced diastolic left ventricular compliance of any cause (including AMI), atrial systole is of greater importance for left ventricular filling. In patients with AMI, atrial systole boosts end-diastolic volume by 15 per cent, end-diastolic pressure by 29 per cent, and stroke volume by 35 per cent.[948]

VENTRICULAR ARRHYTHMIAS

Ventricular Premature Beats (VPBs)
(See also p. 675)

Prior to the widespread use of reperfusion therapy, aspirin, beta blockers, and intravenous nitrates in the management of AMI, it was believed that frequent VPBs (more than five per minute), VPBs with multiform configuration, early coupling (the "R-on-T" phenomenon), and repetitive patterns in the form of couples or salvos (Fig. 37–19) presaged ventricular fibrillation. However, it is now clear that such "warning arrhythmias" are present in as many patients who do not develop fibrillation as those who do.[237] Several reports have shown that primary ventricular fibrillation (see below) occurs without antecedent warning arrhythmias and may even develop in spite of suppression of warning arrhythmias.[949,950] On the other hand, frequent and complex VPBs and R-on-T beats are commonly observed in patients with AMI who never develop ventricular fibrillation.[949,951,952] Campbell et al. have analyzed these observations by pointing out that both primary ventricular fibrillation and VPBs, especially R-on-T beats, all occur during the early phase of AMI when considerable heterogeneity of electrical activity is present.[237,953,954] Although R-on-T beats expose this heterogeneity and can precipitate ventricular fibrillation in a small minority of patients, the ubiquitous nature of VPBs in AMI and the extremely infrequent nature of ventricular fibrillation in the current era of AMI management produces unacceptably low sensitivity and specificity of ECG patterns observed on monitoring systems for identifying patients at risk of ventricular fibrillation.[237]

MANAGEMENT. Given the declining incidence of ventricular fibrillation in AMI seen in CCUs over the last three decades (Fig. 37–43A), the prior practice of prophylactic suppression of VPBs with antiarrhythmic drugs no longer is necessary and may actually be associated with an increased risk of fatal bradycardic and asystolic events[955,956] (Fig. 37–44). Therefore, we pursue a conservative course when VPBs are observed in AMI and do not routinely prescribe antiarrhythmic drugs but instead determine whether recurrent ischemia or electrolyte (Fig. 37–43B) or metabolic disturbances are present.

When, at the very inception of an infarction, VPBs are encountered in the presence of sinus tachycardia, augmented sympathoadrenal stimulation is often a contributing factor and may be treated by beta-adrenoceptor blockade. In fact, early administration of an intravenous beta blocker is effective in reducing the incidence of ventricular fibrillation in evolving MI[957–959] (see p. 1228).

Accelerated Idioventricular Rhythm
(See p. 683)

Commonly defined as a ventricular rhythm with a rate of 60 to 125 beats/min, and frequently called "slow ventricular tachycardia," this arrhythmia is seen in up to 20 per cent of patients with AMI. It occurs frequently during the first 2 days, with about equal frequency in anterior and inferior infarctions, and probably results from enhanced automaticity of Purkinje fibers. Most episodes are of short duration, and the arrhythmia may terminate abruptly, slow

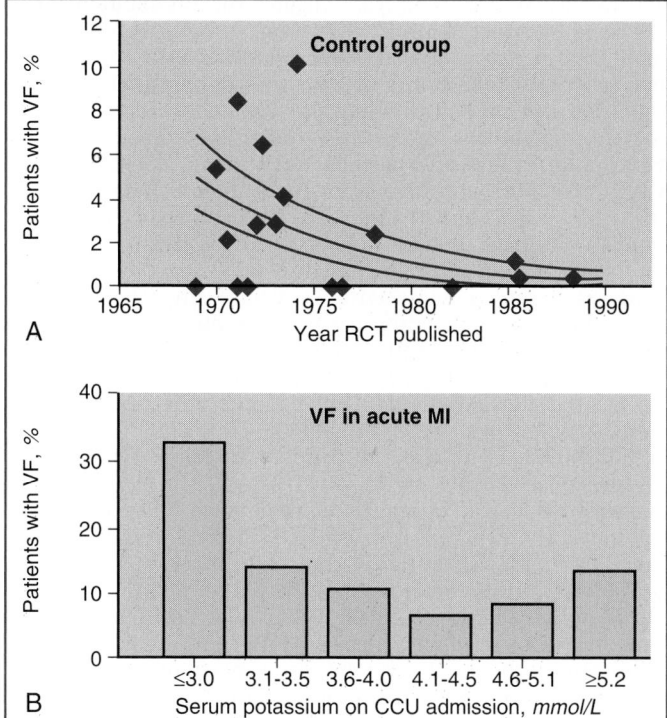

A

B

FIGURE 37–43. *A,* Temporal changes in primary ventricular fibrillation (VF), as shown in this regression analysis of the results of 18 randomized controlled trials (RCTs) in which lidocaine was administered prophylactically to patients with AMI. In 1970, the estimated risk for primary VF in the control group (heavy line) was 4.5 per cent (lighter lines represent 95 per cent confidence intervals). By 1990, this risk was substantially below 1 per cent, probably owing to such factors as the increased use of beta blockers, more aggressive repletion of electrolyte deficits, more effective therapies for left ventricular dysfunction, the decreased use of diuretics, and more effective sedation and anxiolytic therapy. *B,* Importance of electrolyte deficits, as shown in this study in which the risk for VF was strikingly increased in patients who presented to the critical care unit (CCU) with hypokalemia. (*A* adapted from Antman, E. M., and Berlin, J. A.: Declining incidence of ventricular fibrillation in myocardial infarction: Implications for the prophylactic use of lidocaine. Circulation *86:*764, 1992; *B* adapted from Nordrehaug, J. E., and van der Lippe, G.: Hypokalemia and ventricular fibrillation in acute myocardial infarction. Br. Heart J. *50:*525, 1983.)

gradually before termination, or be overdriven by acceleration of the basic cardiac rhythm. Variation of the rate is common.

Accelerated idioventricular rhythm is often observed shortly after successful reperfusion has been established.[960,961] However, the frequent occurrence of these rhythms in patients without reperfusion limits their reliability as markers of restoration of patency of the infarct-related coronary artery.[962,963] In contrast to rapid ventricular

tachycardia, accelerated idioventricular rhythms are thought not to affect prognosis. There is no definitive evidence that this arrhythmia, when left untreated, increases the incidence of either ventricular fibrillation or death.[964] Therefore we do not routinely treat accelerated idioventricular rhythms. In the rare patient with clear-cut hemodynamic compromise or recurrent angina related to accelerated idioventricular rhythms, we attempt to accelerate the sinus rate with atropine or atrial pacing; suppressive antiarrhythmic therapy with lidocaine or procainamide is usually not used unless there is unequivocal precipitation of more serious ventricular tachyarrhythmias.

Ventricular Tachycardia
(See also p. 677)

Nonsustained ventricular tachycardia is usually defined as three or more consecutive ventricular ectopic beats (at a rate > 100 beats/min and lasting < 30 sec; Fig. 37–19); sustained ventricular tachycardia refers to similar rhythms that last longer than 30 seconds or cause hemodynamic compromise *that requires intervention.* (Although most brief runs of ventricular tachycardia cause some reduction in blood pressure that is observed on arterial line pressure tracings, the majority of such episodes are not recognized by the patient[237]). Additional descriptive features of note for sustained ventricular tachycardia are whether the ECG appearance is monomorphic or polymorphic.[965,966] This may be of importance because the former is more likely to be due to a myocardial scar and require aggressive strategies to prevent its recurrence and the latter may be more responsive to measures directed against ischemia. When continuous ECG recordings during the first 12 hours of AMI are analyzed, nonsustained paroxysms of monomorphic or polymorphic ventricular tachycardia may be seen in up to 67 per cent of patients.[954] These *nonsustained* runs of ventricular tachycardia do not appear to be associated with an increased mortality risk, either during hospitalization or over the first year.[966] Episodes of *sustained* ventricular tachycardia during the first 48 hours following AMI are often polymorphic and are associated with a hospital mortality of about 20 per cent.[966] However, the 1-year mortality in patients with sustained ventricular tachycardia who survive to hospital discharge is not increased over that of patients who had only nonsustained runs of ventricular tachycardia or no episodes of ventricular tachycardia during the first 48 hours.[966]

Ventricular tachycardia occurring late in the course of AMI is more common in patients with transmural infarction and left ventricular dysfunction, is likely to be sustained, usually induces marked hemodynamic deterioration, and is associated with both an increased hospital mortality and long-term mortality.[939,967]

MANAGEMENT. Since hypokalemia may increase the risk of developing ventricular tachycardia,[968] low serum potassium should be identified quickly after a patient's admission for AMI and should be treated promptly. The serum

FIGURE 37–44. Pooled results of 14 randomized controlled trials of lidocaine in patients with suspected AMI suggest that the drug increases mortality despite reducing the risk of ventricular fibrillation. Patients received the drug intravenously (nine trials) or by intramuscular injection (five trials) and were followed for roughly the length of treatment (24 to 48 hours of IV administration, a few hours for IM). The narrow vertical bars represent the risk ratio derived from the

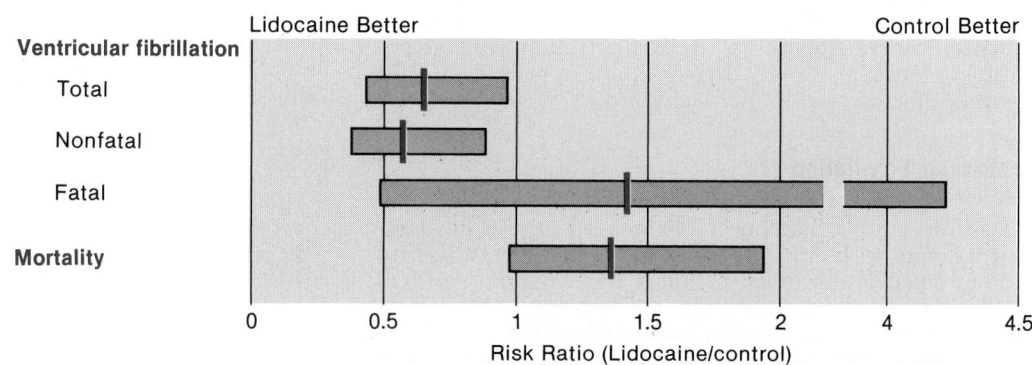

pooled data, and the broad horizontal bars show the 95 per cent confidence limits for these ratios. (Adapted from Antman, E. M., and Braunwald, E.: Acute MI: Management in the 1990s. Hosp. Pract. *25(2):*165, 1990, p. 73. © 1990 The McGraw-Hill Companies, Inc.)

potassium level should be maintained above 4.5 mEq/liter and serum magnesium above 2 mEq/liter.[30]

Rapid abolition of sustained ventricular tachycardia in patients with AMI is mandatory because of its deleterious effect on pump function and because it frequently deteriorates into ventricular fibrillation. When the ventricular rate is rapid (>150/min) and/or there is a decline in arterial pressure, a single attempt at "thumpversion," i.e., striking a sharp blow to the precordium, is indicated (see p. 680). Rapid polymorphic ventricular tachycardia should be managed similar to ventricular fibrillation, with an unsynchronized discharge of 200 joules, whereas monomorphic ventricular tachycardia should be treated with a synchronized discharge of 100 joules.[969] Occasionally lower energy (10 to 20 joules) synchronized discharges can terminate monomorphic ventricular tachycardia.

When the ventricular rate is slower than approximately 150/min and the arrhythmia is well tolerated hemodynamically, antiarrhythmic therapy with one of the following regimens should be attempted[2]:

1. *Lidocaine*—initial bolus of 1.0 to 1.5 mg/kg followed by supplemental boluses of 0.5 to 0.75 mg/kg every 5 to 10 min as needed to a maximum of 3 mg/kg. A maintenance infusion of 20 to 50 μg/kg/min (1 to 4 mg/min) may then be started. It should be recognized that the metabolism of lidocaine is slowed not only in patients with heart failure or hypotension but also in those with diminution of hepatic blood flow due to effects of pharmacological agents such as propranolol.[970] The rate of infusion should be lower in patients with renal failure. Therefore, careful titration is needed to avoid toxicity, manifested primarily by central nervous system hyperactivity, as well as by depression of intraventricular and atrioventricular conduction and cardiac contractility. Saturation of an extravascular pool normally occurs after a continuous infusion of approximately 3 hours, at which time blood levels increase despite maintenance of a constant infusion rate.[971] At this time, it may be desirable to reduce the rate of administration by about 25 per cent (see also p. 605).

2. *Procainamide*—loading infusion of 12 to 17 mg/kg over about 20 to 30 minutes, followed by a maintenance infusion of 1 to 4 mg/min (see also p. 603).

3. *Amiodarone*—loading infusion of 150 mg, followed by a constant infusion of 1.0 mg/min for up to 6 hours and then a maintenance infusion at 0.5 mg/min (see also p. 613).

After reversion to sinus rhythm, every effort should be made to correct underlying abnormalities such as hypoxia, hypotension, acid-base or electrolyte disturbances, and digitalis excess. Although no definitive data are available, it is a common clinical practice to continue maintenance infusions of antiarrhythmic drugs for several days following an index episode of ventricular tachycardia and to discontinue the drug and either observe the patient for recurrence or perform a diagnostic electrophysiology study. Patients with recurrent or refractory ventricular tachycardia should be considered for specialized procedures such as implantation of antitachycardia devices or surgery (see p. 621). Occasionally, urgent attempts at revascularization with angioplasty or coronary artery bypass graft surgery may help control refractory ventricular tachycardia.[965,972]

Ventricular Fibrillation
(See also p. 686)

This arrhythmia may occur in three settings in hospitalized patients with AMI. (Its occurrence as a mechanism of sudden death is discussed in Chap. 24.) *Primary* ventricular fibrillation occurs suddenly and unexpectedly in patients with no or few signs or symptoms of left ventricular failure. Although primary ventricular fibrillation occurred in up to 10 per cent of patients hospitalized with AMI

several decades ago, analyses suggest that its incidence has declined dramatically[955,973,974] (Fig. 37–43A). Approximately 60 per cent of episodes occur within 4 hours and 80 per cent within 12 hours of the onset of symptoms.[954] *Secondary* ventricular fibrillation, on the other hand, is often the final event of a progressive downhill course with left ventricular failure and cardiogenic shock.[237] So-called *late* ventricular fibrillation develops more than 48 hours following AMI and frequently but not exclusively occurs in patients with large infarcts and ventricular dysfunction. Patients with intraventricular conduction defects and anterior wall infarction, patients with persistent sinus tachycardia, atrial flutter, or fibrillation early in the clinical course, and those with right ventricular infarction who require ventricular pacing are at higher risk for suffering late in-hospital ventricular fibrillation than are patients without these features.

PROGNOSIS. The effect of primary ventricular fibrillation on prognosis continues to be debated. The MILIS study suggested that it does not have an adverse effect on hospital mortality, whereas the first GISSI trial suggested that there is an excess mortality due to primary ventricular fibrillation during the hospital phase but not thereafter.[975] On the other hand, secondary ventricular fibrillation occurring in association with marked left ventricular failure or cardiogenic shock clearly entails a poor prognosis, with in-hospital mortality rates of 40 to 60 per cent.[976] With the availability of amiodarone and new antitachycardia devices, the prognosis of late ventricular fibrillation is improving and is probably driven more by residual ventricular function and recurrent ischemia than the arrhythmic risk per se.[977]

PROPHYLAXIS. In the early years of MI care in CCUs, concern about the risk of primary ventricular fibrillation led to aggressive monitoring for warning ventricular arrhythmias (see p.1226) and the initiation of antiarrhythmic therapy when they appeared. Later, when it was shown that warning arrhythmias could not be relied upon to predict the risk of ventricular fibrillation, arrhythmia prophylaxis became routine.[978,979] Lidocaine has been studied most extensively in this regard and has been shown to reduce the incidence of ventricular fibrillation,[980] leading to its widespread routine use in CCUs in patients with known or suspected AMI. However, we no longer endorse that CCU practice for the following reasons:

1. As already noted, the incidence of ventricular fibrillation in patients hospitalized for AMI is decreasing so that the risk for the arrhythmia is now much lower than it was several decades ago (probably under 5 per cent) (Fig. 37–43A). The reasons for this reduction in ventricular fibrillation are not clear but probably include general improvements in the care of AMI patients, greater use of beta blockers, aggressive repletion of electrolytes, prompt treatment of ischemia and congestive heart failure, and reduction in infarct size from reperfusion strategies.[955]

2. There is no evidence that prophylaxis with lidocaine actually reduces mortality in hospitalized patients with AMI because they can almost always be promptly defibrillated. Furthermore, there appear to be trends to excess mortality risk when lidocaine is used on a routine prophylactic basis[956,980] (Fig. 37–44).

3. Beta-adrenoceptor blockers, which should be administered promptly to the majority of patients with AMI (see p. 1211), have been shown to reduce not only ventricular fibrillation[959] but also mortality from AMI.[745]

4. There is an association between hypokalemia and the risk of ventricular fibrillation in the CCU[981,982] (Fig. 37–43B). Although it has not been conclusively shown that correction of hypokalemia to a level of 4.5 mEq/liter actually reduces the incidence of ventricular fibrillation, our experience suggests that this probably is protective and of little risk. The data on magnesium and the risk of ventricu-

lar fibrillation are incomplete at present. Despite the fact that no consistent relationship between hypomagnesemia and ventricular fibrillation has been observed,[982] magnesium deficits may still be involved in the risk of ventricular fibrillation because intracellular magnesium levels are reduced in AMI and are not adequately reflected by serum measurements.[983] For these reasons, plus the fact that it is often difficult to repair a potassium deficit without administering supplemental magnesium, we routinely replete magnesium to a level of 2 mEq/liter.

The only situation in which we might consider prophylactic lidocaine (bolus of 1.5 mg/kg followed by 20 to 50 μg/kg/min) would be the unusual circumstance in which a patient within the first 12 hours of an AMI must be managed in a facility where cardiac monitoring is not available and equipment for prompt defibrillation is not readily accessible.

MANAGEMENT (see also p. 687). The likelihood of successful restoration of an effective cardiac rhythm declines rapidly with time after the onset of uncorrected ventricular fibrillation. Irreversible brain damage may occur within 1 to 2 minutes, particularly in elderly patients. The treatment of ventricular fibrillation is an unsynchronized electrical countershock with at least 200 to 300 joules, implemented as rapidly as possible. This interrupts fibrillation and restores an effective cardiac rhythm in patients under direct medical observation in the CCU. When ventricular fibrillation occurs outside an intensive care unit, resuscitative efforts are much less likely to be successful, primarily because the time interval between the onset of the episode and institution of definitive therapy tends to be prolonged. Because closed-chest cardiopulmonary resuscitation with external cardiac compression provides only a marginal cardiac output even under optimal circumstances, countershock could be implemented as soon as possible after the detection of ventricular fibrillation rather than deferred under the mistaken impression that adequate circulatory and respiratory support can be maintained in the interim. Failure of electrical countershock to restore an effective cardiac rhythm is due almost always to rapidly recurrent ventricular tachycardia or ventricular fibrillation, to electromechanical dissociation, or, very rarely, to electrical asystole.

Ventricular fibrillation often recurs rapidly and repeatedly when the metabolic milieu of the heart has been compromised by severe or prolonged hypoxemia, acidosis, electrolyte abnormalities, or digitalis intoxication. Under these conditions, continued cardiopulmonary resuscitation, prompt implementation of pharmacological and ventilatory maneuvers designed to correct these abnormalities, and rapidly repeated attempts with electrical countershock may be effective. Even though repeated shocks with excessive energy may damage the myocardium and elicit arrhythmias, speed is essential and prompt efforts with high-intensity shocks (generally 300 to 400 watt-seconds) are justified. When ventricular fibrillation persists without documented interruption by electrical countershock, administration of epinephrine either by the intracardiac route (up to 10 ml of a 1:10,000 concentration) or intravenous route (1 mg initially) may facilitate a subsequent defibrillation attempt.

Successful interruption of ventricular fibrillation or prevention of refractory recurrent episodes may also be facilitated by administration of bretylium tosylate, 5 mg/kg intravenously, repeated 5 to 20 minutes later if necessary (see p. 615), or amiodarone (75 to 150 mg bolus). When synchronous cardiac electrical activity is restored by countershock but contraction is ineffective—i.e., during electromechanical dissociation—the usual underlying cause is very extensive myocardial ischemia or necrosis or rupture of the ventricular free wall or septum.[984,985] If rupture has not occurred, intracardiac administration of calcium gluconate

or epinephrine may promote restoration of an effective heartbeat. We do *not* usually administer bicarbonate injections to correct acidosis because of the high osmotic load they impose and the fact that hyperventilation of the patient is probably a more suitable means of clearing the acidosis.

BRADYARRHYTHMIAS

Sinus Bradycardia
(See also p. 645)

Sinus bradycardia is a common arrhythmia occurring during the early phases of AMI, and it is particularly frequent in patients with inferior and posterior infarction.[986] Observations in mobile CCUs indicate that 25 to 40 per cent of patients with AMI have electrocardiographic evidence of sinus bradycardia within the first hour after the onset of symptoms; however, 4 hours after infarction commences, the incidence of sinus bradycardia has declined to 15 to 20 per cent.[938] Stimulation of cardiac vagal afferent receptors (which are more common in the inferoposterior than the anterior or lateral portions of the left ventricle), with resulting efferent cholinergic stimulation of the heart, produces vagotonia with resultant bradycardia and hypotension. This is a manifestation of the Bezold-Jarisch reflex[987] that is mediated by the vagus nerves and occurs during reperfusion, particularly of the right coronary artery.[483,529,530,988] Often sinus bradycardia is a component of vasovagal or vasodepressor response, which may be intensified by severe pain as well as by morphine, and may be related to vasovagal syncope (see p. 863).[989]

On the basis of data obtained in experimental infarction and from some clinical observations, it appears that the increased vagal tone that produces sinus bradycardia during the early phase of AMI may actually be protective, perhaps because it reduces myocardial oxygen demands.[986] Thus, the acute mortality rate appears to be as low in patients with sinus bradycardia as in patients without this arrhythmia.

MANAGEMENT. Isolated sinus bradycardia, unaccompanied by hypotension or ventricular ectopy, should be observed rather than treated initially. In the first 4 to 6 hours following infarction, if the sinus rate is extremely slow (under 40 to 50 bpm), administration of intravenous atropine in aliquots of 0.3 to 0.6 mg every 3 to 10 minutes (with a total dose not exceeding 2 mg) to bring heart rate up to approximately 60 beats/min often abolishes the VBPs commonly associated with this degree of sinus bradycardia. Atropine often contributes to restoration of arterial pressure and hence coronary perfusion and should be employed if hypotension accompanying any degree of sinus bradycardia is present. The favorable effects of atropine may be accompanied by regression of ST-segment elevation. Elevation of the lower extremities also often elevates arterial pressure by redistributing blood from the systemic venous bed to the thorax, thereby augmenting ventricular preload, cardiac output, and arterial pressure.

Sinus bradycardia occurring more than 6 hours after the onset of the AMI is often transitory, is caused by sinus node dysfunction or atrial ischemia rather than vagal hyperactivity, is usually not accompanied by hypotension, and does not usually predispose to ventricular arrhythmias. Treatment is not required unless ventricular performance is compromised or the administration of a beta-adrenoceptor blocker or high doses of antiarrhythmic drugs (which may slow the sinus rate further) is planned. When atropine is ineffective and the patient is symptomatic and/or hypotensive, electrical pacing is indicated (see Chap. 23). In patients with depressed ventricular performance, who require the atrial contribution to ventricular filling, atrial pacing or atrioventricular sequential pacing is superior to simple ventricular pacing.[892]

ATRIOVENTRICULAR AND INTRAVENTRICULAR BLOCK

Ischemic injury can produce conduction block at any level of the AV or intraventricular conduction system. Such blocks may occur in the atrioventricular node and the bundle of His, producing various grades of AV block; in either main bundle branch, producing right or left bundle branch block; and in the anterior and posterior divisions of the left bundle, producing left anterior or left posterior (fascicular) divisional blocks. Disturbances of conduction can, of course, occur in various combinations. The mechanisms and recognition of intraventricular and atrioventricular conduction disturbances are discussed in Chapter 22.

First-Degree AV Block (see also p. 688)

First-degree AV block (Fig. 22–49, p. 688) occurs in less than 15 per cent of patients with AMI admitted to CCUs. His bundle electrocardiographic studies have shown that almost all patients with first-degree AV block have disturbances in conduction above the bundle of His, i.e., intranodal. The localization of the site of block is important because development of complete heart block and ventricular asystole is restricted almost exclusively to those patients with first-degree block in whom the conduction disturbance is *below* the bundle of His; this occurs more commonly in patients with anterior infarction and those with associated bifascicular block.[990]

First-degree AV block generally does not require specific treatment. However, if digitalis intoxication is suspected as the cause, this drug should be discontinued. Beta blockers and calcium antagonists (other than nifedipine) prolong AV conduction and may be responsible for first-degree AV block as well. However, discontinuation of these drugs in the setting of AMI has the potential of increasing ischemia and ischemic injury. Therefore, it is our practice not to decrease the dosage of these drugs unless the PR interval is greater than 0.24 sec. Only if higher-degree block or hemodynamic impairment occurs should these agents be stopped. If the block is a manifestation of excessive vagotonia and is associated with sinus bradycardia and hypotension, administration of atropine, as already outlined, may be helpful. Continued electrocardiographic monitoring is important in such patients in view of the possibility of progression to higher degrees of block.[991]

Second-Degree AV Block

MOBITZ TYPE I OR WENCKEBACH (Fig. 22–51, p. 689). Mobitz type I block occurs in up to 10 per cent of patients with AMI admitted to CCUs and accounts for about 90 per cent of all patients with AMI and second-degree AV block. This type of block (1) generally occurs within the AV node, (2) is usually associated with narrow QRS complexes, (3) is presumably secondary to ischemic injury, (4) occurs more commonly in patients with inferior than anterior myocardial infarction, (5) is usually transient and does not persist for more than 72 hours after infarction, (6) may be intermittent, and (7) rarely progresses to complete AV block (Table 37–13). First-degree and type I second-degree AV blocks do not appear to affect survival, are most commonly associated with occlusion of the right coronary artery, and are caused by ischemia of the AV node.

Specific therapy is not required in patients with second-degree AV block of the Mobitz type I variety when the ventricular rate exceeds 50 beats/min and ventricular irritability, heart failure, and bundle branch block are absent. However, if these complications develop or if the heart rate falls below approximately 50 beats/min and the patient is symptomatic, immediate treatment with atropine (0.3 to 0.6 mg) is indicated; temporary pacing systems are almost never needed in the management of this arrhythmia.

MOBITZ TYPE II (Fig. 22–52, p. 689). This is a rare conduction defect following AMI, occurring in only 10 per cent of all cases of second-degree block.[992] Thus, the overall incidence of Mobitz type II block after infarction is less than 1 per cent. In contrast to Mobitz type I block, type II second-degree block (1) usually originates from a lesion in the conduction system below the bundle of His, (2) is associated with a wide QRS complex, (3) often but not invariably reflects trifascicular block with impaired conduction distal to the bundle of His, (4) often progresses suddenly to complete AV block, and (5) is almost always associated with anterior rather than inferior infarction (Table 37–13).

Because of its potential for progression to complete heart block, Mobitz type II second-degree AV block should be treated with a temporary external or transvenous demand pacemaker with the rate set at approximately 60 beats/min.

Complete (Third-Degree) AV Block (see also p. 691)

The AV conduction system has a dual blood supply, the AV branch of the right coronary artery and the septal perforating branch from the left anterior descending coronary artery.[993] Therefore, complete AV block can occur in patients with either anterior or inferior infarction. Complete AV block develops in 5 to 15 per cent of patients with AMI[994,995]; the incidence may be even higher in patients with right ventricular infarction.[105] As with other forms of AV block, the prognosis depends on the anatomical location of the block in the conduction system and the size of the infarction.[996]

Complete heart block in patients with inferior infarction usually results from an intranodal or supranodal lesion[997] and develops gradually, often progressing from first-degree or type I second-degree block (Table 37–13). The escape rhythm is usually stable without asystole and often junctional, with a rate exceeding 40 beats/min and a narrow QRS complex in 70 per cent of cases and a slower rate and wide QRS in the others. This form of complete AV block is often transient, may be responsive to pharmacological antagonism of adenosine with methylxanthines,[998] and resolves in the majority of patients within a few days.[999] The mortality may approach 15 per cent unless right ventricular infarction is present, in which case the mortality associated with complete AV block may be more than doubled.[1000]

In patients with anterior infarction, third-degree AV block often occurs suddenly, 12 to 24 hours after the onset of infarction, although it is usually preceded by intraventricular block and often Mobitz type II (not first-degree or Mobitz type I) AV block (Table 37–13). Such patients have unstable escape rhythms with wide QRS complexes and rates less than 40 beats/min; ventricular systole may occur quite suddenly. The mortality in this group of patients is extremely high, approximately 70 to 80 per cent.[1001]

PROGNOSIS. This depends on the extent and secondarily on the anatomical site of the myocardial injury.[999,1002] Patients with inferior infarction often have concomitant ischemia or infarction of the AV node secondary to hypoperfusion of the AV node artery. However, the His-Purkinje system usually escapes injury in such individuals. Patients with inferior MI who develop AV block usually have lesions in both the right and left anterior descending coronary arteries.[1003] Likewise, patients with inferior MI and AV block have larger infarcts and more depressed right ventricular and left ventricular function than do patients with inferior infarct and no AV block. As already noted, junctional escape rhythms with narrow QRS complexes occur commonly in this setting. In patients with anterior infarction, AV block usually develops as a result of extensive septal necrosis that involves the bundle branches. The high mortality in this group of patients with slow idioventricular rhythm and wide QRS complexes is the consequence of extensive myocardial necrosis resulting in severe left ventricular failure and often shock.

Although data suggest that complete AV block is *not* an

	LOCATION OF AV CONDUCTION DISTURBANCE	
	Proximal	**Distal**
Site of block	Intranodal	Intranodal
Site of infarction	Inferoposterior	Anteroseptal
Compromised arterial supply	RCA (90%), LCX (10%)	Septal perforators of LAD
Pathogenesis	Ischemia, necrosis, hydropic cell swelling, excess parasympathetic activity	Ischemia, necrosis, hydropic cell swelling
Predominant type of AV nodal block	First-degree (PR > 200 ms) Mobitz type I second-degree	Mobitz type II second-degree Third-degree
Common premonitory features of third-degree AV block	(a) First–second-degree AV block (b) Mobitz I pattern	(a) Intraventricular conduction block (b) Mobitz II pattern
Features of escape rhythm following third-degree block		
(a) Location	(a) Proximal conduction system (His bundle)	(a) Distal conduction system (bundle branches)
(b) QRS width	(b) <0.12/sec*	(b) >0.12/sec
(c) Rate	(c) 45–60/min but may be as low as 30/min	(c) Often <30/min
(d) Stability of escape rhythm	(d) Rate usually stable; asystole uncommon	(d) Rate often unstable with moderate to high risk of ventricular asystole
Duration of high-grade AV block	Usually transient (2–3 days)	Usually transient but some form of AV conduction disturbance and/or intraventricular defect may persist
Associated mortality rate	Low unless associated with hypotension and/or congestive heart failure	High because of extensive infarction associated with power failure or ventricular arrhythmias
Pacemaker therapy		
(a) Temporary	(a) Rarely required; may be considered for bradycardia associated with left ventricular power failure, syncope, or angina	(a) Should be considered in patients with anteroseptal infarction and acute bifascicular block
(b) Permanent	(b) Almost never indicated because conduction defect is usually transient	(b) Indicated for patients with high-grade AV block with block in His–Purkinje system and those with transient advanced AV block and associated bundle branch block

Modified from Antman, E. M. and Rutherford, J. D.: Coronary Care Medicine: A Practical Approach. Boston: Martinus Nijhoff, 1986; Dreifus, L. S., et al.: Guidelines for implantation of cardiac pacemakers and antiarrhythmia devices. Reprinted with permission from the American College of Cardiology. J. Am. Coll. Cardiol. *18*:1, 1991.

* Some studies suggest that a wide QRS escape rhythm (>0.12 sec) following high-grade AV block in inferior infarction is associated with a worse prognosis.

RCA = right coronary artery; LCX = left circumflex coronary artery; LAD = left anterior descending coronary artery.

independent risk factor for mortality,[1004] whether temporary transvenous pacing per se improves survival of patients with anterior AMI remains controversial. Some investigators contend that ventricular pacing is useless when employed to correct complete AV block in patients with anterior infarction in view of the poor prognosis in this group regardless of therapy. We agree with others,[993,1005] however, that ventricular or AV sequential pacing is indicated in essentially all patients with AMI with complete AV block. Pacing is likely to protect against transient hypotension with its attendant risks of extending infarction and precipitating malignant ventricular tachyarrhythmias. Also pacing protects against asystole, a particular hazard in patients with anterior infarction and infranodal block. Improved survival with pacing probably occurs in only a small fraction of patients with complete AV block and anterior wall infarcts because the extensive destruction of the myocardium that almost invariably accompanies this condition results in a very high mortality rate, even in paced patients.

Given these considerations, an extremely large series of patients would be required to demonstrate the small reduction of mortality that might be achieved by pacing. The absence of data supporting such an effect, however, by no means excludes the possibility that it may be present. Although it is generally agreed that pacing is indicated in patients with inferior wall infarction and complete AV block, it is of particular importance if the ventricular rate is very slow (<40 to 50 beats/min), if ventricular irritability or hypotension is present, or if pump failure develops;

atropine is only rarely of value in these patients. Only when complete heart block develops in less than 6 hours after the onset of symptoms is atropine likely to abolish the AV block or cause acceleration of the escape rhythm.[1006] In such cases the AV block is more likely to be transient and related to increases in vagal tone rather than the more persistent block seen later in the course of MI, which generally requires cardiac pacing.

Intraventricular Block

In the prethrombolytic era studies of intraventricular conduction disturbances, i.e., block within one or more of the three subdivisions (fascicles) of the His-Purkinje system (the anterior and posterior divisions of the left bundle and the right bundle, p. 121), had been reported to occur in 5 to 10 per cent of patients with AMI.[1005,1007–1009] The right bundle branch and the left posterior division have a dual blood supply from the left anterior descending and right coronary arteries, whereas the left anterior division is supplied by septal perforators originating from the left anterior descending coronary artery. Not all conduction blocks observed in patients with AMI can be considered to be complications of infarcts because almost half are already present at the time the first ECG is recorded, and they may represent antecedent disease of the conduction system.[1007]

ISOLATED LEFT ANTERIOR DIVISIONAL BLOCK (see p. 121). This occurs in 3 to 5 per cent of patients with AMI[1010] and in an additional 5 per cent of patients with associated right bundle branch block. Isolated left anterior divisional block is unlikely to progress to complete AV block.[1005,1009,1011] Mortality is increased in these patients, although not as much as in patients with other forms of conduction block.

LEFT POSTERIOR DIVISIONAL BLOCK. This occurs in only 1 to 2 per cent of patients with AMI admitted to coronary care units. The posterior fascicle is larger than the anterior fascicle, and, in general, a larger infarct is required to block it. As a consequence, mortality is markedly increased.[1012] Complete AV block is not a frequent complication of either form of isolated divisional block.[1005,1009,1011,1012]

RIGHT BUNDLE BRANCH BLOCK. This defect alone occurs in approximately 2 per cent of patients with AMI and frequently leads to AV block because it is often a new lesion, associated with anteroseptal infarction.[1007,1012] Isolated right bundle branch block is associated with an increased mortality risk in patients with anterior MI even if complete AV block does not occur, but this appears to be the case only if it is accompanied by congestive heart failure.[1007,1009,1010,1012–1015]

BIFASCICULAR BLOCK. The combination of right bundle branch block with either left anterior or posterior divisional block or the combination of left anterior and posterior divisional blocks (i.e., left bundle branch block) is known as bidivisional or bifascicular block (see p. 123). If new block occurs in two of the three divisions of the conduction system, the risk of developing complete AV block is quite high. Mortality is also high because of the occurrence of severe pump failure secondary to the extensive myocardial necrosis required to produce such an extensive intraventricular block.[1011] Left bundle branch block occurs in approximately 5 per cent of patients with AMI. Although the latter defect progresses to complete AV block only half as frequently as does right bundle branch block, it is associated with as high a mortality as right bundle branch block and the other two forms of bifascicular block[939,1009,1012,1013] and with a high late mortality. Patients with intraventricular conduction defects, particularly right bundle branch block,[1016] account for the majority of patients who develop ventricular fibrillation late in their hospital stay. However, the high mortality in these patients occurs even in the absence of high-grade AV block and appears to be related to cardiac failure and massive infarction rather than to the conduction disturbance.

Preexisting bundle branch block or divisional block is less often associated with the development of complete heart block in patients with AMI than are conduction defects acquired during the course of the infarct.[1009] Bidivisional block in the presence of prolongation of the P-R interval (first-degree AV block) may indicate disease of the third subdivision rather than of the AV node. In such cases, termed trifascicular block, nearly 40 per cent progress to complete heart block, a risk that is considerably greater than the risk of complete heart block without first-degree AV block.[1005]

Complete bundle branch block (either left or right), the combination of right bundle branch block and left anterior divisional (fascicular) block, and any of the various forms of trifascicular block are all more often associated with anterior than inferoposterior infarction. All these forms are more frequent with large infarcts and in older patients and have a higher incidence of other accompanying arrhythmias than is seen in patients without bundle branch block.[1013]

Use of Pacemakers in AMI
(See also p. 1964)

TEMPORARY PACING. Just as is the case for complete AV block, transvenous ventricular pacing has not resulted in statistically demonstrable improvement in prognosis among patients with AMI who develop intraventricular conductions defects. However, temporary pacing is advisable in some of these patients because of the high risk of developing complete AV block. This includes patients with new bilateral (bifascicular) bundle branch block, i.e., right bundle branch block with left anterior or posterior divisional block and alternating right and left bundle branch block; first-degree AV block adds to this risk. Isolated new block in only one of the three fascicles even with P-R prolongation and preexisting bifascicular block and normal P-R interval poses somewhat less risk; these patients should be monitored closely, with insertion of a temporary pacemaker deferred unless higher-degree AV block occurs.

It has been proposed on the basis of results of an analysis of several large series of well-characterized patients that the risk of developing complete heart block following AMI can be predicted.[1011] The presence (new or preexisting) of any of the following conduction disturbances is considered a risk factor: first-degree AV block, Mobitz type I second-degree AV block, Mobitz type II second-degree AV block, left anterior hemiblock, left posterior hemiblock, right bundle branch block, and left bundle branch block. Each risk factor was assigned a score of 1, and the risk score was calculated as the sum of these electrocardiographic risk factors. The incidence of complete heart block occurred as follows: risk score 0, 1.2 to 6.8 per cent incidence; risk score 1, 7.8 to 10.4 per cent incidence; risk score 2, 25.0 to 30.1 per cent incidence; and risk score 3, 36 per cent or greater incidence.[1011] Some authorities have pointed out deficiencies in this scoring system in that Mobitz type II AV block is assigned a score of only 1 point but appears to carry more significance; also there is no differentiation between preexisting and newly appearing bundle branch block.[1017]

We believe that failure to demonstrate improved prognosis statistically does not belie the potential value of pacemaker therapy; it probably reflects the overriding impact on mortality of the extensive infarction responsible for the development of the conduction abnormality and the large number of patients required to permit statistical documentation of reduction of mortality.

In assessing the need for temporary pacing (Table 37–13), the clinician must keep in mind that between 10 and 20 per cent of patients develop pacemaker-related complications.[1018] A pericardial friction rub develops in approximately 5 per cent of patients but does not necessarily indicate cardiac perforation, nor is such a finding an indication for withdrawal of the pacemaker electrode. Arrhythmias requiring cardioversion, right ventricular perforation, and local infectious complications occur in 1 to 3 per cent of cases.[1018] Pacemaker malfunction also occurs rather frequently and is, in part, related to the experience of the clinical team in managing the device and its insertion.

Although external temporary cardiac pacing was introduced in 1952,[1019] its widespread clinical use did not occur until relatively recently owing to technical refinements making the technique safe, quickly applicable, and relatively well tolerated. Noninvasive external temporary cardiac pacing is now possible routinely in conscious patients and is acceptable to many but not all patients because of the discomfort.[1020] Used in a standby mode, it is virtually free of complications and contraindications and provides an important alternative to transvenous endocardial pacing. Once it is clinically evident that continuous pacing is required, external pacing, which is generally well tolerated for more than minutes to hours, should be replaced by a temporary transvenous pacemaker (Table 37–13).

PERMANENT PACING. The question of permanent pacing in survivors of AMI associated with conduction defects is still controversial (Table 37–13). Patients with inferior infarction with transient type II second-degree block or complete AV block without an associated intraventricular conduction defect do not appear to require permanent pacing. Some contend that prophylactic pacing makes little difference in the long-term survival of patients with AMI and bundle branch block complicated by transient high-degree block.[1021] On the other hand, in a retrospective multicenter study, survivors of AMI and bundle branch block who experienced transient high-degree (Mobitz type II second-degree, or third-degree) block had a high incidence of recurrent high-degree AV block and sudden death, and this incidence was reduced by insertion of a permanent demand pacemaker.[1005,1009] Thus, these findings suggest a role for prophylactic permanent pacing in patients with AMI and bundle branch block with transient high-degree AV block.

The question of the advisability of permanent pacemaker insertion is complicated by the fact that not all sudden deaths in this population are due to recurrent high-degree block. A high incidence of late in-hospital ventricular fibrillation occurs in CCU survivors with anteroseptal MI complicated by either right or left bundle branch block.[1016] If the propensity for this arrhythmia continued, ventricular fibrillation rather than asystole due to failure of AV conduction and of the infranodal pacemaker could be responsible for late sudden death.

Long-term pacing is often helpful when complete heart block persists throughout the hospital phase in a patient with AMI, when sinus node function is markedly impaired, or when Mobitz II second- or third-degree block occurs intermittently. When high-grade AV block is associated with newly acquired bundle branch block or other criteria of impairment of conduction system function, prophylactic long-term pacing may be justified as well. Thus, despite the difficulty of proving that long-term pacing improves survival after MI because of the high mortality associated with extensive infarction frequently responsible for high degrees of heart block, prophylactic long-term pacing is prudent.

ASYSTOLE. This arrhythmia has been reported to occur in 1 to 14 per cent of patients with AMI admitted to CCUs.[939] This wide variation in incidence reflects differences in the definition of this event. The lower incidence rates include only patients who develop asystole either as a primary event or following abnormalities of AV or intraventricular conduction, whereas the higher rates include patients who develop asystole as a terminal complication. In either event, the mortality is very high.

The presence of apparent ventricular asystole on monitor displays of continuously recorded electrocardiograms may be misleading, because the mechanism may in fact be fine ventricular fibrillation. Because of the predominance of ventricular fibrillation as the cause of cardiac arrest in this setting, initial therapy should include electrical countershock, even if definitive electrocardiographic documentation of this arrhythmia is not available. In the rare instance in which asystole can be documented to be the responsible electrophysiological disturbance, immediate transcutaneous pacing (or stimulation with a transvenous pacemaker if one is already in place) is indicated.[1020]

SUPRAVENTRICULAR TACHYARRHYTHMIAS

SINUS TACHYCARDIA (see also p. 645). This arrhythmia is typically associated with augmented sympathetic activity and may provoke transient hypertension or hypotension. Common causes are anxiety, persistent pain, left ventricular failure, fever, pericarditis, hypovolemia, pulmonary embolism, and the administration of cardioaccelerator drugs such as atropine, epinephrine, or dopamine; rarely it occurs in patients with atrial infarction. Sinus tachycardia is particularly common in patients with anterior infarction, expecially if there is significant accompanying left ventricular dysfunction.[1022] It is an undesirable rhythm in patients with AMI because it results in an augmentation of myocardial oxygen consumption, as well as a reduction in the time available for coronary perfusion, thereby intensifying myocardial ischemia and/or external myocardial necrosis. Persistent sinus tachycardia may signify persistent heart failure and under these circumstances is a poor prognostic sign associated with an excess mortality. An underlying cause should be sought and appropriate treatment instituted, e.g., analgesics for pain, diuretics for heart failure, oxygen, beta blockers and nitroglycerin for ischemia, and aspirin for fever or pericarditis.

Administration of beta-adrenoceptor blocking agents, in the dosage and manner described on page 612, may be helpful in the treatment of sinus tachycardia, particularly when this arrhythmia is a manifestation of a hyperdynamic circulation, which is seen particularly in young patients with an initial MI without extensive cardiac damage. However, beta blockade is contraindicated in patients in whom the sinus tachycardia is a manifestation of hypovolemia or of pump failure, the latter reflected by a systolic arterial pressure below 100 mm Hg, rales involving more than one-third of the lung fields, a pulmonary capillary wedge pressure exceeding 20 to 25 mm Hg, or a cardiac index below approximately 2.2 liters/min/m². A possible exception to this is a patient in whom persistent ischemia is believed to be the cause or the result of tachycardia—cautious administration of an ultrashort-acting beta-adrenoceptor blocker such as esmolol (25 to 200 μg/kg/min) may be tried to ascertain the patient's response to slowing of the heart rate.[416]

ATRIAL PREMATURE CONTRACTIONS (see also p. 650). Atrial premature contractions, and the atrial tachyarrhythmias (paroxysmal supraventricular tachycardia, atrial flutter, and atrial fibrillation) that they often herald, may be caused by atrial distention secondary to increases in left ventricular diastolic pressure, by pericarditis with its associated atrial epicarditis, or, less commonly, by ischemic injury to the atria[1023] and sinus node. Atrial premature beats per se are not associated with an increase in mortality,[1023] and cardiac output is unaffected. No specific therapy is needed, but it should be kept in mind that these beats may indicate excessive autonomic stimulation or the presence of overt or occult heart failure—conditions that may be assessed by physical examination, chest roentgenography, and echocardiography.

PAROXYSMAL SUPRAVENTRICULAR TACHYCARDIA (see also p. 677). This arrhythmia occurs in less than 10 per cent of patients with AMI but requires aggressive management because of the rapid ventricular rate.[1024,1025] Augmentation of vagal tone by manual carotid sinus stimulation may restore sinus rhythm. The drug of choice for paroxysmal supraventricular tachycardia in the non-AMI patient is adenosine (6 to 12 mg).[1025] Few data exist to guide therapy with adenosine in the AMI patient, but we believe that it can be used safely provided that hypotension (systolic pressure <100 mm Hg) is not present prior to its administration. Intravenous verapamil (5 to 10 mg), diltiazem (15 to 20 mg), or metoprolol (5 to 15 mg) are suitable alternatives in patients without significant left ventricular dysfunction. In the presence of congestive heart failure or hypotension, DC countershock or rapid atrial stimulation via a transvenous intraatrial electrode should be utilized. Although digitalis glycosides may be useful in augmenting vagal tone, thereby terminating the arrhythmia, their effect is often delayed.

ATRIAL FLUTTER AND FIBRILLATION (see also pp. 652 and 654). Atrial flutter is the least common major atrial arrhythmia associated with AMI, occurring in less than 5 per cent of patients.[1023] Atrial flutter is usually transient, and in AMI it is typically a consequence of augmented sympathetic stimulation of the atria, often occurring in patients with left ventricular failure or pulmonary emboli in whom the arrhythmia intensifies hemodynamic deterioration.[938,939,1026]

Atrial fibrillation is far more common than flutter, occurring in 10 to 15 per cent of patients with AMI.[1027,1027a] As with atrial premature contractions and atrial flutter, fibrillation is usually transient and tends to occur in patients with left ventricular failure but is also observed in patients with pericarditis and ischemic injury to the atria and right ventricular infarction.[105,1028] The increased ventricular rate and the loss of the atrial contribution to left ventricular filling result in a significant reduction in cardiac output. Atrial fibrillation during AMI is associated with increased mortality and stroke, particularly in patients with anterior wall infarction.[1024,1027,1029] However, because it is more common in patients with clinical and hemodynamic manifestations of extensive infarction and a poor prognosis, atrial fibrillation is probably a marker of poor prognosis, with only a small independent contribution to increased mortality.[1023]

Management. Atrial flutter and fibrillation in patients with AMI are treated in a manner similar to these conditions in other settings (see pp. 654 and 656). Because of the possibility that the rapid ventricular rate and hypotension associated with these arrhythmias can increase infarct size and because of the important role played by atrial contraction in the support of cardiac output in patients with AMI, treatment must be prompt, especially when the ventricular rate exceeds 100 beats/min. When hemodynamic decompensation is prominent, electrical cardioversion is indicated, beginning with 25 to 50 joules for atrial flutter and 50 to 100 joules for atrial fibrillation, with gradual increase if the initial shock is not successful. For patients without hemodynamic compromise, the first maneuver should be to slow the ventricular rate. Ideally, a beta-adrenoceptor blocker (e.g., metoprolol in 5-mg intravenous boluses every 5 to 10 minutes to a total dose of 15 to 20 mg, followed by 25 to 50 mg orally every 6 hours) should be used because of the combined effects of ischemia and sympathetic tone that are usually present in patients with atrial fibrillation. If there is concern about the patient's ability to tolerate beta blockade, esmolol may be used (see p. 610). Intravenous doses of verapamil or diltiazem (see p. 616) are attractive alternatives because of their ability to slow the ventricular rate promptly, but they should be used with caution if at all in patients with pulmonary congestion. In patients with congestive heart failure, digitalis is the principal agent used to slow the ventricular response, although the onset of its effect may be delayed for several hours. Digitalis may be supplemented by small intravenous doses of a beta blocker, which also prolongs the AV nodal refractory period: 1 to 4 mg of propranolol in divided doses is often quite effective in reducing the ventricular rate and is well tolerated, even in patients with mild heart failure and a rapid ventricular rate. An additional important option for the treatment of atrial flutter is the use of rapid atrial stimulation via a transvenous intraatrial electrode (see p. 624).[1030] Because of the increased risk of embolism in atrial fibrillation, intravenous anticoagulation with heparin should be instituted in the absence of any contraindications.

Attention should be directed to the management of the underlying cause, usually heart failure, and then a decision must be made about the advisability of antiarrhythmic therapy to restore and maintain sinus rhythm. In patients who have acute atrial flutter or fibrillation without a history of atrial fibrillation and in whom congestive symptoms are either absent or easily controlled, we usually administer intravenous procainamide (2 to 4 mg/min) for 24 to 48 hours. The goal is to achieve pharmacological cardioversion or secondarily to establish a therapeutic concentration of the drug in preparation for DC cardioversion.[1031]

In view of the mounting evidence of an increased risk of proarrhythmia from antiarrhythmic drugs prescribed for atrial fibrillation, as well as an adverse interaction between recurrent ischemia and antiarrhythmic drugs, we are reluctant to prescribe type I antiarrhythmic agents over the intermediate or long term in patients with AMI.[1032-1035] Amiodarone appears to be an increasingly attractive antiarrhythmic drug for suppression of recurrences of atrial fibrillation.[1036,1037] This drug is also useful for prevention of ventricular arrhythmias and can block the AV node should atrial fibrillation recur—all desirable features following AMI. It may be prescribed in a low dose (200 mg/day), thereby reducing the risk of toxicity. Although experience is limited, we agree with the suggestion that amiodarone is probably the most logical choice of drugs for suppression of atrial fibrillation following AMI[387,1036,1037]; often only a short course of treatment (6 weeks) is needed because the risk of atrial fibrillation decreases as time passes following infarction.

Patients with recurrent episodes of atrial fibrillation should be treated with oral anticoagulants (to reduce the risk of stroke), even if sinus rhythm is present at the time of hospital discharge, because no antiarrhythmic regimen can be relied upon to be completely effective in suppressing atrial fibrillation. In the absence of contraindications,

the majority of patients should receive a beta blocker after AMI; in addition to their several other beneficial effects in MI and post-MI patients, these agents are helpful in slowing the ventricular rate should atrial fibrillation recur.

JUNCTIONAL RHYTHMS (see also p. 659). These arrhythmias are often transient, occur during the first 48 hours of the infarction, typically develop and terminate gradually, and are characterized by QRS complexes that resemble those of normally conducted beats. Retrograde P waves may be evident, or AV dissociation may occur, with the junctional rate slightly in excess of the underlying sinus rate. Junctional rhythms fall into two categories:

1. AV junctional rhythm at a rate of 35 to 60 beats/min in which the AV junctional tissue simply assumes the role of the dominant pacemaker when the sinus node is depressed. This arrhythmia is generally a benign protective escape rhythm that is commonly seen among patients with a slow sinus rate in the presence of inferior myocardial infarction. When there is hemodynamic impairment, transvenous sequential AV pacing may be required to facilitate ventricular performance and maintain adequate peripheral perfusion.

2. Accelerated junctional rhythm (nonparoxysmal junctional tachycardia) is less common and occurs when there is increased automaticity of the junctional tissue, which usurps the role of pacemaker, usually appearing at a rate of 70 to 130 beats/min. This arrhythmia is seen more commonly with inferior than anterior AMI and may also appear in patients with digitalis intoxication. In studies conducted during the prethrombolytic era, the appearance of accelerated junctional rhythm in the setting of anterior infarction was associated with a poor prognosis, but this was not observed when it occurred in patients with inferior infarction.[1038]

OTHER COMPLICATIONS

Recurrent Chest Discomfort

Evaluation of postinfarction chest discomfort may be complicated by previous abnormalities on the ECG and a vague description of the discomfort by the patient who either may be exquisitely sensitive to fleeting discomfort or may deny a potential recrudescence of symptoms. The critical task for clinicians is to distinguish recurrent angina or infarction from nonischemic causes of discomfort that might be caused by infarct expansion (see p. 1195), pericarditis, pulmonary embolism, and noncardiac conditions. Important diagnostic maneuvers include a repeat physical examination, repeat ECG, and assessment of the response to sublingual nitroglycerin, 0.4 mg. (The use of noninvasive diagnostic evaluation for recurrent ischemia in patients whose symptoms only appear with moderate levels of exertion is discussed on page 1295.)

RECURRENT ISCHEMIA AND INFARCTION. The incidence of postinfarction angina without reinfarction is between 20 and 30 per cent.[641] It does not appear to be reduced by the use of thrombolytic therapy as the management strategy during the acute phase,[33,1039] but has been reported to be lower in patients who undergo primary PTCA for AMI.[606] When accompanied by ST and T-wave changes in the same leads where Q waves have appeared, it may be due to occlusion of an initially patent vessel, reocclusion of an initially recanalized vessel,[626] or coronary spasm.[1040]

Extension of the original zone of necrosis or *reinfarction* in a separate myocardial zone can be a difficult diagnosis, especially within the first 24 hours after the index event.[173] It is more convenient to refer to both extension and reinfarction collectively under the more general term *recurrent infarction*.[387] Serum cardiac markers may still be elevated from the initial infarction, and it may not be possible to distinguish the ECG changes that are part of the normal evolution after the index infarction (see p. 1205) from those due to recurrent infarction. Because the cardiac-specific troponins (see p. 1203) remain elevated for more than 1 week following the index event, they are of less value for diagnosing recurrent infarction than are more rapidly rising and falling markers such as CK-MB. Within the first 18 to 24 hours following the initial infarction, when serum cardiac markers may not have returned to the normal range, recurrent infarction should be strongly considered when there is repeat ST-segment elevation on the ECG. Although pericarditis remains a possibility in such patients, the two can usually be distinguished by the presence of a rub and lack of responsiveness to nitroglycerin in patients with pericardial discomfort.

Beyond the first 24 hours, when serum cardiac markers such as CK-MB have usually returned to the normal range (see p. 1203), recurrent infarction may be diagnosed either by re-elevation of the CK-MB above the upper limit of normal and increased by at least 50 per cent of the previous value or the appearance of new Q waves on the ECG.[641,1041] Because of variations in patient populations and definitions of recurrent infarction, estimates of the incidence of this complication of AMI range from about 5 per cent to as high as 20 per cent within the first 6 weeks and may be somewhat higher in patients who have received thrombolytic therapy.[33,641,1042–1044] Marmor reported that recurrent infarction occurred frequently in obese females and was most common in patients with nontransmural infarction.[1045] It is apparently more common in patients with diabetes mellitus, those with a previous MI, and those with an early peaking CK-MB curve (<15 hours), but it is not predictable from the angiographic appearance of the coronary artery early after infarction—at least when thrombolytic therapy has been given.[1043]

Regardless of whether postinfarction angina is persistent or limited, its presence is important because short-term morbidity is higher among such patients; mortality may be increased if the recurrent ischemia is accompanied by ECG changes and hemodynamic compromise.[1046–1050] Recurrent infarction (due in many cases to reocclusion of the infarct-related coronary artery) carries serious adverse prognostic information because it is associated with a two to fourfold higher rate of in-hospital complications (congestive heart failure, heart block) and mortality.[626,1044,1051,1052] The mortality rate at 1 to 3 years following the initial infarction is higher in those patients who suffered from recurrent infarction during their index hospitalization.[1053,1054] Presumably, the higher mortality is related to the larger mass of myocardium whose function becomes compromised.

Of the standard therapies that are routinely prescribed during the acute phase of AMI, aspirin and beta blockers have been associated with a reduction in the incidence of recurrent infarction.[641,746,1055] The data on heparin are less convincing.[2]

Management. As with the acute phase of treatment of AMI, algorithms for management of patients with recurrent ischemic discomfort at rest center on the 12-lead ECG[387,1056] (Fig. 37–45). Those patients with ST-segment reelevation should either receive repeat thrombolysis[1057–1059] or be referred for urgent catheterization and PTCA.[1060] Insertion of an intraaortic balloon pump (see p. 1232) may help stabilize the patient while other procedures are being arranged. For patients believed to have recurrent ischemia who do not have evidence of hemodynamic compromise, an attempt should be made to control symptoms with sublingual or intravenous nitroglycerin and intravenous beta blockade to slow the heart rate to 60 beats/min.[387] When hypotension, congestive heart failure, or ventricular arrhythmias develop during recurrent ischemia, urgent catheterization and revascularization are indicated.

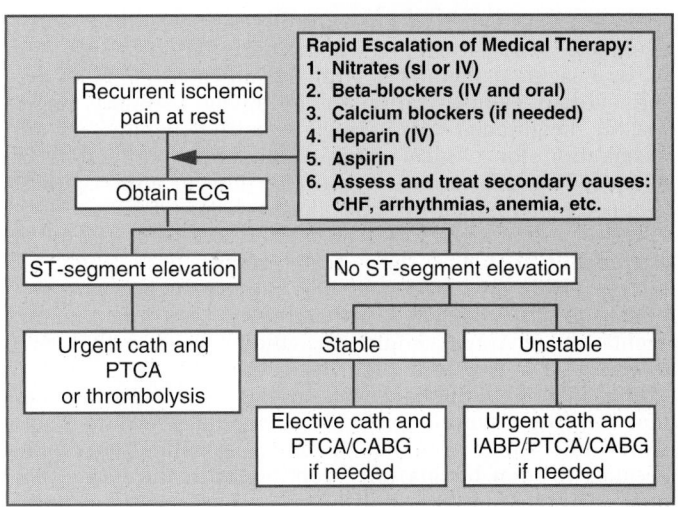

FIGURE 37–45. Treatment of recurrent ischemic events. (From Cannon, C. P., Ganz, L. I., and Stone, P. H.: Complicated myocardial infarction. *In* Rippe, J. M., Irwin, R. S., Fink, M. P., and Cerra, F. B. [eds.]: Intensive Care Medicine. 3rd ed. Boston, Little, Brown & Company, 1995.)

Pericardial Effusion and Pericarditis
(See also pp. 1481 and 1485)

PERICARDIAL EFFUSION. Effusions are generally detected echocardiographically, and their incidence varies with technique, criteria, and laboratory expertise. They occur in approximately 25 per cent of patients after MI.[244] Effusions are more common in patients with anterior MI and with larger infarcts and when congestive failure is present.[1061] The majority of pericardial effusions that are seen following AMI do not cause hemodynamic compromise; when tamponade occurs, it is usually due to ventricular rupture or hemorrhagic pericarditis.[233,1062]

The reabsorption rate of a postinfarction pericardial effusion is slow, with resolution often taking several months. The presence of an effusion does not indicate that pericarditis is present; although they may occur together, the majority of effusions occur without other evidence of pericarditis.[1063]

PERICARDITIS. When secondary to transmural AMI, pericarditis may produce pain as early as the first day and as late as 6 weeks after MI. The pain of pericarditis may be confused with that resulting from postinfarction angina, recurrent infarction, or both. An important distinguishing feature is the radiation of the pain to either trapezius ridge, a finding that is nearly pathognomonic of pericarditis and rarely seen with ischemic discomfort.[233] Transmural myocardial infarction, by definition, extends to the epicardial surface and is responsible for local pericardial inflammation. An acute fibrinous pericarditis (pericarditis epistenocardica) occurs commonly after transmural infarction,[1064] but the majority of patients do not report any symptoms from this process.[233] Although transient pericardial friction rubs are relatively common among patients with transmural infarction within the first 48 hours, pain or electrocardiographic changes occur much less often.[1065] However, the development of a pericardial rub appears to be correlated with a larger infarct and greater hemodynamic compromise.[1066] The discomfort of pericarditis usually becomes worse during a deep inspiration, but it may be relieved or diminished when the patient sits up and leans forward (see Chap. 43).

Although anticoagulation clearly increases the risk for hemorrhagic pericarditis early after MI, this complication has not been reported with sufficient frequency during heparinization or following thrombolytic therapy to warrant absolute prohibition of such agents when a rub is present, but the detection of a pericardial effusion on echocardio-

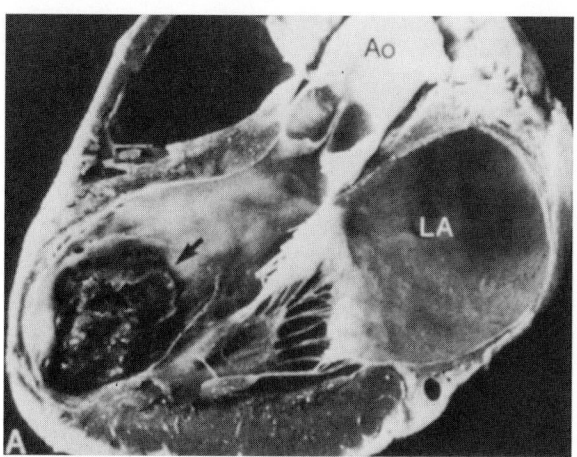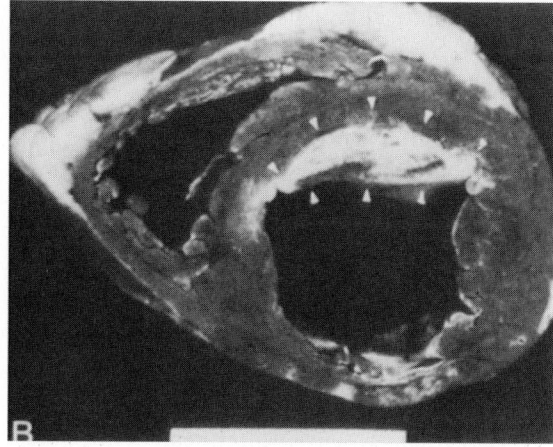

FIGURE 37–46. Postinfarction left ventricular mural thrombus. *A,* Recent thrombus (arrow) with central ulceration. Systemic embolization occurred in this patient. *B,* Old organized thrombus (arrowheads) adjacent to area of infarction. (From Edwards, W. D.: Pathology of myocardial infarction and reperfusion. *In* Gersh, B. J., and Rahimtoola, S. H. [eds.]: Acute Myocardial Infarction. New York, Chapman & Hall, 1991, p. 29.)

may overlie infarcted myocardium in both ventricles. Prospective studies have suggested that patients who develop a mural thrombus early (within 48 to 72 hours of infarction) have an extremely poor early prognosis,[912,1091] with a high mortality from the complications of a large infarction (shock, reinfarction, rupture, and ventricular tachyarrhythmia), rather than emboli from the left ventricular thrombus.[1092]

Although a mural thrombus adheres to the endocardium overlying the infarcted myocardium, superficial portions of it can become detached and produce systemic arterial emboli. Although estimates vary based on patient selection, about 10 per cent of mural thrombi result in systemic embolization.[1088,1093,1094] Echocardiographically detectable features that suggest a given thrombus is more likely to embolize include increased mobility and protrusion into the ventricular chamber, visualization in multiple views, and contiguous zones of akinesis and hyperkinesis.[1090,1095,1096]

MANAGEMENT. About two decades ago three trials involving 3500 patients showed a reduction in the incidence of *systemic embolism* in AMI from 3 per cent to 1 per cent.[668,669,1097] Over the past decade six randomized trials involving only 560 patients tested whether anticoagulant therapy reduced the incidence of *left ventricular thrombus formation.*[675,1093,1098–1101] Collectively these smaller trials showed that anticoagulation (intravenous heparin or high-dose subcutaneous heparin) reduced the development of *thrombi* by 50 per cent, but, because of the low event rate, it was not possible to demonstrate a reduction in the inci-

dence of *systemic embolism.* Additional data from thrombolytic trials suggest that thrombolysis reduces the rate of thrombus formation and the character of the thrombi so that they are less protuberant.[675,686,1102] Of note, however, the data from thrombolytic trials are difficult to interpret because of the confounding effect of antithrombotic therapy with heparin.[1093,1098,1101] Recommendations for anticoagulation vary considerably,[1103–1106] and thrombolysis has precipitated fatal embolization.[1107] Nevertheless, anticoagulation for 3 to 6 months with warfarin is advocated for many patients with demonstrable mural thrombi[1089,1106] (see p. 1265).

Based on the available data, it is our practice to recommend anticoagulation (intravenous heparin to elevate the aPTT to 1.5 to 2.0 times control, followed by a minimum of 3 to 6 months of warfarin) in the following clinical situations: (1) an embolic event has already occurred or (2) the patient has a large anterior infarction whether or not a thrombus is visualized echocardiographically. We are also inclined to follow the same anticoagulation practice in patients with infarctions other than in the anterior distribution if a thrombus or large wall motion abnormality is detected.

Aspirin, although probably not capable of affecting thrombus size in most patients, may prevent further platelet deposition on existing thrombi[1108] and also is protective against recurrent ischemic events (see p. 1264). It should be prescribed in conjunction with warfarin to patients who are candidates for long-term anticoagulation therapy based on the indications discussed above.

CONVALESCENCE, DISCHARGE, AND POST–MYOCARDIAL INFARCTION CARE

Prolonged hospitalization and enforced bed rest for any illness may lead to complications (particularly in elderly patients) such as constipation, decubitus ulcers, excessive resorption of bone with formation of renal calculi, atelectasis, thrombophlebitis, pulmonary emboli, urinary retention, mild anemia due to repetitive blood sampling for diagnostic tests, impaired oral intake of fluids, bleeding from the gastrointestinal tract due to stress ulcers, and deconditioning of cardiovascular reflex responses to postural changes. Because of the precarious status of the heart recovering from AMI, avoidance of such complications is of primary

importance. For example, constipation may lead to straining, transitory reduction of venous return and diminution of cardiac output, impaired coronary perfusion, and ventricular arrhythmias, occasionally culminating in ventricular fibrillation. Early use of a bedside commode, stool softeners, and a bed-chair regimen appear to be useful in avoiding many of the difficulties encountered previously among patients with AMI confined to bed for several weeks.

Although concern has been raised from studies in animals[1109] that early physical activity might unfavorably influence ventricular remodeling, perhaps by causing infarct extension, no evidence indicates that this concern is relevant to patients, and early mobilization appears to be warranted in most stable AMI patients. For the patient with an uncomplicated AMI, washing and personal care may begin within the first 24 hours. If the convalescence continues uneventfully, limited ambulation within the room can be begun on the second or third day (Table 37–6). Once early ambulatory activities are begun, advancement in the activity should depend on the patient's condition. A shower may be allowed some time after the third day.

TIMING OF HOSPITAL DISCHARGE. The time of discharge from the hospital is variable. As noted earlier (see p. 1227), patients who have undergone aggressive reperfusion protocols and have no significant ventricular arrhythmias, recurrent ischemia, or congestive heart failure have been safely discharged in less than 5 days. More commonly discharge occurs 5 or 6 days after admission for patients who experience no complications, who can be followed readily at home, and whose family setting is conducive to convalescence. Most complications that would preclude early discharge occur within the first day or two of admission; therefore, patients suitable for early discharge can be identified early during the hospitalization.[733,1110–1112] Several controlled trials and many uncontrolled trials of early discharge after AMI have failed to show any increase in risk in patients appropriately selected for early discharge.[736,1113]

For patients who have experienced a complication, discharge is deferred until their condition has been stable for several days and it is clear that they are responding appropriately to necessary medications such as antiarrhythmic agents, vasodilators, or positive inotropic agents or that they have undergone the appropriate work-up for recurrent ischemia.

COUNSELING. Before discharge from the hospital, all patients should receive detailed instruction concerning physical activity. Initially, this should consist of ambulation at home but avoidance of isometric exercise such as lifting; several rest periods should be taken daily. In addition, the patient should be given fresh nitroglycerin tablets and instructed in their use and should receive careful instructions about the use of any other medications prescribed. As convalescence progresses, graded resumption of activity should be encouraged. Many approaches have been utilized, ranging from formal rigid guidelines to general advice advocating moderation and avoidance of any activity that evokes symptoms. Sexual counseling is often overlooked during recovery from MI and should also be included as part of the educational process.[1114] Such counseling should begin early after AMI and should include the recommendation that sexual activity be resumed after successful completion of either early submaximal or later symptom-limited exercise stress testing.[1115]

Some evidence indicates that behavioral alteration is possible after recovery from MI and that this may improve prognosis.[1116] A cardiac rehabilitation program with supervised physical exercise and an educational component has been recommended for most MI patients following discharge.[1117] Although the overall clinical benefit of such programs continues to be debated,[1118] there is little question that most people derive considerable knowledge and psychological security from such interventions and they continue to be endorsed by experienced clinicians.[1081,1119] Meta-analyses of randomized trials of medically supervised rehabilitation programs versus usual care that were conducted in an era before widespread use of beta-adrenoceptor blockers and thrombolytics have shown a reduction in cardiovascular death but no change in the incidence of nonfatal reinfarction.[1118–1120] The physical and psychological aspects of rehabilitation of patients convalescing from AMI are discussed in Chapter 40.

RISK STRATIFICATION

The process of risk stratification following AMI occurs in three stages—initial presentation, in-hospital course (CCU, intermediate care unit), and at the time of hospital discharge. The tools used to form an integrated assessment of the patient consist of baseline demographic information, serial electrocardiograms and serum cardiac marker measurements, hemodynamic monitoring data, a variety of noninvasive tests, and, if performed, the findings at cardiac catheterization.

INITIAL PRESENTATION. Certain demographic and historical factors are associated with a poor prognosis in patients with AMI, including female gender,[56,1121] age greater than 70 years,[10,1122,1123] a history of diabetes mellitus,[1124] prior angina pectoris, and previous MI[1125–1127] (Fig. 37–47). Diabetes mellitus, in particular, appears to confer a three- to fourfold increase in risk.[1128,1129] Whether this is due to accelerated atherosclerosis or some other characteristic induced by the diabetic state (such as a larger infarct size[1130]) is unclear.[1131] (Surviving diabetic patients also experience a more complicated post–myocardial infarction course, including a greater incidence of postinfarction angina, infarct extension, and heart failure.[1124])

In addition to playing a central role in the decision pathway for management of patients with AMI based on the presence or absence of ST-segment elevation (see p. 1205), the 12-lead electrocardiogram carries important prognostic information. Mortality is greater in patients experiencing anterior wall MI than after inferior MI, even when corrected for infarct size.[1132,1133] Patients with right ventricular infarction complicating inferior infarction, as suggested by ST-segment elevation in V_4R, have a greater mortality rate than patients sustaining an inferior infarction without right ventricular involvement.[541] Patients with multiple leads showing ST elevation and a high sum of ST-segment elevation have an increased mortality, especially if their infarct is anterior in location.[10,365,1134] Patients whose ECG demonstrates persistent advanced heart block (e.g., Mobitz type II, second-degree, or third-degree AV block) or new intraventricular conduction abnormalities (bifascicular or trifascicular) in the course of an AMI have a worse prognosis than do patients without these abnormalities. The influence of high degrees of heart block is particularly important in patients with right ventricular infarction, for such patients have a markedly increased mortality.[1000] Other electrocardiographic findings that augur poorly are persistent horizontal or downsloping ST-segment depression,[1135] Q waves in multiple leads, evidence of right ventricular infarction accompanying inferior infarction,[105] ST-segment depressions in anterior leads in patients with inferior infarction,[332,540,1136] and atrial arrhythmias (especially atrial fibrillation).[538,1137]

Data from the thrombolytic era have confirmed that important determinants of short- and long-term prognosis appear to be similar in patients who have received thrombolytic therapy compared with those who did not.[538,542,1138] A constellation of clinical factors can be detected at the time of presentation to help select patients at particularly high risk of death in the first 4 to 6 weeks following AMI[538,542] (Table 37–4).

HOSPITAL COURSE. Recurrent ischemia and infarction following AMI, either in the same location as the index infarction or "at a distance" (see p. 1205), influence prognosis adversely.[330] Poor prognosis comes from the loss of viable myocardium, with the resulting larger area of infarction creating a greater compromise in ventricular function. Postinfarction angina generally connotes a less favorable prognosis because it indicates the presence of jeopardized myocardium.[1139] In the current era of aggressive revascularization, early postinfarction angina often

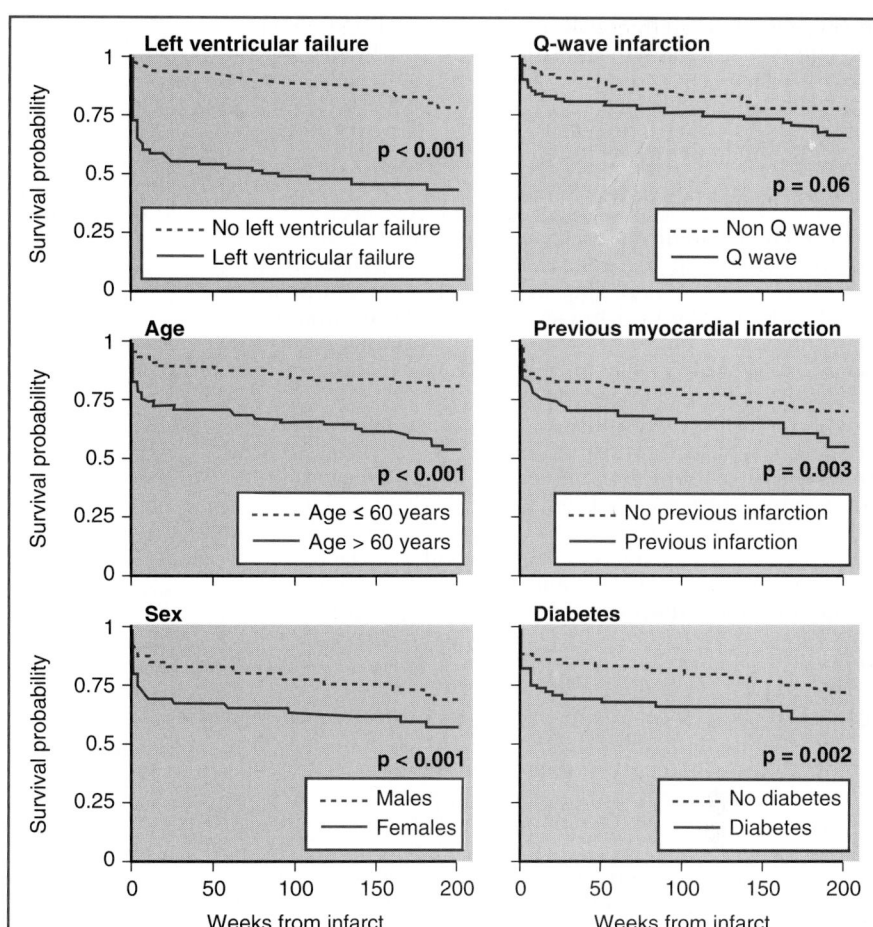

FIGURE 37–47. Kaplan-Meier survival curves illustrating the effects on prognosis after infarction or left ventricular failure, Q-wave infarction, age, gender, diabetes, and history of myocardial infarction. (From Stevenson, R., Ranjadayalan, K., Wilkinson, P., et al.: Short and long term prognosis of acute myocardial infarction since introduction of thrombolysis. BMJ *307:*349, 1993.)

leads to early interventions that tend to improve outcome, diminishing the long-term impact and significance of angina early after AMI. Silent postinfarction ischemia detected by ambulatory monitoring is associated with the same unfavorable prognosis as asymptomatic ischemia after AMI.[1140]

Patients with non-Q-wave AMI are a heterogeneous group presenting with a variety of ECG abnormalities, including ST-segment depression, T-wave inversion, or even no clear abnormality on the standard 12-lead tracing. Nevertheless, non-Q-wave AMI can be viewed as a distinct clinical entity that is due in most patients to a subtotal occlusion of the culprit coronary vessel.[1141] It appears to be increasing in frequency,[329] probably owing to a combination of factors, including more widespread use of antiischemic therapies in the population (e.g., aspirin), the increasing age of the population,[1142,1143] and more sensitive assays for serum markers that may detect smaller infarctions, altering a patient's diagnosis from unstable angina to non-Q-wave MI.[282,289] Following thrombolysis, the classification of infarcts into Q-wave and non-Q-wave categories should be deferred to the period of convalescence because of the tendency of Q waves to both appear and regress after the first 24 hours.[1141a]

Patients with non-Q-wave infarction tend to have smaller infarcts initially and a lower incidence of heart failure early after infarction.[82,1144] However, the higher incidence of subtotal occlusion of the infarct-related artery results in more frequent angina (related to the presence of preserved myocardium with marginal blood supply),[82,1144] leading to the notion that non-Q-wave AMI is an "incomplete" infarction.[1144] The hospital mortality in patients with non-Q-wave infarcts is lower than that in patients with Q-wave infarct,[82,1144] but an increased risk of reinfarction results in long-term mortality similar to that seen in patients with

Q-wave AMI[1145] (Fig. 37–47). In addition to recurrent infarction, other factors associated with a higher risk of morbidity and mortality in patients with non-Q-wave infarction include advanced age, pulmonary congestion associated with infarction, persistent ST-segment depression, and easily provoked ischemic changes on a predischarge exercise test or ambulatory ECG monitor.[82,1146,1147]

The recognition of differences between the early natural histories of these two forms of infarction suggests the need for a more aggressive diagnostic approach, including a careful noninvasive search for ischemia. Often coronary arteriography followed by early coronary angioplasty or coronary bypass surgery is advised in patients who have sustained an acute non-Q-wave infarction.[82,1144]

Despite the logic inherent in this approach, no firm evidence indicates that an early invasive strategy decreases the risk of death or nonfatal infarction compared with a more conservative approach, as reported by the TIMI-IIIB investigators.[395] However, those patients in TIMI-IIIB who were randomized to early diagnostic catheterization and revascularization had lower rates of rehospitalization and a reduced need for antiischemic medications. The majority of patients in the conservative arm ultimately crossed over to a revascularization strategy within the next 12 months. These observations led us to recommend early use of angiography and, if the coronary anatomy is appropriate, either angioplasty or coronary bypass surgery in non-Q-wave AMI patients who have no contraindications to these procedures and who have access to a high-quality tertiary care center capable of performing revascularization with a low risk of complications.

Soon after CCUs were instituted, it became apparent that left ventricular function is an important early determinant of survival. Hospital mortality from AMI depends directly on the severity of left ventricular dysfunction.[240] Risk stratification via clinical findings and invasive hemodynamic monitoring in the CCU (see p. 1226) may also identify important abnormalities such as mitral regurgitation that conveys an adverse long-term prognosis even in the era of reperfusion therapy for AMI.

Assessment at Hospital Discharge

An attempt should be made before hospital discharge to identify patients at higher-than-average risk of reinfarction or cardiac death.[1148,1149] This usually involves noninvasive testing, which may lead to cardiac catheterization and coronary arteriography and, if indicated, to coronary revascularization. Much can be said for accomplishing these procedures before hospital discharge.[1150,1151]

Both short-term and long-term survival after AMI depends on three factors: resting left ventricular function, residual potentially ischemic myocardium, and susceptibility to serious ventricular arrhythmias.[538,542,1150,1152] The most important of these factors is the state of left ventricular function[1152,1153] (Fig. 37–47). The second risk factor is related to how the severity and extent of the obstructive lesions in the coronary vascular bed perfusing residual viable myocardium impacts the risk of recurrent infarction, additional myocardial damage, and serious ventricular arrhythmias.[1153–1156] Thus, survival relates to the quantity of myocardium that has become necrotic and the quantity at risk of becoming necrotic. At one extreme, the prognosis is best for the patient with normal intrinsic coronary vessels whose completed infarction constitutes a small fraction (< 5 per cent) of the left ventricle as a consequence of a coronary embolus and who has no jeopardized myocardium. At the other extreme is the patient with a massive infarct with left ventricular failure whose residual viable myocardium is perfused by markedly obstructed vessels. Obviously, progression of atherosclerosis or lowering of perfusion pressure in these vessels impairs the function and viability of the residual myocardium on which left ventricular function depends. The situation may not be hopeless even in such a patient, however, because revascularization may reduce the threat to the jeopardized myocardium. The third risk factor, the susceptibility to serious arrhythmias, is reflected in ventricular ectopic activity and other indicators of electrical instability such as reduced heart rate variability or baroreflex sensitivity and an abnormal signal-averaged electrocardiogram. All of these identify patients at increased risk of death.[1157–1161]

In addition, as noted earlier, patients with an occluded infarct-related artery late (e.g., 1 to 2 weeks) after AMI have a higher long-term mortality.[162] Persistent occlusion of the culprit artery is associated with an increased incidence of abnormal late potentials on the ECG (Fig. 37–48)[1162] and appears to have an adverse prognostic effect independent of the level of ventricular function (Fig. 37–49).[499]

ASSESSMENT OF LEFT VENTRICULAR FUNCTION. Left ventricular ejection fraction may be the most easily assessed measurement of left ventricular function, and this measurement is extremely useful for risk stratification (Fig. 37–36). Further prognostic information can be obtained by the accurate assessment of end-systolic volume, which is superior to ejection fraction for prediction of survival following AMI.[160,1163] In patients with low left ventricular ejection fraction, the measurement of exercise capacity is useful for further identifying those patients at particularly high risk and also for establishing safe exercise limits following discharge.[1164] Patients with a good exercise capacity despite a reduced ejection fraction have a better long-term outcome than those who cannot perform more than modest exercise.[1165]

Because impaired ventricular function generally is a manifestation of the cumulative extent of myocardial damage sustained, one important determinant of prognosis is

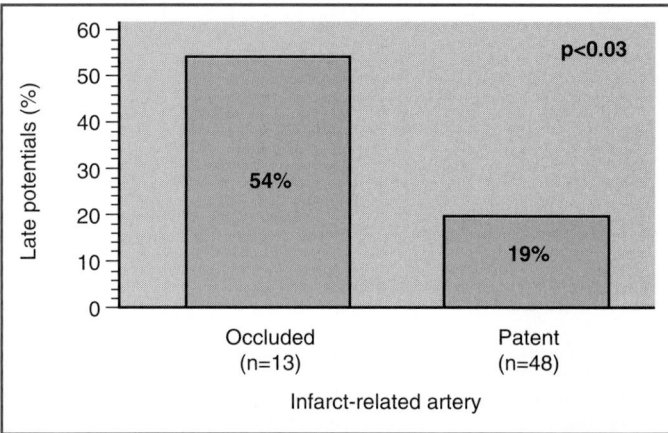

FIGURE 37–48. The frequency of late potentials is significantly greater in patients with an occluded versus patent infarct-related vessel (*P* < 0.03). (From Aguirre, F. V., Kern, M. J., Hsia, J., et al.: Importance of myocardial infarct artery patency on the prevalence of ventricular arrhythmias and late potentials after thrombolysis in acute myocardial infarction. Am. J. Cardiol. *68*:1410, 1991.)

infarct size. This may be estimated from serial measurements of serum cardiac markers,[97] rest echocardiography, or a variety of nuclear cardiology imaging techniques (e.g., radionuclide ventriculography, perfusion scans). However, imaging of the left ventricle at rest may not distinguish adequately between infarcted, irreversibly damaged myocardium and stunned or hibernating myocardium.[1166] To circumvent this difficulty, a variety of techniques has been investigated to assess the extent of residual viable myocardium, including exercise[1167] and pharmacological stress echocardiography,[348,1168–1172] stress radionuclide ventricular angiography,[1173] perfusion imaging in conjunction with pharmacological stress,[1174] and positron emission tomogra-

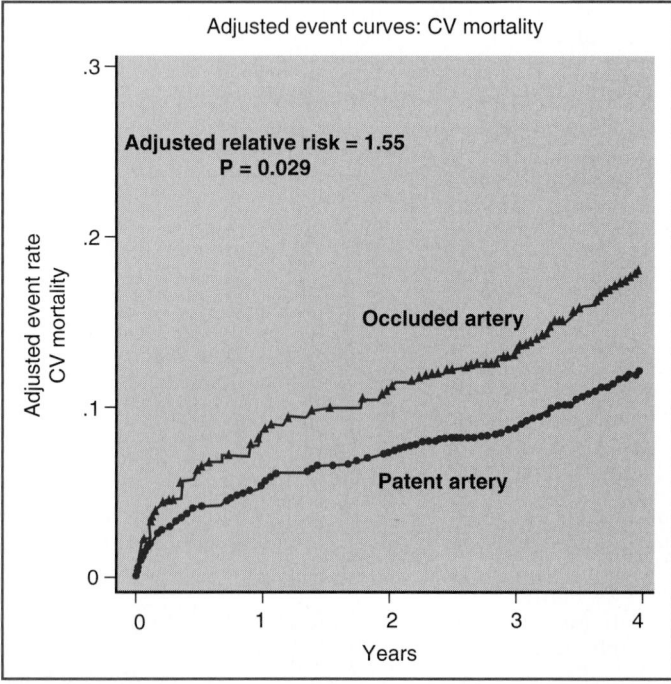

FIGURE 37–49. Impact of patency of the infarct-related artery on long-term mortality. In patients with a patent infarct-related coronary artery at 2 weeks following infarction, the long-term mortality is significantly reduced compared with that of patients with an occluded infarct-related vessel. The beneficial effect of infarct-related artery patency was independent of the number of obstructed coronary arteries or of left ventricular function. (From Lamas, G. A., Flaker, G. C., Mitchell, G., et al.: Effect of infarct artery patency on prognosis after acute myocardial infarction. Circulation *92*:1101, 1995. Copyright 1995 American Heart Association.)

phy[1175] (see p. 305). All of these techniques can be performed safely in postinfarction patients. Clinicians should be guided in their selection of ventricular imaging technique by the availability and level of expertise with a given modality at their local institution. It is our current practice to perform a dobutamine stress echocardiography for assessment of regional myocardial viability in patients who are being evaluated for revascularization but are at above-average risk because of a depressed global ejection fraction (e.g., < 30 per cent).

ASSESSMENT OF MYOCARDIAL ISCHEMIA. Because of the potent adverse consequences of recurrent MI following AMI, it is important to assess a patient's risk for future ischemia and infarction.[1054] Given the increasing array of pharmacological, interventional catheterization, and surgical options available to modify the likelihood of developing recurrent episodes of myocardial ischemia, most clinicians find it helpful to identify patients at risk for provocable myocardial ischemia prior to discharge. A predischarge evaluation for ischemia allows clinicians to select patients who might benefit from catheterization and revascularization following AMI and to assess the adequacy of medical therapy for those patients who are suitable for a more conservative management strategy. Although it may be argued that coronary arteriography for risk stratification after AMI has the advantage of permitting simultaneous identification and treatment (angioplasty) of coronary obstructions, important limitations of this strategy should be noted.[1150] As discussed previously (see p. 1186), the coronary artery plaques that are most likely to rupture (and produce future events) are those that are lipid-laden and have a thin fibrous cap. These cannot be adequately identified with arteriography because they may be associated with less than a 75 per cent stenosis of the coronary artery lumen at the time of angiography after an index AMI.[1176] Furthermore, coronary arteriography does not provide information on the functional significance of coronary lesions. This is most readily accomplished by increasing myocardial oxygen demand in the form of an exercise tolerance test.[1164] The DANAMI (Danish Acute MI) investigators reported that when patients with provokable ischemia after infarction were randomized to catheterization and revascularization versus conservative medical therapy, they experienced a lower requirement for antianginal medications, less unstable angina, and fewer nonfatal infarctions.[1176a]

An exercise test also offers the clinician an opportunity to formulate a more precise exercise prescription and is helpful in boosting patients' confidence in their ability to conduct their daily activities following discharge. Patients who are unable to exercise may be evaluated using a pharmacological stress protocol such as an infusion of dobutamine or dipyridamole with echocardiography or perfusion imaging.[1150,1172]

Treadmill exercise testing following AMI has traditionally utilized a submaximal protocol that requires the patient to exercise until symptoms of angina appear, electrocardiographic evidence of ischemia is seen, or a target workload (approximately 5 METS) has been reached (see Chap. 5).[1164] It has been proposed that symptom-limited exercise tests may be safely performed prior to discharge in patients with an uncomplicated postinfarction course in hospital.[1177,1178] Variables derived from exercise tests following AMI that have been evaluated for their ability to predict the occurrence of death or recurrent nonfatal infarction include the development and magnitude of ST-segment depression, the development of angina, exercise capacity, and the systolic blood pressure response during exercise.[1153,1155,1156,1179]

Myocardial perfusion with thallium-201 or sestamibi during exercise or pharmacological (e.g., dipyridamole, adenosine, or dobutamine) stress increases the sensitivity for detection of patients at risk for death or recurrent infarction.[1180] Similar results have been reported for dipyrida-

mole stress echocardiography.[1172] Although perfusion imaging may be helpful for risk stratification in patients with uninterpretable ECGs or the inability to exercise, the regular use of these more expensive procedures in patients with interpretable ECGs and the ability to exercise has been questioned.[362] An increasing number of patients are treated with thrombolysis, angioplasty, or surgery and have a more favorable natural history than that reported in patients who have not undergone aggressive reperfusion and revascularization for AMI.[362,1181] Until clinical trials relating the findings of a postinfarction perfusion imaging test to long-term outcome in cohorts of patients receiving contemporary therapy for AMI are available, we do not advocate the *routine* use of perfusion imaging for risk stratification following AMI. At present its use should be restricted to patients who are candidates for further revascularization procedures and have physical limitations preventing them from exercising to an adequate workload or those with conduction abnormalities, significant resting ST and T-wave abnormalities, or repolarization abnormalities on the ECG due to ventricular hypertrophy or digitalis therapy.[2,1182] We have also used perfusion imaging studies when a conventional exercise electrocardiogram is mildly abnormal and there is uncertainty about the significance of the finding or uncertainty about the potential culprit vessel or vessels. In such cases perfusion imaging may help guide decisions following catheterization if multiple coronary vessels have important stenoses.

ASSESSMENT FOR ELECTRICAL INSTABILITY. Following AMI, patients are at greatest risk for the development of sudden cardiac death due to malignant ventricular arrhythmias over the course of the first 1 to 2 years.[1183–1187] Several techniques have been devised to stratify patients into those who are at increased risk of sudden death following AMI: measurement of Q-T dispersion (variability of Q-T intervals between ECG leads), ambulatory electrocardiographic recordings for detection of ventricular arrhythmias (Holter monitoring, p. 578), invasive electrophysiological testing,[1188,1188a] recording a signal-averaged electrocardiogram (a measure of delayed, fragmented conduction in the infarct zone), and measuring heart rate variability (beat-to-beat variability in R-R intervals) or baroreflex sensitivity (slope of a line relating beat-to-beat change in sinus rate in response to alteration of blood pressure).[1159,1189,1190]

Given the risks associated with routine use of type I antiarrhythmics prescribed to suppress VPBs that are detected on ambulatory ECG recordings, we do not recommend routine Holter monitoring to determine which patients should receive antiarrhythmic therapy after AMI. The value of empirical administration of the type III antiarrhythmic drug amiodarone following infarction is discussed below (see p. 1265).

The presence of a filtered QRS duration greater than 120 msec and abnormal late potentials recorded on a signal-averaged ECG following AMI have a positive predictive value between 8 and 27 per cent and a negative predictive value of over 95 per cent for serious arrhythmic events.[1158,1159] When viewed in isolation, the signal-averaged ECG suffers from a high false-positive rate, which may be improved by combining it with other variables such as left ventricular ejection fraction.[1158,1190a] Electrophysiological testing also appears to suffer from a high false-positive rate and has the additional disadvantage of being invasive.[1191] The ability of electrophysiological testing to identify patients at risk for arrhythmic events following AMI appears to be improved if it is performed in patients who also have an ejection fraction less than 40 per cent, an abnormal signal-averaged ECG, and VPBs.[1192] Depressed heart rate variability is an independent predictor of mortality and arrhythmic complications following AMI, especially if cutoffs of SDNN (standard deviation of the average interval between normal beats) below 50 msec and HRV triangular index (a geometric method for integrating the distribution of intervals between normal beats) less than 15 are used.[1161,1190] The ATRAMI (Autonomic Tone and Reflexes After Myocardial Infarction) study has reported that among 1284 postinfarction patients, the finding of a depressed baroreflex sensitivity value (< 3.0 msec/mm Hg) was associated with about a threefold increase in the risk of mortality.[1160]

Despite the increased risk of arrhythmic events following AMI in patients who are found to have abnormal results on one or more of the noninvasive tests described above, several points should be emphasized. The low positive predictive value (< 30 per cent) for the noninvasive screening tests limits their usefulness when viewed in isolation. Although the predictive value of screening tests can be improved by combining several of them together, the therapeutic implications of an increased risk profile for arrhythmic events have not been established. In the face of mortality reductions achievable with the general use of beta blockers, ACE inhibitors, aspirin, and revascularization when appropriate following infarction, it is unclear whether interventions such as amiodarone or implantable defibrillators targeted for high-risk asymptomatic patients reduce mortality.[1193] Until the results of ongoing randomized trials evaluating therapy with amiodarone following

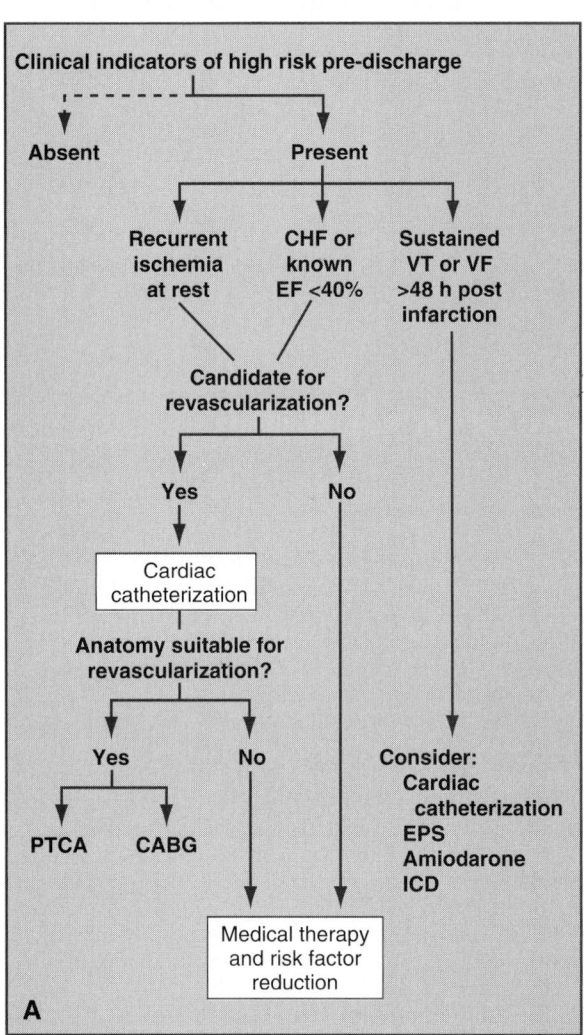

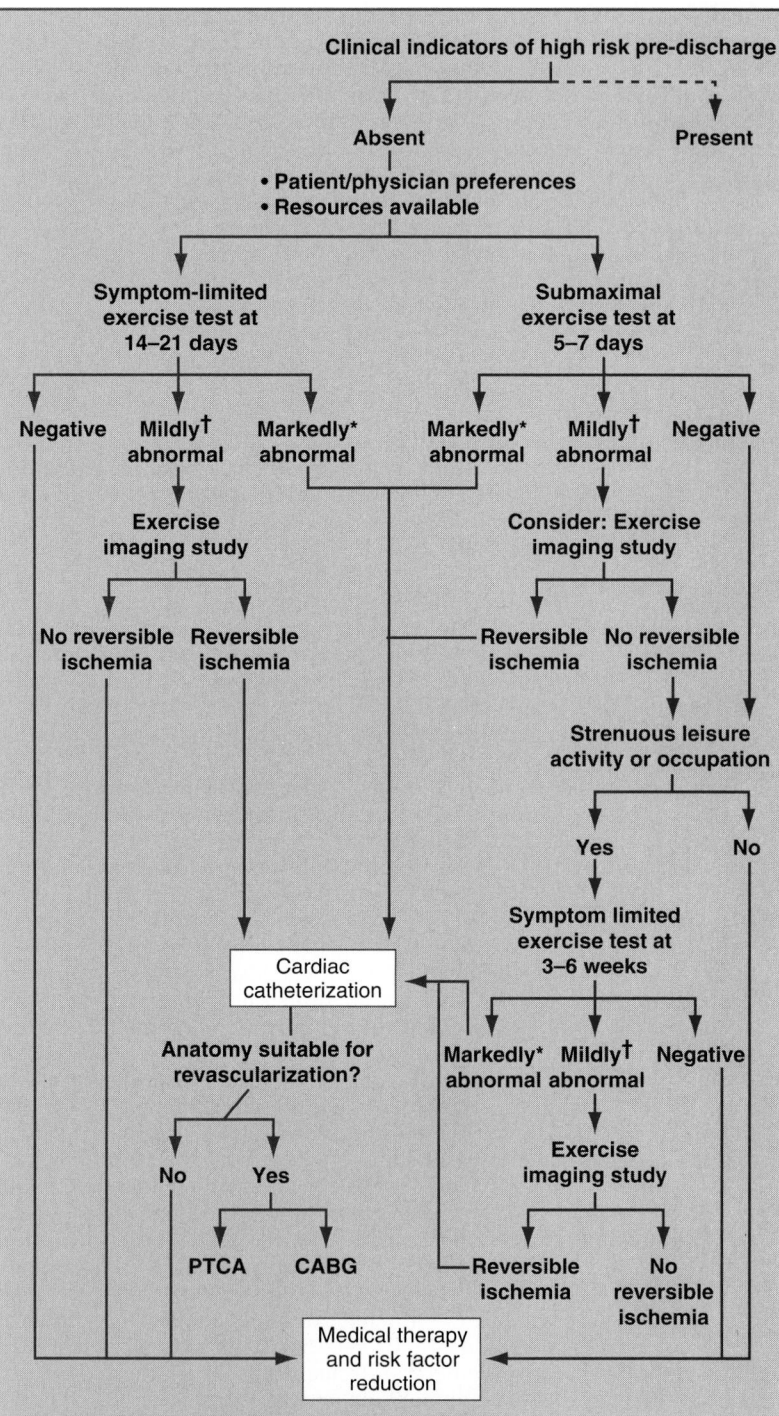

FIGURE 37–50. Management algorithm for risk stratification following acute myocardial infarction. *A,* Patients with clinical indicators of high risk at hospital discharge such as recurrent ischemia at rest or depressed left ventricular function should be considered candidates for revascularization and referral to cardiac catheterization for ultimate triage to either angioplasty/coronary artery bypass graft surgery or medical therapy and risk factor reduction. Patients with life-threatening arrhythmias such as sustained ventricular tachycardia (VT) or ventricular fibrillation (VF) should be considered for diagnostic cardiac catheterization, electrophysiology study (EPS), and management with either amiodarone or an implantable cardioconverter-defibrillator (ICD) or both. *B,* Patients without indicators of high risk at hospital discharge can be evaluated either with a submaximal exercise test prior to discharge (at 5 to 7 days) or with a symptom-limited exercise test at 14 to 21 days. Patients with either a markedly abnormal exercise test or evidence of reversible ischemia on an exercise imaging study should be referred for cardiac catheterization. Patients with a negative exercise test or no evidence of reversible ischemia on an exercise imaging study can be managed with medical therapy and risk factor reduction.

* High risk (≥2 mm ST segment depression, hypotension at peak exercise, low working capacity)

† Positive, not high risk (≤1 mm ST segment depression, good working capacity)

AMI (EMIAT, CAMIAT) and management strategies for patients at risk for sudden death (CABG-PATCH, MUSTT, MADIT) are available, we do not recommend the routine use of noninvasive screening measures for electrical instability. At present such tests should be considered research tools that require additional data on patient outcomes when clinicians act on the results of an abnormal finding.[2,1194]

Recommendations for Predischarge Management

An algorithm for predischarge management of patients at varying levels of risk following infarction is outlined in Figure 37-50. Initially, a judgment is made as to the presence of clinical variables indicative of high risk for future cardiac events. Patients with spontaneous episodes of ischemia or depressed left ventricular function who are considered suitable candidates for revascularization based on their overall medical condition should be referred for cardiac catheterization (Fig. 37–50A). The former group of patients is at increased risk of recurrent infarction (and subsequent increased mortality risk[1054]), whereas the latter group may benefit from revascularization surgery if multivessel coronary artery disease is identified at catheterization (see Chap. 38). Patients with sustained ventricular tachycardia or ventricular fibrillation that occurs more than 48 hours after the acute event (Fig. 37–50A) are at increased risk of sudden cardiac death and should be considered for diagnostic electrophysiology study and treatment as outlined in Chapter 22.

In the absence of high-risk clinical indicators, two management strategies are possible, and the choice between them may be influenced by patient and physician preferences and the availability of resources in the patient's local community for the necessary follow-up procedures (Fig. 37–50B). Initial exercise testing can use conventional electrocardiography with supplementation by a perfusion imaging study for patients with uninterpretable resting ECGs or an equivocal (i.e., mildly abnormal) initial electrocardiographic result. Submaximal exercise testing can be performed before discharge to triage patients to an early catheterization strategy or medical therapy strategy. Plans for a follow-up symptom-limited exercise test in patients without clear indications for catheterization are formulated based on the patient's life style and occupation. Patients who undergo aggressive reperfusion therapy and have an uncomplicated course in the CCU may be suitable candidates for early hospital discharge with plans for a symptom-limited exercise test 2 to 3 weeks later. Subsequent decisions about continued medical therapy or referral for cardiac catheterization can then be made as outlined in Figure 37–50B.

SECONDARY PREVENTION OF ACUTE MYOCARDIAL INFARCTION

(See also p. 1184)

The concept of secondary prevention of reinfarction and death after recovery from an AMI has been investigated actively for several decades. Problems in proving the efficacy of various interventions have been related both to the ineffectiveness of certain strategies and to the difficulty in proving a benefit as mortality and morbidity have improved following AMI. Nevertheless, patients who survive the initial course of AMI are at increased risk because of coronary artery disease and its complications; therefore, it is imperative that efforts be made to reduce this risk.[7,1195–1197] Although secondary prevention drug trials generally have tested one form of therapy against placebo in an attempt to demonstrate a benefit of that therapy, the physician must remember that disciplined clinical care of the individual patient is far more

important than rote use of an agent found beneficial in the latest drug trial.[17]

LIFE STYLE MODIFICATION. Efforts to improve survival and the quality of life after MI that relate to life style modification of known risk factors are considered in Chapter 35. Of these, cessation of smoking and control of hypertension are probably most important. It has been shown that within 2 years of quitting smoking, the risk of a nonfatal MI in these former smokers falls to a level similar to that in patients who never smoked.[1198] Being hospitalized for an AMI is a powerful motivation for patients to cease cigarette smoking, and this is an ideal time to encourage that clearly beneficial and highly cost-effective life style change.[1199,1200] It is also an ideal time to begin to treat hypertension, to counsel patients to achieve optimal body weight, and to consider various strategies to improve the patient's lipid profile (see below).

Physicians caring for patients following an AMI need to be sensitive to the fact that some patients experience major depression following infarction, and the development of this problem is an independent risk factor for mortality.[1201] In addition, lack of an emotionally supportive network in the patient's environment following discharge is associated with an increased risk of mortality and recurrent cardiac events.[1202,1203] The precise mechanisms relating depression and lack of social support to worse prognosis after AMI are not clear, but one possibility is lack of adherence to prescribed treatments, a behavior that has been shown to be associated with increased risk of mortality following infarction.[1204] Evidence exists that a comprehensive rehabilitation program utilizing primary health care personnel who counsel patients and make home visits favorably impacts the clinical course of patients following infarction and reduces the rate of rehospitalization for recurrent ischemia and infarction.[1205] A supportive physician attitude can also have a positive impact on the rate of return to work after AMI.[1206]

MODIFICATION OF LIPID PROFILE. Compelling evidence now exists that an increased cholesterol level, and most importantly an increased LDL cholesterol level, is associated with an increased risk of coronary heart disease.[310,1207] Based on this observation and the finding in the CARE trial that lowering cholesterol reduces the risk of coronary heart disease,[1208] the Adult Treatment Panel II Guidelines recommend a target LDL cholesterol of less than 100 mg/dl in patients with clinically evident coronary heart disease.[310] This recommendation clearly applies to patients with AMI, and it is therefore important to obtain a lipid profile on admission in all patients admitted with acute infarction.[2] (It should be recalled that cholesterol levels may fall 24 to 48 hours following infarction.[307,308])

Surveys of physician practice in the past have revealed a disappointingly low rate of treatment of hypercholesterolemia in patients with proven coronary artery disease, indicating considerable room for improvement in this aspect of secondary prevention following AMI.[1209] Perhaps the most dramatic evidence favoring reduction of cholesterol in patients with clinically overt coronary heart disease is the 30 per cent reduction in total mortality and 42 per cent reduction in coronary heart disease–related deaths over 5.4 years in patients receiving simvastatin for an elevated cholesterol in the Scandinavian Simvastatin Survival Study(4S).[1210] Of particular interest was the relatively constant 35 per cent reduction in coronary death and nonfatal infarction with simvastatin across a wide range of baseline cholesterol levels.[1211]

Recommendations. All patients recovering from AMI should be considered potential candidates for modification of their lipid profile. Initial therapy should consist of an AHA Step II diet (< 7 per cent of total calories as saturated fat and cholesterol < 200 mg/day). We strongly advise adherence to a target LDL cholesterol of less than 125 mg/dl. This requires drug therapy in the majority of patients, and our preference at present is to prescribe an HMG CoA reductase inhibitor prior to hospital discharge (see Chap. 35) in patients with an LDL cholesterol greater than 130 on admission (Fig. 37–18).

ANTIPLATELET AGENTS. On the basis of 11 randomized trials in 20,000 patients with a prior infarction, the Antiplatelet Trialists' Collaboration reported a 25 per cent reduction in the risk of recurrent infarction, stroke, or vascular death in patients receiving prolonged antiplatelet therapy (36 fewer events for every 1000 patients treated).[9] No antiplatelet therapy proved superior to aspirin, and daily doses of aspirin between 80 and 325 mg appear to be effective.[2] Data from the Worcester Heart Attack Study suggest that when an AMI occurs in chronic users of aspirin, it is likely to be smaller and non-Q-wave in nature.[1212] Experimental data on late reperfusion in a rat model of coronary occlusion suggest that aspirin treatment following AMI increases the patency of the microvasculature in the infarcted area, resulting in less infarct expansion and thicker myocardial walls in the infarct zone.[1213] The compelling arguments cited above serve as the basis for the recommendation that all patients recovering from AMI should, in the absence of contraindications, remain on aspirin for an indefinite period.[2,17] Patients with true aspirin allergy should be treated with sulfinpyrazone (400 mg twice daily) or ticlopidine (250 mg twice daily),[9] although the data indicating that these agents reduce mortality following AMI are not nearly as robust as those for aspirin, and some recommend treating aspirin-intolerant patients with warfarin.[671]

ACE INHIBITORS. The rationale for the acute use of ACE inhibitors following AMI has been discussed earlier (see p. 1229). To prevent late remodeling of the left ventricle and also to decrease the likelihood of recurrent ischemic events,[749,758] we advocate indefinite therapy with an ACE inhibitor to all patients with clinically evident congestive heart failure, a moderate decrease in global ejection fraction, or a large regional wall motion abnormality, even in the face of a normal global ejection fraction. A decision-analytic model that tested strategy of prescription of ACE inhibitors to hypothetical 50- to 80-year-old patients with an ejection fraction of 40 per cent or less following AMI reported incremental cost-effectiveness ratios of $4,000 to $10,000 per quality-adjusted life-year (QALY).[1214] These calculations compare quite favorably with the costs of other commonly accepted medical procedures such as angioplasty for one- or two-vessel coronary artery disease ($8,000 to $111,000 per QALY).[1214]

BETA-ADRENOCEPTOR BLOCKERS. Meta-analyses of trials from the prethrombolytic era involving over 20,000 patients who received beta-adrenoceptor blockers in the convalescent phase of AMI have shown a 20 per cent reduction in long-term mortality.[7,744,748] When beta blockade is initiated early (<6 hours) in the acute phase of infarction and continued in the chronic phase of treatment, some of the benefit may result from a reduction in infarct size.[748,1215] However, in the majority of patients who have beta blockade initiated during the convalescent phase of AMI, reduction in long-term mortality is probably due to a combination of an antiarrhythmic effect (prevention of sudden death) and prevention of reinfarction.[414,745,748,1186,1216,1217]

Overviews of the results of trials of beta-adrenoceptor blockers with agonist activity have not shown a beneficial effect on mortality compared with more convincing evidence of a beneficial effect and little evidence of harm for trials of beta blockers without agonist activity (odds ratio 0.69[0.61–0.79]).[414] No differences are seen when cardioselective and noncardioselective agents are compared. The greatest mortality benefit from chronic beta blockade following AMI is seen in patients with the greatest baseline risk—those with compromised ventricular function and ventricular arrhythmias.[1186,1218] The results of the Beta-Blocker Pooling Project, in which data were examined from nine separate studies involving more than 10,000 patients, suggest a highly significant reduction in overall mortality among treated patients with pump failure.[1219]

Recommendations. Although some controversy exists regarding their utility in patients with a non-Q-wave infarction,[1219a] we remain persuaded of the benefits of immediate intravenous beta-adrenoceptor blockade (to reduce infarct size and cardiac rupture—see p. 1211) and long-term therapy with beta blockers, including patients who undergo thrombolysis or angioplasty (see below). Therefore, we begin therapy as early as possible (see p. 1228), continue treatment during hospitalization, and prescribe beta blockers at discharge, as long as contraindications (see p. 1978) are not present. Patients with a relative contraindication to beta blockade (moderate heart failure, bradyarrhythmias) undergo a monitored trial of therapy in the hospital. The dosage should be sufficient to blunt the heart rate response to stress or exercise. Much of the impact of beta blockers in preventing mortality occurs in the first weeks; treatment should commence as soon as possible.[748]

Some controversy exists as to how long patients should be treated.[1220,1221] The collective data from five trials providing information on long-term follow-up of beta-adrenoceptor blockers following infarction suggest that therapy should be continued for at least 2 to 3 years[32,1222,1223] (Fig. 37–51). At that time, if the beta blocker is well tolerated and if there is no reason to discontinue therapy, such therapy probably should be continued in most patients.

Not all patients derive the same benefit from beta blocker therapy. The cost-effectiveness of treatment in medium- or high-risk persons compares very favorably with that of many other accepted interventions such as coronary bypass surgery, angioplasty, and lipid-lowering therapy.[1221] In patients with an extremely good prognosis (first AMI, good ventricular function, no angina, negative stress test, and no complex ventricular ectopy) in whom a mortality rate of approximately 1 per cent per year can be anticipated, beta blockers would have a smaller impact on survival. However, it is our preference to prescribe beta blockers to such patients for whatever postinfarction benefit is achieved and also to have them as part of the patient's usual regimen should AMI recur at an unpredictable time in the future.

NITRATES. Although these agents are suitable for management of specific conditions following AMI such as recurrent angina or as part of a treatment regimen for congestive heart failure, little evidence indicates that they reduce mortality when prescribed on a routine basis to all patients with infarction.[757,761]

ANTICOAGULANTS (see also p. 1828). At least three theoretical reasons exist for anticipating that anticoagulants might be beneficial in the long-term management of pa-

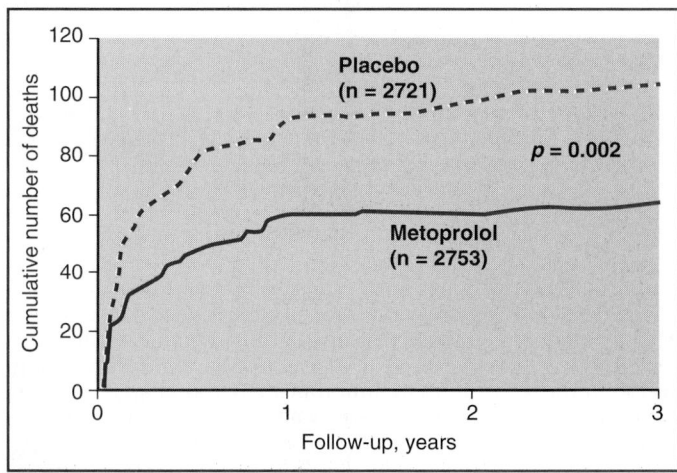

FIGURE 37–51. Prevention of sudden death with long-term beta blockade following MI. Analysis of pooled data from 5 trials in which long-term metoprolol therapy was used after MI revealed a 40 per cent reduction in incidence of sudden cardiac death in both men and women. (From Olsson, G., Wikstrand, J., Warnold, I., et al.: Metoprolol-induced reduction in postinfarction mortality: Pooled results from five double-blind randomized trials. Eur. Heart J. *13:*28, 1992.)

tients after AMI: (1) Because the coronary occlusion responsible for the AMI is often due to a thrombus, anticoagulants might be expected to halt, slow progression, or prevent the development of new thrombi elsewhere in the coronary arterial tree. (2) Anticoagulants might be expected to diminish the formation of mural thrombi and resultant systemic embolization (see p. 1256). (3) Anticoagulants might be expected to reduce the incidence of venous thrombosis and pulmonary embolization.

After several decades of evaluation, the weight of evidence now suggests that anticoagulants have a favorable effect on late mortality, stroke, and reinfarction among patients hospitalized with AMI[7,1224–1226] (Fig. 37–52). Long-term anticoagulant therapy has also been shown to be a cost-effective intervention following AMI, with the major cost savings coming from reductions in the rate of recurrent infarction and related interventions.[1227]

Previous small trials of aspirin versus oral anticoagulation have led to conflicting results, with no clear consensus regarding superiority of either antithrombotic strategy.[1228,1229] The APRICOT Investigators reported that after initially successful thrombolysis, aspirin-treated patients had lower rates of reinfarction, need for revascularization, and mortality than did coumadin-treated patients.[546] As expected, cost-effectiveness calculations show that aspirin is associated with a very favorable economic profile, but its true efficacy compared with or combined with oral anticoagulation remains unknown.[1230] The Coumadin Aspirin Reinfarction Study (CARS) was discontinued prematurely due to lack of evidence of benefit of reduced-dose aspirin (80 mg daily) with either 1 or 3 mg of warfarin daily compared with aspirin 160 mg alone daily. Data on the relative benefits of aspirin versus a combination of aspirin plus warfarin will be forthcoming from the ongoing Combination Hemotherapy and Mortality Prevention (CHAMP) Study.[1230]

Therefore, at present we recommend routine use of aspirin in all AMI patients without contraindications and add warfarin to patients with clear indications for anticoagulation such as deep vein thrombosis, pulmonary embolism, mural thrombus seen at echocardiography, a large

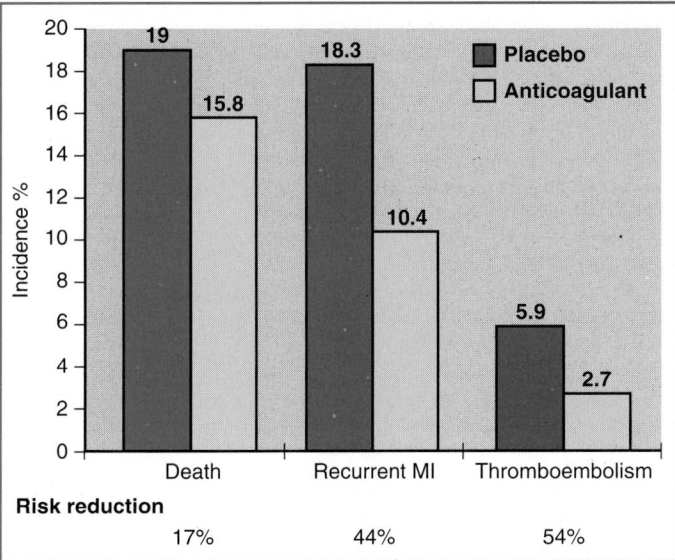

FIGURE 37–52. Meta-analysis of trials of patients who received oral anticoagulant therapy compared with control subjects. These results add to the evidence that long-term warfarin therapy reduces the risks for death, recurrent MI, and thromboembolism. In WARIS, the risk for hemorrhage was 0.6 per cent per year for major hemorrhage and 3.3 per cent for minor hemorrhage; however, it will be of considerable interest to see whether lower levels of anticoagulation (Coumadin, 1 to 3 mg) in conjunction with small amounts of aspirin (80 to 160 mg/d) is safe and effective. This possibility is being tested in the CARS and CHAMP studies. (Adapted from Devine, N., Azarnia, N., Nelson, K., et al.: Long-term anticoagulants in post myocardial infarction patients: A meta-analysis. Circulation 86:I-259, 1992. Copyright 1992 American Heart Association.)

regional wall motion abnormality (especially anterior) seen at echocardiography even in the absence of a visualized thrombus, atrial fibrillation, and a history of embolic cerebrovascular accident.

CALCIUM ANTAGONISTS (see also p. 1231). At present we do not recommend the routine use of calcium antagonists for secondary prevention of infarction. A possible exception is a patient who cannot tolerate a beta-adrenoceptor blocker because of adverse effects on bronchospastic lung disease but who has well-preserved left ventricular function; such patients may be candidates for a rate-slowing calcium antagonist such as diltiazem or verapamil.

ANTIARRHYTHMICS. Although it has been recognized for decades that antiarrhythmic therapy can control atrial and ventricular arrhythmias effectively in many patients, careful reviews of clinical trials following AMI have reported an increased risk of mortality with type I drugs.[1231,1232] The most notable postinfarction trial in this area was the Cardiac Arrhythmia Suppression Trial (CAST), which tested whether encainide, flecainide, or moricizine for suppression of ventricular arrhythmias detected on ambulatory electrocardiographic monitoring would reduce the risk of cardiac arrest and death over the long term. Both the first phase of the trial (encainide or flecainide versus placebo) and the second phase of the trial (moricizine versus placebo) were stopped prematurely because of increased mortality in the active treatment groups.[1232–1234] The mechanism of the increased risk following AMI remains a subject of investigation, but one hypothesis that has been put forth is an adverse interaction between recurrent ischemia and the presence of an antiarrhythmic drug because the risk of death or cardiac arrest was greater in patients with a non-Q-wave AMI than with Q-wave AMI.[1034] Sodium channel blockade by antiarrhythmics may exacerbate electrophysiological differences between subepicardial and subendocardial zones of myocardium, rendering the latter more susceptible to ischemic injury.[1234a]

Subsequent to CAST, another postinfarction prophylactic antiarrhythmic drug trial was undertaken with oral D-sotalol (Survival With ORal D-sotalol = SWORD). This trial was designed to test the hypothesis that prophylactic administration of D-sotalol to patients with depressed left ventricular function (ejection fraction ≤ 40 per cent) and either a recent (6 to 42 days) or remote (>42 days) AMI would reduce total mortality. SWORD also was stopped prematurely after enrollment of only 3121 of a planned 6400 patients because statistical evidence of increased mortality emerged in the active treatment group.[1235]

Four prospective, randomized, placebo-controlled trials compared the empirical prophylactic use of amiodarone versus placebo following AMI (Fig. 37–53). A meta-analysis of these trials revealed an encouraging 55 per cent reduction in sudden death and 46 per cent reduction in total mortality.[1236] The Canadian Amiodarone Myocardial Infarction Trial (CAMIAT) showed that amiodarone reduced VPD frequency in patients with recent MI; this correlated with a reduction in arrhythmic death or resuscitation from ventricular fibrillation. However, 42 per cent of patients discontinued amiodarone during maintenance therapy in CAMIAT because of intolerable side effects. The European Amiodarone Myocardial Infarction Trial (EMIAT) showed a reduction in arrhythmic death following MI in patients with depressed left ventricular function, but there was no reduction in total mortality or other cardiovascular-related mortality.

At the present time, the *routine* use of antiarrhythmic agents (including amiodarone) cannot be recommended. Given the data cited earlier on the protective effects of beta-adrenoceptor blockers against sudden death (see p. 1228) and the ability of aspirin to reduce the risk of reinfarction (see p. 1827), it is unclear that additional mortality reductions would be achieved by the empirical addition of amiodarone in the patient who is convalescing from an AMI and is free of symptomatic sustained ventricular arrhythmias. Whether subgroups of patients with indicators

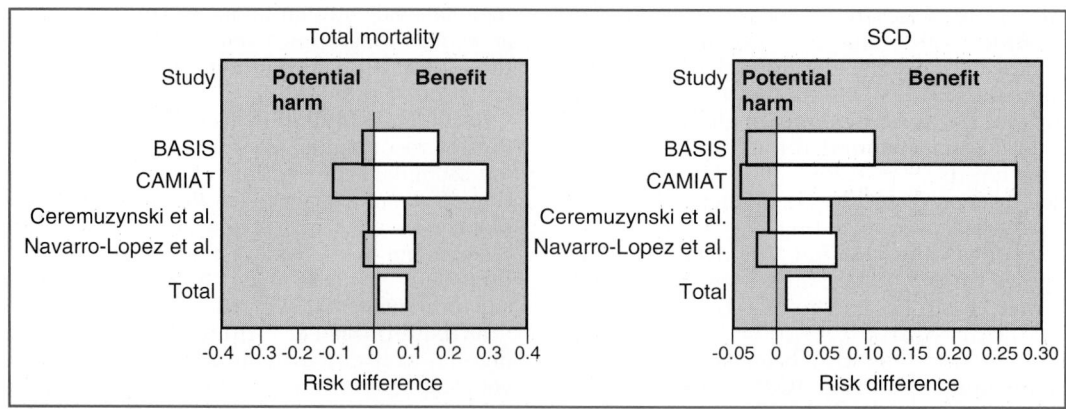

FIGURE 37–53. Amiodarone trials after infarction. Four prospective, randomized, placebo-controlled trials have investigated the benefits of empiric long-term amiodarone prophylaxis following MI. Data from the individual studies are plotted along with the pooled estimate using meta-analytic techniques. The two plots depict the 95 per cent confidence intervals for the risk differences describing the effects of amiodarone on total mortality and sudden cardiac death. Plots of this nature depict benefits from the active therapy (amiodarone) to the right of the vertical line and potential harm to the left. Total mortality in the placebo-treated group was 11.2 per cent, compared with 6.1 per cent in the amiodarone-treated group. This indicates a relative reduction in total mortality of nearly 46 per cent and an absolute reduction ranging from 1.3 per cent to 8.2 per cent, explained almost entirely by the reduction in sudden death from 6.9 per cent in the placebo group to 3.1 per cent in the amiodarone group. (From Zarembski, D. G., Nolan, P. E., Jr., Slack, M. K., et al.: Empiric long-term amiodarone prophylaxis following myocardial infarction: A meta-analysis. Arch. Intern. Med. 153:2661, 1993.)

of high risk of sudden death, such as abnormal heart rate variability or reduced baroreflex sensitivity, should be treated and if so by what strategy remains to be determined.

HORMONE REPLACEMENT THERAPY (see also p. 1708). Estrogen replacement therapy has been reported to be helpful in the primary prevention of coronary heart disease,[1237] improves the coronary artery disease risk factor profile in postmenopausal women,[1238,1238a] and appears to reduce mortality in women with moderate coronary heart disease.[1239] However, the decision to prescribe hormone replacement therapy is often a complex one that involves weighing risks of breast cancer versus modification of a coronary artery disease risk factor profile.[1240] At present we recommend consideration of hormone replacement therapy in postmenopausal women who have suffered an AMI.

Acknowledgment

Drs. Richard Pasternak and Burton Sobel co-authored this chapter with one of the present authors in the third and fourth editions of this textbook. Portions of the chapter appearing in the fourth edition have been retained. The important influence of Drs. Pasternak and Sobel on this chapter is gratefully acknowledged.

REFERENCES

CHANGING PATTERNS IN CLINICAL CARE

1. American Heart Association: Heart and Stroke Facts: 1996 Statistical Supplement. Dallas, American Heart Association, 1996, pp. 1-23.
2. Committee to Develop Guidelines for the Management of Patients with Acute Myocardial Infarction: Guidelines for the management of patients with acute myocardial infarction: A report of the American College of Cardiology/American Heart Association Task Force on Practice Guidelines. J. Am. Coll. Cardiol. *(in press)*.
3. Weinstein, M. C., Coxson, P. G., and Wilman, L.: Forecasting coronary heart disease incidence, mortality, and cost: The Coronary Heart Disease Policy Model. Am. J. Public Health 77:1417, 1987.
4. Goldman, L.: Cost-awareness in medicine. *In* Isselbacher, K. H., Braunwald, E., Wilson, J. D., et al. (eds.): Harrison's Principles of Internal Medicine. New York, McGraw-Hill Book Co., 1994, p. 38.
5. Every, N. R., Fihn, S. D., Maynard, C., et al.: Resource utilization in treatment of acute myocardial infarction: Staff-model health maintenance organization versus fee-for-service hospitals. J. Am. Coll. Cardiol. 26:401, 1995.
5a. The Task Force on the Management of Acute Myocardial Infarction of the European Society of Cardiology: Acute myocardial infarction: prehospital and in-hospital management. Eur. Heart J. 17:43, 1996.
6. Yusuf, S., Sleight, P., Held, P., et al.: Routine medical management of acute myocardial infarction: Lessons from overviews of recent randomized controlled trials. Circulation 82(Suppl. II):117, 1990.

7. Antman, E., Lau, J., Kupelnick, B., et al.: A comparison of results of meta-analyses of randomized control trials and recommendations of clinical experts. JAMA 268:240, 1992.
8. Lau, J., Antman, E. M., Jimenez-Silva, J., et al.: Cumulative meta-analysis of therapeutic trials for myocardial infarction. N. Engl. J. Med. 327:248, 1992.
9. Antiplatelet Trialists' Collaboration: Collaborative overview of randomized trials of antiplatelet therapy. I. Prevention of death, myocardial infarction, and stroke by prolonged antiplatelet therapy in various categories of patients. BMJ 308:81, 1994.
10. Fibrinolytic Therapy Trialists (FTT) Collaborative Group: Indications for fibrinolytic therapy in suspected acute myocardial infarction: Collaborative overview of early mortality and major morbidity results from all randomised trials of more than 1000 patients. Lancet 343:311, 1994.
11. Rogers, W. J.: What is the optimal tool to define appropriate therapy: The randomized clinical trial, meta-analysis, or outcomes research? Commentary. Cur. Opin. Cardiol. 9:401, 1994.
12. Rogers, W., Bowlby, L., Chandra, N., et al.: Treatment of myocardial infarction in the United States (1990 to 1993): Observations from the National Registry of Myocardial Infarction. Circulation 90:2103, 1994.
13. Hlatky, M.: Observational databases. *In* Califf, R. M., Mark, D. B., and Wagner, G. S. (eds.): Acute Coronary Care. 2nd ed. St. Louis, Mosby–Year Book, 1995, p. 145.
14. Kupersmith, J., Holmes-Rovner, M., Hogan, A., et al.: Cost-effectiveness analysis in heart disease. Part I. General principles. Prog. Cardiovasc. Dis. 37:161, 1994.
15. Mark, D. B., Hlatky, M. A., Califf, R. M., et al.: Cost effectiveness of thrombolytic therapy with tissue plasminogen activator as compared with streptokinase for acute myocardial infarction. N. Engl. J. Med. 332:1418, 1995.
16. Goldman, L.: Cost and quality of life: Thrombolysis and primary angioplasty. J. Am. Coll. Cardiol. 25:38S, 1995.
17. Julian, D.: The practical implications of clinical trials: Putting it all together. *In* Julian, D., and Braunwald, E. (eds.): Management of Acute Myocardial Infarction. London, W. B. Saunders Company, 1994, p. 407.
18. Walsh, J. T., Gray, D., Keating, N. A., et al.: ACE for whom? Implications for clinical practice of post-infarct trials. Br. Heart J. 73:470, 1995.
19. Antman, E. M., and Califf, R. M.: Clinical trials and meta-analysis. *In* Smith, T. W. (ed.): Cardiovascular Therapeutics. Philadelphia, W. B. Saunders Company, 1996.
20. Asch, D. A., and Hershey, J. C.: Why some health policies don't make sense at the bedside. Ann. Intern. Med. 122:846, 1995.
21. Rothwell, P. M.: Can overall results of clinical trials be applied to all patients? Lancet 345:1616, 1995.
22. de Vreede, J. J. M., Gorgels, A. P. M., Verstraaten, G. M. P., et al.: Did prognosis after acute myocardial infarction change during the past 30 years? A meta-analysis. J. Am. Coll. Cardiol. 18:698, 1991.
23. Naylor, C. D., and Chen, E.: Population-wide mortality trends among patients hospitalized for acute myocardial infarction: The Ontario experience, 1981 to 1991. J. Am. Coll. Cardiol. 24:1431, 1994.
24. Behar, S., Goldbourt, U., Barbash, G., et al.: Twenty-five-year mortality rate decrease in patients in Israel with a first episode of acute myocardial infarction. Am. Heart J. 130:453, 1995.
24a. Gheorghiade, M., Razumma, P., Borzak, S., et al.: Decline in the rate of hospital mortality from acute myocardial infarction: Impact of changing management strategies. Am. Heart J. 131:250, 1996.
25. Whitney, E. J., Shear, C. L., Mantell, G., et al.: The case for unstable

angina pectoris as a primary endpoint in primary prevention studies. Am. J. Cardiol. 70:738, 1992.

26. Davidson, C.: Cardiac rehabilitation in the district hospital. *In* Jones, D., and West, R. (eds.): Cardiac Rehabilitation. London, BMJ Publishing Group, 1995, p. 144.

27. Pell, S., and Fayerweather, W. E.: Trends in the incidence of myocardial infarction and in associated mortality and morbidity in a large employed population, 1957–1983. N. Engl. J. Med. 312:1005, 1985.

28. Younis, L. T., Miller, D. D., and Chaitman, B. R.: Preoperative strategies to assess cardiac risk before noncardiac surgery. Clin. Cardiol. 18:447, 1995.

29. Mason, J. J., Owens, D. K., Harris, R. A., et al.: The role of coronary angiography and coronary revascularization before noncardiac vascular surgery. JAMA 273:1919, 1995.

30. Antman, E. M.: General hospital management. *In* Julian, D. G., and Braunwald, E. (eds.): Management of Acute Myocardial Infarction. Philadelphia, W. B. Saunders Company, 1994, p. 29.

31. Rentrop, K. P.: Restoration of anterograde flow in acute myocardial infarction: The first 15 years. J. Am. Coll. Cardiol. 25:1S, 1995.

32. Yusuf, S., Wittes, J., and Friedman, L.: Overview of results of randomized clinical trials in heart disease. I. Treatments following myocardial infarction. JAMA 260:2088, 1988.

33. The GUSTO Investigators: An international randomized trial comparing four thrombolytic strategies for acute myocardial infarction. N. Engl. J. Med. 329:673, 1993.

34. Madsen, J. K., and Hansen, J. F.: Mortality of patients excluded from the Danish Verapamil Infarction Trial II: The DAVIT-II Study Group. Eur. Heart J. 14:377, 1993.

35. Pashos, C. L., Newhouse, J. P., and McNeil, B. J.: Temporal changes in the care and outcomes of elderly patients with acute myocardial infarction, 1987 through 1990. JAMA 270:1832, 1993.

36. Udvarhelyi, I. S., Gatsonis, C., Epstein, A. M., et al.: Acute myocardial infarction in the Medicare population: Process of care and clinical outcomes. JAMA 268:2530, 1992.

37. Maggioni, A., Maseri, A., Fresco, C., et al.: Age-related increase in mortality among patients with first myocardial infarctions treated with thrombolysis. N. Engl. J. Med. 329:1442, 1993.

38. White, H. D., Granger, C., Gore, J., et al.: Older age is associated with a large increase in mortality and total stroke, but not non-fatal disabling stroke: Results of the GUSTO trial. Circulation 90(Suppl. I):563, 1994.

39. McClellan, M., McNeil, B. J., and Newhouse, J. P.: Does more intensive treatment of acute myocardial infarction in the elderly reduce mortality? Analysis using instrumental variables. JAMA 272:859, 1994.

40. Latini, R., Avanzini, F., Zuanetti, G., et al.: Changing patterns of pharmacological treatment after myocardial infarction: The GISSI experience. J. Am. Coll. Cardiol. 23:210A, 1994.

41. Antman, E. M., Cannon, C. P., Mueller, J., et al.: Do clinical trial results influence physician drug use in myocardial infarction? Circulation 90(Suppl. I):167, 1994.

42. Sial, S. H., Malone, M., Freeman, J. L., et al.: Beta blocker use in the treatment of community hospital patients discharged after myocardial infarction. J. Gen. Intern. Med. 9:599, 1994.

43. Kennedy, H. L., and Rosenson, R. S.: Physician use of beta-adrenergic blocking therapy: A changing perspective. J. Am. Coll. Cardiol. 26:547, 1995.

44. Meehan, T. P., Hennen, J., Radford, M. J., et al.: Process and outcome of care for acute myocardial infarction among Medicare beneficiaries in Connecticut: A quality improvement demonstration project. Ann. Intern. Med. 122:928, 1995.

44a. Krumholz, H. M., Radford, M. J., Ellerbeck, E. F., et al.: Aspirin in the treatment of acute myocardial infarction in elderly Medicare beneficiaries. Patterns of use and outcomes. Circulation 92:2841, 1995.

45. Pashos, C. L., Normand, S. T., Garfinkle, J. B., et al.: Trends in the use of drug therapies in patients with acute myocardial infarction: 1988 to 1992. J. Am. Coll. Cardiol. 23:1023, 1994.

46. Ellerbeck, E. F., Jencks, S. F., Radford, M. J., et al.: Quality of care for Medicare patients with acute myocardial infarction: A four-state pilot study from the Cooperative Cardiovascular Project. JAMA 273:1509, 1995.

47. Rouleau, J. L., Moye, L. A., Pfeffer, M. A., et al.: A comparison of management patterns after acute myocardial infarction in Canada and the United States. N. Engl. J. Med. 328:779, 1993.

48. Pilote, L., Racine, N., and Hlatky, M. A.: Differences in the treatment of myocardial infarction in the United States and Canada. Arch. Intern. Med. 154:1090, 1994.

49. Pilote, L., Califf, R. M., Sapp, S., et al.: Regional variation across the United States in the management of acute myocardial infarction. N. Engl. J. Med. 333:565, 1995.

50. Guadagnoli, E., Hauptman, P. J., Ayanian, J. Z., et al.: Variation in the use of cardiac procedures after acute myocardial infarction. N. Engl. J. Med. 333:573, 1995.

51. Ketley, D., and Woods, K. L.: Impact of clinical trials on clinical practice: Example of thrombolysis for acute myocardial infarction. Lancet 342:891, 1993.

52. Ayanian, J., Hauptman, P., Guadagnoli, E., et al.: Knowledge and practices of generalist and specialist physicians regarding drug therapy for acute myocardial infarction. N. Engl. J. Med. 331:1136, 1994.

52a. Mark, D. B., Naylor, C. D., Hlatky, M. A., et al.: Use of medical resources and quality of life after acute myocardial infarction in Canada and the United States. N. Engl. J. Med. 331:1130, 1994.

53. Lincoff, A. M., Califf, R. M., Ellis, S. G., et al.: Thrombolytic therapy for women with myocardial infarction: Is there a gender gap? J. Am. Coll. Cardiol. 22:1780, 1993.

54. Krumholz, H. M., Douglas, P. S., Lauer, M. S., et al.: Selection of patients for coronary angiography and coronary revascularization early after myocardial infarction: Is there evidence for a gender bias? Ann. Intern. Med. 116:785, 1992.

55. Becker, R. C., Terrin, M., Ross, R., et al.: Comparison of clinical outcomes for women and men after acute myocardial infarction. Ann. Intern. Med. 120:638, 1994.

56. Bueno, H., Almazan, A., Lopez-Sendon, J. L., et al.: Influence of sex on the short-term outcome of elderly patients with a first acute myocardial infarction. Circulation 92:1133, 1995.

57. White, H. D., Barbash, G. I., Modan, M., et al.: After correcting for worse baseline characteristics, women treated with thrombolytic therapy for acute myocardial infarction have the same mortality and morbidity as men except for a high incidence of hemorrhagic stroke. Circulation 88:2097, 1993.

58. Peterson, E. D., Wright, S. M., Daley, J., et al.: Racial variation in cardiac procedure use and survival following acute myocardial infarction in the Department of Veterans Affairs. JAMA 271:1175, 1994.

PATHOLOGY OF ACUTE MYOCARDIAL INFARCTION

58a. Fallon, J. T.: Pathology of myocardial infarction and reperfusion. *In* Fuster, V., Ross, R., and Topol, E. J. (eds.): Atherosclerosis and Coronary Artery Disease. Philadelphia, Lippincott-Raven, 1996, pp. 791–796.

59. Constantinides, P.: Plaque fissures in human coronary thrombosis. J. Athero. Res. 6:1, 1966.

60. Davies, M. J., and Thomas, A. C.: Plaque fissuring—the cause of acute myocardial infarction, sudden ischemic death, and crescendo angina. Br. Heart J. 53:363, 1985.

61. Falk, E.: Coronary thrombosis: Pathogenesis and clinical manifestations. Am. J. Cardiol. 68:28B, 1991.

62. Willerson, J. T.: Conversion from chronic to acute coronary heart disease syndromes: Role of platelets and platelet products. Tex. Heart Inst. J. 22:13, 1995.

63. Davies, M. J., Richardson, P. D., Woolf, N., et al.: Risk of thrombosis in human atherosclerotic plaques: Role of extracellular lipid, macrophage, and smooth muscle cell content. Br. Heart J. 69:377, 1993.

64. Falk, E., Shah, P. K., and Fuster, V.: Pathogenesis of plaque disruption. *In* Fuster, V., Ross, R., and Topol, E. J. (eds.): Atherosclerosis and Coronary Artery Disease. Philadelphia, Lippincott-Raven, 1996, pp. 492–510.

65. Falk, E., Shah, P. K., and Fuster, V.: Coronary plaque disruption. Circulation 92:657, 1995.

66. Kragel, A. H., Reddy, S. G., Wittes, J. T., et al.: Morphometric analysis of the composition of atherosclerotic plaques in the four major epicardial coronary arteries in acute myocardial infarction and in sudden coronary death. Circulation 80:1747, 1989.

67. Roberts, W. C.: Preventing and arresting coronary atherosclerosis. Am. Heart J. 130:580, 1995.

67a. Stary, H. C.: The histological classification of atherosclerotic lesions in human coronary arteries. *In* Fuster, V., Ross, R., and Topol, E. J. (eds.): Atherosclerosis and Coronary Artery Disease. Philadelphia, Lippincott-Raven, 1996, pp. 463–474.

68. Libby, P.: Molecular basis of the acute coronary syndromes. Circulation 91:2844, 1995.

69. Falk, E.: Plaque rupture with severe pre-existing stenosis precipitating thrombosis: Characteristics of coronary atherosclerotic plaque underlying fatal occlusion thrombi. Br. Heart J. 50:127, 1983.

70. Wilson, R. F., Holida, M. D., and White, C. W.: Quantitative angiographic morphology of coronary stenoses leading to myocardial infarction or unstable angina. Circulation 73:286, 1986.

71. Weiss, E. J., Bray, P. F., Schulman, S. P., et al.: Fibrinogen receptor polymorphism Pl^{A2}: An inherited platelet risk factor for early coronary thrombotic events. Circulation 92(Suppl.):I-30, 1995.

72. Falk, E.: Morphologic features of unstable atherothrombotic plaques underlying acute coronary syndrome. Am. J. Cardiol. 63:114E, 1989.

73. Galis, Z., Sukhova, G., Lark, M., et al.: Increased expression of matrix metalloproteinases and matrix degrading activity in vulnerable regions of human atherosclerotic plaques. J. Clin. Invest. 94:2493, 1994.

74. Kovanen, P. T., Kaartinen, J., and Paavonen, T.: Infiltrates of activated mast cells at the site of coronary atheromatous erosion or rupture in myocardial infarction. Circulation 92:1084, 1995.

75. Constantinides, P.: Infiltrates of activated mast cells at the site of coronary atheromatous erosion or rupture in myocardial infarction. Circulation 92:1083, 1995.

76. Barger, A., Beeuwkes, I. R., Lainey, L., et al.: Hypothesis: Vasa vasorum and neovascularization of human coronary arteries. N. Engl. J. Med. 310:175, 1984.

77. Cheng, G. C., Loree, H. M., Kamm, R. D., et al.: Distribution of circumferential stress in ruptured and stable atherosclerotic lesions: A structural analysis with histopathologic correlation. Circulation 87:1179, 1993.

78. Waxman, S., and Muller, J. E.: Risk factors for an acute ischemic event. *In* Califf, R. (ed.): Acute Myocardial Infarction and Other Acute Ischemic Syndromes. Vol 8 of Braunwald, E. (series ed.): Atlas of Heart Diseases. Philadelphia, Current Science, 1996, pp. 2–2.14.

79. Braunwald, E.: Morning resistance to thrombolytic therapy. Circulation *91*:1604, 1995.
80. Danchin, N.: Is myocardial revascularization for tight coronary stenoses always necessary? Viewpoint. Lancet *342*:224, 1993.
81. Schoen, F. J.: The heart. *In* Cotran, R. S., Kumar, V., and Robbins, S. L. (eds.): Pathologic Basis of Disease. Philadelphia, W. B. Saunders Company, 1994, p. 517.
82. Piérard, L. A.: Non-Q-wave, incomplete infarction. *In* Julian, D., and Braunwald, E. (eds.): Management of Acute Myocardial Infarction. London, W. B. Saunders Ltd., 1994, p. 315.
83. Pfeffer, M. A., and Braunwald, E.: Ventricular remodeling after myocardial infarction: Experimental observations and clinical implications. Circulation *81*:1161, 1990.
84. Vaughan, D. E., and Pfeffer, M. A.: Ventricular remodeling following myocardial infarction and angiotensin-converting enzyme and ACE inhibitors. *In* Fuster, V., Ross, R., and Topol, E. J. (eds.): Atherosclerosis and Coronary Artery Disease. Philadelphia, Lippincott-Raven, 1996, pp. 1193–1205.
85. Freifeld, A. G., Schuster, E. H., and Bulkley, B. H.: Nontransmural versus transmural myocardial infarction. Am. J. Med. *75*:423, 1983.
86. Ambrose, J. A., Tannenbaum, M. A., Alexopoulos, D., et al.: Angiographic progression of coronary artery disease and the development of myocardial infarction. J. Am. Coll. Cardiol. *12*:56, 1988.
87. Jain, D., Crawley, J. C., Lahiri, A., et al.: Indium-111 antimyosin images compared with triphenyl tetrazolium chloride staining in a patient six days after myocardial infarction. J. Nucl. Med. *31*:231, 1990.
88. Ytrehus, K., and Downey, J. M.: Experimental models assessing the physiology of myocardial ischemia. Curr. Opin. Cardiol. *8*:581, 1993.
89. Vivaldi, M. T., Kloner, R. A., and Schoen, F. J.: Triphenyltetrazolium staining of irreversible ischemic injury following coronary artery occlusion in rats. Am. J. Pathol. *121*:522, 1985.
90. Buja, L. M., and McAllister, H. A., Jr.: Coronary artery disease: Anatomic abnormalities. *In* Willerson, J. T., and Cohn, J. N. (eds.): Cardiovascular Medicine. New York, Churchill Livingstone, 1995, p. 316.
91. Kloner, R. A., Ellis, S. G., Lange, R., et al.: Studies of experimental coronary artery reperfusion: Effects on infarct size, myocardial function, biochemistry, ultrastructure and microvascular damage. Circulation *68*:1, 1983.
92. Matsuda, M., Fujiwara, J., Onodera, T., et al.: Quantitative analysis of infarct size, contraction band necrosis, and coagulation necrosis in human autopsied hearts with acute myocardial infarction after treatment with selective intracoronary thrombolysis. Circulation *76*:981, 1987.
93. Schlesinger, M. J., and Reiner, L.: Focal myocytolysis of the heart. Am. J. Physiol. *31*:443, 1955.
94. Buja, L. M., and Willerson, J. T.: Clinicopathologic correlates of acute ischemic heart disease syndromes. Am. J. Cardiol. *47*:343, 1981.
95. Gasser, R. N. A., and Klein, W.: Contractile failure in early myocardial ischemia: Models and mechanisms. Cardiovasc. Drugs Ther. *8*:813, 1994.
96. Gertz, S. D., Kalan, J. M., Kragel, A. N., et al.: Cardiac morphologic findings in patients with acute myocardial infarction treated with tissue plasminogen activator. Am. J. Cardiol. *65*:953, 1990.
97. Adams, J., III, Abendschein, D., and Jaffe, A.: Biochemical markers of myocardial injury: Is MB creatine kinase the choice for the 1990s? Circulation *88*:750, 1993.
98. Roberts, W. C., Potkin, B. N., Solus, D. E., et al.: Mode of death, frequency of healed and acute myocardial infarction, number of major epicardial coronary arteries severely narrowed by atherosclerotic plaque, and heart weight in fatal atherosclerotic coronary artery disease: Analysis of 889 patients studied at necropsy. J. Am. Coll. Cardiol. *15*:196, 1990.
99. Betriu, A., Castaner, A., Sanz, G. A., et al.: Angiographic finding 1 month after myocardial infarction: A prospective study of 259 survivors. Circulation *65*:1099, 1982.
100. DeWood, M. A., Spores, J., Notske, R. N., et al.: Prevalence of total coronary artery occlusion during the early hours of transmural myocardial infarction. N. Engl. J. Med. *303*:897, 1980.
101. Ong, L., Reiser, P., Coromilas, J., et al.: Left ventricular function and rapid release of creatine kinase MB in acute myocardial infarction: Evidence for spontaneous reperfusion. N. Engl. J. Med. *309*:1, 1983.
102. DeWood, M. A., Notske, R. N., Simpson, C. S., et al.: Prevalence and significance of spontaneous thrombolysis in transmural myocardial infarction. Eur. Heart J. *6*:33, 1985.
103. Ellis, S., Alderman, E. L., Cain, K., et al.: Morphology of left anterior descending coronary territory lesions as a predictor of anterior myocardial infarction: A CASS registry study. J. Am. Coll. Cardiol. *13*:1481, 1989.
104. Little, W. C., Constantinescu, M., Applegate, R. J., et al.: Can coronary angiography predict the site of a subsequent myocardial infarction in patients with mild-to-moderate coronary artery disease? Circulation *78*:1157, 1988.
105. Kinch, J. W., and Ryan, T. J.: Right ventricular infarction. N. Engl. J. Med. *330*:1211, 1994.
106. Mittal, S. R.: Isolated right ventricular infarction. Int. J. Cardiol. *46*:53, 1994.
107. Rackley, C. E., Russell, R. O., Jr., Mantle, J. A., et al.: Right ventricular infarction and function. Am. Heart J. *101*:215, 1981.
108. Setaro, J. F., and Cabin, H. S.: Right ventricular infarction. Cardiol. Clin. *10*:69, 1992.
109. Nielsen, F. E., Andersen, H. H., Gram-Hansen, P., et al.: The relationship between ECG signs of atrial infarction and the development of supraventricular arrhythmias in patients with acute myocardial infarction. Am. Heart J. *123*:69, 1992.
110. Ventura, T., Colantonio, D., Leocata, P., et al.: Isolated atrial myocardial infarction: Pathological and clinical features in 10 cases. Cardiologia *36*:345, 1991.
111. Alonso-Orcajo, N., Izquierdo-Garcia, F., and Simarro, E.: Atrial rupture and sudden death following atrial infarction. Int. J. Cardiol. *46*:82, 1994.
112. Iga, K., Konishi, T., and Kusukawa, R.: Intracardiac thrombi in both the right atrium and right ventricle after acute inferior-wall myocardial infarction. Int. J. Cardiol. *46*:169, 1994.
113. Yasuda, S., Nonogi, H., Miyazaki, S., et al.: Hyposecretion of atrial natriuretic peptide due to associated right atrial infarction in a patient with acute right ventricular infarction? Eur. Heart J. *15*:718, 1994.
114. Conti, C. R.: Myocardial infarction: Thoughts about pathogenesis and the role of coronary artery spasm. Am. Heart J. *110*:187, 1985.
115. Vincent, G. M., Anderson, J. L., and Marshall, H. W.: Coronary spasm producing coronary thrombosis and myocardial infarction. N. Engl. J. Med. *309*:220, 1983.
116. Christian, T. F., Gibbons, R. J., Clements, I. P., et al.: Estimates of myocardium at risk and collateral flow in acute myocardial infarction using electrocardiographic indexes with comparison to radionuclide and angiographic measures. J. Am. Coll. Cardiol. *26*:388, 1995.
117. Hirai, T., Fujita, M., Nakajima, H., et al.: Importance of collateral circulation for prevention of left ventricular aneurysm formation in acute myocardial infarction. Circulation *79*:791, 1989.
118. Markis, J. E., Brewer, C. C., Alderman, J., et al.: Myocardial infarction without early coronary angiographic evidence of occlusion: The NHLBI thrombolysis in myocardial infarction trial (TIMI). Circulation *72*(Suppl. III):56S, 1985.
119. Schwartz, H., Leiboff, R. H., Bren, G. B., et al.: Temporal evolution of the human coronary collateral circulation after myocardial infarction. J. Am. Coll. Cardiol. *4*:1088, 1984.
119a. Harrison, D. C.: Nonatherosclerotic coronary disease. *In* Fuster, V., Ross, R., and Topol, E. J. (eds.): Atherosclerosis and Coronary Artery Disease. Philadelphia, Lippincott-Raven, 1996, pp. 757–772.
120. Dollar, A. L., Pierre-Louis, M. L., McIntosh, C. L., et al.: Extensive multifocal myocardial infarcts from cloth emboli after replacement of mitral and aortic valves with cloth-covered caged-ball prostheses. Am. J. Cardiol. *64*:410, 1989.
121. Ackermann, D. M., Hyma, B. A., and Edwards, W. D.: Malignant neoplastic emboli to the coronary arteries. Hum. Pathol. *18*:955, 1987.
122. Obarski, T. P., Loop, F. D., Cosgrove, D. M., et al.: Frequency of acute myocardial infarction in valve repairs versus valve replacement for pure mitral regurgitation. Am. J. Cardiol. *65*:887, 1990.
123. Parrillo, J. E., and Fauci, A. S.: Necrotizing vasculitis, coronary angiitis, and the cardiologist. Am. Heart J. *99*:547, 1980.
124. Spodick, D. H.: Inflammation and the onset of myocardial infarction. Ann. Intern. Med. *99*:547, 1985.
125. Miklozek, C. L., Crumpacker, C. S., Royal, H. D., et al.: Myocarditis presenting as acute myocardial infarction. Am. Heart J. *115*:768, 1988.
126. Connolley, J. E., Eldridge, F. L., Calvin, J. W., et al.: Proximal coronary artery obstruction. N. Engl. J. Med. *271*:213, 1964.
127. Roberts, W. C., MacGregor, R. R., DeBlanc, H. J., et al.: The prepulseless phase of pulseless disease, or pulseless disease with pulses. Am. J. Med. *46*:313, 1969.
128. Pick, R. A., Glover, M. U., and Vieweg, W. V. R.: Myocardial infarction in a young woman with isolated coronary arteritis. Chest *82*:378, 1982.
129. van Camp, G., Deschamps, P., Mestrez, F., et al.: Adult onset Kawasaki disease diagnosed by the echocardiographic demonstration of coronary aneurysms. Eur. Heart J. *16*:1155, 1995.
130. Lie, J. L., Failoni, D. D., and Davis, D. C. J.: Temporal arteritis with giant cell aortitis, coronary arteritis, and myocardial infarction. Arch. Pathol. Lab. Med. *110*:857, 1986.
131. Joensuu, H.: Acute myocardial infarction after heart irradiation in young patients with Hodgkin's disease. Chest *95*:388, 1989.
132. Huang, S., Kumar, G., Steele, H. D., et al.: Cardiac involvement in pseudoxanthoma elasticum. Am. Heart J. *74*:680, 1967.
133. Isner, J. M., and Chokshi, S. K.: Cardiac complications of cocaine abuse. Annu. Rev. Med. *42*:133, 1991.
134. Kloner, R. A., Hale, S., Alker, K., et al.: The effects of acute and chronic cocaine use on the heart. Circulation *85*:407, 1992.
135. Chakko, S., and Myerburg, R. J.: Cardiac complications of cocaine abuse. Clin. Cardiol. *18*:67, 1995.
136. Ashchi, M., Wiedemann, H. P., and James, K. B.: Cardiac complication from use of cocaine and phenylephrine in nasal septoplasty. Arch. Otolaryngol. Head Neck Surg. *121*:681, 1995.
137. Bulbul, Z. R., Rosenthal, D. N., and Kleinman, C. S.: Myocardial infarction in the perinatal period secondary to maternal cocaine abuse: A case report and literature review. Arch. Pediatr. Adoles. Med. *148*:1092, 1994.
138. Lange, R. A., and Willard, J. E.: The cardiovascular effects of cocaine. Heart Dis. Stroke *2*:136, 1993.
139. Killam, A. L.: Cardiovascular and thrombosis pathology associated with cocaine use. Hematol. Oncol. Clin. North Am. *7*:1143, 1993.
140. Alpert, J. S.: Myocardial infarction with angiographically normal coronary arteries. Arch. Intern. Med. *154*:265, 1994.
141. Glover, M. V., Kuber, M. T., Warren, S. E., et al.: Myocardial infarction before age 36: Risk factor and arteriographic analysis. Am. J. Cardiol. *49*:1600, 1982.

142. Ciraulo, D. A., Bresnahan, G. F., Frankel, P. S., et al.: Transmural myocardial infarction with normal coronary angiograms and with single vessel coronary obstruction: Clinical-angiographic features and five-year follow-up. Chest 83:196, 1983.

143. Braunwald, E.: Coronary spasm and acute myocardial infarction—New possibility for treatment and prevention. N. Engl. J. Med. 299:1301, 1978.

144. Makino, H., and Al-Saidr, H.: Myocardial infarction in patients with mitral valve prolapse and normal coronary arteries. J. Am. Coll. Cardiol. 1:661, 1983.

145. Yeager, S. B., and Freed, M. D.: Myocardial infarction as a manifestation of polycythemia in cyanotic heart disease. Am. J. Cardiol. 53:952, 1984.

146. Martin, C. R., Cobb, C., Tatter, D., et al.: Acute myocardial infarction in sickle cell anemia. Arch. Intern. Med. 143:830, 1983.

147. Bergeron, G. A., Goldsmith, R., and Schiller, N. B.: Myocardial infarction, severe, reversible ischemia, and shock following excess thyroid administration in a woman with normal coronary arteries. Arch. Intern. Med. 148:1450, 1988.

148. Carson, P., Oldroyd, K., and Phadke, K.: Myocardial infarction due to amphetamine. BMJ 294:1525, 1987.

149. Pecora, M. J., Roubin, G. S., Cobbs, B. W., et al.: Presentation and late outcome of myocardial infarction in the absence of angiographically significant coronary artery disease. Am. J. Cardiol. 62:363, 1988.

150. Raymond, R., Lynch, J., Underwood, D., et al.: Myocardial infarction and normal coronary aortography: A 10 year clinical and risk analysis of 74 patients. J. Am. Coll. Cardiol. 11:471, 1988.

PATHOPHYSIOLOGY OF ACUTE MYOCARDIAL INFARCTION

151. Tennant, R., and Wiggins, C. J.: The effect of coronary occlusion on myocardial contraction. Am. J. Physiol. 112:351, 1935.

152. Theroux, P., Franklin, D., Ross, J., Jr., et al.: Regional myocardial function during acute coronary artery occlusion and its modification by pharmacologic agents in the dog. Circ. Res. 35:896, 1974.

153. Herman, M. V., Heinle, R. A., Klein, M. D., et al.: Localized disorders in myocardial contraction. N. Engl. J. Med. 227:222, 1967.

154. Swan, H. J. C., Forrester, J. S., Diamond, G., et al.: Hemodynamic spectrum of myocardial infarction and cardiogenic shock. Circulation 45:1097, 1972.

155. Forrester, J. S., Wyatt, H. L., Daluz, P. L., et al.: Functional significance of regional ischemic contraction abnormalities. Circulation 54:64, 1976.

156. Low, W. Y., Chen, Z., Guth, B., et al.: Mechanisms of augmented segment shortening in nonischemic areas during acute ischemia of the canine left ventricle. Circ. Res. 56:351, 1985.

157. Bourdillon, P. D. V., Broderick, T. M., Williams, E. S., et al.: Early recovery of regional left ventricular function after reperfusion in acute myocardial infarction assessed by serial two-dimensional echocardiography. Am. J. Cardiol. 63:641, 1989.

158. Schuster, E. H., and Bulkley, B. H.: Ischemia at a distance after acute myocardial infarction: A cause of early postinfarction angina. Circulation 62:509, 1980.

159. Cortina, A., Ambrose, J. A., Prieto-Granada, J., et al.: Left ventricular function after myocardial infarction: Clinical and angiographic correlations. J. Am. Coll. Cardiol. 5:619, 1985.

160. White, H. D., Norris, R. M., Brown, M. A., et al.: Left ventricular end-systolic volume as the major determinant of survival after recovery from myocardial infarction. Circulation 76:44, 1987.

161. Braunwald, E., and Pfeffer, M. A.: Ventricular enlargement and remodeling following acute myocardial infarction: Mechanisms and management. Am. J. Cardiol. 68:1D, 1991.

162. Braunwald, E., and Kim, C. B.: Late establishment of patency of the infarct-related artery. In Julian, D., and Braunwald, E. (eds.): Acute Myocardial Infarction. London, W. B. Saunders Ltd., 1994, p. 147.

163. Pfeffer, M. A., Lamas, G. A., Vaughan, D. E., et al.: Effect of captopril on progressive ventricular dilatation after anterior myocardial infarction. N. Engl. J. Med. 319:80, 1988.

164. Jeremy, R. W., Hackworthy, R. A., Bautovich, G., et al.: Infarct artery perfusion and changes in left ventricular volume in the month after acute myocardial infarction. J. Am. Coll. Cardiol. 9:989, 1987.

165. Hirsch, A. T., Talsnecs, C. E., Schunkert, H., et al.: Tissue specific activation of cardiac angiotensin converting enzyme in experimental heart failure. Circ. Res. 69:475, 1991.

166. Rackley, C. E., Russell, R. O., Jr., et al.: Modern approach to the patient with acute myocardial infarction. Curr. Probl. Cardiol. 1:49, 1977.

167. Waters, D. D., DaLuz, P., Wyatt, H. L., et al.: Early changes in regional and global left ventricular function induced by graded reduction in regional coronary perfusion. Am. J. Cardiol. 39:537, 1977.

168. Pfeffer, J. M., Pfeffer, M. A., Fletcher, P. J., et al.: Progressive ventricular remodeling in rat with myocardial infarction. Am. J. Physiol. 260:H1406, 1991.

169. Weisman, H. F., Bush, D. E., Mannisi, J. A., et al.: Cellular mechanisms of myocardial infarct expansion. Circulation 78:186, 1988.

170. Pirolo, J. S., Hutchins, G. M., and Moore, G. W.: Infarct expansion: Pathologic analysis of 204 patients with a single myocardial infarct. J. Am. Coll. Cardiol. 7:349, 1986.

171. Pfeffer, M. A.: Left ventricular remodeling after acute myocardial infarction. Annu. Rev. Med. 46:455, 1995.

172. Picard, M. H., Wilkins, G. T., Gillam, L. D., et al.: Immediate regional endocardial surface expansion following coronary occlusion in the canine left ventricle: Disproportionate effects of anterior versus inferior ischemia. Am. Heart J. 121:753, 1991.

173. Weisman, H. F., and Healy, B.: Myocardial infarct expansion, infarct extension, and reinfarction: Pathophysiologic concepts. Prog. Cardiovasc. Dis. 30:73, 1987.

174. Jugdutt, B. I., and Michorowski, B. L.: Role of infarct expansion in rupture of the ventricular septum after acute myocardial infarction: A two-dimensional echocardiographic study. Clin. Cardiol. 10:641, 1987.

175. Schuster, E. H., and Bulkley, B. H.: Expansion of transmural myocardial infarction: A pathophysiologic feature in cardiac rupture. Circulation 60:1532, 1979.

176. Abernathy, M., Sharpe, N., Smith, H., et al.: Echocardiographic prediction of left ventricular volume after myocardial infarction. J. Am. Coll. Cardiol. 17:1527, 1991.

177. McKay, R. G., Pfeffer, M. A., Pasternak, R. C., et al.: Left ventricular remodeling after myocardial infarction: A corollary. Circulation 74:693, 1986.

178. Dambrink, J.-H. E., Sippens Groenewegen, A., van Gilst, W. H., et al.: Association of left ventricular remodeling and nonuniform electrical recovery expressed by nondipolar QRST integral map patterns in survivors of a first anterior myocardial infarction. Circulation 92:300, 1995.

179. Ginzton, L. E., Conant, R., Rodrigues, D. M., et al.: Functional significance of hypertrophy of the noninfarcted myocardium after myocardial infarction in humans. Circulation 80:816, 1989.

180. Lavie, C. J., O'Keefe, J. H., Jr., Chesebro, J. H., et al.: Prevention of late ventricular dilatation after acute myocardial infarction by successful thrombolytic reperfusion. Am. J. Cardiol. 66:31, 1990.

181. Braunwald, E.: The open-artery theory is alive and well—again. N. Engl. J. Med. 329:1650, 1993.

182. Hammerman, H., Kloner, R. A., Hale, S., et al.: Dose-dependent effects of short-term methylprednisone on myocardial infarct extent, scar formation, and ventricular function. Circulation 68:446, 1983.

183. Cortese, D., and Viggiano, R. W.: The lungs in acute myocardial infarction. In Gersh, B. J., and Rahimtoola, S. H. (eds.): Acute Myocardial Infarction. New York, Elsevier, 1991, p. 398.

184. Biddle, T. L., Yu, P. N., Hodges, M., et al.: Hypoxemia and lung water in acute myocardial infarction. Am. Heart J. 92:692, 1976.

185. Hales, C. A., and Kazemi, H.: Clinical significance of pulmonary function tests: Pulmonary function after uncomplicated myocardial infarction. Chest 72:350, 1977.

186. Hales, C. A., and Kazemi, H.: Small-airways function in myocardial infarction. N. Engl. J. Med. 290:761, 1974.

187. Gray, B. A., Hyde, R. W., Hodges, M., et al.: Alterations in lung volume and pulmonary function in relation to hemodynamic changes in acute myocardial infarction. Circulation 59:551, 1979.

188. Kazemi, H., Parsons, E. F., Valenca, L. M., et al.: Distribution of pulmonary blood flow after myocardial ischemia and infarction. Circulation 41:1025, 1970.

189. DaLuz, P. L., Cavanilles, J. M., Michaels, S., et al.: Oxygen delivery, anoxic metabolism and hemoglobin-oxygen affinity (P50) in patients with acute myocardial infarction and shock. Am. J. Cardiol. 36:148, 1975.

190. Vetter, N. J., Adams, W., Strange, R. C., et al.: Initial metabolic and hormonal response to acute myocardial infarction. Lancet 1:284, 1974.

191. Ceremuzynski, L.: Hormonal and metabolic reactions evoked by acute myocardial infarction. Circ. Res. 48:767, 1981.

192. Taegtmeyer, H.: Metabolic support of the postischaemic heart. Lancet 345:1552, 1995.

193. Opie, L. H.: Glucose and the metabolism of ischaemic myocardium. Lancet 345:1520, 1995.

194. Zuanetti, G., Latini, R., Maggioni, A. P., et al.: Influence of diabetes on mortality in acute myocardial infarction: Data from the GISSI-2 study. J. Am. Coll. Cardiol. 22:1788, 1993.

195. Rouleau, J. J., Dagerais, G.-R., Packer, M., et al.: Selective activation of neurohormonal systems in post-infarction left ventricular dysfunction. J. Am. Coll. Cardiol. 17:21A, 1991.

196. Karlsberg, R. P., Cryer, P. E., and Roberts, R.: Serial plasma catecholamine response early in the course of clinical acute myocardial infarction: Relationship to infarct extent and mortality. Am. Heart J. 102:24, 1981.

197. Dzau, V. J., Gibbons, G. H., Cooke, J. P., et al.: Vascular biology and medicine in the 1990s: Scope, concepts, potentials, and perspectives. Circulation 87:705, 1993.

198. Pitt, B.: The role of angiotensin-converting enzyme inhibitors during the early phase. In Julian, D., and Braunwald, E. (eds.): Management of Acute Myocardial Infarction. London, W. B. Saunders Ltd., 1994, p. 253.

199. Hall, C., Cannon, C. P., Forman, S., et al.: Prognostic value of N-terminal proatrial natriuretic factor plasma levels measured within the first 12 hours after myocardial infarction. J. Am. Coll. Cardiol. 26:1452, 1995.

200. Morita, E., Yause, H., Yoshimura, M., et al.: Increased plasma levels of brain natriuretic peptide in patients with acute myocardial infarction. Circulation 88:82, 1993.

201. Bain, R. J., Fox, J. P., Jagger, J., et al.: Serum cortisol levels predict infarct size and patient mortality. Int. J. Cardiol. 37:145, 1992.

202. Wiersinga, W. M., Lie, K. I., and Touber, J. L.: Thyroid hormones in acute myocardial infarction. Clin. Endocrinol. 14:367, 1981.

203. Kahana, L., Keidar, S., Sheinfeld, M., et al.: Endogenous cortisol and thyroid hormone levels in patients with acute myocardial infarction. Clin. Endocrinol. 19:131, 1983.

204. Tomoda, H.: Atrial natriuretic peptide in acute myocardial infarction. Am. J. Cardiol. 62:1122, 1988.

205. Robalino, B. D., Petrella, R. W., Jubran, F. Y., et al.: Atrial natriuretic factor in patients with right ventricular infarction. J. Am. Coll. Cardiol. 15:546, 1990.

206. Willerson, J. T., Golino, P., Eidt, J., et al.: Platelet mediators and unstable coronary artery disease. Circulation 80:198, 1989.

207. Frishman, W. H., Burns, B., Atac, B., et al.: Novel antiplatelet therapies for treatment of patients with ischemic heart disease: Inhibitors of the platelet glycoprotein IIb/IIIa integrin receptor. Am. Heart J. 130:877, 1995.

208. Fitzgerald, D. J., Roy, L., Catella, F., et al.: Platelet activation in unstable coronary disease. N. Engl. J. Med. 315:983, 1986.

209. Fuster, V.: Lewis A. Conner Memorial Lecture: Mechanisms leading to myocardial infarction: Insights from studies of vascular biology. Circulation 90:2126, 1994.

210. Tracey, R. P., and Bovill, E. G.: The coagulation system. In Califf, R. M. (ed.): Acute Myocardial Infarction and Other Acute Ischemic Syndromes. Philadelphia, Current Medicine, 1996.

211. Freudenberger, R., and Fuster, V.: Acute coronary syndromes: Thrombosis and thrombolysis. In Smith, T. W. (ed.): Cardiovascular Therapeutics. Philadelphia, W. B. Saunders Company, 1996.

212. Engler, R. L., Dahlgren, M. D., Morris, D. D., et al.: Role of leukocytes in response to acute myocardial ischemia and reflow in dogs. Am. J. Physiol. 251:H314, 1986.

213. Koenig, W., and Erns, E.: The possible role of hemorheology in atherothrombogenesis. Atherosclerosis 94:93, 1992.

214. Hershberg, P. I., Wells, R. E., and McGandy, R. B.: Hematocrit and prognosis in patients with acute myocardial infarction. JAMA 219:855, 1972.

CLINICAL FEATURES

214a. Braunwald, E.: Acute myocardial infarction—the value of being prepared. N. Engl. J. Med. 334:51, 1996.

215. Mittleman, M. A., Maclure, M., Sherwood, J. B., et al.: Triggering of acute myocardial infarction onset by episodes of anger. Circulation 92:1720, 1995.

215a. Muller, J. E., Tofler, G. H., and Mittleman, M.: Triggering of onset of myocardial infarction and sudden cardiac death. In Fuster, V., Ross, R., and Topol, E. J. (eds.): Atherosclerosis and Coronary Artery Disease. Philadelphia, Lippincott-Raven, 1996, pp. 819–834.

216. Rahe, R. H., Romo, M., Bennett, L., et al.: Recent life changes, myocardial infarction, and abrupt coronary death. Arch. Intern. Med. 133:221, 1974.

216a. Muller, J. E., Tofler, G. H., and Mittleman, M.: Triggering of onset of myocardial infarction and sudden cardiac death. In Fuster, V., Ross, R., and Topol, E. J. (eds.): Atherosclerosis and Coronary Artery Disease. Philadelphia, Lippincott-Raven, 1996, pp. 819–834.

217. Allison, T. G., Williams, D. E., Miller, T. D., et al.: Medical and economic costs of psychologic distress in patients with coronary artery disease. Mayo Clin. Proc. 70:734, 1995.

218. Pasternak, R. C.: Psychologic factors and course after myocardial infarction: Maturing of a risk factor. Mayo Clin. Proc. 70:809, 1995.

219. Hlatkly, M. A., Lam, L. C., Lee, K. L., et al.: Job strain and the prevalence and outcome of coronary artery disease. Circulation 92:327, 1995.

220. Maseri, A., L'Abbate, A., Baroldi, G., et al.: Coronary vasospasm as a possible cause of myocardial infarction. N. Engl. J. Med. 299:1271, 1978.

221. Lange, R. L., Reid, M. S., Tresch, D. D., et al.: Nonatheromatous ischemic heart disease following withdrawal from chronic industrial nitroglycerin exposure. Circulation 46:666, 1972.

222. Psaty, B. M., Heckbert, S. R., Koepsell, T. D., et al.: The risk of myocardial infarction associated with antihypertensive drug therapies. JAMA 274:620, 1995.

223. Lenfant, C.: The calcium channel blocker scare: Lessons for the future. Circulation 91:2855, 1995.

224. Buring, J. E., Glynn, R. J., and Hennekens, C. H.: Calcium channel blockers and myocardial infarction: A hypothesis formulated but not yet tested. JAMA 274:654, 1995.

225. Muller, J. E., Stone, P. H., Turi, Z. G., et al.: Circadian variation in the frequency of onset of acute myocardial infarction. N. Engl. J. Med. 313:1315, 1985.

226. Willich, S. N., Linderer, T., Wegscheider, K., et al.: Increasing morning incidence of myocardial infarction in the ISAM study: Absence with prior β-adrenergic blockade. Circulation 80:853, 1989.

227. Ridker, P. M., Manson, J. E., Buring, J. E., et al.: Circadian variation of acute myocardial infarction and the effect of low-dose aspirin in a randomized trial of physicians. Circulation 82:897, 1990.

228. Willerson, J. T., Cohen, L. S., and Maseri, A.: Coronary artery disease: Pathophysiology and clinical recognition. In Willerson, J. T., and Cohn, J. N. (eds.): Cardiovascular Medicine. New York, Churchill Livingstone, 1995, p. 333.

228a. Huggins, G. S., and O'Gara, P. T.: Clinical presentation and diagnostic evaluation. In Fuster, V., Ross, R., and Topol, E. J. (eds.): Atherosclerosis and Coronary Artery Disease. Philadelphia, Lippincott-Raven, 1996.

229. Harper, R. W., Kennedy, G., DeSanctis, R. W., et al.: The incidence and pattern of angina prior to acute myocardial infarction: A study of 577 cases. Am. Heart J. 97:178, 1979.

230. Muller, R., Gould, L., Betu, R., et al.: Painless myocardial infarction in the elderly. Am. Heart J. 119:202, 1990.

231. Malliani, A., and Lombardi, F.: Consideration of the fundamental mechanisms eliciting cardiac pain. Am. Heart J. 103:575, 1982.

232. Ingram, D. A., Fulton, R. A., Portal, R. W., et al.: Vomiting as a diagnostic aid in acute ischemic cardiac pain. BMJ 281:636, 1980.

233. Spodick, D. H.: Pericardial complications of myocardial infarction. In Francis, G. S., and Alpert, J. S. (eds.): Coronary Care. Boston, Little, Brown and Co., 1995, p. 333.

234. Yano, K., and MacLean, C. J.: The incidence and prognosis of unrecognized myocardial infarction in Honolulu, Hawaii, Heart Program. Arch. Intern. Med. 149:1528, 1989.

235. Sigurdsson, E., Thorgeirsson, G., Sigvaldason, H., et al.: Unrecognized myocardial infarction: Epidemiology, clinical characteristics, and the prognostic role of angina pectoris: The Reykjavik study. Ann. Intern. Med. 122:96, 1995.

236. Bean, W. B.: Masquerade of myocardial infarction. Lancet 1:1044, 1977.

237. Campbell, R. W. F.: Arrhythmias. In Julian, D., and Braunwald, E. (eds.): Management of Acute Myocardial Infarction. London, W.B. Saunders Ltd., 1994, p. 223.

238. Chadda, K. D., Lichstein, E., Gupta, P. K., et al.: Bradycardia-hypotension syndrome in acute myocardial infarction: Reappraisal of the overdrive effects of atropine. Am. J. Med. 59:158, 1975.

239. Webb, S. W., Adgey, A. A., and Pantridge, J. F.: Autonomic disturbance at onset of acute myocardial infarction. BMJ 818:89, 1982.

240. Killip, T., and Kimball, J. T.: Treatment of myocardial infarction in a coronary care unit: A two year experience with 250 patients. Am. J. Cardiol. 20:457, 1967.

241. Gadsboll, N., Hoilund-Carlsen, P. F., et al.: Symptoms and signs of heart failure in patients with myocardial infarction: Reproducibility and relationship to chest x-ray, radionuclide venticulography and right heart catheterization. Eur. Heart J. 10:1017, 1989.

242. Manson, A. L., Nudelman, S. P., Hagley, M. T., et al.: Relationship of the third heart sound to transmitral flow velocity deceleration. Circulation 92:388, 1995.

243. Riley, C. P., Russell, R. O. J., and Rackley, C. E.: Left ventricular gallop sound and acute myocardial infarction. Am. Heart J. 86:598, 1973.

244. Galve, E., Garcia Del Castillo, H., Evangelista, A., et al.: Pericardial effusion in the course of myocardial infarction: Incidence, natural history, and clinical relevance. Circulation 73:294, 1986.

245. Thompson, P. L., and Robinson, J. S.: Stroke after acute myocardial infarction: Relation to infarct size. BMJ 2:457, 1978.

246. Duryee, R.: The efficacy of inpatient education after myocardial infarction. Heart Lung 21:217, 1992.

LABORATORY EXAMINATIONS

247. Pedoe-Tunstall, H., Kuulasmaa, K., Amouyel, P., et al.: Myocardial infarction and coronary deaths in the World Health Organization MONICA Project. Circulation 90:583, 1994.

248. Goldberg, R., Gore, J., Alpert, J., et al.: Incidence and case fatality rates of acute myocardial infarction (1975–1984): The Worcester Heart Attack Study. Am. Heart J. 115:761, 1988.

249. Kannel, W.: Prevalence and clinical aspects of unrecognized myocardial infarction and sudden unexpected death. Circulation 75(Suppl. II):II, 1987.

250. Grimm, R., Tillingshast, S., Daniels, K., et al.: Unrecognized myocardial infarction: Experience in the multiple risk factor intervention trial (MRFIT). Circulation 75(Suppl. II):6, 1987.

251. Gibler, W., Lewis, L., Erb, R., et al.: Early detection of acute myocardial infarction in patients presenting with chest pain and nondiagnostic ECGs: Serial CKMB sampling in the emergency department. Ann. Emerg. Med. 19:1359, 1990.

252. Hedges, J. R., Young, G. P., Henkel, G. F., et al.: Serial ECGs are less accurate than serial CK-MB results for emergency department diagnosis of myocardial infarction. Ann. Emerg. Med. 21:1445, 1992.

253. Gibler, W. B., Young, G. P., Hedges, J. R., et al.: Acute myocardial infarction in chest pain patients with nondiagnostic ECGs: Serial CK-MB sampling in the emergency department: The Emergency Medicine Cardiac Research Group. Ann. Emerg. Med. 21:504, 1992.

254. Sacks, D. B.: Troponin T: A cardiac specific-marker. In Goldman, L., and Katus, H. A. (eds.): Cardiac Troponin T for the Diagnosis of Myocardial Injury. Deerfield, IL, Discovery International, 1994, p. 3.

255. Murray, C., and Alpert, J. S.: Diagnosis of acute myocardial infarction. Curr. Opin. Cardiol. 9:465, 1994.

256. Ellis, A. K.: Serum protein measurements and the diagnosis of acute myocardial infarction. Circulation 83:1107, 1991.

257. Mair, J., Dienstl, F., and Puschendorf, B.: Cardiac troponin T in the diagnosis of myocardial injury. Crit. Rev. Clin. Lab. Sci. 29:31, 1992.

258. Collinson, P. O., Ramhamadamy, E. M., Stubbs, P. J., et al.: Rapid enzyme diagnosis of patients with acute chest pain reduces patient stay in the coronary care unit. Ann. Clin. Biochem. 30:17, 1993.

259. Puleo, P. R., Meyer, D., Wathen, C., et al.: Use of a rapid assay of subforms of creatine kinase MB to diagnose or rule out acute myocardial infarction. N. Engl. J. Med. 331:561, 1994.

260. Antman, E. M., Grudzien, C., and Sacks, D.: Evaluation of a rapid bedside assay for detection of serum cardiac troponin T. JAMA 273:1279, 1995.

261. Roberts, R.: Enzymatic estimation of infarct size: Thrombolysis induced its demise: Will it now rekindle its renaissance? Circulation 81:707, 1990.

262. Lee, T. H., and Goldman, L.: Serum enzyme assays in the diagnosis of acute myocardial infarction. Ann. Intern. Med. 105:221, 1986.

263. Adams, J. E., Bodor, G. S., Davila-Roman, V. G., et al.: Cardiac troponin I: A marker with high specificity for cardiac injury. Circulation 88:101, 1993.

264. Tsung, J. S., and Tsung, S. S.: Creatine kinase isoenzymes in extracts of various human skeletal muscles. Clin. Chem. 32:1568, 1986.

265. Roberts, R., and Sobel, B. E.: Isoenzymes of creatine phosphokinase and diagnosis of myocardial infarction. Ann. Intern. Med. 79:741, 1973.

266. Jaffe, A. S., Garfinkel, B. T., Ritter, C. S., et al.: Plasma MB creatine kinase after vigorous exercise in professional athletes. Am. J. Cardiol. 53:856, 1984.

267. Apple, F.: Creatine kinase-MB. Lab. Med. 23:298, 1992.

268. Vaidya, H. C., Maynard, Y., Dietzler, D. N., et al.: Direct measurement of creatine-kinase MB activity in serum after extraction with a monoclonal antibody specific to the MB isoenzyme. Clin. Chem. 32:657, 1986.

269. Bakker, A. J., Gorgels, J. P. M. C., van Vlies, B., et al.: Contribution of creatine kinase mass concentration at admission to early diagnosis of myocardial infarction. Br. Heart J. 72:112, 1994.

270. El Allaf, M., Chapelle, J., El Allaf, D., et al.: Differentiating muscle damage from myocardial injury by means of the serum creatine kinase (CK) isoenzyme MB mass measure/total CK activity ratio. Clin. Chem. 32:291, 1986.

271. Yusuf, S., Collins, R., Lin, L., et al.: Significance of elevated MB isoenzyme with normal creatine kinase in acute myocardial infarction. Am. J. Cardiol. 59:245, 1987.

272. Roberts, R., and Kleiman, N.: Earlier diagnosis and treatment of acute myocardial infarction necessitates the need for a "new diagnostic mind-set." Circulation 89:872, 1994.

273. Puleo, P. R., Guadagno, P. A., Roberts, R., et al.: Early diagnosis of acute myocardial infarction based on assay for subforms of creatine kinase-MB. Circulation 82:759, 1990.

274. Puleo, P. R., and Perryman, B.: Noninvasive detection of reperfusion in acute myocardial infarction based on plasma activity of creatine kinase MB subfractions. J. Am. Coll. Cardiol. 17:1047, 1991.

275. Ohman, E. M., Casey, C., Bengston, J. R., et al.: Early detection of acute myocardial infarction: Additional diagnostic information from serum concentrations of myoglobin in patients without ST elevation. Br. Heart J. 63:335, 1990.

276. Zabel, M., Hohnloser, S. H., Koster, W., et al.: Analysis of creatine kinase, CK-MB, myoglobin, and troponin T time-activity curves for early assessment of coronary artery reperfusion after intravenous thrombolysis. Circulation 87:1542, 1993.

277. Abendschein, D. R., Ellis, A. K., Eisenberg, P. R., et al.: Prompt detection of coronary recanalization by analysis rates of change of concentrations of macromolecular markers in plasma. Coron. Artery Dis. 2:201, 1991.

278. Yamashita, T., Abe, S., Arima, S., et al.: Myocardial infarct size can be estimated from serial plasma myoglobin measurements within 4 hours of reperfusion. Circulation 87:1840, 1993.

279. Katus, H., Scheffold, T., Remppis, A., et al.: Proteins of the troponin complex. Lab. Med. 23:311, 1992.

280. Katus, H. A., Remppis, A., Scheffold, T., et al.: Intracellular compartmentation of cardiac troponin T and its release kinetics in patients with reperfused and nonreperfused myocardial infarction. Am. J. Cardiol. 67:1360, 1991.

281. Adams, J. E., Schechtman, K. B., Landt, Y., et al.: Comparable detection of acute myocardial infarction by creatine kinase MB isoenzyme and cardiac troponin I. Clin. Chem. 40:1291, 1994.

282. Hamm, C. W.: New serum markers for acute myocardial infarction. N. Engl. J. Med. 331:607, 1994.

283. Katus, H. A., Looser, S., Hallermayer, K., et al.: Development and in vitro characterization of a new immunoassay of cardiac troponin T. Clin. Chem. 38:386, 1992.

284. Wu, A. H. B., Valdes, R., Jr., Apple, F. S., et al.: Cardiac troponin-T immunoassay for diagnosis of acute myocardial infarction. Clin. Chem. 40:900, 1994.

285. Bodor, G. S., Porter, S., Landt, Y., et al.: Development of monoclonal antibodies for an assay of cardiac troponin-I and preliminary results in suspected cases of myocardial infarction. Clin. Chem. 38:2203, 1992.

286. Adams, J. E., Sicard, G. A., Allen, B. T., et al.: Diagnosis of perioperative myocardial infarction with measurement of cardiac troponin I. N. Engl. J. Med. 330:670, 1994.

287. Mair, J., Morandell, D., Genser, N., et al.: Equivalent early sensitivities of myoglobin, creatine kinase MB mass, creatine kinase isoform ratios, and cardiac troponins I and T for acute myocardial infarction. Clin. Chem. 41:1266, 1995.

288. Newby, L. K., Gibler, W. B., Ohman, W. M., et al.: Biochemical markers in suspected acute myocardial infarction: The need for early assessment. Clin. Chem. 41:1263, 1995.

288a. Müller-Bardorff, M., Freitag, H., Scheffold, T., et al.: Development and characterization of a rapid assay for bedside determinations of cardiac troponin T. Circulation 92:2869, 1995.

289. Hamm, C., Ravkilde, J., Gerhardt, W., et al.: The prognostic value of serum troponin T in unstable angina. N. Engl. J. Med. 327:146, 1992.

290. Guest, T. M., Ramanathan, A. V., Tuteur, P. G., et al.: Myocardial injury in critically ill patients: A frequently unrecognized complication. JAMA 273:1945, 1995.

291. Larue, C., Calzolari, C., Bertinchant, J. P., et al.: Cardiac-specific immunoenzymometric assay of troponin I in the early phase of acute myocardial infarction. Clin. Chem. 39:972, 1993.

292. Katus, H. A., Remppis, A., Neumann, F. J., et al.: Diagnostic efficiency of troponin T measurements in acute myocardial infarction. Circulation 83:902, 1991.

293. Remppis, A., Scheffold, T., Karrer, O., et al.: Assessment of reperfusion of the infarct zone after acute myocardial infarction by serial cardiac troponin T measurements in serum. Br. Heart J. 71:242, 1994.

294. Abe, S., Arima, S., Yamashita, T., et al.: Early assessment of reperfusion therapy using cardiac troponin T. J. Am. Coll. Cardiol. 23:1382, 1994.

295. Ravkilde, J., Horder, M., Gerhardt, W., et al.: Diagnostic performance and prognostic value of serum troponin T in suspected acute myocardial infarction. Scand. J. Clin. Lab. Invest. 53:677, 1993.

296. Ravkilde, J., Nissen, H., Horder, M., et al.: Independent prognostic value of serum creatine kinase isoenzyme MB mass, cardiac troponin T and myosin light chain levels in suspected acute myocardial infarction: Analysis of 28 months of follow-up in 196 patients. J. Am. Coll. Cardiol. 25:574, 1995.

297. Hamm, C. W., and Katus, H. A.: New biochemical markers for myocardial cell injury. Curr. Opin. Cardiol. 10:355, 1995.

298. Ohman, E. M., Armstrong, P., Califf, R. M., et al.: Risk stratification in acute ischemic syndromes using serum troponin T. J. Am. Coll. Cardiol. (Special Issue):148A, 1995.

299. Antman, E. M., Tanasijevic, M. J., Cannon, C. P., et al.: Cardiac troponin I on admission predicts death by 42 days in unstable angina and improved survival with an early invasive strategy: Results from TIMI IIIB. Circulation 92(Suppl.): I-663, 1995.

300. Marshall, T., Williams, J., and Williams, K. M.: Electrophoresis of serum enzymes and proteins following acute myocardial infarction. J. Chromatogr. 569:323, 1991.

301. Rabitzsch, G., Mair, J., Lechleitner, P., et al.: Immunoenzymometric assay of human glycogen phosphorylate isoenzyme BB in diagnosis of ischemic myocardial injury. Clin. Chem. 41:966, 1995.

302. Apple, F. S.: Glycogen phosphorylase BB and other cardiac proteins: Challenges to creatine kinase MB as the marker for detecting myocardial injury. Clin. Chem. 41:963, 1995.

303. Vaananen, H. K., Syrjala, H., Rahkila, P., et al.: Serum carbonic anhydrase III and myoglobin concentrations in acute myocardial infarction. Clin. Chem. 36:635, 1990.

304. Vuori, J., Rasi, S., Takala, T., et al.: Dual-label time-resolved fluoroimmunoassay for simultaneous detection of myoglobin and carbonic anhydrase III in serum. Clin. Chem. 37:2087, 1991.

305. Eikvar, L., Pillgram-Larsen, J., Skjaeggestad, Ø., et al.: Serum cardio-specific troponin T after open heart surgery in patients with and without perioperative myocardial infarction. Scand. J. Clin. Lab. Invest. 54:329, 1994.

306. Franz, W. M., Remppis, A., Scheffold, T., et al.: Serum troponin T: A diagnostic marker for acute myocarditis? Circulation 90(Suppl. I):67, 1994.

307. Gore, J. M., Goldberg, R. J., Matsumoto, A. S., et al.: Validity of serum total cholesterol level obtained within 24 hours of acute myocardial infarction. Am. J. Cardiol. 54:722, 1984.

308. Ryder, R., Hayes, T., Mulligan, I., et al.: How soon after myocardial infarction should plasma lipid values be assessed? BMJ 289:1651, 1984.

309. Ronnemaa, T., Viikari, J., Irjala, K., et al.: Marked decrease in serum HDL cholesterol level during acute myocardial infarction. Acta Med. Scand. 207:161, 1980.

310. Expert Panel on Detection, Evaluation and Treatment of High Blood Cholesterol in Adults: Summary of the second report of the National Cholesterol Education Program (NCEP) Expert Panel on Detection, Evaluation, and Treatment of High Blood Cholesterol in Adults (Adult Treatment Panel II). JAMA 269:3015, 1993.

311. Thomson, S. P., Gibbons, R. J., Smars, P. A., et al.: Incremental value of the leukocyte differential and the rapid creatine kinase-MB isoenzyme for the early diagnosis of myocardial infarction. Ann. Intern. Med. 122:335, 1995.

312. Eastham, R. D., and Morgan, E. H.: Plasma-fibrinogen levels in coronary-artery disease. Lancet 2:1196, 1963.

312a. Parker, A. B. III., Waller, B. F., and Gering, L. E.: Usefulness of the 12-lead electrocardiogram in detection of myocardial infarction: Electrocardiographic-anatomic correlations—Part I. Clin. Cardiol. 19:55, 1996.

312b. Sgarbossa, E. B., Pinski, S. L., Barbagelata, A., et al.: Electrocardiographic diagnosis of evolving acute myocardial infarction in the presence of left bundle-branch block. N. Engl. J. Med. 334:481, 1996.

313. Cooksey, J. D., Dunn, M., and Massie, E.: Clinical Vectorcardiography and Electrocardiography. 2nd ed. Chicago, Year Book Medical Publishers, 1977, p. 361.

314. Shen, W. F., Tribouilloy, C., Mirode, A., et al.: Isolated circumflex coronary artery occlusion as a cause of myocardial infarction. Am. J. Noninvas. Cardiol. 7:204, 1993.

315. Ben-Haim, S. A., Gil, A., and Edoute, Y.: Beat-to-beat morphologic variability of the electrocardiogram for the evaluation of chest pain in the emergency room. Am. J. Cardiol. 70:1139, 1992.

316. Kornreich, F., Montague, T. J., and Rautaharju, P. M.: Body surface potential mapping of ST segment changes in acute myocardial infarction. Circulation 87:773, 1993.

317. Lundin, P., Eriksson, S. V., Erhardt, L., et al.: Continuous vectorcar-

diography in patients with chest pain indicative of acute ischemic heart disease. Cardiology 81:145, 1992.

318. Selker, H. P., Griffith, J. L., and Beshansky, J. R.: The Acute Cardiac Ischemia Time-Insensitive Predictive Instrument (ACI-TIPI): A Decision Aid for Emergency Department Triage and a Measure of Appropriateness of Coronary Care Unit Use. In Califf, R. M., Mark, D. B., and Wagner, G. S. (eds.): Acute Coronary Care. St. Louis, Mosby, 1995, p. 201.

319. Coll, S., Betriu, A., De Flores, T., et al.: Significance of Q-wave regression after transmural acute myocardial infarction. Am. J. Cardiol. 61:739, 1988.

320. Taussig, A. S., et al.: Misleading ECGs: Patterns of infarction. J. Cardiovasc. Med. 9:1147, 1983.

321. Phibbs, B.: "Transmural" versus "subendocardial" myocardial infarction: An electrocardiographic myth. J. Am. Coll. Cardiol. 1:561, 1983.

322. Levine, H. D.: Subendocardial infarction in retrospect: Pathologic, cardiographic, and ancillary features. Circulation 72:790, 1985.

323. Dacanay, S., Kennedy, H. L., Uretz, E., et al.: Morphological and quantitative angiographic analyses of progression of coronary stenoses: A comparison of Q-wave and non-Q-wave myocardial infarction. Circulation 90:1739, 1994.

324. Keen, W. D., Savage, M. P., Fischman, D. L., et al.: Comparison of coronary angiographic findings during the first six hours of non-Q-wave and Q-wave myocardial infarction. Am. J. Cardiol. 74:324, 1994.

325. Kudenchuk, P. J., Ho, M. T., Weaver, W. D., et al.: Accuracy of computer-interpreted electrocardiography in selecting patients for thrombolytic therapy: MITI Project Investigators. J. Am. Coll. Cardiol. 17:1486, 1991.

326. Weaver, W. D., Litwin, P. E., Martin, J. S., et al.: Effect of age on use of thrombolytic therapy and mortality in acute myocardial infarction: The MITI Project Group. J. Am. Coll. Cardiol. 81:657, 1991.

327. Spodick, D. H.: Q-wave infarction versus S-T infarction: Non-specificity of electrocardiographic criteria for differentiating transmural and non-transmural lesions. Am. J. Cardiol. 51:913, 1983.

328. Zema, M. J.: Q wave, S-T segment, and T wave myocardial infarction. Am. J. Med. 78:391, 1985.

329. Goldberg, R. J., Gore, J. M., Alpert, J. S., et al.: Non-Q wave myocardial infarction: Recent changes in occurrence and prognosis—a community-wide perspective. Am. Heart J. 113:273, 1987.

330. Schuster, E. H., and Bulkley, B. H.: Early post-infarction angina: Ischemia at a distance and ischemia in the infarct zone. N. Engl. J. Med. 305:1101, 1981.

331. Ferguson, D. W., Pandian, N., Kioschos, J. M., et al.: Angiographic evidence that reciprocal ST-segment depression during acute myocardial infarction does not indicate remote ischemia: Analysis of 23 patients. Am. J. Cardiol. 53:55, 1984.

332. Mukharji, J., Murray, S., Lewis, S. E., et al.: Is anterior ST depression with acute transmural inferior infarction due to posterior infarction? J. Am. Coll. Cardiol. 4:28, 1984.

333. Mirvis, D. M.: Physiologic bases for anterior ST segment depression in patients with acute inferior wall myocardial infarction. Am. Heart J. 116:1308, 1988.

334. Muller, D. W. M., Topol, E. J., Califf, R. M., et al.: Relationship between antecedent angina pectoris and short-term prognosis after thrombolytic therapy for acute myocardial infarction. Am. Heart J. 119:224, 1990.

335. Lopez-Sendon, J., Coma-Canella, I., Alcasena, S., et al.: Electrocardiographic findings in acute right ventricular infarction: Sensitivity and specificity of electrocardiographic alterations in right precordial leads V4R, V3R, V1, V2, and V3. J. Am. Coll. Cardiol. 6:1273, 1985.

336. Kulbertus, H. E.: Right ventricular infarction. In Julian, D., and Braunwald, E. (eds.): Management of Acute Myocardial Infarction. London, W. B. Saunders Ltd., 1994, p. 331.

337. Geft, I. L., Shah, P. K., Rodriguez, L., et al.: ST elevations in leads V1 to V5 may be caused by right coronary artery occlusion and acute right ventricular infarction. Am. J. Cardiol. 53:991, 1984.

338. Lew, A. S., Maddahi, J., Shah, P. K., et al.: Factors that determine the direction and magnitude of precordial ST-segment deviations during inferior wall acute myocardial infarction. Am. J. Cardiol. 55:883, 1985.

339. Robalino, B. D., Whitlow, P. L., Underwood, D. A., et al.: Electrocardiographic manifestations of right ventricular infarction. Am. Heart J. 118:138, 1989.

340. Silvertssen, E., Hoel, B., Bay, G., et al.: Electrocardiographic atrial complex and acute atrial myocardial infarction. Am. J. Cardiol. 31:450, 1973.

341. Brattler, A., Karliner, J. S., Higgins, C. B., et al.: The initial chest x-ray in acute myocardial infarction: Prediction of early and late mortality and survival. Circulation 61:1004, 1980.

342. Katz, A. S., Harrigan, P., and Parisi, A. F.: The value and promise of echocardiography in acute myocardial infarction and coronary artery disease. Clin. Cardiol. 15:401, 1992.

342a. Nishimura, R. A.: Acute myocardial infarction: The role of echocardiography. In Fuster, V., Ross, R., and Topol, E. J. (eds.): Atherosclerosis and Coronary Artery Disease. Philadelphia, Lippincott-Raven, 1996, pp. 855–876.

343. Berning, J., and Steensgard-Hansen, F.: Early estimation of risk by echocardiographic determination of wall motion index in an unselected population with acute myocardial infarction. Am. J. Cardiol. 65:567, 1990.

344. Sabia, P., Abbott, R. D., Afrookteh, A., et al.: Importance of two-dimensional echocardiographic assessment of left ventricular function

in patients presenting to the emergency room with cardiac-related symptoms. Circulation 84:1615, 1991.

345. Hepner, A. M., and Armstrong, W. F.: Echocardiography in acute myocardial infarction. In Francis, G. S., and Alpert, J. S. (eds.): Coronary Care. Boston, Little, Brown and Co., 1995, p. 473.

346. Segar, D. S., Brown, S. E., Sawada, S. G., et al.: Dobutamine stress echocardiography: Correlation with coronary lesion severity as determined by quantitative angiography. J. Am. Coll. Cardiol. 19:1197, 1992.

347. Kuhn, M. B., Egeblad, H., Hojberg, S., et al.: Prognostic value of echocardiography compared to other clinical findings: Multivariate analysis based on long-term survival in 456 patients. Cardiology 86:157, 1995.

348. Salustri, A., Elhendy, A., Garyfallydis, P., et al.: Prediction of improvement of ventricular function after first acute myocardial infarction using low-dose dobutamine stress echocardiography. Am. J. Cardiol. 74:853, 1994.

349. Camarano, G., Ragosta, M., Gimple, L. W., et al.: Identification of viable myocardium with contrast echocardiography in patients with poor left ventricular systolic function caused by recent or remote myocardial infarction. Am. J. Cardiol. 75:215, 1995.

350. Takeuchi, M., Araki, M., Nakashima, Y., et al.: The detection of residual ischemia and stenosis in patients with acute myocardial infarction with dobutamine stress echocardiography. J. Am. Soc. Echocardiogr. 7:242, 1994.

351. Finkelhor, R. S., Sun, J. P., Castellanos, M., et al.: Predicting left heart failure after a myocardial infarction: A preliminary study of the value of echocardiographic measures of left ventricular filling and wall motion. J. Am. Soc. Echocardiogr. 4:215, 1991.

352. Tice, F. D., and Kisslo, J.: Echocardiographic assessment and monitoring of the patient with acute myocardial infarction: Prospects for the thrombolytic era. In Califf, R. M., Mark, D. B., and Wagner, G. S. (eds.): Acute Coronary Care. St. Louis, Mosby-Year Book, 1994, p. 469.

353. Pearson, A. C., Castello, R., and Labovitz, A. J.: Safety and utility of transesophageal echocardiography in the critically ill patient. Am. Heart J. 119:1083, 1990.

354. Harrison, J. K., and Bashore, T. M.: Assessment and management of the critically ill patient with valvular heart disease. In Califf, R. M., Mark, D. B., and Wagner, G. S. (eds.): Acute Coronary Care. St. Louis, Mosby-Year Book, 1995, p. 719.

355. Smyllie, J. H., Sutherland, G. R., Geuskens, R., et al.: Doppler color flow mapping in the diagnosis of ventricular septal rupture and acute mitral regurgitation after myocardial infarction. J. Am. Coll. Cardiol. 15:1449, 1990.

356. Hirose, K., Reed, J. E., and Rumberger, J. A.: Serial changes in regional right ventricular free wall and left ventricular septal wall lengths during the first 4 to 5 years after index anterior wall myocardial infarction. J. Am. Coll. Cardiol. 26:394, 1995.

357. Foster, C. J., Sekiya, T., Love, H. G., et al.: Identification of intracardiac thrombus: Comparison of computed tomography and cross-sectional echocardiography. Br. J. Radiol. 60:327, 1987.

358. Baer, F. M., Theissen, P., Voth, E., et al.: Morphologic correlate of pathologic Q waves as assessed by gradient-echo magnetic resonance imaging. Am. J. Cardiol. 74:430, 1994.

359. Johnston, D. L., Gupta, V. K., Wendt, R. E., et al.: Detection of viable myocardium in segments with fixed defects on thallium-201 scintigraphy: Usefulness of magnetic resonance imaging early after acute myocardial infarction. Magn. Reson. Imaging 11:949, 1993.

360. Holman, E. R., van Jonbergen, H. P., van Dijkman, P. R., et al.: Comparison of magnetic resonance imaging studies with enzymatic indexes of myocardial necrosis for quantification of myocardial infarct size. Am. J. Cardiol. 71:1036, 1993.

360a. Kantor, H. L., and Toussaint, J. F.: Acute myocardial infarction: The role of magnetic resonance. In Fuster, V., Ross, R., and Topol, E. J. (eds.): Atherosclerosis and Coronary Artery Disease. Philadelphia, Lippincott-Raven, 1996, pp. 905–920.

361. Yokota, C., Nonogi, H., Miyazaki, S., et al.: Gadolinium-enhanced magnetic resonance imaging in acute myocardial infarction. Am. J. Cardiol. 75:577, 1995.

362. Committee on Radionuclide Imaging: ACC/AHA Task Force Report: Guidelines for clinical use of cardiac radionuclide imaging. J. Am. Coll. Cardiol. 25:521, 1995.

363. Miller, T. D., Christian, T. F., Hopfenspirger, M. R., et al.: Infarct size after acute myocardial infarction measured by quantitative tomographic ^{99m}Tc sestamibi imaging predicts subsequent mortality. Circulation 92:334, 1995.

363a. Beller, G. A.: Acute myocardial infarction: The role of radionuclide imaging. In Fuster, V., Ross, R., and Topol, E. J. (eds.): Atherosclerosis and Coronary Artery Disease. Philadelphia, Lippincott-Raven, 1996, pp. 877–894.

364. Hasche, E. T., Fernandes, C., Freedman, S. B., et al.: Relation between ischemia time, infarct size, and left ventricular function in humans. Circulation 92:710, 1995.

365. Mauri, F., Gasparini, M., Barbonaglia, L., et al.: Prognostic significance of the extent of myocardial injury in acute myocardial infarction treated by streptokinase (the GISSI trial). Am. J. Cardiol. 63:1291, 1989.

366. Zaret, B. L., and Wackers, F. J.: Nuclear cardiology. N. Engl. J. Med. 329:775, 1993.

367. Antunes, M. L., Tresgallo, M. E., Seldin, D. W., et al.: Effect of infarct size measured from antimyosin single-photon emission computed tomographic scans on left ventricular remodeling. J. Am. Coll. Cardiol. 18:1263, 1991.

368. Johnson, L. L., Seldin, D. W., Keller, A. M., et al.: Dual isotope thallium and indium antimyosin SPECT imaging to identify acute infarct patients at further ischemic risk. Circulation *81*:37, 1990.

369. Lima, J. A. C., Judd, R. M., Bazille, A., et al.: Regional heterogeneity of human myocardial infarcts demonstrated by contrast-enhanced MRI: Potential mechanisms. Circulation *92*:1117, 1995.

MANAGEMENT OF ACUTE MYOCARDIAL INFARCTION

370. Topol, E. J.: Mechanical interventions for acute myocardial infarction. *In* Topol, E. J. (ed.): Textbook of Interventional Cardiology. Philadelphia, W. B. Saunders Company, 1994, p. 292.

371. Zahger, D., and Gotsman, M. S.: Thrombolysis in the era of randomized trials. Curr. Opin. Cardiol. *10*:372, 1995.

372. Holmes, D. R., Califf, R. M., and Topol, E. J.: Lessons we have learned from the GUSTO trial. J. Am. Coll. Cardiol. *25*:10S, 1995.

373. Smith, S. M.: Current management of acute myocardial infarction. Dis. Mon. *41*:363, 1995.

374. van de Werf, F., Califf, R. M., Armstrong, P. W., et al.: Clinical perspective: Progress culminating from ten years of clinical trials on thrombolysis for acute myocardial infarction. Eur. Heart J. *16*:1024, 1995.

PREHOSPITAL CARE

375. National Heart Attack Alert Program Coordinating Committee—60 Minutes to Treatment Working Group: Emergency department: Rapid identification and treatment of patients with acute myocardial infarction. Ann. Emerg. Med. *23*:311, 1994.

376. Gibler, W. B., Kereiakes, D. J., Dean, E. N., et al.: Prehospital diagnosis and treatment of acute myocardial infarction: A north-south perspective: The Cincinnati Heart Project and the Nashville Prehospital TPA Trial. Am. Heart J. *121*:1, 1991.

377. GISSI-Avoidable Delay Study Group: Epidemiology of avoidable delay in the care of patients with acute myocardial infarction in Italy. Arch. Intern. Med. *155*:1481, 1995.

378. National Heart Attack Alert Program: Patient/bystander recognition and action: Rapid identification and treatment of acute myocardial infarction (NIH Publication 93-3303). Bethesda, MD, National Heart, Lung, and Blood Institute, 1994, p. 1.

379. Reilly, A., Dracup, K., and Dattolo, J.: Factors influencing prehospital delay in patients experiencing chest pain. Am. J. Crit. Care. *3*:300, 1994.

380. Lombardi, G., Gallagher, J., and Gennis, P.: Outcome of out-of-hospital cardiac arrest in New York City: The Pre-Hospital Arrest Survival Evaluation (PHASE) Study. JAMA *271*:678, 1994.

381. National Heart Attack Alert Program: 9-1-1: Rapid identification and treatment of acute myocardial infarction (NIH Publication 94-3302). Bethesda, MD, National Heart, Lung, and Blood Institute, 1994, p. 1.

382. Weaver, W. D., Cerqueira, M., Hallstrom, A. P., et al.: Prehospital-initiated vs. hospital-initiated thrombolytic therapy: The Myocardial Infarction Triage and Intervention Trial. JAMA *270*:1211, 1993.

383. Castaigne, A., Herve, C., Duval-Moulin, A., et al.: Prehospital use of APSAC: Results of a placebo-controlled study. Am. J. Cardiol. *64*:30A, 1989.

384. Schofer, J., Buttner, J., Geng, G., et al.: Prehospital thrombolysis in acute myocardial infarction. Am. J. Cardiol. *66*:1429, 1990.

385. GREAT Group: Feasibility, safety, and efficacy of domicillary thrombolysis by general practitioners: Grampian region early anistreplase trial. BMJ *305*:548, 1992.

386. The European Myocardial Infarction Project Group: Prehospital thrombolytic therapy in patients with suspected acute myocardial infarction. N. Engl. J. Med. *329*:383, 1993.

387. Califf, R. M.: Acute myocardial infarction. *In* Smith, T. W. (ed.): Cardiovascular Therapeutics. Philadelphia, W. B. Saunders Company, 1996.

388. National Heart Attack Alert Program: Emergency medical dispatching: Rapid identification and treatment of acute myocardial infarction (NIH Publication 94-3287). Bethesda, MD, National Heart, Lung, and Blood Institute, 1994, p. 1.

389. National Heart Attack Alert Program: Staffing and equipping emergency medical services systems: Rapid identification and treatment of acute myocardial infarction (NIH Publication 93-3304). Bethesda, MD, National Heart, Lung, and Blood Institute, 1994, p. 1.

390. Vincent, R.: Pre-hospital management. *In* Julian, D., and Braunwald, E. (eds.): Management of Acute Myocardial Infarction. London, W. B. Saunders Ltd., 1994, p. 3.

MANAGEMENT IN THE EMERGENCY DEPARTMENT

391. National Heart Attack Alert Program: Emergency Department: Rapid identification and treatment of patients with acute myocardial infarction (NIH Publication 93-3278). Bethesda, MD, National Heart, Lung, and Blood Institute, 1993.

392. Kaul, S., and Abbott, R. D.: Evaluation of chest pain in the Emergency Department. Ann. Intern. Med. *121*:976, 1994.

393. Karlson, B. W., Herlitz, J., Wiklund, O., et al.: Early prediction of acute myocardial infarction from clinical history, examination, and electrocardiogram in the emergency room. Am. J. Cardiol. *68*:171, 1991.

394. Karlsson, J. E., Berglund, U., Bjorkholm, A., et al.: Thrombolysis with recombinant human tissue-type plasminogen activator during instability in coronary artery disease: Effect on myocardial ischemia and need for coronary revascularization: TRIC Study Group. Am. Heart J. *124*:1419, 1992.

395. The TIMI IIIB Investigators: Effects of tissue plasminogen activator

396. Granger, C. B.: Early management of acute coronary syndromes: Need for better understanding and treatment strategies. Clinician *13*:44, 1995.

397. Cragg, D., Friedman, H., Bonema, J., et al.: Outcome of patients with acute myocardial infarction who are ineligible for thrombolytic therapy. Ann. Intern. Med. *115*:173, 1991.

398. Granger, C., Christopher, D., Stebbins, A., et al.: Thrombolytic therapy treats the tip of the MI iceberg: Results from the GUSTO MI registry. Circulation *90*(Suppl. I):663, 1994.

399. Goldman, L., Cook, E., Brand, D., et al.: A computer protocol to predict myocardial infarction in emergency department patients with chest pain. N. Engl. J. Med. *318*:797, 1988.

399a. Baxt, W. G., and Skora, J.: Prospective validation of artificial neural network trained to identify acute myocardial infarction. Lancet *347*:12, 1996.

400. Fuchs, R., and Scheidt, S.: Improved criteria for admission to cardiac care units. JAMA *246*:2037, 1985.

401. Peels, C. H., Visser, C. A., Funke Kupper, A. J., et al.: Usefulness of two-dimensional echocardiography for immediate detection of myocardial ischemia in the emergency room. Am. J. Cardiol. *65*:687, 1990.

402. Armstrong, W.: Echocardiography in acute myocardial infarction. *In* Francis, G., and Alpert, J. (eds.): Modern Coronary Care. Boston, Little, Brown and Co., 1990, p. 455.

403. Wackers, F., Kie, K., Liem, K., et al.: Potential value of thallium-201 scintigraphy as a means of selecting patients for the coronary care unit. Br. Heart J. *41*:111, 1979.

404. Nelson, M.: Critical pathways in the emergency department. J. Emerg. Nurs. *19*:110, 1993.

405. Lyle, K.: Enhancing early cardiac care: Critical pathways and practice guidelines in the ED and CPED. Clinician *13*:60, 1995.

406. Gaspoz, J. M., Lee, T. H., Weinstein, M. C., et al.: Cost-effectiveness of a new short-stay unit to "rule out" acute myocardial infarction in low risk patients. J. Am. Coll. Cardiol. *24*:1249, 1994.

407. Barish, R. A., and Doherty, R. J.: Establishing a chest pain center in an academic medical center: The University of Maryland experience. Clinician *13*:39, 1995.

408. Stein, B., and Fuster, V.: Clinical pharmacology of platelet inhibitors. *In* Fuster, V., and Verstraete, M. (eds.): Thrombosis in Cardiovascular Disorders. Philadelphia, W. B. Saunders Company, 1992, p. 99.

409. Meyer, B. J., and Chesebro, J. H.: Aspirin and anticoagulants. *In* Julian, D., and Braunwald, E. (eds.): Management of Acute Myocardial Infarction. London, W. B. Saunders Ltd., 1994, p. 163.

410. Reilly, I. A. G., and Fitzgerald, G. A.: Inhibition of thromboxane formation *in vivo* and *ex vivo*: Implications for therapy with platelet inhibitory drugs. Blood *69*:180, 1987.

411. Fuster, V., Dyken, M. L., Voonas, P. S., et al.: Aspirin as a therapeutic agent in cardiovascular disease: Special Writing Group. Circulation *87*:659, 1993.

412. Herlitz, J.: Analgesia in myocardial infarction. Drugs *37*:939, 1989.

413. Kock, M., Blomberg, S., Emanuelsson, H., et al.: Thoracic epidural anesthesia improves global and regional left ventricular function during stress-induced myocardial ischemia in patients with coronary artery disease. Anesth. Analg. *71*:625, 1990.

414. Chamberlain, D.: β-Blockers and calcium antagonists. *In* Julian, D., and Braunwald, E. (eds.): Management of Acute Myocardial Infarction. London, W. B. Saunders Ltd., 1994, p. 193.

415. Hjalmarson, A., Elmfeldt, D., Herlitz, J., et al.: Effect on mortality of metoprolol in acute myocardial infarction, a double-blind randomized trial. Lancet *2*:823, 1981.

416. Kirshenbaum, J. M., Kloner, R. F., McGowan, N., et al.: Use of an ultrashort-acting beta receptor blocker (esmolol) in patients with acute myocardial ischemia and relative contraindications to beta-blockade therapy. J. Am. Coll. Cardiol. *12*:773, 1988.

417. Yusuf, S., Held, P., and Furberg, C.: Update of effects of calcium antagonists in myocardial infarction or angina in light of the second Danish Verapamil Infarction Trial (DAVIT-II) and other recent studies. Am. J. Cardiol. *67*:1295, 1991.

418. Furberg, C. D., Psaty, B. M., and Meyer, J. V.: Nifedipine: Dose-related increase in mortality in patients with coronary heart disease. Circulation *92*:1236, 1995.

419. Maroko, P., Radvany, P., Braunwald, E., et al.: Reduction of infarct size by oxygen inhalation following acute coronary occlusion. Circulation *52*:360, 1975.

420. Madias, J. E., and Hood, W. B., Jr.: Reduction of precordial ST-segment elevation in patients with anterior myocardial infarction by oxygen breathing. Circulation *53*:198, 1976.

421. Gersh, B. J., and Anderson, J. L.: Thrombolysis and myocardial salvage: Results of clinical trials and the animal paradigm—paradoxic or predictable? Circulation *88*:296, 1993.

422. Califf, R. M., and Bengtson, J. R.: Cardiogenic shock. N. Engl. J. Med. *330*:1724, 1994.

423. O'Gara, P. T.: Primary pump failure. *In* Fuster, V., Ross, R., and Topol, E. (eds.): Atherosclerosis and Coronary Artery Disease. New York, Raven Press, 1995, p. 1051.

424. Gaudron, P., Eilles, C., Kugler, I., et al.: Progressive left ventricular dysfunction and remodeling after myocardial infarction. Circulation *87*:755, 1993.

425. Pfeffer, M.: ACE inhibition in acute myocardial infarction. N. Engl. J. Med. *332*:118, 1995.

426. Maroko, P. R., and Braunwald, E.: Modification of myocardial infarct size after coronary occlusion. Ann. Intern. Med. *79*:720, 1973.

427. Martin, G. V., and Kennedy, J. W.: Choice of thrombolytic agent. *In* Julian, D., and Braunwald, E. (eds.): Management of Acute Myocardial Infarction. London, W. B. Saunders Ltd., 1994, p. 71.

428. Iliceto, S., Scrutinio, D., Bruzzi, P., et al.: Effects of L-carnitine administration on left ventricular remodeling after acute anterior myocardial infarction: The L-Carnitine Ecocardiografia Digitalizzata Infarto Miocardico (CEDIM) Trial. J. Am. Coll. Cardiol. *26*:380, 1995.

429. Hahn, R., Wond, S. C., Brown, E., et al.: Early benefits of late coronary reperfusion on reducing myocardial infarct expansion: Echo findings and ultrastructural basis. J. Am. Coll. Cardiol. *21*:301A, 1993.

430. Rude, R. E., Muller, J. E., and Braunwald, E.: Efforts to limit the size of myocardial infarcts. Ann. Intern. Med. *95*:736, 1981.

431. Kubler, W., and Doorey, A.: Reduction of infarct size: An attractive concept: Useful or possible in human? Br. Heart J. *53*:5, 1985.

432. Christian, T. F., Schwartz, R. S., and Gibbons, R. J.: Determinants of infarct size in reperfusion therapy for acute myocardial infarction. Circulation *86*:81, 1992.

433. Taegtmeyer, H.: Energy metabolism of the heart: From basic concepts to clinical applications. Curr. Probl. Cardiol. *19*:57, 1994.

434. Kusuoka, H., and Marban, E.: Role of altered calcium homeostasis in stunned myocardium. *In* Kloner, R. A., and Przyklenk, K. (eds.): Stunned Myocardium. New York, Marcel Dekker, 1993, p. 197.

435. Bolli, R.: Oxygen-derived free radicals and postischemic myocardial dysfunction ("stunned myocardium"). J. Am. Coll. Cardiol. *12*:239, 1988.

436. Bolli, R.: Myocardial "stunning" in man. Circulation *86*:1671, 1992.

437. Weglicki, W. B., Phillips, T. M., Mak, I. T., et al.: Cytokines, neuropeptides, and reperfusion injury during magnesium deficiency. Ann. N. Y. Acad. Sci. *723*:246, 1994.

438. Airaghi, L., Lettino, M., Manfredi, M. G., et al.: Endogenous cytokine antagonists during myocardial ischemia and thrombolytic therapy. Am. Heart J. *130*:204, 1995.

439. Przyklenk, K., and Kloner, R. A.: Oxygen radical scavenging agents as adjuvant therapy with tissue plasminogen activator in a canine model of coronary thrombolysis. Cardiovasc. Res. *27*:925, 1993.

440. Kloner, R. A., and Yellon, D.: Does ischemic preconditioning occur in patients? J. Am. Coll. Cardiol. *24*:1133, 1994.

441. Przyklenk, K., Bauer, B., Ovize, M., et al.: Regional ischemic "preconditioning" protects remote virgin myocardium from subsequent sustained coronary occlusion. Circulation *87*:893, 1993.

442. Kloner, R. A., Shook, T., Przyklenk, K., et al.: Previous angina alters in-hospital outcome in TIMI 4: A clinical correlate to preconditioning? Circulation *91*:37, 1995.

443. Kloner, R. A., Muller, J., and Davis, V.: Effects of previous angina pectoris in patients with first acute myocardial infarction not receiving thrombolytics: MILIS Study Group: Multicenter Investigation of the Limitation of Infarct Size. Am. J. Cardiol. *75*:615, 1995.

444. Anzai, T., Yoshikawa, T., Asakura, Y., et al.: Preinfarction angina as a major predictor of left ventricular function and long-term prognosis after a first Q wave myocardial infarction. J. Am. Coll. Cardiol. *26*:319, 1995.

REPERFUSION OF MYOCARDIAL INFARCTION

445. Morgan, C. D., Roberts, R. S., Haq, A., et al.: Coronary patency, infarct size and left ventricular function after thrombolytic therapy for acute myocardial infarction: Results from the tissue plasminogen activator: Toronto (TPAT) placebo-controlled trial: TPAT Study Group. J. Am. Coll. Cardiol. *17*:1451, 1991.

446. Cerqueira, M. D., Maynard, C., and Ritchie, J. L.: Radionuclide assessment of infarct size and left ventricular function in clinical trials of thrombolysis. Circulation *84*:100, 1991.

447. Bassand, J. P., Machecourt, J., Cassagnes, J., et al.: Multicenter trial of intravenous anisoylated plasminogen streptokinase activator complex (APSAC) in acute myocardial infarction: Effects on infarct size and left ventricular function. J. Am. Coll. Cardiol. *13*:988, 1989.

448. Ritchie, J. L., Cerqueira, M., Maynard, C., et al.: Ventricular function and infarct size: The Western Washington Intravenous Streptokinase in Myocardial Infarction Trial. J. Am. Coll. Cardiol. *11*:689, 1988.

449. Althouse, R., Maynard, C., Cerqueira, M. D., et al.: The Western Washington Myocardial Infarction Registry and Emergency Department Tissue Plasminogen Activator Treatment Trial. Am. J. Cardiol. *66*:1289, 1990.

449a. Andreotti, F., Pasceri, V., Hackett, D. R., et al.: Preinfarction angina as a predictor of more rapid coronary thrombolysis in patients with acute myocardial infarction. N. Engl. J. Med. *334*:7, 1995.

450. van der Laarse, A., van Leeuwen, F. T., Krul, R., et al.: The size of infarction as judged enzymatically in 1974 patients with acute myocardial infarction: Relation with symptomatology, infarct localization and type of infarction. Int. J. Cardiol. *19*:191, 1988.

451. Topol, E. J., and Ellis, S. G.: Coronary collaterals revisited: Accessory pathway to myocardial preservation during infarction. Circulation *83*:1084, 1991.

452. Virmani, R., et al.: Reperfusion injury in the ischemic myocardium. Cardiovasc. Pathol. *1*:117, 1992.

453. Kloner, R. A., and Przylenk, K.: Understanding the jargon: A glossary of terms used (and misused) in the study of ischaemia and reperfusion. Cardiovasc. Res. *27*:162, 1993.

454. Kloner, R. A.: Does reperfusion injury exist in humans? J. Am. Coll. Cardiol. *21*:537, 1993.

455. Ito, H., Tomooka, T., Sakai, N., et al.: Lack of myocardial perfusion immediately after successful thrombolysis: A predictor of poor recovery of left ventricular function in anterior myocardial infarction. Circulation *85*:1699, 1992.

456. Gottlieb, R. A., Burleson, K. O., Kloner, R. A., et al.: Reperfusion injury induces apoptosis in rabbit cardiomyocytes. J. Clin. Invest. *94*:1621, 1994.

457. Herzog, W. R., Schlossberg, M. L., MacMurdy, K. S., et al.: Timing of magnesium therapy affects experimental infarct size. Circulation *92*:2622, 1995.

458. Christensen, C. W., Rieder, M. A., Silverstein, E. L., et al.: Magnesium sulfate reduces myocardial infarct size when administered prior to but not after coronary reperfusion in a canine model. Circulation *92*:2617, 1995.

459. Antman, E. M.: Magnesium in acute MI: Timing is critical. Circulation *92*:2367, 1995.

460. Kloner, R. A., Ganote, C. E., and Jennings, R. B.: The "no-reflow" phenomenon after temporary coronary occlusion in the dog. J. Clin. Invest. *54*:1496, 1974.

461. Entman, M. L., Michael, L., Rossen, R. D., et al.: Inflammation in the course of early myocardial ischemia. FASEB J. *5*:2529, 1991.

462. Waller, B. F., Rothbaum, D. A., Pinkerton, C. A., et al.: Status of the myocardium and infarct-related coronary artery in 19 necropsy patients with acute recanalization using pharmacologic (streptokinase, r-tissue plasminogen activator), mechanical (percutaneous transluminal coronary angioplasty) or combined types of reperfusion therapy. J. Am. Coll. Cardiol. *9*:785, 1987.

463. Ohnishi, Y., Butterfield, M. C., Saffitz, J. E., et al.: Deleterious effects of a systemic lytic state on reperfused myocardium: Minimization of reperfusion injury and enhanced recovery of myocardial function by direct angioplasty. Circulation *92*:500, 1995.

464. Gertz, S. D., Kragel, A. H., Kalan, J. M., et al.: Comparison of coronary and myocardial morphologic findings in patients with and without thrombolytic therapy during fatal first acute myocardial infarction. Am. J. Cardiol. *66*:904, 1990.

465. Ferrari, R., Albertini, A., Curello, S., et al.: Myocardial recovery during post-ischaemic reperfusion: Effects of nifedipine, calcium, and magnesium. J. Mol. Cell. Cardiol. *18*:487, 1986.

466. Steenbergen, C., Murphy, E., Levy, L., et al.: Elevation in cytosolic free calcium concentration early in myocardial ischemia in perfused rat heart. Circ. Res. *60*:700, 1987.

467. Werns, S. W., Shea, M. J., Driscoll, E. M., et al.: The independent effects of oxygen radical scavengers on canine infarct size reduction by superoxide dismutase but not catalase. Circ. Res. *56*:895, 1985.

468. Flaherty, J. T., Pitt, B., Gruber, J. W., et al.: Recombinant human superoxide dismutase (h-SOD) fails to improve recovery of ventricular function in patients undergoing coronary angioplasty for acute myocardial infarction. Circulation *89*:1982, 1991.

469. Neumann, F.-J., Ott, I., Gawaz, M., et al.: Cardiac release of cytokines and inflammatory responses in acute myocardial infarction. Circulation *92*:748, 1995.

470. du Toit, E. F., and Opie, L. H.: Modulation of severity of reperfusion stunning in the isolated rat heart by agents altering calcium flux at reperfusion. Circ. Res. *70*:960, 1992.

471. Silver, M. J., Sutton, J. M., Hook, S., et al.: Adjunctive selectin blockade successfully reduces infarct size beyond thrombolysis in the electrolytic canine coronary artery model. Circulation *92*:492, 1995.

472. Smalling, R. W., Feld, S., Ramanna, N., et al.: Infarct salvage with liposomal prostaglandin E$_1$ administered by intravenous bolus immediately before reperfusion in a canine infarction-reperfusion model. Circulation *92*:935, 1995.

473. Klein, H. H., Pich, S., Bohle, R. M., et al.: Myocardial protection by Na$^+$-H$^+$ exchange inhibition in ischemic, reperfused porcine hearts. Circulation *92*:912, 1995.

474. TIMI Study Group: Comparison of invasive and conservative strategies after treatment with intravenous tissue plasminogen activator in acute myocardial infarction: Results of the Thrombolysis in Myocardial Infarction (TIMI) Phase II Trial. N. Engl. J. Med. *302*:618, 1989.

475. Roberts, R., Rogers, W. J., Mueller, H. S., et al.: Immediate versus deferred beta-blockade following thrombolytic therapy in patients with acute myocardial infarction: Results of the Thrombolysis in Myocardial Infarction (TIMI) II-B Study. Circulation *83*:422, 1991.

476. Murry, C. E., Jennings, R. B., and Reimer, K. A.: What is ischemic preconditioning? *In* Przylenk, K., Kloner, R. A., and Yellon, D. M. (eds.): Ischemic Preconditioning: The Concept of Endogenous Cardioprotection. Norwell, MA, Kluwer Academic, 1994, p. 3.

477. Gross, G. J., and Auchampach, J. A.: Blockade of ATP-sensitive potassium channels prevents myocardial preconditioning in dogs. Circ. Res. *70*:222, 1992.

478. Mizumura, T., Nithipatikom, K., and Gross, G. J.: Bimakalim, an ATP-sensitive potassium channel opener, mimics the effects of ischemic preconditioning to reduce infarct size, adenosine release, and neutrophil function in dogs. Circulation *92*:1236, 1995.

479. Hearse, D. J.: Activation of ATP-sensitive potassium channels: A novel pharmacological approach to myocardial protection? Cardiovasc. Res. *30*:1, 1995.

480. Wolfe, C. L., Stevens, R. E., Vissern, F. L. J., et al.: Loss of myocardial protection after preconditioning correlates with the time course of

glycogen recovery within the preconditioned segment. Circulation *87*:881, 1993.

480a. Barbosa, V., Sievers, R. E., Zaugg, C. E., and Wolfe, C. L.: Preconditioning ischemia time determines the degree of glycogen depletion and infarct size reduction in rat hearts. Am. Heart J. *131*:224, 1996.

480b. Sandhu, R., Thomas, U., Diaz, R. J., and Wilson, G. J.: Effect of ischemic preconditioning of the myocardium on cAMP. Circ Res. *78*:137, 1996.

481. Marber, M. S., Latchman, D. S., Walker, M., et al.: Cardiac stress protein elevation 24 hours after brief ischemia or heat stress is associated with resistance to myocardial infarction. Circulation *88*:1264, 1993.

482. Chen, W., Gabel, S., Steenbergen, C., et al.: A redox-based mechanism for cardioprotection induced by ischemic preconditioning in perfused rat heart. Circ. Res. *77*:424, 1995.

483. Wei, J. Y., Markis, J. E., Malagold, M., et al.: Cardiovascular reflexes stimulated by reperfusion of ischemic myocardium in acute myocardial infarction. Circulation *67*:796, 1983.

484. Vera, Z., Pride, H. P., and Zipes, D. P.: Reperfusion arrhythmias: Role of early afterdepolarizations studied by monophasic action potential recordings in the intact canine heart during autonomically denervated and stimulated sites. J. Cardiovasc. Electrophysiol. *6*:532, 1995.

485. Goldberg, S., Greenspon, A. J., Urban, P. L., et al.: Reperfusion of arrhythmia: A marker of restoration of antegrade flow during intracoronary thrombolysis for acute myocardial infarction. Am. Heart J. *105*:26, 1983.

486. Califf, R. M., O'Neill, W., Stack, R. S., et al.: Failure of simple clinical characteristics to predict perfusion status after intravenous thrombolysis. Ann. Intern. Med. *108*:658, 1988.

487. Solomon, S. D., Ridker, P. M., and Antman, E. M.: Ventricular arrhythmias in trials of thrombolytic therapy for acute myocardial infarction: A meta-analysis. Circulation *88*:2575, 1993.

488. Kim, C., and Braunwald, E.: Potential benefits of late reperfusion of infarcted myocardium: The open artery hypothesis. Circulation *88*:2426, 1993.

489. Hochman, J. S., and Choo, H.: Limitation of myocardial infarct expansion by reperfusion independent of myocardial salvage. Circulation *75*:299, 1987.

489a. Alhaddad, A. I., Kloner, R. A., Hakim, I., et al.: Benefits of late coronary artery reperfusion on infarct expansion progressively diminish over time: Relation to viable islets of myocytes within the scar. Am. Heart J. *131*:451, 1996.

490. Braunwald, E.: Coronary artery patency in patients with myocardial infarction. J. Am. Coll. Cardiol. *16*:1550, 1990.

491. Schroder, R., Neuhaus, K. L., Linderer, T., et al.: Impact of late coronary artery reperfusion on left ventricular function one month after acute myocardial infarction (results from the ISAM study). Am. J. Cardiol. *64*:878, 1989.

492. Lavie, C. J., O'Keefe, J. H., Chesebro, J. H., et al.: Prevention of late ventricular dilatation after acute myocardial infarction by successful thrombolytic reperfusion. Am. J. Cardiol. *66*:31, 1990.

493. Topol, E. J., Califf, R. M., Vandormael, M., et al.: A randomized trial of late reperfusion therapy for acute myocardial infarction: Thrombolysis and Angioplasty in Myocardial Infarction-6 Study Group. Circulation *85*:2090, 1992.

494. Golia, G., Marino, P., Rametta, F., et al.: Reperfusion reduces left ventricular dilatation without infarct size limitation by late reperfusion in the acute and chronic phases after myocardial infarction. Am. Heart J. *127*:499, 1994.

495. Nidorf, S. M., Siu, S. C., Galambos, G., et al.: Benefit of late coronary reperfusion on ventricular morphology and function after myocardial infarction. J. Am. Coll. Cardiol. *21*:683, 1993.

496. Zaman, A. G., Morris, J. L., Smylie, J. H., et al.: Late potentials and ventricular enlargement after myocardial infarction. Circulation *88*:905, 1993.

497. Hii, J. T. Y., Traboulsi, M., Mitchell, L. B., et al.: Infarct artery patency predicts outcome of serial electropharmacological studies in patients with malignant ventricular arrhythmias. Circulation *87*:764, 1993.

498. Steinberg, J. S., Hochman, J. S., Morgan, C. D., et al.: The effects of thrombolytic therapy administered 6–24 hours after myocardial infarction on the signal-averaged ECG: Results of a multicenter randomized trial. J. Am. Coll. Cardiol. *21*:225A, 1993.

499. Lamas, G. V., Flaker, G. C., Mitchell, G., et al.: Effects of infarct artery patency on prognosis after acute myocardial infarction. Circulation *92*:1101, 1995.

500. White, H. D., Cross, D. B., Elliott, J. M., et al.: Long-term prognostic importance of patency of the infarct-related coronary artery after thrombolytic therapy for acute myocardial infarction. Circulation *89*:61, 1994.

501. Pirzada, F. A., Weiner, J. M., and Hood, W. B. J.: Experimental myocardial infarction: Accelerated myocardial stiffening related to coronary reperfusion following ischemia. Chest *74*:190, 1978.

502. Richard, V., Murry, C. E., and Reimer, K. A.: Healing of myocardial infarcts in dogs: Effects of late reperfusion. Circulation *92*:1891, 1995.

503. Montalescot, G., Faraggi, M., Drobinski, G., et al.: Myocardial viability in patients with Q wave myocardial infarction and no residual ischemia. Circulation *86*:47, 1992.

504. Boehrer, J. D., Glamann, D. B., Lange, R. A., et al.: Effect of coronary angioplasty on late potentials one to two weeks after acute myocardial infarction. Am. J. Cardiol. *70*:1515, 1992.

505. Gang, E. S., Lew, A. S., Hong, M., et al.: Decreased incidence of ven-

tricular late potentials after successful thrombolytic therapy for acute myocardial infarction. N. Engl. J. Med. *321*:712, 1989.

506. Horvitz, L. L., Pietrolungo, J. F., Suri, R. S., et al.: An open infarct-related artery is associated with a lower risk of lethal arrhythmias in patients with a left ventricular aneurysm. Circulation *86*:I, 1992.

CORONARY THROMBOLYSIS

507. Fletcher, A. P., Alkjaersig, N., Smyrniotis, F. E., et al.: The treatment of patients suffering from early myocardial infarction with massive and prolonged streptokinase therapy. Trans. Assoc. Am. Physicians *71*:287, 1958.

508. Gruppo Italiano Per Lo Studio Della Streptochinasi Nell'Infarct Miocardico (GISSI): Effectiveness of intravenous thrombolytic treatment in acute myocardial infarction. Lancet *1*:397, 1986.

509. van de Werf, F., Ludbrook, P. A., Bergmann, S. R., et al.: Coronary thrombolysis with tissue-type plasminogen activator in patients with evolving myocardial infarction. N. Engl. J. Med. *310*:609, 1984.

510. Kennedy, J., Ritchie, J., Davis, K., et al.: The Western Washington randomized trial of intracoronary streptokinase in acute myocardial infarction: A 12-month follow-up report. N. Engl. J. Med. *312*:1073, 1985.

511. Tiefenbrunn, A. J., and Sobel, B. E.: Thrombolysis and myocardial infarction. Fibrinolysis *5*:1, 1991.

512. Tiefenbrunn, A. J.: Clinical benefits of thrombolytic therapy in acute myocardial infarction. Am. J. Cardiol. *69*:3, 1992.

512a. Lincoff, A. M., and Topol, E. J.: Acute myocardial infarction: Acute management: thrombolytic therapy. *In* Fuster, V., Ross, R., and Topol, E. J. (eds.): Atherosclerosis and Coronary Artery Disease. Philadelphia, Lippincott-Raven, 1996, pp. 955–978.

513. Granger, C. B., Califf, R. M., and Topol, E. J.: Thrombolytic therapy for acute myocardial infarction: A review. Drugs *44*:293, 1992.

514. Topol, E.: Thrombolytic intervention. *In* Topol, E. (ed.): Textbook of Interventional Cardiology. 2nd ed. Philadelphia, W. B. Saunders Company, 1994, p. 68.

515. TIMI Study Group: The Thrombolysis in Myocardial Infarction (TIMI) Trial: Phase I findings. N. Engl. J. Med. *312*:932, 1985.

516. Chesebro, J. H., Knatterud, G., Roberts, R., et al.: Thrombolysis in Myocardial Infarction (TIMI) Trial, Phase 1: A comparison between intravenous tissue plasminogen activator and intravenous streptokinase. Circulation *76*:142, 1987.

517. Gold, H. K., Leinbach, R. C., Garabedian, H. D., et al.: Acute coronary reocclusion after thrombolysis with recombinant human tissue-type plasminogen activator: Prevention by a maintenance infusion. Circulation *73*:347, 1986.

518. Langer, A., Krucoff, M. W., Klootwijk, P., et al.: Noninvasive assessment of speed and stability of infarct-related artery reperfusion: Results of the GUSTO ST segment monitoring study: Global Utilization of Streptokinase and Tissue Plasminogen Activator for Occluded Coronary Arteries. J. Am. Coll. Cardiol. *25*:1552, 1995.

519. The GUSTO Angiographic Investigators: The comparative effects of tissue plasminogen activator, streptokinase, or both on coronary artery patency, ventricular function and survival after acute myocardial infarction. N. Engl. J. Med. *329*:1615, 1993.

520. Lenderink, T., Simoons, M. L., Van Es, G.-A., et al.: Benefits of thrombolytic therapy is sustained throughout five years and is related to TIMI perfusion grade 3 but not grade 2 flow at discharge. Circulation *92*:1110, 1995.

521. Karagounis, L., Sorensen, S. G., Menlove, R. L., et al.: Does Thrombolysis in Myocardial Infarction (TIMI) perfusion grade 2 represent a mostly patent artery or a mostly occluded artery? Enzymatic and electrocardiographic evidence from the TEAM-2 study. J. Am. Coll. Cardiol. *19*:1, 1992.

522. Clemmensen, P., Ohman, E. M., Sevilla, D. C., et al.: Impact of infarct artery patency on the relationship between electrocardiographic and ventriculographic evidence of acute myocardial ischaemia. Eur. Heart J. *15*:1356, 1994.

523. Vogt, A., von Essen, R., Tebbe, U., et al.: Impact of early perfusion status of the infarct-related artery on short-term mortality after thrombolysis for acute myocardial infarction: Retrospective analysis of four German multicenter studies. J. Am. Coll. Cardiol. *21*:1391, 1993.

524. Gibson, C. M., Cannon, C. P., Baim, D. S., et al.: TIMI frame count: A new standardization of infarct-related artery flow grade, and its relationship to clinical outcomes in the TIMI-4 trial. Circulation *90*(Suppl I):220, 1994.

525. Lincoff, A. M., and Topol, E. J.: Illusion of reperfusion: Does anyone achieve optimal reperfusion during acute myocardial infarction? Circulation *87*:1792, 1993.

526. Abendschein, D. R., Meng, Y. Y., Torr-Brown, S., et al.: Maintenance of coronary patency after fibrinolysis with tissue factor pathway inhibitor. Circulation *92*:944, 1995.

527. Yao, S.-K., Akhtar, S., Scott-Burden, T., et al.: Endogenous and exogenous nitric oxide protect against intracoronary thrombosis and reocclusion after thrombolysis. Circulation *92*:1005, 1995.

528. Weaver, W. D.: Time to thrombolytic treatment: Factors affecting delay and their influence on outcome. J. Am. Coll. Cardiol. *25*:3S, 1995.

529. ISIS-2 (Second International Study of Infarct Survival) Collaborative Group: Randomised trial of intravenous streptokinase, oral aspirin, both, or neither among 17,187 cases of suspected acute myocardial infarction: ISIS-2. Lancet *2*:349, 1988.

530. ISAM (Intravenous Streptokinase in Acute Myocardial Infarction)

Study Group: A prospective trial of intravenous streptokinase in acute myocardial infarction (ISAM). N. Engl. J. Med. *314*:1465, 1986.

531. AIMS Trial Study Group: Effect of intravenous APSAC on mortality after acute myocardial infarction: Preliminary report of a placebo-controlled clinical trial. Lancet *1*:545, 1988.

532. Wilcox, R. G., von der Lippe, G., Olsson, C. G., et al.: Trial of tissue plasminogen activator for mortality reduction in acute myocardial infarction: Anglo-Scandinavian Study of Early Thrombolysis (ASSET). Lancet *1*:525, 1988.

533. LATE (Late Assessment of Thrombolytic Efficacy) Study Group: Late Assessment of Thrombolytic Efficacy (LATE) study with alteplase 6–24 hours after onset of acute myocardial infarction. Lancet *342*:759, 1993.

534. EMERAS (Estudio Multicentrico Estreptoquinasa Republicas de America del Sur) Collaborative Group: Randomized trial of late thrombolysis in acute myocardial infarction. Lancet *342*:767, 1993.

535. ISIS-3 (Third International Study of Infarct Survival) Collaborative Group: ISIS-3: A randomized trial of streptokinase vs tissue plasminogen activator vs anistreplase and of aspirin plus heparin vs aspirin alone among 41,299 cases of suspected acute myocardial infarction. Lancet *339*:753, 1992.

536. Krumholz, H. M., Pasternak, R. C., Weinstein, M. C., et al.: Efficacy and cost-effectiveness of thrombolytic therapy in elderly patients with suspected acute myocardial infarction. N. Engl. J. Med. *327*:7, 1992.

537. Topol, E. J., and Califf, R. M.: Thrombolytic therapy for elderly patients. N. Engl. J. Med. *327*:45, 1992.

538. Hillis, L. D., Forman, S., Braunwald, E., et al.: Risk stratification before thrombolytic therapy in patients with acute myocardial infarction. J. Am. Coll. Cardiol. *16*:313, 1990.

539. Zehender, M., Kasper, W., Kauder, E., et al.: Right ventricular infarction as an independent predictor of prognosis after acute inferior myocardial infarction. N. Engl. J. Med. *328*:981, 1993.

540. Peterson, E. G., Hathaway, W. R., Zabel, K. M., et al.: The prognostic importance of anterior ST-segment depression in inferior myocardial infarctions: Results in 16,185 patients. J. Am. Coll. Cardiol. *25*:342A, 1995.

541. Berger, P. B., and Ryan, T. J.: Inferior myocardial infarction: High-risk subgroups. Circulation *81*:401, 1990.

542. Lee, K. L., Woodlief, L. H., Topol, E. J., et al.: Predictors of 30-day mortality in the era of reperfusion for acute myocardial infarction: Results from an international trial of 41,021 patients. Circulation *91*:1659, 1995.

543. Serruys, P. W., Simoons, M. L., Suryapranata, H., et al.: Preservation of global and regional left ventricular function after early thrombolysis in acute myocardial infarction. J. Am. Coll. Cardiol. *7*:729, 1986.

544. Van de Werf, F., Arnold, A. E. R., and for the European Cooperative Study Group for Recombinant Tissue Type Plasminogen Activator: Intravenous tissue plasminogen activator and size of infarct, left ventricular function, and survival in acute myocardial infarction. BMJ *297*:1374, 1988.

545. Gruppo Italiano Per Lo Studio Della Streochi and Nasi Nell'Infarto Miocardico: Long-term effects of intravenous thrombolysis in acute myocardial infarction: Final report of the GISSI study. Lancet *2*:871, 1987.

546. Meijer, A., Verheugt, F. W. A., Werter, C. J. P. J., et al.: Aspirin versus coumadin in the prevention of reocclusion and recurrent ischemia after successful thrombolysis: a prospective placebo-controlled angiographic study: Results of the APRICOT Study. Circulation *87*:1524, 1993.

547. Schroder, R., Neuhaus, K. L., Leizorovicz, A., et al.: A prospective placebo-controlled double-blind multicenter trial of intravenous streptokinase in acute myocardial infarction (ISAM): Long-term mortality and morbidity. J. Am. Coll. Cardiol. *9*:197, 1987.

547a. Collen, D.: Fibrin-selective thrombolytic therapy for acute myocardial infarction. Circulation *93*:857, 1996.

548. The International Study Group: In-hospital mortality and clinical course of 20,891 patients with suspected acute myocardial infarction randomised between alteplase and streptokinase with or without heparin. Lancet *2*:71, 1990.

549. Cannon, C. P., McCabe, C. H., Diver, D. J., et al.: Comparison of front-loaded recombinant tissue-type plasminogen activator, anistreplase and combination thrombolytic therapy for acute myocardial infarction: Results of the Thrombolysis in Myocardial Infarction (TIMI) 4 trial. J. Am. Coll. Cardiol. *24*:1602, 1994.

550. Califf, R. M., Harrelson-Woodlief, L., and Topol, E. J.: Left-ventricular ejection fraction may not be useful as an end point of thrombolytic therapy comparative trials. Circulation *82*:1847, 1990.

551. White, H. D., Norris, R. M., Brown, M. A., et al.: Effect of intravenous streptokinase on left ventricular function and early survival after acute myocardial infarction. N. Engl. J. Med. *317*:850, 1987.

552. St. John Sutton, M., Pfeffer, M. A., Plappert, T., et al.: Quantitative two-dimensional echocardiographic measurements are major predictors of adverse cardiovascular events after acute myocardial infarction: The protective effects of captopril. Circulation *89*:68, 1994.

553. Sheehan, F. H.: Measurement of left ventricular function as an endpoint in trials of thrombolytic therapy. Coronary Art. Dis. *1*:13, 1990.

554. Lavie, C. J., Gersh, B. J., and Chesebro, J. H.: Reperfusion in acute myocardial infarction. Mayo Clin. Proc. *65*:549, 1990.

555. Wackers, F. J. T., Terrin, M. L., Kayden, D. S., et al.: Quantitative radionuclide assessment of regional ventricular function after thrombolytic therapy for acute myocardial infarction: Results of Phase I Thrombolysis in Myocardial Infarction (TIMI) Trial. J. Am. Coll. Cardiol. *13*:998, 1989.

556. Gruppo Italiano per lo Studio della Sopravvivenza nell'Infarto Miocardico: GISSI-2: A factorial randomised trial of alteplase versus streptokinase and heparin versus no heparin among 12,490 patients with acute myocardial infarction. Lancet *336*:65, 1990.

557. Califf, R. M., Fortin, D. F., Tenaglia, A. N., et al.: Clinical risks of thrombolytic therapy. Am. J. Cardiol. *69*:3, 1992.

558. Antman, E. M., for the TIMI 9A Investigators: Hirudin in acute myocardial infarction: Safety report from the Thrombolysis and Thrombin Inhibition in Myocardial Infarction (TIMI) 9A trial. Circulation *90*:1624, 1994.

559. The Global Use of Strategies to Open Occluded Coronary Arteries (GUSTO) IIa Investigators: A randomized trial of intravenous heparin versus recombinant hirudin for acute coronary syndromes. Circulation *90*:1631, 1994.

560. Sane, D. C., Califf, R. M., Topol, E. J., et al.: Bleeding during thrombolytic therapy for acute myocardial infarction: Mechanisms and management. Ann. Intern. Med. *111*:1010, 1989.

561. Gore, J. M., Granger, C. B., Simoons, M. L., et al.: Stroke after thrombolysis: Mortality and functional outcomes in the GUSTO-I Trial. Circulation *92*:2811, 1995.

562. Maggioni, A. P., Franzosi, M. G., Santoro, E., et al.: The risk of stroke in patients with acute myocardial infarction after thrombolytic and antithrombotic treatment. N. Engl. J. Med. *327*:1, 1992.

563. De Jaegere, P. P., Arnold, A. A., Balk, A. H., et al.: Intracranial hemorrhage in association with thrombolytic therapy: Incidence and clinical predictive factors. J. Am. Coll. Cardiol. *19*:289, 1992.

564. Simoons, M., Maggioni, A., Knatterud, G., et al.: Individual risk assessment for intracranial hemorrhage during thrombolytic therapy. Lancet *342*:1523, 1993.

565. Simoons, M. L., Arnold, A. E. R., Betriu, A., et al.: Thrombolysis with tissue plasminogen activator in acute myocardial infarction: No additional benefit from immediate percutaneous coronary angioplasty. Lancet *1*:197, 1988.

566. Mauri, F., DeBiase, A. M., Franzosi, M. G., et al.: In-hospital causes of death in the patients admitted to the GISSI study. G. Ital. Cardiol. *17*:37, 1987.

567. Honan, M. B., Harrell, F. E., Reimer, K. A., et al.: Cardiac rupture, mortality and the timing of thrombolytic therapy: A meta-analysis. J. Am. Coll. Cardiol. *16*:359, 1990.

568. Maynard, C., Weaver, D., Litwin, P. E., et al.: Hospital mortality in acute myocardial infarction in the era of reperfusion therapy (the Myocardial Infarction Triage and Intervention Project). Am. J. Cardiol. *72*:877, 1993.

569. Ohman, E. M., Topol, E. J., Califf, R. M., et al.: An analysis of the cause of early mortality after administration of thrombolytic therapy: The Thrombolysis Angioplasty in Myocardial Infarction Study Group. Coronary Art. Dis. *4*:957, 1993.

570. Becker, R. C., Charlesworth, A., Wilcox, R. G., et al.: Cardiac rupture associated with thrombolytic therapy: Impact of time to treatment in the late assessment of thrombolytic efficacy (LATE) study. J. Am. Coll. Cardiol. *25*:1063, 1995.

571. Kleiman, N., White, H., Ohman, E., et al.: Mortality within 24 hours of thrombolysis for myocardial infarction: The importance of early reperfusion. Circulation *90*:2658, 1994.

572. Kleiman, N. S., Terrin, M., Mueller, H., et al.: Mechanisms of early death despite thrombolytic therapy: Experience from the Thrombolysis in Myocardial Infarction Investigation Phase II (TIMI II) Study. J. Am. Coll. Cardiol. *19*:1129, 1992.

573. Weiner, M. D., and Ong, L. S.: Streptokinase and splenic rupture. Am. J. Med. *86*:249, 1989.

574. Blankenship, J. C., and Almquist, A. K.: Cardiovascular complications of thrombolytic therapy in patients with a mistaken diagnosis of acute myocardial infarction. J. Am. Coll. Cardiol. *14*:1579, 1989.

575. Queen, M., Biem, J., Moe, G. W., et al.: Development of cholesterol embolization syndrome after intravenous streptokinase for acute myocardial infarction. Am. J. Cardiol. *65*:1042, 1990.

576. Wall, T. C., Phillips, H. R., Stack, R. S., et al.: Results of high dose intravenous urokinase for acute myocardial infarction. Am. J. Cardiol. *65*:124, 1990.

577. Tennant, S. N., Dixon, J., Venable, T. C., et al.: Intracoronary thrombolysis in patients with acute myocardial infarction: Comparison of the efficacy of urokinase with streptokinase. Circulation *69*:756, 1984.

578. Neuhaus, K.-L., Von Essen, R., Tebbe, U., et al.: Improved thrombolysis in acute myocardial infarction with front-loaded administration of alteplase: Results of the rt-PA-APSAC Patency Study (TAPS). J. Am. Coll. Cardiol. *19*:885, 1992.

579. Anderson, J. L.: Review of anistreplase (APSAC) for acute myocardial infarction. *In* Anderson, J. L. (ed.): Modern Management of Acute Myocardial Infarction in the Community Hospital. New York, Marcel Dekker, 1991, p. 149.

580. Tebbe, U., Windeler, J., Boesl, I., et al.: Thrombolysis with recombinant unglycosylated single-chain urokinase-type plasminogen activator (saruplase) in acute myocardial infarction: Influence of heparin on early patency rate (LIMITS Study). J. Am. Coll. Cardiol. *26*:365, 1995.

581. Weaver, W. D., Hartmann, J. R., Anderson, J. L., et al.: New recombinant glycosylated prourokinase for treatment of patients with acute myocardial infarction: Prourokinase Study Group. J. Am. Coll. Cardiol. *24*:1242, 1994.

582. Zarich, S. W., Kowalchuk, G. J., Weaver, W. D., et al.: Sequential combination thrombolytic therapy for acute myocardial infarction: Re-

sults of the pro-urokinase and t-PA enhancement of thrombolysis (PATENT) trial. J. Am. Coll. Cardiol. *16*:374, 1995.

583. Califf, R. M., Topol, E. J., Stack, R. S., et al.: Evaluation of combination thrombolytic therapy and timing of cardiac catheterization in acute myocardial infarction: Results of Thrombolysis and Angioplasty in Myocardial Infarction—Phase 5 randomized trial. Circulation *83*:1543, 1991.

584. Urokinase and Alteplase in Myocardial Infarction Collaborative Group: Combination of urokinase and alteplase in the treatment of myocardial infarction. Coronary Art. Dis. *2*:225, 1991.

585. Grines, C. L., Nissen, S. E., Booth, D. C., et al.: A prospective, randomized trial comparing combination half-dose tissue-type plasminogen activator and streptokinase with full-dose tissue-type plasminogen activator: Kentucky Acute Myocardial Infarction Trial (KAMIT) Group. Circulation *84*:540, 1991.

586. Verstraete, M., and Lijnen, H. R.: Novel thrombolytic agents. Cardiovasc. Drugs Ther. *8*:801, 1994.

587. Neuhaus, K. L., von Essen, R., Vogt, A., et al.: Dose finding with a novel recombinant plasminogen activator (BM 06.022) in patients with acute myocardial infarction: Results of the German Recombinant Plasminogen Activator Study: A study of the Arbeitsgemeinschaft Leitender Kardiologischer Krankenhausarzte (ALKK). J. Am. Coll. Cardiol. *24*:55, 1994.

588. Bode, C., Smalling, R. W., Sen, S., et al.: Recombinant plasminogen activator angiographic phase II international dose finding study (RAPID): Patency analysis and mortality endpoints. Circulation *88*(Suppl. I):292, 1993.

589. Weaver, W. D., Bode, C., Burnett, C., et al.: Reteplase vs. Alteplase Patency Investigation During Myocardial Infarction Trial (RAPID 2). J. Am. Coll. Cardiol. (Special Issue):87A, 1995.

590. International Joint Efficacy Comparison of Thrombolytics: Randomised, double-blind comparison of reteplase double-bolus administration with streptokinase in acute myocardial infarction (INJECT): Trial to investigate equivalence. Lancet *346*:329, 1995.

591. Keyt, B. A., Paoni, N. F., Refino, C. J., et al.: A faster-acting and more potent form of tissue plasminogen activator. Proc. Natl. Acad. Sci. U.S.A. *91*:3670, 1994.

592. Meeting Highlights: AHA 68th Scientific Sessions, "TIMI 10A: TNK for acute myocardial infarction." Circulation *93*:843, 1996.

593. Collen, D., and Lijnen, H. R.: Staphylokinase, a fibrin-specific plasminogen activator with therapeutic potential? Blood *84*:680, 1994.

594. Montoney, M., Gardell, S. J., and Marder, V. J.: Comparison of the bleeding potential of vampire bat salivary plasminogen activator versus tissue plasminogen activator in an experimental rabbit model. Circulation *91*:1540, 1995.

595. Fendrick, A., Ridker, P., and Bloom, B.: Improved health care benefits of increased use of thrombolytic therapy. Arch. Intern. Med. *154*:1605, 1994.

596. Simoons, M. L.: Another coronary reperfusion regimen. Lancet *346*:324, 1995.

597. Ridker, P. M., O'Donnell, C., Marder, V. J., et al.: Large-scale trials of thrombolytic therapy for acute myocardial infarction: GISSI-2, ISIS-3, and GUSTO-1. Ann. Intern. Med. *119*:530, 1993.

598. Lee, K. L., Califf, R. M., Simes, J., et al.: Holding GUSTO up to the light. Ann. Intern. Med. *120*:876, 1994.

599. Ridker, P. M., O'Donnell, C. J., Marder, V. J., et al.: A response to "Holding GUSTO up to the light." Ann. Intern. Med. *120*:882, 1994.

600. Ridker, P. M., O'Donnell, C. J., Marder, V. J., et al.: More on the GUSTO trial. Ann. Intern. Med. *120*:818, 1994.

601. Lee, K. L., Califf, R. M., and Topol, E. J.: The last word on GUSTO, for now. Ann. Intern. Med. *120*:970, 1994.

602. Hennekens, C. H., O'Donnell, C. J., Ridker, P. M., et al.: Current issues concerning thrombolytic therapy for acute myocardial infarction. J. Am. Coll. Cardiol. *25*:18S, 1995.

603. Lee, T. H.: Cost effectiveness of tissue plasminogen activator. N. Engl. J. Med. *332*:1443, 1995.

604. Simoons, M. L., and Arnold, A. E.: Tailored thrombolytic therapy: A perspective. Circulation *88*:2556, 1993.

605. Brodie, B. R., Stuckey, T. D., Hansen, C., et al.: Benefit of late coronary reperfusion in patients with acute myocardial infarction and persistent ischemic chest pain. Am. J. Cardiol. *74*:538, 1994.

CORONARY ANGIOPLASTY IN ACUTE MYOCARDIAL INFARCTION

606. Grines, C. L., Browne, K. F., Marco, J., et al.: A comparison of immediate angioplasty with thrombolytic therapy for acute myocardial infarction. N. Engl. J. Med. *328*:673, 1993.

607. Zijlstra, F., de Boer, M. J., Hoorntje, J. C. A., et al.: A comparison of immediate coronary angioplasty with intravenous streptokinase in acute myocardial infarction. N. Engl. J. Med. *328*:680, 1993.

608. Gibbons, R. J., Holmes, D. R., Reeder, G. S., et al.: Immediate angioplasty compared with the administration of a thrombolytic agent followed by conservative treatment for myocardial infarction: The Mayo Coronary Care Unit and Catheterization Laboratory Groups. N. Engl. J. Med. *328*:685, 1993.

609. Lange, R. A., and Hillis, L. D.: Immediate angioplasty for acute myocardial infarction. N. Engl. J. Med. *328*:726, 1993.

610. Stewart, R. E., and O'Neill, W. W.: Direct angioplasty for acute myocardial infarction. Curr. Opin. Cardiol. *10*:367, 1995.

610a. King, S. B. III., and Holmes, D. R. III: Coronary angioplasty for acute myocardial infarction. *In* Fuster, V., Ross, R., and Topol, E. J. (eds.): Atherosclerosis and Coronary Artery Disease. Philadelphia, Lippincott-Raven, 1996, pp. 1143–1156.

611. Topol, E. J.: Coronary angioplasty for acute myocardial infarction. Ann. Intern. Med. *109*:970, 1988.

612. Eckman, M. H., Wong, J. B., Salem, D. N., et al.: Direct angioplasty for acute myocardial infarction: A review of outcomes in clinical subsets. Ann. Intern. Med. *117*:667, 1992.

613. De Franco, A. C., and Topol, E. J.: Angiography and angioplasty. *In* Julian, D., and Braunwald, E. (eds.): Management of Acute Myocardial Infarction. London, W. B. Saunders Ltd., 1994, p. 107.

614. Grines, C. L., and O'Neill, W. W.: Primary angioplasty: The optimal reperfusion strategy in the United States. Br. Heart J. *73*:405, 1995.

615. O'Neill, W. W., Brodie, B. R., Ivanhoe, R., et al.: Primary coronary angioplasty for acute myocardial infarction (the Primary Angioplasty Registry). Am. J. Cardiol. *73*:627, 1994.

616. Brodie, B. R., Grines, C. L., Ivanhoe, R., et al.: Six-month clinical and angiographic follow-up after direct angioplasty for acute myocardial infarction: Final results from the Primary Angioplasty Registry. Circulation *90*:156, 1994.

617. de Boer, M. J., Hoorntje, J. C. A., Ottervanger, J. P., et al.: Immediate coronary angioplasty versus intravenous streptokinase in acute myocardial infarction: Left ventricular ejection fraction, hospital mortality and reinfarction. J. Am. Coll. Cardiol. *23*:1004, 1994.

618. Michels, K. B., and Yusuf, S.: Does PTCA in acute myocardial infarction affect mortality and reinfarction rates? A quantitative overview (meta-analysis) of the randomized clinical trials. Circulation *91*:476, 1995.

619. Vaitkus, P. T.: Percutaneous transluminal coronary angioplasty versus thrombolysis in acute myocardial infarction: A meta-analysis. Clin. Cardiol. *18*:35, 1995.

620. O'Neill, W., Timmis, G. C., Bourdillon, P. D., et al.: A prospective randomized clinical trial of intracoronary streptokinase versus coronary angioplasty for acute myocardial infarction. N. Engl. J. Med. *314*:812, 1986.

621. DeWood, M. A., Fisher, M. J., and for the Spokane Heart Research Group: Direct PTCA versus intravenous rtPA in acute myocardial infarction: Preliminary results from a prospective randomized trial. Circulation *80*(Suppl. II):418, 1989.

622. Ribeiro, E. E., Silva, L. A., Carneiro, R., et al.: Randomized trial of direct coronary angioplasty versus intravenous streptokinase in acute myocardial infarction. J. Am. Coll. Cardiol. *22*:376, 1993.

623. Elizaga, J., Garcia, E. J., Delcan, J. L., et al.: Primary coronary angioplasty versus systemic thrombolysis in acute anterior myocardial infarction: In-hospital results from a prospective randomized trial. Circulation *88*(Suppl. I):411, 1993.

624. Zijlstra, F.: Primary angioplasty is the most effective treatment for an acute myocardial infarction. Br. Heart J. *73*:403, 1995.

625. Himbert, D., Juliard, J. M., Steg, P. G., et al.: Primary coronary angioplasty for acute myocardial infarction with contraindication to thrombolysis. Am. J. Cardiol. *71*:377, 1993.

626. Ohman, E. M., Califf, R. M., Topol, E. J., et al.: Consequences of reocclusion after successful reperfusion therapy in acute myocardial infarction. Circulation *82*:781, 1990.

627. Stone, G. W., Grines, C. L., Browne, K. F., et al.: Implications of recurrent ischemia after reperfusion therapy in acute myocardial infarction: A comparison of thrombolytic therapy and primary angioplasty. J. Am. Coll. Cardiol. *26*:66, 1995.

628. Leung, W. H., and Lau, C. P.: Effects of severity of the residual stenosis of the infarct-related coronary artery on left ventricular dilation and function after acute myocardial infarction. J. Am. Coll. Cardiol. *20*:307, 1992.

629. American Heart Association: Facilities and services in the United States, In hospital statistics 1992–1993. Chicago, AHA, 1992, p. 208.

630. de Jaegere, P. P., and Simoons, M. L.: Immediate angioplasty: A conservative view from Europe: Cost effectiveness needs to be considered. Br. Heart J. *73*:407, 1995.

631. Bedotto, J. B., Kahn, J. K., Rutherford, B. D., et al.: Failed direct coronary angioplasty for acute myocardial infarction: In-hospital outcome and predictors of death. J. Am. Coll. Cardiol. *22*:690, 1993.

632. Vaitkus, P. T.: Limitations of primary angioplasty in acute myocardial infarction: Effectiveness depends on the clinical and operational context. Br. Heart J. *73*:409, 1995.

633. Boyle, R. M.: Immediate angioplasty in the United Kingdom. Br. Heart J. *73*:413, 1995.

634. Ellis, S. G., van de Werf, F., Ribeiro-da Silva, E., et al.: Present status of rescue coronary angioplasty: Current polarization of opinion and randomized trials. J. Am. Coll. Cardiol. *19*:681, 1992.

635. Belenkie, I., Traboulsi, M., Hall, C. A., et al.: Rescue angioplasty during myocardial infarction has a beneficial effect on mortality: A tenable hypothesis. Can. J. Cardiol. *8*:357, 1992.

636. Ellis, S. G., da Silva, E. R., Heyndrickx, G., et al.: Randomized comparison of rescue angioplasty with conservative management of patients with early failure of thrombolysis for acute anterior myocardial infarction. Circulation *90*:2280, 1994.

637. Topol, E. J., Califf, R. M., George, B. S., et al.: A randomized trial of immediate versus delayed elective angioplasty after intravenous tissue plasminogen activator in acute myocardial infarction. N. Engl. J. Med. *317*:581, 1987.

638. Rogers, W. J., Baim, D. S., Gore, J. M., et al.: Comparison of immediate invasive, delayed invasive, and conservative strategies after tissue-type plasminogen activator: Results of the Thrombolysis in Myocardial Infarction (TIMI) Phase II-A Trial. Circulation *81*:1457, 1990.

639. Holmes, D., and Topol, E. J.: Reperfusion momentum: Lessons from the randomization trials of immediate coronary angioplasty for myocardial infarction. J. Am. Coll. Cardiol. *14*:1572, 1989.

640. The TIMI Research Group: Immediate vs delayed catheterization and angioplasty following thrombolytic therapy for acute myocardial infarction: TIMI II A results. JAMA *260*:2849, 1988.

641. The TIMI Study Group: Comparison of invasive and conservative strategies after treatment with intravenous tissue plasminogen activator in acute myocardial infarction: Results of the Thrombolysis in Myocardial Infarction (TIMI) Phase II Trial. N. Engl. J. Med. *320*:618, 1989.

642. SWIFT (Should We Intervene Following Thrombolysis?) Trial Study Group: SWIFT trial of delayed elective intervention v. conservative treatment after thrombolysis with anistreplase in acute myocardial infarction. BMJ *302*:555, 1991.

643. Özbeck, C., Dyckmans, J., Sen, S., et al.: Comparison of invasive and conservative strategies after treatment with streptokinase in acute myocardial infarction: Results of a randomized trial (SIAM). J. Am. Coll. Cardiol. *15*:63A, 1990.

644. Ellis, S. G., Mooney, M. R., George, B. S., et al.: Randomized trial of late elective angioplasty versus conservative management for patients with residual stenoses after thrombolytic treatment of myocardial infarction: Treatment of Post-Thrombolytic Stenoses (TOPS) study group. Circulation *86*:1400, 1992.

645. Holmes, D. R., Bates, E. R., Kleiman, N. S., et al.: Contemporary reperfusion therapy for cardiogenic shock: The GUSTO-1 trial experience. J. Am. Coll. Cardiol. *26*:668, 1995.

646. Hochman, J. S., Boland, J., Sleeper, L. A., et al.: Current spectrum of cardiogenic shock and effect of early revascularization on mortality: Results of an International Registry: SHOCK Registry Investigators. Circulation *91*:873, 1995.

647. Aguirre, F. V., Meritt, R. F., and Carollo, S. C.: The role of coronary angiography after thrombolysis. Curr. Opin. Cardiol. *10*:381, 1995.

648. Vaitkus, P. T.: The continuing evolution of percutaneous transluminal coronary angioplasty in the treatment of coronary artery disease. Coronary Art. Dis. *6*:429, 1995.

649. Ellis, S. G., da Silva, E. R., Heyndrickx, G., et al.: Randomized comparison of rescue angioplasty with conservative management of patients with early failure of thrombolysis for acute anterior myocardial infarction. Circulation *90*:2280, 1994.

650. Erbel, R., Pop, T., Diefenbach, C., et al.: Long-term results of thrombolytic therapy with and without percutaneous transluminal coronary angioplasty. J. Am. Coll. Cardiol. *14*:276, 1989.

651. Guerci, A. D., and Ross, R. S.: TIMI II and the role of angioplasty in acute myocardial infarction. N. Engl. J. Med. *320*:663, 1989.

652. Ishihara, M., Sato, H., Tateishi, H., et al.: Intraaortic balloon pumping as the postangioplasty strategy in acute myocardial infarction. Am. Heart J. *122*:385, 1991.

653. Ohman, E. M., Califf, R. M., George, B. S., et al.: The use of intraaortic balloon pumping as an adjunct to reperfusion therapy in acute myocardial infarction: The Thrombolysis and Angioplasty in Myocardial Infarction (TAMI) study group. Am. Heart J. *121*:895, 1991.

654. Ohman, E. M., George, B. S., White, C. J., et al.: Use of aortic counterpulsation to improve sustained coronary artery patency during acute myocardial infarction: Results of a randomized trial: The Randomized IABP study group. Circulation *90*:792, 1994.

655. DeWood, M. A., Notske, N., Berg, R., et al.: Medical and surgical management of early Q wave myocardial infarction. I. Effects of surgical reperfusion on survival, recurrent myocardial infarction, sudden death and functional class at 10 or more years of follow-up. J. Am. Coll. Cardiol. *14*:65, 1989.

656. Schaff, H. V.: Myocardial infarction: The role of bypass surgery. In Fuster, V., Ross, R., and Topol, E. J. (eds.): Atherosclerosis and Coronary Artery Disease. Philadelphia, Lippincott-Raven, 1996, pp. 1157–1166.

656a. Verstraete, M., Chesebro, J., and Fuster, V.: Acute myocardial infarction: Antithrombotic therapy. In Fuster, V., Ross, R., and Topol, E. J. (eds.): Atherosclerosis and Coronary Artery Disease. Philadelphia, Lippincott-Raven, 1996, pp. 979–994.

657. Kereiakes, D. J., Topol, E. J., George, B. S., et al.: Favorable early and long-term prognosis following coronary bypass surgery therapy for myocardial infarction: Results of a multicenter trial: TAMI Study Group. Am. Heart J. *118*:199, 1989.

658. Schaff, H. V.: The role of bypass surgery in acute myocardial infarction. In Gersh, B. J., and Rahimtoola, S. H. (eds.): Acute Myocardial Infarction. New York, Elsevier, 1991, p. 386.

659. Montoya, A., Mulet, J., Pifarre, R., et al.: Hemorrhagic infarct following myocardial revascularization. J. Thorac. Cardiovasc. Surg. *75*:206, 1978.

660. Kagen, L., Scheidt, S., and Butt, A.: Serum myoglobin in myocardial infarction: The "staccato phenomenon": Is acute myocardial infarction in man an intermittent event? Am. J. Med. *62*:86, 1977.

661. Gersh, B. J., Chesebro, J. H., Braunwald, E., et al.: Coronary artery bypass surgery after thrombolytic therapy in the Thrombolysis in Myocardial Infarction Trial, Phase II (TIMI II). J. Am. Coll. Cardiol. *25*:395, 1995.

662. Tardiff, B. E., Califf, R. M., Morris, D., et al.: Coronary revascularization surgery following myocardial infarction: Effect of bypass surgery on survival following thrombolysis. *(In press).*

663. Naunheim, K. S., Kesler, K. A., Kanter, K. R., et al.: Coronary artery bypass for recent infarction: Predictors of mortality. Circulation *78*(Suppl. I):122, 1988.

664. Kennedy, J. W., Ivey, T. D., Misbach, G., et al.: Coronary artery bypass graft surgery early after acute myocardial infarction. Circulation *79*(Suppl. I):73, 1989.

665. Kalan, J. M., and Roberts, W. C.: Morphologic findings in patients undergoing coronary artery bypass grafting for acute myocardial infarction. Am. J. Cardiol. *62*:144, 1988.

666. Kay, P., Ahmad, A., Floten, S., et al.: Emergency coronary artery bypass surgery after intracoronary thrombolysis for evolving myocardial infarction. Int. J. Cardiol. *7*:281, 1985.

ANTITHROMBOTIC AND ANTIPLATELET THERAPY

667. Report of the Working Party on Anticoagulant Therapy in Coronary Thrombosis to the Medical Research Council: Assessment of short-term anticoagulant administration after cardiac infarction. BMJ *1*:335, 1969.

668. Drapkin, A., and Merskey, C.: Anticoagulant therapy after acute myocardial infarction: Relation of therapeutic benefit to patient's age, sex, and severity of infarction. JAMA *222*:541, 1972.

669. Veterans Administration Cooperative Study: Anticoagulants in acute myocardial infarction. Results of a cooperative clinical trial. JAMA *225*:724, 1973.

670. Chalmers, T. C., Matta, R. J., Smith, H., et al.: Evidence favoring the use of anticoagulants in the hospital phase of acute myocardial infarction. N. Engl. J. Med. *297*:1091, 1977.

671. Cairns, J. A., Hirsh, J., Lewis, H. D., et al.: Antithrombotic agents in coronary artery disease. Chest *108*(Suppl.):3805, 1995.

672. O'Donnell, C. J., Ridker, P. M., Hebert, P. R., et al.: Antithrombotic therapy for acute myocardial infarction. J. Am. Coll. Cardiol. *25*:23S, 1995.

673. Ridker, P. M., Hebert, P. R., Fuster, V., et al.: Are both aspirin and heparin justified as adjuncts to thrombolytic therapy for acute myocardial infarction? Lancet *341*:1574, 1993.

674. Hennekens, C. H., O'Donnell, C. J., and Ridker, P. M.: Current and future perspectives on antithrombotic therapy of acute myocardial infarction. Eur. Heart J. *16*(Suppl.):2, 1995.

675. The SCATI Group: Randomised controlled trial of subcutaneous calcium-heparin in acute myocardial infarction. Lancet *1*:182, 1989.

676. Bleich, S. D., Nichols, T., Schumacher, R. R., et al.: Effect of heparin on coronary patency after thrombolysis with tissue plasminogen activator in acute myocardial infarction. Am. J. Cardiol. *66*:1412, 1990.

677. Hsia, J., Hamilton, W. P., Kleiman, N., et al.: A comparison between heparin and low-dose aspirin as adjunctive therapy with tissue plasminogen activator for acute myocardial infarction. N. Engl. J. Med. *323*:1433, 1990.

678. de Bono, D. P., Simoons, M. I., Tijssen, J., et al.: Effect of early intravenous heparin on coronary patency, infarct size, and bleeding complications after alteplase thrombolysis: Results of a randomized double blind European Cooperative Study Group trial. Br. Heart J. *67*:122, 1992.

679. Topol, E. J., George, B. S., Kereiakes, D. J., et al.: A randomized controlled trial of intravenous tissue plasminogen activator and early intravenous heparin in acute myocardial infarction. Circulation *79*:281, 1989.

680. Col, J., Decoster, O., Hanique, G., et al.: Infusion of heparin conjunct to streptokinase accelerates reperfusion of acute myocardial infarction: Results of a double blind randomized study (OSIRIS). Circulation *86*(Suppl. I):259, 1992.

681. O'Connor, C. M., Meese, R., Carney, R., et al.: A randomized trial of intravenous heparin in conjunction with anistreplase (anisoylated plasminogen streptokinase activator complex) in acute myocardial infarction: The Duke University Clinical Cardiology Study (DUCCS). J. Am. Coll. Cardiol. *23*:11, 1994.

682. Bassand, J. P., Machecourt, J., Cassagnes, J., et al.: A multicenter double-blind trial of intravenous APSAC versus heparin in acute myocardial infarction: Final report of the APSIM study. J. Am. Coll. Cardiol. *11*:232A, 1988.

683. Verheugt, F. W. A., Marsh, R. C., Veen, G., et al.: Megadose bolus heparin as primary reperfusion therapy for acute myocardial infarction: The HEAP pilot study. Eur. Heart J. *16*(Suppl.):176, 1995.

684. Vaitkus, P. T., and Barnathan, E. S.: Usefulness of echocardiography in managing left ventricular thrombi after acute myocardial infarction. Am. J. Cardiol. *66*:387, 1990.

685. Vaitkus, P., and Barnathan, E.: Embolic potential, prevention and management of mural thrombus complicating anterior myocardial infarction: A meta-analysis. J. Am. Coll. Cardiol. *22*:1004, 1993.

686. Vecchio, C., Chiarella, F., Lupi, G., et al.: Left ventricular thrombus in anterior acute myocardial infarction after thrombolysis: A GISSI-2 connected study. Circulation *84*:512, 1991.

687. Warkentin, T. E.: Heparin-induced thrombocytopenia. Annu. Rev. Med. *40*:31, 1989.

687a. Warkentin, T. E., Levine, M. N., Hirsh, J., et al.: Heparin-induced thrombocytopenia in patients treated with low-molecular-weight heparin or unfractionated heparin. N. Engl. J. Med. *332*:1330, 1995.

688. Becker, R. C., Cyr, J., Corrao, J. M., et al.: Bedside coagulation monitoring in heparin-treated patients with active thromboembolic disease: A coronary care unit experience. Am. Heart J. *128*:719, 1994.

689. Cruikshank, M. K., Levine, M. N., Hirsh, J., et al.: A standard nomogram for the management of heparin therapy. Arch. Intern. Med. *151*:333, 1991.

690. Verstraete, M., and Zoldhelyi, P.: Novel antithrombotic drugs in development. Drugs *49*:856, 1995.

691. Meeting Highlights: AHA 68th Scientific Sessions, "TIMI 9B: Heparin

versus hirudin as adjunctive therapy for thrombolysis in acute myocardial infarction." Circulation 93:843, 1996.

691a. Topol, E. The GUSTO IIB Trial. Presentation, Am. Coll. Cardiol., 1996.

692. MacMahon, S., Collins, R., Knight, C., et al.: Reduction in major morbidity and mortality by heparin in acute myocardial infarction. Circulation 78(Suppl. II):98, 1988.

693. Vaitkus, P. T., Berlin, J. A., Schwartz, J. S., et al.: Stroke complicating acute myocardial infarction: A meta-analysis of risk modification by anticoagulation and thrombolytic therapy. Arch. Intern. Med. 152:2020, 1992.

694. Granger, C. B., Hirsch, J., Califf, R. M., et al.: Activated partial thromboplastin time and outcome after thrombolytic therapy for acute myocardial infarction. Circulation 93:870, 1996.

695. Hassan, W. M., Flaker, G. C., Feutz, C., et al.: Improved anticoagulation with a weight adjusted heparin nomogram in patients with acute coronary syndromes: A randomized trial. J. Thromb. Thrombol. 2:245, 1996.

695a. White, H. D., and Yusuf, S.: Issues regarding the use of heparin following streptokinase therapy. J. Thromb. Thrombol. 2:5, 1995.

696. Ward, S. R., and Topol, E. J.: How best to use heparin in MI patients given thrombolysis. J. Crit. Illness 10:385, 1995.

697. Theroux, P., Waters, D., Lam, J., et al.: Reactivation of unstable angina after the discontinuation of heparin. N. Engl. J. Med. 327:141, 1992.

698. Granger, C. B., Miller, J. M., Bovill, E. G., et al.: Rebound increase in thrombin generation and activity after cessation of intravenous heparin in patients with acute coronary syndromes. Circulation 91:1929, 1995.

699. Fuster, V., Badimon, L., Badimon, J. J., et al.: The pathophysiology of coronary artery disease and the acute coronary syndromes. N. Engl. J. Med. 326:242, 1992.

699a. Weitz, J. I., Califf, R. M., Ginsberg, J.S., et al.: New antithrombotics. Chest 108(Suppl.):471S, 1995.

700. Jang, I. K., Gold, H. K., Ziskind, A. A., et al.: Differential sensitivity of erythrocyte-rich and platelet-rich arterial thrombi to lysis with recombinant tissue-type plasminogen activator: A possible explanation for resistance to coronary thrombolysis. Circulation 79:920, 1989.

701. Coller, B. S.: Platelets and thrombolytic therapy. N. Engl. J. Med. 322:33, 1990.

702. Antiplatelet Trialists' Collaboration: Collaborative overview of randomised trials of antiplatelet therapy. II. Maintenance of vascular graft or arterial patency by antiplatelet therapy. BMJ 308:159, 1994.

703. Antiplatelet Trialists' Collaboration: Collaborative overview of randomised trials of antiplatelet therapy. III. Reduction in venous thrombosis and pulmonary embolism by antiplatelet prophylaxis among surgical and medical patients. BMJ 308:235, 1994.

704. Patrono, C.: Aspirin as an antiplatelet drug. N. Engl. J. Med. 330:1287, 1994.

705. Buerke, M., Pittroff, W., Melyer, J., et al.: Aspirin therapy: Optimized platelet inhibition with different loading and maintenance doses. Am. Heart J. 130:465, 1995.

706. Yao, S.-K., Ober, J. C., Ferguson, J. J., et al.: Combination of inhibition of thrombin and blockade of thromboxane A$_2$ synthetase and receptors enhances thrombolysis and delays reocclusion in canine coronary arteries. Circulation 86:1993, 1992.

707. Golino, P., Buja, M., Ashton, J. H., et al.: Effect of thromboxane and serotonin receptor antagonists on intracoronary platelet deposition in dogs with experimental stenosed coronary arteries. Circulation 78:701, 1988.

708. Yasuda, T., Gold, H. K., Yaotia, H., et al.: Antithrombotic effects of ridogrel, a combined thromboxane A$_2$ synthetase inhibitor and prostaglandin endoperoxide-receptor antagonist, in a platelet-mediated coronary artery occlusion preparation in the dog. Coronary Art. Dis. 2:1103, 1991.

709. The RAPT Investigators: Randomized trial of ridogrel, a combined thromboxane A$_2$ synthase inhibitor and thromboxane A$_2$/prostaglandin endoperoxide receptor antagonist, versus aspirin as adjunction to thrombolysis in patients with acute myocardial infarction: The Ridogrel Aspirin Patency Trial (RAPT). Circulation 89:588, 1994.

710. Lefkovits, J., Plow, E. F., and Topol, E. J.: Platelet glycoprotein IIb/IIIa receptors in cardiovascular medicine. N. Engl. J. Med. 332:1553, 1995.

711. Ohman, E. M., Kleiman, N. S., Talley, J. D., et al.: Simultaneous platelet glycoprotein IIb/IIIa integrin blockade with accelerated tissue plasminogen activator in acute myocardial infarction. Circulation 90(Suppl. I):564, 1994.

712. Krucoff, M. W., Ohman, E. M., Trollinger, K. M., et al.: Beneficial impact of a platelet inhibitor, integrelin, on parameters of continuous 12-lead ST-segment recovery from myocardial infarction. Circulation 92(Suppl.):I-416, 1995.

713. Lee, T. H., and Goldman, L.: The coronary care unit turns 25: Historical trends and future directions. Ann. Intern. Med. 108:887, 1988.

714. Davison, G., Suchman, A. L., and Goldstein, B. J.: Reducing unnecessary coronary care unit admissions: A comparison of three decision aids. J. Gen. Intern. Med. 5:474, 1990.

715. Lee, T. H., Cook, E. F., Weisberg, M. C., et al.: Impact of the availability of a prior electrocardiogram on the triage of the patient with acute chest pain. J. Gen. Intern. Med. 5:381, 1990.

716. Lee, T. H.: Chest pain in the emergency department: Uncertainty and the test of time. Mayo Clin. Proc. 66:963, 1991.

717. Bell, M. R., Montarello, J. K., and Steele, P. M.: Does the emergency room electrocardiogram identify patients with suspected acute myocardial infarction who are at low risk of acute complications? Aust. N. Z. J. Med. 20:564, 1990.

718. Brush, J. E., Brand, D. A., Acampora, D., et al.: Use of the initial electrocardiogram to predict in-hospital complications of acute myocardial infarction. N. Engl. J. Med. 312:1137, 1985.

719. Lee, T. L., Cook, E. F., Weisberg, M., et al.: Acute chest pain in the emergency ward: Identification and evaluation of low risk patients. Arch. Intern. Med. 145:65, 1985.

720. Aase, O., Jonsbu, J., Liestøl, K., et al.: Decision support by computer analysis of selected case history variables in the emergency room among patients with acute chest pain. Eur. Heart J. 14:441, 1993.

721. Mirvis, D., Berson, A., Goldberger, A., et al.: Instrumentation and practice standards for electrocardiographic monitoring in special care units. Circulation 79:464, 1989.

722. Romhilt, D., Bloomfield, S., Chou, T., et al.: Unreliability of conventional electrocardiographic monitoring for arrhythmia detection in coronary care units. Am. J. Cardiol. 31:457, 1973.

723. Fineberg, H., Scadden, D., and Goldman, L.: Management of patients with a low probability of acute myocardial infarction: Cost-effectiveness of alternatives to coronary care unit admission. N. Engl. J. Med. 310:1301, 1984.

724. Stern, T. A.: Psychiatric management of acute myocardial infarction in the coronary care unit. Am. J. Cardiol. 60:59J, 1987.

725. Kirchhoff, K. T., Holm, K., Foreman, M. D., et al.: Electrocardiographic response to ice water ingestion. Heart Lung 19:41, 1990.

726. Sortur, S. V., and Khadilkar, S. V.: Worsening of cardiac arrhythmia following drinking chilled water in a patient of acute myocardial infarction. J. Assoc. Phys. India 35:311, 1987.

727. Gross, L., and Malaya, R.: Extrinsically induced arrhythmia in acute myocardial infarction. JAMA 228:1021, 1974.

728. Lynn, L. A., and Kissinger, J. F.: Coronary precautions: Should caffeine be restricted after myocardial infarction? Heart Lung 21:365, 1992.

729. Kirchhoff, K. T.: An examination of the physiologic basis for coronary precautions. Heart Lung 10:874, 1981.

730. Bauer, W. C., and Dracup, K. A.: Physiologic effects of back massage in patients with acute myocardial infarction. Focus Crit. Care. 14:42, 1987.

731. Winslow, E. H., Lane, L., and Gaffney, A.: Oxygen uptake and cardiovascular response in patients with acute myocardial infarction. J. Cardiopul. Rehabil. 4:348, 1984.

732. Levine, S. A., and Lown, B.: "Armchair" treatment of acute coronary thrombosis. JAMA 148:1365, 1952.

733. Krone, R.: The role of risk stratification in the early management of a myocardial infarction. Ann. Intern. Med. 116:223, 1992.

734. Weinberg, S. L.: Intermediate coronary care—observations on the validity of the concept. Chest 73:154, 1978.

735. Topol, E. J., Burek, K., O'Neill, W. W., et al.: A randomized controlled trial of early hospital discharge three days after myocardial infarction in the era of reperfusion. N. Engl. J. Med. 318:1083, 1988.

736. Mark, D. B., Sigmon, K., Topol, E. J., et al.: Identification of acute myocardial infarction patients suitable for early hospital discharge after aggressive interventional therapy: Results from the Thrombolysis and Angioplasty in Acute Myocardial Infarction Registry. Circulation 83:1186, 1991.

736a. Frishman, W. H.: Acute myocardial infarction: Role of β-adrenergic blockers. In Fuster, V., Ross, R., and Topol, E. J. (eds.): Atherosclerosis and Coronary Artery Disease. Philadelphia, Lippincott-Raven, 1996, pp. 1205–1214.

PHARMACOLOGICAL THERAPY

737. Waagstein, F., and Hjalmaarson, A. C.: Double-blind study of the effect of cardioselective beta-blockade on chest pain in acute myocardial infarction. Acta Med. Scand. 587(Suppl.):201, 1975.

738. Norris, R. M., Clarke, E. D., Sammel, N. L., et al.: Protective effect of propranolol in threatened myocardial infarction. Lancet 2:907, 1978.

739. Mueller, H. S., and Ayres, S. M.: The role of propranolol in the treatment of acute myocardial infarction. Prog. Cardiovasc. Dis. 19:405, 1977.

740. The MIAMI Trial Research Group: Metoprolol in acute myocardial infarction: Arrhythmias. Am. J. Cardiol. 56:35G, 1985.

741. Gold, H. K., Leinbach, C., and Maroko, P. R.: Propranolol-induced reduction of signs of ischemic injury during acute myocardial infarction. Am. J. Cardiol. 38:689, 1976.

742. The MIAMI Trial Research Group: Metoprolol in acute myocardial infarction: Enzymatic estimation of infarct size. Am. J. Cardiol. 56:27G, 1985.

743. The International Collaborative Study Group: Reduction of infarct size with the early use of timolol in acute myocardial infarction. N. Engl. J. Med. 310:9, 1984.

744. Held, P. H., and Yusuf, S.: Effects of beta-blockers and calcium channel blockers in acute myocardial infarction. Eur. Heart J. 14:18, 1993.

745. ISIS-1 (First International Study of Infarct Survival) Collaborative Group: Randomized trial of intravenous atenolol among 16,027 cases of suspected acute myocardial infarction. Lancet 2:57, 1986.

746. Yusuf, S.: The use of beta-blockers in the acute phase of myocardial infarction. In Califf, R. M., and Wagner, G. S. (eds.): Acute Coronary Care 1986. Boston, Martinus Nijhoff, 1985, p. 73.

747. ISIS-1 (First International Study of Infarct Survival) Collaborative Group: Mechanisms for the early mortality reduction produced by beta-blockade started early in acute myocardial infarction: ISIS-1. Lancet 1:921, 1988.

748. Yusuf, S., Peto, R., Lewis, J., et al.: Beta blockade during and after myocardial infarction: An overview of the randomized trials. Prog. Cardiovasc. Dis. 27:335, 1985.

749. Pfeffer, M. A., Braunwald, E., Moye, L. A., et al.: Effect of captopril on mortality and morbidity in patients with left ventricular dysfunction after myocardial infarction. N. Engl. J. Med. 327:669, 1992.

750. Pfeffer, J. M., Pfeffer, M. A., and Braunwald, E.: Influence of chronic captopril therapy on the infarcted left ventricle of the rat. Circ. Res. 57:84, 1985.

751. Latini, R., Maggioni, A. P., Flather, M., et al.: "ACE-inhibitor use in patients with myocardial infarction": Summary of evidence from clinical trials. Circulation 32:3132, 1995.

752. The Acute Infarction Ramipril Efficacy (AIRE) Study Investigators: Effect of ramipril on mortality and morbidity of survivors of acute myocardial infarction with clinical evidence of heart failure. Lancet 342:821, 1993.

753. Ambrosioni, E., Borghi, C., Magnani, B., et al.: Effects of the early administration of zofenopril on mortality and morbidity in patients with anterior myocardial infarction: Results of the Survival of Myocardial Infarction Long-Term Evaluation Trial. N. Engl. J. Med. 332:280, 1995.

754. Køber, L., Torp-Pedersen, C., Carlsen, J. E., et al.: A clinical trial of the angiotensin-converting-enzyme inhibitor trandolapril in patients with left ventricular dysfunction after myocardial infarction. N. Engl. J. Med. 333:1670, 1995.

755. Swedberg, K., Held, P., Kjekshus, J., et al.: Effects of early administration of enalapril on mortality in patients with acute myocardial infarction: Results of the Cooperative North Scandinavian Enalapril Survival Study II (CONSENSUS II). N. Engl. J. Med. 327:678, 1992.

756. Chinese Cardiac Study Collaborative Group: Oral captopril versus placebo among 13,634 patients with suspected myocardial infarction: Interim report from the Chinese Cardiac Study (CCS-1). Lancet 345:686, 1995.

757. Gruppo Italiano per lo Studio della Sopravvivenza nell'Infarto Miocardico: GISSI-3: Effects of lisinopril and transdermal glyceryl trinitrate singly and together on 6-week mortality and ventricular function after acute myocardial infarction. Lancet 343:1115, 1994.

758. Rutherford, J. D., Pfeffer, M. A., Moye, L. A., et al.: Effects of captopril on ischemic events after myocardial infarction: Results of the Survival and Ventricular Enlargement Trial. Circulation 90:1731, 1994.

759. Lindsay, H. S. J., Zaman, A. G., and Cowan, J. C.: ACE inhibitors after myocardial infarction: Patient selection or treatment for all? Br. Heart J. 73:397, 1995.

760. Coats, A. J. S.: ACE inhibitors after myocardial infarction: Selection and treatment for all. Br. Heart J. 73:395, 1995.

761. ISIS-4 Collaborative Group: ISIS-4: A randomized factorial trial assessing early oral captopril, oral mononitrate, and intravenous magnesium sulphate in 58,050 patients with suspected acute myocardial infarction. Lancet 345:669, 1995.

762. Horowitz, L. D., Gorlin, R., Taylor, W. J., et al.: Effects of nitroglycerin in regional myocardial blood flow in coronary artery disease. J. Clin. Invest. 50:1578, 1971.

763. Loscalzo, J.: Antiplatelet and antithrombotic effects of organic nitrates. Am. J. Cardiol. 70:18B, 1992.

764. Wilhelmsen, L.: Nitrates. In Julian D., and Braunwald, E. (eds.): Management of Acute Myocardial Infarction. London, W. B. Saunders Ltd., 1994, p. 241.

765. Jugdutt, B. I.: Nitrates in myocardial infarction. Cardiovasc. Drugs Ther. 8:635, 1994.

766. Abrams, J.: The role of nitrates in coronary heart disease. Arch. Intern. Med. 155:357, 1995.

767. Bussmann, W. D., Passek, D., Seidel, W., et al.: Reduction of CK and CK-MB indexes of infarct size by intravenous nitroglycerin. Circulation 63:615, 1981.

768. Jugdutt, B. I., and Warnica, J. W.: Intravenous nitroglycerin therapy to limit myocardial infarct size, expansion, and complications: Effect of timing, dosage, and infarct location. Circulation 78:906, 1988.

769. Yusuf, S., Collins, R., MacMahon, S., et al.: Effect of intravenous nitrates on mortality in acute myocardial infarction: An overview of the randomized trials. Lancet 1:1088, 1988.

770. Chatterjee, K., and Parmley, W. W.: Vasodilator therapy for acute myocardial infarction and chronic congestive heart failure. J. Am. Coll. Cardiol. 1:133, 1983.

771. Ferguson, J. J., Diver, D. J., Boldt, M., et al.: Significance of nitroglycerin-induced hypotension with inferior wall acute myocardial infarction. Am. J. Cardiol. 64:311, 1989.

772. Osuna, P. B., Moreno, M. G., Jimenez, A. A., et al.: Isosorbide dinitrate sublingual therapy for inferior myocardial infarction: Randomized trial to assess infarct size limitation. Am. J. Cardiol. 55:330, 1985.

773. Kaplan, K. J., Taber, M., Teagarden, J. R., et al.: Association of methemoglobinemia and intravenous nitroglycerin administration. Am. J. Cardiol. 55:181, 1985.

774. Jugdutt, B. I., and Warnica, J. W.: Tolerance with low dose intravenous nitroglycerin therapy in acute myocardial infarction. Am. J. Cardiol. 64:581, 1989.

775. Levy, W. E., Katz, R. J., Ruffalo, R. L., et al.: Potentiation of the hemodynamic effects of acutely administered nitroglycerin by methionine. Circulation 78:640, 1988.

776. Opie, L. H., Frishman, W. H., and Thandani, U.: Calcium channel antagonists (Calcium entry blockers). In Opie, L. H. (ed.): Drugs for the Heart. Philadelphia, W. B. Saunders Co., 1995, p. 50.

777. Messerli, F. H.: "Cardioprotection"—Not all calcium antagonists are created equal. Am. J. Cardiol. 66:855, 1990.

777a. Moss, A. J.: Acute myocardial infarction: Role of calcium channel blockers. In Fuster, V., Ross, R., and Topol, E. J. (eds.): Atherosclerosis and Coronary Artery Disease. Philadelphia, Lippincott-Raven, 1996, pp. 1215–1222.

778. Muller, J., Morrison, J., Stone, P. H., et al.: Nifedipine therapy for patients with threatened and acute myocardial infarction: A randomized, double-blind, placebo-controlled comparison. Circulation 69:740, 1984.

779. Sirnes, P. A., Overskeid, K., Pederson, T. R., et al.: Evolution of infarct size during the early use of nifedipine in patients with acute myocardial infarction: The Norwegian Nifedipine Multicenter Trial. Circulation 70:738, 1984.

780. Branagan, J. P., Walsh, K., Kelly, P., et al.: Effect of early treatment with nifedipine in suspected acute myocardial infarction. Eur. Heart J. 7:859, 1986.

781. Gottlieb, S. O., Becker, L. C., Weiss, J. L., et al.: Nifedipine in acute myocardial infarction: An assessment of left ventricular function, infarct size, and infarct expansion: A double blind, randomised, placebo controlled trial. Br. Heart J. 59:411, 1988.

782. Skolnick, A. E., and Frishman, W. H.: Calcium channel blockers in myocardial infarction. Arch. Intern. Med. 149:1669, 1989.

783. Yusuf, S.: Calcium antagonists in coronary artery disease and hypertension: Time for reevaluation? Circulation 92:1079, 1995.

784. Opie, L. H., and Messerli, R. H.: Nifedipine and mortality: Grave defects in the dossier. Circulation 92:1068, 1995.

785. Kloner, R. A.: Nifedipine in ischemic heart disease. Circulation 92:1074, 1995.

786. Erbel, R., Pop, T., Meinertz, T., et al.: Combination of calcium channel blocker and thrombolytic therapy in acute myocardial infarction. Am. Heart J. 115:529, 1988.

787. Report of the Holland Interuniversity Nifedipine/Metoprolol Trial Research Group: Early treatment of unstable angina in the coronary care unit: A randomised, double-blind, placebo-controlled comparison of recurrent ischaemia and thrombolytic therapy in patients treated with nifedipine or metoprolol or both. Br. Heart J. 56:400, 1986.

788. The Danish Study Group on Verapamil in Myocardial Infarction: Verapamil in acute myocardial infarction. Eur. Heart J. 54:516, 1984.

789. Gibson, R. S., Boden, W. E., Theroux, P., et al.: Diltiazem and reinfarction in patients with non-Q wave myocardial infarction: Results of a double-blind, randomized, multicenter trial. N. Engl. J. Med. 315:423, 1986.

790. Hansen, J. F.: Treatment with verapamil after an acute myocardial infarction: Review of the Danish studies on verapamil in myocardial infarction (DAVIT I and II). Drugs 2:43, 1991.

791. Hansen, J. F.: Calcium antagonists and myocardial infarction. Cardiovasc. Drugs Ther. 5:665, 1991.

792. The Multicenter Diltiazem Postinfarction Trial Research Group: The effect of diltiazem on mortality and reinfarction after acute myocardial infarction. N. Engl. J. Med. 319:385, 1988.

793. The Danish Study Group on Verapamil in Myocardial Infarction: Effect of verapamil on mortality and major events after acute infarction (the Danish Verapamil Infarction Trial II-DAVIT II). Am. J. Cardiol. 66:779, 1990.

794. Arsenian, M. A.: Magnesium and cardiovascular disease. Prog. Cardiovasc. Dis. 35:271, 1993.

795. Flink, E. B., Brick, J. E., and Shane, S. R.: Alterations of long-chain free fatty acid and magnesium concentrations in acute myocardial infarction. Arch. Intern. Med. 141:441, 1981.

796. Antman, E.: Randomized trials of magnesium for acute myocardial infarction: Big numbers do not tell the whole story. Am. J. Cardiol. 75:391, 1995.

797. Woods, K. L.: Possible pharmacological actions of magnesium in acute myocardial infarction. Br. J. Clin. Pharmacol. 32:3, 1991.

798. Shechter, M., Kaplinsky, E., and Rabinowitz, B.: The rationale of magnesium supplementation in acute myocardial infarction: A review of the literature. Arch. Intern. Med. 152:2189, 1992.

799. Teo, K. K., and Yusuf, S.: Role of magnesium in reducing mortality in acute myocardial infarction: A review of the evidence. Drugs 46:347, 1993.

800. Woods, K. L., and Fletcher, S.: Long-term outcome after intravenous magnesium sulphate in suspected acute myocardial infarction: The second Leicester Intravenous Magnesium Intervention Trial (LIMIT-2). Lancet 343:816, 1994.

801. Woods, K. L.: Mega-trials and management of acute myocardial infarction. Lancet 346:611, 1995.

802. Antman, E., Lau, J., Berkey, C., et al.: Large versus small trials of magnesium for acute myocardial infarction: Big numbers do not tell the whole story. Circulation 90(Suppl. I):325, 1994.

803. Shechter, M., Hod, H., Kaplinsky, E., et al.: Magnesium therapy in acute myocardial infarction when patients are not candidates for thrombolytic therapy. Am. J. Cardiol. 75:321, 1995.

804. Mantle, J. A., Rogers, W. J., McDaniel, H. G., et al.: Metabolic support of mechanical performance in myocardial infarction in man—a randomized clinical trial of glucose-insulin-potassium. Am. J. Cardiol. 43:395, 1979.

805. Rogers, W. J., Segall, P. H., McDaniel, H. G., et al.: Prospective randomized trial of glucose-insulin-potassium in acute myocardial infarction. Am. J. Cardiol. 43:801, 1979.

806. Heng, M. K., Norris, R. M., Singh, B. N., et al.: Effects of glucose and glucose-insulin-potassium on haemodynamics and enzyme release after acute myocardial infarction. Br. Heart J. 39:748, 1977.

807. Malmberg, K., Ryden, L., Efendic, S., et al.: Randomized trial of insu-

lin-glucose infusion followed by subcutaneous insulin treatment in diabetic patients with acute myocardial infarction (DIGAMI Study): Effects on mortality at 1 year. J. Am. Coll. Cardiol. 26:57, 1995.

808. Leinbach, R. C., Gold, H. K., Harper, R. W., et al.: Early intraaortic balloon pumping for anterior myocardial infarction without shock. Circulation 58:204, 1978.

809. Alderman, J. D., Gabliani, G. I., McCabe, C. H., et al.: Incidence and management of limb ischemia with percutaneous wire-guided intraaortic balloon catheters. J. Am. Coll. Cardiol. 9:524, 1987.

810. Herbaczynska-Cedro, K., Klosiewicz-Wasek, B., Cedro, K., et al.: Supplementation with vitamins C and E suppresses leukocyte oxygen free radical production in patients with myocardial infarction. Eur. Heart J. 16:1044, 1995.

811. Guarnieri, C., Giordano, E., Muscari, C., et al.: Vitamin E can protect myocardium against oxidative damage. Cardiovasc. Res. 30:153, 1995.

812. Klein, H. H.: Vitamin E cannot protect myocardium against oxidative damage. Cardiovasc. Res. 30:156, 1995.

813. Williams, M. W., Taft, C. S., Ramnauth, S., et al.: Endogenous nitric oxide (NO) protects against ischaemia-reperfusion injury in the rabbit. Cardiovasc. Res. 30:79, 1995.

HEMODYNAMIC DISTURBANCES

814. Rackley, C. E., Satler, L. F., Pearle, D. L., et al.: Use of hemodynamic measurements for management of acute myocardial infarction. In Rackley, C. E. (ed.): Advances in Critical Care Cardiology. Philadelphia, F. A. Davis Co., 1986, p. 3.

815. Gewirtz, H., Gold, H. K., Fallon, J. T., et al.: Role of right ventricular infarction in cardiogenic shock associated with inferior myocardial infarction. Br. Heart J. 42:719, 1979.

816. Swan, H. J. C., Ganz, W., Forrester, J. S., et al.: Catheterization of the heart in man with use of a flow-directed balloon-tipped catheter. N. Engl. J. Med. 283:447, 1970.

817. Forrester, J. S., Diamond, G., Chatterjee, K., et al.: Medical therapy of acute myocardial infarction by application of hemodynamic subsets. N. Engl. J. Med. 295:1356, 1976.

818. Paglairello, G.: The Pulmonary Artery (Swan-Ganz) Catheter. Int. J. Technol. Assess. Health Care 9:202, 1993.

818a. Ganz, W., Shah, P. K., and Forrester, J. S.: Acute myocardial infarction: The role of hemodynamic assessment. In Fuster, V., Ross, R., and Topol, E. J. (eds.): Atherosclerosis and Coronary Artery Disease. Philadelphia, Lippincott-Raven, 1996, pp. 895–904.

819. Goldenheim, P. D., and Kazemi, H.: Cardiopulmonary monitoring of critically ill patients. N. Engl. J. Med. 311:776, 1984.

820. Eisenberg, P. R., Jaffe, A. S., and Schuster, D. P.: Clinical evaluation compared to pulmonary artery catheterization in the hemodynamic assessment of critically ill patients. Crit. Care Med. 12:549, 1984.

821. Robin, E. D.: The cult of the Swan-Ganz catheter. Ann. Intern. Med. 103:445, 1985.

822. Robin, E. D.: Death by pulmonary artery flow-directed catheter: Time for a moratorium? Chest 92:727, 1987.

823. Gore, J. M., Goldberg, R. J., Spodick, D. H., et al.: A community-wide assessment of the use of pulmonary artery catheters in patients with acute myocardial infarction. Chest 92:721, 1987.

824. Noble, R. J.: Myocardial infarction with hypotension. Chest 99:1012, 1991.

825. Coma-Canella, I. L.-S. J., and Gamallo, C.: Low output syndrome in right ventricular infarction. Am. Heart J. 98:613, 1979.

826. Rasanen, J., Nikki, O. P., and Heikkila, J.: Acute myocardial infarction complicated by respiratory failure: The effects of mechanical ventilation. Chest 85:21, 1984.

827. Cohn, J. N., Franciosa, J. A., Francis, G. S., et al.: Effect of short-term infusion on sodium nitroprusside in mortality rate in acute myocardial infarction complicated by left ventricular failure: Results of a Veterans Administration Cooperative Study. N. Engl. J. Med. 306:1129, 1982.

828. Passamani, E. R.: Nitroprusside in myocardial infarction. N. Engl. J. Med. 306:1168, 1982.

829. Chiariello, M., Gold, H. K., Leinbach, R. C., et al.: Comparison between the effects of nitroprusside and nitroglycerin on ischemic injury during acute myocardial infarction. Circulation 54:766, 1976.

830. Flaherty, J. T.: Intravenous nitroglycerin. Johns Hopkins Med. J. 151:36, 1982.

831. Rabinowitz, B., Tamari, I., Elazar, E., et al.: Intravenous isosorbide dinitrate in patients with refractory pump failure and acute myocardial infarction. Circulation 65:771, 1982.

832. Cohn, J. N.: Editorial—Progress in vasodilator therapy for heart failure. N. Engl. J. Med. 302:1414, 1980.

833. Franciosa, J. A., Mikulic, E., Cohn, J. N., et al.: Hemodynamic effects of orally administered isosorbide dinitrate in patients with congestive heart failure. Circulation 50:1020, 1974.

834. Chiariello, M., Gold, H. K., Leinbach, R. C., et al.: Comparison between the effects of nitroprusside and nitroglycerin on ischemic injury during acute myocardial infarction. Circulation 54:766, 1976.

835. Derrida, J. P., Sal, R., and Chiche, P.: Favorable effects of prolonged nitroglycerin infusion in patients with acute myocardial infarction. Am. Heart J. 96:833, 1978.

836. Covell, J. W., Braunwald, E., and Ross, J., et al.: Studies on digitalis XVI: Effects on myocardial oxygen consumption. J. Clin. Invest. 45:1535, 1966.

837. Ross, J. J., Waldhausen, J. S., and Braunwald, E.: Studies on digitalis.

I. Direct effects on peripheral vascular resistance. J. Clin. Invest. 39:930, 1960.

838. Marchionni, N., Pini, R., Vanucci, A., et al.: Hemodynamic effects of digoxin in acute myocardial infarction in man: A randomized controlled trial. Am. Heart J. 109:63, 1985.

839. Bonaduce, D., Petretta, M., Arrichiello, P., et al.: Effects of captopril treatment on left ventricular remodeling and function after anterior myocardial infarction: Comparison with digitalis. J. Am. Coll. Cardiol. 19:858, 1992.

840. Moss, A. J., Davis, H. T., Conard, D. L., et al.: Digitalis-associated cardiac mortality after myocardial infarction. Circulation 64:1150, 1981.

841. Ryan, T. J., Bailey, K. R., McCabe, C. H., et al.: The effects of digitalis on survival in high-risk patients with coronary artery disease. Circulation 67:735, 1983.

842. Digitalis Subcommittee of the Multicenter Post-Infarction Research Group: The mortality risk associated with digitalis treatment after myocardial infarction. Cardiovasc. Drugs Ther. 1:125, 1987.

843. Mølstad, P., and Abdelnoor, M.: Digitoxin-associated mortality in acute myocardial infarction. Eur. Heart J. 12:65, 1991.

844. Køber, L., Torp-Pedersen, C., Hildebrandt, C., et al.: Digoxin is an independent risk factor for long term mortality after acute myocardial infarction. Eur. Heart J. 13(Suppl.):1897, 1992.

845. Bigger, J. T., Fleiss, J. L., Rolnitzky, L. M., et al.: Effect of digitalis treatment on survival after acute myocardial infarction. Am. J. Cardiol. 55:623, 1985.

846. Muller, J. E., Turi, Z. G., Stone, P. H., et al.: Digoxin therapy and mortality after myocardial infarction: Experience in the MILIS Study. N. Engl. J. Med. 314:265, 1986.

847. Mølstad, P.: Digitalis in patients after myocardial infarction. Herz 18:118, 1993.

848. Mueller, H., Ayres, S. M., Giannelli, S., et al.: Effect of isoproterenol, 1-norepinephrine, and intra-aortic counterpulsation on hemodynamics and myocardial metabolism in shock following acute myocardial infarction. Circulation 45:335, 1972.

849. Shell, W. E., and Sobel, B. E.: Deleterious effects of increased heart rate on infarct size in the conscious dog. Am. J. Cardiol. 31:474, 1973.

850. Ichard, C., Ricome, J. L., Rimailho, A., et al.: Combined hemodynamic effects of dopamine and dobutamine in cardiogenic shock. Circulation 67:620, 1983.

851. Holzer, J., Karliner, J. S., O'Rourke, R. A., et al.: Effectiveness of dopamine in patients with cardiogenic shock. Am. J. Cardiol. 32:79, 1973.

852. Tuttle, R. R., and Mills, J.: Development of a new catecholamine to selectively increase cardiac contractility. Circ. Res. 36:185, 1975.

853. Maekawa, K., Liang, C. S., Hood, W. B. J., et al.: Comparison of dobutamine and dopamine in acute myocardial infarction: Effects of systemic hemodynamics, plasma catecholamines, blood flows and infarct size. Circulation 67:750, 1983.

854. DiBianco, R.: Acute positive inotropic intervention: The phosphodiesterase inhibitors. Am. Heart J. 121:1871, 1991.

855. Sherry, K. M., and Locke, T. J.: Use of milrinone in cardiac surgical patients. Cardiovasc. Drugs Ther. 7:671, 1993.

856. Wynands, J. E.: The role of amrinone in treating heart failure during and after coronary artery surgery supported by cardiopulmonary bypass. J. Cardiac Surg. 9:453, 1994.

857. Verma, S. P., Silke, B., Reynolds, G. W., et al.: Modulation of inotropic therapy by venodilation in acute heart failure: A randomised comparison of four inotropic agents, alone and combined with isosorbide dinitrate. J. Cardiovasc. Pharmacol. 19:24, 1992.

858. Taylor, S. H., Verma, S. P., Hussain, M., et al.: Intravenous amrinone in left ventricular failure complicated by acute myocardial infarction. Am. J. Cardiol. 56:29B, 1985.

859. Verma, S. P. S. B., and Taylor, S. H.: Hemodynamic dose-response effects of amrinone in left ventricular failure complicating myocardial infarction. Br. J. Clin. Pharmacol. 19:540P, 1985.

860. Colucci, W. S., Wright, R. F., and Braunwald, E.: New positive inotropic agents in the treatment of congestive heart failure. N. Engl. J. Med. 314:349, 1986.

860a. O'Gara, P. T.: Acute myocardial infarction: Primary pump failure. In Fuster, V., Ross, R., and Topol, E. J. (eds.): Atherosclerosis and Coronary Artery Disease. Philadelphia, Lippincott-Raven, 1996, pp. 1051–1064.

CARDIOGENIC SHOCK

861. Scheidt, S., Ascheim, R., and Killip, T.: Shock after acute myocardial infarction: A clinical and hemodynamic profile. Am. J. Cardiol. 26:556, 1970.

862. Goldberg, R. J., Gore, J. M., Alpert, J. S., et al.: Cardiogenic shock after acute myocardial infarction: Incidence and mortality from a community-wide perspective, 1975 to 1988. N. Engl. J. Med. 325:1117, 1991.

863. Hochman, J. S., and LeJemetel, T.: Management of cardiogenic shock. In Julian, D. G., and Braunwald, E. (eds.): Management of Acute Myocardial Infarction. London, W. B. Saunders Ltd., 1994, p. 267.

864. Hands, M. E., Rutherford, J. D., Muller, J. E., et al.: The in-hospital development of cardiogenic shock after myocardial infarction: Incidence, predictors of occurrence, outcome and prognostic factors. J. Am. Coll. Cardiol. 14:40, 1989.

865. Wackers, F. J., Lie, K. I., Becker, A. E., et al.: Coronary artery disease in patients dying from cardiogenic shock or congestive heart failure in the setting of acute myocardial infarction. Br. Heart J. 38:906, 1976.

866. Page, D. L., Caulfield, J. B., Kastor, J. A., et al.: Myocardial changes associated with cardiogenic shock. N. Engl. J. Med. 285:133, 1971.

867. Alonso, D. R., Scheidt, S., Post, M., et al.: Pathophysiology of cardiogenic shock: Quantification of myocardial necrosis, clinical, pathologic and electrocardiographic correlation. Circulation 48:588, 1973.

868. Mueller, H., Ayres, S. M., Gregory, J. J., et al.: Hemodynamics, coronary blood flow, and myocardial metabolism in coronary shock: Response to L-norepinephrine and isoproterenol. J. Clin. Invest. 49:1885, 1970.

869. Mueller, H., Ayres, S. M., Conklin, E. F., et al.: The effects of intraaortic counterpulsation on cardiac performance and metabolism in shock associated with acute myocardial infarction. J. Clin. Invest. 50:1885, 1971.

870. Johnson, S. A., Scanlon, P. J., Loeb, H. S., et al.: Treatment of cardiogenic shock in myocardial infarction by intraaortic balloon counterpulsation and surgery. Am. J. Med. 62:687, 1977.

871. O'Rourke, M. F., Norris, R. M., Campbell, T. J., et al.: Randomized controlled trial of intraaortic balloon counterpulsation in early myocardial infarction with acute heart failure. Am. J. Cardiol. 47:815, 1981.

872. Corral, C. H., and Vaughn, C. C.: Intraaortic balloon counterpulsation: An eleven-year review and analysis of determinants of survival. Texas Heart Inst. J. 13:39, 1986.

873. Goldberg, M. J., Rubenfire, M., Kantrowitz, A., et al.: Intraaortic balloon pump insertion: A randomized study comparing percutaneous and surgical techniques. J. Am. Coll. Cardiol. 9:515, 1987.

874. Isner, J. M., Cohen, S. J., Viruari, R., et al.: Complications of the intraaortic balloon counterpulsation device: Clinical and morphologic observations in 45 necropsy patients. Am. J. Cardiol. 45:260, 1980.

875. Bates, E. R., and Topol, E. J.: Limitations of thrombolytic therapy for acute myocardial infarction complicated by congestive heart failure and cardiogenic shock. J. Am. Coll. Cardiol. 18:1077, 1991.

876. Eltchaninoff, H., Simpfendorfer, C., Franco, I., et al.: Early and 1-year survival rates in acute myocardial infarction complicated by cardiogenic shock: A retrospective study comparing coronary angioplasty with medical treatment. Am. Heart J. 130:459, 1995.

877. Danis, M., Patrick, D. L., Southerland, L. I., et al.: Patients' and families' preferences for medical intensive care. JAMA 260:797, 1988.

878. Champagnac, D., Claudel, J. P., Chevalier, P., et al.: Primary cardiogenic shock during acute myocardial infarction: Results of emergency cardiac transplantation. Eur. Heart J. 14:925, 1993.

879. Pae, W. E., Jr., and Pierce, W. S.: Temporary left ventricular assistance in acute myocardial infarction and cardiogenic shock: Rationale and criteria for utilization. Chest 79:692, 1981.

880. Shawl, F. A., Domanski, M. J., Hernandez, T. J., et al.: Emergency percutaneous cardiopulmonary bypass support in cardiogenic shock from acute myocardial infarction. Am. J. Cardiol. 64:967, 1989.

RIGHT VENTRICULAR INFARCTION

881. Shah, P. K., Maddahi, J., Berman, D. S., et al.: Scintigraphically detected predominant right ventricular dysfunction in acute myocardial infarction: Clinical and hemodynamic correlates and implications for therapy and prognosis. J. Am. Coll. Cardiol. 6:1264, 1985.

882. O'Rourke, R. A., and Dell'Italia, L. J.: Right ventricular myocardial infarction. In Fuster, V., Ross, R., and Topol, E. J. (eds.): Atherosclerosis and Coronary Artery Disease. Philadelphia, Lippincott-Raven, 1996, pp. 1079–1096.

883. Forman, M. B., Goodin, J., Phelan, B., et al.: Electrocardiographic changes associated with isolated right ventricular infarction. J. Am. Coll. Cardiol. 4:640, 1984.

884. Roberts, N., Harrison, D. G., Reimer, K. A., et al.: Right ventricular infarction with shock but without significant left ventricular infarction: A new clinical syndrome. Am. Heart J. 110:1047, 1985.

885. Bansal, R. C., Marsa, R. J., Holland, D., et al.: Severe hypoxemia due to shunting through a patent foramen ovale: A correctable complication of right ventricular infarction. J. Am. Coll. Cardiol. 5:188, 1985.

886. Candell-Riera, J., Figueras, J., Valle, V., et al.: Right ventricular infarction: Relationships between ST segment elevation in V4$_R$ and hemodynamic, scintigraphic, and echocardiographic findings in patients with acute inferior myocardial infarction. Am. Heart J. 101:281, 1981.

887. Braat, S. H., Brugada, P., De Zwaan, C., et al.: Value of electrocardiogram in diagnosing right ventricular involvement in patients with an acute inferior wall myocardial infarction. Br. Heart J. 49:368, 1983.

888. Lopez-Sendon, J., Garcia-Fernandez, M. A., Coma-Canella, I., et al.: Segmental right ventricular function after acute myocardial infarction: Two-dimensional echocardiographic study in 63 patients. Am. J. Cardiol. 51:390, 1983.

889. Arditti, A., Lewin, R. F., Hellman, C., et al.: Right ventricular dysfunction in acute inferoposterior myocardial infarction: An echocardiographic isotopic study. Chest 87:307, 1985.

890. Starling, M. R., Dell'Italia, L. J., Chaudhuri, T. K., et al.: First transit and equilibrium radionuclide angiography in patients with inferior transmural myocardial infarction: Criteria for the diagnosis of associated hemodynamically significant right ventricular infarction. J. Am. Coll. Cardiol. 4:923, 1984.

891. Dell'Italia, L. J., Starling, M. R., Crawford, M. H., et al.: Right ventricular infarction: Identification by hemodynamic measurements before and after volume loading and correlation with noninvasive techniques. J. Am. Coll. Cardiol. 4:931, 1984.

892. Topol, E. J., Goldshlager, N., Ports, T. A., et al.: Hemodynamic benefit of atrial pacing in right ventricular myocardial infarction. Ann. Intern. Med. 96:594, 1982.

893. Marmor, A., Geltman, E. M., Biello, D. R., et al.: Functional response

of the right ventricle to myocardial infarction: Dependence on the site of left ventricular infarction. Circulation 64:1005, 1981.

894. Lorell, B., Leinbach, R. C., Pohost, G. M., et al.: Right ventricular infarction: Clinical diagnosis and differentiation from cardiac tamponade and pericardial constriction. Am. J. Cardiol. 43:465, 1979.

MECHANICAL CAUSES OF HEART FAILURE

895. Reeder, G. S.: Identification and treatment of complications of myocardial infarction. Lancet 70:880, 1995.

895a. Kuhn, F. E., and Gersh, B. J.: Acute myocardial infarction: Mechanical complications. In Fuster, V., Ross, R., and Topol, E. J. (eds.): Atherosclerosis and Coronary Artery Disease. Philadelphia, Lippincott-Raven, 1996, pp. 1065–1079.

896. Pohjola-Sintonen, S., Muller, J. E., Stone, P. H., et al.: Ventricular septal and free wall rupture complicating acute myocardial infarction: Experience in the Multicenter Limitation of Infarct Size. Am. Heart J. 117:809, 1989.

897. Reddy, S. G., and Roberts, W. C.: Frequency of rupture of the left ventricular free wall or ventricular septum among necropsy cases of fatal acute myocardial infarction since introduction of coronary care units. Am. J. Cardiol. 63:906, 1989.

898. Pappas, P. J., Cernaianu, A. C., Baldino, W. A., et al.: Ventricular free-wall rupture after myocardial infarction. Chest 99:892, 1991.

899. Bulkley, B. H., and Roberts, W. C.: Steroid therapy during acute myocardial infarction: A cause of delayed healing and of ventricular aneurysm. Am. J. Med. 56:244, 1974.

900. Silverman, H. W., and Pfeifer, M. P.: Relation between use of anti-inflammatory agents and left ventricular free wall rupture during acute myocardial infarction. Am. J. Cardiol. 59:363, 1987.

901. Shapira, I., Isakov, A., Burke, M., et al.: Cardiac rupture in patients with acute myocardial infarction. Chest 92:219, 1987.

902. Becker, R., Charlesworth, A., Wilcox, R., et al.: Late thrombolysis accelerates the onset of cardiac rupture. Circulation 90(Suppl. I):563, 1994.

903. Edmondson, H. A., and Hoxie, H. J.: Hypertension and cardiac rupture: Clinical and pathological study of 72 cases, in 13 of which rupture of the interventricular septum occurred. Am. Heart J. 24:719, 1942.

904. London, R. E., and London, S. B.: Rupture of the heart: A critical analysis of 47 consecutive autopsy cases. Circulation 31:202, 1965.

905. Kassis, E., Vogelsang, M., and Lyngoborg, K.: Cardiac rupture complicating myocardial infarction: A study concerning early diagnosis and possible management. Dan. Med. Bull. 48:164, 1981.

906. Mann, J. M., and Roberts, W. C.: Rupture of the left ventricular free wall during acute myocardial infarction: Analysis of 138 necropsy patients and comparison with 50 necropsy patients with acute myocardial infarction without rupture. Am. J. Cardiol. 62:847, 1988.

907. Schuster, E. H., and Bulkley, B. H.: Expansion of transmural myocardial infarction: A pathophysiologic factor in cardiac rupture. Circulation 60:1532, 1979.

908. Oliva, P. B., Hammill, S. C., and Edwards, W. D.: Cardiac rupture, a clinically predictable complication of acute myocardial infarction: Report of 70 cases with clinicopathologic correlations. J. Am. Coll. Cardiol. 22:720, 1993.

909. Vlodaver, Z., Coe, J. L., and Edwards, J. E.: True and false left ventricular aneurysms. Circulation 51:567, 1975.

910. Lascault, G., Reeves, F., and Drobinski, G.: Evidence of the inaccuracy of standard echocardiographic and angiographic criteria used for the recognition of true and "false" left ventricular inferior aneurysms. Br. Heart J. 60:125, 1988.

911. Lundberg, S., and Soderstrom, J.: Perforation of the interventricular septum in myocardial infarction. Acta Med. Scand. 172:413, 1962.

912. Held, A. C., Cole, P. L., Lipton, B., et al.: Rupture of the interventricular septum complicating acute myocardial infarction: A multicenter analysis of clinical findings and outcome. Am. Heart J. 116:1330, 1988.

913. Camacho, M. T., Muehrcke, D. D., and Loop, F. D.: Mechanical complications. In Julian, D., and Braunwald, E. (eds.): Management of Acute Myocardial Infarction. London, W. B. Saunders Ltd., 1994, p. 291.

914. Westaby, S., Parry, A., Ormerod, O., et al.: Thrombolysis and postinfarction ventricular septal rupture. J. Thorac. Cardiovasc. Surg. 104:1506, 1992.

915. Edwards, B. S., Edwards, W. D., and Edwards, J. E.: Ventricular septal rupture complicating acute myocardial infarction: Identification of simple and complex types in 53 autopsied hearts. Am. J. Cardiol. 54:1201, 1984.

916. Mann, J. M., and Roberts, W. C.: Acquired ventricular septal defect during acute myocardial infarction: Analysis of 38 unoperated necropsy patients and comparison with 50 unoperated necropsy patients without rupture. Am. J. Cardiol. 62:8, 1988.

917. Lemery, R., Smith, H. C., Giuliani, E. R., et al.: Prognosis in rupture of the ventricular septum after acute myocardial infarction and role of early surgical intervention. Am. J. Cardiol. 70:147, 1992.

918. Cummings, R. G., Reimer, K. A., Califf, R., et al.: Quantitative analysis of right and left ventricular infarction in the presence of postinfarction ventricular septal defect. Circulation 77:33, 1988.

919. Radford, M. J., Johnson, R. A., Daggett, W. M., Jr., et al.: Ventricular septal rupture: A review of clinical and physiologic features and an analysis of survival. Circulation 64:545, 1981.

920. Moore, C. A., Nygaard, T. W., Kaiser, D. L., et al.: Postinfarction ventricular septal rupture: The importance of location of infarction and

right ventricular function in determining survival. Circulation 74:45, 1986.

921. Bansal, R. C., Eng, A. K., and Shakudo, M.: Role of two-dimensional echocardiography, pulsed, continuous wave and color flow Doppler techniques in the assessment of ventricular septal rupture after myocardial infarction. Am. J. Cardiol. 65:852, 1990.

922. Helmcke, F., Mahan, E. F., Nanda, N. C., et al.: Two-dimensional echocardiography and Doppler color flow mapping in the diagnosis and prognosis of ventricular septal rupture. Circulation 81:1775, 1990.

923. Fortin, D. G., Sheikh, K.H., and Kisslo, J.: The utility of echocardiography in the diagnostic strategy of postinfarction ventricular septal rupture: A comparison of two-dimensional echocardiography versus Doppler color flow imaging. Am. Heart J. 121:25, 1991.

924. Lock, J. E., Block, P. C., McKay, R. G., et al.: Transcatheterization closure of ventricular septal defects. Circulation 78:361, 1988.

925. Chwa, E., Gonzalez, A., Bahr, R. D., et al.: Papillary muscle rupture: A reversible cause of cardiogenic shock. Maryland Med. J. 41:893, 1992.

926. Manning, W. J., Waksmonski, C. A., and Boyle, N. G.: Papillary muscle rupture complicating inferior myocardial infarction: Identification with transesophageal echocardiography. Am. Heart J. 129:191, 1995.

927. Barbour, D. J., and Roberts, W. C.: Rupture of a left ventricular papillary muscle during acute myocardial infarction: Analysis of 22 necropsy patients. J. Am. Coll. Cardiol. 8:588, 1986.

928. Coma-Canella, I., Gamallo, C., Onsurve, P. M., et al.: Anatomic findings in acute papillary muscle necrosis. Am. Heart J. 118:1188, 1989.

929. Nishimura, R. A., Schaff, H. V., Shub, C., et al.: Papillary muscle rupture complicating acute myocardial infarction. Am. J. Cardiol. 51:373, 1983.

930. Lader, E., Colvin, S., and Tunick, P.: Myocardial infarction complicated by rupture of both ventricular septum and right ventricular papillary muscle. Am. J. Cardiol. 52:424, 1983.

931. Come, P. C., Riley, M. F., Weintraub, R., et al.: Echocardiographic detection of complete and partial papillary muscle rupture during acute myocardial infarction. Am. J. Cardiol. 56:787, 1985.

932. Buda, A. J.: The role of echocardiography in the evaluation of mechanical complications of acute myocardial infarction. Circulation 84:1109, 1991.

933. Sharma, S. K., Seckler, J., Israel, D. H., et al.: Clinical, angiographic and anatomic findings in acute severe ischemic mitral regurgitation. Am. J. Cardiol. 70:277, 1992.

934. Shah, P. K., and Francis, G. S.: Pump failure, shock, and cardiac rupture in acute myocardial infarction. In Francis, G. S., and Alpert, J. S. (eds.): Coronary Care. Boston, Little, Brown and Company, 1995, p. 289.

935. Goldman, A. P., Glover, M. U., Mick, W., et al.: Role of echocardiography/Doppler in cardiogenic shock: Silent mitral regurgitation. Ann. Thorac. Surg. 52:296, 1991.

936. Jones, M. T., Schofield, P. M., Dark, J. F., et al.: Surgical repair of acquired ventricular septal defects: Determinants of early and late outcome. J. Thorac. Cardiovasc. Surg. 93:680, 1987.

937. Dresdale, A. R., and Paone, G.: Surgical treatment of acute myocardial infarction. Henry Ford Hosp. Med. J. 39:245, 1991.

VENTRICULAR ARRHYTHMIAS

938. Pantridge, J. F., and Adgey, A. A. J.: Pre-hospital coronary care: The mobile coronary care unit. Am. J. Cardiol. 24:666, 1969.

939. Meltzer, L. E., and Cohen, H. E.: The incidence of arrhythmias associated with acute myocardial infarction. In Meltzer, L. E., and Dunning, A. J. (eds.): Textbook of Coronary Care. Philadelphia, Charles Press, 1972.

940. Norris, N. M.: Myocardial Infarction. New York, Churchill-Livingstone, 1982, p. 322.

940a. Kidwell, G. A., and Chung, M. K.: Ischemic ventricular arrhythmias. In Fuster, V., Ross, R., and Topol, E. J. (eds.): Atherosclerosis and Coronary Artery Disease. Philadelphia, Lippincott-Raven, 1996, pp. 995–1012.

941. Corr, P. B., and Gillis, R. A.: Autonomic neural influences on the dysrhythmias resulting from myocardial infarction. Circ. Res. 43:1, 1978.

942. Barber, M. J., Mueller, T. M., Davies, B. G., et al.: Interruption of sympathetic and vagal-mediated afferent responses by transmural myocardial infarction. Circulation 72:623, 1985.

943. Bloor, C. M., Ehsani, A., White, F. C., et al.: Ventricular fibrillation threshold in acute myocardial infarction and its relation to myocardial infarct size. Cardiovasc. Res. 9:468, 1975.

944. Geltman, E. M., Ehsani, A. A., Campbell, M. K., et al.: The influence of location and extent of myocardial infarction on long-term ventricular dysrhythmia and mortality. Circulation 60:805, 1979.

945. Roque, F., Amuchastegui, L. M., Lopez Morillos, M. A., et al.: Beneficial effects of timolol on infarct size and late ventricular tachycardia in patients with myocardial infarction. Circulation 76:610, 1987.

946. Lassers, B. E., Anderton, J. L., George, M., et al.: Hemodynamic effects of artificial pacing in complete heart block complicating acute myocardial infarction. Circulation 38:308, 1968.

947. Ruskin, J., McHale, P. A., Harley, A., et al.: Pressure-flow studies in man: Effects of atrial systole on left ventricular function. J. Clin. Invest. 49:472, 1970.

948. Rahimtoola, S. H., Ehsani, A., Sinno, M. Z., et al.: Left atrial transport function in myocardial infarction: Importance of its booster function. Am. J. Med. 59:686, 1975.

949. El-Sherif, N., Myerburg, R. J., Scherlag, B. J., et al.: Electrocardiographic antecedents of primary ventricular fibrillation: Value of the R-on-T phenomenon in myocardial infarction. Br. Heart J. 38:415, 1976.

950. Weinberg, B., and Zipes, D.: Strategies to manage the post-MI patient with ventricular arrhythmias. Clin. Cardiol. 12:86, 1989.

951. Lee, K. J., Wellens, H. J. J., Dorsnar, E., et al.: Observations on patients with primary ventricular fibrillation complicating acute myocardial infarction. Circulation 52:755, 1975.

952. Surawicz, B.: R on T phenomenon: Dangerous and harmless. J. Appl. Cardiol. 1:39, 1986.

953. Campbell, R. W. F., Murray, A., and Julian, D. G.: Relation of ventricular arrhythmias to ventricular fibrillation. Br. Heart J. 43:109, 1980.

954. Campbell, R. W. F., Murray, A., and Julian, D. G.: Ventricular arrhythmias in first 12 hours of acute myocardial infarction: Natural history study. Br. Heart J. 46:351, 1981.

955. Antman, E. M., and Berlin, J. A.: Declining incidence of ventricular fibrillation in myocardial infarction: Implications for the use of lidocaine. Circulation 84:764, 1992.

956. Hine, L. K., Laird, N., Hewitt, P., et al.: Meta-analytic evidence against prophylactic use of lidocaine in acute myocardial infarction. Arch. Intern. Med. 149:2694, 1989.

957. Hjalmarson, A., Herlitz, J., Holmberg, S., et al.: The Goteborg metoprolol trial: Effects on mortality and morbidity in acute myocardial infarction. Circulation 67:26, 1983.

958. Yusuf, S., Sleight, P., Rossi, P., et al.: Reduction in infarct size, arrhythmias and chest pain by early intravenous beta blockade in suspected acute myocardial infarction. Circulation 67:12, 1983.

959. Norris, R. M., Barnaby, P. F., Brown, M. A., et al.: Prevention of ventricular fibrillation during acute myocardial infarction by intravenous propranolol. Lancet 2:883, 1984.

960. Gressin, V., Gorgels, A., Louvard, Y., et al.: ST-segment normalization time and ventricular arrhythmias as electrocardiographic markers of reperfusion during intravenous thrombolysis for acute myocardial infarction. Am. J. Cardiol. 71:1436, 1993.

961. Gressin, V., Gorgels, A. P., Louvard, Y., et al.: Is arrhythmogenicity related to the speed of reperfusion during thrombolysis for myocardial infarction? Eur. Heart J. 14:516, 1993.

962. Six, A. J., Louwerenburg, J. H., Kingma, J. H., et al.: Predictive value of ventricular arrhythmias for patency of the infarct-related coronary artery after thrombolytic therapy. Br. Heart J. 66:143, 1991.

963. Maggioni, A. P., Zuanetti, G., Franzosi, M. G., et al.: Prevalence and prognostic significance of ventricular arrhythmias after acute myocardial infarction in the fibrinolytic era: GISSI-2 results. Circulation 87:312, 1993.

964. Bigger, J. T., Jr., Dresdale, R. J., Heissenbuttel, R. H., et al.: Ventricular arrhythmias in ischemic heart disease: Mechanism, prevalence, significance, and management. Prog. Cardiovasc. Dis. 19:255, 1977.

965. Wolfe, C. L., Nibley, C., Bhandari, A., et al.: Polymorphous ventricular tachycardia associated with acute myocardial infarction. Circulation 84:1543, 1991.

966. Eldar, M., Sievner, Z., Goldbourt, U., et al.: Primary ventricular tachycardia in acute myocardial infarction: Clinical characteristics and mortality: The SPRINT Study Group. Ann. Intern. Med. 117:31, 1992.

967. Kleiman, R. B., Miller, J. M., Buxton, A. E., et al.: Prognosis following sustained ventricular tachycardia occurring early after myocardial infarction. Am. J. Cardiol. 62:528, 1988.

968. Nordrehaug, J. E., Johannessen, K. A., and von der Lippe, G.: Serum potassium concentration as a risk factor of ventricular arrhythmias early in acute myocardial infarction. Circulation 71:654, 1985.

969. Emergency Cardiac Care Committee and Subcommittees, American Heart Association: Guidelines for cardiopulmonary resuscitation and emergency cardiac care. III. Adult advanced cardiac life support. JAMA 268:2172, 1992.

970. Feely, J., Wade, D., McAllister, C. B., et al.: Effect of hypotension on liver blood flow and lidocaine disposition. N. Engl. J. Med. 307:866, 1982.

971. LeLorier, J., Grenon, D., Latour, Y., et al.: Pharmacokinetics of lidocaine after prolonged intravenous infusions in uncomplicated myocardial infarction. Ann. Intern. Med. 87:700, 1977.

972. Bhaskaran, A., Seth, A., Kumar, A., et al.: Coronary angioplasty for the control of intractable ventricular arrhythmia. Clin. Cardiol. 18:480, 1995.

973. Volpi, A., Maggioni, A., Franzosi, M. G., et al.: In-hospital prognosis of patients with acute myocardial infarction complicated by primary ventricular fibrillation. N. Engl. J. Med. 317:257, 1987.

974. Chiriboga, D., Yarzebski, J., Goldberg, R. J., et al.: Temporal trends (1975 through 1990) in the incidence and case-fatality rate of primary fibrillation complicating acute myocardial infarction: A community wide perspective. Circulation 89:998, 1994.

975. Volpi, A., Cavalli, A., Franzosi, M. G., et al.: One-year prognosis of primary ventricular fibrillation complicating acute myocardial infarction. Am. J. Cardiol. 63:1174, 1989.

976. Behar, S., Reicher Ress, H., Schechter, M., et al.: Frequency and prognostic significance of secondary ventricular fibrillation complicating acute myocardial infarction. Am. J. Cardiol. 71:152, 1993.

977. Jensen, G. V. H., Torp-Pedersen, C., Kober, L., et al.: Prognosis of late versus early ventricular fibrillation in acute myocardial infarction. Am. J. Cardiol. 66:10, 1990.

978. Lown, B., Fakhro, A. M., Hood, W. B., et al.: The coronary care unit: New perspectives and directions. JAMA 199:188, 1967.

979. Harrison, D. C.: Should lidocaine be administered routinely to all patients after acute myocardial infarction? Circulation 58:581, 1978.

980. MacMahon, S., Collins, R., Peto, R., et al.: Effects of prophylactic lidocaine in suspected acute myocardial infarction: An overview of results from the randomized, controlled trials. JAMA 260:1910, 1988.

981. Nordrehaug, J. E., and Lippe, G. V. D.: Hypokalemia and ventricular fibrillation in acute myocardial infarction. Br. Heart J. 50:525, 1983.

982. Higham, P. D., Adams, P. C., Murray, A., et al.: Plasma potassium, serum magnesium and ventricular fibrillation: A prospective study. Q. J. Med. 86:609, 1993.

983. Haigney, M. C. P., Silver, B., Tanglao, E., et al.: Noninvasive measurement of tissue magnesium and correlation with cardiac levels. Circulation 92:2190, 1995.

984. Bellotto, F., Forman, R., and Buja, G.: Electromechanical dissociation in the acute myocardial infarction: A review of the literature shows the need for a codified definition. J. Electrophysiol. 2:517, 1988.

985. Charlap, S., Kahlam, S., Lichstein, E., et al.: Electromechanical dissociation: Diagnosis, pathophysiology, and management. Am. Heart J. 118:355, 1989.

BRADYARRHYTHMIAS

986. Graner, L. E., Gershen, B. J., Orlando, M. M., et al.: Bradycardia and its complications in the pre-hospital phase of acute myocardial infarction. Am. J. Cardiol. 32:607, 1973.

987. Mark, A. L.: The Bezold-Jarisch reflex revisited: Clinical implications of inhibitory reflexes originating in the heart. J. Am. Coll. Cardiol. 1:90, 1983.

988. Koren, G., Weiss, A. T., Ben-David, J., et al.: Bradycardia and hypotension following reperfusion with streptokinase (Bezold-Jarish reflex): A sign of coronary thrombolysis and myocardial salvage. Am. Heart J. 112:468, 1986.

989. Come, P. C., and Pitt, B.: Nitroglycerin-induced severe hypotension and bradycardia in patients with acute myocardial infarction. Circulation 54:624, 1976.

990. Rotman, M., Wagner, G. S., and Wallace, A. G. P.: Bradyarrhythmias in acute myocardial infarction. Circulation 45:703, 1972.

991. Norris, R. M., and Mercer, C. J.: Significance of idioventricular rhythms in acute myocardial infarction. Prog. Cardiovasc. Dis. 16:455, 1974.

992. Bhandari, A. K., and Sager, P. T.: Management of peri-infarctional ventricular arrhythmias and conduction disturbances. In Naccarelli, G. V. (ed.): Cardiac Arrhythmias: A Practical Approach. Mt. Kisco, NY, Futura Publishing, 1991, p. 283.

993. Fisch, J. R., Zipes, D. P., and Fisch, C.: Bundle branch block in sudden death. Prog. Cardiovasc. Dis. 23:187, 1980.

994. Berger, P. B., Ruocco, N. A., Jr., Ryan, T. J., et al.: Incidence and prognostic implications of heart block complicating inferior myocardial infarction treated with thrombolytic therapy: Results from TIMI II. J. Am. Coll. Cardiol. 20:533, 1992.

995. McDonald, K., O'Sullivan, J. J., Conroy, R. M., et al.: Heart block as a predictor of in-hospital death in both acute inferior and acute anterior myocardial infarction. Q. J. Med. 74:277, 1990.

996. Goldberg, R. J., Zevallos, J. C., Yarzebski, J., et al.: Prognosis of acute myocardial infarction complicated by complete heart block (the Worcester Heart Attack Study). Am. J. Cardiol. 69:1135, 1992.

997. Bilbao, F. J., Zabalza, I. E., Vilanova, J. R., et al.: Atrioventricular block in posterior acute myocardial infarction: A clinicopathologic correlation. Circulation 75:733, 1987.

998. Bertolet, B. D., McMurtrie, E. B., Hill, J. A., et al.: Theophylline for the treatment of atrioventricular block after myocardial infarction. Ann. Intern. Med. 123:509, 1995.

999. Clemmensen, P., Bates, E. R., Califf, R. M., et al.: Complete atrioventricular block complicating inferior wall acute myocardial infarction treated with reperfusion therapy: TAMI Study Group. Am. J. Cardiol. 67:225, 1991.

1000. Mavric, Z., Zaputovic, L., Matana, A., et al.: Prognostic significance of complete atrioventricular block in patients with acute inferior myocardial infarction with and without right ventricular involvement. Am. Heart J. 119:823, 1990.

1001. Kostuk, W. J., and Beanlands, D. S.: Complete heart block associated with acute myocardial infarction. Am. J. Cardiol. 26:380, 1970.

1002. Lilavie, C. J., and Gersh, P. J.: Mechanical and electrical complication of acute myocardial infarction. Mayo Clin. Proc. 65:709, 1990.

1003. Bassan, R., Maia, I. G., Bozza, A., et al.: Atrioventricular block in acute inferior wall myocardial infarction: Harbinger of associated obstruction of the left anterior descending coronary artery. J. Am. Coll. Cardiol. 8:773, 1986.

1004. Nicod, P., Gilpin, E., Dittrich, H., et al.: Long-term outcome in patients with inferior myocardial infarction and complete atrioventricular block. J. Am. Coll. Cardiol. 12:589, 1988.

1005. Hindman, M. C., Wagner, G. S., Jaro, M., et al.: The clinical significance of bundle branch block complicating acute myocardial infarction. 2. Indications for temporary and permanent pacemaker insertion. Circulation 58:689, 1978.

1006. Feigl, D., Ashkenazy, J., and Kishon, Y.: Early and late atrioventricular block in acute inferior myocardial infarction. J. Am. Coll. Cardiol. 4:35, 1984.

1007. Klein, R. C., Vera, Z., and Mason, D. T.: Intraventricular conduction defects in acute myocardial infarction: Incidence, prognosis and therapy. Am. Heart J. 108:1007, 1984.

1008. Hollander, G., Nadiminti, V., Lichstein, E., et al.: Bundle branch block in acute myocardial infarction. Am. Heart J. 105:738, 1983.

1009. Hindman, M. C., Wagner, G. S., Jaro, M., et al.: The clinical significance of bundle branch block complicating acute myocardial infarction. 1. Clinical characteristics, hospital mortality, and one-year follow-up. Circulation 58:679, 1978.

1010. Scheinman, M. M., and Gonzalez, R. P.: Fascicular block and acute myocardial infarction. JAMA 244:2646, 1980.

1011. Lamas, G. A., Mueller, J. E., Turi, A. G., et al.: A simplified method to predict occurrence of complete heart block during acute myocardial infarction. Am. J. Cardiol. 57:1213, 1986.

1012. Mullins, C. B., and Atkins, J. M.: Prognoses and management of ventricular conduction blocks in acute myocardial infarction. Mod. Concepts Cardiovasc. Dis. 45:129, 1976.

1013. Dubois, C., Pierard, L. A., Smeets, J.-P., et al.: Short- and long-term prognostic importance of complete bundle-branch complicating acute myocardial infarction. Clin. Cardiol. 11:292, 1988.

1014. Ricou, F., Nicod, P., Gilpin, E., et al.: Influence of right bundle branch block on short- and long-term survival after acute anterior myocardial infarction. J. Am. Coll. Cardiol. 17:858, 1991.

1015. Ricou, F., Nicod, P., Gilpin, E., et al.: Influence of right bundle branch block on short- and long-term survival after inferior Q-wave myocardial infarction. Am. J. Cardiol. 67:1143, 1991.

1016. Lie, K. I., Liem, K. L., Schuilenburg, R. M., et al.: Early identification of patients developing late in-hospital ventricular fibrillation after discharge from the coronary care unit. Am. J. Cardiol. 41:674, 1978.

1017. DeGuzman, M., Cawanish, D. T., and Rahimtoola, S. H.: AV node–His Purkinje system disease: AV block (acute). In Bogan, E., and Wilcoff, K. (eds.): Clinical Cardiac Pacing. Philadelphia, W. B. Saunders Company, 1995, p. 321.

1018. Hynes, J. K., Holmes, D. R., Jr., and Harrison, C. E.: Five-year experience with temporary pacemaker therapy in the coronary care unit. Mayo Clin. Proc. 58:122, 1983.

1019. Zoll, P.: Resuscitation of the heart in ventricular standstill by external electrical stimulation. N. Engl. J. Med. 247:768, 1952.

1020. Zoll, P. M., Zoll, R. H., Falk, R. H., et al.: External non-invasive temporary cardiac pacing: Clinical trials. Circulation 71:937, 1985.

1021. Ginks, W. R., Sutton, R., Oh, W., et al.: Long-term prognosis after acute inferior infarction with atrioventricular block. Br. Heart J. 39:186, 1977.

SUPRAVENTRICULAR TACHYARRHYTHMIAS

1022. Crimm, A., Severance, H. W., Coffey, K., et al.: Prognostic significance of isolated sinus tachycardia during the first three days of acute myocardial infarction. Am. J. Med. 76:983, 1984.

1023. Berisso, M. Z., Carratino, L., Ferroni, A., et al.: Frequency, characteristics and significance of supraventricular tachyarrhythmias detected by 24-hour electrocardiographic recording in the late hospital phase of acute myocardial infarction. Am. J. Cardiol. 65:1064, 1990.

1024. Serrano, C. V., Ramires, J. A. F., Mansur, A. P., et al.: Importance of the time of onset of supraventricular tachyarrhythymias on prognosis of patients with acute myocardial infarction. Clin. Cardiol. 18:84, 1995.

1025. Ganz, L. I., and Friedman, P. L.: Supraventricular tachycardia. N. Engl. J. Med. 332:162, 1995.

1026. DeSanctis, R. W., Block, P., and Hutter, A. M.: Tachyarrhythmias in myocardial infarction. Circulation 45:681, 1972.

1027. Behar, S., Zahavi, Z., Goldbourt, U., et al.: Long-term prognosis of patients with paroxysmal atrial fibrillation complicating acute myocardial infarction. Eur. Heart J. 13:45, 1992.

1027a. Madias, J. E., Patel, D. C., and Singh, D.: Atrial fibrillation in acute myocardial infarction. A prospective study based on data from a consecutive series of patients admitted to the coronary care unit. Clin. Cardiol. 19:180, 1996.

1028. Hod, H., Lew, A. S., Heltai, M., et al.: Early atrial fibrillation during evolving myocardial infarction: A consequence of impaired left atrial perfusion. Circulation 75:146, 1987.

1029. Crenshaw, B. S., Ward, S. R., Stebbins, A. L., et al.: Risk factors and outcomes in patients with atrial fibrillation following acute myocardial infarction. Circulation 92(Suppl.):I-777, 1995.

1030. Kirkorian, G., Moncada, E., Chevalier, P., et al.: Radiofrequency ablation of atrial flutter: Efficacy of an anatomically guided approach. Circulation 90:2804, 1994.

1031. Suttorp, M. J., Kingma, J. H., Jessurun, E. R., et al.: The value of class IC antiarrhythmic drugs for acute conversion of paroxysmal atrial fibrillation or flutter to sinus rhythm. J. Am. Coll. Cardiol. 16:1722, 1990.

1032. Hine, L., Laird, N., Hewitt, P., et al.: Meta-analysis of empirical long-term antiarrhythmic therapy after myocardial infarction. JAMA 262:3037, 1989.

1033. Coplen, S., Antman, E., Berlin, J., et al.: Efficacy and safety of quinidine therapy for maintenance of sinus rhythm after cardioversion: A meta-analysis of randomized control trials. Circulation 82:1106, 1990.

1034. Akiyama, T., Pawitan, Y., Greenberg, H., et al.: Increased risk of death and cardiac arrest from encainide and flecainide in patients after non-Q-wave acute myocardial infarction in the Cardiac Arrhythmia Suppression Trial: CAST Investigators. Am. J. Cardiol. 68:1551, 1991.

1035. Cowan, J. C.: Antiarrhythmic drugs in the management of atrial fibrillation. Br. Heart J. 70:304, 1993.

1036. Middlekauff, H. R., Wiener, I., and Stevenson, W. G.: Low-dose amiodarone for atrial fibrillation. Am. J. Cardiol. 72:26, 1993.

1037. Podrid, P. J.: Amiodarone: Reevaluation of an old drug. Ann. Intern. Med. 122:689, 1995.

1038. Fishenfeld, J., Desser, K. B., and Benchimol, A.: Non-paroxysmal A-V junctional tachycardia associated with acute myocardial infarction. Am. Heart J. 86:754, 1973.

OTHER COMPLICATIONS

1039. Simoons, M. L., Brand, M., de Zwaan, C., et al.: Improved survival after early thrombolysis in acute myocardial infarction. Lancet 2:578, 1985.
1040. Koiwaya, Y., Torii, S., Takeshita, A., et al.: Postinfarction angina caused by coronary arterial spasm. Circulation 65:275, 1982.
1041. Cannon, C. P., McCabe, C. H., Henry, T. D., et al.: A pilot trial of recombinant desulfatohirudin compared with heparin in conjunction with tissue-type plasminogen activator and aspirin for acute myocardial infarction: Results of the Thrombolysis in Myocardial Infarction (TIMI) 5 trial. J. Am. Coll. Cardiol. 23:993, 1994.
1042. Cohen, L. S.: Managing patients after myocardial infarction. Hosp. Prac. 25:49, 1990.
1043. Ellis, S. G., Topol, E. J., George, B. S., et al.: Recurrent ischemia without warning: Analysis of risk factors for in-hospital ischemic events following successful thrombolysis with intravenous tissue plasminogen activator. Circulation 80:1159, 1989.
1044. Ohman, E. M., Armstrong, P. M., Guerci, A. D., et al.: Reinfarction after thrombolytic therapy: Experience from the GUSTO trial. Circulation 88(Suppl. I):490, 1993.
1045. Marmor, A., Sobel, B. E., and Roberts, E.: Factors presaging early recurrent myocardial infarction ("extension"). Am. J. Cardiol. 48:603, 1981.
1046. Benhorin, J., Andrews, M. L., Carleen, E. D., et al.: Occurrence, characteristics, and prognostic significance of early postacute myocardial infarction angina pectoris. Am. J. Cardiol. 62:679, 1988.
1047. Mueller, H. S., Cohen, L. S., Braunwald, E., et al.: Predictors of early morbidity and mortality after thrombolytic therapy of acute myocardial infarction: Analyses of patient subgroups in the Thrombolysis in Myocardial Infarction (TIMI) trial, phase II. Circulation 85:1254, 1992.
1048. Silva, P., Galli, M., Campolo, L., et al.: Prognostic significance of early ischemia after acute myocardial infarction in low-risk patients. Am. J. Cardiol. 71:1142, 1993.
1049. Barbagelata, A., Granger, C. B., Topol, E. J., et al.: Isolated recurrent ischemia after thrombolytic therapy: Incidence, importance, and cost. Am. J. Cardiol. 76:1007, 1995.
1050. Betriu, A., Califf, R. M., Granger, C., et al.: Importance of clinical findings during post-infarction angina in determining prognosis: Results from the GUSTO trial. J. Am. Coll. Cardiol. 23:27A, 1994.
1051. Muller, J. E., Rude, R. E., Braunwald, E., et al.: Myocardial infarct extension: Occurrence, outcome, and risk factors in the Multicenter Investigation of Limitation of Infarct Size. Ann. Intern. Med. 108:1, 1988.
1052. Maisel, A. S., Ahnve, S., Gilpin, E., et al.: Prognosis after extension of myocardial infarct: The role of Q wave or non-Q wave infarction. Circulation 71:211, 1985.
1053. Cannon, C. P., McCabe, C. H., Schweiger, M. J., et al.: Prospective validation of a composite end point for evaluation of new thrombolytic regimens for acute MI: Results from the TIMI 4 trial. Circulation 88(Suppl. I):60, 1993.
1054. Mueller, H. S., Forman, S. A., Menegus, M. A., et al.: Prognostic significance of nonfatal reinfarction during 3-year follow-up: Results of the Thrombolysis in Myocardial Infarction (TIMI) Phase II Clinical Trial. J. Am. Coll. Cardiol. 26:900, 1995.
1055. Roux, S., Christeller, S., and Ludin, E.: Effects of aspirin on coronary reocclusion and recurrent ischemia after thrombolysis: A meta-analysis. J. Am. Coll. Cardiol. 19:671, 1992.
1056. Cannon, C. P., Ganz, L. I., and Stone, P. H.: Complicated myocardial infarction. In Rippe, J. M., Irwin, R. S., Fink, M. P., et al. (eds.): Intensive Care Medicine. Boston, Little, Brown and Company, 1995, p. 477.
1057. Barbash, G. I., Hod, H., Roth, A., et al.: Repeat infusions of recombinant tissue-type plasminogen activator in patients with acute myocardial infarction and early recurrent myocardial ischemia. J. Am. Coll. Cardiol. 16:779, 1990.
1058. Purvis, J. A., McNeil, A. J., Roberts, M. J. D., et al.: First-year follow-up after repeat thrombolytic therapy with recombinant-tissue plasminogen activator for myocardial reinfarction. Coronary Artery Dis. 3:713, 1992.
1059. Simoons, M. L., Arnout, J., van den Brand, M., et al.: Retreatment with alteplase for early signs of reocclusion after thrombolysis: The European Cooperative Study Group. Am. J. Cardiol. 71:524, 1993.
1060. Topol, E. J., Holmes, D. R., and Rogers, W. J.: Coronary angiography after thrombolytic therapy for acute myocardial infarction. Ann. Intern. Med. 114:877, 1991.
1061. Sugiura, T., Iwasaka, T., Takayama, Y., et al.: Factors associated with pericardial effusion in acute Q wave myocardial infarction. Circulation 81:477, 1990.
1062. Barrington, W., Smith, J. E., and Himmelstein, S. I.: Cardiac tamponade following treatment with tissue plasminogen activator: An atypical hemodynamic response to pericardiocentesis. Am. Heart J. 121:1227, 1991.
1063. Clemmensen, P., Grande, P., Saunamäki, K., et al.: Evolution of electrocardiographic and echocardiographic abnormalities during the 4 years following first myocardial infarction. Eur. Heart J. 16:1063, 1995.
1064. Erhardt, L.: Clinical and pathological observations in different types of acute myocardial infarction: A study of 84 patients deceased after treatment in a coronary care unit. Acta Med. Scand. 560(Suppl.):1, 1974.
1065. Krainin, F. M., Flessas, A. P., and Spodick, D. H.: Infarction-associated pericarditis: Rarity of diagnostic electrocardiogram. N. Engl. J. Med. 311:1211, 1984.
1066. Wall, T. C., Califf, R. M., Harrelson-Woodlief, L., et al.: Usefulness of a pericardial friction rub after thrombolytic therapy during acute myocardial infarction in predicting amount of myocardial damage. Am. J. Cardiol. 66:1418, 1990.
1067. Karim, A. H., and Salomon, J.: Constrictive pericarditis after myocardial infarction: Sequela of anticoagulant-induced hemopericardium. Am. J. Med. 79:389, 1985.
1068. Kloner, R., Fishbein, M., Lew, H., et al.: Mummification of the infarcted myocardium by high dose corticosteroids. Circulation 57:56, 1978.
1069. Dressler, W.: The post-myocardial infarction syndrome: A report of forty-four cases. Arch. Intern. Med. 103:28, 1959.
1070. Lichtstein, E., Arsura, E., Hollander, G., et al.: Current incidence of postmyocardial infarction (Dressler's) syndrome. Am. J. Cardiol. 50:1269, 1982.
1071. Khan, A. H.: The postcardiac injury syndromes. Clin. Cardiol. 15:67, 1992.
1072. Dressler, W., Yurkovsky, J., and Starr, M. C.: Hemorrhagic pericarditis, pleurisy, and pneumonia complicating recent myocardial infarction. Am. Heart J. 54:42, 1957.
1073. Northcote, R. J., Hutchinson, S. J., and McGuinness, J. B.: Evidence for the continued existence of the postmyocardial infarction (Dressler's syndrome). Am. J. Cardiol. 53:1201, 1984.
1074. Lichstein, E., Liu, H. M., and Gupta, P.: Pericarditis complicating acute myocardial infarction: Incidence of complications and significance of electrocardiogram on admission. Am. Heart J. 87:246, 1974.
1075. Uuskiula, M. M., Lamp, K. M., and Martin, S. I.: Relationship between the clinical course of acute myocardial infarction and specific sensitization of lymphocytes and lymphotoxin production. Kardiologiia 26:57, 1987.
1076. Brown, E. J., Jr., Kloner, R. A., Schoen, F. J., et al.: Scar thinning due to ibuprofen administration after experimental myocardial infarction. Am. J. Cardiol. 51:877, 1983.
1077. Eppinger, E. C., and Kennedy, J. A.: The cause of death in coronary thrombosis, with special reference to pulmonary embolism. Am. J. Med. Sci. 195:104, 1938.
1078. Hellerstein, H. K., and Martin, J. W.: Incidence of thromboembolic lesions accompanying myocardial infarction. Am. Heart J. 33:443, 1947.
1079. Gueron, M., Wanderman, K. L., Hirsch, M., et al.: Pseudoaneurysm of the left ventricle after myocardial infarction: A curable form of myocardial rupture. J. Thorac. Cardiovasc. Surg. 69:736, 1975.
1080. Kahn, J., and Fisher, M. R.: MRI of cardiac pseudoaneurysm and other complications of myocardial infarction. Magn. Reson. Imaging. 9:159, 1991.
1081. Schoen, F. J.: Ischemic heart disease. In Schoen, F. J. (ed.): Interventional and Surgical Cardiovascular Pathology. Clinical Correlations and Basic Principles. Philadelphia, W. B. Saunders Company, 1989, p. 58.
1082. Forman, M. B., Collins, H. W., Kopelman, H. A., et al.: Determinants of left ventricular aneurysm formation after acute anterior myocardial infarction: A clinical and angiographic study. J. Am. Coll. Cardiol. 8:1256, 1986.
1083. Hirai, T., Fujita, M., Nakajima, H., et al.: Importance of collateral circulation for prevention of left ventricular aneurysm formation in acute myocardial infarction. Circulation 79:791, 1989.
1084. Abrams, D. L., Edelist, A., Luria, M. H., et al.: Ventricular aneurysm: A reappraisal based on a study of 65 consecutive autopsied cases. Circulation 27:164, 1963.
1085. Meizlish, J. L., Berger, H. J., Plankey, M., et al.: Functional left ventricular aneurysm formation after acute anterior transmural myocardial infarction: Incidence, natural history, and prognostic implications. N. Engl. J. Med. 311:1001, 1984.
1086. Lindsay, J., Jr., Dewey, D. C., Talesnick, B. S., et al.: Relation of ST-segment elevation after healing of acute myocardial infarction to the presence of left ventricular aneurysm. Am. J. Cardiol. 54:84, 1984.
1087. Brawley, R. K., Magovern, G. J., Jr., Gott, V. L., et al.: Left ventricular aneurysmectomy: Factors influencing postoperative results. J. Thorac. Cardiovasc. Surg. 85:712, 1983.
1088. Keeley, E. C., and Hillis, L. D.: Left ventricular mural thrombus after acute myocardial infarction. Clin. Cardiol. 19:83, 1996.
1089. Halperin, J. L., and Fuster, V.: Left ventricular thrombi and cerebral embolism. N. Engl. J. Med. 320:392, 1989.
1090. Halperin, J. L., and Petersen, P.: Thrombosis in the cardiac chambers: Ventricular dysfunction and atrial fibrillation. In Fuster, V., and Verstraete, M. (eds.): Thrombosis in Cardiovascular Disorders. Philadelphia, W. B. Saunders Company, 1992, p. 215.
1091. Funke Kupper, A. J., Verheugt, F. W. A., Peels, C. H., et al.: Left ventricular thrombus incidence and behavior studied by serial two-dimensional echocardiography in acute anterior myocardial infarction: Left ventricular wall motion, systemic wall motion, systemic embolism and oral anticoagulation. J. Am. Coll. Cardiol. 13:1514, 1989.
1092. Stein, B., Halperin, J. L., and Fuster, V.: Prevention of left ventricular mural thrombosis and arterial embolism during and after myocardial infarction. Coronary Artery Dis. 1:180, 1990.
1093. Gueret, P., Dubourg, O., Ferrier, A., et al.: Effects of full-dose heparin anticoagulation on the development of left ventricular thrombosis in acute myocardial infarction. J. Am. Coll. Cardiol. 8:419, 1986.
1094. Fernandez-Ortiz, A., Jand, I.-K., and Fuster, V.: Anticoagulant and platelet inhibitory agents for myocardial infarction. In Francis, G. S.,

and Alpert, J. S. (eds.): Coronary Care. Boston, Little, Brown and Company, 1995, p. 569.

1095. Stratton, J. R., and Resnick, A. D.: Increased embolic risk in patients with left ventricular thrombi. Circulation 75:1004, 1987.

1096. Jugdutt, B. I., Sivaram, C. A., Wortman, C., et al.: Prospective two-dimensional echocardiographic evaluation of left ventricular thrombus and embolism after myocardial infarction. J. Am. Coll. Cardiol. 13:554, 1989.

1097. Working Party on Anticoagulant Therapy in Coronary Thrombosis to the Medical Research Council: An assessment of long-term anticoagulant administration after cardiac infarction: BMJ 2:837, 1964.

1098. Nordrehaug, J. E., Johannessen, K. A., and von der Lippe, G.: Usefulness of high-dose anticoagulants in preventing left ventricular thrombus in acute myocardial infarction. Am. J. Cardiol. 55:1941, 1985.

1099. Davis, M. J. E., and Ireland, M. A.: Effect of early anticoagulation on the frequency of left ventricular thrombi after anterior wall acute myocardial infarction. Am. J. Cardiol. 57:1244, 1986.

1100. Arvan, S., and Boscha, K.: Prophylactic anticoagulation for left ventricular thrombi after acute myocardial infarction: A prospective randomized trial. Am. Heart J. 113:688, 1987.

1101. Turpie, A. G. G., Robinson, J. G., Doyle, D. J., et al.: Comparison of high-dose with low-dose subcutaneous heparin to prevent left ventricular mural thrombosis in patients with acute transmural anterior myocardial infarction. N. Engl. J. Med. 320:352, 1989.

1102. Held, A. C., Gore, J. M., Paraskos, J., et al.: Impact of thrombolytic therapy on left ventricular mural thrombi in acute myocardial infarction. Am. J. Cardiol. 62:310, 1988.

1103. Halperin, J. L., and Fuster, V.: Left ventricular thrombus and stroke after myocardial infarction: Toward prevention or perplexity? J. Am. Coll. Cardiol. 14:912, 1989.

1104. Nihoyannopoulos, P., Smith, G. C., Maseri, A., et al.: The natural history of left ventricular thrombus in myocardial infarction: A rationale in support of masterly inactivity. J. Am. Coll. Cardiol. 14:903, 1989.

1105. Stein, B., Fuster, V., Halperin, J. L., et al.: Antithrombitic therapy in cardiac disease: An emerging approach based on pathogenesis and risk. Circulation 80:1501, 1989.

1106. Kouvaras, G., Chronopoulos, G., Soufras, G., et al.: The effects of long-term antithrombotic treatment on left ventricular thrombi in patients after an acute myocardial infarction. Am. Heart J. 119:73, 1990.

1107. Keren, A., Goldberg, S., Gottlieb, S., et al.: Natural history of left ventricular thrombi: Their appearance and resolution in the posthospitalization period of acute myocardial infarction. J. Am. Coll. Cardiol. 15:790, 1990.

1108. Stratton, J. R., and Ritchie, J. L.: The effects of antithrombotic drugs in patients with left ventricular thrombi: Assessment with indium-111 platelet imaging and two-dimensional echocardiography. Circulation 69:561, 1984.

CONVALESCENCE, DISCHARGE, AND POST–MYOCARDIAL INFARCTION CARE

1109. Hammerman, H., Kloner, R. A., Alker, K. J., et al.: Effects of transient increased afterload during experimentally induced acute myocardial infarction in dogs. Am. J. Cardiol. 55:566, 1985.

1110. Gheorghiade, M., Anderson, J., Rosman, H., et al.: Risk identification at the time of admission to coronary care unit in patients with suspected myocardial infarction. Am. Heart J. 116:1212, 1988.

1111. Parsons, R. W., Jamrozik, K. D., Hobbs, M. S., et al.: Early identification of patients at low risk of death after myocardial infarction and potentially suitable for early hospital discharge. BMJ 308:1006, 1994.

1112. Newby, L. K., Califf, R. M., Guerci, A., et al.: Early discharge in the thrombolytic era: An analysis of criteria for uncomplicated infarction from the Global Utilization for Streptokinase and t-PA for Occluded Coronary Arteries (GUSTO) trial. J. Am. Coll. Cardiol. 1996 (in press).

1113. Pryor, D. B., Hindman, M. C., Wagner, G. S., et al.: Early discharge after acute myocardial infarction. Ann. Intern. Med. 99:528, 1983.

1114. Ockene, I. S., Clemow, L. P., and Ockene, J. K.: Psychosocial and behavioral factors during recovery from myocardial infarction. In Francis, G. S., and Alpert, J. S. (eds.): Coronary Care. Boston, Little, Brown and Company, 1995, p. 595.

1115. Tardif, G. S.: Sexual activity after a myocardial infarction. Arch. Phys. Med. Rehabil. 70:763, 1989.

1116. Mendes de Leon, C. F., Powell, L. H., and Kaplan, B. H.: Changes in coronary-prone behaviors in the Recurrent Coronary Prevention Project. Psychosom. Med. 53:407, 1991.

1117. Squires, R. W., Gau, G. T., Miller, T. D., et al.: Cardiovascular rehabilitation: Status, 1990. Mayo Clin. Proc. 65:731, 1990.

1118. O'Connor, G. T., Buring, J. E., Yusuf, S., et al.: An overview of randomized trials of rehabilitation with exercise after myocardial infarction. Circulation 80:234, 1989.

1119. Dennis, C. A.: Rehabilitation following acute myocardial infarction. In Francis, G. S., and Alpert, J. S. (eds.): Coronary Care. Boston, Little, Brown and Company, 1995, p. 629.

1120. Balady, G. J., Fletcher, B. J., Froelicher, E. S., et al.: Cardiac rehabilitation programs: A statement for healthcare professionals from the American Heart Association. Circulation 90:1602, 1994.

1121. Tofler, G. H., Stone, P. H., Muller, J. E., et al.: Effects of gender and race on prognosis after myocardial infarction: Adverse prognosis for women, particularly black women. J. Am. Coll. Cardiol. 9:473, 1987.

1122. Tofler, G. H., Muller, J. E., Stone, P. H., et al.: Factors leading to

shorter survival after acute myocardial infarction in patients aging 65 to 75 years compared with younger patients. Am. J. Cardiol. 62:860, 1988.

1123. Marcus, F. I., Friday, K., McCans, J., et al.: Age-related prognosis after acute myocardial infarction (the Multicenter Diltiazem Postinfarction Trial). Am. J. Cardiol. 65:559, 1990.

1124. Stone, P. H., Muller, J. E., Hartwell, T., et al.: The effect of diabetes mellitus on prognosis and serial left ventricular function after acute myocardial infarction: Contribution of both coronary disease and diastolic left ventricular dysfunction to the adverse prognosis. J. Am. Coll. Cardiol. 14:49, 1989.

1125. DeBusk, R. F., Kraemer, H. C., and Nash, E.: Stepwise risk stratification soon after acute myocardial infarction. Am. J. Cardiol. 52:1161, 1983.

1126. Merrilees, M. A., Scott, P. J., and Norris, R. M.: Prognosis after myocardial infarction: Results of 15 year follow-up. BMJ 288:356, 1984.

1127. Benhorin, J., Moss, A. J., Oakes, D., et al.: Prognostic significance of nonfatal myocardial reinfarction. J. Am. Coll. Cardiol. 15:253, 1990.

1128. Smith, J. W., Marcus, F. I., Serokman, R., et al.: Prognosis of patients with diabetes mellitus after acute myocardial infarction. Am. J. Cardiol. 54:718, 1984.

1129. Abbott, R. D., Donaue, R. P., Kannel, W. B., et al.: The impact of diabetes on survival following myocardial infarction in men vs women: The Framingham Study. JAMA 260:3456, 1988.

1130. Rennert, G., Saltz-Rennerts, H., Wanderman, K., et al.: Size of acute myocardial infarcts in patients with diabetes mellitus. Am. J. Cardiol. 55:1629, 1985.

1131. Gwilt, D. J. G., Petri, M., Lewis, P. W., et al.: Myocardial infarct size and mortality in diabetic patients. Br. Heart J. 54:466, 1985.

1132. Maisel, A. S., Gilpin, E., Holt, B., et al.: Survival after hospital discharge in matched populations with inferior or anterior myocardial infarction. J. Am. Coll. Cardiol. 6:731, 1985.

1133. Hands, M. E., Lloyd, B. L., Robinson, J. S., et al.: Prognostic significance of electrocardiographic site of infarction after correction for enzymatic size of infarction. Circulation 73:885, 1986.

1134. Zabel, K. M., Hathaway, W. R., Peterson, E. D., et al.: Baseline electrocardiogram predicts 30-day mortality among 32,182 patients with acute myocardial infarction treated with thrombolysis. J. Am. Coll. Cardiol. 25:342A, 1995.

1135. Bates, E. R., Clemmensen, P. M., Califf, R. M., et al.: Precordial ST segment depression predicts a worse prognosis in inferior infarction despite reperfusion therapy: The Thrombolysis and Angioplasty in Myocardial Infarction (TAMI) Study Group. J. Am. Coll. Cardiol. 16:1538, 1990.

1136. Wong, C. K., Freedman, S. B., Bautovich, G., et al.: Mechanism and significance of precordial ST-segment depression during inferior wall acute myocardial infarction associated with severe narrowing of the dominant right coronary artery. Am. J. Cardiol. 71:1025, 1993.

1137. Goldberg, R. J., Seeley, D., Becker, R. C., et al.: Impact of atrial fibrillation on the in-hospital and long-term survival of patients with acute myocardial infarction: A community-wide perspective. Am. Heart J. 119:996, 1990.

1138. Chaitman, B. R., Thompson, B. W., Kern, M. J., et al.: Tissue plasminogen activator followed by percutaneous transluminal coronary angioplasty: One year TIMI phase II pilot results. Am. Heart J. 119:213, 1990.

1139. Bosch, X., Théroux, P., Walters, D., et al.: Early postinfarction ischemia: Clinical, angiographic, and prognostic significance. Circulation 75:988, 1987.

1140. Tzivoni, D., Gavish, A., Zin, D., et al.: Prognostic significance of ischemic episodes in patients with previous myocardial infarction. Am. J. Cardiol. 62:661, 1988.

1141. DeWood, M. A., Stifter, W. F., Simpson, C. S., et al.: Coronary arteriographic findings soon after non-Q wave myocardial infarction. N. Engl. J. Med. 315:417, 1986.

1141a. Matetzky, S., Barabash, G. I., Rabinowitz, B., et al.: Q wave and non-Q wave myocardial infarction after thrombolysis. J. Am. Coll. Cardiol. 26:1445, 1995.

1142. Devlin, W., Cragg, D., Jacks, M., et al.: Comparison of outcome in patients with acute myocardial infarction aged > 75 years with that in younger patients. Am. J. Cardiol. 75:573, 1995.

1143. Krikorian, R. K., and Vacek, J. J.: Non-Q-wave myocardial infarction in the elderly: Clinical characteristics and management. Am. J. Ger. Cardiol. 4:41, 1995.

1144. Gibson, R. S.: Non-Q-wave myocardial infarction. In Fuster, V., Ross, R., and Topol, E. J. (eds.): Atherosclerosis and Coronary Artery Disease. Philadelphia, Lippincott-Raven, 1996, pp. 1097–1124.

1145. Berger, C. J., Murabito, J. M., Evans, J. C., et al.: Prognosis after first myocardial infarction: Comparison of Q wave and non-Q wave myocardial infarction in the Framingham Heart Study. JAMA 268:1545, 1992.

1146. Krone, R. J., Greenberg, J., Dwyer, E. M., et al.: Long-term prognostic significance of ST segment depression during acute myocardial infarction. J. Am. Coll. Cardiol. 22:361, 1993.

1147. Mickley, H., Pless, P., Nielsen, J. R., et al.: Residual myocardial ischemia in first non-Q versus Q wave infarction: Maximal exercise testing and ambulatory ST segment monitoring. Eur. Heart J. 14:18, 1993.

1148. Johnston, T. S., and Wenger, N. K.: Risk stratification after myocardial infarction. Curr. Opin. Cardiol. 8:621, 1993.

1149. Pitt, B.: Evaluation of the postinfarct patient. Circulation 91:1855, 1995.

1150. Figueredo, V., and Cheitlin, M. D.: Risk stratification. In Julian, D., and Braunwald, E. (eds.): Management of Acute Myocardial Infarction. London, W. B. Saunders Ltd., 1994, p. 361.

1151. Wolff, A. A., and Karliner, J. S.: Overall risk stratification and management strategies for patients with acute myocardial infarction. In Francis, G. S., and Alpert, J. S. (eds.): Coronary Care. Boston, Little, Brown and Company, 1995, p. 741.

1152. Multicenter Postinfarction Research Group: Risk stratification and survival after myocardial infarction. N. Engl. J. Med. 309:331, 1983.

1153. Volpi, A., De Vita, C., Franzosi, M. G., et al.: Determinants of 6-month mortality in survivors of myocardial infarction after thrombolysis: Results of the GISSI-2 data base: The Ad Hoc Working Group of the Gruppo Italiano per lo Studio della Sopravvivenza nell'Infarto Miocardico (GISSI)-2 Data Base. Circulation 88:416, 1993.

1154. Stevenson, R., Ranjadayalan, K., Wilkinson, P., et al.: Short and long term prognosis of acute myocardial infarction since introduction of thrombolysis. BMJ 307:349, 1993.

1155. Jereczek, M., Andresen, D., Schroder, J., et al.: Prognostic value of ischemia during Holter monitoring and exercise testing after acute myocardial infarction. Am. J. Cardiol. 72:8, 1993.

1156. Myers, M. G., Baigrie, R. S., Charlat, M. L., et al.: Are routine non-invasive tests useful in prediction of outcome after myocardial infarction in elderly people? Lancet 342:1069, 1993.

1157. Ruberman, W., Weinblatt, E., Goldberg, J. D., et al.: Ventricular premature complexes and sudden death after myocardial infarction. Circulation 64:297, 1981.

1158. Gomes, J. A., Winters, S. L., Ip, J.: Post myocardial infarction stratification and signal-averaged electrocardiogram. Prog. Cardiovasc. Dis. 35:263, 1993.

1159. McClements, B. M., Adgey, A. A.: Value of signal-averaged electrocardiography, radionuclide ventriculography, Holter monitoring and clinical variables for prediction of arrhythmic events in survivors of acute myocardial infarction in the thrombolytic era. J. Am. Coll. Cardiol. 21:1419, 1993.

1160. La Rovere, M. T., Bigger, J. T., Marcus, F. I., et al.: Prognostic value of depressed baroreflex sensitivity: The ATRAMI Study. Circulation 92(Suppl.):I-777, 1995.

1161. Task Force of the European Society of Cardiology and The North American Society of Pacing and Electrophysiology: Heart rate variability—standards of measurement, physiological interpretation, and clinical use. Circulation 93:1043, 1996.

1162. Aguirre, F. V., Kern, M. J., Hsia, J., et al.: Importance of myocardial infarct artery patency on the prevalence of ventricular arrhythmia and late potentials after thrombolysis in acute myocardial infarction. Am. J. Cardiol. 68:1410, 1991.

1163. Morris, K. G.: Use of radionuclide angiography following acute myocardial infarction. In Califf, R. M., Mark, D. B., and Wagner, G. S. (eds.): Acute Coronary Care. St. Louis, Mosby, 1995, p. 797.

1164. Fletcher, G. F., Balady, G., Froelicher, V. F., et al.: Exercise standards: A statement for healthcare professionals from the American Heart Association. Circulation 91:580, 1995.

1165. Pilote, L., Silberberg, J., Lisbona, R., et al.: Prognosis in patients with low left ventricular ejection fraction after myocardial infarction. Circulation 80:1636, 1989.

1166. Dilsizian, V., and Bonow, R. O.: Current diagnostic techniques of assessing myocardial viability in patients with hibernating and stunned myocardium. Circulation 87:1, 1993.

1167. Crawford, M. H.: Risk stratification after myocardial infarction with exercise and Doppler echocardiography. Circulation 84(Suppl. I):163, 1991.

1168. Bach, D. S., and Armstrong, W. F.: Dobutamine stress echocardiography. Am. J. Cardiol. 69:18, 1992.

1169. Previtali, M., Poli, A., Lanzarini, L., et al.: Dobutamine stress echocardiography for assessment of myocardial viability and ischemia in acute myocardial infarction treated with thrombolysis. Am. J. Cardiol. 72:16, 1993.

1170. Watada, H., Ito, H., Oh, H., et al.: Dobutamine stress echocardiography predicts reversible dysfunction and quantitates the extent of irreversibly damaged myocardium after reperfusion of anterior myocardial infarction. J. Am. Coll. Cardiol. 24:624, 1994.

1171. Pellikka, P. A., Roger, V. L., Oh, J. K., et al.: Stress echocardiography. Part II. Dobutamine stress echocardiography: Techniques, implementation, clinical applications, and correlations. Mayo Clin. Proc. 70:16, 1995.

1172. Picano, E., Pingitore, A., Sicari, R., et al.: Stress echocardiographic results predict risk reinfarction early after uncomplicated acute myocardial infarction: Large-scale multicenter study. J. Am. Coll. Cardiol. 26:908, 1995.

1173. Coma-Canella, I., del Val Gomez Martinez, M., Rodigro, F., et al.: The dobutamine stress test with thallium-201 single-photon emission computed tomography and radionuclide angiography: Postinfarction study. J. Am. Coll. Cardiol. 22:399, 1993.

1174. Sansoy, V., Glover, D. K., Watson, D. D., et al.: Comparison of thallium-201 resting redistribution with technetium-99m sestamibi uptake and functional response to dobutamine for assessment of myocardial viability. Circulation 92:994, 1995.

1175. Yoshida, K., and Gould, K. L.: Quantitative relation of myocardial infarct size and myocardial viability by positron emission tomography to left ventricular ejection fraction and 3-year mortality with and without revascularization. J. Am. Coll. Cardiol. 22:984, 1993.

1176. Mark, W. I., Webster, M. B., Chesebro, J. H., et al.: Myocardial infarction and coronary artery occlusion: A prospective 5-year angiographic study. J. Am. Coll. Cardiol. 15:218A, 1990.

1176a. Meeting Highlights: AHA 68th Scientific Sessions, "Invasive Versus Medical Treatment of Postinfarction Ischemia" (DANAMI Study). Circulation 93:846, 1996.

1177. Juneau, M., Colles, P., Theroux, P., et al.: Symptom-limited versus low level exercise testing before hospital discharge after myocardial infarction. J. Am. Coll. Cardiol. 20:927, 1992.

1178. Jain, A., Myers, G. H., Sapin, P. M., et al.: Comparison of symptom-limited and low level exercise tolerance tests early after myocardial infarction. J. Am. Coll. Cardiol. 22:1816, 1993.

1179. Stevenson, R., Umachandran, V., Ranjadayalan, K., et al.: Reassessment of treadmill stress testing for risk stratification in patients with acute myocardial infarction treated by thrombolysis. Br. Heart J. 70:415, 1993.

1180. Gibson, R. S., and Beller, G. A.: Value of predischarge myocardial perfusion scintigraphy. In Fuster, V., Ross, R., and Topol, E. J. (eds.): Atherosclerosis and Coronary Artery Disease. Philadelphia, Lippincott-Raven, 1996, pp. 1167–1192.

1181. Lavie, C. J., Gibbons, R. J., Zinsmeister, A. R., et al.: Interpreting results of exercise studies after acute myocardial infarction altered by thrombolytic therapy, coronary angioplasty or bypass. Am. J. Cardiol. 67:116, 1991.

1182. Moss, A. J., Goldstein, R. E., Hall, W. J., et al.: Detection and significance of myocardial ischemia in stable patients after recovery from an acute coronary event. JAMA 269:2379, 1993.

1183. Moss, A. J., Davis, H. T., DeCamilla, J., et al.: Ventricular ectopic beats and their relation to sudden and nonsudden cardiac death after myocardial infarction. Circulation 60:998, 1979.

1184. Bigger, J. T., Fleiss, J. L., Kleiger, R., et al.: The relationships between ventricular arrhythmias, left ventricular dysfunction, and mortality in the 2 years after myocardial infarction. Circulation 69:250, 1984.

1185. Mukharji, J., and MILIS Study Group: Risk factors for sudden death after acute myocardial infarction. Am. J. Cardiol. 54:31, 1984.

1186. Kostis, J. B., Byington, R., Friedman, L. M., et al.: Prognostic significance of ventricular ectopic activity in survivors of acute myocardial infarction. J. Am. Coll. Cardiol. 10:231, 1987.

1187. Morganroth, J., and Bigger, J. T., Jr.: Pharmacologic management of ventricular arrhythmias after the Cardiac Arrhythmia Suppression Trial. Am. J. Cardiol. 65:1497, 1990.

1188. Richards, D. A., Byth, K., Ross, D. L., et al.: What is the best predictor of spontaneous ventricular tachycardia and sudden death after myocardial infarction? Circulation 83:756, 1991.

1188a. Prystowsky, E. N.: Acute myocardial infarction: Role of electrophysiologic testing prior to hospital discharge. In Fuster, V., Ross, R., and Topol, E. J. (eds.): Atherosclerosis and Coronary Artery Disease. Philadelphia, Lippincott-Raven, 1996, pp. 1257–1266.

1189. Hohnloser, S. H., Franck, P., Klingenheben, T., et al.: Open infarct artery, late potentials, and other prognostic factors in patients after acute myocardial infarction in the thrombolytic era: A prospective trial. Circulation 90:1747, 1994.

1190. Farrell, T. G., Bashir, Y., Cripps, T., et al.: Risk stratification for arrhythmic events in postinfarction patients based on heart rate variability, ambulatory electrocardiographic variables and the signal-averaged electrocardiogram. J. Am. Coll. Cardiol. 18:687, 1991.

1190a. Gomes, J. A.: Acute myocardial infarction: Role of signal averaging. In Fuster, V., Ross, R., and Topol, E. J. (eds.): Atherosclerosis and Coronary Artery Disease. Philadelphia, Lippincott-Raven, 1996, pp. 1245–1256.

1191. Bourke, J. P., Richards, D. A. B., Ross, D. L., et al.: Routine programmed electrical stimulation in survivors of acute myocardial infarction for prediction of spontaneous ventricular tachyarrhythmias during follow-up: Results, optimal stimulation protocol, and cost-effective screening. J. Am. Coll. Cardiol. 18:780, 1991.

1192. Pedretti, R., Etro, M. D., Laporta, A., et al.: Prediction of late arrhythmic events after acute myocardial infarction from combined use of noninvasive prognostic variables and inducibility of sustained monomorphic ventricular tachycardia. Am. J. Cardiol. 71:1131, 1993.

1193. Gilman, J. K., Jalal, S., and Naccarelli, G. V.: Predicting and preventing sudden death from cardiac causes. Circulation 90:1083, 1994.

1194. Pieper, S. J., and Hammill, S. C.: Heart rate variability: Technique and investigational application in cardiovascular medicine. Mayo Clin. Proc. 70:955, 1995.

1195. Moss, A. J., and Benhorin, J.: Prognosis and management after a first myocardial infarction. N. Engl. J. Med. 322:743, 1990.

1196. Schoenberger, J. A.: Advances in the primary and secondary prevention of coronary heart disease. Curr. Opin. Cardiol. 8:557, 1993.

1197. Hinstridge, V., and Speight, T. M.: An overview of therapeutic interventions in myocardial infarction: Emphasis on secondary prevention. Drugs 2:8, 1991.

1198. Rosenberg, L., Kaufman, D. W., Helmrich, S. P., et al.: The risk of myocardial infarction after quitting smoking in men under 55 years of age. N. Engl. J. Med. 313:1511, 1985.

1199. Rigotti, N. A., Singer, D. E., Mulley, A. G., Jr., et al.: Smoking cessation following admission to a coronary care unit. J. Gen. Intern. Med. 6:305, 1991.

1200. Krumholz, H. M., Cohen, B. J., Tsevat, J., et al.: Cost-effectiveness of a smoking cessation program after myocardial infarction. J. Am. Coll. Cardiol. 22:1697, 1993.

1201. Frasure-Smith, N., Lesperance, F., and Talajic, M.: Depression following myocardial infarction: Impact on 6-month survival. JAMA *270*:1819, 1993.

1202. Berkman, L. F., Leo-Summers, L., and Horwitz, R. I.: Emotional support and survival after myocardial infarction. Ann. Intern. Med. *117*:1003, 1992.

1203. Bucher, H. C.: Social support and prognosis following first myocardial infarction. J. Gen. Intern. Med. *9*:409, 1994.

1204. Gallagher, E. J., Viscoli, C. M., and Horwitz, R. I.: The relationship of treatment adherence to the risk of death after myocardial infarction in women. JAMA *270*:742, 1993.

1205. Bondestam, E., Breikss, A., and Hartford, M.: Effects of early rehabilitation on consumption of medical care during the first year after acute myocardial infarction in patients > or = 65 years of age. Am. J. Cardiol. *75*:767, 1995.

1206. Dennis, C., Houston-Miller, N., Schwartz, R. G., et al.: Early return to work after uncomplicated myocardial infarction: Results of a randomized trial. JAMA *260*:214, 1988.

1207. Wong, N. D., Wilson, P. W. F., and Kannel, W. B.: Serum cholesterol as a prognostic factor after myocardial infarction: The Framingham Study. Ann. Intern. Med. *115*:687, 1991.

1208. Braunwald, E., Pfeffer, M., and Sacks, F.: The CARE Trial: Presented at American College of Cardiology, 1996.

1209. Cohen, M., Byrne, M., Levine, B., et al.: Low rate of treatment of hypercholesterolemia by cardiologists in patients with suspected and proven coronary artery disease. Circulation *83*:1294, 1991.

1210. Scandinavian Simvistatin Survival Study Group: Randomised trial of cholesterol lowering in 4444 patients with coronary heart disease: The Scandinavian Simvastatin Survival Study (4S). Lancet *344*:1383, 1994.

1211. Scandinavian Simvistatin Survival Study Group: Baseline serum cholesterol and treatment effect in the Scandinavian Simvastatin Survival Study (4S). Lancet *345*:1274, 1995.

1212. Col, N. F., Yarzebski, J., Gore, J. M., et al.: Does aspirin consumption affect the presentation or severity of acute myocardial infarction? Arch. Intern. Med. *155*:1386, 1995.

1213. Alhaddad, I. A., Tkaczevski, L., Siddiqui, F., et al.: Aspirin enhances the benefits of late reperfusion on infarct shape: A possible mechanism of the beneficial effects of aspirin on survival after acute myocardial infarction. Circulation *91*:2819, 1995.

1214. Tsevat, J., Duke, D., Goldman, L., et al.: Cost-effectiveness of captopril therapy after myocardial infarction. J. Am. Coll. Cardiol. *26*:914, 1995.

1215. Herlitz, J., Elmfeldt, D., Holmberg, S., et al.: Goteborg metoprolol trial: Mortality and causes of death. Am. J. Cardiol. *53*:9D, 1984.

1216. Olsson, G., Rehnqvist, N., Sjögren, A., et al.: Long-term treatment with metoprolol in acute myocardial infarction: Effect on 3 year mortality and morbidity. J. Am. Coll. Cardiol. *5*:1428, 1985.

1217. The Norwegian Multicenter Study Group: Timolol-induced reduction in mortality and reinfarction in patients surviving acute myocardial infarction. N. Engl. J. Med. *304*:801, 1981.

1218. Chadda, K., Goldstein, S., Byington, R., et al.: Effect of propranolol after acute myocardial infarction in patients with congestive heart failure. Circulation *73*:503, 1986.

1219. Beta-Blocker Pooling Project Research Group: The Beta-Blocker Pooling Project (BBPP): Subgroup findings from randomized trials in postinfarction patients. Eur. Heart J. *9*:8, 1988.

1219a. O'Rourke, R. A.: Are beta-blockers really underutilized in postinfarction patients? J. Am. Coll. Cardiol. *26*:1437, 1995.

1220. Olsson, G., Levin, L.-A., and Rehnqvist, N.: Economic consequences of postinfarction prophylaxis with β blockers: Cost effectiveness of metoprolol. Br. Heart J. *294*:339, 1987.

1221. Goldman, L., Sia, S. T. B., Cook, E. F., et al.: Costs and effectiveness of routine therapy with long-term beta-adrenergic antagonists after acute myocardial infarction. N. Engl. J. Med. *319*:152, 1988.

1222. Brand, D. A., Newcomer, L. N., Freiburger, A., et al.: Cardiologists'

practices compared with practice guidelines: use of beta-blockade after myocardial infarction. J. Am. Coll. Cardiol. *26*:1432, 1995.

1223. Goldstein, S.: Review of beta blocker myocardial infarction trials. Clin. Cardiol. *12*:54, 1989.

1224. Smith, P., Arnesen, H., and Holme, I.: The effect of warfarin on mortality and reinfarction after myocardial infarction. N. Engl. J. Med. *323*:147, 1990.

1225. Devine, N., Azarnia, N., Nelson, K., et al.: Long-term anticoagulants in post myocardial infarction patients: A meta-analysis. Circulation *86*(Suppl. I):259, 1992.

1226. Anticoagulants in the Secondary Prevention of Events in Coronary Thrombosis (ASPECT) Research Group: Effect of long-term oral anticoagulant treatment on mortality and cardiovascular morbidity after myocardial infarction. Lancet *343*:499, 1994.

1227. van Bergen, P. F. M. M., Jonker, J. J. C., van Hout, B. A., et al.: Costs and effects of long-term oral anticoagulant treatment after myocardial infarction. JAMA *273*:925, 1995,

1228. Breddin, K., Loew, D., Lechner, K., et al.: The German-Austrian aspirin trial: A comparison of acetylsalicylic acid, placebo, and phenprocoumon in secondary prevention of myocardial infarction. Circulation *62*(Suppl. V):V63, 1980.

1229. The EPSIM Research Group: A controlled comparison of aspirin and oral anticoagulants in prevention of death after myocardial infarction. N. Engl. J. Med. *307*:701, 1982.

1230. Cairns, J. A., and Markham, B. A.: Economics and efficacy in choosing oral anticoagulants or aspirin after myocardial infarction. JAMA *273*:965, 1995.

1231. Teo, K. K., Yusuf, S., and Furberg, C. D.: Effects of prophylactic antiarrhythmic drug therapy in acute myocardial infarction. JAMA *270*:1589, 1993.

1232. Epstein, A. E., Hallstrom, A. P., Rogers, W. J., et al.: Mortality following ventricular arrhythmia suppression by encainide, flecainide, and moricizine after myocardial infarction: The original design concept of the Cardiac Arrhythmia Suppression Trial (CAST). JAMA *270*:2451, 1993.

1233. Echt, D. S., Liebson, P. R., Mitchell, L. B., et al.: Mortality and morbidity in patients receiving encainide, flecainide, or placebo: The Cardiac Arrhythmia Suppression Trial. N. Engl. J. Med. *324*:781, 1991.

1234. The Cardiac Arrhythmia Suppression Trial II Investigators: Effects of the antiarrhythmic agent moricizine on survival after myocardial infarction. N. Engl. J. Med. *327*:227, 1992.

1234a. Krishnan, S. C., Shivkumar, K., Garan, H., et al.: Increased vulnerability of the subendocardium to ischaemic injury: An electrophysiological explanation. Lancet *346*:1612, 1995.

1235. Waldo, A. L., Camm, A. J., de Ruyter, H., et al.: Preliminary mortality results from the Survival with Oral D-Sotalol (SWORD) Trial. J. Am. Coll. Cardiol. *25*(Special Issue):15A, 1995.

1236. Zarembski, D. G., Nolan, P. E., Slack, M. K., et al.: Empiric long-term amiodarone prophylaxis following myocardial infarction: A meta-analysis. Arch. Intern. Med. *153*:2661, 1993.

1237. Stevenson, J. C., Crook, D., Godsland, I. F., et al.: Hormone replacement therapy and the cardiovascular system: Nonlipid effects. Drugs *47*(Suppl. 2):35, 1994.

1238. The Writing Group for the PEPI Trial: Effects of estrogen or estrogen/progestin regimens on heart disease risk factors in postmenopausal women: The postmenopausal estrogen/progestin interventions (PEPI) trial. JAMA *273*:199, 1995.

1238a. Samaan, S. A., and Crawford, M.H.: Estrogen and cardiovascular function after menopause. J. Am. Coll. Cardiol. *26*:1403, 1995.

1239. Lobo, R. A., and Speroff, L.: International consensus conference on postmenopausal hormone therapy and the cardiovascular system. Fertil. Steril. *61*:592, 1994.

1240. Colditz, G. A., Hankinson, S. E., Hunter, D. J., et al.: The use of estrogens and progestins and the risk of breast cancer in postmenopausal women. N. Engl. J. Med. *332*:1589, 1995.

Chapter 38
Chronic Coronary Artery Disease

BERNARD J. GERSH, EUGENE BRAUNWALD, JOHN D. RUTHERFORD

Chronic coronary artery disease (CAD) is most commonly due to obstruction of the coronary arteries by atheromatous plaques[1]; the pathogenesis of atherosclerosis is described in Chap. 34. Factors that predispose to this condition are discussed in Chap. 35, the control of coronary blood flow in Chap. 36, and acute myocardial infarction in Chap. 37; sudden cardiac death, another significant consequence of CAD is presented in Chap. 24.

The importance of CAD in contemporary society is attested to by the almost epidemic number of persons afflicted[2-3a]—especially when this number is compared with the anecdotal reports of its occurrence in the medical literature before this century. More than 11 million Americans have CAD, which causes more deaths, disability, and economic loss in industrialized nations than any other group of diseases. About 6.3 million persons in the United

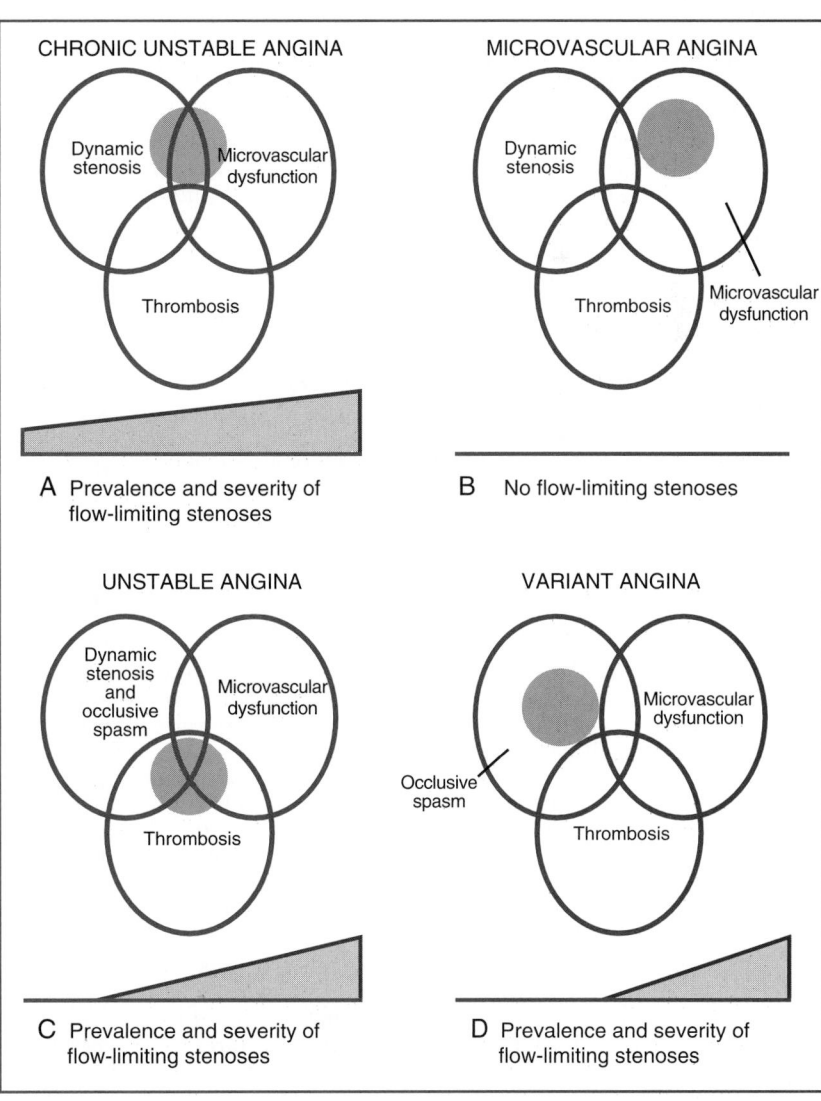

FIGURE 38–1. Pathogenetic components of various anginal syndromes. Chronic stable angina (A) is caused by flow-limiting coronary artery stenoses of variable severity and number, but residual coronary flow reserve can be modulated by dynamic changes in peristenotic smooth muscle tone (dynamic stenoses) or by microvascular dysfunction. Microvascular angina (B) is caused by coronary microvascular dysfunction. Unstable angina (C) is caused by a variable combination of thrombosis, dynamic stenoses, occlusive spasm, and microvascular dysfunction occurring not only in the presence of flow-limiting coronary artery stenoses, but also in their absence. Variant angina (D) is caused by occlusive epicardial coronary artery spasm, which may occur not only at the site of flow-limiting stenoses of variable severity but also in angiographically normal segments. (From Maseri, A.: Ischemic Heart Disease. New York, Churchill Livingstone, 1995, pp. 454–455.)

States have a history of CAD, and the estimated cost for the treatment of heart disease is $56 billion annually. The direct and indirect costs have been estimated at $14 billion per year. Given the current magnitude of the problem and the increasing prevalence of CAD which is anticipated because of the aging of the population, the recognition, management, and prevention of CAD are of major public health importance.[2] However, in the past three decades, encouraging reductions in the consequences of CAD have been noted (see p. 1126).[4] For example, between 1961 and 1991, the age-adjusted death rate for CAD declined by 52 per cent, more so in men than in women.[1] Similar trends have been observed in many industrialized nations with different health care systems. Multiple causes may have contributed to this favorable trend. These include the impact of reduction of risk factors (Chap. 35), improvements in socioeconomic circumstances including enhanced access to care, and new methods of diagnosis and treatment.

There is no uniform presenting syndrome for CAD. Chest discomfort is usually the predominant symptom in chronic (stable) angina (see p. 1291), unstable angina (p. 1334), Prinzmetal's (variant) angina (p. 1340), microvascular angina (p. 1343) (Fig. 38–1), and acute myocardial infarction (p. 1198). However, syndromes of CAD also occur in which ischemic chest discomfort is absent or not prominent. These include asymptomatic (silent) myocardial ischemia (p. 1344), congestive heart failure, cardiac arrhythmias, and sudden death (p. 747). There are also nonatherosclerotic causes of obstructive CAD[6] (p. 1349). Myocardial ischemia may also occur in the *absence* of obstructive CAD, as in the case of aortic valve disease, hypertrophic cardiomyopathy, idiopathic dilated cardiomyopathy, and luetic aortitis. Moreover, CAD may coexist with these other forms of heart disease. It may also be present in patients with noncardiac disease, e.g., esophageal disorders (p. 1291), confusing the differential diagnosis of chest discomfort.

STABLE ANGINA PECTORIS

CLINICAL MANIFESTATIONS

CHARACTERISTICS OF ANGINA (see also p. 4). Angina pectoris is a discomfort in the chest or adjacent areas caused by myocardial ischemia brought on by exertion and associated with a disturbance of myocardial function but without myocardial necrosis.[7] Heberden's initial description of the chest discomfort as conveying a sense of "strangling and anxiety" is still remarkably pertinent, although adjectives frequently used to describe this distress include "vise-like," "constricting," "suffocating," "crushing," "heavy," and "squeezing." In other patients, the quality of the sensation is more vague and is described as a mild pressure-like discomfort or an uncomfortable numb sensation. The site of the discomfort is usually retrosternal, but radiation is common and usually occurs down the ulnar surface of the left arm; the right arm and the outer surfaces of both arms may also be involved[7-9] (Fig. 1-1, p. 6). Anginal discomfort above the mandible or below the epigastrium is rare. Anginal "equivalents" (i.e., symptoms of myocardial ischemia other than angina), such as dyspnea, faintness, fatigue, and eructations, are common, particularly in the elderly. A history of abnormal exertional dyspnea may be an early indicator of CAD even when angina is absent or when there is no electrocardiographic evidence of ischemic heart disease.[10] Dyspnea at rest or with exertion may be a manifestation of very severe ischemia leading to elevation of the left ventricular filling pressure.

A careful clinical history is the key to the correct diagnosis and is particularly important in this era of cost-conscious practice of medicine, when it may obviate the need for more expensive testing. If the quality of the pain, its duration, precipitating factors, and associated symptoms are taken into consideration, it is usually possible to arrive at a correct diagnosis (Table 1-3, p. 5). The typical episode of angina pectoris usually begins gradually and reaches its maximum intensity over a period of minutes before dissipating. It is unusual for angina pectoris to reach its maximum severity within seconds, and it is characteristic that patients with angina usually prefer to rest, sit, or stop walking during episodes.[7]

Typical angina pectoris is relieved within minutes by rest or by the use of nitroglycerin. The response to the latter is often a useful diagnostic tool, although it should be remembered that esophageal pain and other syndromes

may also respond to nitroglycerin.[11] A delay of more than 5 to 10 minutes before relief is obtained suggests that the symptoms are either not due to ischemia or, alternatively, due to severe ischemia. The phenomenon of "first effort" or "warm-up" angina is used to describe the ability of some patients who develop angina with exertion to subsequently continue at the same level of exertion without symptoms after an intervening period of rest. It has been postulated that this may be due to ischemic preconditioning.[12]

The fact that the anginal discomfort varies considerably among patients and that other entities can mimic it often makes the differential diagnosis of chest pain difficult.[7,8,13] (Table 1–1, p. 3). Characteristics that are *not* suggestive of angina are fleeting, momentary chest pains described as "needle jabs" or "sticking pains," discomfort that is aggravated or precipitated by breathing or by a single movement of the trunk or arm, pain that is relieved within a few seconds of lying horizontally, discomfort relieved within a few seconds by one or two swallows of food or water and that is localized to a very small area (e.g., an area the size of the tip of a finger). Pain that is associated with or reproduced by pressure on the chest wall is unlikely to be angina pectoris, as is the syndrome of constant, aching pain that is present for hours at a time. In general, anginal discomfort does not last for more than 30 minutes unless the patient is having a myocardial infarction or an arrhythmia.

MECHANISM. The mechanisms of cardiac pain and the neural pathways remain poorly understood.[14] It is presumed that the discomfort arises from sensory endplates of the intracardiac sympathetic nerves. The afferent fibers traverse the nerves that connect to the upper five thoracic sympathetic ganglia and upper five distal thoracic roots of the spinal cord. Impulses are transmitted by the spinal cord to the thalamus and hence to the neocortex. Within the spinal cord, cardiac sympathetic afferent impulses may converge with impulses from somatic thoracic structures, which may provide a basis for referred cardiac pain (e.g., to the chest).[15] The contribution of vagal afferents to ischemic pain is unclear. Using positron emission tomography to examine changes in regional cerebral blood flow associated with angina pectoris, it was proposed that cortical activation is necessary for the sensation of pain, but that the thalamus may act as a gate to afferent pain signals.[16]

Triggers. The specific substances or triggers that stimulate the sensory nerve endings and begin the series of interactions that culminate in chest discomfort have not been identified. Attention has been paid to a variety of substances, including peptides that are released from cells as a result of transient ischemia, such as adenosine, bradykinin, histamine, and serotonin.[17] In one study, adenosine administered intravenously reproduced the symptom in over 90 per cent of patients with angina. Another hypothesis has suggested that mechanical stretching of a coronary artery may be the cause of pain.[17] Thus, the link between ischemic events at a tissue level and the perception of pain remains a subject of investigation.[17]

Differential Diagnosis of Chest Pain
(see Table 1–2, p. 3 and Fig. 1–2, p. 6)

The differentiation of various disorders from CAD is challenging because the severity of the chest pain and the seriousness of the underlying disorder are not necessarily related. Compounding the difficulty in differential diagnosis is the common myth that pain in the left arm or left side of the chest is an ominous sign signifying the presence of CAD. However, a host of disorders can cause discomfort in these locations.

ESOPHAGEAL DISORDERS. The common painful esophageal disorders that may simulate or coexist with angina pectoris are gastroesophageal reflux and disorders of esophageal motility, including diffuse spasm as well as "nutcracker" esophagus characterized by high-amplitude peristaltic contractions and vigorous achalasia.[19] Symptomatic esophageal reflux is common and is estimated to occur in 7 to 14 per cent of an otherwise "healthy" United States population. The typical characteristics of esophageal and cardiac pain are shown in Table 38–1. The classic presentation of esophageal pain is "heartburn," particularly in relationship to changes in posture and meals and in association with dysphagia. Esophageal spasm also may cause constant retrosternal discomfort of uniform intensity or severe spasmodic pain during or after swallowing.

There is no simple way to diagnose esophageal disease as the cause of chest pain, and the predictive value of each of the standard tests is poor. In one series of 200 patients with esophageal pain, heartburn was the presenting feature in 85 per cent, 21 per cent described pain radiating to the arms, and 5 per cent to the fingers, and 22 per cent experienced pain initiated by exertion.[20] To further compound the difficulty in distinguishing between angina and esophageal pain, both may be relieved by nitroglycerin.[21] However, esophageal pain is often relieved by milk, antacids, foods, or occasionally warm liquids.

GASTROESOPHAGEAL REFLUX. The esophageal acid perfusion, or Bernstein test, may be helpful in its use of alternate infusions of dilute acid and normal saline by a nasal gastric catheter, placing the tip at the level of the midesophagus.[22] Infusion of acid produces pain in over 90 per cent of patients with subjective and objective evidence of gastroesophageal acid reflux, but it is particularly useful if the patient's symptoms are reproduced.[23] Acid reflux into the esophagus can also be recognized by recording the pH from an electrode at the tip of a catheter inserted into the distal esophagus.

ESOPHAGEAL MOTILITY DISORDERS. These are not uncommon in patients with retrosternal chest pain of unclear cause and should be specifically excluded or confirmed, if possible. In addition to chest pain, the majority of such patients have dysphagia. Although barium studies may reveal motility problems, esophageal manometry may show diffuse esophageal spasm, increased pressure at the lower esophageal sphincter, and other motility disorders. Provocative pharmacological agents such as methacholine may provoke esophageal

pain and manometric signs of spasm. Surgical or medical therapy of esophageal reflux improves symptoms in patients whose chest pain coincides with documented episodes of reflux.[24]

CHEST PAIN AND NORMAL CORONARY ARTERIES. It is important to distinguish between chest pain due to esophageal disease and chest pain secondary to ischemia with normal coronary arteries. This condition, also known as *syndrome X*, is discussed later in this chapter (see p. 1343). The incidence of esophageal disease is substantial among patients with nonischemic chest pain and normal coronary arteries. In one study of patients with "angina-like pain" believed to be noncardiac in origin (most of whom had undergone coronary angiography), the combination of esophageal motility and distal esophageal pH monitoring showed evidence of symptomatic esophageal disease in 24 per cent.[25] A more complex problem is determining if part or all of the symptoms in patients with *known* CAD is due to esophageal disease. Both CAD and esophageal disease are common clinical entities that may coexist. A diagnostic evaluation for an esophageal disorder may be indicated in patients with CAD who have a poor symptomatic response to antianginal therapy in the absence of documentation of severe ischemia or in patients with persistent symptoms despite adequate coronary revascularization.

BILIARY COLIC. This symptom is sometimes confused with angina pectoris. It is usually caused by a rapid rise in biliary pressure due to obstruction of the cystic or bile duct. The pain is steady, usually lasts 2 to 4 hours, and subsides spontaneously without any symptoms between attacks. It is generally most intense in the right upper abdomen but may also be felt in the epigastrium or precordium. This discomfort is often referred to the scapula, may radiate around the costal margin to the back, or rarely may be felt in the shoulder, suggesting diaphragmatic irritation. Although nausea and vomiting are common, the relationship of the pain to meals is variable. Although a history of dyspepsia, flatulence, fatty food intolerance, and indigestion may be associated with cholelithiasis, these symptoms are also commonly experienced by the general population. Ultrasonography is accurate in diagnosing gallstones and allows determination of gallbladder size, thickness, and whether or not the bile ducts are dilated. Failure to opacify the gallbladder on oral cholecystography may indicate nonfunction due to disease.

COSTOSTERNAL SYNDROME. In 1921, Tietze first described a syndrome of local pain and tenderness, usually limited to the anterior chest wall, associated with swelling of the costal cartilages. This condition causes pain that can resemble angina pectoris. The full-blown Tietze syndrome, i.e., pain associated with tender swelling of the costochondral junctions, is uncommon, whereas costochondritis causing tenderness of the costochondral junctions (without swelling) is relatively common.[26] Pain on palpation of these joints is a useful clinical sign. Local pressure should be applied routinely to the anterior chest wall during the examination of the patient. Treatment of costochondritis usually consists of reassurance and anti-inflammatory agents.

CERVICAL RADICULITIS. This may occur as a constant ache, sometimes resulting in a sensory deficit. The pain may be related to motion of the neck, just as motion of the shoulder triggers attacks of pain due to bursitis. A hyperalgesic area of skin, noted by running the finger down the back and exerting pressure, may lead to the suspicion of thoracic root pain. Occasionally, pain mimicking angina can be due to compression of the brachial plexus via cervical ribs. Physical examination may also detect pain brought about by movement of an arthritic shoulder, a calcified shoulder tendon, and the like. The musculoskeletal disorders that can mimic angina include subacromial bursitis and costochondritis.

OTHER CAUSES OF ANGINA-LIKE PAIN. *Acute myocardial infarction* is usually associated with prolonged ($>$30 min-

TABLE 38–1 SIMILARITIES AND DIFFERENCES BETWEEN ESOPHAGEAL AND CARDIAC PAIN

	SIMILARITIES OF CARDIAC AND ESOPHAGEAL PAIN	DISTINGUISHING FEATURES OF ESOPHAGEAL PAIN
Location	Mid or lower retrosternal. May be a severe epigastric pain with radiation up to neck.	High epigastric, behind xiphoid process or in low retrosternal area.
Nature	Heaviness, squeezing, tightness, or burning. Can be associated with weakness, diaphoresis, and anxiety.	Often burning or perceived as spasm. Heartburn is frequent association. Can be associated with increased salivation. Dysphagia occurs.
Radiation	Upward toward throat. May radiate to left neck, shoulder, or arm.	Tends to ascend but not radiate to left side. Radiation to both shoulders and/or arms is less frequent. When pain begins in lower retrosternal area it often radiates down to epigastrium.
Precipitants	After eating. Angina is more likely with physical activity after eating.	After eating certain foods—alcohol, coffee, spices. Less likely to be brought on by exertion. Can be precipitated by change in posture, e.g., by lying down.
Duration	Can last a short duration (2 to 10 min).	May last hours; may wax and wane.
Relieving factors	May be relieved or released by nitroglycerin, standing, and relaxing.	

Modified from Miller, A. J.: Diagnosis of Chest Pain. New York, Raven Press, 1988, pp. 74–76.

utes), severe pain that, apart from duration and intensity, may be similar to angina pectoris (see p. 1198). It is associated with characteristic electrocardiographic and enzyme findings.

Severe pulmonary hypertension may be associated with exertional chest pain with the characteristics of angina pectoris, and, indeed, this pain is thought to be due to right ventricular ischemia which develops during exertion (see p. 788). Other associated symptoms include exertional dyspnea, dizziness, and syncope. Associated findings on physical examination, such as a parasternal lift, palpable and loud pulmonary component of the second sound, and right ventricular hypertrophy on the electrocardiogram usually are readily recognized.

Pulmonary embolism presents with dyspnea as the cardinal symptom, but chest pain may be associated (see p. 1587). Pleuritic pain suggests pulmonary infarction, and a history of exacerbation of the pain with inspiration, along with a pleural friction rub, usually helps to distinguish it from angina pectoris.

The pain of *acute pericarditis* (see p. 1481) at times may be difficult to distinguish from angina pectoris. However, pericarditis tends to occur in younger patients than does angina, and the diagnosis depends on chest pain, a pericardial friction rub, and electrocardiographic changes. The chest pain usually is sudden in onset, severe and persistent and is intensified by coughing, swallowing, and inspiration. Relief may be obtained by sitting up and leaning forward; palpation of the trapezius ridge often causes discomfort. A pericardial friction rub can be detected in most patients if listened for carefully, at different times, and with the patient in different positions. Early, widespread ST-segment elevations may be present. Some patients with pericardial disease describe a vague retrosternal discomfort without the characteristics of pleuropericarditis, but a relationship to exertion is not present. Pain due to hepatic congestion may complicate the clinical history.

In many of the disorders just mentioned, angina pectoris can usually be excluded by a careful history and physical examination. It must be emphasized, however, that chronic CAD can and frequently does coexist with any of these other disorders and that noncardiac disease can trigger a true angina attack in a patient with CAD. For example, among patients with severe, disabling angina, obstructive sleep apnea may be a common precipitant of nocturnal angina, which may respond dramatically to the initiation of continuous positive airway pressure.[27]

Physical Examination

GENERAL EXAMINATION. The physical examination has often been considered relatively unhelpful in patients with chronic CAD and stable angina, and, indeed, it is often entirely normal. Nonetheless, a diligently performed physical examination can provide useful clues to the diagnosis and in the identification of patients with risk factors for CAD. The value of the examination is enhanced when performed during and soon after an episode of angina pectoris. Not only should the examination be directed at the cardiovascular system, but particular attention should be directed to the presence of comorbid conditions that exert a major impact on prognosis and on the risks and expectations of coronary revascularization procedures.

Inspection of the eyes may reveal a *corneal arcus,* and examination of the skin may show xanthomas (Fig. 2–2, p. 17). The size of the corneal arcus appears to correlate positively with age and levels of cholesterol and low-density lipoproteins.[28] *Xanthelasma,* in which lipid deposits are intracellular, appear to be promoted by increased levels of triglycerides and a relative deficiency of high-density lipoproteins. In the Lipid Research Clinic study,[29] the incidence of both xanthelasma and corneal arcus increased with age and was highest in patients with type II hyperli-

poproteinemia and usually low in those with the type IV phenotype. Retinal arteriolar changes (see p. 15) are common in patients with CAD and diabetes mellitus or hypertension.

There appears to be some correlation between CAD and *diagonal earlobe crease* (except in native American Indians and Asians). There is often a unilateral diagonal earlobe crease in younger persons with CAD that becomes bilateral with advancing age.[30]

The *blood pressure* may be chronically elevated or may rise acutely (along with heart rate) during an angina attack. Changes in blood pressure may precede (and precipitate) or follow (and be caused by) angina.

Other important features of the general physical examination are abnormalities of the arterial pulses and of the venous system. The association between peripheral vascular disease and CAD is strong and well documented.[31,32] This is not confined to patients with symptomatic or clinically overt peripheral vascular or carotid artery disease but is seen also in asymptomatic subjects with a reduced ankle-brachial blood pressure index or evidence of early carotid disease on ultrasonography.[33] The presence of carotid and peripheral arterial disease on palpation and auscultation increases the likelihood that chest discomfort of unclear origin is caused by CAD. Evaluation of the patient's venous system, particularly in the legs, may have an important bearing on the type of grafting procedure employed in subsequent coronary bypass surgery.

CARDIAC EXAMINATION. The presence of murmurs of hypertrophic cardiomyopathy or aortic valve disease suggests that angina may be due to conditions other than (or in addition to) CAD. It is often helpful to examine the heart *during* an episode of pain because ischemia may produce transient left ventricular dysfunction with a third heart sound and pulmonary rales detectable on physical examination. A softening of the mitral component of the first heart sound due to ischemic left ventricular dysfunction may also be demonstrated during angina. Paradoxical splitting of the second heart sound (see p. 33) may occur transiently during an angina attack and appears to be related to asynergy and prolongation of left ventricular contraction, resulting in delayed closure of the aortic valve. If other obvious cardiac diseases are absent, a third or loud fourth heart sound suggests ischemia as the basis for the chest pain. These sounds are common in patients with angina at rest, and their frequency is increased during handgrip exercise[34] even if the latter does not precipitate angina pectoris. A sustained apical cardiac impulse is common in patients with moderate or severe left ventricular dysfunction.

When patients with CAD lie in the left lateral recumbent position, dyskinetic bulges at the apex may be palpable. These bulges correspond to dyskinetic areas and often complement the auscultatory findings of diastolic filling sounds.[35,36] Transient apical systolic murmurs are quite common in CAD and have been attributed to reversible papillary muscle dysfunction secondary to transient myocardial ischemia. When persistent, such murmurs may be due to papillary muscle fibrosis, often a manifestation of subendocardial infarction or a regional wall motion abnormality altering the alignment of the papillary muscles in relation to other components of the mitral valve apparatus. These murmurs are more prevalent in patients with extensive CAD, especially those with prior myocardial infarction and left ventricular dysfunction. The systolic murmurs may assume a variety of configurations (early, late, or holosystolic) and may be accentuated by exertion or during angina. A midsystolic click, often followed by a late systolic murmur produced by mitral valve prolapse (see p. 1032), also occurs in patients with CAD. A diastolic murmur or a continuous murmur is a rare finding in CAD and has been attributed to turbulent flow across a proximal coronary artery stenosis.[37]

PATHOPHYSIOLOGY

Angina pectoris results from myocardial ischemia, which is caused by an imbalance between myocardial oxygen requirements (MVO_2) and oxygen supply.[37a] The former may be elevated by increases in heart rate, left ventricular wall stress, and contractility (see p. 1161); the latter is determined by coronary blood flow and the coronary arterial oxygen content (Figs. 38–1 and 38–2).

ANGINA DUE TO INCREASED MYOCARDIAL OXYGEN DEMAND. In this condition, sometimes termed "demand angina," MVO_2 increases in the face of a constant oxygen supply. The increased MVO_2 commonly stems from norepinephrine release by adrenergic nerve endings, a physiological response to exertion, emotion, or mental stress. Of great importance to MVO_2 is the *rate* at which any task is carried out. Hurrying is particularly likely to precipitate angina, as are efforts involving motion of the hands over the head. The effects of emotion on the ratio of oxygen supply and demand are complex. Mental stress may increase adrenergic tone, reduce vagal activity, and increase blood pressure.[38] Anger may produce constriction in coronary arteries with preexisting narrowing without necessarily affecting oxygen demand.[39] Other factors causing angina due to an increase in MVO_2 in patients with obstructive CAD include exercise after eating and the excessive metabolic demands imposed by chills, fever, thyrotoxicosis, tachycardia from any cause, and hypoglycemia. Among patients with stable, fixed obstructive CAD, several studies using ambulatory electrocardiographic monitoring have documented the importance of increases in MVO_2 and, in particular, heart rate as a precipitant of ischemia. In these patients, in contrast to those with unstable angina (see p. 1331), ischemic episodes are preceded by significant increases in heart rate, and the likelihood of developing ischemia is proportional to both the magnitude and the duration of the heart rate increase.[11,40]

In all of these conditions, underlying fixed coronary artery obstruction is usually present, and the other factors (e.g., exertion, emotion, or fever) precipitate ischemia and chest discomfort by stimulating myocardial oxygen needs in the presence of a fixed and limited myocardial oxygen supply.

ANGINA DUE TO TRANSIENT DECREASED OXYGEN SUPPLY. There is increasing evidence that not only unstable angina but chronic stable angina may also be caused by transient reductions of oxygen supply as a consequence of coronary vasoconstriction,[1,41,42] a condition sometimes termed "supply angina." The coronary arterial bed is well innervated, and a variety of stimuli alter coronary tone (see p. 1163). Nonocclusive intracoronary thrombi are another cause of reduced oxygen supply and myocardial ischemia, usually causing angina at rest (unstable angina, p. 1331) rather than chronic stable angina.

Patients with angina precipitated by a transient reduction in myocardial oxygen supply comprise a spectrum based upon the severity of the underlying fixed defect and the degree of the dynamic change in coronary arterial tone. In the typical patient with stable angina, the degree of fixed obstruction is sufficient to result in an inadequate coronary flow rate to cope with the increased oxygen demands of exercise. However, superimposed upon this, episodes of transient coronary vasoconstriction may cause additional limitations to coronary flow reserve in many patients.[43]

In rare patients without organic obstructing lesions, severe dynamic obstruction alone can cause myocardial ischemia and resultant angina (Prinzmetal's angina, p. 1340). On the other hand, in patients with severe fixed obstruction to coronary flow, only a minor increase in dynamic obstruction is necessary for blood flow to fall below a critical level and cause myocardial ischemia (Fig. 38–3).

FIXED COMPARED WITH VARIABLE-THRESHOLD ANGINA. The variability of the threshold for angina differs widely among patients with chronic angina. In patients with fixed-threshold angina precipitated by increased oxygen demands, with few if any dynamic (vasoconstrictor) components, the level of physical activity required to precipitate angina is relatively constant. Characteristically, these patients can predict the amount of physical activity that will precipitate angina, e.g., walking up exactly two flights of stairs at a customary pace. When these patients are tested on a treadmill or bicycle, the pressure-rate product that elicits angina and/or electrocardiographic evidence of ischemia is constant or almost so.

Changes in the blood pressure–heart rate product (the double product) provide an approximation of alterations of myocardial oxygen requirements. In patients with fixed-threshold, demand angina,

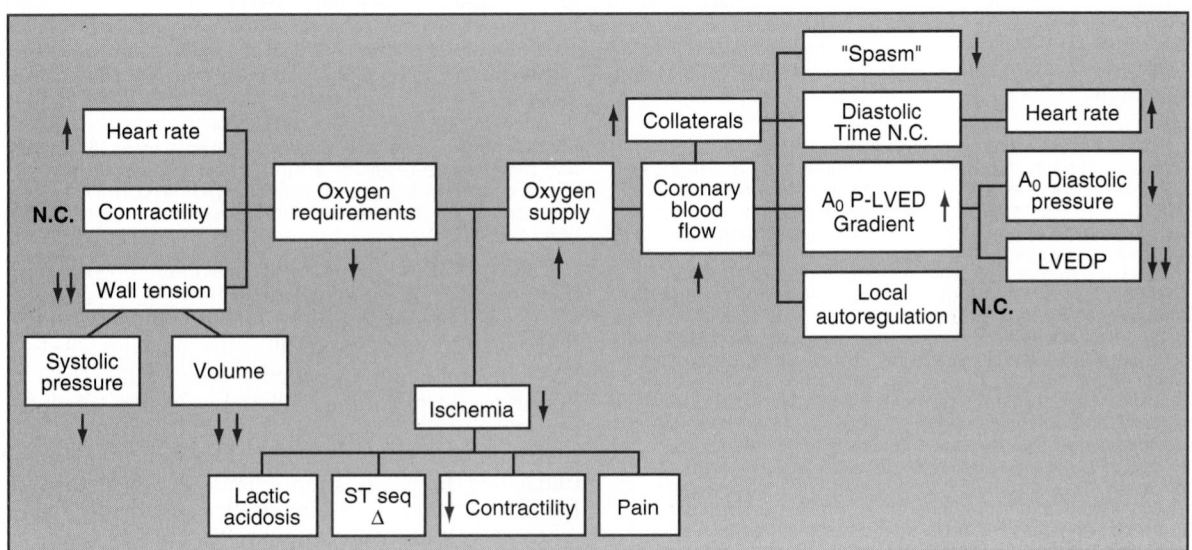

FIGURE 38–2. Factors influencing balance between myocardial oxygen requirements *(left)* and supply *(right).* Arrows indicate effects of nitrates. In relieving angina pectoris, nitrates exert favorable effects by reducing oxygen requirements and increasing supply. Although a reflex increase in heart rate would tend to reduce the time for coronary flow, dilation of collaterals and enhancement of the pressure gradient for flow to occur as the LVEDP falls tend to increase coronary flow. A_0P = aortic pressure; LVEDP = left ventricular end-diastolic pressure; NC = no change. (From Frishman, W. H.: Pharmacology of the nitrates in angina pectoris. Am. J. Cardiol. *56*:81, 1985.)

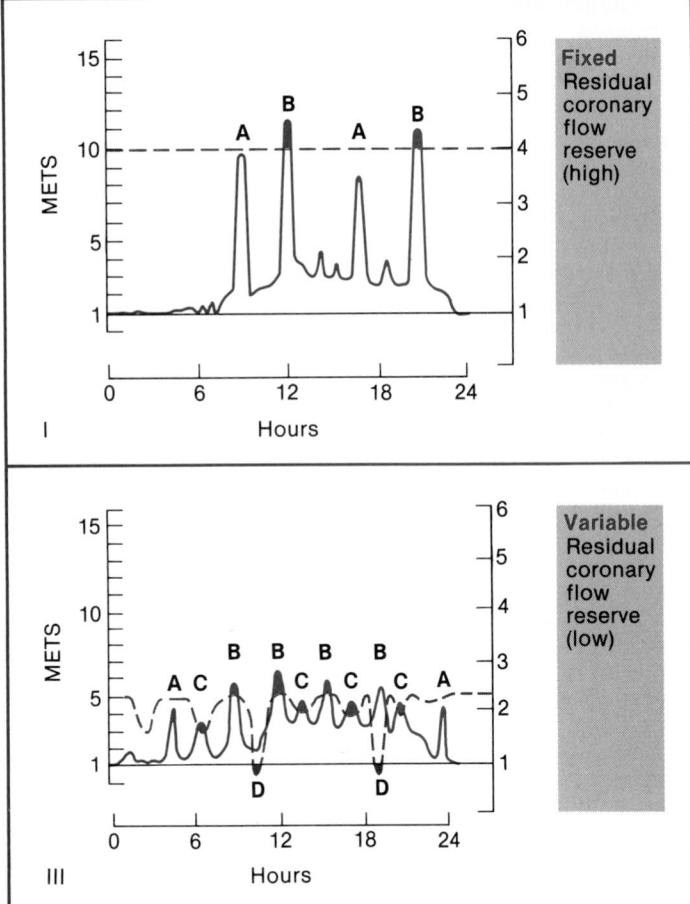

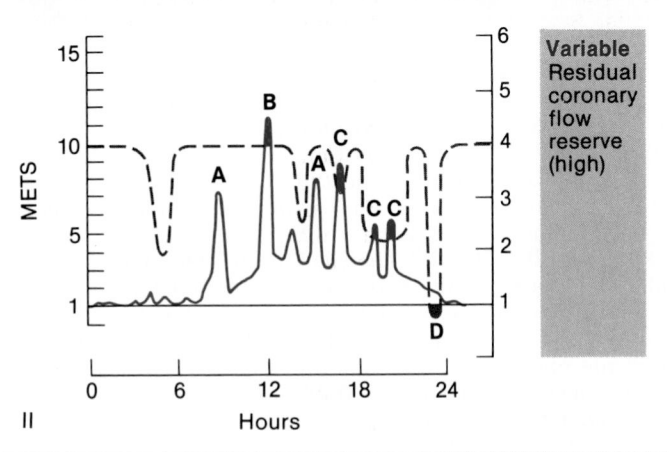

FIGURE 38–3. Schematic illustration of the relation between physical activity (during 24 hours) expressed as METS (multiple of basal metabolic oxygen consumption) and coronary flow reserve. Normally, during resting conditions, coronary flow reserve exactly matches the metabolic demand. However, when metabolic demands increase to a maximum of 16 METS, coronary flow reserve increases up to six times the resting value to match the increased demand for flow by the myocardium so that no ischemia occurs.

I. In this situation, a patient has a moderately severe fixed coronary artery obstruction that reduces coronary flow reserve to four times the resting value. *A*, The patient can exercise up to approximately 10 METS without developing ischemia; *B*, however, exercise above approximately 10 METS triggers ischemia.

II. In this situation, the patient has a moderately severe stenosis that fixes the coronary reserve at four times resting levels as in I. In addition, there is a variable stenosis. Therefore, residual coronary flow reserve has an upper limit that is fixed but that can decrease because of the presence of the mechanisms that transiently interfere with coronary blood flow. Thus, the residual coronary flow reserve can vary throughout the day. Under these conditions, if the patient exercises beyond the maximal residual coronary flow reserve, ischemia will always develop (*B*). However, the patient may also develop ischemia on other occasions after smaller degrees of exercise, when residual coronary flow reserve is decreased by these functional factors (*C*). Occasionally, coronary flow reserve decreases so that resting flow is impaired and ischemia occurs at rest (*D*). At other times of the day, this patient can exercise below the level of his maximal residual coronary flow reserve without experiencing ischemia (*A*).

III. In this situation, the patient has a very severe fixed stenosis and also variable stenosis. Maximal residual coronary flow reserve is reduced to little more than two times the resting value of coronary flow, thus allowing the patient to exercise up to a level of about 5 METS in the absence of any transient impairment of coronary flow. The combination of markedly reduced coronary flow reserve and of transient impairment of coronary flow results in frequent occurrences of ischemic episodes caused by excessive increase of demand above the maximal residual coronary flow (*B*) or by transient impairment of flow during exertion (*C*) or at rest (*D*). However, in the absence of transient impairment of flow, the patient can tolerate activities below 5 METS (*A*). (Modified from Maseri, A., Chierchia, S., and Kaski, J. C.: Mixed angina pectoris. Am. J. Cardiol., 56:31E and 32E, 1985.)

the specific threshold at which ischemia develops (as reflected in angina and/or ST-segment depression) is a function of the myocardial oxygen requirements. As the activity of the left ventricle (and therefore its oxygen requirements) increases, a point is reached at which perfusion distal to a critical coronary arterial obstruction cannot supply sufficient oxygen to the myocardium perfused by the obstructed artery; ischemia and angina ensue. This relationship is, however, modified by the effects of coronary vasomotor tone upon myocardial oxygen supply (Fig. 38–3).[44]

The majority of patients with variable-threshold angina have atherosclerotic coronary arterial narrowing, but dynamic obstruction caused by vasoconstriction plays an important role in causing myocardial ischemia.[45] These patients typically have "good days," when they are capable of substantial physical activity, and "bad days," when even minimal activity can cause clinical and/or electrocardiographic evidence of myocardial ischemia or when angina occurs even at rest. Often, even in the course of a single day, they may be capable of substantial physical activity at one time, while minimal activity results in angina at another. Patients with variable-threshold angina often complain of a circadian variation of angina which is more common in the morning. Angina on exertion and sometimes even at rest may be precipitated by cold temperatures,[46,47] emotion, and mental stress. A cold environment has been shown to increase peripheral resistance,[48–51] both at rest and during exercise. The rise in arterial pressure, by augmenting myocardial oxygen requirements, lowers the threshold for the development of angina. An alternative or additional explanation is the development of cold-induced coronary vasoconstriction.

Worsening of exercise tolerance after a meal is well documented and may be the result of a more rapid increase in MVO₂ when exercise is carried out postprandially. A dynamic coronary vasoconstrictor component to the pathophysiology of postprandial angina has also been suggested.[58]

MIXED ANGINA. This term has been proposed by Maseri to describe the many patients who fall between the two extremes of fixed-threshold and variable-threshold angina[53] (Fig. 38–3II). The pathophysiological and clinical correlations of ischemia in patients with stable CAD may have important implications for the selection of anti-ischemic agents, as well as for their timing. The greater the contribution from increased myocardial oxygen requirements to the imbalance between supply and demand, the greater the likelihood that beta-blocking agents will be effective, whereas nitrates and calcium channel blocking agents, at least on theoretical grounds, are likely to be especially effective in episodes due primarily to vasoconstriction. The finding that in most patients with chronic stable angina an increase in MVO₂ precedes episodes of ischemia, i.e., that they have demand angina, argues in favor of beta-blockers as essential therapeutic agents.[54]

GRADING OF ANGINA PECTORIS. A system of grading the

severity of angina pectoris proposed by the Canadian Cardiovascular Society has gained widespread acceptance.[55] The system is a modification of the New York Heart Association functional classification but allows patients to be categorized in more specific terms. Other grading systems include the specific activity scale developed by Goldman[56] and an anginal "score" developed by Califf et al.[57] The latter integrates the clinical features and "tempo" of angina together with electrocardiographic ST- and T-wave changes and offers independent prognostic information above that provided by age, gender, left ventricular function, and the coronary angiographic anatomy. A limitation of all of these grading systems is their dependence on accurate patient observation and patients' widely varying tolerance for symptoms.[58]

CORRELATION BETWEEN HISTORICAL FEATURES AND CORONARY ANGIOGRAPHY. Diamond and Forrester estimated the presence of angiographic CAD to be 90 per cent, 50 per cent, and 15 per cent, respectively, in middle-aged adults with histories of typical angina, atypical angina, or nonanginal chest pain, respectively, but only 3 to 4 per cent among asymptomatic middle-aged adults.[59] Although the clinical manifestations of CAD, including rest angina and nocturnal and postprandial angina, tend to be more severe among patients with multivessel than with single-vessel disease, neither the severity, duration, nature of the pain, nor its precipitating factors correlate with the extent of disease at angiography. Perhaps the most striking example of the lack of historical-arteriographic correlations is in two subgroups of patients—those with advanced obstructive CAD who are asymptomatic with "silent ischemia" (see p. 1344) and those with Prinzmetal's or variant angina who may have episodes of very severe anginal discomfort, yet with minimal or no underlying coronary atherosclerosis (see p. 1341).

The presentation of CAD and angina differs in men and women. These differences are discussed in Chap. 51.

NONINVASIVE TESTING

Resting Electrocardiogram

This is normal in approximately one-half of patients with chronic stable angina pectoris (Chap. 4). Patients with normal tracings at rest may have severe angina, but they usually have not previously suffered extensive infarction. The most common electrocardiographic abnormalities are nonspecific ST-T changes with or without evidence of prior transmural infarction. There are numerous pitfalls in the use of the *resting* electrocardiogram in the diagnosis of myocardial ischemia. ST-T wave abnormalities are common in the general population, with an overall prevalence of 8.5 per cent for men and 7.7 per cent for women in the Framingham Heart Study.[60] The prevalence increases with increasing age and in subjects with hypertension or diabetes mellitus, in cigarette smokers, and in women.[61] In addition to myocardial ischemia, other conditions that can produce ST-T wave abnormalities include left ventricular hypertrophy and dilatation, electrolyte abnormalities, neurogenic effects, and antiarrhythmic drugs.[61] In patients with CAD, however, the occurrence of ST-T wave abnormalities in the resting electrocardiogram may correlate with the severity of the underlying heart disease, including the number of vessels involved and the presence of left ventricular dysfunction.[62] This may explain the adverse impact of ST-T wave changes upon prognosis in these patients. In contrast, a normal resting electrocardiogram is a more favorable long-term prognostic sign in patients with suspected or definite CAD.[63] However, both the sensitivity and specificity of such electrocardiographic changes in patients with chronic stable angina are low.

A variety of conduction disturbances, most frequently

left bundle branch block and left anterior fascicular block, occur in patients with chronic stable angina, and they are often associated with marked impairment in left ventricular function,[64] reflecting multivessel disease and previous myocardial damage. In patients with chronic stable angina, abnormal Q waves are relatively specific but insensitive indicators of prior myocardial infarction. A variety of arrhythmias, especially ventricular premature beats, may be present on the electrocardiogram, but they too have low sensitivity and specificity for CAD.

Interval electrocardiograms may reveal the development of Q-wave infarctions that have gone unrecognized clinically. The increasing use of ambulatory electrocardiographic monitoring has shown that many patients with symptomatic myocardial ischemia also have episodes of silent ischemia that would otherwise go unrecognized during normal daily activities (see p. 1344).

Left ventricular hypertrophy on the electrocardiogram in patients with chronic stable angina should suggest the presence of underlying hypertension, aortic stenosis, or hypertrophic obstructive cardiomyopathy. This finding is a poor prognostic factor in patients with angina.[65]

Noninvasive Stress Testing

Noninvasive stress testing can provide useful and often indispensable information required to establish the diagnosis and estimate the prognosis in patients with chronic stable angina.[65] However, several studies have emphasized that the indiscriminate use of such tests may provide limited *incremental* information provided by noninvasive testing in patients with stable CAD, over and above that provided by the physicians' detailed and thoughtful clinical assessment.[66–69b] The appropriate application of noninvasive tests requires consideration of Bayesian principles (Fig. 5–11, p. 162). These state that the reliability of any test is defined by its sensitivity and specificity, and its predictive accuracy depends upon the prevalence of disease in the population under study. In an era of emphasis on cost-effectiveness, optimal utilization requires an assessment of the *incremental* amount of information provided by a test, over and above that which can be obtained from the standard clinical variables alone (Chap. 53).

Prior to undertaking noninvasive testing, it is appropriate to ask the question: What will be the response to the test if it is positive or if it is negative? If the answer is the same, the need for the test should be reconsidered.

Exercise Electrocardiography
(See also Chap. 5)
DIAGNOSIS OF CORONARY ARTERY DISEASE. As a screening test for CAD, the exercise electrocardiogram is useful in that it is relatively simple and inexpensive. It is particularly helpful in patients with chest pain syndromes who are considered to have moderate probability of CAD, and in whom the resting electrocardiogram is normal, provided that they are capable of achieving an adequate workload.[69a,70] Although the incremental value of exercise testing in diagnosing CAD is limited to patients in whom the estimated prevalence of CAD is either high or low, the test provides useful, additional information about the severity of ischemia, and the degree of functional limitation as well as the prognosis.[66,69a,71,72]

Certain symptomatic, electrocardiographic, and hemodynamic responses to treadmill exercise testing suggest the presence of significant obstruction in one or more coronary arteries. The most useful exercise electrocardiographic variable for the detection of CAD, and in particular multivessel disease, is the ST-segment shift during exercise and recovery (see p. 157).[73] The predictive value for the detection of CAD is 90 per cent, if typical chest discomfort occurs during exercise with ST horizontal or downward sloping depression of 1 mm or more. ST-segment depression of 2 mm or more accompanied by typical chest discomfort is virtually diagnostic of significant CAD.[72,73] In the absence of typical angina pectoris, downsloping or horizontal ST-segment depression of 1 mm or more has a predictive value of 70 per cent for the detection of significant coronary stenosis, but this increases to 90 per cent with ST-segment depression of 2 mm or more. The early onset of ST-segment depression during exercise, its long persistence following discontinuation of exercise, a downsloping or horizontal depression, and a low work capacity or exercise duration are all strongly associated with multivessel disease. Exercise-induced QRS prolongation also appears to be a function of exercise-induced ischemia[74] and is related to the extent of exercise-induced segmental contraction abnormalities.

In view of the relatively low overall sensitivity (approximately 75 per cent) of exercise stress electrocardiography in CAD, a negative result does not exclude this diagnosis. However, the likelihood of three-vessel or left main disease is markedly reduced by a negative test.

A major limitation of the sensitivity of the end exercise electrocardiogram is that it cannot be interpreted in many patients. This includes patients who are incapable of reaching the level of exercise required for near maximal effort (85 per cent or more of maximal predicted heart rate), particularly those receiving beta-adrenergic blockers, or those who develop fatigue, leg cramps, or dyspnea, and patients with abnormalities in the baseline electrocardiogram including those taking digitalis. In these patients, noninvasive imaging with exercise or pharmacological stress testing or diagnostic coronary angiography may be indicated.

INFLUENCE OF ANTIANGINAL THERAPY. Antianginal pharmacological therapy reduces the sensitivity of exercise testing as a screening tool. Beta blockade increases the exercise duration and suppresses, diminishes, or delays the appearance of ST-segment depression and thus obscures the diagnostic interpretation of exercise testing.[75] Because beta blockade reduces the sensitivity of the test, a negative exercise test in patients receiving antianginal drugs does *not* exclude significant and possibly life-threatening myocardial ischemia. Therefore, if the purpose of the exercise test is to *diagnose* ischemia, it should be performed, if possible, in the absence of antianginal medications. The advisability of withdrawing medications in an individual patient before exercise testing is a matter of judgment. Two or 3 days are required for patients receiving long-acting beta blockers. Unless the patient has severe angina, sublingual nitroglycerin for 1 or 2 days is likely to be sufficient to control symptoms if other therapy is withdrawn. For long-acting nitrates, calcium antagonists, and short-acting beta blockers, discontinuing the medications the day before testing usually suffices. If the purpose of the exercise test is to identify safe levels of daily activity or the extent of functional disability, the test should be carried out while the patient is taking the usual medications.

Nuclear Cardiology Techniques
(See Chap. 9)

STRESS MYOCARDIAL PERFUSION IMAGING (see also p. 288). In this technique, the radionuclide is injected at peak exercise or at symptom-limited endpoints, such as angina pectoris or dyspnea; the patient is encouraged to exercise for another 30 to 45 seconds to ensure that the initial myocardial uptake of the tracer reflects a perfusion pattern at peak stress[76,77] and the images are obtained several minutes later when the patient is at rest. Important advances in the assessment of myocardial viability and ischemia include both 24-hour delayed redistribution imaging and rest thallium-201 reinjection protocols[78–80] as well as the use of technetium-99m (Tc-99m)–labeled perfusion agents (isonitriles).

Exercise thallium (or isonitrile) scintigraphy, simultaneous with electrocardiography, is superior to exercise electrocardiography alone in the detection of CAD, in the identification of multivessel disease, in localizing diseased vessels, and in the detection of myocardial viability in regions of abnormal wall motion with or without Q-waves,[81] both in patients with and without normal resting electrocardiograms.[82] The published results using visual analysis

of exercise-redistribution images include more than 4000 patients with angiographic documentation of the presence or absence of coronary disease. In these studies, the sensitivity averaged 82 per cent and the specificity 88 per cent. In these same patients, conventional ECG exercise stress testing had a sensitivity ranging from 50 to 80 per cent.[83]

Stress myocardial scintigraphy is particularly helpful in the diagnosis of CAD in patients with abnormal resting electrocardiograms, such as those with left ventricular hypertrophy and strain and left bundle branch block. Among homogeneous populations of symptomatic patients, the magnitude of ST-segment depression on symptom-limited exercise testing correlates well with the extent of ischemia as assessed by quantitative thallium-201 scintigraphy. In *mixed* populations in which the proportion of false-positive ST-segment responses increases, greater reliance is placed upon thallium scintigraphy to assess the presence and magnitude of ischemia.[84] Thallium-201 scintigraphy provides important information in regard to prognosis (p. 274).[85–88]

Because stress myocardial scintigraphy is a relatively expensive test (three to four times the cost of an exercise electrocardiogram), certain issues should be considered: (1) a regular exercise electrocardiogram should always be obtained first in patients with chest pain and a normal resting electrocardiogram for screening and detection of CAD; (2) stress myocardial perfusion scintigraphy should *not* be used as a screening test in patients in whom the prevalence of coronary disease is low or moderate; (3) stress myocardial perfusion scintigraphy is more sensitive in detecting CAD, especially in patients with single-vessel coronary artery disease, than exercise electrocardiography.[89]

Pharmacological Nuclear Stress Testing (see also p. 289). For patients unable to exercise adequately, especially the elderly and patients with peripheral vascular disease and those limited by dyspnea, pharmacological stimulation with dipyridamole and adenosine prior to scintigraphic imaging may be employed.[90–95a] In a comparison of 2000 patients undergoing adenosine and dipyridamole pharmacological stress testing, adenosine was shown to cause a slightly greater degree of systemic vasodilation than dipyridamole. Although adverse effects occurred less often with dipyridamole than with adenosine, these were more difficult to manage and necessitated more monitoring time as well as the fairly frequent intravenous use of aminophylline for reversal.[90] In patients with asthma, dobutamine thallium scintigraphy is a useful and safe alternative to dipyridamole and adenosine.[92] A promising new pharmacological stress agent still under investigation is arbutamine, a sympathomimetic agent designed to simulate exercise, that is delivered via a closed-loop delivery device controlled by hemodynamic feedback. It is potentially superior to dobutamine, dipyridamole, and adenosine, but further studies are needed.[95b,95c]

EXERCISE RADIONUCLIDE ANGIOGRAPHY. The use of exercise radionuclide angiography in the detection and estimation of prognosis in CAD has fallen out of favor. Failure to increase the ejection fraction by 5 per cent or more was proposed as a diagnostic test for CAD.[77] However, this is a nonspecific finding that may occur in other conditions that compromise left ventricular function as well as in some healthy women. Although a combination of clinical and exercise variables, including peak ejection fraction, has been shown to be helpful in the identification of patients with severe CAD, the addition of radionuclide ventriculography in patients with normal electrocardiograms at rest adds little to the diagnostic information provided by clinical and other exercise variables.[85]

Echocardiography
(See also p. 89)

Two-dimensional echocardiography is useful in the evaluation of patients with chronic CAD, by assessing global and regional left ventricular function in the absence and presence of ischemia, as well as in establishing left ventricular hypertrophy and associated valve disease. Echocardiography is relatively inexpensive and safe. Rarely, coronary artery occlusion can be diagnosed by transesophageal echocardiography.[96] Stress echocardiography, in which imaging is carried out immediately after exercise, allows the detection of regional ischemia by identifying new areas of wall motion disorders. Adequate images can be obtained in more than 85 per cent of patients, and the test is highly reproducible. The inability to image at peak exercise is only a minor disadvantage because most wall motion abnormalities do not normalize immediately upon cessation of exercise. Several studies have shown that exercise echocardiography can *detect* the presence of CAD with an accuracy similar to that of stress thallium scintigraphic imaging and is superior to exercise electrocardiography alone.[97-99a]

PHARMACOLOGICAL STRESS ECHOCARDIOGRAPHY (see also p. 86). Among patients unable to exercise or those in whom the quality of the echocardiographic images during or immediately after exercise is poor, alternative echocardiographic approaches are available. These include transesophageal pacing with transesophageal echocardiography,[100] high-dose dipyridamole infusion, adenosine infusion, or dobutamine stress echocardiography. Arbutamine is a promising alternative agent.[100a] Whereas exercise echocardiography is the stress test of choice in patients able to achieve an adequate level, pacing and dobutamine stress echocardiography are more sensitive than dipyridamole.[101,102] Atropine increases the accuracy of dobutamine echocardiography, especially in patients taking beta blockers.[103] In one of the few direct comparisons in the same patients of exercise echocardiography, dobutamine echocardiography, and dipyridamole echocardiography, the sensitivity of exercise or dobutamine echocardiography was similar and was significantly higher than that of dipyridamole echocardiography. Specificity did not differ significantly among the tests. Moreover, in patients with known CAD, exercise and dobutamine echocardiography were superior to dipyridamole echocardiography in the assessment of the extent of disease.[101]

Several reports attest to the accuracy of dobutamine stress echocardiography in the detection of significant CAD.[104,105] Transesophageal dobutamine stress echocardiography has been shown to be feasible, safe, and accurate for the detection of myocardial ischemia. This may allow extension of dobutamine stress testing to patients with inadequate transthoracic echocardiographic imaging.[106] Although it has been shown that dobutamine stress echocardiography and exercise echocardiography are superior to exercise electrocardiographic testing alone and that these techniques are an excellent alternative to scintigraphic imaging, it has not been established that stress echocardiography is preferable or necessary in all patients who are otherwise suitable for exercise electrocardiographic testing. It is usually not cost-effective to utilize both techniques, and the choice of which stress to use and when is determined in part by the characteristics of the patients and the level of expertise and experience in any particular laboratory in addition to direct costs.

Clinical Application of Noninvasive Testing

GENDER DIFFERENCES IN THE DIAGNOSIS OF CAD (see also Chap. 51). Based upon earlier studies that documented a very high frequency of false-positive stress tests in women compared to men,[107] it is now generally accepted that electrocardiographic stress testing is not as reliable in women as it is in men. However, the prevalence of CAD among women in the patient populations under study was low, and the major explanation for the lower positive predictive value of exercise electrocardiography in women can be ac-

counted for on the basis of Bayesian principles.[108,109] Once men and women are stratified appropriately according to the pretest prevalence of disease, the results of stress testing are similar.[110]

Soft tissue attenuation artifacts, especially those caused by breast tissue in women, may reduce the diagnostic accuracy of myocardial perfusion scintigraphy in women.[111] Exercise radionuclide ventriculography has little if any place in the *diagnosis* of CAD in women, because a fall or no increase in ejection fraction at higher rates of exercise has been noted to occur in healthy women. However, among women without a prior history of myocardial infarction, exercise echocardiography was superior to exercise electrocardiography in the detection of CAD.[111a]

IDENTIFICATION OF PATIENTS AT HIGH RISK. When applying noninvasive tests to the diagnosis and management of CAD, it is useful to grade the results as negative, indeterminate, positive—not high risk, and positive—high risk. The criteria for high-risk positivity are shown in Table 38–2.

Regardless of the severity of symptoms, patients with high-risk noninvasive tests have a very high likelihood of CAD and, if they have no obvious contraindications to revascularization, should undergo coronary arteriography. Such patients, even if asymptomatic, are at risk of having left main or three-vessel CAD with impaired left ventricular function. They are at high risk of experiencing coronary events, and their prognosis may often be improved by coronary bypass surgery. In contrast, patients with clearly negative exercise tests, regardless of symptoms, have an excellent prognosis which cannot usually be improved by revascularization. If they do not have serious symptoms, they usually do not require coronary arteriography.

ASYMPTOMATIC PERSONS. In asymptomatic persons or in those with chest pain not likely to be angina, who are being screened for CAD, i.e., patients in whom the pretest likelihood of coronary disease is low (less than 15 per cent), a negative exercise electrocardiogram excludes, for practical purposes, ischemic heart disease. However, if in such a patient there is an abnormal exercise electrocardiographic test, several alternatives exist. If the test is positive but not high risk and the patient demonstrates excellent exercise capacity (i.e., to stage IV of a Bruce protocol or the equivalent), the likelihood of left main coronary disease or multivessel CAD is low, the prognosis is excellent, and the

TABLE 38–2 CRITERIA FOR HIGH RISK ON NONINVASIVE TESTING

HIGH-RISK EXERCISE ELECTROCARDIOGRAPHIC VARIABLES
≥ 2.0 mm ST-segment depression
≥ 1 mm ST-segment depression in stage I
ST-segment depression in multiple leads
ST-segment depression for greater than 5 minutes during the recovery period
Achievement of a workload of less than 4 METS or a low exercise maximal heart rate
Abnormal blood pressure response
Ventricular arrhythmias

HIGH-RISK THALLIUM-201 SCINTIGRAPHIC VARIABLES
Multiple perfusion defects (total plus reversible defects) in more than one vascular supply region (e.g., defects in coronary supply regions of the left anterior descending and left circumflex vessels)
Increased lung thallium-201 uptake reflecting exercise-induced left ventricular dysfunction
Postexercise transient left ventricular cavity dilation

From Beller, G. A.: Current status of nuclear cardiology techniques. Curr. Probl. Cardiol. *16*:463, 1991.

patient may usually be observed without further testing. If, on the other hand, such a patient has a high-risk positive exercise electrocardiogram (see p. 1295), coronary angiography is usually indicated to determine whether or not left main CAD or severe multivessel disease with left ventricular dysfunction is present. If the patient falls into an intermediate category (a positive but not high-risk exercise test), then a stress imaging study (echocardiography or perfusion scintigraphy) may provide further information. If both studies are abnormal but not high risk, the likelihood of CAD approaches 90 per cent.

PATIENTS WITH ATYPICAL ANGINA. In these patients, the pretest probability of CAD is approximately 50 per cent. If two noninvasive tests are abnormal, the likelihood of CAD exceeds 95 per cent; if both tests are normal, it falls below 5 per cent. When test results are discordant, they should be evaluated in the light of the exercise level achieved, the presence of accompanying symptoms, and whether or not one of the tests is positive with high risk. Thus, for example, a patient with atypical angina and a normal exercise electrocardiogram who develops multiple large perfusion defects on a stress thallium-201 scintigram at a heart rate of 130 beats/min has a much greater likelihood of having CAD than one who has a normal exercise electrocardiogram and develops a single small perfusion defect without chest pain at a heart rate of 185 beats/min.

PATIENTS WITH TYPICAL ANGINA. In patients with high pretest likelihood of disease of approximately 90 per cent, noninvasive testing is most valuable for estimating the extent and severity of CAD and thereby the prognosis. The development of a high-risk positive stress test points to multivessel disease and a high risk of subsequent coronary events, and unless there are contraindications to revascularization, coronary angiography is indicated.

OTHER TESTS

BIOCHEMICAL TESTS. Serum levels of cardiac enzymes are normal in patients with chronic stable angina, which serves to differentiate them from patients with acute myocardial infarction. There are more relevant discriminators in patients with unstable angina (see p. 1332), in whom elevations in serum creatine phosphokinase (CPK) and a newer marker, serum troponin T (see p. 1335), may be a useful prognostic indicator.[111]

In younger patients (<45 years) with chronic stable angina, metabolic abnormalities that are risk factors for the development of CAD are frequently detected. These include hypercholesterolemia and other dyslipidemias (Chap. 35), carbohydrate intolerance, and insulin resistance.[112,113] All patients with established or suspected CAD warrant biochemical evaluation of total cholesterol, low-density lipoprotein cholesterol, high-density lipoprotein cholesterol, triglycerides, and fasting blood sugar.

CHEST ROENTGENOGRAM. This is usually within normal limits in patients with chronic stable angina, particularly if they have a normal resting electrocardiogram and have not experienced a myocardial infarction. If cardiomegaly is present, it is indicative of either severe CAD with prior myocardial infarction, preexisting hypertension, concomitant valvular heart disease, or an associated nonischemic condition such as cardiomyopathy. The presence of coronary calcification on fluoroscopy is indicative of underlying CAD (see p. 223). In patients with CAD who are scheduled to undergo an invasive procedure, the additional benefit of chest radiography is in the identification of other conditions that could alter or complicate therapy, e.g., chronic obstructive lung disease, chest infections, or neoplasms.[114]

ELECTRON BEAM OR ULTRAFAST COMPUTED TOMOGRAPHY (CT) (see also p. 336). Noninvasive detection of CAD has long been possible through detecting calcification associated with plaques by fluoroscopy. Such calcific deposits are diagnostic of coronary atherosclerosis.[115] Electron beam cardiac CT as a screening technique for coronary atherosclerosis is now available in a number of centers.[115a] However, the relationship of a positive test to subsequent cardiac events in asymptomatic patients has not been established.[116,117] The absence of calcium on CT is strongly predictive of the absence of significant atherosclerotic disease.[118] An analysis by a committee of the American Heart Association on the potential value of electron beam CT or ultrafast CT concluded that, while the technique is highly predictive for the presence of atherosclerosis, the degree of atherosclerosis cannot be predicted and the prognostic importance has not yet been established. Although this modality was considered to have great potential, it was not recommended for routine screening of patients.[119,120]

CATHETERIZATION, ANGIOGRAPHY, AND CORONARY ARTERIOGRAPHY

The clinical examination and noninvasive techniques described above are extremely valuable in establishing the diagnosis of CAD and are indispensable to an overall assessment of patients with this condition. However, the definitive diagnosis of CAD and a precise assessment of its anatomical severity and its effects upon cardiac performance require cardiac catheterization, coronary arteriography, and left ventricular angiography[120a] (Chaps. 7 and 9). Among patients with chronic stable angina pectoris referred for coronary arteriography, approximately 25 per cent of patients each have one-, two-, or three-vessel disease (i.e., >70 per cent luminal diameter narrowing). Five to 10 per cent have obstruction of the left main coronary artery, and in approximately 15 per cent no critical obstruction is detectable. Coronary angiographic findings differ between patients whose first presentation is acute myocardial infarction and chronic stable angina. Patients with unheralded myocardial infarction have fewer diseased vessels, fewer stenoses and chronic occlusions, and less diffuse disease than do chronic stable angina patients, suggesting that the pathophysiological substrate and the propensity to thrombosis differ between the two groups of patients.[121] In patients with chronic angina who have a history of prior infarction, total occlusion of at least one major coronary artery is more common than in those without such a history.

Coronary artery ectasia, i.e., patulous, aneurysmal dilatation involving most of the length of a major epicardial coronary artery, is present in approximately 1 to 3 per cent of patients with obstructive CAD at autopsy or angiography. This angiographic lesion does not appear to affect symptoms, survival, or the incidence of myocardial infarction.[122,123] Coronary ectasia should be distinguished from discrete *coronary artery aneurysms*, which are almost never found in arteries without severe stenoses, are most common in the left anterior descending coronary artery, and are usually associated with extensive CAD.[124] These discrete atherosclerotic coronary artery aneurysms do not appear to rupture, and their resection is not warranted.

Coronary collateral vessels (see p. 1174) may protect against myocardial infarction when total occlusion occurs, provided that they are of adequate size.[125] In patients with abundant collateral vessels, myocardial infarct size is smaller than in patients without collaterals and total occlusion of a major epicardial artery may not lead to left ventricular dysfunction.[126] In patients with chronic occlusion of a major coronary artery but without infarction, collateral-dependent myocardial segments show nearly normal baseline blood flow and oxygen consumption but severely limited flow reserve. This provides an explanation for the ability of collaterals to protect against resting ischemia but not exercise-induced angina.[127]

Myocardial bridging of coronary arteries (Fig. 8–23, p. 258) is observed in angiographically normal coronary arteries and normally does not constitute a hazard. Occasionally, compression of a portion of a coronary artery by a myocardial bridge can be associated with clinical manifestations of myocardial ischemia during strenuous physical activity and may even initiate malignant ventricular arrhythmias.[128,129]

LEFT VENTRICULAR FUNCTION. *Ventricular relaxation*, as reflected in the early diastolic ventricular filling rate, may be impaired at rest in patients with chronic CAD. Diastolic filling becomes even more abnormal (slowed) during exercise, when ischemia intensifies. In patients with chronic stable angina, the frequency of elevation of left ventricular end-diastolic pressure and reduced cardiac output at rest, generally attributed to abnormal left ventricular dynamics, increases with the number of vessels exhibiting critical narrowing and with the number of prior infarctions.[130] However, there is a great deal of overlap among individual patients so that the severity of coronary arterial disease cannot be predicted from these two measurements. The left ventricular end-diastolic pressure may be elevated secondary to reduced ventricular compliance, left ventricular systolic failure, or a combination of these two processes.[131] Both impaired systolic and diastolic function may occur as a consequence of acute, reversible ischemia and/or chronic scar formation. In many patients with normal hemodynamics in the resting state, abnormalities of left ventricular function can be elicited by dynamic or isometric exercise. Elevations of left ventricular end-diastolic pressure usually occur *before* the patient develops angina and before there is electrocardiographic ST-segment depression.

Left ventricular function can be assessed by means of biplane contrast ventriculography. Global abnormalities of left ventricular function are reflected in elevations of left ventricular end-diastolic and end-systolic volumes and depression of the ejection fraction (see p. 425). These changes, are, however, quite nonspecific. Abnormalities of *regional* wall motion (hypokinesis, akinesia, or dyskinesia) are more characteristic of CAD because the latter is usually regional in distribution. Also, hyperkinetic contraction of nonischemic myocardium, detected by left ventriculography, may compensate for hypokinetic or akinetic ischemic or necrotic myocardium, thereby maintaining normal or nearly normal global left ventricular function, despite marked depression of function in one region of the ventricle.[133]

Left ventricular function (global or regional) may be normal at rest in patients with chronic CAD without previous myocardial infarction but may become abnormal during or after stress. Abnormalities of left ventricular function detected angiographically may signify irreversible damage, i.e., prior infarction, or it may indicate acute ischemia or chronic hypoperfusion sufficient to maintain the viability but not the contractility of the myocardium, i.e., "myocardial hibernation"[133–135] (see pp. 388 and 1176). Reversibility of this form of left ventricular dysfunction in patients with CAD and chronic stable angina is reflected in improved contraction assessed angiographically by an inotropic stimulus (postextrasystolic potentiation[136] or the infusion of a sympathomimetic amine[137]) or in long-term improvement after myocardial revascularization.

In addition to demonstrating areas of asynergy, left ventriculography may also show mitral valve prolapse, which occurs in approximately 20 per cent of patients with obstructive CAD[138] and probably results from impaired contractility of the ventricular myocardium and papillary muscles. Mitral regurgitation secondary to left ventricular dilatation may be observed in patients with chronic stable angina and ischemic cardiomyopathy.

CORONARY BLOOD FLOW AND MYOCARDIAL METABOLISM. Cardiac catheterization can also document abnormal myocardial metabolism in patients with chronic stable angina. With a catheter in the coronary sinus, arterial and coronary venous lactate measurements are obtained at rest and after suitable stresses, such as the infusion of isoproterenol[139] or pacing-induced tachycardia.[140] Because lactate is a byproduct of anaerobic glycolysis, its production by the heart and subsequent appearance in coronary sinus blood is a reliable sign of myocardial ischemia (see p. 1204). When combined with coronary arteriography, this technique may be helpful in localizing significant coronary obstructive lesions and myocardial ischemia.[141]

Studies of coronary flow reserve (maximum flow divided by resting flow) and of endothelial function are frequently abnormal in patients with CAD and chronic stable angina. They are discussed on pp. 200 and 1166.

MEDICAL MANAGEMENT

There are five aspects to the comprehensive management of chronic, stable angina: (1) identification and treatment of associated diseases, which can precipitate or worsen angina; (2) reduction of coronary risk factors; (3) general and nonpharmacological methods, with particular attention toward adjustments of lifestyle; (4) pharmacological management; and (5) revascularization by percutaneous transluminal angioplasty (or other catheter-based techniques) or by coronary bypass surgery.[141a] Although discussed individually, all five of these approaches must be considered,

often simultaneously, in each patient. Among the medical therapies only two—aspirin and effective lipid lowering—have been convincingly shown to reduce mortality and morbidity in patients with chronic stable angina. Other therapies such as nitrates, beta blockers, and calcium antagonists have been shown to improve symptomatology and exercise performance, but their effect, if any, on survival has not been demonstrated.

TREATMENT OF ASSOCIATED DISEASES

A number of common medical conditions that can increase myocardial oxygen demands or reduce oxygen delivery may present with new angina pectoris or the exacerbation of previously stable angina. These include anemia, marked weight gain, occult thyrotoxicosis, fever, infections, and tachycardia. Drugs such as amphetamines and isoproterenol all increase myocardial oxygen demands, as do other agents that stimulate the sympathetic nervous system. Cocaine, which can cause acute coronary spasm and myocardial infarction, is discussed on p. 1340. Congestive heart failure, by causing cardiac dilatation and tachyarrythmias including sinus tachycardia, can increase myocardial oxygen needs with an increase in the frequency and severity of angina. Identification and treatment of these conditions is critical to the management of chronic stable angina.

Reduction of Coronary Risk Factors

HYPERTENSION (see also Chaps. 26 and 27). The epidemiological links between an elevated blood pressure and CAD mortality and severity are well established.[142,143] Hypertension increases myocardial oxygen demands and intensifies ischemia in patients with preexisting obstructive coronary vascular disease. Increased left ventricular mass due to left ventricular hypertrophy is a stronger predictor of myocardial infarction and coronary heart disease death than is the actual degree of blood pressure elevation.[144] A meta-analysis of clinical trials of treatment for mild to moderate hypertension showed a statistically significant 16 per cent reduction of CAD events and mortality in patients receiving antihypertensive therapy.[145] It is logical to extend these observations on the benefits of antihypertensive therapy to patients with established CAD. Therefore, blood pressure control is an essential aspect of management of patients with chronic stable angina.

In conjunction with antihypertensive therapy, attainment of an ideal body weight is particularly important in obese patients in whom weight reduction, in addition to aiding blood pressure control, raises the threshold for and may even abolish angina pectoris.

CIGARETTE SMOKING. This is one of the most powerful risk factors for the development of CAD in all age groups (see p. 1147), and cardiac events occur at a younger age in smokers. In a study of Australian men and women with premature CAD, smoking and lipid abnormalities were the two variables most relevant to the *severity* of CAD.[143] Among patients with angiographically documented CAD, cigarette smokers have a higher 5-year mortality and relative risk of infarction or sudden death than those who have stopped smoking,[146] and smoking cessation lessens the risks of adverse coronary events in patients with established CAD.[147] In patients who have undergone coronary bypass surgery, the cessation of cigarette smoking has been shown to decrease substantially both morbidity and mortality.[148,149]

Cigarette smoking may be responsible for aggravating angina pectoris other than through the progression of atherosclerosis. It may increase myocardial oxygen demands and reduce coronary blood flow[150,150a] by means of an alpha-adrenergically mediated increase in coronary artery tone and thereby cause acute ischemia.[151] Cigarette smoking also appears to interfere with the efficacy of antianginal drugs; improvements in exercise tolerance and a reduction in angina pectoris occur when cigarette smoking is discontinued in patients with angina receiving a beta blocker or calcium antagonist.[152] Smoking cessation is one of the most effective and certainly the least expensive approaches to the prevention of disease progression in native vessels and bypass grafts. Techniques for smoking cessation are discussed on p. 1148.

Passive cigarette smoking,[153] the inhalation of smog and carbon monoxide, and ascent to high altitude all lower the threshold for angina, and their avoidance represents an important aspect of therapy. Symptoms may also be aggravated or exercise performance impaired in patients with chronic stable angina who encounter some specific environmental situations (traffic tunnels, houses with defective gas furnaces, and closed automobiles during heavy highway traffic).[154] The mechanism is probably decreased oxygen delivery to the myocardium. Every effort must be made to avoid these aggravating stimuli.[155]

MANAGEMENT OF DYSLIPIDEMIA (see also Chap. 35). Cholesterol lowering by diet and drugs has been shown to reduce the incidence of CAD in primary prevention trials. Among men with moderate hypercholesterolemia in the West of Scotland trial, treatment with pravastatin significantly reduced the incidence of myocardial infarction and death without adversely affecting the risk of death from non-cardiovascular causes.[155a] In patients with *established* CAD, lipid-lowering therapy has demonstrated a significant reduction in disease progression and in subsequent cardiovascular events.[156-159,159b] Angiographic trials of cholesterol lowering in patients with chronic CAD, many of whom had chronic stable angina, have shown that the effects on coronary obstruction are modest whereas the reduction in cardiovascular events is quite impressive. Two studies have shown that aggressive lipid-lowering drugs significantly improve endothelium-mediated responses in the coronary arteries of patients with atherosclerosis.[160,161] These findings may explain the disproportionate reduction in coronary events in patients treated with cholesterol-lowering therapy, despite very small degrees of anatomical regression of atherosclerotic stenoses. The results from the Scandinavian Simvastatin Survival Study (4S) of patients with a history of angina or prior myocardial infarction provide convincing evidence that lipid-lowering therapy significantly improves overall survival and reduces cardiovascular mortality in patients with coronary heart disease.[159]

The revised National Cholesterol Education Program Guidelines (see p. 1990) advocate cholesterol-lowering therapy in *all* patients with coronary heart disease or extracardiac atherosclerosis to LDL levels below 100 mg/dl.

ESTROGEN REPLACEMENT THERAPY (see also p. 1707). The male gender and, in women, the postmenopausal state, are risk factors for the development and progression of CAD. Epidemiological studies have shown that the favorable cardiovascular risk profile in premenopausal women changes after the menopause, in that the levels of total cholesterol, low-density lipoprotein cholesterol (LDL-C), apolipoprotein B, and triglycerides all increase while high-density lipoprotein cholesterol (HDL-C) decreases slightly or remains unchanged.[162,163] Several long-term studies have identified reduced HDL-C and increased triglyceride levels as powerful predictors of CAD risk among postmenopausal women.[164,165] Moreover, numerous, large cross-sectional studies and a randomized trial[166] strongly suggest that postmenopausal hormone replacement therapy with estrogens, alone or in combination with medroxyprogesterone acetate, has a favorable effect upon the cardiovascular risk factor lipid profile (by increasing HDL-C and lowering LDL-C and triglyceride levels[167,168]) and upon the incidence of cardiovascular events[169,170] and the extent of atherosclerosis as determined by carotid ultrasonography.[171]

The beneficial effect of estrogen replacement therapy is probably not limited to altering favorably the lipid profile. It may also involve the interaction between estrogen and estrogen receptors in blood vessels, the maintenance of normal endothelial function (see p. 1166) and their direct modulating effects upon vascular tone. Estrogen replacement therapy may reduce LDL oxidation and uptake by the arterial wall and alter favorably the hemostatic profile.[172,172a] One study of estrogen replacement therapy suggested that the greatest benefit was in women with established CAD and least in those with normal coronary vessels.[173] Thus, the case for estrogen replacement therapy as secondary prevention of CAD is strong[174] (as it is in the primary prevention in women with multiple risk factors for CAD). The National Cholesterol Education Program (NCEP) has tentatively endorsed estrogen therapy as a method of lowering lipid levels in postmenopausal women with *established* CAD.[175]

ANTIOXIDANTS. Oxidized LDL particles are strongly linked to the pathophysiology of atherogenesis (see p. 1116), and epidemiological data support an association between low levels of beta-carotene and myocardial infarction, at least among smokers.[176-178] Other studies imply that a high dietary intake of antioxidants, including flavonoids (polyphenolic antioxidants) naturally present in vegetables, fruits, tea, and wine and vitamin E, is associated with a decline in coronary heart disease events.[177-179] Large randomized trials evaluating the effects of antioxidant supplementation, as well as probucol, a lipid-lowering agent with additional antioxidant properties, are under way. Until the results are available, no firm recommendations can be made regarding antioxidant intake in patients with chronic stable angina. Nonetheless, in a subgroup analysis of patients who had undergone previous coronary bypass surgery, coronary artery lesion progression was less in subjects with a supplementary vitamin E intake of 100 IU per day or more compared with patients with a lower intake.[178]

EXERCISE (see also Chap. 40). The conditioning effect of exercise on skeletal muscles allows a greater workload at any level of total body oxygen consumption. By decreasing the heart rate at any level of exertion, a higher cardiac output can be achieved at any level of myocardial oxygen consumption. The combination of these two effects of exercise conditioning permits the patient with chronic stable angina to increase physical performance substantially following institution of a continuing exercise program.[180]

Most of the information about the physiological effects of exercise and their effect on prognosis in patients with CAD is derived from studies in patients entered into cardiac rehabilitation programs,[181,182] many of whom have sustained a prior myocardial infarction. There is less information on the benefits of exercise in patients with chronic stable CAD, but one study has confirmed a striking and direct relationship between the intensity of exercise and favorable changes in the morphology of obstructive lesions on angiography.[183]

Other studies in patients with known coronary heart disease have demonstrated the beneficial effects of prolonged exercise training on cardiac performance, effort tolerance, quality of life, and stress-induced myocardial ischemia.[184,185] The question of whether or not exercise accelerates the development of collateral vessels in patients with chronic CAD remains unsettled.

Thus, the available evidence suggests that regular, supervised physical exercise should be recommended for most patients with documented CAD and chronic stable angina. It is safe if begun under supervision[186] and, if survivors of a myocardial infarction can be used as a yardstick, it is probably cost-effective.[187] The psychological benefits of exercise are difficult to evaluate. However, exercise conditioning programs may be quite helpful in increasing the self-confidence of patients with chronic CAD (as they are in patients recovering from acute myocardial infarction). Patients who are involved in exercise programs usually are also more likely to be health conscious, to pay attention to diet and weight, and to discontinue cigarette smoking. Thus, in addition to a conditioning effect on skeletal and cardiac muscle, regular dynamic exercise provides the patient with a feeling of well-being, an important consideration in the management of any chronic disease.

For all of the aforementioned reasons, patients should be urged to participate in regular exercise programs—usually walking (see below)—in conjunction with their drug therapy.

ASPIRIN (see also p. 1827). Although platelet hyperaggregability is not considered to be a risk factor for myocardial infarction, reduction of platelet aggregability with aspirin reduces the risk of development of this complication. Moreover, in patients with stable CAD, enhanced thrombin-induced platelet aggregation is strongly associated with angiographic progression of the disease, and a higher incidence of clinical events. The platelet abnormalities may be a marker of increased risk in addition to playing a causative role in the development of coronary events.[188] A meta-analysis on 140,000 patients comprising 300 studies confirmed the prophylactic benefit of aspirin in both male and female patients with angina pectoris, prior myocardial infarction, or prior stroke and after bypass surgery.[189] In a Swedish trial of both men and women with chronic stable angina, 75 mg of aspirin, in conjunction with the beta blocker sotalol, caused a 34 per cent reduction in acute myocardial infarction and sudden death.[190] In a smaller study confined to men with chronic stable angina but without a history of myocardial infarction, 325 mg aspirin on alternate days reduced the risk of myocardial infarction during 5 years of follow-up by 87 per cent.[191] Therefore, 75 to 325 mg of aspirin daily is advisable in patients with chronic stable angina without contraindications to this drug.

Although coumadin has proven beneficial in postinfarct patients, no data support the use of chronic anticoagulation in patients with stable angina.

BETA BLOCKERS. The value of beta blockers in reducing death and recurrent myocardial infarction in patients who have experienced a myocardial infarction is well established[192,193] (see p. 1228), as is their usefulness in the treatment of angina (see p. 1304). Whether these drugs are also of value in preventing infarction and sudden death in patients with chronic stable angina is not clear. However, there is no reason to assume that the favorable effects of beta blockers on ischemia and perhaps upon arrhythmias should not apply to patients with chronic stable angina pectoris. Therefore, it is sensible to use these drugs when angina or hypertension or both are present in patients with chronic CAD and when these drugs are well tolerated.

ANGIOTENSIN-CONVERTING ENZYME (ACE) INHIBITORS. Several small studies that evaluated the effect of ACE inhibitors on the severity of angina pectoris and ischemia have provided conflicting results but were limited by small sample size and brief duration of therapy.[194-198]

A surprising and perhaps far-reaching finding from recent randomized trials of ACE inhibitors in postinfarct and other patients with ischemic and nonischemic causes of left ventricular dysfunction was a striking reduction in the subsequent incidence of ischemic events such as myocardial infarction, unstable angina, and the need for coronary revascularization procedures.[199-203] Data from four trials including approximately 11,000 patients showed a statistically significant risk reduction in myocardial infarction of 21 per cent and in subsequent unstable angina of 15 per cent.[203] The potentially beneficial effects of ACE inhibitors include a reduction in left ventricular hypertrophy, vascular hypertrophy, progression of atherosclerosis, plaque rupture, and thrombosis, in addition to a potentially favorable influence on myocardial oxygen supply/demand relationships, cardiac hemodynamics, and a reduction of sympathetic activity.[203]

Despite these intriguing observations, prospective randomized trials showing the effects of these drugs in patients with chronic stable angina without left ventricular dysfunction have not been completed. Therefore, as of this writing, ACE inhibitors are *not* recommended in patients with chronic stable angina pectoris in the absence of other conditions that would warrant treatment with this class of drugs, i.e., hypertension, heart failure, or asymptomatic left ventricular dysfunction.

Counseling and Changes in Life Style

The psychosocial issues faced by the patient who develops chronic stable angina for the first time are similar to, although usually less intense, than those experienced by

the patient with an acute myocardial infarction. Many patients have an unrealistically gloomy perception of their prognosis; they should be offered a realistic appraisal, together with an understandable explanation of the pertinent clinical features of the disease.

An important aspect of the physician's role is to counsel patients in the kinds of work they can do and in their leisure activities, eating habits, vacation plans, and the like. Certain changes in life style may be helpful, such as modifying strenuous activities if they constantly and repeatedly produce angina. These changes may be minor in many instances. For example, golfing could be modified to include use of a golf cart instead of walking. A history of CAD and stable angina is not inconsistent with the ability to continue to perform vigorous exertion. This is important not only in regard to recreational activities and life style but also for patients in whom physical exertion is required in their employment. Isometric activities such as weight lifting[204] and other activities such as snow shoveling, which involves an energy expenditure between 60 and 65 per cent of peak oxygen consumption,[205] and cross-country or downhill skiing[206] are undesirable. In addition, some activities expose the individual to the detrimental effects of cold on the oxygen demand/supply relationship,[48,49,207] and these too should be avoided if possible.

Thoughtful counseling, which may include supervised exercise sessions simulating the particular activity in question, can play a vital role in maintaining a productive and enjoyable life style in patients with chronic stable angina. Many activities, such as shopping or climbing stairs, need not be discontinued by the patient with chronic angina; often it is necessary merely to perform them more slowly or to pause for brief periods of rest. The patient with chronic stable angina should avoid excessive fatigue and exhaustion. Although it is desirable to minimize the number of bouts of angina, an occasional episode is not to be feared. Indeed, unless patients occasionally reach their angina threshold, they may not appreciate the extent of their exercise capacity. The vast majority of patients with chronic stable angina should not be treated as invalids. Often the propensity for angina actually declines, perhaps as a result of the development of collaterals and/or because of training effects.

Eliminating or reducing the factors that precipitate anginal episodes is of obvious importance. Patients learn their usual threshold by trial and error. Because many anginal episodes are precipitated by increases in the mechanical activity of the heart (owing to increases in myocardial oxygen consumption), patients should avoid sudden bursts of activity, particularly after long periods of rest or after meals and in cold weather. Chronic and unstable angina exhibit a circadian rhythm characterized by a lower angina threshold shortly after arising.[208,208a] Therefore, morning activities such as showering, shaving, and dressing should be done at a slower pace, and if necessary with use of prophylactic nitroglycerin. The stress of sexual intercourse is approximately equal to that of climbing one flight of stairs at a normal pace or to any activity that induces a heart rate of approximately 120 beats/min. With proper precautions, i.e., commencing more than 2 hours postprandially and taking an additional dose of a short-acting beta blocker 1 hour before and nitroglycerin 15 minutes before, the majority of patients with chronic stable angina are able to continue satisfactory sexual activity.

Just as there is a role for exercise in the management of CAD, so is there a role for rest, especially in situations in which angina has become frequent or severe. Marked restriction of activity or even complete bed rest, in addition to drug therapy, may be necessary to control symptoms. In less critical situations, merely reducing the amount of time spent working or increasing the rest periods has a beneficial effect. For example, a long lunch break including a short nap may be beneficial. It may be helpful for the patient to use a face mask or scarf to cover the mouth or nose in cold weather. A hot, humid environment may also precipitate angina, and air conditioning may be a necessity rather than a luxury for patients with chronic angina. Large meals can have a similar effect if they are followed by exertion. An effort should be made to minimize emotional outbursts because they too increase myocardial oxygen requirements and sometimes induce coronary vasoconstriction. Occasionally, antianxiety drugs and sedatives or relaxation techniques using biofeedback mechanisms may be useful. Hostility is an adverse risk factor in CAD.

Nitrates

(See also pp. 1336 and 1342)

Mechanism of Action

Although the clinical effectiveness of amyl nitrite in angina pectoris was first described in 1867 by Brunton, organic nitrates are still the drugs most commonly used in the treatment of patients with this condition. The action of these agents is to relax vascular smooth muscle.[208b] The vasodilator effects of nitrates are evident in both systemic (including coronary) arteries and veins in normal subjects and in patients with ischemic heart disease, but they appear to be predominant in the venous circulation. The venodilator effect reduces ventricular preload,[209] which in turn reduces myocardial wall tension and oxygen requirements. The actions of nitrates to reduce both preload and afterload make them useful in the treatment of heart failure (Fig. 38–2) as well as angina pectoris.

Posture is important in evaluating the hemodynamic effects of nitrates. In a patient in the supine position, venous return is normally greater but exercise tolerance and the angina threshold are lower than in the upright position. The hemodynamic and angina-relieving effects of nitrates are most marked when patients are sitting or standing, i.e., when the preload-reducing effects of these drugs are most prominent. By reducing the heart's mechanical activity, volume, and oxygen consumption, nitrates increase exercise capacity in patients with ischemic heart disease, thereby allowing a greater total body workload to be achieved before the angina threshold is reached.

EFFECTS ON THE CORONARY CIRCULATION. Conductance

Vessels (see Table 38–6, p. 1306). There is evidence, obtained from quantitative, computer-assisted measurements of coronary arterial diameter, that nitroglycerin causes dilatation of epicardial stenoses. These are often eccentric lesions, and nitroglycerin causes relaxation of smooth muscle in the wall of the coronary artery that is not encompassed by the plaque. Even a small increase in the narrowed arterial lumen can produce a significant reduction in resistance to blood flow across obstructed regions (Fig. 36–7, p. 1165).[210] Nitrates may also exert a beneficial effect in patients with an impaired coronary flow reserve by alleviating vasoconstriction due to endothelial dysfunction.[211]

REDISTRIBUTION OF BLOOD FLOW. Studies in experimental animals with coronary obstruction have shown that nitroglycerin causes redistribution of blood flow from normally perfused to ischemic areas, particularly in the subendocardium.[212] This may be mediated in part by an increase in collateral blood flow and in part by a lowering of ventricular diastolic pressure, thereby reducing subendocardial compression. In patients with chronic stable angina responsive to nitroglycerin, topical nitroglycerin under resting conditions alters myocardial perfusion by preferentially increasing flow to areas of reduced perfusion with little or no change in global myocardial perfusion.[213]

The results of studies of nitroglycerin on coronary blood flow in patients have been conflicting. Some studies have reported increased blood flow after sublingual or intravenous nitroglycerin,[213,214] but most report no change or reduced flow.[215] However, because myocardial oxygen demand fell, the net effect on oxygen balance became favorable in the latter studies. Using intracoronary injection of xenon-133 (as well as in retrograde perfusion studies performed during coronary bypass surgery), it was shown that blood flow in regions of myocardium perfused by stenotic coronary arteries rose after administration of nitroglycerin when well-developed collaterals supplying those regions were present.[216] In patients with chronic stable angina, topical nitroglycerin alters myocardial perfusion by preferentially increasing flow to areas of reduced perfusion with little or no change in global myocardial perfusion.[213]

The presence of well-developed collaterals may be an important determinant of a good therapeutic response to nitrates.[216–218] After systemic nitroglycerin, the heart can be paced to higher rates before angina occurs. But this is not the case after intracoronary administration, implying that the systemic effects of nitrates may predominate in patients with pure effort angina.[215] The nitrates have also been shown to improve ventricular wall motion in patients with CAD, as demonstrated by contrast ventriculography,[219] echocardiography, and radionuclide ventriculography, both at rest and during exercise. They also reduce the extent of myocardial ischemia, as reflected in exercise-thallium tomographic perfusion defect therapy.[220]

ANTITHROMBOTIC EFFECTS. The stimulation of guanylate cyclase by nitric oxide (NO) results in inhibitory actions on platelets in addition to vasodilation. Although the antithrombotic effects of intravenous nitroglycerin have been demonstrated both in patients with unstable angina and those with chronic stable angina,[221–223] the clinical significance of these actions is not clear.

CELLULAR MECHANISM OF ACTION. Nitrates have the ability to cause vasodilation whether or not the endothelium is intact.[224] After entering the vascular smooth muscle cell, nitrates are converted to reactive (NO) or S-nitrosothiols, which activate intracellular guanylate cyclase to produce cyclic guanosine monophosphate (GMP),[224,225] which in turn triggers smooth muscle relaxation and antiplatelet aggregatory effects (Fig. 38–4). Sulfhydryl (SH) groups are required for both the formation of NO and the stimulation of guanylate cyclase, and nitroglycerin-induced vasodilation can be enhanced by prior administration of N-acetylcysteine, an agent that increases the availability of SH groups.[226] This action of N-acetylcysteine potentiates the peripheral hemodynamic responses[226] and the coronary vasodilator effect of nitroglycerin[216] and reverses the partial tolerance to the coronary vasodilator effect of nitroglycerin.

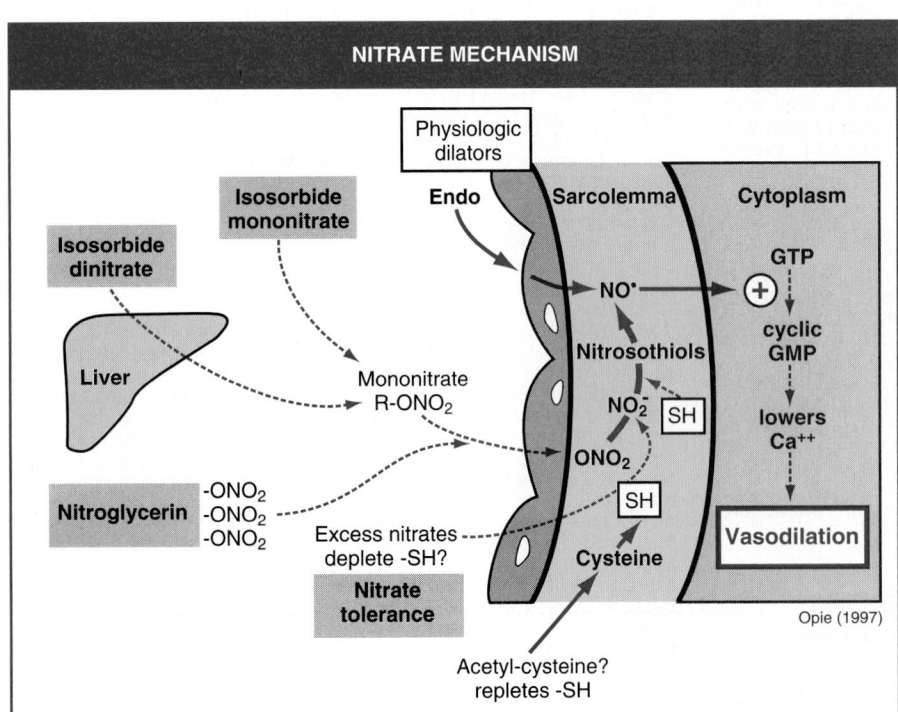

FIGURE 38–4. Mechanisms of the effects of nitrates in the generation of nitric oxide (NO) and the stimulation of guanylate cyclase cyclic GMP, which mediates vasodilation. Sulfhydryl (SH) groups are required for the formation of NO and the stimulation of guanylate cyclase. Isosorbide dinitrate is metabolized by the liver, whereas this is bypassed by the mononitrates. Abbreviations are as follows: SH = sulfhydryl; GTP = guanosine triphosphate; GMP = guanosine monophosphate. (Redrawn from Opie, L. H.: Drugs for the Heart. 4th ed. Philadelphia, W. B. Saunders Company, 1995, p. 33. Figure copyright L. H. Opie.)

TABLE 38–3 RECOMMENDED DOSING REGIMENS FOR LONG-TERM NITRATE THERAPY

PREPARATION OF AGENT	DOSE	SCHEDULE
Nitroglycerin		
Ointment	0.5–2 inches	2–3 times/d
Buccal or transmucosal	1–3 mg	3 times/d
Transdermal patch	0.4–1.2 mg/h for 12 to 14 hours, after which patch is removed	
Oral sustained release	9.0–13.5 mg	2–3 times/d*
Isosorbide dinitrate		
Oral	10–60 mg	2–3 times/d
Oral sustained release	80–120 mg	Once daily
Isosorbide-5-mononitrate		
Oral	20–30 mg	Twice daily given 7–8 h apart
Oral sustained release	60–240 mg	Once daily

* Very limited data available on efficacy.
From Abrams, J.: Medical therapy of stable angina pectoris. *In* Beller, G.: Chronic Ischemic Heart Disease. Atlas of Heart Diseases, vol. 5. Braunwald, E. (ed.). Philadelphia, Current Medicine, 1995, p. 7.18.

Types of Preparations and Routes of Administration
(Table 38–3)

Nitroglycerin administered sublingually remains the drug of choice for the treatment of acute angina episodes and for the prevention of angina. Because sublingual administration avoids first-pass hepatic metabolism, a transient but effective concentration of the drug rapidly appears in the circulation. The half-life of nitroglycerin itself is brief, and it is rapidly converted to two inactive metabolites, both of which are found in the urine after nitroglycerin administration. The liver possesses large amounts of hepatic glutathione organic nitrate reductase, the enzyme that breaks down nitroglycerin, but there is also evidence that blood vessels (veins and arteries) may metabolize nitrates directly. Within 30 to 60 minutes, hepatic breakdown has abolished the hemodynamic and clinical effects.

The usual sublingual dose is 0.3 to 0.6 mg, and most patients respond within 5 minutes to one or two 0.3-mg tablets. If symptoms are not relieved by a single dose, additional doses of 0.3 mg may be taken at 5-minute intervals, but no more than 1.2 mg should be used within a 15-minute period. The development of tolerance (see below) is rarely a problem with intermittent usage. Sublingual nitroglycerin is especially useful when it is taken *prophylactically* shortly before physical activities that are likely to cause angina are undertaken. Used for this purpose, it may prevent angina for up to 40 minutes.

ADVERSE REACTIONS. These are common and include headache, flushing, and hypotension (Table 38–4). The latter is rarely severe, but in some patients, particularly in the face of an unstable ischemic syndrome, volume depletion, and the upright posture, nitrate-induced hypotension is accompanied by a paradoxical bradycardia, consistent with a vasovagal or vasodepressor response. This reaction is more common in the elderly, who are less able to tolerate hypovolemia. The administration of nitrates before a meal, particularly in patients with a tendency toward postprandial hypotension, may enhance venous pooling, preload reduction, and the extent of the fall in blood pressure after the meal.[228] In addition, the partial pressure of oxygen in arterial blood may fall after large doses of nitroglycerin because of a *ventilation-perfusion imbalance* caused by inability of the pulmonary vascular bed to constrict in areas of alveolar hypoxia, thereby leading to perfusion of less hypoxic tissues.[229] *Methemoglobinemia* is a rare complication of very large doses of nitrates; commonly used doses of nitrates cause small elevations of methemoglobin that probably are not of clinical significance.

PREPARATIONS (Table 38–3). **Nitroglycerin Tablets.** These tend to lose their potency, especially if exposed to light, and should be kept in dark containers. Other nitrate preparations are available in sublingual, buccal, oral, spray, and ointment form. An oral nitroglycerin spray that dispenses metered, aerosolized doses of 0.4 mg may be better absorbed than the sublingual form in patients with dry mucosal membranes.[230] It can also be quickly sprayed onto, or under, the tongue. For prophylaxis, the spray should be used 5 to 10 minutes before angina-provoking activities.

Isosorbide Dinitrate. This is an effective antianginal agent but with low bioavailability after oral administration. It undergoes rapid hepatic metabolism, and there are marked variations in plasma concentrations after oral administration. It has two metabolites (one has a potent vasodilator action) that are cleared less rapidly than the parent drug and are excreted unchanged in the urine. It is available in tablets for sublingual use, in chewable form, in tablets for oral use, and in sustained-release capsules.

Partial or complete nitrate tolerance (see below) develops with regimens of isosorbide dinitrate when it is administered as 30 mg three or four times daily.[231] A dosage schedule should be adopted that allows a 10- to 12-hour nitrate-free interval. If the drug is administered on a three-times-daily schedule (e.g., at 8:00 A.M., 1 P.M., and 6 P.M.), the antianginal benefit lasts for approximately 6 hours, and the magnitude of the antianginal benefit decreases with each successive dose.[231]

Isosorbide-5-Mononitrate. This active metabolite of the dinitrate is completely bioavailable with oral administration, because it does not undergo first-pass hepatic metabolism[232] and is efficacious in the treatment of chronic stable angina.[233] Plasma levels of isosorbide-5-mononitrate reach their peak between 30 minutes and 2 hours after ingestion, and the drug has a plasma half-life of 4 to 6 hours. A single

TABLE 38–4 SIDE EFFECTS OF ANTIANGINAL DRUGS*

	HYPOTENSION FLUSHING, HEADACHE	LEFT VENTRICULAR DYSFUNCTION	DECREASED HEART RATE ATRIOVENTRICULAR BLOCK†	GASTROINTESTINAL SYMPTOMS	BRONCHOCONSTRICTION‡	EDEMA
Beta blockers	0	++	+++	+	+++	0
Nitrates	+++	0	0	0	0	0
Diltiazem	+	+	+	0	0	+
Nifedipine	+++	0	0	0	0	+++
Verapamil	+	+	++	++	0	+
Amlodipine	+	0	0	0	0	+++
Bepridil	+	+	+	0	0	0

* 0 = absent; + = mild; ++ = moderate; +++ = sometimes severe.
† In patients with sick sinus node syndrome or conduction system disease.
‡ In patients with obstructive lung disease.
Reprinted by permission from Braunwald, E.: Mechanism of action of calcium channel blocking agents. N. Engl. J. Med. *307*:1618, 1982. Copyright Massachusetts Medical Society.

20-mg tablet still exhibits activity 8 hours after administration. Tolerance has not been demonstrated using once-a-day or eccentric dosing intervals but does occur with a twice-daily dosing regimen at 12-hour intervals. The only sustained-release preparation of isosorbide-5-mononitrate is *Imdur,* which is given once daily in a dose of 30 to 240 mg. Presumably this preparation provides a sufficiently low level of nitrates for a long enough period of time to avoid tolerance, because the duration of activity is estimated to be 12 hours or less.

Topical Nitroglycerin. OINTMENT. Nitroglycerin ointment (15 mg/inch) is efficacious when applied (most commonly to the chest) in strips of 0.5 to 2.0 inches. Delay in the onset of action is approximately 30 minutes. Because it is effective for 4 to 6 hours, this form of the drug is particularly useful in patients with severe angina or unstable angina who are confined to bed and chair. Nitroglycerin ointment also may be used prophylactically after retiring by patients with nocturnal angina. Skin permeability increases with increased hydration, and absorption is also enhanced if the paste is covered with plastic whose edges are taped to the skin.

TRANSDERMAL PATCHES. A silicone gel or polymer matrix impregnated with nitroglycerin results in absorption for 24 to 48 hours at a rate determined by various methods of preparation of the patch, including a semipermeable membrane placed between the drug reservoir and the skin. The release rate of the patches varies from 2.5 to 15 mg per 24 hours. Relatively low doses (2.5 mg to 5 mg per 24 hours) may not produce sufficient plasma and tissue concentrations to sustain consistent, effective antianginal effects. Transdermal nitroglycerin therapy has been shown to increase exercise duration and maintains anti-ischemic effects for 12 hours after patch application throughout 30 days of therapy, without significant evidence of nitrate tolerance or rebound phenomenon,[234] provided that the patch is not applied for more than 12 out of 24 hours.

NITRATE TOLERANCE

This phenomenon has been demonstrated with all forms of nitrate administration which maintain continuous blood levels of the drug.[231,234-236] Although nitrate tolerance is rapid in onset, renewed responsiveness is easily established after a short nitrate-free interval. The problem of tolerance applies to all nitrate preparations and is particularly important in patients with chronic stable angina pectoris, as opposed to those receiving short-acting courses of nitrates (e.g., unstable angina and myocardial infarction).[237,238] Nitrate tolerance appears to be limited to the capacitance and resistance vessels in that it has not been noted in the large conductance vessels, including the epicardial coronary arteries and radial arteries, despite continuous administration of nitroglycerin for 48 hours.[239]

A meta-analysis of randomized clinical trials of nitroglycerin patches suggested that in doses of 5 to 10 mg, exercise duration was improved early after administration but by 24 hours the effect of nitroglycerin on exercise performance was attenuated by the development of nitrate tolerance.[235] However, a regimen in which transdermal nitroglycerin was applied for 12 hours and removed for 12 hours improved exercise performance for 8 to 12 hours after application of the patch. After 1 month of such therapy, responsiveness to transdermal nitroglycerin remained virtually unchanged. Therefore, after application of a transdermal nitroglycerin patch one can expect therapeutic efficacy (improved exercise performance) for 8 to 12 hours. Provided a substantial nitrate-free interval (of 10 to 12 hours) exists every 24-hour period, sustained improvement in exercise performance may be maintained. If a state of tolerance is induced, a nitrate-free interval restores responsiveness. If large intermittent doses of transdermal or oral nitrates are employed (equivalent to 20 mg per 24 hours of a transdermal patch), it is possible that rebound angina may occur during the nitrate-free period.

MECHANISMS. Several mechanisms of nitrate tolerance have been proposed.[219] Their relative importance has not been defined.

Depletion of Sulfhydryl (SH) Groups. Perhaps the most widely accepted explanation of nitrate tolerance is that a depletion of intracellular SH cofactors occurs and that these are a crucial component of the metabolic conversion of nitroglycerin to nitric oxide or S-nitrosothiols, a conversion necessary for the activation of guanylate cyclase.[240]

Neurohormonal Activation. There may be nonspecific activation of neurohormonal mechanisms in response to the hypotensive effects of nitrates with a resultant increase in plasma catecholamines, plasma renin activity, and arginine vasopressin causing sodium reten-

tion and weight gain.[241] It has been suggested that angiotensin-converting enzyme inhibitors modify nitrate tolerance by blunting the neurohormonal responses to nitrate therapy.[242]

Plasma Volume Expansion. Plasma volume expansion occurs during continuous nitrate administration,[241] even in the absence of neurohormonally mediated sodium retention.[242] It may be the result of a fluid shift from the extravascular to the intravascular space in response to the vasodilating or hemodynamic actions of nitrates.[243]

Downregulation of Nitrate Receptors. It has been proposed that high-affinity receptors, which respond to low concentrations of nitrates, are downregulated during the development of tolerance. The activity of low-affinity receptors is maintained and these continue to respond but to increasing concentrations of nitrate.[244]

MANAGEMENT. The only practical strategy is to provide a "nitrate-free" interval. The optimal interval is unknown, but with patches or ointment of nitroglycerin or preparations of isosorbide dinitrate or isosorbide-5-mononitrate, *a 12-hour off period is recommended.*[244-248] The timing of administration should be adapted to the pattern of symptoms, e.g., whether angina is predominantly exercise-related during the day or nocturnal.

NITRATE WITHDRAWAL. A common form of nitrate withdrawal (rebound) is observed in patients whose angina is intensified after discontinuation of large doses of long-acting nitrates.[249] The potential for rebound can be modified by adjusting the dose and timing of administration in addition to the use of other antianginal drugs. Moreover, nitroglycerin administered by the sublingual route does not result in tolerance, and even after 2 weeks of therapy there is no reduction in efficacy when sublingual nitroglycerin is administered two or three times daily.[250]

Because of the possibility of nitrate dependence, nitrate therapy should be withdrawn carefully. In individuals exposed to industrial doses of nitroglycerin, nitrate tolerance, nitrate dependence, and withdrawal symptoms may cause serious problems. During the manufacture of dynamite, substantial levels of nitrates are often present in the atmosphere and can be absorbed through the skin and lungs. After an acute response of headache, hypotension, palpitations, and gastrointestinal disturbances, adaptation occurs.[251] Withdrawal from this environment may result in angina unrelated to exertion or emotion. In fact, spontaneous coronary vasospasm and acute myocardial infarction have been documented during a period of withdrawal.

Beta-Adrenoceptor Blocking Agents
(See also p. 853)

Four beta-adrenoceptor blocking drugs have been approved for the treatment of angina in the United States, and this class of agents constitutes a cornerstone of therapy of this condition. In addition to their anti-ischemic properties, beta blockers are effective antihypertensives (see p. 854) and antiarrhythmics (p. 610). Also, they have been shown to reduce mortality and reinfarction in post–myocardial infarct patients (p. 1264). This combination of actions makes them extremely useful in the management of chronic stable angina. A number of studies have shown that beta-adrenoceptor blockers, in doses that are generally well tolerated, reduce the frequency of anginal episodes and raise the anginal threshold, both when given alone and when added to other antianginal agents.

The salutary action of these drugs (which have a chemical structure resembling that of beta-adrenoceptor agonists) depends on their ability to cause competitive inhibition of the effects of neuronally released and circulating catecholamines on beta adrenoceptors[252-254] (Table 38–5). Beta blockade reduces myocardial oxygen consumption primarily by slowing heart rate; the slower heart rate in turn increases the fraction of the cardiac cycle occupied by diastole with a corresponding increase in the time available for coronary perfusion (Fig. 38–5; Table 38–6). These drugs also reduce exercise-induced rises in blood pressure and limit exercise-induced increases in contractility. Thus, beta blockers reduce myocardial oxygen demands primarily during activity or excitement or when surges of increased sympathetic activity occur.[255] Thus, in the face of impaired myocardial perfusion, the effects of beta blockers on myocardial oxygen demands may critically and favorably alter the imbalance between supply and demand, resulting in the elimination of ischemia.

Beta blockers reduce blood flow to most organs by means of the combination of unopposed alpha-adrenergic vasoconstriction and blockade of the beta$_2$ receptors. Complications are relatively minor, but in patients with peripheral

TABLE 38–5 PHYSIOLOGICAL ACTIONS OF β-ADRENERGIC RECEPTORS

ORGAN	RECEPTOR TYPE	RESPONSE TO STIMULUS
Heart		
SA node	β_1	Increased heart rate
Atria	β_1	Increased contractility and conduction velocity
AV node	β_1	Increased automaticity and conduction velocity
His-Purkinje system	β_1	Increased automaticity and conduction velocity
Ventricles	β_1	Automaticity, contractility, and conduction velocity
Arteries		
Peripheral	β_2	Dilatation
Coronary	β_2	Dilatation
Carotid	β_2	Dilatation
Other	β_1	Increased insulin release
		Increased liver and muscle glycogenolysis
Lungs	β_2	Dilatation of bronchi
Uterus	β_2	Smooth muscle relaxation

From Abrams, J.: Medical therapy of stable angina pectoris. In Beller, G.: Chronic Ischemic Heart Disease. Atlas of Heart Diseases, vol. 5. Braunwald, E. (ed.). Philadelphia, Current Medicine, 1995, p. 7.19.

vascular disease, the reduction in blood flow to skeletal muscles with the use of the nonselective beta blockers may reduce maximal exercise capacity. In patients with preexisting left ventricular dysfunction, beta blockade may increase ventricular volume and thereby enhance oxygen demands.

Characteristics of Different Beta Blockers
(Table 38–7)

SELECTIVITY. Two major subtypes of beta receptors, designated beta$_1$ and beta$_2$, are present in different proportions in different tissues. Beta$_1$ receptors predominate in the heart, and their stimulation leads to an increase in heart rate, AV conduction and contractility, the release of renin from juxtaglomerular cells in the kidneys, and lipolysis in adipocytes. Beta$_2$ stimulation causes bronchodilation, vasodilation, and glycogenolysis. *Nonselective* beta-blocking

drugs (propranolol, nadolol, penbutolol, pindolol, sotalol, timolol, carteolol) block both beta$_1$ and beta$_2$ receptors, whereas *cardioselective* beta blockers (acebutolol, atenolol, betaxolol, bisoprolol, esmolol, and metoprolol) block beta$_1$ receptors while having lesser effects on beta$_2$ receptors. Thus, cardioselective beta blockers reduce myocardial oxygen demands while tending not to block bronchodilation, vasodilation, or glycogenolysis. However, as the doses of these drops are increased, this cardioselectivity diminishes. Because cardioselectivity is only relative, the use of cardioselective beta blockers in doses sufficient to control angina may still cause bronchoconstriction in some susceptible patients.

Some beta blockers also cause vasodilatation. These include labetalol (an alpha-adrenergic blocking agent and beta$_2$ agonist, p. 487), and two investigational drugs, carvedilol (with alpha- and beta$_1$-blocking activity) and bucindolol (a nonselective beta blocker that causes direct [non–alpha-adrenergic mediated] vasodilation).[256,257]

ANTIARRHYTHMIC ACTIONS (see also p. 610). Beta blockers have antiarrhythmic properties as a direct effect of their ability to block sympathoadrenal myocardial stimulation, which in certain situations may be arrhythmogenic.[258] Sotalol (see p. 615) has combined class II (beta-blocking) and class III antiarrhythmic activities; it is an attractive drug when it is desired to treat angina and suppress ventricular tachyarrhythmias.[259,260]

INTRINSIC SYMPATHOMIMETIC ACTIVITY (ISA). Beta blockers with ISA (acebutolol, carteolol, celiprolol, penbutolol, pindolol) are partial beta agonists that also produce blockade by shielding beta receptors from more potent beta agonists. Pindolol and acebutolol produce low-grade beta stimulation when sympathetic activity is low (at rest), whereas these partial agonists behave more like conventional beta blockers when sympathetic activity is high. Agents with ISA may not be as effective as those without this property at reducing heart rate or the frequency, duration, and magnitude of ambulatory ST-segment changes or increasing the duration of exercise in patients with severe angina.[261–263]

POTENCY. This can be measured by the ability of beta blockers to inhibit the tachycardia produced by isoproterenol. All drugs are considered in reference to propranolol, which is given a value of 1.0 (Table 38–7). Timolol and pindolol are the most potent agents, and acebutolol and labetalol are the least.

LIPID SOLUBILITY. The hydrophilicity or lipid solubility of beta blockers is a major determination of their absorption and metabolism. The lipid-soluble (lipophilic) beta blockers, propranolol, metoprolol, and pindolol, are readily absorbed from the gastrointestinal tract, are metabolized predominantly by the liver, have a relatively short half-life, and usually require administration twice or more daily to achieve continuing pharmacological effects. The water-soluble (hydrophilic) beta blockers (atenolol, sotalol, and nadolol) are not as

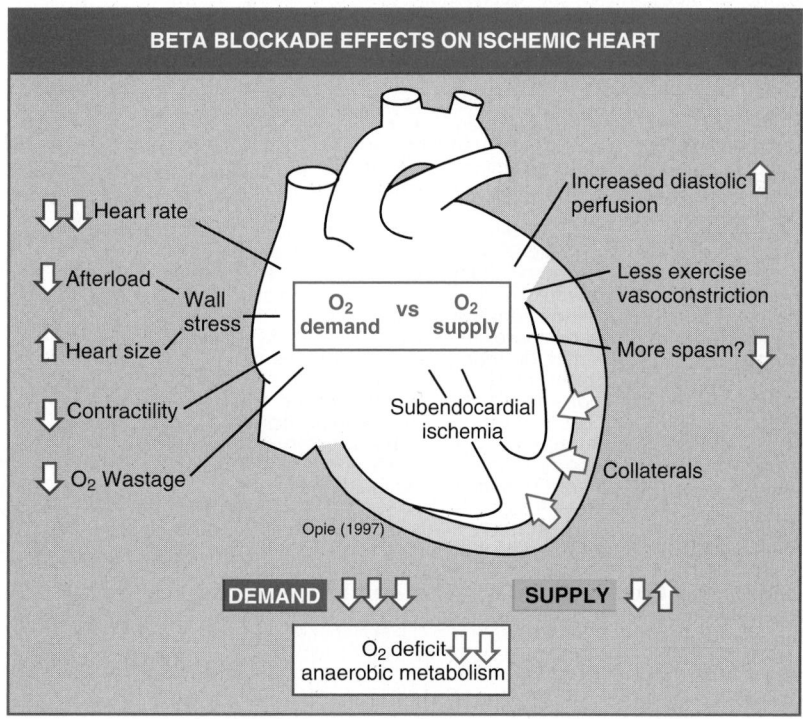

FIGURE 38–5. Effects of beta blockade on the ischemic heart. Beta blockade has a beneficial effect on the ischemic myocardium, unless (1) the preload rises substantially as in left heart failure or (2) there is vasospastic angina when spasm may be promoted in some patients. Note recent proposal that beta blockade diminishes exercise-induced vasoconstriction. (Redrawn from Opie, L. H.: Drugs for the Heart. 4th ed. Philadelphia, W. B. Saunders Company, 1995. Figure copyright L. H. Opie.)

TABLE 38–6 EFFECTS OF ANTIANGINAL AGENTS ON INDICES OF MYOCARDIAL OXYGEN SUPPLY AND DEMAND*

INDEX	NITRATES	BETA-ADRENOCEPTOR BLOCKERS ISA† No	ISA† Yes	Cardio-Selective No	Cardio-Selective Yes	CALCIUM ANTAGONISTS Nifedipine	Verapamil	Diltiazem
Supply								
Coronary resistance								
Vascular tone	↓↓	↑	0	↑	0↑	↓↓↓	↓↓↓	↓↓↓
Intramyocardial diastolic tension	↓↓↓	↑	0	↑	↑	↓↓	0↑	0
Coronary collateral circulation	↑	0	0	0	0	↑	0	↑
Duration of diastole	0(↓)	↑↑↑	0↓	↑↑↑	↑↑↑	0↑(↓↓)	↑↑↑(↓)	↑↑(↓)
Demand								
Intramyocardial systolic tension								
Preload	↓↓↓	↑	0	↑	↑	↓0	↑0↓	0↓
Afterload (peripheral vascular resistance)	↓	↑	↑	↑↑	↑	↓↓	↓	↓
Contractility	0(↑)	↓↓↓	↓	↓↓↓	↓↓↓	↓(↑↑)‡	↓↓(↑)‡	↓(↑)‡
Heart rate	0(↑)	↓↓↓	0↓	↓↓↓	↓↓↓	0(↑↑)	↓↓(↑)	↓↓(↑)

* ↑ = increase, ↓ = decrease, 0 = little or no definite effect. Number of arrows represents relative intensity of effect. Symbols in parentheses indicate reflex-mediated effects.

† ISA = intrinsic sympathomimetic activity.

‡ Effect of calcium entry on left ventricular *contractility*, as assessed in the intact animal model. The net effect on *left ventricular performance* is variable, being influenced by alterations in afterload, reflex cardiac stimulation, and the underlying state of the myocardium.

From Shub, C., et al.: Selection of optimal drug therapy for the patient with angina pectoris. Mayo Clin. Proc. 60:539, 1985.

readily absorbed from the gastrointestinal tract, are not as extensively metabolized, have relatively long plasma half-lives, and can be administered once daily. If either metoprolol or propranolol is administered intravenously, a much higher concentration reaches the bloodstream, and therefore intravenous dosing has much greater potency than oral dosing.

ALPHA-ADRENOCEPTOR BLOCKING ACTIVITY. The alpha-blocking potency of labetalol is approximately 20 per cent of its beta-blocking potency, and it is also one of the weaker beta blockers compared with propranolol,[264] although it possesses significant ISA (Table 38–7). Its combined alpha- and beta-blocking effects make it a particularly useful antihypertensive agent (see p. 487), and it is especially so in patients with hypertension and angina. The major side effects of labetalol are postural hypotension and retrograde ejaculation.[254]

OXIDATION PHENOTYPE. Metoprolol and propranolol are lipid-soluble beta blockers noted for the variability of their pharmacokinetics, drug metabolism, and pharmacodynamics. The oxidative metabolism of metoprolol exhibits the debrisoquin type of genetic polymorphism; poor hydroxylators, or metabolizers (up to 10 per cent of Caucasians), have significant prolongation of the elimination half-life of the drug compared with extensive hydroxylators or metabolizers. Thus, angina might be controlled by a single daily dose of metoprolol in poor metabolizers, whereas extensive metabolizers require the same dose two or three times a day.[265] If a patient exhibits an exaggerated clinical response (e.g., extreme bradycardia) following administration of metoprolol, propranolol, or other lipid-soluble beta blockers, it may be the result of prolongation of the elimination half-life due to slow oxidative metabolism.

EFFECTS ON SERUM LIPIDS. Beta-blocker therapy (with agents lacking ISA) usually cause no significant changes in total or LDL cholesterol but they increase triglycerides and reduce HDL cholesterol.[266] The most commonly studied drug has been propranolol, which can increase plasma triglyceride concentrations by up to 50 per cent and reduce HDL cholesterol by approximately 15 per cent. Adverse effects upon the lipid profile may be more frequent with the nonselective than with beta₁-selective blockers. Two drugs possessing ISA— acebutolol and pindolol—do not significantly change total cholesterol, triglyerides, or LDL cholesterol, and pindolol *increases* serum HDL cholesterol. The effects of these changes in serum lipids after long-term administration of beta blockers for either hypertension or angina must be considered in patients begun and maintained on this therapy.[267]

MEMBRANE-STABILIZING ACTIVITY. This property refers to the "quinidine-like" effect of certain beta blockers that reduces the rate of rise of the cardiac action potential (see p. 612). The clinical relevance of this effect is negligible (except perhaps in cases of overdose) because it is observed only at concentrations far exceeding therapeutic levels.[268]

DOSAGE. For optimal results, the dosage of beta blocker should be carefully adjusted. In the case of propranolol, it

is useful to start with 80 mg of propranolol daily (20 mg four times a day) or comparable doses of other blockers. Twenty-four to 48 hours are required for the drug to achieve an antianginal effect. Efficacy is determined by drug effects on heart rate and symptoms, and, when these are unclear, their effect on exercise performance on a stress test can be evaluated. Resting heart rate should be reduced to between 50 and 60 beats/min, and an increase of less than 20 beats/min should be seen with modest exercise (e.g., climbing one flight of stairs).[269] The usual dosage of propranolol ranges from 80 to 320 mg/day, but some patients require (and tolerate) much higher doses. Therapy needs to be individualized and requires repeated checking of the patient during the initial period of drug administration.

ADVERSE EFFECTS AND CONTRAINDICATIONS. Most of the adverse reactions are a consequence of their beta-blocking properties and include cardiac effects (severe sinus bradycardia, sinus arrest, AV block, reduced left ventricular contractility), bronchoconstriction, fatigue, mental depression, nightmares, gastrointestinal upset, sexual dysfunction, intensification of insulin-induced hypoglycemia, and cutaneous reactions (Tables 38–4 and 38–8). Lethargy, weakness, and fatigue may be caused by reduced cardiac output or may arise from a direct effect on the central nervous system. Bronchoconstriction results from a blockade of beta₂ receptors in the tracheobronchial tree. As a consequence, asthma and chronic obstructive lung disease are contraindications to beta blockers, even to beta₁-selective agents.[270]

In patients who already have impaired left ventricular function, congestive heart failure may be intensified, an effect that can be counteracted, in part, by the use of digitalis or diuretics. Beginning therapy with a very low dose (e.g., metoprolol 10 mg daily for the first week and then gradually raising it has been shown to be beneficial in selected patients with idiopathic dilated cardiomyopathy and, to a lesser extent, in patients with heart failure due to ischemic heart disease) (see p. 1264).[271]

Beta blockers should be used with *great caution* in patients with cardiac conduction disease involving either the sinus node or the AV conduction system. In patients with

TABLE 38–7 PHARMACOKINETICS AND PHARMACOLOGY OF SOME BETA-ADRENOCEPTOR BLOCKERS

	ATENOLOL	METOPROLOL	NADOLOL	PINDOLOL	PROPRANOLOL	TIMOLOL	PROPRANOLOL HCl	ACEBUTOLOL	LABETALOL	BISOPROLOL	BETAXOLOL	CARTEOLOL	PENBUTOLOL
Extent of absorption (%)	≈50	>95	≈30	>90	90	>90	>90	≈70	>90	>90	>90	>90	100
Extent of bioavailability (% of dose)	≈40	≈50	≈30	≈90	≈30	75	≈30	≈50	≈25	80	90	85	100
Beta-blocking plasma concentration	0.2–0.5 µg ml	50–100 ng ml	50–100 ng ml	50–100 ng ml	50–100 ng ml	50–100 ng ml	50–100 ng ml	0.2–2.0 µg ml	0.7–3.0 µg ml	16–70	20–50		
Protein binding (%)	<5	12	≈30	57	93	≈10	93	30–40	≈50	30	50–60	23–30	80–98
Lipophilicity*	Low	Moderate	Low	Moderate	High	Low	High	Low	Low	Moderate	Moderate	Low	High
Elimination half-life (hr)	6 to 9	3 to 4	14 to 25	3 to 4	3.5 to 6.0	3 to 4	3–4	3–4‡	≈6	7–15	12–22	5–7	
Drug accumulation in renal disease	Yes	No	Yes	No	No	No	No	Yes§	No	Yes	Yes	Yes	Yes
Predominant route of elimination†	RE (mostly unchanged)	HM	RE	RE (≈40% unchanged) and HM	HM	RE (≈20% unchanged) and HM	HM	HM§	HM	HM 50% RE 50%	HM	RE	HM
β1-blocker potency ratio (propranolol = 1)	1.0	1.0	1.0	6.0	1.0	6.0	1.0	0.3	0.3	10	4	10	1
Relative β1 sensitivity	+	+	0	0	0	0	0	Yes	0	+	+	0	0
Intrinsic sympathetic activity	0	0	0	+	0	0	0	+	0	0	0	+	+
Membrane-stabilizing activity	0	0	0	+	++	0	++	+	0	0	0	0	0
Usual maintenance dose	50–100 mg qd	50–100 mg qid	40–80 mg qd	5–20 mg tid	60 mg qid	20 mg bid	60 mg qid	200–600 mg bid	100–600 mg/day	5–20 mg qd	5–20 mg qd	2.5–10 mg qd	20 mg qd
FDA-approved indications													
Hypertension	Yes	Yes	Yes	Yes	Yes	Yes	—	Yes	Yes	Yes	Yes	Yes	Yes
Angina	Yes	Yes	Yes	No	Yes	No	—	No	No	No	No	No	No
Post myocardial infarction	Yes	Yes	No	No	Yes	Yes	—	No	No	No	No	No	No

* Determined by the distribution ratio between octanol and water.
† RE = renal excretion; HM = hepatic metabolism.
‡ Half-life of the active metabolite, diacetolol, is 12 to 15 hours.
§ Acebutolol is mainly eliminated by the liver, but its major metabolite, diacetolol, is excreted by the kidney.
Modified from Frishman, W. H., et al.: Antianginal agents, Part 2: β-Blockers. Hosp. Formul. 21:62, 1986.

TABLE 38–8   CANDIDATES FOR USE OF β-BLOCKING AGENTS FOR ANGINA

Ideal Candidates
  Prominent relationship of physical activity to attacks of angina
  Coexistent hypertension
  History of supraventricular or ventricular arrhythmia
  Postmyocardial infarction angina
  Prominent anxiety state
Poor Candidates
  Asthma or reversible airway component in chronic lung patients
  Diabetes
  Severe left ventricular dysfunction
  Congestive heart failure resulting from systolic impairment
  History of depression
  Raynaud's phenomenon
  Peripheral vascular disease
  Bradyarrhythmia

From Abrams, J.: Medical therapy of stable angina pectoris. *In* Beller, G.: Chronic Ischemic Heart Disease. Atlas of Heart Diseases, vol. 5, Braunwald, E. (ed.). Philadelphia, Current Medicine, 1995, p. 7.14.

symptomatic conduction disease, beta blockers are contraindicated unless a pacemaker is in place. In patients with asymptomatic sinus node dysfunction or first degree AV block, beta blockers may be tolerated, but their administration requires careful observation. Pindolol, because of its ISA activity, may be preferable in this situation. Blockade of noncardiac beta$_2$ receptors inhibits catecholamine-induced glycogenolysis so that noncardioselective beta blockers can impair the defense to insulin-induced hypoglycemia.[272] Blockade of beta$_2$ receptors also inhibits the vasodilating effects of catecholamines in peripheral blood vessels and leaves the constrictor (alpha-adrenergic) receptors unopposed and thereby enhances vasoconstriction. Noncardioselective beta blockers may precipitate episodes of Raynaud's phenomenon in patients with this condition and may cause uncomfortable coldness of the distal extremities. Reduced flow to the limbs may occur in patients with peripheral vascular disease.[273]

Abrupt withdrawal of beta-adrenoceptor blocking agents after prolonged administration can result in increased total ischemic activity in patients with chronic stable angina. This may be caused by a return to the previously high levels of myocardial oxygen demand while the underlying atherosclerotic process has progressed.[274] Occasionally such withdrawal can precipitate unstable angina and rarely even provoke myocardial infarction. If abrupt withdrawal of beta blockers is required, patients should be instructed to reduce exertion, manage angina episodes with sublingual nitroglycerin, and/or substitute a calcium antagonist.

Calcium Antagonists
(See also p. 855)

The critical role played by calcium ions in the normal contraction of cardiac and vascular smooth muscle is discussed on p. 366. Calcium antagonists are a heterogeneous group of compounds that inhibit calcium ion movement through slow channels in cardiac and smooth muscle membranes by noncompetitive blockade of voltage-sensitive L-type calcium channels (Fig. 12–10, p. 367).[275–278] There are three major classes of calcium antagonists—the dihydropyridines (of which nifedipine is the prototype), the phenylalkylamines (of which verapamil is the prototype), and the modified benzothiazepines (of which diltiazem is the prototype). The two predominant effects of calcium antagonists result from blocking entry of calcium ions and slowing the recovery of the channel.[275,276] The phenylalkylamines have a marked effect upon the recovery of the channel and thereby exert depressant effects on cardiac pacemakers and conduction, whereas the dihydropyridines,

which do not impair channel recovery, have little effect on the conduction system.

The efficacy of calcium antagonists in patients with angina pectoris is related to the reduction in myocardial oxygen demand, together with an increase in oxygen supply which they induce (Table 38–6)[208a]; the latter is particularly important in patients in whom a prominent vasospastic or vasoconstrictor component may be present (i.e., Prinzmetal's variant angina [see p. 1340], patients with variable threshold angina [p. 1293], and patients with abnormal small coronary arteries and impaired vasodilator reserve[279]). Calcium antagonists may be effective on their own in combination with beta-adrenoceptor blockers and nitrates in patients with chronic stable angina.[280–282a]

Six calcium antagonists—verapamil, nifedipine, diltiazem, nicardipine, amlodipine, and bepridil—have been approved by the Food and Drug Administration (FDA) in the United States for the treatment of angina pectoris (Table 38–9). All of these agents are effective in causing relaxation of vascular smooth muscle in both the systemic arterial and coronary arterial beds. In addition, blockade of the entry of calcium into myocytes results in a negative inotropic effect, which is counteracted to some extent by peripheral vascular dilation and by activation of the sympathetic nervous system in response to drug-induced hypotension.[283] However, the negative inotropic effect must be considered in patients with significant left ventricular dysfunction.

Calcium antagonists have a rapid onset of action and are metabolized by the liver, resulting in a limited bioavailability of between 13 and 52 per cent and a half-life of between 3 and 12 hours. Amlodipine and bepridil are exceptions in that both drugs have long half-lives and may be administered once daily. In the case of some of the other calcium antagonists, sustained-release preparations have been shown to be effective.

ANTIATHEROGENIC ACTION. Studies in experimental animals, both primates and nonprimates, have suggested that calcium antagonists might have an antiatherogenic effect, and human studies support this.[284–286] In multicenter, randomized trials utilizing quantitative coronary arteriography, patients showing mild coronary artery disease developed significantly fewer new lesions taking nifedipine than did patients taking placebo. However, preexisting lesions did not appear to be affected. Prolonged follow-up is necessary to determine whether these angiographic observations are accompanied by clinical benefits. In patients undergoing cardiac transplantation, diltiazem has been reported to be beneficial in reducing the frequency and severity of coronary arteriopathy in the transplanted heart[287] (see p. 526).

NIFEDIPINE. This dihydropyridine is a particularly effective dilator of vascular smooth muscle and is a more potent vasodilator than either diltiazem or verapamil. Although its in vitro actions on myocardium and specialized cardiac tissue are similar to those of other agents, the concentration required to reproduce effects on these tissues is not reached in vivo because of the early appearance of its powerful vasodilating effects. Thus, in clinical practice the potential negative chronotropic, inotropic, and dromotropic (on AV conduction) effects of nifedipine are seldom a problem, although even nifedipine can worsen heart failure in patients with preexisting chronic congestive heart failure.[288]

In contrast to beta blockers, which reduce heart rate and the rate pressure product at rest and during exercise, nifedipine reduces only systolic pressure.[289,290] Thus, the beneficial effects of nifedipine in the treatment of angina result from its capacity to reduce myocardial oxygen needs resulting from its afterload-reducing effect and to increase myocardial oxygen delivery consequent to its dilating action on the coronary vascular bed (Table 38–6). In patients without heart failure, nifedipine causes modest reflex increases in ejection fraction, velocity of circumferential fiber

TABLE 38–9 PHARMACOKINETICS OF CALCIUM ANTAGONISTS USED COMMONLY FOR ANGINA PECTORIS*

	DILTIAZEM	NICARDIPINE	NIFEDIPINE	NIFEDIPINE GITS	VERAPAMIL	AMLODIPINE	FELODIPINE	ISRADIPINE	BEPRIDIL
Usual adult dose	IV: 0.25 mg/kg bolus then 0.15 mg/kg/hr Oral: 30–90 mg tid or qid	IV: 10–15 mg/hr for 30 min then 3–5 mg/hr Oral: 20–30 mg tid	SL: 10–30 mg tid or qid Oral: 10–30 mg tid or qid	Oral: 30–60 mg daily	IV: 0.075 to 0.015 mg/kg Oral: 80–120 mg tid or qid	2.5–10 mg qd	5–20 mg qd	2.5–5.0 mg bid	200–400 mg qd
Extent of absorption (%)	80–90	~100	90	>90	90	>90	>90	>90	>90
Extent of bioavailability (% of dose)	40–70	30	65–75	45–75	20–35	60–65	20	15–24	>80
Onset of action	Oral: <15 min	<20 min	SL: <3 min Oral: <20 min	Approximately 6 hr	IV: 2 min Oral: 2 hr	1–2 hr	2 hr	20 min	2–3 hr
Peak effect	Oral: 30 min	1 hr	Oral: 1–2 hr	After 6 hr	IV 3–5 min Oral 3–4 hr	6–12 hr	2–5 hr	1.5 hr	8 h
Therapeutic serum levels (ng/ml)	50–200	30–50	25–100	25–100	80–300	5–20	1–5	2–10	500–2000
Elimination half-life (hr)	3.5–6.0	2.0–4.0	2.0–5.0	2.0–5.0	3.0–7.0†	30–50	9	8	26–64
Elimination	60% metabolized by liver; remainder excreted by kidneys	High first-pass hepatic metabolism	High first-pass hepatic metabolism	High first-pass hepatic metabolism	85% eliminated by first-pass hepatic metabolism	Hepatic	High first-pass hepatic metabolism	High first-pass hepatic metabolism	Hepatic
Heart rate	↓	↑	↑↑	↑	↓	0	↑	0	→
Peripheral vasc. resistance	↓	↓	↓↓↓	↓↓↓	↓	↓↓↓	↓↓↓	↓↓↓	→
FDA approved indications									
Hypertension	Yes	Yes	Yes	Yes	Yes	Yes	Yes	Yes	Yes
Angina	Yes	Yes	Yes	Yes	Yes	Yes	No	No	Yes
Coronary spasm	Yes	No	Yes	Yes	Yes	Yes	No	No	No

* All agents approved by FDA for treatment of angina pectoris.
† 4.5–12 hr with multiple dosing.
GITS, gastrointestinal therapeutic system; IV, intravenous; SL, sublingual.

shortening, heart rate, and cardiac index; these increases can be blocked by beta-adrenoceptor blockade.

The dose is 10 mg orally every 8 hours, increased stepwise to 20 mg every 6 hours, guided by the blood pressure response to a minimal dose of 160 mg. An extended-release formulation utilizing the gastrointestinal therapeutic system (GITS) of drug delivery (Table 38–9) is designed to deliver 30, 60, or 90 mg of nifedipine in a single daily dose at a relatively constant rate over a 24-hour period and is useful for the treatment of chronic stable angina, Prinzmetal's angina, and hypertension.[291] The efficacy of the extended-release preparation, either alone or in conjunction with beta blockers, in reducing episodes of angina and of ischemia on ambulatory monitoring has been documented.[292]

Adverse Effects. These occur in 15 to 20 per cent of patients and require discontinuation of medication in about 5 per cent. Most adverse effects are related to the systemic vasodilation and include headache, dizziness, palpitations, flushing, hypotension, and leg edema (unrelated to heart failure). Gastrointestinal side effects, including nausea, epigastric pressure, and vomiting, are noted in approximately 5 per cent of patients. Rarely, in patients with extremely severe, fixed coronary obstructions, nifedipine aggravates angina, presumably by lowering arterial pressure excessively with subsequent reflex tachycardia. For this reason, combined therapy of angina with nifedipine and a beta blocker is particularly effective and superior to nifedipine alone.[281,282] Most of the adverse effects are reduced by the use of the extended-release preparations. Review of multiple clinical trials has revealed that short-acting nifedipine may cause an increase in mortality.[292a] There are no firm data that this risk applies to extended-release nifedipine or to other calcium antagonists.[292b,292c] Clearly, insufficient data are available to assess the long-term risks (if any) of calcium antagonists in chronic CAD. As of this writing it is recommended that patients with CAD—especially those with acute coronary syndromes—not receive short-acting nifedipine. Instead, they may be placed on extended-release nifedipine or on another calcium antagonist.

A comparison of the side effects of nifedipine with those of other calcium antagonists is shown in Table 38–4. Because of its potent vasodilator effects, nifedipine is *contraindicated* in patients who are hypotensive or who have severe aortic valve stenosis and in patients with unstable angina who are *not* simultaneously receiving a beta blocker and in whom reflex-mediated increases in heart rate may be harmful. Nifedipine (or one of the second-generation dihydropyridines) is the calcium antagonist of choice in patients with mild left ventricular dysfunction, sinus bradycardia, sick sinus syndrome, and AV block (particularly if a beta-adrenoceptor blocking agent is concurrently administered and additional drug therapy of angina is indicated).[281] This is because in the dosages used clinically these agents have fewer negative effects on myocardial contractility or on the specialized automatic and conduction systems than does verapamil or diltiazem. Nonetheless, in patients with more serious left ventricular dysfunction, all calcium antagonists—even nifedipine—can precipitate heart failure.[288]

Nifedipine interacts significantly with prazosin (resulting in excessive hypotension), cimetidine, and phenytoin (resulting in increased bioavailability of nifedipine and increased quinidine clearance). Nifedipine increases blood levels of propranolol and when the two drugs are used together there is a risk of an added negative inotropic and hypotensive effect.[290] In patients with Prinzmetal's variant angina, abrupt cessation of nifedipine therapy may result in a rebound increase in the frequency and duration of attacks (see p. 1343).

VERAPAMIL (see also p. 616). Verapamil dilates systemic and coronary resistance vessels and large coronary conductance vessels. It slows heart rate and reduces myocardial contractility. This combination of actions results in a reduction of the myocardial oxygen demands, the basis for the drug's efficacy in the management of chronic stable angina. Thrombus formation and whole blood platelet aggregation levels in response to thrombin are decreased by verapamil (as well as to transdermal nitroglycerin). To what extent the clinical benefits of verapamil and nitrates are related to their effects on platelet aggregation and thrombus formation is uncertain.[293]

Verapamil accelerates left ventricular diastolic filling at rest and during exercise in patients with chronic stable angina, whereas beta blockade does not have this effect.[294] Despite the marked negative inotropic effects of verapamil in isolated cardiac muscle preparations, changes in contractility are modest in patients with normal cardiac function. However, in patients with cardiac dysfunction, verapamil, like beta blockers, may reduce cardiac output, elevate left ventricular filling pressure, and cause clinical heart failure. In clinically useful doses, verapamil inhibits calcium influx into specialized cardiac cells, sometimes causing slowing of heart rate and AV conduction. Therefore, it is contraindicated in patients with preexisting atrioventricular nodal disease or sick sinus syndrome, congestive heart failure, and suspected digitalis or quinidine toxicity. In the treatment of effort-related angina, verapamil is comparable to propranolol, causing dose-dependent reductions in the frequency of anginal episodes, although the combination results in better exercise capacity than either alone.[294]

The usual starting dose of verapamil for oral administration is 40 to 80 mg three times daily to a maximum dose of 480 mg/day (Table 38–9). Sustained-release capsules of verapamil are available (60 mg, 90 mg, and 120 mg), and starting doses are 60 to 120 mg twice daily with a usual optimal dose range of 240 to 360 mg/day.

Verapamil interacts significantly with a number of other drugs. *Intravenous* verapamil should not be used together with a beta blocker (given intravenously *or* orally), nor should a beta blocker be administered intravenously in patients receiving oral verapamil. The bioavailability of verapamil is increased by cimetidine and carbamazepine, whereas verapamil may increase plasma levels of cyclosporine and digoxin and may be associated with excessive hypotension in patients receiving quinidine or prazosin. Hepatic enzyme inducers such as phenobarbital may reduce the effects of verapamil.

Adverse effects of verapamil are noted in approximately 10 per cent of patients and relate to systemic dilation (hypotension and facial flushing), gastrointestinal symptoms (constipation and nausea), and central nervous system reactions such as headache and dizziness. A rare side effect is gingival hyperplasia appearing after 1 to 9 months of therapy.[283]

DILTIAZEM. Diltiazem's actions are intermediate between those of nifedipine and verapamil. In clinically useful doses its vasodilator effects are less profound than nifedipine's, and its cardiac depressant action (on the sinoatrial and AV nodes and myocardium) less than those of verapamil. This profile may explain the remarkably low incidence of adverse effects of diltiazem. This drug is a systemic vasodilator, lowering arterial pressure at rest and during exertion and increasing the workload required to produce myocardial ischemia, but it may also increase myocardial oxygen delivery. Although diltiazem causes little vasodilation of epicardial coronary arteries under basal conditions, it may enhance perfusion of the subendocardium distal to a flow-limiting coronary stenosis[295]; it also blocks exercise-induced coronary vasoconstriction.[291] In patients with ischemic heart disease, diltiazem reduces afterload and depresses myocardial systolic function but improves left ventricular relaxation.[296] In patients with chronic stable angina receiving maximally tolerated doses of diltiazem there is a significant reduction in heart rate at rest, but there is no effect on peak blood pressure achieved during exercise, and the duration of symptom-limited treadmill exercise is prolonged.

The dose of diltiazem is 30 to 60 mg four times daily, although higher doses are sometimes needed. A sustained-release formulation (Diltiazem CD) has been approved for the once-daily treatment of systemic hypertension and angina pectoris and is available in capsules of 120 mg, 180 mg, 240 mg, and 300 mg.[297]

Diltiazem is a highly effective antianginal agent. Both atenolol and diltiazem are of similar efficacy in increasing nonischemic exercise duration in patients with variable-threshold angina and act primarily by slowing the resting heart rate.[298] High doses (mean dose 340 mg) have been shown to be a relatively safe addition to maximally tolerated doses of isosorbide dinitrate and a beta blocker, causing increases in exercise tolerance and resting and exercise left ventricular ejection fraction.[297] Major side effects are similar to those of the other calcium channel blockers and related to vasodilatation, but these are relatively infrequent, particularly if the dose does not exceed 240 mg/day.[283] As is the case with verapamil, diltiazem should be used with caution in patients with sick sinus syndrome and AV block. In patients with preexisting left ventricular dysfunction, diltiazem may exacerbate or precipitate heart failure.[283]

Diltiazem interacts with other drugs, including beta-adrenergic blocking agents (causing enhanced negative inotropic, chronotropic, and dromotropic effects), flecainide, and cimetidine (which increases the bioavailability of diltiazem), and diltiazem has been associated with increased plasma levels of cyclosporine, carbamazepine, and lithium carbonate. Diltiazem may cause excess sinus node depression if administered with disopyramide and reduce digoxin clearance, especially in patients with renal failure.[299]

Second-Generation Calcium Antagonists

The "second-generation" calcium antagonists (nicardipine, isradipine, amlodipine, and felodipine) are mainly dihydropyridine derivatives, with nifedipine, the prototypical agent. There is also considerable experience with nimodipine, hisoldipine, and nitrendipine, which, however, are not licensed in the United States. These agents differ in potency, tissue specificity, and pharmacokinetics and in general are potent vasodilators due to greater vascular selectivity than with the "first generation" antagonists, i.e., verapamil, nifedipine, and diltiazem.

AMLODIPINE. This agent, which is less lipid soluble than nifedipine, has a slow, smooth onset and ultralong duration of action (plasma half-life = 36 hours). It causes marked coronary and peripheral dilatation and may be useful in the treatment of patients with angina accompanied by hypertension. It may be used as a once-daily hypotensive or antianginal agent.[300] In a series of randomized placebo-controlled studies in patients with stable exercise-induced angina pectoris, amlodipine has been shown to be effective and well tolerated.[301] It has little, if any, negative inotropic action and may be especially useful in patients with chronic angina and left ventricular dysfunction. It has been suggested that amlodipine may be useful in the treatment of heart failure, but definitive proof awaits the outcome of current ongoing trials.[302,303] Preliminary data from the placebo-controlled Prospective Randomized Amlodipine Survival Evaluation (PRAISE) study demonstrated no increase in mortality or hospitalization for life-threatening cardiovascular events in patients with New York Heart Class III-IV failure and a mean ejection fraction of 21 per cent when amlodipine was added to a full regimen of digoxin, diuretic, and ACE inhibitor therapy. In patients with nonischemic dilated cardiomyopathy, all-cause mortality was 21.5 per cent in those assigned to amlodipine versus 34.5 per cent in those assigned to placebo; a 45 per cent reduction in relative risk ($P = 0.001$). No significant difference in survival was observed in patients with ischemic cardiomyopathy. These data *suggest* that in patients with congestive heart failure due to ischemic heart disease, who need a calcium channel antagonist for hypertension or angina, survival is not adversely affected by amlodipine.[302]

NICARDIPINE. This drug has a similar half-life to nifedipine (2 to 4 hours), but intravenous administration is easier because it is water soluble without associated light sensitivity.[283] It also appears to have greater vascular selectivity. Nicardipine may be used as an antianginal and antihypertensive agent requiring thrice-daily administration, although a sustained-release formulation is available for twice-daily dosing in hypertension. For chronic stable angina pectoris, it appears to be as effective as verapamil or diltiazem, and its efficacy is enhanced when combined with a beta blocker.

FELODIPINE AND ISRADIPINE. In the United States, both drugs are approved by the FDA for the treatment of hypertension but not angina pectoris.[283] A recent study documented similar efficacy between felodipine and nifedipine in patients with chronic stable angina.[304] *Felodipine* has also been reported to be more vascular selective than nifedipine and to have a mild *positive* inotropic effect due to calcium channel agonist properties. *Isradipine* has a longer half-life than nifedipine and demonstrates greater vascular sensitivity.

BEPRIDIL. This calcium antagonist interacts with the dihydropyridine binding site and has a sodium channel blocking effect.[283] It markedly prolongs the atrial refractory period and may be useful in the treatment of patients with angina and arrhythmias, although it is also arrhythmogenic and causes Q-T prolongation and *torsades de pointes*.[305] Although chemically unrelated to the other calcium channel blockers, bepridil has been shown to be an effective antianginal agent. Nonetheless, because of its potential to prolong the Q-T interval and cause torsades de pointes, the drug should be reserved for patients in whom other antianginal drugs have failed.[283] Interactions with antiarrhythmic agents, tricyclic antidepressants, and cardiac glycosides are potentially hazardous.

Medical Management of Angina Pectoris

RELATIVE ADVANTAGES OF BETA BLOCKERS AND CALCIUM ANTAGONISTS. The choice between a beta blocker and a calcium channel antagonist as initial therapy in patients with chronic stable angina is controversial because both classes of agents are effective in relieving symptoms and reducing ischemia.[141a,283a,283b] Because long-term administration of beta blockers has been found to prolong life in patients after acute myocardial infarction and in the treatment of hypertension, many have extrapolated these findings to patients with angina and prefer these agents to calcium antagonists. The authors of this chapter consider this extrapolation to be a reasonable one. In addition, a possible risk of short-acting nifedipine in CAD has been raised (see p. 1310), although this possibility is unresolved. However, it must be recognized that beta blockers (without intrinsic sympathomimetic activity) increase serum triglyerides and decrease HDL cholesterol with uncertain long-term consequences.[266,267] In contrast, the long-term administration of calcium antagonists has *not* been shown to improve long-term survival following acute myocardial infarction, although diltiazem apparently is effective in preventing severe angina and early reinfarction after non-Q-wave infarction[306] and verapamil reduces reinfarction rates,[307] while nifedipine has been associated with the development of fewer new coronary artery lesions[284,285] in patients with established CAD.

The choice of the drug with which to initiate therapy is influenced by a number of clinical factors (Table 38–10).

1. Calcium antagonists are the preferable agents in patients with a history of asthma or chronic obstructive lung disease and/or with wheezing on clinical examination, in whom beta blockers, even relatively selective agents, are contraindicated.

TABLE 38–10 RECOMMENDED DRUG THERAPY (CALCIUM ANTAGONIST VS BETA BLOCKER) IN PATIENTS WHO HAVE ANGINA IN CONJUNCTION WITH OTHER MEDICAL CONDITIONS*

CLINICAL CONDITION	RECOMMENDED DRUG (ALTERNATIVE DRUG)
Cardiac arrhythmias and conduction abnormalities	
Sinus bradycardia	Nifedipine**
Sinus tachycardia (not due to cardiac failure)	Beta blocker
Supraventricular tachycardia	Verapamil or beta blocker
Atrioventricular block	Nifedipine**
Rapid atrial fibrillation (with digitalis)	Verapamil or beta blocker
Ventricular arrhythmias	Beta blocker (± group 1 antiarrhythmic agent)
Left ventricular dysfunction	
Congestive heart failure	
Mild (LVEF ≥ 40%)	Nifedipine** (verapamil, diltiazem, or beta blockers cautiously)
Moderate to severe (LVEF < 40%)	Nifedipine** (cautiously, in combination with other therapy)
Left-sided valvular heart disease†	
Aortic stenosis (mild)‡	Beta blocker
Aortic insufficiency	Nifedipine**
Mitral regurgitation	Nifedipine**
Mitral stenosis§	Beta blocker
Miscellaneous medical conditions	
Systemic hypertension	Beta blocker (calcium antagonists)
Severe preexisting headaches	Beta blockers (verapamil or diltiazem)
COPD with bronchospasm or asthma	Nifedipine,** verapamil, or diltiazem
Hyperthyroidism	Beta blocker
Raynaud's syndrome	Nifedipine**
Claudication	Nifedipine,** verapamil, or diltiazem (low-dose beta$_1$ blocker or beta-ISA)
Depression	Nifedipine,** verapamil, or diltiazem
Neurasthenia or fatigue states	Nifedipine,** verapamil, or diltiazem
Insulin-dependent diabetes mellitus	Nifedipine,** verapamil, or diltiazem (low-dose beta$_1$ blocker or beta-ISA)

* From Shub, C., et al.: Selection of optimal drug therapy for the patient with angina pectoris. Mayo Clin. Proc. *60*:539, 1985.

Beta-ISA = beta blocker with intrinsic sympathomimetic activity such as pindolol or acebutolol; COPD = chronic obstructive pulmonary disease; LVEF = left ventricular ejection fraction.

† Surgical therapy should be considered for patients with severe valvular heart disease; beta blockers are not routinely used in patients with valvular heart disease and left ventricular failure.

‡ Vasodilators may increase aortic valve gradient, and beta blockers can cause left ventricular failure. Any of these drugs should be used with extreme caution in patients with severe aortic stenosis.

§ If congestive heart failure (associated with normal left ventricular function) occurs in a patient with angina, severe mitral stenosis, and rapid atrial fibrillation, a beta blocker (in combination with digitalis) may be used to decrease the heart rate.

** Long-acting slow-release nifedipine.

2. Nifedipine (long-acting) or nicardipine is the calcium antagonist of choice in patients with sick sinus syndrome, sinus bradycardia, or significant AV conduction disturbances, whereas beta blockers and verapamil should be used only with great caution in such patients. In patients with symptomatic conduction disease, neither a beta blocker nor a calcium blocker should be used unless a pacemaker is in place. If a beta blocker is required in patients with asymptomatic evidence of conduction disease, pindolol, which has the greatest intrinsic sympathomimetic activity, is useful. In the case of calcium channel blockers, nifedipine or nicardipine is preferable to verapamil and diltiazem, but careful observation for deterioration of conduction is mandatory.

3. Calcium antagonists are clearly preferred in patients suspected of having Prinzmetal's variant angina; beta blockers may even aggravate angina under these circumstances.

4. Calcium antagonists may be preferred over beta blockers in patients with significant, symptomatic peripheral arterial disease because the latter may cause peripheral vasoconstriction.

5. Beta blockers should usually be avoided in patients with histories of significant depressive illness, sexual dysfunction, sleep disturbance, nightmares, fatigue, or lethargy.

6. The presence of moderate to severe left ventricular dysfunction in patients with angina limits the therapeutic options. Obviously, cardiac failure may be controlled with diuretics, digitalis, and angiotensin-converting enzyme inhibitors, and nitrates can be used for the management of angina. However, when cardiac failure is treated and angina persists, other agents may be required. Verapamil and beta blockers are more likely to be associated with adverse effects under these circumstances. Nifedipine and diltiazem are reasonable choices if the left ventricular ejection fraction is greater than 30 per cent and overt cardiac failure does not exist.[308] Whether amlodipine or a highly vascular-selective calcium antagonist, such as felodipine, will prove to be superior in such patients remains to be seen, but initial results with amlodipine are encouraging.[302].

7. Nifedipine should *not* be used as the initial and only agent in patients with unstable angina (see p. 1337), but treatment should be initiated with nitrates and beta blockers to avoid the reflex-mediated tachycardia associated with nifedipine alone that may aggravate unstable angina.[309] However, long-acting nifedipine may be helpful when added to a beta blocker.

8. Hypertensive patients with angina pectoris do well with either beta blockers or calcium antagonists because both agents have antihypertensive effects.

9. Patients with ischemia (symptomatic and asymptomatic) detected by ambulatory electroardiography are improved by both classes of agents. A combination is more effective than either alone.[310]

10. A beta blocker is usually considered first when there is a relatively fixed anginal threshold and myocardial ischemia is caused primarily by an increase in myocardial oxygen demand in the face of a fixed supply. Conversely, in patients with variable-threshold angina in whom reductions of myocardial blood supply may be caused by alterations in coronary vasomotor tone, a calcium antagonist has been presumed to be preferable to a beta blocker. However, although this is a logical approach, its validity remains to be proven.

COMBINATION THERAPY. The combination of a beta-adrenoreceptor blocker, calcium antagonist, and long-acting nitrate is widely used in the management of chronic stable angina. When adrenergic blockers and calcium antagonists are used together in the treatment of angina pectoris, a number of issues should be considered:

1. The addition of a beta blocker enhances the clinical effect of nifedipine and other dihydropyridines.

2. In patients with moderate or severe left ventricular dysfunction, sinus bradycardia, or AV conduction disturbances, combination therapy with calcium antagonists and beta blockers either should be avoided or should be initiated with caution.[311] In patients with AV conduction system disease, the preferred combination is long-acting nifedipine or another dihydropyridine and a beta blocker. The negative inotropic effects of calcium antagonists are not usually a problem in combined therapy with low doses of beta blockers but can become significant with higher doses. With such doses, nifedipine and nicardipine are the calcium antagonists of choice, but they should be used cautiously.

3. The combination of a dihydropyridine and a long-acting nitrate (without a beta blocker) is not an optimal combination because both are vasodilators.

Approach to the Patient with Chronic Stable Angina

1. Identify and treat precipitating factors, such as anemia, uncontrolled hypertension, thyrotoxicosis, tachyarrhythmias, uncontrolled congestive heart failure, and concomitant valvular heart disease.

2. Initiate risk factor modification, physical exercise, and life style counseling.

3. Initiate pharmacotherapy with aspirin and sublingual nitroglycerin. Employ the latter for the alleviation of symptoms and prophylactically (see p. 1302).

4. In many patients, sublingual nitroglycerin is the only anti-ischemic agent required, but if episodes occur more than two or three times per week, the next step is the addition of *either* a beta blocker or a calcium antagonist; the choice is discussed above. The decision to add a beta blocker or calcium antagonist to a nitrate is not based entirely on the frequency and severity of symptoms. The need to treat concomitant hypertension or the presence of a prior myocardial infarction may indicate the use of one of these agents even in patients in whom episodes of symptomatic angina are infrequent.

5. If angina persists, add a long-acting nitrate using eccentric dosing schedules to prevent nitrate tolerance. An assessment of the pattern and the timing of angina often helps govern the timing of drug administration.

6. If angina persists despite two antianginal agents (a long-acting nitrate preparation with either a beta blocker *or* calcium antagonist), add the third antianginal agent.

7. Coronary angiography, with a view to considering coronary revascularization, is indicated in patients with refractory symptoms or ischemia despite optimal medical therapy; it should also be carried out in patients with "high-risk" noninvasive tests (see p. 165) and in those with occupations or life styles that indicate a more aggressive approach.

PERCUTANEOUS TRANSLUMINAL CORONARY ANGIOPLASTY AND RELATED CATHETER-BASED TECHNIQUES

(See also Chap. 39)

Percutaneous transluminal coronary angioplasty (PTCA) and other catheter-based techniques represent a major therapeutic advance in the management of chronic stable angina.[312,313] Their importance to the management of CAD in the United States is reflected by a performance of approximately 360,000 procedures in 1993, a more than 10-fold increase during the last decade.[314] This increase has not been accompanied by a reduction in the number of patients undergoing coronary bypass surgery.[315]

PATIENT SELECTION (Table 63–8, p. 1955). Improved technology and increasing operator experience have expanded the pool of patients with both single and multivessel disease who are candidates for PTCA (and other catheter-based techniques for revascularization). Factors that need to be taken into account in patient selection include the following:

1. The need for revascularization (surgical or catheter-based) as opposed to medical therapy

2. The likelihood of a successful catheter-based revascularization based upon angiographic characteristics of the lesion—type A, B, or C lesions,[316] which characterize complexity as mild, moderate, or severe, respectively (Table 39–3, p. 1370)

3. The risk and potential consequences of acute PTCA failure

4. The likelihood of restenosis

5. The need for complete revascularization

6. The presence of comorbid conditions and the suitability of the patient for surgery

7. Patient preference

The patient with chronic stable angina who is ideal for PTCA, i.e., who is at low risk for complications and in whom the likelihood of technical success is high, is a male with chronic stable angina less than 70 years of age, with single-vessel and single-lesion CAD, the anatomical characteristics of a type A lesion with less than 90 per cent stenosis, no history of congestive heart failure, and an ejection fraction greater than 40 per cent.

Features associated with increased risk for PTCA include advanced age, female gender, a history of congestive heart failure, the presence of left ventricular dysfunction,[317–319] left main coronary artery equivalent disease, unstable angina, recent thrombolytic therapy, and type B or C lesions. However, it has been suggested that the classification of type A, B, and C lesions may be simplistic in the light of increasing operative experience and new technologies.[320] The presence of the aforementioned features does not necessarily contraindicate PTCA but should raise the threshold for performing the procedure. Lower procedural volumes in individual laboratories have also been shown to correlate with increased complications.[320a]

ACUTE OUTCOME. Continued improvements in the technical aspects of PTCA as well as increasing operator experience have had a favorable impact on the rate of primary success (usually defined as an increase of diameter narrowing > 20 per cent and a final diameter obstruction < 50 per cent) and a reduction in complications. This has occurred despite a broadening of the selection criteria for PTCA to include older and sicker patients with more complex anatomy.[312,319,321] Current expectations for angioplasty are an overall success rate in excess of 90 per cent with an acute complication rate of under 5 per cent, particularly in patients with single-vessel disease.

ABRUPT CLOSURE. This refers to a sustained and significate reduction in flow in the target vessel, which is usually recognized prior to leaving the laboratory.[322] In addition to clinical signs and symptoms of ischemia, the angiographic appearance of extensive dissection or thrombus is strongly associated with subsequent total occlusion. The incidence of abrupt closure ranges from 2 to 11 per cent, depending, in part, upon the definitions used; subsequent morbidity and mortality are high. Clinical risk factors for acute closure include advanced age, female gender, unstable angina pectoris, diabetes, chronic hemodialysis, and recent thrombolytic therapy.[323-325] Angiographic correlates of abrupt closure include proximity of the lesion to a branch vessel, lesion length greater than 10 mm, the presence of thrombus, diffuse disease, angulated lesions, diameter stenosis of 80 to 90 per cent, and calcified lesions.[326,327]

Management. The treatment objectives of abrupt closure are to establish adequate coronary perfusion as a bridge to coronary bypass surgery, or, in some patients, as a definitive strategy. Newer therapeutic options have reduced the morbidity of acute vessel closure and include prolonged balloon inflations, stent placement (Fig. 39–10, p. 1380); the use of autoperfusion catheters (Fig. 39–2, p. 1367), adjunctive hemodynamic support, and in some patients the administration of a thrombolytic agent.[312,321,328-331] A reduction in distal flow without apparent dissection or distal embolization occurs in about 2 per cent of patients undergoing PTCA and is frequently reversed by intracoronary verapamil or diltiazem, suggesting that microvascular spasm is responsible.[332,333]

A randomized trial of a monoclonal antibody to the platelet glycoprotein IIb/IIIa receptor in patients considered at "high risk" of complications after coronary angioplasty has documented a reduction in periprocedural adverse outcome[334] (Table 39–2, p. 1370), but with increased bleeding complications.[335]

Long-Term Results. For the majority of patients undergoing PTCA, the intermediate and late outcomes can be characterized by a low mortality or nonfatal myocardial infarction rate. Long-term prognosis after an initially successful PTCA is similar between men and women.[336]

COMPARISON BETWEEN PTCA AND MEDICAL THERAPY. The first major randomized trial involving PTCA was the Veterans Administration Comparison of Angioplasty with Medical Therapy in the treatment of single-vessel coronary artery disease.[337] Eighty-six per cent of the patients had stable angina, all were male, and the duration of follow-up was 6 months. PTCA was distinctly superior to medical therapy in the relief of angina and in the improvement in exercise tolerance, although repeat PTCA or CABG was required in 15 per cent of patients by 6 months (Fig. 38–6). A conclusion that can be drawn from this study is that a trial of medical therapy followed by PTCA in the event of treatment failure is a reasonable initial strategy for patients with stable angina and single-vessel disease. Nonetheless, indices of quality of life, including functional capacity and the patient's perception of well-being, were significantly better among patients treated with PTCA.[337a] In a small randomized trial of PTCA, medical therapy and coronary bypass surgery in patients with a proximal stenosis of the left anterior descending coronary artery, there was no difference in the combined endpoint of cardiac death, myocardial infarction, or refractory angina requiring revascularization between PTCA and medical therapy. Coronary bypass surgery, however, was superior to the other two therapeutic modalities.[337b]

The Duke University data base provides important information on the relative benefits of bypass surgery, PTCA, and medical therapy upon survival in 9263 patients referred for cardiac catheterization between 1984 and 1990.[338] Adjusted 5-year survival for patients with single-vessel disease was similar—95 per cent with PTCA and 94 per cent with medical therapy; in patients with two-vessel disease, this was 91 per cent versus 86 per cent, respectively; and in patients with three-vessel disease, it was 81 per cent versus 72 per cent. These trends suggest that PTCA is superior to medical management in patients with multivessel disease (Fig. 38–7). The 10-year follow-up of the first series of patients who underwent PTCA performed by Gruentzig is encouraging, with a survival rate of 95 per cent in patients with single-vessel disease and 81 per cent in patients with multivessel disease.[339] In the NHLBI Registry, 5-year survival was 93.2 per cent in patients with single-vessel disease, 88.8 per cent in patients with two-vessel disease, and 86 per cent in three-vessel disease. Both early and late outcomes appear to be improving.[340] Restenosis, the Achilles heel of angioplasty (see below), continues to exert the major influence upon long-term outcome.[321] The recurrence of angina is frequent,[341-350] leading to the need for coronary bypass surgery in approximately 20 per cent of patients after 1 to 3 years and of repeat PTCA in approximately 40 per cent by 3 years.[351]

PTCA IN PATIENTS WITH LEFT VENTRICULAR DYSFUNCTION. Several studies of PTCA in patients with left ventricular dysfunction have documented a high initial procedural success rate with successful dilatation of one lesion in 88 per cent and of 76 per cent for all lesions. However, long-term results were less favorable. Two-year survival among

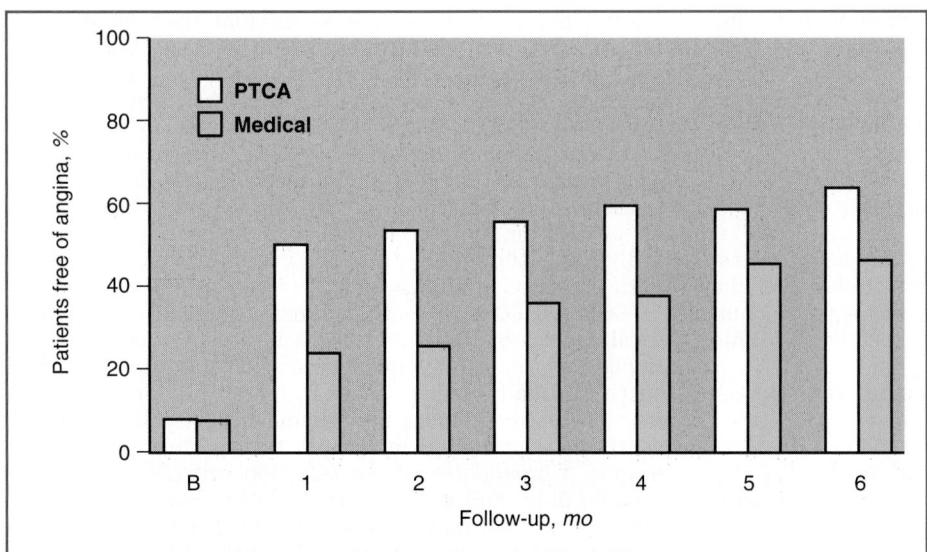

FIGURE 38–6. The percentage of patients free of angina at 1-month intervals after randomization in the Veterans Administration ACME trial. The horizontal axis shows the month after randomization (baseline B) in clinic visits at months 1 through 6 for each treatment group. PTCA = percutaneous transluminal coronary angioplasty. (From Gersh, B. J.: Natural history of chronic coronary artery disease. *In* Beller, G. A. [ed.]: Chronic Ischemic Heart Disease. Atlas of Heart Diseases, vol. 5. Philadelphia, Current Medicine, 1995, p. 1.21. Adapted from Parisi, A. F., et al.: A comparison of angioplasty with medical therapy in the treatment of single-vessel coronary artery disease. N. Engl. J. Med. *326:*10, 1992. Copyright Massachusetts Medical Society.)

FIGURE 38–7. Hazard ratios for percutaneous transluminal coronary angioplasty (PTCA) versus medicine, calculated from the Cox regression model to evaluate relative survival differences. Points indicate hazard ratios for each level of the coronary artery disease index; bars indicate 99 per cent confidence intervals. Horizontal line at ratio 1.0 indicates point of prognostic equivalence between treatments. Hazard ratios below the line favor PTCA; those above the line favor medicine. VD = vessel disease; Prox LAD = proximal left anterior descending coronary artery. (Reproduced with permission from Mark, D. B., Nelson, C. L., Califf, R. M., et al.: Continuing evaluation of therapy for coronary artery disease: Initial results from the era of coronary angioplasty. Circulation 89:2015, 1994. Copyright American Heart Association.)

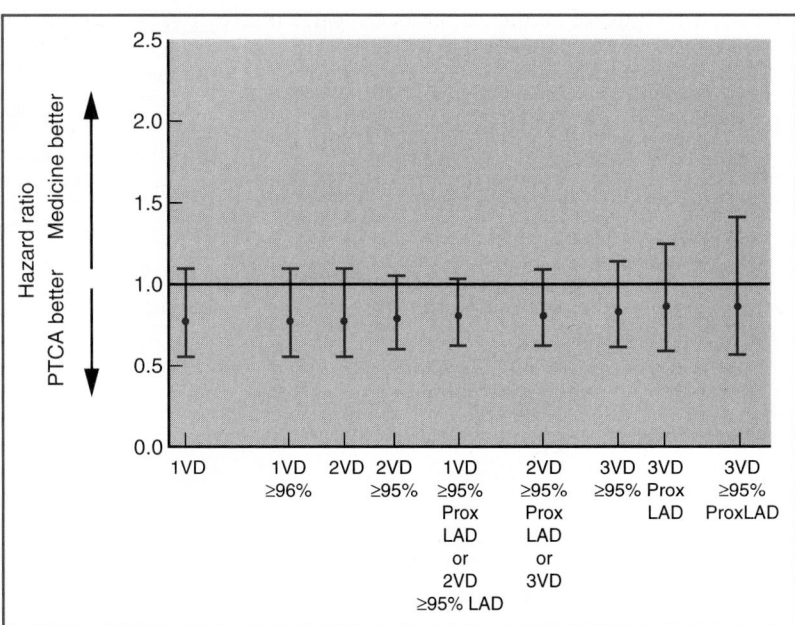

patients with an ejection fraction of 0.40 or less and multivessel disease was only approximately 75 per cent.[352] In another series, 23 per cent of patients with an ejection fraction of 0.35 or less died during a 21-month mean follow-up.[353] In a recent report from the National Heart, Lung and Blood Institute registry, the 4-year survival in patients with very poor left ventricular function in whom the ejection fraction was less than 0.25 was only 45 per cent.[341] Another recent study demonstrated similar results with a 3-year survival of 83 per cent and 92 per cent in patients with ejection fractions of 0.31 to 0.35 and 0.36 to 0.40, respectively, but only 69 per cent in patients with an ejection fraction of 0.30 or less.[341,354] To achieve a good outcome in patients with multivessel disease and left ventricular dysfunction, particularly if angina or ischemia is severe, revascularization should be complete.[342] This is often difficult to achieve with PTCA and other catheter-based revascularization techniques, particularly in the presence of chronic total occlusions. This limitation of angioplasty in the achievement of complete revascularization is an important factor contributing to the relatively disappointing results of this procedure in patients with significant left ventricular dysfunction and multivessel disease.[317]

RESTENOSIS. Although a striking improvement has occurred in the initial results of PTCA during the past 15 years, restenosis continued to dominate late events. The most frequently used definition is a greater than 50 per cent diameter stenosis and/or greater than 50 per cent late loss of the acute luminal gain,[344,347] but there is no clear consensus regarding the optimal angiographic definition.[355] The incidence is approximately 30 to 40 per cent, occurs within 6 months of the procedure, and depends on the patient population, the complexity of the lesion, and the definition of restenosis,[344] but it does not appear to have declined despite a plethora of therapeutic approaches directed toward its prevention. The use of stenting has been found, however, to reduce this complication (Table 39–10, p. 1380). Neither the development of symptoms[355a] nor an abnormal exercise stress electrocardiogram is particularly reliable in the recognition of restenosis, but both are helpful in guiding subsequent therapy.[344]

MECHANISMS OF AND RISK FACTORS FOR RESTENOSIS. The pathogenesis of restenosis in response to mechanical injury is incompletely understood and multifactorial. Traditionally, restenosis has been considered to be due to the development of neointimal thickening as a result of migration and stimulation of smooth muscle by growth factors (see p. 1372). The elastic properties of the vessel undergoing PTCA and its recoil in the development of restenosis have also received attention. Clinical variables that appear to be associated with increased rates of restenosis include diabetes, severe angina, male sex, smoking, and older age.[347] Anatomical factors include total occlusion, left anterior descending coronary artery location, saphenous vein graft lesions, long lesions, and multivessel or multilesion PTCA.[349,350] Procedural variables include a greater residual stenosis, following PTCA, severe dissection, the absence of an intimal tear, the use of inappropriately sized balloons, and the presence of thrombus.

PREVENTION OF RESTENOSIS. A plethora of pharmacological agents of different categories has been evaluated for the prevention of restenosis after coronary angioplasty, with generally disappointing results. None has shown unequivocal success. The EPIC trial of a monoclonal blocking antibody to the platelet glycoprotein IIb/IIIa receptor documented a reduction in clinical endpoints at 6 months, which may, in part, be related to a decline in the incidence of restenosis.[34,355a]

The frequency of restenosis after PTCA and the desire to expand the pool of patients with chronic CAD amenable to transcatheter techniques have spawned the development of a variety of other devices, described in Chap. 39. Two randomized trials of directional coronary atherectomy versus standard balloon angioplasty, however, have failed to document any clinically relevant superiority of one form of therapy over the other,[356,357] but these trials have been criticized on the basis that the optimal results with directional coronary atherectomy were not attained.[358] Two randomized trials demonstrated a reduction in the rate of restenosis and in clinical events in patients receiving balloon-expandable stents compared with patients undergoing standard balloon angioplasty (Table 39–8, p. 1374).[358a] However, this benefit was achieved at a cost of a significantly higher risk of vascular complications and a longer hospital stay and costs.[359–360a] Although rapidly gaining in popularity, the long-term effects of stents have not yet been well defined, and their exact place remains to be defined.

MANAGEMENT OF RESTENOSIS. Restenosis is amenable to repeat PTCA, but it is not entirely clear whether lesions that have developed restenosis are more likely to develop restenosis after a subsequent percutaneous intervention.[361] Among patients with stable or unstable angina and restenosis, a 93 per cent anatomical success rate after repeat angioplasty has been reported, and most patients experienced significant long-term clinical improvement. However, the likelihood of recurrent angina requiring subsequent bypass surgery was greater than in patients undergoing PTCA for the first time.[362] In patients undergoing a third PTCA for restenosis at the same site, an interval of less than 3 months between the second and third procedures was strongly associated with further restenosis, suggesting that such patients should be considered for coronary bypass surgery.[363]

CHRONIC TOTAL OCCLUSION. This poses a formidable obstacle to PTCA success, particularly in the presence of bridging collaterals, an estimated duration of occlusion of more than 3 months, and a vessel diameter of 3 mm.[364–366,366a] After initially successful elective coronary angioplasty of total occlusions, the restenosis rate was 45 per cent in vessels with total occlusions, compared with 34 per cent in those with subtotal obstruction ($P < 0.001$). This is due primarily to an increased number of total occlusions at follow-up angiography (19.2 per cent compared with 5.0 per cent for stenoses, $P < 0.001$).[365] The role of stents is under evaluation.[365a] Explanations for the higher reocclusion rate are speculative, but a major potential contributor could be an increased collateral circulation around previously occluded arteries, a higher incidence of previous myocardial infarction, and more myocardial fibrosis in the distribution of the totally occluded arteries, leading to a reduction in total demand for flow to

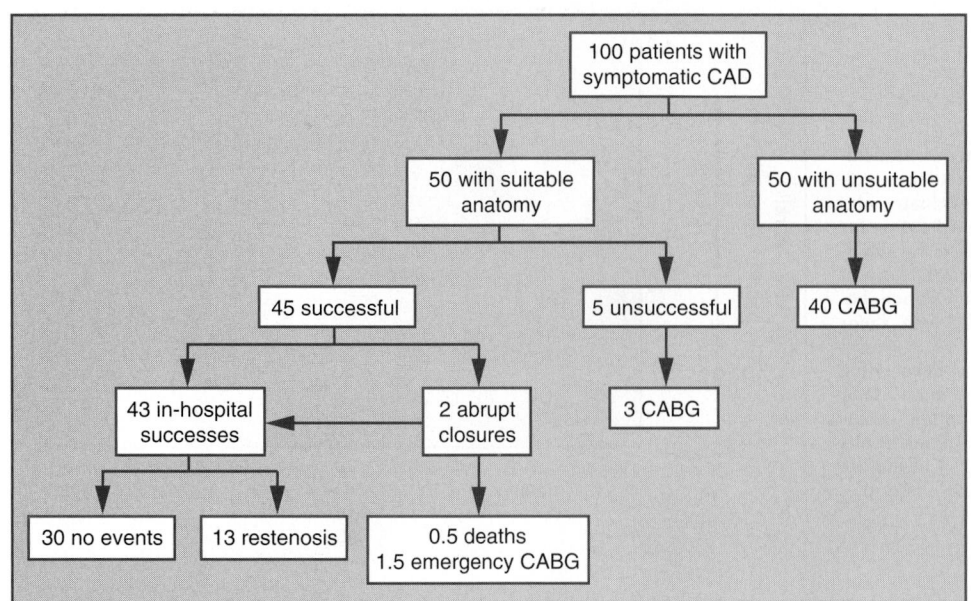

FIGURE 38–8. The limitations of balloon PTCA. Approximately one-half of patients who present with symptomatic coronary artery disease (CAD) and are in need of revascularization are candidates for PTCA. The remaining patients are ineligible because of unfavorable coronary anatomy, which most commonly results from chronic total occlusion more than 3 months in duration. Of the suitable candidates, a small percentage have an unsuccessful procedure and subsequently require CABG. A small percentage of patients who have a successful procedure develop abrupt vessel closure, and 20 to 30 per cent of patients develop restenosis that necessitates a repeat procedure. Thus, approximately 30 per cent of all patients who need myocardial revascularization are successfully treated and free of complications after PTCA. (From Faxon, D. P.: Coronary angioplasty for stable angina pectoris. In Beller, G. A. and Braunwald, E. [eds.]: Chronic Ischemic Heart Disease. Atlas of Heart Diseases, vol. 5. Philadelphia, Current Medicine, 1995, p. 9.16.)

the distal bed. Slow flow across the previously occluded lesion is likely to cause reocclusion consequent to thrombosis rather than fibrointimal hyperplasia or vascular recoil.

PTCA IN WOMEN (see p. 1704).

PTCA IN THE ELDERLY. The mortality and rate of periprocedural complications is increased in elderly patients undergoing PTCA.[367,368] Among hospital survivors, the late recurrence of angina appears to be higher in the elderly than in younger patients. On the other hand, PTCA may be more appropriate than coronary bypass surgery for the frail elderly with comorbid conditions who require revascularization but in whom the risks of surgery are higher.[368a]

PTCA IN CORONARY BYPASS GRAFTS. Coronary artery bypass surgery and PTCA are often considered to be competitive procedures, but it is more appropriate to view them as complementary. Patients who have undergone prior coronary bypass surgery, in whom repeat revascularization is under consideration, may be amenable to PTCA of native vessels or of bypass grafts.[369–372] This application of angioplasty and other transcatheter techniques is increasing rapidly and is particularly helpful in elderly patients, who would otherwise be facing a second or third coronary bypass operation. However, the initial and late success rates of PTCA in bypass grafts, particularly in saphenous vein conduits, are lower than in native vessels.[369] Results are

better with dilatation of distal graft lesions; angiographic success rates approach 90 per cent at the distal site of the graft insertion, 70 per cent in the mid portion, and 55 per cent proximally.

Multiple factors increase the likelihood of *unfavorable* results of PTCA of vein grafts[370]; these include a graft age of 4 to 6 years, diffuse graft disease, chronic total occlusions, vein graft thrombus, and the site of the stenosis (i.e., proximal, mid, or distal). Until new techniques for maintaining long-term vein graft patency after PTCA are shown to be effective, balloon angioplasty should be considered only as a palliative procedure for patients with severe symptoms.[370]

COMPARISON OF PTCA AND CORONARY ARTERY BYPASS SURGERY (see p. 1374).

CONCLUSION. PTCA represents a major advance in the management of chronic stable angina. However, its limitations must be recognized. Only approximately half of all patients with symptomatic CAD are suitable candidates for this procedure, and of this half, only about 60 per cent have successful procedures *and* escape restenosis (Fig. 38–8).

OTHER CATHETER-BASED TECHNIQUES. Lasers, stents, rotablaters and atherectomy[372] are discussed in Chap. 39.

CORONARY ARTERY BYPASS SURGERY

In 1964 Garrett, Dennis, and DeBakey first used coronary artery bypass grafting (CABG) as a "bailout" procedure.[373] This was followed by the widespread use of the technique by Favoloro and Johnson and their respective collaborators in the late 1960s.[374,375] The use of the internal mammary artery (IMA) graft was pioneered by Kolesov in 1966 and Green in 1968.[376,377]

The number of coronary bypass operations in the United States has increased substantially from 180,000 in 1983 to approximately 300,000 in 1993.[314] The advent of PTCA may have blunted the growth of coronary artery bypass surgery somewhat. Nevertheless, CABG remains one of the most frequently performed operations in the United States; approximately 1 in every 1000 persons undergoes CABG on an annual basis, and this procedure results in the expenditure of almost $50 billion annually.[378]

The appropriate use of invasive cardiovascular procedures is undergoing increasing scrutiny. It is, therefore, reassuring to note that in studies of coronary angiography and bypass surgery in New York State and Canada, only 6 per cent and 4 per cent of bypass procedures, respectively, were considered inappropriate.[379] Patients with chronic stable angina represented 48 per cent of those undergoing bypass surgery in the United States and 61 per cent of those in Canada.

Technical Considerations

When the decision has been reached to proceed with coronary bypass surgery, administration of beta-adrenoreceptor blockers, nitrates, and calcium antagonists is continued until operation. It is crucial to minimize perioperative damage and to protect the myocardium. The most commonly used method involves a single period of aortic cross-clamping with intermittent infusion of cold cardioplegia.[380] Continued low-flow normothermic cardioplegic infusion may be equally effective in maintaining cardiac arrest and minimizing cardiac damage.[315] Cardioplegic solutions may be sanguinous, involving high concentrations of potassium with or without added substances, such as oxygen, buffers, and free radical scavengers.[381] Retrograde cardioplegia through the coronary sinus facilitates a more uniform distribution of cardioplegic solution. Many surgeons now use a combination of antegrade and retrograde perfusion[382] as well as topical hypothermia with cold saline or ice slush as an adjunct. Renewed interest in coronary bypass surgery without cardiopulmonary bypass has been stimulated by the desire to avoid blood transfusions, by economic issues, and by the wish to avoid the damaging effects of bypass, particularly in the elderly and in patients with heavily calcified aortas.[383]

VENOUS CONDUITS. The saphenous vein is used mainly for distal branches of the right and circumflex coronary arteries and for sequential grafts to these vessels and diagonal branches (Figs. 38–9 and 38–10). In emergency situations, many surgeons prefer the saphenous vein, which can be harvested and grafted more rapidly, to the internal mammary artery. Arm vein grafts are not as effective as either saphenous veins or internal mammary artery grafts.

Eight to 12 per cent of saphenous vein grafts become occluded during the early perioperative period. Trauma to the vein during surgical preparation can denude the endothelium, impair the intrinsic fibrinolytic activity of saphenous vein, and damage the vessel wall, predisposing to early thrombosis.[384] Careful harvesting of the graft, with particular attention to the avoidance of overdistention and the use of modified storage solutions, has been shown to

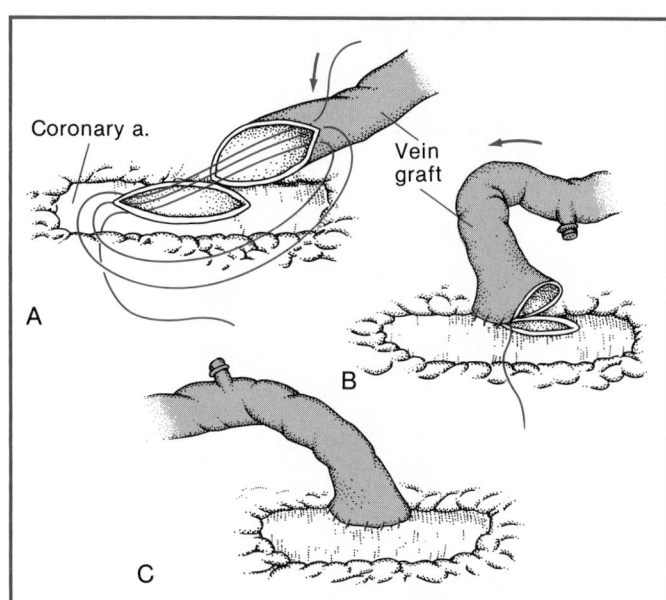

FIGURE 38–10. The venocoronary anastomosis to the proximal portion of the arteriotomy. (From Cohn, L. H.: Surgical techniques of emergency coronary revascularization. *In* Cohn, L. H. [ed.]: The Treatment of Acute Myocardial Ischemia: An Integrated Medical-Surgical Approach. Mt. Kisco, N.Y., Futura Publishing Co., 1979, p. 87.)

improve patency and preserve the integrity of the graft in both animal models and the clinical setting.[380]

INTERNAL MAMMARY ARTERY BYPASS GRAFTS. The internal mammary artery (IMA), also known as the internal thoracic artery, usually is remarkably free of atheroma, especially in patients under the age of 65 years. When it is grafted to a coronary artery (Figs. 38–11 and 38–12), it appears to be virtually immune to the development of intimal hyperplasia, which is almost universally seen in aortocoronary vein grafts.[384a] Atherosclerotic changes in the IMA develop in only a small percentage of patients after coronary bypass surgery. The IMA is delicate, and great care has to

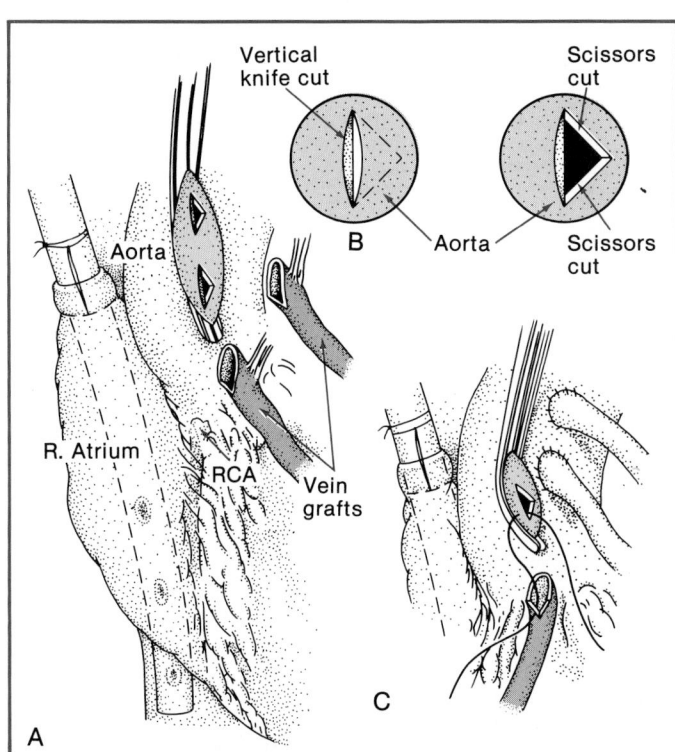

FIGURE 38–9. The aorticovenous anastomosis in a coronary arterial–saphenous vein bypass graft. *A* shows the direction of the anastomotic site for left-sided grafts; *B* shows details of aortic orifices; *C* shows the direction of right coronary artery (RCA) grafts. (From Cohn, L. H.: Surgical techniques of emergency coronary revascularization. *In* Cohn, L. H. [ed.]: The Treatment of Acute Myocardial Ischemia: An Integrated Medical-Surgical Approach. Mt. Kisco, N.Y., Futura Publishing Co., 1979, p. 87.)

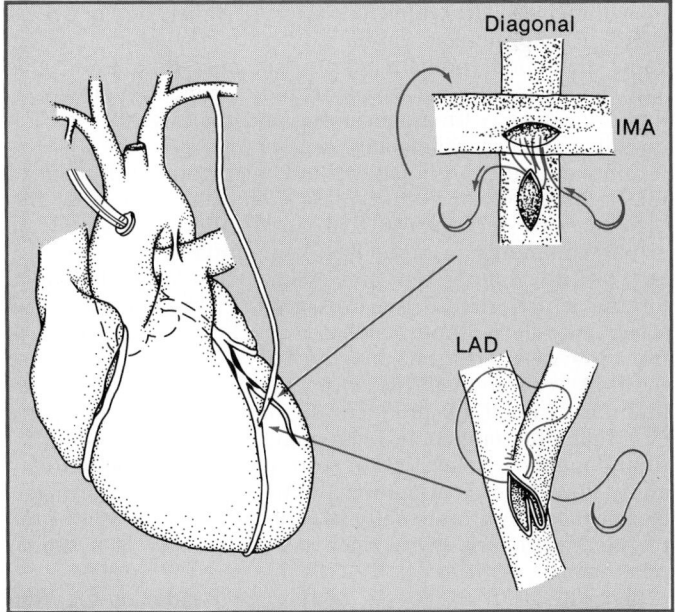

FIGURE 38–11. Internal mammary grafting: In situ left internal mammary artery (IMA) graft to the left anterior descending artery (end-to-side) and diagonal branch (side-to-side) employing the diamond anastomotic technique to the latter. The details show the IMA pedicle rolled up over the diagonal coronary artery to facilitate exposure and use of continuous suture. (From Jones, E. L.: Extended use of the internal mammary coronary artery bypass. J. Cardiac Surg. *1:*13, 1986.)

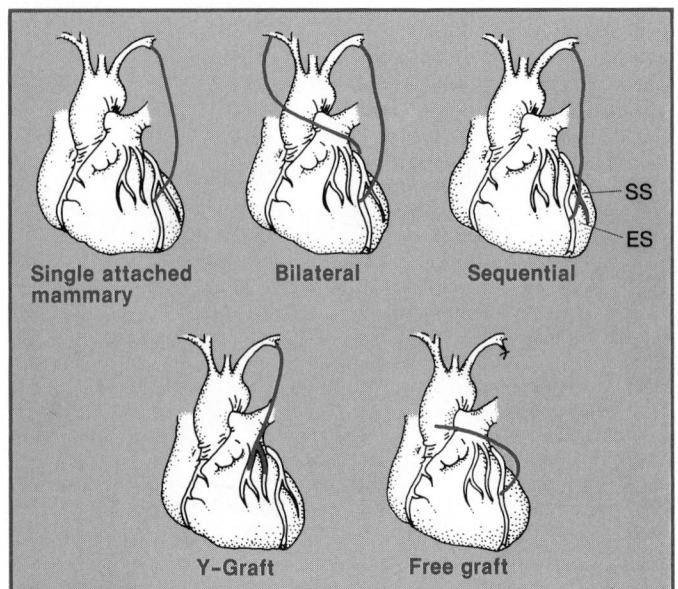

FIGURE 38–12. Different types of internal mammary artery grafts. A single attached internal mammary artery graft (either the right or left) remains attached proximally to the subclavian artery and is connected to the coronary arteries. Bilateral internal mammary artery grafts (right and left) are joined end to side to coronary arteries. Sequential internal mammary artery grafts consist of an attached or free internal mammary artery with one or more side-to-side anastomoses and one end-to-side anastomosis. The internal mammary artery Y graft has two terminal branches of either the attached or free internal mammary artery sutured to two coronary arteries. A free internal mammary graft is placed by transecting the right or left internal mammary artery near its origin in the subclavian artery, and the proximal artery is anastomosed to the aorta with the distal end to the coronary artery. (From Tector, A. J., et al.: Expanding the use of the internal mammary artery to improve patency in coronary artery bypass grafting. J. Thorac. Cardiovasc. Surg. *91*:9, 1986.)

be taken to mobilize the vessel without traumatizing it.[385] This prolongs the operative time and often requires entry into the pleural space. The "skeletonization" technique of IMA dissection, in which the artery is taken down with a strip of endothoracic fascia containing internal thoracic veins and endolymphatic tissue, achieves high flow rates and the pleural space is not usually opened.[380] However, this procedure is time consuming and the IMA therefore is not often used for emergency surgery.

Comparative morphological and angiographic studies of IMA and saphenous vein bypass grafts that have been implanted long term show that accelerated atherosclerosis occurs commonly in saphenous vein grafts but is extremely rare in IMA grafts. There are several potential explanations for the superiority of the IMA graft.[380] The media of the artery may derive nourishment from the lumen as well as from the vasa vasorum, and the internal elastic lamina of the IMA is uniform.[386] Moreover, the finding that the endothelium of the IMA produces significantly more prostacyclin than the saphenous vein may explain why endothelium-dependent relaxation is more pronounced, which may allow flow-dependent autoregulation to occur.[387] The diameter of the IMA graft usually is a closer match to that of the recipient coronary artery than is the diameter of a saphenous vein.

In contrast to the 40 to 60 per cent patency for vein grafts at 10 to 12 years following coronary surgery, that of IMA grafts exceeds 90 per cent.[315] Long-term patency rates were 95 per cent to the left anterior descending coronary artery, 88 per cent to the left circumflex, and 76 per cent to the right coronary artery and were higher for left than for right IMA grafts, and higher for in situ than for free IMA grafts. However, fibrointimal proliferation may occasionally

develop in IMA grafts and cause narrowing and may be a factor in late graft closure.[380]

Loop et al. described improved 10-year survival in patients who received an IMA graft to the anterior descending coronary artery alone, or combined with one or more saphenous vein grafts, compared with survival in patients who had only saphenous vein bypass grafts (Fig. 38–13).[388,389a,389b] This important observation has been confirmed.[389] Patients receiving the IMA graft have a decreased risk of late death, myocardial infarction, cardiac events, and reoperations, and this clinical advantage persists for up to 20 years.[388,390,391] Most surgeons now believe that whenever it is technically feasible, IMA grafting is the preferable treatment, at least for lesions of the anterior descending coronary artery.

Although the benefits of the single IMA graft over the saphenous vein graft alone are not in dispute, it is unclear whether bilateral IMA grafts are superior to a single IMA graft to the left anterior descending coronary artery.[389] The use of bilateral grafts is technically more demanding, but late reoperation rates are reduced in patients receiving bilateral IMA grafts.

Complications of Arterial Conduits. Inadequate flow rates with evidence of myocardial ischemia in the perioperative period are rare after IMA grafts to the left anterior descending coronary artery or its diagonal branches.[380] Perioperative spasm is the presumed cause and can be managed by the administration of sodium nitroprusside or a combination of glyceryl trinitrate and verapamil.[392] Other complications include an increased incidence of sternal wound infections, which is more frequent in obese patients and in diabetics and after bilateral IMA implants.[390]

Other Conduits. The right gastroepiploic artery is increasingly used as a conduit in patients in whom the IMA and saphenous veins have been exhausted and in younger patients, particularly among those with hyperlipidemia.[315,380] The graft is most frequently placed to the right coronary artery.[391] Initial results suggested that patency rates were inferior to those for the IMA, but this may have been part of a "learning curve," with recent data suggesting

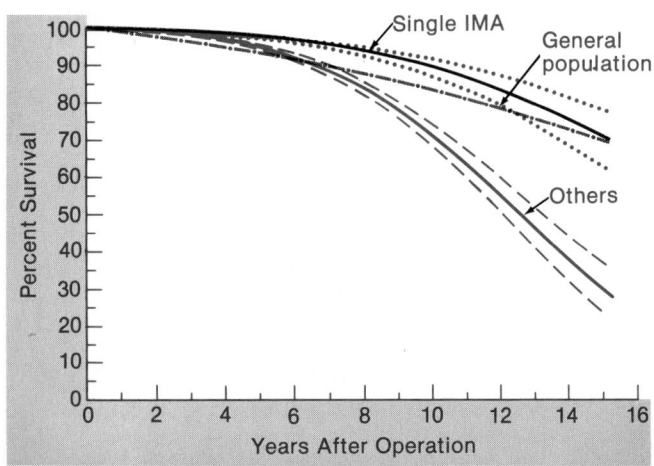

FIGURE 38–13. Survival of patients with extensive three-vessel disease according to whether or not a single internal mammary artery graft (IMA) to the left anterior descending coronary artery was used as a conduit in addition to whatever vein grafts were necessary. "General population" refers to an age, race, and gender-matched general population from government statistics and "Others" refers to patients revascularized without a single IMA graft applied to the left anterior descending coronary artery. These data strongly suggest that having a single IMA graft applied to the left anterior descending coronary artery is beneficial to survival in patients with extensive three-vessel coronary artery disease. (Modified from Kirklin, J. W., et al.: Summary of a consensus concerning death and ischemic events after coronary artery bypass grafting. Circulation *79*[Suppl. I]:81, 1989, copyright American Heart Association.)

that patency rates are equal. Other conduits that have been employed include the radial artery and the inferior epigastric artery.[393]

MILD NATIVE VESSEL OBSTRUCTION. Intraoperative studies have shown that native arteries with less than 50 per cent luminal diameter obstruction often have minimal, if any, pressure gradients across the lesions and little difference in blood flow through the artery distal to the graft when the bypass graft is opened. Patients with higher grade obstructions usually have greater pressure gradients across the lesions. Patency rates of IMA grafts to vessels with less than 50 per cent stenosis are lower than to vessels with more significant lesions.

THE DISTAL VASCULATURE. The state of the distal coronary vasculature is important for the fate of bypass grafts. Late patency of grafts is related to coronary arterial runoff as determined by the diameter of the coronary artery into which the graft is inserted, the size of the distal vascular bed, and the severity of coronary atherosclerosis distal to the site of insertion of the graft. The highest graft patency rates are found when the lumina of the vessels distal to the graft insertion are greater than 1.5 mm in diameter, perfuse a large vascular bed, and are free of atheroma obstructing more than 25 per cent of the vessel lumen.

FLOW RATES. When measured at the time of operation, flow rates through saphenous vein grafts average nearly 70 ml/min. Those in which the flow is less than 45 ml/min— and especially less than 25 ml/min—are more frequently associated with graft closure than those with flow rates exceeding 45 ml/min.[394] The possible causes for reduced flow include (1) subcritical obstruction of the coronary artery, (2) a technically poor anastomosis, with narrowing of the lumen due to kinking of the vessel or pinching at the site of anastomosis, (3) a small myocardial mass perfused by the graft, and (4) a diseased distal vascular bed.

OTHER SURGICAL PROCEDURES FOR ISCHEMIC HEART DISEASE. Coronary bypass surgery may be combined with surgical procedures aimed at correction of atherosclerotic disease elsewhere in the cardiovascular system, with correction of mechanical complications of myocardial infarction (mitral regurgitation at ventricular septal defect), left ventricular aneurysmectomy, and concomitant valvular heart disease.[395,396] Not unexpectedly, morbidity and mortality are correspondingly increased owing to the added complexity of the procedure and, in many patients who require these other procedures, the presence of underlying left ventricular dysfunction.

Outcome of Surgery

OPERATIVE MORTALITY. As Kirklin et al. have pointed out, risk factors for death following coronary artery surgery may be considered in five categories: (1) preoperative factors related to CAD, including recent acute myocardial infarction, hemodynamic instability, left ventricular dysfunction, extensive CAD, the presence of left main coronary artery disease, and severe or unstable angina; (2) preoperative factors related to the aggressiveness of the arteriosclerotic process, as reflected in associated carotid peripheral vascular disease; (3) preoperative biological factors (older age at operation, diabetes mellitus, and perhaps female gender); (4) intraoperative factors (intraoperative ischemic damage and failure to use IMA grafts)[397]; and (5) environmental or institutional factors, including the specific surgeon and treatment protocols used.[398]

The patient population undergoing coronary bypass surgery has been changing over time, particularly with the wider use of PTCA and other catheter-based procedures. In comparison with the 1970's, patients undergoing coronary bypass surgery today are older, include a higher percentage of women, are "sicker," in that a greater proportion have

unstable angina, three-vessel disease, prior coronary revascularization with either coronary bypass surgery or PTCA, left ventricular dysfunction, and comorbid conditions, including hypertension, diabetes, and peripheral vascular disease.[399]

In-hospital mortality after isolated coronary bypass surgery was characterized by a steady decline from 1967 to the early 1980's. Overall mortality for elective first bypass procedures in the United States from 1980 to 1990 was 2.2 per cent in 58,384 patients in the Society of Thoracic Surgeons data base. It was 2.6 per cent in elective patients without IMA grafts and 1.3 per cent in patients receiving such an implant.[399] More recently there has been a stabilization or even a slight overall increase in morbidity and mortality, which reflects the changing characteristics toward an older and sicker population of patients undergoing operation.[400,400a]

Changing Late Results of Coronary Bypass Surgery. Two competing influences warrant a reevaluation of the late results of coronary bypass surgery in the contemporary era. Improved surgical and perioperative techniques, including the use of IMA grafts, improve long-term outcome. On the other hand, the survival to discharge of high-risk patients, who may have died during the perioperative period during an earlier era, may have an opposite effect upon late outcome. In addition, as already noted, the patient population undergoing CABG has shifted toward a greater proportion of older, higher risk patients with a worse prognosis. This trend may substantially alter downward the expectations of late outcome.

PERIOPERATIVE COMPLICATIONS. Perioperative morbidity (see also Chap. 52) has also increased because of a larger fraction of higher risk patients.

PERIOPERATIVE MYOCARDIAL INFARCTION. The diagnosis of perioperative myocardial infarction is hampered by the lack of specificity of repolarization abnormalities and enzyme changes during the perioperative period. Predictors of perioperative myocardial infarction in the Coronary Artery Surgery Study (CASS) were female gender, severe perioperative angina pectoris, severe stenosis of the left main coronary artery, and three-vessel disease.[401] Unstable angina and prolonged cardiopulmonary bypass times are also risk factors.[402] Perioperative myocardial infarction, particularly if it is associated with hemodynamic or arrhythmic complications or preexisting left ventricular dysfunction, has a major adverse effect upon early and late prognosis.[403]

RESPIRATORY COMPLICATIONS. Postoperative changes in pulmonary function after coronary bypass surgery are frequent and troublesome, but rarely serious, except in patients with preexisting chronic lung disease or the elderly.

BLEEDING. Impaired hemostasis and bleeding complications are an inherent risk of coronary bypass surgery. Reoperation for bleeding is required in 2 to 5 per cent of patients.[404] Cardiopulmonary bypass causes derangements of the intrinsic coagulation and fibrinolytic systems in addition to platelet function. The risk of bleeding is increased with age, a smaller surface area, reoperation, bilateral internal thoracic artery grafts, and the preoperative use of heparin, aspirin, and thrombolytic agents. The prophylactic use of epsilon-aminocaproic acid (aprotinin), which may prevent degradation of platelet function, is associated with a significant reduction in both blood loss and transfusion requirements.[405]

WOUND INFECTIONS. Major perioperative wound complications, especially mediastinitis and/or wound dehiscence, occur in approximately 1 per cent of patients.[406] These are associated with a markedly increased in-hospital mortality, morbidity, and length of stay. This risk is substantially increased by the use of double IMA grafts, particularly in diabetics.[406]

POSTOPERATIVE HYPERTENSION. This complication can occur in up to one-third of all patients after coronary bypass surgery (see p. 830). The mechanism is unclear, but it may be related to increased levels of circulating catecholamines and renin. It is important to control postoperative hypertension to prevent myocardial ischemia, cardiac failure, and excessive perioperative bleeding. Postoperative hypertension rarely presents a problem with the use of drugs such as calcium antagonists[407] or nitrates.[408] Esmolol, a short-acting beta-blocking agent (see p. 487), appears to be equally effective in reducing arterial pressure and also slows heart rate.[409]

CEREBROVASCULAR COMPLICATIONS. These include stroke, the incidence of which is 1 to 5 per cent and is age related.[410] Delayed returns of a normal level of consciousness occurs in approximately 3 per cent of patients,[411] and intellectual dysfunction in the early postoperative period, as assessed by a battery of neurocognitive tests, has been noted in approximately 75 per cent of patients.[412] Transient mild visual deficits are common.[410] Fortunately, major long-term sequelae are uncommon. Mild degrees of confusion, agitation, and delusional behavior are frequent and usually transient. The elderly are particularly vulnerable.

ATRIAL FIBRILLATION. This is one of the most frequent complications of coronary bypass surgery. It occurs in up to 40 per cent of patients, primarily within 2 to 3 days.[413,414] In the early postoperative period, rapid ventricular rates and loss of atrial transport may compromise systemic hemodynamics and increase the risk of embolization. Beta blockers are useful in the treatment of the condition once established, and trials have suggested a benefit for the prophylactic value of these drugs.[413]

CONDUCTION DISTURBANCES AND BRADYARRHYTHMIAS. The incidence of postoperative bradyarrhythmias requiring permanent pacemaker implantation was 0.8 per cent in a series of 1614 consecutive patients discharged from the hospital after coronary bypass surgery.[415] Predictive factors were preoperative left bundle branch block, concomitant left ventricular aneurysmectomy, and older age. The majority of patients continued to require permanent pacemaker support during follow-up.[415] Patients with CAD who develop fascicular conduction disturbances often have diffuse myocardial disease and an unfavorable prognosis. The causes of death are ventricular arrhythmias and cardiac failure.

COMPLICATION IN THE OBESE. While obesity per se does not appear to increase significantly the operative mortality,[416] it is associated with a higher incidence of complications, including sternotomy dehiscence, impaired leg wound healing following saphenous vein excision,[417] postoperative hypertension, and bronchoconstriction.

SYMPTOMATIC RESULTS. Major relief of angina pectoris occurs in more than 90 per cent of appropriately selected patients after coronary bypass surgery.[416a] Approximately three-quarters of patients are free from ischemic events, sudden death, occurrence of a myocardial infarction, or return of angina for 5 years after coronary artery surgery and nearly half for at least 10 years.[398] However, by 15 years only about 15 per cent of patients can be expected to be alive and free of an ischemic event.

In the bypass surgery arms of recent randomized trials of PTCA and CABG (see p. 1375), recurrent angina pectoris was reported in 21.5 per cent to 34 per cent of patients at a follow-up ranging from 2 to 3 years, but (Canadian Classification) grade III or IV angina was present in only 6 per cent at 2.5 years in the RITA trial.[418] Only 12 per cent of patients in the Emory Angioplasty Surgery Study (EAST) reported class II, III, or IV angina after 3 years of follow-up (see p. 1375).[351]

RETURN TO EMPLOYMENT. Return to full employment has been disappointing in some series. Among participants in the surgical arm of EAST, whose mean age was 61 years at entry, only 38.5 per cent were gainfully employed at 3 years.[351] In contrast, in a study of patients under the age of 65 years who were employed at the time of revascularization, 79 per cent of patients who had bypass surgery were working at 1 year, and, after adjustment for baseline characteristics, the 1-year employment rates were the same among patients treated with surgery, angioplasty, or medical therapy.[419] Factors that affect adversely the prospects of patients returning to work include advanced age, postoperative angina, and a period of either unemployment or disability before surgery.[420,421] Forty-seven per cent of patients undergoing bypass surgery in the EAST trial were able to engage in moderate or strenuous activity 3 years after the procedure.[351] However, with time there is a fall off in symptomatic benefit, and there is a suggestion that by 10 years after coronary vein graft surgery the relief of symptoms and improved exercise performance noted at 5 years have decreased to levels seen in medically treated patients.[422]

GRAFT PATENCY. Experimental studies and observations in patients suggest that there are several phases of disease development in venous aortocoronary artery bypass grafts. The occlusion rate, which is high in the first year, decreases substantially between the first and sixth years. Between 6 and 10 years after operation the attrition rate for grafts increases again. Early occlusion (prior to hospital discharge) occurs in 8 to 12 per cent of venous grafts, and by 1 year 15 to 30 per cent of vein grafts have become

occluded.[423,424] After the first year, the annual occlusion rate is 2 per cent per year and rises to approximately 4 per cent per year between years 6 and 10. At 10 years, approximately one-third of vein grafts which are patent at 1 year have become occluded, one-third demonstrate significant atherosclerosis, and one-third appear to be unchanged.[423] Moreover, 20 to 40 per cent of grafts that are patent at 10 years after surgery are stenotic.[315,380]

Early Phase (First Month). Technical factors that may cause thrombotic closure at the proximal or distal anastomoses include kinking due to excessive length, tension due to insufficient length, poor graft flow, and inadequate distal runoff. Atheroma at the arteriotomy site may predispose to early thrombotic occlusion. Surgical manipulation of the saphenous vein during harvesting and preparation prior to grafting play key roles in initiating the sequence of endothelial damage with subsequent platelet and fibrin deposition, leading to thrombosis.[384,424,425] Interruption of the nutrient blood flow to the vein wall may also be involved.[423]

Intermediate Phase (1 Month to 1 Year). In vein grafts that have been implanted in the arterial circulation for 1 month to 1 year, there is substantial endothelial denudation and proliferation and migration of medial cells to the intima. Even in the face of endothelial continuity, progressive migration of vascular smooth muscle cells through the internal elastic lamina into the intima may occur.[384,426] The initial phase of rapid proliferation is followed after several months by a marked increase in the connective tissue matrix, which further increases intimal and medial thickness. These events are promoted by aggregation of platelets and secretion of growth factors. This accelerated process of intimal hyperplasia and thickening is an early stage of atherosclerotic plaque formation and is believed to occur because of interaction between platelets and macrophages and endothelial damage. If the proliferation is severe and localized, as may occur at the site of the anastomosis between the grafts and the recipient artery, total occlusion can occur within 1 year. Histological studies of grafts that occlude within 1 year often show either substantial thrombosis with minimal intima-medial changes or marked intimal hyperplasia or superimposed thrombus.[427]

Late Phase (Beyond 1 Year). Some investigators believe that the development of atherosclerosis in vein grafts, as in native arteries, is a continuum starting from platelet deposition and advancing to smooth muscle cell proliferation and finally to lipid incorporation into the plaque. By 10 years, nearly one-half of venous grafts patent at 5 years have become occluded.[428] Beyond the first year, particularly after 3 to 5 years, the histological appearance of occluded or obstructed coronary bypass grafts is consistent with atherosclerosis. There is clear evidence of mature lipid-laden plaques, foam cells, cholesterol clefts, ulceration, and areas of calcification with disruption of the medial layer.[429] Although there are similarities to the atherosclerotic lesions of arterial disease, vein graft atherosclerosis is more diffuse circumferentially.[430] Marked friability of the atherosclerotic lesions may cause intermittent coronary embolization,[431] which complicates revascularization procedures, such as reoperation or PTCA of vein grafts.

DETERMINATION OF GRAFT PATENCY. Although determination of graft patency usually involves postoperative angiography, radionuclide techniques, which assess myocardial perfusion, may also indicate graft patency.[432] Contrast-enhanced computed tomography has been used to assess patency of saphenous vein grafts (Fig. 10–36, p. 338).

PROGRESSION OF DISEASE IN NONGRAFTED ARTERIES. Disease progression, defined as a worsening of a preexisting lesion or appearance of a new diameter narrowing of 50 per cent or greater, can occur at a rate of 20 to 40 per cent over 5 to 10 years in nongrafted native vessels.[433] The rate of disease progression appears highest in arterial segments already showing evidence of disease,[434] and it is between three and six times higher in grafted native coronary arteries than in ungrafted native vessels. Disease progression is also greater in arteries with patent grafts than in arteries with occluded grafts[435] and usually occurs proximal to the site of graft insertion.[433,434] These data suggest that bypassing an artery with minimal disease, even if initially successful, may ultimately be harmful to the patient who incurs both the risk of graft closure and the increased risk of accelerated obstruction of the native vessels.

EFFECTS OF THERAPY ON VEIN GRAFT OCCLUSION AND NATIVE VESSEL PROGRESSION. A meta-analysis of clinical trials suggests that antiplatelet or anticoagulant therapy after coronary artery bypass surgery may prevent graft occlusion.[436]

ANTIPLATELET THERAPY (see also p. 1225). In a prospective randomized double-blind trial, dipyridamole (started 48 hours before operation) plus aspirin (started 7 hours after operation) was compared with placebo treatment. Within 1 month of operation 3 per cent of vein-graft distal anastomoses were occluded in the treated patients, compared with 10 per cent in the placebo group.[437] At angiography performed 1 year after operation, 11 per cent of vein-graft distal anastomoses were occluded in the treated group and 25 per cent in the placebo group.[438] There was no significant increase in blood loss, transfusions, or reoperations in the treated group during the perioperative period. Subsequent studies suggested that dipyridamole is *not* an essential component and that low doses of aspirin (40 to 80 mg/day) may be sufficient.[439]

A Veterans Administration Cooperative Study Group has also examined the effect of specific antiplatelet therapy on vein graft after coronary artery bypass grafting.[440] Early graft patency rates were 92 per cent for aspirin (with or without dipyridamole) compared with 85 per cent for placebo. At 1 year the graft occlusion rate in all of the aspirin groups combined was 16 per cent compared with 23 per cent for the placebo group.[440] Aspirin started 6 hours after surgery appears to be as effective in preventing vein graft complications as is aspirin begun 12 hours preoperatively, but the former has the added benefit of reducing bleeding complications.[441] A meta-analysis of 17 trials of prevention of vein graft occlusion suggested that 100 mg to 325 mg of daily aspirin was more effective than a high dosage (975 mg).[439] Aspirin should be continued indefinitely following coronary bypass surgery. However, aspirin does not affect patency of an internal mammary artery graft.[442]

THERAPY OF HYPERLIPIDEMIA AND OTHER RISK FACTORS. Several studies have drawn attention to the relationship between vein graft atherosclerosis and elevated levels of LDL cholesterol, Lp(a), and reduced HDL cholesterol levels.[424,443–447] The randomized Cholesterol Lowering Atherosclerosis Study (CLAS) of hyperlipidemic men who had undergone coronary bypass surgery demonstrated a significant reduction in disease progression in native vessels and in bypass grafts with lipid-lowering pharmacotherapy.[444] It is essential to maintain ideal body weight, reduce total and LDL cholesterol levels, and permanently cease smoking following coronary artery surgery.[446] In patients randomized to bypass surgery in the Coronary Artery Surgery Study (CASS), mortality and morbidity were lower among men who quit smoking than those who continued to smoke after entry.[148]

Selection of Patients for Coronary Bypass Surgery

The indications for coronary bypass surgery consist of the need for improvement of the quality or quantity of life. Patients whose angina is not controlled by medical management or who have unacceptable side effects with such management should be considered for coronary revascularization. If, on the basis of the coronary anatomy, the patient is a suitable candidate for PTCA and is not in a subgroup that requires operation (such as three-vessel disease with left ventricular dysfunction), angioplasty is ordinarily the procedure of choice.[447a] If the patient is a failure of medical therapy and is not a good candidate for PTCA, then coronary bypass surgery should be considered. This procedure is also indicated in patients with CAD, regardless of symptoms, in whom survival is likely to be prolonged.[448]

In making the critical decision regarding revascularization, it is important to assess the patient's prognosis (Table 38–11) and how it may be affected by operation. The key

TABLE 38–11   DETERMINANTS OF ADVERSE PROGNOSIS IN CORONARY ARTERY DISEASE

Cardiac Determinants
  Left ventricular dysfunction
  Extent of myocardial jeopardy—extent of ischemia at rest and on exercise and number of large vessels diseased
  Extent of myocardium in jeopardy
  Abnormal arrhythmic substrate

Clinical and Electrocardiographic Modifying Factors
  Advanced age
  History of congestive heart failure
  Diabetes
  Rapidly accelerating angina
  Resting electrocardiographic abnormalities
  Left ventricular hypertrophy and hypertension
  Peripheral vascular disease
  Hyperlipidemia

initial step is to stratify patients into categories of risk with continued medical therapy, based upon an analysis of clinical, noninvasive, and, in some patients, angiographic variables. This process defines the *indications* for revascularization over medical therapy; more recent randomized trial data are helpful in defining which *modality* of revascularization (PTCA or surgery) is preferable (see p. 1374).

Natural History of Angina Pectoris

CLINICAL AND ELECTROCARDIOGRAPHIC CRITERIA. Data from the Framingham Study, obtained prior to the widespread use of aspirin, beta blockers, and aggressive modification of risk factors, showed that the average annual mortality rate of patients with chronic stable angina was 4 per cent.[449] The combination of these treatments has improved prognosis. Remission of angina may occur in up to one-third of patients with angina of recent onset, but this is unusual if the condition has been present for several years. Numerous studies attest to the adverse prognostic impact of congestive heart failure (based upon a clinical history of cardiomegaly on chest radiography), prior myocardial infarction, hypertension, and advanced age in patients with stable angina pectoris.[449–451] A third heart sound is a useful clinical predictor of an abnormal left ventricular ejection fraction and an adverse prognosis in patients with CAD. The severity of angina, especially the tempo of intensification, is also an important predictor of outcome.

On the other hand, a normal resting electrocardiogram in patients with stable angina pectoris speaks in favor of well-preserved left ventricular function and a favorable long-term prognosis (see p. 1295).[351,452] Left ventricular hypertrophy, as determined on the electrocardiogram or echocardiogram, is associated with an increased mortality secondary to the effects of hypertension and left ventricular dysfunction.[453]

ANGIOGRAPHIC CRITERIA. The independent impact of multivessel disease and left ventricular dysfunction, and their interaction upon the prognosis of patients with CAD, has been well documented[454–456] (Fig. 38–14). These two risk factors are synergistic in that the adverse effects on prognosis of impaired ventricular function are more pronounced as the number of stenotic vessels increases.[455] When all of the other factors are held constant, the number of coronary arteries with significant stenoses is one of the most powerful prognostic factors. More elaborate classifications of the extent of disease have not provided much additional information, other than the greater the extent of jeopardized myocardium, the worse the prognosis. Among medically treated patients in CASS, 12-year survival was 91 per cent in patients with chronic angina and angiographically normal vessels. In the presence of single-vessel disease, it was 86 per cent in patients with at least one obstruction of 30 to 50 per cent; 79 per cent in patients with at least one stenosis of 50 to 70 per cent, and 74 per

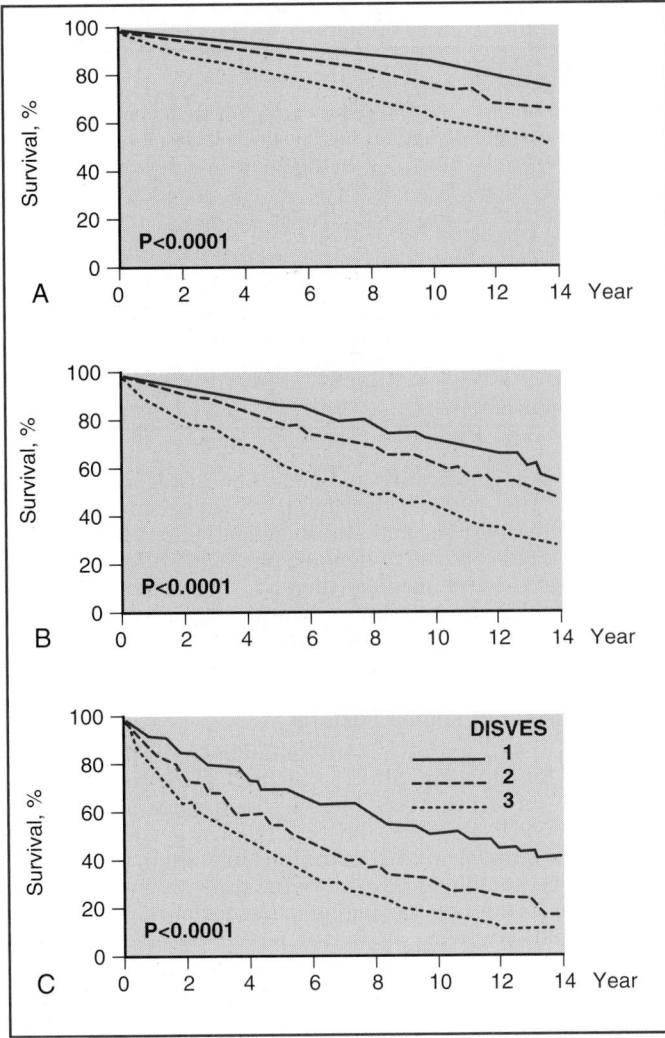

FIGURE 38–14. Graphs showing survival for medically treated CASS patients. *A,* Patients with one-, two-, or three-vessel disease and ejection fraction 50 to 100 per cent by number of diseased vessels (DISVES). *B,* Patients with one-, two-, or three-vessel disease and ejection fraction 35 to 49 per cent by number of diseased vessels. *C,* Patients with one-, two-, or three-vessel disease and ejection fraction 0 to 34 per cent by number of diseased vessels. (Reproduced with permission from Emond, M., et al.: Long-term survival of medically treated patients in the Coronary Artery Surgery Study [CASS] registry. Circulation *90:*2645, 1994. Copyright American Heart Association.)

cent in patients with single-vessel disease and a stenosis of 70 per cent or more.[455]

Studies in symptomatic patients have revealed that if only one of the three major coronary arteries has more than 50 per cent stenosis, the annual mortality rate is approximately 2 per cent.[457] The importance to survival of the quantity of myocardium that is jeopardized is reflected in the observation that an obstructive lesion proximal to the first septal perforating branch of the left anterior descending coronary artery was associated with a 5-year survival of 90 per cent, compared with 98 per cent in patients with more distal lesions.[457] The survival rate of patients with isolated right CAD at 5 years appeared to be higher (96 per cent) than in patients with disease of the left anterior descending coronary artery (92 per cent). The overall survival of medically treated patients with left anterior descending and left circumflex CAD was not significantly different, but both were less than the survival of patients with isolated right CAD.[457]

In symptomatic patients (or in asymptomatic survivors of myocardial infarction, if two of the major arteries exhibit severe stenosis, the 5-year mortality is approximately 9 per cent, and if all three vessels are stenotic it rises to approxi-

mately 15 per cent.[458,459] In an observational study of patients with obstructive CAD who initially were treated medically, 15-year survival rates were 48, 28, 18, and 9 per cent for patients with single-, double-, triple-, and left main vessel disease, respectively.[454] In addition to the number of vessels involved, the severity of obstruction is also important. Prognosis in patients with 50 to 75 per cent narrowing is better than in those with more than 75 per cent narrowing.[460]

High-grade lesions of the left main coronary artery or its "equivalents" are particularly life threatening (Fig. 38–15).[461] Mortality among medically treated patients has been reported as 29 per cent at 18 months, 39 per cent at 2 years, and 43 per cent at 5 years.[462,463] Survival is better for patients having a 50 to 70 per cent stenosis (1- and 3-year survivals of 91 per cent and 66 per cent, respectively) than for patients with a greater than 70 per cent left main coronary artery stenosis (1- and 3-year survivals of 72 and 41 per cent).[464] Furthermore, a number of characteristics found at catheterization or on noninvasive examination are predictors of an adverse prognosis in patients with 70 per cent or greater left main coronary artery stenosis; these include chest pain at rest, ST-T wave changes on the resting electrocardiogram, cardiomegaly on the chest roentgenogram, a history of congestive heart failure, findings of left ventricular dysfunction at catheterization, and elevation of the arterial–mixed venous oxygen difference.[464]

The severity of symptoms is a useful prognostic factor in conjunction with arteriographic findings and left ventricular function. In asymptomatic or mildly symptomatic patients who have one- or two-vessel disease, the prognosis is excellent, and the annual mortality is approximately 1.5 per cent. Even in patients with three-vessel disease who have good exercise capacity (achievement of 85 per cent predicted heart rate or workload of 100 watts or more), the annual mortality rate also is relatively low, 4 per cent.[465]

LIMITATIONS OF ANGIOGRAPHY. The pathophysiological significance of coronary stenoses lies in their impact upon resting and exercise-induced blood flow, in addition to their potential for plaque rupture with superimposed thrombotic occlusion. It is generally accepted that a stenosis of greater than 60 per cent of the luminal diameter is hemodynamically significant, in that it may be responsible for a reduction in exercise-induced myocardial blood flow causing angina and ischemia[466] (see p. 1293). The functional significance of obstruction of "intermediate" severity (approximately 50 per cent diameter stenosis)[467] is less well established.

Another limitation to the routine use of coronary angiography for prognosis in patients with chronic stable angina is its inability to identify which coronary lesions can be considered to be at high risk for future events, such as myocardial infarction or sudden death. Although it is widely accepted that myocardial infarction is the result of thrombotic occlusion at the site of a plaque rupture[468] (see p. 1188), a growing body of evidence suggests that it is not necessarily the plaque causing the most severe stenosis which subsequently ruptures. Several studies of patients undergoing serial coronary angiograms indicate that myocardial infarction often arises from rupture of the plaque which did *not* cause critical obstruction (see p. 1192). Mild lesions can rupture, thrombose, and occlude, leading to myocardial infarction and sudden death.[469–472] In contrast, arteries with severe preexisting stenoses may proceed to clinically silent complete occlusion, often without infarction, presumably due to the formation of collaterals.

In summary, angiographic documentation of the extent of CAD is an indispensable step in the selection of patients for coronary revascularization, particularly if the interaction between the anatomical extent of disease, left ventricular function, and the severity of ischemia is taken into account. However, angiography is not helpful in predicting the site of subsequent occlusions which could cause myo-

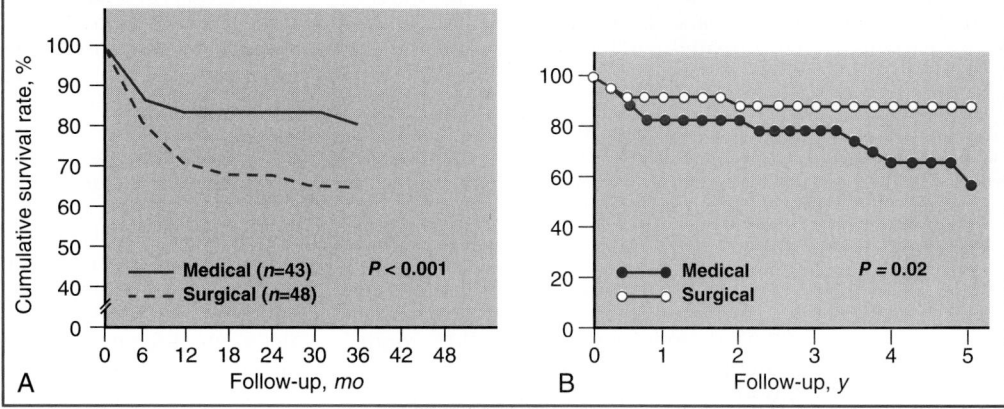

FIGURE 38-15. Cumulative survival with medical and surgical therapy in patients with symptomatic left main coronary disease greater than 50% from the Veterans Administration Cooperative Study (A) and the Coronary Artery Surgery Study patients with left main coronary artery disease (B). (From Gersh, B. J.: Natural history of chronic coronary artery disease. *In* Beller, G. A., and Braunwald, E. [eds.]: Chronic Ischemic Heart Disease. Atlas of Heart Diseases. Philadelphia, Current Medicine, 1995. Adapted from Takaro, T., Hultgren, H. N., Lipton, M. J., et al.: The VA cooperative randomized study of surgery for coronary arterial occlusive disease. II. Subgroup with significant left main lesions. Circulation 51[Suppl. III]: 107, 1976. Copyright American Heart Association.)

cardial infarction or sudden cardiac death, particularly in the individual patient.

NONINVASIVE TESTING (see p. 1295). In the estimation of prognosis in patients with chronic stable angina pectoris, stress testing with or without imaging may provide useful information (Table 38-2)[71,451] (Chaps. 3, 5, and 9). Depending upon the nature of the study, the patient's functioning status, the severity of ischemia, the extent of "jeopardized" myocardium, and ventricular function can all be assessed by these tests. In patients in whom left ventricular function and coronary anatomy have already been defined, stress testing may provide additional prognostic information regarding the functional significance of specific angiographic lesions.

From a clinical standpoint, the initial approach to a patient with chronic stable angina and a normal resting electrocardiogram is to perform a standard exercise electrocardiogram. In patients with major electrocardiographic conduction abnormalities (left or right bundle branch block) or in patients with resting ST-segment changes, in whom the response to exercise may be difficult to interpret, it is reasonable to proceed directly to a stress imaging study. The latter can be determined by nuclear techniques or echocardiography. The choice depends on the expertise available to any individual institution.

One of the most important prognosticators derived from exercise stress testing is exercise duration or capacity.[473] In an 8-year follow-up of medically treated patients with angiographically confirmed CAD and a positive exercise test, the duration of exercise correlated significantly with survival.[71] Patients reaching stage 4 of a Bruce protocol had a survival rate of 93 per cent, compared to only 45 per cent in patients who terminated exercise in stage 1.[71] This relationship between exercise duration and long-term survival was independent of whether the exercise was terminated because of dyspnea, fatigue, or angina. In a 16-year follow-up study from the CASS registry, exercise capacity was shown to be an extremely powerful predictor of survival, particularly among men, and to be helpful in the identification of patients likely to benefit from coronary revascularization.[474] Other factors identified with a poor prognosis in individual series of patients with chronic stable angina are described in Table 38-2.

Prognostic Scores. Mark et al. have incorporated exercise test results into a prognostic score, which stratified patients with stable CAD into three risk groups with 5-year mortality rates of 3 per cent, 9 per cent, and 28 per cent, respectively, and then showed that this score contained information beyond that provided by clinical and catheterization data.[475] Similar studies at the Long Beach Veterans Administration Medical Center considered both clinical and exercise predictors of cardiovascular mortality. A simple score based upon a history of congestive heart failure,

ST-segment depression on the resting electrocardiogram, and a fall in systolic blood pressure below rest during exercise identified three categories of risk with annual cardiac mortality rates of 1 per cent, 7 per cent, and 12 per cent, respectively.[476]

Stress Thallium-201 Myocardial Perfusion Imaging. The value of thallium scintigraphy in the stratification of patients with stable CAD is based upon the documentation of scintigraphic variables, indicative of patients at high risk (see p. 1296) (Table 38-2). Among patients presenting with chest pain, and including patients with angiographically proven CAD, a normal stress perfusion study was associated with a cardiac event rate of less than 1 per cent per year.[477,478]

Pharmacological Perfusion Imaging. Pharmacological stress perfusion imaging techniques with dipyridamole, adenosine, or dobutamine have an established place as an alternative to exercise perfusion imaging in establishing prognosis in patients with stable CAD.[69a,69b,91,93,479,480,480a] These techniques have been particularly useful in patients with peripheral vascular disease and in the elderly.[95,481,482]

Pharmacological (Stress) Echocardiography. There is increasing evidence that echocardiography with exercise[483a] or pharmacological stress (dobutamine, arbutamine, or dipyridamole) can also be useful for risk stratification.[483a,484,485]

Results

Relief of Angina Pectoris

As early as 1972, a committee of the American Heart Association indicated that the most widely accepted indication for surgical revascularization was "significant disability from moderate to severe angina pectoris, unresponsive to optimal medical care."[486] Two and a half decades later, angina pectoris despite medical management remains the principal indication. However, coronary bypass surgery is now being carried out in increasing numbers of patients with multivessel coronary disease and either mild to moderate symptoms, left ventricular dysfunction, or poor exercise tolerance, because of the improved survival in these groups. Patients with unstable angina and left ventricular dysfunction as well as survivors of acute myocardial infarction are also undergoing revascularization with increasing frequency.

Relief of angina pectoris occurs in up to 95 per cent of patients with chronic stable angina following coronary artery bypass surgery. More than half of the patients become totally asymptomatic, at least initially. Most of the others experience substantial symptomatic relief. The major randomized trials have all demonstrated greater relief of angina, better exercise performance, and a lower requirement for antianginal medications for surgically compared with medically treated patients 5 years postoperatively.[448,487,488,498] After 5 years, differences in symptoms between patients initially treated medically and surgically are diminished, owing in part to the high "cross-over" rate from medical to surgical therapy in patients with continued symptoms, and a progression of disease in vein grafts and non-bypassed vessels in the surgical group.[487,488] The reoperation rate for recurrence of symptoms has been reported to be in the range of 6 to 8 per cent per year.[489]

For patients with persistent angina despite adequate medical therapy and for those who cannot tolerate the usual antianginal medications and who are not ideal candidates for PTCA, coronary bypass surgery provides excellent symptomatic relief.[490] With increasing use of IMA grafts, long-term relief of angina and freedom from subsequent cardiac events are improved, compared with previous patient populations who have received coronary artery vein grafts alone.

In summary, after 5 years, approximately three fourths of surgically treated patients can be predicted to be free from an ischemic event, sudden death, occurrence of myocardial infarction, or return of angina; about half remain free for approximately 10 years, and about 15 per cent for 15 or more years.[398,491,492] Symptomatic improvement is best maintained in patients with the most complete revascularization.[420]

Effects of Surgery on Survival in Patients with Chronic Stable Angina

Current clinical practice has been shaped by three major randomized trials into which patients were enrolled between 1972 and 1979, The Veterans Administration (VA), European Cardiac Society Study (ECSS), and the NIH-supported CASS.[493–499] These trials antedated the widespread use of the IMA for revascularization, as well as of aspirin and coronary angioplasty. Only CASS included women and only the VA trial included patients over the age of 65 years. High-risk patients, defined in terms of symptoms, severity of ischemia, age, extent of CAD, and left ventricular dysfunction, were generally excluded from the ECCS and CASS, even though such patients benefit the most from revascularization. The VA trial included a larger number of high-risk patients, and in the ECSS 42 per cent of patients had class III angina (Canadian Cardiovascular Society Criteria). In contrast, in CASS, all patients had either mild angina (Class I-II) or were asymptomatic after myocardial infarction.

In the VA study, there was no significant difference in overall survival between the groups initially assigned to medical and surgical treatment after 11 years of follow-up. However, higher risk subsets, including patients with left main coronary disease and patients who had three-vessel disease with impaired left ventricular function, initially had a significant survival advantage with surgery, although the magnitude of the difference decreased between 7 and 11 years. On retrospective analysis, a higher risk subset, with two or more of the following risk factors —New York Heart Association class III or IV angina; a history of hypertension; a history of prior myocardial infarction; and ST-segment depression on the resting electrocardiogram—experienced a survival benefit from operation.[497] Patients randomized to an initial surgical approach also experienced an overall survival advantage in the ECSS[498] (Fig. 38–16). The benefits of surgery were greater in patients at higher risk, including patients with multivessel disease, which included the proximal left anterior descending coronary artery, older patients, those with evidence of ischemia or infarction on the resting electrocardiogram, patients with peripheral vascular disease, and those with a markedly positive stress test. There was no significant difference in survival between medical and surgical treatment in patients with one-vessel disease and those with two-vessel disease without critical stenosis of the proximal left anterior descending coronary artery. In the CASS randomized trial, there was no difference in overall survival between the medically and surgically treated groups.[493,499] However, survival of patients at higher risk, with a left ventricular ejection fraction between 35 and 50 per cent was improved by surgery.[493]

The results of the ECCS suggest that in patients with moderately severe angina pectoris and normal ventricular function, if several risk factors, such as age greater than 50 years, an abnormal electrocardiogram at rest, ST-segment depression greater than 1.5 mm during exercise, and peripheral arterial disease are present, coronary angiography should be performed. If three-vessel disease (coronary artery diameter stenoses > 75 per cent) or obstruction of the proximal left anterior descending coronary artery and one other major vessel is present, surgery appears to be superior to medical therapy.[448] Other clinical risk factors in patients with three-vessel disease and normal ventricular function that might lead to surgical rather than medical therapy include severe angina pectoris (class III or IV), a

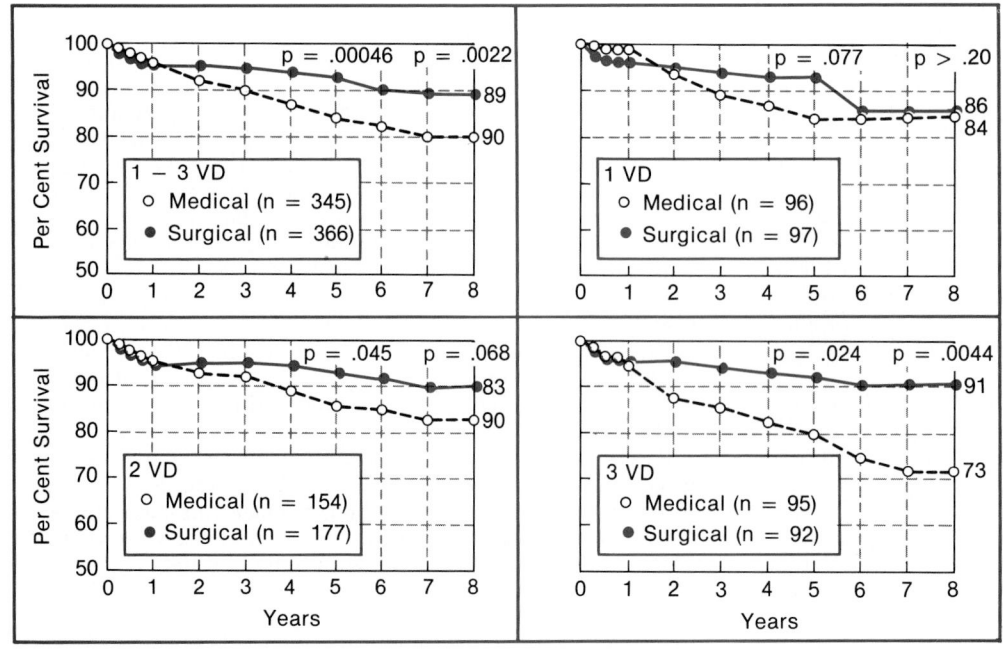

FIGURE 38–16. Cumulative survival curves for patients in the European Coronary Surgery Study. To compare the European prospective randomized coronary surgery study with other studies, a cohort of 711 patients was identified as having greater than 75 per cent obstruction in one, two, or three vessels. A significant improvement in survival with surgery was found in the total cohort and in the subgroup with three-vessel disease; however, there was no significant difference in survival between the two treatments in patients with one-vessel disease and those with two-vessel disease without proximal left anterior descending stenosis. (Reproduced with permission from Varnauskas, E., and the European Coronary Surgery Study Group: Survival, myocardial infarction, and employment status in a prospective, randomized study of coronary bypass surgery. Circulation *72*[Suppl. V]:90, 1985. Copyright American Heart Association.)

history of myocardial infarction, and resulting ST-segment depression.

LEFT MAIN CORONARY ARTERY STENOSIS. There is general agreement that surgical treatment improves survival in patients with left main coronary artery obstruction[500] or its "equivalent" (Fig. 38–15). The CASS registry demonstrated that the superiority of revascularization was equivalent in both symptomatic and asymptomatic patients with disease affecting the left main coronary artery.[462] Although coronary bypass surgery appears to confer the most benefit on patients with severe degrees of left main coronary artery disease and/or those patients with impaired left ventricular function, it is still beneficial in *all* patients with left main coronary stenoses greater than 60 per cent, which has recently been confirmed in a 16-year follow-up study from the CASS registry.[463]

There is continuing debate about whether there is a "left main equivalent" anatomy, which has a natural history similar to that of left main coronary disease. The condition in question may consist of disease in the proximal portions of both the left anterior descending and left circumflex coronary arteries. We believe that the ominous nature of significant left main coronary disease exists because a single event (rupture of a single plaque) can cause infarction of a very large quantity of myocardium. While combined disease of the proximal left anterior descending and circumflex coronary arteries does identify a subgroup of high-risk patients, the prognosis is not as poor as it is for patients with left main coronary artery disease.[502] Nevertheless, patients with combined stenoses of 70 per cent or greater in the left anterior descending coronary artery, before the first septal perforating branch, and in the proximal circumflex coronary artery before the first obtuse marginal branch, who have impaired ventricular function, also have improved survival and less angina following surgical revascularization than if they are treated medically, particularly in the face of left ventricular dysfunction.[503]

OVERVIEW OF THE RANDOMIZED TRIALS. A systematic overview of the seven randomized trials (the three aforementioned large trials and four smaller trials) which compared coronary bypass surgery with medical therapy between 1972 and 1984 yielded 2649 patients (Table 38–12).[448] Patients undergoing coronary bypass surgery had a significantly lower mortality at 5, 7, and 10 years, but by 10 years 41 per cent of the patients initially randomized to medical treatment had undergone CABG. The advantage for surgery was greatest in patients with left main coronary artery disease. An improvement in survival was also noted with surgical treatment in patients with one- or two-vessel disease and stenosis of the proximal left anterior descending coronary artery. In this published meta-analysis, the results for single- versus double-vessel disease in patients with left anterior descending coronary artery disease were not presented separately but it is likely that the majority of the benefit was in the patients with double-vessel disease.[448] Among patients without obstruction of the proximal left anterior descending coronary artery, the reduction in mortality was confined to those with left main coronary artery or three-vessel disease. Patients were further stratified into high-, moderate-, and low-risk subgroups using criteria developed by the Veterans Administration Cooperative Study.[495] These were based upon clinical criteria, including the severity of angina, history of hypertension, prior myocardial infarction, and ST-segment depression at rest. Low-risk patients had none of the four risk factors aside from ST-segment depression, whereas those with two or three risk factors were considered to be at high risk. In patients at high risk, the mortality reduction was 29 per cent at 10 years versus 10 per cent in patients at moderate risk. In low-risk patients, there was a nonsignificant trend toward a greater mortality with bypass surgery.

The results of all the trials and registries[496] taken together indicate that the "sicker" the patient (based upon the se-

TABLE 38–12   EFFECTS OF CORONARY ARTERY BYPASS GRAFT SURGERY ON SURVIVAL*

SUBGROUP	MEDICAL TREATMENT MORTALITY RATE (%)	p FOR CABG SURGERY VS MEDICAL TREATMENT
Vessel disease		
One vessel	9.9	0.18
Two vessels	11.7	0.45
Three vessels	17.6	<0.001
Left main artery	36.5	0.004
No LAD disease		
One or two vessels	8.3	0.88
Three vessels	14.5	0.02
Left main artery	45.8	0.03
Overall	12.3	0.05
LAD disease present		
One or two vessels	14.6	0.05
Three vessels	19.1	0.009
Left main artery	32.7	0.02
Overall	18.3	0.001
LV function		
Normal	13.3	<0.001
Abnormal	25.2	0.02
Exercise test status		
Missing	17.4	0.10
Normal	11.6	0.38
Abnormal	16.8	<0.001
Severity of angina		
Class O, I, II	12.5	0.005
Class III, IV	22.4	0.001

* Systematic overview of coronary artery bypass graft surgery upon survival in comparison with medical therapy based on data from the 7 randomized trials comparing a strategy of initial coronary artery bypass graft surgery with one of initial medical therapy; illustrates subgroup results at 5 years.

From Yusuf, S., Zucker, D., Peduzzi, P., et al.: Effect of coronary artery bypass graft surgery on survival. Overview of 10 year results from randomized trials by the Coronary Artery Bypass Graft Surgery Trialists Collaboration, Lancet *344*:563, 1994.

verity of symptoms or ischemia, age, the number of vessels diseased, and the presence of left ventricular dysfunction), the greater the benefit of surgical over medical therapy on survival (Table 38–12; Fig. 38–17).[338] Among low-risk patients and patients with single-vessel disease, no trial has demonstrated any benefit upon survival.

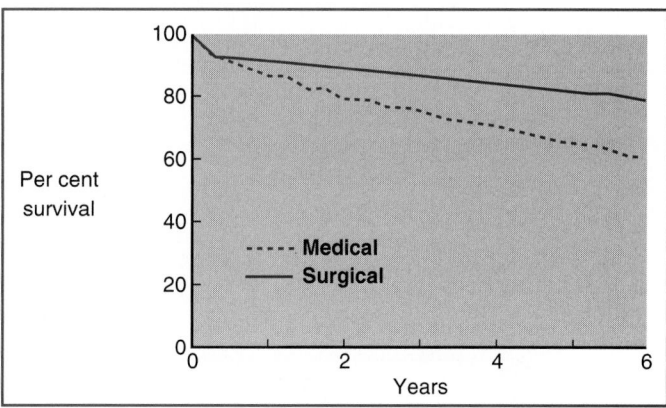

FIGURE 38–17. Cumulative 6-year survival rates in surgical and medical groups in the coronary artery surgery study (CASS) registry of 1491 patients 65 years or older. In addition to improved survival, at 5 years chest pain was absent in 62 per cent of the surgical group and 29 per cent of the medical group (*P* < 0.0001). Benefit of surgical treatment was greatest in the "high-risk" patients and was not observed in a subgroup at "low risk" who had mild angina, good ventricular function, and absence of left main CAD. (From Gersh, B. J., Kronmal, R. A., and Schaff, H. V.: Comparison of coronary artery bypass surgery and medical therapy in patients 65 years of age or older. N. Engl. J. Med. *313*:217, 1985. Copyright Massachusetts Medical Society.)

Thus, coronary bypass surgery prolongs survival in patients with significant left main coronary artery disease irrespective of symptoms, in patients with multivessel disease and impaired left ventricular function, and in patients with three-vessel disease that includes the proximal left anterior descending coronary artery (irrespective of left ventricular function).[448,490] Surgical therapy also has been demonstrated to prolong life in patients with *two-vessel disease* and left ventricular dysfunction, particularly in those with a critical stenosis of the proximal left anterior descending coronary artery. Although no study has documented a survival benefit with surgical treatment in patients with *single-vessel disease,* there is some evidence that such patients who have impaired left ventricular function have a poor long-term survival.[504] Such patients with angina and/or evidence of ischemia at a low or moderate level of exercise, especially those with obstruction of the proximal left anterior descending coronary artery, may benefit from coronary revascularization by either angioplasty or bypass surgery.

EFFECT OF SURGERY ON SUBSEQUENT MYOCARDIAL INFARCTION. The major randomized trials of patients with mild to moderate angina suggested that the likelihood of occurrence of myocardial infarction after 5 to 10 years of follow-up was similar in medically and surgically treated patients.[495–498,505,506] In the CASS, the reported annual risk of nonfatal Q wave myocardial infarction was 2.2 per cent per year with medical treatment compared with 2.8 per cent per year with surgical treatment.[506] However, in an observational study carried out in patients at higher risk for ischemic events (i.e., those with severe angina and three-vessel disease), a benefit of surgical treatment on the incidence of infarction was demonstrated.[507,508]

Patients with Depressed Left Ventricular Function

Over the last two decades, left ventricular dysfunction has changed from a relative contraindication to a strong indication for coronary revascularization.[509,510] Patients with impaired left ventricular function may demonstrate enhancement of left ventricular function and an improved long-term survival after coronary revascularization compared with medical treatment (Fig. 38–18).[511–514] Indeed, the most striking survival advantage as well as symptomatic and functional improvement is displayed by patients with the most impaired ventricular function in whom the prognosis with medical therapy is poor. In patients with a history of heart failure and three-vessel coronary artery disease, coronary bypass surgery may also reduce the incidence of sudden death.[514]

In one study which examined the late results of surgical and medical therapy for patients with CAD and resting left ventricular ejection fraction of 35 per cent or less, 7-year survival and freedom from nonfatal infarction were greater in the surgically than in the medically treated patients.[515] In other studies surgical treatment was shown to prolong survival in patients with ejection fractions of 25 per cent or less.[451] When these observations are taken together with the results of the Duke data base, it appears that if operative mortality is lower than approximately 7 per cent, surgery is likely to offer an advantage over medical therapy in patients with viable ischemic myocardium and severely depressed left ventricular function.[516]

However, congestive heart failure remains a powerful predictor of perioperative mortality and a poorer long-term outcome.[510,511] In the CASS registry, there was an increasing operative mortality with more severe degrees of left ventricular dysfunction[517] (Fig. 38–14). Patients with nor-

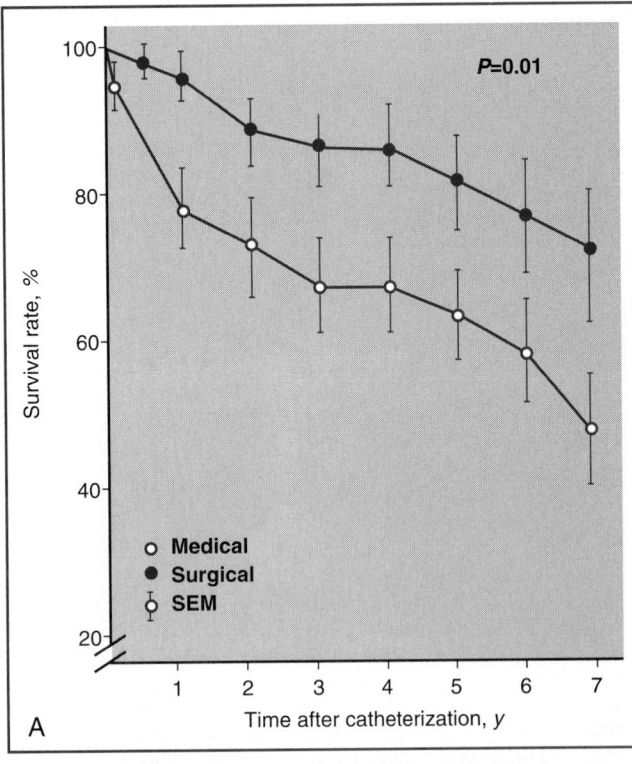

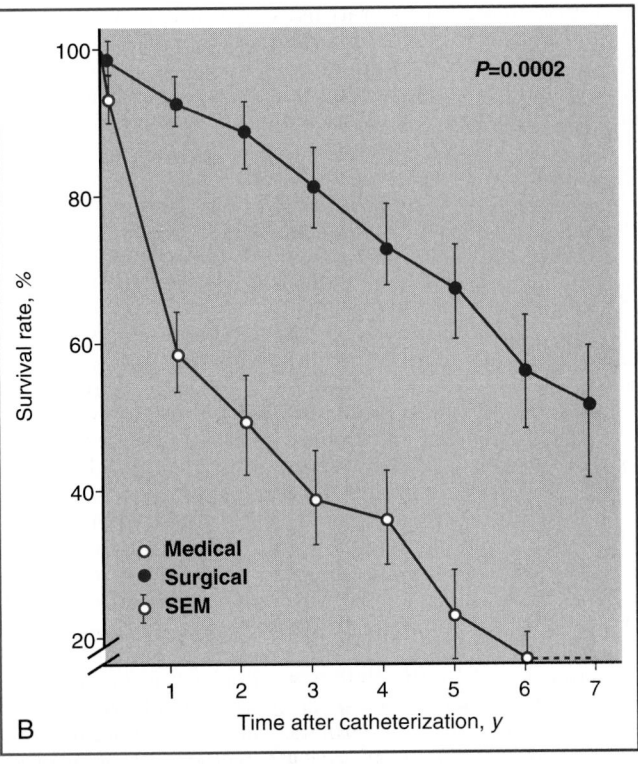

FIGURE 38–18. *A,* Cumulative survival of 47 patients treated surgically and 62 treated medically. All patients had an ejection fraction between 26 and 35 per cent. Seven-year survival rates were 73 and 50 per cent, respectively. *B,* Cumulative survival of 30 patients treated surgically and 53 treated medically. All patients had an ejection fraction of 25 per cent or less. Seven-year survival rates were 46 per cent and 15 per cent, respectively. (From Gersh, B. J.: Natural history of chronic coronary artery disease. *In* Beller, G. A. and Braunwald, E. [eds.]: Chronic Ischemic Heart Disease. Atlas of Heart Diseases, vol. 5. Philadelphia, Current Medicine, 1995, p. 1.16. Adapted from Piggott, J. D., et al.: Late results of surgical and medical therapy for patients with coronary artery disease and depressed left ventricular function. J. Am. Coll. Cardiol. *5:*1036, 1985.)

mal or nearly normal left ventricular function had an operative mortality rate of 2 per cent and a 5-year survival of 92 per cent. Patients with moderate impairment (ejection fraction 0.35 to 0.49) had an operative mortality of 4.2 per cent and a 5-year survival of 80 per cent, and in those with poor ventricular function (ejection fraction < 0.35) the operative mortality was 6.2 per cent and 5-year survival 65 per cent. More recent data on patients with an ejection fraction of 30 per cent or less demonstrated an in-hospital surgical mortality rate of 8.4 per cent.[511]

MYOCARDIAL HIBERNATION. Improvement in survival and left ventricular function following CABG depends on successful reperfusion of viable but noncontractile or poorly contracting "hibernating" myocardium (see p. 388 and 1215). Two related pathophysiological conditions, myocardial *stunning* (prolonged but temporary postischemic ventricular dysfunction without myocardial necrosis) and myocardial *hibernation* (persistent left ventricular dysfunction when myocardial perfusion is chronically reduced but sufficient to maintain the viability of tissue) have been described. The reduction in myocardial contractility in hibernating myocardium conserves metabolic demands and may be protective.

Hibernating myocardium can cause abnormal systolic and/or diastolic ventricular function.[518,519] The predominant clinical feature of myocardial ischemia in these patients may not be angina, but dyspnea secondary to elevation of left ventricular diastolic pressure. Symptoms resulting from chronic left ventricular dysfunction may be inappropriately ascribed to myocardial necrosis and scarring when the symptoms may, in fact, be reversed when the chronic ischemia is relieved by coronary revascularization.

DETECTION OF HIBERNATING MYOCARDIUM. A reduction in *diastolic* wall thickness of dysfunctional left ventricular segments is indicative of scarring. On the other hand, akinetic or dyskinetic segments with preserved diastolic wall thickness may represent a mixture of scarred and viable myocardium. Diastolic wall thickness and segmental function can be assessed by echocardiography, magnetic reso-

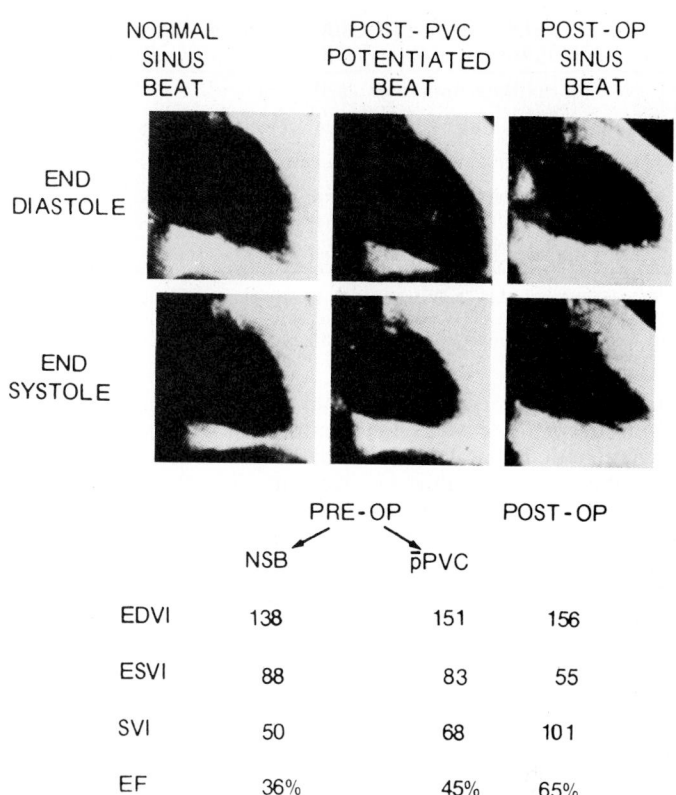

		PRE-OP	POST-OP
	NSB	p̄PVC	
EDVI	138	151	156
ESVI	88	83	55
SVI	50	68	101
EF	36%	45%	65%

FIGURE 38–20. Examples of the ventriculographic analysis performed to evaluate the effects of an inotropic stimulus, including some of the calculations made. p̄PVC = premature ventricular contraction; PRE-OP = preoperative; POST-OP = postoperative; NSB = normal sinus beat; p̄PVC = after premature ventricular contraction; EDVI = end-diastolic volume index (ml/m²); ESVI = end-systolic volume index (ml/m²); SVI = stroke volume index (ml/m²); EF = ejection fraction. (From Popio, K. A., et al.: Post extrasystolic potentiation as a predictor of potential myocardial viability. Am. J. Cardiol. *39*:944, 1977.)

nance imaging, fast computed tomography, and angiocardiography. A useful strategy for the assessment of dysfunctional segments has been developed by Maseri (Fig. 38–19).

The term *contractile reserve* is used to describe the ability of wall segments of hibernating myocardium to exhibit augmented contractility, often causing an improvement in global ejection fraction in response to a suitable stimulus (Fig. 38–20). The demonstration of contractile reserve and of improvement in contractility after revascularization results from the fact that many hypokinetic (and even akinetic) areas of the ventricular wall are composed entirely or in part of viable, hibernating myocardium or of a mixture of the latter and fibrous scar. The viable muscle is capable of responding to a sympathomimetic agent or postextrasystolic potentiation and its contractile state may also respond to improved perfusion after operation. In contrast, necrotic tissue obviously cannot be stimulated to contract by any pharmacological or hemodynamic intervention or by improved perfusion. In patients with poor left ventricular function and poor contractile reserve (< 10 per cent increase in ejection fraction with inotropic stimulation), perioperative mortality is high and long-term survival is poorer than in patients with equally depressed left ventricular function but normal contractile reserve.[137]

Positron emission tomography (PET) has evolved as the noninvasive "gold standard" for assessing viability, with a positive predictive value of 78 to 85 per cent and a negative predictive value of 78 to 92 per cent[520–522a] (Fig. 9–40, color plate 7). The high cost, technical difficulty, and need for a cyclotron limit this technique's widespread applicability. In 1991, a committee of the American Heart Association indicated that "201-thallium imaging may provide

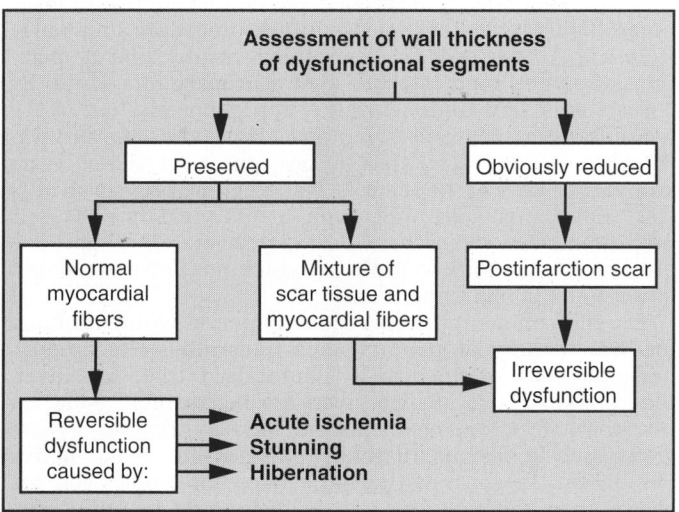

FIGURE 38–19. Flow diagram for the practical assessment of noncontractile segments of myocardial wall potentially recoverable by revascularization procedures. An obviously reduced wall thickness is indicative of postinfarction scar. The absence of contractile function in segments of the ventricular wall with preserved wall thickness may be caused by different mechanisms. An acute ischemic cause can be excluded by administration of sublingual nitrates. Stunning can be excluded by repeating the ventricular wall motion study several days after the last ischemic episode. Hibernating myocardium should be distinguished from a mixture of scar tissue and viable myocardial cells. (From Maseri, A.: Ischemic Heart Disease. New York, Churchill Livingstone, 1995, p. 642.)

TABLE 38–13 CRITERIA FOR DETERMINING MYOCARDIAL VIABILITY FROM THALLIUM SCANS

1. Normal thallium uptake on early scan
2. Complete thallium redistribution on delayed images
3. Defect fill-in following thallium reinjection
4. Partial redistribution of an initial defect on delayed images if defect cts > 50% peak counts
5. Mild fixed defect with defect cts > 50% peak cts

From Johnson, L. L.: Thallium-201 to assess myocardial viability. *In* Iskandrian, A. S., and van der Wall, E. E. (eds.): Myocardial Viability. Dordrecht, The Netherlands, Kluwer, 1994, pp. 19–37. cts = counts.

most of the clinical relevant data regarding viable myocardium in patients with left ventricular dysfunction'' and recommended that PET be used in patients in whom the identification of viable myocardium is a key issue that would change patient management in respect to revascularization. This was considered particularly appropriate if the results from thallium-201 scintigraphy performed were equivocal.[523]

In the last 5 years, there have been further refinements to thallium scintigraphic techniques, including reinjection, rest-redistribution imaging, and quantitative analysis.[524–526] (Fig. 9–1, p. 275; Table 38–13). These new developments have enhanced considerably the sensitivity and specificity for thallium in the prediction of viability in apparently "fixed" defects. New tracers, such as the radiolabeled long-chain fatty acid, 123-iodine-iodophenylpentadecanoic acid (IPPA), in conjunction with thallium SPECT and sestamibi imaging appear to be promising in the assessment of viability as well.[527]

Dobutamine echocardiography may also be useful in the detection of myocardial ischemia. Increasing doses of dobutamine, up to a maximum of 40 μg/kg/min, are used (see p. 1297). On the other hand, low-dose dobutamine (5 to 20 μg/kg/min)[528,528a] can provide information regarding *reversibility* of segmental dysfunction. In patients with chronic CAD, this has been shown to be a promising, easily accessible, and less costly alternative to PET in the prediction of recovery of left ventricular function after revascularization.[528,528a] Myocardial contrast echocardiography during cardiac catheterization is also a promising investigation technique for defining myocardial segments with poor left ventricular function, which are viable and amenable to improvement following revascularization.[529]

Surgical Treatment in Special Groups

WOMEN (see also Ch. 51). It is clear that there are marked differences in the utilization rates of coronary bypass surgery between men and women.[530,531] However, it is unclear whether these differences represent an overutilization in men or underutilization in women or both. Compared with men, women who undergo coronary bypass surgery are "sicker" as defined by age, comorbidity, the severity of angina, and history of congestive heart failure.[531]

Many series have demonstrated a higher morbidity and mortality in coronary surgery in women. The Society of Thoracic Surgeons data base provides a broad perspective of outcomes in the United States.[399] Mortality was almost double in women compared with men, 4.6 per cent and 2.8 per cent, respectively. Perioperative morbidity, including myocardial infarction, respiratory failure, and stroke, was also significantly higher in women. Most of these differences can be accounted for by the "sicker" preoperative status of women, the higher rate of nonelective procedures, and perhaps by the smaller coronary arteries. However, a small independent detrimental effect of female gender persists in most multivarate analyses.[532,533] Despite the increased perioperative mortality and morbidity in women, late survival is similar in men and women,[531,534,535] but the relief of anginal symptoms appears to be less in women.[536]

YOUNGER PATIENTS. Patients aged 35 or younger usually have hyperlipidemia and other major risk factors for CAD.[537] Despite the severity of the underlying disease and the rapidity of the atherosclerotic process, coronary bypass surgery is associated with excellent actuarial survival rates of 94 per cent at 5 years and 85 per cent at 10 years in these patients.[537] However, during longer follow-up, atherosclerosis of the venous grafts becomes an increasingly important problem in these patients,[538] which underlies the current trend to use bilateral IMA grafts and other arterial conduits in younger patients.

THE ELDERLY. The presence of CAD increases strikingly among the elderly, as does morbidity and mortality. In the United States, the utilization of noninvasive cardiovascular procedures in the elderly is extensive, and approximately half of all such procedures are performed in patients over the age of 65 years. Even though hospital mortality with CABG in the elderly has declined steadily,[538–540] age remains an important risk factor for mortality and morbidity and costs, although relief of angina is similar.[541,541a] The increase in perioperative mortality and morbidity in the elderly is, in part, due to diffuse atherosclerotic emboli (see p. 1696).[541b] Predictors of an adverse outcome include the presence and number of comorbid conditions and the presence of noncardiac vascular disease.

Evaluation of the elderly for coronary bypass surgery should take into account other less tangible factors related to quality of life and the potential ability to benefit from the operation. These include not only the chronological age of the patient, but also the estimated physiological age, comorbid conditions, the patient's attitude, including his/her understanding of the risks and expectations of the procedure, as well as an assessment of the patient's level of activity and current life style.

PATIENTS REQUIRING REOPERATION. At least 10 per cent of coronary artery procedures are now reoperations. This percentage is rising rapidly,[399,489,542] and in some centers exceeds 20 per cent. The indications for reoperation include progression of atherosclerosis in native vessels, incomplete revascularization at the time of the first operation, and both early and late graft failure.

Operative mortality rates for reoperations are two to three times higher than that of the initial procedure and range from 2 to 10 per cent.[543] The clinical results after reoperation are not as good as those after a primary procedure. By 5 years after reoperation surgery, approximately half of the patients have recurrent symptoms. However, late survival results are excellent, with a 90 per cent survival at 5 years and 75 per cent at 10 years.[544] Nonetheless, late survival is less than for patients undergoing a first procedure. This is understandable given the older age, severe CAD, and frequency of comorbid conditions, which comprise the population undergoing reoperation.[545]

The indications for reoperation compared with continued medical therapy or percutaneous transcatheter techniques have not been defined in a randomized trial. Moreover, they are subject to change given the increasingly wide application of percutaneous techniques to diseased bypass grafts and to lesions that have progressed in the native circulation. In general, the indications for reoperation are based upon the same principles that apply to initial disease, although the higher risk and poorer late outcome of reoperation than for initial operation need to be taken into account.

OTHER HIGH-RISK SUBGROUPS. Patients with *familial hyperlipidemia* have long been considered to be at particular risk for an adverse late outcome after coronary bypass surgery. More encouraging results have been reported after the use of an IMA or other arterial conduit, in conjunction with aggressive lipid-lowering therapy.[546] The risks of cardiac surgery in patients with *end-stage renal disease* are markedly increased. Nonetheless, the reported results (63 per cent cumulative survival over 5 years in patients with

NYHA class II-III symptoms) justify treating symptomatic patients on dialysis, but before the onset of severe congestive heart failure.[547] Elderly *diabetics* with angiographically proven coronary artery disease are more likely to be female, with evidence of peripheral vascular disease and a higher number of coronary occlusions compared with age-matched nondiabetic patients.[548] In a cohort of CASS registry patients, diabetes was an independent predictor of mortality. However, the relative survival benefit of coronary bypass surgery versus medical therapy was comparable in diabetic and nondiabetic patients, with a significant reduction in mortality of 44 per cent provided by surgery over medical therapy in the former.[548]

Summary of Indications for Coronary Revascularization

1. Certain anatomical subsets of patients are candidates for coronary bypass surgery, irrespective of the severity of symptoms or left ventricular dysfunction. These include patients with significant left main coronary artery disease and most patients with three-vessel disease, which includes the proximal left anterior descending coronary artery, especially those with left ventricular dysfunction.

2. The benefits of coronary bypass surgery are well documented in patients with left ventricular dysfunction and multivessel disease, irrespective of symptoms. In patients whose dominant symptom is heart failure without severe angina, the benefits of coronary revascularization are less well defined, but this approach should be considered in patients with evidence of significant contractile reserve.

3. The primary objective of coronary revascularization in patients with one-vessel disease is the relief of significant symptoms or objective evidence of severe ischemia. For the majority of these, PTCA is the revascularization modality of choice.

4. In patients with angina who are *not* considered to be at high risk, survival is similar in surgically and medically treated patients.

5. All of the indications discussed above relate to the potential benefits of surgery over medical therapy on *survival*. Coronary revascularization using angioplasty or bypass surgery is highly efficacious in relieving symptoms and may be considered for patients with moderate to severe ischemic symptoms who are dissatisfied with medical therapy, even if they are not in a high-risk subset. In such patients the optimal method of revascularization is selected on the basis of arteriographic findings.

OBSERVATIONAL STUDIES. Comparisons between angioplasty and coronary bypass surgery in patients with multivessel disease indicate that mortality and nonfatal myocardial infarction rates are similar between the two groups. The relief of angina is greater and the need for repeat revascularization is substantially lower after surgery. Among patients with left ventricular dysfunction, survival after surgery appears to be better than after angioplasty, probably because of the ability to achieve more complete revascularization with the former.[549] Indeed, complete revascularization is achieved by PTCA in only 25 to 50 percent of patients with two-vessel disease and in 10 to 25 per cent of patients with three-vessel disease.[342,343] In the future, improvements in transcatheter techniques, particularly in the ability to treat chronic total occlusions, may improve the results of this approach in patients with left ventricular dysfunction.

Outcome data 1 year after PTCA in patients (most of whom had single-vessel disease) indicate that approximately 20 per cent of patients undergo CABG; recurrence of symptoms and/or the need for repeat revascularization procedures is high (approximately 40 per cent). Bypass surgery provided a clear survival benefit over angioplasty in the Duke University data base in patients with severe two-vessel disease which included 95 per cent or greater obstruction of the proximal left anterior descending coronary artery and in all forms of three-vessel disease[338] (Fig. 38–21). On the other hand, the effect on survival of the methods of revascularization was equal in patients with two-vessel disease, without proximal left anterior descending coronary artery obstruction.

RANDOMIZED TRIALS. Four randomized trials comparing PTCA with coronary bypass surgery in patients with multivessel disease have been published[314,351,418,550–551c] and are described in Table 39–7, p. 1374. Two randomized trials have compared PTCA with CABG in patients confined to those with single-vessel disease, and the RITA trial included patients with single as well as multivessel disease.[337b,418,551b] An appreciation of the baseline characteristics of the patients entered into these trials is critical to the placement of these trials into a clinical context. Approximately two-thirds of the patients who were eligible clinically were excluded on angiographic grounds, including the presence of chronic total occlusions, complex stenoses, left main coronary artery disease, and the inability to achieve functionally adequate revascularization with angioplasty as well as by recent myocardial infarction and

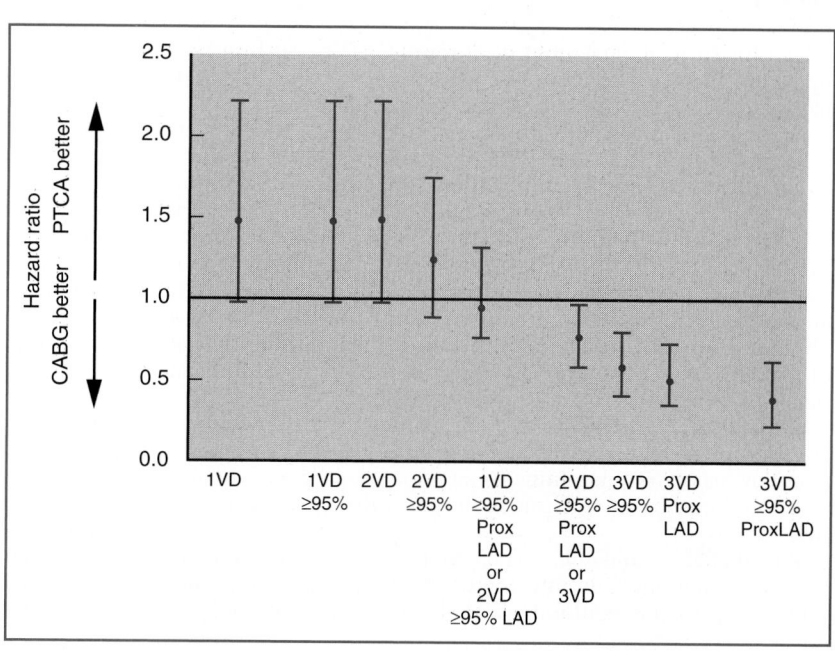

FIGURE 38–21. Hazard ratios for coronary artery bypass graft surgery (CABG) versus percutaneous transluminal coronary angioplasty (PTCA). Points below 1.0 favor CABG. VD = vessel disease; Prox LAD = proximal left anterior descending coronary artery. (Reproduced with permission from Mark, D. B., Nelson, C. L., Califf, R. M., et al.: Continuing evaluation of therapy for coronary artery disease: Initial results from the era of coronary angioplasty. Circulation *89*:2015, 1994. Copyright American Heart Association.)

previous revascularization. In the RITA and ERACI trials, the ability to achieve "equivalent" degrees of revascularization in the two groups was an inclusion criterion.[351,418] Moreover, the majority of patients entered into the trials had well-preserved left ventricular function with a mean ejection fraction exceeding 50 per cent. Patients with significant left ventricular dysfunction and multivessel disease were underrepresented in these trials.

The BARI trial (Bypass Angioplasty Revascularization Investigation), which was carried out in North America in patients with multivessel disease, is the largest of the randomized trials of coronary bypass surgery and PTCA and the only trial with sufficient statistical power to detect differences in mortality. Preliminary data demonstrate a significant difference in 5-year survival in favor of coronary bypass surgery in the approximately 300 diabetic patients receiving therapy for diabetes; no difference in mortality was noted among the remaining approximately 1500 patients (nondiabetics or diabetics not receiving treatment). It should be emphasized that these data are preliminary, but a recent meta-analysis of the randomized trials of CABG and PTCA in patients with multivessel disease (excluding the BARI data) demonstrated a trend toward an overall adverse outcome after hospital discharge in patients treated with PTCA.[314a]

Given the differences between the studies, it is reassuring that the results are remarkably consistent among the trials and with observational data.[551a] In this highly selected group of patients, after 1 to 3 years of follow-up, there were no significant differences in mortality or in the rate of myocardial infarction between patients treated with angioplasty and coronary bypass surgery.[551a] Moreover, as anticipated from observational data, the rate of subsequent revascularization procedures as well as the recurrence of angina were considerably higher in the angioplasty group.[551a] For example, in the EAST study, at 3 years only 13 per cent of patients in the CABG group required additional revascularization (surgery or angioplasty), compared with 54 per cent of the patients in the PTCA group.[351] Another consistent but predictable finding was the lower in-hospital cost in patients undergoing angioplasty. However, the need for recurrent hospitalizations and repeat revascularization procedures over the subsequent period of follow-up contributed to an increase in postdischarge costs in the angioplasty group[552,552a] and almost equal expenditures over a 3-year time span.

The Choice Between Coronary Angioplasty and Bypass Surgery
(Table 38–14)

The medical management of chronic CAD as outlined on pp. 1299 to 1313 involves the reduction of reversible risk factors, life style alterations counseling, the treatment of conditions that intensify angina, and the pharmacological management of ischemia. When an unacceptable level of angina persists, and/or the patient experiences troubling side effects from the anti-ischemic drugs, the coronary anatomy should be defined to allow selection of the appropriate technique for revascularization. In patients in whom the angina is controlled, noninvasive testing is carried out and coronary arteriography is carried out in those having a "high-risk" result (see p. 1297). Following the elucidation of the coronary anatomy, the selection of the technique of revascularization is made as follows:

SINGLE-VESSEL DISEASE. Among patients with single-vessel disease in whom revascularization is deemed necessary and the lesion is anatomically suitable, angioplasty or another catheter-based technique is generally preferred over bypass surgery.

MULTIVESSEL DISEASE. The first step is to decide whether a patient falls into the category of those who were included into the randomized trials comparing angioplasty

TABLE 38–14 COMPARISON OF REVASCULARIZATION STRATEGIES IN MULTIVESSEL DISEASE

	ADVANTAGES	DISADVANTAGES
PTCA	Less invasive	Restenosis
	Shorter hospital stay	High incidence of incomplete revascularization
	Lower initial cost	Relative inefficacy in patients with severe LV dysfunction
	Easily repeated	Uncertain long-term outcome (> 10 y)
	Effective in relieving symptoms	Limited to specific anatomic subsets
CABG	Effective in relieving symptoms	Cost
	Improved survival in certain subsets	Increased risk of a repeat procedure due to late graft closure
	Ability to achieve complete revascularization	
	Wider applicability	Morbidity

Modified from Faxon, D. P.: Coronary angioplasty for stable angina pectoris. In Beller, G. and Braunwald, E. (eds.): Chronic Ischemic Heart Disease. Atlas of Heart Diseases, vol. 5. Philadelphia, Current Medicine, 1995.

and bypass surgery. Patients were included in the trials only if it was believed that equivalent degrees of revascularization were achieved by both techniques and most patients with occluded coronary arteries were excluded. The majority of patients had double-vessel disease and well-preserved left ventricular function.[551a] The lack of any difference in late mortality and in myocardial infarction between the two groups in such patients indicates that angioplasty is a reasonable *initial* strategy, provided that the patient accepts the distinct possibility of symptom recurrence and need for a repeat revascularization procedure. Patients with a single, localized lesion in each affected vessel and preserved left ventricular function fare best with angioplasty. The BARI trial results in diabetics raise additional questions in this subgroup of patients, but further analyses are needed before definitive conclusions can be drawn.[314a]

NEED FOR COMPLETE REVASCULARIZATION. Complete revascularization is an important goal in patients with left ventricular dysfunction and/or multivessel disease. The major advantage of bypass surgery over PTCA is the ability to achieve complete revascularization, particularly in patients with three-vessel disease. In the majority of such patients, particularly those with chronic total coronary occlusion, left ventricular dysfunction, or left main coronary artery disease, coronary bypass surgery is the procedure of choice.[312] Among patients with borderline left ventricular function (ejection fraction between 45 per cent and 50 per cent) and milder degrees of ischemia, PTCA may provide adequate revascularization, even if it is not anatomically complete.

Many patients fall into a gray zone in which either method of revascularization is suitable. Other factors that come into consideration include (1) access to a high quality team and operator with an excellent record of success; (2) patient preference; some patients are made anxious by the idea that following angioplasty they are at high risk of symptom recurrence and may require reintervention. Such patients are better candidates for surgical treatment; (3) patient's age and comorbidity; frail, very elderly patients and those with comorbid conditions, such as cancer or serious hepatic disease with a limited life span, who have disabling angina are often better candidates for angioplasty; (4) angioplasty is often preferable in younger patients (< 50 years) with the expectation that they may require surgery some time in the future and that angioplasty will postpone the need for operation; this sequence may be preferable to two operations.

Coronary Bypass Surgery in Patients with Associated Vascular Disease

The management of patients with combined CAD and peripheral vascular disease, involving the carotid arteries, the abdominal aorta, or the vessels of the lower extremities, presents many challenges.[553] Combined disease is becoming increasingly important as the population of patients under consideration for CABG ages and as technical improvements allow the application of coronary revascularization to ever more complex cases.

IMPACT OF CAD IN PATIENTS WITH PERIPHERAL VASCULAR DISEASE. Clinically apparent CAD occurs frequently in patients with peripheral vascular disease.[31] The prevalence of clinically unrecognized CAD, as documented by angiographic studies, is even higher.[553] Among patients undergoing peripheral vascular surgery, the late outcomes are dominated by cardiac causes of morbidity and mortality.[553-555] Conversely, in patients with CAD the presence of peripheral vascular disease, even if it is asymptomatic, is associated with an adverse prognosis.[556]

If coronary revascularization is performed prior to the vascular surgery in patients with combined peripheral vascular and CAD, the perioperative mortality of the vascular procedure is reduced.[31,557] In seven series totaling 1237 patients undergoing vascular surgical procedures, the mean operative mortality was 1.5 per cent among patients with prior coronary bypass surgery, similar to the 1.3 per cent mortality rate in patients without clinically apparent CAD, and substantially lower than the 6.8 per cent mortality rate in patients with clinically suspected but uncorrected CAD.[31] Late mortality in patients with peripheral vascular disease is also reduced among those who have undergone prior coronary bypass surgery.[558,559] However, because patients with CAD with peripheral atherosclerosis tend to be older and to have more widespread vascular disease and end-organ damage than patients without peripheral atherosclerosis, the perioperative mortality and morbidity consequent to CABG are high and the late outcome not as favorable.[31,540,541,560] Diffuse *atheroembolism* (see p. 1320) is a particularly serious complication of coronary bypass surgery in patients with peripheral vascular disease and aortic atherosclerosis.[541] It is a major cause of perioperative death, stroke, neurocognitive dysfunction, and multiple organ dysfunction after bypass surgery.

It is important to identify CAD and to estimate its severity in patients who are candidates for peripheral vascular surgery. The diagnostic problem is intensified by the fact that these patients often have limited walking capacity and therefore may not develop effort angina. Pharmacological stress myocardial perfusion scintigraphy or echocardiography can be employed. The identification of "high risk" patients using these techniques (see p. 1297) should lead to coronary angiography and, depending on the anatomic findings, to coronary revascularization, often prior to peripheral vascular surgery.

Thus, the presence of peripheral vascular disease suggests that the patient may also have high-risk CAD, with potential benefit from bypass surgery in the long term. In the ECSS, patients with CAD and peripheral vascular disease treated surgically had a much better survival than did medically treated patients.[498] In the CASS registry, patients with peripheral vascular disease and three-vessel CAD who received surgical treatment also exhibited a major reduction in late mortality and morbidity compared with those who managed medically.[31] Observations such as these argue for consideration of coronary revascularization in patients with peripheral vascular disease who have significant CAD. The major indication for coronary revascularization prior to vascular surgery in patients with known chronic coronary artery disease is the intention of improving *long-term* prognosis as opposed to perioperative outcomes alone, because the latter have markedly improved in the current era of sophisticated pre- and perioperative care.[31]

CAROTID ARTERY DISEASE (see also p. 1879). In patients with stable CAD and *carotid artery disease* in whom endarterectomy is planned, exercise stress testing and consideration of coronary revascularization can ordinarily be performed postoperatively.[31] Although the presence of asymptomatic carotid bruits increases the risk of stroke after coronary bypass surgery,[561] there is little to suggest that prophylactic carotid endarterectomy reduces the risk of perioperative stroke in such patients.[562,563]

MANAGEMENT. Patients with severe or unstable coronary disease can be categorized into two groups according to the severity and instability of the accompanying vascular disease.[31] When the noncoronary vascular procedures are elective, they can generally be postponed until the cardiac symptoms have stabilized, either by intensive medical therapy or by revascularization. A combined procedure is necessary in patients with both unstable CAD and an unstable vascular condition, e.g., frequent recurrent transient ischemic attacks or a rapidly expanding abdominal aortic aneurysm.[562,564,565] In some patients in this category, PTCA offers the potential for stabilizing the patient from a cardiac standpoint, prior to proceeding with a definitive vascular repair.[566]

UNSTABLE ANGINA

Coronary artery disease represents a spectrum of conditions, with acute transmural infarction at one end of the spectrum, ranging successively through nontransmural infarction, unstable angina, and chronic stable angina, to silent ischemia at the other. Unstable angina (previously also known as preinfarction angina, crescendo angina, acute coronary insufficiency, and intermediate coronary syndrome) is at the center of this spectrum. This condition is frightening and disabling in nature and may herald acute myocardial infarction. In 1991, the US National Center for Health Statistics reported 570,000 hospitalizations carrying a diagnosis of unstable angina, resulting in 3.1 million hospital days, making it one of the most common serious cardiovascular disorders.[567]

DEFINITION. In addition to the absence of clear-cut electrocardiographic and cardiac enzyme changes diagnostic of a myocardial infarction, the currently used definition of unstable angina pectoris depends on the presence of one or more of the following three historical features: (1) crescendo angina (more severe, prolonged, or frequent) superimposed on a preexisting pattern or relatively stable, exertion-related angina pectoris; (2) angina pectoris of new onset (usually within 1 month), which is brought on by minimal exertion; or (3) angina pectoris at rest as well as with minimal exertion. In some patients, the ischemic episode of unstable angina pectoris can be related to obvious precipitating factors, such as anemia, infection, thyrotoxicosis, or cardiac arrhythmias, and the condition is then called *secondary unstable angina*.[568] Prinzmetal's ("variant") angina is also characterized by angina at rest and may be considered to be a form of unstable angina, but it is pathogenetically distinct and is discussed on p. 1340.

CLASSIFICATION. The syndrome of unstable angina describes a broad population of patients.[568a] They may be patients with single-vessel or multivessel coronary artery disease; a minority have no critically severe obstruction on coronary arteriography. They may or may not have a history of prior myocardial infarction or chronic angina, may have unstable angina while receiving no medical therapy, or may be suffering severe, transient episodes of ischemia despite a combination of medications including full doses of nitrates, calcium antagonists, beta blockers, aspirin, and intravenous heparin.

To categorize this heterogeneous population, one of the authors of this chapter proposed a classification that focuses on three important issues[568] (Table 38–15): (1) the severity of the clinical manifestations, (2) the clinical circumstances in which the unstable angina occurs, and (3) whether or not the symptomatic ischemic episodes are accompanied by transient electrocardiographic changes. This classification notes whether or not rest pain is present, whether rest pain has occurred within the preceding 48 hours, and whether the unstable angina is provoked by conditions such as anemia, fever, infection, and tachyarrhythmias. It is also proposed that the amount of therapy administered be taken into account.[568a]

Severity of Unstable Angina. The severity is graded according to whether or not rest pain has occurred and, if so, its timing. Class I is defined as the onset of severe, accelerated angina, occurring within 2 months of presentation, *without* rest pain. Also included in this class are patients with chronic stable angina who have developed angina that is distinctly more frequent, severe, longer in duration, or precipitated by substantially less exertion than previously. Class II refers to patients with a history of rest angina during the preceding 2 months, but not the preceding 48 hours. Class III refers to patients who have experienced one or more episodes of angina at rest within the preceding 48 hours.

In contrast to unstable angina, Class I, chronic exertional angina is by definition stable, and although it may have developed recently, it is not severe or frequent, as defined above. Angina that is severe and/or frequent and remains unchanged for more than 2 months is also *not* considered to be unstable. Patients with prolonged (> 30 min) chest discomfort accompanied by ST-segment *elevation* are *not* considered to have unstable angina.

Clinical Circumstances in Which Unstable Angina Occurs. Unstable angina is also classified according to the clinical circumstances in which it occurs. Class A (secondary unstable angina) refers to patients, usually with underlying obstructive CAD, in whom the imbalance between myocardial oxygen supply and demand causing the instability results from conditions that are *extrinsic* to the coronary vascular bed. This includes patients in whom reductions of myocardial oxygen supply result from anemia or hypoxemia, while increases in myocardial oxygen demand which precipitate unstable angina may be caused by such conditions as fever, infection, uncontrolled hypertension, aortic stenosis, tachyarrhythmia, unusual emotional stress, and thyrotoxicosis. Class B (primary unstable angina) occurs in the *absence* of an identifiable extracoronary condition responsible for intensifying ischemia and in patients who have not suffered a myocardial infarction within the preceding 2 weeks. This is the most common form of unstable angina and includes a large majority of patients with underlying coronary atherosclerosis and an unstable plaque that has caused subtotal coronary occlusion. Class C (postinfarction unstable angina) is present in patients who develop unstable angina within 2 weeks of a documented acute myocardial infarction; it occurs in approximately 20 per cent of patients following infarction.

This is a clinical classification, which can be related to underlying disease. For example, Class III patients (with recent rest angina) are more likely to have intracoronary thrombus, and heparin may be of greater value in such patients than in patients in Classes I and II. A clinical score based upon this classification is an important predictor of intracoronary thrombus and lesion complexity.[569] Two prospective studies of patients admitted for suspected unstable angina demonstrated that this classification is an appropriate instrument to predict survival, infarct-free survival, and infarct free-survival without intervention.[570,571]

Pathophysiology

As already pointed out, the majority of patients with unstable angina have severe obstructive CAD, and episodes of myocardial ischemia can be precipitated by either an increase in myocardial oxygen demands and/or a reduction in supply.[572] Episodes of spontaneous (rest) angina can be preceded by a reduction of myocardial oxygen supply due to a further reduction in lumen diameter consequent to transient vasoconstrictor influences, and/or platelet thrombi (Fig 38–1C). Elevations of arterial pressure and/or tachycardia, which lead to increases in myocardial oxygen requirements, can also provoke episodes of unstable angina.

In many patients with unstable angina and episodes of rest pain who are continuously monitored, an interesting sequence of events has been demonstrated. First, there is a reduction of coronary sinus oxygen saturation (which, in the presence of constant myocardial oxygen needs, signifies a reduction of coronary blood flow). This is followed by ST-segment depression, and only then does chest discomfort appear. Blood pressure and/or heart rate may rise secondary to the latter.[573] Thus, in many patients with unstable angina, ischemia appears to be precipitated by a reduction in oxygen supply, rather than an increase in oxygen demand, the latter being the most common precipitant of chronic stable angina. It is also likely that in some episodes of unstable angina an increase in myocardial oxygen demand and a reduction in supply occur simultaneously. In a patient with critical coronary obstruction, a mild increase in myocardial oxygen demand and a small reduction in supply could act in concert to produce critical ischemia and unstable angina. Such a sequence could explain the

TABLE 38–15   CLASSIFICATION OF UNSTABLE ANGINA

SEVERITY	
Class I	New-onset, severe, or accelerated angina. Patients with angina of less than 2 months' duration, severe or occurring three or more times per day, or angina that is distinctly more frequent and precipitated by distinctly less exertion. No rest pain in the last 2 months.
Class II	Angina at rest. Subacute. Patients with one or more episodes of angina at rest during the preceding month but not within the preceding 48 hours.
Class III	Angina at rest. Acute. Patients with one or more episodes at rest within the preceding 48 hours.
CLINICAL CIRCUMSTANCES	
Class A	Secondary unstable angina. A clearly identified condition extrinsic to the coronary vascular bed that has intensified myocardial ischemia, e.g., anemia, infection, fever, hypotension, tachyarrhythmia, thyrotoxicosis, hypoxemia secondary to respiratory failure.
Class B	Primary unstable angina.
Class C	Postinfarction unstable angina (within 2 weeks of documented myocardial infarction).
INTENSITY OF TREATMENT	
1. Absence of treatment or minimal treatment.	
2. Occurring in presence of standard therapy for chronic stable angina (conventional doses of oral beta blockers, nitrates, and calcium antagonists).	
3. Occurring despite maximally tolerated doses of all three categories of oral therapy, including intravenous nitroglycerin.	

From Braunwald, E.: Unstable angina: A classification. Circulation *80*:410, 1989. Copyright 1989 American Heart Association.

circadian variation in the distribution of ischemic events in patients with unstable angina in which patients with a low coronary reserve exhibited a higher incidence of severe ischemia in the morning.[208a,574]

Evidence indicates that the development of unstable angina may be preceded by marked recent progression in the extent and severity of CAD.[575,575a] Other important mechanisms contributing to the reduction of oxygen supply, and therefore to the precipitation of ischemic episodes in patients with unstable angina with severe underlying obstructive CAD, include the platelet aggregation, thrombosis, and coronary vasoconstriction, which are discussed below.

PLATELET AGGREGATION. There is substantial evidence to support the role of platelet aggregation either as a primary phenomenon or secondary to plaque rupture or fissure in the precipitation of ischemic episodes in patients with unstable angina as well as myocardial infarction (Fig. 37–7, p. 1188). It is likely that other factors may also be operative, such as increases in sympathetic vascular tone, elevated circulating catecholamine levels, hypercholesterolemia, leukocyte activation,[575b] and impaired fibrinolysis. These may be manifested by increased serum concentrations of plasminogen activator inhibitor type-I, (PAI-1) in addition to the activation of alpha$_2$-adrenergic and serotonergic platelet receptors, which may promote platelet aggregation.[576–578]

Platelets and the coronary vascular endothelium interact in a complex manner; platelets produce thromboxane A$_2$, a proaggregatory and vasoconstrictor substance (see p. 1165), whereas the normal endothelium produces the antiaggregatory vasodilator prostacyclin (prostaglandin I$_2$), as well as tissue plasminogen activator (t-PA) and endothelium-derived relaxing factor (see p. 1164). It has been speculated that the abrupt conversion from chronic stable angina to unstable angina may result from the more intense myocardial ischemia initiated by platelet aggregation,[578] from coronary vasoconstriction resulting from the local accumulation of thromboxane A$_2$ and serotonin, and also from reductions in the local concentrations of endothelially derived vasodilators and inhibitors of platelet aggregation.[579]

In patients with unstable angina who have had pain within the preceding 24 hours, the finding of elevated metabolites of thromboxane A$_2$ derived from aggregating platelets in plasma and urine suggests that local release of thromboxane may be associated with the episodes of unstable angina.[578] The reductions in coronary blood flow in canine preparations with marked coronary obstruction appear to be abolished by platelet inhibitors, including aspirin, sulfinpyrazone, prostacyclin, ibuprofen, and indomethacin but *not* by heparin, nitroglycerin, or papaverine.[580] This finding suggests that these reductions are mediated by platelet aggregation rather than by vasospasm or fibrin deposition. Furthermore, four separate clinical trials have now shown that aspirin can protect against death and nonfatal acute myocardial infarction in patients with unstable angina[581–584] (p. 1829). The beneficial impact of a GP-IIb/IIIa platelet receptor blocker (see p. 1629), which is a potent inhibitor of platelet aggregation, upon recurrent ischemic events in patients with unstable angina, provides further evidence in support of a major role of platelet aggregation in the pathophysiology of unstable angina.[585,586] Finally, in patients with unstable angina who suffer sudden death, aggregates of platelet emboli have been found in small intramyocardial vessels in segments of myocardium immediately downstream from a major epicardial coronary artery containing an atheromatous plaque that has undergone fissuring and on which mural thrombus had developed.[587]

THROMBOSIS. In addition to platelet aggregation, the presence of an active thrombotic process in patients with unstable angina is suggested by increased serum concentrations of fibrin-related antigen and D-dimer (the principal breakdown fragment of fibrin), tissue plasminogen activator and tissue plasminogen activator inhibitor-I,[588,589] pro-

thrombin fragment 1+2, and fibrinopeptide-A.[590,591] These changes do not occur in patients with chronic stable angina and suggest that a hypercoagulable state is not just a marker of the acute thrombotic episode, but persists after clinical stabilization.[590] In patients with unstable angina pectoris, intracoronary thrombus formation is associated with a hypercoagulable state in association with diminished fibrinolytic activity.[592] Several studies in patients with unstable angina have shown intracoronary filling defects having the appearance of thrombi at angiography[593,594] (Fig. 38–22), and this finding has been confirmed by coronary angioscopy.[595,596] Furthermore, when thrombolytic therapy is administered to patients with unstable angina and recent pain, dissolution of intracoronary filling defects has been observed.[593,594,597] Finally, postmortem observations in many patients with unstable angina have suggested an ongoing thrombotic process in a major coronary artery. This process may accumulate in total occlusion, which is responsible for infarction and/or sudden death.[598]

CORONARY CONSTRICTION. Quantitative angiography has shown vasomotor hyperreactivity localized to regions of preexisting coronary atheroma in patients with unstable angina.[599] Postmortem studies have shown that in the majority of significantly diseased coronary arteries a portion of the circumference is circumscribed by normal arterial walls.[600] Therefore, it is likely that a normal pliable muscular elastic arc of vessel wall provides a mechanism whereby normal (vasoconstriction) or abnormally intense (vasospasm) increases in vasomotor tone may narrow lumen caliber and thus flow resistance.[601]

Endothelial dysfunction may lead to vasoconstriction by promoting the release of physiological mediators of vasoconstriction such as endothelin-I, or by inhibiting the release of vasodilator substances, such as prostacyclin and endothelium-derived relaxing factor (see p. 1164).[602,603] Endothelial dysfunction may also impair fibrinolysis in the acute ischemic syndromes because functioning endothe-

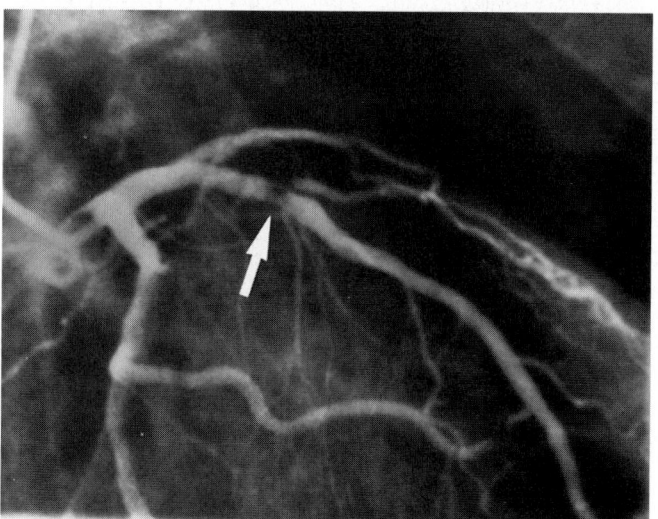

FIGURE 38–22. Coronary artery thrombus in a patient with unstable angina. A 60-year-old man was admitted to the hospital with a history of crescendo angina and prolonged rest pain. He had electrocardiographic T-wave inversions in leads V$_2$-V$_5$, I, aV$_L$ and no abnormalities of serial cardiac enzymes. After 72 hours of hospital treatment with aspirin, heparin, and beta blocker therapy he had a further episode of rest pain associated with 5- to 8-mm anterior ST-segment elevations. Coronary angiography was performed, and the left coronary artery (right anterior oblique caudal projection) is shown. In the left anterior descending coronary artery, at the level of the second diagonal branch, an irregular hazy filling defect is present (arrow). It is surrounded by angiographic contrast medium and extends into the diagonal branch itself. After 4 further days of heparin and antianginal therapy, a repeat coronary angiogram was obtained, and the size of the intracoronary filling defect had decreased, confirming that it was a coronary thrombus.

lium is required to secrete and bind tissue plasminogen activator and plasminogen. Thromboxane A_2, which is released and synthesized by aggregating platelets, is a powerful local vasoconstrictor.[604]

It is likely that progression of atherosclerosis, platelet aggregation, thrombus formation, and changes in vasomotor tone may operate either alone or together at different times in individual patients to produce unstable angina. Alterations in coronary artery tone at the site of plaques may initiate and/or be exacerbated by local formation of platelet thrombi with resulting ischemia. In addition, growth factors, in particular fibroblast growth factor, may be involved in the transformation from stable to unstable angina by causing enhanced smooth muscle proliferation in preexisting atherosclerotic lesions.[605] Thus, unstable angina is a complex, dynamic syndrome that perhaps is often a precursor of myocardial infarction; both conditions share a common patholophysiological link.

Clinical and Laboratory Findings

SYMPTOMS. The chest discomfort in unstable angina is similar in *quality* to that of classic effort-induced angina, although it is often more intense, is usually described as pain, may persist for as long as 30 minutes, and occasionally awakens the patient from sleep.[606] Several clues should alert the physician to a changing pattern of angina and the development of unstable angina. These include an abrupt and persistent reduction in the threshold of physical activity that provokes angina; an increase in the frequency, severity, and duration of angina; the development of rest angina or nocturnal angina, radiation of the discomfort to an additional or new site; and the onset of new associated features such as diaphoresis, nausea, vomiting, palpitation, or dyspnea. The usual regimen of rest and sublingual nitroglycerin administration which controls chronic stable angina, often provides only temporary or incomplete relief in unstable angina.

PHYSICAL EXAMINATION. This may reveal transient diastolic (third and fourth) heart sounds and a dyskinetic apical impulse suggesting left ventricular dysfunction, or a transient systolic murmur of mitral regurgitation during or immediately after an ischemic episode. These findings are nonspecific, because they may also be present in patients with chronic stable angina or acute myocardial infarction. Nonetheless, physical examination may provide important clues to adverse prognosis based upon evidence of acute congestive heart failure or systemic hypotension during an episode of pain.

ELECTROCARDIOGRAM. Transient ST-segment deviations (depression or elevation) and/or T-wave inversions occur commonly, but not universally, in unstable angina. Dynamic shifts in the ST-segment (≥ 1 mm of ST-depression or elevation) or T-wave inversions that resolve at least partially when symptoms are relieved, are important markers of an adverse prognosis, i.e., subsequent acute myocardial infarction or death.[606,607] An unusual, subtle electrocardiographic manifestation of unstable angina is the presence of transient, inverted U waves.[608] Patients with ST changes in the anteroseptal leads, often associated with significant stenosis of the left anterior descending coronary artery, appear to be a particularly high-risk group (Fig. 38–23).[609] The diagnostic accuracy of an abnormal electrocardiogram is enhanced if a prior tracing is available for comparison.[610]

Usually these electrocardiographic changes clear completely or partially with the relief of pain. Persistence for more than 12 hours may suggest that a non–Q-wave infarction has occurred.

If patients have a typical history of chronic stable angina pectoris or established CAD (previous myocardial infarction, abnormal coronary arteriogram, or a history of a positive noninvasive stress test), the diagnosis of unstable angina may be based on clinical symptoms even in the absence of electrocardiographic changes. It is in the subgroup of patients without evidence of previous CAD and no electrocardiographic changes associated with pain that the diagnosis may be inaccurate.

CONTINUOUS ELECTROCARDIOGRAPHIC MONITORING. Ischemic chest pain is not a reliable or sensitive marker of transient acute myocardial ischemia. Episodes of primary reduction in coronary blood flow may be associated with variable and minor electrocardiographic changes that precede symptoms of pain or discomfort.[573] Investigations using continuous electrocardiographic monitoring, which were conducted before the widespread use of aspirin and heparin, documented that up to 60 per cent of patients with unstable angina experienced asymptomatic episodes of ST-segment depression.[611] More recent studies on patients treated with aspirin and heparin have demonstrated that the incidence of transient ST-segment deviation has decreased to between 5 and 20 per cent. More than 85 to 90 per cent of the ischemic episodes detected by Holter monitoring techniques are not associated with chest pain.[612] Furthermore, the presence of ischemia, detected by Holter monitoring, serves as a predictor of unfavorable outcome during hospital admission[613] and follow-up.[561,612] Asymptomatic ischemic electrocardiographic changes are frequently accompanied by transient reductions in myocar-

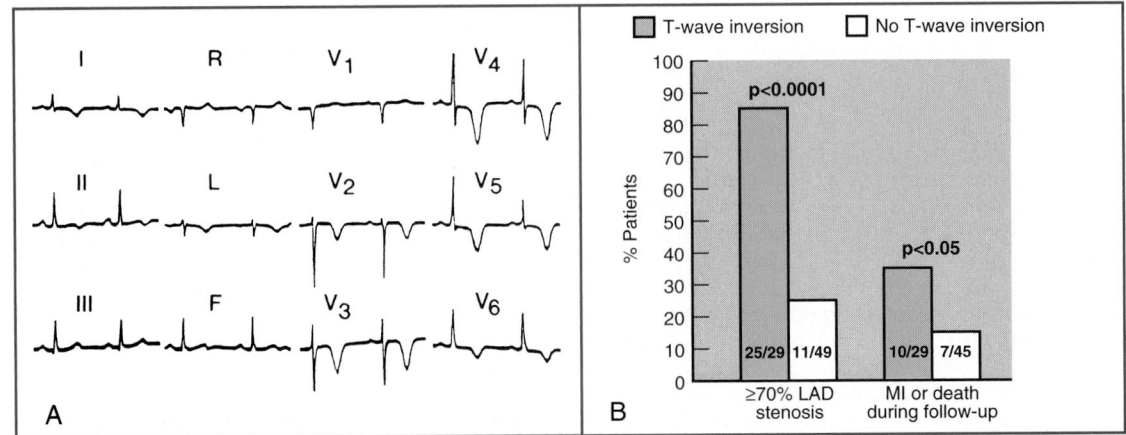

FIGURE 38–23. Unstable angina. *A,* Symmetrical anterior T-wave inversion with isoelectric ST segment frequently associated with critical stenosis of the left anterior descending coronary artery. *B,* Prevalence of significant stenosis of the left anterior descending coronary artery (LAD) and the incidence of cardiac events in patients with and without new T-wave inversion. MI = myocardial infarction. (From Haines, D. E., Raabe, D. S., Gundel, W., and Wackers, F. J.: Anatomic and prognostic significance of new T-wave inversion in unstable angina. Am. J. Cardiol. *52:*14, 1983.)

dial perfusion and abnormalities of ventricular function.[614] More evidence is needed to determine the prognostic significance not only of silent ischemia but of the "total ischemic burden" based upon ambulatory or continuous electrocardiographic monitoring in patients with unstable angina pectoris.[615]

OTHER LABORATORY TESTS. Findings on chest roentgenogram, serum cholesterol level, and carbohydrate tolerance are similar to those observed in patients with chronic stable angina (see p. 1295). Unlike acute myocardial infarction, nonspecific indicators of tissue necrosis, such as leukocytosis and fever, are usually absent. Cardiac enzymes are not abnormally elevated; when cardiac specific enzymes are elevated, by definition the diagnosis is acute myocardial infarction and not unstable angina.

Cardiac troponin-T is a regulatory protein that is a specific marker of myocardial cell injury (see p. 407). In patients with unstable angina, it appears to be a more sensitive indicator of myocardial cell injury than is serum creatine kinase MB activity.[117] Recent evidence suggests a relationship between unstable angina (and other acute ischemic syndromes) and markers of an active inflammatory response. Two circulating acute-phase reactants, C-reactive protein and serum amyloid-A protein, which are sensitive indicators of inflammation, have been shown to be elevated in patients with unstable angina even when creatine kinase and cardiac troponin-T levels were normal, and these proteins are markers of an adverse prognosis.[616]

Coronary Anatomy

CORONARY ARTERIOGRAPHIC FINDINGS. These vary according to the population under study and are dependent upon the patient's history and mode of presentation.[617,618,618a] Patients in whom unstable angina is superimposed on longstanding, stable angina often have multivessel disease, whereas patients with new onset of rest pain may have disease involving only a single coronary artery. Among all patients with unstable angina, three-vessel disease is found in approximately 40 per cent, two-vessel disease in 20 per cent, left main coronary artery disease in approximately 20 per cent, single-vessel disease in about 10 per cent, and no critical obstruction in the remaining 10 per cent. In contrast, in patients in whom unstable angina is the *initial* presentation of CAD (approximately half of all patients with unstable angina), the distribution of CAD is different in that approximately 50 per cent have single-vessel disease (the majority with left anterior descending coronary artery involvement), and less than 20 per cent have three-vessel disease.[619,620]

Among the subset of patients with unstable angina with normal coronary arteriograms or nonobstructive disease are some in whom the diagnosis of angina pectoris is probably incorrect. In the remainder, coronary spasm, the spontaneous lysis of a coronary thrombus, abnormalities of the microvascular circulation, or the presence of a lesion overlooked on coronary arteriography may be responsible. Fourteen per cent of patients with unstable angina enrolled into the TIMI IIIA trial had no luminal diameter stenosis of a major coronary artery of 60 per cent or greater on the baseline arteriogram. In half of these, no visually detectable coronary stenosis was noted. Nearly one-third of the patients without critical coronary stenoses had impaired angiographic filling, suggesting a pathophysiological role for coronary microvascular dysfunction.[621] The short-term prognosis in patients with unstable angina and no critical obstruction of an epicardial coronary artery is excellent.

Postmortem angiograms, histological examinations, and coronary arteriograms typically display eccentric stenoses with scalloped or overhanging edges more frequently in patients with unstable angina than in patients with chronic stable angina (see p. 256).[622] In contrast, lesions with concentric, symmetrical narrowing or asymmetrical narrow-

ing with smooth borders and a broad neck are more common in patients with stable angina. Acute progression had occurred from a previously insignificant lesion in many patients with known coronary anatomy and stable angina pectoris who were restudied after an episode of acute unstable angina.[622] Eccentric lesions with a narrow neck due to one or more overhanging edges or irregular, scalloped borders, or both are the most common morphological feature of disease progression. This finding may represent either a disrupted atherosclerotic plaque, a partially lysed thrombus, or the combination.[623]

When comparing the angiographic findings in patients with chronic stable angina with those having unstable angina, the latter exhibited a higher frequency of complex lesions and thrombus (Fig. 38–22).[569,575a] Coronary arteriography has shown a 40 per cent incidence of coronary thrombi in patients presenting early after the onset of rest angina.[624] Cardiac events (death, myocardial infarction, and the need for urgent revascularization) were more frequent in patients with coronary thrombus (73 per cent), complex coronary morphology (55 per cent), or multivessel disease (58 per cent) than in patients without these angiographic features (17 per cent, 31 per cent, and 7 per cent, respectively). Similarly, intracoronary thrombi were present in 75 per cent of patients requiring urgent coronary arteriography for persistent angina later during admission.[624]

AUTOPSY STUDIES. These suggest that patients with unstable angina have more severe and extensive coronary obstruction than other patients with CAD.[623] Such studies also have shown that about 70 per cent of specimens of diseased arterial segments with significant narrowings (greater than or equal to 50 per cent diameter) have an eccentric, residual arterial lumen that is partially circumscribed by an arc of at least 60 degrees of normal arterial wall which could be responsible for vasoconstriction.[600]

Plaque fissuring has been implicated in acute coronary syndromes, including acute myocardial infarction (Fig. 37–7, p. 1187) and unstable angina.[625] The type of plaque most likely to undergo fissuring is one with an eccentrically situated pool of extracellular lipid contained within the intima. This pool is separated from the blood in the lumen of the artery by a cap of fibrous tissue covered by endothelium. The cap seems most likely to tear at its lateral margin where it is attached to more normal intima. Blood enters the lipid cavity from the lumen, and because of the thrombogenicity of the subendothelial tissues that are exposed, thrombus develops within the plaque itself. This thrombus can expand the volume of the plaque, but subsequently the tear may reseal, restabilize, and heal. Pathological as well as coronary arteriographic studies have suggested the presence of subtotally occlusive coronary arterial thrombi in patients with unstable angina.[626] Plaque fissures heal by the proliferation of smooth muscle, which can contribute to an increase in the severity of chronic obstruction. Some episodes of plaque fissuring are followed by the development of thrombus within the coronary arterial lumen.

CORONARY ANGIOSCOPY. This technique has also revealed complex plaques or thrombi that may not be detected by coronary angiography in patients with unstable angina.[595] The frequency and characteristics of coronary artery thrombi have been evaluated using percutaneous transluminal coronary angioscopy by Mizuno and associates.[596] Patients with unstable angina were frequently observed to have grayish-white (platelet) thrombi, whereas reddish (fibrin) thrombi were more commonly observed in patients with acute myocardial infarction. Moreover, occlusive thrombi occurred frequently in patients with acute myocardial infarction but were not present in patients with unstable angina.

VENTRICULAR FUNCTION. This is usually well preserved in patients with unstable angina, except in those who have had prior myocardial infarction. However, during and following episodes of acute ischemia, localized areas of asynergy are present and stroke volume and ejection fraction decline, whereas left ventricular end-systolic and end-diastolic volumes rise, as does left ventricular filling pressure. Nitroglycerin may restore both global and regional left ventricular function in patients with unstable angina. More recent data demonstrate that angina at rest may be followed by prolonged depression of contractile function in the territory supplied by the "culprit lesion"; this may persist for up to 24 hours or longer[627,628] and represents myocardial stunning (see p. 1176).

Natural History

Unstable angina and acute myocardial infarction are closely related pathogenetically and clinically. Whereas approximately half of patients with acute myocardial infarction report a prodrome of unstable angina shortly before infarction, the opposite is not the case; i.e., only a minority of patients with unstable angina pectoris develop early infarction. Although patients with unstable angina may present difficult management problems, approximately 95 per cent do not in fact develop myocardial infarction over the short term, although recurrent unstable ischemic events are common.[575a] Among patients presenting with unstable angina, who stabilized on standard medical therapy and who were on a waiting list for elective coronary angiography, 57 per cent developed an adverse event (acute coronary syndrome or angiographic total coronary occlusion) during an average follow-up of 8 months.[629] Documentation of all cardiac admissions to coronary and intensive care units in Hamilton, Ontario, over the 1-year period 1979–1980 revealed that in 811 patients admitted with unstable angina, hospital mortality was 1.5 per cent (compared with 17 per cent for acute myocardial infarction), 1-year mortality was 9.2 per cent (compared with 27 per cent for acute myocardial infarction), and only 16 per cent of the patients who died with unstable angina did so during the initial hospitalization. Repeat hospital admission occurred in 28 per cent of patients with unstable angina.[630] In the TIMI III registry of 3318 patients with unstable angina, 21 per cent "ruled in" for a non-Q-wave myocardial infarction on the initial hospitalization; 62 per cent underwent coronary angiography, 22 per cent angioplasty, and 13 per cent coronary bypass surgery. In the subsequent 42 days, 2.4 per cent died and 2.9 per cent experienced a new myocardial infarction.[631]

EXERCISE TESTING. After stabilization of symptoms and before discharge from the hospital, exercise testing can be performed safely in patients admitted with unstable angina who have become asymptomatic.[567,632,633] A normal resting electrocardiogram and an exercise test negative for ischemia in such patients is associated with a 5-year survival greater than 95 per cent. On the other hand, a high-risk exercise stress test (Table 38–2) identifies patients at high risk for subsequent morbid and fatal events.

Exercise thallium scintigraphy after clinical stabilization of unstable angina has demonstrated that the size of the myocardial perfusion defect is a useful predictor of the extent of coronary artery disease[634] and of patients at higher risk for subsequent fatal and morbid events.[635] Exercise electrocardiography, exercise thallium scintigraphy, and dipyridamole thallium scintigraphy showed a similar accuracy in dichotomizing patients with unstable angina into low- and high-risk subgroups for future cardiac events.[567] Two-dimensional echocardiography often reveals transient abnormalities of ventricular wall motion. When persistent, these too are associated with an adverse prognosis.[636]

Data from the Duke Cardiovascular Data Bank demonstrate that the diagnosis of unstable angina at the time of hospital admission carries a risk of death which is intermediate between that of stable angina and that of acute myocardial infarction. The mortality risk in the acute ischemic

syndromes is time-dependent, and by 2 months mortality rates were similar in all three populations. Patients with unstable angina who appear to have a worse prognosis and to be at high risk for adverse events while in the hospital are older,[631] have continuing rest pain despite medical therapy, and demonstrate thrombi, complex coronary morphology, or multivessel disease at coronary arteriography. Ischemia detected by Holter monitoring and significant ST-T wave changes on the electrocardiogram at presentation also suggest an unfavorable outcome.[611–613]

Management

Medical Management

APPROACH. Unstable angina pectoris is a serious, potentially dangerous condition, and its management must be approached with this in mind. The pivotal first step in the management of suspected unstable angina is a prompt evaluation and triage in the emergency room and the immediate initiation of anti-ischemic therapy.[636a] In patients in whom the diagnosis is uncertain and in those considered to be at low-risk (see below), outpatient management may be appropriate. In selected low-risk patients (Table 63–17, p. 1982), an exercise test after a period of observation in the emergency department, which is positive but not "high risk," may identify those who can be discharged on medical therapy.[567] However, the majority of patients with unstable angina should be admitted to the hospital, generally to a coronary care unit or a monitored step-down bed depending upon severity and acuity of the clinical presentation.

The patient should be immediately placed at bed rest. Removal from an emotionally taxing situation, the presence of a quiet atmosphere, physical and emotional rest, the physician's reassurance, mild sedation, and antianxiety drugs are all helpful and by themselves diminish or relieve episodes of rest pain in perhaps half of all patients. Placing the bed into the reverse Trendelenburg position (feet down) is a simple measure that may be helpful, as may the inhalation of 100 per cent oxygen during periods of pain. A vigorous effort must be undertaken immediately to diagnose and treat conditions that may be responsible for transient increases in myocardial oxygen demands, such as infection, fever, thyrotoxicosis, anemia, arrhythmias, exacerbation of preexisting heart failure, concurrent illness (particularly of the pulmonary tract, leading to coughing and hypoxemia, and acute gastrointestinal disturbances, causing vomiting, retching, or diarrhea), tachyarrhythmias (which increase myocardial oxygen demand), and severe bradyarrhythmias (which reduce myocardial perfusion). Control of these aggravating factors is helpful in an additional 10 to 15 per cent of patients.

The electrocardiogram should be monitored continuously; diagnostic tests to rule out a myocardial infarction should include serial CK-MB enzymes. The routine use of other laboratory measurements such as serum troponin-T is under investigation.[117] Invasive monitoring is usually not necessary unless the patient exhibits hemodynamic instability.

NITRATES (see p. 1302). These are a mainstay of therapy. In addition to frequently relieving and preventing recurrence of ischemic pain, nitrates have been shown to improve global and regional left ventricular function. Nitrates may be given sublingually, orally, topically, or intravenously, and they may be of the short- or long-acting variety (Table 38–3). Intravenous nitroglycerin offers the advantage of more consistent control of ischemic episodes during the first 24 hours of treatment. An additional advantage of intravenous nitroglycerin in patients already receiving standard therapy of oral or topical nitrates and beta-blocking drugs is that it reduces the number of anginal episodes, and the need for sublingual nitroglycerin and analgesics. Intravenous nitroglycerin should be started in a dose of 5 to 10 μg/min by continuous infusion and increased by 10 μg/min every 5 to 10 minutes until relief of symptoms or limiting side effects (headache or hypotension with a systolic blood pressure of 90 mm Hg, or more than 30 per cent below starting mean arterial pressure).[408,567] It is recommended that patients on intravenous nitroglycerin be switched to an oral or topical nitrate once they have been symptom-free for 24 hours. Tolerance to continuous intravenous nitroglycerin therapy develops within 24 to 48 hours (p. 1304).

BETA-ADRENOCEPTOR BLOCKERS (see p. 1304). Beta blockers should be administered to all patients with unstable angina, without contraindications to these drugs (Table 38–4).[567] In patients who have not previously received these drugs, the addition of a beta blocker[637,638] or the combination of a beta blocker and nitrates[639] reduces episodes of recurrent ischemia and the occurrence of myocardial infarction.[633,639] In patients already receiving nitrates and/or calcium antagonists who develop unstable angina, the addition of beta blockers reduces the frequency and duration of both symptomatic and silent ischemic episodes. When rapid beta blockade is desired, intravenous esmolol is efficacious and safe, even in patients with compromised left ventricular function.[640] Resolution of drug effect occurs within 20 minutes of discontinuing this drug.

In patients who are already taking a beta blocker at the time unstable angina develops, the drug should be continued unless contraindications are present. The dosage of beta blockers should be adjusted so that the resting heart rate is reduced to between 50 and 60 beats/min. Beta blockade may improve pulmonary congestion if the elevated pulmonary venous pressure is due to an ischemia-induced reduction of left ventricular compliance or left ventricular systolic failure. Rarely, heart failure may be precipitated by beta blockade in patients with previous infarction.

CALCIUM ANTAGONISTS (see also p. 1308). These drugs are as effective as beta blockers in relieving symptoms.[633,637–639] However, an overview of all randomized trials of calcium antagonists in unstable angina suggests that they do *not* prevent the development of acute myocardial infarction or reduce mortality.[641] One randomized, double-blind comparison of recurrent ischemia in patients with unstable angina treated with nifedipine or metoprolol, or both, was terminated prematurely because it appeared that nifedipine therapy alone might have been associated with more nonfatal myocardial infarctions within the first 48 hours of treatment than therapy with metoprolol alone or with a combination of nifedipine and metoprolol.[639] Studies of patients with unstable angina have suggested that the addition of nifedipine to beta blocker therapy or to a combination of nitrates and beta blockers is useful in relieving angina and reducing the subsequent short-term risk of death, myocardial infarction, or the need for urgent coronary artery surgery.[639,642] The possible risks of short-acting nifedipine are discussed on p. 1310. It is therefore recommended that calcium antagonists be used as *second-line* therapy in patients with continued ischemia, despite nitrates and beta blockers. Particular caution should be used in adding a calcium antagonist to a beta blocker in patients with left ventricular dysfunction.

ASPIRIN AND TICLOPIDINE. The potential importance of platelet activation and thrombus formation in the pathogenesis of unstable angina (see p. 1333) has established an important role for aspirin in the management of these patients. Indeed, several randomized trials of aspirin have shown that aspirin reduces the incidence of myocardial infarction and death from cardiac causes by approximately 50 per cent.[581–584,643] Therefore, there is now widespread agreement that aspirin should be started as soon as the diagnosis of unstable angina is established and should then be continued indefinitely (Fig. 38–24). The recommended doses are 160 to 325 mg/day, although lower doses have

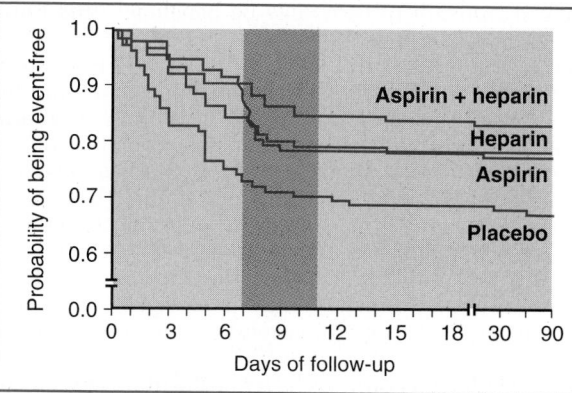

FIGURE 38–24. Kaplan-Meier event-free curves for patients in the four study groups. The curves cover the study period of 7 days, which included the double-blind administration of the study drugs; a 96-hour period early after drug discontinuation, from day 7 to day 11 (indicated by the rectangle); and a follow-up period extending through 3 months. The time of drug discontinuation was adjusted to day 7 for all patients for comparability. The rate of attrition in the heparin group after the discontinuation of the study drug was important, but not when aspirin was administered concomitantly with heparin. (Modified from Theroux, P., Waters, O., Lam, J., et al.: Reactivation of unstable angina after the discontinuation of heparin. N. Engl. J. Med. *327*:141, 1992. Copyright Massachusetts Medical Society.)

proven beneficial. The only contraindications are ongoing major hemorrhage, a recent history of life-threatening bleeding, or a clear-cut history of hypersensitivity to aspirin.[567,644,677]

For the minority of patients with unstable angina with these contraindications, *ticlopidine* in a dose of 250 mg twice daily is a suitable alternative. A multicenter randomized trial of ticlopidine in unstable angina reported a 47% reduction in cardiovascular death and a 46% reduction in nonfatal myocardial infarction at 6 months.[644,645,677]

HEPARIN (see also p. 1823). Intravenous heparin is effective in patients with unstable angina.[583,584] Several trials have suggested that intravenous heparin may be superior to aspirin[646] or that the combination is superior to either drug alone (Fig. 38–24).[584,647] The case for using the combination is strengthened further by the demonstration that rebound angina may be precipitated by discontinuation of heparin in patients who are not taking aspirin.[647–649] There is evidence that this is due to a true "rebound" phenomenon secondary to an increase in thrombin activity after a cessation of heparin.[649a] The more gradual discontinuation of heparin might attenuate this response, and has been recommended in recently published guidelines,[567] but remains unproven. The recommended initial dose of heparin is an 80 units/kg intravenous bolus followed by a constant intravenous infusion of 18 units/kg/hour. An activated partial thromboplastin time (aPTT) is obtained 6 hours after beginning the infusion or 6 hours after any dosage change, and the heparin infusion is adjusted to an aPTT of between 45 and 70 seconds, using a nomogram[650,651] both in patients treated with thrombolytics alone or in combination with PTCA.[655a]

THROMBOLYTIC THERAPY. The initial promise of thrombolytic therapy in acute myocardial infarction raised expectations that this would also be a useful form of therapy in unstable angina, a closely related condition pathogenetically. Despite strong evidence implicating platelet aggregation and thrombosis in unstable angina, these expectations have not been met. Thrombolytic agents have *not* been beneficial, and there is a trend toward a detrimental effect.[567,652–655] The combination of aspirin plus a high dose of low molecular weight heparin has been shown in one trial to be associated with fewer recurrent ischemic events than aspirin alone or aspirin plus unfractionated heparin.[651a] There is some evidence, however, that low-dose, prolonged infusion of t-PA may be beneficial; this remains to be confirmed.[656]

INVESTIGATIVE ANTITHROMBOTIC AGENTS. Despite the proven benefits of both aspirin and heparin in the acute ischemic syndromes, both drugs have their limitations. Aspirin interferes with only one of several pathways which lead to platelet aggregation. Heparin requires a cofactor for its action; it is ineffective against clot-bound thrombin and may be inactivated by a number of substances, which are generated by platelet aggregation and thrombosis. Given these limitations, the attraction of the newer antithrombotic (see p. 1817) and antiplatelet agents (see p. 1818) is understandable. These drugs are currently under intensive study in patients with unstable angina.[585,657]

INTRAAORTIC BALLOON COUNTERPULSATION (see also p. 1232). The large majority of patients with unstable angina respond to therapy with heparin, aspirin, nitrates, calcium antagonists, and beta blockers, and true refractory unstable angina is uncommon. In a series of patients referred to a tertiary care center for "refractory" unstable angina, almost all were rendered chest pain–free with a more aggressive medical regimen, and only 9 per cent were considered to be truly refractory.[658] Intraaortic balloon counterpulsation is considered when medical therapy has failed, and it is usually effective in stabilizing the patient's condition, both symptomatically and hemodynamically. Intraaortic balloon counterpulsation is usually initiated either before or during coronary arteriography with a view to continuing it through revascularization.[659] This technique is useful primarily because it allows the safe performance of coronary arteriography and ensures that the patient goes to coronary bypass surgery or PTCA under optimal conditions. Although there has never been a randomized trial of the efficacy of intraaortic balloon counterpulsation in patients with unstable angina, it is an extremely effective method for the control of ischemia in this setting. However, local complications related to intraaortic balloon placement are common in the elderly, women, and diabetics.[660]

INDICATIONS FOR CATHETERIZATION AND ANGIOGRAPHY. After initial therapy with bed rest, oxygen, analgesics, aspirin, heparin, nitrates, beta-adrenoreceptor blocking drugs, and/or calcium antagonists, more than 80 per cent of patients who are hospitalized with unstable angina become asymptomatic within 48 hours, and their electrocardiographic signs of transient ischemia disappear. During this period, serial electrocardiographic and enzyme evaluations confirm that no infarction has taken place, thereby differentiating them from patients with acute myocardial infarction.

In patients in whom medical therapy fails with recurrent angina or electrocardiographic changes of recurrent ischemia, the initial diagnostic approach may be to proceed with cardiac catheterization in order to evaluate them for revascularization.[660a] In such patients, noninvasive testing is unlikely to provide sufficient incremental information so as to alter the proposed treatment strategy. In patients who respond to initial medical therapy and those in whom the indications for intervention are less clear-cut, noninvasive evaluation is indicated for further risk stratification.[567]

The approach to patients who have stabilized on medical therapy was comprehensively addressed by the AHCPR Clinical Practice Guidelines (Table 63–17, p. 1983) and is based, in part, on the results of the TIMI-IIIB trial.[567,652] This trial suggested that early coronary arteriography followed by revascularization may be the most appropriate approach for patients admitted to a center with facilities for high-quality PTCA and bypass surgery, provided that there are no contraindications to revascularization and the coronary anatomy is suitable. An initially more conservative strategy of continuing medical therapy at home in patients who have stabilized on intensive medical management in the hospital is appropriate for patients with unstable angina who do not have access to a tertiary care center, those with contraindications to revascularization, those who

refuse it, and those who are considered to be at extremely low risk for cardiac events on continued medical therapy. The latter includes patients with unstable angina who have not experienced rest pain, patients with new-onset angina with an onset more than 2 weeks earlier, and those with a normal or unchanged electrocardiogram during pain. If such patients become asymptomatic on medical management and do *not* exhibit a "high-risk" stress test (see p. 1297), they may be followed *without* angiography with a very low incidence of an adverse cardiac outcome, i.e., death or myocardial infarction.

Catheterization and arteriography are helpful in the majority of patients with unstable angina in that they identify several subgroups of patients and can thus be used to guide therapy: (1) patients with left main coronary artery disease —the most life-threatening form of disease—in whom urgent surgery is indicated; (2) patients with multivessel obstructive disease without a clear "culprit" lesion who are not suitable for PTCA; unless there are contraindications, we recommend that in such patients coronary artery bypass surgery be planned on a semiurgent basis (within 10 days) after the patient's hemodynamic condition has stabilized; (3) patients with multivessel disease and left ventricular dysfunction who should also be revascularized; (4) patients with single-vessel or double-vessel disease with normal left ventricular function and a discrete narrow proximal lesion (i.e., "culprit" lesion) amenable to PTCA or other catheter-based revascularization (see p. 1313); (5) a small number of patients (about 10 per cent of all patients with unstable angina) with no demonstrable CAD, in whom the prognosis appears to be excellent with medical management and in whom revascularization is obviously not necessary. In some of these patients, coronary spasm is responsible for the angina, and this can be established by provocative testing at the time of coronary arteriography (see p. 264); intensification of therapy with nitrates and calcium antagonists would then be indicated; and (6) patients with diffuse distal CAD unsuitable for angioplasty or bypass grafting.

Maximal medical therapy and heparinization should be maintained up to and continued through the time of cardiac catheterization. The risks of coronary arteriography are slightly greater in patients with unstable than in those with chronic stable angina.[661] This risk is increased further in patients who continue to have symptoms despite optimal medical management.

Revascularization

PERCUTANEOUS TRANSLUMINAL CORONARY ANGIOPLASTY (PTCA). In patients with unstable angina, successful PTCA results in the immediate cessation of ischemic episodes as well as in improvement in both regional and global ischemic left ventricular dysfunction.[662] The initial success rate of dilation of significant stenoses is 83 to 93 per cent.[663-666] Although the acute complications of PTCA are slightly higher in patients with unstable as opposed to stable angina,[663-667] late outcomes are similar.[668,669] Patients with unstable angina appear to be at a somewhat higher risk of developing a myocardial infarction at the time of PTCA than patients with chronic stable angina.[663] The risk factors for a procedure-related complication include very severe degrees of stenosis, the presence of thrombus, ST-segment elevations, or persistent T-wave inversions and the number of lesions attempted.[664] The incidence of ischemic complications in patients with unstable angina undergoing PTCA was reduced by treatment with the chimeric monoclonal anti-IIb/IIIa antibody 7E3 in the randomized EPIC trial[670] (see p. 1369).

If angioplasty is performed immediately after the onset of unstable angina, the complication rate is higher and the success rate is lower. Some have therefore advocated deferring angioplasty for 4 to 7 days in patients with an intraluminal filling defect with the appearance of thrombus, thus allowing time for continued therapy with aspirin and intravenous heparin to be effective. It appears that delayed angioplasty in such patients is safe and effective, although it does increase the length of hospitalization.[671]

The incidence of restenosis following PTCA is generally similar in patients with unstable angina and chronic stable angina, although in some analyses the presence of unstable angina emerges as an independent predictor of a higher rate of restenosis.[664,666] The risk factors for restenosis in patients with unstable angina appear to be multifactorial and include poor perfusion beyond the "culprit" lesion, multiple irregularities in the vessel being dilated, the presence of intraluminal thrombus, involvement of the left anterior descending coronary artery, and the presence of collateral vessels. In patients with medically refractory rest angina who are also considered at high risk for coronary bypass surgery, the 2-year mortality after PTCA was comparable to that in a similar group of "high-risk" patients undergoing coronary bypass surgery at the same institution.[671]

Despite the aforementioned problems, angioplasty and related catheter-based techniques[672] are now a cornerstone in the treatment of unstable angina. The 5-year survival rate exceeds 90 per cent, and approximately three-fourths of patients remain free of angina following successful angioplasty.[663–666,673] The incidence of myocardial infarction during long-term follow-up does not differ substantially from that following PTCA for chronic stable angina.[673]

CORONARY BYPASS SURGERY. In patients with *refractory* unstable angina who have not suffered recent myocardial infarction, the operative mortality for coronary artery surgery is 3.7 per cent, approximately twice that observed in patients with chronic stable angina pectoris, and the incidence of perioperative myocardial infarction is 10 per cent. The later mortality rate is approximately 2 per cent per year, and the rate of nonfatal infarction is 3 to 4 per cent per year.

The Veterans Administration Cooperative Study compared medical with surgical management in 468 patients with unstable angina. No difference in two-year mortality was observed overall, although in patients with left ventricular dysfunction surgical therapy conferred a survival advantage that was sustained for 5 years[676,677] (Fig. 38–25). Subsequent follow-up has demonstrated that the survival advantage of surgery after 5 and 8 years of follow-up did not reach statistical significance at 10 years when patients were analyzed according to the "intention to treat" principle. But if patients who "crossed over" to surgical therapy were censored, there remained a highly significant advantage to surgical treatments.[677] In addition, the cumulative rate of repeat hospitalizations was lower in patients treated with surgery, and the quality of their life appeared to be better.[678] Rahimtoola et al. assessed the late results of bypass surgery performed for unstable angina in more than 1000 patients between 1970 and 1982. The actuarial 5- and 10-year survival rates were 92 per cent and 83 per cent, respectively.[679]

The results of coronary bypass surgery compared with medical therapy in patients with unstable angina are consistent with the findings in patients with chronic stable angina (see p. 1959) in that the major benefit of surgical over medical therapy is in the "sickest" patients, characterized by the presence of multivessel disease, severe symptoms, and left ventricular dysfunction.[679a] Thus, operation appears to be the treatment of choice for patients with unstable angina pectoris, abnormal left ventricular function, and extensive CAD.[677] Risk factors for increased operative mortality in patients undergoing coronary artery bypass grafting for unstable angina are also similar to those for chronic stable angina and include advanced age, clinical and laboratory evidence of left ventricular dysfunction, and the need for an intraaortic balloon for preoperative control of angina.[680] In patients who have postinfarction unstable angina, the independent predictors of perioperative mortality include the presence of an anterior transmural myocardial infarction and the need for preoperative intraaortic

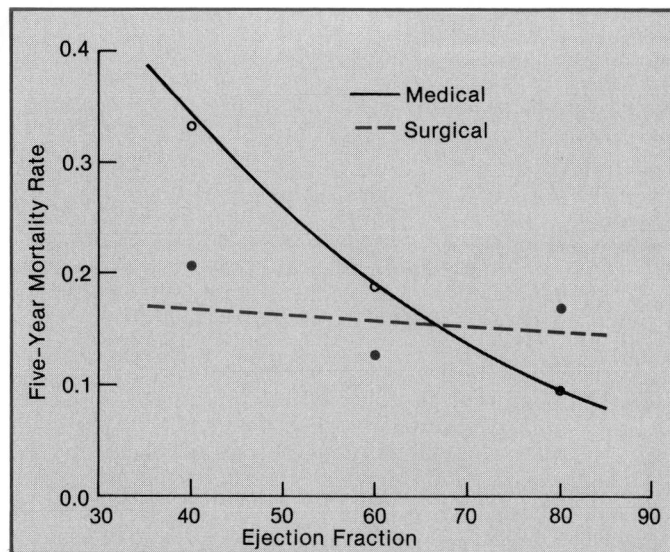

FIGURE 38–25. Mortality following medical and surgical treatment of unstable angina using ejection fraction as a continuous variable. Curves computed by logistic regression analysis based on 5-year mortality of 468 patients with unstable angina randomized to medical (open circles) and surgical (closed circles) therapy. The mean observed per cent mortality is illustrated for ejection fraction intervals 0.30–0.49, 0.50–0.69, and >0.70. The worse the ejection fraction, the poorer the survival in medically treated patients; thus, surgery should be recommended for patients with unstable angina and reduced ejection fraction for three-vessel coronary artery disease suitable for surgical revascularization because it offers improved 5-year survival. (Reproduced with permission from Parisi, A. F., et al.: Medical compared with surgical management of unstable angina: 5-year mortality and morbidity in the Veterans Administration Study. Circulation 80:1176, 1989. Copyright American Heart Association.)

balloon pumping for either continuing angina or congestive heart failure.[674] In patients who have undergone coronary bypass grafting and later develop unstable angina, the risk of subsequent death and myocardial infarction is higher because they are less suitable candidates for further revascularization.[681]

Management: A Summary

The role of coronary arteriography and reperfusion and the timing of such therapy remain controversial in patients with unstable angina. Patients with unstable angina who respond to intensive medical therapy may be managed by either an aggressive approach with early angiography or more conservatively based upon the results of the TIMI-IIIB trial.[652] One can make a strong case, however, for routine coronary angiography in all patients with unstable angina and evidence of left ventricular dysfunction and in patients with adverse prognostic features, such as a recent myocardial infarction, persistent T-wave inversion in the anterior leads, or significant ST-segment depression during episodes of angina.[682] In patients with unstable angina and multivessel disease, the approach to PTCA, other catheter-based techniques, or coronary bypass surgery must be individualized, as in patients with chronic stable angina (see p. 1298).

If a patient has received intensive medical therapy for a 48-hour period and there is persistent evidence of continuing ischemia, it is our policy to proceed with catheterization and coronary arteriography. Intraaortic balloon counterpulsation is often instituted either before or during cardiac catheterization if the patient exhibits hemodynamic instability or continued rest pain. If the patient has single-vessel disease and well-maintained left ventricular function, then PTCA is performed, if technically feasible. On the other hand, in patients in whom there is evidence of left main coronary disease, ventricular dysfunction, or multivessel disease and the anatomy is suitable for bypass grafting, operation is performed immediately.

In 1959, Prinzmetal et al. described an unusual syndrome of cardiac pain secondary to myocardial ischemia that occurs almost exclusively at rest, is usually not precipitated by physical exertion or emotional stress, and is associated with electrocardiographic ST-segment elevations.[683] This syndrome, now known as *Prinzmetal's* or *variant angina,* may be associated with acute myocardial infarction and severe cardiac arrhythmias, including ventricular tachycardia and fibrillation, as well as sudden death.

Mechanisms

Variant angina pectoris has been demonstrated convincingly to be due to coronary artery spasm.[1,684,684a] (Fig. 38–11). The latter causes a transient, abrupt, marked reduction in the diameter of an epicardial (or large septal) coronary artery resulting in myocardial ischemia. This occurs in the absence of any preceding increases in myocardial oxygen demand, as reflected in elevations of heart rate or blood pressure. The reduction in diameter can usually be reversed by nitroglycerin, sometimes requiring large doses, and can occur in either normal or diseased coronary arteries. The striking reduction in luminal diameter is usually focal and involves a single site. Measurements of great cardiac vein flow and left anterior descending coronary artery diameters in patients with vasospastic angina suggest that not only epicardial but also the resistance coronary arteries are affected by the coronary vasomotion disorder.[685] This focal, severe vasospasm should not be confused with vasoconstriction of both the large and small coronary vessels, a *normal* response to stimuli such as cold exposure. The latter response is much less intense and occurs diffusely throughout the coronary vascular bed.

In patients with Prinzmetal's angina, basal coronary artery tone may be increased. Although responses to ergonovine, acetylcholine, and nitrates are greater in spastic segments of the coronary arteries, there is also hypersensitivity to vasoconstrictor stimuli throughout the entire coronary artery tree.[686] Sites of spasm in Prinzmetal's angina may be adjacent to atheromatous plaques. It has been suggested that in this subgroup of patients the basic abnormality may be hypercontractility of the arterial wall associated with the atherosclerotic process itself. Other suggested mechanisms include endothelial injury (which reverses the dilator response to a variety of stimuli, e.g., acetylcholine [see p. 1342]) and hypercontractility of vascular smooth muscle due to vasoconstrictor mitogens, leukotrienes, serotonin,[687] and higher local concentrations of blood-borne vasoconstriction in areas adjacent to neovascularized atherosclerotic plaques.

Iodine-123 metaiodobenzylguanidine (^{123}I MIBG) positron emission–computed tomography (PET) (see p. 307) has been carried out in patients with Prinzmetal's angina in whom coronary vasospasm has been provoked by the intracoronary administration of acetylcholine. This technique has demonstrated regional myocardial sympathetic dysinnervation, which was not observed in patients with significant obstructive CAD disease and in subjects with normal coronary arteries. The region of myocardial sympathetic dysinnervation was usually located in the area of distribution of the vessel developing vasospasm.[688]

Coronary spasm in patients with variant angina may induce stasis and result in the conversion of fibrinogen to fibrin in the coronary vessels, with elevated levels of plasma fibrinopeptide A, an index of fibrin formation.[689] The latter displays significant circadian variation in plasma concentration, with the peak levels occurring from midnight to early morning, in parallel with the frequency of the ischemic attacks in these patients.[690] In addition, these patients also demonstrate a morning peak in the values of plasminogen activator antigen and free plasminogen activa-

tor inhibitor activity.[691] The possibility that vasospasm may induce leukocyte adhesion in the coronary circulation in the initiation of an inflammatory process has been suggested.[691a]

Cigarette smoking is an important risk factor for Prinzmetal's angina.[692,693] *Magnesium sulfate* has been shown to terminate cold pressor–induced anginal attacks, to prevent induction of further attacks,[694] and to suppress attacks induced by hyperventilation[695] and exercise in these patients.[696]

Cocaine, which blocks the presynaptic uptake of the neurotransmitters norepinephrine and dopamine, causes alpha-adrenergically mediated coronary constriction when taken intranasally.[697] There is a high incidence of spontaneous, silent myocardial ischemia detected by Holter monitoring in cocaine abusers during the early stages of withdrawal.[698] The possibility that coronary vasoconstriction may be mediated by therapeutic or illicit cocaine use in patients with suspected coronary artery spasm should always be considered. Spasm causing total occlusion of a coronary vessel, in response to intracoronary ergonovine, has been demonstrated after blunt thoracic trauma.[699] Both *hyperinsulinemia* and *insulin resistance* may be risk factors for variant angina, in the causation of early atheromatous lesions and the subsequent development of occlusive lesions.[699a]

Clinical Manifestations

Patients with variant angina tend to be younger than patients with chronic stable angina or unstable angina, and many do not exhibit classic coronary risk factors except that they are often heavy cigarette smokers.[693] The anginal discomfort is often extremely severe, is generally referred to as "pain," and may be accompanied by syncope, the latter presumably caused by arrhythmias. Attacks of Prinzmetal's angina tend to be clustered between midnight and 8 A.M.[690] Patients studied by means of ambulatory electrocardiography, even those without clinically apparent angina pectoris, show more frequent abnormalities in the morning. In contrast to the situation in patients with unstable angina, the rest pain in patients with Prinzmetal's angina has usually not progressed from a period of chronic stable angina. Although exercise capacity is usually well preserved in patients with Prinzmetal's angina, some patients experience typical pain and ST-segment elevations not only at rest but during or after exertion as well.

Clinical features do not reliably differentiate patients with Prinzmetal's angina with normal or mildly abnormal coronary arteriograms from those with this syndrome and severe coronary obstruction.[699b] However, the latter may have a combination of fixed-threshold, exertion-induced angina with ST-segment depression, as well as episodes of rest angina with ST-segment elevation. Rarely, Prinzmetal's angina develops following coronary artery bypass surgery,[700] and occasionally it appears to be a manifestation of a generalized vasospastic disorder associated with attacks of migraine and Raynaud's phenomenon; it has also been reported in association with aspirin-induced asthma.[701] Some patients appear to demonstrate a distinct relationship between emotional distress and episodes of coronary vasospasm. Alcohol withdrawal may precipitate variant angina,[702] and alcohol ingestion may prevent coronary spasm.[703] Variant angina has been reported to be provoked by 5-fluorouracil[704] and by cyclophosphamide (see p. 1803).[705]

Cardiac examination is usually normal in the absence of ischemia (unless the patient has suffered a previous myocardial infarction) but often reveals signs of dyskinesis and impaired left ventricular function during episodes of myocardial ischemia.

ELECTROCARDIOGRAM. The key to the diagnosis of variant angina lies in the detection of ST-segment elevation with pain (Fig. 38–26). In some patients, episodes of ST-segment depression follow episodes of ST-segment elevation and are associated with T-wave changes. ST-segment and T-wave alternans[706] is the result of ischemic conduction delay and may be associated with potentially lethal ventricular arrhythmias.[707] R-wave "growth" may also be associated with the occurrence of ventricular arrhythmias.[708] Many patients exhibit multiple episodes of asymptomatic ST-segment elevation (silent ischemia). The ST-segment deviations may be present in any leads; the concurrent presence of ST-segment elevations in both the inferior and anterior leads (reflecting extensive ischemia) is associated with an increased risk of sudden death.[709]

Transient conduction disturbances may occur during episodes of ischemia.[710] Ventricular ectopic activity is more frequent during longer episodes of ischemia, is often associated with ST-segment T-wave alternans,[708] and is of ominous prognostic import.

In survivors of out-of-hospital cardiac arrest without flow-limiting coronary stenoses, spontaneous or induced focal coronary spasm has been found to be associated with life-threatening ventricular arrhythmias. In some patients, reperfusion rather than ischemia itself correlates with the onset of ventricular arrhythmias (Fig. 38–27).[711] Myocardial cell damage, as reflected by the release of small quantities of CK-MB, may occur in the absence of persistent electrocardiographic changes in patients with prolonged attacks of variant angina; transient Q waves have been observed.[712] Transmural myocardial infarction due to coronary artery

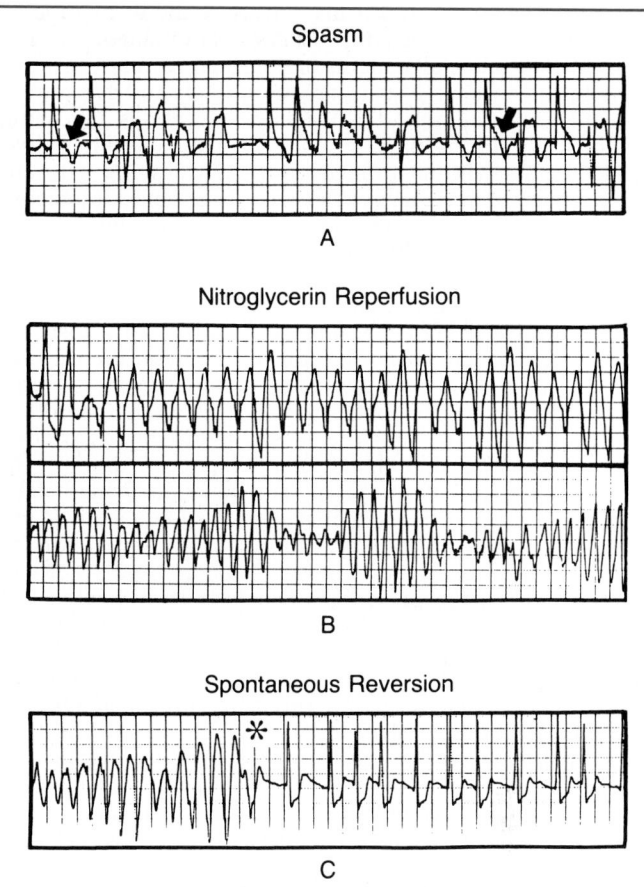

FIGURE 38–27. Arrhythmia during silent ischemia and reperfusion. Selected strips from a 2.5-minute continuous recording (lead II) in Patient 2 during an angiographically documented spasm of the right coronary artery are shown. Tracing A began 24 seconds after the onset of ST-segment elevations (arrows) and demonstrates premature ventricular contractions and salvos. The top strip of tracing B was recorded 70 seconds after onset, immediately after the sublingual administration of nitroglycerin (1/150 grain); the bottom strip of tracing B was recorded 36 seconds later. Tracing C was recorded 130 seconds after onset and shows spontaneous reversion (asterisk) and atrial fibrillation. (From Myerburg, R. J., Kessler, K. M., Mallon, S. M., et al.: Life-threatening ventricular arrhythmias in patients with silent myocardial ischemia due to coronary artery spasm. N. Engl. J. Med. 326:1451, 1992. Copyright Massachusetts Medical Society.)

spasm in the absence of angiographically demonstrable obstructive coronary artery disease has been described.[713]

Exercise testing in patients with variant angina is of limited value because the response is so variable. Approximately equal numbers of patients show ST-segment depression, no change in ST segments during exercise, or ST-segment elevation, reflecting the presence of underlying fixed CAD in some patients, the absence of significant lesions in others, and the provocation of spasm by exercise in the remainder.

Hemodynamic and Arteriographic Studies

Spasm of a proximal coronary artery with resultant transmural ischemia has been convincingly documented arteriographically and is the diagnostic hallmark of Prinzmetal's angina.[714] Echocardiographic studies performed during episodes of spontaneous variant angina have demonstrated abnormalities in ventricular function that precede the onset of symptoms of angina and electrocardiographic changes.[715]

Significant fixed proximal coronary obstruction of at least one major vessel occurs in the majority of patients, and in them spasm usually occurs within 1 cm of the obstruction. The remainder have normal coronary arteries in the absence of ischemia. Spasm is most common in the

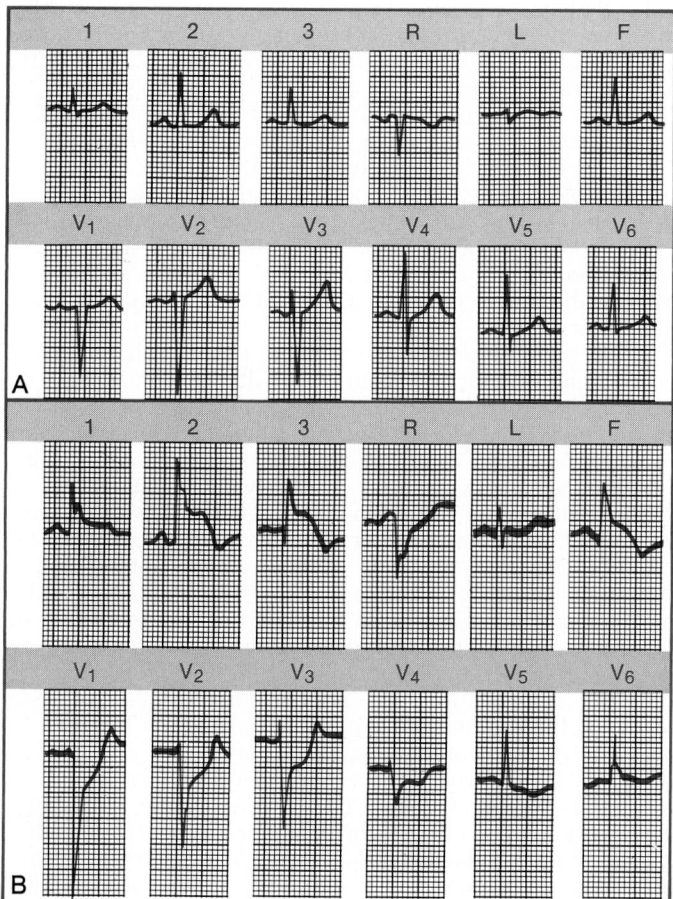

FIGURE 38–26. ECG (A) prior to an episode of Prinzmetal's angina and (B) during an episode of Prinzmetal's angina. ST segments are now markedly elevated in the inferior leads, with reciprocal depression in the anterior leads. After nitroglycerin was given, the electrocardiogram returned to baseline. (From Berman, N. D., et al.: Prinzmetal's angina with coronary artery spasm. Angiographic, pharmacologic, metabolic and radionuclide perfusion studies. Am. J. Med. 60:727, 1976.)

right coronary artery, and it may occur at one or more sites in one artery or in multiple arteries simultaneously. Patients with Prinzmetal's angina and normal coronary arteriograms in the absence of pain are more likely to have purely nonexertional angina and ST-segment elevations involving inferior leads during pain. In contrast, patients with Prinzmetal's angina who have fixed obstructive lesions with superimposed coronary artery spasm often have associated effort-induced angina and ischemia in anterolateral leads. Patients with no or mild fixed coronary obstruction tend to experience a more benign course than do patients with associated severe obstructive lesions.

THE ERGONOVINE TEST. A number of provocative tests for coronary spasm have been developed. Of these, the ergonovine test is the most sensitive. Ergonovine maleate, an ergot alkaloid that stimulates both alpha-adrenergic and serotonergic receptors and therefore exerts a direct constrictive effect on vascular smooth muscle,[716] has been used to induce coronary artery spasm in patients with Prinzmetal's angina. Coronary arteries that constrict spontaneously appear to be abnormally sensitive to this agent. When administered intravenously in doses ranging from 0.05 to 0.40 mg, ergonovine provides a sensitive and specific test for provoking coronary artery spasm. There is an inverse correlation between the dose of ergonovine required to induce a positive test and the frequency of spontaneous attacks.[717] In low doses and in carefully controlled clinical situations, ergonovine is a relatively safe drug, but prolonged coronary artery spasm precipitated by ergonovine may cause myocardial infarction. Because of this hazard, it is recommended that ergonovine be administered only to patients in whom coronary arteriography has demonstrated normal or nearly normal coronary arteries and in gradually increasing doses, beginning with a very low dose.

The ergonovine test should be carried out only in a setting where appropriate resuscitative equipment, drugs, and personnel are readily available, usually in the cardiac catheterization laboratory, and with a catheter poised to enter the coronary arteries, so that the angiographic diagnosis of spasm can be made and intracoronary nitroglycerin administered to abolish the spasm.

The response of the *normal* coronary arterial bed to larger doses (≥ 0.40 mg) of ergonovine is a diffuse reduction in arterial caliber. In patients with atypical chest pain who do not have Prinzmetal's angina, sequential intravenous bolus injections of ergonovine maleate result in progressive diffuse reductions in coronary dimensions. These vasoconstrictor responses appear to be accentuated in women and in patients with intimal coronary arteriographic irregularities, suggesting the existence of minor atherosclerotic disease. This dose-dependent phenomenon differs from the abnormal response in Prinzmetal's angina, which is characterized by severe focal spasm, usually at much lower doses of the agent. The sensitivity of the ergonovine test is high in patients with active disease (who have at least one attack daily) and lower in patients with sporadic episodes of variant angina.[718]

HYPERVENTILATION. This stimulus has also been demonstrated to provoke some episodes of intense angina,[719] electrocardiographic ST-segment elevations, angiographic evidence of coronary artery spasm, and ventricular arrhythmias.[718] In patients with active disease who have at least one daily attack of Prinzmetal's angina, the sensitivity of hyperventilation was 95 per cent, compared with 100 per cent for ergonovine. However, in patients with less frequent attacks of angina, hyperventilation has a lower sensitivity than ergonovine and, therefore, is of more limited diagnostic value.[718]

ACETYLCHOLINE. Intracoronary injections of acetylcholine have been shown to induce severe coronary spasm in patients with variant angina. This spasm should not be confused with the mild diffuse constriction that acetylcholine induces in patients with abnormal coronary endothelium.

Because this method allows induction of spasm separately in the left and right coronary arteries, it is useful in patients with known multivessel disease or spasm. In such patients, the use of intracoronary acetylcholine has been shown to be sensitive, reliable, and safe.[720] Indeed, the sensitivity (95 per cent) and the specificity (99 per cent) of acetylcholine for induction of coronary spasm[720,721] are comparable to those of ergonovine.

Methacholine, a parasympathomimetic drug, histamine,[712] and dopamine[722] also can induce coronary artery spasm. Like ergonovine and acetylcholine, these agents are capable of causing marked coronary artery spasm in patients with variant angina who have severe underlying arteriosclerotic coronary artery narrowing and in those without such fixed stenoses. Exercise, the cold pressor test, and induced alkalosis all can cause coronary spasm in patients with variant angina, but none of these tests is as sensitive as ergonovine or acetylcholine.

MYOCARDIAL PERFUSION SCINTIGRAPHY. Localization of the myocardial perfusion defect to an area perfused by a coronary artery in which spasm can be demonstrated by arteriography has been reported using thallium-201 scintigraphy,[723] and a reduction in coronary sinus flow during episodes of spasm has also been noted. These studies support the relationship between coronary spasm and the resultant myocardial perfusion and ischemia.

Management

There are several important differences between the optimal management of Prinzmetal's variant angina and classic (stable and unstable) angina.

1. Patients with both variant and classic angina usually respond well to nitrates; sublingual or intravenous nitroglycerin often abolishes attacks of variant angina promptly, and long-acting nitrates are useful in preventing attacks.[724] However, the mechanism of action of the drugs may differ in the two types of angina. As already discussed (see p. 1302), in chronic (effort-induced) stable angina, as well as in unstable angina, one important action of the nitrates is to reduce myocardial oxygen needs and the second is to cause coronary vasodilation. In Prinzmetal's angina, nitrates abolish or prevent myocardial ischemia *exclusively* by exerting a direct vasodilating effect on the spastic coronary arteries.

2. In patients with classic angina (stable and unstable), beta-adrenoreceptor blockade is usually beneficial, but the response in patients with Prinzmetal's angina to these agents is variable. Some, particularly those with associated fixed lesions, exhibit a reduction in the frequency of exertion-induced angina caused primarily by augmentation of myocardial oxygen requirements. In others, however, nonselective beta-adrenoreceptor blockers may actually be detrimental, because blockade of the beta$_2$ receptors, which subserve coronary dilation, allows unopposed alpha receptor–mediated coronary vasoconstriction to occur; in these patients, the duration of episodes of vasotonic angina may be prolonged by propranolol.[725]

3. In contrast to the variable effectiveness of beta blockers, the calcium antagonists are extremely effective in preventing the coronary artery spasm of variant angina,[726,727] and they should ordinarily be prescribed in maximally tolerated doses. These drugs, along with long- and short-acting nitrates, are the mainstay of therapy. Because calcium antagonists act through a different mechanism than do nitrates, the vasodilatory actions of these two classes of drugs may be additive. Similar efficacy rates have been noted for nifedipine, diltiazem, and verapamil. Rarely, a patient responds to only one of these three agents, and even less commonly simultaneous administration of two or even three antagonists is required.[728] Slow-release nifedipine has been shown to be highly effective in suppressing not only symptomatic but also asymptomatic myocardial ischemia in patients with variant angina.[729] Once-

daily felodipine has also been shown to be highly effective in preventing ergonovine-induced myocardial ischemia in patients with variant angina.[730] Reports have suggested a rebound of symptoms when calcium antagonists are discontinued.[731]

4. Prazosin, a selective alpha-adrenoreceptor blocker (see p. 852), has also been found to be of value in patients with Prinzmetal's angina.[732] Aspirin, helpful in unstable angina (see p. 1337), may actually *increase* the severity of ischemic episodes in patients with Prinzmetal's angina because it inhibits biosynthesis of the naturally occurring coronary vasodilator prostacyclin.[733]

5. Coronary angioplasty and occasionally coronary artery bypass surgery may be helpful in patients with variant angina with discrete, proximal fixed obstructive lesions.[734] Calcium antagonists should be continued for at least 6 months following successful revascularization. PTCA and coronary artery bypass surgery are *contraindicated* in patients with isolated coronary artery spasm without accompanying obstructive disease.

Prognosis

Many patients with Prinzmetal's angina pass through an acute, active phase, with frequent episodes of angina and cardiac events during the first 6 months after presentation. Long-term survival at 5 years is excellent (89 to 97 per

cent).[735] The extent and severity of CAD and the activity of the disease have an adverse influence on long-term survival free of myocardial infarction. Nonfatal myocardial infarction occurs in up to 20 per cent of patients and death in up to 10 per cent during this period. Patients with variant angina who develop serious arrhythmias (ventricular tachycardia, ventricular fibrillation, high-degree atrioventricular block, or asystole) during spontaneous episodes of pain are at a higher risk for sudden death.[736] Patients with Prinzmetal's angina and severe obstructive coronary artery lesions are at greater risk for persistent anginal symptoms, acute myocardial infarction, and death.[737] In most patients who survive an infarction or the initial 3- to 6-month period of frequent episodes, the condition stabilizes and there is a tendency for symptoms and cardiac events to diminish with time. In patients who experience such remissions, cautious tapering of calcium antagonists may be attempted. For reasons that are not clear, some patients, after a relatively quiescent period of months or even years, experience a recrudescence of vasospastic activity with frequent and severe episodes of ischemia.[738] Fortunately, these patients respond to re-treatment with calcium antagonists and nitrates. Most patients in whom symptoms recur after a pain-free period demonstrate spasm on provocative testing at the same location as previously demonstrated and respond once more to treatment with nitrates and calcium antagonists.

OTHER MANIFESTATIONS OF CORONARY ARTERY DISEASE

CHEST PAIN WITH NORMAL CORONARY ARTERIOGRAM

The syndrome of angina or angina-like chest pain with a normal coronary arteriogram, often referred to as *syndrome X,* is an important clinical entity that should be differentiated from classic ischemic heart disease caused by CAD. In this condition the prognosis is usually excellent,[739–741] in contrast to the variable outcome in patients with angina caused by coronary atherosclerosis. Patients with chest pain with normal coronary arteriograms may constitute as many as 10 to 20 per cent of those undergoing coronary arteriography because of the clinical suspicion of angina. The cause(s) of the syndrome is unclear. True myocardial ischemia, reflected in the production of lactate by the myocardium during exercise or pacing, is present in some of these patients.[742]

It is postulated that the syndrome of angina pectoris with normal coronary arteries reflects a number of conditions. Included in syndrome X are patients with microvascular dysfunction in whom angina may be the result of ischemia.[743] This condition is frequently referred to as *microvascular angina* (Fig. 38–1B). In others, chest discomfort without ischemia may be due to abnormal pain perception or sensitivity. This may result in an awareness of chest pain in response to stimuli such as arterial stretch or changes in heart rate, rhythm, or contractility.[744] A sympathovagal imbalance with sympathetic predominance in some of these patients has also been postulated. At the time of cardiac catheterization, some patients with syndrome X are unusually sensitive to intracardiac instrumentation, with typical chest pain being consistently produced by direct right atrial stimulation and saline infusion.[744] Other patients appear to have a combination of microvascular dysfunction and abnormal pain sensitivity (Fig. 38–23B). Studies with intravascular ultrasound have demonstrated the anatomical and physiological heterogeneity of syndrome X, with a spectrum ranging from normal coronary arteries to vessels with intimal thickening and atheromatous plaque.[744a]

MICROVASCULAR DYSFUNCTION OR INADEQUATE VASODILATOR RESERVE (see also p. 1173). Patients with chest pain and angiographically normal coronary arteries and no evidence of large vessel spasm even after an acetylcholine challenge may demonstrate an abnormally reduced capacity to reduce coronary resistance and increase coronary flow in response to stimuli such as exercise, dipyridamole, and atrial pacing. These patients also have an exaggerated response of small coronary vessels to vasoconstrictor stimuli and an impaired response to intracoronary papavarine[745] (Fig. 36–20, p. 1173). This abnormality appears to affect the smaller resistance vessels that are not visible angiographically, while the large proximal conductance vessels are normal.[745a] The reduced vasodilator reserve in the microcirculation may be associated with exercise-induced regional wall-motion abnormalities as well as abnormalities of diastolic function.[746] The reduced coronary flow reserve may cause abnormalities of myocardial perfusion which are detectable by means of positron emission tomography.[747] It has been reported that these patients also have an impairment of vasodilator reserve in forearm vessels[748] and airway hyperresponsiveness,[749] suggesting that, in addition to their coronary circulation, smooth muscle in their systemic arteries and other organs may be affected.

A link between coronary microvascular dysfunction and ischemia in response to exercise is an attractive concept that could explain abnormal left ventricular function resulting from exercise in some patients with chest pain and normal coronary arteries.[747,750,751] Abnormal endothelial function and increased sympathetic drive or responsiveness have been reported.[752,753]

EVIDENCE FOR ISCHEMIA. Despite general acceptance that microvascular and/or endothelial dysfunction is present in many patients with syndrome X, whether ischemia is in fact the putative cause of the symptoms in these patients is not at all clear.[750,751] The development of left ventricular dysfunction and of electrocardiographic or scintigraphic abnormalities during exercise in some of these patients supports an ischemic etiology. On the other hand, support for a noncardiac cause for the pain is provided by several reports of behavioral or psychiatric disorders in patients with chest pain and normal coronary angiograms.[754,755]

The absence of definitive evidence of ischemia in some patients with syndrome X has focused attention upon alternative nonischemic causes of cardiac-related pain, including a reduced threshold for pain perception—the so-called sensitive heart syndrome.[744,751,756] Esophageal dysmotility and the reproduction of pain with the infusion of hydrochloric acid into the esophagus (Bernstein test) or intraesophageal balloon distention have been reported in some of these patients.[757] These observations suggest that some patients with this syndrome may not have cardiac disease at all.

CLINICAL FEATURES. The syndrome of angina or angina-like chest pain with normal epicardial arteries occurs more frequently in women,[758] many of whom are premenopausal, whereas obstructive CAD is found more commonly in men and postmenopausal women. Fewer than half of the patients with syndrome X have typical angina pectoris; the majority have a variety of forms of atypical chest pain. Although the features are frequently atypical, the chest pain may nonetheless be severe and disabling.[758] The condition may be benign in regard to survival, but it may have adverse effects on the quality of life, employment, and increased use of health care resources.

In some patients with minimal or no coronary disease, an exaggerated preoccupation with personal health is associated with the chest pain, and panic disorder may be responsible in a proportion of such patients.[754] Potts and Bass found that two-thirds of patients with chest pain and normal coronary arteries have predominantly psychiatric disorders.[758a] Others have reported that the incidence of obstructive CAD is extremely low in patients with atypical chest pain who are anxious and/or depressed.[759,760] The association between syndrome X and insulin resistance warrants further study.

FINDINGS ON PHYSICAL AND LABORATORY EXAMINATION. Abnormal physical findings reflecting ischemia, such as a precordial bulge, gallop sound, and the murmur of mitral regurgitation, are uncommon in syndrome X. The resting electrocardiogram may be normal, but nonspecific ST-T wave abnormalities are often observed, sometimes occurring in association with the chest pain. Approximately 20 per cent of patients with chest pain and normal coronary arteriograms have positive exercise tests. However, many of the patients with this syndrome fail to complete the exercise test, discontinuing because of fatigue or mild chest discomfort. Left ventricular function is usually normal at rest and during stress,[746] unlike the situation in obstructive CAD in which function often becomes impaired during stress. A small percentage of patients with syndrome X exhibit lactate production and ST-segment depression during exercise, signifying significant ischemia. Some patients show abnormal myocardial perfusion reserve, but there is no consistent pattern of abnormal myocardial blood flow.

PROGNOSIS. Important prognostic information on patients with angina and either normal or nearly normal coronary arteriograms has been obtained from the CASS registry.[761] In patients with an ejection fraction of 50 per cent or more, the 7-year survival rate was 96 per cent for patients with a normal arteriogram and 92 per cent for those whose arteriographic study revealed mild disease (< 50 per cent luminal stenosis). In such patients, an ischemic response to exercise was not associated with increased mortality, although a history of smoking or hypertension was. Thus, long-term survival of patients with anginal chest pain and normal coronary angiograms is excellent, markedly better than in patients with obstructive CAD and no different from that in an age-matched general population.[750,751,762,763] Nonetheless, the symptoms are persistent, and most patients continue to experience chest pain leading to repeated cardiac catheterizations and hospital admissions.[750,764]

MANAGEMENT. In patients with angina-like chest pain

syndrome and normal epicardial coronary arteries, esophageal abnormalities should be considered (see p. 1291). Such patients may show either motility disorders of the esophagus or abnormal reflux. Exercise electrocardiography and/or myocardial perfusion scintigraphy are often helpful in excluding obstructive CAD. When a noninvasive stress test is positive, or even in patients with serious disability and multiple hospital admissions in whom it is negative, the documentation of normal coronary arteries by coronary angiography provides an objective basis for firm reassurance.

In patients with the syndrome in whom ischemia can be demonstrated by noninvasive stress testing, a trial of anti-ischemic therapy with nitrates and beta blockers is logical, but the response to this therapy is often poor.[751] In contrast to patients with organic coronary artery disease, sublingual nitrates are ineffective in improving exercise tolerance in patients with syndrome X, and, in some, exercise tolerance may further deteriorate.[765] Calcium antagonists are effective in reducing the frequency and severity of angina and improving exercise tolerance in some patients. When these conditions are present, the treatment of esophageal reflux and dysmotility may be effective.

Estrogen has been shown to attenuate normal coronary vasomotor responses to acetylcholine, to increase coronary blood flow, and to potentiate endothelium-dependent vasodilation in postmenopausal women.[766,767] Although estrogen would therefore seem to be a logical treatment for postmenopausal women with syndrome X, its clinical effectiveness in these patients has yet to be documented. Imipramine (50 mg) has been reported to be helpful in some patients.[755]

SILENT MYOCARDIAL ISCHEMIA

Two forms of silent myocardial ischemia are recognized. The first and less common form, designated type I silent ischemia, occurs in patients with obstructive CAD, sometimes severe, who *do not experience angina at any time;* some type I patients do not even experience pain in the course of myocardial infarction. Epidemiological studies of sudden death (Chap. 24), as well as clinical and postmortem studies of patients with silent myocardial infarction, and studies of patients with chronic angina pectoris suggest that many patients with extensive coronary artery obstruction never experience angina pectoris in any of its recognized forms (stable, unstable, or variant).[768] These patients with type I silent ischemia may be considered to have a defective anginal warning system. Both the patient and physician may be unaware of the presence of ischemic heart disease until a fatal event ensues or an infarction is detected on routine electrocardiogram.

In the Framingham Study, one-quarter of patients who developed myocardial infarction had unrecognized infarctions, detected only by pathological Q waves on routine 2-year electrocardiogram, and of these approximately half were truly silent.[769] This important observation has been confirmed.[770] In other patients, symptomatic myocardial infarction is the first clinical manifestation of CAD, although postmortem or angiographic studies indicate that severe coronary artherosclerosis must have existed prior to the infarction yet the patient had never complained of angina. Such patients with silent ischemia may be identified prior to such an event by an abnormal electrocardiogram (occasionally at rest, more commonly during exercise), by the presence of arrhythmias, or by means of coronary arteriography performed as a result of a positive exercise test.

The second and much more frequent form, designated type II silent ischemia, occurs in patients with the usual forms of chronic stable angina, unstable angina, and Prinzmetal's angina. When monitored, patients with this form of silent ischemia exhibit some episodes of ischemia that are associated with chest discomfort and other episodes that are not—i.e., episodes of silent (asymptomatic) ischemia. The "total ischemic burden" in these patients refers to the total period of ischemia, both symptomatic and asymptomatic.

AMBULATORY ELECTROCARDIOGRAPHY. The extensive use of ambulatory electrocardiographic monitoring has led to a greater appreciation of the high frequency of type II "silent" ischemia (Fig. 38–28).[768] It has become apparent that anginal pain is a poor indicator and an underestimator of the frequency of significant cardiac ischemia.[771–773] Exercise-induced hemodynamic changes indicative of myocardial ischemia (increasing left ventricular end-diastolic pressure and decreasing left ventricular ejection fraction) occur in patients with CAD, irrespective of the development of ischemic discomfort.[774] Ambulatory studies in patients with type II silent ischemia have demonstrated that, although increases in myocardial oxygen demand often lead to ischemia, many episodes of ischemia, both symptomatic and asymptomatic, are not preceded by an acceleration of heart rate or a rise in arterial pressure. This suggests that reductions in myocardial oxygen supply make an important contribution to the initiation of both symptomatic and asymptomatic ischemic episodes in these patients.[775]

Transient ST-segment depression of 0.1 mV or more that lasts for more than 30 seconds is a very rare finding in normal subjects.[776] Patients with known CAD show a strong correlation between such transient ST-segment depression and independent measurements of impaired regional myocardial perfusion and ischemia using rubidium-82 uptake measured by positron-emission tomography.[777,778] In patients with type II silent ischemia, perfusion defects occur in the same myocardial regions during symptomatic and asymptomatic episodes of ST-segment depression.

Type II silent ischemia is extremely common. Thus, analyses of ambulatory electrocardiograms in patients with exertion-induced angina suggest that the majority of ischemic episodes occurring during normal daily activities are, in fact, asymptomatic. Their frequency is such that it has been suggested that overt angina pectoris is merely the "tip of the ischemic iceberg." Episodes of silent ischemia have

been estimated to be present in approximately half of all patients with angina, although a higher prevalence has been reported in diabetics.[768–770] Episodes of ST-segment depression, both symptomatic and asymptomatic, exhibit a circadian rhythm and are more common in the morning.[773] Asymptomatic nocturnal ST-segment changes are almost invariably an indicator of two- or three-vessel CAD or left main coronary artery stenosis.

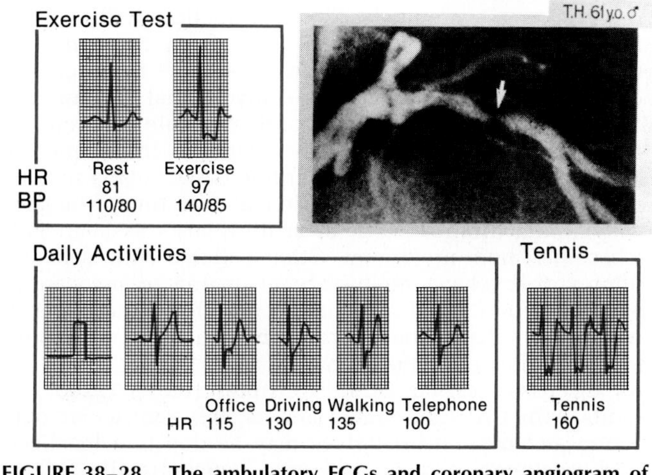

Pharmacological agents that reduce or abolish episodes of symptomatic ischemia, i.e., nitrates, beta blockers, and calcium antagonists, also reduce or abolish episodes of silent ischemia.[771,779]

MECHANISMS OF SILENT ISCHEMIA. It is not clear why some patients with unequivocal evidence of ischemia do not experience chest pain whereas others are symptomatic. Maseri has proposed that silent ischemia results from a variable combination of an increased sensitivity to painful stimuli and coronary microvascular dysfunction[1] (Fig. 38–29). Investigation into the causes of silent ischemia has focused primarily upon four areas: (1) The association between diabetes and both silent ischemia and "painless infarctions" has been attributed to an autonomic neuropathy.[781–784] (2) Patients with silent ischemia have been shown to have a high threshold for other forms of pain such as that resulting from electrical shocks or limb ischemia.[785,786] (3) These patients produce an excessive quantity of endogenous opioids (endorphins), which raise the pain threshold.[787,788] (4) In patients with type II silent ischemia, the asymptomatic episodes may result from a less severe ischemia than the symptomatic episodes. In some of these patients, shorter periods of ischemia on Holter electrocardiography tend to be asymptomatic, whereas longer periods are accompanied by angina.[788–790a] It is not clear which of these four possibilities or a combination plays a dominant role in the production of silent ischemia.

PROGNOSIS. Irrespective of the mechanism(s) responsible, ample evidence supports the view that myocardial ischemia, regardless of whether it is symptomatic or asymptomatic, is of prognostic importance in patients with CAD. The presence of frequent and accelerating episodes of ST-segment depression on ambulatory electrocardiography, whether silent or symptomatic, identifies a group of patients with CAD at higher risk of subsequent events than patients with fewer or no such episodes.[779,791] In asymptomatic patients, the presence of exercise-induced ST-segment depression has been shown to predict a four- to fivefold increase in cardiac mortality compared with those without this finding.[792] It has been reported that multiple episodes of asymptomatic ischemia detected by ambulatory electrocardiography are a predictor of an adverse outcome,[793] but it is not clear that the detection of such episodes contributes *independent* prognostic information.[780,780a]

Whereas the adverse prognosis of asymptomatic but electrocardiographically abnormal stress tests is clear, the clinical value of the detection of silent ischemia by ambulatory electrocardiographic monitoring has not been established. Exercise electrocardiography can identify the majority of patients likely to have significant ischemia during their daily activities[791] and remains the most important screening test for significant CAD. Many patients with type I silent ischemia have been identified because of an asymptomatic positive exercise electrocardiogram obtained following a myocardial infarction. In such patients with a defective anginal warning system, it is reasonable to assume that asymptomatic ischemia has a significance similar to symptomatic ischemia and that their management with respect to coronary angiography and revascularization should be similar.

MANAGEMENT. Drugs that are effective in preventing episodes of symptomatic ischemia (nitrates, calcium antagonists, and beta blockers) are effective in reducing or eliminating episodes of silent ischemia as well[794,795] (Fig. 38–

FIGURE 38–28. The ambulatory ECGs and coronary angiogram of a severe left anterior descending stenosis in a patient with fatigue (but not angina) during a tennis match. In stage II of a treadmill exercise test (Bruce protocol), 4 mm of ST-segment depression were seen in lead V_5. Ambulatory Holter monitoring of lead V_5 demonstrates ischemic ST-segment depressions during a number of ordinary activities, e.g., walking, telephoning. During a game of tennis, marked ST-segment depression was recorded when the patient was asymptomatic. (Reproduced with permission from Nabel, E. G., et al.: Characteristics and significance of ischemia detected by ambulatory electrocardiographic monitoring. Circulation 75[Suppl. II]:74, 1987. Copyright American Heart Association.)

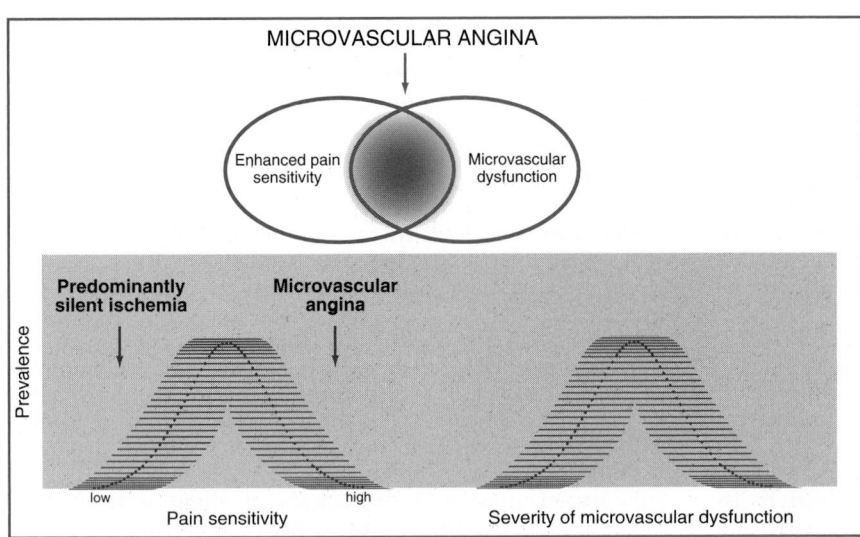

FIGURE 38–29. Proposed pathogenetic mechanisms of microvascular angina. The syndrome results from a variable combination of two components: an increased sensitivity to painful stimuli associated with a coronary microvascular dysfunction (indicated by recurring ST-segment depression), both of which have a bell-shaped prevalence in the population. Furthermore, within any individual, either component may vary in time (indicated by the horizontal lines). In patients with a markedly enhanced sensitivity to pain, even a minimal microvascular dysfunction can cause angina. Conversely, some patients with severe microvascular dysfunction (indicated by recurring ST-segment depression) may not come to medical attention if they have a normal or a low sensitivity to pain. (From Maseri, A.: Ischemic Heart Disease. New York, Churchill Livingstone, 1995, p. 522.)

30). In one randomized study, metoprolol was superior to diltiazem in reducing the mean number of ischemic episodes and mean duration of ischemia.[796] Nitrates are helpful. A combination of a beta blocker and a calcium antagonist is superior to either class of drug alone in suppressing ischemia detected by ambulatory electrocardiography. Although the suppression of ischemia in patients with asymptomatic ischemia is a worthwhile objective, whether treatment should be guided by symptoms or by ischemia as reflected in ambulatory electrocardiography has not been established. The Asymptomatic Cardiac Ischemia Pilot (ACIP) study demonstrated that cardiac ischemia can be suppressed in 40 to 55 per cent of patients with either medication or revascularization, but the outcomes were similar between patients assigned to an "ischemia-guided" strategy as opposed to an "angina-guided" strategy.[797–797d] These data have provided the foundation for a prospective, large randomized trial, including coronary revascularization as one of the therapeutic modalities.

HEART FAILURE

Manifestations of congestive heart failure are common in patients with chronic CAD. Heart failure may be the dominant clinical feature in some patients, especially those who have sustained prior myocardial infarction(s), in whom ischemic areas have become replaced with a fibrous scar, leading to disappearance or reduction of the angina. The three most common causes of congestive heart failure are (1) an inadequate quantity of normally contracting myocardium, (2) left ventricular aneurysm, and (3) mitral regurgitation due to papillary muscle dysfunction. The first is the most common of the three.

Ischemic Cardiomyopathy

In 1970 Burch and colleagues first used the term *ischemic cardiomyopathy* to describe the condition in which CAD results in severe myocardial dysfunction, with clinical manifestations often indistinguishable from those of primary dilated cardiomyopathy (see p. 1407).[798] Symptoms of heart failure, caused by ischemic myocardial dysfunction (hibernation), diffuse fibrosis, and multiple infarctions, alone or in combination, may dominate the clinical picture of CAD. In some patients with chronic CAD, angina may be the principal clinical manifestation at one time, but later this symptom diminishes or even disappears as heart failure becomes more prominent. Other patients with ischemic cardiomyopathy have no history of angina or myocardial infarction (type I silent ischemia, see p. 1344), and it is in this subgroup that ischemic cardiomyopathy is often confused with dilated cardiomyopathy.

As discussed earlier in this chapter (see p. 1293), in patients with CAD and stable angina, left ventricular dysfunction and overt heart failure may be due to a localized infarct, scattered fibrosis, ischemic noncontractile (hibernating) myocardium, or some combination of these. A similar situation exists in patients without angina who present with heart failure and little or no angina as their primary manifestation of CAD. It is important to recognize hibernating myocardium in patients with ischemic cardiomyopathy because symptoms resulting from chronic left ventricular dysfunction may be incorrectly thought to result from necrotic and scarred myocardium rather than from a reversible ischemic process. Hibernating myocardium may be present in patients with known or suspected CAD with a

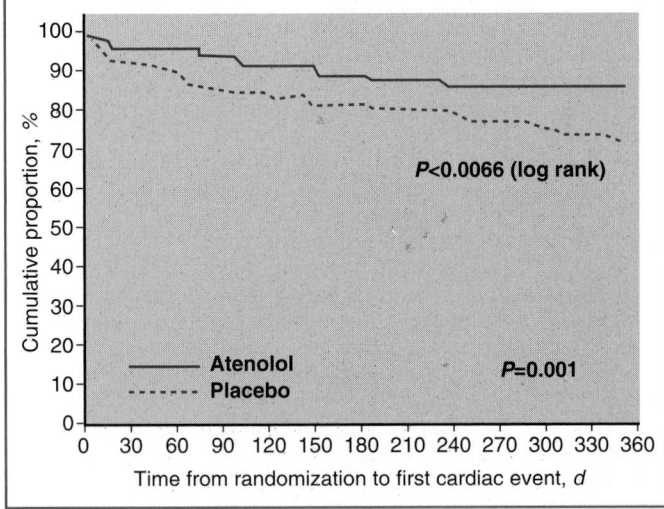

FIGURE 38–30. Atenolol in silent ischemia trial (ASIST). The recently reported ASIST is the first controlled trial to demonstrate modification of cardiac risk through treatment of silent myocardial ischemia (SMI). A total of 306 asymptomatic or minimally symptomatic patients with coronary artery disease, positive exercise tests, and ambulatory electrocardiographic (ECG episodes) of SMI were randomized to receive atenolol or placebo. Ambulatory ECG monitoring was repeated at 4 weeks, and outcome was assessed after 1 year. At 4 weeks, atenolol was associated with a significant reduction in SMI. After 1 year, a significant (56 per cent) relative reduction in adverse events (death, resuscitated ventricular tachycardia and fibrillation, nonfatal myocardial infarction, and unstable or worsening angina) was found when patients given atenolol were compared with those given placebo. The presence of ischemia at 4 weeks was the most important independent factor associated with adverse outcomes after 1 year. (From Bertolet, B. D., and Pepine, C. J.: Silent Myocardial Ischemia. *In* Beller, G. A. and Braunwald, E. [eds.]: Chronic Ischemic Heart Disease. Atlas of Heart Diseases, vol. 5. Philadelphia, Current Medicine, 1995, p. 8.9.)

degree of cardiac dysfunction or heart failure not readily accounted for by prior myocardial infarctions.

The outlook for patients with ischemic cardiomyopathy treated medically is quite poor, and revascularization or cardiac transplantation may be considered.[799] The prognosis is particularly poor in patients in whom the ischemic cardiomyopathy is secondary to multiple myocardial infarctions and in those with associated ventricular arrhythmias. On the other hand, patients whose heart failure, even if severe, is secondary to large segments of reversibly injured but viable (hibernating) myocardium have a better prognosis following revascularization. Thus, the key to the management of patients with ischemic cardiomyopathy is to assess the extent of residual viable myocardium with a view to coronary revascularization. Techniques for detecting hibernating myocardium are described on p. 1327.

Left Ventricular Aneurysm

This is usually defined as a segment of the ventricular wall that exhibits paradoxical (dyskinetic) systolic expansion. Chronic fibrous aneurysms interfere with ventricular performance principally through loss of contractile tissue. Aneurysms made up largely of a mixture of scar tissue and viable myocardium or of thin scar tissue also cause a mechanical disadvantage by a combination of paradoxical expansion and loss of effective contraction. *False aneurysms* (pseudoaneurysms) represent localized myocardial rupture, in which the hemorrhage is limited by pericardial adhesions, and have a mouth that is considerably smaller than the maximal diameter (Fig. 38–31).

The frequency of ventricular aneurysms depends on the incidence of transmural myocardial infarction and congestive heart failure in the population studied. Left ventricular aneurysm can also result from myocardial infarction secondary to blunt chest trauma.[800] More than 80 per cent of left ventricular aneurysms are located anterolaterally near the apex. They are often associated with total occlusion of the left anterior descending coronary artery and a poor collateral blood supply.[801] Approximately 5 to 10 per cent of aneurysms are located posteriorly. Three-quarters of patients with aneurysms have multivessel CAD.[802]

Almost half of the patients with moderate or large aneurysms have symptoms of heart failure (with or without associated angina), a third have severe angina alone, and approximately 15 per cent have symptomatic ventricular arrhythmias, which may be intractable and life threatening.[803] Mural thrombi are found in almost half of patients with chronic left ventricular aneurysms and can be detected by angiography and two-dimensional echocardiography (Fig. 3–93, p. 88). Systemic embolic events in patients with thrombi in left ventricular aneurysms tend to occur within the initial 4 to 6 months after infarction.

DETECTION. Clues to the presence of aneurysm include persistent ST-segment elevations on the resting electrocardiogram (in the absence of chest pain) and a characteristic bulge of the silhouette of the left ventricle on a chest roentgenogram (see p. 228). These findings, when clear-cut, are relatively specific, but they have limited sensitivity. Radionuclide ventriculography and two-dimensional echocardiography can demonstrate ventricular aneurysm more readily; the latter is also helpful in distinguishing between true and false aneurysms, based upon the demonstration of a narrow neck in relationship to cavity size in the latter.[804] Color-flow echocardiographic imaging is useful in establishing the diagnosis because flow "in and out" of the aneurysm as well as abnormal flow within the aneurysm can be detected, and subsequent pulsed Doppler imaging can reveal a "to-and-fro" pattern with characteristic respiratory variation of the peak systolic velocity.[804] Computed

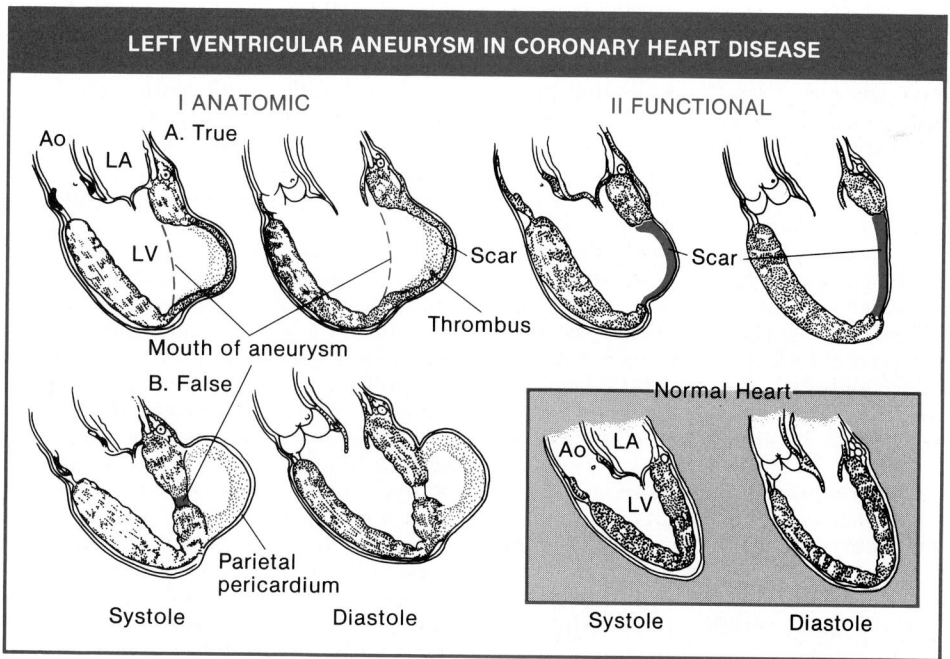

FIGURE 38–31. Hearts in systole and diastole with true and false anatomical and functional left ventricular aneurysms and healed myocardial infarction. A normal heart in systole and diastole is shown for comparison. The true anatomical left ventricular aneurysm protrudes during both systole and diastole, has a mouth that is as wide as or wider than the maximal diameter, has a wall that was formerly the wall of the left ventricle, and is composed of fibrous tissue with or without residual myocardial fibers. A true aneurysm may or may not contain thrombus and almost never ruptures once the wall is healed. The false anatomical left ventricular aneurysm protrudes during both systole and diastole, has a mouth that is considerably smaller than the maximal diameter of the aneurysm and represents a myocardial rupture site, has a wall made up of parietal pericardium, virtually always contains thrombus, and often ruptures. The functional left ventricular aneurysm protrudes during ventricular systole but not during diastole and consists of fibrous tissue with or without myocardial fibers. (From Cabin, H. S., and Roberts, W. C.: Left ventricular aneurysm, intraaneurysmal thrombus and systemic embolus in coronary heart disease. Chest 77:586, 1980.)

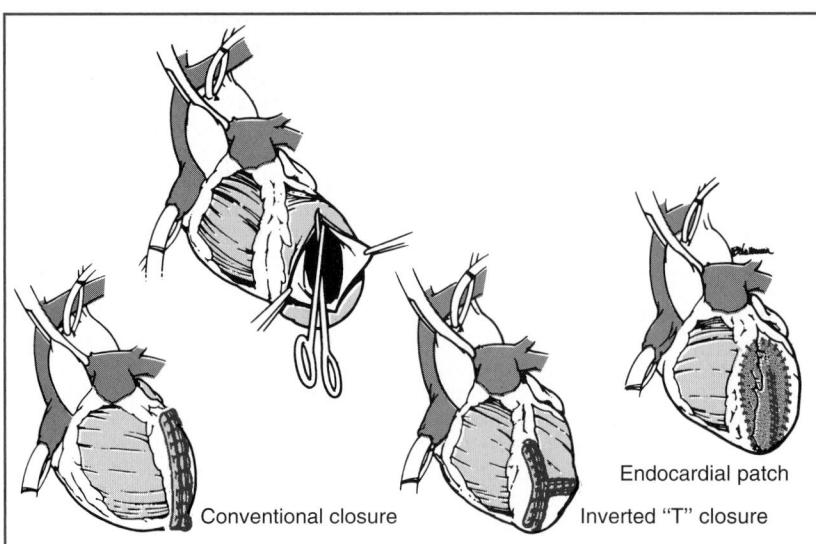

FIGURE 38–32. Operative techniques used in left ventricular aneurysm repair. The figure depicts resection of the ventricular aneurysm enclosure by one of three methods. The conventional closure is illustrated on the left. The "T" closure and the endocardial patch techniques were developed in an attempt to restore normal left ventricular geometry. (From Komeda, M., David, T. E., Malik, A., et al.: Operative risks and long-term results of operation for left ventricular aneurysm. Ann. Thorac. Surg. *53:*22, 1992.)

tomography and magnetic resonance imaging are reliable noninvasive techniques for the identification of left ventricular aneurysms (Fig. 10–34, p. 337) and screening for resectability.[805] However, biplane left ventriculography remains the most precise method available for outlining a true left ventricular aneurysm, assessing septal motion, and determining the quantity of functioning residual myocardium.

LEFT VENTRICULAR ANEURYSMECTOMY. True ventricular aneurysms do not rupture, and operative excision is carried out to improve the clinical manifestations, most often heart failure, but sometimes also angina, embolization, and life-threatening tachyarrhythmias.[803,806] Coronary revascularization is frequently carried out along with aneurysmectomy, especially in patients in whom angina accompanies heart failure.

A large left ventricular aneurysm in a patient with symptoms of heart failure, particularly if angina pectoris is also present, is an indication for operation. The operative mortality rate for left ventricular aneurysmectomy is approximately 10 per cent (ranging from 2 to 19 per cent).[806,807] Risk factors for early death include poor left ventricular function, recent myocardial infarction, the presence of mitral regurgitation, and intractable ventricular arrhythmias.[807–809] Operation carries a particularly high risk in patients with severe heart failure, a low-output state, and akinesis of the interventricular septum, as assessed echocardiographically.[810] Akinesis or dyskinesia of the posterior basal segment of the left ventricle and significant right coronary artery stenoses are additional risk factors.[810] Pseudoaneurysms rupture frequently and should therefore be resected on an urgent basis as soon as the diagnosis is established.[811]

Risk factors for late mortality following survival from operation include incomplete revascularization, impaired systolic function of the basal segments of the ventricle and of the septum not involved by the aneurysm, the presence of a large aneurysm with a small quantity of residual viable myocardium, and the presence of severe cardiac failure as the presenting feature.

Improvement in left ventricular function has been reported in survivors of resection of left ventricular aneurysms complicated by cardiac failure.[808,809] A concomitant improvement in exercise performance may also occur, particularly in patients who have undergone complete revascularization. In patients carefully selected for surgical treatment, 70 to 80 per cent of survivors are in NYHA Class I or II after 5 years, with a 10-year actuarial survival of 69 per cent in patients undergoing left ventricular aneurysmectomy and revascularization, compared with 57 per cent in those undergoing left ventricular aneurysmectomy alone.[812]

New surgical approaches to the repair of left ventricular aneurysms are designed to restore normal left ventricular geometry by using an alternative method of epicardial closure and/or an endocardial patch to divide the area of the aneurysm from the remainder of the ventricular cavity (Fig. 38–32).[813–815]

Mitral Regurgitation Secondary to Coronary Artery Disease

Mitral regurgitation is an important cause of heart failure in some patients with CAD. Rupture of a papillary muscle, or of the head of a papillary muscle, usually causes severe acute mitral regurgitation in the course of acute myocardial infarction (Fig. 37–40, p. 1243). Chronic mitral regurgitation in patients with CAD is most commonly caused by papillary muscle dysfunction due to ischemia or fibrosis[816] in concert with a wall motion abnormality in the region of the papillary muscle (Fig. 32–10, p. 1019) and/or by dilatation of the mitral annulus; many of the latter patients have ventricular aneurysms. Most patients with chronic CAD and mitral regurgitation have suffered a prior myocardial infarction.

Clinical features that help to identify mitral regurgitation due to papillary muscle dysfunction as the cause of acute pulmonary edema or of milder symptoms of left-sided failure include a loud systolic murmur and demonstration of a flail mitral valve leaflet on echocardiography. The latter is the preferred diagnostic technique because the timing and duration of the murmur are variable. Instead of being only mid to late systolic, as was originally thought, murmurs may be holosystolic or early systolic. Doppler echocardiography is helpful in assessing the severity of the regurgitation (see p. 72).

As in mitral regurgitation of other causes, the left atrium is usually not greatly enlarged unless mitral regurgitation has been present for more than 6 months (Fig. 32–14, p. 1021). The electrocardiogram is nonspecific, and most patients have angiographic evidence of multivessel CAD. In patients with ischemic mitral regurgitation, in addition to the severity of regurgitation, advanced age, comorbid disorders (renal failure or pulmonary dysfunction), ventricular dysfunction, the need for intensive care management, and the extent of CAD all influence long-term survival adversely.[316]

In patients with posterior papillary muscle dysfunction resulting from acute myocardial infarction, reperfusion therapy with thrombolysis or PTCA may be attempted initially because urgent surgery is often accompanied by a very high hospital mortality. In patients with rupture of a papillary muscle, or, more frequently, one or more heads of a papillary muscle, immediate surgery is required provided that there is a chance of satisfactory outcome.[817] The procedure of choice, when possible, is mitral valve repair rather than replacement. The decision is based upon the anatomical characteristics of the structures comprising the mitral valve apparatus, the urgency of the need for surgery, and individual expertise.

Ischemic mitral regurgitation secondary to dilatation of the mitral annulus is common in patients with ischemic cardiomyopathy and can intensify the severity of the left ventricular failure. Improvement of left ventricular function by medical therapy with reduction of left ventricular volume and the annular diameter reduces the severity of mitral regurgitation (see p. 1026). Direct surgical treatment of the mitral valve is not indicated in these patients, although if other indications are present multivessel myocardial revascularization may be helpful.

CARDIAC ARRHYTHMIAS

Various degrees and forms of ventricular ectopic activity are the most common arrhythmias in patients with chronic CAD. In some patients with CAD, cardiac arrhythmias are the dominant clinical manifestation of the disease. That there is a substantial subgroup of patients with CAD and occult arrhythmias is suggested by the frequency with which sudden death is the first manifestation of this condition. The frequency and severity of ventricular arrhythmias induced during exercise tests and ambulatory monitoring correlate, in general, with the degree of arteriographically documented CAD. Patients with severe left ventricular dysfunction associated with multivessel disease have more high-grade ectopic activity than do those with normal ventricular function and single-vessel disease.

The recognition and management of patients with malignant ventricular arrhythmias and/or sudden cardiac death due to chronic CAD are discussed in detail in Chap. 24.

NONATHEROMATOUS CORONARY ARTERY DISEASE

Although atherosclerosis is, by far, the most important cause of CAD, a number of other conditions may also be responsible.[818,818a] The most common causes of nonatheromatous CAD resulting in myocardial ischemia are the syndrome of angina-like pain with normal coronary arteriograms, i.e., so-called syndrome X, and Prinzmetal's angina, both of which have been discussed earlier in this chapter (see pp. 1343 and 1340).

Nonatheromatous CAD may also result from diverse abnormalities. These include congenital abnormalities in the origin or distribution of the coronary arteries (see pp. 908 and 967). The most important of these are anomalous origin of a coronary artery (usually the left) from the pulmonary artery, origin of both coronary arteries from either the right or left sinus of Valsalva, and coronary arteriovenous fistula. Anomalous origin of either the left main coronary artery or right coronary artery from the aorta with subsequent coursing between the aorta and pulmonary trunk is a rare and sometimes fatal coronary arterial anomaly.[819]

In an autopsy study of 150 cases of sudden death in persons 35 years or younger, death was attributed to CAD in 48. In 16 of these, the disease was not atherosclerosis but attributable to abnormalities in the origin and course of the coronary arteries, including a deep intramyocardial course, ostial obstruction, an abnormal origin of the right or left coronary artery, or spontaneous dissection of a coronary artery. In one patient, effort-induced acute myocardial infarction was noted in the presence of an intramural coronary arterial trunk.[820]

A number of inherited connective tissue disorders are associated with myocardial ischemia. These include the Marfan syndrome (causing aortic and coronary artery dissection; p. 1671), Hurler syndrome (causing coronary obstruction), homocystinuria (causing coronary artery thrombosis; p. 1673), Ehlers-Danlos syndrome (coronary artery dissection; p. 1672), and pseudoxanthoma elasticum (causing accelerated CAD; p. 1673). Kawasaki disease (the mucocutaneous lymph node syndrome) may cause coronary artery aneurysms and ischemic heart disease in children (p. 994).

Spontaneous dissection of a coronary artery can cause unheralded myocardial infarction and sudden death and is often discovered first at postmortem examination. Two-thirds of the described cases have occurred in women, and one-half of these were associated with the postpartum state.[821] In patients who survive spontaneous coronary artery dissection, there is a 20 per cent mortality over the subsequent 3 years. In general, coronary revascularization is recommended, particularly in patients who have ongoing ischemia.

Coronary vasculitis due to connective tissue diseases or autoimmune forms of vasculitis, including polyarteritis nodosum,[822] giant-cell [temporal] arteritis,[823] and scleroderma,[824] is well described (Chap. 56). Coronary arteritis is seen at autopsy in about 20 per cent of patients with rheumatoid arthritis but is rarely associated with clinical manifestations.[825] The incidence of CAD is increased in women

with systemic lupus erythematosus.[826] In patients with systemic lupus erythematosus CAD has been attributed to a vasculitis, immune complex–mediated endothelial damage, and coronary thrombosis due to antiphospholipid antibodies,[826–828] as well as to accelerated atherosclerosis (see p. 1779). The antiphospholipid syndrome, which presents with arterial and venous thrombosis and is associated with the presence of antiphospholipid antibodies, may be associated with myocardial infarction, angina, and diffuse left ventricular dysfunction.[828]

Rarely, *Takayasu's arteritis* (see p. 1572) is associated with angina, myocardial infarction, and cardiac failure in patients under the age of 40 years.[829] Coronary blood flow may be decreased by involvement of the ostia or proximal segments of the coronary arteries, but disease of distal coronary segments is rare.[830,831] The average age of onset of symptoms is 24 years, and event-free survival at 10 years after diagnosis is approximately 60 percent.[829] Luetic aortitis may also produce myocardial ischemia by causing obstruction of coronary ostia (see p. 1441).

An unusual cause of nonatherosclerotic coronary artery disease, but one that is well described, is radiation-induced coronary stenosis following radiation therapy[832] (see p. 1799). Radiation injury may be latent and may not be manifest clinically for many years after therapy, and it has been suggested that hypercholesterolemia may exacerbate the process.[833]

Myocardial ischemia not caused by coronary atherosclerosis can also result from embolism, infective endocarditis (Chap. 33), implanted prosthetic cardiac valves (Chap. 32), calcified aortic valves, mural thrombi, and primary cardiac tumors (Chap. 42).

An interesting nonatherosclerotic myocardial ischemic syndrome has been described in workers in the nitrate industry who apparently experience nitrate withdrawal symptoms on weekends. It is presumed to be secondary to coronary spasm when there is no counterstimulation to the vasoconstriction that they undergo as an adaptation to the vasodilating actions of the high concentrations of nitrates to which they have been exposed (see p. 1302).[834]

Cocaine use is a well-documented cause of chest pain and in particular acute myocardial infarction.[834a]

CARDIAC TRANSPLANT–ASSOCIATED CORONARY ARTERIOPATHY (see p. 525). This condition is frequently observed in cardiac transplant survivors. It is a rapidly evolving, diffuse, concentric arteriosclerosis involving epicardial and intramural coronary vessels.[835,836] It is presumed to be caused by chronic immune injury to the coronary endothelium of the donor heart, but the precise mechanism and risk factors have not been clarified. Other suggested etiologic factors include opportunistic infections (cytomegalovirus infection), immunosuppressive therapy, cyclosporine-induced endothelial injury, and elevated lipid levels. Acute myocardial infarction can result, and this complication is usually not accompanied by chest pain or typical electrocardiographic changes. Infarction in these patients is associated with a high mortality rate, and, at anatomical examination, there is diffuse disease of the coronary arteries and multiple foci of nontransmural cardiac infarction. The management of this form of CAD is difficult, usually requires a second cardiac transplantation, and is discussed on p. 526.

REFERENCES

1. Maseri, A.: Ischemic Heart Disease. New York, Churchill Livingstone, 1995, 713 pp.
2. Centers for Disease Control and Prevention: National Center for Health Statistics, National Vital Statistics and The United States Bureau of the Census. Health, United States 1993, p. 31.
3. AHA: Heart and Stroke Facts: 1995 Statistical Supplement. Dallas, American Heart Association, 1995.
3a. Kannel, W. B.: Incidence, prevalence, and mortality of coronary artery disease. In Fuster, V., Ross, R., and Topol, E. J. (eds.): Atherosclerosis and Coronary Artery Disease. Philadelphia, Lippincott, 1996, pp. 13–24.
4. Goldberg, R. J., Gorak, E. J., Yarzebski, J., et al.: A community-wide perspective of sex differences and temporal trends in the incidence and survival rates after acute myocardial infarction out-of-hospital deaths caused by coronary heart disease. Circulation 87:1947, 1993.
5. Davis, D. L., Dinse, G. E., and Hoeld, G.: Decreasing cardiovascular disease and increasing cancer among whites in the U.S.A. from 1972 through 1987. JAMA 271:431, 1994.
6. Virmani, R., and Forman, M. B.: Nonatherosclerotic Ischemic Heart Disease. 1st ed. New York, Raven Press, 1989.

STABLE ANGINA PECTORIS

7. Matthews, M. B., and Julian, D. G.: Angina pectoris: Definition and description. In Julian, D. G. (ed.): Angina Pectoris, 2nd ed. New York, Churchill Livingstone, 1985, p. 2.
8. Christie, L. G., Jr., and Conti, C. R.: Systematic approach to evaluation of angina-like chest pain: Pathophysiology and clinical testing with emphasis on objective documentation of myocardial ischemia. Am. Heart J. 102:897, 1981.
8a. DeServi, S., Arbustini, E., Marsico, F., et al.: Correlation between clinical and morphologic findings in unstable angina. Am. J. Cardiol. 77:128, 1996.
9. Angina pectoris. In Fowler, N. O. (ed.): Diagnosis of Heart Disease. New York, Springer-Verlag, 1991, pp. 187–206.
10. Cook, D. G., and Shaper, A. G.: Breathlessness, angina pectoris, and coronary artery disease. Am. J. Cardiol. 63:921, 1989.

11. Andrews, T. C., Fenton, T., Toyosaki, N., et al.: Subsets of ambulatory myocardial ischemia based on heart rate activity: Circadian distribution and response to anti-ischemic medication. Circulation 88:92, 1993.

12. Marber, M. S., Joy, M. D., and Yellond, M.: Is warm-up in angina ischemic preconditioning? Br. Heart J. 72(Edit.):213, 1994.

13. Constant, J.: The clinical diagnosis of nonanginal chest pain: The differentiation of angina from nonanginal chest pain by history. Clin. Cardiol. 6:11, 1983.

14. Maseri, A., Crea, F., Kaski, J. C., and Davies, G.: Mechanisms and significance of cardiac ischemic pain. Prog. Cardiovasc. Dis. 35:1, 1992.

15. Janes, R. D., Brandys, J. C., Hopkins, D. A., et al.: Anatomy of human extrinsic cardiac nerves and ganglia. Am. J. Cardiol. 57:299, 1986.

16. Rosen, S. D., Paulesu, E., and Frith, C. D.: Central nervous pathways mediating angina pectoris. Lancet 344:147, 1994.

17. Crea, F., Pupita, G., Galassi, A. R., et al.: Role of adenosine in pathogenesis of anginal pain. Circulation 81:164, 1990.

18. Lam, H. G., Dekker, W., Kan, G., et al.: Esophageal dysfunction as a cause of angina pectoris ("linked angina"): Does it exist? Am. J. Med. 96:359, 1994.

19. Davies, H. A., Jones, D. B., Rhodes, J., and Newcombe, R. G.: Angina-like esophageal pain: Differentiation from cardiac pain by history. J. Clin. Gastroenterol. 7:477, 1985.

20. Henderson, R. D., Wigle, E. D., Sample, K., and Marryatt, G.: Atypical chest pain of cardiac and esophageal origin. Chest 73:24, 1978.

21. Brand, D. L., Ilves, R., and Pope, C. E.: Evaluation of esophageal function in patients with central chest pain. Acta Med. Scand. 644(Suppl.):53, 1981.

22. Bernstein, L. M., Fruin, R. C., and Pacini, R.: Differentiation of esophageal pain from angina pectoris: Role of the esophageal acid perfusion test. Medicine 41:143, 1962.

23. Henderson, R. D., and Maryatt, G.: Characteristics of esophageal pain. Acta Med. Scand. 544(Suppl.):49, 1981.

24. DeMeester, T. R., O'Sullivan, G. C., Bermudez, G., et al.: Esophageal function in patients with angina-type chest pain and normal coronary angiograms. Ann. Surg. 196:488, 1982.

25. Brand, D. L., Martin, D., and Pope, C. E.: Esophageal manometrics in patients with angina-like chest pain. Am. J. Dig. Dis. 22:300, 1977.

26. Epstein, S. E., Gerber, L. H., and Borer, J. S.: Chest wall syndrome: A common cause of unexplained cardiac pain. JAMA 241:2793, 1979.

27. Franklin, K. A., et al.: Sleep apnea and nocturnal angina. Lancet 345:1085, 1995.

28. Winder, A. F.: Relationship between corneal arcus and hyperlipidemia is clarified by studies in familial hypercholesterolaemia. Br. J. Ophthalmol. 67:789, 1983.

29. Segal, P., Insull, W., Chambless, L. E., et al.: The association of dyslipoproteinemia with corneal arcus and xanthelasma: The Lipid Research Clinic's Program Prevalence Study. Circulation 73:108, 1986.

30. Tranchesi, B., Jr., Barbosa, V., de Albuquerque, C. P., et al.: Diagonal earlobe crease as a marker of the presence and extent of coronary atherosclerosis. Am. J. Cardiol. 70:1417, 1992.

31. Gersh, B. J., Rihal, C. S., Rooke, T. W., and Ballard, D. J.: Evaluation and management of patients with both peripheral vascular and coronary artery disease. J. Am. Coll. Cardiol. 18:203, 1991.

32. Eagle, K. A., Rihal, C. S., Foster, E. D., et al.: Long-term survival in patients with coronary artery disease: Importance of peripheral vascular disease. J. Am. Coll. Cardiol. 23:1091, 1994.

33. Ogren, M., Hedblad, B., Isacsson, S. O., et al.: Non-invasively detected carotid stenosis and coronary heart disease in men with leg arteriosclerosis. Lancet 342:1138, 1993.

34. Cohn, P. F., Thompson, S., Strauss, W., et al.: Diastolic heart sounds during static (handgrip) exercise in patients with chest pain. Circulation 47:1217, 1973.

35. Heckerling, P. S., Weiner, S. L., Wolfkiel, C. J., et al.: Accuracy and reproducibility of precordial percussion and palpation for detecting increased left ventricular end-diastolic volume and mass: A comparison of physical findings and ultrafast computed tomography of the heart. JAMA 270:1943, 1993.

36. Ranganathan, N., Juma, Z., and Sivaciyan, V.: The apical impulse in coronary heart disease. Clin. Cardiol. 8:20, 1985.

37. Sangster, J. F., and Oakley, C. M.: Diastolic murmur of coronary artery stenosis. Br. Heart J. 35:840, 1973.

37a. Schwartz, G. G., and Karliner, J. S.: Pathophysiology of chronic stable angina. In Fuster, V., Ross, R., and Topol, E. J. (eds.): Atherosclerosis and Coronary Artery Disease. Philadelphia, J. B. Lippincott, 1996, pp. 1389–1400.

38. Jiang, W., Hayano, J., Coleman, E. R., et al.: Relation of cardiovascular responses to mental stress and cardiac vagal activity in coronary artery disease. Am. J. Cardiol. 72:551, 1993.

39. Boltwood, M. D., Taylor, C. B., Burke, M. B., et al.: Anger report predicts coronary artery vasomotor response to mental stress and atherosclerotic segments. Am. J. Cardiol. 72:1361, 1993.

40. Panza, J. A., Diodati, J. G., Callahan, T. S., et al.: Role of increase in heart rate in determining the occurrence and frequency of myocardial ischemia during daily life in patients with stable coronary artery disease. J. Am. Coll. Cardiol. 20:1092, 1992.

41. Hillis, L. D., and Braunwald, E.: Coronary artery spasm. N. Engl. J. Med. 299:695, 1978.

42. Ganz, P., Abben, R. P., and Barry, W. H.: Dynamic variations in resistance of coronary arterial narrowings in angina pectoris at rest. Am. J. Cardiol. 59:66, 1987.

43. Tousoulis, D., Davies, G., McFadden, E., et al.: Coronary vasomotor effects of serotonin in patients with angina. Circulation 88:1518, 1993.

44. Epstein, S. E., and Talbot, T. L.: Dynamic coronary tone in precipitation, exacerbation and relief of angina pectoris. Am. J. Cardiol. 48:797, 1981.

45. Maseri, A.: Medical therapy of chronic stable angina pectoris. Circulation 82:2258, 1990.

46. Benhorin, J., Banai, S., Moriel, M., et al.: Circadian variations in ischemic threshold and their relation to occurrence of ischemic episodes. Circulation 87:808, 1993.

47. Juneau, M., Johnstone, M., Dempsey, E., and Waters, D. D.: Exercise-induced myocardial ischemia in a cold environment: Effect of antianginal medications. Circulation 79:1015, 1989.

48. Epstein, S. E., Stampfer, M., Beiser, G. D., et al.: Effects of a reduction in environmental temperature on the circulatory response to exercise in man: Implications concerning angina pectoris. N. Engl. J. Med. 280:7, 1969.

49. Marchant, B., Donaldson, G., Mridha, K., et al.: Mechanisms of cold intolerance in patients with angina. J. Am. Coll. Cardiol. 23:630, 1994.

50. Gottdiener, J. S., Krantz, D. S., Howell, R. H., et al.: Induction of silent myocardial ischemia with mental stress testing: Relation to the triggers of ischemia during daily life activities and to ischemia's functional severity. J. Am. Coll. Cardiol. 24:1645, 1994.

51. Dodds, P. A., Bellamy, C. M., Muirhead, R. A., and Perry, R. A.: Vasoconstrictor peptides and cold intolerance in patients with stable angina pectoris. Br. Heart J. 73:25, 1995.

52. Colles, P., Juneau, M., Gregoire, J., et al.: Effect of a standardized meal on the threshold of exercise-induced myocardial ischemia in patients with stable angina. J. Am. Coll. Cardiol. 21:1052, 1993.

53. Maseri, A., Chierchia, S., and Keski, J. C.: Mixed angina pectoris. Am. J. Cardiol. 56:30E, 1985.

54. Parker, J. D., Testa, M. A., Jimenez, A. H., et al.: Morning increase and ambulatory ischemia in patients with stable coronary artery disease: Importance of physical activity in increased cardiac demand. Circulation 89:604, 1994.

55. Campeau, L.: Grading of angina pectoris. Circulation 54:522, 1976.

56. Goldman, L., Hashimoto, B., Cook, E. F., and Loscalzo, A.: Comparative reproducibility and validity of systems for assessing cardiovascular functional class: Advantages of a new specific activity scale. Circulation 64:1227, 1981.

57. Califf, R. M., Mark, D. B., Harrell, F. E., et al.: Importance of clinical measures of ischemia in the prognosis of patients with documented coronary artery disease. J. Am. Coll. Cardiol. 11:20, 1988.

58. Cox, J. L., Naylor, D., Johnstone, D. E., et al.: Limitations of Canadian Cardiovascular Society classification of angina pectoris. Am. J. Cardiol. 74:276, 1994.

59. Diamond, G. A., and Forrester, J. S.: Analysis of probability as an aid in the clincial diagnosis of coronary artery disease. N. Engl. J. Med. 300:1350, 1979.

60. Kannel, W. B., Anderson, K., and McGee, D. L.: Nonspecific electrocardiographic abnormality as a predictor of coronary heart disease: The Framingham Study. Am. Heart J. 113:370, 1987.

61. Mirvis, D. M., El-Zeky, F., Vander Zwaag, R., et al.: Clinical and pathophysiologic correlates of ST-T wave abnormalities in coronary artery disease. Am. J. Cardiol. 66:699, 1990.

62. Miranda, C. P., Lehmann, K. G., and Froehlicher, V. F.: Correlation between resting ST segment depression, exercise testing, coronary angiography, and long-term prognosis. Am. Heart J. 122:1617, 1991.

63. Crenshaw, J. H., Mirvis, D. M., El-Zeky, F., et al.: Interactive effects of ST-T wave abnormalities on survival of patients with coronary artery disease. J. Am. Coll. Cardiol. 18:1413, 1991.

64. Hamby, R. I., Weissman, R. H., Prakash, M. N., and Hoffman, L.: Left bundle branch block: A predictor of poor left ventricular function in coronary artery disease. Am. Heart J. 106:471, 1983.

65. Hammermeister, K. E., DeRouen, T. A., and Dodge, H. T.: Variables predictive of survival in patients with coronary disease: Selection by univariate and multivariate analyses from the clinical, electrocardiographic, exercise, arteriographic, and quantitative angiographic evaluations. Circulation 59:421, 1979.

65a. Pattillo, R. W., Fuchs, S., Johnson, J., et al.: Predictors of prognosis by quantitative assessment of coronary angiography, single photon emission computed tomography thallium imaging, and treadmill exercise testing. Am. Heart J. 131:582, 1996.

66. Chang, J. A., and Froelicher, V. F.: Clinical and exercise test markers of prognosis in patients with stable coronary artery disease. Curr. Probl. Cardiol. 19:533, 1994.

67. Peterson, M. C., Holbrook, J. H., Hales, D., et al.: Contributions of the history, physical examination and laboratory investigation in making medical diagnoses. West. J. Med. 156:163, 1992.

68. Marantz, P. R., Tobin, J. N., Wassertheil-Smoller, S., et al.: Prognosis in ischemic heart disease: Can you tell as much at the bedside as in the nuclear laboratory? Arch. Intern. Med. 152:2433, 1992.

69. Pryor, D. B., Shore, L., McCants, C. B., et al.: Value of the history and physical in identifying patients at increased risk for coronary artery disease. Ann. Intern. Med. 118:81, 1993.

69a. Christian, T. F., Miller, T. D., Bailey, K.R., and Gibbons, R.J.: Exercise tomographic thallium-201 imaging in patients with severe coronary artery disease and normal electrocardiograms. Ann. Intern. Med. 121:825, 1994.

69b. Berman, D.S., Hachamovitch, R., Kiat, H., et al.: Incremental value of prognostic testing in patients with known or suspected ischemic heart disease: A basis for optimal utilization of exercise technetium-99m Sestamibi myocardial perfusion single-photon emission computed tomography. J. Am. Coll. Cardiol. 26:639, 1995.

70. Wilson, R. F., Marcus, M. L., Christensen, B. V., et al.: Accuracy of exercise electrocardiography in detecting physiologically significant coronary arterial lesions. Circulation 83:412, 1991.

71. Bogaty, P., Dagenais, G. R., Cantin, B., et al.: Prognosis in patients with a strongly positive exercise electrocardiograph. Am. J. Cardiol. 64:1284, 1989.

72. Weiner, D. A., McCabe, C., Hueter, D. C., et al.: The predictive value of anginal chest pain as an indicator of coronary disease during exercise testing. Am. Heart J. 96:458, 1978.

73. Ribisl, P. M., Morris, C. K., Kawaguchi, T., et al.: Angiographic patterns and severe coronary artery disease: Exercise test correlates. Arch. Intern. Med. 152:1618, 1992.

74. Michaelides, A., Ryan, J. M., VanFossen, D., et al.: Exercise-induced QRS prolongation in patients with coronary artery disease: A marker of myocardial ischemia. Am. Heart J. 126:1320, 1993.

75. Ho, S. W., McComish, M. J., and Taylor, R. R.: Effect of beta adrenergic blockade on the results of exercise testing related to the extent of coronary artery disease. Am. J. Cardiol. 55:258, 1985.

76. Coyne, E. P., Belvedere, D. A., Vande Streek, P. R., et al.: Thallium-201 scintigraphy after intravenous infusion of adenosine compared with exercise thallium testing in the diagnosis of coronary artery disease. J. Am. Coll. Cardiol. 17:1289, 1991.

77. Gibbons, R. J., Fyke, F. E., Clements, I. P., et al.: Noninvasive identification of severe coronary artery disease using exercise radionuclide angiography. J. Am. Coll. Cardiol. 11:28, 1988.

78. Dilsizian, V., Smeltzer, W. R., Freedman, N. M., et al.: Thallium reinjection after stress-redistribution imaging: Does 24-hour delayed imaging after reinjection enhance detection of viable myocardium? Circulation 83:1247, 1991.

79. Bonow, R. O., Dilsizian, V., Cuocolo, A., and Bacharach, S. L.: Identification of viable myocardium in patients with chronic coronary artery disease and left ventricular dysfunction: Comparison of thallium scintigraphy with reinjection and PET imaging with ^{18}F-fluorodeoxyglucose. Circulation 83:26, 1991.

80. Dilsizian, V., Perone-Filardi, P., Arrighi, J. A., et al.: Concordance and discordance between stress-redistribution-reinjection and rest-redistribution thallium imaging for assessing viable myocardium: Comparison with metabolic activity by PET. Circulation 88:941, 1993.

81. Brown, K. A.: Prognostic value of thallium-201 myocardial perfusion imaging: A diagnostic tool comes of age. Circulation 83:363, 1991.

82. European Coronary Surgery Study Group (ECSSG): Long-term results of prospective randomized study of coronary artery bypass surgery and stable angina pectoris. Lancet 2:1173, 1982.

83. Assessment of myocardial perfusion and viability. In Cerqueira, M. D. (ed.): Nuclear Cardiology. Cambridge, MA, Blackwell Scientific Publications, 1994, p. 160.

84. Taylor, A. J., Sackett, M. C., and Beller, G. A.: The degree of ST-segment depression on symptom-limited exercise testing: Relation to the myocardial ischemia burden as determined by thallium-201 scintigraphy. Am. J. Cardiol. 75:228, 1995.

85. Beller, G. A.: Current status of nuclear cardiology techniques: Curr. Probl. Cardiol. 16:451, 1991.

86. Kotler, T. S., and Diamond, G. A.: Exercise thallium-201 scintigraphy in the diagnosis and prognosis of coronary artery disease. Ann. Intern. Med. 113:684, 1990.

87. Christian, T. F., Miller, T. D., Bailey, K. R., and Gibbons, R. J.: Noninvasive identification of severe coronary artery disease using exercise tomographic thallium-201 imaging. Am. J. Cardiol. 70:14, 1992.

88. Kaul, S., Lilly, D. R., Gascho, J. A., et al.: Prognostic utility of the exercise thallium-201 test in ambulatory patients with chest pain: Comparison with cardiac catheterization. Circulation 77:745, 1988.

89. Port, S. C., Oshima, M., Ray, G., et al.: Assessment of single-vessel coronary artery disease: Results of exercise electrocardiography, thallium-201 myocardial perfusion imaging and radionuclide angiography. J. Am. Coll. Cardiol. 6:75, 1985.

90. Johnston, D. L., Daley, J. R., Hodge, D. O., et al.: Hemodynamic responses and adverse effects associated with adenosine and dipyridamole pharmacological stress testing: A comparison of 2,000 patients. Mayo Clin. Proc. 70:331, 1995.

91. Iskandrian, A. S., Heo, J., Lemek, J., et al.: Identification of high risk patients with left main and three vessel coronary artery disease by adenosine-single photon emission computed tomographic thallium imaging. Am. Heart J. 125:1130, 1993.

92. Pennell, D. J., Underwood, S. R., and Ell, P. J.: Safety of dobutamine stress for thallium-201 myocardial perfusion tomography in patients with asthma. Am. J. Cardiol. 71:1346, 1993.

93. Gupta, N. C., Esterbrooks, D. J., Hilleman, B. E., and Mohiuddin, S. M.: Multicenter Adenosine Study Group: Comparison of adenosine in exercise thallium-201 single-photon emission computed tomography (SPECT) myocardial perfusion imaging. J. Am. Coll. Cardiol. 19:248, 1992.

94. Nishimura, S., Mahmarian, J. J., Boyce, T. M., and Verani, M. S.: Equivalence between adenosine and exercise thallium-201 myocardial tomography: A multicenter, prospective, crossover trial. J. Am. Coll. Cardiol. 20:265, 1992.

95. Shaw, L., Chaitman, B. R., Hilton, T. C., et al.: Prognostic value of dipyridamole thallium-201 imaging in elderly patients. J. Am. Coll. Cardiol. 19:1390, 1992.

95a. Dagianti, A., Penco, M., Agati, L., et al.: Stress echocardiography: Comparison of exercise, dipyridamole and dobutamine in detecting and predicting the extent of coronary artery disease. J. Am. Coll. Cardiol. 26:1180, 1995.

95b. Kiat, H., Iskandrian, A. S., Villegas, B.J., et al.: Arbutamine stress thallium-201 single-photon emission computed tomography using a computerized closed-loop delivery center system multicenter trial for evaluation and safety of diagnosis accuracy. J. Am. Coll. Cardiol. 26:1159, 1995.

95c. Dennis, C. A., Poole, P. E., Perrins, E.J., et al.: Stress testing with closed-loop arbutamine as an alternative to exercise. J. Am. Coll. Cardiol. 26:1151, 1995.

96. Decker, P. J., Scott, C. H., and Fishman, L. S.: A rare case of coronary artery occlusion diagnosed by echocardiography. Am. J. Cardiol. 75:104, 1995.

97. Marwick, T. H., Nemec, J. J., Pashkow, F. J., et al.: Accuracy and limitations of exercise echocardiography in a routine clinical setting. J. Am. Coll. Cardiol. 19:74, 1992.

98. Quinones, M. A., Verani, M. S., Haichin, R. M., et al.: Exercise echocardiography versus 201 Tl single-photon emission computed tomography in evaluation of coronary artery disease: Analysis of 292 patients. Circulation 85:1026, 1992.

99. Roger, V. L., Pellikka, P. A., Oh, J. K., et al.: Identification of multivessel coronary artery disease by exercise echocardiography. J. Am. Coll. Cardiol. 24:109, 1994.

99a. Marwick, T. H., Torelli, J., Harka, K., et al.: Influence of left ventricular hypertrophy and detection of coronary artery disease using exercise echocardiography. J. Am. Coll. Cardiol. 26:1180, 1995.

100. Iliceto, S., Galiuto, L., Marangelli, V., and Rizzon, P.: Clinical use of stress echocardiography: Factors affecting diagnostic accuracy. Eur. Heart J. 15:672, 1994.

100a. Cohen, J. L., Chan, K. L., Jaarsman, W., et al.: Arbutamine echocardiography: Efficacy and safety of a new pharmacologic stress agent to induce myocardial ischemia and to detect coronary artery disease. J. Am. Coll. Cardiol. 26:1168, 1995.

101. Dagianti, A., Penco, N., Agati, L., et al.: Stress echocardiography: Comparison of exercise dipyridamole and dobutamine in detecting and predicting the extent of coronary artery disease. J. Am. Coll. Cardiol. 26:18, 1995.

102. Marangelli, V., Iliceto, S., Piccinni, G., et al.: Detection of coronary artery disease by digital stress echocardiography: Comparison of exercise, transesophageal atrial pacing and dipyridamole echocardiography. J. Am. Coll. Cardiol. 24:117, 1994.

103. Fioretti, P. M., Poldermans, D., Salustri, A., et al.: Atropine increases the accuracy of dobutamine stress echocardiography in patients taking beta-blockers. Eur. Heart J. 15:355, 1994.

104. Marwick, T., Willemart, B., D'Hondt, A. M., et al.: Selection of the optimal nonexercise stress for the evaluation of ischemic regional myocardial dysfunction and malperfusion. Circulation 87:345, 1993.

105. Beleslin, B. D., Ostojic, M., Stepanovic, J., et al.: Stress echocardiography in the detection of myocardial ischemia: Head-to-head comparison of exercise, dobutamine and dipyridamole tests. Circulation 90:1168, 1994.

106. Frohwein, S., Klein, L., Lane, A., et al.: Transesophageal dobutamine stress echocardiography in the evaluation of coronary artery disease. J. Am. Coll. Cardiol. 25:823, 1995.

107. Sketch, M. H., Mohiuddin, S. M., Lynch, J. D., et al.: Significant sex differences in the correlation of electrocardiographic exercise testing in coronary arteriograms. Am. J. Cardiol. 36:169, 1975.

108. Proceedings of an N.H.L.B.I. Conference: Exercise ECG testing with and without radionuclide studies. In Cardiovascular Health and Disease in Women. Greenwich, CT, Le Jacq Communications, Inc., 1993, p. 74.

109. Pryor, D. B., Shaw, L., and Harrell, F. E.: Estimating the likelihood of severe coronary artery disease. Am. J. Med. 90:553, 1991.

110. Shaw, L. J., Miller, D. D., Romeis, J. C., et al.: Gender differences in the noninvasive evaluation and management of patients with suspected coronary artery disease. Ann. Intern. Med. 120:559, 1994.

111. Hamm, C. W., Ravkilde, J., Gerhardt, W., et al.: The prognostic value of serum troponin T in unstable angina. N. Engl. J. Med. 327:146, 1992.

111a. Marwick, T. H., Anderson, T., Williams, J., et al.: Exercise electrocardiography is an accurate and cost-efficient technique for detection of coronary artery disease in women. J. Am. Coll. Cardiol 26:335, 1995.

112. French, J. K., Elliott, J. M., Williams, B. F., et al.: Association of angiographically detected coronary artery disease with low levels of high-density lipoprotein cholesterol and systemic hypertension. Am. J. Cardiol. 71:505, 1993.

113. NIH Consensus Development Panel: Triglyceride, high-density lipoprotein, and coronary heart disease. JAMA 269:505, 1993.

114. Pearson, M., and Layton, C.: Value of the chest radiograph before cardiac catheterization in adults. Br. Heart J. 72:505, 1994.

115. Chae, S. C., Heo, J., Iskandrian, A. S., et al.: Identification of extensive coronary artery disease in women by exercise single-photon emission computed tomographic (SPECT) thallium imaging. J. Am. Coll. Cardiol. 21:1305, 1993.

115a. Kajinami, K., Seki, H., Takekoshi, N., et al.: Noninvasive prediction of coronary atherosclerosis by quantification of coronary artery calcification using electron beam computed tomography. Comparison with electrocardiographic and thallium exercise stress test results. J. Am. Coll. Cardiol. 26:1209, 1995.

116. Loecker, T. H., Schwartz, R. S., Cottac, W., et al.: Fluoroscopic coronary artery calcification and associated coronary disease in asymptomatic young men. J. Am. Coll. Cardiol. 19:1167, 1992.

117. Rumberger, J. A., Sheedy, P. F., III, Breen, J. F., et al.: Coronary calcium as determined by electron beam computer tomography and coronary disease on arteriograms: Effects of patients' sex on diagnosis. Circulation 91:1363, 1995.

118. Detrano, R., Wong, N., Tang, W., et al.: Prognostic significance of cardiac cinefluoroscopy for coronary calcific deposits in asymptomatic, high risk subjects. J. Am. Coll. Cardiol. 24:354, 1994.

119. Simons, D. B., Schwartz, R. S., Edwards, W. D., et al.: Noninvasive definition of anatomic coronary artery disease by ultrafast computed tomographic scanning: A quantitative pathological comparison study. J. Am. Coll. Cardiol. 20:1118, 1992.

120. Committee on Advanced Cardiac Imaging and Technology, Council on Clinical Cardiology, American Heart Association: Potential value of ultrafast computed tomography to screen for coronary artery disease. Circulation 87:2071, 1993.

120a. Ellis, S. G.: Chronic stable angina: Role of coronary angiography. In Fuster, V., Ross, R., and Topol, E. J. (eds): Atherosclerosis and Coronary Artery Disease. Philadelphia, J. B. Lippincott, 1996, pp. 1433–1450.

121. Bogaty, P., Brecker, S. J., White, S. E., et al.: Comparison of coronary angiographic findings in acute and chronic first presentation of ischemic heart disease. Circulation 87:1938, 1993.

122. Stajduhar, K. C., Laird, J. R., Rogan, K. M., and Wortham, D. C.: Coronary arterial ectasia: Increased prevalence in patients with abdominal aortic aneurysm as compared to occlusive atherosclerotic peripheral vascular disease. Am. Heart J. 125:86, 1993.

123. Hartnell, G. G., Parnell, B. M., and Pridie, R. B.: Coronary artery ectasia: Its prevalence and clinical significance in 4993 patients. Br. Heart J. 54:392, 1985.

124. Tunick, P. A., Slater, J., Kronzon, I., and Glassman, E.: Discrete atherosclerotic coronary artery aneurysms: A study of 20 patients. J. Am. Coll. Cardiol. 15:279, 1990.

125. Agarwal, J. B., and Helfant, R. H.: Functional importance of coronary collateral circulation. Int. J. Cardiol. 4:94, 1983.

126. Newman, P. E.: The coronary collateral circulation: Determinants and functional significance in ischemic heart disease. Am. Heart J. 102:431, 1981.

127. Vanoverschelde, J. L., Winjns, W., Depre, C., et al.: Mechanisms of chronic regional postischemic dysfunction in humans: New insights from the study of noninfarcted collateral-dependent myocardium. Circulation 87:1513, 1993.

128. Kracoff, O. G., Ovsyshcher, I., and Gueron, M.: Malignant course of a benign anomaly: Myocardial bridging. Chest 92:1113, 1987.

129. Bestetti, R. B., Costa, R. S., Kazava, D. K., and Oliviera, J. S.: Can isolated myocardial bridging of the left anterior descending coronary artery be associated with sudden death during exercise? Acta Cardiol. 46:27, 1991.

130. Moraski, R. E., Russell, R. O., Jr., Smith, M., and Rackley, C. E.: Left ventricular function in patients with and without myocardial infarction and one, two or three-vessel coronary artery disease. Am. J. Cardiol. 35:1, 1975.

131. Mann, T., Brodie, B. R., Grossman, W., and McLaurin, L. P.: Effect of angina on the left ventricular diastolic pressure-volume relationship. Circulation 35:761, 1977.

132. Stack, R. S., Phillips, H. R., 3d., Grierson, D. S., et al.: Functional improvement of jeopardized myocardium following intracoronary streptokinase infusion in acute myocardial infarction. J. Clin. Invest. 72:84, 1983.

133. Rahimtoola, S. H.: The hibernating myocardium. Am. Heart J. 117:211, 1989.

134. Braunwald, E., and Rutherford, J. D.: Reversible ischemic left ventricular dysfunction: Evidence for the "hibernating myocardium." J. Am. Coll. Cardiol. 8:1467, 1986.

135. Marban, E.: Myocardial stunning and hibernation: The physiology behind the colloquialisms. Circulation 83:681, 1991.

136. Popio, K. A., Gorlin, R., Bechtel, D., and Levine, J. A.: Postextrasystolic potentiation as a predictor of potential myocardial viability: Preoperative analyses compared with studies after coronary bypass surgery. Am. J. Cardiol. 39:944, 1977.

137. Nesto, R. W., Cohn, L. H., Collins, J. J., Jr., et al.: Inotropic contractile reserve: A useful predictor of increased 5-year survival and improved postoperative left ventricular function in patients with coronary artery disease and reduced ejection fraction. Am. J. Cardiol. 50:39, 1982.

138. Verani, M. S., Carroll, R. J., and Falsetti, H. L.: Mitral valve prolapse in coronary artery disease. Am. J. Cardiol. 37:1, 1976.

139. Herman, M. V., Elliott, W. C., and Gorlin, R.: An electrocardiographic, anatomic, and metabolic study of zonal myocardial ischemia in coronary heart disease. Circulation 35:834, 1967.

140. Gertz, E. W., Wisneski, J. A., Neese, R., et al.: Myocardial lactate metabolism: Evidence of lactate release during net chemical extraction in man. Circulation 63:1273, 1981.

141. Cannon, P. J., Weiss, M. B., and Sciacca, R. R.: Myocardial blood flow in coronary artery disease: Studies at rest and during stress with inert gas washout techniques. Prog. Cardiovasc. Dis. 20:95, 1977.

141a. Rutherford, J. D.: Chronic stable angina: Medical management. In Fuster, V., Ross, R., and Topol, E. J. (eds): Atherosclerosis and Coronary Artery Disease. Philadelphia, J. B. Lippincott, 1996, pp. 1419–1432.

142. Stamler, J., Stamler, R., and Neaton, J. D.: Blood pressure, systolic and diastolic, and cardiovascular risks. Arch. Intern. Med. 153:598, 1993.

143. Wang, X. L., Tam, C., McCredie, R. M., and Wilcken, D. E.: Determinants of severity of coronary artery disease in Australian men and women. Circulation 89:1974, 1994.

144. Devereux, R. B., and Roman, M. J.: Inter-relationships between hypertension, left ventricular hypertrophy and coronary heart disease. J. Hypertens. 11(Suppl. 4):S3, 1993.

145. Hebert, P. R., Moser, M., Mayer, J., et al.: Recent evidence on drug therapy of mild to moderate hypertension and decreased risk of coronary heart disease. Arch. Intern. Med. 153:578, 1993.

146. Vliestra, R. E., Kronmal, R. E., Oberman, A., et al.: Effect of cigarette smoking on survival of patients with angiographically documented coronary artery disease: Report from CASS Registry. JAMA 255:1023, 1986.

147. Hermanson, B., Omenn, G. S., Kronmal, R. A., and Gersch, B. J.: Beneficial six-year outcome of smoking cessation in older men and women with coronary artery disease: Results from the CASS Registry. N. Engl. J. Med. 319:1365, 1988.

148. Cavender, J. B., Rogers, W. J., Fisher, L. D., et al.: Effects of smoking on survival and morbidity in patients randomized to medical or surgical therapy in the Coronary Artery Surgery Study (CASS): Ten-year follow-up. J. Am. Coll. Cardiol. 20:287, 1992.

149. Pearson, T., Rapaport, E., Criqui, M., et al.: Optimal risk factor management in the patient after coronary revascularization: A statement for healthcare professionals from an American Heart Association Writing Group. Circulation 90:3125, 1994.

150. Nicod, P., Rehr, R., Winniford, M. D., et al.: Acute systemic and coronary hemodynamic and serologic responses to cigarette smoking in long-term smokers with atherosclerotic coronary artery disease. J. Am. Coll. Cardiol. 4:964, 1984.

150a. Czernin, J., Sun, K., Bruken, R., et al.: Effect of acute and long-term smoking on myocardial blood flow and flow reserve. Circulation 91:2891, 1995.

151. Winniford, M. D., Wheelan, K. R., Kremers, M. S., et al.: Smoking-induced coronary vasoconstriction in patients with atherosclerotic coronary artery disease: Evidence for adrenergically mediated alterations in coronary artery tone. Circulation 73:662, 1986.

152. Deanfield, J., Wright, C., Kirkler, S., et al.: Cigarette smoking and the treatment of angina with propranolol, atenolol, and nifedipine. N. Engl. J. Med. 310:951, 1984.

153. Aronow, W. S.: Effect of passive smoking on angina pectoris. N. Engl. J. Med. 299:21, 1978.

154. Allred, E. N., Bleecker, E. R., Chaitman, B. R., et al.: Short-term effects of carbon monoxide exposure on the exercise performance of subjects with coronary artery disease. N. Engl. J. Med. 321:1426, 1989.

155. Adams, K. F., Koch, G., Chatterjee, B., et al.: Acute elevation of blood carboxyhemoglobin to 6% impairs exercise performance and aggravates symptoms in patients with ischemic heart disease. J. Am. Coll. Cardiol. 12:900, 1988.

155a. Shepherd, J., Cobbe, S. W., Ford, I., et al.: Prevention of coronary heart disease with pravastatin in men with hypercholesterolemia. N. Engl. J. Med. 16:333, 1995.

156. Pitt, B., Mancini, G. B. J., Ellis, S. G., et al.: Pravastatin limitation of atherosclerosis in the coronary arteries (PLACI): Reduction of atherosclerosis progression in clinical events. J. Am. Coll. Cardiol. 26:1133, 1995.

157. Rubins, H. B., Robins, S. J., Collins, D., et al.: Distribution of lipids in 8500 men with coronary artery disease. Am. J. Cardiol. 175:1196, 1995.

158. Blankenhorn, D. H., Azen, S. P., Kramsch, D. M., et al.: Coronary angiographic changes with lovastatin therapy: The Monitored Atherosclerosis Regression Study (MARS). Ann. Intern. Med. 119:969, 1993.

159. Scandinavian Simvastatin Survival Study Group: Randomised trial of cholesterol lowering in 4444 patients with coronary heart disease: the Scandinavian Simvastatin Survival Study (4S). Lancet 344:1383, 1994.

160. Anderson, T. J., Meredith, I. T., Yeung, A. C., et al.: The effect of cholesterol-lowering and antioxidant therapy on endothelium-dependent coronary vasomotion. N. Engl. J. Med. 332:488, 1995.

161. Treasure, C. B., Klein, J. L., Weintraub, W. S., et al.: Beneficial effects of cholesterol-lowering therapy on the coronary endothelium in patients with coronary artery disease. N. Engl. J. Med. 332:481, 1995.

162. Bonithon-Kopp, C., Scarabin, P. Y., Darne, B., et al.: Menopause-related changes in lipoproteins and some other cardiovascular risk factors. Int. J. Epidemiol. 19:42, 1990.

163. van Beresteijn, E. C., Korevaar, J. C., Huijbregts, P. C., et al.: Perimenopausal increase in serum cholesterol: A 10-year longitudinal study. Am. J. Epidemiol. 137:383, 1993.

164. Bass, K. M., Newschaffer, C. J., Klage, M. J., and Bush, T. L.: Plasma lipoprotein levels as predictors of cardiovascular death in women. Arch. Intern. Med. 153:2209, 1993.

165. Stensvold, I., Tverdal, A., Urdal, P., and Graff-Iversen, S.: Non-fasting serum triglyceride concentration and mortality from coronary heart disease and any cause in middle aged Norwegian women. Br. Med. J. 307:1318, 1993.

166. The Post Menopausal Estrogen/Progestin Interventions (PEPI) Trial, the writing group for the PEPI trial: Effects of estrogen or estrogen/progestin regimens on heart disease, risk factors in post menopausal women. JAMA 273:199, 1995.

167. Vaziri, S. M., Evans, J. C., Larson, M. J., and Wilson, P. W.: The impact of female hormone usage on the lipid profile. Arch. Intern. Med. 153:2200, 1993.

168. Nabulsi, A. A., Folsom, A. R., White, A., et al.: Association of hormone-replacement therapy with various cardiovascular risk factors in post-menopausal women. N. Engl. J. Med. 328:1069, 1993.

169. Grady, D., Rubin, S. M., Petitti, D. B., et al.: Hormone therapy to prevent disease and prolong life in postmenopausal women. Ann. Intern. Med. 117:1016, 1992.

170. Rosenberg, L., Palmer, J. R., and Shapiro, S.: A case-control study of myocardial infarction in relation to use of estrogen supplements. Am. J. Epidemiol. *137*:54, 1993.

171. Manolio, T. A., Furberg, C. D., Shemanski, L., et al.: Associations of post-menopausal estrogen use with cardiovascular disease and its risk factors in older women. Circulation *88*:2163, 1993.

172. LaRosa, J. C.: Estrogen: Risk versus benefit for the prevention of cardiovascular disease. Cor. Art. Dis. *4*:588, 1993.

172a. Gebara, O. C. E., Mittleman, M. A., Sutherland, P., et al.: Association between increased estrogen status and increased fibrinolytic potential in the Framingham offspring study. Circulation *91*:1952, 1995.

173. Sullivan, J. M.: Hormone replacement in the secondary prevention of cardiovascular disease. *In* Wenger, N. K., Speroff, T., and Packad, B. (eds.): Proceedings of a NHLBI Conference: Cardiovascular Health and Disease in Women. Greenwich, CT, Le Jacq Communications, Inc., 1993, p. 189.

174. Sullivan, J. M., Vander Zwaag, R., Hughes, J. P., et al.: Estrogen replacement and coronary artery disease: Effect on survival in postmenopausal women. Arch. Intern. Med. *150*:2557, 1990.

175. Expert Panel on Detection, Evaluation and Treatment of High Blood Cholesterol in Adults: Summary of the second report of the National Cholesterol Education Program (NCEP): Expert panel on detection, evaluation and treatment of high blood cholesterol in adults (adult treatment panel II). JAMA *269*:3015, 1993.

176. Kardinaal, A. F., Kok, F. J., Ringstad, J., et al.: Antioxidants in adipose tissue and risk of myocardial infarction: The EURAMIC study. Lancet *342*:1379, 1993.

177. Jha, P., Flather, M., Lonn, E., et al.: The antioxidant vitamins and cardiovascular disease: a critical review of epidemiologic and clinical trial data. Ann. Intern. Med. *123*:816, 1995.

178. Hodis, H. N., Mack, W. G., LaBree, L., et al.: Serial coronary angiographic evidence that antioxidant vitamin intake reduces progression of coronary artery atherosclerosis. JAMA *273*:1849, 1995.

179. Stampfer, M. J., Hennekens, C. H., Manson, J. E., et al.: Vitamin E consumption and the risk of coronary disease in women. N. Engl. J. Med. *328*:1444, 1993.

180. Ferguson, R. J., Taylor, A. W., Cote, P., et al.: Skeletal muscle and cardiac changes with training in patients with angina pectoris. Am. J. Physiol. *243*:H830, 1982.

181. Bittner, V., and Oberman, A.: Efficacy studies in coronary rehabilitation. Cardiol. Clin. *11*:333, 1993.

182. Hedback, B., Perk, J., and Wodlin, P.: A long-term reduction of cardiac mortality after myocardial infarction: 10-Year results of a comprehensive rehabilitation program. Eur. Heart J. *14*:831, 1993.

183. Hambrecht, R., Niebauer, J., Marburger, C., et al.: Various intensities of leisure time physical activity in patients with coronary artery disease: Effects of coronary respiratory fitness and progression of coronary atherosclerotic lesions. J. Am. Coll. Cardiol. *22*:468, 1993.

184. Shuler, G., Hambrecht, R., Schlierf, G., et al.: Myocardial perfusion and regression of coronary artery disease in patients on a regimen of intensive physical exercise and low-fat diet. J. Am. Coll. Cardiol. *19*:34, 1992.

185. Ades, P. A., Waldmann, M. L., Poehlman, E. T., et al.: Exercise conditioning in older coronary patients: Submaximal lactate response and endurance capacity. Circulation *88*:572, 1993.

186. Stratton, J. R., Levy, W. C., Cerqueira, M. D., et al.: Cardiovascular responses to exercise: Effects of aging and exercise training in healthy men. Circulation *89*:1648, 1994.

187. Oldridge, N., Furlong, W., Feeny, D., et al.: Economic evaluation of cardiac rehabilitation soon after acute myocardial infarction. Am. J. Cardiol. *72*:154, 1993.

188. Lam, J. Y. T., Latour, J., Lesperance, J., et al.: Platelet aggregation, coronary artery disease, progression in future coronary events. Am. J. Cardiol. *73*:333, 1994.

189. Antiplatelet Trialists' Collaboration: Collaborative overview of randomized trial of antiplatelet therapy. I. Prevention of death, myocardial infarction and stroke by prolonged antiplatelet therapy in various categories of patients. Br. Med. J. *308*:81, 1994.

190. SAPAT (Swedish Angina Pectoris Aspirin Trial) Group, Juul-Moller, S., Edvardsson, N., Jahnmatz, B., et al.: Double-blind trial of aspirin in primary prevention of myocardial infarction in patients with stable chronic angina pectoris. Lancet *340*:1421, 1992.

191. Ridker, P. M., Manson, J. E., Gaziano, J. M., et al.: Low-dose aspirin therapy for chronic stable angina: A randomized, placebo-controlled clinical trial. Ann. Intern. Med. *114*:835, 1991.

192. The Beta-Blocker Pooling Project Research Group: The Beta-blocker Pooling Project (BBPP): Subgroup findings from randomized trials in post-infarction patients. Eur. Heart J. *9*:8, 1988.

193. Goldman, L., Sia, S. T., Cook, E. F., et al.: Costs and effectiveness of routine therapy with long-term beta-adrenergic antagonists after acute myocardial infarction. N. Engl. J. Med. *319*:152, 1988.

194. Daly, P., Mettauer, B., Rouleau, J. L., et al.: Lack of reflex increase in myocardial sympathetic tone after captopril: Potential anti-anginal effect. Circulation *71*:317, 1985.

195. Strozzi, C., Portaluppi, F., Cocco, G., and Urso, L.: Ergometric evaluation of the effects of enalapril maleate in normotensive patients with stable angina. Clin. Cardiol. *11*:246, 1988.

196. Simon, J., Gibbs, R., Crean, P. A., et al.: The variable effects of angiotensin converting enzyme inhibition on myocardial ischemia in chronic stable angina. Br. Heart J. *62*:112, 1989.

197. Cleland, J. G., Henderson, E., McLenachan, J., et al.: Effect of captopril, an angiotensin-converting enzyme inhibitor, in patients with angina pectoris and heart failure. J. Am. Coll. Cardiol. *17*:733, 1991.

198. Sogaard, P., Gotzsche, C. O., Ravkilde, J., and Thygesen, K.: Effects of captopril on ischemia and dysfunction of the left ventricle after myocardial infarction. Circulation *87*:1093, 1993.

199. Pfeffer, M. A., Braunwald, E., Moye, L. A., et al.: Effect of captopril on mortality and morbidity in patients with left ventricular dysfunction after myocardial infarction. N. Engl. J. Med. *327*:669, 1992.

200. SOLVD Investigators: Effects of enalapril on survival in patients with reduced left ventricular ejection fractions and congestive heart failure. N. Engl. J. Med. *325*:293, 1991.

201. SOLVD Investigators: Effect of enalapril on mortality and the development of heart failure in asymptomatic patients with reduced left ventricular ejection fractions. N. Engl. J. Med. *327*:685, 1992.

202. The Acute Infarction Ramipril Efficacy (AIRE) Study Investigators: Effect of ramipril on mortality and morbidity of survivors of acute myocardial infarction with clinical evidence of heart failure. Lancet *342*:821, 1993.

203. Lonn, E. M., Yusuf, S., Jha, P., et al.: Emerging role of angiotensin-converting enzyme inhibitors in cardiac and vascular protection. Circulation *90*:2056, 1994.

204. Featherstone, J. F., Holly, R. G., and Amsterdam, E. A.: Physiologic responses to weight lifting in coronary artery disease. Am. J. Cardiol. *71*:287, 1993.

205. Franklin, B. A., Hogan, P., Bonzheim, K., et al.: Cardiac demands on heavy snow shoveling. JAMA *273*:880, 1995.

206. Kahn, J. F., Jouanin, J. C., Espirito-Santo, J., and Monod, H.: Cardiovascular responses to leisure alpine skiing in habitually sedentary middle-aged men. J. Sports Sci. *11*:31, 1993.

207. Luurila, O. J., Karjalainen, J., Viitasalo, N., and Toivonen, L.: Arrhythmias and ST segment deviation during prolonged exhaustive exercise (ski marathon) in healthy, middle-aged men. Eur. Heart J. *15*:507, 1994.

208. Rocco, M. B., Barry, J., Campbell, S., et al.: Circadian variation of transient myocardial ischemia in patients with coronary artery disease. Circulation *75*:395, 1987.

208a. Figueras, J., and Lidon, R. M.: Early morning reduction in ischemic threshold in patients with unstable angina and significant coronary disease. Circulation *92*:1737, 1995.

208b. Robertson, R. M., and Robertson, D.: Drugs used for the treatment of myocardial ischemia. *In* Hardman, J. G., et al. (eds): Goodman & Gilman's The Pharmacological Basis of Therapeutics. 9th ed. New York, McGraw-Hill, 1996, pp. 759–780.

209. Williams, J. F., Jr., Glick, G., and Braunwald, E.: Studies on cardiac dimensions in intact unanesthetized man. V. Effects of nitroglycerin. Circulation *32*:767, 1965.

210. Brown, B. G., Bolson, E., Petersen, R. B., et al.: The mechanisms of nitroglycerin action: Stenosis vasodilatation as a major component of the drug response. Circulation *64*:1089, 1981.

211. Parker, J. O.: Nitrates and angina pectoris. Am. J. Cardiol. *72*:3C, 1993.

212. Bache, R. J., Ball, R. M., Cobb, F. R., et al.: Effects of nitroglycerin on transmural myocardial blood flow in the unanesthetized dog. J. Clin. Invest. *55*:1219, 1975.

213. Fallen, E. L., Nahmias, C., Scheffel, A., et al.: Redistribution of myocardial blood flow with topical nitroglycerin in patients with coronary artery disease. Circulation *91*:1381, 1995.

214. Sudhir, K., MacGregor, J. S., Barbant, S. D., et al.: Assessment of coronary conductance and resistive vessel reactivity in response to nitroglycerine, ergonovine and adenosine: In vivo studies with simultaneous intravascular two-dimensional and Doppler ultrasound. J. Am. Coll. Cardiol. *21*:1261, 1993.

215. Ganz, W., and Marcus, H. S.: Failure of intracoronary nitroglycerin to alleviate pacing-induced angina. Circulation *46*:880, 1972.

216. Dove, J. T., Shah, P. M., and Schreiner, B. F.: Effect of sublingually administered nitroglycerin on left ventricular wall motion in coronary artery disease. Circulation *49*:682, 1974.

217. Ohno, A., Fujita, M., Miwa, K., et al.: Importance of coronary collateral circulation for increased treadmill exercise capacity by nitrates in patients with stable effort angina pectoris. Cardiology *78*:323, 1991.

218. Cohen, M. V., Downey, J. M., Sonnenblick, E. H., and Kirk, E. S.: The effects of nitroglycerin on coronary collaterals and myocardial contractility. J. Clin. Invest. *52*:2836, 1973.

219. Dove, J. T., Shah, P. M., Schreiner, B. F.: Effects of nitroglycerin on left ventricular wall motion in coronary artery disease. Circulation *49*:662, 1974.

220. Mahmarian, J. J., Fenimore, N. L., Marks, G. F., et al.: Transdermal nitroglycerin patch therapy reduces the extent of exercise-induced myocardial ischemia: Results of a double-blind, placebo-controlled trial using quantitative thallium-201 tomography. J. Am. Coll. Cardiol. *24*:25, 1994.

221. Chirkov, Y. Y., Naukalis, J. I., Sage, E., and Horowitz, J. D.: Antiplatelet effects of nitroglycerin in healthy subjects and in patients with stable angina pectoris. J. Cardiovasc. Pharmacol. *21*:384, 1993.

222. Lacoste, L. L., Theroux, P., Lidon, R. M., et al.: Antithrombotic properties of transdermal nitroglycerin in stable angina pectoris. Am. J. Cardiol. *73*:1058, 1994.

223. Andrews, R., May, J. A., Vickers, J., and Heptinstall, S.: Inhibition of platelet aggregation by transdermal glyceryl trinitrate. Br. Heart J. *72*:575, 1994.

224. Murad, F.: Cyclic guanosine monophosphate as a mediator of vasodilation. J. Clin. Invest. *78*:1, 1986.

225. Anderson, T. J., Meredith, I. T., Ganz, P., et al.: Nitric oxide and nitro-

vasodilators: Similarities, differences and potential interactions. J. Am. Coll. Cardiol. *24*:555, 1994.

226. Horowitz, J. D., Antman, E. M., Lorell, B. H., et al.: Potentiation of the cardiovascular effects of nitroglycerin by N-acetylcysteine. Circulation *68*:1247, 1983.

227. Winniford, M. D., Kennedy, P. L., Wells, P. J., and Hillis, L. D.: Potentiation of nitroglycerin-induced coronary dilatation by N-acetylcysteine. Circulation *73*:138, 1986.

228. Jansen, R. W., and Lipsitz, L. A.: Postprandial hypotension: Epidemiology, pathophysiology and clinical management. Ann. Intern. Med. *122*:286, 1995.

229. Hales, C. A., and Westphal, D.: Hypoxemia following the administration of sublingual nitroglycerin. Am. J. Med. *65*:911, 1978.

230. Parker, J. O., Vankoughnett, K. A., and Farrell, B.: Nitroglycerin lingual spray: Clinical efficacy and dose-response relation. Am. J. Cardiol. *57*:1, 1986.

231. Bassan, M. M.: The daylong pattern of the antianginal effect of long-term three times daily administered isosorbide dinitrate. J. Am. Coll. Cardiol. *16*:936, 1990.

232. de Belder, M. A., Schneeweiss, A., and Camm, A. J.: Evaluation of the efficacy and duration of action of isosorbide mononitrate in angina pectoris. Am. J. Cardiol. *65*:6J, 1990.

233. Nordlander, R., and Walter, M.: Once- versus twice-daily administration of controlled-release isosorbide-5-mononitrate 60 mg in the treatment of stable angina pectoris: A randomized, double-blind, cross-over study: The Swedish Multicenter Group. Eur. Heart J. *15*:108, 1994.

234. Parker, J. O., Amies, M. H., Hawkinson, R. W., et al.: Intermittent transdermal nitroglycerin therapy in angina pectoris: Clinically effective without tolerance or rebound. Circulation *91*:1368, 1995.

235. Munzel, T., Heitzer, T., Kurz, S., et al.: Dissociation of coronary vascular tolerance and neurohormonal adjustments during long-term nitroglycerin therapy in patients with stable coronary artery disease. J. Am. Coll. Cardiol. *27*:297, 1996.

236. Mangione, N. J., and Glasser, S. P.: Phenomenon of nitrate tolerance. Am. Heart J. *128*:137, 1994.

237. Demots, H., and Glasser, S. P.: Intermittent transdermal nitroglycerin therapy in the treatment of chronic stable angina. J. Am. Coll. Cardiol. *13*:786, 1989.

238. Abrams, J.: Clinical aspects of nitrate tolerance. Eur. Heart J. *12*:42, 1991.

239. Jeserich, M., Munzel, T., Pape, L., et al.: Absence of vascular tolerance in conductance vessels after 48 hours of intravenous nitroglycerin in patients with coronary artery disease. J. Am. Coll. Cardiol. *26*:50, 1995.

240. Packer, M.: What causes tolerance to nitroglycerin? The 100 year old mystery continues. J. Am. Coll. Cardiol. *16*:932, 1990.

241. Parker, J. D., Farrell, B., Fenton, T., et al.: Counter-regulatory responses to continuous and intermittent therapy with nitroglycerin. Circulation *84*:2336, 1991.

242. Parker, J. D., and Parker, J. O.: Effect of therapy with an angiotensin-converting enzyme inhibitor of hemodynamic and counter-regulatory responses during continuous therapy with nitroglycerin. J. Am. Coll. Cardiol. *21*:1445, 1993.

243. Dupuis, J., Lalonde, G., Lemieux, R., and Rouleau, J. L.: Tolerance to intravenous nitroglycerin in patients with congestive heart failure: Rate of increased intravascular volume, neurohumoral activation and task of prevention with N-acetylcysteine. J. Am. Coll. Cardiol. *16*:923, 1990.

244. Watanabe, H., Kakihana, M., Ohtsuka, S., et al.: Platelet cyclic GNP: A potentially useful indicator to evaluate the effects of nitroglycerin on nitrate tolerance. Circulation *88*:29, 1993.

245. Schaer, D. F., Buff, L. A., and Katz, R. J.: Sustained antianginal efficacy of transdermal nitroglycerin patches using an overnight 10-hour nitrate-free interval. Am. J. Cardiol. *61*:46, 1988.

246. Fox, K. M., Dargie, H. J., Deanfield, J., and Maseri, A., on behalf of the Transdermal Nitrate Investigators: Avoidance of tolerance and lack of rebound with intermittent dose titrated transdermal glyceral trinitrate. Br. Heart J. *66*:151, 1991.

247. DeMots, H., and Glasser, S. P.: Intermittent transdermal nitroglycerin therapy in the treatment of chronic stable angina. J. Am. Coll. Cardiol. *13*:786, 1989.

248. de Belder, M. A., Schneeweiss, A., and Camm, A. J.: Evaluation of the efficacy and duration of action of isosorbide mononitrate in angina pectoris. Am. J. Cardiol. *65*:6J, 1990.

249. Przybojewski, J. Z., and Heyns, M. H.: Acute coronary vasospasm secondary to industrial nitroglycerin withdrawal. S. Afr. Med. J. *63*:158, 1983.

250. May, D. C., Popma, J. J., Black, W. H., et al.: In vivo induction and reversal of nitroglycerin tolerance in human coronary arteries. N. Engl. J. Med. *317*:805, 1987.

251. Schwartz, A.: The cause, relief, and prevention of headaches arising from contact with dynamite. N. Engl. J. Med. *235*:541, 1948.

252. Hoffman, B. B., and Lefkowitz, R. J.: Catecholamines, sympathomimetic drugs, and adrenergic receptor antagonists. *In* Hardman, J. G., et al. (eds.): Goodman & Gilman's The Pharmacological Basis of Therapeutics. 9th ed. New York, McGraw-Hill, 1996, pp. 199–248.

253. Lefkowitz, R. J., and Caron, M. G.: Adrenergic receptors: Models for the study of receptors coupled to guanine nucleotide regulatory proteins. J. Biol. Chem. *263*:4993, 1988.

254. Opie, L. H., Sonnenblick, E. H., Kaplan, N. M., et al.: Beta-blocking agents. *In* Opie, L. H. (ed.): Drugs for the Heart. 4th ed. Philadelphia, W. B. Saunders Company, 1995, pp. 1–3.

255. Parker, J. D., Testama, A., Jimenez, A. H., et al.: Morning increase in ambulatory ischemia in patients with stable coronary artery disease:

Importance of physical activity in increased cardiac demand. Circulation *89*:604, 1994.

256. Bristow, M. R., O'Connell, J. B., Gilbert, E. M., et al.: Dose-response of chronic beta-blocker treatment in heart failure from either idiopathic dilated or ischemic cardiomyopathy. Circulation *89*:1632, 1994.

257. Olse, S. L., Gilbert, E. M., Renlund, D. G., et al.: Carvedilol improves left ventricular function and symptoms in chronic heart failure: A double-blind randomized study. J. Am. Coll. Cardiol. *25*:1225, 1995.

258. Steinbeck, G., Andresen, D., Bach, P., et al.: A comparison of electrophysiologically guided anti-arrhythmic drug therapy with beta-blocker therapy in patients with symptomatic, sustained ventricular tachyarrhythmias. N. Engl. J. Med. *327*:987, 1992.

259. Anastasiou-Nana, M. I., Gilbert, E. M., Miller, R. H., et al.: Usefulness of d,I Sotalol for suppression of chronic ventricular arrhythmias. Am. J. Cardiol. *67*:511, 1991.

260. Singh, B. N., Deedwania, P., Nademanee, K., et al.: Sotalol: A review of its pharmacodynamic and pharmacokinetic properties and therapeutic use. Drugs *34*:311, 1987.

261. Frishman, W. H.: Pindolol: A new β-adrenoceptor antagonist with partial agonist activity. N. Engl. J. Med. *308*:940, 1983.

262. Kostis, J. B., Frishman, W., Hosler, M. H., et al.: Treatment of angina pectoris with pindolol: The significance of intrinsic sympathomimetic activity of beta blockers. Am. Heart J. *104*:496, 1982.

263. Quyyumi, A. A., Wright, C., Mockus, L., and Fox, K. M.: Effect of partial agonist activity in beta blockers in severe angina pectoris: A double-blind comparison of pindolol and atenolol. Br. Med. J. *289*:951, 1984.

264. Frishman, W., and Halprin, S.: Clincial pharmacology of the new beta-adrenergic blocking drugs. VII. New horizons in beta-adrenoceptor blockade therapy—labetolol. Am. Heart J. *98*:660, 1979.

265. Lennard, M. S.: The polymorphic oxidation of beta-adrenoceptor antagonists. Pharmacol. Ther. *41*:461, 1989.

266. Lehtonen, A.: Effect of beta blockers and blood lipid profile. Am. Heart J. *109*:1192, 1985.

267. Northcote, R. J., Todd, I. C., and Ballantyne, D.: Beta blockers and lipoproteins: A review of current knowledge. Scott. Med. J. *31*:220, 1986.

268. Henry, J. A., and Cassidy, S. L.: Membrane stabilizing activity: A major cause of fatal poisoning. Lancet *1*:1414, 1986.

269. Borzak, S., Fenton, T., Glasser, S. P., et al. for the Angina and Silent Ischemia Study Group (ASISG): Discordance between effects of anti-ischemic therapy on ambulatory ischemia, exercise performance and anginal symptoms in patients with stable angina pectoris. J. Am. Coll. Cardiol. *21*:1605, 1993.

270. Opie, L. H., Sonnenblick, E. H., Kaplan, N. M., et al.: Beta-agents. *In* Opie, L. H. (ed.): Drugs for the Heart. 4th ed. Philadelphia, W. B. Saunders Company, 1995, pp. 20–23.

271. Waagstein, F., Bristow, M. R., Swidberg, K., et al.: Beneficial effects of metoprolol in idiopathic dilated cardiomyopathy. Lancet *342*:1441, 1993.

272. Deacon, S. P., Karunanayake, A., and Barnett, D.: Acebutolol, atenolol and propranolol and metabolic responses to acute hypoglycemia in diabetes. Br. Med. J. *2*:1255, 1977.

273. Hiatt, W. R., Stoll, S., and Nies, A. S.: Effect of beta-adrenergic blockers on the peripheral circulation in patients with peripheral vascular disease. Circulation *72*:1226, 1985.

274. Miller, R. R., Olsen, H. G., Amsterdam, E. A., and Mason, D. T.: Propranolol withdrawal rebound phenomenon: Exacerbation of coronary events after abrupt cessation of antianginal therapy. N. Engl. J. Med. *293*:416, 1975.

275. Katz, A. M.: Cardiac ion channels. N. Engl. J. Med. *328*:1244, 1993.

276. Hurwitz, L., Partridge, L. D., and Leach, J. D. (eds.): Calcium Channels: Their Properties, Functions, Regulation and Clinical Relevance. Boca Raton, FL, CRC Press, 1991.

277. Opie, L. H.: Calcium channel antagonists. Part I. Fundamental properties: Mechanisms, classification, sites of action. Cardiovasc. Drugs Ther. *1*:411, 1987.

278. Wood, A. J.: Calcium antagonists: Pharmacologic differences and similarities. Circulation *80*(Suppl. IV):184, 1989.

279. Cannon, R. O., Watson, R. M., Rosing, D. R., and Epstein, S. E.: Efficacy of calcium channel blocker therapy for angina pectoris resulting from small-vessel coronary artery disease and abnormal vasodilator reserve. Am. J. Cardiol. *56*:242, 1985.

280. Braunwald, E.: Mechanisms of action of calcium-channel blocking agents. N. Engl. J. Med. *307*:1618, 1982.

281. Strauss, W. E., and Parisi, S. F.: Combined use of calcium-channel and beta-adrenergic blockers for the treatment of chronic stable angina. Ann. Intern. Med. *109*:570, 1988.

282. Packer, M.: Combined beta-adrenergic and calcium-entry blockade in angina pectoris. N. Engl. J. Med. *320*:709, 1989.

282a. Opie, L. H.: Calcium channel antagonists in the treatment of coronary artery disease: Fundamental pharmacological properties relevant to clinical use. Prog. Cardiovasc. Dis. *38*:273, 1996.

283. Frishman, W. H.: Current Cardiovascular Drugs. 2nd ed. Philadelphia, Current Medicine, 1995, pp. 129–148.

283a. Ryden, L., and Malmberg, K.: Calcium channel blockers or beta receptor antagonists for patients with ischaemic heart disease. What is the best choice? Eur. Heart J. *17*:1, 1996.

283b. Fox, K. M., Mulcahy, D., Findlay, I., et al.: The Total Ischaemic Burden European Trial (TIBET): Effects of atenolol, nifedipine SR and their combination on the exercise test and the total ischaemic burden in 608 patients with stable angina. Eur. Heart J. *17*:96, 1996.

284. Lichtlen, P. R., Hugenholtz, P. G., Raffenbeul, W., et al.: Retardation of angiographic progression of coronary artery disease by nifedipine: Results of the International Nifedipine Trial on Antiatherosclerotic Therapy (INTACT). Lancet 335:1109, 1990.

285. Loaldi, A., Polese, A., Montorsi, P., et al.: Comparison of nifedipine, propranolol and isosorbide dinitrate on angiographic progression and regression of coronary arterial narrowings in angina pectoris. Am. J. Cardiol. 64:433, 1989.

286. Waters, D., and Lesperance, J.: Interventions that beneficially influence the evolution of coronary atherosclerosis: The case for calcium channel blockers. Circulation 86(Suppl. III):111, 1992.

287. Schroeder, J. S., Gao, S. Z., Alderman, E. L., et al.: A preliminary study of diltiazem in the prevention of coronary artery disease in heart transplant recipients. N. Engl. J. Med. 328:164, 1993.

288. Elkayam, U., Amin, J., Mehra, A., et al.: A prospective, randomized, double-blind, crossover study to compare the efficacy and safety of chronic nifedipine therapy with that of isosorbide dinitrate and their combination in the treatment of chronic congestive heart failure. Circulation 82:1954, 1990.

289. Vetrovec, G. W.: Hemodynamic and electrophysiologic effects of first- and second-generation calcium antagonists. Am. J. Cardiol. 73:34a, 1994.

290. Opie, L. H., Frishman, W. H., and Thadani, U.: Calcium channel antagonists (calcium entry blockers). In Opie, L. H. (ed.): Drugs for the Heart. 4th ed. Philadelphia, W. B. Saunders Company, 1995, p. 53.

291. Wallace, W. A., Willington, K. L., Chess, M. A., et al.: Comparison of nifedipine gastrointestinal therapeutic system and atenolol on anti-anginal efficacies and exercise hemodynamic responses in stable angina pectoris. Am. J. Cardiol. 73:23, 1994.

292. Parmley, W. W., Nestor, W., Singh, B. N., et al.: Attenuation of the circadian patterns of myocardial ischemia with nifedipine GITS in patients with chronic stable angina. J. Am. Coll. Cardiol. 19:1380, 1992.

292a. Furberg, C. D., Psaty, B. M., and Meyer, J. V.: Nifedipine: Dose related increase in mortality in patients with coronary heart disease. Circulation 92:1737, 1995.

292b. Opie, L. H., and Messerli, F. H.: Nifedipine and mortality: Grave defects in the dossier. Circulation 92:1068, 1995.

292c. Yusuf, S.: Calcium antagonists in coronary artery disease and hypertension. Time for reevaluation. Circulation 92:1079, 1995.

293. LaCoste, L., Lamb, J. Y. T., Hung, J., et al.: Oral verapamil inhibits platelet thrombus formation in humans. Circulation 89:630, 1994.

294. Leon, M. B., Rosing, D. R., Bonow, R. O., et al.: Clinical efficacy of verapamil alone and combined with propranolol in treating patients with chronic stable angina pectoris. Am. J. Cardiol. 48:131, 1981.

295. Bache, R. J.: Effects of calcium entry blockade on myocardial blood flow. Circulation 80(Suppl. IV):40, 1989.

296. Murakami, T., Hess, O. M., and Krayenbuehl, H. P.: Left ventricular function before and after diltiazem in patients with coronary artery disease. J. Am. Coll. Cardiol. 5:723, 1985.

297. Klinke, W., Baird, M., Juneau, M., et al.: Anti-anginal efficacy and safety of control-delivery diltiazem QD versus an equivalent dose of immediate-release diltiazem. Cardiovasc. Drugs Ther. 9:319, 1995.

298. Nadazin, A., and Davies, G. J.: Investigation of therapeutic mechanisms of atenolol and diltiazem in patients with variable-threshold angina. Am. Heart J. 127:312, 1994.

299. Piepho, R. W., Culbertson, V. L., and Rhodes, R. S.: Drug interactions with the calcium-entry blockers. Circulation 75(Suppl. V):V181, 1987.

300. Abernethy, D. R.: An overview of the pharmacokinetics and pharmacodynamics of amlodipine in elderly persons with systemic hypertension. Am. J. Cardiol. 73:10A, 1994.

301. Ezekowitz, M. D., Hossack, K., Metta, J. L., et al.: Amlodipine in chronic stable angina: Results of a multicenter double-blind crossover trial. Am. Heart J. 129:527, 1995.

302. Packer, M., For the Prospective Randomized Amlodipine Survival Evaluation [PRAISE] Investigators: Presented at the Annual Scientific Sessions of the American College of Cardiology, New Orleans, LA, March 1995.

303. Landau, A. G., Gentilucci, M., Cavusoglu, E., and Frishman, W. H.: Calcium antagonists for the treatment of congestive heart failure. Cor. Art. Dis. 5:37, 1994.

304. Ekelund, L. G., Ulvenstam, G., Walldius, G., and Aberg, A.: Effects of felodipine versus nifedipine on exercise tolerance in stable angina pectoris. Am. J. Cardiol. 73:658, 1994.

305. Frishman, W. H.: Comparative efficacy and concomitant use of bepridil and beta-blockers in the management of angina pectoris. Am. J. Cardiol. 69:50D, 1992.

306. Multicentre Diltiazem Postinfarction Trial Research Group: The effect of diltiazem on mortality and reinfarction after myocardial infarction. N. Engl. J. Med. 319:385, 1988.

307. The Danish Study Group on Verapamil in Myocardial Infarction: Effect of verapamil on mortality and major events after acute myocardial infarction: The Danish Verapamil Infarction Trial II-DAVIT II. Am. J. Cardiol. 66:779, 1990.

308. Boden, W. E., Bough, E. W., Reichman, M. J., et al.: Beneficial effects of high-dose diltiazem in patients with persistent effort angina on beta blockers and nitrates: A randomized, double-blind, placebo-controlled cross-over study. Circulation 71:1197, 1985.

309. HINT Research Group: Early treatment of unstable angina in the coronary care unit: A randomised, double-blind, placebo-controlled comparison of recurrent ischaemia in patients treated with nifedipine or metoprolol or both: Report of the Holland Interuniversity Nifedipine/Metoprolol Trial (HINT). Br. Heart J. 56:400, 1986.

310. White, H. D., Polak, J. F., Wynne, J., et al.: Addition of nifedipine to maximal nitrate and beta-adrenoreceptor blocker therapy in coronary artery disease. Am. J. Cardiol. 55:1303, 1985.

311. Packer, M., Meller, J., Medina, N., et al.: Hemodynamic consequences of combined beta-adrenergic and slow calcium channel blockade in men. Circulation 65:660, 1982.

PERCUTANEOUS TRANSLUMINAL CORONARY ANGIOPLASTY

312. Gersh, B. J.: Coronary revascularization in the 1990's: A cardiologist's perspective. Can. J. Cardiol. 10:661, 1994.

313. King, S. B. III., and Holmes, D. J., Jr.: Chronic stable angina: Role of coronary intervention. In Fuster, V., Ross, R., and Topol, E. J. (eds): Atherosclerosis and Coronary Artery Disease. Philadelphia, J. B. Lippincott, 1996, pp. 1485–1504.

314. National Heart, Lung and Blood Institute Alert, No. 21, 1995.

315. Lytle, B. W., and Cosgrove, D. M.: Coronary artery bypass surgery. Curr. Probl. Surg. 29:756, 1992.

316. Ryan, T. J., Bauman, W. B., Kennedy, J. W., et al.: ACC/AHA Task Force Report: Guidelines for percutaneous transluminal coronary angioplasty: A report of the American College of Cardiology/American Heart Association Task Force on assessment of diagnostic and therapeutic cardiovascular procedures [Committee on Percutaneous Transluminal Angioplasty]. J. Am. Coll. Cardiol. 22:2033, 1993.

317. Kimmel, S. C., Berlin, J. A., Strom, B. L., et al.: Development and validation of a simplified predictive index for major complications in contemporary percutaneous transluminal coronary angioplasty practice. J. Am. Coll. Cardiol. 26:931, 1995.

318. Serota, H., Deligonul, U., Lee, W-H., et al.: Predictors of cardiac survival after percutaneous transluminal coronary angioplasty in patients with severe left ventricular dysfunction. Am. J. Cardiol. 67:367, 1991.

319. Holmes, D. R., Holubkov, R., Vlietstra, R. E., and the coinvestigators of the NHLBI Transluminal Coronary Angioplasty Registry: Comparison of complications during percutaneous transluminal coronary angioplasty from 1977 to 1981 and from 1985 to 1986. J. Am. Coll. Cardiol. 12:1149, 1988.

320. Faxon, D. P., Holmes, D. R., Hartzler, G., et al.: ABCs of coronary angioplasty: Have we simplified it too much? Cathet. Cardiovasc. Diagn. 25:1, 1992.

320a. Jollis, J. G., Peterson, E. D., DeLong, E. R., et al.: The relation between the volume of coronary angioplasty procedures in hospitals treating Medicare beneficiaries and short-term mortality. N. Engl. J. Med. 331:1625, 1994.

321. Landau, C., Lange, R. A., and Hillis, L. D.: Percutaneous transluminal coronary angioplasty (review). N. Engl. J. Med. 330:981, 1994.

322. Lincoff, A. M.: Patients at high risk for ischemic complications. J. Invest. Cardiol. 6(Suppl. A):13A, 1994.

323. Kuntz, R. E., Piana, R., Pomerantz, R. M., et al.: Changing incidence and management of abrupt closure following coronary intervention in the new device era. Cathet. Cardiovasc. Diagn. 27:183, 1992.

324. Lincoff, A. M., Popma, J. J., Ellis, S. G., et al.: Abrupt vessel closure complicating coronary angioplasty: Clinical, angiographic and therapeutic profile. J. Am. Coll. Cardiol. 19:926, 1992.

325. deFeyter, P. J., deJaegere, P. P., and Serruys, P. W.: Incidence, predictors and management of acute coronary occlusion after coronary angioplasty. Am. Heart J. 127:643, 1994.

326. Reeder, G. S., Bryant, S. C., Suman, V. J., et al.: Intracoronary thrombus: Still a risk factor for PTCA failure? Cathet. Cardiovasc. Diagn. 34:191, 1995.

327. Tan, K., Sulke, N., Taub, N., and Sowton, E.: Clinical and lesion morphologic determinants of coronary angioplasty success and complications: Current experience. J. Am. Coll. Cardiol. 24:855, 1995.

328. Lincoff, A. M., Topol, E. J., Chapekis, A. T., et al.: Intracoronary stenting compared with conventional therapy for abrupt vessel closure complicating coronary angioplasty: A matched case-control study. J. Am. Coll. Cardiol. 21:866, 1993.

329. Sutton, J. M., Ellis, S. G., Roubin, G. S., et al.: Major clinical events after coronary stenting: The multicentre registry of acute and elective Gianturco-Roubin stent placement: Gianturco-Roubin Intracoronary Stent Investigator Group. Circulation 89:1126, 1994.

330. Gibbs, J. S., Sigwart, U., and Buller, N. P.: Temporary stent as a bail-out device during percutaneous transluminal coronary angioplasty: Preliminary clinical experience. Br. Heart J. 71:372, 1994.

331. Schomig, A., Kastrati, A., Dietz, R., et al.: Emergency coronary setting for dissection during percutaneous transluminal coronary angioplasty: Angiographic follow-up after stenting and after repeat angioplasty of the stent segment. J. Am. Coll. Cardiol. 23:1053, 1994.

332. Piana, R. N., Paik, G. Y., Moscucci, M., et al.: Incidence and treatment of "no-reflow" after percutaneous coronary intervention. Circulation 89:2514, 1994.

333. Weyrens, F. J., Mooney, J., Lesser, J., and Mooney, M. R.: Intracoronary diltiazem for microvascular spasm after interventional therapy. Am. J. Cardiol. 75:849, 1995.

334. The EPIC Investigators: Use of a monoclonal antibody directed against the platelet glycoprotein IIb/IIIa receptor in high-risk coronary angioplasty. N. Engl. J. Med. 330:956, 1994.

335. Aguirre, F. V., Topol, E. J., Ferguson, J. J., et al.: Bleeding complications with a chimeric antibody to platelet glycoprotein IIb/IIIa integrin in patients undergoing percutaneous coronary intervention. Circulation 91:282, 1995.

336. Detre, K., Yeh, W., Kelsey, S., et al.: Has improvement in PTCA inter-

vention affected long-term prognosis? The NHLBI PTCA Registry Experience. Circulation 91:2868, 1995.

336a. Weintraub, W., King, S. B., Douglas, J. S., et al.: Percutaneous transluminal coronary angioplasty as a first revascularization procedure in single-, double-, and triple-vessel coronary artery disease. J. Am. Coll. Cardiol. 26:142, 1995.

337. Parisi, A. F., Folland, E. D., and Hartigan, P., for the Veterans Affairs ACME Investigators: A comparison of angioplasty with medical therapy and the treatment of single-vessel coronary artery disease. N. Engl. J. Med. 326:10, 1992.

337a. Strauss, W. E., Fortin, T., Hartigan, P., et al.: A comparison of quality of life scores in patients with angina pectoris after angioplasty compared with after medical therapy outcomes of a randomized clinical trial. Circulation 92:1710,1995.

337b. Hueb, W. A., Bellotti, G., Almeida, S., et al.: The Medicine, Angioplasty or Surgery Study (MASS). A prospective randomized trial of medical therapy, balloon angioplasty or bypass surgery for single proximal left anterior descending artery stenosis. J. Am. Coll. Cardiol. 26:1600, 1995.

338. Mark, D. B., Nelson, C. L., Califf, R. M., et al.: Continuing evaluation of therapy for coronary artery disease: Initial results from the era of coronary angioplasty. Circulation 89:2015, 1994.

339. King, S. B., and Schlumpf, N.: 10-year completed follow-up of percutaneous transluminal coronary angioplasty: The early Zurich experience. J. Am. Coll. Cardiol. 22:353, 1993.

340. Ellis, S. G., Cowley, M. J., Whitlow, P., et al.: Prospective case-control comparison of percutaneous transluminal coronary revascularization in patients with multivessel disease treated in 1986–1987 versus 1991: Improved in-hospital and 12-month results. J. Am. Coll. Cardiol. 25:1137, 1995.

341. Holmes, D. R., Jr., Detre, K. M., Williams, D. O., et al.: Long-term outcome of patients with depressed left ventricular function undergoing percutaneous transluminal coronary angioplasty: The NHLBI PTCA Registry. Circulation 87:21, 1993.

342. Bell, M. R., Bailey, K. R., Reeder, G. S., et al.: Percutaneous transluminal angioplasty in patients with multivessel coronary disease: How important is complete revascularization for cardiac event-free survival? J. Am. Coll. Cardiol. 16:553, 1990.

343. Bourassa, M. G., Holubkov, R., Yeh, W., et al.: Strategy of complete revascularization in patients with multivessel coronary artery disease (a report from the 1985–86 NHLBI PTCA Registry). Am. J. Cardiol. 70:174, 1992.

344. Kuntz, R. E., and Baim, D. S.: Defining coronary restenosis. Circulation 88:1310, 1993.

345. Kuntz, R. E., Gibson, C. M., Nobuyoshi, M., and Baim, D. S.: Generalized model of restenosis after conventional balloon angioplasty, stenting and directional atherectomy. J. Am. Coll. Cardiol. 21:15, 1993.

346. Cameron, J., Mahanonda, N., Aroney, C., et al.: Outcome 5 years after percutaneous transluminal coronary angioplasty or coronary artery bypass grafting for significant narrowing limited to the left anterior descending coronary artery. Am. J. Cardiol. 74:544, 1994.

347. Weintraub, W. S., Kosinski, A. S., Brown, C. L., and King, S. B.: Can restenosis after coronary angioplasty be predicted from clinical variables. J. Am. Coll. Cardiol. 21:6, 1993.

348. Buffet, T., Colasante, B., Feldmann, L., et al.: Long-term follow-up after coronary angioplasty in patients younger than 40 years of age. Am. Heart J. 127:509, 1994.

349. LeFeuvre, C., Bonan, R., Lesperance, J., et al.: Predictor factors of restenosis after multivessel percutaneous transluminal coronary angioplasty. Am. J. Cardiol. 73:840, 1994.

350. Wilson, W. S., and Stone, G. W.: Late results of percutaneous transluminal coronary angioplasty of two or more major native coronary arteries. Am. J. Cardiol. 73:1041, 1994.

351. King, S. B., Lembo, N. J., Weintraub, W. S., et al.: A randomized trial comparing coronary angioplasty with coronary bypass surgery: Emory Angioplasty versus Surgery Trial (EAST). N. Engl. J. Med. 33:1044, 1994.

352. Ellis, S. G., Cowley, M. J., DiSciascio, G., et al.: Determinants of two-year outcome after coronary angioplasty in patients with multivessel disease on the basis of comprehensive preprocedural evaluation: Implications for patient selection. Circulation 83:1905, 1991.

353. Kohli, R. S., DiSciascio, G., Cowley, M. J., et al.: Coronary angioplasty in patients with severe left ventricular dysfunction. J. Am. Coll. Cardiol. 16:807, 1990.

354. Eitchaninoff, H., Franco, I., Whitlow, P. L., et al.: Late results of coronary angioplasty in patients with left ventricular ejection fraction of less than or equal to 40%. Am. J. Cardiol. 73:1047, 1994.

355. Hillegass, W. B., Ohma, E. M., Leinberger, J. D., et al.: A meta-analysis of randomized trials of calcium antagonists to reduce restenosis after coronary angioplasty. Am. J. Cardiol. 73:835, 1994.

355a. Pratt, R. E., and Dzau, V. J.: Pharmacological strategies to prevent restenosis. Lessons learned from blockade of the renin-angiotensin system. Circulation 93:848, 1996.

356. CAVEAT Study Group: A comparison of directional atherectomy with coronary angioplasty in patients with coronary artery disease. N. Engl. J. Med. 329:221, 1993.

357. Adelman, A. G., Cohen, E. A., Kimball, B. P., et al.: A comparison of directional atherectomy with balloon angioplasty for lesions of the left anterior descending coronary artery. N. Engl. J. Med. 329:228, 1993.

358. Violaris, A. G., and Serruys, P. W.: New technologies in interventional cardiology. Curr. Opin. Cardiol. 9:493, 1994.

358a. Serruys, P. W., Emanuelsson, H., van der Giessen, W., et al.: Heparin-

coated Palmaz-Schatz stents in human coronary arteries. Early outcome of the Benestent II Pilot Study. Circulation 93:412, 1996.

359. Fischman, D. L., Leon, M. B., Baim, D. S., et al.: A randomized comparison of coronary-stent placement in balloon angioplasty in the treatment of coronary artery disease: Stent Restenosis Study Investigators (SRSI). N. Engl. J. Med. 331:496, 1994.

360. Serruys, P. W., deJaegere, P., Kiemeneij, F., et al.: A comparison of balloon-expandable-stent implantation with balloon angioplasty in patients with coronary artery disease: Benestent Study Group. N. Engl. J. Med. 321:489, 1994.

361. Moscucci, M., Piana, R. N., Kuntz, R. E., et al.: Effective prior coronary restenosis on the risk of subsequent restenosis after stent placement or directional atherectomy. Am. J. Cardiol. 73:1147, 1994.

362. Piessens, J. H., Stammen, F., Desmet, W., et al.: Immediate and 6-month follow-up results of coronary angioplasty for restenosis: Analysis of factors predicting recurrent clinical restenosis. Am. Heart J. 126:565, 1993.

363. Bauters, C., McFadden, E. P., Lablanche, J. H., et al.: Restenosis rate after multiple percutaneous transluminal coronary angioplasty procedures at the same site. Circulation 88:969, 1993.

364. Puma, J. A., Sketch, M. H., Tcheng, J. E., et al.: Percutaneous revascularization of chronic coronary occlusion. An overview. J. Am. Coll. Cardiol. 26:1, 1995.

364a. Goldberg, S. L., Colomba-Maiello, L., et al.: Intracoronary stent insertion after balloon angioplasty of chronic total occlusions. J. Am. Coll. Cardiol. 26:713, 1995.

365. Violaris, A. G., Melkert, R., and Serruys, P. W.: Long-term luminal renarrowing after successful elective coronary angioplasty of total occlusion: A quantitative angiographic analysis. Circulation 91:2140, 1995.

366. Harrington, R. A., Lincoff, A. M., Califf, R. M., et al.: Characteristics and consequences of myocardial infarction after percutaneous coronary intervention: Insights from the Coronary Angioplasty Versus Excisional Atherectomy Trial (CAVEAT). J. Am. Coll. Cardiol. 25:1693, 1995.

366a. Berger, P. B., Holmes, D. R., Jr., Ohman, E. M., et al.: Restenosis, reocclusion and adverse cardiovascular events after successful balloon angioplasty of occluded versus nonoccluded coronary arteries: Results from the Multicenter American Research Trial with Cilazapril after Angioplasty to Prevent Transluminal Coronary Obstruction and Restenosis (MARCATOR). J. Am. Coll. Cardiol. 27:1, 1996.

367. Thompson, R. C., Holmes, D. R., Jr., Gersh, B. J., et al.: Percutaneous transluminal coronary angioplasty in the elderly: Early and long-term results. J. Am. Coll. Cardiol. 17:1245, 1991.

368. Thompson, R. C., Holmes, D. R., Jr., Gersh, B. J., and Bailey, K. R.: Predicting early and intermediate-term outcome of coronary angioplasty in the elderly. Circulation 88:1579, 1993.

368a. Kaul, T. K., Fields, B. L., Wyatt, D. A., et al.: Angioplasty versus coronary artery bypass in octogenarians. Ann. Thorac. Surg. 58:1419, 1994.

369. Lau, K.-W., and Sigwart, U.: Angioplasty, stenting, atherectomy and laser treatment after coronary artery bypass grafting. Curr. Opin. Cardiol. 8:951, 1993.

370. de Feyter, P. J., van Suylen, R. J., de Jaegere, P. P., et al.: Balloon angioplasty for the treatment of lesions in saphenous vein bypass grafts. J. Am. Coll. Cardiol. 21:1539, 1993.

371. Morrison, D. A., Crowley, S. T., Veerakul, G., et al.: Percutaneous transluminal angioplasty of saphenous vein grafts for medically refractory unstable angina. J. Am. Coll. Cardiol. 23:1066, 1994.

372. Baim, D. S., and Leon, M. B.: The use of new angioplasty devices for the treatment of stable angina. In Fuster, V., Ross, R., and Topol, E. J. (eds): Atherosclerosis and Coronary Artery Disease. Philadelphia, J. B. Lippincott, 1966, pp. 1527–1542.

CORONARY ARTERY BYPASS SURGERY

373. Garrett, H. E., Dennis, E. W., and DeBakey, M. E.: Aortocoronary bypass with saphenous vein graft: Seven-year follow-up. JAMA 223:792, 1973.

374. Favaloro, R. G.: Saphenous vein autograft replacement of severe segmental coronary artery occlusion: Operative technique. Ann. Thorac. Surg. 5:334, 1968.

375. Johnson, W. D., Flemma, R. J., Lepley, D., Jr., and Ellison, E. H.: Extended treatment of severe coronary artery disease: A total surgical approach. Ann. Surg. 170:460, 1969.

376. Kolessov, V. I.: Mammary artery–coronary artery anastomosis as a method of treatment of angina pectoris. J. Thorac. Cardiovasc. Surg. 54:535, 1967.

377. Green, G. E., Spencer, F. C., Tice, D. A., and Stertzer, S. H.: Arterial and venous microsurgical bypass grafts for coronary artery disease. J. Thorac. Cardiovasc. Surg. 60:491, 1970.

378. Marwick, C.: Coronary bypass grafting economics, including rehabilitation. Curr. Opin. Cardiol. 9:635, 1994.

379. McGlynn, E. A., Naylor, D., Anderson, G. M., et al.: Comparison of the appropriateness of coronary angiography and coronary artery bypass graft surgery between Canada and New York state. JAMA 272:934, 1994.

380. Turina, M.: Coronary artery surgical technique. Curr. Opin. Cardiol. 8:919, 1993.

381. Hearse, D. J., Stewart, D. A., and Baimbridge, M. V.: Hypothermic arrest and potassium arrest, metabolic and myocardial protection during elective cardiac arrest. Circ. Res. 36:481, 1975.

382. Ikonomidis, J. S., Yau, T. M., Weisel, R. D., et al.: Optimal flow rates for retrograde warm cardioplegia. J. Thorac. Cardiovasc. Surg. 107:510, 1994.

383. Westaby, S.: Coronary surgery without cardiopulmonary bypass. Br. Heart J. 73:203, 1995.

384. Bryan, A. J., and Angelini, G. D.: The biology of saphenous vein graft occlusion: Etiology and strategies for prevention. Curr. Opin. Cardiol. 9:641, 1994.

384a. Loop, F. D.: Internal-thoracic-artery grafts—Biologically better coronary arteries. N. Engl. J. Med. 334:263, 1996.

385. Green, G. E.: Use of internal thoracic artery for coronary artery grafting. Circulation 79(Suppl. I):30, 1989.

386. Ferro, M., Conti, M., Novero, D., et al.: The thin intima of the internal mammary artery as the possible reason for freedom from atherosclerosis and success in coronary bypass. Am. Heart J. 122:1192, 1991.

387. Chaikhouni, A., Crawford, F. A., Kochel, P. J., et al.: Human internal mammary artery produces more prostacyclin than saphenous vein. J. Thorac. Cardiovasc. Surg. 92:88, 1986.

388. Loop, F. D., Lytle, B. W., Cosgrove, D. M., et al.: Influence of the internal mammary artery graft on 10-year survival and other cardiac events. N. Engl. J. Med. 314:1, 1986.

389. Naunheim, K. S., Barner, H. B., and Fiore, A. C.: Results of internal thoracic artery grafting over 15 years: Single versus double graft: 1992 Update. Ann. Thorac. Surg. 53:716, 1992.

389a. Boylan, M. J., Lytle, B. W., Loop, F. D., et al.: Surgical treatment of isolated left anterior descending coronary stenosis. A comparison of left internal mammary artery and venous autograft at 18–20 years of follow-up. J. Thorac. Cardiovasc. Surg. 107:657, 1994.

389b. Cameron, A., Davis, K. B., Green, G., and Schaff, H. V.: Coronary bypass surgery with internal-thoracic-artery grafts—Effects on survival over a 15-year period. N. Engl. J. Med. 334:216, 1996.

390. He, G. W., Ryan, W. H., and Acuff, T. E.: Risk factors for operative mortality and sternal wound infection in bilateral mammary artery grafting. J. Thorac. Cardiovasc. Surg. 107:196, 1994.

391. Boylan, M. J., Lytle, B. W., Loop, F. D., et al.: Surgical treatment of isolated left anterior descending coronary stenosis: Comparison of left internal mammary artery and venous autograft at 18–20 years of follow-up. J. Thorac. Cardiovasc. Surg. 107:657, 1994.

392. He, G. W., Buxton, B. F., Rosenfeldt, F. L., et al.: Pharmacologic dilatation of internal mammary artery during coronary bypass grafting. J. Thorac. Cardiovasc. Surg. 107:1440, 1994.

393. Jones, E. L.: Conduits for coronary artery bypass. Ann. Thorac. Surg. 55:194, 1993.

394. Grondin, C. M., Lepage, G., Castonguay, Y. R., et al.: Aortocoronary bypass graft: Initial blood flow through the graft, and early postoperative patency. Circulation 44:815, 1971.

395. Carrel, T., Stillhard, G., and Turina, M.: Combined carotid and coronary artery surgery: Early and late results. Cardiology 80:118, 1992.

396. Vermeulen, F. E., Hamerlijnck, P. H., DeFauw, J. J., and Ernst, S. M.: Synchronous operation for ischemic cardiac and cerebral vascular disease: Early results and long-term follow-up. Ann. Thorac. Surg. 53:381, 1992.

397. Edwards, F. H., Clark, R. E., and Schwartz, M.: Impact of internal mammary artery conduits and operative mortality in coronary revascularization. Ann. Thorac. Surg. 56:27, 1994.

398. Kirklin, J. W., Naftel, D. C., Blackstone, E. H., and Pohost, G. M.: Summary of a consensus concerning death and ischemic events after coronary artery byass grafting. Circulation 79(Suppl. I):I81, 1989.

399. Edwards, F. H., Clark, R. E., and Schwartz, M.: Coronary artery bypass grafting: The Society of Thoracic Surgeons National Database Experience. Ann. Thorac. Surg. 57:12, 1994.

400. Naunheim, K. S., Fiore, A. C., Wadley, J. J., et al.: The changing profile of the patient undergoing coronary artery bypass surgery. J. Am. Coll. Cardiol. 11:494, 1988.

400a. Treasure, T.: Risks and results of surgery. Br. Heart J. 74:1112, 1995.

401. Schaff, H. V., Gersh, B. J., Fisher, L. D., et al.: Detrimental effect of perioperative myocardial infarction on late survival after coronary artery bypass. J. Thorac. Cardiovasc. Surg. 88:972, 1984.

402. Craddock, D., Iyer, V. S., and Russell, W. J.: Factors influencing mortality and myocardial infarction after coronary artery bypass grafting. Curr. Opin. Cardiol. 9:664, 1994.

403. Force, T., Hibberd, P., Weeks, G., et al.: Perioperative myocardial infarction after coronary artery bypass surgery: Clinical significance and approach to risk stratification. Circulation 82:903, 1990.

404. Shainoff, J. R., Estafanous, F. G., Yared, J. P., et al.: Low factor XIIIA levels are associated with increased blood loss after coronary artery bypass grafting. J. Thorac. Cardiovasc. Surg. 108:437, 1994.

405. Havel, M., Grabenwoger, F., Schneider, J., et al.: Aprotinin does not decrease early graft patency after coronary artery bypass grafting despite reducing postoperative bleeding and the use of donated blood. J. Thorac. Cardiovasc. Surg. 107:807, 1994.

406. Loop, F. D., Lytle, B. W., Cosgrove, D. M., et al.: Sternal wound complications after isolated coronary artery bypass grafting: Early and late mortality, morbidity and cost of care. Ann. Thorac. Surg. 49:179, 1990.

407. Mullen, J. C., Miller, D. R., Weisel, R. D., et al.: Postoperative hypertension: A comparison of diltiazem, nifedipine, and nitroprusside. J. Thorac. Cardiovasc. Surg. 96:122, 1988.

408. Durkin, M. A., Thys, D., Morris, R. B., et al.: Control of perioperative hypertension during coronary artery surgery: A randomized double-blind study comparing isosorbide dinitrate and nitroglycerin. Eur. Heart J. 9(Suppl. A):181, 1988.

409. Gray, R. J., Bateman, T. M., Czer, L. S., et al.: Use of esmolol in hypertension after cardiac surgery. Am. J. Cardiol. 56:49F, 1985.

410. Hornick, P., Smith, P. L., and Taylor, K. M.: Cerebral complications after coronary artery bypass grafting. Curr. Opin. Cardiol. 9:670, 1994.

411. Shaw, P. J., Bates, D., Cartlidge, N. E., et al.: Neurological complications of coronary artery bypass graft surgery. Br. Med. J. 293:165, 1986.

412. Shaw, P. J., Bates, D., Cartlidge, N. E., et al.: Early intellectual dysfunction following coronary bypass surgery. J. Med. 58:59, 1986.

413. Frost, L., Molgaard, H., Christiansen, E. H., et al.: Atrial fibrillation and flutter after coronary artery bypass surgery: Epidemiology, risk factors and preventive trials. Int. J. Cardiol. 36:253, 1992.

414. Campbell, R. W. F.: Post operative arrhythmias in the role of implantable cardioverter-defibrillators. Curr. Opin. Cardiol. 8:932, 1993.

415. Emlein, G., Huang, S. K., Pires, L. A., et al: Prolonged bradyarrhythmias after isolated coronary artery bypass graft surgery. Am. Heart J. 126:1084, 1993.

416. Koshal, A., Hendry, P., Raman, S. V., and Keon, W. J.: Should obese patients not undergo coronary artery surgery? Can. J. Surg. 28:331, 1985.

416a. Cameron, A. A. C., Davis, K. B., and Rogers, W. J.: Recurrence of angina after coronary bypass surgery. Predictors and prognosis (CASS Registry). J. Am. Coll. Cardiol. 26:895, 1995.

417. Utley, J. R., Thomason, M. E., Wallace, D. J., et al.: Preoperative correlates of impaired wound healing after saphenous vein excision. J. Thorac. Cardiovasc. Surg. 98:147, 1989.

418. RITA Trial Participants: Coronary angioplasty versus coronary artery bypass surgery: The Randomized Intervention Treatment of Angina (RITA) Trial. Lancet 341:573, 1993.

419. Mark, D. B., Lam, L. C., Lee, K. L., et al.: Effects of coronary angioplasty, coronary bypass surgery, and medical therapy on employment in patients with coronary artery disease: A prospective comparison study. Ann. Intern. Med. 120:111, 1994.

420. Hymowitz, Z., Freiman, I., Borman, J., et al.: Work status before and after coronary artery bypass surgery. Public Health 99:367, 1985.

421. Hall, R. J., Elayda, M. A., Gray, A., et al.: Coronary artery bypass: Long-term follow-up of 22,284 consecutive patients. Circulation 68(Suppl. II):20, 1983.

422. Peduzzi, P., Hultgren, H., Thomsen, J., and Detre, K.: Ten-year effect of medical and surgical therapy on quality of life: Veterans Administration Cooperative Study of Coronary Artery Surgery. Am. J. Cardiol. 59:1017, 1987.

423. Bourassa, M. G.: Long-term vein graft patency. Curr. Opin. Cardiol. 9:685, 1994.

424. Pelletier, L. C.: The saphenous vein graft: What have we learned from the past 25 years? In Carrier, M., Pelletier, L. C. (eds.): Conduits for Myocardial Revascularization. Austin, TX, R. G. Landes Co., 1993, p. 3.

425. Underwood, M. J., More, R., Weerasena, N., et al.: The effect of surgical preparation and in vitro distension on the intrinsic fibrinolytic activity of human saphenous vein. Eur. J. Vasc. Surg. 7:518, 1993.

426. Angelini, G. D., Bryan, A. J., Williams, H. M., et al.: Time course of medial and intimal thickening in pig venous arterial grafts: Relationship to endothelial injury and cholesterol accumulation. J. Thorac. Cardiol. Surg. 103:1093, 1992.

427. Vlodaver, Z., and Edwards, J. E.: Pathologic changes in aortic coronary arterial saphenous vein grafts. Circulation 44:719, 1971.

428. FitzGibbon, G. M., Leach, A. J., Kafka, H. P., and Keon, W. J.: Coronary bypass graft fate: Long-term angiographic study. J. Am. Coll. Cardiol. 17:1075, 1991.

429. Cox, J. L., Chiasson, D. A., and Gotlieb, A. I.: Stranger in a strange land: The pathogenesis of saphenous vein grafts stenosis with emphasis on structural and functional differences between veins and arteries. Prog. Cardiovasc. Dis. 34:45, 1991.

430. Fitzmaurice, M., and Ratliff, N. B.: Immunoglobulin deposition in atherosclerotic aortocoronary saphenous vein grafts. Arch. Pathol. Lab. Med. 114:388, 1990.

431. Keon, W. J., Heggtveit, H. A., and Leduc, J.: Perioperative myocardial infarctions caused by atheroembolism. J. Thorac. Cardiovasc. Surg. 84:849, 1982.

432. Rasmussen, S. L., Nielsen, S. L., Amtorp, O., et al.: 201-Thallium imaging as an indicator of graft patency after coronary artery bypass surgery. Eur. Heart J. 5:494, 1984.

433. Hwang, M. H., Meadows, W. R., Palac, R. T., et al.: Progression of native coronary artery disease at 10 years: Insights from a randomized study of medical versus surgical therapy for angina. J. Am. Coll. Cardiol. 16:1066, 1990.

434. Goldman, S., Copeland, J., Moritz, T., et al.: Saphenous vein graft patency 1 year after coronary artery bypass surgery and effects of antiplatelet therapy: Results of a Veterans Administration Cooperative Study. Circulation 80:1190, 1989.

435. Kroncke, G. M., Kosolcharoen, P., Clayman, J. A., et al.: Five-year changes in coronary arteries of medical and surgical patients of the Veterans Administration randomized study of bypass surgery. Circulation 78(Suppl. I):144, 1988.

436. Henderson, W. G., Goldman, S., Copeland, J. G., et al.: Antiplatelet or anticoagulant therapy after coronary artery bypass surgery: A meta-analysis of clinical trials. Ann. Intern. Med. 111:743, 1989.

437. Chesebro, J. H., Clements, I. P., Fuster, V., et al.: A platelet-inhibitor drug trial in coronary artery bypass operations: Benefit of perioperative dipyridamole and aspirin therapy on early post-operative vein-graft patency. N. Engl. J. Med. 307:73, 1982.

438. Chesebro, J. H., Fuster, V., Elveback, L. R., et al.: Effect of dipyridamole and aspirin on late vein-graft patency after coronary bypass operations. N. Engl. J. Med. 310:209, 1984.

439. Fremes, S. E., Levinton, C., Naylor, C. D., et al.: Optimal antithrombotic therapy following aortocoronary bypass: A meta-analysis. Eur. J. Cardiothorac. Surg. 7:169, 1993.

440. Goldman, S., Copeland, J., Moritz, T., et al.: Improvement in early saphenous vein graft patency after coronary artery bypass surgery with

antiplatelet therapy: Results of a Veterans Administration cooperative study. Circulation 77:1324, 1988.

441. Goldman, S., Copeland, J., Moritz, T., et al.: Long-term graft patency (3 years) after coronary artery surgery: Effects of aspirin: Results of a Veterans Administration cooperative study. Circulation 89:1138, 1994.

442. Goldman, S., Copeland, J., Moritz, T., et al.: Internal mammary and saphenous vein graft patency. Circulation 82(Suppl. IV): 237, 1990.

443. Hoff, H. F., Beck, G. J., Skibinski, C. I., et al.: Serum Lp(a) level as a predictor of vein graft stenosis after coronary artery bypass surgery in patients. Circulation 77:1238, 1988.

444. Blankenhorn, D. H., Nessim, S. A., Johnson, R. L., et al.: Beneficial effects of combined colestipol-niacin therapy on coronary atherosclerosis and coronary venous bypass grafts. JAMA 257:3233, 1987.

445. Barbir, M., Hunt, B. J., Galloway, D., et al.: A randomized pilot trial of low-dose combination lipid-lowering therapy following coronary artery bypass grafting. Clin. Cardiol. 17:59, 1994.

446. Rigotti, N. A., McKool, K. N., and Shiffman, S.: Predictors of smoking cessation after coronary artery bypass graft surgery: Results of the randomized trial with 5-year follow-up. Ann. Intern. Med. 120:287, 1994.

447. Solymoss, B. C., Nadeau, P., Millette, D., and Campeau, L.: Late thrombosis of saphenous vein coronary bypass grafts related to risk factors. Circulation 78(Suppl. I):140, 1988.

447a. McGiffin, D. J., and Kirklin, J. K.: Role of bypass surgery. In Fuster, V., Ross, R., and Topol, E. J. (eds): Atherosclerosis and Coronary Artery Disease. Philadelphia, J. B. Lippincott, 1996, pp. 1543–1560.

448. Yusuf, S., Zucker, D., Peduzzi, P., et al.: Effect of coronary artery bypass graft surgery on survival: Overview of 10 year results from randomized trials by the Coronary Artery Bypass Graft Surgery Trialists Collaboration. Lancet 344:563, 1994.

449. Kannel, W. B., and Feinlieb, M.: Natural history of angina pectoris in the Framingham study: Progress and survival. Am. J. Cardiol. 29:154, 1972.

450. Gandhi, M. M., Lampe, F. C., and Wood, D. A.: Incidence, clinical characteristics, and short-term prognosis of angina pectoris. Br. Heart J. 73:193, 1995.

451. Chang, J. A., and Froelicher, V. F.: Clinical and exercise test markers of prognosis in patients with stable coronary artery disease. Curr. Probl. Cardiol. 9:533, 1994.

452. O'Keefe, J. H., Jr., Zinmeister, A. R., and Gibbons, R. J.: Value of normal electrocardiographic findings in predicting resting left ventricular function in patients with chest pain and suspected coronary artery disease. Am. J. Med. 86:658, 1989.

453. Galderisi, M., Lauer, M. S., and Levy, D.: Echocardiographic determinants of clinical outcome in subjects with coronary artery disease (the Framingham Heart Study). Am. J. Cardiol. 70:971, 1992.

454. Proudfit, W. J., Bruschke, A. V. G., MacMillan, J. P., et al.: Fifteen-year survival study of patients with obstructive coronary artery disease. Circulation 68:986, 1983.

455. Emond, M., Mark, M. B., Davis, K. B., et al.: Long-term survival of medically treated patients in the Coronary Artery Surgery Study (CASS) registry. Circulation 90:2645, 1994.

456. Weiner, D. A., Ryan, T. J., McCabe, C. H., et al.: Comparison of coronary artery bypass surgery and medical therapy in patients with exercise-induced silent myocardial ischemia: A report from the Coronary Artery Surgery Study (CASS) registry. J. Am. Coll. Cardiol. 12:595, 1988.

457. Califf, R. M., Tomabechi, Y., Lee, K. L., et al.: Outcome in one-vessel coronary artery disease. Circulation 67:283, 1983.

458. Proudfit, W. L., Kramer, J. R., Goormastic, M., and Loop, F. D.: Survival of patients with mild angina or myocardial infarction without angina: A comparison of medical and surgical treatment. Br. Heart J. 59:641, 1988.

459. Humphries, J. O., Kuller, L., Ross, R. S., et al.: Natural history of ischemic heart disease in relation to angiographic findings. Circulation 49:489, 1974.

460. Harris, P. J., Behar, V. S., Conley, J. J., et al.: The prognostic significance of 50 per cent coronary stenosis in medically treated patients with coronary artery disease. Circulation 62:240, 1980.

461. Conti, C. R., Selby, J. H., Christie, L. G., et al.: Left main coronary artery stenosis: Clinical spectrum, pathophysiology and management. Prog. Cardiovasc. Dis. 22:73, 1979.

462. Taylor, H. A., Deumite, N. J., Chaitman, B. R., et al.: Asymptomatic left main coronary artery disease in the Coronary Artery Surgery Study (CASS) registry. Circulation 79:1171, 1989.

463. Caracciolo, E. A., Davis, K. B., Sopko, G., et al.: Comparison of surgical and medical group survival in patients with left main coronary artery disease: Long-term CASS experience. Circulation 91:2325, 1995.

464. Conley, M. J., Ely, R. L., Kisslo, J., et al.: The prognostic spectrum of left main stenosis. Circulation 57:947, 1978.

465. Kent, K. M., Rosing, D. R., Ewels, C. J., et al.: Prognosis of asymptomatic or mildly symptomatic patients with coronary artery disease. Am. J. Cardiol. 49:1823, 1982.

466. Vogel, R. A.: Coronary stenosis significance: Lessons learned from recent trials. Curr. Opin. Cardiol. 9:705, 1994.

467. Folland, E. D., Vogel, R. A, Hartigan, P., et al.: Relation between coronary artery stenosis assessed by visual, caliper and computer methods and exercise capacity in patients with single-vessel coronary artery disease. Circulation 89:2005, 1994.

468. Ellis, S., Alderman, E., Cain, K., et al.: Prediction of risk of arterial myocardial infarction by lesion severity and measurement method of stenoses in the left anterior descending coronary distribution: A CASS registry study. J. Am. Coll. Cardiol. 11:908, 1988.

469. Little, W. C., Downes, T. R., and Applegate, R. J.: The underlying coronary lesion in myocardial infarction: Implications for coronary angiography. Clin. Cardiol. 14:868, 1991.

470. Giroud, D., Li, J. M., Urban, P., et al.: Relation of the site of acute myocardial infarction to the most severe coronary arterial stenosis at prior angiography. Am. J. Cardiol. 69:729, 1992.

471. Little, W. C., Constantinescu, M., Applegate, R. J., et al.: Can coronary angiography predict the site of a subsequent myocardial infarction in patients with mild to moderate coronary artery disease? Circulation 78:1157, 1988.

472. Ambrose, J. A., Winters, S. L., Arora, R. R., et al.: Coronary angiographic morphology in myocardial infarction: A link between the pathogenesis of unstable angina and myocardial infarction. J. Am. Coll. Cardiol. 6:1233, 1985.

473. Vanhees, L., Fagard, R., Thijs, L., et al.: Prognostic significance of peak exercise capacity in patients with coronary artery disease. J. Am. Coll. Cardiol. 23:358, 1994.

474. Weiner, D. A., Ryan, T. I., Parsons, L., et al.: Long-term prognostic value of exercise testing in men and women from the Coronary Artery Surgery Study (CASS) registry. Am. J. Cardiol. 75:865, 1995.

475. Mark, D. B., Shaw, L., Harrell, F. E., et al.: Prognostic value of a treadmill exercise score in patients with suspected coronary artery disease. N. Engl. J. Med. 325:849, 1991.

476. Morrow, K., Morris, C. K., Froelicher, V. E., et al.: Prediction of cardiovascular death in men undergoing noninvasive evaluation for coronary artery disease. Ann. Intern. Med. 118:689, 1993.

477. Marie P-Y, Danchin, N., Durand, J. F., et al.: Long-term prediction of major ischemic events by exercise thallium-201 single-photon emission computer tomography. Incremental prognostic value compared with clinical, exercise testing, catheterization and radionuclide angiographic data. J. Am. Coll. Cardiol. 26:879, 1995.

478. Hilton, T. C., Shaw, L. J., Chaitman, B. R., et al.: Prognostic significance of exercise thallium-201 testing in patients aged greater than or equal to 70 years with known or suspected coronary artery disease. Am. J. Cardiol. 69:45, 1992.

479. Herman, S. D., LaBresh, K. A., Santos-Ocampo, C. D., et al.: Comparison of dobutamine and exercise using technetium-99m sestamibi imaging for the evalution of coronary artery disease. Am. J. Cardiol. 73:164, 1994.

480. Verani, M. S.: Pharmacologic stress myocardial perfusion imaging. Curr. Probl. Cardiol. 18:481, 1993.

480a. Heller, G. V., Herman, S. D., Travin, M. I., et al.: Independent prognostic value of intravenous dipyridamole technetium with 99-m sestamibi tomographic imaging in predicting cardiac events and cardiac-related hospital admissions. J. Am. Coll. Cardiol. 26:1202, 1995.

481. Stratmann, H. G., Tamesis, B. R., Younis, L. T., et al.: Prognostic value of dipyridamole technetium-99m sestamibi myocardial tomography in patients with stable chest pain who are unable to exercise. Am. J. Cardiol. 73:647, 1994.

482. Shaw, L., Miller, D. D., Kong, B. A., et al.: Determination of perioperative cardiac risk by adenosine thallium-201 myocardial imaging. Am. Heart J. 124:861, 1992.

483. Williams, M. J., Marwick, T. H., O'Gorman, D., and Foale, R. A.: Comparison of exercise echocardiography with an exercise score to diagnose coronary artery disease in women. Am. J. Cardiol. 74:435, 1994.

483a. Panza, J. A., Curiel, R. V., Laurienzo, J. M., et al.: Relation between ischemic threshold measured during dobutamine stress echocardiography and known indices of poor prognosis in patients with coronary artery disease. Circulation 92:2095, 1995.

484. Poldermans, D., Irnese, M., Fioretti, P. M., et al.: Improved cardiac risk stratification in major vascular surgery with dobutamine-atropine stress echocardiography. J. Am. Coll. Cardiol. 26:648, 1995.

485. Coletta, C., Galati, A., Greco, G., et al.: Prognostic value of high dose dipyridamole echocardiography in patients with chronic coronary artery disease and preserved left ventricular function. J. Am. Coll. Cardiol. 26:887, 1995.

486. Report of Inter-Society Commission for Heart Disease Resources: Optimal resources for coronary artery surgery. Circulation 46:A-325, 1972.

487. Rogers, W. J., Coggin, C. J., Gersh, B. J., et al.: Ten-year follow-up of quality of life in patients randomized to receive medical therapy or coronary artery bypass graft surgery: The Coronary Artery Surgery Study (CASS). Circulation 82:1647, 1990.

488. The VA Coronary Artery Bypass Surgery Cooperative Study Group: 18-year follow-up in the Veterans Affairs Cooperative Study of Coronary Artery Bypass Surgery for Stable Angina. Circulation 86:121, 1992.

489. Cameron, A., Kemp, H. G., Jr., and Green, G. E.: Reoperation for coronary artery disease: 10 years of clinical follow-up. Circulation 78(Suppl. I):158, 1988.

490. American College of Cardiology/American Heart Association Task Force on Assessment of Diagnostic and Therapeutic Cardiovascular Procedures (Subcommittee on Coronary Artery Bypass Graft Surgery): Guidelines and indications for coronary artery bypass graft surgery. J. Am. Coll. Cardiol. 17:543, 1991.

491. van Brussel, B. L., Plokker, H. W., Ernst, S. M., et al.: Venous coronary artery bypass surgery: A 15-year follow-up study. Circulation 88:II87, 1993.

492. Rosenfeldt, T. F. L., and Wong, J.: Current expectations for survival and complications in coronary artery bypass grafting. Curr. Opin. Cardiol. 8:910, 1993.

493. Passamani, E., Davis, K. B., Gillespie, M. J., and Killip, T.: A randomized trial of coronary artery bypass surgery: Survival of patients with a low ejection fraction. N. Engl. J. Med. 312:1685, 1985.

494. Detre, K. M., Takaro, T., Hultgren, H., and Peduzzi, P.: Long-term mortality and morbidity results of the Veterans Administration randomized

trial of coronary artery bypass surgery. Circulation 72(Suppl. V):84, 1985.

495. The Veterans Administration Coronary Artery Bypass Surgery Cooperative Study Group: Eleven-year survival in the Veterans Administration randomized trial of coronary bypass surgery for stable angina. N. Engl. J. Med. 311:1333, 1984.

496. Gersh, B. J., Kronmal, R. A., and Schaff, H. V.: Comparison of coronary artery bypass surgery and medical therapy in patients 65 years of age or older. N. Engl. J. Med. 313:217, 1985.

497. Detre, K., Peduzzi, P., Scott, S. M., and Davies, B.: Long-term survival results in medically and surgically randomized patients. Progr. Cardiovasc. Dis. 28:235, 1986.

498. Varnauskas, E.: Survival, myocardial infarction, and employment status in a prospective randomized study of coronary bypass surgery. Circulation 72(Suppl. V):90, 1985.

499. Alderman, E. L., Bourassa, M. G., Cohen, L. S., et al.: Ten-year follow-up of survival and myocardial infarction in the randomized Coronary Artery Surgery Study (CASS). Circulation 82:1629, 1990.

500. Takaro, T., Pifarre, R., and Fish, R.: Left main coronary artery disease. Prog. Cardiovasc. Dis. 28:229, 1985.

501. Carraciolo, E. A., Davis, K. B., Sopko, G., et al.: Comparison of surgical and medical group survival in patients with left main equivalent coronary artery disease: Long-term CASS experience. Circulation 91:2335, 1995.

502. Califf, R. M., Conley, M. J., Behar, V. S., et al.: Left main coronary artery disease: Its clinical presentation and prognostic significance with nonsurgical therapy. Am. J. Cardiol. 53:1489, 1984.

503. Caracciolo, E. A., Davis, K. B., Sopko, G., et al.: Comparison of surgical and medical group survival in patients with left main coronary artery disease: Long-term CASS experience. Circulation 91:2325, 1995.

504. Emond, M., Mock, M. B., and Davis, K. B.: Long-term survival of medically treated patients in the Coronary Artery Surgery Study (CASS registry). Circulation 90:2645, 1994.

505. Murphy, M. L., Meadows, W. R., Thomsen, J., et al.: The effect of coronary artery bypass surgery on the incidence of myocardial infarction and hospitalization. Prog. Cardiovasc. Dis. 28:309, 1986.

506. CASS Principal Investigators and Their Associates: Myocardial infarction and mortality in the Coronary Artery Surgery Study (CASS) randomized trial. N. Engl. J. Med. 310:750, 1984.

507. Myers, W. O., Schaff, H. V., Fisher, L. D., et al.: Time to first new myocardial infarction in patients with severe angina and three-vessel disease comparing medical and early surgical therapy: A CASS registry study of survival. J. Thorac. Cardiovasc. Surg. 95:382, 1988.

508. Davis, K. B., Alderman, E. L., Kosinski, A. S., et al.: Early mortality of acute myocardial infarction in patients with and without prior coronary revascularization surgery. Circulation 85:2100, 1992.

509. Jones, E. L., Craver, J. M., Kaplan, J. A., et al.: Criteria for operability and reduction of surgical mortality in patients with severe left ventricular ischemia and dysfunction. Ann. Thorac. Surg. 25:413, 1978.

510. Christakis, G. T., Weisel, R. D., Fremes, S. E., et al.: Coronary artery bypass grafting in patients with poor ventricular function. J. Thorac. Cardiovasc. Surg. 103:1083, 1992.

511. Elefteriades, J. A., Tolis, G., Jr., Levi, E., et al.: Coronary artery bypass grafting in severe left ventricular dysfunction: Excellent survival with improved ejection fraction and functional state. J. Am. Coll. Cardiol. 22:1411, 1993.

512. Alfieri, O.: Coronary artery bypass grafting for left ventricular dysfunction. Curr. Opin. Cardiol. 9:658, 1994.

513. Balu, V., Szmedra, L., Dean, D., and Bhayana, J.: Long-term survival of patients with low ejection fraction. Texas Heart Inst. J. 15:44, 1988.

514. Holmes, D. R., Davis, K. B., Mock, M. B., et al.: The effect of medical and surgical treatment on subsequent sudden cardiac death in patients with coronary artery disease: A report from the Coronary Artery Surgery Study (CASS). Circulation 73:1254, 1986.

515. Pigott, J. D., Kouchoukos, N. T., Oberman, A., and Cutter, G. R.: Late results of surgical and medical therapy for patients with coronary artery disease and depressed left ventricular function. J. Am. Coll. Cardiol. 5:1036, 1985.

516. Bounous, E. P., Mark, D. B., Pollock, B. G., et al.: Surgical survival benefits for coronary disease patients with left ventricular dysfunction. Circulation 78(Suppl. I):151, 1988.

517. Myers, W. O., Davis, K., Foster, E. D., et al.: Surgical survival in the Coronary Artery Surgery Study (CASS) registry. Ann. Thorac. Surg. 40:245, 1985.

518. Ross, J., Jr.: Myocardial perfusion–contraction matching: Implications for coronary heart disease and hibernation. Circulation 83:1076, 1991.

519. Lewis, S. J., Sawada, S. G., Ryan, T., et al.: Segmental wall motion abnormalities in the absence of clinically documented myocardial infarction: Clinical significance and evidence of hibernating myocardium. Am. Heart J. 121:1088, 1991.

520. Eitzman, D., Al-Aouar, Z., Kanter, H. L., et al.: Clinical outcome of patients with advanced coronary artery disease after viability studies with positron emission tomography. J. Am. Coll. Cardiol. 20:559, 1992.

521. Tillisch, J., Brunken, R., Marshall, R., et al.: Reversibility of cardiac wall-motion abnormalities predicted by positron tomography. N. Engl. J. Med. 314:884, 1986.

522. Tamaki, N., Kawamoto, M., Tadamura, E., et al.: Prediction of reversible ischemia after revascularization: Perfusion and metabolic studies with positron emission tomography. Circulation 91:1697, 1995.

522a. Conversano, A., Walsh, J. F., Geltman, E. M., et al.: Delineation of myocardial stunning and hibernation by positron emission tomography in advanced coronary artery disease. Am. Heart J. 131:440, 1996.

523. Bonow, R. O., Burman, D. S., Givens, R. J., et al.: Cardiac positron emission tomography: A report for health professionals from the Committee on Advanced Cardiac Imaging and Technology of the Council of Clinical Cardiology, American Heart Association. Circulation 84:447, 1991.

524. Sansoy, V., Glover, D. K., Watson, D. D., et al.: Comparison of thallium-201 resting redistribution with technetium-99m sestamibi uptake and functional response to dobutamine for assessment of myocardial viability. Circulation 92:994, 1995.

525. Ragosta, M., Beller, G. A., Watson, D. D., et al.: Quantitative planar rest-redistribution 201 Tl imaging in detection of myocardial viability and prediction of improvement in left ventricular function after coronary bypass surgery in patients with severely depressed left ventricular function. Circulation 87:1630, 1993.

526. Gioia, G., Powers, J., Heo, J, and Iskandrian, A. S.: Prognostic value of rest-redistribution tomographic thallium-201 imaging in ischemic cardiomyopathy. Am. J. Cardiol. 75:759, 1995.

527. Murray, G., Schad, N., Lad, W., et al.: Metabolic cardiac imaging in severe coronary disease: Assessment of viability with I-123 iodo phenylpentadecanoic acid and multicrystal gamma camera, and correlation with biopsy. J. Nucl. Med. 33:1269, 1992.

528. Chen, C., Chen, L., Prada, J. V., et al.: Incremental doses of dobutamine induce a biphasic response in dysfunctional left ventricular regions subtending coronary stenoses. Circulation 92:756, 1995.

529. Camarano, G., Ragosta, M., Gimple, L. W., et al.: Identification of viable myocardium with contrast echocardiography in patients with poor left ventricular systolic functions caused by recent or previous myocardial infarction. Am. J. Cardiol. 75:215, 1995.

530. Ayanian, J. Z., and Epstein, A. M.: Differences in the use of procedures between women and men hospitalized for coronary heart disease. N. Engl. J. Med. 325:221, 1991.

531. Cosgrove, D. M.: Coronary artery surgery in women. In Proceedings of an N.H.L.B.I. Conference: Cardiovascular Health and Disease in Women. Greenwich, CT, Le Jacq Communications, Inc., 1993, p. 117.

532. Disch, D. L., O'Connor, G. T., Birkmeyer, J. D., et al.: Changes in patients undergoing coronary artery bypass grafting 1987–1990. Ann. Thorac. Surg. 57:416, 1994.

533. Barbir, M., Lazem, F., Ilsley, C., et al.: Coronary artery surgery in women compared with men: Analysis of coronary risk factors and in-hospital mortality in a single centre. Br. Heart J. 71:408, 1994.

534. Findlay, I. N.: Coronary bypass surgery in women. Curr. Opin. Cardiol. 9:650, 1994.

535. Davis, K. B., Chaitman, B., Ryan, T., et al.: Comparison of 15 year survival for men and women after initial medical or surgical treatment for coronary artery disease: A CASS Registry study. J. Am. Coll. Cardiol. 25:1000, 1995.

536. Rahimtoola, S. H., Bennett, A. J., Grunkemeier, G. L., et al.: Survival at 15 to 18 years after coronary bypass surgery for angina in women. Circulation 88:II71, 1993.

537. Lytle, B. W., Kramer, J. R., Golding, L. R., et al.: Young adults with coronary atherosclerosis: 10-year results of surgical myocardial revascularization. J. Am. Coll. Cardiol. 4:445, 1984.

538. FitzGibbon, G. M., Hamilton, M. G., Leach, A. J., et al.: Coronary artery disease and coronary bypass grafting in young men: Experience with 138 subjects 39 years of age and younger. J. Am. Coll. Cardiol. 9:977, 1987.

539. Peterson, E. D., Jollis, J. G., Bebchuk, J. D., et al.: Changes in mortality after myocardial revascularization in the elderly: The national Medicare experience. Ann. Intern. Med. 121:919, 1994.

540. Mullany, C. J., Darling, G. E., Pluth, J. R., et al.: Early and late results after isolated coronary artery bypass surgery in 159 patients aged 80 years and older. Circulation 82(Suppl. IV):IV-229, 1990.

541. Ricou, F. J., Suilen, C., Rothmeier, C., et al.: Coronary angiography in octogenarians. Results and implications for revascularization. Am. J. Med. 99:16, 1995.

541a. Tsai, T. P., Chaux, A., Matloff, J. M., et al.: Ten-year experience of cardiac surgery in patients aged 80 years and over. Ann. Thorac. Surg. 58:445, 1994.

541b. Blauth, C. I., Cosgrove, D. M., Webb, B. W., et al.: Atheroembolism from the ascending aorta: An emerging problem in cardiac surgery. J. Thorac. Cardiovasc. Surg. 103:1104, 1992.

542. Loop, F. D., Lytle, B. W., Cosgrove, D. M., et al.: Reoperation for coronary atherosclerosis: Changing practice in 2509 patients. Ann. Surg. 212:378, 1990.

543. Rosengart, T. K.: Risk analysis of primary versus reoperative coronary artery bypass grafting. Ann. Thorac. Surg. 56(Suppl.):S-74, 1993.

544. Noppeney, T., Eberlein, U., Langhans, L., and von der Emde, J.: The influence of age and other risk factors on the results of coronary reoperation. Thorac. Cardiovasc. Surg. 41:43, 1993.

545. Akie, S., Ozdogan, E., Ohri, S. K., et al.: Early and long-term results of re-operation for coronary artery disease. Br. Heart J. 68:176, 1992.

546. Takahashi, T., Nakano, S., Shimazaki, Y., et al.: Long-term appraisal of coronary bypass operations in familial hypercholesterolemia. Ann. Thorac. Surg. 56:499, 1993.

547. Kaul, T. K., Fields, M. A., Reddy, D. R., and Kahn, D. R.: Cardiac operations in patients with end-stage renal disease. Ann. Thorac. Surg. 57:691, 1994.

548. Barzilay, J. I., Kronmall, R. A., Bittner, V., et al.: Coronary artery disease and coronary artery bypass grafting in diabetic patients age ≥65 years (Report from the Coronary Artery Surgery Study [CASS] registry). Am. J. Cardiol. 74:334, 1994.

549. O'Keefe, J. H., Jr., Sutton, M. B., McCallister, B. D., et al.: Coronary

angioplasty versus bypass surgery in patients >70 years old matched for ventricular function. J. Am. Coll. Cardiol. 24:425, 1994.

550. Hamm, C., Reimers, J., Ischinger, T., et al.: A randomized study of coronary angioplasty compared with bypass surgery in patients with symptomatic multivessel coronary disease: German Angioplasty Bypass Surgery Investigation (GABI). N. Engl. J. Med. 331:1037, 1994.

551. CABRI Trial Participants: First-year results of CABRI (Coronary Angioplasty versus Bypass Revascularization Investigation). Lancet 346:1179, 1995.

551a. Pocock, S. J., Henderson, R. A., Rickards, A. F., et al.: Meta-analysis of randomized trials comparing coronary angioplasty with bypass surgery. Lancet 346:1184, 1995.

551b. Sim, I., Gupta, M., McDonald, K., et al.: A meta-analysis of randomized trials comparing coronary artery bypass grafting with percutaneous transluminal coronary angioplasty in multivessel coronary artery disease. Am. J. Cardiol. 76:1025, 1995.

551c. Goy, J-J, Eeckhout, E., Bernand, B., et al.: Coronary angioplasty versus internal mammary grafting for isolated proximal left anterior descending coronary artery stenosis. Lancet 343:1449, 1994.

552. Sculpher, M. J., Seed, P., Henderson, R. A., et al.: Health service costs of coronary angioplasty and coronary artery bypass surgery: The Randomized Intervention Treatment of Angina (RITA trial). Lancet 344:927, 1994.

552a. Weintraub, W. S., Mauldin, P. D., Becker, E., et al.: A comparison of the costs and quality of life after coronary angioplasty or coronary surgery for multivessel coronary artery disease. Circulation 92:2831, 1995.

553. Rihal, C. S., Eagle, K. A., Mickel, M. C., et al.: Surgical therapy for coronary artery disease among patients with combined coronary artery and peripheral vascular disease. Circulation 91:46, 1995.

554. Farkouh, M. E., Rihal, C. S., Gersh, B. J., et al.: Influence of coronary heart disease on morbidity and mortality after lower extremity revascularization surgery: A population-based study in Olmsted County, Minnesota (1970–1987). J. Am. Coll. Cardiol. 24:1290, 1994.

555. Langer, R. D., Criqui, M. H., Fronek, A., et al.: Isolated small vessel peripheral arterial disease is associated with future cardiovascular events. Circulation 81:724, 1990.

556. Smith, G. D., Shipley, M. J., and Rose, G.: Intermittent claudication, heart disease risk factors, and mortality: The Whitehall study. Circulation 82:1925, 1990.

557. Mangano, D. T.: Perioperative cardiac morbidity. Anesthesiology 72:153, 1990.

558. Hertzer, N. R., Young, J. R., Beven, E. G., et al.: Late results of coronary bypass in patients with peripheral vascular disease. I. Five-year survival according to age and clinical cardiac status. Cleve. Clin. J. Med. 53:133, 1986.

559. European Coronary Surgery Study Group: Prospective randomized study of coronary artery bypass surgery in stable angina pectoris: Second interim report. Lancet 2:491, 1980.

560. Shaw, P. J., Bates, D., Cartlidge, N. E., et al.: Neurologic and neuropsychological morbidity following major surgery: Comparison of coronary artery bypass and peripheral vascular surgery. Stroke 18:700, 1987.

561. Ballantyne, C. M., Verani, M. S., Short, H. D., et al.: Delayed recovery of severely "stunned" myocardium with the support of a left ventricular assist device after coronary bypass graft surgery. J. Am. Coll. Cardiol. 10:710, 1987.

562. Barnett, H. J., Eliasziw, M., and Meldrum, H. E.: Drugs and surgery in the prevention of ischemic stroke. N. Engl. J. Med. 332:238, 1995.

563. Beebe, H. G., Clagett, G. P., DeWesse, J. A., et al.: Assessing risk associated with carotid endarterectomy. Circulation 79:472, 1989.

564. Hertzer, N. R., Loop, F. D., Beven, E. G., et al.: Surgical staging for simultaneous coronary and carotid disease: A study including prospective randomization. J. Vasc. Surg. 9:455, 1989.

565. Babu, S. C., Shah, P. M., Singh, B. M., et al.: Coexisting carotid stenosis in patients undergoing cardiac surgery: Indications and guidelines for simultaneous operations. Am. J. Surg. 150:207, 1985.

566. Huber, K. C., Evans, M. A., Bresntan, J. F., et al.: Outcome of non-cardiac surgery in patients with severe coronary disease treated preoperatively with coronary angioplasty. Mayo Clin. Proc. 67:15, 1992.

UNSTABLE ANGINA

567. Braunwald, E., Mark, D. B., Jones, R. H., et al.: Unstable Angina: Diagnosis and management: Clinical Practice Guideline. Rockville, MD, Agency for Healthcare Policy and Research and the National Heart, Lung and Blood Institute, Public Health Service, U.S. Department of Health and Human Services. AHCPR Publication No. 94-0602:154, 1994, pp. 28, 92.

568. Braunwald, E.: Unstable angina: A classification. Circulation 80:410, 1989.

568a. Braunwald, E., and Fuster, V.: Unstable angina. Definition, pathogenesis, and classification. In Fuster, V., Ross, R., and Topol, E. J. (eds.): Atherosclerosis and Coronary Artery Disease. Philadelphia, J. B. Lippincott, 1996, pp. 1285–1298.

569. Ahmed, W. H., Bittl, J. A., and Braunwald, E.: Relation between clinical presentation and angiographic findings in unstable angina pectoris, and comparison with that in stable angina. Am. J. Cardiol. 72:544, 1993.

570. van Miltenburg-van Zijl, A. J., Simoons, M. L., Veerhoek, R. J., and Bossuyt, P. M.: Incidence and follow-up of Braunwald subgroups in unstable angina pectoris. J. Am. Coll. Cardiol. 25:1286, 1995.

571. Calvin, J. E., Klein, L. W., VandenBurg, B. J., et al.: Risk stratification in unstable angina: Prospective validation of the Braunwald classification. J.A.M.A. 273:136, 1995.

572. Bugiardini, R., Borghi, A., Pozzati, A., et al.: Relation of severity of

symptoms to transient myocardial ischemia and prognosis in unstable angina. J. Am. Coll. Cardiol. 25:597, 1995.

573. Chierchia, S., Brunelli, C., Simonetti, I., et al.: Sequence of events in angina at rest: Primary reduction in coronary flow. Circulation 61:759, 1980.

574. Figueras, J., and Lidon, R. M.: Circadian rhythm of angina in patients with unstable angina: Relationship with extent of coronary disease, coronary reserve and ECG changes during pain. Eur. Heart J. 15:753, 1994.

575. Moise, A., Theroux, P., Taeymans, Y., et al.: Unstable angina and progression of coronary atherosclerosis. N. Engl. J. Med. 309:685, 1983.

575a. Kaski, J. C., Chester, M. R., Chen, L., et al.: Rapid angiographic progression of coronary disease in patients with unstable angina pectoris. The role of complex stenosis morphology. Circulation 92:2058, 1995.

575b. DeServi, S., Mazzone, A., Ricevuti, G., et al.: Clinical and angiographic correlates of leukocyte activation in unstable angina. J. Am. Coll. Cardiol. 26:1151, 1995.

576. MacIsaac, A., Thomas, J., and Topol, E.: Toward the quiescent coronary plaque. J. Am. Coll. Cardiol. 22:1228, 1993.

577. Osborne, J. A., and Stone, P. H.: Recent advances in the understanding and management of stable and unstable angina pectoris and asymptomatic myocardial ischemia. Curr. Opin. Cardiol. 9:448, 1994.

578. Grande, P., Grauholt, A. M., and Madsen, J. K.: Unstable angina pectoris: Platelet behavior and prognosis in progressive angina and intermediate coronary syndrome. Circulation 81(Suppl. I):16, 1990.

579. Willerson, J. T., Golino, P., Eidt, J., et al.: Specific platelet mediators and unstable coronary artery lesions: Experimental evidence and potential clinical implications. Circulation 80:198, 1989.

580. Folts, J. D., Gallagher, K., and Rowe, G. G.: Blood flow reductions in stenosed canine coronary arteries: Vasospasm or platelet aggregation? Circulation 65:248, 1982.

581. Lewis, H. D., Jr., Davis, J. W., Archibald, D. G., et al.: Protective effects of aspirin against acute myocardial infarction and death in men with unstable angina. N. Engl. J. Med. 309:396, 1983.

582. Cairns, J. A., Gent, M., Singer, J., et al.: Aspirin, sulfinpyrazone, or both in unstable angina: Results of a Canadian multicenter trial. N. Engl. J. Med. 313:1369, 1985.

583. Theroux, P., Ouimet, H., McCans, J., et al.: Aspirin, heparin, or both to treat acute unstable angina. N. Engl. J. Med. 319:1105, 1988.

584. The RISC Group: Risk of myocardial infarction and death during treatment with low-dose aspirin and intravenous heparin in men with unstable coronary artery disease. Lancet 336:827, 1990.

585. Simoons, M. L., deBoer, M. J., van den Brand, M. J., et al.: Randomized trial of a GP-IIb/IIIa platelet receptor blocker in refractory unstable angina—European Cooperative Study Group. Circulation 89:596, 1994.

586. Theroux, P., White, H., David, D., et al.: A heparin-controlled study of MK-383 in unstable angina. Circulation 90(Abs.):I-231, 1994.

587. Falk, E.: Unstable angina with fatal outcome: Dynamic coronary thrombosis leading to infarction and/or sudden death. Circulation 71:699, 1985.

588. Chesebro, J. H., and Fuster, V.: Thrombosis in unstable angina. N. Engl. J. Med. 327:192, 1992.

589. Gurfinkel, E., Altman, R., Scazziota, A., et al.: Importance of thrombosis and thrombolysis in silent ischemia: Comparison of patients with acute myocardial infarction and unstable angina. Br. Heart J. 71:151, 1994.

590. Merlini, P. A., Bauer, K. A., Oltrona, L., et al.: Persistent activation of coagulation mechanism in unstable angina and myocardial infarction. Circulation 90:61, 1994.

591. Kruskal, J. B., Commerford, P. J., Franks, J. J., et al.: Fibrin and fibrinogen related antigens in patients with stable and unstable coronary artery disease. N. Engl. J. Med. 317:1361, 1987.

592. Hoffmeister, H. M., Jur, M., Wendell, H. P., et al.: Alterations of coagulation in fibrinolytic and kallikrein-kinin systems in the acute and post acute phases in patients with unstable angina pectoris. Circulation 91:2520, 1995.

593. Zalewski, A., Shi, Y., Nardone, D., et al.: Evidence for reduced fibrinolytic activity in unstable angina at rest: Clinical, biochemical and angiographic correlates. Circulation 83:1685, 1991.

594. The TIMI IIIA Investigators, Braunwald, E., Chairman: Early effects of tissue-type plasminogen activator added to conventional therapy on the culprit coronary lesion in patients presenting with ischemic cardiac pain at rest. Circulation 87:38, 1993.

595. Sherman, C. T., Litvack, F., Grundfest, W., et al.: Coronary angioscopy in patients with unstable angina pectoris. N. Engl. J. Med. 315:913, 1986.

596. Mizuno, K., Satomura, K., Miyamoto, A., et al.: Angioscopic evaluation of coronary-artery thrombi in acute coronary syndromes. N. Engl. J. Med. 326:287, 1992.

597. Gold, H. K., Johns, J. A., Leinbach, R. C., et al.: A randomized, blinded, placebo-controlled trial of recombinant human tissue-type plasminogen activator in patients with unstable angina pectoris. Circulation 75:1192, 1987.

598. Falk, E.: Unstable angina with fatal outcome: Dynamic coronary thrombosis leading to infarction and/or sudden death. Circulation 71:699, 1985.

599. Brown, B. G., Bolson, E. L., and Dodge, H. T.: Dynamic mechanisms in human coronary stenosis. Circulation 70:917, 1984.

600. Saner, H. E., Gobel, F. L., Salomonowitz, E., et al.: The disease-free wall in coronary atherosclerosis: Its relation to degree of obstruction. J. Am. Coll. Cardiol. 6:1096, 1985.

601. Kaski, J. C., Tousoulis, D., Haider, A. W., et al.: Reactivity of eccentric and concentric coronary stenosis in patients with chronic stable angina. J. Am. Coll. Cardiol. 17:627, 1991.

602. Aoyama, T., Yui, Y., Morishita, H., and Kawai, C.: Prostaglandin I₂, half-life regulated by high density lipoprotein is decreased in acute myocardial infarction and unstable angina pectoris. Circulation 81:1784, 1990.

603. Qiu, S., Theroux, P., Marcil, M., and Solymoss, B. C.: Plasma endothelin-1 levels in stable and unstable angina. Cardiology 82:12, 1993.

604. Hirsh, P. D., Hillis, L. D., Campbell, W. B., et al.: Release of prostaglandins and thromboxane into the coronary circulation in patients with ischemic heart disease. N. Engl. J. Med. 304:685, 1981.

605. Flugelman, M. Y., Virmani, R., Correa, R., et al.: Smooth muscle cell abundance and fibroblast growth factors in coronary lesions of patients with nonfatal unstable angina: A clue to the mechanism of transformation from the stable to the unstable clinical state. Circulation 88:2493, 1993.

606. Califf, R. M., and Mark, D. B.: Unstable angina. Clinical presentation and diagnostic techniques. In Fuster, V., Ross, R., and Topol, E. J. (eds.): Atherosclerosis and Coronary Artery Disease. Philadelphia, J. B. Lippincott, 1996, pp. 1299–1314.

607. Bosch, X., Theroux, P., Pelletier, G. B., et al.: Clinical and angiographic features and prognostic significance of early post infarction angina with and without electrocardiographic signs of transient ischemia. Am. J. Med. 91:493, 1991.

608. Jaffe, N. D., and Boden, W. E.: Spontaneous transient, inverted U waves as initial electrocardiographic manifestation of unstable angina. Am. Heart J. 129:1028, 1995.

609. Haines, D. E., Raabe, D. S., Gundel, W., and Wackers, F. J.: Anatomic and prognostic significance of new T-wave inversion in unstable angina. Am. J. Cardiol. 52:14, 1983.

610. Lee, T. H., Cook, E. F., Weisberg, M. C., et al.: Impact of the availability of a prior electrocardiogram on the triage of the patient with acute chest pain. J. Gen. Intern. Med. 5:381, 1990.

611. Gottlieb, S. O., Weisfeldt, M. L., Ouyang, P., et al.: Silent ischemia predicts infarction and death during 2 years follow-up of unstable angina. J. Am. Coll. Cardiol. 10:756, 1987.

612. Nademanee, K., Intarachot, V., Josephson, M. A., et al.: Prognostic significance of silent myocardial ischemia in patients with unstable angina. J. Am. Coll. Cardiol. 10:1, 1987.

613. Kaski, J. C.: Silent ischemia in unstable angina: Prognosis. In Fuster, V., Ross, R., and Topol, E. J. (eds.): Atherosclerosis and Coronary Artery Disease. Philadelphia, J. B. Lippincott, 1996, pp. 1377–1388.

614. Chierchia, S., Lazzari, M., Freedman, B., et al.: Impairment of myocardial perfusion and function during painless myocardial ischemia. J. Am. Coll. Cardiol. 1:924, 1983.

615. Romeo, F., Rosano, G. M., Martuscelli, E., et al.: Unstable angina: Role of silent ischemia and total ischemia time (silent plus painful ischemia), a six-year follow-up. J. Am. Coll. Cardiol. 19:1173, 1992.

616. Liuzzo, G., Biasucci, L. M., Gallimore, J. R., et al.: The prognostic value of C-reactive protein and serum amyloid-A protein in severe unstable angina. N. Engl. J. Med. 331:417, 1994.

617. Bugiardini, R., Pozzati, A., Borghi, A., et al.: Angiographic morphology in unstable angina and its relation to transient myocardial ischemia and hospital outcome. Am. J. Cardiol. 67:460, 1991.

618. Califf, R. M., and Mark, D. B.: Unstable angina: Clinical presentation and diagnostic techniques. In Fuster, V., Ross, R., and Topol, E. J.: (eds.): Atherosclerosis and Coronary Artery Disease. Philadelphia, Lippincott-Raven, 1996, pp. 1299–1314.

619. Victor, M. F., Likoff, M. J., Mintz, G. S., et al.: Unstable angina pectoris of new onset. A prospective clinical and arteriographic study of 75 patients. Am. J. Cardiol. 47:228, 1981.

620. Roberts, K. B., Califf, R. M., Harrell, F. E., Jr., et al.: The prognosis for patients with new-onset angina who have undergone cardiac catheterization. Circulation 68:970, 1983.

621. Diver, D. J., Bier, J. D., Ferreira, P. E., et al.: Clinical and arteriographic characterization of patients with unstable angina without critical coronary arterial narrowing (from the TIMI-IIIA trial). Am. J. Cardiol. 74:531, 1994.

622. Fuster, V., Stein, B., Ambrose, J. A., et al.: Atherosclerotic plaque rupture and thrombosis: Evolving concepts. Circulation 82(Suppl. II):47, 1990.

623. Roberts, W. C.: Qualitative and quantitative comparison of amounts of narrowing by atherosclerotic plaques in the major epicardial coronary arteries at necropsy in sudden coronary death, transmural acute myocardial infarction, transmural healed myocardial infarction and unstable angina pectoris. Am. J. Cardiol. 64:324, 1989.

624. Freeman, M. R., Williams, A. E., Chisholm, R. J., et al.: Intracoronary thrombus and complex morphology and unstable angina: Relation to timing of angiography and in-hospital cardiac events. Circulation 80:17, 1989.

625. Falk, E., Shah, P. K., and Fuster, V.: Pathogenesis of plaque disruption. In Fuster, V., Ross, R., and Topol, E. J. (eds.): Atherosclerosis and Coronary Artery Disease. Philadelphia, J. B. Lippincott, 1996, pp. 492–511.

626. Davies, M. J., Thomas, A. C., Knapman, P. A., and Hangartner, J. R.: Intramyocardial platelet aggregation in patients with unstable angina suffering sudden ischemic cardiac death. Circulation 73:418, 1986.

627. Jeroudi, M. O., Cheirif, J., Habib, G., and Bolli, R.: Prolonged wall motion abnormalities after chest pain at rest in patients with unstable angina: A possible manifestation of myocardial stunning. Am. Heart J. 127:1241, 1994.

628. Warner, M., DiSciascio, G., Kohli, R., et al.: Frequency and predictors of left ventricular segmental dysfunction in patients with recent rest angina. Am. J. Cardiol. 69:1521, 1992.

629. Chester, M., Chen, L., and Kaski, J. C.: Identification of patients at high risk for adverse coronary events while awaiting routine coronary angioplasty. Br. Heart J. 73:216, 1995.

630. Cairns, J. A., Singer, J., Gent, M., et al.: One year mortality outcomes of all coronary intensive care unit patients with acute myocardial infarction, unstable angina or other chest pain in Hamilton, Ontario, a city of 375,000 people. Can. J. Cardiol. 5:239, 1989.

631. Stone, P. H., Thompson, B., Anderson, H. V., et al.: The influence of race, gender and age on the natural history and management of patients with unstable angina and non-Q-wave myocardial infarction: The TIMI III Registry. JAMA (in press).

632. Swahn, E., Areskog, M., Berglund, U., et al.: Predictive importance of clinical findings and a predischarge exercise test in patients with suspected unstable coronary artery disease. Am. J. Cardiol. 59:208, 1987.

633. Theroux, P., Taeymans, Y., Morissette, D., et al.: A randomized study comparing propranolol and diltiazem in the treatment of unstable angina. J. Am. Coll. Cardiol. 5:717, 1985.

634. Freeman, M. R., Chisholm, R. J., and Armstrong, P. W.: Usefulness of exercise electrocardiography and thallium scintigraphy in unstable angina pectoris in predicting the extent and severity of coronary artery disease (erratum published in Am. J. Cardiol. 63:392, 1989). Am. J. Cardiol. 62:1164, 1988.

635. Brown, K. A.: Prognostic value of thallium-201 myocardial perfusion imaging in patients with unstable angina who respond to medical treatment [published erratum J. Am. Coll. Cardiol. 18:889, 1991]. J. Am. Coll. Cardiol. 17:1053, 1991.

636. Bixon, J. V., Brown, C. N., and Smitherman, T. C.: Identification of transient and persistent segmental wall motion abnormalities in patients with unstable angina by two-dimensional echocardiography. Circulation 65:1497, 1982.

636a. Mark, D. B., and Braunwald, E.: Medical management of unstable angina. In Fuster, V., Ross, R., and Topol, E. J. (eds.): Atherosclerosis and Coronary Artery Disease. Philadelphia, Lippincott-Raven, 1996, pp. 1315–1326.

637. HINT Research Group: Early treatment of unstable angina in the coronary care unit: A randomized, double-blind, placebo-controlled comparison of recurrent ischemia in patients treated with nifedipine or metoprolol or both. Br. Heart J. 56:400, 1986.

638. Tijssen, J. G., and Lubsen, J.: Early treatment of unstable angina with nifedipine or metoprolol—the HINT trial. J. Cardiovasc. Pharmacol. 12:S71, 1988.

639. Muller, J. E., Turi, Z. G., Pearle, D. L., et al.: Nifedipine and conventional therapy for unstable angina pectoris: A randomized double-blind comparison. Circulation 69:728, 1984.

640. Wallis, D. E., Pope, C., Littman, W. J., and Scanlon, P. J.: Safety and efficacy of esmolol for unstable angina pectoris. Am. J. Cardiol. 62:1033, 1988.

641. Held, P. H., Yusuf, S., and Furberg, C. D.: Calcium channel blockers in acute myocardial infarction and unstable angina: An overview. Br. Med. J. 299:1187, 1989.

642. Gerstenblith, G., Ouyang, P., Achuff, S. C., et al.: Nifedipine in unstable angina: A double-blind, randomized trial. N. Engl. J. Med. 306:885, 1982.

643. Wallentin, L. C.: Aspirin (75 mg/day) after an episode of unstable coronary artery disease: Long term effects on the risk of myocardial infarction, occurrence of severe angina and the need for revascularization: Research Group on Instability and Coronary Artery Disease in Southeast Sweden. J. Am. Coll. Cardiol. 18:1587, 1991.

644. Willard, J. E., Langer, R. A., and Hillis, L. D.: The use of aspirin in ischemic heart disease. N. Engl. J. Med. 327:175, 1992.

645. Balsano, F., Rizzon, P., Violi, F., et al.: Antiplatelet treatment with triclopidine in unstable angina: A controlled multicenter clinical trial: The Studio Della Ticlopidina Nell'Angina Instabile Group. Circulation 82:17, 1990.

646. Theroux, P., Waters, D., Qiu, S., et al.: Aspirin versus heparin to prevent myocardial infarction during the acute phase of unstable angina. Circulation 88:2045, 1993.

647. Holdright, D., Patel, D., Cunningham, D., et al.: Comparison of the effect of heparin and aspirin versus aspirin alone on transient myocardial ischemia and in-hospital prognosis in patients with unstable angina. J. Am. Coll. Cardiol. 24:39, 1994.

648. Cohen, M., Adams, P. C., Parry, G., et al.: Combination antithrombotic therapy in unstable rest angina and non–Q-wave infarction in nonprior aspirin users: Primary end points analysis from the ATACS Trial: Antithrombotic Therapy in Acute Coronary Syndromes Research Group. Circulation 89:81, 1994.

649. Theroux, P., Waters, D., Lam, J., et al.: Reactivation of unstable angina after the discontinuation of heparin. N. Engl. J. Med. 327:141, 1992.

649a. Granger, C. B., Miller, J. M., Bovill, E. G., et al.: Rebound increase in thrombin generation and activity after cessation of intravenous heparin in patients with acute coronary syndrome. Circulation 91:1929, 1995.

650. Raschke, R. A., Reilly, B. M., Guidry, J. R., et al.: The weight-based heparin dosing nomogram compared with "standard care" nomogram. Ann. Intern. Med. 119:874, 1993.

651. Flaker, G. C., Bartolozzi, J., Davis, V., et al.: Use of the standardized nomogram to achieve therapeutic anticoagulation after thrombolytic therapy in myocardial infarction. Arch. Intern. Med. 154:1492, 1994.

651a. Gurfinkel, E. P., Manos, E. J., Mejail, R. I., et al.: Low-molecular weight heparin versus regular heparin of aspirin in the treatment of unstable angina and silent ischemia. J. Am. Coll. Cardiol. 26:313, 1995.

652. TIMI-IIIB investigators: Effects of tissue-plasminogen activator and a comparison of early invasive and conservative strategies in unstable

angina and non–Q-wave myocardial infarction: Results of the TIMI-IIIB trial. Circulation 89:1545, 1994.

653. Schreiber, T. L., Rizik, D., White, C., et al.: Randomized trial of thrombolysis versus heparin in unstable angina. Circulation 86:1407, 1992.

654. Bar, F. W., Verheugt, F. W., Cohl, J., et al.: Thrombolysis in patients with unstable angina improves the angiographic, but not the clinical outcome: Results of UNASEM, a multicenter, randomized, placebo-controlled clinical trial with anistreplase. Circulation 86:150, 1992.

655. Freeman, M. R., Langer, A., Wilson, R. F., et al.: Thrombolysis in unstable angina: Randomized double-blind trial of t-PA and placebo. Circulation 85:150, 1992.

655a. Mehran, R., Ambrose, J. A., Bongu, R. M., et al.: Angioplasty of complex lesions and ischemic rest angina. Results of the thrombolysis and angioplasty in unstable angina (TAUSA) trial. J. Am. Coll. Cardiol. 26:961, 1995.

656. Romeo, F., Rosano, G. M., Martuscelli, E., et al.: Effectiveness of prolonged low dose recombinant tissue-type plasminogen activator for refractory unstable angina. J. Am. Coll. Cardiol. 25:1295, 1995.

657. Fuchs, J., Cannon, C. P., and the TIMI VII Investigators: Hirulog in the treatment of unstable angina. Results of the thrombin inhibition in myocardial ischemia (TIMI) VII trial. Circulation 92:727, 1995.

658. Grambow, D. W., and Topol, E. J.: Effect of maximal medical therapy on refractoriness of unstable angina pectoris. Am. J. Cardiol. 70:577, 1992.

659. Szatmary, L. J., Marco, J., Fajadet, J., and Caster, L.: The combined use of diastolic counterpulsation and coronary dilation in unstable angina due to multivessel disease under unstable hemodynamic conditions. Int. J. Cardiol. 19:59, 1988.

660. Makhoul, R. G., Cole, C. W., and McCann, R. L.: Vascular complications of the intra-aortic balloon pump: An analysis of 436 patients. Am. Surg. 59:564, 1993.

660a. Willerson, J. T.: Management of the patient with unstable angina after the initial therapy. In Fuster, V., Ross, R., and Topol, E. J. (eds.): Atherosclerosis and Coronary Artery Disease. Philadelphia, J. B. Lippincott, 1996, pp. 1327–1338.

661. Kennedy, J. W.: Complications associated with cardiac catheterization and angiography. Cathet. Cardiovasc. Diagn. 8:5, 1982.

662. DeFeyter, P. J., Suryapranata, H., Serruys, P. W., et al.: Effects of successful percutaneous transluminal coronary angioplasty on global and regional left ventricular function in unstable angina pectoris. Am. J. Cardiol. 60:993, 1987.

663. Kamp, O., Beatt, K. J., deFeyter, P. J., et al.: Short-, medium-, and long-term follow-up after percutaneous transluminal coronary angioplasty for stable and unstable angina pectoris. Am. Heart J. 117:991, 1989.

664. DeFeyter, P. J., and Serruys, P. W.: Unstable angina. Role of coronary interventions. In Fuster, V., Ross, R., and Topol, E. J. (eds.): Atherosclerosis and Coronary Artery Disease. Philadelphia, Lippincott-Raven, 1996, pp. 1351–1358.

665. Grassman, E. D., Leya, F., Johnson, S. A., et al.: Percutaneous transluminal coronary angioplasty for unstable angina: Predictors of outcome in a multicenter study. J. Thrombosis Thrombolysis 1:73, 1994.

666. Halon, D. A., Merdler, A., Shefer, A., et al.: Identifying patients at high risk for restenosis after percutaneous transluminal coronary angioplasty for unstable angina pectoris. Am. J. Cardiol. 64:289, 1989.

667. Tenaglia, A. N., and Stack, R. S.: Angioplasty for acute coronary syndromes. Annu. Rev. Med. 44:465, 1993.

668. Stammen, F., DeScheerder, I., Glazier, J. J., et al.: Immediate and follow-up results of the conservative coronary angioplasty strategy for unstable angina pectoris. Am. J. Cardiol. 69:1533, 1992.

669. Ruygrok, P., deJaegere, P., Van Domburg, R., et al.: Unstable angina patients fare no worse than stable patients 10 years after balloon angioplasty. J. Am. Coll. Cardiol. 25(Abs.):249-A, 1995.

670. The EPIC Investigators: Use of a monoclonal antibody directed against the platelet glycoprotein IIb/IIIa receptor in high-risk coronary angioplasty. N. Engl. J. Med. 330:956, 1994.

671. Morrison, D. A., Sacks, J., Grover, F., et al.: Effectiveness of percutaneous transluminal coronary angioplasty for patients with medically refractory rest angina pectoris and high risk of adverse outcomes with coronary artery bypass grafting. Am. J. Cardiol. 75:237, 1995.

672. Abdelmeguid, A. E., Ellis, S. G., Sapp, S. K., et al.: Directional coronary atherectomy in unstable angina. J. Am. Coll. Cardiol. 24:46, 1994.

673. Talley, J. D., Hurst, J. W., King, S. B., III, et al.: Clinical outcome 5 years after attempted percutaneous transluminal coronary angioplasty in 427 patients. Circulation 77:820, 1988.

674. Gardner, T. J., Stuart, R. S., Greene, P. S., and Baumgartner, W. A.: The risk of coronary bypass surgery for patients with postinfarction angina. Circulation 79(Suppl., I):I79, 1989.

675. Kaiser, G. C., Schaff, H. V., and Killip, T.: Myocardial revascularization for unstable angina pectoris. Circulation 79(Suppl. I):I60, 1989.

676. Luchi, R. J., Scott, S. M., and Deupree, R. H.: Comparison of medical and surgical treatment for unstable angina pectoris: Results of a Veterans Administration Cooperative Study. N. Engl. J. Med. 316:977, 1987.

677. Scott, S. N., Deupree, R. H., Sharma, G. V., et al.: VA study of unstable angina: 10-year results show duration of surgical advantage for patients with impaired ejection fraction. Circulation 90(Suppl.):II-120, 1994.

678. Booth, D. C., Deupree, R. H., Hultgren, H. N., et al.: Quality of life after bypass surgery for unstable angina: 5-year follow-up results of a Veterans Affairs Cooperative Study. Circulation 83:87, 1991.

679. Rahimtoola, S. H., Nunley, D., Grunkemeier, G., et al.: Ten-year survival after coronary bypass surgery for unstable angina. N. Engl. J. Med. 308:676, 1983.

679a. Schoff, H. V.: Unstable angina. Role of bypass surgery. In Fuster, V.,

Ross, R., and Topol, E. J. (eds.): Atherosclerosis and Coronary Artery Disease. Philadelphia, J. B. Lippincott, 1996, pp. 1359–1366.

680. Naunheim, K. S., Fiore, A. C., Arango, D. C., et al.: Coronary artery bypass grafting for unstable angina pectoris: Risk analysis. Ann. Thorac. Surg. 47:569, 1989.

681. Waters, D. D., Walling, A., Roy, D., and Theroux, P.: Previous coronary artery bypass grafting as an adverse prognostic factor in unstable angina pectoris. Am. J. Cardiol. 58:465, 1986.

682. Murphy, J. G., and Gersh, B. J.: Pros and cons of revascularization versus a conservative approach. In Rutherford, J. D. (ed.): Unstable Angina. New York, Marcel Dekker, 1992, p. 247.

PRINZMETAL'S VARIANT ANGINA

683. Prinzmetal, M., Kennamer, R., Merliss, R., et al.: A variant form of angina pectoris. Am. J. Med. 27:375, 1959.

684. Cohen, M.: Variant angina pectoris. In Fuster, V., Ross, R., and Topol, E. J. (eds.): Atherosclerosis and Coronary Artery Disease. Philadelphia, J. B. Lippincott, 1996, pp. 1367–1376.

684a. Crea, F., Kaski, J. C., Masori, A., et al.: Key references on coronary artery spasm. Circulation 89:2442, 1994.

685. Nakamura, Y., Yamaguro, T., Inoki, I., et al.: Vasomotor response to ergonovine of epicardial and resistance coronary arteries in the nonspastic vascular bed in patients with vasospastic angina. Am. J. Cardiol. 74:1006, 1994.

686. Hoshio, A., Kotake, H., and Mashiba, H.: Significance of coronary artery tone in patients with vasospastic angina. J. Am. Coll. Cardiol. 14:604, 1989.

687. McFadden, E. P., Clarke, J. G., Davies, G. J., et al.: Effect of intracoronary serotonin on coronary vessels in patients with stable angina and patients with variant angina. N. Engl. J. Med. 324:648, 1991.

688. Takano, H., Nakamura, T., Satou, T., et al.: Regional myocardial sympathetic dysinnervation in patients with coronary vasospasm. Am. J. Cardiol. 75:324, 1995.

689. Irie, T., Imaizumi, T., Matuguchi, T., et al.: Increased fibrinopeptide A during anginal attacks in patients with variant angina. J. Am. Coll. Cardiol. 14:589, 1989.

690. Ogawa, H., Yasue, H., Oshima, S., et al.: Circadian variation of plasma fibrinopeptide A level in patients with variant angina. Circulation 80:1617, 1989.

691. Masuda, T., Ogawa, H., Miyao, Y., et al.: Circadian variation in fibrinolytic activity in patients with variant angina. Br. Heart J. 71:156, 1994.

692. Nobuyoshi, M., Abe, M., Nosaka, H., et al.: Statistical analysis of clinical risk factors for coronary artery spasm: Identification of the most important determinant. Am. Heart J. 124:32, 1992.

693. Sugiishi, M., and Takatsu, F.: Cigarette smoking is a major risk factor for coronary spasm. Circulation 87:76, 1993.

694. Cohen, L., and Kitzes, R.: Prompt termination and/or prevention of cold-pressor-stimulus–induced vasoconstriction of different vascular beds by magnesium sulfate in patients with Prinzmetal's angina. Magnes. Trace Elem. 5:144, 1986.

695. Miyagi, H., Yasue, H., Okumura, K., et al.: Effect of magnesium on anginal attack induced by hyperventilation in patients with variant angina. Circulation 79:597, 1989.

696. Kugiyama, K., Yasue, H., Okumura, K., et al.: Suppression of exercise-induced angina by magnesium sulfate in patients with variant angina. J. Am. Coll. Cardiol. 12:1177, 1988.

697. Lange, R. A., Cigarroa, R. G., and Yancy, C. W., Jr.: Cocaine-induced coronary-artery vasoconstriction. N. Engl. J. Med. 321:1557, 1989.

698. Nademanee, K., Gorelick, D. A., Josephson, M. A., et al.: Myocardial ischemia during cocaine withdrawal. Ann. Intern. Med. 111:876, 1989.

699. Fourneir, J. A., Sanchez, A. F., and Cortacero, J.-A. P.: Selective ergonovine induced coronary artery spasm and ST-segment alternans after blunt thoracic trauma. Int. J. Cardiol. 47:290, 1995.

699a. Shinozaki, K., Suzuki, M., Ikebuchi, I., et al.: Insulin resistance associated with compensatory hyperinsulinemia as an independent risk factor for vasospastic angina. Circulation 92:1749, 1995.

699b. Onaka, H., Yasue, H., Shimada, S., et al.: Clinical observation of spontaneous anginal attacks and multivessel spasm in variant angina pectoris with normal coronary arteries: Evaluation by 24-hour 12-lead electrocardiography with computer analysis. J. Am. Coll. Cardiol. 27:38, 1996.

700. Waters, D. D., Theroux, P., Crittin, J., et al.: Previously undiagnosed variant angina as a cause of chest pain after coronary artery bypass surgery. Circulation 61:1159, 1980.

701. Habbab, M. A., Szwed, S. A., and Haft, I.: Is coronary arterial spasm part of the aspirin-induced asthma syndrome? Chest 90:141, 1986.

702. Pijls, N. H., and van der Werf, T.: Prinzmetal's angina associated with alcohol withdrawal. Cardiology 75:226, 1988.

703. Matsuguchi, T., Araki, H., Nakamura, N., et al.: Prevention of vasospastic angina by alcohol ingestion: Report of 2 cases. Angiology 39:394, 1988.

704. Kleiman, N. S., Lehane, D. E., Geyer, C. E., Jr., et al.: Prinzmetal's angina during 5-fluorouracil chemotherapy. Am. J. Med. 82:566, 1987.

705. Stefenelli, T., Zielinski, C. C., Mayr, H., and Scoheithauer, W.: Prinzmetal's angina during cyclophosphamide therapy. Eur. Heart J. 9:1155, 1988.

706. Chockalingam, V., Jagnathan, V., Chandrasekar, P. V., et al.: A case of ST-segment and T-wave alternans. Arch. Intern. Med. 143:1792, 1983.

707. Salerno, J. A., Previtali, M., Panciroli, C., et al.: Ventricular arrhythmias during acute myocardial ischaemia in man: The role and significance of R-ST-T alternans and the prevention of ischaemic sudden death by medical treatment. Eur. Heart J. 7(Suppl. A):63, 1986.

708. Bayes de Luna, A., Carreras, F., Cladellias, M., et al.: Holter ECG study of the electrocardiographic phenomena in Prinzmetal angina attacks with emphasis on the study of ventricular arrhythmias. J. Electrocardiol. 18:267, 1985.

709. Yasue, H., Takizawa, A., Nagao, M., et al.: Long-term prognosis for patients with variant angina and influential factors. Circulation 78:1, 1988.

710. Ortega-Carnicer, J., Garcia-Nieto, F., Malillos, M., and Sanchez-Fernandez, A.: Transient left posterior hemiblock during Prinzmetal's angina culminating in acute myocardial infarction. Chest 84:638, 1983.

711. Myerburg, R. J., Kessler, K. M., Mallon, S. M., et al.: Life threatening ventricular arrhythmias in patients with silent myocardial ischemia due to coronary artery spasm. N. Engl. J. Med. 326:1451, 1992.

712. Meller, J., Conde, C. A., Donoso, E., and Dack, S.: Transient Q waves in Prinzmetal's angina. Am. J. Cardiol. 35:691, 1975.

713. Gersh, B. J., Bassendine, M., Forman, R., et al.: Coronary artery spasm and myocardial infarction in the absence of angiographically demonstrable coronary artery disease. Mayo Clin. Proc. 56:700, 1981.

714. Masuda, Y., Ozaki, M., Ogawa, H., et al.: Coronary arteriography and left ventriculography during spontaneous and exercise-induced ST-segment elevation in patients with variant angina. Am. Heart J. 106:509, 1983.

715. Distante, A., Rovai, D., Picano, E., et al.: Transient changes in left ventricular mechanics during attacks of Prinzmetal's angina: An M-mode echocardiographic study. Am. Heart J. 107:465, 1984.

716. Yokoyama, M., Akita, H., Hirata, K., et al.: Supersensitivity of isolated coronary artery to ergonovine in a patient with variant angina. Am. J. Med. 89:507, 1990.

717. Harding, M. B., Leithe, M. E., Mark, D. B., et al.: Ergonovine maleate testing during cardiac catheterization: A 10 year perspective in 3,447 patients without significant coronary artery disease or Prinzmetal's variant angina. (erratum J. Am. Coll. Cardiol. 21:848, 1993). J. Am. Coll. Cardiol. 20:107, 1992.

718. Previtali, M., Ardissino, D., Barberis, P., et al.: Hyperventilation and ergonovine tests in Prinzmetal's variant angina pectoris in men. Am. J. Cardiol. 63:17, 1989.

719. Minoda, K., Yasue, H., Kugiyama, K., et al.: Comparison of the distribution of myocardial blood flow between exercise-induced and hyperventilation-induced attacks of coronary spasm: A study with thallium-201 myocardial scintigraphy. Am. Heart J. 127:1474, 1994.

720. Okumura, K., Yasue, H., Matsuyama, K., et al.: Sensitivity and specificity of intracoronary injection of acetylcholine for the induction of coronary artery spasm. J. Am. Coll. Cardiol. 12:883, 1988.

721. Okumura, K., Yasue, H., Matsuyama, K., et al.: Effect of H1 receptor stimulation on coronary artery diameter in patients with variant angina: Comparison with effect of acetylcholine. J. Am. Coll. Cardiol. 17:338, 1991.

722. Crea, F., Chierchia, S., Kaski, J. C., et al.: Provocation of coronary spasm by dopamine in patients with active variant angina pectoris. Circulation 74:262, 1986.

723. Maseri, A., Parodi, O., Severi, S., and Pesola, A.: Transient transmural reduction of myocardial blood flow, demonstrated by thallium-201 scintigraphy, as a cause of variant angina. Circulation 54:280, 1976.

724. Ginsburg, R., Lamb, I. H., Schroeder, J. S., et al.: Randomized-blind comparison of nifedipine and isosorbide dinitrate therapy in variant angina pectoris due to coronary artery spasm. Am. Heart J. 103:44, 1982.

725. Robertson, R. M., Wood, A. J., Vaughn, W. K., et al.: Exacerbation of vasotonic angina pectoris by propranolol. Circulation 6:281, 1982.

726. Antman, E., Muller, J., Goldberg, S., et al.: Nifedipine therapy for coronary-artery spasm: Experience in 127 patients. N. Engl. J. Med. 302:1269, 1980.

727. Ginsburg, R., Lamb, I. H., Schroeder, J. S., et al.: Randomized double-blind comparison of nifedipine and isosorbide dinitrate therapy in variant angina pectoris due to coronary artery spasm. Am. Heart J. 103:44, 1982.

728. Prida, X. E., Gelman, J. S., Feldman, R. L., et al.: Comparison of diltiazem and nifedipine alone and in combination in patients with coronary artery spasm. J. Am. Coll. Cardiol. 9:412, 1987.

729. Morikami, Y., and Yasue, H.: Efficacy of slow-release nifedipine on myocardial ischemic episodes in variant angina pectoris. Am. J. Cardiol. 68:580, 1991.

730. Chimienti, M., Negroni, M. S., Pusineri, E., et al.: Once daily felodipine in preventing ergonovine-induced myocardial ischemia in Prinzmetal's variant angina. Eur. Heart J. 15:389, 1994.

731. Pesola, A., Lauro, A., Gallo, R., et al.: Efficacy of diltiazem in variant angina: Results of a double-blind crossover study in CCU by Holter monitoring: The possible occurrence of a withdrawal syndrome. G. Ital. Cardiol. 17:329, 1987.

732. Tzivoni, D., Keren, A., Benhorin, J., et al.: Prazosin therapy for refractory variant angina. Am. Heart J. 105:262, 1983.

733. Miwa, K., Kambara, H., and Kawai, C.: Effect of aspirin in large doses on attacks of variant angina. Am. Heart J. 105:351, 1983.

734. Corcos, T., David, P. R., Bourassa, M. G., et al.: Percutaneous transluminal coronary angioplasty for the treatment of variant angina. J. Am. Coll. Cardiol. 5:1046, 1985.

735. Yasue, H., Takizawa, D., Nagao, M., et al.: Long-term prognosis of patients with variant angina and influential factors. Circulation 78:1, 1988.

736. Shimokawa, H., Nagasaw, A. K., Irie, T., et al.: Clinical characteristics and long-term prognosis of patients with variant angina: A comparative study between Western and Japanese populations. Int. J. Cardiol. 18:331, 1988.

737. Mark, D. B., Califf, R. M., Morris, K. G., et al.: Clinical characteristics

and long-term survival of patients with variant angina. Circulation 69:880, 1984.

738. Ozaki, Y., Takatsu, F., Osugi, J., et al.: Long term study of recurrent vasospastic angina using coronary angiograms during ergonovine provocation tests. Am. Heart J. 123:1191, 1992.

CHEST PAIN WITH NORMAL CORONARY ARTERIOGRAM

739. Kemp, H. G., Kronmal, R. A., Vlietstra, R. E., and Frye, R. L.: Seven-year survival of patients with normal and near normal coronary arteriograms: A CASS registry study. J. Am. Coll. Cardiol. 7:479, 1986.

740. Papanicolaou, M. N., Califf, R. M., Hlatky, M. A., et al.: Prognostic implications of angiographically insignificant and insignificantly narrowed coronary arteries. Am. J. Cardiol. 58:1181, 1986.

741. Maseri, A., Crea, F., Kaski, C., and Crake, T.: Mechanisms of angina pectoris in syndrome X. J. Am. Coll. Cardiol. 17:499, 1991.

742. Camici, P. G., Marraccini, P., Lorenzoni, R., et al.: Coronary hemodynamics and myocardial metabolism in patients with syndrome X: Response to pacing stress. J. Am. Coll. Cardiol. 17:1461, 1991.

743. Bortone, A. S., Hess, O. M., Eberli, F. R., et al.: Abnormal coronary vasomotion during exercise in patients with normal coronary arteries and reduced coronary flow reserve. Circulation 79:516, 1989.

744. Shapiro, L. M., Crake, T., and Poole-Wilson, P. A.: Is altered cardiac sensation responsible for chest pain in patients with normal coronary arteries? Clinical observation during cardiac catheterization. Br. Med. J. 296:170, 1988.

744a. Wiederman, J. G., Schwartz, A., Apfelbaum, M., et al.: Anatomic and physiologic heterogeneity in patients with syndrome X. An intravascular ultrasound study. J. Am. Coll. Cardiol. 25:131, 1995.

745. Chauhan, A., Mullens, P. A., Petch, M. C., et al.: Is coronary flow reserve in response to papaverine really normal in syndrome X? Circulation 89:1998, 1994.

745a. Cannon, R. O.: The microcirculation in atherosclerotic coronary artery. In Fuster, V., Ross, R., and Topol, E. J. (eds.): Atherosclerosis and Coronary Artery Disease. Philadelphia, Lippincott-Raven, 1996, pp. 773–790.

746. Cannon, R. O., Bonow, R. O., Bacharach, S. L., et al.: Left ventricular dysfunction in patients with angina pectoris, normal epicardial coronary arteries, and abnormal vasodilator reserve. Circulation 71:218, 1985.

747. Geltman, E. M., Henes, C. G., Senneff, M. J., et al.: Increased myocardial perfusion at rest and diminished perfusion reserve in patients with angina and angiographically normal coronary arteries. J. Am. Coll. Cardiol. 16:586, 1990.

748. Sax, F. L., Cannon, R. O., Hanson, C., and Epstein, S. E.: Impaired forearm vasodilator reserve in patients with microvascular angina. N. Engl. J. Med. 317:1366, 1987.

749. Cannon, R. O., III, Peden, D. B., Berkebile, C., et al.: Airway hyperresponsiveness in patients with microvascular angina: Evidence for a diffuse disorder of smooth muscle responsiveness. Circulation 82:2011, 1990.

750. Cannon, R. O.: Chest pain with normal coronary angiograms. In Fuster, V., Ross, R., and Topol, E. J. (eds.): Atherosclerosis and Coronary Artery Disease. Philadelphia, J. B. Lippincott, 1996, pp. 1577–1590.

751. Cannon, R. O., III: The sensitive heart: A syndrome of abnormal cardiac pain perception. JAMA 273:883, 1995.

752. Vrints, C. J., Bult, H., Hitter, E., et al.: Impaired endothelium-dependent cholinergic coronary vasodilation in patients with angina and normal coronary arteriograms. J. Am. Coll. Cardiol. 19:21, 1992.

753. Bugiardini, R., Pozzati, A., Ottani, F., et al.: A spectrum of ischemic syndromes involving functional abnormalities of the epicardial and microvascular coronary circulation. J. Am. Coll. Cardiol. 22:417, 1993.

754. Carter, C., Maddock, R., and Amsterdam, E.: Panic disorder and chest pain in the coronary care unit. Psychosomatica 23:302, 1992.

755. Cannon, R. O., Quyyumi, A. A., Mincemoyer, R., et al.: Imipramine in patients with chest pain despite normal coronary angiograms. N. Engl. J. Med. 330:1411, 1994.

756. Lagerqvist, B., Sylven, C., and Waldenstrom, A.: Lower threshold for adenosine-induced chest pain in patients with angina and normal coronary angiograms. Br. Heart J. 68:282, 1992.

757. DeMeester, T. R., O'Sullivan, G. C., Bermudez, G., et al.: Esophageal function in patients with angina-type chest pain and normal coronary angiograms. Ann. Surg. 196:488, 1982.

758. Rosen, S. D., Uren, N. G., Kaski, J. C., et al.: Coronary vasodilator reserve, pain perception and sex in patients with syndrome X. Circulation 90:50, 1994.

758a. Potts, S. G., Bass, C. M., et al.: Psychological morbidity in patients with chest pain and normal or near-normal coronary arteries. A long-term follow-up study. Psychol. Med. 25:339, 1995.

759. Kaski, J. C., Rosano, G. M., Collins, P., et al.: Cardiac syndrome X: Clinical characteristics and left ventricular function. J. Am. Coll. Cardiol. 25:807, 1995.

760. Channer, K. S., James, M. A., Papouchado, M., et al.: Anxiety and depression in patients with chest pain referred for exercise testing. Lancet 2:820, 1985.

761. Kemp, H. G., Kronmal, R. A., Vlietstra, R. E., et al.: Seven-year survival of patients with normal or near normal coronary arteriograms: A CASS registry study. J. Am. Coll. Cardiol. 7:479, 1986.

762. Ockene, I. S., Shay, M. J., Alpert, J. S., et al.: Unexplained chest pain in patients with normal coronary arteriograms: A follow-up study of functional status. N. Engl. J. Med. 303:1249, 1980.

763. Pupita, G., Kaski, J. C., Galassi, A. R., et al.: Long-term variability of

angina pectoris and electrocardiographic signs of ischemia in syndrome X. Am. J. Cardiol. 64:139, 1989.

764. Romeo, J., Rosano, G. M., Martuscelli, E., et al.: Long-term follow-up of patients initially diagnosed with syndrome X. Am. J. Cardiol. 71:669, 1993.

765. Lanza, G. A., Manzoli, A., Bia, E., et al.: Acute effects of nitrates in exercise testing in patients with syndrome X: Clinical and pathophysiological implications. Circulation 90:2695, 1994.

766. Gilligan, D. M., Quyyumi, A. A., Cannon, R. O., 3d, et al.: Effects of physiological levels of estrogen on coronary vasomotor function in postmenopausal women. Circulation 89:2545, 1994.

767. Reis, E., Gloth, S. T., Blumenthal, R. S., et al.: Ethinyl estradiol acutely attenuates abnormal coronary vasomotor responses to acetylcholine in postmenopausal women. Circulation 89:52, 1994.

SILENT MYOCARDIAL ISCHEMIA

768. Kellermann, J. J., and Braunwald, E. (eds.): Silent Myocardial Ischemia: A Critical Appraisal. Basel, Karger, 1990.

769. Kannel, W. B., and Abbott, R. D.: Incidence and prognosis of unrecognized myocardial infarction. N. Engl. J. Med. 3:1144, 1984.

769a. Cohn, P. F.: Silent ischemia. In Fuster, V., Ross, R., and Topol, E. J. (eds.): Atherosclerosis and Coronary Artery Disease. Philadelphia, J. B. Lippincott, 1996, pp. 1561–1576.

770. Sigurdsson, E., Thorgeirsson, G., Sigvaldason, H., and Sigfusson, N.: Unrecognized myocardial infarction: Epidemiology, clinical characteristics, and the prognostic role of angina pectoris: The Reykjavik study. Ann. Intern. Med. 122:96, 1995.

771. Mulcahy, D., Keegan, J., Crean, P., et al.: Silent ischemia in chronic stable angina: A study of its frequency and characteristics in 150 patients. Br. Heart J. 60:417, 1988.

772. Epstein, S. E., Quyyumi, A. A., and Bonow, R. A.: Myocardial ischemia: Silent or symptomatic. N. Engl. J. Med. 318:1038, 1988.

773. Rocco, M. B., Barry, J., Campbell, S., et al.: Circadian variation of transient myocardial ischemia in patients with coronary artery disease. Circulation 75:395, 1987.

774. Hirzel, H. O., Leutwyler, R., and Kralyenbuehl, H. P.: Silent myocardial ischemia: Hemodynamic changes during dynamic exercise in patients with proven coronary artery disease despite absence of angina pectoris. J. Am. Coll. Cardiol. 6:275, 1985.

775. Chierchia, S., Gallino, A., Smith, G., et al.: Role of heart rate in pathophysiology of chronic stable angina. Lancet 2:1353, 1984.

776. Deanfield, J. E., Ribiero, P., Oakley, K., et al.: Analysis of ST-segment changes in normal subjects: Implications for ambulatory monitoring in angina pectoris. Am. J. Cardiol. 54:1321, 1984.

777. Deanfield, J., Shea, M., Ribiero, P., et al.: Transient ST-segment depression as a marker of myocardial ischemia during daily life. Am. J. Cardiol. 54:1195, 1984.

778. Quyyumi, A. A., Mockus, L., Wright, C., and Fox, K. M.: Morphology of ambulatory ST-segment changes in patients with varying severity of coronary artery disease. Br. Heart J. 53:186, 1985.

779. Cohn, P. F.: Silent Myocardial Ischemia and Infarction. 3rd ed. New York, Marcel Dekker, Inc., 1993, p. 73.

780. Mulcahy, D., Purcell, H., Patel, D., and Fox, K.: Asymptomatic ischaemia during daily life in stable coronary artery disease: Relevant or redundant? Br. Heart J. 72:5, 1994.

780a. Quyyumi, A. A., Panza, J. A., Diodati, J. G., et al.: Prognostic implications of myocardial ischemia during daily life in low risk patients with coronary artery disease. J. Am. Coll. Cardiol. 21:700, 1993.

781. Aronow, W. S., Mercando, A. D., and Epstein, S.: Prevalence of silent myocardial ischemia detected by 24-hour ambulatory electrocardiography, and its association with new coronary events at 40 month follow-up in elderly diabetic and nondiabetic patients with coronary artery disease. Am. J. Cardiol. 69:555, 1992.

782. Ranjadayalan, K., Umachandran, V., Ambepityia, G., et al.: Prolonged anginal perceptual threshold in diabetes: Effects of exercise capacity and myocardial ischemia. J. Am. Coll. Cardiol. 16:1120, 1990.

783. Nesto, R. W., Philips, R. T., Kett, K. G., et al.: Angina and exertional myocardial ischemia in diabetic and non-diabetic patients: Assessment by exercise thallium scintigraphy. Ann. Intern. Med. 108:170, 1988.

784. Naka, M., Haramatsu, K., Aizawa, T., et al.: Silent myocardial ischemia in patients with non–insulin dependent diabetes mellitus as judged by treadmill exercise testing and coronary arteriography. Am. Heart J. 123:46, 1992.

785. Glazier, J. J., Chierchia, S., Brown, M. J., and Maseri, A.: Importance of generalized defective perception of painful stimuli as a cause of silent myocardial ischemia in chronic stable angina pectoris. Am. J. Cardiol. 58:667, 1986.

786. Droste, C., and Roskamm, H.: Experimental pain measurement in patients with asymptomatic myocardial ischemia. J. Am. Coll. Cardiol. 1:940, 1983.

787. Sheps, D. S., Ballenger, M. N., DeGent, G. E., et al.: Psychophysical responses to a speech stressor: Correlation of plasma-beta endorphin levels at rest and after psychological stress with thermally measured pain threshold in patients with coronary artery disease. J. Am. Coll. Cardiol. 25:1499, 1995.

788. Hikita, H., Kurita, A., Takase, B., et al.: Usefulness of plasma beta-endorphin levels, pain threshold and autonomic function in assessing silent myocardial ischemia in patients with and without diabetes mellitus. Am. J. Cardiol. 72:140, 1993.

789. Marwick, T. H.: Is silent ischemia painless because it is mild? J. Am. Coll. Cardiol. 25:1513, 1995.

790. Nihoyannapoulos, P., Marsonis, A., Joshi, J., et al.: Magnitude of myocardial dysfunction is greater in painful than in painless myocardial ischemia: An exercise echocardiographic study. J. Am. Coll. Cardiol. 25:1507, 1995.

790a. Klein, J., Chaors, Y., Burman, D. S., et al.: Is "silent" myocardial ischemia really as severe as symptomatic ischemia? The analytical effect of patient selection biases. Circulation 89:1958, 1994.

791. Petretta, M., Bonaduce, D., Bianchi, V., et al.: Characteristics and prognostic significance of silent myocardial ischemia or predischarge electrocardiographic monitoring in unselected patients with myocardial infarction. Am. J. Cardiol. 69:579, 1992.

792. Ekelund, L. G., Suchindran, C. M., McMahon, R. P., et al.: Coronary heart disease morbidity and mortality in hypercholesterolemic men predicted from an exercise test: The Lipid Research Clinics Coronary Primary Prevention Trial. J. Am. Coll. Cardiol. 14:556, 1989.

793. Deedwania, P. C.: Comparison of the prognostic values of ischemia during daily life and ischemia induced by treadmill exercise testing. Am. J. Cardiol. 74:15B, 1994.

794. Stern, S., Cohn, P. F., and Pepine, C. J.: Silent myocardial ischemia. Curr. Probl. Cardiol. 18:301, 1993.

795. TIBET Study Group, Total Ischemia Burden European Trial (TIBET): Effective treatment on exercise and Holter ECG and angina. Circulation 86(Suppl. I):I-713, 1992.

796. Portegies, M. C. M., Sijbring, P., Gobel, E. J. A. N., et al.: Efficacy of metoprolol and diltiazem in treating silent myocardial ischemia. Am. J. Cardiol. 74:1095, 1994.

797. Knatterud, G. L., Bourassa, B. M. J., Papine, C. J., et al.: Effective treatment strategies to suppress ischemia in patients with coronary artery disease: Twelve-week results of the Asymptomatic Cardiac Ischemia Pilot (ACIP) study. J. Am. Coll. Cardiol. 24:11, 1994.

797a. Chaitman, B. R., Stone, P. H., Knatterud, G. L., et al.: Asymptomatic Cardiac Ischemia Pilot (ACIP) study: Impact of anti-ischemia therapy and 12-week rest electrocardiogram and exercise test outcomes. J. Am. Coll. Cardiol. 26:585, 1995.

797b. Roberts, W. J., Bourassa, M. G., Andrews, T. C., et al.: Asymptomatic Cardiac Ischemia Pilot (ACIP) study. Outcome at 1-year for patients with asymptomatic cardiac ischemia randomized to medical therapy or revascularization. J. Am. Coll. Cardiol. 26:594, 1995.

797c. Bourassa, M. G., Pepine, C. J., Foreman, S. A., et al.: Asymptomatic Cardiac Ischemia Pilot (ACIP) study. Effects of coronary angioplasty and coronary artery bypass graft surgery on recurrent angina and ischemia. J. Am. Coll. Cardiol. 26:606, 1995.

HEART FAILURE

798. Burch, G. E., Giles, T. D., and Colcolough, H. L.: Ischemic cardiomyopathy. Am. Heart J. 79:291, 1970.

799. Kron, I. L., Flanagan, T. L., Blackbourne, L. H., et al.: Coronary revascularization rather than cardiac transplantation for chronic ischemic cardiomyopathy. Ann. Surg. 210:348, 1989.

800. Grieco, J. G., Montoya, A., Sullivan, H. J., et al.: Ventricular aneurysm due to blunt chest injury. Ann. Thorac. Surg. 47:322, 1989.

801. Hirai, T., Fujita, M., Nakajima, H., et al.: Importance of collateral circulation for prevention of left ventricular aneurysm formation in acute myocardial infarction. Circulation 79:791, 1989.

802. Barratt-Boyes, B. G., White, H. D., Agnew, T. M., et al.: The results of surgical treatment of left ventricular aneurysms: An assessment of the risk factors affecting early and late mortality. J. Thorac. Cardiovasc. Surg. 87:87, 1984.

803. Stephenson, L. W., Hargrove, W. C., Ratcliffe, M. B., et al.: Surgery for left ventricular aneurysm: Early survival with and without endocardial resection. Circulation 79(Suppl. X):1, 1989.

804. Sutherland, G. R., Smyllie, J. H., and Roelandt, J. R.: Advantages of colour flow imaging in the diagnosis of left ventricular pseudoaneurysm. Br. Heart J. 61:59, 1989.

805. Marcus, M. L., Stanford, W., Hajduczok, Z. D., and Weiss, R. M.: Ultrafast computed tomography in the diagnosis of cardiac diseases. Am. J. Cardiol. 64:54E, 1989.

806. Couper, G. S., Bunton, R. W., Birjiniuk, V., et al.: Relative risks of left ventricular aneurysmectomy in patients with akinetic scars versus true dyskinetic aneurysms. Circulation 82(Suppl. IV):248, 1990.

807. Cosgrove, D. M., Lytle, B. W., Taylor, P. C., et al.: Ventricular aneurysm resection. Circulation 79(Suppl. I):97, 1989.

808. Mangschau, A., Forfang, K., Rootwelt, K., and Frysaker, T.: Improvement in cardiac performance and exercise tolerance after left ventricular aneurysm surgery: A prospective study. Thorac. Cardiovasc. Surg. 36:320, 1988.

809. Louagie, Y., Alouini, T., Lesperance, J., and Pelletier, L. C.: Left ventricular aneurysm complicated by congestive heart failure: An analysis of long-term results and risk factors of surgical treatment. J. Cardiovasc. Surg. 30:648, 1989.

810. Barratt-Boyes, B. G., White, H. D., Agnew, T. M., et al.: Results of surgical treatment of left ventricular aneurysm: An assessment of the risk factors affecting early and late mortality. J. Thorac. Cardiovasc. Surg. 87:87, 1984.

811. Ivert, T., Almdahl, S. M., Lunde, P., and Lindblom, D.: Post infarction left ventricular pseudoaneurysm—echocardiographic diagnosis and surgical repair. Cardiovasc. Surg. 2:463, 1994.

812. Olearchyk, A. S., Lemole, G. M., and Spagna, P. M.: Left ventricular aneurysm: Ten years' experience in surgical treatment of 244 cases: Improved clinical status, hemodynamics and long-term longevity. J. Thorac. Cardiovasc. Surg. 88:544, 1984.

813. Prates, P. R., Vitola, D., Sant'anna, J. R., et al.: Surgical repair of ventricular aneurysms: Early results with Cooley's technique. Texas Heart Inst. J. 20:19, 1993.

814. Dor, V., Montiglio, F., Sabatier, M., et al.: Left ventricular shape changes induced by aneurysmectomy with endoventricular circular patch plasty reconstruction. Eur. Heart J. 15:1063, 1994.

815. Komeda, M., David, T. E., Malik, A., et al.: Operative risks and long-term results of operation for left ventricular aneurysm. Ann. Thorac. Surg. 53:22, 1992.

816. Rankin, J. S., Hickey, M. S., Smith, L. R., et al.: Ischemic mitral regurgitation. Circulation 79(Suppl. I):I-116, 1989.

817. Replogle, R. L., and Campbell, C. D.: Surgery for mitral regurgitation associated with ischemic heart disease. Circulation 79(Suppl. I):122, 1989.

818. Drexler, H., and Schroeder, J. S.: Unusual forms of ischemic heart disease. Curr. Opin. Cardiol. 9:457, 1994.

818a. Harrison, D. C.: Nonatherosclerotic coronary disease. In Fuster, V., Ross, R., and Topol, E. J. (eds.): Atherosclerosis and Coronary Artery Disease. Philadelphia, Lippincott-Raven, 1996, pp. 757–772.

819. Kragel, A. H., and Roberts, W. C.: Anomalous origin of either the right or left main coronary artery from the aorta with subsequent coursing between aorta and pulmonary trunk· Analysis of 32 necroscopy cases. Am. J. Cardiol. 62:771, 1988.

820. Corrado, D., Thiene, E. G., Cocco, P., and Frescura, C.: Non-atherosclerotic coronary artery disease and sudden death in the young. Br. Heart J. 68:601, 1992.

821. DeMaio, S. J., Jr., Kinsella, S. H., and Silverman, M. E.: Clinical course and long-term prognosis of spontaneous coronary artery dissection. Am. J. Cardiol. 64:471, 1989.

822. Schrader, M. L., Hochman, J. S., and Bulkley, B. A.: The heart and polyarteritis nodosa: A clinicopathologic study. Am. Heart J. 109:1353, 1985.

823. Saito, S., Arai, H., Kim, K., and Aoki, N.: Acute myocardial infarction in a young adult due to solitary giant cell arteritis of the coronary artery diagnosed antemortemly by primary directional coronary atherectomy. Cathet. Cardiovasc. Diagn. 33:245, 1994.

824. LeRoy, E. C.: The heart in systemic sclerosis. N. Engl. J. Med. 310:188, 1984.

825. Morris, P. B., Imber, M. J., Heinsimer, J. A., et al.: Rheumatoid arthritis and coronary arteritis. Am. J. Cardiol. 57:689, 1986.

826. Bidani, A. K., Roberts, J. L., Schwartz, M. N., and Lewis, E. J.: Immunopathology of cardiac lesions in fatal sytemic lupus erythematosus. Am. J. Med. 69:849, 1980.

827. Korbet, S. M., Schwartz, M. M., and Lewis, E. J.: Immune complex deposition and coronary vasculitis in systemic lupus erythematosus: Report of two cases. Am. J. Med. 77:141, 1984.

828. Leung, W. H., Wong, K. L., Lau, C. P., et al.: Association between anti-phospholipid antibodies and cardiac abnormalities in patients with systemic lupus erythematosus. Am. J. Med. 89:411, 1990.

829. Subramanyan, R., Joy, J., and Balakrishnan, K. G.: Natural history of aortoarteritis (Takayasu's disease). Circulation 80:429, 1989.

830. Kihara, M., Kimura, K., Yakuwa, H., et al.: Isolated left coronary ostial stenosis as the sole arterial involvement in Takayasu's disease. J. Intern. Med. 232:353, 1992.

831. Case records of the Massachusetts General Hospital Case 4-1995: A 26-year-old woman with recurrent angina after a triple-coronary-artery bypass graft. N. Engl. J. Med. 332:380, 1995.

832. Scholz, K. H., Herrmann, C., Tebbe, U., et al.: Myocardial infarction in young patients with Hodgkin's disease: Potential pathogenic role of radiotherapy, chemotherapy and splenectomy. Clin. Invest. 71:57, 1993.

833. Wan, S. K., and Babb, J. D.: Radiation-induced stenosis of the left main coronary artery. Cathet. Cardiovasc. Diagn. 28:225, 1993.

834. Lange, R. L., Reid, M. S., Tresch, D. D., et al.: Nonatheromatous ischemic heart disease following withdrawal from chronic industrial nitroglycerin exposure. Circulation 46:666, 1972.

834a. Hollander, J. E.: The management of cocaine-associated myocardial ischemia. N. Engl. J. Med. 333:1267, 1995.

835. Paavonen, T., Mennander, A., Lautenschlager, I., et al.: Endothelialitis and accelerated arteriosclerosis in human heart transplant coronaries. J. Heart Lung Transpl. 12:117, 1993.

836. Schuler, S., Matschke, K., Loebe, M., et al.: Coronary artery disease in patients with hearts from older donors: Morphologic features and therapeutic implications. J. Heart Lung Transpl. 12:100, 1993.

Chapter 39
Interventional Catheterization Techniques

A. MICHAEL LINCOFF, ERIC J. TOPOL

HISTORY

Interventional cardiology, the application of catheter-based techniques to the treatment of coronary artery, valvular, or congenital cardiac diseases, arose as the culmination of the use of catheters as instruments for the *diagnosis* of heart disease. Cournand and Ranges[1] and others first reported the potential utility of the right-heart catheter in 1941, ushering in a period during which cardiac catheterization was used to evaluate congenital and rheumatic defects and leading ultimately to the development in the late 1950's and 1960's of selective coronary arteriography by Sones and Judkins. The earliest percutaneous *treatment* of a cardiovascular disorder was the Rashkind balloon septostomy to create interatrial defects in patients with transposition of the great vessels.[2]

Dotter and Judkins introduced the therapeutic application of percutaneous "angioplasty" of atherosclerotic peripheral vascular stenoses in 1964,[3] although their cumbersome system of multiple coaxial catheters failed to gain widespread acceptance because of the frequent occurrence of traumatic, hemorrhagic, or embolic vascular complications. The modern era of cardiovascular intervention began as an outgrowth of these ideas, however, with the development by Andreas Gruentzig of a double-lumen balloon catheter, with which dilatation of arterial lesions in the iliac and femoral vessels could be safely achieved with a high rate of procedural success. Miniaturization of this balloon catheter system led to the first percutaneous transluminal coronary angioplasty (PTCA) procedure performed by Gruentzig in September, 1977 in Zurich, where a high-grade narrowing in the proximal left anterior descending coronary artery of a 37-year-old man was successfully dilated,[4] leading to sustained resolution of the stenosis at 1-month angiographic follow-up.

Since the initial application of balloon angioplasty to the treatment of coronary artery disease in humans in 1977, there has been explosive growth in the field of interventional cardiology. While percutaneous revascularization was initially restricted to relatively young patients with stable angina, normal left ventricular function, and proximal, discrete, subtotal, noncalcified concentric stenoses of a single coronary artery, current indications for this procedure have expanded to include unstable angina and acute myocardial infarction, elderly patients and those with depressed left ventricular function, multivessel coronary artery disease, and stenoses with complex morphology or in coronary artery bypass grafts.

A variety of "new devices" for coronary intervention have been developed which allow atherosclerotic plaque to be excised, pulverized, aspirated, ablated by laser or other energy, or supported by metal prosthetic scaffolds, each of which has been advocated to overcome some of the limitations of balloon angioplasty in treating lesions with high-risk characteristics or in reversing the complications of balloon dilatation. The role of adjunctive pharmacological therapy in preventing ischemic complications has been established, with ongoing evaluation of several promising new agents. Novel imaging techniques, including intravascular ultrasonography, fiberoptic angioscopy, and Doppler flow assessment, provide information regarding plaque morphology and physiological function which is complementary to data derived from conventional contrast angiography, facilitating the selection of optimal means of revascularization and assessment of outcome.

Several randomized trials are under way or have been completed to evaluate the efficacy of percutaneous revascularization relative to that of coronary artery bypass surgery in the management of advanced coronary artery disease. Finally, there has been parallel development of new methods for nonsurgical treatment of peripheral vascular and cardiac valve stenoses, as well as transcatheter therapies of congenital cardiac defects.

PERCUTANEOUS TRANSLUMINAL CORONARY ANGIOPLASTY

Since the introduction of coronary balloon angioplasty into clinical practice in 1977,[5] improvements in equipment design and operator experience have permitted this procedure to be applied to the treatment of a broad spectrum of coronary artery disease. More than 400,000 percutaneous revascularization procedures are carried out each year by balloon angioplasty or related "new device" technologies in the United States,[6,7] now exceeding the number of coronary artery bypass surgeries.

ANGIOPLASTY EQUIPMENT. Equipment used during the earliest period of balloon angioplasty was comparatively primitive. Guide catheters were composed of solid Teflon, a material that did not allow adequate retention of shape or torque control. Balloon catheters were bulky and difficult to pass across tight coronary stenoses, with initial designs using no guidewire. Balloon angioplasty was thus confined primarily to proximal lesions in nontortuous vessels.

Wall construction of contemporary guide catheters has evolved into a composite of different layers, conferring improved stability, shape retention, and torque control to catheters with less traumatic distal tips, smaller external diameters, and larger inner lumen dimensions. A variety of preformed shapes are now available, thus optimizing coaxial coronary ostial engagement and support for passage of dilatation catheters. "Over-the-wire" balloon catheter systems have been developed, wherein a freely movable guidewire is passed through the entire length of the central lumen of the angioplasty catheter (Fig. 39–1); such steerable guidewires, with diameters of only 0.009 to 0.018 inch and specialized tips of varying degrees of stiffness, can be precisely shaped, allowing even distal coronary lesions beyond tortuosity to be routinely accessed. Perhaps most remarkable has been the evolution of the balloon angioplasty catheter, with current deflated profiles as small as 1 mm and shaft constructions that optimize trackability and transmission of "push" force. Different polymers are used as balloon materials, permitting accurate sizing, conformability to angulated lesions, and dilatation of rigid lesions with pressures as high as 18 to 20 atmospheres. Specialized catheter designs now include those with the capability of providing distal coronary perfusion during balloon inflation or after abrupt vessel closure (Fig. 39–2) and those with balloons as long as 80 mm intended for diffuse coronary lesions.

Finally, there have been substantial improvements in the quality of radiographic imaging in the cardiac catheterization laboratory. The development of high-resolution fluoroscopy, digital image reconstruction, and on-line com-

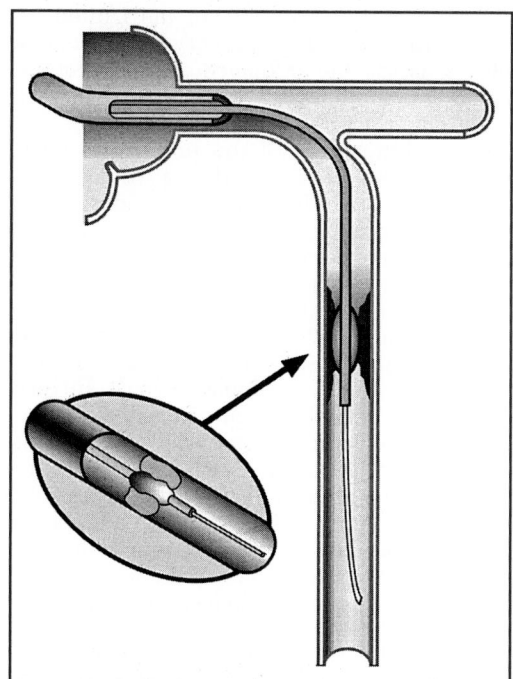

FIGURE 39-1. Diagram of balloon angioplasty catheter with movable guidewire.

puterized quantitative analysis has permitted clear visualization of small-diameter guidewires and catheters within the vasculature, the use of high-definition frozen frames as coronary "road maps," accurate assessment of luminal dimensions before and after revascularization, and improved detection of adverse outcomes such as vascular wall dissection or thrombus formation.

TECHNIQUE. Patients receive antiplatelet therapy with

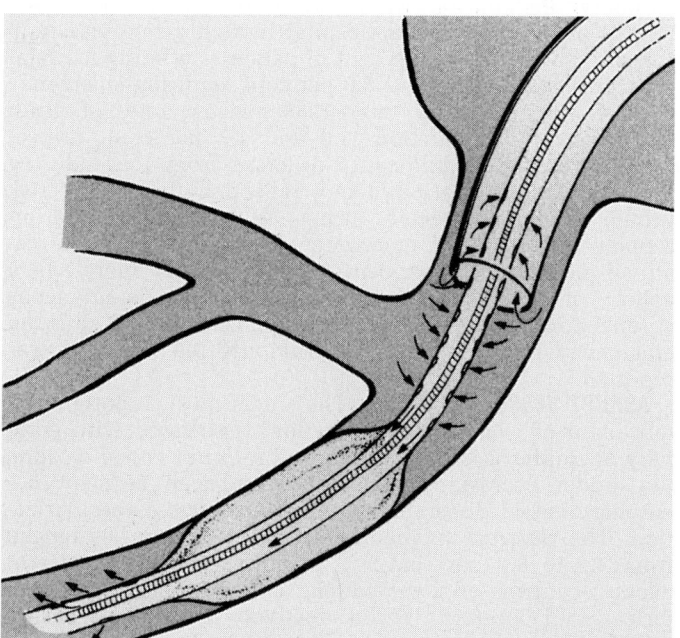

FIGURE 39-2. Schematic diagram of an autoperfusion balloon catheter. Distal coronary perfusion can be maintained during balloon angioplasty using this catheter design (Advanced Cardiovascular Systems, Inc., Mountain View, CA). Once an autoperfusion catheter is inflated across the stenosis, blood enters sideholes proximal to the balloon, flows passively through the central lumen, and exits the catheter via sideholes distal to the coronary occlusion. Flow rates are proportional to proximal arterial perfusion pressure. (From Folland, E. D.: Balloon angioplasty. *In* Topol, E. J., and Serruys, P. [eds.]: Current Review of Interventional Cardiology. Philadelphia, Current Medicine, 1994, p. 1.8.)

aspirin, 80 to 325 mg daily, ideally beginning at least 1 day prior to the coronary angioplasty procedure. Following local anesthesia, vascular access is achieved by percutaneous femoral puncture or, less frequently, brachial puncture or cutdown. At some institutions or in some high-risk patients, a catheter is placed in the pulmonary artery for monitoring of right heart pressures. The coronary vessel is intubated with a No. 7 to 9 French (2.3 to 3.0 mm diameter) guide catheter, and arteriography performed in orthogonal radiographic projections demonstrating unforeshortened views of the target stenosis. Stable coaxial orientation of the guide catheter within the coronary ostium without damping of the pressure waveform must be assured. Systemic heparinization is universally employed, as an initial bolus followed by a continuous infusion or additional periodic boluses, with most laboratories monitoring the adequacy of anticoagulation during the procedure by measurement of activated clotting times (target ≥ 300 seconds). A steerable coronary guidewire, the tip of which has been shaped into a curve appropriate for the specific coronary anatomy, is advanced through the guide catheter into the coronary vessel and manipulated under fluoroscopic guidance across the stenosis by rotation of its distal tip using a manual torquing handle.

A balloon angioplasty catheter of suitable inflated diameter (usually ≤ 110 per cent of the estimated "normal" vessel diameter) is advanced across the guidewire to the stenosis and inflated over a period of seconds or minutes to a pressure at which the balloon appears fully expanded under fluoroscopy (typically at 4 to 8 atmospheres). The duration of balloon inflation may vary from 15 seconds to 2 to 3 minutes or more at the operator's discretion. Some evidence indicates that acute angiographic outcome may be improved by prolongation of balloon inflation time,[8] although the duration of inflation is usually limited primarily by the development of ischemic signs or symptoms due to interruption of distal coronary blood flow. Inadequate improvement in the degree of stenosis may be treated by repeat balloon inflations, exchange over the guidewire for a balloon catheter of larger inflated diameter, or exchange for another percutaneous revascularization device.

After the angioplasty procedure, patients are observed at least overnight in an inpatient cardiology unit for the infrequent development of recurrent myocardial ischemia or hemorrhagic complications; postprocedural ischemia, particularly if prolonged and associated with electrocardiographic changes, usually necessitates urgent repeat angiography and revascularization. If a suboptimal angiographic result is obtained during the angioplasty procedure, particularly if coronary dissection or thrombus is present, heparin anticoagulation is usually continued by infusion for at least several hours. Patients are maintained indefinitely on daily aspirin therapy. Routine long-term follow-up is not uniform but often includes risk factor modification and surveillance for recurrent ischemia by stress testing 3 to 6 months following revascularization.

PATHOPHYSIOLOGY. The mechanisms by which coronary balloon angioplasty may improve vessel luminal dimensions have been characterized by studies in animal models, cadaveric human arterial models, and specimens obtained from patients who died following successful or complicated coronary angioplasty; the recent development of intravascular ultrasound imaging has provided a powerful means of studying the in vivo arterial response during and following percutaneous revascularization[9] (Figs. 3-15, p. 58, and 39-7, p. 1377). The radial force exerted by balloon dilatation within a coronary artery universally produces endothelial denudation with variable degrees of fracture and separation of plaque from the underlying media, stretching of the medial and adventitial layers, and fracture or dissection of the media. Based on these findings, Waller[10] has postulated five different mechanisms for the hemodynamic benefit derived from balloon angioplasty (Fig. 39–3); for any particular lesion, one or more of these mechanisms may be operative. *Plaque compression* appears to play only a minor role in the improvement of the dense fibrocalcific stenoses typically present in advanced coronary artery disease. A major mechanism of balloon angioplasty appears to be *plaque fracture,* with immediate formation of fissures within the atherosclerotic lesion which provide channels for blood flow; the ultimate luminal geometry and extent of enlargement are influenced by subsequent plaque healing and remodeling. An important degree of additional expansion in cross-sectional area is obtained when more extensive arterial injury results in localized *medial dissection* accompanying plaque fracture. *Stretching* with minimal compression of concentric dense fibrocollagenous plaques may also occur, providing an immediate improvement of luminal diameter, which may be partially or completely attenuated, however, by elastic recoil. Similarly, vessels in which an eccentric plaque is dilated may be enlarged simply as a result of *stretching of plaque-free arterial segments* with little or no fracture or compression of plaque, with a propensity for early loss of luminal dimensions due to gradual relaxation of the overstretched segment.

Procedural Outcome and Complications

Gruentzig et al. reported the short-term results among the first 50 patients to undergo balloon angioplasty in 1979.[5] Procedural success was achieved in only 32 of these 50 patients (64 per cent), with the majority of failures due to inability to reach or cross the coronary stenoses using the equipment available at the time.

The National Heart, Lung, and Blood Institute (NHLBI) established a voluntary registry of 3248 consecutive PTCA cases performed at 105 hospitals in the United States between 1977 and 1981. This registry was reopened from 1985–1986 to assess the influence of technological developments and greater operator experience, with 15 of the sites in the original 1977–1981 registry enrolling a total of 2094 patients. Comparison of the procedural results from these two registries[11] has provided a valuable source of data regarding the evolution and expected short-term outcomes of this technique among a diverse population of patients. During the original 1977–1981 NHLBI registry experience, angiographic success (improvement in luminal stenosis by ≥ 20 per cent), as in Gruentzig's first cohort, was achieved in only 67 per cent of stenoses for which angioplasty was attempted,[11] and 21 per cent of patients required urgent or elective coronary bypass surgery during the hospitalization period; 22 per cent of lesions could not be passed by the balloon catheter and an additional 7 per cent could not be dilated. By 1985–1986, however, despite an increased proportion of patients with advanced age, impaired left ventricular function, unstable angina, multivessel coronary disease, total occlusions, and complex stenosis morphology, angiographic success was achieved in 88 per cent of lesions,[11] with elective bypass surgery performed in only 2.2 per cent. More recent reports of data derived during 1989 and 1990–1991 have corroborated the NHLBI findings, with procedural failure rates of only 3.7 per cent and 7.7 per cent, respectively.[12,13]

The majority of patients treated with coronary angioplasty experience substantial immediate relief of symptoms of myocardial ischemia. The procedure has been estimated to be effective in decreasing or eliminating angina in 88 per cent and 76 per cent of patients,[14] respectively, with improvement or resolution of ischemic signs on exercise stress testing following successful balloon dilatation.[15] The extent of improvement in symptom status is better among patients with single-vessel coronary artery disease than among those with multivessel involvement.[16,17]

Major ischemic complications occur infrequently during coronary angioplasty. Even during the early 1977–1981 NHLBI experience, the in-hospital mortality rate was only 1.2 per cent, with 4.9 per cent of patients suffering nonfatal myocardial infarction and 5.8 per cent requiring emergency bypass surgery. In the 1985–1986 registry, rates of death and myocardial infarction (1.0 and 4.3 per cent, respectively) were not significantly different from those during the earlier study period, likely reflecting the greater risk profile of patients treated during the later time period, although the need for emergency bypass surgery had declined modestly (3.4 per cent). Among an even more recent cohort of patients undergoing multivessel percutaneous coronary intervention at five experienced clinical sites, an emergency bypass surgery rate of only 0.9 per cent was reported.[18]

ABRUPT VESSEL CLOSURE. The single most important determinant of ischemic complications associated with coronary angioplasty is the occurrence of *abrupt vessel closure,* the sudden occlusion of the target or adjacent segment of a coronary vessel during or after percutaneous revascularization. The reported incidence of abrupt closure has ranged from 4.2 to 8.3 per cent,[19–22] with roughly one-quarter of events occurring after the patient has left the cardiac catheterization laboratory. While relatively infrequent, abrupt vessel closure has important clinical sequelae (Table 39–1).

The pathophysiological mechanisms of abrupt coronary occlusion are similar to those that produce the therapeutic benefit derived from balloon dilatation. Although plaque and medial fissuring induced by balloon angioplasty usually remains localized, extensive disruption of the medial layer can occur, leading to obstructive dissection flaps or intramural hematoma (Fig. 39–4). Exposure of subendothelial vascular wall components results in platelet deposition and activation with formation of thrombin; occlusive thrombosis may occur, often in association with blood

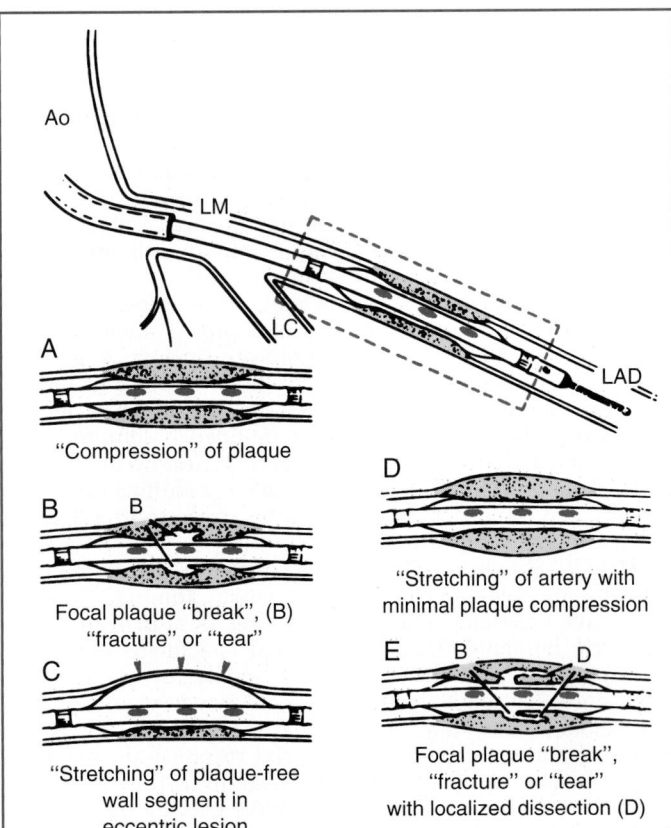

"Compression" of plaque

Focal plaque "break", (B) "fracture" or "tear"

"Stretching" of plaque-free wall segment in eccentric lesion

"Stretching" of artery with minimal plaque compression

Focal plaque "break", "fracture" or "tear" with localized dissection (D)

FIGURE 39–3. Diagram of five possible mechanisms of coronary balloon angioplasty. Ao = aorta; LAD = left anterior descending artery; LC = left circumflex artery; LM = left main artery. (From Waller, B. F.: Coronary luminal shape and the arc of disease free wall: Morphologic observations and clinical relevance. J. Am. Coll. Cardiol. 6:1100, 1985.)

TABLE 39–1 REPORTED CLINICAL SEQUELAE OF ABRUPT VESSEL CLOSURE

SERIES	YEARS	DEATH (%)	MI (%)	CABG (%)
NHLBI Registry I	1979–81	4.9	4.1	7.2
Beth Israel Hospital	1981–86	2.0	3.5	3.3
Emory University	1982–86	2.0	5.4	5.5
Cleveland Clinic	1983–85	0	4.3	4.1
NHLBI Registry II	1985–86	4.9	4.0	4.0
Thoraxcenter	1986–88	6.0	3.6	3.0
University of Michigan	1988–90	8.0	2.0	2.0
Beth Israel Hospital	1989–91	2.5	3.1	2.3

CABG = coronary artery bypass graft surgery; MI = myocardial infarction; NHLBI = National Heart, Lung, and Blood Institute.

From Lincoff, A. M., and Topol, E. J.: Abrupt vessel closure. In Topol, E. J. (ed.): Textbook of Interventional Cardiology. 2nd ed. Philadelphia, W. B. Saunders Company, 1994, p. 207.

stasis produced by medial dissection flaps. In some patients, particularly those with unstable ischemic syndromes, propagation of pre-existent mural thrombus present at the treatment site may be the predominant mechanism of coronary obstruction.

A number of preventive measures may limit the occurrence of abrupt vessel closure during coronary angioplasty. Pharmacological approaches have focused on suppression of both platelet aggregation and thrombus formation at the site of balloon dilatation or on preprocedural resolution of pre-existent mural thrombus. Aspirin, an irreversible inactivator of thromboxane A_2 synthesis and inhibitor of platelet activation, has been demonstrated to reduce the incidence of periprocedural myocardial infarction or occlusive coronary thrombosis.[23]

Although no controlled trials have assessed the efficacy of heparin in the prevention of abrupt closure, observational data suggest that this agent may be useful prior to, during, or after the angioplasty procedure. Among patients with unstable angina or angiographically visible intracoronary thrombus, treatment with aspirin and continuous heparin infusion for 3 to 7 days before percutaneous revascularization has been associated with improved procedural success, diminished risk of periprocedural vessel occlusion,

and angiographic regression of thrombus.[24,25] Although the necessary or target dose for heparin therapy during coronary intervention has never been definitively evaluated, the probability of abrupt vessel closure or ischemic complications appears to be inversely related to the level of anticoagulation[26]; administration of sufficient heparin to achieve an activated coagulation time of 300 to 350 seconds or more prior to initiating coronary angioplasty is thus routinely recommended.[27,28] Finally, although randomized trials have failed to demonstrate a benefit derived from therapy with heparin after uncomplicated angioplasty,[29,30] the temporal relationship noted between discontinuation or inadequate doses of postprocedural heparin suggests that this agent may be useful in preventing closure in selected patients with suboptimal angiographic results following balloon angioplasty.[31]

In contrast to heparin and aspirin, however, adjunctive therapy with thrombolytic agents before balloon angioplasty has *not* been shown to confer clinical benefit, may in fact be detrimental among patients with unstable angina, and is clearly associated with an increased risk of hemorrhagic complications.[32,33] Procedural mechanical factors that may reduce the risk of abrupt closure include selection of appropriately sized balloons to avoid excessive overdilation relative to the normal coronary diameter,[34,35] the use of long (30 to 40 mm) balloons for angulated or diffuse lesions, and gradual and prolonged inflations.[8,36]

A recent large-scale clinical trial, the EPIC trial, demonstrated the efficacy of c7E3Fab (Abciximab, Centocor, Inc., Malvern, PA), a novel monoclonal antibody fragment directed against the platelet membrane glycoprotein IIb/IIIa receptor which binds circulating fibrinogen and cross-links adjacent platelets as the final common pathway to platelet aggregation.[37] Administration of c7E3Fab for 12 hours during and following high-risk coronary angioplasty or atherectomy, in addition to conventional therapy with heparin and aspirin, reduced the incidence of death, myocardial infarction, or urgent repeat revascularization by 35 per cent over the subsequent 30 days[38] (Table 39–2, see also p. 1820).

If abrupt closure occurs, initial management typically consists of repeat prolonged balloon dilatation to induce adhesion of obstructive dissection flaps to the arterial wall or compression of intraluminal thrombus.[22] A number of "new device" technologies, most prominently intracoronary

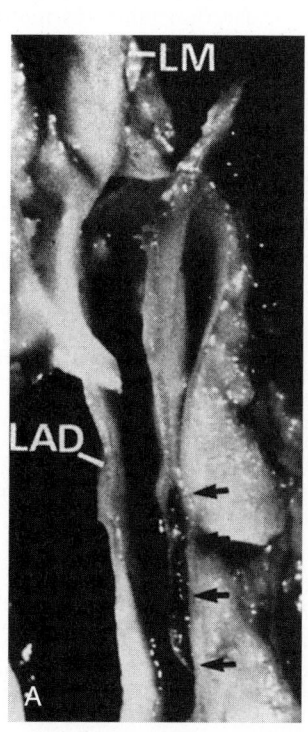
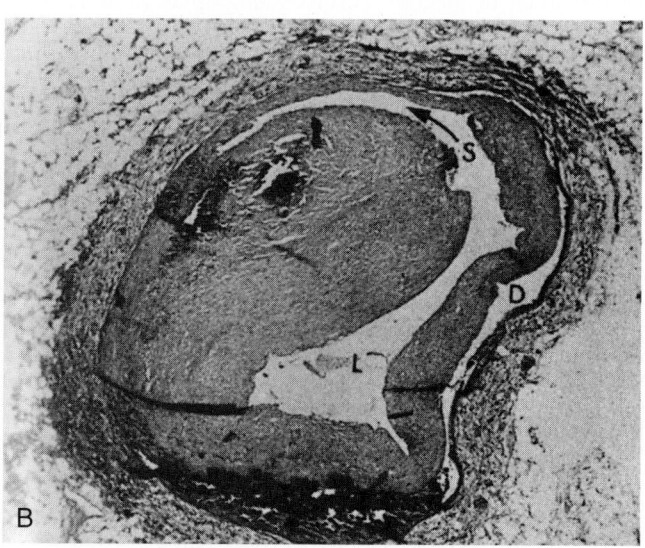

FIGURE 39–4. Pathological findings of coronary dissection following balloon angioplasty. *A,* Localized coronary artery dissection *(arrows)* is present at angioplasty site in left anterior descending artery (LAD). LM = left main coronary artery. (From Waller, B. F.: Early and late morphologic changes in human coronary arteries after PTCA. Clin. Cardiol. *6:*363, 1983.) *B,* Section of left anterior descending artery at site of angioplasty, revealing splitting (S, *arrow*) of the atherosclerotic plaque and dissecting hematoma of the outer media (D). The split has enlarged the original lumen (L). (From Block, P. C., Myler, R. K., Stertzer, S., and Fallon, J. T.: Morphology after transluminal angioplasty in human beings. N. Engl. J. Med. *305:*383, 1981. Copyright 1981, Massachusetts Medical Society.)

TABLE 39–2 OUTCOME IN EPIC TRIAL TESTING AT 30 DAYS AND 6 MONTHS

	PLACEBO (N = 696)	c7E3 FAb BOLUS (N = 695)	c7E3 FAb BOLUS + INFUSION (N = 708)	P VALUE
	\% of Patients			
30-day events				
Composite*	12.8	11.4	8.3	0.009
Death	1.7	1.3	1.7	0.96
Nonfatal MI	8.6	6.2	5.2	0.013
Emergency PTCA	4.5	3.6	0.8	< 0.001
Emergency CABG	3.6	2.3	2.4	0.177
6-month events				
Composite†	35.1	32.6	27.0	0.001
Death	3.4	2.6	3.1	0.832
Nonfatal MI	10.5	8.0	6.9	0.016
PTCA	20.9	19.9	14.4	0.001
CABG	10.9	9.9	9.4	0.343
Target vessel revascularization (PTCA or CABG)	22.3	21.0	16.5	0.007

CABG = coronary artery bypass graft surgery; MI = myocardial infarction; PTCA = coronary angioplasty.

* 30-day composite endpoint = death, myocardial infarction, or emergency PTCA, CABG, stent, or intra-aortic balloon pump placement.

† 6-month composite endpoint = death, myocardial infarction, any PTCA, or any CABG.

Data from EPIC Investigators: Use of a monoclonal antibody directed against the platelet glycoprotein IIb/IIIa receptor in high-risk coronary angioplasty. N. Engl. J. Med. *330*:956, 1994; and Topol, E. J., Califf, R. M., Weisman, H. S., et al.: Reduction of clinical restenosis following coronary intervention with early administration of platelet IIb/IIIa integrin blocking antibody. Lancet *343*:881, 1994.

stents that "scaffold" the disrupted angioplasty site (see p. 1378), also hold promise as means of successfully managing abrupt closure, even in settings where prolonged balloon dilatation has failed. Intracoronary administration of thrombolytic agents has been used successfully in selected patients with thrombotic coronary occlusion,[39] although the preponderance of published data suggest that this strategy is of limited usefulness.[21,22,32]

Notwithstanding the expansion of catheterization laboratory strategies for management of abrupt closure, emergency coronary artery bypass surgery is required in a proportion of patients (Table 39–1) because of failure to achieve stable vessel recanalization. The autoperfusion catheter (Fig. 39–2) can be used to protect jeopardized myocardium while the patient is prepared for operation. Current guidelines issued by the American College of Cardiology and the American Heart Association thus mandate the presence of on-site cardiac surgical facilities for the performance of elective coronary angioplasty.[7] Even at experienced, high-volume surgical centers, however, emergency surgical revascularization performed in this setting does not yield results equivalent to more elective procedures. Perioperative death and myocardial infarction occur more frequently than would be expected for comparable patients managed by primary elective surgery, with published mortality rates ranging from 1.4 to 19 per cent and perioperative Q wave infarction rates from 20 to 57 per cent.[40]

RISK FACTORS FOR ISCHEMIC COMPLICATIONS. Clinical, angiographic, and procedural parameters have been identified which are associated with mortality or morbidity during percutaneous coronary revascularization. Unstable angina has been associated with elevated risks for mortality (up to 5.4 per cent), myocardial infarction (up to 12 per cent), and emergency surgery (up to 12 per cent).[41–43] Interventions performed within 1 to 2 weeks after the onset of unstable ischemic symptoms appear to be associated with a particular hazard,[41,42,44,45] while the complication profile among patients with unstable angina in whom revascularization could be delayed for 2 to 4 weeks may be the same as in patients with stable angina.[44] Other clinical variables associated with ischemic risk include acute myocardial infarction, diabetes mellitus,[46] and possibly female gender[47,48] and advanced age.[49,50]

Multivariate analyses have demonstrated that coronary angiographic assessment provides a powerful means of preprocedural risk stratification. A number of angiographic risk factors have been identified and formally incorporated

TABLE 39–3   AMERICAN COLLEGE OF CARDIOLOGY/AMERICAN HEART ASSOCIATION CLASSIFICATION OF LESION TYPE

Type A Lesions (high success, >85%; low risk)	
Discrete (<10 mm length)	Little or no calcification
Concentric	Less than totally occlusive
Readily accessible	Not ostial in location
Nonangulated segment <45°	No major branch involvement
Smooth contour	Absence of thrombus
Type B Lesions (moderate success, 60–85%; moderate risk)	
Tubular (10–20 mm length)	Moderate to heavy calcification
Eccentric	Total occlusion <3 months old
Moderate tortuosity of proximal segment	Ostial in location
Moderately angulated segment, 45–90°	Bifurcation lesions requiring double guidewires
Irregular contour	Some thrombus present
Type C Lesions (low success, <60%; high risk)	
Diffuse (>2 cm length)	Total occlusion >3 months old
Excessive tortuosity of proximal segment	Inability to protect major sidebranches
Extremely angulated segments >90°	Degenerated vein grafts with friable lesions

From Ryan, T. J., Faxon, D. P., Gunnar, R. M., et al.: Guidelines for percutaneous transluminal coronary angioplasty. A report of the American College of Cardiology/American Heart Association Task Force on assessment of diagnostic and therapeutic cardiovascular procedures (subcommittee on percutaneous transluminal coronary angioplasty). J. Am. Coll. Cardiol. *22*:2033, 1993.

TABLE 39–4 CORRELATES OF MORTALITY AFTER ABRUPT CLOSURE

Female gender

Age > 65–70 years

History of congestive heart failure

Left ventricular ejection fraction ≤ 30%

Unstable angina

Multivessel or left main coronary disease

Collaterals arising from target vessel

Proximal right coronary artery dilation

Jeopardy score

New-onset angina

into a coronary lesion classification by an American College of Cardiology and American Heart Association task force[51] (Table 39–3); this schema defines characteristics of so-called Type A, B, and C lesions based on expected procedural success rates and risks of complications. This scoring system has been independently validated by Ellis and colleagues,[46] among others, who demonstrated that procedural success rates declined from 92 per cent to 61 per cent for Type A versus C lesions, respectively, with an increase in the complication rate from 2 to 21 per cent. Importantly, however, individual angiographic analyses have had inadequate statistical power to accurately estimate the magnitude of risk associated with the various angiographic risk factors,[52] and abrupt closure thus often remains unforeseeable. Nevertheless, in the absence of identifiable angiographic risk factors, procedural success in the hands of skilled operators should exceed 90 to 92 per cent.[12,13,46]

A suboptimal angiographic result following angioplasty may also portend an increased risk of subsequent abrupt closure. The most important procedural correlate of abrupt closure is the occurrence of coronary dissection (Fig. 39–4) during balloon angioplasty. Dissections detectable by angiography likely represent the most extreme of the spectrum of intimal/medial disruptions which occur during all balloon angioplasty procedures. Ischemic risk following dissection is related to the length of the dissection, residual stenosis and luminal diameter.[20,48,53,54]

If abrupt closure occurs during coronary angioplasty, the risk of mortality is influenced by several clinical and angiographic factors (Table 39–4). Most of the clinical predictors likely portend an inadequate myocardial or systemic reserve to compensate for an acute ischemic insult, whereas the angiographic parameters reflect the amount of myocardium in jeopardy for ischemia or infarction.[55–59]

Long-Term Outcome

Among patients who have undergone initially successful coronary angioplasty, outcome over the first 6 to 12 months is influenced primarily by the development of recurrent stenoses at treated sites ("restenosis"), while events over the longer term appear to depend on progression of atherosclerotic disease. Several groups have obtained outcome data for up to 10 years following percutaneous revascularization. Reported rates of survival have been excellent by 1, 5, and 10 years of follow-up, at 97 per cent,[60,61] 88 to 97 per cent,[60–63] and 78 to 90 per cent,[64,65] respectively. Survival free from myocardial infarction or coronary bypass surgery has been somewhat less favorable, however, ranging from 81 to 90 per cent at 1 year,[60,61] 79 per cent at 5 years,[63] and 65 per cent at 10 years.[64]

Recurrence of ischemic signs or symptoms among patients treated with coronary angioplasty appears to occur primarily over the first year following the procedure. The 1985–1986 NHLBI Registry reported that 72 per cent of

treated patients were alive and free of anginal symptoms by 1 year follow-up,[60] although intercurrent coronary artery bypass surgery or repeat percutaneous revascularization had been performed during that time period in 6.4 per cent and 20.7 per cent of patients in that Registry, respectively. By 5-year follow-up, clinical status was essentially the same, with 73 per cent of patients reported alive and free of symptoms in the NHLBI series[66] and 85 per cent in the Emory report.[63] Of the 119 patients surviving for 10 years in the original cohort of 133 successfully treated by Gruentzig in Zurich, 75 per cent were symptom-free, with repeat angioplasty or coronary bypass surgery each carried out in 31 per cent of patients.[64]

Long-term outcome following percutaneous revascularization is clearly inferior among patients with multivessel rather than single-vessel coronary disease.[60,62,64,65] Rates of mortality, myocardial infarction, coronary bypass surgery, and repeat percutaneous intervention were all significantly worse among patients with multivessel disease than those with single-vessel disease at 1-, 5-, or 10-year follow-up in reports of the Emory,[65] NHLBI,[60] or Zurich[64] experience. Signs and symptoms of myocardial ischemia have also been more frequent among patients with multivessel disease in several reports.[16,17,64] The apparently less favorable long-term prognosis for patients with multivessel disease treated by balloon angioplasty may be related in part to the completeness of revascularization. Patients undergoing coronary artery bypass surgery usually achieve complete revascularization. In contrast, complete revascularization is achieved in only a minority of patients with multivessel disease undergoing coronary angioplasty.

In a report of the 1985–1986 NHLBI Registry experience,[67] complete revascularization was attempted in only 33 per cent and 15 per cent of patients with two-vessel and three-vessel disease, respectively, and was successful in 23 per cent and 9 per cent. Similarly in the Mayo Clinic series, complete revascularization was accomplished in 41 per cent.[68] The reason for failure to attempt or accomplish complete revascularization by percutaneous techniques was the presence, most commonly, of a chronic total occlusion, but also of complex or diffuse atherosclerosis or a stenosis of only intermediate severity (50 to 69 per cent diameter stenosis).[67,68] Moreover, particularly among patients with unstable angina, a strategy of dilatation of only the "culprit lesion" has been advocated and demonstrated to provide symptomatic relief in many patients.[69]

The impact of complete revascularization on clinical outcome among patients with multivessel coronary disease treated percutaneously, however, remains unresolved. Although the extent of revascularization appears to influence prognosis among patients undergoing coronary bypass surgery,[70] the relative ease with which repeat procedures may be carried out by percutaneous methods and the risk of restenosis following dilatation of even those lesions of intermediate severity may diminish the importance of complete revascularization among patients undergoing balloon angioplasty. In fact, results of different published studies have varied considerably regarding the outcome among patients with complete versus incomplete revascularization. Although some series have suggested that patients with incomplete revascularization are more symptomatic and more likely to require subsequent coronary bypass surgery,[71] others have failed to demonstrate a significant difference in long-term outcome between the groups of patients defined by the extent of revascularization.[68,72,73] In the Mayo Clinic series,[68] for example, differences in baseline clinical and angiographic features appeared to account entirely for the apparent excess risk for mortality, coronary bypass surgery, or the development of severe angina among patients with incomplete revascularization. Faxon and colleagues have suggested that patients with incomplete revascularization that is nevertheless *functionally adequate* (defined as successful dilatation of all stenoses in bypassable vessels subserving viable myocardium) have a prognosis at 1 year that is equivalent to those with complete revascularization.[72]

Restenosis

The principal factor limiting the long-term benefit of coronary angioplasty is restenosis, the angiographic renarrowing of the vessel lumen following successful balloon dilatation of a vascular lesion. The incidence of restenosis has remained largely unchanged since the introduction of coronary angioplasty, with reported rates ranging from 30 to 50 per cent or more depending upon the method of follow-up and the criteria used to define restenosis. A recent analysis using a private insurance claims data base of 2101 patients treated with coronary angioplasty has provided an estimate of the economic cost of restenosis; surgery or PTCA was required in 30 per cent of these patients within the subsequent 1 year, at a projected total of 1.6 billion dollars in charges within the United States.[6]

Restenosis has traditionally been an angiographic diagnosis, defined most commonly as greater than 50 per cent diameter stenosis at follow-up angiography.[74,75] The most common clinical manifestation of restenosis is recurrence of anginal chest pain.[34,76] Myocardial infarction as the first indication of restenosis is extremely rare, and it has been speculated that the fibroproliferative restenotic lesion is less likely than the lipid-laden native atherosclerotic plaque to undergo plaque rupture.[77] The presence of angiographic restenosis has only limited predictive value for the occurrence of clinical events, however, with up to 30 per cent of patients with restenosis found to be asymptomatic.[76,78,79] Hillegass and colleagues have estimated that the positive predictive value of symptoms for the occurrence of angiographic restenosis is approximately 60 per cent, whereas the likelihood that asymptomatic patients are free from angiographic restenosis (negative predictive value) is approximately 85 per cent.[80] The apparent discordance between clinical outcome and angiographic restenosis is likely related to the influence of collateral vessels,[78] incomplete revascularization, or progression of atherosclerotic disease in other arteries, as well as to the limitations of a dichotomous definition of restenosis, in which intermediate narrowings of 50 to 70 per cent are classified together with more severe lesions as restenotic but are unlikely to produce ischemic symptoms. Moreover, estimation of the true *functional* severity of stenoses by angiography may be problematic, as has been suggested by intravascular ultrasound and Doppler flow studies.

The time course of angiographic restenosis has been elucidated by important serial angiographic studies performed by Serruys and colleagues[81] and Nobuyoshi and associates.[82] Taken together, these two studies suggested an immediate loss of luminal diameter over the first 24 hours after angioplasty, stabilization or slight improvement in the lesion appearance during the first month, progressive loss of luminal diameter over the period between 1 and 4 months, and a relative plateau after 4 months. Restenosis rates were 12.7 per cent, 43.0 per cent, 49.4 per cent, and 52.5 per cent at 1, 3, 6, and 12 months, respectively, in the Nobuyoshi report.[82] At any given time following percutaneous revascularization, changes in luminal diameter appear to occur in nearly all patients, but with the extent of renarrowing normally distributed and only a proportion of patients satisfying dichotomous criteria for restenosis.[83] Typically, ischemic symptoms due to restenosis develop within 6 months of the coronary angioplasty procedure[76,83a]; patients presenting with angina after 6 months more frequently have progression of coronary disease in other vessels than restenosis.[84]

The pathogenesis of restenosis is complex (see p. 1315) and likely multifactorial. Pathological studies of the limited numbers of patients undergoing necropsy following successful balloon angioplasty have suggested that there may be two important subgroups of restenosis lesions: those exhibiting "atherosclerotic plaque only" without morphological evidence of previous balloon angioplasty (approximately 30 per cent of patients), and those with intimal fibrous hyperplasia superimposed upon previous intimal-medial fractures and dissections.[85,86] Restenosis within lesions that do not show evidence of prior balloon injury or intimal hyperplasia likely results from stretching of disease-free arterial wall (in eccentric lesions) or of atherosclerotic plaque (in concentric stenoses) during initial balloon dilatation, followed by "chronic elastic recoil" of the stretched arterial segments.[85] Recent studies have also suggested that shrinkage or remodeling of arterial cross-sectional area may occur following balloon dilatation, with pathological findings in animal models demonstrating structural changes extending throughout the arterial wall.[87,88] Serial intravascular ultrasound studies in humans have also supported the concept that remodeling may be an important mechanism of restenosis following coronary intervention.[89]

In lesions exhibiting intimal fibrous hyperplasia following balloon angioplasty, restenosis appears to be the result of an excessive arterial response to injury.[89a] The magnitude

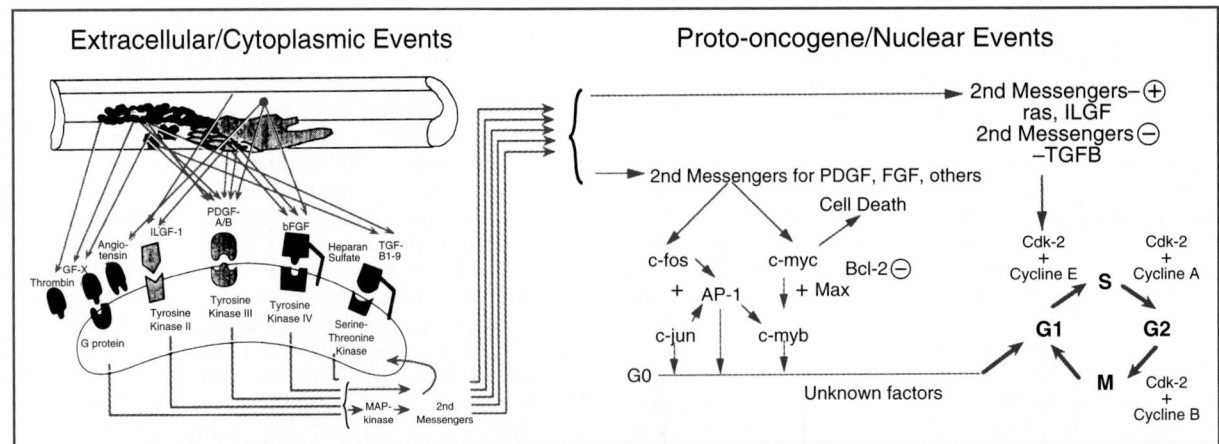

FIGURE 39–5. Possible pathways leading to neointimal hyperplasia component of restenosis. Fundamental pathways have been demonstrated, but not all are known to exist in arterial smooth muscle cells. ILGF = insulin-like growth factor; PDGF = platelet-derived growth factor; bFGF = basic fibroblast growth factor; TGFβ = transforming growth factor β; GFX = growth factor "X" (unknown growth factors); MAPkinase = mitogen activated kinase. (From Lincoff, A. M., Topol, E. J., and Ellis, S. G.: Local drug delivery for the prevention of restenosis. Fact, fancy, and future. Circulation 90:2070, 1994. Copyright American Heart Association.)

of this response, and hence the amount of proliferative tissue, has been noted in animal models and human pathological studies to be proportional to the degree of arterial injury during percutaneous revascularization.[85,90] The cascade of events leading to the formation of the neointimal proliferative lesion in response to arterial injury is not completely understood but has been characterized to some extent in animal models and in vitro systems[91-97] (Fig. 39–5). Balloon angioplasty produces endothelial denudation, plaque disruption, and exposure of subendothelial components, leading to platelet deposition and activation, thrombus formation, and release of mitogens from activated platelets and endothelium. Circulating monocytes, macrophages, and polymorphonuclear leukocytes are recruited by endothelial and platelet migratory factors to the site of arterial injury. Growth and chemotactic factors released from platelets, inflammatory cells, endothelium, and smooth muscle cells induce proliferation and migration of vascular smooth muscle cells from the arterial media to intima and synthesis of extracellular collagen and proteoglycan matrix. Excessive fibrocellular accumulation results in luminal narrowing and restenosis.

Several retrospective studies have identified clinical, anatomical, and procedural factors that may influence the risk of restenosis following coronary angioplasty (Table 39–5). Owing to differences in definitions, angiographic follow-up, and patient populations in these studies, however, the associations between many of these features and restenosis have been variable. Among the clinical factors, only the presence of unstable angina (new or recent onset, accelerating, occurring at rest),[74-76,98-100] variant angina,[101-103] and diabetes mellitus[75,76,99,104] has consistently predicted an elevated incidence of restenosis. The anatomical factors listed in Table 39–5 may predict elevated restenosis risk due to excessive plaque burden or excessive dilatation forces required to achieve an acceptable angiographic result. Similarly, procedural variables associated with restenosis tend to be related to inadequacy of the initial procedural result, with quantitative angiographic studies demonstrating that the extent of postprocedural enlargement in luminal diameter is a potent predictor of angiographic outcome.[105]

Research into means of diminishing or preventing restenosis following coronary angioplasty has thus far been largely unsuccessful. A number of pharmacological agents have been tested which, by virtue of their effects in vitro or

TABLE 39–5 CLINICAL, ANATOMICAL, AND PROCEDURAL CORRELATES OF RESTENOSIS

Clinical Factors
  Unstable angina
  Variant angina
  Diabetes mellitus
  Male gender
  Cigarette smoking
  Hypercholesterolemia
  End-stage renal disease

Anatomical Factors
  Severe preangioplasty stenosis
  Proximal stenosis
  Left anterior descending artery stenosis
  Long stenosis
  Saphenous vein graft stenosis
  Chronic total occlusion
  Lesion calcification
  Bend stenosis
  Bifurcation stenosis
  Ostial stenosis
  Presence of collaterals

Procedural Factors
  Postangioplasty stenosis > 30%
  Use of undersized balloon
  Small residual minimal luminal diameter

Adapted from Popma, J. J., and Topol, E. J.: Factors influencing restenosis after coronary angioplasty. Am. J. Med. 88:1, 1990; with permission.

TABLE 39–6 PHARMACOLOGICAL AGENTS TESTED IN CLINICAL TRIALS FOR PREVENTION OF RESTENOSIS

Antiplatelet Agents
  Aspirin (± dipyridamole)
  Ticlopidine
  Thromboxane A_2 inhibitors
  Serotonin receptor antagonist
  Prostacyclin analogs

Anticoagulants
  Warfarin
  Heparin
  Enoxaparin (low molecular weight heparin)
  Hirudin

Calcium Channel Antagonists
  Diltiazem
  Nifedipine
  Verapamil

Antiproliferative Agents
  Colchicine
  Trapidil
  Corticosteroids

Angiotensin-converting Enzyme Inhibitor
  Cilazapril

Lipid-lowering Agents
  Lovastatin
  Fish oil

Adapted from Hillegass, W. B., Ohman, E. M., and Califf, R. M.: Restenosis: The clinical issues. In Topol, E. J. (ed.): Textbook of Interventional Cardiology. 2nd ed. Philadelphia, W. B. Saunders Company, 1994, p. 415.

in animal models, might be expected to favorably influence different components of the arterial response to injury (Table 39–6).[105a] Unfortunately, clinical trials have failed to demonstrate an unequivocal reduction in the incidence of angiographic restenosis with any of these agents.[80] Although many of these negative clinical studies have accurately reflected the failure of the pharmacological therapy under evaluation to control the restenotic response, some of the trials have been flawed by overly restrictive entry criteria, inadequate sample sizes, or poor rates of angiographic follow-up.[80,106] One promising agent may be the c7E3 Fab antibody fragment against the platelet membrane glycoprotein IIb/IIIa receptor, which reduced the need for repeat coronary revascularization by 28 per cent over 6 months in a large-scale clinical trial (Table 39–2), although systematic angiographic follow-up was not performed to determine the mechanism of this benefit.[107] One of the "new device" technologies for percutaneous revascularization, intracoronary stenting (see p. 1378), has been demonstrated in randomized controlled angiographic trials to be useful in the prevention of restenosis (Table 39–10, p. 1380), albeit in a relatively select group of patients and with a significant risk of hemorrhagic or thrombotic complications.[108,109]

Repeat revascularization of patients with angiographic restenosis is generally reserved for those with clinical symptoms or demonstrable ischemia, as the prognosis in asymptomatic patients is quite favorable.[78,110] Although restenosis may recur following subsequent dilatations, sustained patency can ultimately be achieved in most patients by repeat angioplasty procedures.[111,112]

Comparative Trials of Coronary Angioplasty

Only one randomized trial has been performed evaluating the efficacy of PTCA relative to medical therapy, the Angioplasty Compared to Medicine (ACME) study carried out within the Veterans Administration.[113] Among 212 patients with single-vessel coronary disease and stable angina, an abnormal stress test, or recent myocardial infarction, treatment with coronary angioplasty resulted in a greater likelihood of freedom from angina and better performance during treadmill testing than did intensification of medical therapy over 6 months follow-up; patients

TABLE 39–7 RANDOMIZED TRIALS OF BYPASS SURGERY VERSUS CORONARY ANGIOPLASTY IN PATIENTS WITH MULTIVESSEL CORONARY DISEASE

TRIAL	NUMBER	STUDY ENDPOINTS		ENTRY CRITERIA		FOLLOW-UP PERIOD
		Primary	Secondary	Clinical	Angiographic	
RITA[115]	1011	Death + MI	Repeat revascularization, angina severity, exercise tolerance, employment status	Revascularization appropriate by PTCA or CABG	1, 2, 3 vessels >50% stenosis, equivalent revascularization feasible by CABG or PTCA	5 years
GABI[117]	359	Freedom from angina	Death, MI, repeat revascularization	Revascularization appropriate by PTCA or CABG, Class III angina	2 or 3 vessels >70% stenosis, no total occlusions	1 year
EAST[118]	392	Death + QMI + large ischemic burden on thallium	Repeat revascularization, angina severity, angiographic status	Revascularization appropriate by PTCA or CABG	2 or 3 vessels >50% stenosis	3 years
ERACI[116]	127	Death + MI + repeat revascularization + angina	In-hospital complications, completeness of revascularization	Revascularization appropriate by PTCA or CABG	2 or 3 vessel disease, complete revascularization feasible	5 years
CABRI	1054	Angina, functional capacity	Death, MI, repeat revascularization, angiography, L function	Revascularization appropriate by PTCA or CABG	2 or 3 vessels >50% stenosis	5 years
BARI	1829	Death	MI, angina, repeat revascularization, treadmill performance, angiography, L function	Revascularization appropriate by PTCA or CABG	2 or 3 vessels >50% stenosis	5 years

CABG = Coronary artery bypass graft surgery; L = left ventricle; MI = myocardial infarction; N = number of enrolled patients; PTCA = coronary angioplasty; BARI = Bypass Angioplasty Revascularization Investigation; CABRI = Coronary Angioplasty Bypass Revascularization Investigation; EAST = Emory Angioplasty versus Surgery Trial; ERACI = Argentine Randomized Trial of Percutaneous Transluminal Coronary Angioplasty Versus Coronary Artery Bypass Surgery in Multivessel Disease; GABI = German Angioplasty Bypass Surgery Investigation; RITA = Randomized Intervention Treatment of Angina; QMI = Q-wave MI.

Adapted from Gersh, B. J.: Efficacy of percutaneous transluminal coronary angioplasty (PTCA) in coronary artery disease: Why we need randomized trials. In Topol, E. J. (ed.): Textbook of Interventional Cardiology. 2nd ed. Philadelphia, W. B. Saunders Company, 1994, p. 251.

within the angioplasty group more frequently required coronary artery bypass surgery than those randomized to medicine (6.7 versus 0 per cent, $P < 0.01$), however, and 15 per cent underwent repeat PTCA. Among 101 patients with double-vessel disease in the same trial, the benefit of angioplasty compared with medical therapy appeared to be less marked than for those with single-vessel disease.[114] A large-scale prospective nonrandomized analysis of more than 9000 patients treated at Duke University over a 7-year period observed a trend toward a 20 per cent reduction in long-term mortality by PTCA relative to medicine for patients with single-vessel coronary disease or less severe forms of double-vessel disease, although for double-vessel disease with proximal left anterior descending artery involvement or for triple-vessel disease, the effects of PTCA and medical therapy on survival appeared to be equivalent.[62]

Six randomized clinical trials have been performed or are under way comparing coronary angioplasty with bypass surgery in patients with multivessel coronary disease (Table 39–7), and interim or final results have been reported for five[115–118] (Table 39–8, see also p. 1330). At one year follow-up, the ERACI,[116] GABI,[117] and CABRI[119] trials reported no difference between angioplasty and surgery with respect to in-hospital or 1-year mortality. Myocardial infarction rates were equivalent between the two therapies in the ERACI and CABRI studies, although in-hospital infarction rates were higher among surgically treated patients in GABI (8.1 versus 2.3 per cent, $P = 0.022$).

In all three studies, substantially more patients required repeat coronary revascularization following initial PTCA (44 per cent versus 6 per cent in GABI and 40 per cent versus 8.6 per cent in CABRI). The RITA[115] and EAST[118] trials have reported outcome among patients followed for

TABLE 39–8 PTCA VERSUS CABG TRIALS: CLINICAL OUTCOME

	RITA		ERACI		GABI		CABRI		EAST	
	PTCA	CABG	PTCA	CABG	PTCA	CABG	PTCA	CABG	PTCA	CABG
Randomized	510	501	63	64	182	177	541	513	198	194
Early Outcome	In-hospital		In-hospital		In-hospital		30 days		In-hospital	
Death (%)	0.8	1.2	1.5	4.6	1.1	2.3	1.7	0.9	1.0	1.0
MI (%)	3.5	2.4	6.3	6.2	2.3*	8.1*	3.1	2.9	2.0	10.3*
Reintervention (%)	6.7	NA	1.5	1.5	11.0	1.7*	10.1	1.6*	10.1	0*
Late Outcome	2–2.5 years		1 year		1 year		1 year		3 years	
Death (%)	3.1	3.6	4.8	4.6	2.2	5.1	3.9	2.1	7.1	6.2
MI (%)	6.7	5.2	9.5	7.8	3.8	7.3	2.9	3.3	14.6	19.6
PTCA (%)	18.2	0.8	14.2	3.3	27.5	1.1	20.1	7.2	40	13
CABG (%)	18.8	3.2†	17.5	0†	22.5	4.0†	20.2	1.4†	21.2	0.5†
Angina-free (%)	69*	7	62	86	71	74	85	91	80	88
Event-free survival (%)	62*	8	64	84	56	94	60	85*	46	70*

* Statistically significant difference
† Statistically significant difference for all reinterventions (CABG + PTCA)
CABG = Coronary artery bypass graft surgery; MI = myocardial infarction; NA = not available; PTCA = coronary angioplasty.
Trials: RITA = Randomized Intervention Treatment of Angina; ERACI = Argentine Randomized Trial of Percutaneous Transluminal Coronary Angioplasty versus Coronary Bypass Surgery in Multivessel Disease; GABI = German Angioplasty versus Bypass Surgery Investigation; CABRI = Coronary Angioplasty versus Bypass Revascularization Investigation; EAST = Emory Angioplasty Surgery Trial.
From Moliterno, D. J., Elliott, J. M., and Topol, E. J.: Randomized trials of myocardial revascularization. Curr. Probl. Cardiol. 20:171, 1995, with permission.

2.5 and 3 years, respectively. Both studies found no differences between patients treated with surgery or PTCA in the incidence of death or myocardial infarction over this follow-up period, nor was there a difference between treatment groups with regard to the prevalence of large ischemic defects on thallium scanning in EAST. As with ERACI and GABI, however, RITA and EAST observed a 3- to 4-fold higher rate of repeat coronary revascularization among patients who were initially treated with balloon angioplasty. Similar results were reported for 134 patients with isolated proximal left anterior descending artery disease followed for 2.5 years after randomization to PTCA or internal mammary artery bypass grafting.[120] The results of the large-scale BARI trial, with primary endpoints at 5 years follow-up, have yet to be reported.

The existing randomized data can be summarized as demonstrating equivalent clinical outcome with regard to "hard" endpoints of death and myocardial infarction among patients managed with initial strategies of either coronary angioplasty or bypass surgery, although with a somewhat greater periprocedural morbidity following treatment with surgery and a greater need for repeat revascularization in patients undergoing angioplasty. It is important to recognize, however, that only a minor proportion of patients screened at the institutions participating in these trials were actually randomized (4 per cent in GABI and 8 per cent in EAST), with many patients excluded from enrollment due to clinical or anatomical factors that were thought to render them unsuitable for PTCA (such as left main disease or chronically occluded vessels). Thus, the results of these randomized trials must be interpreted within the context of the patient populations examined and cannot necessarily be extrapolated to the patients with more complex or severe coronary disease. Moreover, these trials were carried out prior to the widespread use of new device technologies for coronary intervention, and thus, particularly in view of the impact of coronary stenting, may not accurately reflect the current state of the art of percutaneous coronary revascularization.

Indications for Coronary Angioplasty
(See also pp. 1313 and 1954)

Despite the growing body of data regarding the risk factors for acute and long-term complications and the efficacy of coronary angioplasty compared with medical therapy or surgical revascularization, a consensus on firm indications for the procedure has not been established. Coronary angioplasty is effective in relieving symptoms in patients with single-vessel and multivessel coronary disease, even when applied to stenoses with relative high-risk characteristics; although the need for repeat revascularization is the most common adverse outcome, repeat procedures can usually be performed without significant morbidity. Selection of patients for PTCA involves careful consideration of the extent of symptoms or ischemic myocardium, the response to medical therapy, the risk of abrupt vessel closure, the likelihood of fatal or serious morbid outcomes in the event of abrupt closure, the prospects for complete or "functionally complete" revascularization, the expected incidence of restenosis, and the suitability of the patient for coronary artery bypass surgery.

The only "absolute contraindications" to angioplasty are the absence of a hemodynamically significant coronary stenosis, significant (>50 per cent stenosis) left main coronary disease unprotected by at least one patent bypass graft, and (in the United States, at least) absence of on-site cardiac surgical support.[7] In general, angioplasty is considered the revascularization procedure of choice for patients with angina or an ischemic response on exercise testing who have single-vessel or double-vessel coronary disease without proximal left anterior descending artery involvement,[121] although the usefulness of medical therapy in this setting must not be disregarded. Among patients who are candidates for surgical revascularization, the benefits of coronary artery bypass appear clear in the setting of severe symptoms and multivessel coronary disease that either cannot be completely revascularized or that is poorly amenable to angioplasty due to the presence of diffuse coronary involvement, a severely degenerated saphenous vein graft target, or a single remaining conduit for myocardial circulation.[7,14,62]

CORONARY ANGIOPLASTY FOR ACUTE MYOCARDIAL INFARCTION (see also p. 1221). Several randomized trials have examined the role of coronary angioplasty as primary or adjunctive therapy for patients with acute myocardial infarction. Given the known limitations of thrombolytic therapy in this setting, including delayed reperfusion, failed or incomplete reperfusion, and reocclusion, balloon angioplasty has intuitive appeal as a means of restoring infarct vessel patency or treating residual stenoses following thrombolysis to prevent recurrent ischemia or reocclusion. Five different strategies for percutaneous revascularization for acute infarction have thus been advocated: (1) *primary angioplasty* to achieve acute infarct vessel reperfusion without prior administration of thrombolytic agents, (2) *urgent adjunctive coronary angioplasty* performed routinely within a few hours after successful thrombolytic reperfusion to treat an underlying stenosis, (3) *deferred adjunctive coronary angioplasty* of the infarct-related artery carried out routinely within the first week of thrombolysis to prevent recurrent ischemia, (4) *conservative adjunctive coronary angioplasty* applied selectively to patients who demonstrate spontaneous recurrent or inducible ischemia following thrombolysis for myocardial infarction, and (5) *rescue coronary angioplasty* performed immediately in patients for whom thrombolytic agents have failed to achieve infarct vessel reperfusion.

Several observational reports have suggested that primary PTCA may be as effective as thrombolytic therapy in reducing mortality and salvaging left ventricular function during acute myocardial infarction.[122,123] Importantly, many of the patients treated with angioplasty in these series would have been considered ineligible for thrombolytic therapy because of excessive risk for hemorrhage or other exclusionary criteria. Four small-scale randomized trials have compared direct angioplasty to intravenous thrombolytic therapy for acute infarction,[124-127] the largest of which, the Primary Angioplasty in Myocardial Infarction (PAMI) study,[124] randomized 395 patients to PTCA or tissue plasminogen activator (t-PA). PAMI demonstrated a lower incidence of death or reinfarction by hospital discharge and during 6 months follow-up among patients treated with PTCA compared with thrombolysis. Although the data regarding the use of acute angioplasty as primary therapy for acute infarction appear quite promising, the limitations of these studies, including the small numbers of patients tested and the failure to compare with accelerated t-PA, must be surmounted before the efficacy of direct balloon angioplasty relative to optimal thrombolytic therapy can be firmly established.

Three large randomized trials have examined the strategy of immediate adjunctive coronary angioplasty following successful thrombolysis with t-PA.[128-130] Despite differences in design, the findings of these studies were concordant: urgent PTCA in this setting offers no clinical benefit, with a trend toward greater mortality, reocclusion, and recurrent ischemia in the immediate angioplasty arm of each trial and no differences in ventricular function. The failure of angioplasty to improve outcome following successful thrombolysis may be due to a diminished likelihood of procedural success and increased risk of thrombotic occlusion when balloon dilatation is performed within recently lysed clot. Similarly, two major trials examining the strategy of "deferred" routine percutaneous revascularization in the days following successful thrombolysis also failed to detect a clinical benefit from the more aggressive approach,[131,132] again with a slight trend toward more frequent death or reinfarction among patients undergoing PTCA. Thus, the conservative approach of reserving percutaneous revascularization for situations of spontaneous or demonstrable ischemia appears to be most suitable for the majority of stable patients following apparently successful thrombolysis for acute infarction. In contrast to the routine adjunctive strategy, however, the application of PTCA as a mode of "rescue" for failed thrombolysis may offer significant benefit, at least for patients with large myocardial infarctions. In a controlled trial of 150 patients with anterior infarction and persistently occluded infarct arteries after thrombolysis,[133] randomization to rescue PTCA resulted in a substantial reduction in the endpoints of death or severe congestive heart failure (16.6 versus 6.4 per cent for PTCA and conservative therapy, respectively, $P = 0.05$).

NEW DEVICES FOR PERCUTANEOUS CORONARY REVASCULARIZATION

The development of new devices for percutaneous revascularization has been motivated by the recognition that despite improvements in equipment design and operator experience, balloon angioplasty remains substantially limited by the risk of procedural complications, difficulties in achieving an adequate angiographic result, and the persistently high incidence of restenosis when this technique is applied to certain patient or coronary lesion subsets. Stenoses that are complex, calcified, long, bulky, eccentric, totally occluded, within saphenous vein grafts, or associated with thrombus are particularly challenging to treat with conventional methods of balloon dilatation. In part, the limitations of coronary angioplasty in this regard are thought to be related to the uncontrolled plaque disruption and vessel stretching induced by balloon dilatation, leading unpredictably to coronary dissection and excessive vascular trauma (Fig. 39–4) and the resultant sequelae of acute ischemic events or late restenotic "response to injury." The potential efficacy of new devices relative to PTCA may be twofold. First, these techniques have been purported to produce a more predictable degree of arterial trauma, thereby reducing the risk of abrupt coronary closure; additionally, the mechanical support of the arterial wall afforded by one class of devices, stents, appears to successfully reverse vascular disruption induced by other methods of revascularization and to prevent ischemic complications. Second, in that plaque is actually removed or elastic recoil eliminated by new devices interventions, these techniques may achieve a better improvement in luminal dimensions than does PTCA, thereby potentially leading to a larger residual lumen at long-term follow-up and less restenosis ("bigger is better").[105]

Following the introduction into investigational use of directional atherectomy for the treatment of coronary stenoses in 1986, six new devices have been approved by the Food and Drug Administration (FDA) since 1990 and a number of others are in various stages of review. Interventional cardiologists have embraced these techniques with great enthusiasm, yet few of these methods have been compared in controlled clinical trials to balloon angioplasty. Observational data, in the form of single-center or multicenter registries, are useful in assessing safety and efficacy during the early stages of clinical testing of new devices but are limited by selection bias and the frequent requirement for adjunctive balloon angioplasty to obtain an acceptable final angiographic result. Thus, the most appropriate indications and limitations of most new devices remain to be defined. Table 39–9 summarizes the potential "niches" for new devices for percutaneous coronary interventions.[133a]

TABLE 39–9 POTENTIAL "NICHES" FOR NEW DEVICES FOR PERCUTANEOUS CORONARY INTERVENTION: EFFICACY RELATIVE TO BALLOON ANGIOPLASTY SUGGESTED BY PUBLISHED OBSERVATIONAL AND RANDOMIZED TRIAL DATA

INDICATION	STENT	ROTO	TEC	LASER	DCA
Acute Outcome					
Treat abrupt vessel closure	++	NA	NA	NA	+
Complex lesion morphology					
Calcification	–	++	– –	+	– –
Thrombus	– –	–	+	+	+
Saphenous vein graft	++	–	+	+	+
Degenerated saphenous vein graft	0	– –	++	+	0
Eccentric	+	+	–	–	++
Ostial	+	++	–	+	+
Long	+	++	0	+	–
"Undilatable" (rigid) stenosis	–	++	–	+	– –
Long-term Outcome					
Reduce restenosis	++	0	0	0	0

DCA = directional coronary atherectomy; Roto = rotational atherectomy (Rotablator); TEC = transluminal extraction catheter.

Assessment of efficacy is for use of new device alone or in combination with balloon angioplasty only. Some devices may be more effective than balloon angioplasty when used in combination with other devices, such as rotational atherectomy followed by stenting for undilatable or calcified stenoses.

NA   Data regarding efficacy relative to balloon angioplasty not available.
++   Appears to be substantially more effective than balloon angioplasty
+   Possibly more effective than balloon angioplasty
0   Appears equivalent to balloon angioplasty
–   Possibly less effective (or associated with higher complication risk) than balloon angioplasty
– – Appears to be substantially less effective (or associated with higher complication risk) than balloon angioplasty

Coronary Atherectomy

Three different devices that remove atheromatous material from coronary lesions have been approved for clinical use. Two of these, the directional and extraction atherectomy catheters, operate on the principle of physically cutting the stenosis using a spinning blade, while rotational atherectomy abrades and pulverizes the plaque. Each technique has been extensively evaluated in patients and advocated for particular coronary lesion subsets.

DIRECTIONAL CORONARY ATHERECTOMY. The directional coronary atherectomy catheter (Simpson Coronary Atherocath, Devices for Vascular Intervention, Inc., Redwood City, CA) consists of a metal cylinder at its distal end, which houses a coaxial rotating cup-shaped blade (Fig. 39–6A).

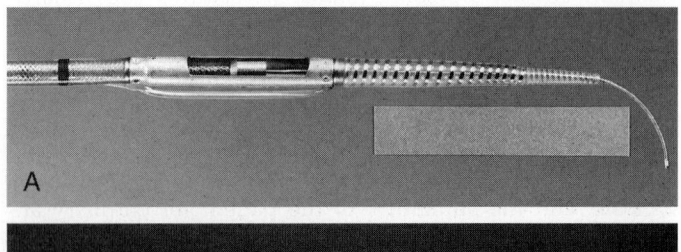

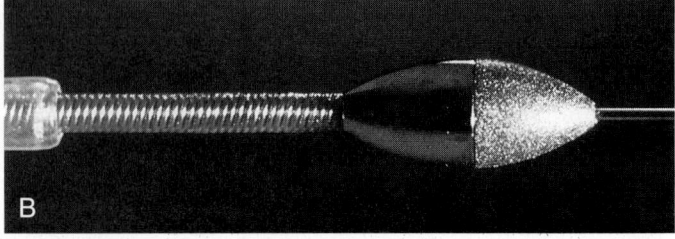

FIGURE 39–6. Atherectomy devices. A, Directional atherectomy. (Courtesy of Devices for Vascular Interventions, Redwood City, CA.) B, Rotational atherectomy. (Courtesy of Heart Technology, Seattle, WA.)

One side of the cylindrical housing contains a window 9 mm in length over a 120-degree arc, with a noncompliant balloon attached to the metal housing opposite the window. A flexible conical nosecone at the distal tip of the housing serves as a collecting chamber for excised atheromatous tissue. Once passed over a guidewire to the coronary stenosis, the eccentric balloon is inflated to low pressure (1 to 2 atmospheres), pressing the window against the plaque and invaginating the atherosclerotic tissue into the cutting chamber. The cutter within the housing, connected by a drive cable through the shaft of the catheter to an external drive unit, is activated and slowly pushed forward through the housing as it spins at approximately 2000 rpm; tissue prolapsing into the catheter is excised and pushed forward into the hollow nosecone collecting chamber. The balloon is deflated and the catheter torqued to reorient the window to other diseased quadrants. Following multiple cuts, some of which may be performed with the balloon inflated to higher pressures (2 to 4 atmospheres), the catheter is withdrawn and fragments of excised plaque are retrieved from the distal nosecone. Many patients require adjunctive balloon angioplasty following atherectomy to achieve an optimal angiographic result.

The mechanism of enlargement of luminal diameter by directional atherectomy appears to be twofold. Clearly, plaque excision reduces the obstructive bulk of atheroma (Fig. 39–7), but intravascular ultrasound studies and geometric calculations suggest that the majority of improvement in luminal dimensions is a result of dilatation by the atherectomy catheter balloon.[134,135] Atherectomy into the plaque, arterial media, and even adventitia may change the compliance of the artery and allow selective and sustained stretching of the arterial wall.

Observational registry experience demonstrated directional atherectomy to be effective and safe for treating a wide variety of coronary stenoses,[136] with an overall procedural success rate of 85 per cent following atherectomy, increasing to 92 per cent with adjunctive balloon angioplasty. Rates of in-hospital death, nonfatal Q wave myocardial infarction, and emergency coronary bypass surgery were similar to those associated with PTCA: 0.5 per cent, 0.9 per cent, and 4.0 per cent, respectively. Plaque removal by directional atherectomy may produce an angiographic result superior to that obtainable by balloon angioplasty, particularly for lesions that are eccentric, ostial, restenotic, or associated with intraluminal thrombus.[137,138] Failures of atherectomy are most frequently due to inability to pass the bulky catheter to or across the coronary stenosis, although other complications include coronary occlusion, embolization, and perforation. As with balloon angioplasty, outcome using this technique is influenced by clinical and coronary morphological features.

Three multicenter randomized trials have evaluated the hypothesis that directional atherectomy can reduce restenosis rates relative to balloon angioplasty.[139–141] In the Coronary Angioplasty Versus Excisional Atherectomy Trial[139] (CAVEAT-1), immediate angiographic success rates and postprocedural luminal diameters were greater among the 512 patients with de novo native coronary artery stenoses allocated to directional atherectomy than the 500 undergoing balloon angioplasty, although only a nonsignificant trend toward reduced restenosis rates in the atherectomy group was observed (50 versus 57 per cent, $P = 0.06$). Importantly, however, acute procedural ischemic complications (death, myocardial infarction, emergency bypass surgery, and abrupt closure) occurred significantly more frequently among patients randomized to atherectomy than to PTCA (11 versus 5 per cent, $P < 0.001$), as did the actuarial incidence of death or myocardial infarction by 6 months follow-up (9.4 versus 3.6 per cent, $P = 0.0002$). Moreover, atherectomy resulted in higher hospital costs, longer procedure times, and longer fluoroscopy times than balloon angioplasty. Notably, 1-year follow-up of the CAVEAT-1 cohort demonstrated a higher mortality for patients treated with atherectomy than with angioplasty (2.2 versus 0.6 per cent, $P = 0.035$), although the explanation for this observation is thus far elusive.[142]

The Canadian Coronary Atherectomy Trial (CCAT)[140] focused on patients undergoing revascularization of de novo proximal left anterior descending artery stenoses, an anatomical location believed to be particularly well suited for atherectomy owing to its large luminal diameter and the relatively high risk for restenosis following balloon angioplasty. As with CAVEAT-1, acute procedural success rates and luminal dimensions were superior following atherectomy, but no difference in restenosis rates was observed (46 versus 43 per cent for atherectomy and angioplasty, respectively, $P = 0.71$). Finally, CAVEAT-2[141] compared the two techniques among patients with saphenous vein graft stenoses, with no significant difference in the rates of 6-month restenosis (45.6 per cent and 50.5 per cent following atherectomy and angioplasty, respectively, $P = 0.49$), although there was a trend toward fewer repeat target vessel revascularization procedures in atherectomy-treated patients (18.6 versus 26.2 per cent, $P = 0.09$).

Some authors,[143] citing the thesis of "bigger is better," have attributed the absence of demonstrable long-term advantage of atherectomy over angioplasty in these three trials to the failure of the interventional operators to perform atherectomy to obtain a residual stenosis close to 0

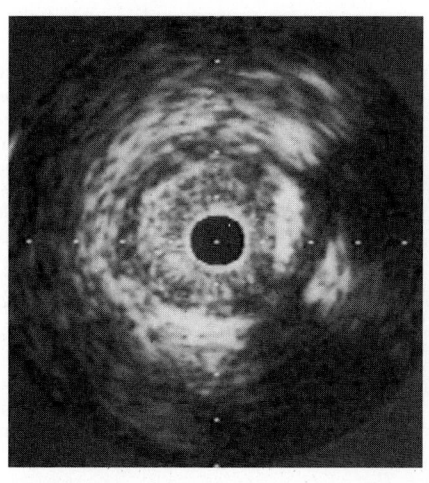 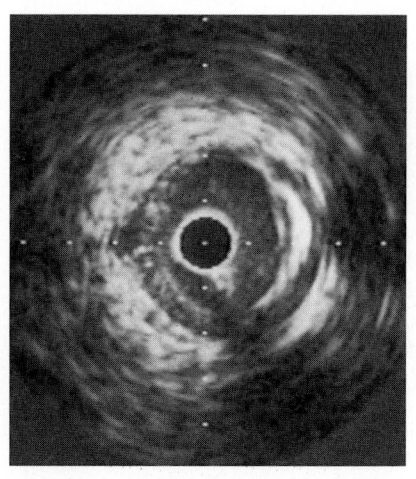

FIGURE 39–7. Intravascular ultrasound images before and after directional coronary atherectomy. *Left,* Circumferential atheromatous plaque with severe luminal compromise prior to atherectomy. Arc of calcification with ultrasound shadowing is visible between 1 and 4 o'clock. *Right,* Following directional atherectomy, there is nearly complete removal of atherosclerotic plaque material with an excellent residual lumen. The arc of calcium is still present. (From Nissen, S. E., Tuzcu, E. M., and DeFranco, A. C.: Coronary intravascular ultrasound: Diagnostic and interventional applications. *In* Topol, E. J. [ed.]: Textbook of Interventional Cardiology. Update 14. Philadelphia, W. B. Saunders Company, 1994, p. 219.)

per cent.[144] Whether such an approach of "aggressive" atherectomy will reduce the incidence of restenosis compared to angioplasty, without an unacceptably high incidence of acute ischemic complications, is being tested in an ongoing randomized trial. Until results of this trial become available, the settings in which directional atherectomy may lead to a convincingly better clinical or long-term angiographic outcome remain unclear.

ROTATIONAL ATHERECTOMY. The rotational atherectomy catheter (Rotablator, Heart Technology, Inc., Bellevue, WA) uses a rapidly spinning abrasive tip welded to the end of a flexible metal drive shaft to grind or "polish" the internal lumen of an atherosclerotic plaque. The distal end of the catheter consists of an elliptical burr coated with 10- to 40-μm diamond chips (Fig. 39–6B) which rotates at 170,000 to 200,000 rpm while slowly advanced across the atherosclerotic plaque. Rotational atherectomy produces abraded atheromatous particles of less than 10 to 12 μm in diameter which typically pass downstream without obstruction of the microcirculation,[145] although larger debris may be formed by rotablation of heavily calcified stenoses. Multiple passes of the Rotablator are typically performed until no resistance is encountered; progressively larger burrs ranging in size from 1.25 to 2.5 mm may be used.

Rotational atherectomy theoretically operates on the principle of "differential cutting," where rigid material such as calcium or fibrotic plaque is preferentially pulverized rather than the elastic components of the arterial wall.[146] As such, this technique has been particularly advocated for heavily calcified, inelastic or "nondilatable," eccentric, and diffuse coronary lesions (Fig. 39–8). Intravascular ultrasound studies of heavily calcified lesions treated with rotational atherectomy appear to confirm that the primary mechanism of improvement of luminal dimension is selective removal of calcified plaque, with little or no stretching of the vessel itself.[147] Adjunctive balloon angioplasty, however, required in most cases because of the relatively small diameters of available Rotablator burrs,[148] further increases the luminal area by vessel stretching and plaque fracture.

A recent report from the multicenter rotational atherectomy registry of 709 patients treated at 17 institutions with the Rotablator demonstrated a high rate of procedural success (94.7 per cent), which appeared unrelated to traditional high-risk characteristics.[149] Rates of death, Q-wave myocardial infarction, non-Q-wave infarction, and emergency bypass surgery were 0.8 per cent, 0.9 per cent, 5.2 per cent, and 1.7 per cent, respectively; restenosis at 6 months was documented in 37.7 per cent of patients who returned for angiographic follow-up. Other analyses have generally confirmed these findings,[148,150] also identifying delayed coronary runoff ("slow reflow"), possibly resulting from distal embolization of microparticulate debris or microcavitation bubbles, as an important contributor to the incidence of periprocedural myocardial infarction. Although observational data thus suggest that rotational atherectomy may be useful in treating certain lesion subsets that appear poorly suited for balloon angioplasty, randomized trials comparing this technique with other forms of percutaneous coronary revascularization have yet to be performed.

TRANSLUMINAL EXTRACTION ATHERECTOMY. The transluminal extraction catheter (TEC, InterVentional Technologies, Inc., San Diego, CA) was designed to excise and extract atheromatous material and has been applied primarily to diffusely degenerated saphenous vein grafts and to thrombus-containing lesions. It consists of a flexible, hollow torque tube, the distal end of which consists of two blades oriented in a conical configuration. Once activated within the coronary vasculature, the torque tube spins at 750 rpm with vacuum applied through its lumen; this design is intended to aspirate plaque and thrombus cut by the rotating blades through the hollow tube into an external vacuum bottle.

The multicenter observational TEC registry experience reported a procedural success rate of 88 per cent,[151] with major complications occurring in 5.7 per cent of patients, including death, myocardial infarction following occlusion or embolization, emergency bypass surgery, and vessel perforation in 2.2 per cent, 1.3 per cent, 2.3 per cent, and 1 per cent, respectively.[152] The relatively high rate of complications observed in this registry may be related in part to the prevalence of high-risk characteristics among patients treated with this device, such as degenerated saphenous vein grafts or acute myocardial infarction.[151] In contrast to balloon angioplasty, in which vein graft age has been associated with the risk of ischemic complications,[153] procedural success with TEC in bypass grafts appears to be unrelated to graft age[151]; distal embolization may occur in up to 23 per cent of patients nonetheless,[154] particularly from diffusely degenerated grafts and following adjunctive balloon angioplasty. Restenosis rates among different subsets of patients treated with the TEC catheter have not been better than those obtained with PTCA, ranging from 45 to 51 per cent in native coronary arteries and 46 to 53 per cent in vein grafts.[151]

Intracoronary Stents

As an alternative to the removal of plaque material by atherectomy, intravascular stents may be used to support and maintain stretch of a diseased segment of artery, thus eliminating acute or chronic recoil, scaffolding disrupted or friable atherosclerotic tissue, minimizing contact between blood and thrombogenic subintimal arterial wall components, and optimizing coronary blood flow dynamics. There has been a broad observational experience with the use of stents as a means of treating abrupt closure or im-

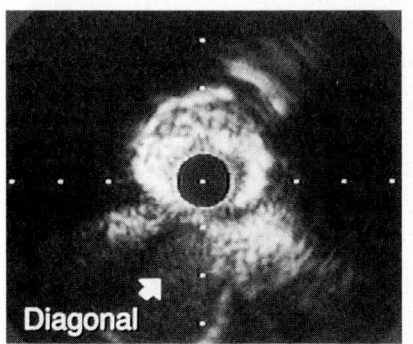 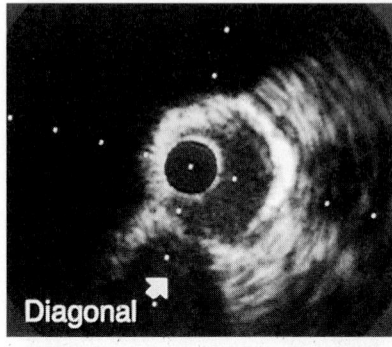

FIGURE 39–8. Intravascular ultrasound images before and after rotational atherectomy (Rotablator). Presence of a visible diagonal branch of the left anterior descending artery in both images documents matching of location and orientation within the artery. *Left,* Densely calcified atherosclerotic plaque with severe compromise of vessel lumen prior to rotational atherectomy; deep vascular structures are obscured by nearly complete shadowing of ultrasound beam by calcification. *Right,* Following rotational atherectomy, there is significant removal of calcified plaque with marked improvement in vascular lumen. More deep wall structures are visible after removal of calcium. (From DeFranco, A. C., Tuzcu, E. M., and Nissen, S. E.: Diagnostic and interventional applications of coronary intravascular ultrasound. *In* Topol, E. J., and Serruys, P. [eds.]: Current Review of Interventional Cardiology. Philadelphia, Current Medicine, 1995, pp. 174–191.)

proving an inadequate angiographic result during percutaneous revascularization, and two randomized trials have demonstrated efficacy in reducing the incidence of restenosis.

Stents currently in clinical use are composed of various metals that have been demonstrated to possess adequate radial hoop strength and to be biocompatible without degradation. The major disadvantage of metallic stents is their potential for thrombogenicity at the blood-tissue interface, with the resultant risk of acute thrombotic closure or distal embolization. Stents have thus been designed with various mesh or coil configurations to minimize the surface area of exposed metal; nevertheless, early experience with most of these designs indicated that intensive anticoagulation was required for the 2 to 3 months following stent placement before re-endothelialization occurs. Such vigorous anticoagulation regimens, consisting of aspirin, heparin, warfarin, and often dipyridamole and dextran, are associated with a substantial risk of hemorrhagic complications, particularly from vascular access sites. Recent data, however, suggest that *optimal* stent implantation with enhanced antiplatelet therapy may obviate the need for long-term warfarin in many patients.

WALLSTENT. The Wallstent (Medinvent, Schneider Europe, Zurich, Switzerland) was the first stent to be used in humans and is the only self-expanding stent design in clinical use. It consists of a flexible woven stainless steel mesh tube available in a number of lengths, which is delivered to the stenosis site on a catheter in a constrained form and deployed by withdrawal of an overlying membrane (Fig. 39–9A). By virtue of its self-expanding properties, the Wallstent does not require balloon dilatation for implantation and maintains a residual radial expansion force on the arterial wall.

The outcome of the initial clinical experience with the Wallstent by a group of European investigators (antedating all other stent projects) highlighted both the promise and risks associated with the use of stents in coronary arteries.[155,156] A total of 265 patients, many of whom had relatively complex pathology including saphenous vein graft stenoses, were treated with the Wallstent at different institutions with widely varying anticoagulation regimens. A limited number of stents were subsequently retrieved from patients undergoing coronary artery bypass surgery, demonstrating deposition of platelets, fibrin, and leukocytes during the first 3 to 7 days following implantation, with subsequent ingrowth of varying degrees of neointima by 3 to 10 months. Although the restenosis rate following placement of the Wallstent in this series was an encouraging 27 per cent (18 per cent in native coronary vessels, 39 per cent in saphenous vein grafts), enthusiasm for this device was dampened by the prohibitively high subacute thrombotic occlusion rate of 15 per cent. Eleven of the 265 patients (4.1 per cent) died during the hospitalization period, the majority due either to myocardial infarction sustained during thrombotic stent closure (seven patients) or to intracranial hemorrhage (three patients) related to the intensive anticoagulation regimen. Other hemorrhagic complications, including femoral hematomas or gastrointestinal and genitourinary bleeding, were observed more frequently than in balloon angioplasty series. It is likely that the high incidence of adverse events in this first stenting experience was related to the "learning curve" for proper patient and lesion selection and the management of anticoagulation; after withdrawal of the coronary Wallstent from the market in 1990, this device is undergoing renewed clinical investigation in the United States and is commonly used in Europe.

GIANTURCO-ROUBIN STENT. The Gianturco-Roubin Flexstent (Cook, Inc., Bloomington, IN) was the first coronary stent approved by the FDA for the indication of abrupt or threatened closure. It consists of a single 0.006-inch diameter stainless steel wire wrapped into an interdigitating ser-

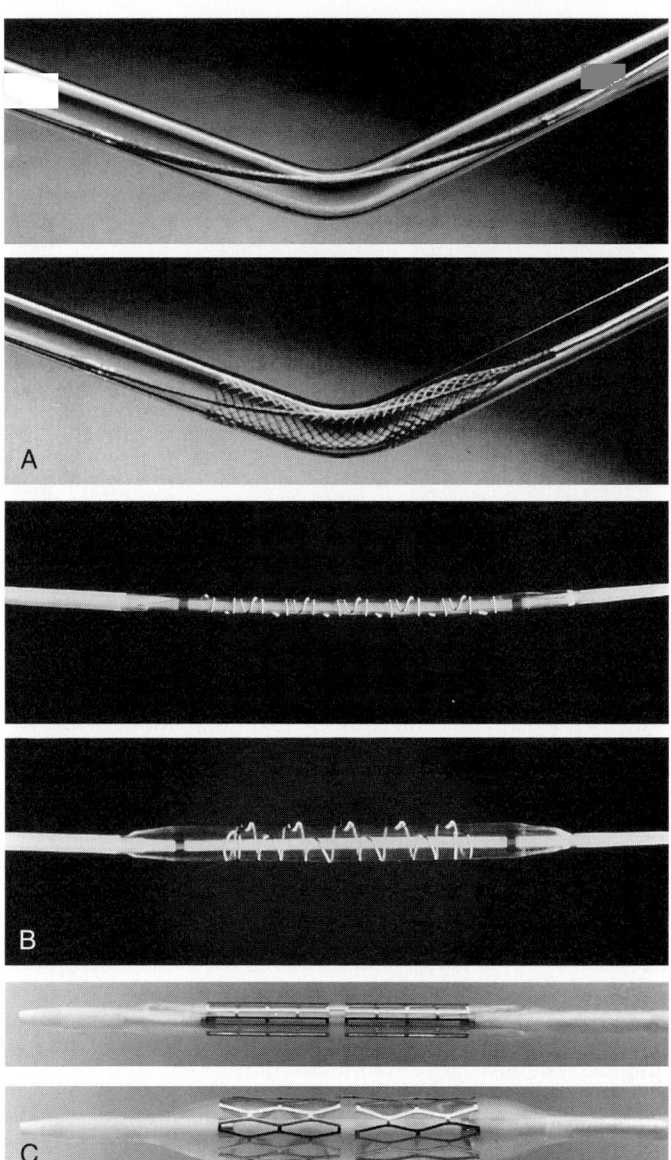

FIGURE 39–9. Intracoronary stents. *A,* Self-expanding Wallstent. *Top,* Prior to deployment. *Bottom,* Nearly completely deployed by withdrawal of constraining membrane. (Courtesy of Schneider, USA, Minneapolis, MN.) *B,* Gianturco-Roubin balloon-expandable coil stent. *Top,* Undeployed, wrapped around delivery balloon. *Bottom,* Deployed by expansion of delivery balloon. (Courtesy of Cook, Inc., Bloomington, IN.) *C,* Palmaz-Schatz balloon-expandable slotted tube stent. *Top,* Undeployed, wrapped around delivery balloon. *Bottom,* Deployed by expansion of delivery balloon. (Courtesy of Johnson and Johnson Interventional Systems, Warren, NJ.)

pentine coil and mounted on a balloon catheter (Fig. 39–9B); this flexible, low-profile system is placed across a coronary lesion and the stent deployed by balloon inflation. During preclinical animal studies, placement of the Gianturco-Roubin stent was followed by early nonocclusive thrombus deposition, with subsequent reconstitution of an endothelial layer by 2 weeks that appeared morphologically normal by 6 months.[157]

An extensive registry experience has demonstrated the effectiveness of the Gianturco-Roubin stent in reversing abrupt or threatened coronary closure (Fig. 39–10), although randomized controlled trials have not been reported. In the largest single-center series,[158] 115 patients had the stent placed as either primary or bailout therapy for severe dissection or vessel closure with a 93 per cent rate of angiographic resolution. Among this group of patients who would have been expected to be at very high risk for ischemic events with conventional therapy (Table

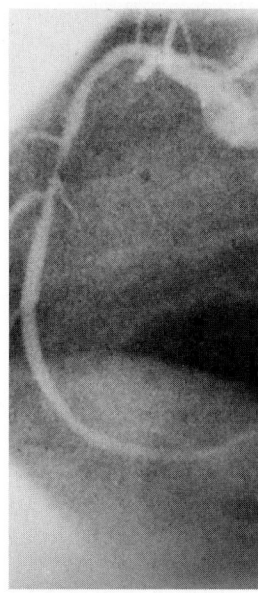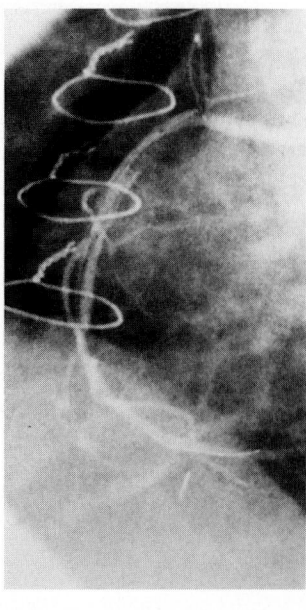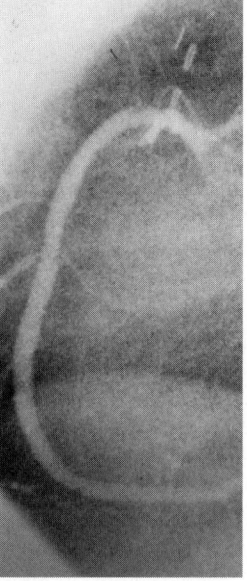

FIGURE 39–10. Angiographic efficacy of stenting for treating coronary dissection. *Left,* Stenosis in mid-right coronary artery prior to intervention. *Middle,* Extensive spiral dissection extending from the tip of the guide catheter to the acute margin of the vessel. *Right,* Final appearance of the vessel after the insertion of three overlapping Gianturco-Roubin stents. The vessel is widely patent with brisk distal flow. (From Muller, D. W. M., and Ellis, S. G.: Advances in coronary angioplasty: Endovascular stents. Coron. Artery Dis. *1:*438, 1990.)

39–1), complications following stent implantation were infrequent; death occurred in 1.7 per cent, emergency bypass surgery in 4.2 per cent, and Q-wave and non-Q-wave infarction in 7 per cent and 9 per cent, respectively. Similarly, in a larger multicenter registry experience of 415 patients treated for abrupt closure, rates of death, myocardial infarction, and coronary bypass surgery were 3 per cent, 5 per cent, and 12 per cent, respectively.[152] Despite anticoagulation with aspirin, dipyridamole, heparin, dextran, warfarin, and occasionally urokinase, however, stent thrombosis has been reported to occur in 6 to 12 per cent of these patients[158–160]; bleeding complications associated with anticoagulation have ranged from 11 to 25 per cent.[158,159] Placement of the Gianturco-Roubin stent has not yet been documented to appreciably affect restenosis risk, with angiographic restenosis rates within 6 months ranging from 40 to 45 per cent.[158,159]

PALMAZ-SCHATZ STENT. The Palmaz-Schatz stainless steel slotted tube stent (Johnson and Johnson Interventional Systems, Warren, NJ) is deployed by balloon expansion within a coronary lesion, assuming a meshwork of adjacent parallelograms (Fig. 39–9C). The advantage of this design over wire coil stents appears to be its greater radial support strength; longitudinal flexibility of this somewhat stiff stent was improved by incorporation of a single filament articulation point at its center. As with the Gianturco-Roubin stent, preclinical studies with this device documented early thrombus deposition (usually nonocclusive), followed by endothelialization within 3 weeks.[161]

During the initial clinical experience with the Palmaz-Schatz stent, with only aspirin and dipyridamole administered during the posthospitalization period, a subacute thrombosis rate of 18 per cent was observed.[162] This thrombosis risk was reduced to 4 to 5 per cent following elective implantation by the addition of warfarin therapy for 1 to 3 months.[162,163] Noncomparative reports suggested that use of this stent might lead to a reduced incidence of restenosis.[164a] Among 206 patients in whom Palmaz-Schatz stents were placed in native coronary arteries, restenosis occurred in only 16.3 per cent of de novo and 35 per cent of restenotic lesions.[164] Similarly, among 200 focal saphenous vein graft lesions, for which restenosis rates following balloon angioplasty approaching 70 per cent have been reported,[165] treatment with the Palmaz-Schatz stent was associated with angiographic restenosis in only 17 per cent of patients.[166]

Two randomized trials comparing Palmaz-Schatz stent placement to conventional balloon angioplasty have confirmed that this device can reduce the frequency of re-

stenosis following percutaneous revascularization in patients with de novo native coronary stenoses.[108,109] In the Belgium and Netherlands Stent Study[109,109a] (BENESTENT), angiographic restenosis at 6 months follow-up was present in 22 per cent and 32 per cent of patients in the stent and PTCA groups, respectively, while in the Stent Restenosis Study[108] (STRESS), restenosis rates were 31 per cent and 42 per cent among lesions treated with stents or balloon angioplasty (Table 39–10). The mechanism by which stents reduced the incidence of restenosis in these trials was acute improvement in the immediate angiographic result relative to balloon angioplasty, not a reduction in neointimal hyperplasia. Postprocedural luminal diameters were substantially greater following stenting than after PTCA, which, despite *significantly more loss* in luminal diameter over the subsequent 6 months, translated to greater luminal

TABLE 39–10 OUTCOME IN BENESTENT AND STRESS TRIALS OF STENTING VERSUS CORONARY ANGIOPLASTY

	BENESTENT		STRESS	
	Stent (N = 259)	PTCA (N = 257)	Stent (N = 205)	PTCA (N = 202)
Early Events	In-hospital		14 days	
Death (%)	0	0	0	1.5
Myocardial infarction (%)	3.4	3.1	5.4	5.0
CABG (%)	3.1	1.6	2.4	4.0
Repeat PTCA (%)	0.4	1.2	2.0	1.0
Late Events	7 months		240 days	
Death (%)	0.8	0.4	1.5	1.5
Myocardial infarction (%)	4.2	4.6	6.3	6.9
CABG (%)	6.2	4.4	4.9	8.4
Repeat PTCA (%)	13.5*	23.3	11.2	12.4
Target vessel revascularization (%)	NR	NR	10.2	15.4
Restenosis Rate† (%)	22*	32	32*	42

* Statistically significant difference

† >50% diameter stenosis on follow-up angiography

CABG = coronary artery bypass graft surgery; NR = not reported; PTCA = coronary angioplasty.

Data from Serruys, P. W., de Jaegere, P., Kiemeneij, F., et al.: A comparison of balloon-expandable-stent implantation with balloon angioplasty in patients with coronary artery disease. N. Engl. J. Med. *331:*489, 1994; and Fischman, D. L., Leon, M. B., Baim, D. S., et al.: A randomized comparison of coronary-stent placement and balloon angioplasty in the treatment of coronary artery disease. N. Engl. J. Med. *331:*496, 1994. Copyright Massachusetts Medical Society.

two trials led to approval of the Palmaz-Schatz stent by the FDA in 1994 for the prevention of restenosis in de novo atherosclerotic lesions.

The Palmaz-Schatz stent has also been successfully employed as a "bailout" procedure following abrupt or threatened vessel closure or for suboptimal results following other forms of percutaneous revascularization (Fig. 39–11). Preliminary results of a small randomized trial have confirmed that stent placement for failed angioplasty results in more frequent resolution and fewer ischemic complications than do other forms of therapy such as prolonged repeat balloon inflations.[167]

OTHER STENT DESIGNS. Various other balloon-expandable stent designs are currently under clinical investigation. The Wiktor sinusoidal coil[168] (Medtronic Interventional Vascular, Minneapolis, MN) and Strecker wire mesh[169] (Boston Scientific, Watertown, MA) stents are composed of tantalum, a radiopaque metal that renders these stents particularly simple to position precisely within coronary vessels. Early results derived from human implantations appear to be similar to those obtained with earlier stent designs. A nickel-titanium alloy (nitinol) with "thermal memory" properties has been used to construct a balloon-expandable stent that can be removed within several days of implantation; heated fluid administered through a specialized intracoronary catheter causes the stent to collapse around the catheter into its predeployment configuration.[170] This and other temporary stent designs may be useful in situations where only transient mechanical support is required. Various coatings, including polymers, pharmacological agents, and endothelial cells, have been applied to stent surfaces and tested in animal models with the intent of reducing thrombosis or limiting neointimal hyperplasia. A heparin-coated Palmaz-Schatz stent is currently under pilot-phase clinical investigation, with early results suggesting that systemic anticoagulation can be markedly diminished without an increased risk for thrombotic complications.

OPTIMAL STENT IMPLANTATION AND REDUCED ANTICOAGULATION. Intravascular ultrasound studies performed after implantation of the Palmaz-Schatz and other stents have demonstrated that despite the angiographic appearance of complete stent expansion, most stents are in fact inadequately deployed by traditional balloon inflation pressures (6 to 8 atmospheres) with poor apposition of stent struts to the arterial wall.[171] Repeat balloon inflations within the stents using larger balloons or higher pressures (up to 16 atmospheres) result in improved luminal dimensions with complete implantation of the stent struts within the plaque material (Fig. 39–12). Based upon these findings and the hypothesis that stent thrombosis may arise primarily at sites of poorly supported arterial plaque or stent struts protruding into the arterial lumen, several groups of investigators have recently evaluated outcome *without* warfarin

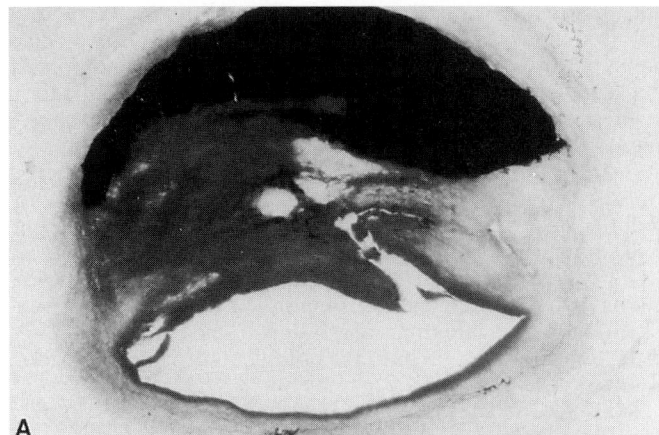

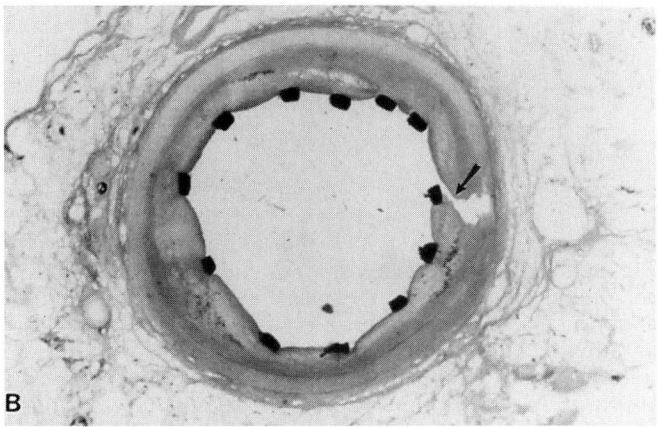

FIGURE 39–11. Pathological efficacy of stenting for treating coronary dissection. *A,* Micrograph of dilated but not stented human cadaver coronary artery with a typical intimal and medial dissection and luminal collapse. *B,* Dilated and stented human cadaver coronary artery with a large intimal and medial tear "tacked up" by the stent struts *(arrow).* (Reproduced with permission from Schatz, R. A.: A view of vascular stents. Circulation *79:*445, 1989. Copyright American Heart Association.)

diameters at follow-up. The decrease in angiographic restenosis documented in these two trials was accompanied by clinical benefit as well, with significant reductions in the need for repeat target vessel revascularization (13.5 per cent versus 23.3 per cent in BENESTENT, 10.2 per cent versus 15.4 per cent in STRESS). Bleeding and vascular complications, however, developed more frequently among patients treated with stents who had received heparin, aspirin, dextran, dipyridamole, and warfarin (13.5 per cent versus 3.1 per cent in BENESTENT and 7.3 per cent versus 4.0 per cent in STRESS), although subacute stent closure occurred in only 3.4 to 3.5 per cent. The findings of these

FIGURE 39–12. Intravascular ultrasound images after intracoronary stent placement. *Left,* Following deployment of a Palmaz-Schatz intracoronary stent using a 4.0-mm-diameter balloon, echogenic stent struts between 3 and 7 o'clock can be seen to be incompletely apposed to the underlying vascular wall. *Right,* Following inflations of a 5.0-mm balloon within the stent, complete apposition of all stent struts against the arterial wall is visible. (From Defranco, A. C., Tuzcu, E. M., and Nissen, S. E.: Diagnostic and interventional applications of coronary intravascular ultrasound. *In* Topol, E. J., and Serruys, P. [eds.]: Current Review of Interventional Cardiology. Philadelphia, Current Medicine, 1995, pp. 174–191.)

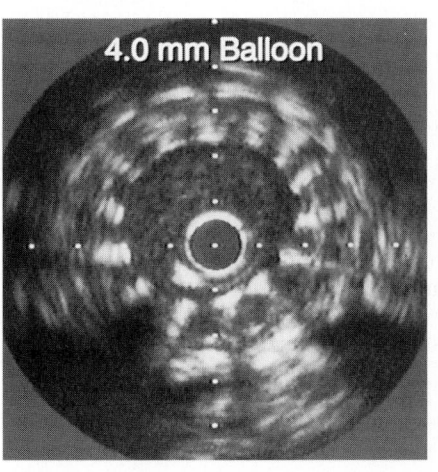

4.0 mm Balloon

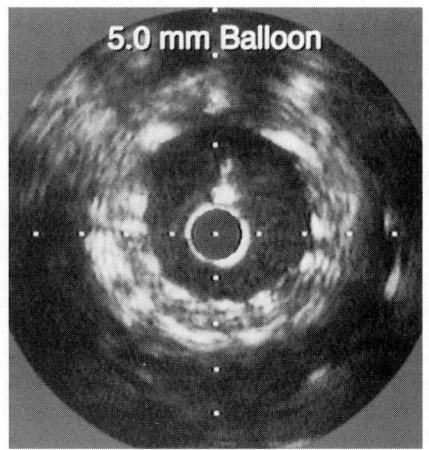

5.0 mm Balloon

therapy following "optimal" stent implantation.[164a,172,173] Initial series uniformly employed intravascular ultrasonography to demonstrate that stent struts were completely expanded following high-pressure balloon inflations, although subsequent reports have suggested that ultrasonography may not routinely be necessary.[174] Enhanced antiplatelet therapy with ticlopidine in addition to aspirin for several weeks has usually been considered a key component of this reduced anticoagulation regimen, with some groups using low molecular weight heparin as well. The incidence of subacute thrombosis during antiplatelet therapy without warfarin following optimal stent implantation has been surprisingly low, usually less than 2 to 3 per cent, with rates of vascular and hemorrhagic complications equivalent to those for coronary balloon angioplasty.[174a] Observational reports have suggested that this method of stenting may also result in lower rates of late restenosis than traditional stenting techniques, by virtue of the improved postprocedural angiographic result.[175]

If the strategy of optimal stent implantation by high-pressure balloon inflations, with or without intravascular ultrasound guidance, proves to eliminate the need for intensive anticoagulation while preserving or enhancing the benefits of stenting in reducing the incidence of restenosis and treating abrupt or threatened coronary closure, a major transformation in the practice of interventional cardiology may follow. Without the thrombotic or hemorrhagic risks traditionally associated with stent placement, this technique may be applied to a wide variety of coronary lesions that would otherwise be considered at "high risk" for acute complications or subsequent restenosis, with a consequent broadening of the indications for percutaneous coronary revascularization. Importantly, however, widespread acceptance of stenting should await the acquisition of long-term follow-up (5 years or more) experience in patients with this prosthesis.

Lasers and Other Ablative Energy

Other new devices for percutaneous coronary intervention have been developed with mechanisms of action similar to those of atherectomy catheters or stents. Instead of mechanical excision of atherosclerotic material, thermal, photochemical, or acoustic energy is used to ablate coronary plaque. Additionally, compliance and other physical properties of the arterial wall may be modified by these devices, resulting in decreased elastic recoil and sealing of disrupted dissection flaps. Although several types of ablative techniques are currently under investigation, only the excimer laser has been approved by the FDA for coronary revascularization.

THERMAL BALLOON ANGIOPLASTY. Laser, radiofrequency, and microwave energy have all been used to deliver heat to coronary stenoses during balloon inflations. Heating of the vascular wall occurs either by direct radiation (laser and microwave) or conduction of heat from the fluid within the balloon (radiofrequency). Preclinical studies in animal models have indicated that each of these devices may reduce elastic recoil, weld disrupted tissue planes, desiccate intraluminal thrombus, and produce a better postprocedural luminal enlargement than conventional balloon angioplasty, with varying degrees of necrosis of the arterial wall, medial thinning, straightening of the elastic laminae, and protein coagulation.

A laser balloon catheter employs an Nd:YAG near-infrared laser source that is transmitted through a fiberoptic to a diffusing silica fiber within the angioplasty balloon. Although experience with laser balloon angioplasty following conventional PTCA demonstrated this technique to be effective in improving the angiographic result in many patients with relatively high-risk coronary lesions and reversing severe dissections or acute or threatened closure,[176,177] this device was withdrawn from clinical use because of the

high incidence of restenosis and major clinical events.[177] A radiofrequency balloon catheter has been used in a technique of physiologically controlled low stress angioplasty (PLOSA), based on the concept that thermal modification of the arterial wall at moderate temperatures (approximately 60°C) during balloon inflations with pressures as low as 2 atmospheres may allow vascular distention without disruption, thus minimizing elastic recoil and the restenotic healing response. In pilot-phase clinical experience, immediate clinical and angiographic results following PLOSA were similar to those that would be expected following conventional balloon angioplasty[178]; an intravascular ultrasound evaluation has failed to detect a difference in the mechanisms of luminal enlargement by PLOSA and PTCA.[179]

LASER ANGIOPLASTY. Laser angioplasty devices directly ablate atherosclerotic plaque by three different mechanisms, the relative contributions of which depend upon the wavelength and intensity of laser energy, the mode of operation (continuous or pulsed), the lasing media (blood, saline, or radiographic contrast), the degree of tissue contact, and the absorption characteristics of different components of vascular tissue. *Thermal* effects melt or vaporize tissue and denature proteins. The precision or selectivity of thermal plaque ablation may be optimized by use of ultraviolet or infrared laser energy delivered in pulses of short duration, operating characteristics that minimize diffusion of heat away from the target zone and injury of adjacent tissue. *Acoustic* pressure transients arise from plasma or vapor bubble formation during pulsed, high-energy laser operation, producing plaque and tissue disruption and likely playing a major role in the development of ischemic complications during laser angioplasty. *Photodissociation* occurs when absorption of laser energy leads to direct rupture of intramolecular bonds within a tissue without appreciable heating, an effect that is highly specific to the absorption characteristics of individual tissue components. Although photodissociation is thus the ideal objective of laser angioplasty, thermal and acoustic mechanisms appear to predominate under clinical conditions.

Pulsed lasers currently used for vascular applications operate with wavelengths in the ultraviolet (excimer), mid-infrared (holmium), or visible (dye) range. Despite the initial excitement surrounding the use of "high technology" lasers for coronary revascularization, clinical expectations of exceptional efficacy, selectivity, and safety have been inadequately fulfilled. Immediate results of laser angioplasty have proven to be unpredictable and not clearly different from those obtained by conventional balloon dilatation, even for complex lesion subsets thought to be most suited for laser ablation. Moreover, laser angioplasty has been associated with an increased risk for procedural complications, including dissection, abrupt closure, and perforation. Registry studies have thus far failed to detect a reduction in the incidence of restenosis using this technique.

Excimer Laser. This has been the most extensively evaluated coronary laser system. High-intensity, short-duration (100 to 200 nsec) pulses of 308-nm ultraviolet light are transmitted through a fiberoptic bundle catheter to the coronary stenosis, where the laser energy is absorbed by proteins within the plaque. Histopathological changes resulting from excimer laser ablation in animal models have included focal crater formation without charring and localized intimal disruption. In two large clinical series[180,181] of over 3500 patients undergoing excimer laser coronary angioplasty, immediate procedural success was achieved in approximately 90 per cent, despite the high prevalence of complex morphological features, with adjunctive balloon angioplasty required in up to 95 per cent of patients to improve the narrow lumen achieved by laser ablation alone. Although rates of in-hospital death, myocardial infarction, and emergency bypass surgery were similar to those expected for balloon angioplasty, coronary dissection and perforation appeared to occur more frequently, in 16 to 22 per cent and 1.6 to 2.4 per cent of treated lesions, respectively. Angiographic restenosis occurred in 46 per cent of patients following successful excimer laser angioplasty.[182] Two recent randomized trials comparing excimer laser to conventional balloon angioplasty for the treatment of long[183] or totally occluded[184] lesions failed to demonstrate a difference between these two techniques in long-term clinical or angiographic outcome. The development of directional laser catheters may improve the safety and outcome of excimer laser angioplasty in certain lesion subsets.

Other lasers under clinical investigation include the *holmium* and *pulsed dye* lasers. The holmium infrared laser energy is absorbed by water within atherosclerotic and vascular tissue. Early clinical results using this device have been similar to those obtained with excimer, with no apparent reduction in restenosis. The visible light produced by the pulsed dye laser is absorbed primarily by hemoglobin, and the energy threshold for ablation of thrombus is 100-fold lower than that for arterial tissue. This device may thus find a "niche" as a means of thrombolysis during myocardial infarction or acute ischemic syndromes.

THERAPEUTIC ULTRASOUND. The ablative effects of high-intensity, low-frequency ultrasound have been attributed primarily to mechanical vibration and cavitation. Tissues containing a heavy matrix of collagen or elastin, such as arterial wall, are resistant to ultrasound, while those without elastic support, such as thrombus or atherosclerotic plaque, are disrupted by ultrasonic energy. Ultrasound ablation of atherosclerotic plaque or thrombi may thus be accomplished at energy levels below that required to damage normal arterial wall structures. Preclinical studies have demonstrated the potential efficacy of catheter-based ultrasound devices in recanalizing resistant, totally or subtotally occluded arterial segments or dissolving intravascular thrombus.[185] Pilot-phase human investigation is currently under way.

INTRAVASCULAR IMAGING TECHNIQUES

Despite improvements in the resolution of coronary radiographic imaging and the development of computerized angiographic digital reconstruction, several inherent limitations remain to the use of angiography as a means of assessing coronary lesion morphology and the results of percutaneous revascularization. Coronary angiography visualizes only the opacified lumen of the artery, rendering this technique inadequate to evaluate pathological structures within the vascular wall. Substantial atherosclerosis may develop before reduction in luminal dimensions,[186] a proc-

ess that cannot be discerned by angiographic assessment. The two-dimensional view provided by the coronary angiogram is often inadequate to appreciate the severity of eccentric or complex lesions and underestimates the degree of stenosis in the presence of diffuse coronary disease extending into adjacent "normal" segments. Three new modalities have thus been applied clinically in the setting of percutaneous coronary intervention to more precisely visualize the arterial wall and vascular lumen or assess the functional significance of a coronary stenosis.

INTRAVASCULAR ULTRASONOGRAPHY (see also Fig. 3–15, p. 58). There has been rapid evolution of technology for miniaturization of high-frequency transducers to permit ultrasound imaging from within the coronary vasculature. Ultrasound energy emitted from an intraluminal probe penetrates into the vascular wall, with reflections formed at the interfaces between tissue components with different acoustic properties. Intravascular ultrasonography (IVUS) thus produces high-resolution cross-sectional images that not only delineate absolute luminal dimensions, but also the extent and structure of the atherosclerotic plaque and the arterial wall (Fig. 39–5). Images produced by this technique correlate well with histological findings.[187,188]

Two types of intravascular ultrasound catheters have been developed. *Solid state* designs consist of multiple transducers located circumferentially around the tip of the catheter, which are electronically activated in sequence to produce a 360-degree image; *mechanical scanners* employ a rotating transducer (or a rotating reflector with a fixed transducer) at the tip of the catheter. Cross-sectional images are formed by computerized analysis of ultrasound energy reflected from the tissue to the transducer. Serial cross-sectional images obtained throughout a vessel segment may be integrated to form a three-dimensional computerized reconstruction.[189] Current ultrasound catheters used for coronary arteries have distal tips ranging in diameter from 0.9 to 1.7 mm, allowing interrogation of distal coronary segments.

Intravascular ultrasonography has been employed clinically to identify angiographically inapparent atherosclerotic plaque, quantify luminal dimensions, and characterize the composition of stenotic lesions ("soft" plaque, "hard" plaque, calcification [Figs. 39–7, 39–8, 39–12, and 39–13], thrombus). Several groups have demonstrated that diffuse atherosclerotic disease is frequently detectable by IVUS in arteries that appear to be angiographically normal, particularly in segments adjacent to stenotic lesions,[190] due in part to the Glagov phenomenon of arterial remodeling[186]; the true plaque burden within a coronary vessel is thus often much more extensive than would be expected from its an-

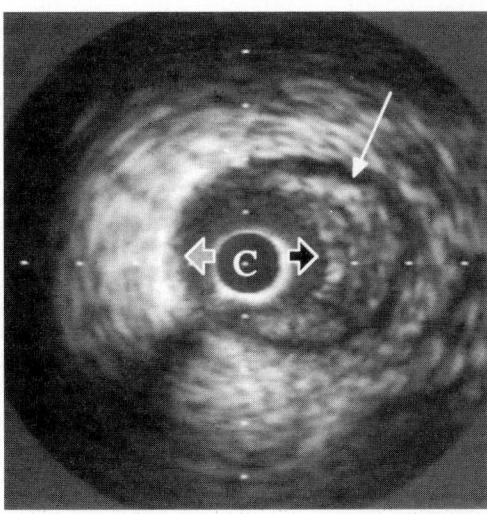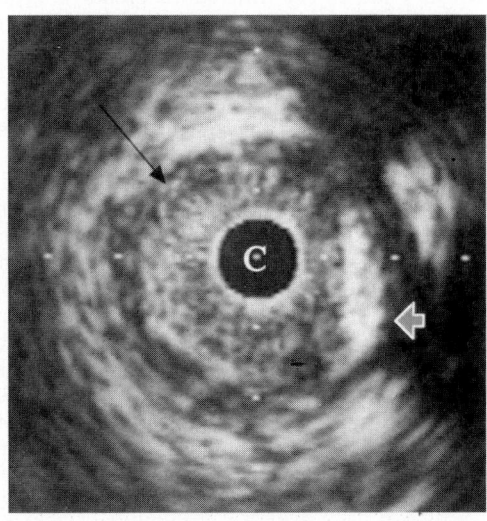

FIGURE 39–13. Examples of intracoronary ultrasound images. C designates ultrasound transducer catheter (1.3 mm diameter) in center of each vessel. Tick marks represent 1 mm distance. *Left,* Eccentric atheromatous lesion. Wide gray arrow denotes undiseased arterial intima, wide black arrow denotes soft crescentic atherosclerotic plaque, narrow white arrow indicates hypoechoic arterial media. *Right,* Circumferential atheromatous lesion with severe compromise of arterial lumen. Wide gray arrow denotes arc of calcification, with dropout of structural features located deep to calcium due to shadowing of ultrasound beam. Narrow black arrow indicates arterial media. (Courtesy of S. Nissen, M.D., Cleveland Clinic Foundation.)

giographic appearance. Similarly, ultrasonography has been useful in assessing the degree of luminal compromise in lesions that appear to be equivocal or indeterminate by angiography due to tortuosity, foreshortening, or vessel overlap, such as in the left main coronary artery.[191,192] IVUS has been shown to be significantly more sensitive than angiography in detecting the presence of calcium within an atherosclerotic lesion,[193] and some investigators have also suggested this modality may be useful in differentiating thrombus from other plaque components.[194]

Intravascular ultrasound studies have contributed markedly to our understanding of the mechanisms of balloon angioplasty[9] and new device interventions[134,147,195] (Figs. 39–7, 39–8, and 39–12); this technique has been employed clinically to guide the application and assess the results of percutaneous revascularization techniques. Identification of certain morphological features by ultrasonography may predict the outcome of percutaneous intervention[196] and aid selection of the best device to obtain an optimal angiographic result.[197] For example, localized deposits of calcium may predispose to medial dissection during balloon angioplasty.[198] Superficial calcium may be considered an indication for the use of rotational atherectomy, bulky eccentric noncalcified lesions for directional atherectomy, intraluminal thrombus for extraction atherectomy or thrombolysis, and fibrotic plaque for stenting or balloon angioplasty.[197] Serial IVUS examinations may also be performed during the revascularization procedure to assess interim results and guide further interventional therapy (Fig. 39–12). Prototype devices have been developed in which an ultrasound transducer is integrated into a balloon angioplasty catheter or directional atherectomy device, optimizing the coronary intervention by concurrent IVUS imaging. Following percutaneous revascularization, intravascular ultrasonography provides a more accurate estimation of luminal dimensions than does angiography,[199] owing to the irregular luminal contour produced by most interventional techniques. IVUS also appears to be the most sensitive method for evaluating the completeness of lesion dilatation, plaque removal, or stent deployment and for detecting plaque disruption or medial dissection, observations that may be correlated with subsequent ischemic complications or restenosis.

CORONARY ANGIOSCOPY. Direct visualization of the lumen of a coronary artery in living patients was made practical by the development of low-profile, flexible, fiberoptic imaging catheters with sufficient fiber density to provide high-resolution images. The most advanced angioscope design currently in clinical use (Baxter Edwards, Irvine, CA) is passed into the coronary artery over a standard angioplasty guidewire, a soft latex occlusion balloon is inflated proximal to the area of interest, and warm Ringer's lactate is infused to create a blood-free field for imaging. The movable imaging bundle containing 5000 fibers (pixels) can be advanced distally as much as 5 cm beyond the occlusion balloon to visualize the arterial segment under high-intensity illumination, with images transmitted through the fiberoptic to a video camera and monitor.

Coronary angioscopy can be performed safely during diagnostic cardiac catheterization or percutaneous revascularization procedures. Pathological structures in the lumen and on the surface of the vascular wall can often be more clearly delineated by angioscopy than by angiography or even intravascular ultrasonography. Stable atheromatous lesions appear as white fibrotic or yellow lipid-laden plaques within the arterial wall with smooth or slightly irregular surfaces.[200] Saphenous vein graft stenoses often appear more complex, with friable plaque components and diffuse disease.[201] In the setting of unstable ischemic syndromes, however, most "culprit lesion" plaques are found by angioscopy to have visible clefts or dissections, with up to 94 per cent associated with white (platelet-rich) or red (eryth-

rocyte- and fibrin-rich) thrombi.[202,203] In the setting of coronary intervention, angioscopy appears to be valuable as a more sensitive means than angiography of identifying intraluminal thrombus, elucidating the mechanism of abrupt or threatened closure, or assessing the completeness of stent deployment[204] or plaque removal by atherectomy.[205]

INTRACORONARY DOPPLER. Measurement of blood flow velocity using the Doppler principle was until recently a complex procedure reserved largely for research applications. The development of piezoelectric crystals that may be mounted at the distal tip of a coronary guidewire has enabled intracoronary Doppler to be used routinely in the clinical evaluation of stenosis severity and the results of coronary intervention. As intracoronary Doppler allows assessment of the *physiological* significance of a coronary lesion, this technique provides data that are complementary to the structural and geometric information derived from other forms of imaging in the catheterization laboratory.

The Doppler guidewire currently in widespread use has the dimensions, flexibility, and handling characteristics of a typical 0.018-inch-diameter angioplasty guidewire. The small cross-sectional area of this wire produces minimal disturbance of the flow profile across a vascular stenosis, thus enabling accurate measurement of blood flow velocities beyond tight coronary lesions. Three alterations in the normal intracoronary velocity patterns have been identified by the Doppler technique which are associated with hemodynamically significant coronary lesions: reduced diastolic/systolic velocity ratio, reduced distal/proximal flow velocity ratio, and blunted hyperemic response.[206]

Clinical applications of intracoronary Doppler include evaluation of the functional significance of intermediate lesions (50 to 70 per cent stenosis) by coronary angiography, diagnosis of abnormalities in coronary vasodilatory reserve, and the assessment of outcome, complications, collateral flow, and additional lesions during percutaneous coronary revascularization. The extent to which continuous Doppler flow measurements in the distal vessel normalize during coronary intervention provides an immediate indication of the adequacy of luminal enlargement, while deterioration in flow parameters appears to be an early signal of impending coronary closure. Cyclical variations in intracoronary Doppler flow velocities may signal the presence of platelet aggregation and intraluminal thrombus formation in an artery with a satisfactory angiographic result following percutaneous intervention, with the potential for late thrombotic coronary occlusion.

NONCORONARY ARTERIAL REVASCULARIZATION

Techniques for percutaneous noncoronary arterial revascularization have been developed in parallel with those for coronary intervention, with increasing application to lesions that would previously have been treated by reconstructive vascular surgery. Although balloon angioplasty has been the traditional mainstay of peripheral arterial revascularization, the role of new device technologies, particularly stents, as a means of improving procedural results and decreasing restenosis has expanded.

PERIPHERAL BALLOON ANGIOPLASTY. Percutaneous transluminal angioplasty (PTA) has proven highly effective in treating claudication, rest pain, ischemic ulcers, and poor wound healing due to ileofemoral and runoff vessel disease. Percutaneous revascularization techniques are associated with less morbidity and shorter recovery periods than surgery and allow preservation of venous conduits in patients who may require future surgery for coronary, cerebrovascular, or peripheral vascular disease. Alternatively, PTA may be used as an adjunct to surgical revascularization, to improve in-flow or outflow to a graft, or to treat anastomotic stenoses arising from prior surgery. Initial success rates for balloon angioplasty of aortic bifurcation occlusive disease have been reported as high as 92 per cent, with 81 per cent and 72 per cent patency rates at 3 and 5 years.[207]

A randomized trial comparing surgery to angioplasty among patients with lower extremity arterial disease demonstrated no difference in long-term outcome following initially successful results by either of the two treatment techniques[208]; initial procedural failure occurred more frequently in patients treated with balloon angioplasty but did not increase the risk of limb loss or subsequent surgical failure. Femoropopliteal disease more commonly presents as diffuse or occluded lesions than does iliac atherosclerosis, yet outcome following treatment of femoropopliteal disease in recent series has largely been favorable, with initial success rates of approximately 90 per cent[209] and 5-year patency rates of nearly 60 per cent.[210] The infrapopliteal and distal tibial circulation are also approached with improving technical success.

Balloon angioplasty has become the preferred procedure for revascularization of renal artery stenoses due to fibromuscular dysplasia, with acute success rates in excess of 90 per cent.[207,211] Atherosclerotic disease of the renal arteries is somewhat more difficult to treat percutaneously, particularly if diffuse or ostial. Balloon dilatation has also been successfully applied in recent years to aortic and mesenteric vessels. Early work using balloon angioplasty to treat stenoses of the subclavian or extracranial carotid and vertebral arteries has proceeded cautiously owing to major concern regarding the risk of distal embolization from these vessels.[207,212] Despite the effectiveness of surgical carotid endarterectomy, however, percutaneous revascularization may prove to be preferable for patients with severe medical comorbidities or lesions within the intrathoracic or distal carotid vessels which are not easily accessible by surgery.

NEW DEVICES FOR PERIPHERAL REVASCULARIZATION. Directional atherectomy, rotational atherectomy, transluminal extraction atherectomy, and excimer laser have all been evaluated for peripheral arterial revascularization. These devices may be particularly useful for debulking total occlusions or eccentric lesions but in general are associated with acute success and restenosis rates similar to those of balloon angioplasty. Intraluminal stenting, however, may prove to be a substantial advance over balloon angioplasty in many situations. When implanted in large vessels, such as ileofemoral arteries, chronic anticoagulation is not required. Stents appear to limit the restenosis risk in nonrandomized reports[213] and are useful in lesions that are less amenable to balloon angioplasty, such as ostial renal stenoses[214] or total occlusions. Early experience has suggested that stents may also limit the embolic risk during treatment of ulcerated carotid or vertebral artery lesions. Recently, repair of abdominal aortic aneurysms has been reported using percutaneously deployed prosthetic grafts anchored to the arterial wall by proximal and distal metallic stents.[215] Endovascular stent grafts have also been used in carotid and other peripheral arteries and represent a promising alternative to surgical revascularization.

PERCUTANEOUS BALLOON VALVULOPLASTY

AORTIC VALVULOPLASTY (see also p. 1044). Although surgical valve replacement has proven to be highly effective treatment for aortic valve stenosis, surgical mortality and morbidity may be elevated in some patients, particularly the elderly or those with other comorbidities. Percutaneous balloon valvuloplasty has thus been proposed as a less invasive means of treating aortic stenosis. Although early experience with this procedure demonstrated encouraging acute procedural results, short-lived hemodynamic benefit and high rates of restenosis were subsequently documented. Percutaneous treatment of aortic stenosis is now reserved primarily for patients who are either (1) not candidates for surgical valve replacement, but in whom balloon valvuloplasty would be expected to palliate severe symptoms or stabilize cardiogenic shock, or (2) potentially suitable for definitive surgical treatment in the future but first require stabilization of aortic stenosis for urgent noncardiac surgery.

Both anterograde and retrograde approaches have been described, the latter performed via puncture of the interatrial septum. The aortic valve is crossed with an extra stiff guidewire, over which a dilation balloon measuring 15 to 23 mm in diameter is passed; correct sizing of the balloon is accomplished by either echocardiographic or radiographic measurements or by increasing balloon sizes until inflation produces transient hypotension. Multiple inflations are performed until the properly sized balloon is fully inflated. If results of dilatation are suboptimal (aortic valve area less than 0.5 cm²) despite full inflation, a double balloon technique may be employed. Balloon dilatation improves the valvular cross-sectional area primarily by fracture of calcific deposits, although to a lesser extent, splitting of fused commissures or stretching of the valvular

annulus also occurs. Acute complications of aortic valvuloplasty include aortic regurgitation, leaflet avulsion or aortic rupture, ventricular perforation, systemic embolization or stroke, and peripheral vascular injury from the large-bore catheters and sheaths.

Acutely following aortic balloon valvuloplasty, the aortic valve area is typically doubled and the transvalvular gradient halved.[216,217] Most patients experience an improvement in functional status,[216,217] and subsequent mortality risk is likely reduced if the valve area has been increased to greater than 0.7 cm². Long-term outcome appears to be best among patients with preserved left ventricular function[219] and those in whom echocardiography performed several days after the procedure demonstrates sustained improvement in valve area and gradient (thus, minimal annular recoil).[218] Overall, however, more than half of patients develop recurrence of symptoms during the first 6 months and the vast majority within 1 year following successful aortic valvuloplasty, although symptomatic improvement may persist despite evidence of valvular restenosis by cardiac catheterization.[216,217]

MITRAL VALVULOPLASTY (see also p. 1016). In contrast to aortic valvuloplasty, percutaneous mitral balloon valvuloplasty has been shown to provide substantial and sustained clinical benefit in selected patients with rheumatic mitral stenosis. Immediate hemodynamic results are usually excellent and procedural complications uncommon, with long-term outcome among suitable patients similar to that among patients treated with open surgical commissurotomy.[220]

There is no one standard technique of balloon mitral valvuloplasty. The valve is usually approached in an anterograde direction via an interatrial septal puncture, although a retrograde technique has been reported. One or two tubular balloons or a specialized nylon-rubber (Inoue) balloon is advanced across the mitral valve and repetitive inflations performed until the balloons have fully expanded (Fig. 39–14). The Inoue technique is less cumbersome and as effective as valvuloplasty performed using single or double tubular balloons, and generally results in a smaller atrial septal puncture. The mechanism of improvement in the valve area is via splitting of fused commissures. Acute complications include leaflet tears or chordal or papillary rupture leading to mitral regurgitation, ventricular perforation, tamponade resulting from transseptal puncture, and systemic embolization.

Hemodynamic improvement following mitral valvuloplasty occurs immediately, with valve area increasing on average by 1.0 cm², with a prompt drop in pulmonary pres-

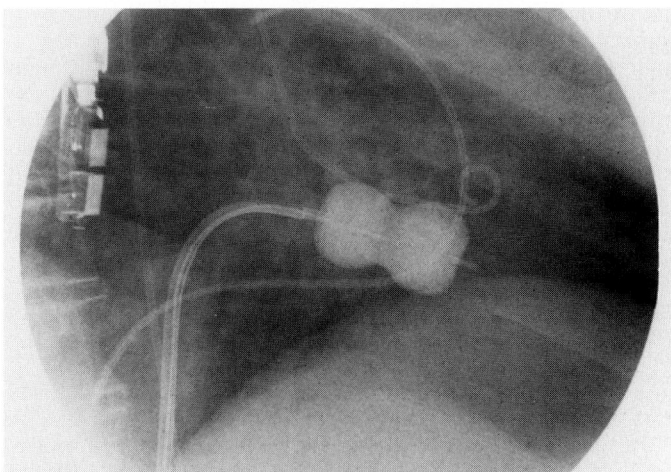

FIGURE 39–14. Cineangiogram frame during mitral valvuloplasty using Inoue balloon. The "waist" of the inflating balloon is within the stenotic mitral valve. A pigtail catheter within the left ventricle and a pulmonary artery catheter are also visible.

sures (Fig. 32–8, p. 1016).[221] Echocardiographic criteria have been developed to identify which patients with symptomatic mitral stenosis are most likely to derive benefit from this procedure[222]; these criteria have been shown to be the most important predictors of procedural outcome. The valve is assessed on the basis of four characteristics, each of which is graded on a scale of 0 to 4 (favorable to unfavorable): leaflet mobility, valvular thickening, subvalvular thickening, and valvular calcification. A good procedural result (valve area >1.5 cm²) was obtained in 91 per cent of patients with a cumulative score of 8 or less but only 33 per cent of those with echocardiographic scores greater than 12 in a large single center experience.[221] Outcome by 4 years follow-up was generally good, with 91 per cent of patients alive and 67 per cent free from mitral valve replacement or severe (NYHA Class III–IV) heart failure.[221] Long-term outcome in this cohort was best among patients with lower echocardiographic scores, no mitral calcification on fluoroscopy, no atrial fibrillation, good functional class prior to valvuloplasty, and a large immediate postprocedural valve area. A randomized trial comparing mitral balloon valvuloplasty to open surgical commissurotomy among patients with favorable valvular anatomy demonstrated comparable initial hemodynamic results and clinical outcome among patients treated with either technique, although hemodynamic findings at 3 years were more favorable in the balloon valvuloplasty group.[220]

INTERVENTIONS FOR CONGENITAL HEART DISEASE

(See also Chap. 29)

Since the origin of the field of interventional cardiology in 1966 with balloon atrial septostomy,[2] a procedure directed at congenital heart disease, pediatric interventional cardiologists have developed percutaneous techniques for relieving congenital valvular and great vessel stenoses and transcatheter closure of aberrant vascular channels. Some of these methods, such as pulmonary balloon valvuloplasty, have gained widespread acceptance, whereas others are in early stages of clinical investigation.

BALLOON VALVULOPLASTY. Percutaneous balloon dilation of isolated congenital semilunar valvular stenoses has proven to be highly effective in providing long-term hemodynamic and symptomatic benefit in neonatal, pediatric, and adult patients. The pathology of congenital pulmonic and aortic stenosis consists of variable degrees of valvular deformity and commissural fusion, but, in contrast to acquired forms of valvular heart disease, severe thickening and calcification are less frequently present. Balloon valvuloplasty in these patients thus substantially reduces the extent of ventricular outflow obstruction, primarily through splitting along the lines of commissural fusion, although tearing of the valve leaflets may occur as well.

Kan and associates described the first clinical application of balloon valvuloplasty[223] in 1982, in which excellent acute improvement in transvalvular gradient was achieved in five children with *pulmonary valve stenosis.* In the report of the Pediatric Valvuloplasty Registry[224] in which 784 children underwent this procedure, mean gradient decreased acutely from 71 to 28 mm Hg, with the least benefit observed among patients with pulmonary valve dysplasia. Procedural mortality was only 0.2 per cent. Pulmonary valvuloplasty may be particularly challenging in neonates with severe stenosis or pulmonary atresia, in whom catheterization of the pulmonary artery may be difficult and require graded dilatation (see p. 926). Among the limited number of patients for whom long-term (2 to 5 years) follow-up is available, late results of pulmonic valvuloplasty appear to be excellent.[225,226] Valve gradients have on average been even lower than those immediately following val-

vuloplasty,[225,226] with less frequent development of pulmonic regurgitation or ventricular arrhythmias than in matched patients treated surgically.[226] Balloon pulmonary valvuloplasty may therefore be curative for patients with pulmonary stenosis and is considered the procedure of choice.

Unlike pulmonary valve stenosis, *congenital aortic stenosis* tends to be progressive over time, with a substantial rate of restenosis over 5 to 20 years following surgical valvotomy. Balloon aortic valvuloplasty can be performed in this group of patients with a satisfactory acute outcome (see p. 918); among 204 patients in the Pediatric Valvuloplasty Registry,[224] mean transvalvular gradient decreased from 77 to 30 mm Hg. Mortality risk was 2.4 per cent, confined entirely to patients 3 months old or less, with 10.2 per cent of patients exhibiting some increase in aortic regurgitation. Although long-term follow-up data are not yet available, no restenosis was observed in one series by a mean of 1.7 years after aortic valvuloplasty.[227]

OTHER PERCUTANEOUS INTERVENTIONS FOR CONGENITAL HEART DISEASE. Pulmonary artery stenosis or hypoplasia may be effectively treated by catheter-based technologies (see p. 924). Success rates following balloon dilatation of these vessels have ranged from 50 to 60 per cent, with failures due primarily to elastic recoil.[228] The use of balloon-expandable intraluminal stents is under investigation, with very encouraging immediate and short-term results in the limited number of patients studied thus far.[229] Long-term effectiveness and management strategies following stent placement in growing children must be evaluated. There has also been a limited experience with balloon angioplasty or stent placement for management of aortic coarctation, venous obstruction, or stenoses of Fontan shunts.

A variety of devices for transcatheter closure of the atrial septal defect, patent ductus arteriosus (PDA), or anomalous systemic-pulmonary collateral vessels are under preclinical or clinical evaluation. Current implants for closure of atrial septal defects are based on a double-disc design, in which part of the device lies in the right and left atria on either side of the defect. Small to moderate-size atrial septal defects have been effectively closed using clamshell or buttoned occluder devices in early clinical trials, although deployment failures, residual interatrial shunting, or late embolic events or device failures have been reported in a sizeable proportion of patients.[230,231] The Rashkind PDA Occluder, another double-disc design, has been investigated for closure of the persistently patent ductus arteriosus in over 650 patients, with low mortality risk and a 5 to 10 per cent rate of residual ductus murmur.[232] Embolization coils and a modified buttoned occluder are also under evaluation for patent ductus arteriosus closure.

QUALITY OF CARE AND CREDENTIALING

Advances in the technology for percutaneous coronary revascularization have been accompanied by a dramatic increase in the number of procedures carried out in the United States as well as a proliferation in the number of operators and sites performing these interventions. In a survey by the American College of Cardiology, fully 43 per cent of members stated that they performed coronary angioplasty.[233] Several studies have highlighted considerable variability in practice patterns and outcome associated with percutaneous revascularization procedures. An examination of a private insurance data base, for example, demonstrated substantial differences between geographical regions and types of hospitals with respect to per capita rates of coronary angioplasty, utilization of preprocedural functional testing, hospital charges and length of stay, and crossover to bypass surgery.[6] Indications for coronary revascularization in studies conducted in New York state were found to be much more frequently "uncertain" or "inappropriate" for angioplasty[234] than for coronary bypass surgery.[235]

Operator and institutional experience and caseload appear to substantially influence angioplasty practice and outcome. The number of cases per interventional operator per year in the United States has been estimated to range widely from 1 to 700, but with a median of only 22 to 35.[236] Similarly, a recent Medicare data base analysis revealed that the annual volume of angioplasty procedures per hospital carried out in Medicare beneficiaries ranged from 1 to 987, with half of patients treated at centers that performed 54 or fewer angioplasties in this patient population per year.[237] Two large-scale studies have demonstrated that mortality and complications occur more frequently among patients treated at low-volume centers. In a state-wide survey of angioplasty procedures performed among nearly 25,000 patients in California,[238] the risk of death or emergency coronary bypass surgery was 43 to 49 per cent higher at centers performing less than 200 cases per year than at centers with annual institutional volumes of more than 400 cases. A larger analysis of more than 217,000 Medicare patients treated throughout the United States confirmed the association between outcome and institutional volume, noting a fall in 30-day mortality from 4.2 per cent among patients treated at lowest volume sites to 2.7 per cent at high-volume centers.[237]

Based upon recognition of the consistent association between operator skill and experience and efficacy of percutaneous revascularization, the American College of Cardiology and American Heart Association have promulgated guidelines for minimal levels of training and experience.[7] The American Board of Internal Medicine is considering a Certificate of Added Qualification for interventional cardiology equivalent to that for cardiac electrophysiology. For the time being, however, credentialing in interventional cardiology is at the discretion of individual institutions. Nevertheless, it is recommended that interventional operators have undergone a formal angioplasty training program, during which a minimum of 125 procedures, including 75 as the primary operator, were performed. It should be noted that these guidelines for operator volume were derived empirically without prospective validation.[7] Further, in order to maintain privileges to carry out coronary angioplasty, a minimum of 75 procedures should be performed each year as primary operator. Finally, it is recommended that an institutional minimum of 200 cases annually is "essential for maintenance of quality and safe care."[7] The issue of institutional and operator procedural volume is even more problematic when new devices for percutaneous revascularization are considered; assessment of competence is complex owing to the steep "learning curves" associated with many of these devices, their relatively infrequent use at many centers, and the absence of validated mechanisms of teaching operators who are not part of training programs.

FUTURE DIRECTIONS

The remarkable development of new and enhanced techniques for percutaneous coronary revascularization over the last 15 years has led to considerable expansion in the list of candidates for the procedure and improvements in immediate and long-term outcome. Continued progress is certain. While the technology for balloon angioplasty may remain relatively stable, the development of new devices for percutaneous revascularization will continue, with somewhat more enlightened and realistic expectations of the biological responses within the coronary artery. Indications and methods for existing modalities will be refined, with randomized trials playing a key role in defining the specific settings for their use. Novel technologies will be introduced and developed, directed at the efficient removal or

modification of arterial plaque with minimal arterial trauma or at site-specific drug delivery to inhibit thrombosis and restenosis. Concurrently, as intravascular ultrasound and angioscopy will be further refined and integrated into revascularization devices, allowing precise guidance and optimization of plaque ablation or remodeling while limiting associated coronary injury. Finally, understanding of the vascular biology of percutaneous revascularization, thrombosis, and restenosis will improve, leading to pharmacological therapies designed to ameliorate adverse thrombotic, proliferative, and remodeling responses. It is realistic to expect that both acute-phase results and long-term outcome of percutaneous revascularization can be markedly improved, with further extension of these techniques in the management of obstructive coronary artery disease.

REFERENCES

HISTORY

1. Cournand, A. F., and Ranges, H. S.: Catheterization of the right auricle in man. Proc. Soc. Exp. Biol. Med. 46:462, 1941.
2. Rashkind, W. J., and Miller, W. W.: Creation of an atrial septal defect without thoracotomy: Palliative approach to complete transposition of the great vessels. JAMA 196:991, 1966.
3. Dotter, C. T., and Judkins, M. P.: Transluminal treatment of arteriosclerotic obstruction: Description of a new technique and preliminary report of its application. Circulation 30:654, 1964.
4. Gruentzig, A. R.: Transluminal dilatation of coronary artery stenosis (letter). Lancet 1:263, 1978.

PERCUTANEOUS TRANSLUMINAL CORONARY ANGIOPLASTY

5. Gruentzig, A. R., Senning, A., and Siegenthaler, W. E.: Nonoperative dilatation of coronary-artery stenosis. Percutaneous transluminal coronary angioplasty. N. Engl. J. Med. 301:61, 1979.
6. Topol, E. J., Ellis, S. G., Cosgrove, D. M., et al.: Analysis of coronary angioplasty practice in the United States with an insurance-claims data base. Circulation 87:1489, 1993.
7. Ryan, T. J., Bauman, W. B., Kennedy, J. W., et al.: Guidelines for percutaneous transluminal coronary angioplasty. A report of the American College of Cardiology/American Heart Association Task Force on Assessment of Diagnostic and Therapeutic Cardiovascular Procedures (Committee on Percutaneous Transluminal Coronary Angioplasty). J. Am. Coll. Cardiol. 22:2033, 1993.
8. Ohman, E. M., Marquis, J. F., Ricci, D. R., et al.: A randomized comparison of the effects of gradual prolonged versus standard primary balloon inflation on early and late outcome. Results of a multicenter clinical trial. Circulation 89:1118, 1994.
9. Honye, J., Mahon, D. J., Jain, A., et al.: Morphological effects of coronary balloon angioplasty in vivo assessed by intravascular ultrasound imaging. Circulation 85:1012, 1992.
10. Waller, B. F.: Coronary luminal shape and the arc of disease free wall: Morphologic observations and clinical relevance. J. Am. Coll. Cardiol. 6:1100, 1985.
11. Detre, K., Holubkov, R., Kelsey, S., et al.: Percutaneous transluminal coronary angioplasty in 1985-1986 and 1977-1981. The National Heart, Lung, and Blood Registry. N. Engl. J. Med. 318:265, 1988.
12. Kahn, J. K., and Hartzler, G. O.: Frequency and causes of failure with contemporary balloon coronary angioplasty and implications for new technologies. Am. J. Cardiol. 66:858, 1990.
13. Myler, R. K., Shaw, R. E., Stertzer, S. H., et al.: Lesion morphology and coronary angioplasty: Current experience and analysis. J. Am. Coll. Cardiol. 19:1641, 1992.
14. Wong, J. B., Sonnenberg, F. A., Salem, D. N., and Pauker, S. G.: Myocardial revascularization for chronic stable angina. Analysis of the role of percutaneous transluminal coronary angioplasty based on data available in 1989. Ann. Intern. Med. 113:852, 1990.
15. Rosing, D. R., Cannon, R. D., Watson, R. M., et al.: Three year anatomic, functional, and clinical follow-up after successful percutaneous transluminal coronary angioplasty. J. Am. Coll. Cardiol. 9:1, 1987.
16. Faxon, D. P., Ruocco, N., and Jacobs, A. K.: Long-term outcome of patients after percutaneous transluminal coronary angioplasty. Circulation 81:IV-9, 1990.
17. Gruentzig, A. R., King, S. B., Schlumpf, M., and Siegenthaler, W.: Long-term follow-up after percutaneous transluminal coronary angioplasty. The early Zurich experience. N. Engl. J. Med. 316:1127, 1987.
18. Ellis, S. G., Cowley, M. J., Whitlow, P. L., et al.: Prospective case-control comparison of percutaneous transluminal coronary revascularization in patients with multivessel disease treated in 1986-1987 versus 1991: Improved in-hospital and 12-month results. Multivessel Angioplasty Prognosis Study (MAPS) Group. J. Am. Coll. Cardiol. 25:1137, 1995.
19. Kuntz, R. E., Piana, R., Pomerantz, R. M., et al.: Changing incidence and management of abrupt closure following coronary intervention in the new device era. Cathet. Cardiovasc. Diagn. 27:189, 1992.

20. Detre, K. M., Holmes, D. R., Holubkov, R., et al.: Incidence and consequences of periprocedural occlusion. The 1985–1986 National Heart, Lung, and Blood Institute percutaneous transluminal coronary angioplasty registry. Circulation 82:739, 1990.

21. de Feyter, P. J., van den Brand, M., Jaarman, G. J., et al.: Acute coronary artery occlusion during and after percutaneous transluminal coronary angioplasty. Frequency, prediction, clinical course, management, and follow-up. Circulation 83:927, 1991.

22. Lincoff, A. M., Popma, J. J., Ellis, S. G., et al.: Abrupt vessel closure complicating coronary angioplasty: Clinical, angiographic, and therapeutic profile. J. Am. Coll. Cardiol. 19:926, 1992.

23. Schwartz, L., Bourassa, M. G., Lesperance, J., et al.: Aspirin and dipyridamole in the prevention of restenosis after percutaneous transluminal coronary angioplasty. N. Engl. J. Med. 318:1714, 1988.

24. Laskey, M. A., Deutsch, E., Barnathan, E., et al.: Influence of heparin therapy on percutaneous transluminal coronary angioplasty outcome in unstable angina pectoris. Am. J. Cardiol. 65:1425, 1990.

25. Laskey, M. A., Deutsch, E., Hirshfeld, J. W. J., et al.: Influence of heparin therapy on percutaneous transluminal coronary angioplasty outcome in patients with coronary arterial thrombus. Am. J. Cardiol. 65:179, 1990.

26. McGarry, T. F., Gottlieb, R. S., Morganroth, J., et al.: The relationship of anticoagulation level and complications after successful percutaneous transluminal coronary angioplasty. Am. Heart J. 123:1445, 1992.

27. Dougherty, K. G., Gaos, C. M., Bush, H. S., et al.: Activated clotting times and activated partial thromboplastin times in patients undergoing coronary angioplasty who receive bolus doses of heparin. Cathet. Cardiovasc. Diagn. 26:260, 1992.

28. Bowers, J., and Ferguson, J. J.: The use of activated clotting times to monitor heparin therapy during and after interventional procedures. Clin. Cardiol. 17:357, 1994.

29. Ellis, S. G., Roubin, G. S., Wilentz, J., et al.: Effect of 18- to 24-hour heparin administration for prevention of restenosis after uncomplicated coronary angioplasty. Am. Heart J. 117:777, 1989.

30. Friedman, H. Z., Cragg, D. R., Glazier, S. M., et al.: Randomized prospective evaluation of prolonged versus abbreviated intravenous heparin therapy after coronary angioplasty. J. Am. Coll. Cardiol. 24:1214, 1994.

31. Gabliani, G., Deligonul, U., Kern, M. J., and Vandormael, M.: Acute coronary occlusion occurring after successful percutaneous transluminal coronary angioplasty: Temporal relationship to discontinuation of anticoagulation. Am. Heart J. 116:696, 1988.

32. Vaitkus, P. T., and Laskey, W. K.: Efficacy of adjunctive thrombolytic therapy in percutaneous transluminal coronary angioplasty. J. Am. Coll. Cardiol. 24:1415, 1994.

33. Ambrose, J. A., Almeida, O. D., Sharma, S. K., et al.: Adjunctive thrombolytic therapy during angioplasty for ischemic rest angina. Results of the TAUSA Trial. Circulation 90:69, 1994.

34. Roubin, G. S., Douglas, J. S., King, S. B., et al.: Influence of balloon size on initial success, acute complications, and restenosis after percutaneous transluminal coronary angioplasty. A prospective randomized study. Circulation 78:557, 1988.

35. Nichols, A. B., Smith, R., Berke, A. D., et al.: Importance of balloon size in coronary angioplasty. J. Am. Coll. Cardiol. 13:1094, 1989.

36. Tenaglia, A. N., Quigley, P. J., Kereiakes, D. J., et al.: Coronary angioplasty performed with gradual and prolonged inflation using a perfusion balloon catheter: Procedural success and restenosis rate. Am. Heart J. 124:585, 1992.

37. Phillips, D. R., Charo, I. F., Parise, L. V., and Fitzgerald, L. A.: The platelet membrane glycoprotein IIb/IIIa complex. Blood 71:831, 1988.

38. EPIC Investigators: Use of a monoclonal antibody directed against the platelet glycoprotein IIb/IIIa receptor in high-risk coronary angioplasty. N. Engl. J. Med. 330:956, 1994.

39. Schieman, G., Cohen, B. M., Kozina, J., et al.: Intracoronary urokinase for intracoronary thrombus accumulation complicating percutaneous transluminal coronary angioplasty in acute ischemic syndromes. Circulation 82:2052, 1990.

40. Lincoff, A. M., and Topol, E. J.: Abrupt vessel closure. In Topol, E. J. (ed.): Textbook of Interventional Cardiology. 2nd ed. Philadelphia, W. B. Saunders Company, 1994, p. 207.

41. de Feyter, P. J., Serruys, P. W., Soward, A., et al.: Coronary angioplasty for early postinfarction unstable angina. Circulation 74:1365, 1986.

42. de Feyter, P. J., Suryapranata, H., Serruys, P. W., et al.: Coronary angioplasty for unstable angina: Immediate and late results in 200 consecutive patients with identification of risk factors for unfavorable early and late outcome. J. Am. Coll. Cardiol. 12:324, 1988.

43. de Feyter, P. J.: Coronary angioplasty in unstable angina. Am. Heart J. 118:860, 1989.

44. Myler, R. K., Shaw, R. E., Stertzer, S. H., et al.: Unstable angina and coronary angioplasty. Circulation 82:II-88, 1990.

45. Stammen, F., De Scheerder, I., Glazier, J. J., et al.: Immediate and follow-up results of the conservative coronary angioplasty strategy for unstable angina pectoris. Am. J. Cardiol. 69:1533, 1995.

46. Ellis, S. G., Vandormael, M. G., Cowley, M. J., et al.: Coronary morphologic and clinical determinants of procedural outcome with angioplasty for multivessel coronary disease. Implications for patient selection. Circulation 82:1193, 1990.

47. Cowley, M. J., Dorros, G., Kelsey, S. F., et al.: Acute coronary events associated with percutaneous transluminal coronary angioplasty. Am. J. Cardiol. 53:12, 1984.

48. Ellis, S. G., Roubin, G. S., King, S. B., et al.: Angiographic and clinical predictors of acute closure after native vessel coronary angioplasty. Circulation 77:372, 1988.

49. Kern, M. J., Deligonul, U., Galan, K., et al.: Percutaneous transluminal coronary angioplasty in octogenarians. Am. J. Cardiol. 61:457, 1988.

50. Kelsey, S. F., Miller, D. P., Holubkov, R., et al.: Results of percutaneous transluminal coronary angioplasty in patients ≥ 65 years of age (from the 1985 to 1986 National Heart, Lung, and Blood Institute's coronary angioplasty registry). Am. J. Cardiol. 66:1033, 1990.

51. Ryan, T. J., Faxon, D. P., Gunnar, R. M., et al.: Guidelines for percutaneous transluminal coronary angioplasty. A report of the American College of Cardiology/American Heart Association Task Force on assessment of diagnostic and therapeutic cardiovascular procedures (subcommittee on percutaneous transluminal coronary angioplasty). J. Am. Coll. Cardiol. 12:529, 1988.

52. Tenaglia, A. N., Fortin, D. F., Frid, D. J., et al.: A simple scoring system to predict PTCA abrupt closure. J. Am. Coll. Cardiol. 19(Abs.):139, 1992.

53. Black, A. J. R., Namay, D. L., Niederman, A. L., et al.: Tear of dissection after coronary angioplasty—morphologic correlates of an ischemic complication. Circulation 79:1035, 1989.

54. Huber, M. S., Mooney, J. F., Madison, J., and Mooney, M. R.: Use of a morphologic classification to predict clinical outcome after dissection from coronary angioplasty. Am. J. Cardiol. 68:467, 1991.

55. Ellis, S. G., Myler, R. K., King, S. B., et al.: Causes and correlates of death after unsupported coronary angioplasty: Implications for use of angioplasty and advanced support techniques in high-risk settings. Am. J. Cardiol. 68:1447, 1991.

56. Ellis, S. G., Roubin, G. S., King, S. B., et al.: In-hospital cardiac mortality after acute closure after coronary angioplasty: Analysis of risk factors from 8,207 procedures. J. Am. Coll. Cardiol. 11:211, 1988.

57. Califf, R. M., Phillips, H. R., Hindman, M. C., et al.: Prognostic value of a coronary artery jeopardy score. J. Am. Coll. Cardiol. 5:1055, 1985.

58. Holmes, D. R. J., Holubkov, R., Vlietstra, R. E., et al.: Comparison of complications during percutaneous transluminal coronary angioplasty from 1977 to 1981 and from 1985 to 1986: The National Heart Lung, and Blood Institute Percutaneous Transluminal Coronary Angioplasty Registry. J. Am. Coll. Cardiol. 12:1149, 1988.

59. Bergelson, B. A., Jacobs, A. K., Cupples, L. A., et al.: Prediction of risk for hemodynamic compromise during percutaneous transluminal coronary angioplasty. Am. J. Cardiol. 70:1540, 1992.

60. Detre, K., Holubkov, R., Kelsey, S., et al.: One-year follow up results of the 1985–1986 National Heart, Lung, and Blood Institute's percutaneous transluminal coronary angioplasty registry. Circulation 80:421, 1989.

61. O'Keefe, J. H. Jr., Rutherford, B. D., McConahay, D. R., et al.: Multivessel coronary angioplasty from 1980 to 1989: Procedural results and long-term outcome. J. Am. Coll. Cardiol. 16:1097, 1990.

62. Mark, D. B., Nelson, C. L., Califf, R. M., et al.: Continuing evolution of therapy for coronary artery disease. Initial results from the era of coronary angioplasty. Circulation 89:2015, 1994.

63. Talley, J. D., Hurst, J. W., King, S. B., et al.: Clinical outcome 5 years after attempted percutaneous transluminal coronary angioplasty in 427 patients. Circulation 77:820, 1988.

64. King, S. B. I., and Schlumpf, M.: Ten-year completed follow-up of percutaneous transluminal coronary angioplasty: The early Zurich experience. J. Am. Coll. Cardiol. 22:353, 1993.

65. Weintraub, W. S., Douglas, J. S., Morris, D. C., et al.: Long term follow-up after PTCA in patients with single and multivessel coronary artery disease. J. Am. Coll. Cardiol. 23(Abs.):352, 1994.

66. Kent, K., Cowley, M., Detre, K., et al.: Report of five-year outcome for 1977–81 and 1985–86 cohorts of the NHLBI PTCA registry. J. Am. Coll. Cardiol. 86(Abs.):I-55, 1992.

67. Bourassa, M. G., Holubkov, R., Yeh, W., et al.: Strategy of complete revascularization in patients with multivessel coronary artery disease (a report from the 1985–1986 NHLBI PTCA Registry). Am. J. Cardiol. 70:174, 1992.

68. Bell, M. R., Bailey, K. R., Reeder, G. S., et al.: Percutaneous transluminal angioplasty in patients with multivessel coronary disease: How important is complete revascularization for cardiac event-free survival? J. Am. Coll. Cardiol. 16:553, 1990.

69. Wohlgelernter, D., Cleman, M., Highman, H. A., and Zaret, B. L.: Percutaneous transluminal coronary angioplasty of the "culprit lesion" for management of unstable angina pectoris in patients with multivessel coronary disease. Am. J. Cardiol. 56:460, 1986.

70. Jones, E. L., Craver, J. M., Guyton, R. A., et al.: Importance of complete revascularization in performance of the coronary bypass operation. Am. J. Cardiol. 51:7, 1983.

71. Deligonul, U., Vandormael, M. G., Kern, M. J., et al.: Coronary angioplasty: A therapeutic option for symptomatic patients with two and three vessel coronary disease. J. Am. Coll. Cardiol. 11:1173, 1988.

72. Faxon, D. P., Ghalilli, K., Jacobs, A. K., et al.: The degree of revascularization and outcome after multivessel coronary angioplasty. Am. Heart J. 123:854, 1992.

73. Reeder, G. S., Holmes, D. R. J., Detre, K., et al.: Degree of revascularization in patients with multivessel coronary disease: A report from the National Heart, Lung, and Blood Institute percutaneous transluminal coronary angioplasty registry. Circulation 77:638, 1988.

74. Leimgruber, P., Roubin, G. S., Hollman, J., et al.: Restenosis after successful coronary angioplasty in patients with single-vessel disease. Circulation 73:710, 1986.

75. Ellis, S. G., Roubin, G. S., King, S. B., et al.: Importance of stenosis morphology in the estimation of restenosis risk after elective per-

cutaneous transluminal coronary angioplasty. Am. J. Cardiol. 63:30, 1989.

76. Holmes, D. R., Vlietstra, R. E., Smith, H. C., et al.: Restenosis after percutaneous transluminal coronary angioplasty: A report of the PTCA Registry of the National Heart, Lung, and Blood Institute. Am. J. Cardiol. 53:77, 1984.

77. Nobuyoshi, M., Kimura, T., Ohishi, H., et al.: Restenosis after percutaneous transluminal coronary angioplasty: Pathologic observations in 20 patients. J. Am. Coll. Cardiol. 17:433, 1991.

78. Popma, J. J., VanDenBerg, E. K., and Dehmer, G.: Long-term outcome of patients with asymptomatic restenosis after percutaneous transluminal coronary angioplasty. Am. J. Cardiol. 62:1298, 1988.

79. Bengtson, J. R., Mark, D. B., Honan, M. B., et al.: Detection of restenosis after elective percutaneous transluminal coronary angioplasty using the exercise treadmill test. Am. J. Cardiol. 65:28, 1990.

80. Hillegass, W. B., Ohman, E. M., and Califf, R. M.: Restenosis: the clinical issues. In Topol, E. J. (ed.): Textbook of Interventional Cardiology. 2nd ed. Philadelphia, W. B. Saunders Company, 1993, p. 415.

81. Serruys, P. W., Liujten, H. E., Beatt, K. J., et al.: Incidence of restenosis after successful coornary angioplasty: A time-related phenomenon. A quantitative angiographic study in 342 consecutive patients at 1, 2, 3, and 4 months. Circulation 77:361, 1988.

82. Nobuyoshi, M., Kimura, T., Nosaka, H., et al.: Restenosis after successful percutaneous transluminal coronary angioplasty: Serial angiographic follow-up of 229 patients. J. Am. Coll. Cardiol. 12:616, 1988.

83. Rensing, B. J., Hermans, W. R. M., Deckers, J. W., et al.: Lumen narrowing after percutaneous transluminal coronary balloon angioplasty follows a near gaussian distribution: A quantitative angiographic study in 1445 successfully dilated lesions. J. Am. Coll. Cardiol. 19:939, 1992.

83a. Moliterno, D. J., and Topol, E. J.: Clinical evaluation of restenosis. In Fuster, V., Ross, R., and Topol, E. J. (eds.): Atherosclerosis and Coronary Artery Disease. Philadelphia, Lippincott-Raven, 1996, pp. 1505–1526.

84. Joelson, J. M., Most, A. S., and Williams, D. O.: Angiographic findings when chest pain recurs after successful percutaneous transluminal coronary angioplasty. Am. J. Cardiol. 60:792, 1987.

85. Waller, B. F., Pinkerton, C. A., Orr, C. M., et al.: Restenosis 1 to 24 months after clinically successful coronary balloon angioplasty: A necropsy study of 20 patients. J. Am. Coll. Cardiol. 17:58, 1991.

86. Waller, B. F., Pinkerton, C. A., Orr, C. M., et al.: Morphologic observations late (>30 days) after clinically successful coronary balloon angioplasty: An analysis of 20 necropsy patients and review of 41 necropsy patients with coronary angioplasty restenosis. Circulation 83:I-28, 1991.

87. Post, M. J., Borst, C., and Kuntz, R. E.: The relative importance of arterial remodeling compared with intimal hyperplasia in lumen renarrowing after balloon angioplasty. A study in the normal rabbit and the hypercholesterolemic Yucatan micropig. Circulation 89:2816, 1994.

88. Kakuta, T., Currier, J. W., Haudenschild, C. C., et al.: Differences in compensatory vessel enlargement, not intimal formation, account for restenosis after angioplasty in the hypercholesterolemic rabbit model. Circulation 89:2809, 1994.

89. Mintz, G. S., Kovach, J. A., Javier, S. P., et al.: Geometric remodeling is the predominant mechanism of late lumen loss after coronary angioplasty. Circulation 88(Abs.):I-654, 1993.

89a. Falk, E., and Nobuyoshi, M.: Differences between atherosclerosis and restenosis. Harrison, D.C.: Nonatherosclerotic coronary disease. In Fuster, V., Ross, R., and Topol, E. J. (eds.): Atherosclerosis and Coronary Artery Disease. Philadelphia, Lippincott-Raven, 1996, pp. 683–700.

90. Schwartz, R. S., Huber, K. C., Murphy, J. G., et al.: Restenosis and the proportional neointimal response to coronary artery injury: Results in a porcine model. J. Am. Coll. Cardiol. 19:267, 1992.

91. Ip, J. H., Fuster, V., Badimon, L., et al.: Syndromes of accelerated atherosclerosis: Role of vascular injury and smooth muscle cell proliferation. J. Am. Coll. Cardiol. 15:1667, 1990.

92. Clowes, A. W., Reidy, M. A., and Clowes, M. M.: Mechanisms of stenosis after arterial injury. Lab. Invest. 49:208, 1983.

93. Clowes, A. W., and Schwartz, S. M.: Significance of quiescent smooth muscle migration in the injured rat carotid artery. Circ. Res. 56:139, 1985.

94. Forrester, J. S., Fishbein, M., Helfant, R., and Fagin, J.: A paradigm for restenosis based on cell biology: Clues for the development of new preventive therapies. J. Am. Coll. Cardiol. 17:758, 1991.

95. Glagov, S.: Intimal hyperplasia, vascular modeling, and the restenosis problem. Circulation 89:2888, 1994.

96. Schwartz, R. S., Holmes, D. R., and Topol, E. J.: The restenosis paradigm revisited: An alternative proposal for cellular mechanisms. J. Am. Coll. Cardiol. 20:1284, 1992.

97. Lindner, V., Lappi, D. A., Baird, A., et al.: Role of basic fibroblast growth factor in vascular lesion formation. Circ. Res. 68:106, 1991.

98. Hirshfeld, J. W., Schwartz, J. S., Jugo, R., et al.: Restenosis after coronary angioplasty: A multivariate statistical model to relate lesion and procedure variables to restenosis. J. Am. Coll. Cardiol. 18:647, 1991.

99. Lambert, M., Bonan, R., Cote, G., et al.: Multiple coronary angioplasty: A model to discriminate systemic and procedural factors related to restenosis. J. Am. Coll. Cardiol. 12:310, 1988.

100. Guiteras, V. P., Bourassa, M. G., David, P. R., et al.: Restenosis after successful percutaneous transluminal coronary angioplasty: The Montreal Heart Institute experience. Am. J. Cardiol. 60:50, 1987.

101. Bertrand, M. E., Lablanche, J. M., Fourrier, J. L., et al.: Relation to restenosis after percutaneous transluminal coronary angioplasty to vasomotion of the dilated coronary arterial segment. Am. J. Cardiol. 63:277, 1989.

102. Bertrand, M. E., LaBlanche, J. M., Thieuleux, F. A., et al.: Comparative results of percutaneous transluminal coronary angioplasty in patients with dynamic versus fixed coronary stenosis. J. Am. Coll. Cardiol. 8:504, 1986.

103. Corcos, T., David, P. R., Bourassa, M. G., et al.: Percutaneous transluminal coronary angioplasty for the treatment of variant angina. J. Am. Coll. Cardiol. 5:1046, 1985.

104. Austin, G. E., Lynn, M., and Hollman, J.: Laboratory test results as predictors of recurrent coronary artery stenosis following angioplasty. Arch. Pathol. Lab. Med. 111:1158, 1987.

105. Kuntz, R. E., Gibson, C. M., Nobuyoshi, M., and Baim, D. S.: Generalized model of restenosis after conventional balloon angioplasty, stenting, and directional atherectomy. J. Am. Coll. Cardiol. 21:15, 1993.

105a. Pratt, R. E., and Dzau, V. J.: Pharmacological strategies to prevent restenosis. Lessons learned from blockade of the renin-angiotensin system. Circulation 93:848, 1996.

106. Popma, J. J., Califf, R. M., and Topol, E. J.: Clinical trials of restenosis after coronary angioplasty. Circulation 84:1426, 1991.

107. Topol, E. J., Califf, R. M., Weisman, H. S., et al.: Reduction of clinical restenosis following coronary intervention with early administration of platelet IIb/IIIa integrin blocking antibody. Lancet 343:881, 1994.

108. Fischman, D. L., Leon, M. B., Baim, D. S., et al.: A randomized comparison of coronary-stent placement and balloon angioplasty in the treatment of coronary artery disease. N. Engl. J. Med. 331:496, 1994.

109. Serruys, P. W., de Jaegere, P., Kiemeneij, F., et al.: A comparison of balloon-expandable-stent implantation with balloon angioplasty in patients with coronary artery disease. N. Engl. J. Med. 331:489, 1994.

109a. Macaya, C., Serruys, P. W., Ruygrok, P., et al.: Continued benefit of coronary stenting versus balloon angioplasty: One-year clinical follow-up of Benestent trial. J. Am. Coll. Cardiol. 27:255, 1996.

110. Hernandez, R. A., Macaya, C., Iniguez, A., et al.: Midterm outcome of patients with asymptomatic restenosis after coronary balloon angioplasty. J. Am. Coll. Cardiol. 19:1402, 1992.

111. Teirstein, P. S., Hoover, C. A., Ligon, R. W., et al.: Repeat coronary angioplasty: Efficacy of a third angioplasty for a second restenosis. J. Am. Coll. Cardiol. 13:291, 1989.

112. Black, A. J. R., Anderson, V., Roubin, G. S., et al.: Repeat coronary angioplasty: Correlates of a second restenosis. J. Am. Coll. Cardiol. 11:714, 1988.

113. Parisi, A. F., Folland, E. D., Hartigan, P., and Veterans Affairs ACME Investigators: A comparison of angioplasty with medical therapy in the treatment of single-vessel coronary artery disease. N. Engl. J. Med. 326:10, 1992.

114. Folland, E. D., Parisi, A. F., Hartigan, P., for the VA ACME Investigators: PTCA vs medicine for double vessel disease: Initial results of the randomzied VA ACME trial. Circulation 84(Abs.):II-252, 1991.

115. RITA Trial Participants: Coronary angioplasty versus coronary artery bypass surgery: The Randomized Intervention Treatment of Angina (RITA) trial. Lancet 335:1315, 1993.

116. Rodriguez, A., Boullon, F., Perez-Balino, N., et al.: Argentine randomized trial of percutaneous transluminal coronary angioplasty versus coronary artery bypass surgery in multivessel disease (ERACI): In-hospital results and 1-year follow up. J. Am. Coll. Cardiol. 22:1060, 1993.

117. Hamm, C. W., Reimers, J., Ischinger, T., et al.: A randomized study of coronary angioplasty compared with bypass surgery in patients with symptomatic multivessel coronary disease. N. Engl. J. Med. 331:1037, 1994.

118. King, S. B., Lembo, N. J., Weintraub, W. S., et al.: A randomized trial comparing coronary angioplasty with coronary bypass surgery. N. Engl. J. Med. 331:1044, 1994.

119. Moliterno, D. J., Elliott, J. M., and Topol, E. J.: Randomized trials of myocardial revascularization. In O'Rourke, R. A. (ed.): Current Problems in Cardiology. Vol. XX. Linn, MO, C. V. Mosby, 1995, p. 121.

120. Goy, J. J., Eeckhout, E., Burnand, B., et al.: Coronary angioplasty versus left internal mammary artery grafting for isolated proximal left anterior descending artery stenosis. Lancet 343:1449, 1994.

121. Mark, D. B., Lam, L. C., Lee, K. L., et al.: Effects of coronary angioplasty, coronary bypass surgery, and medical therapy on employment in patients with coronary artery disease. A prospective comparison study. Ann. Intern. Med. 120:111, 1994.

122. Eckman, M. H., Wong, J. B., Salem, D. N., and Pauker, S. G.: Direct angioplasty for acute myocardial infarction. A review of outcomes in clinical subsets. Ann. Intern. Med. 117:667, 1992.

123. O'Keefe, J. H., Rutherford, B. D., McConahay, D. D. R., et al.: Early and late results of coronary angioplasty without antecedent thrombolytic therapy for acute myocardial infarction. Am. J. Cardiol. 64:1221, 1989.

124. Grines, C. L., Browne, K. F., Marco, J., et al.: A comparison of immediate angioplasty with thrombolytic therapy for acute myocardial infarction. N. Engl. J. Med. 328:673, 1993.

125. de Boer, M. J., Hoorntje, J. C. A., Ottervanger, J. P., et al.: Immediate coronary angioplasty versus intravenous streptokinase in acute myocardial infarction: Left ventricular ejection fraction, hospital mortality and reinfarction. J. Am. Coll. Cardiol. 23:1004, 1994.

126. Gibbons, R. J., Holmes, D. R., Reeder, G. S., et al.: Immediate angioplasty compared with the administration of a thrombolytic agent followed by conservative treatment for myocardial infarction. N. Engl. J. Med. 328:685, 1993.

127. Ribeiro, E. E., Silva, L. A., Carneiro, R., et al.: A randomized trial of direct PTCA vs intravenous streptokinase in acute myocardial infarction. J. Am. Coll. Cardiol. 17:152, 1991.

128. TIMI Research Group: Immediate vs. delayed catheterization and angio-

plasty following thrombolytic therapy for acute myocardial infarction. TIMI IIA results. JAMA 260:2849, 1988.

129. Topol, E. J., Califf, R. M., George, B. S., et al.: A randomized trial of immediate versus delayed elective angioplasty after intravenous tissue plasminogen activator in acute myocardial infarction. N. Engl. J. Med. 317:581, 1987.

130. Simoons, M. L., Betriu, A., Col, J., et al.: Thrombolysis with tissue plasminogen activator in acute myocardial infarction: No additional benefit from immediate percutaneous coronary angioplasty. Lancet 1:197, 1988.

131. TIMI Study Group: Comparison of invasive and conservative strategies after treatment with intravenous tissue plasminogen activator in acute myocardial infarction. Results of the thrombolysis in myocardial infarction (TIMI) phase II trial. N. Engl. J. Med. 320:618, 1989.

132. SWIFT: SWIFT trial of delayed elective intervention v conservative treatment after thrombolysis with anistreplase in acute myocardial infarction. Br. Med. J. 302:555, 1991.

133. Ellis, S. G., da Silva, E. R., Heyndrickx, G., et al.: Randomized comparison of rescue angioplasty with conservative management of patients with early failure of thrombolysis for acute anterior myocardial infarction. Circulation 90:2280, 1994.

133a. Baim, D. S., and Leon, M. B.: The use of new angioplasty devices for the treatment of stable angina. In Fuster, V., Ross, R., and Topol, E. J. (eds.): Atherosclerosis and Coronary Artery Disease. Philadelphia, Lippincott-Raven, 1996, pp. 1527–1542.

NEW DEVICES FOR PERCUTANEOUS CORONARY REVASCULARIZATION

134. Tenaglia, A. N., Buller, C. E., Kisslo, K. B., et al.: Mechanisms of balloon angioplasty and directional coronary atherectomy as assessed by intracoronary ultrasound. J. Am. Coll. Cardiol. 20:682, 1992.

135. Penny, W. F., Schmidt, D. A., Safian, R. D., et al.: Insights into the mechanism of luminal improvement after directional coronary atherectomy. Am. J. Cardiol. 67:435, 1991.

136. Baim, D. S., Hinohara, T., Holmes, D., et al.: Results of directional coronary atherectomy during multicenter preapproval testing. The US Directional Coronary Atherectomy Investigator Group. Am. J. Cardiol. 72:6, 1993.

137. Hinohara, T., Rowe, M. H., Robertson, G. C., et al.: Effect of lesion characteristics on outcome of directional coronary atherectomy. J. Am. Coll. Cardiol. 17:1112, 1991.

138. Ellis, S. G., DeCesare, N. B., Pinkerton, C. A., et al.: Relation of stenosis morphology and clinical presentation to the procedural results of directional coronary atherectomy. Circulation 84:644, 1991.

139. Topol, E. J., Leya, F., Pinkerton, C. A., et al.: A comparison of coronary angioplasty with directional atherectomy in patients with coronary artery disease. N. Engl. J. Med. 329:221, 1993.

140. Adelman, A. G., Cohen, E. A., Kimball, B. P., et al.: A comparison of directional atherectomy with balloon angioplasty for lesions of the left anterior descending coronary artery. N. Engl. J. Med. 329:228, 1993.

141. Holmes, D. R., Topol, E. J., Califf, R. M., et al.: A multicenter, randomized trial of coronary angioplasty versus directional atherectomy for patients with saphenous vein bypass graft lesions. Circulation 91:1966, 1995.

142. Elliott, J. M., Berdan, L. G., Holmes, D. R., et al.: One-year follow-up in the coronary angioplasty versus excisional atherectomy trial (CAVEAT I). Circulation 91:2158, 1995.

143. Kuntz, R. E., Safian, R. D., Carrozza, J. P., et al.: The importance of acute luminal diameter in determining restenosis after coronary atherectomy or stenting. Circulation 86:1827, 1992.

144. Baim, D. S., and Kuntz, R. E.: Directional coronary atherectomy: How much lumen enlargement is optimal? Am. J. Cardiol. 72:65, 1993.

145. Hansen, D. D., Auth, D. C., Vrocko, R., and Ritchie, J. L.: Rotational atherectomy in atherosclerotic rabbit iliac arteries. Am. Heart J. 115:160, 1988.

146. Ahn, S. S., Auth, D., Marcus, D. R., and Moore, W. S.: Removal of focal atheromatous lesions by angioscopically guided high-speed rotary atherectomy. J. Vasc. Surg. 7:292, 1988.

147. Kovach, J. A., Mintz, G. S., Pichard, A. D., et al.: Sequential intravascular ultrasound characterization of the mechanisms of rotational atherectomy and adjunct balloon angioplasty. J. Am. Coll. Cardiol. 22:1024, 1993.

148. Ellis, S. G., Popma, J. J., Buchbinder, M., et al.: Relation of clinical presentation, stenosis morphology, and operator technique to the procedural results of rotational atherectomy and rotational atherectomy-facilitated angioplasty. Circulation 89:882, 1994.

149. Warth, D. C., Leon, M. B., O'Neill, W., et al.: Rotational atherectomy multicenter registry: Acute results, complications, and 6-month angiographic follow-up in 709 patients. J. Am. Coll. Cardiol. 24:641, 1994.

150. Teirstein, P. S., Warth, D. C., Haq, N., et al.: High speed rotational coronary atherectomy for patients with diffuse coronary artery disease. J. Am. Coll. Cardiol. 18:1694, 1991.

151. Sketch, M. H., Labinaz, M., and Stack, R. S.: Extraction atherectomy. In Topol, E. J. (ed.): Textbook of Interventional Cardiology. 2nd ed. Philadelphia, W. B. Saunders Company, 1994, p. 668.

152. Sutton, J. M., Ellis, S. G., Roubin, G. S., et al.: Major clinical events after coronary stenting. The multicenter registry of acute and elective Gianturco-Roubin stent placement. Circulation 89:1126, 1994.

153. Platko, W. P., Hollman, J., Whitlow, P. L., and Franco, I.: Percutaneous transluminal angioplasty of saphenous vein graft stenosis: Long-term follow-up. J. Am. Coll. Cardiol. 14:1645, 1989.

154. Popma, J. J., Leon, M. B., Mintz, G. S., et al.: Results of coronary angioplasty using the transluminal extraction catheter. Am. J. Cardiol. 70:1526, 1992.

155. Strauss, B. H., Serruys, P. W., Bertrand, M. E., et al.: Quantitative angiographic follow-up of the coronary wallstent in native vessels and bypass grafts (European experience—March 1986 to March 1990). Am. J. Cardiol. 69:475, 1992.

156. Serruys, P. W., Strauss, B. H., Beatt, K. J., et al.: Angiographic follow-up after placement of a self-expanding coronary-artery stent. N. Engl. J. Med. 324:13, 1991.

157. Roubin, G. S., Robinson, K. A., King, S. B., et al.: Early and late results of intracoronary arterial stenting after coronary angioplasty in dogs. Circulation 76:891, 1987.

158. Roubin, G. S., Cannon, A. D., Agrawal, S. K., et al.: Intracoronary stenting for acute and threatened closure complicating percutaneous transluminal coronary angioplasty. Circulation 85:916, 1992.

159. Cannon, A. D., and Roubin, G. S.: The Gianturco-Roubin stent. In Topol, E. J. (ed.): Textbook of Interventional Cardiology. 2nd ed. Philadelphia, W. B. Saunders Company, 1994, p. 712.

160. Agrawal, S. K., Ho, D. S. W., Liu, M. W., et al.: Predictors of thrombotic complications after placement of the flexible coil stent. Am. J. Cardiol. 73:1216, 1994.

161. Schatz, R. A., Palmaz, J. C., Tio, F. O., et al.: Balloon-expandable intracoronary stents in the adult dog. Circulation 76:450, 1987.

162. Schatz, R. A., Baim, D. S., Leon, M., et al.: Clinical experience with the Palmaz-Schatz coronary stent. Initial results of a multicenter study. Circulation 83:148, 1991.

163. Savage, M. P., Fischman, D. L., Schatz, R. A., et al.: Long-term angiographic and clinical outcome after implantation of a balloon-expandable stent in the native coronary circulation. J. Am. Coll. Cardiol. 24:1207, 1994.

164. Ellis, S. G., Savage, M., Fischman, D., et al.: Restenosis after placement of Palmaz-Schatz stents in native coronary arteries. Initial results of a multicenter experience. Circulation 86:1836, 1992.

164a. Fernandez-Aviles, F., Alonso, J. J., Duran, J. M., et al.: Subacute occlusion, bleeding complications, hospital stay and restenosis after Palmaz-Schatz coronary stenting under a new antithrombotic regimen. J. Am. Coll. Cardiol. 27:22, 1996.

165. de Feyter, P. J., van Suylen, R. J., de Jaegere, P. P. T., et al.: Balloon angioplasty for the treatment of lesions in saphenous vein bypass grafts. J. Am. Coll. Cardiol. 21:1539, 1993.

166. Piana, R. N., Moscucci, M., Cohen, D. J., et al.: Plamaz-Schatz stenting for treatment of focal vein graft stenosis: Immediate results and long-term outcome. J. Am. Coll. Cardiol. 23:1296, 1994.

167. Ricci, D. R., Buller, C. E., O'Neill, B., et al.: Coronary stent versus prolonged perfusion balloon for failed coronary angioplasty—a randomized trial. Circulation 90(Abs.):I-651, 1994.

168. Burger, W., Sievert, H., Steinmann, J., et al.: Acute and mid-term experiences with the Wiktor stent in acute complications and restenosis after coronary angioplasty. J. Intervent. Cardiol. 5:147, 1992.

169. Reifart, N., Langer, A., Storger, H., et al.: Strecker stent as a bailout device following percutaneous transluminal coronary angioplasty. J. Intervent. Cardiol. 5:79, 1992.

170. Lambert, T. L., Dev, V., Rechavia, E., et al.: Localized arterial wall drug delivery from a polymer-coated removable metallic stent. Kinetics, distribution, and bioactivity of forskolin. Circulation 90:1003, 1994.

171. Mudra, H., Klauss, V., Blasini, R., et al.: Ultrasound guidance of Palmaz-Schatz intracoronary stenting with a combined intravascular ultrasound balloon catheter. Circulation 90:1252, 1994.

172. Morice, M. C., Bourdonnec, C., Lefevre, T., et al.: Coronary stenting without coumadin, Phase III. Circulation 90(Abs.):I-125, 1994.

173. Colombo, A., Hall, P., Nakamura, S., et al.: Intracoronary stenting without anticoagulation accomplished with ultrasound guidance. Circulation 91:1676, 1995.

174. Barragan, P., Silvestri, M., Sainsous, J., et al.: Prevention of subacute occlusion after coronary stenting with ticlopidine regimen without intravascular ultrasound guided stenting. J. Am. Coll. Cardiol. 25(Abs.):182, 1995.

174a. Mak, K-H, Belli, G., Ellis, S. G., and Moliterno, J.: Subacute stent thrombosis: Evolving issues and current concepts. J. Am. Coll. Cardiol. 27:494, 1996.

175. Colombo, A., Hall, P., Nakamura, S., et al.: Angiographic follow up and restenosis results after Palmaz-Schatz intracoronary stenting without anticoagulation. Circulation 90(Abs.):I-124, 1994.

176. Spears, J. R., Reyes, V. P., Wynne, J., et al.: Percutaneous coronary laser balloon angioplasty: Initial results of a multicenter experience. J. Am. Coll. Cardiol. 16:293, 1990.

177. Spears, J. R., Safian, R. D., Douglas, J. S., et al.: Multicenter acute and chronic results of laser balloon angioplasty for refractory abrupt closure after PTCA. Circulation 84(Abs.):II-517, 1991.

178. Deutsch, E.: Physiologically controlled low-stress angioplasty. In Topol, E. J. (ed.): Textbook of Interventional Cardiology. 2nd ed. Philadelphia, W. B. Saunders Company, 1994, p. 947.

179. Goicolea, J., Arganda, L., Alfonso, F., et al.: Mechanisms of radiofrequency thermal balloon angioplasty. A study with intracoronary ultrasound. J. Am. Coll. Cardiol. 25(Abs.):143, 1995.

180. Baumbach, A., Bittl, J. A., Fleck, E., et al.: Acute complications of excimer laser coronary angioplasty: A detailed analysis of multicenter results. J. Am. Coll. Cardiol. 23:1305, 1994.

181. Litvack, F., Eigler, N., Margolis, J., et al.: Percutaneous excimer laser

coronary angioplasty: Results in the first consecutive 3,000 patients. J. Am. Coll. Cardiol. 23:323, 1994.

182. Bittl, J. A., Sanborn, T. A., Tcheng, J. E., et al.: Clinical success, complications and restenosis rates with excimer laser coronary angioplasty. Am. J. Cardiol. 70:1533, 1992.

183. Appelman, Y. E. A., Piek, J. J., de Feyter, P. J., et al.: Excimer laser coronary angioplasty versus balloon angioplasty used in long coronary lesions: The long-term results of the AMRO trial. J. Am. Coll. Cardiol. 25(Abs.):329, 1995.

184. Appelman, Y. E. A., Koolen, J. J., de Feyter, P. J., et al.: Long term outcome of excimer laser angioplasty versus balloon angioplasty in functional and total coronary occlusions. J. Am. Coll. Cardiol. 25(Abs.):330, 1995.

185. Siegel, R. J., Gunn, J., Ahsan, A., et al.: Use of therapeutic ultrasound in percutaneous coronary angioplasty. Experimental in vitro studies and initial clinical experience. Circulation 89:1587, 1994.

INTRAVASCULAR IMAGING TECHNIQUES

186. Glagov, S., Weisenberg, E., Zarins, C., et al.: Compensatory enlargement of various human atherosclerotic arteries. N. Engl. J. Med. 316:1371, 1987.

187. Nishimura, R., Edwards, W., Warnes, C., et al.: Intravascular ultrasound imaging: In vitro validation and pathologic correlation. J. Am. Coll. Cardiol. 16:145, 1990.

188. Bartorelli, A., Neville, R., Keren, G., et al.: In vitro and in vivo intravascular ultrasound imaging. Eur. Heart J. 13:102, 1992.

189. Roelandt, J. R. T. C., di Mario, C., Pandian, N. G., et al.: Three-dimensional reconstruction of intracoronary ultrasound images. Rationale, approaches, problems, and directions. Circulation 90:1044, 1994.

190. Nissen, S., Gurley, J., Grines, C., et al.: Intravascular ultrasound assessment of lumen size and wall morphology in normal subjects and patients with coronary artery disease. Circulation 84:1087, 1991.

191. White, C., Ramee, S., Collins, T., et al.: Ambiguous coronary angiography: Clinical utility of intravascular ultrasound. Cathet. Cardiovasc. Diagn. 26:200, 1992.

192. Isner, J., and Rosenfield, K.: Enough with the fantastic voyage: Will IVUS play in Peoria? Cathet. Cardiovasc. Diagn. 26:192, 1992.

193. Mintz, G., Douek, P., Pichard, A., et al.: Target lesion calcification in coronary artery disease: An intravascular ultrasound study. J. Am. Coll. Cardiol. 20:1149, 1992.

194. Pandian, N., Kreis, A., and Brockway, B.: Detection of intraarterial thrombus by intravascular high frequency two-dimensional ultrasound imaging in in vitro and in vivo studies. Am. J. Cardiol. 65:1280, 1990.

195. Honye, J., Mahon, D., Nakamura, S., et al.: Intravascular ultrasound imaging after excimer laser angioplasty. Cathet. Cardiovasc. Diagn. 32:213, 1994.

196. Hodgson, J., Reddy, K., Suneja, R., et al.: Intracoronary ultrasound imaging: Correlation of plaque morphology with angiography, clinical syndrome and procedural results in patients undergoing coronary angioplasty. J. Am. Coll. Cardiol. 21:35, 1993.

197. Mintz, G., Pichard, A., Kovach, J., et al.: Impact of preintervention intravascular ultrasound imaging on transcatheter treatment strategies in coronary artery disease. Am. J. Cardiol. 73:423, 1994.

198. Fitzgerald, P., Ports, T., and Yock, P.: Contribution of localized calcium deposits to dissection after angioplasty. An observational study using intravascular ultrasound. Circulation 86:64, 1992.

199. De Sheerder, I., De Man, F., Herregods, M., et al.: Intravascular ultrasound versus angiography for measurement of luminal diameters in normal and diseased coronary arteries. Am. Heart J. 127:243, 1994.

200. Mizuno, K., Arai, T., Satomura, K., et al.: New percutaneous transluminal coronary angioscope. J. Am. Coll. Cardiol. 13:363, 1989.

201. White, C., Ramee, S., Collins, T., et al.: Percutaneous angioscopy of saphenous vein coronary bypass grafts. J. Am. Coll. Cardiol. 21:1180, 1993.

202. Ramee, S., White, C., Collins, T., et al.: Percutaneous angioscopy during coronary angioplasty using a steerable microangioscope. J. Am. Coll. Cardiol. 17:100, 1991.

203. Mizuno, K., Satomura, K., Miyamoto, A., et al.: Angioscopic evaluation of coronary-artery thrombi in acute coronary syndromes. N. Engl. J. Med. 326:287, 1992.

204. Strumpf, R., Heuser, R., and Eagan, J.: Angioscopy: A valuable tool in the deployment and evaluation of intracoronary stents. Am. Heart J. 126:1204, 1993.

205. Hofling, A., Polnitz, A., Bauriedel, G., et al.: Use of angioscopy to assess the results of percutaneous atherectomy. Am. J. Cardiac Imaging 3:20, 1989.

206. Donohue, T. J., Kern, M. J., Aguirre, F. V., et al.: Assessing the hemodynamic significance of coronary artery stenoses: Analysis of translesional pressure-flow velocity relations in patients. J. Am. Coll. Cardiol. 22:449, 1993.

NONCORONARY ARTERIAL REVASCULARIZATION

207. Becker, G. J., Katzen, B. T., and Dake, M. D.: Noncoronary angioplasty. Radiology 170:921, 1989.

208. Wilson, S. E., Wolf, G. L., and Cross, A. P.: Percutaneous transluminal angioplasty versus operation for peripheral arteriosclerosis. J. Vasc. Surg. 9:1, 1989.

209. Morgenstern, B. R., Getrajdman, G. I., Laffey, K. J., et al.: Total occlusions of the femoropopliteal artery: High technical success rate of conventional balloon angioplasty. Radiology 172:937, 1989.

210. Capek, P., McLean, G. K., and Berkowitz, H. D.: Femoropopliteal angioplasty: Factors influencing long-term success. Circulation 83:I-70, 1991.

211. Miller, G. A., Ford, K. K., Braun, S. D., et al.: Percutaneous transluminal angioplasty vs surgery for renovascular hypertension. Am. J. Roentgenol. 144:447, 1985.

212. Kachel, R., Basche, S., Heerklotz, I., et al.: Percutaneous transluminal angioplasty (PTA) of supra-aortic arteries, especially the internal carotid artery. Neuroradiology 33:191, 1991.

213. Palmaz, J. C., Laborde, J. C., Rivera, F. J., et al.: Stenting of the iliac arteries with the Palmaz stent: Experience from a multicenter trial. Cardiovasc. Intervent. Radiol. 15:291, 1992.

214. Joffre, F., Rousseau, H., Bernadet, P., et al.: Midterm results of renal artery stenting. Cardiovasc. Intervent. Radiol. 15:313, 1992.

215. Dake, M. D., Miller, D. C., Semba, C. P., et al.: Transluminal placement of endovascular stent-grafts for the treatment of descending thoracic aortic aneurysms. N. Engl. J. Med. 331:1729, 1994.

PERCUTANEOUS BALLOON VALVULOPLASTY

216. Safian, R. D., Berman, A. D., Diver, D. J., et al.: Balloon aortic valvuloplasty in 170 consecutive patients. N. Engl. J. Med. 319:125, 1988.

217. Block, P. C., and Palacios, I. F.: Clinical and hemodynamic follow-up after percutaneous aortic valvuloplasty in the elderly. Am. J. Cardiol. 62:760, 1988.

218. Palacios, I. F.: Aortic and mitral balloon valvuloplasty: The United States experience. In Topol, E. J. (ed.): Textbook of Interventional Cardiology. Philadelphia, W. B. Saunders Company, 1994, p. 1189.

219. Lewin, R. F., Dorros, G., King, J. F., and Mathiak, L.: Percutaneous transluminal aortic valvuloplasty: Acute outcome and follow-up of 125 patients. J. Am. Coll. Cardiol. 14:1210, 1989.

220. Reyes, V. P., Raju, B. S., Wynne, J., et al.: Percutaneous balloon valvuloplasty compared with open surgical commissurotomy for mitral stenosis. N. Engl. J. Med. 331:961, 1994.

221. Block, P. C., and Palacios, I. F.: Aortic and mitral valvuloplasty: The United States experience. In Topol, E. J. (ed.): Textbook of Interventional Cardiology. Philadelphia, W. B. Saunders Company, 1994, p. 1189.

222. Wilkins, G. T., Weyman, A. E., Abascal, V. M., et al.: Percutaneous mitral valvotomy: An analysis of echocardiographic variables related to outcome and the mechanism of dilatation. Br. Heart J. 60:299, 1988.

INTERVENTIONS FOR CONGENITAL HEART DISEASE

223. Kan, J. S., White, R. I. J., Mitchell, S. E., and Gardner, T. J.: Percutaneous balloon valvuloplasty: A new method for treating congenital pulmonary valve stenosis. N. Engl. J. Med. 307:540, 1982.

224. Stanger, P., Cassidy, S. C., Girod, D. A., et al.: Balloon pulmonary valvuloplasty: Results of the valvuloplasty and angioplasty of congenital anomalies registry. Am. J. Cardiol. 65:775, 1990.

225. McCrindle, B. W., and Kan, J. S.: Long-term results after balloon pulmonary valvuloplasty. Circulation 83:1915, 1991.

226. O'Connor, B. K., Beekman, R. H., Lindauer, A., and Rocchini, A.: Intermediate-term outcome after pulmonary balloon valvuloplasty: Comparison to a matched surgical control group. J. Am. Coll. Cardiol. 20:169, 1992.

227. O'Connor, B. K., Beekman, R. H., Rocchini, A. P., and Rosenthal, A.: Intermediate-term effectiveness of balloon valvuloplasty for congenital aortic stenosis: A prospective follow-up study. Circulation 84:732, 1991.

228. Kan, J. S., Marvin, W. J., Bass, J. L., et al.: Balloon angioplasty for branch pulmonary artery stenosis. Results from the valvuloplasty and angioplasty of congenital anomalies registry. Am. J. Cardiol. 65:798, 1990.

229. O'Laughlin, M. P., Perry, S. B., Lock, J. E., and Mullins, C. E.: Use of endovascular stents in congenital heart disease. Circulation 83:1923, 1991.

230. Lloyd, T. R., Mendelsohn, A. M., Beekman, R. H., et al.: Atrial septal occlusion with the buttoned device: Early FDA trial results. Circulation 86(Abs.):I-633, 1992.

231. Latson, L. A., Benson, L. N., Hellenbrand, W. E., et al.: Transcatheter closure of ASD—early results of multicenter trial of the Bard clamshell septal occluder. Circulation 84(Abs.):II-544, 1991.

232. Latson, L. A.: Residual shunts after transcatheter closure of patent ductus arteriosus: A major concern of benign "technomalady"? Circulation 84:2591, 1991.

QUALITY OF CARE AND CREDENTIALING

233. ACC Survey: American College of Cardiology Fellowship and Members. On file, Heart House, Bethesda, Maryland, 1991.

234. Hilborne, L. H., Leape, L. L., Bernstein, S. J., et al.: The appropriateness of use of percutaneous transluminal coronary angioplasty in New York state. JAMA 269:761, 1993.

235. Leape, L. L., Hilborne, L. H., Park, R. E., et al.: The appropriateness of use of coronary artery bypass graft surgery in New York state. JAMA 269:753, 1993.

236. Topol, E. J., and Califf, R. M.: Scorecard cardiovascular medicine. Its impact and future directions. Ann. Intern. Med. 120:65, 1994.

237. Jollis, J. G., Peterson, E. D., DeLong, E. R., et al.: The relation between the volume of coronary angioplasty procedures at hospitals treating medicare beneficiaries and short-term mortality. N. Engl. J. Med. 331:1625, 1994.

238. Ritchie, J. L., Phillips, K. A., and Luft, H. S.: Coronary angioplasty. Statewide experience in California. Circulation 88:2735, 1993.

Chapter 40
Rehabilitation of Patients With Coronary Artery Disease

CHARLES DENNIS

Cardiac rehabilitation is traditionally provided to low-risk patients with coronary artery disease. The rapid evolution of management of coronary disease has changed the process of rehabilitation. Aggressive medical and revascularization therapies are now delivered earlier in the course of illness. Physical disability is less common in patients with uncomplicated coronary disease. Changes in diet and life style in combination with drug therapy slow progression or cause regression of coronary atherosclerosis. Higher-risk subsets of patients, such as those with congestive heart failure, benefit from modified programs of physical training. Although the scope of services has increased, only a minority of patients who might benefit from cardiac rehabilitation actually receive it.[1]

Cardiac rehabilitation has both short- and long-term goals. The former include physical reconditioning sufficient for the resumption of customary activities, education of patients and family about the disease process, and psychological support during the early recovery phase of the illness. The latter include identifying and treating risk factors that influence the progression of disease, teaching and reinforcing the health behaviors that improve prognosis, optimizing physical conditioning, and facilitating a return to occupational and avocational activities. Cardiac rehabilitation must be both comprehensive and individualized. The most important factors to consider when developing a program of rehabilitation are severity of disease, medical and surgical therapy, risk factors, physical condition, vocational status, and emotional state.

EXERCISE IN CARDIAC REHABILITATION

Physical Conditioning

FACTORS INFLUENCING PHYSICAL CAPACITY. Peak exercise capacity is defined as the maximal ability of the cardiovascular system to deliver oxygen to exercising skeletal muscle and of the ability of exercising muscle to extract oxygen from the blood. The most accurate measure of exercise capacity is the maximal oxygen uptake ($\dot{V}O_{2\,max}$), representing the liters of oxygen transported from the lungs per minute and used by skeletal muscle at peak effort (see also Fig. 5-1, p. 154 and 14-29, p. 440). Because measurement of $\dot{V}O_{2\,max}$ is cumbersome, multiples of resting oxygen consumption (METs) are used clinically in most uncomplicated cases. One MET equals 3.5 ml oxygen uptake/kg body weight/min, representing the approximate metabolic cost to stand quietly. Exercise tests are calibrated to approximate MET requirements at each stage, although treadmill testing usually overestimates the $\dot{V}O_{2\,max}$ for cardiac patients.[2] Complicated cases, such as patients with congestive heart failure, can be assessed more accurately using cardiopulmonary stress testing.[3–5]

The degree of physical incapacity following a cardiac event is related to several factors: physical capacity prior to the event; treatments such as bed rest and medications; intravascular volume depletion; left ventricular dysfunction; residual myocardial ischemia; age; autonomic function; skeletal muscle performance; peripheral vascular abnormalities; respiratory function; other noncardiac medical problems; and symptoms experienced by the patient during physical activity. Distinguishing the influence of each factor can be difficult, but recognizing their potential effects on physical capacity is paramount to minimizing iatrogenic effects and developing a conditioning program.

IATROGENIC AND PHYSIOLOGICAL FACTORS. Early mobilization and shorter hospitalizations have become standard care for coronary disease. Bed rest remains the most important iatrogenic cause of physical deconditioning. Left ventricular dysfunction is the most important physiological cause. Deconditioning, caused by bed rest or secondary to left ventricular dysfunction, shares some features. Sympathetic hyperactivity with concomitant diminished parasympathetic tone, and decreased skeletal muscle fiber size and oxidative enzyme content are common to both processes.[6] Pulmonary function abnormalities, such as diminished lung volumes and vital capacity and increased respiratory exchange ratio, occur in both.[7] Clinical manifestations are similar in both, including intolerance to exercise, postural hypotension, resting tachycardia, and diminished capacity for exercise.[8] Vigorous exercise training in the supine position fails to prevent the deterioration in upright exercise capacity.[9] As little as 3 hours of daily upright posture significantly diminishes the deconditioning effects of bed rest.[8] However, even limited bed rest will cause some decrement in $\dot{V}O_{2\,max}$.

Chronotropic incompetence, the inability to achieve the age-predicted maximal heart rate response to exercise, is common in patients with coronary disease.[10] The cause is not clearly defined but appears to be related to a loss of normal vagal reflexes during exercise.[11] Peak heart rate can decrease by as much as 25 percent in the first few weeks after myocardial infarction. Because heart rate is quantitatively the most important contributor to cardiac output, chronotropic incompetence is an important predictor of intolerance to exercise.[12] Chronotropic incompetence improves spontaneously over the first 3 to 8 weeks following myocardial infarction, leading to increases in $\dot{V}O_{2\,max}$, even in the absence of formal exercise training.[13]

LEFT VENTRICULAR DYSFUNCTION. Some physiological changes related to left ventricular dysfunction differ from those caused by bed rest. Skeletal muscle fiber type and distribution are altered in the former,[14] whereas leg blood flow is reduced and leg vascular tone is increased.[15] Higher rates of lactate production and reduced consumption of skeletal muscle oxygen occur despite heightened oxygen extraction, supporting the hypothesis that skeletal muscle hypoperfusion is a primary cause of intolerance to exercise in patients with left ventricular dysfunction[15] (Fig. 40-1).

These differences explain, in part, the longstanding observations that most measures of ventricular performance at rest and with exercise correlate poorly with exercise capacity, including left ventricular end-diastolic dimension, velocity of circumferential fiber shortening, systolic time intervals, and ejection fraction.[16] In addition, the results of exercise testing do not predict an individual patient's potential for an exercise training effect.[17] However, central hemodynamic factors beyond ventricular performance negatively influence peak exercise cardiac output, including diminished exercise stroke volume, impaired diastolic relaxation, pulmonary hypoperfusion, and mitral regurgita-

tion. The relative role of each has not been defined, but all are associated with lower $\dot{V}O_{2\,max}$.[18]

MYOCARDIAL ISCHEMIA. If large areas of myocardium become ischemic with exercise, patients may be limited by symptoms of angina, dyspnea, or fatigue. Dyspnea and fatigue in the absence of angina may reflect fixed left ventricular dysfunction or exercise-induced ischemic left ventricular dysfunction, leading to elevated pulmonary vascular pressures or inadequate cardiac output. Angina may also limit exercise performance in the absence of exercise-induced left ventricular dysfunction. Because angina is perceived differently, the same degree of myocardial ischemia may limit some patients and be tolerated by others.[19] Amelioration of symptomatic and asymptomatic ischemia by medication may improve capacity for exercise and myocar-

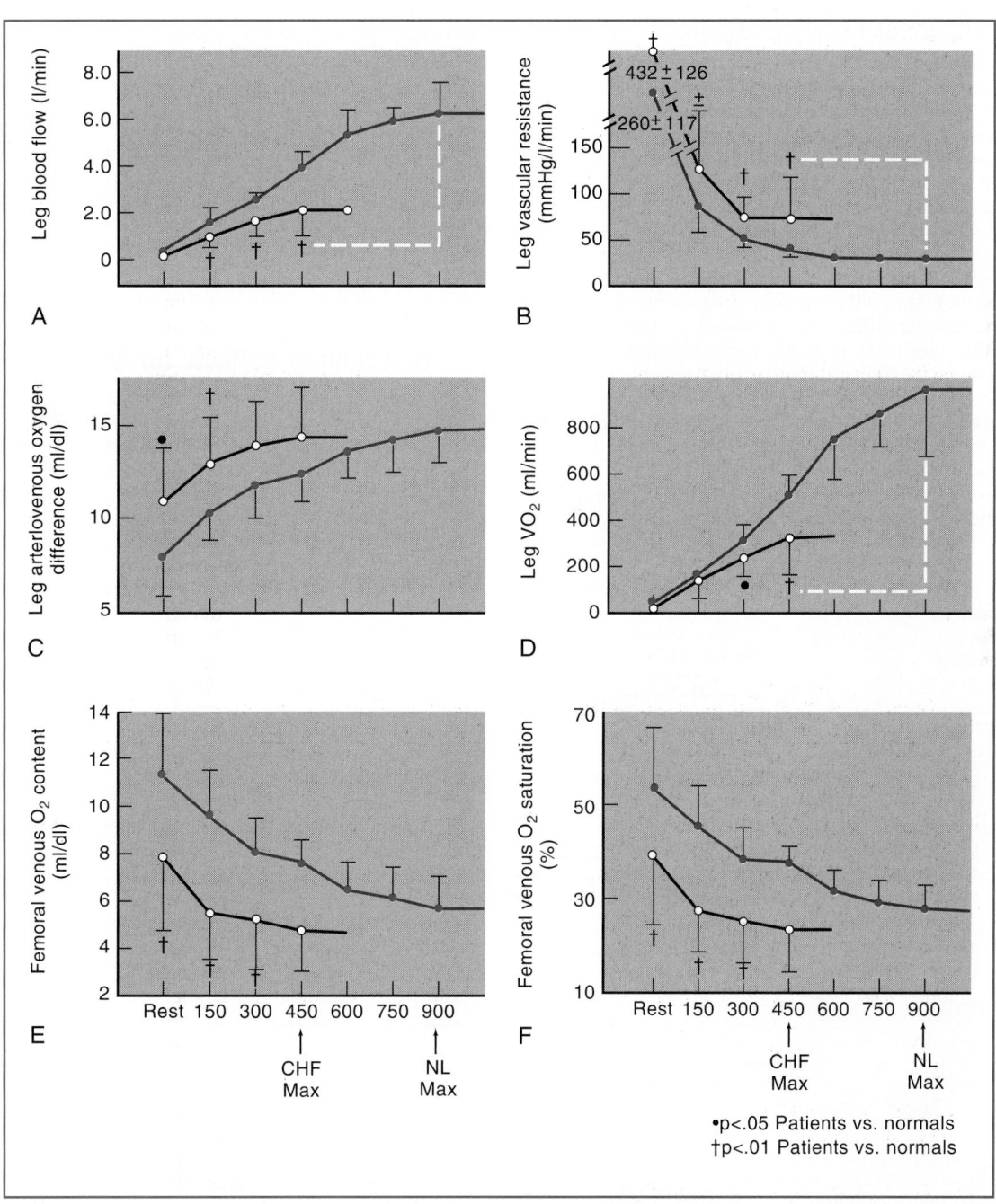

FIGURE 40–1. Resting and exercise single leg blood flow, leg vascular resistance, single leg VO₂, femoral venous O₂ content, and femoral venous O₂ saturation in patients with chronic heart failure (n = 30) (○) and normal subjects (n = 12) (·); *p < 0.05, †p < 0.01, patients versus normal subjects. Dashed lines indicate intergroup comparisons of maximal data. (Reproduced with permission from Sullivan, M. J., Knight, D. J., Higginbotham, M. B., and Cobb, F. R.: Relation between central and peripheral hemodynamics during exercise in patients with chronic heart failure: muscle blood flow is reduced with maintenance of arterial perfusion pressure. Circulation 80:769, 1989. Copyright American Heart Association.)

dial perfusion even in the absence of formal exercise training.[19,20]

OTHER FACTORS. Concomitant illnesses, such as chronic obstructive pulmonary disease and peripheral vascular disease, can limit the capacity for exercise before the effects of ischemia or left ventricular dysfunction are manifested. The common cardiovascular drugs, including nitrates, beta blockers, and calcium channel blockers, increase the exercise capacity by increasing coronary blood flow, decreasing myocardial oxygen demand, or improving hemodynamics during exercise.[21–23] Angiotensin-converting enzyme inhibitors appear to be particularly beneficial for increasing capacity for exercise in patients with congestive heart failure, probably because of their effects on peripheral circulation.[24–26]

Effects of Exercise Training

SKELETAL MUSCLE. The primary physiological improvements from exercise training are on skeletal muscle performance and are directly related to increases in capillary density, oxidative enzyme content, myoglobin concentration,[6,14] and increased numbers and size of mitochondria.[27] These changes increase skeletal muscle perfusion and the efficiency of extraction of oxygen.

MYOCARDIAL PERFORMANCE. Current evidence suggests that myocardial performance may improve in patients with coronary disease subjected to training programs that are either of a higher intensity, greater frequency, or longer duration than those traditionally provided in cardiac rehabilitation.[28,29] In contrast to low- and moderate-intensity programs, patients in high-intensity programs have shown improvements in myocardial oxygenation using electrocardiographic and perfusion measures.[29,30] The minimal intensity, frequency, and duration required for such effects have not been established.

Exercise training lowers heart rate and blood pressure at rest and, at submaximal exercise, increases peak MET capacity and increases both endurance and strength. The lower the initial MET capacity, the greater the benefit in most patients.[31,32] Patients with a combination of myocardial ischemia and resting left ventricular dysfunction are less likely to benefit from short-term exercise training.[33] Treatment with beta blockers does not prevent a training effect in patients with coronary heart disease although the training effect may be blunted.[22] Other benefits of exercise, include reduction of weight, improved glucose tolerance in patients with diabetes, raised high-density lipoprotein (HDL) cholesterol levels, and psychological benefits including a greater confidence to resume customary activities more quickly.[31,34]

MORBIDITY AND MORTALITY. Exercise training has not been definitively shown to improve morbidity and mortality in patients with coronary heart disease. Only one of 22 randomized trials of cardiac rehabilitation with exercise training demonstrated a statistically significant cardiovascular mortality benefit.[35] However, all other studies were limited by inadequate sample size, short follow-up or crossovers after randomization. Two meta-analyses showed that overall mortality and cardiovascular mortality, defined as fatal reinfarction or sudden death, were reduced by 20 per cent to 25 per cent in patients randomized to exercise training. Rates of nonfatal reinfarction were similar in exercise and control groups[36,37] (Fig. 40–2). The magnitude of benefit is similar to that seen in the randomized trials of prophylactic beta blockade after myocardial infarction,[38] suggesting that exercise training may be equally beneficial.

Selection of Patients for Exercise Testing and Training

PATIENTS ELIGIBLE FOR EXERCISE TRAINING. The indications for exercise training have been expanded to include higher-risk patients in recent years. The safety and efficacy of training in patients previously considered to be at high risk, particularly those with congestive heart failure, has

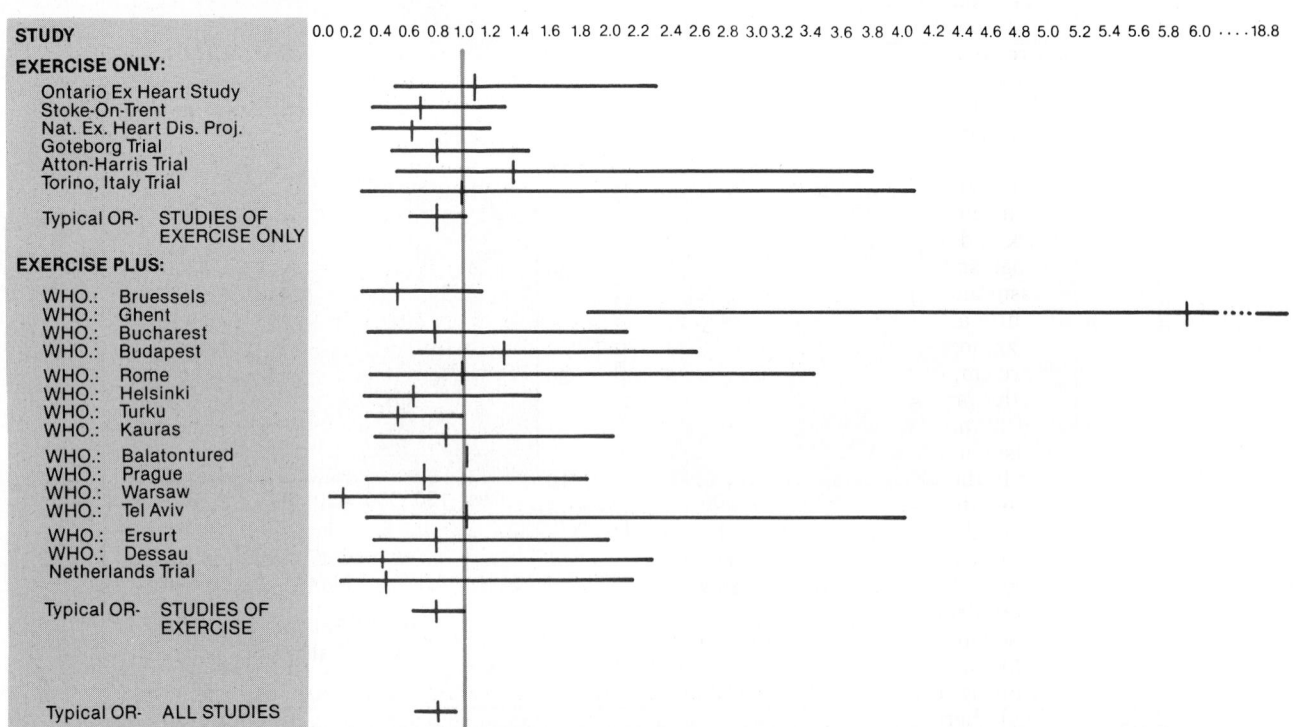

FIGURE 40–2. Chart of effects of pooling from randomized trials of cardiac rehabilitation on the estimate of mortality 3 years after randomization. Short vertical lines indicate the point estimates; horizontal lines depict the 95 per cent confidence intervals. "Exercise Plus" usually refers to life style and dietary modifications in both the exercise and control groups. (Reproduced with permission from O'Connor, G. T., Buring, J. E., Yusuf, S., et al.: An overview of randomized trials of rehabilitation with exercise after myocardial infarction. Circulation *80*:234, 1989. Copyright American Heart Association.)

been demonstrated. Exercise training benefits patients recovering from myocardial infarction, coronary artery bypass graft surgery, coronary angioplasty, valve surgery and cardiac transplantation, and those with stable angina and compensated congestive heart failure.[31,34,39,40] Prescription for exercise should be based upon the results of exercise tests. Cardiopulmonary stress testing may provide additional information helpful for prescribing exercise training in patients with congestive heart failure.[27,41] Patients ineligible for exercise testing because of severe angina, uncompensated congestive heart failure, and uncontrolled arrhythmias are not candidates for exercise training. Other limiting noncardiac illnesses such as chronic obstructive pulmonary disease, peripheral vascular disease, stroke, and orthopedic disease do not necessarily obviate exercise testing and training because specialized techniques, such as arm-crank ergometry, can be used.[42]

EXERCISE TESTING. Exercise testing to a symptom or sign limit should be performed as soon after a cardiac event as the patient's condition permits. In uncomplicated cases, testing can be performed 7 to 21 days after myocardial infarction,[43] 3 to 10 days following coronary angioplasty,[44] and 14 to 28 days following cardiac surgery. Exercise testing is performed later in patients who have undergone cardiac surgery to minimize the detrimental effects of wound healing and pulmonary dysfunction on performance of exercise.

Submaximal exercise testing is commonly used prior to or soon after discharge from hospital because of the perceived safety of such testing compared with maximal testing (see also Chap. 5). Maximal testing is then performed at 6 to 8 weeks following discharge from hospital. However, there is no evidence that submaximal testing is safer than symptom-limited testing in properly selected patients,[43] and there are disadvantages to submaximal testing. Prognostically important signs of myocardial ischemia, left ventricular dysfunction and arrhythmias, may not be elicited by submaximal testing. Patients may be inappropriately limited in their customary activities and in exercise training if submaximal testing is used to evaluate physical capacity.[45,46] Return to work may be significantly delayed.[47,48]

Because capacity for exercise is reduced in patients recovering from a cardiac event, a modified treadmill protocol should be used. Table 40-1 compares the standard Bruce protocol with a modified Naughton protocol. The Bruce protocol increases by 2 to 3 METs at each stage and quickly surpasses the average capacity of patients recovering from a cardiac event. The modified Naughton protocol starts at a lower MET workload and increases at 1-MET increments. This gradual progression is better tolerated and provides a more accurate assessment of MET capacity. The usual symptomatic endpoints are dyspnea and fatigue, whereas moderate angina, dizziness, and claudication occur less commonly. Signs that are important endpoints include high-grade ventricular arrhythmias (such as triplets), a fall in systolic blood pressure of 20 mm Hg compared with the previous stage, and marked ischemia.

Although the exercise test is the basis of the prescription for exercise, certain test results contraindicate exercise training. Severe exercise-induced ischemia, arrhythmias, or left ventricular dysfunction must be corrected before patients can be allowed to exercise. Exercise testing should be repeated after treatment to confirm that the abnormalities, in fact, have resolved. Less severe abnormalities that occur at high heart rates and workloads are not necessarily contraindications to exercise training, especially if patients are being given maximal medical therapy, and no other treatment options are available. In some instances, the exercise prescription is modified as discussed below, and more intensive surveillance is used during exercise training. The advisability of early testing and training after anterior myocardial infarction has been questioned because of experimental and clinical evidence showing formation of abnor-

TABLE 40–1 COMPARISON OF THE MODIFIED NAUGHTON AND BRUCE PROTOCOLS FOR TREADMILL EXERCISE TESTING

Min	METs	MODIFIED NAUGHTON Stage	Speed (mph)	Grade (%)	BRUCE Stage	Speed (mph)	Grade (%)
3	3	1	2.0	3.5			
3	4	2	2.0	7.0			
3	5	3	2.0	10.5	1	1.7	10.0
3	6	4	2.0	14.0			
3	7	5	2.0	17.5	2	2.5	12.0
3	8	6	3.0	12.5			
3	9	7	3.0	15.0			
3	10	8	3.0	17.0	3	3.4	14.0

mal myocardial scars.[49,50] However, evaluation of patients recovering from anterior myocardial infarction found that moderate exercise training was not associated with worsening left ventricular topography or function.[51]

The prognostic value of exercise testing after myocardial infarction has been questioned.[45,52] For purposes of rehabilitation, the absence of exercise-induced ischemic abnormalities with preserved exercise capability identifies a group of patients at very low risk for a recurrent cardiac event, irrespective of the use of a thrombolytic agent at the time of infarction.[53,54] Issues related to exercise testing are more completely developed in Chapter 5.

Exercise Prescription

INDIVIDUALIZED PRESCRIPTION IN UNCOMPLICATED CASES. The exercise prescription is individualized, based on the results of the symptom-limited exercise test. The components of the prescription are summarized by the acronym *FIT*: *f*requency, *i*ntensity, and *t*ime. The minimum frequency needed to improve cardiovascular fitness is three times weekly. Intensity is most easily prescribed as a target heart rate. The time or duration of exercise is usually 30 to 60 minutes for each session but is also individually determined. Thresholds for frequency, intensity, and duration have not been established, and the guidelines suggested reflect recommendations of national organizations.[31,32,34,39,55] Modifications of the prescription for complicated cases are described below.

The conditioning effect is a balance between the intensity and duration of exercise. The intensity of exercise is based upon the peak heart rate achieved during exercise testing. A low intensity is prescribed initially to allow the patient to complete 1-hour sessions without excessive fatigue. A target heart rate of 65 per cent of peak heart rate is a common starting point. In some instances, especially after cardiac surgery, the resting pulse is high, and 65 per cent of the peak heart rate places the target rate near the resting pulse. In those cases, a slightly higher initial target of 75 per cent may be used. Alternatively, 40 to 50 per cent of the difference between the peak and the resting heart rate may be calculated and added to the resting pulse to determine the target. For convenience, the target is given as a 10-second count.

COMPONENTS OF EXERCISE SESSIONS. Exercise sessions, whether performed individually or in a group, should last 1 hour. Each session includes a warm-up period, a period of aerobic and muscular conditioning, and a cool-down period. A 10-minute warm-up includes stretching and light calisthenics to prevent musculoskeletal injury and gradually increase the heart rate. A 40-minute conditioning period is best spent in aerobic exercise, such as walking, jogging, and bicycling, during the first several weeks of training. Swimming is excellent aerobic exercise but creates problems with surveillance, pulse monitoring, and response in the event of a cardiovascular emergency. The exercise session is concluded with a 10-minute cool-down using stretching exercises similar to those in the warm-up period. This is especially important for coronary patients in whom ventricular arrhythmias are commonly precipitated by the abrupt cessation of moderate or high-intensity exercise.[56,57]

Aerobic conditioning, rather than strength training, is emphasized in the first several weeks of exercise training. Arm training, especially isometric exercise, is usually proscribed in the early training period because it causes a disproportionate increase in blood pressure compared with heart rate[58] and may compromise sternal wound healing in the first 4 to 6 weeks after cardiac surgery. Standard exercise programs emphasizing dynamic leg training by walking, jogging, and bicycling also increase arm strength and endurance even without specific arm training.[59] If arm and shoulder strength training is important, patients can begin using light hand weights during walk-jog exercises early in the exercise program. Circuit and strength training emphasizing muscular conditioning in both upper and lower extremities may be advantageous to some patients later in their training program.[60–63] This is especially true of patients who perform a significant amount of upper extremity work in their jobs.

ADVANCING THE PRESCRIPTION. The Borg scale of rate of perceived exertion (RPE)[64] is a useful tool for advancing the exercise prescription during training. As shown in Table 40-2, the RPE scale gives a numeric value to a perceived level of exertion. Patients should exercise at an RPE of 13 to 15. As patients become more fit, the RPE will fall, and the intensity of exercise may then be increased. The target is usually increased by 5 per cent to 10 per cent of the peak heart rate. Ultimately, patients should be able to exercise at 85 per cent of their peak heart rate for the entire session, and most patients reach this intensity within eight to 12 sessions.

Follow-up treadmill testing should be performed 4 to 8 weeks after beginning training. Many patients will achieve significantly higher heart rates on subsequent testing. Higher achieved heart rates are related to improvements in chronotropic competence in some patients and the ability to achieve a maximal cardiovascular effort in others previously limited by severe skeletal muscle deconditioning.[13] The follow-up treadmill test can be used to advance the exercise prescription for most patients and to allow some to graduate to lower levels of surveillance during exercise.

PATIENTS WITH MYOCARDIAL ISCHEMIA. Patients with exercise-induced myocardial ischemia should receive optimal therapy to eliminate or ameliorate the problem. Some patients will still show evidence of ischemia. Assuming that ischemia does not occur at extremely low workloads, these patients may still exercise safely as long as their target heart rate remains well below that at which ischemia occurs.[65] Limiting the maximal target heart rate to 10 beats/min below that at which ischemic abnormalities occur is clinically useful. Increased surveillance during exercise, such as with continuous electrocardiographic monitoring, is also recommended in the initial stages of exercise training.[31,34,39]

PATIENTS WITH HEART FAILURE. These patients are at higher risk for complications related to exercise but also tend to have the most significant improvements from exercise training. Supervised exercise training has been shown to be safe in patients with heart failure.[3,27,66,67] The exercise prescription often must be modified for patients with heart failure because of their limited endurance. Shorter periods of aerobic training, lower target heart rates, and intermittent rest periods can all be used to limit the degree of fatigue felt by these patients.[27] The ultimate target heart rate should also be kept 10 beats/min below that at which significant symptoms of dyspnea and fatigue occur on exercise testing.

In patients with heart failure, the presence of inducible ischemia generally predicts a poor response to exercise training. These patients are less likely to show a training effect with the usual duration of training[19,65] and are more likely to have complications related to coronary disease during follow-up.[4,65]

PATIENTS WITH ARRHYTHMIAS. These patients present a significant challenge to the clinician because of controversies regarding therapy and the uncertainty of the safety of exercise. No definitive data are available regarding the safety of exercise in patients with arrhythmias. Patients with exercise-induced ventricular arrhythmias and coronary disease are at high risk for both fatal events and nonfatal ischemic complications.[56] The usual clinical approach in cardiac rehabilitation is to exclude patients with severe exercise-induced arrhythmias from exercise training until suppression of the arrhythmia has been achieved. Higher levels of surveillance are recommended during exercise using continuous electrocardiographic monitoring. It is unknown whether exercise training affects arrhythmias.[68] One study has shown a reduction in ventricular arrhythmia frequency with training, perhaps due to modulation of sympathetic response during exercise.[69] Stable patterns of arrhythmia during electrocardiogram-monitored exercise training are often used as evidence to allow patients to begin supervised, unmonitored exercise. However, the safety of this approach has not been documented.

Risks of Exercise Training

Exercise training is not without risks. The greatest risk lies in patients with untreated or unrecognized left ventricular dysfunction, myocardial ischemia, and ventricular arrhythmias. In patients receiving optimal therapy, the greatest risk lies in exercising at or above the level at which the abnormalities can be elicited by exercise testing.[70] For this reason, the maximum target heart rate used in exercise training must be lower than the heart rate at which abnormalities become evident on testing.

PATIENT SELECTION AND SURVEILLANCE. Safe exercise training is best assured by proper selection of patients and adequate surveillance during exercise. Guidelines to stratify risk of exercise training have been published by several professional organizations.[31,39,40,55] Patients at high risk for cardiovascular complications during exercise have one or more of the characteristics listed in Table 40-3.[39,71] Every attempt should be made to ameliorate or correct high-risk conditions before recommending exercise. If the abnormality cannot be corrected, the risks and benefits of exercise training should be carefully considered and the highest level of surveillance during exercise recommended. Patients in whom the risks of exercise outweigh the benefits despite optimal medical therapy should be informed of the risks and counseled not to exercise. Because the natural history of conditions such as congestive heart failure limits

TABLE 40–2 BORG SCALE OF RATE OF PERCEIVED EXERTION (RPE)

	6
Very, very light	7
	8
Very light	9
	10
Light	11
	12
Somewhat hard	13
	14
Hard	15
	16
Very hard	17
	18
Very, very hard	19
	20

From Borg, G.: Perceived exertion as an indicator of somatic stress. Scand. J. Rehabil. Med. *2:*92, 1970.

TABLE 40–3 INDICATIONS FOR CONTINUOUS ELECTROCARDIOGRAPHIC MONITORING DURING EXERCISE TRAINING

CLINICAL INDICATION	OBJECTIVE SIGNS

Severe left ventricular dysfunction
    Congestive heart failure
    History of cardiogenic shock
	Ejection fraction <30%

Severe exercise-induced ischemia	ST-segment depression ≥ 0.2 mV Angina at a workload ≤ 5 METs Multiple perfusion defects (Exercise nuclear study) Multiple dyskinetic segments (Exercise echocardiography study)

Complex ventricular arrhythmia
    (at rest or exercise-induced)
    Previous cardiac arrest
	Nonsustained ventricular tachycardia

Hypotensive response to exercise	Systolic drop of 20 mm Hg or more at increasing load
Low functional capacity Inability to self-monitor heart rate	Peak workload ≤ 5 METs

prognosis, patients and physicians should be aware of the need for close medical follow-up beyond that available in supervised exercise programs.

The highest level of surveillance is supervised group exercise with continuous electrocardiographic monitoring. Approximately 15 per cent to 25 per cent of patients eligible for exercise training have one or more of the characteristics in Table 40–3 and require continuous electrocardiographic monitoring.[31,34,39] The next level of surveillance is unmonitored group exercise training supervised by health professionals with advanced cardiac life-support certification. Patients without high-risk characteristics, and those who improve during electrocardiogram-monitored training can participate in supervised, unmonitored group training.[72] Very low-risk patients can safely exercise independently after learning the principles of pulse monitoring and recognition of symptoms. In general, low-risk patients have an exercise capacity of eight METs or more without symptoms or signs of left ventricular dysfunction, myocardial ischemia, or ventricular arrhythmias. These criteria may be used to graduate patients from supervised programs.[73]

All patients should be taught to monitor their pulse and recognize symptoms during exercise. The concepts of the target heart rate and RPE are conveyed and reinforced during group exercise sessions. These principles and concepts guide patients in independent, safe, and effective exercise after completion of a formal exercise program. Patients who are unable or unwilling to follow the exercise prescription should receive higher levels of surveillance.

SAFETY OF SUPERVISED PROGRAMS. Despite the potential for cardiovascular complications during exercise, supervised programs have an extremely good safety record. In a survey of 167 programs, the incidence rate per million patient hours of exercise for fatal events was 1.3, for myocardial infarction 3.4, and for resuscitated cardiac arrests 8.9. There were no significant differences in rates for continuous electrocardiogram-monitored compared with intermittently monitored programs.[71] The event rates in this study were significantly lower than in a survey performed a decade earlier[74] and were reconfirmed in a more recent study.[75] The reasons for improvement are speculative. Improved risk stratification, improved revascularization and medical therapies, more rigorous standards for cardiac rehabilitation programs, and increased awareness of the necessity of monitoring high-risk patients may have contributed to the improved safety record.

Comprehensive cardiac rehabilitation includes an aggressive approach to treatment of risk factors. Lipid lowering is discussed in Chapter 35, treatment of hypertension in Chapter 27, and control of diabetes mellitus in Chapter 61. In this chapter, attention is directed on cessation of cigarette smoking in secondary prevention.

RISKS. Cigarette smoking is an established risk factor for the development of angina and myocardial infarction[76] and increases the risk for recurrent infarction and death.[77] Survivors of myocardial infarction who continue to smoke have twice the rate of recurrent infarction and cardiac death compared with patients who quit smoking. The risk of a second cardiac event declines rapidly after cessation of smoking. Within 3 years of myocardial infarction, former smokers have approximately the same risk for reinfarction as survivors of myocardial infarction who never smoked.[78,79] Patients who continue to smoke after coronary bypass surgery have two to six times the expected mortality compared with nonsmokers or those who quit smoking after surgery.[80,81]

PATHOPHYSIOLOGY. The pathophysiology underlying the increased risk for death and reinfarction is uncertain. Platelet aggregation, thrombosis, coronary spasm, and diminished coronary and collateral flow reserve have all been implicated.[76,82,83] Fibrinogen levels are significantly higher in smokers than nonsmokers and increase the primary risk of myocardial infarction.[77] Although the degree of coronary atherosclerosis is not closely correlated with smoking habits, the risk for myocardial infarction in smokers is strongly correlated with the extent of coronary artery disease and plasma cholesterol levels.[84]

ETIOLOGY OF TOBACCO DEPENDENCE. Smoking is a complex behavior with physiological, psychological, and sociological roots. There are several theories regarding the etiology, although no single theory is adequate to explain all aspects of smoking behavior. Physiological dependence on nicotine causes acute craving for cigarettes with abrupt cessation of smoking. Smoking is a habit that appears to minimize negative emotions such as distress, anger, and fear and counteracts feelings of insecurity. It may also be used as a coping mechanism to transfer such negative emotions into a socially acceptable behavior. Finally, a smoking habit may have deep sociological origins such as modeling behavior after parents and peers.[85]

PROGRAMS FOR CESSATION OF SMOKING. Demographic and psychological factors identify patients who are more likely to continue smoking after a cardiac event. Lower occupational and educational levels, smoking of a larger number of cigarettes, increasing age, and higher rates of consumption of alcohol are demographic factors associated with continued smoking.[86] Psychological factors, such as a less negative attitude regarding smoking, higher anxiety levels, and a low sense of personal control over life events, identify those smokers who are less likely to quit after a cardiac event.[76]

Myocardial infarction, coronary surgery, and coronary angioplasty are sufficient impetus to stop smoking in 20 per cent to 60 per cent of patients.[87,88] Patients who receive strong advice to stop smoking from health professionals are more likely to quit and remain abstinent compared with those who do not receive such advice.[89–91] This is particularly true of patients who believe that they are at personal risk if they continue smoking. Unfortunately, high acute rates of cessation are associated with high rates of recidivism in the absence of interventions to maintain abstinence.

Cessation of smoking is facilitated by treating both the physiological and psychological aspects of the habit. Hospital confinement for myocardial infarction or coronary surgery usually provides sufficient time for the physiological manifestations of nicotine withdrawal, such as irritability, emotionality, inability to concentrate, nausea, and headache, to resolve. In patients who continue to crave cigarettes, nicotine dependence is strong, and more gradual nicotine withdrawal may be necessary.[76]

Nicotine withdrawal can be managed by tapering cigarette smoking, gradually changing to lower-nicotine cigarettes, or using nicotine-replacement therapy. Transdermal nicotine patches and oral nicotine polacrilex raise serum nicotine levels to 30 per cent to 60 per cent of the level obtained with cigarette smoking[92,93] which is sufficient to significantly blunt the craving for cigarettes.[94,95] Smokers using nicotine replacement therapy are twice as likely to be abstinent from cigarettes 1 year following treatment compared with those not using nicotine replacement therapy.[96,97] Although prescription of nicotine polacrilex alone does not decrease the long-term rate of abstinence,[98] there is evidence that transdermal nicotine patches increase rates of abstinence, even in the absence of adjuvant behavioral therapy.[97]

Behavioral therapy, with or without nicotine replacement, increases long-term rates of abstinence. Such therapy can be provided by physicians, nurses, or other trained personnel.[94] Using techniques of self-control or substitution of healthful behaviors for smoking assist the patient in abstinence. Role-playing cigarette refusal and enlisting social support of family, friends, and coworkers reinforces nonsmoking behavior. Long-term rates of abstinence up to 70 per cent have been achieved with formal programs, particularly with patients who have recently diagnosed coronary disease.[99] Behavioral interventions are best targeted to the period immediately after cessation of smoking, as relapse in the first 2 to 3 weeks is highly predictive of continued smoking.[93,99]

PSYCHOLOGICAL FACTORS

COMMON PSYCHIATRIC PROBLEMS. Severe psychological stress or major depression complicate myocardial infarction in approximately 15 per cent of cases and have been associated with significantly higher rates of morbidity and mortality.[100,101] Although most professionals providing cardiac rehabilitation believe that exercise training and related services provide significant psychological benefits, severe stress or major depression require specific therapy. There is evidence that specific therapy for severe stress can influence outcome positively, although comparable data for major depression are lacking.[102] The more common and less disabling problems of delirium in the acute care setting and anxiety and minor depression during early recovery are generally transient and easily treated.[103,104]

SELF-EFFICACY. Acute cardiac illnesses have many psychosocial sequelae including medical restrictions on even the most routine of activities. These restrictions are reinforced by family, friends, and coworkers who perceive a poor prognosis and are concerned that physical and emotional stress can further damage the heart. If patients have a poor understanding of their illness, fear of recurrent cardiac problems leads to a sense of loss of control and a lack of confidence to resume customary activities. This lack of confidence can be a significant impediment to the resumption of a full and active life.

Self-efficacy is a psychological term describing how a person's judgment regarding the capacity for performance of a task or action is an important determinant of whether that person will attempt the task or action.[105] Self-efficacy reflects confidence and is highly predictive of action. Self-efficacy for specific tasks can be rated on 0 to 100 per cent confidence scales. For example, self-efficacy scales have been validated for physical activity that predicts whether a coronary patient will be successful with a regular exercise program.[106–108] The most common areas of low self-efficacy

for coronary patients are physical exertion, emotional stress, and sexual activity.[105]

Self-efficacy can be increased in coronary patients by four methods: persuasion, information, vicarious experience, and enactive techniques. Using exercise as an example, physicians can persuade patients that they are capable of exercising. Patients can be informed about what sensations to expect with exercise, so they do not misread normal physiological responses, such as tachycardia, as grave symptoms. Vicarious experiences can be shared by other patients who have successfully undertaken exercise programs. The most powerful method for increasing exercise self-efficacy is the performance of a supervised exercise test.[105,108]

Self-efficacy is a useful measure for predicting potential success for other important behavioral changes such as cessation of smoking and dietary modification.[108,109] In circumstances of low self-efficacy, informative, persuasive, vicarious and enactive techniques to raise self-efficacy are helpful for increasing the rate of success for behavioral change. Spousal perceptions are equally important. Self-efficacy scales that rate spouses' perceptions of the patients' potential for success with a particular task are also highly predictive of success or failure. Support and encouragement by the spouse in change of behavior are extremely important for success. Spousal self-efficacy can be raised using similar techniques as for patients.[110]

TYPE A BEHAVIOR. Although Type A behavior is recognized as a risk factor for the development of coronary artery disease,[111] its effect on prognosis is unknown. Conflicting results are reported in several studies, although there are limitations in each. The major limitations are the populations studied, the instruments used to classify behavior, the duration of follow-up, and the endpoints studied. One of the most important concepts that has emerged from the Type A controversy is recognition that the construct probably reflects a collection of behaviors, not all of which are related to either the development or prognosis of coronary disease. Of the three primary characteristics of Type A behavior—competitive striving for achievement, time urgency, and hostility—only the latter appears to be independently related to outcomes of coronary disease, but there is continued controversy in this area.[112–114] There is limited evidence that modification of Type A behavior can change prognosis of coronary disease.[115] Further investigation is needed before such therapy can be recommended.

VOCATIONAL REHABILITATION

The cost of cardiovascular disability is high. The direct costs of care for patients with heart disease are estimated at $85 billion annually in the United States.[116] Indirect costs, due to goods and services not provided because of cardiovascular illness, are several times greater. Indirect costs can be significantly reduced by increasing the numbers of patients who return to work and shortening the interval between a cardiac event and return to work.

FACTORS RELATED TO EMPLOYMENT. Employment after a cardiac event is related to demographic, medical, and psychosocial factors. Patients unemployed at the time of a cardiac event, those over the age of 60, and those with blue-collar jobs are significantly less likely to work after the event.[117] Retirement and disability benefits are more easily obtained after age 60, encouraging patients to leave the work force. Blue-collar workers, especially those who are unskilled, are easily replaced in the work force and consequently lose their jobs more commonly after a cardiac event.[118]

After a cardiac event, the medical condition of the patient and the advice provided by the physician regarding return to work are the most important factors influencing the rate of reemployment in previously employed patients.[47,48] In the absence of demographic and psychosocial impediments, the physician must first ensure that the risk of a cardiovascular complication is low and will not be increased by returning to work. The physician must then determine if the patient has the physical capacity to perform occupational work. Finally, the physician must provide explicit advice regarding the timing of return to work and any work restrictions that the patient and employer must follow.

FACILITATING REEMPLOYMENT. In the majority of patients recovering from cardiac surgery and myocardial infarction, a careful clinical evaluation and a symptom-limited treadmill test are sufficient to guide the physician in the return-to-work decision. Accurate methods to stratify the risk of recurrent coronary events rely on clinical information obtained during hospitalization and specialized testing performed during or shortly after hospitalization.[46] More than half of patients surviving myocardial infarction have no symptoms or signs of congestive heart failure or myocardial ischemia. Their risk of cardiac death, myocardial infarction, or unstable angina in the year following the primary event is less than 10 per cent. A symptom-limited exercise capacity on treadmill testing of 7 METs or more without ischemia lowers the risk to under 3 per cent.[119]

The treadmill test also establishes peak physical capacity that can be related to the patient's occupational work. Individuals can sustain 6 to 8 hours of continuous effort at 40 per cent of their peak MET capacity. Continuous tolerance for work declines at higher levels, averaging 4 hours at 60 per cent of peak capacity and 2 hours above 60 per cent of peak capacity.[120] The average job has an energy requirement well under 5 METs, which means that a peak capacity of 7 to 10 METs is sufficient for most individuals to perform their occupational work.[120] There is evidence that with increasing levels of automation, current guidelines overestimate the work requirements for household and occupational activities.[121,122] Only 16 per cent of Americans perform jobs requiring manual labor, and that percentage declines rapidly with age.[123] Most manual labor jobs require only intermittent high-energy expenditure, which significantly prolongs tolerance for work.

Intensive physical reconditioning is not necessary for the average patient to return to work. In patients with very low functional capacity and those with higher occupational physical requirements, an exercise training program can hasten their return to work. Unless the patient's job requires lifting and carrying of moderate to heavy loads, the standard aerobic training previously described is sufficient to expedite return to work. In specialized circumstances, exercise programs that include upper extremity isometric training can be provided. Work simulation and specialized training programs may be helpful in unusual circumstances. In the particular circumstance of jobs affecting public safety, such as with pilots, police, and fire fighters, more stringent requirements regarding return to work are legislated.[124]

The average interval between uncomplicated myocardial infarction and return to work is 70 to 90 days; it averages 15 to 30 days after coronary angioplasty and 50 to 100 days after uncomplicated coronary surgery.[47,117,120] These intervals can be shortened substantially with a coordinated approach using risk stratification, treadmill testing, and explicit physician advice regarding the timing of return to work. In employed patients without high-risk clinical characteristics or severe treadmill ischemia, the time from myocardial infarction was shortened from 75 to 51 days in a randomized trial of an early return-to-work intervention. Recurrent cardiac events averaged 3.5 per cent in the 6 months after infarction and were no higher in patients returning to work earlier compared with those returning to work later.[47] Similar results were obtained in a subsequent study that also demonstrated very low-risk patients without evidence of ischemia on treadmill testing could return to work safely approximately 1 month after myocardial infarction.[48] Although these studies did not include a special program for patients performing manual labor, the intervention was as successful in the 11 to 17 per cent of the population performing manual labor as it was in the sedentary workers. Higher-risk patients with evidence of congestive heart failure or myocardial ischemia accounted for 23 per cent of all employed patients under the age of 60 and were specifically excluded from study. Return-to-work decisions in such patients must be individualized.[47,48]

BENEFITS OF REEMPLOYMENT. The benefits of an early return to work are financial and psychological. In the trial discussed above,[47] patients randomized to the return to work intervention earned $2100 more than patients randomized to usual care in the 6 months following myocardial infarction. Although not specifically examined, financial benefits to employers probably accrued including increased productivity and reduced costs of temporary employees and disability insurance payments.[125] Interventions that increase the numbers of patients returning to work and shorten the interval between the illness and reemployment will have the greatest impact on reducing the economic burden of cardiovascular disability.

⊙ ORGANIZATION OF CARDIAC REHABILITATION SERVICES

For most patients, cardiac rehabilitation begins in the hospital following a cardiac event and continues for several months thereafter. Traditionally, cardiac rehabilitation has been provided in phases with activity guidelines based upon the time from the cardiac event. Although phased rehabilitation provides a framework, individual patients will progress more slowly or quickly depending upon their age, condition prior to their cardiac event, the severity of illness, and motivation. The rehabilitation program should be individualized to facilitate a rate of recovery commensurate with the patient's status.[39]

Inpatient Rehabilitation

Hospitalization has been significantly shortened for patients recovering from myocardial infarction and cardiac surgery. Therefore, inpatient rehabilitation must make patients self-sufficient in the activities of daily living in a short period of time. The behavioral changes required for secondary prevention may be introduced in the hospital but are mainly deferred until patients are at home.

EARLY MOBILIZATION. Early mobilization reduces the detrimental effects of bed rest as discussed previously[7–9] and maximizes the rate at which customary activities can be resumed. In the coronary care unit, assisted range of motion exercises can be initiated in the first 24 to 48 hours for most patients. Patients in stable condition should be encouraged to sit in a chair for increasing periods each day to minimize depletion of intravascular volume, deconditioning of skeletal muscle, and orthopedic impairment. Self-care activities, such as shaving, oral hygiene, and sponge bathing, should be encouraged as soon as the patient's condition is stable.

GRADUATED PHYSICAL ACTIVITY. On transfer of the patient from the intensive care unit, a graduated program of physical and self-care activities can begin. Upright posture should be encouraged as much as tolerated. Patients should walk with assistance at least twice daily. Although some inpatient programs suggest walking specific distances each day, ambulation can be based on the patient's tolerance. In that way, patients are neither pushed beyond their tolerance nor held back in their recovery. The target heart rate and RPE scale can be used to individualize the intensity and time of activity. For each session, standing heart rate and blood pressure are obtained, followed by 5 minutes of range of motion and flexibility exercises. Patients are then assisted with walking at a rate that keeps the pulse within the range of resting pulse plus 20 beats per minute and the RPE less than 14. Most patients will tolerate a minimum of 5 minutes of walking the first day. As long as the pulse and RPE remain within prescribed limits, walking time can be increased until patients are walking at least 30 minutes twice daily. At that point, the walking sessions should include stair climbing to ensure that patients can perform that task at home. Patients able to walk unassisted for 30 minutes and climb stairs have sufficient strength and endurance for most activities of daily living.

EDUCATION AND COUNSELING. During the periods of assisted ambulation, the nurse or physical therapist teaches patients how to count their pulse, use the RPE scale, and recognize important symptoms. Before discharge from the hospital, patients are taught how to access emergency medical care; learn the names, dosages, effects, and side-effects of their medications; and have specific questions regarding their cardiac status answered. During these or other times, basic information regarding the risk factors for coronary disease should be presented with emphasis on those that affect the patient.

At the time of hospital discharge, patients should receive very specific advice about resumption of activities at home. Even common-sense knowledge should not be presumed by the health professionals caring for the patient. The spouse should receive the advice with the patient because the retention of information by hospitalized patients is limited, and most disagreements between patient and spouse in the early recovery period are related to perceptions of medical advice given.[126–129] A simple approach to providing guidelines for physical activities is to treat them as forms of exercise. Patients can use the resting pulse plus 20 beats-per-minute rule for most household activities. The patient quickly will learn the heart rate response to each activity and be confident in undertaking such activities at home. Patients should be told what restrictions are placed on common activities such as climbing stairs, lifting, driving, socializing with visitors, shopping, and walking outdoors.

Activities that involve more mental than physical stress, such as driving, socializing, and shopping, concern patients and family at the time of discharge from the hospital. Mental stress has been shown to affect cardiac performance negatively.[130–133] However, in studies directly comparing the physiological stress of exercise with formal methods of psychological stress, the hemodynamic response was always significantly greater with exercise than mental stress.[134–137] The pathophysiology of mental stress and its influence on prognosis are incompletely understood.[135,136,138,139] It appears unlikely that mental stress, unless severe, will precipitate a cardiac event soon after myocardial infarction or in the setting of stable coronary disease.

Early Postdischarge Exercise Testing and Rehabilitation

ACTIVITIES BEFORE EXERCISE TESTING. The interval between hospital discharge and formal cardiac rehabilitation should be as brief as possible. During this period, patients can continue their walking program as prescribed in the hospital. They should walk a minimum of 30 minutes twice daily at a target heart rate within the resting pulse plus 20 beats/min range at an RPE of less than 14. Patients able to tolerate the duration of walking should be encouraged to add a third session or increase the two sessions to 45 minutes each. Secondary prevention efforts can begin as patients are motivated and have time to begin behavioral changes. Initial visits with a dietitian may be scheduled if weight loss or reduction of cholesterol is necessary.[140] A smoking abstinence program may begin during this pe-

riod.[99] Patients should be provided with resources to teach them about coronary disease and risk-factor management.[141]

RECOMMENDATIONS FOLLOWING EXERCISE TESTING. A postdischarge exercise test is a good focal point for the subsequent rehabilitation effort. The formal exercise prescription may then be given. Goals for weight loss, reduction of serum cholesterol, cessation of smoking, and return to work may be established. In the absence of significant abnormalities on the treadmill test, patients may begin most customary activities such as driving, sexual activity, and light lifting. Although lifting is often proscribed for 6 to 8 weeks after myocardial infarction and cardiac surgery, studies suggest that lifting and carrying of moderate loads is not dangerous after uncomplicated myocardial infarction and cardiac surgery. In patients with coronary disease, including those recovering from myocardial infarction, static lifting and combined static lifting and dynamic treadmill walking were associated with similar or lower double products compared with dynamic treadmill walking alone. In these studies, there was no evidence of myocardial ischemia induced by static lifting alone.[142–144]

SEXUAL ACTIVITY. The most common sexual problems of coronary patients are reduced or absent libido, avoidance of sexual activity even if libido has recovered, impotence, and premature or delayed ejaculation in men. The causes of sexual dysfunction include preexisting conditions, fear of precipitating a cardiac event, depression, and medications, especially beta blockers and diuretics. In addition, the sexual partner may believe that sexual activity could precipitate a cardiac event and therefore may avoid sexual activity. Because patients are reluctant to discuss sexual dysfunction, the physician should address issues of sexuality and consider the effects of medications on sexual drive.[129,145–148]

The hemodynamic response to sexual intercourse has been evaluated in patients recovering from myocardial infarction. The maximal heart rate during sexual intercourse averages 120 beats/min, which approximates maximal heart rates attained in the performance of other customary activities.[147] The hemodynamic response to sexual activity is far greater with an unfamiliar compared with a familiar partner, in unfamiliar settings, and after excessive eating and consumption of alcohol.[145] The exercise test can be used to gauge the potential cardiac stress of sexual activity. Patients without significant treadmill abnormalities can be advised to resume sexual activity gradually. Cardiac work associated with sexual intercourse can be minimized by adopting relaxed positions such as side-to-side rather than top-to-bottom postures that increase the isometric work.[145,147] Patients should be told to report symptoms such as angina, prolonged dyspnea, excessive fatigue, or tachycardia lasting more than 10 minutes after intercourse. In sedentary individuals, such symptoms may be the only manifestation of exercise-induced ischemia or left ventricular dysfunction.

Outpatient Rehabilitation Programs

Formal cardiac rehabilitation programs typically have both medical and program directors. The medical director is a physician, whereas the program director may be trained in a variety of disciplines. The rehabilitation team is multidisciplinary and includes nurses, physical therapists, exercise physiologists, dietitians, vocational counselors, and psychologists. When smaller programs cannot support the broad range of services, a referral network that includes all the disciplines is necessary. Adequate facilities for outpatient exercise training are needed. If high-risk patients are included, continuous electrocardiographic monitoring must be available. Equipment and training for cardiopulmonary resuscitation is mandatory.

EXERCISE TRAINING. Exercise training guidelines have

been presented earlier. Most patients can benefit from group exercise programs. The standard group training program provides three sessions weekly for 8 to 12 weeks. Some patients require more prolonged training, whereas others may progress to independent exercise more quickly. In such groups, proper techniques of exercise training can be reinforced, and patients can learn how to perform safe and effective exercise independently. The group setting is also an opportunity for patients to receive reliable information from health professionals regarding coronary disease and risk-factor modification. Although difficult to quantitate, there is an obvious benefit of the social support provided by interactions with other patients in various stages of recovery from coronary illness. Group exercise sessions are often the focal point for the development of educational programs and support groups.

RISK FACTOR MODIFICATION. A comprehensive program of cardiac rehabilitation should combine exercise training with risk factor modification (Chap. 35). Smoking abstinence programs and dietary counseling are the two most important additional services a program should provide. Continued reinforcement of the principles of risk-factor modification improves compliance with behavioral programs.[89,106,108,149]

Current evidence suggests that cardiac rehabilitation programs offering exercise training, smoking abstinence, and cholesterol treatment programs can improve the rates of morbidity and mortality of patients with coronary artery disease.[36,37] Cardiac rehabilitation programs can also facilitate functional recovery.[150-152] Early risk stratification, including treadmill testing, can identify patients requiring further treatment and hasten the resumption of customary activities of low-risk patients. Education and counseling can improve psychosocial outcomes. Significant economic benefits can be realized when vocational rehabilitation is included in a cardiac rehabilitation program.[47,48] Participation in a cardiac rehabilitation program may decrease subsequent costs of care through reductions in numbers of rehospitalizations and use of other medical services.[107,125,153-155] As the principles of cardiac rehabilitation become more broadly applied, larger numbers of patients with coronary disease will benefit medically, socially, and psychologically.

REFERENCES

EXERCISE IN CARDIAC REHABILITATION

1. DeBusk, R. F.: Why is cardiac rehabilitation not widely used? (Editorial). West. J. Med. 156:206, 1992.
2. Roberts, J. M., Sullivan, M., Froelicher, V. F., et al.: Predicting oxygen uptake from treadmill testing in normal subjects and coronary artery disease patients. Am. Heart J. 108:1454, 1984.
3. Coats, A. J.: Exercise rehabilitation in chronic heart failure. J. Am. Coll. Cardiol. 22:172A–177A, 1993.
4. Sullivan, M. J., Higginbotham, M. B., and Cobb, F. R.: Exercise training in patients with severe left ventricular dysfunction. Circulation 78:506, 1988.
5. Sullivan, M. J., Higginbotham, M. B., and Cobb, F. R.: Exercise training in patients with chronic heart failure delays ventilatory anaerobic threshold and improves submaximal exercise performance. Circulation 79:324, 1989.
6. Adamopoulos, S., Coats, A. J., Brunotte, F., et al.: Physical training improves skeletal muscle metabolism in patients with chronic heart failure. J. Am. Coll. Cardiol. 21:1101, 1993.
7. Teasell, R., and Dittmer, D. K.: Complications of immobilization and bed rest. Part 2: Other complications. Can. Fam. Physician 39:1440, 1445, 1993.
8. Dittmer, D. K., and Teasell, R.: Complications of immobilization and bed rest. Part 1: Musculoskeletal and cardiovascular complications. Can. Fam. Physician 39:1428, 1435, 1993.
9. Hughson, R. L., Yamamoto, Y., Blabler, A. P., et al.: Effect of 28-day head-down bed rest with countermeasures on heart rate variability during LBNP. Aviat. Space Environ. Med. 65:293, 1994.
10. Weins, R. D., Lafia, P., Marder, C. M., et al.: Chronotropic incompetence in clinical exercise testing. Am. J. Cardiol. 54:74, 1984.
11. Thoren, P. N.: Activation of left ventricular receptors with non-medulated vagal afferent fibers during occlusion of a coronary artery in the cat. Am. J. Cardiol. 37:146, 1976.
12. Wetherbee, S., Franklin, B. A., Hollingsworth, V., et al.: Relationship

between arm and leg training work loads in men with heart disease: Implications for exercise prescription. Chest 99:1271, 1991.
13. Haskell, W. L., and DeBusk, R. F.: Cardiovascular responses to repeated treadmill testing soon after myocardial infarction. Circulation 60:1247, 1979.
14. Sullivan, M. J., Green, H. J., and Cobb, F. R.: Skeletal muscle biochemistry and histology in ambulatory patients with long-term heart failure. Circulation 81:518, 1990.
15. Sullivan, M. J., Knight, D. J., Higginbotham, M. B., and Cobb, F. R.: Relation between central and peripheral hemodynamics during exercise in patients with chronic heart failure: Muscle blood flow is reduced with maintenance of arterial perfusion pressure. Circulation 80:769, 1989.
16. McKelvie, R. S., Teo, K. K., McCartney, N., et al.: Effects of exercise training in patients with congestive heart failure: A critical review. J. Am. Coll. Cardiol. 25:789, 1995.
17. Smith, R. F., Johnson, G., Ziesche, S., et al.: Functional capacity in heart failure. Comparison of methods for assessment and their relation to other indexes of heart failure. The V-HeFT VA Cooperative Studies Group. Circulation 87(Suppl. 6):VI88, 1993.
18. Sullivan, M. J., and Cobb, F. R.: Central hemodynamic response to exercise in patients with chronic heart failure. Chest 101:340S, 1992.
19. Ades, P. A., Grunvald, M. H., and Weiss, R. M.: Usefulness of myocardial ischemia as a predictor of training effect in cardiac rehabilitation after acute myocardial infarction or coronary artery bypass grafting. Am. J. Cardiol. 63:1032, 1989.
20. Rice, K. R., Gervino, E., Jarisch, W. R., and Stone P. H.: Effects of nifedipine on myocardial perfusion during exercise in chronic stable angina pectoris. Am. J. Cardiol. 65(16):1097, 1990.
21. Stone, P. H., Gibson, R. S., Glasser, S. P., et al.: Comparison of propranolol, diltiazem, and nifedipine in the treatment of ambulatory ischemia in patients with stable angina: Differential effects on ambulatory ischemia, exercise performance, and anginal symptoms. The ASIS Study Group. Circulation 82:1962, 1990.
22. Gordon, N. F., and Duncan J. J.: Effect of beta-blockers on exercise physiology: implications for exercise training. Med. Sci. Sports Exerc. 23:668, 1991.
23. MacGowan, G. A., O'Callaghan, D., Webb, H., and Horgan, J. H.: The effects of verapamil on training in patients with ischemic heart disease. Chest 101:141, 1992.
24. Mancini, D. M., Davis, L., Wexler, J. P., et al.: Dependence of enhanced maximal exercise performance on increased peak skeletal muscle perfusion during long-term captopril therapy in heart failure. J. Am. Coll. Cardiol. 10:845, 1987.
25. Drexler, H., Banhardt, U., Meinertz, T., et al. Contrasting peripheral short-term effects of converting enzyme inhibition in patients with congestive heart failure: A double blind, placebo-controlled trial. Circulation 79:491, 1989.
26. Dickstein, K., and Aarsland, T.: Effect on exercise performance of enalapril therapy initiated early after myocardial infarction. Nordic Enalapril Exercise Trial. J. Am. Coll. Cardiol. 22:975, 1993.
27. Hanson, P.: Exercise testing and training in patients with chronic heart failure. Med. Sci. Sports Exerc. 26:527, 1994.
28. Hagberg, J. M.: Physiologic adaptations to prolonged high-intensity exercise training in patients with coronary artery disease. Med. Sci. Sports Exerc. 23:661, 1991.
29. Rogers, M. A., Yamamotao, C., Hagberg, J. M., et al.: The effect of 7 years of intense training in patients with coronary artery disease. J. Am. Coll. Cardiol. 10:321, 1987.
30. Laslett, L. J., Paumer, L., and Amsterdam, E. A.: Increase in myocardial oxygen consumption indexes by exercise training at onset of ischemia in patients with coronary artery disease. Circulation 71:958, 1985.
31. American College of Sports Medicine. Position stand. Exercise for patients with coronary artery disease. Med. Sci. Sports Exerc. 26:1, 1994.
32. Cox, M. H.: Exercise training programs and cardiorespiratory adaptation. Clin. Sports Med. 10:19, 1991.
33. Squires, R. W., Lavie, C. J., Brandt, T. R. et al.: Cardiac rehabilitation in patients with severe ischemic left ventricular dysfunction. Mayo Clin. Proc. 62:997, 1987.
34. Statement on exercise: A position statement for health professionals by the Committee on Exercise and Cardiac Rehabilitation of the Council on Clinical Cardiology, American Heart Association. Circulation 81:396, 1990.
35. Kallio,V., Hamalainen, H., Hakkila, J., et al.: Reduction in sudden deaths by a multifactorial intervention programme after acute myocardial infarction. Lancet 2:1091, 1979.
36. O'Connor, G. T., Buring, J. E., Yusuf, S., et al.: An overview of randomized trials of rehabilitation with exercise after myocardial infarction. Circulation 80:234, 1989.
37. Oldridge, N. B., Guyatt, G. H., Fischer, M. E., et al.: Cardiac rehabilitation after myocardial infarction: Combined experience of randomized clinical trials. JAMA 260:945, 1988.
38. Yusuf, S., Peto, R., Lewis, J., et al.: Beta blockade during and after myocardial infarction: An overview of randomized trials. Prog. Cardiovasc. Dis. 27:335, 1985.
39. American Association for Cardiovascular and Pulmonary Rehabilitation. Guidelines for Cardiac Rehabilitation Programs. Ed. 2 Champaign, Ill., Human Kinetics, 1995.
40. Fletcher, G. F., Froelicher, V. F., Hartley, L. H., et al.: Exercise standards: A statement for health professionals from the American Heart Association. Circulation 82:228, 1990.

41. Weber, K. T., and Janicki, J. S.: Cardiopulmonary exercise testing for the evaluation of heart failure. Am. J. Cardiol. 55:22A, 1985.
42. Levandoski, S. G., Sheldahl, L. M., Wilke, N. A., et al.: Cardiopulmonary responses of coronary artery disease patients to arm and leg cycle ergometry. J. Cardiopulm. Rehabil. 10:39, 1990.
43. Juneau, M., Colles, P., Theroux, P., et al.: Symptom-limited versus low level exercise testing before hospital discharge after myocardial infarction. J. Am. Coll. Cardiol. 20:927, 1992.
44. Ben-Ari, E., and Rothbaum, D. Clinical and exercise considerations for the percutaneous transluminal coronary angioplasty patient. J. Cardiopulm. Rehabil. 11:145, 1991.
45. Lavie, C. J., Gibbons, R. J., Zinsmeister, A. R., and Gersh, B. J.: Interpreting results of exercise studies after acute myocardial infarction altered by thrombolytic therapy, coronary angioplasty or bypass. Am. J. Cardiol. 67:116, 1991.
46. Krone, R. J.: The role of risk stratification in the early management of a myocardial infarction. Ann. Intern. Med. 116:223, 1992.
47. Dennis, C., Houston-Miller, N., Schwartz, R. G., et al.: Early return to work after uncomplicated myocardial infarction: Results of a randomized trial. JAMA 260:214, 1988.
48. Pilote, L., Thomas, R. J., Dennis, C., et al.: Return to work after uncomplicated myocardial infarction: A trial of practice guidelines in the community. Ann. Intern. Med. 117:383, 1992.
49. Gaudron, P., Hu, K., Schamberger, R., et al.: Effect of endurance training early or late after coronary artery occlusion on left ventricular remodeling, hemodynamics, and survival in rats with chronic transmural myocardial infarction. Circulation 89:402, 1994.
50. Jugdutt, B. S., Michorowski, B. L., Kappagoda, C. T., et al.: Exercise training after anterior Q-wave myocardial infarction: Importance of regional left ventricular function or topography. J. Am. Coll. Cardiol. 12:362, 1988.
51. Giannuzzi, P., Tavazzi, L., Temporelli, P. L., et al.: Long-term physical training and left ventricular remodeling after anterior myocardial infarction: Results of the Exercise in Anterior Myocardial Infarction (EAMI) trial. EAMI Study Group. J. Am. Coll. Cardiol. 22:1821, 1993.
52. Moss, A. J., Goldstein, R. E., Hall, W. J., et al.: Detection and significance of myocardial ischemia in stable patients after recovery from an acute coronary event. Multicenter Myocardial Ischemia Research Group. JAMA 269:2379, 1993.
53. Sacknoff, D. M., and Coplan, N. L.: Exercise testing for stratifying cardiac risk following thrombolytic therapy for acute myocardial infarction [Editorial]. Am. Heart J. 124:1400, 1992.
54. Piccalo, G., Pirelli, S., Massa, D., et al.: Value of negative predischarge exercise testing in identifying patients at low risk after acute myocardial infarction treated by systemic thrombolysis. Am. J. Cardiol. 70:31, 1992.
55. American College of Sports Medicine: Position Stand. Physical activity, physical fitness, and hypertension. Med. Sci. Sports Exerc. 25:1, 1993.
56. Marieb, M. A., Beller, G. A., Gibson, R. S., et al.: Clinical relevance of exercise-induced ventricular arrhythmias in suspected coronary artery disease. Am. J. Cardiol. 66:172, 1990.
57. Sparks, K. E., Shaw, D. K., Eddy, D., et al.: Alternatives for cardiac rehabilitation patients unable to return to a hospital-based program. Heart Lung 22:298, 1993.
58. Bertagnoli, K., Hanson, P., and Ward, A.: Attenuation of exercise-induced ST depression during combined isometric and dynamic exercise in coronary artery disease. Am. J. Cardiol. 65:314, 1990.
59. Ben-Ari, E., Kellermann, J. J., Rothbaum, D. A., et al.: Effects of prolonged intensive versus moderate leg training on the untrained arm exercise response in angina pectoris. Am. J. Cardiol. 59:231, 1987.
60. Haennel, R. G., Quinney, H. A., and Kappagoda, C. T.: Effects of hydraulic circuit training following coronary artery bypass surgery. Med. Sci. Sports Exerc. 23:158, 1991.
61. Sparling, P. B., Cantwell, J. D., Dolan, C. M., and Niederman, R. K.: Strength training in a cardiac rehabilitation program: A six-month follow-up. Arch. Phys. Med. Rehabil. 71:148, 1990.
62. Faigenbaum, A. D., Skrinar, G. S., Cesare, W. F., et al.: Physiologic and symptomatic responses of cardiac patients to resistance exercise. Arch. Phys. Med. Rehabil. 71:395, 1990.
63. McCartney, N., McKelvie, R. S., Haslam, D. R., and Jones, N. L.: Usefulness of weightlifting training in improving strength and maximal power output in coronary artery disease. Am. J. Cardiol. 67:939, 1991.
64. Borg, G.: Perceived exertion as an indicator of somatic stress. Scand. J. Rehabil. Med. 2:92, 1970.
65. Arvan, S.: Exercise performance of the high-risk acute myocardial infarction patient after cardiac rehabilitation. Am. J. Cardiol. 62:197, 1988.
66. Coats, A. J., Adamopoulos, S., Radaelli, A., et al.: Controlled trial of physical training in chronic heart failure: Exercise performance, hemodynamics, ventilation, and autonomic function. Circulation 85:2119, 1992.
67. Rossi, P.: Physical training in patients with congestive heart failure. Chest 101:350S, 1992.
68. O'Hara, G. E., Brugada, P., Rodriguez, L. M., et al.: Incidence, pathophysiology and prognosis of exercise-induced sustained ventricular tachycardia associated with healed myocardial infarction. Am. J. Cardiol. 70:875, 1992.
69. Hertzeanu, H. L., Shemesh, J., Aron, L. A., et al.: Ventricular arrhythmias in rehabilitated and nonrehabilitated post-myocardial infarction patients with left ventricular dysfunction. Am. J. Cardiol. 71:24, 1993.
70. Van Camp, S. P., and Peterson, R. A.: Identification of the high-risk cardiac rehabilitation patient. J. Cardiopulm. Rehabil. 9:103, 1989.
71. Van Camp, S. P., and Peterson, R. A.: Cardiovascular complications of outpatient cardiac rehabilitation programs. JAMA 256:1160, 1986.
72. Greenland, P., and Chu, J. S.: Efficacy of cardiac rehabilitation services: With emphasis on patients after myocardial infarction. Ann. Intern. Med. 109:650, 1988.
73. DeBusk, R. F., Haskell, W. L., Miller, N. H., et al.: Medically directed at-home rehabilitation soon after clinically uncomplicated acute myocardial infarction. Am. J. Cardiol. 55:251, 1985.
74. Haskell, W. L.: Cardiovascular complications during exercise training of cardiac patients. Circulation 57:920, 1978.
75. Hossack, J. M., and Hartwig, R.: Cardiac arrest associated with supervised cardiac rehabilitation. J. Cardiac Rehabil. 2:402, 1992.

SECONDARY PREVENTION

76. Lakier, J. B.: Smoking and cardiovascular disease. Am. J. Med. 93:8S, 1992.
77. Dobson, A. J., Alexander, H. M., Heller, R. F., and Lloyd D. M. How soon after quitting smoking does risk of heart attack decline? J. Clin. Epidemiol. 44:1247, 1991.
78. Kawachi, I., Colditz, G. A., Stampfer, M. J., et al.: Smoking cessation in relation to total mortality rates in women: A prospective cohort study. Ann. Intern. Med. 119:992, 1993.
79. Kawachi, I., Colditz, G. A., Stampfer, M. J., et al.: Smoking cessation and time course of decreased risks of coronary heart disease in middle-aged women. Arch. Intern Med 154:169, 1994.
80. Cavender, J. B., Rogers, W. J., Fisher, L. D., et al.: Effects of smoking on survival and morbidity in patients randomized to medical or surgical therapy in the Coronary Artery Surgery Study (CASS): 10-year follow-up. CASS Investigators. J. Am. Coll. Cardiol. 20:287, 1992.
81. Ramanathan, K. B., Vander Zwaag, R., Maddock, V., et al.: Interactive effects of age and other risk factors on long-term survival after coronary artery surgery. J. Am. Coll. Cardiol. 15:1493, 1990.
82. Caralis, D. G., Deligonul, U., Kern, M. J., and Cohen, J. D.: Smoking is a risk factor for coronary spasm in young women. Circulation 85:905, 1992.
83. Terres, W., Weber, K., Kupper, W., and Bleifeld, W.: Age, cardiovascular risk factors and coronary heart disease as determinants of platelet function in men: A multivariate approach. Thromb. Res. 62:649, 1991.
84. Robinson, J. G., and Leon, A. S.: The prevention of cardiovascular disease: Emphasis on secondary prevention. Med. Clin. North Am. 78:69, 1994.
85. Sherman, C. B.: Health effects of cigarette smoking. Clin. Chest Med. 12:643, 1991.
86. Freund, K. M., D'Agostino, R. B., Belanger, A. J., et al.: Predictors of smoking cessation: The Framingham Study. Am. J. Epidemiol. 135:957, 1992.
87. Crouse, J. D., and Hagaman, A. P.: Smoking cessation in relation to cardiac procedures. Am. J. Epidemiol. 134:699, 1991.
88. Rigotti, N. A., McKool, K. M., and Shiffman, S.: Predictors of smoking cessation after coronary artery bypass graft surgery: Results of a randomized trial with 5-year follow-up. Ann. Intern. Med. 120:287, 1994.
89. Schwartz, J. L.: Methods of smoking cessation. Med. Clin. North Am. 76:451, 1992.
90. Rigotti, N. A., Singer, D. E., Mulley, A. G., Jr., and Thibault, G. E.: Smoking cessation following admission to a coronary care unit. J. Gen. Intern. Med. 6:305, 1991.
91. Frank, E., Winkleby, M. A., Altman, D. G., et al.: Predictors of physician's smoking cessation advice. JAMA 266:3139, 1991.
92. Hurt, R. D., Dale, L. C., Offord, K. P., et al.: Serum nicotine and cotinine levels during nicotine-patch therapy. Clin. Pharmacol. Ther. 54:98, 1993.
93. Kenford, S. L., Fiore, M. C., Jorenby, D. E., et al.: Predicting smoking cessation: Who will quit with and without the nicotine patch. JAMA 271:589, 1994.
94. Hurt, R. D., Dale, L. C., Fredrickson, P. A., et al.: Nicotine patch therapy for smoking cessation combined with physician advice and nurse follow-up: One-year outcome and percentage of nicotine replacement. JAMA 271:595, 1994.
95. Tonnesen, P., Norregaard, J., Simonsen, K., and Sawe U. A double-blind trial of a 16-hour transdermal nicotine patch in smoking cessation. N. Engl. J. Med. 325:311, 1991.
96. Silagy, C., Mant, D., Fowler, G., and Lodge, M.: Meta-analysis on efficacy of nicotine replacement therapies in smoking cessation. Lancet 343:139, 1994.
97. Fiore, M. C., Smith, S. S., Jorenby, D. E., and Baker, T. B.: The effectiveness of the nicotine patch for smoking cessation: A meta-analysis. JAMA 271:1940, 1994.
98. Tsevat, J.: Impact and cost-effectiveness of smoking interventions. Am. J. Med. 93:43S, 1992.
99. Taylor, C. B., Houston-Miller, N., Killen, J. D., and DeBusk, R. F.: Smoking cessation after acute myocardial infarction: Effects of a nurse-managed intervention. Ann. Intern. Med 113:118, 1990.

PSYCHOLOGICAL FACTORS

100. Frasure-Smith, N.: In-hospital symptoms of psychological stress as predictors of long-term outcome after acute myocardial infarction in men. Am. J. Cardiol. 67:121, 1991.
101. Frasure-Smith, N., Lesperance, F., and Talajic, M.: Depression following myocardial infarction. Impact on 6-month survival. JAMA 270:1819, 1993.

102. Brown, M. A., Munford, A. M., and Munford, P. R.: Behavior therapy of psychological distress in patients after myocardial infarction or coronary bypass. J. Cardiopulm. Rehabil. *13*:201, 1993.

103. Kavan, M. G., Elsasser, G. N., and Hurd, R. H.: Depression after acute myocardial infarction: The role of primary care physicians in rehabilitation. Postgrad. Med. *89*:83, 1991.

104. Ladwig, K. H., Roll, G., Breithardt, G., et al.: Post-infarction depression and incomplete recovery 6 months after acute myocardial infarction. Lancet *343*:20, 1994.

105. Bandura, A.: Self-efficacy mechanism in human agency. Am. Psychol. *37*:122, 1982.

106. Damrosch, S.: General strategies for motivating people to change their behavior. Nurs. Clin. North Am. *26*:833, 1991.

107. Oldridge, N. B., and Rogowski, B. L.: Self-efficacy and in-patient cardiac rehabilitation. Am. J. Cardiol. *66*:362, 1990.

108. Robertson, D., and Keller, C.: Relationships among health beliefs, self-efficacy, and exercise adherence in patients with coronary artery disease. Heart Lung *21*:56, 1992.

109. Vidmar, P. M., and Rubinson, L.: The relationship between self-efficacy and exercise compliance in a cardiac population. J. Cardiopulm. Rehabil. *14*:246, 1994.

110. Ewart, C. K., Taylor, B., Reese, L. B., et al.: Exercise testing to enhance wives' confidence in their husbands' cardiac capability soon after uncomplicated acute myocardial infarction. Am. J. Cardiol. *55*:635, 1985.

111. The review panel on coronary-prone behavior and coronary heart disease. Coronary-prone behavior and coronary heart disease: A critical review. Circulation *63*:1199, 1981.

112. Dembroski, T., MacDougall, J., Costa, P., and Grandits, C.: Components of hostility as predictors of sudden death and myocardial infarction in the multiple risk factor intervention trial. Psychosom. Med. *51*:514, 1989.

113. Helmer, D. C., Ragland, D. R., and Syme, S. L.: Hostility and coronary artery disease. Am. J. Epidemiol. *133*:112, 1991.

114. Maruta, T., Hamburgen, M. E., Jennings, C. A., et al.: Keeping hostility in perspective: Coronary heart disease and the Hostility Scale on the Minnesota Multiphasic Personality Inventory. Mayo Clin. Proc. *68*:109, 1993.

115. Friedman, M., Thoresen, C. E., Gill, J. J., et al.: Alteration of Type A behavior and its effect on cardiac recurrences in post myocardial infarction patients: Summary results of the recurrent coronary prevention project. Am. Heart J. *112*:653, 1986.

VOCATIONAL REHABILITATION

116. Wittels, E. H., Hay, J. W., and Gotto, A. M.: Medical costs of coronary artery disease in the United States. Am. J. Cardiol. *65*:432, 1990.

117. Mark, D. B., Lam, L. C., Lee, K. L., et al.: Identification of patients with coronary disease at high risk for loss of employment: A prospective validation study. Circulation *86*:1485, 1992.

118. Guillette, W., Judge, R. D., Koehn, E., et al.: Committee report on economic, administrative, and legal factors influencing the insurability and employability of patients with ischemic heart disease: 20th Bethesda conference. J. Am. Coll. Cardiol. *14*:1010, 1989.

119. Pryor, D. B., Bruce, R. A., Chaitman, B. R., et al.: Task force I: Determination of prognosis in patients with ischemic heart disease: 20th Bethesda conference. J. Am. Coll. Cardiol. *14*:1016, 1989.

120. Haskell, W. L., Brachfeld, N., Bruce, R. A., et al.: Task force II: Determination of occupational working capacity in patients with ischemic heart disease: 20th Bethesda conference. J. Am. Coll. Cardiol. *14*:1025, 1989.

121. Wilke, N. A., Sheldahl, L. M., Dougherty, S. M., et al.: Baltimore Therapeutic Equipment work simulator: Energy expenditure of work activities in cardiac patients. Arch. Phys. Med. Rehabil. *74*:419, 1993.

122. Wilke, N. A., Sheldahl, L. M., Dougherty, S. M., et al.: Energy costs of household tasks in women with coronary artery disease. Am. J. Cardiol. *75*:670, 1995.

123. Bureau of Labor Statistics. Handbook of Labor Statistics. Washington, D.C.: U.S. Department of Labor, 1993.

124. DeBusk, R. F.: Determination of cardiac impairment and disability: 20th Bethesda conference. J. Am. Coll. Cardiol. *14*:1043, 1989.

125. Picard, M. H., Dennis, C., Schwartz, R. G., et al.: Cost-benefit of early return to work after uncomplicated myocardial infarction. Am. J. Cardiol. *63*:1308, 1989.

126. Cupples, S. A.: Effects of timing and reinforcement of preoperative education on knowledge and recovery of patients having coronary artery bypass graft surgery. Heart Lung *20*:654, 1991.

127. Duryee, R.: The efficacy of inpatient education after myocardial infarction. Heart Lung *21*:217, 1992.

128. Nyamathi, A., Jacoby, A., Constancia, P., and Ruvevich, S.: Coping and adjustment of spouses of critically ill patients with cardiac disease. Heart Lung *21*:160, 1992.

129. Beach, E. K., Maloney, B. H., Plocica, A. R., et al.: The spouse: A factor in recovery after acute myocardial infarction. Heart Lung *21*:30, 1992.

130. Burg, M. M., Jain, D., Soufer, R., et al.: Role of behavioral and psychological factors in mental stress-induced silent left ventricular dysfunction in coronary artery disease. J. Am. Coll. Cardiol. *22*:440, 1993.

131. Coumel, P., and Leenhardt, A. Mental activity, adrenergic modulation, and cardiac arrhythmias in patients with heart disease. Circulation *83*:1158, 1991.

132. Follick, M. J., Ahern, D. K., Gorkin, L., et al.: Relation of psychosocial and stress reactivity variables to ventricular arrhythmias in the Cardiac Arrhythmia Pilot Study (CAPS). Am. J. Cardiol. *66*:63, 1990.

133. Ironson, G., Taylor, C. B., Boltwood, M., et al.: Effects of anger on left ventricular ejection fraction in coronary artery disease. Am. J. Cardiol. *70*:281, 1992.

ORGANIZATION OF CARDIAC REHABILITATION SERVICES

134. Specchia, G., Falcone, C., Traversi, E., et al.: Mental stress as a provocative test in patients with various clinical syndromes of coronary heart disease. Circulation *83*(Suppl. 4):II108, 1991.

135. Specchia, G., Falcone, C., Traversi, E., et al.: Mental stress as provocative test in patients with various clinical syndromes of coronary heart disease. Circulation *83*:108, 1991.

136. Rozanski, A., Krantz, D. S., and Bairey, C. N.: Ventricular responses to mental stress testing in patients with coronary artery disease: Pathophysiological implications. Circulation *83*:137, 1991.

137. Gottdiener, J. S., Krantz, D. S., Howell, R. H., et al.: Induction of silent myocardial ischemia with mental stress testing: Relation to the triggers of ischemia during daily life activities and to ischemic functional severity. J. Am. Coll. Cardiol. *24*:1645, 1994.

138. L'Abbate, A., Simonetti, I., Carpeggiani, C., and Michelassi, C.: Coronary dynamics and mental arithmetic stress in humans. Circulation *83*:94, 1991.

139. Grignani, G., Soffiantino, F., Zucchella, M., et al.: Platelet activation by emotional stress in patients with coronary artery disease. Circulation *83*:128, 1991.

140. Montgomery, D. A., and Amos, R. J.: Nutritional information needs during cardiac rehabilitation: Perceptions of the cardiac patient and spouse. J. Am. Diet Assoc. *91*:1078, 1991.

141. Squires, R. W., Gau, G. T., Miller, T. D., et al.: Cardiovascular rehabilitation: Status, 1990. Mayo Clin. Proc. *65*:731, 1990.

142. DeBusk, R. F., Valdez, R., Houston, N., and Haskell, W.: Cardiovascular responses to dynamic and static effort soon after myocardial infarction. Circulation *58*:368, 1978.

143. Wilke, N. A., Sheldahl, S. G., Levandoski, S. G., et al.: Weight carrying versus handgrip exercise testing in men with coronary artery disease. Am. J. Cardiol. *64*:736, 1989.

144. Featherstone, J. F., Holly, R. G., and Amsterdam, E. A.: Physiologic responses to weight lifting in coronary artery disease. Am. J. Cardiol. *71*:287, 1993.

145. Cooper, A. J.: Myocardial infarction and advice on sexual activity. Practitioner *229*:575, 1985.

146. Hamilton, G. A., and Seidman, R. N.: A comparison of the recovery period for women and men after an acute myocardial infarction. Heart Lung *22*:308, 1993.

147. Tardif, G. S.: Sexual activity after a myocardial infarction. Arch. Phys. Med. Rehabil. *70*:763, 1989.

148. Froelicher, E. S., Kee, L. L., Newton, K. M., et al.: Return to work, sexual activity and other activities after acute myocardial infarction. Heart Lung *23*:423, 1994.

149. van Dixhoorn, J., Duivenvoorden, H. J., and Pool J.: Success and failure of exercise training after myocardial infarction: Is the outcome predictable? J. Am. Coll. Cardiol. *15*:974, 1990.

150. Allen, J. K.: Physical and psychosocial outcomes after coronary artery bypass graft surgery: Review of the literature. Heart Lung *19*:49, 1990.

151. Bethell, H. J., and Mullee, M. A.: A controlled trial of community-based coronary rehabilitation. Br. Heart J. *64*:370, 1990.

152. Juneau, M., Geneau, S., Marchand, C., and Brosseau, R.: Cardiac rehabilitation after coronary bypass surgery. Cardiovasc. Clin. *21*:25, 1991.

153. Ades, P. A., Huang, D., and Weaver, S. O.: Cardiac rehabilitation participation predicts lower rehospitalization costs. Am. Heart J. *123*:916, 1992.

154. Levin, L. A., Perk, J., and Hedback, B.: Cardiac rehabilitation: A cost analysis. J. Intern. Med. *230*:427, 1991.

155. Oldridge, N. B.: Cardiac rehabilitation services: What are they and are they worth it? Compr. Ther. *17*:59, 1991.

Chapter 41
The Cardiomyopathies and Myocarditides

JOSHUA WYNNE and EUGENE BRAUNWALD

The cardiomyopathies constitute a group of diseases, outlined in Table 41–1, in which the dominant feature is involvement of the heart muscle itself. They are distinctive because they are not the result of pericardial, hypertensive, congenital, valvular, or ischemic diseases. The term *ischemic cardiomyopathy* (see p. 1346) refers to the condition in which coronary artery disease causes multiple infarctions or diffuse fibrosis and leads to left ventricular dilatation with congestive heart failure; it may or may not be associated with angina pectoris.[1,2] Although the diagnosis of cardiomyopathy requires the exclusion of these etiological factors, the features of cardiomyopathy are often sufficiently distinctive—both clinically and hemodynamically—to allow a positive diagnosis to be made.[3] With increasing awareness of this condition, along with improvements in diagnostic techniques, cardiomyopathy is being recognized as a significant cause of morbidity and mortality.[4] Whether the result of improved recognition or of other factors, the incidence and prevalence of cardiomyopathy appear to be increasing.[4,5]

A variety of schemes has been proposed for classifying the cardiomyopathies. The most widely recognized classification is that promulgated by the World Health Organization (WHO) (Fig. 41–1),[5a] although there have been objections to this scheme[6–8] (Tables 41–1 and 41–2). In the WHO classification, the term *cardiomyopathy* is restricted to diseases solely involving the heart muscle that are of unknown cause; other diseases that affect the myocardium but are of known cause or are part of a generalized systemic disorder are termed *specific heart muscle diseases*. Although conceptually sound, this classification system may be overly rigid for the clinician, because the *clinical* features of a given cardiomyopathy are often identical to those of one of the specific heart muscle diseases. We prefer to use the term *secondary cardiomyopathy* to identify those patients with a specific heart muscle disease that clinically closely simulates an idiopathic or *primary* cardiomyopathy.

Three basic types of functional impairment have been described (Table 41–2): (1) *dilated* (formerly called congestive), the most common form, characterized by ventricular dilatation, contractile dysfunction, and often symptoms of congestive heart failure; (2) *hypertrophic,* recognized by inappropriate left ventricular hypertrophy, often with asymmetrical involvement of the interventricular septum, usually with preserved or enhanced contractile function; and (3) *restrictive,* the most common form in western countries, marked by impaired diastolic filling, in some cases with endocardial scarring of the ventricle. Most forms of secondary cardiomyopathy are characterized by the dilated cardiomyopathy pattern. The distinction between these three

functional categories is not absolute, and often there is overlap[6]; in particular, patients with hypertrophic cardiomyopathy also have increased wall stiffness (as a consequence of the myocardial hypertrophy) and thus present some of the features of a restrictive cardiomyopathy. It is difficult to fit a few conditions (such as arrhythmogenic right ventricular dysplasia, early or "latent" cardiomyopathy, and the entity of mildly dilated cardiomyopathy) neatly into the traditional functional classification scheme.[6–9]

Endomyocardial Biopsy

Evaluation of some patients suspected of suffering from a cardiomyopathy has been facilitated by the use of endo-

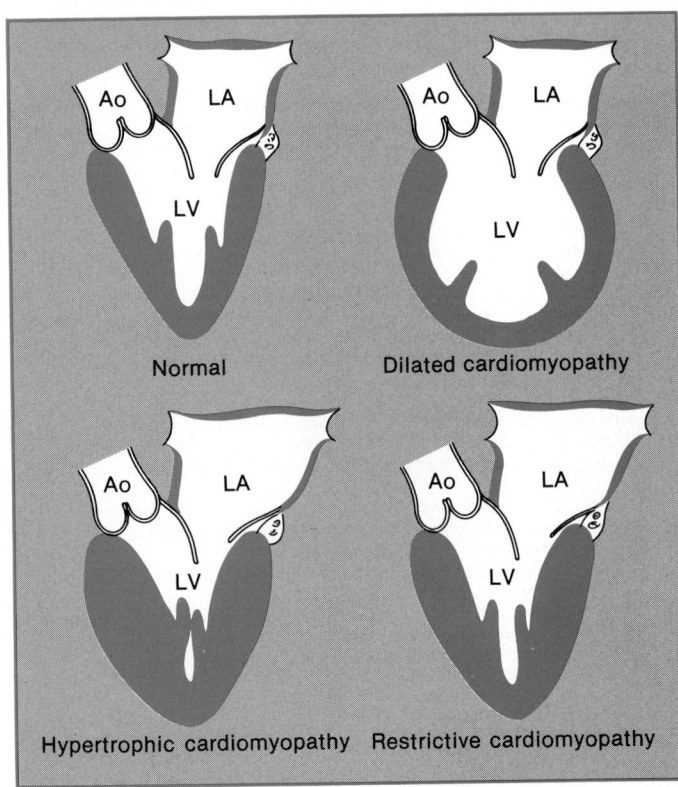

FIGURE 41–1. Diagram comparing three morphologic types of cardiomyopathies of unknown cause. Ao = Aorta, LA = left atrium, LV = left ventricle. (From Waller, B. F.: Pathology of the cardiomyopathies. J. Am. Soc. Echocardiog. *1:*4, 1988.)

1. **Inflammatory**
   a. Infective
      Viral
      Rickettsial
      Bacterial
      Mycobacterial
      Spirochetal
      Fungal
      Parasitic
   b. Noninfective
      Collagen diseases
      Granulomatous
      Kawasaki

2. **Metabolic**
   a. Nutritional
      Thiamine
      Kwashiorkor
      Pellagra
      Scurvy
      Hypervitaminosis D
      Obesity
      Selenium deficiency
      Carnitine deficiency
   b. Endocrine
      Acromegaly
      Thyrotoxicosis
      Myxedema
      Uremia
      Cushing's disease
      Pheochromocytoma
      Diabetes mellitus
   c. Altered metabolism
      Gout
      Oxalosis
      Porphyria
   d. Electrolyte imbalance

3. **Toxic**
   a. Cobalt
   b. Alcohol
   c. Bleomycin
   d. Adriamycin
   e. Phenothiazines and anti-
      depressants
   f. Antimony compounds
   g. Carbon monoxide
   h. Lead
   i. Emetine and dehydroeme-
      tine
   j. Chloroquine
   k. Lithium
   l. Cyclophosphamide
   m. Hydrocarbons
   n. Catecholamines
   o. Phosphorus
   p. Mercury
   q. Insect stings
   r. Snake bites
   s. Paracetamol
   t. Reserpine
   u. Corticosteroids
   v. Cocaine
   w. Methysergide

4. **Infiltrative**
   a. Amyloidosis
   b. Hemochromatosis
   c. Neoplastic
   d. Glycogen storage disorders
   e. Sarcoidosis
   f. Mucopolysaccharidosis
   g. Fabry disease

   h. Whipple disease
   i. Gaucher disease
   j. Sphingolipidoses

5. **Fibroplastic**
   a. Endomyocardial fibrosis
   b. Endocardial fibroelastosis
   c. Löffler's fibroplastic endo-
      carditis
   d. Carcinoid

6. **Hematological**
   a. Sickle cell anemia
   b. Polycythemia vera
   c. Thrombotic thrombocyto-
      penic purpura
   d. Leukemia

7. **Hypersensitivity**
   a. Methyldopa
   b. Penicillin
   c. Sulfonamides
   d. Tetracycline
   e. Phenindione
   f. Phenylbutazone
   g. Antituberculous drugs
   h. Giant cell myocarditis
   i. Cardiac transplant rejec-
      tion

8. **Genetic**
   a. Hypertrophic cardiomyop-
      athy
      With gradient
      Without gradient

   b. Neuromuscular
      Duchenne muscular
      dystrophy
      Facioscapulohumeral
      muscular dystrophy
      Limb-girdle dystrophy
      of Erb
      Myotonia dystrophica
      Friedreich's ataxia
      Kearns-Sayre syndrome
      Nemaline cardiomyop-
      athy
      Multicore cardiomyop-
      athy

9. **Miscellaneous acquired**
   a. Postpartum cardiomyopa-
      thy
   b. Obesity

10. **Idiopathic**
    a. Idiopathic dilated cardio-
       myopathy
    b. Idiopathic restrictive car-
       diomyopathy
    c. Idiopathic hypertrophic
       cardiomyopathy
    d. Idiopathic arrhythmo-
       genic right ventricular
       dysplasia

11. **Physical agents**
    a. Heat stroke
    b. Hypothermia
    c. Radiation
    d. Tachycardia

myocardial biopsy (see p. 186).[10,11] Using a flexible bioptome, the clinician easily and safely may obtain tissue samples from the right (and occasionally left) ventricle via a transvenous (or transarterial) approach (Fig. 41–2). The availability of disposable transfemoral bioptomes has further facilitated endomyocardial biopsy. Two-dimensional echocardiography may help guide the placement of the bioptome and reduce or eliminate radiation exposure.[12–15] Endomyocardial biopsy results in a small tissue sample (average size 1 to 2 mm), and multiple samples (usually four or more) are required because pronounced topographic variations may be found within the myocardium. Which

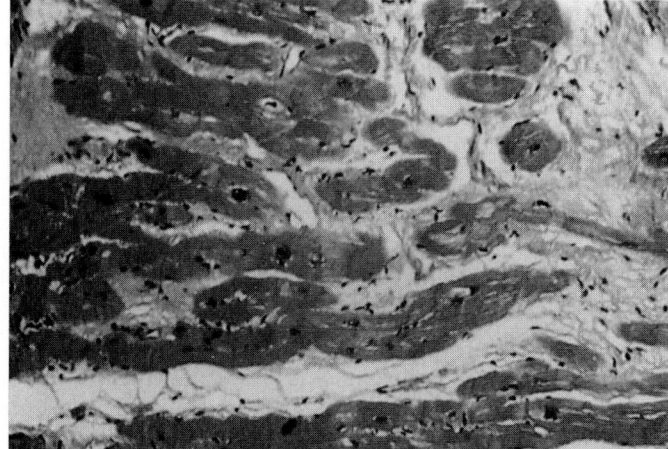

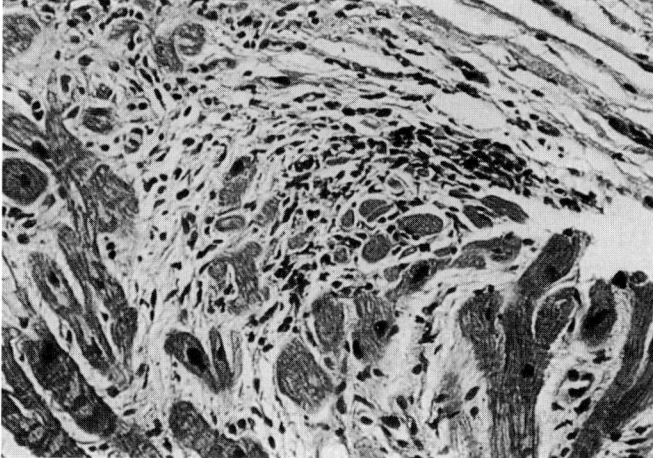

FIGURE 41–2. Histological specimens obtained by right ventricular endomyocardial biopsy. *A,* Idiopathic dilated cardiomyopathy with varying degrees of interstitial fibrosis and myocyte hypertrophy (trichrome stain, ×210). *B,* Myocarditis with dense focal area of mononuclear cell infiltrate adjacent to necrotic and degenerating myocytes, with irregular myocytic hypertrophy and dense interstitial fibrosis (hematoxylin and eosin, ×210). (From Dec, G. W., and Fuster, V.: Idiopathic dilated cardiomyopathy. N. Engl. J. Med. *331:*1564, 1994. Copyright Massachusetts Medical Society.)

TABLE 41–2 FUNCTIONAL CLASSIFICATION OF THE CARDIOMYOPATHIES

	DILATED	RESTRICTIVE	HYPERTROPHIC
Symptoms	Congestive heart failure, particularly left-sided Fatigue and weakness Systemic or pulmonary emboli	Dyspnea, fatigue Right-sided congestive heart failure Signs and symptoms of systemic disease: amyloidosis, iron storage disease, etc.	Dyspnea, angina pectoris Fatigue, syncope, palpitations
Physical Examination	Moderate to severe cardiomegaly; S_3 and S_4 Atrioventricular valve regurgitation, especially mitral	Mild to moderate cardiomegaly: S_3 or S_4 Atrioventricular valve regurgitation; inspiratory increase in venous pressure (Kussmaul's sign)	Mild cardiomegaly Apical systolic thrill and heave; brisk carotid upstroke S_4 common Systolic murmur that increases with Valsalva maneuver
Chest Roentgenogram	Moderate to marked cardiac enlargement, especially left ventricular Pulmonary venous hypertension	Mild cardiac enlargement Pulmonary venous hypertension	Mild to moderate cardiac enlargement Left atrial enlargement
Electrocardiogram	Sinus tachycardia Atrial and ventricular arrhythmias ST-segment and T-wave abnormalities Intraventricular conduction defects	Low voltage Intraventricular conduction defects AV conduction defects	Left ventricular hypertrophy ST-segment and T-wave abnormalities Abnormal Q waves Atrial and ventricular arrhythmias
Echocardiogram	Left ventricular dilatation and dysfunction Abnormal diastolic mitral valve motion secondary to abnormal compliance and filling pressures	Increased left ventricular wall thickness and mass Small or normal-sized left ventricular cavity Normal systolic function Pericardial effusion	Asymmetrical septal hypertrophy (ASH) Narrow left ventricular outflow tract Systolic anterior motion (SAM) of the mitral valve Small or normal-sized left ventricle
Radionuclide Studies	Left ventricular dilatation and dysfunction (RVG)	Infiltration of myocardium (^{201}Tl) Small or normal-sized left ventricle (RVG) Normal systolic function (RVG)	Small or normal-sized left ventricle (RVG) Vigorous systolic function (RVG) Asymmetrical septal hypertrophy (RVG or ^{201}Tl)
Cardiac Catheterization	Left ventricular enlargement and dysfunction Mitral and/or tricuspid regurgitation Elevated left- and often right-sided filling pressures Diminished cardiac output	Diminished left ventricular compliance "Square root sign" in ventricular pressure recordings Preserved systolic function Elevated left- and right-sided filling pressures	Diminished left ventricular compliance Mitral regurgitation Vigorous systolic function Dynamic left ventricular outflow gradient

RVG = Radionuclide ventriculogram; ^{201}Tl = thallium-201.

patients should be subjected to biopsy remains controversial, but there is general agreement that biopsy may be of benefit in certain specific situations; there is little debate

TABLE 41–3 CLINICAL INDICATIONS FOR ENDOMYOCARDIAL BIOPSY

DEFINITE
Monitoring of cardiac allograft rejection Monitoring of anthracycline cardiotoxicity

POSSIBLE
Detection and monitoring of myocarditis Diagnosis of secondary cardiomyopathies Differentiation between restrictive and constrictive heart disease

UNCERTAIN
Unexplained, life-threatening ventricular tachyarrhythmias AIDS Formulation of prognosis in idiopathic dilated cardiomyopathy

From Mason, J. W., and O'Connell, J. B.: Clinical merit of endomyocardial biopsy. Circulation *79*:971, 1989. Copyright American Heart Association.

as to its clinical utility in detecting infiltrative disorders of the myocardium and in monitoring for anthracycline cardiotoxicity and cardiac transplant rejection (Table 41–3).[10,11]

Although on occasion endomyocardial biopsy may identify a specific etiological agent in an individual patient with cardiac disease of uncertain cause (Table 41–4), the clinical utility of routine biopsy in cardiomyopathy is limited (particularly because no definitive pattern has been found in dilated cardiomyopathy) (Table 41–5).[5] It has been estimated that a specific etiologic diagnosis is obtained by biopsy in less than 10 per cent of patients with cardiomyopathy, and a treatable disease is found in only about 2 per cent.[10,11]

Dallas Criteria. Interpretation of biopsy specimens had been plagued by a high degree of interobserver variability; the adoption of a generally accepted set of histological definitions,[16] the *Dallas criteria,* appears to have substantially improved agreement. It is hoped that newer immunohistochemical and molecular biological techniques (such as the polymerase chain reaction or in situ hybridization techniques to detect viral infection of the heart) may expand further the diagnostic utility of endomyocardial biopsy.[16–21]

TABLE 41–4   SPECIFIC DIAGNOSES THAT CAN BE CONFIRMED BY MYOCARDIAL BIOPSY

Cardiac allograft rejection	Fabry disease of the heart	Henoch-Schönlein purpura
Myocarditis	Carcinoid disease	Rheumatic carditis
Giant cell myocarditis	Irradiation injury	Chagasic cardiomyopathy
Doxorubicin cardiotoxicity	Glycogen storage disease	Chloroquine cardiomyopathy
Cardiac amyloidosis	Cardiac tumors of cardiac origin	Lyme carditis
Cardiac sarcoidosis	Cardiac tumors of noncardiac origin	Carnitine deficiency cardiomyopathy
Cardiac hemochromatosis	Kearns-Sayre syndrome	Right ventricular lipomatosis
Endocardial fibrosis	Cytomegalovirus infection	Hypereosinophilic syndrome
Endocardial fibroelastosis	Toxoplasmosis	

From Mason, J. W., and O'Connell, J. B.: Clinical merit of endomyocardial biopsy. Circulation *79:*971, 1989, reprinted by permission of the American Heart Association, Inc.

TABLE 41–5   ENDOMYOCARDIAL BIOPSY CHARACTERISTICS

DILATED CARDIOMYOPATHY
  Light Microscopy
    Increase in myofiber size
    Attenuation of cells
    Hyperchromatic, irregular shaped nuclei
    Interstitial, focal, perivascular fibrosis

  Electron Microscopy
    Hypertrophic changes
    Increased number of sarcomeres and mitochondria
    Large, lobulated nuclei
    Z-band abnormalities
    Irregular invaginations of sarcolemma
    Widened, convoluted, intercalated discs

  Degenerative Changes
    Myofilament loss
    Aggregation of glycogen and mitochondria
    Pleomorphic mitochondria
    Myelin figures, lipid vacuoles

HYPERTROPHIC CARDIOMYOPATHY
  Light Microscopy
    Endocardial thickening and fibrosis
    Marked myocardial hypertrophy
    Large, bizarre nuclei
    Myofiber disorganization
    Interstitial fibrosis

  Electron Microscopy
    Myofibrillar disarray
    Increased side-to-side junctions
    Increased cell branching
    Increased glycogen

MYOCARDITIS
  Light and Electron Microscopy
    Inflammatory infiltrate, usually lymphocytic
    Necrosis or degeneration of adjacent myocytes
    Uninvolved, normal myocardium
    Absence of severe chronic myocardial changes

From Leatherbury, L., Chandra, R. S., Chapiro, S. R., and Perry, L. W.: Value of endomyocardial biopsy in infants, children, and adolescents with dilated or hypertrophic cardiomyopathy and myocarditis. Reprinted from the American College of Cardiology. J. Am. Coll. Cardiol. *12:*1547, 1988.

DILATED CARDIOMYOPATHY

IDIOPATHIC DILATED CARDIOMYOPATHY

Dilated cardiomyopathy (DCM) is a syndrome characterized by cardiac enlargement and impaired systolic function of one or both ventricles (Fig. 41–3). Although it was formerly called congestive cardiomyopathy, the term *dilated cardiomyopathy* is now preferred because the earliest abnormality usually is ventricular enlargement and systolic contractile dysfunction, with congestive heart failure often (but not invariably) developing later. In an occasional patient, the predominant finding is that of contractile dysfunction with only a mildly dilated left ventricle.[22,23]

The incidence of DCM is reported to be about 5 to 8 cases per 100,000 population per year and appears to be increasing, although the true figure likely is higher as a consequence of underreporting of mild or asymptomatic cases.[5,24] It occurs almost three times more frequently in blacks and males than in whites and females, and this difference does not appear to be related solely to differing degrees of hypertension, cigarette smoking, or alcohol use[4,5,25–27]; furthermore, survival in blacks appears to be worse than in whites.[23,28]

Although the cause is not definable in many cases, more than 75 specific diseases of heart muscle can produce the clinical manifestations of DCM. It is likely that this condition represents a final common pathway that is the end result of myocardial damage produced by a variety of cytotoxic, metabolic, immunological, familial, and infectious mechanisms.[24] Alcohol, for example, may lead to severe

cardiac dysfunction and may produce clinical, hemodynamic, and pathological findings identical to those present in idiopathic dilated cardiomyopathy (see p. 1412).

The natural history of DCM is not well established. Many

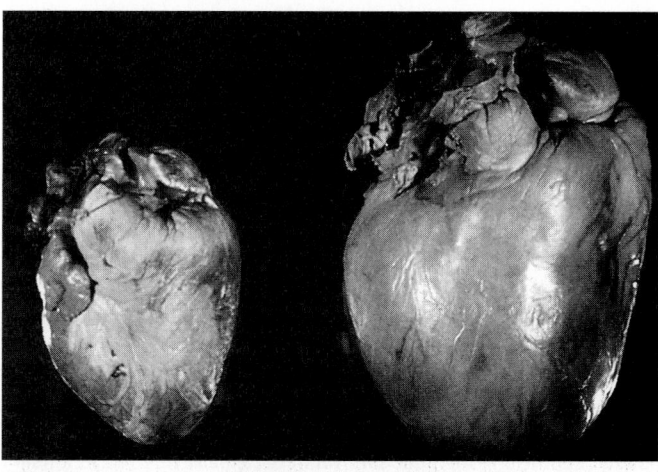

FIGURE 41–3. Gross pathology of normal heart *(left)* and heart in idiopathic dilated cardiomyopathy *(right),* characterized by biventricular hypertrophy and four-chamber enlargement. (From Kasper, E. K., Hruban, R. H., and Baughman, K. L.: Idiopathic dilated cardiomyopathy. *In* Abelmann, W. H., and Braunwald, E., [eds.]: Cardiomyopathies, Myocarditis, and Pericardial Disease. Atlas of Heart Diseases. Vol. 2. Philadelphia, Current Medicine, 1995, pp. 3.1–3.18.)

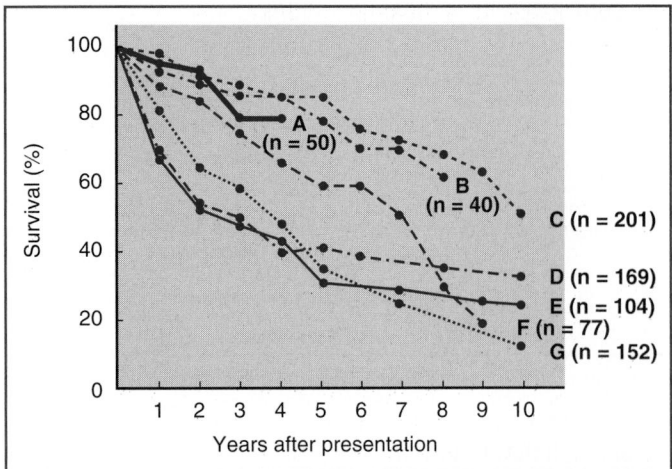

FIGURE 41–4. Survival of patients with idiopathic dilated cardiomyopathy in seven published series (A to G). n = number of patients studied. To identify each specific series, see article by Dec and Fuster. (From Dec, G. W., and Fuster, V.: Idiopathic dilated cardiomyopathy. N. Engl. J. Med. *331:*1564, 1994. Copyright Massachusetts Medical Society.)

patients have minimal or no symptoms and the progression of the disease in these patients is unclear, although there is some evidence that the long-term prognosis is not good.[29] Nevertheless, in symptomatic patients the course usually is one of progressive deterioration, with a quarter of newly diagnosed patients referred to major medical centers dying within a year, and half dying within 5 years, although a minority improve, with a reduction in cardiac size and longer survival (Fig. 41–4).[22,24] Recent data suggest that in patients with mild dilatation not referred to a medical center the prognosis may be more favorable, reflecting earlier diagnosis and better treatment (Fig. 41–5).[3,5,24] About a quarter of patients with recent onset DCM improve spontaneously, even some sick enough initially to be considered for cardiac transplantation.[30,31] In some patients clinical and functional improvements may occur years after initial presentation. A variety of clinical predictors of patients at enhanced risk of death in DCM have been identified (Table 41–6).[32] However, the predictive reliability of any single feature is not high.[33] It may be difficult to predict with any accuracy the clinical course and outcome in an individual

TABLE 41–6   FACTORS ASSOCIATED WITH REDUCED SURVIVAL IN DILATED CARDIOMYOPATHY

S_3
Left ventricular conduction delay
Elevation of filling pressures
Absence of left ventricular thickening
Age > 55 years
Cardiac enlargement
Depressed cardiac output
Depressed ejection fraction
Depressed serum sodium levels
Elevated serum norepinephrine levels
Functional class
Ventricular arrhythmias
Large thallium defects
Myocardial biopsy findings
Ventricular shape (more spherical)

patient.[5,24] Nevertheless, greater ventricular enlargement and worse dysfunction tend to correlate with poorer prognosis.[24,32,34–36] Cardiopulmonary exercise testing also can provide prognostic information (see p. 153). Marked limitation of exercise capacity manifested by reduced maximal systemic oxygen uptake (especially when below 10 to 12 ml/kg/min) is a reliable predictor of mortality and is used widely as an indicator for consideration of cardiac transplantation.[24] It has been suggested that specific endomyocardial biopsy morphological findings (such as loss of intracellular myofilaments) may offer some predictive information regarding prognosis[24,37,38] (Table 41–5).

Pathology

POSTMORTEM EXAMINATION. This reveals enlargement and dilatation of all four chambers; the ventricles are more dilated than the atria (Fig. 41–3). Although the thickness of the ventricular wall is increased in some cases, the degree of hypertrophy often is less than might be expected given the severe dilatation present.[24] The development of left ventricular hypertrophy appears to have a protective or beneficial role in dilated cardiomyopathy, presumably because it reduces systolic wall stress and thus protects against further cavity dilatation.[39,40] The cardiac valves are intrinsically normal, and intracavitary thrombi, particularly in the ventricular apex, are common.[24,41] The coronary arteries usually are normal. The right ventricle is preferentially involved in some cases of dilated cardiomyopathy, sometimes on a familial basis.

HISTOLOGICAL EXAMINATION. Microscopic study reveals extensive areas of interstitial and perivascular fibrosis, particularly involving the left ventricular subendocardium (Fig. 41–2). Small areas of necrosis and cellular infiltrate are seen on occasion, but these typically are not prominent features.[41] There is marked variation in myocyte size; some myocardial cells are hypertrophied and others are atrophied.[41] Cardiac biopsy specimens obtained during life demonstrate a variety of similar abnormalities, including interstitial fibrosis, cellular infiltrates, myocyte hypertrophy, and myocardial cell degeneration.[42] No viruses or other etiological agents have been identified with any regularity in tissue from patients with DCM. Particularly disappointing has been the failure to identify any immunological, histochemical, morphological, ultrastructural, or microbiological marker that might be used to establish the diagnosis of idiopathic dilated cardiomyopathy or to clarify its cause.

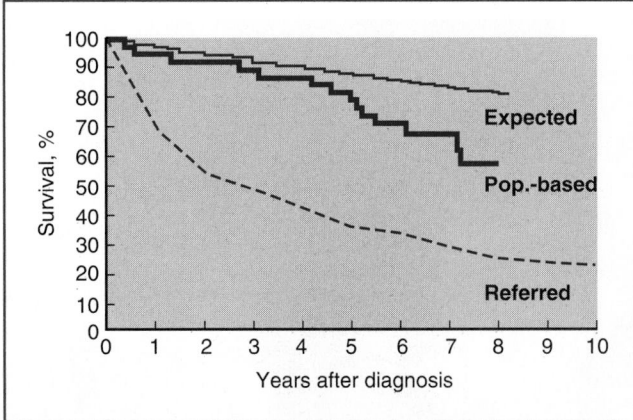

FIGURE 41–5. Survival of patients with idiopathic dilated cardiomyopathy, contrasting the poor survival in the cohort referred to a major medical center (Referred) with the much better survival in the nonreferred population-based cohort (Pop.-based). Both survival curves are compared with the expected survival of a 1980 Minnesota white cohort (Expected). (From Sugrue, D. D., Rodeheffer, R. J., Codd, M. B., et al.: The clinical course of idiopathic dilated cardiomyopathy. A population-based study. Ann. Intern. Med. *117:*117, 1992.)

Etiology

It is likely that idiopathic DCM represents a common expression of myocardial damage that has been produced by a variety of as yet unestablished myocardial insults. Although the cause(s) remain unclear,[43] interest has centered on three possible basic mechanisms of damage: familial and genetic factors; viral myocarditis and other cytotoxic insults; and immunological abnormalities (Fig. 41–6).[23,24,44]

Familial linkage of DCM occurs more commonly than often appreciated. In 20 per cent of patients, a first-degree relative also shows evidence of DCM, suggesting that familial transmission is relatively frequent.[5,23,45–48,48a] Most familial cases demonstrate autosomal dominant transmission[23,48] (see p. 1665), but the disease is genetically quite heterogeneous, and autosomal recessive[49] and X-linked inheritance[46,50,51] has been found. One form of familial X-linked dilated cardiomyopathy is due to a deletion in the promotor region and the first exon of the gene that codes for the protein dystrophin, a component of the cytoskeleton of myocytes.[50] This has fueled speculation that a resulting deficiency of cardiac dystrophin is the cause of the dilated cardiomyopathy.[46] Mutations involving mitochondrial DNA have been reported as well.[52–55] Whether any of the patients without apparent familial linkage have a genetic predisposition to DCM remains unknown.[46] There is great interest in using molecular genetic techniques to identify markers of disease susceptibility in asymptomatic carriers at risk for the eventual development of overt clinical DCM.[51,56,56a] An example of such a marker may be the angiotensin-converting enzyme DD genotype that is found with increased frequency in DCM patients.[57] One intriguing familial metabolic deficiency is that of carnitine, with improvement occurring in the myopathy with carnitine repletion.[58,59]

There has been wide speculation that an episode of subclinical viral myocarditis initiates an autoimmune reaction that culminates in the development of full-blown DCM.[60–62] Although this hypothesis is inviting, it remains largely unsupported[63]; it has been estimated that only 15 per cent of patients with myocarditis progress to DCM.[64] In some patients who exhibit the clinical features of DCM, endomyocardial biopsy reveals evidence of an inflammatory myocarditis. The reported frequency of finding evidence of an inflammatory infiltrate in DCM varies widely and undoubtedly depends largely on patient selection and the criteria used for diagnosis; using rigorous criteria, only about 10 per cent (or less) of patients with DCM have biopsy evidence of myocarditis.[10,11] Other evidence favoring the concept that DCM is a postviral disorder includes the presence of high antibody viral titers,[60,65] viral-specific RNA sequences,[66,67] and apparent viral parti-

cles[64] in patients with "idiopathic" dilated cardiomyopathy. On the other hand, the more rigorous technique of polymerase chain reaction generally has not confirmed the presence of viral remnants in the myocardium of most cardiomyopathy patients,[68–71] although data are conflicting.[72–74]

Abnormalities of both humoral and cellular immunity have been found in patients with DCM,[23,44,75–77] although the findings have not been completely reproducible. There is speculation that antibodies might be the *result* of myocardial damage, rather than the cause.[78] There appears to be an association with specific HLA Class II antigens (such as DR4 and DQw4), suggesting that abnormalities of immunoregulation may play a role in DCM.[56,79] Circulating antimyocardial antibodies to a variety of antigens (including the myosin heavy chain, the beta-adrenoreceptor, the muscarinic receptor, laminin, and mitochondria) have been identified.[44,45,76,80–84] Abnormalities of various T cells, including cytotoxic T cells, suppressor T lymphocytes, and natural killer cells have been found in some but not all studies.[24,85] It has been suggested that these putative immunological abnormalities may be the consequence of prior viral myocarditis.[85] It is thought that viral components may be incorporated into the cardiac sarcolemma, only to serve as an antigenic source that directs the immune response to attack the myocardium. Nevertheless, the precise role of either humoral or cellular immunomodulation in the pathogenesis of DCM remains unestablished.[24]

A variety of other possible causes has been proposed, although none is accepted as *the* cause of DCM. Thus, endocrine abnormalities as well as the effects of chemicals or toxins have been suggested as possible etiological factors. It has been suggested that microvascular hyperreactivity (spasm) may lead to myocellular necrosis and scarring, with resultant heart failure, although this remains speculative.[1,39] From a clinical standpoint, the more important causes of secondary DCM include alcohol and cocaine abuse, human immunodeficiency virus,[86] metabolic abnormalities, and the cardiotoxicity of anticancer drugs (especially doxorubicin).

ABNORMALITIES OF THE SYMPATHETIC NERVOUS SYSTEM. Several abnormalities of the sympathetic nervous system have been demonstrated in DCM, but they appear to be more the result than the cause of the disease.[24,87] A reduction in density of membrane-associated beta-adrenoceptors[88–90] is believed to be a consequence of the development of anti–beta-adrenoceptor autoantibodies.[76,82] An alteration in the signal transmission pathway by which the beta-receptors stimulate the contractile apparatus (the G-protein system) has been found as well. Inhibition of this system is enhanced in DCM patients, perhaps accounting for their depressed contractile function. An increase of the α subunits of the inhibitory guanine nucleotide–binding protein ($G_{I\alpha}$) has been reported to occur in the membranes of myocytes from failing hearts.[91–93] This abnormality has been shown to be more profound in myocardial membranes from hearts with dilated than in those with ischemic cardiomyopathy.[94] This increase in $G_{I\alpha}$ is associated with a striking reduction of basal adenylate cyclase activity and of the positive inotropic effects of isoproterenol and of the phosphodiesterase inhibitor milrinone (see p. 484). These findings suggest that the increase of $G_{I\alpha}$ might contribute to the reduced effects of endogenous catecholamines in DCM. The precise cause of contractile dysfunction at the cellular level in patients with DCM remains unclear. Although there are demonstrable abnormalities of cellular metabolism and calcium handling by cardiomyopathic tissue,[1,95–99] the significance of these findings is not yet clear.

Clinical Manifestations
(Fig. 41–7)

HISTORY. Symptoms usually develop gradually in patients with DCM. Some patients are asymptomatic and yet have left ventricular dilatation for months or even years which is clinically recognized only later when symptoms develop or when routine chest roentgenography demonstrates cardiomegaly.[100] Other patients, after recovery from what appears to be a systemic viral infection, develop symptoms of heart failure for the first time. In still others, severe heart failure develops acutely during an episode of myocarditis; although some recovery occurs, chronic manifestations of diminished cardiac reserve persist and heart failure reappears months or years later. It is important to carefully question the patient and family about alcohol consumption, because excessive alcohol consumption is a major cause of secondary DCM, and its cessation may result in substantial clinical improvement.[24] Although patients of any age may be affected, the disease is most common in middle age and is more frequent in men than in women.

The most striking symptoms are those of left ventricular failure. Fatigue and weakness due to diminished cardiac output are common. Exercise intolerance is common and

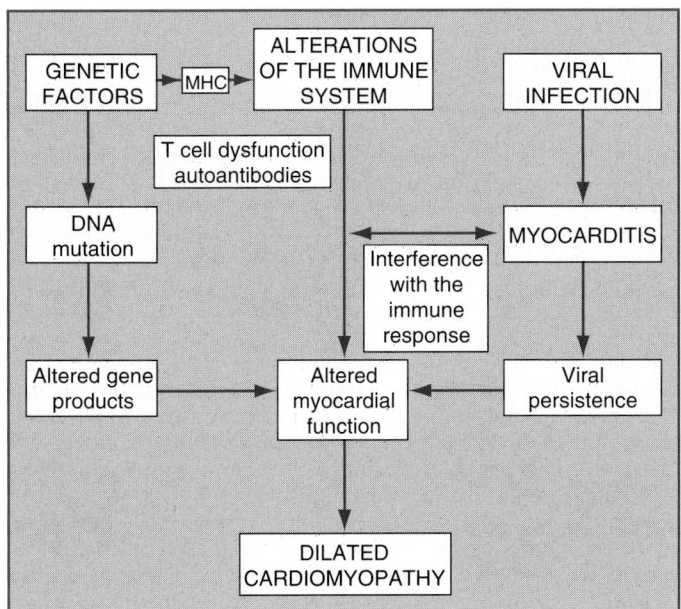

FIGURE 41–6. Hypotheses to explain the pathogenesis of dilated cardiomyopathy. (From Mestroni, L., Krajinovic, M., Severini, G. M., et al.: Familial dilated cardiomyopathy. Br. Heart J. 72:S35, 1994.)

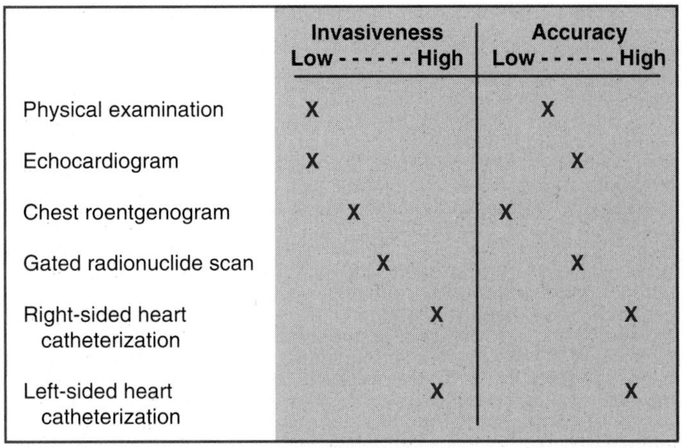

	Invasiveness Low - - - - - - High		Accuracy Low - - - - - - High	
Physical examination	X		X	
Echocardiogram	X			X
Chest roentgenogram		X	X	
Gated radionuclide scan		X		X
Right-sided heart catheterization		X		X
Left-sided heart catheterization		X		X

FIGURE 41–7. Assessment of utility of diagnostic techniques in idiopathic dilated cardiomyopathy. (From Manolio, T. A., Baughman, K. L., Rodeheffer, R., et al.: Prevalence and etiology of idiopathic dilated cardiomyopathy [summary of a National Heart, Lung, and Blood Institute workshop]. Am. J. Cardiol. 69:1458, 1992.)

relates, at least in part, to reduced skeletal muscle perfusion as well as histological and biochemical alterations in the exercising muscle groups.[101] Right heart failure is a late and ominous sign and is associated with a particularly poor prognosis. Chest pain occurs in about one-third of patients and may suggest concomitant ischemic heart disease.[3,24,102] A reduction in the vasodilator reserve of the coronary microvasculature in DCM suggests that subendocardial ischemia may play a role in the genesis of chest pain despite angiographically normal coronary arteries.[103] Chest pain secondary to pulmonary embolism and abdominal pain secondary to congestive hepatomegaly are frequent in the late stages of illness.

PHYSICAL EXAMINATION. This usually reveals variable degrees of cardiac enlargement and findings of congestive heart failure. The systolic blood pressure is usually normal or low, and the pulse pressure is narrow, reflecting a diminished stroke volume. *Pulsus alternans* (see p. 22) is common when severe left ventricular failure is present. The jugular veins are distended when right heart failure appears, but on initial presentation most patients do not have evidence of this.[24] Prominent *a* and *v* waves are visible, the latter a late manifestation of the presence of tricuspid valvular regurgitation. The liver may be engorged and pulsatile. Peripheral edema and ascites are present when right heart failure is advanced. Wheezing resulting from bronchospasm may be found, apparently as a consequence of bronchial hyperresponsiveness.[104]

The precordium usually reveals left and, occasionally, right ventricular impulses, but the heaves are not sustained, as they are in patients with ventricular hypertrophy. The apical impulse is usually displaced laterally, reflecting left ventricular dilatation. A presystolic *a* wave may be palpable. The second heart sound is usually normally split, although paradoxical splitting (see p. 33) may be detected in the presence of left bundle branch block, an electrocardiographic finding that is not unusual in dilated cardiomyopathy. If pulmonary hypertension is present, the pulmonary component of the second heart sound may be accentuated, and the splitting may be narrow. Presystolic gallop sounds (S₄) are almost universally present and often precede the development of overt congestive heart failure.[24] Ventricular gallops (S₃) are the rule once cardiac decompensation occurs, and a summation gallop is heard when there is concomitant tachycardia. Systolic murmurs are common and are usually due to mitral or, less commonly, tricuspid valvular regurgitation.[24] Mitral regurgitation results from enlargement and abnormal motion of the mitral annulus; ventricular dilatation with resultant distortion of the geometry of the subvalvular apparatus ("papillary mus-

cle dysfunction") plays a lesser role.[105] Gallop sounds and regurgitant murmurs can often be elicited or intensified by isometric handgrip exercise with its attendant enhancement of systemic vascular resistance and impedance to left ventricular outflow (see p. 48). Systemic emboli resulting from dislodgment of intracardiac thrombi from the left atrium and ventricle and pulmonary emboli that originate in the venous system of the legs are common late complications.

NONINVASIVE LABORATORY EXAMINATIONS. To identify potentially reversible secondary causes of dilated cardiomyopathy, several basic screening biochemical tests are indicated, including determination of serum phosphorus (hypophosphatemia), serum calcium (hypocalcemia), serum creatinine and urea nitrogen (uremia), thyroid function studies (hypo- and hyperthyroidism), and iron studies (hemochromatosis). It is prudent to test for the human immunodeficiency virus (HIV) as well, as this infection is an important and often unrecognized cause of congestive heart failure.[86] The *chest roentgenogram* usually reveals generalized cardiomegaly and pulmonary vascular redistribution; interstitial and alveolar edema are less common on initial presentation.[24] Pleural effusions may be present, and the azygos vein and superior vena cava may be dilated when right heart failure supervenes.

Electrocardiography. The electrocardiogram often shows sinus tachycardia when heart failure is present. The entire spectrum of atrial and ventricular tachyarrhythmias may be seen. Poor R-wave progression and intraventricular conduction abnormalities, especially left bundle branch block, are common.[24] Anterior Q waves may be present when there is extensive left ventricular fibrosis, even without a discrete myocardial scar.[24,106] ST-segment and T-wave abnormalities are common, as are P-wave changes, especially left atrial abnormality.[106] Ambulatory monitoring demonstrates the ubiquity of ventricular arrhythmias, with about half of monitored patients with DCM exhibiting nonsustained ventricular tachycardia.[24] There is no consensus that complex or frequent ventricular arrhythmias predict sudden (presumably arrhythmic) death, although they do appear to predict total mortality.[106–108] Perhaps ventricular arrhythmias as detected on ambulatory monitoring are a marker for the extent of myocardial damage in DCM and therefore are *associated* with sudden death without necessarily being its *cause*. In occasional cases, particularly in children, recurrent and/or incessant supraventricular or ventricular tachyarrhythmias may actually be the *cause* (rather than the result) of ventricular dysfunction.[109–112] In those cases, restoration of sinus rhythm or slowing of the heart rate may be therapeutic.

Echocardiography. Two-dimensional and Doppler forms of echocardiography are useful in assessing the degree of impairment of left ventricular function and for excluding concomitant valvular or pericardial disease (Chap. 3).[5] In addition to examining all four cardiac valves for evidence of structural or functional abnormalities, echocardiography allows evaluation of the size of the ventricular cavity and thickness of the ventricular walls. A pericardial effusion may be demonstrated on occasion. Doppler studies are useful in delineating the severity of mitral (and tricuspid) regurgitation.[76,82] Patients with a pattern of left ventricular filling on Doppler studies which simulates that seen with restrictive cardiomyopathy appear to have more advanced disease.[113] Combining echocardiography with dobutamine infusion may identify patients with left ventricular dysfunction due to coronary artery disease by demonstrating provocable regional differences in wall motion and thus distinguish them from patients with idiopathic DCM.[114,114a] It has been suggested that *thallium-201* imaging may be helpful in distinguishing left ventricular enlargement caused by DCM from that caused by coronary artery disease,[115,116] although there is not complete agreement on this point.[24,117] Scanning with *gallium* or *antimyosin antibody* (see p. 296) may help to identify patients more likely to have evidence of myocarditis on biopsy, although whether this finding is useful clinically is not yet established.[24,118-120]

Radionuclide Ventriculography. Like echocardiography, radionuclide ventriculography reveals increased end-diastolic and end-systolic left ventricular volumes, reduced ejection fractions in both ventricles, and wall-motion abnormalities; it is used most commonly when echocardiography is technically suboptimal.[24] Like echocardiography, it may demonstrate segmental wall motion abnormalities in DCM even in the absence of coronary artery disease, the disease process that most commonly produces regional dysfunction. In most patients it is not necessary to carry out serial studies or batteries of noninvasive tests in order to follow patients with DCM and evaluate their response to treatment.

CARDIAC CATHETERIZATION AND ANGIOCARDIOGRAPHY. Only select patients with DCM require cardiac catheterization[24] (particularly those with chest pain and a suspicion of ischemic disease, or patients thought to have a treatable systemic disease such as sarcoidosis or hemochromatosis). When cardiac catheterization is done, the left ventricular end-diastolic, left atrial, and pulmonary artery wedge pressures are usually elevated. Modest degrees of pulmonary arterial hypertension are common. Advanced cases may demonstrate right ventricular dilatation and failure as well, with resultant elevation of the right ventricular end-diastolic, right atrial, and central venous pressures.

Left ventriculography demonstrates enlargement of this chamber, typically with diffuse reduction in wall motion. Segmental wall motion abnormalities are not uncommon and may simulate the angiographic findings in ischemic heart disease.[121] However, prominent localized wall disorders are more characteristic of ischemic heart disease, whereas diffuse global dysfunction is more typical of DCM. The ejection fraction is reduced and the end-systolic volume is increased as a result of the impairment of left ventricular contractility. Sometimes left ventricular thrombi may be visualized within the left ventricle as intracavitary filling defects. Mild mitral regurgitation is often present. On occasion, it may be difficult to distinguish left ventricular dilatation secondary to severe mitral regurgitation due to intrinsic mitral valve disease from DCM with secondary mitral regurgitation.

Coronary arteriography usually reveals normal vessels, although coronary vasodilatory capacity may be impaired[103,122,123]; in some cases this may relate to marked elevation of the left ventricular filling pressures.[124] This examination may be of particular value in excluding coronary artery disease in patients with abnormal Q waves on the electrocardiogram or regional left ventricular wall motion abnormalities on noninvasive testing. Coronary arteriography thus helps to distinguish between myocardial infarction as a result of obstructive coronary artery disease, and extensive localized myocardial fibrosis secondary to severe DCM in the absence of coronary artery obstruction.

Management

Because the cause of idiopathic dilated cardiomyopathy is unknown, specific therapy is not possible. Treatment, therefore, is for heart failure, as discussed in Chapter 17.[125] Physical, dietary, and pharmacological interventions may help to control symptoms; only cardiac transplantation[125a] (Chap. 18) and specific pharmacological therapy (the vasodilators enalapril or hydralazine plus nitrates, and the beta-adrenoceptor blocker carvedilol) have been shown to prolong life (Table 41-7).[24,125-128,128a] Although the demonstrated benefits of vasodilator therapy are more equivocal in asymptomatic patients, we favor their use when not contraindicated in hopes of limiting progressive ventricular dilatation and preventing or delaying symptomatic deterioration.

Because of evidence that activation of the sympathetic nervous system may have deleterious cardiac effects (rather

Initiate conventional management with digoxin, diuretics, and angiotensin-converting enzyme inhibitors or hydralazine/isosorbide dinitrate.

Consider beta-adrenergic blockade if symptoms persist.

Add anticoagulation for ejection fraction less than 0.30, history of thromboembolic phenomena, or detection of mural thrombi.

If symptomatic at rest despite above measures, add intravenous dobutamine and/or phosphodiesterase inhibitor and consider cardiac transplantation.

Adapted from O'Connell, J. B., Moore, C. K., and Waterer, H. C.: Treatment of end stage dilated cardiomyopathy. Br. Heart J. *72*:S52, 1994.

than being an important compensatory mechanism as traditionally thought), beta-adrenoceptor blockade (usually with metoprolol) has been suggested as treatment for DCM[24] (see p. 487). Results to date generally have been favorable, with evidence of improved symptoms, exercise capacity, and left ventricular function, and a suggestion that survival has been improved.[24,129-136] Beta-adrenoceptor blockade has been surprisingly well tolerated, with infrequent aggravation of heart failure (which, on occasion, may be profound). The mechanism of beneficial action of beta-adrenoceptorblockers is unknown[125] but may relate to: (1) negative chronotropic effect with reduced myocardial oxygen demand, (2) reduced myocardial damage due to catecholamines, (3) improved diastolic relaxation, (4) inhibition of sympathetically mediated vasoconstriction, (5) increase ("upregulation") in myocardial beta-adrenoceptor density,[137] or (6) improved calcium handling at slower rates.[88,138-141] Despite the encouraging data, the use of beta-adrenoceptor blockade in DCM still is considered investigational. Recent data indicate that carvedilol (a beta-adrenoceptor blocker with alpha-adrenoceptor blocking and antioxidant effects) substantially reduces mortality in DCM.[128a]

Because of the possible link between DCM, microvascular circulatory abnormalities, and abnormal myocardial calcium handling, there has been interest in the use of calcium antagonists. Diltiazem in particular appears to be safe and preliminary results regarding clinical utility are encouraging, although myocardial depression is an important potential side effect of the calcium antagonists as a group. Combining a calcium antagonist with a vasodilator does not appear to have any additional beneficial effects on reducing mortality in DCM.[141a] At present, the use of calcium antagonists in DCM is considered investigational and not yet first-line therapy.[125,142]

Although there is no definitive evidence that antiarrhythmic agents prolong life or prevent sudden death in DCM,[24,125,142a] it may be appropriate to use them in the treatment of symptomatic arrhythmias. Because of the adverse effects of most available agents, many of which depress myocardial contractility and have a proarrhythmic effect (see Chap. 21), treatment should be individualized, with both efficacy and toxicity carefully monitored. Unfortunately, electrophysiological testing is of limited utility in DCM because it is positive in a minority of patients at risk[24,143]; the lack of inducibility of ventricular tachyarrhythmias does not identify a low-risk group, and pharmacological suppression of provoked arrhythmias does not necessarily predict freedom from recurrences.[144] The recording of late potentials by the signal-averaged electrocardiogram appears to be of benefit in assessing the risk of death,[145-147] although this has not been a universal finding and awaits further confirmation.[148,149] Implantation of the internal defibrillator (see p. 732) should be considered in appropriate candidates with symptomatic ventricular tachyarrhythmias.[125,143,150,151]

Even in the absence of controlled clinical trials demonstrating their efficacy,[152,153] anticoagulants are recommended in patients with DCM and heart failure (particularly in the presence of atrial fibrillation or a prior stroke) (see p. 509).[24] Anticoagulants should be used even without direct clinical or echocardiographic evidence of thrombus formation if there are no specific contraindications to these agents with a target prolongation of the prothrombin time to 2.0 to 3.0 (international normalized ratio [INR]).[24] In those patients with chronic heart failure secondary to DCM and lymphocytic infiltrate on myocardial biopsy, treatment with corticosteroids and immunosuppressive agents has been advocated. Prednisone therapy does not appear to have a clinically important effect on symptoms, exercise performance, or ejection fraction (in more than just the short term) and is associated with significant complications in half the patients so treated.[154,155] Routine clinical use of immunosuppressive therapy thus cannot be recommended at present.[24,125]

Surgical treatment (such as with mitral annuloplasty) or replacement of regurgitant valves has been attempted in some patients with prominent atrioventricular valvular regurgitation. The results of operation are usually less than satisfactory because of the degree of pre-existing cardiac dysfunction and damage. In appropriate patients, cardiac transplantation may be an alternative (Chap. 18), with a 5-year survival rate of over 70 per cent.[24] Surgical translocation of the latissimus dorsi muscle to wrap around the heart and augment cardiac performance (dynamic cardiomyoplasty) appears to have benefited some patients who are not otherwise suitable candidates for cardiac transplantation.[156-162]

ALCOHOLIC CARDIOMYOPATHY

Chronic excessive consumption of alcohol may be associated with congestive heart failure, hypertension, cerebrovascular accidents, arrhythmias, and sudden death; it is the major cause of secondary, nonischemic dilated cardiomyopathy in the Western world and accounts for upwards of one-third of all cases of DCM.[163-165] It is estimated that two-thirds of the adult population use alcohol to some extent, and more than 10 per cent are heavy users.[166] Therefore, it is not surprising that alcoholic cardiomyopathy is a major problem. Ceasing alcohol consumption early in the course of alcoholic cardiomyopathy may halt the progression or even reverse left ventricular contractile dysfunction, unlike nonalcoholic cardiomyopathy that often is marked by progressive clinical deterioration.[39]

The consumption of alcohol may result in myocardial damage by three basic mechanisms: (1) a presumed direct toxic effect of alcohol or its metabolites; (2) nutritional effects, most commonly in association with thiamine deficiency that leads to beriberi heart disease (see p. 461); and (3) rarely, toxic effects due to additives in the alcoholic beverage (cobalt)[167] (see p. 1413). There had been speculation that alcohol caused myocardial damage only through dietary deficiencies, but it is now clear that alcoholic cardiomyopathy occurs in the absence of nutritional deficiencies.[163,166,168]

Typical Oriental beriberi may coexist with alcoholic cardiomyopathy, although it is no longer seen with any frequency.[169] The distinguishing features of each include peripheral vasodilatation and high-output heart failure, often right-sided, in the former and reduced contractility with typically left-sided low-output failure in the latter.[163,169]

Alcohol results in acute as well as chronic depression of myocardial contractility and may produce reversible cardiac dysfunction even when ingested by normal nonalcoholic individuals.[170] What is responsible for the transition from the reversible acute effects to permanent myocardial damage remains unclear.[171]

The precise mechanisms of cardiac depression produced by alcohol is undetermined,[172] but a direct toxic effect on striated muscle is likely (particularly because alcoholics often demonstrate concomitant skeletal myopathy and cardiomyopathy).[163,166] In acute studies, alcohol and its metabolite acetaldehyde have been shown to interfere with a number of membrane and cellular functions that involve the transport and binding of calcium, mitochondrial respiration, myocardial

lipid metabolism, myocardial protein synthesis, and signal transduction.[166,170,171] Studies in isolated ferret papillary muscles have shown that ethanol in concentrations similar to those occurring in intoxicated humans depresses myocardial contractility by interfering with excitation-contraction coupling through inhibition of the interaction between calcium and the myofilaments.[170] The accumulation of metabolites of ethanol in the myocardium may interfere with normal myocardial lipid metabolism and may play a role in the pathogenesis of alcohol-induced myocardial damage.[171] The role that other associated electrolyte imbalances (hypokalemia, hypophosphatemia, hypomagnesemia) may play in alcohol-mediated damage has not been settled.[168]

PATHOLOGY. The gross and microscopic pathological findings are nonspecific and similar to those observed in idiopathic DCM, with interstitial fibrosis, myocytolysis, evidence of small vessel coronary artery disease, and myocyte hypertrophy.[163,173,174] Electron microscopy shows enlarged and disorganized mitochondria, with large glycogen-containing vacuoles.[168]

Clinical Manifestations

Alcoholic cardiomyopathy most commonly occurs in men 30 to 55 years of age who have been heavy consumers of whisky, wine, or beer, usually for more than 10 years.[164,174] Although alcoholic cardiomyopathy may be observed in the homeless, malnourished, "skid row" alcoholic man, many patients are well-nourished individuals of middle and even upper socioeconomic status without liver disease or peripheral neuropathy. Accordingly, unless a high index of suspicion is maintained, it may be easy to miss a history of alcohol abuse. Persistent questioning of the patient and particularly the relatives of patients with unexplained cardiomegaly or cardiomyopathy is often required to elicit a history of alcoholism.

It is frequently possible to demonstrate mild depression of cardiac function in chronic alcoholics even before cardiac dysfunction becomes clinically manifest.[164,175] Abnormalities of both systolic function (reduced ejection fraction) and diastolic function (increased myocardial wall stiffness) have been demonstrated in alcoholic patients without cardiac symptoms by a variety of invasive and noninvasive techniques.[176] Although overt alcoholic liver disease and cardiac involvement usually do not occur together, even cirrhotic patients without signs or symptoms of heart disease have demonstrable evidence of asymptomatic myocardial disease.[164]

The development of symptoms may be insidious, although some patients have acute and florid left-sided congestive heart failure. A paroxysm of atrial fibrillation is a relatively frequent initial presenting finding.[164] More advanced cases demonstrate findings of biventricular failure, with left ventricular dysfunction usually dominating. Dyspnea, orthopnea, and paroxysmal nocturnal dyspnea frequently are observed. Palpitations and syncope due to tachyarrhythmias, usually supraventricular, occasionally are present. Angina pectoris does not occur unless there is concomitant coronary artery disease or aortic stenosis, although atypical chest pain may be seen.

PHYSICAL EXAMINATION. The cardiac findings resemble those seen in idiopathic dilated cardiomyopathy. Examination usually reveals a narrow pulse pressure, often with an elevated diastolic pressure secondary to excessive peripheral vasoconstriction. There is cardiomegaly, and protodiastolic (S_3) and presystolic (S_4) gallop sounds are common.[164] An apical systolic murmur of mitral regurgitation often is found. The severity of right heart failure varies, but jugular venous distention and peripheral edema are common. A concomitant skeletal muscle myopathy involving the shoulder and pelvic girdle is a frequent finding, and the degree of muscle weakness and histological abnormality in the skeletal muscles parallels that in the heart.[163,168]

LABORATORY EXAMINATION. The *chest roentgenogram* in the advanced case demonstrates considerable cardiac enlargement, pulmonary congestion, and pulmonary venous hypertension (see p. 219). Pleural effusions often are seen. *Electrocardiographic abnormalities* are common and frequently are the only indication of alcoholic heart disease during the preclinical phase. Alcoholic patients without other evidence of heart disease often are seen after developing palpitations, chest discomfort, or syncope, typically following a binge of alcohol consumption on a weekend, particularly during the year-end holiday season. This is dubbed the "holiday heart syndrome." The most common arrhythmia observed is atrial fibrillation, followed by atrial flutter and frequent ventricular premature contractions.[164] Alcohol consumption may predispose to atrial flutter or fibrillation, even in nonalcoholics.[168] Hypokalemia may play a role in the genesis of some of these arrhythmias. Supraventricular arrhythmias are also frequently observed in patients with overt alcoholic cardiomyopathy. Sudden, unexpected death is not uncommon in young adult alcoholics, and it is likely that ventricular fibrillation is responsible.[164]

Atrioventricular conduction disturbances (most commonly first-degree heart block), bundle branch block, left ventricular hypertrophy, poor R-wave progression across the precordium, and repolarization abnormalities are common electrocardiographic findings.[164] Prolongation of the Q-T interval is noted frequently. ST-segment and T-wave changes are often restored to normal within several days after cessation of alcohol consumption.

The hemodynamic findings observed at cardiac catheterization and the assessment of left ventricular function by noninvasive methods (echocardiography and isotope angiography) resemble those found in idiopathic DCM.

MANAGEMENT. The *natural history* of alcoholic cardiomyopathy depends on the drinking habits of the patient. Total abstinence in the early stages of the disease may lead to resolution of the manifestations of congestive heart failure and a return of heart size toward normal, although patients with severe heart failure may show no improvement in function or prognosis.[164] Continued alcohol consumption leads to further myocardial damage and fibrosis, with the development of refractory congestive heart failure. Death may also be due to arrhythmia, heart block, and systemic or pulmonary embolism.

The key to the long-term treatment of alcoholic cardiomyopathy is *immediate and total abstinence* as early in the course of the disease as possible.[164] This may be quite effective in improving the signs and symptoms of congestive heart failure.[177,177a] The reversibility of alcoholic myocardial

depression is supported by the demonstration of a reduction of myocardial uptake of labeled monoclonal antimyosin antibodies (a marker of myocyte damage) in alcoholics who stop drinking.[120] The prognosis in patients who continue to drink, particularly if they have been symptomatic for a long time, is poor. In the overall population of patients with alcoholic cardiomyopathy, between 40 and 50 per cent succumb within a 3- to 6-year period, especially if they continue to drink.[164] Prolonged bed rest is thought to result in functional improvement, although its major benefit may simply be the decreased alcohol consumption.[164]

The management of acute episodes of congestive heart failure is similar to that of idiopathic DCM (see p. 1411 and Table 41–7). For patients with severe congestive heart failure, it is prudent to administer thiamine on the chance that beriberi may be contributing to the heart failure.[169] Whether to use chronic anticoagulation (as is usually recommended for idiopathic DCM) is a difficult question; we usually do not prescribe warfarin because of the risk of bleeding due to noncompliance, trauma, and overanticoagulation due to hepatic dysfunction.

COBALT CARDIOMYOPATHY

A previously unrecognized syndrome of severe congestive heart failure appeared in the mid-1960s, first in Canada and subsequently in the United States and Europe.[167] The disease was found in people who drank a particular brand of beer to which cobalt sulfate had been added as a foam stabilizer. Since cobalt was removed from the process, no more cases of the disease have been reported. On very rare occasions occupational exposure to cobalt may result in myocardial damage and attendant congestive heart failure.[167,178]

ARRHYTHMOGENIC RIGHT VENTRICULAR DYSPLASIA
(See also p. 324)

This unique cardiomyopathy (which is also called right ventricular cardiomyopathy) is marked by partial or total replacement of right ventricular muscle by adipose and fibrous tissue (Fig. 41–8) and may be associated with reentrant ventricular tachyarrhythmias of right ventricular origin (left bundle branch block configuration of the QRS complex).[179–182] The cause of the myocardial changes is unclear, but in about one-third of the cases there is autosomal dominant inheritance of the disease.[182–184] It appears to be distinct from Uhl's disease, which is marked by extreme thinning of the ventricular wall. The diagnosis is based on a constellation of clinical, electrocardiographic, histological, and echocardiographic findings.[182,185] Typical clinical features include male predominance, normal physical examination, inverted T waves in the right precordial electrocardiographic leads, symptoms of palpitations and syncope, and a risk of sudden

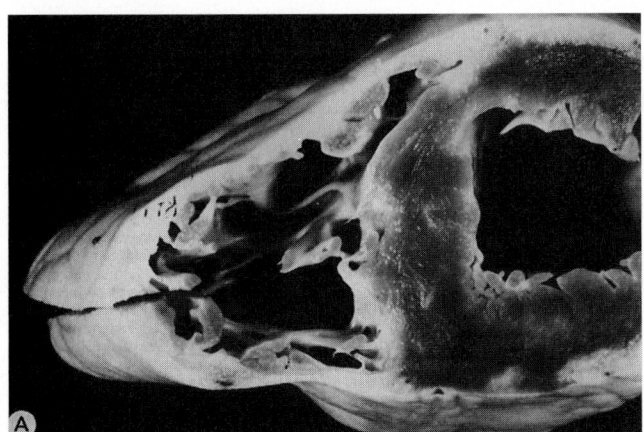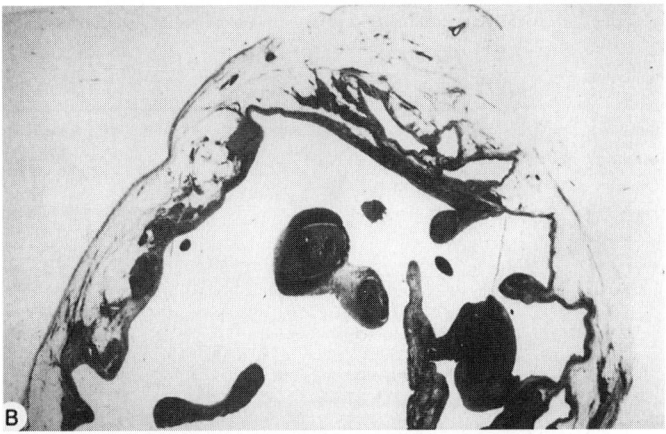

FIGURE 41–8. Pathological findings in a 39-year-old man with arrhythmogenic right ventricular dysplasia and a family history of sudden death. *A,* Cross-section of the heart showing pronounced adipose infiltration of the right ventricular free wall and nearly normal left ventricle and ventricular septum. *B,* Histological view of the right ventricular free wall showing myocardial atrophy and massive fibrofatty replacement. (Azan, × 1). (From McKenna, W. J., Thiene, G., Nava, A., et al.: Diagnosis of arrhythmogenic right ventricular dysplasia/cardiomyopathy. Task Force of the Working Group Myocardial and Pericardial Disease of the European Society of Cardiology and of the Scientific Council on Cardiomyopathies of the International Society and Federation of Cardiology. Br. Heart J. *71:*215, 1994.)

death.[182,184,186-188] In some patients with ventricular arrhythmias of no evident cause, clinically subtle right ventricular dysplasia may be etiologic.[189-192]

Noninvasive and invasive evaluation demonstrate a dilated, poorly contractile right ventricle, usually with a normal left ventricle, although some degree of left ventricular dysfunction has been seen.[193,194] Magnetic resonance imaging (MRI) shows promise for iden-

tifying patients with this condition.[195] Antiarrhythmic therapy, especially with beta-adrenoceptor blockers, often is effective in controlling the arrhythmias.[190,192] The arrhythmias appear to be related to abnormalities of regional right ventricular sympathetic innervation, as demonstrated by noninvasive scintigraphy.[180] Cryoablation of the presumed arrhythmogenic focus has been successful in resolving the ventricular arrhythmia in some patients.[196]

HYPERTROPHIC CARDIOMYOPATHY

Although first described about a century ago, the unique features of hypertrophic cardiomyopathy (HCM) were not studied systematically until the late 1950s.[197,198] The characteristic finding was inappropriate myocardial hypertrophy that occurred in the absence of an obvious cause for the hypertrophy (such as aortic stenosis or systemic hypertension), often predominantly involving the interventricular septum of a nondilated left ventricle that showed hyperdynamic ventricular function (Fig. 41-9).[198] A distinctive clinical feature was soon recognized in some patients with HCM—a dynamic pressure gradient in the subaortic area that divided the left ventricle into a high-pressure apical region and a lower-pressure subaortic region (Fig. 41-10). Although subsequent studies have shown that only a minority of patients (perhaps a quarter)[199] demonstrate this outflow gradient, its unique features attracted much attention and led to a myriad of terms (more than 75) used to describe the disease (among the more popular terms were *idiopathic hypertrophic subaortic stenosis (IHSS)* and *mus-*

cular subaortic stenosis). The term *hypertrophic cardiomyopathy* is now preferred because most patients do not have an outflow gradient or "stenosis" of the left ventricular outflow tract. Because hypertrophy typically occurs in the absence of a pressure gradient, the characteristic distinguishing feature of HCM is myocardial hypertrophy that is out of proportion to the hemodynamic load.

The physiological characteristics of HCM differ substantially from those of DCM (Table 41-8). The most characteristic pathophysiological abnormality in HCM is *diastolic*

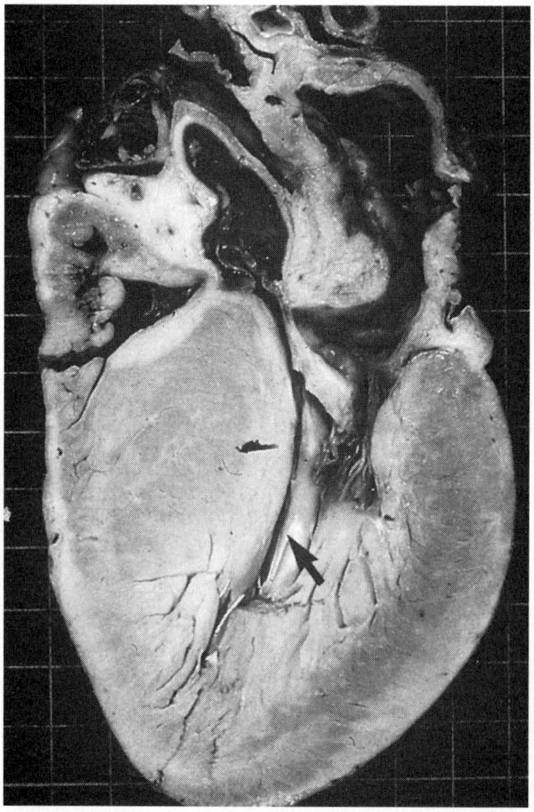

FIGURE 41-9. Pathological findings in a patient with hypertrophic cardiomyopathy with a left ventricular outflow tract gradient during life. The heart is opened in the longitudinal plane. This patient had mitral regurgitation that was partially due to abnormal insertion of an anomalous papillary muscle (arrow) onto the ventricular surface of the anterior mitral leaflet. (Modified from Wigle, E. D., Sasson, Z., Henderson, M. A., et al.: Hypertrophic cardiomyopathy. The importance of the site and the extent of hypertrophy: A review. Prog. Cardiovasc. Dis. 28:1, 1985.)

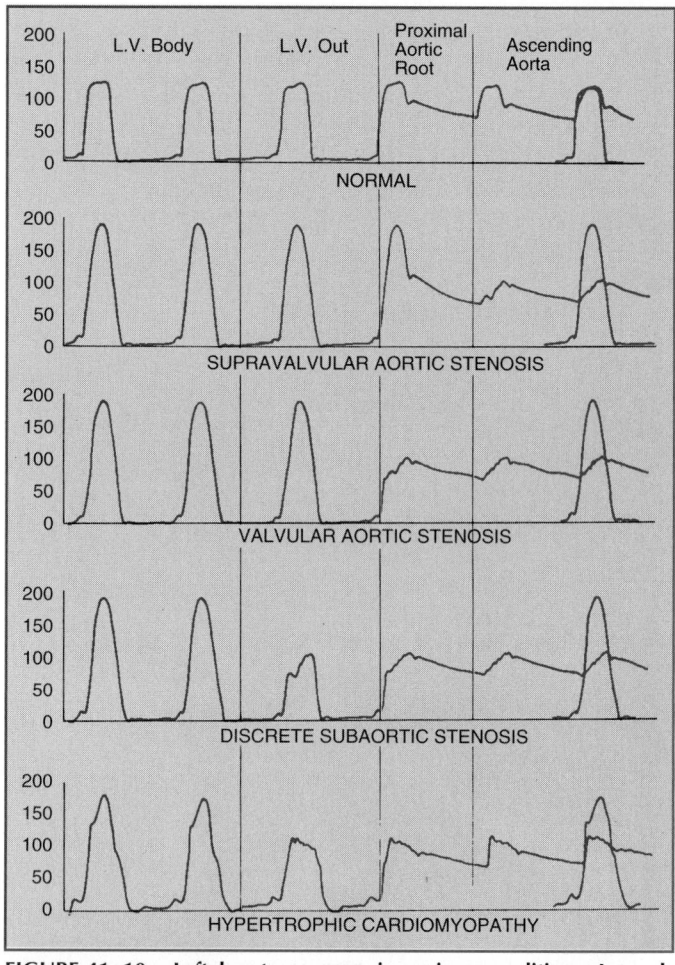

FIGURE 41-10. Left heart pressures in various conditions. In each horizontal panel there is an idealized depiction of the pressure tracing that would be obtained as a catheter is withdrawn from the left ventricular body through the left ventricular outflow tract into the proximal aortic root. On the far right is a superimposition of the pressures in the left ventricular body and in the aorta. The vertical lines bound the regional catheter position within the heart during withdrawal. All forms of discrete stenosis (supravalvular, valvular, and subvalvular) have delayed aortic upstroke rates downstream from the stenosis. Only in hypertrophic cardiomyopathy is the aortic upstroke rate rapid and parallel to the left ventricular pressure. LV = Left ventricular, Out = outflow tract. (From Criley, J. M., and Siegel, R. J.: Subaortic stenosis revisited: The importance of the dynamic pressure gradient. Medicine [Baltimore] 72:412, 1993.)

TABLE 41–8 DIFFERENCES IN SYSTOLIC AND DIASTOLIC FUNCTION IN DILATED (CONGESTIVE) AND HYPERTROPHIC CARDIOMYOPATHY

	DILATED CARDIOMYOPATHY	HYPERTROPHIC CARDIOMYOPATHY
Left ventricular volume		
End-diastolic	Increased	Normal
End-systolic	Markedly increased	Decreased
Left ventricular mass	Increased	Markedly increased
Mass/volume ratio	Decreased	Increased
Systolic function		
Ejection fraction	Decreased	Normal or increased
Myocardial shortening	Decreased	Increased
Wall stress	Increased	Decreased
Diastolic function		
Chamber stiffness	Decreased	Increased
Myocardial stiffness	Increased	Increased

From Chatterjee, K.: Pathophysiology of cardiomyopathy. *In* Giles, T. D., and Sander, G. E. (eds.): Cardiomyopathy. Middleton, MA, PSG Publishing Co., 1988, p. 65.

rather than systolic dysfunction (see also pp. 402 and 447).[197] Thus, HCM is characterized by abnormal stiffness of the left ventricle with resultant impaired ventricular filling. This abnormality in diastolic relaxation produces increased left ventricular end-diastolic pressure with resulting pulmonary congestion and dyspnea, the most common symptoms in HCM, despite typically hyperdynamic left ventricular systolic function. The disease appears to be genetically transmitted in about half the patients as an autosomal dominant trait with disease loci on one of at least four different chromosomes (chromosomes 1, 11, 14, and 15).[200,201] The cause of HCM (see p. 1417) in the remainder of patients is unknown. Morphological evidence of the disease is found in about one-fourth of the first-degree relatives of a patient with HCM; in many of the relatives the disease is milder than in the propositus, the degree of hypertrophy is less and is more localized, and outflow gradients usually are lacking. Symptoms often are absent or minimal, and the disease is detected only by echocardiography. The overall prevalence of HCM is low and has been estimated to occur in 0.02 to 0.2 per cent of the population.[202,202a] It is found in 0.5 per cent of unselected patients referred for an echocardiographic examination.[203]

Pathology

MACROSCOPIC EXAMINATION. This typically discloses a marked increase in myocardial mass, and the ventricular cavities are small (Fig. 41–9).[198] The left ventricle is usually more involved with the hypertrophic process than is the right.[204] The atria are dilated and often hypertrophied, reflecting the high resistance to filling of the ventricles caused by diastolic dysfunction and the effects of atrioventricular valve regurgitation. The pattern and extent of left ventricular hypertrophy in HCM vary greatly from patient to patient, and a characteristic feature is heterogeneity in the amount of hypertrophy evident in different regions of the left ventricle.[198] A typical feature found in most patients with HCM is disproportionate involvement of the interventricular septum and anterolateral wall compared with the posterior segment of the free wall of the left ventricle.[198] When hypertrophy is largely localized to the septum, the process has been called asymmetrical septal hypertrophy (ASH). Other patterns of hypertrophy may be seen on occasion, including concentric left ventricular hypertrophy, with symmetrical thickening of the left ventricle involving the septum and free wall equally. This variant may occasionally be seen in patients with the genetically

transmitted as well as the sporadic forms of HCM. The differentiation of the "physiological" hypertrophy that occurs in some highly trained male athletes from that seen in HCM may be difficult; athletes may demonstrate left ventricular wall thicknesses up to 16 mm in the absence of HCM (normal < 12 mm) (Fig. 41–11).[205–207] Some patients with HCM have substantial hypertrophy in unusual locations, such as the posterior portion of the septum, the posterobasal free wall, and the midventricular level.[198] One unusual variant demonstrates marked posterior wall hypertrophy and virtually no septal hypertrophy; patients with this form of HCM tend to be young and severely symptomatic.[208]

An inverse relationship exists between the extent of hypertrophy and age. Whether this is due to premature death of younger patients with greater hypertrophy or progressive reduction in the extent of hypertrophy is unknown.[198]

Apical HCM. A variant with predominant involvement of the apex is common in Japan and is estimated to represent a quarter of Japanese HCM patients.[209] In other parts of the world, apical HCM is much less common. Typical features include a characteristic spade-like configuration of the left ventricle during angiographic study (although some patients with this variant do not demonstrate this abnormality),[210] giant negative T waves in the precordial electrocardiographic leads, the absence of an intraventricular pressure gradient, mild symptoms, and a generally benign course.[198,211,212]

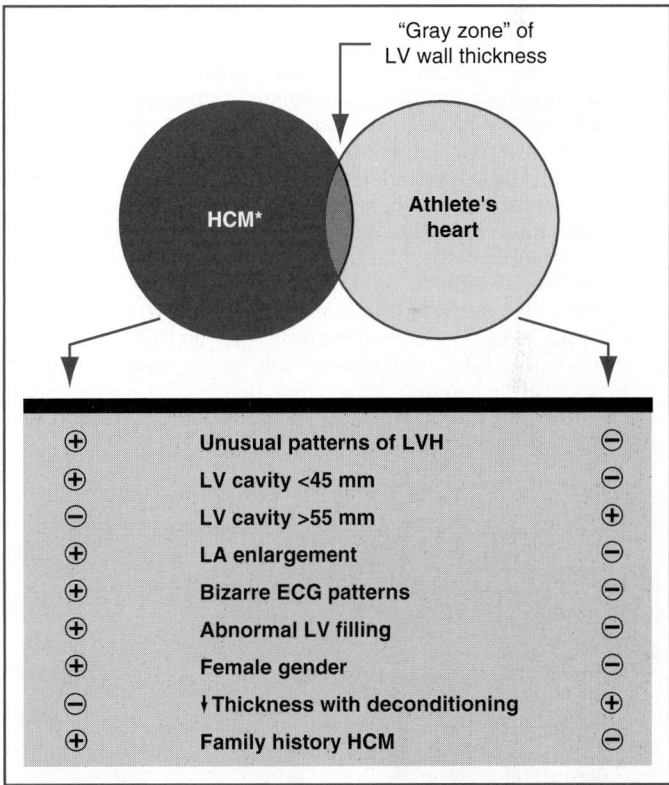

FIGURE 41–11. Criteria used to distinguish hypertrophic cardiomyopathy from athlete's heart. The shaded area (gray zone) indicates that there can be overlap between the two diagnoses, and the criteria listed below indicate which diagnosis would be favored (+) or less likely (−) for each criterion. ↓ = Decreased, HCM = hypertrophic cardiomyopathy, LA = left atrial, LV = left ventricular, LVH = left ventricular hypertrophy. * = Assumes that systolic anterior motion of the mitral valve is absent because its presence would indicate the presence of hypertrophic cardiomyopathy even in an athlete. (Reproduced by permission from Maron, B. J., Pelliccia, A., and Spirito, P.: Cardiac disease in young trained athletes. Insights into methods for distinguishing athlete's heart from structural heart disease, with particular emphasis on hypertrophic cardiomyopathy. Circulation 91: 1596, 1995. Copyright 1995 American Heart Association.)

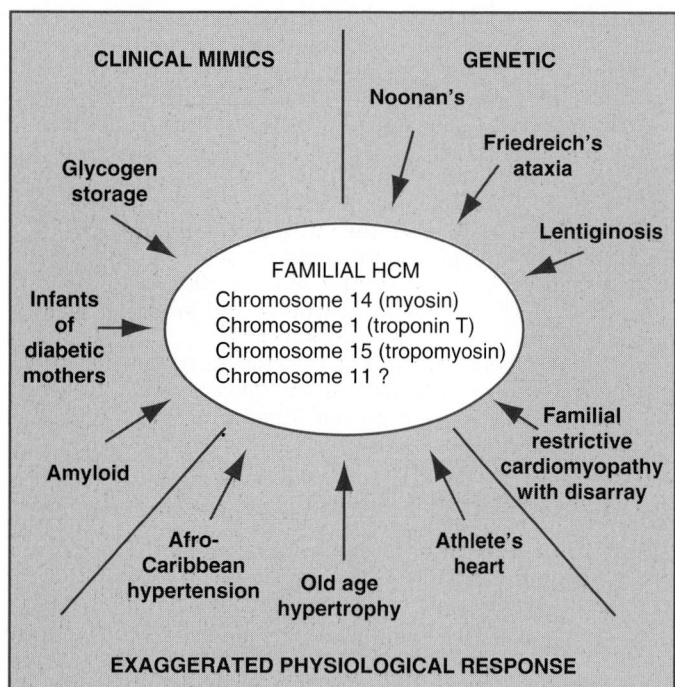

CLINICAL MIMICS   GENETIC

Noonan's

Friedreich's ataxia

Glycogen storage

Lentiginosis

FAMILIAL HCM
Chromosome 14 (myosin)
Chromosome 1 (troponin T)
Chromosome 15 (tropomyosin)
Chromosome 11 ?

Infants of diabetic mothers

Familial restrictive cardiomyopathy with disarray

Amyloid

Afro-Caribbean hypertension   Old age hypertrophy   Athlete's heart

EXAGGERATED PHYSIOLOGICAL RESPONSE

FIGURE 41–12. Classification of the causes of myocardial hypertrophy that can be confused with or may be related to familial hypertrophic cardiomyopathy. (From Davies, M. J., and McKenna, W. J.: Hypertrophic cardiomyopathy: An introduction to pathology and pathogenesis. Br. Heart J. 72:S2, 1994.)

Two variants of HCM are seen particularly in elderly women. The first, termed *hypertensive hypertrophic cardiomyopathy of the elderly,* is characterized by severe concentric left ventricular hypertrophy and small left ventricular cavity size, and is associated with hypertension.[213,214] The second presentation also is marked by an especially small left ventricular cavity but with relatively mild hypertrophy; other findings include marked anterior displacement of the mitral valve, extensive submitral (annular) calcification, a left ventricular outflow gradient, and the late appearance of severe and progressive symptoms.[215] In contrast to young patients with HCM, the elderly patient is more likely to show a localized septal bulge just below the aortic valve and is less likely to have marked abnormalities in the orientation and curvature of the septum.[216]

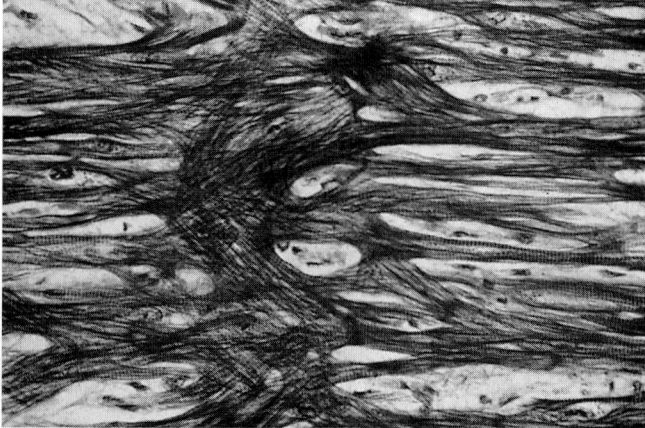

FIGURE 41–13. Histological specimen of a patient with hypertrophic cardiomyopathy showing myofibrillar disarray. In the central area the myofibrils cross each other in a disorganized manner, but in adjacent areas on each side the appearance is more normal, with parallel arrays of myofibrils. (PTHA stain, × 240). (From Davies, M. J., and McKenna, W. J.: Hypertrophic cardiomyopathy: An introduction to pathology and pathogenesis. Br. Heart J. 72:S2, 1994.)

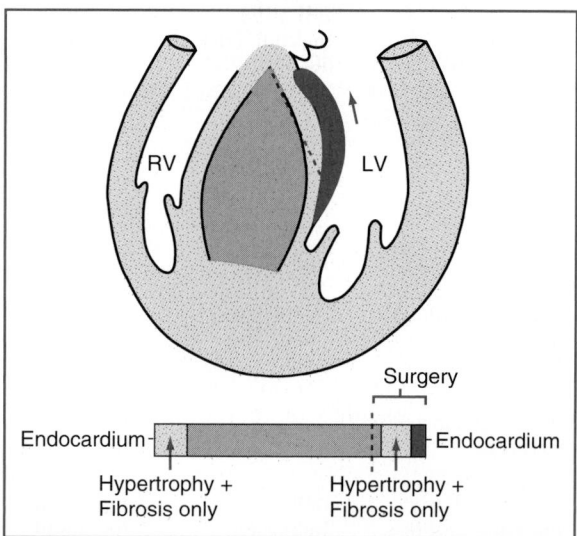

RV   LV

Surgery

Endocardium —   — Endocardium

Hypertrophy + Fibrosis only   Hypertrophy + Fibrosis only

FIGURE 41–14. Diagrammatic representation showing usual location of myocyte disarray in interventricular septum in hypertrophic cardiomyopathy. This explains why disarray is usually deep or absent in septectomy specimen, and why endomyocardial biopsy (3-mm maximum dimension) is also unlikely to sample zone of disarray. RV = Right ventricle, LV = left ventricle. (From Tazelaar, H. D., and Billingham, M. E.: The surgical pathology of hypertrophic cardiomyopathy. Arch. Pathol. Lab. Med. 111:257, 1987.)

A variety of disparate conditions may present similar gross morphological features as HCM, including hyperparathyroidism, infants of diabetic mothers, neurofibromatosis, generalized lipodystrophy, lentiginosis, pheochromocytoma, Friedreich's ataxia, and Noonan syndrome (Fig. 41–12).[217,218] Rarely, the findings may be simulated by amyloid, glycogen storage disease, or tumor involvement of the septum.[219,220]

HISTOLOGY. Microscopic findings in HCM are distinctive, with myocardial hypertrophy and gross disorganization of the muscle bundles resulting in a characteristic whorled pattern; abnormalities are found in the cell-to-cell arrangement (disarray) and disorganization of the myofibrillar architecture within a given cell (Fig. 41–13).[198] Fibrosis is usually prominent[221] and may be extensive enough to produce grossly visible scars. Foci of disorganized cells are often interspersed between areas of hypertrophied but otherwise normal-appearing muscle cells. Interstitial (matrix) connective tissue elements are increased.[198] Disarray in HCM patients is found in grossly hypertrophied myocardial segments as well as relatively normal segments.[222] Although abnormally arranged cardiac muscle cells initially were considered specific for HCM, it is now recognized that they may be found in a variety of acquired and congenital heart conditions.[198] What is unique about the disarray in HCM is its ubiquity and frequency. Findings in almost all HCM patients have some degree of disarray, and most have involvement of 5 per cent or more of the myocardium; in contrast, disarray findings in non-HCM patients (when they occur) usually involve only about 1 per cent of the myocardium[198] (Fig. 41–14).

Abnormal intramural coronary arteries, with a reduction in the size of the lumen and thickening of the vessel wall, are common in HCM, occurring in more than 80 per cent of patients.[198,199] This abnormality occurs most frequently in the ventricular septum; it also has been observed in infants who died of this condition and could represent a congenital component of the condition. The prominence of abnormal intramural coronary arteries in areas of extensive myocardial fibrosis is consistent with the hypothesis that these abnormalities may be responsible for the development of myocardial ischemia.[198]

Etiology

The cause of the myocardial hypertrophy in HCM remains unknown.[223] Suggestive data link abnormal myocardial calcium kinetics[224] and specific features of HCM, particularly the abnormalities of diastolic function.[197] Abnormal calcium fluxes with a resultant increase in intracellular calcium concentration appear to occur as a consequence of an increase in the number of calcium channels.[225,226] This in turn may produce (in an as yet undefined process) hypertrophy and cellular disarray.

Other suggested causes of HCM include (1) abnormal sympathetic stimulation because of heightened responsiveness of the heart to or excessive production of circulating catecholamines[227] or reduced neuronal uptake of cardiac norepinephrine[228]; (2) abnormally thickened intramural coronary arteries that do not dilate normally and lead to myocardial ischemia, with resultant fibrosis and abnormal compensatory hypertrophy; (3) subendocardial ischemia, possibly related to abnormalities of the microcirculation, that depletes the energy stores essential for the sequestration of calcium during diastole, resulting in persistent interaction of the contractile elements during diastole and attendant increased diastolic stiffness; and (4) structural abnormalities, including a catenoid configuration of the septum, that lead to myocardial cell hypertrophy and disarray.

GENETICS OF HYPERTROPHIC CARDIOMYOPATHY (see also pp. 1664 to 1665). Familial HCM occurs as an autosomal dominant mendelian-inherited disease about 50 per cent of the time.[200,229] It is thought that some if not all of the sporadic forms of the disease may be due to spontaneous mutations.[229,230] At least five different genes on at least four chromosomes are associated with HCM, with over three dozen different mutations discovered thus far (Fig. 41–15).[200,223] The proteins encoded by three of the genes have been identified. Familial HCM thus is a genetically heterogeneous disease (i.e., it can be caused by genetic defects at more than one locus).[231,232] However, the genetic heterogeneity does *not* appear to explain the clinical variability. The genetic basis of HCM was first reported in 1989 by Seidman and her collaborators, who reported the existence of a disease gene located on 14 q1 (i.e., the long arm of the 14th chromosome in the band closest to the centromere) and termed it *FHC-1* (for familial hypertrophic cardiomyopathy).[233,234] Subsequently they found this to be the gene encoding for beta cardiac myosin heavy chain (βMHC); it is now known as CMH1 (cardiomyopathy, hypertrophic, 1).[200] Sequencing of this gene in one family with HCM revealed that the abnormality was caused by a gene duplication in which the alpha and beta MHC genes were fused and present in an extra copy. In the second family, there was a point mutation in the beta MHC sequence that alters the myosin's arginine to glutamine. Both of these mutations affect the polypeptides crucial to the structure of myofibrils and might be responsible for the myocyte and myofibrillar disarray characteristic of familial HCM. Other disease loci that have been identified include CMH2 on chromosome 1 g3 (encoding for troponin T); CMH3 on chromosome 15 q2 (encoding for α tropomyosin); CMH4 on chromosome 11, and an additional gene that is not yet localized.[200,201,235] It is estimated that about 30 per cent of familial HCM is due to mutations of the cardiac myosin heavy chain gene, 15 per cent is caused by mutations of the cardiac troponin T gene, less than 3 per cent is due to mutations of the α tropomyosin gene, and the remainder to mutations of other unidentified genes.[235a]

There is wide variation in the phenotypic expression of a given mutation of a given gene, with variability in clinical symptoms and degree of hypertrophy expressed.[200,236–238] Of particular interest are mutations of the troponin T gene that typically result in only modest hypertrophy but indicate a poor prognosis and a high risk of sudden death.[235a] Conversely, certain genes and mutations are associated with more favorable prognoses (Fig. 41–16).[239,240] It is possible to detect the CMH1 gene in DNA extracted from blood lymphocytes, so the disease can be detected in childhood even before it becomes clinically evident.[241] It is likely that soon it may be possible to screen for all or most of the genes associated with HCM.[200,201] In some patients with an abnormal gene and no echocardiographic evidence of HCM, the electrocardiogram is abnormal.[242] Therefore, otherwise unexplained abnormalities of the electrocardiogram in first-degree relatives of patients with HCM may be indicative of a carrier or preclinical state.[242]

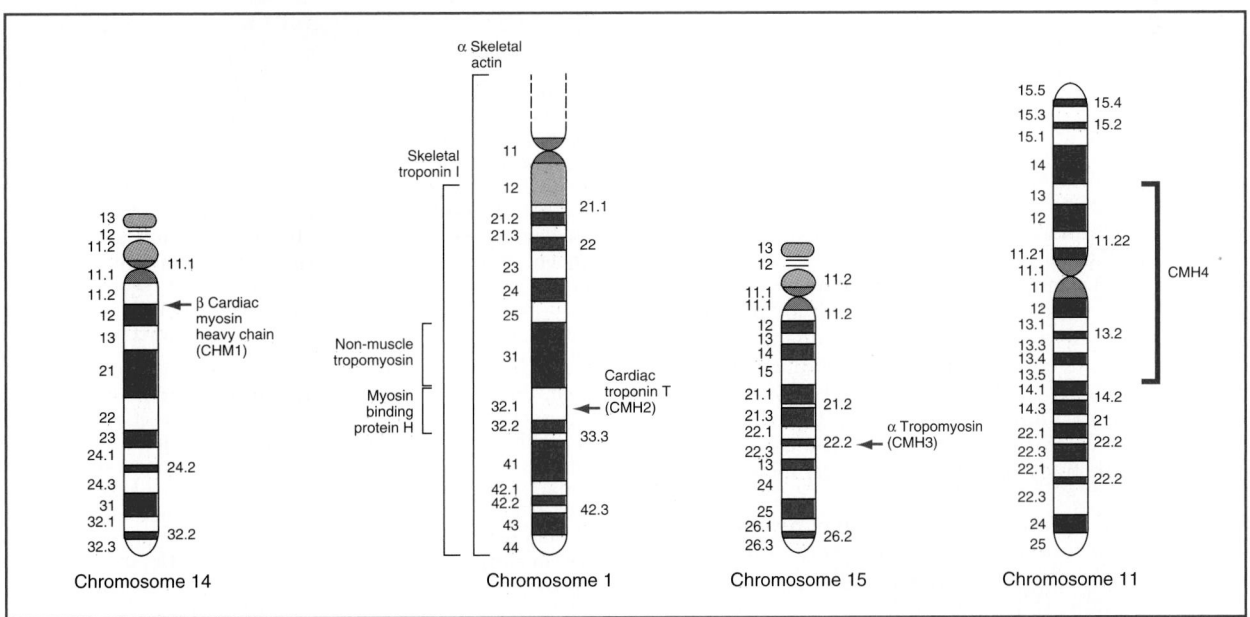

FIGURE 41–15. Diagrammatic depiction of the four chromosomes containing known disease gene loci for hypertrophic cardiomyopathy. The disease loci (designated CMH1-4) and relevant genes are identified by arrows (where the gene itself is known) or by square brackets showing the range of possible map locations. The positions of four other contractile protein genes, previously considered gene candidates for CMH2 on chromosome 1, are also shown by square brackets. (From Watkins, H.: Multiple disease genes cause hypertrophic cardiomyopathy. Br. Heart J. 72:S4, 1994.)

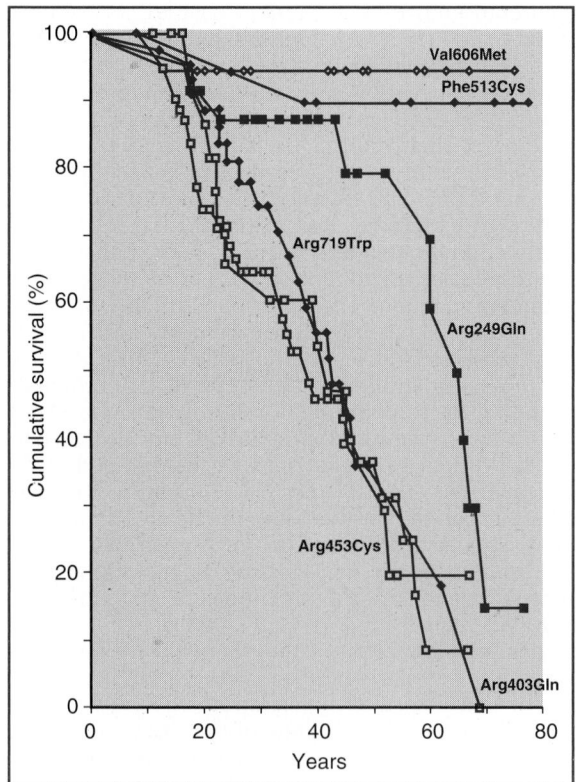

FIGURE 41–16. Kaplan-Meier curves showing the survival of affected individuals with different mutations for hypertrophic cardiomyopathy. (From Watkins, H.: Multiple disease genes cause hypertrophic cardiomyopathy. Br. Heart J. *72:*S4, 1994.)

Pathophysiology

SYSTOLE. Since the initial descriptions of HCM, the feature that has attracted the greatest attention is the dynamic pressure gradient (Fig. 41–10). Although this pressure gradient was initially thought to be due to a muscular sphincter action in the subaortic region or was an artifact, it appears to be related to further narrowing of an already small outflow tract (narrowed by the prominent septal hypertrophy and possibly abnormal location of the mitral valve) by systolic anterior motion (SAM) of the mitral valve against the hypertrophied septum.[198]

There continues to be considerable controversy about the cause and significance of the outflow gradient.[243,244] Central to the disagreement is whether there is true obstruction to left ventricular ejection or whether the pressure gradient is simply the consequence of vigorous ventricular emptying.[243] Most now favor the view that a true mechanical impediment to left ventricular ejection occurs when outflow gradients are present and is the result of distal portions of the mitral valve apparatus moving anteriorly across the outflow tract and contacting the ventricular septum in midsystole. It is likely that the mitral valve is displaced anteriorly because of Venturi effects and as a result of the increased ejection velocities produced by the abnormal left ventricular outflow tract orientation and geometry[245] (Fig. 41–17).

DIASTOLE. Most patients with HCM demonstrate abnormalities of diastolic function (see pp. 402 and 447) whether or not a pressure gradient is present and whether or not they are symptomatic (Fig. 41–18).[246,247] These abnormalities of global diastolic filling are largely independent of the extent and distribution of myocardial hypertrophy; patients with mild and apparently localized hypertrophy may demonstrate prominent diastolic dysfunction, suggesting that the myopathic process occurs in ventricular regions that are not macroscopically hypertrophied.[248] Others have found that diastolic filling varies in different regions of the left ventricle and is influenced by the thickness of the septum.[249] Diastolic dysfunction in turn leads to increased filling pressure despite a normal or small left ventricular cavity and appears to result from abnormalities of left ventricular relaxation and distensibility.[250] Early diastolic filling is impaired when relaxation is prolonged, perhaps related to abnormal calcium kinetics, subendocardial ischemia, or the abnormal loading conditions found in HCM.[225,251] Late diastolic filling is altered when left ventricular distensibility is impaired; as a consequence, filling pressures rise. HCM may cause abnormal distensibility of the ventricle because of fibrosis or cellular disorganization.[221,225]

MYOCARDIAL ISCHEMIA. Myocardial ischemia is common and multifactorial in HCM (Table 41–9). Major causes include impaired vasodilator reserve (perhaps related to the thickened and narrowed small intramural coronary arteries found in HCM)[252–254]; increased oxygen demand, especially in patients with outflow gradients; and elevated filling pressures with resultant subendocardial ischemia.[198]

Clinical Manifestations

SYMPTOMS. The majority of patients with HCM are asymptomatic or only mildly symptomatic[255] and often are

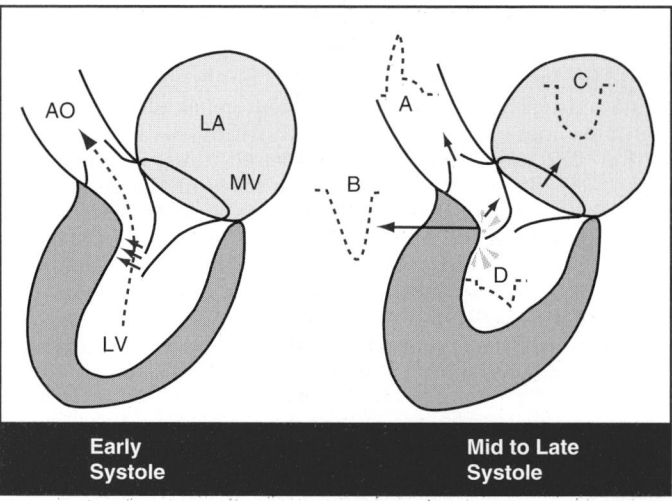

| **Early Systole** | **Mid to Late Systole** |

FIGURE 41–17. *Left,* Proposed mechanism of mitral leaflet systolic anterior motion (SAM) in early systole in hypertrophic cardiomyopathy (HCM). Ventricular septal hypertrophy causes narrowed outflow tract, as result of which ejection velocity is rapid and path of ejection *(dashed line)* is closer to mitral leaflets (MV) than is normal. This results in Venturi forces (three short oblique arrows in outflow tract) drawing anterior and/or posterior mitral leaflets toward septum. Subsequent mitral leaflet-septal contact results in obstruction to left ventricular (LV) outflow and concomitant mitral regurgitation as seen on right panel. By midsystole, SAM-septal contact is well established, causing marked narrowing of LV outflow tract with obstruction to outflow. LA = Left atrium.

Right, Proximal to level of SAM-septal contact, converging lines indicate acceleration of jet just proximal to obstruction and narrowing of jet width that occurs. Distal to obstruction, arrow and diverging lines indicate high-velocity flow that emanates from site of SAM-septal contact, directed posterolaterally at considerable angle from normal path of aortic outflow. In late systole, although forward flow continues into outflow tract and aorta (AO), the volume of flow is much less than in early nonobstructed systole. Typical Doppler flow patterns are shown.

A, Integrated Doppler flow signal in ascending aorta; *B,* high outflow tract velocity recorded by continuous wave (CW) Doppler at site of SAM-septal contact; *C,* presence of mitral regurgitation recorded by CW Doppler; *D,* late systolic velocity peak that can be recorded in apical region of LV. (Reproduced with permission from Wigle, E. D.: Hypertrophic cardiomyopathy: A 1987 viewpoint. Circulation *75:*312, 1987. Copyright 1987 American Heart Association.)

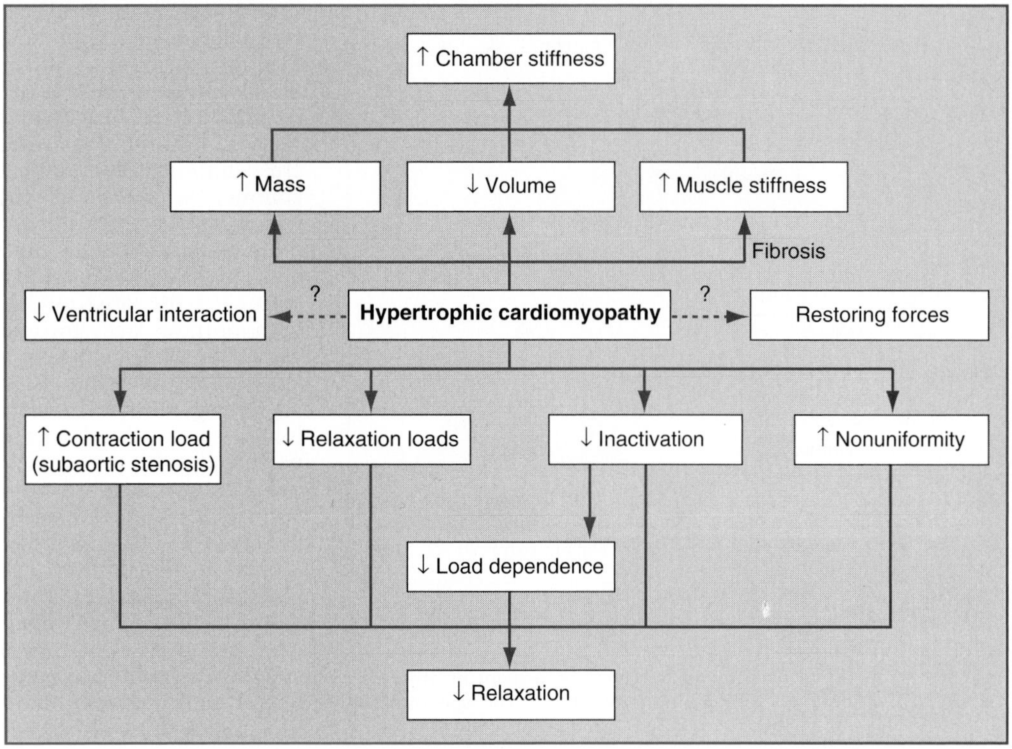

FIGURE 41-18. Diastolic dysfunction in HCM. There is increased chamber stiffness or decreased compliance as a result of increased muscle mass and the resulting decreased ventricular volume. Increased muscle stiffness from myocardial fibrosis also occurs. Thus, all three factors that affect the stiffness or compliance of the ventricle are altered in a way that increases chamber stiffness. Left ventricular relaxation in HCM is impaired because of changes in loading conditions, decreased inactivation, and increased nonuniformity. The subaortic stenosis in obstructive HCM represents a contraction load on the ventricle, which delays and impairs relaxation. Coronary and ventricular filling loads, which aid in relaxation, are reduced in HCM because of the degree of hypertrophy and other reasons. High myoplasmic calcium results in decreased inactivation, which impairs relaxation both directly and indirectly by reducing the load dependence of the relaxation process. Finally, much nonuniformity exists in HCM, which also impairs relaxation. Thus all three factors controlling relaxation are altered to impair it in HCM. (From Wigle, E. D., Kitching, A. D., Rakowski, H.: Hypertrophic cardiomyopathy. *In* Abelmann, W. H., and Braunwald, E. [eds.]: Cardiomyopathies, Myocarditis, and Pericardial Disease. Atlas of Heart Diseases. Vol. 2. Philadelphia, Current Medicine, 1995.)

identified during screening of relatives of a patient with HCM. Unfortunately, the first clinical manifestation of the disease in such individuals may be sudden death. The disease is identified most often in adults in their 30s and 40s; it occurs more often than commonly suspected in elderly patients. The condition has been observed at necropsy in stillborns and both clinically and pathologically in octogenarians. The importance of recognizing this disorder in children at the earliest possible time is highlighted by the higher mortality rate in younger patients; death is often sudden and unexpected. When HCM is first diagnosed in older patients, several features are distinctive and are in contrast to findings in younger patients: generally mild degrees of left ventricular hypertrophy; frequent demonstration of outflow gradients; and appearance of marked symptoms only after age 55.[256] A particularly high index of suspicion of this condition must be maintained to make the clinical diagnosis in the elderly because their symptoms may easily be confused with those of coronary artery or aortic valve disease. Because syncope and sudden death have been associated with competitive sports and severe exertion in patients with HCM, it is important to diagnose this condition so that these activities may be proscribed. The disease is slightly more common in men, although women may be more likely to be severely disabled and may initially present at a younger age than men.[257]

The clinical picture varies considerably, ranging from the asymptomatic relative of a patient with recognized HCM who has a slightly abnormal echocardiogram but no other manifestation of the illness to the patient with incapacitating symptoms. A general relationship exists between the extent of hypertrophy and the severity of symptoms, but the relationship is not absolute, and some patients have severe symptoms with only mild and apparently localized hypertrophy, and vice versa.[198] A complex interaction occurs between left ventricular hypertrophy, the left ventricular pressure gradient, diastolic dysfunction, and myocardial ischemia, which accounts for the great variability in symptoms from patient to patient (Fig. 41-19).

The most common symptom is *dyspnea,* occurring in up to 90 per cent of symptomatic patients, which is largely a consequence of the elevated left ventricular diastolic (and therefore left atrial and pulmonary venous) pressure, which results principally from impaired ventricular filling owing to diastolic dysfunction.[198] Angina pectoris (found in about three-fourths of symptomatic patients), fatigue, and presyncope and syncope are also common. Palpitations, paroxysmal nocturnal dyspnea, overt congestive heart failure, and dizziness are found less frequently, although severe congestive heart failure culminating in death may be seen. Exertion tends to exacerbate many of the symptoms.[258] A variety of mechanisms may contribute to the production of angina pectoris (Table 41-9). It is at least in part the result of an imbalance between oxygen supply and demand as a consequence of the greatly increased myocardial mass. Transmural infarction may occur in the absence of narrowing of the extramural coronary arteries.[198] Abnormalities of the small coronary arteries may contribute to myocardial ischemia, particularly during exertion, and perhaps 20 per cent of older patients with hypertrophic cardiomyopathy may have concurrent atheromatous obstructive coronary artery disease. Impaired diastolic relaxation may produce subendocardial ischemia as a result of prolonged maintenance of wall tension with a concomitant slower-than-normal decrease in the impedance to coronary blood flow. Syncope may result from inadequate cardiac output with exertion or from cardiac arrhythmias. It occurs

TABLE 41-9 PROPOSED CAUSES OF ISCHEMIA IN HCM DESPITE NORMAL EPICARDIAL CORONARY ARTERIES

Increased muscle mass

Inadequate capillary density

Elevated diastolic filling pressures

Abnormal intramural coronary arteries

Impaired vasodilatory reserve

Systolic compression of arteries

Enhanced myocardial oxygen demand (increased wall stress)

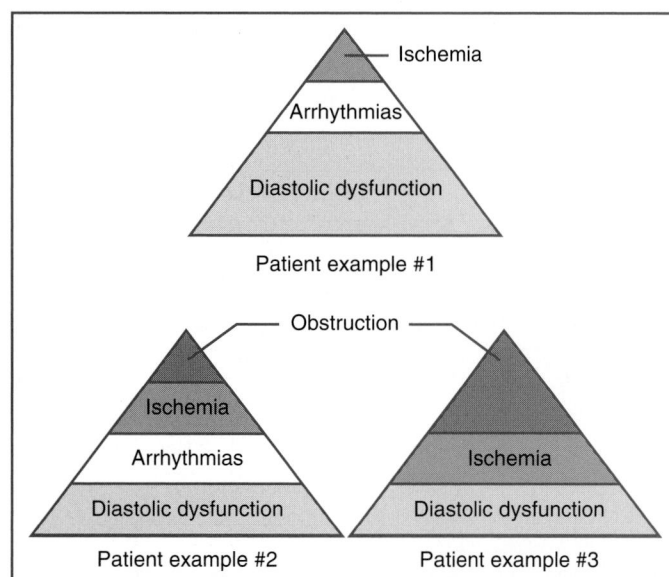

FIGURE 41–19. The pathological basis for symptoms in hypertrophic cardiomyopathy, shown as triangles from three hypothetical patients. A variety of other potential combinations and relative contributions of the four pathophysiological components may be present in other patients not represented here. (From Maron, B. J.: The spectrum of prognosis and treatment strategies in hypertrophic cardiomyopathy. *In* Sekiguchi, M., and Richardson, P. J. [eds.]: Prognosis and Treatment of Cardiomyopathies and Myocarditis. Tokyo, University of Tokyo Press, 1994, pp. 3–32.)

most commonly in young patients with small left ventricular chamber size and evidence of ventricular tachycardia on ambulatory monitoring.[259] Near-syncopal ("graying out") spells that occur in the erect posture and that can be relieved by immediately lying down are common. However, in contrast to valvular aortic stenosis, syncope or near-syncope may not be an ominous finding in adult patients with HCM; some patients have a history of such episodes dating back many years without deterioration. In children and adolescents, however, presyncope and syncope identify patients at increased risk of sudden death (see Natural History below).

PHYSICAL EXAMINATION. This may be normal in asymptomatic patients without gradients, particularly those with the apical variant of HCM, save for a left ventricular lift and a loud fourth heart sound, but findings are usually prominent in patients with a left ventricular outflow tract pressure gradient. The apical precordial impulse is often displaced laterally and is usually abnormally forceful and enlarged.[257] Because of decreased left ventricular compliance, a prominent presystolic apical impulse that results from forceful atrial systole often is present. This may result in a double apical impulse as a result of the prominent *a* wave. A more characteristic but less frequently recognized abnormality is a triple apical beat, the third impulse being a late systolic bulge that occurs when the heart is almost empty and is performing near-isometric contraction.[257] The jugular venous pulse may demonstrate a prominent *a* wave, reflecting diminished right ventricular compliance secondary to massive hypertrophy of the ventricular septum. The carotid pulse typically rises briskly and then declines in midsystole as the gradient develops, followed by a secondary rise.[257] This may be appreciated on physical examination but can be demonstrated more clearly by means of indirect pulse tracings (Fig. 2–8E, p. 21).

The first heart sound is normal and is often preceded by a fourth heart sound that corresponds to the apical presystolic impulse.[257] The second heart sound usually is normally split. In some patients, however, it is narrowly split and in others, particularly those with severe outflow gradients, paradoxical splitting may be noted. A third heart sound may be present but does not have the same ominous significance as in patients with valvular aortic stenosis. Systolic ejection sounds relating to rapid acceleration of blood flow may be found on occasion. The auscultatory hallmark of HCM associated with an outflow gradient is a systolic murmur that typically is harsh and crescendo-decrescendo in configuration (Fig. 2–12, p. 27); it usually commences well after the first heart sound and is best heard between the apex and the left sternal border.[257] It often radiates well to the lower sternal border, the axillae, and base of the heart but not into the neck vessels. In patients with large gradients, the murmur usually reflects both outflow tract turbulence and concomitant mitral regurgitation.[243] Accordingly, the murmur is often more holosystolic and blowing at the apex and in the axillae (due to mitral regurgitation) and midsystolic and harsher along the lower sternal border (due to turbulent flow across the narrowed outflow tract).[257]

The murmur is labile in intensity and duration, and a variety of maneuvers may be used to augment or suppress it (Table 41–10). A diastolic rumbling murmur, reflecting increased transmitral flow, may occur in patients with marked mitral regurgitation. The murmur of aortic regurgitation is observed in about 10 per cent of patients, although mild aortic regurgitation can be demonstrated by Doppler echocardiography in one-third.[260] It may develop after operation to correct the outflow gradient[261] or following infective endocarditis.

It is important to emphasize the features of physical examination that permit differentiation of HCM from fixed orifice obstruction, most commonly due to valvular aortic stenosis (see p. 1041). The character of the carotid pulse and features of the murmur are most useful in this regard. Because there is obstruction to left ventricular emptying from the beginning of systole with fixed valvular stenosis, the carotid upstroke is slowed and of low amplitude (pulsus parvus et tardus). With HCM, initial ejection of blood from the left ventricle is actually enhanced, and therefore the arterial upstroke is brisk. The murmur of HCM, as opposed to that of aortic stenosis, can be reliably identified by its increase with the Valsalva maneuver and during standing from a squatting position, and its decrease during squatting from a standing position, passive leg elevation, and handgrip (Table 41–10).[257] Other features that

TABLE 41–10 EFFECTS OF INTERVENTIONS ON OUTFLOW GRADIENT AND SYSTOLIC MURMUR IN HCM

	CONTRACTILITY	PRELOAD	AFTERLOAD
Increase in Gradient and Murmur			
Valsalva maneuver (during strain)	—	↓	↓
Standing	—	↓	—
Postextrasystole	↑	↑	—
Isoproterenol	↑	↓	↓
Digitalis	↑	↓	—
Amyl nitrite	— then ↑	↓ then ↑	↓
Nitroglycerin	—	↓	↓
Exercise	↑	↑	↑
Tachycardia	↑	↓	—
Hypovolemia	↑	↓	↓
Decrease in Gradient and Murmur			
Mueller maneuver	—	↑	↑
Valsalva overshoot	—	↑	↑
Squatting	—	↑	↑
Alpha-adrenocepter stimulation (phenylephrine)	—	—	↑
Beta-adrenocepter blockade	↓	↑	—
General anesthesia	↓	↑	—
Isometric handgrip	—	—	↑

↑ = increase; ↓ = decrease; — = no major change.

may be helpful but are of considerably less significance are the location of the murmur (it radiates along the carotid arteries in valvular aortic stenosis but not in HCM), and the location of the systolic thrill when present (most prominent in the second right intercostal space in valvular aortic stenosis and in the fourth interspace along the left sternal border in HCM).

ELECTROCARDIOGRAM. This is usually abnormal in HCM[198] and invariably so in symptomatic patients with left ventricular outflow gradients. Entirely normal electrocardiograms are seen in only about 15 per cent of patients and usually are found in the presence of only localized left ventricular hypertrophy. The most common abnormalities are ST-segment and T-wave abnormalities, followed by evidence of left ventricular hypertrophy, with QRS complexes that are tallest in the midprecordial leads.[198] Progressive electrocardiographic evidence of hypertrophy may develop over time. Giant negative T waves in the midprecordial leads of Japanese patients are characteristic of HCM involving the apex,[262] but such a pattern in the west may be found with HCM involving segments other than the apex.[263] Prominent Q waves are relatively common, occurring in 20 to 50 per cent of patients. The Q-wave abnormalities often involve the inferior (II, III, aV_F) and/or precordial (V_2-V_6) leads.[264] The cause of the Q waves remains unestablished[265]; although they do not correlate simply with the degree of septal hypertrophy,[198] they may relate to the balance of electrical forces emanating from the left versus the right ventricle.[264] A variety of other electrocardiographic abnormalities may occur, including abnormal electrical axis (usually left-axis deviation) and P-wave abnormalities (usually left atrial abnormality). Accessory atrioventricular pathways have been found in HCM, although they are uncommon.[266] Clinically significant abnormalities of atrioventricular conduction are uncommon but may cause syncope.[266]

Although hemodynamic or ischemic mechanisms may play roles in the death of patients with HCM (particularly the young), many deaths, particularly those that are known to have been sudden, likely are due to an arrhythmia.[267–273] Because of the systolic and diastolic abnormalities in this disorder, rhythm disturbances are less well tolerated.

Ventricular arrhythmias are common in patients with HCM, occurring in more than three-fourths of patients undergoing continuous ambulatory electrocardiographic monitoring.[274] Runs of nonsustained ventricular tachycardia are found in about one-fourth of HCM patients, although sustained monomorphic tachycardia is uncommon.[267,275] In some it is a harbinger of subsequent sudden death; however, its overall predictive value in identifying patients at high risk for sudden death is limited.[268] Treadmill testing may expose arrhythmias that are not present at rest, although continuous ambulatory monitoring is superior in detecting repetitive ventricular tachyarrhythmias.

Supraventricular tachycardia may be found in one-fourth to one-half of patients.[267,274] Atrial fibrillation occurs in about 10 per cent of patients (often those with no gradient and mild hypertrophy), and the resultant loss of the atrial contribution to the filling of a hypertrophied, stiff ventricle may result in clinical deterioration.[198,276,277] Treatment is often effective in controlling symptoms and restoring sinus rhythm; if this is done, long-term survival usually is not jeopardized.[277] The signal-averaged electrocardiogram has not proved to be helpful in identifying patients at increased risk of sustained or lethal ventricular arrhythmia, although additional studies are necessary.[278] Reduced heart rate variability on ambulatory monitor recordings, a predictor of increased sudden death risk after myocardial infarction, appears to be less useful in risk stratification in HCM patients.[279,280]

ELECTROPHYSIOLOGICAL TESTING. The role of electrophysiological studies in identifying HCM patients at increased risk of sudden death is controversial.[198] These studies iden-

tify a variety of abnormalities in HCM patients, but most important is their ability to induce ventricular tachycardia (often polymorphic) in two-thirds of patients with syncope or aborted sudden death,[273] compared with 10 per cent in other HCM patients.[266] However, unlike its utility in ischemic heart disease, the predictive value of inducible sustained ventricular arrhythmias during electrophysiological testing is low in HCM.[205,281] Aggressive stimulation protocols are required to induce a sustained arrhythmia in high-risk HCM patients, often resulting in arrhythmias in low-risk patients as well.[269] Tilt-table testing has not been particularly useful in identifying the cause of syncope in HCM; neurally mediated syncope is uncommon in this setting and true positive tests are uncommon, but false positive tests are frequent and significantly limit the utility of the test.[282]

CHEST ROENTGENOGRAM. The findings on radiographic examination are variable; the cardiac silhouette may range from normal to markedly increased, and in most cases of apparent "cardiomegaly" the enlarged cardiac silhouette is the result of left ventricular hypertrophy and/or left atrial enlargement.[198] Left atrial enlargement is observed frequently, especially when significant mitral regurgitation is present. Aortic root enlargement and valvular calcification are not seen unless associated diseases are present, although calcification of the mitral annulus is common in HCM.

ECHOCARDIOGRAPHY. Because echocardiography combines the attributes of high resolution and no known risk, it has been widely utilized in the evaluation of HCM (Figs. 3–99, 3–100, 3–101, pp. 91–92). It is useful in the study of patients with suspected HCM and also in the screening of relatives of HCM patients. The echocardiogram is of value in identifying and quantifying morphological features (i.e., distribution of septal hypertrophy), functional aspects (e.g., hypercontractile left ventricle), and (when combined with Doppler recordings) hemodynamic findings (e.g., magnitude of outflow gradient).

The cardinal echocardiographic feature of HCM is left ventricular hypertrophy. Although the characteristic feature is hypertrophy of the septum and anterolateral free wall, the echocardiogram is useful in identifying involvement of other left ventricular locations, including portions of the free wall and the apex.[198,222,283] Considerable variability exists in the degree and pattern of hypertrophy; in most patients, there is variation in the extent of hypertrophy from one left ventricular region to another.[198] Maximal hypertrophy of the septum often occurs midway between the base and apex of the left ventricle. The finding of a thickened septum that is at least 1.3 to 1.5 times the thickness of the posterior wall when measured in diastole just prior to atrial systole has been the time-honored criterion for the diagnosis of ASH. The septum not only is relatively thicker than the posterior wall but is typically at least 15 mm in thickness (normal ≤ 11 mm). Although the average wall thickness detected on echocardiography is about 20 mm (i.e., almost twice normal), there is great variation, ranging from very mild hypertrophy (13 to 15 mm) to massive hypertrophy (50 mm).[207]

An unusual echocardiographic pattern consisting of a ground-glass appearance has been noted in portions of the hypertrophied myocardium in some patients with HCM. Even when abnormalities are not apparent on visual inspection, quantitative texture analysis often identifies them in both nonhypertrophied (but presumably abnormal) and hypertrophied regions of the ventricle[284] and can be used to distinguish HCM patients from those with secondary hypertrophy.[285] It has been speculated that this pattern may be related to the abnormal cellular architecture and myocardial fibrosis that has been noted in pathological studies.[284]

A second echocardiographic feature often found in HCM in addition to left ventricular hypertrophy is narrowing of the left ventricular outflow tract, which is formed by the interventricular septum anteriorly and the anterior leaflet of the mitral valve posteriorly. The mitral valve leaflets are abnormally large and elongated and are associated with abnormal left ventricular outflow tract geometry and production of a pressure gradient.[283,286–289] When HCM is associated with a pressure gradient, there is abnormal systolic anterior motion (SAM) of the anterior leaflet, and occasionally the posterior leaflet of the mitral valve (see Fig. 4–95A, p. 91).[283] Although the role of SAM in *producing* the gradient is controversial, a close relationship exists between the degree of SAM and the magnitude of the outflow gradient. Prolonged interventricular septal contact of the mitral apparatus is limited to HCM with resting pressure gradients, and a close temporal relationship exists between the onset of the pressure gradient and the onset of septal apposition of the mitral apparatus.

Three explanations have been offered for SAM: (1) the mitral valve is *pulled* against the septum by contraction of the papillary muscles, because of the abnormal location and orientation of these muscles resulting from septal hypertrophy[290]; (2) the mitral valve is *pushed* against the septum (perhaps by the left ventricular posterior wall) because of its abnormal position in the outflow tract; and (3) the mitral valve is drawn toward the septum because of the lower pressure that occurs as blood is ejected at a high velocity through a narrowed outflow tract (Venturi effect).[291] In a minority of cases (less than 15 per cent), one or both papillary muscles insert anomalously directly into the anterior mitral leaflet, causing a long area of midventricular narrowing that results in an intraventricular pressure gradient.[292] SAM of the mitral valve and dynamic left ventricular gradients are not pathognomonic of HCM but may be found in a variety of other conditions, including hypercontractile states, left ventricular hypertrophy, transposition of the great arteries, and infiltration of the septum. Even mild degrees of left ventricular hypertrophy may be associated with SAM and outflow gradients, particularly under conditions of enhanced sympathetic tone. In many cases in conditions other than HCM, SAM is due to buckling of the chordae tendineae rather than to movement of the anterior mitral valve leaflet as occurs in HCM (although the chordae tendineae and papillary muscles may contribute to SAM in HCM).

Several other echocardiographic findings may be present: (1) a small left ventricular cavity; (2) reduced septal motion and thickening during systole, particularly of the upper septum (presumably because of the disarray of the myofibrillar architecture and abnormal contractile function)[293,294]; (3) normal or increased motion of the posterior wall; (4) a reduced rate of closure of the mitral valve in mid-diastole secondary to a decrease in left ventricular compliance or abnormal transmitral flow during diastole; (5) mitral valve prolapse; and (6) partial systolic closure or, more commonly, coarse systolic fluttering of the aortic valve related to turbulent blood flow in the outflow tract. MRI studies have shown that regional left ventricular function and the degree of local hypertrophy are inversely related, and the hypertrophied septum typically is hypokinetic.[293,295,296] The echocardiographic findings that accompany a left ventricular outflow tract gradient (SAM and aortic valve partial closure) may be quite labile, and provocative measures such as the Valsalva maneuver, pharmacologically induced vasodilatation with amyl nitrite, stimulation of contractility with isoproterenol, or an induced premature ventricular contraction may be required to precipitate the findings.

Abnormalities of diastolic function (see p. 402) may be demonstrated by echocardiography and Doppler recordings in about 80 per cent of patients with HCM, independent of the presence or absence of a systolic pressure gradient.[198] Because the septum is typically hypokinetic, the rate of left ventricular filling is determined primarily by the rate of free wall thinning. Little relationship exists between the extent of hypertrophy and the severity of abnormalities of diastolic function.[248] Doppler ultrasonography has confirmed the virtual ubiquity of mitral regurgitation when an outflow gradient is present[198] and has accurately measured the magnitude of the outflow tract gradient.[199] Doppler color flow imaging reveals mitral regurgitation, most prominent in late systole, accompanying the appearance of turbulent flow in the left ventricular outflow tract. Recordings

from the left ventricular outflow tract support the concept that true obstruction to flow occurs and accounts for the pressure gradient.[199]

RADIONUCLIDE SCANNING. *Thallium-201* myocardial imaging, particularly when tomographic imaging (SPECT) is performed (see p. 282), permits direct determination of the relative thicknesses of the septum and free wall and may be of particular value when technical constraints limit the reliability of echocardiographic evaluation in a given patient with presumed HCM. Reversible thallium defects, presumably indicative of ischemia, are common findings in HCM in the absence of obstructive coronary artery disease.[297] They are common in adult patients with HCM and in those young patients with a history of sudden death or syncope, suggesting that myocardial ischemia is an important factor and probably a mechanism of demise in younger patients.[298] Fixed defects, probably indicative of myocardial scarring, occur primarily in patients with impaired systolic function. *Gated radionuclide ventriculography* with blood pool labeling permits the evaluation of not only the size but also the motion of the septum and left ventricle. As with the echocardiogram, abnormal diastolic filling of the ventricle has been observed in patients with HCM (both with and without gradients) by computer analysis of the blood pool scan.[299] Because of the ease and availability of transthoracic and transesophageal echocardiography, this technique is not widely used in the evaluation of HCM.

Hemodynamics and Angiography

CARDIAC CATHETERIZATION. This discloses diminished diastolic left ventricular compliance and in some patients a systolic pressure gradient within the body of the left ventricle, which is separated from a subaortic chamber by the thickened septum and the anterior leaflet of the mitral valve that abuts the septum (Fig. 41–10, p. 1414).[199] The pressure gradient may be quite labile and may vary between 0 and 175 mm Hg in the same patient under different conditions (see below). The arterial pressure tracing may demonstrate a "spike and dome" configuration similar to the carotid pulse recording.[199] As a consequence of diminished left ventricular compliance, the mean and particularly the *a* wave in the left atrial pressure pulse and the left ventricular end-diastolic pressures are usually elevated. Artifactual outflow gradients may occur if the left ventricular catheter becomes entrapped in the trabeculae of a markedly hypertrophied left ventricle.[243] Proper technique and choice of catheters with side holes should clarify the mechanism of such gradients. Cardiac output may be depressed in patients with longstanding severe gradients. In the majority of patients it is normal; occasionally it is elevated.

Hemodynamic abnormalities in HCM are not limited to the left heart. Approximately one-fourth of patients demonstrate pulmonary hypertension, which is usually mild but in some cases may be moderate to severe. This is due (at least in part) to elevated mean left atrial pressures as a consequence of diminished left ventricular compliance. A pressure gradient in the right ventricular outflow tract occurs in approximately 15 per cent of patients who have obstruction to left ventricular outflow[257] and appears to result from markedly hypertrophied right ventricular tissue.[300] Right atrial and right ventricular end-diastolic pressures may be slightly elevated.

LABILITY OF GRADIENT. A feature characteristic of HCM is the variability and lability of the left ventricular outflow gradient (Table 41–10). A given patient may demonstrate a large outflow gradient on one occasion but have none at another time. In some patients without a resting gradient, it may be temporarily provoked. Three basic mechanisms are involved in the production of dynamic gradients, all of which act by reducing ventricular volume and presumably accentuate the apposition of the anterior mitral leaflet against the septum: (1) increased contractility, (2) decreased preload, and (3) decreased afterload. In a minority of patients with HCM, the gradient is midventricular and may be intensified by increased contractility, which exerts a direct muscular sphincteric action.[199,243] The stimuli that provoke or intensify left ventricular outflow tract gradients in HCM generally improve myocardial performance in normal subjects and in patients with most other forms of heart disease. Conversely, reductions in contractility or increases in preload or afterload, which increase left ventricular dimensions, reduce or abolish the left ventricular outflow gradient.

Alterations in the magnitude of the gradient are reflected by changes in the findings on physical examination, noninvasive tests, and left heart catheterization. *This dynamic characteristic of HCM distinguishes it from the discrete forms of obstruction to ventricular outflow.* An increase in the gradient usually results in a louder murmur, a longer ejection period with a more characteristic spike and dome configuration in the carotid pulse, and more flagrant echocardiographic evidence of SAM of the anterior mitral leaflet. In some patients, the intensity of the murmur may *not* track with the gradient, perhaps because in many cases the murmur reflects mitral regurgitation (at least in part).[243]

A number of bedside procedures may be useful in the evaluation of suspected HCM.[301] Perhaps the most helpful is sudden standing from a squatting position. Squatting results in an increase in venous return and an increase in aortic pressure, which increases ventricular volume, diminishing the gradient and decreasing the intensity of the murmur. Sudden standing has the opposite effects and results in accentuation of the gradient and the murmur. The Valsalva maneuver is another useful bedside technique for eliciting or exacerbating the gradient. Following a transient increase in arterial pressure that usually lasts for four or five cardiac cycles after the onset of the strain and coincident with an increase in heart rate, the arterial systolic and pulse pressures and ventricular volume decline, and the gradient (and murmur) increases. Following release of the strain, a compensatory overshoot of arterial pressure and venous return with cardiac slowing occur, all of which increase ventricular volume and reduce the magnitude of the gradient and the murmur. Occasional patients may show paradoxical attenuation of the systolic murmur despite an increase in the pressure gradient, presumably related to a critical reduction in stroke volume. Inhalation of amyl nitrite[302] also intensifies the murmur and the abnormality of the arterial pulse. The murmur of HCM is attenuated by passive leg elevation, handgrip, and sudden squatting from a standing position.[301]

One of the most potent stimuli for enhancing the gradient is *postextrasystolic potentiation* (see p. 380), which may occur following a spontaneous premature contraction or be induced by mechanical stimulation with a catheter. The resultant increase in contractility in the beat following the extrasystole is so marked that it outweighs the otherwise salutary effect of increased ventricular filling caused by the compensatory pause and produces an increase in the gradient and often of the murmur as well. A characteristic change often occurs in the directly recorded arterial pressure tracing, which, in addition to displaying a more marked spike and dome configuration, exhibits a pulse pressure that fails to increase as expected or actually decreases (the so-called Brockenbrough-Braunwald phenomenon).[243] This is one of the more reliable signs of dynamic obstruction of the left ventricular outflow tract. In some patients, the postextrasystolic murmur is attenuated despite an increase in the outflow gradient, apparently because in this setting the murmur (a hybrid of outflow tract turbulence and mitral regurgitation) is mirroring to a greater degree changes in the severity of mitral regurgitation rather than changes in the outflow tract gradient.[243]

Digitalis glycosides and the beta-adrenoceptor agonist isoproterenol augment the gradient because they increase myocardial contractility, whereas nitroglycerin and amyl nitrite exaggerate the gradient by decreasing arterial pressure and ventricular volume.[303] Hypovolemia (as a result of hemorrhage or overly aggressive diuresis) may also provoke overt obstruction to left ventricular outflow. The intensity of the murmur and the left ventricular outflow gradient may be decreased by beta-adrenoceptor blockade, although the effect of the latter is often not dramatic and is of most hemodynamic benefit in protecting against the *increase* in the gradient that may be provoked by exercise. In most patients the severity of mitral regurgitation and the intensity of the apical blowing regurgitant murmur vary with the degree of obstruction of left ventricular outflow.

ANGIOGRAPHY. Left ventriculography shows a hypertrophied ventricle; when an outflow gradient is present, the anterior leaflet of the mitral valve moves anteriorly during systole and encroaches upon the outflow tract. Associated with this motion of the leaflet is mitral regurgitation, which appears to be a constant finding in patients with gradients. The left ventricular cavity is often small, and systolic ejection is typically vigorous, resulting in virtual obliteration of the cavity at end-systole, although the apparent hypercontractile state may relate more to reduced afterload (end-systolic wall stress) than to enhanced inotropy. The papillary muscles are often prominent and may fill the left ventricular cavity in late systole. In patients with apical involvement, the extensive hypertrophy may convey a spade-like configuration to the left ventricular angiogram.[212]

It may be helpful to supplement angiographic evaluation of the left ventricle with simultaneous right ventriculography in a cranially angulated left anterior oblique (LAO) projection in order to obtain optimal visualization of the size, shape, and configuration of the interventricular septum. The left septal surface either is flat or bulges into the left ventricular cavity at its mid or lower portion, in contrast to the normal findings of the septum curving toward the right ventricle.

In patients over 45 years of age, obstructive coronary artery disease is rather common, although the symptoms of ischemic pain are indistinguishable from those of patients with normal coronary angiograms and HCM. The left anterior descending and septal perforator coronary arteries may demonstrate phasic narrowing and associated abnormalities of flow during systole.[304]

Natural History

The clinical course in HCM is varied; in many patients symptoms are absent or mild, remain stable, and in some instances improve over a period of 5 to 10 years. The annual mortality is about 3 per cent in adults seen in large referral centers[305] but probably is closer to 1 per cent when all patients with HCM are included.[255,306,307] The risk of sudden death is higher in children, perhaps as high as 6 per cent per year.[229] Clinical deterioration (aside from sudden death) usually is slow. Although symptoms are unrelated to the severity or even the presence of a gradient,[198] the percentage of severely symptomatic patients does increase with age.[308] The onset of atrial fibrillation may lead to an increase in symptoms, although often it is well tolerated.[277] Conversion to sinus rhythm by pharmacological or electrical cardioversion should be attempted, although maintenance of sinus rhythm may be difficult.[198] Patients who develop atrial fibrillation ordinarily are started on long-term therapy with oral anticoagulants.

Progression of HCM to left ventricular dilatation and dysfunction without a gradient, i.e., dilated cardiomyopathy, occurs in 10 to 15 per cent of patients.[198,309] It appears to result, at least in part, from wall thinning and scar formation as a consequence of myocardial ischemia caused by small vessel coronary artery disease.[198,221] It is more likely to occur in patients with marked septal hypertrophy and is

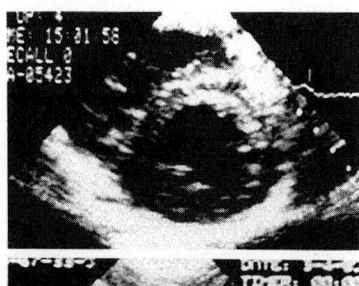
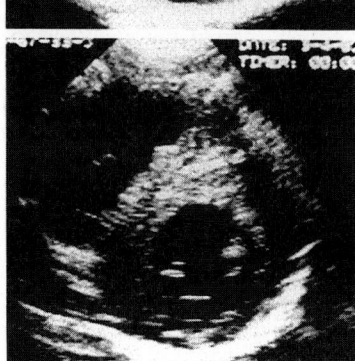
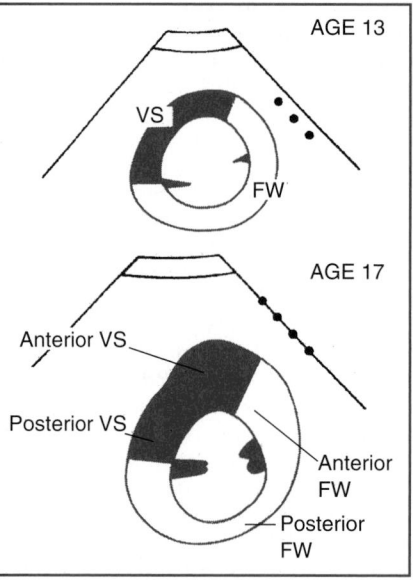

FIGURE 41–20. Two-dimensional echocardiographic study at end diastole obtained in a girl with a family history of hypertrophic cardiomyopathy. *Top*, At age 13, the left ventricular wall was of normal thickness. *Bottom*, At age 17, there is now pronounced hypertrophy of the anterior ventricular septum and contiguous regions of the anterior free wall and posterior septum. FW = Free wall, VS = ventricular septum. (From Spirito, P., and Bellone, P.: Natural history of hypertrophic cardiomyopathy. Br. Heart J. 72:S10, 1994.)

associated with a generally poor prognosis.[305,310] The extent of left ventricular hypertrophy in adults usually remains stable over time, although a majority of children demonstrate increasing degrees of hypertrophy (often considerable).[309] In some children, the findings of HCM may develop despite a previous normal echocardiogram (Fig. 41–20); this does not appear to occur in adults.[205] Its occurrence does emphasize that a single normal echocardiogram does *not* exclude HCM in a child or adolescent; cellular disarray and the attendant risk of sudden death may be present even in the absence of left ventricular hypertrophy.[205] A marker for the later appearance of clinical HCM may be an initially abnormal electrocardiogram demonstrating increased QRS voltage.[311]

SUDDEN DEATH. Death is most often sudden in HCM and may occur in previously asymptomatic patients, in individuals who were unaware they had the disease, and in patients with an otherwise stable course.[281] There is great difficulty in identifying those patients at particular risk of sudden death; nevertheless, the features that most reliably identify high-risk patients include young age (< 30 years) at diagnosis, a family history of HCM with sudden death (so-called malignant family history), and genetic abnormalities associated with increased prevalence of sudden death (Table 41–11, Fig. 41–16).[281,305] The presence or severity of an outflow tract gradient,[268] the degree of functional limitation, and symptoms in general do not correlate with the risk of death.[205,269,305] A history of syncope is ominous in children, less so in adults.[259,281,312,313] In the latter, nonsustained ventricular tachycardia (NSVT) on 48-hour electrocardiographic monitoring has some predictive value for subsequent sudden death, although most patients (over 75 per cent) with NSVT do *not* die suddenly.[314] The absence of NSVT is a stronger predictor of a good prognosis than is the presence of NSVT of a bad one.[267] The combination of NSVT and inducible arrhythmias during electrophysiological testing appears to have reasonable positive and negative predictive value.[269] It is presumed, but not established, that sudden death is due to a ventricular arrhythmia, although atrial arrhythmias may play a role in sensitizing the heart so that ventricular arrhythmias appear subsequently.

In children, the mechanism of death may be different because spontaneous ventricular arrhythmias and inducibility on electrophysiological testing are much less common.[273] It is thought that ischemia may play a prominent role in these patients.[298,315–318] Hemodynamic mechanisms may also be involved, as younger patients are more likely to demonstrate abnormal changes in peripheral vascular resistance in response to exercise.[319] Sudden death often occurs during exercise but also demonstrates a circadian distribution, with clustering of deaths in the morning and early evening.[320] Guidelines for participation in competitive sports have been developed; strenuous exertion should probably be proscribed in all patients with HCM whether or not symptoms are prominent, especially if high-risk clinical characteristics are present (Table 41–12).[205] Unsuspected HCM is the most common abnormality found at

TABLE 41–11 PROBABLE RISK FACTORS ASSOCIATED WITH SUDDEN CARDIAC DEATH IN HYPERTROPHIC CARDIOMYOPATHY

Youth

"Malignant" family history of sudden death

Gene abnormalities associated with increased prevalence of sudden death

Aborted sudden cardiac death

Sustained ventricular or supraventricular tachyarrhythmias

Recurrent syncope in the young

Nonsustained ventricular tachycardia (Holter monitoring)

Bradyarrhythmias (occult conduction disease)

Adapted from Maron, B. J., Cecchi, F., and McKenna, W. J.: Risk factors and stratification for sudden death in patients with hypertrophic cardiomyopathy. Br. Heart J. 72:S13, 1994.

TABLE 41–12 RECOMMENDATIONS FOR ATHLETIC ACTIVITY OF PATIENTS WITH HYPERTROPHIC CARDIOMYOPATHY (HCM)

1. Athletes with HCM should not ordinarily participate in most competitive sports (whether or not symptoms and/or outflow gradient are present).

2. In selected low-risk older patients (> 30 years of age) with HCM, consideration may be given to athletic participation if all of the following are absent:
   a. Ventricular tachycardia on Holter monitoring
   b. Family history of sudden death due to HCM
   c. History of syncope or episode of impaired consciousness
   d. Severe hemodynamic abnormalities, including a left ventricular outflow gradient ≥ 50 mm Hg
   e. Exercise-induced hypotension
   f. Moderate or severe mitral regurgitation
   g. Enlarged left atrium (≥ 50 mm)
   h. Paroxysmal atrial fibrillation
   i. Abnormal myocardial perfusion

Adapted from Maron, B. J., Isner, J. M., and McKenna, W. J.: Task force 3: Hypertrophic cardiomyopathy, myocarditis and other myopericardial diseases and mitral valve prolapse. Reprinted by permission of the American College of Cardiology. J. Am. Coll. Cardiol. 24:845–899, 1994.

autopsy in young competitive athletes who die suddenly.[205] Why some athletes with HCM die suddenly and others are able to continue to compete without limitation or death is not known.[321] It has been speculated that the extent and severity of myocardial disarray may play an important role in determining prognosis.[281] Although patients with marked hypertrophy are at increased risk, the degree of left ventricular hypertrophy does not appear to correlate well with prognosis; patients with massive hypertrophy are often no more than minimally symptomatic and appear to have no more malignant courses than do patients with moderate hypertrophy.[281,322] Sudden death is unlikely, however, in asymptomatic or mildly symptomatic patients with mild hypertrophy.[323] Bradyarrhythmias and conducting system disease may play a role as well in sudden death.[281]

Management

Management of patients with HCM is directed toward alleviation of symptoms, prevention of complications, and reduction in the risk of death. Whether asymptomatic patients should receive drug therapy is not established because no adequate controlled studies are available.[198] However, reversible thallium perfusion defects develop during exercise in half of the asymptomatic patients with HCM, and most of these defects can be improved by the use of verapamil.[324] *Digitalis glycosides* should generally be avoided unless atrial fibrillation or systolic dysfunction develops. *Diuretics* were previously thought to be contraindicated to avoid precipitating or worsening the outflow gradient. More recent experience indicates that cautious use of diuretics often helps reduce symptoms of pulmonary congestion, particularly when combined with beta-adrenergic blockers or calcium antagonists.[325] *Beta-adrenergic agonists* may improve diastolic filling but should not be used because they may produce ischemia and usually worsen the outflow gradient.[326]

BETA-ADRENOCEPTOR BLOCKERS. These drugs are the mainstay of medical therapy. With their use, angina, dyspnea, and presyncope may all be improved.[268] Beta-adrenoceptor blockade may prevent the increase in outflow obstruction that accompanies exercise, although resting gradients are largely unchanged.[327] It decreases the determinants of myocardial oxygen consumption and thus angina pectoris and perhaps exerts an antiarrhythmic action. Angina pectoris generally responds more favorably to treatment with a beta-adrenoceptor blocker than does dyspnea. It has been suggested that beta-adrenoceptor blockade may prevent sudden death (and accordingly some use prophylactic beta-adrenoceptor blockade therapy in asymptomatic patients), but its efficacy for this purpose has not been established.[199,229,268] Beta-adrenoceptor blockade also blunts the chronotropic response, thus limiting the demand for increased myocardial oxygen delivery. Beta-adrenoceptor blockade previously was thought to have a beneficial effect on diastolic ventricular filling, but it now appears that any benefit is simply the consequence of a slower heart rate.[199] The overall clinical response to beta-adrenoceptor blockade is variable, however, because only about one-third to two-thirds of patients experience symptomatic improvement.[199] One small blinded trial of beta-adrenoceptor blocker therapy found that nadolol improved symptoms better than a placebo or a calcium antagonist, but did not improve exercise capacity.[328] If beta-adrenoceptor blockers are discontinued, they should be withdrawn slowly to avoid rebound adrenergic hypersensitivity.[329]

CALCIUM ANTAGONISTS. These are an alternative to beta-adrenoceptor blockade in the management of HCM; most of the experience has been with verapamil, with more limited use of nifedipine and diltiazem.[198,199] No clear consensus exists as to whether therapy should be initiated first with a beta-adrenoceptor blocker or a calcium antagonist, although verapamil often is effective in improving symptoms in patients who have failed beta-adrenoceptor blockade therapy.[198] Exercise performance in particular may be improved when patients are changed from a beta-adrenoceptor blocker to verapamil. Both the hypercontractile systolic function and the abnormalities of diastolic filling may be related to abnormal calcium kinetics, and drugs that block the inward transport of calcium across the myocardial cell membrane may be able to rectify both abnormalities.

Verapamil has been the most widely utilized calcium antagonist in this condition.[198] Its use was suggested, at least in part, by the observation that it produces a protective and beneficial effect in the hereditary cardiomyopathy of the Syrian hamster, a condition marked by intracellular calcium overload, in which propranolol is ineffective.[95] Although the vasodilator effects of verapamil should not be helpful in HCM, it appears that by depressing myocardial contractility, verapamil can decrease the left ventricular outflow gradient when given intravenously or orally. Perhaps more important from a symptomatic point of view, verapamil improves diastolic filling in HCM, at least in part by reducing asynchronous regional diastolic performance.[198,199,225] It also improves regional myocardial blood flow in some patients, which may contribute to the improvement in diastolic behavior.[330] Verapamil appears to improve diastolic filling by improving relaxation rather than by changing left ventricular diastolic stiffness; at any given diastolic volume, filling pressure is reduced.[225] Although variable clinical responses have been reported with verapamil, about two-thirds or more of patients show increased exercise capacity and an improved symptomatic status.[198,199] Sustained symptomatic improvement has been noted with the long-term administration of verapamil in ambulatory patients,[331] although important adverse effects, including sudden death, have been observed in a small fraction of patients so treated. Complications with verapamil include suppression of sinus node automaticity and inhibition of atrioventricular conduction, vasodilatation, and negative inotropic effects. These side effects may culminate in hypotension, pulmonary edema, and death; antiarrhythmic agents, especially quinidine, may exacerbate the deleterious hemodynamic effects of verapamil. Because of these adverse effects, it has been suggested that verapamil should not be used, or should be used only with extreme caution, in patients with high left ventricular filling pressure or symptoms of paroxysmal nocturnal dyspnea or orthopnea. Unfortunately, these are usually the patients in greatest need of therapy.

Nifedipine has also been used in HCM, and it may have theoretical advantages over verapamil because it causes less depression of atrioventricular conduction. This may be counteracted by its more potent vasodilator action. Reports of its effect on diastolic function have shown inconsistent results.[199,332,333] Nifedipine may alleviate the chest pain in HCM patients. Combined administration of nifedipine and propranolol may be of benefit in some patients, particularly those with outflow gradients. However, it should be recognized that the potent vasodilator effects of nifedipine may lead to systemic hypotension and an increase in the outflow gradient,[333] and in high doses it may depress left ventricular function.[334] *Diltiazem* has also shown beneficial effects in HCM, producing improved diastolic function.[199]

The combination of a beta-adrenoceptor blocker and a calcium antagonist may be efficacious in patients responding inadequately to monotherapy.[335]

OTHER NONSURGICAL MEASURES. *Disopyramide,* an antiarrhythmic drug that alters calcium kinetics, has produced symptomatic improvement and abolition of the pressure gradient in patients with HCM, presumably as a consequence of depression of left ventricular systolic performance as well as a peripheral vasoconstrictor effect.[336,337] It does not appear to have significant effects on diastolic function,[336,338] although this issue is not entirely resolved.[339] Long-term experience with disopyramide is limited, particularly in asymptomatic patients and those without outflow gradients.

Beta-adrenoceptor blockers, calcium antagonists, and the conventional antiarrhythmic agents do not appear to suppress serious ventricular arrhythmias or reduce the frequency of supraventricular arrhythmias. However, *amiodarone* is effective in the treatment of both supraventricular and ventricular tachyarrhythmias in HCM.[314] Although there is some belief that amiodarone improves prognosis in HCM,[340] only limited and inconclusive data are available. Amiodarone may also improve symptoms and exercise capacity, although its putative beneficial effects on diastolic ventricular function are controversial.[199,271] Experience with *sotalol*, although limited, has been generally favorable; in addition to its antiarrhythmic effects on supraventricular and ventricular arrhythmias, its beta-adrenoceptor blocking effects are beneficial.[341] We do not favor empirical use of amiodarone (or other antiarrhythmic agents for that matter) and share the concern about possible proarrhythmic effects and potential toxicity, including sudden death.[229,268,271,342]

Strenuous exercise should be avoided because of the risk of sudden death; although more deaths in HCM occur during rest or mild activity, almost half the deaths occur during or just after strenuous physical activity.[281] Even though many individuals with subclinical HCM exercise vigorously, the threat of sudden death is sufficiently real that competitive sports are proscribed in patients with marked hypertrophy or other factors believed to be associated with increased risk (Table 41–11).[205] Atrial fibrillation should usually be pharmacologically or electrically converted because of the hemodynamic consequences of the loss of the atrial contribution to ventricular filling in this disorder. Anticoagulants should be given to patients with chronic atrial fibrillation when no contraindication exists. Infective endocarditis may occur in about 5 per cent of patients, and antibiotic prophylaxis is indicated.[198] The infection usually occurs on the aortic valve or mitral apparatus, on the endocardium, or at the site of the contact lesion on the septum; thus, chronic endocardial trauma may provide a nidus for subsequent infection.

DDD PACING. Insertion of a dual-chamber DDD pacemaker may be useful in some patients with an outflow gradient and severe symptoms,[343–348,348a] but it is likely that no more than 10 per cent of HCM patients are candidates. Symptoms generally are improved, and the gradient is reduced by an average of about 50 per cent.[198] Benefits have been described even after termination of pacing, suggesting a modification of myocardial properties.[345,347] The long-term utility of pacing, however, is not known at present.[349,349a,349b] The benefit of its use in patients without a resting outflow gradient is even more equivocal; it usually improves symptoms and exercise capacity, but there is no improvement or even worsening of various hemodynamic variables and pharmacological therapy usually needs to be reinstituted.[350] Therefore, its use in this setting generally is not recom-

mended at present. In high-risk patients or those surviving a cardiac arrest, insertion of an implantable cardioverter-defibrillator should be considered.[273] A few patients have benefited from intentional infarction of a portion of the interventricular septum by the infusion of alcohol into a selectively catheterized septal artery.[350a]

SURGICAL TREATMENT. A variety of surgical procedures aimed at reducing the outflow gradient have been developed and are most commonly used in the markedly symptomatic patient with a gradient above 50 mm Hg who has not responded well to medical management.[198,261,351,352,352a] The most popular operation for HCM consists of excising a portion of the hypertrophied septum. A transaortic approach with septal myotomy-myectomy is the most widely used procedure, although left transventricular as well as combined transaortic and left ventricular approaches have also been used successfully. Operative management is facilitated by intraoperative echocardiography, and operative mortality is now less than 5 per cent[268,352–354]; large centers have reported series of patients with mortalities under 3 per cent.[198,261] Operation often relieves the obstruction as well as the mitral regurgitation. The reduction in left ventricular systolic pressure produced by the operation leads to reduced evidence of postoperative myocardial ischemia on thallium stress testing.[355] Patients over the age of 65 as well as under the age of 10 years have undergone successful operations; the operative risk is higher in older patients.[349]

Surgery results in long-term improvement in symptoms and exercise capacity in most patients.[356,357] Occasional patients experience myocardial damage and fibrosis as a consequence of the procedure.[355] Significant aortic regurgitation is an uncommon complication of the transaortic valve approach, occurring in less than 4 per cent of patients.[261] Myotomy-myectomy may be combined with other necessary operative procedures (particularly coronary artery bypass grafting), although the risk is increased.[354] There has been recent enthusiasm for combining septal myotomy-myectomy with plication of the anterior leaflet of the mitral valve.[358] Although mitral valve replacement or repair is performed in fewer centers than myotomy-myectomy, the long-term results also have been favorable, with symptomatic benefit and an improvement in hemodynamics.[359] The rationale for this operation is that it abolishes obstruction by preventing SAM of the mitral valve (see p. 91). It appears to be of particular value in patients with less than severe (<18 mm) hypertrophy of the upper septum or other atypical septal morphology, in those with previous myotomy-myectomy with persistent severe symptoms and obstruction, and in patients with intrinsic mitral valve disease.[360] In appropriate candidates not responding to maximal standard medical and surgical therapy, cardiac transplantation may be an option; this usually is required only for patients who have entered the dilated phase of HCM and have intractable symptoms of congestive heart failure.[361]

RESTRICTIVE AND
INFILTRATIVE CARDIOMYOPATHIES

Of the three major functional categories of the cardiomyopathies (dilated, hypertrophic, and restrictive), the restrictive are the least common in Western countries, although secondary forms of restrictive cardiomyopathy such as endomyocardial disease (see p. 1431) are common in specific geographical regions.[362,363] The hallmark of the restrictive cardiomyopathies is abnormal diastolic function; the ventricular walls are excessively rigid and impede ventricular filling. Contractile function, on the other hand, often is unimpaired, even in many cases of extensive infiltration of the myocardium.[6,364] Thus, restrictive cardiomyopathy bears

some functional resemblance to constrictive pericarditis, which is also characterized by normal or nearly normal systolic function but abnormal ventricular filling.[365,366] Differentiation of the two conditions is mandatory because of the potential for successful surgical treatment of constriction (Table 43–8, p. 1503).[219,363,363a]

A variety of specific pathological processes may result in restrictive cardiomyopathy, although the cause often remains unknown. Myocardial fibrosis, infiltration, or endomyocardial scarring is usually responsible for the abnormal diastolic behavior; there often is histological evidence of

TABLE 41-13 CLASSIFICATION OF THE RESTRICTIVE CARDIOMYOPATHIES

MYOCARDIAL
Noninfiltrative
Idiopathic
Scleroderma

Infiltrative
Amyloid
Sarcoid
Gaucher disease
Hurler disease

Storage Diseases
Hemochromatosis
Fabry disease
Glycogen storage diseases

ENDOMYOCARDIAL
Endomyocardial fibrosis
Hypereosinophilic syndrome
Carcinoid
Metastatic malignancies
Radiation
Anthracycline toxicity

myocyte hypertrophy.[366,367] Myocardial involvement with amyloid is a common cause of secondary restrictive cardiomyopathy, although it can be caused by a variety of other conditions (Table 41-13).[363]

Some patients may manifest the clinical features of a restrictive cardiomyopathy and yet exhibit the pathological findings of left ventricular hypertrophy and fibrosis[6]; certainly ventricular hypertrophy, especially HCM, can cause diminished ventricular compliance, but not restrictive cardiomyopathy per se. Restrictive cardiomyopathy on occasion is inherited; in those cases there may be an associated skeletal muscle myopathy.[367,368]

HEMODYNAMICS. The clinical and hemodynamic features of restrictive heart disease simulate those of chronic constrictive pericarditis; endomyocardial biopsy, CT scanning (Fig. 10-40, p. 340), MRI (Fig. 10-14, p. 325) and radionuclide angiography (Fig. 43-28, p. 1504) may be particularly useful in differentiating the two diseases by demonstrating myocardial scarring or infiltration (biopsy) or thickening of the pericardium (CT and MRI).[362,363,369,370] With the use of these modalities, exploratory thoracotomy should rarely be required; nevertheless, if the differentiation between constriction and restrictive cardiomyopathy cannot be established with certainty, surgical exploration is in order.[219] The characteristic hemodynamic feature in both conditions is a deep and rapid early decline in ventricular pressure at the onset of diastole, with a rapid rise to a plateau in early diastole (although this finding is absent in some patients with restrictive cardiomyopathy).[365,367] This dip and plateau has been termed the "square root" sign (Fig. 43-19, p. 1502) and is manifested in the atrial pressure tracing as a prominent y descent followed by a rapid rise and plateau.[219] The x descent may also be rapid, and the combination results in the characteristic M or W waveform in the atrial pressure tracing. The a wave is prominent and often is of the same amplitude as the v wave. Both systemic and pulmonary venous pressures are elevated, although patients with restrictive heart disease typically have left ventricular filling pressures that exceed right ventricular filling pressure by more than 5 mm Hg[366]; this difference is accentuated by exercise, fluid challenge, and Valsalva maneuver (although not all patients demonstrate this finding).[219,371] In this respect they differ from patients with constrictive pericarditis, in whom diastolic pressures are similar in both ventricles, usually differing by no more than 5 mm Hg.[365] The pulmonary artery systolic pressure is often greater than 50 mm Hg in patients with restrictive cardiomyopathy but is lower in constrictive pericarditis.[362,365] Furthermore, the plateau of the right ventricular

diastolic pressure is usually at least one-thrd of the peak right ventricular systolic pressure in patients with constrictive pericarditis, whereas it is frequently less in restrictive cardiomyopathy.[365] Patients who demonstrate all three typical hemodynamic features (difference of biventricular diastolic pressures, pulmonary artery systolic pressure, ratio of right ventricular diastolic to systolic pressure) can be classified correctly, although in one-fourth the differentiation between constriction and restriction cannot be made on hemodynamic grounds.[365]

CLINICAL MANIFESTATIONS. Exercise intolerance is frequent because of the inability of patients with restrictive cardiomyopathy to increase their cardiac output by tachycardia without further compromising ventricular filling. Weakness and dyspnea are often prominent. Exertional chest pain may be prominent in some patients but is usually absent. Particularly in advanced cases, the central venous pressure is elevated, with attendant peripheral edema, enlarged liver, ascites, and anasarca. *Physical examination* may reveal jugular venous distention, and an S_3, S_4, or both. An inspiratory increase in venous pressure (Kussmaul sign, p. 1497) may be seen. However, in contrast to constrictive pericarditis, the apex impulse is usually palpable in restrictive cardiomyopathy.

Various ancillary laboratory findings in addition to endomyocardial biopsy, CT scanning, and MRI[369] may be useful in distinguishing between constrictive and restrictive disease. While pericardial calcification is neither absolutely sensitive nor specific for constrictive pericarditis (see p. 1499), its presence in a patient in whom the differential diagnosis rests between restrictive cardiomyopathy and constrictive pericarditis lends strong support to the latter diagnosis.[219] The *echocardiogram* may demonstrate thickening of the left ventricular wall and an increase of left ventricular mass in patients with infiltrative disease causing restrictive cardiomyopathy (Fig. 41-21).[362] The pattern of filling of the left ventricle differs in the two conditions, as can be demonstrated by digitized echocardiograms,[372] transthoracic[373-375] and transesophageal[376,377] Doppler ultrasonography, and radionuclide ventriculography.[378,379] In patients with constrictive pericarditis, respiratory variations in left ventricular isovolumic relaxation time and peak mitral valve velocity in early diastole are prominent; however, this finding is not present in patients with restrictive cardiomyopathy (nor in normal subjects).[375]

The prognosis in restrictive cardiomyopathy is quite variable; usually it is one of relentless symptomatic progression and high mortality.[219] No specific therapy (other than symptomatic) is available (excepting the secondary restrictive cardiomyopathy due to iron overload which is improved by removal of the iron), although there is speculation that calcium antagonists may be of some value.[362]

· AMYLOIDOSIS

ETIOLOGY AND TYPES. Amyloidosis is a disease complex that results from deposition of unique twisted B-pleated sheet fibrils formed from various proteins by several different pathogenic mechanisms.[363,380,381] Amyloid may be found in almost any organ, but clinically evident disease does not appear unless infiltration is extensive. Several classification systems have been used to characterize the different clinical presentations of amyloidosis. The condition with the traditional designation of primary amyloidosis is now known to be caused by the production of an amyloid protein composed of portions of immunoglobulin light chain (designated AL) by a monoclonal population of plasma cells, often as a consequence of multiple myeloma.[382] Secondary amyloidosis is due to the production of a nonimmunoglobulin protein termed AA.[380]

Familial amyloidosis, inherited as an autosomal dominant trait, results from the production of a variant prealbumin protein termed transthyretin; more than 50 different point mutations have been described so far.[383-385] It generally occurs in one of three clinical presentations: progressive neuropathy, cardiomyopathy, or nephropathy.[381] Senile systemic amyloidosis is due to the production of either an atrial natriuretic-like protein or transthyretin[380,386] and is becoming

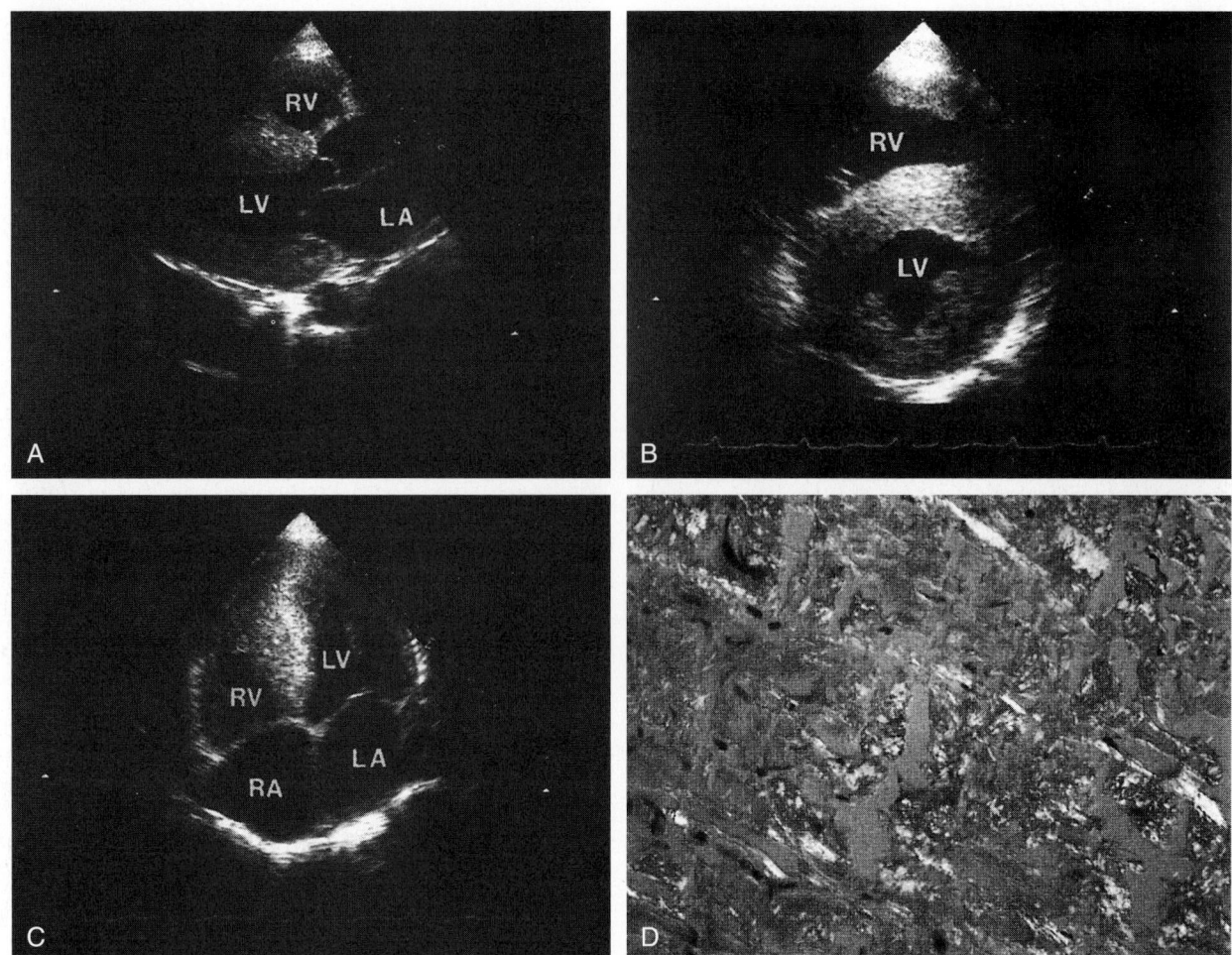

FIGURE 41–21. Two-dimensional echocardiogram in various orientations (A to C) and cardiac biopsy specimen (D) of a 68-year-old man with cardiac amyloidosis. A, Parasternal long-axis view shows marked increase of wall thickness of the left ventricle and thickening of both the mitral and aortic valves. B, Parasternal short-axis view of the left ventricle shows an increase in wall thickness and a prominent speckled pattern of the myocardium that is characteristic of infiltrative cardiomyopathy. C, Apical four-chamber view shows hypertrophy of both ventricles and thickening of both the mitral and tricuspid valves and the interatrial septum. D, Endomyocardial biopsy specimen demonstrates amyloid protein showing apple-green birefringence when viewed under polarized light (Congo red stain, ×3). LA = Left atrium; LV = left ventricle; RA = right atrium; RV = right ventricle. (From Douglas, P. S.: Images in clinical medicine. N. Engl. J. Med. 327:1574, 1992. Copyright Massachusetts Medical Society.)

increasingly common as the average age of the population increases. Scattered deposits of amyloid localized to the aorta or atria are virtually ubiquitous in individuals over the age of 80.[363,380] Small deposits of amyloid may often be found in the pulmonary vessels or the vessels of other organs as well.

Cardiac Amyloidosis

Involvement of the heart is a common finding and is the most frequent cause of death in amyloidosis associated with an immunocyte dyscrasia.[387] Clinically apparent heart disease is present in one-third of patients, although the heart is virtually always involved when studied pathologically.[381] In secondary amyloidosis, on the other hand, clinically significant cardiac involvement is uncommon[388]; the myocardial deposits are typically small and perivascular and usually do not result in significant myocardial dysfunction.[380] Familial amyloidosis is associated with overt cardiac involvement in about one-quarter of the afflicted patients, usually late in the course of the disease.[389] The clinical course is usually dominated by neurological or renal dysfunction, although death is due to heart failure or arrhythmia about half the time.[389] Cardiac involvement in senile amyloidosis varies from small atrial deposits that do not result in functional impairment to extensive ventricular involvement with resultant cardiac failure.[385]

Cardiac amyloidosis occurs more commonly in men than in women, and it is rare before the age of 30 years.[381] Even in the familial form, the onset of clinical cardiac disease usually does not occur before the age of 35 years and generally occurs much later in life.[388]

PATHOLOGY. The pathological findings often include mild atrial enlargement, usually without significant ventricular dilatation. The walls of both ventricles are typically firm, rubbery, noncompliant, and thickened. Amyloid is present between the myocardial fibers (Fig. 41–21D), with extensive deposition in the papillary muscles occurring commonly. Endocardial involvement of the atria[382] and ventricles is frequent. Amyloidosis often results in focal thickening of or deposits on the cardiac valves, but these abnormalities do not appear to interfere with valvular function other than to produce murmurs. The intramural coronary arteries and veins frequently contain amyloid deposits in the media and adventitia, occasionally compromising the lumina of the vessels.[364,384]

CLINICAL MANIFESTATIONS. Involvement of the cardiovascular system by amyloidosis occurs in four general forms:

1. The most common presentation of cardiac amyloidosis is that of *restrictive cardiomyopathy*.[219] Right-sided findings dominate the clinical presentation; peripheral

edema is a prominent finding, whereas paroxysmal nocturnal dyspnea and orthopnea are absent.[363] Amyloid infiltration of the myocardium results in increased stiffness of the myocardium, producing the characteristic diastolic dip and plateau (square root sign) in the ventricular pressure pulse that may simulate constrictive pericarditis. In contrast to the accelerated early left ventricular diastolic filling found in constrictive pericarditis, cardiac amyloidosis is marked by an impaired rate of early diastolic filling.

2. A second common presentation is congestive heart failure due to systolic dysfunction.[219,385] Hemodynamic evidence of restriction of ventricular filling may not be prominent in these patients. In some patients amyloid deposition in the atrium may be responsible for loss of atrial transport function despite the maintenance of electrical "sinus" rhythm and the precipitation of congestive heart failure.[382] The course of this form of the disease is often relentless progression, usually poorly responsive to treatment. Angina pectoris occurs on occasion despite angiographically normal coronary arteries.[364]

3. Orthostatic hypotension is the third mode of presentation, occurring in about 10 per cent of cases. Although most likely due to amyloid infiltration of the autonomic nervous system or of blood vessels, amyloid deposition in the heart and adrenals may contribute to this manifestation. Hypovolemia as a result of the nephrotic syndrome secondary to renal amyloidosis may aggravate the postural hypotension.[389]

4. An abnormality of cardiac impulse formation and conduction is the fourth and least common mode of presentation and may result in arrhythmias and conduction disturbances.[380] Sudden death, presumably arrhythmic in origin, is relatively common.[389]

Physical Examination. This often reveals congestive heart failure, especially right-sided[363]; a systolic murmur due to atrioventricular valvular regurgitation may be present. Jugular venous distention, a protodiastolic gallop, hepatomegaly, peripheral edema, and a narrow pulse pressure are found in patients presenting with restrictive cardiomyopathy. A fourth heart sound is uncommon, presumably due to amyloid infiltration of the atrium. Patients typically are normotensive or hypotensive; even previously hypertensive individuals usually have a fall in blood pressure as the disease progresses.

Noninvasive Testing. The *chest roentgenogram* usually shows cardiomegaly in patients with systolic dysfunction, although heart size may be normal in patients with the restrictive form.[363] Pulmonary congestion may be prominent in patients with congestive heart failure. The *electrocardiogram* is often abnormal; the most characteristic feature (but often absent) is diffusely diminished voltage.[363] Myocardial infarction is often simulated because of small or absent R waves in right precordial leads or, less frequently, by Q waves in the inferior leads.[380] Arrhythmias, particularly atrial fibrillation, are common, although they rarely are the presenting feature of cardiac amyloidosis. Complex ventricular arrhythmias are found frequently in patients with cardiac amyloidosis, and in some may be a harbinger of sudden death.[384] Various forms of AV conduction defects are often seen.[389] Abnormalities of AV conduction appear to be particularly common in familial amyloidosis with polyneuropathy.[389] Sinus node involvement is common, and the clinical and electrocardiographic features of the sick sinus syndrome may be present (see p. 648).

Echocardiography (Fig. 3–102, p. 92) in advanced cases most commonly reveals increased thickness of the walls of the ventricles, small ventricular chambers, dilated atria, and thickening of the interatrial septum,[380] although the findings are more prominent in the familial than in the primary (AL) form (Fig. 41–21).[364] Left ventricular dysfunction may be seen, especially in advanced cases, but systolic

function often is surprisingly normal.[364] Early preclinical unsuspected cardiac involvement may be detectable only by echocardiography or Doppler ultrasonography.[390] Although the cardiac valves may be thickened, they usually move normally.[385] A pericardial effusion is common but rarely results in tamponade. The appearance of the thickened cardiac walls is often distinctive on two-dimensional echocardiography, demonstrating a granular sparkling texture, presumably due to the amyloid deposit.[219,391] In some cases the pattern of increased wall thickness is nonuniform and may resemble HCM.[219] Echocardiographic demonstration of thick left ventricular walls with concomitant low voltage on the electrocardiogram appears to distinguish cardiac amyloidosis from pericardial disease or left ventricular hypertrophy, and this distinctive voltage/mass ratio is characteristic of myocardial infiltration by amyloid.[391] Doppler ultrasonography[392] and radionuclide ventriculography[393] routinely demonstrate abnormalities of diastolic function, and by estimating the degree of cardiac involvement by amyloid, provide prognostic information.[394]

Scintigraphy with technetium-99m pyrophosphate is often strongly positive with prominent amyloid involvement,[395] although in a minority of cases it is falsely negative.[219,391] Positive scans tend to correlate with extensive cardiac involvement. Scanning with indium-labeled antimyosin antibody may also detect cardiac amyloid involvement.[396]

DIAGNOSIS. Whereas two or three decades ago the clinical diagnosis of systemic amyloidosis was made correctly antemortem only 25 per cent of the time, with more recent clinical awareness of the disease and the utilization of *biopsy techniques,* the diagnosis is now made before death in the majority of cases. An abdominal fat aspirate has been the single most useful diagnostic procedure, combining the attributes of ease of performance, sensitivity, and safety.[363] Biopsy of rectum, gingiva, bone marrow, liver, kidney, and various other tissues has also been used. Endomyocardial biopsy of the right or left ventricles may be helpful in establishing the diagnosis of cardiac amyloidosis if the abdominal fat aspirate is negative.[363]

MANAGEMENT. The treatment of cardiac amyloidosis is generally unsatisfactory and ineffective, although it is speculated that alkylating agents may have some role in primary (AL) amyloidosis.[363,385,397] Digitalis glycosides should be used with caution because patients with cardiac amyloidosis appear to be particularly sensitive to digitalis preparations, and the use of ordinary doses may lead to serious arrhythmias; this may relate to selective binding of digoxin to amyloid fibrils in the myocardium.[363] Similarly, nifedipine binds to amyloid fibrils; its use and that of the other calcium antagonists may lead to exacerbation of congestive heart failure symptoms due to an enhanced negative inotropic effect.[363,398] Insertion of a permanent pacemaker may be beneficial in the short term in patients with symptomatic conducting system disease. Careful use of low doses of diuretics and vasodilators may afford some symptomatic benefit,[381] but there is a real risk of hypotension with use of these agents. In patients with atrial standstill due to amyloid infiltration, anticoagulation may be appropriate even in the absence of atrial arrhythmias, as there is some risk of thrombus formation, presumably as a consequence of stasis in the atrium.[382] A few patients have undergone cardiac transplantation, with inferior long-term results (39 per cent survival at 4 years in one study) due to progressive amyloidosis in other organs; accordingly, cardiac transplantation is not recommended in these patients.[399] An heroic alternative approach for the familial form of cardiac amyloidosis is simultaneous heart and liver transplantation because the circulating transthyretin in these patients is produced in the liver and can be corrected with liver transplantation.[384,385] No therapy is effective for the senile form.[385]

INHERITED INFILTRATIVE DISORDERS CAUSING CARDIOMYOPATHY

The intramyocardial accumulation or infiltration of an abnormal metabolic product typically produces a restrictive picture with impaired diastolic ventricular filling. Systolic impairment may be seen as well but is not invariably found. A variety of infiltrative diseases, often inherited, may result in this hemodynamic picture, including the glycogenoses, the mucopolysaccharidoses, Fabry disease, and Gaucher disease.

FABRY DISEASE

Fabry disease (angiokeratoma corporis diffusum universale) is an X-linked recessive disorder of glycosphingolipid metabolism due to a deficiency of the lysosomal enzyme α-galactosidase A as a consequence of one of more than four dozen mutations.[400–402] Some mutations result in no detectable α-galactosidase A activity and widespread manifestations throughout the body, whereas others produce some degree of enzyme activity with attendant atypical variants of Fabry disease with involvement limited solely to the myocardium.[403,404,404a] The disease is characterized by an intracellular accumulation of a neutral glycolipid, with prominent involvement of the skin and kidneys as well as the myocardium in the classic form. *Histological examination* often reveals widespread involvement of the myocardium, vascular endothelium, conducting tissues, and valves, particularly the mitral valve (Fig. 41–22).[403] The major clinical manifestations of the disease result from the accumulation of the glycolipid substrate in endothelial cells, with eventual occlusion of small arterioles. The accumulation of the glycolipid occurs in the lysosomes of the cardiac tissues and is responsible for the multiple cardiovascular manifestations of Fabry disease.

CARDIAC FINDINGS. These typically include angina and myocardial infarction despite angiographically normal coronary arteries (due to accumulation of lipid moieties in coronary endothelial cells, increased left ventricular wall thickness simulating HCM (due to accumulation in myocytes), left ventricular dysfunction and failure, and mitral regurgitation (due to deposition in valvular fibroblasts).[403] Symptomatic cardiovascular involvement occurs eventually in most affected males, whereas female carriers usually are asymptomatic or only minimally symptomatic. Systemic hypertension, mitral valve prolapse, and congestive heart failure are common clinical manifestations. *Electrocardiographic* abnormalities include AV block or a short P-R interval, and ST-segment and T-wave abnormalities.[405] The *echocardiogram* usually reveals increased left ventricular wall thickness as a result of glycolipid deposition, which may simulate HCM.[403] Differentiation from other hypertrophic or restrictive processes (such as cardiac amyloidosis) may not be possible on echocardiographic grounds but may be possible with nuclear MRI. *Endomyocardial biopsy* may be of considerable value in making a definitive diagnosis, as is low plasma α-galactosidase A activity.[403]

GAUCHER DISEASE

Gaucher disease is an uncommon inherited disorder of glycosyl ceramide metabolism. It is secondary to a deficiency of the enzyme β-glucosidase and results in accumulation of cerebrosides in the spleen, liver, bone marrow, lymph nodes, brain, and myocardium.

Diffuse interstitial infiltration of the left ventricle by cells laden with cerebroside occurs, with attendant reduced left ventricular compliance and cardiac output. Clinical evidence of cardiac involvement is uncommon, but when present it is characterized by left ventricular dysfunction, hemorrhagic pericardial effusion, increased left ventricular mass, and thickening of the left-sided valves.[406–408] Liver transplantation may produce a reduction in tissue infiltration by cerebrosides.[409]

HEMOCHROMATOSIS
(See also p. 1674)

Hemochromatosis is characterized by excessive deposition of iron in a variety of parenchymal tissues (heart, liver, gonads, and pancreas). It may occur (1) as a familial (autosomal recessive)[410] or idiopathic disorder, (2) in association with a defect in hemoglobin synthesis resulting in ineffective erythropoiesis, (3) in chronic liver disease, and (4) with excessive oral or parenteral intake of iron (or blood transfusions) over many years.[411–413] Although patients who have iron deposits in the myocardium almost always have deposits in other organs (e.g., liver, spleen, pancreas, bone marrow), the severity of myocardial involvement varies widely and only roughly parallels that in other organs. Cardiac involvement leads to a mixed dilated/ restrictive cardiomyopathic presentation with both systolic and diastolic dysfunction, often with associated arrhythmias.[411,414,415] Myocardial damage is thought to be due to direct tissue toxicity of the free iron moiety rather than simply to tissue infiltration.[411] Although cirrhosis and hepatocellular carcinoma are the most common causes of death, cardiac mortality is an important additional concern (especially in the group of patients—usually men—who present at a young age).[413,416]

PATHOLOGICAL FINDINGS. These consist of a dilated heart with thickened ventricular walls.[417] Myocardial iron deposits are found within the sarcoplasmic reticulum and are most common in the subepicardial region, followed by the subendocardial region, and are least common in the midmyocardial wall.[418] They are more extensive in ventricular than in atrial myocardium. Involvement of the cardiac conducting system is common. Myocardial degeneration and fibrosis may also occur (Fig. 57–5, p. 1791).

The severity of myocardial dysfunction is proportional to the quantity of iron present in the myocardium.[417] Extensive deposits of cardiac iron (particularly those grossly visible at postmortem examination) are invariably associated with cardiac dysfunction.

CLINICAL MANIFESTATIONS. These vary widely, depending on the extent of myocardial involvement. Some patients remain asymptomatic despite echocardiographic evidence of myocardial involvement, which is expressed initially as increased left ventricular wall thickness and later as chamber enlargement and contractile dysfunction.[417] In such cases, a variety of noninvasive techniques (CT and especially MRI) may demonstrate early subclinical myocardial involvement in which treatment is most effective.[411,419] Symptomatic cardiac involvement is usually associated with electrocardiographic abnormalities, including ST-segment and T-wave abnormalities, as well as supraventricular arrhythmias[417,420]; these electrocardiographic changes correlate with the degree of iron deposit in the heart.

Cardiac involvement usually is evident from the clinical and echocardiographic features; endomyocardial biopsy may be useful to confirm (but not exclude) the diagnosis.[413] The diagnosis is aided by finding an elevated plasma iron level, a normal or low total iron-binding capacity, and markedly elevated values for serum ferritin, urinary iron, liver iron, and especially saturation of transferrin.[413] Repeated phlebotomies or the use of the chelating agent desferrioxamine may be clinically beneficial[410,411] (see p. 1791).

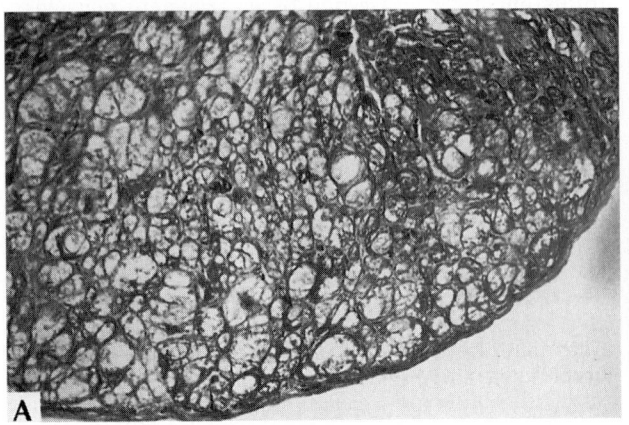 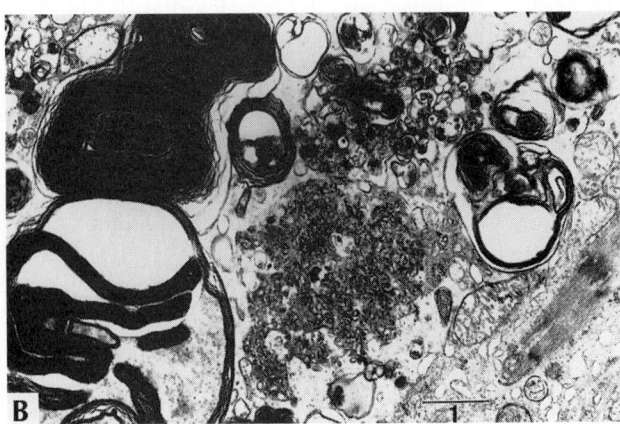

FIGURE 41–22. Histological findings in Fabry disease. *A,* Endomyocardial biopsy showing markedly vacuolated myocytes. *B,* Transmission electron microscopic appearance of the characteristic intracellular deposits of whorled membrane-bound glycoproteins. Bar = 1 μm. (From Butany, J., and Schoen, F. J.: Endomyocardial biopsy. *In* Abelmann, W. H., and Braunwald, E. [eds.]: Cardiomyopathies, Myocarditis, and Pericardial Disease. Atlas of Heart Diseases. Vol. 2. Philadelphia, Current Medicine, 1995, pp. 12.1–12.17.)

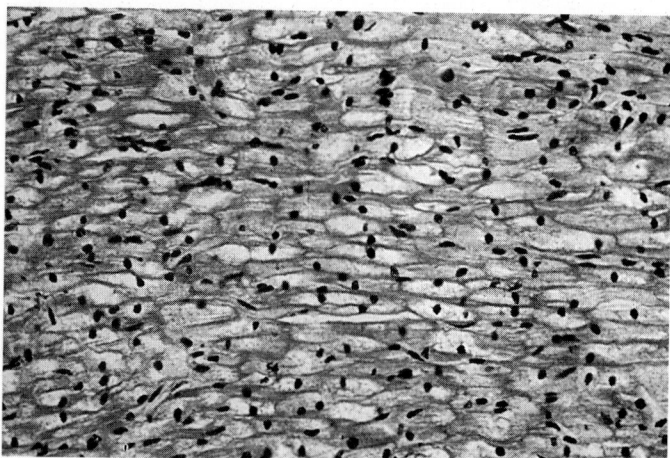

FIGURE 41–23. Endomyocardial biopsy specimen from a patient with glycogen storage disease. The intracytoplasmic lucency is caused by accumulation of glycogen. (From Kasper, E. K., Hruban, R. H., and Baughman, K. L.: Idiopathic dilated cardiomyopathy. *In* Abelmann, W. H., and Braunwald, E. [eds.]: Cardiomyopathies, Myocarditis, and Pericardial Disease. Atlas of Heart Diseases. Vol. 2. Philadelphia, Current Medicine, 1995, pp. 3.1–3.18.)

GLYCOGEN STORAGE DISEASES

Adult patients may demonstrate cardiac involvement in these diseases (Fig. 41–23); in Type III (glycogen debranching enzyme deficiency), cardiac involvement is found only in patients with deficient enzyme in muscle tissue.[421] Cardiac involvement is marked most commonly by apparent left ventricular hypertrophy on the electrocardiogram and echocardiogram.[220,421]

SARCOIDOSIS

Sarcoidosis is a granulomatous disorder of unknown cause, characterized by multisystem involvement. Infiltration of the lungs, reticuloendothelial system, and skin usually dominates the clinical picture, but virtually any tissue may be affected. The most important manifestation results from pulmonary involvement. This often leads to diffuse fibrosis that may result in fatal right heart failure. Primary cardiac involvement is not often recognized clinically, although it may be demonstrated at autopsy in 20 to 30 per cent of cases, most of which demonstrate generalized sarcoidosis.[422–426]

Clinical manifestations of sarcoid heart disease are present in less than 5 per cent of patients, although myocardial involvement may result in heart block, congestive heart failure, ventricular arrhythmias, and sudden death.[423] Myocardial sarcoidosis may have restrictive as well as congestive features because cardiac infiltration by sarcoid granulomas results not only in increased stiffness of the ventricular wall but in diminished systolic contractile function as well. Myocardial sarcoidosis typically affects young or middle-aged adults of either gender; there usually is evidence of generalized sarcoidosis.[422–424,427]

PATHOLOGY. The typical pathological feature of sarcoidosis is the presence of noncaseating granulomas, which occur in many organs. They infiltrate the myocardium and may eventually become fibrotic scars.[423] The granulomas may involve any region of the heart, although the left ventricular free wall and the interventricular septum are the most common sites, and extensive granulomas and scar tissue in the cephalad portion of the interventricular septum is a constant finding in patients with abnormalities of the conduction system.[428] Cardiac infiltration may range from a few scattered lesions to extensive involvement.[423] Because of the variable cardiac involvement, myocardial biopsy may be positive in only about half of the patients, and therefore a negative biopsy by no means excludes the diagnosis.[423] Transmural involvement is common, and large portions of the ventricular wall may be replaced by scar tissue, which may lead to aneurysm formation. Although involvement of small coronary artery branches may be found in sarcoidosis, the larger conductance vessels are uninvolved.[423]

CLINICAL MANIFESTATIONS. Sudden death is the most feared and unfortunately one of the more common manifestations of cardiac sarcoidosis.[423,429–432] Conduction disturbances and congestive heart failure are common manifestations of symptomatic involvement in nonfatal cases, but many patients are asymptomatic despite extensive cardiac involvement.[425] Syncope is common and may reflect paroxysmal arrhythmias or conduction disturbances.[423] Atrial and ventricular arrhythmias, especially ventricular tachycardia, are observed frequently.[423,429–432] Although cor pulmonale as a consequence of pulmonary sarcoidosis accounts for some of the symptoms of heart failure, many symptoms are caused by direct myocardial involvement by granulomas and scar tissue, and the patients show the clinical features of restrictive and/or dilated cardiomyopathy.[423] Symptoms of myocardial sarcoid may be present for variable lengths of time; however, the disease may progress rapidly to death, and in some patients the interval from the onset of the cardiac symptoms to death is measured in months. Survival may be considerably longer, however.[423]

Cardiac dysfunction is often severe and progressive. Occasionally, patients with extensive involvement develop overt left ventricular aneurysms.[423] Pericardial effusions are not uncommon in patients with sarcoidosis.[433]

The *physical examination* may reveal findings of extracardiac sarcoid or may be totally normal. A systolic murmur reflecting mitral regurgitation is common. This appears to be more the result of left ventricular dilatation than of direct sarcoid involvement of the papillary muscles.

The *electrocardiogram* frequently is abnormal in patients with known sarcoid and most commonly demonstrates T-wave abnormalities. Sarcoidosis appears to have an affinity for involvement of the AV junction and bundle of His, and thus varying degrees of intraventricular or AV block are common.[423] With extensive myocardial involvement, pathological Q waves may appear and simulate myocardial infarction. Characteristic features of *echocardiography* include left ventricular dilatation and dysfunction, often with regional wall motion abnormalities suggestive of ischemic heart disease[423,434]; a small to moderate-sized pericardial effusion is seen in about 20 per cent.[433]

DIAGNOSIS. In many cases the diagnosis may be suspected in patients with bilateral hilar lymphadenopathy on chest roentgenogram in whom there is clinical or electrocardiographic evidence of myocardial disease. *Endomyocardial biopsy* may be useful in establishing the diagnosis, although the nonuniform involvement of the heart by sarcoidosis means that a negative biopsy does not exclude the diagnosis.[426] The *echocardiogram* demonstrates diffuse and often regional left ventricular wall motion abnormalities in patients with clinical cardiac involvement.[435] *Myocardial imaging* with *thallium-201* may be helpful in demonstrating segmental perfusion defects that result from sarcoid infiltration of the myocardium.[436–440] Imaging may also indicate the presence of right ventricular hypertrophy in patients with right ventricular overload due to pulmonary fibrosis and pulmonary hypertension. Uptake of technetium pyrophosphate, gallium, and labeled antimyosin antibody may aid in the diagnosis, as may nuclear MRI.[423,437,438,441–443]

MANAGEMENT. The treatment of myocardial sarcoidosis is difficult. Arrhythmias are often refractory to antiarrhythmic drugs.[430] Permanent pacing may be helpful in patients with conducting system involvement.[426] Although the matter is not settled, corticosteroids may be of some benefit in treating the conduction disturbances, arrhythmias, and myocardial dysfunction of sarcoidosis.[422,423,426,444–448] Because the risk of sudden death appears to be greatest in patients with extensive myocardial involvement, it may be reasonable to attempt to halt the progression of the disease with steroids before irreversible fibrosis occurs. Insertion of an implantable cardioverter-defibrillator may be considered in appropriate patients at high risk of sudden death.[430,449] Heart or heart-lung transplantation has been used in selected patients with intractable heart failure.[426,450]

ENDOMYOCARDIAL DISEASE

DEFINITION AND PATHOGENESIS. Endomyocardial disease (EMD) is a common form of secondary restrictive cardiomyopathy in equatorial

Africa and is encountered with less frequency in South America, Asia, and nontropical countries, including the United States.[362,451,452] It is marked by intense endocardial fibrotic thickening of the apex and subvalvular regions of one or both ventricles that results in obstruction to inflow of blood into the respective ventricle, thus producing restrictive physiology. For many years it had been thought that there are two variants of the disease, one occurring principally in tropical countries (termed endomyocardial fibrosis, EMF, or Davies disease) and the other in temperate countries (Löffler endocarditis parietalis fibroplastica, or hypereosinophilic syndrome).[363] This conclusion was reached in part because the pathological findings in advanced cases are identical.[453,454] Despite the pathological similarities, differences occur in clinical presentation. In addition to the geographical differences, the temperate form of the disease (Löffler endocarditis) acts as a more aggressive and rapidly progressive disorder, affecting principally males, and is associated with hypereosinophilia, thromboembolic phenomena, and generalized arteritis.[363] EMF, conversely, shows no gender predilection, occurs in younger patients, and is not associated with an intense eosinophilia.[363,455]

It has also been postulated that Löffler endocarditis and EMF are different phases in a single disease that results from the toxic effect of eosinophils on the heart.[454,456–458] Under this formulation, an initial hypereosinophilia of whatever cause results in damage to the myocardium that produces the first phase of EMD: a necrotic phase, marked by an intense myocarditis, rich in eosinophils, and with an associated arteritis (i.e., Löffler endocarditis).[457,459] This initial phase occurs within the first few months of illness. It appears to be followed by a thrombotic stage, occurring about a year after initial presentation, during which the myocarditis has receded, nonspecific thickening of the myocardium is beginning, and there is a variable degree of superimposed thrombus formation.[457] The last stage is one of fibrosis, presenting all of the features of EMF.[454] The three stages —necrotic, thrombotic, and fibrotic—have been defined on the basis of postmortem material, and it is not suggested that each patient with advanced disease (manifested by EMF) has necessarily passed through the earlier phases.

There is now, however, increasing speculation that this continuum occurs only in the temperate countries, and the endemic EMF found in tropical countries is a distinct and separate disease, as a link with eosinophilia has been virtually impossible to document.[363,460,461] The fibrosis of tropical EMF has been linked to the higher levels of cerium and lower concentrations of magnesium that apparently are found in endemic areas.[460,461]

The possible role of *eosinophils* in the production of the cardiac abnormalities has intrigued investigators for years.[454,457,462] Eosinophils may damage tissues by direct invasion or by the release of toxic substances.[456] The presence of degranulated peripheral eosinophils in patients with Löffler endocarditis suggests that the protein constituents of the eosinophil's granule may be cardiotoxic,[463] first producing the necrotic phase of EMD, followed by the thrombotic and fibrotic phases after the disappearance of the initial eosinophilia.[454]

Because the clinical manifestations of EMD demonstrate geographical and clinical differences, Löffler endocarditis and EMF are discussed separately, even though they could be part of the same disease continuum.

Löffler Endocarditis: The Hypereosinophilic Syndrome

Marked eosinophilia of any cause may be associated with endomyocardial disease (Fig. 41–24). The typical patient who presents with Löffler endocarditis is a man in his fourth decade who lives in a temperate climate and has the hypereosinophilic syndrome (i.e., persistent eosinophilia with ≥ 1500 eosinophils/mm³ for at least 6 months or until death, with evidence of organ involvement).[362,363,457,464] Cardiac involvement in the hypereosinophilic syndrome is the rule, occurring in more than three-fourths of patients.[454,465] Hypereosinophilia and cardiac involvement are also seen in the Churg-Strauss syndrome, which is differentiated by asthma or allergic rhinitis and a necrotizing vasculitis.[363,466] The cause of the eosinophilia in most patients with Löffler endocarditis is unknown, although in some it may be the result of leukemia, or it may be reactive (i.e., secondary to various parasitic, allergic, granulomatous, hypersensitivity, or neoplastic disorders).[459,462,465]

PATHOLOGY. In the hypereosinophilic syndrome, a variety of organs are usually involved besides the heart, including the lungs, bone marrow, and brain.[362,454,457] Cardiac involvement is often biventricular, with mural endocardial thickening of the inflow portions and apex of the ventricles.[363] Histological findings include variable degrees of (1) an acute inflammatory eosinophilic myocarditis involving the myocardium and endocardium; (2) thrombosis, fibrinoid change, and inflammatory reaction involving small intramural coronary vessels; (3) mural thrombosis, often containing eosinophils; and (4) fibrotic thickening of up to several millimeters.[363,457]

CLINICAL MANIFESTATIONS. The principal clinical features include weight loss, fever, cough, skin rash, and congestive heart failure. Although early cardiac involvement may be asymptomatic, overt cardiac dysfunction occurs in more than half the patients and may be right- and/or left-sided.[454] Cardiomegaly, often without overt symptoms of congestive heart failure, may be present, and the murmur of mitral regurgitation is common.[457] Systemic embolism is frequent and may lead to neurological and renal dysfunction. Death is usually due to congestive heart failure, often with associated renal, hepatic, or respiratory dysfunction.[363]

LABORATORY EXAMINATION. The *chest roentgenogram* may reveal cardiomegaly and pulmonary congestion or, less commonly, pulmonary infiltrates. The *electrocardiogram* most commonly shows nonspecific ST-segment and T-wave abnormalities.[363,465] Arrhythmias, especially atrial fibrillation, and conduction defects, particularly right bundle branch block, may also be present.

The *echocardiogram* commonly demonstrates localized thickening of the posterobasal left ventricular wall, with absent or markedly limited motion of the posterior leaflet of the mitral valve.[362,363] There may be obliteration of the apex by thrombus. Enlargement of the atria may be seen,

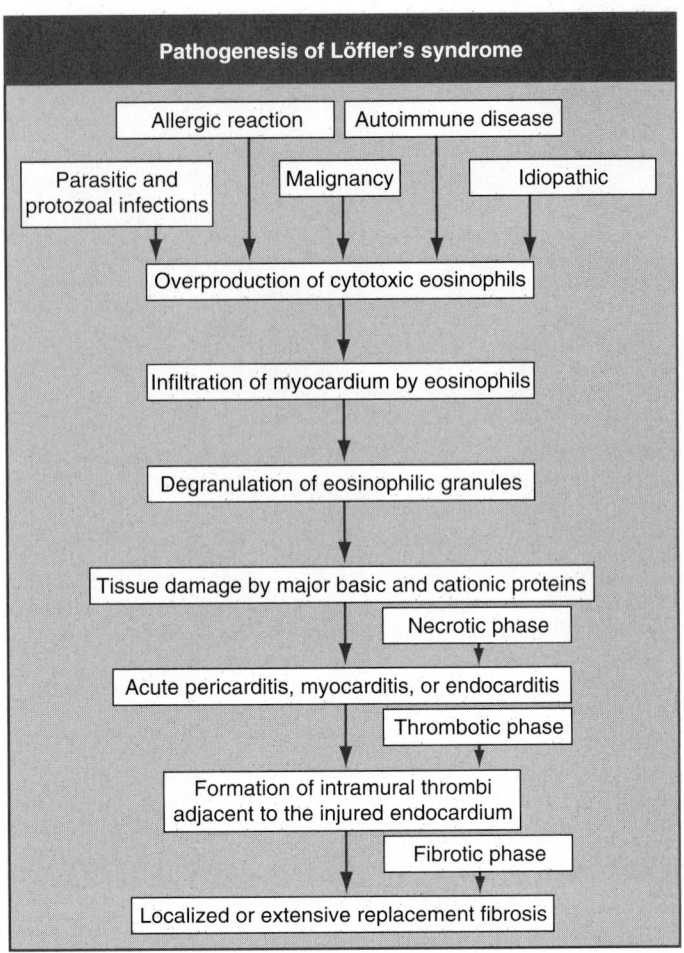

FIGURE 41–24. The pathogenesis of Löffler's syndrome. Tissue damage is caused by major basic and cationic proteins derived from cytotoxic eosinophils. These cytotoxic proteins may stay in the myocardium for a prolonged period and produce continuous tissue damage. In the fibrotic phase, various types of heart diseases, such as endomyocardial fibrosis, dilated cardiomyopathy, AV block, or valvular regurgitation can be seen according to the difference of the most dominantly involved site. (From Hirota, Y.: Restrictive cardiomyopathy, cardiac amyloidosis, and hypereosinophilic heart disease. *In* Abelmann, W. H., and Braunwald, E. [eds.]: Cardiomyopathies, Myocarditis and Pericardial Disease. Atlas of Heart Diseases. Vol. 2. Philadelphia, Current Medicine, 1995.)

along with Doppler ultrasound evidence of atrioventricular valve regurgitation.[363] Systolic function often is well preserved, in keeping with the restrictive picture seen in this condition.[454]

The *hemodynamic* consequences of the dense endocardial scarring seen in Löffler endocarditis are those of a restrictive cardiomyopathy, with abnormal diastolic filling due to increased stiffness of the ventricles and a reduction in the size of the ventricular cavity by organized thrombus.[454,457] Atrioventricular valvular regurgitation may occur because of involvement of the supporting apparatus of the mitral or tricuspid valves.[454] *Cardiac catheterization* reveals markedly elevated ventricular filling pressures, and there may be evidence of tricuspid or mitral regurgitation. A characteristic feature on angiocardiography is largely preserved systolic function with obliteration of the apex of the ventricles.[457] The diagnosis is often confirmed by percutaneous endomyocardial biopsy,[457] but the biopsy is not invariably positive.[462]

MANAGEMENT. Medical therapy during the course of early Löffler endocarditis and surgical therapy during the later phases of fibrosis may have a positive effect on symptoms and survival. Corticosteroids appear to have a beneficial effect on acute myocarditis,[459] and together with cytotoxic drugs (hydroxyurea in particular), may improve survival substantially.[454,457,465] A limited number of patients not responding to standard therapy have responded to treatment with interferon.[462,464] Routine cardiac therapy with digitalis, diuretics, afterload reduction, and anticoagulation as indicated are adjuncts in the management of these patients.[454,457] Surgical therapy (see Management of EMF, p. 1434) appears to offer significant palliation of symptoms once the fibrotic stage has been reached.[363,457,465]

Endomyocardial Fibrosis

EMF occurs most commonly in tropical and subtropical Africa, particularly Uganda and Nigeria.[461] It is typified by fibrous endocardial lesions of the inflow portion of the right or left ventricle or both and often involves the AV valves, resulting in regurgitation.[452,460] It is a relatively frequent cause of heart failure and death in equatorial Africa, accounting for 10 to 20 per cent of deaths due to heart disease.[362,363]

Although most prominent in Africa, it is also found in tropical and subtropical regions in the rest of the world, including India,[452] Brazil, Colombia, and Sri Lanka. EMF is most common in specific ethnic groups, notably the Rwanda tribe in Uganda, and in people of low socioeconomic status.[461] The disease is equally frequent in both genders, and, although most common in children and young adults, its reported age range is 4 to 70 years.[362,455] It is most common in blacks, but cases have been reported occasionally in whites in temperate climates, rarely in the absence of prior residence in tropical areas.

PATHOLOGY

A pericardial effusion, which may be quite large, may be present.[461] The heart is normal in size or slightly enlarged, but massive cardiomegaly does not occur. The right atrium is often dilated, and in patients with severe right ventricular involvement there may be massive enlargement of this chamber. Indentation of the right border of the heart above the apex as a result of apical scarring may occur.[461]

Combined right and left ventricular disease occurs in about half the cases, with pure left ventricular involvement occurring in 40 per cent and pure right ventricular involvement in the remaining 10 per cent of patients who are examined post mortem.[362,453] When affected, the right ventricle exhibits extensive, dense, fibrous thickening of the inflow tract and apex, with involvement of the papillary muscles and chordae tendineae. Involvement of the right ventricle may lead to obliteration of the apex, with a mass of thrombus and fibrous tissue filling the cavity.[453] The tricuspid valve is often pulled down and distorted by the fibrous process involving the supporting structures. Right atrial thrombi occur commonly. Left ventricular involvement is similar, with fibrosis extending from the apex up the inflow portion of the left ventricle to the posterior mitral valve leaflet. The anterior leaflet of the mitral valve and the outflow portion of the left ventricle are usually spared. Thrombi often overlie the endocardial lesions, and widely distributed endocardial calcific deposits may occur. The coronary arteries are uninvolved, as is the remainder of the body.[362]

HISTOLOGIC FINDINGS. Microscopically, the involved endocardium demonstrates a thick layer of collagen tissue on top of a layer of loosely arranged connective tissue.[467] Septa composed of fibrous and granulation tissue extend for variable distances into the myocardium.[362,467] Interstitial edema is often present, but there is no prominent cellular infiltration. Small patches of fibroelastosis may occur in both ventricular outflow tracts beneath the semilunar valves but are thought to be a secondary phenomenon due to local trauma rather than a result of the basic pathological process.

CLINICAL MANIFESTATIONS

As already noted, EMF may involve both ventricles or either ventricle selectively; left-sided involvement results in symptoms of pulmonary congestion, whereas predominant right-sided disease may present features of a restrictive cardiomyopathy and therefore simulate constrictive pericarditis. There is often regurgitation of one or both AV valves. The onset of the disease is usually insidious, but it is sometimes ushered in by an acute febrile illness. Rarely, the disease appears to stabilize; although survival for up to 12 years has been observed, EMF is usually relentlessly progressive.[363] Death is due to progressive myocardial failure, often associated with pulmonary congestion, infection, or infarction, or sudden, unexpected cardiovascular collapse, presumably arrhythmic in origin.[362] Survival appears to be unrelated to site of predominant involvement (right or left ventricle), although patients presenting in advanced right-sided failure have a worse prognosis than other patients.[363,455]

RIGHT VENTRICULAR EMF. Pure or predominant right ventricular involvement is characterized by fibrous obliteration of the right ventricular apex that diminishes the capacity of this chamber.[453] The fibrosis often extends to the supporting apparatus of the tricuspid valve,[468,469] resulting in tricuspid regurgitation.[470] Clinical manifestations in patients with right-sided involvement include an elevated jugular venous pressure, a prominent v wave, and a rapid y descent. A protodiastolic gallop sound may be heard along the lower sternal border, reflecting right ventricular dysfunction.[453] The liver is usually large and pulsatile, and ascites, splenomegaly, and peripheral edema are common. Pulmonary congestion is not present in the absence of left-sided involvement, and the pulmonary artery and pulmonary capillary wedge pressures are normal. A pericardial effusion, which is sometimes quite large, may be present. The right atrium is often enlarged, sometimes massively so.

Laboratory Findings. The *electrocardiogram* is usually abnormal, with diminished QRS voltage (probably resulting from the presence of a pericardial effusion), ST-segment and T-wave abnormalities, and findings of right atrial enlargement, especially a qR pattern in lead V_1.[471] The *chest roentgenogram* demonstrates cardiac enlargement, usually with gross prominence of the right atrium and a pericardial effusion. Calcification in the walls of the right or, less commonly, the left ventricle may be seen.[452] *Echocardiography* may demonstrate right ventricular thickening, obliteration of the apex, dilated atrium, strong echoes emanating from the endocardial surface, and abnormal septal motion in patients with tricuspid regurgitation.[453,461,472] At *angiography* the right ventricular apex is characteristically not visualized because of obliteration by the fibrous endocardium, but tricuspid regurgitation, right atrial enlargement, and filling defects in the right atrium due to intraatrial thrombi are sometimes seen.[362] Early angiographic changes that may be present before advanced disease develops include a change in the endocardial appearance, small apical filling defects, and mild tricuspid regurgitation.

LEFT VENTRICULAR EMF. With predominant *left-sided* involvement, the endomyocardial fibrosis invades the apex of the ventricle and usually the chordae tendineae or the posterior mitral valve leaflet as well, leading to mitral regurgitation.[473] The murmur may be confined to late systole, as is characteristic of the papillary muscle dysfunction type of murmur, or it may be pansystolic. Findings of pulmonary hypertension may be prominent. A protodiastolic gallop is commonly heard.

Laboratory Findings. The *electrocardiogram* usually shows T-wave abnormalities and diminished QRS voltage in the presence of a pericardial effusion, although left ventricular hypertrophy may be present.[362,363] There may be findings of left atrial abnormality. As with right-sided involvement, atrial fibrillation often is present. *Echocardiographic* features include thickening and reduced motion of the posterobasal wall and posterior mitral leaflet, increased echoreflectivity of the endocardium, preserved systolic wall motion in the presence of apical obliteration, dilated atrium, and Doppler ultrasound evidence of mitral regurgitation.[363] *Cardiac catheterization* often reveals pulmonary hypertension, with elevated left ventricular filling pressures and a reduced cardiac index.[473] The left ventriculogram usually shows mitral regurgitation, and a filling defect due to an intracavitary thrombus within the ventricle may be seen on occasion.[362] Coronary arteriography does not reveal obstructive disease.

BIVENTRICULAR EMF. This form of EMF occurs more frequently than either isolated right- or left-sided disease.[474] If there is more than minimal right ventricular involvement, severe pulmonary hypertension does not occur, and the right-sided findings dominate the clinical presentation. Typical patients with biventricular involvement may have the features of right ventricular EMF, with only a mitral regurgitant murmur to suggest left ventricular involvement. Systemic embolization may occur in up to 15 per cent of patients; infective endocarditis is even less frequent and is found in less than 2 per cent.

This is based on the presence in an individual of the typical clinical and laboratory features, particularly angiography, from the appropriate geographical area. Eosinophilia is usually not a prominent feature and when present may reflect associated parasitic infestation. *Endomyocardial biopsy* may occasionally be helpful in establishing the diagnosis. However, this risks dislodging a mural thrombus, with resultant embolization, and left-sided biopsy is *not* recommended. In addition, because the disease is often focal, the biopsy may miss the pathological process, particularly if a right ventricular biopsy is performed in a patient with isolated left-sided disease.[461]

MANAGEMENT

The medical treatment of EMF is often difficult and not particularly effective.[473] In patients with advanced disease, the outlook is poor, with a 35 to 50 per cent 2-year mortality.[455,474] Substantially better survival may be seen in less symptomatic patients who have milder forms of the disease.[474,475] Digitalis glycosides may be helpful in controlling the ventricular rate in patients with atrial fibrillation,[363] but the response of congestive symptoms is disappointing. Diuretics are not particularly helpful in the treatment of ascites.[363] Once endomyocardial disease has reached the fibrotic stage, surgery offers the possibility of symptomatic improvement and is the treatment of choice.[362] Operative excision of the fibrotic endocardium and replacement of the mitral and/or tricuspid valves have led to substantial symptomatic improvement, especially with predominant left-sided involvement.[461,475,476] Mitral valve repair, rather than replacement, can be accomplished in some patients.[477] Postoperative catheterization has provided objective evidence of hemodynamic improvement with a reduction in ventricular filling pressures, an increase in cardiac output, and normalization of the angiographic appearance.[476] Operative mortality has been high, running between 15 and 25 per cent in the larger series,[363,461,471,475] although it appears to be lower if replacement of valves can be avoided.[476,477]

Endocardial Fibroelastosis
(See p. 991)

Carcinoid Heart Disease

ETIOLOGY AND PATHOLOGY. The carcinoid syndrome is caused by a metastasizing carcinoid tumor and is characterized by cutaneous flushing, diarrhea, bronchoconstriction, and endocardial plaques composed of a unique type of fibrous tissue. The vasomotor, bronchoconstrictor, and cardiac manifestations are undoubtedly related to circulating humoral substances secreted by the tumor,[478,479] although the precise substance(s) responsible remains to be elucidated.[480,481] Virtually all patients develop diarrhea and flushing, and cardiac abnormalities are found on echocardiography in more than half; clinically apparent and severe right-sided disease is seen in a quarter of patients.[478,479]

Sixty to 90 per cent of tumors arise in the small bowel and appendix, and the rest originate in other areas of the gastrointestinal tract and bronchus.[478] Carcinoid tumors of the ileum are the most likely to metastasize, with involvement of the regional lymph nodes and liver. Usually only carcinoid tumors that invade the liver result in carcinoid heart disease.[478] The cardiac lesions may be related to large circulating quantities of serotonin, bradykinin, or other substances secreted by the tumor, which usually are inactivated by the liver, lungs, and brain.[481a] Hepatic metastases apparently allow large quantities of tumor products to reach the heart without being inactivated by the liver. The preferential right-sided involvement presumably is related to inactivation of the offending humoral substance(s) by the lungs. In 5 to 10 per cent of cases, significant left-sided valvular disease develops,[482] related in most to passage of blood directly from the right to the left side of the heart through a patent foramen ovale, or less commonly by tumor involvement of the lungs.[478]

The characteristic *pathological* findings are fibrous plaques that involve the "downstream" aspect of the tricuspid and pulmonic valves, the endocardium of the cardiac chambers, and the intima of the venae cavae, pulmonary artery, and coronary sinus. The fibrous tissue in the plaques results in distortion of the valves, leading to both stenosis and regurgitation.[478] Histologically, the plaques consist of deposits of fibrous tissue located superficially on the endocardium, often with extension into the underlying layers.[479,481] Ultrastructural and immunohistochemical studies have demonstrated that the plaques are composed of smooth muscle cells embedded in a stroma rich in acid mucopolysaccharides and collagen.[481] Metastatic involvement of the myocardium itself is rare.[478]

CLINICAL MANIFESTATIONS. *Physical examination* usually reveals a systolic murmur along the left sternal border, produced by tricuspid regurgitation; in some cases, there may be a concomitant murmur of pulmonic stenosis and/or regurgitation.[478]

The *chest roentgenogram* is normal in half the patients, but may reveal enlargement of the heart, and pleural effusions or nodules[478]; the pulmonary artery trunk is typically of normal size, without evidence of post-stenotic dilatation as occurs in congenital pulmonic stenosis. No specific *electrocardiographic pattern* is diagnostic of carcinoid heart disease.[478] Right atrial enlargement may be seen on occasion, but electrocardiographic evidence of right ventricular hypertrophy usually is lacking. Nonspecific ST-segment and T-wave abnormalities and sinus tachycardia are the most common findings,[478] although severely symptomatic patients usually have low QRS voltage.[483] *Echocardiography* may reveal evidence of tricuspid and/or pulmonary valve thickening, along with right atrial and right ventricular dilatation; small pericardial effusions are present in a minority.[478,479,484]

The *hemodynamic findings* most commonly encountered are those of tricuspid regurgitation (see p. 1058) and occasionally pulmonic stenosis. A rare patient with the carcinoid syndrome demonstrates a hyperkinetic state (which may lead to high-output heart failure) but without the typical cardiac lesions; in one patient this was caused by profound vasodilatation by substance P.[485]

MANAGEMENT. In patients with mild congestive heart failure this consists of digitalis and diuretics. Symptomatic improvement and improved survival have been noted with the use of somatostatin analogs.[483] Balloon valvuloplasty of the right-sided valves has produced symptomatic improvement in a few patients with stenotic tricuspid or pulmonary valves,[486] although others have developed recurrent symptoms despite "successful" valvuloplasty.[487] Surgical replacement of the tricuspid valve and pulmonic valvotomy or valvectomy may result in symptomatic improvement in severely symptomatic patients with serious valvular dysfunction, although the operative mortality is high (35 per cent in one series).[483] Surgery may improve the functional status and survival of patients with carcinoid heart disease, but patients over the age of 60 years have a very high surgical mortality (reportedly over 50 per cent).[482] The long-term mortality remains high regardless of treatment modality, with half the patients dead within 1 to 2 years.[478,483]

Obesity and Heart Disease
(See p. 1152)

Diabetic Cardiomyopathy
(See p. 1150)

Myocarditis is said to be present when the heart is involved in an inflammatory process, often caused by an infectious agent. The inflammation may involve the myocytes, interstitium, vascular elements, and/or pericardium; involvement of the latter structure is discussed in Chapter 43.

Myocarditis has been described during and following a wide variety of viral, rickettsial, bacterial, protozoal, and metazoal diseases; indeed, virtually any infectious agent may produce cardiac inflammation (Table 41–14).[488] Infectious agents cause myocardial damage by three basic mechanisms: (1) invasion of the myocardium; (2) production of a myocardial toxin, e.g., diphtheria; and (3) immunologically mediated myocardial damage.[489–491] The principal mechanism of heart involvement in viral myocarditis is believed to be a cell-mediated immunological reaction to new cell surface changes or a new antigen related to the virus, and not merely the result of cell damage caused by viral replication.[492–494] Additional evidence for an immune-mediated mechanism is the demonstration of a marked increase in major histocompatibility complex antigen expression in the biopsy specimens from patients with myocarditis.[495] Antibodies against intracellular components may also play a role.[496] Patients with ongoing myocarditis (unlike those with resolved myocarditis) have myocytes that express the intercellular adhesion molecule termed ICAM-1, and it is speculated that the persistent expression of ICAM-1 may play a role in continued myocardial inflammation.[494] Although often mistakenly limited to inflammation due to an infective agent, myocarditis may also be caused by allergic reactions and pharmacological agents, as well as occurring during the course of some systemic diseases such as vasculitis.

Myocarditis may be an acute or a chronic process and may occur during the peripartum period (see p. 1851). In North America, viruses (especially enteroviruses) are presumed to be the most common agents producing myocarditis,[497,498] whereas in South America, Chagas' disease (produced by *Trypanosoma cruzi*) is far more common.[499] The identification of the specific etiological agent responsible for infectious myocarditis usually rests on the associated extracardiac findings because the cardiovascular signs and symptoms are often nonspecific.[490] The histological findings vary, depending on the stage of the disease, the mechanism of myocardial damage, and the specific etiological agent. Myocardial involvement may be focal or diffuse, but the myocardial lesions are generally randomly distributed in the heart, and thus the clinical consequences depend to a large extent on the size and number of the lesions. However, a single small lesion may have profound consequences if it is located within the cardiac conducting system. The histological findings are usually nonspecific (except for some parasitic and granulomatous forms of myocarditis), and with certain exceptions (Table 41–4), myocardial biopsy seldom elucidates the specific etiological agent.

The natural history of myocarditis is varied, as shown in Figure 41–25.

CLINICAL MANIFESTATIONS. The clinical expression of myocarditis ranges from the asymptomatic state secondary to focal inflammation to fulminant fatal congestive heart failure due to diffuse myocarditis.[488] An initial episode of viral myocarditis, perhaps unrecognized and forgotten, may be the initial event that eventually culminates in an "idiopathic" DCM.[16] In experimental animals, the structural and functional myocardial alterations that follow viral myocarditis may persist well beyond the stage of viral replication and myocardial inflammatory response, and the late changes resemble those of DCM.[500]

The outcome after viral myocarditis is quite variable,[488] perhaps related to differing genetic susceptibility of individual patients. In most patients, the event is entirely self-limited and often unrecognized.[498,501] More overt myocarditis may result in acute congestive heart failure.[488,502] In others, unrecognized myocarditis may be the cause of arrhythmias in what appears to be a structurally normal heart.[503] Some patients with chest pain and angiographically normal coronary arteries may have had subclinical myocarditis at some point in the past. Most intriguing is the possibility that viral myocarditis may culminate in DCM, presumably as a consequence of viral-mediated immunological cardiac damage.[501]

Although transient electrocardiographic abnormalities suggesting myocardial involvement are noted in many patients with infectious disease, most patients do not have other clinical manifestations of myocarditis.[504,505] It is postulated that these electrocardiographic changes reflect subclinical myocardial involvement. That unrecognized myocardial involvement occurs with systemic infections is supported by histological evidence of unsuspected myocarditis during routine postmortem examinations; this occurs about 1 per cent of the time.[506] Some degree of myocardial involvement, often subepicardial in location, also frequently occurs in patients with acute pericarditis.

Because myocardial involvement is subclinical in most acute infectious diseases, the majority of patients have no specific complaints referable to the cardiovascular system[504]; the presence of myocarditis is often inferred from ST-segment and T-wave abnormalities on the electrocardiogram.[488] From a clinical viewpoint, myocardial involvement

TABLE 41–14 PRINCIPAL INFECTIOUS ETIOLOGICAL AGENTS ASSOCIATED WITH MYOCARDITIS

BACTERIAL INFECTIONS

Streptococcal	Brucellosis
Staphylococcal	Diphtheria
Pneumococcal	Salmonellosis
Meningococcal	Tuberculosis
Haemophilus	Tularemia
Gonococcal	

SPIROCHETAL INFECTIONS

Leptospirosis	Relapsing fever
Lyme disease	Syphilis

FUNGAL INFECTIONS

Aspergillosis	Coccidiodomycosis
Actinomycosis	Cryptococcosis
Blastomycosis	Histoplasmosis
Candidiasis	

PARASITIC INFECTIONS

Cysticercosis	Trichinosis
Schistosomiasis	Trypanosomiasis
Toxoplasmosis	Visceral larva migrans

RICKETTSIAL INFECTIONS

Rocky Mountain spotted fever	Scrub typhus
Q fever	Typhus

VIRAL INFECTIONS

Adenovirus	*Mycoplasma pneumoniae*
Arbovirus	Poliomyelitis
Coxsackievirus	Psittacosis
Cytomegalovirus	Respiratory syncytial virus
Echovirus	Rabies
Encephalomyocarditis virus	Rubella
Hepatitis	Rubeola
Human immunodeficiency virus	Vaccina
Infectious mononucleosis	Varicella
Influenza	Variola
Mumps	Yellow fever

Adapted from Marboe, C. C., and Fenoglio, J. J.: Pathology and natural history of human myocarditis. Pathol. Immunopathol. Res. 7:226, 1988.

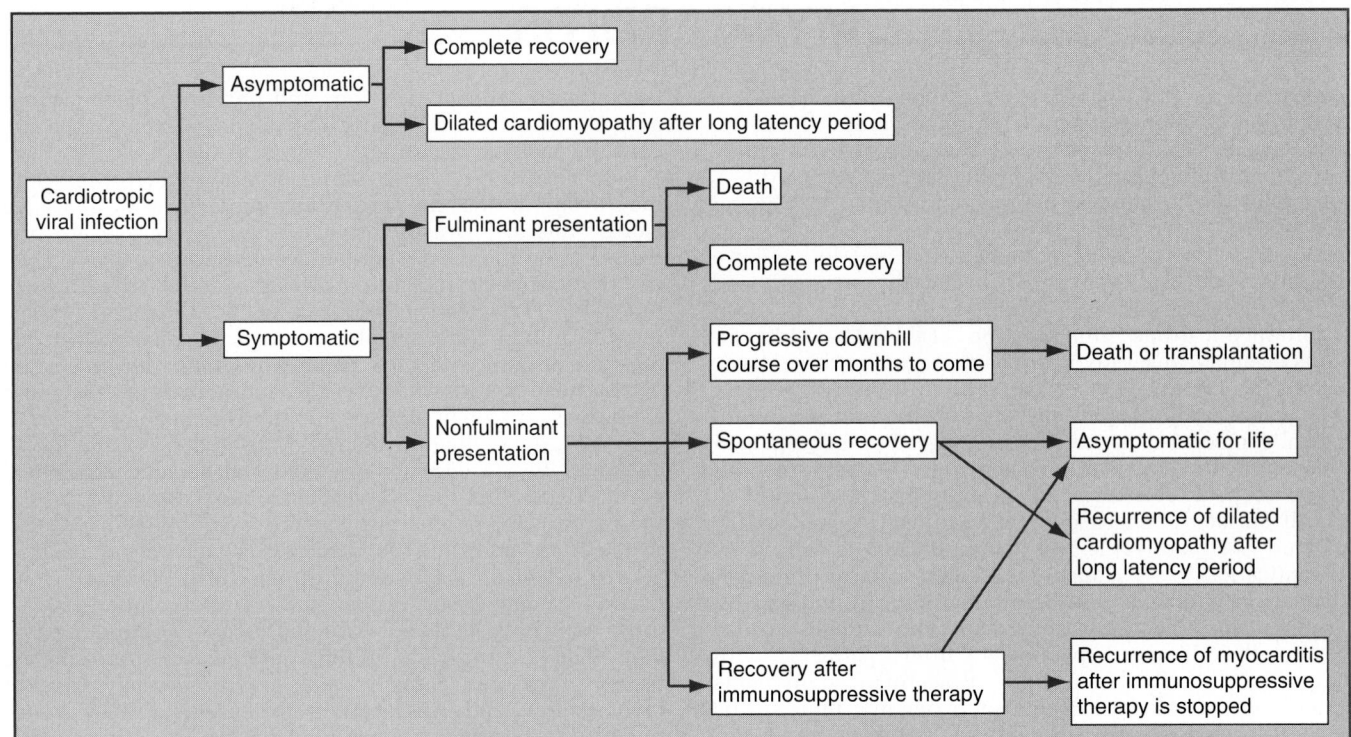

FIGURE 41–25. The natural history of human myocarditis. Most patients with mild symptoms of acute myocarditis are not seen by cardiologists and most of these patients appear to recover fully. Of the patients with symptomatic heart disease typically seen by cardiologists, a small number have fulminant presentations and either die in the acute stage or appear to recover fully. Of the remaining patients with myocarditis, a few are characterized by a progressive downhill course over a period of months to years that ends in death from heart failure or intractable arrhythmias. Some spontaneously recover and remain asymptomatic for life, and others have an asymptomatic period followed by development of dilated cardiomyopathy. (From Herskowitz, A., and Ansari, A. A.: Myocarditis. *In* Abelmann, W. H., and Braunwald, E. [eds.]: Cardiomyopathies, Myocarditis, and Pericardial Disease. Atlas of Heart Diseases. Vol. 2. Philadelphia, Current Medicine, 1995.)

is associated with nonspecific symptoms, including fatigue, dyspnea, palpitations, and precordial discomfort.[119,488] Chest pain usually reflects associated pericarditis, but precordial discomfort suggestive of myocardial ischemia is occasionally observed.[119] In some cases, the clinical presentation (with chest pain, electrocardiographic abnormalities, increased muscle enzyme levels, and regional wall motion abnormalities) may simulate an acute myocardial infarction.[507,508]

Physical Examination. Tachycardia is usual and may be out of proportion to the temperature elevation.[488] The first heart sound is often muffled, and a protodiastolic gallop may be present. A transient apical systolic murmur may appear,[488] but diastolic murmurs are rare. Clinical evidence of congestive heart failure occurs only in the more severe cases.[488] The heart is usually normal in size in the clinically silent cases, but it may be dilated in patients with congestive heart failure. Pulmonary and systemic emboli may occur.

Laboratory Findings. *Electrocardiographic* abnormalities are usually transient and occur far more frequently than does clinical myocardial involvement. The most common changes are abnormalities of the ST segment and T wave, but atrial and in particular ventricular arrhythmias, AV and intraventricular conduction defects, and, rarely, Q waves may be seen.[488] Complete AV block is usually transient and resolves without sequelae, but it is occasionally a cause of sudden death in patients with myocarditis.[509] Intraventricular conduction abnormalities are associated with more severe myocardial damage and a worse prognosis.[509,510] On *radiological examination,* heart size may range from normal to markedly enlarged, and pulmonary congestion may be present in patients with fulminant disease.[488] *Echocardiography* demonstrates some degree of left ventric-

ular dysfunction (surprisingly often regional in nature) in many patients with clinical myocarditis, although wall motion may be normal. Often findings may include increased wall thickness, left ventricular thrombi, and abnormal diastolic filling despite normal systolic function.[511] *Radionuclide scanning* after the administration of gallium-67, indium-111 antimyosin antibody, or technetium-99m pyrophosphate may identify inflammatory and necrotic changes characteristic of myocarditis, as may nuclear MRI.[119,488,512–514]

DIAGNOSIS. This is often predicated on the identification of the associated systemic illness and its characteristic features.[16] The diagnosis of viral myocarditis is supported by the identification of the virus in stool, throat washings, blood, myocardium, or pericardial fluid, or by a distinct (usually fourfold) increase in virus-neutralizing antibody, complement-fixation, or hemagglutination inhibition titers, but cultures usually are negative and serological tests nondiagnostic.[490,498] Even in fatal cases, isolation of virus from the myocardium at necropsy is unusual.[488,515] *Endomyocardial biopsy* frequently is used to confirm the diagnosis of myocarditis (Fig. 41–2).[16] A borderline or negative biopsy does not exclude the diagnosis,[516,517] and, if clinically indicated, a repeat biopsy may be appropriate and diagnostic.[518] Molecular biological techniques (using tissue obtained by endomyocardial biopsy) offer promise as a way of rapidly and confidently diagnosing acute myocarditis.[20]

PATHOLOGY. Patients with myocarditis demonstrate a wide spectrum of gross and histological changes, reflecting the range of disease seen clinically. Grossly, the hearts in acute cases are flabby, with focal hemorrhages; in chronic cases, the heart is enlarged and hypertrophied.[500] The histological hallmark of myocarditis is an inflammatory myocardial infiltrate, with associated evidence of myocyte damage (Fig. 41-2).[488,500] The inflammatory infiltrate may be composed of a variety of cell types, including polymorphonuclear cells, lymphocytes, macrophages, plasma cells, eosinophils, and/or giant cells.[500] In bacterial myocarditis, polymorphonuclear cells predominate; in viral infections, lymphocytes predominate; and in hypersensitivity myocarditis, eosinophils are seen in abundance.[500] Routine histological examination of the heart rarely provides a specific diagnosis, although in some instances electron microscopic and immunofluorescent techniques may allow elucidation of a specific cause.

MANAGEMENT. Therapy is often supportive and is usually directed at the more prominent systemic manifestations of the disease.[488] The demonstration of a particular predilection for involvement of the AV conducting system in some forms of myocarditis suggests that patients with suspected myocarditis should be observed closely for any evidence of conduction abnormality. Bed rest (or at least restricted activity) is advisable[488,505] because exercise in experimental animals with myocarditis is deleterious.[490,500] Because myocarditis often occurs in young adults, it is important to limit their athletic activities; it is recommended that athletes abstain from sports for a 6-month convalescent period, and until heart size and function have returned to normal.[205] Congestive heart failure responds to routine management,[488] including digitalization and diuresis, although patients with myocarditis appear to be particularly sensitive to digitalis, and toxicity should be watched for. Significant symptomatic arrhythmias should be treated with antiarrhythmic agents, although beta-adrenoceptor blockers are probably best avoided in view of their negative inotropic action[519]; participation in athletic and sporting activities should be proscribed until arrhythmias have resolved.[205]

The use of corticosteroids is controversial.[491,520-522] Although these agents were previously thought to be proscribed in acute viral myocarditis (because increased tissue necrosis and viral replication have been demonstrated following their use in experimental myocarditis), their use in a small number of patients has not been associated with similar dire short-term consequences.[500,501] A randomized trial of immunosuppression in myocarditis found no improvement in left ventricular ejection fraction or survival.[522a] Nonsteroidal anti-inflammatory agents—indomethacin, salicylates, and ibuprofen,[523] along with cyclosporine[524,525]—are contraindicated during the acute phase of viral myocarditis (the first 2 weeks) because they increase myocardial damage.[488,491,505] On the other hand, nonsteroidal anti-inflammatory agents appear to be safe in the late phase of myocarditis.[523] At least in children, high-dose intravenous gamma globulin appears to be associated with more rapid resolution of left ventricular dysfunction, and perhaps improved survival.[526] In experimental models of myocarditis, the converting enzyme inhibitor captopril has beneficial effects in the acute phase of myocarditis; human data are not yet available.[527,528]

It is hoped that effective antiviral agents,[522,529] immunosuppressive agents,[490] or antilymphocyte monoclonal antibodies for treating viral myocarditis will be available soon for clinical use.[488,505,530] It may also be possible, in the future, to treat patients with myocarditis with agents that stimulate production of interferon because this substance affords protection against the effects of viral myocarditis, at least in experimental animals.[490,531] Antibiotics may also be employed with benefit in infections caused by atypical pneumonia and psittacosis.

VIRAL MYOCARDITIS

Approximately two dozen viruses may be associated with clinical evidence of myocarditis (Table 41-14).[500] The myocarditis characteristically develops after a lag period of several weeks following the initial systemic infection, suggesting involvement of an immunological mechanism. In animals, a variety of factors appears to enhance susceptibility to myocardial damage, including radiation, malnutrition, steroids, exercise, and previous myocardial injury. Viral myocarditis may be particularly virulent in infants[498] and in pregnant women.

COXSACKIEVIRUS. Both Coxsackie viruses A and B may produce myocarditis, although infection with Coxsackie B is more common; this agent is the most frequent cause of viral myocarditis, causing more than half the cases.[490,532-534] The myocardium appears to be particularly susceptible to the effects of this virus because of the apparent affinity of myocardial membrane receptors for the viral particles. Necropsy often demonstrates a pericardial effusion, pericarditis, cardiac enlargement, and a predominantly mononuclear inflammatory infiltrate, with necrosis of the atrial and ventricular myocardium. In some cases, focal myocardial necrosis simulating myocardial infarction is seen, despite normal coronary arteries.[535]

Although most infections are benign, self-limited, and subclinical, Coxsackie myocarditis appears to be particularly virulent in the neonate and child.[502,536] In most infections in adults, the other clinical manifestations of viral involvement, such as pleurodynia, myalgia, upper respiratory tract symptoms, and arthralgias, predominate.[532] Severe cases in the adult are characterized by myopericardial involvement with pleuritic or pericarditic chest pain, palpitations, and fever. Many patients with overt myocardial involvement develop congestive heart failure with cardiomegaly and pulmonary edema.[502,536]

The *electrocardiogram* is virtually always abnormal, with ST-segment and T-wave abnormalities and arrhythmias, often ventricular in origin; AV conduction disturbances are common.[536,537] Blood levels of myocardial enzymes (serum transaminases, creatine kinase) may be normal or elevated, reflecting the absence or presence of variable degrees of clinically detectable myocardial necrosis.[502] *Echocardiography* may reveal diffuse and regional left ventricular wall motion abnormalities that usually improve or disappear over time.[533,538]

Most patients recover completely within weeks,[502] although the electrocardiogram and ventricular function may require months to return to normal. Rarely, Coxsackie myocarditis is fatal in adults.[537] Some patients become symptomatic following resolution of the infection, and they may present years later with dilated cardiomyopathy.[533]

Treatment is symptomatic, and despite occasional postmortem evidence of intracardiac thrombi, anticoagulation should probably be avoided because of the risk of a hemorrhagic pericardial effusion. Bed rest is indicated during the acute course of myocarditis, but no convincing evidence exists that a period of prolonged rest after apparent resolution of the acute process is useful. Heart failure and cardiac arrhythmias are treated in the usual fashion.

CYTOMEGALOVIRUS. Unrecognized infection with cytomegalovirus (CMV) is extremely common in childhood, and the majority of the adult population have antibodies to CMV.[539] Primary infection after the age of 35 years is uncommon, and generalized infection usually occurs only in immunosuppressed patients with neoplastic disease, after transplantation, and with HIV infection.[540-542] The cardiovascular manifestations in adults are generally limited to asymptomatic and transient electrocardiographic abnormalities. Symptomatic cardiac involvement is rare, although a hemorrhagic pericardial effusion or myocarditis with left ventricular dysfunction and attendant congestive heart failure may occur.[541-543] The diagnosis of CMV myocarditis may be suggested by the presence of viral inclusions in myocardial biopsy specimens and confirmed by the detection of viral DNA in the myocardium.[540,544] Although fatalities are unusual, when they do occur, histological examination of the heart may reveal focal lymphocytic infiltration and fibrosis.

DENGUE. Although previous dengue epidemics often were associated with symptomatic cardiac involvement, more recent outbreaks have been associated with fewer apparent cardiac complications.[545] Nonspecific electrocardiographic repolarization abnormalities are common but typically benign and transient.[545,546] Transient ventricular arrhythmias may be seen on occasion.

HEPATITIS. Clinical cardiac involvement in hepatitis is rare; an occasional patient may develop fulminant myocarditis with congestive heart failure, hypotension, and death.[547,548] The characteristic *pathological changes* in the myocardium associated with viral hepatitis are minute foci of necrosis of isolated muscle bundles, often surrounded by lymphocytes and a diffuse serous inflammation.[548] The ventricles may be dilated, with petechial hemorrhages. Hemorrhage into the myocardium may be a conspicuous finding.[548] Myocardial damage may be produced indirectly through an immune-mediated mechanism or directly by viral invasion of the heart.[548]

Symptomatic myocarditis is generally observed in the first to third week of illness. Patients may have dyspnea, palpitations, and anginal chest pain; fatalities have been reported.[548,549] *Electrocardiographic changes*, including bradycardia, ventricular premature beats, and ST-segment and T-wave abnormalities, may be seen during the course of hepatitis.[548] These abnormalities are usually transient and asymptomatic, although congestive heart failure, cardiomegaly, and sudden death have been reported.[547,548]

Heart involvement in the acquired immunodeficiency syndrome (AIDS) may consist of metastatic involvement from Kaposi's sarcoma, a wide variety of infective and nonspecific forms of myocarditis, pericarditis with or without an effusion, endocarditis (especially nonbacterial thrombotic endocarditis), and dilated cardiomyopathy (Table 41–15).[550-552] Cardiac involvement occurs in about one-quarter to one-half of patients (on the basis of echocardiographic, endomyocardial biopsy, and autopsy findings) (Fig. 41–26 and 41–27)[552-554]; however, it leads to clinically apparent heart disease in only approximately 10 per cent.[555-560] When there are clinical manifestations, congestive heart failure is the most common finding and is due to left ventricular dilatation and dysfunction, simulating a dilated cardiomyopathy.[86,550] Because of the frequency of opportunistic pulmonary infections, dyspnea may be attributed incorrectly to lung disease rather than congestive heart failure; echocardiography may be useful in identifying left ventricular dysfunction as the cause of the dyspnea.[550,551] Particular surveillance for cardiac toxoplasmosis in HIV infection should be maintained, as it may be the precipitant for symptomatic congestive heart failure and is potentially treatable.[561] Other common clinical and echocardiographic

TABLE 41–15   CARDIAC LESIONS IN AIDS

MYOCARDITIS
  Opportunistic infections
    Pneumocystis carinii
    Mycobacterium tuberculosis
    Mycobacterium avium-intracellulare
    Cryptococcus neoformans
    Aspergillus fumigatus
    Candida albicans
    Histoplasma capsulatum
    Coccidioides immitis
    Toxoplasma gondii
    Herpes simplex
  Viral agents
    Cytomegalovirus
    Human immunodeficiency virus (HIV)
    Herpes simplex
  Lymphocytic myocarditis
  Noninflammatory myocardial necrosis
    Microvascular spasm?

ENDOCARDITIS
  Marantic endocarditis (nonbacterial thrombotic endocarditis)
  Bacterial endocarditis
  Aspergillus endocarditis

PERICARDITIS
  Infectious
    Tuberculous
    Herpes simplex
    Histoplasmosis
    Cryptococcus
  Noninfectious
  Pericardial effusion

CARDIOMEGALY
  Right ventricular hypertrophy or dilation
  Biventricular dilation (dilated cardiomyopathy)

VASCULAR LESIONS
  Arteriopathy
  Myocardial infarction

MALIGNANCY
  Kaposi's sarcoma
  Malignant lymphoma

TOXIC LESIONS
  Drug-induced
    Drugs used in combating opportunistic infections
    Anti-HIV drugs

Modified from Acierno, L. J.: Cardiac complications in acquired immunodeficiency syndrome (AIDS): A review. Reprinted by permission of the American College of Cardiology. J. Am. Coll. Cardiol. *13*:1144, 1989.

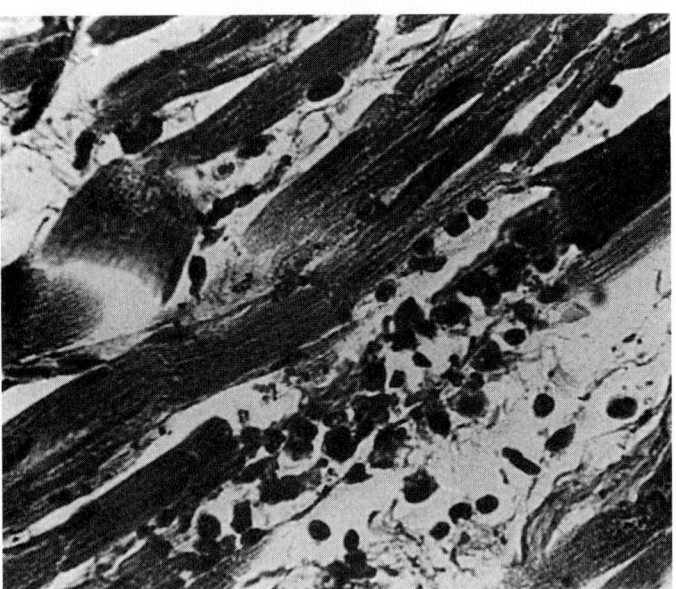

FIGURE 41–26. Example of lymphocytic myocarditis showing myocyte necrosis in AIDS patient (× 400, reduced by 5 per cent). (From Baroldi, G., Corallo, S., Moroni, M., et al.: Focal lymphocytic myocarditis in acquired immunodeficiency syndrome (AIDS): A correlative morphologic and clinical study in 26 consecutive fatal cases. Reprinted by permission from the American College of Cardiology. J. Am. Coll. Cardiol. *12*:463, 1988.)

findings that result in symptoms in a minority of patients include pericardial effusion (usually but not invariably without cardiac tamponade), ventricular arrhythmias, repolarization changes on the electrocardiogram, marantic endocarditis, and right ventricular dilatation and hypertrophy.[551,552,555,559,560]

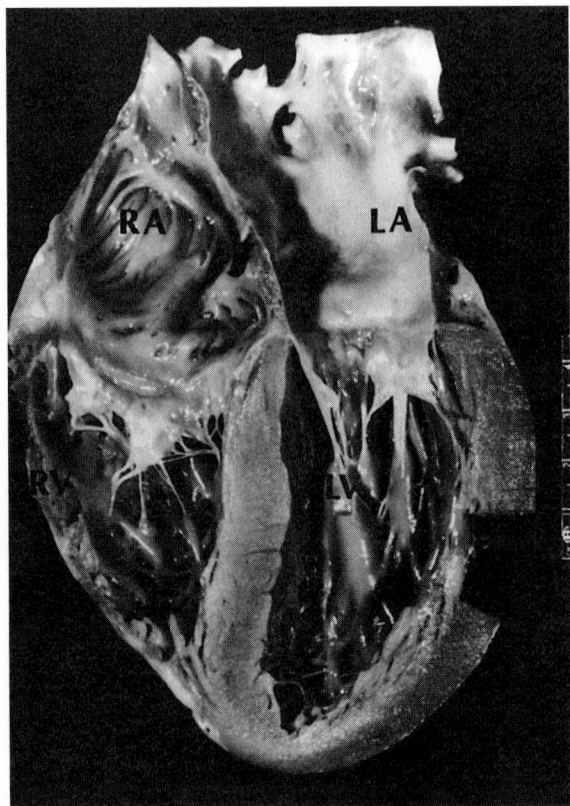

FIGURE 41–27. Marked dilatation of all four chambers of the heart in a patient with AIDS. LA = Left atrium, RA = right atrium. (Reproduced by permission from Cohen, I. S., Anderson, D. W., Virmani, R., et al.: Congestive cardiomyopathy in association with the acquired immunodeficiency syndrome. N. Engl. J. Med. *315*:628, 1986. Copyright Massachusetts Medical Society.)

The cause of myocardial damage in HIV infection is not clearly established and likely is multifactorial.[562] Although some of the cardiac effects are due to the commonly associated opportunistic infections, damage as a consequence of the HIV virus itself and/or through activation of the immune system is thought to be likely.[550,555,556,563,564] Whether agents used to treat AIDS (such as zidovudine [AZT]) may be cardiotoxic themselves has not been resolved.[564a]

Pathological cardiac findings in AIDS patients are common, with myocarditis the most frequent.[552] Although opportunistic infections caused by a wide variety of viral, fungal (Fig. 41–28, p. 1441), parasitic, and bacterial pathogens account for some cases of myocarditis, most are unexplained but are suspected to be related to the HIV itself.[552,556,565] Isolation of HIV from the myocardium has added further credence to this speculation.[556] It has been speculated that the HIV-related myocarditis may result in the dilated cardiomyopathy found in some patients.[550] Other important postmortem findings include pericardial effusions, right and/or left ventricular dilatation, and nonbacterial thrombotic endocarditis.[552,555]

Treatment of AIDS-associated heart disease may afford some degree of symptomatic improvement.[552,566] Relief of cardiac tamponade, therapy for infective myocarditis, and treatment of congestive heart failure have resulted in at least short-term palliation.[552,567]

INFECTIOUS MONONUCLEOSIS. Evident cardiac involvement in infectious mononucleosis is extremely rare, although nonspecific ST-segment and T-wave abnormalities may be seen. In rare cases, pericarditis and myocarditis (even simulating a myocardial infarction) may be present.[568]

INFLUENZA. Although clinically apparent myocarditis is rare in influenza, the presence of preexisting cardiovascular disease greatly increases the risk of morbidity and mortality.[569] During epidemics, 5 to 10 per cent of infected patients may experience cardiac symptoms.[16] Postmortem findings in fatal cases include biventricular dilatation,[522] with evidence of a mononuclear infiltrate,[570] especially in perivascular areas.

Cardiac involvement typically occurs within 1 to 2 weeks of the onset of the illness and may be severe, sometimes contributing to mortality.[522] The *clinical manifestations* include dyspnea, palpitations, anginal chest pain, arrhythmia, and heart failure; there may be concomitant involvement of the pericardium.[522] Sinus tachycardia or, less commonly, sinus bradycardia may be seen. The *electrocardiogram* may show transient ST-segment and T-wave abnormalities, conduction defects, and even complete AV block; death may be associated with massive hemorrhagic pulmonary edema due to viral or bacterial involvement of the lungs.[571]

LASSA FEVER. Lassa fever, a major cause of death in West Africa that is caused by an arenavirus, often is associated with electrocardiographic abnormalities[572] that may represent subclinical myocardial involvement. More than half the patients demonstrate nonspecific repolarization changes and low voltage.[572] Pericardial involvement may occur.[573] *Pathological findings* include myocardial congestion, edema, and a mononuclear cellular infiltrate. In most cases, however, the putative cardiac involvement does not appear to play a major clinical role.[572]

MUMPS. Myocardial involvement during the course of mumps is rarely recognized.[574,575] The hearts of only a few patients with mumps have come to postmortem examination, and they have been found to be both dilated and hypertrophied. Histologically, there is diffuse interstitial fibrosis, with infiltration of mononuclear cells and areas of focal necrosis.[574]

Cardiac involvement is usually unrecognized clinically, and the diagnosis of myocarditis is based on nonspecific electrocardiographic changes.[574] Transient ST-segment and T-wave abnormalities are most common, but extrasystoles and atrioventricular conduction block may occur.[574–576] Tachycardia, a transient apical systolic murmur, and protodiastolic gallop may be present.[574–576]

POLIOMYELITIS. Myocarditis occurs about 5 to 10 per cent of the time during epidemics and is a frequent finding in fatal cases of poliomyelitis, occurring in half or more of all patients dying with this disease; death may be sudden.[16] Although myocardial involvement is usually focal and minimal in extent, some patients with bulbar disease succumb early in the course of the illness, often with cardiovascular collapse.[577,578] These patients all have viral infection of the medulla and severe systemic vasoconstriction that leads to pulmonary edema. Myocarditis appears to contribute to the heart failure.[577] The *electrocardiogram* is frequently abnormal, with ST-segment and T-wave abnormalities, prolongation of the P-R and Q-T intervals,[579] premature contractions, tachycardia, and atrial fibrillation. *Treatment* is symptomatic, with aggressive support of pulmonary function; tracheostomy and prolonged mechanical ventilatory support may be required. Fortunately, this disease has been largely eliminated by immunization.

RESPIRATORY SYNCYTIAL VIRUS. Although respiratory syncytial virus is an important cause of respiratory disease, particularly in children, it rarely results in cardiac involvement.[580] Congestive heart failure and complete heart block have been seen on occasion.[581]

RUBELLA AND RUBEOLA. Congenital cardiovascular lesions may develop in the offspring when *rubella* is contracted by the mother during the first trimester of pregnancy, with persistent ductus arteriosus and pulmonary artery maldevelopment as prominent anomalies.[498] Rare cases of postgestational myocarditis occur, with attendant conduction defects and heart failure.[582,583]

Overt myocarditis is quite rare in *rubeola*,[534] although transient electrocardiographic abnormalities, including prolongation of the P-R interval, ST-segment and T-wave changes, AV conduction abnormalities, and ventricular tachycardia, have been reported.[584] Congestive heart failure occurs on rare occasions, and its appearance is a poor prognostic sign, often indicating a fatal outcome.[585] Histological examination of the heart in fatal cases has revealed evidence of myocarditis characterized predominantly by a perivascular lymphocytic infiltrate.[584]

VARICELLA. Clinical myocarditis is a rare finding in varicella, although unsuspected myocarditis is common in fatal varicella.[586] Occasionally a patient may develop overt clinical evidence of myocarditis with congestive heart failure.[586–588] Histological findings include rare but characteristic intranuclear inclusion bodies within the myocardial cells, along with interstitial edema, cellular infiltrates, and myonecrosis.[587] The electrocardiogram may show conduction abnormalities, including complete heart block; sudden death occurs rarely.[589]

VARIOLA AND VACCINIA. Cardiac involvement following smallpox is rare, although several cases of myocarditis associated with acute cardiac failure and death have been reported. Myocarditis with pericardial effusion and congestive heart failure has also been observed as a complication of smallpox vaccination[590]; an immunological mechanism has been suggested, and dramatic responses to steroids have been reported. The histological changes include a mixed mononuclear infiltrate, with interstitial edema and occasional degenerating or necrotic muscle bundles.[591]

RICKETTSIAL MYOCARDITIS

The rickettsial diseases frequently are associated with evidence of myocardial involvement, but usually it is subclinical. Transient ST-segment and T-wave alterations in particular are observed commonly. The circulatory collapse that may accompany these diseases is largely a manifestation of abnormalities of the peripheral vascular bed, but a myocardial component may also be present. The basic histopathological process is a vasculitis, with a periarterial interstitial infiltrate.

Q FEVER. Endocarditis is the most common cardiac manifestation of infection with *R. burnettii* (Q fever).[592] Myocarditis is not a prominent feature,[593] although dyspnea and chest pain, perhaps reflecting associated pericarditis, occur frequently. The electrocardiogram may demonstrate transient ST-segment and T-wave changes as well as paroxysmal ventricular arrhythmias. Abnormalities of the immune system have been implicated in the pathogenesis of the disease.[594]

ROCKY MOUNTAIN SPOTTED FEVER. Clinical evidence of myocarditis is more common than often appreciated in Rocky Mountain spotted fever (caused by *R. rickettsii*), and the heart is often involved in the multisystem damage that occurs as the result of a widespread vasculitis.[595–597] Unsuspected left ventricular dysfunction is common, and echocardiographic evidence of dysfunction may persist in some patients.[595]

SCRUB TYPHUS. Myocarditis is common during the course of scrub typhus (tsutsugamushi disease, caused by *R. tsutsugamushi*), especially in fatal cases.[598,599] The histological findings are those of a focal panvasculitis involving the small blood vessels. Myocardial necrosis is unusual, but hemorrhage into the heart and subepicardial petechiae may occur.[599] Clinical evidence of myocardial involvement typically is not severe and is usually not associated with residual cardiac damage.[598] The electrocardiogram may show nonspecific ST-segment and T-wave abnormalities, as well as first-degree AV block.[599] A protodiastolic gallop and apical systolic murmur suggestive of mitral regurgitation are occasionally found.[598]

BACTERIAL MYOCARDITIS

BRUCELLOSIS. Cardiac involvement in the course of brucellosis is uncommon, usually consisting of endocarditis. Myocardial involvement, when it occurs, is manifested by T-wave abnormalities and prolongation of AV conduction.[600] An occasional patient develops fulminant myocarditis, with a lymphocytic and polymorphonuclear infiltrate.[600]

CLOSTRIDIA. Cardiac involvement is common in patients with clostridial infections with multiple organ involvement.[601] The myocardial damage results from the toxin elaborated by the bacteria, but the precise actions of the toxin remain to be elucidated.[602] The *pathological findings* are distinctive, with gas bubbles usually present in the myocardium. Areas of degenerated muscle fibers are apparent, but an inflammatory infiltrate is usually absent.[601] *C. perfringens* may cause myocardial abscess formation, with myocardial perforation and resultant purulent pericarditis.[603]

DIPHTHERIA. Myocardial involvement is one of the more serious complications of diphtheria and occurs in up to one-quarter of cases.[604,605] Indeed, myocardial involvement is the most common cause of death in this infection, and half of the fatal cases demonstrate cardiac involvement.[605] Cardiac damage is due to the liberation by the diphtheria bacillus of a toxin that inhibits protein synthesis by interfering with the transfer of amino acids from soluble RNA to polypeptide chains under construction. The toxin has a particular affinity for the cardiac conducting system.[604]

Pathological findings include a flabby and dilated heart with a myocardium that has a "streaky" appearance. Microscopic examination reveals characteristic fatty infiltration of the myocytes,[605] often with an interstitial inflammatory infiltrate, myocytolysis, and hyaline necrosis of muscle fibers. With time, fibrosis and hypertrophy of the remaining myocardial cells develop. The conduction system is often involved.

Clinical signs of cardiac dysfunction typically appear at the end of the first week of the illness. Cardiomegaly and severe congestive heart failure are often present. A protodiastolic gallop and pulmonary congestion may be prominent features. Elevation of the serum transaminase levels may be seen; a high level is associated with a poor prognosis. Sudden circulatory failure and death may occur. Many patients develop ST-segment and T-wave abnormalities, but atrial and ventricular arrhythmias and conduction defects may also occur.[605] Persistently abnormal electrocardiograms are common following diphtheritic myocarditis, as are cardiomegaly and symptoms of reduced cardiac reserve. Some patients recover fully.

Because of the serious effects of the toxin on the myocardium, antitoxin should be administered as rapidly as possible.[605] Antibiotic therapy is of less urgency. Overt congestive heart failure may be resistant to therapy with cardiac glycosides. The development of complete AV block is an ominous complication, and mortality is high despite insertion of a transvenous pacemaker.[604]

LEGIONNAIRES' DISEASE. Although pneumonia, rhabdomyolysis, renal failure, and hepatic as well as central nervous system involvement are common with *Legionella pneumophila*, overt cardiac involvement is not.[606] Occasional electrocardiographic changes may be noted, consisting primarily of ST-segment and T-wave abnormalities; ventricular arrhythmias may be seen. Rarely, pericardial effusion, myocarditis with evidence of myocardial necrosis, or congestive heart failure may be seen.[606,607]

MENINGOCOCCUS. Myocardial involvement is common during the course of fatal meningococcal infections but is less commonly recognized in the usual case.[608,609] *Pathological* findings include hemorrhagic myocardial lesions, occasionally associated with intracellular organisms.[608] An interstitial myocarditis composed of lymphocytes, plasma cells, and polymorphonuclear leukocytes may be observed, occasionally with myonecrosis.[608]

Meningococcal myocarditis may result in congestive heart failure as well as in pericardial effusion with tamponade.[609] Death may occur suddenly and be associated with involvement of the atrioventricular node.[608]

MYCOPLASMA PNEUMONIAE. Electrocardiographic abnormalities are common during the course of atypical pneumonia, although clinically apparent myocarditis is not.[534] When carditis occurs, it may be serious, and, rarely, fatal.[610] Nonspecific ST-segment and T-wave abnormalities are the most common manifestations of cardiac involvement; a rare patient may develop complete heart block.[610] The electrocardiographic findings usually resolve within 1 to 2 weeks. A cell-mediated autoimmune myocarditis has been postulated as the cause of the changes.[534] Pericarditis may be a prominent finding, and congestive heart failure is occasionally seen.[611] A protodiastolic gallop[612] and pericardial friction rub may be noted in occasional cases. Complete recovery is the rule in most patients,[612] although occasional patients may have persistent sequelae, including arrhythmias.[611]

PSITTACOSIS. Myocarditis complicating psittacosis is a relatively common occurrence and is characterized by congestive heart failure and acute pericarditis.[613,614] *Pathological changes* include fibrinous pericarditis as well as endocarditis and myocarditis. Fever, chest pain, electrocardiographic changes, cardiomegaly, systemic emboli, tachycardia, and hypotension may occur. Although most patients recover completely, fatalities have been reported.[613] The systemic infection may be treated effectively with tetracycline, but the effect of the antibiotic on the myocardium is unknown.

SALMONELLA. Symptomatic myocardial involvement during salmonella infections is rare,[615–617] although electrocardiographic abnormalities are often seen, suggesting subclinical myocarditis.[618] Other cardiovascular complications include infected mural thrombi, occasionally resulting in pulmonary and systemic emboli, and mycotic aneurysms.[619] Myocardial abscesses may rupture, producing fatal cardiac tamponade. Myocarditis with congestive heart failure occurs most commonly in children who are severely ill with salmonellosis, and it is associated with a high mortality.[620] When myocarditis occurs, it often develops rapidly, with evidence of biventricular failure, tachycardia, a protodiastolic gallop, an apical systolic murmur of mitral regurgitation, and peripheral edema.[620]

Electrocardiographic abnormalities include ST-segment and T-wave changes, prolonged P-R or Q-T intervals, and low QRS voltage.[618,621]

STREPTOCOCCUS. The most commonly detected cardiac finding following beta-hemolytic streptococcal infection is acute rheumatic fever, which is discussed in detail in Chapter 55.

Involvement of the heart by the streptococcus may produce a myocarditis that is distinct from acute rheumatic carditis.[622,623] It is characterized by an interstitial infiltrate composed of mononuclear cells with occasional polymorphonuclear leukocytes[624]; the infiltrate may be focal or diffuse and may be localized to the subendocardial or perivascular region. There may be small areas of myocardial necrosis.[624] *Electrocardiographic abnormalities*, including prolongation of the P-R and Q-T intervals, occur frequently. Although these abnormalities are rarely associated with other clinical manifestations of myocardial involvement, sudden death, conduction disturbances, and arrhythmias may occur.[622,624]

TUBERCULOSIS. Tuberculous involvement of the myocardium (not as a complication of tuberculous pericarditis) is extremely rare, particularly since the introduction of drugs effective against tuberculosis.[625,626] Most cases of myocardial tuberculosis are clinically silent and are diagnosed only at autopsy.[625] Tuberculous involvement of the myocardium occurs via hematogenous or lymphatic spread, or directly from contiguous structures; it may lead to arrhythmias, including atrial fibrillation and ventricular tachycardia, complete atrioventricular block, congestive heart failure, left ventricular aneurysms, and sudden death.[625–627]

WHIPPLE DISEASE

Intestinal lipodystrophy, or Whipple disease, may be associated with myocardial involvement, and PAS-positive macrophages may be found in the myocardium, pericardium, and heart valves of patients with this disorder.[628,629] Coronary artery lesions, with smooth muscle necrosis, panarteritis, and medial scarring, are not rare.[630] Electron microscopy has demonstrated rod-shaped structures in the myocardium similar to those found in the small intestine, and it has been suggested that they are the causative agent of the myocardial abnormalities. There may be an associated inflammatory infiltrate and foci of fibrosis.[628] The valvular fibrosis may be severe enough to result in aortic regurgitation and mitral stenosis.[630] Although asymptomatic, nonspecific electrocardiographic changes are most common; systolic murmurs, pericarditis, and even overt congestive heart failure may occur.[629] Antibiotic therapy appears to be effective in treating the basic disease; however, relapses can occur, often more than 2 years after initial diagnosis.[631,632]

SPIROCHETAL INFECTIONS

LEPTOSPIROSIS (WEIL DISEASE). Most patients with leptospiral infections have mild or subclinical disease and little evidence of heart involvement. Cardiac involvement in severe or fatal leptospirosis is common, however, with 50 to 100 per cent of fatal cases demonstrating evidence of myocarditis.[633] Many patients with severe systemic disease demonstrate first-degree heart block and transient ST-segment and T-wave abnormalities, presumably reflecting myocarditis.[633,634] Bradycardia despite fever, ventricular premature depolarizations, congestive heart failure, and pericarditis may be seen as well.[633,634] The *pathological findings* in the occasional fatal case include petechiae or large foci of hemorrhage (often located in the epicardium), an interstitial myocardial infiltration (often subendocardial in location), aortitis, and coronary arteritis.[633]

LYME CARDITIS. Lyme disease is caused by a tickborne spirochete *(Borrelia burgdorferi)*.[635] It usually begins during the summer months with a characteristic skin rash (erythema chronicum migrans), followed in weeks to months by neurologic, joint, or cardiac involvement; some clinical manifestations may persist for years.[636]

About 10 per cent of patients with Lyme disease develop evidence of transient cardiac involvement, the most common manifestation being variable degrees of AV block.[636–639] The location of the block appears to be at the level of the AV node.[635] Syncope due to complete heart block is frequent with cardiac involvement because often there is an associated depression of ventricular escape rhythms.[635,640] Ventricular tachycardia occurs uncommonly.[638] Diffuse ST-segment and T-wave abnormalities and transient, usually asymptomatic, left ventricular dysfunction may be found in some patients, although cardiomegaly or symptoms of congestive heart failure are rare.[639,641] A positive gallium or indium antimyosin antibody scan may point to suspected cardiac involvement in this disease.[635,642,643] The demonstration of spirochetes in myocardial biopsies of some patients with Lyme carditis suggests that the cardiac manifestations are due to a direct toxic effect, although there is speculation that immune-mediated mechanisms may be involved as well.[635]

The value of specific therapy in Lyme carditis remains uncertain,[644] and even without therapy the disease usually is self-limited with complete recovery the rule; nevertheless, it is thought that treating the early manifestations of the disease may prevent development of late complications.[645] Patients with second-degree or complete heart block should be hospitalized and undergo continuous electrocardiographic monitoring.[644] Temporary transvenous pacing may be required for up to a week or longer in patients with high-grade block.[635] Although the efficacy of antibiotics is not established, they are utilized routinely in Lyme carditis. Intravenous antibiotics (ceftriaxone, 2 gm, or penicillin G, 20 million units daily for 14 days) are suggested, although oral antibiotics (doxycycline, 100 mg twice daily, or amoxicillin, 500 mg three times daily for 14 to 21 days) may be used when there is only mild cardiac involvement (first-degree AV block of less than 40 msec duration).[645] Whether anti-inflammatory agents (salicylates, corticosteroids) can ameliorate heart block is not clear.[640]

RELAPSING FEVER. Many infections are currently observed in Ethiopia. During pandemics, mortality may be particularly high, reaching 70 per cent, although sporadic cases are often more benign.[646] Cardiac involvement is said to be a common complication and is often implicated as a cause of death, although one report involving 63 children did not find evidence of cardiac involvement.[647] AV conduction defects occur frequently and may be responsible for sudden death, although tachyarrhythmias have also been implicated.[646] Numerous petechiae are observed with a diffuse histiocytic interstitial infiltrate, particularly around small arterioles in the left ventricle.

SYPHILIS. Aortitis is the most common manifestation of luetic involvement of the cardiovascular system.[648] Aortic regurgitation and coronary ostial narrowing are associated findings. Syphilitic involvement of the myocardium itself in the form of gumma formation is uncommon and usually unsuspected clinically.[648] Involvement of the base of the interventricular septum may result in damage to the conduction system and AV block.[648] In one case a ruptured left ventricular aneurysm was found as a result of syphilitic endarteritis.[649]

FUNGAL INFECTIONS OF THE HEART

Cardiac fungal infections occur most frequently in patients with malignant disease and/or those receiving chemotherapy, steroids, radiation, or immunosuppressive therapy. Cardiac surgery, intravenous drug abuse, and infection with HIV are also predisposing factors for fungal cardiac involvement.

ACTINOMYCOSIS. Myocarditis is a rare complication of actinomycotic infection, occurring in less than 2 per cent of patients.[650] However, cardiac involvement is quite serious when it does occur. Involvement of the heart most commonly is the result of direct extension of disease within the thorax.[650,651] Initially the pericardium is invaded, with eventual obliteration of the pericardial space. The myocardium may be involved by extension of the pericardial process. Myocardial seeding is less common.[650] The myocardial lesion is a suppurative, necrotizing abscess containing the organism, surrounded by granulation tissue. Both right- and left-sided failure are common manifestations. A pericardial rub may be heard, sometimes associated with clinical evidence of a pericardial effusion or constriction.[650,651]

ASPERGILLOSIS. Myocardial involvement is not uncommon in generalized aspergillosis, and when it occurs it is usually fatal.[652] It is being encountered increasingly in the immunocompromised patient.[653–655] On pathologic examination, myocardial necrosis and infarction caused by thrombosis of vessels that contain fungal mycelia are commonly seen, along with myocardial abscesses and pericardial involvement (Fig. 41–28).[654,656] The electrocardiogram may be normal in the face of significant myocardial damage, but T-wave changes may be present. The *diagnosis* of aspergillus infection is often diffi-

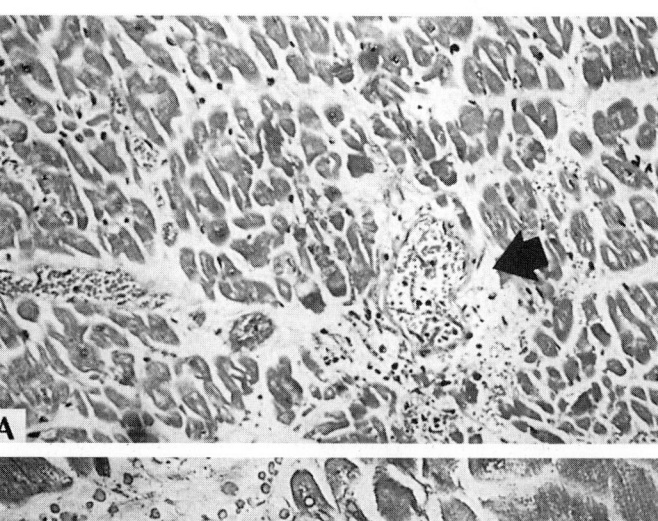

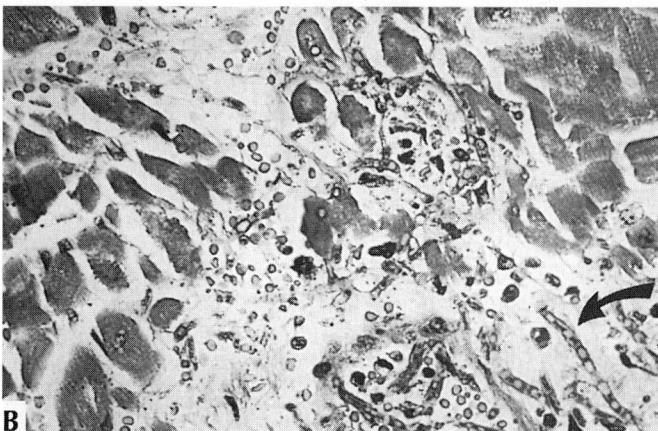

FIGURE 41–28. Aspergillus myocarditis in a patient with AIDS. *A,* Section of heart with blood vessel and mild inflammation (arrow) (×330). *B,* High-powered examination of this area reveals fungal hyphae invading through a blood vessel wall and into the myocardium (arrow) (×825). (Courtesy of G. K. Haines, Northwestern University, Chicago, IL.)

cult.[655] Identification of aspergillus through open lung biopsy, aspiration lung biopsy, transtracheal aspiration, or bronchial brush technique may be successful.[654,657] Treatment is difficult and usually unsuccessful.[654]

BLASTOMYCOSIS. Involvement of the heart by the fungus is quite uncommon, even in the immunocompromised heart. When involvement occurs, it is most often by direct extension from the pericardium.

CANDIDIASIS. Disseminated monilial infections are common opportunistic infections, particularly in the compromised host.[658] Endocarditis is the most frequent manifestation of cardiac involvement (see p. 1082), occurring most commonly in cardiac surgical patients or drug addicts, although multiple abscesses of the myocardium may occur as associated or independent findings.[659] Complete heart block may be caused by microabscesses of the conduction system.[658]

COCCIDIOIDOMYCOSIS. Involvement of the heart is rare in patients with generalized coccidioidomycosis.[660] The hearts may be grossly normal, although epicardial lesions with resultant pericarditis are common, and progression to constrictive pericarditis may occur (p. 1498). A nonspecific, focal interstitial, and perivascular cellular infiltrate with associated muscle fiber degeneration and interstitial edema is commonly found, although granulomas containing fungi are also seen sometimes.

CRYPTOCOCCOSIS. Cryptococcal infection of the myocardium occurs most commonly in immunocompromised patients with disseminated malignancy or HIV infection.[661] *Pathological examination* may show cardiac dilatation, with epithelial granulomas, giant cells, and an inflammatory infiltrate.[661] When congestive heart failure occurs, pulmonary congestion and muffled heart sounds may be found on physical examination, and cardiomegaly on the chest roentgenogram.[661] The *electrocardiogram* may show first-degree AV block and T-wave inversions; ventricular arrhythmias have been observed.

HISTOPLASMOSIS. Cardiac involvement in histoplasmosis is rare and usually is related to mediastinal fibrosis, the most serious complication of histoplasmosis.[662,663] Pericarditis with effusion may occur (see p. 1510), and superior vena caval obstruction has been observed.[663]

Myocardial involvement is uncommon, although atrial arrhythmias and T-wave abnormalities have been reported.

MUCORMYCOSIS. Cardiac involvement in the setting of disseminated mucormycosis occurs in about 20 per cent of patients and is characterized by fungal invasion of the coronary arteries with resultant areas of myocardial infarction.[664] Valvular and pericardial involvement may be seen as well. Clinical manifestations are nonspecific, and cardiac involvement often is not suspected but may include congestive heart failure, arrhythmias, conduction defects, and endocarditis.[664]

PROTOZOAL MYOCARDITIS

Trypanosomiasis (Chagas' Disease)

Chagas' disease is caused by the protozoan *Trypanosoma cruzi.* The major cardiovascular manifestation is an extensive myocarditis that typically becomes evident years after the initial infection. The disease is prevalent in Central and South America, particularly in Brazil, Argentina, and Chile, where it is a major public health problem (Fig. 41–29). Upwards of 20 million people are thought to be infected with the parasite, and an estimated 100 million are at risk of infection.[499,665,666] In rare cases, the disease may be found in nonendemic areas as a consequence of transfusion with contaminated blood products[667]; somewhat more common is that patients with the disease emigrate to nonendemic areas.[499]

The natural history of Chagas' disease is characterized by three phases: acute, latent, and chronic. During the *acute phase,* the disease is transmitted to humans (usually below the age of 20 years)[668,669] through the bite of a reduviid bug (subfamily Triatominae), which harbors the parasite in its gastrointestinal tract.[670] This insect acquires the disease from feeding on infected animals, including the armadillo, raccoon, opossum, and skunk as well as domestic dogs and cats. The reduviid bug, popularly known in Argentina as "vinchuca," meaning "to let oneself drop," lives in the walls and roofs of houses and, during nocturnal feedings, drops from the ceiling onto the sleeping person below. The

bug then often bites the person around the eyes, and infection of the human host occurs when the trypanosomes in the animal's feces gain entry through abraded skin or through the conjunctivae. Occasionally, this results in unilateral periorbital edema and swelling of the eyelid, termed *Romaña's sign,*[499] while entry through the skin may result in a lesion called a *chagoma.* Transmission may occur through blood transfusions as well as congenitally, although this appears to be uncommon.[668]

ACUTE TRYPANOSOMIASIS. Following inoculation, the protozoa multiply and then migrate widely throughout the body. In less than 10 per cent of cases an acute illness occurs[666,669]; the latter is fatal in about 10 per cent of patients.[499]

Pathological examination during the acute phase often reveals parasites in the cardiac fibers with a marked cellular infiltrate, particularly around cardiac cells that have ruptured and released the parasites.[671] Involvement may extend into the endocardium, resulting in thrombus formation, and into the epicardium, resulting in pericardial effusion. The pathogenesis of the myocardial lesions of acute Chagas' disease appears to relate in large part to immune lysis by antibody and cell-mediated immunity directed against antigens released from *T. cruzi*–infected cells, which become adsorbed onto the surface of infected and noninfected host cells.[670]

Clinical Manifestations. These include fever, muscle pains, sweating, hepatosplenomegaly, myocarditis with congestive heart failure, and, occasionally, meningoencephalitis.[666] Most patients recover, and their symptoms resolve over several months. Young children most commonly develop clinical acute disease and generally are more seriously ill than adults.

CHRONIC TRYPANOSOMIASIS. The disease then enters a *latent phase* without clinical symptoms; however, there is evidence of early and progressive subclinical cardiomyopathy. Electrocardiographic changes often appear at this stage and are a marker for the eventual clinical heart disease and increased mortality to become evident later. At an average of 20 years after the initial (and usually unrecognized) infestation, approximately 30 per cent of infected individuals develop findings of *chronic Chagas' disease,* the manifestations of which cover a wide spectrum from asymptomatic but seropositive patients through those with electrocardiographic abnormalities to those with advanced disease characterized by cardiomegaly, congestive heart failure, arrhythmias, thromboembolic phenomena, atypical chest pain, right bundle branch block, and sudden death.[672–675] In the advanced stage, cardiac dilatation typically involves all the cardiac chambers, although right-sided enlargement may predominate.[676]

The central paradox in the pathogenesis of this disorder is the negative correlation between the severity of disease and the level of parasitemia. It is not unusual to be unable to detect parasites in patients dying of Chagas' disease.[665,677] An autoimmune mechanism has been proposed.[499,678–680] It appears (at least in an animal model) that self-reactive cytotoxic T lymphocytes develop following the initial infection, and these lymphocytes are able to lyse normal host cells, perhaps related to cross-reacting antigens of *T. cruzi* and striated muscle.[39] A variety of antibodies against myocyte sarcoplasmic reticulum, laminin, and other constituents have also been implicated in the pathogenesis of Chagas' myocarditis.[679] It is thought that the acute phase results in the release from parasite-modified host cells of self-components that are immunogenic.[670] Another hypothesis suggests that cardiac parasympathetic denervation leads to eventual chronic Chagas' disease.[499,665]

Pathology. Nerves and autonomic ganglia are frequently abnormal, and megaesophagus and megacolon may occur; less commonly, there is dilatation of the stomach, duodenum, ureter, and bronchi. Different strains of *T. cruzi* may account for the geographical differences in the expression

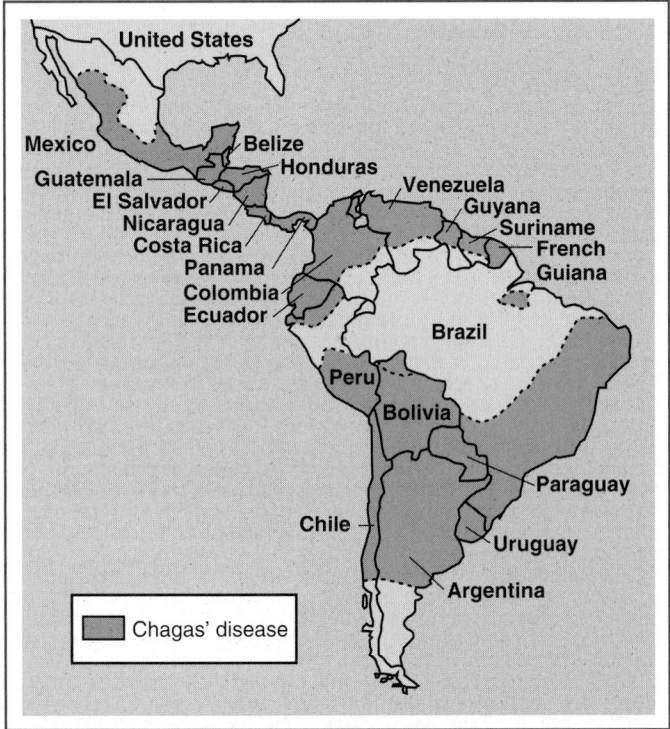

FIGURE 41–29. Distribution of Chagas' disease in the Americas. (From Acquatella, H.: Chagas' disease. *In* Abelmann, W. H., and Braunwald, E. [eds.]: Cardiomyopathies, Myocarditis, and Pericardial Disease. Atlas of Heart Diseases. Vol. 2. Philadelphia, Current Medicine, 1995, pp. 8.1–8.18.)

of Chagas' disease; in Brazil, megaesophagus and megacolon are common, but these conditions are unusual in Venezuela.[681] Lesions of the cardiac nerves are routinely found in patients with chronic Chagas' disease, with evidence of cardiac parasympathetic denervation.[666] Pathological cardiac findings include cardiac enlargement, with dilatation and hypertrophy of all cardiac chambers. In more than half the patients, the left (and occasionally right) ventricular apex is thin and bulging, resembling an aneurysm (Fig. 41–30).[499,665,672] Thrombus formation is frequent and may fill much of the apex; the right atrium also frequently contains thrombus. It has been suggested that this characteristic apical aneurysm may be the result of intravascular platelet aggregation leading to focal myocardial necrosis.[682]

The microscopic findings are principally those of extensive fibrosis, particularly of the left ventricle.[668] A chronic cellular infiltrate composed of lymphocytes, plasma cells, and macrophages often is present.[666] Preferential involvement of the right bundle branch and the anterior fascicle of the left bundle branch by inflammatory and fibrotic changes explains the frequent occurrence of right bundle branch and left anterior fascicular block.[499] The basement membranes of capillaries, vascular smooth muscle cells, and myocytes are thickened.[679] It is unusual to be able to find parasites in the myofibers of autopsied patients.[665]

Clinical Manifestations. These include anginal chest pain, symptomatic conducting system disease, and sudden death[499]; chronic progressive heart failure, often predominantly right-sided, is the rule in advanced cases. Thus, although pulmonary congestion is occasionally noted, the usual findings include fatigue due to diminished cardiac output, peripheral edema, ascites, and hepatic congestion.[672] Tricuspid regurgitation is often present, particularly in patients with severe right-sided heart failure, although mitral regurgitation is frequently present as well. The second heart sound is widely split, often with an accentuated pulmonic component, reflecting the combined effects of right bundle branch block and pulmonary hypertension. Autonomic dysfunction is common, with marked abnormalities in the expected reflex changes in heart rate produced by various maneuvers.

The *chest roentgenogram* often demonstrates severe cardiomegaly, with or without pulmonary venous hypertension.[672] *Electrocardiographic abnormalities* are the rule late in the course of the disease,[674] particularly in patients who are seroreactive to *T. cruzi* antigen. Right bundle branch block, left anterior hemiblock, atrial fibrillation, and ventricular premature depolarizations are the most common findings in patients with chronic Chagas' disease.[499,666,672,683,684] ST-segment and T-wave abnormalities also are common,[683] as are Q waves; P-wave abnormalities

and AV block are seen less frequently.[499] Early in the disease, the electrocardiogram may be normal or nearly so.[674,676] Administration of the antiarrhythmic agent ajmaline may precipitate the appearance of electrocardiographic abnormalities and thus identify patients with as yet clinically silent cardiac involvement. Furthermore, electrophysiological testing of asymptomatic patients, even those with normal electrocardiograms, may demonstrate abnormalities of the conducting system in many.

Ventricular arrhythmias are a prominent feature of chronic Chagas' disease.[666] Frequent ventricular premature depolarizations, often with multiple morphologies, are seen frequently, and bouts of ventricular tachycardia may occur.[673,683] Ventricular arrhythmias are particularly common during and following exercise,[666] occurring in the majority of patients subjected to stress electrocardiographic testing (including some without any clinical evidence of cardiac involvement). Ventricular tachycardia induced by electrophysiological testing[685] is most common in patients with evidence of conduction abnormalities on the electrocardiogram, low ejection fraction, and apical left ventricular aneurysm.[670] Syncope and sudden death due to ventricular fibrillation are constant threats and may develop even before cardiomegaly or heart failure.[499,666,686,687] Sinus bradycardia may also be seen, even in patients with severe heart failure when a tachycardia would be expected, presumably related to cardiac autonomic dysfunction.[666] Atrial arrhythmias, including atrial fibrillation (often with a slow ventricular response), also may occur.[666] Thromboembolic phenomena are a frequent complication, occurring in more than 50 per cent of the patients.

The *echocardiographic findings* in advanced cases are those of a dilated cardiomyopathy with increased end-diastolic and end-systolic volumes and reduced ejection fraction, often with enlargement of the left atrium and right ventricle.[666] Diastolic filling of the left ventricle is frequently abnormal, even in those without other clinical or echocardiographic evidence of cardiac involvement. In the majority of advanced cases, the echocardiographic appearance is distinctive, with left ventricular posterior wall hypokinesis and relatively preserved interventricular septal motion; an apical aneurysm is often seen on two-dimensional echocardiography. Ten to 15 per cent of asymptomatic patients demonstrate apical dyskinesis.

Radionuclide ventriculography may, like echocardiography, demonstrate right or left ventricular wall motion abnormalities in the absence of an overall depression of global ventricular function.[688] Perfusion scanning with thallium-201 may show fixed defects (corresponding to areas of fibrosis) as well as evidence of reversible ischemia.[499,689]

Left ventricular cineangiography in advanced cases shows a dilated, hypokinetic left ventricle with a large api-

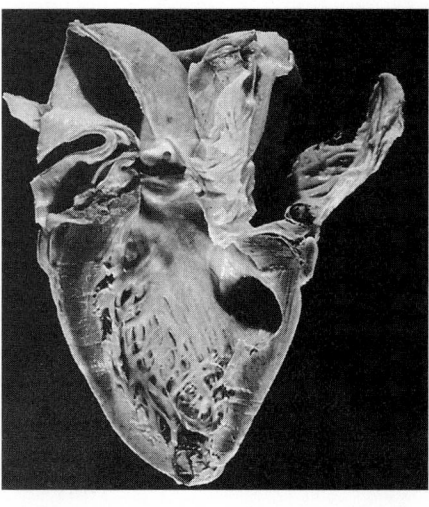
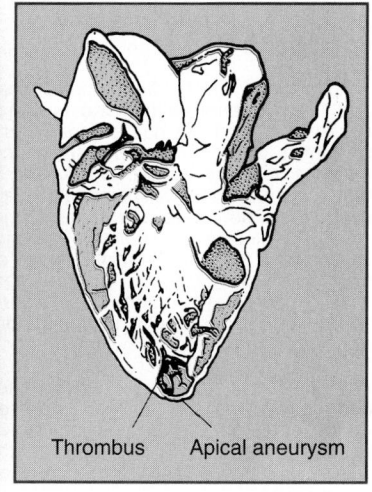

FIGURE 41–30. The heart from a patient who died suddenly with Chagas' disease. The narrow-necked left ventricular apical aneurysm is typical of Chagas' disease. (From Acquatella, H.: Chagas' disease. *In* Abelmann, W. H., and Braunwald, E. [eds.]: Cardiomyopathies, Myocarditis, and Pericardial Disease. Atlas of Heart Diseases. Vol. 2. Philadelphia, Current Medicine, 1995, pp. 8.1–8.18.)

Thrombus   Apical aneurysm

cal aneurysm[499] containing intracavitary thrombus, often with evidence of mitral regurgitation. *Coronary angiography* is usually normal,[499] although abnormalities of the coronary microcirculation have been suggested as a cause of the clinical manifestations of Chagas' disease.

The *complement-fixation test* (Machado-Guerreiro test) is useful in diagnosis; it has high sensitivity and specificity for the identification of chronic Chagas' disease.[499] Also used in diagnosis are the indirect immunofluorescent antibody, the enzyme-linked immunosorbent assay (ELISA), and the hemagglutination tests.[499,690] Another test that is occasionally useful is the detection of parasites in the blood of patients with chronic Chagas' disease (which occurs in 30 to 40 per cent of cases) by means of *xenodiagnosis*.[669] The patient is bitten by reduviid bugs bred in the laboratory; the subsequent identification of parasites in the intestine of the insect is proof of infection in the human host.

MANAGEMENT. The treatment of Chagas' disease remains difficult; although slowly progressive at first, once cardiac decompensation develops there is usually a rapid and inexorable progression to death, which is usually due to arrhythmia, although congestive failure and systemic thromboembolism account for additional mortality.[499,691] Patients at greatest risk of mortality are those with left ventricular enlargement and especially those with impaired left ventricular function.[684,686] Major efforts are aimed at interrupting transmission of the parasite to humans; such vector control methods have been generally successful.[499,667,668] They may prevent not only the initial infection but also reinfection that may play a role in determining the severity of the resulting cardiomyopathy. *Amiodarone* appears to be particularly effective in controlling the ubiquitous ventricular arrhythmias seen in Chagas' disease, although whether this translates into improved survival remains to be established.[669] Anticoagulation may be of some benefit in preventing recurrent thromboembolic episodes. Although antiparasitic agents such as nifurtimox and benzimidazole are effective in reducing parasitemia, no evidence indicates that they are efficacious in curing the disease.[499,690] A promising avenue of approach appears to be immunoprophylaxis, although a clinically useful vaccine is not yet available. Insertion of an implantable cardioverter-defibrillator,[692] use of the latissimus dorsi muscle wrap around the heart (dynamic cardiomyoplasty),[693,694] and heart transplantation have been performed in a few patients[695] but are not practical options for the vast majority of patients.

AFRICAN TRYPANOSOMIASIS. African sleeping sickness, caused by *Trypanosoma gambiense* or *T. rhodesiense*, may be associated with myocardial abnormalities, although they are usually of less functional significance than in Chagas' disease.[696] *T. rhodesiense*, in particular, may lead to cardiac failure,[696] although the central nervous system findings (excessive somnolence) usually dominate the clinical picture.

Pathological examination often reveals pericardial fluid.[696] The heart is not as greatly dilated and hypertrophied as it is in Chagas' disease and may appear grossly to be normal. There is often epicardial thickening with a cellular exudate composed of lymphocytes, plasma cells, and histiocytes. The myocardium typically displays a diffuse interstitial infiltrate, often with zones of patchy fibrosis and interstitial edema.[697]

Nonspecific *electrocardiographic* changes, commonly ST-segment and T-wave abnormalities and prolongation of the Q-T interval, are observed in at least half the patients.[696] Unlike Chagas' disease, arrhythmias and conduction disturbances are usually not prominent features, and the arterial pressure is usually normal. Some patients have asymptomatic cardiomegaly,[696] although both pulmonary congestion and peripheral edema have been reported.

TOXOPLASMOSIS. *Toxoplasma* infections are caused by an obligate intracellular parasite (*T. gondii*); both congenital and acquired forms may occur. Symptomatic acquired toxoplasmic infections involving the heart are uncommon. They occur most commonly in immunosuppressed patients with malignant diseases and occasionally in patients with AIDS and following cardiac or bone marrow transplantation.[561,698] An inflammatory infiltrate, often with eosinophils and variable degrees of edema and degeneration of the muscle bundles, and pericardial effusion are often present.[698]

Most adult cases are asymptomatic, but *Toxoplasma* infections may produce a severe, fatal disease with multisystem involvement.[561] Toxoplasmic myocarditis, often with pericarditis, may occur as an iso-

lated disease process or as part of a multisystem disseminated disease.[561] Manifestations may include arrhythmias (atrial and ventricular), sudden death, AV block, pericarditis, and heart failure.[561] Large pericardial effusions may be seen on occasion.[698] Diagnosis may be aided by endomyocardial biopsy.[567]

Treatment is with a combination of pyrimethamine and triple sulfonamides, but the response to therapy is variable[567]; it appears to have no effect on the cyst form.[561]

MALARIA. Although myocardial changes may be demonstrated during the course of malaria, particularly with *Plasmodium falciparum*, clinical findings to indicate cardiac involvement are rare.[699,700] The heart generally demonstrates few gross abnormalities. The principal findings are histological. The capillaries are often filled and even distended with an accumulation of parasites, sometimes totally occluding the lumen of the vessels. Thrombosis of the capillaries and ischemic myocardial changes may be seen.[700] Focal myocardial damage may be present, along with an interstitial infiltrate composed of lymphocytes, plasma cells, and macrophages.[700] In rare cases, cardiac failure may contribute to or even cause death.[700] ST-segment and T-wave changes on the electrocardiogram may be the only clinical indications of myocardial involvement.[699]

METAZOAL MYOCARDIAL DISEASE

ECHINOCOCCUS (HYDATID CYST). *Echinococcus* is endemic in many sheep-raising areas of the world, particularly Argentina, Uruguay, New Zealand, Greece, North Africa, and Iceland, but cardiac involvement in hydatid disease is uncommon, occurring in less than 2 per cent of cases.[701–703] The usual host of *Echinococcus granulosus* is the dog, but human beings may serve as intermediate hosts (rather than the sheep, the usual intermediate host) if they accidentally ingest ova from contaminated dog feces.

When cardiac involvement is present, the cysts usually are intramyocardial in the interventricular septum or left ventricular free wall; involvement of the right ventricle or atrium may occur.[702–704] Involvement of the tricuspid valve may be seen on occasion,[702] and pericardial involvement with compression of the heart is not uncommon.[702,704] In most cases, a single cardiac cyst is present.[701,702]

A myocardial cyst may degenerate and calcify, develop daughter cysts, or rupture. Rupture of the cyst is the most dreaded complication; rupture into the pericardium may result in acute pericarditis, which may progress to chronic constrictive pericarditis. Rupture into the cardiac chambers may result in systemic or pulmonary emboli.[705,706] Rapidly progressive pulmonary hypertension may occur with rupture of right-sided cysts, with subsequent embolization of hundreds of scolices into the pulmonary circulation.[702] The liberation of hydatid fluid into the circulation may produce profound, fatal circulatory collapse due to an anaphylactic reaction to the protein constituents of the fluid.[702]

Symptoms depend on the location, size, and integrity of the cyst; patients may be asymptomatic or in profound circulatory collapse.[701,702] The *electrocardiogram* may reflect the location of the cyst; T-wave changes and loss of QRS voltage may occur with left ventricular involvement, while AV conduction defects or right bundle branch block may be seen with involvement of the interventricular septum. Chest pain is usually due to rupture of the cyst into the pericardial space with resultant pericarditis. Large cystic masses may sometimes produce right-sided obstruction.[701,702]

Diagnosis. Recognition of an echinococcal cyst of the heart is a relatively simple matter if there is evidence of cysts in other organs, particularly the liver and lung. However, a cardiac cyst may be an isolated, solitary finding. The *chest roentgenogram* frequently shows an abnormal cardiac silhouette or a calcified lobular mass adjacent to the left ventricle. Although CT and nuclear MRI may aid in the detection and localization of heart cysts, two-dimensional echocardiography is thought to be the best choice.[702,704,707] *Eosinophilia*, present in some patients, is a useful adjunctive finding. The *Casoni skin test* is not very helpful because both false-positive and false-negative results occur. Serological tests, including hemagglutination and complement fixation, are more useful.

Management. Until recently, treatment for hydatid disease was limited to surgical excision.[704,708] Because of the significant risk of rupture of the cyst and its attendant serious and sometimes fatal consequences, surgical excision is generally recommended, even for asymptomatic patients. The surgical results have been generally favorable. Experience suggests that the benzimidazole derivative mebendazole may be somewhat useful in the medical management of this disease.[709]

VISCERAL LARVA MIGRANS. People are occasional accidental hosts of the roundworm infestations of dogs due to *Toxocara canis*, but cardiac involvement is rare. Most cases occur in children 1 to 3 years of age.[710] Myocarditis may occur in association with invasion of the myocardium by larvae.[710] The myocardial lesions include granulomas or extensive inflammatory infiltrates (often with eosinophils) with foci of muscle necrosis.[710] Congestive heart failure and death may occur, although asymptomatic cardiac involvement may be seen as well.[710]

SCHISTOSOMIASIS AND RELATED DISEASE. Direct cardiac involvement in schistosomiasis, heterophyiasis, and cysticercosis is distinctly unusual. The principal cardiovascular manifestation of schistosomiasis is right heart overload as a consequence of embolization of the ova to the pulmonary vasculature, with attendant pulmonary hypertension.

TRICHINOSIS. Infestation with *Trichinella spiralis* is a common human finding. Mild myocarditis is frequent, but symptomatic involvement is uncommon and may be responsible for the majority of fatalities.[711,712] Less frequently, death is due to pulmonary embolism secondary to venous thrombosis, or encephalitis.[712]

Although the parasite may invade the heart, it does not usually encyst there, and it is rare to find larvae or larval fragments in the myocardium. Nonetheless, *pathological findings* at autopsy may be impressive. The heart may be dilated and flabby and a pericardial effusion may be present. A prominent focal infiltrate composed of lymphocytes and eosinophils is commonly found, with occasional microthrombi in the intramural arterioles.[712] Areas of muscle degeneration and necrosis are present. The actual cause of the myocardial lesions is debated; whether they bear any relationship to the ubiquitous eosinophilia is uncertain.[712]

Clinical Manifestations. Myocarditis usually is mild and goes unnoticed, but in occasional cases it is manifested by congestive heart failure and chest pain, usually appearing around the third week of the disease, when the general constitutional symptoms are abating.[713] Physical examination may be normal, or there may be gross cardiomegaly with severe congestive heart failure. Sudden death may occur, usually in the fourth to eighth week of the illness.

Electrocardiographic abnormalities may be detected in one-fourth of patients with trichinosis and parallel the time course of clinical cardiac involvement, initially appearing in the second or third week and usually resolving by the seventh week of the illness.[714] The most common electrocardiographic abnormalities are repolarization abnormalities and conduction defects.[714] The electrocardiographic changes usually resolve completely.

The definitive *diagnosis* is based on the demonstration of larval forms in tissue biopsy samples, usually of the gastrocnemius muscle.[714] Eosinophilia, when present, is a supportive finding. The skin test is usually but not invariably positive. Treatment is with corticosteroids; dramatic improvement in cardiac function has been reported following their use.[714]

TOXIC, CHEMICAL, IMMUNE, AND PHYSICAL DAMAGE TO THE HEART

A wide variety of substances other than infectious agents may act on the heart and damage the myocardium. In some cases, the damage is acute, transient, and associated with evidence of an inflammatory infiltrate with myocyte necrosis (such as with arsenicals and lithium); in other cases, a hypersensitivity reaction occurs, without evidence of necrosis (as with sulfonamides). Other agents that damage the myocardium may lead to chronic changes with resulting histological evidence of fibrosis and a clinical picture of a dilated cardiomyopathy. Furthermore, many offending stimuli may be associated with both acute and chronic phases (e.g., alcohol, doxorubicin). The response often is related to the dose and rate of exposure.

Numerous chemicals and drugs (both industrial and therapeutic) may lead to cardiac damage and dysfunction. Several physical agents (e.g., radiation and excessive heat) may also result in myocardial damage. Furthermore, myocardial involvement may be evident in a variety of systemic disease, which are described in Part V of this book.

COCAINE. The illicit use of this drug has increased dramatically recently. It has been associated with a variety of cardiovascular complications, including myocardial ischemia and infarction (unassociated with obstructive coronary artery disease in about one-third), accelerated atherosclerosis, arrhythmias and sudden death, electrophysiological effects, coronary vasoconstriction, myocarditis, dilated cardiomyopathy, rupture of the aorta, cerebrovascular events, increased platelet aggregation, arterial thrombosis, and an apparent predisposition to the development of endocarditis[715-733] (Fig. 41-31). The actual frequency of these complications is in some dispute[734]; the number of adverse events reported in the literature is far less than the casual impression of medical caregivers in inner-city hospitals would suggest.[735] In one study of cocaine abusers who presented to the hospital with chest pain, the frequency of documented myocardial infarction was low.[736] The effects of cocaine on the myocardium itself include transient depression of ventricular function whether the drug is taken acutely or chronically (Fig. 41-32),[720,737,738] scattered areas of myocardial necrosis and myocarditis unrelated to coronary artery disease (which in some cases include contraction band necrosis), and fibrosis.[739,740] In a few cases there has been evidence of dilated cardiomyopathy.[723,737] Even asymptomatic cocaine abusers may have clinically silent myocardial depression.[738]

The cardiovascular effects of cocaine likely are related to its principal pharmacological effects: blocking the reuptake of catecholamines in the presynaptic neurons; blocking sodium channels, leading to local anesthetic, membrane-stabilizing effects; and reducing spontaneous sympathetic activity as a result of effects on the brain stem.[729,739] It has been speculated that the myocardial damage seen with cocaine relates to excess catecholamines damaging myocytes because their reuptake is blocked; this may lead to calcium overload of the cells, or perhaps to local vasoconstriction with subsequent ischemic damage.[724] Vasoconstriction has also been shown as a direct effect of cocaine itself.[741] The monocellular infiltrate (myocarditis) that has been found may merely be a reaction to the associated myocyte death or could be a hypersensitivity reaction to the cocaine, a metabolite,[724] or a contaminant.

Treatment is empirical; nitrates, alpha-adrenoceptor blockers, calcium antagonists, and thrombolytic therapy (for acute myocardial infarctions) have been advocated but without any definite demonstration of their efficacy.[723,742] Beta-adrenoceptor blockers probably should be avoided, as they have been shown to further reduce coronary blood flow and increase coronary vascular resistance during cocaine use, and may predispose to cocaine-mediated cardiac conduction defects.[719,723,739,743]

DAUNORUBICIN AND DOXORUBICIN (See pp. 1800 to 1803)

INTERFERON-ALPHA. Interferon-alpha is a leukocyte-derived protein used therapeutically to treat malignancies and HIV infections.

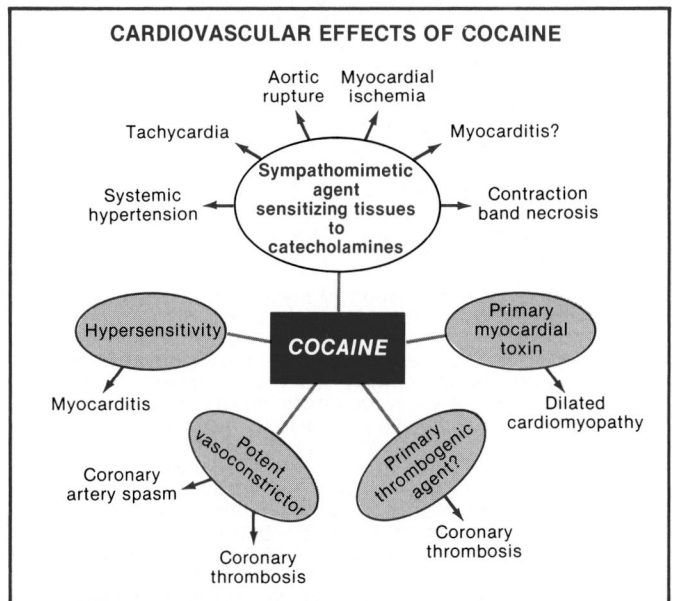

FIGURE 41-31. Diagram showing the effects of cocaine on the heart. (From Waller, B. F.: Cocaine and the heart. Indiana Med. 81:956, 1988.)

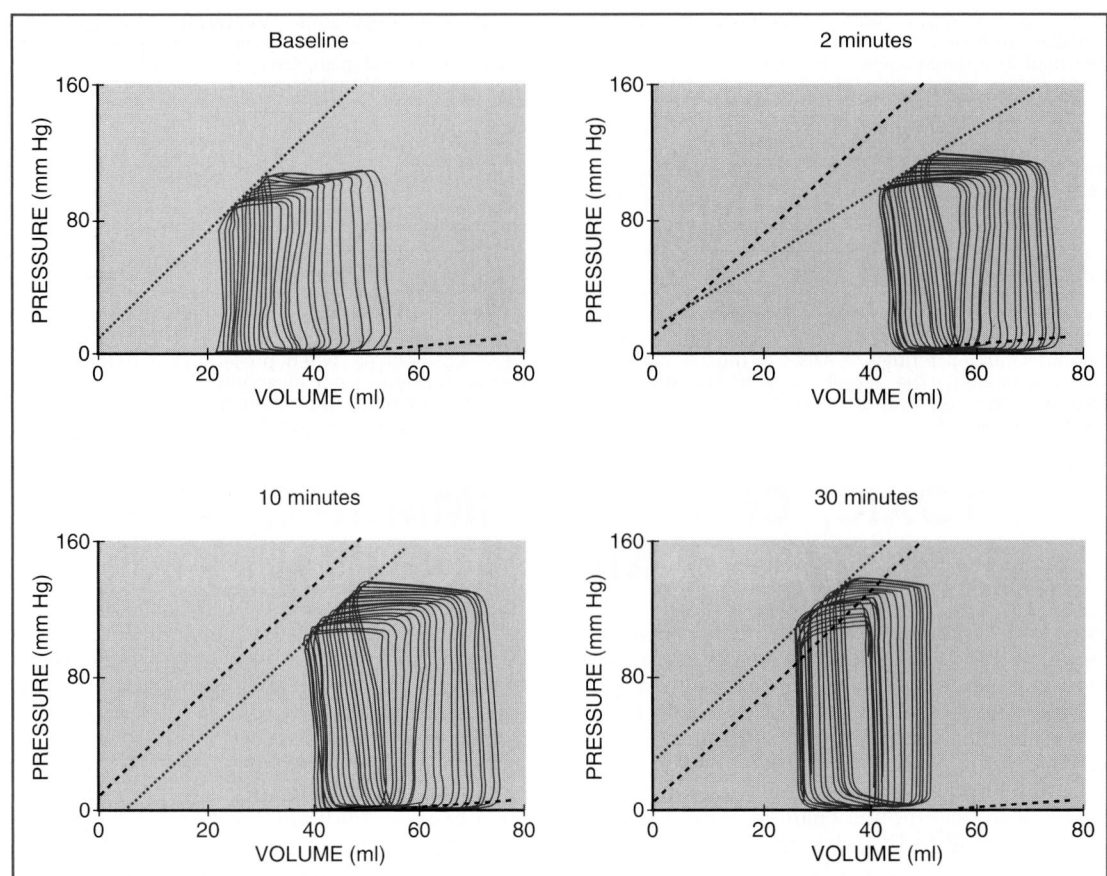

FIGURE 41–32. Left ventricular pressure-volume loops in canine subjected to injection of cocaine. The dashed line at the left upper boundary is the end-systolic pressure-volume relationship that defines the contractile state of the ventricle. There is evidence of contractile depression *(dotted line)* at 2 minutes, with partial resolution at 10 minutes. By 30 minutes there has been complete recovery of the transient myocardial depression. (From Liu, C. P., Tunin, C., and Kass, D. A.: Transient time course of cocaine-induced cardiac depression versus sustained peripheral vasoconstriction. Reprinted by permission of the American College of Cardiology. J. Am. Coll. Cardiol. 21:260, 1993.)

Cardiotoxicity, usually consisting of hypotension, tachycardia, and transient arrhythmias, occurs in a minority of patients (perhaps up to 10 per cent).[744,745] Several patients have developed congestive heart failure and the clinical picture of a dilated cardiomyopathy during interferon-alpha therapy; in at least some patients, cardiomyopathy resolves rapidly with discontinuation of interferon.[745]

TRICYCLIC ANTIDEPRESSANTS. Although sudden death, disturbances in rhythm, and abnormalities of atrioventricular conduction may be seen with the tricyclic antidepressants, particularly when taken as an overdose,[746] important depression of left ventricular function is usually not seen, even in patients with pre-existing heart disease. Particular caution is indicated when using tricyclic antidepressants in patients with prior myocardial infarction and/or pre-existing ventricular arrhythmias, as these agents have a class I antiarrhythmic effect and might be proarrhythmic in these settings.[746] A rare case of hypersensitivity myocarditis has been reported.[747]

INTERLEUKIN-2 (see also p. 1803). The lymphokine interleukin-2, an antineoplastic agent, has significant cardiovascular toxicity, the most prominent of which is a diffuse capillary leak syndrome with hypotension and oliguria.[748] In about 5 per cent of patients, additional cardiotoxicity is seen, consisting of myocardial ischemia, infarction, injury, arrhythmias, and eosinophilic myocarditis.[748–750]

PHENOTHIAZINES. The phenothiazines may be associated with a variety of cardiac disturbances, including electrocardiographic changes, atrial and ventricular arrhythmias, and sudden death.[751] Postural hypotension may also be seen. The cardiac effects are largely dose-dependent. Electrocardiographic abnormalities may be seen with as little as 200 mg of thioridazine per day and consist of lengthening of the Q-T interval and T-wave changes. Prolongation of the Q-T interval may set the stage for the emergence of ventricular arrhythmias, particularly torsades de pointes (p. 685).[751] Higher doses may lead to frank T-wave inversion and increased amplitude of the U wave. Changes in the P wave, QRS complex, and ST segment are usually absent. The electrocardiographic abnormalities and arrhythmias resolve with discontinuation of the drug, usually within 48 hours.

Pathological changes in the hearts of patients who have received psychotropic drugs and who have died suddenly include the deposition of acid mucopolysaccharide between muscle bundles in periarteriolar regions as well as the conduction system, with myofibrillar

degeneration, and endothelial proliferation in the smaller blood vessels, although a direct causal relationship between drug administration and cardiomyopathic changes is only inferential.[752] A variety of explanations have been invoked for the apparent cardiac damage, including direct toxic effects of the phenothiazines on the myocardium, stimulation of higher autonomic centers, and changes in circulating or myocardial levels of catecholamines.

EMETINE. Cardiovascular changes are said to be common with the chronic use of emetine, a drug often employed in the treatment of amebiasis and schistosomiasis as well as the active ingredient in ipecac syrup (used for childhood poisoning).[753] Myocardial lesions may be observed in some but not all patients at autopsy, and similar cardiac damage is noted in experimental animals given emetine.[753,754] The myocardial lesions consist of myofibrillar degeneration and necrosis,[754] with an interstitial infiltrate of mononuclear cells and histiocytes.

The *electrocardiogram*, which may be abnormal in 50 per cent of treated patients, most commonly shows reduced T-wave amplitude or inversion. Prolongation of the Q-T interval and ST-segment shifts may also be seen, although abnormalities of the P wave, P-R segment, and QRS complex are infrequent. The electrocardiographic changes usually resolve within weeks or months after cessation of treatment. Sinus tachycardia and hypotension may also be seen, although clinical evidence of myocardial toxicity is usually lacking. Only rare fatalities have been reported.[755] *Dehydroemetine* results in electrocardiographic abnormalities similar to those of emetine, but they are less prominent and of shorter duration.

METHYSERGIDE. The widespread fibrotic reactions seen with this drug can also involve the heart. Up to 1 per cent of patients treated long term may develop typically left-sided valvular lesions, resulting in stenosis and regurgitation.[752] Fibrotic endocardial and pericardial lesions are also seen on occasion, producing a hemodynamic picture of restrictive and constrictive disease.[756]

CHLOROQUINE. This drug has been widely used in the prophylaxis and treatment of a variety of parasitic and other diseases, including collagen and dermatologic disorders.[757] Electrocardiographic changes may be seen with its use, along with conduction disturbances and features of a restrictive cardiomyopathy.[757] In toxic doses, chloroquine may result in depressed cardiac output, bradycardia, arrhythmias, heart block, and death. Characteristic histological changes are found by electron microscopy (Fig. 41–33).[757]

ANTIMONY COMPOUNDS. Various antimony compounds, such as stibophen and tartar emetic, have been widely used in the treatment of schistosomiasis; less toxic agents are now becoming available. The antimony compounds are associated with electrocardiographic changes in almost all patients.[758] Typical *electrocardiographic changes* include prolongation of the Q-T interval with flattening or inversion of T waves.[758] ST-segment shifts and P-wave changes may be seen, although the QRS complex usually demonstrates no abnormality. The majority of patients do not demonstrate cardiac findings, although chest pain, bradycardia, hypotension, ventricular arrhythmias (including paroxysmal ventricular tachycardia), and sudden death may occur.[758]

LITHIUM. Lithium carbonate, used in the treatment of bipolar disorders, is associated with T-wave changes in one-fourth or more of patients who receive the drug.[759] Clinical evidence of myocardial involvement is usually lacking, although intoxication with lithium may be associated with ventricular arrhythmias, symptomatic sinus node abnormalities, AV conduction disturbances, congestive heart failure, and in rare cases, death.[759] In fatal lithium toxicity, the heart is said to be dilated, with evidence of myofibrillar degeneration associated with a lymphocytic interstitial infiltrate and fibrosis, although no definite proof is available that these changes are due to lithium.[759]

HYDROCARBONS. Ingestion of hydrocarbons may result in fragmentation and vacuolization of the muscle fibers with loss of cross-striations.[760] Electrocardiographic changes, arrhythmias, and cardiomegaly may occur. Involvement of the central nervous, renal, hepatic, and pulmonary systems may dominate the clinical presentation and obscure the myocardial damage, which may well contribute to the mortality of hydrocarbon ingestion.[760]

The *fluorinated hydrocarbons,* commonly used as aerosol propellants, appear to be cardiac toxins, contrary to their reputation of being inert. In animal preparations at least, the aerosol propellants cause ventricular tachyarrhythmias, depress myocardial contractility, and lower systemic vascular resistance and arterial pressure.[761] These cardiovascular effects may be involved in the sudden deaths seen in individuals who abuse aerosols for their psychotropic effect.[761]

CATECHOLAMINES. A severe reversible dilated cardiomyopathy has been observed in conjunction with pheochromocytoma, and the myocardial damage has been attributed to high levels of circulating catecholamines (see p. 829).[762-764] Similar changes have been demonstrated in experimental animals treated with prolonged infusions of L-norepinephrine.[763,764] Catecholamines also may produce acute myocarditis, with focal myocardial necrosis, inflammation, epicardial hemorrhages, tachycardia, and arrhythmias.[765] Similar findings have been described with excessive use of beta-adrenoceptor agonist inhalants and methylxanthines in the treatment of decompensated pulmonary disease.[766] The cardiomyopathy associated with pheochromocytoma is one of the conditions that should be considered when heart failure suddenly appears without other obvious explanation.[763,764]

A variety of mechanisms of myocardial damage have been suggested.[767] A direct toxic effect may be involved, or the damage may be secondary to relative tissue hypoxia because of heightened metabolic demands. Alternatively, the damage may result from changes in autonomic tone, enhanced lipid mobility, calcium overload, damaging effects of catecholamine oxidation products (free radicals), or increased sarcolemmal permeability.[765,767,768] Catecholamine-induced vasospasm also may play a role.[764]

LEAD. The prominent features in lead poisoning generally center on the gastrointestinal and central nervous systems. However, myocardial involvement may contribute to or be the principal cause of death in some cases.[769] Electrocardiographic changes, atrioventricular conduction defects, and overt congestive heart failure may occur.[769] The electrocardiographic and myocardial changes appear to be reversible with chelation therapy.[769]

CARBON MONOXIDE. Both acute and chronic carbon monoxide toxicity can occur. Although central nervous system findings usually dominate the clinical presentation, significant and occasionally fatal cardiac abnormalities may be present.[770] Because carbon monoxide has a higher affinity for hemoglobin than does oxygen, reduced amounts of oxygen are delivered to the tissues. Thus, the cardiac toxicity may be partially caused by myocardial hypoxia, but a direct toxic effect of the gas on myocardial mitochondria may play an even more important role.[771,772] The *histological features* include focal areas of necrosis, most marked in the subendocardium. Focal perivascular infiltrates and punctate hemorrhages are also seen.[772]

Cardiac involvement may appear promptly after exposure, or it may be delayed for up to several days. Palpitations, sinus tachycardia, and various arrhythmias, including ventricular extrasystoles and atrial fibrillation, are common in more severe cases.[773] Bradycardia and AV block may occur in patients with ischemic heart disease, angina pectoris and myocardial infarction may be precipitated. Electrocardiographic ST-segment and T-wave abnormalities are quite common. Transient right and/or left ventricular wall motion abnormalities may be present.[772] Administration of 100 per cent oxygen, bed rest, and surveillance for serious rhythm or conduction abnormalities usually permit rapid recovery.

HYPOCALCEMIA. In rare patients with chronic hypocalcemia (often due to hypoparathyroidism), congestive heart failure may occur and resolve only when the serum calcium level is raised.[774] Rapid transfusion of citrated blood can produce hypocalcemia and reversible myocardial depression, as can ambulatory peritoneal dialysis in patients with chronic renal failure.[775]

HYPOPHOSPHATEMIA. A form of reversible left ventricular dysfunction may be seen with severe hypophosphatemia. Restoration of the serum phosphate level to normal results in hemodynamic recovery.

HYPOMAGNESEMIA. Focal cardiac necrosis is found in experimental magnesium deficiency and may account for the supraventricular and ventricular arrhythmias and electrocardiographic changes that are seen clinically. In addition to arrhythmias, coronary spasm and acute myocardial infarction may be seen.[776] A rare case of fatal cardiomyopathy has been reported.[776,777]

TAURINE DEFICIENCY. A deficiency of taurine, an amino acid found in high concentration in cardiac and retinal tissue, produces a dilated cardiomyopathy in cats that is reversible with oral taurine supplementation.[778] Whether a similar condition exists in humans is not known; this has been the subject of speculation.[779]

CARNITINE DEFICIENCY. Carnitine, an essential cofactor for the oxidation of fatty acids, produces a hypertrophic or dilated cardiomyopathy in children when deficient.[780-783] Carnitine supplementation can lead to symptomatic and functional improvement[780,783-785]; determination of carnitine levels therfore is important in children with unexplained cardiomyopathy.[780] Myocardial carnitine levels are reduced in the hearts of patients with dilated cardiomyopathy, but the significance of this observation is not known at present.[781]

SELENIUM DEFICIENCY. Dietary deficiency of the trace element selenium appears to be one of the principal factors responsible for a form of dilated cardiomyopathy endemic to certain rural areas in China,[786] although the etiological role played by selenium has been

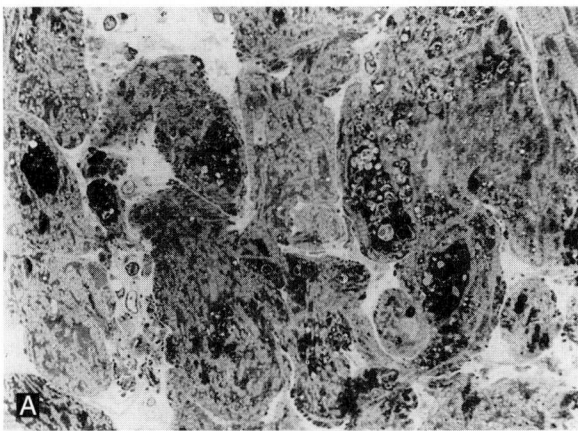
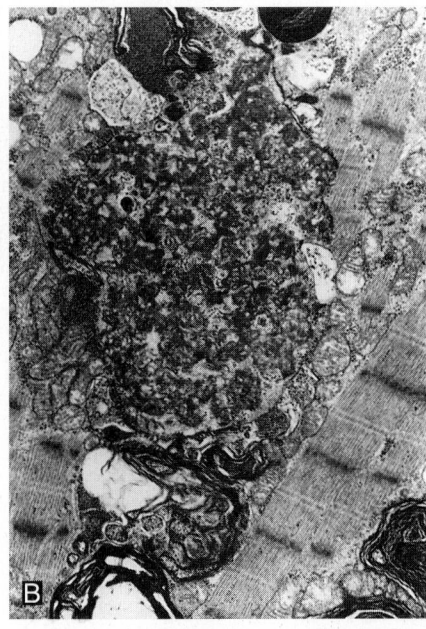

FIGURE 41–33. Endomyocardial biopsy specimen from a patient with chloroquine cardiomyopathy. *A,* 1-μm-thick section demonstrating numerous cytoplasmic inclusions that occupy the central area of myocytes (alkaline toluidine blue stain, ×700). *B,* Electron micrograph demonstrating that the cytoplasmic inclusions are composed of irregularly arranged electron-dense concentric lamellae and curvilinear bodies (×30,000). (Reproduced by permission from Ferrans, V. J., Hall, R. J., and McAllister, H. A. Jr.: Chloroquine-induced cardiomyopathy. Circulation *88:*785, 1993; copyright, 1993 American Heart Association.)

questioned.[787,788] Termed *Keshan disease,* it affects mainly children and young women and apparently is prevented by the prophylactic administration of sodium selenite tablets.[787,789] A similar cardiomyopathy may be found in Occidentals subjected to prolonged parenteral hyperalimentation; supplementation with oral selenium may reverse the cardiomyopathy.[788,790,791]

SCORPION STING. The venom of the scorpion is mainly neurotoxic, but cardiac findings may be prominent and even fatal, particularly in children.[792-795] Electrocardiographic changes and myocardial damage with elevated serum cardiac enzyme levels are common findings.[795] Hearts are normal on gross examination, with prominent microscopic changes usually but not invariably present, particularly in the subendocardial region and papillary muscles. Degeneration and necrosis of muscle fibers are noted, with interstitial edema and a mononuclear infiltrate.[795] The histological features of scorpion sting suggest high levels of circulating catecholamines and are similar to those seen with experimental catecholamine infusion and in pheochromocytoma.[792] The parasympathetic system appears to be stimulated as well.[792]

The *electrocardiogram* often initially shows tall, peaked T waves that progress to inversions and ST-segment shifts. Q waves may appear, and the Q-T interval is usually prolonged.[796] Atrial, junctional, and ventricular arrhythmias may occur. Tachycardia, hypertension, anxiety, diaphoresis, and pulmonary edema—findings resembling those of a massive catecholamine effect—are striking in many patients.[796] A smaller number of patients are in shock with peripheral vascular collapse. Most deaths are due to pulmonary edema, presumably the result of left ventricular dysfunction.[797] Occasionally, sudden and unexpected deaths occur in a smaller percentage of patients, presumably as a consequence of arrhythmias. Adrenergic blocking agents and the use of specific antivenom appear to be useful in the management of the cardiovascular manifestation of scorpion stings.[794]

WASP AND SPIDER STINGS. Stings by the vespine wasps may lead to anaphylaxis, with hypotension, circulatory collapse, and cyanosis.[798] Occasional patients may have chest pain and clinical findings compatible with acute myocardial infarction.[798] The mechanism of myocardial damage is unclear; perhaps it merely reflects necrosis from profound hypotension, although a direct toxic effect on the myocardium or an indirect effect on the coronary arteries may be involved.[798]

SNAKE BITE. Cardiac complications are not prominent features of snake bites, and the clinical picture is usually dominated by the neurological, hematological, and vascular damage produced by the snakebite toxin.[799,800] Myocardial involvement is seen on occasion and may rarely contribute to morbidity and mortality. T-wave abnormalities are the most common manifestation of myocardial involvement, although ST-segment depression, QRS prolongation, and AV conduction defects may also be seen.[751] The electrocardiographic changes are usually transient, but when persistent they are attributed to direct myocardial damage due to the toxin. Death may occur from circulatory collapse, myocardial depression, or myocardial infarction due to hypotension and coronary artery thrombosis. Coronary artery vasospasm may also be involved.[801,802]

ARSENIC. Myocardial involvement may be seen in both acute and chronic arsenical poisoning, usually from pesticides; the heart may be dilated, with accumulation of pericardial fluid.[803] Multiple local and confluent areas of subepicardial and subendocardial hemorrhage are characteristic findings. The myocardium is usually abnormal, with evidence of a perivascular mononuclear infiltrate.[803]

Clinically unrecognized interstitial myocarditis is manifested by T-wave inversions and ST-segment depressions, along with prolongation of the Q-T interval.[803] The electrocardiographic changes usually revert to normal within 2 to 4 weeks. The electrocardiographic abnormalities appear to resolve more rapidly when BAL (British antilewisite, dimercaprol) is used in therapy.[803]

CYCLOPHOSPHAMIDE (see also p. 1803). High doses of cyclophosphamide have been associated with electrocardiographic changes, congestive heart failure, and death from hemorrhagic myocarditis.[804] In the majority of patients treated, a reversible decrease of QRS voltage and systolic function is seen, often asymptomatic, although more than 20 per cent may succumb as a consequence of myopericarditis.[805] The myocardial damage appears to result from direct endothelial damage and resultant fibrin microthrombi in the capillaries.[805]

AZIDE. Sodium azide, a chemical preservative that interferes with oxidative phosphorylation, may produce fatal acute cardiotoxicity when accidentally ingested.[806,807] Pathological findings include marked interstitial edema and myofibrillar degeneration. Clinical features include arrhythmias, myocardial ischemia, left ventricular dysfunction, and hypotension.[806]

PARACETAMOL. Paracetamol, a phenacetin metabolite, may result in massive liver necrosis. On occasion it also results in fatty degeneration and focal necrosis of the myocardium after an overdose.[808]

5-FLUOROURACIL. This antineoplastic agent has been associated with cardiotoxicity manifested by chest pain, electrocardiographic changes, and arrhythmia.[809,810] Swelling of myocardial fibers without an inflammatory infiltrate has been found at necropsy.[811]

PACLITAXEL. The most common cardiac effect of paclitaxel is sinus bradycardia, usually asymptomatic, which occurs in about one-fourth of patients.[812] A variety of other findings (ischemia, arrhythmias, conduction defects) have been noted on occasion, but usually in patients with pre-existing cardiac pathology; the etiologic role of paclitaxel is not established.[812]

HYPERSENSITIVITY

Hypersensitivity to a variety of agents may result in allergic reactions that involve the myocardium. A variety of drugs (most commonly the sulfonamides, the penicillins, and methyldopa) or other sensitizers may lead to an allergic myocarditis (Table 41–16),[813] characterized by peripheral eosinophilia and a perivascular infiltration of the myocardium by eosinophils, lymphocytes, and histiocytes; necrosis is seen on occasion.[814,815] Hypersensitivity myocarditis is rarely recognized clinically and is often first discovered at postmortem examination, although it is occasionally diagnosed on endomyocardial biopsy.[815,816] Most patients who have hypersensitivity myocarditis are not critically ill, but die suddenly, presumably the consequence of an arrhythmia. An occasional patient has intense eosinophilic infiltration of the myocardium of no obvious cause, with prominent necrosis evident and findings of hemodynamic collapse; some of these patients may have undiagnosed hypersensitivity myocarditis.[463,814,816] Because of the potential for significant deleterious effects, a high index of suspicion for this condition should be maintained; in one unusual case, penicillin residue in pet food led to hypersensitivity myocarditis in a young child.[817] Therapy includes discontinuation of the offending agent and corticosteroids and/or immunosuppression therapy in severe cases.[814,816]

METHYLDOPA. Although hepatitis is the most frequently encountered serious adverse reaction to methyldopa, sudden and unexpected death has been reported in a number of patients found at necropsy to have had an unsuspected myocarditis.[815,816] The *histological findings* have the characteristics of an allergic myocarditis, showing an interstitial inflammatory infiltrate with abundant eosinophils,[815] a vasculitis, and focal myocardial necrosis. Electrocardiographic changes include sinus bradycardia, sinus pauses, and first- and second-degree AV block.[818]

PENICILLIN. Allergic reactions to penicillin are fairly common, but myocardial involvement is rare.[819] *Histological findings* consist of a perivascular and interstitial infiltrate composed of eosinophils and mononuclear cells.[815] Both myocardial infarction and pericarditis may occur and account for some of the electrocardiographic changes.[817,820] Transient electrocardiographic changes may be the only manifestation of cardiac involvement, with sinus tachycardia, ST-segment elevation, and T-wave inversion.[817]

SULFONAMIDES. Sulfonamides may result in myocardial damage owing to a hypersensitivity vasculitis as well as a myocarditis.[820] In fatal cases eosinophilic myocarditis,[815] sometimes with granulomas, usually can be demonstrated. Although usually clinically silent, myocardial involvement may produce severe and even fatal congestive heart failure.[816] Electrocardiographic changes are usually absent, but nonspecific ST-segment and T-wave abnormalities may be seen.

TETRACYCLINE. Allergic reactions to antibiotics of the tetracycline class include fever, tachycardia, and first-degree AV block. Postmortem findings include cardiac dilatation, fibrinoid muscle cell degeneration, and a diffuse interstitial and perivascular infiltrate.[815]

TABLE 41–16 PRINCIPAL DRUGS CAPABLE OF CAUSING HYPERSENSITIVITY MYOCARDITIS

Antibiotics	**Anti-inflammatory**
Amphotericin B	Indomethacin
Ampicillin	Oxyphenbutazone
Chloramphenicol	Phenylbutazone
Penicillin	
Tetracycline	**Diuretics**
Streptomycin	Acetazolamide
	Chlorthalidone
Sulfonamides	Hydrochlorothiazide
Sulfadiazine	Spironolactone
Sulfisoxazole	
	Others
Anticonvulsants	Amitriptyline
Phenindione	Methyldopa
Phenytoin	Sulfonylureas
Carbamazepine	Tetanus toxoid
Antituberculous	
Isoniazid	
Paraaminosalicylic acid	

From Kounis, N. G., Zavras, G. M., Soufras, G. D., and Kitrou, M. P.: Hypersensitivity myocarditis. Ann. Allergy 62:71, 1989.

ANTITUBERCULOUS DRUGS. Most reactions to antituberculous drugs consist of a fever, rash, or both, but serious and fatal cardiac reactions may occur on rare occasions. *Paraaminosalicylic acid* may lead to the development of interstitial edema, acute inflammatory infiltrate, refractory congestive heart failure, hypotension, and ventricular irritability.[821]

Streptomycin has been implicated as an unusual cause of myocarditis. Pathological findings may include cardiac dilatation, myocarditis with necrosis, hemorrhage, and a fibrinous pericardial effusion.[821] Clinically, it may be associated with chest pain, dyspnea, fever, and rash, followed by collapse and death.

GIANT CELL MYOCARDITIS

Giant cell myocarditis is a rare disease of unknown cause characterized by the presence of multinucleated giant cells in the myocardium. (It is included here because of the possibility that it may be of immune or autoimmune origin.) Also called granulomatous myocarditis, this condition is typically a rapidly fatal disease, often of young to middle-aged adults.[822] *Pathological findings* are usually impressive. The ventricles are dilated, and mural thrombi may be present. A serpiginous area of myocardial necrosis may be seen involving the right as well as the left ventricle.[822] Multinucleated giant cells are found, particularly at the margins of the areas of myocardial necrosis; the giant cells appear to be of macrophage rather than myocyte origin.[823]

Giant cell myocarditis occurs on occasion in association with systemic diseases such as sarcoidosis, systemic lupus erythematosus, drug hypersensitivity, infections (especially syphilis and tuberculosis), and thyrotoxicosis, but the cause of the disease remains obscure.[822] In many ways the clinical features suggest a viral myocarditis except for the rapid and virulent course. However, despite careful investigation there has been no serological or bacteriological evidence of an infectious cause.[822,823] It has been suggested that the cause is an autoimmune reaction, although little evidence aside from the histological findings supports this view.[822,823]

Both genders are equally affected; the onset typically is rapid, with dyspnea, chest pain, orthopnea, and hypotension. Fever is usually present, with electrocardiographic evidence of widespread myocardial involvement. Conduction defects, ventricular arrhythmias, and AV block are common.[822] Overt congestive heart failure and sudden death may occur.[824] Therapy (other than cardiac transplantation[825,826]) often is unsuccessful, although corticosteroids and immunosuppressive agents appear to have benefited some patients. Because the prognosis in general is poor, empirical immunosuppressive therapy probably is warranted.[822,823,827–829] Occasional patients have had long-term survival.[825]

PHYSICAL AGENTS

HEAT STROKE. This condition results from failure of the thermoregulatory center following exposure to high ambient temperature and is manifested principally by hyperpyrexia and central nervous system dysfunction. However, cardiovascular abnormalities (usually electrocardiographic) appear to be common; pulmonary edema and right ventricular dysfunction may occur,[830] along with hypotension and circulatory collapse. *Pathological changes* include dilatation of the right side of the heart, particularly the right atrium. Hemorrhages of the subendocardium and the subepicardium are frequently seen at necropsy and often involve the interventricular septum and posterior wall of the left ventricle.[830] Histological findings include degeneration and necrosis of muscle fibers as well as interstitial edema.[830] Possible factors responsible for myocardial damage include direct thermal injury, myocardial hypoxia secondary to circulatory collapse, decreased coronary blood flow, and metabolic abnormalities resulting from widespread injury to other organs.

Sinus tachycardia is invariably present, whereas atrial and ventricular arrhythmias are usually absent. Transient prolongation of the Q-T interval may be seen, along with ST-segment and T-wave abnormalities. It may take up to several months for these repolarization abnormalities to resolve. Serum enzyme levels may be elevated and may reflect myocardial damage, at least in part.[830]

HYPOTHERMIA. Low temperature may also result in myocardial damage. Cardiac dilatation may occur with epicardial petechiae and subendocardial hemorrhages. Microinfarcts are found in the ventricular myocardium, presumably related to abnormalities in the microcirculation.[831] The lesions are not due to the low temperature per se but appear to be the result of the circulatory collapse, hemoconcentration, capillary slugging, and depressed cellular metabolism that accompany hypothermia. Clinical manifestations of hypothermia include sinus bradycardia, conduction disturbances, atrial (and occasionally ventricular) fibrillation, hypotension, a fall in cardiac output, reversible myocardial depression, and a characteristic deflection of the terminal portion of the QRS pattern (Osborn wave).[831,832] Treatment includes core warming, cardiopulmonary resuscitation, and management of pulmonary, hematological, and renal complications.[832]

RADIATION. The use of ionizing radiation during radiation therapy (or less commonly after radiation accidents) may result in a variety of occasionally acute but usually chronic cardiac complications, including pericarditis with effusion, tamponade, or constriction; coronary artery fibrosis and myocardial infarction; valvular abnormalities; myocardial fibrosis; and conduction disturbances.[833–835] Although the heart has been regarded as one of the organs more resistant to the effects of radiation, the clinical significance of radiation-induced heart disease is greater than usually thought.[834] Although radiation probably results in some degree of tissue damage in all patients, clinically significant cardiac involvement occurs in the minority of patients, usually long after the radiation treatment has ended.[834] Radiation-induced cardiac damage is related to the dose of radiation, the mass of heart irradiated, and the dose schedule of the radiation.

The late cardiac damage that may follow irradiation appears to result from a long-lasting injury of the capillary endothelial cells, which leads to cell death, capillary rupture, and microthrombi.[834] Because of this damage to the microvasculature, ischemia results and is followed by myocardial fibrosis. In addition to microvascular damage, the major epicardial coronary arteries may become narrowed, especially at the ostia.[835,836]

Only an occasional patient manifests acute cardiac abnormality clinically with radiation therapy; typically this consists of acute pericarditis. A mild, transient, asymptomatic depression of left ventricular function may be seen early after radiation therapy.[837] The more common clinical expressions of radiation heart disease occur months or years after the exposure. The pericardium is the most common site of clinical involvement, with findings of chronic pericardial effusion or pericardial constriction.[834] Myocardial damage occurs less frequently and is characterized by myocardial fibrosis with or without endocardial fibrosis or fibroelastosis. Left and/or right ventricular dysfunction at rest or with exercise appears to be a common, albeit usually asymptomatic, finding 5 to 20 years after radiation therapy, especially in those in whom the now-outmoded technique of a single anteroposterior port was used.[834,838,839] Occasional patients may develop usually asymptomatic left-sided (and rarely right-sided) valvular regurgitation (or on occasion stenosis) that rarely requires valve replacement; often there is a latent period of a decade or more between the radiation exposure and the development of valvular deformity.[833,839–842] Electrocardiographic abnormalities, heart block, and a variety of arrhythmias may be seen months or years after therapeutic radiation, although usually they are of limited clinical significance.[840,843,844]

REFERENCES

1. Siu, S. C., and Sole, M. J.: Dilated cardiomyopathy. Curr. Opin. Cardiol. *9*:337, 1994.
2. Hare, J. M., Walford, G. D., Hruban, R. H., et al.: Ischemic cardiomyopathy: Endomyocardial biopsy and ventriculographic evaluation of patients with congestive heart failure, dilated cardiomyopathy and coronary artery disease. J. Am. Coll. Cardiol. *20*:1318, 1992.
3. Sugrue, D. D., Rodeheffer, R. J., Codd, M. B., et al.: The clinical course of idiopathic dilated cardiomyopathy. A population-based study. Ann. Intern. Med. *117*:117, 1992.

4. Coughlin, S. S., Comstock, G. W., and Baughman, K. L.: Descriptive epidemiology of idiopathic dilated cardiomyopathy in Washington County, Maryland, 1975–1991. J. Clin. Epidemiol. 46:1003, 1993.

5. Manolio, T. A., Baughman, K. L., Rodeheffer, R., et al.: Prevalence and etiology of idiopathic dilated cardiomyopathy (summary of a National Heart, Lung, and Blood Institute workshop). Am. J. Cardiol. 69:1458, 1992.

5a. Richarrdson, P., McKenna, W., Bristow, M., et al.: Report of the 1995 World Health Organization/International Society and Federation of Cardiology Task Force on the Definition and Classification of Cardiomyopathies. Circulation 93:841, 1996.

6. Keren, A., and Popp, R. L.: Assignment of patients into the classification of cardiomyopathies. Circulation 86:1622, 1992.

7. Boffa, G. M., Thiene, G., Nava, A., and Dalla Volta, S.: Cardiomyopathy: A necessary revision of the WHO classification. Int. J. Cardiol. 30:1, 1991.

8. Abelmann, W. H.: Introduction. In Abelmann W. H. (ed.): Cardiomyopathies, Myocarditis, and Pericardial Disease. Current Medicine 1:2, 1995.

9. Goodwin, J. F.: Cardiomyopathies and specific heart muscle diseases. Definitions, terminology, classifications and new and old approaches. Postgrad. Med. J. 68(Suppl. 1):S3, 1992.

10. Kasper, E. K., Agema, W. R., Hutchins, G. M., et al.: The causes of dilated cardiomyopathy: A clinicopathologic review of 673 consecutive patients. J. Am. Coll. Cardiol. 23:586, 1994.

11. Mason, J. W.: Endomyocardial biopsy and the causes of dilated cardiomyopathy. J. Am. Coll. Cardiol. 23:591, 1994.

12. Pytlewski, G., Georgeson, S., Burke, J., et al.: Endomyocardial biopsy under transesophageal echocardiographic guidance can be safely performed in the critically ill cardiac transplant recipient. Am. J. Cardiol. 73:1019, 1994.

13. Balzer, D., Moorhead, S., Saffitz, J. E., et al.: Pediatric endomyocardial biopsy performed solely with echocardiographic guidance. J. Am. Soc. Echocardiogr. 6:510, 1993.

14. Blomstrom-Lundqvist, C., Noor, A. M., Eskilsson, J., and Persson, S.: Safety of transvenous right ventricular endomyocardial biopsy guided by two-dimensional echocardiography. Clin. Cardiol. 16:487, 1993.

15. Bell, C. A., Kern, M. J., Aguirre, F. V., et al.: Superior accuracy of anatomic positioning with echocardiographic-over fluoroscopic-guided endomyocardial biopsy. Cathet. Cardiovasc. Diagn. 28:291, 1993.

16. Herskowitz, A., Campbell, S., Deckers, J., et al.: Demographic features and prevalence of idiopathic myocarditis in patients undergoing endomyocardial biopsy. Am. J. Cardiol. 71:982, 1993.

17. Kyu, B., Matsumori, A., Sato, Y., et al.: Cardiac persistence of cardioviral RNA detected by polymerase chain reaction in a murine model of dilated cardiomyopathy. Circulation 86:522, 1992.

18. Archard, L. C., Bowles, N. E., Cunningham, L., et al.: Molecular probes for detection of persisting enterovirus infection of human heart and their prognostic value. Eur. Heart J. 12(Suppl. D):56, 1991.

19. Jin, O., Sole, M. J., Butany, J. W., et al.: Detection of enterovirus RNA in myocardial biopsies from patients with myocarditis and cardiomyopathy using gene amplification by polymerase chain reaction. Circulation 82:8, 1990.

20. Martin, A. B., Webber, S., Fricker, F. J., et al.: Acute myocarditis. Rapid diagnosis by PCR in children. Circulation 90:330, 1994.

21. Okada, I., Matsumori, A., and Kyu, B.: Detection of viral RNA in experimental coxsackievirus B3 myocarditis of mice using the polymerase chain reaction. Int. J. Exp. Pathol. 73:721, 1992.

DILATED CARDIOMYOPATHY

22. Keren, A., Gottlieb, S., Tzivoni, D., et al.: Mildly dilated congestive cardiomyopathy. Use of prospective diagnostic criteria and description of the clinical course without heart transplantation. Circulation 81:506, 1990.

23. Mestroni, L., Krajinovic, M., Severini, G. M., et al.: Familial dilated cardiomyopathy. Br. Heart J. 72:S35, 1994.

24. Dec, G. W., and Fuster, V.: Medical progress: Idiopathic dilated cardiomyopathy. N. Engl. J. Med. 331:1564, 1994.

25. Coughlin, S. S., Neaton, J. D., Sengupta, A., and Kuller, L. H.: Predictors of mortality from idiopathic dilated cardiomyopathy in 356,222 men screened for the Multiple Risk Factor Intervention Trial. Am. J. Epidemiol. 139:166, 1994.

26. Coughlin, S. S., Labenberg, J. R., and Tefft, M. C.: Black-white differences in idiopathic dilated cardiomyopathy: The Washington DC Dilated Cardiomyopathy Study. Epidemiology 4:165, 1993.

27. Coughlin, S. S., Szklo, M., Baughman, K., and Pearson, T. A.: The epidemiology of idiopathic dilated cardiomyopathy in a biracial community. Am. J. Epidemiol. 131:48, 1990.

28. Coughlin, S. S., Gottdiener, J. S., Baughman, K. L., et al.: Black-white differences in mortality in idiopathic dilated cardiomyopathy: The Washington DC Dilated Cardiomyopathy Study. J. Natl. Med. Assoc. 86:583, 1994.

29. Redfield, M. M., Gersh, B. J., Bailey, K. R., and Rodeheffer, R. J.: Natural history of incidentally discovered, asymptomatic idiopathic dilated cardiomyopathy. Am. J. Cardiol. 74:737, 1994.

30. Steimle, A. E., Stevenson, L. W., Fonarow, G. C., et al.: Prediction of improvement in recent onset cardiomyopathy after referral for heart transplantation. J. Am. Coll. Cardiol. 23:553, 1994.

31. Semigran, M. J., Thaik, C. M., Fifer, M. A., et al.: Exercise capacity and systolic and diastolic ventricular function after recovery from acute dilated cardiomyopathy. J. Am. Coll. Cardiol. 24:462, 1994.

32. Fruhwald, F. M., Dusleag, J., Eber, B., et al.: Long-term outcome and prognostic factors in dilated cardiomyopathy. Preliminary results. Angiology 45:763, 1994.

33. Anguita, M., Arizon, J. M., Bueno, G., et al.: Clinical and hemodynamic predictors of survival in patients aged <65 years with severe congestive heart failure secondary to ischemic or nonischemic dilated cardiomyopathy. Am. J. Cardiol. 72:413, 1993.

34. Borggrefe, M., Block, M., and Breithardt, G.: Identification and management of the high risk patient with dilated cardiomyopathy. Br. Heart J. 72:S42, 1994.

35. De Maria, R., Gavazzi, A., Recalcati, F., et al.: Comparison of clinical findings in idiopathic dilated cardiomyopathy in women versus men. The Italian Multicenter Cardiomyopathy Study Group (SPIC). Am. J. Cardiol. 72:580, 1993.

36. Saxon, L. A., Stevenson, W. G., Middlekauff, H. R., et al.: Predicting death from progressive heart failure secondary to ischemic or idiopathic dilated cardiomyopathy. Am. J. Cardiol. 72:62, 1993.

37. Pelliccia, F., d'Amati, G., Cianfrocca, C., et al.: Histomorphometric features predict 1-year outcome of patients with idiopathic dilated cardiomyopathy considered to be at low priority for cardiac transplantation. Am. Heart J. 128:316, 1994.

38. Yamada, T., Fukunami, M., Ohmori, M., et al.: Which subgroup of patients with dilated cardiomyopathy would benefit from long-term beta-blocker therapy? A histologic viewpoint. J. Am. Coll. Cardiol. 21:628, 1993.

39. Abelmann, W. H., and Lorell, B. H.: The challenge of cardiomyopathy. J. Am. Coll. Cardiol. 13:1219, 1989.

40. Kuroda, T., Shiina, A., Suzuki, O., et al.: Prediction of prognosis of patients with idiopathic dilated cardiomyopathy: A comparison of echocardiography with cardiac catheterization. Jpn. J. Med. 28:180, 1989.

41. Ferrans, V. J.: Pathologic anatomy of the dilated cardiomyopathies. Am. J. Cardiol. 64:9C, 1989.

42. Schaper, J., Froede, R., Hein, S., et al.: Impairment of the myocardial ultrastructure and changes of the cytoskeleton in dilated cardiomyopathy. Circulation 83:504, 1991.

43. Bender, J. R.: Idiopathic dilated cardiomyopathy. An immunologic, genetic, or infectious disease, or all of the above? Circulation 83:704, 1991.

44. Neumann, D. A.: Autoimmunity and idiopathic dilated cardiomyopathy. Mayo Clin. Proc. 69:193, 1994.

45. Michels, V. V., Moll, P. P., Rodeheffer, R. J., et al.: Circulating heart autoantibodies in familial as compared with nonfamilial idiopathic dilated cardiomyopathy. Mayo Clin. Proc. 69:24, 1994.

46. Michels, V. V.: Progress in defining the causes of idiopathic dilated cardiomyopathy. N. Engl. J. Med. 329:960, 1993.

47. Zachara, E., Caforio, A. L., Carboni, G. P., et al.: Familial aggregation of idiopathic dilated cardiomyopathy: Clinical features and pedigree analysis in 14 families. Br. Heart J. 69:129, 1993.

48. Michels, V. V., Moll, P. P., Miller, F. A., et al.: The frequency of familial dilated cardiomyopathy in a series of patients with idiopathic dilated cardiomyopathy. N. Engl. J. Med. 326:77, 1992.

48a. Goerss, J. B., Michels, V. V., Burnett, J., et al.: Frequency of familial dilated cardiomyopathy. Eur. Heart J. 16 (Suppl O):2, 1996.

49. Kelly, D. P., and Strauss, A. W.: Inherited cardiomyopathies. N. Engl. J. Med. 330:913, 1994.

50. Muntoni, F., Cau, M., Ganau, A., et al.: Brief report: Deletion of the dystrophin muscle-promoter region associated with X-linked dilated cardiomyopathy. N. Engl. J. Med. 329:921, 1993.

51. Towbin, J. A., Hejtmancik, J. F., Brink, P., et al.: X-linked dilated cardiomyopathy. Molecular genetic evidence of linkage to the Duchenne muscular dystrophy (dystrophin) gene at the Xp21 locus. Circulation 87:1854, 1993.

52. Remes, A. M., Hassinen, I. E., Ikaheimo, M. J., et al.: Mitochondrial DNA deletions in dilated cardiomyopathy: A clinical study employing endomyocardial sampling. J. Am. Coll. Cardiol. 23:935, 1994.

53. Silvestri, G., Santorelli, F. M., Shanske, S., et al.: A new mtDNA mutation in the tRNA(Leu(UUR)) gene associated with maternally inherited cardiomyopathy. Hum. Mutat. 3:37, 1994.

54. Tranchant, C., Mousson, B., Mohr, M., et al.: Cardiac transplantation in an incomplete Kearns-Sayre syndrome with mitochondrial DNA deletion. Neuromuscul. Disord. 3:561, 1993.

55. Anan, R., Nakagawa, M., Miyata, M., et al.: Cardiac involvement in mitochondrial diseases. A study on 17 patients with documented mitochondrial DNA defects. Circulation 91:955, 1995.

56. Carlquist, J. F., Menlove, R. L., Murray, M. B., et al.: HLA class II (DR and DQ) antigen associations in idiopathic dilated cardiomyopathy. Validation study and meta-analysis of published HLA association studies. Circulation 83:515, 1991.

56a. Mestroni, L., Krajinovic, M., Severini, G. M., et al.: Molecular genetics of dilated cardiomyopathies. Eur. Heart J. 16 (Suppl O):5, 1996.

57. Raynolds, M. V., Bristow, M. R., Bush, E. W., et al.: Angiotensin-converting enzyme DD genotype in patients with ischaemic or idiopathic dilated cardiomyopathy. Lancet 342:1073, 1993.

58. Bakker, H. D., Scholte, H. R., Luyt-Houwen, I. E., et al.: Neonatal cardiomyopathy and lactic acidosis responsive to thiamine. J. Inherit. Metab. Dis. 14:75, 1991.

59. Bratton, S. L., Garden, A. L., Bohan, T. P., et al.: A child with valproic acid-associated carnitine deficiency and carnitine-responsive cardiac dysfunction. J. Child Neurol. 7:413, 1992.

60. Muir, P., Nicholson, F., Tilzey, A. J., et al.: Chronic relapsing pericarditis and dilated cardiomyopathy: Serological evidence of persistent enterovirus infection. Lancet 1:804, 1989.

61. Shabetai, R.: Myocarditis and dilated cardiomyopathy: Twins or distant relatives? Cardiology 76:332, 1989.

62. Sole, M. J., and Liu, P.: Viral myocarditis: A paradigm for understand-

ing the pathogenesis and treatment of dilated cardiomyopathy. J. Am. Coll. Cardiol. 22:99A, 1993.

63. Keeling, P. J., Lukaszyk, A., Poloniecki, J., et al.: A prospective case-control study of antibodies to coxsackie B virus in idiopathic dilated cardiomyopathy. J. Am. Coll. Cardiol. 23:593, 1994.

64. O'Connell, J. B.: Immunosuppression for dilated cardiomyopathy. N. Engl. J. Med. 321:1119, 1989.

65. Tracy, S., Chapman, N. M., McManus, B. M., et al.: A molecular and serologic evaluation of enteroviral involvement in human myocarditis. J. Mol. Cell Cardiol. 22:403, 1990.

66. Why, H. J., Meany, B. T., Richardson, P. J., et al.: Clinical and prognostic significance of detection of enteroviral RNA in the myocardium of patients with myocarditis or dilated cardiomyopathy. Circulation 89:2582, 1994.

67. Bowles, N. E., Rose, M. L., Taylor, P., et al.: End-stage dilated cardiomyopathy. Persistence of enterovirus RNA in myocardium at cardiac transplantation and lack of immune response. Circulation 80:1128, 1989.

68. Grasso, M., Arbustini, E., Silini, E., et al.: Search for Coxsackievirus B3 RNA in idiopathic dilated cardiomyopathy using gene amplification by polymerase chain reaction. Am. J. Cardiol. 69:658, 1992.

69. Keeling, P. J., Jeffery, S., Caforio, A. L., et al.: Similar prevalence of enteroviral genome within the myocardium from patients with idiopathic dilated cardiomyopathy and controls by the polymerase chain reaction. Br. Heart J. 68:554, 1992.

70. Weiss, L. M., Liu, X. F., Chang, K. L., and Billingham, M. E.: Detection of enteroviral RNA in idiopathic dilated cardiomyopathy and other human cardiac tissues. J. Clin. Invest. 90:156, 1992.

71. Giacca, M., Severini, G. M., Mestroni, L., et al.: Low frequency of detection by nested polymerase chain reaction of enterovirus ribonucleic acid in endomyocardial tissue of patients with idiopathic dilated cardiomyopathy. J. Am. Coll. Cardiol. 24:1033, 1994.

72. Martino, T. A., Liu, P., and Sole, M. J.: Viral infection and the pathogenesis of dilated cardiomyopathy. Circ. Res. 74:182, 1994.

73. Schwaiger, A., Umlauft, F., Weyrer, K., et al.: Detection of enteroviral ribonucleic acid in myocardial biopsies from patients with idiopathic dilated cardiomyopathy by polymerase chain reaction. Am. Heart J. 126:406, 1993.

74. Satoh, M., Tamura, G., Segawa, I., et al.: Enteroviral RNA in dilated cardiomyopathy. Eur. Heart J. 15:934, 1994.

75. Caforio, A. L., Keeling, P. J., Zachara, E., et al.: Evidence from family studies for autoimmunity in dilated cardiomyopathy. Lancet 344:773, 1994.

76. Limas, C., Limas, C. J., Boudoulas, H., et al.: Anti-beta-receptor antibodies in familial cardiomyopathy: Correlation with HLA-DR and HLA-DQ gene polymorphisms. Am. Heart J. 127:382, 1994.

77. Carlquist, J. F., Ward, R. H., Husebye, D., et al.: Major histocompatibility complex class II gene frequencies by serologic and deoxyribonucleic acid genomic typing in idiopathic dilated cardiomyopathy. Am. J. Cardiol. 74:918, 1994.

78. Barry, W. H.: Mechanisms of immune-mediated myocyte injury. Circulation 89:2421, 1994.

79. Limas, C., Limas, C. J., Boudoulas, H., et al.: HLA-DQA1 and -DQB1 gene haplotypes in familial cardiomyopathy. Am. J. Cardiol. 74:510, 1994.

80. Neumann, D. A., Burek, C. L., Baughman, K. L., et al.: Circulating heart-reactive antibodies in patients with myocarditis or cardiomyopathy. J. Am. Coll. Cardiol. 16:839, 1990.

81. Limas, C. J., and Limas, C.: Immune-mediated modulation of sarcoplasmic reticulum function in human dilated cardiomyopathy. Basic Res. Cardiol. 87(Suppl. 1):269, 1992.

82. Magnusson, Y., Wallukat, G., Waagstein, F., et al.: Autoimmunity in idiopathic dilated cardiomyopathy. Characterization of antibodies against the beta 1-adrenoceptor with positive chronotropic effect. Circulation 89:2760, 1994.

83. Fu, L. X., Magnusson, Y., Bergh, C. H., et al.: Localization of a functional autoimmune epitope on the muscarinic acetylcholine receptor-2 in patients with idiopathic dilated cardiomyopathy. J. Clin. Invest. 91:1964, 1993.

84. Caforio, A. L., Grazzini, M., Mann, J. M., et al.: Identification of alpha- and beta-cardiac myosin heavy chain isoforms as major autoantigens in dilated cardiomyopathy. Circulation 85:1734, 1992.

85. Caforio, A. L. P.: Role of autoimmunity in dilated cardiomyopathy. Br. Heart J. 72:S30, 1994.

86. Herskowitz, A., Vlahov, D., Willoughby, S., et al.: Prevalence and incidence of left ventricular dysfunction in patients with human immunodeficiency virus infection. Am. J. Cardiol. 71:955, 1993.

87. Tomita, T., Murakami, T., Iwase, T., et al.: Chronic dynamic exercise improves a functional abnormality of the G stimulatory protein in cardiomyopathic BIO 53.58 Syrian hamsters. Circulation 89:836, 1994.

88. Gilbert, E. M., Olsen, S. L., Renlund, D. G., and Bristow, M. R.: Beta-adrenergic receptor regulation and left ventricular function in idiopathic dilated cardiomyopathy. Am. J. Cardiol. 71:23C, 1993.

89. Merlet, P., Delforge, J., Syrota, A., et al.: Positron emission tomography with 11C CGP-12177 to assess beta-adrenergic receptor concentration in idiopathic dilated cardiomyopathy. Circulation 87:1169, 1993.

90. Bristow, M. R., Anderson, F. L., Port, J. D., et al.: Differences in beta-adrenergic neuroeffector mechanisms in ischemic versus idiopathic dilated cardiomyopathy. Circulation 84:1024, 1991.

91. Feldman, A. M., Jackson, D. G., Bristow, M. R., et al.: Immunodetectable levels of the inhibitory guanine nucleotide-binding regulatory proteins in failing human heart: Discordance with measurements of adenylate cyclase activity and levels of pertussis toxin substrate. J. Mol. Cell Cardiol. 23:439, 1991.

92. Bristow, M. R., and Feldman, A. M.: Changes in the receptor-G protein-adenylyl cyclase system in heart failure from various types of heart muscle disease. Basic Res. Cardiol. 87(Suppl. 1):15, 1992.

93. Feldman, A. M., Tena, R. G., Kessler, P. D., et al.: Diminished beta-adrenergic receptor responsiveness and cardiac dilation in hearts of myopathic Syrian hamsters (BIO 53.58) are associated with a functional abnormality of the G stimulatory protein. Circulation 81:1341, 1990.

94. Bohm, M., Gierschik, P., Jakobs, K. H., et al.: Increase of Gi alpha in human hearts with dilated but not ischemic cardiomyopathy. Circulation 82:1249, 1990.

95. Wikman-Coffelt, J., Stefenelli, T., Wu, S. T., et al.: [Ca²⁺]i transients in the cardiomyopathic hamster heart. Circ. Res. 68:45, 1991.

96. Hasenfuss, G., Reinecke, H., Studer, R., et al.: Relation between myocardial function and expression of sarcoplasmic reticulum Ca(2+)-ATPase in failing and nonfailing human myocardium. Circ. Res. 75:434, 1994.

97. Studer, R., Reinecke, H., Bilger, J., et al.: Gene expression of the cardiac Na(+)-Ca²⁺ exchanger in end-stage human heart failure. Circ. Res. 75:443, 1994.

98. Jeck, C. D., Zimmermann, R., Schaper, J., and Schaper, W.: Decreased expression of calmodulin mRNA in human end-stage heart failure. J. Mol. Cell Cardiol. 26:99, 1994.

99. Go, L. O., Moschella, M. C., Watras, J., et al.: Differential regulation of two types of intracellular calcium release channels during end-stage heart failure. J. Clin. Invest. 95:888, 1995.

100. Stewart, R. A., McKenna, W. J., and Oakley, C. M.: Good prognosis for dilated cardiomyopathy without severe heart failure or arrhythmia. Q. J. Med. 74:309, 1990.

101. Caforio, A. L., Rossi, B., Risaliti, R., et al.: Type 1 fiber abnormalities in skeletal muscle of patients with hypertrophic and dilated cardiomyopathy: Evidence of subclinical myogenic myopathy. J. Am. Coll. Cardiol. 14:1464, 1989.

102. Komajda, M., Jais, J. P., Reeves, F., et al.: Factors predicting mortality in idiopathic dilated cardiomyopathy. Eur. Heart J. 11:824, 1990.

103. Treasure, C. B., Vita, J. A., Cox, D. A., et al.: Endothelium-dependent dilation of the coronary microvasculature is impaired in dilated cardiomyopathy. Circulation 81:772, 1990.

104. Cabanes, L. R., Weber, S. N., Matran, R., et al.: Bronchial hyperresponsiveness to methacholine in patients with impaired left ventricular function. N. Engl. J. Med. 320:1317, 1989.

105. Feldman, M. D., and Beller, G. A.: Is secondary mitral regurgitation in congestive heart failure a marker of clinical importance? J. Am. Coll. Cardiol. 15:181, 1990.

106. Wilensky, R. L., Yudelman, P., Cohen, A. I., et al.: Serial electrocardiographic changes in idiopathic dilated cardiomyopathy confirmed at necropsy. Am. J. Cardiol. 62:276, 1988.

107. Keogh, A. M., Baron, D. W., and Hickie, J. B.: Prognostic guides in patients with idiopathic or ischemic dilated cardiomyopathy assessed for cardiac transplantation. Am. J. Cardiol. 65:903, 1990.

108. De Maria, R., Gavazzi, A., Caroli, A., et al.: Ventricular arrhythmias in dilated cardiomyopathy as an independent prognostic hallmark. Italian Multicenter Cardiomyopathy Study (SPIC) Group. Am. J. Cardiol. 69:1451, 1992.

109. Corey, W. A., Markel, M. L., Hoit, B. D., and Walsh, R. A.: Regression of a dilated cardiomyopathy after radiofrequency ablation of incessant supraventricular tachycardia. Am. Heart J. 126:1469, 1993.

110. Cruz, F. E., Cheriex, E. C., Smeets, J. L., et al.: Reversibility of tachycardia-induced cardiomyopathy after cure of incessant supraventricular tachycardia. J. Am. Coll. Cardiol. 16:739, 1990.

111. Yoshimura, H., Ishikawa, T., Kuji, N., et al.: Two cases of dilated cardiomyopathy associated with incessant supraventricular tachycardia who showed a favorable response to beta-blockade. Heart Vessels 5(Suppl.):88, 1990.

112. Katritsis, D., Leatham, E., Pumphrey, C., et al.: Low-energy DC catheter ablation of left atrial ectopic tachycardia that had resulted in reversible cardiomyopathy. PACE Pacing Clin. Electrophysiol. 16:1345, 1993.

113. Pinamonti, B., Di Lenarda, A., Sinagra, G., and Camerini, F.: Restrictive left ventricular filling pattern in dilated cardiomyopathy assessed by Doppler echocardiography: Clinical, echocardiographic and hemodynamic correlations and prognostic implications. Heart Muscle Disease Study Group. J. Am. Coll. Cardiol. 22:808, 1993.

114. Sharp, S. M., Sawada, S. G., Segar, D. S., et al.: Dobutamine stress echocardiography: Detection of coronary artery disease in patients with dilated cardiomyopathy. J. Am. Coll. Cardiol. 24:934, 1994.

114a. Vigna, C., Russo, A., De Rito, V., et al.: Regional wall motion analysis by dobutamine stress echocardiography to distinguish between ischemic and nonischemic dilated cardiomyopathy. Am. Heart J. 131:537, 1996.

115. Tauberg, S. G., Orie, J. E., Bartlett, B. E., et al.: Usefulness of thallium-201 for distinction of ischemic from idiopathic dilated cardiomyopathy. Am. J. Cardiol. 71:674, 1993.

116. Doi, Y. L., Chikamori, T., Tukata, J., et al.: Prognostic value of thallium-201 perfusion defects in idiopathic dilated cardiomyopathy. Am. J. Cardiol. 67:188, 1991.

117. Glamann, D. B., Lange, R. A., Corbett, J. R., and Hillis, L. D.: Utility of various radionuclide techniques for distinguishing ischemic from nonischemic dilated cardiomyopathy. Arch. Intern. Med. 152:769, 1992.

118. Werner, G. S., Figulla, H. R., Munz, D. L., et al.: Myocardial indium-111 antimyosin uptake in patients with idiopathic dilated cardiomyopathy: Its relation to haemodynamics, histomorphometry, myocardial enteroviral infection, and clinical course. Eur. Heart J. 14:175, 1993.

119. Dec, G. W., Palacios, I., Yasuda, T., et al.: Antimyosin antibody cardiac

imaging: Its role in the diagnosis of myocarditis. J. Am. Coll. Cardiol. *16*:97, 1990.

120. Obrador, D., Ballester, M., Carrio, I., et al.: Presence, evolving changes, and prognostic implications of myocardial damage detected in idiopathic and alcoholic dilated cardiomyopathy by ^{111}In monoclonal antimyosin antibodies. Circulation *89*:2054, 1994.

121. Sunnerhagen, K. S., Bhargava, V., and Shabetai, R.: Regional left ventricular wall motion abnormalities in idiopathic dilated cardiomyopathy. Am. J. Cardiol. *65*:364, 1990.

122. Inoue, T., Sakai, Y., Morooka, S., et al.: Vasodilatory capacity of coronary resistance vessels in dilated cardiomyopathy. Am. Heart J. *127*:376, 1994.

123. Inoue, T., Sakai, Y., Morooka, S., et al.: Coronary flow reserve in patients with dilated cardiomyopathy. Am. Heart J. *125*:93, 1993.

124. Shannon, R. P., Komamura, K., Shen, Y. T., et al.: Impaired regional subendocardial coronary flow reserve in conscious dogs with pacing-induced heart failure. Am. J. Physiol. *265*:H801, 1993.

125. O'Connell, J. B., Moore, C. K., and Waterer, H. C.: Treatment of end stage dilated cardiomyopathy. Br. Heart J. *72*:S52, 1994.

125a. O'Connell, J. B., Breen, T. J., and Hosenpud, J. D.: Heart transplantation in dilated heart muscle disease and myocarditis. Eur. Heart J. *16* (Suppl O):137, 1996.

126. The SOLVD Investigators.: Effect of enalapril on survival in patients with reduced left ventricular ejection fraction and congestive heart failure. N. Engl. J. Med. *325*:293, 1991.

127. The CONSENSUS Trial Study Group.: Effects of enalapril on mortality in severe congestive heart failure. Results of the Cooperative North Scandinavian Enalapril Survival Study. N. Engl. J. Med. *316*:1429, 1987.

127a. Cohn, J. N.: ACE inhibitors in non-ischaemic heart failure: Results from the MEGA trials. Eur. Heart J. *16* (Suppl O):133, 1996.

128. Cohn, J. N., Johnson, G., Ziesche, S., et al.: A comparison of enalapril with hydralazine-isosorbide dinitrate in the treatment of chronic congestive heart failure. N. Engl. J. Med. *325*:303, 1991.

128a. Packer, M., Bristow, M. R., Cohn, J. N., et al.: Effect of carvedilol on the survival of patients with chronic heart failure. Circulation *92*(Suppl. I):142, 1995

129. Andersson, B., Hamm, C., Persson, S., et al.: Improved exercise hemodynamic status in dilated cardiomyopathy after beta-adrenergic blockade treatment. J. Am. Coll. Cardiol. *23*:1397, 1994.

130. Waagstein, F., Bristow, M. R., Swedberg, K., et al.: Beneficial effects of metoprolol in idiopathic dilated cardiomyopathy. Metoprolol in Dilated Cardiomyopathy (MDC) Trial Study Group. Lancet *342*:1441, 1993.

131. Marino, P., Prioli, A. M., Destro, G., et al.: The left atrial volume curve can be assessed from pulmonary vein and mitral valve velocity tracings. Am. Heart J. *127*:886, 1994.

132. Eichhorn, E. J., Heesch, C. M., Barnett, J. H., et al.: Effect of metoprolol on myocardial function and energetics in patients with nonischemic dilated cardiomyopathy: A randomized, double-blind, placebo-controlled study. J. Am. Coll. Cardiol. *24*:1310, 1994.

133. Andersson, B., Blomstrom-Lundqvist, C., Hedner, T., and Waagstein, F.: Exercise hemodynamics and myocardial metabolism during long-term beta-adrenergic blockade in severe heart failure. J. Am. Coll. Cardiol. *18*:1059, 1991.

134. Waagstien, F.: Adrenergic beta-blocking agents in congestive heart failure due to idiopathic dilated cardiomyopathy. Eur. Heart J. *16* (Suppl O):128, 1996.

135. Hjalmarson, A., and Waagstein, F.: The role of beta-blockers in the treatment of cardiomyopathy and ischaemic heart failure. Drugs *47*(Suppl. 4):31, 1994.

136. Metra, M., Nardi, M., Giubbini, R., and Dei Cas, L.: Effects of short- and long-term carvedilol administration on rest and exercise hemodynamic variables, exercise capacity and clinical conditions in patients with idiopathic dilated cardiomyopathy. J. Am. Coll. Cardiol. *24*:1678, 1994.

137. Ishida, S., Makino, N., Masutomo, K., et al.: Effect of metoprolol on the beta-adrenoceptor density of lymphocytes in patients with dilated cardiomyopathy. Am. Heart J. *125*:1311, 1993.

138. Asseman, P., McFadden, E., Bauchart, J. J., et al.: Why do beta-blockers help in idiopathic dilated cardiomyopathy—frequency mismatch? Lancet *344*:803, 1994.

139. Sato, H., Hori, M., Ozaki, H., et al.: Exercise-induced upward shift of diastolic left ventricular pressure-volume relation in patients with dilated cardiomyopathy. Effects of beta-adrenoceptor blockade. Circulation *88*:2215, 1993.

140. Swedberg, K.: Initial experience with beta blockers in dilated cardiomyopathy. Am. J. Cardiol. *71*:30C, 1993.

141. Fowler, M. B.: Controlled trials with beta blockers in heart failure: Metoprolol as the prototype. Am. J. Cardiol. *71*:45C, 1993.

141a. Cohn, J. N., Ziesche, S. M., Loss, L. E., Anderson, G. F., and the V-HeFT Study Group: Effect of felodipine on short-term exercise and neurohormone and long-term mortality in heart failure: Results of V-HeFT III. Circulation *92*(Suppl. I):143, 1995.

142. Figulla, H. R., Rechenberg, J. V., Wiegand, V., et al.: Beneficial effects of long-term diltiazem treatment in dilated cardiomyopathy. J. Am. Coll. Cardiol. *13*:653, 1989.

142a. Singh, S. N., Fletcher, R. D., Fisher, S. G., et al.: Amiodarone in patients with congestive heart failure and asymptomatic ventricular arrhythmia. N. Engl. J. Med. *333*:77, 1995.

143. Chen, X., Shenasa, M., Borggrefe, M., et al.: Role of programmed ventricular stimulation in patients with idiopathic dilated cardiomyopathy and documented sustained ventricular tachyarrhythmias: Inducibility and prognostic value in 102 patients. Eur. Heart J. *15*:76, 1994.

144. Kulick, D. L., Bhandari, A. K., Hong, R., et al.: Effect of acute hemodynamic decompensation on electrical inducibility of ventricular arrhythmias in patients with dilated cardiomyopathy and complex nonsustained ventricular arrhythmias. Am. Heart J. *119*:878, 1990.

145. Turitto, G., Ahuja, R. K., Bekheit, S., et al.: Incidence and prediction of induced ventricular tachyarrhythmias in idiopathic dilated cardiomyopathy. Am. J. Cardiol. *73*:770, 1994.

146. Mancini, D. M., Wong, K. L., and Simson, M. B.: Prognostic value of an abnormal signal-averaged electrocardiogram in patients with nonischemic congestive cardiomyopathy. Circulation *87*:1083, 1993.

147. Yi, G., Keeling, P. J., Goldman, J. H., et al.: Prognostic significance of spectral turbulence analysis of the signal-averaged electrocardiogram in patients with idiopathic dilated cardiomyopathy. Am. J. Cardiol. *75*:494, 1995.

148. Turitto, G., Ahuja, R. K., Caref, E. B., and el-Sherif, N.: Risk stratification for arrhythmic events in patients with nonischemic dilated cardiomyopathy and nonsustained ventricular tachycardia: Role of programmed ventricular stimulation and the signal-averaged electrocardiogram. J. Am. Coll. Cardiol. *24*:1523, 1994.

149. Winters, S. L., Goldman, D. S., and Banas, J. S. Jr.: Prognostic impact of late potentials in nonischemic dilated cardiomyopathy. Potential signals for the future. Circulation *87*:1405, 1993.

150. Borggrefe, M., Chen, X., Martinez-Rubio, A., et al.: The role of implantable cardioverter defibrillators in dilated cardiomyopathy. Am. Heart J. *127*:1145, 1994.

151. Lessmeier, T. J., Lehmann, M. H., Steinman, R. T., et al.: Outcome with implantable cardioverter-defibrillator therapy for survivors of ventricular fibrillation secondary to idiopathic dilated cardiomyopathy or coronary artery disease without myocardial infarction. Am. J. Cardiol. *72*:911, 1993.

152. Cheng, J. W., and Spinler, S. A.: Should all patients with dilated cardiomyopathy receive chronic anticoagulation? Ann. Pharmacother. *28*:604, 1994.

153. Falk, R. H.: A plea for a clinical trial of anticoagulation in dilated cardiomyopathy. Am. J. Cardiol. *65*:914, 1990.

154. Latham, R. D., Mulrow, J. P., Virmani, R., et al.: Recently diagnosed idiopathic dilated cardiomyopathy: Incidence of myocarditis and efficacy of prednisone therapy. Am. Heart J. *117*:876, 1989.

155. Parrillo, J. E., Cunnion, R. E., Epstein, S. E., et al.: A prospective, randomized, controlled trial of prednisone for dilated cardiomyopathy. N. Engl. J. Med. *321*:1061, 1989.

156. Lalinde, E., Sanz, J., Bazan, A., et al.: The use of latissimus dorsi muscle flap in reconstructive heart surgery. Plast. Reconstr. Surg. *94*:490, 1994.

157. Bocchi, E. A., Bellotti, G., Moreira, L. F., et al.: Prognostic indicators of one-year outcome after cardiomyoplasty for idiopathic dilated cardiomyopathy. Am. J. Cardiol. *73*:604, 1994.

158. Bellotti, G., Moraes, A., Bocchi, E., et al.: Late effects of cardiomyoplasty on left ventricular mechanics and diastolic filling. Circulation *88*:II304, 1993.

159. Lorusso, R., Zogno, M., La Canna, G., et al.: Dynamic cardiomyoplasty as an effective therapy for dilated cardiomyopathy. J. Card. Surg. *8*:177, 1993.

160. Moreira, L. F., Bocchi, E. A., Stolf, N. A., et al.: Current expectations in dynamic cardiomyoplasty. Ann. Thorac. Surg. *55*:299, 1993.

161. Chiu, R. C.: Dynamic cardiomyoplasty for heart failure (editorial). Br. Heart J. *73*:1, 1995.

162. Bocchi, E. A., Moreira, L. F., de Moraes, A. V., et al.: Arrhythmias and sudden death after dynamic cardiomyoplasty. Circulation *90*:II107, 1994.

163. Fernandez-Sola, J., Estruch, R., Grau, J. M., et al.: The relation of alcoholic myopathy to cardiomyopathy. Ann. Intern. Med. *120*:529, 1994.

164. Regan, T. J.: Alcohol and the cardiovascular system. JAMA *264*:377, 1990.

165. Piano, M. R., and Schwertz, D. W.: Alcoholic heart disease: A review. Heart Lung *23*:3, 1994.

166. Preedy, V. R., Atkinson, L. M., Richardson, P. J., and Peters, T. J.: Mechanisms of ethanol-induced cardiac damage. Br. Heart J. *69*:197, 1993.

167. Jarvis, J. Q., Hammond, E., Meier, R., and Robinson, C.: Cobalt cardiomyopathy. A report of two cases from mineral assay laboratories and a review of the literature. J. Occup. Med. *34*:620, 1992.

168. Urbano-Marquez, A., Estruch, R., Navarro-Lopez, F., et al.: The effects of alcoholism on skeletal and cardiac muscle. N. Engl. J. Med. *320*:409, 1989.

169. Djoenaidi, W., Notermans, S. L., and Dunda, G.: Beriberi cardiomyopathy. Eur. J. Clin. Nutr. *46*:227, 1992.

170. Guarnieri, T., and Lakatta, E. G.: Mechanism of myocardial contractile depression by clinical concentrations of ethanol. A study in ferret papillary muscles. J. Clin. Invest. *85*:1462, 1990.

171. Diamond, I.: Alcoholic myopathy and cardiomyopathy. N. Engl. J. Med. *320*:458, 1989.

172. Rubin, E., and Urbano-Marquez, A.: Alcoholic cardiomyopathy. Alcohol. Clin. Exp. Res. *18*:111, 1994.

173. Teragaki, M., Takeuchi, K., and Takeda, T.: Clinical and histologic features of alcohol drinkers with congestive heart failure. Am. Heart J. *125*:808, 1993.

174. Cerqueira, M. D., Harp, G. D., Ritchie, J. L., et al.: Rarity of preclinical alcoholic cardiomyopathy in chronic alcoholics < 40 years of age. Am. J. Cardiol. *67*:183, 1991.

175. Fabrizio, L., and Regan, T. J.: Alcoholic cardiomyopathy. Cardiovasc. Drugs Ther. *8*:89, 1994.

176. Kupari, M., Koskinen, P., and Suokas, A.: Left ventricular size, mass and function in relation to the duration and quantity of heavy drinking in alcoholics. Am. J. Cardiol. *67*:274, 1991.

177. Nethala, V., Brown, E. J. Jr., Timson, C. R., and Patcha, R.: Reversal of alcoholic cardiomyopathy in a patient with severe coronary artery disease. Chest *104*:626, 1993.

178. Seghizzi, P., D'Adda, F., Borleri, D., et al.: Cobalt myocardiopathy. A critical review of literature. Sci. Total Environ. *150*:105, 1994.

179. Mehta, D., Davies, M. J., Ward, D. E., and Camm, A. J.: Ventricular tachycardias of right ventricular origin: Markers of subclinical right ventricular disease. Am. Heart J. *127*:360, 1994.

180. Wichter, T., Hindricks, G., Lerch, H., et al.: Regional myocardial sympathetic dysinnervation in arrhythmogenic right ventricular cardiomyopathy. An analysis using 123I-meta-iodobenzylguanidine scintigraphy. Circulation *89*:667, 1994.

181. Ricci, C., Longo, R., Pagnan, L., et al.: Magnetic resonance imaging in right ventricular dysplasia. Am. J. Cardiol. *70*:1589, 1992.

182. McKenna, W. J., Thiene, G., Nava, A., et al.: Diagnosis of arrhythmogenic right ventricular dysplasia/cardiomyopathy. Task Force of the Working Group Myocardial and Pericardial Disease of the European Society of Cardiology and of the Scientific Council on Cardiomyopathies of the International Society and Federation of Cardiology. Br. Heart J. *71*:215, 1994.

183. Rampazzo, A., Nava, A., Danieli, G. A., et al.: The gene for arrhythmogenic right ventricular cardiomyopathy maps to chromosome 14q23-q24. Hum. Mol. Genet. *3*:959, 1994.

184. Nava, A., Thiene, G., Canciani, B., et al.: Familial occurrence of right ventricular dysplasia: A study involving nine families. J. Am. Coll. Cardiol. *12*:1222, 1988.

185. Angelini, A., Thiene, G., Boffa, G. M., et al.: Endomyocardial biopsy in right ventricular cardiomyopathy. Int. J. Cardiol. *40*:273, 1993.

186. Metzger, J. T., de Chillou, C., Cheriex, E., et al.: Value of the 12-lead electrocardiogram in arrhythmogenic right ventricular dysplasia, and absence of correlation with echocardiographic findings. Am. J. Cardiol. *72*:964, 1993.

187. Buja, G. F., Nava, A., Martini, B., et al.: Right ventricular dysplasia: A familial cardiomyopathy? Eur. Heart J. *10*(Suppl. D):13, 1989.

188. Thiene, G., Nava, A., Corrado, D., et al.: Right ventricular cardiomyopathy and sudden death in young people. N. Engl. J. Med. *318*:129, 1988.

189. Scognamiglio, R., Fasoli, G., Nava, A., et al.: Relevance of subtle echocardiographic findings in the early diagnosis of the concealed form of right ventricular dysplasia. Eur. Heart J. *10*(Suppl. D):27, 1989.

190. Nava, A., Canciani, B., Daliento, L., et al.: Juvenile sudden death and effort ventricular tachycardias in a family with right ventricular cardiomyopathy. Int. J. Cardiol. *21*:111, 1988.

191. Nava, A., Thiene, G., Canciani, B., et al.: Clinical profile of concealed form of arrhythmogenic right ventricular cardiomyopathy presenting with apparently idiopathic ventricular arrhythmias. Int. J. Cardiol. *35*:195, 1992.

192. Martini, B., Nava, A., Thiene, G., et al.: Monomorphic repetitive rhythms originating from the outflow tract in patients with minor forms of right ventricular cardiomyopathy. Int. J. Cardiol. *27*:211, 1990.

193. Pinamonti, B., Sinagra, G., Di Lenarda, A., et al.: Left ventricular involvement in right ventricular cardiomyopathy. Postgrad. Med. J. *68*(Suppl. 1):S36, 1992.

194. Martini, B., Nava, A., and Buja, G. F.: Complex arrhythmias in a patient with predominantly right ventricular cardiomyopathy. Int. J. Cardiol. *19*:268, 1988.

195. Blake, L. M., Scheinman, M. M., and Higgins, C. B.: MR features of arrhythmogenic right ventricular dysplasia. A.J.R. *162*:809, 1994.

196. Misaki, T., Watanabe, G., Iwa, T., et al.: Surgical treatment of arrhythmogenic right ventricular dysplasia: Long-term outcome. Ann. Thorac. Surg. *58*:1380, 1994.

HYPERTROPHIC CARDIOMYOPATHY

197. Braunwald, E.: Hypertrophic cardiomyopathy—continued progress. N. Engl. J. Med. *320*:800, 1989.

198. Maron, B. J.: Hypertrophic cardiomyopathy. Curr. Probl. Cardiol. *18*:639, 1993.

199. Louie, E. K., and Edwards, L. C. 3rd.: Hypertrophic cardiomyopathy. Prog. Cardiovasc. Dis. *36*:275, 1994.

200. Davies, M. J., and Krikler, D. M.: Genetic investigation and counselling of families with hypertrophic cardiomyopathy. Br. Heart J. *72*:99, 1994.

201. Watkins, H.: Multiple disease genes cause hypertrophic cardiomyopathy. Br. Heart J. *72*:S4, 1994.

202. Codd, M. B., Sugrue, D. D., Gersh, B. J., and Melton, L. J. 3rd.: Epidemiology of idiopathic dilated and hypertrophic cardiomyopathy. A population-based study in Olmsted County, Minnesota, 1975–1984. Circulation *80*:564, 1989.

202a. Maron, B. J., Gardin, J. M., Flack, J. M., et al.: Prevalence of hypertrophic cardiomyopathy in a general population of young adults. Echocardiographic analysis of 4111 subjects in the CARDIA Study. Circulation *92*:785, 1995.

203. Maron, B. J., Peterson, E. E., Maron, M. S., and Peterson, J. E.: Prevalence of hypertrophic cardiomyopathy in an outpatient population referred for echocardiographic study. Am. J. Cardiol. *73*:577, 1994.

204. McKenna, W. J., Kleinebenne, A., Nihoyannopoulos, P., and Foale, R.: Echocardiographic measurement of right ventricular wall thickness in hypertrophic cardiomyopathy: Relation to clinical and prognostic features. J. Am. Coll. Cardiol. *11*:351, 1988.

205. Maron, B. J., Isner, J. M., and McKenna, W. J.: 26th Bethesda conference: recommendations for determining eligibility for competition in athletes with cardiovascular abnormalities. Task Force 3: Hypertrophic

cardiomyopathy, myocarditis and other myopericardial diseases and mitral valve prolapse. J. Am. Coll. Cardiol. *24*:880, 1994.

206. Maron, B. J., Pelliccia, A., Spataro, A., and Granata, M.: Reduction in left ventricular wall thickness after deconditioning in highly trained Olympic athletes. Br. Heart J. *69*:125, 1993.

207. Maron, B. J., Pelliccia, A., and Spirito, P.: Cardiac disease in young trained athletes. Insights into methods for distinguishing athlete's heart from structural heart disease, with particular emphasis on hypertrophic cardiomyopathy. Circulation *91*:1596, 1995.

208. Lewis, J. F., and Maron, B. J.: Hypertrophic cardiomyopathy characterized by marked hypertrophy of the posterior left ventricular free wall: Significance and clinical implications. J. Am. Coll. Cardiol. *18*:421, 1991.

209. Maron, B. J.: Apical hypertrophic cardiomyopathy: The continuing saga. J. Am. Coll. Cardiol. *15*:91, 1990.

210. Suzuki, J., Watanabe, F., Takenaka, K., et al.: New subtype of apical hypertrophic cardiomyopathy identified with nuclear magnetic resonance imaging as an underlying cause of markedly inverted T waves. J. Am. Coll. Cardiol. *22*:1175, 1993.

211. Webb, J. G., Sasson, Z., Rakowski, H., et al.: Apical hypertrophic cardiomyopathy: Clinical follow-up and diagnostic correlates. J. Am. Coll. Cardiol. *15*:83, 1990.

212. Smolders, W., Rademakers, F., Conraads, V., and Snoeck, J.: Apical hypertrophic cardiomyopathy. Acta Cardiol. *48*:369, 1993.

213. Shapiro, L. M.: Hypertrophic cardiomyopathy in the elderly. Br. Heart J. *63*:265, 1990.

214. Karam, R., Lever, H. M., and Healy, B. P.: Hypertensive hypertrophic cardiomyopathy or hypertrophic cardiomyopathy with hypertension? A study of 78 patients. J. Am. Coll. Cardiol. *13*:580, 1989.

215. Lewis, J. F., and Maron, B. J.: Elderly patients with hypertrophic cardiomyopathy: A subset with distinctive left ventricular morphology and progressive clinical course late in life. J. Am. Coll. Cardiol. *13*:36, 1989.

216. Lever, H. M., Karam, R. F., Currie, P. J., and Healy, B. P.: Hypertrophic cardiomyopathy in the elderly. Distinctions from the young based on cardiac shape. Circulation *79*:580, 1989.

217. Davies, M. J.: Hypertrophic cardiomyopathy: One disease or several? Br. Heart J. *63*:263, 1990.

218. Davies, M. J., and McKenna, W. J.: Hypertrophic cardiomyopathy: An introduction to pathology and pathogenesis. Br. Heart J. *72*:S2, 1994.

219. Wilmshurst, P. T., and Katritsis, D.: Restrictive cardiomyopathy. Br. Heart J. *63*:323, 1990.

220. Carvalho, J. S., Matthews, E. E., Leonard, J. V., and Deanfield, J.: Cardiomyopathy of glycogen storage disease type III. Heart Vessels *8*:155, 1993.

221. Factor, S. M., Butany, J., Sole, M. J., et al.: Pathologic fibrosis and matrix connective tissue in the subaortic myocardium of patients with hypertrophic cardiomyopathy. J. Am. Coll. Cardiol. *17*:1343, 1991.

222. Maron, B. J., Wolfson, J. K., and Roberts, W. C.: Relation between extent of cardiac muscle cell disorganization and left ventricular wall thickness in hypertrophic cardiomyopathy. Am. J. Cardiol. *70*:785, 1992.

223. Roberts, R.: Molecular genetics. Therapy or terror? Circulation *89*:499, 1994.

224. Sapp, J. L., and Howlett, S. E.: Density of ryanodine receptors is increased in sarcoplasmic reticulum from prehypertrophic cardiomyopathic hamster heart. J. Mol. Cell Cardiol. *26*:325, 1994.

225. Bonow, R. O.: Left ventricular diastolic function in hypertrophic cardiomyopathy. Herz *16*:13, 1991.

226. Wagner, J. A., Sax, F. L., Weisman, H. F., et al.: Calcium-antagonist receptors in the atrial tissue of patients with hypertrophic cardiomyopathy. N. Engl. J. Med. *320*:755, 1989.

227. Lefroy, D. C., de Silva, R., Choudhury, L., et al.: Diffuse reduction of myocardial beta-adrenoceptors in hypertrophic cardiomyopathy: A study with positron emission tomography. J. Am. Coll. Cardiol. *22*:1653, 1993.

228. Brush, J. E. Jr., Eisenhofer, G., Garty, M., et al.: Cardiac norepinephrine kinetics in hypertrophic cardiomyopathy. Circulation *79*:836, 1989.

229. Clark, A. L., and Coats, A. J.: Screening for hypertrophic cardiomyopathy. B.M.J. *306*:409, 1993.

230. Watkins, H., Thierfelder, L., Hwang, D. S., et al.: Sporadic hypertrophic cardiomyopathy due to de novo myosin mutations. J. Clin. Invest. *90*:1666, 1992.

231. Keating, M.: The devil's in the details: Progress in familial hypertrophic cardiomyopathy. J. Clin. Invest. *93*:2, 1994.

232. Solomon, S. D., Jarcho, J. A., McKenna, W., et al.: Familial hypertrophic cardiomyopathy is a genetically heterogeneous disease. J. Clin. Invest. *86*:993, 1990.

233. Jarcho, J. A., McKenna, W., Pare, J. A., et al.: Mapping a gene for familial hypertrophic cardiomyopathy to chromosome 14q1. N. Engl. J. Med. *321*:1372, 1989.

234. MacRae, C. A., Watkins, H. C., Jarcho, J. A., et al.: An evaluation of ribonuclease protection assays for the detection of beta-cardiac myosin heavy chain gene mutations. Circulation *89*:33, 1994.

235. Thierfelder, L., Watkins, H., MacRae, C., et al.: Alpha-tropomyosin and cardiac troponin T mutations cause familial hypertrophic cardiomyopathy: A disease of the sarcomere. Cell *77*:701, 1994.

235a. Watkins, H., McKenna, W. J., Thierfelder, L., et al.: Mutations in the genes for cardiac troponin T and α-tropomyosin in hypertrophic cardiomyopathy. N. Engl. J. Med. *332*:1058, 1995.

236. Okamoto, S., Ozaki, M., Konishi, T., and Nakano, T.: A case report of

siblings with hypertrophic cardiomyopathy that progressed to dilated cardiomyopathy—case reports. Angiology 44:406, 1993.

237. Solomon, S. D., Wolff, S., Watkins, H., et al.: Left ventricular hypertrophy and morphology in familial hypertrophic cardiomyopathy associated with mutations of the beta-myosin heavy chain gene. J. Am. Coll. Cardiol. 22:498, 1993.

238. Hecht, G. M., Klues, H. G., Roberts, W. C., and Maron, B. J.: Coexistence of sudden cardiac death and end-stage heart failure in familial hypertrophic cardiomyopathy. J. Am. Coll. Cardiol. 22:489, 1993.

239. Watkins, H., Rosenzweig, A., Hwang, D. S., et al.: Characteristics and prognostic implications of myosin missense mutations in familial hypertrophic cardiomyopathy. N. Engl. J. Med. 326:1108, 1992.

240. Anan, R., Greve, G., Thierfelder, L., et al.: Prognostic implications of novel beta cardiac myosin heavy chain gene mutations that cause familial hypertrophic cardiomyopathy. J. Clin. Invest. 93:280, 1994.

241. Rosenzweig, A., Watkins, H., Hwang, D. S., et al.: Preclinical diagnosis of familial hypertrophic cardiomyopathy by genetic analysis of blood lymphocytes. N. Engl. J. Med. 325:1753, 1991.

242. Al-Mahadawi, S., Chamberlain, S., Chojnowska, L., et al.: The electrocardiogram is more sensitive than echocardiography of hypertrophic cardiomyopathy in families with a mutation in the MYH7 gene. Br. Heart J. 72:105, 1994.

243. Criley, J. M., and Siegel, R. J.: Subaortic stenosis revisited: The importance of the dynamic pressure gradient. Medicine (Baltimore) 72:412, 1993.

244. Kramer, D. S., French, W. J., and Criley, J. M.: The postextrasystolic murmur response to gradient in hypertrophic cardiomyopathy. Ann. Intern. Med. 104:772, 1986.

245. Sherrid, M. V., Chu, C. K., Delia, E., et al.: An echocardiographic study of the fluid mechanics of obstruction in hypertrophic cardiomyopathy. J. Am. Coll. Cardiol. 22:816, 1993.

246. Betocchi, S., Hess, O. M., Losi, M. A., et al.: Regional left ventricular mechanics in hypertrophic cardiomyopathy. Circulation 88:2206, 1993.

247. Hayashida, W., Kumada, T., Kohno, F., et al.: Left ventricular regional relaxation and its nonuniformity in hypertrophic nonobstructive cardiomyopathy. Circulation 84:1496, 1991.

248. Spirito, P., and Maron, B. J.: Relation between extent of left ventricular hypertrophy and diastolic filling abnormalities in hypertrophic cardiomyopathy. J. Am. Coll. Cardiol. 15:808, 1990.

249. Losi, M. A., Betocchi, S., Grimaldi, M., et al.: Heterogeneity of left ventricular filling dynamics in hypertrophic cardiomyopathy. Am. J. Cardiol. 73:987, 1994.

250. Wigle, E. D.: Impaired left ventricular relaxation in hypertrophic cardiomyopathy: Relation to extent of hypertrophy. J. Am. Coll. Cardiol. 15:814, 1990.

251. Gwathmey, J. K., Warren, S. E., Briggs, G. M., et al.: Diastolic dysfunction in hypertrophic cardiomyopathy. Effect on active force generation during systole. J. Clin. Invest. 87:1023, 1991.

252. Perrone-Filardi, P., Bacharach, S. L., Dilsizian, V., et al.: Regional systolic function, myocardial blood flow and glucose uptake at rest in hypertrophic cardiomyopathy. Am. J. Cardiol. 72:199, 1993.

253. Tomochika, Y., Tanaka, N., Wasaki, Y., et al.: Assessment of flow profile of left anterior descending coronary artery in hypertrophic cardiomyopathy by transesophageal pulsed Doppler echocardiography. Am. J. Cardiol. 72:1425, 1993.

254. Memmola, C., Iliceto, S., Napoli, V. F., et al.: Coronary flow dynamics and reserve assessed by transesophageal echocardiography in obstructive hypertrophic cardiomyopathy. Am. J. Cardiol. 74:1147, 1994.

255. Spirito, P., Chiarella, F., Carratino, L., et al.: Clinical course and prognosis of hypertrophic cardiomyopathy in an outpatient population. N. Engl. J. Med. 320:749, 1989.

256. Lewis, J. F., and Maron, B. J.: Clinical and morphologic expression of hypertrophic cardiomyopathy in patients > or = 65 years of age. Am. J. Cardiol. 73:1105, 1994.

257. Frank, S., and Braunwald, E.: Idiopathic hypertrophic subaortic stenosis. Clinical analysis of 126 patients with emphasis on the natural history. Circulation 37:759, 1968.

258. Chikamori, T., Counihan, P. J., Doi, Y. L., et al.: Mechanisms of exercise limitation in hypertrophic cardiomyopathy. J. Am. Coll. Cardiol. 19:507, 1992.

259. Nienaber, C. A., Hiller, S., Spielmann, R. P., et al.: Syncope in hypertrophic cardiomyopathy: Multivariate analysis of prognostic determinants. J. Am. Coll. Cardiol. 15:948, 1990.

260. Kar, A. K., Roy, S., and Panja, M.: Aortic regurgitation in hypertrophic cardiomyopathy. J. Assoc. Physicians India 41:576, 1993.

261. Brown, P. S. Jr., Roberts, C. S., McIntosh, C. L., and Clark, R. E.: Aortic regurgitation after left ventricular myotomy and myectomy. Ann. Thorac. Surg. 51:585, 1991.

262. Usui, M., Inoue, H., Suzuki, J., et al.: Relationship between distribution of hypertrophy and electrocardiographic changes in hypertrophic cardiomyopathy. Am. Heart J. 126:177, 1993.

263. Alfonso, F., Nihoyannopoulos, P., Stewart, J., et al.: Clinical significance of giant negative T waves in hypertrophic cardiomyopathy. J. Am. Coll. Cardiol. 15:965, 1990.

264. Lemery, R., Kleinebenne, A., Nihoyannopoulos, P., et al.: Q waves in hypertrophic cardiomyopathy in relation to the distribution and severity of right and left ventricular hypertrophy. J. Am. Coll. Cardiol. 16:368, 1990.

265. Maron, B. J.: Q waves in hypertrophic cardiomyopathy: A reassessment. J. Am. Coll. Cardiol. 16:375, 1990.

266. Fananapazir, L., Tracy, C. M., Leon, M. B., et al.: Electrophysiologic abnormalities in patients with hypertrophic cardiomyopathy. A consecutive analysis in 155 patients. Circulation 80:1259, 1989.

267. Stewart, J. T., and McKenna, W. J.: Management of arrhythmias in hypertrophic cardiomyopathy. Cardiovasc. Drugs Ther. 8:95, 1994.

268. DeRose, J. J. Jr., Banas, J. S. Jr., and Winters, S. L.: Current perspectives on sudden cardiac death in hypertrophic cardiomyopathy. Prog. Cardiovasc. Dis. 36:475, 1994.

269. Fananapazir, L., Chang, A. C., Epstein, S. E., and McAreavey, D.: Prognostic determinants in hypertrophic cardiomyopathy. Prospective evaluation of a therapeutic strategy based on clinical, Holter, hemodynamic, and electrophysiological findings. Circulation 86:730, 1992.

270. McAreavey, D., and Fananapazir, L.: Suppression of incessant ventricular tachycardia in hypertrophic cardiomyopathy associated with improvement of severe left ventricular dysfunction. PACE Pacing Clin. Electrophysiol. 15:1642, 1992.

271. Fananapazir, L., Leon, M. B., Bonow, R. O., et al.: Sudden death during empiric amiodarone therapy in symptomatic hypertrophic cardiomyopathy. Am. J. Cardiol. 67:169, 1991.

272. Fananapazir, L., and Epstein, S. E.: Value of electrophysiologic studies in hypertrophic cardiomyopathy treated with amiodarone. Am. J. Cardiol. 67:175, 1991.

273. Fananapazir, L., and Epstein, S. E.: Hemodynamic and electrophysiologic evaluation of patients with hypertrophic cardiomyopathy surviving cardiac arrest. Am. J. Cardiol. 67:280, 1991.

274. Lazzeroni, E., Domenicucci, S., Finardi, A., et al.: Severity of arrhythmias and extent of hypertrophy in hypertrophic cardiomyopathy. Am. Heart J. 118:734, 1989.

275. Alfonso, F., Frenneaux, M. P., and McKenna, W. J.: Clinical sustained uniform ventricular tachycardia in hypertrophic cardiomyopathy: Association with left ventricular apical aneurysm. Br. Heart J. 61:178, 1989.

276. Spirito, P., Lakatos, E., and Maron, B. J.: Degree of left ventricular hypertrophy in patients with hypertrophic cardiomyopathy and chronic atrial fibrillation. Am. J. Cardiol. 69:1217, 1992.

277. Robinson, K., Frenneaux, M. P., Stockins, B., et al.: Atrial fibrillation in hypertrophic cardiomyopathy: A longitudinal study. J. Am. Coll. Cardiol. 15:1279, 1990.

278. Kulakowski, P., Counihan, P. J., Camm, A. J., and McKenna, W. J.: The value of time and frequency domain, and spectral temporal mapping analysis of the signal-averaged electrocardiogram in identification of patients with hypertrophic cardiomyopathy at increased risk of sudden death. Eur. Heart J. 14:941, 1993.

279. Ajiki, K., Murakawa, Y., Yanagisawa-Miwa, A., et al.: Autonomic nervous system activity in idiopathic dilated cardiomyopathy and in hypertrophic cardiomyopathy. Am. J. Cardiol. 71:1316, 1993.

280. Counihan, P. J., Fei, L., Bashir, Y., et al.: Assessment of heart rate variability in hypertrophic cardiomyopathy. Association with clinical and prognostic features. Circulation 88:1682, 1993.

281. Maron, B. J., Cecchi, F., and McKenna, W. J.: Risk factors and stratification for sudden death in patients with hypertrophic cardiomyopathy. Br. Heart J. 72:S13, 1994.

282. Sneddon, J. F., Slade, A., Seo, H., et al.: Assessment of the diagnostic value of head-up tilt testing in the evaluation of syncope in hypertrophic cardiomyopathy. Am. J. Cardiol. 73:601, 1994.

283. Klues, H. G., Roberts, W. C., and Maron, B. J.: Morphological determinants of echocardiographic patterns of mitral valve systolic anterior motion in obstructive hypertrophic cardiomyopathy. Circulation 87:1570, 1993.

284. Lattanzi, F., Spirito, P., Picano, E., et al.: Quantitative assessment of ultrasonic myocardial reflectivity in hypertrophic cardiomyopathy. J. Am. Coll. Cardiol. 17:1085, 1991.

285. Naito, J., Masuyama, T., Tanouchi, J., et al.: Analysis of transmural trend of myocardial integrated ultrasound backscatter for differentiation of hypertrophic cardiomyopathy and ventricular hypertrophy due to hypertension. J. Am. Coll. Cardiol. 24:517, 1994.

286. Klues, H. G., Proschan, M. A., Dollar, A. L., et al.: Echocardiographic assessment of mitral valve size in obstructive hypertrophic cardiomyopathy. Anatomic validation from mitral valve specimen. Circulation 88:548, 1993.

287. Mautner, S. L., Klues, H. G., Mautner, G. C., et al.: Comparison of mitral valve dimensions in adults with valvular aortic stenosis, pure aortic regurgitation and hypertrophic cardiomyopathy. Am. J. Cardiol. 71:949, 1993.

288. Klues, H. G., Maron, B. J., Dollar, A. L., and Roberts, W. C.: Diversity of structural mitral valve alterations in hypertrophic cardiomyopathy. Circulation 85:1651, 1992.

289. Grigg, L. E., Wigle, E. D., Williams, W. G., et al.: Transesophageal Doppler echocardiography in obstructive hypertrophic cardiomyopathy: Clarification of pathophysiology and importance in intraoperative decision making. J. Am. Coll. Cardiol. 20:42, 1992.

290. Cape, E. G., Simons, D., Jimoh, A., et al.: Chordal geometry determines the shape and extent of systolic anterior mitral motion: In vitro studies. J. Am. Coll. Cardiol. 13:1438, 1989.

291. Lin, C. S., Chen, K. S., Lin, M. C., et al.: The relationship between systolic anterior motion of the mitral valve and the left ventricular outflow tract Doppler in hypertrophic cardiomyopathy. Am. Heart J. 122:1671, 1991.

292. Klues, H. G., Roberts, W. C., and Maron, B. J.: Anomalous insertion of papillary muscle directly into anterior mitral leaflet in hypertrophic cardiomyopathy. Significance in producing left ventricular outflow obstruction. Circulation 84:1188, 1991.

293. Kramer, C. M., Reichek, N., Ferrari, V. A., et al.: Regional heterogeneity of function in hypertrophic cardiomyopathy. Circulation 90:186, 1994.
294. Young, A. A., Kramer, C. M., Ferrari, V. A., et al.: Three-dimensional left ventricular deformation in hypertrophic cardiomyopathy. Circulation 90:854, 1994.
295. Dong, S. J., MacGregor, J. H., Crawley, A. P., et al.: Left ventricular wall thickness and regional systolic function in patients with hypertrophic cardiomyopathy. A three-dimensional tagged magnetic resonance imaging study. Circulation 90:1200, 1994.
296. Arrive, L., Assayag, P., Russ, G., et al.: MRI and cine MRI of asymmetric septal hypertrophic cardiomyopathy. J. Comput. Assist. Tomogr. 18:376, 1994.
297. Cannon, R. O. 3rd, Dilsizian, V., O'Gara, P. T., et al.: Myocardial metabolic, hemodynamic, and electrocardiographic significance of reversible thallium-201 abnormalities in hypertrophic cardiomyopathy. Circulation 83:1660, 1991.
298. Dilsizian, V., Bonow, R. O., Epstein, S. E., and Fananapazir, L.: Myocardial ischemia detected by thallium scintigraphy is frequently related to cardiac arrest and syncope in young patients with hypertrophic cardiomyopathy. J. Am. Coll. Cardiol. 22:796, 1993.
299. Chikamori, T., Dickie, S., Poloniecki, J. D., et al.: Prognostic significance of radionuclide-assessed diastolic function in hypertrophic cardiomyopathy. Am. J. Cardiol. 65:478, 1990.
300. Maron, B. J., McIntosh, C. L., Klues, H. G., et al.: Morphologic basis for obstruction to right ventricular outflow in hypertrophic cardiomyopathy. Am. J. Cardiol. 71:1089, 1993.
301. Lembo, N. J., Dell-Italia, L. J., Crawford, M. H., and O'Rourke, R. A.: Bedside diagnosis of systolic murmurs. N. Engl. J. Med. 318:1572, 1988.
302. Hadjimiltiades, S., Panidis, I. P., McAllister, M., et al.: Dynamic changes in left ventricular outflow tract flow velocities after amyl nitrite inhalation in hypertrophic cardiomyopathy. Am. Heart J. 121:1143, 1991.
303. Sheikh, K. H., Pearce, F. B., and Kisslo, J.: Use of Doppler echocardiography and amyl nitrite inhalation to characterize left ventricular outflow obstruction in hypertrophic cardiomyopathy. Chest 97:389, 1990.
304. Akasaka, T., Yoshikawa, J., Yoshida, K., et al.: Phasic coronary flow characteristics in patients with hypertrophic cardiomyopathy: A study by coronary Doppler catheter. J. Am. Soc. Echocardiogr. 7:9, 1994.
305. Vassalli, G., Seiler, C., and Hess, O. M.: Risk stratification in hypertrophic cardiomyopathy. Curr. Opin. Cardiol. 9:330, 1994.
306. Maron, B. J., and Spirito, P.: Impact of patient selection biases on the perception of hypertrophic cardiomyopathy and its natural history. Am. J. Cardiol. 72:970, 1993.
307. Kofflard, M. J., Waldstein, D. J., Vos, J., and ten Cate, F. J.: Prognosis in hypertrophic cardiomyopathy observed in a large clinic population. Am. J. Cardiol. 72:939, 1993.
308. McKenna, W. J.: The natural history of hypertrophic cardiomyopathy. Cardiovasc. Clin. 19:135, 1988.
309. Spirito, P., and Bellone, P.: Natural history of hypertrophic cardiomyopathy. Br. Heart J. 72:S10, 1994.
310. Bingisser, R., Candinas, R., Schneider, J., and Hess, O. M.: Risk factors for systolic dysfunction and ventricular dilatation in hypertrophic cardiomyopathy. Int. J. Cardiol. 44:225, 1994.
311. Panza, J. A., and Maron, B. J.: Relation of electrocardiographic abnormalities to evolving left ventricular hypertrophy in hypertrophic cardiomyopathy during childhood. Am. J. Cardiol. 63:1258, 1989.
312. Romeo, F., Cianfrocca, C., Pelliccia, F., et al.: Long-term prognosis in children with hypertrophic cardiomyopathy: An analysis of 37 patients aged less than or equal to 14 years at diagnosis. Clin. Cardiol. 13:101, 1990.
313. Brandenburg, R. O.: Syncope and sudden death in hypertrophic cardiomyopathy. J. Am. Coll. Cardiol. 15:962, 1990.
314. Almendral, J. M., Ormaetxe, J., Martinez-Alday, J. D., et al.: Treatment of ventricular arrhythmias in patients with hypertrophic cardiomyopathy. Eur. Heart J. 14(Suppl. J):71, 1993.
315. Botvinick, E. H., Dae, M. W., Krishnan, R., and Ewing, S.: Hypertrophic cardiomyopathy in the young: Another form of ischemic cardiomyopathy? J. Am. Coll. Cardiol. 22:805, 1993.
316. Nienaber, C. A., Gambhir, S. S., Mody, F. V., et al.: Regional myocardial blood flow and glucose utilization in symptomatic patients with hypertrophic cardiomyopathy. Circulation 87:1580, 1993.
317. Takata, J., Counihan, P. J., Gane, J. N., et al.: Regional thallium-201 washout and myocardial hypertrophy in hypertrophic cardiomyopathy and its relation to exertional chest pain. Am. J. Cardiol. 72:211, 1993.
318. Pedrinelli, R., Spessot, M., Chiriatti, G., et al.: Evidence for a systemic defect of resistance-sized arterioles in hypertrophic cardiomyopathy. Coron. Artery Dis. 4:67, 1993.
319. Counihan, P. J., Frenneaux, M. P., Webb, D. J., and McKenna, W. J.: Abnormal vascular responses to supine exercise in hypertrophic cardiomyopathy. Circulation 84:686, 1991.
320. Maron, B. J., Kogan, J., Proschan, M. A., et al.: Circadian variability in the occurrence of sudden cardiac death in patients with hypertrophic cardiomyopathy. J. Am. Coll. Cardiol. 23:1405, 1994.
321. Maron, B. J., and Klues, H. G.: Surviving competitive athletics with hypertrophic cardiomyopathy. Am. J. Cardiol. 73:1098, 1994.
322. McKenna, W. J., and Camm, A. J.: Sudden death in hypertrophic cardiomyopathy. Assessment of patients at high risk. Circulation 80:1489, 1989.
323. Spirito, P., and Maron, B. J.: Relation between extent of left ventricular hypertrophy and occurrence of sudden cardiac death in hypertrophic cardiomyopathy. J. Am. Coll. Cardiol. 15:1521, 1990.
324. Udelson, J. E., Bonow, R. O., O'Gara, P. T., et al.: Verapamil prevents silent myocardial perfusion abnormalities during exercise in asympto-matic patients with hypertrophic cardiomyopathy. Circulation 79:1052, 1989.
325. Gilligan, D. M., Chan, W. L., Stewart, R., et al.: Cardiac responses assessed by echocardiography to changes in preload in hypertrophic cardiomyopathy. Am. J. Cardiol. 73:312, 1994.
326. Udelson, J. E., Cannon, R. O. 3rd, Bacharach, S. L., et al.: Beta-adrenergic stimulation with isoproterenol enhances left ventricular diastolic performance in hypertrophic cardiomyopathy despite potentiation of myocardial ischemia. Comparison to rapid atrial pacing. Circulation 79:371, 1989.
327. Bonow, R. O., Maron, B. J., Leon, M. B., et al.: Medical and surgical therapy of hypertrophic cardiomyopathy. Cardiovasc. Clin. 19:221, 1988.
328. Gilligan, D. M., Chan, W. L., Joshi, J., et al.: A double-blind, placebo-controlled crossover trial of nadolol and verapamil in mild and moderately symptomatic hypertrophic cardiomyopathy. J. Am. Coll. Cardiol. 21:1672, 1993.
329. Gilligan, D. M., Chan, W. L., Stewart, R., and Oakley, C. M.: Adrenergic hypersensitivity after beta-blocker withdrawal in hypertrophic cardiomyopathy. Am. J. Cardiol. 68:766, 1991.
330. Gistri, R., Cecchi, F., Choudhury, L., et al.: Effect of verapamil on absolute myocardial blood flow in hypertrophic cardiomyopathy. Am. J. Cardiol. 74:363, 1994.
331. Shaffer, E. M., Rocchini, A. P., Spicer, R. L., et al.: Effects of verapamil on left ventricular diastolic filling in children with hypertrophic cardiomyopathy. Am. J. Cardiol. 61:413, 1988.
332. Yamakado, T., Okano, H., Higashiyama, S., et al.: Effects of nifedipine on left ventricular diastolic function in patients with asymptomatic or minimally symptomatic hypertrophic cardiomyopathy. Circulation 81:593, 1990.
333. Richardson, P. J.: Calcium antagonists in cardiomyopathy. Br. J. Clin. Pract. Symp. 60(Suppl.):33, 1988.
334. Betocchi, S., Bonow, R. O., Cannon, R. O. 3rd, et al.: Relation between serum nifedipine concentration and hemodynamic effects in nonobstructive hypertrophic cardiomyopathy. Am. J. Cardiol. 61:830, 1988.
335. Dimitrow, P. P., and Dubiel, J. S.: Effects on left ventricular function of pindolol added to verapamil in hypertrophic cardiomyopathy. Am. J. Cardiol. 71:313, 1993.
336. Fifer, M. A., O'Gara, P. T., McGovern, B. A., and Semigran, M. J.: Effects of disopyramide on left ventricular diastolic function in hypertrophic cardiomyopathy. Am. J. Cardiol. 74:405, 1994.
337. Duncan, W. J., Tyrrell, M. J., and Bharadwaj, B. B.: Disopyramide as a negative inotrope in obstructive cardiomyopathy in children. Can. J. Cardiol. 7:81, 1991.
338. Millaire, A., Goullard, L., Decoulx, E., et al.: Efficiency of disopyramide in hypertrophic cardiomyopathy during stress states. Am. J. Cardiol. 69:423, 1992.
339. Sumimoto, T., Hamada, M., Ohtani, T., et al.: Effect of disopyramide on left ventricular diastolic function in patients with hypertrophic cardiomyopathy: Comparison with diltiazem. Cardiovasc. Drugs Ther. 6:425, 1992.
340. Counihan, P. J., and McKenna, W. J.: Low-dose amiodarone for the treatment of arrhythmias in hypertrophic cardiomyopathy. J. Clin. Pharmacol. 29:436, 1989.
341. Tendera, M., Wycisk, A., Schneeweiss, A., et al.: Effect of sotalol on arrhythmias and exercise tolerance in patients with hypertrophic cardiomyopathy. Cardiology 82:335, 1993.
342. Gilligan, D. M., Missouris, C. G., Boyd, M. J., and Oakley, C. M.: Sudden death due to ventricular tachycardia during amiodarone therapy in familial hypertrophic cardiomyopathy. Am. J. Cardiol. 68:971, 1991.
343. McAreavey, D., and Fananapazir, L.: Altered cardiac hemodynamic and electrical state in normal sinus rhythm after chronic dual-chamber pacing for relief of left ventricular outflow obstruction in hypertrophic cardiomyopathy. Am. J. Cardiol. 70:651, 1992.
344. Jeanrenaud, X., Goy, J. J., and Kappenberger, L.: Effects of dual-chamber pacing in hypertrophic obstructive cardiomyopathy. Lancet 339:1318, 1992.
345. Fananapazir, L., Cannon, R. O. 3rd, Tripodi, D., and Panza, J. A.: Impact of dual-chamber permanent pacing in patients with obstructive hypertrophic cardiomyopathy with symptoms refractory to verapamil and beta-adrenergic blocker therapy. Circulation 85:2149, 1992.
346. McDonald, K. M., and Maurer, B.: Permanent pacing as treatment for hypertrophic cardiomyopathy. Am. J. Cardiol. 68:108, 1991.
347. McDonald, K., McWilliams, E., O'Keeffe, B., and Maurer, B.: Functional assessment of patients treated with permanent dual chamber pacing as a primary treatment for hypertrophic cardiomyopathy. Eur. Heart J. 9:893, 1988.
348. Kappenberger, L.: Pacing for obstructive hypertrophic cardiomyopathy. Br. Heart J. 73:107, 1995.
348a. Slade, A. K. B., Sadoul, N., Shapiro, L., et al.: DDD pacing in hypertrophic cardiomyopathy: A multicentre clinical experience. Heart 75:44, 1996.
349. Nishimura, R. A., and Danielson, G. K.: Dual chamber pacing for hypertrophic obstructive cardiomyopathy: Has its time come? Br. Heart J. 70:301, 1993.
349a. Nishimura, R., Hayes, D. L., Ilstrup, D. M., et al.: Effect of dual-chamber pacing on systolic and diastolic function in patients with hypertrophic cardiomyopathy: Acute Doppler echocardiographic and catheterization hemodynamic study. J. Am. Coll. Cardiol. 27:421, 1996.
349b. Maron, B.: Appraisal of dual-chamber pacing therapy in hypertrophic cardiomyopathy. Too soon for a rush to judgment? J. Am. Coll. Cardiol. 27:431, 1996.
350. Cannon, R. O. 3rd, Tripodi, D., Dilsizian, V., et al.: Results of perma-

nent dual-chamber pacing in symptomatic nonobstructive hypertrophic cardiomyopathy. Am. J. Cardiol. 73:571, 1994.

350a. Sigwart, U.: Nonsurgical myocardial reduction for hypertrophic obstructive cardiomyopathy. Lancet 346:211, 1995.

351. Delahaye, F., Jegaden, O., de Gevigney, G., et al.: Postoperative and long-term prognosis of myotomy-myomectomy for obstructive hypertrophic cardiomyopathy: Influence of associated mitral valve replacement. Eur. Heart J. 14:1229, 1993.

352. Seiler, C., Hess, O. M., Schoenbeck, M., et al.: Long-term follow-up of medical versus surgical therapy for hypertrophic cardiomyopathy: A retrospective study. J. Am. Coll. Cardiol. 17:634, 1991.

352a. Nakatani, S., Schwammenthal, E., Lever, H. M., et al.: New insights into the reduction of the mitral valve systolic anterior motion after ventricular septal myectomy in hypertrophic obstructive cardiomyopathy. Am. Heart J. 131:294, 1996.

353. Blanchard, D. G., and Ross, J. Jr.: Hypertrophic cardiomyopathy: Prognosis with medical or surgical therapy. Clin. Cardiol. 14:11, 1991.

354. Schulte, H. D., Bircks, W. H., Loesse, B., et al.: Prognosis of patients with hypertrophic obstructive cardiomyopathy after transaortic myectomy. Late results up to twenty-five years. J. Thorac. Cardiovasc. Surg. 106:709, 1993.

355. Cannon, R. O. 3rd, Dilsizian, V., O'Gara, P. T., et al.: Impact of surgical relief of outflow obstruction on thallium perfusion abnormalities in hypertrophic cardiomyopathy. Circulation 85:1039, 1992.

356. Diodati, J. G., Schenke, W. H., Waclawiw, M. A., et al.: Predictors of exercise benefit after operative relief of left ventricular outflow obstruction by the myotomy-myectomy procedure in hypertrophic cardiomyopathy. Am. J. Cardiol. 69:1617, 1992.

357. ten Berg, J. M., Suttorp, M. J., Knaepen, P. J., et al.: Hypertrophic obstructive cardiomyopathy. Initial results and long-term follow-up after Morrow septal myectomy. Circulation 90:1781, 1994.

358. McIntosh, C. L., Maron, B. J., Cannon, R. O. 3rd, and Klues, H. G.: Initial results of combined anterior mitral leaflet plication and ventricular septal myotomy-myectomy for relief of left ventricular outflow tract obstruction in patients with hypertrophic cardiomyopathy. Circulation 86:II60, 1992.

359. Joyce, F. S., Lever, H. M., and Cosgrove, D. M. 3rd: Treatment of hypertrophic cardiomyopathy by mitral valve repair and septal myectomy. Ann. Thorac. Surg. 57:1025, 1994.

360. Krajcer, Z., Leachman, R. D., Cooley, D. A., and Coronado, R.: Septal myotomy-myomectomy versus mitral valve replacement in hypertrophic cardiomyopathy. Ten-year follow-up in 185 patients. Circulation 80:157, 1989.

361. Shirani, J., Maron, B. J., Cannon, R. O. 3rd, et al.: Clinicopathologic features of hypertrophic cardiomyopathy managed by cardiac transplantation. Am. J. Cardiol. 72:434, 1993.

RESTRICTIVE AND INFILTRATIVE CARDIOMYOPATHIES

362. Child, J. S., and Perloff, J. K.: The restrictive cardiomyopathies. Cardiol. Clin. 6:289, 1988.

363. Spyrou, N., and Foale, R.: Restrictive cardiomyopathies. Curr. Opin. Cardiol. 9:344, 1994.

363a. Garcia, M. J., Rodriguez, L., Ares, M., et al.: Differentiation of constrictive pericarditis from restrictive cardiomyopathy: Assessment of left ventricular diastolic velocities in longitudinal axis by Doppler tissue imaging. J. Am. Coll. Cardiol. 27:108, 1996.

364. Benson, M. D.: Hereditary amyloidosis and cardiomyopathy. Am. J. Med. 93:1, 1992.

365. Vaitkus, P. T., and Kussmaul, W. G.: Constrictive pericarditis versus restrictive cardiomyopathy: A reappraisal and update of diagnostic criteria. Am. Heart J. 122:1431, 1991.

366. Hirota, Y., Shimizu, G., Kita, Y., et al.: Spectrum of restrictive cardiomyopathy: Report of the national survey in Japan. Am. Heart J. 120:188, 1990.

367. Katritsis, D., Wilmshurst, P. T., Wendon, J. A., et al.: Primary restrictive cardiomyopathy: Clinical and pathologic characteristics. J. Am. Coll. Cardiol. 18:1230, 1991.

368. Fitzpatrick, A. P., Shapiro, L. M., Rickards, A. F., and Poole-Wilson, P. A.: Familial restrictive cardiomyopathy with atrioventricular block and skeletal myopathy. Br. Heart J. 63:114, 1990.

369. Masui, T., Finck, S., and Higgins, C. B.: Constrictive pericarditis and restrictive cardiomyopathy: Evaluation with MR imaging. Radiology 182:369, 1992.

370. Schoenfeld, M. H.: The differentiation of restrictive cardiomyopathy from constrictive pericarditis. Cardiol. Clin. 8:663, 1990.

371. Gasperetti, C. M., Sarembock, I. J., and Feldman, M. D.: Usefulness of dynamic hand exercise for developing maximal separation of left and right ventricular pressures at end-diastole and usefulness in distinguishing restrictive cardiomyopathy from constrictive pericardial disease. Am. J. Cardiol. 69:1508, 1992.

372. Morgan, J. M., Raposo, L., Clague, J. C., et al.: Restrictive cardiomyopathy and constrictive pericarditis: Non-invasive distinction by digitised M mode echocardiography. Br. Heart J. 61:29, 1989.

373. Acquatella, H., Rodriguez-Salas, L. A., and Gomez-Mancebo, J. R.: Doppler echocardiography in dilated and restrictive cardiomyopathies. Cardiol. Clin. 8:349, 1990.

374. Mancuso, L., D'Agostino, A., Pitrolo, F., et al.: Constrictive pericarditis versus restrictive cardiomyopathy: The role of Doppler echocardiography in differential diagnosis. Int. J. Cardiol. 31:319, 1991.

375. Hatle, L. K., Appleton, C. P., and Popp, R. L.: Differentiation of con-

strictive pericarditis and restrictive cardiomyopathy by Doppler echocardiography. Circulation 79:357, 1989.

376. Schiavone, W. A., Calafiore, P. A., and Salcedo, E. E.: Transesophageal Doppler echocardiographic demonstration of pulmonary venous flow velocity in restrictive cardiomyopathy and constrictive pericarditis. Am. J. Cardiol. 63:1286, 1989.

377. Klein, A. L., Cohen, G. I., Pietrolungo, J. F., et al.: Differentiation of constrictive pericarditis from restrictive cardiomyopathy by Doppler transesophageal echocardiographic measurements of respiratory variations in pulmonary venous flow. J. Am. Coll. Cardiol. 22:1935, 1993.

378. Gerson, M. C., Colthar, M. S., and Fowler, N. O.: Differentiation of constrictive pericarditis and restrictive cardiomyopathy by radionuclide ventriculography. Am. Heart J. 118:114, 1989.

379. Aroney, C. N., Ruddy, T. D., Dighero, H., et al.: Differentiation of restrictive cardiomyopathy from pericardial constriction: Assessment of diastolic function by radionuclide angiography. J. Am. Coll. Cardiol. 13:1007, 1989.

380. Hesse, A., Altland, K., Linke, R. P., et al.: Cardiac amyloidosis: A review and report of a new transthyretin (prealbumin) variant. Br. Heart J. 70:111, 1993.

381. Gertz, M. A., and Kyle, R. A.: Primary systemic amyloidosis—a diagnostic primer. Mayo Clin. Proc. 64:1505, 1989.

382. Plehn, J. F., Southworth, J., and Cornwell, G. G. 3rd: Brief report: Atrial systolic failure in primary amyloidosis. N. Engl. J. Med. 327:1570, 1992.

383. Skinner, M.: Familial amyloidotic cardiomyopathy. J. Lab. Clin. Med. 117:171, 1991.

384. Booth, D. R., Tan, S. Y., Hawkins, P. N., et al.: A novel variant of transthyretin, $59^{Thr \rightarrow Lys}$, associated with autosomal dominant cardiac amyloidosis in an Italian family. Circulation 91:962, 1995.

385. Kyle, R. A.: Amyloidosis. Circulation 91:1269, 1995.

386. Nichols, W. C., Liepnieks, J. J., Snyder, E. L., and Benson, M. D.: Senile cardiac amyloidosis associated with homozygosity for a transthyretin variant (ILE-122). J. Lab. Clin. Med. 117:175, 1991.

387. Gertz, M. A., Kyle, R. A., and Noel, P.: Primary systemic amyloidosis: A rare complication of immunoglobulin M monoclonal gammopathies and Waldenstrom's macroglobulinemia. J. Clin. Oncol. 11:914, 1993.

388. Gertz, M. A., and Kyle, R. A.: Secondary systemic amyloidosis: Response and survival in 64 patients. Medicine (Baltimore) 70:246, 1991.

389. Gertz, M. A., Kyle, R. A., and Thibodeau, S. N.: Familial amyloidosis: A study of 52 North American–born patients examined during a 30-year period. Mayo Clin. Proc. 67:428, 1992.

390. Kinoshita, O., Hongo, M., Yamada, H., et al.: Impaired left ventricular diastolic filling in patients with familial amyloid polyneuropathy: A pulsed Doppler echocardiographic study. Br. Heart J. 61:198, 1989.

391. Simons, M., and Isner, J. M.: Assessment of relative sensitivities of noninvasive tests for cardiac amyloidosis in documented cardiac amyloidosis. Am. J. Cardiol. 69:425, 1992.

392. Hongo, M., Kono, J., Yamada, H., et al.: Doppler echocardiographic assessments of left ventricular diastolic filling in patients with amyloid heart disease. J. Cardiol. 21:391, 1991.

393. Hongo, M., Fujii, T., Hirayama, J., et al.: Radionuclide angiographic assessment of left ventricular diastolic filling in amyloid heart disease: A study of patients with familial amyloid polyneuropathy. J. Am. Coll. Cardiol. 13:48, 1989.

394. Klein, A. L., Hatle, L. K., Taliercio, C. P., et al.: Prognostic significance of Doppler measures of diastolic function in cardiac amyloidosis. A Doppler echocardiography study. Circulation 83:808, 1991.

395. Hartmann, A., Frenkel, J., Hopf, R., et al.: Is technetium-99m-pyrophosphate scintigraphy valuable in the diagnosis of cardiac amyloidosis? Int. J. Card. Imaging 5:227, 1990.

396. Lekakis, J., Nanas, J., Moustafellou, C., et al.: Cardiac amyloidosis detected by indium-111 antimyosin imaging. Am. Heart J. 124:1630, 1992.

397. Gertz, M. A., Kyle, R. A., and Greipp, P. R.: Response rates and survival in primary systemic amyloidosis. Blood 77:257, 1991.

398. Pollak, A., and Falk, R. H.: Left ventricular systolic dysfunction precipitated by verapamil in cardiac amyloidosis. Chest 104:618, 1993.

399. Hosenpud, J. D., DeMarco, T., Frazier, O. H., et al.: Progression of systemic disease and reduced long-term survival in patients with cardiac amyloidosis undergoing heart transplantation. Follow-up results of a multicenter survey. Circulation 84:III-338, 1991.

400. Eng, C. M., and Desnick, R. J.: Molecular basis of Fabry disease: Mutations and polymorphisms in the human alpha-galactosidase A gene. Hum. Mutat. 3:103, 1994.

401. Ishii, S., Kase, R., Sakuraba, H., and Suzuki, Y.: Characterization of a mutant alpha-galactosidase gene product for the late-onset cardiac form of Fabry disease. Biochem. Biophys. Res. Commun. 197:1585, 1993.

402. Eng, C. M., Resnick-Silverman, L. A., Niehaus, D. J., et al.: Nature and frequency of mutations in the alpha-galactosidase A gene that cause Fabry disease. Am. J. Hum. Genet. 53:1186, 1993.

403. von Scheidt, W., Eng, C. M., Fitzmaurice, T. F., et al.: An atypical variant of Fabry's disease with manifestations confined to the myocardium. N. Engl. J. Med. 324:395, 1991.

404. Elleder, M., Bradova, V., Smid, F., et al.: Cardiocyte storage and hypertrophy as a sole manifestation of Fabry's disease. Report on a case simulating hypertrophic non-obstructive cardiomyopathy. Virchows Arch. A. Pathol. Anat. Histopathol. 417:449, 1990.

404a. Nakao, S., Takenaka, T., Maeda, M., et al.: An atypical variant of Fabry's disease in men with left ventricular hypertrophy. N. Engl. J. Med. 333:288, 1995.

405. Pochis, W. T., Litzow, J. T., King, B. G., and Kenny, D.: Electrophysio-

logic findings in Fabry's disease with a short PR interval. Am. J. Cardiol. *74*:203, 1994.

406. Mester, S. W., and Weston, M. W.: Cardiac tamponade in a patient with Gaucher's disease. Clin. Cardiol. *15*:766, 1992.

407. Uyama, E., Takahashi, K., Owada, M., et al.: Hydrocephalus, corneal opacities, deafness, valvular heart disease, deformed toes and leptomeningeal fibrous thickening in adult siblings: A new syndrome associated with β-glucocerebrosidase deficiency and a mosaic population of storage cells. Acta Neurol. Scand. *86*:407, 1992.

408. Saraclar, M., Atalay, S., Kocak, N., and Ozkutlu, S.: Gaucher's disease with mitral and aortic involvement: Echocardiographic findings. Pediatr. Cardiol. *13*:56, 1992.

409. Starzl, T. E., Demetris, A. J., Trucco, M., et al.: Chimerism after liver transplantation for type IV glycogen storage disease and type 1 Gaucher's disease. N. Engl. J. Med. *328*:745, 1993.

410. Crawford, D. H., and Halliday, J. W.: Current concepts in rational therapy for haemochromatosis. Drugs *41*:875, 1991.

411. Liu, P., and Olivieri, N.: Iron overload cardiomyopathies: New insights into an old disease. Cardiovasc. Drugs Ther. *8*:101, 1994.

412. Hauser, S. C.: Hemochromatosis and the heart. Heart Dis. Stroke *2*:487, 1993.

413. Porter, J., Cary, N., and Schofield, P.: Haemochromatosis presenting as congestive heart failure. Br. Heart J. *73*:73, 1995.

414. Westra, W. H., Hruban, R. H., Baughman, K. L., et al.: Progressive hemochromatotic cardiomyopathy despite reversal of iron deposition after liver transplantation. Am. J. Clin. Pathol. *99*:39, 1993.

415. Wang, T. L., Chen, W. J., Liau, C. S., and Lee, Y. T.: Sick sinus syndrome as the early manifestation of cardiac hemochromatosis. J. Electrocardiol. *27*:91, 1994.

416. Fargion, S., Mandelli, C., Piperno, A., et al.: Survival and prognostic factors in 212 Italian patients with genetic hemochromatosis. Hepatology *15*:655, 1992.

417. Cecchetti, G., Binda, A., Piperno, A., et al.: Cardiac alterations in 36 consecutive patients with idiopathic haemochromatosis: Polygraphic and echocardiographic evaluation. Eur. Heart J. *12*:224, 1991.

418. Olson, L. J., Edwards, W. D., McCall, J. T., et al.: Cardiac iron deposition from idiopathic hemochromatosis: Histologic and analytic assessment of 14 hearts from autopsy. J. Am. Coll. Cardiol. *10*:1239, 1987.

419. Blankenberg, F., Eisenberg, S., Scheinman, M. N., and Higgins, C. B.: Use of cine gradient echo (GRE) MR in the imaging of cardiac hemochromatosis. J. Comput. Assist. Tomogr. *18*:136, 1994.

420. Milman, N.: Hereditary haemochromatosis in Denmark 1950–1985. Clinical, biochemical and histological features in 179 patients and 13 preclinical cases. Dan. Med. Bul. *38*:385, 1991.

421. Coleman, R. A., Winter, H. S., Wolf, B., et al.: Glycogen storage disease type III (glycogen debranching enzyme deficiency): Correlation of biochemical defects with myopathy and cardiomyopathy. Ann. Intern. Med. *116*:896, 1992.

422. Anonymous: Case records of the Massachusetts General Hospital. Weekly clinicopathological exercises. Case 11-1993. A 52-year-old man with cardiomyopathy and pulmonary disease. N. Engl. J. Med. *328*:792, 1993.

423. Sharma, O. P., Maheshwari, A., and Thaker, K.: Myocardial sarcoidosis. Chest *103*:253, 1993.

424. Sharma, O. P.: Sarcoidosis. Disease a Month. *36*:469, 1990.

425. Gibbons, W. J., Levy, R. D., Nava, S., et al.: Subclinical cardiac dysfunction in sarcoidosis. Chest *100*:44, 1991.

426. Sharma, O. P.: Myocardial sarcoidosis. A wolf in sheep's clothing. Chest *106*:988, 1994.

427. Alton, M., Juhlin-Dannfelt, A., Pehrsson, S. K., and Ryden, L.: Sarcoid heart disease. Sarcoidosis *9*:147, 1992.

428. Bohle, W., and Schaefer, H. E.: Predominant myocardial sarcoidosis. Pathol. Res. Pract. *190*:212, 1994.

429. Shammas, R. L., and Movahed, A.: Sarcoidosis of the heart. Clin. Cardiol. *16*:462, 1993.

430. Winters, S. L., Cohen, M., Greenberg, S., et al.: Sustained ventricular tachycardia associated with sarcoidosis: Assessment of the underlying cardiac anatomy and the prospective utility of programmed ventricular stimulation, drug therapy and an implantable antitachycardia device. J. Am. Coll. Cardiol. *18*:937, 1991.

431. Huang, P. L., Brooks, R., Carpenter, C., and Garan, H.: Antiarrhythmic therapy guided by programmed electrical stimulation in cardiac sarcoidosis with ventricular tachycardia. Am. Heart J. *121*:599, 1991.

432. Jain, A., Starek, P. J., and Delany, D. L.: Ventricular tachycardia and ventricular aneurysm due to unrecognized sarcoidosis. Clin. Cardiol. *13*:738, 1990.

433. Angomachalelis, N., Hourzamanis, A., Salem, N., et al.: Pericardial effusion concomitant with specific heart muscle disease in systemic sarcoidosis. Postgrad. Med. J. *70*(Suppl. 1):S8, 1994.

434. Klein, A. L., Oh, J. K., Miller, F. A., et al.: Two-dimensional and Doppler echocardiographic assessment of infiltrative cardiomyopathy. J. Am. Soc. Echocardiogr. *1*:48, 1988.

435. Burstow, D. J., Tajik, A. J., Bailey, K. R., et al.: Two-dimensional echocardiographic findings in systemic sarcoidosis. Am. J. Cardiol. *63*:478, 1989.

436. Yamamoto, N., Gotoh, K., Yagi, S., et al.: Thallium-201 myocardial SPECT findings at rest in sarcoidosis. Ann. Nucl. Med. *7*:97, 1993.

437. Tawarahara, K., Kurata, C., Okayama, K., et al.: Thallium-201 and gallium 67 single photon emission computed tomographic imaging in cardiac sarcoidosis. Am. Heart J. *124*:1383, 1992.

438. Taki, J., Nakajima, K., Bunko, H., et al.: Cardiac sarcoidosis demonstrated by Tl-201 and Ga-67 SPECT imaging. Clin. Nucl. Med. *15*:636, 1990.

439. Fields, C. L., Ossorio, M. A., Roy, T. M., et al.: Thallium-201 scintigra-

phy in the diagnosis and management of myocardial sarcoidosis. South. Med. J. *83*:339, 1990.

440. Kinney, E. L., and Caldwell, J. W.: Do thallium myocardial perfusion scan abnormalities predict survival in sarcoid patients without cardiac symptoms? Angiology *41*:573, 1990.

441. Hirose, Y., Ishida, Y., Hayashida, K., et al.: Myocardial involvement in patients with sarcoidosis. An analysis of 75 patients. Clin. Nucl. Med. *19*:522, 1994.

442. Knapp, W. H., Bentrup, A., and Ohlmeier, H.: Indium-111-labelled antimyosin antibody imaging in a patient with cardiac sarcoidosis. Eur. J. Nucl. Med. *20*:80, 1993

443. Kurata, C., Sakata, K., Taguchi, T., et al.: SPECT imaging with Tl-201 and Ga-67 in myocardial sarcoidosis. Clin. Nucl. Med. *15*:408, 1990.

444. Shammas, R. L., and Movahed, A.: Successful treatment of myocardial sarcoidosis with steroids. Sarcoidosis *11*:37, 1994.

445. Schaedel, H., Kirsten, D., Schmidt, A., et al.: Sarcoid heart disease—results of follow-up investigations. Eur. Heart J. *12*(Suppl D):26, 1991.

446. Shiotani, H., Miyazaki, T., Matsunaga, K., and Kado, T.: Improvement of severe heart failure with corticosteroid therapy in a patient with myocardial sarcoidosis. Jpn. Circ. J. *55*:393, 1991.

447. Fujita, N., Hiroe, M., Suzuki, Y., et al.: A case with cardiac sarcoidosis. Significance of the effect of steroids on the reversion of advanced atrioventricular block and myocardial scintigraphic abnormalities. Heart Vessels *5*(Suppl.):16, 1990.

448. Okamoto, M., Hashimoto, M., Sueda, T., et al.: Polymorphic ventricular tachycardia with cardiac sarcoidosis: Treatment with low-dose metoprolol and cibenzoline. Intern. Med. *33*:296, 1994.

449. Paz, H. L., McCormick, D. J., Kutalek, S. P., and Patchefsky, A.: The automated implantable cardiac defibrillator. Prophylaxis in cardiac sarcoidosis. Chest *106*:1603, 1994.

450. Scott, J., and Higenbottam, T.: Transplantation of the lungs and heart and lung for patients with severe pulmonary complications from sarcoidosis. Sarcoidosis *7*:9, 1990.

451. Valiathan, S. M., and Kartha, C. C.: Endomyocardial fibrosis—the possible connexion with myocardial levels of magnesium and cerium. Int. J. Cardiol. *28*:1, 1990.

452. Vijayaraghavan, G., Balakrishnan, M., Sadanandan, S., and Cherian, G.: Pattern of cardiac calcification in tropical endomyocardial fibrosis. Heart Vessels *5*(Suppl.):4, 1990.

453. Ribeiro, P. A., Muthusamy, R., and Duran, C. M.: Right-sided endomyocardial fibrosis with recurrent pulmonary emboli leading to irreversible pulmonary hypertension. Br. Heart J. *68*:326, 1992.

454. Parrillo, J. E.: Heart disease and the eosinophil. N. Engl. J. Med. *323*:1560, 1990.

455. Gupta, P. N., Valiathan, M. S., Balakrishnan, K. G., et al.: Clinical course of endomyocardial fibrosis. Br. Heart J. *62*:450, 1989.

456. Shah, A. M., Brutsaert, D. L., Meulemans, A. L., et al.: Eosinophils from hypereosinophilic patients damage endocardium of isolated feline heart muscle preparations. Circulation *81*:1081, 1990.

457. Weller, P. F., and Bubley, G. J.: The idiopathic hypereosinophilic syndrome. Blood *83*:2759, 1994.

458. Seshadri, S., Narula, J., and Chopra, P.: Asymptomatic eosinophilic myocarditis: 2 + 2 = 4 or 5. Int. J. Cardiol. *31*:348, 1991.

459. Uetsuka, Y., Kasahara, S., Tanaka, N., et al.: Hemodynamic and scintigraphic improvement after steroid therapy in a case with acute eosinophilic heart disease. Heart Vessels *5*(Suppl.):8, 1990.

460. Shaper, A. G.: What's new in endomyocardial fibrosis? Lancet *342*:255, 1993.

461. Valiathan, M. S.: Endomyocardial fibrosis. Natl. Med. J. India *6*:212, 1993.

462. Felice, P. V., Sawicki, J., and Anto, J.: Endomyocardial disease and eosinophilia. Angiology *44*:869, 1993.

463. deMello, D. E., Liapis, H., Jureidini, S., et al.: Cardiac localization of eosinophil-granule major basic protein in acute necrotizing myocarditis. N. Engl. J. Med. *323*:1542, 1990.

464. Butterfield, J. H., and Gleich, G. J.: Interferon-alpha treatment of six patients with the idiopathic hypereosinophilic syndrome. Ann. Intern. Med. *121*:648, 1994.

465. Arnold, M., McGuire, L., and Lee, J. C.: Loeffler's fibroplastic endocarditis. Pathology *20*:79, 1988.

466. Anonymous: Case records of the Massachusetts General Hospital. Weekly clinicopathological exercises. Case 47-1993. Presentation of case. A 28-year-old man with recurrent ventricular tachycardia and dysfunction of multiple organs. N. Engl. J. Med. *329*:1639, 1993.

467. Chopra, P., Narula, J., Talwar, K. K., et al.: Histomorphologic characteristics of endomyocardial fibrosis: An endomyocardial biopsy study. Hum. Pathol. *21*:613, 1990.

468. D'Silva, S. A., Kohli, A., Dalvi, B. V., and Kale, P. A.: MRI in right ventricular endomyocardial fibrosis. Am. Heart J. *123*:1390, 1992.

469. Chopra, P., and Dave, T. H.: Right-sided endomyocardial fibrosis: An unusual morphological type. Int. J. Cardiol. *27*:383, 1990.

470. Mady, C., Barretto, A. C., Oliveira, S. A., et al.: Evolution of the endocardial fibrotic process in endomyocardial fibrosis. Am. J. Cardiol. *68*:402, 1991.

471. Martinez, E. E., Venturi, M., Buffolo, E., et al.: Operative results in endomyocardial fibrosis. Am. J. Cardiol. *63*:627, 1989.

472. Saraclar, M., Ozer, S., Oztunc, F., and Celiker, A.: Echocardiographic findings in endomyocardial fibrosis. Turk. J. Pediatr. *34*:47, 1992.

473. Mady, C., Barretto, A. C., Mesquita, E. T., et al.: Maximal functional capacity in patients with endomyocardial fibrosis. Eur. Heart J. *14*:240, 1993.

474. Barretto, A. C., da Luz, P. L., de Oliveira, S. A., et al.: Determinants of survival in endomyocardial fibrosis. Circulation *80*:I177, 1989.

475. Mady, C., Pereira Barretto, A. C., de Oliveira, S. A., et al.: Effectiveness of operative and nonoperative therapy in endomyocardial fibrosis. Am. J. Cardiol. 63:1281, 1989.

476. de Oliveira, S. A., Pereira Barreto, A. C., Mady, C., et al.: Surgical treatment of endomyocardial fibrosis: A new approach. J. Am. Coll. Cardiol. 16:1246, 1990.

477. Uva, M. S., Jebara, V. A., Acar, C., et al.: Mitral valve repair in patients with endomyocardial fibrosis. Ann. Thorac. Surg. 54:89, 1992.

477a. La Vecchia, L., Bedogni, F., Bozzola, L., et al.: Prediction of recovery after abstinence in alcoholic cardiomyopathy: Role of hemodynamic and morphometric parameters. Clin. Cardiol. 19:45, 1996.

478. Pellikka, P. A., Tajik, A. J., Khandheria, B. K., et al.: Carcinoid heart disease. Clinical and echocardiographic spectrum in 74 patients. Circulation 87:1188, 1993.

479. Lundin, L.: Carcinoid heart disease. A cardiologist's viewpoint. Acta Oncol. 30:499, 1991.

480. Waltenberger, J., Lundin, L., Oberg, K., et al.: Involvement of transforming growth factor-beta in the formation of fibrotic lesions in carcinoid heart disease. Am. J. Pathol. 142:71, 1993.

481. Lundin, L., Funa, K., Hansson, H. E., et al.: Histochemical and immunohistochemical morphology of carcinoid heart disease. Pathol. Res. Pract. 187:73, 1991.

481a. Robiolio, P. A., Rigolin, V. H., Wilson, J. S., et al.: Carcinoid heart disease. Correlation of high serotonin levels with valvular abnormalities detected by cardiac catheterization and echocardiography. Circulation 92:790, 1995.

482. Robiolio, P. A., Rigolin, V. H., Harrison, J. K., et al.: Predictors of outcome of tricuspid valve replacement in carcinoid heart disease. Am. J. Cardiol. 75:485, 1995.

483. Connolly, H. M., Nishimura, R. A., Smith, H. C., et al.: Outcome of cardiac surgery for carcinoid heart disease. J. Am. Coll. Cardiol. 25:410, 1995.

484. Lundin, L., Landelius, J., Andren, B., and Oberg, K.: Transoesophageal echocardiography improves the diagnostic value of cardiac ultrasound in patients with carcinoid heart disease. Br. Heart J. 64:190, 1990.

485. Yun, D., and Heywood, J. T.: Metastatic carcinoid disease presenting solely as high-output heart failure. Ann. Intern. Med. 120:45, 1994.

486. Onate, A., Alcibar, J., Inguanzo, R., et al.: Balloon dilation of tricuspid and pulmonary valves in carcinoid heart disease. Tex. Heart Inst. J. 20:115, 1993.

487. Grant, S. C., Scarffe, J. H., Levy, R. D., and Brooks, N. H.: Failure of balloon dilatation of the pulmonary valve in carcinoid pulmonary stenosis. Br. Heart J. 67:450, 1992.

MYOCARDITIS

488. Peters, N. S., and Poole-Wilson, P. A.: Myocarditis—continuing clinical and pathologic confusion. Am. Heart J. 121:942, 1991.

489. Herzum, M., and Maisch, B.: Humoral and cellular immune reactions to the myocardium in myocarditis. Herz 17:91, 1992.

490. See, D. M., and Tilles, J. G.: Viral myocarditis. Rev. Infect. Dis. 13:951, 1991.

491. Olinde, K. D., and O'Connell, J. B.: Inflammatory heart disease: Pathogenesis, clinical manifestations, and treatment of myocarditis. Annu. Rev. Med. 45:481, 1994.

492. Leslie, K. O., Schwarz, J., Simpson, K., and Huber, S. A.: Progressive interstitial collagen deposition in Coxsackievirus B3-induced murine myocarditis. Am. J. Pathol. 136:683, 1990.

493. Seko, Y., Matsuda, H., Kato, K., et al.: Expression of intercellular adhesion molecule-1 in murine hearts with acute myocarditis caused by coxsackievirus B3. J. Clin. Invest. 91:1327, 1993.

494. Toyozaki, T., Saito, T., Takano, H., et al.: Expression of intercellular adhesion molecule-1 on cardiac myocytes for myocarditis before and during immunosuppressive therapy. Am. J. Cardiol. 72:441, 1993.

495. Herskowitz, A., Ahmed-Ansari, A., Neumann, D. A., et al.: Induction of major histocompatibility complex antigens within the myocardium of patients with active myocarditis: A nonhistologic marker of myocarditis. J. Am. Coll. Cardiol. 15:624, 1990.

496. Rose, N. R., Neumann, D. A., and Herskowitz, A.: Coxsackievirus myocarditis. Adv. Intern. Med. 37:411, 1992.

497. McNulty, C. M.: Active viral myocarditis: Application of current knowledge to clinical practice. Heart Dis. Stroke 1:135, 1992.

498. Hyypia, T.: Etiological diagnosis of viral heart disease. Scand. J. Infect. Dis. 88(Suppl.):25, 1993.

499. Hagar, J. M., and Rahimtoola, S. H.: Chagas' heart disease in the United States. N. Engl. J. Med. 325:763, 1991.

500. Marboe, C. C., and Fenoglio, J. J. Jr.: Pathology and natural history of human myocarditis. Pathol. Immunopathol. Res. 7:226, 1988.

501. Davies, M. J., and Ward, D. E.: How can myocarditis be diagnosed and should it be treated? Br. Heart J. 68:346, 1992.

502. Gowrishankar, K., and Rajajee, S.: Varied manifestations of viral myocarditis. Indian J. Pediatr. 61:75, 1994.

503. Friedman, R. A., Kearney, D. L., Moak, J. P., et al.: Persistence of ventricular arrhythmia after resolution of occult myocarditis in children and young adults. J. Am. Coll. Cardiol. 24:780, 1994.

504. Abelmann, W. H.: Myocarditis and dilated cardiomyopathy. West. J. Med. 150:458, 1989.

505. Peters, N. S., and Poole-Wilson, P. A.: Myocarditis—a controversial disease. J. R. Soc. Med. 84:1, 1991.

506. Gravanis, M. B., and Sternby, N. H.: Incidence of myocarditis. A 10-year autopsy study from Malmo, Sweden. Arch. Pathol. Lab. Med. 115:390, 1991.

507. Narula, J., Khaw, B. A., Dec, G. W. Jr., et al.: Brief report: Recognition of acute myocarditis masquerading as acute myocardial infarction. N. Engl. J. Med. 328:100, 1993.

508. Dec, G. W. Jr., Waldman, H., Southern, J., et al.: Viral myocarditis mimicking acute myocardial infarction. J. Am. Coll. Cardiol. 20:85, 1992.

509. Morgera, T., Di Lenarda, A., Dreas, L., et al.: Electrocardiography of myocarditis revisited: Clinical and prognostic significance of electrocardiographic changes. Am. Heart J. 124:455, 1992.

510. Matsuura, H., Palacios, I. F., Dec, G. W., et al.: Intraventricular conduction abnormalities in patients with clinically suspected myocarditis are associated with myocardial necrosis. Am. Heart J. 127:1290, 1994.

511. James, K. B., Lee, K., Thomas, J. D., et al.: Left ventricular diastolic dysfunction in lymphocytic myocarditis as assessed by Doppler echocardiography. Am. J. Cardiol. 73:282, 1994.

512. Memel, D. S., DeRogatis, A. J., and William, D. C.: Ga-67 citrate myocardial uptake in a patient with AIDS, toxoplasmosis, and myocarditis. Clin. Nucl. Med. 16:315, 1991.

513. Matsumori, A., Yamada, T., Tamaki, N., et al.: ^{111}In monoclonal antimyosin antibody imaging: Imaging of myocardial infarction and myocarditis. Jpn. Circ. J. 54:333, 1990.

514. Matsouka, H., Hamada, M., Honda, T., et al.: Evaluation of acute myocarditis and pericarditis by Gd-DTPA enhanced magnetic resonance imaging. Eur. Heart J. 15:283, 1994.

515. Huber, S. A.: Viral myocarditis—a tale of two diseases. Lab. Invest. 66:1, 1992.

516. Hauck, A. J., Kearney, D. L., and Edwards, W. D.: Evaluation of postmortem endomyocardial biopsy specimens from 38 patients with lymphocytic myocarditis: Implications for role of sampling error. Mayo Clin. Proc. 64:1235, 1989.

517. Chow, L. H., Radio, S. J., Sears, T. D., and McManus, B. M.: Insensitivity of right ventricular endomyocardial biopsy in the diagnosis of myocarditis. J. Am. Coll. Cardiol. 14:915, 1989.

518. Dec, G. W., Fallon, J. T., Southern, J. F., and Palacios, I.: "Borderline" myocarditis: An indication for repeat endomyocardial biopsy. J. Am. Coll. Cardiol. 15:283, 1990.

519. Rezkalla, S., Kloner, R. A., Khatib, G., et al.: Effect of metoprolol in acute coxsackievirus B3 murine myocarditis. J. Am. Coll. Cardiol. 12:412, 1988.

520. Maisch, B., Schonian, U., Crombach, M., et al.: Cytomegalovirus associated inflammatory heart muscle disease. Scand. J. Infect. Dis. 88(Suppl.):135, 1993.

521. Jones, S. R., Herskowitz, A., Hutchins, G. M., and Baughman, K. L.: Effects of immunosuppressive therapy in biopsy-proved myocarditis and borderline myocarditis on left ventricular function. Am. J. Cardiol. 68:370, 1991.

522. Chan, K. Y., Iwahara, M., Benson, L. N., et al.: Immunosuppressive therapy in the management of acute myocarditis in children: A clinical trial. J. Am. Coll. Cardiol. 17:458, 1991.

522a. Mason, J. W., O'Connell, J. B., Herskowitz, A., et al.: A clinical trial of immunosuppressive therapy for myocarditis. N. Engl. J. Med. 333:269, 1995.

523. Rezkalla, S. H., and Kloner, R. A.: Management strategies in viral myocarditis. Am. Heart J. 117:706, 1989.

524. Kishimoto, C., and Abelmann, W. H.: Absence of effects of cyclosporine on myocardial lymphocyte subsets in Coxsackievirus B3 myocarditis in the aviremic stage. Circ. Res. 65:934, 1989.

525. Kishimoto, C., Thorp, K. A., and Abelmann, W. H.: Immunosuppression with high doses of cyclophosphamide reduces the severity of myocarditis but increases the mortality in murine Coxsackievirus B3 myocarditis. Circulation 82:982, 1990.

526. Drucker, N. A., Colan, S. D., Lewis, A. B., et al.: Gamma-globulin treatment of acute myocarditis in the pediatric population. Circulation 89:252, 1994.

527. Rezkalla, S., Kloner, R. A., Khatib, G., and Khatib, R.: Beneficial effects of captopril in acute coxsackievirus B3 murine myocarditis. Circulation 81:1039, 1990.

528. Rezkalla, S., Kloner, R. A., Khatib, G., and Khatib, R.: Effect of delayed captopril therapy on left ventricular mass and myonecrosis during acute coxsackievirus murine myocarditis. Am. Heart J. 120:1377, 1990.

529. Ray, C. G., Icenogle, T. B., Minnich, L. L., et al.: The use of intravenous ribavirin to treat influenza virus-associated acute myocarditis. J. Infect. Dis. 159:829, 1989.

530. Kishimoto, C., and Abelmann, W. H.: Monoclonal antibody therapy for prevention of acute coxsackievirus B3 myocarditis in mice. Circulation 79:1300, 1989.

531. Kishimoto, C., Crumpacker, C. S., and Abelmann, W. H.: Prevention of murine coxsackie B3 viral myocarditis and associated lymphoid organ atrophy with recombinant human leucocyte interferon alpha A/D. Cardiovasc. Res. 22:732, 1988.

532. Hingorani, A. D.: Postinfectious myocarditis. BMJ 304:1676, 1992.

533. Remes, J., Helin, M., Vaino, P., and Rautio, P.: Clinical outcome and left ventricular function 23 years after acute coxsackie virus myopericarditis. Eur. Heart J. 11:182, 1990.

534. Saiman, L., and Prince, A.: Infections of the heart. Adv. Pediatr. Infect. Dis. 4:139, 1989.

535. Frustaci, A., and Maseri, A.: Localized left ventricular aneurysms with normal global function caused by myocarditis. Am. J. Cardiol. 70:1221, 1992.

536. Wolfgram, L. J., and Rose, N. R.: Coxsackievirus infection as a trigger of cardiac autoimmunity. Immunol. Res. 8:61, 1989.

537. Joy, J., Rao, Y. Y., Raveendranath, M., et al.: Coxsackie viral myocarditis: A clinical and echocardiographic study. Indian Heart J. 42:441, 1990.

538. Pinamonti, B., Alberti, E., Cigalotto, A., et al.: Echocardiographic findings in myocarditis. Am. J. Cardiol. 62:285, 1988.

539. Lowry, R. W., Adam, E., Hu, C., et al.: What are the implications of cardiac infection with cytomegalovirus before heart transplantation? J. Heart Lung Transplant. 13:122, 1994.

540. Partanen, J., Nieminen, M. S., Krogerus, L., et al.: Cytomegalovirus myocarditis in transplanted heart verified by endomyocardial biopsy. Clin. Cardiol. 14:847, 1991.

541. Gonwa, T. A., Capehart, J. E., Pilcher, J. W., and Alivizatos, P. A.: Cytomegalovirus myocarditis as a cause of cardiac dysfunction in a heart transplant recipient. Transplantation 47:197, 1989.

542. Shabtai, M., Luft, B., Waltzer, W. C., et al.: Massive cytomegalovirus pneumonia and myocarditis in a renal transplant recipient: Successful treatment with DHPG. Transplant. Proc. 20:562, 1988.

543. Schindler, J. M., and Neftel, K.: Simultaneous primary infection with HIV and CMV leading to severe pancytopenia, hepatitis, nephritis, perimyocarditis, myositis, and alopecia totalis. Klin. Wochenschr. 68:237, 1990.

544. Powell, K. F., Bellamy, A. R., Catton, M. G., et al.: Cytomegalovirus myocarditis in a heart transplant recipient: Sensitive monitoring of viral DNA by the polymerase chain reaction. J. Heart Lung Transplant. 8:465, 1989.

545. George, R.: Dengue haemorrhagic fever in Malaysia: A review. Southeast Asian J. Trop. Med. Public Health 18:278, 1987.

546. Songco, R. S., Hayes, C. G., Leus, C. D., and Manaloto, C. O. R.: Dengue fever/dengue haemorrhagic fever in Filipino children: Clinical experience during the 1983–1984 epidemic. Southeast Asian J. Trop. Med. Public Health 18:284, 1987.

547. Singh, D. S., Gupta, P. R., Gupta, S. S., et al.: Cardiac changes in acute viral hepatitis in Varanasi (India): Case reports. J. Trop. Med. Hyg. 92:243, 1989.

548. Ursell, P. C., Habib, A., Sharma, P., et al.: Hepatitis B virus and myocarditis. Hum. Pathol. 15:481, 1984.

549. Mahapatra, R. K., and Ellis, G. H.: Myocarditis and hepatitis B virus. Angiology 36:116, 1985.

550. Jacob, A. J., and Boon, N. A.: HIV cardiomyopathy: A dark cloud with a silver lining? Br. Heart J. 66:1, 1991.

551. Francis, C. K.: Cardiac involvement in AIDS. Curr. Probl. Cardiol. 15:569, 1990.

552. Kaul, S., Fishbein, M. C., and Siegel, R. J.: Cardiac manifestations of acquired immune deficiency syndrome: A 1991 update. Am. Heart J. 122:535, 1991.

553. Anderson, D. W., Virmani, R., Reilly, J. M., et al.: Prevalent myocarditis at necropsy in the acquired immunodeficiency syndrome. J. Am. Coll. Cardiol. 11:792, 1988.

554. Baroldi, G., Corallo, S., Moroni, M., et al.: Focal lymphocytic myocarditis in acquired immunodeficiency syndrome (AIDS): A correlative morphologic and clinical study in 26 consecutive fatal cases. J. Am. Coll. Cardiol. 12:463, 1988.

555. Akhras, F.: HIV and opportunistic infections: which makes the heart vulnerable? Br. J. Clin. Pract. 47:232, 1993.

556. Grody, W. W., Cheng, L., and Lewis, W.: Infection of the heart by the human immunodeficiency virus. Am. J. Cardiol. 66:203, 1990.

557. Acierno, L.: Cardiac complications in acquired immunodeficiency syndrome (AIDS): A review. J. Am. Coll. Cardiol. 13:1144, 1989.

558. Blanchard, D. G., Hagenhoff, C., Chow, L. C., et al.: Reversibility of cardiac abnormalities in human immunodeficiency virus (HIV)-infected individuals: A serial echocardiographic study. J. Am. Coll. Cardiol. 17:1270, 1991.

559. Levy, W. S., Simon, G. L., Rios, J. C., and Ross, A. M.: Prevalence of cardiac abnormalities in human immunodeficiency virus infection. Am. J. Cardiol. 63:86, 1989.

560. Himelman, R. B., Chung, W. S., Chernoff, D. N., et al.: Cardiac manifestations of human immunodeficiency virus infection: A two-dimensional echocardiographic study. J. Am. Coll. Cardiol. 13:1030, 1989.

561. Hofman, P., Drici, M. D., Gibelin, P., et al.: Prevalence of toxoplasma myocarditis in patients with the acquired immunodeficiency syndrome. Br. Heart J. 70:376, 1993.

562. Herskowitz, A., Willoughby, S., Wu, T. C., et al.: Immunopathogenesis of HIV-1-associated cardiomyopathy. Clin. Immunol. Immunopathol. 68:234, 1993.

563. Beschorner, W. E., Baughman, K., Turnicky, R. P., et al.: HIV-associated myocarditis. Pathology and immunopathology. Am. J. Pathol. 137:1365, 1990.

564. Herskowitz, A., Wu, T. C., Willoughby, S. B., et al.: Myocarditis and cardiotropic viral infection associated with severe left ventricular dysfunction in late-stage infection with human immunodeficiency virus. J. Am. Coll. Cardiol. 24:1025, 1994.

564a. Lipshultz, S. E., Orav, E. J., Sanders, S. P., et al.: Cardiac structure and function in children with human immunodeficiency virus infection treated with zidovudine. N. Engl. J. Med. 327:1260, 1992.

565. Cox, J. N., di Dio, F., Pizzolato, G. P., et al.: Aspergillus endocarditis and myocarditis in a patient with the acquired immunodeficiency syndrome (AIDS). A review of the literature. Virchows Arch. A. Pathol. Anat. Histopathol. 417:255, 1990.

566. Grange, F., Kinney, E. L., Monsuez, J. J., et al.: Successful therapy for Toxoplasma gondii myocarditis in acquired immunodeficiency syndrome. Am. Heart J. 120:443, 1990.

567. Albrecht, H., Stellbrink, H. J., Fenske, S., et al.: Successful treatment of Toxoplasma gondii myocarditis in an AIDS patient. Eur. J. Clin. Microbiol. Infect. Dis. 13:500, 1994.

568. Tyson, A. A. Jr., Hackshaw, B. T., and Kutcher, M. A.: Acute Epstein-Barr virus myocarditis simulating myocardial infarction with cardiogenic shock. South. Med. J. 82:1184, 1989.

569. Sprenger, M. J., Van Naelten, M. A., Mulder, P. G., and Masurel, N.: Influenza mortality and excess deaths in the elderly, 1967–1982. Epidemiol. Infect. 103:633, 1989.

570. Agnholt, J., Sorensen, H. T., Rasmussen, S. N., et al.: Cardiac hypersensitivity to 5-aminosalicylic acid. Lancet 1:1135, 1989.

571. Ruben, F. L., and Cate, T. R.: Influenza pneumonia. Semin. Respir. Infect. 2:122, 1987.

572. Cummins, D., Bennett, D., Fisher-Hoch, S. P., et al.: Electrocardiographic abnormalities in patients with Lassa fever. J. Trop. Med. Hyg. 92:350, 1989.

573. McCormick, J. B., King, I. J., Webb, P. A., et al.: Lassa fever: A case-control study of the clinical diagnosis and course of Lassa fever. J. Infect. Dis. 155:445, 1987.

574. Ozkutlu, S., Soylemezoglu, O., Calikoglu, A. S., et al.: Fatal mumps myocarditis. Jpn. Heart J. 30:109, 1989.

575. Ward, S. C., Wiselka, M. J., and Nicholson, K. G.: Still's disease and myocarditis associated with recent mumps infection. Postgrad. Med. J. 64:693, 1988.

576. Chaudary, S., and Jaski, B. E.: Fulminant mumps myocarditis. Ann. Intern. Med. 110:569, 1989.

577. Hildes, J. A., Schaberg, A., and Alcock, A. U. W.: Cardiovascular collapse in acute poliomyelitis. Circulation 12:986, 1955.

578. Teloh, H. A.: Myocarditis in poliomyelitis. Arch. Pathol. 55:408, 1953.

579. Weinstein, L., and Shelokov, A.: Cardiovascular manifestations of acute poliomyelitis. N. Engl. J. Med. 244:281, 1951.

580. Pahl, E., and Gidding, S. S.: Echocardiographic assessment of cardiac function during respiratory syncytial virus infection. Pediatrics 81:830, 1988.

581. Martin, J. T., Kugler, J. D., Gumbiner, C. H., et al.: Refractory congestive heart failure after ribavirin in infants with heart disease and respiratory syncytial virus. Nebr. Med. J. 75:23, 1990.

582. Hoyer, S., Berglin, E., Pettersson, G., et al.: Cardiac transplantation in patients with active myocarditis. Transplant. Proc. 22:1450, 1990.

583. Frustaci, A., Abdulla, A. K., Caldarulo, M., and Buffon, A.: Fatal measles myocarditis. Cardiologia 35:347, 1990.

584. Degen, J. A. Jr.: Visceral pathology in measles: A clinicopathologic study of 100 fatal cases. Am. J. Med. Sci. 194:104, 1937.

585. Weinstein, L.: Cardiovascular manifestations in some of the common infectious diseases. Mod. Concepts Cardiovasc. Dis. 23:229, 1954.

586. Lorber, A., Zonis, Z., Maisuls, E., et al.: The scale of myocardial involvement in varicella myocarditis. Int. J. Cardiol. 20:257, 1988.

587. Tsintsof, A., Delprado, W. J., and Keogh, A. M.: Varicella zoster myocarditis progressing to cardiomyopathy and cardiac transplantation. Br. Heart J. 70:93, 1993.

588. Waagner, D. C., and Murphy, T. V.: Varicella myocarditis. Pediatr. Infect. Dis. J. 9:360, 1990.

589. Rich, R., and McErlean, M.: Complete heart block in a child with varicella. Am. J. Emerg. Med. 11:602, 1993.

590. Matthews, A. W., and Griffiths, I. D.: Post-vaccinal pericarditis and myocarditis. Br. Heart J. 36:1043, 1974.

591. Finlay-Jones, L. R.: Fatal myocarditis after vaccinations for smallpox. N. Engl. J. Med. 270:41, 1964.

592. Chevalier, P., Moncada, E., Kirkorian, G., et al.: Q fever-induced EMF. Am. Heart J. 125:1818, 1993.

593. Gur, H., Gefel, D., and Tur-Kaspa, R.: Transient electrocardiographic changes during two episodes of relapsing brucellosis. Postgrad. Med. J. 60:544, 1984.

594. Maisch, B.: Rickettsial perimyocarditis—a follow-up study. Heart Vessels 2:55, 1986.

595. Marin-Garcia, J., and Barrett, F. F.: Myocardial function in Rocky Mountain spotted fever: Echocardiographic assessment. Am. J. Cardiol. 51:341, 1983.

596. Marin-Garcia, J., and Mirvis, D. M.: Myocardial disease in Rocky Mountain spotted fever: Clinical, functional, and pathologic findings. Pediatr. Cardiol. 5:149, 1984.

597. Marin-Garcia, J.: Left ventricular dysfunction in Rocky Mountain spotted fever. Clin. Cardiol. 6:501, 1983.

598. Ganjoo, R. K., Sharma, S. N., and Roy, A. K.: Typhus myocarditis. J. Assoc. Physicians India 37:357, 1989.

599. Yotsukura, M., Aoki, N., Fukuzumi, N., and Ishikawa, K.: Review of a case of tsutsugamushi disease showing myocarditis and confirmation of Rickettsia by endomyocardial biopsy. Jpn. Circ. J. 55:149, 1991.

600. Jubber, A. S., Gunawardana, D. R., and Lulu, A. R.: Acute pulmonary edema in Brucella myocarditis and interstitial pneumonitis. Chest 97:1008, 1990.

601. Roberts, W. C., and Beard, G. W.: Gas gangrene of the heart in clostridial septicemia. Am. Heart J. 74:482, 1967.

602. Stevens, D. L., Troyer, B. E., Merrick, D. T., et al.: Lethal effects and cardiovascular effects of purified alpha- and theta-toxins from Clostridium perfringens. J. Infect. Dis. 157:272, 1988.

603. Guneratne, P.: Gas gangrene (abscess) of heart. N. Y. State J. Med. 75:1766, 1975.

604. Stockins, B. A., Lanas, F. T., Saavedra, J. G., and Opazo, J. A.: Prognosis in patients with diphtheric myocarditis and bradyarrhythmias: Assessment of results of ventricular pacing. Br. Heart J. 72:190, 1994.

605. Havaldar, P. V., Patil, V. D., Siddibhavi, B. M., et al.: Fulminant diphtheritic myocarditis. Indian Heart J. 41:265, 1989.

606. Armengol, S., Domingo, C., and Mesalles, E.: Myocarditis: A rare complication during Legionella infection. Int. J. Cardiol. 37:418, 1992.

607. Devriendt, J., Staroukine, M., Schils, E., et al.: Legionellosis and "torsades de pointes." Acta Cardiol. 45:329, 1990.

608. Sandler, M. A., Pincus, P. S., Weltman, M. D., et al.: Meningococcaemia complicated by myocarditis. A report of 2 cases. S. Afr. Med. J. 75:391, 1989.

609. Ejlertsen, T., Vesterlund, T., and Schmidt, E. B.: Myopericarditis with cardiac tamponade caused by Neisseria meningitidis serogroup W135. Eur. J. Clin. Microbiol. Infect. Dis. 7:403, 1988.

610. Agarwala, B. N., and Ruschhaupt, D. G.: Complete heart block from mycoplasma pneumoniae infection. Pediatr. Cardiol. 12:233, 1991.

611. Murray, B. J.: Nonrespiratory complications of M. pneumoniae infection. Am. Fam. Physician 37:127, 1988.

612. Karjalainen, J.: A loud third heart sound and asymptomatic myocarditis during Mycoplasma pneumoniae infection. Eur. Heart J. 11:960, 1990.

613. Page, S. R., Stewart, J. T., and Bernstein, J. J.: A progressive pericardial effusion caused by psittacosis. Br. Heart J. 60:87, 1988.

614. Odeh, M., and Oliven, A.: Chlamydial infections of the heart. Eur. J. Clin. Microbiol. Infect. Dis. 11:885, 1992.

615. Lerner, A. M.: A new continuing fatigue syndrome following mild viral illness. A proscription to exercise. Chest 94:901, 1988.

616. Delapenha, R. A., Greaves, W. L., Mani, V., and Frederick, W. R.: Typhoid fever with unusual clinical features. South. Med. J. 81:417, 1988.

617. Burt, C. R., Proudfoot, J. C., Roberts, M., and Horowitz, R. H.: Fatal myocarditis secondary to Salmonella septicemia in a young adult. J. Emerg. Med. 8:295, 1990.

618. Wander, G. S., Khurana, S. B., and Puri, S.: Salmonella myopericarditis presenting with acute pulmonary oedema. Indian Heart J. 44:55, 1992.

619. Utley, J. R., Story, J. R., and Dandilides, P. C.: Resection of infected ventricular aneurysm (Salmonella) following saddle embolus. J. Card. Surg. 8:143, 1993.

620. Singh, S., and Singhi, S.: Cardiovascular complications of enteric fever. Indian Pediatr. 29:1319, 1992.

621. Kovoor, P., Mathew, M., Abraham, T., and Taneja, P. K.: Enteric fever complicated by myocarditis, hepatitis and shock. J. Assoc. Physicians India 36:353, 1988.

622. Putterman, C., Caraco, Y., and Shalit, M.: Acute nonrheumatic perimyocarditis complicating streptococcal tonsillitis. Cardiology 78:156, 1991.

623. Maher, D., and Ostrowski, J.: Highly virulent Streptococcus pyogenes rheumatic pancarditis and fatal septicaemia with septic shock. J. Infect. 26:195, 1993.

624. Karjalainen, J.: Streptococcal tonsillitis and acute nonrheumatic myopericarditis. Chest 95:359, 1989.

625. Bali, H. K., Wahi, S., Sharma, B. K., et al.: Myocardial tuberculosis presenting as restrictive cardiomyopathy. Am. Heart J. 120:703, 1990.

626. O'Neill, R. G., Rokey, R., Greenberg, S., and Pacifico, A.: Resolution of ventricular tachycardia and endocardial tuberculoma following antituberculous therapy. Chest 100:1467, 1991.

627. Chan, A. C., and Dickens, P.: Tuberculous myocarditis presenting as sudden cardiac death. Forensic Sci. Int. 57:45, 1992.

628. Southern, J. F., Moscicki, R. A., Magro, C., et al.: Lymphedema, lymphocytic myocarditis, and sarcoidlike granulomatosis. Manifestations of Whipple's disease. JAMA 261:1467, 1989.

629. Sossai, P., DeBoni, M., and Cielo, R.: The heart and Whipple's disease. Int. J. Cardiol. 23:275, 1989.

630. James, T. N., and Bulkley, B. H.: Abnormalities of the coronary arteries in Whipple's disease. Am. Heart J. 105:481, 1983.

631. Keinath, R. D., Merrell, D. E., Vlietstra, R., and Dobbins, W. O. III: Antibiotic treatment and relapse in Whipple's disease. Long-term follow-up of 88 patients. Gastroenterology 88:1867, 1985.

632. Feldman, M.: Whipple's disease. Am. J. Med. Sci. 291:56, 1986.

633. Dixon, A. C.: The cardiovascular manifestations of leptospirosis. West. J. Med. 154:331, 1991.

634. Watt, G., Padre, L. P., Tuazon, M., and Calubaquib, C.: Skeletal and cardiac muscle involvement in severe, late leptospirosis. J. Infect. Dis. 162:266, 1990.

635. McAlister, H. F., Klementowicz, P. T., Andrews, C., et al.: Lyme carditis: An important cause of reversible heart block. Ann. Intern. Med. 110:339, 1989.

636. van der Linde, M. R., Crijns, H. J., De Koning, J., et al.: Range of atrioventricular conduction disturbances in Lyme borreliosis: A report of four cases and review of other published reports. Br. Heart J. 63:162, 1990.

637. van der Linde, M. R.: Lyme carditis: Clinical characteristics of 105 cases. Scand. J. Infect. Dis. (Suppl.)77:81, 1991.

638. Haywood, G. A., O'Connell, S., and Gray, H. H.: Lyme carditis: A United Kingdom perspective. Br. Heart J. 70:15, 1993.

639. Asch, E. S., Bujak, D. I., Weiss, M., et al.: Lyme disease: an infectious and postinfectious syndrome. J. Rheumatol. 21:454, 1994.

640. Vlay, S. C., Dervan, J. P., Elias, J., et al.: Ventricular tachycardia associated with Lyme carditis. Am. Heart J. 121:1558, 1991.

641. Rees, D. H., Keeling, P. J., McKenna, W. J., and Axford, J. S.: No evidence to implicate Borrelia burgdorferi in the pathogenesis of dilated cardiomyopathy in the United Kingdom. Br. Heart J. 71:459, 1994.

642. Stanek, G., Klein, J., Bittner, R., and Glogar, D.: Isolation of Borrelia burgdorferi from the myocardium of a patient with longstanding cardiomyopathy. N. Engl. J. Med. 322:249, 1990.

643. Kimball, S. A., Janson, P. A., and LaRaia, P. J.: Complete heart block as the sole presentation of Lyme disease. Arch. Intern. Med. 149:1897, 1989.

644. Cox, J., and Krajden, M.: Cardiovascular manifestations of Lyme disease. Am. Heart J. 122:1449, 1991.

645. Rahn, D. W., and Malawista, S. E.: Lyme disease: Recommendations for diagnosis and treatment. Ann. Intern. Med. 114:472, 1991.

646. Wengrower, D., Knobler, H., Gillis, S., and Chajek-Shaul, T.: Myocarditis in tick-borne relapsing fever. J. Infect. Dis. 149:1033, 1984.

647. Mekasha, A.: Louse-borne relapsing fever in children. J. Trop. Med. Hyg. 95:206, 1992.

648. Jackman, J. D. Jr., and Radolf, J. D.: Cardiovascular syphilis. Am. J. Med. 87:425, 1989.

649. Chino, M., Minami, T., and Nishikawa, K.: Ruptured ventricular aneurysm in secondary syphilis. Lancet 342:935, 1993.

650. Nahass, R. G., Scholz, P., Mackenzie, J. W., and Gocke, D. J.: Chronic constrictive pericarditis. A case report and review of the literature. Arch. Intern. Med. 149:1200, 1989.

651. Slutzker, A. D., and Claypool, W. D.: Pericardial actinomycosis with cardiac tamponade from a contiguous thoracic lesion. Thorax 44:442, 1989.

652. Berarducci, L., Ford, K., Olenick, S., and Devries, S.: Invasive intracardiac aspergillosis with widespread embolization. J. Am. Soc. Echocardiogr. 6:539, 1993.

653. Russack, V.: Aspergillus terreus myocarditis: Report of a case and review of the literature. Am. J. Cardiovasc. Pathol. 3:275, 1990.

654. Hori, M. K., Knight, L. L., Carvalho, P. G., and Stevens, D. L.: Aspergillar myocarditis and acute coronary artery occlusion in an immunocompromised patient. West. J. Med. 155:525, 1991.

655. Massin, E. K., Zeluff, B. J., Carrol, C. L., et al.: Cardiac transplantation and aspergillosis. Circulation 90:1552, 1994.

656. Rogers, J. G., Windle, J. R., McManus, B. M., and Easley, A. R. Jr.: Aspergillus myocarditis presenting as myocardial infarction with complete heart block. Am. Heart J. 120:430, 1990.

657. McCalmont, T. H., Silverman, J. F., and Geisinger, K. R.: Cytologic diagnosis of aspergillosis in cardiac transplantation. Arch. Surg. 126:394, 1991.

658. Hall, J. C., and Giltman, L. I.: Candida myocarditis in a patient with chronic active hepatitis and macronodular cirrhosis. J. Tenn. Med. Assoc. 79:473, 1986.

659. Atkinson, J. B., Connor, D. H., Robinowitz, M., et al.: Cardiac fungal infections: Review of autopsy findings in 60 patients. Hum. Pathol. 15:935, 1984.

660. Vartivarian, S. E., Coudron, P. E., and Markowitz, S. M.: Disseminated coccidioidomycosis. Unusual manifestations in a cardiac transplantation patient. Am. J. Med. 83:949, 1987.

661. Lafont, A., Wolff, M., Marche, C., et al.: Overwhelming myocarditis due to Cryptococcus neoformans in an AIDS patient. Lancet 2:1145, 1987.

662. Garrett, H. E. Jr., and Roper, C. L.: Surgical intervention in histoplasmosis. Ann. Thorac. Surg. 42:711, 1986.

663. Loyd, J. E., Tillman, B. F., Atkinson, J. B., and Des Prez, R. M.: Mediastinal fibrosis complicating histoplasmosis. Medicine (Baltimore) 67:295, 1988.

664. Jackman, J. D. Jr., and Simonsen, R. L.: The clinical manifestations of cardiac mucormycosis. Chest 101:1733, 1992.

665. Rossi, M. A.: Comparison of Chagas' heart disease to arrhythmogenic right ventricular cardiomyopathy. Am. Heart J. 129:626, 1995.

666. Hagar, J. M., and Rahimtoola, S. H.: Chagas' heart disease. Curr. Probl. Cardiol. 20:825, 1995.

667. Grant, I. H., Gold, J. W. M., Wittner, M., et al.: Transfusion-associated acute Chagas' disease acquired in the United States. Ann. Intern. Med. 111:849, 1989.

668. Mota, E. A., Guimaraes, A. C., Santana, O. O., et al.: A nine year prospective study of Chagas' disease in a defined rural population in northeast Brazil. Am. J. Trop. Med. Hyg. 42:429, 1990.

669. Morris, S. A., Tanowitz, H. B., Wittner, M., and Bilezikian, J. P.: Pathophysiological insights into the cardiomyopathy of Chagas' disease. Circulation 82:1900, 1990.

670. Sadigursky, M., von Kreuter, B. F., Ling, P. Y., and Santos-Buch, C. A.: Association of elevated anti-sarcolemma, anti-idiotype antibody levels with the clinical and pathologic expression of chronic Chagas myocarditis. Circulation 80:1269, 1989.

671. Palacios-Pru, E., Carrasco, H., Scorza, C., and Espinoza, R.: Ultrastructural characteristics of different stages of human chagasic myocarditis. Am. J. Trop. Med. Hyg. 41:29, 1989.

672. Bestetti, R. B., Freitas, O. C., Muccillo, G., and Oliveira, J. S.: Clinical and morphological characteristics associated with sudden cardiac death in patients with Chagas' disease. Eur. Heart J. 14:1610, 1993.

673. Carrasco, H. A., Guerrero, L., Parada, H., et al.: Ventricular arrhythmias and left ventricular myocardial function in chronic chagasic patients. Int. J. Cardiol. 28:35, 1990.

674. Casado, J., Davila, D. F., Donis, J. H., et al.: Electrocardiographic abnormalities and left ventricular systolic function in Chagas' heart disease. Int. J. Cardiol. 27:55, 1990.

675. Rossi, M. A.: Microvascular changes as a cause of chronic cardiomyopathy in Chagas' disease. Am. Heart J. 120:233, 1990.

676. Espinosa, R. A., Pericchi, L. R., Carrasco, H. A., et al.: Prognostic indicators of chronic chagasic cardiopathy. Int. J. Cardiol. 30:195, 1991.

677. Jones, E. M., Colley, D. G., Tostes, S., et al.: Amplification of a Trypanosoma cruzi DNA sequence from inflammatory lesions in human chagasic cardiomyopathy. Am. J. Trop. Med. Hyg. 48:348, 1993.

678. Reis, D. D., Jones, E. M., Tostes, S., et al.: Expression of major histocompatibility complex antigens and adhesion molecules in hearts of patients with chronic Chagas' disease. Am. J. Trop. Med. Hyg. 49:192, 1993.

679. Sanchez, J. A., Milei, J., Yu, Z. X., et al.: Immunohistochemical localization of laminin in the hearts of patients with chronic chagasic cardiomyopathy: Relationship to thickening of basement membranes. Am. Heart J. *126*:1392, 1993.

680. Mengel, J. O., and Rossi, M. A.: Chronic chagasic myocarditis pathogenesis: Dependence on autoimmune and microvascular factors. Am. Heart J. *124*:1052, 1992.

681. Oliveira, J. S. M., and Marin-Neto, J. A.: Parasympathetic impairment in Chagas' heart disease: Cause or consequence? Int. J. Cardiol. *21*:153, 1988.

682. Abelmann, W. H.: The dilated cardiomyopathies: Experimental aspects. Cardiol. Clin. *6*:219, 1988.

683. Bestetti, R. B., Santos, C. R., Machado-Junior, O. B., et al.: Clinical profile of patients with Chagas' disease before and during sustained ventricular tachycardia. Int. J. Cardiol. *29*:39, 1990.

684. Bestetti, R. B., Dalbo, C. M., Freitas, O. C., et al.: Noninvasive predictors of mortality for patients with Chagas' heart disease: A multivariate stepwise logistic regression study. Cardiology *84*:261, 1994.

685. Giniger, A. G., Retyk, E. O., Laino, R. A., et al.: Ventricular tachycardia in Chagas' disease. Am. J. Cardiol. *70*:459, 1992.

686. Carrasco, H. A., Parada, H., Guerrero, L., et al.: Prognostic implications of clinical, electrocardiographic and hemodynamic findings in chronic Chagas' disease. Int. J. Cardiol. *43*:27, 1994.

687. de Paola, A. A. V., Gomes, J. A., Miyamoto, M. H., and Fo, E. E.: Transcoronary chemical ablation of ventricular tachycardia in chronic chagasic myocarditis. J. Am. Coll. Cardiol. *20*:480, 1992.

688. Marin-Neto, J. A., Marzullo, P., Sousa, A. C., et al.: Radionuclide angiographic evidence for early predominant right ventricular involvement in patients with Chagas' disease. Can. J. Cardiol. *4*:231, 1988.

689. Marin-Neto, J. A., Marzullo, P., Marcassa, C., et al.: Myocardial perfusion abnormalities in chronic Chagas' disease as detected by thallium-201 scintigraphy. Am. J. Cardiol. *69*:780, 1992.

690. Kirchhoff, L. V.: Is *Trypanosoma cruzi* a new threat to our blood supply? Ann. Intern. Med. *111*:773, 1989.

691. de Paola, A. A. V., Horowitz, L. N., Miyamoto, M. H., et al.: Angiographic and electrophysiologic substrates of ventricular tachycardia in chronic chagasic myocarditis. Am. J. Cardiol. *65*:360, 1990.

692. de Paola, A. A. V., Horowitz, L. N., Miyamoto, M. H., et al.: Automatic implantable defibrillator with VVI pacemaker in a patient with chronic Chagas myocarditis and total atrioventricular block. Am. Heart J. *118*:415, 1989.

693. Bocchi, E. A., Moreira, L. F., Bellotti, G., et al.: Hemodynamic study during upright isotonic exercise before and six months after dynamic cardiomyoplasty for idiopathic dilated cardiomyopathy or Chagas' disease. Am. J. Cardiol. *67*:213, 1991.

694. Jatene, A. D., Moreira, L. F., Stolf, N. A., et al.: Left ventricular function changes after cardiomyoplasty in patients with dilated cardiomyopathy. J. Thorac. Cardiovasc. Surg. *102*:132, 1991.

695. Bocchi, E. A., Bellotti, G., Uip, D., et al.: Long-term follow-up after heart transplantation in Chagas' disease. Transplant. Proc. *25*:1329, 1993.

696. Tsala Mbala, P., Blackett, K., and Mbonifor, C. L.: Functional and immunologic involvement in human African trypanosomiasis caused by *Trypanosoma gambiense*. Bull. Soc. Pathol. Exot. Filiales *81*:490, 1988.

697. Holmes, P. H.: Pathophysiology of parasitic infections. Parasitology *94*:S29, 1987.

698. Adair, O. V., Randive, N., and Krasnow, N.: Isolated toxoplasma myocarditis in acquired immune deficiency syndrome. Am. Heart J. *118*:856, 1989.

699. Franzen, D., Curtius, J. M., Heitz, W., et al.: Cardiac involvement during and after malaria. Clin. Investig. *70*:670, 1992.

700. Sharma, S. N., Mohapatra, A. K., and Machave, Y. V.: Chronic falciparum cardiomyopathy. J. Assoc. Physicians India *35*:251, 1987.

701. Russo, G., Tamburino, C., Cuscuna, S., et al.: Cardiac hydatid cyst with clinical features resembling subaortic stenosis. Am. Heart J. *117*:1385, 1989.

702. Oliver, J. M., Sotillo, J. F., Dominguez, F. J., et al.: Two-dimensional echocardiographic features of echinococcosis of the heart and great blood vessels. Clinical and surgical implications. Circulation *78*:327, 1988.

703. Akhtar, M. J.: Hydatid disease of the right ventricle and role of tomographic scanning in its diagnosis. Int. J. Cardiol. *33*:432, 1991.

704. Abid, A., Khayati, A., and Zargouni, N.: Hydatid cyst of the heart and pericardium. Int. J. Cardiol. *32*:108, 1991.

705. Bayezid, O., Ocal, A., Isik, O., et al.: A case of cardiac hydatid cyst localized on the interventricular septum and causing pulmonary emboli. J. Cardiovasc. Surg. (Torino) *32*:324, 1991.

706. Benomar, A., Yahyaoui, M., Birouk, N., et al.: Middle cerebral artery occlusion due to hydatid cysts of myocardial and intraventricular cavity cardiac origin. Two cases. Stroke *25*:886, 1994.

707. Cantoni, S., Frola, C., Gatto, R., et al.: Hydatid cyst of the interventricular septum of the heart: MR findings. A.J.R. *161*:753, 1993.

708. Miralles, A., Bracamonte, L., Pavie, A., et al.: Cardiac echinococcosis. Surgical treatment and results. J. Thorac. Cardiovasc. Surg. *107*:184, 1994.

709. Urbanyi, B., Rieckmann, C., Hellberg, K., et al.: Myocardial echinococcosis with perforation into the pericardium. J. Cardiovasc. Surg. (Torino) *32*:534, 1991.

710. Dao, A. H., and Virmani, R.: Visceral larva migrans involving the myocardium: Report of two cases and review of literature. Pediatr. Pathol. *6*:449, 1986.

711. Compton, S. J., Celum, C. L., Lee, C., et al.: Trichinosis with ventilatory failure and persistent myocarditis. Clin. Infect. Dis. *16*:500, 1993.

712. Fourestie, V., Douceron, H., Brugieres, P., et al.: Neurotrichinosis. A cerebrovascular disease associated with myocardial injury and hypereosinophilia. Brain *116*:603, 1993.

713. Ursell, P. C., Habib, A., Babchick, O., et al.: Myocarditis caused by *Trichinella spiralis*. Arch. Pathol. Lab. Med. *108*:4, 1984.

714. Lopez-Lozano, J. J., Garcia Merino, J. A., and Liano, H.: Bilateral facial paralysis secondary to trichinosis. Acta Neurol. Scand. *78*:194, 1988.

TOXIC, CHEMICAL, IMMUNE AND PHYSICAL DAMAGE TO THE HEART

715. Sauer, C. M.: Recurrent embolic stroke and cocaine-related cardiomyopathy. Stroke *22*:1203, 1991.

716. Henzlova, M. J., Smith, S. H., Prchal, V. M., and Helmcke, F. R.: Apparent reversibility of cocaine-induced congestive cardiomyopathy. Am. Heart J. *122*:577, 1991.

717. Eisenberg, M. J., Mendelson, J., Evans, G. T. Jr., et al.: Left ventricular function immediately after intravenous cocaine: A quantitative two-dimensional echocardiographic study. J. Am. Coll. Cardiol. *22*:1581, 1993.

718. Pilati, C. F., Espinal, A. R., and Pukys, T. F.: Persistent left ventricular dysfunction after cocaine treatment in rabbits. Proc. Soc. Exp. Biol. Med. *203*:100, 1993.

719. Clarkson, C. W., Chang, C., Stolfi, A., et al.: Electrophysiological effects of high cocaine concentrations on intact canine heart. Evidence for modulation by both heart rate and autonomic nervous system. Circulation *87*:950, 1993.

720. Liu, C. P., Tunin, C., and Kass, D. A.: Transient time course of cocaine-induced cardiac depression versus sustained peripheral vasoconstriction. J. Am. Coll. Cardiol. *21*:260, 1993.

721. Om, A.: Cardiovascular complications of cocaine. Am. J. Med. Sci. *303*:333, 1992.

722. Kimura, S., Bassett, A. L., Xi, H., and Myerburg, R. J.: Early afterdepolarizations and triggered activity induced by cocaine. A possible mechanism of cocaine arrhythmogenesis. Circulation *85*:2227, 1992.

723. Kloner, R. A., Hale, S., Alker, K., and Rezkalla, S.: The effects of acute and chronic cocaine use on the heart. Circulation *85*:407, 1992.

724. Brogan, W. C. 3rd, Lange, R. A., Glamann, D. B., and Hillis, L. D.: Recurrent coronary vasoconstriction caused by intranasal cocaine: Possible role for metabolites. Ann. Intern. Med. *116*:556, 1992.

725. Minor, R. L. Jr., Scott, B. D., Brown, D. D., and Winniford, M. D.: Cocaine-induced myocardial infarction in patients with normal coronary arteries. Ann. Intern. Med. *115*:797, 1991.

726. Tracy, C. M., Bachenheimer, L., Solomon, A., et al.: Evidence that cocaine slows cardiac conduction by an action on both AV nodal and His-Purkinje tissue in the dog. J. Electrocardiol. *24*:257, 1991.

727. Moliterno, D. J., Lange, R. A., Gerard, R. D., et al.: Influence of intranasal cocaine on plasma constituents associated with endogenous thrombosis and thrombolysis. Am. J. Med. *96*:492, 1994.

728. Jennings, L. K., White, M. M., Sauer, C. M., et al.: Cocaine-induced platelet defects. Stroke *24*:1352, 1993.

729. Hageman, G. R., and Simor, T.: Attenuation of the cardiac effects of cocaine by dizocilpine. Am. J. Physiol. *264*:H1890, 1993.

730. Stewart, G., Rubin, E., and Thomas, A. P.: Inhibition by cocaine of excitation-contraction coupling in isolated cardiomyocytes. Am. J. Physiol. *260*:H50, 1991.

731. Isner, J. M., and Chokshi, S. K.: Cardiac complications of cocaine abuse. Annu. Rev. Med. *42*:133, 1991.

732. Petty, G. W., Brust, J. C., Tatemichi, T. K., and Barr, M. L.: Embolic stroke after smoking "crack" cocaine. Stroke *21*:1632, 1990.

733. Majid, P. A., Patel, B., Kim, H. S., et al.: An angiographic and histologic study of cocaine-induced chest pain. Am. J. Cardiol. *65*:812, 1990.

734. Lange, R. A., and Willard, J. E.: The cardiovascular effects of cocaine. Heart Dis. Stroke *2*:136, 1993.

735. Chakko, S., and Myerburg, R. J.: Cardiac complications of cocaine abuse. Clin. Cardiol. *18*:67, 1995.

736. Gitter, M. J., Goldsmith, S. R., Dunbar, D. N., and Sharkey, S. W.: Cocaine and chest pain: clinical features and outcome of patients hospitalized to rule out myocardial infarction. Ann. Intern. Med. *115*:277, 1991.

737. Chokshi, S. K., Moore, R., Pandian, N. G., and Isner, J. M.: Reversible cardiomyopathy associated with cocaine intoxication. Ann. Intern. Med. *111*:1039, 1989.

738. Chakko, S., Fernandez, A., Mellman, T. A., et al.: Cardiac manifestations of cocaine abuse: A cross-sectional study of asymptomatic men with a history of long-term abuse of "crack" cocaine. J. Am. Coll. Cardiol. *20*:1168, 1992.

739. Kloner, R. A., and Hale, S.: Unraveling the complex effects of cocaine on the heart. Circulation *87*:1046, 1993.

740. Virmani, R., Robinowitz, M., Smialek, J. E., and Smyth, D. F.: Cardiovascular effects of cocaine: an autopsy study of 40 patients. Am. Heart J. *115*:1068, 1988.

741. Egashira, K., Morgan, K. G., and Morgan, J. P.: Effects of cocaine on excitation contraction coupling of aortic smooth muscle from the feret. J. Clin. Invest. *87*:1322, 1991.

742. Hale, S. L., Alker, K. J., Rezkalla, S. H., et al.: Nifedipine protects the

heart from the acute deleterious effects of cocaine if administered before but not after cocaine. Circulation 83:1437, 1991.

743. Lange, R. A., Cigarroa, R. G., Flores, E. D., et al.: Potentiation of cocaine-induced coronary vasoconstriction by beta-adrenergic blockade. Ann. Intern. Med. 112:897, 1990.

744. Karch, S. B., and Billingham, M. E.: The pathology and etiology of cocaine-induced heart disease. Arch. Pathol. Lab. Med. 112:225, 1988.

745. Deyton, L. R., Walker, R. E., Kovacs, J. A., et al.: Reversible cardiac dysfunction associated with interferon alfa therapy in AIDS patients with Kaposi's sarcoma. N. Engl. J. Med. 321:1246, 1989.

746. Glassman, A. H., Roose, S. P., and Bigger, J. T. Jr.: The safety of tricyclic antidepressants in cardiac patients. JAMA 269:2673, 1993.

747. Morrow, P. L., Hardin, N. J., and Bonadies, J.: Hypersensitivity myocarditis and hepatitis associated with imipramine and its metabolite, desipramine. J. Forensic Sci. 34:1016, 1989.

748. Schuchter, L. M., Hendricks, C. B., Holland, K. H., et al.: Eosinophilic myocarditis associated with high-dose interleukin-2 therapy. Am. J. Med. 88:439, 1990.

749. Goel, M., Flaherty, L., Lavine, S., and Redman, B. G.: Reversible cardiomyopathy after high-dose interleukin-2 therapy. J. Immunother. 11:225, 1992.

750. Samlowski, W. E., Ward, J. H., Craven, C. M., and Freedman, R. A.: Severe myocarditis following high-dose interleukin-2 administration. Arch. Pathol. Lab. Med. 113:838, 1989.

751. Raehl, C. L., Patel, A. K., and LeRoy, M.: Drug-induced torsade de pointes. Clinical Pharmacy 4:675, 1985.

752. Horowitz, J. D.: Drugs that induce heart problems. Which agents? What effects? J. Cardiovasc. Med. 8:308, 1983.

753. Combs, A. B., and Acosta, D.: Toxic mechanisms of the heart: a review. Toxicol. Pathol. 18:583, 1990.

754. Khan, M. Y., Haider, B., and Thind, I. S.: Emetine-induced cardiomyopathy in rabbits. J. Submicrosc. Cytol. Pathol. 15:495, 1983.

755. Day, L., Kelly, C., Reed, G., et al.: Fatal cardiomyopathy: Suspected child abuse by chronic ipecac administration. Vet. Hum. Toxicol. 31:255, 1989.

756. Harbin, A. D., Gerson, M. C., and O'Connell, J. B.: Simulation of acute myopericarditis by constrictive pericardial disease with endomyocardial fibrosis due to methylsergide therapy. J. Am. Coll. Cardiol. 4:196, 1984.

757. Iglesias Cubero, G., Rodriguez Reguero, J. J., and Rojo Ortega, J. M.: Restrictive cardiomyopathy caused by chloroquine. Br. Heart J. 69:451, 1993.

758. Chulay, J. D., Spencer, H. C., and Mugambi, M.: Electrocardiographic changes during treatment of leishmaniasis with pentavalent antimony (sodium stibogluconate). Am. J. Trop. Med. Hyg. 34:702, 1985.

759. Brady, H. R., and Horgan, J. H.: Lithium and the heart: Unanswered questions. Chest 93:166, 1988.

760. James, F. W., Kaplan, S., and Benzig, G. 3rd: Cardiac complications following hydrocarbon ingestion. Am. J. Dis. Child. 121:431, 1971.

761. Cunningham, S. R., Dalzell, G. W., McGirr, P., and Khan, M. M.: Myocardial infarction and primary ventricular fibrillation after glue sniffing. BMJ 294:739, 1987.

762. Elian, D., Harpaz, D., Sucher, E., et al.: Reversible catecholamine-induced cardiomyopathy presenting as acute pulmonary edema in a patient with pheochromocytoma. Cardiology 83:118, 1993.

763. Anonymous: Phaeochromocytoma still surprises. Lancet 335:1189, 1990.

764. Sardesai, S. H., Mourant, A. J., Sivathandon, Y., et al.: Phaeochromocytoma and catecholamine induced cardiomyopathy presenting as heart failure. Br. Heart J. 63:234, 1990.

765. Jiang, J. P., and Downing, S. E.: Catecholamine cardiomyopathy: Review and analysis of pathogenetic mechanisms. Yale J. Biol. Med. 63:581, 1990.

766. Raper, R., Fisher, M., and Bihari, D.: Profound, reversible, myocardial depression in acute asthma treated with high-dose catecholamines. Crit. Care Med. 20:710, 1992.

767. Jiang, J. P., Chen, V., and Downing, S. E.: Modulation of catecholamine cardiomyopathy by allopurinol. Am. Heart J. 122:115, 1991.

768. Frustaci, A., Loperfido, F., Gentiloni, N., et al.: Catecholamine-induced cardiomyopathy in multiple endocrine neoplasia. A histologic, ultrastructural, and biochemical study. Chest 99:382, 1991.

769. Kopp, S. J., Barron, J. T., and Tow, J. P.: Cardiovascular actions of lead and relationship to hypertension: A review. Environ. Health Perspect. 78:91, 1988.

770. Kurppa, K., Hietanen, E., and Klockars, M.: Chemical exposures at work and cardiovascular morbidity. Atherosclerosis, ischemic heart disease, hypertension, cardiomyopathy and arrhythmias. Scand. J. Work Environ. Health 10:381, 1984.

771. Penney, D. G.: A review: Hemodynamic response to carbon monoxide. Environ. Health Perspect. 77:121, 1988.

772. McMeekin, J. D., and Finegan, B. A.: Reversible myocardial dysfunction following carbon monoxide poisoning. Can. J. Cardiol. 3:118, 1987.

773. Marius-Nunez, A. L.: Myocardial infarction with normal coronary arteries after acute exposure to carbon monoxide. Chest 97:491, 1990.

774. Kudoh, C., Tanaka, S., Marusaki, S., et al.: Hypocalcemic cardiomyopathy in a patient with idiopathic hypoparathyroidism. Intern. Med. 31:561, 1992.

775. Feldman, A. M., Fivush, B., Zahka, K. G., et al.: Congestive cardiomyopathy in patients on continuous ambulatory peritoneal dialysis. Am. J. Kidney Dis. 11:76, 1988.

776. Kurnik, B. R., Marshall, J., and Katz, S. M.: Hypomagnesemia-induced cardiomyopathy. Magnesium 7:49, 1988.

777. Riggs, J. E., Klingberg, W. G., Flink, E. B., et al.: Cardioskeletal mitochondrial myopathy associated with chronic magnesium deficiency. Neurology 42:128, 1992.

778. Lake, N.: Effects of taurine deficiency on arrhythmogenesis and excitation-contraction coupling in cardiac tissue. Adv. Exp. Med. Biol. 315:173, 1992.

779. Tenaglia, A., and Cody, R.: Evidence for a taurine-deficiency cardiomyopathy. Am. J. Cardiol. 62:136, 1988.

780. Rodrigues Pereira, R., Scholte, H. R., Luyt-Houwen, I. E., and Vaandrager-Verduin, M. H.: Cardiomyopathy associated with carnitine loss in kidneys and small intestine. Eur. J. Pediatr. 148:193, 1988.

781. Regitz, V., Shug, A. L., and Fleck, E.: Defective myocardial carnitine metabolism in congestive heart failure secondary to dilated cardiomyopathy and to coronary, hypertensive and valvular heart diseases. Am. J. Cardiol. 65:755, 1990.

782. Unsigned Editorial: Carnitine deficiency. Lancet 335:631, 1990.

783. Bautista, J., Rafel, E., Martinez, A., et al.: Familial hypertrophic cardiomyopathy and muscle carnitine deficiency. Muscle Nerve 13:192, 1990.

784. Ino, T., Sherwood, W. G., Benson, L. N., et al.: Cardiac manifestations in disorders of fat and carnitine metabolism in infancy. J. Am. Coll. Cardiol. 11:1301, 1988.

785. Taillard, F., Mundler, O., Tillous-Borde, I., et al.: Value of radionuclide assessment with thallium 201 scintigraphy in carnitine deficiency cardiomyopathy. Eur. Heart J. 9:811, 1988.

786. Yang, F. Y., Lin, Z. H., Li, S. G., et al.: Keshan disease—an endemic mitochondrial cardiomyopathy in China. J. Trace Elem. Electrolytes Health Dis. 2:157, 1988.

787. Yang, G. Q., Ge, K. Y., Chen, J. S., and Chen, X. S.: Selenium-related endemic diseases and the daily selenium requirement of humans. World Rev. Nutr. Diet. 55:98, 1988.

788. Bunker, V. W., and Clayton, B. E.: Selenium status in disease: The role of selenium as a therapeutic agent. Br. J. Clin. Pract. 44:401, 1990.

789. Cheng, Y. Y., and Qian, P. C.: The effect of selenium-fortified table salt in the prevention of Keshan disease on a population of 1.05 million. Biomed. Environ. Sci. 3:422, 1990.

790. Levy, J. B., Jones, H. W., and Gordon, A. C.: Selenium deficiency, reversible cardiomyopathy and short-term intravenous feeding. Postgrad. Med. J. 70:235, 1994.

791. Abrams, C. K., Siram, S. M., Galsim, C., et al.: Selenium deficiency in long-term total parenteral nutrition. Nutr. Clin. Pract. 7:175, 1992.

792. Murthy, K. R., Zolfagharian, H., Medh, J. D., et al.: Disseminated intravascular coagulation & disturbances in carbohydrate & fat metabolism in acute myocarditis produced by scorpion (Buthus tamulus) venom. Indian J. Med. Res. 87:318, 1988.

793. Brand, A., Keren, A., Kerem, E., et al.: Myocardial damage after a scorpion sting: long-term echocardiographic follow-up. Pediatr. Cardiol. 9:59, 1988.

794. Murthy, K. R. K., Vakil, A. E., Yeolekar, M. E., and Vakil, Y. E.: Reversal of metabolic and electrocardiographic changes induced by Indian red scorpion (Buthus tamulus) venom by administration of insulin, alpha blocker and sodium bicarbonate. Indian J. Med. Res. 88:450, 1988.

795. Sofer, S., Shahak, E., Slonim, A., and Gueron, M.: Myocardial injury without heart failure following envenomation by the scorpion Leiurus quinquestriatus in children. Toxicon 29:382, 1991.

796. Sinha, A. K.: Cardiovascular manifestations of scorpion sting in a case of congenital complete atrioventricular block. J. Indian Med. Assoc. 87:237, 1989.

797. Amaral, C. F. S., Lopes, J. A., Magalhaes, R. A., and de Rezende, N. A.: Electrocardiographic, enzymatic and echocardiographic evidence of myocardial damage after Tityus serrulatus scorpion poisoning. Am. J. Cardiol. 67:655, 1991.

798. Jones, E., and Joy, M.: Acute myocardial infarction after a wasp sting. Br. Heart J. 59:506, 1988.

799. Moore, R. S.: Second-degree heart block associated with envenomation by Vipera berus. Arch. Emerg. Med. 5:116, 1988.

800. Burch, J. M., Agarwal, R., Mattox, K. L., et al.: The treatment of crotalid envenomation without antivenin. J. Trauma 28:35, 1988.

801. Tibballs, J., Sutherland, S., and Kerr, S.: Studies on Australian snake venoms. Part 1: The haemodynamic effects of brown snake (Pseudonaja) species in the dog. Anaesth. Intensive Care 17:466, 1989.

802. Than-Than, Francis, N., Tin-Nu-Swe, et al.: Contribution of focal haemorrhage and microvascular fibrin deposition to fatal envenoming by Russell's viper (Vipera russelli siamensis) in Burma. Acta Trop. (Basel) 46:23, 1989.

803. Hall, J. C., and Harruff, R.: Fatal cardiac arrhythmia in a patient with interstitial myocarditis related to chronic arsenic poisoning. South. Med. J. 82:1557, 1989.

804. Kantrowitz, N. E., and Bristow, M. R.: Cardiotoxicity of antitumor agents. Prog. Cardiovasc. Dis. 27:195, 1984.

805. Cazin, B., Gorin, N. C., Laporte, J. P., et al.: Cardiac complications after bone marrow transplantation. A report on a series of 63 consecutive transplantations. Cancer 57:2061, 1986.

806. Judge, K. W., and Ward, N. E.: Fatal azide-induced cardiomyopathy presenting as acute myocardial infarction. Am. J. Cardiol. 64:830, 1989.

807. Howard, J. D., Skogerboe, K. J., Case, G. A., et al.: Death following accidental sodium azide ingestion. J. Forensic Sci. 35:193, 1990.

808. Fagan, E., Forbes, A., and Williams, R.: Toxic myocarditis in paracetamol poisoning. BMJ 296:63, 1988.
809. Misset, B., Escudier, B., Leclercq, B., et al.: Acute myocardiotoxicity during 5-fluorouracil therapy. Intensive Care Med. 16:210, 1990.
810. Sasson, Z., Morgan, C. D., Wang, B., et al.: 5-Fluorouracil related toxic myocarditis: case reports and pathological confirmation. Can. J. Cardiol. 10:861, 1994.
811. Martin, M., Diaz-Rubio, E., Furio, V., et al.: Lethal cardiac toxicity after cisplatin and 5-fluorouracil chemotherapy. Report of a case with necropsy study. Am. J. Clin. Oncol. 12:229, 1989.
812. Rowinsky, E. K., Eisenhauer, E. A., Chaudhry, V., et al.: Clinical toxicities encountered with paclitaxel (Taxol). Semin. Oncol. 20:1, 1993.
813. Gravanis, M. B., Hertzler, G. L., Franch, R. H., et al.: Hypersensitivity myocarditis in heart transplant candidates. J. Heart Lung Transplant. 10:688, 1991.
814. Getz, M. A., Subramanian, R., Logemann, T., and Ballantyne, F.: Acute necrotizing eosinophilic myocarditis as a manifestation of severe hypersensitivity myocarditis. Antemortem diagnosis and successful treatment. Ann. Intern. Med. 115:201, 1991.
815. Burke, A. P., Saenger, J., Mullick, F., and Virmani, R.: Hypersensitivity myocarditis. Arch. Pathol. Lab. Med. 115:764, 1991.
816. Kounis, N. G., Zavras, G. M., Soufras, G. D., and Kitrou, M. P.: Hypersensitivity myocarditis. Ann. Allergy 62:71, 1989.
817. Markus, C. K., Chow, L. H., Wycoff, D. M., and McManus, B. M.: Pet food−derived penicillin residue as a potential cause of hypersensitivity myocarditis and sudden death. Am. J. Cardiol. 63:1154, 1989.
818. Sadjadi, S. A., Lehari, R. U., and Berger, A. R.: Prolongation of the PR interval induced by methyldopa. Am. J. Cardiol. 54:675, 1984.
819. Garty, B. Z., Offer, I., Livni, E., and Danon, Y. L.: Erythema multiforme and hypersensitivity myocarditis caused by ampicillin. Ann. Pharmacother. 28:730, 1994.
820. Taliercio, C. P., Olney, B. A., and Lie, J. T.: Myocarditis related to drug hypersensitivity. Mayo Clin. Proc. 60:463, 1985.
821. Nariman, S.: Adverse reactions to drugs used in the treatment of tuberculosis. Adverse Drug React. Toxicol. Rev. 7:207, 1988.
822. Davidoff, R., Palacios, I., Southern, J., et al.: Giant cell versus lymphocytic myocarditis. A comparison of their clinical features and long-term outcomes. Circulation 83:953, 1991.
823. Mason, J. W.: Distinct forms of myocarditis. Circulation 83:1110, 1991.
824. Khoury, Z., Keren, A., Benhorin, J., and Stern, S.: Aborted sudden death in a young patient with isolated granulomatous myocarditis. Eur. Heart J. 15:397, 1994.
825. Ren, H., Poston, R. S. Jr., Hruban, R. H., et al.: Long survival with giant cell myocarditis. Mod. Pathol. 6:402, 1993.
826. Laruelle, C., Vanhaecke, J., van de Werf, F., et al.: Cardiac transplantation in giant cell myocarditis. A case report. Acta Cardiol. 49:279, 1994.
827. Desjardins, V., Pelletier, G., Leung, T. K., and Waters, D.: Successful treatment of severe heart failure caused by idiopathic giant cell myocarditis. Can. J. Cardiol. 8:788, 1992.
828. Kong, G., Madden, B., Spyrou, N., et al.: Response of recurrent giant cell myocarditis in a transplanted heart to intensive immunosuppression. Eur. Heart J. 12:554, 1991.
829. Nieminen, M. S., Salminen, U. S., Taskinen, E., et al.: Treatment of serious heart failure by transplantation in giant cell myocarditis diagnosed by endomyocardial biopsy. J. Heart Lung Transplant. 13:543, 1994.
830. Zahger, D., Moses, A., and Weiss, A. T.: Evidence of prolonged myocardial dysfunction in heat stroke. Chest 95:1089, 1989.
831. Maaravi, Y., and Weiss, A. T.: The effect of prolonged hypothermia on cardiac function in a young patient with accidental hypothermia. Chest 98:1019, 1990.
832. Weinberg, A. D.: Hypothermia. Ann. Emerg. Med. 22:370, 1993.
833. Carlson, R. G., Mayfield, W. R., Normann, S., and Alexander, J. A.: Radiation-associated valvular disease. Chest 99:538, 1991.
834. Loyer, E. M., and Delpassand, E. S.: Radiation-induced heart disease: Imaging features. Semin. Roentgenol. 28:321, 1993.
835. Om, A., Ellahham, S., and Vetrovec, G. W.: Radiation-induced coronary artery disease. Am. Heart J. 124:1598, 1992.
836. Cosset, J. M., Henry-Amar, M., and Meerwaldt, J. H.: Long-term toxicity of early stages of Hodgkin's disease therapy: The EORTC experience. EORTC Lymphoma Cooperative Group. Ann. Oncol. 2(Suppl 2):77, 1991.
837. Lagrange, J.-L., Darcourt, J., Benoliel, J., et al.: Acute cardiac effects of mediastinal irradiation: assessment by radionuclide angiography. Int. J. Radiat. Oncol. Biol. Phys. 22:897, 1992.
838. Savage, D. E., Constine, L. S., Schwartz, R. G., and Rubin, P.: Radiation effects on left ventricular function and myocardial perfusion in long term survivors of Hodgkin's disease. Int. J. Radiat. Oncol. Biol. Phys. 19:721, 1990.
839. Gustavsson, A., Eskilsson, J., Landberg, T., et al.: Late cardiac effects after mantle radiotherapy in patients with Hodgkin's disease. Ann. Oncol. 1:355, 1990.
840. Glanzmann, C., Huguenin, P., Lutolf, U. M., et al.: Cardiac lesions after mediastinal irradiation for Hodgkin's disease. Radiother. Oncol. 30:43, 1994.
841. Horimoto, M., Igarashi, K., Takenaka, T., and Batra, S.: Pulmonary infundibular stenosis, coronary artery disease, and aortic regurgitation caused by mediastinal radiation. Am. Heart J. 126:1002, 1993.
842. Jones, R. A., Hall, R. J. C., and Fraser, A. G.: Severe mitral regurgitation caused by immobile posterior leaflet after radiotherapy. J. Am. Soc. Echocardiogr. 8:207, 1995.
843. Larsen, R. L., Jakacki, R. I., Vetter, V. L., et al.: Electrocardiographic changes and arrhythmias after cancer therapy in children and young adults. Am. J. Cardiol. 70:73, 1992.
844. Orzan, F., Brusca, A., Gaita, F., et al.: Associated cardiac lesions in patients with radiation-induced complete heart block. Int. J. Cardiol. 39:151, 1993.

Chapter 42
Primary Tumors of the Heart
WILSON S. COLUCCI, FREDERICK J. SCHOEN, EUGENE BRAUNWALD

With an incidence of 0.0017 to 0.28 per cent in autopsy series,[1-5] primary tumors of the heart* are far less common than metastatic tumors to the heart.[6] The diagnosis is further complicated by the fact that the most common cardiac tumor, myxoma, causes a variety of nonspecific clinical signs and symptoms that often masquerade as many other more common cardiovascular and systemic diseases (Tables 42–1 and 42–2). Prior to the advent of modern cardiopulmonary bypass surgical techniques, the correct antemortem diagnosis of an intracardiac tumor was largely academic, since effective therapy was not possible. However, now that many cardiac tumors are curable by operation, it is critically important to establish this diagnosis whenever possible. During the last decade, major advances in noninvasive cardiovascular diagnostic techniques—especially echocardiography (see p. 94), computed tomography (see p. 341), and magnetic resonance imaging (see p. 325)—have greatly facilitated this task, and it is now possible safely and readily to screen patients suspected of having a cardiac tumor, in many cases arriving at a definitive diagnosis preoperatively. Nevertheless, a high index of suspicion remains the most important element in diagnosing a cardiac tumor.

TABLE 42–1   SYMPTOMS AND SIGNS OF CARDIAC MYXOMA

SYMPTOMS	INCIDENCE %
Dyspnea on exertion	>75
Paroxysmal dyspnea	~25
Fever	~50
Weight loss	~25
Severe dizziness/syncope	~20
Sudden death	~15
Hemoptysis	~15
SIGNS	**INCIDENCE %**
Mitral diastolic murmur	~75
Mitral systolic murmur	~50
Pulmonary hypertension	~70
Right heart failure	~70
Pulmonary emboli	~25
Anemia	>33
Elevated ESR	>33
Third heart sound (tumor plop)	>33
Atrial fibrillation	~15
Elevated globulins	~10
Clubbing	~5
Raynaud's phenomenon	<5

ESR = Erythrocyte sedimentation rate.
From Fisher, J.: Cardiac myxoma. Cardiovasc. Rev. Rep. *9*:1195, 1983.

---

* Tumors arising elsewhere in the body and metastasizing to the pericardium and heart are discussed in Chap. 43 (Pericardial Disease) and Chap. 57 (Hematologic-Oncologic Disorders and Heart Disease).

CLINICAL PRESENTATION

SYSTEMIC FINDINGS. Cardiac tumors, particularly cardiac myxoma, can produce a broad array of systemic (i.e., noncardiac) findings including fever, cachexia, malaise, arthralgias, Raynaud's phenomenon, rash, clubbing, and episodic bizarre behavior,[7,8] as well as systemic and pulmonary emboli. A variety of laboratory findings has been reported, including hypergammaglobulinemia, elevated erythrocyte sedimentation rate, thrombocytosis, thrombocytopenia, polycythemia, leukocytosis, and anemia. Systemic signs and symptoms frequently resolve when the tumor is removed.

Role of Interleukin-6. The association of constitutional symptoms with cardiac myxoma is likely to be due to the tumor's constitutive synthesis and secretion of interleukin-

TABLE 42–2   CONDITIONS OFTEN CONFUSED WITH ATRIAL MYXOMA

LEFT ATRIUM
Rheumatic mitral valve disease (MS, MR)
Pulmonary hypertension (primary, or secondary to mitral valve disease or LV failure)
Intrinsic lung disease
Cerebrovascular disease (CVA, TIA)
Endocarditis
Rheumatic fever
Myocarditis
Vasculitis (polyarteritis, lupus erythematosus)

RIGHT ATRIUM
Rheumatic tricuspid valve diseae (TS, TR)
Ebstein's anomaly
Atrial septal defect
Pulmonary hypertension
Pulmonary emboli
Constrictive pericarditis
Pleuropericarditis (rub)
Carcinoid heart disease
Cardiomyopathy

RIGHT VENTRICLE
Pulmonic stenosis
Infundibular stenosis
Pulmonary emboli
Pulmonary hypertension

LEFT VENTRICLE
Aortic stenosis
Subaortic stenosis
Cerebrovascular disease
Mural thrombus

MS = mitral stenosis; MR = mitral regurgitation; LV = left ventricular; CVA = cerebrovascular accident; TIA = transient ischemic attack; TS = tricuspid stenosis; TR = tricuspid regurgitation.
From Fisher, J.: Cardiac myxoma. Cardiovasc. Rev. Rep. *9*:1195, 1983.

6 (IL-6),[9–16] an inflammatory cytokine thought to be a major inducer of the acute phase response, which is associated with fever, leukocytosis, and activation of the complement and clotting cascades.[10] In vitro, IL-6 induces the synthesis of C-reactive protein, serum amyloid A, alpha-2-macroglobulin, and fibrinogen by human hepatocytes.[10] High levels of myxoma cell production of IL-6 may be accompanied by elevated serum concentration in patients with cardiac myxoma who have symptoms characteristic of autoimmune diseases.[14] In some cases, serum IL-6 levels become undetectable and the immunological features resolve upon removal of the tumor.[15] Increased titers of antibodies to myocardium[16] and neutrophils[17] have also been found in patients with myxoma and were shown to fall after removal of the tumor. A case of multiple myeloma has been attributed to continuous immunological stimulation by a left atrial myxoma.[18] Because the cardiac findings are nonspecific and may be subtle or absent, it is not unusual for these systemic findings to lead to a diagnosis of collagen vascular disease, infection, or noncardiac malignant disease.[19–21] Rarely, myxomas may be superinfected by bacteria or fungi.[22,23]

EMBOLIC PHENOMENA. The embolization of tumor fragments or of thrombi from the surface of a tumor is a frequent and often dramatic clinical occurrence.[24–28] Although myxomas are the source of most tumor emboli because of the combination of their friable consistency and intracavitary location (Fig. 42–1), other types of cardiac tumors occasionally may embolize.

The distribution of tumor emboli depends upon the location of the tumor and the presence or absence of intracardiac shunts. Left-sided tumors embolize to the systemic circulation, resulting in infarction and hemorrhage of viscera, including the heart,[24] as well as peripheral limb ischemia and vascular aneurysms. The diagnosis of an intracardiac tumor may be made after histological examination of systemic embolic material,[29,30] and therefore it is of critical importance to make every effort to recover and examine embolic material. In some cases, particularly when petechiae are present, biopsy of skin or muscle[28] may demonstrate intravascular tumor emboli.

Multiple systemic emboli may mimic systemic vasculitis[28] or infective endocarditis, especially when associated with other manifestations of a systemic illness such as fever, weight loss, arthralgias, elevated erythrocyte sedimentation rate, and elevated serum gamma globulins. The finding at angiography of multiple vascular aneurysms secondary to tumor emboli in the cerebral, renal, femoral, and coronary arteries is not infrequent[31] and may lead to the mistaken diagnosis of polyarteritis nodosa.[19] The neurological consequences of embolization include transient ischemic attacks, seizures, syncope, and cerebral, cerebellar, brain stem, spinal cord, or retinal infarction.[32] The neurological event may occasionally be the first or only clinical manifestation of a cardiac tumor. An embolic stroke in a young person without evidence of cerebrovascular disease, particularly in the presence of sinus rhythm, should raise the possibility of intracardiac myxoma, as well as infective endocarditis and prolapse of the mitral valve.

Right-sided cardiac tumors, and left-sided cardiac tumors proximal to left-to-right intracardiac shunts, may result in pulmonary emboli.[25,26] Indeed, serious pulmonary hypertension and secondary cor pulmonale due to chronic recurrent pulmonary emboli from a right atrial myxoma have been noted.[33] Clinically, the findings may be indistinguishable from pulmonary emboli secondary to venous thromboembolism (Chap. 46). Although the findings on chest roentgenogram are nonspecific, perfusion lung scanning in such patients may be atypical of pulmonary embolism in two respects: (1) The tumor-produced perfusion defects may remain static for long periods, as opposed to typical pulmonary embolic disease in which the defects usually resolve over the course of a few weeks; and (2) there may be complete absence of flow to one lung in the presence of com-

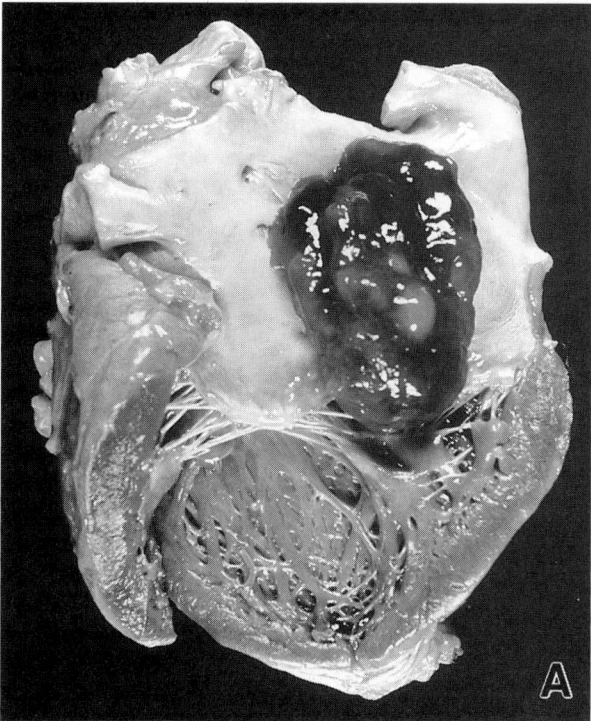
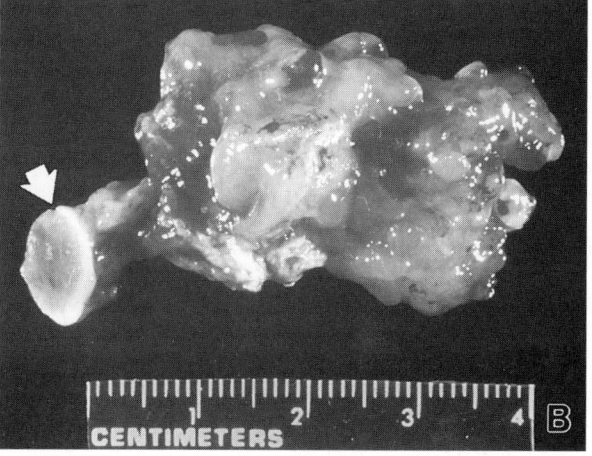

FIGURE 42–1. Photographs of the two most frequent gross appearances of cardiac myxomas. *A*, Polypoid, smooth, round, hemorrhagic left atrial myxoma, noted at autopsy. The tumor mass nearly fills the left atrium and extends into the mitral valve orifice. *B*, Irregular gelatinous, friable myxoma mass, surgically removed. The resection margin that surrounds the proximal portion of the stalk is indicated by an arrow. (*A* from Cotran, R. S., et al.: Robbins' Pathologic Basis of Disease. 5th ed. Philadelphia, W. B. Saunders Company, 1994. *B* from Schoen, F. J.: Interventional and Surgical Cardiovascular Pathology: Clinical Correlations and Basic Principles. Philadelphia, W. B. Saunders Company, 1989.)

pletely normal perfusion of the opposite lung, a pattern unusual with typical pulmonary emboli.

Cardiac Manifestations

The specific signs and symptoms produced by tumors are more closely related to their precise anatomical location than to their histological types.[34] Thus, it is useful to consider the constellation of findings typical of each location. The presentation of *pericardial tumors* is considered on page 1522 and will not be discussed here except to point out that primary tumors of the myocardium and endocardium may extend into the pericardial space and produce many of the clinical manifestations of pericardial tumors, including hemorrhagic pericardial effusion and compression of the heart by the effusion or the tumor itself.

MYOCARDIAL TUMORS. When clinically apparent, myocardial tumors most commonly result in disturbances of conduction or rhythm,[35-38] the precise nature of which is determined by the location of the tumor. Thus, tumors in the area of the atrioventricular node, typically angiomas and mesotheliomas, may produce atrioventricular (AV) conduction disturbances, including complete heart block and asystole, and can lead to sudden death.[35-38] A wide variety of arrhythmias may be produced, including atrial fibrillation or flutter, paroxysmal atrial tachycardia with or without block, nodal rhythm, ventricular premature beats, ventricular tachycardia, and ventricular fibrillation.[34,38] Intramural tumors may also produce symptoms by virtue of their size and location. Impairment of ventricular performance may simulate congestive, restrictive, or hypertrophic cardiomyopathy (Chap. 41). Tumor infiltration of the myocardial wall occasionally causes myocardial rupture.[39]

LEFT ATRIAL TUMORS. Mobile, pedunculated, left atrial tumors may prolapse to variable degrees into the mitral valve orifice, resulting in obstruction to atrioventricular blood flow and, frequently, mitral regurgitation. The resultant signs and symptoms often mimic those of mitral valve disease[1,5,39] (Table 42–2), especially mitral stenosis (see p. 1011)[40] and include dyspnea, orthopnea, paroxysmal nocturnal dyspnea, pulmonary edema, cough, hemoptysis, chest pain, peripheral edema, and fatigue. However, weight loss, pallor, syncope, and sudden death—manifestations that are uncommon with mitral valve disease—also occur. It is not unusual for the symptoms to be sudden in onset, intermittent, and related to the patient's body position.[5,34] Although the majority of symptoms produced by left atrial tumors are nonspecific, the occurrence of paroxysmal symptoms that arise characteristically in a particular body position and are out of proportion to the clinical findings should raise suspicion of a left atrial tumor. The most common primary cardiac tumor presenting in the left atrium is the benign myxoma, which, in the large majority of cases, is solitary (see p. 1467).

Physical Examination. This may disclose signs of pulmonary congestion, an S_4, a loud S_1 which is often widely split, a holosystolic murmur which is loudest at the apex and resembles mitral regurgitation, and a diastolic murmur resulting from obstruction to flow through the mitral orifice produced by the tumor. The loud S_1 that occurs in patients with left atrial myxoma may be due to the late onset of mitral valve closure resulting from prolapse of the tumor through the mitral valve orifice.[41] Consequently the left ventricular–left atrial pressure crossover occurs at a higher pressure, as in patients with mitral stenosis or a short P-R interval. It has been suggested that the finding of a loud S_1 in the absence of a short P-R interval or a mitral diastolic murmur should raise the suspicion of a left atrial tumor.[41] In many cases an early diastolic sound, termed a tumor plop, can be identified. It is thought to be produced as the tumor strikes the endocardial wall or as its excursion is abruptly halted. Although in most cases the tumor plop occurs later than the opening snap of the mitral valve and

earlier than the S_3, it is not surprising that this sound is frequently confused with the opening snap or the S_3.

RIGHT ATRIAL TUMORS. Right atrial tumors frequently produce symptoms of right heart failure, including fatigue, peripheral edema, ascites, hepatomegaly, and prominent *a* waves in the jugular venous pulse.[34,42–44a] The average time interval from the symptomatic presentation to the correct diagnosis of right atrial tumor may be years. The development of right heart failure may be rapidly progressive and is often associated with new systolic or diastolic murmurs or both. The murmurs are generally the result of tumor obstruction to tricuspid valve flow or of tricuspid regurgitation caused by tumor interference with valve closure or valve destruction caused directly or indirectly by the tumor.[45] It is not surprising that right atrial tumors have been misdiagnosed as Ebstein's anomaly of the tricuspid valve, constrictive pericarditis, tricuspid stenosis, carcinoid syndrome, superior vena caval syndrome, and cardiomyopathy (Table 42–2). Pulmonary embolism and pulmonary hypertension occur and may simulate classic thromboembolic disease.[43] Right atrial hypertension may cause right-to-left shunting through a patent foramen ovale, with systemic hypoxia, cyanosis, clubbing, and polycythemia.[44a] Whereas myxomas occur much more commonly in the left atrium than in the right atrium, sarcomas occur more commonly in the right atrium.

Physical Examination. This may reveal peripheral edema, evidence of superior vena caval obstruction, hepatomegaly, and ascites. An early diastolic rumbling murmur, alone or in combination with a holosystolic murmur secondary to tricuspid regurgitation, may demonstrate respiratory or positional variation. Because of the rarity of *isolated* rheumatic tricuspid valvular disease, the lack of other valvular findings should raise the question of a right atrial tumor. A protodiastolic tumor plop has been described and is thought to be similar in etiology to that produced by left atrial tumors.[46] The jugular venous pressure may be elevated, and a prominent *a* wave and steep *y* descent may be present.

RIGHT VENTRICULAR TUMORS. Right ventricular tumors often present with right heart failure as a result of obstruction to right ventricular filling or outflow. Clinical manifestations include peripheral edema, hepatomegaly, ascites, shortness of breath, syncope, and sudden death.

A systolic ejection murmur at the left sternal border is usually found on physical examination. A presystolic murmur and a diastolic rumble[34] have been noted and are thought to be due to obstruction of the tricuspid valve. An S_3 may be audible, and a low-pitched diastolic sound that coincides with the maximal anterior excursion of the tumor has been ascribed either to tumor or to late closure of the pulmonary valve.[47] P_2 is often delayed, and its intensity may be normal, decreased, or increased. Tumor emboli to the pulmonary arteries may result in pulmonary hypertension, and the presence of tumor in the pulmonic valve orifice may lead to pulmonary regurgitation. The jugular veins are frequently distended with a prominent *a* wave and may demonstrate Kussmaul's sign (see p. 19).

The cardiac findings often lead to a diagnosis of pulmonic stenosis, restrictive cardiomyopathy, or tricuspid regurgitation. Whereas pulmonic stenosis is often asymptomatic and slowly progressive, the symptoms of right ventricular tumors are often rapidly progressive, and there is no poststenotic dilatation or systolic ejection click.

LEFT VENTRICULAR TUMORS. When left ventricular tumors are predominantly intramural in location, they are often asymptomatic, or they may present as conduction disturbances or arrhythmias, or they may interfere with ventricular function. However, when the tumor also has a significant intracavitary component, there may be obstruction to left ventricular outflow, resulting in syncope and findings consistent with left ventricular failure. Atypical chest pain has also been reported and, in some cases, may

TABLE 42–3 RELATIVE INCIDENCE OF BENIGN TUMORS OF THE HEART

BENIGN TUMOR	% OF GROUP		
	Adults	Children	Infants
Myxoma	46	15	0
Lipoma	21	0	0
Papillary fibroelastoma	16	0	0
Rhabdomyoma	2	46	65
Fibroma	3	15	12
Hemangioma	5	5	4
Teratoma	1	13	18
Mesothelioma of the AV node	3	4	2
Granular cell tumor	1	0	0
Neurofibroma	1	1	0
Lymphangioma	1	0	0
Hamartoma	0	1	0

Data representing the extensive investigations of the Armed Forces Institute of Pathology as well as the cumulative experience of other researchers. A total of 265, 82, and 49 benign tumors were found in adults (aged >16 years), children (aged 1 to 16 years), and infants (aged <1 year), respectively. Myxomas were the most common reported benign tumors in adults, whereas rhabdomyomas were the most common benign tumors in both children and infants; benign teratomas also occurred frequently in children and infants.

From Allard, M. F. et al.: Primary cardiac tumors. *In* Goldhaber, S., and Braunwald, E. (eds): Atlas of Heart Diseases. Philadelphia, Current Medicine, 1995, pp. 15.1–15.22.

reflect obstruction of a coronary artery either directly by tumor involvement or as a result of a tumor embolus to the coronary artery.

Physical Examination. This reveals a systolic murmur, and both the murmur and the blood pressure may vary with position. Left ventricular tumors may simulate the findings of aortic stenosis, subaortic stenosis, hypertrophic cardiomyopathy, endocardial fibroelastosis, and coronary artery disease.

Benign Versus Malignant Tumors

The types of benign and malignant mesenchymal tumors that may develop in the heart are typical of those occurring in any mass of striated muscle and connective tissue. Although the exact incidence of each specific tumor type cannot be stated, about 75 per cent of all cardiac tumors are benign histologically and the remainder are malignant.[1] The majority of benign cardiac tumors are myxomas, followed in frequency by a wide variety of other tumors (Table 42–3). Almost all malignant cardiac tumors are sar-

TABLE 42–4 RELATIVE INCIDENCE OF PRIMARY MALIGNANT TUMORS OF THE HEART

TUMOR TYPE	% OF GROUP		
	Adults	Children	Infants
Angiosarcoma	33	0	0
Rhabdomyosarcoma	21	33	66
Mesothelioma	16	0	0
Fibrosarcoma	11	11	33
Malignant lymphoma	6	0	0
Extraskeletal osteosarcoma	4	0	0
Thymoma	3	0	0
Neurogeic sarcoma	3	11	0
Leiomyosarcoma	1	0	0
Liposarcoma	1	0	0
Synovial sarcoma	1	0	0
Malignant teratoma	0	44	0

A total of 117, nine, and three malignant tumors were found in adults (aged >16 years), children (aged 1 to 16 years), and infants (aged <1 year), respectively. Angiosarcomas were the most commonly reported malignant tumors in adults, but rhabdomyosarcomas and mesotheliomas were also relatively common. Malignant teratomas were the most common tumors in children. Rhabdomyosarcomas were the most frequently reported malignant tumors in infants, with fibrosarcomas the second most common.

From Allard, M. F., et al.: Primary cardiac tumors. *In* Goldhaber, S., and Braunwald, E. (eds): Atlas of Heart Diseases, Philadelphia, Current Medicine, 1995, pp. 15.1–15.22.

comas, and of these the angiosarcoma and rhabdomyosarcoma are the most common forms (Table 42–4).

Although it is often difficult or impossible to differentiate histologically benign from malignant tumors prior to operation, certain findings may be helpful. Characteristics suggestive of malignancy include the presence of distant metastases, local mediastinal invasion, evidence of rapid growth in tumor size, hemorrhagic pericardial effusion, precordial pain, location of the tumor on the right side of the heart or on the atrial free wall, evidence of combined intramural and intracavitary location, and extension into the pulmonary veins. Benign tumors are more likely to occur on the left side of the interatrial septum and to grow slowly. Although benign tumors do not metastasize, distant tumor emboli may mimic peripheral or pulmonary metastases.[48] The preoperative differentiation between benign and malignant tumors may occasionally be made by examination of peripheral tumor emboli recovered by arteriotomy or by biopsy of skin or muscle.[5,27,29,30]

SPECIFIC CARDIAC TUMORS

Benign Tumors

Myxomas

As already pointed out, myxomas are the most common type of primary cardiac tumor, comprising 30 to 50 per cent of the total in most pathological series.[1–6] The mean age of patients with sporadic myxoma is 56 years, and 70 per cent are females. However, myxomas have been described in patients ranging in age from 3 to 83 years and are now not infrequently diagnosed in elderly patients in whom the symptoms and signs of cardiac tumor may have been attributed to other causes for a substantial time. Approximately 86 per cent of myxomas occur in the left atrium, and over 90 per cent are solitary[5,6] (Fig. 42–1). In the left atrium, the usual site of attachment is in the area of the fossa ovalis. Myxomas also may occur in the right atrium and, less often, in the right or left ventricle. Multiple tumors may occur in the same chamber or in a combination of chambers. Although myxomas may occasionally be found on the posterior left atrial wall, tumors presenting in this location should raise the suspicion of malignancy. Myxomas of the mitral and tricuspid valves have been reported.[44,48]

The clinical signs and symptoms produced by cardiac myxomas include nonspecific manifestations as already discussed, embolization, and mechanical interference with cardiac function (Table 42–1). Not surprisingly, the symptoms produced by cardiac myxomas may simulate a wide variety of other cardiac and noncardiac conditions (Table 42–2).

FAMILIAL MYXOMAS. Familial cardiac myxomas constitute approximately 10 per cent or less of all myxomas and appear to have an autosomal dominant transmission.[1,49,50,50a] Some patients with cardiac myxoma have a syndrome, frequently called "syndrome myxoma" or "Carney syndrome," that also consists of: (1) myxomas in other locations (breast or skin), (2) spotty pigmentation (lentigines, pigmented nevi, or both) (Fig. 42–2), and (3) endocrine overactivity (pituitary adenoma, primary pigmented nodular adrenocortical disease, or testicular tumors involving the endocrine components).[51–53] Patients with the Carney syndrome tend to be younger (mean age, 20's), are more likely to have myxomas in locations other than the left atrium, sometimes have bilateral tumors, and are more likely to develop recurrences (Table 42–5).

Although the etiology of the syndrome myxoma is unknown, it has been proposed to result from a widespread abnormality resulting in excessive proliferation of certain mesenchymal cells, and excessive glycosaminoglycans

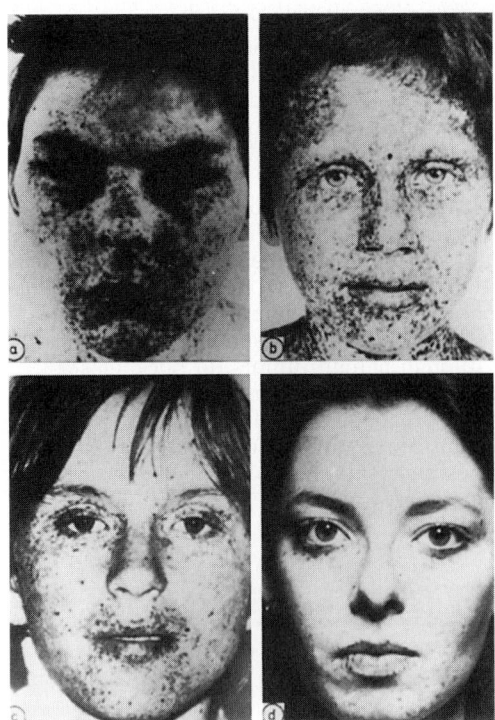

FIGURE 42–2. Four patients with extensive facial freckling, a finding that is associated with "syndrome myxoma." Patients with this syndrome tend to be younger than patients with sporadic myxoma and have a substantially higher incidence of ventricular, multiple, biatrial, recurrent, and familial myxomas of the heart. In addition, these patients, in contrast to patients with sporadic myxoma, may have noncardiac myxomas and endocrine neoplasms. (From Vidaillet, H. J., Jr., et al.: "Syndrome myxoma": a subset of patients with cardiac myxoma associated with pigmented skin lesions and peripheral and endocrine neoplasms. Br. Heart J. *57:* 247, 1987.)

(GAG) production by them, possibly analogous to the neural masses in von Recklinghausen's neurofibromatosis.[54] Patients may have two or more components of this complex, and generally the first component is diagnosed at a relatively young age (mean age, 18 years). Some patients have been said to have the NAME syndrome (*n*evi, *a*trial myxoma, *m*yxoid neurofibroma, *e*phelides)[50a,55] or the LAMB syndrome (*l*entigines, *a*trial *m*yxoma, and *b*lue nevi).[56]

Because cardiac myxomas may be familial, routine echocardiographic screening of first-degree relatives is appropriate, particularly if the patient is young or has multiple tumors. In one recent study, screening of families of six patients with familial myxoma yielded four close relatives with cardiac myxoma.[57] Moreover, in patients with a familial history or other components of the syndrome described

TABLE 42–5 COMPARISON OF THE CLINICAL FEATURES OF SPORADIC MYXOMA AND SYNDROME MYXOMA

FEATURE	SPORADIC	SYNDROME
Age (yr) (range)	56 (39–82)	25 (10–56)
Female/male ratio	2.7 : 1	1.8 : 1
Patients (No.)	70	44
Cardiac myxomas (No.)	72	103
Distributions of myxomas (%)		
Atrial/ventricular	100/0	87/13
Single/multiple	99/1	50/50
Biatrial	0	23
Recurrent	0	18
Familial	0	27
Freckling (%)	0	68
Noncardiac tumors (%)	0	57
Endocrine neoplasm (%)	0	30

Vidaillet, H. J., Jr., et al.: "Syndrome myxoma": A subset of patients with cardiac myxoma associated with pigmented skin lesions and peripheral and endocrine neoplasms. Br. Heart J. *57:*247, 1987.

above who are undergoing resection, a careful search should be made preoperatively for multiple cardiac myxomas. Postoperatively, these patients should be observed closely for the development of other tumors; this occurs in 12 to 22 per cent of such patients.[58] The pathological features of familial myxomas do not differ from those occurring sporadically (see below).[59]

PATHOLOGY. Most cardiac myxomas are received by the pathologist as surgically excised specimens that have been removed for clinical symptomatology. Rarely, cardiac myxomas are encountered incidentally at autopsy. The pathological characteristics of myxomas are well described and are independent of location.[1,48,60–62]

Gross Pathology. Myxomas are gelatinous (often termed myxoid), smooth and round with a glistening surface, or variably friable, and either irregular or polypoid (Fig. 42–2). They are either sessile or pedunculated with a distinct stalk, which may be narrow or broad. In approximately 90 per cent of cases arising in the atria, the base of attachment is the atrial septum, usually in the region of the limbus of the fossa ovalis. In approximately 10 per cent of cases, the point of origin is the posterior or anterior atrial wall or atrial appendage; valvular myxomas are rare. Cardiac myxomas can be multicentric. Areas of hemorrhage are frequent. The tumors average 4 to 8 cm in diameter but range from less than 1 cm to 15 cm or greater.

Histology. The diagnosis of myxoma is made by the observation of characteristic patterns of cells (often called "lipidic" cells) embedded in a myxoid stroma rich in glycosaminoglycans (GAGs) (Fig. 42–3).[60–62] Myxoma cells have a round, elongated or polyhedral shape, scant pink cytoplasm, and an ovoid nucleus with an open chromatin pattern; they are occasionally multinuclear. Although they may be present individually, myxoma cells are typically present as cords, rings, or florets, sometimes as multiple layers surrounding vascular structures. Diagnosis of myxoma requires the presence of characteristic isolated or clustered collections of myxoma cells. Hemorrhages, macrophages, often containing iron pigment, and lymphocytes and plasma cells are variably present. Calcification is present in approximately 10 to 20 per cent of cardiac myxomas. Extramedullary hematopoiesis, glandular structures lined by mucin-filled goblet cells,[63] and cellular atypia may be present in a minority of cases; these features may simulate malignancy. Since emboli from myxomas usually derive from the most superficial portions, they may have less definitive histologic features than the intracardiac lesion from which they originated.

Ultrastructural and Immunohistochemical Findings. Myxoma cells have abundant fine cytoplasmic filaments similar to those of smooth muscle cells.[62] The cells most resemble embryonic mesenchymal cells with multipotential capabilities for cellular differentiation, including vasoformative activity, and are especially similar to embryonic endocardial cushion tissue.[64] *Immunohistochemical studies* demonstrate variable positivity for the endothelial cell markers Factor VIII–related antigen and *Ulex europaeus.* More consistent positivity is obtained when myxomas are stained for *vimentin,* indicative of the mesenchymal derivation of the cells, as well as some neuroendocrine markers and smooth muscle cell antigens. Analysis by immunohistochemistry has not been useful for either diagnostic purposes or elucidation of histogenesis.

Embolization. Although myxomas or other benign cardiac tumors can cause death from coronary or cerebral embolization,[65] metastatic tumor implantation with wasting is rare. Occasional reports suggest that myxomas may have a malignant counterpart, with local invasion of the interatrial septum, recurrence, or metastasis. However, some cases of purported malignancy probably represent malignant tumors of other types with extensive areas of myxoid degeneration or of multicentricity that was not appreciated, inadequate excision, or embolization of benign lesions.

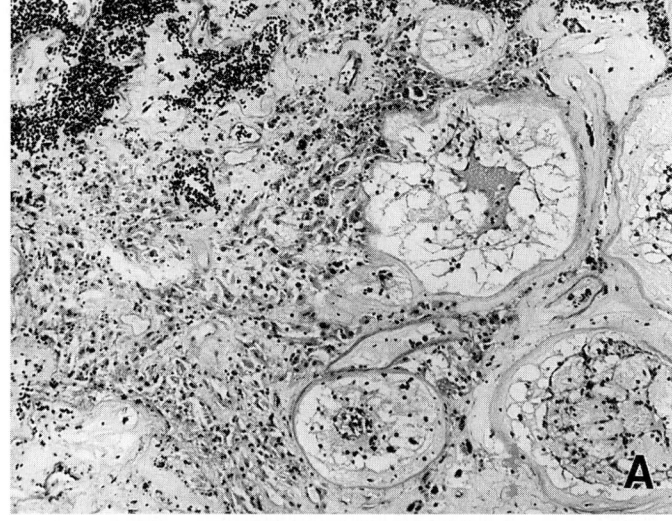

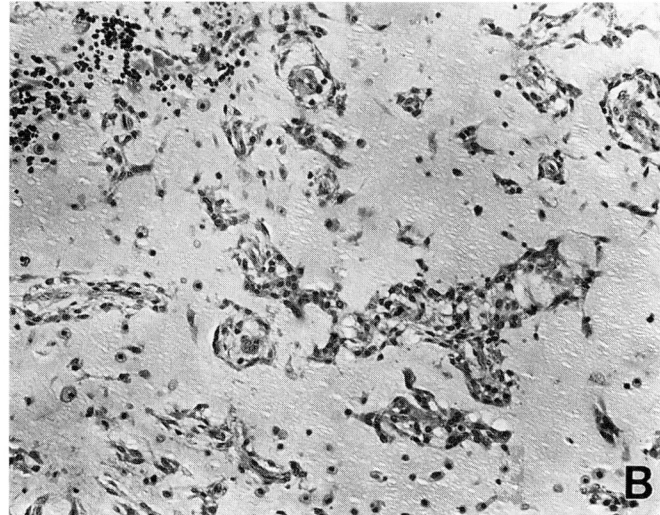

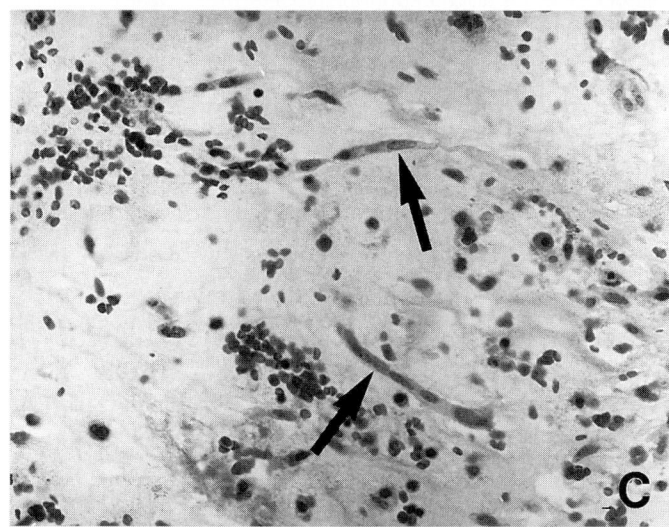

FIGURE 42–3. Characteristic histological features of myxoma. *A*, Low-power view demonstrating individual tumor cells, clusters, and islands scattered throughout the characteristic pale-staining granular extracellular matrix. Hemorrhage is present at upper left. Scattered inflammatory cells are also present. *B*, Medium-power view, demonstrating groups of polygonal myxoma cells. *C*, High-magnification view, showing individual variably rounded to elongated myxoma cells, some arranged in cords (arrows). *A*, 50×; *B*, 175×; *C*, 400×; all stained with hematoxylin and eosin.

Many of the morphological features of organizing mural thrombi resemble those of myxoma, including abundant loose amorphous extracellular matrix, connective tissue cells, and small vascular channels. It is difficult to distinguish between some myxomas and mural thrombi in various stages of organization; indeed, cellular intracardiac thrombi and peripheral thromboemboli occasionally erroneously receive a diagnosis of myxoma. The resemblance to organizing/organized thrombi has been put forth as evidence that myxomas have a thrombotic origin,[66] but most investigators currently find this notion untenable.[60,64]

Histogenesis. The histogenesis of cardiac myxomas is uncertain, but the weight of evidence favors benign neoplasia, with the tumor probably originating from subendocardial nests of primitive mesenchymal cells that may differentiate into several cell types, including endothelial and lipidic cells. Cytogenetic analyses demonstrating clonal chromosomal abnormalities provide the best support for this concept. One study of the cytogenetics of eight cases[67] yielded three with telomeric associations involving chromosome 2 (one with Carney's syndrome); in the same study, four other cases had nonclonal rearrangements involving the short arm of chromosome 12. In an additional recently reported myxoma from a patient with Carney's syndrome, clonal telomeric associations between chromosomes 13 and 15 were demonstrated, and similar nonclonal associations between chromosomes 12 and 17 and others were observed.[68] Nevertheless, the most convincing case of clonal structural aberrations was recently reported by Dijkhuizen,[69] in which a cardiac myxoma from a 48-year-old man had normal chromosome number but a complex clonal rearrangement, which included a breakpoint at 12p12, the

location of the *Ki-ras* oncogene. The authors speculated that *Ki-ras* might play a role in the origin of cardiac myxoma. The presence of aneuploidy in some cardiac myxomas provides additional support for the concept of a neoplastic origin.[70]

Before the discussion of nonmyxomatous cardiac tumors is continued below, it should be noted that peculiar microscopic-sized cellular cardiac lesions have been noted incidentally as part of endomyocardial biopsy or surgically removed tissue specimens or at cardiac surgery, free-floating or loosely attached to a valvular or endocardial mass.[71,72] Not neoplastic, they have been termed *M*esothelial/monocytic *I*ncidental *C*ardiac *E*xcrescences ("MICE"). Histologically, such lesions are composed largely of clusters and ribbons of mesothelial cells and entrapped erythrocytes and leukocytes, embedded within a fibrin mesh. Previously considered to be a reactive mesothelial and/or monocytic (histiocytic) hyperplasia, they are now considered to be common artefacts—formed by compaction of mesothelial strips (likely from the pericardium) or other tissue debris and fibrin which are transported via catheters or around an operative site on a cardiotomy suction tip.[73] Such tissue fragments are of importance only in that they should not be confused with metastatic carcinoma.

PAPILLARY TUMORS OF HEART VALVES (PAPILLARY FIBROELASTOMA). The most common tumors of the cardiac valves, papillary fibroelastomas of the cardiac valves and adjacent endocardium, are found not uncommonly postmortem and may be identified during life by two-dimensional echocardiography.[74,75] Although many are clinically insignificant, they have the potential to embolize to vital structures or cause valvular dysfunction, and those on the aortic valve can partially obstruct a coronary arterial orifice.[76] These lesions have a characteristic frond-like appearance resembling a sea anemone, may be single or multiple up to 3 or 4 cm in diameter, and may occur on any valve or on papillary muscle, chordae tendineae, or endocardium, usually attached by a short pedicle (Fig. 42–4). Most often, the ventricular surface of semilunar valves and the atrial surface of atrioventricular valves are affected. The tricuspid valve is most commonly involved in children and the mitral and aortic valves in adults. Histologically, the tumor is covered by endothelium that surrounds a core of loose connective tissue rich in GAGs, collagen, and elastic fibers and containing smooth muscle cells (often as a fine meshwork surrounding a central collagen or dense elastic fiber core).

Pathogenesis. The pathogenesis of these lesions is unsettled, but it appears that they may originate secondary to endocardial trauma and/or the organization of mural thrombi.[66] Papillary tumors are generally distinguished from Lambl's excrescences, which are acellular deposits of thrombus and connective tissue covered by a single layer of endothelium and are found on heart valves at the site of endothelial damage in many adults, particularly along the closure margins of the aortic valve cusps. In contrast, papillary fibroelastomas are unusually found at valvular contact areas.

RHABDOMYOMAS. These are the most common cardiac tumors of infants and children; approximately three-fourths occur in patients younger than 1 year.[77,78] They occur with equal frequency in the left and right ventricular and septal myocardium; nearly all are multiple. Approximately one-third also involve either one or both atria. In approximately half of affected patients, at least one of the tumors is intracavitary and obstructive. Nonspecific clinical manifestations, including cardiomegaly, right or left ventricular failure or both, an S_3, S_4, and systolic or diastolic murmurs, may mimic mitral stenosis, mitral atresia, aortic stenosis, subaortic stenosis, or infundibular pulmonic stenosis.

Association with Tuberous Sclerosis. Rhabdomyomas are strongly associated with tuberous sclerosis, a familial syndrome characterized by hamartomas in several organs, epilepsy, mental deficiency, and adenoma sebaceum.[79–81] A recent study indicated that at least 80 per cent of patients with cardiac rhabdomyomas have tuberous sclerosis, and 60 per cent of patients with tuberous sclerosis less than 18 years old have cardiac rhabdomyomas.[81] Conversely, approximately 50 per cent or more of patients having tuberous sclerosis but no signs or symptoms of cardiac disease have been shown to have findings on echocardiography that are consistent with one or more rhabdomyomas. Rhabdomyomas causing significant intracavity obstruction may result in death within the first 24 hours of life, whereas patients with less severe involvement may either remain asymptomatic or have difficulty during infancy or early childhood.

Pathology. Rhabdomyomas are yellow-gray and range from 1 mm to several centimeters in diameter. They are circumscribed but not encapsulated; microscopically, they are easily distinguished from the surrounding myocardium as clusters of abnormal cells. The microscopic hallmark, termed the "spider cell," is a large (up to 80 mm diameter) cell containing a central cytoplasmic mass that is suspended by fine fibrillar processes radiating to the periphery, thus giving the appearance of a spider hanging in a net. Such cells are sufficiently characteristic that the tumor may be diagnosed by fine-needle aspiration.[82] The cytoplasm is rich in glycogen and stains positively with periodic acid–Schiff reagent. Electron microscopy demonstrates myofibrils, cytoplasmic and mitrochondrial glycogen, and apparent intercellular junctions similar to intercalated discs. Immunohistochemistry reveals diffuse positivity for myoglobin, actin, desmin and vimentin, and the absence of neuroendocrine markers, similar to the staining pattern of the adjacent cardiac muscle. Evidence suggests that rhabdomyomas are actually myocardial hamartomas or malformations rather than true neoplasms. In support of this concept is their multiple occurrence and preponderance in children, especially in those with tuberous sclerosis.

FIBROMAS. Fibromas are benign connective tissue tumors that occur predominantly in children and constitute the second most common type of primary cardiac tumor occurring in the pediatric age group.[83] The majority occur before the age of 10 years, and about 40 per cent are diagnosed in infants less than 1 year of age. Males and females appear to be equally affected. Derived from fibroblasts and considered low-grade connective tissue tumors, cardiac fibromas resemble and have the same biological behavior as soft tissue fibromatoses at other sites.

Pathology. Almost all cardiac fibromas occur within the ventricular myocardium, most frequently within the anterior free wall of the left ventricle or the interventricular septum and much less often in the posterior left ventricular wall or right ventricle. Typically, they are gray, firm, circumscribed, not encapsulated, and range in size from 3 to 10 cm. Grossly, they exhibit a whorled appearance on cut sections. Microscopically, cardiac fibromas consist of elongated fibroblasts admixed with fibrous tissue consisting mostly of collagen. Their cellularity is variable, and mitotic figures are rarely, if ever, seen. Fibrous tissue is intermingled with adjacent myocardial fibers at the margins of the lesion. Calcification and islands of bone formation may be seen microscopically and occasionally radiographically. The *Gorlin syndrome*, the main features of which are multiple nevoid basal cell carcinomas, cysts of the jaw, and skeletal abnormalities, may be associated in some cases with cardiac tumors, either fibromas or fibrous histiocytomas.[84]

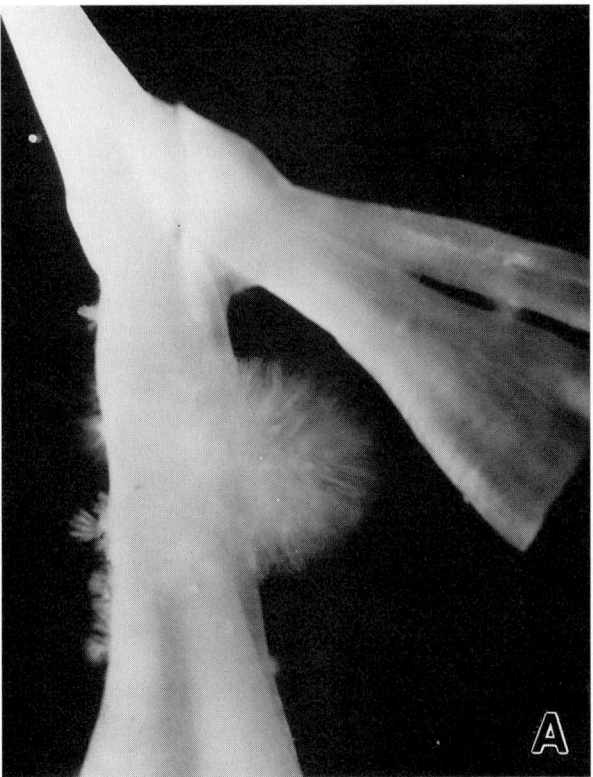 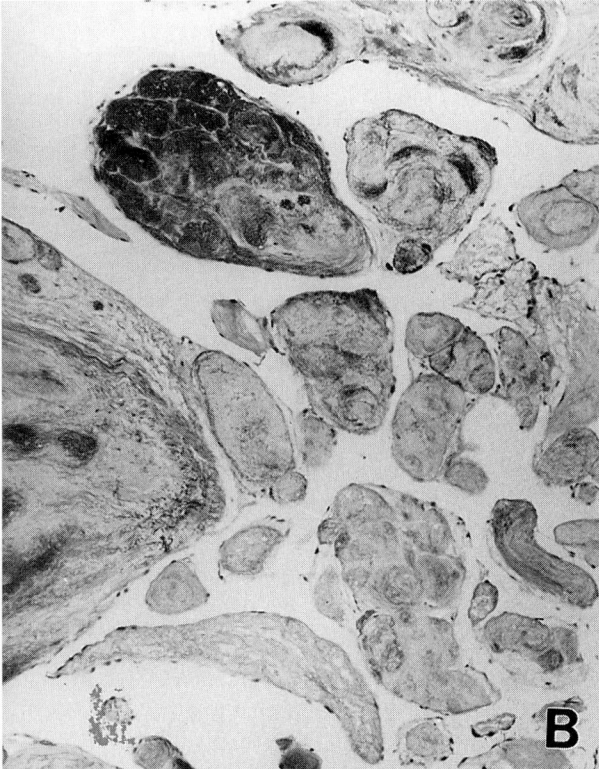

FIGURE 42–4. Papillary fibroelastoma. *A*, Gross photograph demonstrating resemblance of this lesion to a sea anemone, with myriad papillary fronds, arising from the chordae tendineae near the mitral leaflet. In this case, multiple lesions were present, all associated with the mitral valve apparatus. *B*, Histological appearance of papillary fibroelastoma, demonstrating the multiple papillary fronds consisting of a collagen core surrounded by elastic fibers and loose connective tissue, all covered by endocardial endothelium. 100×; stained with elastica van Gieson stain (elastin black).

Clinical Manifestations. Although fibromas may be incidental findings at postmortem examination, approximately 70 per cent at some time cause mechanical interference with intracardiac flow, ventricular contraction abnormalities, or conduction disturbances. Clinical manifestations are protean and include murmurs, atypical chest pain, congestive heart failure and signs of subaortic stenosis, valvular or infundibular pulmonic stenosis with right ventricular hypertrophy, tricuspid stenosis, conduction disturbances, ventricular tachycardia, and sudden death. As in the case of rhabdomyomas, the increased usage of echocardiography has rarely resulted in the detection of cardiac fibromas in patients without cardiac signs or symptoms. Surgical excision of cardiac fibromas may be possible.[85,86]

LIPOMAS AND LIPOMATOUS HYPERTROPHY OF THE ATRIAL SEPTUM. Lipomas occur at all ages and with equal frequency in both sexes. Most range in diameter from 1 to 15 cm, although some have been reported to weigh more than 2 kg. Most tumors are sessile or polypoid and occur in the subendocardium or subpericardium, although about one-fourth are completely intramuscular. Subendocardial tumors with intracavity extension produce symptoms that are characteristic of their location, whereas subepicardial tumors may cause compression of the heart and pericardial effusion. The most common chambers affected are the left ventricle, right atrium, and interatrial septum. Intramural tumors may be asymptomatic or result in arrhythmias, AV or intraventricular conduction disturbances, or mechanical interference. However, many tumors are clinically silent and are found only at autopsy or become apparent on a routine chest roentgenogram.

Microscopically, the lesions are usually well encapsulated, composed of typical mature fat cells, and occasionally contain fibrous connective tissue (fibrolipoma), muscular tissue (myolipoma), or vacuolated brown (fetal) fat resembling a hibernoma.

Whereas lipomas are true neoplasms, a condition termed *lipomatous hypertrophy of the interatrial septum* represents the occurrence of a nonencapsulated hyperplastic accumulation of mature and fetal adipose tissue within the interatrial septum. These lesions range from 1 to 7 cm in dimension, most often protrude into the right atrium, and are more common in obese, elderly, or female patients.[87] A variety of atrial arrhythmias have been attributed to these lesions, but a cause-and-effect relationship has been difficult to establish.[87] Since this lesion may occasionally be detected by cineangiography, echocardiography, computed tomography, or other diagnostic techniques, the major clinical dilemma is the differential diagnosis and treatment of an intraatrial filling defect.

ANGIOMAS. Composed of benign proliferations of endothelial cells, hemangiomas and lymphangiomas are extremely rare.[88] Anatomically, they may occur in any part of the heart, but usually they are intramural, often in the interventricular septum or AV node, where they may cause complete heart block and sudden death. Cardiac tamponade due to hemopericardium may be the presenting clinical syndrome. More commonly found in the right heart chambers, hemangiomas are red, hemorrhagic, generally sessile or polypoid subendocardial nodules, ranging from 2 to 4 cm in diameter. Histologically, the tumors consist of endothelium-lined spaces which may contain blood, lymph, or thrombi; they are classified according to the predominant type of proliferating vascular channel. Dilated, often thrombosed, subendocardial blood vessels (varices) are frequently mistaken for hemangiomas; they are usually found incidentally.

TERATOMAS. These tumors, which contain elements of all three germ cell layers, occur within the heart less frequently than in the anterior mediastinum.[89] Teratomas are generally observed in children, and when located within the heart, they occur predominantly within the right atrium, right ventricle, or the interatrial or interventricular septum.

CYSTIC TUMOR ("MESOTHELIOMA") OF THE ATRIOVENTRICULAR NODE. Of controversial histogenesis, these small tumors (usually less than 15 mm in largest dimension) frequently cause death by complete heart block, ventricular fibrillation,[36] or cardiac tamponade.[90] They occur in patients of virtually any age as poorly circumscribed, often multicystic nodules in the atrial septum, immediately cephalad to the commissure of the septal and anterior leaflets of the tricuspid valve, in the region of the AV node. These lesions are characterized by tubules and cysts lined by flat or cuboidal cells that are devoid of mitotic activity, but may have secretory function. Although often considered to be derived from mesothelial rests, similar to the adenomatoid tumors of the ovary and testis that they resemble histologically, recent studies have suggested an endodermal rather than mesothelial origin.[91,92]

ENDOCRINE TUMORS OF THE HEART. Approximately 2 per cent of *paragangliomas* are intrathoracic, and of these, most are located in the posterior mediastinum. However, these tumors can also occur in close association with the left atrial or left ventricular epicardium, where they are thought to have arisen from sympathetic fibers to the heart or from ectopic chromaffin cells. More rarely still, paragangliomas may arise within the interatrial septum. Tumors in any of these locations may secrete catecholamines and therefore can be associated with signs and symptoms characteristic of pheochromocytoma.[93]

Rarely, benign *thyroid tumors* arise within the heart, presumably from ectopic rests of thyroid tissue. These tumors most often arise from the interventricular septum and present, not infrequently, as obstruction to right ventricular outflow.

About one-fourth of all cardiac tumors exhibit malignant histological characteristics and invasive or metastatic behavior. Nearly all of these are sarcomas, thus making these tumors second only to myxomas in overall frequency. Sarcomas may occur at any age but are most common between the third and fifth decades, are distinctly unusual in infant and children, and show no sex preference. In decreasing order of frequency the sites involved are the right atrium, left atrium, right ventricle, left ventricle, and interventricular septum.

Sarcomas derive from mesenchyme and therefore may display a wide variety of morphological types, including angiosarcoma, rhabdomyosarcoma, fibrosarcoma, osteosarcoma, and others.[94–96]

From a clinical viewpoint, sarcomas characteristically display a rapid downhill course. Death most often occurs from a few weeks to 2 years after the onset of symptoms. These tumors proliferate rapidly and generally cause death through widespread infiltration of the myocardium, obstruction of flow within the heart, or distant metastases. About 75 per cent of all patients with cardiac sarcomas have pathological evidence of distant metastases at the time of death.[1,97,98] The most frequent sites are the lungs, thoracic lymph nodes, mediastinum, and vertebral column; less often the liver, kidneys, adrenals, pancreas, bone, spleen, and bowel are involved.

The cardiac findings are determined primarily by the location of the tumor and by the extent of intracavitary obstruction. Typical presentations include progressive, unexplained, congestive heart failure, particularly of the right side; precordial pain; pericardial effusion; tamponade; arrhythmias; conduction disturbances; obstruction of the venae cavae; and sudden death. Tumors limited to the myocardium without intracavitary extension may produce no cardiac symptoms or may cause arrhythmias and conduction disturbances. Because of the rapid growth potential of sarcomas, they commonly extend into the cardiac chambers, the pericardial space, or both. In about 20 per cent of cases, the tumor is sessile or polypoid. When there is extension into the pericardial space, hemorrhagic pericardial effusion is common and tamponade may occur. Because the right side of the heart is most commonly affected, sarcomas frequently cause signs of right heart failure as a result of obstruction of the right atrium, right ventricle, or tricuspid or pulmonic valves. In addition, obstruction of the superior vena cava may result in swelling of the face and upper extremities, whereas obstruction of the inferior vena cava may result in visceral congestion.

ANGIOSARCOMAS. Included within this category are angiosarcomas and Kaposi's sarcomas.[99,100] All 40 patients in one series were adults. In distinction to most other cardiac sarcomas, in which the sex distribution is equal, there appears to be a 2:1 male-to-female ratio among patients with angiosarcomas. These tumors have a striking predilection for the right atrium (Fig. 42–5) and may be infiltrative or polypoid in nature. Microscopically, angiosarcomas are characterized by ill-defined but variable anastomotic vascular channels lined with atypical, often heaped-up, endothelial cells. By electron microscopy, immature endothelial cells, primitive pericytes, and undifferentiated mesenchymal cells may be identified.[101]

RHABDOMYOSARCOMAS. These are tumors of striated muscle which often diffusely infiltrate the myocardium but which may also, on occasion, form a polypoid extension into the cardiac chambers and therefore have been clinically mistaken for myxoma.[102] Rhabdomyoblasts (cross-striations by light microscopy; thick and thin filaments and Z-band material by electron microscopy) are the histological hallmark of this tumor, and 20 to 30 per cent of the tumors have cross-striations.

FIBROSARCOMAS AND MALIGNANT FIBROUS HISTIOCYTOMAS. Fibrosarcomas of the heart have a whitish, soft "fish flesh" consistency characteristic of these tumor types elsewhere in the body.[101a] Fibroblastic in differentiation, they are composed of spindle-shaped cells with elongated blunt-ended nuclei, and frequent mitoses. They may contain areas of hemorrhage and necrosis and extensively infiltrate the heart, often involving more than one cardiac chamber. A thrombus may form in an obstructed pulmonary vein, in the vena cava, or over the mural surface of the tumor.

LYMPHOMAS. Although cardiac involvement of a systemic lym-

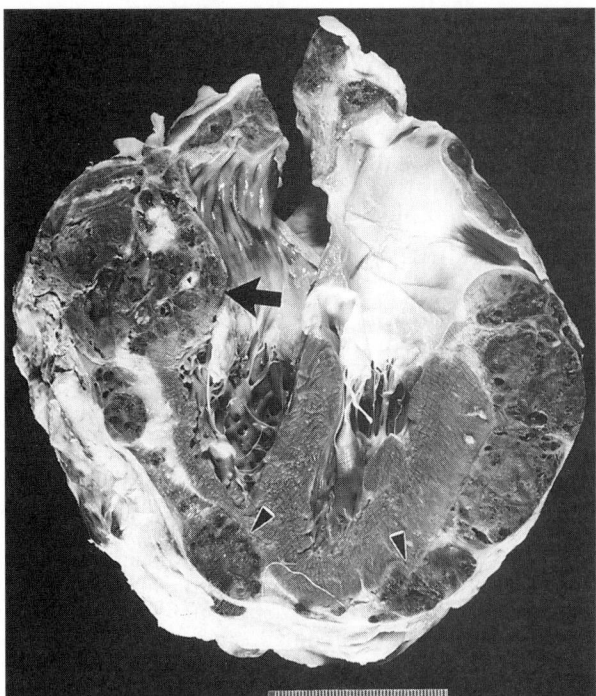

FIGURE 42–5. Massive pericardial angiosarcoma, with deep myocardial invasion at multiple sites (arrowheads), particularly at right atrium (arrow). (From Schoen, F. J.: Interventional and Surgical Cardiovascular Pathology: Clinical Correlations and Basic Principles. Philadelphia, W. B. Saunders Company, 1989.)

phoma has been reported in 25 to 36 per cent of cases, primary lymphoma involving only the heart or pericardium is much less common.[102,103] Myocardial infiltration by lymphoma may be nodular or diffuse, and the clinical syndrome of hypertrophic cardiomyopathy has been mimicked. Some of these tumors are predominantly intracavitary.

PULMONARY ARTERY SARCOMAS. Sarcomas of the pulmonary artery trunk, main branches, or pulmonic valves may present as tumor emboli to the lungs or as right ventricular outflow obstruction.[104] These tumors usually present after the fourth decade, show a 2:1 female predominance, and may originate from undifferentiated tissue of the bulbis cordis. Typical symptoms include dyspnea, chest pain, cough, and hemoptysis and may be associated with radiographic findings of a pulmonary hilar mass or cardiomegaly. Right ventricular injection of contrast material helps to delineate the tumor. Although most reported cases were previously diagnosed at autopsy, it is likely that early diagnosis, surgical resection, and possibly chemotherapy may have an impact on survival of future patients with this tumor.[105]

Although certain clinical manifestations may be suggestive of a cardiac tumor, no clinical finding or set of findings is pathognomonic. Furthermore, the majority of cardiac tumors produce signs and symptoms typical of the common forms of heart disease. The development of modern diagnostic methods has had a major impact on the diagnosis and hence the natural history of cardiac tumors. It is not unusual for cardiac tumors to be diagnosed and cured in patients who are totally asymptomatic or without signs of cardiovascular disease.[106] Although cardiac catheterization made possible the definitive preoperative diagnosis of cardiac tumors, it was not until the advent of echocardiography that it was feasible to evaluate all patients suspected of this diagnosis. Both M-mode and two-dimensional echocardiography are effective screening techniques. However, two-dimensional echocardiography, and particularly transesophageal imaging (Fig. 42–6), is more sensitive and provides considerably more information regarding the site of tumor attachment, pattern of tumor movement, and size. In many centers, the information provided by two-dimensional echocardiography, computed tomography (CT), or magnetic resonance imaging (MRI) (Fig. 42–7) is considered sufficient to proceed directly to surgery without cardiac catheterization and angiography. However, catheterization and angiography should not be omitted in the absence of a technically adequate two-dimensional echocardiographic study, CT, or MRI that has visualized all four cardiac chambers.

It is imperative that noninvasive evaluation, preferably by two-dimensional echocardiography (or CT or MRI), be performed before cardiac catheterization whenever the diagnosis of cardiac tumor is considered. When left atrial myxoma is suspected, it is safest to visualize the left atrium by injecting the contrast agent into the pulmonary artery and film during the levophase. It is particularly important to avoid the transseptal approach, since this risks dislodgment of fragments of tumor that may be attached in the region of the fossa ovalis. Furthermore, since cardiac tumors may be multiple and present in more than one chamber, all four chambers should be visualized noninvasively prior to cardiac catheterization whenever possible.

Clinical and Noninvasive Methods

CLINICAL EXAMINATION. When valvular or myocardial disease is suspected on clinical grounds, certain atypical

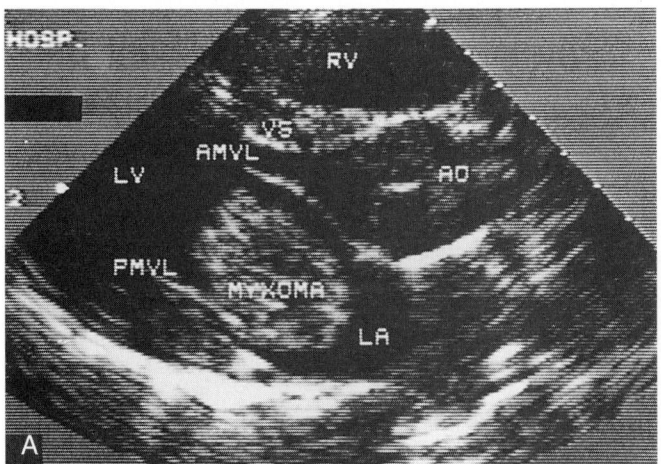

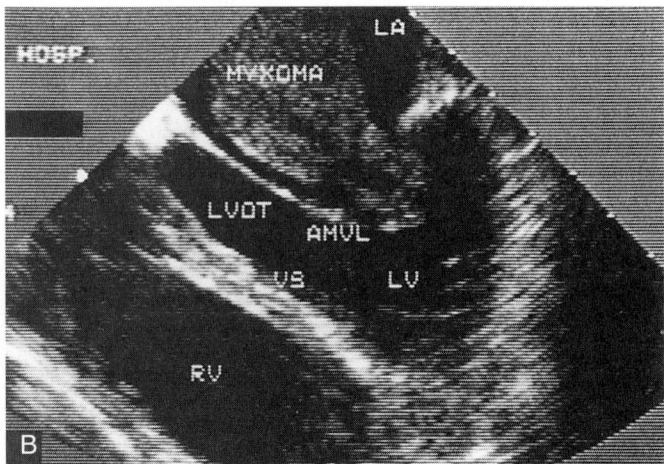

FIGURE 42–6. Transthoracic two-dimensional echocardiogram (*A*) and transesophageal two-dimensional echocardiogram (*B*) showing a left atrial (LA) mass prolapsing into and obstructing the mitral valve orifice. Note the superior resolution of the transesophageal echocardiogram. Although not visible here, the myxoma was attached to the mid-portion of the atrial septum. (From Allard, M. F., et al.: Primary cardiac tumors. *In* Goldhaber, S. Z., and Braunwald, E. (eds.): Cardiopulmonary Diseases and Cardiac Tumors. Atlas of Heart Diseases. Vol. 3. Philadelphia, Current Medicine, 1995, pp. 15.1–15.22.)

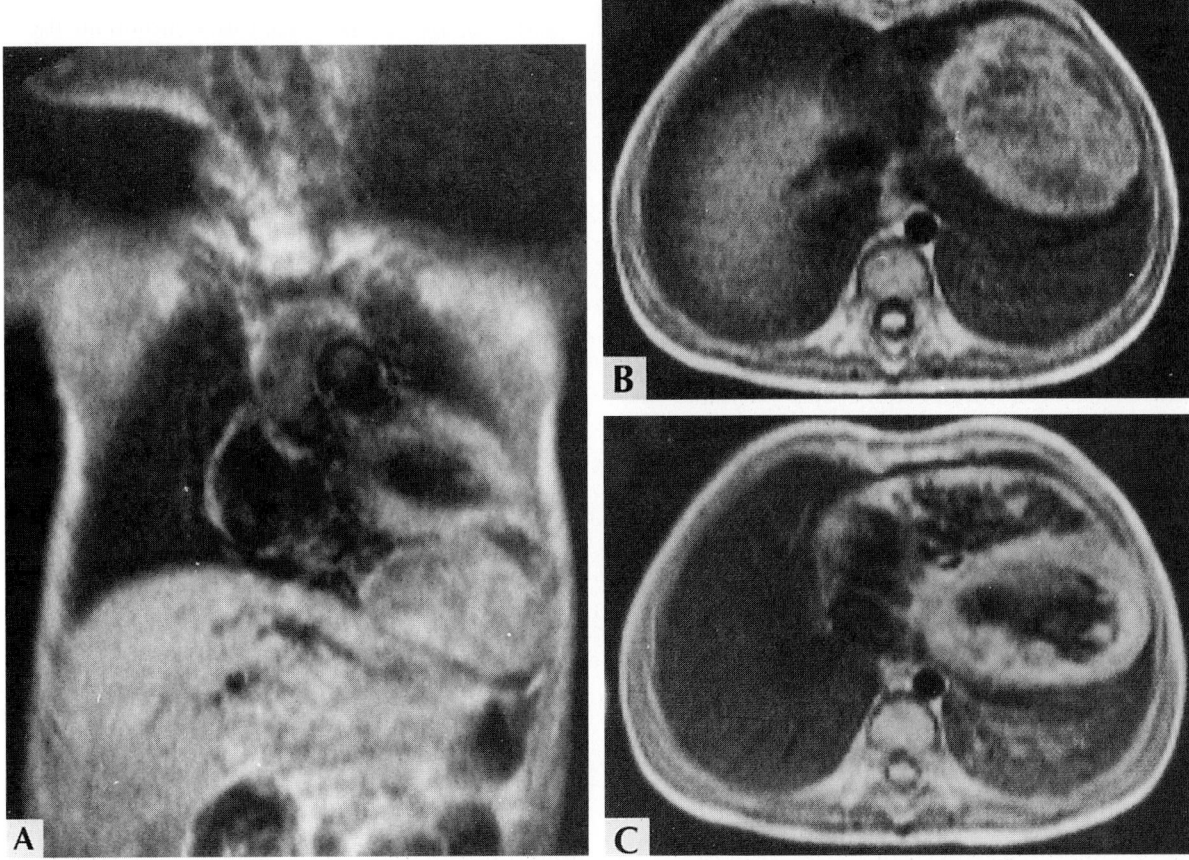

FIGURE 42–7. Magnetic resonance images illustrating a large tumor in the right ventricular apex, impinging on the apical septum. In the coronal view, the prominent mass indents the septum *(A)*. In the axial views, the tumor shows areas of tissue inhomogeneity *(B)* and indents the ventricular septum *(C)*. (From Allard, M. F., et al.: Primary cardiac tumors. *In* Goldhaber, S. Z., and Braunwald, E. (eds.): Cardiopulmonary Diseases and Cardiac Tumors. Atlas of Heart Disease. Vol. 3. Philadelphia, Current Medicine, 1995, pp. 15.1–15.22.)

findings may raise the question of cardiac tumor. The intensity of the systolic or diastolic murmur caused by a left atrial myxoma is often exquisitely sensitive to positional change, a finding atypical of valvular heart disease. S_1 may be delayed as a consequence of an elevated left atrial pressure, as in mitral stenosis. It is often intense and widely split, and an early systolic sound may occur, representing tumor movement toward the atrium during systole. In addition, a tumor "plop" may be present about 100 msec after S_2, which appears to result from the sudden tension of the tumor stalk as it prolapses into the left ventricle during diastole or from the tumor striking the myocardium. The tumor plop *precedes* the end of the rapid filling wave of the apexcardiogram and can thereby be differentiated from an S_3; as noted, it usually occurs later than an opening snap. Systolic time intervals are usually consistent with a reduced stroke volume. Apexcardiography often shows a deep notch on the upstroke, which occurs at the time of extrusion of the tumor through the mitral valve in early systole.

Right atrial tumors may also result in a widely split S_1 and an early systolic sound. The S_2 may be paradoxically split as a result of early pulmonic valve closure. A tumor plop and systolic and diastolic murmurs, which are increased by inspiration, may also occur with right atrial tumors. The jugular venous pulse tracing may reflect obstruction of the tricuspid orifice, demonstrating an accentuated *a* wave, attenuation of the *x* descent, or an early, broad *v* wave.

RADIOLOGICAL EXAMINATION

Cardiac tumors may display several findings on plain chest roentgenograms. These include alterations in cardiac contour, changes in overall cardiac size, specific chamber enlargement, alterations in pulmonary vascularity, and intracardiac calcification (Chap. 7). The cardiac contour may be normal, may display generalized or specific chamber enlargement that mimics virtually any type of valvular heart disease, or may demonstrate a bizarre appearance. Pericardial effusions are rather common and generally indicate invasion of the pericardial space by a malignant tumor. Mediastinal widening, due to hilar and paramediastinal adenopathy, may indicate spread of a malignant cardiac tumor. A bumpy, irregular, or fuzzy cardiac border may be seen when the pericardium is involved. Cardiac enlargement may reflect rapid tumor growth, particularly in the case of sarcomas, whereas specific chamber enlargement is frequently due to intracavitary obstruction, particularly by pedunculated tumors such as myxomas. Thus, left atrial myxoma may produce the radiological pattern characteristic of mitral stenosis. Occasionally a large tumor mass displaces the heart and may simulate enlargement of a specific chamber.

Calcification visible by roentgenographic methods may occur with several types of cardiac tumor, including rhabdomyomas, fibromas, hamartomas, teratomas, myxomas, and angiomas. Visualization of intracardiac calcium in an infant or a child is unusual and should immediately raise the question of an intracardiac tumor. Cardiac fluoroscopy and laminography may be helpful in differentiating calcification of cardiac tumor from that of other structures, such as cardiac valves, coronary arteries, pericardium, and mural thrombus. Occasionally, calcified atrial polypoid tumors may be seen to prolapse into the ventricle during diastole. Fluoroscopy is also useful in differentiating cardiac tumor from ventricular aneurysm, both of which may result in a localized protrusion on plain chest roentgenograms. However, on fluoroscopic examination, cardiac tumors do not display the paradoxical motion during ventricular contraction that is characteristic of ventricular aneurysm.

ECHOCARDIOGRAPHY (see Fig. 3–105, p. 94). Two-dimensional echocardiography provides substantial advantages over conventional M-mode echocardiography for the diagnosis and preoperative evaluation of intracardiac tumors.[5] In the majority of cases of cardiac tumors, the information provided by two-dimensional echocardiography provides adequate information regarding tumor size, attachment, and mobility to allow operative resection without preoperative angiography. This technique is sensitive for detection of small tumors and is especially useful for detection of left ventricular tumors and tumors that do not prolapse through the mitral or tricuspid valve orifices.

Left atrial myxomas have been classified by their echocardiographic appearance as follows: Class I tumors are small and prolapse through the mitral valve; Class II tumors are small and nonprolapsing; Class III tumors are large and prolapse; and Class IV tumors are large and nonprolapsing.[107] The increased sensitivity of two-dimensional echocardiography makes possible the diagnosis of cardiac tumors in neonates and in utero.[108] The improved diagnostic power and widespread use of two-dimensional echocardiography have resulted in an increase in the detection of primary cardiac tumors,[106] in many cases prior to the onset of clinical signs or symptoms.

Two-dimensional echocardiography may facilitate the differentiation between left atrial thrombus and myxoma, because the former typically produces a layered appearance and is generally situated in the posterior portion of the atrium, whereas the latter is often mottled in appearance and rarely occurs in the posterior portion of the atrium. In some atrial myxomas, areas of echolucency may be seen within the tumor mass, corresponding to areas of hemorrhage within the tumor. Since these areas of echolucency are not found in thrombotic or infective lesions, this finding may be of value in the differential diagnosis of an intraatrial mass. Continuous-mode Doppler ultrasonography may be useful for evaluating the hemodynamic consequences of valvular obstruction or incompetence caused by cardiac tumors.[109]

Transesophageal Echocardiography (see Fig. 3–106, p. 95). This approach provides an unimpeded view of both atria and the atrial septum, and appears to be superior to transthoracic echocardiography in many patients.[110] The potential advantages of transesophageal echocardiography include improved resolution of the tumor and its attachment (Fig. 42–6), the ability to detect some masses not visualized by transthoracic echocardiography, and improved visualization of right atrial tumors. In 17 patients suspected of having a cardiac tumor, transthoracic echocardiography yielded four false-positives and two false-negatives, whereas transesophageal echocardiography resulted in only one false-positive and no false-negatives.[111] In the same series, transesophageal echocardiography proved to be superior for visualizing anatomic details such as tumor contour, cysts, and calcification, and identified a stalk in 10 or 11 tumors subsequently shown to have a stalk at surgery, whereas transthoracic echocardiography identified a stalk in only 5 of the 11 tumors. Transesophageal echocardiography has been used to guide the percutaneous biopsy of a right atrial myxoma.[112] Although transesophageal echocardiography does not appear warranted on a routine basis, it should be considered when the transthoracic study is suboptimal or confusing.

RADIONUCLIDE IMAGING. Gated blood pool scanning has been used to identify atrial, ventricular, and intramural tumors.[113] Radionuclide ventriculography generally has a lower rate of resolution than does echocardiography or contrast injection angiography and therefore may be less sensitive for the detection of small filling defects. In some cases in which the cardiac tumor was not evident by routine static or dynamic radionuclide imaging, it has been possible to delineate the tumor and its movement during a cardiac cycle by use of a computer-generated composite functional image.[113]

COMPUTED TOMOGRAPHY. CT of the heart has been used to demonstrate cardiac tumors.[114] Although more experience will be necessary to establish its role, certain advantages are apparent. These include a high degree of tissue discrimination, which may allow definition of the degree of intramural tumor extension; evaluation of the extracardiac structures; and the ability to construct images in any plane.

Resolution appears to be improved substantially by gating the computed tomographic acquisition to the cardiac cycle. Currently, CT appears to be most useful in the evaluation of suspected tumors of the heart to determine the degree of myocardial invasion and the involvement of pericardial and extracardiac structures. Ultrafast CT, a technique that uses electron beam technology, has a short scanning acquisition time that eliminates the motion artifacts occurring with conventional CT and appears to be useful for assessment of intracardiac masses.[114]

MAGNETIC RESONANCE IMAGING. MRI may be of considerable value in the detection and delineation of cardiac tumors and in some cases may depict the size, shape, and surface characteristics of the tumor more clearly than two-dimensional echocardiography[115] (Fig. 10–18, p. 326). The larger field of view with MRI (Fig. 42–7) provides better definition of tumor prolapse, secondary valve obstruction, and cardiac chamber size than does two-dimensional echocardiography. Contrast enhancement with Gd-DTPA and multislice imaging in the transaxial, sagittal, and long axes can provide precise three-dimensional information. MRI can also provide information regarding tissue composition that can help to differentiate tumors from thrombi.[116]

Angiography

Cardiac catheterization and selective angiocardiography are not necessary in all cases of cardiac tumors, since, as already discussed, in many cases adequate preoperative information may be obtained by echocardiography, CT, or MRI. However, several circumstances exist in which the risk and expense of cardiac catheterization are outweighed by the supplemental information it may provide. These situations include cases in which (1) noninvasive evaluation has not been adequate in defining fully tumor location or attachment; (2) all four cardiac chambers have not been adequately visualized noninvasively; (3) a malignant cardiac tumor is considered likely; or (4) other cardiac lesions may coexist with a cardiac tumor and possibly dictate a different surgical approach. For instance, when a malignant cardiac tumor is suspected, cardiac angiography may provide valuable information regarding the degree of myocardial, vascular, and/or pericardial invasion. Likewise, in certain cases, such as the presence of pulmonary hypertension or the coexistence of significant valvular or coronary artery lesions, cardiac catheterization and angiography may provide information that significantly affects the surgical approach.[117]

The major angiographic findings in patients with cardiac tumors include (1) compression or displacement of cardiac chambers or large vessels, (2) deformity of cardiac chambers, (3) intracavitary filling defects, (4) marked variations in myocardial thickness, (5) pericardial effusion, and (6) local alterations in wall motion. Displacement of the cardiac chambers or the great vessels without deformation of the internal contour may be observed in both benign and malignant tumors, whereas deformation of a cardiac chamber usually indicates an infiltrating malignant lesion. The most frequent angiographic findings are intracavitary filling defects, which may be either fixed or mobile. Fixed defects may be lobulated or appear as a coarse nodularity of the myocardium often difficult to distinguish from a mural thrombus. Such defects may reflect endocardial tumors with broad attachments or intramural tumors with intracavitary extension. Mobile intracavitary defects are usually pedunculated tumors, typically myxomas, although the stalk may be difficult to visualize. Such tumors may prolapse into the AV valve orifice during diastole or, in the case of ventricular tumors, into the left ventricular outflow tract during systole. An atrial ball thrombus may mimic a pedunculated tumor, but is more likely to be associated with clot in the atrial appendage.

A localized increase in myocardial wall thickness, especially when accompanied by a pericardial effusion, suggests an infiltrating malignant tumor. It is often difficult to differentiate myocardial thickening from pericardial effusion, but this may be aided by observation of the thickness of the right atrial wall. Since the right atrial wall is seldom infiltrated by tumor, the finding of right atrial thickening to greater than 5 mm suggests a pericardial effusion.[117] In myocardial infiltration, localized areas of disordered wall motion may also be noted by cineangiography. Coronary arteriography may in some cases allow visualization of the vascular supply of the tumor, thus demarcating the extent of tumor invasion, the source of its blood supply, and its relation to the coronary arteries.[118,119] However, the vascular pattern of cardiac tumors has not proved to be a useful sign of malignancy.

False-negative angiographic studies generally occur when the diagnosis is not suspected prior to catheterization. False-positive studies are most often the result of thrombus, but may also be produced by many entities, such as streaming of nonopaque venous blood, a hematoma in the atrial septum, an aneurysm of the muscular or membranous ventricular septum, Bernheim syndrome, congenital septal dysplasia, and hydatid cysts of the interventricular septum.

The major risk of angiography is peripheral embolization due to dislodgement of a fragment of tumor or of an associated thrombus. Therefore, the thorough evaluation of all cardiac chambers by noninvasive methods prior to catheterization is recommended in patients suspected of having cardiac tumors so that contrast material can be injected into the chamber proximal (upstream) to the location of the tumor. The transseptal approach to the left atrium (see p. 186) is particularly hazardous because of the frequent occurrence of left atrial myxomas in the region of the fossa ovalis.[120]

TREATMENT AND PROGNOSIS

Benign Tumors

Operative excision is the treatment of choice for most benign cardiac tumors and in many cases results in a complete cure.[5,121-123] Although many tumors are histologically benign, all cardiac tumors are potentially lethal as a result of intracavitary or valvular obstruction, peripheral embolization, and disturbances of rhythm or conduction. Unfortunately, it is not unusual for patients to die or experience a major complication while awaiting operation, and therefore it is mandatory to carry out the operation promptly after the diagnosis has been established.

Although some epicardial tumors may be removed without the aid of extracorporeal circulation, most intramural and intracavitary tumors must be excised under direct vision, requiring use of the heart-lung machine. Closed approaches are not now recommended because of increased risk of dislodging tumor fragments. In addition, excision cannot be as complete, and adequate inspection of the other cardiac chambers for additional tumors is not possible.

The dislodgment of tumor fragments constitutes a major risk of operation and may result in peripheral emboli or the dispersion of micrometastases, which may seed peripherally. To reduce this risk, manipulation of the heart prior to cardiopulmonary bypass should be minimized. Some surgeons recommend that venous cannulation for cardiopulmonary bypass be performed via the femoral or azygos vein rather than through the right atrium to avoid dislodging an unsuspected right atrial tumor. In addition, the tumor should be removed en bloc when possible, and the chamber then irrigated well with saline.

ATRIAL MYXOMAS. Numerous reports document complete cure of left and right atrial myxomas with follow-up periods of 10 to 15 years.[124,125] In about 1 to 5 per cent of cases a recurrence or second cardiac myxoma has been reported following resection of the initial myxoma.[126,127] Possible causes of the second tumor include incomplete excision of the original tumor with regrowth, growth from a second "pretumorous" focus, i.e., metasynchronous, or intracardiac implantation from the original tumor. Because of the first two possibilities, some surgeons have advocated excision of the entire region of the fossa ovalis and repair of the resultant atrial septal defect to remove presumably high concentrations of "pretumor" cells thought to be located in that region. In one case, the large size of a myxoma, together with its location on the posterior left atrial wall, necessitated complete removal of the heart, followed by autotransplantation, i.e., reimplantation of the patient's excised heart.[127a] Laser photocoagulation of a 1-cm area around the stalk attachment site has also been suggested as a way of eradicating pretumorous cells without the necessity of creating an atrial septal defect.[128] Other surgeons have reported equally successful long-term recurrence-free periods with simple excision of the tumor and a small rim at the

base. It now appears that in approximately 7 per cent of patients with (1) a familial history of cardiac myxoma, (2) features of the complex of lentigines and other abnormalities described on page 1467, or (3) synchronous tumor appearance (i.e., multiple tumors at the time of presentation), the incidence of a second tumor occurring at some time in the future is in the range of 12 to 22 per cent, as compared to approximately 1 per cent for patients with sporadic atrial myxoma.[127] It is believed that tumor recurrence in these cases is from a second pretumorous focus of cells. In these high-risk patients, a careful search for multiple tumors preoperatively and more extensive resection of the underlying endocardium, atrial septum, or both is recommended. Careful echocardiographic follow-up for detection of metasynchronous tumors is recommended[127] in all patients following resection of a myxoma.

OTHER BENIGN TUMORS. Successful excision has also been reported for ventricular myxomas, as well as most other types of benign cardiac tumor, including rhabdomyoma, hamartoma, fibroma, lipoma, hemangioma, and papillary fibroelastoma.[129-131] The major surgical considerations in excision of ventricular tumors include preservation of adequate ventricular myocardium, maintenance of proper atrioventricular valve function, and preservation of as much of the conduction system as possible. Often, however, papillary muscles, chordae tendineae, or the AV conduction system must be sacrificed during the resection of a tumor, thereby necessitating replacement of the atrioventricular valve, implantation of a pacemaker, or both.

Malignant Tumors

Operation is not an effective treatment for the great majority of primary malignant tumors of the heart because of the large mass of cardiac tissue involved or the presence of metastases. The major role for surgery in such cases is to establish a diagnosis in order to exclude the possibility of a curable benign tumor. Nevertheless, in some cases palliation of hemodynamics and/or constitutional symptoms and extension of life may be achieved by aggressive therapy. Survivals of 1 to 3 years have been reported following partial resection, chemotherapy, radiation therapy, orthotopic cardiac transplantation or various combinations of these modalities.[132-136] In some instances, localized recurrences have been eliminated by multiple operations. Some success in palliation of symptoms has been reported following the combination of chemotherapy and radiation therapy[137] and radiation therapy alone.[136] Lymphosarcoma of the heart frequently responds to chemotherapy, radiation therapy, or both.[138,139] Unfortunately, many other reports indicate a failure to alter the course of cardiac sarcomas despite various combinations of surgery, chemotherapy, and radiation therapy.

REFERENCES

CLINICAL PRESENTATION

1. Allard, M. F., Taylor, G. P., Wilson, J. E., and McManus, B. M.: Primary cardiac tumors. In Goldhaber, S. Z. and Braunwald, E. (eds.): Cardiopulmonary Diseases and Cardiac Tumors. Atlas of Heart Diseases. vol. 3. Philadelphia, Current Medicine, 1995, pp. 15.1–15.22.
2. Reynan, K.: Frequency of primary tumors of the heart. Am. J. Cardiol. 77:107, 1996.
3. Lam, K. Y. L., Dickens, P., and Chan, A. C. L.: Tumors of the heart. Arch. Pathol. Lab. Med. 117:1027, 1993.
4. Tazelaar, H. D., Locke, T. J., and McGregir, C. G. A.: Pathology of surgically excised primary cardiac tumors. Mayo Clin. Proc. 67:957, 1992.
5. Salcedo, E. E., Cohen, G. I., White, R. D., and Davison, M. B.: Cardiac tumors: Diagnosis and treatment. Curr. Probl. Cardiol. 17:73, 1992.
6. Hanson, E. C.: Cardiac tumors: A current perspective. N. Y. State J. Med. 92:41, 1992.
7. Goodwin, J. F.: Symposium on cardiac tumors. The spectrum of cardiac tumors. Am. J. Cardiol. 21:307, 1968.
8. St. John Sutton, M. G., Mercier, L., Guliani, E. R., and Lie, J. T.: Atrial myxomas: A review of clinical experience in 40 patients. Mayo Clin. Proc. 55:371, 1980.
9. Hirano, T., Taga, T., and Yasukawa, K.: Human B-cell differentiation

factor defined by an anti-peptide antibody and its possible role in autoantibody production. Proc. Natl. Acad. Sci. USA *84*:228, 1987.

10. Borden, E. C., and Chin, P.: Interleukin-6: A cytokine with potential diagnostic and therapeutic roles. J. Lab. Clin. Med. *123*:824, 1994.

11. Wada, A., Kanda, T., Hayashi, R., et al.: Cardiac myxoma metastasized to the brain: Potential role of endogenous interleukin-6. Cardiology *83*:208, 1993.

12. Takahara, H., Mori, A., Tabata, R., et al.: Left atrial myxoma with production of interleukin-6. J. Jpn. Assoc. Thorac. Surg. *40*:326, 1992.

13. Seino, Y., Ikeda, U., and Shimada, K.: Increased expression of interleukin-6 mRNA in cardiac myxomas. Br. Heart J. *69*:565, 1993.

14. Seguin, J. R., Beigbeder, J.-Y., Hvass, U., et al.: Interleukin-6 production by cardiac myxomas may explain constitutional symptoms. J. Thorac. Cardiovasc. Surg. *103*:599, 1992.

15. Jourdan, M., Bataille, R., Sequin, J., et al.: Constitutive production of interleukin-6 and immunologic features in cardiac myxomas. Arthritis Rheum. *33*:398, 1990.

16. Curry, H. L. F., Matthews, J. A., and Robinson, J.: Right atrial myxoma mimicking a rheumatic disorder. Br. Med. J. *1*:542, 1967.

17. Savige, J. A., Yeung, S. P., Davis, D. J., et al.: Anti-neutrophil cytoplasmic antibodies associated with atrial myxoma. Am. J. Med. *85*:755, 1988.

18. Graham, S. L., and Sellers, A. L.: Atrial myxoma with multiple myeloma. Arch. Intern. Med. *139*:116, 1979.

19. Leonhardt, E. T. G., and Kullenberg, K. P. G.: Bilateral atrial myxomas with multiple arterial aneurysms. A syndrome mimicking polyarteritis nodosa. Am. J. Med. *62*:792, 1977.

20. Byrd, W. E., Matthews, O. P., and Hunt, R. E.: Left atrial myxoma presenting as a systemic vasculitis. Arthritis Rheum. *23*:240, 1980.

21. Feldman, A. R., and Keeling, J. H.: Cutaneous manifestation of atrial myxoma. J. Am. Acad. Dermatol. *21*:1080, 1989.

22. Quinn, T. J., Condini, M. A., and Harris, A. A.: Infected cardiac myxoma. Am. J. Cardiol. *53*:381, 1984.

23. Whitman, M. S., Rovito, M. A., Klions, D., and Tunkel, A. R.: Infected atrial myxoma: Case report and review. Clin. Infect. Dis. *18*:657, 1994.

24. Hashimoto, H., Takahashi, H., Fujiwara, Y., et al.: Acute myocardial infarction due to coronary embolization from left atrial myxoma. Jpn. Circ. J. *57*:1016, 1993.

25. De Carli, S., Sechi, L. A., Ciani, R., et al.: Right atrial myxoma with pulmonary embolism. Cardiology *84*:368, 1994.

26. Miyauchi, Y., Endo, T., Kuroki, S., and Hayakawa, H.: Right atrial myxoma presenting with recurrent episodes of pulmonary embolism. Cardiology *81*:178, 1992.

27. Eriksen, U. H., Baandrup, U., and Jensen, B. S.: Total disruption of left atrial myxoma causing a cerebral attack and a saddle embolus in the iliac bifurcation. Int. J. Cardiol. *35*:127, 1992.

28. Boussen, K., Moalla, M., Blondeau, P., et al.: Embolization of cardiac myxomas masquerading as polyarteritis nodosa. J. Rheumatol. *18*:283, 1991.

29. Weerasena, N. A., Groome, D., Pollock, J. G., and Pollock, J. C.: Atrial myxoma as the cause of acute lower limb ischemia in a teenager. Scott. Med. J. *34*:440, 1989.

30. Reed, R. J., Utz, M. P., and Terezakis, N.: Embolic and metastatic cardiac myxoma. Am. J. Dermatopathol. *11*:157, 1989.

31. Michael, A. S., Mikhael, M. A., and Christ, M.: Myxoma of the heart presenting with recurrent episodes of hemorrhagic cerebral infarction: MR findings. J. Comput. Assist. Tomogr. *13*:123, 1989.

32. Knepper, L. E., Biller, J., Adams, H. P., Jr., and Bruno, A.: Neurologic manifestations of atrial myxoma. A 12-year experience and review. Stroke *19*:1435, 1988.

33. Heath, D., and Mackinnon, J.: Pulmonary hypertension due to myxoma of the right atrium. With special reference to the behavior of emboli of myxoma in the lung. Am. Heart J. *68*:227, 1964.

34. Harvey, W. P.: Clinical aspects of cardiac tumors. Am. J. Cardiol. *21*:328, 1968.

35. Kawano, H., Okada, R., Kawano, Y., et al.: Mesothelioma in the atrioventricular node. Case report. Jpn. Heart J. *35*:255, 1994.

36. Balasundaram, S., Halees, S. A., and Duran, C.: Mesothelioma of the atrioventricular node: First successful follow-up after excision. Eur. Heart J. *13*:718, 1992.

37. James, T. N., and Galakhov, I.: De subitaneis mortibus XXVI. Fatal electrical instability of the heart associated with benign congenital polycystic tumor of the atrioventricular node. Circulation *56*:667, 1977.

38. Strauss, W. E., Asinger, R. W., and Hodges, M.: Mesothelioma of the AV node: Potential utility of pacing. PACE *11*:1296, 1988.

39. Lantz, D. A., Dougherty, T. H., and Lucca, M. J.: Primary angiosarcoma of the heart causing cardiac rupture. Am. Heart J. *118*:186, 1989.

40. Mitral stenosis and left atrial myxoma. In Fowler, N. O.: Diagnosis of Heart Disease. New York, Springer-Verlag, 1991, pp. 146–159.

41. Gershlick, A. H., Leech, G., Mills, P. G., and Leatham, A.: The loud first heart sound in left atrial myxoma. Br. Heart J. *52*:403, 1984.

42. Teoh, K. H., Mulji, A., Tomlinson, C. W., and Lobo, F. V.: Right atrial myxoma originating from the eustachian tube. Can. J. Cardiol. *9*:441, 1993.

43. Heck, H. A., Jr., Gross, C. M., and Houghton, J. L.: Long-term severe pulmonary hypertension associated with right atrial myxoma. Chest *102*:301, 1992.

44. Pessotto, R., Santini, F., Piccin, C., et al.: Cardiac myxoma of the tricuspid valve: Description of a case and review of the literature. J. Heart Valve Dis. *3*:344, 1994.

44a. Savino, J. S., and Weiss, S. J.: Right atrial tumor. N. Engl. J. Med. *333*:1608, 1995.

45. Waxler, E. B., Kawai, N., and Kasparian, H.: Right atrial myxoma: Echocardiographic, phonocardiographic and hemodynamic signs. Am. Heart J. *82*:251, 1972.

46. Keren, A., Chenzbruna, A., Schuger, L., et al.: The etiology of tumor plop in a patient with huge right atrial myxoma. Chest *95*:1147, 1989.

47. Hada, Y., Wolfe, C., Murry, C. F., and Craige, E.: Right ventricular myxoma. Case report and review of phonocardiographic auscultatory manifestations. Am. Heart J. *100*:871, 1980.

48. Gosse, P., Herpin, D., Roudant, R., et al.: Myxoma of the mitral valve diagnosed by echocardiography. Am. Heart J. *111*:803, 1986.

SPECIFIC CARDIAC TUMORS

49. Carney, J. A., Hruska, L. S., Beauchamp, G. D., and Gordon, H.: Dominant inheritance of the complex of myxomas, spotty pigmentation and endocrine overactivity. Mayo Clin. Proc. *61*:165, 1986.

50. Van Gelder, H. M., O'Brien, D. J., Staples, E. D., and Alexander, J. A.: Familial cardiac myxoma. Ann. Thorac. Surg. *53*:419, 1992.

50a. Koopman, R. J., and Happle, R.: Autosomal dominant transmission of the NAME syndrome (nevi, atrial myxoma, mucinosis of the skin and endocrine overactivity). Hum. Genet. *86*:300, 1991.

51. Carney, J. A., Gordon, J., Carpenter, P. C., et al.: The complex of myxomas, spotty pigmentation and endocrine overactivity. Medicine *64*:270, 1985.

52. Vidaillet, H. J., Jr., Seward, J. B., Fyke, F. E., et al.: "Syndrome myxoma": A subset of patients with cardiac myxoma associated with pigmented skin lesions and peripheral and endocrine neoplasms. Br. Heart J. *57*:247, 1987.

53. Bennett, W. S., Skelton, T. N., and Lehan, P. H.: The complex of myxomas, pigmentation and endocrine overactivity. Am. J. Cardiol. *65*:399, 1990.

54. Carney, J. A., and Behnaz, C. T.: Myxoid fibroadenoma and allied conditions (myxomatosis) of the breast. Am. J. Surg. Pathol. *15*:713, 1991.

55. Vidaillet, H. J., Jr., Seward, J. B., Fyke, E., and Tajik, A. J.: NAME syndrome (nevi, atrial myxoma, myxoid neurofibroma, ephelides): A new and unrecognized subset of patients with cardiac myxoma. Minn. Med. *67*:695, 1984.

56. Rhodes, A. R., Silverman, R. A., Harrist, T. J., and Perez-Atayde, A. R.: Mucocutaneous lentigines, cardiomucocutaneous myxoma, and multiple blue nevi: The "LAMB" syndrome. Am. Acad. Dermatol. *10*:72, 1984.

57. Farah, M. G.: Familial cardiac myxoma. A study of relatives of patients with myxoma. Chest *105*:65, 1994.

58. McCarthy, P. M., Piehler, J. M., Schaff, H. V., et al.: The significance of multiple, recurrent, and "complex" cardiac myxomas. Thorac. Cardiovasc. Surg. *91*:389, 1986.

59. Carney, J. A.: Differences between nonfamilial and familial cardiac myxoma. Am. J. Surg. Pathol. *9*:53, 1985.

60. McAllister, H. A., Jr.: Tumors of the heart and pericardium. In Silver, M. D. (ed.): Cardiovascular Pathology. 2nd ed. New York, Churchill Livingstone, 1991, p. 1297.

61. Burke, A. P., and Virmani, R.: Cardiac myxoma. A clinicopathologic study. Am. J. Clin. Pathol. *100*:671, 1993.

62. Ferrans, V. J., and Roberts, W. L.: Structural features of cardiac myxomas. Histology, histochemistry and electron microscopy. Hum. Pathol. *4*:111, 1973.

63. Goldman, B. I., Frydman, C., Harpaz, N., et al.: Glandular cardiac myxomas. Cancer *59*:1767, 1987.

64. Lie, J. T.: The identity and histogenesis of cardiac myxomas: A controversy put to rest. Arch. Pathol. Lab. Med. *113*:724, 1989.

65. Hashimoto, H., Takahashi, H., Fujiwara, Y., et al.: Acute myocardial infarction due to coronary embolization from left atrial myxoma. Jpn. Circ. J. *57*:1016, 1993.

66. Salyer, W. R., Page, D. L., and Hutchins, G. M.: The development of cardiac myxomas and papillary endocardial lesions from mural thrombus. Am. Heart J. *89*:4, 1975.

67. Dewald, G. W., Dahl, R. J., Spurbeck, B. S., et al.: Chromosomally abnormal clones and non-random telomeric translocations in cardiac myxomas. Mayo Clin. Proc. *62*:558, 1987.

68. Richkind, K. E., Wason, D., and Vidaillet, H.: Cardiac myxoma characterization by clonal telomeric association. Genes Chrom. Cancer *9*:68, 1994.

69. Dijkhuizen, T., van den Berg, E., and Molenaar, W. M.: Cytogenetics of a case of cardiac myxoma. Cancer Genet. Cytogenet. *73*:73, 1992.

70. Seidman, J. D., Berman, J. J., Hitchcock, C. L., et al.: DNA analysis of cardiac myxomas: Flow cytometry and image analysis. Hum. Pathol. *22*:494, 1991.

71. Luthringer, D. J., Virmani, R., Weiss, S. W., and Rosai, J.: A distinctive cardiovascular lesion resembling histiocytoid (epithelioid) hemangioma. Am. J. Surg. Pathol. *14*:993, 1990.

72. Veinot, J. P., Tazelaar, H. D., Edwards, W. D., and Colby, T. V.: Mesothelial/monocytic incidental cardiac excrescences: Cardiac MICE. Mod. Pathol. *7*:9, 1994.

73. Courtice, R. W., Stinson, W.A., and Walley, V. M.: Tissue fragments recovered at cardiac surgery masquerading as tumoral proliferations. Am. J. Surg. Pathol. *18*:167, 1994.

PAPILLARY TUMORS OF HEART VALVES

74. Shahian, D. W., Labib, S. B., and Chang, G.: Cardiac papillary fibroelastoma. Ann. Thorac. Surg. *59*:538, 1995.

75. LiMandri, G., Homma, S., Di Tullio, M. R., et al.: Detection of multiple papillary fibroelastomas of the tricuspid valve by transesophageal echocardiography. J. Am. Soc. Echo. 7:315, 1994.

76. Pomerance, A.: Papillary "tumours" of the heart valves. J. Pathol. Bacteriol. 87:135, 1981.

77. Fenoglio, J. J., McAllister, H. A., and Ferrans, V. J.: Cardiac rhabdomyoma: A clinicopathologic and electron microscopic study. Am. J. Cardiol. 38:241, 1976.

78. Burke, A. P., and Virmani, R.: Cardiac rhabdomyoma: A clinicopathologic study. Mod. Pathol. 4:70, 1991.

79. Bass, J. L., Breningstall, G. N., and Swaiman, K. F.: Echocardiographic incidence of cardiac rhabdomyoma in tuberous sclerosis. Am. J. Cardiol. 55:137, 1985.

80. Gibbs, J. L.: The heart and tuberous sclerosis. An echocardiographic and electrocardiographic study. Br. Heart J. 54:596, 1985.

81. Webb, D. W., Thomas, R. D., and Osborne, J. P.: Cardiac rhabdomyomas and their association with tuberous sclerosis. Arch. Dis. Child. 68:367, 1993.

82. Moriarty, A. T., Nelson, W. A., and McGahey, B.: Fine-needle aspiration of rhabdomyosarcoma of the heart. Acta Cytologica. 34:74, 1990.

83. Van der Hauwaert, L. G.: Cardiac tumours in infancy and childhood. Br. Heart J. 33:125, 1971.

84. Jones, K. L., Wolf, P. L., Jensen, P., et al.: The Gorlin syndrome: A genetically determined disorder associated with cardiac tumor. Am. Heart J. 111:1013, 1986.

85. Miralles, A., Bracamonte, L., Soncul, H., et al.: Cardiac tumors: Clinical experience and surgical results in 74 patients. Ann. Thorac. Surg. 52:886, 1991.

86. Tazelaar, H. D., Locke, T. J., and McGregor, C. G. A.: Pathology of surgically excised primary cardiac tumors. Mayo Clin. Proc. 67:957, 1992.

87. Prior, J. T.: Lipomatous hypertrophy of cardiac interatrial septum. Arch Pathol. 78:11, 1964.

88. Chao, J. C., Reyes, C. V., and Hwang, M. H.: Cardiac hemangioma. South. Med. J. 83:44, 1990.

89. Cox, J. N., Friedli, B., Mechmeche, M., et al.: Teratoma of the heart. Virchows Arch. (A) 402:163, 1983.

90. Meysman, M., Noppen, M., Demeyer, G., and Vincken, W.: Malignant epithelial mesothelioma presenting as cardiac tamponade. Eur. Heart J. 14:1576, 1993.

91. Monma, N., Satodate, R., Tashiro, A., and Segawa, I.: Origin of so-called mesothelioma of the atrioventricular node. Arch. Pathol. Lab. Med. 115:1026, 1991.

92. Burke, M. A. P., Anderson, P. G., Virmani, R., et al.: Tumor of the atrioventricular nodal region. Arch. Pathol. Lab. Med. 114:1057, 1990.

93. David, T. E., Lenkei, S. C., Marquez-Julio, A., et al.: Pheochromocytoma of the heart. Ann. Thorac. Surg. 41:98, 1986.

MALIGNANT CARDIAC TUMORS

94. Putnam, J. B., Sweeney, M. S., Colon, R., et al.: Primary cardiac sarcomas. Ann. Thorac. Surg. 51:906, 1991.

95. Burke, A. P., Cowan, D., and Virmani, R.: Primary sarcoma of the heart. Cancer 69:387, 1992.

96. Thomas, C. R., Johnson, G. W., Stoddard, M. F., and Clifford, S.: Primary malignant cardiac tumors: Update 1992. Med. Pediatr. Oncol. 20:519, 1992.

97. Whorton, C. M.: Primary malignant tumor of the heart. Cancer 2:245, 1949.

98. Burke, A. P., and Virmani, R.: Osteosarcomas of the heart. Am. J. Surg. Pathol. 15:289, 1991.

99. Klima, U., Wimmer-Greinecker, G., Harringer, W., et al.: Cardiac angiosarcoma—a diagnostic dilemma. Cardiovasc. Surg. 1:674, 1993.

100. Herrmann, M. A., Shankerman, R. A., Edwards, W. D., et al.: Primary cardiac angiosarcoma: A clinicopathologic study of six cases. J. Thorac. Cardiovasc. Surg. 103:655, 1992.

101. Keohane, M. E., Lazzam, C., Halperin, J. L., et al.: Angiosarcoma of the left atrium mimicking myxoma. Case report. Hum. Pathol. 20:599, 1989.

101a. Basso, C., Stefani, A., Calabrese, F., et al.: Primary right atrial fibrosarcoma diagnosed by endocardial biopsy. Am. Heart J. 131:399, 1996.

102. Proctor, M. S., Tracy, G. P., and Von Koch, L.: Primary cardiac B-cell lymphoma. Am. Heart J. 118:179, 1989.

103. Kasai, K., Kuwao, S., Sato, Y., et al.: Case report of primary cardiac lymphoma. The applications of PCR to the diagnosis of primary cardiac lymphoma. Acta Pathol. Jpn. 42:667, 1992.

104. Marvasti, M. A., Obeid, A. I., Potts, J. L., and Parker, F. B.: Approach in the management of atrial myxoma with long-term follow-up. Ann. Thorac. Surg. 38:53, 1984.

105. Bleisch, N., Kraus, F.: Polypoid sarcoma of the pulmonary trunk. Cancer 46:314, 1980.

DIAGNOSIS, TREATMENT, PROGNOSIS

106. Lane, G. E., Kapples, E. J., Thompson, R. C., et al.: Quiescent left atrial myxoma. Am. Heart J. 127:1629, 1994.

107. Charuzi, Y., Bolger, A., Beeder, C., and Lew, A. S.: A new echocardiographic classification of left atrial myxoma. Am. J. Cardiol. 55:614, 1985.

108. Dennis, M. A., Appareti, K., Manco-Johnson, M. L., et al.: The echocardiographic diagnosis of multiple fetal cardiac tumors. Ultrasound Med. 4:327, 1985.

109. Panidis, I. P., Mimtz, G. S., and McAllisterm M.: Hemodynamic consequences of the left atrial myxomas as assessed by Doppler ultrasound. Am. Heart J. 111:927, 1986.

110. Edwards, L. C. III, and Louie, E. K.: Transthoracic and transesophageal echocardiography for the evaluation of cardiac tumors, thrombi, and valvular vegetations. Am. J. Card. Imag. 8:45, 1994.

111. Shyu, K-G., Chen, J-J., Cheng, J-J., et al.: Comparison of transthoracic and transesophageal echocardiography in the diagnosis of intracardiac tumors in adults. J. Clin. Ultrasound 22:381, 1994.

112. Azuma, T., Ohira, A., Akagi, H., et al.: Transvenous biopsy of a right atrial tumor under transesophageal echocardiographic guidance. Am. Heart J. 131:402, 1996.

113. Bough, E., Bodem, W., Gandsman, E., et al.: Radionuclide diagnosis of left atrial myxoma with computer-generated functional images. Am. J. Cardiol. 52:1365, 1986.

114. Bleiweis, M. S., Georgiou, D., and Brundage, B. H.: Detection of intracardiac masses by ultrafast computed tomography. Am. J. Card. Imag. 8:63, 1994.

115. Fujita, N., Caputo, G. R., and Higgins, C. B.: Diagnosis and characterization of intracardiac masses by magnetic resonance imaging. Am. J. Card. Imag. 8:69, 1994.

116. Reddy, D. B., Jena, Col. A., and Venugopal, P.: Magnetic resonance imaging (MRI) in evaluation of left atrial masses: An in vitro and in vivo study. J. Cardiovasc. Surg. 35:289, 1994.

117. Fueredi, G. A., Knetchtges, T. E., and Czarnecki, D. J.: Coronary angiography in atrial myxoma: Findings in nine cases. Am. J. Roentgenol. 152:737, 1989.

118. Singh, R. N., Burkholder, J. A., and Magovern, G. J.: Coronary arteriography as an aid in left atrial myxoma diagnosis. Cardiovasc. Intervent. Radiol. 7:40, 1984.

119. Weyne, A. E., Heyndrickx, G. R., Cavelier, C. C., et al.: Cardiac imaging techniques in the diagnosis of angiosarcoma of the heart: Report of two cases. Postgrad. Med. J. 61:271, 1985.

120. Pendyck, F., Pierce, E. C., Baron, M. G., and Lukban, S. B.: Embolization of left atrial myxoma after transseptal cardiac catheterization. Am. J. Cardiol. 30:569, 1972.

121. Wiatrowska, B. A., Walley, V. M., Masters, R. G., et al.: Surgery for cardiac tumors: The University of Ottawa Heart Institute experience (1980–1991). Can. J. Cardiol. 9:65, 1993.

122. MacGowan, S. W., Sidhu, P., Aherne, T., et al.: Atrial myxoma: National incidence, diagnosis and surgical management. Ir. J. Med. Sci. 162:223, 1993.

123. Aru, G. M., Falchi, S., Cardu, G., et al.: The role of transesophageal echocardiography in the monitoring of cardiac mass removal: A review of 17 cases. J. Card. Surg. 8:554, 1993.

124. Larsson, S., Lepore, V., and Kennergren, C.: Atrial myxomas: Results of 25 years' experience and review of the literature. Surgery 105:695, 1989.

125. Bortolotti, U., Maraglino, G., Rubino, M., et al.: Surgical excision of intracardiac myxomas: A 20-year follow-up. Ann. Thorac. Surg. 49:449, 1990.

126. Waller, D. A., Ettles, D. F., Saunders, N. R., and Williams, G.: Recurrent cardiac myxoma: The surgical implications of two distinct groups of patients. Thorac. Cardiovasc. Surg. 37:226, 1989.

127. McCarthy, P. M., Piehler, J. M., Schaff, H. V., et al.: The significance of multiple, recurrent, and "complex" cardiac myxomas. Thorac. Cardiovasc. Surg. 91:389, 1986.

127a. Scheid, H. H., Nestle, H. W., Kling, D., et al.: Resection of a heart tumor using autotransplantation. Thorac. Cardiovasc. Surg. 36:40, 1988.

128. Mesnildrey, P., Bloch, G., Cachera, J. P., and Piwicna, A.: Atrial myxoma: A new surgical approach using neodynium:yttrium-aluminum-garnet laser photocoagulation. J. Thorac. Cardiovasc. Surg. 98:313, 1989.

129. Goldman, S., Lortscher, R., and Pappas, G.: Surgical treatment for rhabdomyoma of the right atrium causing arrhythmias. J. Thorac. Cardiovasc. Surg. 89:802, 1985.

130. Corno, A., deSimone, G., Catena, G., and Marcelletti, C.: Cardiac rhabdomyoma: Surgical treatment in the neonate. Thorac. Cardiovasc. Surg. 87:725, 1984.

131. Orringer, M. B., Sisson, J. C., Glazer, G., et al.: Surgical treatment of cardiac pheochromocytomas. J. Thorac. Cardiovasc. Surg. 89:753, 1985.

132. Aufiero, T. X., Pae, W. E. Jr., Clemson, B. S., et al.: Heart transplantation for tumor. Ann. Thorac. Surg. 56:1174, 1993.

133. Yuh, D. D., Kubo, S. H., Francis, G. S., et al.: Primary cardiac lymphoma treated with orthotopic heart transplantation: A case report. J. Heart Lung Transplant. 13:538, 1994.

134. Baay, P., Karawande, S. V., Kushner, J. P., et al.: Successful treatment of a cardiac angiosarcoma with combined modality therapy. J. Heart Lung Transplant. 13:923, 1994.

135. Crespo, M. G., Pulpon, L. A., Pradas, G., et al.: Heart transplantation for cardiac angiosarcoma: Should its indication be questioned? J. Heart Lung Transplant. 12:527, 1993.

136. Baay, P., Karwande, S. V., Kushner, J. P., et al.: Successful treatment of a cardiac angiosarcoma with combined modality therapy. J. Heart Lung Transplant. 13:923, 1994.

137. Hollingworth, J. H., and Sturgill, B. C.: Treatment of primary angiosarcoma of the heart. Am. Heart J. 78:254, 1969.

138. Terry, L. N., and Kilgerman, M. M.: Pericardial and myocardial involvement by lymphomas and leukemias. The role of radiotherapy. Cancer 25:1003, 1970.

139. Gerfein, O. B.: Lymphosarcoma of the right atrium. Angiographic and hemodynamic documentation of response to chemotherapy. Arch. Intern. Med. 135:325, 1975.

Chapter 43
Pericardial Diseases
BEVERLY H. LORELL

ANATOMY

The pericardium forms a strong flask-shaped sac with short tubelike extensions that enclose the origins of the aorta and its junction with the aortic arch, the pulmonary artery where it branches, the proximal pulmonary veins, and venae cavae. Fibrous tissue of the pericardium actually blends with adventitia of the great arteries to form very strong attachments. In addition, the pericardium has firm ligamentous attachments anteriorly to the sternum and xiphoid process, posteriorly to the vertebral column, and inferiorly to the diaphragm.[1,2] The human pericardium receives its arterial blood supply from small branches of the aorta and internal mammary and musculophrenic arteries. The pericardium is innervated by the vagus, left recurrent laryngeal nerve, and esophageal plexus and also has rich sympathetic innervation from the stellate and first dorsal ganglia and the cardiac, aortic, and diaphragmatic plexuses. The phrenic nerves course over the pericardium en route to the diaphragm. The afferent nerves responsible for pain perception appear to be transmitted via the phrenic nerve entering the spinal cord at C4–C5.[2] Peripheral sensory fibers that enter the dorsal root ganglia at C8–T2 supply both the brachial plexus and the pericardium, which provides a possible morphological explanation for referred pericardial pain.[3]

THE TWO LAYERS OF THE PERICARDIUM. The pericardium is composed of a fibrous outer layer and an inner serous membrane composed of a single layer of mesothelial cells. The inner serous layer is intimately attached to the surface of the heart and epicardial fat to form the visceral pericardium, and this inner serous membrane reflects back on itself to line the outer fibrous layer to form the parietal pericardium.

The pericardium has two major serosal tunnels: the transverse sinus, which lies posterior to the great arteries and anterior to the atria and superior vena cava, and the oblique sinus, which lies posterior to the left atrium so that the posterior left atrial wall is actually separated from the pericardial space. The serous visceral pericardium is attached to the parietal pericardium by delicate connective tissue with elastin fibers. The parietal pericardium is composed of collagen fibers interlaced with extensive elastic fibers, which are wavy during childhood and become progressively straighter with age, suggesting that young pericardia are more compliant than those of the elderly.

ELECTRON MICROSCOPY. This reveals that exuberant microvilli and long, single cilia project from the serous mesothelium composing the visceral pericardium and the inner lining of the parietal pericardium,[4] which increase markedly the surface area available for fluid transport. Both microvilli and cilia provide a specialized surface to permit movement of the pericardial membranes over each other during each cardiac cycle and to permit the pericardium to accommodate changes in cardiac shape during contraction. In addition, numerous small fenestrations or pores less than 50 μ in diameter provide direct communication between the pericardial and pleural cavities in mammals.[5]

PERICARDIAL FLUID. The human pericardium normally contains up to 50 ml of clear fluid. The visceral pericardium is believed to be the source of normal pericardial fluid and excessive fluid in disease states. Normal pericardial fluid appears to be an ultrafiltrate of plasma because electrolytes are present in pericardial fluid in concentrations compatible with such an ultrafiltrate; protein concentrations are about one-third those of the plasma, and albumin is present in a higher ratio in pericardial fluid, reflecting its lower molecular weight. Current data suggest that drainage of the pericardial space occurs both by the thoracic duct via the parietal pericardium and by the right lymphatic duct via the right pleural space.

Pericardial fluid also contains phospholipids that serve as a lubricant to reduce friction between the surfaces of the parietal pericardium and the visceral pericardium.[6] The pericardium appears to produce prostaglandins in response to physiological stimuli that may modulate efferent cardiac sympathetic stimulation and alter cardiac electrophysiological properties.[7] The clinical implications of this potential regulatory effect of the pericardium on electrical conduction of the heart are not yet known.

FUNCTIONS OF THE PERICARDIUM

The pericardium's ligamentous attachments help to fix the heart anatomically and prevent excessive motion with changes in body position. The pericardium also reduces friction between the heart and surrounding organs and provides a barrier against the extension of infection and malignancy from contiguous organs to the heart itself. The role of the pericardium in the regulation of the circulation is controversial because congenital absence of the pericardium is not associated with overt disturbances of cardiac function. However, observations in both dogs and humans indicate that the pericardium may play a role in (1) the distribution of hydrostatic forces on the heart, (2) the prevention of acute cardiac dilatation, and (3) diastolic coupling of the two ventricles.

The normal pericardium is relatively stiff, and the relationship between pressure within the pericardium and total intrapericardial volume, which is the sum of the volume of the heart itself and the reserve volume of the surrounding pericardial sac, appears as a steep curve when plotted on a graph.[1] Once the pericardium is filled, intrapericardial pressure rises sharply as volume is increased (Fig. 43–1). Thus, the stiffness of the pericardium increases when the load is increased, and then it becomes almost inextensible. Although much of our knowledge regarding the physiological role of the pericardium has been derived from experimental studies in dogs, it is important to recognize that the human pericardium is about three times as thick and much less distensible than canine pericardium.[8] Usually, the pericardial sac is filled with a thin film of fluid distributed throughout the pericardial space in such a way that the pericardial reserve volume is not exceeded. This permits respiratory and postural changes in cardiac volume and total intrapericardial volume to occur without significant changes in intrapericardial pressure. When measured with a fluid-filled or micromanometer-tipped catheter, pericardial pressure is nearly equal to intrapleural pressure and varies from −5 to +5 cm H_2O during the respiratory cycle.[9]

INTRAPERICARDIAL PRESSURE. Normal intrapericardial pressure is zero or negative. This has major implications for our understanding of the influence of pericardial pressure on the transmural distending pressure of the cardiac chambers and the operation of the Frank-Starling mechanism in the beat-to-beat regulation of stroke volume.[10] The transmural distending pressure of either vehicle is the difference between intracardiac and intrapericardial pressures and is independent of gravity. When intrapericardial pressure is assumed to be negative, normally a substantial transmural distending pressure would be expected to exist across both ventricles. For example, when left ventricular end-diastolic pressure is +8 mm Hg and intrapericardial pressure is −2 mm Hg relative to atmosphere, the actual left ventricular distending pressure would be 8 − (−2) = 10 mm Hg, and when right ventricular end-diastolic pressure is 4 mm Hg and intrapericardial pressure is −2 mm Hg relative to the atmosphere, the actual right ventricular distending pressure would be 4 − (−2) = 6 mm Hg.

Studies using micromanometer pressure measurements support the view that pericardial pressure is usually very low and thus exerts only a small influence on the average transmural distending pressure of the heart as long as pericardial reserve volume is not exceeded by volume loading.[9] Under normal conditions, it is clear that the pericardium does influence the pattern of venous return and ventricular filling that occurs in every cardiac cycle. Ventricular ejection is accompanied by abrupt descent of the atrioventricular junction (the "base" of the heart) and a reduction in right atrial pressure, manifest by the x descent* in the right atrial pressure pulse as well as by a decline in intrapericardial pressure. These changes result in a surge of venous return during systole, particularly when ventricular and pericardial pressures are increased. This acceleration of

---

*It is recognized that the descent in venous pressure after the *a* wave is usually termed the x descent and, after the *c* wave, the x′ descent. In this chapter, the major systolic venous pressure descent after the *a* and *c* waves is termed the x descent.

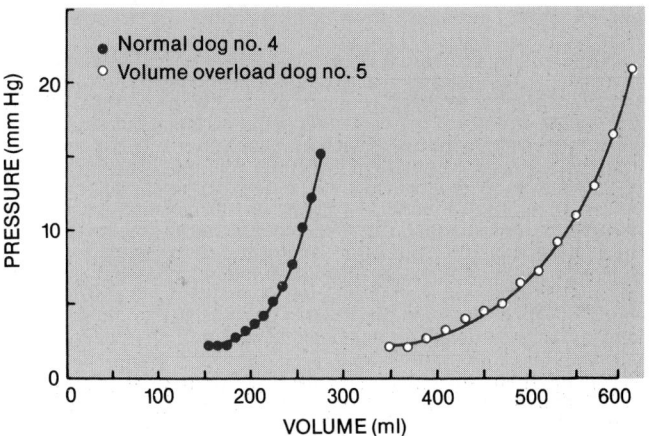

FIGURE 43–1. Pericardial pressure-volume curves from a normal dog *(left)* and from a dog with chronic volume overload *(right)*. Note that the normal pressure-volume curve *(right)* is initially flat but becomes extremely steep as total volume within the pericardium increases. In response to chronic cardiac dilatation, the pericardium enlarges in size and mass such that the pericardium can accommodate a large volume of low pressure *(right curve)*. (Reproduced by permission from Freeman, G. L., and LeWinter, M. M.: Pericardial adaptations during chronic dilation in dogs. Circ. Res. *54*:294, 1984. Copyright American Heart Association.)

venous return during systolic ejection is diminished by opening of the pericardium.

When the volume of the heart or other contents of the pericardial sac increase and exceed the elastic limits of the pericardium during diastole, the heart operates on the steep portion of the curve relating intrapericardial pressure and volume, resulting in marked increases in intrapericardial and intracardiac pressures. However, the difference between the two pressures, i.e., the transmural pressure, usually declines. In the extreme case of cardiac tamponade, in which both intrapericardial and intracardiac pressures are markedly increased, the transmural pressure distending the ventricles may fall precipitously toward zero, resulting in decreased ventricular diastolic volumes and preload. These findings, taken together, support the classic view that the pericardium is a distensible "loosely fitting" sac that modestly affects stroke volume by changes in intrapericardial pressure and transmural pressure and exerts a substantial influence only at higher ventricular and pericardial pressures.

CHALLENGES TO THE "CLASSIC VIEW." This classic view has been seriously challenged by Smiseth and coworkers,[11] who contend that the use of either fluid-filled or micromanometer catheters underestimates pericardial pressure and its influence on transmural distending pressures in normal hearts. They have shown in dogs that the measurement of the *surface contact pressure* of the pericardium against the heart using a flat balloon is more accurate than a fluid-filled catheter in estimating the actual pericardial pressure (the fall in left ventricular pressure observed immediately after opening the pericardium in the absence of any change in chamber volume). Observations from dogs and from humans indicate that when the amount of fluid in the pericardial sac is small, pericardial pressure measured in this way is much higher than intrathoracic pressure or pericardial pressure measured with a fluid-filled or micromanometer catheter, whereas pericardial pressures measured by either a balloon or fluid-filled catheter are similar when a substantial volume of pericardial fluid (40 to 50 ml) is present.[12,13] Thus the controversy regarding the concept of pericardial surface contact pressure does not detract from the accuracy or the clinical utility of measuring intrapericardial pressure with a catheter in patients with large pericardial effusions and cardiac tamponade.

However, these arguments profoundly challenge classic views regarding the normal physiology of the heart and the accurate measurement of the transmural pressure of each ventricle. These studies have emphasized that intrapericardial surface contact pressure is not zero or negative and, to the contrary, is virtually equal to right atrial pressure.[11,12] A further assumption is that differences in pericardial surface contact pressure do not exist over different chambers of the heart. This analysis indicates that left ventricular transmural pressure in normal hearts should be estimated by subtracting right atrial pressure rather than intrathoracic pressure. It also carries the remarkable implication that the transmural distending pressure of the normal right ventricle is extremely small, and negligible or zero at end-diastole.

Experiments by Santamore et al.[14] and Slinker et al.[15] have modified this concept and indicate that closed flat-balloon catheters probably exaggerate the constraining pressure exerted by the normal pericardium on the surface of the heart. Recent experiments in dogs before and after pericardiectomy, as well as observations in patients, suggest that pericardial constraint accounts for about 96 per cent of right atrial intracavitary pressure in the dog, and about 90 per cent in humans when central venous pressure is 10 mm Hg.[16] In addition, experiments indicate that the pressure exerted by the pericardium on the surface of the heart is not uniform over different regions of the heart.[17] Measurements by Chew et al.[18] of in situ regional pericardial strain in dogs show that the normal pericardium is strained by the underlying heart, even during vena caval occlusion. These studies indicate that a completely unloaded state cannot be achieved in the presence of an intact pericardium.

Taken together, these experiments suggest that right atrial pressure cannot be used to estimate precisely the pericardial constraint or to calculate transmural pressures of either ventricle in the normal heart. Furthermore, pericardial catheter measurements tend to underestimate while pericardial balloons tend to overestimate pericardial pressure, which appears to be within the range of 0.2 to 3 mm Hg under normal physiological conditions. Finally, these experiments confirm that the pericardium modifies the filling and intracavitary pressures of both ventricles, particularly when cardiac distention occurs.

LIMITATIONS OF CARDIAC DISTENTION

The relatively nondistensible pericardium may help to limit acute distention of the heart. This was appreciated as early as 1898 by Bernard, who used a pump to increase pressure in excised hearts with and without the pericardium and noted that hearts unsupported by the pericardium ruptured at lower pressures than did hearts with intact pericardia.[19] Subsequent studies in dogs demonstrated that the pericardium restrains right and left ventricular filling, so that ventricular volume is greater at any given ventricular pressure with the pericardium removed than with the pericardium intact. Thus, acute changes in intracardiac and total intrapericardial volume result in an upward shift of both the left and right ventricular pressure-volume relationships, which is in part mediated by the restraining effect of the pericardium and an increase in intrapericardial pressure.[15,20,21] As ventricular volumes increase, the proportional contribution of the pericardium to end-diastolic pressure of the thin-walled right ventricle increases relative to that of the left ventricle.[15] Thus, as the heart is distended, the pericardium makes a greater contribution to right ventricular end-diastolic pressure than to left ventricular end-diastolic pressure.

EFFECTS OF ACUTE VOLUME LOADING. The hemodynamic effects of acute volume loading and vasodilators are in part mediated by pericardial constraint. Shirato et al.[22] demonstrated that acute volume loading with dextran in dogs with intact pericardia resulted in an upward shift in the left ventricular pressure–segment length relation; i.e., left ventricular pressure was higher at any given segment length, whereas the reduction of venous return and cardiac volume by means of nitroprusside administration shifted the curves downward toward control levels. This occurred because nitroprusside and other vasodilators that decrease right heart filling reduce the total volume occupied by the heart within the pericardial space and thus reduce the restraining of the left ventricle by the pericardium; in turn, this causes a downward shift of the left ventricular pressure-volume relation so that a given left ventricular volume is associated with lower left ventricular diastolic pressure.

After pericardiectomy, volume loading results in a rightward shift in the pressure-segment length relation and, after nitroprusside, a leftward shift along a single curve.[22] When the effect of the pericardium is eliminated by plotting left ventricular transmural pressure versus segment length, the points during all interventions fall along a single curve. Smiseth et al.[23] have extended these findings and have shown that the opposite effects of angiotensin (upward shift) and nitroprusside (downward shift) of the left ventricle pressure-volume relation depend on changes in intrapericardial pressure mediated by shifts in blood volume from the heart to systemic vascular beds.

EFFECTS OF CHRONIC VOLUME LOADING. A restraining effect of the pericardium has been observed early in the course of chronic volume overloading induced by formation of arteriovenous shunts in dogs prior to enlargement of the pericardium by stretch or hypertrophy. However, this restraining effect was not apparent in dogs studied late during the course of chronic volume overload.[24] This occurs because chronic left ventricular enlargement and hypertrophy are accompanied by an increase in the compliance of the pericardial chamber and an increase in total pericardial volume due to the addition of new pericardial tissue.[25] In addition to its effects on ventricular filling, pericardial pressure also appears to influence indices of isovolumic relaxation of the left ventricle. Frais et al.[26] showed that alterations in the asymptote and time constant of left ventricular pressure decay (tau) in dogs subjected to volume loading vary with changes in intrapericardial pressure.

These observations suggest that shifts in the left and right ventricular diastolic pressure-volume relations following volume loading or

vasodilator administration are largely due to changes in intrapericardial pressure. However, the pericardium does not affect *intrinsic* myocardial compliance; neither does it account for changes in the left ventricular diastolic pressure-volume relationship observed during ischemia.[27]

VENTRICULAR INTERDEPENDENCE. The pericardium also contributes to diastolic coupling between the two ventricles. The distention of one ventricle alters the distensibility of the other, even in the absence of the pericardium.[28] This effect appears to be mediated in part by shared encircling muscle bands and by the interventricular septum, which tends to bulge into the left ventricle, causing a change in the shape of the left ventricle when the right ventricle is distended.[29] In the absence of the pericardium, large increases in right ventricular volume and pressure are required to cause an appreciable increase in left ventricular filling pressure.[30] In contrast, the presence of an intact pericardium markedly accentuates the coupling between ventricular diastolic pressures.[31] When right ventricular volume and pressure are increased with the normal pericardium intact, right and left ventricular filling pressures are closely correlated, and left ventricular volume is smaller than in the absence of the pericardium. In the absence of the pericardium, cardiac distensibility is primarily related to properties of the myocardium. This effect of the pericardium on the interaction between the two ventricles is accentuated in experimental constrictive pericarditis when the distensibility of the pericardium is decreased.[32] This effect of the pericardium on diastolic ventricular interaction is present at normal filling pressures and becomes of increasing importance at high right ventricular filling pressures. During volume loading in normal conscious dogs, it has been shown that pericardial pressure exerts a disproportionately greater effect on the thin-walled right ventricle, which suggests that the pericardium couples diastolic function of the two ventricles via its influence on right ventricular filling and geometry.[9,15]

Although normal pericardium does not appear to contribute importantly to the interaction of the ventricles during systole at normal filling pressures,[33] it does influence global and regional systolic function during conditions of acute distention of the heart.[34,35] Kanazawa et al.[34] showed that removal of the pericardium in dogs caused insignificant changes in stroke volume, whereas removal of the pericardium during volume loading caused a substantial increase in stroke volume associated with an increase in end-diastolic segment length and systolic excursion. Although pericardial pressure was not measured, it is likely that this increase in stroke volume was due to the Frank-Starling mechanism via an increase of the transmural distending pressure of the ventricle following removal of the pericardium. Furthermore, during volume overload, the pericardium caused an upward shift in the left ventricular end-systolic pressure-volume relationship in the absence of a change in inotropic state. Pericardial constraint also appears to modify regional systolic function during acute right ventricular pressure overload and distention. Goto et al.[35] found that acute right ventricular loading in dogs results in nonuniform decreases in regional left ventricular shortening, an effect that is enhanced by the presence of the pericardium.

The pericardium also appears to limit maximal body oxygen consumption by limiting stroke volume and cardiac output during maximal exercise in conscious dogs.[36] These observations suggest that the normal pericardium exerts a restraining effect and modifies ventricular interaction during systole at high ventricular filling pressures.

In *summary*, there is experimental evidence from canine studies that the pericardium limits acute distention of the heart, enhances the effect that distention of one ventricle has on the diastolic pressure-volume relations and systolic function of the contralateral ventricle, and modifies cardiac growth.

FUNCTIONS OF THE PERICARDIUM IN HUMANS. There is substantial evidence that the restraining effects of the pericardium are clinically relevant. For example, in humans after pericardiotomy, there is a downward shift of the left ventricular pressure-volume curve that is increasingly prominent as left ventricular volume increases.[37] Similarly, routine pericardial closure after open-heart surgery has been shown to result in an increase in right heart filling pressure associated with a reduction in left ventricular diastolic cavity dimension and cardiac output, whereas open-

FIGURE 43–2. Left ventricular pressure-volume curves in man *(A)* before and after nitroglycerin (NG) and *(B)* before and after amyl nitrite (AN). Nitroglycerin, which causes venodilation and reduces total intrapericardial volume, shifts the curve downward and leftward. In contrast, the curves before and after amyl nitrite, which causes arterial dilation, can be superimposed. (Reproduced by permission from Ludbrook, P. A., et al.: Influence of right ventricular hemodynamics on left ventricular diastolic pressure-volume relations in man. Circulation *59:*21, 1979. Copyright American Heart Association.)

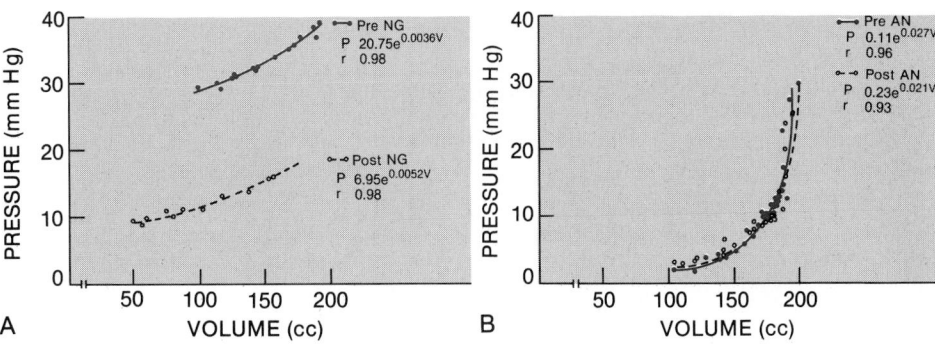

ing of the pericardium causes the opposite effects.[38] In addition, angiotensin, nitroprusside, and nitroglycerin infusions, which alter intracardiac volume, cause acute shifts in the left ventricular diastolic pressure-volume relation in humans,[39] an effect that has been shown in animal studies to depend on the presence of the constraint of the pericardium.[23] Ludbrook demonstrated in humans that the downward shift in the left ventricular pressure-volume curve that occurs during nitroglycerin administration is not observed with amyl nitrite, which alters aortic pressure but has little acute effect on intrapericardial volumes (Fig. 43–2).[39,40] After pericardiotomy and loss of the restraining effect of the pericardium, the human left ventricular pressure-volume curve is not altered by nitroprusside administration.[41] These observations indicate that the beneficial effects of interventions such as nitroprusside infusion, in which an augmentation of stroke volume may be observed at a lower ventricular filling pressure, are in part due to an alteration of apparent cardiac distensibility mediated by reducing the restraining effect of the pericardium.[42]

The pericardium may also provide a significant restraining effect on acute cardiac dilatation during acute volume loading in humans.[43] Extrapolating the findings of dog experiments may underestimate the restraining effect of the human pericardium during acute volume loading because normal human pericardium is thicker and shows much greater viscous responses than canine pericardium.[8] In patients, volume overload due to acute mitral regurgitation is sometimes associated with striking elevation and equilibration of diastolic pressures in all four cardiac chambers similar to that observed in constrictive pericardial disease (see p. 1501), but these findings do not appear to be present in patients with chronic volume overload.[44] Similarly, acute right ventricular infarction is sometimes associated with

elevation and equilibration of diastolic right and left ventricular pressures[45] that have been shown experimentally to be related to the elevation of intrapericardial pressure.[46]

EFFECTS ON MYOCARDIAL GROWTH. The restraining effect of the pericardium also appears to modulate chronic changes in cardiac volume and physiological growth of the human heart. Because animal studies have suggested that left ventricular mass increases after pericardiectomy, Tischler et al.[47] used quantitative two-dimensional echocardiography to examine changes in left ventricular volume and mass in 25 patients with normal left ventricular ejection fraction 1 day before and 6 weeks and 7 months after elective bypass surgery with the pericardium left widely open. Both left ventricular end-diastolic volume and left ventricular mass were significantly increased by 6 weeks after surgery, and by 7 months after surgery, left ventricular end-diastolic volume had increased by 29 per cent and left ventricular mass had increased by 20 per cent in the absence of changes in systemic arterial blood pressure, left ventricular end-systolic wall stress, or end-systolic volume. It is likely that these effects on left ventricular mass were mediated by an increase in the transmural distending pressure following opening of the pericardium. These observations support the notion that the relief of pericardial constraint in humans results in a stimulus for myocardial growth and an increase in left ventricular mass.

ROLE IN HEART FAILURE. The role of the pericardium in the pathogenesis of chronic heart failure in patients is controversial and not yet well understood. Although compensatory enlargement and increased capacitance of the pericardium are likely to occur in humans with chronic cardiac enlargement, it is feasible that acute increases in venous return in patients with heart failure could accentuate the effects of the pericardium on ventricular diastolic and systolic function. Consistent with this hypothesis, Janicki studied the effects of the augmentation of venous return by exercise in 61 patients with chronic heart failure and deduced that pericardial constraint became evident when stroke volume abruptly became invariant and a similar increment in right and left heart filling pressures occurred during progressive exercise.[48] In this study, pericardial constraint became evident during exercise in half of the patients. Thus, it appears that the pericardium can be an important determinant of the limits of systolic pump function and result in the coupling of right and left ventricular diastolic pressures in patients with heart failure.

ACUTE PERICARDITIS

Acute pericarditis is a syndrome due to inflammation of the pericardium characterized by chest pain, a pericardial friction rub, and serial electrocardiographic abnormalities. The incidence of pericardial inflammation detected in several autopsy series ranges from 2 to 6 per cent, whereas pericarditis is diagnosed clinically in only about 1 of 1000 hospital admissions. This suggests that pericarditis is frequently inapparent clinically, although it may occur in the presence of a vast number of medical and surgical disorders (Table 43–1). The most common causes of the syndrome of acute pericarditis include idiopathic or viral pericarditis, uremia, bacterial infection, acute myocardial infarction, pericardiotomy associated with cardiac surgery, tuberculosis, neoplasm, and trauma. All types of pericarditis are more common in men than in women, and in adults compared with young children. The relative frequency of causes of pericarditis depend on the clinical setting. Presumed viral or idiopathic pericarditis is common in an outpatient setting, whereas pericarditis related to trauma,

neoplasm, and uremia is seen more frequently in tertiary hospitals.

The *pathological changes* of acute pericarditis are those of acute inflammation, including the presence of polymorphonuclear leukocytes, increased pericardial vascularity, and deposition of fibrin. Inflammation may also involve the superficial myocardium, and fibrinous adhesions may form between the pericardium and epicardium and between the pericardium and adjacent sternum and pleura. The visceral pericardium may also react to acute injury by exudation of fluid. The pathological and clinical features of specific causes of pericarditis are discussed later in this chapter. This section focuses on clinical features common to acute pericarditis of many causes.

HISTORY. *Chest pain* is frequently the chief complaint of patients with acute pericarditis; its quality and location are variable. Pain is often localized to retrosternal and left precordial regions and frequently radiates to the trapezius ridge and neck (Table 43–2). Occasionally it may be local-

TABLE 43–1 CAUSES OF PERICARDITIS

1. **Idiopathic (nonspecific)**

2. **Viral Infections:** Coxsackie A virus, Coxsackie B virus, echovirus, adenovirus, mumps virus, infectious mononucleosis, varicella, hepatitis B, AIDS (acquired immunodeficiency syndrome)

3. **Tuberculosis**

4. **Acute Bacterial Infection:** pneumococcus, staphylococcus, streptococcus, gram-negative septicemia, *Neisseria meningitidis*, *Neisseria gonorrhoeae*, tularemia, *Legionella pneumophila*

5. **Fungal Infections:** histoplasmosis, coccidioidomycosis, *Candida*, blastomycosis

6. **Other Infections:** toxoplasmosis, amebiasis, mycoplasma, *Nocardia*, actinomycosis, echinococcosis, Lyme disease

7. **Acute Myocardial Infarction**

8. **Uremia:** untreated uremia; in association with hemodialysis

9. **Neoplastic Disease:** lung cancer, breast cancer, leukemia, Hodgkin's disease, lymphoma

10. **Radiation**

11. **Autoimmune Disorders:** acute rheumatic fever, systemic lupus erythematosus, rheumatoid arthritis, scleroderma, mixed connective tissue disease, Wegener's granulomatosis, polyarteritis nodosa

12. **Other Inflammatory Disorders:** sarcoidosis, amyloidosis, inflammatory bowel disease, Whipple disease, temporal arteritis, Behçet disease

13. **Drugs:** hydralazine, procainamide, phenytoin, isoniazid, phenylbutazone, dantrolene, doxorubicin, methysergide, penicillin (with hypereosinophilia)

14. **Trauma:** including chest trauma; hemopericardium following thoracic surgery; pacemaker insertion; cardiac diagnostic procedures; esophageal rupture; pancreatic-pericardial fistula

15. **Delayed Postmyocardial-Pericardial Injury Syndromes:**
    a. Postmyocardial infarction (Dressler) syndrome
    b. Postpericardiotomy syndrome

16. **Dissecting Aortic Aneurysm**

17. **Myxedema**

18. **Chylopericardium**

ized to the epigastrium, mimicking an "acute abdomen," or have a dull or oppressive quality, with radiation to the left arm similar to the ischemic pain of myocardial infarction. The pain is often aggravated by lying supine, coughing, deep inspiration, and swallowing and is eased by sitting up and leaning forward. Sometimes it is noted with each heartbeat. The pain associated with pericarditis may arise from inflammation of both the pericardium and the adjacent pleura, accounting for the pleuritic nature of the discomfort. Pericardial pain may also be provoked by stretch of the pericardial sac due to the presence of intrapericardial fluid. The inspiratory and positional aggravation of pericardial pain may be confused with chest pain caused by acute pulmonary embolism. It is important also to recognize that acute pericarditis may develop in about 4 per cent of patients a few days after acute pulmonary embolism.[49]

Acute pericarditis may also cause *dyspnea*. This symptom is related in part to the need to breathe shallowly to avoid pericardiopleuritic chest pain. Dyspnea may be aggravated by the presence of fever or by the development of a large pericardial effusion that compresses adjacent bronchi and pulmonary parenchyma. Additional symptoms such as cough, sputum production, or weight loss may be due to an underlying systemic disease such as tuberculosis or uremia. The classic clinical features of chest pain and dyspnea are more subtle in elderly patients with pericardi-

tis and are easily confused with other causes of chest pain.[50]

PHYSICAL EXAMINATION: THE FRICTION RUB. The *pericardial friction rub* (p. 45) is the pathognomonic physical finding of acute pericarditis. It is a scratching, grating, high-pitched sound, described by Laennec's associate Victor Collin as "the squeak of leather of a new saddle under the rider." Although the sound is believed to arise from friction between the roughened pericardial and epicardial surfaces, a loud pericardial rub may also be heard in the presence of scant or large pericardial effusions.[51] The pericardial friction rub is classically described as having three components that are related to cardiac motion during atrial systole (presystole), ventricular systole, and rapid ventricular filling in early diastole. Spodick's prospective analysis of the pericardial friction rub revealed that the presystolic component is present in about 70 per cent of cases, while a ventricular systolic component is the loudest and most easily heard component, present in almost all cases.[52] The rapid diastolic filling component is detected less frequently and may be slurred into that of atrial contraction, resulting in a biphasic "to-and-fro" rub. In this series, a true three-component rub was detected about half the time and at the lower left sternal border. The single-component rub is the least common but is likely to be the auscultatory finding in patients with atrial fibrillation.

An important feature of the pericardial friction rub is that it is often evanescent and may change in quality from one examination to the next. Detection of the rub is aided by listening with the stethoscope diaphragm applied firmly to the chest at the lower left sternal border during inspiration and full expiration with the patient sitting up and leaning forward. Occasionally, rubs may be detected with the patient lying supine with arms extended above the head during inspiration or suspended respiration. The single-component pericardial friction rub may be mistaken for a systolic murmur or tricuspid or mitral regurgitation. A pericardial rub may also be confused with the crunch of air in the mediastinum or the artifact of skin scratching against the stethoscope. Pericardial friction rubs may be differentiated from murmurs by (1) the use of exercise to permit detection of a classic three-component rub, (2) the failure of a rub to radiate widely or to vary in timing and duration with inspiration or a change in posture in a manner characteristic of regurgitant murmurs, and (3) by the confirmatory finding of typical electrocardiographic and echocardiographic changes of pericarditis.

TABLE 43–2 PERICARDIAL VERSUS ISCHEMIC PAIN

	ISCHEMIA	PERICARDITIS
Location	Retrosternal; left shoulder, arm	Precordium; left trapezius ridge
Quality	Pressure, burning, buildup	Sharp, pleuritic; or dull, oppressive
Thoracic motion	No effect	Increased by breathing, rotating thorax
Duration	Angina; 1 or 2 to 15 min Unstable angina: ½ hr to hours	Hours or days
Effort	Stable angina: usually Unstable angina or infarction: usually not	No relation
Posture	No effect; may sit, belch, use Valsalva or knee-chest position for relief	Leaning forward for relief; aggravated by recumbency

From Fowler, N. O.: Acute pericarditis. *In* Fowler, N. O. (ed.): The Pericardium in Health and Disease. Mt. Kisco, NY, Futura Publishing Co., 1985, p. 158.

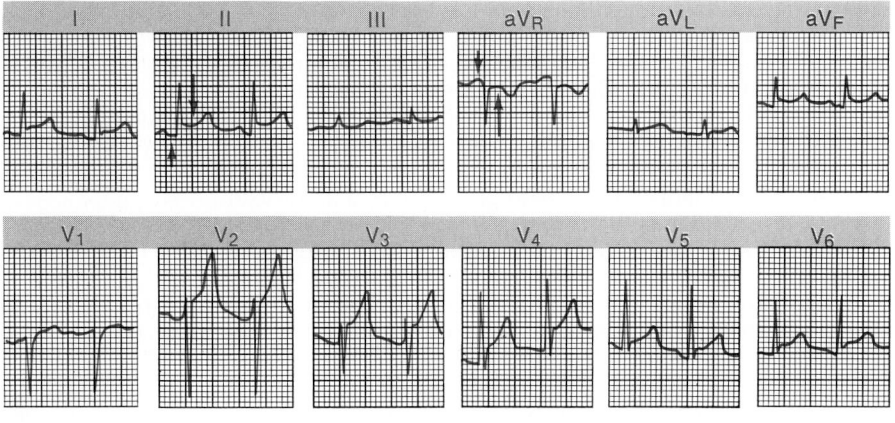

FIGURE 43–3. Stage I electrocardiographic changes from a patient with acute pericarditis. Diffuse ST-segment elevation, which is concave upward, is present in all leads except aV$_R$ and V$_1$. (A short P-R interval unrelated to acute pericarditis is also present.) Depression of the PR segment, an electrocardiographic abnormality that is common in patients with acute pericarditis, is not evident because of the short P-R interval.

ELECTROCARDIOGRAM. Serial electrocardiograms are extremely helpful in confirming the diagnosis of acute pericarditis. Electrocardiographic changes can occur a few hours or days after the onset of pericardial pain, and the electrocardiographic diagnosis of acute pericarditis is made by detecting the serial appearance of four stages of abnormalities of the ST segments and T waves (Fig. 43–3).[53] These changes are believed to be related to an actual current of injury caused by superficial myocardial inflammation or epicardial injury. There are four stages in the evolution of acute pericarditis (Table 43–3). Stage I electrocardiographic changes accompany the onset of chest pain and are virtually diagnostic of acute pericarditis. These comprise ST-segment elevation, which, unlike the pattern of ST-segment elevation in acute myocardial infarction, is concave upward and usually present in all leads except aVr and V1. The T waves are usually upright in the leads with ST-segment elevation. The ST-segment axis in the frontal plane also differs in these two conditions and is reported to range from 30 to 60 degrees in acute pericarditis, unlike acute anterior myocardial infarction in which the ST-segment axis varies from 100 to 120 degrees.[54]

Recent studies of body surface potential mapping in patients with acute pericarditis suggest that the mechanism of ST elevation is a current flowing from the epicardial surface out into the thorax and back into the heart through the atria and great vessels.[55] Stage II occurs several days later and represents the return of ST segments to baseline, accompanied by T-wave flattening. This change in the ST segments usually occurs prior to the appearance of T-wave inversion. In contrast, T waves in acute myocardial infarction often become inverted before the ST segments return to baseline. Stage III is characterized by inversion of the T waves so that the T-wave vector becomes directed opposite to the ST-segment vector. T-wave inversion is generally present in most leads and is not associated with the loss of R-wave voltage or the appearance of Q waves. These features help to differentiate this stage of nonspecific T-wave inversion from changes associated with the evolution of transmural or subendocardial myocardial infarction. Stage

IV represents the reversion of T-wave changes to normal, which may occur up to weeks or months later. T-wave inversion may occasionally persist indefinitely in patients with chronic pericardial inflammation due to tuberculosis, uremia, or neoplastic pericardial disease.

Electrocardiographic abnormalities appear in about 90 per cent of cases of acute pericarditis,[53,56] and the finding of typical Stage I changes or a classic evolution of all four stages can be diagnostic even when other clinical features of pericarditis are misleading. All four stages are detected in about 50 per cent of patients with acute pericarditis. In addition, depression of the PR segment occurs in about 80 per cent of patients with acute pericarditis.[53] Depression of the PR segment occurs during the early stages of ST-segment elevation or T-wave inversion, is usually present in both limb and precordial leads, and may reflect abnormal atrial repolarization due to atrial inflammation.

Variations of the patterns already described are present in slightly less than 50 per cent of patients with pericarditis and include (1) isolated PR-segment depression, (2) the absence of one or more stages of the ST-segment and T-wave changes, (3) evolution of Stage I (ST-segment elevation) directly to Stage IV (reversion of T waves to normal), (4) persistence of T-wave inversion, (5) appearance of ST-segment changes in only a few leads, (6) the appearance of marked T-wave inversion before the ST segments returned to baseline, and (7) the absence of any serial electrocardiographic changes whatsoever.[57]

Regional ST-segment deviation may be confused with electrocardiographic changes of regional myocardial ischemia. ST-segment elevation in the right precordial leads has been described in acute pericarditis.[58] The frequency of acute right precordial ST-segment elevation in acute pericarditis has not been systematically studied, and this finding could cause confusion with acute right ventricular infarction.

In addition to the features already described that help to distinguish the ST-segment changes of pericarditis from those of acute myocardial infarction, the changes of Stage I must also be differentiated from the electrocardiographic

TABLE 43–3   FOUR-STAGE ("TYPICAL") ECG EVOLUTION OF ACUTE PERICARDITIS

SEQUENCE	LEADS OF "EPICARDIAL" DERIVATION (I, II, aV$_L$, aV$_F$, V$_{3-6}$)			LEADS REFLECTING "ENDOCARDIAL" POTENTIAL aV$_R$, OFTEN V$_1$, SOMETIMES V$_2$		
Stage	J-ST*	T Waves	PR Segment	ST Segment	T Waves	PR Segment
I	Elevated	Upright	Depressed or isoelectric	Depressed	Inverted	Elevated or isoelectric
II early	Isoelectric	Upright	Isoelectric or depressed	Isoelectric	Inverted	Isoelectric or elevated
II late	Isoelectric	Low to flat to inverted	Isoelectric or depressed	Isoelectric	Shallow to flat to upright	Isoelectric or elevated
III	Isoelectric	Inverted	Isoelectric	Isoelectric	Upright	Isoelectric
IV	Isoelectric	Upright	Isoelectric	Isoelectric	Inverted	Isoelectric

* J-ST = junction of S (or T) wave with the end of the QRS complex.
Modified from Spodick, D. H.: Electrocardiographic changes in acute pericarditis. Am. J. Cardiol. *33*:470, 1974.

variant of normal early repolarization (see p. 109).[59] This pattern is usually seen in young males, in whom the clinical syndrome of pain and dyspnea suggesting acute pericarditis is absent; PR-segment depression is occasionally present but is uncommon, and most importantly, the electrocardiogram does not evolve through a pattern of the return of ST segments to baseline followed by T-wave inversion. An ST-segment/T wave ratio greater than 0.25 in lead V_6 also appears to discriminate patients with acute pericarditis from those with the normal variant of early repolarization.[60]

Sinus tachycardia is common and may be present in the absence of other contributing factors, such as fever or hemodynamic compromise.[61] Other atrial arrhythmias are infrequent in uncomplicated acute pericarditis and suggest the presence of underlying heart disease.[62] Atrioventricular block, bundle branch block, and ventricular tachycardia are not features of acute pericarditis, and these findings suggest the presence of extensive myocardial inflammation, fibrosis, or acute ischemia.

ECHOGARDIOGRAM. The echocardiogram is at present the most sensitive and accurate tool in the detection and quantification of pericardial fluid and is discussed on pages 93 to 94 and is illustrated in Figures 3–103 and 3–104.

THE CHEST ROENTGENOGRAM. This is of relatively little diagnostic value in uncomplicated acute pericarditis. If acute pericarditis is complicated by the appearance of a large pericardial effusion, the chest roentgenogram may show both enlargement and changes in configuration of the cardiac silhouette. The chest roentgenogram may provide clues to the underlying cause of the pericarditis, as in the case of pericarditis secondary to tuberculosis, or malignant disease. Pleural effusions occur in about one-fourth of patients with pericarditis and are usually left-sided, in contrast to patients with heart failure in whom right pleural effusions predominate.[56,63]

RADIONUCLIDE SCANS. Technetium-99m pyrophosphate scans,[64] gallium radionuclide scans, and Gd-DTPA enhanced nuclear magnetic resonance imaging scans have also been reported to be useful in detecting acute pericarditis.[65,66] However, their sensitivity and specificity have not been clearly established.

BLOOD TESTS. Acute pericarditis is often associated with nonspecific indicators of inflammation, including leukocytosis and elevation of the sedimentation rate. Cardiac isoenzymes are usually normal, but modest elevation of the MB fraction of creatine phosphokinase may occur in the presence of epicardial inflammation accompanying acute pericarditis.[67] For this reason, cardiac isoenzymes cannot always be used to differentiate between acute pericarditis and acute myocardial infarction, particularly non-Q-wave infarction.

Based on the history, including recent travel, physical examination, and clinical setting, some patients may require more extensive diagnostic tests to clarify the possibility of an underlying systemic disease. Because of the serious consequences of missing the diagnosis of tuberculosis pericarditis, screening for tuberculosis with a tuberculin skin test and a control skin test to exclude anergy is reasonable for patients with acute pericarditis in geographical areas and in patient populations with a low pretest risk of having a positive tuberculin skin test.

Other diagnostic tests that may be indicated in individual patients are based on the clinical presentation: (1) blood cultures to exclude associated possible infective endocarditis and bacteremia; (2) acute and convalescent cultures of blood, urine, throat, and feces, if available from the hospital laboratory, to evaluate a suspected viral etiology; (3) HIV test to evaluate the possibility of acquired immunodeficiency syndrome and unusual pathogens in patients with a compatible clinical syndrome; (4) fungal serological tests to evaluate a suspected fungal cause in patients from endemic areas or in immunocompromised patients; (5) ASO titer in children with suspected rheumatic fever; (6) cold agglutinins to exclude a mycoplasmal cause; (7) heterophile antibody test to exclude mononucleosis; (8) immunofluorescent antibody titers for toxoplasmosis; (9) TSH, T_4, and T_3 to exclude hypothyroidism; (10) BUN and creatinine to exclude uremia; and (11) antinuclear antibody titer (ANA) and rheumatoid factor, to exclude systemic lupus erythematosus and rheumatoid arthritis.

AORTIC DISSECTION. In middle-aged and elderly patients, close attention should be paid to the history, chest roentgenogram, and echocardiogram for evidence of prior aortic dissection (see p. 1568) because subacute inflammatory pericarditis following the slow penetration of blood into the pericardial space can be the initial presentation of aortic dissection.[68]

PERICARDIOCENTESIS AND PERICARDIAL BIOPSY. The issue of the additional diagnostic yields of pericardiocentesis or pericardial biopsy has been addressed by a prospective study of 231 patients with acute pericarditis of inapparent cause.[69] Noninvasive clinical and laboratory studies as described above were done in all patients, whereas diagnostic pericardiocentesis was done if clinical illness and an effusion lasted more than 1 week, and diagnostic biopsy was done if clinical illness lasted more than 3 weeks. This strategy yielded a diagnosis in 14 per cent of patients, which in the majority warranted specific therapy (bacterial pericarditis, tuberculosis, toxoplasmosis, unsuspected malignant disease). The diagnostic yield was substantial when pericardiocentesis or pericardiectomy with biopsy was done to relieve cardiac tamponade (39 and 54 per cent, respectively), and only 5 per cent when these procedures were done for diagnostic reasons. This experience suggests that there is a higher likelihood of establishing an etiologic diagnosis in patients who develop cardiac tamponade than in those with uncomplicated acute pericarditis, and therapeutic pericardiocentesis or pericardiectomy should always be accompanied by a rigorous examination of fluid or tissue for occult malignant disease or infection. In the immunocompetent patient with uncomplicated acute pericarditis who does not have cardiac tamponade, diagnostic pericardiocentesis or biopsy has a very low yield and is not justified. Pericardiocentesis should be performed for diagnostic reasons in the absence of cardiac tamponade only in patients in whom there is an urgent need to confirm a diagnosis of suspected purulent pericarditis.

MANAGEMENT. The first step in the management of acute pericarditis consists of establishing whether the pericarditis is related to an underlying problem that requires specific therapy. Nonspecific therapy of an initial episode of pericarditis should include bed rest until pain and fever have disappeared, because activity may cause worsening of symptoms. Initial observation in the hospital is warranted for almost all patients with acute pericarditis to exclude an associated myocardial infarction or a pyogenic process and to watch for the development of tamponade, which occurs in about 15 per cent of patients with acute pericarditis.[69]

The *pain of* pericarditis usually responds to nonsteroidal antiinflammatory agents such as aspirin (650 mg orally every 3 or 4 hours) or indomethicin (25 to 50 mg orally four times daily). When pain is severe and does not respond to this therapy within 48 hours, corticosteroids may be employed. If prednisone is used, large doses, such as 60 to 80 mg daily in divided doses, should be given. After 5 to 7 days, if the patient has been free of symptoms for several days, antiinflammatory agents should be tapered. Owing to the adverse consequence of long-term steroid therapy, it is desirable to avoid their use for pain control whenever possible. When long-term steroid administration is needed to control pain and other evidence of inflammation, alternate-day therapy should be attempted. Patients in whom steroids cannot be discontinued may tolerate tapering of steroids and weaning to nonsteroidal antiinflammatory agents. The rapid resolution of symptomatic acute pericarditis has also been reported in response to ketorolac tromethamine, a parenteral nonsteroidal antiinflammatory drug, but experience with this agent is limited.[70]

Antibiotics should be used to treat only documented purulent pericarditis. Oral anticoagulants should not be administered during the acute phase of pericarditis of any cause. If anticoagulants must be continued owing to the presence of a mechanical prosthetic heart valve, we recommend use of intravenous heparin, the action of which can be promptly reversed with protamine, and both physical examination and echocardiography should be performed at regular intervals to watch closely for the development of a pericardial effusion under pressure.

NATURAL HISTORY. Viral pericarditis, idiopathic pericarditis, post–myocardial infarction pericarditis, or the postpericardiotomy syndrome are usually self-limited; clinical and laboratory signs of inflammation abate after 2 to 6 weeks. Sagrista-Sauleda et al.[71] have observed, by physical examination and noninvasive readings, that about 9 per cent of patients with acute idiopathic pericarditis and pericardial effusion develop signs of mild cardiac constriction within the first 30 days after onset of the illness when signs of acute pericarditis and the effusion have already abated. These findings spontaneously disappear within 3 months and indicate that the development of transient constrictive physiology may occur during the resolution of acute pericardial inflammation.

RECURRENT PERICARDITIS. The most troublesome complication is the development of recurrent episodes of pericardial inflammation at intervals of weeks or months after the initial episode. In two series of patients with acute pericarditis, between 20 and 28 per cent of patients experienced recurrent episodes of pericarditis with severe chest pain.[56,71] The majority of patients can be managed by reinstitution of high-dose nonsteroidal anti-inflammatory agents and very gradual tapering over several months to discontinuation or alternate-dose therapy. In rare patients, disabling chest pain associated with fever may recur over a period of years and require steroid administration for pain relief.[72] Intravenous methylprednisolone given as pulse therapy may be useful in the management of severe recurrent acute idiopathic pericarditis.[73] Pericardiectomy has been proposed for the relief of refractory relapsing pericarditis,[74] but pericardiectomy is not always followed by relief of pain.[72,75]

A new, promising approach for the treatment of symptomatic recurrent pericarditis before using corticosteroids is the chronic administration of colchicine. In a series of 19 consecutive patients with recurrent idiopathic pericarditis occurring at a mean interval of 7 months, chronic colchicine therapy at a dose of 1 mg daily was associated with no recurrence in 14 of 19 patients (74 per cent) during a mean follow-up time of 37 months.[76] Similar observations have been reported in other small series of patients,[77,78] but these results have not yet been collaborated in a prospective, double-blind study.

Pericarditis can also be complicated by the development of disabling or life-threatening hemodynamic complications due to cardiac compression. These include (1) the development of pericardial effusion under pressure, resulting in cardiac tamponade; (2) the development of fibrosis and/or calcification of the pericardium, resulting in chronic constrictive physiology; and (3) a combination of both effusive and constrictive pericardial disease.

PERICARDIAL EFFUSION

Pericardial effusion may develop as a response to injury of the parietal pericardium with all cases of acute pericarditis. It may be clinically silent, but if the accumulation of fluid causes intrapericardial pressure to increase, resulting in cardiac compression, the symptoms of cardiac tamponade develop. The development of increased intrapericardial pressure secondary to pericardial effusion depends on several factors: (1) the absolute volume of the effusion, (2) the rate of fluid accumulation, and (3) the physical characteristics of the pericardium itself. The pericardial space in humans normally contains between 15 and 50 ml of fluid. If additional fluid accumulates slowly, the pericardium stretches; the pericardial sac can accommodate up to 2 liters without elevation of intrapericardial pressure. However, the normal unstretched pericardial sac can accommodate the rapid addition of only 80 to 200 ml of fluid and still remain on the flat portion of the curve relating intrapericardial pressure and volume (Fig. 43–1). If additional fluid is rapidly added to a volume exceeding about 150 to 200 ml, a marked rise of intrapericardial pressure occurs. Intrapericardial pressure may also increase markedly after the accumulation of a smaller amount of fluid if the pericardium is excessively stiff because of fibrosis or tumor infiltration.

PERICARDIAL EFFUSION WITHOUT CARDIAC COMPRESSION

HISTORY. Patients who develop pericardial effusion without elevation of intrapericardial pressure may have no symptoms whatsoever. Occasionally these patients complain of a constant oppressive dull ache or pressure in the chest. Large pericardial effusions may cause symptoms by mechanical compression of adjacent structures, including dysphagia from esophageal compression, cough due to bronchial/tracheal compression, dyspnea from lung compression with subsequent atelectasis, hiccups due to phrenic nerve compression, or hoarseness due to recurrent laryngeal nerve compression. Nausea and a sense of abdominal fullness may be present from pressure on adjacent abdominal viscera.

PHYSICAL EXAMINATION. A small pericardial effusion in the absence of an increase in intrapericardial pressure may result in no specific physical findings, whereas a large effusion may produce several characteristic physical findings. The heard sounds may be muffled owing to the interposition of fluid between the chest wall and the cardiac chambers. Compression of the base of the left lung by pericardial fluid produces Ewart's sign, i.e., a patch of dullness on auscultation beneath the angle of the left scapula. Rales

may be heard over the lung fields secondary to compression of lung parenchyma. Abnormalities of the arterial pulse, systemic blood pressure, and jugular venous pulse do not occur when a large pericardial effusion is present without significant elevation of the intrapericardial pressure.

CHEST ROENTGENOGRAM. Enlargement of the cardiac silhouette usually does not occur until at least 250 ml of fluid have accumulated in the pericardial space. Therefore, a normal or unchanged chest roentgenogram does not exclude the presence of a hemodynamically important pericardial effusion. This examination may suggest the presence of a pericardial effusion if there is a rapid increase in the size of the cardiac silhouette in the presence of clear lung fields. In some cases the heart may assume a globular or water bottle shape, blurring the contours along the left cardiac border and obscuring the hilar vessels. Loculated effusions may have a cyst-like appearance (Fig. 43–4).

The parietal pericardial and epicardial fat layers are normally separated by 1 to 2 mm. The presence of effusion may result in more marked separation of the pericardial fat lines, apparent on high-quality frontal or lateral chest films in about 25 per cent of patients with pericardial effusions.[79] Fluoroscopy may reveal the absence of or weak pulsations and the absence of any changes in the size and shape of the cardiac silhouette during inspiration. These findings

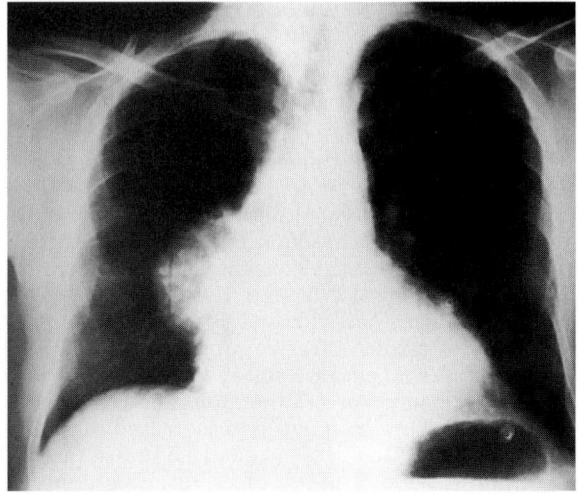

FIGURE 43–4. Posteroanterior chest roentgenogram from a patient with recurrent pericarditis and a loculated pericardial effusion that was subsequently drained surgically. In this patient, the loculated pericardial effusion simulated the roentgenographic appearance of a pericardial cyst.

are especially useful in the cardiac catheterization laboratory when perforation of the heart is suspected. Computed tomography (CT) (see p. 340) has also been used to image pericardial effusions, and magnetic resonance imaging (MRI) (see p. 324) can identify effusions, characterize an effusion as hemorrhagic, differentiate fluid from epicardial fat, and delineate other pathology including pericardial thickening and intrapericardial masses (Fig. 10–41, p. 341).[80]

ELECTROCARDIOGRAM. The electrocardiogram may reveal the nonspecific findings of a reduction in QRS voltage and flattening of the T waves as a fluid accumulates within the pericardial space. Electrical alternans suggests the presence of massive pericardial effusion and cardiac tamponade.

ECHOCARDIOGRAM (see also p. 93). This is the most accurate, rapid, and widely used technique for evaluating pericardial effusion, in following the accumulation or resolution of fluid over time, and in assessing the functional status of the cardiac valves and myocardium. Recognition of pericardial fluid depends on the acoustical differences among the pericardium, cardiac muscle, and pericardial fluid. Accumulation of pericardial fluid results in the appearance of an echo-free space between the posterior left ventricular wall and posterior parietal pericardium and between the anterior wall of the right ventricle and adjacent echoes of the parietal pericardium and chest wall (Figs. 3–103 and 3–104, p. 93). Posterior and anterior epicardial fat can simulate this echocardiographic appearance of pericardial effusion. M-mode echocardiography appears to be sufficiently sensitive to detect as little as 20 ml of pericardial fluid.[81]

The incidence of small pericardial effusions detected by echocardiography in asymptomatic subjects ranges between 8 and 15 per cent.[82,83] In normal pregnant women, a substantial subset (43 per cent) has been found to have asymptomatic pericardial effusions that resolve within the first weeks after delivery.[83]

Although the quantification of pericardial effusions by echocardiography is not precise, several guidelines of assessment are helpful. Very small effusions are likely to be imaged only posteriorly, with separation of the pericardial and epicardial echoes only in systole. Small-to-moderate-sized effusions are likely to be imaged only posteriorly, with the presence of an echo-free space throughout the cardiac cycle. Pericardial effusions of approximately 300 ml can usually be imaged both anteriorly and posteriorly. Moderate to large effusions may be associated with excessive swinging motion of the heart and the false-positive appearance of mitral valve prolapse and anterior septal motion. Usually, the echo-free space representing a pericardial effusion disappears behind the left atrium owing to the absence of fluid in the oblique pericardial sinus. However, in massive effusions, fluid may also collect in the oblique sinus, resulting in an echo-free space behind the left atrium as well as the left ventricle.

Two-dimensional echocardiography is now the gold standard for identifying circumferential pericardial effusions and in identifying a loculated pericardial effusion.[84] Blood in the pericardial space can often be differentiated from an effusion of lower acoustical density, and two-dimensional echocardiography is useful in identifying rapidly the presence of hemopericardium with or without thrombus formation secondary to cardiac invasive procedures.

MANAGEMENT. The clinical significance of any pericardial effusion depends on (1) the presence or absence of hemodynamic embarrassment due to increased intrapericardial pressure and (2) the presence and nature of the underlying systemic disease. The use of echocardiography to establish the diagnosis of pericardial effusion is warranted in suspected cases of acute pericarditis because the presence of effusion is suggestive, although not diagnostic, of pericardial inflammation. Pericardiocentesis (see p. 1505) is not indicated unless there is evidence of cardiac compression

due to cardiac tamponade or analysis of pericardial fluid is necessary to establish a diagnosis such as acute bacterial pericarditis.

Chronic Pericardial Effusion

Chronic pericardial effusions persisting for more than 6 months may occur in any form of pericardial disease. Often they are surprisingly well tolerated, with no symptoms of cardiac compression, and are discovered when a routine chest roentgenogram discloses an unexpectedly large cardiac silhouette. Chronic pericardial effusions are particularly likely to be found in patients with previous idiopathic or viral pericarditis, uremic pericarditis, and pericarditis secondary to myxedema or neoplasm. Chronic pericardial effusions can also occur in association with ascites and pleural effusions in the setting of chronic salt and water retention of many causes, including chronic heart failure, nephrotic syndrome, and hepatic cirrhosis. Massive idiopathic chronic pericardial effusion is reported to be the initial presentation in about 3 per cent of patients with primary pericardial disease, with predominance in women.[85] The management of chronic pericardial effusion depends in part on the cause, and occult hypothyroidism should always be excluded. Stable and apparently idiopathic effusions in asymptomatic patients usually require no specific treatment except for avoidance of anticoagulants.

CARDIAC TAMPONADE

An increase in intrapericardial pressure secondary to fluid accumulation within the pericardial space results in cardiac tamponade, which is characterized by (1) elevation of intracardiac pressures, (2) progressive limitation of ventricular diastolic filling, and (3) reduction of stroke volume and cardiac output.

Pathophysiology

When intrapericardial pressure is measured using a conventional fluid-filled catheter, usually it is quite close to intrapleural pressure and several millimeters of mercury lower than right and left ventricular diastolic pressures. As already noted (see p. 1480), recent studies using special catheters with closed flat balloons indicate that the *constraint* pressure exerted by the normal pericardium is very close to right atrial pressure.[14] However, this controversy regarding the accurate measurement of normal pericardial pressure does not limit the use of fluid-filled catheters in patients with cardiac tamponade, because intrapericardial pressure can be accurately measured by either technique once about 50 ml of free fluid is present in the pericardial space. When the addition of fluid into the pericardial space causes intrapericardial pressure to rise to the level of the right atrial and right ventricular diastolic pressures, the transmural pressure distending these chambers declines to close to zero and cardiac tamponade occurs. The rise of right atrial and intrapericardial pressures is less marked in the presence of hypovolemia, and therefore cardiac tamponade may be masked when hypovolemia is present. Further accumulation of intrapericardial fluid causes both intrapericardial and right ventricular diastolic pressures to rise together to the level of left ventricular diastolic pressure, and all three pressures subsequently rise together in association with a fall in systemic atrial pressure. If left ventricular diastolic pressure is markedly elevated owing to preexisting left ventricular disease, cardiac tamponade occurs when right atrial and right ventricular diastolic and pericardial pressure equalize but at a lower level than the left ventricular diastolic pressure.[86]

CONSEQUENCES OF CARDIAC TAMPONADE. Equalization of intrapericardial and ventricular filling pressures results in markedly diminished transmural distending pressures and diastolic volumes of both ventricles and a fall in stroke volume (Fig. 43–5).[87] During cardiac tamponade, normal regional variations in intrapericardial pressure over different regions of the heart are lost and ventricular coupling is enhanced such that small change in intraventricular volume or pressure in one ventricle markedly increase pressure and diminish filling of the contralateral ventricle.[88,89] The reduction in stroke volume is initially compensated for by reflex increases in adrenergic tone; both tachycardia and increases in ejection fraction initially help to maintain forward cardiac output. The increase in efferent sympathetic nerve activation of the heart is accompanied by sustained excitation of the adrenal gland, brain, and liver and vagal-mediated inhibition of sympathetic nerve activity to the kidney.[90] Cardiac sympathetic nerve activation also mediates the acceleration of left ventricular relaxation during tamponade, which helps to maintain diastolic filling.[91] The importance of the adrenergic support of the heart is reflected in the finding that when beta-adrenergic blockade is carried out in cardiac tamponade, ejection fraction and stroke volume decline, and ventricular relaxation slows.[91,92]

Systemic vascular resistance increases so that, at first, systemic arterial pressure is maintained at the expense of cardiac output. Acute increases in pericardial volume and

pressure also reflexly induce a marked decrease in urinary sodium excretion, associated with the inhibition of release of atrial natriuretic factor and secretion of arginine vasopressin.[93–95]

With severe cardiac tamponade, as cardiac output declines, compensatory mechanisms are no longer sufficient to maintain systemic arterial pressure, and perfusion of vital organs becomes impaired; reduced coronary perfusion causes selective hypoperfusion of the subendocardium.[96] The superimposition of myocardial ischemia during cardiac tamponade could further compromise left ventricular stroke volume. In extreme cardiac tamponade, transmural diastolic ventricular pressures may actually be less than zero, suggesting that ventricular filling occurs by diastolic suction. Sinus bradycardia, mediated by the cardiac depressor branches of the vagus nerve and by the nonvagal mechanism of sinoatrial node ischemia, may also occur during severe cardiac tamponade.[97] Profound bradycardia often occurs during severe hypotension and precedes the development of electrical-mechanical dissociation and death.

Cardiac tamponade also alters the dynamics of systemic venous return and cardiac filling. Normally, one surge of systemic venous return occurs during ventricular ejection coincident with the systolic x descent of the venous pressure pulse, and a second surge occurs during right atrial emptying with the opening of the tricuspid valve in diastole, corresponding to the y descent. In cardiac tamponade, the heart is compressed throughout the cardiac cycle.

During ejection, intracardiac volume decreases, resulting in a transient fall in both intrapericardial and right atrial pressures, manifest as the x descent, which is accompanied by a surge of systemic venous return into the right atrium. However, in early diastole the total volume within the pericardial space remains elevated despite opening of the tricuspid valve; intrapericardial pressure remains elevated and equal to or exceeds early diastolic right atrial pressure so that transmural distending pressure is close to zero or negative. As a result, the usual surge of systemic venous return during early diastole is abolished, right atrial emptying is impeded, and the right atrium is compressed or partially collapsed during diastole. These events are graphically reflected in the right atrial or systemic venous waveform in cardiac tamponade, in that the systolic x descent is prominent while the early diastolic y descent is usually completely absent or attenuated.

REGIONAL TAMPONADE. The individual chambers of the heart resist external compressive force differently, and the magnitude of hemodynamic deterioration during cardiac tamponade crucially depends on the specific region of the heart that is compressed during diastole. Fowler and Gable[98] studied regional cardiac tamponade in dogs and showed that isolated tamponade of the right or left ventricle has little hemodynamic effect and that a substantial fall in cardiac output and aortic pressure occurs only when the atria (and intrapericardial veins) are also compressed. A subsequent study of regional tamponade in dogs has shown that right atrial and right ventricular compression causes greater depression of cardiac output and aortic pressure than does left heart compression.[99]

In patients with cardiac tamponade, compression of the right heart chambers is likely to be more important than left atrial compression because pericardial fluid is often not present behind the left atrium during cardiac tamponade, and the presence of left atrial and left ventricular diastolic collapse is variable. For the normal thin-walled right atrium and right ventricle, the critical buckling pressure consists of a negative transmural pressure of only 0.05 to 0.1 mm Hg.[13] This critical difference between pericardial and right atrial or right ventricular diastolic pressure can occur when pericardial pressure is lower than that of the thick-walled left ventricle, whereas right ventricular collapse may be absent in the presence of severe right ventricular hypertrophy. Localized left ventricular tamponade can occur in the setting of cardiac tamponade after cardiac surgery (see p. 1727). Schwartz et al. simulated this situation in dogs with regional left heart tamponade.[100] Left ventricular diastolic collapse occurred when left pericardial pressure exceeded left ventricular diastolic pressure by about 3 mm Hg in association with a fall in cardiac output, and this occurred before the development of arterial hypotension.

RIGHT ATRIAL AND VENTRICULAR COLLAPSE. During the development of tamponade, collapse of the right atrium and right ventricle occurs only in early diastole in association with delayed diastolic filling of the right ventricle and a modest fall in cardiac output without hypotension or overt hemodynamic deterioration.[101] Pandiastolic right atrial and ventricular buckling occurs when pericardial pressure equals or exceeds right atrial and ventricular pressures throughout diastole so that the ventricles may fill only during atrial systole. This stage is accompanied by a severe reduction in ventricular volumes, a failure of compensatory mechanisms, and hypotension. In this setting, pulsus alternans may occur because of beat-to-beat variation in right ventricular output and left ventricular filling.

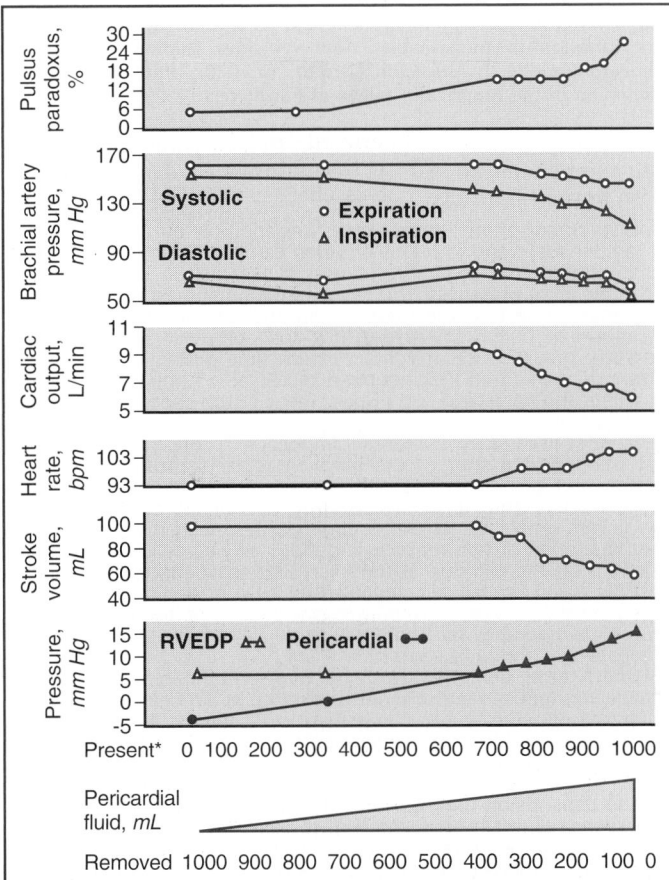

FIGURE 43–5. Hemodynamic changes during serial fluid withdrawals in a 22-year-old man with tamponade due to uremic pericarditis. Pulsus paradoxus is expressed as a percentage fall in systolic arterial pressure with inspiration. Note that significant pulsus paradoxus (> 9 per cent inspiratory fall in systolic blood pressure) and changes in cardiac output, heart rate, and stroke volume occur at the point of equilibrium of right ventricular diastolic pressure (RVEDP) and pericardial pressure. Asterisk indicates the predicted values, assuming complete withdrawal. (From Fowler, N.: Pericardial disease. In Abelmann, W. H. [ed.]: Cardiomyopathies, Myocarditis, and Pericardial Disease, in Braunwald, E. (series ed.): Atlas of Heart Diseases. Philadelphia, Current Medicine, 1995. Adapted from: Reddy, P. S.: Hemodynamics of cardiac tamponade in man. In Reddy, P. S. et al. [eds.]: Pericardial Disease. New York, Raven Press, 1982, pp. 161–177.)

During hypovolemia with low right heart pressures, right ventricular collapse occurs at low intrapericardial pressures while volume expansion delays the development of right ventricular diastolic collapse and hemodynamic deterioration until a higher intrapericardial pressure is achieved.[101,102] Singh et al.[103] have obtained simultaneous hemodynamics and two-dimensional echocardiographic measurements in patients undergoing pericardiocentesis and have shown that hemodynamic improvement first occurs at the point of disappearance of right ventricular diastolic collapse, which is followed by the subsequent disappearance of right atrial collapse and further improvement in cardiac output during continued pericardiocentesis.

MECHANISM OF PULSUS PARADOXUS. Inspiration and the transmission of negative intrathoracic pressure to the pericardial space further alter the dynamics of right and left ventricular filling and are responsible for pulsus paradoxus, the inspiratory fall of aortic systolic pressure greater than 10 mm Hg. The finding of weakening of the arterial pulse during inspiration was described by Kussmaul in 1873 as the apparent *paradox* of the disappearance of the pulse during inspiration despite persistence of the heartbeat. It should be emphasized that pulsus paradoxus is in fact an exaggeration of the normal inspiratory decline of left ventricular stroke volume by about 7 per cent and of systemic arterial pressure by 3 per cent.[104] Inspiration is normally accompanied by an increase in diastolic dimensions of the right ventricle, a small decrease in left ventricular dimension, and increased velocity of flow from the

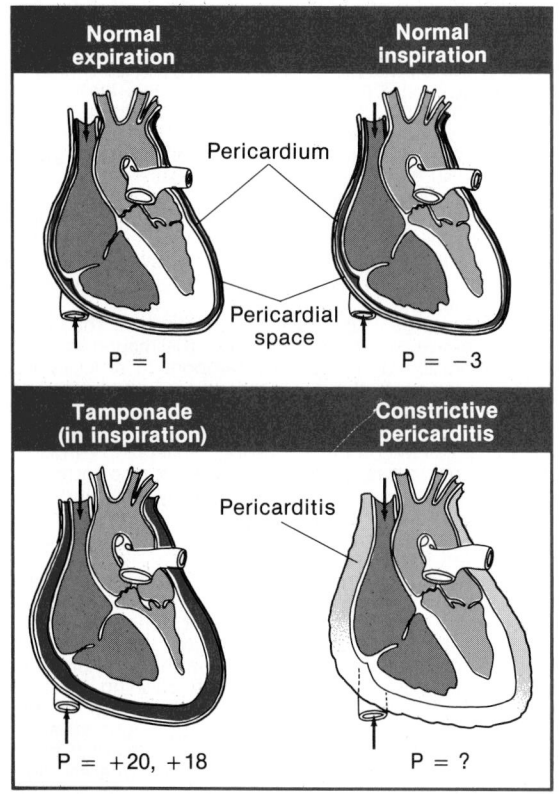

FIGURE 43–6. The hemodynamic effects of respiration. In the normal heart *(upper panel)*, inspiration results in a fall in intrathoracic and intrapericardial pressure from +1 to −3 mm Hg, which causes an increase in venous return (heavy black arrows) and a slight increase in right ventricular size at the expense of a slight decrease in left ventricular size due to displacement of the interventricular septum from right to left. During cardiac tamponade *(lower left panel)*, inspiration causes a fall in the elevated intrapericardial pressure from +20 to +18 mm Hg. Although both the right and left heart volumes are diminished owing to compression by the pericardial effusion, the inspiratory fall in intrapericardial pressure results in an increase in venous return (heavy black arrows), an increase in right heart volume due to septal bulging, and a further decrease in left heart volume. In constrictive pericarditis *(lower right panel)*, the inspiratory fall in intrathoracic pressure is not transmitted to the heart because the pericardial space is obliterated. For this reason, there is minimal or no increase in venous return (light black arrows) during inspiration. (From Shabetai, R.: The Pericardium. New York, Grune and Stratton, 1981, p. 244.)

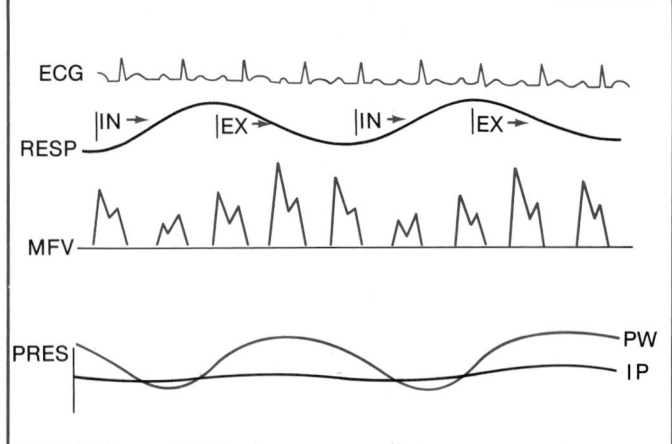

FIGURE 43–7. Relation between mitral flow velocity (MFV) and pericardial and pulmonary wedge pressures. The first beat after the onset of inspiration is associated with a reduced pressure gradient between the pulmonary venous circulation and intrapericardial (and left ventricular diastolic) pressures, which results in an abrupt reduction in mitral flow velocity, as shown, and an increase in tricuspid flow velocity. Opposite changes occur with the onset of expiration. ECG = electrocardiogram, RESP = respiratory phase determined by a nasal thermistor, IN = inspiration, EX = expiration, PRES = pressure, PW = pulmonary capillary wedge, IP = intrapericardial. (From Appleton, C. P., et al.: Cardiac tamponade and pericardial effusion: Respiratory variation in transvalvular flow velocities studied by Doppler echocardiography. J. Am. Coll. Cardiol. *11*:1020, 1988; reprinted by permission of the American College of Cardiology.)

venae cavae into the right atrium. Pulsus paradoxus in cardiac tamponade appears to result from an exaggeration of these normal findings.

Measurement of intracardiac pressures and flow during experimental tamponade[105] and in humans during cardiac tamponade[104,106] have demonstrated that inspiration causes a decrease in intrapericardial and right atrial pressures. This results in augmentation of flow from the venae cavae into the right atrium and right ventricle and augmentation of pulmonary artery flow and pulmonary artery systolic pressure. The increase in venous return flow during inspiration results in a marked and exaggerated increase in right ventricular dimensions and flattening and displacement of the septum toward the left ventricle.

Recent studies of experimental tamponade in conscious dogs show that this leftward shift of the intraventricular septum unloads the septum and eliminates the septal contribution to left ventricular stroke work.[107] Thus, inspiration during tamponade causes a reduction in left ventricular stroke volume via the mechanisms of a transient reduction of left ventricular preload as well as impaired septal function. On the left side of the heart, left atrial and left ventricular diastolic pressures fall, accompanied by a fall in aortic flow and systolic arterial pressure. Thus, *pulsus paradoxus in cardiac tamponade is critically dependent on the inspiratory augmentation of systemic venous return and right ventricular filling.*

Shabetai et al. demonstrated that when experimental cardiac tamponade was induced in dogs, pulsus paradoxus did not develop when either the right heart was bypassed or right ventricular volume was strictly controlled.[105] These experiments also demonstrated that traction on the heart by the diaphragm was not an essential mechanism. These observations indicate that pulsus paradoxus in cardiac tamponade depends on the inspiratory expansion of right-heart filling at the expense of left-heart filling (Fig. 43–6).

The importance of respiratory preload variation is supported by recent observations in patients with cardiac tamponade that showed that left ventricular transmural diastolic pressure falls to or below zero during inspiration.[13] An additional factor that may contribute to the inspiratory fall of left ventricular stroke volume and systolic arterial pressure is a transient reduction in the gradient between the pulmonary venous circulation and the left heart during inspiration causing inspiratory pooling of blood in the lungs (Fig. 43–7).[108] Also the underfilled left ventricle may be operating on the steep ascending limb of the Starling curve so that any inspiratory reduction of left ventricular filling results in marked depression of left ventricular stroke volume and systolic pressure. Pulsus paradoxus is occasionally observed in constrictive pericarditis and restrictive heart disease, and the latter mechanisms may account for its presence in these disorders.

THE NONSPECIFICITY OF PULSUS PARADOXUS. Pulsus paradoxus has also been observed in severe lung disease and massive pulmonary embolism.[109] Under these circumstances, pulsus paradoxus is probably related to the transmission of excessively negative intrathoracic pressure during inspiration to the aorta, inspiratory pooling of right ventricular stroke volume in the lungs, and exaggerated right-heart filling with an associated decrease in left-heart filling during inspiration.

Pulsus paradoxus may be absent in cardiac tamponade when left ventricular hypertrophy or heart failure causes a marked elevation of left ventricular diastolic pressure so that the two ventricles are unequally compressed. This may occur in atrial septal defect when the increase in systemic venous return during inspiration is shared between the two sides of the heart, and in aortic regurgitation when there is a major component of left ventricular filling that is independent of respiratory variation.[86,110] Pulsus paradoxus may also be absent in the presence of pulmonary hypertension and right ventricular hypertrophy that impedes the inspiratory increase in right ventricular filling; in this unusual clinical situation, the depression of left ventricular diastolic filling and cardiac outcome may depend on regional compression of the left ventricle.[111]

Etiology

Cardiac tamponade may occur with almost any cause of pericarditis and may exist in either an acute or a chronic form. The distributions of the causes of acute cardiac tamponade in a city hospital between 1963 and 1980 and at our institution between 1984 and 1988 are noted in Table 43–4. In these series the most frequent causes of cardiac tamponade were neoplasm, idiopathic or viral pericarditis, and uremia, followed by pericarditis associated with myocardial infarction, invasive cardiac diagnostic procedures, purulent bacterial infection, and tuberculosis.

Clinical Manifestations

The physical findings in cardiac tamponade are shown in Table 43–5. The triad of (1) a decline in systemic arterial pressure; (2) elevation of systemic venous pressure; and (3) a small, quiet heart was described by the thoracic surgeon Claude S. Beck in 1935.[113] These three features are typical of cardiac tamponade from sudden intraperitoneal hemorrhage due to penetrating heart wounds from trauma or invasive diagnostic cardiac procedures, aortic dissection, and intrapericardial rupture of an aortic or cardiac aneurysm. This syndrome develops when the pericardium is not enlarged or stretched, so that the addition of less than 200 ml of fluid or blood causes intrapericardial pressure to rise abruptly to above 20 to 30 mm Hg. In cases that are not immediately fatal, both cardiac output and arterial pressure fall, accompanied by tachycardia and tachypnea. The pa-

TABLE 43–4   COMMON CAUSES OF CARDIAC TAMPONADE

DISORDER	1980 (%)	1988 (%)
Malignant disease	32	58
Idiopathic pericarditis	14	14
Uremia	9	14
Acute cardiac infarction (receiving heparin)	9	
Diagnostic procedures with cardiac perforation	7.5	
Bacterial	7.5	5
Tuberculosis	5	1
Radiation	4	
Myxedema	4	
Dissecting aortic aneurysm	4	
Postpericardiotomy syndrome	2	
Systemic lupus erythematosus	2	2
Cardiomyopathy (receiving anticoagulants)	2	6

Modified from Guberman, B. A., et al.: Cardiac tamponade in medical patients. Circulation 64:633, 1981; copyright American Heart Association; and from Levine, M. J., et al.: Implications of echocardiographically-assisted diagnosis of pericardial tamponade in contemporary medical patients. J. Am. Coll. Cardiol. 17:59, 1991.

TABLE 43–5   PHYSICAL FINDINGS IN CARDIAC TAMPONADE   **1489**

Ch 43

TABLE 43–5   PHYSICAL FINDINGS IN CARDIAC TAMPONADE

FINDING	n(%)
Elevated systemic venous pressure	56(100)
Paradoxical pulse	55(98)
Respiratory rate > 20/min	45(80)
Heart rate ≥ 100/min	43(77)
Systolic blood pressure ≥ 100 mm Hg	36(64)
Diminished heart sounds	19(34)
Pericardial friction rub	16(29)
Rapidly declining blood pressure	14(25)

Modified from Guberman, B. A., et al.: Cardiac tamponade in medical patients. Circulation 64:633, 1981; copyright American Heart Association.

tient may be stuporous or agitated and restless, and the additional important finding of pulsus paradoxus may be difficult to appreciate when profound hypotension is present. Jugular venous pressure is usually markedly elevated. Precordial heart activity is usually not palpable, and heart sounds are distant or inaudible. Cold, clammy extremities and anuria may be present.

Patients in whom cardiac tamponade develops slowly differ from those with cardiac tamponade due to cardiac penetration or rupture. In the setting of more slowly developing cardiac tamponade, patients usually appear acutely ill but not in extremis, and the major complaint is usually dyspnea.[112] Studies of acute cardiac tamponade in dogs have shown that the elevation of intrapericardial pressure results in the accumulation of interstitial fluid without the development of alveolar edema or hypoxemia.[114] Thus the sensation of dyspnea experienced by many patients with cardiac tamponade may be due to lung stiffening from increased interstitial fluid that increases the work of breathing. Chest pain may also be present. In patients with chronic development of tamponade, additional systemic symptoms may include weight loss, anorexia, and profound weakness.

PHYSICAL EXAMINATION. Jugular venous distention was the most common physical finding in a series of 56 medical patients whose cardiac tamponade was diagnosed at the bedside.[112] In addition to absolute elevation of the systemic venous pressure, a characteristic waveform consisting of a prominent systolic x descent and absence of diastolic y descent can often be appreciated at the bedside. Other common physical findings include tachypnea (80 per cent), tachycardia (77 per cent), pulsus paradoxus (77 per cent), pulsus paradoxus with total inspiratory disappearance of the brachial pulse and Korotkoff sounds (23 per cent), pericardial friction rub (29 per cent), hypatomegaly (55 per cent), and diminished heart sounds (34 per cent). It is noteworthy that systolic arterial hypotension, consisting of a systolic pressure less than 100 mm hg, was present in a minority (36 per cent), and the majority of patients were alert, with warm extremities and preservation of urine output.[112] Elevated systemic arterial pressure may occur in patients with cardiac tamponade who have preexisting hypertension.[115]

Pulsus Paradoxus (see p. 23). The finding of pulsus paradoxus is crucial in making the diagnosis of cardiac tamponade because most patients with slowly developing cardiac tamponade do not have the classical physical findings of a small, quiet heart and severe hypotension. Pulsus paradoxus can be detected on physical examination as an inspiratory decrease in the amplitude of the palpated pulse in the femoral or carotid arteries. Total paradox, i.e., complete disappearance of the palpated pulse during inspiration, occurs during very severe cardiac tamponade or tamponade combined with hypovolemia. The magnitude of the paradoxical pulse can be accurately quantified by means of an intraarterial catheter but may be estimated by cuff sphygmomanometry. The cuff should be inflated 20 mm Hg above systolic pressure and slowly deflated until the Korotkoff sounds are heard only during expiration. The cuff should then be deflated to the point at which Korotkoff sounds are heard equally well in inspiration and expiration. The difference between these pressures is the estimated magnitude of pulsus paradoxus.

Other disorders with systemic venous distention, pulsus paradoxus, and clear lungs that can be confused with cardiac tamponade include obstructive pulmonary disease, constrictive pericarditis, restrictive cardiomyopathy, and massive pulmonary embolism. Pulsus paradoxus is occasionally noted during severe hypovolemia due to hemorrhagic shock, but jugular venous distention is usually absent. Cardiac tamponade may be confused with shock due to right ventricular infarction with jugular venous distention and clear lungs.[45] However, the hemodynamics of right ventricular infarction are more like those of pericardial constriction than of tamponade (see p. 1496).

LOW-PRESSURE TAMPONADE. The clinical findings may be further modified in patients with so-called *low-pressure cardiac tamponade* in whom jugular venous distention is absent and the right atrial pressure is low. This syndrome, which occurs in the setting of hypovolemia, represents an early stage in the development of cardiac tamponade in which accumulation of a pericardial effusion causes intrapericardial pressure to rise and equilibrate with low right heart diastolic filling pressures.[116] Pericardiocentesis reduces intrapericardial pressure and causes the separation of right atrial and intrapericardial pressures. Low-pressure cardiac tamponade tends to occur in patients with tuberculosis and neoplastic pericarditis complicated by severe dehydration.

TENSION PNEUMOPERICARDIUM. This condition causes hemodynamic changes similar to those of acute hemorrhagic cardiac tamponade. It is being increasingly recognized as a cause of cardiac tamponade with high mortality in infants during mechanical ventilation and in adults as a result of penetrating chest trauma, gastric and esophageal rupture, carcinomatous bronchopericardial fistula, gas production from contiguous infection, and diagnostic procedures such as sternal bone marrow aspiration.[117] Characteristic clinical findings include muffled heart sounds, bradycardia, and shifting tympany over the precordium. Unique auscultatory findings can be detected, including a metallic cracking sound, and the bruit de moulin, which was described in

the first report of pneumopericardium in 1844 by Bricheteau as "the noise made by floats of a mill wheel as they strike the water,"[118] and which indicates the presence of both air and fluid in the pericardial space.

Laboratory Studies

CHEST ROENTGENOGRAM. There are no roentgenographic features diagnostic of cardiac tamponade. The heart may appear completely normal in size in cardiac tamponade that develops from acute hemopericardium due to cardiac rupture or laceration. On the other hand, if an effusion that accumulates more slowly to more than approximately 250 ml is responsible, the cardiac silhouette may be enlarged with a water bottle configuration (Fig. 7–47, p. 234). This finding suggests the presence of a large pericardial effusion but supplies no information about its hemodynamic significance. In patients with cardiac tamponade due to tension pneumopericardium, the chest roentgenogram usually shows that the heart is surrounded by air delineated by a strip of soft tissue extending up the aorta consisting of the pericardium.

ELECTROCARDIOGRAM. The electrocardiographic abnormalities seen in acute cardiac tamponade include those of acute pericarditis and pericardial effusion per se. The development of electrical alternans is a more specific indicator of pericardial tamponade and reflects pendular swinging of the heart within the pericardial space (Fig. 43–8).[119] Electrical alternans may also be related to a beat-to-beat alteration of right and left ventricular filling.

Electrical alternans may also occur in constrictive pericarditis, in tension pneumothorax, after myocardial infarction, and with severe cardiac muscle dysfunction. However, the appearance of electrical alternans in a patient with a known pericardial effusion is highly suggestive of cardiac tamponade—a finding that has been confirmed in experimental cardiac tamponade.[120] Electrical alternans of the QRS complex may occur in a 2:1 or 3:1 pattern. Alternans is usually limited to the QRS complex, but alternans of the P wave, QRS complex, and T wave may rarely occur in extreme cardiac tamponade. Both the abnormal heart motion within the pericardial sac and electrical alternans disappear when pericardial fluid is aspirated.

ECHOCARDIOGRAM (see also p. 93). In patients with jugular venous distention and the possibility of cardiac tamponade, echocardiography is extremely useful and should be performed prior to consideration of pericardiocentesis (Table 43–6). In a rare patient who is in extremis from the

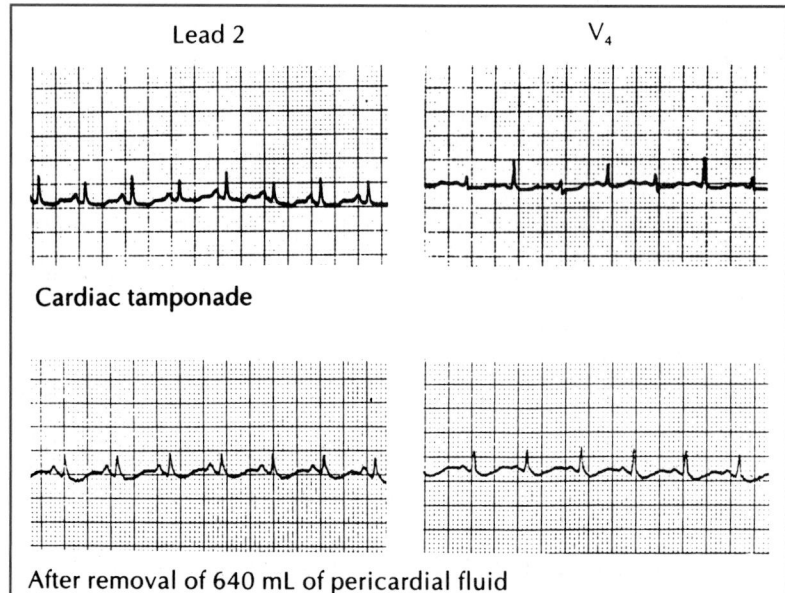

FIGURE 43–8. Electrical alternans of the QRS complex in a patient with cardiac tamponade. Electrical alternans of the QRS complex may also occur with pericarditis without tamponade, with supraventricular or ventricular tachycardia, and with coronary artery disease. Total alternans, involving P, QRS, and T complexes, is almost diagnostic of cardiac tamponade. (From Fowler, N.: Pericardial disease. *In* Abelmann, W. H. [ed.]: Cardiomyopathies, Myocarditis, and Pericardial Disease, in Braunwald, E. (series ed.): Atlas of Heart Diseases. Philadelphia, Current Medicine, 1995.)

TABLE 43–6 ECHOCARDIOGRAPHIC FINDINGS IN CARDIAC TAMPONADE

Right atrial diastolic collapse

Right ventricular early diastolic collapse

Left atrial collapse

Abnormal inspiratory increase in tricuspid valve flow and >15% inspiratory decrease of mitral valve flow

Abnormal inspiratory increase of right ventricular dimension with abnormal inspiratory decrease of left ventricular dimension

Inspiratory decrease of mitral valve DE excursion and EF slope

Inferior vena caval plethora (failure to decrease proximal diameter by ≥50% on sniff or deep inspiration)

Left ventricular pseudohypertrophy

Swinging heart

extremely rapid development of cardiac tamponade, the physician may have to rely on the history and physical findings to make a judgment about the need for pericardiocentesis. If echocardiography is readily available and the patient with suspected cardiac tamponade is not moribund, obtaining an echocardiogram increases the likelihood of diagnosing cardiac tamponade correctly and prevents inappropriate and potentially lethal attempts at pericardiocentesis or pericardiotomy. First, the echocardiogram helps to document the presence and magnitude of pericardial effusion (Fig. 3–104, p. 93). The absence of echocardiographic evidence of pericardial effusion virtually excludes the diagnosis of cardiac tamponade, *with the exception of the postoperative cardiac surgery patient in whom loculated fluid or thrombus may cause cardiac compression.* Second, the echocardiogram can rapidly differentiate cardiac tamponade from other causes of systemic venous hypertension and arterial hypotension, including constrictive pericarditis, cardiac muscle dysfunction, and right ventricular infarction. The appearance of dense echoes in the pericardial space or extrinsic to the pericardium suggests the presence of compression by material other than free fluid. Echocardiograms can often detect both massive extracardiac hematoma and extrinsic compression of the heart by tumor, which can cause cardiac compression with the physiology of cardiac constriction or cardiac tamponade.

Two-dimensional and Doppler echocardiography can provide additional clues that pericardial effusion is associated with cardiac tamponade. The presence of pulsus paradoxus is associated with sudden leftward motion of the septum during inspiration and an exaggerated increase in right ventricular size.[108,121] This characteristic respiratory variation in ventricular preload can also be detected by the Doppler ultrasound findings of exaggerated tricuspid and pulmonic flow velocities and reduction of peak mitral flow velocity with the onset of inspiration and the opposite changes after the onset of expiration (Fig. 43–7).[122,123] When the inspiratory reduction in left ventricular filling is extreme, the aortic valve may close prematurely or fail to open[124] and mitral valve opening may be delayed until atrial systole. Recent combined hemodynamic and echocardiographic-Doppler studies in patients with tamponade before and during pericardiocentesis show that the presence and magnitude of respiratory variation in mitral flow velocity are *not* predictive of the magnitude of hemodynamic compromise.[125] Cardiac tamponade is also associated with "pseudohypertrophy" (an increase in left ventricular diastolic wall thickness), which correlates inversely with the decrease in cavity volume, but the independent prognostic value of this sign is not known.[126] Diastolic right atrial and right ventricular compression or collapse occur early during the development of cardiac tamponade[101,102,103] (Fig. 43–9). Left atrial and left ventricular diastolic collapse can occur when regional left heart compression is present.[100,127]

Right ventricular diastolic collapse appears to be more predictive of cardiac tamponade than pulsus paradoxus, particularly during hypovolemia, and these echocardiographic signs may be reversed by volume expansion.[128,129] Right ventricular diastolic collapse may be absent in the presence of right ventricular hypertrophy and can occur when a large pleural effusion causes elevation of intrapericardial pressure by external compression.[130] Thus, the echocardiographic findings of pericardial effusion, an inspiratory increase in right ventricular dimensions, and right atrial and ventricular diastolic collapse strongly suggest the diagnosis of cardiac tamponade, but these changes are not 100 per cent sensitive or specific. Experimental studies confirm that a single echocardiogram cannot always predict the presence or severity of cardiac tamponade.[131]

Furthermore, hemodynamic observations at our institution in a consecutive series of 50 patients with suspected cardiac tamponade and echocardiographic evidence of right atrial and ventricular diastolic collapse showed that these echocardiographic findings were uniformly associated with elevation of pericardial pressure and the near equilibration of right atrial and right ventricular pressures.[132] However,

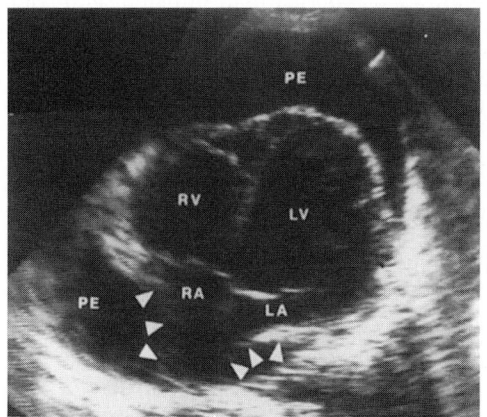

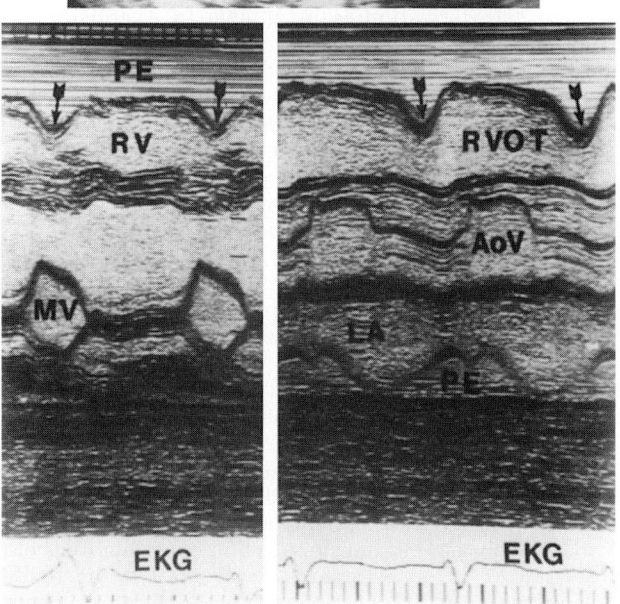

FIGURE 43–9. Two-dimensional *(upper panel)* and M-mode *(lower panels)* echocardiograms from a patient with a malignant pericardial effusion and cardiac tamponade. The two-dimensional image shows a large pericardial effusion (PE) adjacent to the borders of the right ventricle (RV), right atrium (RA), and left ventricle (LV). The effusion is sufficiently large that fluid is also present behind the left atrium (LA). Diastolic compression (white arrowheads) of both the right and left atria is present. The M-mode images also show striking diastolic compression (dark arrows) of the right ventricle during diastole when the mitral valve (MV) is open and compression of the right ventricular outflow tract (RVOT) in early to mid diastole after aortic valve (AoV) closure.

right heart diastolic collapse was associated with a wide spectrum of hemodynamic derangement, including a subset of patients with minimal elevation of right atrial pressure and the preservation of a normal cardiac output and systemic arterial pressure. Eisenberg et al. have examined the prognostic value of echocardiography in 187 hospitalized patients with pericardial effusion, of whom 16 (9 per cent) subsequently required pericardiocentesis or surgical drainage.[133] This study concluded that the size of the pericardial effusion was the most powerful predictor of outcome, whereas right heart diastolic collapse, distention of the superior vena cava, and altered response to respiration added little prognostic information. Thus, the recognition of patients with cardiac tamponade by echocardiography requires complementary clinical and hemodynamic assessment to distinguish patients with milder degrees of cardiac compression from those with hemodynamic decompensation who require urgent drainage of pericardial fluid.

We agree with Fowler's recent suggestion that in most patients, cardiac tamponade requiring pericardial drainage should be diagnosed by a clinical examination showing elevated systemic venous pressure, tachycardia, dyspnea, and pulsus paradoxus.[87] Many patients with echocardiographic findings of pericardial effusion and right heart compression who do not have these clinical findings may be observed closely, and pericardial drainage may not be necessary. In contrast, in patients with suspected cardiac perforation or rupture who have echocardiographic signs of pericardial effusion and right heart compression, urgent pericardial drainage by pericardiocentesis or surgery is almost always needed. Cardiac tamponade is a *clinical*, not an echocardiographic or a radionuclide, diagnosis that is established definitively by documentation of the elevation and equilibration of intrapericardial and right atrial pressures and the reversal of these findings by evacuation of pericardial fluid.

Cardiac Catheterization

Cardiac catheterization is invaluable in establishing the hemodynamic importance of pericardial effusion. Except in extreme emergencies, such as when the patient is moribund, we prefer to catheterize the right heart and pericardial space in conjunction with pericardiocentesis. Cardiac catheterization (1) provides absolute confirmation of the diagnosis of cardiac tamponade; (2) quantitates the hemodynamic compromise; (3) guides pericardiocentesis by documenting that pericardial aspiration is associated with hemodynamic improvement; and (4) permits the detection of coexisting hemodynamic problems, including left ventricular failure, effusive-constrictive pericarditis (see p. 1505), and unsuspected pulmonary hypertension in patients with malignant effusions.

Cardiac catheterization typically demonstrates elevation of right atrial pressure with a characteristic preserved systolic *x* descent and absence of or a diminutive diastolic *y* descent. When intrapericardial and right atrial pressures are recorded simultaneously, both are elevated and virtually identical (Fig. 43–10); both pressures fall during inspiration, and intrapericardial pressure may fall slightly below right atrial pressure during systolic ejection at the time of the *x* descent. If intrapericardial pressure is not elevated, and if right atrial and intrapericardial pressures are not virtually identical, the diagnosis of cardiac tamponade must be reconsidered.

Right ventricular mid-diastolic pressure is elevated and equal to right atrial and intrapericardial pressures and lacks the dip-and-plateau configuration characteristic of constrictive pericarditis. Because right ventricular and pulmonary artery systolic pressures are equal to the sum of the pressure developed by the right ventricle plus the intrapericardial pressure, right ventricular and pulmonary artery systolic pressures are usually moderately elevated, in the

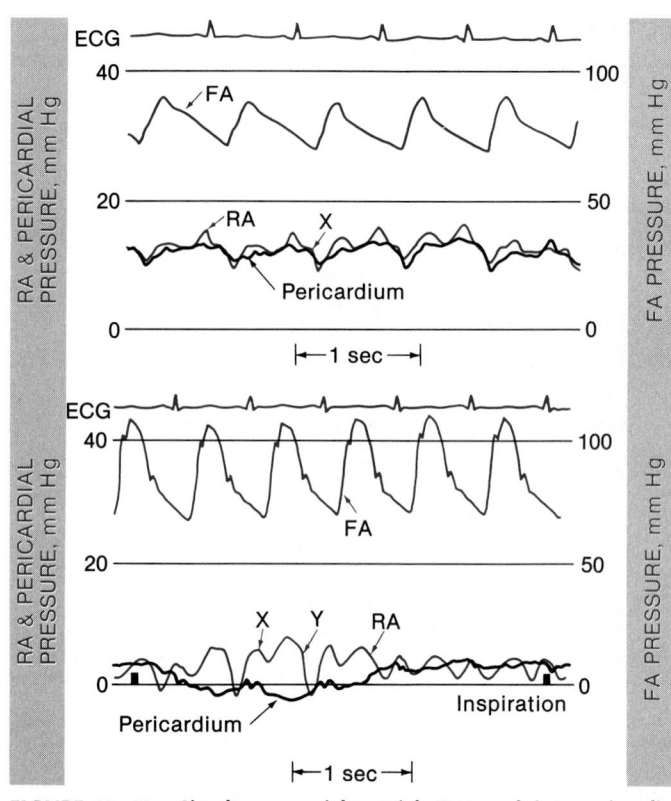

FIGURE 43–10. Simultaneous right atrial (RA) and intrapericardial pressures (scale 0 to 40 mm Hg) and femoral artery pressure (scale 0 to 100 mm Hg) from a patient with decompensated cardiac tamponade. Before pericardiocentesis *(upper panel)*, systemic hypotension is present, and there is elevation and equalization of right atrial and intrapericardial pressures. Note that a systolic *x* descent is present, but the diastolic *y* descent is absent, suggesting that right atrial emptying is impeded by compression of the right ventricle in early diastole. After aspiration of about 300 ml of pericardial fluid *(lower panel)*, cardiac tamponade is relieved, as shown by the restoration of intrapericardial pressure to zero, the restoration of right atrial pressure to a normal level, and the improvement in systemic arterial pressure. The right atrial tracing shows the appearance of a diastolic *y* descent, which indicates the relief of cardiac compression and restoration of normal right atrial emptying in early diastole. Although this degree of fluid aspiration relieved tamponade physiology, an additional 1500 ml of fluid was subsequently aspirated from the pericardial space. (Modified from Lorell, B. H., and Grossman, W.: Profiles in constrictive pericarditis, restrictive cardiomyopathy, and cardiac tamponade. *In* Grossman, W., and Baim, D. S. [eds.]: Cardiac Catheterization, Angiography and Intervention. Philadelphia, Lea and Febiger, 1991, p. 644.)

range of 35 to 50 mm Hg. In the case of severe cardiac compression, right ventricular systolic pressure may be reduced and only slightly higher than right ventricular diastolic pressure.

Usually the pulmonary capillary wedge pressure and left ventricular diastolic pressure are elevated and equal to intrapericardial pressure when recorded simultaneously. During expiration, the pulmonary capillary wedge pressure is usually slightly higher than intrapericardial pressure, resulting in a pressure gradient that promotes left-heart filling. During inspiration, the pulmonary capillary wedge pressure may transiently decrease more than intrapericardial pressure such that the pressure gradient between the pulmonary venous circulation and the left heart is reduced or absent. In patients with severe underlying left ventricular dysfunction or hypertrophy and elevation of the left ventricular diastolic pressure, cardiac tamponade can be present when intrapericardial and right atrial pressures are equal but lower than left ventricular diastolic pressure. Depending on the severity of cardiac compression, left ventricular systolic and aortic pressures may be normal or reduced.

Pulsus paradoxus can be easily documented by intraarterial catheterization and pressure measurement. Simultaneous recording of systemic arterial and right ventricular pressures shows that the inspiratory pressure variation is out of phase. Stroke volume is usually markedly depressed. Cardiac output may be normal, owing to the compensatory effect of tachycardia, or it may be markedly reduced when cardiac tamponade is severe; systemic vascular resistance is usually elevated.

Angiographic studies add no additional information if echocardiographic findings suggestive of cardiographic tamponade were obtained prior to cardiac catheterization. In an otherwise normal heart, right and left ventricular end-diastolic volumes are usually reduced with normal or increased ejection fractions.

Aspiration of pericardial fluid results initially in the lowering of the identical intrapericardial, right atrial, right ventricular, and left ventricular diastolic pressures, followed by a fall of intrapericardial pressure below right atrial pressure and reappearance of the y descent in the right atrial waveform (Fig. 43–10). Further aspiration causes intrapericardial pressure to fall to a mean level of zero and to fluctuate with changes in intrathoracic pressure. Because the pressure-volume curve of the pericardium is steep, the initial aspiration of 50 to 100 ml of pericardial fluid usually leads to striking reduction in intrapericardial pressure, marked improvement in systemic arterial pressure and cardiac output, and abolition of pulsus paradoxus. The reduction of intrapericardial pressure is often followed by diuresis, related both to the augmentation of cardiac output and the release of atrial natriuretic factor.[93-95]

If intrapericardial pressure falls to zero or becomes negative and right atrial pressure remains elevated, *effusive-constrictive pericarditis* (see p. 1505) should be strongly considered, especially in patients with underlying neoplasm or prior radiation. Other causes of continued elevation of right atrial pressure after successful pericardiocentesis include the coexistence of cardiac tamponade and preexisting left ventricular dysfunction, causing, in turn, pulmonary hypertension and right atrial hypertension, tricuspid valve disease, and restrictive cardiomyopathy. In patients with suspected malignant disease, pulmonary hypertension due to pulmonary microvascular tumor is an important cause of persistent elevation of right atrial pressure and the failure to relieve dyspnea after complete drainage of the pericardial space.[132]

The distinction between cardiac tamponade and the superior vena cava syndrome must always be made in patients with neoplastic disease in whom these lesions may occur singly or together. In patients with obstruction of the superior vena cava, cardiac tamponade may be suspected from the presence of elevated jugular venous pressure and pulsus paradoxus due to respiratory distress. In this condition (without accompanying cardiac tamponade), pressure in the superior vena cava is markedly elevated, with dampened pulsations, and exceeds right atrial and inferior vena cava pressures. Two-dimensional and Doppler echocardiography may not be successful in distinguishing between these conditions because cardiac tamponade as well as other causes of elevated central venous pressure may modify the appearance and respiratory fluctuation of flow in the venae cavae.[123,133] If elevation of jugular venous pressure persists after relief of cardiac tamponade in patients with neoplastic disease, obstruction of the superior vena cava, as reflected in a pressure gradient between the superior vena cava and right atrium, should be sought. Superior vena caval obstruction may be amenable to radiation therapy.

Pericardiocentesis

Hemodynamic support during preparation of the patient for pericardiocentesis or pericardiotomy should include ad-

ministration of intravenous fluid, blood, plasma, or saline. The rationale for volume expansion is that it has been shown to delay the appearance of right ventricular diastolic collapse and hemodynamic deterioration.[102] In experimental cardiac tamponade, administration of norepinephrine and dobutamine has produced an increase in cardiac output, whereas dobutamine appears to delay the onset of tissue hypoxia by promoting a greater augmentation of cardiac output and oxygen delivery at any level of intrapericardial pressure.[134] The vasodilators hydralazine and nitroprusside have also been employed in experimental cardiac tamponade to promote an increase in cardiac output secondary to the reduction of elevated systemic resistance.[135] The administration of vasodilators in conjunction with volume expansion must be done with extreme caution in patients with cardiac tamponade, because it may be hazardous in patients with borderline or frank hypotension. Beta-adrenergic blockade should be avoided because increased adrenergic activity helps to maintain cardiac output. Positive-pressure ventilation should be avoided whenever possible because it has been shown to depress cardiac output further in patients with cardiac tamponade.[136]

Pericardial fluid under pressure causing tamponade can be evacuated by (1) percutaneous pericardiocentesis using a needle or catheter, (2) pericardiotomy via a subxiphoid incision, or (3) partial or extensive surgical pericardiectomy. Considerable controversy exists regarding the exact indications for pericardiocentesis, although the procedure has been performed extensively since its initial demonstration in 1840 by the Viennese physician Franz Schuh. The benefits of pericardiocentesis include the rapid relief of cardiac tamponade and the opportunity to obtain accurate hemodynamic measurements before and after pericardial aspiration. The major risk of percutaneous pericardiocentesis is laceration of the heart, coronary arteries, or lung. Prior to the 1970s, pericardiocentesis was usually performed blindly at the bedside using a sharp needle without hemodynamic or echocardiographic monitoring, and the risk of death or life-threatening complications appeared to be as high as 20 per cent.[137]

TECHNIQUE. The modern approach is exemplified by the Stanford experience in 123 patients.[138] In the majority of patients, pericardiocentesis was performed by a cardiologist in the cardiac catheterization laboratory using a subxiphoid approach under fluoroscopic guidance with hemodynamic and electrocardiographic monitoring. In this experience, five deaths occurred in association with pericardiocentesis; nonfatal hemopericardium developed in an additional five patients. Pericardiocentesis in this study was successful in obtaining pericardial fluid in 106 of 123 patients. Importantly, the probability of success in safely obtaining fluid was directly related to the size of the pericardial effusion because fluid was obtained in 93 per cent of patients with large effusions located both anteriorly and posteriorly on echocardiogram but in only 58 per cent with a small posterior pericardial effusion. In 23 patients a specific etiological diagnosis was possible from analysis of the pericardial fluid. Cardiac tamponade was successfully relieved by pericardiocentesis in 61 per cent, whereas the remainder required subsequent surgical drainage owing either to failure to relieve tamponade or to recurrence after pericardiocentesis. Surgery was most frequently required in patients with acute traumatic hemopericardium (see p. 1536). An unsuspected physiological cause of increased systemic venous pressure other than simple cardiac tamponade was documented in 40 per cent of the patients studied, including effusive-constrictive pericarditis in 17 per cent, congestive heart failure in 16 per cent, and coexisting neoplastic superior vena caval obstruction in 5 per cent. Similar experiences regarding the efficacy and safety of pericardiocentesis have been reported by ourselves in a consecutive series of 50 patients[132] and others.[139,140]

Two-dimensional echocardiography is useful in guiding

pericardiocentesis. Callahan et al.[141] have reported their experience in 132 consecutive pericardiocenteses guided by two-dimensional echocardiography. Pericardiocentesis was successful in obtaining pericardial fluid in 95 per cent of the procedures. There were no deaths, one pneumothorax, and three minor complications. Partial or complete surgical pericardiectomy was subsequently required in 25 per cent of patients for recurrent effusion, chronic relapsing pericarditis, or effusive-constrictive disease. Two-dimensional echocardiographic guidance is particularly helpful in percutaneous pericardiocentesis in patients with loculated pericardial effusion after cardiac surgery.

RISKS AND COMPLICATIONS. Thus, pericardiocentesis is now safer than it was a decade ago, and when the procedure is performed by an experienced operator, the risk of developing a life-threatening complication is generally less than 5 per cent.[132,138–142] The procedure is most likely to be successful and uncomplicated when performed in patients with clear-cut echocardiographic evidence of a large effusion with an anterior clear space of 10 mm or more. These recent experiences with pericardiocentesis indicate that the procedure should usually be performed in conjunction with hemodynamic measurements, including right heart and intrapericardial pressures, to (1) document the presence of the physiological changes of cardiac tamponade prior to attempted pericardiocentesis and (2) exclude other important coexisting causes of elevated jugular venous pressure, such as effusive-constrictive disease, superior vena caval obstruction, and left ventricular failure. There is rarely justification for performing blind needle pericardiocentesis at the bedside in the absence of optimal hemodynamic monitoring or of a prior echocardiogram documenting the presence of a large anterior and posterior effusion.

Pericardiocentesis is likely to be either complicated or unsuccessful in improving hemodynamics in patients with (1) acute traumatic hemopericardium in which blood enters the pericardial space as rapidly as it can be aspirated, (2) a small pericardial effusion judged to be less than 200 ml in size, (3) absence of an anterior effusion based on echocardiogram, (4) a loculated effusion, or (5) clot and fibrin as well as fluid filling the mediastinal or pericardial space postoperatively. Acute hemopericardium secondary to laceration, puncture of the heart, or leaking left ventricular or aortic aneurysm is likely to recur rapidly after pericardiocentesis. This procedure should be used only as an emergency temporizing measure prior to surgical pericardial exploration in which repair of the heart or aorta may be necessary. Surgical drainage is also usually preferred in patients with tamponade caused by purulent pericarditis to permit extensive drainage and in patients with suspected or known tuberculous pericarditis to permit bacteriological and histological examination of pericardial biopsy specimens. A rare but important complication that may occur after the relief of cardiac tamponade is the development of sudden ventricular dilatation and acute pulmonary edema.[143,144] The mechanism is probably a sudden increase in pulmonary venous blood flow following the relief of pericardial compression in the presence of underlying ventricular dysfunction.

COMBINED CATHETERIZATION AND PERICARDIOCENTESIS

We prefer the following method of combined catheterization and pericardiocentesis, which allows documentation of increased intrapericardial pressure and assessment of hemodynamic improvement after pericardiocentesis.[145] In contrast to traditional bedside sharp-needle pericardiocentesis, this method utilizes a soft catheter for pericardial aspiration and eliminates the prolonged presence of a sharp needle in the pericardial sac, thereby minimizing the risk of cardiac laceration. If possible, pericardiocentesis should be performed in a cardiac procedure laboratory where radiographic and hemodynamic monitoring facilities are optimal and by cardiologists experienced with hemodynamic measurements and the procedure itself. Before the procedure, the patient's blood should be typed and crossmatched and the cardiac surgery team alerted.

Pericardiocentesis is performed after the recording of baseline right atrial, right ventricular, pulmonary artery, and pulmonary capillary wedge pressures using a balloon-tipped catheter and cardiac output. Before pericardiocentesis, the transducer system that will be used to record intrapericardial pressure should be leveled with the other transducers, calibrated, and connected to a short length of fluid-filled tubing and a stopcock. Care should be taken to use equisensitive transducers and to avoid an underdamped catheter-transducer system.

PATIENT POSITION AND ROUTE. Pericardiocentesis is carried out with the patient's thorax and head tilted up, which enhances the pooling of the effusion anteriorly and inferiorly. Although multiple sites have been advocated for pericardiocentesis, we strongly prefer the subxiphoid route because it is extrapleural and avoids the coronary, pericardial, and internal mammary arteries. The skin is shaved, cleansed, and prepared in aseptic fashion, and the skin and subcutaneous tissue are anesthetized with 1 per cent lidocaine. The skin is pierced with a No. 11 blade, 0.5 cm below and to the left of the xiphoid process, and the subcutaneous tissues are spread with a small curved clamp.

NEEDLE INSERTION. A long, 8-inch, thin-walled No. 18-gauge pointed needle (pericardiocentesis kit, Mansfield Scientific, Inc., Mansfield, MA) is attached via a stopcock to a hand-held syringe containing 1 per cent lidocaine. One port of the stopcock is connected to the short length of fluid-filled tubing and the transducer that will be used to measure pericardial pressure (Fig. 43–11). The thin-walled needle commonly used for lumbar puncture is not adequate because its long sharp bevel poses some hazard. The metal hub of the needle may be attached by a sterile connector to the V lead of an electrocardiographic machine, and the electrocardiogram should be continuously recorded. *It is essential that the electrocardiographic apparatus have equipotential grounding with no chance of a current wave that could induce ventricular fibrillation.* If this condition cannot be assured, it is safer to omit electrocardiographic monitoring from the needle.

The needle is directed posteriorly until the tip passes posterior to the bony cage. The hub of the needle is then pressed toward the diaphragm, and the needle is advanced with a 15-degree posterior tilt, either directly toward the patient's head or toward the right or left shoulder. As the needle is smoothly and slowly advanced, the operator periodically attempts to aspirate fluid and then injects a small amount of lidocaine to clear the needle and to provide anesthesia of the deep tissues. The needle is advanced until the pericardial membrane is felt to "give" and pericardial fluid is aspirated or until ST-segment elevation and ventricular premature beats appear on the electrocardiogram, indicating that the needle has reached the

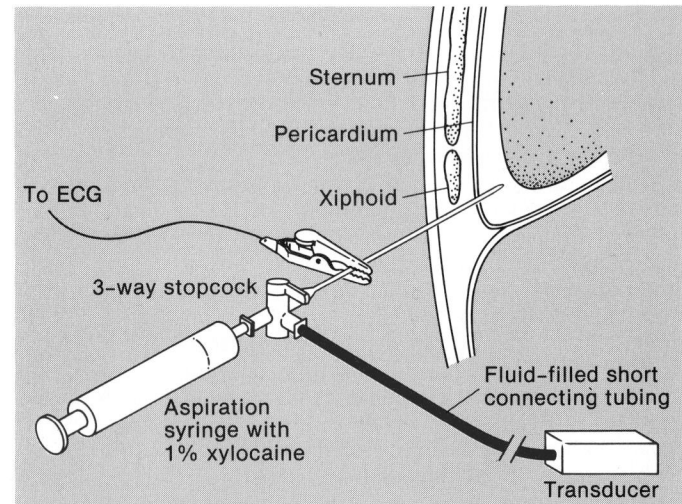

FIGURE 43–11. Pericardiocentesis using the subxiphoid approach, which avoids the major epicardial vessels. A hollow needle, which is attached via a stopcock to an aspiration syringe and to a short length of connecting tubing to a transducer, is used to enter the pericardial space. When fluid is initially aspirated, the pressure waveform at the needle tip should be briefly examined to confirm that the needle tip is in the pericardial space. A floppy-tipped guidewire is then passed through the hollow needle, the needle is exchanged for a soft flexible catheter with end and side holes to facilitate safe and thorough drainage of the pericardial sac. (Modified from Lorell, B. H., and Grossman, W.: Profiles in constrictive pericarditis, restrictive cardiomyopathy, and cardiac tamponade. *In* Grossman, W., and Baim, D. S. [eds.]: Cardiac Catheterization, Angiography and Intervention. Philadelphia, Lea and Febiger, 1991, p. 643.)

epicardium. In the latter case, the needle is promptly and smoothly withdrawn while the operator attempts to aspirate pericardial fluid until the needle lies within the fluid-filled pericardial space and the ECG changes disappear. If fluid cannot be freely aspirated, the needle is slowly withdrawn out of the body, avoiding lateral motion; the needle is flushed and the procedure repeated.

If hemorrhagic fluid is freely aspirated and it is not clear whether the needle is in the ventricle, atrium, or pericardial space, a few milliliters of contrast medium may be injected under fluoroscopic observation. If the contrast medium instantly swirls and disappears, the needle is within a cardiac chamber; in contrast, the appearance of sluggish layering of contrast medium inferiorly indicates that the needle is correctly positioned. When fluid can be freely aspirated, the stopcock is turned into its transducer and needle tip, and phasic right atrial pressures are simultaneously displayed. If the needle tip is in the pericardial space, pericardial and right atrial pressures should be equal with identical waveforms. A soft floppy-tip 0.038-inch guidewire is then passed through the hollow needle so that its tip lies within the pericardial space, as confirmed by fluoroscopy. A soft tampered large-bore lumen No. 6 French or 7 French catheter with multiple sideholes and an end hole is advanced over the guidewire, the guidewire is removed, and a few milliliters of fluid are aspirated. The catheter is then promptly connected to the prepared transducer, and intrapericardial pressure is recorded simultaneously with right atrial and systemic arterial pressure to document the presence of cardiac tamponade.

THE PERICARDIAL FLUID. Fluid samples are then aspirated from the catheter and sent for analysis of protein, amylase, glucose, and cholesterol content; hematocrit and white blood cell count; and bacteriological culture for aerobic and anaerobic bacteria, tuberculosis, and fungi. In most cases, a generous sample of fluid should also be sent in a heparinized container for cytological examination. Right atrial, systemic arterial, and intrapericardial pressures should then be recorded periodically as aliquots of fluid are removed—not only until intrapericardial pressure falls to zero but until no further fluid can be aspirated; intrapericardial pressure may return to normal levels after removal of only 50 to 100 ml of fluid in the presence of an effusion of 1 to 2 liters. *In our experience, extremely thorough drainage can be accomplished by connecting the intrapericardial catheter via sterile noncollapsible tubing to a stoppered sterile glass bottle with a vacuum.* This should be done only when a soft catheter is in the pericardial space because vacuum suction would be hazardous with sharp needle drainage. When no further fluid can be aspirated or drained, cardiac output and systemic arterial pressure as well as right atrial, right ventricular, and pulmonary capillary wedge pressures should be recorded, the last three simultaneously. The jugular veins should also be examined.

COMPLETION OF DRAINAGE. Successful relief of cardiac tamponade is documented by (1) the fall of intrapericardial pressure to levels of −3 and +3 mm Hg, (2) the fall of elevated right atrial pressure and separation between right- and left-heart filling pressures, (3) augmentation of cardiac output, and (4) disappearance of pulsus paradoxus. The presence of continued elevation and equilibration of right and left ventricular diastolic pressures with the appearance of a prominent y descent in the right atrial pressure tracing strongly suggests the presence of constricting pericardium due to effusive-constrictive pericarditis (see p. 1505). Jugular venous distention despite a fall in right atrial pressure should raise the question of coexisting superior vena caval obstruction, particularly in patients with known or suspected malignant disease.

Some cardiologists advocate the routine injection of a small volume of CO_2 or air into the pericardial space to outline the pericardium at the end of the procedure. This procedure has not been shown to be of aid in identifying unsuspected tumor masses,[138] and we do not advocate it. When the pericardial space is nearly obliterated, there is also the risk of injecting gas into a pleural cavity or cardiac chamber or the production of air tamponade.

POSTASPIRATION MANAGEMENT. It is often desirable to leave the intrapericardial catheter in place for several hours to permit repeated aspiration of fluid if cardiac tamponade recurs or to allow instillation of a nonabsorbable corticosteroid or antineoplastic agent in special cases. The catheter may be sutured securely to the skin and attached via a three-way stopcock to a closed drainage system. If the fluid is hemorrhagic or rich in fibrin, the catheter must be cleared frequently with a few millimeters of fluid. Dilute heparin may be instilled into the catheter to prevent clotting. The catheter should usually be removed after 24 to 48 hours because of the risk of introducing infection and producing iatrogenic purulent pericarditis. However, in some patients, continuous catheter drainage for several days has been reported to be necessary and effective in relieving cardiac tamponade.[141,146]

Percutaneous pericardial drainage in infants and children can be done without complications using a modification of this approach in which a catheter is inserted over a curved guidewire into the pericardial space under fluoroscopic control.[146]

Following pericardiocentesis, the majority of patients should be observed for about 24 hours in an intensive care setting for recurrence of cardiac tamponade. It is frequently helpful to obtain an echocardiogram soon after pericardiocentesis to establish the appearance of the heart and pericardium following aspiration.

PERCUTANEOUS BALLOON PERICARDIOTOMY. The technique of percutaneous balloon pericardiotomy was proposed by Palacios et al.,[147] and the experience of the first 50 patients with either larger pericardial effusions or tamponade undergoing this procedure as part of a multicenter registry has been recently reported.[148] In this series, the majority (88 per cent) had large pericardial effusions and a history of malignancy. Balloon pericardiotomy is performed as part of percutaneous pericardiocentesis with measurement of pericardial fluid and sampling of fluid for cytology and other studies. Approximately 200 ml of fluid is then left within the pericardial sac. After further dilation of the pericardial tract, a 20-mm diameter, 3-cm-long dilating balloon (Mansfield) is advanced over a guidewire to straddle the parietal pericardium, and the balloon is manually inflated to create a tear ("window") in the pericardium (Fig. 43–12). Sometimes additional punctures and balloon-induced rents in the pericardium are performed. After the pericardiotomy, the pericardial catheter is reinserted over a guidewire and all remaining fluid is drained. Postprocedure echocardiography and chest radiography (to monitor accumulation of left pleural effusion) should be done 24 hours later and at monthly follow-up.

This procedure was successful in 46 patients (92 per cent) in relieving tamponade with a short follow-up of 3 months, whereas two patients required early operation and

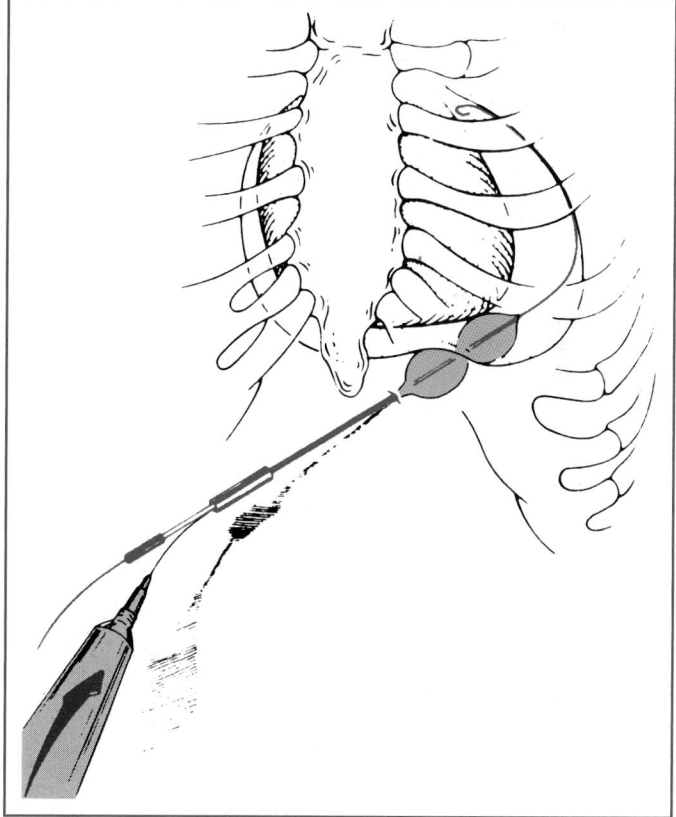

FIGURE 43–12. Illustration of the percutaneous balloon pericardiotomy technique. After partial drainage of the pericardium using a pericardial catheter, an 0.038-inch stiff J-tip wire is introduced into the pericardial space. A 3-cm-long dilating balloon is then advanced over the guidewire to "straddle" the parietal pericardial membrane and manually inflated to create a rent in the pericardium. (Modified from Ziskind, A. A., et al.: Percutaneous balloon pericardiotomy for the treatment of cardiac tamponade and large pericardial effusions: Description of technique and report of the first 50 cases. J. Am. Coll. Cardiol. *21*:1, 1993; reprinted by permission of the American College of Cardiology.)

two patients required late operation for recurrent tamponade. Complications included coronary artery laceration in 2 per cent, fever in 12 per cent, and the development of pleural effusion (presumably due to pericardial drainage) requiring thoracentesis or chest tube placement within 30 days in 16 per cent. Thus, this procedure is a novel and promising option for the management of large pericardial effusion with tamponade. However, the early postprocedure morbidity was significantly higher than we have observed in a prospective series of 50 patients managed with percutaneous catheter pericardiocentesis with complete drainage assisted by vacuum suction, as described above.[132] The long-term efficacy of percutaneous catheter pericardiocentesis, balloon pericardiotomy, and surgical subxiphoid pericardiotomy in the management of large pericardial effusions with hemodynamic compromise have not yet been compared in a prospective trial.

SURGICAL PERICARDIOTOMY. Surgical evacuation of pericardial fluid under pressure can be accomplished for patients who do not require extensive pericardial excision with the subxiphoid limited pericardiotomy. Subxiphoid pericardiotomy can usually be performed under local anesthesia. In patients who are not in extremis, the procedure is usually done without initial palliative pericardiocentesis so that the pericardial sac is distended. After a small longitudinal incision is made below the xiphoid process through the linea alba, the diaphragm and pericardium are dissected away from the sternum, and the diaphragm is retracted inferiorly to permit direct exposure of the anterior pericardium. The tense parietal pericardium is visualized, a small incision is made in the pericardium, a small segment of pericardium is resected for drainage, and a tube is inserted into the pericardial space for extrathoracic drainage by gravity into a sterile container.

PERICARDIECTOMY. The use of the term *subxiphoid pericardial window* for the procedure just described should probably be avoided because it creates confusion with a limited pericardiectomy, which is often referred to as a pleuropericardial window or pericardial window. A limited pericardiectomy via a left hemithorax drains the pericardial cavity into the left hemithorax, and all accessible pericardial tissue is not excised. In a complete pericardiectomy the pericardium is resected from the right phrenic nerve to the left pulmonary veins (sparing the left phrenic nerve) and from the great vessels to the mid-diaphragm, while a partial pericardiectomy is limited by the great vessels.

OUTCOME. The relative efficacy of these surgical approaches has been reviewed in three large series.[149–151] The overall 30-day surgical mortality ranged from 12.0 to 15.5 per cent, and was higher in patients with malignant than benign effusions. The subxiphoid pericar-diotomy has some advantages over extensive formal pericardiectomy in that it is simpler and shorter, permits both drainage of pericardial fluid and examination of a small pericardial biopsy specimen, and can usually be performed safely using local anesthesia in critically ill patients.[151]

A prospective series of 57 patients managed with subxiphoid pericardial biopsy and pericardiotomy reported that the procedure was performed with local anesthesia in 81 per cent.[151] At 1-year follow-up, seven patients (12 per cent) had recurrent effusions, and only four patients (7 per cent) needed reoperation.[151] This suggests that the less invasive subxiphoid pericardiotomy should be chosen as a palliative procedure in patients who are critically ill with limited expected survival. The left thoracotomy partial pericardiectomy appears to offer none of the advantages of the subxiphoid pericardiotomy and is associated with higher operative mortality.[150] Complete pericardiectomy is usually recommended for the surgical treatment of patients with effusive-constrictive pericardial disease or loculated effusion who are in good general condition and who are expected to survive more than a few months.

PERICARDIOSCOPY AND BIOPSY. With use of a flexible fiberoptic bronchoscope or endoscope, this procedure has been reported as an adjunct to subxiphoid pericardiotomy following the drainage of the effusion.[152,153] Pericardioscopy permits visualization of the parietal pericardium and epicardium on the anterior, posterior, and inferior surfaces of the heart and allows selective biopsies beyond the small region of pericardium that is usually accessible with a subxiphoid incision.

PERCUTANEOUS PERICARDIAL BIOPSY. Endrys et al.[154] described a technique for percutaneous pericardial biopsy using an endomyocardial bioptome inserted via a curved sheath after percutaneous pericardiocentesis and distention of the pericardial space with air. Maisch et al.[155] have recently described a modification of this technique in which a No. 9 French sheath is introduced into the pericardial effusion over a guidewire under echocardiographic or fluoroscopic guidance, the pericardial effusion is aspirated and replaced by about 150 ml of body-temperature clear saline solution, and a flexible endoscope is then introduced. Pericardioscopy with optically guided epicardial biopsy offers the potential for analysis of small tissue samples for viral, tuberculous, and malignant myopericarditis using conventional histology as well as new molecular techniques of polymerase chain reaction and in situ hybridization.[156] Percutaneous pericardial biopsy has also been described as an adjunct to pericardiocentesis and cytological fluid examination using a pericardial bioptome to sample the posterolateral visceral pericardium under simple fluoroscopic guidance.[157] Particularly in patients with suspected but undocumented malignancy, pericardial biopsy appears to increase the yield of a positive diagnosis of malignancy compared with pericardial fluid cytology alone.[155–157] These techniques offer new approaches for obtaining diagnostic information in patients with suspected malignant or infectious pericardial disease, but the efficacy and safety of these approaches in comparison with surgical subxiphoid pericardiotomy under local anesthesia, and pericardial biopsy are not yet established.

CONSTRICTIVE PERICARDITIS

Constrictive pericarditis is present when a fibrotic, thickened, and adherent pericardium restricts diastolic filling of the heart. It usually begins with an initial episode of acute pericarditis, which may not be detectable clinically, characterized by fibrin deposition, often with a pericardial effusion. This then slowly progresses to a subacute stage of organization and resorption of the effusion, followed by a chronic stage consisting of fibrous scarring and thickening of the pericardium with obliteration of the pericardial space. In the majority of cases, the visceral and parietal layers become completely fused, but in a few cases, the constricting process is produced primarily by the visceral pericardium (epicardium). In the chronic stage of constrictive pericarditis, calcium deposition may contribute to thickening and stiffening of the pericardium. Constrictive pericarditis is usually a symmetrical scarring process that produces uniform restriction of the filling of all heart chambers. Rare cases of strictly localized pericardial thickening have been reported, including constricting bands in the atrioventricular groove surrounding the semilunar valve rings, or in the aortic groove, right ventricular outflow tract, and venae cavae.[158]

Pathophysiology

In classic constrictive pericarditis, the heavily fibrosed or calcified pericardium restricts diastolic filling of all chambers of the heart and determines the diastolic volume of the heart. The symmetrical constricting effect of the pericardium results in elevation and equilibrium of diastolic pressures in all four cardiac chambers (as well as of pulmonary capillary wedge pressures). In early diastole when intracardiac volume is less than that defined by the stiff pericardium, diastolic filling is unimpeded, and early diastolic filling occurs abnormally rapidly because venous pressure is elevated. Rapid early diastolic filling is abruptly halted when the intracardiac volume reaches the limit set by the noncompliant pericardium.

Instantaneous plots of ventricular volume versus time in patients with constrictive pericarditis have shown that virtually all filling of the ventricle occurs very early in diastole. This abnormal pattern of diastolic filling is reflected in the characteristic dip-and-plateau waveforms in both right and left ventricles (Fig. 43–13). The early diastole dip corresponds to the period of excessively rapid diastolic filling, while the plateau phase corresponds to the period of mid and late diastole when there is little additional ventricular volume expansion. Because the atria are equilibrated with the ventricles in early diastole, the jugular venous waveform and right and left atrial waveforms show a prominent and deep diastolic y descent. The systolic x descent is usually also present, and the venous waveform may therefore exhibit a characteristic M or W configuration.

A bimodal pattern of systemic venous return occurs in

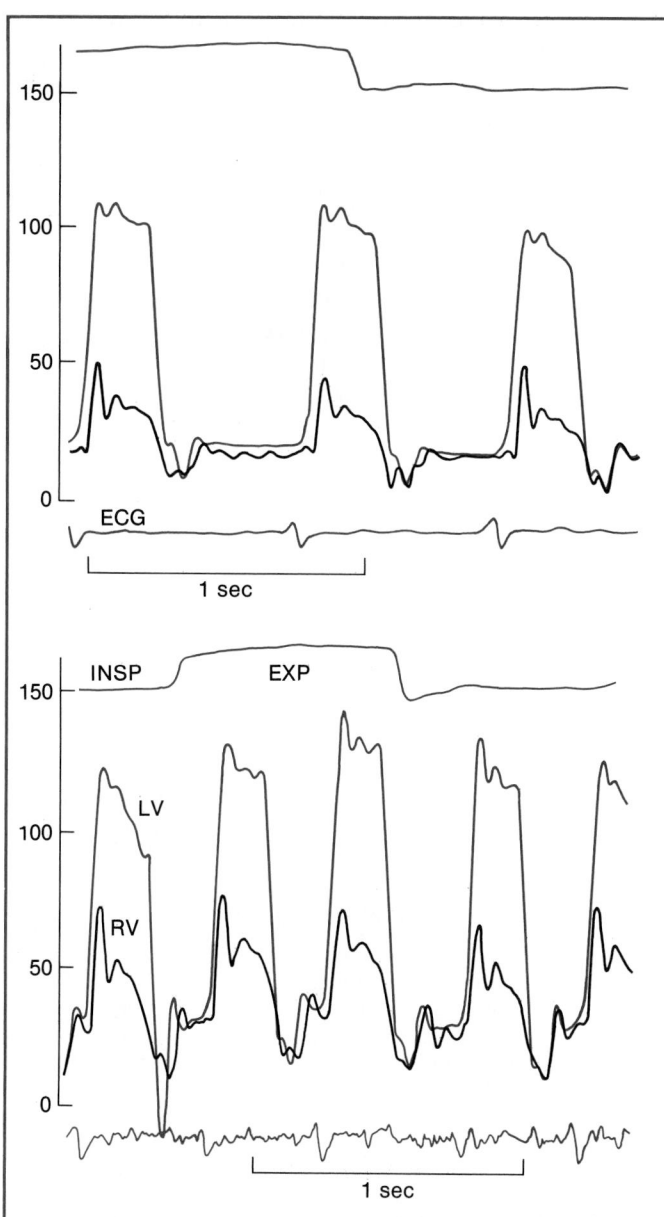

FIGURE 43–13. Left (LV) and right ventricular (RV) pressure recordings from a patient with constrictive pericarditis illustrating that the presence of tachycardia partially obscures evaluation of the diastolic waveforms. The long diastole following a premature beat allows recognition of equilibrium of ventricular diastolic pressures before the *a* wave, as well as detection of a dip-and-plateau configuration of the waveforms. (From Lorell, B. H., and Grossman, W.: Profiles in constrictive pericarditis, restrictive cardiomyopathy, and cardiac tamponade. *In* Grossman, W. [ed.]: Cardiac Catheterization and Angiography. Philadelphia, Lea and Febiger, 1986, p. 430.)

KUSSMAUL'S SIGN. Another striking abnormality of constrictive pericarditis is the failure of intrathoracic pressure changes during respiration to be transmitted to the pericardial space and intracardiac chambers. As a consequence, during inspiration, systemic venous and right arterial pressures do not fall and venous flow into the right atrium does not increase, in contrast to the situation in normal subjects and patients with cardiac tamponade. In some patients, systemic venous pressure may actually increase with inspiration, i.e., *Kussmaul's sign.*[160] This finding may occur in other disorders such as chronic right ventricular failure and restrictive cardiomyopathy, in which right atrial and systemic venous pressures also are markedly elevated. However, Kussmaul's sign does *not* occur in acute cardiac tamponade, in which the inspiratory fall in intrathoracic pressure is transmitted to the fluid-filled pericardial space. Pulsus paradoxus (see p. 1488) is also less common in constrictive pericarditis than in cardiac tamponade, in which the exaggerated increase in right ventricular filling during inspiration at the expense of left ventricular filling is more prominent. The presence of an inspiratory fall in arterial pressure greater than 10 mm Hg suggests the presence of a tense pericardial effusion or coexisting pulmonary disease with an exaggerated inspiratory fall in intrathoracic pressure.

Restriction of diastolic filling ultimately results in compensatory renal retention of sodium and water that contributes further to the increase in systemic venous pressure and initially serves to maintain diastolic filling of the ventricles despite pericardial compression. The inhibition of the release of atrial natriuretic factor may contribute to renal fluid retention.[161] In some cases, the pericardial scar is so dense that diastolic ventricular volumes are reduced, which may cause stroke volume and then cardiac output to fall despite compensatory tachycardia. The presence of reduced cardiac output, tachycardia, and elevated right and left heart filling pressures may simulate myocardial failure, and classic ventricular performance curves may show reduced left ventricular stroke volume relative to elevated left ventricular filling pressure. However, systolic contraction of the ventricles and the intrinsic contractile state of the myocardium are usually normal or nearly so. Because stroke volume is relatively fixed and most ventricular filling occurs in early diastole, cardiac output depends on heart rate and mild tachycardia improves cardiac output in patients with severe constrictive pericarditis. Chandrashekhar et al. showed that increasing heart rate with atrial pacing augmented the cardiac output, whereas stroke volume and ventricular filling pressures were unchanged up to heart rates of 140 beats per minute.[162] These effects of atrial pacing were no longer present after surgical pericardiectomy. In severe cases of constrictive pericarditis, myocardial systolic function may also be depressed, owing to myocardial atrophy, fibrosis, or obliteration of epicardial coronary arteries in the fibrotic pericardium resulting in myocardial ischemia.[163,164] Although the presence of coexisting cardiomyopathy is usually a factor predictive of a poor outcome after pericardiectomy (see p. 1505), a striking improvement of left ventricular ejection fraction may occasionally occur after stripping of a fibrotic and thick pericardium.

SUBACUTE NONCALCIFIC PERICARDITIS. Pathophysiological and hemodynamic findings in patients with subacute noncalcific pericarditis may differ from those in patients with chronic constrictive pericarditis in whom the pericardium resembles a rigid shell. Hancock has suggested that the presence of a thick fluid-fibrin layer in the process of organization leads to relatively elastic compression of the heart, which may be compared to "wrapping the heart tightly with rubber bands."[165] The pathophysical disturbance caused by this nonrigid fibroelastic form of constrictive pericarditis is similar to that in cardiac tamponade because fibroelastic constriction compresses the heart continuously

constrictive pericarditis with an acceleration of systemic venous blood flow from the venae cavae into the right atrium during both ventricular systolic ejection and early diastole. The greatest acceleration of venous blood flow occurs during early diastole simultaneous with the *y* descent. This contrasts with the normal filling pattern, in which a bimodal pattern of systolic venous return also is present, but the major surge of venous return occurs during systole. The pattern of systemic venous return in constrictive pericarditis also contrasts with that in cardiac tamponade. Cardiac compression is present throughout diastole in cardiac tamponade, so that the diastolic surge of venous return is blunted or abolished such that the atria fill during ventricular ejection in early systole[159] and the venous pressure tracing shows absence of or blunted diastolic *y* descent and a preserved *x* descent.

TABLE 43–7   CLINICAL AND HEMODYNAMIC COMPRESSIVE PERICARDIAL DISEASE

	CARDIAC TAMPONADE	SUBACUTE "ELASTIC" CONSTRICTION	CHRONIC "RIGID" CONSTRICTION
Duration of symptoms	Hours to days	Weeks to months	Months to years
Chest pain, friction rub	Usual	Recent past	Remote
Pulsus paradoxus	Prominent	Usually prominent	Slight or absent
Kussmaul's sign	Absent	Usually absent	Often present
Early diastolic knock	Absent	Usually absent	Often present
Heart size on chest roentgenogram	Usually enlarged	Usually enlarged	Usually normal, sometimes enlarged
Pericardial calcification	Absent	Rare	Often present
Abnormal P waves or atrial fibrillation	Absent	Absent	Often present
Venous (right atrial) waveform	X or Xy	Xy or XY	XY or xY
Pericardial effusion	Always present	Often present	Absent

X and Y = prominent *x* and *y* descents, respectively; *x* and *y* = inconspicuous *x* and *y* descents.
Modified from Hancock, E. W.: On the elastic and rigid forms of constrictive pericarditis. Am. Heart J. *100*:917, 1980.

throughout the cardiac cycle, and respiratory changes in intrathoracic pressure usually are transmitted to the cardiac chambers.[165] Thus, patterns of ventricular filling and waveforms in the subacute form of fibroelastic compression tend to resemble those of cardiac tamponade rather than of constrictive pericarditis and include a systemic venous waveform with a predominant *x* descent or equal *x* and *y* descents, an inconspicuous early diastolic dip in the ventricular waveform, an inspiratory fall in systemic venous and right atrial pressures, and the presence of pulsus paradoxus (Table 43–7).

Etiology

Tuberculosis was formerly the leading cause of constrictive pericarditis in Western nations as reported in the classic series of Paul[166] and Andrews[167] and their coworkers. In disadvantaged nations, this is still true, whereas with the advent of antituberculosis therapy this disease now accounts for 15 per cent or less of cases in developed nations.[168,169] The largest number of cases of constrictive pericarditis today are of unknown cause (42 per cent) and are attributed to earlier clinically inapparent viral pericarditis.[169] In the past decade, constrictive pericarditis after cardiac surgery has emerged as an important cause (see p. 1734). In a series of 84 consecutive patients with constrictive pericarditis seen from 1979 to 1989, the largest numbers of cases were of unknown and presumed viral origin (55 per cent).[170] Postsurgical pericarditis accounted for 4 per cent of all cases, tuberculosis accounted for 12 per cent, and prior mediastinal radiation therapy accounted for 5 per cent of cases.[170] Other nontubercular causes include chronic renal failure treated with hemodialysis (see p. 1935); connective tissue disorders, including rheumatoid arthritis and systemic lupus erythematosus (p. 1776); and neoplastic pericardial infiltration or encasement of the heart due most commonly to lung cancer, breast cancer, Hodgkin's disease, and lymphoma. Constrictive pericarditis can develop after incomplete drainage of purulent pericarditis (p. 1509) and as a complication of fungal infections (p. 1510) and parasitic infections (p. 1511). It may occasionally follow pericarditis associated with acute myocardial infarction and the postpericardiotomy syndrome, (p. 1520), and in association with pulmonary asbestosis.[171]

CONSTRICTIVE PERICARDITIS IN CHILDREN (see also p. 1509). Constrictive pericarditis is far less common in children than in adults and may rarely occur following a viral syndrome in a child mistakenly thought to have hepatitis or a protein-losing enteropathy. When constrictive pericarditis occurs in young children, tuberculosis should be strongly considered because it was a proved or highly likely cause of 56 per cent of 84 children with constrictive pericarditis reported in the literature.[172] Nontraumatic he-

mopericardium has been reported in children and young adults with congenital bleeding disorders complicated by a second process such as endocarditis or viral syndrome, and constrictive pericarditis has occurred following pericardial bleeding due to congenital afibrinogenemia.[173] The newly described familial syndrome of pericarditis, arthritis, and camptodactyly (flexion contractures) is a rare cause of constrictive pericarditis in children and young adults.[174] A rare congenital cause of constrictive pericarditis is *mulibrey nanism,* an autosomal recessive disorder characterized by dwarfism, constrictive pericarditis, abnormal fundi, and fibrous dysplasia of the long bones.[175]

Clinical Features

In patients in whom systemic venous and right atrial pressures are modestly elevated (10 to 15 mm Hg), left ventricular filling pressure is also usually only modestly elevated. In this setting, symptoms secondary to systemic venous congestion such as edema, abdominal swelling, and discomfort due to ascites and passive hepatic congestion may predominate. Vague abdominal symptoms such as postprandial fullness, dyspepsia, flatulence, and anorexia may also be present. When both right and left heart filling pressures are elevated to the level of 15 to 30 mm Hg, symptoms of pulmonary venous congestion, such as exertional dyspnea, cough, and orthopnea, are present. Pleural effusions and elevation of the diaphragm due to ascites may also contribute to dyspnea. Severe platypnea, the symptom of dyspnea in the upright position, whose mechanism is not understood, is noted occasionally in chronic constrictive pericarditis.[176] Severe fatigue, weight loss, and muscle wasting suggest the presence of fixed or reduced cardiac output. Chest pain typical of angina may be related to underperfusion of the coronary arteries or compression of an epicardial coronary artery by the thickened pericardium.[164]

PHYSICAL EXAMINATION. The single most important finding is elevation of jugular venous pressure. If the neck is examined casually, or if the patient is examined supine so that jugular venous pressure is measured above the angle of the jaw, this important clue to the presence of constrictive pericarditis may be missed. A prominent feature of the elevated jugular venous pressure is the rapidly collapsing negative wave of the diastolic *y* descent. In patients in sinus rhythm, both *x* and *y* descents can be distinguished; the *x* descent is synchronous with the carotid pulse while the diastolic *y* descent is out of phase with the carotid pulse. These features may be difficult to detect in patients with tachycardia, tachypnea, or arrhythmia. It may also be difficult to distinguish between right heart failure due to tricuspid regurgitation and chronic constrictive pericarditis by neck vein examination at the bedside. The finding of

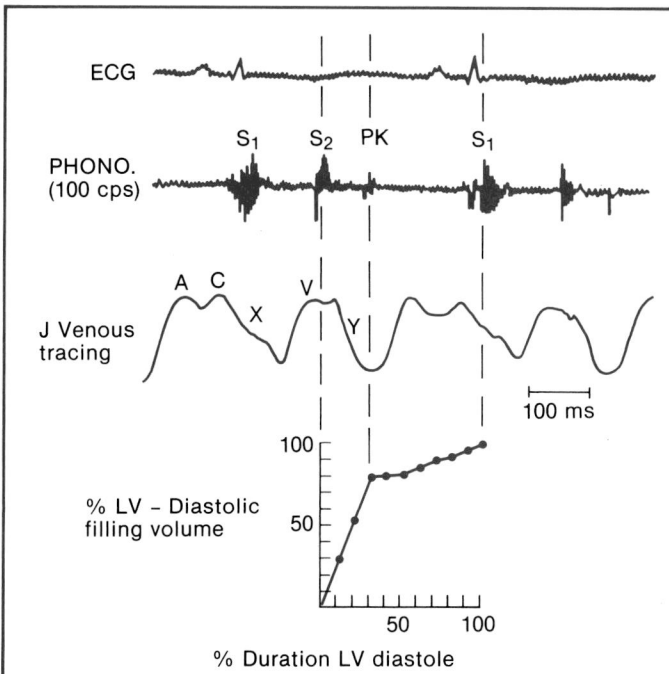

FIGURE 43–14. The electrocardiogram (ECG), phonocardiogram (PHONO), jugular venous pulse tracing, and left ventricular (LV) diastolic filling curve in a patient with constrictive pericarditis and pericardial knock (PK). The pericardial knock (PK) occurs simultaneously with the nadir of the diastolic *y* descent and sudden plateau of the LV filling curve. (From Tyberg, T. I., et al.: Genesis of pericardial knock in constrictive pericarditis. Am. J. Cardiol. *46:*570, 1980.)

Kussmaul's sign (an inspiratory increase in systemic venous pressure) is difficult to appreciate at the bedside and may be confused with exaggerated amplitude of the venous waves during inspiration.

The arterial pulse may be normal or show diminished pulse pressure. Severe pulsus paradoxus is uncommon in rigid constrictive pericarditis and rarely exceeds 10 mm Hg unless pericardial fluid under pressure is also present. Systolic retraction of the apical impulse occurs in the majority of patients and usually consists of an unobtrusive diffuse precordial movement. The most impressive abnormality during auscultation is the diastolic pericardial knock, an early diastolic sound that is often heard along the left sternal border in rigid constrictive pericarditis, infrequently heard in subacute constrictive pericarditis of the fibroelastic variety, and not heard in pure cardiac tamponade. The pericardial knock usually occurs 0.09 to 0.12 second after A_2 and corresponds in timing to the sudden cessation of ventricular filling and the premature diastolic plateau of the diastolic ventricular volume curve[177] (Fig. 43–14). The pericardial knock tends to occur earlier and to have a higher acoustic frequency than the typical S_3 gallop sound, and therefore it may be confused with the opening snap of mitral stenosis. Widening of the split between the aortic and pulmonic components of the second heart sound may occur in constrictive pericarditis. This is attributed to (1) a fixed right ventricular stroke volume during inspiration due to pericardial compression and (2) premature aortic valve closure due to a transitory inspiratory decrease in left ventricular stroke volume.

Hepatomegaly is usually present, and prominent hepatic pulsations that conform to the jugular venous pulse can be detected in 70 per cent of patients.[178] Other evidence of hepatic dysfunction secondary to passive liver congestion and diminished cardiac output may include ascites, icterus, spider angiomas, and palmar erythema. Constrictive pericarditis may rarely have the presenting feature of hepatic coma.[179] In young patients with competent venous valves, edema of the extremities may be noticeably absent in the

presence of marked abdominal distention. Older patients with long-standing constrictive pericarditis may have enormous ascites and massive edema of the scrotum, thighs, and calves.[180] In contrast, the upper torso and arms may show evidence of marked muscle wasting and cachexia. The volume overload of pregnancy can occasionally promote the development of symptoms and signs of severe constriction in women who were asymptomatic with pericardial disease prior to pregnancy.[181]

CHEST ROENTGENOGRAM (see also p. 235). The cardiac silhouette may be small, normal, or enlarged. Cardiac enlargement may be apparent because of coexisting pericardial effusion, the contribution of an enormously thickened pericardium, or preexisting cardiac chamber enlargement or hypertrophy. The right superior mediastinum may be prominent as a result of engorgement of the superior vena cava, and left atrial enlargement is common.[182] Extensive calcification of the pericardium is present in approximately half the patients and raises the possibility of a tubercular etiology. The location of calcification is helpful in distinguishing between pericardial and myocardial aneurysm calcium because pericardial calcification is predominantly located over the right heart chambers and in the atrioventricular grooves, whereas isolated calcification of the left ventricular apex or posterior wall suggests left ventricular aneurysm. However, this finding is not specific for constrictive pericarditis in that *a calcified pericardium is not necessarily a constricted one.* The lateral chest film is particularly useful for the detection of pericardial calcium in the atrioventricular groove or along the anterior and diaphragmatic surfaces of the right ventricle (Fig. 43–15). Fluoroscopy may be helpful in distinguishing pericardial calcification from calcium within the wall of a myocardial aneurysm or thrombus or within the mitral or aortic valves, mitral annulus, or coronary arteries. Pleural effusions are present in about 60 per cent of patients, and unexplained persistent pleural effusion can be the presenting manifesta-

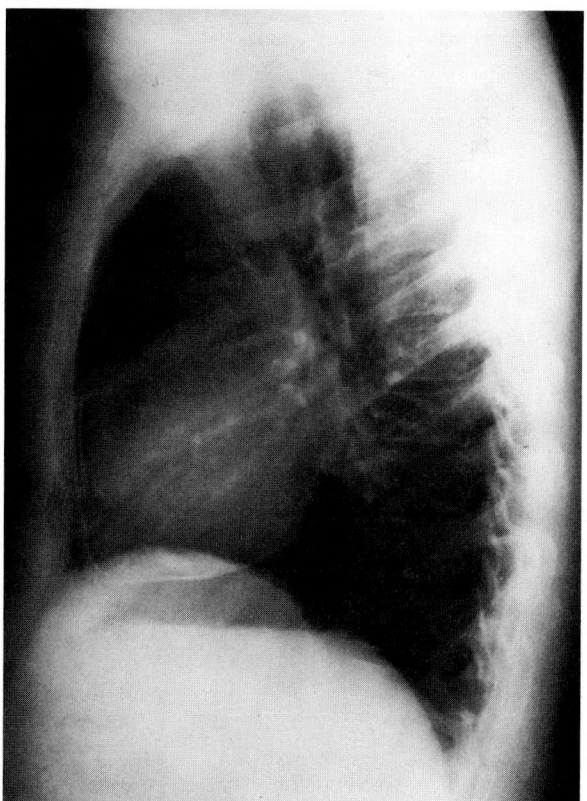

FIGURE 43–15. Lateral chest roentgenogram showing calcification of the pericardium in a patient with chronic constrictive pericarditis of idiopathic (postviral) etiology. The eggshell rim of pericardial calcification is often best appreciated in the lateral projection.

T.D. CONSTRICTIVE PERICARDITIS

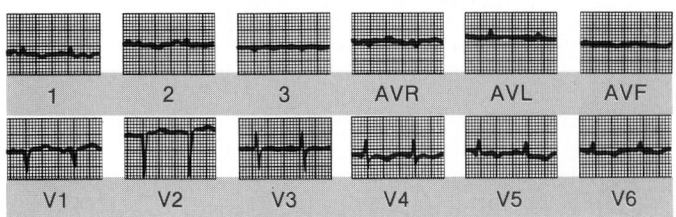

FIGURE 43–16. Electrocardiogram from a patient with surgically proven constrictive pericarditis and normal coronary arteries who had symptoms of chronic fatigue, dyspnea, and chest pain. The electrocardiogram is notable for the presence of a wide, notched P wave and diffuse T-wave inversion. These changes were initially mistakenly thought to be related to coronary insufficiency.

tion.[183] Because left atrial pressure is commonly elevated to 15 to 30 mm Hg, there may be evidence of redistribution of blood flow, but Kerley's B lines or infiltrates suggestive of frank pulmonary edema are rare.

ELECTROCARDIOGRAM. Electrocardiographic findings include low QRS voltage, generalized T-wave inversion or flattening, and left atrial abnormalities suggestive of P mitrale (Fig. 43–16). Atrial fibrillation occurs in less than half the patients with constrictive pericarditis and is thought to be related to longstanding elevation of atrial pressures and atrial enlargement. In a postmortem study of constrictive pericarditis, Levine noted that atrioventricular block, intraventricular conduction defects, and pseudoinfarction patterns with deep wide Q waves seemed to be related to an extension of calcification into the myocardium and around the coronary arteries, compromising coronary blood flow.[163] An unusual pattern that simulates right ventricular hypertrophy with right-axis deviation may be present in about 5 per cent of patients and due to dense pericardial scar overlying the right ventricle in association with compensatory dilation and hyperkinesis of the outflow tract.[184]

ECHOCARDIOGRAM. One distinct M-mode echocardiographic pattern of pericardial thickening in constrictive pericarditis consists of two parallel lines representing the visceral and parietal pericardia separated by a clear space of at least 1 mm; another consists of multiple dense echoes.[185] Other M-mode echocardiographic abnormalities include abrupt posterior motion of the interventricular septum in early diastole, coinciding with the pericardial knock, abrupt posterior motion during atrial systole, reduced amplitude of left ventricular posterior wall motion, and premature pulmonic valve opening secondary to a high right ventricular early diastolic pressure. These changes are also seen in other disorders with high right ventricular early diastolic pressure, such as tricuspid and pulmonic regurgitation. Engle et al.[186] reviewed M-mode echocardiograms from 40 patients with proven constrictive pericarditis and 40 normal subjects. They observed that normal left ventricular size, left atrial enlargement, flattened diastolic ventricular wall motion, and abnormal septal motion were found in most patients, but no single feature was diagnostic of constrictive pericarditis. Left atrial dilatation as well as abnormalities of wall motion tend to normalize after successful pericardiectomy.[187]

Two-dimensional echocardiography in constrictive pericarditis shows an immobile and dense appearance of the pericardium, abrupt displacement of the interventricular septum during early diastolic filling ("septal bounce"), prominent early diastolic filling, and an abnormal contour of the junction of the left ventricle and left atrial posterior wall.[188] Dilatation of the hepatic veins and inferior vena cava, intense and spontaneous contrast in the inferior vena cava, and distention of the inferior vena cava with blunted respiratory fluctuations in diameter ("plethora") are also observed in patients with constrictive pericarditis. Himelman et al.[189] reviewed the diagnostic value of pericardial

adhesions, septal bounce, and vena cava plethora and noted that false-positive findings occurred in patients with pacemakers or bundle branch block after pericardiotomy, and with other causes of right heart failure. Studies in an experimental dog model and in patients have confirmed that two-dimensional echocardiography can demonstrate abnormal early diastolic filling but greatly overestimates pericardial thickness.[190]

Doppler echocardiography of the engorged hepatic vein has been reported to show a W-wave pattern that corresponds to the characteristic pattern of right atrial filling and consists of rapid forward flow during early diastole, abrupt deceleration and subsequent reverse flow before the *a* wave, and a second wave of rapid forward flow during early systolic ejection with reverse flow in late systole.[191] Constrictive pericarditis is also associated with characteristic Doppler patterns of transvalvular and central venous flow velocities during respiration.[192,193] In constrictive pericarditis, the pericardial shell isolates the heart from changes in intrathoracic pressure. Because the thickened pericardium isolates the heart from the lungs, inspiration causes a decrease in the pressure gradient between the pulmonary capillaries and the left heart, resulting in an inspiratory decrease in diastolic mitral inflow and pulmonary venous flow velocities. This decrease in left ventricular filling results in a leftward shift of the interventricular septum, allowing augmented diastolic inspiratory inflow into the right ventricle manifest as increased early diastolic tricuspid inflow and hepatic vein flow velocities during inspiration. Opposite changes occur during early expiration (Fig. 43–17). The marked limitation of right heart filling during expiration also causes exaggeration of the normal pattern of expiratory reversal of hepatic vein flow during diastole.

In a study of 28 patients who underwent exploratory thoracotomy, 22 of 23 patients with Doppler findings of constrictive pericarditis were found to have this diagnosis at operation, whereas Doppler features consistent with restriction were found in four patients, three of whom were found to have constriction and one a restrictive myopathy.[193] In two patients with a normal pericardium, one patient had a normal Doppler study whereas one patient had

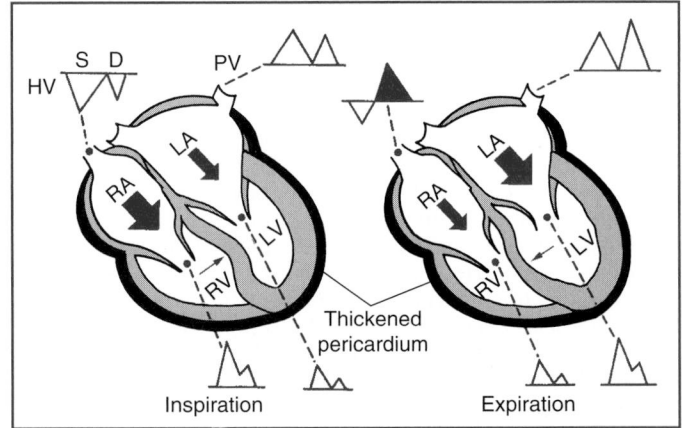

FIGURE 43–17. The effects of respiration on transvalvular flow in constrictive pericarditis. Because the pericardial shell isolates the heart from inspiratory pressure changes in the lungs, early inspiration causes a reduction in the driving pressure gradient between the pulmonary capillaries and the left atrium (LA), which leads to a decrease in pulmonary venous (PV) and mitral valve velocities. This reduction in left ventricular (LV) filling causes a slight leftward bowing of the septum associated with an inspiratory increase in right heart filling manifest as increased tricuspid inflow and diastolic hepatic venous (HV) flow velocities *(left panel)*. The opposite changes are seen during expiration. (Adapted from Oh, J. K., et al.: Diagnostic role of Doppler echocardiography in constrictive pericarditis. J. Am. Coll. Cardiol. **23**:154, 1994; reprinted by permission of the American College of Cardiology.)

Doppler findings of constriction related to chronic pulmonary disease with a normal pericardium. These observations illustrate that respiratory Doppler flow patterns suggestive of constriction are highly sensitive but also occur in conditions in which a dilated right ventricle is constrained by the normal pericardium, such as chronic lung disease, pulmonary embolism, and right ventricular infarction. Transient findings of "constrictive" respiratory changes in Doppler flow velocities have also been observed during the resolution of acute pericarditis with pericardial effusion, presumably related to transient stiffening and thickening of the inflamed pericardium.[194]

CT AND MRI. CT has also emerged as a valuable tool in the evaluation of suspected constrictive pericarditis. The technique is especially useful in identifying pericardial thickening and in identifying other findings compatible with constrictive pericarditis, including dilation of the venae cavae and deformation of the right ventricle, and increased filling fraction of the ventricles in early diastole.[195,196] Nonvisualization of the left ventricular posterolateral wall by CT suggests coexisting myocardial fibrosis or atrophy and may predict a poor outcome following pericardiectomy.[197]

Experience with MRI in patients with constrictive pericarditis suggests that it can also detect pericardial thickening, dilation of the venae cavae and hepatic veins, narrowing of the right ventricle, and dilatation of the right atrium[198,199] (Figs. 43–18 and Fig. 16–14, p. 325). MRI is probably the most sensitive imaging technique currently available for delineating the thickness of the pericardium, the morphology of regional or annular thickening or calcification, and the relationship of extracardiac masses to the pericardium and surface of the heart.[198,199] Both CT scanning and MRI have the potential to identify patients with a thickened pericardium and associated myocardial atrophy and fibrosis. Although the number of patients reported to date is relatively small, the identification of myocardial atrophy and/or fibrosis may have prognostic value in patients subjected to pericardial exploration. In a series of 7 patients with severe atrophy or fibrosis and pericardial thickening who underwent pericardiectomy, 100 per cent died of acute heart failure, whereas 4 (9 per cent) of 43 patients without myocardial atrophy died following pericardiectomy.[199] In assessing the role of these expensive imaging technologies, it must be emphasized that severe constrictive physiology can occur in the presence of a diseased but minimally thickened pericardium, whereas *pericardial thickening or calcification alone is not diagnostic of hemodynamically significant constrictive pericarditis.*[196]

The use of noninvasive imaging techniques, especially two-dimensional echocardiography, to assist in discrimination between constrictive pericarditis and restrictive cardiomyopathy is discussed below.

OTHER LABORATORY FINDINGS. Other abnormal laboratory findings may be present as a result of chronic elevation of right atrial pressure causing passive congestion of the liver, kidneys, and gastrointestinal tract. These include depressed serum albumin, elevated serum globulin, elevated conjugated and unconjugated serum bilirubin, and abnormal hepatocellular function tests. In patients with hepatomegaly and ascites, liver biopsy may show histological features similar to the Budd-Chiari syndrome, including hepatic venule thrombi and ductular proliferation.[200] Chylous ascites may occur because of impedance of lymphatic drainage due to central venous hypertension.[201] Protein-losing enteropathy may be evident from the presence of albumin in the stool and lymphangiectasis on small-bowel biopsy.[202] Elevated systemic venous pressure may also produce variable degrees of albuminuria as well as pronounced protein loss consistent with the nephrotic syndrome.[203] Nonspecific evidence of the presence of chronic disease such as normocytic and normochromic anemia may be found.

DIFFERENTIAL DIAGNOSIS. Constrictive pericarditis should be suspected in patients with jugular venous distention, unexplained pleural effusion, hepatomegaly, systemic edema, or ascites. It must be distinguished from superior vena caval obstruction, nephrotic syndrome, hepatic and intra-abdominal disease due to malignancy, and other cardiac causes of right atrial hypertension, including restrictive cardiomyopathy, tricuspid stenosis, tricuspid regurgitation, hypertrophic cardiomyopathy, and right atrial myxoma. It may be extremely difficult to distinguish patients with constrictive pericarditis from those with restrictive physiology due to amyloidosis, sarcoidosis, radiation injury, hemochromatosis, and the hypereosinophilic syndrome, which may involve pericardium as well as the myocardium.[204–207] Both constrictive pericarditis and restrictive cardiomyopathy may show the electrocardiographic changes of atrial fibrillation, left atrial abnormalities, and diffuse low QRS voltage with T-wave flattening. The presence of atrioventricular block and conduction disturbances simulating myocardial infarction favors the diagnosis of restrictive cardiomyopathy. Echocardiography in some patients with restrictive cardiomyopathy may show abnormal thickening of the ventricular myocardium or a peculiar "sparkling" appearance when amyloidosis is present. The simultaneous use of electrocardiography and echocardiography to demonstrate a reduction of the voltage/mass ratio has been described in patients with amyloid

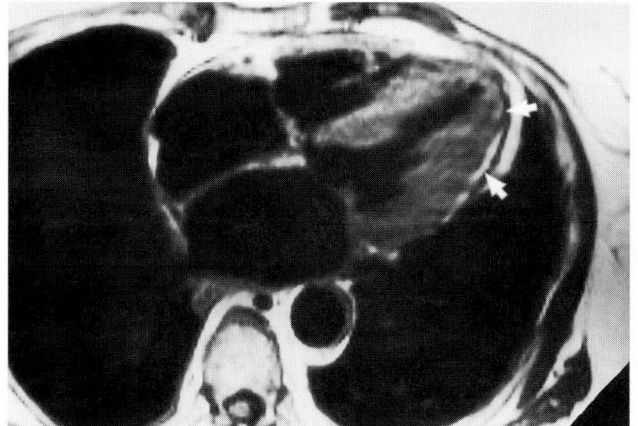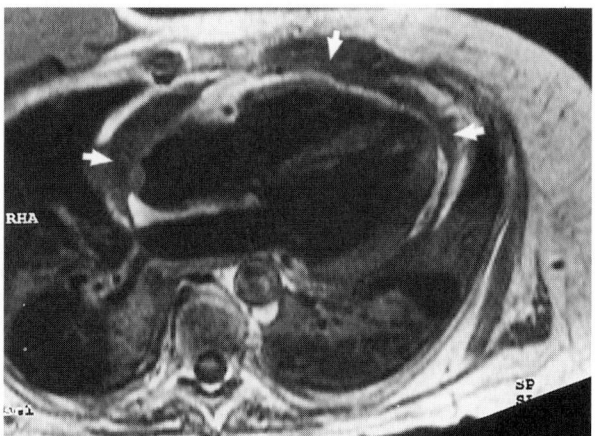

FIGURE 43–18. *Left,* Spin-echo magnetic resonance image in the transverse plane of a normal heart and thin pericardium (≤3 mm) of a normal adult. *Right,* Spin-echo magnetic resonance image (transverse plane) of the heart of a patient with a thickened pericardium (white arrows) and hemodynamic documentation of constrictive pericarditis at cardiac catheterization.

restrictive cardiomyopathy in whom diffuse low QRS voltage is associated with increased thickness of the left ventricular wall due to amyloid deposition.[208]

In the presence of findings suggestive of constrictive pericarditis, right- and left-heart catheterization should be performed to document the presence of constrictive physiology and to exclude other causes of right atrial hypertension. Diuresis should be avoided prior to catheterization because hypovolemia may obscure the characteristic hemodynamic findings. MRI, cardiac catheterization, and angiography, often with endomyocardial biopsy, are usually decisive in discriminating between constrictive pericarditis and restrictive cardiomyopathy in many patients, but in a small minority exploratory thoracotomy may be required.

Cardiac Catheterization and Angiography

Cardiac catheterization is useful in the assessment of patients suspected of having constrictive pericarditis to (1) document the presence of elevation and equilibration of actually diastolic filling pressures, (2) assess the effect of constrictive pericarditis on stroke volume and cardiac output, (3) evaluate myocardial systolic function, (4) assist in the difficult discrimination between constrictive pericarditis and restrictive cardiomyopathy, and (5) exclude compression of the coronary arteries or regional outflow tract compression by the fibrotic pericardium.

Catheterization of both the right and left ventricles should be performed to permit simultaneous recording of right and left heart filling pressures. Typical findings include the elevation and virtual identity (within 5 mm Hg) of right atrial, right ventricular diastolic, left atrial (pulmonary capillary wedge), and left ventricular diastolic pressures before the *a* wave. Right atrial pressure is characterized by a preserved systolic *x* descent, a prominent early diastolic *y* descent, and *a* and *v* waves that are small and equal in height and result in the typical M or W configurations (Fig. 43–19). Both the right and left ventricular diastolic pressures show an early diastolic dip followed by a plateau. This sign may be obscured by the presence of tachycardia, although the equilibration of diastolic pressures persists during exercise (Fig. 43–20), and by the damping effect of connecting tubes or bubbles within the catheters and transducers. Right ventricular and pulmonary artery systolic pressures are usually modestly elevated, in the range of 35 to 40 mm Hg, and rarely exceed 60 mm Hg. When hemodynamics in the baseline state are unremarkable, the rapid infusion of about 1000 ml of warmed saline over 6 to 8 minutes may unmask these findings in the rare patient with occult constrictive pericarditis.[209]

Careful recordings during respiration show that mean right atrial pressure fails to decrease normally or actually rises during inspiration. Because inspiration is associated with transient pooling of blood within the pulmonary bed and reduction in right ventricular afterload, inspiration causes a fall in pulmonary artery and right ventricular systolic pressures, pulmonary capillary wedge pressure, and left ventricular diastolic pressure. Because constrictive pericarditis is associated with inspiratory swings in right ventricular filling which are less marked than those observed in cardiac tamponade, pulsus paradoxus is usually absent or less prominent than that observed in cardiac tamponade. Both cardiac output and stroke volume are low-normal or depressed. When they are depressed, compensatory tachy-

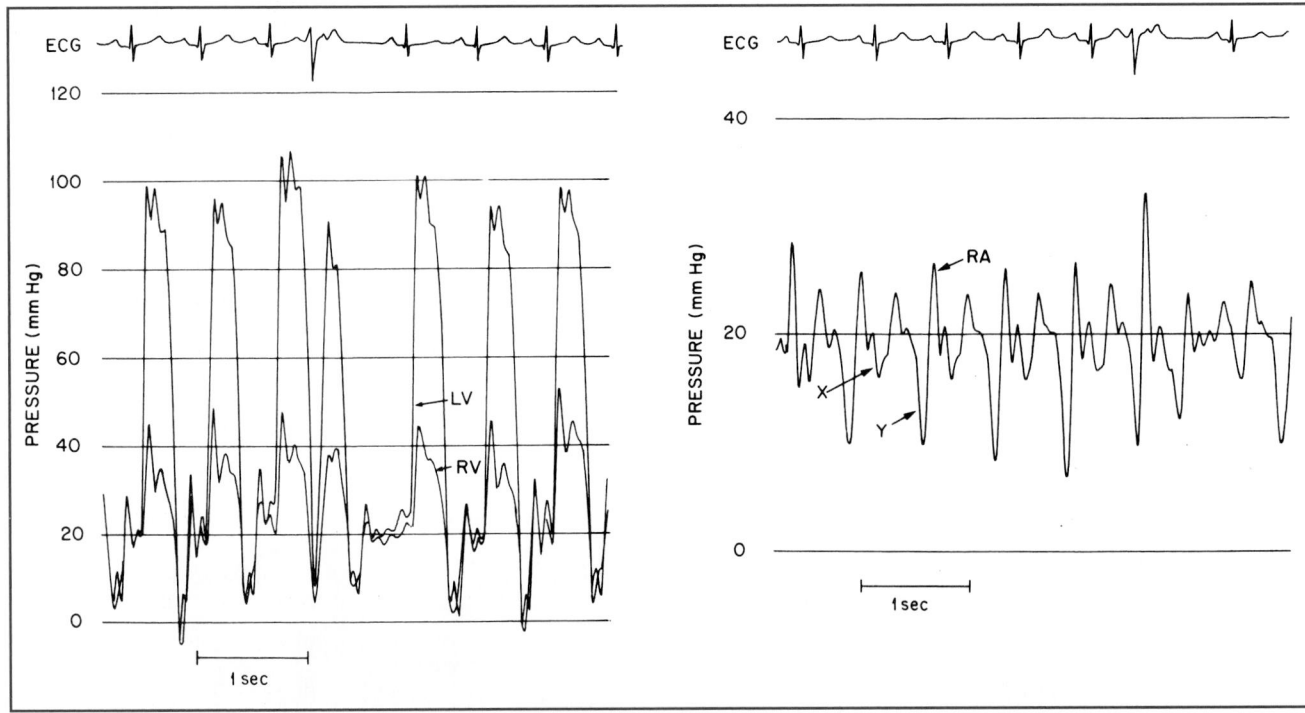

FIGURE 43–19. *Left,* Left (LV) and right (RV) ventricular pressures recorded simultaneously in the same patient with constrictive pericarditis illustrate that the presence of resting tachycardia partially obscures evaluation of the diastolic waveforms, and underdamping of the left ventricular pressure-transducer system accentuates an undershoot of left ventricular pressure in early diastole and an overshoot during atrial contraction. A long diastole following a premature beat permits the recognition of equilibrium of left and right ventricular diastolic pressures and the appreciation of a dip-and-plateau component of the ventricular waveform. *Right,* Right atrial (RA) pressure recording from a patient with constrictive pericarditis, illustrating that the pressure is elevated and equal throughout diastole. Note the prominent Y descent in the right atrial waveform, which indicates that the right atrial emptying is rapid and unimpeded in early diastole. The nadir of the Y descent corresponds with the abrupt cessation of early diastolic ventricular filling. The prominent X and Y descents give the right atrial waveform its characteristic M- or W-shaped appearance in constrictive pericarditis. (From Lorell, B. H., and Grossman, W.: Profiles in constrictive pericarditis, restrictive cardiomyopathy, and cardiac tamponade. *In* Grossman, W., and Baim, D. S. [eds.]: Cardiac Catheterization and Angiography. Philadelphia, Lea and Febiger, 1995).

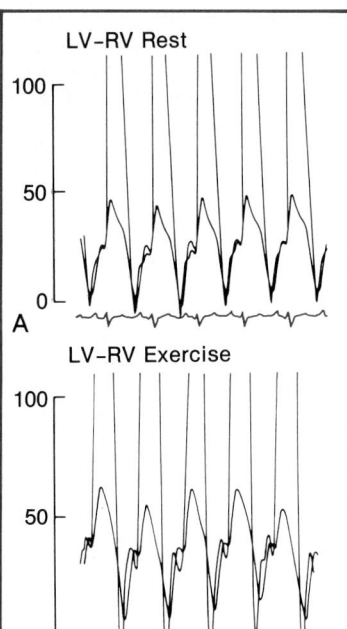

FIGURE 43–20. Representative left (LV) and right ventricular (RV) pressure tracings obtained at rest *(A)* and during exercise *(B)* from a patient with constrictive pericarditis. The diastolic equalization of pressures that is present at rest persists during exercise when the diastolic pressure of both ventricles is substantially higher. (From Robbins, M. A., et al.: Resting and exercise hemodynamics in constrictive pericarditis and a case of cardiac amyloidosis mimicking constriction. Cathet. Cardiovasc. Diagn. *9:*463, 1983.)

cardia and an elevation of systemic vascular resistance may be found.

The left ventricular angiogram usually demonstrates that left ventricular end-systolic and end-diastolic volumes are normal or decreased. In the absence of myocardial fibrosis or inflammation, both isovolumic and ejection phase indices of systolic function are normal. Venous angiography or simple fluoroscopy may demonstrate dilatation of the superior vena cava and straightening of the right heart border; pericardial thickening may be detectable. These findings contrast with those of cardiac tamponade in which diastolic compression of the superior vena cava and right atrium is present. Coronary angiography may demonstrate that the coronary arteries are within the coronary silhouette rather than on the surface of the heart, and rarely, diastolic pinching or external compression of the coronary arteries may be detected.[164,210] In rare patients, careful hemodynamic measurements may demonstrate the presence of regional pericardial constriction causing pulmonary outflow tract obstruction, which can be confirmed by right ventricular angiography or noninvasive echocardiography or CT imaging.

HEMODYNAMIC DIFFERENTIATION AMONG CONSTRICTIVE PERICARDITIS, CARDIAC TAMPONADE, AND RESTRICTIVE CARDIOMYOPATHY

Although both constrictive pericarditis and tamponade are characterized by elevation and equilibrium of right and left ventricular diastolic pressures, several hemodynamic features differ. In contrast with patients with constrictive pericarditis, patients with cardiac tamponade demonstrate (1) marked pulsus paradoxus, (2) a fall in right atrial pressure during inspiration, (3) elevation of intrapericardial pressure, (4) a right atrial pressure tracing with a predominant x descent and absence of or an attenuated y descent, and (5) lack of a prominent dip-and-plateau pattern in the right and left ventricular pressure pulses.

The findings of cardiac catheterization help to differentiate some but not all patients with constrictive pericarditis from those with restrictive cardiomyopathy (Table 43–8) due to amyloidosis, radiation injury, hemochromatosis, or other causes. In both conditions, right

TABLE 43–8 CONSTRICTIVE PERICARDITIS VERSUS RESTRICTIVE CARDIOMYOPATHY

	CONSTRICTIVE PERICARDITIS	RESTRICTIVE CARDIOMYOPATHY
S_3 gallop	Absent	May be present
Pericardial knock	May be present	Absent
Palpable systolic apical impulse	Absent	May be present
Pericardial calcification	Present 50%	Absent
Pulsus paradoxus	May be present	May be present
Equal RV and LV diastolic pressures	Usually present	LV > RV
Rate of LV filling	80% in first half of diastole	40% in first half of diastole
PEP/LVET	Av. 0.31	Av. 0.48 (congestive failure)
CAT scan, echo, MRI	Thickened pericardium	Normal pericardium

Modified from Fowler, N. O.: Constrictive pericarditis. *In* Fowler, N. O. (ed.): The Pericardium in Health and Disease. Mt. Kisco, NY, Futura Publishing Co., 1985, p. 319.

and left ventricular diastolic pressures are elevated, stroke volume and cardiac output are depressed, left ventricular end-diastolic volume is normal or decreased, and diastolic filling is impaired. A diagnosis of restrictive cardiomyopathy is more likely when marked right ventricular systolic hypertension is present (pressure > 60 mm Hg) and left ventricular diastolic pressure exceeds right ventricular diastolic pressure at rest or during exercise by more than 5 mm Hg.[211] However, in some patients with restrictive cardiomyopathy, hemodynamics at rest and during exercise may be indistinguishable from constrictive pericarditis, with equilibration of right and left ventricular diastolic pressures and a predominant dip-and-plateau pattern in the ventricular waveforms.[145,212–214]

Angiographically, straightening of the right heart border may be present in both conditions, and thickening of the heart border may be detected as a result of either pericardial or myocardial thickening. The finding of a depressed left ventricular ejection fraction in the presence of a small heart has been suggested as a discriminating feature of restrictive cardiomyopathy. However, the left ventricular ejection fraction may be normal in some patients with restrictive cardiomyopathy and, conversely, is occasionally reduced in patients with constrictive pericarditis.[212,213]

ANALYSIS OF VENTRICULAR FILLING. Frame-by-frame analysis of left ventricular filling using left ventricular angiograms has been suggested as a method for distinguishing between constrictive pericarditis and restrictive cardiomyopathy.[215] In constrictive pericarditis, early diastolic filling tends to be excessively rapid in contrast to restrictive cardiomyopathy, in which early diastolic filling is slower than normal with greater dependence on the atrial contribution to filling. The discrimination between these patterns of left ventricular filling in constrictive pericarditis versus restrictive cardiomyopathy has also been accomplished using noninvasive methods, including the assessment of diastolic filling by radionuclide angiography[216] (Fig. 43–21), and Doppler echocardiography.[192,217]

ANALYSIS OF FLOW VELOCITIES. The use of transthoracic Doppler echocardiography for the analysis of respiratory changes in transvalvular flow velocities and the use of transesophageal Doppler echocardiography to analyze patterns of pulmonary venous flow velocity during respiration have been proposed to distinguish between these conditions.[192,217,218]

Recent clinical studies suggest that the marked respiratory variations in transvalvular, hepatic, and pulmonary flow velocities which are characteristic of constrictive pericarditis can correctly identify about 85 per cent of patients with constrictive pericarditis.[193,219,220] False-positive patterns of constrictive respiratory variations in flow velocities can occur in patients with chronic pulmonary disease and pulmonary embolism, and these respiratory flow velocity patterns can be more difficult to distinguish in patients with constrictive pericarditis and atrial fibrillation. This marked respiratory variation in Doppler flow velocities is not usually observed in restrictive cardiomyopathy (Fig. 43–22). In contrast, restrictive cardiomyopathy, including amyloid heart disease, is characterized by a spectrum of echo-Doppler abnormalities, including slowed left ventricular relaxation associated with a reduced transmitral early diastolic pressure gradient which is evident as a reduced peak velocity of early transmitral diastolic flow (E wave) and enhanced flow velocity during atrial contraction (A wave). More severe restrictive myopathy may progress to "pseudonormalization" of Doppler flow velocity patterns and to the advanced stage of "restrictive" flow patterns characterized by a short isovolumic relaxation time, increase in E wave peak velocity

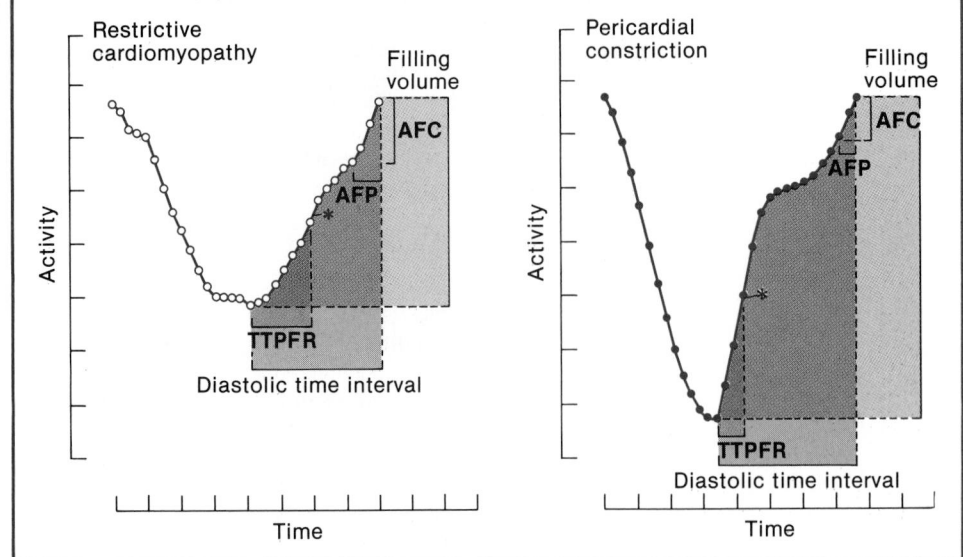

FIGURE 43–21. Time-activity curves obtained using first-pass radionuclide angiography in a patient with restrictive cardiomyopathy *(left panel)* and a patient with constrictive pericarditis *(right panel)*. The curve for the patient with constrictive pericarditis is characterized by an increased peak filling rate and an increased extent of ventricular filling, which occurs in early diastole, in contrast to the curve for the patient with restrictive cardiomyopathy that shows a "sluggish" pattern of diastolic filling with slower peak filling rate, a longer time to peak filling rate, and an enhanced atrial contribution to total left ventricular filling volume. * = peak filling rate; AFC = atrial filling contribution; TTPFR = time to peak filling rate. (From Aroney, C. N., et al.: Differentiation of restrictive cardiomyopathy from pericardial constriction: Assessment of diastolic function by radionuclide angiography. J. Am. Coll. Cardiol. *13*:1007, 1989; reprinted by permission of the American College of Cardiology.)

with shortened deceleration time, and reduced A wave peak velocity[193,220] (Fig. 3–103, p. 93, and p. 356). The presence of restrictive Doppler flow velocity patterns does not exclude constriction in a patient with clinical and hemodynamic findings of constriction.[193] In this setting, CT or MRI may be helpful to document pericardial thickening and/or the presence of myocardial atrophy or fibrosis before consideration of pericardiectomy. However, value of the assessment of filling patterns is also not clarified in the patient with suspected restrictive cardiomyopathy and mildly thickened pericardium who has a dip-and-plateau ventricular waveform that simulates constrictive physiology and itself suggests a pattern of rapid and abruptly attenuated diastolic filling.

ENDOMYOCARDIAL BIOPSY. This technique is very useful in documenting the presence of specific causes of restrictive physiology such as amyloidosis or myocarditis in patients in whom constrictive pericarditis and restrictive cardiomyopathy cannot be differentiated at cardiac catheterization.[212,221] However, normal biopsy findings do not exclude the presence of restrictive cardiomyopathy.[213] Furthermore, pericardial involvement may coexist with several causes of restrictive physiology, including amyloid heart disease, radiation-induced myopathy, and hypereosinophilic syndrome.[204–207,222] In a minority of patients, exploratory thoracotomy with careful examination of both pericardial and myocardial biopsy specimens is warranted. These examinations differentiate constrictive pericarditis, a condition that is usually treatable surgically, from restrictive cardiomyopathy, in which treatment is usually expectant.

Management

Chronic constrictive pericarditis is a progressive disease without spontaneous reversal of either pericardial thickening or abnormal symptoms and hemodynamics. A minority of patients may survive for many years with modest jugular venous distention and peripheral edema that is controlled by the judicious use of diet and diuretics. Drugs that slow the heart rate, such as beta-blockers and calcium channel blockers, should usually be avoided because mild sinus tachycardia is a compensatory mechanism.[162] The majority of patients who are symptomatic and come to medical attention, however, become progressively more disabled by weakness, ascites, and peripheral edema and subsequently suffer the complications of severe cardiac cachexia. Treatment for constrictive pericarditis is complete resection of the pericardium, which achieves excision of the pericardium from the anterior and inferior surfaces of the right ventricle and the diaphragmatic and anterolateral surfaces of the left ventricle extending to the great vessels and to or across the atrioventricular grooves. Attention must also be paid to the presence of right atrial thrombosis in association with constrictive pericarditis, which can partially obstruct the tricuspid valve and should be managed with thrombectomy at the time of pericardiectomy.[223,224] Changes in technique have included the use of median sternotomy rather than left thoracotomy, cardiopulmonary bypass to permit greater mobilization of the heart,[225] and performance of pericardiectomy earlier in the course of the disease prior to the appearance of cardiac cachexia and dense pericardial calcification. Ultrasonic debridement using an ultrasonic surgical aspiration device has been reported to be a useful adjunct to the complete surgical removal of densely calcified and adherent pericardium.[226]

RESULTS OF PERICARDIECTOMY. In 1980, Culliford et al. reported an operative mortality of 15 per cent with a range of 6 to 25 per cent in over 300 reported cases of pericardiectomy.[227] In over 800 cases reported in surgical series since 1981, the average operative mortality ranged from 5.6 to 19 per cent.[149,169,170,228–234] A low-output syndrome occurs in 14 to 28 per cent of patients in the immediate postoperative period, and risk factors predictive of in-hospital mortality and low-output syndrome include the degree of preoperative disability (functional Class III or IV) and severity of constriction as indicated by marked elevation of right ventricular end-diastolic pressure or right atrial pressure.[228,229,232]

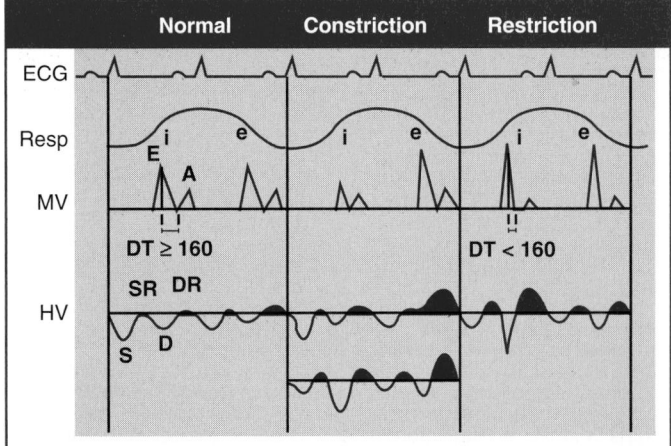

FIGURE 43–22. Representative Doppler velocity patterns of mitral valve (MV) inflow and hepatic vein (HV) inflow in normal humans, and patients with constriction or restriction. E = Peak velocity of early rapid filling; A = peak velocity of filling during atrial contraction; DT = deceleration time of early diastolic transmittal flow velocity; e = expiration; i = inspiration. (Adapted from Oh, J. K., et al.: Diagnostic role of Doppler echocardiography in constrictive pericarditis. J. Am. Coll. Cardiol. *23*:154, 1994; reprinted by permission of the American College of Cardiology.)

Among patients who survive the operation, symptomatic improvement can be expected in about 90 per cent and complete relief of symptoms in about 50 per cent of patients.[228-234]

Actuarial analysis of long-term survival has been available in large series from the Mayo Clinic,[229] Stanford,[232] Erlangen,[228] and Paris[170] which have reported a 5-year survival ranging from 74 to 87 per cent. Long-term survival and symptomatic relief do not appear to be influenced by age, choice of median sternotomy or left thoracotomy, or transient low-output syndrome postoperatively. However, overall outcome is unfavorably influenced by the presence of severe preoperative functional disability (NYHA Class III or IV, diuretic use), renal insufficiency in the preoperative state, the presence of extensive nonresectable calcifications, incomplete pericardial resection, and the presence of radiation pericarditis, which is commonly complicated by myocardial fibrosis and restrictive myocardial disease. These considerations indicate that pericardiectomy should be performed early in the course of constrictive pericarditis in symptomatic patients because the development of severe clinical disability is associated with a poor surgical outcome.

Pericardiectomy should probably not be routinely attempted in very elderly patients with severe liver dysfunction, cachexia, densely calcified pericardium, and massive cardiac enlargement indicative of underlying myocardial damage or in patients with limited life expectancy. Patients with known or suspected tubercular pericarditis should be treated with multidrug antituberculosis therapy for 2 to 4 weeks before operation; if the diagnosis is confirmed, these drugs should be continued for 6 to 12 months after pericardiectomy.

Striking hemodynamic and symptomatic improvement is apparent in some patients immediately after operation. In others, symptomatic improvement and resolution of elevated jugular venous pressure and abnormal filling patterns may be delayed for weeks to months. This delayed or inadequate response to pericardiectomy has been attributed to incomplete pericardial resection, myocardial atrophy or fibrosis caused by the inflammatory process,[233] and the development of recurrent cardiac compression by mediastinal inflammation and fibrosis.[199,232,235] The role of unrecognized constriction by an epicardial peel (visceral pericardium) as a cause for a poor response to pericardiectomy was described by Harrington in 1944[236] and subsequently confirmed.[237] The importance of visceral constriction has also been underscored by the Stanford experience in which 59 per cent of cases had involvement of the visceral pericardium (epicardium) and required visceral decortication.[232] When there is little change in size of the heart or fall in intracardiac pressures after removal of the parietal pericardial layer, considerations should be given to epicardial dissection. The worsening of underlying tricuspid or mitral regurgitation can also cause hemodynamic deterioration after pericardiectomy.[238,239]

Effusive-constrictive pericarditis is the condition of a tense pericardial effusion in the presence of visceral pericardial constriction.[240,241] *The hallmark of this condition is continued elevation of right atrial pressure after the aspiration of pericardial fluid and restoration of intrapericardial pressure to zero.* This entity may represent a stage in the development of classic constrictive pericarditis. The most common causes of effusive-constrictive pericarditis are the same as for chronic constrictive pericarditis (see p. 1498) and include idiopathic or presumed viral pericarditis, tuberculosis, neoplastic infiltration of the pericardium, and mediastinal irradiation.[240] Symptoms are nonspecific and include atypical chest pain and a heavy sensation over the precordium; in advanced cases, exertional dyspnea may be present.

The physical findings usually resemble those of cardiac tamponade, including pulsus paradoxus, normal or diminished pulse pressure, and jugular venous distention with a predominant x descent and absence of y descent. The chest roentgenogram usually shows cardiac enlargement consistent with the presence of pericardial effusion, and the electrocardiogram may show nonspecific ST- and T-wave abnormalities or diffuse low QRS voltage. Both M-mode and two-dimensional echocardiograms may show a pericardial effusion sandwiched between thickened pericardial membranes with fibrinous pericardial bands.[242]

Although effusive-constrictive pericarditis can be suspected on clinical grounds, the diagnosis is made by recording right heart and intrapericardial pressure both before and after pericardiocentesis.[240,241] Before pericardiocentesis, the physiology of cardiac tamponade may be present (see p. 1486) with elevation and equilibrium of intrapericardial, right atrial, right ventricular, and left ventricular diastolic pressures. The right atrial pressure tracing usually shows a prominent x descent and an inspiratory fall in right heart filling pressure. Pericardiocentesis with restoration of intrapericardial pressure to zero may reduce pulsus paradoxus and improve cardiac output, but it does not restore the hemodynamics entirely to normal. After pericardiocentesis, there is persistent elevation and equilibration of right atrial and right and left ventricular diastolic pressures. The waveforms convert to a pattern like that in constrictive pericarditis, with a prominent y descent in the right atrial pressure tracing, a dip-and-plateau pattern in the right ventricular pressure, and the absence of respiratory variation in right heart filling pressures.

Pericardiocentesis may be useful in transiently improving systemic arterial pressure and cardiac output. However, persistent constriction after successful pericardiocentesis indicates the presence of a thickened, constrictive visceral pericardium and the need for further intervention. Treatment consists of total parietal and visceral pericardiectomy.[232,237,240]

SPECIFIC FORMS OF PERICARDITIS

A variety of infectious organisms may be responsible for pericarditis (Table 43-9).

VIRAL PERICARDITIS

ETIOLOGY AND PATHOGENESIS. The viruses that most commonly cause acute pericarditis are coxsackievirus group B and echovirus type 8.[243,244] There are no clinical features that distinguish acute viral pericarditis from idiopathic pericarditis, and it is likely that the majority of cases of community-acquired idiopathic pericarditis are due to unrecognized viral infections. The seasonal peak incidence of idiopathic pericarditis is in the spring and fall, whereas the peak incidence of acute myocarditis with heart failure is in late winter.[245] Other viruses responsible for acute pericarditis include those that cause mumps, influenza, infectious mononucleosis, poliomyelitis, varicella, rubella, and hepatitis B, as well as vaccination against hepatitis B.[246-252] Infectious mononucleosis may cause acute myopericarditis with the complications of cardiac tamponade, constrictive pericarditis, and severe chest pain, and this cause can be confirmed by a positive heterophile test.[247] The Epstein-Barr virus genome has been demonstrated in pericar-

TABLE 43–9   ETIOLOGY OF INFECTIOUS PERICARDITIS

Viral diseases (coxsackie A and B viruses, echovirus, influenza, adenovirus, Epstein-Barr virus, chickenpox, psittacosis, AIDS, mumps, infectious mononucleosis)

Mycobacterial infections *(Mycobacterium tuberculosis, M. avium, M. intracellulare)*

Protozoa (toxoplasmosis, *Entamoeba histolytica, Trypanosoma cruzi)*

Fungal infections (histoplasma, coccidioides, blastomycosis, candida, aspergillus)

Bacterial infections *(Staphylococcus, Streptococcus,* gram-negative bacilli, meningococcus, pneumococcus, *Salmonella* species, *Brucella, Legionella, Campylobacter, Haemophilus influenzae,* Lyme disease)

Rickettsial infections

Parasitic infections (trichinosis, microfilaria, echinococcus disease)

Anaerobic organisms *(Clostridium,* anaerobic streptococci)

Miscellaneous infections *(Nocardia, Actinomyces, Mycoplasma,* psittacosis-lymphopathia venereum group)

dial tissue of a patient with pericarditis by polymerase chain reaction (PCR) and in situ hybridization.[248] Varicella (chickenpox) may be associated with the complications of severe viral pneumonia, arthritis, and/or acute pericarditis.[250] *Coxiella burnetii,* the rickettsial agent that causes tick-borne Q fever (fever, headache, pneumonitis), is also a cause of pericarditis in endemic areas.[252] Rarely, *Mycoplasma pneumoniae,* an important cause of nonbacterial pneumonia, causes myopericarditis.[254]

Cytomegalovirus may cause pericarditis in otherwise healthy adults with cytomegalovirus mononucleosis[255] and in immunocompromised patients.[256] Acute pericarditis is now being recognized with increasing frequency in the early stage of acquired immunodeficiency syndrome (AIDS) and may be idiopathic or related to specific viral pathogens.[257] However, two recent series characterizing pericarditis and pericardial effusions in patients with AIDS underscore the importance of infectious causes other than viral pathogens. In a series of 37 consecutive patients with cardiac tamponade seen at an inner-city New York hospital, 13 patients (35 per cent) had HIV infection, 2 of whom had acute purulent bacterial pericarditis and 2 had tuberculous pericarditis.[258] In another series of 50 consecutive patients with acute pericarditis and large pericardial effusion at an inner-city hospital who underwent pericardiocentesis, AIDS was present in 14 patients (28 per cent), 1 of whom had bacterial pericarditis, 1 pericardial lymphoma, and 8 (57 per cent) tuberculous pericarditis.[259] In those patients with pericarditis of "idiopathic" etiology who also have AIDS, it is not yet known if the underlying pathogens are the enteroviruses that most commonly cause pericarditis or HIV itself.

PATHOLOGY. Viral pericarditis causes inflammation of the visceral and parietal pericardial membranes, with infiltration first of polymorphonuclear leukocytes and then of lymphocytes around small vessels. Fibrin is deposited in the pericardial space, giving the pericardium a shaggy, reddened appearance. In some cases the inflammation may result in a serous, serofibrinous, suppurative, or hemorrhagic effusion with a predominance of lymphocytes. Both echoviruses and coxsackieviruses may produce suppurative effusions that resolve by organization, formation of thick adhesions, calcification, and a thickening of the pericardium, resulting in constrictive pericarditis.[260]

CLINICAL FINDINGS. A prodromal syndrome of an upper respiratory tract infection that may be described as a "cold" or "the flu" within the preceding weeks is frequently reported by patients with viral pericarditis. The clinical features of viral pericarditis are similar to those of acute pericarditis of many causes, which were described earlier (see p. 1482). Viral or idiopathic pericarditis should be suspected in young or otherwise healthy adults with a characteristic prodromal illness and a syndrome of acute pericardial pain. It must be differentiated from pericarditis due to trauma, purulent pericardial infection, myocarditis, and systemic lupus erythematosus. HIV infection is common in young patients who present with pericarditis and large pericardial effusions at inner-city hospitals.[258,259] In young patients who present with acute pericarditis with effusions in urban settings in which HIV is endemic, the coexistence of pulmonary infiltrates and fever is suggestive of underlying HIV infection and an increased risk of purulent bacterial or tuberculous pericarditis. In older patients, the possibility that pericarditis may be due to rheumatoid disorders, myocardial infarction, tuberculosis, or neoplasm should be investigated before one presumes a viral etiology.

The diagnosis of viral infection is strongly supported by the finding of a greater than fourfold rise in serial neutralizing viral antibody titers during the initial 3 weeks of illness. It is rarely productive to attempt to isolate virus from blood, pericardial fluid, pleural fluid, or stool. The development of reverse immunoassays (RIA) of antibodies to enteroviruses holds promise for studies of the role of these viruses in acute pericarditis. Frisk et al. evaluated the incidence of positive coxsackie B-specific IgM RIA titers that were detected in 97 per cent of 30 patients with proven enterovirus infections and in 49 per cent of 37 patients with idiopathic myopericarditis, while positive responses were rare in control specimens from normal subjects.[261] A similar incidence (44 per cent) of acute group B coxsackie viral infection has been reported in a cohort of 95 patients with acute myopericarditis.[262] It is of interest that enterovirus-specific IgM and IgA titers indicative of persistent enterovirus infection have been shown in a series of patients with chronic relapsing pericarditis in whom the persistence of chronically high levels of antibody differed from a cohort of patients with a single episode of acute pericarditis.[263]

Recent advances in pericardioscopy and optically directed pericardial and epicardial biopsy offer the potential for the diagnosis of both viral and tuberculous pericarditis using molecular techniques of in situ hybridization and PCR.[156,248,256] However, in the case of common viral pathogens such as Coxsackievirus, echovirus, and Epstein-Barr virus, the prevalence of viral genome which can be detected in the heart by sensitive PCR technology in the general population versus patients with acute or chronic pericarditis is not yet known.

The diagnosis of acute pericarditis of probable viral etiology is confirmed clinically by the finding of a characteristic pericardial friction rub. Serial electrocardiographic changes of acute pericarditis (see p. 1483) are not specific for either viral or idiopathic pericarditis; however, the appearance of characteristic electrocardiographic changes may lead to the recognition of pericardial involvement in patients with a viral upper respiratory tract infection. Echocardiographic documentation of substantial pericardial effusion is also supportive evidence of pericardial inflammation in a patient with a viral upper respiratory tract infection and chest pain. Other laboratory findings suggestive of inflammation but not diagnostic of pericarditis include elevation of the sedimentation rate and leukocytosis. Cardiac isoenzymes are frequently abnormally elevated and suggest the presence of extensive associated epicarditis or myocarditis.[67]

NATURAL HISTORY. Acute viral or idiopathic pericarditis is usually a short, dramatic, self-limited illness lasting 1 to 3 weeks. Important complications of acute viral or idiopathic pericarditis include (1) associated myocarditis, (2) recurrent pericarditis, (3) pericardial effusion with cardiac tamponade, and (4) the late development of constrictive pericarditis (see p. 1494). Acute myocarditis, which may develop in association with pericarditis due to coxsackieviruses and echoviruses, may result in acute congestive heart failure, arrhythmias, or conduction disturbances, and cardiac enlargement that usually resolves completely or rarely leads to the development of a chronic congestive cardiomyopathy. Pericarditis may recur several weeks later in about 20 to 30 per cent of patients, and a small number of patients develop disabling recurrences over months to years that are extremely difficult to manage. It is unclear whether recurrences of pericardial pain in patients with enterovirus pericarditis are due to an immunological response to the initial viral injury, recurrent viral infections of the pericardium, or relapsing chronic viral infection.[263]

MANAGEMENT. Treatment is directed against symptoms, with close observation for the development of cardiac tamponade for myocarditis early in the course of the disease. The management of patients with acute viral pericarditis has already been discussed (see p. 1484).

TUBERCULOUS PERICARDITIS

ETIOLOGY AND PATHOGENESIS. In industrialized nations, the incidence of tuberculosis pericarditis has decreased within the past four decades as a result of effective chemotherapy and public health surveillance. In this setting, it is now a very uncommon cause of acute pericarditis except in patients with AIDS. In a series of 231 consecutive patients whose disease was evaluated prospectively using a rigorous protocol that included pericardiocentesis and biopsy, tuberculosis was diagnosed in only 4 per cent of patients and in 7 per cent of the subset of patients who developed cardiac tamponade.[69] Similarly, tuberculous pericarditis was reported in none of 145 patients who required pericardial drainage[150] and in only 6 per cent of 231 patients who underwent pericardiectomy for chronic constriction[229] at the Mayo Clinic. The incidence of tuberculous pericarditis among patients with pulmonary tuberculosis ranges from about 1 to 8 per cent.[264] The disease continues to be important in immunosuppressed patients and in patients with AIDS.[258,259] Pericarditis can also be caused by atypical mycobacteria in association with AIDS. It is also a major cause of pericarditis among the underprivileged, including South and West African blacks, the black poor of the United States, and Asian and African immigrants.[265-268] For example, in Transkei, South Africa, tuberculous pericarditis with secondary constriction is the second most common cause of "heart failure" after rheumatic heart disease.[266]

Tuberculous pericarditis usually develops by retrograde spread from peribronchial, peritracheal, or mediastinal lymph nodes or by early hematogenous spread from the primary tuberculous infection. Less commonly, the pericardium is involved by the breakdown and contiguous spread of a necrotic tuberculous lesion in the lung, pleura, or spine or by hematogenous spread from distant secondary genitourinary or skeletal infections.[269,270]

PATHOLOGY. Tuberculous pericarditis usually begins with diffuse fibrin deposits, granuloma formation, and the presence of viable acid-fast bacilli.[269] A pericardial effusion then develops, which may be serous but more often contains some blood with a protein content exceeding 2.5 gm/dl. Although polymorphonuclear leukocytes are present early in the development of the effusion, they are later replaced by lymphocytes, monocytes, and plasma cells. Both complement-fixing antimyolemmal and antimyosin types of antibodies have been demonstrated in about 75 per cent of patients with acute tuberculous pericarditis, in contrast to the much lower incidence in patients with viral pericarditis or constrictive pericarditis due to tuberculosis, which suggests that cytolysis mediated by antimyolemmal antibodies may contribute to the development of exudative tuberculous pericarditis.[271] When a tuberculous pericardial effusion accumulates rapidly, even a small effusion may produce cardiac tamponade. As the effusion is absorbed, the pericardium thickens, granulomas proliferate, and a thick coat of fibrin is deposited on the parietal pericardium. At this stage, viable acid-fast bacilli may no longer be present, but caseation may develop and penetrate the myocardium. Finally, fibrous pericarditis develops as the granulomatous reaction is replaced by fibrous tissue and collagen. These changes are followed by the accumulation of cholesterol crystals and the development of pericardial calcification. Constrictive pericarditis develops ultimately in almost all patients with untreated tuberculous pericarditis and in about half or less of the patients who receive antituberculosis chemotherapy.[267,272-275]

CLINICAL MANIFESTATIONS. Tuberculous pericarditis is usually detected clinically either in the effusive stage or late, i.e., after the development of constrictive pericarditis. It usually develops slowly, with nonspecific systemic symptoms such as fever, night sweats, fatigue, and dyspnea.[266,272,273] In South Africa, right upper abdominal aching

due to liver congestion is common in patients with effusive tuberculous pericarditis.[266,272] A torpid course is not invariably present, and an acute illness of less than 2 weeks' duration was described in four of nine patients in whom tuberculous pericarditis was diagnosed during a prospective evaluation of acute pericarditis.[69] Severe pericardial pain of acute onset characteristic of viral and idiopathic pericarditis is uncommon in tuberculous pericarditis.[273,276,277] Heavy sputum production, cough, and hemoptysis—clues to the presence of cavitary pulmonary tuberculosis—are usually absent.

Abnormalities of *physical examination* usually include fever, sinus tachycardia, and pericardial friction rub. In South African patients with tuberculous pericardial effusion, evidence of chronic cardiac compression that mimics heart failure is by far the most common presentation. In one series of 88 patients with effusive tuberculous pericarditis, jugular venous distention was present in 88 per cent, hepatomegaly in 95 per cent, and ascites in 73 per cent, whereas a pericardial friction rub was heard in only 18 per cent.[266] If the complications of cardiac tamponade or effusive-constrictive pericarditis are present, the physical examination may reveal edema, jugular venous distention, pulsus paradoxus, distant heart sounds, hepatomegaly, and ascites. The chest roentgenogram usually shows an enlarged cardiac silhouette, and pleural effusions may be detected in about half the patients. However, the apices and hila of the lung are usually normal, and pulmonary infiltrates or calcification is present in a minority of the patients.

The clinical presentation of patients with tuberculous pericarditis who develop chronic constrictive pericarditis differs from those with acute or subacute effusive tuberculous pericarditis. Dramatic symptoms such as high fever, night sweats, and precordial pain are uncommon. Findings compatible with severe chronic systemic venous congestion with low output predominate, including jugular venous distention, hypotension with a low pulse pressure, abdominal distention, edema, and muscle wasting. Dyspnea related to large pleural effusions is common.[266,272]

During the transition from effusion to constrictive pericarditis, dense, frond-like echoes or transient masses may be appreciated in the pericardial space.[278] Gallium-67 uptake in the pericardium is a nonspecific indicator of pericardial inflammation and can occur in tuberculous, purulent, and acute nonspecific pericarditis.[279]

DIAGNOSIS. Tuberculous pericarditis should be suspected in patients with fever and unexplained cardiomegaly, particularly those who are susceptible to tuberculosis, i.e., the underprivileged or immunosuppressed, and those at risk for underlying HIV infection. In a minority of patients with pericarditis, a definitive diagnosis of a tuberculous origin may be made by culture or histological demonstration of tuberculosis outside the pericardium (sputum, gastric wash, pleural fluid, liver or bone marrow biopsy). A definitive diagnosis can be made by isolation of the bacillus from the pericardial fluid or pericardial biopsy. It is difficult to establish a definitive bacteriological diagnosis because of (1) the low yield of the bacillus when pericardial fluid is examined by acid-fast stain on microscopy, (2) the failure of the bacillus to grow on appropriate media or in guinea pigs, even in patients with known tuberculous pericardial effusion, and (3) the need to observe bacterial cultures for at least 8 weeks. The probability of obtaining a definitive diagnosis is greatest if both pericardial fluid and a pericardial biopsy specimen are examined early in the effusive stage,[277,280] and may be enhanced by the one of the new techniques of pericardioscopy and optically guided pericardial biopsy (see p. 1496).[156] However, it must be emphasized that a normal pericardial biopsy result does not exclude tuberculous pericarditis because in some patients examination of the entire pericardium removed at pericardiectomy or autopsy is required to demonstrate clear-cut evidence of tuberculosis.[277,281] Furthermore, the finding of granulomas and caseous material without viable bacilli is also not diagnostic of tuberculous pericarditis because these findings can be present in chronic pericardial disease due to rheumatoid arthritis and sarcoidosis. The measurement of a high level of adenosine deaminase activity (>40 units/liter) in pleural or pericardial fluid, although not diagnostic, is supportive of a diagnosis of tuberculous pericarditis.[282] In a prospective study of 26 patients with large pericardial effusion who underwent therapeutic pericardioscopy with drainage and biopsy, a level of adenosine deaminase activity of 40 units/liter or higher in pericardial fluid had a sensitivity of 93 per cent and specificity of 97 per cent for the diagnosis of tuberculous pericarditis.[282] Furthermore, the combined measurement of adenosine deaminase and carcinoembryonic antigen in pericardial effusion discriminated patients with tuberculous pericarditis from those with malignant effusion. Tuberculous pericarditis has also been presumptively diagnosed by PCR in pericardial biopsy specimen.[283]

It may be necessary to make a presumptive clinical diagnosis of tuberculous pericarditis in severely ill patients with a large hemorrhagic pericardial effusion, a positive tuberculin skin test, and systemic symptoms such as weight loss and anorexia, even when examinations of the pericardial fluid and biopsy do not reveal tuberculosis. In such patients, clinical improvement may occur after initiation of antituberculosis chemotherapy. It should be emphasized that the tuberculin skin test alone is not a reliable indicator of tuberculous pericarditis because it may be negative in as many as 30 per cent of patients with documented tuberculosis due to anergy, and is positive in about 30 to 40 per cent of patients with acute idiopathic pericarditis and benign natural history.[69,168] Making a presumptive clinical diagnosis of tuberculous pericarditis requires careful judgment because; on the one hand, treatment should not be withheld from seriously ill patients, while, on the other, it is not prudent to commit patients with nontuberculous effusions to a prolonged course of multiple-drug antituberculosis therapy. The systematic approach suggested by Permanyer-Miralda et al. (see p. 1484) appears to have a high likelihood of identifying patients with tuberculous pericarditis with very low risk of either missing active tuberculosis or inappropriately applying blind antituberculous therapy.[69] This strategy remains to be validated in other populations, such as patients at high risk for HIV infection.

MANAGEMENT. In the era before antituberculosis chemotherapy, tuberculous pericarditis was rapidly fatal, with an early mortality rate greater than 80 per cent; the remaining patients had a protracted course of months to years with frequently fatal outcome due to miliary tuberculosis or constrictive pericarditis. Since the introduction of early chemotherapy, mortality from acute tuberculous pericarditis has fallen to less than 50 per cent, but the effectiveness of antituberculosis chemotherapy in preventing the development of constrictive pericarditis is controversial.[273,274] In a recent series of 294 consecutive patients with acute pericarditis, 13 patients were shown to have tuberculous pericarditis and 7 of these (54 per cent) developed constrictive pericarditis requiring pericardiectomy.[277]

Treatment of tuberculous pericarditis includes hospitalization with bedrest and particular attention to findings of physical examination, electrocardiography, and echocardiography that suggest the development of an enlarging pericardial effusion and tamponade or constrictive pericarditis. Initial chemotherapy should usually consist of a three-drug regimen, such as oral isoniazid, oral ethambutol, and intramuscular streptomycin. The use of corticosteroids has been advocated to reduce pericardial inflammation and enhance resorption of pericardial effusion.

In a controlled trial in South Africa, 143 patients with tuberculous pericarditis and clinical signs of constrictive physiology were randomized to receive antitubercular drug therapy with prednisolone or placebo added during the first 11 weeks of treatment.[284] In this trial, clinical improvement occurred more rapidly, and there was a lower mortality at 24 months (4 versus 11 per cent) and a lower requirement for pericardiectomy (21 versus 30 per cent) in the prednisolone versus placebo-treated cohort. The use of steroids earlier in the course of tuberculous pericarditis before the development of constrictive physiology has not been studied in a clinical trial. We believe that corticosteroids should be reserved for critically ill patients with recurrent large effusion who do not respond to pericardial drainage and antituberculosis drugs alone.

In patients with documented cardiac tamponade or with a large pericardial effusion seen on the echocardiogram, the effusion should be drained initially by percutaneous pericardiocentesis with continued catheter drainage. Pericardiectomy should be performed after 4 to 6 weeks of antituberculosis drug therapy if patients develop large recurrent effusions or cardiac compression due to effusive-constrictive disease or early constrictive pericarditis.[273,284] Pericardiectomy should be performed early in the course in patients with clinical and hemodynamic evidence of chronic cardiac compression with anticipation of a good outcome. In a South African study of 113 patients with severe constrictive tuberculous pericarditis who underwent pericardiectomy, 97 per cent were discharged from the hospital; in the majority, hepatomegaly and edema promptly resolved, whereas resolution of venous congestion required 2 to 3 months in some patients.[285] Mortality is higher among patients who undergo pericardiectomy at the late stage of calcific pericardial constriction.[265,285]

BACTERIAL (PURULENT) PERICARDITIS

Although the clinical spectrum of bacterial purulent pericarditis has changed over the past five decades, mortality remains high. Since the introduction of antibiotics in the 1940's, the overall incidence as well as the incidence of bacterial pericarditis detected at autopsy have decreased.[286,287] Purulent pericarditis continues to occur primarily as a complication of pneumonia or empyema due to staphylococci, pneumococci, and streptococci.[287,288] Acute self-limited pericarditis has also been observed in young adults with acute streptococcal tonsillitis in the absence of rheumatic fever.[289] The incidence of hospital-acquired penicillin-resistant staphylococcal pericarditis in post-thoracotomy patients has increased, and there is a widened spectrum of organisms responsible for bacterial pericarditis, including non-group A streptococcus[290] the gram-negative bacilli (*Proteus, Escherichia coli, Pseudomonas, Klebsiella*),[286] *Brucella melitensis*,[291] *Salmonella* species,[292,293] *Neisseria gonorrhoeae*,[294] *Haemophilus influenzae*,[295] *Francisella tularensis*,[296] and other unusual pathogens.[297-301]

Purulent pericarditis is rarely caused by anaerobic bacteria, and a recent review of 30 cases showed that isolated anaerobic bacteria were identified in 57 per cent and with a mixture of facultative or aerobic bacteria in 43 per cent of cases.[302] Infection usually occurs from a contiguous source of infection or via hematogenous seeding related to subdiaphragmatic or intrapulmonary abscess, gastrointestinal malignancy or rupture, and rarely in association with gas gangrene due to *Clostridium septicemia*.[297,302-305] It is now established that *Neisseria meningitidis*, particularly from serogroup C and W, can cause either a primary infection of the pericardium in the absence of meningitis, or secondary pericarditis complicating meningitis and sepsis.[306] *Legionella pneumophila*, the causative organism in legionnaire's disease, has been reported as a cause of purulent pericarditis associated with pneumonia and as a primary infection.[307] Important predisposing factors for the development of purulent pericarditis include a preexisting pericardial effusion as in uremic pericarditis, as well as immunosuppression due to burns, immunotherapy, lymphoma, leukemia, or AIDS (see p. 1506).

The routes of pericardial infection have also changed. Direct pulmonary extension of bacterial pneumonia or empyema now accounts for between 20 and 50 per cent of cases of purulent pericarditis.[287,297] Today, purulent pericarditis tends to occur in adults via (1) contiguous spread from an early postoperative infection after thoracic surgery or trauma, (2) infection related to infective endocarditis, (3) extension from a subdiaphragmatic suppurative source, and (4) hematogenous spread during bacteremia.

In patients with endocarditis, bacterial pericarditis is a life-threatening complication that is detected ante mortem in about 1 of 25 patients with endocarditis,[308] in about 1 of 8 patients with endocarditis studied at autopsy, and in a higher percentage of those with staphylococcal endocarditis.[286] In such patients, bacterial pericarditis may develop (1) by extension from a valve ring abscess, (2) by rupture of an aneurysm, (3) by extension from a myocardial abscess, or (4) from a septic coronary embolus.[309] An infected myocardial infarction or aortic aneurysm may also be a source for the development of purulent bacterial pericarditis. In patients with AIDS, the high rate of skin and nasal colonization and use of intravenous catheters contribute to the development of *Staphylococcus aureus* pericarditis.[310] Extension of a subdiaphragmatic abscess into the pericardial space is a rare source of purulent pericarditis.[302,305]

BACTERIAL PERICARDITIS IN CHILDREN. In children, the most common organisms include *Staphylococcus aureus* followed by *Haemophilus influenzae* and *Neisseria meningitis*.[311,312] *H. influenzae* pericarditis has been increasingly recognized in young children and is usually characterized by a mild prodromal illness followed by the rapid development of cardiac compression and death due to pericardial effusion.[313,314] Pediatric illnesses associated with the development of bacterial pericarditis include pharyngitis, pneumonia, meningitis, otitis media, impetigo, endocarditis, and bacterial arthritis. The development of bacterial pericarditis in infants and children carries a high mortality—approaching 70 per cent, depending on the organism, and the risk of extremely rapid early development of constrictive pericarditis, if it is not diagnosed early.[311,315] The high mortality in children appears to be reduced by early diagnosis and combined treatment with parenteral antibiotics and open surgical pericardial drainage, if effusion recurs after initial pericardiocentesis. Following this contemporary approach for parenteral antibiotics and early drainage of purulent fluid, a recent series of purulent pericarditis in children reported a mortality of 2 per cent without late development of constriction.[311]

PATHOLOGY. Bacterial pericarditis is usually frankly suppurative by the time it is detected clinically. The inflammation may result in organization and dense adhesions with a loculated pericardial effusion followed by obliteration of the pericardial space, thickening, and eventual calcification of the pericardium. In some patients, the inflammation may involve the adjacent sternum, pleura, and diaphragm with formation of dense adhesions between the parietal pericardium and contiguous structures. The evolution of this inflammatory process has been studied in an animal model of pericarditis caused by the injection of heat-killed staphylococci into the pericardial space.[316]

CLINICAL FEATURES. Bacterial pericarditis is usually an acute fulminant illness of only a few days' duration. In one series,[297] the mean duration of symptoms prior to hospitalization was only 3 days. High fevers, shaking chills, night sweats, and dyspnea are common. In most patients the symptom of typical pericardial chest pain is absent. Tachycardia is present in nearly all patients, but a pericardial friction rub is present in less than half. In many cases the pericarditis remains unsuspected because of the dominant presence of symptoms and signs related to an underlying known infection, such as pneumonia or mediastinitis following complicated thoracic surgery or trauma. The appearance of new jugular venous distention and pulsus paradoxus may be the first evidence of pericardial involvement, and these ominous signs reflect the development of cardiac tamponade due to the acute accumulation of suppurative fluid under pressure. In one series, cardiac tamponade developed acutely in 38 per cent of patients with previously unsuspected purulent pericarditis and contributed to death in the majority.[297]

LABORATORY FINDINGS. These usually include a leukocytosis with a marked leftward shift. The chest roentgenogram usually shows enlargement of the cardiac shadow and, less commonly, widening of the mediastinitis. In the majority of cases the roentgenogram shows evidence of underlying pneumonia, empyema, or mediastinitis. Electrocardiographic changes typically include ST-segment and T-wave changes characteristic of pericarditis in the majority of patients. The appearance of electrical alternans suggests the possibility of cardiac tamponade. In patients with suspected infective endocarditis, the appearance of a prolonged P-R interval, atrioventricular dissociation, or bundle branch block is strong evidence of extension of infection from the valve ring into the adjacent myocardium. The latter is an important predisposing factor for the development of pericarditis, especially in patients with staphylococcal endocarditis.[297]

PERICARDIAL FLUID. This usually shows polymorphonuclear leukocytosis and sometimes frank pus. Pericardial glucose levels are usually depressed, and the protein content is increased; lactate dehydrogenase values may also be markedly elevated.

Purulent bacterial pericarditis should be suspected in a debilitated patient with unexplained high spiking fevers, dyspnea, markedly elevated white blood cell count, and an increase in the size of the cardiac silhouette on chest roentgenogram. The key to the diagnosis, which unfortunately is frequently not made before death, is a high index of suspicion. An echocardiogram should be promptly obtained to look for evidence of a new pericardial effusion and/or loculation of fluid with adhesions. Spontaneous contrast echoes in a patient with suspected purulent pericarditis raise the possibility of a gas-producing bacterial infection.[317] Both indium and gallium scintigraphy have been reported to show a "halo sign" of increased pericardial tracer uptake in bacterial pericarditis, but this finding can also be seen in viral, tuberculous, and other forms of pericarditis.[279,318,319]

NATURAL HISTORY. Despite the lower incidence of purulent bacterial pericarditis in the antibiotic era, overall survival continues to be extremely poor, averaging about 30 per cent in modern series.[297,320] The poor prognosis stems in large part from failure of clinical diagnosis before death. In patients treated only with antibiotics without pericardial drainage, the rapid unsuspected development of a large pericardial effusion may result in sudden cardiovascular collapse and death due to cardiac tamponade. The high mortality from purulent pericarditis can be reduced substantially through the institution of both appropriate parenteral antibiotic therapy and early complete surgical drainage.[287,297,320,321] Early surgical drainage of the pericardium may help to prevent the complication of constrictive pericarditis. In a recent surgical series of pericardiectomy with antibiotic treatment, the surgical mortality was 8 per cent, with a 5-year survival of 91 per cent and no late cases of pericardial constriction.[321] Successful treatment of bacterial endocarditis with long-term simple catheter drainage of the pericardial space has been reported, but experience with this approach is limited.[322,323] The instillation of intrapericardial urokinase in three patients with purulent fibrinous pericarditis has also been reported.[323]

Meningococcal Pericarditis. The pericardium may become infected early during meningococcal sepsis (in the presence or absence of meningitis), causing purulent pericarditis with cardiac tamponade, as described earlier. In these cases the pericardial fluid is frankly purulent, and viable organisms can usually be isolated. In addition, sterile pericarditis may occur late in the convalescent period in association with arthritis, pleuritis, and ophthalmitis. This syndrome appears to have an immunological cause, does not require further antibiotic therapy if the primary infection has been adequately treated, and responds to antiinflammatory agents. Febrile, self-limited polyserositis with pericarditis has also been reported after effective treatment of sepsis due to *Staphylococcus aureus*,[324] and in young adults with acute streptococcal tonsillitis in the absence of rheumatic fever.[289]

MANAGEMENT. Suspicion of the presence of purulent pericardial fluid is an indication to explore the pericardial space. This may be done by percutaneous pericardiocentesis only if there is echocardiographic evidence of a large anterior and posterior pericardial effusion that may be safely tapped or, preferably, by a generous subxiphoid pericardiotomy with thorough pericardial drainage. Both pericardial fluid and pericardial tissue should be immediately studied by means of Gram-stained, acid-fast, and fungal smears by an experienced examiner. The fluid should then be cultured for aerobic and anaerobic bacteria with appropriate antibiotic sensitivity testing and for fungi and tuberculosis. Pericardial fluid should also be examined; the number of white blood cells, the differential count, hematocrit, and glucose and protein content should be determined. Cultures of blood, sputum, and recent surgical wounds should also be obtained.

Results of Gram staining of the pericardial fluid should be used in the selection of antibiotic therapy. If the effusion is purulent but no organisms can be easily identified and tuberculosis is not considered likely, therapy should be initiated with both a semisynthetic antistaphylococcal antibiotic and an aminoglycoside. Depending on the results of the cultures of the pericardial fluid and blood, antibiotic therapy may then be modified. High concentrations of antibiotics can be achieved in pericardial fluid, so that instillation of antibiotics into the pericardial space is not warranted.[325] However, systemic antibiotics alone are inadequate treatment, and prompt and thorough surgical drainage of the pericardium is essential in almost all patients with bacterial pericarditis.[297,313,321] Percutaneous aspiration of a large effusion may be extremely helpful in making an initial bacteriological diagnosis and initiating therapy, and percutaneous aspiration followed by catheter drainage is sometimes effective in preventing recurrent effusion.[322,323,326] However, purulent pericardial effusions are likely to recur, and more extensive surgical drainage may be needed in some patients after antibiotic therapy has been initiated. Open drainage, through creation of a subxiphoid pericardiotomy, is usually adequate when the diagnosis is made early and when the pericardial fluid is thin and the pericardium minimally thickened. This procedure is also the preferred route of drainage in severely disabled patients because it can be performed under local anesthesia and avoids the pleural cavities. In a patient with a thick purulent effusion and dense adhesions with loculation, extensive pericardiectomy is needed to achieve adequate drainage and to prevent development of constrictive pericarditis,[286,297,315,321] which can occur very early after presentation.[327]

FUNGAL PERICARDITIS

ETIOLOGY AND PATHOPHYSIOLOGY. Histoplasmosis is the most common cause of fungal pericarditis. This diagnosis should be considered in young and otherwise healthy patients suspected of having acute viral or tuberculous pericarditis who live in the Ohio or Mississippi River Valley or the Western Appalachians, where the fungus is endemic.[328] In these areas, histoplasmosis is acquired by inhalation of spores during small rural outbreaks from bird or bat droppings and during major urban outbreaks related to excavation and building demolition. Coccidioidomycosis pericarditis occurs in patients who have inhaled chlamydospores from soil or dust in areas of the American Southwest, particularly the San Joaquin Valley, and Argentina, where it is endemic.[329,330] Other fungal infections responsible for pericarditis include aspergillosis, blastomycosis, and those caused by *Candida albicans* and *Candida tropicalis*.[331–334] Groups at increased risk for the development of fungal pericarditis consequent to disseminated infection include drug addicts, patients who are immunosuppressed or who have received potent broad-spectrum antibiotics, and patients recovering from complicated open-heart surgery.

Histoplasmosis pericarditis most commonly develops as a noninfectious inflammatory response to infection confined to adjacent mediastinal lymph nodes and rarely by direct or hematogenous infection in patients with disseminated infection.[328,335] The isolation of organisms from pericardial fluid is unusual, and its predilection for young immunocompetent males suggests that self-limited histoplasmosis pericarditis usually represents a sterile immune reaction. Pericarditis due to fungi other than histoplasmosis may occur as a complication of open-heart surgery in adults and children as a result of spread from contiguous infected lymph nodes or pulmonary lesions or hematogenous dissemination in immunosuppressed patients with fungal sepsis.

PATHOLOGY. Pericardial fluid may accumulate extremely rapidly and to massive quantities in patients with histoplasmosis. The fluid can be serous or hemorrhagic with increased protein content and polymorphonuclear leukocytosis. In cases of fungal pericarditis due to agents other than *Histoplasma*, exudative pericardial effusions may accumulate more slowly, so that an effusion may be present for months. Histoplasmosis and other fungal pericardial effusions occasionally become organized, with pericardial thickening, the appearance of granulomas and multinucleated giant cells, and the development of a constricting, calcified pericardium.[328,335]

Histoplasmosis in patients with disseminated infection may rarely cause infection of the myocardium and endocardium as well as of the pericardium.[335] Similarly, aspergillosis, candidiasis, and coccidioidomycosis may cause pericarditis in the context of pulmonary infection, endocarditis, and myocardial abscess.[329–332] Therefore, cardiac decompensation in patients with fungal pericarditis may be due either to the presence of cardiac compression from a pericardial effusion or a constricting pericardium or to an underlying myocardial infection.

CLINICAL FEATURES. The clinical course of histoplasmosis pericarditis is now better understood from two large urban outbreaks in which 6.3 per cent of 712 patients with clinically recognized histoplasmosis had acute pericarditis.[328] Almost all of the patients had a preceding respiratory illness, and pericardial pain and typical electrocardiographic changes at presentation. The chest roentgenogram was always abnormal, an enlarged cardiac silhouette was present in 95 per cent, and pleural effusions and intrathoracic adenopathy were present in two-thirds of the patients. Notably, the "classic" manifestations of histoplasmosis—acute self-limited disseminated infection or severe cavitary pulmonary infection—were absent. However, more than 40 per cent of patients had hemodynamic compromise or frank cardiac tamponade consistent with other reports.[328,335] Histoplasmosis pericarditis can rarely occur in the less common setting of severe prolonged disseminated infection evident by fever, anemia, leukopenia, and the syndrome of pneumonitis progressing to pulmonary cavitation, massive hepatomegaly, meningitis, myocarditis, or endocarditis. Severe disseminated infections are especially likely to occur in young infants, elderly males, and immunosuppressed patients.

Coccidioidomycosis Pericarditis. This condition does not occur in the brief self-limited influenza-like form of the infection but is instead a complication of the progressive disseminated form of coccidioidomycosis.[329,330] Blacks, Filipinos, and Chicanos appear to be especially vulnerable to the development of disseminated coccidioidomycosis. These patients are usually chronically ill and debilitated, with fever, weight loss, and the complications of pulmonary cavitations with lymphadenopathy, osteomyelitis, and meningitis. In immunocompromised patients, the insidious appearance of symptoms of fungal pericarditis and underlying myocardial infection may initially be overlooked because attention is focused on symptoms related to underlying lymphoma, leukemia, or known valvular endocarditis. Physical findings suggestive of cardiac compression (jugular venous distention, hypotension, pulsus paradoxus) may be the first clues to the diagnosis of fungal pericarditis.

DIAGNOSIS. **Histoplasmosis Pericarditis.** In young and otherwise healthy adults with evidence of pericarditis, a presumptive clinical diagnosis of histoplasmosis pericarditis can be made on the basis of (1) residence or travel in an endemic area, (2) an elevated complement fixation titer of at least 1:32, and (3) a positive immunodiffusion test.[328] Most patients do not show a progressive rise in titer, because pericarditis usually occurs after initial mild or asymptomatic pneumonitis such that titers are high when first measured. Histoplasmin skin tests are not helpful, and their use may falsely elevate antibody titers.[328] *Histoplasma* may be isolated from specimens from invasive biopsies of mediastinal nodes, but cultures or methenamine silver stains rarely identify the organism in extrapulmonary sites such as the liver, bone marrow, and pericardium in patients with benign, self-limited forms of pericarditis. Histoplasmosis pericarditis that occurs in the setting of severe disseminated infection must be differentiated from sarcoidosis, tuberculosis, Hodgkin's disease, and brucellosis. Histological tissue examination and culture are important in disseminated progressive histoplasmosis, and in this setting the organism may be isolated from extrapericardial sites such as the bone marrow, exudate from ulcers, or sputum by inoculation on Sabouraud's medium or by guinea pig inoculation with subsequent subculture of the spleen.

Coccidioidomycosis Pericarditis. A presumptive diagnosis of coccidioidomycosis pericarditis is made in a patient with pericarditis who has (1) a history of dust exposure in an endemic area in the American Southwest, California Central Valley, or South America, (2) a characteristic clinical picture of disseminated coccidioidomycosis involving the lungs and other organs, (3) the appearance of a positive serum precipitin test early in the infection followed by a rising positive complement-fixation antibody titer, and (4) microscopic evidence of the characteristic spherule in biopsy material. A definitive diagnosis is made by culture identification of the organism on Sabouraud's medium. Coccidioidin skin tests are often negative in the presence of progressive disseminated disease.

Other Fungal Pericarditis. If pericarditis due to other fungal organisms is suspected, appropriate complement-fixing antibody titers should be measured. Serology and precipitin tests for *Candida* are not sensitive or specific, and the diagnosis of candida pericarditis depends on growth of the fungus from several sites other than superficially contaminated catheters in association with immunosuppression or complicated cardiac surgery.[332] Depending on the clinical setting, it may be important to obtain pericardial fluid and a pericardial biopsy specimen. It must be emphasized that the microscopic finding of granulomas alone is nonspecific and may occur in tuberculosis, fungal and parasitic infections, and sarcoid involvement of the pericardium. Therefore, histological documentation of the characteristic appearance of the fungus and subsequent culture identification are important.

MANAGEMENT. *Histoplasmosis pericarditis* is generally a benign illness that resolves within 2 weeks and does not require treatment with amphotericin.[328] Nonsteroidal anti-inflammatory drugs or steroids appear to shorten the duration of chest pain, fever, pericardial friction rub, and effusion.[328] Patients should always be hospitalized because histoplasmosis may cause the rapid development of massive effusions with acute cardiac tamponade that require emergency pericardiocentesis or pericardiectomy.[328,335] Although pericardial calcification and pericardial constriction have been reported in histoplasmosis pericarditis, these complications are uncommon. Intravenous amphotericin B is required only for patients with histoplasmosis pericarditis and severe disseminated systemic disease.

In *nonhistoplasmosis fungal pericarditis* the diagnosis is rarely made before death. Spontaneous remissions do not occur; infection progresses until the patient dies either of the underlying disease or of fungal pericardial and myocardial involvement. Survival from nonhistoplasmosis fungal pericarditis has been reported in occasional patients treated with parenteral antifungal therapy and surgical drainage by pericardiectomy.[332,336] Drug therapy for pericarditis associated with disseminated coccidioidomycosis, aspergillosis, and blastomycosis consists of prolonged intravenous therapy with amphotericin B. The South American form of blastomycosis may require the addition of a sulfonamide. Candida pericarditis associated with fungal sepsis and disseminated infection is treated with amphotericin B, in addition to pericardiectomy.[332] Candida pericarditis has been successfully treated with antifungal therapy and drainage of pericardiocentesis, but there is little experience with this approach.[333] In many cases of nonhistoplasmosis fungal pericarditis, chronic pericardial fungal infection progresses to severe pericardial constriction or, less commonly, cardiac tamponade. Therefore, depending on the patient's underlying medical condition, pericardiectomy is usually indicated. Intrapericardial instillation of antifungal agents has not proved helpful in these diseases. The serious toxicity associated with prolonged amphotericin B administration underscores the importance of making a definitive diagnosis after histological examination or culture.

Pericarditis complicated by the development of cardiac tamponade and chronic constrictive pericarditis may also be caused by *Actinomyces israelii* and *Nocardia asteroides*, which are intermediate forms between fungi and bacteria.[337–339] These organisms may cause indolent infections and invasion of the pericardium from thoracic, abdominal, or cervicofascial abscesses.

OTHER INFECTIOUS PERICARDITIS

The mycoplasmas, fastidious organisms that cause pulmonary and urogenital disease, are newly recognized as pathogens that can cause pericarditis in association with large pericardial effusions.[340] Mycoplasma pericarditis appears to occur in patients who are immunocompromised or have undergone cardiac surgery. The parasite *Toxoplasma gondii*, which is usually acquired by accidental cyst ingestion in endemic areas, is a cause of myocarditis, acute pericarditis with tamponade, and chronic pericardial effusion.[341–343] The prevalence of *Toxoplasma* as a cause of acute pericarditis of unknown origin may be underestimated.[69] Toxoplasmosis pericarditis can occur in the setting of fever of unknown origin with lymphadenopathy in both normal and immunosuppressed patients.[342–344] It is presumptively diagnosed by documenting high IgM or rising IgG antibodies, and definitively diagnosed by inoculation of infected pericardial fluid into mice, and it is usually treated with sulfadiazine and pyrimethamine antibiotic therapy in addition to drainage of pericardial fluid.

Other parasitic causes include amebiasis,[345–347] schistosomiasis,[348] and echinococcosis.[349,350] The diagnosis of amebic pericarditis is facilitated by the demonstration of multiple cystic lesions in the region of the pericardium by chest roentgenography and two-dimensional echocardiography.[347] Uncommon causes of parasitic pericarditis include dracunculosis,[351] cysticercosis, and filariasis.[352] These unusual infections rarely cause acute cardiac tamponade but may cause chronic constrictive pericarditis. The spirochetes *Borrelia burgdorferi* and *Babesia microti* are increasingly recognized as causes of pericarditis with tamponade and myocarditis in association with tick-borne Lyme disease.[353,354] The diagnosis can be made by the demonstration of IgM and IgG antibodies in pericardial fluid by indirect immunofluorescence and identification of spirochetes in pericardial or myocardial biopsies or synovial biopsies. Lyme pericarditis is usually treated by a 14-day course of intravenous ceftriaxone, and pericardial drainage if needed. The psittacosis agent, *Chlamydia psittaci*, an obligate intracellular parasite-like bacterium that causes a febrile pneumonitis via bird-to-human transmission; and the recently discovered respiratory pathogen *Chlamydia pneumoniae* are also rare causes of effusive pericarditis.[355,356]

(See also p. 1255)

Pericarditis is a common occurrence during the first few days after acute myocardial infarction.[357,358] The incidence of early postmyocardial infarction pericarditis varies from 28 to 40 per cent of fatal transmural infarctions studied at autopsy.[359] In a review by Oliva et al. of 14 reports of postinfarction pericarditis, the mean incidence of postinfarction pericarditis detected by a friction rub alone was 14 per cent, whereas the mean incidence was 25 per cent if the symptom of classic positional chest pain or a rub or both were used as diagnostic criteria.[359] The recent use of thrombolytic therapy in acute myocardial infarction appears to have caused about a 50 per cent reduction in the incidence of early postinfarction pericarditis.[359–363] Furthermore, observations from the GISSI trial have shown that the earlier the thrombolytic treatment is initiated, the lower is the incidence of pericarditis, and that pericardial involvement is strongly associated with several indices of infarct size.[362] The late development of Dressler syndrome is now exceedingly rare in patients who have received thrombolytic therapy with successful reperfusion.[364] In a prospective study of 703 patients with acute myocardial infarction, pericarditis, defined by the detection of a pericardial friction rub, occurred in 25 per cent of patients with transmural infarction and in 9 per cent of patients with non-Q-wave infarction.[365]

Fibrinous pericarditis is detected in about 10 per cent of patients with non-Q-wave infarction at autopsy.[366] Pericarditis is more prevalent in anterior than in inferior infarction[365] and also occurs following lateral and predominant right ventricular infarction. Other forms of pericardial involvement after myocardial infarction include acute pericardial hemorrhage secondary to cardiac rupture and the late occurrence of Dressler syndrome (see p. 1256).

CLINICAL FEATURES. Pericarditis is recognized clinically by the appearance of a pericardial friction rub within 12 hours to 10 days after acute myocardial infarction. In most patients with postinfarction pericarditis, a pericardial friction rub appears on the first, second, or third day after infarction.[358,359,365] In about 70 per cent of patients, the presence of a pericardial rub is accompanied by pleuritic or positional chest pain.[365] There is usually a slight temperature elevation, but pneumonitis is uncommon. Appearance of a new friction rub more than 10 days after acute infarction probably represents the onset of Dressler syndrome or pericarditis complicating a second infarction. Because pericardial friction rubs are notoriously evanescent, serial auscultatory evaluation of the patient in various positions in a quiet room is important for detection. Pericardial rubs with a single systolic component heard near the apex may be confused with a new murmur of mitral regurgitation due to papillary muscle dysfunction or rupture. Postinfarction pericarditis does not directly cause hemodynamic deterioration unless pericardial effusion under pressure develops, causing cardiac tamponade.

In a series of patients with acute infarction and pericardial effusion,[367] the use of heparin did not appear to be associated with increased risk. However, hemorrhagic cardiac tamponade related to the use of anticoagulants has been reported as a rare complication in patients with postinfarction pericarditis.[368] Constrictive pericarditis has been reported as a sequel of hemopericardium after infarction.[369]

The typical diagnostic electrocardiographic changes of acute pericarditis are extremely rare in early postinfarction pericarditis.[358] Two types of atypical T-wave evolution have been observed in patients with regional postinfarction pericarditis preceding myocardial rupture. These two patterns of T-wave evolution consist of T waves that remain persistently positive 48 hours or more after infarction, or the pattern of premature reversal of initially inverted T waves to positive deflections.[370] A recent study of 200 patients with acute infarction without rupture, of whom 43 had postinfarction pericarditis, confirmed that the sensitivity and specificity of these patterns of T-wave evolution for postinfarction pericarditis is 100 and 77 per cent, respectively.[371] The other processes that can cause these patterns of T-wave evolution are cardiopulmonary resuscitation, reinfarction, and very small infarcts. Thrombolytic therapy with clinically evident reperfusion accelerates both the appearance of maximum T-wave negativity and evolution of T-wave changes.[371] Depression of the PQ segment in acute anterior infarction occurs with a higher incidence in patients with postinfarction pericarditis and correlates with larger infarct size.[372] The finding of a small pericardial effusion in a post–myocardial infarction patient in the absence of hemodynamic compromise is not pathognomonic of acute postinfarction pericarditis. Galve et al. found that a small pericardial effusion could be detected in 28 per cent of patients early after acute infarction in comparison with 8 per cent of asymptomatic patients with unstable angina and 5 per cent of normal subjects.[367] In a recent study of 303 consecutive patients with myocardial infarction, a pericardial effusion was detected in 41 per cent of the subset of 65 patients with a pericardial rub.[373] The presence of pericardial effusion correlates highly with the presence of extensive infarction and congestive failure, but not with clinical pericarditis reflected in the appearance of a pericardial rub or pain.[367,373]

Patients who develop pericarditis after infarction experience a more complicated hospital course and more extensive myocardial damage than do patients without pericarditis, as evidenced by higher myocardial MB-CK enzyme levels and lower ejection fraction.[362,365] The development of congestive heart failure and a high Killip class are more common in patients with postinfarction pericarditis.[357,365] The development of atrial tachyarrhythmias is also more common in patients with pericarditis following infarction.[365,374,375] The appearance of acute postinfarction pericarditis *per se* does not appear to affect the in-hospital mortality as an independent risk factor, but it does appear to be associated with an increase in 12-month mortality, which is probably accounted for by its association with larger infarct size and lower ejection fraction.[357,358,362,365]

Postinfarction pericarditis without cardiac compression must be differentiated from acute pulmonary embolism, and, most importantly, from recurrent myocardial ischemia. Myocardial ischemia pain can usually be differentiated from the pain of postinfarction pericarditis by (1) obvious amelioration of the pain by nitroglycerin, (2) the appearance of new regional ST-segment and T-wave changes with reciprocal changes, characteristic of recurrent ischemia, and (3) the typical evolutionary pattern of T-wave changes characteristic of postinfarction pericarditis.[370,371]

CARDIAC TAMPONADE. The development of cardiac tamponade in patients with myocardial infarction may be related to pericardial hemorrhage secondary to pericarditis or to myocardial rupture within the first 3 days after infarction. Both situations may be associated with cardiovascular collapse, the appearance of dense echoes in the pericardial space or two-dimensional echocardiogram, and an abrupt increase in heart size on the chest roentgenogram. Pericardiocentesis may successfully relieve postinfarction hemorrhagic cardiac tamponade with rupture in occasional patients.[376] Massive cardiac hemorrhage secondary to cardiac rupture is usually followed by the rapid development of electromechanical dissociation and death, although survivors have been reported after subacute rupture managed with pericardiocentesis and surgical repair.[377,378] Postinfarction pericarditis can rarely cause localized tamponade of the right heart chambers with hypoxemia due to right-to-left shunting.[379] The development of a chronic myocardial rupture (pseudoaneurysm) with effusive-constrictive pericarditis is a rare complication of extensive silent infarction with postinfarction pericarditis.[380]

Acute cardiac tamponade secondary to postinfarction pericarditis must also be differentiated from cardiogenic shock without intrapericardial hemorrhage due to an acute ventricular septal defect or mi-

tral regurgitation. In the setting of an inferior myocardial infarction, the appearance of hypotension, pulsus paradoxus, and jugular venous distension may be related to massive right ventricular infarction rather than to cardiac tamponade. Echocardiographic findings of right ventricular enlargement without a significant pericardial effusion and catheterization findings suggestive of constrictive physiology (right atrial waveform with steep y descent) rather than cardiac tamponade (right atrial waveform with attenuated y descent) help to differentiate these entities and prevent possibly disastrous attempts at pericardiocentesis. In patients who have received thrombolytic therapy, acute tamponade developing within hours after administration must also be differentiated from inadvertent administration of thrombolytic therapy in the setting of aortic dissection misdiagnosed as acute infarction. There are now several reports of this complication in young patients; although some patients can be salvaged by emergency surgical evacuation and aortic repair, this complication is usually fatal.[381-383] The development of cardiac tamponade due to erroneous administration of thrombolytic therapy in the setting of idiopathic pericarditis is extremely rare.[384]

MANAGEMENT. Postinfarction pericarditis may produce mild symptoms that require no specific therapy or severe chest pain that persists for several days. If the pain is severe, high-dose aspirin relieves pain within 48 hours in most patients. A short course of prednisone may be required in patients whose pain does not improve after a 48-hour trial of nonsteroidal anti-inflammatory agents.[385]

There is experimental evidence that indomethacin, ibuprofen, and multiple large doses of corticosteroids interfere with the conversion of the myocardial infarct into a scar, so that thinning of the myocardial wall occurs. Myocardial rupture has been observed in patients during ibuprofen and corticosteroid use for postinfarction pericarditis,[386,387] and there is evidence of a higher incidence of pericardial rupture in postmyocardial infarction patients who receive nonsteroidal anti-inflammatory drugs. Therefore, these drugs should be employed with great caution in patients with acute myocardial infarction. Fortunately, aspirin does not appear to cause any of these adverse effects, and postinfarction pericarditis usually responds well to aspirin. Accordingly, we favor use of this drug.

UREMIC PERICARDITIS

Pericarditis is a frequent and serious complication of chronic renal failure (see also p. 1928). Before the advent of dialysis, uremic pericarditis was detected in about half of the patients with untreated chronic renal failure and was usually a harbinger of death. Uremic pericarditis is now detected clinically in up to 20 per cent of uremic patients who require chronic dialysis.[388] Uremic pericarditis tends to be a complication that occurs either prior to initiation of dialysis or during the first few months of therapy.

ETIOLOGY. The etiology of uremic pericarditis is unknown. Viral causes have been proposed, but there is no consistent evidence to suggest a viral etiology in the majority of cases of uremic pericarditis. The occasional observation of a seasonal clustering of episodes of pericarditis in uremic patients is consistent with a viral etiology. Specific etiological factors, including purulent bacterial infections, are common in patients with uremic pericarditis, and it is unwise to assume that pericarditis in a patient with severe renal disease is simply related to uremia. Toxic catabolic nitrogen metabolites and secondary hyperparathyroidism have been suggested mechanisms responsible for uremic pericarditis. This suggestion is supported by the observations that uremic pericarditis is rare in patients with acute mild renal failure and that uremic pericarditis often improves with initiation of dialysis in previously untreated patients. However, there is no clear correlation between the development of pericarditis and the levels of catabolic metabolites in uremic patients.

It has also been proposed that pericarditis in dialysis patients may reflect an immunological response. Some support for this hypothesis comes from Maisch and Kochsiek's observations that 64 per cent of 25 patients with chronic uremia and pericarditis had complement-fixing antimyolemmal antibodies with cytolytic properties for cardiac tissue, whereas antimyocardial antibodies were rarely detected in patients with acute renal failure due to surgery or trauma.[389] It is possible that etiological factors in nondialyzed patients differ from those in patients undergoing regular dialysis. In the latter group, systemic and regional heparinization during dialysis itself may exacerbate uremic pericarditis by promoting the tendency of vascular pericardial granulation tissue to bleed into the pericardial space. Nafamostat mesylate as a substitute for heparin anticoagulation has been proposed for patients with hemorrhagic pericarditis during continuous hemofiltration, but its role in lowering the incidence of uremic pericarditis has not been studied.[390]

Acute uremic pericarditis is characterized by the appearance of shaggy, hemorrhagic, fibrinous exudate on both parietal and visceral pericardial surfaces with little acute inflammatory cellular reaction. In some patients, the friable pericardial surface may bleed, giving rise to hemorrhagic pericardial effusion. Subacute or chronic constrictive pericarditis may develop, coincident with organization of the effusion and formation of thick adhesions within the pericardial space.[391] Uremic pericarditis is usually found in association with additional cardiac pathology, including left ventricular hypertrophy, coronary atherosclerosis, and myocardial fibrosis.[391]

CLINICAL FEATURES. The development of pericarditis in patients undergoing dialysis is of clinical importance because it may (1) cause disability or life-threatening cardiac tamponade in patients who are otherwise well compensated when undergoing dialysis, (2) compromise the status of patients who are candidates for renal transplantation, and (3) cause hemodynamic complications during routine dialysis. Patients with uremic pericarditis usually come to attention because of the development of chest pain. A pericardial friction rub is present on initial presentation in nearly 90 per cent of patients. Fever, leukocytosis, and tachycardia are frequent but nonspecific findings. Dyspnea and cardiac enlargement on the chest roentgenogram are common, but these findings can be related to underlying myocardial dysfunction and volume overload. Uremic pericarditis with a large pericardial effusion may first come to clinical attention when an otherwise asymptomatic patient becomes hypotensive and confused upon fluid removal during ultrafiltration. This occurs because volume depletion may cause an abrupt fall in systemic blood pressure when ventricular filling is already compromised by the presence of a large, tense pericardial effusion. Uremic pericarditis can also present as acute or subacute tamponade with the findings of jugular venous distention, hypotension, and pulsus paradoxus. In a study of 1058 patients undergoing dialysis over a 14-year period, acute cardiac tamponade developed in 17 per cent of 161 episodes of uremic pericarditis.[388]

ECHOCARDIOGRAPHY. The presence of a small pericardial effusion is common in uremic patients, and in the absence of typical pericardial pain and friction rubs it is not diagnostic of pericarditis. Asymptomatic pericardial effusions of small to moderate size occur in 36 to 62 per cent of uremic patients who require dialysis and appear to be related to volume overload and clinical congestive heart failure.[392,393] On the other hand, the presence of a large anterior and posterior pericardial effusion in patients with uremic pericarditis that persists after about 10 days of intensive dialysis is associated with a high likelihood of requiring intervention to relieve tamponade.[388,392,394] The presence of a large pericardial effusion in association with echocardiographic findings of right atrial and right ventricular collapse is highly suggestive of cardiac tamponade in a patient with uremic pericarditis. Prior to consideration of pericardiostomy or pericardiectomy, it is important to document that these clinical findings are indeed related to the hemodynamics of cardiac tamponade (elevation and equilibration of pericardial, right and left heart filling pressures) rather than to underlying congestive cardiomyopathy, ischemic heart disease, or excessively vigorous ultrafiltration. It must be remembered that pulsus paradoxus may be absent in uremic patients with cardiac tamponade and coexisting left ventricular failure and elevated left ventricular filling pressures.

MANAGEMENT. Uremic patients who develop symptomatic pericarditis prior to the initiation of dialysis almost always respond to the initiation of vigorous dialysis.[392] In patients with acute uremic pericarditis with a large pericardial effusion, a period of 10 days to 3 weeks is usually required for resolution of the effusion after initiation of intensive dialysis.[392,395] In contrast, less than half of pa-

tients with asymptomatic pericardial effusions show resolution of effusion after initiation of dialysis.[392] No treatment is required for small, asymptomatic pericardial effusions that can be followed simply by serial echocardiography.[393,395]

Treatment of symptomatic uremic pericarditis that develops in patients more than 3 months after the initiation of chronic dialysis is controversial, and multiple approaches have been advocated. About two-thirds of the patients who develop effusive uremic pericarditis following the initiation of dialysis respond to a program of intensification of dialysis and regional heparinization. The remainder are likely to require operative drainage of the pericardium.

Factors that predict that the strategy of intensive dialysis is likely to fail include the presence of large anterior and posterior effusions, high fever, leukocytosis with left shift, and clinical evidence of the development of cardiac tamponade, such as hypotension and jugular venous distention.[395] Nonsteroidal anti-inflammatory drugs have been widely advocated as therapy for patients with uremic pericarditis. A randomized, double-blind comparison of indomethacin versus placebo in symptomatic patients with uremic pericarditis showed that indomethacin reduced the duration of fever, but it had no significant effect on the duration of chest pain, pericardial rub, pericardial effusion, or need for relief of tamponade, which occurred in 20 per cent of patients.[398] The complications of long-term steroid administration limit its usefulness in the treatment of recurrent uremic pericarditis.

Pericardiocentesis with an indwelling catheter followed by instillation of a nonresorbable steroid into the epicardial space has also been advocated, but this procedure has been complicated by the development of purulent pericarditis.[399] A single pericardiocentesis followed by a one-time instillation of triamcinolone appears to be effective and may eliminate the need for prolonged catheter drainage.[400] There are reports of repetitive pericardiocenteses with low morbidity and mortality in uremic patients.[395,401] Subxiphoid pericardiocentesis for the management of pericardial effusion in patients undergoing peritoneal dialysis can be complicated by development of a fistula between the pericardial and peritoneal cavities.[402] The presence of a friable visceral pericardium may increase the risk of traumatic intrapericardial hemorrhage in uremic pericarditis, and the status of many patients is also compromised by the presence of left ventricular dysfunction. These considerations warrant special caution during the performance of pericardiocentesis in uremic patients, and this procedure probably should be carried out only by experienced personnel in an optimal environment.

Surgical Treatment. The surgical treatment of uremic patients with pericardial effusions with a subxiphoid pericardiostomy or limited pericardiectomy (window) performed through a left thoracotomy is effective in relieving cardiac tamponade. These approaches do not appear to be associated with an appreciable risk of developing recurrent effusions or constriction.[403,404] The intrapericardial instillation of steroids during surgical drainage has also been advocated,[395] although there is no evidence that this offers any advantage over thorough drainage alone. There is little experience yet with the use of percutaneous balloon pericardiotomy for the management of large hemorrhagic effusions in uremic patients.

Early surgical intervention in uremic patients with a large pericardial effusion has been advocated as a prophylactic measure to prevent the development of cardiac tamponade and to allow the procedures to be carried out at a time when the patient's condition is clinically stable. We believe that this approach is excessively aggressive because many symptomatic uremic patients with pericardial effusions respond well to intensification of dialysis.

We advocate that patients with hemodynamic instability and with hemodynamic evidence of cardiac tamponade and echocardiographic evidence of a large anterior and posterior effusion be treated by percutaneous catheter pericardiocentesis with continued catheter drainage of the pericardial sac for 24 to 48 hours. Subxiphoid pericardiotomy or limited pericardiectomy is reserved for patients with hemodynamic instability associated with recurrent pericardial effusions following pericardiocentesis or with loculated pericardial effusions.

NEOPLASTIC PERICARDITIS

(See also p. 1796)

PATHOLOGY. At autopsy, the pericardium is involved in 5 to 15 per cent of patients with malignant neoplasm.[405] Lung cancer, breast cancer, leukemia, Hodgkin's disease, and non-Hodgkin's lymphoma account for about 80 per cent of reported cases of malignant pericarditis.[405–410] Other neoplastic diseases reported to lead to pericardial involvement include gastrointestinal cancer, ovarian cancer, cervical cancer, sarcoma, leiomyosarcoma, multiple myeloma, mediastinal teratoma, thymoma, and melanoma[410–416] (Table 43–10). In children the most common etiologic factors are non-Hodgkin's lymphoma, neuroblastoma, sarcomas, and Wilms' tumor,[417] whereas

TABLE 43–10   CAUSES OF TUMORS METASTATIC TO THE PERICARDIUM

PRIMARY MALIGNANT NEOPLASM	FREQUENCY (%)
Lung carcinoma	40
Breast carcinoma	22
Gastrointestinal carcinoma	3
Other carcinomas	6
Leukemia and lymphoma	15
Melanoma	3
Sarcoma	4
Other (including malignant mesothelioma, germ cell tumors)	7

Relative frequency of neoplasms metastatic to the pericardium in 1315 patients.

Data from Goodie, R. B.: Secondary tumors of the heart and pericardium. Br. Heart J. *17*:183, 1955; and Scott, R. W., and Garvin, C. F.: Tumors of the heart and pericardium. Am. Heart J. *17*:431, 1939.

pericardial teratomas are a rare cause of hydrops fetalis in utero and in neonates.[418]

PRIMARY PERICARDIAL TUMORS. Primary malignant neoplasms of the pericardium are rare and are predominantly due to mesothelioma, including that arising after asbestos and fiber glass exposure,[419,420] and, less frequently, to benign localized fibrous mesothelioma, malignant fibrosarcoma, angiosarcoma, lipomas and liposarcomas, and benign and primary malignant teratomas.[421–424] Rare primary neoplasms of the pericardium occasionally have been reported in association with congenital developmental disorders such as tuberous sclerosis.[425] Catecholamine-secreting pheochromocytoma is a rare primary neoplasm of the pericardium.[426] In patients with AIDS, an increasing number of patients have been reported with malignant involvement of the pericardium and heart due to Kaposi's sarcoma and cardiac lymphoma.[258,259,427,428] Pericardial tamponade can be an early presentation of HIV infection, and purulent pericarditis as well as malignancy must always be excluded in these patients.[258,259]

PERICARDIAL METASTASES. These may involve the heart in several ways: (1) extension and attachment to the pericardium of a malignant mediastinal mass, (2) nodular tumor deposits from hematogenous or lymphatic spread (Fig. 43–23), (3) diffuse pericardial thickening and infiltration with tumor, and (4) local infiltration of the pericardium.[408]

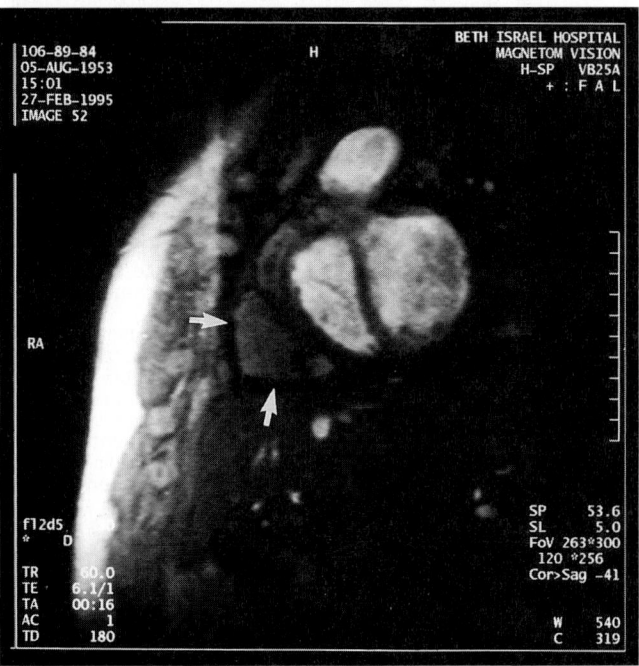

FIGURE 43–23.   Spin-echo magnetic resonance image of the heart and pericardium from a patient with non-Hodgkin's lymphoma and elevation of right atrial and right ventricular diastolic pressures. The scan showed a discrete large mass (white arrows) within the pericardial sac which overlaid and compressed the right ventricle. Biopsy of the mass confirmed the presence of intrapericardial lymphoma. (Courtesy of W. Manning, M.D.)

In the majority of cases, the epicardium and myocardium are *not* involved.

EFFUSION IN NEOPLASTIC PERICARDITIS. Neoplastic pericarditis may cause several syndromes of cardiac compression. Neoplastic involvement of the pericardium may result in serosanguineous or hemorrhagic effusions, which may develop extremely rapidly, causing acute or subacute cardiac tamponade.[428a] Pericardial involvement by tumors such as sarcomas, mesotheliomas, and melanomas can also erode the cardiac chamber or intrapericardial blood vessels, causing acute pericardial distention and abrupt fatal cardiac tamponade. A rare cause of hemorrhagic effusion and cardiac tamponade is intrapericardial extramedullary hematopoiesis associated with preleukemic conditions and during blast crisis with Philadelphia chromosome–positive chronic myeloid leukemia and chronic myelomonocytic leukemia.[429,430] Cardiac compression may also occur as a consequence of the development of both thickened pericardium and pericardial effusion under pressure (effusive-constrictive pericarditis), or it may be caused by thickening of the pericardium produced by tumor encasement of the heart, causing the physiology of constrictive pericarditis.

Not all pericardial effusions associated with mediastinal cancer are malignant. Asymptomatic pericardial effusions are common in patients with mediastinal lymphoma and Hodgkin's disease.[431] These evanescent effusions are frequently detected during staging procedures and presumably develop as a result of impaired lymphatic drainage. Transient effusions may also occur in association with mediastinal thymoma and primary cardiac tumors.[432,433] Fracp et al. have observed that small, clinically unsuspected pericardial effusions detectable by echocardiography are common in women with metastatic breast cancer.[434] In a prospective study of 38 women with metastatic breast cancer in whom echocardiography was done on a routine basis, 53 per cent were found to have small pericardial effusions that did not progress to cause hemodynamic embarrassment in any patient. It is uncertain whether small pericardial effusions in asymptomatic women with metastatic breast cancer are due to indolent malignant pericardial involvement or impaired lymphatic drainage.

CLINICAL FEATURES. Neoplastic pericarditis is often totally asymptomatic and detected only as an incidental finding at autopsy. However, it is the most common specific cause of acute pericarditis in developed countries. In a prospective series of patients with acute pericarditis of unknown cause, a diagnostic protocol revealed an unsuspected malignant etiology in 5 per cent of patients.[68] In patients with undiagnosed cancer, leukemia, or primary pericardial tumors, cardiac tamponade can be the initial manifestation.[408,415,421] In patients with known malignancy, symptoms resulting from pericardial involvement may be incorrectly attributed to the underlying neoplasm, so that malignant pericarditis is not suspected until symptoms and signs of severe cardiac compression appear.

In patients with malignant pericarditis, dyspnea is by far the most common symptom.[408,410,435] Other frequent symptoms and physical findings include chest pain, cough, orthopnea, and hepatomegaly. Distant heart sounds and a pericardial friction rub are rarely detected, which is in part probably due to a low index of suspicion.[408,435] In the majority of patients the diagnosis is made only when there is evidence of cardiac compression or frank cardiac tamponade, manifest as jugular venous distention, pulsus paradoxus, and hypotension.[436]

The *chest roentgenogram* is abnormal in more than 90 per cent of patients with malignant pericarditis and may show pleural effusion, cardiac enlargement, mediastinal widening, a hilar mass, or, less commonly, an irregular nodular contour of the cardiac silhouette. The *electrocardiogram* is usually abnormal but nonspecific, showing tachycardia, ST- and T-wave changes, low QRS voltage, and occasionally atrial fibrillation. In occasional patients, persistent tachycardia or electrocardiographic changes are the initial findings that lead to the diagnosis. Electrocardiographic findings that are rarely seen in pericarditis, such as atrioventricular conduction disturbances, suggest malignant invasion of the myocardium and conduction system.

DIAGNOSIS. Patients with cancer and pericarditis benefit from a systematic evaluation, and these patients should not be summarily assumed to have a preterminal condition. The diagnosis of malignant pericarditis depends on both documentation of pericardial inflammation and substantiation that pericarditis is due to neoplasm. It is often not appreciated that in approximately half the patients with symptomatic pericarditis and neoplastic disease there is a nonmalignant cause; most commonly the condition is due to prior radiation or to idiopathic causes.[138,408] Many patients with advanced neoplastic disease are immunosuppressed as a consequence of their malignant disease and/or therapy and are therefore also at risk for tuberculous and fungal pericarditis. Acute pericarditis has also been rarely reported as a complication of intravenous administration of the chemotherapeutic agents doxorubicin and daunorubicin. Sudden tamponade during chemotherapy for bone marrow transplantation for malignancy and thalassaemia has been described. This complication accounted for 29 per cent of all deaths within 1 month of treatment in a series of 400 consecutive transplant patients.[437] The mechanism is not yet understood but may be related to the drug-conditioning regimen.

Neoplastic pericarditis with cardiac compression must be differentiated from other causes of jugular venous distention, hepatomegaly, and peripheral edema in cancer patients. The most important of these are (1) underlying left ventricular dysfunction secondary to prior cardiac disease or doxorubicin cardiac toxicity, (2) superior vena caval obstruction, (3) malignant hepatic involvement with portal hypertension, and (4) microvascular tumor spread in the lungs with secondary pulmonary hypertension.

Echocardiography often provides critical information about the presence and size of a pericardial effusion and the thickness and motion of the pericardium and may suggest the presence of abnormal diastolic filling of the heart due to cardiac compression. Two-dimensional echocardiography may be helpful in the detection of irregular undulating masses that protrude into the pericardial space and define the presence of pericardial space-occupying lesions.[438] *CT* and *MRI* (Fig. 43–23) can also detect the presence of pericardial effusions and, in some instances, may give added information regarding the presence and location of space-occupying masses within the pericardium and adjacent mediastinum and lungs.[423,439]

PERICARDIOCENTESIS AND CARDIAC CATHETERIZATION. We recommend that pericardiocentesis using the catheter drainage technique (see p. 1493) be performed in conjunction with cardiac catheterization in cancer patients with suspected cardiac tamponade in whom a large pericardial effusion is documented by echocardiography. Two additional diagnoses should always be systematically evaluated during cardiac catheterization in these patients: (1) Superior vena caval obstruction may coexist with malignant cardiac tamponade and contribute to the development of facial edema and jugular venous distention and should be systematically excluded at cardiac catheterization in cancer patients. (2) Cyanosis, hypoxemia, and elevation of the pulmonary vascular resistance are not features of cardiac tamponade, and pulmonary microvascular tumor (lymphangitic tumor) should be strongly suspected in a patient with these findings, hypoxemia, or persistent dyspnea following pericardiocentesis. Support for this diagnosis can be obtained at the same setting as pericardiocentesis and right-heart catheterization by obtaining a sample of blood from the pulmonary capillary wedge position for cytological analysis using the right-heart catheter.[440]

The appearance of the pericardial fluid does not differentiate among neoplastic, radiation, or idiopathic causes. Because treatment strategies differ, it is necessary to carry out a meticulous cytological examination of pericardial fluid in an attempt to differentiate malignant pericarditis from radiation-induced or idiopathic pericarditis. Cytological examination of pericardial fluid is diagnostic of a malignant neoplasm in about 85 per cent of the cases of malignant pericarditis.[138,408,441] False-negative cytological diagnoses are uncommon in carcinomatous pericarditis but occur more

commonly with involvement by lymphoma or mesothelioma.[441] The measurement of carcinoembryonic antigen (CEA) may add to the diagnostic yield of the examination of pericardial fluid in patients with suspected neoplastic pericarditis[282]; open pericardial biopsy may be required if the results of cytological examination of pericardial fluid are normal. If a sufficiently large biopsy specimen is obtained, open pericardial biopsy should provide a histological diagnosis in up to 90 per cent of cases. However, false-negative diagnoses may occur if only a small tissue sample is obtained, and in critically ill patients open pericardial biopsy is not without risk. Optically guided percutaneous pericardioscopy with biopsy is a new and alternative approach for the diagnosis of suspected neoplastic pericardial involvement.[155,156]

In patients with echocardiographic evidence of a thickened pericardium and the physical findings of cardiac compression (jugular venous distention, edema, ascites, and hepatomegaly), cardiac catheterization is useful for documenting the presence of constrictive physiology before a decision is made to proceed with aggressive surgical intervention, i.e., extensive pericardiectomy.

NATURAL HISTORY. If cardiac tamponade can be avoided or successfully treated, the mere presence of neoplastic pericarditis does not imply that death is imminent. Because lung cancer and breast cancer are by far the most common causes of malignant pericarditis with cardiac tamponade, both the management strategy and subsequent natural history usually depend on the type of underlying malignant disease. The natural history of neoplastic pericarditis in patients treated for cardiac tamponade was studied using a Kaplan-Meier analysis in two series.[150,408] In both series, the mean survival was 4 months with 25 per cent surviving 1 year. We studied the outcome of a consecutive series of 29 patients with malignant pericardial effusion and tamponade managed with pericardiocentesis in whom the 1-year survival rate was 17 per cent compared with 91 per cent for 21 patients with nonmalignant effusion.[132] These series indicate that a subset of about 25 per cent of patients with cardiac tamponade due to malignant pericarditis who are managed surgically or with pericardiocentesis survive 1 year or longer.

The outcome in patients with malignant pericarditis due to breast cancer is strikingly better than that in patients with lung cancer or other metastatic carcinomas. Following surgical treatment of cardiac tamponade in lung cancer patients, Piehler et al. reported that the mean survival was only 3.5 months, in contrast with breast cancer patients in whom mean survival was 9 months with survivorship extending to more than 5 years.[150] Similarly, Stewart et al. reported that the median survival following surgical treatment of malignant effusion in lung cancer patients was 2 months, compared with a survival of 8.4 months for breast cancer.[406] In one series of breast cancer patients with malignant pericarditis managed with pericardiectomy or pericardiotomy, the overall median survival was 17 months.[434] A similar prolonged survival in patients with malignant effusion due to breast cancer has been reported by others.[408,441,442]

MANAGEMENT. Decisions about the management of neoplastic pericardial effusion depend on the underlying condition of the patient, the presence or absence of clinical manifestations related to cardiac compression, and the prognosis and treatment options available for the specific histology and stage of the underlying malignant disease. At one end of the spectrum are debilitated patients with end-stage malignant disease for whom there is no promising treatment option for the underlying malignant disease and for whom the prognosis is bleak. In this setting, diagnostic procedures should be as brief and painless as possible, and intervention should be directed toward alleviation of symptoms with a goal of improving the quality of the remaining days or weeks of life. In these patients, pericardiocentesis with catheter drainage is indicated for immediate relief of severe dyspnea, chest pain, or orthopnea. Our experience[132] and that of other centers experienced in catheter pericardiocentesis shows that neoplastic cardiac tamponade can be safely relieved with pericardiocentesis in 90 to 100 per cent of cases with a low (<2 per cent) risk of major complications.[407,444] At centers with a high complication rate with pericardiocentesis or if cardiac tamponade recurs, palliation can be achieved with an equally high success rate and low morbidity by a subxiphoid pericardiotomy, which can usually be performed under local anesthesia.[150,151,406,445,446] The more invasive and debilitating partial pericardiectomy (window) done via a left thoracotomy has also been advocated, but this procedure appears to have no advantage as a palliative procedure over a subxiphoid pericardiectomy and should rarely be done in patients with end-stage malignancy.[150,406]

The new percutaneous technique of balloon pericardiotomy (Fig. 43–12) is a promising new technique for the management of malignant pericardial effusion. Although this technique was successful in relieving tamponade in 92 per cent of a recent series of 50 patients, it was associated with higher morbidity than reported in a recent series of catheter pericardiocentesis, including the requirement for urgent surgery in 4 per cent and chest tube or thoracentesis in about 20 per cent of the patients.[147,148] Thus, the morbidity of this technique may be higher than percutaneous catheter pericardiocentesis with vacuum-assisted drainage of the pericardial sac.[132] To date, there has not been a prospective trial comparing efficacy and outcome of catheter pericardiocentesis, percutaneous balloon pericardiotomy, and subxiphoid pericardiotomy in the management of malignant effusion.

When the general prognosis of the patient is better, several more aggressive treatment options are available, the goals of which are (1) relief of cardiac tamponade, (2) prevention of recurrence of the malignant effusion, and (3) treatment or prevention of constrictive pericardial disease.

In patients with asymptomatic pericardial effusion who have a treatment option of effective chemotherapy or hormonal therapy directed against the underlying malignant disease, treatment with systemic agents alone can be attempted while progression of the effusion is observed by means of echocardiography. In patients with cardiac tamponade and large effusions secondary to neoplastic pericarditis, pericardiocentesis with thorough catheter drainage in combination with systemic chemotherapy can be attempted. Based on small series of patients, the instillation of tetracycline and other chemotherapeutic agents into the pericardial space following pericardiocentesis or surgical drainage has been advocated, with the aim being sclerosis of the pericardial membranes and obliteration of the pericardial space.[444–447] However, in comparison with complete catheter or surgical pericardial drainage by subxiphoid pericardiotomy, there is no convincing evidence to date from either a large collective experience or prospective trial to indicate that instillation of drugs into the pericardial space alters the outcome. Side effects of instillation of intrapericardial agents include chest pain, nausea, high fever, atrial arrhythmias, and the rapid development of pericardial constriction.[448]

External-beam radiation therapy is an important option for patients with radiosensitive tumors who have not yet received extensive mediastinal or cardiac radiation as a treatment modality. Approximately half the patients with malignant pericarditis due to a variety of radiosensitive tumors respond to this form of treatment.[449] In one series, malignant pericardial effusion improved significantly in 11 of 16 patients with breast cancer, whereas 6 of 7 patients with malignant pericarditis secondary to leukemia or lymphoma improved with cardiac radiation.[449]

In cancer patients whose overall condition is good and who develop recurrent symptomatic effusions after pericardiocentesis, a limited subxiphoid pericardiotomy should probably not be chosen when the goal is definitive therapy. The procedure has a much higher likelihood of being followed by recurrent tamponade, constriction, or reoperation than does extensive pericardiectomy, and tamponade almost always recurs in less than 1 year after operation.[150] Because one of four patients with malignant effusive pericarditis is likely to survive at least 1 year, extensive surgical pericardiectomy should be strongly considered in cancer patients with recurrent effusions or pericardial constriction who have (1) potential response to systemic cancer therapy or (2) 1 or more years of expected survival.

RADIATION PERICARDITIS

ETIOLOGY. Radiation injury to the heart and pericardium is an important complication of radiation therapy used in breast carcinoma, Hodgkin's disease, and non-Hodgkin's lymphoma. Factors that influence the development of radiation-induced heart disease include (1) the radiation dose; (2) the duration and fractionation of therapy; (3) the volume of the heart included in the radiation field; (4) the use of a ^{60}Co source, with inhomogeneous dose distribution, in comparison with a linear accelerator source; and (5) anterior weighting of the radiation dose.[450,451] When at least 60 per cent of the cardiac silhouette is included within the treatment beam, as occurs in mantle field therapy of patients with Hodgkin's disease, the risk of radiation-induced pericarditis is about 5 to 7 per cent when a dose less than 4000 rads is delivered over 4 weeks and rises sharply in incidence above this dose.[450–453] When the whole pericardium is included in the field, the incidence of pericarditis is about 20 per cent, while the use of a subcarinal block that shields the heart decreases the risk to about 2.5 per cent.[454] The observation has been confirmed in a contemporary series of 590 patients who received mantle irradiation as initial treatment for Hodgkin's disease at the Joint Center for Radiation Therapy; 2.2 per cent of patients developed postirradiation pericarditis.[452]

In patients with Hodgkin's disease who receive radiation therapy using a ^{60}Co source or anterior weighting of the beam, which results in a higher dose to the pericardium, the incidence of pericarditis rises to about 20 per cent.[455] It approaches 50 per cent when a fluid challenge is used to unmask occult constrictive pericarditis.[456] In breast cancer radiation therapy, in which the volume of the heart included in the field is usually less than 30 per cent, the incidence of radiation-induced pericarditis is less than 5 per cent, with a tolerance for up to 6000 rads given over 6 weeks.[450] In a series of 831 women with early-stage breast cancer who received radiation therapy to the left breast on a linear accelerator following conservative surgery, pericarditis requiring hospitalization occurred in only 0.4 per cent.[457] The incidence of pericarditis with effusion is higher (15 per cent) in patients with esophageal cancer undergoing contemporary treatment with radiation as an adjunct to surgery.[458]

Pericardial injury may occur during the course of treatment or, more commonly, months later. In one series, 92 per cent of cases in patients presenting with pericardial effusions occurred within 12 months after completion of the course of radiation therapy.[459] However, it is now recognized that radiation pericarditis manifesting as chronic pericardial effusion or constrictive pericarditis may become apparent many years after radiation therapy.[450,453,455–459] In a series of patients with postirradiation constrictive pericarditis referred for pericardiectomy at Stanford, recent cases appeared to have a longer latent period between radiation therapy and presentation with constrictive pericarditis (4.7 years for cases during 1970 to 1980, versus 11 years for cases in 1980 to 1985).[169] The risk and latency period for the later development of constrictive pericarditis in children undergoing mediastinal irradiation is not known. In a study of 17 children observed for 72 months after radiation therapy for Hodgkin's disease, 47 per cent had prominent pericardial thickening on echocardiograms without overt evidence of cardiac constriction.[460]

PATHOLOGY. Radiation pericarditis is associated with fibrin deposition and pericardial fibrosis. The acute inflammatory stage may be accompanied by a pericardial effusion that can be serous, serosanguineous, or hemorrhagic with a high protein and lymphocyte content.[450] The inflammation and initial effusion may resolve spontaneously. Alternatively, the effusion may organize and progress to a stage of dense fibrinous adhesions with gradual obliteration of the pericardial space, thickening of the pericardium, and proliferation of small blood vessels within the pericardium associated with a chronic pericardial effusion or a constricting pericardium. The visceral pericardium may also become fibrotic and thickened, and radiation pericarditis is a common cause of effusive-constrictive pericardial disease. Depending on the radiation dose and fractionation, recent studies in animals have shown that myocardial degeneration with secondary fibrosis and endothelial cell injury with myointimal cell proliferation can also occur over a late and progressive time course.[461]

RADIATION-INDUCED DAMAGE OF THE MYOCARDIUM. It is important to recognize that radiation may occasionally injure the heart itself, causing interstitial myocardial fibrosis, valvular thickening with regurgitation, endothelial proliferation, aortitis, and fibrotic thickening of small intramyocardial arteries. Radiation may also cause premature atherosclerosis of the epicardial coronary arteries, including ostial narrowing.[450,462,463] The presence of radiation-induced coronary artery disease has important implications for its surgical management. The internal mammary artery often cannot be used as a conduit due to vessel friability and associated mediastinal fibrosis, and there is an increased risk of severe pericardial inflammation causing graft closure and constriction.[462]

The most important consequence of radiation-induced myocardial fibrosis is the development of restrictive cardiomyopathy, which may coexist with constrictive pericarditis and contribute to inadequate relief of symptoms of pulmonary and venous congestion and poor survival after pericardiectomy.

CLINICAL FEATURES. The *acute* form of pericarditis is seldom evident clinically. It usually occurs in the context of irradiation of bulky mediastinal tumor adjacent to the pericardium, which suggests that acute pericarditis is largely related to inflammatory necrosis of the adjacent tumor. Patients may have a syndrome of acute pericarditis consisting of fever, pericardial pain, anorexia, malaise, a pericardial friction rub, and electrocardiographic abnormalities. Acute pericarditis that occurs during radiation therapy usually abates rapidly, does not preclude completion of planned treatment, and correlates poorly with the risk of late pericardial damage.

In the *delayed* form of pericardial injury, the onset of symptoms is usually within 12 months but varies from 4 months to more than 20 years. It may present as the syndrome of acute idiopathic pericarditis or as an asymptomatic pericardial effusion with a coexisting pleural effusion on the chest roentgenogram. In about half of the patients, there is some degree of cardiac compression associated with dyspnea, jugular venous distention, and pulsus paradoxus due to delayed chronic pericarial effusion. The importance of this mode of presentation is underscored by the fact that radiation-induced pericardial effusion now accounts for 10 per cent of patients who undergo surgical drainage of the pericardium.[149,150] In the Stanford experience,[450] about 20 per cent of patients with delayed pericardial injury progress to development of chronic pericarditis that requires pericardiectomy. These patients may present years after radiation therapy with the insidious onset of fatigue, dyspnea, systemic edema, and jugular venous distention due to the development of constrictive pericarditis. The clinical recognition and consequences of this delayed form of pericardial injury have become increasingly important as patients with breast cancer and Hodgkin's disease have prolonged survival and cures.

DIAGNOSIS. Radiation-induced pericarditis with pericardial effusion is most often confused with pericarditis due to the underlying malignant disease. However, patients with malignant pericardial effusion are more likely to have massive effusions and cardiac tamponade, and cytological examination of pericardial fluid can identify a malignant origin in about 85 per cent of cases.[408] When symptoms referable to the pericardium occur years after apparently successful treatment of Hodgkin's disease or lymphoma, the pericarditis is much more likely to be related to radiation injury than to recurrent mediastinal malignant disease. Similarly, the development of pericarditis with effusion in women with treated breast cancer with no evidence of metastatic disease is likely to be related to prior radiation, radiation-induced hypothyroidism, or idiopathic (viral) inflammation.[434] Occasionally, histological examination of the pericardium or pericardial fluid may be required to differentiate between radiation-induced pericarditis and recurrent metastatic disease in the pericardium.

MANAGEMENT. Patients in whom an asymptomatic pericardial effusion develops after radiation therapy may be followed up by physical examination and serial echocardiography without the institution of specific therapy. Percutaneous pericardiocentesis by skilled operators should be limited to the treatment of cardiac tamponade or to drainage of a large pericardial effusion when cytological examination is required for management. Radiation-induced thyroid dysfunction occurs in about 25 per cent of patients who undergo mantle irradiation,[452] and hypothyroidism should always be excluded as a cause of effusive pericarditis following radiation therapy. Systemic corticosteroids should be reserved for patients with severe intractable pain or life-threatening effusive disease because of the well-documented risk of unmasking latent radiation-induced lung or heart injury when steroids are withdrawn.[464]

Surgical Treatment. Pericardiectomy is required for that small number of symptomatic patients with a large recurrent pericardial effusion or severe effusive-constrictive or constrictive pericarditis. The surgical experience at the Mayo Clinic has shown that late constriction developed in 75 per cent of patients with radiation-induced pericarditis who underwent drainage with a limited left thoracic partial pericardiectomy (window).[150] These data are supported by others[149,232] and suggest that extensive pericardiectomy should be performed in patients with severe effusive or effusive-constrictive radiation-induced pericarditis whose prognosis is otherwise favorable. Operative mortality for pericardiectomy in patients after radiation therapy is 21 per cent, compared with a rate of about 8 per cent in patients with idiopathic constrictive pericarditis.[169] Actuarial analysis has shown that the 5-year survival rate of patients after pericardiectomy for postirradiation pericarditis is 51 per cent, which is inferior to the 83 per cent 5-year survival rate of other patients who underwent pericardiectomy.[232] Factors that contribute to a poor outcome include failure to resect constricting visceral pericardium (epicardium), and underlying myocardial injury and fibrosis causing advanced restrictive cardiomyopathy.[232,450,451,465,466] Prospective studies are needed to elucidate the potential role of endomyocardial biopsy and nuclear MRI for the assessment of myocardial atrophy and fibrosis to aid in discriminating patients with radiation-induced constrictive pericarditis with a high probability of experiencing a good outcome following pericardiectomy from those with a low probability.

PERICARDITIS RELATED TO HYPERSENSITIVITY OR AUTOIMMUNITY

ACUTE RHEUMATIC FEVER
(See also p. 1770)

During the 19th century, acute rheumatic fever was believed to be the most common cause of pericarditis, and it was recognized that rheumatic pericarditis could occur independently of overt rheumatic endocarditis.[467] The condition is now uncommon, but occasionally the development of a pericardial friction rub or effusion is the initial clue to the presence of rheumatic carditis.

PATHOPHYSIOLOGY. Rheumatic pericarditis is characterized by fibrin deposition that can be accompanied by a fibrinous, serofibrinous, or purulent exudate.[467,468] The pericardial reaction usually resolves spontaneously. The deposition of IgG, IgM, and complement on the pericardial surface during active pericarditis has been reported,[468] but it is still unclear whether pericarditis occurs as an immune-mediated mechanism or simply as nonspecific inflammation associated with underlying myocarditis. The development of chronic calcification and constrictive pericarditis, although reported, is very rare.[469]

CLINICAL FEATURES. Rheumatic pericarditis usually occurs at the onset of the initial episode of acute rheumatic fever and may be asymptomatic or associated with typical pericardial pain and other symptoms of acute rheumatic fever, including fever, malaise, and arthralgias (see p. 1771). When present, pericarditis usually indicates extensive pancarditis. The diagnosis of rheumatic pericarditis is based on the presence of pericardial chest pain, a pericardial friction rub, or echocardiographic evidence of pericardial effusion in association with the revised Jones clinical criteria for acute rheumatic fever and serological evidence of antecedent Group A streptococcal infection[470] (see p. 1770). In children, the onset of pericarditis, which is otherwise rare in this age group, should prompt a rigorous search for evidence of acute rheumatic fever.[469] The combination of pericarditis, fever, arthralgias, and rash in a child or young adult may be mistaken for a viral exanthem, Lyme disease, infectious endocarditis, juvenile rheumatoid arthritis, systemic lupus erythematosus, Henoch-Schönlein purpura, Crohn's disease, or sickle cell crisis.

MANAGEMENT. The treatment of rheumatic pericarditis is that of acute rheumatic fever and includes bed rest and penicillin as well as digoxin if myocardial failure is present. Chest pain associated with rheumatic pericarditis should be treated with aspirin, as described on page 1772. Rarely, corticosteroids are required. Small or moderate-sized pericardial effusions usually resolve spontaneously, and pericardiocentesis should not be performed solely for diagnostic reasons in a patient with documented acute rheumatic fever.

SYSTEMIC LUPUS ERYTHEMATOSUS
(See also p. 1778)

Pericarditis usually occurs during flare-ups of disease activity in patients with systemic lupus erythematosus (SLE) and is the most common cardiovascular manifestation of the disease.[471] Pericarditis is detected clinically in about 20 to 45 per cent of these patients during the course of their disease.[471-473] Echocardiographic abnormalities can be detected in a higher percentage of these patients, but the clinical significance of this is unclear.[474] The inflammatory process may cause fibrinous or effusive pericarditis with the rare occurrence of pathognomic hematoxylin bodies in the visceral pericardium. Pericardial fluid may be serous or grossly hemorrhagic with a high protein content, low glucose content, and white cell count below 10,000/mm³ (composed primarily of polymorphonuclear leukocytes). Low pericardial fluid complement levels relative to normal serum values have been reported, but caution must be used in interpreting this finding, because total hemolytic complement levels appear to be normally low in pericardial fluid.[471]

CARDIAC TAMPONADE. This occurs in less than 10 per cent of patients with SLE and clinically recognized pericarditis, while the development of constrictive pericarditis has been reported but is rare.[471-473] Occasionally, cardiac tamponade is the presenting manifestation of SLE.[473,475] Pericarditis due to SLE may be accompanied by other cardiac lesions, including verrucous endocarditis, inflammation and necrosis involving the conduction system, and coronary artery vasculitis.[471]

CLINICAL FEATURES. Pericarditis should be suspected when patients with SLE develop pleuritic chest pain, a pericardial rub, or an enlarging cardiac silhouette on the chest roentgenogram. *Electrocardiographic abnormalities* are those characteristics of acute pericarditis. Because pericarditis usually occurs during periods of active disease and frequently in association with nephritis, there is typically evidence of increased disease activity on blood tests for complement fixation levels, antinuclear antibodies, lupus erythematosus cell preparations, and sedimentation rate.[473,476] The *chest roentgenogram* may show enlargement of the cardiac silhouette, pleural effusions, and parenchymal infiltrates. The *echocardiogram* may show evidence of a new pericardial effusion, suggesting the presence of pericardial inflammation. Because many patients with SLE are treated with immunosuppressive drugs, corticosteroids, and cytotoxic agents, a careful physical examination, blood cultures, and tuberculin skin test should be obtained to search for evidence of purulent, fungal, or tuberculous pericarditis. Except when purulent pericarditis is strongly suspected, it is not necessary to confirm the clinical diagnosis of SLE pericarditis by performing pericardiocentesis.

MANAGEMENT. In the majority of patients, pericarditis subsides when the systemic disease becomes inactive following treatment with corticosteroids or immunotherapy. The unusual complication of cardiac tamponade can ordinarily be treated with pericardiocentesis or subxiphoid pericardiotomy, but recurrent effusions and pericardial thickening with constriction may occur in as many as 40 per cent of these patients.[473] Because the development of acute cardiac tamponade is unpredictable, symptomatic patients with SLE pericarditis should be hospitalized and under close observation.

RHEUMATOID ARTHRITIS
(See also p. 1776)

Although pericarditis is detected at autopsy in up to 50 per cent of patients with rheumatoid arthritis, the clinical incidence of symptomatic pericarditis is between 10 and 25 per cent.[472,477] Based on echocardiographic criteria for the presence of a pericardial effusion, possible effusive pericarditis has been detected in 50 per cent of patients with chronic nodular rheumatoid arthritis, in 15 per cent of patients with typical non-nodular rheumatoid arthritis, and in no patients of comparable age with osteoarthritis.[478] Pericarditis tends to appear in patients with other evidence of severe rheumatoid arthritis, including extensive joint deformity, subcutaneous rheumatoid nodules, pneumonitis, and positive serum rheumatoid factor. On rare occasions, rheumatoid pancarditis with pericarditis can occur in patients with seronegative rheumatoid arthritis.[479]

Rheumatoid pericarditis in adults can cause cardiac tamponade and has been recognized as a cause of effusive-constrictive pericarditis and constrictive pericarditis.[477,479,480] Pericarditis, and the complication of cardiac tamponade, may occur with or without evidence of active joint involvement in about 6 per cent of children with juvenile rheumatoid arthritis.[481] Males predominate among these patients, and pericarditis frequently occurs in association with myocarditis. Pericarditis complicated by tamponade may also occur in adult Still's disease.[482]

PATHOLOGY. Typical pathological changes in the pericardium are those of pericardial vasculitis nonspecific fibrous thickening of the visceral and parietal pericardium with adhesions. Rarely, small, necrotic granulomatous nodules are detected on the epicardial surface that are histologically identical to the subcutaneous, rheumatoid nodule. Pericardial effusions, whose characteristics are similar to those of pleural effusions associated with rheumatoid arthritis pericarditis, are usually serous or hemorrhagic, with greater than 5 gm/dl of protein, glucose levels less than 45 mg/dl, high cholesterol levels, and white blood cell counts ranging from 20,000 to 90,000/mm³.[477] Soluble immune complexes, positive latex fixation titers, and low complement levels in the pericardial fluid as well as immune complex and complement deposits with CD8+ T-cell infiltration in the pericardium have also been described.[479,483,484] Acute pericarditis may progress to cause diffusely constricting fibrotic pericarditis and can coexist with other cardiac lesions, including granulomatous aortic and mitral valve deformity causing chronic aortic or mitral insufficiency.[485]

CLINICAL FEATURES. Rheumatoid arthritis is often associated with fever, precordial chest pain, and dyspnea in association with a pericardial friction rub. Pericarditis commonly coexists with exacerbation of joint inflammation and pleuritis, manifest on the chest roentgenogram as a unilateral or bilateral pleural effusion at about 65 per cent of cases. The *ECG* usually shows nonspecific ST-segment and T-wave changes. The presence of atrioventricular block in patients with rheumatoid pericarditis probably reflects rheumatoid myocardial involvement. On *echocardiography* a pericardial effusion is present in approximately half of patients with nodular rheumatoid arthritis,[477,478,485] but its presence does not always correlate with the presence of symptomatic pericarditis. In some patients, two-dimensional echocardiography can demonstrate the presence of dense fibrinous strands in the pericardial space.[486]

CARDIAC TAMPONADE AND CONSTRICTION. Although rheumatoid pericarditis is usually self-limited and benign, cardiac tamponade may develop abruptly in 3 to 25 per cent of patients[477]; it has been reported as a complication of sudden steroid withdrawal[487] and in association with intravenous anticoagulant therapy.[488] An uncommon but major complication is the rapid onset of subacute effusive-constrictive pericarditis.[477,483] The development of chronic constrictive pericarditis is a well-recognized complication that is more prevalent in men than in women.[240,477,480,489]

MANAGEMENT. Patients with symptomatic pericarditis may be treated with aspirin or other nonsteroidal anti-inflammatory agents, as described on page 1772. Suppression of recurrent rheumatoid pericarditis with effusion has been reported in response to colchicine treatment, but experience with this therapy is limited.[490]

Pericardiocentesis is indicated for relief of a large anterior-posterior effusion causing cardiac tamponade. Although intrapericardial steroid instillation has been advocated, there is no clear evidence that steroids alter the natural history of effusions or prevent the development of the constrictive pericarditis. There is now an extensive experience in the *surgical management* of rheumatoid pericarditis, and patients with connective tissue disorders (predominantly rheumatoid arthritis) now constitute between 4 and 20 per cent of patients undergoing pericardiectomy.[169,230,231] In patients with documented effusive-constrictive or constrictive rheumatoid pericarditis, pericardiectomy can provide gratifying hemodynamic and symptomatic improvement.[169,230,231,477,480,489]

PROGRESSIVE SYSTEMIC SCLEROSIS
(See also p. 1781)

Pericardial involvement is found at autopsy in about 50 per cent of patients with progressive systemic sclerosis (scleroderma), while pericarditis is detected clinically in about 10 per cent.[472,491-493] Although the pathogenesis of scleroderma pericarditis is unknown, it has been suggested that increased collagen formation by fibroblasts, in combination with tissue hypoxia, may result in aberrant collagen metabolism. Histological changes include nonspecific fibrotic pericardial thickening with adhesions and perivascular inflammatory cells. Pericardial effusions can be detected by means of echocardiography in about 40 per cent of patients with scleroderma, but in the majority of patients a small pericardial effusion is not associated with symptoms.

When present, the pericardial effusion is straw colored and characterized by a protein content greater than 5 gm/dl, low cell count, and—in contrast to the characteristics of pericardial effusions in SLE and rheumatoid arthritis—the absence of autoantibodies, low complement levels, and immune complexes. Pericardial involvement is often associated with sclerodermatous infiltration of the heart, causing restrictive cardiomyopathy, arrhythmias, and conduction abnormalities.[492]

Scleroderma pericardial disease may present as an acute syndrome resembling viral myocarditis, with fever, chest pain, and pericardial friction rub, and nonspecific electrocardiographic ST- and T-wave changes. In other cases, patients develop a chronic pericardial effusion or pericardial constriction with symptoms of right and left atrial hypertension, cardiomegaly, and pleural effusions on the chest roentgenogram, and low QRS voltage on the electrocardiogram.

MANAGEMENT. There is no definitive treatment for scleroderma pericarditis. Patients with the syndrome of acute pericarditis may be treated with aspirin, as described on pages 1484 and 1513. Rarely, pericardial effusions with cardiac tamponade may develop.[494] Patients with constrictive pericarditis may require pericardiectomy. Severe recurrent constrictive pericarditis has also been reported as a complication of idiopathic retroperitoneal and mediastinal fibrosis, which are regional expressions of a systemic sclerosing disease.[495] It is important to perform cardiac catheterization in patients with scleroderma and suspected cardiac tamponade or constrictive pericarditis because dyspnea and systemic venous hypertension may be related to sclerodermatous cardiac involvement or to pulmonary hypertension secondary to pulmonary fibrosis. The development of symptomatic pericarditis in patients with scleroderma is ominous because the 5-year survival rate is about 25 per cent when isolated pericardial or other cardiac involvement is present and about 75 per cent in patients with heart, lung, or kidney involvement.[496]

PERICARDITIS IN OTHER CONNECTIVE TISSUE DISORDERS

Pericarditis is rarely the initial presentation of mixed connective tissue disease, and the diagnosis can be supported by documentation of a high antibody titer against ribonuclease-sensitive ribonucleoprotein.[497,498] Pericardial involvement, including tamponade, develops in about 11 per cent of patients with dermatomyositis.[472,499,500]

Pericarditis may rarely develop in other connective tissue disorders, including Sjögren's syndrome,[501] ankylosing spondylitis,[502] Wegener's granulomatosis,[503] Reiter's syndrome,[504] severe serum sickness,[505] and Felty's syndrome.[506] Pericarditis associated with polyarteritis nodosa may occur in patients who are hepatitis B antigen–positive. It also occurs in disorders of possible autoimmune etiology, including temporal arteritis,[507] inflammatory bowel disease,[508] Kawasaki's disease,[509] familial Mediterranean fever,[510] Whipple's disease,[511] celiac disease,[512] eosinophilic fasciitis,[513] giant lymph node hyperplasia (Castleman's disease),[514] Behçet's disease, and myasthenia gravis.[515] Amyloidosis is well known as a cause of infiltrative restrictive myopathy, the hemodynamics of which may mimic constrictive pericarditis (p. 1427), but it may also involve the pericardium.[206,207,222] Pericarditis with tamponade has been reported as a complication of rhabdomyolysis.[516]

Cardiac involvement is present at autopsy in about 25 per cent of patients with sarcoidosis and can involve the pericardium in the absence of significant myocardial infiltration.[517] Sarcoidosis can be a rare cause of cardiac tamponade and constrictive pericarditis[518,519]; in the latter case, the findings of pericardial thickening with noncaseating granulomas may cause confusion with tuberculous or fungal pericarditis (Fig. 43–24).

DRUG- AND TOXIN-RELATED PERICARDITIS

Pericarditis occurs in about 25 per cent of patients with procainamide-related and 2 per cent of those with hydralazine-related development of the SLE syndrome.[520] In these patients, pericarditis may occasionally be complicated by the development of cardiac tamponade or the rapid development of pericardial constriction.[521] Other drugs that may produce pericarditis in association with the drug-in-

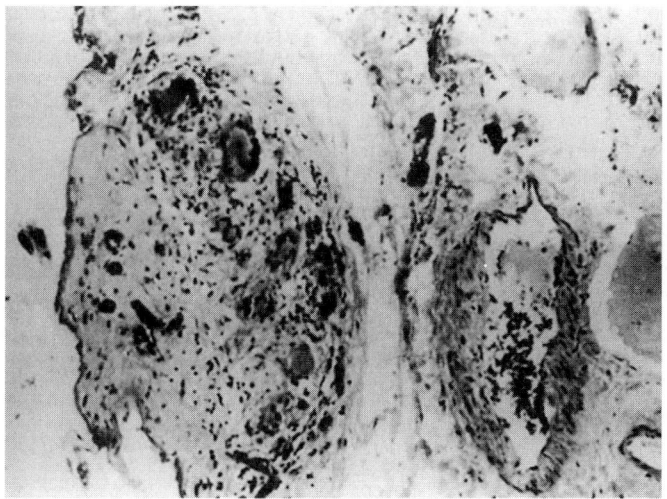

FIGURE 43–24. Photomicrograph of a pericardial biopsy specimen from a patient with cardiac tamponade secondary to cardiac sarcoidosis showing a noncaseating granuloma with several giant cells (250 ×). (From Verkleeren, J. L., et al.: Cardiac tamponade secondary to sarcoidosis. Am. Heart J. *106:*601, 1983.)

duced syndrome of SLE include reserpine, methyldopa, isoniazid, and phenytoin and mesalazine.[520,522–524]

Other drugs appear to produce pericarditis through separate mechanisms. Pericarditis has been reported as a complication of a hypersensitivity reaction with peripheral eosinophilia after administration of penicillin,[525] cromolyn sodium,[526] and tryptophan.[527] The mechanisms of drug-induced pericarditis following administration of 6-amino-9-D-psicofuranosylpurine,[528] minoxidil,[529] dantrolene sodium,[530] and practolol[531] are not understood. Pericarditis has also been observed in association with polymer fume fever, a syndrome of pleuritis and noncardiogenic pulmonary edema that occurs following inhalation of fumes from the burning of polytetrafluoroethylene (Teflon).[532] Methysergide is well recognized as a cause of constrictive pericarditis as part of a generalized process of mediastinal fibrosis.[533] The anthracycline neoplastic agents doxorubicin and daunorubicin may cause acute pericarditis as well as myocardial inflammation,[534] and pericarditis has also been reported in association with the use of cytosine arabinoside.[535] Pericarditis has similarly been noted as a foreign body reaction to the presence of silicone[536] and talc[537] within the pericardial space, in association with cardiac iron deposition and pericardial fibrosis in thalassemia,[538] in association with chronic asbestos exposure,[539] and as a toxic response to scorpionfish sting.[540]

Acute drug-related pericarditis usually resolves when the offending drug is discontinued, and improvement may be accelerated by administration of corticosteroids. The rare development of chronic constrictive pericarditis may be treated by pericardiectomy.

Postmyocardial Infarction (Dressler) Syndrome
(See also p. 1511)

Dressler syndrome is an acute illness with fever, pericarditis, and pleuritis, possibly of autoimmune origin, that occurs weeks to months after an acute myocardial infarction.[541,542] A similar syndrome of fever and pericarditis has been reported in six patients following pulmonary embolism with infarction.[543] Today, a distinction is usually made between acute postinfarction pericarditis, which occurs during the first week after infarction (p. 1256), and Dressler syndrome, which usually appears 2 to 3 weeks after infarction, with a range of 1 week to several months. Dressler estimated that this syndrome occurred in up to 4 per cent of patients after acute myocardial infarction[544]; however, a more recent series from the same hospital indicates that the incidence of the Dressler syndrome has markedly decreased.[545] Dressler syndrome is extremely rare in patients following thrombolytic therapy with successful reperfusion.[364]

The cause of Dressler syndrome is unknown. The association of symptoms and the appearance of antimyocardial antibodies has led to the hypothesis that an autoimmune mechanism, with or without a latent viral infection, is the etiologic factor,[545] whereas some workers have concluded that the development of antimyocardial antibodies is not specific for the presence of Dressler syndrome.[545,546] Leakage of blood into the pericardial space is another proposed mechanism, and the current lower incidence of the syndrome may reflect less use of oral anticoagulants in the postinfarction period.[545] It is likely that there are common factors in the pathogenesis of Dressler syndrome and the postpericardiotomy syndrome, both of which have the following features: (1) an initial insult of endothelial cell injury and entry of blood into the pericardial space; (2) a delayed response after the initial insult, consisting of fever and inflammation of the pericardial surfaces; (3) development of antiheart antibodies; (4) a dramatic response to antiinflammatory agents; and (5) a tendency for recurrence.

PATHOLOGY. The histology of the pericardium usually reveals a nonspecific inflammation with fibrin deposition. In contrast to acute pericarditis following myocardial infarction in which pericardial inflammation is often patchy, overlying the regions of infarction, the pericarditis in Dressler syndrome is usually diffuse.

CLINICAL FEATURES. Patients characteristically have severe malaise, fever, chest pain, and pleurisy.[544,547] The chest pain may be severe enough initially to cause both patient and physician to consider that it is caused by a second myocardial infarction or postinfarction angina.

Dressler syndrome is occasionally the initial presentation of a previously undiagnosed infarction. *Physical examination* often discloses a pericardial friction rub and sometimes a pleural friction rub as well. The chest roentgenogram commonly reveals an enlarged cardiac silhouette secondary to pericardial effusion associated with pleural effusions[544,547] and, occasionally, transient pulmonary infiltrates. The *echocardiographic* evidence of pericardial effusion in the absence of other symptoms is not diagnostic of Dressler syndrome, because asymptomatic small pericardial effusions occur in about one of four patients after myocardial infarction. *Electrocardiographic* abnormalities usually consist of serial ST-segment and T-wave changes strongly suggestive of acute pericarditis, but the electrocardiogram may not be helpful in patients with persistent repolarization abnormalities following infarction. Blood tests usually reveal the nonspecific findings of an increased erythrocyte sedimentation rate and peripheral leukocytosis. Tests for antimyocardial antibodies are not established as a means of confirming the diagnosis. Gallium scanning has been reported to be ineffective in identifying patients with pericarditis due to Dressler syndrome.[548]

Dressler syndrome can usually be discriminated from recurrent myocardial infarction by (1) the characteristics of the chest pain and its failure to improve with nitroglycerin; (2) the absence of new Q waves on the ECG; and (3) the absence of a marked rise in the CK-MB band. Small increases in cardiac enzyme levels may occur in pericarditis when the underlying epicardium is involved. Dressler syndrome must also be distinguished from hemorrhagic pericarditis secondary to chronic systemic anticoagulation.

MANAGEMENT. A single episode of Dressler syndrome is usually self-limited, but the syndrome does tend to recur. The onset of severe pericarditis usually warrants hospital admission and observation for the development of cardiac tamponade.[547] Oral anticoagulants should be discontinued because of the risk of pericardial hemorrhage. As in other patients with acute pericarditis, patients with severe symptoms with fever and chest pain usually benefit from bed rest and treatment with aspirin or a nonsteroidal anti-inflammatory agent. Recurrent episodes of Dressler syndrome may respond only to corticosteroids and occasionally require complete pericardiectomy for relief of intractable pericardial pain or prevention of recurrence. Colchicine therapy has been reported to be successful in the treatment of recurrent steroid-dependent pericarditis in Dressler syndrome.[549] Cardiac tamponade in the absence of anticoagulant therapy can usually be managed with pericardiocentesis. Constrictive pericarditis is a well-recognized complication of Dressler syndrome that may be treated by pericardiectomy.[550,551]

Postpericardiotomy Syndrome

ETIOLOGY. The postpericardiotomy syndrome is identified by the appearance of fever, pericarditis, and pleuritis more than 1 week after a cardiac operation in which the pericardium has been opened and manipulated. This syndrome was first recognized in patients after mitral commisurotomy for rheumatic heart disease, and it was initially believed to represent reactivation of rheumatic fever.[552] Subsequently, it was realized that the syndrome could occur following cardiac operations in patients without rheumatic heart disease and that the common denominator appeared to be wide incision and manipulation of the pericardium.[553] An identical clinical syndrome has been reported following cardiac perforation by pacemaker implantation, blunt chest trauma, percutaneous diagnostic left ventricular puncture, and epicardial pacemaker implantation, and coronary perforation due to balloon angioplasty.[554,555]

The incidence of postpericardiotomy syndrome following cardiac surgery ranges from 10 to 40 per cent in various series and is higher in children than in adults.[556-558] The observation of a 31 per cent incidence of postpericardiotomy syndrome in patients undergoing cardiac surgery for the Wolff-Parkinson-White syndrome clearly indicates that pericardial damage prior to surgery is not a contributing factor.[558] Furthermore, pericardial drainage techniques do not appear to affect the frequency of development of the syndrome after cardiac surgery.[559]

Analogous to the Dressler syndrome, the cause of postpericardio-tomy syndrome is hypothesized to be an autoimmune reaction directed against the epicardium, possibly in concert with a new or reactivated viral infection. Studies by Engle and colleagues have demonstrated that antiheart antibodies appear in the serum of some patients who undergo pericardiotomy and that there is a positive correlation between the level of the titers and the incidence of the syndrome.[557] Approximately 70 per cent of patients with the postpericardiotomy syndrome and high antiheart antibody titers also develop a fourfold or higher rise in titer against one or more viral antigens, whereas in patients without the postpericardiotomy syndrome, a rise in viral titers occurs in only 8 per cent of those with normal antiheart antibody titers and in only 19 per cent of those with low levels of antiheart antibody titers; these findings suggest that viral infection may be a triggering or permissive factor. The posperi-cardiotomy syndrome is rare in children under 2 years of age who undergo cardiac surgery, a finding that may be related to the short exposure time to viruses or to protective maternal antibodies transmitted via the placenta. The development of pleuritis and pleural effusions is believed to reflect involvement of the pleura adjacent to the inflamed pericardium; involvement of serous membranes distant from the heart is uncommon.

PATHOLOGY. There are no pathognomonic histological features of postpericardiotomy syndrome. The presence of blood in the pericardial space adjacent to an injured epicardium may result in later development of pericardial adhesions, thickening of the pericardial membranes, and occasionally fibrinous obliteration of the pericardial space, causing pericardial constriction. Recent observations during open heart surgery in patients demonstrate that the pericardium produces tissue-type plasminogen activator and that prolonged operation time is associated with increasing pericardial mesothelial damage and inflammation and a reduction in pericardial fibrinolytic activity which may contribute to the development of postoperative pericardial inflammation and adhesions.[560] Pericardial effusions in patients with postpericardiotomy syndrome may be straw colored, serosanguineous, or frankly hemorrhagic, with a protein content greater than 4.5 gm/dl and a white blood cell count between 3,000 and 8,000/mm^3 (composed of both lymphocytes and granulocytes).[561]

CLINICAL FEATURES. Patients typically develop an acute illness characterized by fever, malaise, and chest pain that usually begins during the second or third postoperative week. In some cases, the fever may reflect a continuation of the more common problem of fever in the first week after operation. The chest pain is typical of acute pericarditis (p. 1481) and usually has a pleuritic quality. Nonspecific signs of inflammation, including an elevated sedimentation rate and polymorphonuclear leukocytosis, may also be present. Noncardiac pulmonary edema may also occur.[562]

Physical examination often reveals a pericardial friction rub. It should be noted that the friction rub present in almost all patients during the first few days after cardiac surgery disappears in most patients who do not develop postpericardiotomy syndrome by the end of the first postoperative week. The *chest roentgenogram* demonstrates left-sided or bilateral pleural effusions in about two-thirds of patients, pulmonary infiltrates in about one-tenth, and transient enlargement of the cardiac silhouette in half.[558] The *ECG* shows nonspecific ST-segment and T-wave changes and episodic atrial tachyarrhythmias. *Echocardiography* is useful in monitoring the appearance and size of a pericardial effusion and in detecting evidence of cardiac compression such as right atrial collapse. However, it should be noted that pericardial effusions are extremely common after cardiac surgery, occurring in 56 to 84 per cent of patients within the first 10 days.[563] Thus, the diagnosis of postpericardiotomy syndrome is made on clinical grounds based on recognition of the distinctive features of the syndrome in the postoperative patient. Other causes of postoperative fever, including infection, as well as the viral-induced postperfusion syndrome of atypical lymphocytosis, fever, and hepatosplenomegaly, must be excluded.

MANAGEMENT. The postpericardiotomy syndrome is a self-limited but often prolonged and disabling illness. Fever and severe chest pain are usually relieved by aspirin or nonsteroidal anti-inflammatory drugs. Corticosteroids should be reserved for patients in whom fever and chest pain are not relieved within 48 hours by other anti-inflammatory agents. Recurrences tend to appear during the first 6 months after surgery.

Cardiac Tamponade. This is an important and well-recognized complication of the postpericardiotomy syndrome.[561,564] In one large series of adult patients who survived cardiac surgery, almost 1 per cent developed cardiac tamponade an average of 49 days after surgery, in association with fever, a pericardial friction rub, and pericardial chest pain typical of the postpericardiotomy syndrome.[561] In contrast to the important role of anticoagulation in early postoperative bleeding after cardiac surgery, the use of anticoagulants did not appear to be a prerequisite for the development of cardiac tamponade in association with the postpericardiotomy syndrome. Cardiac tamponade can be managed conservatively by pericardiocentesis followed by the administration of anti-inflammatory agents.[561] Patients with recurrent tamponade require surgical drainage and pericardiectomy. Percutaneous pericardiocentesis should not be attempted in patients with echocardiographic evidence of only a small posterior effusion, a loculated effusion, or an effusion with dense echoes suggesting the presence of both thrombus and free fluid. Constrictive pericarditis is a rare complication that may occur months to years after the postpericardiotomy syndrome.

Postoperative and Postcatheterization Hemopericardium

Acute cardiac tamponade and pericardial constriction in the absence of typical features of the postpericardiotomy syndrome also occur secondary to hemopericardium following cardiac surgery. In a review of 510 consecutive patients who underwent cardiac surgery, 2 per cent developed cardiac tamponade within 1 to 30 days (average 8 days) after operation.[565] A similar incidence has been reported in other series.[566,567] Although small pericardial effusions can be detected by echocardiography in at least 50 per cent of patients after cardiac surgery,[563,568] the development of large pericardial effusions with tamponade is 10 times more common in anticoagulated patients than in patients receiving aspirin therapy.[569] Postoperative tamponade accounts for about 10 per cent of cases of unexplained hypotension after surgery and may be confused with hypovolemia or ventricular failure.[570] Hepatic congestion secondary to right heart compression can simulate acute postoperative hepatitis or present as a pulsatile epigastric mass[571,572] and superior vena cava syndrome.[573]

Transesophageal echocardiography at the bedside is an indispensible diagnostic tool for identification of postoperative global or regional tamponade.[565,568,570,574] Selective compression of the left ventricle, right ventricle, and atria is common, in association with absence of anterior pericardial fluid and tethering of the right ventricle to the anterior chest wall.[565] The clinical and echocardiographic signs of circumferential versus regional tamponade differ. In a recent study of 29 patients with tamponade after cardiac surgery, only 34 per cent had circumferential effusion which was associated with pulsus paradoxus, typical echocardiographic signs of right atrial and ventricular collapse in 70 per cent, and the elevation and equalization of diastolic pressures in 71 per cent.[575] In contrast, the majority of patients had regional tamponade which was associated with left ventricular diastolic collapse in 89 per cent, whereas right ventricular diastolic collapse was rare (5 per cent). In this group, elevation and equalization of diastolic pressures was present in 86 per cent of patients.[575] In patients with circumferential or large localized effusion, cardiac tamponade can be managed by two-dimensional echocardiographically guided percutaneous catheter pericardiocentesis at centers with expertise in this technique.[576] In patients with loculated posterior effusions or regional thrombus, patients should be managed by surgical removal in the operating room.[565]

The incidence of cardiac perforation and acute cardiac tamponade during cardiac catheterization was reviewed in 11,845 consecutive patients seen during a 6-year period at our institution.[577] Cardiac tamponade due to perforation occurred during mitral balloon valvuloplasty (4.7 per cent), aortic balloon valvuloplasty (1.5 per cent), pericardiocentesis (1 per cent), temporary pacing (0.06 per cent), and diagnostic catheterization (0.01 per cent). Pericardiocentesis was effective in managing half of the cases, whereas the remaining patients required surgical repair of the perforation. Cardiac perforation and/or tamponade occurs in about 1.5 per cent of transvenous right ventricular endomyocardial biopsies,[578] and it is a rare complication following transseptal left heart catheterization,[579] percutaneous coronary angioplasty (0.02 per cent),[580,581] intracoronary stent implantation,[582] and laser-assisted valve dilatation in children.[583] Other invasive procedures that have been reported to cause hemopericardium and cardiac tamponade include sternal bone marrow aspiration,[584] esophagoscopy,[585] and mediastinoscopy.[586] Endoscopic sclerotherapy for esophageal varices is a new cause of both acute hemopericardium and the later development of pericarditis associated with chest pain and the development of cardiac tamponade.[587]

Acute symptomatic pericarditis with effusion requiring antiinflammatory therapy has also been observed in 5 per cent of patients undergoing pacemaker implantation with an endocardial active fixation screw-in atrial lead.[588]

Aortic Dissection. Cardiac tamponade can also occur due to acute hemopericardium in patients suffering acute aortic dissection (see p. 1565), and this complication is associated with a mortality of about 60 per cent. Recent observations suggest that attempts to stabilize such patients with pericardiocentesis before emergency aortic repair may contribute to subsequent electrical-mechanical dissociation and death.[589] The potentially harmful effect of pericardiocentesis in some patients with tamponade complicating aortic dissection may be related to inadvertent loss of compression of the leak between the aorta and the pericardial sac by the pressurized hemopericardium as well as surgical delay.

POST-SURGICAL CONSTRICTIVE PERICARDITIS

This condition is being increasingly recognized as a complication of cardiac surgery and may occur in patients in whom the pericardium is left open but in situ.[590,591] The time from cardiac surgery to definitive diagnosis is usually about 1 year but ranges from less than 1 month to more than 15 years. In one review of 5207 adults who underwent cardiac surgery, 0.2 per cent (11 patients) developed constrictive pericarditis, documented by cardiac catheterization, an average of 82 days after operation,[590] similar to other series.[591] Delayed pericardial effusion and constriction can also occur in up to 12 per cent of patients following cardiac transplantation and may be confused with the development of myopathy due to chronic rejection.[592,593]

ETIOLOGY. Povidone-iodine irrigation of the heart is postulated to be a triggering factor in some patients. This factor has been absent in most reports, and it is likely that intrapericardial hemorrhage and serosal injury are major contributing factors.[590] In the series of 45 patients reported by Killian et al., transient postpericardiotomy syndrome may have been a contributing factor in about 60 per cent of the patients.[594] There is now strong evidence that postoperative constrictive pericarditis can involve bypass grafts and can contribute to premature graft closure as well as damage to grafts during pericardiectomy.[595] The development of constrictive pericarditis, possibly related to both occult hemopericardium and the development of a foreign body reaction or localized infection involving the epicardial patch electrodes, has been observed several months after the placement of automatic implantable cardioverter-defibrillators (AICD).[596,597]

Important clinical features in patients with postsurgical constrictive pericarditis include dyspnea, chest pain, jugular venous distention, pedal edema, and increased roentgenographic heart size, while echocardiographic evidence of pericardial thickening with a posterior pericardial effusion is present in the majority. MR and CT are useful in showing pericardial thickening in some patients.

MANAGEMENT. In patients in whom this syndrome is suspected, the diagnosis of constrictive pericarditis should be confirmed at cardiac catheterization before the pericardium is explored (p. 1502). The majority of these patients are found to have hemorrhage-induced fibrosis of the pericardium, often associated with a posterior organized hematoma and about 85 per cent improve after undergoing extensive pericardiectomy.[591,594] The operative mortality for pericardiectomy in these patients is high, ranging from 5 to 14 per cent.[591]

OTHER FORMS OF PERICARDIAL DISEASE

MYXEDEMA PERICARDIAL DISEASE
(See also page 1894)

Myxedema is frequently associated with myopathy; pericardial effusion also occurs in up to one-third of patients.[598,599] Because myxedematous patients frequently have ascites, pleural effusions, and uveal edema, it has been suggested that pericardial effusion may be related to a combination of sodium of water retention, slow lymphatic drainage, and increased capillary permeability with protein extravasation.[600] The pericardial fluid is usually clear or straw-colored, with elevated protein and cholesterol concentrations and few leukocytes or red blood cells. Pericardial fluid usually accumulates very slowly and may achieve enormous volumes—as much as 5 to 6 liters. Occasionally, the pericardial effusion may resemble a viscous jelly rather than a clear fluid. Myxedematous pericardial effusions usually do not cause symptoms. Often attention is called to the heart by the finding of unsuspected marked cardiomegaly on a chest roentgenogram, and a large pericardial effusion is occasionally the presenting feature of hypothyroidism.[601]

Because infants and elderly patients with hypothyroidism may be asymptomatic, this etiologic factor should always be excluded in these patients with pericardial effusion of unknown cause. Hypothyroidism should always be considered as the cause of pericardial effusion in patients following mediastinal radiation therapy, in whom 25 per cent develop radiation-induced thyroid dysfunction.[452] The *ECG* often shows nonspecific abnormalities, including low QRS voltage and flattened or inverted T waves, due to either myxedematous heart disease or pericardial effusion. In myxedematous patients with cardiac compression from a pericardial effusion, the expected compensatory tachycardia may be absent. Massive macroglossia has been reported as a feature of hypothyroidism and pericardial effusion with elevated venous pressure.[602]

Myxedematous pericardial effusions tend to regress slowly and ultimately disappear over a period of months after patients have been treated with thyroid replacement and have returned to the euthyroid state.[598,601] Cardiac tamponade has been reported, but it is a rare complication.[601,603,604]

CHOLESTEROL PERICARDITIS

Cholesterol pericarditis results from pericardial injury associated with deposition of cholesterol crystals and a mononuclear cell inflammatory reaction consisting of foam cells, macrophages, and giant cells. The presence of cholesterol crystals in the pericardial space is believed to provoke a chronic inflammatory response that results in effusion and may ultimately lead to the development of constrictive pericarditis. A pericardial effusion that contains microscopic cholesterol crystals typically has a glittering "gold" appearance. The similarities in the lipid and cholesterol contents of pericardial fluid and serum in some patients with cholesterol pericarditis suggest that simple transudation may explain the high cholesterol content in the pericardial space.

MANAGEMENT. The management of patients with cholesterol pericarditis includes detection and treatment of an underlying predisposing condition associated with the development of cholesterol pericarditis, such as tuberculous, rheumatoid, or myxedematous pericarditis or hypercholesterolemia. However, in the majority of cases, cholesterol pericarditis occurs in the absence of a clear underlying disease.[605] Cholesterol pericardial effusions are usually large, but because they develop slowly, cardiac tamponade is an unusual complication.[606] Pericardiectomy is indicated in the unlikely event of cardiac tamponade as well as in the treatment of massive cholesterol pericardial effusion, which may cause dyspnea and chest pain.[607] The development of constrictive pericarditis requiring pericardiectomy has been reported but is extremely rare.[608]

CHYLOPERICARDIUM

Idiopathic chylopericardium is rare, and chylopericardium is usually associated with mechanical obstruction of the thoracic duct or its drainage into the left subclavian vein resulting from (1) surgical or traumatic rupture of the thoracic duct or (2) lymphatic blockage by neoplasms, tuberculosis, or congenital lymphangiomatosis.[609,610] Thoracic duct obstruction with failure of adequate collateral drainage then results in the reflux of chyle through lymphatics draining the pericardium. Most patients with chylopericardium are asymptomatic and come to clinical attention when a large, slowly accumulating pericardial effusion is detected on chest roentgenogram or echocardiogram.

The presence of a connection between a damaged thoracic duct and the pericardial space can be established by lymphangiography and radionuclide lymphangiography with technetium-99m antimony sulfur colloid, as well as by the recovery of ingested Sudan III, a lipophilic dye, from pericardial aspirate.[609,610] CT may demonstrate density compatible with fat in the pericardial space.[611] The pericardial fluid is usually milky white in a high cholesterol and triglyceride content, protein content greater than 3.5 gm/dl, and microscopic fat droplets demonstrated with a Sudan III stain.[610] Lymphopericardium, which is due to pericardial angiomas as part of generalized lymphangiectasis, is characterized by clear pericardial fluid.

Cardiac tamponade and constrictive pericarditis are rare complications.[610,611] Chylopericardium has been reported as a rare cause of cardiac tamponade after cardiac surgery.[612,613] The management of symptomatic chylopericardium consists of efforts to reduce the likelihood of recurrence. These include ingestion of a diet rich in medium-chain triglycerides or, if this is unsuccessful, in ligation of the thoracic duct and parietal pericardiectomy to evacuate chylous fluid and prevent reaccumulation.[610,613]

TRAUMATIC PERICARDITIS

(See also p. 1536)

In addition to penetrating or nonpenetrating cardiac trauma (Chap. 44), other important causes of traumatic pericarditis include rupture of the esophagus into the pericardial space, which may occur from esophageal erosion secondary to esophageal carcinoma or sudden rupture of the esophageal contents into the pericardial space in Boerhaave's syndrome, or as a complication of esophagogastrectomy. Pericarditis with tamponade and late constriction has also followed esophageal perforation by accidental ingestion of tooth picks and fish bones.[614,615] Traumatic pericarditis due to esophageal rupture

is usually followed by intense erosive pericardial inflammation and infection. Esophageal rupture or perforation may also be followed by the development of an esophagopericardial fistula.[616] These disorders usually require immediate surgical intervention and are associated with a high mortality, although medical management with spontaneous fistula closure has been reported.[616] Pericarditis may also occur secondary to pancreatitis associated with a pericardial effusion with high amylase content and, rarely, the development of cardiac tamponade or a pancreatic-pericardial fistula.[617] The incidence of occult pericardial effusion in patients with acute alcoholic pancreatitis is significantly higher (47 per cent) than in control subjects (11 per cent).[617] The development of fistulas to the pericardium in response to ulcer formation, malignant disease, or surgery may occur from other sites, including the stomach,[618] biliary tract,[619] colon,[620] and bronchi.[621]

Pericardial trauma may also give rise to unusual traumatic syndromes, including cardiovascular collapse following herniation of the heart through a rent in the pericardium caused by trauma, or prior pericardiotomy mimicking congenital partial absence of the pericardium with cardiac subluxation,[622] and intrapericardial diaphragmatic hernia.[623] Diagnosis of cardiac herniation can be made by CT and MRI.[624] Life-threatening cardiac herniation may also occur following radical left pneumonectomy with partial pericardial resection.[625] Intrapericardial herniation of loops of bowel following manual reduction of an umbilical hernia is a rare complication that can be diagnosed by echocardiography.[626]

PERICARDIAL CYSTS

Pericardial cysts are rare developmental anomalies and are typically located at the right costophrenic angle.[627] Unusual locations include the left costophrenic angle, hilum, and superior mediastinum at the level of the aortic arch. They are usually unilocular and filled with clear liquid, giving rise to the term *springwater cysts.*

Pericardial cysts usually do not cause symptoms or unusual physical findings. Rarely, chest pain may occur owing to torsion of the cyst. These lesions typically come to medical attention as an unsuspected finding of a round, sharply defined mass along the right cardiac border on a chest roentgenogram. The size of the cyst in asymptomatic patients may vary over time.[627,628] In most cases, a cyst can be differentiated from solid tumor or aneurysm by two-dimensional echocardiography or CT (Fig. 43-25).[628] When a suspected pericardial cyst is in an unusual location, angiography may occasionally be needed to discriminate a cyst from an aneurysm or pseudoaneurysm. Pericardial cysts located at the right costophrenic angle can be accurately diagnosed and treated by percutaneous aspiration under fluoroscopic guidance.[629] Because long-term follow-up studies have shown that most asymptomatic patients do not develop symptoms, most patients should be managed conservatively, without surgical exploration.[630]

Other benign developmental abnormalities of the pericardium include benign intrapericardial teratomas and intrapericardial bronchial cysts, which can be identified by CT.[631]

CONGENITAL ABSENCE AND DEFECTS OF THE PERICARDIUM

Congenital absence of the pericardium was first described anatomically by Realdus Columbus in 1559, but its antemortem detection did not occur until 1959.[632] In patients with pericardial agenesis, the anomaly usually involves a partial defect of the left-sided pericardium, which is potentially lethal, in 70 per cent; total absence in 9 per cent; partial absence of the right-sided pericardium, in 11 per cent; and absence of the inferior pericardium, in 17 per cent.[633] There is a 3:1 male/female predominance among patients with pericardial defects, and about 30 per cent have other congenital anomalies, including atrial septal defect, bicuspid aortic valve, bronchogenic cysts, or pulmonic sequestration. A familial occurrence of congenital absence of the pericardium has been reported.[634]

Total absence of the pericardium is not usually associated with symptoms. Occasionally the patient may complain of chest discomfort and palpitations. The cause of these symptoms is unknown, but they may be related to torsion of the great vessels due to excess mobility of the heart. Most asymptomatic patients come to attention because of an unexplained heart murmur or abnormal chest roentgenogram. The extremely rare complication of acute chest pain due to strangulation of the heart between the diaphragm and the pulmonary ligament has been reported.[635]

TOTAL ABSENCE OF THE LEFT PERICARDIUM. Patients with total absence of the left pericardium often have widened splitting of the second heart sound, a hyperdynamic precordial impulse, leftward displacement of the apical impulse, and a systolic murmur at the upper left sternal border that may be related to turbulent blood flow in an unusually mobile heart. ECG abnormalities include right-axis deviation due to levoposition of the heart, incomplete right bundle branch block, clockwise displacement of the QRS transition zone of the precordial leads, and tall and peaked P waves in the right precordial leads.[636]

The standard posteroanterior view of the chest roentgenogram re-

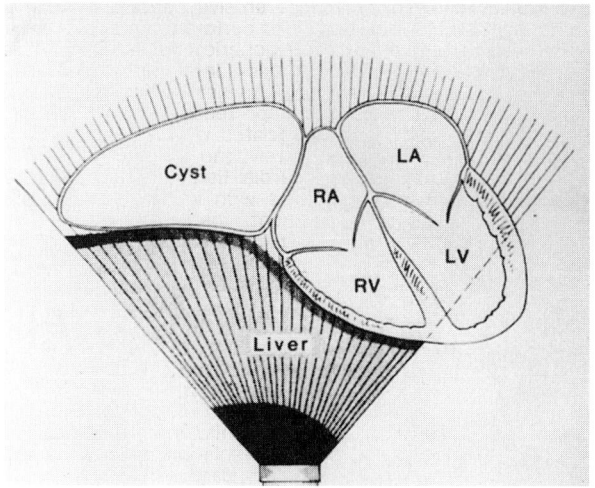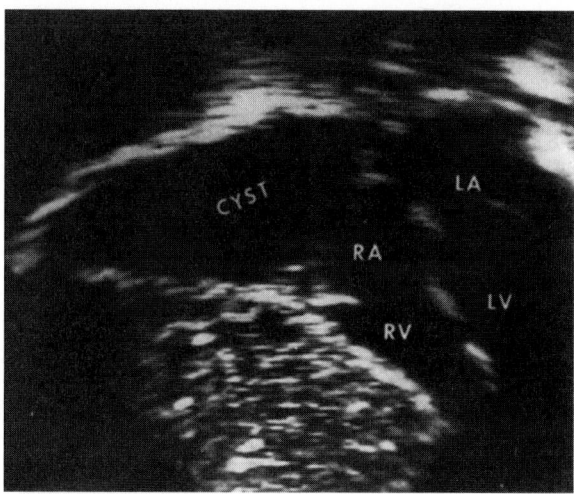

FIGURE 43–25. Two-dimensional subcostal echocardiographic appearance of a well-demarcated benign pericardial cyst adjacent to the right atrial (RA) wall. (From Hynes, J. K., et al.: Two-dimensional echocardiographic diagnosis of pericardial cyst. Mayo Clin. Proc. *58*:60, 1983.)

veals marked leftward displacement of the cardiac silhouette, prominence of the main pulmonary artery, and interposition of radiolucent lung tissue between the aorta and main pulmonary artery or between the left hemidiaphragm and inferior cardiac border. This anomaly must be differentiated from other conditions that cause prominence of the left hilum or pulmonary artery on the standard chest film, including pulmonic valve stenosis, atrial septal defect, idiopathic dilatation of the pulmonary artery, and hilar adenopathy.

M-mode *echocardiographic findings* simulate those seen in right ventricular volume overload, including dilatation of the right ventricle and paradoxical anterior motion of the septum in systole, which is an artifact related to exaggerated cardiac rotation. Two-dimensional echocardiography can demonstrate localized bulging of the left ventricular contour and the drop-off of pericardial echoes.[637] Radionuclide perfusion imaging can be used to confirm the diagnosis by demonstration of a wedge of lung tissue between the heart and left hemidiaphragm[638]; CT and MRI can also be used to detect absence of the left pericardium by demonstrating visibility of the right pericardium and absence of the left pericardium, absence of the preaortic recess, and the abnormal presence of a wedge of lung between the aorta and pulmonary artery.[639]

Findings at catheterization are usually normal. Cardiac catheterization with angiography is indicated only if there is a strong suspicion of associated congenital anomalies requiring surgical correction. Usually no specific therapy is required for management of complete absence of the left-sided pericardium.

PARTIAL ABSENCE OF THE PERICARDIUM. Partial left-sided pericardial defects may be complicated by herniation of the left atrial appendage, atrium, or left ventricle through the defect, associated with

chest pain, syncope, and sudden death from cardiac strangulation.[640–642] The chest roentgenogram usually shows the nonspecific finding of prominence of the second arch of the left heart border, which must be distinguished from pulmonary artery dilation or aneurysm of the left atrial appendage.[643] Two-dimensional echocardiography and MRI are helpful in demonstrating dilation of the left atrial appendage that extends beyond the pulmonary artery[643,644] (Fig. 43–26). Pulmonary artery angiography with follow-through of contrast opacification to the left heart is the standard method of definitively demonstrating herniation of the left atrium or left atrial appendage beyond the left heart border.[643,644] Partial herniation of the heart and diastolic collapse and compression of the coronary arteries through the defect is a complication of this anomaly that uncommonly may contribute to the development of chest pain and coronary artery strictures.[642,645]

The even rarer anomaly of partially right-sided pericardial defect may be associated with inspiratory right-sided chest pain secondary to herniation of the right atrium and right ventricle through the defect or herniation of lung into the pericardial cavity. The chest roentgenogram may show an unusual protuberance of the right heart border, and technetium-99m cardiac blood pool imaging may demonstrate that the abnormal contour of the right heart border fills simultaneously with the right atrium.[646] Right atrial angiography in the left anterior oblique projection is helpful in documenting herniation of the right atrium and right ventricle through the pericardial defect. Surgical treatment of partial left- or right-sided pericardial defects is usually indicated to relieve symptoms and prevent cardiac strangulation. The defect may be approached by excision of the atrial appendage, pericardioplasty, or pericardiotomy.[647]

FIGURE 43–26. Noninvasive diagnostic features of partial absence of the left pericardium. The chest roentgenogram (A) shows knoblike prominence of the left atrial appendage (arrow). The short-axis cross-sectional two-dimensional echocardiogram (B) shows an enlarged left atrial appendage (arrow) extending beyond the pulmonary artery. The frontal plane magnetic resonance image (C) shows enlargement and lateral protuberance of the left atrial appendage (arrow). A contrast cineangiogram (D) with the catheter positioned across a patent foramen ovale in the left atrial appendage shows a characteristic wedge of lung between the aorta and pulmonary artery and confirms the herniation of the left atrial appendage (arrow). (From Altman, C. A., et al.: Noninvasive diagnostic features of partial absence of the pericardium. Am. J. Cardiol. *63*:1536, 1989.)

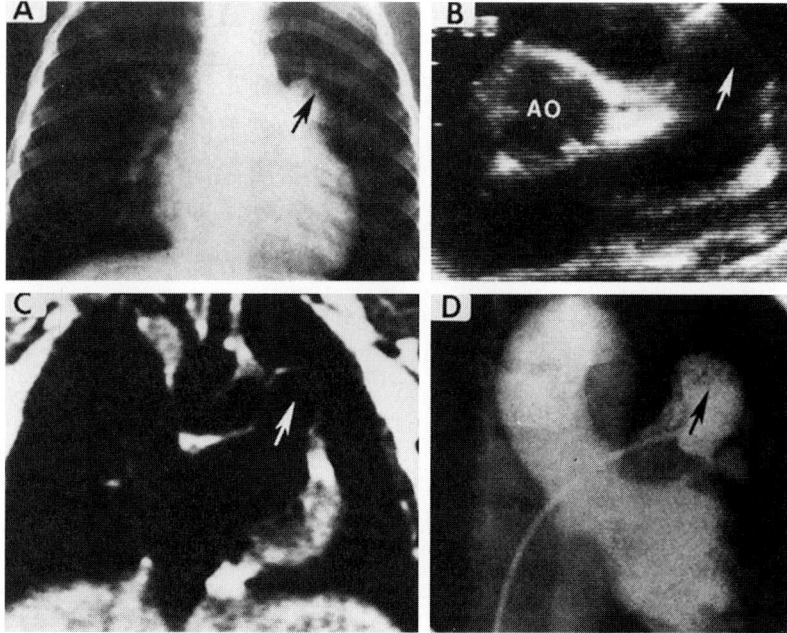

REFERENCES

ANATOMY AND FUNCTIONS

1. Fowler, N. O.: Pericardial diseases. *In* Diagnosis of Heart Disease. New York, Springer-Verlag, 1991, pp. 292–313.
2. Holt, J. P.: The normal pericardium. Am. J. Cardiol. *26*:455, 1970.
3. Alles, A., and Dom, R. M.: Peripheral sensory nerve fibers that dichotomize to supply the brachium and the pericardium in the rat. Brain Res. *342*:382, 1970.
4. Ishihara, T., Ferrans, V. J., Jones, M., et al.: Histologic and ultrastructural features of a normal human parietal pericardium. Am. J. Cardiol. *46*:744, 1980.
5. Fukuo, Y., Nakatani, T., Shinohara, H., and Matsuda, T.: Pericardium of rodents: Pores connect the pericardial and pleural cavities. Anat. Res. *220*:132, 1988.
6. Hills, B. A., and Butler, B. D.: Phospholipids identified on the pericardium and their ability to impart boundary lubrication. Ann. Biomed. Eng. *13*:573, 1985.
7. Miyazaki, T., Pride, H. P., and Zipes, D. P.: Prostaglandins in the pericardial fluid modulate neural regulation of cardiac electrophysiological properties. Circ. Res. *66*:163, 1990.
8. Lee, M. D., Fung, Y. C., Shabetai, R., and LeWinter, M. M.: Biaxial mechanical properties of human pericardium and canine comparisons. Am. J. Physiol. *253*:H75, 1987.
9. Tyson, G. S., Jr., Maier, G. W., Olsen, C. O., et al.: Pericardial influences on ventricular filling in the conscious dog. Circ. Res. *54*:173, 1984.
10. Shabetai, R.: Pericardial and cardiac pressure. Circulation *77*:1, 1988.
11. Smiseth, O. A., Frais, M. A., Kingma, I., et al.: Assessment of pericardial constraint in dogs. Circulation *71*:158, 1985.
12. Smiseth, O. A., Frais, M. A., Kingma, I., et al.: Assessment of pericardial constraint: The relation between right ventricular filling pressure and pericardial pressure measured after pericardiocentesis. J. Am. Coll. Cardiol. *7*:307, 1986.
13. Boltwood, C. M., Jr.: Ventricular performance related to transmural filling pressure in clinical tamponade. Circulation *73*:428, 1987.
14. Santamore, W. P., Constantinesco, M., and Little, W. C.: Direct assessment of right ventricular transmural pressure. Circulation *75*:744, 1987.
15. Slinker, B. K., Ditchey, R. V., Bell, S. P., and LeWinter, M. M.: Right heart pressure does not equal pericardial pressure in the potassium chloride arrested canine heart in situ. Circulation *7G*:357, 1987.
16. Hamilton, D. R., Dani, R. S., Semlacher, R. A., et al: Right atrial and right ventricular transmural pressures in dogs and humans. Effects of the pericardium. Circulation *90*:2492, 1994.
17. Hoit, B. D., Lew, W. Y., and LeWinter, M.: Regional variation in pericardial contact pressure in the canine ventricle. Am. J. Physiol. *255*:H1370, 1988.
18. Chew, P. H., Humphrey, J. D., and Yin, F. C.: Regional finite deformations of the in situ canine pericardium. Am. J. Physiol. *264*:H97, 1993.
19. Bernard, H. L.: The functions of the pericardium. J. Physiol. *22*:43, 1898.
20. Junemann, M., Smiseth, O. A., Refsum, H., et al.: Quantification of effect of pericardium on LV diastolic PV relation in dogs. Am. J. Physiol. *252*:H963, 1987.
21. Gilbert, J. C., and Glantz, S. A.: Determinants of ventricular filling and of the diastolic pressure-volume relation. Circ. Res. *64*:827, 1989.
22. Shirato, K., Shabetai, R., Bhargave, V., et al.: Alteration of the left ventricular diastolic pressure-segment length relation produced by the pericardium. Circulation *57*:1191, 1978.
23. Smiseth, O. A., Manyari, D. E., Lima, J. A., et al.: Modulation of vascular capacitance by angiotensin and nitroprusside: A mechanism of changes in pericardial pressure. Circulation *76*:875, 1987.
24. LeWinter, M. M., and Pavelec, R.: Influence of the pericardium on left ventricular end-diastolic pressure-segment relations during early and later stages of experimental chronic volume overload in dogs. Circ. Res. *50*:501, 1982.
25. Freeman, G. L., and LeWinter, M. M.: Pericardial adaptations during chronic cardiac dilation in dogs. Circ. Res. *54*:294, 1984.
26. Frais, M. A., Bergman, D. W., Kingma, I., et al.: The dependence of the time constant of left ventricular isovolumic relaxation (tau) on pericardial pressure. Circulation *81*:1071, 1990.
27. Serizawa, T., Carabello, B. A., and Grossman, W.: Effect of pacing induced ischemia on left ventricular diastolic pressure-volume relations in dog with coronary stenosis. Circ. Res. *46*:430, 1980.
28. Armoore, J. N., Santamore, W. P., Coring, W. J., and George, D. T.: Computer simulation of the effects of ventricular interdependence on indices of left ventricular systolic function. J. Biomed. Eng. *14*:257, 1992.
29. Brinker, J. A., Weiss, J. L., Lappe, D. L., et al.: Leftward septal displacement during right ventricular loading in man. Circulation *61*:626, 1980.
30. Lorell, B. H., Palacios, I., Daggett, W. M., et al.: Right ventricular distention and left ventricular compliance. Am. J. Physiol. *240*:H87, 1981.
31. Hoit, B. D., Dalton, N., Bhargava, V., and Shabetai, R.: Pericardial influences on right and left ventricular filling dynamics. Circ. Res. *68*:197, 1991.
32. Santamore, W. P., Bartlett, R., Van Buren, S. J., et al.: Ventricular coupling in constrictive pericarditis. Circulation *74*:597, 1986.
33. Mangano, D. T.: The effect of the pericardium on ventricular systolic function in man. Circulation *61*:352, 1980.
34. Kanazawa, M., Shirato, K., Ishikawa, K., et al.: The effect of pericardium on the end-systolic pressure-segment length relationship in the

canine left ventricle in acute volume overload. Circulation *68*:1290, 1983.
35. Goto, Y., Slinker, B. K., and LeWinter, M. M.: Nonhomogeneous left ventricular regional shortening during acute right ventricular pressure overload. Circ. Res. *65*:43, 1989.
36. Stray-Gendersen, J., Musch, T. I., Haidet, G. C., et al.: The effect of pericardiectomy on maximal oxygen consumption and maximal cardiac output in untrained dogs. Circ. Res. *58*:523, 1986.
37. Ringertz, H. G., Misbach, G. A., and Tyberg, J. V.: Effect of the normal pericardium on the left ventricular diastolic pressure-volume relationship. Acta Radiol. *22*:529, 1981.
38. Jarvinen, A., Peltola, K., Rasanen, J., and Heikkila, J.: Immediate hemodynamic effects of pericardial closure after open-heart surgery. Scand. J. Thorac. Cardiovasc. Surg. *21*:131, 1987.
39. Ludbrook, P. A., Byrne, J. D., Kurnik, P. B., and McKnight, R. C.: Influence of reduction of preload and afterload by nitroglycerin on left ventricular diastolic pressure-volume relations and relaxation in man. Circulation *56*:937, 1977.
40. Ludbrook, P. A., Byrne, J. D., and McKnight, R. C.: Influence of right ventricular hemodynamics on left ventricular diastolic pressure-overload relations in man. Circulation *59*:21, 1979.
41. Wong, C. Y., and Spotnitz, H. M.: Effect of nitroprusside on end-diastolic pressure-diameter relations of the human left ventricle after pericardiectomy. J. Thorac. Cardiovasc. Surg. *82*:350, 1981.
42. Ross, J., Jr.: Acute displacement of the diastolic pressure-volume curve of the left ventricle: Role of the pericardium and the right ventricle. Circulation *59*:32, 1979.
43. Lee, M. J., and Boughner, D. R.: Mechanical properties of human pericardium. Circ. Res. *57*:475, 1985.
44. Bartle, S. H., and Hermann, H. J.: Acute mitral regurgitation in man. Hemodynamic evidence and observations indicating an early role for the pericardium. Circulation *36*:839, 1967.
45. Lorell, B. H., Leinbach, R. C., Pohost, G. M., et al.: Right ventricular infarction. Am. J. Cardiol. *43*:465, 1979.
46. Goldstein, J. A., Vlahakes, G. H., Verrier, E. D., et al.: The role of right ventricular systolic dysfunction and elevated intrapericardial pressure in the genesis of low output in experimental right ventricular infarction. Circulation *65*:513, 1982.
47. Tischler, M. D., Rowan, M., and LeWinter, M. M.: Increased left ventricular mass after thoracotomy and pericardiectomy. A role for the relief of pericardial constraint? Circulation *87*:1921, 1993.
48. Janicki, J. S.: Influence of the pericardium and ventricular interdependence of left ventricular diastolic and systolic function in patients with heart failure. Circulation *81*(Suppl. II):15, 1990.

ACUTE PERICARDITIS

49. Garty, I., Mader, R., and Schonfeld, S.: Post pulmonary embolism pericarditis. Clin. Nucl. Med. *19*:519, 1994.
50. Wenger, N. K.: Pericardial disease in the elderly. Cardiovasc. Clin. *22*:97, 1992.
51. Markiewicz, W., Brik, A., Brook, G., et al.: Pericardial rub in pericardial effusion: Lack of correlation with amount of fluid. Chest *77*:643, 1980.
52. Spodick, D. H.: Pericardial rub: Prospective, multiple observer investigation of pericardial friction rub in 100 patients. Am. J. Cardiol. *35*:357, 1975.
53. Spodick, D. H.: Diagnostic electrocardiographic sequences in acute pericarditis: Significance of PR segment and PR vector changes. Circulation *48*:575, 1973.
54. Kouvaras, G., Soufras, G., Chronopoulos, G., et al.: The ST segment as a different diagnostic feature between acute pericarditis and acute inferior myocardial infarction. Angiology *41*:207, 1990.
55. Teh, B. S., Walsh, J., Bell, A. J., et al.: Electrical current paths in acute pericarditis. J. Electrocardiol. *26*:291, 1993.
56. Toriya Martinez, R. N., and Gonzalez Hermosillo, J. A.: Acute nonspecific pericarditis. Arch. Inst. Cardiol. Mex. *57*:307, 1987.
57. Bruce, M. A., and Spodick, D. H.: Atypical electrocardiogram in acute pericarditis: Characteristics and prevalence. J. Electrocardiol. *13*:61, 1980.
58. Carson, W.: Maximal spatial ST vector of ST segment elevation in the right praecordial leads on electrocardiogram due to acute pericarditis. Eur. Heart. J. *9*:665, 1988.
59. Wanner, W. R., Schaal, S. F., Bashore, T. M., et al.: Repolarization variant vs. acute pericarditis. A prospective electrocardiographic and echocardiographic evaluation. Chest *83*:180, 1983.
60. Ginzton, L. E., and Laks, M. M.: The differential diagnosis of acute pericarditis. Circulation *65*:1004, 1982.
61. Dressler, N.: Sinus tachycardia complicating and outlasting pericarditis. Am. Heart J. *72*:422, 1966.
62. Spodick, D. H.: Frequency of arrhythmias in acute pericarditis determined by Holter monitoring. Am. J. Cardiol. *53*:842, 1984.
63. Weiss, J. M., and Spodick, D. H.: Association of left pleural effusion with pericardial disease. N. Engl. J. Med. *308*:696, 1983.
64. Olson, H. G., Lyons, K. P., Aronow, W. S., et al.: Technetium-99m stannous pyrophosphate myocardial scintigrams in pericardial disease. Am. Heart J. *99*:459, 1980.
65. Kodama, K., Igase, M., Funada, J., et al.: Gallium-67 citrate scintigraphy in idiopathic pericarditis: Report of a case. Jpn. Circ. J. *58*:298, 1994.

66. Matsouka, H., Hamada, M., Honda, T., et al.: Evaluation of acute myocarditis and pericarditis by Gd-DTPA enhanced magnetic resonance imaging. Eur. Heart J. 15:283, 1994.

67. Karjalainen, J., and Heikkila, J.: Acute pericarditis: Myocardial enzyme release as evidence for myocarditis. Am. Heart J. 111:546, 1986.

68. Saner, H. E., Gobel, F. L., Nicoloff, D. M., and Edwairds, J. E.: Aortic dissection presenting as pericarditis. Chest 91:71, 1987.

69. Permanyer-Miralda, G., Sagrista-Sauleda, J., and Soler-Soler, J.: Primary acute pericardial disease: A prospective series of 231 consecutive patients. Am. J. Cardiol. 56:623, 1985.

70. Arunsalam, S., and Siegel, R. J.: Rapid resolution of symptomatic acute pericarditis with ketorolac tromethamine: A parenteral nonsteroidal anti-inflammatory agent. Am. Heart J. 125:1455, 1993.

71. Sagrista-Sauleda, J., Permanyer-Miralda, G., Candell-Riera, J., et al.: Transient cardiac constriction: An unrecognized pattern of evolution in effusive acute idiopathic pericarditis. Am. J. Cardiol. 59:961, 1987.

72. Fowler, N. O., and Harbin, A. D.: Recurrent pericarditis: Follow-up of 31 patients. J. Am. Coll. Cardiol. 7:300, 1986.

73. Melchior, T. M., Ringsdal, V., Hildebrandt, P., and Torp-Pedersen, C.: Recurrent acute idiopathic pericarditis treated with intravenous methylprednisone given as pulse therapy. Am. Heart J. 123:1086, 1992.

74. Hatcher, C. R., Logue, R. B., Logan, W. D., et al.: Pericardiectomy for recurrent pericarditis. J. Thorac. Cardiovasc. Surg. 62:371, 1971.

75. Permanyer-Miralda, G., Sagrista-Sauleda, J., Shabetai, R., et al.: Acute pericardial disease: An approach to etiologic diagnosis and treatment. In Soler-Soler, J., Permanyer-Miralda, G., and Sagrista-Sauleda, J. (eds.): Pericardial Disease: New Insights and Old Dilemmas. Dordrecht, The Netherlands, Kluwer Academic Publishers, 1990, pp. 193–214.

76. Millaire, A., deGroote, P., Decoulx, E., et al.: Treatment of recurrent pericarditis with colchicine. Eur. Heart J. 15:120, 1994.

77. Adler, Y., Zandman-Goddard, G., Ravid, M., et al.: Usefulness of colchicine in preventing recurrences of pericarditis. Am. J. Cardiol. 73:916, 1994.

78. Guindo, J., Rodriguez de la Serna, A., Ramio, J., et al.: Recurrent pericarditis. Relief with colchicine. Circulation 82:1117, 1990.

PERICARDIAL EFFUSION

79. Carsky, E. W., Mauceri, R. A., and Azimi, F.: The epicardial fat pad sign: Analysis of frontal and lateral chest radiographs in patients with pericardial effusion. Radiology 137:303, 1980.

80. Miller, S. W.: Imaging pericardial disease. Radiol. Clin. North Am. 27:1113, 1989:

81. Horowitz, M. S., Schultz, C. S., and Stinson, E. B.: Sensitivity and specificity of echocardiographic diagnosis of pericardial effusion. Circulation 50:239, 1974.

82. Berger, M., Bobak, K., Jelveh, M., and Goldberg, E.: Pericardial effusion diagnosed by echocardiography. Clinical and electrocardiographic findings. Chest 74:174, 1978.

83. Enein, M., Zina, A. A., Kassem, M., and el-Tabbakh, G.: Echocardiography of the pericardium in pregnancy. Obstet. Gynecol. 69:851, 1987.

84. Friedman, M. J., Sahn, D. J., and Haber, K.: Two-dimensional echocardiography and B-mode ultrasonography for the diagnosis of loculated pericardial effusion. Circulation 60:1644, 1979.

85. Soler-Soler, J.: Massive chronic idiopathic pericardial effusion. In Soler-Soler, J., Permanyer-Miralda, G., and Sagrista-Sauleda, J. (eds.): Pericardial Disease: New Insights and Old Dilemmas. Dordrecht, The Netherlands, Kluwer Academic Publishers, 1990, pp. 153–165.

86. Reddy, P. S., Curtiss, E. I., O'Toole, J. D., and Shaver, J. A.: Cardiac tamponade: Hemodynamic observations in man. Circulation 58:265, 1978.

87. Fowler, N. O.: Cardiac tamponade. A clinical or an echocardiographic diagnosis? Circulation 87:1738, 1993.

88. Harasawa, H., Li, K. S., Nakamoto, T., et al.: Ventricular coupling via the pericardium: Normal versus tamponade. Cardiovasc. Res. 27:1470, 1993.

89. Nakamoto, T., Li, K. S., Johnston, W. E., and Santamore, W. P.: Differential effects of positive end expiratory pressure and cardiac tamponade on left-right ventricular mechanical function in the dog. Cardiovasc. Res. 26:148, 1992.

90. Shibamoto, T., Hayashi, T., Jr., Saeki, Y., et al.: Differential control of sympathetic outflow to kidney, heart, adrenal gland, and liver during systemic hypotension produced by cardiac tamponade in anesthetized dogs. Circ. Shock 39:114, 1993.

91. Nishikawa, Y., Roberts, J. P., Talcott, M. R., et al.: Accelerated myocardial relaxation in conscious dogs during acute tamponade. Am. J. Physiol. 266:H1953, 1994.

92. Pegram, B. L., Kardon, M. B., and Bishop, V. S.: Changes in left ventricular internal diameter with increasing pericardial pressure. Cardiovasc. Res. 9:707, 1975.

93. Mancini, G. B. J., McGillem, M. J., Bates, E. R., et al.: Hormonal responses to cardiac tamponade: Inhibition of release of atrial natriuretic factor despite elevation of atrial pressures. Circulation 76:884, 1987.

94. Stokhof, A. A., Overduin, L. M., Mol, J. A., and Rijnberk, A.: Effects of pericardiocentesis on circulating concentrations of atrial natriuretic hormone and arginine vasopressin in dogs with spontaneous pericardial effusion. Eur. J. Endocrinol. 130:357, 1994.

95. Casale, P. N., Fifer, M. A., Graham, R. M., and Palacios, I. F.: Relation of atrial pressure and plasma levels of atrial natriuretic factor in cardiac tamponade. Am. J. Cardiol. 73:610, 1994.

96. Wechsler, A. S., Auerbach, B. J., Graham, T. C., and Sabiston, D. C.: Distribution of intramyocardial blood flow during pericardial tamponade: Correlation with microscopic anatomy and intrinsic myocardial contractility. J. Thorac. Cardiovasc. Surg. 68:847, 1974.

97. Kostreva, D. R., Castaner, A., Pedersen, D. H., and Kampine, J. P.: Nonvagally mediated bradycardia during tamponade or severe hemorrhage. Cardiology 68:65, 1981.

98. Fowler, N. O., and Gabel, M.: The hemodynamic effects of cardiac tamponade: Mainly the result of atrial, not ventricular, compression. Circulation 71:154, 1985.

99. Fowler, N. O., Gabel, M., and Buncher, C. R.: Cardiac tamponade: A comparison of right versus left heart compression. J. Am. Coll. Cardiol. 12:187, 1988.

100. Schwartz, S. L., Pandian, N. G., Cao, Q. L., et al.: Left ventricular diastolic collapse in regional left heart cardiac tamponade. An experimental echocardiographic and hemodynamic study. J. Am. Coll. Cardiol. 22:907, 1993.

101. Leimgruber, P. P., Klopfenstein, H. S., Wann, L. S., and Brooks, H. L.: The hemodynamic derangement associated with right ventricular diastolic collapse in cardiac tamponade: An experimental echocardiographic study. Circulation 68:612, 1983.

102. Klopfenstein, H. S., Cogswell, T. L., Bernath, G. A., et al.: Alternations in intravascular volume affect the relation between right ventricular diastolic collapse and the hemodynamic severity of cardiac tamponade. J. Am. Coll. Cardiol. 6:1057, 1985.

103. Singh, S., Wann, L. S., Schuchard, G. H., et al.: Right ventricular and right atrial collapse in patients with cardiac tamponade—a combined echocardiographic and hemodynamic study. Circulation 70:966, 1984.

104. Ruskin, J., Bache, R. J., Rembert, J. C., and Greenfield, J. C., Jr.: Pressure-flow studies in man: Effect of respiration on left ventricular stroke volume. Circulation 48:79, 1973.

105. Shabetai, R., Fowler, N. O., Fenton, J. C., and Masangkay, M.: Pulsus paradoxus. J. Clin. Invest. 44:1882, 1965.

106. Shabetai, R., Fowler, N. O., and Gueron, M.: The effects of respiration on aortic pressure and flow. Am. Heart J. 65:525, 1963.

107. Savitt, M. A., Tyson, G. S., Elbeery, J. R., et al.: Physiology of cardiac tamponade and paradoxical pulse in conscious dogs. Am. J. Physiol. 265:H1996, 1993.

108. Gonzales, M. S., Basnight, M. A., Appleton, C. P., et al.: Experimental pericardial effusion: Relation of abnormal respiratory variation in mitral flow velocity to hemodynamics and diastolic right heart collapse. J. Am. Coll. Cardiol. 17:239, 1991.

109. Settle, H. P., Jr., Engel, P. J., Fowler, N. O., et al.: Echocardiographic study of the paradoxical arterial pulse in chronic obstructive lung disease. Circulation 62:1297, 1980.

110. Winer, H. E., and Krozon, I.: Absence of paradoxical pulse in patients with cardiac tamponade and atrial septal defects. Am. J. Cardiol. 44:378, 1979.

111. Cunningham, M. J., Safian, R. D., Come, P. C., and Lorell, B. H.: Absence of pulsus paradoxus in a patient with cardiac tamponade and coexisting pulmonary artery obstruction. Am. J. Med. 83:973, 1987.

112. Guberman, B. A., Fowler, N. O., Engel, P. J., et al.: Cardiac tamponade in medical patients. Circulation 64:633, 1981.

113. Beck, C. S.: Two cardiac compression triads. JAMA 104:714, 1935.

114. Sznajder, J. I., Evander, E., Pollak, E. R., et al.: Pericardial effusion causes interstitial pulmonary edema in dogs. Circulation 76:843, 1987.

115. Brown, J., MacKinnon, D., King, A., and Vanderbush, E.: Elevated arterial blood pressure in cardiac tamponade. N. Engl. J. Med. 327:463, 1992.

116. Labib, S. B., Udelson, J. E., and Pandian, N. G.: Echocardiography in low pressure cardiac tamponade. Am. J. Cardiol. 63:1156, 1989.

117. Katzir, D., Klinovsky, E., Kent, V., et al.: Spontaneous pneumopericardium: Case report and review of the literature. Cardiology 76:305, 1989.

118. Bricheteau: Observat d'hydropneumopercarde accompane d'un fluctuation perceptible a l'orielle. Arch. Gen. Med. 4:334, 1844.

119. Usher, B. W., and Popp, R. L.: Electrical alternans: Mechanism in pericardial effusion. Am. Heart J. 83:459, 1972.

120. Friedman, H. S., Lajam, F., Calderon, J., et al.: Electrocardiographic features of experimental cardiac tamponade in closed-chest dogs. Eur. J. Cardiol. 6:311, 1977.

121. D'Cruz, I. A., Cohen, H. C., Prabhus, R., and Glick, G.: Diagnosis of cardiac tamponade by echocardiography (changes in mitral valve motion and ventricular dimensions with special reference to paradoxical pulse). Circulation 52:460, 1975.

122. Appleton, C. P., Hatle, L. K., and Popp, R. L.: Cardiac tamponade and pericardial effusion: Respiratory variation in transvalvular flow velocities studied by Doppler echocardiography. J. Am. Coll. Cardiol. 11:1020, 1988.

123. Burstow, D. J., Jae, K. O., Baileys, K. R., et al.: Cardiac tamponade: Characteristic Doppler observations. Mayo Clin. Proc. 64:312, 1989.

124. Shindler, D. M., Reddy, S., Shindler, O. I., and Kostis, J. B.: Failure of the aortic valve to open during inspiration in cardiac tamponade. Chest 82:797, 1982.

125. Simeonidou, E., Hamouratidis, N., Tzimas, K., et al.: Respiratory variation in mitral flow velocity in pericardial effusion and cardiac tamponade. Angiology 45:213, 1994.

126. DiSegni, E., Feinberg, M. S., Sheinowitz, M., et al.: Left ventricular

pseudohypertrophy in cardiac tamponade: An echocardiographic study in a canine model. J. Am. Coll. Cardiol. *21:*1286, 1993.

127. Chuttani, K., Pandian, N. G., Mohanty, P. K., et al.: Left ventricular diastolic collapse: An echocardiographic sign of regional cardiac tamponade. Circulation *83:*1999, 1991.

128. Cogswell, T. L., Bernath, G. A., Wann, L. S., et al.: Effects of intravascular volume on the value of pulsus paradoxus and right ventricular diastolic collapse in predicting cardiac tamponade. Circulation *72:*1076, 1985.

129. Tunick, P. A., Nachamie, M., and Kronzon, I.: Reversal of echocardiographic signs of pericardial tamponade by transfusion. Am. Heart J. *119:*199, 1990.

130. Vaska, K., Wann, L. S., Sagar, K., and Klopfenstein, H. S.: Pleural effusion as a cause of right ventricular diastolic collapse. Circulation *86:*609, 1992.

131. Martins, J. B., and Kerber, R. E.: Can cardiac tamponade be diagnosed by echocardiography? Circulation *60:*737, 1979.

132. Levine, M. J., Lorell, B. H., Diver, D. J., and Come, P. C.: Implications of echocardiographically-assisted diagnosis of pericardial tamponade in contemporary medical patients: Detection prior to hemodynamic embarrassment. J. Am. Coll. Cardiol. *17:*59, 1991.

133. Eisenberg, M. J., Oken, K., Guerrero, S., et al.: Prognostic value of echocardiography in hospitalized patients with pericardial effusion. Am. J. Cardiol. *70:*934, 1992.

134. Zhang, H., Spapen, H., and Vincent, J. L.: Effects of dobutamine and norepinephrine on oxygen availability in tamponade-induced stagnant hypoxia: A prospective, randomized controlled study. Crit. Care Med. *22:*299, 1994.

135. Kerber, R. E., Jascho, J. A., Litchfield, R., et al.: Hemodynamic effects of volume expansion and nitroprusside compared with the pericardiocentesis in patients with cardiac tamponade. N. Engl. J. Med. *307:*929, 1982.

136. Moller, C. T., Schoonbee, C. G., and Rosendorff, C.: Hemodynamics of cardiac tamponade during various modes of ventilation. Br. J. Anaesth. *51:*409, 1979.

137. Kilpatrick, Z. M., and Chapman, C. B.: On pericardiocentesis. Am. J. Cardiol. *16:*722, 1965.

138. Krikorian, J. G., and Hancock, E. W.: Pericardiocentesis. Am. J. Med. *65:*808, 1978.

139. Kaiser, E., and Loewenneck, H.: Pericardial puncture. The most favorable anatomical approach. Munch. Med. Wochenschr. *123:*1697, 1981.

140. Heilerh, B., Anderes, U., and Follath, F.: Diagnosis and therapy of cardiac tamponade. An analysis of 50 patients. Schweiz. Med. Wochenschr. *111:*735, 1981.

141. Callahan, J. A., Seward, J. B., Nishimura, R. A., et al.: Two-dimensional echocardiographically guided pericardiocentesis: Experience in 117 consecutive patients. Am. J. Cardiol. *55:*476, 1985.

142. Morgan, C. D., Marshall, S. A., and Ross, J. R.: Catheter drainage of the pericardium: Its safety and efficacy. Can. J. Surg. *32:*331, 1989.

143. Armstrong, N. F., Feigenbaum, H., and Dillon, J. C.: Acute right ventricular dilation and echocardiographic volume overload following pericardiocentesis for relief of cardiac tamponade. Am. Heart J. *107:*1266, 1984.

144. Glasser, F., Fein, A. M., Feinsilver, S. H., et al.: Non-cardiogenic pulmonary edema after pericardial drainage for cardiac tamponade. Chest *94:*869, 1988.

145. Lorell, B. H., and Grossman, W.: Profiles in constrictive pericarditis, restrictive cardiomyopathy, and cardiac tamponade. *In* Grossman, W., and Baim, D. S. (eds.): Cardiac Catheterization, Angiography, and Intervention. 5th ed. Philadelphia, Lea & Febiger, 1996, pp. 787–800.

146. Lock, J. E., Bass, J. L., Kulif, F. J., and Fuhrman, B. P.: Chronic percutaneous pericardial drainage with modified pigtail catheters in children. Am. J. Cardiol. *53:*1179, 1984.

147. Palacios, I. F., Tuzcu, E. M., Ziskind, A. A., et al.: Percutaneous pericardial window for patients with malignant pericardial effusions and tamponade. Cathet. Cardiovasc. Diagn. *22:*244, 1991.

148. Ziskind, A. A., Pearce, A. C., Lemmon, C. C., et al.: Percutaneous balloon pericardiotomy for the treatment of cardiac tamponade and large pericardial effusions: Description of technique and report of the first 50 cases. J. Am. Coll. Cardiol. *21:*1, 1993.

149. Palatianos, G. M., Thurer, R. J., and Kaiser, G. A.: Comparison of effectiveness and safety of operations on the pericardium. Chest *88:*30, 1985.

150. Piehler, J. M., Pluth, J. R., Schaff, H. V., et al.: Surgical management of effusive pericardial disease. J. Thorac. Cardiovasc. Surg. *90:*506, 1986.

151. Wall, T. C., Campbell, P. T., O'Connor, C. M., et al.: Diagnosis and management (by subxiphoid pericardiotomy) of large pericardial effusions causing cardiac tamponade. Am. J. Cardiol. *69:*1075, 1992.

152. Little, A. G., and Ferguson, M. K.: Pericardioscopy as adjunct to pericardial window. Chest *89:*53, 1986.

153. Wurtz, A., Chambon, J. P., Millaire, A., et al.: Pericardioscopy: Techniques, indications and results. Apropos of an experience with 70 cases. Ann. Chir. *46:*188, 1992.

154. Endrys, J., Simo, M., Shafie, M. Z., et al.: New nonsurgical technique for multiple pericardial biopsies. Cathet. Cardiovasc. Diag. *15:*92, 1988.

155. Maisch, B., and Druge, L.: Pericardioscopy—a new window to the heart in inflammatory heart disease. Herz *17:*71, 1992.

156. Maisch, B.: Pericardial diseases with a focus on etiology, pathogenesis, pathophysiology, new diagnostic imaging methods, and treatment. Curr. Opin. Cardiol. *9:*379, 1994.

157. Ziskind, A. A., Rodriguez, S., Lemmon, C., and Burstein, S.: Percutaneous pericardial biopsy as an adjunctive technique for the diagnosis of pericardial disease. Am. J. Cardiol. *74:*288, 1994.

CONSTRICTIVE PERICARDITIS

158. Nishimura, R. A., Kazmier, F. J., Smith, H. C., and Danielson, G. K.: Right ventricular outflow obstruction caused by constrictive pericardial disease. Am. J. Cardiol. *55:*1447, 1985.

159. Beloucif, S., Takata, M., Shimada, M., and Robotham, J. L.: Influence of pericardial constraint on atrioventricular interactions. Am. J. Physiol. *263:*H125, 1992.

160. Meyer, T. E., Sareli, P., Marcus, R. H., et al.: Mechanism underlying Kussmaul's sign in chronic constrictive pericarditis. Am. J. Cardiol. *64:*1069, 1989.

161. Wolozin, M. W., Ortola, F. V., Spodick, D. H., and Seifter, J. L.: Release of atrial natriuretic factor after pericardiectomy for chronic constrictive pericarditis. Am. J. Cardiol. *62:*1323, 1988.

162. Chandrashekhar, Y., Anand, I. S., Kalra, G. S., and Wander, G. S.: Rate-dependent hemodynamic responses during incremental atrial pacing in chronic constrictive pericarditis before and after surgery. Am. J. Cardiol. *72:*615, 1993.

163. Levine, H. D.: Myocardial fibrosis in constrictive pericarditis. Electrocardiographic and pathologic observations. Circulation *48:*1268, 1973.

164. Topaz, O., Nair, R., and MacKall, J. A.: Observations of angina and myocardial infarction in constrictive pericarditis. Int. J. Cardiol. *39:*121, 1993.

165. Hancock, E. W.: On the elastic and rigid forms of constrictive pericarditis. Am. Heart J. *100:*917, 1980.

166. Paul, O., Castleman, B., and White, P. D.: Chronic constrictive pericarditis: A study of 53 cases. Am. J. Med. Sci. *216:*361, 1948.

167. Andrews, G. W. S., Pickering, G. W., and Sellors, T. H.: The aetiology of constrictive pericarditis with special reference to tuberculous pericarditis, together with a note on polyserositis. Q. J. Med. *17:*291, 1948.

168. Blake, S., Bonar, S., O'Neill, H., et al.: Aetiology of chronic constrictive pericarditis. Br. Heart J. *50:*273, 1983.

169. Cameron, J., Oesterle, S. N., Baldwin, J. C., and Hancock, E. W.: The etiologic spectrum of constrictive pericarditis. Am. Heart J. *113:*354, 1987.

170. Nataf, P., Cacoub P., Dorent, R., et al.: Results of subtotal pericardiectomy for constrictive pericarditis. Eur. J. Cardiothorac. Surg. *7:*252, 1993.

171. Fischbein, L., Namade, M., Sachs, R. N., et al.: Chronic constrictive pericarditis associated with asbestosis. Chest *94:*646, 1988.

172. Van der Horst, R. L.: Pericardial calcification in childhood. Cardiovasc. Radiol. *1:*265, 1978.

173. Bonische, C. H., and Jaffe, J. P.: Spontaneous severe constrictive pericarditis in congenital afibrinogenemia: Mechanism, evaluation and successful surgical management. Am. Heart J. *101:*503, 1981.

174. Laxer, R. M., Cameron, B. J., Chaisson, D., et al.: The camptodactyly-arthropathy-pericarditis syndrome: Case report and literature review. Arthritis Rheum. *29:*439, 1986.

175. Cotton, J. B., Rebelle, C., Bosnio, A., et al.: Familial intrauterine nanism with constrictive pericarditis: The Mulibrey syndrome. Pediatrics *43:*197, 1988.

176. Mashman, W. E., and Silverman, M. E.: Platypnea related to constrictive pericarditis. Chest *105:*636, 1994.

177. Tyberg, T. I., Goodyer, A. V. N., and Langou, R. A.: Genesis of pericardial knock in constrictive pericarditis. Am. J. Cardiol. *46:*570, 1980.

178. Manga, P., Vythilingum, S., and Mitha, A. S.: Pulsatile hepatomegaly in constrictive pericarditis. Br. Heart J. *52:*465, 1984.

179. Arora, A., Seth, S., Acharya, S. K., and Sharma, M. P.: Hepatic coma as the presenting feature of constrictive pericarditis. Am. J. Gastroenterol. *88:*430, 1993.

180. Anand, I. S., Ferrari, R., Kalra, G. S., et al.: Pathogenesis of edema in constrictive pericarditis. Circulation *83:*1880, 1991.

181. Bakri, Y. N., Martan, A., Amri, A., and Amri, M.: Pregnancy complicating irradiation-induced constrictive pericarditis. Acta Obstet. Gynecol. Scand. *71:*143, 1972.

182. Plus, G. E., Brower, A. J., and Clagett, O. T.: Chronic constrictive pericarditis: Roentgenologic findings in 35 surgically proved cases. Proc. Staff Meet. Mayo Clin. *32:*555, 1957.

183. Tomaselli, G., Gamsu, G., and Stolberg, M. S.: Constrictive pericarditis presenting as pleural effusion of unknown origin. Arch. Intern. Med. *149:*201, 1989.

184. Fukuda, K., Nakamura, Y., Ogawa, S., et al.: Constrictive pericarditis with electrocardiographic evidence of right ventricular hypertrophy. Chest *96:*691, 1989.

185. Schnittger, I., Bowden, R. E., Abrams, J., and Popp, R. L.: Echocardiography: Pericardial thickening and constrictive pericarditis. Am. J. Cardiol. *42:*388, 1978.

186. Engle, P. J., Fowler, N. O., Tei, C. W., et al.: M-mode echocardiography in constrictive pericarditis. J. Am. Coll. Cardiol. *6:*471, 1985.

187. Mantri, R. R., Singh, S., Radhakrishnan, S., and Sinna, N.: Left atrial dilatation in constrictive pericarditis. A pre and post-operative echocardiographic study. Int. J. Cardiol. *45:*69, 1994.

188. D'Cruz, I. A., Dick, A., Gross, C. M., et al.: Abnormal left ventricular–left atrial posterior wall contour: A new two-dimensional echocardiographic sign in constrictive pericarditis. Am. Heart J. 118:128, 1989.

189. Himelman, R. B., Lee, E., and Schiller, N. B.: Septal bounce, vena cava plethora, and pericardial adhesion: Informative two-dimensional echocardiographic signs in the diagnosis of pericardial constriction. J. Am. Soc. Echocardiogr. 1:333, 1988.

190. Pandian, N. G., Skorton, D. J., Kieso, R. A., and Kerber, R. E.: Diagnosis of constrictive pericarditis by two-dimensional echocardiography: Studies in a new experimental model and in patients. J. Am. Coll. Cardiol. 4:1164, 1984.

191. Von Bibra, H., Schober, K., Jenni, R., et al.: Diagnosis of constrictive pericarditis by pulsed Doppler echocardiography of the hepatic vein. Am. J. Cardiol. 63:483, 1989.

192. Hatle, L. K., Appleton, C. P., and Popp, R. L.: Differentiation of constrictive pericarditis and restrictive cardiomyopathy by Doppler echocardiography. Circulation 79:357, 1989.

193. Oh, J. K., Hatle, L. K., Seward, J. B., et al.: Diagnostic role of Doppler echocardiography in constrictive pericarditis. J. Am. Coll. Cardiol. 23:154, 1994.

194. Oh, J. K., Hatle, L. K., Mulvagh, S. L., and Tajik, A. J.: Transient constrictive pericarditis: Diagnosis by two-dimensional Doppler echocardiography. Mayo Clin. Proc. 67:201, 1992.

195. Sutton, F. J., Whitney, N. O., and Applefeld, M. M.: The role of echocardiography and computed tomography in the evaluation of constrictive pericarditis. Am. Heart J. 109:350, 1985.

196. Oren, R. M., Grover-McKay, M., Stanford, W., and Weiss, R. M.: Accurate preoperative diagnosis of pericardial constriction using cine computed tomography. J. Am. Coll. Cardiol. 22:832, 1993.

197. Reinmuller, R., Doppman, J. L., Lossner, J., et al.: Constrictive pericardial disease: Prognostic significance of a nonvisualized left ventricular wall. Radiology 156:753, 1985.

198. Matsui, T., Finck, S., and Higgins, C. B.: Constrictive pericarditis and restrictive cardiomyopathy: Evaluation with MR imaging. Radiology 182:369, 1992.

199. Reinmuller, R., Gurgan, M., Erdmann, E., et al.: CT and MR evaluation of pericardial constriction: A new diagnostic and therapeutic concept. J. Thoracic. Imaging 8:108, 1993.

200. Solano, F. X., Young, E., Talamo, T. S., and Dekker, A.: Constrictive pericarditis mimicking Budd-Chiari syndrome. Am. J. Med. 80:113, 1986.

201. Savage, M. P., Munoz, S. J., Herman, W. M., and Kusiak, V. M.: Chylous ascites caused by constrictive pericarditis. Am. J. Gastroenterol. 82:1088, 1987.

202. Wilkinson, P., Pinto, B., and Senior, J. R.: Reversible protein-losing enteropathy with intestinal lymphangiectasia, secondary to chronic constrictive pericarditis. N. Engl. J. Med. 273:1178, 1965.

203. Pastor, B. H., and Cahn, M.: Reversible nephrotic syndrome resulting from constrictive pericarditis. N. Engl. J. Med. 262:872, 1960.

204. Wasserman, A. J., Richardson, D. W., Baird, C. L., and Wyso, E. M.: Cardiac hemochromatosis simulating constrictive pericarditis. Am. J. Med. 32:316, 1962.

205. Arrillo, J. E., Borer, J. S., Henry, W. L., et al.: The cardiovascular manifestations of the hypereosinophilic syndrome. Am. J. Med. 67:572, 1979.

206. Daubert, J. P., Gaede, J., and Cohen, H. J.: A fatal case of constrictive pericarditis due to a marked, selective pericardial accumulation of amyloid. Am. J. Med. 94:335, 1993.

207. Navarro, J. F., Rivera, M., and Ortuno, J.: Cardiac tamponade as the initial presentation of systemic amyloidosis. Int. J. Cardiol. 36:107, 1992.

208. Carroll, J. D., Gaasch, W. H., and McAdam, K. P. W. J.: Amyloid cardiomyopathy: Characterization by a distinctive voltage/mass ratio. Am. J. Cardiol. 49:9, 1982.

209. Bush, C. A., Stang, J. M., Wooley, C. G., and Kilman, J.: Occult constrictive pericardial disease. Diagnosis by rapid volume expansion and correction by pericardiectomy. Circulation 56:924, 1977.

210. Goldberg, E., Stein, J., Berger, M., and Berdoff, R. L.: Diastolic segmental coronary artery obliteration in constrictive pericarditis. Cath. Cardiovasc. Diag. 7:197, 1981.

211. Meaney, E., Shabetai, R., and Bhargava, V.: Cardiac amyloidosis, constrictive pericarditis and restrictive cardiomyopathy. Am. J. Cardiol. 38:547, 1976.

212. Swanton, R. H., Brooksby, I. A. B., Davies, M. J., et al.: Systolic and diastolic ventricular function in cardiac amyloidosis. Studies in six cases diagnosed with endomyocardial biopsy. Am. J. Cardiol. 39:658, 1977.

213. Benotti, J. R., Grossman, W., and Cohn, P. F.: Clinical profile of restrictive cardiomyopathy. Circulation 61:1206, 1980.

214. Robbins, M. A., Pizzarello, R. A., Stechel, R. P., et al.: Resting and exercise hemodynamics in constrictive pericarditis and a case of cardiac amyloidosis mimicking constriction. Cath. Cardiovasc. Diag. 9:463, 1983.

215. Tyberg, T. I., Goodyer, A. V. N., Hurst, V. W., et al.: Left ventricular filling in differentiating restrictive amyloid cardiomyopathy and constrictive pericarditis. Am. J. Cardiol. 47:791, 1981.

216. Aroney, C. N., Ruddy, T. D., Dighero, H., et al.: Differentiation of restrictive cardiomyopathy from pericardial constriction. J. Am. Coll. Cardiol. 13:1007, 1989.

217. Klein, A. L., Oh, J. K., Miller, F. A., et al.: Two-dimensional and Doppler echocardiographic assessment of infiltrative cardiomyopathy. J. Am. Soc. Echocardiogr. 1:48, 1988.

218. Schiavone, W. A., Calafiore, P. A., and Salcedo, E. E.: Transesophageal Doppler echocardiographic demonstration of pulmonary venous flow velocity in restrictive cardiomyopathy and constrictive pericarditis. Am. J. Cardiol. 63:1286, 1989.

219. Klein, A. L., Cohen, G. I., Pietrolungo, J. F., et al.: Differentiation of constrictive pericarditis from restrictive cardiomyopathy by Doppler transesophageal echocardiographic measurements of respiratory variations in pulmonary venous flow. J. Am. Coll. Cardiol. 22:1935, 1993.

220. Klein, A. L., and Cohen, G. I.: Doppler echocardiographic assessment of constrictive pericarditis, cardiac amyloidosis, and cardiac tamponade. Cleve. Clin. J. Med. 59:278, 1992.

221. Schoenfeld, M. H., Supple, E. W., Dec, G. W., et al.: Restrictive cardiomyopathy versus constrictive pericarditis: Role of endomyocardial biopsy in avoiding unnecessary thoracotomy. Circulation 75:1012, 1987.

222. Kern, M. J., Lorell, B. H., and Grossman, W.: Cardiac amyloidosis masquerading as constrictive pericarditis. Cath. Cardiovasc. Diag. 8:629, 1982.

223. Katagiri, M., Tanabe, Y., Takahashi, M., and Kasuya, S.: Right atrial thrombosis: Association with constrictive pericarditis. Ann. Thorac. Surg. 49:145, 1990.

224. Priestley, K. A., Wallwork, J., and Schofield, P. M.: Right atrial thrombosis in constrictive pericarditis. Int. J. Cardiol. 37:256, 1992.

225. Copeland, J. G., Stinson, E. B., Griepp, R. B., and Shumway, N. E.: Surgical treatment of chronic constrictive pericarditis using cardiopulmonary bypass. J. Thorac. Cardiovasc. Surg. 69:236, 1975.

226. Johnson, R. G., Thurer, R. L., Lorell, B. H., and Weintraub, R. M.: Ultrasonic debridement of calcified pericardium in constrictive pericarditis. Ann. Thorac. Surg. 48:855, 1989.

227. Culliford, A. T., Lipton, M., and Spencer, F. C.: Operation for chronic constrictive pericarditis: Do the surgical approach and degree of pericardial resection influence the outcome significantly? Ann. Thorac. Surg. 29:146, 1980.

228. Tirilomis, T., Unverdorben, S., and von der Emde, J.: Pericardiectomy for chronic constrictive pericarditis: Risks and outcome. Eur. J. Cardiothorac. Surg. 8:487, 1994.

229. McCaughlin, B. C., Schaff, H. V., Piehler, J. M., et al.: Early and late results of pericardiectomy for constrictive pericarditis. J. Thorac. Cardiovasc. Surg. 89:340, 1985.

230. Robertson, J. M., and Mulder, D.G.: Pericardiectomy: A changing scene. Am. J. Surg. 148:86, 1984.

231. Aagaard, M. T., and Haraldsted, V. Y.: Chronic constrictive pericarditis treated with total pericardiectomy. Thorac. Cardiovasc. Surg. 32:311, 1984.

232. Siefert, F. C., Miller, C. D., Oesterle, S. N., et al.: Surgical treatment of constrictive pericarditis: Analysis of outcome and diagnostic error. Circulation 72(Suppl. 2):264, 1985.

233. Astrudillo, R., and Ivert, T.: Late results after pericardiectomy for constrictive pericarditis via left thoracotomy. Scand. J. Thorac. Cardiovasc. Surg. 23:115, 1989.

234. Bashi, I., Ravikumar, J. S., Jairaj, P. S., et al.: Early and late results of pericardiectomy in 118 cases of constrictive pericarditis. Thorax 43:637, 1988.

235. Pick, R. A., Joswig, B. C., and Bloor, C. M.: Recurrent cardiac constriction after pericardiectomy. Arch. Intern. Med. 144:2061, 1984.

236. Harrington, S. W.: Chronic constrictive pericarditis. Partial pericardiectomy and epicardiolysis in 24 cases. Ann. Surg. 120:468, 1944.

237. Walsh, T. J., Baughman, K. L., Gardner, T. J., and Bulkley, B. H.: Constrictive epicarditis as a cause of delayed or absent response to pericardiectomy. J. Thorac. Cardiovasc. Surg. 83:126, 1982.

238. Johnson, T. L., Bauman, W. B., and Josephson, R. A.: Worsening tricuspid regurgitation following pericardiectomy for constrictive pericarditis. Chest 104:79, 1993.

239. Buckingham, R. E., Jr., Furnary, A. P., Weaver, M. T., et al.: Mitral insufficiency after pericardiectomy for constrictive pericarditis. Ann. Thorac. Surg. 58:1171, 1994.

240. Hancock, E. W.: Subacute effusive constrictive pericarditis. Circulation 43:183, 1971.

241. Kern, M. J., and Aguirre, F. V.: Interpretation of cardiac pathophysiology from pressure waveform analysis: Pericardial compressive hemodynamics. Part III. Cathet. Cardiovasc. Diagn. 26:152, 1992.

242. Martin, R. P., Bowden, R., Filly, K., and Popp, R. L.: Intrapericardial abnormalities in patients with pericardial effusion. Circulation 61:568, 1980.

SPECIFIC FORMS OF PERICARDITIS

Viral Pericarditis

243. Brodie, H. R., and Marchessault, V.: Acute benign pericarditis caused by Coxsackie virus group B. N. Engl. J. Med. 262:1278, 1960.

244. Friman, G., and Fohlman, J.: The epidemiology of viral heart disease. Scand. J. Infect. Dis. (Suppl.) 88:7, 1993.

245. Herskowitz, A., Campbell, S., Deckers, J., et al.: Demographic features and prevalence of idiopathic myocarditis in patients undergoing endomyocardial biopsy. Am. J. Cardiol. 71:982, 1993.

246. Kleinfeld, M., Milles, S., and Lidsky, M.: Mumps pericarditis: Review of the literature and report of a case. Am. Heart J. 55:153, 1958.

247. Cheng, T. C.: Severe chest pain due to infectious mononucleosis. Postgrad. Med. 73:149, 1983.

248. Satoh, T., Kojima, M., and Ohshima, K.: Demonstration of the Epstein-Barr genome by polymerase chain reaction and in situ hybridization in a patient with viral pericarditis. Br. Heart J. 69:563, 1993.

249. Adler, R., Takahashi, M., and Wright, H. T., Jr.: Acute pericarditis associated with hepatitis B infection. Pediatrics 61:716, 1978.

250. Williams, A. J., Freemont, A. J., and Barnett, D. B.: Pericarditis and arthritis complicating chicken pox. Br. J. Clin. Pract. 37:226, 1983.

251. Fink, C., Schaad, V. B., and Stocker, F. P.: Pericarditis as a complication of rubella. Schweiz. Med. Wochenschr. 117:28, 1987.

252. Bensaid, J., and Denis, F.: Benign acute pericarditis after vaccination against hepatitis B. Presse Med. 22:269, 1993.

253. Beaman, M. H., and Hung, J.: Pericarditis associated with tick-borne Q fever. Aust. N. Z. J. Med. 19:254, 1989.

254. Balaguer, A., Boronat, M., and Carrascosa, A.: Successful treatment of pericarditis associated with Mycoplasma pneumoniae infection. Pediatr. Infect. Dis. J. 9:141, 1990.

255. Biton, A., and Herman, J.: Perimyocarditis. Report on an unusual cause. Postgrad. Med. 85:77, 1989.

256. Saatci, V., Ozen, S., Ceyhan, M., and Secmeer, G.: Cytomegalovirus disease in a renal transplant manifesting with pericarditis. Int. Urol. Nephrol. 25:617, 1993.

257. Acierno, L. J.: Cardiac complications in acquired immune deficiency syndrome (AIDS): A review. J. Am. Coll. Cardiol. 13:1144, 1990.

258. Kwan, T., Karve, M. M., and Emerole, O.: Cardiac tamponade in patients infected with HIV. A report from an inner-city hospital. Chest 104:1059, 1993.

259. Reynolds, M. M., Hecht, S. R., Berger, M., et al.: Large pericardial effusions in the acquired immunodeficiency syndrome. Chest 102:1746, 1992.

260. Cooper, D. K. C., and Sturridge, M. F.: Constrictive pericarditis following Coxsackie virus infection. Thorax 31:472, 1976.

261. Frisk, G., Torfason, E. G., and Diderholm, H.: Reverse immunoassays of IgM and IgG antibodies to Coxsackie B viruses in patients with acute myopericarditis. J. Med. Virol. 14:191, 1984.

262. Riecansky, I., Schreinerova, Z., Egnerova, A., et al.: Incidence of Coxsackie virus infection in patients with dilated cardiomyopathy. Cor Vasa 31:325, 1989.

263. Muir, P., Nicholson, F., Tilzey, A. J., et al.: Chronic relapsing pericarditis and dilated cardiomyopathy: Serologic evidence of persistent enterovirus infection. Lancet 1:804, 1989.

Tuberculous Pericarditis

264. Larneu, A. J., Tyers, G. F., Williams, E. H., and Derrick, J. R.: Recent experience with tuberculous pericarditis. Ann. Thorac. Surg. 29:464, 1980.

265. Desai, H. N.: Tuberculous pericarditis: A review of 100 cases. S. Afr. Med. J. 55:877, 1979.

266. Strang, J. I. G.: Tuberculous pericarditis in Transkei. Clin. Cardiol. 5:667, 1984.

267. Hugo-Hamman, C. T., Scher, H., and DeMoor, M. M.: Tuberculous pericarditis in children: A review of 44 cases. Pediatr. Infect. Dis. J. 13:13, 1994.

268. Gooi, H. C., and Smith, J. M.: Tuberculous pericarditis in Birmingham. Thorax 33:94, 1978.

269. Peel, A. A. F.: Tuberculous pericarditis. Br. Heart J. 10:195, 1948.

270. Auerbach, O.: Pleural, peritoneal, and pericardial tuberculosis. Am. Rev. Tuberc. 61:845, 1950.

271. Maisch, B., Maisch, S., and Kocksiek, K.: Immune reactions in tuberculous and chronic constrictive pericarditis. Am. J. Cardiol. 50:1007, 1982.

272. Schrire, V.: Experience with pericarditis of Groote Schuur Hospital, Cape Town: An analysis of one hundred and sixty cases over a six-year period. S. Afr. Med. J. 33:810, 1959.

273. Hageman, J. H., D'Esopo, N. D., and Glenn, W. W. L.: Tuberculosis of the pericardium: A long-term analysis of forty-four cases. N. Engl. J. Med. 270:327, 1964.

274. Long, E., Younes, M., Patton, N., and Hershfield, E.: Tuberculous pericarditis: Long-term outcome in patients who received medical therapy alone. Am. Heart J. 117:1133, 1989.

275. Komsuoglu, B., Goldeli, O., Kulan, K., and Gedik, Y.: Tuberculous pericarditis in north-east Turkey. An echocardiographic study. Acta Cardiol. 49:157, 1994.

276. Quale, J. M., Lipschik, G. Y., and Heurich, A. E.: Management of tuberculous pericarditis. Ann. Thorac. Surg. 43:653, 1987.

277. Sagrista-Sauleda, J., Permanyer-Miralda, G., and Soler-Soler, J.: Tuberculous pericarditis: Ten-year experience with a prospective protocol for diagnosis and treatment. J. Am. Coll. Cardiol. 11:724, 1988.

278. Agrawal, S., Radhakrishnan, S., and Sinha, N.: Echocardiographic demonstration of resolving intrapericardial mass in tuberculous pericardial effusion. Int. J. Cardiol. 26:240, 1990.

279. Schmidt, V., and Rebarber, I. F.: Tuberculous pericarditis identified with gallium-67 and indium-111 leukocyte imaging. Clin. Nucl. Med. 19:146, 1994.

280. Barr, J. F.: The use of pericardial biopsy in establishing etiologic diagnosis in acute pericarditis. Arch. Intern. Med. 96:693, 1955.

281. Cheitlin, M. D., Serfos, L. J., Sbar, S. S., and Glosser, S. P.: Tuberculous pericarditis: Is limited pericardial biopsy sufficient for diagnosis? Am. Rev. Resp. Dis. 98:287, 1968.

282. Koh, K. K., Kim, E. J., Cho, C. H., et al.: Adenosine deaminase and carcinoembryonic antigen and pericardial effusion diagnosis, especially in suspected tuberculous pericarditis. Circulation 89:2728, 1994.

283. Seino, Y., Ikeda, U., Kawaguchi, K., et al.: Tuberculous pericarditis presumably diagnosed by polymerase chain reaction analysis. Am. Heart J. 126:249, 1993.

284. Strang, J. I., Kakaza, H. H., Gibson, D. G., et al.: Controlled trial of prednisolone as adjuvant in the treatment of tuberculous constrictive pericarditis in Transkei. Lancet 2:1418, 1987.

285. Fennell, W. M. P.: Surgical treatment of constrictive tuberculous pericarditis. S. Afr. Med. J. 62:353, 1982.

Bacterial (Purulent) Pericarditis

286. Klacsmann, P. B., Bulkley, B. H., and Hutchins, G. M.: The changed spectrum of purulent pericarditis. An 86 year autopsy experience in 200 patients. Am. J. Med. 63:666, 1977.

287. Sagrista-Sauleda, J., Barrabes, J. A., Permanyer-Miralda, G., and Soler-Soler, J.: Purulent pericarditis: Review of a 20-year experience in a general hospital. J. Am. Coll. Cardiol. 22:1661, 1993.

288. Park, S., and Bayer, A. S.: Purulent pericarditis. Curr. Clin. Top. Infect. Dis. 12:56, 1992.

289. Karjalainen, J.: Streptococcal tonsillitis and acute nonrheumatic myopericarditis. Chest 95:359, 1989.

290. Marsa, R. J., Blomquist, I. K., Bansal, R. C., et al.: Acute pericarditis due to group C Streptococcus: Report of a medically treated case. Am. J. Med. 86:474, 1989.

291. Rivera, J. M., Garcia-Bragado, F., Gomez, F. A., et al.: Brucellar pericarditis. Infection 16:254, 1988.

292. Verghese, S. L., Annapurna, E. M., and Bhave, G. G.: Purulent pericarditis caused by Salmonella typhimurium. Indian J. Med. Sci. 47:75, 1993.

293. Sanchez-Guerrero, J., and Alarcon-Segovia, D.: Salmonella pericarditis with tamponade in systemic lupus erythematosis. Br. J. Rheumatol. 29:69, 1990.

294. Vietzke, W. M.: Gonococcal arthritis with pericarditis. Arch. Intern. Med. 117:270, 1966.

295. Welikovitch, L., Knight, J. L., Burggraf, G. W., and Sanfilippo, A. J.: Cardiac tamponade secondary to hemophilus pericarditis: A case report. Can. J. Cardiol. 8:303, 1992.

296. Evans, M. E., Gregory, D. W., Schaffner, W., and McGee, Z. A.: Tularemia: A 30-year experience with 88 cases. Medicine 64:251, 1985.

297. Rubin, R. H., and Moellering, R. C., Jr.: Clinical, microbiologic, and therapeutic aspects of purulent pericarditis. Am. J. Med. 59:68, 1975.

298. Ferguson, R., Yee, S., Finkle, H., et al.: Listeria-associated pericarditis in an AIDS patient. J. Natl. Med. Assoc. 85:225, 1993.

299. Zollner, B., Sobottka, I., von der Lippe, G., et al.: Perimyocarditis caused by Yersinia enterocolitica serotype 0:3. Dtsch. Med. Wochenschr. 117:1794, 1992.

300. Kahn, M. Y.: Subacute constrictive pericarditis from Serratia marcescens. Hum. Pathol. 14:1089, 1983.

301. Lieber, I. H., Rensimer, E. R., and Ericsson, C. D.: Campylobacter pericarditis in hypothyroidism. Am. Heart J. 102:462, 1981.

302. Skiest, D. J., Steiner, D., Werner, M., and Garner, J. G.: Anaerobic pericarditis: Case report and review. Clin. Infect. Dis. 19:435, 1994.

303. Francois, B., Delaire, L., Vignon, P., et al.: Gas gangrene and purulent pericarditis during Clostridium septicemia revealing a cecal carcinoma. Intens. Care Med. 20:309, 1994.

304. Epstein, S. K., Winslow, C. J., Brecher, S. M., and Faling, L. J.: Polymicrobial bacterial pericarditis after transbronchial needle aspiration. Case report with an investigation on the risk of bacterial contamination during fiberoptic bronchoscopy. Am. Rev. Respir. Dis. 146:523, 1992.

305. Wesley Farr, R., Khakoo, R. A., Maxwell, L. P., and Hill, R. C.: Citrobacter pericarditis secondary to a subphrenic abscess. Clin. Infect. Dis. 18:838, 1994.

306. Blaser, M. J., Reingold, A. L., Alsever, R. N., and Hightower, A.: Primary meningococcal pericarditis: A disease of adults associated with serogroup C Neisseria meningitidis. Rev. Infect. Dis. 6:625, 1984.

307. Luck, P. C., Helbig, J. H., Wunderlich, E., et al.: Isolation of Legionella pneumophila serogroup 3 from pericardial fluid in a case of pericarditis. Infection 17:388, 1989.

308. Pititalot, J. P., Allal, J., Thomas, P., et al.: Cardiac complications of infectious endocarditis. Ann. Med. Interne (Paris) 136:539, 1985.

309. Weinstein, L.: Life-threatening complications of infective endocarditis and their management. Arch. Intern. Med. 146:953, 1986.

310. Decker, C. F., and Tuazon, C. V.: Staphylococcus aureus pericarditis in HIV-infected patients. Chest 105:615, 1994.

311. Dupuis, C., Gronnier, P., Kachaner, J., et al.: Bacterial pericarditis in infancy and childhood. Am. J. Cardiol. 74:807, 1994.

312. Moss, W., and Prince, A.: Pericarditis complicating meningococcal meningitis in a 7-month old boy. Clin. Pediatr. 33:169, 1994.

313. Fyfe, D. A., Hagler, D. J., Puga, F. J., and Driscoll, D. J.: Clinical and therapeutic aspects of Hemophilus influenzae pericarditis in pediatric patients. Mayo Clin. Proc. 59:415, 1984.

314. St. John, M. A., Noah, P. K., Talma, T. E., et al.: Acute purulent pericarditis in children caused by Haemophilus influenzae. West Indian Med. J. 42:161, 1993.

315. Chun, P. K., and Rocchini, A. P.: Occult constrictive pericarditis in infancy. Chest 78:648, 1980.

316. Leak, L. V., Ferrans, V. J., Cohen, S. R., et al.: Animal model of acute pericarditis and its progression to pericardial fibrosis and adhesions: Ultrastructural studies. Am. J. Anat. *180*:373, 1987.

317. Matan, A., Marvric, Z., Vukas, D., and Beg-Zec, Z.: Spontaneous contrast echoes in pericardial effusion: Sign of gas-producing infection. Am. Heart J. *124*:521, 1992.

318. Desai, S. P., and Yuille, D. L.: The unsuspected complications of bacterial endocarditis imaged by gallium-67 scanning. J. Nucl. Med. *34*:955, 1993.

319. Copeland, D. B., Tarriff, B., Fung, A. Y., and Sartori, C.: The "hot halo" sign: Pyogenic pericarditis on In-111 leukocyte scintigraphy. Clin. Nucl. Med. *17*:579, 1992.

320. Gould, K., Barnett, J. A., and Sanford, J. P.: Purulent pericarditis in the antibiotic era. Arch. Intern. Med. *134*:923, 1974.

321. Niederhauser, U., Vogt, M., von Segesser, L. K., et al.: Pericardiectomy and acute infectious pericarditis. Schweiz Med. Wochenschr. *122*:158, 1992.

322. Thavendrarajah, V., Ghia, P. S., Kozinn, W., and Little, T.: Catheter lavage and drainage of pneumococcal pericarditis. Cathet. Cardiovasc. Diagn. *29*:322, 1993.

323. Winkler, W. B., Karnik, R., and Slany, J.: Treatment of exudative fibrinous pericarditis with intraperitoneal urokinase. Lancet *344*:1541, 1994.

324. Miller, G. C., and Witham, A. C.: Delayed febrile pleuropericarditis after sepsis. Ann. Intern. Med. *79*:194, 1973.

325. Tan, J. S., Holmes, J. C., Fowler, N. O., et al.: Antibiotic levels in pericardial fluid. J. Clin. Invest. *53*:7, 1974.

326. Karim, M. A., Bach, R. G., Dressler, F., et al.: Purulent pericarditis caused by group B streptococcus with pericardial tamponade. Am. Heart J. *126*:727, 1993.

327. Laaban, J. P., d'Orbcastel, O. R., Prudent, J., et al.: Primary pneumococcal pericarditis complicated by acute constriction. Intensive Care Med. *10*:155, 1984.

328. Wheat, L. J., Stein, L., Corya, B. C., et al.: Pericarditis as a manifestation of histoplasmosis during two large urban outbreaks. Medicine *62*:110, 1983.

329. Chapman, M. G., and Kaplan, L.: Cardiac involvement in coccidioidomycosis. Am. J. Med. *23*:87, 1957.

330. Amundson, D.E.: Perplexing pericarditis caused by coccidioidomycosis. South Med. J. *86*:694, 1993.

331. van Ede, A. E., Meis, J. F., Koot, R. A., et al.: Pneumopericardium complicating invasive pulmonary aspergillosis: Case report and review. Infection *22*:102, 1994.

332. Kraus, W. E., Valenstein, P. N., and Corey, G. R.: Purulent pericarditis caused by Candida: Report of three cases and identification of high-risk populations as an aid to early diagnosis. Rev. Infect. Dis. *10*:34, 1988.

333. Karp, R., Meldahl, R., and McCabe, R.: *Candida albicans* purulent pericarditis treated successfully without surgical drainage. Chest *102*:953, 1992.

334. Pancorvo, C., and Cohen, I.: Candida pericarditis in a child. J. La. State Med. Soc. *145*:53, 1993.

335. Prager, R. L., Burney, D. P., Waterhouse, G., and Bender, H. W., Jr.: Pulmonary, mediastinal, and cardiac presentations of histoplasmosis. Ann. Thorac. Surg. *30*:385, 1980.

336. Kaufman, L. D., Seifert, F. C., Eilbott, D. J., et al.: Candida pericarditis and tamponade in a patient with systemic lupus erythematosus. Arch. Intern. Med. *148*:715, 1988.

337. Clenney, T. L., Hammond, M. D., McKeown, P. P., et al.: Cardiac tamponade due to *Nocardia asteroides*. Chest *103*:641, 1993.

338. Tabrizi, S. J.: Nocardia pericarditis. Br. Med. J. *309*:1495, 1994.

339. Zijlstra, E. E., Swart, G. R., Godfroy, F. J., and Degener, J. E.: Pericarditis, pneumonia and brain abscess due to a combined Actinomyces-Actinobacillus actinomycetemcomitans infection. J. Infect. *25*:83, 1992.

340. Kenney, R. T., Li, J. S., Clyde, W. A., Jr., et al.: Mycoplasma pericarditis: Evidence of invasive disease. Clin. Infect. Dis. *558* (Suppl. 1):17, 1993.

341. Sagrista-Sauleda, J., Permanyer-Miralda, G., Juste-Sanchez, C., et al.: Huge chronic pericardial effusion caused by *Toxoplasma gondii*. Circulation *66*:895, 1992.

342. Lyngbye, K. K., Vennervald, B. J., Bygbjerg, I. C., et al.: Toxoplasma pericarditis mimicking systemic lupus erythematosus. Ann. Med. *24*:337, 1992.

343. Zweiker, R., Eber, B., Samonigg, H., et al.: Toxoplasmosis peri-myocarditis as initial manifestation of highly malignant non-Hodgkin's lymphoma. J. Kardiol. *83*:234, 1994.

344. Guerot, E., Assayag, P., Morgant, C., et al.: Pericardial manifestations of toxoplasmosis. Arch. Mal. Coeur Vaiss. *85*:109, 1992.

345. Gomersall, L. N., Currie, J., and Jeffrey, R.: Amoebiasis: A rare cause of cardiac tamponade. Br. Heart J. *71*:368, 1994.

346. Perna, A. M., and Montesi, G. F.: Cardiac tamponade secondary to intrapericardial rupture of a hepatic amoebic abscess. Eur. J. Cardiothorac. Surg. *8*:106, 1994.

347. Strang, J. I.: Two-dimensional echocardiography in the diagnosis of amoebic pericarditis. S. Afr. Med. J. *71*:328, 1987.

348. van der Horst, R.: Schistosomiasis of the pericardium. J. R. Soc. Tropical Med. Hygiene *73*:243, 1979.

349. Chens, W.: Hydatid cysts in the pericardium—a new case and review of the literature. J. Thorac. Cardiovasc. Surg. *30*:56, 1982.

350. Umut, S., Tosun, C. A., and Mihmanh, A.: Hydatidosis with pericardial involvement. Chest *102*:1916, 1992.

351. Kinare, S. G., Parulkar, G. B., and Sen, P. K.: Constrictive pericarditis resulting from dracunculosis. Br. Med. J. *1*:845, 1962.

352. Charon, A., and Sinha, K.: Constrictive pericarditis following filiariasis. Indian Heart J. *25*:213, 1973.

353. Bruyn, G. A., DeKoning, J., Reijsoo, F. J., et al.: Lyme pericarditis leading to tamponade. Br. J. Rheumatol. *33*:862, 1994.

354. Bergler-Klein, J., Sochor, H., Stanek, G., et al.: Indium 111-monoclonal antimyosin antibody and magnetic resonance imaging in the diagnosis of acute Lyme myopericarditis. Arch. Intern. Med. *153*:2696, 1993.

355. Page, S. R., Stewart, J. T., and Bernstein, J. J.: A progressive pericardial effusion caused by psittacosis. Br. Heart J. *60*:87, 1988.

356. Oden, M., and Oliven, A.: Chlamydial infections of the heart. Eur. J. Clin. Microbiol. Infect. Dis. *11*:885, 1992.

Pericarditis Following Acute Myocardial Infarction

357. Dubois, C., Smeets, J. P., Demoulin, J. C., et al.: Frequency and clinical significance of pericardial friction rubs in the acute phase of myocardial infarction. Eur. Heart J. *6*:766, 1985.

358. Krainin, F. M., Flessas, A. P., and Spodick, D. H.: Infarction-associated pericarditis. N. Engl. J. Med. *311*:1211, 1984.

359. Oliva, P. B., Hammill, S. C., and Talano, J. V.: Effect of definition on incidence of postinfarction pericarditis. Is it time to redefine postinfarction pericarditis? Circulation *90*:1537, 1994.

360. Simoons, M. L., Brand, M. V. D., de Zwaan, C., et al.: Improved survival after early thrombolysis in acute myocardial infarction: A randomized trial by the Interuniversity Cardiology Institute in the Netherlands. Lancet *2*:578, 1985.

361. Van de Wert, F., and the European Cooperative Study Group: Lessons from the European Cooperative Recombinant Tissue-type Plasminogen Activator (rt-PA) versus Placebo Trial. J. Am. Coll. Cardiol. *12*:14A, 1988.

362. Correale, E., Maggioni, A. P., Romano, S., et al.: Comparison of frequency, diagnostic and prognostic significance of pericardial involvement in acute myocardial infarction treated with and without thrombolytics. Gruppo Italiano per lo Studio della Sopravvivenza nell'Infarto Miocardico (GISSI). Am. J. Cardiol. *71*:1377, 1993.

363. Oliva, P. B., and Hammill, S. C.: The clinical distinction between regional postinfarction pericarditis and other causes of postinfarction chest pain: Ancillary observations regarding the effect of lytic therapy upon the frequency of postinfarction pericarditis, postinfarction angina, and reinfarction. Clin. Cardiol. *17*:471, 1994.

364. Sahar, A., Hod, H., Barabash, G. M., et al.: Disappearance of a syndrome: Dressler's syndrome in the era of thrombolysis. Cardiology *85*:255, 1994.

365. Tofler, G. H., Muller, J. A., Stone, P. H., et al.: Pericarditis in acute myocardial infarction: Characterization and clinical significance. Am. Heart J. *117*:86, 1990.

366. Levine, H. D.: Subendocardial infarction in retrospect: Pathologic, cardiographic, and ancillary features. Circulation *72*:790, 1985.

367. Galve, E., Garcia-del-Castillo, H., Evangelista, A., et al.: Pericardial effusion in the course of myocardial infarction: Incidence, natural history, and clinical relevance. Circulation *73*:294, 1986.

368. Aarseth, S., and Lange, H. F.: The influence of anticoagulant therapy on the occurrence of cardiac rupture and hemopericardium following heart infarction. I. A study of 89 cases of hemopericardium. Am. Heart J. *56*:250, 1958.

369. Karim, A. M., and Solomon, J.: Constrictive pericarditis after myocardial infarction. Am. J. Med. *79*:389, 1985.

370. Oliva, P. B., Hammill, S. C., and Edwards, W. D.: Cardiac rupture, a clinically predictable complication of acute myocardial infarction: A report of 70 cases with clinico-pathologic correlations. J. Am. Coll. Cardiol. *22*:720, 1993.

371. Oliva, P. B., Hammill, S. C., and Edwards, W. D.: Electrocardiographic diagnosis with postinfarction regional pericarditis. Ancillary observations regarding the effect of reperfusion on the rapidity and amplitude of T wave inversion after acute myocardial infarction. Circulation *88*:896, 1993.

372. Nagahama, Y., Sugiura, T., Takehana, K., et al.: Clinical significance of PQ segment depression in acute Q wave anterior myocardial infarction. J. Am. Coll. Cardiol. *23*:885, 1994.

373. Sigiura, T., Iwasaka, T., Takehana, K., et al.: Clinical significance of pericardial effusion associated with pericarditis in acute Q-wave anterior myocardial infarction. Chest *104*:415, 1993.

374. Liberthson, R. R., Salisbury, K. W., and Hutter, A. M., Jr.: Atrial tachyarrhythmias in acute myocardial infarction. Am. J. Med. *60*:956, 1976.

375. Widimsky, P., and Gregor, P.: Recent atrial fibrillation in acute myocardial infarction: A sign of pericarditis. Cor Vasa *35*:230, 1993.

376. Proli, J., and Laufer, N.: Left ventricular rupture following myocardial infarction treated with streptokinase: Successful resuscitation in the cardiac catheterization laboratory using pericardiocentesis and autotransfusion. Cathet. Cardiovasc. Diag. *29*:257, 1993.

377. Stryjer, D., Friedensohn, A., and Hendler, A.: Myocardial rupture in acute myocardial infarction: Urgent management. Br. Heart J. *59*:73, 1988.

378. Pollak, H., Diez, W., Spiel, R., et al.: Early diagnosis of subacute free

wall rupture complicating acute myocardial infarction. Eur. Heart J. *14*:640, 1993.

379. Musselman, D. R., Dehmer, G. J., Hoffman, B. J., Jr., and Hinderliter, A. L.: Localized right atrial tamponade and right-to-left shunting as a complication of pericarditis after myocardial infarction. Am. Heart J. *125*:241, 1993.

380. Sehgal, E., Sherman, W., Isom, O. W., et al.: Left ventricular pseudoaneurysm causing superior vena caval obstruction and effusive-constrictive pericarditis. J. Nucl. Med. *28*:918, 1987.

381. Eriksen, V. H., Molgaard, H., Ingerslev, J., and Nielsen, T. T.: Fatal hemostatic complications due to thrombolytic therapy in patients falsely diagnosed as acute myocardial infarction. Eur. Heart J. *13*:840, 1992.

382. Mertens, D., Herregods, M. C., and van de Werf, F.: Thrombolytic therapy and acute aortic dissection. Acta Cardiol. *47*:501, 1992.

383. Martin, A. J., Harris, S. L., Pickett, J. D., et al.: Inadvertent administration of rtPA to a patient with type 1 aortic dissection and subsequent tamponade. Am. J. Emerg. Med. *11*:613, 1993.

384. Heymann, T. D., and Culling, W.: Cardiac tamponade after thrombolysis. Postgrad. Med. J. *70*:455, 1995.

385. Berman, J., Haffajee, C. I., and Alpert, J. S.: Therapy of symptomatic pericarditis after myocardial infarction: Retrospective and prospective studies of aspirin, indomethacin, prednisone, and spontaneous resolution. Am. Heart J. *101*:750, 1981.

386. Boden, W. E., and Sadaniantz, A.: Ventricular septal rupture during ibuprofen therapy for pericarditis after acute myocardial infarction. Am. J. Cardiol. *55*:1631, 1985.

387. Sakai, K., Hosoda, S., and Shimamoto, K.: Late rupture of left ventricular true aneurysm after acute myocardial infarction. Clin. Cardiol. *16*:573, 1993.

Uremic Pericarditis

388. Rutsky, E. A., and Rostand, S. G.: Treatment of uremic pericarditis and pericardial effusion. Am. J. Kidney Dis. *10*:2, 1987.

389. Maisch, B., and Kochsiek, K.: Humoral immune reactions in uremic pericarditis. Am. J. Nephrol. *3*:264, 1983.

390. Hiraide, A., Tazaki, O., Fujii, N., et al.: Cardiac tamponade secondary to hemorrhagic pericarditis during continuous hemofiltration for renal failure. The role of anticoagulant. Renal Failure *16*:299, 1994.

391. Ansari, A., Kaupke, C. J., Vaziri, N. D., et al.: Cardiac pathology in patients with end stage renal disease maintained on hemodialysis. Int. J. Artif. Organs *16*:31, 1993.

392. Frommer, J. P., Young, J. B., and Ayus, J. C.: Asymptomatic pericardial effusion in uremic patients: Effect of long-term dialysis. Nephron *39*:296, 1985.

393. Yoshida, K., Shiina, A., Asano, Y., and Hosoda, S.: Uremic pericardial effusion: Detection and evaluation of uremic pericardial effusion by echocardiography. Clin. Nephrol. *13*:260, 1980.

394. Leehey, D. J., Daugirdas, J. T., Popli, S., et al.: Predicting need for surgical drainage of pericardial effusion in patients with end-stage renal disease. Int. J. Artif. Organs *12*:618, 1989.

395. Morlans, M.: Pericardial involvement in end stage renal disease. *In* Soler-Soler, J., Permanyer-Miralda, G., and Sagrista-Sauleda, J.: Pericardial Disease: New Insights and Old Dilemmas. Dordrecht, The Netherlands, Kluwer Academic Publishers, 1990, pp. 123–139.

396. Masson, J. F., Maes, M. L., and Zilberman, C.: Pericarditis in chronic renal insufficiency treated by periodic hemodialysis. Rev. Med. Intern. *2*:447, 1981.

397. Kwasnik, E. M., Koster, J. K., Lazarus, J. M., et al.: Conservative management of uremic pericardial effusions. J. Thorac. Cardiovasc. Surg. *76*:629, 1978.

398. Spector, D., Alfred, H., Seidlecki, M., and Briefel, G.: A controlled study of the effect of indomethacin in uremic pericarditis. Kidney Int. *24*:663, 1983.

399. Feinroth, M. V., Goldstein, E. J., Josephson, A., and Friedman, E. A.: Infection complicating intrapericardial steroid instillation in uremic pericarditis. Clin. Nephrol. *15*:331, 1981.

400. Quigg, R. J., Idelson, B. A., Yoburn, D. C., et al.: Local steroids in dialysis-associated pericardial effusion. Arch. Intern. Med. *145*:2249, 1985.

401. Beaudry, C., Nakamoto, S., and Koloff, W. J.: Uremic pericarditis and cardiac tamponade in chronic renal failure. Ann. Intern. Med. *64*:990, 1966.

402. Hou, C. H., Tsai, T. J., and Hsu, K. L.: Peritoneal-pericardial communication after pericardiocentesis in a patient on continuous ambulatory peritoneal dialysis with dialysis pericarditis. Nephron *68*:125, 1994.

403. Frame, J. R., Lucas, S. K., Pederson, J. A., and Elkins, R. C.: Surgical treatment of pericarditis in the dialysis patient. Am. J. Surg. *146*:300, 1983.

404. Prager, R. L., Wilson, C. H., and Bender, H. W., Jr.: The subxiphoid approach to pericardial disease. Ann. Thor. Surg. *34*:6, 1982.

Neoplastic Pericarditis

405. Mukai, K., Shinkai, T., Tominaga, K., and Shimosato, Y.: The incidence of secondary tumors of the heart and pericardium: A ten-year study. Jpn. J. Clin. Oncol. *18*:195, 1988.

406. Stewart, J. R., DeBoer, D. A., Merrill, W. H., et al.: Results of surgical treatment of malignant pericardial disease. Proceedings of Society of Surgical Oncology, 46th Annual Cancer symposium in conjunction with Society of Head and Neck Surgeons, 1993, p. 29.

407. Caldas, C., and El-Deiry, W.: Favorable outcome of cancer patients with

408. Posner, M. R., Cohen, G. I., and Skarin, A. T.: Pericardial disease in patients with cancer. Am. J. Med. *71*:407, 1981.

409. Roberts, W. C., Bodey, G. P., and Wertlake, P. T.: The heart in acute leukemia: A study of 420 autopsy cases. Am. J. Cardiol. *21*:388, 1968.

410. Thurber, D. L., Edwards, J. E., and Achor, R. W.: Secondary malignant tumors of the pericardium. Circulation *26*:228, 1962.

411. Prayson, R. A., and Biscotti, C. V.: Recurrent cervical squamous cell carcinoma presenting with cardiac tamponade. Am. J. Cardiovasc. Pathol. *4*:69, 1992.

412. Susuki, M., Hamada, M., Abe, M., et al.: Accurate diagnosis of metastatic cardiac leiomyosarcoma with infundibular stenosis and cardiac tamponade by transesophageal echocardiography and Gd-DTPA magnetic resonance imaging—report of a case. Jpn. Circ. J. *58*:222, 1994.

413. Santaya, O., Vivas, P. H., Ramos, A., et al.: Multiple myeloma involving the pericardium associated with cardiac tamponade and constrictive pericarditis. Am. Heart J. *126*:737, 1993.

414. Tsukamoto, S., Omori, K., Kitamura, K., et al.: A case report of mediastinal teratoma complicated with cardiac tamponade. Nippon Kyobu Geka Gakkai Zasshi *41*:688, 1993.

415. Chow, W. H., Chow, T. C., and Chiu, S. W.: Pericardial metastasis and effusion as the initial manifestation of malignant thymoma: Identification by cross-sectional echocardiography. Int. J. Cardiol. *37*:258, 1992.

416. Wilding, G., Green, H. L., Longo, D. L., and Urba, W. J.: Tumors of the heart and pericardium. Cancer Treat. Rev. *15*:165, 1988.

417. Chan, H. S., Sonley, M. J., Moes, C. A., et al.: Primary and secondary tumors of childhood involving the heart, pericardium, and great vessels. Cancer *56*:825, 1985.

418. Skyggebjerg, K. D.: Hydrops fetalis caused by intrapericardial teratoma. Acta Obstet. Gynecol. Scand. *67*:653, 1988.

419. Lund, O., Hansen, O. K., Ardest, S., and Baandrup, V.: Primary malignant pericardial mesothelioma mimicking left atrial myxoma. Scand. J. Thorac. Cardiovasc. Surg. *21*:273, 1987.

420. Rose, D. S., Vigneswaren, W. T., Bovill, B. A., et al.: Primary pericardial mesothelioma presenting as tuberculous pericarditis. Postgrad. Med. J. *68*:137, 1992.

421. Can, C., Arpaci, F., Celasun, B., et al.: Primary pericardial liposarcoma presenting with cardiac tamponade and multiple organ metastases. Chest *103*:328, 1993.

422. Eng, J., Ruiz, K., and Kay, P. H.: Giant epicardial lipoma. Int. J. Cardiol. *37*:115, 1992.

423. Kim, E. E., Wallace, S., Abello, R., et al.: Malignant cardiac fibrous histiosarcomas and angiosarcomas: MR features. J. Comput. Assist. Tomagr. *13*:627, 1989.

424. Meissner, A., Kirch, W., Regensburger, D., et al.: Intrapericardial teratoma in an adult. Am. J. Med. *84*:1089, 1988.

425. Naramoto, A., Itoh, N., Nakano, M., and Shigematsu, H.: An autopsy case of tuberous sclerosis associated with primary pericardial mesothelioma. Acta Pathol. Jpn. *39*:400, 1989.

426. Shimoyama, Y., Kawada, K., and Imamura, H.: A functioning intrapericardial paraganglioma (pheochromocytoma). Br. Heart J. *57*:380, 1987.

427. Remick, S. C., Hoisington, S. A., and Migliozzi, J. A.: Epidemic Kaposi's sarcoma presenting with pleuropericarditis. N. Y. State J. Med. *92*:359, 1992.

428. Just, M., Raventos, A., Romeu, J., et al.: Cardiac tamponade and Kaposi's sarcoma. Med. Clin. (Barc.) *102*:495, 1994.

428a. Laham, R. J., Cohen, D. J., Kuntz, R. E., et al.: Pericardial effusion in patients with cancer: outcome with contemporary management strategies. Heart *75*:67, 1996.

429. Bradford, C. R., Smith, S. R., and Wallis, J. P.: Pericardial extramedullary hematopoesis in chronic myelomonocytic leukemia. J. Clin. Pathol. *46*:674, 1993.

430. Mann, S., and Duffy, T. P.: Pericardial tamponade in chronic myelomonocytic leukemia. Chest *106*:967, 1994.

431. Markiewicz, W., Gladstein, E., London, E. J., and Popp, R. L.: Echocardiographic detection of pericardial effusion and pericardial thickening in malignant lymphoma. Radiology *123*:161, 1977.

432. Shisedo, M., Yano, K., Ichiki, H., and Yano, M.: Pericarditis as the initial manifestation of malignant thymoma. Disappearance of pericardial effusion with corticosteroid therapy. Chest *106*:313, 1994.

433. Galve, E., Permanyer-Miralda, G., Tornas, M. P., et al.: Self-limited acute pericarditis as the initial manifestation of primary cardiac tumor. Am. Heart J. *123*:1690, 1992.

434. Fracp, M. B., Ingle, J. N., Giuliani, E. R., et al.: Pericardial effusion in women with breast cancer. Cancer *60*:263, 1987.

435. Theologides, A.: Neoplastic cardiac tamponade. Semin. Oncol. *5*:181, 1978.

436. Markman, M.: Common complications and emergencies associated with cancer and its therapy. Cleve. Clin. J. Med. *61*:105, 1994.

437. Angelucci, E., Mariotti, E., Lucarelli, G., et al.: Sudden cardiac tamponade after chemotherapy for bone marrow transplantation in thalassaemia. Lancet *339*:287, 1992.

438. Engberding, R., Schulze-Waltrup, N., Grosse-Heitmeyer, W., and Stoll, V.: Transthoracic and transesophageal 2-D echocardiography in the diagnosis of peri- and paracardiac tumors. Dtsch. Med. Wochenschr. *112*:49, 1987.

439. Brown, J. J., Barakos, J. A., and Higgins, C. B.: Magnetic resonance

imaging of cardiac and paracardiac masses. J. Thorac. Imaging 4:58, 1989.

440. Safian, R. D., Come, S. E., Kadin, M., and Lorell, B. H.: Use of pulmonary capillary wedge aspirates for the antemortem diagnosis of pulmonary microvascular tumor. Cathet. Cardiovasc. Diag. 17:112, 1989.

441. King, D. T., and Nieberg, R. K.: The use of cytology to evaluate pericardial effusions. Ann. Clin. Lab. Sci. 9:18, 1979.

442. Yancik, R., Reis, L. G., and Yates, J. W.: Breast cancer in aging women. A population-based study of contrasts in stage, surgery, and survival. Cancer 63:976, 1989.

443. Carter, C. L., Allen, C., and Henson, D. E.: Relation of tumor size, lymph node status, and survival in 24,740 breast cancer cases. Cancer 63:181, 1989.

444. Vaitkus, P. T., Herrmann, H. C., and LeWinter, M. M.: Treatment of malignant pericardial effusion. JAMA 272:59, 1994.

445. Campbell, P. T., Van Trigt, P., Wall, T. C., et al.: Subxiphoid pericardiotomy in the diagnosis and management of large percardial effusions associated with malignancy. Chest 101:938, 1992.

446. Okamoto, H., Shinkai, T., Yamakido, M., and Saijo, N.: Cardiac tamponade caused by primary lung cancer and the management of pericardial effusion. Cancer 71:93, 1993.

447. Grau, J. J., Estape, J., Palombo, H., et al.: Intracavitary oxytetracycline in malignant pericardial tamponade. Oncology 49:489, 1992.

448. Lin, M. T., Yang, P. C., and Luh, K. T.: Constrictive pericarditis after sclerosing therapy with mitomycin C for malignant pericardial effusion: Report of a case. J. Formos. Med. Assoc. 93:250, 1994.

449. Cham, W. C., Freiman, A. H., and Carstens, P. H. B.: Radiation therapy of cardiac and pericardial mestatases. Ther. Radiol. 114:701, 1975.

Radiation Pericarditis

450. Stewart, J. R., and Fajardo, L. F.: Radiation-induced heart disease: An update. Prog. Cardiovasc. Dis. 27:173, 1984.

451. Cosset, J. M., Henry-Amar, M., Girinski, T., et al.: Late toxicity of radiotherapy in Hodgkin's disease. The role of fraction size. Acta. Oncol. 27:123, 1988.

452. Tarbell, N. J., Thompson, L., and Mauch, P.: Thoracic irradiation in Hodgkin's disease: Disease control and long-term complications. Int. J. Radiat. Oncol. Biol. Phys. 18:275, 1990.

453. Mill, S. B., Baglan, R. J., Kurichety, P., et al.: Symptomatic radiation-induced pericarditis in Hodgkin's disease. Int. J. Radiat. Oncol. Biol. Phys. 10:2061, 1984.

454. Carmel, R. J., and Kaplan, H. S.: Mantle irradiation in Hodgkin's disease. Cancer 37:2813, 1976.

455. Coltart, R. S., Roberts, J. T., Thom, C. H., and Petch, M. C.: Severe constrictive pericarditis after single 16 MeV anterior mantle irradiation for Hodgkin's Disease. Lancet 1:488, 1985.

456. Applefeld, M. M., Slawson, R. G., Spicer, K. M., and Singleton, R. T.: Long-term cardiovascular evaluation of patients with Hodgkin's disease treated by thoracic mantle radiation therapy. Cancer Treat. Rep. 66:1003, 1982.

457. Pierce, S. M., Recht, A., Lingos, T. I., et al.: Long-term radiation complications following conservative surgery and radiation therapy in patients with early stage breast cancer. Int. J. Radiat. Oncol. Biol. Phys. 23:915, 1992.

458. Cwikiel, M., Albertsson, M., and Hambraeus, G.: Acute and delayed effects of radiotherapy in patients with oesophageal squamous cell carcinoma treated with chemotherapy, surgery, and pre- and postoperative radiotherapy. Acta Oncol. 33:49, 1994.

459. Martin, R. G., Ruckdeschel, J. C., Chang, P., et al.: Radiation-related pericarditis. Am. J. Cardiol. 35:216, 1975.

460. Green, D. M., Gingell, R. L., Pearce, J., et al.: The effect of mediastinal irradiation on cardiac function of patients treated during childhood and adolescence for Hodgkin's disease. J. Clin. Oncol. 5:239, 1987.

461. Schultz-Hector, S.: Radiation-induced heart disease: Review of experimental data on dose response and pathogenesis. Int. J. Radiat. Biol. 61:149, 1992.

462. Hicks, G. L., Jr.: Coronary artery operation in radiation-associated atherosclerosis: Long-term follow-up. Ann. Thorac. Surg. 53:670, 1992.

463. Orzan, F., and Brusca, A.: Radiation-induced constrictive pericarditis. Associated cardiac lesions, therapy, and follow-up. G. Ital. Cardiol. 24:817, 1994.

464. Castellino, R. A., Gladstein, E., and Turbow, M. M.: Latent radiation injury of lungs or heart activated by steroid withdrawal. Ann. Intern. Med. 80:593, 1974.

465. Ni, Y., von Segesser, L. K., and Turina, M.: Futility of pericardiectomy for postirradiation constrictive pericarditis? Ann. Thorac. Surg. 49:445, 1990.

466. Karram, T., Rinkevitch, D., and Markiewicz, W.: Poor outcome in radiation-induced constrictive pericarditis Int. J. Radiat. Oncol. Biol. Phys. 25:329, 1993.

Pericarditis Related to Hypersensitivity or Autoimmunity

467. Osler, W.: The Principles and Practice of Medicine. New York, D. Appleton and Company, 1892, p. 273.

468. Persellin, S. T., Ramirez, G., and Moatamed, F.: Immunopathology of rheumatic pericarditis. Arthritis Rheum. 25:1054, 1982.

469. Przybojewski, J. Z.: Rheumatic constrictive pericarditis. A case report and review of the literature. S. Afr. Med. J. 59:682, 1981.

470. Special Writing Group of the Committee on Rheumatic Fever, Endocar-

ditis, and Kawasaki Disease, of the Council on Cardiovascular Disease in the Young, of the American Heart Association: Guidelines for the diagnosis of rheumatic fever. Jones Criteria, 1992 Update. JAMA 268:2069, 1992.

471. Ansari, A., Larson, P. H., and Bates, H. D.: Cardiovascular manifestations of systemic lupus erythematosus: Current perspective. Prog. Cardiovasc. Dis. 27:421, 1985.

472. Langley, R. L., and Treadwell, E. L.: Cardiac tamponade and pericardial disorders in connective tissue diseases: Case report and literature review. J. Natl. Med. Assoc. 86:149, 1994.

473. Kahl, L. E.: The spectrum of pericardial tamponade in systemic lupus erythematosus. Arthritis Rheum. 35:1343, 1992.

474. Chang, R. W.: Cardiac manifestation of systemic lupus erythematosus. Clin. Rheum. Dis. 8:197, 1982.

475. Gulati, S., and Kumar, L.: Cardiac tamponade as an initial manifestation of systemic lupus erythematosus in early childhood. Ann. Rheum. Dis. 51:279, 1992.

476. Morono, G., Banfi, G., and Ponticelli, C.: Clinical status of patients after 10 years of lupus nephritis. Q. J. Med. 84:681, 1992.

477. Thadani, U., Iveson, J. M., and Wright, V.: Cardiac tamponade, constrictive pericarditis and pericardial resection in rheumatoid arthritis. Medicine 54:261, 1975.

478. Kirk, J., and Cosh, J.: The pericarditis of rheumatoid arthritis. Q. J. Med. 38:397, 1969.

479. Bologna, C., Poirier, J. L., Herlsson, C., and Simon, L.: Constrictive pericarditis in severe seronegative rheumatoid arthritis. Rev. Med. Interne 13:64, 1992.

480. Hakala, M., Pettersson, T., Tarkka, M., et al.: Rheumatoid arthritis as a cause of cardiac compression. Favourable long-term outcome of pericardiectomy. Clin Rheumatol. 12:199, 1993.

481. Goldenberg, J., Ferraz, M. B., Pessoa, A. P., et al.: Symptomatic pericardial involvement in juvenile rheumatoid arthritis. Int. J. Cardiol. 34:57, 1992.

482. Jamieson, T. W.: Adult Still's disease complicated by cardiac tamponade. JAMA 249:2065, 1983.

483. Butman, S., Espinoza, L. R., Carpio, J. D., and Osterland, C. K.: Rheumatoid pericarditis. Rapid deterioration with evidence of local vasculitis. JAMA 238:2394, 1977.

484. Travaglio-Encinoza, A., Anaya, J. M., Dupuy D'Angeac, A. D., et al.: Rheumatoid pericarditis: New immunopathologic aspects. Clin. Exp. Rheumatol. 12:313, 1994.

485. Parkash, R., Atassi, A., Poske, R., and Rosen, K. M.: Prevalence of pericardial effusion and mitral valve involvement in patients with rheumatoid arthritis without cardiac symptoms. N. Engl. J. Med. 289:597, 1973.

486. Lam, D., and Rapaport, E.: Two-dimesional echocardiographic demonstration of intrapericardial fibrinous strands in rheumatoid pericarditis. Am. Heart J. 114:442, 1987.

487. Mathew, P. K.: Pericardial tamponade secondary to sudden steroid withdrawal in chronic rheumatoid arthritis. Chest 75:532, 1977.

488. Cotton, D. W., Cooper, C., Searle, M., et al.: Fatal cardiac tamponade complicating anticoagulant therapy in rheumatoid arthritis. Clin. Exp. Rheumatol. 5:367, 1987.

489. Thould, A. K.: Constrictive pericarditis in rheumatoid arthritis. Ann. Rheum. Dis. 45:89, 1986.

490. Fernandez-Muixi, J., Vidal, F., Bardaji, A., and Richart, C.: Recurrent pericarditis and cardiac tamponade in rheumatoid arthritis: Effectiveness of colchicine. Br. J. Rheumatol. 33:596, 1994.

491. Nassar, W. K., Miskin, M. E., and Rosenbaum, D.: Pericardial and myocardial disease in progressive systemic sclerosis. Am. J. Cardiol. 22:538, 1968.

492. Janosik, D. L., Osborn, T. G., Moore, T. L., et al.: Heart disease in systemic sclerosis. Semin. Arthritis Rheum. 19:191, 1989.

493. Smith, J. W., Clements, P. J., Levisman J., et al.: Echocardiographic features of progressive systemic sclerosis. Am. J. Med. 66:28, 1979.

494. Lawrence, M. R., Robinson, J. C., and Terry, E. E.: Progressive systemic sclerosis causing rapidly progressive myocardial disease and death. South Med. J. 85:770, 1992.

495. Hanley, P. C.: Constrictive pericarditis associated with combined retroperitoneal and mediastinal fibrosis. Mayo Clin. Proc. 59:300, 1984.

496. Medsger, T. A., Jr., Masi, A. T., and Rodnan, G. P.: Survival with systemic sclerosis (scleroderma). A life-table analysis of clinical and demographic factors in 309 patients. Ann. Intern. Med. 75:369, 1971.

497. Alpert, M. A., Goldberg, S. H., Singsen, B. H., et al.: Cardiovascular complications of mixed connective tissue disease in adults. Circulation 69:1182, 1983.

498. Beier, J. M., Nielsen, H. L., and Neilsen, D.: Pleuritis-pericarditis—an unusual initial manifestation of mixed connective tissue disease. Europ. Heart J. 13:859, 1992.

499. Yale, S. H., Adlakha, A., and Stanton, M. S.: Dermatomyositis with pericardial tamponade and polymyositis with pericardial effusion. Am. Heart J. 126:997, 1993.

500. Peieira, R. M., Lerner, S., Maeda, W. T., et al.: Pericardial tamponade in juvenile dermatomyositis. Clin. Cardiol. 15:301, 1992.

501. Rantapaa-Dahlquist, S., Backman, C., Sandgren, H., and Ostberg, Y.: Echocardiographic findings in patients with primary Sjogren's syndrome. Clin. Rheumatol. 12:214, 1993.

502. Shah, A., and Askari, A. D.: Pericardial changes and left ventricular function in ankylosing spondylitis. Am. Heart J. 113:1529, 1987.

503. Grant, S. C., Levy, R. D., Venning, M. C., et al.: Wegener's granulomatosis and the heart. Br. Heart J. *71*:82, 1994.

504. Csonka, G. W., and Oates, J. K.: Pericarditis and electrocardiographic changes in Reiter's syndrome. Br. Med. J. *1*:866, 1957.

505. Goldman, M. J., and Lau, F. Y. K.: Acute pericarditis associated with serum sickness. N. Engl. J. Med. *250*:278, 1954.

506. Shapiro, L., and Buckingham, R. B.: Septic rheumatoid pericarditis complicating Felty's syndrome. Arthritis Rheum. *24*:1435, 1981.

507. Sonnenblick, M., Nesher, G., and Rosin, A.: Nonclassical organ involvement in temporal arteritis. Semin. Arthritis Rheum. *19*:183, 1989.

508. Sarrouj, B. J., Zampino, D. J., and Cilurso, A. M.: Pericarditis as the initial manifestation of inflammatory bowel disease. Chest *106*:1911, 1994.

509. Cullen, S., Duff, D. F., Denham, B., and Ward, O. C.: Cardiovascular manifestations in Kawasaki disease. Ir. J. Med. Sci. *158*:253, 1989.

510. Zimand, S., Tauber, T., Hegesch, T., and Aladjem, M.: Familial Mediterranean fever presenting with massive cardiac tamponade. Clin. Exp. Rheumatol. *12*:67, 1994.

511. Crake, T., Sandie, G. I., Crisp, A. J., and Record, C. O.: Constrictive pericarditis and intestinal hemorrhage due to Whipple's disease. Postgrad. Med. J. *59*:194, 1983.

512. Dawes, P. T., and Atherton, S. T.: Coeliac disease presenting as recurrent pericarditis. Lancet *1*:1021, 1981.

513. Naschitz, J. E., Yeshurun, D., Miselevich, I., and Boss, J. H.: Colitis and pericarditis in a patient with eosinophilic fasciitis. A contribution to the multisystem nature of eosinophilic fasciitis. J. Rheumatol. *16*:688, 1989.

514. Nicolosi, A. C., Almassi, G. H., and Komorowski, R.: Cardiac tamponade secondary to giant lymph node hyperplasia (Castleman's disease). Chest *105*:637, 1994.

515. Wanner, W. R., Williams, T. E., Fulkerson, P. K., et al.: Postoperative pericarditis following thymectomy for myasthenia gravis. A prospective study. Chest *83*:647, 1983.

516. King, D. L.: Rhabdomyolysis with pericardial tamponade. Ann. Emerg. Med. *23*:583, 1994.

517. Silverman, K. J., Hutchins, G. M., and Bulkley, B. H.: Cardiac sarcoid: A clinicopathologic study of 84 unselected patients with systemic sarcoidosis. Circulation *58*:1204, 1978.

518. Garrett, J., O'Neill, H., and Blake, S.: Constrictive pericarditis associated with sarcoidosis. Am. Heart J. *107*:394, 1984.

519. Diderholm, E., Eklund, A., Orinius, E., and Widstrom, O.: Exudative pericarditis in sarcoidosis. Sarcoidosis *6*:60, 1989.

520. Alarcon-Segovia, D.: Drug-induced lupus syndromes. Mayo Clin. Proc. *44*:664, 1969.

521. Browning, C. A., Bishop, R. L., Heilpern, R. J., et al.: Accelerated constrictive pericarditis in procainamide-induced systemic lupus erythematosus. Am. J. Cardiol. *53*:376, 1984.

522. Harrington, T. M., and Davis, D. E.: Systemic lupus–like syndrome induced by methyldopa therapy. Chest *79*:696, 1981.

523. Lim, A. G., and Hine, K. R.: Fever, vasculitic rash, arthritis, pericarditis, and pericardial effusion after mesalazine. Br. Med. J. *308*:113, 1994.

524. Pent, M. T., Ganapathy, S., Holdsworth, C. D., and Channer, K. C.: Mesalazine induced lupus-like syndrome. Br. Med. J. *308*:113, 1994.

525. Schoenwetter, A. H., and Silber, E. N.: Penicillin hypersensitivity, acute pericarditis and eosinophilia. JAMA *191*:136, 1965.

526. Slater, E. E.: Cardiac tamponade and peripheral eosinophilia in a patient receiving cromolyn sodium. Chest *73*:878, 1978.

527. Dell-Isola, B, Rezgui, N., Thiollieres, J. M., et al.: Acute pericarditis with eosinophilia after ingestion of tryptophan. Rev. Prat. *43*:2563, 1993.

528. Yates, R. C., and Olson, K. B.: Drug-induced pericarditis. Report of three cases due to 6-amino-9-D-psicofuranosylpurine. N. Engl. J. Med. *265*:274, 1961.

529. Krehlik, J. M., Hindson, D. A., Crowley, J. J., Jr., and Knight, L. L.: Minoxidil-associated pericarditis and fatal cardiac tamponade. West. J. Med. *143*:527, 1985.

530. Miller, D. H., and Haas, L. F.: Pneumonitis, pleural effusion and pericarditis following treatment with dantrolene. J. Neurol. Neurosurg. Psych. *47*:553, 1984.

531. Lipworth, B. J., and Oakley, D. G.: Surgical treatment of constrictive pericarditis due to practolol. A case report. J. Cardiovasc. Surg. *29*:408, 1988.

532. Haugtomt, H., and Haerem, J.: Pulmonary edema and pericarditis after inhalation of Teflon fumes. Tidsskr. Nor. Laegeforen *109*:584, 1989.

533. Harbin, A. D., Gerson, M. C., and O'Connell, J. B.: Simulation of acute myopericarditis by constrictive pericardial disease with endomyocardial fibrosis to methysergide therapy. J. Am. Coll. Cardiol. *4*:196, 1984.

534. Bristow, M. R., Thompson, P. D., Martin, R. P., et al.: Early anthracycline toxicity. Am. J. Med. *65*:823, 1978.

535. Cazin, B., Gorin, N. C., Laporte, J. P., et al.: Cardiac complications after bone marrow transplantation. Cancer *57*:2061, 1986.

536. Ratliff, N. B., McMahon, J. T., Shirey, E. K., and Groves, L. K.: Silicone pericarditis. Cleve. Clin. Q. *51*:185, 1984.

537. Fraker, T. D., Jr., Walsh, T. E., Morgan, R. J., and Kim, K.: Constrictive pericarditis after the Beck operation. Am. J. Cardiol. *54*:931, 1984.

538. Sonakul, D., Thakerngpol, K., and Pocaree, P.: Cardiac pathology in 76 thalassemic patients. Birth Defects *23*:177, 1988.

539. Cordioli, E., Tondini, C., Pizzi, C., and Bugiardini, R.: Exudative pericarditis with pleural plaques caused by exposure to asbestos, resolved with steroidal treatment. Minerva Med. *85*:555, 1994.

540. Abdun Nur, D., Marcus, C. S., and Russell, F. E.: Pericarditis associated with scorpionfish (Scorpaena buttata) sting. Toxicon *19*:579, 1981.

541. Dressler, W.: A postmyocardial infarction syndrome. Preliminary report of a complication resembling idiopathic recurrent benign pericarditis. JAMA *160*:1379, 1956.

542. Lichstein, E., Arsura, E., Hollander, G., et al.: Current incidence of postmyocardial infarction (Dressler's) syndrome. Am. J. Cardiol. *50*:1269, 1982.

543. Jerjes-Sanchez, C., Ibarra-Perez, C., Ramirez-Rivera, A., et al.: Dressler-like syndrome after pulmonary embolism and infarction. Chest *92*:115, 1987.

544. Dressler, W.: The post-myocardial infarction syndrome. A report of forty-four cases. Arch. Intern. Med. *103*:28, 1959.

545. Van der Geld, H.: Anti-heart antibodies in the post-pericardiotomy and the post-myocardial infarction syndrome. Lancet *2*:617, 1964.

546. Liem, K. L., ten Veen, J. H., Lie, K. I., et al.: Incidence and significance of heart muscle antibodies in patients with acute myocardial infarction and unstable angina. Acta Med. Scand. *206*:473, 1971.

547. Khan, A. H.: The postcardiac delayed injury syndromes. Clin. Cardiol. *15*:67, 1992.

548. Hutchison, S. J., McKillop, J. H., and Hutton, I.: Failure of gallium-67 citrate imaging to diagnose post-myocardial infarction (Dressler's) syndrome. Eur. J. Nucl. Med. *13*:52, 1987.

549. Madsen, S. M., and Jakobsen, T. J.: Colchicine treatment of recurrent steroid-dependent pericarditis in a patient with post-myocardial-infarction syndrome (Dressler's syndrome). Ugeskr. Laeger *154*:3427, 1992.

550. Goldhaber, S. Z., Lorell, B. H., and Green, L. H.: Constrictive pericarditis. A case requiring pericardiectomy following Dressler's postmyocardial infarction syndrome. J. Thorac. Cardiovasc. Surg. *81*:793, 1981.

551. Kanawaty, D. S., Burggraf, G. W., and Abdollah, H.: Constrictive pericarditis and anemia post myocardial infarction. Can. J. Cardiol. *5*:147, 1989.

552. Soloff, L. A., Zatuchni, J., Janton, D. H., et al.: Reactivation of rheumatic fever following mitral commisurotomy. Circulation *8*:481, 1953.

553. Engle, M. A., and Ito, T.: The postpericardiotomy syndrome. Am. J. Cardiol. *7*:73, 1961.

554. Peters, R. W., Scheinman, M. M., Raskin, S., and Thomas, A. N.: Unusual complications of epicardial pacemakers. Am. J. Cardiol. *45*:1088, 1980.

555. Escaned, J., Ahmad, R. A., and Shiu, M. F.: Pleural effusion following coronary perforation during balloon angioplasty: An unusual presentation of the postpericardiotomy syndrome. Eur. Heart J. *13*:716, 1992.

556. Livelli, F. D., Jr., Johnson, R. A., McEnany, M. T., et al.: Unexplained in-hospital fever following cardiac surgery: Natural history, relationship to postpericardiotomy syndrome and a prospective study of therapy with indomethacin versus placebo. Circulation *57*:968, 1978.

557. Engle, M. A., Gay, W. A., Jr., Zabriskie, J. B., and Senterfit, L. B.: The postpericardiotomy syndrome: 25 years' experience. J. Cardiovasc. Med. *4*:321, 1984.

558. Kaminsky, M. E., Rodan, B. A., Osborne, D. R., et al.: Postpericardiotomy syndrome. Am. J. Radiol. *138*:503, 1982.

559. DeSaulniers, D., Gervais, N., and Rouleau, J.: Does pericardial drainage decrease the frequency of the postpericardiotomy syndrome? Can. J. Surg. *24*:265, 1981.

560. Nkere, U. U., Whawell, S. A., Thompson, J. N., and Taylor, E. M.: Changes in pericardial morphology and fibrinolytic activity during cardiopulmonary bypass. J. Thorac. Cardiovasc. Surg. *106*:339, 1993.

561. Ofori-Krakye, S. K., Tyberg, T. I., Geha, A. S., et al.: Late cardiac tamponade after open heart surgery: Incidence, role of anticoagulants in its pathogenesis and its relationship to the postpericardiotomy syndrome. Circulation *63*:1323, 1981.

562. Kassanoff, A. H., and Martirossian, M. G.: Postpericardiotomy and post-myocardial infarction syndrome presenting as noncardiac pulmonary edema. Chest *99*:1410, 1991.

563. Weitzman, L. B., Tinkler, W. P., Kronzon, I., et al.: The incidence and natural history of pericardial effusion after cardiac surgery—an echocardiographic study. Circulation *69*:506, 1984.

564. King, T. E., Jr., Stelzner, T. J., and Sahn, S. A.: Cardiac tamponade complicating the postpericardiotomy syndrome. Chest *83*:500, 1983.

565. Russo, A. M., O'Connor, W. H., and Waxman, H. L.: Atypical presentations and echocardiographic findings in patients with cardiac tamponade occurring early and later after cardiac surgery. Chest *104*:71, 1993.

566. Terada, Y., Saitoh, T., Shimoyama, Y., et al.: Late cardiac tamponade after open heart surgery. Kyobu Geka *47*:128, 1994.

567. Carrel, T., Jennl, R., Ritter, M., and Turina, M.: Late pericardial tamponade: A dangerous complication of postoperative anticoagulation following heart surgery. Schweiz. Med. Wochenschr. *123*:2401, 1993.

568. D'Cruz, I. A., Overton, D. H., and Pai, G. M.: Pericardial complications of cardiac surgery: Emphasis on the diagnostic role of echocardiography. J. Card. Surg. *7*:257, 1992.

569. Malour, J. F., Alam, S., Gharzeddine, W., and Stefadouros, M. A.: The role of anticoagulation in the development of pericardial effusion and late tamponade after cardiac surgery. Eur. Heart J. *15*:583, 1994.

570. Reichert, C. L., Visser, C. A., Koolen, J. J., et al.: Transesophageal echocardiography in hypotensive patients after cardiac operations. Comparison with hemodynamic parameters. J. Thorac. Cardiovasc. Surg. *104*:321, 1992.

571. Rex, D. K., Rogers, D. W., Mohammed, Y., and Williams, E. S.: Post-cardiac surgery tamponade mimicking acute hepatitis. J. Clin. Gastroenterol. *14*:136, 1992.

572. Battle, R. W., and Tischler, M. D.: Late postoperative cardiac tamponade presenting as a pulsatile epigastric mass. Scand. J. Thorac. Cardiovasc. Surg. *27*:183, 1993.

573. Maggiano, H. J., Higgins, T. L., Lobo, W., et al.: Superior vena cava syndrome after open heart surgery. Cleve. Clin. J. Med. 59:93, 1992.

574. Berge, K. H., Lanier, W. L., and Reeder, G. S.: Occult cardiac tamponade detected by transesophageal echocardiography. Mayo Clin. Proc. 67:667, 1992.

575. Chuttani, K., Tischler, M. D., Pandian, N. G., et al.: Diagnosis of cardiac tamponade after cardiac surgery: Relative value of clinical, echocardiographic, and hemodynamic signs. Am. Heart J. 127:913, 1994.

576. Susini, G, Pepi, M., Sisillo, E., et al.: Percutaneous pericardiocentesis versus subxiphoid pericardiotomy in cardiac tamponade due to postoperative pericardial effusion. J. Cardiothorac. Vasc. Anesthesia 7:178, 1993.

577. Friedrich, S. P., Berman, A. D., Baim, D. S., and Diver, D. J.: Myocardial perforation in the cardiac catheterization laboratory: Incidence, presentation, diagnosis, and management. Cathet. Cardiovasc. Diagn. 32:99, 1994.

578. Deckers, J. W., Hare, J. M., and Baughman, K. L.: Complications of transvenous right ventricular endomyocardial biopsy in adult patients with cardiomyopathy: A seven-year survey of 546 consecutive diagnostic procedures in a tertiary referral center. J. Am. Coll. Cardiol. 19:43, 1992.

579. B-Lundqvist, C., Olsson, S. B., and Varnauskas, E.: Transseptal left heart catheterization: A review of 278 studies. Clin. Cardiol. 9:21, 1986.

580. Goldbaum, T. S., Jacob, A. S., Smith, D. F., et al.: Cardiac tamponade following percutaneous transluminal coronary angioplasty. Cath. Cardiovasc. Diag. 11:413, 1985.

581. Seggewiss, H., Schmidt, H. K., Mellwig, K. P., et al.: Acute pericardial tamponade after percutaneous transluminal coronary angioplasty (PTCA). Z. Kardiol. 82:721, 1993.

582. Gunther, H. V., Strupp, G., Volmar, J., et al.: Coronary stent implantation: Infarction and abscess with fatal outcome. Z. Kardiol. 82:521, 1993.

583. Rosenthal, E., Qureshi, S. A., Sakadekar, A. P., et al.: Technique of percutaneous laser-assisted valve dilatation for valvar atresia in congenital heart disease. Br. Heart J. 69:556, 1993.

584. Bichel, J.: Serious complications of sternal puncture. Ugeskr. Laeger 151:442, 1989.

585. Mellon, J. K., Galvin, J. F., Bowe, P. C., et al.: Oesophago-pericardial fistula and cardiac tamponade after oesophagoscopy. Eur. J. Cardiothorac. Surg. 2:282, 1988.

586. Puhakka, H. J.: Complications of mediastinoscopy. J. Laryngol. Otol. 103:312, 1989.

587. Brown, D. L., and Luchi, R. J.: Cardiac tamponade and constrictive pericarditis complicating endoscopic sclerotherapy. Arch. Intern. Med. 147:2169, 1987.

588. Greene, T. O., Portnow, A. S., and Huang, S. K.: Acute pericarditis resulting from an endocardial active fixation screw-in atrial lead. Pacing Clin. Electrophysiol. 17:21, 1994.

589. Isselbacher, E. M., Cigarroa, J. E., and Eagle, K. A.: Cardiac tamponade complicating proximal aortic dissection. Is pericardiocentesis harmful? Circulation 90:2375, 1994.

590. Ng, A. S. H., Dorosti, K., and Sheldon, W. C.: Constrictive pericarditis following cardiac surgery—Cleveland Clinic Experience: Report of 12 cases and review. Cleve. Clin. Q. 50:39, 1984.

591. Cimino, J. J., and Kogan, A. D.: Constrictive pericarditis after cardiac surgery: Report of three cases and review of the literature. Am. Heart J. 118:1292, 1989.

592. Carrier, M., Hudson, G., Paquet, E., et al.: Mediastinal and pericardial complications after transplantation. Not-so-unusual postoperative problems? Cardiovasc. Surg. 2:395, 1994.

593. Hinkamp, T. J., Sullivan, H. J., Montoya, A., et al.: Chronic cardiac rejection masking as constrictive pericarditis. Ann. Thorac. Surg. 57:1579, 1994.

594. Killian, D. M., Furiasse, J. G., Scanlon, P. J., et al.: Constrictive pericarditis after cardiac surgery. Am. Heart J. 118:563, 1989.

595. Kabbani, S. S., Bashour, T., Ellertson, D. G., et al.: Constrictive pericarditis following myocardial revascularization: A possible cause of graft occlusion. Am. Heart J. 110:493, 1985.

596. Almassi, G. H., Chapman, R. D., Troup, P. J., et al.: Constrictive pericarditis associated with patch electrodes of the automatic implantable cardioverter-defibrillator. Chest 92:369, 1987.

597. Kassanoff, A. H., Levin, C. B., Wyndham, C. R., and Mills, L. J.: Implantable cardioverter defibrillator infection causing constrictive pericarditis. Chest 102:960, 1992.

OTHER FORMS OF PERICARDIAL DISEASE

598. Kerber, R. E., and Sherman, B.: Echocardiographic evaluation of pericardial effusion in myxedema. Incidence and biochemical and clinical correlations. Circulation 52:823, 1975.

599. Hardisty, C. A., Naik, D. R., and Munro, D. S.: Pericardial effusion in hypothyroidism. Clin. Endocrinol. 13:349, 1980.

600. Parving, H., Hansen, J. M., Nielsen, S. V., et al.: Mechanisms of edema formation in myxedema-increased protein extravasation and relatively slow lymphatic drainage. N. Engl. J. Med. 301:460, 1981.

601. Zimmerman, J., Yahalom, J., and Bar-On, H.: Clinical spectrum of pericardial effusion as the presenting feature of hypothyroidism. Am. Heart J. 106:770, 1983.

602. Meares, N., Brande, S., and Burgess, K.: Massive macroglossia as a presenting feature of hypothyroid-associated pericardial effusion. Chest 104:1632, 1993.

603. Manolis, A. S., Varriale, P., and Ostrowski, R. M.: Hypothyroid cardiac tamponade. Arch. Intern. Med. 147:1167, 1987.

604. Rubillon, J. F., Sanchez, B., Vuolo-Figaud, A. M., et al.: Cardiac tamponade in severe hypothyroidism. A rare cause. Presse Med. 22:1221, 1993.

605. Rosenbau, D. L., and Yu, P. N.: Idiopathic cholesterol pericarditis with effusion. Am. Heart J. 70:515, 1965.

606. Van Buren, P. C., and Roberts, W. C.: Cholesterol pericarditis and cardiac tamponade with congenital hypothyroidism in adulthood. Am. Heart J. 119:697, 1990.

607. Ridenhouse, C. E., and Kiphart, R. J.: Idiopathic cholesterol pericarditis treatment with pericardiectomy. Ann. Thorac. Surg. 4:360, 1967.

608. Stanley, R. J., Subramanian, R., and Lie, J. T.: Cholesterol pericarditis terminating as constrictive calcific pericarditis. Follow-up study of patient with 40-year history of disease. Am. J. Cardiol. 46:511, 1980.

609. Bhatti, M. A., Ferrante, J. W., Gielchinsky, I., and Norman, J. C.: Pleuropulmonary and skeletal lymphangiomatosis with chylothorax and chylopericardium. Ann. Thorac. Surg. 40:398, 1985.

610. Rose, D. M., Colvin, S. B., Danilowicz, D., and Isom, O. W.: Cardiac tamponade secondary to chylopericardium following cardiac surgery: Case report and review of the literature. Ann. Thorac. Surg. 34:333, 1982.

611. Morishita, Y., Taira, A., Furoi, A., et al.: Constrictive pericarditis secondary to primary chylopericardium. Am. Heart J. 109:373, 1985.

612. Pereira, W. M., Kalil, R. A., Prates, P. R, and Nesralla, I. A.: Cardiac tamponade due to chylopericardium after cardiac surgery. Ann. Thorac. Surg. 46:572, 1988.

613. Bar-El, Y., Smolinsky, A., and Yellin, A.: Chylopericardium as a complication of mitral valve replacement. Thorax 44:74, 1989.

614. Meyns, B. P., Faveere, B. C., Van de Werf, F. J., et al.: Constrictive pericarditis due to ingestion of a toothpick. Ann. Thorac. Surg. 57:489, 1994.

615. Sharland, M. G., and McCaughan, B. C.: Perforation of the esophagus by a fish bone leading to cardiac tamponade. Ann. Thorac. Surg. 56:969, 1993.

616. Naggar, C. Z., Daly, P. A., Burke, M. J., and Swartz, M. R.: Successful medical management of esophagopericardial fistula. Heart Lung 16:47, 1987.

617. Variyam, E. P., and Shah, A.: Pericardial effusion and left ventricular function in patients with acute alcoholic pancreatitis. Arch. Intern. Med. 147:923, 1987.

618. Letoquart, J. P., Fasquel, J. L., L'Huillier, J. P., et al.: Gastropericardial fistula. Review of the literature apropos of an original case. J. Chir. (Paris) 127:6, 1990.

619. Song, Z. L.: Cholangiothoracic fistulae. Chung Hua Wai Ko Tsa Chih 27:269, 1989.

620. Isolauri, J., and Markkula, H.: Recurrent ulceration and colopericardial fistula as late complications of colon interposition. Ann. Thorac. Surg. 44:84, 1987.

621. Ali, I., and Beg, M. H.: Traumatic bronchopericardial fistula presenting as cardiac tamponade. J. Thorac. Cardiovasc. Surg. 95:740, 1988.

622. Aho, A. J., Vanttinen, E. A., and Nelimarkka, O. I.: Rupture of the pericardium with luxation of the heart after blunt trauma. J. Trauma 27:560, 1987.

623. Callejas, M. A., Mestres, C. A., Catalan, M., and Sanchez-Lloret, J.: Traumatic intrapericardial diaphragmatic rupture. Thorac. Cardiovasc. Surg. 32:376, 1984.

624. Kirsch, J. D., and Escarous, A.: CT diagnosis of traumatic pericardium rupture. J. Comput. Assist. Tomogr. 13:523, 1989.

625. Cassorla, L., and Katz, J. A.: Management of cardiac herniation after intrapericardial pneumonectomy. Anesthesiology 60:362, 1984.

626. DuBroft, R. J., and Hoffman, I.: Intestinal tamponade: Cardiac compression by intestinal contents. J. Am. Soc. Echocardiogr. 7:89, 1994.

627. Feigin, D. S., Fenoglio, J. J., McAllister, H. A., and Madewell, J. E.: Pericardial cysts: A radiologic-pathologic correlation and review. Radiology 125:15, 1977.

628. Hynes, J. K., Tajik, A. J., Osborn, M. J., et al.: Two-dimensional echocardiographic diagnosis of pericardial cyst. Mayo Clin. Proc. 58:60, 1983.

629. Klatte, E. C., and Yune, H. Y.: Diagnosis and treatment of pericardial cysts. Radiology 104:541, 1972.

630. Unverferth, D. V., and Wooley, C. F.: The different diagnosis of paracardiac lesions: Pericardial cysts. Cath. Cardiovasc. Diag. 5:31, 1979.

631. Moncada, R., Baglia, K., Moguillansky, S. J., et al.: CT diagnosis of congenital intrapericardial masses. J. Comput. Assist. Tomogr. 9:56, 1985.

632. Ellis, K., Leeds, N. E., and Himmelstein, A.: Congenital deficiencies in partial pericardium: Review of two new cases including successful diagnosis by plain roentgenography. Am. J. Roentgenol. 82:125, 1959.

633. Letanche, G., Gayet, C., Souguet, P. J., et al.: Agenesis of the pericardium: Clinical, echocardiographic and MRI aspects. Rev. Pneumol. Clin. 44:105, 1988.

634. Taysi, K., Hartmann, A. F., Shackelford, G. D., and Sundarum, V.: Congenital absence of the pericardium in a family. Am. J. Med. Genet. 21:77, 1985.

635. Gehlmann, H. R., and van Ingen, G. J.: Symptomatic congenital complete absence of the left pericardium. Case report and review of the literature. Eur. Heart J. 10:670, 1989.

636. Inoue, H., Fujii, J., Mashima, S., and Marao, S.: Pseudo right atrial overloading pattern in complete defect of the left pericardium. J. Electrocardiol. *14*:413, 1981.

637. Candan, I., Erol, C., and Sonel, A.: Cross sectional echocardiographic appearance in presumed congenital absence of the left pericardium. Br. Heart J. *55*:405, 1986.

638. D'Altoria, R. A., and Caro, J. Y.: Congenital absence of the left pericardium detected by imaging of the lung: Case report. J. Nucl. Med. *18*:267, 1977.

639. Gutierrez, F. R., Shackelford, G. D., McKnight, R. C., et al.: Diagnosis of congenital absence of left pericardium by MR imaging. J. Comput. Assist. Tomogr. *9*:551, 1985.

640. Saito, R., and Hotta, F.: Congenital pericardial defect associated with cardiac incarceration: Case Report. Am. Heart J. *100*:866, 1980.

641. Jones, J. W., and McManus, B. M.: Fatal cardiac strangulation by congenital partial pericardial defect. Am. Heart J. *107*:183, 1984.

642. Auch-Schweik, W., Bonzel, T., Krause, T., et al.: Differential diagnosis of chest pain and diagnostic findings in pericardial defects combined with coronary artery disease. Clin. Cardiol. *11*:650, 1988.

643. Altman, C. A., Ettedgui, J. A., Wozney, P., and Beerman, L. B.: Noninvasive diagnostic features of partial absence of the pericardium. Am. J. Cardiol. *63*:1536, 1989.

644. Ruys, F., Paulus, W., Stevens, C., and Brutsaert, D.: Expansion of the left atrial appendage is a distinctive cross-sectional echocardiographic feature of congenital defect of the pericardium. Eur. Heart J. *4*:738, 1983.

645. Wolff, F., Fritz, A., Dumeny, P., and Eisenmann, B.: Diastolic coronary prolapse in partial left pericardial agenesis. Arch. Mal. Coeur. *80*:206, 1987.

646. Minocha, G. K., Falicov, R. E., and Nijensohn, E.: Partial right-sided congenital pericardial defect with herniation of the right atrium and right ventricle. Chest *76*:484, 1979.

647. Bernal, J. M., Lepiedra, J. O., Gonzalez, I., et al.: Angiocardiographic demonstration of partial defect of the pericardium with herniation of the left atrium and ventricle. J. Cardiovasc. Surg. *27*:344, 1986.

Chapter 44
Traumatic Heart Disease
PETER F. COHN, EUGENE BRAUNWALD

Violent injury accounts for the majority of deaths in persons under 40 years of age in the United States, and among these victims cardiac trauma is one of the leading causes of death.[1,2] For example, chest injuries are directly responsible for more than 25 per cent of the 50,000 to 60,000 deaths that result annually from automobile accidents and contribute significantly to another 25 per cent of these deaths.[3] The increasing frequency of physical violence has also resulted in a corresponding increase in the incidence of traumatic heart disease, especially in *young adult males*. These are the most frequent victims, because they are more likely to have automobile and motorcycle accidents, to incur injuries while performing heavy labor, and, as the daily headlines attest, to be involved in or victims of acts of physical violence.

The frequency of these mishaps is increasing. In Houston,[4] a 30-year analysis of 4459 patients with cardiovascular injuries (86 per cent of whom were males) showed a steady rise between 1958 (averaging 27 patients/yr) and 1988 (213 patients/yr) (Table 44–1). In addition, the incidence of medically-related cardiac trauma is also rising, such as increased use of intravascular and intracardiac catheters leading to penetrating injuries of the heart and great vessels, and resuscitative cardiac massage causing a variety of nonpenetrating injuries of these organs.

The two principal, immediate consequences of cardiac injury are *exsanguinating hemorrhage* and *cardiac tamponade*. Effective treatment has resulted in an increasing number of immediate survivors, and later sequelae— including myocardial infarction, ventricular aneurysm and pseudoaneurysm, ventricular septal defect, valvular damage, recurrent pericarditis, and constrictive pericarditis—are becoming far more common. Serious cardiac trauma is frequently overlooked in patients with nonpenetrating injury, particularly when other structures such as the thoracic cage and lungs are obviously damaged. Such oversight can be tragic, because the lethal consequences of cardiac injury may suddenly emerge after the superficial injuries have been attended to. Clearly, a much higher index of suspicion of this possibility is necessary if the increasing magnitude of this problem is to be halted and reversed.

NONPENETRATING CARDIAC INJURY

Nonpenetrating injuries result from the effects of external physical forces, but it is important to recognize that these forces need not necessarily be applied directly to the chest, because injuries to the heart and great vessels may also occur with trauma to other parts of the body.

The most common cause of nonpenetrating injury in civilian life is probably that directly related to *vehicular impact,*[5] either by direct compression, usually with the steering wheel squeezing the heart between the sternum and the spine, or by indirect compression. Causes of nonpenetrating injuries other than automobile and motorcycle accidents include direct blows to the chest by any kind of blunt object or missile, such as a clenched fist and various kinds of sporting equipment, as well as by the kicks of animals, falls, and cardiac resuscitative procedures. Fractures of the bony structures of the chest wall *are not* necessary accompaniments of cardiac injury in any of these situations. This point is of crucial importance, because *the absence of such obvious injuries following trauma should by no means exclude the possibility of nonpenetrating injury to the heart.* The clinical manifestations may not be apparent for days or even weeks after the accident.

Pathological findings following nonpenetrating cardiac injury usually include some degree of *pericarditis,* which may be associated with the late development of *pericardial constriction.* Changes in the heart itself range from minute ecchymotic areas in the subepicardium or subendocardium to transmural contusions with edematous, fragmented, or necrotic muscle fibers, surrounded at first by red blood cells and invaded soon thereafter by polymorphonuclear leukocytes. The external appearance of the heart may be misleading in the case of nonpenetrating injury, as large areas of intramural contusion, including involvement of the interventricular septum, may not be apparent.[6] In patients who survive the injury, healing is by scar formation resembling that following acute myocardial infarction, and posttraumatic aneurysms resembling postinfarction aneurysms may develop.[7] The types of cardiac injury resulting from blunt (nonpenetrating) trauma are listed in Table 44–2, the

TABLE 44–1 ETIOLOGY OF PATIENT CARDIOVASCULAR INJURIES: 1958–1988

ETIOLOGY	1958–63	1964–69	1970–73	1974–78	1979–83	1984–88	TOTAL
Gunshot wound	42	236	436	501	625	456	2296
Stab/laceration	64	110	161	229	362	463	1389
Blunt trauma	1	17	58	90	62	76	304
Shotgun wound	1	15	45	55	61	37	214
Iatrogenic	1	1	0	0	4	25	31
Other/unknown	54	20	111	25	3	12	225
Total	163	399	811	900	1117	1069	4459

From Mattox, K. L., et al.: Five thousand seven hundred sixty cardiovascular injuries in 4459 patients: Epidemiologic evaluation 1958 to 1988. Ann. Surg. *209*:698, 1989.

TABLE 44–2   TYPES OF CARDIAC INJURY FROM BLUNT TRAUMA

A. **MYOCARDIUM**
  1. Contusion
  2. Laceration
  3. Rupture
  4. Septal perforation
  5. Aneurysm, pseudoaneurysm
  6. Hemopericardium, tamponade
  7. Thrombosis, systemic embolism

B. **PERICARDIUM**
  1. Pericarditis
  2. Postpericardiotomy syndrome
  3. Constrictive pericarditis
  4. Pericardial laceration
  5. Hemorrhage
  6. Cardiac herniation

C. **ENDOCARDIAL STRUCTURES**
  1. Rupture of papillary muscle
  2. Rupture of chordae tendineae
  3. Rupture of atrioventricular and semilunar valves

D. **CORONARY ARTERY**
  1. Thrombosis
  2. Laceration
  3. Fistula

From Jackson, D. H., and Murphy, G. W.: Nonpenetrating cardiac trauma. Mod. Conc. Cardiovasc. Dis. *45*:123, 1976. Copyright 1976 American Heart Association.

most severe forms being rupture of the aortic or mitral valve and rupture of the interventricular septum or even of the free wall of a cardiac chamber. The relative incidences of the various consequences of nonpenetrating cardiac trauma are shown in Table 44–3.

TABLE 44–3   NONPENETRATING CARDIAC TRAUMA

TYPE AND/OR SITE OF INJURY	NO. OF CASES	CASES COMBINED WITH AORTIC RUPTURE	TOTAL
Rupture	273	80	353
Right ventricle	56	10	66
Left ventricle	46	13	59
Right atrium	35	6	41
Left atrium	24	2	26
IV septum	25(20*)	7(4*)	32(24*)
IA septum	18(10*)	5(3*)	23(13*)
Multiple chamber ruptures	69	37	106
Contusion/laceration	105	24	129
Pericardial laceration	18	18	36
Hemopericardium	13	12	25
Valvular laceration/rupture	1(2†)	0(4†)	1(6†)
Aortic valve	1(1†)	0(2†)	1(3†)
Pulmonic valve	0(4†)	0	0(4†)
Tricuspid valve	0(8†)	0	0(8†)
Mitral valve	0(8†)	0(1†)	0(9†)
Mitral and tricuspid valves	0(1†)	0(1†)	0(2†)
Coronary artery laceration/rupture	0(7†)	1(2†)	1(9†)
Papillary muscle laceration/rupture	1(23†)	0	1(23†)
TOTAL	411	135	546

Numbers in parentheses indicate more significant associated cardiac injuries (tabulated in another column).
* Associated with other sites of cardiac rupture.
† Combined with cardiac rupture or other cardiac injury.
From Parmley, L. F., et al.: Nonpenetrating traumatic injury of the heart. Circulation *18*:371, 1958. Copyright 1958 American Heart Association.

Pericardium

Injury to the pericardium in blunt trauma may range from contusion to laceration or rupture. Whether the pericardium tears or not, some degree of traumatic pericarditis is found at autopsy or operation in most patients sustaining severe blunt trauma of the chest, especially of the precordial area. In their classic study Parmley et al. reported pericardial laceration or rupture in 249 of 546 autopsy cases of nonpenetrating trauma to the heart[8]; however, it should be noted that this rarely occurs as an isolated lesion (Table 44–3) and is usually associated with cardiac contusion and even more serious cardiac injury. On the basis of a series of landmark experiments in a canine model, in which 14 of 18 dogs receiving sublethal blunt chest trauma developed pericardial rents, DeMuth et al. suggested that a higher frequency of pericardial tears than is generally appreciated occurs in survivors of chest trauma.[9] Clinically, a tear in the pericardium can occur as a consequence of blunt trauma, and delayed herniation of the heart through the rent may then compromise circulatory function acutely.

CLINICAL FEATURES AND DIAGNOSIS. Traumatic pericarditis is manifested by the development of a typical pericardial friction rub and ST–T-wave changes on the electrocardiogram characteristic of pericarditis (see p. 1482). During and immediately following the acute episode, the major problem is not the pericarditis itself but its most common complications, i.e., hemopericardium and resultant tamponade, discussed on page 1486. Commonly, the patient is restless, with hypotension, oliguria or anuria, distant heart sounds, and pulsus paradoxus. There is usually diffuse low voltage on the electrocardiogram. Pericardial fluid on the echocardiogram (see p. 1486) is a key finding.[10]

TREATMENT AND PROGNOSIS. As a rule, uncomplicated pericarditis secondary to cardiac trauma simply resolves. Tamponade, however, requires emergency operative treatment, as discussed below. Recurrent pericardial effusions sometimes associated with chest pain and fever, i.e., the so-called postpericardiotomy syndrome, occur in a small number of patients. The cause of this syndrome is not clear (see p. 1520). Although patients with recurrent effusion usually respond to aspirin or nonsteroidal antiinflammatory agents, occasionally glucocorticosteroids are necessary. *Constrictive pericarditis* (see p. 1496) occurs as a rare complication of traumatic pericarditis, with or without recurrent effusions.

Myocardium

CONTUSION. Myocardial contusion usually produces no significant symptoms and often goes unrecognized. At times, manifestations of the injury are masked by injury to the chest wall or other organs.[6,11,12] This is important because as many as 75 per cent of patients with myocardial contusion can have signs of external chest injury.[13] Thus there is a higher frequency of diagnosis of cardiac contusion associated with increasing awareness of the lesion.

Clinical Features and Diagnosis. The most common symptom of myocardial contusion is precordial pain resembling that of myocardial infarction, but the pain from other sites of chest trauma can confuse the clinical picture.[12,13] As with myocardial infarction, nitroglycerin and related drugs have little effect in relieving the pain. The *electrocardiogram* probably represents one of the most helpful tools for recognizing contusion of the left ventricle. Either nonspecific ST–T abnormalities or the classic findings of pericarditis are the most common changes noted. Initially, electrocardiographic signs of deeper injury to the myocardium, i.e., pathological Q waves, may be dwarfed by pericardial inflammation; only as the latter subsides does injury to the myocardium become more evident. However, because the possibility of cardiac trauma is often not considered in trauma victims, an electrocardiogram is often not recorded immediately on patients with chest injuries and

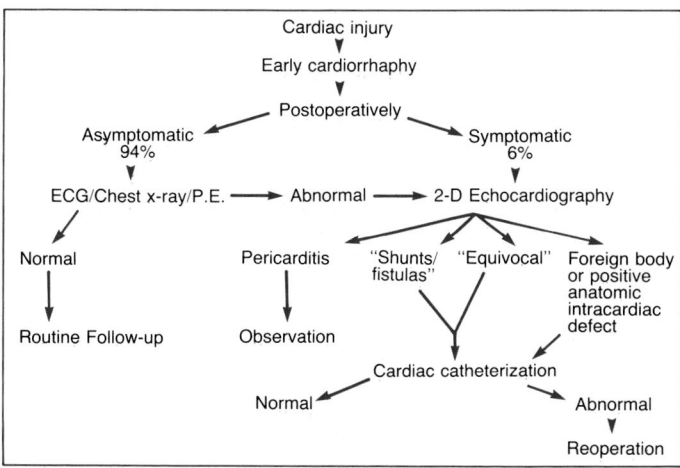

```
                    Cardiac injury
                         ↓
                 Early cardiorrhaphy
                         ↓
                   Postoperatively
                    ↙         ↘
        Asymptomatic              Symptomatic
            94%                       6%
             ↓                         ↓
    ECG/Chest x-ray/P.E. ──→ Abnormal ──→ 2-D echocardiography
       ↙                                  ↙    ↓    ↘
    Normal         Pericarditis    "Shunts/  "Equivocal"  Foreign body
      ↓                ↓           fistulas"              or positive
  Routine Follow-up  Observation                          anatomic
                                        ↘    ↓    ↙       intracardiac
                                                          defect
                                   Cardiac catheterization
                                      ↙            ↘
                                   Normal          Abnormal
                                                      ↓
                                                  Reoperation
```

FIGURE 44-1. A recommended decision schema for post-traumatic cardiac evaluation. Following cardiac injury, repair is generally carried out by simple cardiorrhaphy. This algorithm shows a suggested approach to detect residual damage following emergency cardiorrhaphy. (From Mattox, K. L., et al.: Cardiac evaluation following heart injury. J. Trauma 25:758, © by Williams and Wilkins, 1985.)

the diagnosis may be missed. Just as in acute myocardial infarction, serial findings, i.e., the evolution of Q waves and the subsidence of the ST-segment and T-wave abnormalities, are crucial. The sensitivity and specificity of electrocardiographic findings are less than 100 per cent, however; hence the need for additional tests.

A recommended decision schema for evaluating cardiac injury immediately after early cardiorrhaphy (suturing of the heart) is depicted in Figure 44-1.

SERUM ENZYMES. Because *enzyme levels* may be elevated by trauma to noncardiac as well as to cardiac tissue, they too are of limited diagnostic value. With the widespread availability of reliable measurements of the MB band of creatine kinase (CK), the presence or absence of cardiac necrosis can be better documented in patients with blunt trauma. Indeed, with the electrocardiogram and CK-MB as screening tests, the detection of myocardial contusion has increased from 7 to 17 per cent in patients with blunt chest trauma entering the Henry Ford Hospital.[14] Similarly, at the Mayo Clinic 58 of 291 such patients (20 per cent) had elevations of CK-MB.[15] However, false-positive elevations of the CK-MB isoenzyme can also be seen if the total CK is greater than 20,000 units; this can occur after massive injury to skeletal muscle.

RADIONUCLIDE IMAGING (see Chap. 9). Myocardial perfusion is reduced in areas of myocardial contusion. Contused myocardium concentrates [99mTc]-pyrophosphate in amounts comparable to those observed in ischemic injury. Scanning following injection of radioactive thallium to detect areas of reduced perfusion and of labeled pyrophosphate to locate areas of recent necrosis may be expected to identify patients with myocardial damage following blunt trauma, to localize this damage, and to indicate the extent of the damage. Radionuclide ventriculography often shows a reduced ventricular ejection fraction in such patients. These tests show changes similar to those observed in patients with acute myocardial infarction (Chap. 37). Sutherland et al.[16] used radionuclide ventriculography to define focal defects in ventricular wall motion. They subgrouped the 43 patients whom they studied into those with right ventricular abnormalities (18), left ventricular abnormalities (4), biventricular abnormalities (6), and neither kind (15). They described the state of right ventricular pump function using modified ventricular function curves and found it to be surprisingly well preserved. Schamp et al. also found a high (83 per cent) frequency of right ventricular abnormalities in the 40 patients they studied.[17]

ECHOCARDIOGRAPHY. In addition to identifying pericardial effusion, *two-dimensional echocardiography* is also useful in evaluating cardiac injuries, including myocardial contusion. Such findings as abnormal wall motion and chamber enlargement can be detected with this technique. Echocardiography is useful when the patient with suspected cardiac injury first undergoes testing, as well as after emergency thoracotomy and cardiac repair in an effort to detect residual cardiac damage. When confirmed with pulsed-Doppler echocardiography, intracardiac shunts and regurgitant lesions can be demonstrated.

Because patients with severe chest wall injuries often have suboptimal transthoracic echocardiographic results, the development of the transesophageal approach has significantly added to the value of echocardiography in diagnosing cardiac injury. For example, Karalis et al.[10] reported that 20 of 105 whose transthoracic echocardiographic results were nondiagnostic had wall motion abnormalities on

transesophageal echocardiography. The spectrum of myocardial injury detected by the combined techniques in their study is depicted in Figure 44-2.

ARRHYTHMIAS. A wide variety of arrhythmias is common with areas of extensive contusion, and ventricular tachycardia that degenerates into ventricular fibrillation represents a frequent cause of death in these patients, although atrial fibrillation is also commonly associated with a poor outcome.[6] The precise mechanism responsible for these arrhythmias has not been defined. In addition, both atrioventricular and intraventricular conduction defects, as well as sinus node dysfunction, are seen.[19,20] Blunt impact to the chest can also lead to cardiac arrest *without* obvious signs of structural injury.[20a] In contrast to acute myocardial infarction, cardiac contusion rarely leads to severe *heart failure* unless massive damage to a valve or rupture of the interventricular septum has occurred.[21,22] However, some impairment of right and/or left ventricular function, as reflected in depressed ejection fractions and ventricular function (myocardial performance) curves, may be found.[16] In the animal model, alcohol ingestion potentiates the effect of blunt trauma on the myocardium.[23] This gives added strength to the warning not to mix drinking and driving.

Treatment and Prognosis. In this era of progressively earlier ambulation of patients with acute myocardial infarction, a similar approach appears to be reasonable after several days of close observation for myocardial contusion. Several groups have concluded that in trauma patients in stable condition, contusion neither increases the complication rate nor necessitates intensive care unit monitoring.[24,25] In a study from the Boston City Hospital, Cachecho et al.[11] prospectively divided 336 patients admitted to the surgical intensive care unit with possible myocardial contusion into three groups: (1) those with a normal electrocardiogram, (2) those with an abnormal one, and (3) those with either normal or abnormal electrocardiograms but with many associated thoracic or extrathoracic injuries. Noninvasive studies were most abnormal in the latter group (Table 44-4), who were also the oldest (mean age 40). Cardiac complications were absent in Groups 1 and 2 as opposed to 19/138 in Group 3. The authors concluded that young patients with minor blunt trauma and a normal or slightly abnormal electrocardiogram do not benefit from cardiac monitoring. From the point of view of physical activity, we recommend treating these patients in a manner similar to that for those with acute myocardial infarction with comparable extent of myocardial damage (Chap. 37). However, treatment with *anticoagulants and obviously with thrombolytics* is con-

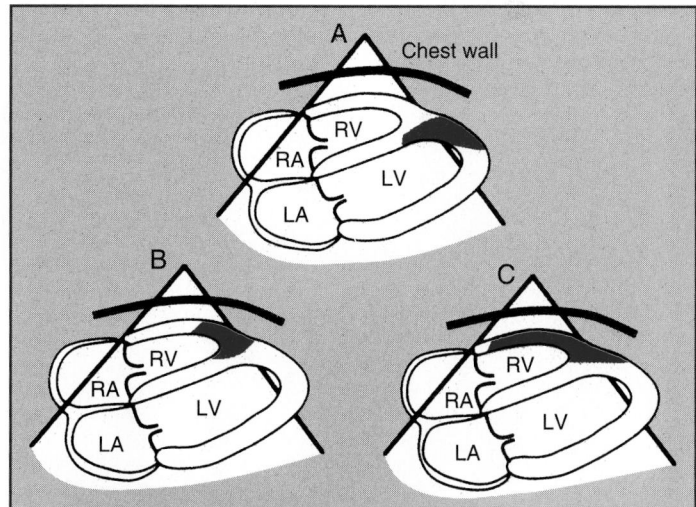

FIGURE 44-2. Spectrum of myocardial injury detected by echocardiography among 105 patients. When the left ventricle (LV) was injured, the myocardial contusion was limited to a small area of the LV spectrum and apex (A). When the right ventricle (RV) was injured, the myocardial contusion in 72 per cent of patients (B) was limited to a small area of the RV anteroapical wall; however, in the other 28 per cent (C) the myocardial contusion was extensive, involving most of the anterior RV wall and apex. LA = left atrium, RA = right atrium. (From Karalis, D. G., et al.: The role of echocardiography in blunt chest trauma: A transthoracic and transesophageal echocardiographic study. J. Trauma 36:53, © by Williams and Wilkins, 1994.)

TABLE 44-4   RESULTS OF NONINVASIVE STUDIES IN 36 PATIENTS WITH MYOCARDIAL CONTUSION

	GROUP 1		GROUP 2		GROUP 3	
	NO. OF STUDIES	NO. POSITIVE (%)	NO. OF STUDIES	NO. POSITIVE (%)	NO. OF STUDIES	NO. POSITIVE (%)
CPK-MB*	155	1 (0.6)	43	0 (0)	138	2 (1.4)
2D-Echo†	56	0 (0)	28	0 (0)	56	3 (5.3)
GBP‡	65	3 (4.6)	30	2 (6.6)	66	10 (15)
ECG§	155	0 (0)	43	43 (100)	138	44 (32)

All group 2 patients had an abnormal trauma floor ECG; % positive in parentheses.
* CPK-MB = Creatine phosphokinase myocardial band.
† Echo = two-dimensional echocardiography.
‡ GBP = gated blood pool scan.
§ ECG = serial electrocardiograms.
From Cachecho, R., et al.: The clinical significance of myocardial contusion. J. Trauma 33:68–73, 1992. © by Williams and Wilkins, 1992.

traindicated, because intramyocardial or intrapericardial hemorrhage may be precipitated or exacerbated. Atrial fibrillation, when present, usually reverts to sinus rhythm spontaneously. If it does not, digitalis glycosides may be used to slow the ventricular rate and may also cause reversion to sinus rhythm. Chest pain is best treated with analgesics; nonsteroidal antiinflammatory agents are not advised because they might interfere with myocardial healing (see p. 1210). When the postcardiac injury syndrome occurs, corticosteroids have proved helpful.[26]

As already noted, the prognosis for complete or partial recovery is generally excellent, but these patients require careful follow-up to observe for late complications, ranging from ventricular arrhythmias to cardiac rupture. Coronary occlusion,[27–29] aorto–right atrial fistula,[30] and ventricular aneurysms (Fig. 44–3)[7] are occasional sequelae, and there is no agreement about whether or not surgical resection of the last-named is required. It is our policy to use the presence of heart failure as an indication for operation of aneurysms analogous to that in patients with postinfarct aneurysms (see p. 1256). Pseudoaneurysms, however, require immediate repair (see p. 1242).

Although many analogies can be drawn between the cardiac necrosis caused by trauma and that caused by ischemic heart disease, a number of crucial differences must be emphasized. Patients with acute myocardial infarction secondary to coronary artery disease generally have diffuse, obstructive, gradually progressive coronary atherosclerosis, are frequently middle-aged or elderly, and may have underlying heart disease such as that secondary to prolonged hypertension or diabetes mellitus; patients with traumatic myocardial contusion generally have normal coronary vessels and only a discrete area of myocardial damage; most often, they are young and without underlying cardiovascular illness. Hence, the long-term prognosis in surviving patients with myocardial necrosis secondary to trauma tends to be far better than in patients with myocardial infarction secondary to atherosclerotic coronary artery disease.

CARDIAC RUPTURE. There appear to be two mechanisms of cardiac rupture: (1) acute laceration due to compression of the heart by direct force, and (2) contusion and hemorrhage leading to necrosis, softening, and rupture several days following the trauma.[31] Rupture of a cardiac chamber usually, but not always, results in immediate death. It is this minority of patients who survive the initial trauma that must be assessed and treated immediately in the emergency department setting.[32]

Clinical Features and Diagnosis. In the patient who survives the first few minutes of cardiac rupture, the clinical picture of cardiac tamponade described above is common. Although ventricular rupture is far more common than is atrial rupture, the latter occurs particularly following automobile accidents, as detailed in a series of 63 patients reported from Tokyo (Fig. 44–4).[33] Wearing a seatbelt does not necessarily prevent this complication of motor vehicle accidents, as noted in a large series from Helsinki.[34] Rupture of the interventricular septum should be suspected in patients who develop severe congestive heart failure immediately or within several days of the trauma, together with a new holosystolic murmur along the left sternal border; however, trauma to the mitral valve apparatus, which may be manifested with a similar picture clinically, must be excluded. On the basis of a series of 546 autopsy cases of nonpenetrating injury to the heart, the incidence of rupture of the ventricular septum has been estimated by Parmley et al. to be almost 10 per cent, with a similar number of patients experiencing rupture of the atrial septum (Table 44–3).[8] These lesions may occur without other serious cardiac injuries, but occasionally other abnormalities are present, including valve cusp perforations and a variety of intracardiac shunts. Although the predilection for perforation of the ventricular septum is highest at the apex, any portion of the muscular septum may be involved, and multiple perforations are not uncommon. The diagnosis of ventricular septal defect and of damage to the mitral valve apparatus can be confirmed by means of catheterization, demonstration of an oxygen step-up in the right ventricle, left ventricular angiography, as well as by color-flow Doppler echocardiography[10,18] (see p. 1541).

Treatment and Prognosis. Patients with external rupture of the heart obviously require emergency surgery if they are to have any chance of survival. Although operation should not be postponed, pericardiocentesis and expansion of the intravascular volume can be carried out while the most rapid preparations possible for operation are undertaken. Successful surgical treatment of external

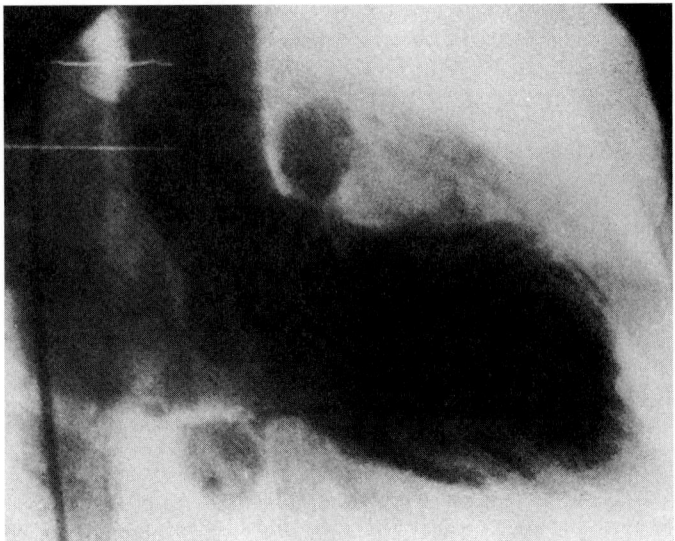

FIGURE 44–3. Right anterior oblique left ventriculogram. Submitral aneurysms appear as saccular narrow-necked structures at superior and inferior portions of mitral annulus during diastole. Top of inferior aneurysm is compressed by left atrium. (From Matthews, R. V., et al.: Chest trauma and subvalvular left ventricular aneurysms. Chest 95:474, 1989.)

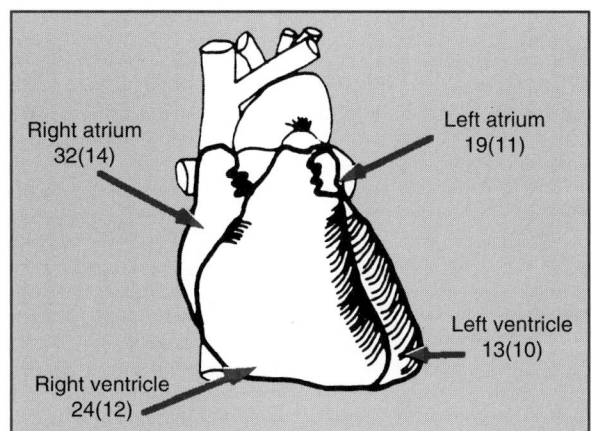

FIGURE 44–4. Location of cardiac rupture. There were 20 cases with multiple chamber injuries. Fourteen had two chambers ruptured, five had three chambers ruptured, and one had four chambers ruptured. In parentheses are numbers of multiple chamber injuries. (From Kato, K., et al.: Blunt traumatic rupture of the heart: An experience in Tokyo. J. Trauma 36:859, © by Williams and Wilkins, 1994.)

cadiac rupture has been reported in a small number of cases.[33–35] In contrast, patients with rupture of the interventricular septum do not always require emergency operation. Indeed, many defects are small, with minimal left-to-right shunts, and may even heal spontaneously. If heart failure develops subsequently, as occurs in many patients, surgical correction should be carried out promptly and is often successful.[36]

Complications of Cardiac Resuscitation

Closed-chest (external) cardiac massage (see p. 763) is generally thought to be safe and simple—so much so that it is included as part of the cardiopulmonary resuscitation technique taught to lay persons. What is not sufficiently appreciated is that the procedure itself can result in serious complications, which may go unrecognized because many of the patients succumb to the cardiac arrest itself.[37] Even at postmortem examination, the complications may be improperly attributed to the underlying cardiac disease.

Rupture of the left ventricle is a more common complication of cardiac massage than is rupture of the right ventricle. However, rupture of either chamber may occur and may be life-threatening if the patient survives the arrhythmia that necessitated massage in the first place. Because in most instances external resuscitation is performed for patients with myocardial infarction, it may not always be clear whether the left ventricular rupture preceded the massage or occurred as a consequence of it.

Rupture of right ventricular papillary muscles with acute tricuspid regurgitation has also been reported as a complication of closed-chest cardiac massage, as has rupture of the atria and aorta and dissecting hematoma of a coronary artery.[38] A variety of noncardiovascular traumatic lesions, such as fracture of the sternum, hemothorax, pneumothorax, and laceration of abdominal organs may occur. Because of the efficacy of cardiopulmonary resuscitation and its increasing use by paramedical personnel and lay people, an increasing number of such complications may be anticipated in the future. This increased incidence will be stemmed only by educational programs for all individuals likely to employ this technique.

PENETRATING CARDIAC INJURY

Penetrating cardiac injuries occurring in civilian life are due to a variety of objects, such as bullets, knives, ice picks, and the like. The demographics of penetrating cardiac trauma in Jefferson County, Alabama were reviewed

by Naughton, et al.[39] As with blunt trauma, male victims predominated and gunshot wounds were the major mechanism of injury. Penetrating injuries may also be due to the inward displacement of ribs or sternal fragments accompanying chest injuries. The chamber most commonly involved in this type of injury is the right ventricle because of its anterior position, followed, in descending order of frequency, by the left ventricle, the right atrium, and the left atrium. However, penetrating wounds of the precordium are not the only types of wounds that may result in cardiac injury. Occasionally, wounds of other areas of the chest, as well as of the neck and upper abdomen, are associated with penetration of the heart. In addition, intravenous or intracardiac catheters may fracture and become impaled within the walls of a great vessel or cardiac chamber (Chap. 6). Migration of an indwelling venous catheter into the pulmonary artery, which may ultimately lead to perforation of this vessel, is another complication that has increased in frequency with its widespread use in intensive care units. Formerly, thoracotomy was necessary to remove these catheter fragments, but catheters with snares and other devices are now available for this purpose.[40,44]

Perforation of the right ventricle with a transvenous pacing electrode is not uncommon, but tamponade is rare. During cardiac catheterization, perforation of the thin-walled right atrium or outflow tract of the right ventricle has been reported. Such patients usually require only careful observation, but when tamponade occurs, immediate drainage is mandatory. Coronary angioplasty[42] and endomyocardial biopsy[43,44] can also result in tamponade. Dissection of the aorta or arch vessels has been reported as a complication of retrograde arterial catheterization and occasionally is also severe enough to require operative intervention.

Penetrating wounds of the heart often result in laceration of the pericardium, sometimes occurring alone but usually associated with laceration of the myocardium itself. One or more chambers but also the cardiac valves and their accessory structures, as well as the interventricular and interatrial septa, may be perforated. Occasionally, low-velocity missiles may penetrate the cardiac chambers but may be retained within the myocardium.

The most common penetrating injuries resulting from physical violence are stab and gunshot wounds.[2,39,45] The former do not necessarily cause extensive cellular destruction adjacent to the wound; they resemble surgical incisions, and transmural wounds in the thick-walled left ventricle may actually seal quickly without disastrous consequences. In contrast, bullet wounds are associated with bleeding that is not usually self-limited and extensive cellular destruction in and adjacent to the path of the bullet. When a coronary artery is lacerated or perforated, myocardial infarction may ensue.

CLINICAL FEATURES AND DIAGNOSIS. The clinical picture of a penetrating wound of the heart depends on several factors, including the object responsible for the injury (e.g., bullet, knife, ice pick), the size of the wound, and the precise location of the structures injured. Pericardial laceration occurring by itself is uncommon and of relatively little significance unless infection supervenes. Rather, the injuries to underlying cardiac structures usually determine the clinical presentation, course, and choice of treatment. However, the nature of the pericardial wound is important, i.e., whether or not the wound is open and allows free drainage of intrapericardial blood. If the pericardium remains open and extravasated blood can pass freely into the pleural cavities or mediastinum, cardiac tamponade will not develop, at least initially, and the presenting signs and symptoms will be those of hemorrhage and hemothorax. On the other hand, if the pericardium does *not* permit free drainage because its opening has been obliterated by a blood clot, adjacent lung tissue, or other structures, or because a flap develops in the pericardial rent, immediate exsanguination may be averted, but tamponade may occur

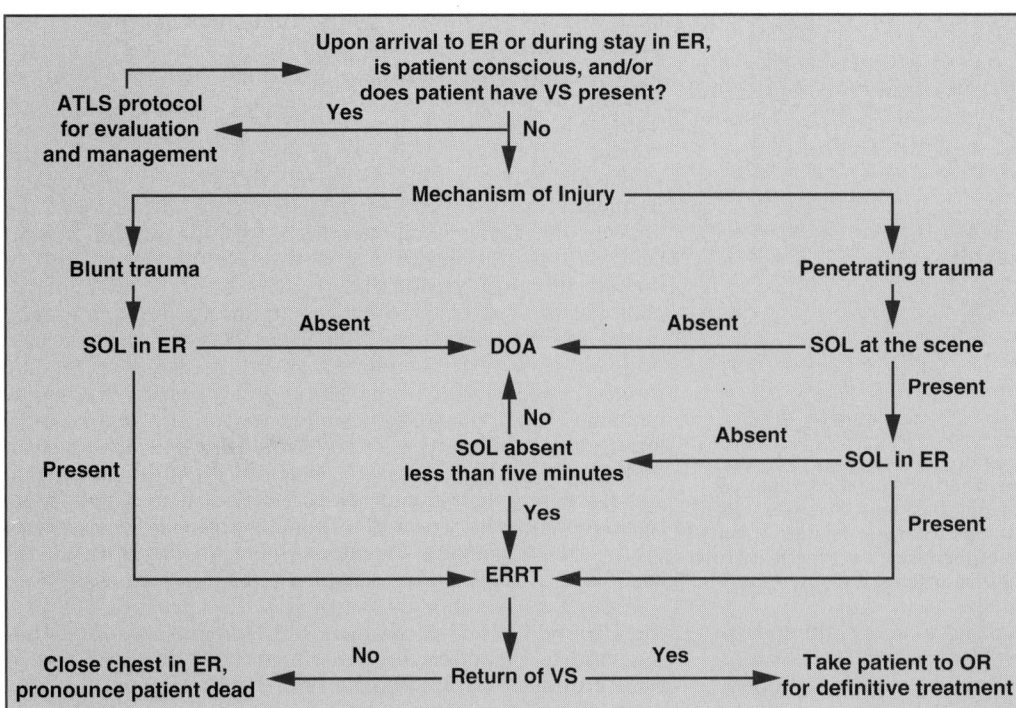

FIGURE 44–5. Emergency room resuscitative thoracotomy algorithm. ER = emergency room, ATLS = advanced trauma life support, SOL = signs of life, DOA = dead on arrival, ERRT = emergency room resuscitative thoracotomy, VS = vital signs. (From Boyd, M., et al.: Emergency room resuscitative thoracotomy: When is it indicated? J. Trauma *33*:714, © by Williams and Wilkins, 1994.)

minutes or hours later. In some instances, blood accumulates both intra- and extrapericardially.

Whether the hemorrhage is intra- or extrapericardial, its severity can often be surmised from the clinical picture. Traumatic penetrating lesions of the heart are usually associated with injuries to the lungs and other organs, which may predominate at first; a high index of suspicion of cardiac penetration is necessary when patients are evaluated following thoracic or upper abdominal trauma. Although extensive injuries to the pericardium and underlying heart are usually immediately fatal or result in shock, delayed clinical manifestations of cardiac injury as a result of hemorrhage, infection, retained foreign bodies, or arrhythmias may become apparent after the other bodily injuries have been attended to. Failure to give serious consideration to the possibility that *cardiac* damage has occurred in a patient with obvious noncardiac trauma may lead to an unanticipated catastrophe.

Although echocardiography is extremely valuable in the recognition of pericardial effusion[10,18,20,46] (see p. 93), foreign bodies in the heart,[47] and intracardiac shunts,[10,18,48,49] it is not always readily available in an emergency setting. When agitation, cool and clammy skin, neck vein distention, pulsus paradoxus, and other classic findings of tamponade (considered earlier) are present, the diagnosis can be relatively simple; in patients without such typical findings, the clinical picture may be attributed to blood loss, especially since volume expansion can improve the hemodynamic state, at least temporarily. Whether or not pericardiocentesis should be performed as a diagnostic test is controversial. If nonclotting blood is obtained, the diagnosis of hemopericardium is confirmed, and the accompanying decompression may constitute effective, albeit temporary, initial treatment. If the pericardiocentesis is negative, however, cardiac tamponade cannot be ruled out. Because, as discussed later, the primary management in any event is thoracotomy, it seems pointless to waste valuable time with pericardial aspiration unless there is doubt regarding the diagnosis.

MANAGEMENT. The definitive treatment of cardiac wounds *accompanied by severe hemorrhage* is immediate thoracotomy and cardiorrhaphy.[50] Although multiple pericardiocenteses are no longer considered a substitute for thoracotomy in the treatment of cardiac wounds associated with cardiac tamponade, there may still be a role for peri-

cardial aspiration *while the patient is being prepared for operation.* The availability in many hospitals of surgical teams and equipment for cardiopulmonary bypass has permitted the safe and effective repair of many penetrating injuries of the heart.

Emergency department resuscitative thoracotomy has also been advocated in selected instances. (Figure 44–5 illustrates one proposed algorithm).[51,52] The best survival rate is in those patients with penetrating wounds and signs of life present in the emergency department. It is therefore not surprising that successful prehospital resuscitative measures can increase the success of a hospital emergency procedure.[53] A novel approach to hospital emergency thoracotomy cardiac stapling was successfully used in 28 patients with penetrating cardiac injuries at the San Francisco General Hospital[54] between 1987 and 1992. This technique also prevents the surgeon from exposure to contaminated needle sticks while suturing the heart. Operative treatment includes repair of the pericardium, myocardium, aorta, and valves as well as of any lacerations of the coronary arteries. At operation, the heart and great vessels should be thoroughly examined for the presence of multiple wounds. When the bullet has penetrated the anterior wall of the heart, the posterior wall should always be inspected for an exit wound before the chest is closed. Many victims of penetrating cardiac injury, young and other-

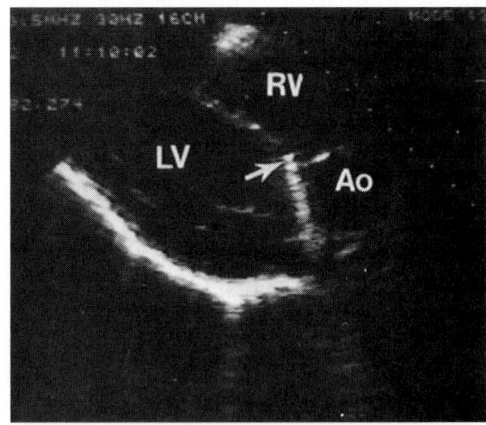

FIGURE 44–6. Two-dimensional echocardiographic image in the left parasternal long-axis view. A bullet fragment (arrow) is located high in the interventricular septum and has the typical appearance of such missiles with dense trailing reverberations. Ao = aortic root; LV = left ventricle; RV = right ventricle. (From Hassett, A., et al.: Utility of echocardiography in the management of patients with penetrating missile wounds of the heart. Reprinted with permission of the American College of Cardiology. J. Am. Coll. Cardiol. *7*:1151, 1986.)

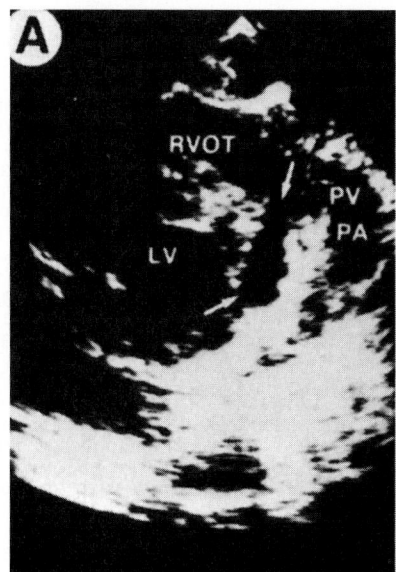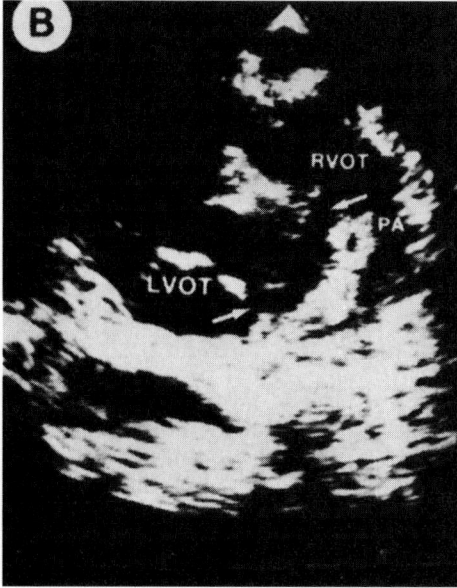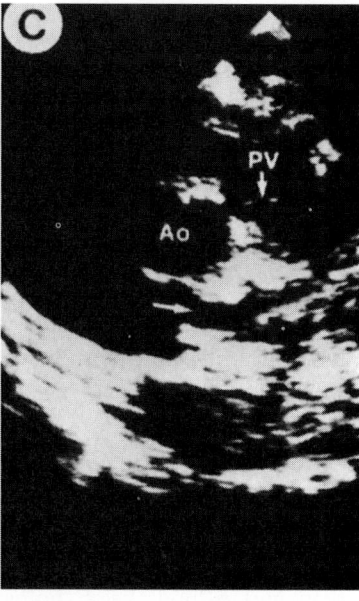

FIGURE 44–7. Two-dimensional echocardiogram from the parasternal short-axis position in a patient with a ventricular septal defect caused by knife stabbing. *A,* A defect is seen in the interventricular septum (arrows) between the left ventricle (LV) and the right ventricular outflow tract (RVOT) just proximal to the pulmonary valve (PV). *B,* At a slightly higher level the defect originates in the left ventricular outflow tract (LVOT) and exits in the distal right ventricular outflow tract. *C,* At an even higher level, but just below the aorta (Ao) and left atrium, a portion of the defect is seen (arrow). PA = pulmonary artery. (From Goldfarb, M. S., et al.: Two-dimensional Doppler echocardiographic diagnosis of a traumatic intracardiac shunt. Am. J. Cardiol. *57:*494, 1986.)

wise in good health, can withstand relatively long periods of hypoperfusion without irreversible brain, renal, or cardiac damage. Therefore, one should err on the side of aggressive attempts at resuscitation in patients who arrive moribund in the operating room. Retained foreign bodies in the heart are less of a problem in civilian than in military injuries, because shootings in civilian life usually occur at short range and thus result in through-and-through wounds.

There is disagreement concerning whether or not retained foreign bodies should be removed. Certainly, if the projectile is accessible, it should be removed; echocardiography (Fig. 44–6) can be helpful in locating foreign bodies.[47,55] If deemed not dangerous, they can probably be left in place (as has been done in the pulmonary arteries[56]), although there is some risk of later infection, pain, aneurysm formation, or migration of the foreign body.[55] In addition, dealing with a patient who is preoccupied with the knowledge that he or she has a foreign body retained in or close to the heart may present some difficulty; indeed, anxiety can become excessive, impairing the patient's function more than the physical damage and, occasionally, becoming an indication for reoperation and extraction of the object. The serious consequences of a foreign body embolus from the left ventricle also encourage a more aggressive surgical policy toward foreign bodies lodged in that chamber than in the right ventricle. Foreign bodies embedded at strategic points in great vessels may erode the vessel and cause potentially severe hemorrhage or may embolize[55] and should, if possible, be removed.

Late complications of penetrating wounds of the heart are quite common and include post-traumatic pericarditis and infection as well as arrhythmias, ventricular septal defect, and ventricular aneurysm.

PROGNOSIS. The outlook following a penetrating injury depends, first and foremost, on the extent of the injury. Gunshot wounds of the heart are more often fatal than are stab wounds, while among the latter, knife wounds are more serious than are ice pick wounds. Salvage rates are lower in patients with extrapericardial hemorrhage compared with tamponade and also with penetrating wounds involving thin-walled structures such as the atria or the pulmonary artery, since they rarely seal off spontaneously, whereas injury to the ventricles is associated with distinctly higher survival.

The state of consciousness and the extent of damage, if any, to the central nervous system at the time the patient is brought to the hospital also affect prognosis. It is clear that delay in performing the initial thoracotomy also adversely influences the chances for survival.

Rupture of the interventricular septum (Fig. 44–7) is often a late complication of penetrating injury as it is with blunt injury. Asfaw et al. described 12 patients with stab wounds who presented with cardiac tamponade and who had epicardial and pericardial wounds that were repaired at thoracotomy.[57] Days to years later, septal defects were diagnosed, but only four patients were symptomatic enough to warrant subsequent reoperation for closure of the defect. Residual injuries requiring reoperation can often be detected with color-flow Doppler echocardiography.[10,18]

INJURIES TO CARDIAC VALVES, PAPILLARY MUSCLES, AND CHORDAE TENDINEAE

Patients with preexisting valvular heart disease may be at higher risk than those with normal valves for the development of valvular injury following blunt trauma. Parmley et al. cited a 9 per cent incidence of valvular injury in their report of 546 cases of nonpenetrating chest trauma (Table 44–3).[8] In most series (although not in Parmley's) damage to the aortic valve is by far the most common of these lesions (Fig. 44–8). Indeed, sustained damage of the aortic

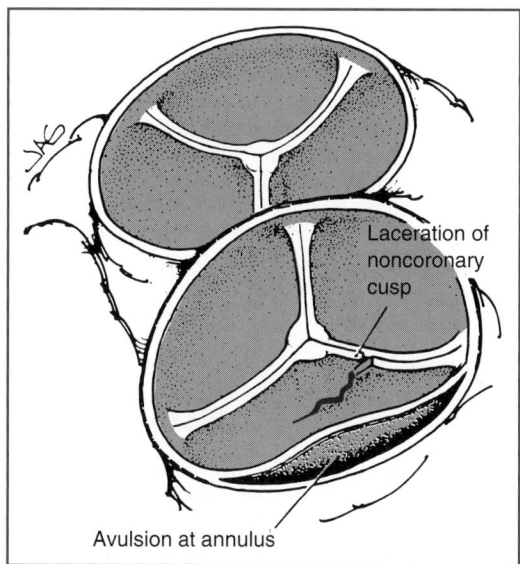

FIGURE 44–8. Diagram showing laceration of noncoronary cusp and avulsion at annulus of aortic valve following blunt trauma. (From German, D. S., et al.: Acute aortic valvular incompetence following blunt thoracic deceleration injury: Case report. J. Trauma *30:*1411, © by Williams and Wilkins, 1990.)

valve should be suspected in any patient without a history of heart disease who has a heart murmur after severe blunt trauma to the chest. Damage to cardiac valves may also occur as a consequence of penetrating wounds of the heart, but, in contrast to the damage caused by nonpenetrating injury, these are rarely solitary lesions.[58,59] Blunt chest trauma has also been reported to cause bioprosthetic valve dysfunction.[60]

CLINICAL FEATURES AND DIAGNOSIS. New, loud, musical murmurs are characteristic of injury to the valves and their supporting structures. The combination of a high-pitched diastolic blowing murmur with a widened pulse pressure following blunt trauma to the chest suggests rupture of the *aortic valve*. The murmur and the hemodynamic consequences of the rupture may not appear for several days following the trauma. Aortic regurgitation may also occur transiently owing to perivalvular edema or hemorrhage.

Rupture of the *mitral valve* or of a papillary muscle appears to occur as a consequence of sudden obstruction of left ventricular outflow due to blunt injury in early diastole.[61] It is usually associated with the development of precordial pain and a loud, harsh holosystolic murmur that radiates to the apex. Fulminant pulmonary edema quickly develops; compensation in those patients with lesser degrees of regurgitation due to torn leaflets or chordae tendineae may remain for longer periods of time, although they may eventually show signs of decompensation.

Rupture of the *tricuspid valve* is not as rare as previously thought[62] and is more benign than mitral valve rupture, with symptoms ranging from fatigue to ascites and edema. Physical findings can be striking, with prominent systolic venous pulsations, hepatic pulsations, and a typical holosystolic murmur with inspiratory accentuation.

TREATMENT AND PROGNOSIS. The prognosis depends largely on the severity of the regurgitation. Because the lesion usually develops suddenly, the ventricle does not have the opportunity to adapt to this burden, as it does in most forms of chronic valvular regurgitation. Obviously, the baseline condition of the ventricle prior to the trauma, the presence of other injuries occurring simultaneously, and the severity of the regurgitation affect the heart's ability to tolerate the insult. When effective surgical treatment is not possible, survival without the need for operation is not uncommon in patients with mild or moderate regurgitation. With severe left ventricular failure due to a ruptured mitral valve or papillary muscle, however, early surgery is mandatory.

The diagnosis of acute left ventricular failure may be difficult immediately after serious trauma, because fractured ribs and pulmonary contusions may be blamed for the shortness of breath and dyspnea. When left ventricular failure develops slowly or the lesion is not hemodynamically significant, as with lesser degrees of injury, medical therapy may suffice. Hemorrhage into a papillary muscle may cause late necrosis and delayed rupture, and these patients must be observed carefully.

INJURIES TO THE CORONARY ARTERIES AND GREAT VESSELS

CORONARY ARTERIES. Transmural myocardial infarctions have been reported following blunt trauma (including trauma to the head),[63] but angiographic confirmation of coronary obstruction is uncommon, and, when found, its relationship to preexisting coronary atherosclerosis may be difficult to determine. When infarction occurs, it may not be clear whether it results directly from myocardial contusion, from trauma to a coronary artery, or from some combination of these two processes. In many cases of myocardial infarction, preexisting coronary artery disease has been present, and it is reasonable to postulate that the injury dislodges a plaque, which then obstructs the vessel completely. However, it is also possible that a normal coronary artery becomes occluded, by either a traumatically induced intimal tear or hemorrhage.[64] Indeed, coronary arteriography has provided strong evidence that myocardial infarction follows blunt chest trauma in previously asymptomatic persons with normal vessels except for complete obstruction of the vessel supplying the infarcted area.[29] The complications of myocardial infarction—arrhythmias, pump failure, and late development of aneurysms—are similar when the lesion has an atherosclerotic basis, and treatment is similar as well. However, it may be anticipated that *following survival from the initial episode, the long-term prognosis will be more favorable in patients with traumatic damage of a coronary artery*, because the remaining vessels are usually normal. There are exceptions, however.[65]

ANEURYSM. Left ventricular *aneurysm and pseudoaneurysm* following injury to the coronary arteries can lead to ventricular rupture, cardiac failure, embolism, or arrhythmia. Operative intervention is indicated in the presence of a pseudoaneurysm, in which the myocardium has actually ruptured but in which a thrombus, fibrous tissue, and/or pericardium prevent exsanguination, because external rupture—an event that is usually fatal—is likely to occur ultimately if the condition is left untreated. Pseudoaneurysm can often be differentiated from true aneurysm by contrast or radionuclide angiography (see p. 1347).

FISTULA. Formation of an *arteriovenous fistula* is an unusual complication of traumatic damage of a coronary artery.[66] Injury to the right coronary artery is more commonly followed by an arteriovenous fistula than is injury to the left. The venous side of the fistula may be the coronary sinus, the great cardiac vein, the right atrium, or the right ventricle; in the last instance, the fistula should be termed an "arteriocameral fistula." The murmur in traumatic coronary arteriovenous or arteriocameral fistula is usually loud, widely radiating, and continuous; the electrocardiogram frequently shows transmural myocardial infarction, and the roentgenogram exhibits cardiomegaly with increased pulmonary vascularity. In patients who do not undergo surgical repair, symptoms of congestive heart failure and chest pain are frequent unless the shunt is minimal.

The left anterior descending coronary artery is the vessel most commonly involved, and at operation, the treatment of choice is suture-ligation of the cut vessel with coronary artery bypass grafting if the lacerated vessel is large and the lesion is a proximal one. Not all patients will require cardiopulmonary bypass during surgery.[67] Angiography is not advised in the emergency setting, as it is with nonpenetrating trauma. However, postoperative angiography is useful in

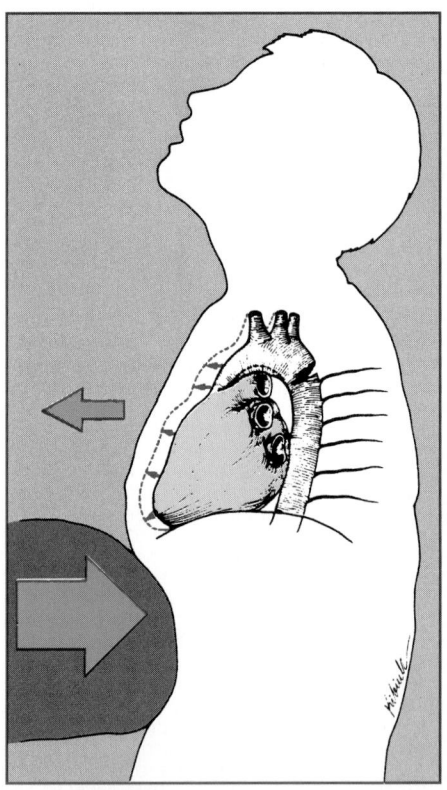

FIGURE 44–9. When the body is suddenly arrested against an obstacle, the heart and horizontal portion of the aortic arch continue their forward movement, while the descending aorta is fixed to the spine by the intercostal arteries ("deceleration" mechanism of injury). The aortic tear is posterior in this example, but it can also be anteromedial if there is upward displacement of the heart. (From Maggisano, R., and Cina, C.: Traumatic rupture of the thoracic aorta. *In* McMurtry, R. Y. and McLellan, B. A. [eds.]: *Management of Blunt Trauma.* Baltimore, Williams and Wilkins, 1990, pp. 206–226.)

localizing the presence of possible residual injuries such as a coronary arteriocameral fistula.

GREAT VESSELS. Rupture of the aorta is one of the most common traumatic lesions involving the heart or great vessels. It is most common after automobile accidents[68-70] but can also occur after falls from heights or other types of crushing injuries.[71] In automobile accidents, most commonly rupture occurs at the isthmus (Fig. 44–9), whether the collisions are head-on or broadside.[68]

It has been estimated that 10 to 20 per cent of patients with ruptured aortas live long enough to be treated successfully under ideal circumstances, which include a high level of awareness of the possibility of aortic rupture in victims of automobile accidents as well as a well-coordinated team approach.[70] As with cardiac injury, rupture of the aorta may be overshadowed by injuries to other organs, and the diagnosis may be overlooked.[71] Common clinical and radiological findings are listed in Table 44–5. Patients with aortic rupture often complain of pain in the back in addition to the chest, as do patients with aortic dissection (see p. 1556). If the expanding mediastinal hematoma or false aneurysm narrows the aortic lumen, or if the torn intima and media cause partial aortic obstruction, ischemia of the spinal cord and kidneys may ensue. A systolic murmur may be heard in the midscapular region, and widening of the superior mediastinum is visible on the chest roentgenogram (Fig. 45–9, p. 1558) along with other findings.[72,73]

A diagnostic triad that occurs in well over half the cases of ruptured aorta was initially reported by Symbas et al.[74] It consists of (1) increased arterial pressure and pulse amplitude in the upper extremities, (2) decreased pressure and pulse amplitude in the lower extremities, and (3) radiological evidence of widening of the superior medi-

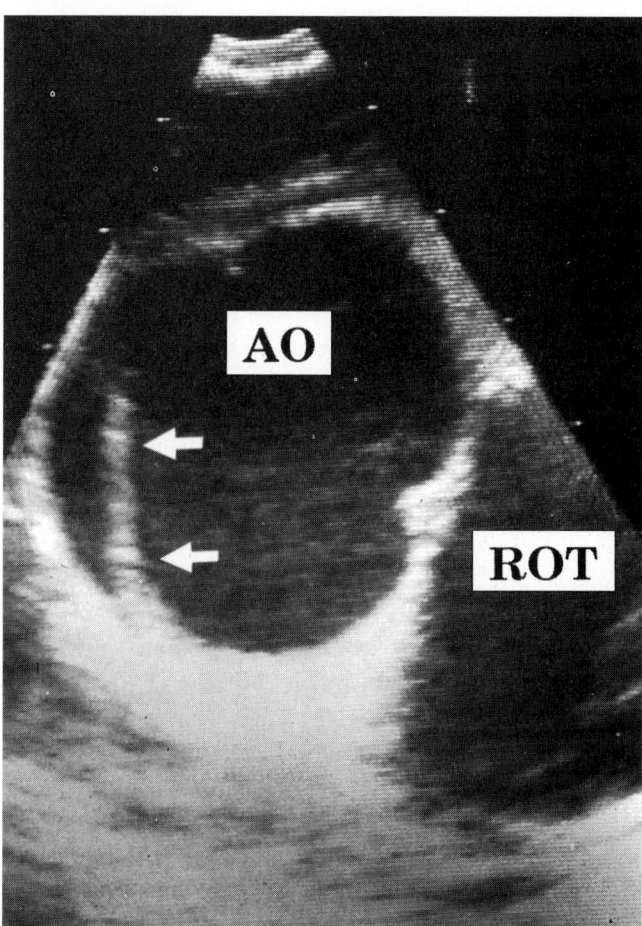

FIGURE 44–10. Transesophageal echocardiographic view of the aortic root (AO) just above the origin of the right coronary artery. White arrows indicate an intimal flap on the right aortic wall. ROT, right outflow tract. (From Catoire, P., et al.: Traumatic laceration of the ascending aorta detected by transesophageal echocardiography. Ann. Emerg. Med. *23*:356, 1994.)

TABLE 44–5 CLINICAL AND RADIOGRAPHIC CHARACTERISTICS OF 93 PATIENTS EVALUATED FOR AORTIC TRAUMA

CHARACTERISTIC	RUPTURE (N = 11)	NO RUPTURE (N = 82)
Age—yr		
Mean ± SD	42.9 ± 15.1	44.5 ± 19.2
Range	17–66	13–87
Sex—M/F	7/4	62/20
Mechanism of injury—no. (%)		
Motor vehicle accident (unrestrained)	7 (63.6)	48 (58.5)
Motor vehicle accident (restrained)	2 (18.2)	12 (14.6)
Pedestrian hit by car	0	8 (9.8)
Motorcycle accident	1 (9.1)	6 (7.3)
Fall	1 (9.1)	5 (6.1)
Gunshot	0	1 (1.2)
Crushed by car	0	2 (2.4)
External chest trauma—no. (%)	2 (18.2)	16 (19.5)
Intubation—no. (%)	5 (45.5)	30 (36.6)
Systolic blood pressure—mm Hg		
Mean ± SD	118.8 ± 33.4	130.6 ± 26.5
Range	70–170	76–198
Heart rate—beats/min		
Mean ± SD	115.7 ± 30.3	103.8 ± 22.9
Range	62–167	60–178
Glasgow coma score		
Mean ± SD	12.1 ±3.8	12.3 ± 3.8
Range	6–15	3–15
Injury-severity score*		
Mean ± SD	51.1 ± 15.2	26.7 ± 13.3
Range	25–75	5–75
Chest-film findings		
No. of signs/patient		
Mean	2.70	2.48
Range	0–6	1–6
Wide mediastinum—no. (%)	10 (90.9)	74 (90.2)
Normal—no (%)	1 (9.1)	0
Death—no. (%)	4 (36.4)	9 (11.0)

* P < 0.001 for the comparison between the groups.

None of the deaths were due to aortic injury.

From Smith, M. D., et al.: Transesophageal echocardiography in the diagnosis of traumatic rupture of the aorta. N. Engl. J. Med. *332*:356, 1995. Copyright 1995 by the Massachusetts Medical Society.

astinum. CT scanning is *not* a useful screening procedure,[75] but transesophageal echocardiography has become increasingly useful in documenting aortic lacerations (Fig. 44–10).[76-79] Despite these advances the procedure is not infallible,[80,81] and Vlahakes and Warren[82] recommend that "at each institution results of transesophageal echocardiography be calibrated against the existing gold standard of aortography." When equivocal echocardiography results are obtained —or a negative study is obtained in patients strongly suspected of aortic rupture—an aortogram should be obtained. The entire thoracic aorta and its branches should be visualized so as not to overlook a rupture occurring at an unusual site or multiple sites of rupture.

PENETRATING TRAUMA TO THE GREAT VESSELS. This is usually the result of bullet or stab wounds and occurs most commonly in conjunction with cardiac wounds. Cardiac tamponade is a frequent complication of injury to the intrapericardial segment of one of the great vessels, but when it is extrapericardial, massive hemothorax is usually the presenting finding. The superior vena cava, trachea, or esophagus or some combination of these structures may be compressed if a large mediastinal hematoma forms as a result of bleeding. Injury to the innominate or carotid arteries may compress these vessels, with resultant neurological signs. An arteriovenous fistula may develop with symptoms of congestive heart failure accompanied by a systolic or, more commonly, a continuous murmur. These fistulous connections may also involve the systemic and pulmonary vessel. Blunt trauma has also been reported to cause transection of the inferior vena cava.[83]

Penetrating injury to the great vessels should be suspected in any patient in whom a projectile traverses the mediastinum and is suggested by radiological evidence of a widened mediastinum. Aortography should be performed immediately, provided that emergency thoracotomy for shock or tamponade can be deferred briefly. Immediate operation, sometimes using a heparinized shunt between the ascending and descending aorta, should be carried out as soon as the diagnosis of thoracic aortic disruption has been established whether by blunt or penetrating injury.[84] Camp et al.[70] described their experience with 75 patients with lacerations of the descending thoracic aorta secondary to blunt trauma who reached the hospital alive. There was a significantly higher mortality rate in patients over 55 than in younger patients, 82.4 vs. 12 per cent $p < 0.001$. The authors concluded that elderly patients may be better candidates for *nonsurgical* management.

Antiadrenergic agents such as guanethidine, reserpine, and propranolol, which have been utilized in the treatment of spontaneous dissection of the aorta (see p. 1565), may also have a role in treatment of patients with aortic rupture if, for logistical reasons, operation must be deferred.

REFERENCES

1. Cheitlin, M. D.: Cardiovascular trauma. Circulation *65:*1529; *66:*244, 1982.
2. Henderson, V. J., Smith, R. S., Fry, W. R., et al.: Cardiac injuries: Analysis of an unselected series of 251 cases. J. Trauma *36:*341, 1994.
3. Sherman, M. M., Saini, U. K., Yarnoz, M. D., et al.: Management of penetrating heart wounds. Am. J. Surg. *135:*553, 1978.
4. Mattox, K. L., Feliciano, D. V., Burch, J., et al.: Five thousand seven hundred sixty cardiovascular injuries in 4459 patients: Epidemiologic evolution 1958 to 1987. Ann. Surg. *209:*698, 1989.

NONPENETRATING CARDIAC INJURY

5. Glock, Y., Massabuau, P., and Puel, P.: Cardiac damage in nonpenetrating chest injuries. J. Cardiovasc. Surg. *30:*27, 1989.
6. McLean, R. F., Devitt, J. H., McLellan, B. A., et al.: Significance of myocardial contusion following blunt chest trauma. J. Trauma *33:*240, 1992.
7. Matthews, R. V., French, W. J., and Criley, J. M.: Chest trauma and subvalvular left ventricular aneurysms. Chest *95:*474, 1989.
8. Parmley, L. F., Manion, W. C., and Mattingly, T. W.: Nonpenetrating traumatic injury of the heart. Circulation *18:*371, 1958.
9. DeMuth, W. E., Lerner, E. H., and Liedtke, A. J.: Nonpenetrating injury of the heart: An experimental model. J. Trauma *13:*639, 1973.
10. Karalis, D. G., Victor, M. F., Davis, G. A., et al.: The role of echocardiography in blunt chest trauma: A transthoracic and transesophageal echocardiographic study. J. Trauma *36:*53, 1994.
11. Cachecho, R., Grindlinger, G. A., and Lee, V. W.: The clinical significance of myocardial contusion. J. Trauma *33:*68, 1992.
12. Tenzer, M. L.: The spectrum of myocardial contusion: A review. J. Trauma *25:*620, 1985.
13. Snow, N., Richardson, J. D., and Flint, L. M., Jr.: Myocardial contusion: Implications for patients with multiple traumatic injuries. Surgery *92:*744, 1982.
14. Torres-Mirabal, P., Gruenberg, J. C., Brown, R. S., and Obeid, F. N.: Spectrum of myocardial contusion. Am. Surg. *48:*383, 1982.
15. Frazee, R. C., Mucha, P., Jr., Farnell, M. B., and Miller, F. A., Jr.: Objective evaluation of blunt cardiac trauma. J. Trauma *26:*510, 1986.
16. Sutherland, G. R., Cheung, H. W., Holliday, R. L., et al.: Hemodynamic adaptation to acute myocardial contusion complicating blunt chest injury. Am. J. Cardiol. *57:*291, 1986.
17. Schamp, D. J., Plotnick, G. D., Croteau, D., et al.: Clinical significance of radionuclide angiographically-determined abnormalities following acute blunt chest trauma. Am. Heart J. *116:*500, 1988.
18. Mattox, K. L., Limacher, M. C., Feliciano, D. V., et al.: Cardiac evaluation following heart injury. J. Trauma *25:*758, 1985.
19. Cooperman, Y., Low, S., and Laniado, S.: Traumatic heart block. PACE *12:*25, 1989.
20. Bognolo, D. A., Rabow, F. I., Vijayanagar, R. R., and Eckstein, P. F.: Traumatic sinus node dysfunction. Ann. Emerg. Med. *11:*319, 1982.
20a. Maron, B. J., Poliac, L. C., Kaplan, J. A. and Mueller, F. O.: Blunt impact to the chest leading to sudden death from cardiac arrest during sports activities. N. Engl. J. Med. *333:*337, 1995.
21. Évora, P. R. B., Ribeiro, P. J. F., Brasil, J. C. F., et al.: Late surgical repair of ventricular septal defect due to nonpenetrating chest trauma: Review and report of two contrasting cases. J. Trauma *25:*1007, 1985.
22. German, D. S., Shapiro, M. I., and Willman, V. L.: Acute aortic valvular incompetence following blunt thoracic deceleration injury: Case report. J. Trauma *30:*1411, 1990.
23. Desiderio, M. A.: The potentiation of the response to blunt cardiac trauma by ethanol in dogs. J. Trauma *26:*467, 1986.
24. Dubrow, T. J., Mihalka, J., Eisenhauer, D. M., et al.: Myocardial contusion in the stable patient: What level of care is appropriate? Surgery *106:*267, 1989.
25. Soliman, M. H., and Waxman, K.: Value of a conventional approach to the diagnosis of traumatic cardiac contusion after chest injury. Crit. Care Med. *15:*218, 1987.
26. Wiegand, L., and Zwillich, C. W.: The post-cardiac injury syndrome following blunt chest trauma: Case report. J. Trauma *34:*445, 1993.
27. Watt, A. H., and Stephens, M. R.: Myocardial infarction after blunt chest trauma incurred during rugby football that later required cardiac transplantation. Br. Heart J. *55:*408, 1986.
28. Espinosa, R., Badui, E., Castaño, R., and Madrid, R.: Acute posterior wall myocardial infarction secondary to football chest trauma. Chest *88:*928, 1985.
29. Unterberg, C., Buchwald, A., and Viegand, V.: Traumatic thrombosis of the left main coronary artery and myocardial infarction caused by blunt chest trauma. Clin. Cardiol. *12:*672, 1989.

30. Chang, H., Chu, S-H., and Lee, Y-T.: Traumatic aorto-right atrial fistula after blunt chest injury. Ann. Thorac. Surg. *45:*778, 1989.
31. Getz, B. S., Davies, E., Steinberg, S. M., et al.: Blunt cardiac trauma resulting in right atrial rupture. J. A. M. A. *255:*761, 1986.
32. Brathwaite, C. E. M., Rodriguez, A., Turney, S. Z., et al.: Blunt traumatic cardiac rupture: A 5-year experience. Ann. Surg. *212:*701, 1990.
33. Kato, K., Kushimoto, S., Mashiko, K., et al.: Blunt traumatic rupture of the heart: An experience in Tokyo. J. Trauma *36:*859, 1994.
34. Santavirta, S., and Arajarvi, E.: Ruptures of the heart in seatbelt wearers. J. Trauma *32:*275, 1992.
35. Leavitt, B. J., Meyer, J. A., Morton, J. R., et al.: Survival following non-penetrating traumatic rupture of cardiac chambers. Ann. Thorac. Surg. *44:*532, 1987.
36. End, A., Rodler, S., Oturanlar, D., et al.: Elective surgery for blunt cardiac trauma. J. Trauma *37:*798, 1994.
37. Eisenberg, M. S., Horwood, B. T., Cummins, R. O., et al.: Cardiac arrest and resuscitation: A tale of 29 cities. Ann. Emerg. Med. *19:*179, 1990.
38. Baker, P. B., Keyhani-Rofagha, S., Graham, R. L., and Sharma, H. M.: Dissecting hematoma (aneurysm) of coronary arteries. Am. J. Med. *80:*317, 1986.

PENETRATING CARDIAC INJURY

39. Naughton, M. J., Brissie, R. M., Bessey, P. Q., et al.: Demography of penetrating cardiac trauma. Ann. Surg. *209:*676, 1989.
40. Auge, J. M., Oriol, A., Serra, C., and Crexells, C.: The use of pigtail catheters for retrieval of foreign bodies from the cardiovascular system. Cathet. Cardiovasc. Diagn. *10:*625, 1984.
41. McIvor, M. E., Kaufman, S. L., Satre, R., et al.: Search and retrieval of a radiolucent foreign object. Cath. Cardiovasc. Diagn. *16:*19, 1989.
42. Goldbaum, T. S., Jacob, A. S., Smith, D. F., et al.: Cardiac tamponade following percutaneous transluminal coronary angioplasty: Four case reports. Cathet. Cardiovasc. Diagn. *11:*413, 1985.
43. Przybojewski, J. Z.: Endomyocardial biopsy: A review of the literature. Cathet. Cardiovasc. Diagn. *11:*287, 1985.
44. Anastasious-Nana, M. I., O'Connell, J. B., Nanas, J. N., et al.: Relative efficiency and risk of endomyocardial biopsy: Comparisons in heart transplant and nontransplant patients. Cath. Cardiovasc. Diagn. *16:*7, 1989.
45. Shirani, J., Zafari, A. M., Hill, V. E., et al.: Long asymptomatic survival with a bullet adjacent to the left main coronary artery, the only site of atherosclerotic plaque in the coronary tree. Am. Heart J. *128:*1043, 1994.
46. Nagy, K. K., Lohmann, C., Kim, D. O., and Barrett, J.: Role of echocardiography in the diagnosis of occult penetrating cardiac injury. J. Trauma *38:*859, 1995.
47. Hassett, A., Moran, J., Sabiston, D. C., and Kisslo, J.: Utility of echocardiography in the management of patients with penetrating missile wounds of the heart. J. Am. Coll. Cardiol. *7:*1151, 1986.
48. Miller, J. T., Richards, K. L., Miller, J. F., and Crawford, M. H.: Doppler echocardiographic determination of the cause of a systolic murmur following penetrating chest trauma. Am. Heart J. *111:*988, 1986.
49. Goldfarb, M. S., Walpole, H. T., Jr., Landolt, C. C., et al.: Two-dimensional Doppler echocardiographic diagnosis of a traumatic intracardiac shunt. Am. J. Cardiol. *57:*494, 1986.
50. Martin, L. F., Mavroudis, C., Dyess, D. L., et al.: The first 70 years' experience managing cardiac disruption due to penetrating and blunt injuries at the University of Louisville. Am. Surg. *52:*14, 1986.
51. Lorenz, H. P., Steinmetz, B., Lieberman, J., et al.: Emergency thoracotomy: Survival correlates with physiologic status. J. Trauma *32:*780, 1992.
52. Boyd, M., Vanek, V. W., and Bourguet, C. C.: Emergency room resuscitative thoracotomy: When is it indicated? J. Trauma *33:*714, 1992.
53. Durham, A. A., Richardson, R. J., Wall, M. J., Jr., et al.: Emergency center thoracotomy: Impact of prehospital resuscitation. J. Trauma *32:*775, 1992.
54. Macho, J. R., Markison, R. E., and Schecter, W. P.: Cardiac stapling in the management of penetrating injuries of the heart: Rapid control of hemorrhage and decreased risk of personal contamination. J. Trauma *34:*711, 1993.
55. Bergin, P. J.: Aortic thrombosis and peripheral embolization after thoracic gunshot wound diagnosed by transesophageal echocardiography. Am. Heart J. *119:*688, 1990.
56. Kortbeek, J. B., Clark, J. A., and Carraway, R. C.: Conservative management of a pulmonary artery bullet embolism: Case report and review of the literature. J. Trauma *33:*906, 1992.
57. Asfaw, I., Thoms, N. W., and Arfulu, A.: Interventricular septal defects from penetrating injuries of the heart: A report of 12 cases and review of the literature. J. Thorac. Cardiovasc. Surg. *69:*450, 1975.
58. Rustad, D. G., Hopeman, A. R., Murr, P. C., and VanWay, C. W., III: Aorta-cardiac fistula with aortic valve injury from penetrating trauma. J. Trauma *26:*266, 1986.
59. Werne, C., Sagraves, S. G., and Costa, C.: Mitral and tricuspid valve rupture from blunt trauma sustained during a motor vehicle collision. J. Trauma *29:*15, 1989.
60. Rumisek, J. D., Robonowitz, M., Virmani, R., et al.: Bioprosthetic heart valve rupture associated with trauma. J. Trauma *26:*276, 1986.
61. Cho, M-C., Kim, D-W., Hong, J-M., et al.: Left ventricular and papillary muscle rupture following blunt chest trauma. Am. J. Cardiol. *76:*424, 1995.
62. Gayet, C., Pierre, B., Delahaye, J-P., et al.: Traumatic tricuspid insufficiency: An underdiagnosed disease. Chest *92:*429, 1987.
63. Bashour, T. T., Morelli, R. L., Cunningham, T., and Budge, W. R.: Acute

coronary thrombosis following head trauma in a young man. Am. Heart J. 119:676, 1990.

64. Sabbah, H. N., Mohyi, J., and Stein, P. D.: Coronary arteriography in dogs following blunt cardiac trauma: A longitudinal assessment. Cath. Cardiovasc. Diagn. 15:155, 1988.

65. Watt, A. H., and Stephens, M. R.: Myocardial infarction after blunt chest trauma incurred during rugby football that later required cardiac transplantation. Br. Heart J. 55:408, 1986.

66. Martin, R., Mitchell, A., and Dhalla, N.: Late pericardial tamponade and coronary arteriovenous fistula after trauma. Br. Heart J. 55:216, 1986.

67. Reissman, P., Rivkind, A., Jurim, O., et al.: Simon D: Case Report: The management of penetrating cardiac trauma with major coronary artery injury—is cardiopulmonary bypass essential? J. Trauma 33:773, 1992.

68. Feczko, J. D., Lynch, L., Pless, J. E., et al.: An autopsy case review of 142 nonpenetrating (blunt) injuries of the aorta. J. Trauma 33:846, 1992.

69. Ben-Menachem, Y.: Rupture of the thoracic aorta by broadside impacts in road traffic and other collisions: Further angiographic observations and preliminary autopsy findings. J. Trauma 35:363, 1993.

70. Camp, P. C., Jr., Rogers, F. B., Shackford, S. R., et al.: Blunt traumatic thoracic aortic lacerations in the elderly: An analysis of outcome. J. Trauma 37:418, 1994.

71. Shaikh, K. A., Schwab, C. W., and Camishion, R. C.: Aortic rupture in blunt trauma. Am. Surg. 52:47, 1986.

72. Gundry, S. R., Burney, R. E., Mackenzie, J. R., et al.: Assessment of mediastinal widening associated with traumatic rupture of the aorta. J. Trauma 23:293, 1983.

73. Heystraten, F. M., Rosenbusch, G., Kingma, L. M., et al.: Chest radiography in acute traumatic rupture of the thoracic aorta. Acta Radiol. 29:411, 1988.

74. Symbas, P. N., Tyras, D. H., Ware, R. E., and Hatcher, C. R., Jr.: Rupture of the aorta: A diagnostic triad. Ann. Thorac. Surg 15:405, 1973.

75. Miller, F. B., Richardson, J. D., Thomas, H. A., et al.: Role of CT in diagnosis of major arterial injury after blunt thoracic trauma. Surgery 106:596, 1989.

76. Catoire, P., Bonnet, F., Delaunay, L., et al.: Traumatic laceration of the ascending aorta detecting by transesophageal echocardiography. Ann. Emerg. Med. 23:356, 1994.

77. Smith, M. K., Cassidy, J. M., Souther, S., et al.: Transesophageal echocardiography in the diagnosis of traumatic rupture of the aorta. N. Engl. J. Med. 332:356, 1995.

78. Catoire, P., Orliaguet, G., Liu, N., et al.: Systematic transesophageal echocardiography for detection of mediasternal lesions in patients with multiple injuries. J. Trauma 38:96, 1995.

79. Vignon, P., Gueret, P., Vedrinne, J-M., et al.: Role of transesophageal echocardiography in the diagnosis and management of traumatic aortic disruption. Circulation 92:2959, 1995.

80. Oxorn, D., and Towers, M.: Traumatic aortic disruption: False positive diagnosis on transesophageal echocardiography. J. Trauma 39:386, 1995.

81. Saletta, S., Lederman, E., Fein, S., et al.: Transesophageal echocardiography for the initial evaluation of the widened mediastinum in trauma patients. J. Trauma 39:137, 1995.

82. Vlahakes, G. J., and Warren, R. L.: Traumatic rupture of the aorta. N. Engl. J. Med. 332(Edit.):356, 1995.

83. Peitzman, A. B., Udekwu, A. O., Pevec, W., and Albrink, M.: Transection of the inferior vena cava from blunt thoracic trauma: Case reports. J. Trauma 29:534, 1989.

84. Akins, C. W., Buckley, M. J., Daggett, W., et al.: Acute traumatic disruption of the thoracic aorta: A ten-year experience. Ann. Thorac. Surg. 31:305, 1981.

Chapter 45
Diseases of the Aorta
ERIC M. ISSELBACHER, KIM A. EAGLE, ROMAN W. DESANCTIS

THE NORMAL AORTA

FUNCTION

Appropriately called "the greatest artery" by the ancients, the aorta is admirably suited for its task. In an average lifetime, this thin but large and remarkably tough vessel must absorb the impact of 2.3 to 3 billion heartbeats while carrying roughly 200 million liters of blood through the body. Arteries can be categorized as either *conductance* or *resistance* vessels. Conductance vessels are the conduits for blood, and the aorta is the ultimate conductance vessel.

The aorta is composed of three layers: the thin inner layer, or *intima;* a thick middle layer, or *media;* and a rather thin outer layer, the *adventitia.* The strength of the aorta lies in the media, which is composed of laminated but intertwining sheets of elastic tissue arranged in a spiral manner that affords maximum tensile strength. Indeed, as thin as it is, the aortic wall can withstand the experimental pressure of thousands of millimeters of mercury without bursting. In contrast to the peripheral arteries, the aortic media contains relatively little smooth muscle and collagen between the elastic layers. It is this tremendous accretion of elastic tissue that gives the aorta not only tensile strength but also distensibility and elasticity, which serve a vital circulatory role. The aortic intima is a thin and delicate layer that is lined by endothelium and easily traumatized. The adventitia contains mainly collagen and carries the important vasa vasorum, which nourish the outer half of the aortic wall, including much of the media.

During ventricular systole, the aorta is distended by the force of the blood ejected into it by the left ventricle, and in this manner part of the kinetic energy generated by the contracting left ventricle is converted into potential energy stored in the aortic wall. Then, during diastole, this potential energy is transformed back into kinetic energy as the aortic walls recoil, propelling the blood in the aortic lumen distally into the arterial bed. Thus, the aorta plays an essential role in maintaining forward circulation of the blood in diastole after it is delivered into the aorta by the left ventricle during systole. The pulse wave itself, with its milking effect, is transmitted along the aorta to the periphery at a speed of about 5 m/sec. This is much faster than the velocity of the intraluminal blood itself, which travels at only 40 to 50 cm/sec.

The systolic pressure developing within the aorta is a function of the volume of blood ejected into the aorta, the compliance or distensibility of the aorta, and the resistance to blood flow. This resistance is determined primarily by the tone of the peripheral muscular arteries and arterioles, and to a slight extent by the inertia of the column of blood in the aorta when systole commences.

In addition to its conductance and pumping functions, the aorta also plays a role in indirectly controlling systemic vascular resistance and heart rate. Pressure-responsive receptors, analogous to those in the carotid sinus, lie in the ascending aorta and aortic arch and send afferent signals to the vasomotor center in the brain stem by way of the vagus nerves. Raising the intra-aortic pressure causes reflex bradycardia and reduction of systemic vascular resistance, whereas lowering the pressure increases the heart rate and vascular resistance.

ANATOMICAL CONSIDERATIONS

The aorta is divided anatomically into its thoracic and abdominal components. The thoracic aorta is further divided into the *ascending, arch,* and *descending* segments, while the abdominal aorta consists of *suprarenal* and *infrarenal* segments.

The ascending aorta is 5 cm long and has two distinct segments. The lower segment is the *aortic root,* beginning at the level of the aortic valve and extending to the sinotubular junction. This is the widest portion of the ascending aorta, measuring about 3.3 cm in width. The bases of the aortic leaflets are supported by the aortic root from which the three sinuses of Valsalva bulge outward to allow for the full excursion of aortic valve leaflets during systole. In addition, the two coronary arteries arise from these sinuses of Valsalva. The upper tubular segment of the ascending aorta rises to join the aortic arch. Normally the ascending aorta sits just to the right of midline, with its proximal portion lying within the pericardial cavity. Nearby structures include the pulmonary artery anteriorly and leftward, the left atrium, right pulmonary artery, and right mainstem bronchus posteriorly, and the right atrium and superior vena cava to the right.

The *arch of the aorta* gives rise to all of the brachiocephalic arteries. From the ascending aorta it courses slightly leftward in front of the trachea and then proceeds posteriorly to the left of the trachea and esophagus. The pulmonary artery bifurcation and right pulmonary artery lie inferior to the arch, as does the left lung. The recurrent laryngeal nerve loops underneath the arch distally, and the phrenic and vagus nerves lie to the left.

The *descending thoracic aorta* begins in the posterior mediastinum to the left of the vertebral column and gradually courses in front of the vertebral column as it descends, occupying a position immediately behind the esophagus. Distally it passes through the diaphragm, usually at the level of the twelfth thoracic vertebra.

The point at which the aortic arch joins the descending aorta is called the *aortic isthmus.* The aorta is especially vulnerable to trauma at this site because it is here that the relatively mobile portion of the aorta—the ascending aorta and arch—becomes relatively fixed to the thoracic cage by the pleural reflections, the paired intercostal arteries, and the left subclavian artery. This is also where coarctations of the aorta are located.

The abdominal aorta continues from the thoracic aorta, giving off the important splanchnic arteries and ending at its bifurcation at the level of the fourth lumbar vertebra.

AGING OF THE AORTA

As discussed above, the elastic properties of the aorta are crucial to its normal function. However, it has been well demonstrated that the elasticity and distensibility of the aorta decline with age. Such changes are seen even in normal healthy adults, and for unknown reasons these changes occur earlier and are more progressive among men than women.[1] The loss of elasticity and aortic compliance likely accounts for the increase in pulse pressure commonly seen in the elderly. This progressive loss of aortic elasticity with aging is accelerated among those with hypertension compared with age-matched normotensive controls.[2] Similarly, those with hypercholesterolemia[3] or coronary artery disease show a greater loss of elasticity than do controls.[4] Conversely, among healthy athletes elasticity is higher than among their age-matched controls.[4]

Histologically, the aging aortic wall exhibits fragmentation of elastin with a concomitant increase in collagen, resulting in an increased collagen-to-elastin ratio that contributes to the loss of aortic distensibility observed physiologically.[5] Recent experimental animal data suggest that impairment of vasa vasorum flow to the aortic wall results in stiffening of the aorta with similar histological changes and may therefore be one cause of the degenerative changes seen with age.[6]

In animal models it has been demonstrated that a loss of aortic distensibility directly affects the mechanical performance of the left ventricle, producing increases in left ventricular systolic pressure and wall tension and in end-diastolic pressure and volume.[7] Furthermore, reduced aortic compliance causes a 20 to 40 per cent increase in myocardial oxygen consumption in order to maintain a given stroke volume.[8] It is therefore likely that, over time, the changes in aortic compliance seen with age may cause clinically important alterations in cardiac function.[7]

EXAMINATION OF THE AORTA

Unless the aorta is abnormally enlarged, the only location in which it can be palpated is the abdomen. The ease with which it can be felt depends largely on the body habitus and the pulse pressure: It is readily felt in thin individuals. It may be quite sensitive to palpation. Auscultation usually is unrevealing in aortic diseases, except for occasional bruits at the sites of narrowing of the aorta or its arterial branches. Diseases of the aortic root and proximal ascending aorta sometimes involve the aortic valve, with resultant aortic regurgitation that may be detectable on auscultation. Regurgitant murmurs secondary to root dilatation, rather than primary valvular disease, are often loudest along the right sternal border.

Chest roentgenography and fluoroscopy are valuable and simple procedures for assessing the aorta. Normally, the ascending aorta is not visible on the direct anteroposterior chest roentgenogram. The aorta is seen as a "knob" in the superior mediastinum just to the left of the vertebral column. The lateral border of the descending thoracic aorta can often be distinguished to the left of the spine. On the lateral chest roentgenogram, the aortic root and proximal ascending aorta are visible as an indistinct shadow in the middle of the mediastinum arising from the base of the heart. The ascending aorta and arch are best demonstrated in a left anterior oblique projection—a view that should always be included when disease of the thoracic aorta is suspected (Fig. 7–17, p. 216).

A number of imaging modalities are available for diagnostic examination of the aorta. These include aortography, computed tomographic scanning, magnetic resonance imaging, and both transthoracic and transesophageal echocardiography. The use of intravascular ultrasonography for the diagnosis of aortic pathology is under investigation. The respective utility of these imaging modalities is discussed below in the context of specific aortic diseases.

AORTIC ANEURYSMS

The term *aortic aneurysm* refers to a pathological dilatation of the normal aortic lumen involving one or several segments. Although there is perhaps no universally accepted definition, an aortic aneurysm is best described as a permanent localized dilatation of the aorta having a diameter at least 1.5 times that of the expected normal diameter of that given aortic segment.[9] Aneurysms are usually described in terms of their location, size, morphology, and etiology. The morphology of an aortic aneurysm is typically either *fusiform,* which is the more common shape, or *saccular.* A fusiform aneurysm is fairly uniform in shape, with symmetrical dilatation that involves the full circumference of the aortic wall. The dilatation seen in saccular aneurysms, on the other hand, is more localized, appearing as an outpouching of only a portion of the aortic wall. In addition, there may be a *pseudoaneurysm* or *false aneurysm* of the aorta, which is not actually an aneurysm at all but rather a well-defined collection of blood and connective tissue outside the vessel wall. This may be a consequence of a contained rupture of the aortic wall.

The presence of an aortic aneurysm may be a marker of more diffuse aortic disease. Overall, up to 13 per cent of all patients diagnosed with an aortic aneurysm are found to have multiple aneurysms,[10] with up to 25 to 28 per cent of those with thoracic aortic aneurysms having concomitant abdominal aortic aneurysms.[11,12] For this reason, Crawford and Cohen have recommended that a patient in whom an aortic aneurysm is discovered undergo examination of the entire aorta for the possible presence of other aneurysms.[10]

Abdominal Aortic Aneurysms

Abdominal aortic aneurysms are much more common than are thoracic aortic aneurysms. Age is an important risk factor, as the incidence rises rapidly after 55 years of age in men and 70 years of age in women,[13] and abdominal

aortic aneurysms occur four to five times more frequently in men than in women. The incidence of abdominal aneurysms has increased threefold in recent decades, from 8.7 per 100,000 person-years in 1951 to 1960 to 36.5 per 100,000 person-years in 1971 to 1980.[14] Because the incidence of abdominal aneurysms of all sizes has increased, it is believed that these data at least in part reflect a true increase in the disease incidence. Other factors that may have contributed to the marked rise in the incidence of such aneurysms include the increasing mean age of the population, a greater awareness of the association of aneurysmal disease with other prevalent cardiovascular conditions, and improvements in diagnostic evaluation. The prevalence of abdominal aortic aneurysms in the population 50 years of age and older is at least 3 per cent.[15]

ETIOLOGY AND PATHOGENESIS. Although it is now evident that abdominal aortic aneurysms arise as a consequence of multiple interacting factors, classically atherosclerosis has been considered the common underlying etiology. The infrarenal abdominal aorta is most affected by the atherosclerotic process and is similarly the most common site of abdominal aneurysm formation; only a fraction of abdominal aortic aneurysms are suprarenal, with these tending to arise only as an extension of a thoracic (thoracoabdominal) aneurysm. The atherosclerotic process less often involves the descending thoracic aorta, and involvement of the ascending aorta is distinctly uncommon.

Atherosclerotic disease of the aorta may produce either stenotic obstruction, a process that tends to be confined to the infrarenal abdominal aorta, or aneurysmal dilatation; why one process should predominate over the other in any given individual is unknown.[15] Although the mechanism by which atherosclerosis results in aortic aneurysms is obscure, a recent hypothesis may account for the disease's predilection for the infrarenal abdominal aorta over other segments.[16] The media of the infrarenal aorta in humans has no vasa vasorum, and as a consequence at least the inner media must receive oxygen and nutrients by diffusion from the aortic lumen. Atherosclerotic disease causes thickening of the intima and may thereby compromise the diffusion of such oxygen and nutrients to the medial layer. Exacerbated by increases in aortic wall stress from hypertension, this hypoxemia may lead to ischemic injury of the media, thus initiating a process of degeneration of the media and its elastic elements.[16] The damage produces a weakening of the aortic wall which over time allows the formation of fusiform or, less commonly, saccular dilatation of the aorta. As the aorta then widens, tension in the vessel wall rises in accordance with Laplace's law, which states that tension is proportional to the product of pressure and radius. Further widening results in even greater wall tension, which in turn leads to acceleration of aneurysm enlargement. A vicious circle is thus established in which the dilatation is often rapidly progressive.

Although atherosclerosis certainly contributes to the pathogenesis of abdominal aortic aneurysms, genetic and cellular factors play important roles as well. A genetic predisposition to the development of abdominal aortic aneurysms has been repeatedly suggested by studies of familial incidence, with up to 28 per cent of patients who have an abdominal aortic aneurysm having a first-degree relative similarly affected.[17] A recent report analyzing 313 pedigrees has confirmed the importance of familial factors in the pathogenesis of abdominal aortic aneurysms and supports the hypothesis that abdominal aortic aneurysm might be a predominantly genetic disease.[18] At present, however, no genetic marker has been shown to be definitively related to aneurysm formation, and it appears likely that the genetic factors involved may be heterogeneous.

An area of expanding investigation is the role of the cellular mechanisms in the pathogenesis of aortic aneurysms. Destruction of the media and its elastic tissue is the striking histological feature of aortic aneurysms when compared with the normal aorta. Experimental evidence indicates excessive activity of proteolytic enzymes in the aortas of affected patients which may lead to the deterioration of structural matrix proteins such as elastin and collagen in the aortic media, and thereby promote or perpetuate the formation of aneurysms. Studies have shown that aneurysmal aortas contain elastolytic activity with an active elastase not present in the normal aorta[19] and that other active proteolytic enzymes are present as well. An active inflammatory process may also contribute, given that an abnormal presence of macrophages[20] and elevated levels of cytokines[21] have been demonstrated in aneurysmal aortic tissue.

As a result of flow turbulence through the aneurysmal aortic segment, blood may stagnate along the walls and thus allow the formation of mural thrombus. Such thrombus, as well as atherosclerotic debris, may embolize distally and compromise the circulation of tributary arteries. However, the major risk posed by abdominal aortic aneurysms is that of aneurysm rupture. When rupture does occur, 80 per cent rupture into the left retroperitoneum, which may contain the rupture, whereas most of the remainder rupture into the peritoneal cavity, causing uncontrolled hemorrhage and rapid circulatory collapse.[22] Rarely, an aneurysm may rupture into the inferior vena cava, iliac vein, or renal vein.[23,24]

The majority of abdominal aortic aneurysms are asymptomatic and are discovered incidentally on routine physical examination or on an abdominal roentgenogram[14] or ultrasound scan ordered for other indications. Younger patients (50 years old or less), however, are several times more likely to be symptomatic at the time of diagnosis.[25] Among those who are symptomatic at presentation, pain is the most frequent complaint[14] and is usually located in the hypogastrium or lower back. The pain is usually steady, with a gnawing quality, and may last for hours to days at a time. In contrast to musculoskeletal back pain, aneurysm pain is not affected by movement, although patients may be more comfortable in certain positions, such as with the legs drawn up. Some astute patients may suspect an aneurysm by recognizing an abnormal pulsation of the aorta, as when lying down reading a book perched on the abdomen.

RUPTURED ANEURYSM. Expansion and impending rupture are heralded by the development of new or worsening pain, often of sudden onset. This pain is characteristically constant, severe, and located in the back or lower abdomen, sometimes with radiation into the groin, buttocks, or legs. Actual rupture is associated with abrupt onset of back pain with abdominal pain and tenderness. Most patients have a palpable, pulsatile abdominal mass and many are hypotensive at presentation. However, this familiar triad of abdominal/back pain, a pulsatile abdominal mass, and hypotension—recognized as pathognomonic of ruptured abdominal aortic aneurysm—is seen in as few as one-third of cases.[26] Moreover, a ruptured aneurysm may mimic other acute abdominal conditions, such as renal colic, diverticulitis, or a gastrointestinal hemorrhage and therefore may be initially misdiagnosed in as many as 30 per cent of cases.[27]

Patients who suffer rupture of an abdominal aortic aneurysm are critically ill.[28] Hemorrhagic shock may ensue rapidly and is manifested by hypotension, vasoconstriction, mottled skin, diaphoresis, mental obtundation, oliguria, and terminally by arrhythmias and cardiac arrest.[29] Retroperitoneal hemorrhage may be signaled by hematomas in the flanks and groin. Rupture into the abdominal cavity may result in abdominal distention, whereas rupture into the duodenum presents as massive gastrointestinal hemorrhage.

PHYSICAL EXAMINATION. Many aneurysms can be detected on physical examination, although even large aneurysms may be difficult or impossible to detect in obese individuals. When palpable, a pulsatile mass extending variably from the xiphoid process to the umbilicus may be appreciated. Owing to difficulty in distinguishing the abdominal aorta from surrounding structures by palpation, the size of an aneurysm tends to be overestimated on physical examination. Moreover, it may be difficult to differentiate a tortuous, ectatic aorta from true aneurysmal dilatation. Aneurysms are often sensitive to palpation and may be quite tender if they are rapidly expanding or about to rupture. Aneurysms should always be palpated cautiously, particularly if they are tender.

Associated occlusive arterial disease is sometimes present in the femoral pulses and distal pulses in the legs and feet. Bruits arising from associated narrowed arteries may be heard over the aneurysm. Rarely, an aneurysm may expand in such a way as to occlude the inferior vena cava or one of the iliac veins, resulting in venous congestion and edema in one or both legs. Occasionally an arteriovenous fistula may be formed by spontaneous rupture into the inferior vena cava, iliac vein, or renal vein and a syndrome of hemodynamic collapse and acute high-output cardiac failure.[24,30]

DIAGNOSIS AND SIZING. Several diagnostic imaging modalities are currently used for detecting, sizing, and serially following abdominal aortic aneurysms, as well as for precisely defining the aortic anatomy preoperatively. Abdominal ultrasonography is perhaps the most practical way to screen for abdominal aortic aneurysms. It can visualize an aneurysm in the transverse and longitudinal planes, has a sensitivity of nearly 100 per cent,[31] and can accurately define aneurysm size to within ± 0.3 cm.[32,33] Its major advantages are that it is inexpensive and noninvasive and does not require the use of a contrast agent. However, ultrasonography is limited by its inability to visualize the cephalad or pelvic extent of disease or to define the associated mesenteric and renal arterial anatomy. Therefore it is insufficient for planning operative repair.

Computed tomography (CT) is an extremely accurate method for both diagnosing aortic aneurysms (Fig. 45–1) and sizing them to within ± 0.2 cm.[34,35] CT has the advantage over ultrasonography that it can better define the shape and extent of the aneurysm, as well as the local anatomical relationships of the visceral and renal vessels.[34,36] Disadvantages are that the procedure is more expensive and less widely available than ultrasonography, and it also requires the use of ionizing radiation and intravenous contrast. Although CT may therefore be less practical than ultrasonography as a screening tool, its high accuracy in sizing aneurysms makes it an excellent modality for serially following changes in aneurysm size.[33] It is important to note that CT measurements of aneurysm size tend to be larger than ultrasound measurements by an average of 0.27 cm.[37] At present, CT scanning is limited in the preoperative evaluation of abdominal aortic aneurysms because it does not provide information regarding renal or mesenteric arterial occlusive disease. However, newer techniques such as helical CT with three-dimensional display of the aorta and its branches[38] may overcome this problem.

Aortography has long been the standard imaging modality for the preoperative definition of abdominal aortic aneurysm anatomy. Although it is well recognized that aortography may underestimate aneurysm size in the presence of nonopacified mural thrombus lining the aneurysm walls, it nevertheless remains an excellent technique for defining the suprarenal extent of the aneurysm and any associated iliofemoral disease. It is also excellent for defining renal

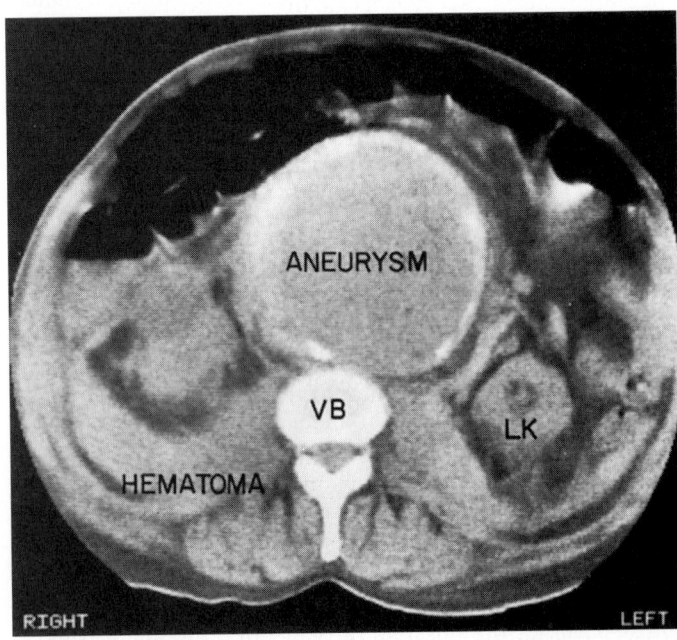

FIGURE 45–1. Abdominal CT scan showing a large, leaking abdominal aortic aneurysm. The aneurysm measures approximately 11 cm in diameter and abuts the vertebral body (VB) posteriorly. The light areas in the periphery of the aneurysm are calcified deposits in the aortic wall. The lower pole of the left kidney is identified (LK); behind the right kidney is a retroperitoneal hematoma. (Courtesy of Jack Wittenberg, M.D., Department of Radiology, Massachusetts General Hospital, Boston.)

and mesenteric arterial anatomy. There is ongoing debate regarding the need for routine preoperative aortography,[39] and in fact many surgeons now use it only selectively.[40] Disadvantages are that it is expensive, it is an invasive procedure with inherent risks, and it requires the use of intraarterial contrast and ionizing radiation.

Most recently, *magnetic resonance (MR) angiography* has been promoted as an alternative to aortography for the preoperative evaluation of aortic aneurysms.[39] Whereas flowing blood appears as a signal void on conventional spin-echo magnetic resonance imaging (MRI), with the use of MR angiography blood has a bright appearance and vessels can be displayed in a projective fashion similar to what is seen with traditional angiography.[41] Moreover, because tomographic images are reconstructed to create a three-dimensional image, the aorta may be visualized from a series of projections, facilitating appreciation of anatomical relationships.[41] MR angiography is extremely accurate in determining aneurysm size, and it correctly defines the proximal extent of disease and iliofemoral involvement in greater than 80 per cent of cases.[39] Nevertheless, it remains limited in its ability to define renal and mesenteric arterial occlusive disease.[39,42] The exact role of MR angiography in the evaluation of abdominal aortic aneurysms continues to be investigated.

An important but unresolved issue regarding the detection of abdominal aortic aneurysms is the potential role, if any, of screening asymptomatic patients for the presence of aneurysms. At present there are no controlled trials of aneurysm screening with outcomes data that might be used in guiding any such recommendations. A recent study based on the existing literature suggests that screening men 60 to 80 years of age by physical examination is cost-effective although of small benefit, whereas screening the same population with ultrasonography is at the upper limit of cost-effectiveness and of modest benefit.[43] Repeated screening was found not to be cost-effective. Many authors currently recommend the use of screening ultrasonography only for those at high risk, in particular those with a family history of abdominal aortic aneurysm.[17]

NATURAL HISTORY. The paramount concern in managing abdominal aortic aneurysms is their tendency to rupture. Mortality from rupture is quite high: 60 per cent die prior to receiving medical attention,[44] and the operative mortality for those reaching the hospital is approximately 50 per cent,[32] yielding an overall mortality from rupture of 80 per cent. In 1950, prior to the introduction of modern surgical repair, Estes first assessed survival rates for those with abdominal aortic aneurysms[45] and found survival at 3 to 5 years to be 49 per cent and 19 per cent, respectively, far lower than for age-matched controls, with two-thirds of deaths due to aneurysm rupture. However, following the introduction of modern surgical repair, it was found that survival among abdominal aortic aneurysm patients undergoing operative repair was significantly higher than among those managed nonoperatively. Surgical repair thus remains the therapy of choice for aneurysms considered to be at risk for rupture.

Darling et al. convincingly demonstrated that the risk of rupture increases with aneurysm size.[46] Present estimates suggest that aneurysms less than 4.0 cm in size have a 0 to 2 per cent risk of rupture,[47,48] whereas those greater than 5.0 cm in size have a 22 per cent risk of rupture within 2 years.[48] Because 80 per cent of abdominal aortic aneurysms expand over time—with as many as 15 to 20 per cent expanding rapidly (>0.5 cm/yr)—the risk of rupture may concomitantly increase with time.

Accordingly, the ability to predict rates of aortic aneurysm expansion would be useful in estimating the risk of future rupture. Although the mean rate of abdominal aortic aneurysm expansion appears to be approximately 0.4 cm per year,[32] the rates of expansion within a population are extremely variable, and expansion rates even vary within

one individual over time. Baseline aneurysm size is perhaps the best predictor of aneurysm expansion rate,[32] with larger aneurysms expanding more rapidly than small ones—probably as a consequence of Laplace's law. A rapid rate of expansion apparently also predicts aneurysm rupture, especially among abdominal aneurysms of 5.0 cm or greater in diameter.[49] Many surgeons therefore consider both large size and rapid expansion to be indications for repair.

Management

SURGICAL TREATMENT. There is ongoing debate as to the optimal timing of surgical repair in asymptomatic abdominal aortic aneurysms. The decision to operate must weigh the natural history of the aneurysm and life expectancy of the patient against the anticipated morbidity and mortality of the proposed surgical procedure. Operative mortality is 4 to 6 per cent overall for elective aneurysm repair and is as low as 2 per cent in low-risk patients. However, operative mortality rises to 19 per cent for urgent aortic repair and reaches 50 per cent for repair of a ruptured aneurysm.[32,50] As of this writing aneurysm size remains the primary indicator for repair of asymptomatic aneurysms, although no clear consensus yet exists as to the minimal aneurysm diameter that necessitates surgery. Whereas all vascular surgeons would operate for an abdominal aortic aneurysm larger than 6.0 cm in diameter and most for aneurysms larger than 5.0 cm in patients who are reasonable surgical risks, few would operate for an asymptomatic aneurysm less than 4.0 cm. The benefit of surgery for asymptomatic aneurysms 4.0 to 5.0 cm in size, however, has not yet been defined. The recommendation of the Society for Vascular Surgery and the International Society for Cardiovascular Surgery is for elective repair of abdominal aortic aneurysms 4.0 cm or larger in diameter,[32] although many other surgeons still consider 5.0 cm or larger to be the indication for surgery. Prospective controlled multicenter trials currently under way in the United States, Canada, and the United Kingdom, from which results are expected by the end of the decade, should help address the optimal timing of surgery based on aneurysm size.[51,52]

Surgical repair of abdominal aortic aneurysms consists of resection of the aneurysm and insertion of a synthetic prosthesis, usually fabricated of Dacron. Sometimes a simple tube graft is all that is necessary, although frequently the operation must be carried distally into one or both of the iliac arteries in order to excise the aneurysm completely. In the case of large aneurysms, much of the aneurysm wall may be left in situ ("intrasaccular approach of Creech"), thereby reducing the need for extensive dissection and thus decreasing aortic cross-clamping time.

A promising new interventional option for the treatment of abdominal aortic aneurysms is the use of percutaneously implanted expanding endovascular stents (see p. 1385). Endovascular stents have been demonstrated to be useful in the treatment of coronary artery disease, renal artery stenosis, and occlusive peripheral vascular disease. For aortic aneurysm repair, the stent serves to bridge the region of the aneurysm, thereby excluding it from the circulation while allowing aortic blood flow to continue distally through the stent lumen. These devices have been shown to be quite effective in animal models of abdominal aortic aneurysm.[53,54] Although the results of early human trials of endovascular stent-grafts suggest a successful outcome in 80 per cent of high-risk subjects with abdominal aortic or aortoiliac aneurysms, this was accompanied by a 10 per cent rate of procedural death.[55]

Assessing Operative Risk. Because patients with abdominal aneurysms, by definition, suffer from vascular disease, there is a high likelihood of concomitant coronary, renal, and cerebrovascular arterial disease that significantly increases the risk of major vascular surgery (see p. 1822). Indeed, Hertzer found that half of all perioperative deaths from aneurysm repair are due to myocardial infarction.[56] In addition, routine coronary arteriography in those undergoing aneurysm repair revealed severe correctable coronary artery disease in 31 per cent of all patients, including an 18 per cent incidence in patients without prior clinical manifestations of coronary disease.[57] Moreover, among those with angiographically significant coronary artery disease, multivessel disease was seen in the majority.[57]

Studies by Boucher et al.[58] and Eagle et al.[59] have suggested that dipyridamole-thallium cardiac scanning (see p. 288) is an effective means of identifying patients at highest risk for perioperative ischemic events. Patients with reversible thallium defects in multiple segments of myocardium are at highest risk,[60] and it is in this subgroup that coronary angiography is likely to be most helpful. The safety of dipyridamole-thallium studies in such patients has been well established. Although exercise thallium scintigraphy is also a useful screening method,[61] many patients with vascular disease fail to achieve an adequate heart rate owing to limited exercise capacity. Other techniques shown to be effective for preoperative evaluation of myocardial ischemia include dobutamine stress echocardiography[62] and electrocardiogram exercise testing in patients with a normal baseline electrocardiogram and adequate exercise tolerance.

Selective preoperative evaluation to identify the presence and severity of coronary artery disease among patients with clinical markers of coronary artery disease has been widely advocated,[63] and some further suggest screening those with strong cardiac risk factors despite the absence of clinical evidence of coronary artery disease.[64,65] Although patients found to have significant correctable coronary artery disease are presumed to benefit from preoperative coronary revascularization with selective coronary artery bypass surgery or angioplasty, at present this conclusion remains unproved.[64] The data available from nonrandomized studies of patients with significant coronary artery disease undergoing vascular surgery do demonstrate a lower mortality for those who have undergone coronary bypass surgery.[66] Furthermore, a recent randomized study demonstrates that the long-term outcome of patients having combined peripheral vascular disease and high-risk coronary artery disease is improved by coronary artery revascularization in those with three-vessel coronary disease.[67] As is the case for coronary artery bypass surgery, there are as yet no available data to confirm that preoperative coronary angioplasty for significant coronary stenoses decreases the risk from major vascular surgery.

In addition to such preoperative screening and potential coronary revascularization, operative risk secondary to cardiac ischemic events may be further reduced through the use of perioperative invasive hemodynamic monitoring and careful perioperative surveillance for evidence of ischemia.[68,69] Furthermore, myocardial ischemia and perhaps myocardial infarction may be prevented by using beta-adrenergic blockers perioperatively.[70]

Late Survival. A review by Kiell and Ernst of late survival following abdominal aortic aneurysm repair among almost 2500 patients revealed 1-, 5-, and 10-year survival rates of 93, 63, and 40 per cent, respectively.[26] The long-term survival of those with concomitant coronary artery disease has been found to be approximately 10 per cent lower than for those without coronary disease.[71]

MEDICAL MANAGEMENT. Risk factor modification is fundamental in the medical management of abdominal aortic aneurysms. Hypercholesterolemia and hypertension should be carefully controlled. Most patients with abdominal aortic aneurysms are cigarette smokers, and smoking must be discontinued. Beta blockers have long been considered an important therapy for reducing the risk of aneurysm expansion and rupture, and both animal and human studies support such a role. Brophy et al.[72] demonstrated that propranolol delays the development of aneurysms in a mouse model prone to develop spontaneous aortic aneurysms. Interestingly, it appears that the drug's efficacy in this model

may have been independent of reductions of blood pressure or dP/dt but rather may have been the result of changes in connective tissue metabolism and the structure of the aortic wall. In humans, a recent study has shown that the mean rate of abdominal aortic aneurysm expansion was slower among patients treated with beta blockers than among those not treated with beta blockers, with the effect most marked among large aneurysms.[49]

Should one elect to observe an abdominal aortic aneurysm of 4.0 cm in size or larger, careful routine follow-up is indicated in order to detect either rapid expansion (≥ 0.5 cm/year) or an increase in size to 5.0 cm or larger, either of which is an indication for surgery.[73] CT scanning every 6 months, and perhaps as frequently as every 3 months for those at higher risk, has been advocated as an effective method of following such patients.[32]

Thoracic Aortic Aneurysms

Thoracic aortic aneurysms are much less common than are aneurysms of the abdominal aorta, and their incidence did not increase over the same 30-year period that saw a marked increase in the incidence of abdominal aortic aneurysms (as noted above).[12] Thoracic aneurysms are classified by the portion of aorta involved, i.e., the ascending, arch, or descending thoracic aorta. This anatomical distinction is important because the etiology, natural history, and therapy of thoracic aneurysms differ for each of these segments. Aneurysms of the descending aorta occur most commonly, followed by aneurysms of the ascending aorta, whereas arch aneurysms occur much less often.[11] In addition, descending thoracic aneurysms may extend distally to involve the abdominal aorta, creating what is known as a *thoracoabdominal aortic aneurysm.* Sometimes the entire aorta may be ectatic, with localized aneurysms seen at sites in both the thoracic and abdominal aorta.

ETIOLOGY AND PATHOGENESIS. Aneurysms of the ascending thoracic aorta most often result from the process of *cystic medial degeneration* (or *cystic medial necrosis*). Histologically cystic medial degeneration has the appearance of smooth muscle cell necrosis and elastic fiber degeneration, with the appearance in the media of cystic spaces filled with mucoid material. Although these changes occur most frequently in the ascending aorta, in some cases the entire aorta may be similarly affected. The histological changes lead to weakening of the aortic wall, which in turn results in the formation of a fusiform aneurysm. Such aneurysms often involve the aortic root and may consequently result in aortic regurgitation. The term *annuloaortic ectasia* is often used to describe this condition (see below).

Cystic medial degeneration is found in virtually all cases of the Marfan syndrome[74] and may be associated with other connective tissue disorders as well, such as Ehlers-Danlos syndrome. The Marfan syndrome (see p. 1669) is an autosomal dominant heritable disorder of connective tissue that has recently been discovered to be due to mutations of one of the genes for fibrillin, a structural protein that helps to direct and orient elastin in the developing aorta.[75] These mutations result in a decrease in the amount of elastin in the aortic wall,[76] together with a loss of the elastin's normally highly organized structure. As a consequence, from an early age the marfanoid aorta exhibits markedly abnormal elastic properties and increased systemic pulse wave velocities, and over time the aorta exhibits progressively increasing degrees of stiffness and dilatation.[77]

In those patients without the Marfan syndrome, however, it is not possible to recognize the histological diagnosis of cystic medial degeneration prospectively (i.e., without surgery or necropsy).[78] This fact has significantly limited our understanding of medial degeneration and its natural history, and it remains unclear to what extent this syndrome may represent an independent disease process versus a manifestation of another disease state. It has long been suspected that some patients who have annuloaortic ectasia and proven cystic medial degeneration without the classic phenotypic manifestations of the Marfan syndrome may, in fact, have a variation or forme fruste of the Marfan syndrome,[79] although this remains unproved. On the contrary, many patients with ascending thoracic aortic aneurysms appear to have nothing more than idiopathic cystic medial degeneration.

ATHEROSCLEROSIS. Atherosclerotic aneurysms infrequently occur in the ascending aorta and, when they do, tend to be associated with diffuse aortic atherosclerosis.

Aneurysms in the aortic arch are often contiguous with aneurysms of the ascending or descending aorta. They may be due to atherosclerotic disease, cystic medial degeneration, syphilis, or other infections. The predominant cause of aneurysms of the descending thoracic aorta is atherosclerosis.[81] These aneurysms tend to originate just distal to the origin of the left subclavian artery and may be either fusiform or saccular.[82] The pathogenesis of such atherosclerotic aneurysms in the thoracic aorta may be similar to that of abdominal aneurysms but has not been extensively examined.

SYPHILIS. This was once a common cause of ascending thoracic aortic aneurysm, but today it has become a rarity in most major medical centers[12,80] as a result of aggressive antibiotic treatment of the disease in its early stages. The latent period from initial spirochetal infection to aortic complications may range from 5 to 40 years but is most commonly 10 to 25 years. During the secondary phase of the disease there is direct spirochetal infection of the aortic media, most commonly involving the ascending aorta. The muscular and elastic medial elements are destroyed by the infection and inflammatory response and replaced by fibrous tissue that frequently calcifies. Weakening of the aortic wall from medial destruction results in progressive aneurysmal dilatation. In addition, the infection may spread into the aortic root, and the subsequent root dilatation may result in aortic regurgitation.

INFECTIOUS AORTITIS. This rare cause of aortic aneurysm may result from a primary infection of the aortic wall, causing aortic dilatation with the formation of fusiform or saccular aneurysms (see p. 1547). More commonly, infected or *mycotic* aneurysms may arise secondarily from an infection occurring in a preexisting aneurysm of another etiology. When an infected aneurysm involves the ascending aorta, it is often the consequence of direct spread from aortic bacterial endocarditis.

Several other causes of thoracic aortic aneurysms are discussed in detail elsewhere in this chapter, including aortic infection (see p. 1575), giant cell arteritis (p. 1573), aortic trauma (p. 1543), and aortic dissection (p. 1554). Note that the clinical presentation, natural history, and therapy of thoracic aneurysms discussed below apply specifically to *nondissecting thoracic aortic aneurysms.*

Clinical Manifestations

Forty per cent of patients with thoracic aortic aneurysms are asymptomatic at the time of diagnosis,[11] with such aneurysms typically discovered as incidental findings on a routine physical examination or chest roentgenogram. When patients do experience symptoms, the symptoms tend to reflect either a vascular consequence of the aneurysm or a local mass effect. Vascular consequences include aortic regurgitation due to dilatation of the aortic root, often associated with secondary congestive heart failure; myocardial ischemia or infarction due to local compression of the coronary arteries by enlarged sinuses of Valsalva; sinus of Valsalva aneurysms that may rupture into the right side of the heart to cause a continuous murmur and congestive heart failure; and thromboembolism causing stroke, lower extremity ischemia, renal infarction, or mesenteric ischemia.

Local mass effect from an ascending or arch aneurysm may cause superior vena cava syndrome due to obstruction of venous return via compression of the superior vena cava or innominate veins. Aneurysms of the arch or descending aorta may compress the trachea (Fig. 45–2) or mainstem bronchus, producing tracheal deviation, wheezing, cough, dyspnea (with symptoms that may be positional), hemoptysis, or recurrent pneumonitis. Compression of the esophagus may produce dysphagia, and compression of the recurrent laryngeal nerve may cause hoarseness. Chest pain and back pain occur in 37 per cent and 21 per cent, respectively, of nondissecting aneurysms[11] and result from direct compression of other intrathoracic structures or from erosion into adjacent bone. Typically such pain is steady, deep, boring, and at times extremely severe.

As with abdominal aortic aneurysms, the most worrisome consequence of thoracic aneurysms is leakage or rupture. Rupture is accompanied by the dramatic onset of excruciating pain, usually in the region where less severe pain had previously existed. Rupture occurs most commonly into the left intrapleural space or the intrapericardial space, presenting as hypotension. The third most common site of rupture is from the descending thoracic aorta into the adjacent esophagus (an aortoesophageal fistula), presenting as life-threatening hematemesis.[83] Acute aneurysm expansion, which may herald rupture, can cause sim-

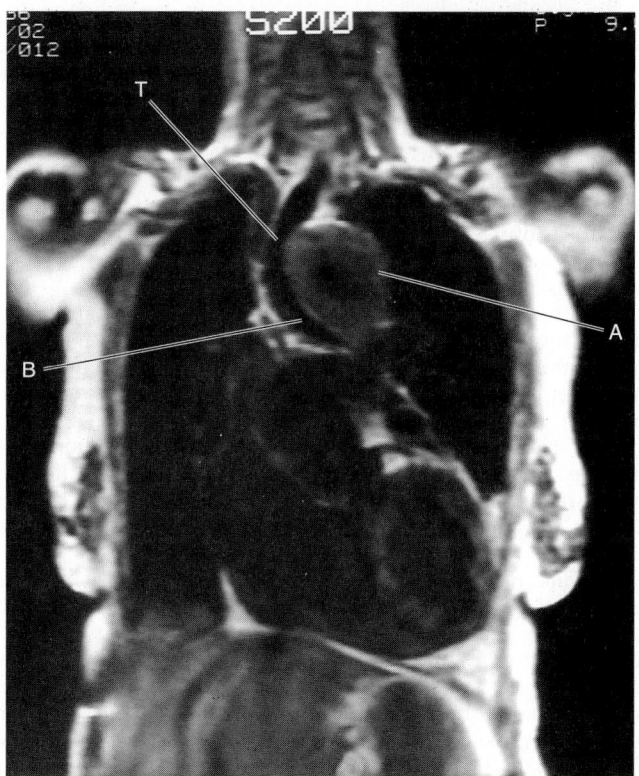

FIGURE 45–2. MRI in the coronal projection of a large thoracic aortic aneurysm in an elderly woman presenting with a complaint of dyspnea and cough. In this view the markedly dilated aortic arch (A) compresses the trachea (T), causing rightward tracheal deviation. The aneurysm also compresses the left mainstem bronchus (B). In addition, all four cardiac chambers are dilated, consistent with the patient's known idiopathic dilated cardiomyopathy.

ilar pain. Thoracic aneurysms may also develop aortic dissection, which is discussed in detail later in this chapter.

DIAGNOSIS AND SIZING. Many thoracic aneurysms are readily visible on chest roentgenogram (Fig. 45–3), presenting as widening of the mediastinal silhouette, enlargement of the aortic knob, or displacement of the trachea from midline. Unfortunately, smaller aneurysms, especially saccular ones, may not be evident on chest roentgenogram; therefore, this technique cannot exclude the diagnosis of aortic aneurysm.

Aortography is still the preferred modality for the preoperative evaluation of thoracic aortic aneurysms and precise

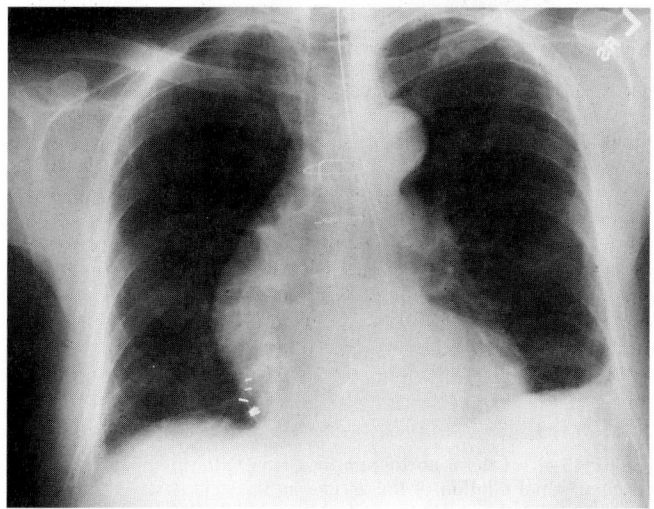

FIGURE 45–3. Chest roentgenogram of a patient with a very large aneurysm of the ascending thoracic aorta. Evident are both marked widening of the mediastinum and an abnormal aortic contour.

definition of the anatomy of the aneurysm and great vessels (Fig. 45–4). As is the case for abdominal aortic aneurysms, contrast-enhanced CT scanning is very accurate in detecting and sizing thoracic aortic aneurysms[84] and is useful as a method to follow aneurysm size. MRI is also useful in defining thoracic aortic anatomy and detecting aneurysms[85] (Fig. 45–2) and is of particular utility in patients with preexisting aortic disease. MR angiography may prove especially useful in defining the anatomy of the aortic branch vessels, but its utility in evaluating thoracic aortic aneurysms has not yet been extensively studied.

Transthoracic echocardiography is not very accurate for diagnosing thoracic aneurysms and is particularly limited in its ability to examine the descending thoracic aorta. Transesophageal echocardiography (TEE), a far more accurate method for assessing the thoracic aorta, has become widely used for detection of aortic dissection. There has been less experience with TEE in evaluation of nondissecting thoracic aneurysms. (The advantages and disadvantages of each imaging modality are discussed in greater detail on p. 356.)

NATURAL HISTORY. Defining the natural history of thoracic aortic aneurysms is complex, given the numerous contributing factors. The cause of an aneurysm may affect both its rate of growth and propensity for rupture. The presence or absence of aneurysm symptoms is another important predictor, as symptomatic patients have a much poorer prognosis than those without symptoms,[81] in large part because the onset of new symptoms is frequently a harbinger of rupture or death. Moreover, the high prevalence of additional cardiovascular diseases in these patients may have a dramatic impact on mortality; in fact, second to aneurysm rupture, the most common causes of death in this population are other cardiovascular diseases.[82,86]

Several small studies of the natural history of thoracic aortic aneurysms have been reported, but the data are far more limited than those available regarding abdominal aortic aneurysms. In the largest modern series, the 1-, 3-, and 5-year survival rates for patients with thoracic aortic aneurysms not undergoing surgical repair were approximately 65, 36, and 20 per cent, respectively.[12,86,87] Aneurysm rupture occurs in 32 to 68 per cent of patients not treated surgically, with rupture accounting for 32 to 47 per cent of all patient deaths.[81,86,87] Fewer than half of the patients with rupture may arrive at the hospital alive,[80] as mortality at 6 hours is 54 per cent and at 24 hours reaches 76 per cent.[80] There is no apparent association between thoracic aneurysm location and the risk of death due to rupture.[86]

Because size is an important predictor of the risk of aneurysm rupture, several studies have examined the rate of expansion of thoracic aortic aneurysms. As with abdominal aneurysms, initial size is the only independent predictor of the rate of thoracic aneurysm growth,[84] although some data also suggest that descending thoracic aneurysms may expand more slowly than others.[88] In a recent report, Dapunt et al. followed 67 patients with thoracic aortic aneurysm using serial CT scanning and found a mean rate of expansion of 0.43 cm/year.[89] The only independent predictor of a rapid expansion (greater than 0.5 cm/year) was an initial aortic diameter larger than 5.0 cm: Those aneurysms that were 5.0 cm or smaller showed mean growth rates of 0.17 cm/year, whereas those larger than 5.0 cm grew by 0.79 cm/year. Unfortunately, even when controlling for initial aneurysm size, there was still substantial variation in individual aneurysm growth rates, making such mean growth rates of little value in predicting aneurysm growth for a given patient. More helpful, however, was the finding that growth rates among small aneurysms were more consistent, with only 1 of 25 aneurysms 4.0 cm or less at baseline showing rapid growth. Two additional findings in this series were that no aneurysm smaller than 5.0 cm ruptured during the follow-up period, and that the only variable predictor of survival was initial aneurysm size.

Management

SURGICAL TREATMENT. The optimal timing of surgical repair of thoracic aortic aneurysms remains uncertain for several reasons. First, as noted above, the available data on the natural history of thoracic aneurysms are limited, especially with respect to the outcomes of surgical intervention. Second, with the high incidence of coexisting cardiovascular disease in this population, many patients die of other cardiovascular causes before their aneurysms ever rupture. Finally, significant risks are associated with thoracic aortic surgery, particularly in the arch and descending aorta, which in many cases may outweigh the potential benefits of aortic repair.

We currently recommend surgery when thoracic aortic aneurysms reach 6.0 cm or larger, or often 7.0 cm or larger in patients at high operative risk. Indications for surgery in smaller aneurysms include rapid rate of expansion, associated significant aortic regurgitation, or the presence of aneurysm-related symptoms. In patients with the Marfan syndrome, given their higher risk of dissection and rupture, we recommend repair of thoracic aneurysms when they reach only 5.5 cm in size.[90] Surgery should be considered even sooner in Marfan patients at especially high risk, such as those with rapid and progressive aortic dilatation, those with a family history of the Marfan syndrome plus aortic dissection, or women planning pregnancy. Of course, the aggressiveness with which surgical repair is undertaken in any case should be appropriately influenced by the general condition of the individual patient.

Thoracic aortic aneurysms are generally resected and replaced with a prosthetic sleeve of appropriate size (Fig. 45–5). Cardiopulmonary bypass is necessary for the removal of ascending aortic aneurysms, and partial bypass to support the circulation distal to the aneurysm is often advisable in resection of descending thoracic aortic aneurysms. A temporary Gott shunt may be used from the proximal aorta to the aorta beyond the aneurysm in order to perfuse the distal circulation while the aortic site being

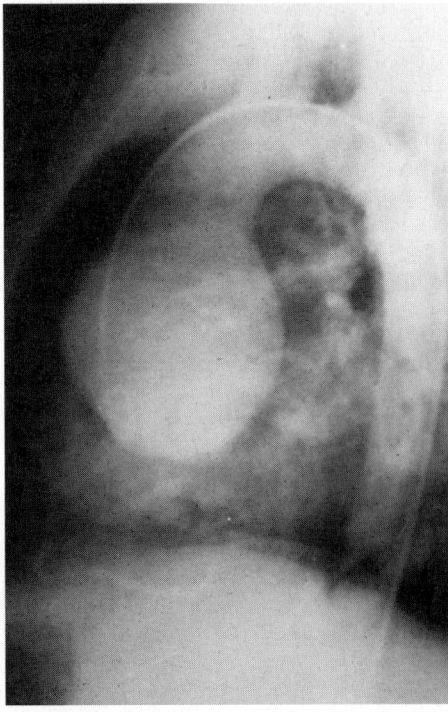

FIGURE 45–4. Lateral aortogram in a man with annuloaortic ectasia and aneurysmal dilation of the ascending thoracic aorta. The bulbous, pear-shaped aortic root can easily be seen. The left ventricle is partially opacified consequent to aortic regurgitation. (Courtesy of Christos Athanasoulis, M.D., and Arthur Waltman, M.D., Section of Vascular Radiology, Massachusetts General Hospital, Boston.)

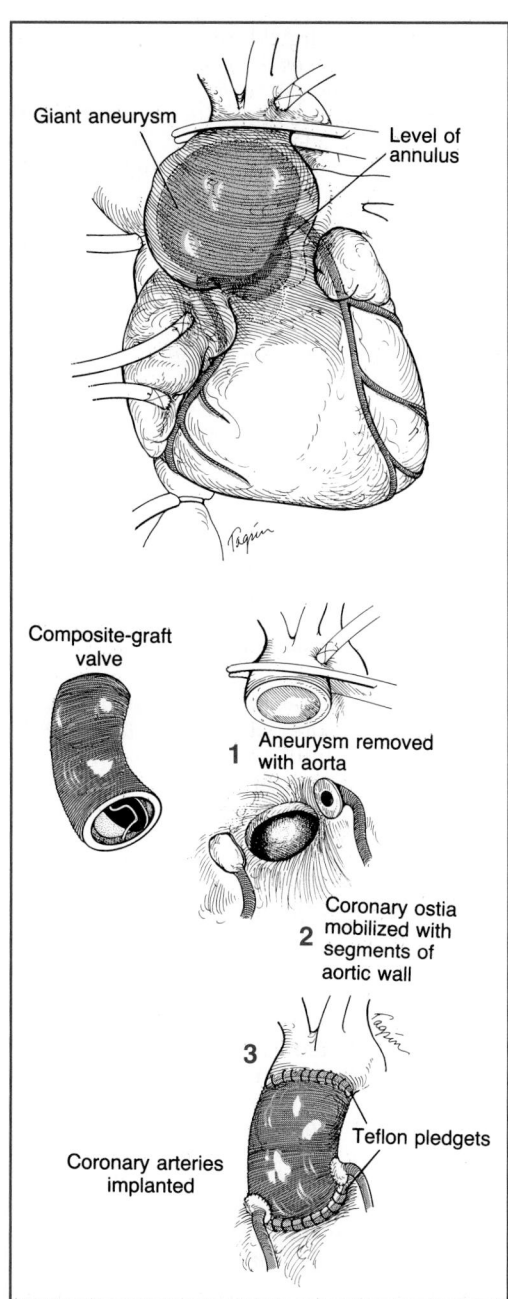

Giant aneurysm

Level of annulus

Composite-graft valve

1 Aneurysm removed with aorta

2 Coronary ostia mobilized with segments of aortic wall

3

Coronary arteries implanted

Teflon pledgets

FIGURE 45–5. Technique for the composite graft replacement of an aneurysm of the ascending aorta. *Top,* The aneurysm is shown, involving the sinuses of Valsalva. The patient is on total cardiopulmonary bypass. *Bottom,* The composite graft is shown, with a low-profile, tilting-disc aortic prosthesis attached to its inferior end. (1) The aneurysm is resected with the native aortic valve. (2) The coronary ostia have been excised and mobilized with a button of aortic wall. (3) The composite graft has been secured in place using Teflon felt reinforcement for the suture line. The coronary artery ostia are then reimplanted directly to the graft.

repaired is cross-clamped.[91] The use of such adjuncts is less important, however, than the nature and extent of the aneurysm in determining the incidence of postoperative complications.[92]

The use of a composite graft consisting of a Dacron tube with a prosthetic aortic valve sewn into one end (Bentall procedure) is generally the method of choice in treating ascending thoracic aneurysms involving the root which are associated with significant aortic regurgitation.[93] The valve and graft are sewn directly into the aortic annulus, and the coronary arteries then reimplanted into the Dacron aortic graft (Fig. 45–5). The operative risk for mortality is about 5 per cent.[93] For those patients with structurally normal aortic valve leaflets whose aortic regurgitation is secondary to

dilatation of the root, David et al. have successfully repaired the native valve by either reimplanting it in a Dacron graft or reconstructing the aortic root. In a recent series, 41 of 45 patients had mild or no aortic regurgitation after this method of aortic valve repair and were stable at a mean of 18 months.[94]

Aneurysms of the aortic arch may be successfully excised surgically, but the procedure may be particularly challenging. The brachiocephalic vessels must be removed from the aortic arch prior to its resection. Then, after interposition of the prosthetic tube graft, the island of native aortic tissue containing the brachiocephalic vessels is reimplanted into the graft and normal cerebral perfusion restored. There is, however, a significantly increased risk of stroke secondary to variable periods of cerebral ischemia. The incidence of stroke in recent series is 3 to 7 per cent.[95,96] The standard method for carrying out this operation today is with the use of profound hypothermic circulatory arrest, as introduced by Griepp et al. in 1974.[97] Some have attempted to add selective cerebral perfusion during aneurysmectomy, but cannulation techniques are difficult. In fact, the incidence of stroke may actually be as high or higher with this method, possibly due to cannulation-induced cerebral emboli.[96,99] A more recent adjunct for cerebral protection during hypothermic arrest is the use of retrograde cerebral perfusion via a superior vena cava cannula.[95] Not only does this technique provide nutrients and oxygen to the brain,[100] but it may also serve to flush out both air and particulate matter from the cerebral and carotid arteries that would otherwise embolize. The results of retrograde cerebral perfusion have thus far been quite encouraging, with trends toward lower stroke rates in recent reports.[95,99]

More than half of the patients undergoing surgical repair of a thoracic aortic aneurysm in Crawford's series had multiple aortic segments involved, and almost three-quarters of those with descending thoracic aneurysms had multiple involvement.[98] Such widespread aneurysmal dilatation of the aorta presents a particular challenge to the surgeon and often precludes operation. However, Crawford et al. have demonstrated that it is possible to successfully replace virtually the entire diseased thoracic and abdominal aorta.[98] A method known as the "elephant trunk" technique, carried out in sequential stages of aortic replacement, has been shown to facilitate such extensive surgical procedures and reduce the associated risks.[101]

Elective surgical repair of ascending and descending thoracic aortic aneurysms has a 90 to 95 per cent early survival rate in most centers.[102,103] Major complications are technical, especially hemorrhage from tearing of the diseased aorta. A catastrophic complication of resection of descending thoracic aortic aneurysms is postoperative paraplegia secondary to interruption of the blood supply to the spinal cord. The incidence of paraplegia ranges from 0 to 17 per cent,[91,92] although most series show an incidence of about 5 to 6 per cent.[92,104] A number of methods have been proposed to reduce the likelihood of paraplegia, although none has proved to be consistently safe and effective. One of the more promising techniques involves maintaining distal aortic perfusion during surgery with the use of the heparinless Gott shunt (aorto-aorta bypass).[91] Although some groups have achieved good success with such techniques,[91] others have had mixed results. Controlled trials might better clarify the efficacy of these techniques.

An alternative approach to the surgical management of descending thoracic aneurysms, as recently reported by Dake et al., is the use of a transluminally placed endovascular stent-graft. This technique has the advantage of being far less invasive than surgery and has the potential of reducing the incidence of paraplegia from surgically induced spinal cord ischemia. The authors report successful device deployment in all 14 of their patients, with documented thrombosis of the residual aneurysm lumen surrounding the stent-graft in 12.[105] Although still experimental at present, such a device may in the future have an important role in the management of patients who are at risk for aortic rupture but are otherwise poor surgical candidates. Unfortunately, the curvilinear nature of the ascending aorta and arch makes application of similar techniques to aneurysms of these proximal aortic segments far more problematic.

Complications of associated atherosclerosis, such as myocardial infarction, cerebrovascular accidents, and renal failure, often become manifested under the massive physiological stress of aortic surgery. The most frequent causes of early postoperative death are myocardial infarction, congestive heart failure, stroke, renal failure, hemorrhage, respiratory failure, and sepsis. Advanced age, emergency operation, prolonged aortic cross-clamp time, extent of the aneurysm, diabetes, prior aortic surgery, aneurysm symptoms, and intraoperative hypotension are the most important factors determining perioperative morbidity and mortality.[106] Many patients with atherosclerotic aneurysms are heavy smokers, and pulmonary complications following surgery are common. The left lung may be severely traumatized by compression during resection of large aneurysms of the descending thoracic aorta, a complication that may seriously jeopardize the patient's survival, particularly in the setting of underlying pulmonary disease.

Late deaths are usually associated with cardiac complications, aneurysm rupture, respiratory failure, or stroke.[102] Aneurysm rupture may be due to aneurysm formation at the graft margins or the appearance of new aneurysms at other aortic sites.[11]

MEDICAL MANAGEMENT. The long-term impact of medical therapy on aneurysm growth and survival in patients with typical atherosclerotic thoracic aneurysms has not been examined. However, in a recent report, Shores et al. examined the efficacy of beta blockers in adult patients with the Marfan syndrome.[107] They randomized 70 patients to treatment with propranolol versus no beta blocker therapy and followed them over a 10-year period. The treated group showed a significantly slower rate of aortic dilatation, fewer adverse clinical endpoints (death, aortic dissection, aortic regurgitation, aortic root >6 cm), and significantly lower mortality from the 4-year point onward.[107] Although this study examined only the effect of beta blockade in the Marfan syndrome, it follows logically that medical therapy to reduce dP/dt and control blood pressure is essential to the treatment of thoracic aortic aneurysm, both for those with smaller aneurysms being followed serially and for patients having undergone aortic aneurysm repair.

Annuloaortic Ectasia

The term *annuloaortic ectasia* was first used by Ellis et al. in 1961 to describe a clinicopathological condition seen in a subset of patients with thoracic aortic aneurysms in whom idiopathic dilatation of the proximal aorta and the aortic annulus leads to pure aortic regurgitation.[108] The entity has subsequently been recognized with increasing frequency and makes up about 5 to 10 per cent of the population undergoing aortic valve replacement for pure aortic regurgitation. Annuloaortic ectasia is more common in men than in women, typically presenting in the fourth, fifth, and sixth decades with progressively more severe aortic regurgitation. Sudden onset of symptoms followed by rapid progression is occasionally seen.

The common pathological feature shared by patients with annuloaortic ectasia is that of cystic medial degeneration of the afflicted aortic wall, leading to progressive dilatation. With widening of the aortic root, the valve annulus dilates and the aortic leaflets are pulled apart, resulting in aortic regurgitation, despite the fact that the aortic valve leaflets themselves are structurally normal. The weakened aortic walls are also prone to dissection. When aortic dissection does occur, the dissection tends to be small, circumscribed, and confined to the ascending aorta.

Clinically, little distinguishes the aortic regurgitation in patients with annuloaortic ectasia from that due to other causes. On physical examination, the diastolic murmur tends to be of greater intensity to the right of the sternum in cases of annuloaortic ectasia and to the left of the sternum in cases of primary aortic regurgitation. Lemon and White found that two features—acute or subacute development of symptoms and the presence of associated chest pain—were more common in patients with annuloaortic ectasia than primary aortic regurgitation.[109]

The chest roentgenogram usually shows a grossly dilated aortic root and ascending aorta with left ventricular enlargement proportional to the degree of aortic regurgitation. Aortographically, annuloaortic ectasia has one of three typical appearances. Most common is a pear-shaped enlargement of the ascending aorta (Fig. 45–4). Also seen are diffuse symmetrical dilatation and dilatation limited to the aortic root.[109]

Surgical correction is usually undertaken for relief of aortic regurgitation when it is severe and responsible for symptoms of left ventricular failure or when the left ventricle or ascending aorta is increasing in size. In such cases, the aortic valve together with the proximal ascending aorta is usually replaced with a composite graft.

AORTIC DISSECTION

Acute aortic dissection is an uncommon but potentially catastrophic illness that occurs with an incidence of at least 2000 cases per year in the United States.[110,111] Early mortality is as high as 1 per cent per hour if untreated,[112] but survival may be significantly improved by the timely institution of appropriate medical and/or surgical therapy. Prompt clinical recognition and definitive diagnostic testing are therefore essential in the management of patients with aortic dissection.

Aortic dissection is believed to begin with the formation of a tear in the aortic intima that directly exposes an underlying diseased medial layer to the driving force (or pulse pressure) of the intraluminal blood (Fig. 45–6A). This blood penetrates the diseased medial layer and cleaves the laminar plane of the media in two, thus dissecting the aortic wall. Driven by persistent intraluminal pressure, the dissection process extends a variable length along the aortic wall, typically antegrade (driven by the forward force of aortic blood flow) but sometimes retrograde from the site of intimal tear. The blood-filled space between the dissected layers of the aortic wall becomes the *false lumen*. Shear forces may lead to further tears in the *intimal flap* (the inner portion of the dissected aortic wall), producing exit sites or additional entry sites for blood flow in the false lumen. The false lumen may become distended with blood, causing the intimal flap to bow into the *true lumen*, thereby narrowing its caliber and distorting its shape.

It has also been suggested that aortic dissection may begin instead with the rupture of the vasa vasorum within the aortic media, i.e., with the development of an intramural hematoma (Fig. 45–6B). Local hemorrhage then secondarily ruptures through the intimal layer, creating the intimal tear and aortic dissection. The fact that in autopsy series as many as 13 per cent of aortic dissections do not have an identifiable intimal tear[113] argues that, at least in this minority of cases, independent medial hemorrhage is the primary cause of dissection. On the other hand, one might argue that the lack of an intimal tear in these patients indicates that they do not, in fact, have classic aortic dissection, but rather suffer intramural hematoma of the aorta, a closely related condition (see below).

CLASSIFICATION. Most classification schemes for aortic dissection are based on the fact that the vast majority of aortic dissections originate in one of two locations: (1) the ascending aorta, within several centimeters of the aortic

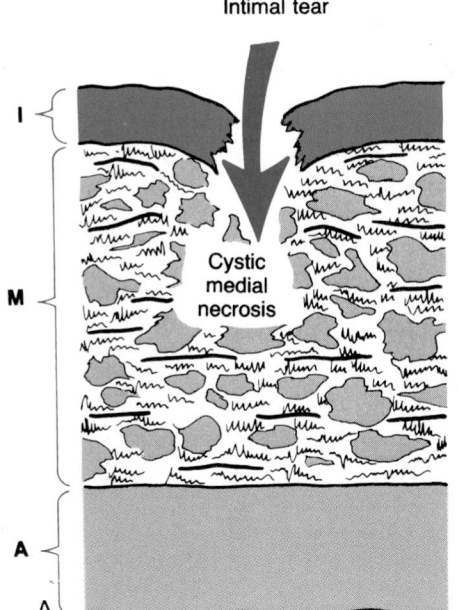
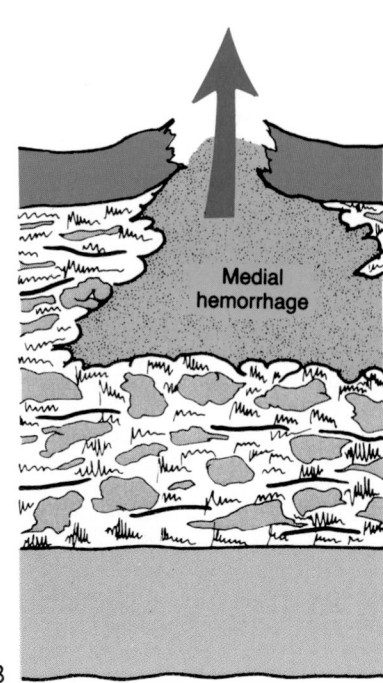

Intimal tear

Cystic medial necrosis

Medial hemorrhage

I = intima; M = media; A = adventitia

A   B

FIGURE 45–6. Proposed mechanisms of initiation of aortic dissection. In both cases, cystic medial necrosis is present. In A, an intimal tear is the initial event, allowing aortic blood to enter the media. In B, the primary event is hemorrhage into the media, with secondary rupture of the overlying intima. I = intima; M = media; A = adventitia.

valve, and (2) the descending aorta, just distal to the origin of the left subclavian artery at the site of the ligamentum arteriosum.[111] Sixty-five per cent of intimal tears occur in the ascending aorta, 20 per cent in the descending aorta, 10 per cent in the aortic arch, and 5 per cent in the abdominal aorta.[98]

There are three major classification systems to define the location and extent of aortic involvement, as defined in Table 45–1 and depicted in Figure 45–7: (1) DeBakey types I, II, and III[114]; (2) Stanford types A and B[115]; and (3) anatomical categories "proximal" and "distal." All three schemes share the same basic principle of distinguishing those aortic dissections with and without ascending aortic involvement for prognostic and therapeutic reasons; in general, surgery is indicated for dissections involving the ascending aorta, whereas medical management is reserved for those dissections without ascending aortic involvement. Accordingly, because both DeBakey types I and II involve the ascending aorta, they are grouped together for simplicity in the Stanford (type A) and anatomical (proximal) classification systems. Aortic dissections confined to the ab-

dominal aorta,[116] although quite uncommon, are best categorized as type B or distal dissections. Proximal or type A dissections occur in about two-thirds of cases, with distal dissections composing the remaining one-third.

In addition to its location, aortic dissection is also classified according to its duration, defined as the length of time from symptom onset to medical evaluation. The mortality from dissection and its risk of progression decrease progressively over time, making therapeutic strategies for long-standing aortic dissections quite different from those for dissections presenting acutely. A dissection present less than 2 weeks is defined as "acute," whereas those present 2 weeks or more are defined as "chronic" because the mortality curve for untreated aortic dissections begins to level off at 75 to 80 per cent at this time.[112] At diagnosis, about two-thirds of aortic dissections are acute and the remaining third are chronic.[117]

ETIOLOGY AND PATHOGENESIS. Medial degeneration, as

TABLE 45–1 COMMONLY USED CLASSIFICATION SYSTEMS TO DESCRIBE AORTIC DISSECTION

TYPE	SITE OF ORIGIN AND EXTENT OF AORTIC INVOLVEMENT
DeBakey	
Type I	Originates in the ascending aorta, propagates at least to the aortic arch and often beyond it distally
Type II	Originates in and is confined to the ascending aorta
Type III	Originates in the descending aorta and extends distally down the aorta or, rarely, retrograde into the aortic arch and ascending aorta
Stanford	
Type A	All dissections involving the ascending aorta, regardless of the site of origin
Type B	All dissections not involving the ascending aorta
Descriptive	
Proximal	Includes DeBakey types I and II or Stanford type A
Distal	Includes DeBakey type III or Stanford type B

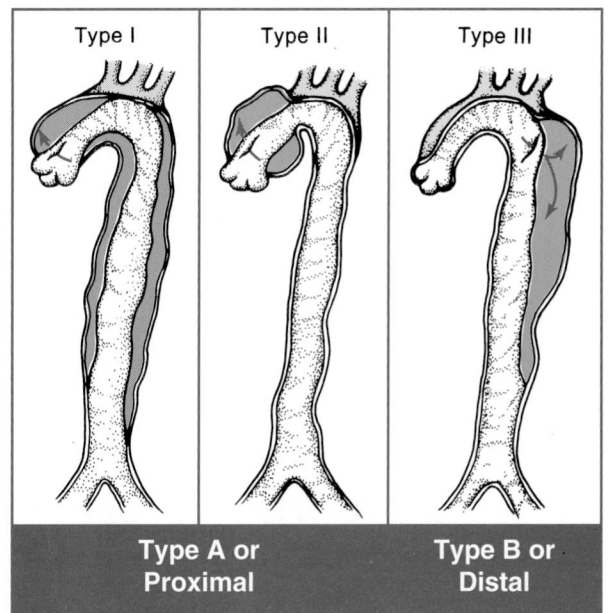

FIGURE 45–7. Commonly used classification systems for aortic dissection. (Refer to Table 45–1 for definitions.)

evidenced by deterioration of the medial collagen and elastin, is considered to be the chief predisposing factor in most nontraumatic cases of aortic dissection.[78,95] Therefore, any disease process or other condition that undermines the integrity of the elastic or muscular components of the media predisposes the aorta to dissection. Cystic medial degeneration is an intrinsic feature of several hereditary defects of connective tissue, most notably the Marfan (see p. 1671) and Ehlers-Danlos (see p. 1672) syndromes. In addition to their propensity to develop thoracic aortic aneurysms, patients with the Marfan syndrome are indeed at high risk of developing aortic dissection—especially proximal dissection—at a relatively young age. In fact, the Marfan syndrome accounts for 6 to 9 per cent of all aortic dissections.[117,118]

In the absence of the Marfan syndrome, histologically classic cystic medial degeneration is identified in only a minority of cases of aortic dissection.[117,118] Nevertheless, the degree of medial degeneration found in most other cases of aortic dissection still tends to be qualitatively and quantitatively much greater than that expected as part of the aging process. Although the cause of such medial degeneration remains unclear, advanced age and hypertension appear to be two of the most important factors.

The peak incidence of aortic dissection is in the sixth and seventh decades of life, with men affected twice as often as women.[117] A coexisting history of hypertension is found in almost 80 per cent of cases in a recent series of 236 cases of aortic dissection from Spittell et al.[117] Bicuspid aortic valve is a well-established risk factor for proximal aortic dissection and historically has been found in 7 to 14 per cent of all aortic dissections.[117,118] Interestingly, the risk of aortic dissection appears to be independent of the severity of the bicuspid valve stenosis.[118] Certain other congenital cardiovascular abnormalities predispose the aorta to dissection, including unicuspid aortic valve and possibly coarctation of the aorta.[118] Aortic dissection has also been reported to occur in association with the Noonan[119] and the Turner syndromes.[117,120] Rarely, aortic dissection complicates arteritis involving the aorta (see p. 1574), particularly giant cell arteritis.[117] A number of reports describe aortic dissection in association with cocaine abuse among younger men,[121] but no direct causal relationship has yet been established.

An unexplained relationship exists between pregnancy and aortic dissection (see p. 1855). About half of all aortic dissections in women under 40 years of age occur during pregnancy, typically in the third trimester[122] and also occasionally in the early postpartum period.[123] Increases in blood volume, cardiac output, and blood pressure seen in late pregnancy may contribute to the risk,[124] although this explanation cannot account for postpartum occurrence. Women with the Marfan syndrome and a dilated aortic root are at particular risk of suffering acute aortic dissection during pregnancy,[125] and in some cases the diagnosis of the Marfan syndrome is first made when such women present with a peripartum aortic dissection.

Direct trauma to the aorta may also cause aortic dissection. Blunt trauma tends to cause localized tears, hematomas, or frank aortic disruption rather than classic aortic dissection (see p. 1543). Iatrogenic trauma, on the other hand, is associated with true aortic dissection. Intraarterial catheterization and the insertion of intraaortic balloon pumps[126] both may induce aortic dissection, probably resulting from direct trauma to the aortic intima. Cardiac surgery is associated with a very small risk of aortic dissection occurring at an aortic incision site or the site of aortic cross-clamping.[127] The majority of these dissections are discovered intraoperatively and repaired at that time, although 20 per cent are detected only after a delay.[128] A distinct group of cardiac surgical patients undergoing aortic valve replacement suffer aortic dissection as a late complication, usually not until several years after the procedure.[129]

Clinical Manifestations

SYMPTOMS. By far the most common presenting symptom of acute aortic dissection is severe pain, found in 74 to 90 per cent of cases,[117,130] whereas the large majority of those presenting without pain are found to have chronic dissections.[117] The pain is typically of sudden onset, and is as severe at its inception as it ever becomes, contrasting with the pain of myocardial infarction, which usually has a crescendo-like onset. In fact, the pain may be all but unbearable in some instances, forcing the patient to writhe in agony, fall to the ground, or pace restlessly in an attempt to gain relief. Several features of the pain should arouse suspicion of aortic dissection. The quality of the pain as described by the patient is often morbidly appropriate to the actual event, with adjectives such as "tearing," "ripping," and "stabbing" frequently used. Another important characteristic of the pain of aortic dissection is its tendency to migrate from its point of origin to other sites, generally following the path of the dissection as it extends through the aorta. Such migratory pain was noted in 70 per cent of our cases.[130]

The location of pain may be quite helpful in suggesting the location of the aortic dissection, because localized symptoms tend to reflect involvement of the underlying aorta. In the series by Spittell et al.,[117] when the location of chest pain was anterior only (or if the most severe pain was anterior), more than 90 per cent had involvement of the ascending aorta. Conversely, when the chest pain was interscapular only (or when the most severe pain was interscapular), more than 90 per cent had involvement of the descending thoracic aorta (i.e., DeBakey type I or III). The presence of any pain in the neck, throat, jaw, or face strongly predicted involvement of the ascending aorta, whereas pain anywhere in the back, abdomen, or lower extremities strongly predicted involvement of the descending aorta.

Less common symptoms at presentation, occurring with or without associated chest pain, include congestive heart failure, syncope, cerebrovascular accident, ischemic peripheral neuropathy, paraplegia, and cardiac arrest or sudden death. The presence of acute congestive heart failure in this setting is almost invariably due to severe aortic regurgitation induced by a proximal aortic dissection (discussed below). The occurrence of syncope without focal neurological signs, in 4 to 5 per cent of aortic dissections,[117,130] may be an ominous sign suggesting a surgical emergency. It is associated most often with a rupture of a proximal aortic dissection into the pericardial cavity with resultant cardiac tamponade, and less often with rupture of the descending thoracic aorta into the intrapleural space.[117]

PHYSICAL FINDINGS. Although extremely variable, the findings on physical examination generally reflect the location of the aortic dissection and extent of associated cardiovascular involvement. In some cases physical findings alone may be sufficient to suggest the diagnosis, whereas in other cases such pertinent findings may be subtle or absent, even in the presence of extensive aortic dissection. Hypertension is seen in more than 80 to 90 per cent of those with distal aortic dissection but is less common in proximal dissection. Hypotension, on the other hand, occurs much more commonly among those with proximal than distal aortic dissection.[130] True hypotension usually is the result of cardiac tamponade, intrapleural rupture, or intraperitoneal rupture. Dissection involving the brachiocephalic vessels may result in "pseudohypotension," an inaccurate measurement of blood pressure due to compromise or occlusion of the brachial arteries.

The physical findings most typically associated with aortic dissection—pulse deficits, the murmur of aortic regurgitation, and neurological manifestations—are more characteristic of proximal than of distal dissection. The presence of *pulse deficits* (diminution or absence) in patients with

PLATE 10

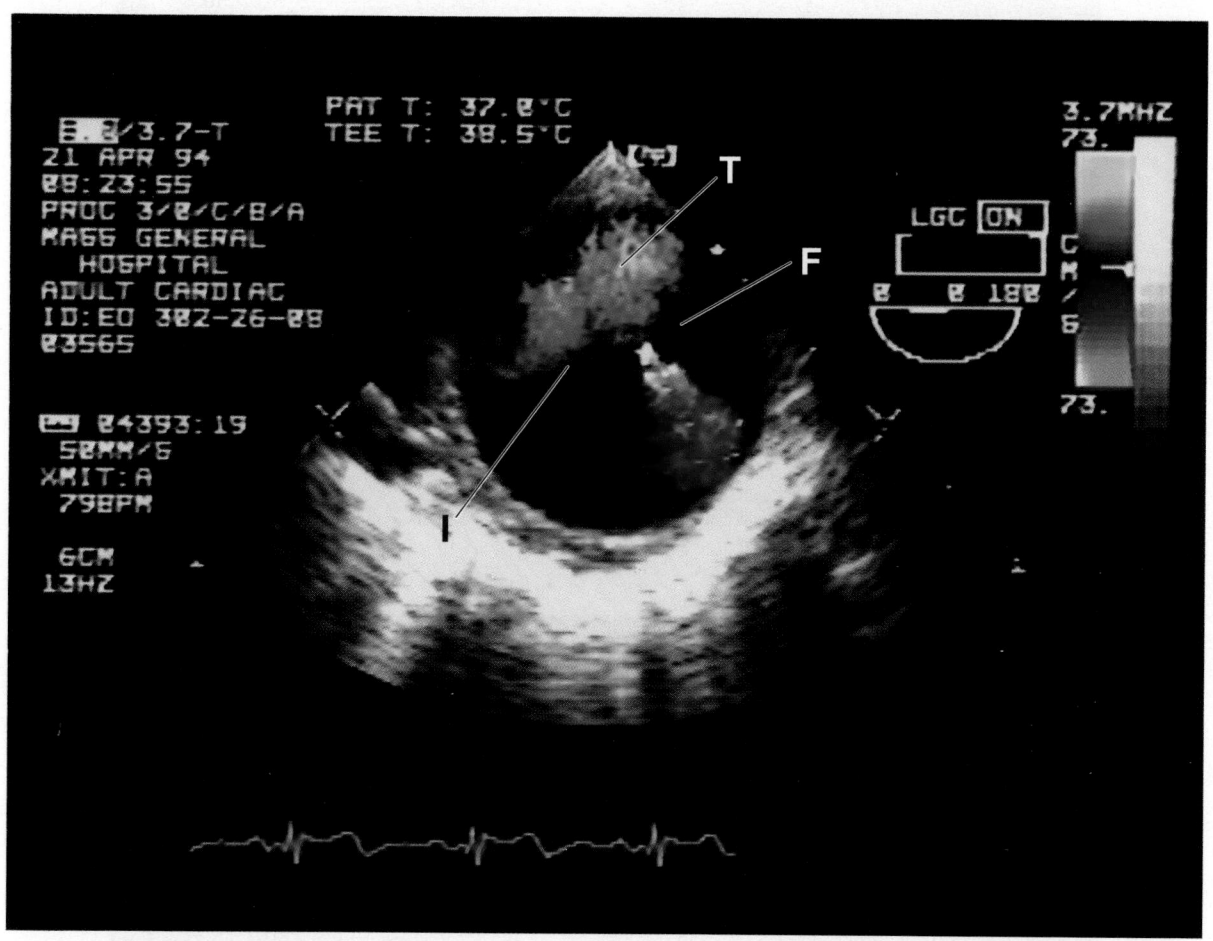

FIGURE 45–16. A cross-sectional transesophageal echocardiogram of a descending aortic dissection demonstrating a site of intimal tear. Blood flow (in orange) is evident in the true lumen (T) during systole, while a narrow jet of high-velocity blood (in blue) crosses into the false lumen (F) through a tear in the intimal flap (I).

PLATE 11

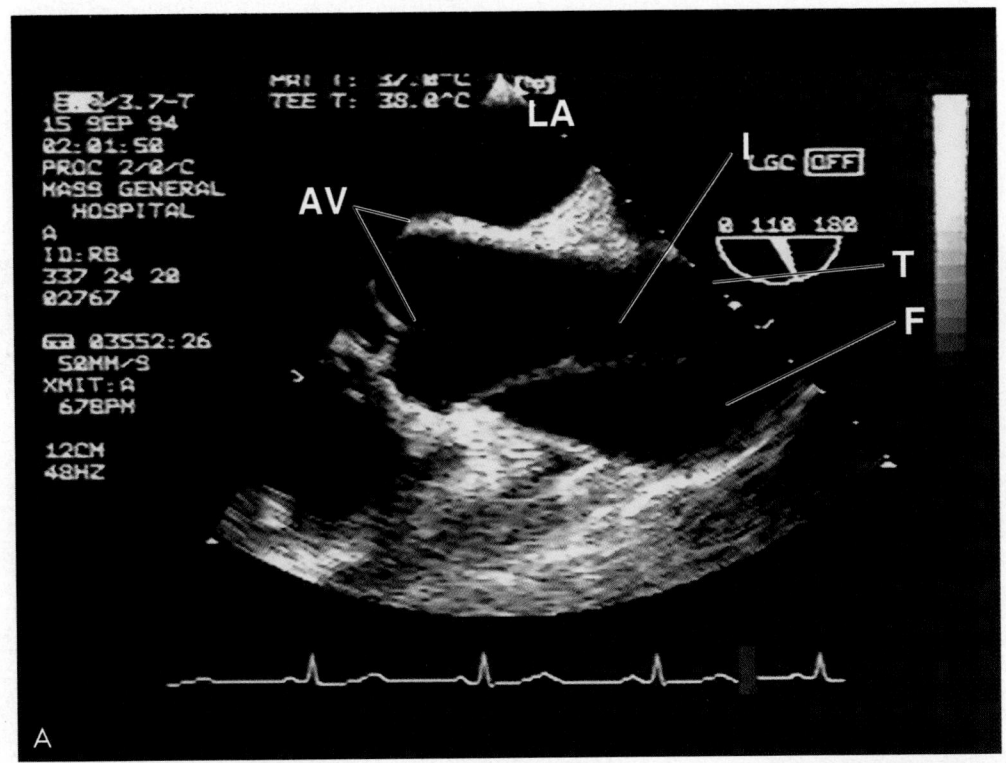

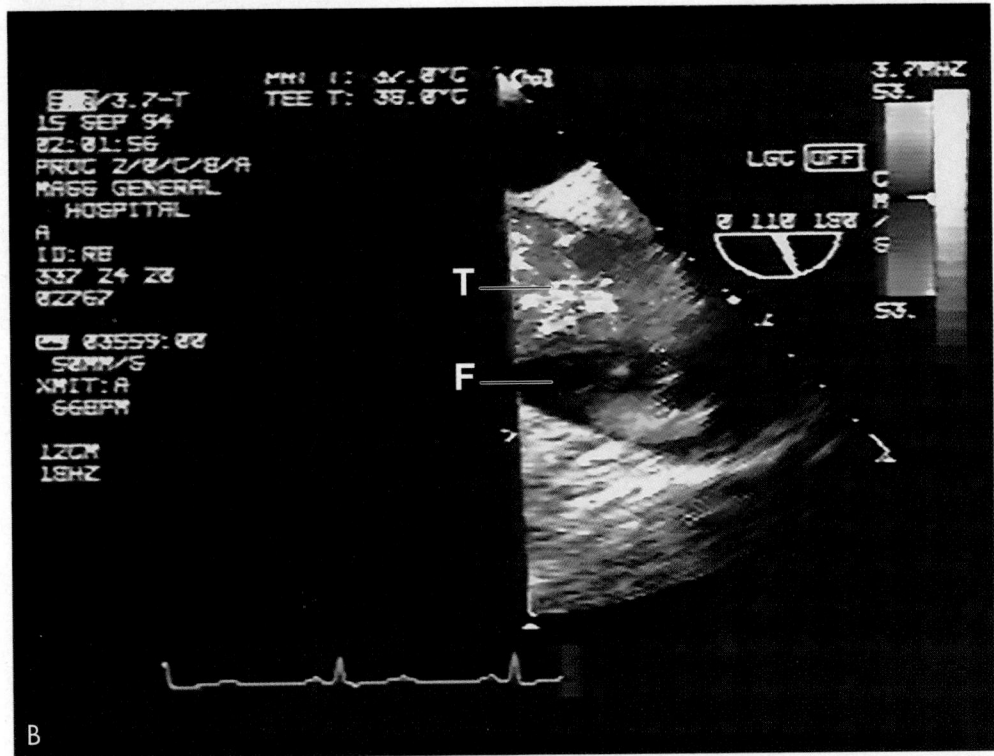

FIGURE 45–17.   A transesophageal echocardiogram of the proximal ascending aorta in long axis in a patient with a proximal aortic dissection. *A,* The left atrium (LA) is closest to the transducer. The aortic valve (AV) is seen on the left in this view, with the ascending aorta extending to the right. Within the proximal aorta is an intimal flap (I), which originates just at the level of the sinotubular junction above the right sinus of Valsalva. The true lumen (T) and the false lumen (F) are separated by the intimal flap. *B,* The addition of color flow Doppler in the same view confirms the presence of two distinct lumens. The true lumen (T) fills completely with brisk blood flow (bright blue color), while at the same time there is minimal retrograde flow (dark orange) in the false lumen (F).

acute chest pain strongly suggests the presence of aortic dissection. Pulse deficits are present in about 50 per cent of proximal aortic dissection and occur throughout the arterial tree but are seen in only 15 per cent of distal dissections, where they usually involve the femoral or left subclavian arteries. Such pulse deficits result from extension of the dissection flap into an artery with compression of the true lumen by the false channel, or from proximal obstruction of flow due to a mobile portion of the intimal flap overlying the vessel's orifice. Whichever the cause, the pulse deficits in aortic dissection may be transient, secondary to decompression of the false lumen by distal reentry into the true lumen or to movement of the intimal flap away from the occluded orifice.

Aortic regurgitation is an important feature of proximal aortic dissection, with the murmur of aortic regurgitation detected in anywhere from 16 to 67 per cent of cases.[117,130] When aortic regurgitation is present in patients with distal dissection, it generally antedates the dissection and may be the result of preexisting dilatation of the aortic root due to the underlying aortic pathology, such as cystic medial degeneration. The murmur of aortic regurgitation associated with proximal dissection often has a musical quality and may be heard better along the right than the left sternal border. It may wax and wane, the intensity varying directly with the height of the arterial blood pressure. Depending on the severity of the regurgitation, other peripheral signs of aortic incompetence may be present, such as collapsing pulses and a wide pulse pressure. However, in some cases congestive heart failure secondary to severe acute aortic regurgitation may occur with little or no murmur and no peripheral signs of aortic runoff.

The aortic regurgitation associated with proximal aortic dissection, occurring in one-half to two-thirds of cases,[131] may result from any of several mechanisms, as depicted in Figure 45–8. First, the dissection may dilate the aortic root, widening the annulus so that the aortic leaflets are unable to coapt properly in diastole. Second, in an asymmetrical dissection, pressure from the dissecting hematoma may depress one leaflet below the coaptation line of the others so as to render the valve incompetent. Third, the annular support of the leaflets or the leaflets themselves may be torn, causing leaflet flail. Lastly, in the setting of an extensive or circumferential intimal tear, the unsupported intimal flap may prolapse into the left ventricular outflow tract,[132] occasionally appearing as frank intimal intussusception,[133] producing severe aortic regurgitation.

Neurological manifestations occur in as many as 6 to 19 per cent of all aortic dissections[117,130,134] but are more common with proximal dissection. Cerebrovascular accidents may occur in 3 to 6 per cent when there is direct involvement of the innominate or left common carotid arteries.[134] Less frequently, patients may present with altered consciousness or even coma. When spinal artery perfusion is compromised (more common in distal dissection[117]), ischemic spinal cord damage may produce paraparesis or paraplegia.[135]

In a small minority, about 1 to 2 per cent of cases,[117,136] a proximal dissection flap may involve the ostium of a coronary artery and cause acute myocardial infarction. The dissection more often affects the right coronary artery than the left, explaining why these myocardial infarctions tend to be inferior in location.[117] Unfortunately, when secondary myocardial infarction does occur, its symptoms may complicate the clinical picture by obscuring the symptoms of the primary aortic dissection. Most worrisome is the possibility that, in the setting of electrocardiographic evidence of myocardial infarction, the underlying aortic dissection may go unrecognized. Moreover, the consequences of such a misdiagnosis can be catastrophic in the era of thrombolytic therapy. In a recent review of the literature, Kamp et al. described an early mortality of 71 per cent (many from cardiac tamponade) among 21 cases of aortic dissection treated with thrombolysis.[137] It thus remains essential that when evaluating patients with acute myocardial infarction—particularly inferior infarctions—one carefully consider the possibility of an underlying aortic dissection before thrombolytic or anticoagulant therapy is instituted. Although some physicians feel reassured that performing a chest roentgenogram prior to the institution of thrombolysis is adequate to exclude the diagnosis of dissection, a blinded study of roentgenogram interpretation in this setting suggests that this is not sufficient.[138]

Extension of aortic dissection into the abdominal aorta may cause other vascular complications. Compromise of one or both renal arteries occurs in about 5 to 8 per cent[134,139] and may lead to renal ischemia or frank infarction, resulting in severe hypertension and acute renal failure. Mesenteric ischemia and infarction are also occasional complications of abdominal dissection, seen in 3 to 5 per cent of cases.[134,139] In addition, aortic dissection may extend into the iliac arteries, causing femoral pulse deficits (12 per cent[134]) and acute lower extremity ischemia. If in such cases the associated chest pain is minimal or absent, the pulse deficit and ischemic peripheral neuropathy may be mistaken for a peripheral embolic event.

Additional clinical manifestations of aortic dissection include the presence of pleural effusions, seen more commonly on the left side. The effusion typically arises secondary to an exudative inflammatory reaction around the involved aorta, but in some cases may result from a hemothorax due to a transient rupture or leak from a descending dissection. Several rarely encountered clinical manifestations of aortic dissection include hoarseness,[117] upper airway obstruction,[140] rupture into the tracheobronchial tree with hemoptysis,[117] dysphagia,[117] hematemesis due to rupture into the esophagus,[141] superior vena cava syndrome,[117] pulsation of the sternoclavicular joint,[142] pulsating neck masses, Horner syndrome, and unexplained fever.[143] Other rare presentations associated with the presence of a continuous murmur include rupture of the aortic dissection into the right atrium,[144] into the right ventricle,[145] or into the left atrium with secondary congestive heart failure.[146]

A variety of conditions may mimic aortic dissection. These include myocardial infarction or ischemia, acute aortic regurgitation without dissection, nondissecting thoracic or abdominal aortic aneurysms, pericarditis, musculoskeletal pain, or mediastinal tumors. Diagnostic confusion may be particularly likely when a patient with chest pain presents coincidentally with another clinical symptom, physical finding, or chest roentgenographic finding typically associated with aortic dissection.[147]

LABORATORY FINDINGS. Chest roentgenography is included in the discussion of clinical manifestations of aortic dissection rather than in the discussion of diagnostic techniques because an abnormal incidental finding on a routine

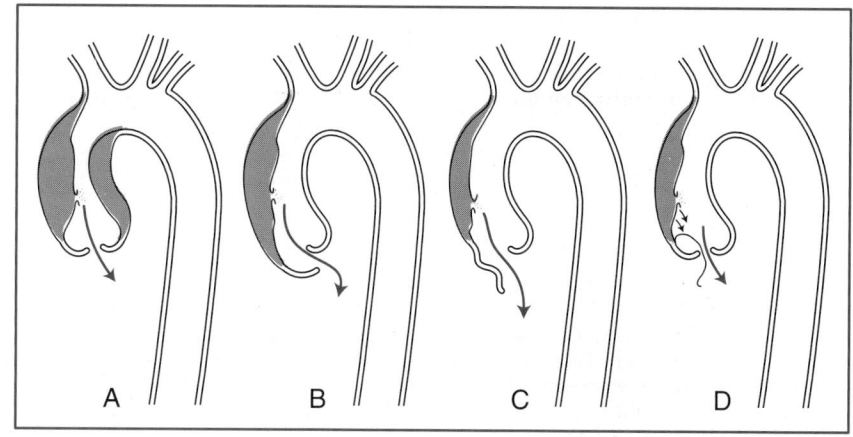

FIGURE 45–8. **Mechanisms of aortic regurgitation in proximal aortic dissection.** *A,* An extensive or circumferential tear dilates the aortic root and annulus, preventing the aortic valve leaflets from coapting. *B,* With asymmetrical dissection, pressure from the false lumen depresses one aortic leaflet below the coaptation line of the other leaflets. *C,* The annular support is disrupted, resulting in a flail aortic leaflet. *D,* Prolapse of a mobile intimal flap through the aortic valve during diastole prevents leaflet coaptation.

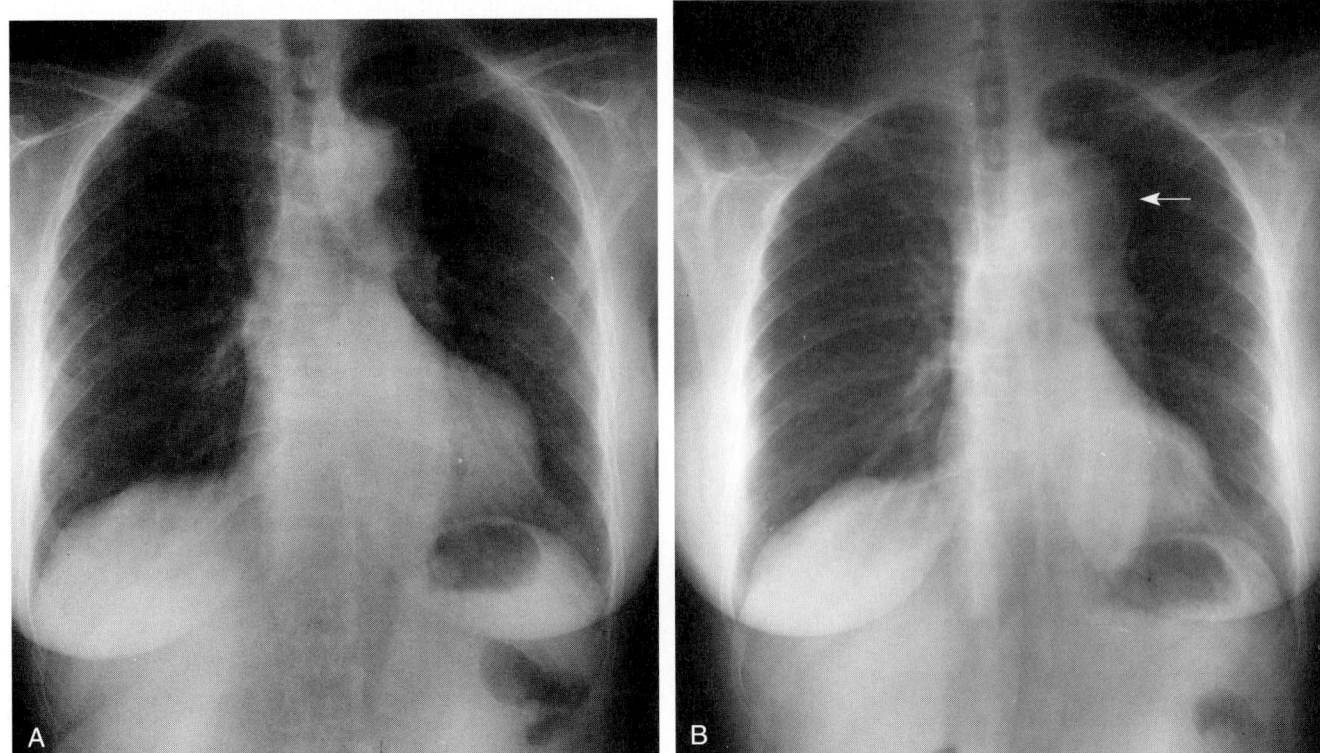

FIGURE 45–9. Chest roentgenogram of a patient with aortic dissection. *A,* The patient's baseline study from 3 years prior to admission, with a normal appearing aorta. *B,* The chest roentgenogram upon admission, which is remarkable for the interval enlargement of the aortic knob (arrow). The patient was found to have a proximal aortic dissection. (From Isselbacher, E. M., Cigarroa, J. E., and Eagle, K. A.: Aortic dissection. *In* Creager, M. (ed.): Vascular Disease. Braunwald, E. [series ed.]: Atlas of Heart Diseases, vol. 7. Philadelphia, Current Medicine, 1996.)

chest roentgenogram may first raise clinical suspicion of aortic dissection. Moreover, although chest roentgenography may help support a diagnosis of suspected aortic dissection, the findings are nonspecific and rarely diagnostic. The findings of chest roentgenography, therefore, add to the other available clinical data used in deciding if suspicion of aortic dissection warrants proceeding to a more definitive diagnostic study.

The most common abnormality seen on chest roentgenogram in aortic dissection is a widening of the aortic silhouette, appearing in 81 to 90 per cent of cases[117,130] and sometimes with a localized bulge overlying the site of origin. Less often, nonspecific widening of the superior mediastinum is seen. If calcification of the aortic knob is present, separation of the intimal calcification from the outer aortic soft tissue border by more than 1.0 cm—the "calcium sign"—is suggestive, although not diagnostic, of aortic dissection (Fig. 45–9). Comparison of the current chest roentgenogram with a previous study may reveal acute changes in the aortic or mediastinal silhouettes that would otherwise have gone unrecognized. Pleural effusions may occasionally be present, typically on the left side and more often associated with dissection involving the descending aorta. Although the majority of patients with aortic dissection have one or more of these roentgenographic abnormalities, the remainder, up to 12 per cent,[117] have chest roentgenograms that appear unremarkable. Therefore, a normal chest roentgenogram can never exclude the presence of aortic dissection.

Electrocardiographic findings in aortic dissection are nonspecific. One-third of electrocardiograms show changes consistent with left ventricular hypertrophy, and another one-third are normal in appearance. Nevertheless, obtaining an electrocardiogram is diagnostically important for two reasons: (1) in aortic dissection patients presenting with nonspecific chest pain, the absence of ischemic ST-segment and T-wave changes on electrocardiogram may argue against the diagnosis of myocardial ischemia and thereby prompt consideration of other chest pain syndromes including aortic dissection; and (2) in patients with proximal dissection, the electrocardiogram may reveal acute myocardial infarction when the dissection flap has involved a coronary artery.

Because of the variable extent of aortic, branch vessel, and cardiac involvement occurring with aortic dissection, the signs and symptoms associated with the condition occur sporadically. Consequently, the presence or absence of aortic dissection cannot be diagnosed accurately in most cases on the basis of symptoms and clinical findings alone. In the series from Spittell et al., of all aortic dissections (presenting without a known diagnosis) the initial clinical diagnosis was aortic dissection in only 62 per cent,[117] and the other 38 per cent were thought initially to have myocardial ischemia, congestive heart failure, nondissecting aneurysms of the thoracic or abdominal aorta, symptomatic aortic stenosis, pulmonary embolism, and so forth. Among this 38 per cent in whom aortic dissection went undiagnosed at presentation, nearly two-thirds had their aortic dissection detected incidentally while undergoing a diagnostic procedure for other clinical questions, and in nearly one-third the aortic dissection remained undiagnosed until necropsy.[117] Given the clinical challenge that detection of aortic dissection presents, physicians should remain vigilant for any risk factors, symptoms, and signs consistent with aortic dissection if a timely diagnosis is to be made.

Diagnostic Techniques

Once the diagnosis of aortic dissection is suspected on clinical grounds, it is essential to confirm the diagnosis both promptly and accurately.[147a] The diagnostic modalities currently available for this purpose include aortography, contrast-enhanced CT, MRI, and transthoracic or transesophageal echocardiography. Each modality has certain advantages and disadvantages with respect to diagnostic accuracy, speed, convenience, risk, and cost, but none is appropriate in all situations.

When comparing the four imaging modalities, one must begin by considering what diagnostic information is needed.[148] First and foremost, the study must confirm or refute the diagnosis of aortic dissection. Second, it must determine whether the dissection involves the ascending aorta (i.e., proximal or type A) or is confined to the descending aorta or arch (i.e., distal or type B). Third, if possible, it should identify a number of the anatomical features of the dissection, including its extent, the sites of entry and reentry, the presence of thrombus in the false lumen, branch vessel involvement by the dissection, the presence and severity of aortic regurgitation, the presence or absence of pericardial effusion, and any coronary artery involvement by the intimal flap. Unfortunately, no single imaging modality provides all of this anatomical detail. Choice of diagnostic modalities should therefore be guided by the clinical scenario and by targeting information that will best assist patient management.

AORTOGRAPHY. Retrograde aortography was the first accurate diagnostic technique for evaluating suspected aortic dissection. The diagnosis of aortic dissection is based on direct angiographic signs, including visualization of two lumens or an intimal flap (considered diagnostic), as in Figure 45–10, or indirect signs (considered suggestive), such as deformity of the aortic lumen, thickening of the aortic walls, branch vessel abnormalities, and aortic regurgitation.[149,150] Earnest et al. showed that the false lumen was visualized in 87 per cent, the intimal flap in 70 per cent, and the site of intimal tear in 56 per cent of dissections.[151]

Aortography had long been considered the diagnostic standard for the evaluation of aortic dissection because for several decades it was the only accurate method for diagnosing aortic dissection ante mortem, although its true sensitivity could not be defined. However, the recent introduction of alternative diagnostic modalities has indicated that aortography is not as sensitive as previously thought. A prospective study by Erbel et al. in 1989 found that for the diagnosis of aortic dissection the sensitivity and specificity of aortography were 88 and 95 per cent, respectively.[152] Furthermore, a recent series by Bansal et al. found that the sensitivity of aortography was only 77 per cent when the definition of aortic dissection included intramural hematoma with noncommunicating dissection[153] (see p. 1568). False-negative aortograms occur because of thrombosis of the false lumen, equal and simultaneous opacification of both the true and false lumens,[154] or the presence of an intramural hematoma.

Important advantages of aortography include its ability to delineate the extent of the aortic dissection, including branch vessel involvement (Figs. 45–11 and 45–12). It is also useful in detecting some of the major complications of aortic dissection, such as thrombus in the false lumen or the presence of aortic regurgitation (Fig. 45–11), and often in revealing the patency of the coronary arteries (Fig. 45–10). Moreover, aortography is widely available and surgeons are very comfortable with its use. In addition to the limited sensitivity of aortography, other disadvantages are the inherent risks of the invasive procedure, the risks associated with the use of contrast material, and the time in completing the study, both in assembling an angiography team and because of the procedure's long duration. Lastly, it requires that potentially unstable patients travel to the angiography suite.

COMPUTED TOMOGRAPHY. In contrast-enhanced CT scanning, aortic dissection is diagnosed by the presence of two distinct aortic lumens, either visibly separated by an inti-

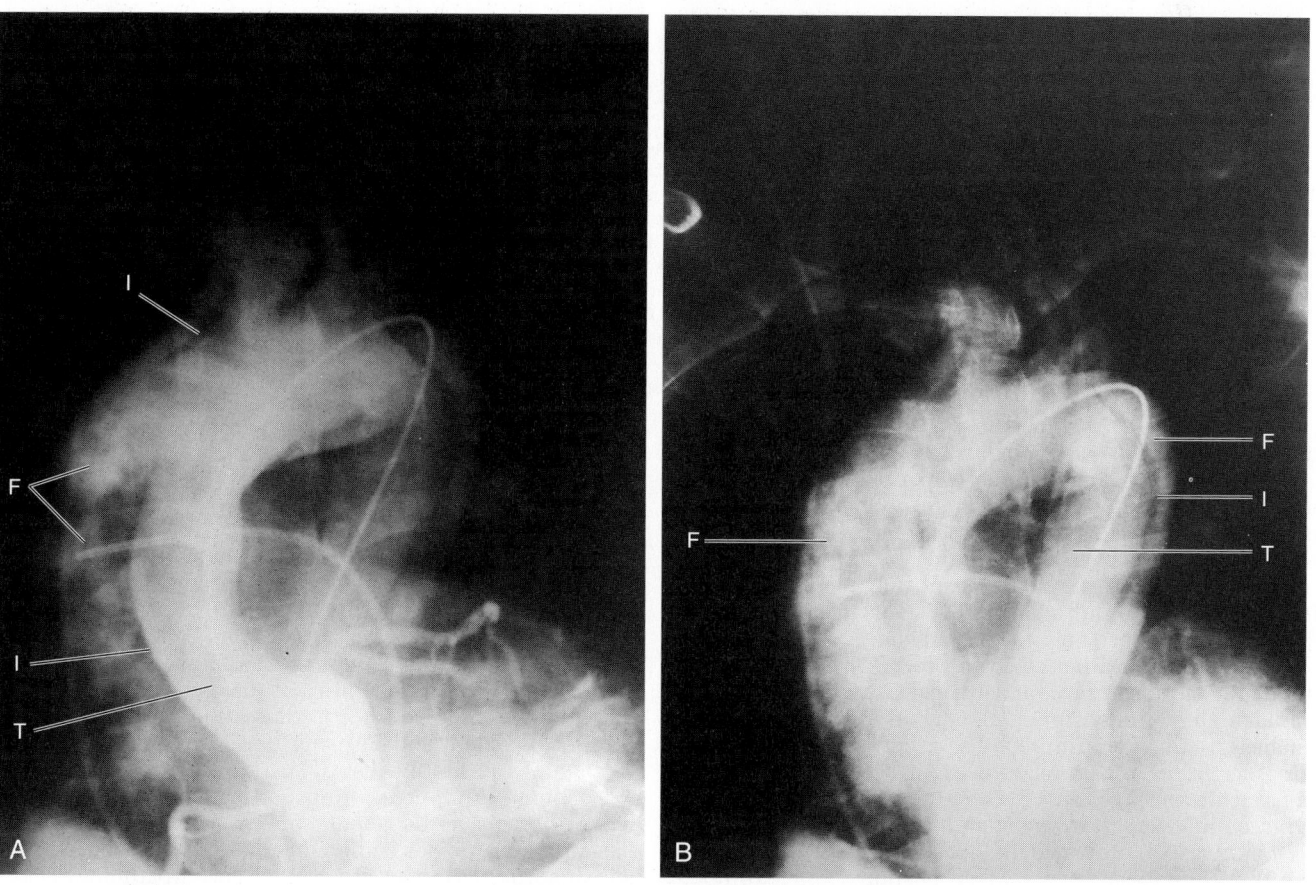

FIGURE 45–10. Thoracic aortogram in the anteroposterior view demonstrating the presence of a proximal aortic dissection. *A,* The well-opacified true lumen (T) and the poorly opacified false lumen (F) are separated by an intimal flap (I), which is visible in the ascending aorta as a thin radiolucent line within the aorta. Additionally, the proximal portions of both coronary arteries are well visualized. *B,* In a subsequent aortographic exposure, the false lumen has filled-in late and the intimal flap is now clearly visible as it courses distally down the descending aorta. (*A* from Cigarroa, J. E., Isselbacher, E. M., DeSanctis, R. W., and Eagle, K. A.: Diagnostic imaging in the evaluation of suspected aortic dissection: Old standards and new directions. N. Engl. J. Med. *328:*35, 1993. *B* from Isselbacher, E. M., Cigarroa, J. E., and Eagle, K. A.: Aortic dissection. *In* Creager, M. (ed.): Vascular Disease. Braunwald, E. [series ed.]: Atlas of Heart Diseases, vol. 7. Philadelphia, Current Medicine, 1996.)

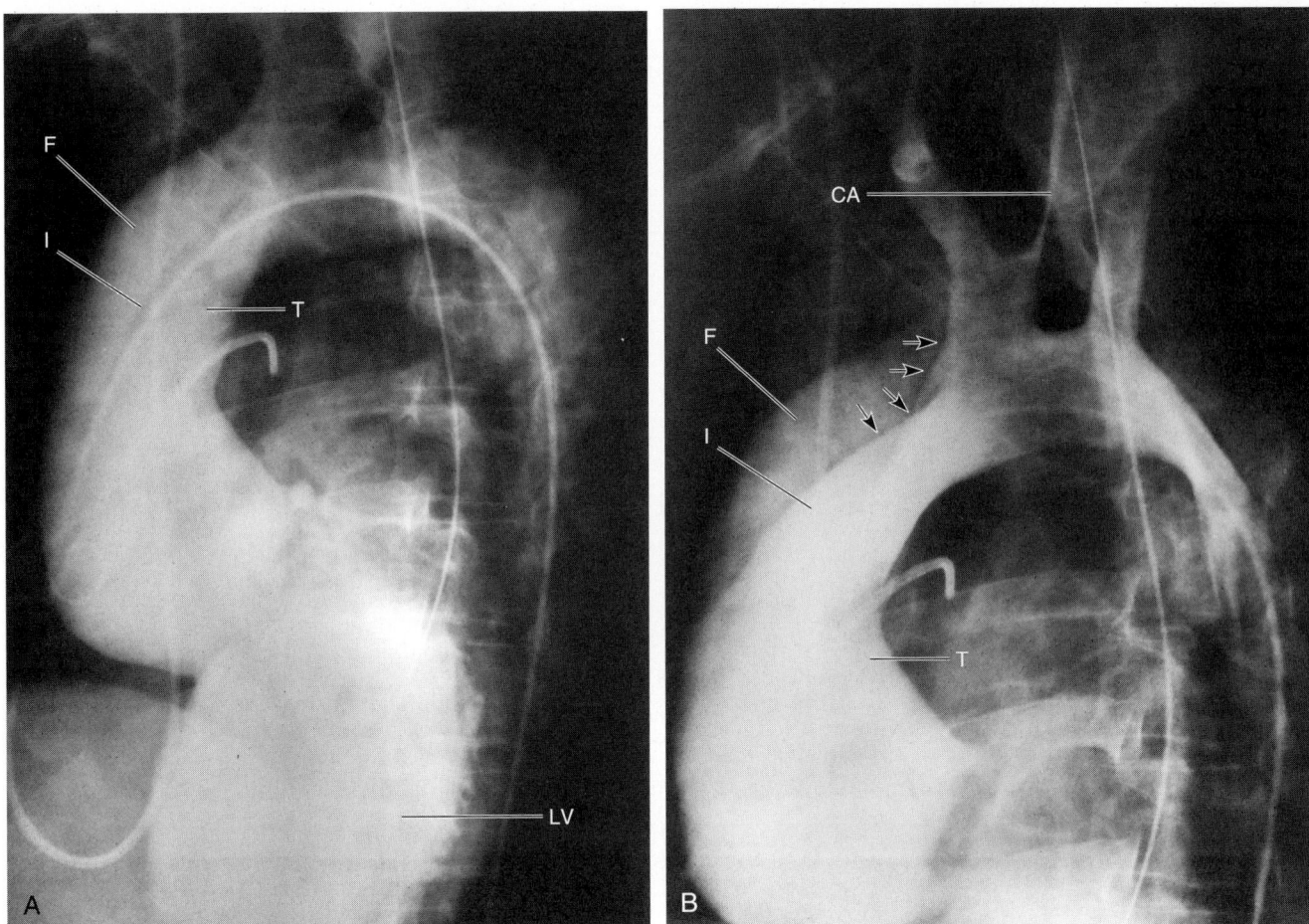

FIGURE 45–11. Aortogram in the left oblique view demonstrating a proximal aortic dissection and its associated cardiovascular complications. *A*, The aortic root is dilated. The true lumen (T) and false lumen (F) are separated by the intimal flap (I), which is faintly visible as a radiolucent line following the contour of the pigtail catheter. The abundance of contrast in the left ventricle (LV) is indicative of significant aortic insufficiency (see Fig. 45–8). *B*, The true lumen is better opacified than the false lumen and two planes of the intimal flap can now be distinguished (arrows). The branch vessels are opacified and there is marked narrowing of the right carotid artery (CA), suggesting that its lumen is compromised by the dissection. (*A* from Cigarroa, J. E., Isselbacher, E. M., DeSanctis, R. W., and Eagle, K. A.: Diagnostic imaging in the evaluation of suspected aortic dissection: Old standards and new directions. N. Engl. J. Med. *328:35*, 1993. *B* from Isselbacher, E. M., Cigarroa, J. E., and Eagle, K. A.: Aortic dissection. *In* Creager, M. (ed.): Vascular Disease. Braunwald, E. [series ed.]: Atlas of Heart Diseases, vol. 7. Philadelphia, Current Medicine, 1996.)

mal flap (Fig. 45–13) or distinguished by a differential rate of contrast opacification. Indirect signs of aortic dissection may also be evident.[148] In two large prospective series of patients with suspected aortic dissection, Erbel et al.[152] found contrast-enhanced CT scanning to have a sensitivity of 83 per cent with a specificity of 100 per cent, while Nienaber et al.[155] found a sensitivity of 94 per cent with a specificity of 87 per cent. Recent advances, such as ultrafast CT scanning with an electron beam,[156] which provides superior image resolution, and helical CT scanning, which permits a three-dimensional display of the aorta and its branches,[38] will likely improve the accuracy of CT in diagnosing aortic dissection as well as in better defining anatomical features.[157]

CT scanning has the advantage that, unlike aortography, it is noninvasive. However, it does require the use of an intravenous contrast agent. Most hospitals are equipped with a readily accessible CT scanner, available on an emergency basis. CT is also helpful in identifying the presence of thrombus in the false lumen and detecting the presence of a pericardial effusion. A disadvantage of CT scanning is that its sensitivity for aortic dissection is lower than that for other available modalities. Moreover, an intimal flap is identified in only two-thirds of cases, and the site of intimal tear is rarely identified.[158] CT scanning also cannot

reliably detect the presence of aortic regurgitation or involvement of the branch vessels.

MAGNETIC RESONANCE IMAGING. The use of MRI has particular appeal for diagnosing aortic dissection in that it is entirely noninvasive and does not require the use of intravenous contrast material or ionizing radiation. Furthermore, MRI produces high-quality images in the transverse, sagittal, and coronal planes, as well as in a left anterior oblique view that displays the entire thoracic aorta in one plane (Fig. 45–14). The availability of these multiple views facilitates the diagnosis of aortic dissection and the determination of its extent and in many cases reveals the presence of branch vessel involvement. MRI is ideal for the evaluation of patients with preexisting aortic disease, such as those with thoracic aortic aneurysms or prior aortic-graft repair because it provides sufficient anatomical detail to distinguish aortic dissection from other aortic pathology.[139]

In the series by Nienaber et al.,[155] MRI was used to evaluate 105 patients with suspected aortic dissection and was found to have both a sensitivity and specificity of 98 per cent, consistent with previous findings.[159,160] MRI had a sensitivity of 88 per cent for identifying the site of intimal tear, 98 per cent for the presence of thrombus, and 100 per cent for the presence of a pericardial effusion. Furthermore, the use of the cine-MRI technique in a subset of these

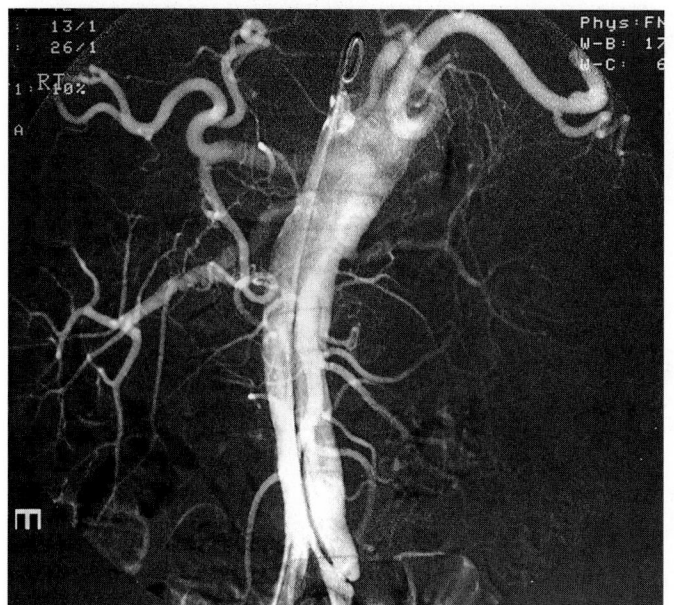

FIGURE 45–12. Digital subtraction angiogram of the abdominal aorta to assess the status of renal perfusion in a patient with a distal thoracic aortic dissection. This study confirmed the presence of an intimal flap extending down into the left common iliac artery. The celiac axis, superior mesenteric artery, and right renal artery are widely patent and fill from the true lumen. The left renal artery fills from the false lumen, with the intimal flap involving the ostium of the artery and impairing distal flow. As a consequence there is minimal contrast excretion by the left kidney compared with the right.

patients showed an 85 per cent sensitivity for detecting aortic regurgitation.

The remarkably high accuracy of MRI has made it the current gold standard for diagnosing the presence or absence of aortic dissection. Still, MRI does have a number of disadvantages. It is contraindicated in patients with pacemakers, certain types of vascular clips, and certain older types of metallic prosthetic heart valves.[161] MRI provides only limited images of the branch vessels and does not consistently identify the presence of aortic regurgitation. MR scanners are not available in many hospitals and, when present, may not be readily available on an emergency basis. Many patients with aortic dissection are hemodynamically unstable, often intubated or receiving intrave-

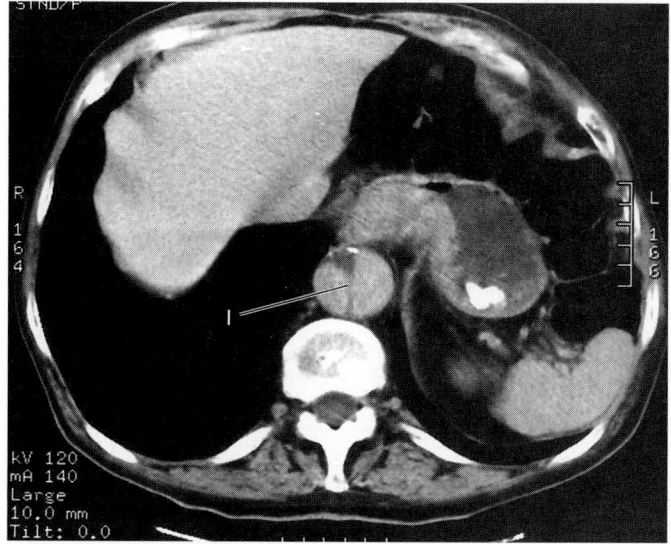

FIGURE 45–13. Contrast-enhanced CT scan of the chest at the level of the diaphragm showing an intimal flap (I) separating the two lumens of an aortic dissection of the descending thoracic aorta.

nous antihypertensive medications with arterial pressure monitoring, but the MR scanners limit the presence of many monitoring and support devices in the imaging suite and also limit patient accessibility during the lengthy study. Understandably, concern for the safety of unstable patients has led many physicians to conclude that the use of MRI is relatively contraindicated for unstable patients. Notably, despite such concerns, in the studies by Nienaber et al.[155,159] no complications occurred among their unstable aortic dissection patients during the performance of MRI.

ECHOCARDIOGRAPHY. Echocardiography is well suited for the evaluation of patients with suspected aortic dissection because it is readily available in most hospitals and is noninvasive and quick to perform, and the full examination can be completed at the bedside. The echocardiographic finding considered diagnostic of an aortic dissection is the presence of an undulating intimal flap within the aortic lumen separating true and false channels. Reverberations and other artifacts can cause linear echodensities within the aortic lumen that mimic aortic dissection; to definitively distinguish an intimal flap from such artifacts, the flap should be identified in more than one view, it should have a motion independent of that of the aortic walls or other cardiac structures, and there should be a differential in color Doppler flow patterns between the two lumens. In cases in which the false lumen is thrombosed, displacement of intimal calcification[152] or thickening of the aortic wall may suggest aortic dissection.

Transthoracic Echocardiography. This technique has a sensitivity of 59 to 85 per cent and specificity of 63 to 96 per cent for the diagnosis of aortic dissection. Its sensitivity is as high as 78 to 100 per cent for dissections involving the ascending aorta but drops to only 31 to 55 per cent for dissections of the descending aorta.[148] Such poor sensitivity, especially in the case of distal dissections, significantly limits the general utility of this technique. Furthermore, image quality is often adversely affected by obesity, emphysema, mechanical ventilation, or small intercostal spaces.

Transesophageal Echocardiography. The proximity of the esophagus to the aorta enables TEE to overcome many of the limitations of transthoracic imaging and permits the use of higher frequency ultrasonography, which provides better anatomical detail (Fig. 45–15). The examination is generally performed at the bedside with the patient under sedation or light general anesthesia and typically requires 10 to 15 minutes to complete.[162,163] The procedure is relatively noninvasive and requires no intravenous contrast or ionizing radiation. Relative contraindications include known esophageal disease (strictures, tumors, and varices), and the required esophageal intubation may not be tolerated in up to 3 per cent of patients. The incidence of important side effects (such as hypertension, bradycardia, bronchospasm, or, rarely, esophageal perforation) is much less than 1 per cent.[163] One important disadvantage of TEE is its limited ability to visualize the distal ascending aorta and proximal arch owing to the interposition of the air-filled trachea and left mainstem bronchus. Although the use of biplane and multiplane probes has helped reduce this problem, a blind spot persists in the proximal aortic arch.[164]

The results of large prospective studies by Erbel et al.[152] and Nienaber et al.[155] demonstrated that the sensitivity of TEE for aortic dissection is 98 to 99 per cent. The sensitivity for detecting an intimal tear was 73 per cent (Fig. 45–16) and for the presence of thrombus in the false lumen, 68 per cent.[155] Furthermore, TEE detected both aortic regurgitation and pericardial effusion in 100 per cent.[155] The specificity of TEE for the diagnosis of aortic dissection is less well defined. Although Erbel et al. found the specificity to be as high as 97 per cent,[152] Nienaber et al. found it to be 77 per cent.[155] However, in the latter study the early inexperience of those performing the examinations and the use of monoplane transducers may have contributed to the incidence of false positives.

Several methods have been suggested to reduce the possibility of false-positive diagnosis by TEE,[148] including the use of biplane or mul-

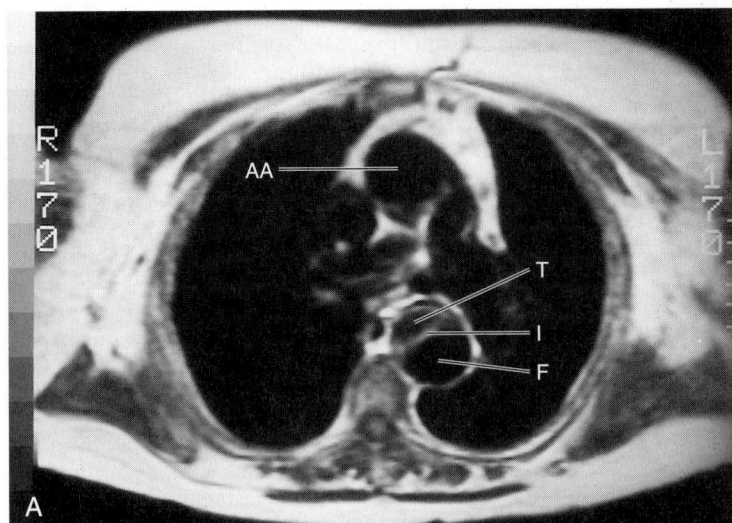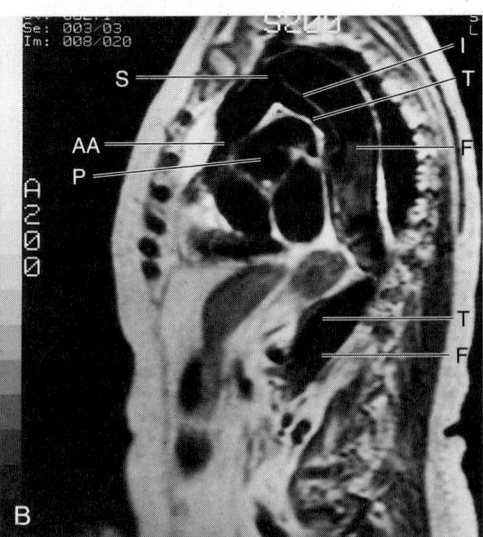

FIGURE 45–14. Magnetic resonance images in two planes in a patient with a distal aortic dissection. *A*, This image in the transverse plane through the upper thorax at the level of the pulmonary artery shows an intact ascending aorta (AA), but in the descending aorta reveals an intimal flap (I) separating the true (T) and false (F) lumens. *B*, This image in the sagittal plane of the aorta shows the site of intimal tear (S) together with the intimal flap (I), which begins just distal to the take-off of the left subclavian artery and spirals distally along the descending aorta. The true (T) and false (F) lumens are identified in both the descending thoracic aorta above as well as in the abdominal aorta below. The ascending aorta (AA) is uninvolved by the dissection. Also seen here is the pulmonary artery (P) at its bifurcation. Notice that in both views the false lumen originates posteriorly and is wider than the true lumen. This pattern is quite typical in distal aortic dissections. (From Isselbacher, E. M., Cigarroa, J. E., and Eagle, K. A.: Aortic dissection. *In* Creager, M. (ed.): Vascular Disease. Braunwald, E. [series ed.]: Atlas of Heart Diseases. Philadelphia, Current Medicine, 1996.)

tiplane ultrasound transducers and confirmation of two lumens by the demonstration of differential color flow patterns (Fig. 45–17). We have proposed[148] that if, in addition to an intimal flap, confirmatory evidence of at least one other echocardiographic feature of aortic dissection is identified, the aortic dissection may be called "definite." If an intimal flap alone is seen (i.e., one that is not considered an artifact) with no other supporting evidence, the diagnosis of dissection should not be considered definitive, and examination with another imaging modality should be sought to exclude the possibility of a false positive. If this conservative approach were applied to the echocardiographic interpretations in the study by Nienaber et al.,[155] the specificity of "definite" aortic dissection would have been 100 per cent.[148]

In addition to its high sensitivity for detecting aortic dissection, TEE may provide other important information useful to the surgeon. Some surgeons wish to know preoperatively if the intimal flap involves the ostia of the coronary arteries, but this determination has traditionally required the performance of coronary angiography.[165]

Ballal et al.[166] performed TEE on 34 patients with aortic dissection, seven of whom had coronary artery involvement confirmed at surgery. In six of these seven patients, TEE identified the intimal flap extending into the coronary ostia. However, TEE delineates only the very proximal portions of the coronary arteries so when the assessment of coronary atherosclerosis is necessary, coronary angiography is still required (see below).

Among patients presenting with suspected aortic dissection, the diagnosis is excluded in 42 to 68 per cent,[159,167,168] yielding a group of patients with a chest pain syndrome of unknown etiology. Granato et al.[168] found that transthoracic echocardiography was helpful in establishing an alternative cause of chest pain in 42 per cent of these cases, by identifying cardiac abnormalities such as left ventricular wall motion abnormalities, aortic stenosis, the presence of pericardial effusion or cardiac tamponade. More recently, Chan[169] found that among patients found not to have dissection, TEE detected other aortic abnormalities in 73 per cent and evidence of acute myocardial infarction or ischemia in 23 per cent.

INTRAVASCULAR ULTRASONOGRAPHY. One of the most recent developments in the echocardiographic evaluation of aortic dissection has been the utilization of intravascular ultrasonography to define the detailed anatomy of the involved aorta and determine the extent of dissection. The intravascular ultrasound catheter is inserted through an introducer in the femoral artery and positioned within the aortic lumen under fluoroscopic guidance. The aorta is then imaged in a transverse plane through its short axis, allowing visualization of the two lumens and the intimal flap.

The most extensive assessment of this technique to date was reported by Yamada et al.,[170] who studied 15 patients with previously known chronic aortic dissection and compared the findings of intravascular ultrasonography with those of other established imaging modalities. Intravascular ultrasonography accurately detected the intimal flap in all segments of the aorta, although it was poor at detecting the sites of intimal tear in the thoracic aorta, probably due to vessel curvature. However, intravascular ultrasonography was quite useful in the evaluation of the abdominal aorta: It demonstrated the origins of the renal arteries and the distal extent of dissection in all cases and identified the site of intimal tear of the abdominal aorta in 78 per cent of cases. Accurate assessment of the abdominal aorta

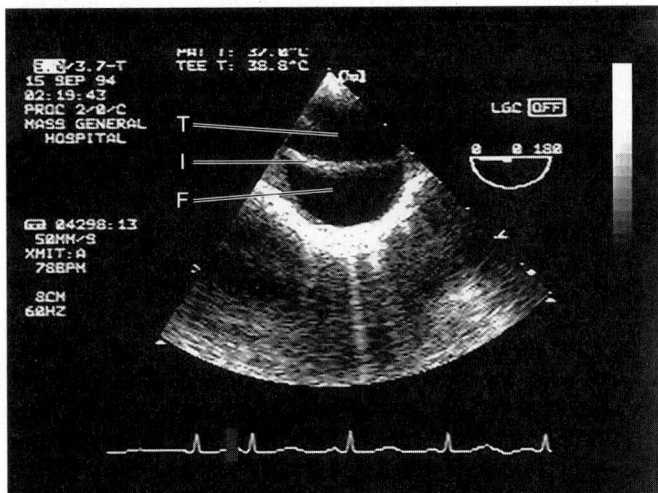

FIGURE 45–15. A cross-sectional transesophageal echocardiogram of the descending thoracic aorta demonstrating an aortic dissection. The aorta is dilated. Evident is an intimal flap (I) dividing the true lumen (T) anteriorly and the false lumen (F) posteriorly. The true lumen fills during systole and therefore is seen bowing slightly into the false lumen in this systolic image.

FIGURE 45–16. See color plate 10.

FIGURE 45–17. See color plate 11.

with this technique may have particular relevance given the inability of TEE to image this portion of the aorta. Furthermore, intravascular ultrasonography may play an important role in the positioning and deployment of endovascular stenting devices[171] (see below). Nevertheless, the potential future role of intravascular ultrasonography in both the evaluation and management of patients with aortic dissection requires further study.

Selecting an Imaging Modality

Each of the four imaging modalities has particular advantages and disadvantages. In selecting among them, one must consider the accuracy as well as the safety and availability of each test. MRI and TEE are the most sensitive of the four studies, but given its unsurpassed specificity, MRI is considered by most to be the present gold standard for evaluating aortic dissection. The four modalities differ in their ability to detect the complications associated with dissection, so the specific diagnostic information sought by the treating physician and/or surgeon should bear upon the procedure chosen. A summary of the diagnostic performance of each of the four imaging modalities is presented in Table 45–2.

Both the accessibility of imaging studies and the time required to complete them are key considerations given the high early mortality of unoperated proximal aortic dissection. Aortography can rarely be performed on an emergency basis, requiring the assembly of an angiography team at night, and carries the risks of an invasive procedure and the use of a contrast agent. MRI, although optimal in its accuracy, is also generally unavailable on an emergency basis and poses the risks of limited patient monitoring and accessibility during the lengthy procedure. CT scanning is more readily available in most emergency rooms and is quickly completed. TEE is also readily available in most larger centers and can be completed quickly at the bedside, making it ideal for evaluating unstable patients. The practical assessment of the four imaging modalities is summarized in Table 45–3.

In the setting in which all of these imaging modalities are available, we believe that TEE should be considered first in the evaluation of suspected aortic dissection, in light of its accuracy, safety, speed, and convenience. In many institutions TEE has indeed become the procedure of choice,[172] with surgeons taking patients to the operating room on the basis of the echocardiographic findings alone.[173,174] In institutions where TEE is not readily available, CT scanning instead serves as an effective screening test for aortic dissection. However, if the diagnosis of aortic dissection is confirmed by CT, after patient transfer to a tertiary care center an additional diagnostic study may be

TABLE 45–2 DIAGNOSTIC PERFORMANCE OF IMAGING MODALITIES IN THE EVALUATION OF SUSPECTED AORTIC DISSECTION

DIAGNOSTIC PERFORMANCE	ANGIO	CT	MRI	TEE
Sensitivity	++	++	+++	+++
Specificity	+++	+++	+++	++/+++
Site of intimal tear	++	+	+++	++
Presence of thrombus	+++	++	+++	+
Presence of aortic insufficiency	+++	−	+	+++
Pericardial effusion	−	++	+++	+++
Branch vessel involvement	+++	+	++	+
Coronary artery involvement	++	−	−	++

Key: +++ excellent, ++ good, + fair, − not detected. Angio = angiography; CT = computed tomography; MRI = magnetic resonance imaging; TEE = transesophageal echocardiography.

Modified from Cigarroa, J.E., Isselbacher, E.M., DeSanctis, R.W., and Eagle, K.A.: Diagnostic imaging in the evaluation of suspected aortic dissection: Old standards and new directions. N. Engl. J. Med. *328*:35, 1993. Copyright by the Massachusetts Medical Society.

TABLE 45–3 PRACTICAL ASSESSMENT OF IMAGING MODALITIES IN THE EVALUATION OF SUSPECTED AORTIC DISSECTION

ADVANTAGES OF STUDY	ANGIO	CT	MRI	TEE
Readily available	Fairly	Quite	Fairly	Very
Quickly performed	Fairly	Quite	Fairly	Very
Performed at bedside	No	No	No	Yes
Noninvasive	No	Yes	Yes	Yes
IV contrast	Yes	Yes	No	No
Cost	High	Reasonable	Moderate	Reasonable

Angio = angiography; CT = computed tomography; MRI = magnetic resonance imaging; TEE = transesophageal echocardiography.

Modified from Cigarroa, J. E., Isselbacher, E. M., DeSanctis, R. W., and Eagle, K. A.: Diagnostic imaging in the evaluation of suspected aortic dissection: Old standards and new directions. N. Engl. J. Med. *328*:35, 1993. Copyright by the Massachusetts Medical Society.

required to more completely define the aortic anatomy prior to surgery. However, in such instances, the patient may be taken directly to the operating room, where a TEE can then be performed to confirm the diagnosis and better define the dissection anatomy without unduly delaying surgery.[173]

Although MRI is less practical than other modalities for the assessment of suspected acute aortic dissection, it is nonetheless well suited for stable or chronic dissections. Given its extraordinary accuracy and its high-quality detailed images, we recommend the use of MRI for following patients with aortic dissection, whether treated medically or surgically, as a means of identifying subsequent aneurysm formation, extension of the dissection, or other complications.

Despite its relative disadvantages, aortography still plays an important role when clear definition of the anatomy of the branch vessels is essential for management. The performance of aortography should also be considered when a definitive diagnosis is not made by one or more of the other imaging modalities.

In the final analysis, each institution must determine its own best diagnostic approach in the evaluation of suspected aortic dissection based on available human and material resources and the speed with which such resources can be mobilized. It must be emphasized that regardless of which of the four imaging modalities are available at a given institution, the levels of skill and experience of those who carry out each diagnostic procedure must, with good reason, also be considerations in deciding the study of choice.

The Role of Coronary Angiography

The importance of assessing the status of coronary artery patency prior to surgical repair of acute aortic dissection continues to be controversial. Some surgeons believe that obtaining this information prior to surgery is essential, whereas others are content to assess the coronaries intraoperatively. Two types of coronary artery involvement must be considered in the setting of aortic dissection. The first is acute proximal coronary narrowing or occlusion as a result of the dissection itself, often due to occlusion of the coronary ostia by the intimal flap. The second is the possible presence of chronic atherosclerotic coronary artery disease which, although generally independent of the dissection process, may complicate its surgical management.

In some cases, coronary involvement by the intimal flap is self-evident if the electrocardiogram shows evidence of acute myocardial ischemia or infarction. However, should this acute process not be clinically evident, TEE can effectively define the patency of the proximal coronaries in a majority of cases.[166] Aortography may also reveal such coronary artery involvement. A more comprehensive evaluation requires the performance of coronary angiography; however, this may be risky in patients with aortic dissection and often prolongs the time to aortic repair by several hours. Moreover, catheterization of the coronary arteries is sometimes unsuccessful in patients with proximal dissections and a dilated root, in which case the added procedural delay gains no potential benefit. In addition, such proximal coronary obstructions can usually be readily identified at the time of surgery.

Chronic coronary artery disease is seen in about one-quarter of patients presenting with aortic dissection. Identifying the presence of this underlying coronary disease is beyond the capability of any of the four imaging modalities discussed above. Furthermore, accurately defining such atherosclerotic disease intraoperatively is challenging, although Rizzo et al. have suggested the use of probing the proximal coronaries, epicardial palpation, and angioscopy as possible means to identify coronary stenoses.[173]

The impact of unrecognized coronary artery disease on outcome is not certain. In a 10-year review examining 54 patients undergoing urgent aortic repair, Kern et al. found that only 1 of 27 patients with a proximal dissection had a perioperative myocardial infarction; this patient had a prior history of coronary artery disease.[165] In addition, Rizzo et al. observed that of those patients in whom unrecognized coronary artery disease was discovered at autopsy, none died of coronary ischemia but several died of aortic rupture.[173] Accordingly, we and others[165] recommend avoiding preoperative coronary angiography unless a specific indication exists, such as a known history of coronary artery disease or the presence of ischemic electrocardiographic changes. Conversely, Creswell et al. report good outcomes when performing combined aortic repair and coronary artery bypass grafting in patients with underlying coronary artery disease, and therefore argue that all stable patients with acute proximal dissection should undergo preoperative coronary angiography.[175] While the debate continues unresolved, the trend in the literature has been a retreat from the routine performance of coronary angiography in acute aortic dissection.

Management

Therapy for aortic dissection is directed at halting the progression of the dissecting hematoma because lethal complications arise not from the intimal tear itself, but rather from the subsequent course taken by the dissecting aorta, e.g., vascular compromise or aortic rupture.[147a] Without treatment, aortic dissection has a high mortality. In a collective review of long-term survival in untreated aortic dissection, more than one-fourth of all patients died within the first 24 hours following onset of dissection, more than one-half died within the first week, more than three-fourths died within 1 month, and more than 90 per cent died within 1 year.[176]

The first surgical approach to aortic dissection was a fenestration procedure in which the dissected aorta was incised and a distal communication created between the true and false channels, thereby decompressing the false lumen.[177] This procedure is, in fact, still used by some surgeons in selected cases of dissection involving the descending aorta to relieve limb, renal, or mesenteric ischemia.[178] Definitive surgical therapy was pioneered by DeBakey et al. in the early 1950's.[179] Its purpose is to excise the intimal tear, obliterate the false channel by oversewing the aortic edges, reconstruct the aorta directly or with the interposition of a synthetic graft, and, in the case of proximal dissection, restore aortic valve competence either by resuspension of the displaced aortic leaflets or by prosthetic aortic valve replacement.

Aggressive medical treatment of aortic dissection was first advocated by Wheat et al.[180] They established the two primary goals for pharmacological therapy as reduction of systolic blood pressure and diminution of the force of left ventricular ejection (dP/dt). This force is thought to be a major stress acting upon the aortic wall, contributing to both the genesis and subsequent propagation of aortic dissection. Originally introduced for patients too ill to withstand surgery, medical therapy is now the initial treatment for virtually all patients with aortic dissection prior to definitive diagnosis and fur-

thermore serves as the primary long-term therapy in a subset of patients, particularly those with distal dissections.

Immediate Medical Management

All patients in whom there is a strong suspicion of acute aortic dissection should immediately be placed in an acute care setting for hemodynamic stabilization and monitoring of blood pressure, cardiac rhythm, and urine output. Two large bore intravenous catheters should be inserted, to be used for intravenous medications and fluid resuscitation if necessary. An arterial line should be placed, preferably in the right arm so that it remains functional during surgery when the aorta is cross-clamped. However, in cases in which the blood pressure is significantly greater on the left than on the right, the arterial line should be placed on the left. In those with a lower likelihood of dissection who are hemodynamically stable, a automatic blood pressure cuff should suffice.

A central venous line or pulmonary arterial line should be considered in patients with hypotension or congestive heart failure, in order to monitor central venous pressure or pulmonary artery wedge pressure and cardiac output. Femoral lines and blood gases should be avoided if possible, in order to conserve these sites for bypass cannulation during a potential aortic repair. If a femoral line must be placed emergently, the opposite groin site should be protected from needle punctures.

BLOOD PRESSURE REDUCTION. Initial therapeutic goals include the elimination of pain and the reduction of systolic blood pressure to 100 to 120 mm Hg (mean 60 to 75 mm Hg), or to the lowest level commensurate with adequate vital organ (cardiac, cerebral, renal) perfusion. Simultaneously, arterial dP/dt, reflecting the force of left ventricular ejection, should be reduced through the use of beta blockade, regardless of whether pain or systolic hypertension is present. The use of long-acting medications should be avoided in patients who are surgical candidates, as this may complicate intraoperative arterial pressure management. Pain, which may itself exacerbate hypertension and tachycardia, should be promptly treated with intravenous morphine sulfate.

For the acute reduction of arterial pressure, the potent vasodilator sodium nitroprusside is very effective. It is initially infused at 20 μg/min with dosage titrated upward, as high as 800 μg/min, according to blood pressure response. When used alone, however, sodium nitroprusside can actually cause an increase in dP/dt, which in turn may potentially contribute to the propagation of the dissection. Therefore, when this drug is used the concomitant administration of adequate beta blockade is essential.

To reduce dP/dt acutely, an intravenous beta blocker should be administered in incremental doses until there is evidence of satisfactory beta blockade, usually indicated by a heart rate of 60 to 80 beats/min in the acute setting. Because propranolol was the first generally available beta blocker, it has been used most widely in treating aortic dissection. However, it is believed that other beta blockers are equally effective. Propranolol should be administered in intravenous doses of 1 mg every 3 to 5 minutes until the desired effect is achieved, although the maximum initial dose should not exceed 0.15 mg/kg (or approximately 10 mg). In order to maintain adequate beta blockade, as evidenced by heart rate, additional propranolol should be given intravenously every 4 to 6 hours, usually in doses somewhat lower than the total initial dose, i.e., 2 to 6 mg.

Labetalol, which acts as both an alpha- and beta-adrenergic receptor blocker, may be especially useful in the setting of aortic dissection[181] because it effectively lowers both dP/dt and arterial pressure. The initial dose of labetalol is 10 mg, administered intravenously over 2 minutes, followed by additional doses of 20 to 80 mg every 10 to 15 minutes (up to a maximum total dose of 300 mg) until heart rate and blood pressure have been controlled. Maintenance dosing may then be achieved with a continuous intravenous infusion, starting at 2 mg/min and titrating up to 5 to 20 mg/min.

The ultra–short-acting beta blocker esmolol may be particularly useful in patients with labile arterial pressure, especially if surgery is planned, as it can be abruptly discontinued if necessary.[182] It is administered as a 30-mg intravenous bolus followed by continuous infusion at 3 mg/min and titrated up to 12 mg/min. Esmolol may also be useful as a means to test beta blocker safety and tolerance in patients with a history of obstructive pulmonary disease who may be at uncertain risk for bronchospasm from beta blockade. In such patients, a cardioselective beta blocker, such as atenolol or metoprolol, may be considered.

When contraindications exist to the use of beta blockers —including sinus bradycardia, second- or third-degree atrioventricular block, congestive heart failure, or bronchospasm—other agents to reduce arterial pressure and dP/dt should be considered. Calcium channel antagonists, proven effective in managing hypertensive crisis,[183] are now used with increasing frequency in the treatment of aortic dissection. Sublingual nifedipine, successfully used in treating refractory hypertension associated with aortic dissection,[184] can be given immediately while other medications are being prepared. A key limitation of nifedipine, however, is that it has little negative chronotropic or inotropic effect. In contrast, the combined vasodilator and negative inotropic effects of both diltiazem and verapamil make these agents well suited for the treatment of aortic dissection. Moreover, both of these agents may be administered intravenously.

Refractory hypertension may result when a dissection flap compromises one or both of the renal arteries, thereby causing the release of large amounts of renin. In this situation the most efficacious antihypertensive may be the intravenous angiotensin-converting enzyme (ACE) inhibitor enalaprilat, which is administered initially in doses of 0.625 mg every 4 to 6 hours and then titrated upward.

If patients are normotensive rather than hypertensive on presentation, beta blockers may be used alone to reduce dP/dt or, if contraindicated, diltiazem or verapamil are alternatives.

In the event that the patient with suspected aortic dissection presents with significant hypotension, rapid volume expansion should be considered, given the possible presence of cardiac tamponade or aortic rupture. Before initiating aggressive treatment of such hypotension, however, the possibility of pseudohypotension, which occurs when the arterial pressure is being measured in an extremity whose circulation is selectively compromised by the dissection, should be carefully excluded. If vasopressors are absolutely required for refractory hypotension, norepinephrine (Levophed) or phenylephrine (Neo-Synephrine) are preferred. Dopamine should be reserved for improving renal perfusion and used only at very low doses, given that it may raise dP/dt.

Once appropriate medical therapy has been initiated and the patient sufficiently stabilized, a definitive diagnostic study should be promptly undertaken. If a patient remains unstable, a TEE is preferred because it can be performed at the bedside in the emergency department or intensive care unit, allowing both monitoring and therapeutic intervention to continue uninterrupted. When a patient with a strongly suspected dissection becomes extremely unstable, there is likely to be aortic rupture or cardiac tamponade and the patient should go directly to the operating room rather than delaying surgery for diagnostic imaging. In such situations an intraoperative TEE can be used both to confirm the diagnosis and to guide surgical repair.

MANAGEMENT OF CARDIAC TAMPONADE. Cardiac tamponade frequently complicates acute proximal aortic dissection and is one of the most common mechanisms of death in these patients. It is often the cause of hypotension when

patients present with aortic dissection, and pericardiocentesis is commonly performed in this setting in an effort to stabilize patients while they await definitive surgical repair. However, in a retrospective series we found that pericardiocentesis may be harmful rather than beneficial in this setting, as it may precipitate hemodynamic collapse and death rather than stabilize the patient as intended.[185] Seven patients in this series were relatively stable at presentation (six hypotensive, one normotensive). Three of four who underwent successful pericardiocentesis died suddenly, secondary to acute electromechanical dissociation, between 5 and 40 minutes following the procedure. In contrast, none of the three patients without pericardiocentesis died prior to surgery. It may be that, in such patients, the increase in intraaortic pressure which follows pericardiocentesis causes a closed communication between the false lumen and pericardial space to reopen, leading to recurrent hemorrhage and lethal cardiac tamponade.

Therefore, when a patient with acute aortic dissection complicated by cardiac tamponade is relatively stable, the risks of pericardiocentesis likely outweigh the benefits and *every effort should be made to proceed as urgently as possible to the operating room for direct surgical repair of the aorta with intraoperative drainage of the hemopericardium.* However, when patients present with electromechanical dissociation or marked hypotension, an attempt to resuscitate the patient with pericardiocentesis is warranted. A prudent strategy in such cases might be to aspirate only enough pericardial fluid to raise blood pressure to the lowest acceptable level.[185]

Definitive Therapy

Despite minor variations from center to center, a reasonable consensus as to the definitive therapy of aortic dissection has evolved over the past several decades. It is universally agreed that surgical therapy is superior to medical therapy for acute proximal dissection.[186,187] With even limited progression of a proximal dissection, patients may suffer the potentially devastating consequences of aortic rupture or cardiac tamponade, acute aortic regurgitation, or neurological compromise. Thus, by controlling this risk, immediate surgical repair promises a better outcome. Occasional patients with proximal dissection who refuse surgery or for whom surgery is contraindicated (e.g., by age or prior debilitating illness) may potentially be treated successfully with medical therapy.[131,187]

Patients suffering acute distal aortic dissection, on the other hand, are generally at lower risk for early death from complications of the dissection than are those with proximal dissection.[131] Furthermore, as patients with distal dissection tend to be older and have a relatively increased prevalence of advanced atherosclerosis or cardiopulmonary disease, their surgical risk is often considerably higher. Early reports showed medical therapy to be as effective as surgery in this group,[115,131] and accordingly many centers advocated treating distal dissections medically. Nevertheless, agreement on this principle was not unanimous. Some investigators, reporting progressive improvement in surgical mortality, advocated surgical treatment of all dissections— both proximal and distal.[188] The debate was perpetuated by the notable absence of controlled prospective data on therapy and outcome. More recently, however, a large retrospective series involving patients from both Duke and Stanford Universities has, using multivariate analysis, suggested that medical therapy does provide an outcome equivalent to surgical therapy in patients with uncomplicated distal dissection.[189] As a consequence, medical therapy for such patients is currently favored by most groups. An important exception is that when a distal dissection is complicated by rupture, expansion, saccular aneurysm formation, vital organ or limb ischemia, or continued pain, the results of medical therapy are poor and surgery is therefore recommended.[178,187] Surgical therapy is also rec-

TABLE 45–4   INDICATIONS FOR DEFINITIVE SURGICAL AND MEDICAL THERAPY IN AORTIC DISSECTION

Surgical
1. Treatment of choice for acute proximal dissection
2. Treatment for acute distal dissection complicated by the following:
   a. Progression with vital organ compromise
   b. Rupture or impending rupture (e.g., saccular aneurysm formation)
   c. Aortic regurgitation (rare)
   d. Retrograde extension into the ascending aorta
   e. Dissection in the Marfan syndrome

Medical
1. Treatment of choice for uncomplicated distal dissection
2. Treatment for stable, isolated arch dissection
3. Treatment of choice for stable chronic dissection (uncomplicated dissection presenting 2 weeks or later after onset)

ommended for patients with the Marfan syndrome with either proximal or distal dissections.

Patients who present with chronic aortic dissection have, through self-selection, survived the early period of highest mortality and, whether treated medically or surgically, their subsequent hospital survival is approximately 90 per cent.[190,191] Accordingly, medical therapy is recommended for the management of all stable patients with chronic proximal and distal dissection, again unless complicated by rupture, aneurysm formation, aortic regurgitation, arterial occlusion, or extension or recurrence of dissection.

SURGICAL MANAGEMENT.   The generally advocated indications for definitive surgical therapy are summarized in Table 45–4. Surgical candidacy should be determined whenever possible at the start of the patient's evaluation because this guides the selection of diagnostic studies. Surgical risk for all patients is increased by: age; comorbid disease (especially pulmonary emphysema); aneurysm leakage; cardiac tamponade; shock; or vital organ compromise as a result of such conditions as myocardial infarction, cerebrovascular accident, and particularly preexisting renal failure.[188]

Preoperative mortality in acute dissection ranges from 3 per cent when surgery is expedited to as high as 20 per cent when the preoperative evaluation is more prolonged.[173] These data reinforce the fact that prompt diagnosis and repair are essential to prevent even minimal progression of the dissection that might lead to further complications.[96]

The usual objectives of definitive surgical therapy include the resection of the most severely damaged segment of the aorta, excision of the intimal tear, and obliteration of entry into the false lumen by suturing the edges of the dissected aorta both proximally and distally. After resecting the diseased segment containing the intimal tear, typically a segment of the ascending aorta in proximal dissections or the proximal descending aorta in distal dissections, aortic continuity is reestablished by interposing a prosthetic sleeve graft between the two ends of the aorta (Fig. 45–18). Less commonly, following resection of the intimal tear, the edges of the aorta may be rejoined as a direct repair without the use of a graft.

Importantly, Miller et al. have found that the immediate and long-term survival of patients treated surgically was not significantly affected by failure to excise the intimal tear.[186,192] Some patients with proximal dissection have an intimal tear located in the aortic arch. Because surgical repair of the arch may increase the morbidity and mortality of the procedure and because resection of the tear may not necessarily improve mortality, many authors have elected not to repair the arch if the sole purpose of surgery is resecting the intimal tear.[192] However, with improvements in surgical technique during the last decade, several groups now suggest that even these challenging lesions can be resected with favorable results.[193,194]

When aortic regurgitation complicates aortic dissection, simple decompression of the false lumen is sometimes all that is required to allow resuspension of the aortic leaflets and restoration of valvular competence. More often, however, preservation of the aortic valve requires approximation of the two layers of dissected aortic wall and resuspension of the commissures with pledgeted sutures. This resuspension technique has had favorable results with a fairly low incidence of recurrent aortic regurgitation in long-term follow-up.[123,195] Preserving the aortic valve in this fashion may avoid the complications associated with pros-

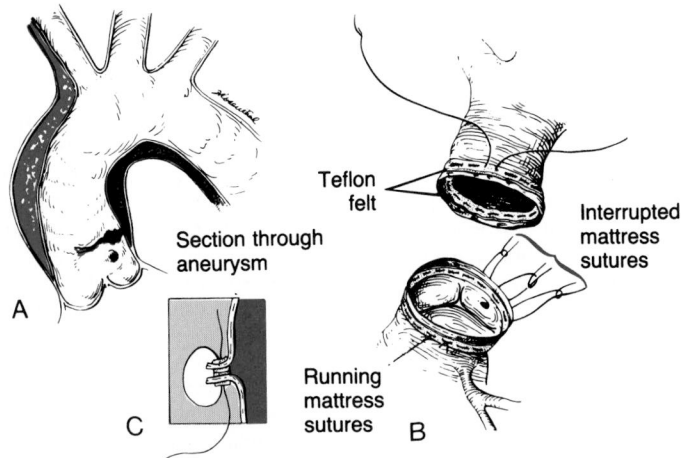

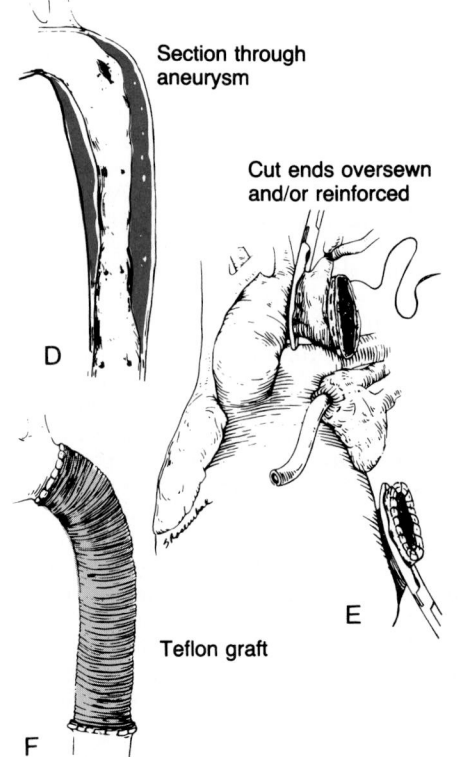

FIGURE 45–18.   Several steps in the surgical repair of a proximal (*A*, *B*, and *C*) and a distal (*D*, *E*, and *F*) aortic dissection. *A* and *D* show the dissections and intimal tears. *B*, The aorta has been transected, and the ends of the aorta have been oversewn to obliterate the false lumen and have been buttressed with Teflon felt to prevent the sutures from tearing through the fragile tissue. *C*, The aortic ends are brought together in such a way that the Teflon is again used to reinforce the suture line between the two ends of the aorta and between the aorta and a sleeve graft, if such a graft is necessary for the reconstitution of the aorta. *E* shows resection of a distal dissection, with a Teflon graft interposed in *F*. (*D*, *E*, and *F* from Austen, W. G., and DeSanctis, R. W.: Surgical treatment of dissecting aneurysm of the thoracic aorta. N. Engl. J. Med. *272*:1314, 1965.)

thetic valve replacement, especially the requirement for oral anticoagulation that may pose an added risk in patients prone to future aortic rupture.

Prosthetic aortic valve replacement is frequently necessary, however, either because attempts at a valve repair are unsuccessful or in the setting of preexisting valvular disease or the Marfan syndrome.[195] Many surgeons are aggressive about replacing the aortic valve if it appears that even moderate aortic regurgitation will remain after the leaflets are resuspended, choosing to avoid the risk of having to replace the aortic valve at some later date in a second operation through a diseased aorta. When the proximal aorta is fragile or badly torn, most use the Bentall procedure, in which a composite prosthetic graft—a prosthetic aortic valve sewn onto the end of a Dacron tube graft—facilitates the replacement of both the ascending aorta and aortic valve together (Fig. 45-5). The coronary arteries are then reimplanted as buttons of aortic tissue into the graft wall.[196]

For repair of a proximal dissection, total cardiopulmonary bypass is necessary. On occasion, because of extensive dissection of the aorta, it may be difficult to find a safe site for placement of a perfusion cannula and, rarely, we have had to abandon plans for surgical repair of a proximal dissection for this reason. In the repair of dissections of the descending thoracic aorta, support of the distal circulation may be necessary and can be achieved either by partial left heart bypass or by use of a bypass conduit that carries blood from the proximal aorta to distal aorta, thereby circumventing the site of the dissection.

The operative procedure in aortic dissection is technically demanding. The wall of the diseased aorta is often friable, and the repair must be performed with meticulous care. The use of Teflon felt to buttress the wall and prevent sutures from tearing through the fragile aorta is essential (Fig. 45-18). An alternative surgical approach involves wrapping an unstable aortic arch dissection with Dacron.[197]

Determining the sources of vital organ perfusion distal to the surgical site by diagnostic imaging studies may be of critical importance. For example, if one or both renal arteries are supplied by the false lumen and are not going to be directly corrected surgically, the surgeon may leave communication between the true and false channel distal to the site of aortic repair so as not to jeopardize renal perfusion.

COMPLICATIONS. Bleeding, infection, pulmonary failure, and renal insufficiency constitute the most common early complications of surgical therapy. Spinal cord ischemia with paraplegia due to inadvertent interruption of blood supply from the anterior spinal or intercostal arteries is an uncommon but dreaded consequence of descending thoracic aortic repair. Late complications include progressive aortic regurgitation if the aortic valve has not been replaced, localized aneurysm formation, and recurrent dissection at the original site or at a secondary site.[192] With modern operative techniques, surgical survival is 80 to 90 per cent for proximal and distal dissections.

NEWER SURGICAL TECHNIQUES. Several innovative techniques for the surgical treatment of aortic dissection have been reported. The thromboexclusion procedure, applied typically in dissections of the descending aorta, consists of bypassing the dissected aorta with a long Dacron sleeve, ligating the aorta at the site of proximal extension of the dissection, and creating reversal of flow in the distal aorta to perfuse the major arterial branches arising from the dissected segment.[178] In most cases gradual thrombosis of the occluded aortic segment occurs, thereby reducing the risk of extension or rupture.[178]

As a modification of more standard operative techniques, several investigators have unified the layers of the dissected aortic wall using either a fibrin sealant[198] or gelatin-resorcine-formaldehyde glue.[199,200] After resection of the diseased aortic segment, this glue is used in place of pledgeted sutures to seal the false lumen of the aortic stumps, prior to implantation of the Dacron prosthesis. The glue not only hardens and reinforces the fragile dissected aortic tissue but also may simplify the operation, facilitate resuspension of the aortic valve, and potentially reduce the incidence of late aortic root aneurysm formation.[198] Another group has used such glue in carrying out direct surgical repair of the aorta without an interposing graft by first suturing the intimal tear, then applying the glue in the false lumen to unify the layers of the dissected aorta, and finally reattaching the free aortic ends. Although early reports show favorable morbidity and mortality with the use of these new techniques,[200,201] direct comparison with standard operative techniques is needed.

ENDOVASCULAR TECHNIQUES. One of the more promising avenues of investigation is the use of endovascular techniques for treating high-risk patients with aortic dissection. For example, because patients with renal or visceral artery compromise from dissection have operative mortality rates exceeding 50 per cent,[202,203] alternative management strategies are desirable. Walker et al. have successfully performed combined renal artery angioplasty and stent placement in five patients with aortic dissection, achieving immediate and sustained improvement in blood pressure control in four.[203] In another case, in order to improve peripheral perfusion, they successfully performed balloon dilation of a preexisting fenestration in the intimal flap, with favorable results.[203]

More definitive endovascular techniques have also been introduced. Sutureless intraluminal prostheses, placed during cardiopulmonary bypass, are intended to improve outcome by decreasing in-

traoperative and postoperative bleeding complications.[204] These devices have been used successfully with good outcomes in two small series of patients with proximal aortic dissections.[205,206] More recently, intraluminal stent-grafts, placed percutaneously by the transfemoral catheter technique, have been introduced as a potential alternative to aortic repair.[207,208] Kato et al. have recently demonstrated the efficacy of their self-expanding stent in an experimental canine model of distal aortic dissection, with angiographically confirmed closure of the entry site and thrombosis of the false lumen within 2 hours of device placement.[208] Again, such nonsurgical procedures may be particularly well suited for high-risk patients, but data on human trials of intraluminal stent-grafts for aortic dissection are not yet available.

DEFINITIVE MEDICAL MANAGEMENT. The indications for definitive medical therapy are summarized in Table 45-4. As discussed above, we prefer medical therapy for stable patients with uncomplicated acute distal dissection. However, surgery must clearly be performed in cases of medical management failure, such as rupture or impending rupture, progression of the dissection with vital organ compromise, aortic regurgitation (which is extremely rare), or an inability to control pain or blood pressure with medicines. Because of the extreme difficulty of surgery to repair the aortic arch when it is involved by the dissection, medical therapy is also usually advocated for distal dissections that either originate in the arch or extend retrograde into the arch. Operative therapy is again reserved for those with serious complications.

Medical therapy is also generally recommended for patients presenting with chronic aortic dissection, whether proximal or distal, unless late complications of the dissection, such as aortic regurgitation or localized aneurysm formation, necessitate surgery. Complications of medical therapy include orthostasis or more severe hypotension secondary to the medications. If unchecked, persistent hypotension may in turn precipitate acute tubular necrosis, cerebrovascular accident, or myocardial infarction.[131]

Long-Term Therapy and Late Follow-Up

Late follow-up of patients leaving the hospital with treated aortic dissection shows an actuarial survival rate not much worse than that of individuals of comparable age without dissection. There are no significant differences among discharged patients when comparing proximal versus distal dissection, acute versus chronic dissection, or medical versus surgical treatment.[131] Five-year survival rates for all of these groups are typically 75 to 82 per cent.[131,186,192] Thus, the initial success of surgical or medical therapy is usually sustained on long-term follow-up. Late complications include aortic regurgitation, recurrent dissection, and aneurysm formation or rupture.

Long-term medical therapy to control hypertension and reduce dP/dt is indicated for all patients who have sustained an aortic dissection, regardless of whether their in-hospital definitive treatment was surgical or medical. Indeed, one study found that late aneurysm rupture following aortic dissection was 10 times more common among patients with poorly controlled hypertension than among those with controlled blood pressure,[209] dramatically demonstrating the importance of aggressive life-long antihypertensive therapy. Systolic blood pressure should be maintained at or below 130 to 140 mm Hg. Preferred agents are beta blockers or other agents with a negative inotropic as well as a hypotensive effect, such as calcium channel antagonists, together with a diuretic if necessary to control blood pressure. Pure vasodilators, such as hydralazine and minoxidil, may cause an increase in dP/dt and should therefore be used only in conjunction with adequate beta blockade. ACE inhibitors are attractive antihypertensive agents for treating aortic dissection and may be of particular benefit in those with some degree of renal ischemia as a consequence of the dissection.

Up to 29 per cent of late deaths following surgery result from rupture of either the dissecting aneurysm or another aneurysm at a remote site. Moreover, the incidence of subsequent aneurysm formation at a site remote from the surgical repair is 17 to 25 per cent,[114,210] with these remote aneurysms accounting for many of the rupture-related deaths. The mean time interval from primary aortic dissection to the appearance of subsequent aneurysms is 18 months, with the majority appearing within 2 years.[210] Many such aneurysms occur from dilatation of the residual false lumen in the more distal aortic segments not resected at the time of surgery. Because the dissected aneurysm wall is relatively thin, consisting of only the outer half of the original aortic wall, these aneurysms rupture more frequently than do typical atherosclerotic thoracic aneurysms.[87,210] Thus, an aggressive approach to treating such late-appearing aneurysms may be indicated.

The high incidence of late aneurysm formation and rupture emphasizes both the diffuse nature of the aortic disease process in this population and the tremendous importance of careful follow-up. The primary goal of long-term surveillance is the early detection of aortic lesions that might require subsequent surgical intervention, such as the appearance of new aneurysms or rapid aneurysm expansion, progression or recurrence of dissection, aortic regurgitation, or peripheral vascular compromise.

Follow-up evaluation of patients after aortic dissection should include careful and repeated physical examinations, periodic chest roentgenograms, and serial aortic imaging with either TEE,[211] CT scanning,[187] or MRI.[178] We generally prefer MRI for serially following these patients because it is completely noninvasive and provides excellent anatomical detail that may be exceedingly helpful in evaluating interval changes.[212] Patients are at highest risk immediately following hospitalization and during the first 2 years, with the risk progressively declining thereafter. It is therefore important to have more frequent follow-up early on; for example, patients may be seen at 3 and 6 months initially, then return every 6 months for 2 years, after which time they may be reevaluated at 6- to 12-month intervals, depending on the given patient's risk.

Atypical Aortic Dissection

In recent years it has become increasingly clear that in addition to aortic dissection as classically described, there are two other closely related diseases of the aorta, *intramural hematoma* of the aorta and *penetrating atherosclerotic ulcer* of the aorta. These two conditions share with aortic dissection many of the predisposing risk factors and presenting symptoms, and indeed both may lead either to classic aortic dissection or to aortic rupture.

INTRAMURAL HEMATOMA. This is essentially a contained hemorrhage within the medial layer of the aortic wall. Although the pathogenesis of intramural hematoma is still uncertain, rupture of the vasa vasorum is believed to be the initiating event, resulting in hemorrhage into the outer media and extending into the adventitia.[213,213a] This may produce a localized or discrete hematoma, but more often the hemorrhage extends for a variable distance by dissecting along the outer media beneath the adventitia.[214] Intramural hematoma is distinguished from typical aortic dissection by the lack of an associated tear in the intima or direct communication between the media and aortic lumen; hence, some have termed it *aortic dissection without intimal rupture*.[213] Previous pathological studies of what were considered clinically to be aortic dissections have found that 3 to 13 per cent[112,113,215] did not have an identifiable intimal tear, and it is possible that such cases were in fact actually intramural hematomas. Moreover, it remains uncertain whether intramural hematoma is a distinct pathological entity or instead represents a reversible precursor of classic aortic dissection.

Clinically, intramural hematoma may be indistinguishable from true aortic dissection. The majority of patients are elderly with a history of hypertension and typically have extensive aortic atherosclerosis.[216,217] Almost all patients have the chest and back pain symptoms typical of classic aortic dissection. Aortic regurgitation and pulse deficits may be present. One-half of patients may have associated left pleural effusion[213,216] that may not appear until several days after the hematoma develops.[213] A pericardial effusion may appear when the ascending aorta is involved.[216]

Intramural hematoma is best diagnosed by CT scanning. On a non-contrast-enhanced CT scan (Fig. 45–19) it appears as a continuous, crescentic, high-attenuation area along the aortic wall without evidence of an intimal tear, false lumen, or associated intimal atherosclerotic ulcer.[214] This study is followed by a contrast-enhanced CT scan, which demonstrates failure of the intramural hematoma to enhance, thereby excluding communication with the aortic lumen. In some cases it may be difficult to distinguish intramural hematoma from aortic dissection with thrombosis of the false lumen or from mural thrombus within an aortic aneurysm.[213] However, with an intramural hematoma the aortic lumen retains its overall size and shape, unlike in aortic dissection.

On MRI, an intramural hematoma appears as a crescentic high-intensity area along the aortic wall.[213] On TEE it is manifested as a continuous crescentic or nearly concentric circular thickening of the aortic wall which, in some cases, may be difficult to distinguish from severe atherosclerotic thickening of the aortic wall.[218] Aortography may fail to detect an intramural hematoma because it does not usually compress the aortic lumen to produce recognizable aortographic signs such as are seen with aortic dissection.[213]

The natural history of intramural hematoma is not well defined. Involvement of the ascending aorta appears to carry a high risk of death or complications requiring surgical repair, whereas hematomas of the descending aorta have a more favorable prognosis. In a recent retrospective series, Nienaber et al. determined that 13 per cent of 195 patients presenting with aortic dissection–like syndromes in fact suffered intramural hematoma.[218] The actuarial survival rates were similar for the groups with intramural hematoma and overt aortic dissection.[218] Of those with proximal intramural hematoma, 30-day mortality was 80 per cent for those treated medically, compared with 0 per cent for those undergoing early repair. On the other hand, early mortality for distal intramural hematoma was 9 per cent and did not differ significantly between medical and surgical treatment.

Intramural hematomas may regress with time or even

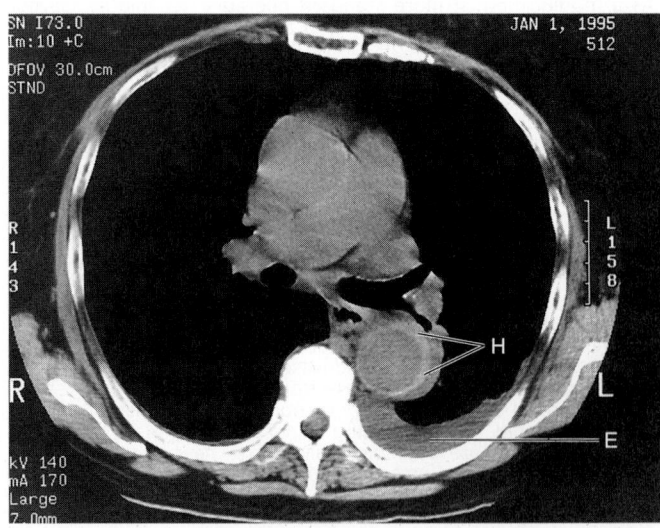

FIGURE 45–19. Intramural hematoma of the aorta. A CT scan without contrast enhancement demonstrates crescentic thickening of the aortic wall which is of increased density (H), consistent with an intramural hematoma of the aorta. A left pleural effusion (E) is also present.

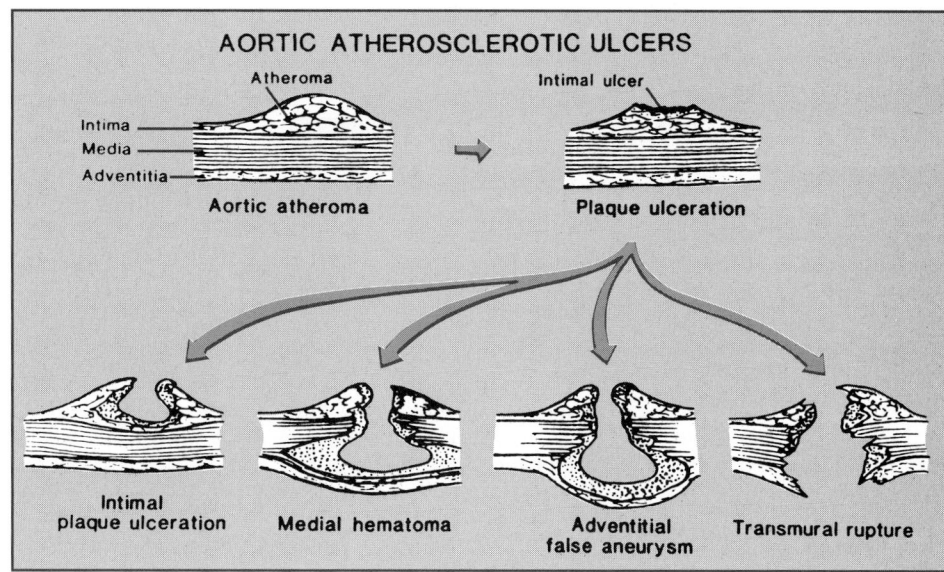

FIGURE 45–20. The evolution of a penetrating atherosclerotic ulcer of the aorta. Once an intimal ulcer has formed, it may then progress to a variable depth. Penetration through the intima causes a medial hematoma, whereas penetration through the media leads to the formation of a pseudoaneurysm and perforation through the adventitial layer results in aortic rupture. (From Stanson, A. W., Kazmier, F. J., Hollier, L. H., et al.: Penetrating atherosclerotic ulcers of the thoracic aorta: Natural history and clinicopathological correlations. Ann. Vasc. Surg. *1:*15, 1986.)

completely resolve on follow-up imaging[213] or, alternatively, may progress to overt aortic dissection within days[218,219] to months of initial presentation.[214] Nienaber et al. found progression to overt dissection, aortic rupture, or cardiac tamponade in one-third of patients.[218]

The limited data on the natural history of intramural hematoma suggest that it behaves very much like classic aortic dissection and should therefore be treated in a similar fashion. Thus surgical therapy is best for proximal hematomas, whereas medical therapy is reasonable for distal hematomas. There should be a low threshold, however, for proceeding to surgery in distal disease if symptoms persist or if there is evidence of progression. Medical management should therefore include serial imaging studies to follow the progression or regression of the intramural hematoma.

PENETRATING ATHEROSCLEROTIC ULCER. Penetrating atherosclerotic ulcer, first defined in the literature in 1986 by Stanson et al.,[220] is an ulceration of an atherosclerotic lesion of the aorta that penetrates the internal elastic lamina and allows hematoma formation within the media of the aortic wall (Fig. 45–20). Although such ulcerations occur almost exclusively in the descending thoracic aorta, with the majority located in its mid to distal portion,[221] they may rarely occur in the ascending aorta or arch.[222,223] The hematoma that results from a penetrating atherosclerotic ulcer usually remains localized or extends several centimeters in length but does not develop a false lumen.[224] These ulcers penetrate through the media in one-quarter of cases to cause aortic pseudoaneurysms, or through the adventitia in 8 per cent to cause transmural aortic rupture[222] (Fig. 45–20). Rarely, a penetrating atherosclerotic ulcer may progress to an extensive classic aortic dissection.[223] Over time, penetrating atherosclerotic ulcers frequently lead to the formation of saccular or fusiform aortic aneurysms.[225]

The patients who develop penetrating atherosclerotic ulcers tend to be elderly, with a history of hypertension and evidence of other atherosclerotic cardiovascular disease.[221] Presenting symptoms include chest and back pain similar to that of aortic dissection, but without associated pulse deficits, neurological deficits, or aortic regurgitation.[220] The majority are hypertensive at presentation.[221,226]

Chest roentgenogram often demonstrates a dilated descending thoracic aorta as well as left-sided or bilateral pleural effusions.[221] Aortography is the diagnostic standard for detecting a penetrating atherosclerotic ulcer, with the lesion appearing as contrast-filled outpouching in the descending aorta in the absence of an intimal flap or false lumen[222] (Fig. 45–21). On CT scanning[221] or MRI[227] the lesion appears as a focal ulceration, with thickening of the aortic wall and inward displacement of intimal calcifica-

tion consistent with intramural hematoma. TEE may identify the presence of a culprit atherosclerotic ulcer in the setting of a visible intramural hematoma,[228] but diagnosis is difficult.[164]

The natural history of penetrating atherosclerotic ulcer remains largely unclear, and at present there is no definitive treatment strategy. Certainly, patients who are hemodynamically unstable or who have evidence of pseudoaneurysm formation or transmural rupture should undergo urgent surgical repair. Continued or recurrent pain, distal embolization, or progressive aneurysmal dilatation are also indications for surgery.[224] Those without such complications should be treated with antihypertensive medications and monitored closely with follow-up imaging studies, similar to the management of a patient with a distal aortic dissection.

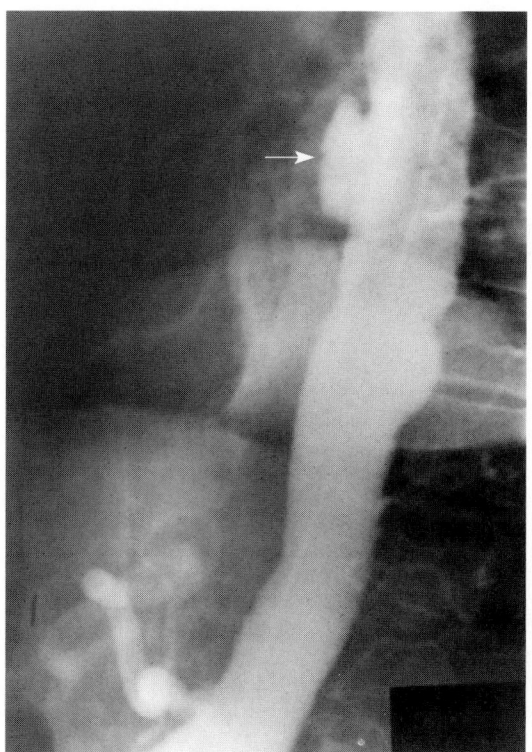

FIGURE 45–21. A thoracic aortogram demonstrating a penetrating atherosclerotic ulcer of the distal descending aorta (arrow). The hematoma of the aortic wall is evident as a localized contrast-filled outpouching of the aorta. The remainder of the aorta is diffusely atherosclerotic.

Aortic Trauma
See discussion on p. 1543.

AORTIC ATHEROMATOUS EMBOLI

AORTOGENIC ATHEROTHROMBOTIC EMBOLI. The clinical importance of atherosclerotic disease of the aorta has long been recognized, as atheromatous or fibrinous material, thrombi, or cholesterol particles dislodged from atherosclerotic plaques may cause cerebral or peripheral embolic phenomena.[229,229a] However, assessing the degree of such atherosclerotic disease ante mortem has been limited by the inability of the several imaging modalities to directly visualize the aortic intima.[230] Aortography demonstrates the aortic lumen rather than the aortic walls themselves and thus can only detect gross atherosclerotic changes, whereas CT scanning or MRI rarely detect protruding atheromas because the normal pulsatile motion of the aorta may limit definition of the aortic wall on the tomographic images. On the other hand, TEE is uniquely suited to assess atherosclerotic disease of the aorta in real time and has been demonstrated to have greater sensitivity for aortic arch atherosclerosis than chest roentgenography, aortography, or CT scanning.[230] On echocardiography, mild atherosclerosis appears as intimal thickening, irregularity, and calcification, whereas more severe disease appears as thick plaques with protruding atheromas (Fig. 45–22). In some cases protruding lesions have highly mobile components that may represent atheroma with superimposed thrombus.[231,232]

Risk factors for aortic atherosclerosis include age, hypertension, diabetes,[233] hyperlipidemia,[234] and other vascular disease.[235] Through the use of TEE, the prevalence and extent of macroscopic atherosclerotic disease have now been documented in a variety of patient populations.[235a] Atheromatous disease is least common in the ascending aorta, more common in the arch, and most common in the descending thoracic aorta.[236] Whereas aortic atheromas are detected in as few as 2 per cent of those without a history of stroke or known aortic disease, they are found in 38 per cent of those with significant carotid artery disease,[237] 60 per cent of those with ischemic stroke,[236] and up to 90 per cent of those with obstructive coronary artery disease.[238]

In an autopsy series Amarenco et al. found that the presence of ulcerated plaques in the aortic arch was a significant independent risk factor for stroke, particularly cryptogenic stroke,[235] and multiple clinical studies using TEE have found an association between aortic atherosclerosis and stroke as well as other peripheral embolic events.[229,234,239] In both retrospective and prospective studies, protruding aortic atheromas are detected in 7 to 8 per cent of patients undergoing routine TEE,[229,240] with about a 33 per cent incidence of embolic vascular events over a 2-year follow-up period.[240] The embolic risk is even higher among those with pedunculated or mobile lesions and those undergoing invasive aortic procedures.[229]

In a recent prospective case-control study, Amarenco et al. found atherosclerotic plaques of 4 mm or more in the ascending aorta or proximal arch in 14 per cent of patients with ischemic stroke, compared with only 2 per cent of controls. After adjustment for atherosclerotic risk factors, the odds ratio for stroke was 9.1 for ischemic stroke and 4.7 for cryptogenic stroke, with an even higher risk ratio for complex atheromas than for simple ones.[236] However, the increased risk of stroke was associated only with the large atheromas involving the ascending aorta and proximal arch, not with atheromas in the distal arch or descending aorta,[236] supporting the hypothesis that atheromas in the ascending aorta and proximal aortic arch embolize directly into the cerebral circulation to cause ischemic strokes in such patients.[241]

Little is known about the natural history of atheromatous lesions[242] of the aorta, and at present therapeutic strategies are limited. Potential approaches for chronic management include the use of antithrombotic[243,244] or antiplatelet[242] therapy to prevent thrombus formation. Some have reported the surgical removal, under hypothermic circulatory arrest, of protruding atheromas detected in patients following embolic events.[239] However, this surgery carries the risk of an early adverse outcome, and at present no controlled data suggest that it actually reduces the incidence of future embolization in this population.[245]

CARDIAC SURGERY AND ATHEROEMBOLISM. Perioperative dislodgment and embolization of atherosclerotic material from the aorta is a well-recognized hazard of cardiac surgery and has been increasingly implicated as an important cause of postoperative strokes and other embolic events in these patients. The incidence of cerebral ischemic events following cardiac surgery typically ranges from 1 to 3 per cent, with an increased risk among the elderly.[233,246] In an autopsy series of patients having undergone cardiac surgery, Blauth et al. identified atheroemboli in 22 per cent of cases.[247] Atheroembolic events occurred in 37 per cent of those with severe atherosclerosis of the ascending aorta, compared with only 2 per cent of those without significant ascending aortic atherosclerosis. Moreover, 96 per cent of patients suffering perioperative atheroemboli had severe atherosclerosis of their ascending aorta.[247] Mobile pedunculated lesions appear more prone to embolize.[229]

Mechanisms by which aortic atherosclerotic debris may be dislodged during cardiac surgery include external manipulation of the aorta during palpation,[246] cross-clamping, cannula placement, anastomosis of the bypass grafts to the aorta,[233] and the "sandblasting" effect of the high-velocity jet of blood that exits the aortic cannula and strikes the atherosclerotic intima of the opposite aortic wall.[246,247] Although surgeons have long relied on direct digital palpation to detect the presence of atherosclerosis in the ascending aorta, this method underestimates the incidence, severity, and extent of atherosclerotic disease.[248,249] In contrast, both TEE and intraoperative epiaortic ultrasonography appear to be superior techniques for delineating the presence and severity of atherosclerotic disease of the ascending aorta.[229]

Several studies have examined the potential role of aortic ultrasonography in identifying patients at highest risk for perioperative atheroemboli. In 8 to 17 per cent of cases, the ultrasonographic findings led to modifications in surgical technique such as changing the sites of aortic cannulation

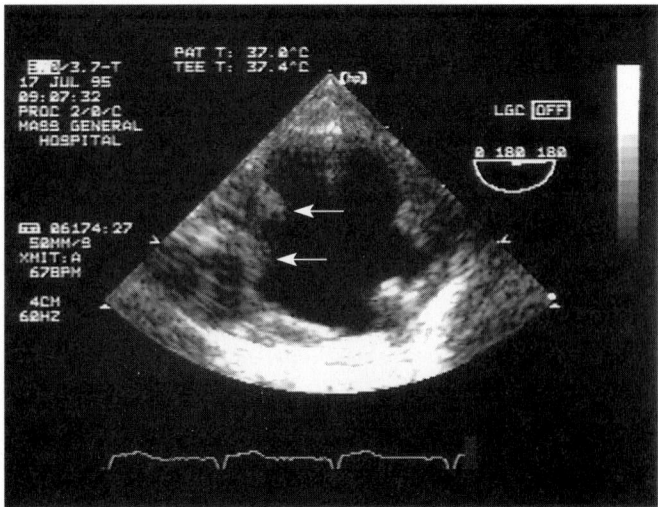

FIGURE 45–22. A cross-sectional transesophageal echocardiogram of the descending thoracic aorta demonstrating extensive atherosclerotic disease. This patient had recently suffered an embolic stoke of uncertain etiology. Multiple atheromatous plaques, up to 7 mm in thickness, protrude into the aortic lumen. When viewed in real-time, two plaques (arrows) had small mobile intraluminal components.

(with cannulation of the distal aorta or femoral artery instead), of cross-clamping, or of anastomosis of vein grafts.[233,246,248,250] The results of such procedural modifications have been promising, with several reports showing a trend toward reduction of stroke rates.

CHOLESTEROL EMBOLIZATION SYNDROME. Cholesterol embolization syndrome is caused by distal showering of cholesterol crystals from ulcerated atheromatous plaques in the aorta or iliac and proximal femoral arteries in patients with diffuse atherosclerosis. These cholesterol crystals then obstruct small peripheral arteries (100 to 300 μm in size), causing local tissue ischemia or necrosis, and frequently induce a local inflammatory reaction that may contribute to the arteriolar occlusive process.[251]

The precise mechanisms that precipitate cholesterol embolization are unclear. The syndrome is most commonly seen following instrumentation of the aorta, such as with cardiac catheterization, PTCA, angiography, or intraaortic balloon pump insertion.[252] The overall incidence following cardiac catheterization was 0.1 per cent in the Coronary Artery Surgery Study.[253] Cholesterol embolization may also complicate aortic surgery or cardiopulmonary bypass. At times, cholesterol embolization syndrome may occur spontaneously. Studies have suggested a causal relationship between warfarin therapy and such spontaneous cholesterol embolization.[254]

The clinical manifestations depend on the organs affected. Cutaneous manifestations, typically of the lower extremities, are most common and include livedo reticularis, gangrene, cyanosis, and ulceration.[255] Acute onset of pain with digital ischemia and small areas of cutaneous gangrene is often referred to as the "blue toe" or "purple toe syndrome."[254,256] The presence of preserved pedal pulses in the setting of peripheral ischemia distinguishes this syndrome from embolic occlusion of larger arteries.

Acute nonoliguric renal failure with or without hypertension is a common consequence of renal emboli, often presenting as a rise in creatinine over several weeks, followed by a slow but progressive worsening of renal function that may become severe and irreversible. Cholesterol embolization to the central nervous system is quite uncommon, but may present as focal neurological deficits, amaurosis fugax from retinal emboli, paralysis from spinal cord emboli, or a diffuse encephalopathy. Mesenteric embolization may present with abdominal pain, gastrointestinal bleeding, or pancreatitis. Finally, multiple organ systems may be simultaneously involved, mimicking vasculitis or bacterial endocarditis.[251]

When the cholesterol embolization syndrome occurs as a consequence of an invasive procedure, the temporal relation of events often suggests the diagnosis. In the case of spontaneous embolization, however, recognizing the syndrome remains extremely challenging, and diagnosis in the absence of cutaneous manifestations is especially difficult. An elevated erythrocyte sedimentation rate, eosinophilia, and a reduced complement level are helpful in suggesting the diagnosis, but making a definitive diagnosis requires a tissue biopsy. Paraffin-fixed sections reveal needle-shaped clefts in the arteriolar lumens, representing the spaces occupied by cholesterol particles prior to fixation.

No specific therapy effectively treats cholesterol embolization syndrome.[251,252] Because cholesterol embolization resembles other atheroembolic phenomena, some have advocated the use of anticoagulant therapy. However, such therapy is typically unsuccessful and may even exacerbate the condition,[257] whereas discontinuing anticoagulation may improve the condition in some cases.[258] Glucocorticoid therapy has also been tried without success. Surgical therapy is generally limited to the amputation of an ischemic or gangrenous extremity. Overall, the prognosis for those suffering cholesterol embolization syndrome is quite poor, with a mortality rate of 38 to 80 per cent.[259,260]

Acute aortic occlusion is an infrequent but potentially catastrophic condition with an early mortality of 31 to 52 per cent.[261-263] It is caused by either embolic occlusion of the infrarenal aorta at the bifurcation, known as a "saddle embolus," or acute thrombosis of the abdominal aorta. At least 95 per cent of aortic emboli originate from the left side of the heart,[262] typically as thrombus from the left atrium secondary to atrial fibrillation, particularly in the setting of rheumatic mitral stenosis, or from the left ventricle secondary to myocardial infarction, aneurysm, or dilated cardiomyopathy. Less common cardiac sources of emboli include atrial myxoma, prosthetic valve thrombus, and acute bacterial or fungal endocarditis.[264] Primary thrombosis accounts for the remaining 35 to 92 per cent[261,262] of acute aortic occlusions. Seventy-five to 80 per cent of thrombotic aortic occlusions occur in the setting of underlying severe aortoiliac occlusive disease, and they are frequently precipitated by a low-flow state secondary to heart failure or dehydration. In those without aortoiliac occlusive disease, a hypercoagulable state may precipitate thrombosis of an abdominal aortic aneurysm, leading to aortic occlusion.[261,262]

Acute aortic occlusion is in most cases heralded by the sudden onset of excruciating bilateral lower extremity pain —usually radiating from the mid-thigh distally—associated with weakness, numbness, and paresthesias. Nonclassic presentations include sudden onset of bilateral lower extremity weakness, severe hypertension from renal artery involvement, and abdominal pain from mesenteric ischemia. Persistent ischemia may lead to myonecrosis with secondary hypotension, hyperkalemia, myoglobinuria, and acute tubular necrosis. If perfusion is not reestablished within hours, death is almost inevitable.

DIAGNOSIS. Physical examination reveals cold pale extremities that are cyanotic and often exhibit a mottled, reticulated, and reddish blue appearance that may progress to the blue-black color of gangrene. Pulses are notably absent below the abdominal aorta, and capillary refill is absent. Signs of ischemic neuropathy are present and include symmetrical weakness, loss of all modalities of sensation (usually with demarcation at the level of the mid-thigh), and diminished or absent deep tendon reflexes. When neurological symptoms predominate, patients are often mistakenly thought to have spinal cord infarction or compression and their ischemic symptoms may initially be overlooked. In fact, as many as 11 to 17 per cent of such patients may initially undergo a neurological or neurosurgical evaluation before the vascular cause is recognized.[261,262]

The diagnosis of acute aortic occlusion is confirmed by aortography. Although some suggest that all stable patients should undergo the procedure,[261] others advise prompt surgical intervention without aortography if the diagnosis is strongly suspected,[262,263] because added delays increase the likelihood of irreversible ischemic damage to the limbs. Aortography is desirable if there is concomitant abdominal pain, hypertension, or anuria, to evaluate the possibility of renal and mesenteric arterial involvement.[262]

MANAGEMENT. Once a clinical diagnosis of acute aortic occlusion is made, intravenous heparin therapy should be initiated while awaiting immediate surgery. A saddle embolus can be removed using Fogarty balloon-tipped catheters inserted through a transfemoral arterial approach under local anesthesia. If the embolus cannot be retrieved with Fogarty catheters, removal by direct transabdominal aortotomy is undertaken. Patients with thrombotic occlusion generally undergo either direct aortic reconstruction or revascularization with aortofemoral or axillofemoral bypass. Operative mortality for acute aortic occlusion is 31 to 40 per cent[262,263] and as high as 85 per cent among those with severe left ventricular dysfunction or a hypercoagulable state.[261] Limb salvage rates are as high as 98 per cent.[262,263] Lifelong anticoagulant therapy is necessary following surgery in almost all cases to prevent recurrent emboli.[265]

AORTOARTERITIS SYNDROMES

Takayasu's Arteritis

Takayasu's arteritis is a chronic inflammatory disease of unknown etiology involving the aorta and its major branches, which was first noted in 1908 by the Japanese ophthalmologist Takayasu. This disease entity has been variously termed "aortic arch syndrome," "pulseless disease," "aortoarteritis," "occlusive thromboaortopathy," "young female arteritis," and "reversed coarctation," in addition to the familiar *Takayasu's arteritis.*

ETIOLOGY AND PATHOPHYSIOLOGY. Takayasu's arteritis occurs worldwide, although the large majority of cases are seen in Asia and Africa. The incidence in North American and European populations is 1.2 to 2.6 per million per year. A specific cause has not been found,[266] although the bulk of evidence favors an autoimmune etiology. It has been linked to rheumatic fever, streptococcal infections, rheumatoid arthritis, and other collagen vascular diseases. An association between the disease and certain HLA subtypes has been reported,[267,268] although it is of unclear significance.[266]

In the early stage of the disease there is active inflammation involving a granulomatous arteritis of the aorta and its branches, with secondary alterations in the media and adventitia. The disease progresses at variable rates to a later sclerotic stage in which there is intimal hyperplasia, medial degeneration, and adventitial fibrosis. The proliferative process leads to obliterative luminal changes in the aorta and other involved arteries.

Takayasu's arteritis most often involves the aortic arch and its major branches, with changes that are usually most marked at branch points in the aorta. It may present as multisegmental aortic disease with areas of normal wall between affected sites, as diffuse involvement of the aorta, or as disease of individual arteries arising from the aorta. The pulmonary artery may also be involved. Lesions are purely stenotic in 85 per cent of patients, purely dilatative in 2 per cent, and mixed in 13 per cent. The coronary arteries are affected in less than 10 per cent of patients. Aortic regurgitation as a consequence of disease of the proximal ascending aorta is seen in about one-quarter of cases. Ueno et al. have subdivided the disease into three types, depending on the predominant site of involvement[269] (Fig. 45–23). Type I involves primarily the aortic arch and its branches; type II spares the aortic arch, involving the thoracoabdominal aorta and its branches; type III combines the features of both. Lupi-Herrera et al. have suggested a fourth category, type IV, in which there is pulmonary arterial involvement.[270]

CLINICAL MANIFESTATIONS. The disease affects women much more frequently than men, in a ratio of 8:1.[271] The mean age at the time of diagnosis is 29 years. In as many as three-fourths of cases, onset is in the teenage years, although cases beginning from infancy to late middle-age have been reported.[271] Because the symptoms of Takayasu's arteritis are generally nonspecific, there may be a delay of months to years between the first appearance of symptoms and the time of diagnosis. In fact, only 6 per cent of the patients in the Mayo Clinic series were suspected of having Takayasu's arteritis at presentation.[272] More than half the patients with Takayasu's arteritis develop initial symptoms suggestive of a systemic inflammatory process, characterized by fever, anorexia, malaise, weight loss, night sweats, arthralgias, pleuritic pain, and fatigue. Localized pain and tenderness may be noted over affected arteries. The disease may occasionally present as fever of unknown origin.[273]

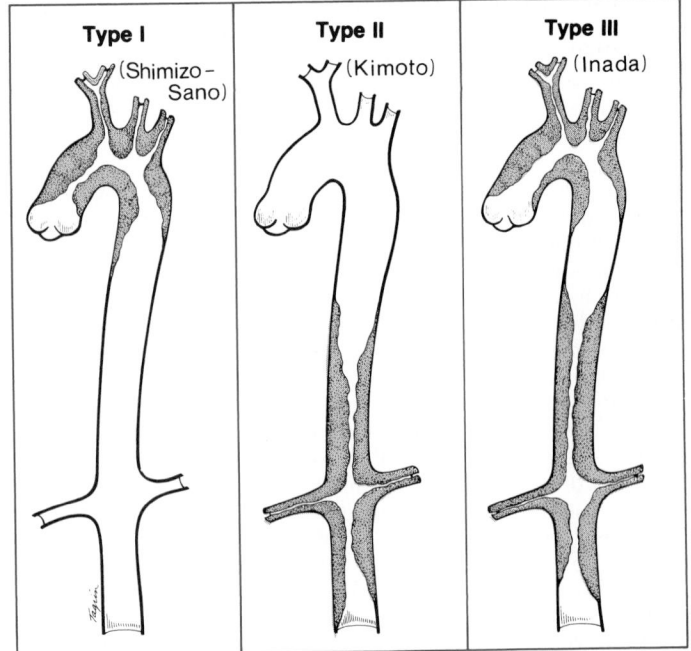

FIGURE 45–23. Types of Takayasu's arteritis. Type I involves primarily the aortic arch and brachiocephalic vessels. Type II affects the thoracoabdominal aorta and particularly the renal arteries. Type III combines features of both types I and II. Types I and III may be complicated by aortic regurgitation. The eponyms for each type are noted.

At the time of diagnosis, 85 to 96 per cent of patients have entered the sclerotic phase of the disease and have symptoms of vascular insufficiency of either the upper extremities or, less commonly, the lower extremities.[270] Patients with types I and III exhibit those findings most typical of the disease, namely "reversed" coarctation of the aorta with absent or diminished upper body pulses and barely detectable blood pressure in the arms, higher blood pressure in the lower extremities, bruits overlying diseased arteries, and manifestations of ischemia at various affected sites. Most have a pulse pressure difference of 30 mm Hg or more between their two arms, and many have postural dizziness or even syncope. The retinopathy originally described by Takayasu is seen in only about one-quarter of patients[271] and is usually associated with carotid artery involvement. Patients with type II arteritis may have abdominal angina and claudication of the limbs but also tend to develop hypertension because of renal artery involvement.

Hypertension complicates this disease in 50 to 60 per cent of cases[271] but may be difficult to recognize because of diminished pulses in the arms. Hypertension typically arises from renal artery stenosis and hemodynamically significant acquired coarctation of the aorta, although decreased aortic distensibility and reduced baroreceptor reactivity may also contribute.[274] Another major complication of Takayasu's arteritis is congestive heart failure, occurring in 28 per cent of cases[270] as a consequence of the systemic hypertension or, more rarely, aortic regurgitation.[275] Coronary artery involvement may cause angina or myocardial infarction.[276]

NATURAL HISTORY. The natural history of this uncommon disease has been best defined in a recent series by Ishikawa and Maetani, who followed 120 patients with Takayasu's arteritis for up to 15 years.[277] The overall 15-year survival was 83 per cent. Death usually resulted from cerebrovascular accidents, congestive heart failure, or myocardial infarction. The authors showed that the survival rate was only 66 per cent among those with major complications—severe hypertension, moderate or severe aortic regurgitation, aortic or arterial aneurysms, and

Takayasu's retinopathy—compared with a 96 per cent survival rate for those without such complications.[277]

DIAGNOSIS. Laboratory abnormalities during the acute systemic phase include an elevated sedimentation rate, a low-grade leukocytosis, and mild anemia of chronic disease. These return toward normal when the systemic phase resolves. IgG and IgM levels are elevated in more than half the patients.[266] Chest roentgenograms are usually unrevealing, although a rim of calcification is sometimes visible in the walls of involved arteries. Arteriography typically reveals findings of an irregular intimal surface, with stenoses of the aorta or its branch vessels, poststenotic dilatation, aortic or arterial aneurysms, and even complete occlusion of vessels (Fig. 45–24). The affected thoracic aorta has been described as having a narrowed, "rat-tail" angiographic appearance (Fig. 45–25).[278]

Proposed criteria for the clinical diagnosis of Takayasu's arteritis are shown in Table 45–5 (p. 1575).[279] An obligatory criterion is age 40 years or less at diagnosis. The two major criteria reflect involvement of either subclavian artery. A high probability of the disease exists if, in addition to age of 40 years or less, a patient meets two major criteria, one major criterion and two minor criteria, or four minor criteria.[279]

MANAGEMENT. Glucocorticoids in high doses (prednisone, 1 mg/kg body weight per day) are well established as the primary therapy of Takayasu's arteritis[266] and often dramatically improve the constitutional symptoms, halt disease progression in patients in the systemic inflammatory stage, and lower the sedimentation rate toward normal.[266,272] In fact, the sedimentation rate, usually an accurate indicator of systemic disease activity, is quite useful in directing therapy. When patients fail to respond to steroid therapy, cyclophosphamide (2 mg/kg/day) has been used with some success.[266] Alternatively, low-dose methotrexate (about 0.3 mg/kg/week) may enhance the efficacy of steroid therapy and facilitate steroid tapering.[280] Although medical therapy has been successful in improving symptoms in a majority of patients, it is not known whether it

prevents the long-term complications of this disease or prolongs life.[266]

The indications for surgery in the treatment of Takayasu's arteritis are not well established. Given the diffuse nature of the arteritis, surgery often requires the bypass or reconstruction of multiple aortic or arterial segments. Surgery is generally performed to correct renovascular hypertension, relieve cerebral ischemia, repair aortic or arterial aneurysms, treat aortic regurgitation, or bypass coronary arteries. Renal artery stenosis is currently the most common indication. Surgery during the active phase of disease carries a significant risk of reocclusion and therefore, whenever possible, should be postponed until the inflammation has subsided. If surgery during the active phase is essential, postoperative steroid therapy is necessary.

One promising advance in the treatment of the obstructive lesions of Takayasu's arteritis is the use of percutaneous transluminal angioplasty. Tyagi et al. performed angioplasty for stenotic lesions of the aorta in a series of patients, with success in 94 per cent as indicated by an increase in aortic diameter, a decline in the pressure gradient across the stenosis, and a decline in blood pressure.[281] All patients with successful angioplasty had marked improvements in their symptoms. Tyagi et al. had similar success with renal artery angioplasty for management of hypertension in Takayasu's arteritis.[282]

Giant Cell Arteritis

Giant cell arteritis is one of the most common forms of vasculitis, occurring predominantly among older people and characteristically involving medium-sized arteries. The aorta and its branches, however, are affected in about 15 per cent of cases.[283] The disease is also referred to as "granulomatous arteritis," "temporal arteritis," and "cranial arteritis."

ETIOLOGY AND PATHOPHYSIOLOGY. Unlike Takayasu's arteritis, the highest incidence of giant cell arteritis is in the

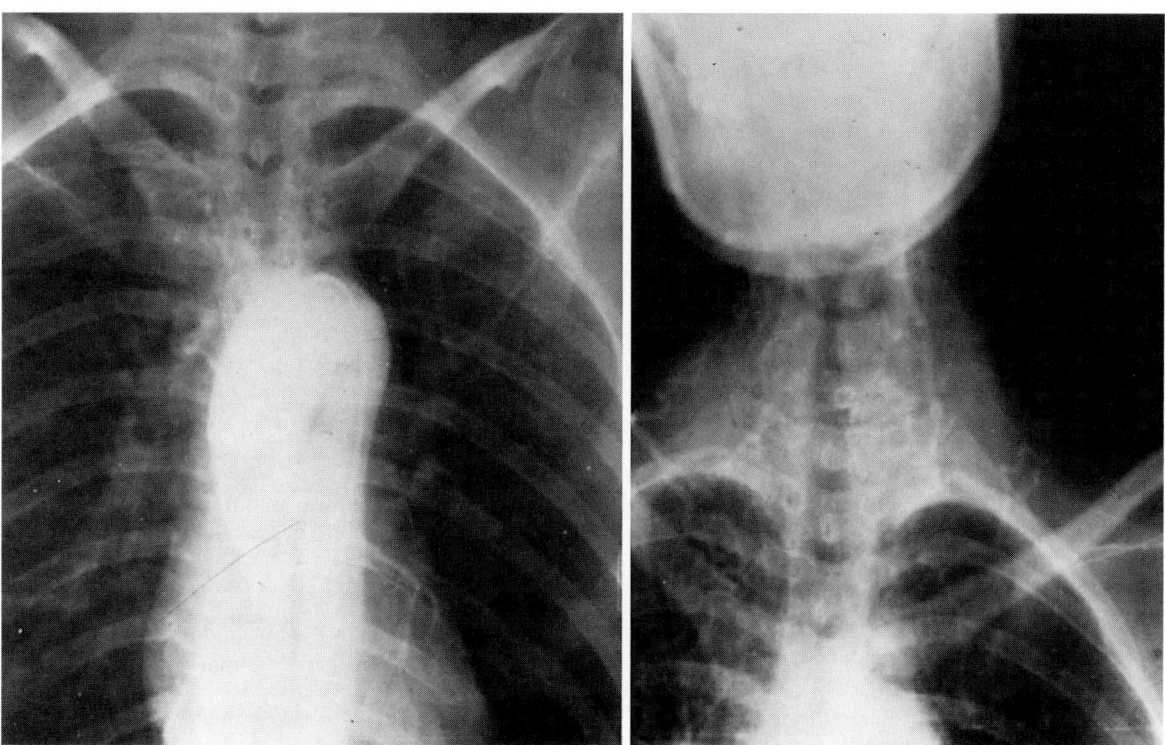

FIGURE 45–24. Thoracic aortogram *(left)* and late films of the head, neck, and upper thorax *(right)* in a 34-year-old Chinese woman with Takayasu's arteritis and no palpable pulses in the upper half of her body. The aortogram shows no direct filling of any of the major arteries arising from the aorta except the coronary arteries. In the delayed film *(right)* collateral channels faintly fill the carotid and vertebral systems.

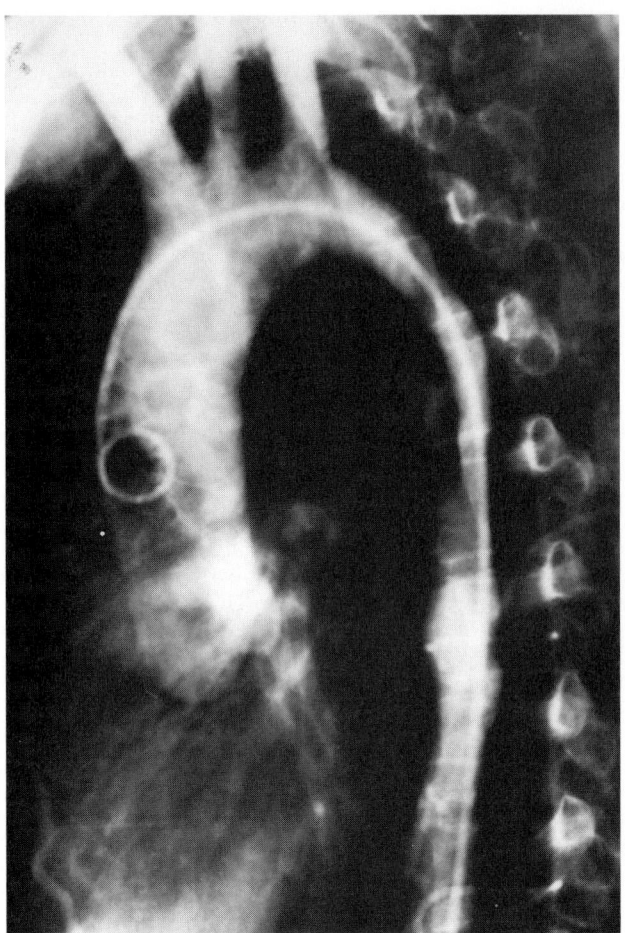

FIGURE 45–25. Thoracic aortogram in a 28-year-old Korean man with the clinical features of coarctation of the aorta that proved to be the result of Takayasu's arteritis. Note the typical "rat-tail" angiographic appearance of the descending aorta.

northern United States and Europe.[284] Its cause is unknown, although the generalized systemic manifestations of the disease and its occasional apparent temporal relationship to prior immunization or viral illness suggest a possible infectious or autoimmune origin.[285] Genetic factors may also play a role.[286]

The characteristic pathological lesion that distinguishes it from other arteritides is the granulomatous inflammation of the media of large and medium-caliber arteries,[287] about the size of the temporal artery. The disease has a special predilection for the branches of the proximal aorta, especially those supplying the head and neck, extracranial structures, and upper extremities.[284] Endarteritis is not an important feature, but the mural involvement can lead to obstruction of involved arteries. Involvement of the aorta[288] and its major branches usually coexists with the more classic and prevalent syndromes of temporal arteritis and polymyalgia rheumatica, although the aorta may rarely serve as the primary target of this disease. Narrowing or occlusions of the aorta are rare in giant cell arteritis.[287] Infrequently, the inflammatory process may weaken the aortic wall, leading to localized aneurysm formation, aortic annular dilatation, and aortic regurgitation.[289]

CLINICAL MANIFESTATIONS. Giant cell arteritis usually affects patients over the age of 50, with a mean age of 67, and occurs predominantly in women. The classic presentation is one of severe headaches, scalp or temporal artery tenderness, and constitutional symptoms. Headaches are often intense and almost unbearable, typically occurring over involved arteries (usually the temporal arteries). The area surrounding these arteries is exquisitely sensitive to pressure, and complaints such as being unable to rest the

head comfortably against a pillow or to comb one's hair are common. Jaw claudication while chewing occurs in up to half of the patients.[271]

On *physical examination,* fever is quite common and patients frequently appear ill. Involved vessels are thickened and very tender. Pulses may be absent or diminished, and bruits may occur over sites of arterial occlusion. Signs of aortic regurgitation are occasionally present. Laboratory tests may be helpful in making the diagnosis. A markedly elevated sedimentation rate is virtually a sine qua non for this disease and is a valuable guide to disease activity. A moderate normochromic, normocytic anemia is the rule. Acute phase reactant levels are often elevated.[290]

The diagnosis is confirmed by biopsy of an involved artery, most often the temporal artery. However, false-negative biopsies occur in about 14 per cent[271] and therefore, if clinical suspicion persists, a second biopsy of another vessel should be performed. The rate of positive biopsies progressively declines after just a few days of glucocorticoid therapy, with as few as 10 per cent being positive after 1 week. Accordingly, biopsies should be performed without delay once the diagnosis is suspected and therapy initiated. In cases of larger vessel and aortic involvement, angiography may serve to differentiate arteritis from atherosclerosis.[283]

A serious complication is the onset of blindness from involvement of the ophthalmic artery. When visual loss occurs, progression to complete blindness is usually rapid and often irreversible. Overall, visual symptoms ranging from blurring to diplopia to vision loss occur in 36 to 58 per cent of patients.[271] In the milder form of giant cell arteritis, patients may complain only of generalized muscle aches and pains and unusual fatigue, the symptoms of polymyalgia rheumatica.

Narrowing or occlusion of the branch vessels of the thoracic aorta—often referred to as *aortic arch syndrome*—may be found in 9 to 14 per cent of cases,[283] producing symptoms similar to those of Takayasu's arteritis, such as decreased upper extremity pulses and blood pressure, arm or leg claudication, Raynaud's phenomenon, transient ischemic attacks, coronary ischemia,[291] and abdominal angina. Interestingly, in contrast with Takayasu's arteritis, renal artery involvement is almost never seen.[283] Aortic aneurysms, aortic regurgitation, and aortic dissection occur less commonly. In a recent series by Evans et al., aortic aneurysms occurred in 15 per cent of patients and at a median of 6 years after the giant cell arteritis was diagnosed.[287] Two-thirds were thoracic aortic aneurysms, with the majority located in the ascending aorta.[292] Almost one-half of those with thoracic aortic aneurysms died suddenly from aortic dissection, and one-third developed symptomatic aortic regurgitation.[287]

MANAGEMENT. High-dose glucocorticoid therapy (prednisone, 40 to 60 mg/day) is recommended in all patients with giant cell arteritis.[284] The goals of therapy are to reverse the disease and to prevent further progression, especially in the ophthalmic arteries in order to prevent blindness. Using constitutional symptoms, vascular symptoms, and the sedimentation rate as guides, the clinician can usually gradually reduce steroids to a maintenance dose for 1 to 2 years. The overall course of the disease is one of progressive improvement and eventual complete resolution, although in some patients it may be protracted for months to years. Methotrexate may be beneficial in patients with steroid-resistant symptoms, and both methotrexate and Dapsone may be useful as glucocorticoid-sparing agents in patients requiring protracted treatment.[286,293] Surgery, ideally performed while the disease is inactive and in the absence of steroid therapy, may be necessary in up to 41 per cent of those with thoracic aortic aneurysms.[292]

OTHER ARTERITIS SYNDROMES. In addition to the acute inflammation of Takayasu's and giant cell arteritis, isolated aortic regurgitation due to dilatation of the aortic annulus may occur during the

TABLE 45–5   PROPOSED CRITERIA FOR THE CLINICAL DIAGNOSIS OF TAKAYASU'S DISEASE*

CRITERION	DEFINITION
Obligatory Criterion	
Age ≤ 40 yr	Age ≤ 40 yr at diagnosis or at onset of "characteristic signs and symptoms"† of 1 month duration in patient history.
Two Major Criteria	
1. Left mid subclavian artery lesion	The most severe stenosis or occlusion present in the mid portion from the point 1 cm proximal to the left vertebral artery orifice to that 3 cm distal to the orifice determined by angiography.
2. Right mid subclavian artery lesion	The most severe stenosis or occlusion present in the mid portion from the right vertebral artery orifice to the point 3 cm distal to the orifice determined by angiography.
Nine Minor Criteria	
1. High ESR	Unexplained persistent high ESR ≥ 20 mm/h (Westergren) at diagnosis or presence of the evidence in patient history.
2. Carotid artery tenderness	Unilateral or bilateral tenderness of common carotid arteries by physician palpation: neck muscle tenderness is unacceptable.
3. Hypertension	Persistent blood pressure ≥ 140/90 mm Hg brachial or ≥ 160/90 mm Hg popliteal at age ≤ 40 yr or presence of the history at age ≤ 40 yr.
4. Aortic regurgitation or	By auscultation or Doppler echocardiography or angiography.
Annuloaortic ectasia	By angiography or two-dimensional echocardiography.
5. Pulmonary artery lesion	Lobar or segmental arterial occlusion or equivalent determined by angiography or perfusion scintigraphy; or presence of stenosis, aneurysm, luminal irregularity, or any combination in pulmonary trunk or in unilateral or bilateral pulmonary arteries determined by angiography.
6. Left mid common carotid lesion	Presence of the most severe stenosis or occlusion in the mid portion of 5 cm in length from the point 2 cm distal to its orifice determined by angiography.
7. Distal brachiocephalic trunk lesion	Presence of the most severe stenosis or occlusion in the distal third determined by angiography.
8. Descending thoracic aorta lesion	Narrowing, dilation or aneurysm, luminal irregularity, or any combination determined by angiography: tortuosity alone is unacceptable.
9. Abdominal aorta lesion	Narrowing, dilation or aneurysm, luminal irregularity, or any combination and absence of lesion in aortoiliac region consisting of 2 cm of terminal aorta and bilateral common iliac arteries determined by angiography; tortuosity alone is unacceptable.

* The proposed criteria consist of one obligatory criterion, two major criteria, and nine minor criteria. In addition to the obligatory criterion, the presence of two major criteria, or one major and two or more minor criteria, or four or more minor criteria suggests a high probability of the presence of Takayasu's disease.

† "Characteristic signs and symptoms" are explained in the reference text. ESR = erythrocyte sedimentation rate.

From Ishikawa, K.: Diagnostic approach and proposed criteria for the clinical diagnosis of Takayasu's arteriopath. J. Am. Coll. Cardiol. *12*:964, 1988.

course of ankylosing spondylitis,[294] psoriatic arthritis,[295] arthritis associated with ulcerative colitis, relapsing polychondritis, polyarteritis nodosa,[296] and Reiter's syndrome.[297] In addition, aneurysms of the aorta, pulmonary artery, and other major vessels can complicate Behçet's disease.[298]

Reported instances of aortitis complicating each of these diseases are rare. For example, aortic regurgitation has been documented in only 1 to 4 per cent of patients with ankylosing spondylitis, 2 per cent of patients with Behçet's disease,[299] and a small number of cases of Reiter's syndrome. Nevertheless, in these uncommon cases the symptoms of aortic regurgitation and ensuing congestive heart failure may eventually dominate the clinical picture.

The pathological features appear to be similar in each of the aforementioned diseases. In the early stage of inflammation there is marked dilatation of the aortic annulus with patchy elastic tissue disruption, an active inflammatory cell infiltrate, and subendothelial fibrosis.[300] These changes are most marked in the aortic root, which typically dilates but without frank aneurysm formation. The aortic valve cusps remain essentially normal in early stages but later become thickened and retracted.

The associated aortic regurgitation shares the clinical features of annuloaortic ectasia. The course of this condition is variable, with some patients exhibiting a rapidly progressive course of cardiac decompensation, whereas others have a more indolent and stable natural history. Thus, the development of aortic regurgitation does not necessarily signify an irreversible downhill course. Treatment is generally directed toward the underlying disease state. Aortic valve replacement should be performed when indicated, although, in contrast to annuloaortic ectasia, replacement of the ascending aorta itself is almost never necessary.

BACTERIAL INFECTIONS OF THE AORTA

Infected aortic aneurysms are rare, with as few as one case per year recently reported from a large medical center.[301] In an effort to avoid confusion with infections truly of fungal origin, the term "infected aneurysm" has gradually replaced the original designation "mycotic aneurysm" used by Osler to define the localized dilatation caused by sepsis in the wall of the aorta. Although saccular aneurysms are seen most commonly, infections can also cause fusiform and false aneurysms. In a minority of cases, infection may arise in a preexistent aortic aneurysm, typically atherosclerotic ones. Rarely, one may encounter nonaneurysmal bacterial aortitis.[301,302]

PATHOGENESIS. Aortic infection may arise by several mechanisms.

Septic emboli from bacterial endocarditis were once the most common cause but have become rare in the era of efficacious antibiotic treatment of septicemia. Contiguous spread of infection from adjacent sites is also infrequently seen. The most common cause of infected aneurysm is the direct deposition of circulating bacteria in a diseased, atherosclerotic, or traumatized aortic intima,[301] after which organisms penetrate the aortic wall through breeches in intimal integrity to cause microbial arteritis. Recent reports suggest that the majority of aortic infections occur in patients with impaired immunity as a consequence of chronic disease, immunosuppressive therapy, or immune deficiency.[301,303]

MICROBIOLOGY. Although virtually any organism may infect the aorta, certain bacteria seem to have a proclivity for this site. *Staphylococcus aureus* and *Salmonella* species are consistently the most frequently identified organisms.[304] *Salmonella* commonly infects atherosclerotic arteries[302] but may also adhere to a normal aortic wall and directly penetrate an intact intima.[305] In fact, as many as one-quarter of patients over the age of 50 who experience *Salmonella* bacteremia may also develop secondary aortic infection.[305] Other gram-positive organisms, particularly pneumococcus, and gram-negative organisms may also cause infected aortic aneurysms. *Pseudomonas, Bacteroides fragilis, Campylobacter fetus, Neisseria gonorrhoeae*, and fungal infections are seen less often.[301,306] Aortic infections with unusual organisms are now seen with increasing frequency in the overtly immunocompromised population.[301]

CLINICAL MANIFESTATIONS. Most patients with infected aortic aneurysm are febrile, with extremely high fevers with rigors being common. Symptoms may arise from localized expansion of an infected aneurysm, which is palpable in as many as 50 per cent of patients and almost always tender.[307] A tender and pulsatile abdominal mass in a febrile patient should therefore be considered an infected aneurysm until proven otherwise.

Leukocytosis and an elevated erythrocyte sedimentation rate are present in most cases. When positive, blood cultures are helpful in suggesting the diagnosis and identifying the pathogen. In any patient with fever of unknown origin and documented *Salmonella* bacteremia, an arterial source of infection should be considered.[302] The absence of positive blood cultures, however, does not exclude the diagnosis of infected aortic aneurysm, as cultures have been found to be negative in one-quarter of cases.

Although abdominal ultrasonography may identify the presence of an aortic aneurysm, CT scanning is superior in demonstrating associated pathological findings suggestive of an infectious cause.[308,309] However, sometimes the aorta is normal in size when bacterial aortitis first presents, so lack of aneurysmal dilatation does not exclude the diagnosis.[304] In such cases, if a patient's fever, leukocytosis, and pain persist, follow-up imaging should be performed, as the aorta may rapidly dilate during the course of the infection. Aortography may also be used to make the diagnosis and is generally performed preoperatively to assist in surgical planning.

The natural history of infected aortic aneurysms is that of expansion and eventual rupture, with extremely rapid progression.[301,304] Salmonella and gram-negative infections have a greater tendency toward early rupture and death.[307] Overall mortality from infected aortic aneurysms is over 50 per cent, despite advances in therapy.[302,310]

MANAGEMENT. Infected aortic aneurysms are treated with intravenous antibiotics and surgical excision. The standard surgical approach involves resection of the infected aneurysm and infected retroperitoneal tissue, oversewing of the native aorta as stumps, and restoration of distal perfusion by placement of an extraanatomical bypass graft tunneled through unaffected tissue planes to avoid placing a graft in a contaminated region. Antibiotic therapy must be continued postoperatively for at least 6 weeks. Several reports suggest that in selected patients with localized infection and no gross pus, an effective and simpler surgical approach is the in situ reconstruction of the aorta with a prosthetic graft.[303,310]

PRIMARY TUMORS OF THE AORTA

Primary tumors of the aorta are quite rare, with only 45 cases reported in the literature from 1873 to the present. The frequency of such reports has increased significantly over the past decade, probably consequent to improvements in noninvasive imaging techniques. Most are diagnosed in the seventh to eighth decade of life. The thoracic and abdominal aorta are involved with equal frequency. In several cases aortic tumors have appeared in association with previously inserted Dacron aortic grafts.[311] Histologically, the majority of primary aortic tumors are classified as sarcomas, with the malignant fibrous histiocytoma subtype especially common.

The majority of primary aortic tumors arise in the intima[312] and grow along the intimal surface and into the aortic lumen to form polypoid masses (often with superimposed thrombus) but tend not to invade the aortic wall. Intimal tumors may present with symptoms of vascular obstruction from narrowing of the aortic lumen or, more typically, with signs and symptoms of peripheral embolization identical to those of atherothrombotic emboli. Emboli are commonly a mixture of tumor and thrombus, and the correct diagnosis may remain obscure until histological analysis of an embolectomy specimen is completed. Less commonly, aortic tumors arise in the medial or adventitial layers of the aortic wall. Such tumors tend not to invade the aortic lumen, but instead behave as aggressive mass lesions and present with constitutional symptoms or back pain.

Because primary aortic tumors are so uncommon and their presentation nonspecific, the diagnosis is rarely considered prior to surgical exploration or necropsy. However, several imaging modalities may be helpful in suggesting the diagnosis. Aortography demonstrates narrowing of the lumen or an intraluminal filling defect in the presence of an intimal tumor but may be negative if the tumor is adventitial.[313] An intraaortic biopsy of an intraluminal aortic mass using intravascular biopsy forceps guided by aortography has been reported.[314] CT scanning can detect intimal tumors but may not easily differentiate these from protruding atheromas.[313] MRI may better de-

fine both the tumor anatomy and the extent of invasion.[315] Lastly, the ability of TEE to image the aortic intima may make it especially useful in the detection of intimal tumors of the thoracic aorta (Fig. 45–26).[316]

Treatment of primary aortic tumors has met with little success. As the majority of patients present with metastatic disease, surgical approaches are often only palliative, i.e., to prevent further embolization. Many die secondary to the consequences of multiple emboli to vital organs. Of those undergoing surgical therapy, the large majority die within days to months postoperatively.

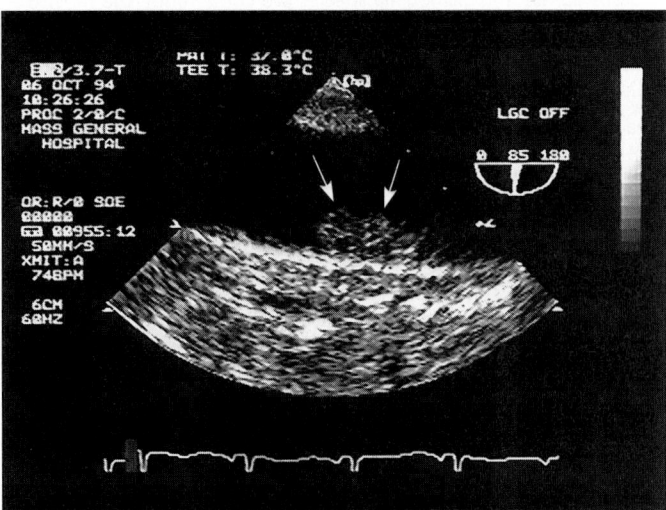

FIGURE 45–26. A transesophageal echocardiogram in long axis of the descending thoracic aorta demonstrating a primary tumor of the aorta (arrows) protruding into the lumen. The tumor, which is 3.5 cm in length, involves the intimal layer but does not appear to invade any further into the aortic wall.

REFERENCES

THE NORMAL AORTA

1. Sonesson, B., Länne, T., Vernersson, E., and Hansen, F.: Sex differences in the mechanical properties of the abdominal aorta in human beings. J. Vasc. Surg. 20:959, 1994.
2. Shimojo, M., Tsuda, N., Iwasaka, T., and Inada, M.: Age-related changes in aortic elasticity determined by gated radionuclide angiography in patients with systemic hypertension or healed myocardial infarcts and in normal subjects. Am. J. Cardiol. 68:950, 1991.
3. Dart, A. M., Lacombe, F., Yeoh, J. K., et al.: Aortic distensibility in patients with isolated hypercholesterolemia, coronary artery disease, or cardiac transplant. Lancet 338:270, 1991.
4. Mohiaddin, R. H., Underwood, S. R., Bogren, H. G., et al.: Regional aortic compliance studied by magnetic resonance imaging: The effects of age, training, and coronary artery disease. Br. Heart J. 62:90, 1989.
5. Schlatmann, T. J. M., and Becker, A. E.: Histologic changes in the normal aging aorta: Implications for dissecting aortic aneurysm. Am. J. Cardiol. 39:13, 1977.
6. Stefanadis, C., Vlachopoulos, C., Karayannacos, P., et al.: Effect of vasa vasorum flow on structure and function of the aorta in experimental animals. Circulation 91:2669, 1995.
7. Urschel, C. W., Covell, J. W., Sonnenblick, E. H., et al.: Effects of decreased aortic compliance on performance of the left ventricle. Am. J. Physiol. 214:298, 1968.
8. Kelly, R. P., Tunin, R., and Kass, D. A.: Effect of reduced aortic compliance on cardiac efficiency and contractile function of in situ canine left ventricle. Circ. Res. 71:490, 1992.

AORTIC ANEURYSMS

9. Johnston, K. W., Rutherford, R. B., Tilson, M.D., et al.: Suggested standards for reporting on arterial aneurysms. J. Vasc. Surg. 13:444, 1991.
10. Crawford, E. S., and Cohen, E. S.: Aortic aneurysm: A multifocal disease. Arch. Surg. 117:1393, 1982.
11. Pressler, V., and McNamara, J. J.: Aneurysm of the thoracic aorta: Review of 260 cases. J. Thorac. Cardiovasc. Surg. 89:50, 1985.
12. Bickerstaff, L. K., Pairolero, P. C., Hollier, L. H., et al.: Thoracic aortic aneurysms: A population based study. Surgery 92:1103, 1982.
13. Bengtsson, H., Bergquist, D., and Sternby, N. H.: Increasing prevalence of abdominal aortic aneurysms: A necropsy study. Eur. J. Surg. 158:19, 1992.
14. Bickerstaff, L. K., Hollier, L. H., Van Peenan, H. J., et al.: Abdominal aortic aneurysms: The changing natural history. J. Vasc. Surg. 1:6, 1984.
15. Anidjar, S., and Kieffer, E.: Pathogenesis of acquired aneurysms of the abdominal aorta. Ann. Vasc. Surg. 6:298, 1992.
16. Holmes, D. R., Liao, S., Parks, W. C., and Thompson, R. W.: Medial neovascularization in abdominal aortic aneurysms: A histopathologic marker of aneurysm degeneration with pathophysiologic implications. J. Vasc. Surg. 21:761, 1995.
17. Webster, M. W., Ferrell, R. F., St. Jean, P. L., et al.: Ultrasound screening of first-degree relatives of patients with abdominal aortic aneurysm. J. Vasc. Surg. 13:9, 1991.
18. Verloes, A., Sakalihassan, L., Koulischer, L., and Limet, R.: Aneurysms of the abdominal aorta: Familial and genetic aspects in three hundred thirteen pedigrees. J. Vasc. Surg. 21:646, 1995.
19. Reilly, J. M., Brophy, C. M., and Tilson, M.D.: Characterization of an elastase from aneurysmal aorta which degrades intact aortic elastin. Ann. Vasc. Surg. 6:499, 1992.
20. Anidjar, S., Dobrin, P. B., Eichorst, M., et al.: Correlation of inflammatory infiltrate with the enlargement of experimental aortic aneurysms. J. Vasc. Surg. 16:139, 1992.
21. Newman, K. M., Jean-Claude, J., Li, H., et al.: Cytokines that activate proteolysis are increased in abdominal aortic aneurysms. Circulation 90(Part 2):II-224, 1994.
22. Darling, R. C.: Ruptured arteriosclerotic abdominal aortic aneurysms. Am. J. Surg. 119:397, 1970.
23. Rantakokko, V., Havia, T., Inberg, M. V., and Vänttinen, E.: Abdominal aortic aneurysms: A clinical and autopsy study of 408 patients. Acta Chir. Scand. 149:151, 1983.
24. Astarita, D., Filippone, D. R., and Cohn, J. D.: Spontaneous major intra-abdominal arteriovenous fistulas: A report of several cases. Angiology 36:656, 1985.
25. Muluk, S. C., Gertler, J. P., Brewster, D. C., et al.: Presentation and patterns of aortic aneurysms in young patients. J. Vasc. Surg. 20:880, 1994.
26. Kiell, C. S., and Ernst, C. B.: Advances in the management of abdominal aortic aneurysm. Adv. Surg. 26:73, 1993.
27. Marston, W. A., Ahlquist, R., Johnson, G., Jr., and Meyer, A. A.: Mis-

diagnosis of ruptured abdominal aortic aneurysms. J. Vasc. Surg. 16:17, 1992.

28. Martinussen, H. J., Lolk, A., Rohr, N., et al.: Ruptured abdominal aortic aneurysm with fistula into the inferior vena cava. J. Cardiovasc. Surg. 27:298, 1986.

29. Crew, J. R., Bashour, T. T., Ellertson, D., et al.: Ruptured abdominal aortic aneurysms: Experience with 70 cases. Clin. Cardiol. 8:433, 1985.

30. Jenkins, A. M., Ruckley, C. V., and Nolan, B.: Ruptured abdominal aortic aneurysm. Br. J. Surg. 73:395, 1986.

31. LaRoy, L. L., Cormier, P. J., Matalon, T. A. S., et al.: Imaging of abdominal aortic aneurysms. A. J. R. 152:785, 1989.

32. Hollier, L. H., Taylor, L. M., and Ochsner, J.: Recommended indications for operative treatment of abdominal aortic aneurysms: Report of a subcommittee of the Joint Council of the Society for Vascular Surgery and of the North American Chapter of the International Society for Cardiovascular Surgery. J. Vasc. Surg. 15:1046, 1992.

33. Ernst, C. B.: Abdominal aortic aneurysm. N. Engl. J. Med. 328:1167, 1993.

34. Todd, G. J., Nowygrod, R., Benvenisty, A., et al.: The accuracy of CT scanning in the diagnosis of abdominal and thoracoabdominal aortic aneurysms. J. Vasc. Surg. 13:302, 1991.

35. Pillari, G., Chang, J. B., Zito, J., et al.: Computed tomography of abdominal aortic aneurysm: An in vivo pathological report with a note on dynamic predictors. Arch. Surg. 123:727, 1988.

36. Gomes, M. N., and Choyke, P. L.: Improved identification of the renal arteries in patients with aortic aneurysms by means of high-resolution computed tomography. J. Vasc. Surg. 6:262, 1987.

37. Lederle, F. A., Wilson, S. E., Johnson, G. R., et al.: Variability in measurement of abdominal aortic aneurysms. J. Vasc. Surg. 21:945, 1995.

38. Gomes, M. N., Davros, W. J., and Zemen, R. K.: Preoperative assessment of abdominal aortic aneurysm: The value of helical and three-dimensional computed tomography. J. Vasc. Surg. 20:367, 1994.

39. Petersen, M. J., Cambria, R. P., Kaufman, J. A., et al.: Magnetic resonance angiography in the preoperative evaluation of abdominal aortic aneurysms. J. Vasc. Surg. 21:891, 1995.

40. Campbell, J. J., Bell, D. D., and Gaspar, M. R.: Selective use of arteriography in the assessment of aortic aneurysm repair. Ann. Vasc. Surg. 4:419, 1990.

41. Edelman, R. R.: MR angiography: Present and future. A. J. R. 161:1, 1993.

42. Kandarpa, K., Piwnica-Worms, D., Chopra, P. S., et al.: Prospective double-blinded comparison of MR imaging and aortography in the preoperative evaluation of abdominal aortic aneurysms. J. Vasc. Intervent. Radiol. 3:83, 1992.

43. Frame, P. S., Fryback, D. G., and Patteson, C.: Screening for abdominal aortic aneurysm in men ages 60 to 80 years: A cost-effectiveness analysis. Ann. Intern. Med. 119:411, 1993.

44. Ingoldby, C. J. H., Wujanto, R., and Mitchell, J. E.: Impact of vascular surgery on community mortality from ruptured aortic aneurysm. Br. J. Surg. 73:551, 1986.

45. Estes, J. E., Jr.: Abdominal aortic aneurysm: A study of one hundred and two cases. Circulation 2:258, 1950.

46. Darling, R. C., Messina, C. R., Brewster, D. C., and Ottinger, L. W.: Autopsy study of unoperated abdominal aortic aneurysms: The case for early resection. Circulation 56(Suppl. II):II-161, 1977.

47. Ouriel, K., Green, R. M., Donayre, C., et al.: An evaluation of new methods of expressing aortic aneurysm size: Relationships to rupture. J. Vasc. Surg. 15:12, 1992.

48. Limet, R., Sakalihassan, N., and Adelin, A.: Determination of the expansion rate and incidence of rupture of abdominal aortic aneurysms. J. Vasc. Surg. 14:540, 1991.

49. Gadowski, G. R., Pilcher, D. B., and Ricci, M. A.: Abdominal aortic aneurysm expansion rate: Effect of size and beta-adrenergic blockade. J. Vasc. Surg. 19:727, 1994.

50. Katz, D. J., Stanley, J. C., and Zelenock, G. B.: Operative mortality rates for intact and ruptured abdominal aortic aneurysms in Michigan: An eleven-year statewide experience. J. Vasc. Surg. 19:804, 1994.

51. Lederle, F. A., Wilson, S. E., Johnson, G. R., et al.: Design of the abdominal aortic aneurysm detection and management study. J. Vasc. Surg. 20:296, 1994.

52. Johnston, K. W., and the Canadian Society for Vascular Surgery Aneurysm Study Group: Non-ruptured abdominal aortic aneurysm: Six-year follow-up results from the multicenter prospective Canadian aneurysm study. J. Vasc. Surg. 20:163, 1994.

53. Parodi, J. C., Palmaz, J. C., and Barone, H. D.: Transfemoral intraluminal graft implantation for abdominal aortic aneurysms. Ann. Vasc. Surg. 5:491, 1991.

54. Ruiz, C. E., Zhang, H. P., Douglas, J. T., et al.: A novel method for treatment of abdominal aortic aneurysms using percutaneous implantation of a newly designed endovascular device. Circulation 91:2470, 1995.

55. Parodi, J. C.: Endovascular repair of abdominal aortic aneurysms and other arterial lesions. J. Vasc. Surg. 21:549, 1995.

56. Hertzer, N. R.: Fatal myocardial infarction following abdominal aortic aneurysm resection: Three hundred forty-three patients followed 6–11 years postoperatively. Ann. Surg. 192:667, 1980.

57. Hertzer, N. R., Beven, E. G., Young, Y. R., et al.: Coronary artery disease in peripheral vascular patients: A classification of 1000 coronary angiograms and results of surgical management. Ann. Surg. 199:223, 1984.

58. Boucher, C. A., Brewster, D. C., Darling, R. C., et al.: Determination of

59. Eagle, K. A., Singer, D. E., Brewster, D. C., et al.: Dipyridamole-thallium scanning in patients undergoing vascular surgery: Optimizing preoperative evaluation of cardiac risk. JAMA 257:2185, 1987.

60. Levinson, J. R., Boucher, C. A., Coley, C. M., et al.: Usefulness of semiquantitative analysis of dipyridamole-thallium 201 redistribution for improving risk stratification before vascular surgery. Am. J. Cardiol. 66:406, 1990.

61. Leppo, J., Plaja, J., Gionet, M., et al.: Noninvasive evaluation of cardiac risk before elective vascular surgery. J. Am. Coll. Cardiol. 9:269, 1987.

62. Lalka, S. G., Sawada, S. G., Dalsing, M. C., et al.: Dobutamine stress echocardiography as a predictor of cardiac events associated with aortic surgery. J. Vasc. Surg. 15:831, 1992.

63. Cambria, R. P., Brewster, D. C., Abbott, W. M., et al.: The impact of selective use of dipyridamole-thallium scans and surgical factors on the current morbidity of aortic surgery. J. Vasc. Surg. 15:43, 1992.

64. Gersh, B. J., Rihal, C. S., Rooke, T. W., and Ballard, D. J.: Evaluation and management of patients with both peripheral vascular and coronary artery disease. J. Am. Coll. Cardiol. 18:203, 1991.

65. Steinberg, J. B., Kresowik, T. F., and Behrendt, D. M.: Prophylactic myocardial revascularization based on dipyridamole-thallium scanning before peripheral vascular surgery. Cardiovasc. Surg. 1:552, 1993.

66. Hertzer, N. R., Young, J. R., Beven, E. G., et al.: Late results of coronary bypass in patients with peripheral vascular disease. II. Five-year survival according to sex, hypertension, and diabetes. Cleve. Clin. J. Med. 54:15, 1987.

67. Rihal, C. S., Eagle, K. A., Mickel, M. C., et al.: Surgical therapy for coronary artery disease among patients with combined coronary artery and peripheral vascular disease. Circulation 91:46, 1995.

68. Pasternack, P. F., Grossi, E. A., Bauman, F. G., et al.: Silent myocardial ischemia monitoring predicts late as well as perioperative cardiac events in patients undergoing vascular surgery. J. Vasc. Surg. 16:171, 1992.

69. Landesberg, G., Luria, M. H., Cotev, S., et al.: Importance of long-duration postoperative ST-segment depression in cardiac morbidity after vascular surgery. Lancet 341:715, 1993.

70. Pasternack, P. F., Grossi, E. A., Bauman, F. G., et al.: Beta blockade to decrease silent myocardial ischemia during peripheral vascular surgery. Am. J. Surg. 158:113, 1989.

71. Reigel, M. M., Hollier, L. H., Kazmier, F. J., et al.: Late survival in abdominal aortic aneurysm patients: The role of selective myocardial revascularization on the basis of clinical symptoms. J. Vasc. Surg. 5:222, 1987.

72. Brophy, C., Tilson, J. E., and Tilson, M. D.: Propranolol delays the formation of aneurysms in the male blotchy mouse. J. Surg. Res. 44:687, 1988.

73. Treiman, R. L., Hartunian, S. L., Cossman, D. V., et al.: Late results of small untreated abdominal aortic aneurysms. Ann. Vasc. Surg. 5:359, 1991.

74. Pyeritz, R. E., and McKusick, V. A.: The Marfan syndrome: Diagnosis and management. N. Engl. J. Med. 300:772, 1979.

75. Milewicz, D. M.: Ultrasonic characterization of the aortic architecture in Marfan patients. Circulation 91(Edit.):1272, 1995.

76. Hollister, D. W., Goodfrey, M., Sakai, L. Y., and Pyeritz, R. E.: Immunohistologic abnormalities of the microfibrillar-fiber system in the Marfan syndrome. N. Engl. J. Med. 323:152, 1990.

77. Jeremy, R. W., Huang, H., Hwa, J., et al.: Relation between age, arterial distensibility, and aortic dilatation in the Marfan syndrome. Am. J. Cardiol. 74:369, 1994.

78. Marsalese, D. L., Moodie, D. S., Lytle, B. W., et al.: Cystic medial necrosis of the aorta in patients without Marfan's syndrome: Surgical outcome and long-term follow up. J. Am. Coll. Cardiol. 16:68, 1990.

79. Emanuel, R., Ng, R. A., Marcomichelakis, J., et al.: Formes frustes of Marfan's syndrome presenting with severe aortic regurgitation: Clinicogenetic study of 18 families. Br. Heart J. 39:190, 1977.

80. Johansson, G., Markström, U., and Swedenborg, J.: Ruptured thoracic aortic aneurysms: A study of incidence and mortality rates. J. Vasc. Surg. 21:985, 1995.

81. Joyce, J. W., Fairbairn, J. F., II, Kincaid, O. W., and Juergens, J. L.: Aneurysms of the thoracic aorta: A clinical study with special reference to prognosis. Circulation 29:176, 1964.

82. McNamara, J. J., and Pressler, V. M.: Natural history of arteriosclerotic thoracic aortic aneurysms. Ann. Thorac. Surg. 26:468, 1978.

83. Bogey, W. M., Jr., Thomas, J. H., and Hermreck, A. S.: Aortoesophageal fistula: Report of a successfully managed case and review of the literature. J. Vasc. Surg. 16:90, 1992.

84. Masuda, Y., Takanashi, K., Takasu, J., et al.: Expansion rate of thoracic aortic aneurysms and influencing factors. Chest 102:461, 1992.

85. Dinsmore, R. E., Liberthson, R. R., Wismer, G. L., et al.: Magnetic resonance imaging of thoracic aortic aneurysms: Comparison with other diagnostic methods. A. J. R. 146:309, 1986.

86. Pressler, V., and McNamara, J. J.: Thoracic aortic aneurysm: Natural history and treatment. J. Thorac. Cardiovasc. Surg. 79:489, 1980.

87. Crawford, E. S., and DeNatale, R. W.: Thoracoabdominal aortic aneurysm: Observations regarding the natural course of disease. J. Vasc. Surg. 3:578, 1986.

88. Hirose, Y., Hamada, S., Takamiya, M., et al.: Aortic aneurysm: Growth rate measured with CT. Radiology 185:249, 1992.

89. Dapunt, O. E., Galla, J. D., Sadeghi, A. M., et al.: The natural history of thoracic aortic aneurysms. J. Thorac. Cardiovasc. Surg. 107:1323, 1994.

90. Treasure, T.: Elective replacement of the aortic root in Marfan's syndrome. Br. Heart J. 69(Edit.):101, 1993.

91. Verdant, A., Cossette, R., Page, A., et al.: Aneurysms of the descending thoracic aorta: Three hundred sixty-six consecutive cases resected without paraplegia. J. Vasc. Surg. 21:385, 1995.

92. Livesay, J. J., Cooley, D. A., Ventemiglia, R. A., et al.: Surgical experience in descending thoracic aneurysmectomy with and without adjuncts to avoid ischemia. Ann. Thorac. Surg. 39:37, 1985.

93. Gott, V. L., Gillinov, A. M., Pyeritz, R. E., et al.: Aortic root replacement: Risk factor analysis of a seventeen-year experience with 270 patients. J. Thorac. Cardiovasc. Surg. 109:536, 1995.

94. David, T. E., Feindel, C. M., and Bos, J.: Repair of the aortic valve in patients with aortic insufficiency and aortic root aneurysm. J. Thorac. Cardiovasc. Surg. 109:345, 1995.

95. Coselli, J. S., Büket, S., and Djukanovic, B.: Aortic arch operation: Current treatment and results. Ann. Thorac. Surg. 59:19, 1995.

96. Svensson, L. G., Crawford, S., Hess, R., et al.: Dissection of the aorta and dissecting aortic aneurysms: Improving early and long-term survival results. Circulation 82(Suppl. IV):IV-24, 1990.

97. Griepp, R. B., Stinson, E. B., Hollingsworth, J. F., and Buehler, D.: Prosthetic replacement of the aortic arch. J. Thorac. Cardiovasc. Surg. 70:1051, 1975.

98. Crawford, E. S., Coselli, J. S., Svensson, L. G., et al.: Diffuse aneurysmal disease (chronic aortic dissection, Marfan, and mega aorta syndromes) and multiple aneurysm. Ann. Surg. 211:521, 1990.

99. Kitamura, M., Hashimoto, A., Akimoto, T., et al.: Operation for type A aortic dissection: Introduction of retrograde cerebral perfusion. Ann. Thorac. Surg. 59:1195, 1995.

100. Usui, A., Hotta, T., Hiroura, M., et al.: Retrograde perfusion through a superior vena caval cannula protects the brain. Ann. Thorac. Surg. 53:47, 1992.

101. Heinemann, M. K., Buehner, B., Jurmann, M. J., and Borst, H.-G.: Use of the "elephant trunk technique" in aortic surgery. Ann. Thorac. Surg. 60:2, 1995.

102. Crawford, E. S., Svensson, L. G., Coselli, J. S., et al.: Surgical treatment of aneurysm and/or dissection of the ascending aorta, transverse aortic arch, and ascending aorta and transverse arch: Factors influencing survival in 717 patients. J. Thorac. Cardiovasc. Surg. 98:659, 1989.

103. Coselli, J. S., and Crawford, E. S.: Composite valve-graft replacement of aortic root using separate Dacron tube for coronary artery reattachment. Ann. Thorac. Surg. 47:558, 1989.

104. Hollier, L. H., Symmonds, J. B., Pairolero, P. C., et al.: Thoracoabdominal aortic aneurysm repair: Analysis of postoperative morbidity. Arch. Surg. 123:871, 1988.

105. Dake, M. D., Miller, D. C., Semba, C. P., et al.: Transluminal placement of endovascular stent-grafts for the treatment of descending thoracic aneurysms. N. Engl. J. Med. 331:1729, 1994.

106. Moreno-Cabral, C. E., Miller, D. C., Mitchell, R. S., et al.: Degenerative and atherosclerotic aneurysms of the thoracic aorta. J. Thorac. Cardiovasc. Surg. 88:1020, 1984.

107. Shores, J., Berger, K. R., Murphy, E. A., and Pyeritz, R. E.: Progression of aortic dilatation and the benefit of long-term β-adrenergic blockade in Marfan's syndrome. N. Engl. J. Med. 330:1335, 1994.

108. Ellis, R. P., Cooley, D. A., and DeBakey, M. E.: Clinical considerations and surgical treatment of annulo-aortic ectasia. J. Thorac. Cardiovasc. Surg. 42:363, 1961.

109. Lemon, D. K., and White, C. W.: Annuloaortic ectasia: Angiographic, hemodynamic, and clinical comparison with aortic valve insufficiency. Am. J. Cardiol. 41:482, 1978.

AORTIC DISSECTION

110. Wheat, M. W., Jr.: Acute dissecting aneurysms of the aorta: Diagnosis and treatment—1979. Am. Heart J. 99:373, 1980.

111. Roberts, W. C.: Aortic dissection: Anatomy, consequences, and causes. Am. Heart J. 101:195, 1981.

112. Hirst, A. E., Johns, V. J., Jr., and Kime, S. W., Jr.: Dissecting aneurysm of the aorta: A review of 505 cases. Medicine 37:217, 1958.

113. Wilson, S. K., and Hutchins, G. M.: Aortic dissecting aneurysms: Causative factors in 204 subjects. Arch. Pathol. Lab. Med. 106:175, 1982.

114. DeBakey, M. E., McCollum, C. H., Crawford, E. S., et al.: Dissection and dissecting aneurysms of the aorta: Twenty-year follow-up of five hundred twenty-seven patients treated surgically. Surgery 92:1118, 1982.

115. Daily, P. O., Trueblood, H. W., Stinson, E. B., et al.: Management of acute aortic dissections. Ann. Thorac. Surg. 10:237, 1970.

116. VanMaele, R. G., De Bock, L., Van Schil, P. E., et al.: Limited acute dissections of the abdominal aorta: Report of five cases. J. Cardiovasc. Surg. 33:298, 1992.

117. Spittell, P. C., Spittell, J. A., Jr., Joyce, J. W., et al.: Clinical features and differential diagnosis of aortic dissection: Experience with 236 cases (1980 through 1990). Mayo Clin. Proc. 68:642, 1993.

118. Larson, E. W., and Edwards, W. D.: Risk factors for aortic dissection: A necropsy study of 161 patients. Am. J. Cardiol. 53:849, 1984.

119. Shachter, N., Perloff, J. K., and Mulder, D. G.: Aortic dissection in Noonan's syndrome. Am. J. Cardiol. 54:464, 1984.

120. Price, W. H., and Wilson, J.: Dissection of the aorta in Turner's syndrome. J. Med. Genet. 20:61, 1983.

121. Om, A., Porter, T., and Mohanty, P. K.: Transesophageal echocardiographic diagnosis of acute aortic dissection complicating cocaine abuse. Am. Heart J. 123:532, 1992.

122. Williams, G. M., Gott, V. L., Brawley, R. K., et al.: Aortic disease associated with pregnancy. J. Vasc. Surg. 8:470, 1988.

123. Mazzucotelli, J.-P., Deleuze, P. H., Baureton, C., et al.: Preservation of the aortic valve in acute aortic dissection: Long-term echocardiographic assessment and clinical outcome. Ann. Thorac. Surg. 55:1513, 1993.

124. Pumphrey, C. W., Fay, T., and Weir, I.: Aortic dissection during pregnancy. Br. Heart J. 55:106, 1986.

125. Elkayam, U., Ostzega, E., Shotan, A., and Mehra, A.: Cardiovascular problems in pregnant women with the Marfan syndrome. Ann. Intern. Med. 123:117, 1995.

126. Jacobs, L. E., Fraifeld, M., Kotler, M. N., and Ioli, A. W.: Aortic dissection following intraaortic balloon insertion: Recognition by transesophageal echocardiography. Am. Heart J. 124:536, 1992.

127. Murphy, D. A., Craver, J. M., Jones, E. L., et al.: Recognition and management of ascending aortic dissection complicating cardiac surgical operations. J. Thorac. Cardiovasc. Surg. 85:247, 1983.

128. Still, R. J., Hilgenberg, A. D., Akins, C. W., et al.: Intraoperative aortic dissection. Ann. Thorac. Surg. 53:374, 1992.

129. Albat, B., and Thevenet, A.: Dissecting aneurysms of the ascending aorta occurring late after aortic valve replacement. J. Cardiovasc. Surg. 33:272, 1992.

130. Slater, E. E., and DeSanctis, R. W.: The clinical recognition of dissecting aortic aneurysm. Am. J. Med. 60:625, 1976.

131. Doroghazi, R. M., Slater, E. E., DeSanctis, R. W., et al.: Long-term survival of patients with treated aortic dissection. J. Am. Coll. Cardiol. 3:1026, 1984.

132. Vilacosta, I., Castillo, J. A., San Román, J. A., et al.: New echo-anatomical correlations in aortic dissection. Eur. Heart J. 16:126, 1995.

133. Hurak, A. M., and Konstadt, S. N.: Aortic intussusception: A rare complication of aortic dissection. Anesthesiology 82:1292, 1994.

134. Fann, J. I., Sarris, G. E., Mitchell, R. S., et al.: Treatment of patients with aortic dissection presenting with peripheral vascular complications. Ann. Surg. 212:705, 1990.

135. Zull, D. N., and Cydula, R.: Acute paraplegia: A presenting manifestation of aortic dissection. Am. J. Med. 84:765, 1988.

136. Glower, D. D., Speier, R. H., White, W. D., et al.: Management and long-term outcome of aortic dissection. Ann. Surg. 214:31, 1991.

137. Kamp, T. J., Goldschmidt-Clermont, P. J., Brinker, J. A., and Resar, J. R.: Myocardial infarction, aortic dissection, and thrombolytic therapy. Am. Heart J. 128:1234, 1994.

138. Hartnell, G. G., Wakeley, C. J., Tottle, A., et al.: Limitations of chest radiography in discriminating between aortic dissection and myocardial infarction: Implications for thrombolysis. J. Thorac. Imaging 8:152, 1993.

139. Cambria, R. P., Brewster, D. C., Moncure, A. C., et al.: Spontaneous aortic dissection in the presence of coexistent or previously repaired atherosclerotic aortic aneurysm. Ann. Surg. 208:619, 1988.

140. Giannoccaro, P. J., Marquis, J.-F., Chan, K.-L., et al.: Aortic dissection presenting as upper airway obstruction. Chest 99:256, 1991.

141. Roth, J. A., and Parekh, M. A.: Dissecting aneurysms perforating the esophagus. N. Engl. J. Med. 299:776, 1978.

142. Logue, R. B., and Sikes, C.: A new sign in dissecting aneurysm of the aorta: Pulsation of a sternoclavicular joint. JAMA 148:1209, 1952.

143. Murray, H. W., Mann, J. J., Genecin, A., and McKusick, V. A.: Fever with dissecting aneurysm of the aorta. Am. J. Med. 61:10, 1976.

144. Hurley, D. V., Nishimura, R. A., Schaff, H. V., and Edwards, W. D.: Aortic dissection with fistula to right atrium: Noninvasive diagnosis by two-dimensional and Doppler echocardiography with successful repair: Case report and review of the literature. J. Thorac. Cardiovasc. Surg. 92:953, 1986.

145. Perryman, R. A., and Gay, W. A.: Rupture of dissecting thoracic aortic aneurysm into the right ventricle. Am. J. Cardiol. 30:277, 1972.

146. Oliveira, J. S. M., Bestetti, R. B., Marin-Neto, J. A., et al.: Ruptured aortic dissection into the left atrium: A rare cause of congestive heart failure. Am. Heart J. 121:936, 1991.

147. Eagle, K. A., Quertermous, T., Kritzer, G. A., et al.: Spectrum of conditions initially suggesting acute aortic dissection but with negative aortograms. Am. J. Cardiol. 57:322, 1986.

147a. O'Gara, P. T., and DeSanctis, R. W.: Acute aortic dissection and its variants: Toward a common diagnostic and therapeutic approach. Circulation 92:1376, 1995.

148. Cigarroa, J. E., Isselbacher, E. M., DeSanctis, R. W., and Eagle, K. A.: Diagnostic imaging in the evaluation of suspected aortic dissection: Old standards and new directions. N. Engl. J. Med. 328:35, 1993.

149. Wilbers, C. R., Carrol, C. L., and Hnilica, M. A.: Optimal diagnostic imaging of aortic dissection. Texas Heart Inst. J. 17:271, 1990.

150. Petasnick, J. P: Radiologic evaluation of aortic dissection. Radiology 180:297, 1991.

151. Earnest, F., IV, Muhm, J. R., and Sheedy, P. F., II: Roentgenographic findings in thoracic aortic dissection. Mayo Clin. Proc. 54:43, 1979.

152. Erbel, R., Daniel, W., Visser, C., et al.: Echocardiography in diagnosis of aortic dissection. Lancet 1:457, 1989.

153. Bansal, R. C., Chandrasekaran, K., Ayala, K., and Smith, D.: Frequency and explanation of false negative diagnosis of aortic dissection by aortography and transesophageal echocardiography. J. Am. Coll. Cardiol. 25:1393, 1995.

154. Mugge, A., Daniel, W. G., Laas, J., et al.: False-negative diagnosis of proximal aortic dissection by computed tomography or angiography and possible explanations based on transesophageal echocardiographic findings. Am. J. Cardiol. 65:527, 1990.

155. Nienaber, C. A., von Kodolitsch, Y., Nicolas, V., et al.: Definitive diagnosis of thoracic aortic dissection: The emerging role of noninvasive imaging modalities. N. Engl. J. Med. *328*:1, 1993.

156. Hamada, S., Takamiya, M., Kimura, K., et al.: Type A aortic dissection: Evaluation with ultrafast CT. Radiology *183*:155, 1992.

157. Zemen, R. K., Berman, P. M., Silverman, P. M., et al.: Diagnosis of aortic dissection: Value of helical CT with multiplanar reformation and three-dimensional rendering. A. J. R. *164*:1375, 1995.

158. White, R. D., Lipton, M. J., Higgins, C. B., et al.: Noninvasive evaluation of suspected thoracic aortic disease by contrast-enhanced computed tomography. Am. J. Cardiol. *57*:282, 1986.

159. Nienaber, C. A., Spielmann, R. P., von Kodolitsch, Y., et al.: Diagnosis of thoracic aortic dissection: Magnetic resonance imaging versus transesophageal echocardiography. Circulation *85*:434, 1992.

160. Kersting-Sommerhoff, B. A., Higgins, C. B., White, R. D., et al.: Aortic dissection: Sensitivity and specificity of MR imaging. Radiology *166*:651, 1988.

161. Shellock, F. G., and Curtis, J. S.: MR imaging and biomedical implants, materials, and devices: An updated review. Radiology *180*:541, 1991.

162. Adachi, H., Omoto, R., Kyo, S., et al.: Emergency surgical intervention of acute aortic dissection with the rapid diagnosis by transesophageal echocardiography. Circulation *84*(Suppl. III):III-14, 1991.

163. Evangelista, A., Garcia-del-Castillo, H., Gonzales-Alujas, T., et al.: Diagnosis of ascending aortic dissection by transesophageal echocardiography: Utility of M-mode in recognizing artifacts. J. Am. Coll. Cardiol. *27*:102, 1996.

164. Blanchard, D. G., Kimura, B. J., Dittrich, H. C., and DeMaria, A. N.: Transesophageal echocardiography of the aorta. JAMA *272*:546, 1994.

165. Kern, M. J., Serota, H., Callicoat, P., et al.: Use of coronary arteriography in the preoperative management of patients undergoing urgent repair of the thoracic aorta. Am. Heart J. *119*:143, 1990.

166. Ballal, R. S., Nanda, N. C., Gatewood, R., et al.: Usefulness of transesophageal echocardiography in assessment of aortic dissection. Circulation *84*:1903, 1991.

167. Erbel, R., Oelert, H., Meyer, J., et al.: Effect of medical and surgical therapy on aortic dissection evaluated by transesophageal echocardiography: Implications for prognosis and therapy. Circulation *87*:1604, 1993.

168. Granato, J. E., Dee, P., and Gibson, R. S.: Utility of two-dimensional echocardiography in suspected ascending aortic dissection. Am. J. Cardiol. *56*:123, 1985.

169. Chan, K.: Usefulness of transesophageal echocardiography in the diagnosis of conditions mimicking aortic dissection. Am. Heart J. *122*:495, 1991.

170. Yamada, E., Matsumura, M., Kyo, S., and Omoto, R.: Usefulness of a prototype intravascular ultrasound imaging in evaluation of aortic dissection and comparison with aortographic study, transesophageal echocardiography, computed tomography, and magnetic resonance imaging. Am. J. Cardiol. *75*:161, 1995.

171. Moon, M. R., Dake, M. D., Pelc, L. R., et al.: Intravascular stenting of acute experimental type B dissections. J. Surg. Res. *54*:381, 1993.

172. Banning, A. P., Ruttley, M. S. T., Musumeci, F., and Fraser, A. G.: Acute dissection of the thoracic aorta: Transesophageal echocardiography is the investigation of choice. Br. Med. J. *310*:72, 1995.

173. Rizzo, R. J., Aranki, S. F., Aklog, L., et al.: Rapid noninvasive diagnosis and surgical repair of acute ascending aortic dissection. J. Thorac. Cardiovasc. Surg. *108*:567, 1994.

174. Simon, P., Owen, A. N., Havel, M., et al.: Transesophageal echocardiography in the emergency surgical management of patients with aortic dissection. J. Thorac. Cardiovasc. Surg. *103*:1113, 1992.

175. Creswell, L. L., Kouchoukos, N. T., Cox, J. L., and Rosenbloom, M.: Coronary artery disease in patients with type A aortic dissection. Ann. Thorac. Surg. *59*:585, 1995.

176. Anagnostopoulos, C. E., Prabhakar, M. J. S., and Kittle, C. F.: Aortic dissections and dissecting aneurysms. Am. J. Cardiol. *30*:263, 1972.

177. Shaw, R. W.: Acute dissecting aortic aneurysms: Treatment by fenestration of the internal wall of the aneurysm. N. Engl. J. Med. *253*:331, 1955.

178. Elefteriades, J. A., Hartleroad, J., Gusberg, R. J., et al.: Long-term experience with descending aortic dissection: The complication-specific approach. Ann. Thorac. Surg. *53*:11, 1992.

179. DeBakey, M. E., Cooley, D. A., and Creech, O., Jr.: Surgical considerations of dissecting aneurysms of the aorta. Ann. Surg. *142*:586, 1955.

180. Wheat, M. W., Jr., Palmer, R. F., Barley, T. D., and Seelman, R. C.: Treatment of dissecting aneurysms of the aorta without surgery. J. Thorac. Cardiovasc. Surg. *50*:364, 1965.

181. Grubb, B. P., Sirio, C., and Zelis, R.: Intravenous labetalol in acute aortic dissection. JAMA *258*:78, 1987.

182. Fenner, S. G., Mahoney, A., and Cashman, J. N.: Repair of traumatic transection of the thoracic aorta: Esmolol for intraoperative control of arterial pressure. Br. J. Anaesth. *67*:483, 1991.

183. Frishman, W. H., Weinberg, P., Peled, H. B., et al.: Calcium entry blockers for the treatment of severe hypertension and hypertensive crisis. Am. J. Med. *77*(Suppl. 2B):35, 1984.

184. White, S. R., and Hall, J. B.: Control of hypertension with nifedipine in the setting of aortic dissection. Chest *88*:781, 1985.

185. Isselbacher, E. M., Cigarroa, J. E., and Eagle, K. A.: Cardiac tamponade complicating proximal aortic dissection: Is pericardiocentesis harmful? Circulation *90*:2375, 1994.

186. Miller, D. C., Stinson, E. B., Oyer, P. E., et al.: Operative treatment of aortic dissections: Experience with 125 patients over a sixteen-year period. J. Thorac. Cardiovasc. Surg. *78*:365, 1979.

187. Masuda, Y., Yamada, Z., Morooka, N., et al.: Prognosis of patients with medically treated aortic dissections. Circulation *84*(Suppl. III):III-7, 1991.

188. Miller, D. C., Mitchell, R. C., Oyer, P. E., et al.: Independent determinants of operative mortality for patients with aortic dissections. Circulation *70*(Suppl. I):153, 1984.

189. Glower, D. D., Fann, J. I., Speier, R. H., et al.: Comparison of medical and surgical therapy for uncomplicated descending aortic dissection. Circulation *82*(Suppl IV):IV-39, 1990.

190. Crawford, E. S., Svensson, L. G., Coselli, J. S., et al.: Aortic dissection and dissecting aortic aneurysms. Ann. Surg. *208*:254, 1988.

191. Cachera, J. P., Vouhe, P. R., Loisance, D. Y., et al.: Surgical management of acute dissections involving the ascending aorta. J. Thorac. Cardiovasc. Surg. *82*:576, 1981.

192. Haverich, A., Miller, D. C., Scott, W. C., et al.: Acute and chronic aortic dissections: Determinants of long-term outcome for operative survivors. Circulation *72*(Suppl. II):II-22, 1985.

193. Crawford, E. S., Kirklin, J. W., Naftel, D. C., et al.: Surgery for acute dissection of the ascending aorta: Should the arch be included? J. Thorac. Cardiovasc. Surg. *104*:46, 1992.

194. Yun, K. L., Glower, D. D., Miller, D. C., et al.: Aortic dissection resulting from tear of transverse arch: Is concomitant arch repair warranted? J. Thorac. Cardiovasc. Surg. *102*:355, 1991.

195. Fann, J. I., Glower, D. D., Miller, D. C., et al.: Preservation of aortic valve in type A aortic dissection complicated by aortic regurgitation. J. Thorac. Cardiovasc. Surg. *102*:62, 1991.

196. Culliford, A. T., Ayvaliotis, B., Shemin, R., et al.: Aneurysms of the descending aorta: Surgical experience in 48 patients. J. Thorac. Cardiovasc. Surg. *85*:98, 1983.

197. Kolff, J., Bates, R. J., Balderman, S. C., et al.: Acute aortic arch dissection: Reevaluation of the indications for medical and surgical therapy. Am. J. Cardiol. *39*:727, 1977.

198. Séguin, J. R., Picard, E., Frapier, J.-M., and Chaptal, P.-A.: Aortic valve repair with fibrin glue for type A acute aortic dissection. Ann. Thorac. Surg. *58*:304, 1994.

199. Weinschelbaum, E. E., Schamun, C., Caramutti, V., et al.: Surgical treatment of acute type A dissecting aneurysm, with preservation of the native valve and the use of biologic glue: Follow-up to 6 years. J. Thorac. Cardiovasc. Surg. *103*:369, 1992.

200. Bachet, J., Goudot, B., Teodori, G., et al.: Surgery of type A acute aortic dissection with gelatine-resorcine-formol biological glue: A twelve-year experience. J. Cardiovasc. Surg. *31*:263, 1990.

201. Séguin, J. R., Frapier, J.-M., Colson, P., and Chaptal, P.-A.: Fibrin sealant improves surgical results of type A acute aortic dissection. Ann. Thorac. Surg. *52*:745, 1991.

202. Cambria, R. P., Brewster, D. C., Gertler, J., et al.: Vascular complications associated with spontaneous aortic dissection. J. Vasc. Surg. *7*:199, 1988.

203. Walker, P. J., Dake, M. D., Mitchell, R. S., and Miller, D. C.: The use of endovascular techniques for the treatment of complications of aortic dissection. J. Vasc. Surg. *18*:1042, 1993.

204. Dureau, G., Villard, J., George, M., et al.: New surgical technique for the operative management of acute dissections of the ascending aorta. J. Thorac. Cardiovasc. Surg. *76*:385, 1978.

205. Liu, D. W., Lin, P. J., and Chang, C. H.: Treatment of acute type A aortic dissection with intraluminal sutureless prosthesis. Ann. Thorac. Surg. *57*:987, 1994.

206. Lemole, G. M., Strong, M. D., Spagna, P. M., and Karmilowicz, M. P.: Improved results for dissecting aneurysms: Intraluminal sutureless prosthesis. J. Thorac. Cardiovasc. Surg. *83*:249, 1982.

207. Yoshida, H., Yasuda, K., and Tanabe, T.: New approach to aortic dissection: Development of an insertable aortic prosthesis. Ann. Thorac. Surg. *58*:806, 1994.

208. Kato, M., Matsuda, T., Kaneko, M., et al.: Experimental assessment of newly devised transcatheter stent-graft for aortic dissection. Ann. Thorac. Surg. *59*:908, 1995.

209. Neya, K., Omoto, R., Kyo, S., et al.: Outcome of Stanford type B acute aortic dissection. Circulation *86*(Suppl. II):II-1, 1992.

210. Heinemann, M., Laas, J., Karck, M., and Borst, H. G.: Thoracic aortic aneurysms after type A aortic dissection: Necessity for follow-up. Ann. Thorac. Surg. *49*:580, 1990.

211. Khandheria, B. K.: Aortic dissection: The last frontier. Circulation *87*(Edit.):1765, 1993.

212. Laissy, J.-P., Blanc, F., Soyer, P., et al.: Thoracic aortic dissection: Diagnosis with transesophageal echocardiography versus MR imaging. Radiology *194*:331, 1995.

213. Yamada, T., Tada, S., and Harada, J.: Aortic dissection without intimal rupture: Diagnosis with MR imaging and CT. Radiology *168*:347, 1988.

213a. Nienaber, C. A., von Kodolitsch, Y., Petersen, B., et al.: Intramural hemorrhage of the thoracic aorta: Diagnostic and therapeutic implications. Circulation *92*:1465, 1995.

214. Lui, R. C., Menkis, A. H., and McKenzie, F. N.: Aortic dissection without intimal rupture: Diagnosis and management. Ann. Thorac. Surg. *53*:886, 1992.

215. Gore, I.: Pathogenesis of dissecting aneurysm of the aorta. Arch. Pathol. *53*:142, 1952.

216. Mohr-Kahaly, S., Erbel, R., Kearney, P., et al.: Aortic intramural hematoma visualized by transesophageal echocardiography: Findings and prognostic implications. J. Am. Coll. Cardiol. *23*:658, 1994.

217. Robbins, R. C., McManus, R. P., Mitchell, R. S., et al.: Management of patients with intramural hematoma of the thoracic aorta. Circulation 88:1, 1993.
218. Nienaber, C. A., von Kodolitsch, Y., Petersen, B., et al.: Intramural hemorrhage of the thoracic aorta. Circulation 92:1465, 1995.
219. Zotz, R. J., Erbel, R., and Meyer, J.: Noncommunicating intramural hematoma: An indication of developing aortic dissection? J. Am. Soc. Echocardiogr. 4:636, 1991.
220. Stanson, A. W., Kazmier, F. J., Hollier, L. H., et al.: Penetrating atherosclerotic ulcers of the thoracic aorta: Natural history and clinicopathological correlations. Ann. Vasc. Surg. 1:15, 1986.
221. Kazerooni, E. A., Bree, R. L., and Williams, D. M.: Penetrating atherosclerotic ulcers of the descending thoracic aorta: Evaluation with CT and distinction from aortic dissection. Radiology 183:759, 1992.
222. Movsowitz, H. D., Lampert, C., Jacobs, L. E., and Kotler, M. N.: Penetrating atherosclerotic aortic ulcers. Am. Heart J. 128:1210, 1994.
223. Benitez, R. M., Gurbel, P. A., Chong, H., and Rajasingh, C.: Penetrating atherosclerotic ulcer of the aortic arch resulting in extensive and fatal dissection. Am. Heart J. 129:821, 1995.
224. Braverman, A. C.: Penetrating atherosclerotic ulcers of the aorta. Curr. Opin. Cardiol. 9:591, 1994.
225. Harris, J. A., Bis, K. G., Glover, J. L., et al.: Penetrating atherosclerotic ulcers of the aorta. J. Vasc. Surg. 19:90, 1994.
226. Hussain, S., Glover, J. L., Bree, R., and Bendick, P. J.: Penetrating atherosclerotic ulcers of the thoracic aorta. J. Vasc. Surg. 9:710, 1989.
227. Yucel, E. K., Steinberg, F. L., Egglin, T. K., et al.: Penetrating atherosclerotic ulcers: Diagnosis with MR imaging. Radiology 177:779, 1990.
228. Movsowitz, H. D., David, M., Movsowitz, C., et al.: Penetrating atherosclerotic ulcers: The role of transesophageal echocardiography in the diagnosis and clinical management. Am. Heart J. 126:745, 1993.

AORTIC ATHEROMATOUS EMBOLI

229. Karalis, D. G., Chandrasekaran, K., Victor, M. F., et al.: Recognition and embolic potential of intraaortic atherosclerotic debris. J. Am. Coll. Cardiol. 17:73, 1991.
229a. Halperin, J. L.: Atherosclerotic diseases of the aorta. In Fuster, V., Ross, R., and Topol, E. J. (eds.): Atherosclerosis and Coronary Artery Disease. Philadelphia, Lippincott-Raven, 1996, pp. 1625–1642.
230. Toyoda, K., Yasaka, M., Nagata, S., and Yamaguchi, T.: Aortogenic embolic stroke: A transesophageal echocardiography approach. Stroke 23:1056, 1992.
231. Culliford, A. T., Colvin, S. B., Rohrer, K., et al.: The atherosclerotic ascending aorta and transverse arch: A new technique to prevent cerebral injury during bypass: Experience with 13 patients. Ann. Thorac. Surg. 41:27, 1986.
232. Tunick, P. A., Perez, J. L., and Kronzon, I.: Protruding atheromas in the thoracic aorta and systemic embolization. Ann. Intern. Med. 115:423, 1991.
233. Davila-Roman, V. G., Barzilai, B., Wareing, T. H., et al.: Intraoperative ultrasonographic evaluation of the ascending aorta in 100 consecutive patients undergoing cardiac surgery. Circulation 84(Suppl. III):III-47, 1991.
234. Mitusch, R., Stierle, U., Tepe, C., et al.: Systemic embolism in aortic arch atheromatosis. Eur. Heart J. 15:1373, 1994.
235. Amarenco, P., Duyckaerts, C., Tzourio, C., et al.: The prevalence of ulcerated plaques in the aortic arch in patients with stroke. N. Engl. J. Med. 326:221, 1992.
235a. Montgomery, D. H., Ververis, J., McGorisk, G., et al.: Natural history of severe atheromatous disease of the thoracic aorta. A transesophageal echocardiographic study. J. Am. Coll. Cardiol. 27:95, 1996.
236. Amarenco, P., Cohen, A., Tzourio, C., et al.: Atherosclerotic disease of the aortic arch and the risk of ischemic stroke. N. Engl. J. Med. 331:1474, 1994.
237. Demopoulos, L. A., Tunick, P. A., Bernstein, N. E., et al.: Protruding atheromas of the aortic arch in symptomatic patients with carotid artery disease. Am. Heart J. 129:40, 1995.
238. Fazio, G. P., Redberg, R. F., Winslow, T., and Schiller, N. B.: Transesophageal echocardiographically detected atherosclerotic aortic plaque is a marker for coronary artery disease. J. Am. Coll. Cardiol. 21:144, 1993.
239. Tunick, P. A., Culliford, A. T., Lamparello, P. J., and Kronzon, I.: Atheromatosis of the aortic arch as an occult source of multiple systemic emboli. Ann. Intern. Med. 114:391, 1991.
240. Tunick, P. A., Rosensweig, B. P., Katz, E. S., et al.: High risk for vascular events in patients with protruding aortic atheromas: A prospective study. J. Am. Coll. Cardiol. 23:1085, 1994.
241. Jones, E. F., Kalman, J. M., Calafiore, P., et al.: Proximal aortic atheroma: An independent risk factor for cerebral ischemia. Stroke 26:218, 1995.
242. Kistler, J. P.: The risk of embolic stroke: Another piece of the puzzle. N. Engl. J. Med. 331(Edit.):1517, 1994.
243. Freedberg, R. S., Tunick, P. A., Culliford, A. T., et al.: Disappearance of a large intraaortic mass in a patient with prior systemic embolization. Am. Heart J. 125:1445, 1993.
244. Bansal, R. C., Pauls, G. L., and Shankel, S. W.: Blue digit syndrome: Transesophageal echocardiographic identification of thoracic aortic plaque–related thrombi and successful outcome with warfarin. J. Am. Soc. Echocardiogr. 6:319, 1993.
245. Culliford, A. T., Tunick, P. A., Katz, E. S., et al.: Initial experience with removal of protruding atheroma from the aortic arch: Diagnosis by

246. Katz, E. S., Tunick, P. A., Rusinek, H., et al.: Protruding atheromas predict stroke in elderly patients undergoing cardiopulmonary bypass: Experience with intraoperative transesophageal echocardiography. J. Am. Coll. Cardiol. 20:70, 1992.
247. Blauth, C. I., Cosgrove, D. M., Webb, B. W., et al.: Thromboembolism from the ascending aorta: An emerging problem in cardiac surgery. J. Thorac. Cardiovasc. Surg. 103:1104, 1992.
248. Wareing, T. H., Davila-Roman, V. G., Barzilai, B., et al.: Management of the severely atherosclerotic aorta during cardiac operation: A strategy for detection and treatment. J. Thorac. Cardiovasc. Surg. 103:453, 1992.
249. Barzilai, B., Marshall, W. G., Safitz, J. E., and Kouchoukos, N. T.: Avoidance of embolic complications by ultrasonic characterization of the ascending aorta. Circulation 80(Suppl. I):I-275, 1989.
250. Duda, A. M., Letwin, L. B., Sutter, F. P., and Goldman, S. M.: Does routine use of aortic ultrasonography decrease the stroke rate in coronary artery bypass surgery? J. Vasc. Surg. 21:98, 1995.
251. Om, A., Ellahham, S., and DiSciascio, G.: Cholesterol embolism: An underdiagnosed clinical entity. Am. Heart J. 124:1321, 1992.
252. Colt, H. G., Begg, R. J., Saporito, J. J., et al.: Cholesterol emboli after cardiac catheterization: Eight cases and a review of the literature. Medicine 67:389, 1988.
253. Davis, K., Kennedy, J. W., Kemp, H. G., Jr., et al.: Complications of coronary arteriography from the collaborative study of coronary artery surgery (CASS). Circulation 59:1105, 1979.
254. Hyman, B. T., Landas, S. K., Ashman, R. F., et al.: Warfarin-related purple toes syndrome and cholesterol microembolization. Am. J. Med. 82:1233, 1987.
255. Falanga, V., Fine, M. J., and Kapoor, W. N.: The cutaneous manifestations of cholesterol crystal embolization. Arch. Dermatol. 122:1194, 1986.
256. Karmody, A. M., Powers, S. R., Monaco, V. J., and Leather, R. P.: "Blue toe" syndrome: An indication for limb salvage surgery. Arch. Surg. 111:1263, 1976.
257. Arora, R. R., Magun, A. M., Grossman, M., and Katz, J.: Cholesterol embolization syndrome after intravenous tissue plasminogen activator for acute myocardial infarction. Am. Heart J. 126:225, 1993.
258. Bruns, F. J., Segel, D. P., and Apler, S.: Control of cholesterol embolization by discontinuation of anticoagulant therapy. Am. J. Med. Sci. 275:105, 1978.
259. Blankenship, J. C., Butler, M., and Garbes, A.: Prospective assessment of cholesterol embolization in patients with acute myocardial infarction treated with thrombolytic vs. conservative therapy. Chest 107:662, 1995.
260. Fine, M. J., Kapoor, W., and Falanga, V.: Cholesterol crystal embolization: A review of 221 cases in the English literature. Angiology 38:769, 1987.

ACUTE AORTIC OCCLUSION

261. Babu, S. C., Shah, P. M., and Nitahara, J.: Acute aortic occlusion: Factors that influence outcome. J. Vasc. Surg. 21:567, 1995.
262. Dossa, C. D., Shepard, A. D., Reddy, D. J., et al.: Acute aortic occlusion: A 40-year experience. Arch. Surg. 129:603, 1994.
263. Tapper, S. S., Jenkins, J. M., Edwards, W. H., et al.: Juxtarenal aortic occlusion. Ann. Surg. 215:443, 1992.
264. Light, J. T., Hendrickson, M., Sholes, W. M., et al.: Acute aortic occlusion secondary to Aspergillus endocarditis in an intravenous drug abuser. Ann. Vasc. Surg. 5:271, 1991.
265. Busuttil, R. W., Keehn, G., Milliken, J., et al.: Aortic saddle embolus: A twenty-two year experience. Ann. Surg. 197:698, 1983.

AORTOARTERITIS SYNDROMES

266. Shelhamer, J. H., Volkman, D. J., Parrillo, J. E., et al.: Takayasu's arteritis and its therapy. Ann. Intern. Med. 103:121, 1985.
267. Volkman, D. J., Mann, D. L., and Fauci, A. S.: Association between Takayasu's arteritis and a B-cell alloantigen in North Americans. N. Engl. J. Med. 306:464, 1982.
268. Numano, F., Isohisa, I., Egami, M., et al.: HLA-DR MT and MB antigens in Takayasu disease. Tissue Antigens 21:208, 1983.
269. Ueno, A., Awane, G., and Wakahayachi, A.: Successfully operated obliterative brachiocephalic arteritis (Takayasu) associated with the elongated coarctation. Jpn. Heart J. 8:538, 1967.
270. Lupi-Herrera, E., Sanchez-Torres, G., Marcushamer, J., et al.: Takayasu's arteritis: Clinical study of 107 cases. Am. Heart J. 93:94, 1977.
271. Procter, C. D., and Hollier, L. H.: Takayasu's arteritis and temporal arteritis. Ann. Vasc. Surg. 6:195, 1992.
272. Hall, S., Barr, W., Lie, J. T., et al.: Takayasu arteritis: A study of 32 North American patients. Medicine 64:89, 1985.
273. Wu, Y. J., Martin, B., Ong, K., et al.: Takayasu's arteritis as a cause of fever of unknown origin. Am. J. Med. 87:476, 1989.
274. Takeshita, A., Tanaka, S., Orita, Y., et al.: Baroreflex sensitivity in patients with Takayasu's aortitis. Circulation 55:803, 1977.
275. Akikusa, B., Kondo, Y., and Muraki, N.: Aortic insufficiency caused by Takayasu's arteritis without usual clinical features. Arch. Pathol. Lab. Med. 105:650, 1981.
276. Hashimoto, Y., Numano, F., Maruyama, Y., et al.: Thallium-201 stress scintigraphy in Takayasu arteritis. Am. J. Cardiol. 67:879, 1991.

277. Ishikawa, K., and Maetani, S.: Long term outcome for 120 Japanese patients with Takayasu's disease. Circulation *90:*1855, 1994.

278. Lande, A., and Rossi, P.: The value of total aortography in the diagnosis of Takayasu's arteritis. Radiology *114:*287, 1975.

279. Ishikawa, K.: Diagnostic approach and proposed criteria for the clinical diagnosis of Takayasu's arteriopathy. J. Am. Coll. Cardiol. *12:*964, 1988.

280. Hoffman, G. S., Leavitt, R. Y., Kerr, G. S., et al.: Treatment of glucocorticoid resistant or relapsing Takayasu arteritis with methotrexate. Arthritis Rheum. *4:*578, 1994.

281. Tyagi, S., Kaul, U. A., Nair, M., et al.: Balloon angioplasty of the aorta in Takayasu's arteritis: Initial and long term results. Am. Heart J. *124:*876, 1992.

282. Tyagi, S., Singh, B., Kaul, U. A., et al.: Balloon angioplasty for renovascular hypertension in Takayasu's arteritis. Am. Heart J. *125:*1386, 1993.

283. Klein, R. G., Hunder, G. G., Stanson, A. W., and Sheps, S. G.: Larger artery involvement in giant cell (temporal) arteritis. Ann. Intern. Med. *83:*806, 1975.

284. Hunder, G. G.: Giant cell (temporal) arteritis. Rheum. Dis. Clin. North Am. *16:*399, 1990.

285. Ghose, M. K., Shensa, S., and Lerner, P. I.: Arteritis of the aged (giant cell arteritis) and fever of unexplained origin. Am. J. Med. *60:*429, 1976.

286. Hunder, G. G., Lie, J. T., Goronzy, J. J., and Weyand, C. M.: Pathogenesis of giant cell arteritis. Arthritis Rheum. *36:*757, 1993.

287. Evans, J. M., O'Fallon, W. M., and Hunder, G. G.: Increased incidence of aortic aneurysm and dissection in giant cell (temporal) arteritis: A population based study. Ann. Intern. Med. *122:*502, 1995.

288. Perruquet, J. L., Davis, D. E., and Harrington, T. M.: Aortic arch arteritis in the elderly: An important manifestation of giant cell arteritis. Arch. Intern. Med. *146:*289, 1986.

289. Austen, W. G., and Blennerhassett, M. B.: Giant cell aortitis causing an aneurysm of the ascending aorta and aortic regurgitation. N. Engl. J. Med. *272:*80, 1965.

290. Malmvall, B. E., and Bengtsson, B. A.: Serum levels of immunoglobulin and complement in giant cell arteritis. JAMA *236:*1876, 1976.

291. Mitnick, H. J., Tunick, P. A., Rotterdam, H., and Esposito, R.: Antemortem diagnosis of giant cell arteritis. J. Rheumatol. *17:*708, 1990.

292. Evans, J. M., Bowles, C. A., Bjornsson, J., et al.: Thoracic aortic aneurysm and rupture in giant cell arteritis. Arthritis Rheum. *37:*1539, 1994.

293. Krall, P. L., Mazanec, D. J., and Wilke, W. S.: Methotrexate for corticosteroid-resistant polymyalgia rheumatica and giant cell arteritis. Cleve. Clin. J. Med. *56:*253, 1989.

294. Townend, J. N., Emery, P., Davies, M. K., and Littler, W. A.: Acute aortitis and aortic incompetence due to systemic rheumatological disorders. Int. J. Cardiol. *33:*253, 1991.

295. Muna, W. F., Roller, D. H., Craft, J., et al.: Psoriatic arthritis and aortic regurgitation. JAMA *244:*363, 1980.

296. Iino, T., Eguchi, K., Sakai, M., et al.: Polyarteritis nodosa with aortic dissection: Necrotizing vasculitis of the vasa vasorum. J. Rheumatol. *19:*1632, 1992.

297. Hoogland, Y. T., Alexander, E. P., Patterson, R. H., and Nashel, D. J.: Coronary artery stenosis in Reiter's syndrome: A complication of aortitis. J. Rheumatol. *21:*757, 1994.

298. González, T., Hernández-Beriain, J. A., Rodríguez-Lozano, B., and Martín-Herrera, A.: Severe aortic regurgitation in Behçet's disease. J. Rheumatol. *20:*10, 1993.

299. Koç, Y., Güllü, I., Akpek, G., et al.: Vascular involvement in Behçet's disease. J. Rheumatol. *19:*402, 1992.

300. Paulus, H. E., Pearson, C. M., and Pitts, W.: Aortic insufficiency in five patients with Reiter's syndrome: A detailed clinical and pathologic study. Am. J. Med. *53:*464, 1972.

301. Gomes, M. N., Choyke, P. L., and Wallace, R. B.: Infected aortic aneurysms: A changing entity. Ann. Surg. *215:*435, 1992.

302. Katz, S. G., Andros, G., and Kohl, R. D.: Salmonella infections of the abdominal aorta. Surg. Gynecol. Obstet. *175:*102, 1992.

303. Pasic, M., Carrel, T., von Segesser, L., and Turina, M.: In situ repair of mycotic aneurysm of the ascending aorta. J. Thorac. Cardiovasc. Surg. *105:*321, 1993.

304. Oz, M. C., Brener, B. J., Buda, J. A., et al.: A ten-year experience with bacterial aortitis. J. Vasc. Surg. *10:*439, 1989.

305. Cohen, O. S., O'Brien, T. F., Schoenbaum, S. C., and Mederos, A. A.: The risk of endothelial infection in adults with Salmonella bacteremia. Ann. Intern. Med. *89:*931, 1978.

306. Byard, R. W., Jimenez, C. L., Carpenter, B. F., and Hsu, E.: Aspergillus-related aortic thrombosis. Can. Med. Assoc. J. *136:*155, 1987.

307. Jarrett, F., Darling, R. C., Mundth, E. D., and Austen, W. G.: The management of infected arterial aneurysms. J. Cardiovasc. Surg. *17:*361, 1977.

308. Vogelzang, R. L., and Sohaey, R.: Infected aortic aneurysms: CT appearance. J. Comput. Assist. Tomogr. *12:*109, 1988.

309. Gomes, M. N., and Choyke, P. L.: Infected aortic aneurysms: CT diagnosis. J. Cardiovasc. Surg. *32:*4, 1991.

310. Robinson, J. A., and Johansen, K.: Aortic sepsis: Is there a role for in situ graft reconstruction? J. Vasc. Surg. *13:*677, 1991.

311. Fyfe, B. S., Quintana, C. S., Kaneka, M., and Griepp, R. B.: Aortic sarcoma four years after Dacron graft insertion. Ann. Thorac. Surg. *58:*1752, 1994.

312. Wright, E. P., Glick, A. D., Virmani, R., and Page, D. L.: Aortic intimal sarcoma with embolic metastases. Am. J. Surg. Pathol. *9:*950, 1985.

313. Navarra, G., Occhionorelli, S., Mascoli, F., et al.: Primary leiomyosarcoma of the aorta: Report of a case and review of the literature. J. Cardiovasc. Surg. *35:*33, 1994.

314. Ronaghi, A. H., Roberts, A. C., and Rosenkrantz, H.: Intraaortic biopsy of a primary aortic tumor. J. Vasc. Intervent. Radiol. *5:*777, 1994.

315. Higgins, R., Posner, M. C., Moosa, H. H., et al.: Mesenteric infarction secondary to tumor emboli from primary aortic sarcoma. Cancer *68:*1622, 1991.

316. Cziner, D. G., Freedberg, R. S., Tunick, P. A., et al.: Transesophageal echocardiographic diagnosis of a primary intraaortic tumor. Am. Heart J. *125:*1189, 1993.

Chapter 46
Pulmonary Embolism

SAMUEL Z. GOLDHABER

Pulmonary embolism (PE) and deep venous thrombosis (DVT) account for hundreds of thousands of hospitalizations annually in the United States and afflict millions of individuals worldwide. The likelihood of survival after PE or DVT is reduced compared with that of controls matched by age, gender, and race (Fig. 46–1A). As the population ages, venous thromboembolism will become more prevalent because the incidence of PE and DVT increases steadily with age (Fig. 46–1B).[1]

Cardiovascular specialists are often consulted to help diagnose unexplained dyspnea, lightheadedness, and chest pain—the three most common presenting symptoms of hemodynamically important PE. Cardiologists must become skilled in risk stratification of patients with established PE. For high-risk patients who have poor prognoses with anticoagulation alone, cardiologists will often be the ones to administer primary therapy for PE—thrombolysis or removal of clot with mechanical interventions in the catheterization laboratory.

Advances in molecular medicine have quickened the pace of progress in the field of venous thrombosis and have renewed interest in improving upon contemporary methods to diagnose, treat, and prevent PE and DVT. Recent discovery of specific genetic mutations that predispose to venous thrombosis will have immediate practical utility in the clinical management of PE.

PATHOPHYSIOLOGY

Hypercoagulable States

In 1856 Rudolf Virchow postulated that a triad of factors led to intravascular coagulation: (1) local trauma to the vessel wall, (2) hypercoagulability, and (3) stasis.[2] Classically, the pathogenesis of PE was dichotomized as due to either unusual "inherited" (primary) or commonly "acquired" (secondary) risk factors. Now, however, it appears likely that many patients who develop PE are genetically predisposed (Tables 46–1 and 46–2) but often require a precipitating stress (Table 46–3) to elicit overt thrombosis.

PRIMARY HYPERCOAGULABLE STATES. The identification of a poor anticoagulant response to activated protein C (aPC) (Fig. 48–6, p. 1634) is the most exciting and far-reaching breakthrough ever to occur in the field of prethrombotic markers. Normally, a specified amount of aPC can be added to plasma and prolongation of the activated partial thromboplastin time (PTT) can be observed (see p. 1817). However, patients with "aPC resistance" have inadequate PTT prolongation. In contrast to classic coagulation protein deficiencies, which are rare (Table 46–

TABLE 46–1 HYPERCOAGULABLE STATES ASSOCIATED WITH VENOUS THROMBOSIS

HYPERCOAGULABLE STATE	CITATION	COMMENTS
Mutation in factor V Gene	Bertina[3]; Ridker;[5]	Replaces arginine 506 with glutamine, rendering factor V resistant to inactivation by activated protein C
Resistance to activated protein C	Zöller[8]	Molecular background for resistance to activated protein C was found to be heterogeneous
Mutation in protein C gene	Allaart[7]	Associated with protein C deficiency
Protein S deficiency	Gladson[9]	Protein S a cofactor for protein C
Antithrombin III deficiency	Hirsh[10]	Autosomal dominant inheritance
Plasminogen deficiency	Hach-Wunderle[11]	Plasminogen that is present functions normally
Antiphospholipid antibodies	Hughes[12]	Encompasses anticardiolipin antibodies and lupus anticoagulant; associated with venous and arterial thrombosis
Elevated concentration of factor VIII	Koster[13]	Relative risk of venous thrombosis is 5-fold; higher among patients with factor V concentrations > 1500 IU/liter

TABLE 46–2A FREQUENCY OF CLASSIC COAGULATION PROTEIN DEFICIENCIES AMONG PATIENTS WITH VENOUS THROMBOSIS

ABNORMAL	GLADSON[9] (N = 141)(%)	HEIJBOER[14] (N = 277)(%)	MALM[15] (N = 439)(%)
Protein C	4	3	2
Protein S	5	2	2
Antithrombin III	3	1	1
Plasminogen	2	1	0.5

TABLE 46–2B FREQUENCY OF ACTIVATED PROTEIN C RESISTANCE AMONG PATIENTS WITH VENOUS THROMBOSIS

ABNORMALITY	SVENSSON[16] (N = 104)(%)	KOSTER[17] (N = 301)(%)
APC Resistance	33	21

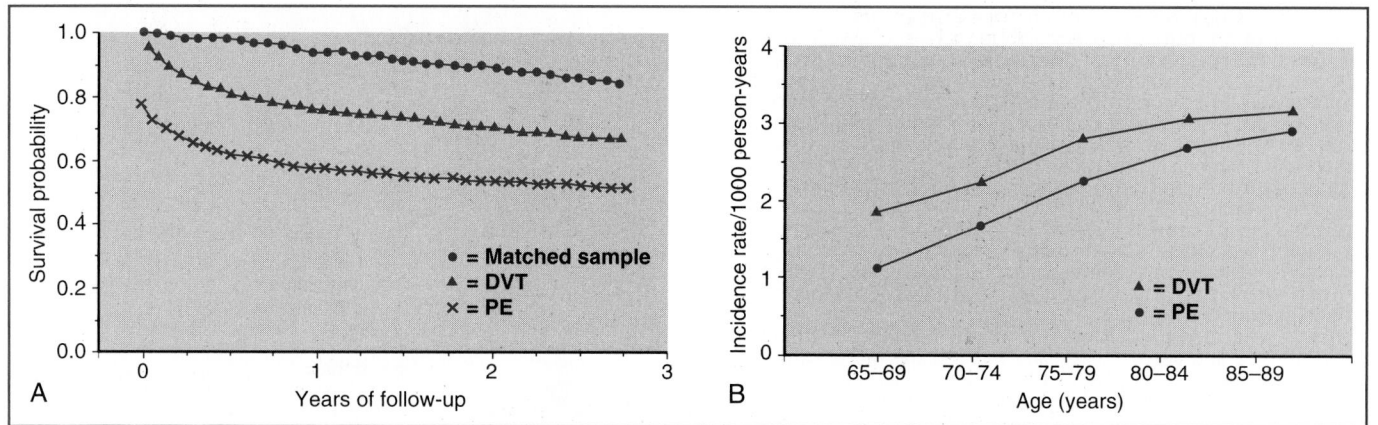

FIGURE 46–1. *A*, Survival for United States Medicare enrollees with pulmonary embolism or deep vein thrombosis compared with a sample of United States Medicare enrollees matched by age, gender, and race. *B*, Incidence of pulmonary embolism and deep venous thrombosis among United States Medicare enrollees according to age. (From Kniffin, W. D., Jr., Baron, J. A., Barrett, J., et al.: The epidemiology of diagnosed pulmonary embolism and deep venous thrombosis in the elderly. Arch. Intern. Med. *154*:861, 1994. Copyright 1994 American Medical Association.)

2*A*), aPC resistance occurs frequently among patients with venous thrombosis (Table 46–2*B*).

The phenotype of aPC resistance is associated with a single point mutation, designated factor V Leiden, in the factor V gene.[3] This mutation results from a single nucleotide substitution of adenine for guanine 1691 that replaces the amino acid arginine with glutamine at position 506. This change eliminates the protein C cleavage site in factor V (Fig. 48–6, p. 1634).[4]

The allelic frequency of this mutation is about 3 per cent in healthy male physicians in the United States. In the Physicians' Health Study, no statistically significant differences were found between the incidence of the mutation among previously healthy men who subsequently developed myocardial infarction or stroke compared with men who remained free of cardiovascular disease. However, the incidence of the factor V mutation was three times higher among men who developed venous thrombosis.[5]

The ramifications of testing for this mutation will become evident over the next decade. For example, in a case-control study of premenopausal women who developed DVT, the risk of thrombosis among users of oral contraceptives was increased fourfold. However, the risk of thrombosis among carriers of the factor V Leiden mutation was eightfold compared with noncarriers. When both oral contraceptive use and the mutation were accounted for, the risk of thrombosis was increased more than 30-fold.[6] The presence of the factor V Leiden mutation among pregnant women appears to increase the risk of first-trimester PE.[6a] The mutation is also associated with a fourfold increased risk of recurrent PE or DVT after completion of a course of anticoagulation.[6b]

Other genetic mutations also predispose to venous thrombosis. One study suggested that half of heterozygotes for a mutation in the protein C gene and 10 per cent of

normal relatives can be expected to have an episode of venous thrombosis by the age of 45.[7]

Although molecular medicine can help elucidate pathogenesis, a careful family history is still the most rapid and cost-effective method of identifying a predisposition to venous thrombosis. Investigation with blood tests (Table 46–1) to detect a hypercoagulable state is best deferred to the outpatient setting because the results of in-hospital work-ups can be misleading. For example, consumption coagulopathy due to venous thrombosis may be misdiagnosed as deficiency of antithrombin III, protein C, or protein S. Heparin administration can depress antithrombin III levels, and use of warfarin will ordinarily cause a mild deficiency of protein C or S.

ACQUIRED CONDITIONS THAT MAY PRECIPITATE VENOUS THROMBOSIS. Conditions that increase venous stasis or cause endothelial damage (Table 46–3) are likely to predispose toward venous thrombosis, especially among patients who already have subclinical hypercoagulable states.

The stasis and immobilization associated with postoperative venous thrombosis may increase after hospital discharge, because many of the patients who are forced to ambulate during hospitalization may become confined to bed upon returning home. PE is increasingly likely to occur *after* hospital discharge because of the contemporary emphasis on minimizing the length of stay after surgery. Among general surgery patients at the University Hospital of Geneva,[18] PE occurred a median of 18 days postoperatively. The rate of postoperative PE increased by 30 per cent when emboli occurring within 30 days of hospital discharge were accounted for, compared with the rate during the initial hospital stay.

Coronary artery bypass grafting has been associated with a 4 per cent risk of PE[19] and a 20 per cent risk of venous thrombosis of the deep leg veins.[20] After *major trauma*, the DVT rate was 58 per cent in a prospective study in which contrast venograms were obtained.[21] Among immobilized *medical intensive care unit patients*, the rate of venous thrombosis detected with ultrasonography was 33 per cent.[22]

OTHER RISK FACTORS FOR PULMONARY EMBOLISM

Among women in both the Framingham Heart Study and Nurses Health Study, marked obesity was a crucial risk factor for PE. In the Framingham Heart Study,[23] multivariate logistic regression showed a strong association (p < 0.001) between increased relative weight in women and major PE at autopsy. In the Nurses Health Study,[24] obese women (Quetelet's index >29.0) compared with lean women had a relative risk of pulmonary embolism of 2.53. These findings suggest that weight reduction in obese women may decrease the likelihood of clinical venous thrombosis.

TABLE 46–3 ACQUIRED CONDITIONS THAT MAY PRECIPITATE VENOUS THROMBOSIS

Surgery/Immobilization/Trauma
Obesity
Increasing age
Oral contraceptives/Pregnancy/Postpartum
Cancer (sometimes occult adenocarcinoma) and cancer chemotherapy
Stroke/Spinal cord injury
Indwelling central venous catheter

In the Nurses Health Study,[25] *current oral contraceptive* users had a relative risk of 3.1, but past users had no increased risk of PE, after adjustment for coronary heart disease risk factors. Third-generation oral contraceptives (which use either desogestrel or gestodene as the progesterone component) are associated with about a doubled risk of venous thrombosis compared with other oral contraceptives.[25a] Postmenopausal estrogen use was not associated with increased risk of venous thrombosis. A case-control study also found no association between estrogen replacement therapy and the risk of venous thrombosis.[26]

PE is the most common medical cause of *maternal mortality* associated with live births.[27] Pregnancy and the puerperium alter the physiological balance between coagulation and fibrinolysis, thus predisposing women to a hypercoagulable state, especially during the first postpartum month.

Cancer is an acquired risk factor for venous thrombosis. The tumor may synthesize and secrete procoagulants. Furthermore, cancer patients often have concomitant predisposing factors for venous thrombosis such as surgery or immobility. Among 145 patients with venographically proven idiopathic venous thrombosis, cancer was diagnosed in 8 per cent during 2 years of follow-up. However, among those with idiopathic venous thrombosis who suffered a recurrence, the cancer incidence during this period was 17 per cent.[28] In a large Swedish case-control study, patients with venographically diagnosed DVT were 2.5 times more likely to develop cancer within the ensuing 6 months compared with controls who had normal venograms.[29] A similar relationship between PE and subsequent cancer risk has also been observed in a cohort study.[30]

Patients receiving *chemotherapy* for metastatic breast cancer are at risk of developing venous thromboembolic disease. In a randomized controlled trial of very low dose warfarin versus placebo, 4 per cent of the placebo group developed venous thrombosis during the average 6-month follow-up period.[31] Hemocysteinemia, which can be hereditary or acquired, appears to be a common risk factor for recurrent venous thrombosis.[31a]

Leg DVT is a common complication of *acute ischemic stroke*, particularly in the paralyzed limb. Even when patients receive 5000 units twice daily of unfractionated heparin for prophylaxis, the venous thrombosis rate is as high as 31 per cent.[32] With spinal cord injury there is also a high rate of venous thrombosis,[33] but devastating complications such as PE tend to occur more often.

Thrombotic complications due to indwelling central venous catheters are common and are often associated with catheter sepsis.[34] Thrombosis can be due to a fibrin sleeve or vascular occlusion. Soon after insertion, most indwelling vascular catheters become engulfed in a thrombin or fibrin sheath that can serve as a nidus for subsequent infection.

RELATIONSHIP BETWEEN DEEP VENOUS THROMBOSIS AND PULMONARY EMBOLISM. Most pulmonary emboli result from thrombi that originate in the pelvic or deep veins of the leg; occasionally, thrombi in the axillary or subclavian veins embolize to the pulmonary arteries. In an autopsy study of patients who died of PE, 83 per cent had leg DVT, but only 19 per cent had symptoms of DVT before death.[35] In a treatment trial of proximal leg DVT, Moser et al. found that nearly 40 per cent of patients had asymptomatic PE, based on concomitantly obtained ventilation–perfusion scans.[36] There is also a small but appreciable risk of asymptomatic PE due to isolated calf vein thrombosis[37] or upper extremity thrombosis.[38]

When venous thrombi become dislodged from their site of formation, they flow through the venous system to the pulmonary arterial circulation. If an embolus is extremely large, it may lodge at the bifurcation of the pulmonary artery, forming a saddle embolus (Fig. 46–2, *top*). More commonly, a major pulmonary vessel is occluded (Fig. 46–2, *bottom*).

RIGHT VENTRICULAR DYSFUNCTION. The extent of pulmonary vascular obstruction is probably the most important factor determining whether right ventricular dysfunction ensues. As obstruction increases, pulmonary artery pressures rise. Moreover, the release of vasoconstricting compounds (e.g., serotonin), reflex pulmonary artery vasoconstriction, and hypoxemia may further increase pulmonary vascular resistance and result in pulmonary hypertension.[39]

VENTRICULAR INTERDEPENDENCY. The sudden rise in pulmonary artery pressure reflects an abrupt increase in right ventricular afterload, with consequent elevation of right ventricular wall tension followed by right ventricular dilatation and dysfunction (Fig. 46–3). As the right ventricle dilates, the interventricular septum shifts toward the left ventricle, which may lead to underfilling of this chamber

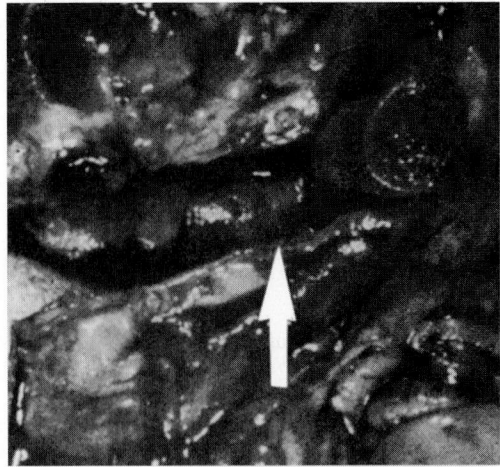

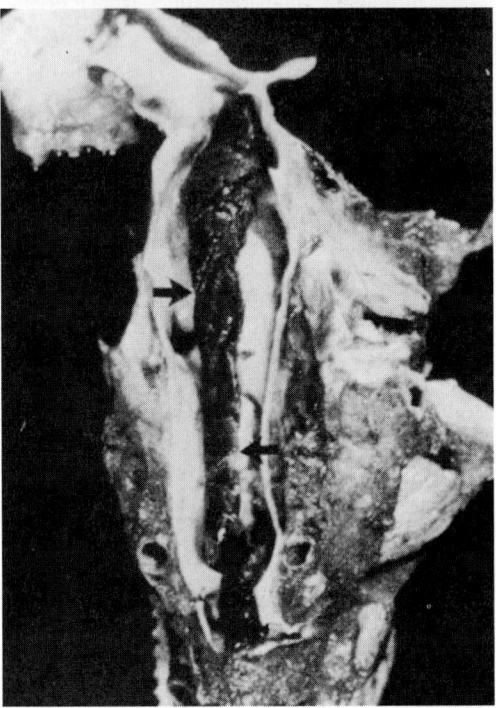

FIGURE 46–2. *Top,* saddle embolus (arrow) at the bifurcation of the pulmonary artery. *Bottom,* Pulmonary embolus in left lower lobe pulmonary artery, with minimal attachment to the wall of the vessel. The embolus was dark red, typical of venous thrombi, and had indentations believed to represent impressions of the venous valves (arrows). (From Godleski, J. J.: Pathology of deep venous thrombosis and pulmonary embolism. *In* Goldhaber, S. Z. [ed.]: Pulmonary Embolism and Deep Venous Thrombosis. Philadelphia, W. B. Saunders Company, 1985, p. 17.)

due to pericardial constraint.[40,41] In addition, right ventricular contractile dysfunction may decrease right ventricular cardiac output and further reduce left ventricular preload. As the right ventricle distends, coronary venous pressure increases and left ventricular diastolic distensibility decreases.[42]

The reduction in left ventricular preload may also lead to interventricular septal shift toward the left ventricle. With underfilling of the left ventricle, systemic cardiac output and pressure both decrease, potentially compromising coronary perfusion and producing myocardial ischemia. Elevated right ventricular wall tension following massive PE reduces right coronary flow and increases right ventricular myocardial oxygen demand, which may result in ischemia and possibly cardiogenic shock. Perpetuation of this cycle can lead to right ventricular infarction, circulatory collapse, and death.

SUMMARY OF PATHOPHYSIOLOGY. Pulmonary embolism can have the following pathophysiological effects: (1) in-

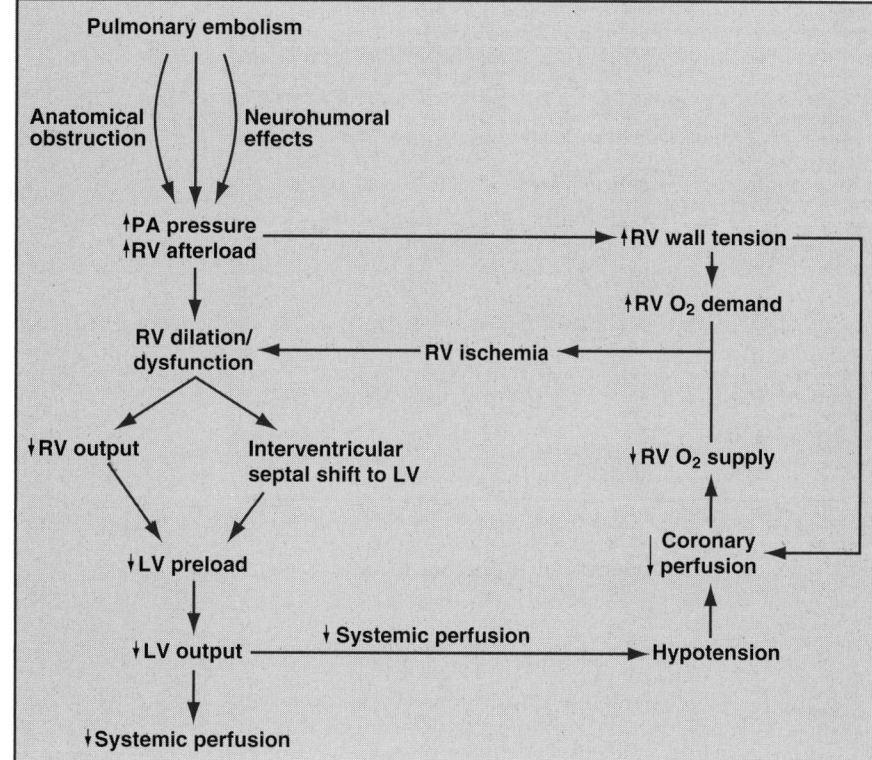

FIGURE 46–3. Pathophysiology of right ventricular dysfunction.

creased pulmonary vascular resistance due to vascular obstruction, neurohumoral agents, or pulmonary artery baroreceptors; (2) impaired gas exchange due to increased alveolar dead space from vascular obstruction and hypoxemia from alveolar hypoventilation, low V/Q units, and right-to-left shunting, as well as impaired carbon monoxide transfer due to loss of gas-exchange surface; (3) alveolar hyperventilation due to reflex stimulation of irritant receptors; (4) increased airway resistance due to bronchoconstriction; and (5) decreased pulmonary compliance due to lung edema, lung hemorrhage, and loss of surfactant.[39]

DIAGNOSIS

Diagnosis of PE is more difficult than treatment or prevention. For patients with PE, the most dangerous period is that preceding the establishment of the correct diagnosis. Fortunately, reliable noninvasive diagnostic approaches have become increasingly available—particularly venous ultrasound, plasma D-dimer ELISA, and echocardiography—and complement the more-established techniques of lung scanning and pulmonary angiography. Furthermore, procedures for pulmonary angiography have been developed that increase patient comfort and safety. The contemporary diagnosis of PE emphasizes a strategy that integrates the clinical findings with a variety of diagnostic methods.[43]

Clinical Presentation

Clinical suspicion of PE is of paramount importance in guiding diagnostic testing. Among patients without prior cardiopulmonary disease, dyspnea appears to be the most frequent symptom and tachypnea the most frequent sign of PE (Table 46–4). In general, dyspnea, syncope, or cyanosis portends a major life-threatening PE. However, pleuritic pain often signifies that the embolism is small and located in the distal pulmonary arterial system, near the pleural lining.

PE should be suspected in hypotensive patients when: (1) there is evidence of, or there are predisposing factors for, venous thrombosis and (2) there is clinical evidence of

acute cor pulmonale (acute right ventricular failure) such as distended neck veins, an S_3 gallop, a right ventricular heave, tachycardia, or tachypnea, especially if (3) there is electrocardiographic evidence of acute cor pulmonale manifested by a new S_1-Q_3-T_3 pattern, new incomplete right bundle branch block, or right ventricular ischemia.[44]

DIFFERENTIAL DIAGNOSIS. The differential diagnosis of PE is broad and covers a spectrum from life-threatening dis-

TABLE 46–4 SYMPTOMS AND SIGNS OF PE IN 117 PATIENTS WITH NO PRIOR CARDIOPULMONARY DISEASE

SYMPTOMS	FREQUENCY (%)
Dyspnea	73
Pleuritic pain	66
Cough	37
Leg swelling	28
Leg pain	26
Hemoptysis	13
Palpitations	10
Wheezing	9
Angina-like pain	4

SIGNS	
Tachypnea (≥20/min)	70
Rales (crackles)	51
Tachycardia (>100/min)	30
Fourth heart sound	24
Increased pulmonary component of second sound	23
Clinically apparent deep venous thrombosis	11
Diaphoresis	11
Temperature > 38.5°C	7
Wheezes	5
Homans' sign	4
Right ventricular lift	4
Pleural friction rub	3
Third heart sound	3
Cyanosis	1

Reprinted with permission from Stein, P. D., Terrin, M. L., Hales, C. A., et al.: Clinical, laboratory, roentgenographic, and electrocardiographic findings in patients with acute pulmonary embolism and no pre-existing cardiac or pulmonary disease. Chest 100:598, 1991.

TABLE 46–5 DIFFERENTIAL DIAGNOSIS OF PULMONARY EMBOLISM

Myocardial infarction
Pneumonia
Congestive heart failure ("left-sided")
Cardiomyopathy (global)
Primary pulmonary hypertension
Asthma
Pericarditis
Intrathoracic cancer
Rib fracture
Pneumothorax
Costochondritis
"Musculoskeletal pain"
Anxiety

ease such as acute myocardial infarction to innocuous anxiety states (Table 46–5). Some patients have concomitant PE and other illnesses. So, for example, if pneumonia or heart failure does not respond to appropriate therapy, the possibility of coexisting PE should be considered.

Distinguishing between PE and primary pulmonary hypertension (Chap. 25) deserves special vigilance (Table 46–6). Although both conditions ordinarily warrant anticoagulation, other advances in management (such as high doses of calcium channel blockers[45] and long-term prostacyclin

TABLE 46–6 PRIMARY PULMONARY HYPERTENSION VS. RECURRENT PULMONARY EMBOLISM

SIMILARITIES	
Symptoms	Fatigue, dyspnea on exertion—most common; chest pain, syncope, hemoptysis, cyanosis—also common
Clinical course	Progressive dyspnea, right-heart failure
Hemodynamics	Elevated right-heart pressures, normal pulmonary capillary wedge pressure
Histology	Thrombotic lesions usually present
Treatment	Includes anticoagulation

DIFFERENCES		
VARIABLE	PPH	RECURRENT PE
Age (years)	20–40	>50
Female/male ratio	4:1	1:1
Clinical course	Continued deterioration	Deterioration, with intermittent stabilization
Perfusion lung scan	No segmental perfusion defects	Segmental or larger perfusion defects
Pulmonary artery systolic pressure	>60 mm Hg	<60 mm Hg
Pulmonary angiogram	"Pruning"	Intraluminal filling defects
Confounding problems with angiogram	Thrombi may occur on or distal to PPH lesions	"Pruning" can also suggest PE
Diagnostic alternatives	Lung biopsy	Pulmonary angioscopy
Therapy	Anticoagulation; high-dose nifedipine or diltiazem; long-term continuous IV prostacyclin	Anticoagulation; IVC interruption; Thromboendarterectomy

Adapted from Goldhaber, S. Z.: Strategies for diagnosis. In Goldhaber, S. Z. (ed.): Pulmonary Embolism and Deep Vein Thrombosis. Philadelphia, W. B. Saunders Company, 1985, p. 89.

infusions to treat primary pulmonary hypertension[46]) require differentiation between these two illnesses. Surprisingly, some patients will have a hybrid condition that is similar to primary pulmonary hypertension but that includes thrombi. Among these patients, large central pulmonary artery thrombi can develop.[47] Often it is impossible to determine whether these thrombi formed in situ or whether they embolized to the pulmonary arteries from a separate site.

Clinical Syndromes of Pulmonary Embolism

Classification of PE into various syndromes (Table 46–7) is useful for prognostication and for deciding on subsequent clinical management.[48]

MASSIVE PULMONARY EMBOLISM. These patients are at risk of developing cardiogenic shock. They have thrombosis often affecting at least half of the pulmonary arterial system. Clot is almost always present bilaterally. Dyspnea is usually the cardinal symptom, and systemic arterial hypotension requiring pressor support is the predominant sign.

MODERATE TO LARGE PULMONARY EMBOLISM. These patients have right ventricular hypokinesis on echocardiography but normal systemic arterial pressure. Usually, perfusion lung scanning indicates that more than 30 per cent of the lung is not perfused. The condition of such patients was previously termed hemodynamically stable. However, this description is misleading because these patients have right ventricular hemodynamic instability that is masked

TABLE 46–7 SIX SYNDROMES OF ACUTE PULMONARY EMBOLISM

SYNDROME	PRESENTATION	RV DYSFUNCTION	THERAPY
Massive	Breathlessness, syncope, and cyanosis with persistent systemic arterial hypotension; typically greater than 50% obstruction of pulmonary vasculature	Present	Heparin plus thrombolytic therapy or mechanical intervention
Moderate to Large	Normal systemic arterial blood pressure; typically greater than 30% perfusion defect on lung scan	Present	Heparin plus thrombolytic therapy or mechanical intervention
Small to Moderate	Normal arterial blood pressure	Absent	Heparin
Pulmonary Infarction	Pleuritic chest pain, hemoptysis, pleural rub, or evidence of lung consolidation; typically small peripheral emboli	Rare	Heparin and NSAIDs
Paradoxical Embolism	Sudden systemic embolic event such as stroke	Rare	Variable*
Non-Thrombotic Embolism	Most commonly air, fat, tumor fragments, or amniotic fluid	Rare	Supportive

Adapted from Goldhaber, S. Z.: Treatment of acute pulmonary embolism. In Goldhaber, S. Z. (ed.): Cardiopulmonary diseases and cardiac tumors. Braunwald, E., Series ed. Atlas of Heart Diseases. Philadelphia, Current Medicine, 1995, vol. III, pp 7.1–7.12.
RV = right ventricular
NSAIDs = nonsteroidal antiinflammatory drugs
* Therapy depends on right ventricular function and presence or absence of contraindications to thrombolysis or heparin.

by normal systemic arterial pressure. Right ventricular dilatation and hypokinesis can be detected echocardiographically. It appears that these patients are at risk for recurrent (and possibly fatal) PE, even with adequate anticoagulation.[49] Therefore, these patients are receiving increasing consideration for primary therapy of PE with thrombolytics or embolectomy.

SMALL TO MODERATE PULMONARY EMBOLISM. This syndrome is characterized by both normal systemic arterial pressure and normal right ventricular function. Patients usually have a good prognosis if anticoagulation or an inferior vena caval filter is used to prevent recurrent PE.

PULMONARY INFARCTION. This syndrome is characterized by unremitting chest pain, occasionally accompanied by hemoptysis. The embolus usually lodges in the peripheral pulmonary arterial tree, near the pleura and close to the diaphragm.[50] Tissue infarction usually occurs 3 to 7 days after embolism. The syndrome at that time often includes fever, leukocytosis, and chest radiologic evidence of infarction.

PARADOXICAL EMBOLISM. This syndrome often presents with a sudden, devastating stroke and concomitant PE. Patients often have abnormally elevated pulmonary arterial pressure with a patent foramen ovale evident on echocardiography.[51] Among patients suspected of paradoxical embolism, occult leg vein thrombosis is frequently present and often is confined to the calves.[52]

NONTHROMBOTIC PULMONARY EMBOLISM. Sources of embolism other than thrombus are less commonly detected than thrombotic PE. Fat embolism syndrome is most often observed after blunt trauma complicated by long-bone fractures.[53] Among cancer patients, tumor embolism is more difficult to diagnose clinically than thrombotic PE because presenting symptoms and signs are similar in both conditions.[54] Air embolus can occur during placement or removal of a central venous catheter.[55] It has also been described from presumed inadvertent pressure placed on a partially empty plastic intravenous infusion bag.[56]

Intravenous drug abusers tend to inject inadvertently a variety of substances that contaminate their drug supply. Commonly found materials at autopsy include hair, talc, and cotton. These patients are also susceptible to septic PE, which may be accompanied by endocarditis of the tricuspid or pulmonic valves.

Nonimaging Diagnostic Methods

PLASMA D-DIMER ELISA. This is the most promising blood test for pulmonary embolism screening. An abnormally elevated level of *ELISA-determined plasma D-dimer* has more than 90 per cent sensitivity for identifying patients with PE proven by lung scan[57] or by angiogram (Fig. 46–4).[58] This test relies on the principle that most patients with PE have ongoing endogenous fibrinolysis that is not effective enough to prevent PE but that does break down some of the fibrin clot to D-dimers. These D-dimers can be assayed by monoclonal antibodies in commercially available kits.

Although elevated plasma concentrations of D-dimers are sensitive for the presence of PE, they are not specific. Levels are elevated in patients for at least 1 week postoperatively and are also increased in patients with myocardial infarction, sepsis, or almost any other systemic illness. Therefore the plasma D-dimer ELISA is best used in patients with suspected PE who have no coexisting acute systemic illness.

The usual D-dimer measurement obtained in hospital laboratories utilizes a latex agglutination assay to detect disseminated intravascular coagulation. Unlike the ELISA, the latex agglutination assay is simply not sensitive enough for reliable PE screening. Alternatively, a two-step approach can be used in which a latex D-dimer is obtained as an initial screening test. If it is elevated, the ELISA will

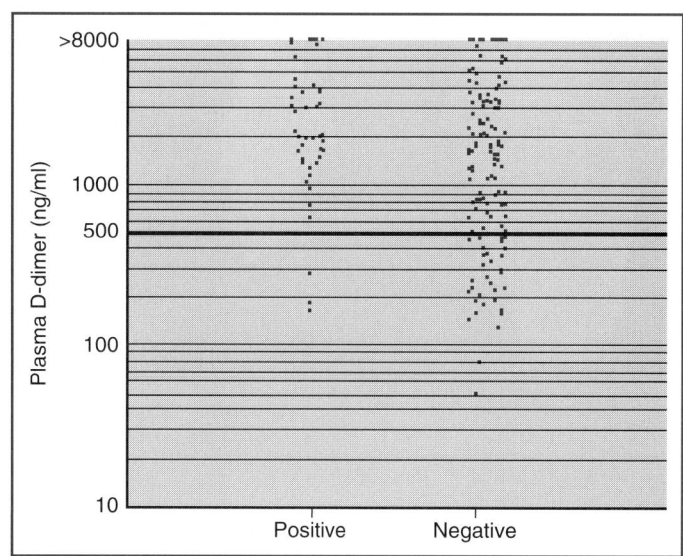

FIGURE 46–4. Distribution of plasma D-dimer levels, sorted according to pulmonary angiographic findings, among 173 patients with suspected acute pulmonary embolism. Plasma D-dimer levels < 500 ng/ml are rarely observed in patients with pulmonary angiographic evidence of PE. (Reprinted with permission from Goldhaber, S. Z., Simons, G. R., Elliott, C. G., et al.: Quantitative plasma D-dimer levels among patients undergoing pulmonary angiography for suspected pulmonary embolism. JAMA *270:*2819, 1993. Copyright 1993 the American Medical Association.)

also be elevated. However, if the latex D-dimer is normal, an ELISA D-dimer is required to help exclude PE.[59]

ARTERIAL BLOOD GASES. Among patients suspected of PE who underwent angiography in the Prospective Investigation of Pulmonary Embolism Diagnosis (PIOPED) (see p. 1589), determination of the partial pressure of oxygen in arterial blood did not discriminate between those with and without PE. There was no difference between the average pO_2 (70 mm Hg) among patients with PE compared with those without PE (72 mm Hg) at angiography. Importantly, among patients with angiographically proven PE who had no prior cardiopulmonary disease, the pO_2 was ≥ 80 mm Hg in 26 per cent.[60] Furthermore, normal values of the alveolar–arterial oxygen gradient did not exclude the diagnosis of acute PE.[61] Therefore, obtaining arterial blood gases should not be part of the diagnostic strategy when investigating suspected PE.

ELECTROCARDIOGRAM (see p. 118). The electrocardiogram is useful not only to help exclude acute myocardial infarction but also for rapidly identifying some patients with large PE, who may have electrocardiographic manifestations of right-heart strain. In a series of 49 consecutive patients with subsequently proven PE, at least three of seven electrocardiographic features suggestive of right ventricular overload (Table 46–8) were identified on 76 per cent of electrocardiograms obtained at hospital admission.[62]

IMPEDANCE PLETHYSMOGRAPHY (IPG). This is a very indi-

TABLE 46–8 ELECTROCARDIOGRAPHIC FINDINGS IN PULMONARY EMBOLISM

Incomplete or complete right bundle branch block
S in Lead I and aVL > 1.5 mm
Transition zone shift to V5
Qs in leads III and aVF, but not in Lead II
QRS axis > 90° or indeterminate axis
Low limb lead voltage
T-wave inversion in leads III and aVF or in leads V1–V4

Modified from Sreeram, N., Cheriex, E. C., Smeets, J. L. R. M., et al.: Value of the 12-lead electrocardiogram at hospital admission in the diagnosis of pulmonary embolism. Am. J. Cardiol. *73:*298, 1994.

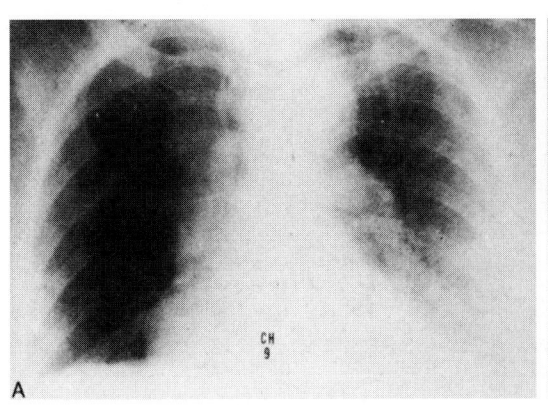
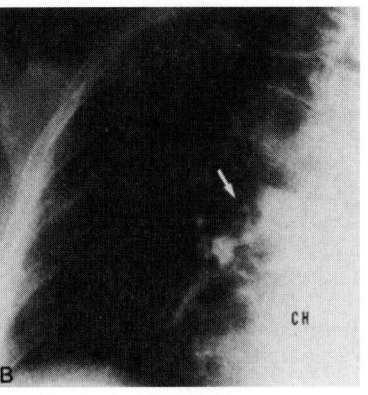

FIGURE 46–5. *A*, Chest film of patient with clinical signs of pulmonary embolism showing marked oligemia (Westermark's sign) in the entire right lobe. *B*, Arteriogram from same patient showing massive saddle embolus in the right main pulmonary artery (arrow). (Courtesy of Jack L. Westcott, M.D., The New York Hospital and Cornell University Medical College.)

rect approach to DVT diagnosis; it measures changes in electric resistance caused by obstruction to venous outflow. IPG was often used to detect DVT but now has only a limited role in special circumstances to help detect recurrence of DVT or to help assess the severity of venous insufficiency. In a study of consecutive patients with suspected DVT who underwent both IPG and contrast venography, IPG failed to detect 35 per cent of patients with proximal leg DVT.[63]

Imaging Methods

Chest Roentgenography

The chest radiograph is usually the first imaging study obtained in patients with suspected PE. Although more than half of patients with PE have an abnormal chest film examination, a near-normal radiograph in the setting of severe respiratory compromise is highly suggestive of massive PE. Classic chest film abnormalities are uncommon but include focal oligemia (Westermark's sign) (Fig. 46–5), indicating massive central embolic occlusion.[64] A peripheral wedge-shaped density above the diaphragm (Hampton's hump) (Fig. 46–6) usually indicates pulmonary infarction.[65] In PIOPED, PE patients with either a prominent central pulmonary artery or cardiomegaly had higher pulmonary arterial mean pressures than did patients with atelectasis, a pulmonary parenchymal abnormality, or pleural effusion.[66]

One should always search for subtle abnormalities such as distention of the descending right pulmonary artery. Often the vessel tapers rapidly after the enlarged portion. The chest radiograph can also help to identify patients with diseases that can mimic PE, such as lobar pneumonia or pneumothorax. Patients with these latter illnesses can also have concomitant PE.[67]

Venous Ultrasonography

The primary diagnostic criterion to establish the presence of DVT by ultrasonography is the loss of vein compressibility (Fig. 46–7). Normally the vein will collapse completely when gentle pressure is applied to the skin overlying it. Generally the applied pressure is kept below what is necessary to collapse the artery. The artery is not as affected because intraarterial pressure is much greater than venous pressure, and the structure of the arterial wall is more resistant to the pressure deformation than the venous wall. Upper extremity DVT may be more difficult to diagnose because the clavicle can hinder attempts to compress the subclavian vein. With acute DVT of either the upper extremity or leg, there is associated passive dilation of the vein.[68]

As many as half of PE patients have no imaging evidence of DVT. Therefore, if clinical suspicion of PE is high, patients without evidence of DVT should still be investigated for PE. For detection of DVT, ultrasound is more accurate than impedance plethysmography.[69] Suspected DVT may be most efficiently evaluated by developing a "critical pathway."[69a]

Ultrasonography is usually reliable in diagnosing proximal leg DVT in *symptomatic outpatients*.[70] The presence of newly detected DVT may sometimes be a useful surrogate for PE. At selected centers with special expertise, ultrasonography may also be dependable for evaluating suspected symptomatic infrapopliteal DVT.[71] Serial ultrasound measurement of thrombus mass after an episode of acute DVT may allow the subsequent correct identification of recurrent DVT.[72] Unfortunately, ultrasonography is unreliable because of its low sensitivity for screening of *asymptomatic patients* with possible DVT after orthopedic surgery[73] or after craniotomy.[74]

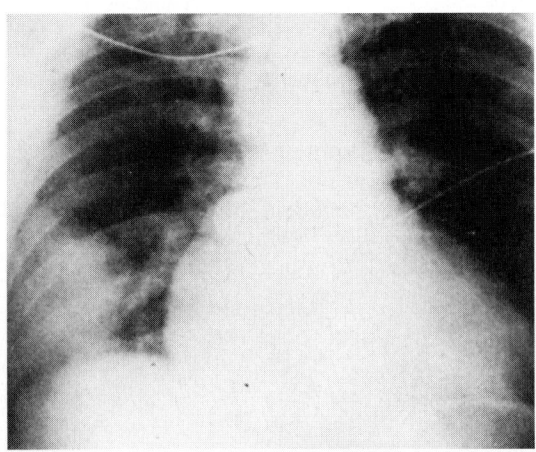

FIGURE 46–6. Posteroanterior chest film of patient with pulmonary embolism showing "Hampton's hump" in right lower lung field, a homogeneous, wedge-shaped density in the peripheral field, convex to the hilum. (Courtesy of Jack L. Westcott, M.D., The New York Hospital and Cornell University Medical College.)

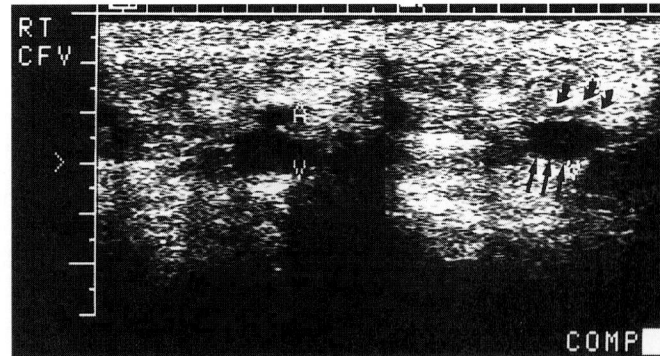

FIGURE 46–7. Right common femoral vein (RT CFV) thrombosis (transverse view) diagnosed by compression ultrasonography. The left half of the image is the baseline ultrasound examination demonstrating the artery (A) superior to the vein (V). During the examination, the artery can be seen to pulsate and appears to "wink" at the examiner. The vein is typically larger than the artery but normally is not several-fold larger. With compression (COMP) in the right half of the image, the artery is deformed (curved upper arrows), but the vein fails to compress (straight lower arrows).

TABLE 46-9 PIOPED: COMPARISON OF SCAN CATEGORY TO ANGIOGRAM FINDINGS

	PULMONARY EMBOLISM			NO ANGIOGRAM	TOTAL N
	Present	Absent	Uncertain		
Scan category					
High	102	14	1	7	124
Intermediate	105	217	9	33	364
Low	39	199	12	62	312
Near-normal/ normal	5	50	2	74	131
Total	251	480	24	176	931

From the PIOPED Investigators: Value of the ventilation/perfusion scan in acute pulmonary embolism. JAMA 263:2756, 1990.
PIOPED = Prospective Investigation of Pulmonary Embolism Diagnosis

CONTRAST PHLEBOGRAPHY. Although contrast phlebography has traditionally been considered the gold standard for DVT diagnosis,[75] venograms are now being obtained with less frequency because of the utility of ultrasonography. Venography is costly, invasive, and occasionally results in contrast allergy or contrast-induced phlebitis. Furthermore, there is considerable disagreement in the interpretation of contrast venograms among experienced readers.[76] Patients with massive leg DVT often have non-diagnostic venograms because the contrast agent simply cannot reach the totally obstructed deep leg veins. Consequently we reserve contrast phlebography for situations in which the ultrasound examination is equivocal or, alternatively, when the ultrasound examination is normal despite a high clinical suspicion for DVT.

LUNG SCANNING. Despite its limitations, lung scanning remains the principal test for diagnosing PE. Perfusion lung scintigraphy is sensitive but not specific for detecting pulmonary perfusion abnormalities. Small particulate aggregates of albumin or microspheres labeled with a gamma-emitting radionuclide are injected intravenously. The particles are trapped in the pulmonary capillary bed, reflecting pulmonary blood flow at the time of injection. Planar views of the chest are then obtained. Ventilation scans improve the specificity of the perfusion scan by indicating abnormal nonventilated lung, which could provide explanations for absence of perfusion other than acute PE.[67] If ventilation scanning cannot be performed, useful information can often be obtained from the perfusion scans alone if the scans either have multiple segmental perfusion defects or are normal or near normal.[77]

The diagnosis of PE is very unlikely in patients with normal and near-normal scans. High-probability scans usually indicate acute PE, but fewer than half of PE patients have a high-probability scan. Scans that fall between these extremes of the spectrum should be called intermediate probability. Many patients with low-probability scans but high clinical suspicion for PE do, in fact, have PE at angiography.[78] Therefore the term low-probability scan is a potentially lethal misnomer.[79]

Under the auspices of the National Heart, Lung, and Blood Institute, a multicenter study was undertaken to determine the diagnostic utility of the ventilation-perfusion lung scan in acute PE.[80] The PIOPED recruited 931 patients, of whom 81 per cent completed mandatory angiography within a day of having an abnormal lung scan. Among the 755 patients who completed angiography, 33 per cent had PE. The most important finding in PIOPED is that of the 251 patients with positive angiograms, only 102 (41 per cent) had high-probability lung scans. Therefore, because of the lung scan's low sensitivity, more than half (59 per cent) of patients with PE would not be recognized if high-probability lung scans were relied upon exclusively to establish the diagnosis of PE.

In PIOPED, the positive predictive value of lung scanning for PE at angiography was as follows: 87 per cent for high, 32 per cent for intermediate, 16 per cent for low, and 9 per cent for near-normal scans (Table 46–9). When the "clinical probability" was factored into the interpretation of the lung scan, it was evident that some patients suspected of PE would not require further work-up prior to making a disposition. For example, among patients who had both high probability lung scans and a clinical suspicion for PE of more than 80 per cent, the likelihood of PE at angiography was 96 per cent. Conversely, among patients who had both a low probability lung scan and a clinical suspicion for PE of less than 20 per cent, the likelihood of PE at angiography was only 4 per cent. Unfortunately, the majority of patients will not fit neatly into either of these categories. For example, patients with a high clinical suspicion of PE and a low probability scan had a 40 per cent likelihood of having PE at angiography (Table 46–10).

Retrospective analysis of the PIOPED data base has led to a slight revision of the initial PIOPED lung scan probability criteria (Table 46–11). For example, scans with a single moderate segmental mismatch are now classified as intermediate rather than low probability.[81]

ECHOCARDIOGRAPHY (see p. 95). Echocardiography is a rapid, practical, and sensitive technique for the identification of right ventricular overload following PE (Fig. 46–8).[82] The frequency of echocardiographic signs of PE (Table 46–12) depends on the population being studied. For example, Kasper et al. reported that the frequency of right ventricular dilatation exceeded 90 per cent when PE was accompanied by pulmonary hypertension; right ventricular free wall asynergy was present in 81 per cent with pulmonary hypertension, but in none with normal pulmonary artery pressures.[83] For those patients in whom transthoracic imaging is unsatisfactory, transesophageal echocardiography can be carried out.[84]

Patients with right ventricular dysfunction after PE have a worse prognosis and may be at increased risk for recurrent PE and death compared with those who have normal right ventricular function. Therefore, detection of right ventricular dysfunction at the time of presentation with PE is useful for risk stratification and prognostication. Echocar-

TABLE 46-10 PIOPED: PULMONARY EMBOLISM STATUS

	CLINICAL PROBABILITY (%)			
	80–100 No. PE/PTS (%)	20–79 No. PE/PTS (%)	0–19 No. PE/PTS (%)	ALL PROBABILITIES No. PE/PTS (%)
Scan category				
High	28/29 (96)	70/ 80 (88)	5/ 9 (56)	103/118 (87)
Intermediate	27/41 (66)	66/236 (28)	11/ 68 (16)	104/345 (30)
Low	6/15 (40)	30/191 (16)	4/ 90 (4)	40/296 (14)
Near-normal/normal	0/ 5 (0)	4/ 62 (6)	1/ 61 (2)	5/128 (4)
Total	61/90 (68)	170/569 (30)	21/228 (9)	252/887 (28)

From the PIOPED Investigators: Value of the ventilation/perfusion scan in acute pulmonary embolism. JAMA 263:2757, 1990.
PIOPED = Prospective Investigation of Pulmonary Embolism Diagnosis.
80–100, 20–79, 0–19 represent the clinical probabilities of PE.
No. PE/PTS (%) represents the number and percentage of patients in each subgroup with PE.

TABLE 46-11 REVISED PIOPED V/Q SCAN CRITERIA

High Probability (≥ 80%)
≥ 2 Large mismatched segmental perfusion defects or the arithmetic equivalent in moderate or large + moderate defects*

Intermediate Probability (20%–79%)
One moderate to two large mismatched segmental perfusion defects or the arithmetic equivalent in moderate or large + moderate defects*
Single matched ventilation/perfusion defect with clear chest radiograph†
Difficult to categorize as low or high, or not described as low or high

Low Probability (≤ 19%)
Nonsegmental perfusion defects (e.g., cardiomegaly, enlarged aorta, enlarged hilum, elevated diaphragm)
Any perfusion defect with a substantially larger chest radiographic abnormality
Perfusion defects matched by ventilation abnormality† provided that there are: (1) clear chest radiograph and (2) some areas of normal perfusion in the lungs
Any number of small perfusion defects with a normal chest radiograph

Normal
No perfusion defects or perfusion outlines exactly the shape of the lungs seen on the chest radiograph (note that hilar and aortic impressions may be seen and the chest radiograph and/or ventilation study may be abnormal)

Reprinted with permission from Gottschalk, A., Sostman, D., Coleman, E., et al.: Ventilation-perfusion scintigraphy in the PIOPED study. Part II. Evaluation of the scintigraphic criteria and interpretations. J. Nucl. Med. *34*:1119, 1993.
PIOPED =.Prospective Investigation of Pulmonary Embolism Diagnosis
* Two large mismatched perfusion defects are borderline for "high probability." Individual readers may correctly interpret individual scans with this pattern as "high probability." In general, it is recommended that more than this degree of mismatch be present for the "high probability" category.
† Very extensive matched defects can be categorized as "low probability." Single V/Q matches are borderline for "low probability" and thus should be categorized as "intermediate" in most circumstances by most readers, although individual readers may correctly interpret individual scans with this pattern as "low probability."

diograms done on normotensive patients with lung perfusion defects of greater than 30 per cent identify more than 90 per cent of patients with right ventricular dysfunction.[49]

Right ventricular dilatation and hypokinesis may occur in chronic pulmonary hypertension of any cause. Long-term elevation of right ventricular afterload is usually accompanied by right ventricular hypertrophy. In patients with chronic pulmonary hypertension, the velocity of the tricuspid regurgitant jet may be elevated to a greater level than in patients with acute PE and no underlying cardiopulmonary disease. Right ventricular infarction, cardiomyopathy, and right ventricular dysplasia may also result in right ventricular hypokinesis and dilatation on the echocardiogram. In these conditions, however, the velocity of tricuspid regurgitation is usually less than in acute PE.

It appears that right ventricular contractile dysfunction following PE has a distinct regional pattern in which wall excursion is hypokinetic from the base through the free wall but remains almost normal at the right ventricular apex (Fig. 46-8B). This pattern of right ventricular contractile dysfunction differs from the global dysfunction observed in primary pulmonary hypertension.[85] A possible explanation is that in PE the left ventricle may tether the right ventricular apex, thereby preserving near-normal wall motion in this region.

PULMONARY ANGIOGRAPHY. Selective pulmonary angiography is the most specific examination available for establishing the clinical diagnosis of PE.[86] Angiography should be undertaken as part of an integrated diagnostic approach that combines the clinical assessment with noninvasive diagnostic methods. Angiography tends to be most useful among patients in whom the clinical likelihood of PE differs substantially from the probability of PE based upon noninvasive testing. It is most often undertaken when the lung scan shows intermediate probability for PE.

Pulmonary angiography also has a role in primary therapy of PE. It is a first and necessary step prior to mechanical intervention in the catheterization laboratory with techniques such as suction catheter embolectomy or mechanical clot fragmentation.

PERFORMANCE OF PULMONARY ANGIOGRAPHY

As with any procedure, there is a learning curve for proper and safe performance of pulmonary angiography. Hospitals that perform fewer than several of these studies per month should probably refer their patients to centers that undertake this procedure more frequently. In PIOPED, complications from angiography resulted in death in five patients (0.5 per cent), two of whom were on ventilators and two of whom had severe heart failure prior to the procedure. Nine patients (1 per cent) had major nonfatal complications; respiratory distress occurred in four, renal failure in three, and hematoma requiring transfusion in two.[87] When a team of physicians and nurses is experienced in managing PE patients, even those with moderate or severe pulmonary hypertension can undergo pulmonary angiography safely. In a consecutive series of 67 such patients, 14 of whom had right ventricular end-diastolic pressure that equaled or exceeded 20 mm Hg, no major rhythm disturbances or systemic hypotension requiring therapy occurred, and there were no deaths.[88]

Contrast agents of lower osmolality are less toxic than conventional angiographic dye in patients with pulmonary hypertension. Furthermore, low osmolar contrast agents virtually abolish the heat sensation and urge to cough.[89] We employ low osmolar contrast agents rather than conventional angiographic dye to maximize patient comfort and to minimize repetition of the procedure because of patient coughing and consequent blurring of the films.

PREPARATION OF THE PATIENT. The rationale for performing pulmonary angiography should be explained carefully to the patient and the patient's family. The patient should be told that the procedure may cause discomfort.

A history of allergy to contrast medium should be sought. If present, high-dose oral corticosteroids should be administered both 12 hours and 2 hours before challenge with contrast agent.[90] Heparin can be discontinued immediately before the procedure, unless the clinical suspicion for PE is very high. Patients should avoid heavy meals for at least 4 hours before angiography.

THE ANGIOGRAPHIC PROCEDURE. The perfusion lung scan serves as a road map to the angiographer, who performs selective angiography rather than injecting into the main pulmonary artery. Obtaining accurate and high-quality recordings of right-heart pressures and waveforms is of paramount importance. If the pressure tracing "dampens" or "wedges" in the proximal pulmonary artery, anatomically massive PE should be suspected prior to injection of contrast agent. If the pulmonary artery systolic pressure exceeds approximately 50 mm Hg, the differential diagnosis should include chronic PE or acute superimposed upon chronic PE. Information gleaned from catheterization may occasionally make angiography unnecessary. For example, unexplained dyspnea might be due to cardiac tamponade or left ventricular failure rather than PE. Patients with dyspnea and pulmonary hypertension might have intracardiac shunting that can be defined most precisely with an oxygen saturation run.

Our preferred approach is via the right femoral vein. Percutaneous cannulation of the femoral vein (located 1 to 2 cm medial to the palpable femoral artery) permits rapid access to a large vessel and avoids the problems of using small brachial veins, which are prone to venospasm. To avoid inadvertent perforation of the right ventricle, a catheter with a pigtail configuration can be used rather than one with a straight end.[91] A pigtail catheter can usually be easily manipulated into the pulmonary artery (Fig. 46-9A).

Once the catheter has been positioned and the patient has been placed in the desired projection, a test dose of 5 to 10 ml of contrast agent is administered. A plain "scout" film is then obtained to ensure satisfactory exposure and field of view. Prior to the major contrast injection, the patient should be instructed carefully about proper breathing technique and should be reminded to try to suppress the urge to cough. Filming is carried out during maximal inspiration. Twenty to 25 ml of contrast medium per second is injected for 2

TABLE 46-12 ECHOCARDIOGRAPHIC SIGNS OF PULMONARY EMBOLISM

Direct visualization of thrombus (rare)

Right ventricular dilatation

Right ventricular hypokinesis (with sparing of the apex)

Abnormal interventricular septal motion

Tricuspid valve regurgitation

Pulmonary artery dilatation

Lack of decreased inspiratory collapse of inferior vena cava

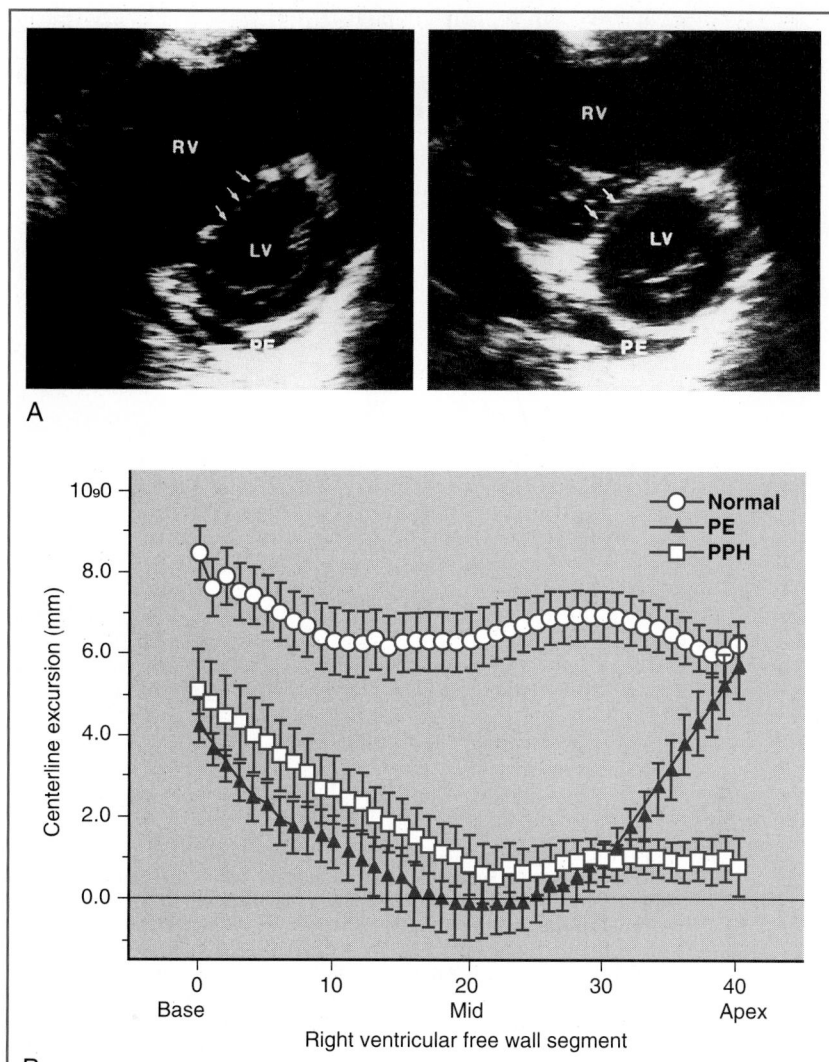

FIGURE 46–8. *A,* Parasternal short-axis views of the right ventricle (RV) and left ventricle (LV) in diastole *(left)* and systole *(right).* There is diastolic and systolic bowing of the interventricular septum (arrows) into the left ventricle compatible with right-ventricular volume and pressure overload, respectively. The right ventricle is appreciably dilated and markedly hypokinetic, with little change in apparent right-ventricular area from diastole to systole. PE = small pericardial effusion. (Reprinted with permission from Come, P. C.: Echocardiographic evaluation of pulmonary embolism and its response to therapeutic interventions. Chest *101:*151S, 1992.)

B, Segmental right ventricular free wall excursion (mean ± SEM) by centerline analysis in patients with acute pulmonary embolism (PE) or primary pulmonary hypertension (PPH) and in normal persons. The acute increase in afterload in PE results in regional right ventricular dysfunction predominantly affecting the mid free wall as it assumes a more spherical shape to equalize wall stress. The right ventricular apex is spared. In contrast, the chronic pressure overload of PPH results in more diffuse right ventricular dysfunction, with limited shape change of the hypertrophied right ventricle. (From McConnell, M. V., Rayan, M. E., Solomon, S. D., et al.: Echocardiographic diagnosis of acute pulmonary embolism: A distinct pattern of abnormal right ventricular wall motion. Am. J. Cardiol. *in press*).

seconds. The exposure rates for this phase are three per second for 3 seconds and then one per second for the pulmonary venous phase, which occurs 5 to 7 seconds after injection. After the selective pulmonary artery injection, pulmonary artery pressures are rechecked to monitor a possible pulmonary hypertensive response, and systemic arterial pressure should be rechecked (with a sphygmomanometer rather than an indwelling arterial cannula) to detect potential hypotension. This "large film" method offers high resolution, clarity of vascular detail, and versatility in field size. An alternative approach utilizes cineangiography.

Interpreting the Angiogram. Standard contrast pulmonary angiography can detect emboli as small as 1 to 2 mm. PE cannot be excluded unless the vasculature appears normal on two different views. Conversely, a definitive diagnosis of PE depends upon visualization of an intraluminal filling defect (Fig. 46–9*B*) in more than one projection. Secondary signs of PE reflect decreased perfusion and consist of abrupt occlusion ("cut off") of vessels, oligemia or avascularity of a segment, a prolonged arterial phase with slow filling and emptying of veins, and tortuous, tapering peripheral vessels.[92]

Not all pulmonary artery filling defects or occlusions are due to acute PE. In chronic PE, arteries may appear "pouched," and thrombus appears organized with a concave edge. Bandlike defects called webs may be present, in addition to intimal irregularities and abrupt narrowing or occlusion of lobar vessels.[93] Other causes of intraluminal filling defects include pulmonary Takayasu's arteritis (see p. 1572), angiosarcoma, and sarcoidosis.[67]

Angiographic methods for quantitating the severity of PE have been problematic. The Walsh scoring system,[94] which is most commonly used in the United States, does not take into account the impairment of peripheral perfusion. The Miller index,[95] which is commonly used in Europe, can overestimate the extent of pulmonary vascular obstruction among patients with massive PE. Both methods fail to differentiate adequately between clot size and the degree of vascular occlusion.

EVOLVING IMAGING METHODS

INTRAVASCULAR ULTRASOUND. Intravascular ultrasound is emerging as a useful technique for identifying patients with acute[96] and chronic[97] PE. Although the main pulmonary artery and large branches can be quickly accessed and examined, cannulation and visualization of peripheral branches are difficult to accomplish rapidly.

PULMONARY ANGIOSCOPY. Percutaneous pulmonary angioscopy using a guiding balloon catheter helps to differentiate among acute PE, chronic PE, and primary pulmonary hypertension.[98] Because aggressive interventional procedures for these three conditions are being undertaken with increasing frequency, the application of pulmonary angioscopy during the diagnostic work-up will probably increase.

SPIRAL COMPUTED TOMOGRAPHY. Spiral computed tomography (CT) allows continuous scanning of organ volumes during a single breath hold by advancing the patient through the roentgenography beam during continuous scanning. In a landmark study, 42 consecutive patients with suspected PE were prospectively evaluated with both spiral CT and selective pulmonary angiography. Patients received between 90 and 120 ml of contrast agent during the CT. All 23 patients with normal spiral CT also had normal pulmonary angiograms. Thromboemboli visualized with spiral CT were almost always seen on standard pulmonary angiography.[99] Spiral CT appears most effective in detecting emboli in the second to fourth division pulmonary vessels but may be ineffective in diagnosing smaller, peripheral PE.[100]

MAGNETIC RESONANCE IMAGING. Magnetic resonance pulmonary angiography provides images similar to catheter angiography, without the necessity of injecting iodinated contrast media.[101] For detecting DVT, magnetic resonance imaging (MRI) already compares favorably with venography and ultrasound. MRI is noninvasive and may be performed in patients with poor venous access, poor renal function, and contraindications to iodinated contrast. MRI is much less operator dependent than ultrasound, and MRI (unlike ultrasound) can provide good images of the inferior vena cava and iliac veins.[102]

Overall Strategy: An Integrated Diagnostic Approach

The diagnosis of PE requires an interdisciplinary effort, commonly involving cardiologist and radiologist. Unfortu-

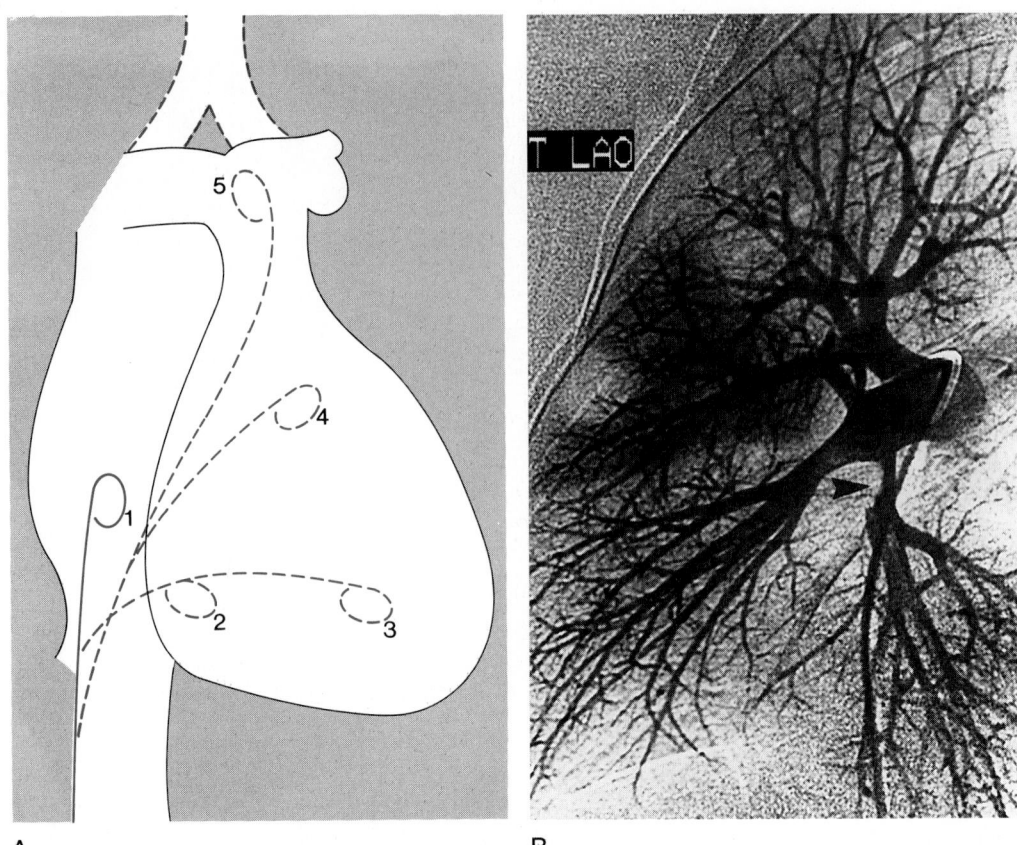

A   B

FIGURE 46–9. *A,* Technique for pulmonary artery catheterization. The pigtail catheter is advanced into the right atrium (1). A deflector guidewire is inserted into the catheter, the tip of the wire lying immediately proximal to the pigtail loop. The guidewire is deflected using the external handle, so that the catheter is curved toward the tricuspid valve (2). With the deflected guidewire fixed, the catheter is stripped off the wire and into the right ventricle (3). After deflection is released, the catheter will assume a straighter course, pointing toward the right ventricular outflow tract (4). As counterclockwise torque is applied, the catheter is advanced into the main pulmonary artery (5). With further advancement, the catheter will usually enter the left pulmonary artery. To select the right pulmonary artery, the deflector wire can be used to deflect the catheter toward the right, just below the level of the tracheal bifurcation. Pressure measurements are obtained in each right-sided cardiac chamber between each of the maneuvers described here. (From Meyerovitz, M.: How to maximize the safety of coronary and pulmonary angiography in patients receiving thrombolytic therapy. Chest *97*:134S, 1990.)

B, Pulmonary angiogram with digital subtraction (left anterior oblique projection) demonstrates a large, acute embolus in the right lower lobar pulmonary artery (arrowhead).

nately, PE may be quite difficult to diagnose despite the availability of an array of noninvasive tests, including lung scanning as well as the more recently popularized plasma D-dimer ELISA, leg ultrasonography, and echocardiography.

With the combination of clinical assessment, lung scanning, and evaluation for DVT, patients who require pulmonary angiography can be more carefully selected than was previously possible.[43] An approach that combines lung scanning and leg ultrasonography reduces by half the number of patients who require pulmonary angiography.[103] Combining the D-dimer ELISA results with leg ultrasonography among patients with intermediate probability lung scans can also reduce substantially the requirement for pulmonary angiography.[104] Among 202 patients with suspected PE and intermediate probability scans, a definitive diagnosis was obtained by combining clinical probability, plasma D-dimer ELISA, leg ultrasonography, and judicious use of pulmonary angiography. This approach appeared to be safe, based on 6-month follow-up of 99 per cent of the cohort, only 1 per cent of whom had a subsequent DVT or PE after the diagnostic protocol had excluded PE.[105] Thus, I advocate an *integrated diagnostic approach* for patients suspected of PE. When this strategy is used, clinical likelihood of PE is combined with the results of noninvasive testing to determine whether pulmonary angiography is warranted (Fig. 46–10).

Overall, for patients suspected of PE, the initial clinical assessment includes the history, physical examination, electrocardiogram, and chest radiograph. Then the initial branch point is deciding between plasma D-dimer ELISA as a blood screening test and lung scanning. If clinical suspicion is low, the plasma D-dimer ELISA can be considered. If the D-dimer is normal, the work-up for PE can be halted at this point. Otherwise, lung scanning is appropriate. If the lung scan is high probability for PE, treatment can be undertaken, often without further diagnostic testing. In contrast, if the lung scan is normal, the work-up for PE can stop. For the many patients who have intermediate or low probability scans, D-dimer ELISA can be obtained at this point. Unless there is high clinical suspicion, the work-up can stop if the D-dimer ELISA is normal. If the D-dimer ELISA is elevated, the investigation of PE can be pursued with leg ultrasonography, echocardiography, and, if these are unrevealing, pulmonary angiography.

MANAGEMENT

The classic "treatment" of PE with heparin constitutes secondary prevention of recurrent PE rather than primary therapy of PE. A contemporary management approach relies on risk stratification of PE patients. The proportion of nonperfused lung on scintigraphy and the presence of right

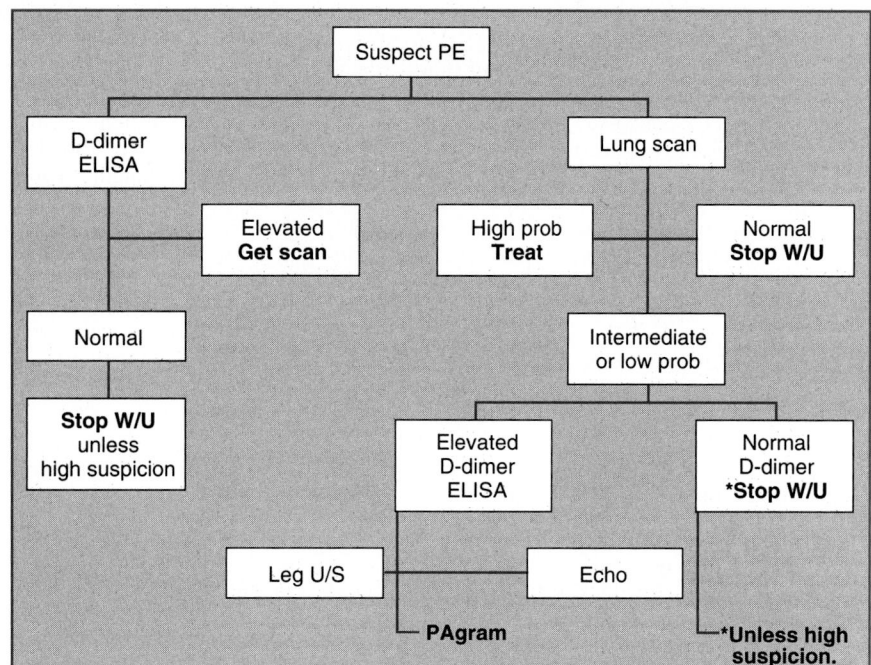

FIGURE 46–10. PE diagnosis strategy: Overall approach. (W/U = work-up.)

ventricular hypokinesis on echocardiography are used to help establish a prognosis. Patients with normal ventricular function with small or moderate-size PE have an excellent outcome if they receive anticoagulation alone.[49] PE patients now undergo more intensive and rapid anticoagulation than previously, with heparin dosing often guided by formal protocols that used fixed[106] or weight-adjusted[107] dosing (Table 46–13). Heparin is ordinarily administered for at least 5 to 7 days, with a target PTT of 1.5 to 2.5 times the upper limit of normal of the control PTT value.

There is an increasing tendency to provide primary treatment with thrombolysis or mechanical intervention (Table 46–14) to PE patients with right ventricular hypokinesis, even if they have normal systemic arterial pressure.[49] Primary therapy to decrease the size and hemodynamic impact of the embolism is combined with anticoagulation, which helps prevent recurrent PE. Another emerging trend is to employ thrombolysis among PE cases that are diagnosed noninvasively rather than with angiography, thus decreasing the rate of bleeding complications, particularly groin hematomas, that would otherwise occur at the site of femoral vein catheterization for pulmonary angiography.[108] Finally, embolectomy, especially in the catheterization la-

TABLE 46–13 THE "RASCHKE" WEIGHT-BASED HEPARIN NOMOGRAM

VARIABLE	HEPARIN DOSE
Initial heparin dose	80 U/kg bolus, then 18 U/kg/h
aPTT < 35 s (< 1.2 × control)	80 U/kg bolus, then increase infusion by 4 U/kg/h
aPTT 35–45 s (1.2–1.5 × control)	40 U/kg bolus, then increase infusion by 2 U/kg/h
aPTT 46–70 s (1.5–2.3 × control)	No change
aPTT 71–90 s (2.3–3 × control)	Decrease infusion by 2 U/kg/h
aPTT > 90 s (> 3 × control)	Hold infusion 1 hr; then decrease infusion rate by 3 U/kg/h

s = seconds.

From Raschke, R. A., Reilly, B. M., Guidry, J. R., et al.: The weight-based heparin dosing nomogram compared with a "standard care" nomogram. A randomized controlled trial. Ann. Intern. Med. 119:874, 1993.

TABLE 46–14 PRIMARY THERAPY FOR PULMONARY EMBOLISM

Medical
  Thrombolytic therapy
  Inotropic and vasoactive agents (e.g., dobutamine)
Catheter Based
  Suction embolectomy
  Local mechanical dispersion (e.g., pulverization or fragmentation)
  Local pharmacological thrombolysis
  Combined mechanical and pharmacological thrombolysis
Surgical Embolectomy

oratory, is enjoying a renaissance, because results are improving as techniques are refined.[109]

ADJUNCTIVE MEASURES. Simple but important measures include provision of adequate pain relief and supplemental oxygenation. Nonsteroidal antiinflammatory agents may be more effective than narcotics in relieving pleuritic chest pain and are usually safe to administer despite concomitant anticoagulation. Temporary mechanical ventilation may be of great utility for hypoxic patients prior to the onset of frank respiratory failure. Dobutamine—a beta-adrenergic agonist with positive inotropic and pulmonary vasodilating effects (see p. 1237)—should be considered a first-line agent to treat right heart failure and cardiogenic shock. In general, volume loading these patients is ill advised because ventricular interdependence can lead to even further reductions in left ventricular output. For patients with pulmonary hypertension and a patent foramen ovale, inhaled nitric oxide may reverse right-to-left shunting and improve oxygenation.[110]

Secondary Prevention: Anticoagulation

Heparin (see also p. 1817)

Standard, unfractionated heparin is a highly sulfated glycosaminoglycan that is partially purified from either porcine intestinal mucosa or bovine lung. Its molecular weight ranges from 3000 to 30,000 daltons and averages 15,000. *Low molecular weight heparins (LMWHs)* are fragments of unfractionated heparin that exhibit less binding to plasma proteins and endothelial cells than unfractionated heparin. Therefore, LMWHs have greater bioavailability, more predictable dose response, and longer half-life than unfractionated heparin. LMWHs have not received Food and Drug Administration approval for PE or DVT treatment.

Heparin acts primarily by binding to antithrombin III (AT III), an enzyme that inhibits the coagulation factors thrombin (factor IIa), Xa, IXa, XIa, and XIIa. Heparin subsequently promotes a conformational change in AT III that accelerates its activity approximately 100- to 1000-fold.[111] This prevents additional thrombus formation and permits endogenous fibrinolytic mechanisms to lyse clot that has already formed. However, heparin does *not* directly dissolve thrombus that already exists.

One placebo-controlled randomized trial of heparin has been carried out in PE patients.[112] The mortality rate was significantly lower among the treated patients, and the trial was discontinued for ethical reasons. Nevertheless, the efficacy of heparin is limited because clot-bound thrombin is protected from heparin–antithrombin III inhibition.[113] Furthermore, heparin resistance can occur because unfractionated heparin binds to plasma proteins.[114]

MONITORING HEPARIN. An activated partial thromboplastin time (PTT) that is at least 1½ times greater than the control value should provide a minimum therapeutic level of heparin. However, there are many different PTT reagent kits and virtually no standardization of PTT levels.[115] Therefore, an individual hospital's target PTT range for heparin anticoagulation should correspond to a plasma heparin level of approximately 0.2 to 0.5 units/ml. At Brigham and Women's Hospital, we quantitatively measure the heparin level by having our chemistry laboratory use a HEPRN pack (Du Pont) in the automated clinical analyzer used for other chemistry tests. The plasma heparin level is a chromogenic assay based on the inhibition of factor X_a by heparin-activated antithrombin III. The HEPRN pack contains excess factor X_a and essentially analyzes the heparin level by means of an anti-factor X_a assay. Blood for this assay should be drawn into a citrated tube, placed on ice, centrifuged within 30 minutes, and analyzed within 4 hours.

The plasma heparin level is particularly useful in two situations: (1) monitoring heparin anticoagulation among patients with baseline elevated PTTs due to a lupus anticoagulant or anticardiolipin antibodies and (2) monitoring heparin among DVT and PE patients who require large daily doses of heparin.[116]

For patients in whom warfarin therapy has failed or who cannot take warfarin (e.g., pregnant women), we treat initially with continuous intravenous heparin and then teach self-administration of full-dose subcutaneous heparin. With subcutaneous injections, peak heparin levels are usually obtained at approximately 3 hours, and the effect may last for 8 to 12 hours if the heparin dose is adequate. To monitor heparin, the target is a midinterval PTT of approximately 50 to 90 seconds.[117] I rarely permit more than 15,000 units of unfractionated heparin per injection because of concern about possible poor absorption. This means that many patients require injections three times daily. If they object to this schedule, or if their heparin dosing regimen is difficult to adjust, I encourage ambulatory management with a continuous intravenous unfractionated heparin infusion.[118]

INITIATING HEPARIN THERAPY. Heparin is the cornerstone of treatment for acute PE. Before heparin therapy is begun, risk factors for bleeding should be considered, such as a prior history of bleeding with anticoagulation, thrombocytopenia, vitamin K deficiency, increasing age, underlying diseases, and concomitant drug therapy. The most frequently overlooked portion of the physical examination is a rectal examination for occult blood.

The Raschke regimen for achieving rapid, effective, and safe heparinization is presented in Table 46–13. In general, heparin infusion rates as high as 1500 to 2000 units per hour are quite commonly required to achieve adequate anticoagulation during the first few days of heparin administration.

Unless a severe bleeding problem such as active gastrointestinal bleeding is detected, heparin can be started prior to lung scanning or pulmonary angiography. In cases of severe bleeding, heparin therapy should be withheld, and nonpharmacological treatment (secondary prevention) with insertion of an inferior vena cava (IVC) filter should be considered if the diagnosis of PE is confirmed.

COMPLICATIONS. The most important adverse effect of heparin is hemorrhage. Major bleeding during anticoagulation may unmask a previously silent lesion, such as bladder or colon cancer. For most cases of moderate bleeding, cessation of heparin therapy will suffice, and the PTT will usually return to normal within 6 hours because the half-life of heparin is only 60 to 90 minutes. Resumption of heparin at a lower dose or implementing alternative therapy will depend on the severity of the bleeding, the risk of recurrent thromboembolism, and the extent to which bleeding may have resulted from excessive anticoagulation (i.e.,

a PTT greater than three times the baseline value). Risk factors for major in-hospital bleeding among anticoagulated patients include the presence of comorbid conditions, age greater than 60 years, or liver dysfunction that worsens during treatment.[119]

In the event of life-threatening or intracranial hemorrhage, protamine sulfate can be administered at the time heparin is discontinued. Protamine, a strongly basic protein, will immediately reverse anticoagulant activity by forming a stable complex with the acidic heparin. For life-threatening hemorrhage, the usual dose is approximately 1 mg/100 units of heparin, administered slowly (e.g., 50 mg over 10 to 30 minutes). Protamine sulfate may cause allergic reactions, particularly in diabetics who have had prior exposure to protamine after using neutral protamine Hagedorn (NPH) insulin.[111]

Heparin-associated thrombocytopenia can occur via two mechanisms. Platelet agglutination and aggregation that is rarely of clinical importance is more common but less ominous than immunologically mediated thrombocytopenia, which promotes platelet aggregation and subsequent destruction. Typically, platelet counts will decline below 100,000 per mm³. This latter form of thrombocytopenia may be associated with either thrombocytopenic bleeding or with life-threatening arterial ("white clot syndrome") and venous thrombosis. Testing for heparin antibodies is specific but not sensitive.[111]

Patients receiving prolonged heparin therapy may develop osteopenia, osteoporosis, or pathological bone fractures. In most cases, asymptomatic osteopenia is the most severe adverse effect on bone metabolism. This finding is most readily assessed with bone densitometry.[120] Among women who have discontinued heparin after pregnancy, the osteopenia usually resolves within a year.[121]

Heparin-associated elevations in transaminase levels occur commonly, have no relation to whether the heparin is of bovine or porcine origin, and are rarely associated with clinical toxicity.[122,123] Heparin causes aldosterone depression by an unknown mechanism within 4 to 8 days after initiation of therapy. In patients with a normally functioning renin-angiotensin-aldosterone axis, this is probably of no clinical significance, although serum sodium levels may drop slightly. However, it may cause clinically important hyperkalemia in certain patients, such as those with diabetes or renal failure.[124]

Dextran

Dextran is a polysaccharide that inhibits erythrocyte aggregation, platelet adhesiveness, and leukocyte plugging. For patients in whom the hemorrhagic or thrombocytopenic risk of heparin is prohibitively high, the use of continuous infusion dextran can in some cases provide safe and immediate anticoagulation.[125] In practice, a test dose of 20 ml of dextran 1 is administered, followed by a continuous infusion of dextran 40 at approximately 20 ml/hr for as long as 5 days. During this period, patients can receive concomitant oral anticoagulation with warfarin.

Warfarin Sodium (see also p. 1818)

Warfarin is a vitamin K antagonist that prevents gamma carboxylation activation of coagulation factors II, VII, IX, and X. The full anticoagulant effect of warfarin may not be apparent for 5 days, even if the prothrombin time, used to monitor warfarin's effect, becomes elevated more rapidly. Elevation in the prothrombin time may initially reflect depletion of coagulation factor VII, which has a half-life of about 6 hours, whereas factor II has a half-life of about 5 days.

OVERLAP WITH HEPARIN. When warfarin therapy is initiated during an active thrombotic state, the levels of protein C and S decline, thus creating a thrombogenic potential. By overlapping heparin and warfarin for 5 days, the procoagulant effect of unopposed warfarin can be counteracted. In a Dutch study, patients with DVT were randomized to oral anticoagulation alone versus heparin plus oral anticoagulation. The recurrent DVT rate was three times higher in the group that received oral anticoagulation alone.[126] This study demonstrates that warfarin should be given with heparin coverage and overlap to patients with an active thrombotic state.

MONITORING WARFARIN. The prothrombin time, utilized to adjust the dose of warfarin, should be reported according to the International Normalized Ratio (INR), not the prothrombin time ratio or the prothrombin time expressed in seconds. Fewer bleeding complications occur when the INR is used to monitor warfarin dosing rather than the prothrombin time ratio.[131]

INTENSITY AND DURATION OF THERAPY. It is our practice to treat with 5 to 7 days of heparin and to initiate warfarin administration on the first hospital day after documenting a PTT within the therapeutic range.[127] It is clear that the recurrence rate after completion of anticoagulation is halved by utilizing 6 months of oral anticoagulation rather than 6 weeks.[127a] In otherwise healthy patients, I usually initiate warfarin therapy with 7.5 to 10 mg and then adjust the warfarin dose to achieve a target INR. Among systemically ill patients, however, vitamin K deficiency[128] may lead to marked overanticoagulation just after a single dose of warfarin. I tend to treat first-time DVT of the calf for 3 months,[130] proximal DVT for 6 months, and PE for 1 year. The target INR for first-time DVT is 2.0 to 3.0, but I tend to treat PE more intensively, with a target INR of at least 3.0. Whenever possible, patients with DVT or PE who also have the antiphospholipid-antibody syndrome should be maintained with a target INR of at least 3.0.[130a]

The optimal duration of therapy is unknown. In a prospective 12-year follow-up study of 58 low-risk DVT patients in Zurich, 14 per cent and 24 per cent suffered recurrent venous thrombosis.[130b] In Padua, Italy, 355 consecutive DVT patients were treated with warfarin for 3 months and then followed long-term. The cumulative incidence of recurrent thrombosis at 2, 5, and 8 years was 18, 25, and 30 per cent, respectively.[129] For patients with recurrent thrombosis or underlying long-term risk factors for thrombosis (e.g., metastatic cancer or massive obesity), I often advise indefinite anticoagulation. Three ongoing trials are randomizing DVT patients to short-term (3 months) versus long-term anticoagulation with 1 to 3 years of warfarin.

COMPLICATIONS. The major toxic effect of warfarin is bleeding. The risk of bleeding increases as the INR increases. Risk factors for hemorrhage include severe hepatic or renal disease, alcoholism, drug interactions, trauma, malignant disease, and known previous bleeding sites in the gastrointestinal tract. Of 130 cases of bleeding in one study, 38 per cent were due to remediable lesions, half of which were occult prior to warfarin administration.[132] Among outpatients who develop intracranial hemorrhage with warfarin treatment, age is the most important risk factor other than the prothrombin time.[133]

Major life-threatening bleeding requires immediate treatment with enough cryoprecipitate or fresh frozen plasma (FFP) (usually 2 units) to normalize the INR and achieve immediate hemostasis. To treat less serious bleeding, vitamin K may be administered parenterally; a dose of 10 mg subcutaneously or intramuscularly will usually reverse the effects of warfarin in 6 to 12 hours. However, this approach will make the patient relatively refractory to warfarin for up to 2 weeks, so that reinstitution of warfarin becomes more difficult. Minor bleeding with a prolonged INR may merely require interruption of warfarin therapy, without administration of FFP, until the INR has returned to the therapeutic range. If bleeding occurs when the INR is within the therapeutic range, occult malignant disease

should be suspected and ruled out. Evaluation of cases of minor bleeding and an INR above the therapeutic range is less productive.

Warfarin-induced skin necrosis[134] is a rare but important complication that may be related to warfarin-induced reduction of protein C. The "purple toes syndrome" is another rare complication of warfarin that appears to be caused by cholesterol microembolization.[135] In this syndrome, crystals are released from ulcerated atherosclerotic plaques. It appears that warfarin may worsen cholesterol microembolic disease by interfering with the healing of ulcerated atherosclerotic plaques.

During pregnancy, heparin should generally be used instead of warfarin because warfarin is associated with a 10-fold higher rate of congenital anomalies.[136] The fetus is particularly susceptible to warfarin embryopathy during the sixth through twelfth week of gestation.[137] The main features are saddle nose, nasal hypoplasia, frontal bossing, short stature, stippled epiphyses, optic atrophy, cataracts, mental retardation, and flexure contractures. Intracranial bleeding may also lead to secondary central nervous system deformities. Women can take warfarin post partum and breast feed safely. The level of warfarin in breast milk is so low (25 ng/ml)[138] that it cannot be detected in the baby's plasma.[138,139]

In the office setting, I routinely assess warfarin dosing with a machine that provides the INR result in 2 minutes by use of a drop of whole blood obtained from a fingertip puncture. Substantial saving of time has resulted, and patients leave the office with greater peace of mind and with a more accurate understanding of their warfarin dosing regimen. This device has the potential for home use,[140] but current Federal Clinical Laboratory Improvement Amendment of 1988 (CLIA) regulations make this approach impractical in the United States. Testing with fingertip puncture is also available for the PTT[141] and is particularly useful in patients (e.g., during pregnancy) who require long-term adjusted-dose heparin.

Aspirin
(see also p. 1818)

Aspirin exerts its antithrombotic effect by eliminating platelet prostaglandin synthesis, thereby blocking thromboxane A_2 formation and causing a moderate decrease in platelet function and a mild hemostatic defect.[142] Consequently, aspirin has at least a modest role in prevention of venous thrombosis.[143] I prescribe low-dose aspirin, usually 80 mg daily, for some patients who have finished their full course of warfarin. This strategy averts an abrupt transition from full anticoagulation to no anticoagulation.

Secondary Prevention: Inferior Vena Caval Interruption

The major indications for placement of an inferior vena caval (IVC) filter are listed in Table 46-15. Of note is that most "free-floating" DVTs rarely embolize and can be managed with heparin anticoagulation alone.[144] An IVC filter prevents PE, not DVT. Therefore, when a filter is inserted, anticoagulation should also be utilized, whenever possible, to prevent further thrombosis.[145] Recently a removable IVC filter has been tested with an infusion port that can be used to deliver thrombolytic therapy; the efficacy appeared promising, and the complication rate was low.[146]

Most IVC filters are placed below the renal veins. For suprarenal vein placement, the largest experience is with

TABLE 46-15 INDICATIONS FOR INFERIOR VENA CAVAL FILTERS

1. Anticoagulation contraindicated and PE is documented
a. Active bleeding that might cause exsanguination (e.g., gastrointestinal)
b. Feared bleeding that might be catastrophic (e.g., postoperative craniotomy)
c. Ongoing complications of anticoagulation (e.g., heparin-associated thrombocytopenia)
d. Planned intensive cancer chemotherapy (with anticipated pancytopenia or thrombocytopenia)
2. Anticoagulation failure despite documentation of adequate therapy (e.g., recurrent pulmonary embolism)
3. Prophylaxis in high-risk patients
a. Extensive or progressive venous thrombosis
b. In conjunction with catheter-based or surgical pulmonary embolectomy
c. Severe pulmonary hypertension or cor pulmonale

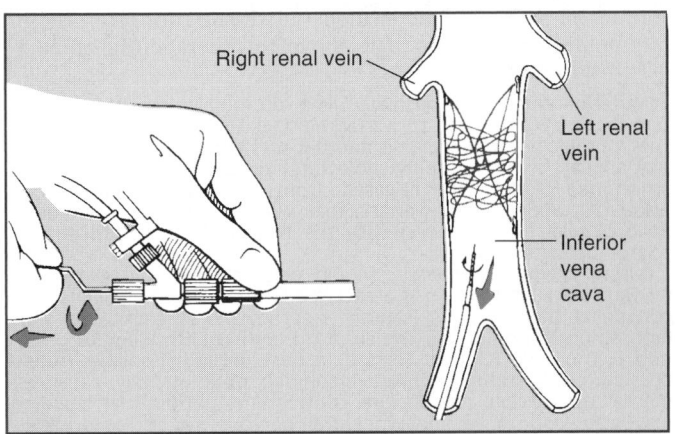

FIGURE 46–11. Inferior vena caval filters. Most filters are placed percutaneously via the right femoral vein. Our current preference is percutaneous placement of a Bird's Nest Filter (Cook Incorporated, Bloomington, IN), which has a low rate of failure, thrombogenicity, and occlusion. The smallness of its sheath may help minimize the risk of bleeding during and after the procedure. To insert the Bird's Nest Filter, the right-angled handle of the wire guide pusher is rotated counterclockwise for 10 to 15 turns to disengage it from the filter. Then the wire guide pusher is removed first, followed by the empty filter catheter. The introducing sheath is left in place so that a post-procedure venacavogram can be obtained. (Reprinted with permission from Goldhaber, S. Z.: Treatment of venous thrombosis. *In* Goldhaber, S. Z. (ed.): Cardiopulmonary Diseases and Cardiac Tumors. Braunwald, E., Series ed. Atlas of Heart Diseases. Philadelphia, Current Medicine, 1995, vol. III, pp. 12.1–12.14.)

the titanium Greenfield filter. Recently, however, unsatisfactory deployment of the titanium Greenfield filter legs has been reported, with wide gaps between the filter legs.[147] This problem has been associated with fatal PE.[48] At Brigham and Women's Hospital, we primarily use the Bird's Nest Filter (Fig. 46–11).

Primary Treatment

Thrombolysis

Thrombolytic therapy (Table 46–16) may be a useful adjunct to heparin in patients who have either systemic arterial hypotension or normal systemic arterial pressure with echocardiographic evidence of right ventricular dysfunction. Rapid improvement of right ventricular function and pulmonary perfusion, accomplished with thrombolytic therapy followed by heparin, may lead to a lower rate of death and recurrent PE.[49] Thrombolysis may (1) prevent the downhill spiral of right heart failure by physical dissolu-

TABLE 46–16 FDA-APPROVED THROMBOLYTIC REGIMENS FOR PULMONARY EMBOLISM

STREPTOKINASE: 250,000 IU as a loading dose over 30 min, followed by 100,000 U/hr for 24 hr—approved in 1977.

UROKINASE: 4400 IU/kg as a loading dose over 10 min, followed by 4400 IU/kg/hr for 12–24 hr—approved in 1978

rt-PA: 100 mg as a continuous peripheral IV infusion administered over 2 hr—approved in 1990

tion of anatomically obstructing pulmonary arterial thrombus (Fig. 46–12); (2) prevent the continued release of serotonin and other neurohumoral factors that might otherwise lead to worsening pulmonary hypertension; and (3) dissolve much of the source of the thrombus in the pelvic or deep leg veins, thereby decreasing the likelihood of recurrent large PE.

The potential benefits of immediately reversing right heart failure and preventing recurrent PE must be balanced by the risk of hemorrhage. Contraindications to thrombolysis, such as intracranial disease, recent surgery, or trauma, preclude its use in some patients who can safely receive heparin alone. There is about a 1 per cent risk of intracranial hemorrhage. Careful patient screening for contraindications to thrombolysis is the best way to minimize bleeding risk (see p. 1218).

The largest thrombolysis-versus-heparin-alone trial was carried out about 30 years ago when urokinase (UK) was compared with heparin alone in the Urokinase Pulmonary Embolism Trial (UPET).[148] Urokinase dissolved pulmonary arterial clot more rapidly than heparin alone and, in certain instances, reversed clinical shock. In UPET, it appeared that thrombolytic therapy followed by heparin might reduce the mortality and recurrent PE rate when compared with heparin alone. However, statistical significance was not demonstrated, possibly because of a relatively small sample size. Furthermore, among PE patients who survived for 1 week, there was no significant difference in lung scan improvement between the two treatments.

At Brigham and Women's Hospital, we have coordinated five trials of PE thrombolysis, including the second largest trial of thrombolysis versus heparin alone: 101 hemodynamically stable patients were randomized to rt-PA 100 mg/2 hours followed by intravenous heparin versus heparin alone.[149] The initial systolic arterial pressure was at least 90 mm Hg in every patient. Qualitative assessment of right ventricular wall motion demonstrated that 39 per cent of the rt-PA patients improved (Figs. 46–13A and 46–13B) and 2.4 per cent worsened, compared with 17 per cent improvement and 17 per cent worsening among those who received heparin alone (p < 0.005). Quantitative assessment showed that rt-PA patients had a significant decrease in right ventricular end-diastolic area during the 24 hours after randomization compared with none among those allocated to heparin alone (p < 0.01). rt-PA patients also had an absolute improvement in pulmonary perfusion of 14.6 per cent at 24 hours (Fig. 46–13C and 13D), compared with 1.5 per cent improvement among heparin-alone patients (p < 0.0001).

Most importantly, no clinical episodes of recurrent PE occurred among rt-PA patients, but there were five (two fatal and three non-

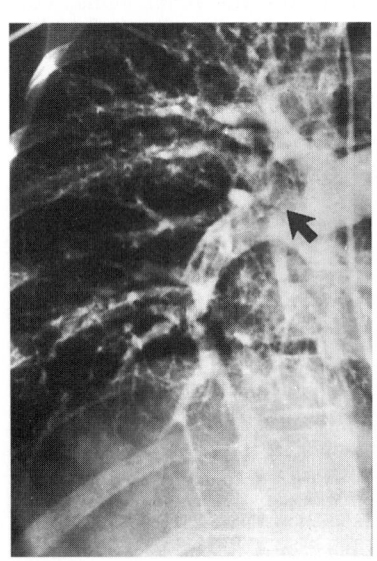
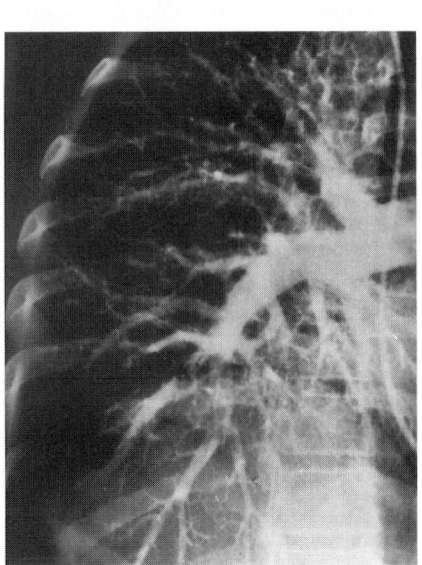

FIGURE 46–12. *Left,* A large embolus in the right pulmonary artery (arrow). *Right,* After a 2-hour infusion of rt-PA through a peripheral vein, there is pronounced resolution, with only a small amount of residual thrombus in segmental branches. (Reprinted with permission from Goldhaber, S. Z., Vaughan, D. E., Markis, J. E., et al.: Acute pulmonary embolism treated with tissue plasminogen activator. Lancet 2:886, 1986.)

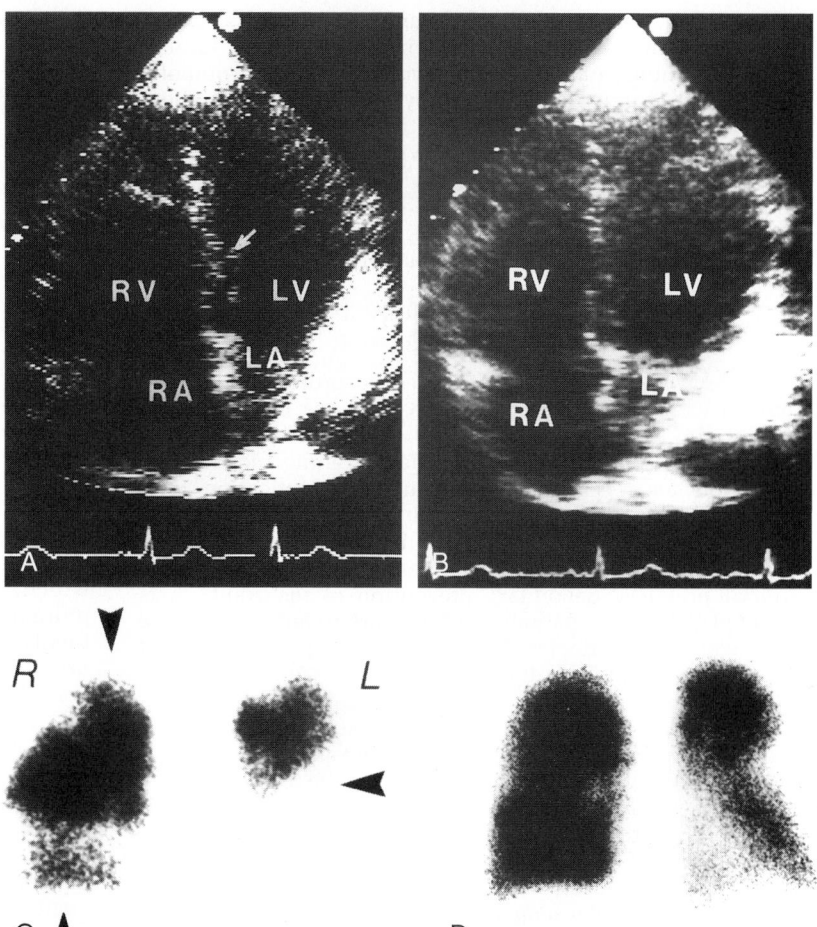

FIGURE 46–13. Echocardiograms (four-chamber view) and perfusion lung scans (anterior view) in a 53-year-old previously healthy man treated with rt-PA for PE. *A*, Right ventricular enlargement before treatment. The right ventricular end-diastolic area was 42.9 cm², and the interventricular septum (arrow) was displaced toward the left ventricle. There was moderately severe right ventricular hypokinesis. *B*, Three hours after initiation of rt-PA therapy, the size of the right ventricle normalized (with a planimetered area of 25.7 cm²), and the interventricular septum resumed its normal configuration. Right ventricular wall motion normalized. *C*, The pretherapy lung scan *(left)* shows absence of perfusion in the right middle lobe (lower arrowhead) and in most of the right upper lobe, particularly the apical segment of the right upper lobe (upper arrowhead). The left lung shows absence of perfusion in the lingula and anterior segment of the left upper lobe (horizontal arrowhead), and irregular perfusion in the apical-posterior segment of the left upper lobe. *D*, The posttherapy scan *(right)* shows marked improvement in perfusion. (Reprinted with permission from Goldhaber, S. Z.: Treatment of acute pulmonary embolism. *In* Goldhaber, S. Z. (ed.): Cardiopulmonary Diseases and Cardiac Tumors. Braunwald, E., Series ed. Atlas of Heart Diseases. Philadelphia, Current Medicine, 1995, vol. III, pp. 3.1–3.25.

fatal) clinically suspected recurrent PEs within 14 days in patients randomized to heparin alone (p < 0.06). All five initially showed right ventricular hypokinesis on echocardiogram. This latter observation suggests that echocardiography may help identify a subgroup of PE patients at high risk of adverse clinical outcomes if treated with heparin alone. Such patients in particular would appear to be excellent candidates for thrombolytic therapy in the absence of contraindications.

There are currently three FDA-approved thrombolytic regimens from which to choose (Table 46–16).[150] We often can make the diagnosis of PE by lung scan without resorting to angiography. This makes PE thrombolysis safer because the risk is avoided of a major groin hematoma at the site of the femoral vein puncture.[108] Unlike myocardial infarction–thrombolysis patients, PE patients have a wide "window" for effective use of thrombolysis. Specifically, patients who receive thrombolysis 6 to 14 days after new symptoms or signs have as effective a response as those patients who receive thrombolytic therapy within 5 days after the onset of PE. Therefore, patients suspected of PE should be considered as potentially eligible for thrombolysis if they have had any new symptoms or signs within the 2 weeks before presentation.

DVT THROMBOLYSIS

Most patients with DVT have contraindications to thrombolysis.[151] Totally occlusive venous thrombosis usually does not lyse if the agent is administered through a peripheral vein.[152] Furthermore, the only FDA-approved regimen for DVT thrombolysis, 250,000 units of streptokinase followed by 100,000 units/hour for 24 to 72 hours, is not satisfactory because of frequent allergic reactions to prolonged streptokinase infusions and because the concentration of streptokinase usually has to be doubled or quadrupled to maintain a systemic lytic state. Newer thrombolytic regimens appear promising, including repeated administration of boluses of UK[153] and pro-UK.[154] For patients with iliofemoral venous thrombosis, catheter-directed thrombolysis[155] or thrombolysis plus venous angioplasty[156] may be successful.

Embolectomy

The results of embolectomy can be optimized if patients are referred for this procedure before the onset of cardiogenic shock. The Greenfield embolectomy device is probably the most frequently used catheter-based method of extracting pulmonary arterial thrombus (Fig. 46–14).[157] It consists of a 10F steerable catheter with a suction cup attached at the tip. Because of the cup's large size, a surgical venotomy is utilized, usually the right internal jugular vein. A steerable handle controls progression of the catheter through the right cardiac chambers and the pulmonary arterial branches.

Alternative catheterization methods include mechanical fragmentation of thrombus with a standard pulmonary artery catheter[158] or clot pulverization with an investigational rotating basket catheter. This 5F Teflon catheter has a distal tip that is divided into four 15-mm bends. The high-speed mechanical rotation of the catheter (about 100,000 revolutions per minute) causes centrifugal force to open the distal bends and form a soft flexible helical spiral that can disintegrate thrombus into microscopic particles within seconds.[159] Another approach is simultaneous mechanical clot fragmentation and pharmacological thrombolysis.[160] Finally, balloon angioplasty has also been utilized to improve pulmonary arterial flow among patients with PE.[161]

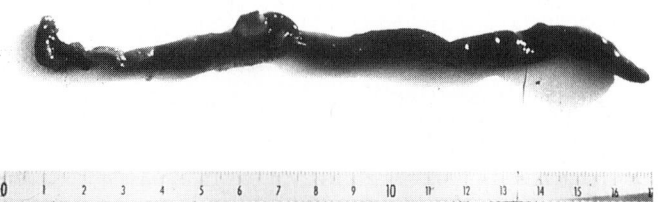

FIGURE 46–14. Philippe Reynaud, M.D., at the Laennec Hospital in Paris, used a Greenfield embolectomy catheter to remove this 17-cm thrombus from a severely compromised PE patient. Rapid hemodynamic improvement ensued. (Reprinted with permission from Meyer, G., Tamiser, D., Reynaud, P., and Sors, H.: Acute pulmonary embolectomy. *In* Goldhaber, S. Z. (ed.): Cardiopulmonary Diseases and Cardiac Tumors. Braunwald, E., Series ed. Atlas of Heart Diseases. Philadelphia, Current Medicine, 1995, vol. III, pp. 7.1–7.12.)

If catheter-based strategies fail, emergency surgical embolectomy with cardiopulmonary bypass can be undertaken.[162] A nonrandomized comparison of rt-PA thrombolysis versus surgical embolectomy indicated that both approaches can be lifesaving in the majority of patients with massive PE.[163] For patients with PE causing systemic arterial hypotension or right heart failure, pulmonary embolectomy in the catheterization laboratory or operating room should be considered when there are contraindications to thrombolysis or when thrombolysis has failed.[164]

Overall Management Approach for Acute Pulmonary Embolism

Therapy for PE should be tailored according to the anatomical extent of the embolus, the presence of underlying cardiopulmonary disease, and the detection of right-heart dysfunction. The echocardiogram is becoming increasingly important for risk stratification and prognostication (Fig. 46–15). Primary therapy frequently is being used for patients with right ventricular dilatation and hypokinesis on echocardiogram, even in the presence of normal systemic arterial pressure. Secondary prevention of recurrent PE is directed toward all patients and appears to suffice in those with small to moderate PE in the absence of right heart abnormalities. After initial treatment but prior to hospital discharge, obtaining a follow-up lung scan is useful to establish a new baseline, in case the patient subsequently complains of symptoms suggesting recurrent PE.

EMOTIONAL SUPPORT. Although PE can be as emotionally devastating as myocardial infarction, the psychological burden for PE patients may be greater. The lay public is not familiar with PE, particularly regarding the possibility of genetic predisposition, long-term disability, and recurrence of disease. By discussing the implications of PE with the patient and family, the emotional burden may be assuaged. We initiated a Pulmonary Embolism Support Group, co-led by a nurse-physician team, and have been gratified by the experience. Although these sessions have an educational component, the major emphasis is discussing the anxieties and living difficulties that occur in the aftermath of PE.

Chronic Pulmonary Embolism

Patients with chronic pulmonary hypertension due to previous PE may be virtually bedridden with breathlessness due to high pulmonary arterial pressures. They should

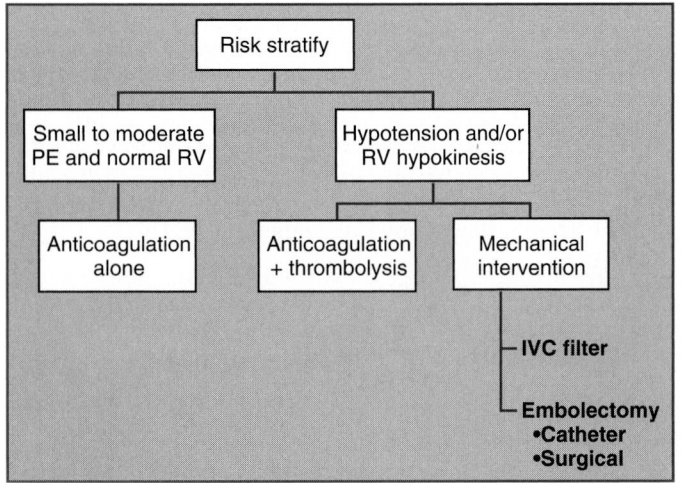

FIGURE 46–15. Proposed strategy for treatment of PE in which risk stratification, usually with echocardiography, is undertaken to assess right ventricular (RV) function. This evaluation helps to determine prognosis as well as appropriateness of aggressive intervention with thrombolysis or mechanical measures to remove thrombus. (From Goldhaber, SZ: Treatment of acute pulmonary embolism. *In* Goldhaber, SZ (ed.): *Cardiopulmonary Diseases and Cardiac Tumors. In* Braunwald, E.: *Atlas of Heart Diseases,* Vol. III. Current Medicine, 1995, pp. 3.1–3.25.)

TABLE 46–17 AVERAGE HEMODYNAMIC VALUES IN 34 PATIENTS BEFORE AND IMMEDIATELY AFTER THROMBOENDARTERECTOMY AND AT FOLLOW-UP

	PREOP	IMMEDIATE POSTOP	FOLLOW-UP*
Mean pulmonary artery pressure (mm Hg)	49	27	24
Mean pulmonary artery systolic pressure (mm Hg)	80	43	38
Cardiac output (liters/min)	3.8	5.9	4.9
Pulmonary vascular resistance (dynes-sec-cm^{-5})	997	230	272

* Follow-up 3 months to 16 years after thromboarterectomy.
Modified from Moser, K. M., Auger, W. R., and Fedullo, P. F.: Chronic major-vessel thromboembolic pulmonary hypertension. Circulation *81*:1735, 1990. Copyright 1990 the American Heart Association.

be considered for pulmonary thromboendarterectomy, which, if successful, can reduce and at times even cure pulmonary hypertension (Table 46–17).[165] The operation involves a median sternotomy, institution of cardiopulmonary bypass, and deep hypothermia with circulatory arrest periods. Incisions are made in both pulmonary arteries into the lower-lobe branches. Pulmonary thromboendarterectomy is always bilateral, with removal of organized thrombus and endarterectomy plane from all involved vessels.

At the University of California at San Diego, 275 patients underwent pulmonary thromboendarterectomy between 1990 and 1993, with a mortality rate of 6 per cent. The two major causes of mortality are: (1) inability to remove sufficient thrombotic material at surgery, resulting in persistent postoperative pulmonary hypertension and right ventricular dysfunction; and (2) severe reperfusion lung injury.[166] Thus, at selected centers, pulmonary thromboendarterectomy can be performed with good results and at an acceptable risk among patients debilitated from chronic pulmonary hypertension due to PE (Fig. 46–16).

Prevention

PE is difficult to diagnose, expensive to treat, and occasionally lethal despite therapy. Therefore, preventive measures are of paramount importance.[167] A variety of mechanical measures and pharmacological agents can be utilized. The most recent innovation has been FDA approval of two different low molecular weight heparins, one (enoxaparin) for use in patients undergoing total hip or knee replacement and another (dalteparin) for patients undergoing high-risk abdominal or pelvic surgery.

In 1986, an NIH Consensus Development Conference strongly recommended prophylaxis against DVT and PE for most surgical patients.[168] Initially, physicians followed the specific guidelines only in a minority of instances. In one survey, two-thirds of high-risk patients did not receive prophylaxis.[169] More recently, however, the concept of prophylaxis has gained much wider acceptance. This is due, at least in part, to the medicolegal liability of physicians who omit prophylaxis among their hospitalized patients with risk factors for venous thrombosis.[170] Furthermore, a policy of prophylaxis is cost-effective. It is estimated that for every 1,000,000 patients undergoing operation who receive prophylaxis against DVT and PE, approximately $60,000,000 can be saved in direct health care costs.[171]

Mechanical Measures

GRADUATED COMPRESSION STOCKINGS. These provide continuous stimulation of blood flow and prevent dilation of the venous system in the legs. Graduated compression stockings (GCS) exert more compression at the ankles (usually 18 mm Hg) than at the popliteal fossa or upper thigh (usually 8 mm Hg). In an overview of 12 trials in moderate-risk surgery, GCS reduced the DVT rate by two-thirds.[172] Thus, GCS should be considered first-line prophylaxis for most hospitalized patients and should suffice for prophylaxis among low-risk patients.

INTERMITTENT PNEUMATIC COMPRESSION. Intermittent pneumatic compression (IPC) devices expel blood from the leg veins and thus prevent venous stasis. The mechanical force of compression appears to enhance systemic fibrinolytic activity.[173] IPC is particularly worthwhile among patients who have an absolute contraindication to anti-mechanical prophylaxis measure that can be implemented is IVC filter placement. Use of an IVC filter might be appropriate for patients with recently diagnosed PE or DVT who must undergo major surgery that places them at high risk for suffering perioperative PE.

1599

Ch 46

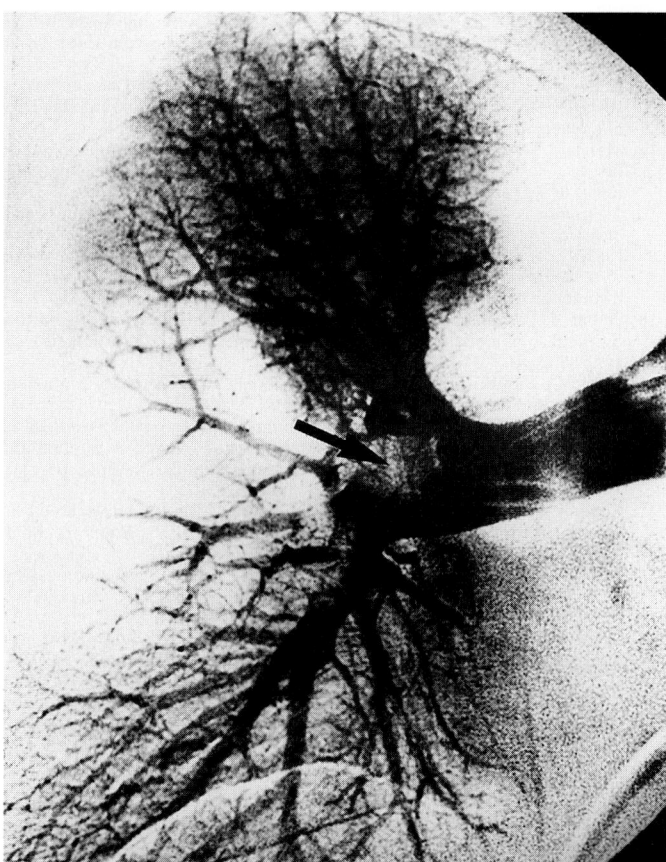

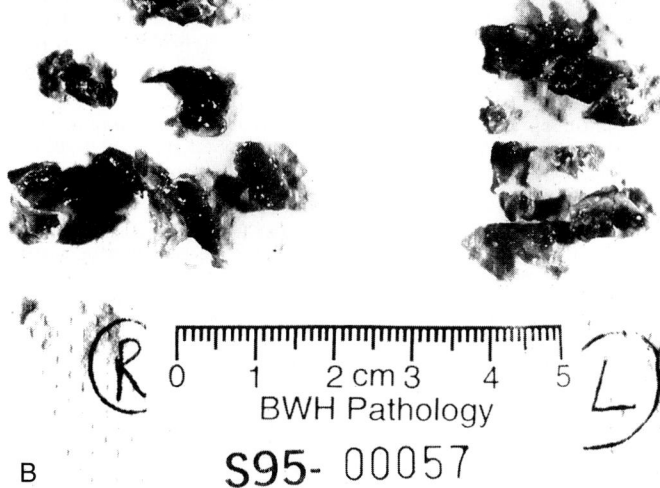

FIGURE 46–16. A 69-year-old woman who underwent pulmonary thromboendarterectomy at Brigham and Women's Hospital had a 1-month history of progressive dyspnea on exertion and recurrent syncope. *A,* Right-heart catheterization demonstrated pulmonary artery systolic pressure of 60 mm Hg. Right pulmonary arteriogram showed multiple filling defects clustered mainly around the hilum (arrow). *B,* At operation, large amounts of thrombus with focal organization were removed from the right and left pulmonary arteries. There were no postoperative complications. The subsequent course has been characterized by marked functional improvement.

coagulation, such as patients undergoing neurosurgery. In addition, for patients receiving postoperative warfarin prophylaxis, IPC devices have special utility because they are immediately useful, whereas warfarin requires 4 to 5 days of administration before it is entirely effective as an anticoagulant. IPC devices are, in general, used properly in intensive care units. However, in one survey, they were either not applied or applied improperly in the majority of patients after transfer from an intensive care to a regular general surgery unit.[174]

INFERIOR VENA CAVAL INTERRUPTION (see p. 1595). The most invasive

Pharmacological Agents

UNFRACTIONATED HEPARIN. The International Multicentre Trial studied pharmacological prophylaxis among 4121 patients undergoing elective major surgery. The intervention group received fixed-dose unfractionated heparin in a dose of 5000 units subcutaneously every 8 hours. The first injection was given 2 hours before the skin incision. Of autopsied subjects, 16 controls died of PE, compared with only 2 patients in the heparin group. Although more patients who received heparin prophylaxis had wound hematomas, the number of deaths due to hemorrhage was not increased among those who received heparin.[175] Collins et al. subsequently pooled data from 78 randomized controlled unfractionated heparin trials with 15,598 patients and confirmed the results of the International Multicentre Trial. Among patients who received heparin prophylaxis, there was a 40 per cent reduction in nonfatal PE and a 64 per cent reduction in fatal PE.[176] In more recent pharmacological prophylaxis trials, at times, prophylaxis has been deferred until the early postoperative period. Any loss of efficacy resulting from deferring prophylaxis until shortly after surgery is unlikely to be marked.[177]

LOW MOLECULAR WEIGHT HEPARIN. Low molecular weight heparin (LMWH) has a more predictable dose-response, more dose-independent mechanisms of clearance, and a longer plasma half-life than unfractionated heparin. LMWHs can achieve higher plasma heparin

TABLE 46–18 STRATEGIES FOR PREVENTION OF PULMONARY EMBOLISM AND DEEP VEIN THROMBOSIS

CONDITION	STRATEGY
Orthopedic surgery*	Coumadin (target INR 2.0–2.5 × 4–6 weeks IPC ± Coumadin Low molecular weight heparin × 5–14 days (e.g., enoxaparin 30 mg SC twice daily)
Nonorthopedic surgery Gynecologic cancer surgery	Coumadin (target INR 2.0–2.5) q IPC Unfractionated heparin 5000 U q8h ± IPC Dalteparin 2500 U SC once daily
Urological surgery	Coumadin (target INR 2.0–2.5) ± IPC
Thoracic surgery	IPC plus unfractionated heparin 5000 U q8h
High-risk general surgery (e.g., prior VTE, current cancer, or obesity)	IPC or graded-compression stockings plus unfractionated heparin 5000 U q8h Dalteparin 2500 U SC once daily
General, gynecological, or urological surgery (without prior VTE) for benign conditions	Graded-compression stockings plus unfractionated heparin 5000 q12h IPC alone
Neurosurgery, eye surgery, or other surgery when pharmacological prophylaxis is contraindicated	Graded-compression stockings ± IPC
Pregnancy Antepartum (with prior VTE)	Graded compression stockings plus daily exercise program plus serial leg examinations Subcutaneous unfractionated heparin
Peripartum (with prior VTE)	IPC ± subcutaneous unfractionated heparin
Postpartum (with prior VTE)	Coumadin (target INR 2.0–3.0) with subcutaneous unfractionated heparin continued until target INR attained
Medical conditions	Graded-compression stockings ± heparin 5000 q 8–12h IPC alone

* Especially total hip or knee replacement.
IPC = intermittent pneumatic compression
VTE = venous thromboembolism
INR = International Normalized Ratio

levels with less bleeding than equivalent doses of unfractionated heparin. A meta-analysis of prophylaxis in patients undergoing orthopedic or general surgery showed that LMWHs are more effective than unfractionated heparin in preventing venous thrombosis, without any difference in the bleeding risk.[178]

ASPIRIN. While aspirin is not a primary perioperative pharmacological prophylaxis, an overview of trials suggests that it does have some efficacy in preventing venous thrombosis.[143]

Prophylaxis Strategies for Specific Conditions

ORTHOPEDIC SURGERY. Universal prophylaxis of total hip replacement patients with adjusted-dose warfarin (Table 46–18) is practical,[179] efficacious,[180] and cost-effective.[181] This approach avoids predischarge leg ultrasonography, which is insensitive in asymptomatic patients after orthopedic surgery.[73] Because warfarin requires 4 to 5 days to be a fully effective anticoagulant, IPC devices can be applied in the early postoperative period. Importantly, fixed minidose warfarin (1 mg/day) does not prevent venous thrombosis after hip replacement.[182] LMWH appears to be more effective than warfarin[183] for prophylaxis after total hip or knee replacement but may be associated with a slight increase in bleeding complications.[184] In the future, direct antithrombin agents may be shown to be even more effective than either warfarin or LMWHs.[185]

NONORTHOPEDIC SURGERY. Strategies for preventing venous thrombosis in nonorthopedic surgery are listed in Table 46–18. The specific regimen that is selected for prophylaxis will depend primarily upon the individual patient's risk of thrombosis and risk of bleeding.

PREGNANCY. For pregnant women who have suffered prior venous thromboembolism, we often employ vascular compression stockings, daily exercise, and serial leg surveillance during the first two trimesters. In the third trimester, we usually switch to subcutaneous unfractionated heparin. Because the risk of venous thrombosis is greatest in the postpartum state, we often treat for 6 weeks post partum with warfarin. Nevertheless, the optimal management of pregnant women at risk for venous thromboembolism has not been well defined.[186]

MEDICAL PATIENTS. In a survey of 152 Medical Intensive Care Unit (MICU) patients, only one-third received any form of prophylaxis.[187] A subsequent study in the same MICU found that one-third of patients had asymptomatic venous thrombosis, even though 60 per cent of this group had received some form of prophylaxis.[22] Therefore, routine surveillance with leg ultrasonography may be appropriate in MICU patients.

REFERENCES

EPIDEMIOLOGY

1. Kniffin, W. D., Baron, J. A., Barett, K., et al.: The epidemiology of diagnosed pulmonary embolism and deep venous thrombosis in the elderly. Arch. Intern. Med. *154*:861, 1994.

HYPERCOAGULABILITY

2. Virchow, R.: Gesammelte Abhandlungen zur Wissenschaftlichen Medizin. Frankfurt, Meidinger Sohn, 1856, p. 219.
3. Bertina, R. M., Koeleman, B. P. C., Koster, T., et al.: Mutation in blood coagulation factor V associated with resistance to activated protein C. Nature *369*:64, 1994.
4. Hajjar, K. A.: Factor V Leiden—an unselfish gene? N. Engl. J. Med. *331*:1585, 1994.
5. Ridker, P. M., Hennekens, C. H., Lindpaintner, K., et al.: Mutation in the gene coding for coagulation factor V and risks of future myocardial infarction, stroke, and venous thrombosis in apparently healthy men. N. Engl. J. Med. *332*:912, 1995.
6. Vandenbroucke, J. P., Koster, T., Briët, E., et al.: Increased risk of venous thrombosis in oral-contraceptive users who are carriers of factor V Leiden mutation. Lancet *344*:1453, 1994.
6a. Hirsch, D. R., Mikkola, K. M., Marks, P. W., et al.: Pulmonary embolism and deep venous thrombosis during pregnancy or oral contraceptive use. Am. Heart J. *(in press)*.
6b. Ridker, P. M., Miletich, J. P., Stempfer, M. J., et al.: Factor V Leiden and risks of recurrent idiopathic venous thromboembolism. Circulation *92*:2800, 1995.
7. Allaart, C. F., Poort, S. R., Rosendaal, F. R., et al.: Increased risk of venous thrombosis in carriers of hereditary protein C deficiency defect. Lancet *341*:134, 1993.
8. Zöller, B., and Dahlbäck, B.: Linkage between inherited resistance to activated protein C and factor V gene mutation in venous thrombosis. Lancet *343*:1536, 1994.
9. Gladson, C. L., Scharrer, I., Hach, V., et al.: The frequency of type I heterozygous protein S and protein C deficiency in 141 unrelated young patients with venous thrombosis. Thromb. Haemost. *59*:18, 1988.
10. Hirsh, J., Piovella, F., and Pini, M.: Congenital antithrombin III deficiency: Incidence and clinical features. Am. J. Med. *87*:34S, 1989.
11. Hach-Wunderle, V., Scharrer, I., and Lottenberg, R.: Congenital deficiency of plasminogen and its relationship to venous thrombosis. Thromb. Haemost. *59*:277, 1988.
12. Hughes, G. R. V.: The antiphospholipid syndrome: Ten years on. Lancet *342*:341, 1993.

13. Koster, T., Blann, A. D., Briët, E., et al.: Role of clotting factor VIII in effect of von Willebrand factor on occurrence of deep-vein thrombosis. Lancet *345*:152, 1995.
14. Heijboer, H., Brandjes, D. P. M., Büller, H. R., et al.: Deficiencies of coagulation-inhibiting and fibrinolytic proteins in outpatients with deep-vein thrombosis. N. Engl. J. Med. *323*:1512, 1990.
15. Malm, J., Laurell, M., Nilsson, I. M., and Dahlbäck, B.: Thromboembolic disease—critical evaluation of laboratory investigation. Thromb. Haemost. *68*:7, 1992.
16. Svensson, P. J., and Dahlbäck, B.: Resistance to activated protein C as a basis for venous thrombosis. N. Engl. J. Med. *330*:517, 1994.
17. Koster, T., Rosendaal, F. R., de Ronde, H., et al.: Venous thrombosis due to poor anticoagulant response to activated protein C: Leiden thrombophilia study. Lancet *342*:1503, 1993.
18. Huber, O., Bounameaux, H., Borst, F., and Rohner, A.: Postoperative pulmonary embolism after hospital discharge: An underestimated risk. Arch. Surg. *127*:310, 1992.
19. Josa, M., Siouffi, S. Y., Silverman, A. B., et al.: Pulmonary embolism after cardiac surgery. J. Am. Coll. Cardiol. *21*:990, 1993.
20. Goldhaber, S. Z., Hirsch, D. R., MacDougall, R. C., et al.: Prevention of venous thrombosis after coronary artery bypass surgery: A randomized trial comparing two mechanical prophylaxis strategies. Am. J. Cardiol. *76*:993, 1995.
21. Geerts, W. H., Code, K. I., Jay, R. M., et al.: A prospective study of venous thromboembolism after major trauma. N. Engl. J. Med. *331*:1601, 1994.
22. Hirsch, D. R., Ingenito, E. P., and Goldhaber, S. Z.: Prevalence of deep venous thrombosis among patients in medical intensive care. JAMA *274*:335, 1995.
23. Goldhaber, S. Z., Savage, D. D., Garrison, R. J., et al.: Risk factors for pulmonary embolism: The Framingham study. Am. J. Med. *74*:1023, 1983.
24. Goldhaber, S. Z., Stampfer, M. J., Manson, J. E., et al.: Prospective study of risk factors for pulmonary embolism in women. J. Am. Coll. Cardiol. *21*(Abs.):318A, 1993.
25. Stampfer, M. J., Goldhaber, S. Z., Manson, J. E., et al.: A prospective study of exogenous hormones and risk of pulmonary embolism in women. Circulation *86*(Abs.):I-767, 1992.
25a. Weiss, N.: Third-generation oral contraceptive: How risky? Lancet *346*:1570, 1995.
26. Devor, M., Barrett-Connor, E., Renvall, M., et al.: Estrogen replacement therapy and the risk of venous thrombosis. Am. J. Med. *92*:275, 1992.
27. Koonin, l. M., Atrash, H. K., Lawson, H. W., and Smith, J. C.: Maternal mortality surveillance, United States, 1979–1986: Centers for Disease Control. CDC Surveillance Summaries, July 1991. M.M.W.R. *40*:1, 1991.
28. Prandoni, P., Lensing, A. W. A., Büller, H. R., et al.: Deep-vein thrombosis and the incidence of subsequent symptomatic cancer. N. Engl. J. Med. *327*:1128, 1992.
29. Nordström, M., Lindblad, B., Anderson, H., et al.: Deep venous thrombosis and occult malignancy: An epidemiological study. BMJ *308*:891, 1994.
30. Monréal, M., Casals, A., Boix, J., et al.: Occult cancer in patients with acute pulmonary embolism: A prospective study. Chest *103*:816, 1993.
31. Levine, M., Hirsch, J., Gent, M., et al.: Double-blind randomised trial of very-low-dose warfarin for prevention of thromboembolism in stage IV breast cancer. Lancet *343*:886, 1994.
31a. den Heijer, M., Blom, H. J., Gerrits, W. B. J., et al.: Is hyperhomocysteinaemia a risk factor for recurrent venous thrombosis? Lancet *345*:882, 1995.
32. Turpie, A. G. G., Gent, M., Côte, R., et al.: A low-molecular-weight heparinoid compared with unfractionated heparin in the prevention of deep vein thrombosis in patients with acute ischemic stroke: A randomized, double-blind study. Ann. Intern. Med. *117*:353, 1992.
33. Green, D., Lee, M. Y., Lim, A. C., et al.: Prevention of thromboembolism after spinal cord injury using low-molecular-weight heparin. Ann. Intern. Med. *113*:571, 1990.
34. Raad, I. I., Luna, M., Khalil, S-A. M., et al.: The relationship between the thrombotic and infectious complications of central venous catheters. JAMA *271*:1014, 1994.
35. Sandler, D. A., and Martin, J. F.: Autopsy proven pulmonary embolism in hospital patients: Are we detecting enough deep vein thrombosis? J. R. Soc. Med. *82*:203, 1989.
36. Moser, K. M., Fedullo, P. F., LitteJohn, J. K., and Crawford, R.: Frequent asymptomatic pulmonary embolism in patients with deep venous thrombosis. JAMA *271*:223, 1994.
37. Huisman, M. V., Büller, H. R., ten Cate, J. W., et al.: Unexpected high prevalence of silent pulmonary embolism in patients with deep venous thrombosis. Chest *95*:498, 1989.
38. Becker, D. M., Philbrick, J. T., and Walker, F. B., IV: Axillary and subclavian venous thrombosis: Prognosis and treatment. Arch. Intern. Med. *151*:1934, 1991.

PATHOPHYSIOLOGY

39. Elliott, C. G.: Pulmonary physiology during pulmonary embolism. Chest *101*:163S, 1992.
39a. Lualdi, J. C., and Goldhaber, S. Z.: Right ventricular dysfunction after acute pulmonary embolism: Pathophysiologic factors, detection, and therapeutic implications. Am. Heart J. *130*:1276, 1995.
40. Jardin, F., Dubourg, O., Guéret, P., et al.: Quantitative two-dimensional

echocardiography in massive pulmonary embolism: Emphasis on ventricular interdependence and leftward septal displacement. J. Am. Coll. Cardiol. *10:*1201, 1987.

41. Belenkie, I., Dani, R., Smith, E. R., and Tyberg, J. V.: The importance of pericardial constraint in experimental pulmonary embolism and volume loading. Am. Heart J. *123:*733, 1992.

42. Watanabe, J., Levine, M. J., Bellotto, F., et al.: Effects of coronary venous pressure on left ventricular diastolic distensibility. Circ. Res. *67:*923, 1990.

43. Stein, P. D., Hull, R. D., Saltzman, H. A., and Pineo, G.: Strategy for diagnosis of patients with suspected acute pulmonary embolism. Chest *103:*1553, 1993.

44. Goldhaber, S. Z., and Morpurgo, M., for the WHO/ISFC Task Force on Pulmonary Embolism: Diagnosis, treatment, and prevention of pulmonary embolism: Report of the WHO/International Society and Federation of Cardiology Task Force. JAMA *268:*1727, 1992.

45. Rich, S., Kaufmann, E., and Levy, P. S.: The effect of high doses of calcium-channel blockers on survival in primary pulmonary hypertension. N. Engl. J. Med. *327:*76, 1992.

46. Cremona, G., and Higenbottam, T.: Role of prostacyclin in the treatment of primary pulmonary hypertension. Am. J. Cardiol. *75:*67A, 1995.

47. Moser, K. M., Fedullo, P. F., Finkbeiner, W. E., and Golden, J.: Do patients with primary pulmonary hypertension develop extensive central thrombi? Circulation *91:*741, 1995.

48. Goldhaber, S. Z.: Treatment of acute pulmonary embolism. *In* Goldhaber, S. Z. (ed.): Cardiopulmonary diseases and cardiac tumors. Braunwald, E., Series ed. Atlas of Heart Diseases. Philadelphia, Current Medicine, Vol. 3, p. 3.1, 1995.

49. Wolfe, M. W., Lee, R. T., Feldstein, M. L., et al.: Prognostic significance of right ventricular hypokinesis and perfusion lung scan defects in pulmonary embolism. Am. Heart J. *127:*1371, 1994.

50. Wagenvoort, C. A.: Pathology of pulmonary thromboembolism. Chest *107:*10S, 1995.

51. Kasper, W., Geibel, A., Tiede, N., and Just, H.: Patent foramen ovale in patients with haemodynamically significant pulmonary embolism. Lancet *340:*561, 1992.

52. Stöllberger, C., Slany, J., Schuster, I., et al.: The prevalence of deep venous thrombosis in patients with suspected paradoxical embolism. Ann. Intern. Med. *119:*461, 1993.

53. Fabian, T. C.: Unraveling the fat embolism syndrome. N. Engl. J. Med. *329:*961, 1993.

54. Goldhaber, S. Z., Dricker, E., Buring, J. E., et al.: Clinical suspicion of autopsy-proven thrombotic and tumor pulmonary embolism in cancer patients. Am. Heart J. *114:*1432, 1987.

55. Phifer, T. J., Bridges, M., and Conrad, S. A.: The residual central venous catheter track—an occult source of lethal air embolism: Case report. J. Trauma *31:*1558, 1991.

56. Rothenberg, F., Schumacher, J. R., and Rosenthal, R. L.: Near-fatal pulmonary air embolus from presumed inadvertent pressure placed on a partially empty plastic intravenous infusion bag. Am. J. Cardiol. *73:*1035, 1994.

DIAGNOSIS

57. Bounameaux, H., de Moerloose, P., Perrier, A., and Reber, G.: Plasma measurement of D-dimer as diagnostic aid in suspected venous thromboembolism: An overview. Thromb. Haemost. *71:*1, 1994.

58. Goldhaber, S. Z., Simons, G. R., Elliott, C. G., et al.: Quantitative plasma D-dimer levels among patients undergoing pulmonary angiography for suspected pulmonary embolism. JAMA *270:*2819, 1993.

59. de Moerloose, P., Minazio, P., Reber, G., et al.: D-Dimer determination to exclude pulmonary embolism: A two-step approach using latex assay as a screening tool. Thromb. Haemost. *72:*89, 1994.

60. Stein, P. D., Terrin, M. L., Hales, C. A., et al.: Clinical, laboratory, roentgenographic, and electrocardiographic findings in patients with acute pulmonary embolism and no pre-existing cardiac or pulmonary disease. Chest *100:*598, 1991.

61. Stein, P. D., Goldhaber, S. Z., and Henry, J. W.: Alveolar-arterial oxygen gradient in the assessment of acute pulmonary embolism. Chest *107:*139, 1995.

62. Sreeram, N., Cheriex, E. C., Smeets, J. L. R. M., et al.: Value of the 12-lead electrocardiogram at hospital admission in the diagnosis of pulmonary embolism. Am. J. Cardiol. *73:*298, 1994.

63. Ginsberg, J., Wells, P. S., Hirsh, J., et al.: Reevaluation of the sensitivity of impedance plethysmography for the detection of proximal deep vein thrombosis. Arch. Intern. Med. *154:*1930, 1994.

64. Westermark, N.: On the roentgen diagnosis of lung embolism. Acta Radiol. *19:*357, 1938.

65. Hampton, A. O., and Castleman, B.: Correlation of postmortem chest teleroentgenograms with autopsy findings with special reference to pulmonary embolism and infarction. AJR *43:*305, 1940.

66. Stein, P. D., Athanasoulis, C., Greenspan, R. H., and Henry, J. W.: Relation of plain chest radiographic findings to pulmonary arterial pressure and arterial blood oxygen levels in patients with acute pulmonary embolism. Am. J. Cardiol. *69:*394, 1992.

67. Skibo, L., Goldhaber, S. Z.: Diagnosis of acute pulmonary embolism. *In* Braunwald, E., and Goldhaber, S. Z. (eds.): Atlas of Heart Diseases. Vol. III, Cardiopulmonary Diseases and Cardiac Tumors. Philadelphia, Current Medicine, 1995, p. 2.1.

68. Polak, J. F.: Diagnosis of venous thrombosis. *In* Goldhaber, S. Z. (ed.): Cardiopulmonary diseases and cardiac tumors. Braunwald, E., Series ed. Atlas of Heart Diseases. Philadelphia, Current Medicine, Vol. 3, pp. 11.1–11.17, 1995.

69. Heijboer, H., Büller, H. R., Lensing, A. W. A., et al.: A comparison of real-time compression ultrasonography with impedance plethysmography for the diagnosis of deep-vein thrombosis in symptomatic outpatients. N. Engl. J. Med. *329:*1365, 1993.

69a. Pearson, S. D., Polak, J. L., Cartwright, S., et al.: A critical pathway to evaluate suspected deep vein thrombosis. Arch. Intern. Med. *155:*1773, 1995.

70. Lensing, A. W. A., Prandoni, P., Brandjes, D., et al.: Detection of deep-vein thrombosis by real-time B-mode ultrasonography. N. Engl. J. Med. *320:*342, 1989.

71. Simons, G. R., Skibo, L. K., Polak, J. F., et al.: Utility of leg ultrasonography in suspected symptomatic isolated calf deep venous thrombosis. Am. J. Med. *99:*43, 1995.

72. Prandoni, P., Cogo, A., Bernardi, E., et al.: A simple ultrasound approach for detection of recurrent proximal-vein thrombosis. Circulation *88:*1730, 1993.

73. Wells, P. S., Lensing, A. W. A., Davidson, B. L., et al.: Accuracy of ultrasound for the diagnosis of deep venous thrombosis in asymptomatic patients after orthopedic surgery: A meta-analysis. Ann. Intern. Med. *122:*47, 1995.

74. Jongbloets, L. M. M., Lensing, A. W. A., Koopman, M. M. W., et al.: Limitations of compression ultrasound for the detection of symptomless postoperative deep vein thrombosis. Lancet *343:*1142, 1994.

75. Rabinov, K., and Paulin, S.: Roentgen diagnosis of venous thrombosis in the leg. Arch. Surg. *104:*134, 1972.

76. Couson, F., Bounameaux, C., Didier, D., et al.: Influence of variability of interpretation of contrast venography for screening of postoperative deep venous thrombosis on the results of a thromboprophylactic study. Thromb. Haemost. *70:*573, 1993.

77. Stein, P. D., Terrin, M. L., Gottschalk, A., et al.: Value of ventilation/perfusion scans versus perfusion scans alone in acute pulmonary embolism. Am. J. Cardiol. *69:*1239, 1992.

78. Hull, R. D., and Raskob, G. E.: Low-probability lung scan findings: A need for change. Ann. Intern. Med. *114:*142, 1991.

79. Bone, R. C.: The low-probability lung scan: A potentially lethal reading. Arch. Intern. Med. *153:*2621, 1993.

80. The PIOPED Investigators: Value of the ventilation/perfusion scan in acute pulmonary embolism: Results of the Prospective Investigation of Pulmonary Embolism Diagnosis (PIOPED). JAMA *263:*2753, 1990.

81. Gottschalk, A., Sostman, H. D., Coleman, R. E., et al.: Ventilation-perfusion scintigraphy in the PIOPED study. Part II. Evaluation of the scintigraphic criteria and interpretations. J. Nucl. Med. *34:*1119, 1993.

82. Cheriex, E. C., Sreeram, N., Eussen, Y. F. J. M., et al.: Cross sectional Doppler echocardiography as the initial technique for the diagnosis of acute pulmonary embolism. Br. Heart J. *72:*52, 1994.

83. Kasper, W., Geibel, A., Tiede, N., et al.: Distinguishing between acute and subacute massive pulmonary embolism by conventional and Doppler echocardiography. Br. Heart J. *70:*352, 1993.

84. Patel, J. J., Chandrasekaran, K., Maniet, A. R., et al.: Impact of the incidental diagnosis of clinically unsuspected central pulmonary artery thromboembolism in treatment of critically ill patients. Chest *105:*986, 1994.

85. McConnell, M. V., Rayan, M. E., Solomon, S. D., et al.: Echocardiographic diagnosis of acute pulmonary embolism: A distinct pattern of abnormal right ventricular wall motion. J. Am. Coll. Cardiol. (Abs.):352a, 1995.

86. Sasahara, A. A., Stein, M., Simon, M., and Littman, D.: Pulmonary angiography in the diagnosis of thromboembolic disease. N. Engl. J. Med. *270:*1075, 1964.

87. Stein, P. D., Athanasoulis, C., Alavi, A., et al.: Complications and validity of pulmonary angiography in acute pulmonary embolism. Circulation *85:*462, 1992.

88. Nicod, P., Peterson, K., Levine, M., et al.: Pulmonary angiography in severe chronic pulmonary hypertension. Ann. Intern. Med. *107:*565, 1987.

89. Hirshfeld, J. W., Jr.: Low-osmolality contrast agents—who needs them? N. Engl. J. Med. *326:*482, 1992.

90. Lasser, E. C., Berry, C. C., Talner, L. B., et al.: Pretreatment with corticosteroids to alleviate reactions to intravenous contrast material. N. Engl. J. Med. *317:*845, 1987.

91. Meyerovitz, M.: How to maximize the safety of coronary and pulmonary angiography in patients receiving thrombolytic therapy. Chest *97:*132S, 1990.

92. Wolfe, M. W., Skibo, L. K., and Goldhaber, S. Z.: Pulmonary embolic disease: Diagnosis, pathophysiologic aspects, and treatment with thrombolytic therapy. Curr. Probl. Cardiol. *18:*585, 1993.

93. Auger, W. R., Fedullo, P. F., Moser, K. M., et al.: Chronic major-vessel thromboembolic pulmonary artery obstruction: Appearance at angiography. Radiology *182:*393, 1992.

94. Walsh, R. N., Greenspan, R. H., Simon, M., et al.: An angiographic severity index for pulmonary embolism. Circulation *47:*2, 1973.

95. Miller, G. A. H., Sutton, G. C., Kerr, I. I. H., et al.: Comparison of streptokinase and heparin in treatment of isolated acute massive pulmonary embolism. B. M. J. *2:*681, 1971.

96. Tapson, V. F., Davidson, C. J., Kisslo, K. B., and Stack, R. S.: Rapid visualization of massive pulmonary emboli utilizing intravascular ultrasound. Chest *105:*888, 1994.

97. Ricou, F., Nicod, P. H., Moser, K. M., and Peterson, K. L.: Catheter-

based intravascular ultrasound imaging of chronic thromboembolic pulmonary disease. Am. J. Cardiol. *67*:749, 1991.

98. Uchida, Y., Oshima, T., Hirose, T., et al.: Angioscopic detection of residual pulmonary thrombin in the differential diagnosis of pulmonary embolism. Am. Heart J. *130*:854, 1995.

99. Remy-Jardin, M., Remy, J., Wattinne, L., and Giraud, F.: Central pulmonary thromboembolism: Diagnosis with spiral volumetric CT with the single-breath-hold technique—comparison with pulmonary angiography. Radiology *185*:381, 1992.

100. Blum, A. G., Delfau, F., Grignon, B., et al.: Spiral-computed tomography versus pulmonary angiography in the diagnosis of acute massive pulmonary embolism. Am. J. Cardiol. *74*:96, 1994.

101. Wielopolski, P. A.: Pulmonary arteriography. M.R.I. Clin. North Am. *1*:295, 1993.

102. Spritzer, C. E., Norconk, J. J., Jr., Sostman, H. D., and Coleman, R. E.: Detection of deep venous thrombosis by magnetic resonance imaging. Chest *104*:54, 1993.

103. Ouderk, M., van Beek, E. J. R., van Putten, W. L. J., and Büller, H. R.: Cost-effectiveness analysis of various strategies in the diagnostic management of pulmonary embolism. Arch. Intern. Med. *153*:947, 1993.

104. Perrier, A., Bounameaux, H., Morabia, A., et al.: Contribution of D-dimer plasma measurement and lower-limb venous ultrasound to the diagnosis of pulmonary embolism: A decision analysis model. Am. Heart J. *127*:624, 1994.

105. Perrier, A., Bounameaux, H., Morabia, A., et al.: Diagnosis of pulmonary embolism by a decision analysis based strategy including clinical probability, D-dimer and ultrasonography: A management study. Personal communication, 1995.

MANAGEMENT

106. Cruickshank, M. K., Levine, M. N., Hirsh, J., et al.: A standard heparin nomogram for the management of heparin therapy. Arch. Intern. Med. *151*:333, 1991.

107. Raschke, R. A., Reilly, B. M., Guidry, J. R., et al.: The weight-based heparin dosing nomogram compared with a "standard care" nomogram: A randomized controlled trial. Ann. Intern. Med. *119*:874, 1993.

108. Stein, P. D., Hull, R. D., and Raskob, G.: Risks for major bleeding from thrombolytic therapy in patients with acute pulmonary embolism: Consideration of noninvasive management. Ann. Intern. Med. *121*:313, 1994.

109. Meyer, G., Tamiser, D., Reynaud, P., and Sors, H.: Acute pulmonary embolectomy. *In* Braunwald, E., and Goldhaber, S. Z. (eds.): Atlas of Heart Diseases. Vol. II, Cardiopulmonary Diseases and Cardiac Tumors. Philadelphia, Current Medicine, 1995, p. 6.1.

110. Estagnasié, P., Le Bourdellès, G., Mier, L., et al.: Use of inhaled nitric oxide to reverse flow through a patent foramen ovale during pulmonary embolism. Ann. Intern. Med. *120*:757, 1994.

111. Kondo, N. I., Maddi, R., Ewenstein, B. M., and Goldhaber, S. Z.: Anticoagulation and hemostasis in cardiac surgical patients. J. Cardiovasc. Surg. *9*:443, 1994.

112. Barritt, D. W., and Jordan, S. C.: Anticoagulant drugs in the treatment of pulmonary embolism: A controlled trial. Lancet *1*:1309, 1960.

113. Weitz, J. I., Hudoba, M., Massel, D., et al.: Clot-bound thrombin is protected from inhibition by heparin–antithrombin III but is susceptible to inactivation by antithrombin III–independent inhibitors. J. Clin. Invest. *86*:385, 1990.

114. Young, E., Prins, M., Levine, M. N., and Hirsh, J.: Heparin binding to plasma proteins, an important mechanism for heparin resistance. Thromb. Haemost. *67*:639, 1992.

115. Brill-Edwards, P., Ginsberg, J. S., Johnston, M., and Hirsh, J.: Establishing a therapeutic range for heparin therapy. Ann. Intern. Med. *119*:104, 1993.

116. Levine, M. N., Hirsh, J., Gent, M., et al.: A randomized trial comparing activated thromboplastin time with heparin assay in patients with acute venous thromboembolism requiring large daily doses of heparin. Arch. Intern. Med. *154*:49, 1994.

117. Hirsh, D. R., Lee, T. H., Morrison, R. B., et al.: Shortened hospitalization by means of adjusted-dose subcutaneous heparin for deep venous thrombosis. Am. Heart J. *131*:276, 1996.

118. Brabeck, M. C.: Ambulatory management of thromboembolic disease during pregnancy with continuous infusion of heparin. J. A. M. A. *257*:1790, 1987.

119. Landefeld, C. S., Cook, E. F., Flatley, M., et al.: Identification and preliminary validation of predictors of major bleeding in hospitalized patients starting anticoagulant therapy. Am. J. Med. *82*:703, 1987.

120. Ginsberg, J. S., Kowalchuk, G., Hirsh, J., et al.: Heparin effect on bone density. Thromb. Haemost. *64*:286, 1990.

121. Dahlman, T., Lindvall, N., and Hellgren, M.: Osteopenia in pregnancy during long-term heparin treatment: A radiological study post partum. Br. J. Obstet. Gynaecol. *97*:221, 1990.

122. Dukes, G. E., Sanders, S. W., Russo, J., et al.: Transaminase elevations in patients receiving bovine or porcine heparin. Ann. Intern. Med. *100*:646, 1984.

123. Goldhaber, S. Z., Meyerovitz, M. F., Green, D., et al.: Randomized controlled trial of tissue plasminogen activator in proximal deep venous thrombosis. Am. J. Med. *88*:235, 1990.

124. Oster, J. R., Singer, I., and Fishman, L. M.: Heparin-induced aldosterone suppression and hyperkalemia. Am. J. Med. *98*:575, 1995.

125. Bergqvist, D.: Dextran. *In* Goldhaber, S. Z. (ed.): Prevention of Venous Thromboembolism. New York, Marcel Dekker, 1993, p. 167.

126. Brandjes, D. P. M., Heijboer, H., Büller, H. R., et al.: Acenocoumarol and heparin compared with acenocoumarol alone in the initial treatment of proximal-vein thrombosis. N. Engl. J. Med. *327*:1485, 1992.

127. Pearson, S. D., Lee, T. H., McCabe-Hassan, S., et al.: A critical pathway to treat proximal lower extremity deep vein thrombosis. Am. J. Med. *100*:283, 1996.

127a. Schulman, S., Rhedin, A-S., Lindmarker, P., et al.: A comparison of 6 weeks with 6 months of oral anticoagulant therapy after a first episode of venous thromboembolism. N. Engl. J. Med. *332*:1661, 1995.

128. Shearer, M. J.: Vitamin K. Lancet *345*:229, 1995.

129. Prandoni, P., Lensing, A. W. A., Cogo, A., et al.: The clinical course of deep-vein thrombosis in symptomatic patients. Personal communication, 1995.

130. Lagerstedt, C. I., Olsson, C.-G., Fagher, B. O., et al.: Need for long-term anticoagulant treatment in symptomatic calf-vein thrombosis. Lancet *2*:515, 1985.

130a. Khamashta, M. A., Cuadrado, M. J., Mujic, F., et al.: The management of thrombosis in the antiphospholipid antibody syndrome. N. Engl. J. Med. *332*:993, 1995.

130b. Franzeck, U. K., Schalch, I., and Jager, K. A.: Prospective 12-year follow-up study of clinical and hemodynamic sequelae after deep vein thrombosis in low-risk patients. (Zurich Study). Circulation *93*:74, 1996.

131. Andrews, T. C., Peterson, D. W., Doeppenschmidt, D., et al.: Complications of warfarin therapy monitored by the international normalized ratio versus the prothrombin time ratio. Clin. Cardiol. *18*:80, 1995.

132. Landefeld, C. S., Rosenblatt, M. W., and Goldman, L.: Bleeding in outpatients treated with warfarin: Relation to the prothrombin time and important remediable lesions. Am. J. Med. *87*:153, 1989.

133. Hylek, E. M., and Singer, D. E.: Risk factors for intracranial hemorrhage in outpatients taking warfarin. Ann. Intern. Med. *120*:897, 1994.

134. Broekmans, A. W., Bertina, R. M., Leoliger, E. A., et al.: Protein C and the development of skin necrosis during anticoagulant therapy. Thromb. Haemost. *49*:251, 1983.

135. Hyman, B. T., Landas, S. K., Ashman, R. F., et al.: Warfarin-related purple toes syndrome and cholesterol microembolization. Am. J. Med. *82*:1233, 1987.

136. Hall, J. G., Pauli, R. M., and Wilson, K. M.: Maternal and fetal sequelae of anticoagulation during pregnancy. Am. J. Med. *68*:122, 1980.

137. Iturbe-Alessio, I., Fonseca, M. D. C., Mutchinick, O., et al.: Risks of anticoagulant therapy in pregnant women with artificial heart valves. N. Engl. J. Med. *315*:1390, 1986.

138. Orme, M. L. E., Lewis, P. J., de Swiet, M., et al.: May mothers given warfarin breast-feed their infants? B. M. J. *1*:1564, 1977.

139. McKenna, R., Cole, E. R., and Vasan, U.: Is warfarin sodium contraindicated in the lactating mother? J. Pediatr. *103*:325, 1983.

140. Anderson, D. R., Harrison, L., and Hirsh, J.: Evaluation of a portable prothrombin time monitor for home use by patients who require long-term oral anticoagulant therapy. Arch. Intern. Med. *153*:1441, 1993.

141. Vacek, J. L., Hibiya, K., Rosamond, T. L., et al.: Validation of a bedside method of activated partial thromboplastin time measurement with clinical range guidelines. Am. J. Cardiol. *68*:557, 1991.

142. Roth, G. J., and Calverley, D. C.: Aspirin, platelets, and thrombosis: Theory and practice. Blood *83*:885, 1994.

143. Antiplatelet Trialists' Collaboration: Collaborative overview of randomised trials of antiplatelet therapy—III: Reduction in venous thrombosis and pulmonary embolism by antiplatelet prophylaxis among surgical and medical patients. B. M. J. *308*:235, 1994.

144. Baldridge, E. D., Martin, M. A., and Welling, R. E.: Clinical significance of free-floating venous thrombi. J. Vasc. Surg. *11*:62, 1990.

145. Becker, D. M., Philbrick, J. T., and Selby, J. B.: Inferior vena cava filters: Indications, safety, effectiveness. Arch. Intern. Med. *152*:1985, 1992.

146. Dievart, F., Lefebvre, J. M., Fourrier, J. L., et al.: New infusion removable inferior vena caval filter catheter (Filcard RF 02) for protected thrombolytic treatment in deep venous thrombosis (DVT) and pulmonary embolism (PE): Results of an international multicentric study. J. Am. Coll. Cardiol. *95A*(Abs.):95a, 1994.

147. Sweeney, T. J., and Van Aman, M. E.: Deployment problems with the titanium Greenfield filter. JVIR *4*:691, 1993.

148. Urokinase Pulmonary Embolism Trial: A National Cooperative Study. Circulation *47* and *48* (Suppl. II):1, 1973.

149. Goldhaber, S. Z., Haire, W. D., Feldstein, M. L., et al.: Alteplase versus heparin in acute pulmonary embolism: Randomised trial assessing right-ventricular function and pulmonary perfusion. Lancet *341*:507, 1993.

150. Goldhaber, S. Z.: Contemporary pulmonary embolism thrombolysis. Chest *107*:45S, 1995.

151. Markel, A., Manzo, R. A., and Strandness, D. E., Jr.: The potential role of thrombolytic therapy in venous thrombosis. Arch. Intern. Med. *152*:1265, 1992.

152. Meyerovitz, M. F., Polak, J. F., and Goldhaber, S. Z.: Short-term response to thrombolytic therapy in deep venous thrombosis: Predictive value of venographic appearance. Radiology *184*:345, 1992.

153. Goldhaber, S. Z., Polak, J. F., Feldstein, M. L., et al.: Efficacy and safety of repeated boluses of urokinase in the treatment of deep venous thrombosis. Am. J. Cardiol. *73*:75, 1994.

154. Moia, M., Mannucci, P. M., Pini, M., et al.: A pilot study of pro-urokinase in treatment of deep vein thrombosis. Thromb. Haemost. *72*:430, 1994.

155. Comerota, A. J., Aldridge, S. C., Cohen, G., et al.: A strategy of aggressive regional therapy for acute iliofemoral venous thrombosis with con-

temporary venous thrombectomy or catheter-directed thrombolysis. J. Vasc. Surg. 20:244, 1994.

156. Marache, P., Asseman, P., Jabinet, J. L., et al.: Percutaneous transluminal venous angioplasty in occlusive iliac vein thrombosis resistant to thrombolysis. Am. Heart J. 125:362, 1993.

157. Greenfield, L. J., Proctor, M. C., Williams, D. M., and Wakefield, T. W.: Long-term experience with transvenous catheter pulmonary embolectomy. J. Vasc. Surg. 18:450, 1993.

158. Brady, A. J. B., Crake, T., and Oakley, C. M.: Percutaneous catheter fragmentation and distal dispersion of proximal pulmonary embolus. Lancet 338:1186, 1991.

159. Dievart, F., Fourrier, J. L., Lefebvre, J. M., et al.: Treatment of severe pulmonary embolism by means of a high speed rotational catheter (Angiocor Thrombolizer): First experience of mechanical thrombolysis in human beings. J. Am. Coll. Cardiol. 474(Abs.):474a, 1994.

160. Essop, M. R., Middlemost, S., Skoularigis, J., and Sareli, P.: Simultaneous mechanical clot fragmentation and pharmacologic thrombolysis in acute massive pulmonary embolism. Am. J. Cardiol. 69:427, 1992.

161. Voorburg, J. A. I., Cats, V. M., Buis, B., and Bruschke, A. V. G.: Balloon angioplasty in the treatment of pulmonary hypertension caused by pulmonary embolism. Chest 94:1249, 1988.

162. Meyer, G., Tamisier, D., Sors, H., et al.: Pulmonary embolectomy: A 20-year experience at one center. Ann. Thorac. Surg. 51:232, 1991.

163. Gulba, D. C., Schmid, C., and Borst, H.-G.: Medical compared with surgical treatment for massive pulmonary embolism. Lancet 343:565, 1994.

164. Meyer, G., Tamisier, D., Reynaud, P., and Sors, H.: Acute pulmonary embolectomy. In Goldhaber, S. Z. (ed.): Cardiopulmonary diseases and cardiac tumors. Braunwald, E., Series ed. Atlas of Heart Diseases. Philadelphia, Current Medicine, Vol. 3, 1995, p. 6.1.

165. Moser, K. M., Auger, W. R., and Fedullo, P. F.: Chronic major-vessel thromboembolic pulmonary hypertension. Circulation 81:1735, 1990.

166. Fedullo, P. F., Auger, W. R., Channick, R. N., et al.: A multidisciplinary approach to chronic thromboembolic pulmonary hypertension. In Braunwald, E., and Goldhaber, S. Z. (eds.): Atlas of Heart Diseases. Vol. III, Cardiopulmonary Diseases and Cardiac Tumors. Philadelphia, Current Medicine, 1995, p. 7.1.

PREVENTION

167. Goldhaber, S. Z. (ed.): Prevention of Venous Thromboembolism. New York, Marcel Dekker, Inc., 1993, 607 pp.

168. NIH Consensus Development Conference: Prevention of venous thrombosis and pulmonary embolism. J. A. M. A. 256:744, 1986.

169. Anderson, F. A., Jr., Wheeler, H. B., Goldberg, R. J., et al.: Physician practices in the prevention of venous thromboembolism. Ann. Intern. Med. 115:591, 1991.

170. Goldhaber, S. Z.: Malpractice claims relation to PE and DVT. Forum. Cambridge, MA, Risk Management Foundation of the Harvard Medical Institutions, Inc., 1994.

171. Landefeld, C. S., and Hanus, P.: Economic burden of venous thromboembolism. In Goldhaber, S. Z. (ed.): Prevention of Venous Thromboembolism. New York, Marcel Dekker, Inc., 1993, p. 69.

172. Wells, P. S., Lensing, A. W. A., and Hirsh, J.: Graduated compression stockings in the prevention of postoperative venous thromboembolism. Arch. Intern. Med. 154:67, 1994.

173. Knight, M. T. N., and Dawson, R.: Effect of intermittent compression of the arms on deep venous thrombosis in the legs. Lancet 2:1265, 1976.

174. Comerota, A. J., Katz, M. L., and White, J. V.: Why does prophylaxis with external pneumatic compression for deep vein thrombosis fail? Am. J. Surg. 164:265, 1992.

175. Prevention of fatal postoperative pulmonary embolism by low doses of heparin: An international multicentre trial. Lancet 2:45, 1975.

176. Collins, R., Scrimgeour, A., Yusuf, S., and Peto, R.: Reduction in fatal pulmonary embolism and venous thrombosis by perioperative administration of subcutaneous heparin: Overview of results of randomized trials in general, orthopedic, and urologic surgery. N. Engl. J. Med. 318:1162, 1988.

177. Kearon, C., and Hirsh, J.: Starting prophylaxis for venous thromboembolism postoperatively. Arch. Intern. Med. 155:366, 1995.

178. Leizorovicz, A., Haugh, M. C., Chapuis, F. R., et al.: Low molecular weight heparin in prevention of perioperative thrombosis. BMJ 305:913, 1992.

179. Reis, S. E., Hirsch, D. R., Wilson, M. G., et al.: Program for the prevention of venous thromboembolism in high-risk orthopaedic patients. J. Arthroplasty 6:S11, 1991.

180. Paiement, G. D., Wessinger, S. J., Hughes, R., and Harris, W. H.: Routine use of adjusted low-dose warfarin to prevent venous thromboembolism after total hip replacement. J. Bone Joint Surg. 75A:893, 1993.

181. Paiement, G. D., Wessinger, S. J., and Harris, W. H.: Cost-effectiveness of prophylaxis in total hip replacement. Am. J. Surg. 161:519, 1991.

182. Fordyce, M. J. F., Baker, A. S., and Staddon, G. E.: Efficacy of fixed minidose warfarin prophylaxis in total hip replacement. BMJ 303:219, 1991.

183. RD Heparin Arthroplasty Group: RD heparin compared with warfarin for prevention of venous thromboembolic disease following total hip or knee arthroplasty. J. Bone Joint Surg. 76A:1174, 1994.

184. Hull, R., Raskob, G., Pineo, G., et al.: A comparison of subcutaneous low-molecular-weight heparin with warfarin sodium for prophylaxis against deep-vein thrombosis after hip or knee implantation. N. Engl. J. Med. 329:1370, 1993.

185. Ginsberg, J. S., Nurmohamed, M. T., Gent, M., et al.: Use of hirulog in the prevention of venous thrombosis after major hip or knee surgery. Circulation 90:2385, 1994.

186. Barbour, L. A., and Pickard, J.: Controversies in thromboembolic disease during pregnancy: A critical review. Obstet. Gynecol. 86:621, 1995.

187. Keane, M. G., Ingenito, E. P., and Goldhaber, S. Z.: Utilization of venous thromboembolism prophylaxis in the medical intensive care unit. Chest 106:13, 1994.

Chapter 47
Cor Pulmonale*

HERBERT P. WIEDEMANN, RICHARD A. MATTHAY

Acute cor pulmonale is defined as right heart strain or overload secondary to acute pulmonary hypertension, often due to massive pulmonary embolism.[1-3] *Chronic cor pulmonale* is characterized by hypertrophy and dilatation of the right ventricle (RV) secondary to the pulmonary hypertension caused by disease of the pulmonary parenchyma and/or pulmonary vascular system between the origins of the main pulmonary artery and the entry of the pulmonary veins into the left atrium.[1-4] In this chapter, the anatomical and pathophysiological correlates of acute and chronic cor pulmonale are reviewed and the relevant principles of clinical management are discussed. Particular emphasis is given throughout the chapter to COPD. Primary pulmonary hypertension and pulmonary thromboembolism, two important causes of cor pulmonale, are discussed in Chapters 27 and 48, respectively.

for this may include endothelial cell edema, diffuse microembolism or thrombosis, and fibrotic microvascular obliteration.[5] Primary disorders of the pulmonary circulation produce pulmonary hypertension through narrowing or obstruction of vessels.[5]

Because the normal pulmonary circulation is a low-resistance, high-compliance system with substantial reserve, considerable abnormality must occur before significant and sustained pulmonary hypertension develops.[5] This explains why the clinical appearance of cor pulmonale heralds a poor prognosis in chronic lung diseases,[9-12] primary pulmonary hypertension,[13] and neuromuscular disorders.[3]

The physiological significance of the muscular left ventricle (LV) and its role in human disease have long been appreciated. The thin-walled right ventricle (RV), however, has sometimes been considered a redundant, almost unnecessary, chamber (Fig. 47–1). This view originated from ani-

ETIOLOGIES

The most frequent cause of *chronic* cor pulmonale in North America is chronic obstructive pulmonary disease (COPD) resulting from chronic obstructive bronchitis or emphysema, whereas the most important cause of *acute* cor pulmonale is pulmonary thromboembolism.[1-5] In addition to COPD and thromboembolic disease, a number of other disorders may cause cor pulmonale (Table 47–1).[5] Although many disorders may lead to cor pulmonale, the major mechanisms resulting in pulmonary hypertension are relatively few.[5] Alveolar hypoxia secondary to hypoventilation is the primary cause of pulmonary hypertension in neuromuscular diseases, thoracic cage deformities, and disorders of ventilatory control. Alveolar hypoxia is a potent stimulus for acute pulmonary vasoconstriction.[5] In addition, sustained vasoconstriction resulting from chronic hypoxia leads to structural alterations in the pulmonary vasculature that contribute to pulmonary hypertension.[6] Lung diseases, such as emphysema and interstitial fibrotic disorders, cause pulmonary hypertension not only through hypoxia but also by frank anatomical destruction of vessels.[5] Pulmonary hypertension frequently is observed in patients with the adult respiratory distress syndrome (ARDS), even after correction of arterial hypoxemia.[7,8] The mechanisms

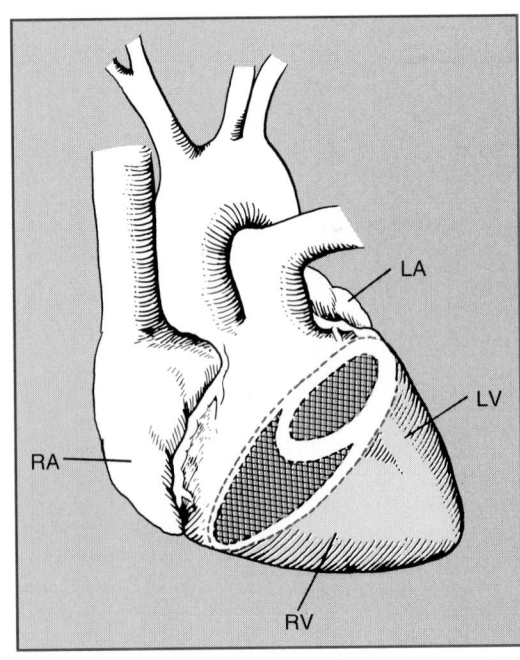

FIGURE 47–1. The anatomical relationship of the right ventricle (RV) to the left ventricle (LV), showing the globular shape of the LV and the half-moon shape of the RV. (Modified from Guyton, A. C.: The pulmonary circulation. *In* Guyton, A. C.: *Human Physiology and Mechanisms of Disease.* 4th ed. Philadelphia, W. B. Saunders Company, 1987, 124.)

---

* Portions of this chapter have been reproduced from the chapter on Cor Pulmonale in the 4th edition of *Heart Disease* with the gracious permission of its authors, McFadden and Braunwald.

TABLE 47-1 ETIOLOGY OF PULMONARY HEART DISEASE

I. DISEASES AFFECTING THE PULMONARY VASCULATURE
  A. Primary diseases of the arterial wall
    (1) Primary pulmonary hypertension
    (2) Granulomatous pulmonary arteritis
    (3) Toxin-induced pulmonary hypertension
       a. Aminorex fumarate
       b. Intravenous drug abuse
    (4) Chronic liver disease
    (5) Peripheral pulmonic stenosis
  B. Thrombotic disorders
    (1) Sickle cell diseases
    (2) Pulmonary microthrombi
  C. Embolic disorders
    (1) Thromboembolism
    (2) Tumor embolism
    (3) Other embolism (amniotic fluid, air)
    (4) Schistosomiasis and other parasitic diseases

II. PRESSURES ON PULMONARY ARTERIES BY MEDIASTINAL TUMORS, ANEURYSMS, GRANULOMATA, OR FIBROSIS

III. DISEASES OF THE NEUROMUSCULAR APPARATUS AND CHEST WALL
  A. Neuromuscular weakness
  B. Kyphoscoliosis
  C. Thoracoplasty
  D. Pleural fibrosis
  E. Sleep apnea syndromes
  F. Idiopathic hypoventilation

IV. DISEASES AFFECTING AIR PASSAGES OF THE LUNG AND ALVEOLI
  A. Chronic obstructive pulmonary diseases
  B. Cystic fibrosis
  C. Congenital developmental defects
  D. Infiltrative or granulomatous diseases
    (1) Idiopathic pulmonary fibrosis
    (2) Sarcoidosis
    (3) Pneumoconiosis
    (4) Scleroderma
    (5) Mixed connective tissue disease
    (6) Systemic lupus erythematosus
    (7) Rheumatoid arthritis
    (8) Polymyositis
    (9) Eosinophilic granuloma
    (10) Malignant infiltration
    (11) Radiation
  E. Upper airways obstruction
  F. Pulmonary resection
  G. High-altitude disease

Adapted from Rubin, L. J.: Introduction. Pulmonary Heart Disease. Boston, Martinus Nijhoff, 1984, p. 1.

mal studies conducted in the 1940's and 1950's, the results of which showed that the contractile function of the free wall of the RV is not required to maintain circulation over the short term, either at rest or under stress. Interest in the structure and function of the RV, however, has revived, primarily because RV dysfunction has been found to be critical in such important cardiopulmonary disorders as pulmonary embolism, COPD, ARDS, and coronary artery disease (RV ischemia or infarction).

ANATOMICAL AND PATHOPHYSIOLOGICAL CORRELATES

RIGHT VENTRICULAR ANATOMY

In humans born at or near sea level, the RV is the dominant chamber for the first 3 months of life. During this time, the RV is larger and heavier and has a greater end-diastolic volume than the LV.[3,14-18] The LV, however, gradually becomes dominant, and in adults, the RV is relatively thin walled and crescent shaped (Fig. 47-1).[3] At high altitude, the degree of RV predominance is greater at birth and after 3 months than that at lower altitude, and the relative RV enlargement may persist through the first decade of life.[17] Among adult natives living above 12,000 feet, 93 per cent showed some degree of RV enlargement in a necropsy series.[19] These morphological findings reflect the hemodynamic characteristics of persons living at high altitude and can be related to the degree of pulmonary artery hypertension.[20]

RIGHT VENTRICULAR HYPERTROPHY. The presence of RV hypertrophy and its severity have traditionally been determined by measuring ventricular weight and wall thickness.[3] However, many investigators believe that measuring the thickness of the ventricular wall is not sufficiently precise. Fulton et al.[21] have proposed widely used weight criteria, according to which the RV is dissected free and weighed, and the LV and the septum are weighed together. Right ventricular weight is then determined absolutely or relative to the weight of the LV plus the septum (S): (LV + S)/RV. By these criteria, a heart is considered normal only if the total ventricular weight is less than 250 gm, the free wall of the RV weighs less than 65 gm in men and 50 gm in women, and the value of (LV + S)/RV is between 2.3 and 3.3. If LV hypertrophy also is present, the ratio may be within normal limits or even raised. Using this method, Mitchell and colleagues[22] found that the upper limits of normal (defined by the mean plus two standard deviations) in men 40 years of age or older at death were 69 gm for the RV and 203 gm for the LV plus the septum. In this study, RV thickness was a relatively poor index of hypertrophy.

Other investigators have determined muscle fiber size morphometrically and found the distribution of myocardial fiber diameters to be uniform, with a distinct bell-shaped distribution for the RV, LV, and septum.[23] In pure RV hypertrophy, the distribution shifts so that the mean diameter of the muscle fibers from the RV exceeds that of the septum or normal LV.[3] An enlarged RV in cor pulmonale is shown in Figure 47-2.

Right Ventricular Function

Because RV hypertrophy is usually associated with long-standing pulmonary hypertension, an analogy often has been made between the LV in systemic hypertension and the RV in pulmonary hypertension.[3] The structure and the pumping action of the two ventricles are essentially the same before birth, and therefore the differences in the adult have been attributed to the flow resistance in the respective circulation.[24] As noted, the normal adult RV is thin walled and crescent shaped (see Fig. 47-1); its pumping action is similar to that of a bellows working in series with a low-pressure circuit in contrast to the concentric contraction of the LV.[25-27] The thin-walled RV is more compliant than the LV[27] and, compared with the LV, is better able to handle an increase in volume than in pressure. This latter finding was derived primarily from animal studies that measured the effects of increasing preload and afterload on RV and LV function.[28-31]

In the left panel of Figure 47-3, stroke volume is plotted as a function of various afterloads produced experimentally by constricting the main pulmonary artery and aorta in the dog.[28,29] Small increases in pulmonary artery pressure are associated with sharp decreases in right ventricular stroke volume. In contrast, the LV, which normally works against high initial pressure, maintains stroke volume despite substantial increases in systemic arterial pressure. The right panel of the figure shows the effects of increasing preload. These ventricular function curves were obtained by volume infusions in the atria of dogs.[31] The respective ventricular stroke work differs markedly as right and left atrial pressures are increased. For a fourfold increase in filling pres-

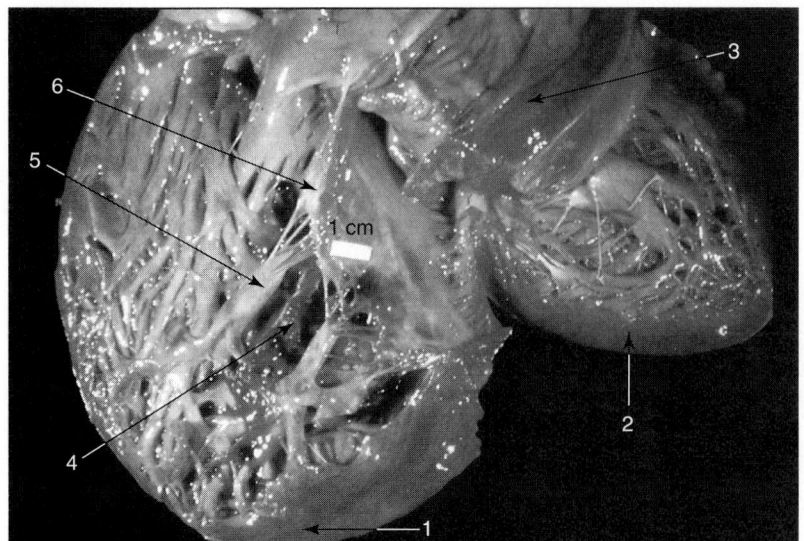

FIGURE 47–2. Heart specimen illustrating right ventricular enlargement and hypertrophy in a patient with cor pulmonale. (Number Key: 1, right ventricular free wall; 2, left ventricular free wall; 3, interventricular septum; 4, right ventricular chamber; 5, right ventricular papillary muscle; and 6, tricuspid valve.) The right ventricular free wall is markedly thickened, approximately 2.5 cm at widest diameter (normal ≤ 5 mm). Also, the right ventricular chamber and papillary muscles are significantly larger than the left ventricular chamber and papillary muscles. (From Matthay, R. A., and Berger, H. J.: Right and left ventricular performance in chronic obstructive pulmonary disease. Med. Clin. North Am. *65*:489, 1981.)

sure (e.g., from 5 to 20 cm H_2O), the increase in left ventricular work was about five times that of the right.

In response to chronic pressure loads, the structure, mass, and functional characteristics of the RV change significantly. The rate of such changes in humans, and the pressure needed to produce them, are unknown. Animal studies show that structure and function can change rapidly after experimental outflow tract obstruction. Spann et al.[32] observed a 71 per cent increase in RV weight in cats 2 days after the pulmonary artery was banded, and, within a month, RV weight had risen by 150 per cent of control. The response may not be as rapid in humans, but it is qualitatively similar.

The lumen of the main pulmonary artery can be reduced acutely by 60 to 80 per cent before aortic pressure declines as a consequence of a fall in cardiac output.[33–35] Because these experiments did not consider the effects of neurohumoral compensation that supports the systemic circulation, the impression has arisen that the acute RV response is abrupt and absolute. However, as suggested in Figure 47–3, RV decompensation is continuous.[28,31] At RV systolic pressures of 60 to 80 mm Hg, RV dilatation and failure occur with systemic hypotension and hypoperfusion.[36] The rate and absolute extent of outflow tract obstruction at which these changes develop can be greatly amplified or attenuated by respectively decreasing or increasing right coronary artery blood flow.[36] The effect of coronary artery blood

flow in acute right heart failure in humans has not been determined.[3]

Pulmonary Vascular Anatomy

WALL STRUCTURE. From the pulmonary artery distally toward the capillaries, four structural regions can be identified: elastic, muscular, partially muscular, and nonmuscular[37] (see Fig. 25–16, p. 798). The main pulmonary artery and the first five generations are elastic, although less so than the aorta and major systemic arteries. These vessels have more than five elastic laminae in their media and in adults are more than 2000 μm in diameter. In the axial pathway, the next three generations are transitional.

Muscular arteries have two to five elastic laminae and a continuous muscle coat. These arteries constitute the majority of vessels in the lung and in adults range from 150 to 2000 μm in diameter. The medial muscle coat is much thinner than the arterioles in the systemic circulation. These vessels give way to partially muscular arteries in which the muscle is arranged in a spiral, so that in cross section it looks like a crescent, with the rest of the wall being like a capillary. Nonmuscular arteries are larger than capillaries, ranging from 30 to 75 μm in diameter in adults. Partially muscular and nonmuscular arteries lie within the alveolar units in adults. The smallest muscular and partially muscular arteries are probably the resistance arteries.[37]

Although the sizes of arteries that accompany conducting airways such as lobar bronchi vary greatly, arteries that follow the respiratory bronchi and alveolar ducts are muscular or partially muscular.[37] The implications for function of these observations are several-fold. Gas exchange occurs in respiratory bronchi and alveolar ducts through the arteries that accompany these structures.[38] In addition, hypoxia

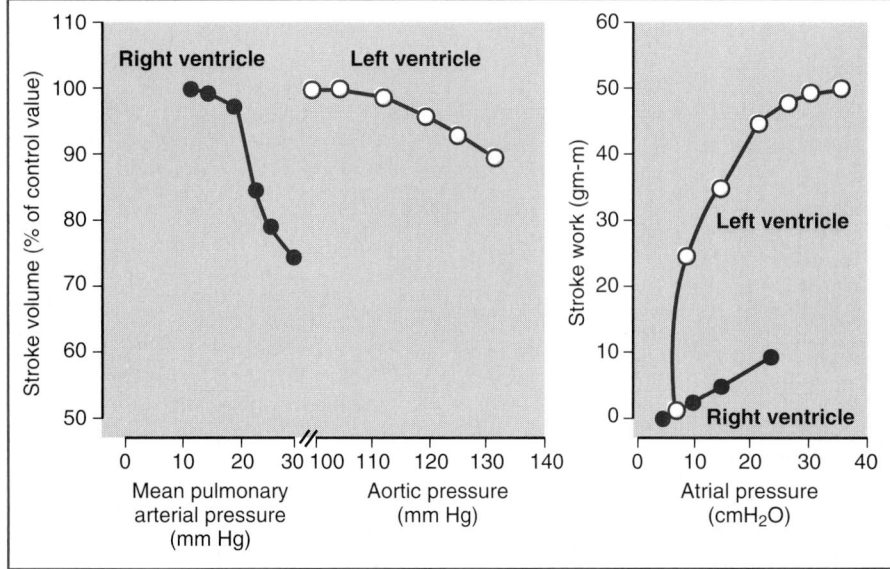

FIGURE 47–3. Effects of increasing preload and afterload on right and left ventricular function. The data in the left panel were obtained by constricting the main pulmonary artery and aorta in dogs. The right panel demonstrates the effect in increasing preloads.

induces constriction of the muscular arteries; therefore, this area of the lung evidently actively controls pulmonary blood flow. Furthermore, because the spiral of muscle in the partially muscular arteries is continuous with the muscle encircling the larger vessels, retrograde propagation of the hypoxic stimulus can occur in the intracellular pathways of the muscle syncytium,[37] thereby producing a wider and more severe response.

INNERVATION. Although the pulmonary circulation has both adrenergic and cholinergic fibers, they are sparse compared with those innervating systemic vessels of similar size, and they tend to be concentrated in the larger vessels at the hilum.[38,39] Evidence suggests that these nerves contain other neurotransmitters such as vasoactive intestinal peptide in parasympathetic fibers; substance P, the neurokinins, and calcitonin gene-related peptide in sensory fibers; and neuropeptide tyrosine in sympathetic fevers.[40] Some studies in children indicate that the predominant neuropeptide transmitter is tyrosine and that, during growth and development, the relative density of nerve fibers increases only in the arteries of the respiratory unit.[40] In this work, pulmonary hypertension in infants was associated with premature innervation of these arteries.

In summary, the structure of the pulmonary circulation conforms to its hemodynamics.[3] The thin-walled, sparsely innervated vessels that contain relatively small amounts of smooth muscle (see Fig. 25–15, p. 797) do not favor the development of marked vasomotor responses, and vasoconstriction alone is not sufficient to overload the RV to the point of producing acute cor pulmonale.[41] Therefore, in acute cor pulmonale, mechanical obstruction of the pulmonary circulation can be inferred, and in chronic cor pulmonale, structural alterations in the pulmonary vascular bed must be present.

PHYSIOLOGY OF THE PULMONARY CIRCULATION

(See also Chap. 25)

Most of the pulmonary vascular bed is contained within the parenchyma of the lung, and therefore the vessels are subject to external distending and compressive forces that are independent of any intrinsic properties of the vessels themselves.[3] In addition, the pulmonary circulation is in series with a pump that can develop only low pressures, yet it must accommodate the entire cardiac output under all states of physical activity.[3] Consequently, it must adjust to wide variations in blood flow without much change in pressure so as not to overload the RV.

PRESSURE–VOLUME RELATIONS. The pulmonary circulation was once thought to be highly elastic in order to accommodate increases in cardiac output, thus preventing an increase in pulmonary artery pressure in high-flow states.[42,43] Measurement of the compliance of the pulmo-

nary vascular bed, however, has shown that it is significantly stiffer than its systemic counterpart[44,45] and that the large pulmonary vessels can accept only small increases in blood volume.[46–49] The increased blood flow and blood volume are primarily accommodated by the recruitment of previously unperfused vessels.[44,50] Morphological evidence suggests that, with an increase in pulmonary blood flow, both recruitment and distention occur and the transmural pressures to which the vessel is subjected determine which one predominates.[51] Recruitment appears to predominate in superior portions of the lung where the vessels are collapsed or where alveolar pressure is greater than pulmonary venous pressure, whereas distention is more important in dependent portions of the lung where pulmonary venous pressure is greater than alveolar pressure.

PRESSURE–FLOW RELATIONS. The pressure–flow relationship of the pulmonary circulation in normal humans is hyperbolic, with large changes in pulmonary blood flow being associated with small elevations in pulmonary artery pressure (Fig. 47–4A). The net result is that as flow increases, pulmonary vascular resistance decreases (Fig. 47–4B).[41] Consequently, whether distention or recruitment occurs, a low-pressure circuit is maintained during increased blood flow.

A U-shaped curve describes pulmonary vascular resistance as a function of lung volume (Fig. 47–4C).[48] At the extremes of lung volume at full inflation and deflation, vascular resistance is high, and it reaches its nadir at about the resting end-expiratory position (i.e., at functional residual capacity).

These findings can be explained by morphological changes in the alveolar and intrapulmonic but extra-alveolar vessels in response to the transmural pressures to which they are exposed.[3] The dimensions of the pulmonary vessels reflect the forces exerted on them by the pulmonary parenchyma. At low lung volumes, the extra-alveolar vessels tend to collapse because radial traction no longer supports them. Simultaneously, the alveolar vessels are pulled open by the increased recoil forces generated by the tendency of the alveoli to become smaller. As the lung is inflated above functional residual capacity, the larger vessels tend to be pulled open, but the resistance of the small vessels progressively increases as they are squeezed and lengthened by enlarging alveoli. In addition, changes in alveolar pressure also can dynamically affect the lumina of small vessels. When alveolar pressure is positive, as it is during expiration or with the Valsalva maneuver, vessels are compressed, whereas when pressure is negative, as it is during inspiration or with the Mueller maneuver, small

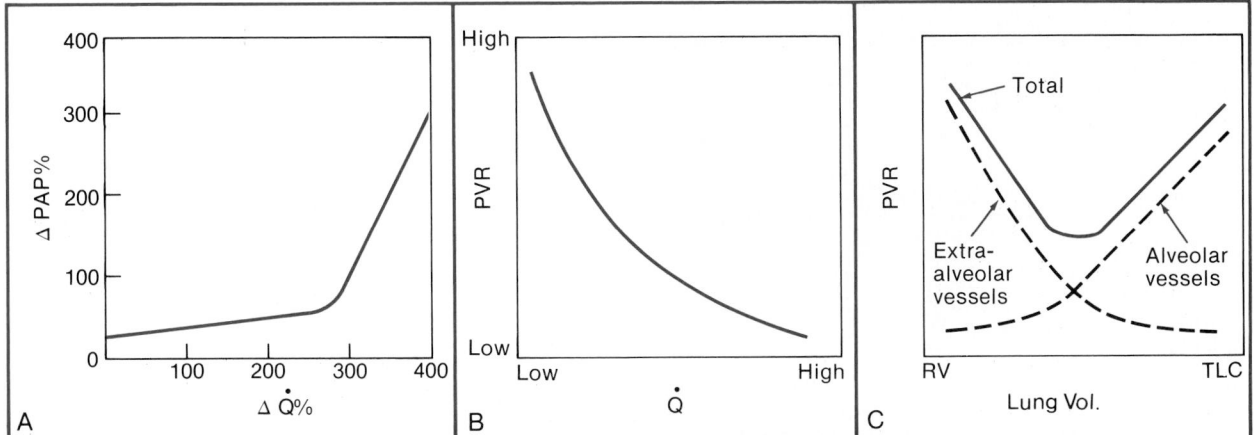

FIGURE 47–4. Some aspects of pulmonary vascular physiology. *A,* Pressure-flow relation. *B,* Resistance-flow relation. *C,* Pulmonary vascular resistance (PVR) as a function of lung volume for the total system and for extraalveolar and alveolar vessels. △PAP = percentage of change in mean pulmonary artery pressure from control; △Q = percentage of change in cardiac output; 100 = normal cardiac output; RV = residual volume; TLC = total lung capacity.

vessels are distended. It is therefore apparent that alveolar pressure can play a crucial role in determining the distribution of pulmonary blood flow and, accordingly, gas exchange.[3]

Effects of Alveolar Gas Tension on the Pulmonary Circulation

HYPOXIA. The most potent stimulus for pulmonary vasoconstriction is alveolar hypoxia[38,52-54] (see Fig. 25–2, p. 782). Although acute vasoconstriction appears when the alveolar pO_2 is 60 mm Hg or lower, this response is found only in about two-thirds of normal subjects.[55] The subjects who respond to hypoxemia with pulmonary vasoconstriction may be prone to chronic cor pulmonale if they develop a disease that interferes with effective alveolar ventilation.[56] The pulmonary constrictor response to hypoxia appears to be locally mediated because it can be elicited in denervated lungs and isolated perfused lungs.

ACIDOSIS. Acidosis significantly increases pulmonary vascular resistance as well as acting synergistically with hypoxia.[57] In contrast, an increase in arterial pCO_2 seems to exert no direct effect but rather to operate by way of the induced increase in hydrogen-ion concentration. Hypoxia and acidemia frequently coexist, and their interaction, which is clinically important, follows a predictable pattern (Fig. 47–5). At minor degrees of oxygen unsaturation, pulmonary artery pressure is relatively insensitive to hydrogen-ion concentration but extremely sensitive to high levels of unsaturation. However, when the pH is high, the pressor effect of hypoxia is blunted.

Most studies indicate that the pulmonary vascular pressor response occurs in partially muscular arteries less than 200 μm in diameter.[37,52,58,59] The mechanism by which hypoxia causes pulmonary artery smooth muscle to constrict is unclear, but the likely alternatives are an indirect effect by which hypoxia causes endothelial cells to release eicosanoids or other cells in the pulmonary parenchyma to release vasoactive substances (e.g., histamine from mast cells) or a direct effect of hypoxia on pulmonary artery smooth muscle. Other influences may enhance hypoxic pulmonary vasoconstriction; for example, extrapulmonic reflexes or the adrenergic neurotransmitter norepinephrine may augment the pressor response.

CONSEQUENCES OF PULMONARY VASOCONSTRICTION. The

mechanism that controls the resting tone of the pulmonary circulation is unknown. The smooth muscle and connective tissue elements in the walls of the vessels certainly contribute. The roles of other potential controlling factors have yet to be explored; these include the neuropeptides of the nonadrenergic noncholinergic nervous system or locally formed or circulating mediators such as the eicosanoids (prostacyclin, thromboxane, leukotrienes), catecholamines (epinephrine, norepinephrine), autocoids (histamine, bradykinin), and endothelial-derived relaxing and contrasting factors.[60]

Pulmonary vasoconstriction produces an acute elevation in pulmonary vascular pressure, and continuing constriction with pulmonary hypertension for even a few days is associated with structural changes in the vessels.[37] The lumen is narrowed by an increase in the thickness of the medial coat, endothelial swelling, muscular hypertrophy, and the appearance of muscle at more peripheral levels than normal. With continued insult, the cross-sectional area of the vascular bed is reduced in association with an increase in RV weight. These structural and functional changes occur with all forms of pulmonary hypertension, but the time sequences of development and ultrastructural patterns vary with different disease processes.

ASSESSMENT OF PATIENTS WITH COR PULMONALE

In patients with cor pulmonale, pulmonary hemodynamics and RV function are assessed by measuring pressure and flow, which requires the use of cardiac catheterization.[1] Because of the variable and irregular shape of the RV, even in normal subjects, measuring RV function and the chamber volumes is difficult.[1,61] Until recently, RV volume could be assessed only by contrast angiography,[1,62] an invasive technique that was not used widely in patients with cor pulmonale.[1] However, experience is now available with various noninvasive techniques including radionuclide ventriculography, echocardiography, and magnetic resonance imaging (MRI).

CLINICAL ASSESSMENT. The physical examination is insensitive for diagnosing cor pulmonale, especially in patients with COPD in whom hyperinflation of the chest usually obscures the typical signs of pulmonary hypertension or RV dysfunction.[1,3,63,64] For example, the intrathoracic pressure varies widely in such patients, making the jugular venous pressure difficult to assess. In addition, peripheral edema may be absent in patients with pulmonary artery hypertension or may be due to other causes such as hypoalbuminemia.[1] Other physical findings characteristic of cor pulmonale but not always present or frequently modified by hyperinflation include a systolic parasternal heave (indicating RV hypertrophy) and extra heart sounds or the murmur of tricuspid regurgitation (both suggesting RV dysfunction). Accentuation of the pulmonary component of the second heart sound, which usually suggests pulmonary hypertension, is also an insensitive finding in patients with COPD.[1]

ELECTROCARDIOGRAPHY (see also Chap. 4). Electrocardiography is highly specific but rather insensitive for detecting right ventricular hypertrophy.[1,65]

Classic electrocardiographic criteria for cor pulmonale (Table 47–2), which were derived from patients with congenital heart disease,[3,66,67] have not been sensitive in patients with COPD,[3,68,69] apparently because moderate RV hypertrophy is a late event in cor pulmonale, occurring only after prolonged dilatation of the RV.[70]

Assessing the effects of dynamic events on the electrocardiogram in 200 patients with COPD, Kilcoyn et al.[69] found that at least one of the following electrocardiographic changes occurred when arterial oxygen saturation fell

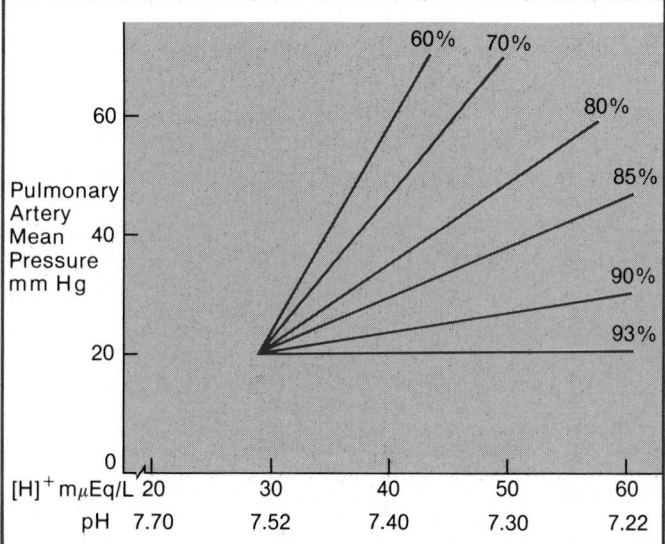

FIGURE 47–5. Relation of arterial oxygen saturation and hydrogen ion concentration to pulmonary artery pressure. (Reproduced from Enson, Y., et al.: The influence of hydrogen ion concentration and hypoxia on the pulmonary circulation. J. Clin. Invest. *43*:1146, 1964, by copyright permission of the American Society for Clinical Investigation.)

TABLE 47–2 ELECTROCARDIOGRAPHIC CHANGES IN COR PULMONALE

ECG CRITERIA FOR COR PULMONALE WITHOUT OBSTRUCTIVE DISEASE OF THE AIRWAYS*

1. Right-axis deviation with a mean QRS axis to the right of +110°
2. R/S amplitude ratio in V_1 > 1
3. R/S amplitude ratio in V_6 < 1
4. Clockwise rotation of the electrical axis
5. P-pulmonale pattern
6. S_1Q_3 or $S_1S_2S_3$ pattern
7. Normal voltage QRS

ECG CHANGES IN CHRONIC COR PULMONALE WITH OBSTRUCTIVE DISEASE OF THE AIRWAYS†

1. Isoelectric P waves in lead I or right-axis deviation of the P vector
2. P-pulmonale pattern (an increase in P-wave amplitude in II, III, AV_f)
3. Tendency for right-axis deviation of the QRS
4. R/S amplitude ratio in V_6 < 1
5. Low-voltage QRS
6. S_1Q_3 or $S_1S_2S_3$ pattern
7. Incomplete (and rarely complete) right bundle branch block
8. R/S amplitude ratio in V_1 > 1
9. Marked clockwise rotation of the electrical axis
10. Occasional large Q wave or QS in the inferior or mid-precordial leads, suggesting healed myocardial infarction

* Any one of the first three criteria suffices to raise suspicion of right ventricular hypertrophy. The diagnosis becomes more certain if two or more of these findings are present (2 and 7). The last four criteria commonly occur in cor pulmonale secondary to primary alveolar hypoventilation, interstitial diseases of the lung, or pulmonary vascular disease.

† The first seven criteria are suggestive but nonspecific; the last three are more characteristic of cor pulmonale in obstructive disease of the airways.

Reproduced with permission from Holford, F. D.: The electrocardiogram in lung disease. In Fishman, A. P. (ed.): Pulmonary Diseases and Disorders. New York, McGraw-Hill Book Co., 1980, p. 140.

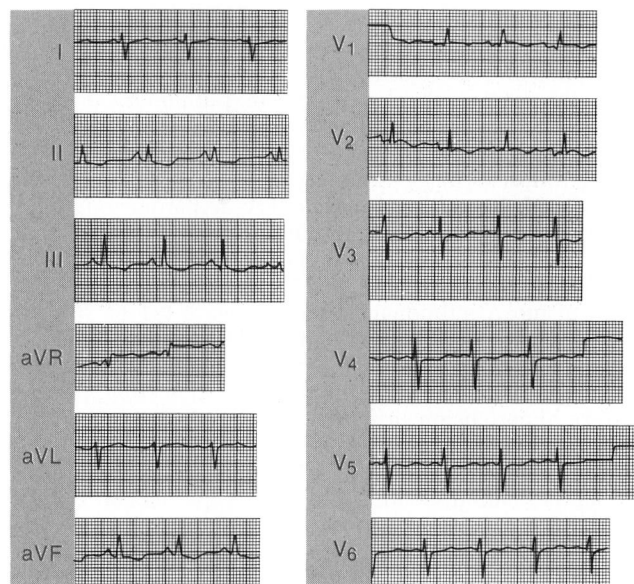

FIGURE 47–6. Electrocardiogram in a patient with emphysema and diffuse lung disease; there is right axis deviation, "P pulmonale," a qR pattern in V_1 and an rS pattern in V_6 (From McGowan, F. X., and Wagner, G. S.: The electrocardiogram in chronic lung disease. In Rubin, L. J. [ed.]: Pulmonary Heart Disease. Boston, Martinus Nijhoff, 1984, p. 117.)

below 85 per cent and mean pulmonary artery pressure rose to 25 mm Hg or greater: a rightward shift of the mean QRS axis of 30 degrees or more from its previous position; inverted, biphasic or flattened T waves in the precordial leads; depressed ST segments in leads II, III, and aV_f; and incomplete or complete right bundle branch block. These changes disappeared when arterial oxygen saturation increased. Transient T-wave changes in the right precordial leads and axis shifts to the right, which developed with only modest elevations in pulmonary artery pressure, persisted if pressure elevations were more severe and recurred frequently. If pulmonary function failed to improve, R-wave voltage increased in the right precordial leads and true right-axis deviation (a frontal plane axis greater than +90 degrees) developed. Increased R-wave voltage in the right precordial leads rarely returned to normal after improvement in arterial blood gases (Fig. 47–6).

In other studies of patients with chronic cor pulmonale, RV hypertrophy has been suggested by clockwise rotation, right-axis deviation, a qR pattern in aV_r, and electrocardiographic evidence of right atrial enlargement (P pulmonale) in that order.[3] In patients with COPD, the mean QRS axis is sometimes directed posteriorly, superiorly, and to the right with an apparent left-axis deviation in the standard limb leads.[3] This pattern, along with low voltage, has been associated most often with emphysema.[3] Electrocardiography is less accurate for detecting RV hypertrophy in patients with COPD than in patients with primary pulmonary artery hypertension. This is because COPD causes flattening of the diaphragm and hyperinflation of the lungs.[3,70]

CHEST RADIOGRAPHY (see also Chap. 7). The heart size may be normal on the plain chest radiograph in patients with cor pulmonale,[71] but in advanced disease, the heart may rotate counterclockwise and the aortic knob become less prominent.[71] Moreover, because the RV extends anteriorly and to the left, it infringes on the retrosternal space.[71,72] In the posteroanterior (PA) projection, the enlarged RV consti-

tutes most of the left-heart border, forcing the LV to the rear and giving the left heart a lobular appearance.[71,72]

On the plain chest radiograph, pulmonary hypertension is indicated by dilatation of the main pulmonary artery and its branches with concurrent underperfusion of the peripheral branches (Fig. 47–7).[71,73] In one study of patients with COPD, measurement of the widest diameter of the right and left descending pulmonary arteries on the plain chest ra-

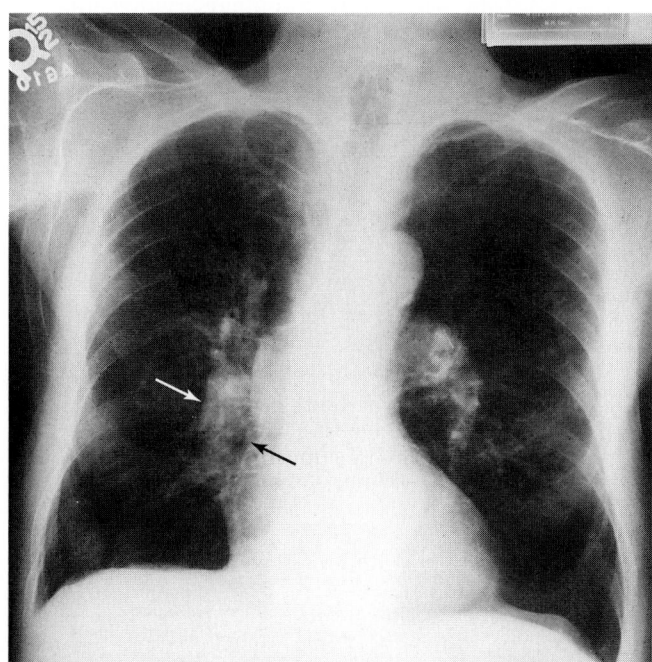

FIGURE 47–7. Upright chest radiograph in the posteroanterior (PA) projection in a man with severe COPD and pulmonary artery hypertension (mean pulmonary artery pressure = 47 mm Hg). The arrows indicate the widest dimensions of the enlarged right-descending pulmonary artery. Note also the enlarged main pulmonary artery in the central left hemithorax. An enlarged right-descending pulmonary artery (>15 mm) and an enlarged main pulmonary artery on the PA projection are indicative of pulmonary artery hypertension in patients with COPD.

diograph provided evidence of pulmonary artery hypertension (mean pulmonary artery pressure >20 mm Hg).[73] The diameter of both arteries was increased in 43 of 46 patients (93 per cent) with elevated mean pulmonary artery pressure. The right descending pulmonary artery was considered enlarged if it was more than 16 mm (Fig. 47–7),[74] and the left descending pulmonary artery if it was more than 18 mm.[73] Of 46 cases of pulmonary hypertension, 45 were correctly diagnosed by combining increased diameter measurements of the right and left descending pulmonary arteries. By these criteria, all 25 patients with a mild elevation of mean pulmonary artery pressure (21 to 30 mm Hg) were identified. Thus, measuring the diameter of right and left descending pulmonary arteries on the plain chest radiograph is a sensitive method for detecting pulmonary artery hypertension in patients with COPD.

In another study of patients with COPD,[75] a ≥20-mm widest diameter of the right-descending pulmonary artery separated patients with pulmonary hypertension from those without it. The hilar cardiothoracic ratio was an even more sensitive index: 95 per cent for pulmonary artery hypertension in patients with COPD.[68] Although these measures can indicate the presence of pulmonary artery hypertension, they cannot predict the precise pressures or the severity.

RADIONUCLIDE VENTRICULOGRAPHY (see also p. 299). Radionuclide ventriculography can measure the volume of the RV despite its variable and irregular shape.[76,77] An intravenous injection of technetium-99m-labeled erythrocytes or human serum albumin is detected in the central circuit by a gamma camera to produce a time-activity curve, either during the first pass of the radiolabeled tracer through the central circulation or by gating counts from several points throughout the cardiac cycle once the radiotracer has equilibrated in the blood pool.[1,76,78] Variation in the shape of the RV does not affect the measurement because radioactive counts are proportional to volume.[1]

Radionuclide ventriculography overcomes the problem of the variation in ventricular shape so problematic with contrast angiography and appears to be ideal for assessing RV function.[1,79–82] In patients with pulmonary hypertension, especially those with COPD, increases in pulmonary vascular resistance and pulmonary artery pressure are fairly accurately reflected in RV performance on radionuclide ventriculography.[76,82,83] In patients with COPD, the pulmonary artery pressure correlates inversely with the RV ejection fraction (RVEF).[82,84] Moreover, in one study, RVEF was abnormal in all patients with cor pulmonale due to COPD.[76] RVEF of less than or equal to 40 per cent on first-pass study indicates pulmonary arterial hypertension in patients with COPD.[76,83] Therefore, abnormal RVEF can help to identify patients with COPD who have pulmonary hypertension. RV performance on radionuclide angiocardiography can also be used to assess the efficacy of therapy (oxygen, vasodilators) in augmenting RVEF.[82]

THALLIUM IMAGING. Thallium-201 myocardial scintigraphy has been used to diagnose RV hypertrophy in patients with pulmonary artery hypertension.[1,85–90] Regional myocardial blood flow as well as myocardial mass determine the distribution of the radiotracer.[80] The large LV can be clearly visualized at rest, but the RV is usually not evident.[80] In one study, thallium imaging was 73 per cent sensitive for diagnosing RV pressure overload in 46 patients with COPD.[89] The clearest image usually occurs in patients with the highest RV systolic pressure and highest pulmonary vascular resistance, suggesting a correlation between RV hypertrophy and the degree of visualization.[80,90] However, thallium-201 scintigraphy is qualitative rather than quantitative, and because it offers no advantage over echocardiography, it has not been widely used clinically.[1]

ECHOCARDIOGRAPHY (see also Chap. 3). Doppler echocardiography has improved the assessment of pulmonary artery pressure.[1,91–99] The mean right atrial pressure and the peak systolic pressure gradient between the RV and the right atrium must be measured and the results added to estimate peak systolic pulmonary artery pressure.[1] The height of the jugular venous pulse is used to estimate the right atrial pressure.[1]

The tricuspid valve regurgitant jet can be assessed by Doppler echocardiography to measure the right ventricular-atrial gradient.[1,100,101] Tricuspid regurgitation occurs in normal subjects[1,102] and in patients with COPD.[1,101,103] By augmenting the signal with an intravenous infusion of saline, the quality of the signal to detect tricuspid regurgitation using continuous-wave Doppler echocardiography can be improved.[1,104,105] With the modified Bernoulli equation ($P = 4V^2$), using the peak velocity of the tricuspid regurgitant jet (V), peak pressure difference between the RV and atrium (P) can be calculated.[1,106] The systolic pulmonary artery pressure can be calculated, as stated above, by adding this pressure gradient to the mean right atrial pressure.[1,106]

Although continuous-wave Doppler echocardiography fails to produce an adequate assessment in 35 per cent of patients, even with intravenous saline contrast,[1,106] pulsed-wave Doppler echocardiography is even more sensitive for detecting tricuspid insufficiency.[1,92] In one study,[92] systolic pulmonary artery pressure could be measured in 91 per cent of patients with COPD. Moreover, the pulsed-wave Doppler echocardiographic technique can be used to assess changes in pulmonary artery pressure during exercise.[1,92] Cardiac catheterization results have been compared with those using echocardiographic measurements of pulmonary artery pressure and showed good correlations,[1,91–99] including in patients with COPD.[1,91]

The difficulty in differentiating the RV wall from its surrounding structures limits the use of echocardiography for detecting RV hypertrophy.[1] Echocardiographically measured RV wall thickness has correlated poorly with RV weight determined at autopsy.[1,107,108]

Unlike radionuclide ventriculography, echocardiography cannot readily show changes in RV function in patients with COPD and pulmonary arterial hypertension.[1] For a qualitative assessment, however, the position and the curvature of the interventricular septum give an indication of RV afterload.[1] Although the interventricular septum moves to the left during systolic ejection and to the right during diastolic filling in the normal heart, in patients with RV volume overload, this pattern reverses during cardiac ejection and filling.[1,109] Moreover, RV pressure overload displaces the septum further toward the LV.[1]

MAGNETIC RESONANCE IMAGING (see also Ch. 10). MRI produces the best images of the RV and is therefore considered by some authorities to be the gold standard for measuring ventricular dimensions.[1,110,111] Although MRI does not impose a radiation burden on the patient and is not invasive, it is expensive and is available only in specialized centers.[1] The RV free-wall volume determined by MRI correlates with both the pulmonary artery pressure (r = 0.72, P < 0.01) and the pulmonary vascular resistance (r = 0.65, P < 0.01) in patients with COPD.[111] In addition to being the best method for measuring RV dimensions,[111,112] MRI can be used to define RV hypertrophy in patients with COPD and to study the effects of therapy.[1,113,114]

ACUTE COR PULMONALE

Pathophysiology

RIGHT VENTRICULAR RESPONSE TO ACUTE PULMONARY HYPERTENSION. The foundation for the study of RV response to acute pulmonary hypertension was primarily established in animal experiments.[115] Figure 47–8 shows changes in mean systemic arterial pressure, mean pulmonary artery pressure, mean RV pressure, and mean right atrial pressure as the pulmonary artery of the dog is progressively constricted during a 4- to 5-minute period.[116] In response, the RV increased pressure and sustained cardiac output until the circulation suddenly and rapidly collapsed. When systemic pressure dropped below a critical value of about 60 mm Hg, progressive circulatory collapse ensued, even if the degree of pulmonary artery constriction remained constant. This finding, which has been reproduced by other investigators, suggests that acute increases in pressure load on the RV progress until a point at which a physiological "vicious circle" produces circulatory collapse.[115]

THE ROLE OF MYOCARDIAL ISCHEMIA. RV ischemia is likely a limiting factor in response to acute pressure

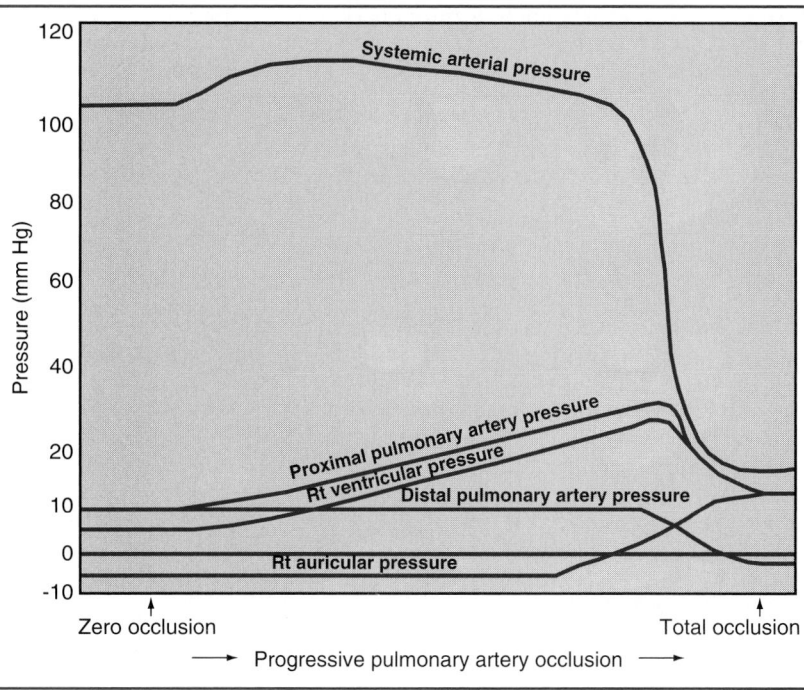

FIGURE 47–8. Mean pressures observed as the main pulmonary artery of the dog is progressively constricted over a 4- to 5-minute period. The right ventricle is unable to generate mean pulmonary artery pressures greater than 40 mm Hg, and sudden circulatory collapse occurs. (Reproduced with permission from Guyton, A. C., Lindsey, A. W., and Gilluly, J. J.: The limits of right ventricular compensation following acute increase in pulmonary circulatory resistance. Circ. Res. 2:326, 1954. Copyright 1954 American Heart Association.)

load.[115,117] The right coronary artery, which supplies the RV free wall and a portion of the interventricular septum, originates in the aorta, and this fact may partially explain the frequent observation that LV function and systemic arterial pressure help determine whether the RV can continue to function despite pulmonary hypertension.[115,117]

Brooks et al.[118] showed that dogs with an acutely occluded right coronary artery had a diminished RV response to increased pressure load. As pulmonary artery pressure was increased above normal, cardiac output and aortic pressure fell and RV pressure rose more rapidly than in normal dogs. Such decompensation was reversible by perfusing the right coronary artery with higher than normal pressures. Spotnitz and colleagues[119] found that occluding the descending aorta with a balloon catheter reversed otherwise inexorable and fatal circulatory collapse in dogs with experimentally induced pulmonary embolism. The circulatory collapse was probably prevented by increased proximal aortic pressure and enhanced right coronary artery perfusion, although coronary blood flow was not measured.

RIGHT CORONARY ARTERY PERFUSION. Other studies in experimental animals directly assessed right coronary perfusion during progressive pulmonary hypertension and subsequent right ventricular failure.[120–123] Fixler et al.[120] and Cooper et al.[122] found that dogs with a degree of RV hypertension that leads to sudden circulatory collapse had inadequate right coronary blood flow relative to myocardial oxygen requirement (estimated from the RV tension-time index). Manohar et al.[121] caused RV pressure overload in pigs by inflating a cuff around the pulmonary artery trunk. By adjusting the degree of pulmonary artery constriction, they maintained a condition of RV dysfunction (a 30 per cent fall in cardiac output and a 15-mm Hg decrease in mean aortic pressure) without inducing sudden progressive circulatory collapse. Total blood flow to the RV free wall was markedly increased (91 per cent) over control conditions, despite a reduction in right coronary driving pressure (mean aortic pressure minus mean right ventricular pressure), indicating compensatory coronary vasodilation. Furthermore, infusion of adenosine (a vasodilator) increased right coronary flow. This occurred despite a further decrease in mean aortic pressure and therefore a decrease in right coronary driving pressure, indicating that there was coronary vasodilator reserve.

In similar experiments, Vlahakes et al.[123] constricted the pulmonary artery beyond the maximum pressure that could be generated by the RV (systolic pressure above 65 mm Hg), and irreversible circulatory collapse occurred. The point of collapse correlated with the sudden development of RV ischemia, manifested by loss of the normal endocardial–epicardial-blood-flow ratio, abnormal myocardial levels of metabolic markers (adenosine triphosphate, creatine kinase, lactate, and pyruvate), and loss of coronary vasodilator reserve. Infusion of phenylephrine after the onset of RV failure improved systolic function and alleviated the manifestations of ischemia. This effect was likely due to an increase in central aortic pressure and therefore a higher right coronary driving pressure.

Other investigators[124,125] showed in the dog that systemic infusion of norepinephrine, which increased aortic pressure, reversed RV failure and shock in acute pulmonary embolism. In these experiments, vasoconstrictor therapy was more effective than either volume ex-

pansion or isoproterenol. The mechanism of the beneficial effect of norepinephrine was presumed to be improved right coronary perfusion and alleviation of myocardial ischemia.

In contrast to these studies, Scharf et al.[126] suggest that ischemia may not be necessary for RV failure secondary to afterload stress. In their study, dogs were subjected to graded occlusion of the pulmonary artery until the circulation failed. Measurement of intramyocardial pH did not indicate myocardial ischemia at either the highest tolerated degree of occlusion or the point of frank circulatory failure. However, occluding the descending aorta, with an increase in central aortic pressure, increased RV load tolerance without any detectable change in right coronary arterial inflow, RV contractility, or intramyocardial pH. The mechanism for this effect on RV function is unexplained, but increased diastolic and systolic tension of the fibers of the LV, which occurs after aortic occlusion, may assist the RV, which shares some fibers with the larger LV.

VENTRICULAR INTERACTION. The RV distension that sometimes occurs abruptly in acute pulmonary hypertension may affect the LV pressure–volume relationship, thus causing the ventricles to compete for space within the pericardium.[115,127–132] The result is a form of LV diastolic "tamponade"[115,133] (Fig. 47–9).

Stool et al.[130] measured the dimensional changes of the LV during acute pulmonary hypertension in the dog and found that LV volume decreased progressively beginning at mean pulmonary artery pressures above 30 mm Hg. The LV became distorted and the septal–lateral wall axis became disproportionately shortened at both end diastole and end systole. Heart rate increased to maintain cardiac output as LV stroke volume decreased with increased pulmonary pressure. At a mean pulmonary artery pressure of 60 mm Hg, end-diastolic volume of the LV was reduced by 30 per cent from control conditions. If mean pulmonary artery pressure was maintained at this level or increased, circulatory collapse occurred, presumably partially because of reduced LV output.

ACUTE RIGHT VENTRICULAR FAILURE. As shown in Figure 47–10, the pathophysiology of acute RV failure can be viewed as a vicious circle. In response to mild or moderate pressure loading, right coronary flow increases despite a decrease in right coronary artery driving pressure because compensatory dilation of the coronary artery reduces resistance to flow.[115,117] Systolic function of the RV may be maintained, in part, by an augmentation of preload or end-diastolic volume; however, marked RV distention has adverse effects including increased wall tension (oxygen demand), decreased LV compliance, and tricuspid regurgitation.[115,117] The latter two effects may decrease cardiac

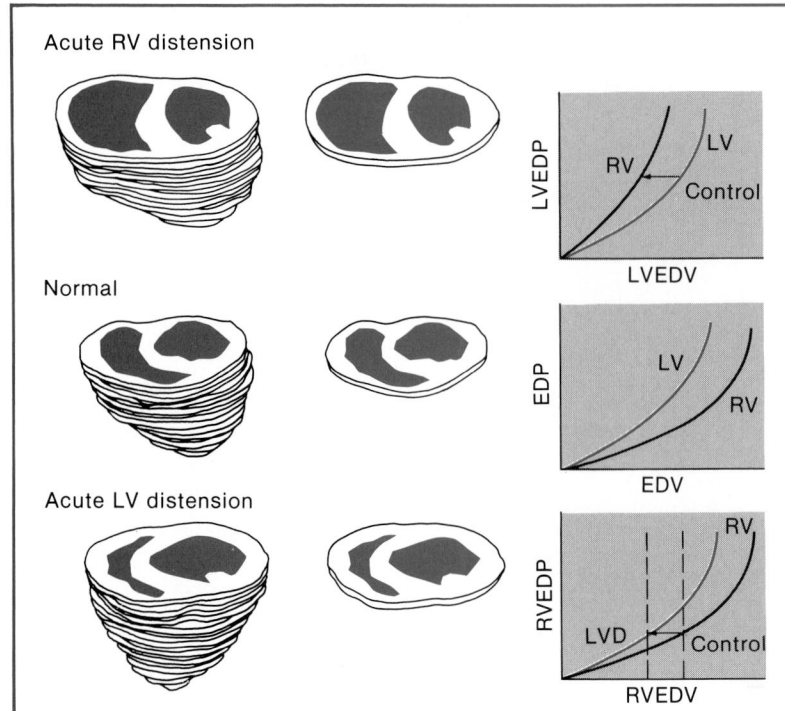

FIGURE 47–9. Alterations in compliance by distention of the contralateral ventricle. Note that acute distention of either ventricle changes not only that ventricle's pressure-volume curve but alters the compliance of the other ventricle as well. The middle graph shows the end-diastolic volume-pressure relationship for the right ventricle (RV) and left ventricle (LV). The top graph shows these relations for the LV with a normal RV *(right curve)* and after the RV has been acutely distended (RVD, *left curve*). The bottom graph shows the relations for the RV with a normal LV *(right curve)* and after the LV has been acutely distended (LVD). (From Weber, K. T., et al.: Contractile mechanics and interaction of the right and left ventricles. Am. J. Cardiol. *47*:686, 1981.)

output and aortic pressure, thereby further reducing right coronary driving pressure when the RV myocardium requires more oxygen. When vasodilatory reserve of the right coronary artery is exhausted, myocardial ischemia may ensue, with a resultant loss of RV function. At the critical point of RV decompensation, the circle irreversibly closes, and circulatory collapse rapidly follows.[115,117]

Treatment

Right Ventricular Preload Augmentation

Intravascular volume expansion helps maintain cardiac output in acute pulmonary hypertension.[115,134–137] For example, augmentation of RV preload enhances the circulation in acute pulmonary artery constriction[116] and in ARDS.[134] As venous volume increases, the systemic mean pressure rises, and peripheral edema is likely to develop.[115] If diuretic therapy is used to alleviate the edema, cardiac

output may decline. Therefore, patients with reduced RV function may have to tolerate peripheral edema to maintain acceptable cardiac output.[115]

The use of RV preload augmentation to maintain cardiac output is theoretically limited. Increased RV volume potentially leads to reduced LV diastolic filling and tricuspid insufficiency. Although the RV is very compliant, increasing the volume also increases the wall tension and oxygen demand. In addition, the high systolic pressure necessary to overcome outflow resistance reduces right coronary artery driving pressure.

A number of studies[138–141] have shown that continued volume expansion against increasing pulmonary vascular resistance in anesthetized and ventilated dogs leads to circulatory deterioration. Molloy et al.[124] showed that volume expansion alone did not resuscitate dogs in shock caused by experimental pulmonary embolism. Sibbald et al.[134] showed that in ARDS patients with high pulmonary vascular resistance and very elevated RV volume, contractility was reduced compared with similar patients with lower pressure load and less chamber enlargement.

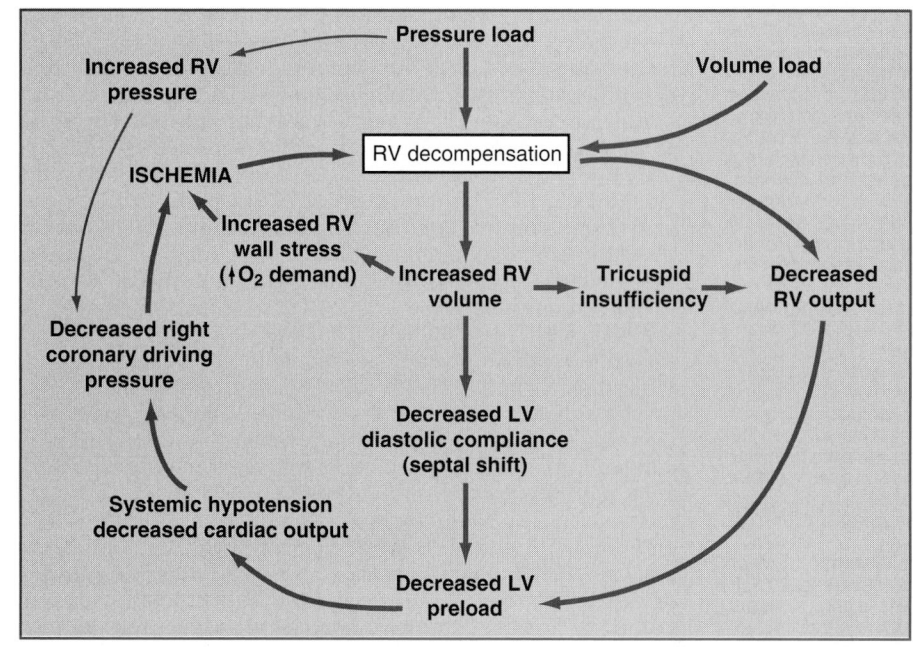

FIGURE 47–10. Pathophysiology of acute right ventricular failure: the vicious circle. (From Wiedemann, H. P., and Matthay, R. A.: Acute right heart failure. Crit. Care Clin. *1*:631, 1985.)

In patients with ARDS who have increased pulmonary capillary permeability,[115] volume loading may aggravate pulmonary edema.[115] If RV volume is increased to the degree that LV diastolic compliance is altered, maintenance of LV preload, or volume, requires a higher filling pressure (wedge pressure); thus pulmonary edema worsens.[115] Therefore, in patients with RV dysfunction, volume expansion usually improves cardiac output initially, but volume expansion beyond a certain amount causes progressive deterioration of the circulation.[115] This condition should be suspected when volume infusion abruptly increases left- or right-sided filling pressure without improving cardiac output.[141]

Right Ventricular Afterload Reduction

OXYGEN THERAPY. Hypoxic pulmonary vasoconstriction may aggravate pulmonary hypertension in acute cor pulmonale, and therefore oxygen therapy may be beneficial by reducing right ventricular afterload. In patients with increased pulmonary vascular resistance due to obliterative anatomical lesions, supplemental oxygen therapy may be the only means of rapidly lowering afterload stress in acute RV failure.[115]

VASODILATOR THERAPY. Defining a beneficial hemodynamic response to pharmacological vasodilation in patients with pulmonary hypertension is complex.[115] Mean pulmonary artery pressure may remain unchanged as calculated pulmonary artery resistance decreases and cardiac output increases. In addition, vasodilator therapy may cause such adverse effects as systemic hypotension and decreased arterial oxygen saturation in patients with pulmonary hypertension.[142,143] Hypotension may result because most vasodilators affect the systemic circulation more than the pulmonary circulation.[115] In many patients with significant pulmonary hypertension and reduced right-sided cardiac output, systemic vasoconstriction helps maintain systemic arterial pressure. In such patients, selective dilation of the systemic vasculature may cause hypotension and precipitate RV failure (caused by decreased right coronary blood flow) and circulatory collapse.[117] Decreased arterial oxygen tension may result because of worsening ventilation-perfusion matching within the lung and increasing physiological shunting.[115,142,144]

Systemic vasodilator therapy for acute RV hypertension has been evaluated primarily in experimental studies of acute lung injury.[145–148] Vasodilators have been evaluated in this setting because patients with ARDS have elevated pulmonary vascular resistance, pulmonary hypertension, increased RV end-diastolic volume, and decreased RVEF.[134,149–152] In addition, in patients who survive ARDS, unlike nonsurvivors, the pulmonary vascular resistance usually progressively normalizes.[149] Nitric oxide (NO), a potent vasodilator, is becoming more widely used clinically. Inhaled NO has a rapid onset of action, and it is quickly inactivated after binding to hemoglobin. As a result, inhaled NO is a selective pulmonary vasodilator, and its vasodilator effect is greatest in well ventilated areas of the lung, thereby improving ventilation-perfusion matching. In patients with ARDS,[153] inhaled NO reduces pulmonary artery pressure and improves gas exchange. Controlled trials are in progress to test whether these physiological benefits improve outcome.

Maintenance of Aortic Pressure

The effective therapies for RV failure, including occlusion of the descending aorta,[115,126,154] intra-aortic balloon counterpulsation,[119] phenylephrine infusion,[155,156] and norepinephrine infusion,[124,140,141] all augment aortic pressure, which may be beneficial by increasing aortic pressure and thereby improving right coronary artery perfusion and alleviating myocardial ischemia.[126]

Therapies that may decrease systemic blood pressure should be used cautiously in patients with acute cor pulmonale.[115] For instance, vasodilators, by lowering aortic pressure, may adversely affect right coronary perfusion, an effect that might explain the instances of death after administration of hydralazine or diazoxide in patients with

severe pulmonary hypertension.[142,143] Conversely, therapies directed at raising aortic pressure, such as norepinephrine infusion, should be considered if they are not contraindicated.

CHRONIC COR PULMONALE

Causes and Pathophysiology

The most common cause of chronic cor pulmonale in North America is COPD (emphysema, chronic obstructive bronchitis). The pathophysiology, natural history, and treatment of cor pulmonale secondary to COPD are discussed in detail in the later sections. Various other disorders associated with chronic cor pulmonale are shown in Table 47–1, and the pathogenetic mechanisms by which these disorders lead to pulmonary hypertension and cor pulmonale are summarized in Table 47–3.

Pulmonary Vascular Disorders
(See also Chap. 25)

Diseases such as primary pulmonary hypertension, which primarily affect the pulmonary vasculature and have little or no parenchymal involvement, clearly represent the pathogenetic progression from increased pulmonary vascular resistance resulting from gradual obliteration of the pulmonary vascular bed to pulmonary hypertension and RV overload. Patients with pulmonary vascular disorders invariably have dyspnea and very high pulmonary artery pressure, even though vital capacity and pulmonary gas exchange may be only minimally impaired.[157]

Disorders of the Neuromuscular Apparatus and Chest Wall

These disorders, which have in common the mechanical failure of the bellows apparatus, through weakness or paralysis of the respiratory muscles or distortion of the geometry of the thorax, can lead to cor pulmonale by failure of

TABLE 47–3 POTENTIAL PATHOGENETIC MECHANISMS LEADING TO PULMONARY ARTERIAL HYPERTENSION AND COR PULMONALE

MECHANISMS	EXAMPLE
Primary	
Anatomical decrease in cross-sectional area (vessel destruction; encroachment on lumen by hypertrophy) of the pulmonary resistance vessels	Interstitial fibrosis and granuloma
Vasoconstriction of pulmonary resistance vessels	Hypoxia and acidosis
Contributory	
Large increments in pulmonary blood flow	Exercise
Increased pressures on the left side of the heart and pulmonary veins	Left ventricular failure or pulmonary venoocclusive disease
Increased viscosity of the blood	Secondary polycythemia or chronic hypoxia
Unproved	
Compression of pulmonary resistance vessels by raised alveolar pressures in their vicinity	Asthmatic bronchitis
Bronchial arterial–pulmonary arterial anastomoses	Expanded bronchial circulation

From Fishman, A. P.: Pulmonary hypertension and cor pulmonale. *In* Fishman, A. P.: Pulmonary Diseases and Disorders, 2nd ed. New York, McGraw-Hill Book Co., 1988, p. 1001.

the neuromuscular apparatus, diaphragmatic paralysis, and distortion of the chest wall.[3]

FAILURE OF THE NEUROMUSCULAR APPARATUS. Weakness of the respiratory muscles can be caused by either generalized muscle diseases, such as myopathic infiltrating diseases or muscular dystrophy, or more commonly by such neurological disorders as a cord lesion at or below the third cervical vertebra, amyotrophic lateral sclerosis, myasthenia gravis, poliomyelitis, or Guillain-Barré syndrome.[3,157,158] These diseases result in *generalized alveolar hypoventilation*. The lungs and airways, although usually not affected primarily, may be injured by retained secretions and multiple aspirations. Cor pulmonale usually develops in response to the hypoxic and hypercapnic stimuli in patients with chronic forms of these disorders; consequently, cor pulmonale tends to be more common in patients with cord lesions than with the other disorders noted. Mechanical ventilatory support is the only therapy for the hypoventilation; a cuirass type of respirator is effective. In addition, vigorous bronchial toilet may alleviate the impaired handling of secretions.[3]

DIAPHRAGMATIC PARALYSIS. Bilateral diaphragmatic paralysis is an uncommon but often unrecognized cause of cor pulmonale.[3,159] When an affected patient is upright, ventilation may be normal or almost so, but when the patient is supine, gas exchange deteriorates. The diagnosis may be suspected in a patient with supine breathlessness, a disturbed sleep pattern, paradoxical (i.e., inward) motion of the abdomen on inspiration, and a low vital capacity in the upright position.[3] Therapy for this disorder consists of assisting ventilation when the patient is supine or during sleep, which is usually done by using a rocking bed; however, electrical pacing of the diaphragm may be necessary.[160] Diaphragmatic fatigue sometimes contributes to the respiratory failure of COPD.[161] Bilateral diaphragmatic paralysis may occur after cardiac surgery.[162] Ice cardioplegia can damage the phrenic nerves and lead to transitory respiratory failure that becomes manifest when the patient is removed from the ventilator. Diaphragmatic function usually returns in such patients.[3]

CHEST WALL DISORDERS. Common congenital or acquired abnormalities that distort the thoracic cage are kyphoscoliosis, pectus excavatum, pectus carinatum, and ankylosing spondylitis: Dyspnea is the major symptom of these disorders, but only kyphoscoliosis is associated with cor pulmonale.[3,163] Kyphosis consists of posterior angulation of the spine and scoliosis anterior angulation. Cor pulmonale may develop in a patient with a kyphotic angle exceeding 100 degrees or a scoliotic angle exceeding 120 degrees.[3,164] These structural abnormalities of the thorax cause repositioning and dysfunction of the respiratory muscles, compression of the lung and pulmonary vasculature, and abnormal gas exchange[163,165] (Fig. 47–11). In addition, scoliosis may interfere with the growth and development of alveoli and pulmonary arteries.[166]

Therapy for chest wall disorders is directed toward preventing infection; acute respiratory failure in such patients is treated with mechanical ventilation.[3] Surgical repair of the thoracic deformity often does not improve cardiorespiratory function.[167]

Disorders of Ventilatory Control

These disorders produce pulmonary hypertension as the result of chronic hypoxemia and hypercapnia due to alveolar hypoventilation (Fig. 47–11). Patients with primary central hypoventilation ("Ondine's curse") have abnormally blunted ventilatory responses to hypercapnic and hypoxic stimulation; the pathogenesis of the congenital form of this disorder is unknown. The acquired disease may follow encephalitis, meningitis, or brain-stem injury or surgery.[168] A form of alveolar hypoventilation also occurs in some obese patients. The so-called pickwickian syndrome consists of the constellation of obesity, hypoventilation, somnolence, and peripheral edema.[169-171]

Treatment consists of weight reduction; respiratory stimulants, such as progesterone, may increase alveolar ventilation and thereby alleviate hypoxemia, hypercapnia, and cor pulmonale.[172,173] Patients with sleep-disordered breathing may have intermittent and repetitive nocturnal hypoxemia that can lead to pulmonary hypertension and cor pulmonale.[172,173] This is true even though most such patients have adequate ventilation and gas exchange while they are awake.

SLEEP APNEA SYNDROMES. These are classified into three general types: (1) central apnea, in which airflow stops in conjunction with cessation of all respiratory muscle effort; (2) obstructive apnea, in which upper airway obstruction causes cessation of airflow despite continuing efforts of the respiratory muscles; and (3) mixed apnea, in which airflow obstruction and respiratory effort both stop initially in the episode, followed first by a resumption of unsuccessful respiratory effort.[3,172,174,175] The upper airway obstruction in patients with sleep-disordered breathing may be due to a combination of such factors as discoordination and relaxation of the buccal and pharyngeal muscles, collapse of the walls of the pharynx and backward movement of the tongue due to inactivity of the genioglossus muscle, and anatomical factors such as enlarged tonsils and adenoids or narrowing due to marked obesity.[3,174]

Patients with sleep apnea may have 40 to 60 apneic episodes per hour,[174] which are associated with phasic hypoxemia and hypercapnia.[3] During the episodes, the pO_2 may fall to as low as 20 to 25 mm Hg, with saturation below 50 per cent.[3] Pulmonary and systemic arterial pressures rise with each episode, and stroke volume, heart rate, and cardiac output fall.[171] The pulmonary artery pressure progressively increases during the night,[171] and pulmonary hypertension is most severe in the morning. The pressure falls during the day but rises with sleep the next night.[3] Hypoxemia, hypercapnia, and pulmonary hypertension eventually become permanent and gradually worsen while the patient is awake.[3]

Patients with sleep apnea also often have severe bradyarrhythmias, which occur during apneic episodes, and tachyarrhythmias, which occur when breathing resumes.[176,177] The arrhythmias consist of sinus bradycardia,

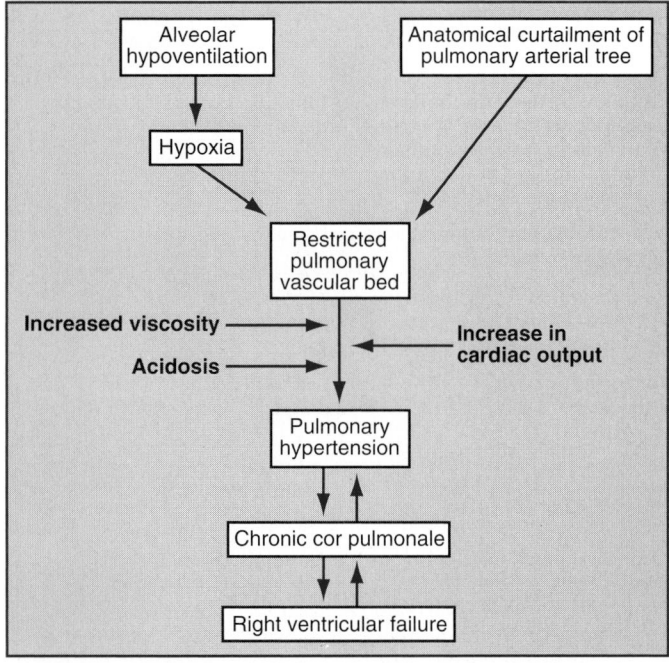

FIGURE 47–11. Pathogenesis of pulmonary hypertension and cor pulmonale in kyphoscoliosis and disorders of ventilatory control. (From Fishman, A. P.: Pulmonary hypertension and cor pulmonale. *In* Fishman, A. P. [ed.]: Pulmonary Diseases and Disorders. 2nd ed. New York, McGraw-Hill Book Co., 1988, p. 1033.)

sinus arrest, long asystolic periods (ranging from 2 to 13 seconds), sinoatrial block, premature atrial contractions, atrial fibrillation, ventricular premature beats with bigeminy and trigeminy, multifocal premature beats, and ventricular tachycardia.[176-179] Pulmonary artery wedge pressure also may increase during episodes of apnea.[180] Clinical effects of apnea differ with the type, frequency, and intensity of the abnormal respiratory pattern.

Patients with sleep apnea rarely reach deep sleep and therefore are chronically sleep deprived.[3,181] Other common clinical manifestations are loud snoring, somnambulism, tremors, myoclonus, altered states of consciousness, nocturnal enuresis, morning headache, daytime hypersomnolence, hypnagogic hallucinations, and systemic hypertension.[3,181,182] Affected patients are usually not obese and breathe normally when awake. Patients with obstructive apnea tend to have milder hypoventilation and fewer hemodynamic abnormalities than patients with central apnea or mixed apnea. The diagnosis of sleep apnea is established by polysomnography.

About 20 per cent of patients with sleep apnea have COPD, and most of these eventually develop pulmonary hypertension.[183-186] Diagnosis of coexisting sleep apnea and COPD can be difficult, and both disorders must be treated to control symptoms.[3]

Etiology. The cause of sleep apnea is not always clear.[3] Obstructive apneas likely occur because of occlusion of the upper airway in the region of the pharynx.[173,187] Central apnea may have multiple mechanisms, including sleep-induced alteration in respiratory muscle drive, depressed central ventilatory output, or a change in the thresholds for sleep or arousal.[173,188]

Management. In patients with sleep apnea, sedatives and antihistamines should be assiduously avoided or withdrawn, and oxygen therapy should be used cautiously.[3] Narcoleptics and uncontrolled oxygen therapy have resulted in death in some patients.[174] Central apnea is treated with respiratory stimulants or nocturnal ventilatory support with respirators.[174,188] Phrenic nerve or diaphragmatic pacing also has been recommended.[159] Obstructive apnea is most often treated with nasal continuous positive airway pressure (CPAP) and far less commonly tracheostomy.[174,182] Tracheostomy bypasses the area of obstruction, whereas CPAP likely acts as a pneumatic splint that prevents upper airway collapse. Obese patients with obstructive apnea who lose weight may not need a permanent tracheal cannula.[3] Surgical removal of enlarged tonsils or adenoids or surgical enlargement of the entrance to the airway may also be efficacious.[3,182] In some patients, nocturnal oxygen therapy may reduce the duration of apneic episodes and decrease

the arrhythmias, but, as noted, oxygen must be used cautiously in these patients.[189]

Upper Airway Obstruction

Obstruction of the upper airways may result in inadequate ventilatory drive, global alveolar hypoventilation, and cor pulmonale.[3] This disorder occurs primarily in children,[190] especially African-American children who have enlarged tonsils and adenoids, but cor pulmonale has been reported as a sequela of acute tonsillitis in adults.[191] Other causes of airway obstruction include vascular ring, macroglossia, micrognathia, laryngotracheomalacia, laryngeal web, Crouzon's disease, Hurler's syndrome, and severe Pierre Robin syndrome,[192,193] but the upper airways can become obstructed during sleep in both children and adults.[194] The mechanism for the hypoventilation is not clear, but an abnormally reactive pulmonary vascular bed, a defect in the central control of respiration, and an interference with normal sleep physiology (as in the sleep apnea syndrome), may alone or in combination have some effect. Ventilatory responsiveness to carbon dioxide is blunted in these patients and it is not normalized by therapy.[195]

The clinical features may mimic asthma, but affected patients usually have somnolence, stridor, and recurrent respiratory tract infection.[3] Treatment consists of surgical removal of the obstruction.[3]

Restrictive Lung Diseases

Pulmonary parenchymal disease, especially when associated with tissue fibrosis and secondary vascular changes, can eventually lead to severe pulmonary hypertension, although significant cor pulmonale usually occurs very late (Table 47-3). In some patients with scleroderma (especially patients with the so-called CREST variant), however, significant pulmonary vascular disease predominates[196,197] (p. 1781). These patients may develop severe pulmonary hypertension and cor pulmonale, even without significant lung fibrosis or restriction of lung mechanics.

Chronic Obstructive Pulmonary Disease

ETIOLOGY AND NATURAL HISTORY OF PULMONARY HYPERTENSION IN COPD. In patients with COPD, pulmonary vasoconstriction may be caused by hypoxia or acidosis, and the pulmonary vascular bed may contract owing to chronic hypoxia-induced structural narrowing and loss of capillaries from emphysema.[1,5] Pulmonary hypertension results as may increased cardiac output, increased pulmonary blood volume, increased blood viscosity, and increased intrathoracic pressure due to expiratory airflow limitation[3,5,198] (see Figs. 47-11, 47-12, and 47-13). Although LV failure cannot be a

FIGURE 47-12. Pathogenesis of cor pulmonale. (From Summer, W. R.: Acute cor pulmonale. In Rubin, L. J. [ed.]: Pulmonary Heart Disease. Boston, Martinus Nijhoff, 1984, p. 285.)

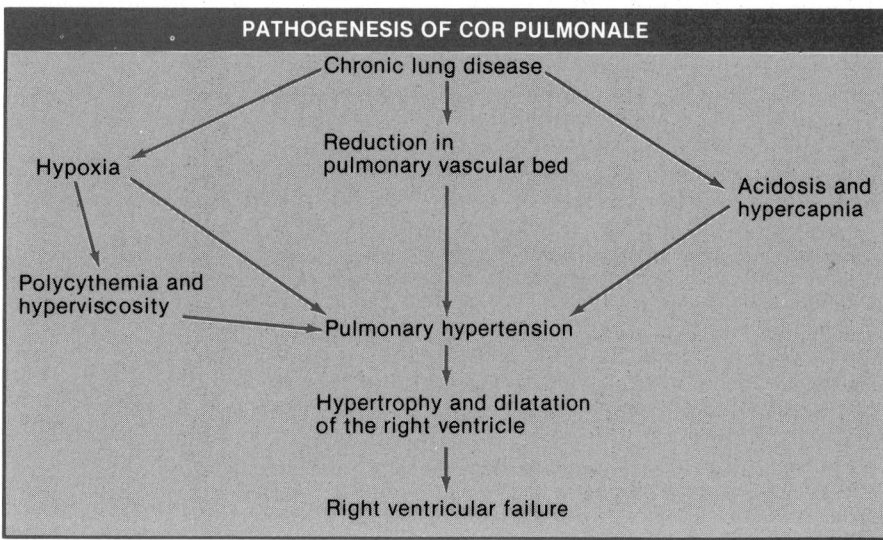

PATHOGENESIS OF COR PULMONALE

Chronic lung disease

Hypoxia

Reduction in pulmonary vascular bed

Acidosis and hypercapnia

Polycythemia and hyperviscosity

Pulmonary hypertension

Hypertrophy and dilatation of the right ventricle

Right ventricular failure

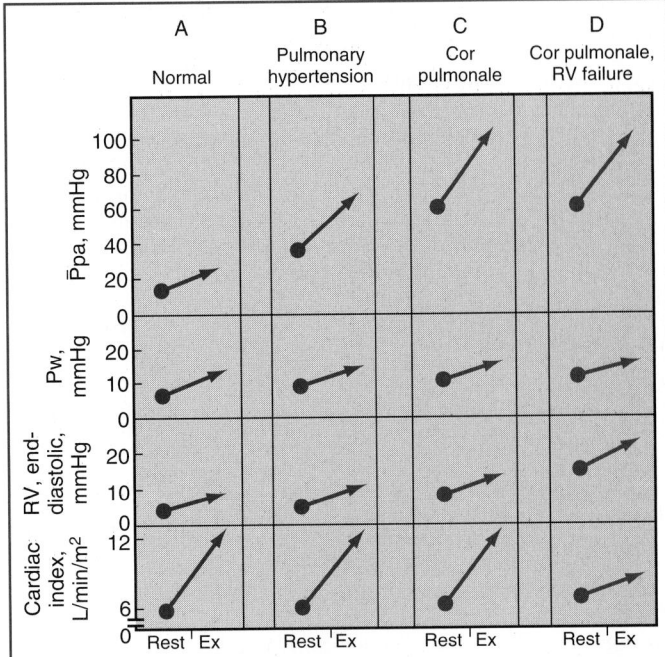

FIGURE 47-13. Schematic representation of evolution of chronic cor pulmonale; hemodynamic studies at rest and during exercise in a normal subject (A). The stage of pulmonary artery hypertension (B) is succeeded by cor pulmonale (C), in which the right ventricle performs normally despite pulmonary artery hypertension but the RV is known to be enlarged from radiographic and electrocardiographic findings. Once RV failure supervenes (D), cardiac output fails to increase normally during exercise, despite an increase of right ventricular filling pressure (end diastolic) to abnormally high levels. (From Fishman, A. P.: Pulmonary hypertension and cor pulmonale. *In* Fishman, A. P. [ed.]: Pulmonary Diseases and Disorders. 2nd ed. New York, McGraw-Hill Book Co., 1988, p. 1010.)

primary cause of cor pulmonale, elevated pulmonary venous pressure nevertheless exacerbates pulmonary hypertension (Table 47-3).

HYPOXIA. This is likely the primary causative factor in the development of pulmonary artery hypertension and RV hypertrophy in patients with COPD.[1,5,199,200] Longitudinal studies show that resting pulmonary artery pressure increases slowly in patients with emphysema or chronic obstructive bronchitis who have mild or moderate arterial hypoxemia.[201-203] Furthermore, patients with COPD who have an accelerated progression of pulmonary hypertension are usually significantly hypoxemic. One large study found that the extent of pulmonary artery hypertension correlated most closely to resting arterial oxygen saturation, measured while the patient was awake.[204,205] In fact, arterial oxygen saturation accounted for 43 per cent of the variance of pulmonary artery pressure among patients, whereas adding FEV_1 in a multiple progression equation that included arterial oxygen saturation accounted for only an additional 1 per cent of the variance. In patients with pure emphysema, however, the FEV_1 and diffusing capacity may correlate more closely with the degree of pulmonary hypertension than arterial blood gases at rest.[206]

As recently reviewed by MacNee,[1] anatomical and radiographic studies also suggest that destruction of the alveolar walls (with the loss of capillary bed) does not itself cause sustained pulmonary hypertension at rest in patients with COPD; however, loss of capillary bed may worsen pulmonary hypertension during exercise[207] (see Fig. 47-13 and Table 47-3). Postmortem studies have shown that RV hypertrophy does not significantly correlate with the extent of emphysema or total alveolar surface area.[208] Furthermore, there is no significant correlation between pulmonary artery pressure and the extent of emphysema as measured by computerized tomography (CT) scanning.[209] Autopsies of patients in the Nocturnal Oxygen Therapy Trial (NOTT) showed that patients with cyanosis and peripheral edema (so-called blue bloaters) had heavier RVs than the "pink puffers," and the degree of RV hypertrophy correlated with the extent of chronic inflammatory changes in the airways.[210]

How hypoxemia and hypoxic pulmonary vasoconstriction lead to sustained pulmonary hypertension is not known, but structural changes in the pulmonary vasculature are undoubtedly important.[1] Chronic hypoxemia causes proliferation of endothelial cells and thickening in the intima of small pulmonary arterioles where vascular smooth muscle cells accumulate.[211-215] Other potential contributing factors include medial hypertrophy in the muscular pulmonary arteries and abnormalities in endothelium-dependent vasodilation, which is thought to be mediated by nitric oxide.[1,216-218] Endothelium-mediated vasodilation is impaired in pulmonary vascular rings from patients with severe COPD undergoing lung transplantation and in experimental animals made chronically hypoxemic.[219,220]

PERIPHERAL EDEMA. Formation of edema in patients with COPD is complex and may not be primarily related to pulmonary hypertension and RV dysfunction; in advanced COPD, abnormalities in sodium and water metabolism instead may contribute to the formation of edema.[221] Many hypoxemic and edematous patients with COPD did not have RV hypertrophy or evidence of RV failure.[222,223] Furthermore, although most edematous patients with COPD are hypoxemic, hypoxemia alone cannot explain the edema. Persons who live at high altitudes and are therefore chronically hypoxemic usually are not edematous,[224] and hypoxemia alone is not associated with abnormal renal sodium or water metabolism.[225,226] However, hypoxemia with coexisting hypercapnia may impair excretion of sodium and water. Moreover, edema is rare in patients with COPD who are not hypercapnic.[221,227]

MacNee[221] proposed the following hypothesis for the formation of edema in patients with COPD (Fig. 47-14). In patients who are hypoxemic, the development of hypercapnia may cause a sodium- and water-retaining state by inducing loss of H^+ ions in exchange for sodium reabsorption and by CO_2-induced peripheral vasodilation that inactivates arterial baroreceptors; this effect leads to an increase in noradrenalin and stimulation of the renin–angiotensin system. Renal blood flow is reduced indirectly by the increase in sympathetic activity and directly by the effect of high $PaCO_2$. With increased renin–angiotensin activity, vasopressin is released. The net effect of these changes is the retention of sodium and water. Extracellular volume expansion, along with pulmonary artery hypertension, leads to atrial distension and release of atrial natriuretic peptide (ANP) that, although protective against edema, may be overwhelmed by the activity of the renin–angiotensin system. Furthermore, ANP-induced pulmonary vasodilation, though potentially beneficial, may induce peripheral vasodilation, further inactivating arterial baroreceptors and continuing the cycle. Infrarenal dopamine, which may also protect against the development of edema in such patients, also eventually fails.

CARDIAC OUTPUT, OXYGEN TRANSPORT, AND MIXED VENOUS OXYGENATION. Kawakami et al.[228] evaluated the relation of the oxygen delivery, mixed venous oxygenation, and pulmonary hemodynamics to prognosis in patients with COPD and found potentially clinically important relationships between mixed venous oxygenation and survival. Fifty patients with COPD underwent a single right-sided cardiac catheterization; 4 years later (without follow-up catheterization), the 23 survivors were compared with the 27 patients who died. The nonsurvivors had a significantly lower PaO_2 and mixed venous pO_2 than the survivors at the time of the initial catheterization but had no significant difference in mean pulmonary artery pressure, right ventricular work, oxygen transport, or coefficient of oxygen delivery (ratio of oxygen transport to oxygen consumption). Hypoxemia had thus reduced survival but not, it appears, through the generally accepted mechanism of cor pulmonale. The results of this study must be interpreted cautiously, however. Longitudinal hemodynamic data were not evaluated, and the patients who died may have had significant progression of pulmonary hypertension or undetected changes in oxygen transport.

Mixed venous oxygen pressure reflects the lowest oxygen pressure in the vasculature and thereby determines the

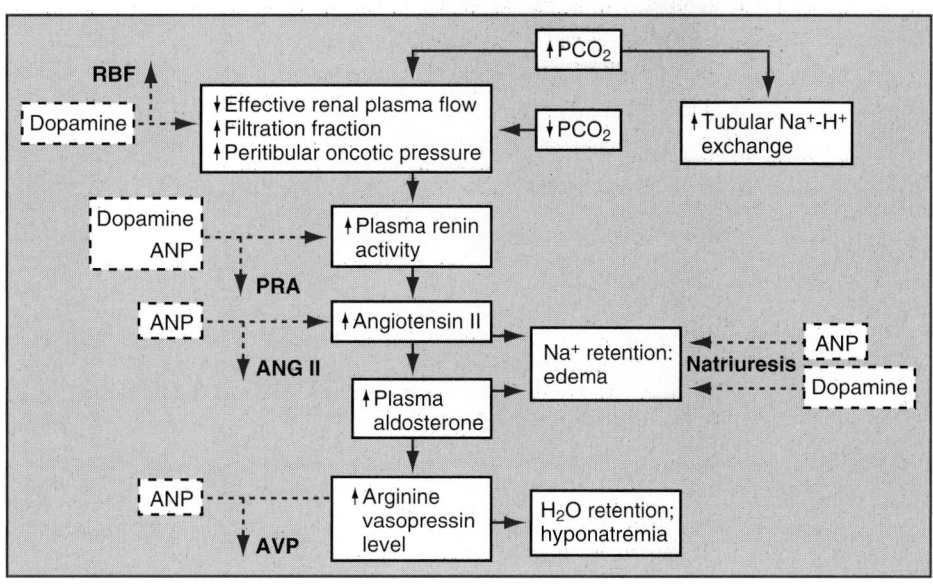

FIGURE 47–14. Mechanisms of salt and water disturbance in patients with COPD. The continuous lines and boxes indicate the abnormalities in renal function, salt water, and hormonal balance. The dotted lines indicate proposed protective mechanisms against this disturbance. RBF = renal blood flow; ANP = atrial natriuretic peptide; ANG II = angiotensin II; Na$^+$ = sodium; H+ = hydrogen ion; AVP = arginine vasopressin; PRA = plasma renin activity. (From Mac-Nee, W.: Pathophysiology of cor pulmonale in chronic obstructive pulmonary disease. Am. J. Respir. Crit. Care Med. *150:*833, 1994.)

driving pressure gradient for diffusion into the tissues.[5] Oxygen transport, which is the product of cardiac output and the arterial oxygen content, must be sufficient to replenish the oxygen consumed in order to prevent significant lowering of venous oxygenation. If consumption remains independent of delivery, the adequacy of oxygen transport largely determines the venous oxygen pressure.[229,230] Oxygen transport can be affected by changes in either cardiac output or arterial oxygen content, and arterial oxygen content is affected by changes in either hemoglobin concentration or saturation.[5] The effect of such changes on mixed venous oxygenation may be quantitatively very different; depending on how hemoglobin concentration or saturation is altered, oxygen delivery may be associated with different values for mixed venous pO_2 (Fig. 47–15).

Tenney and Mithoefer[231] plotted the relation between mixed venous oxygen saturation and the coefficient of oxygen delivery in 68 patients with COPD at rest breathing room air (Fig. 47–16). The coefficient of oxygen delivery is obtained by dividing oxygen transport by oxygen consumption, thus showing a "supply-to-demand" ratio.[232] The coefficient of oxygen delivery varies with age; it is about 5.0 in the third decade, and it falls to 3.5 in the sixth and seventh decades. Tenney and Mithoefer[232] found a close correlation between oxygen delivery and mixed venous oxygenation in patients with COPD (r = 0.84); however, the value varied widely in certain individuals (Fig. 47–16).

The data of Tenney and Mithoefer[231] support the findings of Kawakami et al.,[228] who concluded that lower mixed venous oxygen saturation is an independent indicator of a poor prognosis in untreated patients with similar pulmonary hemodynamics and coefficient of oxygen delivery. It also seems that increasing oxygen capacity by the development of polycythemia to maintain systemic oxygen transport in the face of hypoxic COPD is not a successful long-term adaptation. Rather, cardiac output must increase to maintain mixed venous oxygenation despite lowering arterial saturation.[231] This hypothesis, rather than negating the importance of cardiac output in the prognosis for COPD, suggests that cardiac output is critical to the physiological adaptation to COPD.[233–235] That is, failure to increase cardiac output in the face of significant venous hypoxemia adversely affects survival. Thus, interventions that maintain or enhance cardiac output in patients with COPD and cor pulmonale have great therapeutic importance.[5]

Therapy

In the following discussion, the emphasis is exclusively on therapy for cor pulmonale caused by COPD.

Oxygen

SURVIVAL BENEFIT. In clinical trials sponsored by the United States National Institutes of Health (Nocturnal Oxygen Therapy Trial Group, 1980) and British Medical Research Council (1981), long-term oxygen therapy clearly improved the survival of hypoxemic patients with COPD (Fig. 47–17).[236,237] The British study compared the effects of treatment with oxygen for about 15 hours/day with the effects of no oxygen therapy. The NIH study compared nocturnal oxygen therapy (about 12 hours/day) with "continuous" oxygen therapy (at least 19 hours/day). The studies had similar entry criteria; patients with COPD and a PaO_2 of less than 60 mm Hg and no other major disease.[238] In the NIH study, patients with PaO_2 between 55 and 60 mm Hg were accepted only if they also had polycythemia, edema, or electrocardiographic evidence of cor pulmonale. Only clinically stable patients with persistent hypoxemia during a 3-week observation period were accepted. In most of the British patients, oxygen was administered at 2 liters/min via nasal prongs. The oxygen dose used in the NIH study was that which raised PaO_2 to at least 65 mm Hg and an additional 1 liter/min at night. In each study, the mean baseline PaO_2 when the patient was breathing ambient air was 51 mm Hg; the mean FEV_1 was about 0.7 to 0.8 liters in both. Despite the similarities, the British patients had a higher mean $PaCO_2$ (54.0 versus 43.7 mm Hg), a higher mean hematocrit (53.0 versus 47.5 per cent), a higher mean pulmonary artery pressure (34.4 versus 29.5 mm Hg), and a higher mean cardiac output (6.01 versus 5.07 liters/min).[238]

Oxygen therapy was beneficial in both studies (Fig. 47–17). In the British study, only 19 of 42 (45 per cent) oxygen-treated patients died within 5 years, whereas 30 of 45 (67 per cent) untreated patients died. In the NIH study, the mortality rate after a year was 20.6 per cent in the group receiving nocturnal oxygen and only 11.9 per cent in the group receiving continuous oxygen therapy. After 2 years, mortality was 40.8 per cent and 22.4 per cent respectively. The relative risk of death for nocturnal oxygen therapy compared with continuous oxygen was 1.94. Oxygen therapy is therefore effective, and continuous therapy is more effective than nocturnal therapy only.[239]

Long-term oxygen therapy enhances neuropsychological function as well as improving survival.[238] Improvement was subtle in the NIH study after 6 months of therapy, but after 1 year, the patients receiving continuous oxygen had significantly better neuropsychological performance than patients receiving nocturnal therapy.[240] Short-term oxygen therapy (6 hours/day) fails to reverse information-processing deficits in hypoxic patients with COPD.[241] Neuropsy-

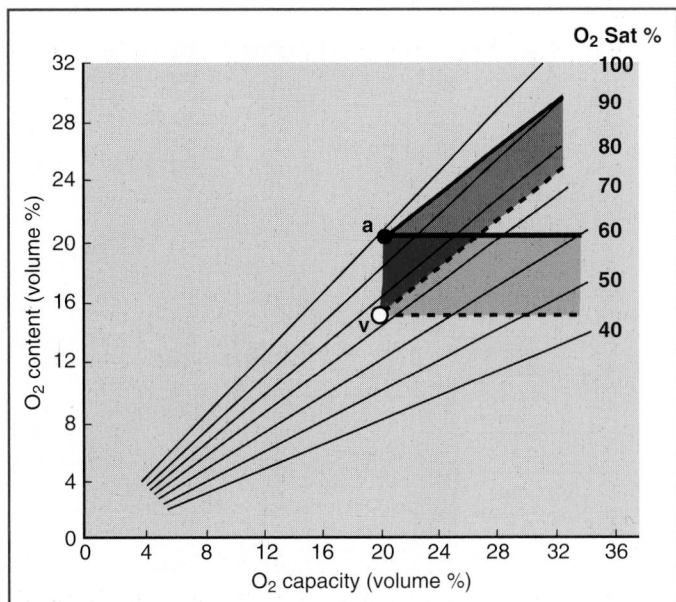

FIGURE 47–15. The relationships among oxygen content (ordinate), oxygen capacity or hemoglobin (Hb) concentration times 1.34 (abscissa), arterial and venous oxygen saturations, and arteriovenous oxygen content difference (CaO$_2$-CvO$_2$). A family of iso-oxygen saturation lines radiates from the origin. The normal arterial and venous points are labeled "a" and "v" (Hb, 15 g/dl blood; normal O$_2$ capacity, 20 ml/dl blood; full saturation is assumed to occur at pO$_2$ = 100 torr; normal CaO$_2$-CvO$_2$ = 5 ml/dl blood). The vertical separation between a pair of arterial and venous points is inversely related to cardiac output. The horizontal shaded band represents the situation in which the arterial oxygen content and the arteriovenous oxygen content difference are maintained constant in the face of progressive hypoxemia and "compensatory" polycythemia (keeping oxygen content stable) as may occur in COPD; i.e., this band represents constant oxygen delivery in the face of decreasing arterial saturation but increasing oxygen capacity. Notice that venous oxygen saturation is markedly decreased despite maintenance of oxygen delivery. The oblique lines extending up and to the right from points "a" and "v" show the degree of polycythemia necessary to maintain normal venous saturation (75 per cent) in the face of hypoxemia. It is clear that a severe degree of polycythemia would be necessary in response to even relatively mild hypoxemia, e.g., at the right end of this band, an arterial oxygen saturation of 90 per cent (PaO$_2$ = 60 mm Hg) would require an arterial oxygen capacity of about 32 volumes per cent (Hb, 24) to maintain normal mixed venous saturation. This is far in excess of what is observed clinically; furthermore, this assumes that cardiac output can be maintained at this high hemoglobin concentration. (From Tenney, S. M., and Mithoefer, J. D.: The relationship of mixed venous oxygenation to oxygen transport: With special reference to adaptations to high altitude and pulmonary disease. Am. Rev. Respir. Dis. *125:*474–479, 1982; with permission. Courtesy of the American Lung Association.)

chological benefits appear to be achieved only after at least 1 month of oxygen therapy.[240]

HEMODYNAMIC EFFECTS OF OXYGEN. How oxygen therapy improves survival is unknown. Two major hypotheses have been proposed: (1) oxygen relieves pulmonary vasoconstriction, decreasing pulmonary vascular resistance and thus enabling the right ventricle to increase stroke volume and (2) oxygen therapy improves arterial oxygen content, providing enhanced oxygen delivery to the heart, brain, and other vital organs.[115,242] These two hypotheses are not mutually exclusive, and each one has supporting evidence. Oxygen therapy clearly alleviates the progressive pulmonary hypertension of untreated COPD. Also, patients who exhibit a significant decrease in pulmonary artery pressure (>5 mm Hg) after acute oxygen therapy (28 per cent oxygen for 1 day) have a much greater rate of survival than patients who do not respond acutely when both groups of patients are subsequently treated with long-term continuous oxygen therapy.[243] In contrast, a study by Morrison and coworkers[242] suggested that enhanced RV performance dur-

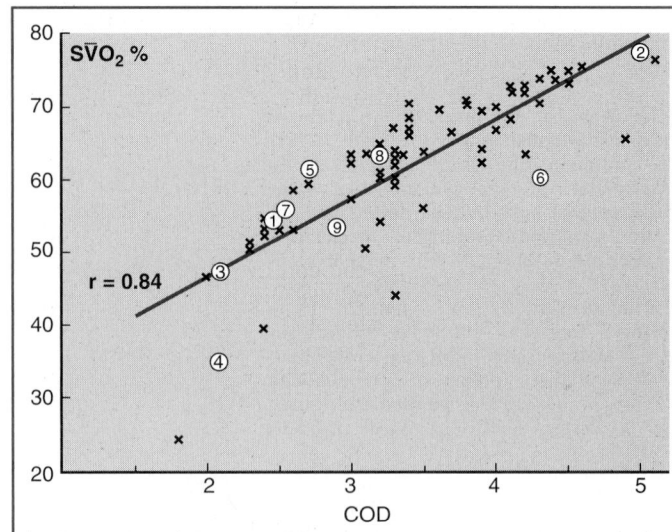

FIGURE 47–16. The relationship between mixed venous oxygen saturation (SV̄O$_2$%) and the coefficient of oxygen delivery (COD) (the product of cardiac output and arterial oxygen content) in 68 patients with COPD at rest, breathing air. (From Tenney, S. M., and Mithoefer, J. C.: The relationship of mixed venous oxygenation to oxygen transport: with special reference to adaptations to high altitude and pulmonary disease. Am. Rev. Respir. Dis. *125:*474–479, 1982; with permission. Courtesy of the American Lung Association.)

ing short-term oxygen therapy may be the direct result of improved tissue (e.g., myocardial) oxygenation rather than decreased pulmonary vascular resistance.

RECOMMENDATIONS. Long-term oxygen therapy is warranted if the resting PaO$_2$ remains less than 55 mm Hg after a 3-week stabilization period on maximal medical therapy (e.g., bronchodilators, antimicrobial agents, diuretics).[115,220,244] Patients with a PaO$_2$ above 55 mm Hg should be considered for oxygen therapy if they are polycythemic[115,221] or have clinical evidence (e.g., electrocardiographic, physical examination) of pulmonary hypertension and cor pulmonale.[115] Hypoxemia should be documented after a stabilization period to avoid the cost of long-term oxygen therapy in patients who do not require it. In the NOTT study,[237] 45 per cent of hypoxemic patients initially selected for study improved enough during 3 to 4 weeks of observation and treatment to suspend plans for long-term oxygen therapy. An even longer observation period of 2 or 3 months may be necessary to exclude patients who eventually achieve acceptable PaO$_2$ values on medical therapy

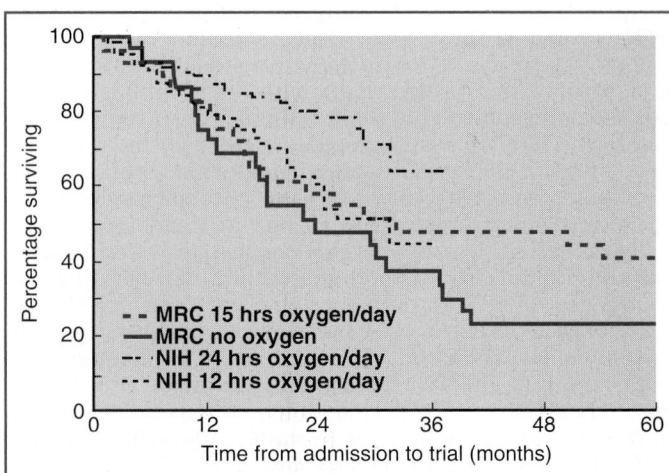

FIGURE 47–17. Survival curves in the MRC (British) and NIH (U.S.) long-term oxygen therapy trials in patients with severe hypoxemia and cor pulmonale. (From Flenley, D. C., and Muir, A. L.: Cardiovascular effects of oxygen therapy for pulmonary arterial hypertension. Clin. Chest Med. *4:*297, 1983.)

alone.[245] Nocturnal oxygen therapy may be important in patients with sleep desaturation.[238,246] Patients with desaturation only during exertion should receive supplemental oxygen during exercise, although the long-term benefits of such therapy remain unproven.[238]

Digitalis

(See also p. 484)

The effect of digitalis on RV function is complex.[5] The cardiac glycosides increase the contractility of the RV myocardium, but they also produce pulmonary vasoconstriction.[247] Furthermore, Sylvester et al.[248] showed that in dogs, digitalis increased the "unstressed reservoir volume" of the circulation through an effect on the peripheral vasculature. This effect reduces venous return and may adversely affect cardiac output.

Digitalis therapy should be used only in patients with cor pulmonale and coexistent LV failure.[200,249–254] For example, Mathur et al.[253] evaluated the effect of 8 weeks of digoxin therapy on resting RV function in patients with severe COPD. All patients were found to have a reduced RVEF at the start of the study. Digoxin therapy did not improve RVEF if the initial LV ejection fraction (LVEF) was normal; only patients with a reduced initial LVEF showed an improvement in RVEF with digoxin. A subsequent study of the effects of 2 weeks of therapy with oral digoxin (0.25 mg per day) in patients with COPD found no improvement in RVEF at rest or during exercise and no increase in maximal exercise performance.[250] Similarly, Mathur et al.[254] also found no improvement in exercise performance in patients with COPD who had had long-term digoxin therapy. Digitalis therapy also causes an increased incidence of adverse side effects (e.g. cardiac arrhythmias) in patients with obstructive lung disease, presumably in part owing to the effect of hypoxia.[255]

Although digoxin is not indicated in the routine hemodynamic management of cor pulmonale, one study indicated that intravenous digoxin improved diaphragm strength and blood flow in patients with COPD who had acute respiratory failure.[256] Therefore, there is a role for digoxin in the management of the acutely decompensated patient.

Theophylline

Theophylline is widely used for its bronchodilator activity.[5] However, sustained-release theophylline reduces dyspnea even in some patients with nonreversible obstructive airways disease.[257] This evidence supports the clinical impression that in some patients with COPD, theophylline may have salutary effects not directly related to bronchodilation.

Theophylline appears to have beneficial cardiovascular effects in patients with COPD with and without cor pulmonale.[221,258,259] Intravenous aminophylline acutely decreases pulmonary artery pressure and increases both RVEF and LVEF. The long-term consequences of oral theophylline therapy on RV function in patients with COPD are also favorable.[260] Eleven patients treated for an average of 4 months had a sustained improvement in RVEF (Fig. 47–18).[260] LVEF also increased slightly.

A combination of reduced afterload (lowered pulmonary and systemic vascular resistance) and enhanced myocardial contractility probably accounts for the improved biventricular pump function with theophylline therapy.[5,258] In isolated papillary muscle preparations, theophylline causes a shift upward and to the right in the force–velocity relationship.[261] In vivo studies in dogs also document an increase in cardiac contractility from aminophylline.[262,263] Other evidence indicates theophylline also probably acts directly to lower vascular resistance.[258,264] In dogs, however, aminophylline does not inhibit acute hypoxic pulmonary vasoconstriction.[265]

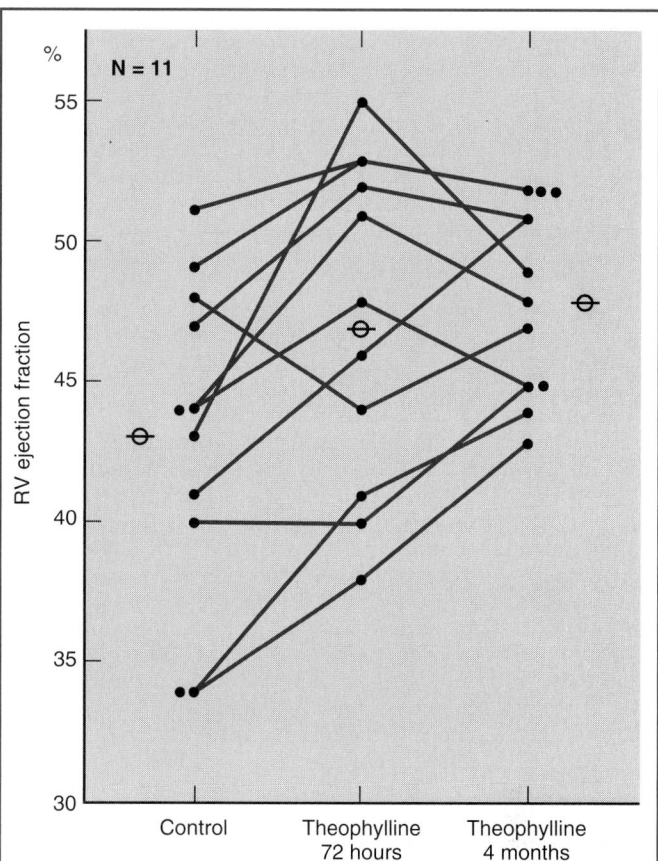

FIGURE 47–18. Oral long-acting theophylline (Theo-Dur) significantly ($p < 0.05$) increased right ventricular ejection fraction (RVEF) after 72 hours and after an average of 4 months of therapy in 11 patients with COPD. (From Matthay, R. A. and Berger, H. J.: Cardiovascular function in cor pulmonale. Clin. Chest Med. 4:269, 1983.)

Beta-Adrenergic Agonists

Although traditionally used as bronchodilators, the selective β_2-adrenergic receptor agonists may have salutary effects in cor pulmonale by causing pulmonary vasodilatation (the human pulmonary circulation contains β-adrenergic receptors) or direct inotropic action on myocardium.[5,221,266–268] In short-term studies, both terbutaline[269–272] and pirbuterol[5,266,273] have been shown to lower pulmonary vascular resistance, increase cardiac output, and increase RVEF and LVEF in most patients with COPD and cor pulmonale. However, these benefits are not sustained during chronic administration (longer than 6 months), especially in patients who are also receiving appropriate supplemental oxygen therapy.[273]

Vasodilators

Assessing the efficacy of vasodilators in COPD is difficult because the hemodynamic changes with therapy are complex, and it has not been established which changes are desirable.[115,221,274,275] Reducing pulmonary hypertension is often the goal of vasodilator therapy, but a fall in vascular resistance may be offset by a rise in cardiac output, leaving the pulmonary artery pressure unchanged.[115] Perhaps this is a beneficial effect (e.g., increased oxygen transport) despite the unrelieved pulmonary hypertension. Conversely, a medication that reduces venous return (nitroglycerin) or depresses RV function (nifedipine) may decrease pulmonary hypertension by lowering cardiac output.[115] This might not be beneficial despite the reduction in pulmonary artery pressure. Long-term studies are needed to evaluate the hemodynamic responses to vasodilators and to assess the overall survival effect of different agents.[115]

Vasodilator therapy may cause such adverse effects as

systemic hypotension and decreased arterial oxygen saturation in patients with pulmonary hypertension.[142,143,276] Most vasodilators affect the systemic circulation more than the pulmonary circulation. In patients with significant pulmonary hypertension and reduced right-sided cardiac output, systemic vasoconstriction may serve as an important protective mechanism to maintain systemic arterial pressure. In these patients, selective dilation of the systemic vasculature may cause hypotension and initiate a vicious circle of right ventricular failure (due to decreased right coronary blood flow) and circulatory collapse.[117] Vasodilators may also lead to arterial hypoxemia by disrupting pulmonary vascular tone, which helps maintain local ventilation-perfusion matching.[5]

The efficacy of various vasodilators has been evaluated in patients with COPD, including nitrates (nitroprusside, nitroglycerin),[266,277] hydralazine,[266,277-287] calcium channel antagonists (verapamil,[288] nifedipine,[289-291] nitrendipine,[292] and felodipine[293]), α-adrenergic antagonists (phentolamine,[294,295] urapidil,[296-298] prazosin[299]), angiotensin-converting enzyme inhibitors (captopril),[300-302] and prostaglandins.[303-305] The results of studies with these agents have been equivocal, and none of these agents is currently used in routine clinical practice. The nitrates appear to have essentially no role because both arterial oxygenation and cardiac index decrease. Therapy with currently available prostaglandins is limited by significant side effects. Some agents (including nifedipine, nitrendipine, urapidil, felodipine, and flosequinan) produce generally favorable short-term benefits, but these benefits are not sustained.

RECOMMENDATIONS. Vasodilator therapy should be considered in patients with COPD only when conventional therapy and oxygen have failed to alleviate signs of RV failure or pulmonary hypertension.[5] Because these agents have potentially adverse consequences,[286] their effects on hemodynamics and oxygenation must be carefully assessed; this usually requires invasive RV catheterization.

Rubin[274,275,306] provides the following guidelines to what constitutes a beneficial hemodynamic response to a vasodilator:

1. Pumonary vascular resistance is reduced by at least 20 per cent, *and*
2. Cardiac output is increased or unchanged, *and*
3. Pulmonary artery pressure is decreased or unchanged, *and*
4. Systemic blood pressure is not significantly reduced (e.g., no side effects.)

If vasodilator therapy produces these benefits, an affected patient should be reassessed after 4 or 5 months of therapy to determine whether the hemodynamic benefits are sustained.

Phlebotomy

Whether phlebotomy is efficacious in polycythemic patients with cor pulmonale is controversial.[5,115] Early studies by Segal and Bishop,[307] using exchange transfusions established that pulmonary artery pressure is more affected by blood volume than blood viscosity. After phlebotomy, in the resting patient, mean pulmonary pressure and pulmonary vascular resistance usually decrease, cardiac output does not significantly change, and systemic oxygen transport falls.[307-310] Despite the decrease in systemic oxygen transport, resting oxygen consumption remained unchanged in most investigations.[308,310] However, Segal and Bishop[307] reported that resting oxygen consumption was lower after phlebotomy, whereas Rakita and coworkers[311] found an increase in oxygen consumption 1 hour after phlebotomy.

The effect of phlebotomy on hemodynamic events during exercise may be more important than the changes observed at rest.[5] Many researchers have found that exercise performance significantly improves in polycythemic patients

subjected to phlebotomy.[307,308,310] Weisse and coworkers[310] studied 12 patients with stable cor pulmonale and hematocrit values above 55 per cent. They were evaluated at baseline (mean hematocrit 61 per cent), after initial phlebotomy (mean hematocrit 50 per cent), and after a second phlebotomy (mean hematocrit 44 per cent). After the first reduction of hematocrit, exercise performance improved; however, no significant changes occurred with the further reduction in hematocrit to normal levels. Similarly, Chetty and colleagues[308] studied 15 patients with moderate to severe COPD (mean FEV$_1$ 970 ml) and marked polycythemia (hematocrit above 55 per cent). Phlebotomy was performed until the hematocrit fell below 52 per cent and was at least five percentage points below the initial value. The mean workload, duration of exercise, and maximal oxygen consumption all increased significantly subsequent to phlebotomy.

In summary, reducing markedly elevated hematocrit to a value of about 50 per cent produces short-term salutary effects on circulatory hemodynamics, especially during exercise.[5] However, whether there are long-term benefits of repeated phlebotomy is unclear. Furthermore, the use of continuous oxygen therapy in appropriately selected patients should reduce the number of patients with COPD who become severely polycythemic. Phlebotomy should be reserved for adjunctive therapy in acute management of the markedly polycythemic patient who has an acute decompensation of cor pulmonale or in the rare patient who remains significantly polycythemic despite appropriate long-term oxygen therapy.[5]

REFERENCES

ETIOLOGIES

1. MacNee, W.: Pathophysiology of cor pulmonale in chronic obstructive pulmonary disease (Part One). Am. J. Respir. Crit. Care Med. *150*:833, 1994.
2. Chronic cor pulmonale: Report of an expert committee. W. H. O. Tech. Rep. Ser. *213*:1, 1961.
3. McFadden, E. R., and Braunwald, E.: Cor pulmonale. *In* Braunwald, E. (ed.): Heart Disease, 4th ed. Philadelphia, W.B. Saunders Company, 1992, pp. 1581–1601.
4. Fowler, N. O.: Chronic cor pulmonale. *In* Fowler, N. O.: Diagnosis of Heart Disease, New York, Springer-Verlag, 1991, pp. 268–282.
5. Wiedemann, H. P., and Matthay, R. A.: Cor pulmonale in chronic obstructive pulmonary disease. Circulatory pathophysiology and management. Clin. Chest Med. *11*:523, 1990.
6. Reid, L. M.: Structure and function in pulmonary hypertension: New perceptions. Chest *89*:279, 1986.
7. Zapol, W., and Snider, M. T.: Pulmonary hypertension in severe acute respiratory failure. N. Engl. J. Med. *296*:476, 1977.
8. Sibbald, W. J., Driedger, A. A., Myers, M. L., et al.: Biventricular function in the adult respiratory distress syndrome: Hemodynamic and radionuclide assessment, with special emphasis on right ventricular function. Chest *84*:126, 1983.
9. Renzetti, Jr., A. D., McClement, J. H., and Litt, B. D.: The Veterans Administration Cooperative Study of Pulmonary Function III. Mortality in relation to respiratory function in chronic obstructive lung disease. Am. J. Med. *41*:115, 1966.
10. Fishman, A. P.: Chronic cor pulmonale. Am. Rev. Respir. Dis. *114*:775, 1976.
11. Stern, R. C., Borkat, G., Hirschfeld, S. S., et al.: Heart failure in cystic fibrosis: Treatment and prognosis of cor pulmonale with failure of the right side of the heart. Am. J. Dis. Child. *134*:267, 1980.
12. Moss, A. J.: The cardiovascular system in cystic fibrosis. Pediatrics *70*:728, 1982.
13. Hughes, J. D., and Rubin, L. J.: Primary pulmonary hypertension: An analysis of 28 cases and a review of the literature. Medicine *65*:56, 1986.

ANATOMICAL AND PATHOPHYSIOLOGICAL CORRELATES

14. Lewis, T.: Observations upon ventricular hypertrophy with special reference to preponderance of one or other chamber. Heart *5*:367, 1914.
15. Emery, J. L., and Mithal, A.: Weight of cardiac ventricles at and after birth. Br. Heart J. *23*:313, 1961.
16. Keen, E. N.: The post-natal development of the human cardiac ventricles. J. Anat. *89*:484, 1955.
17. Arias-Stella, J., and Recavarren, S.: Right ventricular hypertrophy in native children living at high altitude. Am. J. Pathol. *41*:55, 1962.
18. Mathew, R., Thilenius, O. G., and Arcilla, R. A.: Comparative response of right and left ventricles to volume overload. Am. J. Cardiol. *38*:239, 1976.

19. Recavarren, S., and Arias-Stella, J.: Right ventricular hypertrophy in people born and living at high altitudes. Br. Heart J. 26:806, 1964.

20. Penaloza, D., Sime, F., Bancero, N., et al.: Pulmonary hypertension in healthy men born and living at high altitudes. Am. J. Cardiol. 11:150, 1963.

21. Fulton, R. M., Hutchinson, E. C., and Jones, A. M.: Ventricular weight in cardiac hypertrophy. Br. Heart J. 14:413, 1952.

22. Mitchell, R. S., Stanford, R. E., Silvers, G. W., and Dart, G.: The right ventricle in chronic airway obstruction: A clinicopathologic study. Am. Rev. Respir. Dis. 114:147, 1976.

23. Ishikawa, S., Fattal, G. A., Popiewicz, J., and Wyatt, J. P.: Functional morphometry of myocardial fibers in cor pulmonale. Am. Rev. Respir. Dis. 105:358, 1972.

24. Brecher, G. A., and Galletti, P. M.: Functional anatomy of cardiac pumping. In Hamilton, A. F., and Dow, P. (eds.): Handbook of Physiology: Circulation. Vol. II. Washington, D.C., American Physiological Society, 1963, p. 759.

25. Visner, M. S., Arenizen, C. E., O'Connor, M. J., et al.: Alterations in left ventricular three-dimensional dynamic geometry and systolic function during acute right ventricular hypertension in the conscious dog. Circulation 67:353, 1983.

26. Barnard, D., and Alpert, J. S.: Right ventricular function in health and disease. Curr. Prob. Cardiol. 12:417, 1987.

27. Laks, M. M., Garner, D., and Swan, H. J. C.: Volumes and compliances measured simultaneously in the right and left ventricles of the dog. Circ. Res. 20:565, 1967.

28. Abel, F. L., and Waldhausen, J. A.: Effects of alterations in pulmonary vascular resistance on right ventricular function. J. Thorac. Cardiovasc. Surg. 54:886, 1967.

29. Abel, F. L.: Effects of alterations in peripheral resistance on left ventricular function. Proc. Soc. Exp. Biol. Med. 120:52, 1965.

30. Morrison, D., Goldman, S., Wright, A. L., et al.: The effect of pulmonary hypertension on systolic function of the right ventricle. Chest 84:250, 1983.

31. Sarnoff, S. J., and Berglund, E.: Ventricular function. I. Starling's law of the heart studied by means of simultaneous right and left ventricular function curves in the dog. Circulation 8:706, 1954.

32. Spann, J. R., Buccino, R. A., Sonnenblick, E. H., and Braunwald, E. B.: Contractile state of cardiac muscle obtained from cats with experimentally produced ventricular hypertrophy and heart failure. Circ. Res. 21:341, 1967.

33. Haggard, G. E., and Walker, A. M.: The physiology of pulmonary embolism as disclosed by quantitative occlusion of the pulmonary artery. Arch. Surg. 5:763, 1923.

34. Gibbons, J. H., Hopkinson, M., and Churchill, E. D.: Changes in the circulation produced by gradual occlusion of the pulmonary artery. J. Clin. Invest. 11:543, 1932.

35. Fineberg, M. H., and Wiggens, C. J.: Compensation and failure of the right ventricle. Am. Heart J. 11:255, 1936.

36. Brooks, H., Kirk, E. S., Bokonas, P. S., et al.: Performance of the right ventricle under stress: Relation to right coronary flow. J. Clin. Invest. 50:2176, 1971.

37. Meyrick, B., and Reid, L. M.: Pulmonary hypertension: Anatomic and physiologic correlations. Clin. Chest Med. 4:199, 1983.

38. Fishman, A. P.: The normal pulmonary circulation. In Fishman, A. P. (ed.): Pulmonary Diseases and Disorders. 2nd ed. New York, McGraw-Hill, 1991, p. 975–998.

39. Hebb, C.: Motor innervation of the pulmonary blood vessels of mammals. In Fishman, A. P., and Hecht, H. H. (eds.): The Pulmonary Circulation and the Interstitial Space. Chicago, University of Chicago Press, 1969, p. 195.

40. Allen, K. M., Wharton, J., Polak, I. M., and Ghaworth, S. G.: A study of nerves containing peptides in the pulmonary vasculature of healthy infants and children and those with pulmonary hypertension. Br. Heart J. 62:353, 1989.

41. Fishman, A. P.: Dynamics of the pulmonary circulation. In Hamilton, W. F., and Dow, P. (eds.): Handbook of Physiology: Circulation. Vol. II. Washington, D.C., American Physiological Society, 1963, p. 1667.

42. Bard, P.: The pulmonary circulation and respiratory variations in the systemic circulation. In Bard, P. (ed.): Medical Physiology. St. Louis, C. V. Mosby, 1961, p. 231.

43. Brofman, B. L., Charms, B. L., Kohn, P. M., et al.: Unilateral pulmonary artery occlusion in man: Control studies. J. Thorac. Surg. 34:206, 1957.

44. Guyton, A. C.: Circulatory Physiology: Cardiac Output and its Regulation, Philadelphia, W.B. Saunders Company, 1963.

45. Maseri, A., Caldini, P., Howard, P., et al.: Determinants of pulmonary vascular volume-recruitment versus distensibility. Circ. Res. 31:218, 1972.

46. Lanari, A., and Agrest, A.: Pressure-volume relationship in the pulmonary vascular bed. Acta Physiol. Lat. Am. 4:116, 1954.

47. Caro, C. G.: Extensibility of blood vessels in isolated rabbit lung. J. Physiol. (Lond.) 178:193, 1965.

48. Howell, J. B., Permutt, S., Proctor, D. F., and Riley, R. L.: Effect of inflation of the lung on different parts of the pulmonary vascular bed. J. Appl. Physiol. 16:71, 1961.

49. Englebert, J., and DuBois, A. B.: Mechanics of pulmonary circulation in isolated rabbit lungs. Am. J. Physiol. 186:401, 1959.

50. Maseri, A., Calcini, P., Permutt, S., and Zierler, K. L.: Pressure volume relationship in the pulmonary circulation. In Widimsky, J., Daum, S., and Herzog, H. (eds.): Progress in Respiration Research. Vol. 5, Basel, S. Karger, 1970, p. 53.

51. Glazier, J. B., Highes, J. M. B., Maloney, J. E., and West, J. B.: Measurements of capillary dimensions and blood volume in rapidly frozen lungs. J. Appl. Physiol. 26:65, 1969.

52. Grover, R. F.: Chronic hypoxic pulmonary hypertension. In Fishman, A. P. (ed.): The Pulmonary Circulation: Normal and Abnormal. Philadelphia, University of Pennsylvania Press, 1990, pp. 283–299.

53. Fishman, A. P.: Hypoxia and its effects on the pulmonary circulation. Circ. Res. 38:221, 1976.

54. Habb, P. E., and Duranad-Arczynska, W. Y.: Carbon monoxide effects on oxygen transport. In Crystal, R. G., and West, J. B. (eds.): The Lung: Scientific Foundations. New York, Raven Press, 1991, pp. 1267–1276.

55. Fowler, K. T., and Read, J.: Effect of alveolar hypoxia on zonal distribution of pulmonary blood flow. J. Appl. Physiol. 18:244, 1963.

56. Lindsay, D. A., and Reed, L.: Pulmonary vascular responsiveness in the prognosis of chronic obstructive lung disease. Am. Rev. Repair. Dis. 105:242, 1972.

57. Enson, Y., Guintini, C., Lewis, M. L., et al.: The influence of hydrogen ion concentration and hypoxia on the pulmonary circulation. J. Clin. Invest. 43:1146, 1964.

58. Bergofsky, E. H.: Mechanisms underlying vasomotor regulation of regional pulmonary blood flow in normal and disease states. Am. J. Med. 57:378, 1974.

59. Bergofsky, E. H., Haas, F., and Procelli, R. I.: Determination of the sensitive vascular sites from which hypoxia and hypercapnia elicit rises in pulmonary arterial pressure. Fed. Proc. 27:1420, 1968.

60. Bergofsky, E. H.: Humoral control of the pulmonary circulation. Annu. Rev. Physiol. 42:221, 1980.

ASSESSMENT OF PATIENTS WITH COR PULMONALE

61. Arcilla, R. A., Tsai, P., Thilenus, O., and Ranniger, K.: Angiographic method for volume estimation of the right and left ventricles. Chest 60:446–454, 1971.

62. Gentzler, R., Briselli, M., and Gault, J.: Angiographic estimation of right ventricular volume in man. Circulation 4:1, 1974.

63. Fishman, A. P.: State of the art: Chronic cor polmonale. Am. Rev. Respir. Dis. 114:775–794, 1976.

64. Rubin, L. J.: Pulmonary Heart Disease. Boston, Martinus Nijhoff, 1984.

65. Lehtonen, J., Sutinen, S., Ikaheimo, P., and Paako, P.: Electrocardiographic criteria for the diagnosis of right ventricular hypertrophy verified at autopsy. Chest 93:839, 1988.

66. McGowan, F. X., and Wagner, G. S.: The electrocardiogram in chronic lung disease. In Rubin, L. J. (ed.): Pulmonary Heart Disease. Boston, Martinus Nijhoff, 1984, p. 117.

67. Goodwin, J. F., and Abdin, Z. N.: The cardiogram of congenital and acquired right ventricular hypertrophy. Br. Heart. J. 21:523, 1959.

68. Phillips, R. W.: The electrocardiogram in cor pulmonale secondary to pulmonary emphysema: A study of 18 cases proved by autopsy. Am. Heart J. 56:352, 1958.

69. Kilcoyne, M. M., Davis, A. L., and Ferrer, M. I.: A dynamic electrocardiographic concept useful in the diagnosis of cor pulmonale. Circulation 42:903, 1970.

70. Holford, F. D.: The electrocardiogram in pulmonary disease. In Fishman, A. P. (ed.): Pulmonary Diseases and Disorders. 2nd ed. New York, McGraw-Hill, 1991, pp. 471–478.

71. Matthay, R. A., and Shub, C.: Imaging techniques for assessing pulmonary artery hypertension and right ventricular performance with special reference to COPD. J. Thorac. Imaging 5:47, 1990.

72. Matthay, R. A., and Berger, H. J.: Noninvasive assessment of right and left ventricular function in acute and chronic respiratory failure. Crit. Care Med. 11:329, 1983.

73. Matthay, R. A., Schwarz, M. I., Ellis, H., Jr., et al.: Pulmonary artery hypertension in chronic obstructive pulmonary disease: Chest radiographic assessment. Invest. Radiol. 16:95, 1981.

74. Chang, C. H.: The normal roentgenographic measurement of the right descending pulmonary artery in 1,085 cases. Am. J. Roentgenol. 87:929, 1962.

75. Chetty, K. G., Brown, S. E., and Light, R. W.: Identification of pulmonary hypertension in chronic obstructive pulmonary disease from routine chest radiographs. Am. Rev. Respir. Dis. 126:338, 1982.

76. Berger, H. J., Matthay, R. A., Loke, J., et al.: Assessment of cardiac performance with quantitative radionuclide angiography: Right ventricular ejection fraction with reference to findings in chronic obstructive pulmonary disease. Am. J. Cardiol. 41:897, 1978.

77. Oliver, R. M., Fleming, J. S., and Waller, D. G.: Right ventricular function at rest and exercise in chronic obstructive pulmonary disease: Comparison of two radionuclide techniques. Chest 103:74, 1993.

78. Maddahi, J., Bermon, D. S., Matsuoka, D. T., et al.: A new technique for assessing right ventricular ejection fraction using rapid multiple gated equilibrium cardiac blood pool scintigraphy. Circulation 60:581, 1979.

79. Xue, Q. F., MacNee, W., Flenley, D. C., et al.: Can right ventricular performance be assessed by gated equilibrium ventriculography? Thorax 38:486, 1983.

80. Matthay, R. A., and Berger, J. J.: Cardiovascular function in cor pulmonale. Clin. Chest. Med. 4:269, 1983.

81. MacNee, W., Xue, Q. F., Hannan, W. J., et al.: Assessment by radionuclide angiography of right and left ventricular function in chronic bronchitis and emphysema. Thorax 38:494–500, 1983.

82. Jain, D., and Zaret, B. J.: Assessment of right ventricular function: Role of nuclear imaging techniques. Cardiol. Clin. 10:23, 1992.

83. Brent, B. N., Berger, H. J., Matthay, R. A., et al.: Physiologic correlates

of right ventricular ejection fraction in chronic obstructive pulmonary disease: A combined radionuclide and hemodynamic study. Am. J. Cardiol. *50:*255, 1982.

84. Brent, B. N., Mahler, D. A., Matthay, R. A., et al.: Noninvasive diagnosis of pulmonary arterial hypertension in chronic obstructive pulmonary disease: Right ventricular ejection fraction at rest. Am. J. Cardiol. *53:*1349, 1984.

85. Cohen, H. A., Baird, M. G., Rouleau, J. R., et al.: Thallium 201 myocardial imaging in patients with pulmonary hypertension. Circulation *54:*790, 1976.

86. Khaja, F., Alam, M., Goldstein, S., Anbe, D. T., and Marks, D. S.: Diagnostic value of visualization of the right ventricle using Thallium 201 myocardial imaging. Circulation *59:*182, 1979.

87. Ohsuzu, F., Handa, S., Kondo, M., et al.: Thallium 201 myocardial imaging to evaluate right ventricular overloading. Circulation *61:*620, 1980.

88. Berger, H., Wackers, F., Mahler, D., et al.: Right ventricular visualization of Thallium 201 myocardial images in chronic obstructive pulmonary disease: Relationship to right ventricular function and hypertrophy (abstract). Circulation *62:*111, 1980.

89. Weitzenblum, E., Moyses, B., Dickele, M., and Methlin, G.: Detection of right ventricular pressure overloading by Thallium 201 myocardial scintigraphy: Results in 57 patients with chronic respiratory diseases. Chest *85:*164, 1984.

90. Kondo, M., Unbo, A., Yamafaki, H., et al.: Thallium-201 myocardial imaging for evaluation of right ventricular overloading. J. Nucl. Med. *19:*1197, 1978.

91. Shiller, N. B., and Sahn, D. J.: Pulmonary pressure measurement by Doppler and two-dimensional echocardiography in adult and paediatric populations. *In* Weir, E. K., Archer, S. L., and Reeves, J. T. (eds.): The Diagnosis and Treatment of Pulmonary Hypertension. New York, Futura, 1992, pp. 41–59.

92. Migueres, M., Escamilla, R., Coca, F., et al.: Pulsed Doppler echocardiography in the diagnosis of pulmonary hypertension in COPD. Chest *98:*280, 1990.

93. Morpurgo, M., Saviotti, M., Dickele, M. C., et al.: Echocardiographic aspect of pulmonary arterial hypertension in chronic lung disease. Bull. Eur. Physiopathol. Respir. *20:*251, 1984.

94. Macharaoui, A., von Dryander, S., Hinrichsen, M., et al.: Two dimensional echocardiographic assessment of right cardiac pressure overload in patients with chronic obstructive airway disease. Respiration *60:*65, 1993.

95. Trivedi, H. S., Joshi, M. N., and Gamade, A. R.: Echocardiography and pulmonary artery pressure: Correlation in chronic obstructive pulmonary disease. J. Postgrad. Med. *38:*24, 1992.

96. Burghuber, O. C., Brummer, C. H., Schenk, P., and Weissel, M.: Pulsed Doppler echocardiography to assess pulmonary artery hypertension in chronic obstructive pulmonary disease. Monaldi Arch. Chest Dis. *48:*121, 1993.

97. Marangoni, S., Sealvini, S., Schena, M., et al.: Right ventricular diastolic function in chronic obstructive lung disease. Eur. Respir. J. *5:*438, 1992.

98. Yock, P. J., and Popp, R. L.: Non-invasive estimation of right ventricular systolic pressure by Doppler ultrasound in patients with tricuspid regurgitation. Circulation *70:*657, 1984.

99. Masuyama, T., Kodama, K., Kitabatakem, A., et al.: Continuous wave Doppler echocardiographic detection of pulmonary regurgitation and its application to noninvasive estimation of pulmonary arterial pressure. Circulation *74:*484, 1986.

100. Stevenson, G., Kawabori, I., and Guntheroth, W.: The validation of Doppler diagnosis of tricuspid regurgitation. Circulation *64:*255, 1981.

101. Tramarin, R., Torbicki, A., Marchandise, B., et al.: Doppler echocardiographic evaluation of pulmonary artery pressure in chronic obstructive pulmonary disease. A European multicentre study. Eur. Heart J. *12:*103, 1991.

102. Berger, M., Hecht, S., Van Tosh, A., and Lingam, U.: Pulse and continuous wave Doppler echocardiographic assessment of valvular regurgitation in normal subjects. J. Am. Coll. Cardiol. *113:*1540, 1989.

103. Morrison, D. A., Ovitt, T., and Hammermeister, K. E.: Functional tricuspid regurgitation and right ventricular dysfunction in pulmonary hypertension. Am. J. Cardiol. *62:*108, 1988.

104. Himelman, R. B., Stulbarg, K., Kircher, B., et al.: Noninvasive evaluation of pulmonary arterial pressure during exercise by saline enhanced Doppler echocardiography in chronic pulmonary disease. Circulation *79:*683, 1989.

105. Beard, J. T., and Byrd, B. F.: Saline contrast enhancement of trivial tricuspid regurgitation signals for estimating pulmonary artery pressure. Am. J. Cardiol. *62:*486, 1988.

106. Laaban, J. P., Diebold, B., Raffoul, H., et al.: Noninvasive estimation of systolic pulmonary arterial pressure (Pps) using continuous wave Doppler ultrasound in COPD. Am. Rev. Respir. Dis. *137:*150, 1988.

107. Mitchell, R. S., Stanford, R. E., Silvers, G. W., and Dart, G.: The right ventricle in chronic airway obstruction: A clinico-pathologic study. Am. Rev. Respir. Dis. *11:*147, 1976.

108. Murphy, M. L.: The pathology of the right heart in chronic hypertrophy and failure. *In* Fisk, R. L. (ed.): The Right Heart. Philadelphia, F. A. Davis, 1987, pp. 159–167.

109. Konstam, M. A., and Levine, H. A.: Effects of afterload and preload on right ventricular systolic performance. *In* Konstam, M. A., Isner, J. (eds.): The Right Ventricle. Boston, Kluwer Academic, 1988, pp. 17–35.

110. Langmore, D. B., Kerpstein, R. H., Underwood, S. R., et al.: Dimen-

sional accuracy of magnetic resonance studies of the heart. Lancet *1:*1360, 1985.

111. Turnbull, L. W., Ridgeway, J. P., Biernacki, W., et al.: Assessment of the right ventricle by magnetic resonance imaging in chronic obstructive lung disease. Thorax *45:*597, 1990.

112. Wacker, C. M., Schad, L. R., Behling, U., et al.: The pulmonary artery acceleration time determined with the MR-RACE-technique: comparison to pulmonary artery mean pressure in 12 patients. Magn. Reson. Imaging *12:*25, 1994.

113. Saito, H., Dambura, T., Aiba, M., Suzuki, T., and Kira, S.: Evaluation of cor pulmonale on a modified short-axis section of the heart by magnetic resonance imaging. Am. Rev. Respir. Dis. *146:*1576, 1992.

114. Pattynama, P. M., Willems, L. N., Smith, A. H., et al.: Early diagnosis of cor pulmonale with MR imaging of the right ventricle. Radiology *182:*375, 1992.

ACUTE COR PULMONALE

115. Wiedemann, H. P., and Matthay, R. A.: The management of acute and chronic cor pulmonale. *In* Scharf, S. M., and Cassidy, S. S. (eds.): Heart-Lung Interactions in Health and Disease. New York, Marcel Dekker, Inc., 1989, pp. 915–981.

116. Guyton, A. C., Lindsey, A. W., and Gilluly, J. J.: The limits of right ventricular compensation following acute increases in pulmonary circulatory resistance. Circ. Res. *2:*326, 1954.

117. Wiedemann, H. P., and Matthay, R. A.: Acute right heart failure. Crit. Care Clin. *1:*631, 1985.

118. Brooks, H., Holland, R., and Al-Sadir, J.: Right ventricular performance during ischemia: An anatomic and hemodynamic analysis. Am. J. Physiol. *233:*500, 1977.

119. Spotnitz, H. M., Berman, M. A., and Epstein, S. E.: Pathophysiology and experimental treatment of acute pulmonary embolism. Am. Heart J. *82:*511, 1971.

120. Fixler, D. E., Archie, J. P., Ullyot, D. J., et al.: Effects of acute right ventricular systolic hypertension on regional myocardial blood flow in anesthetized dogs. Am. Heart J. *85:*491, 1973.

121. Manohar, M., Tranquilli, W. J., Parks, C. M., et al.: Regional myocardial blood flow and coronary vasodilator reserve during acute right ventricular failure due to pressure overload in swine. J. Surg. Res. *31:*382, 1981.

122. Cooper, N., Brazier, J., and Buckberg, G.: Effects of systemic-pulmonary shunts on regional myocardial blood flow in experimental pulmonary stenosis. J. Thorac. Cardiovasc. Surg. *70:*166, 1975.

123. Vlahakes, G. J., Turley, K., and Hoffman, J. I. E.: The pathophysiology of failure in acute right ventricular hypertension: Hemodynamic and biochemical correlations. Circulation *63:*87, 1981.

124. Molloy, W. D., Lee, K. Y., Girling, L., et al.: Treatment of shock in a canine model of pulmonary embolus. Am. Rev. Respir. Dis. *130:*870, 1984.

125. Ghignone, M., Girling, L., and Prewitt, R. M.: Volume expansion versus norepinephrine in treatment of a low cardiac output complicating an acute increase in right ventricular afterload in dogs. Anesthesiology *60:*132, 1984.

126. Scharf, S. M., Warner, K. G., Josa, M., et al.: Load tolerance of the right ventricle: Effect of increased aortic pressure. J. Crit. Care. *1:*163, 1986.

127. Laks, M. M., Garner, D., and Swan, H. J. C.: Volumes and compliances measured simultaneously in the right and left ventricles of the dog. Circ. Res. *20:*565, 1967.

128. Taylor, R. R., Covell, J. W., Sonnenblick, E. H., and Ross, J., Jr.: Dependence of ventricular distensibility on filling of the opposite ventricle. Am. J. Physiol. *213:*711, 1982.

129. Kelly, D. T., Spotnitz, H. M., Beiser, G. D., et al.: Effects of chronic right ventricular volume and pressure loading on left ventricular performance. Circulation *44:*403, 1971.

130. Stool, E. W., Mullins, C. B., Leshin, S. J., and Mitchell, J. H.: Dimensional changes of the left ventricle during acute pulmonary arterial hypertension in dogs. Am. J. Cardiol. *33:*868, 1974.

131. Weyman, A. E., Warn, S., Feigenbaum, H., and Dillon, J. C.: Mechanism of abnormal septal motion in patients with right ventricular volume overload: A cross-sectional echocardiographic study. Circulation *27:*594, 1963.

132. Goldstein, J. A., Vlahakes, G. J., Verrier, E. D., et al.: The role of right ventricular systolic dysfunction and elevated intrapericardial pressures in the genesis of low output in experimental right ventricular infarction. Circulation *65:*513, 1982.

133. Laver, M. B., Strauss, H. W., and Phost, G. M.: Right and left ventricular geometry: Adjustments during acute respiratory failure. Crit. Care Med. *7:*509, 1979.

134. Sibbald, W. J., Driedger, A. A., Myers, M. L., et al.: Biventricular function in the adult respiratory distress syndrome: Hemodynamic and radionuclide assessment, with special emphasis on right ventricular function. Chest *84:*126, 1983.

135. Guyton, A. C.: Determination of cardiac output by equating venous return curves with cardiac response curves. Physiol. Rev. *35:*123, 1955.

136. Goldberg, H. S., and Rabson, J.: Control of cardiac output by systemic vessels: Circulatory adjustments to acute and chronic respiratory failure and the effect of therapeutic intervention. Am. J. Cardiol. *47:*696, 1981.

137. Rothe, C. F.: Physiology of venous return: An unappreciated boost to the heart. Arch. Intern. Med. *146:*977, 1986.

138. Ghignone, M., Girling, L., Prewitt, R. M.: Effect of increased pulmonary vascular resistance (PVR) and treatment on right ventricular perform-

ance in acute respiratory failure (ARF). Am. Rev. Respir. Dis. *125*:99, 1982.

139. Paetkau, D., Kettner, J., Girling, L., et al.: What is the appropriate therapy to maintain cardiac output as pulmonary vascular resistance increases? Anesthesiology 57:A56, 1982.

140. Prewitt, R. M., and Ghignone, M.: Treatment of right ventricular dysfunction in acute respiratory failure. Crit. Care. Med. 11:346, 1983.

141. Prewitt, R. M., Matthay, M. A., and Ghignone, M.: Hemodynamic management in the adult respiratory distress syndrome. Clin. Chest. Med. *4*:251, 1983.

142. Rubin, L. J.: Cardiovascular effects of vasodilator therapy for pulmonary arterial hypertension. Clin. Chest Med. *4*:309, 1983.

143. Packer, M.: Vasodilator therapy for primary pulmonary hypertension. Ann. Intern. Med. *103*:258, 1985.

144. Melot, C., Hallemans, R., Naeije, R., et al.: Deleterious effect of nifedipine on pulmonary gas exchange in chronic obstructive pulmonary disease. Am. Rev. Respir. Dis. *130*:612, 1984.

145. Harrison, W. D., Raizen, N., Ghignone, M., et al.: Treatment of canine low pressure pulmonary edema. Nitroprusside versus hydralazine. Am. Rev. Respir. Dis. *128*:857, 1983.

146. Benoit, A., Ducas, J., Girling, L., et al.: Acute cardiopulmonary effects of nitroglycerin in canine oleic acid pulmonary edema. Anesthesiology *62*:754, 1985.

147. Ghignone, M., Girling, L., and Prewitt, R. M.: Effects of vasodilators on canine cardiopulmonary function when a decrease in cardiac output complicates an increase in right ventricular afterload. Am. Rev. Respir. Dis. *131*:527, 1985.

148. Bishop, M. J., and Cheney, F. W.: Vasodilators worsen gas exchange in dog oleic-acid lung injury. Anesthesiology *64*:435, 1986.

149. Zapol, W. M., and Snider, M. T.: Pulmonary hypertension in severe acute respiratory failure. N. Engl. J. Med. *296*:476, 1977.

150. Martyn, J. A. J., Snider, M. T., Szyfelbein, S. K., et al.: Right ventricular dysfunction in acute thermal injury. Ann. Surg. *191*:330, 1980.

151. Her, C.: Right ventricular stroke-work: An index of distribution of pulmonary perfusion in acute respiratory failure. Chest *84*:719, 1983.

152. Sibbald, W. J., and Driedger, A. A.: Right ventricular function in acute disease states: Pathophysiologic considerations. Crit. Care Med. *11*:339, 1983.

153. Rossaint, R., Falke, K. J., and Lopez, F.: Inhaled nitric oxide for the adult respiratory distress syndrome. N. Engl. J. Med. *328*:399, 1993.

154. Parr, G. V. S., Pierce, W. S., Rosenberg, G., and Waldhausen, J. A.: Right ventricular failure after repair of left ventricular aneurysm. J. Thorac. Cardiovasc. Surg. *80*:79, 1980.

155. Prewitt, R. M., Girling, L., and Ghignone, M.: Effects of increased pulmonary vascular resistance (PVR) on right ventricular (RV) function in canine acute respiratory failure. Am. Rev. Respir. Dis. *125*:99, 1982.

156. Vlahakes, G. J., Turley, K., and Hoffman, J. I. E.: The pathophysiology of failure in acute right ventricular hypertension: Hemodynamic and biochemical correlations. Circulation *63*:87, 1981.

CHRONIC COR PULMONALE

157. Williams, M. H., Jr., Adler, J. J., and Colp, C.: Pulmonary function studies as an aid in the differential diagnosis of pulmonary hypertension. Am. J. Med. *47*:378, 1969.

158. White, J., Bullock, R. E., Hudgson, P., and Gibson, G. J.: Neuromuscular disease, respiratory failure and cor pulmonale. Postgrad. Med. J. *68*:820, 1992.

159. Davis, J. N., Goldman, M., Loh, L., et al.: Diaphragm function and alveolar hypoventilation. Q. J. Med. *45*:87, 1976.

160. Glenn, W. W. L., Holcomb, W. C., Hogan, J., et al.: Diaphragm pacing by radiofrequency transmission in the treatment of chronic ventilatory insufficiency: Present status. J. Thorac. Cardiovasc. Surg. *66*:606, 1973.

161. Aubier, M., DeTroyer, A., Sampson, M., et al.: Aminophylline improves diaphragmatic contractility. N. Engl. J. Med. *305*:249, 1981.

162. Chandler, K. W., Roxas, C. J., Kory, R. C., and Goldman, A. L.: Bilateral diaphragmatic paralysis complicating local cardiac hypothermia during open heart surgery. Am. J. Med. *77*:243, 1984.

163. Bergofsky, E. H.: Respiratory failure in disorders of the thoracic cage. Am. Rev. Respir. Dis. *119*:643, 1979.

164. Bergofsky, E. H., Turino, G. M., and Fishman, A. P.: Respiratory impairment and airway closure in patients with untreated idiopathic scoliosis. Medicine *38*:263, 1959.

165. Bijure, J., Grimby, G., Kasalicky, J., et al.: Respiratory impairment and airway closure in patients with untreated idiopathic scoliosis. Thorax *25*:451, 1970.

166. Davies, G., and Reid, L.: Effect of scoliosis on growth of alveoli and pulmonary arteries and on the right ventricle. Arch. Dis. Child. *46*:623, 1971.

167. Westgate, H. D., and Moe, J. H.: Pulmonary function in kyphoscoliosis before and after correction by the Harrington instrumentation method. J. Bone Joint Surg. *51*:935, 1969.

168. Mellins, R. B., Balfour, H. H., Jr., Turino, G. M., and Winters, R. W.: Failure of automatic control of ventilation (Ondine's curse). Medicine *49*:487, 1970.

169. Burwell, C. S., Robin, E. D., Whaley, R. D., and Bickelman, A. G.: Extreme obesity associated with alveolar hypoventilation: A pickwickian syndrome. Am. J. Med. *21*:811, 1956.

170. Rochester, D. F., and Enson, Y.: Current concepts in the pathogenesis of the obesity-hypoventilation syndrome. Am. J. Med. *57*:402, 1974.

171. Weil, J. V.: Pulmonary Hypertension and Cor Pulmonale in Hypoventilation. Mount Kisco, N.Y., Futura Publishing Co., 1984, p. 321.

172. Cherniack, N. S.: Respiratory dysrhythmias during sleep. N. Engl. J. Med. *305*:325, 1981.

173. Millman, R. P., and Fishman, A. P.: Sleep apnea syndromes. *In* Fishman, A. P. (ed.): Pulmonary Diseases and Disorders. 2nd ed. New York, McGraw-Hill Book Co., 1991, pp. 1347–1362.

174. Strohl, K. P., Cherniack, N. S., and Gather, B.: Physiologic basis of therapy in sleep apnea. Am. Rev. Respir. Dis. *134*:791, 1986.

175. Khoo, M. C. K.: Periodic breathing. *In* Crystal, R. G., and West, J. B. (eds.): The Lung: Scientific Foundations. New York, Raven Press, 1991, pp. 1419–1432.

176. Burrek, B.: The hypersomina-sleep apnea syndrome: Its recognition in clinical cardiology. Am. Heart J. *107*:543, 1984.

177. Shephard, J. W., Jr.: Hypotension, cardiac arrhythmias, myocardial infarction, and stroke in relation to obstructive sleep apnea. Clin. Chest Med. *13*:437, 1992.

178. Guilleminault, C., Cannally, S. J., and Winkler, R. A.: Cardiac arrhythmia and conduction disturbances during sleep in 400 patients with sleep apnea syndrome. Am. J. Cardiol. *52*:490, 1983.

179. Peiser, J., Ovnat, A., Uwyyed, K., et al.: Cardiac arrhythmias during sleep in morbidly obese sleep-apneic patients before and after gastric bypass surgery. Clin. Cardiol. *8*:519, 1985.

180. Buda, A. J., Schroeder, J. S., and Gulleminault, C.: Abnormalities of pulmonary wedge pressures in sleep-induced apnea. Int. J. Cardiol. *1*:67, 1981.

181. Moldofsky, H.: Evaluation of daytime sleepiness. Clin. Chest Med. *13*:417, 1992.

182. Kryger, M. H.: Management of obstructive sleep apnea. Clin. Chest Med. *13*:481, 1992.

183. Bradley, T. D.: Right and left ventricular functional impairment and sleep apnea. Clin. Chest Med. *13*:459, 1992.

184. Fletcher, E. C., Schaaf, J. W., Miller, J., and Fletcher, J. G.: Long term cardiopulmonary sequelae in patients with sleep apnea and chronic lung disease. Am. Rev. Respir. Dis. *135*:525, 1987.

185. Weitzenblum, E., Krieger, J., Apprill, M., et al.: Daytime pulmonary hypertension in patients with obstructive sleep apnea syndrome. Am. Rev. Respir. Dis. *138*:345, 1988.

186. Weitzenblum, E., Krieger, J., Oswald, M., et al.: Chronic obstructive pulmonary disease and sleep apnea syndrome. Sleep *15*(Suppl. 6):S33, 1992.

187. Hudgel, D. W.: The role of upper airway anatomy and physiology in obstructive sleep apnea. Clin. Chest Med. *13*:383, 1992.

188. Bradley, T. D., and Phillipson, E. A.: Central sleep apnea. Clin. Chest Med. *13*:493, 1992.

189. Martin, R. J., Sanders, M. H., Gray, B. A., and Pennock, B. E.: Acute and long-term ventilatory effects of hyperoxia in adult sleep apnea syndrome. Am. Rev. Respir. Dis. *125*:175, 1982.

190. Bland, J. W., Edwards, F. K., and Brainsfield, D.: Pulmonary hypertension and congestive heart failure in children with chronic upper airway obstruction: New concepts and etiologic factors. Am. J. Cardiol. *23*:830, 1969.

191. Randall, C. S., Braman, S. S., and Millman, R. P.: Rapid development of cor pulmonale following acute tonsillitis in adults. Chest *95*:462, 1989.

192. Noonan, J. A.: Pulmonary heart disease. Pediatr. Clin. North Am. *18*:1255, 1971.

193. Johnson, G. M., and Todd, D. W.: Cor pulmonale in severe Pierre Robin syndrome. Pediatrics *65*:152, 1980.

194. Glenn, W. W. L., Gee, J. B. L., Cole, D. R., et al.: Combined central alveolar hypoventilation and upper airway obstruction. Treatment by tracheostomy and diaphragm pacing. Am. J. Med. *64*:50, 1978.

195. Ingram, R. H., Jr., and Bishop, J. B.: Ventilatory response to carbon dioxide after removal of chronic upper airway obstruction. Am. Rev. Respir. Dis. *102*:645, 1970.

196. Ungerer, R. G., Tashkin, D. P., Furst, D., et al.: Prevalence and clinical correlates of pulmonary arterial hypotension in progressive systemic sclerosis. Am. J. Med. *75*:65, 1983.

197. Young, R. H., and Mark, G. S.: Pulmonary vascular changes in scleroderma. Am. J. Med. *64*:998, 1978.

198. Wright, J. L., Lawson, L., Pare, P. D., et al.: The structure and function of the pulmonary vasculature in mild chronic obstructive pulmonary disease: The effect of oxygen and exercise. Am. Rev. Respir. Dis. *128*:702, 1983.

199. Calverley, P. M., Howatson, R., Flenley, D. C., and Lamb, D.: Clinicopathological correlations in cor pulmonale. Thorax *47*:494, 1992.

200. Arroliga, A. C., Matthay, M. A., and Matthay, R. A.: Pulmonary thromboembolism and other pulmonary vascular diseases. *In* George, R. B., Light, R. W., Matthay, M. A., and Matthay, R. A. (eds.): Chest Medicine: Essentials of Pulmonary and Critical Care Medicine. 3rd ed. Baltimore, Williams and Wilkins, 1995, pp. 271–302.

201. Boushy, J. F., and North, L. B.: Hemodynamic changes in chronic obstructive pulmonary disease. Chest *72*:565, 1977.

202. Weitzenblum, E., Loisceau, A., Hirth, C., et al.: Course of pulmonary hemodynamics in patients with chronic obstructive pulmonary disease. Chest *75*:565, 1979.

203. Weitzenblum, E., Sautegeau, A., Ehrhart, M., et al.: Long-term course of pulmonary arterial pressure in chronic obstructive pulmonary disease. Am. Rev. Respir. Dis. *130*:993–998, 1984.

204. Bishop, J. M., and Cross, K. W.: Use of other physiological variables to predict pulmonary arterial pressure in patients with chronic respiratory disease: Multicenter study. Eur. Heart J. *2*:509, 1981.

205. Bishop, J. M., and Cross, K. W.: Physiological variables and mortality in patients with various categories of chronic respiratory disease: WHO multicenter study. Eur. Heart J. *2*:509, 1981.

206. Oswald-Mammosser, M., Apprill, M., Bachez, P., et al.: Pulmonary hemodynamics in chronic obstructive pulmonary disease of the emphysematous type. Respiration *58*:304, 1991.

207. Mahler, D. A., Brent, B. N., Loke, J., et al.: Right ventricular performance and central circulatory hemodynamics during upright exercise in patients with chronic obstructive pulmonary disease. Am. Rev. Respir. Dis. *130*:722, 1984.

208. Hicken, P., Brewer, D., and Heath, D.: The relation between the weight of the right ventricle of the heart and the internal surface area and the number of alveoli in the human lung in emphysema. J. Pathol. Bacteriol. *92*:529, 1966.

209. Biernacki, W., Gould, G. A., Whyte, K. F., and Flenley, D. C.: Pulmonary hemodynamics, gas exchange and the severity of emphysema as assessed by quantitative CT scan in chronic bronchitis and emphysema. Am. Rev. Respir. Dis. *139*:1509, 1989.

210. Jamal, K., Fleetham, J. A., and Thurlbeck, W. M.: Cor pulmonale: Correlation with central airways lesions, peripheral airways lesions, emphysema, and control of breathing. Am. Rev. Respir. Dis. *141*:1172, 1990.

211. Hasleton, P. S., Heath, D., and Brewer, D. B.: Hypertensive pulmonary vascular disease in states of chronic hypoxia. J. Pathol. Bacteriol. *95*:431, 1968.

212. Lamb, D.; Pathology of COPD. *In* Brewis, R. A. L., Gibson, G. J., and Geddes, D. M. (eds.): Respiratory Medicine. London, Baillière Tindall, 1990, pp. 497–507.

213. Wilkinson, M., Langhorn, C. A., Heath, D., et al.: A pathophysiological study of 10 cases of hypoxic cor pulmonale. Q. J. Med. *66*:65, 1988.

214. Wright, J. L., Lawson, L., Pare, P. D., et al.: The structure and function of pulmonary vasculature in mild chronic obstructive pulmonary disease: the effect of oxygen on exercise. Am. Rev. Respir. Dis. *128*:702, 1983.

215. Magee, F., Wright, J. L., Wiggs, B. R., et al.: Pulmonary vascular structure and function in chronic obstructive pulmonary disease. Thorax *43*:183, 1988.

216. Crawley, D. E., Liu, S. F., Evans, T. W., and Barnes, P. J.: Inhibitory role of endothelium-derived relaxing factor in rat and human pulmonary arteries. Br. J. Pharmacol. *101*:166, 1990.

217. Liu, S. F., Crawley, D. E., Barnes, P. J., and Evans, T. W.: Endothelium-derived relaxing factor inhibits hypoxic pulmonary vasoconstriction in rats. Am. Rev. Respir. Dis. *143*:32, 1991.

218. Dinh-Xuan, A. T.: Endothelial modulation of pulmonary vascular tone. Eur. Respir. J. *5*:757, 1992.

219. Din-Xuan, A. T., Higenbottam, T. W., Clelland, C. A., et al.: Impairment of endothelium-dependent pulmonary artery relaxation in chronic obstructive lung disease. N. Engl. J. Med. *324*:1539, 1991.

220. Adnot, S., Raffestin, B., Addahibi, S., et al.: Loss of endothelium-dependent relaxant activity in the pulmonary circulation of rats exposed to chronic hypoxia. J. Clin. Invest. *87*:155, 1991.

221. MacNee, W.: Pathophysiology of cor pulmonale in chronic obstructive pulmonary disease (Part 2). Am. J. Respir. Crit. Care Med. *150*:1158, 1994.

222. Weitzenblum, E., Apprill, M., Oswald, M., et al.: Pulmonary hemodynamics in patients with chronic obstructive pulmonary disease before and during an episode of peripheral edema. Chest *105*:1377, 1994.

223. Fulton, F. M., Hutchison, E. C., and Jones, A. M.: Ventricular weight in cardiac hypertrophy. Br. Heart J. *14*:413, 1952.

224. Heath, D., and Williams, D. R.: Man at High Altitude. Edinburgh, Churchill Livingstone, 1981.

225. Farber, M. O., Bright, T. P., Strawbridge, R. A., et al.: Impaired water handling in chronic obstructive lung disease. J. Lab. Clin. Med. *85*:41, 1975.

226. Farber, M. O., Kiblawi, S. S. O., Strawbridge, R. A., et al.: Studies on plasma vasopressin and the renin-angiotensin-aldosterone system in chronic obstructive lung disease. J. Lab. Clin. Med. *90*:373, 1977.

227. Campbell, E. J. M., and Short, D. S.: The cause of oedema in 'cor pulmonale.' Lancet *1*:1184, 1960.

228. Kawakami, Y., Kishi, F., Yamamoto, H., et al.: Relation of oxygen delivery, mixed venous oxygenation, and pulmonary hemodynamics to prognosis in chronic obstructive pulmonary disease. N. Engl. J. Med. *308*:1045, 1983.

229. Albert, R. K., Schrijen, F., and Poincelot, F.: Oxygen consumption and transport in stable patients with chronic obstructive pulmonary disease. Am. Rev. Respir. Dis. *134*:678, 1986.

230. Chappell, T. R., Rubin, L. J., Markham, R. V., Jr., et al.: Independence of oxygen consumption and systemic oxygen transport in patients with either stable pulmonary hypertension or refractory left ventricular failure. Am. Rev. Respir. Dis. *128*:30, 1983.

231. Tenney, S. M., and Mithoefer, J. D.: The relationship of mixed oxygenation to oxygen transport, with special reference to adaptations to high altitude and pulmonary disease. Am. Rev. Respir. Dis. *125*:474, 1982.

232. Mithoefer, J. C.: Assessment of tissue oxygenation. *In* Simmons, D. H. (ed.): Current Pulmonology. Vol. 4. New York, John Wiley and Sons, 1982, p. 215.

233. Bergorsky, E. H.: Tissue oxygen delivery and cor pulmonale in chronic obstructive pulmonary disease. N. Engl. J. Med. *308*:1092, 1983.

234. Burrows, B., Kettel, K. J., Niden, A. H., et al.: Patterns of cardiovascular dysfunction in chronic obstructive lung disease. N. Engl. J. Med. *286*:912, 1972.

235. Howard, P.: Drugs or oxygen for hypoxic cor pulmonale? Br. Med. J. *287*:1159, 1983.

236. Medical Research Council Working Party: Long term domiciliary oxygen therapy in chronic hypoxic cor pulmonale complicating chronic bronchitis and emphysema: A clinical trial. Lancet *1*:681, 1981.

237. Nocturnal Oxygen Therapy Trial Group: Continuous or nocturnal oxygen therapy in hypoxemic chronic obstructive lung disease. Ann. Intern. Med. *93*:931, 1980.

238. Anthonisen, N. R.: Long-term oxygen therapy. Ann. Intern. Med. *99*:519, 1983.

239. Flenley, D. C., and Muir, A. L.: Cardiovascular effects of oxygen therapy for pulmonary arterial hypertension. Clin. Chest. Med. *4*:297, 1983.

240. Heaton, R. K., Grant, I., McSweeny, A. J., et al.: Psychologic effects of continuous and nocturnal oxygen therapy in hypoxemic chronic obstructive pulmonary disease. Arch. Intern. Med. *143*:1941, 1983.

241. Wilson, D. K., Kaplan, R. M., Timms, R. M., and Dawson, A.: Acute effects of oxygen treatment upon information processing in hypoxemic COPD patients. Chest *88*:239, 1985.

242. Morrison, D. A., Henry, R., and Goldman, S.: Preliminary study of the effects of low flow oxygen on oxygen delivery and right ventricular function in chronic lung disease. Am. Rev. Respir. Dis. *133*:390, 1986.

243. Ashutosh, K., Mead, G., and Dunsky, M.: Early effects of oxygen administration and prognosis in chronic obstructive pulmonary disease and cor pulmonale. Am. Rev. Respir. Dis. *127*:399–404, 1983.

244. Petty, R. L.: Who needs home oxygen? Am. Rev. Respir. Dis. *131*:930, 1985.

245. Levi-Valensi, P., Weitzenblum, E., Pedinielli, J.-L., et al.: Three-month follow-up of arterial blood gas determination in candidates for long-term oxygen therapy. Am. Rev. Respir. Dis. *133*:547, 1986.

246. Flenley, D. C.: Long-term home oxygen therapy. Chest *87*:99, 1985.

247. Kim, Y. S., and Aviado, D. M.: Digitalis and the pulmonary circulation. Am. Heart J. *62*:680, 1961.

248. Sylvester, J. T., Goldberg, H. S., and Permutt, S.: The role of the vasculature in the regulation of cardiac output. Clin. Chest Med. *4*:222–236, 1983.

249. Berglund, E., Eidimsky, J., and Malmberg, R.: Lack of effect of digitalis in patients with pulmonary disease with and without heart disease. Am. J. Cardiol. *41*:897, 1978.

250. Brown, S. E., Pakron, F. J., Milne, N., et al.: Effects of digoxin on exercise capacity and right ventricular function during exercise in chronic airflow obstruction. Chest *85*:187, 1984.

251. Coates, A. L., Desmond, K., Asher, M. I., et al.: The effect of digoxin on exercise capacity and exercising cardiac function in cystic fibrosis. Chest *82*:543, 1982.

252. Jezek, V., and Schrijen, F.: Hemodynamic effect of deslanoside at rest and during exercise in patients with chronic bronchitis. Br. Heart J. *35*:2, 1973.

253. Mathur, P. N., Powles, A. C. P., Pugsley, S. O., et al.: Effect of long-term administration of digoxin on exercise performance in chronic airflow obstruction. Eur. J. Respir. Dis. *66*:273, 1985.

254. Mathur, P. N., Powles, A. C. P., Pugsley, S. O., et al.: Effect of digoxin on right ventricular function in severe chronic airflow obstruction. Ann. Intern. Med. *95*:283, 1981.

255. Green, L. H., and Smith, T. W.: The use of digitalis in patients with pulmonary disease. Ann. Intern. Med. *87*:459, 1977.

256. Aubier, M., Murciano, D., Viires, N., et al.: Effects of digoxin on diaphragmatic strength generation in patients with chronic obstructive pulmonary disease during acute respiratory failure. Am. Rev. Respir. Dis. *135*:544, 1987.

257. Mahler, D. A., Matthay, R. A., Snyder, P. E., et al.: Sustained-release theophylline reduces dyspnea in nonreversible obstructive airway disease. Am. Rev. Respir. Dis. *131*:22, 1985.

258. Matthay, R. A.: Effects of theophylline on cardiovascular performance in chronic obstructive pulmonary disease. Chest *88*(Suppl.):11S, 1985.

259. Matthay, R. A., and Berger, H. J.: Cardiovascular function in cor pulmonale. Clin. Chest Med. *4*:269, 1983.

260. Matthay, R. A., Berger, H. J., Davies, R., et al.: Improvement in cardiac performance by oral long-acting theophylline in chronic obstructive pulmonary disease. Am. Heart J. *104*:1022, 1982.

261. Marcus, M. L., Skelton, C. L., Grauer, L. E., et al.: Effects of theophylline on myocardial mechanics. Am. J. Physiol. *222*:1361, 1972.

262. DiMarco, A. F., Nochomovitz, M., DiMarco, J.: Comparative effects of aminophylline on diaphragm and cardiac contractility. Am. Rev. Respir. Dis. *132*:800, 1985.

263. Rutherford, J. D., Vatner, S. E., and Braunwald, E.: Effects and mechanisms of action of aminophylline on cardiac function and regional blood flow distribution in conscious dogs. Circulation *63*:378, 1981.

264. Murphy, G. W., Schreiner, B. R., and Yu, P. M.: Effects of aminophylline on the pulmonary circulation and left ventricular performance in patients with valvular heart disease. Circulation *37*:361, 1968.

265. Benumof, J. L., and Trousdale, F. R.: Aminophylline does not inhibit canine hypoxic pulmonary vasoconstriction. Am. Rev. Respir. Dis. *126*:1017, 1982.

266. Brent, B. N., Berger, H. J., Matthay, R. A., et al.: Contrasting acute effects of vasodilators (nitroglycerin, nitroprusside, and hyralazine) on right ventricular performance in patients with chronic obstructive pulmonary disease and pulmonary hypertension: A combined radionuclide-hemodynamic study. Am. J. Cardiol. *51*:1682, 1983.

267. MacNee, W., Walthen, C. G., Hannan, W. J., et al.: Effects of pirbuterol and sodium nitroprusside on pulmonary haemodynamics in hypoxic cor pulmonale. Br. Med. J. *287*:1169–1172, 1983.

268. Whyte, K. F., and Flenley, D. C.: Can pulmonary vasodilators improve survival in cor pulmonale due to hypoxic chronic bronchitis and emphysema? Thorax 43:1, 1988.

269. Brent, B. N., Mahler, D., Berger, H. J., et al.: Augmentation of right ventricular performance in chronic obstructive pulmonary disease by terbutaline. A combined radionuclide and hemodynamic study. Am. J. Cardiol. 50:313, 1982.

270. Stockley, R. A., Finnegan, P., and Bishop, J. M.: Effect of intravenous terbutaline on arterial blood gas tensions, ventilation and pulmonary circulation in patients with chronic bronchitis and cor pulmonale. Thorax 32:601, 1977.

271. Jones, R. M., Stockley, R. A., and Bishop, J. M.: Early effects of intravenous terbutaline on cardiopulmonary function in chronic obstructive bronchitis and pulmonary hypertension. Thorax 37:746, 1982.

272. Teule, G. J. J., and Majid, P. A.: Hemodynamic effects of terbutaline in chronic obstructive airways disease. Thorax 35:536, 1980.

273. Biernacki, W., Pruice, K., Whyte, K., et al.: The effect of six months of daily treatment with the beta-2 agonist oral pirbuterol on pulmonary hemodynamics in patients with chronic hypoxic cor pulmonale receiving long-term oxygen therapy. Am. Rev. Respir. Dis. 139:492, 1989.

274. Rubin, L. J.: Vasodilators and pulmonary hypertension: Where do we go from here? Am. Rev. Respir. Dis. 135:288, 1987.

275. Salvaterra, C. G., and Rubin, L. J.: Investigation and management of pulmonary hypertension in chronic obstructive pulmonary disease. Am. Rev. Respir. Dis. 148:1414, 1993.

276. Packer, M.: Vasodilator therapy for primary pulmonary hypertension. Ann. Intern. Med. 103:258, 1985.

277. Brent, B. N., Matthay, R. A., Mahler, D. A., et al.: Relationship between oxygen uptake and oxygen transport in stable patients with chronic obstructive pulmonary disease: Physiologic effects of nitroprusside and hydralazine. Am. Rev. Respir. Dis. 129:682, 1984.

278. Corriveau, M. L., Minh, V.-D., and Dolan, G. F.: Long-term effects of hydralazine on ventilation and blood gas values in patients with chronic obstructive pulmonary disease hypertension. Am. J. Med. 83:886, 1987.

279. Corriveau, M. L., Rosen, B. J., Keller, C. A., et al.: Effect of posture, hydralazine, and nifedipine on hemodynamics, ventilation, and gas exchange in patients with chronic obstructive pulmonary disease. Am. Rev. Respir. Dis. 138:1494, 1988.

280. Dal Nogare, A. R., and Rubin, L. J.: The effects of hydralazine on exercise capacity in pulmonary hypertension secondary to chronic obstructive pulmonary disease. Am. Rev. Respir. Dis. 133:385, 1986.

281. Keller, C. A., Shepard, J. W., Chun, D. S., et al.: Effects of hydralazine on hemodynamics, ventilation and gas exchange in patients with chronic obstructive pulmonary disease and pulmonary hypertension. Am. Rev. Repair. Dis. 130:606, 1984.

282. Miller, M. J., Chappell, T. R., Cook, W., et al.: Effects of oral hydralazine on gas exchange in patients with cor pulmonale. Am. J. Med. 75:937, 1983.

283. Rubin, L. J., and Peter, R. H.: Hemodynamics at rest and during exercise after oral hydralazine in patients with cor pulmonale. Am. J. Cardiol. 47:116, 1981.

284. Lupi-Herrera, E., Seoane, M., and Verdejo, J.: Hemodynamic effect of hydralazine in advanced, stable chronic obstructive pulmonary disease with cor pulmonale: Immediate and short-term evaluation at rest and during exercise. Chest 85:156, 1984.

285. McGoon, M. D., Seward, J. B., Vliestra, R. E., et al.: Haemodynamic response to intravenous hydralazine in patients with pulmonary hypertension. Br. Heart J. 50:579, 1983.

286. Packer, M.: Greenberg, B., Massie, B., et al.: Deleterious effects of hydralazine in patients with pulmonary hypertension. N. Engl. J. Med. 306:1326, 1982.

287. Tuxen, D. V., Powles, A. C. P., Mathur, P. N., et al.: Detrimental effects of hydralazine in patients with chronic air-flow obstruction and pulmonary hypertension: A combined hemodynamic and radionuclide study. Am. Rev. Respir. Dis. 129:388, 1984.

288. Brown, S. E., Linden, G. S., Kling, R. R., et al.: Effects of verapamil on pulmonary haemodynamics during hypoxaemia, at rest, and during exercise in patients with chronic obstructive pulmonary disease. Thorax 38:840, 1983.

289. Kalra, L., and Bone, M. F.: Effect of nifedipine on physiologic shunting and oxygenation in chronic obstructive pulmonary disease. Am. J. Med. 94:419, 1993.

290. Domenighetti, G. M., and Saglini, V. G.: Short- and long-term hemodynamic effects of oral nifedipine in patients with pulmonary hypertension secondary to COPD and lung fibrosis: Deleterious effects in patients with restrictive disease. Chest 102:708, 1992.

291. Kennedy, T. P., Michael, J. R., Huang, C.-K., et al.: Nifedipine inhibits hypoxic pulmonary vasoconstriction during rest and exercise in patients with chronic obstructive pulmonary disease. Am. Rev. Respir. Dis. 129:544, 1984.

292. Rubin, L. J., and Moser, K.: Long-term effects of nitrendipine on hemodynamics and oxygen transport in patients with cor pulmonale. Chest 89:141–145, 1986.

293. Sajkov, D., McEvoy, R. D., Cowie, R. J., et al.: Felodipine improves pulmonary hemodynamics in chronic obstructive pulmonary disease. Chest 103:1354, 1993.

294. Geggel, R. L., Dozor, A. J., Fyler, D. C., et al.: Effects of vasodilators at rest and during exercise in young adults with cystic fibrosis and chronic cor pulmonale. Am. Rev. Respir. Dis. 131:531, 1985.

295. Gould, L., Zahir, M., DeMartino, A., et al.: Haemodynamic effects of phentolamine in chronic obstructive pulmonary disease. Br. Heart J. 33:445, 1971.

296. Spahn, F., Rottman, B., and Schmidt, U.: Effects of single intravenous administration of urapidil and diltiazem in patients with nonfixed pulmonary hypertension secondary to chronic obstructive lung disease. J. Cardiovasc. Pharmacol. 23:517, 1994.

297. Adnot, S., DeFouilloy, C., Brun-Buisson, C., et al.: Hemodynamic effects of urapidil in patients with pulmonary hypertension: A comparative study with hydralazine. Am. Rev. Respir. Dis. 135:288, 1987.

298. Adnot, S., Anrivet, P., Piquet, J., et al.: The effects of urapidil therapy on hemodynamics and gas exchange in exercising patients with chronic obstructive pulmonary disease and hypertension. Am. Rev. Respir. Dis. 137:1068, 1988.

299. Vik-Mo, H., Walde, N., Jentoft, H., and Halvorsen, F. I.: Improved haemodynamics but reduced arterial oxygen tension at rest and during exercise after long-term oral prazosin therapy in chronic cor pulmonale. Eur. Heart J. 6:1047, 1985.

300. Zielinski, J., Hawrylkiewicz, I., Gorecka, D., et al.: Captopril effects on pulmonary and systemic hemodynamics in chronic cor pulmonale. Chest 90:562, 1986.

301. Burke, C. M., Harte, M., Duncan, J., et al.: Captopril and domiciliary oxygen in chronic airflow obstruction. Br. Med. J. 290:1251, 1985.

302. Kastanos, N., Miro, R. E., and Agusti-Vidal, A.: Captopril in pulmonary hypertension. Br. Heart J. 49:513, 1983.

303. Ishizaki, T., Miyabo, S., Mifune, J., et al.: OP-1206, A prostaglandin E[1] derivative: Effects of oral administration to patients with chronic lung disease. Chest 85:382, 1984.

304. Jones, K., Higgenbottom, T., and Wallwork, J.: Pulmonary vasodilation and prostacyclin in primary and secondary pulmonary hypertension. Chest 96:784, 1989.

305. Dujic, Z., Eterovic, D., Tocilj, J., et al.: About mechanisms of prostaglandin E[1] induced deterioration of pulmonary gas exchange in COPD patients. Clin. Physiol. 13:497, 1993.

306. Rubin, J. J.: Cardiovascular effects of vasodilator therapy for pulmonary arterial hypertension. Clin. Chest Med. 4:309, 1983.

307. Segal, N., and Bishop, J. M.: The circulation in patients with chronic bronchitis and emphysema at rest and during exercise, with special reference to the influence of changes in blood viscosity and blood volume on the pulmonary circulation. J. Clin. Invest. 45:1555–1568, 1966.

308. Chetty, K. G., Brown, S. E., and Light, R. W.: Improved exercise tolerance of the polycythemic lung patient following phlebotomy. Am. J. Med. 74:415, 1983.

309. Dayton, L. M., McCullough, R. E., Scheinhorn, D. J., et al.: Symptomatic and pulmonary response to acute phlebotomy in secondary polycythemia. Chest 68:785, 1975.

310. Weisse, A. B., Moschos, C. B., Frank, M. S., et al.: Hemodynamic effects of staged hematocrit reduction in patients with stable cor pulmonale and severely elevated hematocrit levels. Am. J. Med. 58:92, 1975.

311. Rakita, L., Gillespie, D. G., and Sancetta, S.: The acute and chronic effects of phlebotomy on general hemodynamics and pulmonary functions of patients with secondary polycythemia associated with pulmonary emphysema. Am. Heart. J. 70:466, 1965.

Part IV

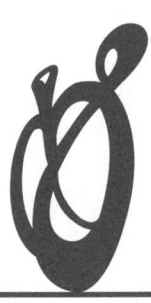

Broader Perspectives on Heart Disease and Cardiologic Practice

Chapter 48

Principles of Cardiovascular Molecular and Cellular Biology

KENNETH R. CHIEN, ANDREW A. GRACE

The past two decades of cardiovascular biology and medicine have been based largely upon the consideration of the heart and vasculature as an integrated physiological system, a view that has resulted in major therapeutic advances. With the advent of developments in gene transfer, mouse and human genetics, genetic engineering of intact animals, and molecular and cellular technology, cardiovascular medicine is now on the threshold of a molecular therapeutic era.[1] Major steps have been taken toward unraveling the molecular determinants of complex, integrative, and polygenic cardiovascular disease states, including atherosclerosis, hypertension, cardiac hypertrophy and failure, congenital heart disease, and coronary restenosis following balloon angioplasty. Our improved understanding of the fundamental basis of these important cardiovascular disease processes has established a scientific foundation for diagnostic, prognostic, and therapeutic advances in the mainstream of cardiovascular medicine.

This chapter provides a few selected examples that highlight the breadth and growing impact of the molecular sciences on the practice of cardiovascular medicine. A primer of basic molecular biology can also be found in a number of specialized texts and reviews devoted to molecular and cellular biology.[2–4] Although the scope of this chapter does not allow for a comprehensive analysis of this rapidly expanding area, a companion text[5] provides further background to the themes underlying the impact of molecular advances in cardiovascular medicine.

RECOMBINANT PROTEIN THERAPY

The production of clinically valuable recombinant proteins and their subsequent manipulation using protein engineering are among the major medical applications of recombinant DNA technology and have given rise to the biotechnology industry, which has been based upon the need for large-scale protein isolation and purification.[6] In medical applications, the recombinant protein can be the therapeutic agent, designed for replacement therapy where disease is based upon an acquired or genetic deficiency of a specific protein, as in diabetes mellitus or hemophilia. Alternatively, the therapeutic application may be based upon the promotion or inhibition of a specific biological pathway, e.g., stimulating erythrocytosis in chronic renal failure.[7] At present, a number of recombinant proteins have documented clinical utility, including insulin, factor VIII, erythropoietin, and hemopoietic growth factors.[7,8] Tissue plasminogen activator was the first product of protein engineering designed for clinical use in the cardiovascular field,[9,10] and a number of other potentially valuable proteins will be tested in the next few years.[11,12]

The techniques for large-scale production of proteins have necessitated industrial-scale approaches, but they fundamentally rely on conventional molecular technology utilizing gene cloning, expression, and mutagenesis to manipulate and match protein structure to particular tasks. Producing a recombinant protein first requires the cloning of the gene encoding the protein of interest, construction of an expression vector, and transfer of the gene construct into a surrogate cell system that is programmed for large-scale synthesis.[3]

Tissue Plasminogen Activators (t-PA)

CLONING OF THE t-PA GENE. Identification of a tissue source of t-PA[13] was followed only many years later by protein isolation from a human Bowes melanoma cell line[14] and subsequent purification and characterization of the enzyme.[15] The initial samples of t-PA for intracoronary thrombolysis came from this source, although conventional protein purification from the melanoma cell line was inadequate for purposes beyond small-scale clinical use.[10]

The therapeutic potential of thrombolytic agents and the availability of recombinant technology led to considerable efforts to genetically engineer t-PA[3,9] and has provided a paradigm for the industrial application of molecular technology. The project was initially pursued by two independent groups, using similar strategies to isolate and clone the t-pA gene.[16,17] The protein was isolated from the human melanoma cell line and the molecular weight identified at approximately 63,000 kDa. The amino acid sequence of a small stretch of the t-PA protein was determined, allowing the synthesis of oligonucleotides complementary to the DNA nucleotide sequence which encode defined portions of the molecule. The oligonucleotides were utilized as probes to isolate the t-PA cDNA from a library of sequences derived from Bowes melanoma cells.[3] The isolation of a full-length t-PA cDNA that followed served as the source for the recombinant t-PA that is currently used for thrombolytic therapy[10,18] (see pp. 1220 and 1907).

PRODUCTION OF RECOMBINANT t-PA IN CELL SYSTEMS. The techniques for the production of recombinant proteins harness the endogenous capacity of a surrogate cell system to be programmed to express the desired gene product and require the stable integration of an amplified expression vector.[3] A variety of bacterial, yeast, and mammalian cell systems have been used for this purpose. *Escherichia coli* is commonly used and displays several advantages of simplicity, short generation time, large yields, and relatively low cost.[3] Although this prokaryotic system is still standard for the production of recombinant products in the laboratory, the large-scale production of biologically active material usually requires more sophisticated methods, as the bacterial system can introduce folding defects and is unable to incorporate appropriate post-translational modifications (acetylation, glycosylation, phosphorylation), which can lead to functionally impaired products.[3]

The size, complexity, and maintenance of the proper folding of the t-PA protein provide a point of contrast with less complex proteins, such as insulin and growth hormone. The necessity for maintaining proper processing of t-PA led to the development of the Chinese hamster ovary (CHO) expression system, which has become standard in the field.[3] Transfection of a t-PA cDNA into these cells leads to the efficient generation of t-PA protein, which can be adapted to culture in large-scale fermenters (Fig. 48-1). Although the first mammalian expression systems displayed relatively low capacity, a novel modification increased expression of t-PA by gene amplification.[19] Resistance of cancer cells to methotrexate is associated with the rapid amplification of the dihydrofolate reductase *(dhfr)* gene. By fusing the t-PA gene to that of *dhfr* and exposing the CHO cells to serial increases in methotrexate, one can select for a CHO cell line displaying an increase in *dhfr* gene copy number with coamplification of the t-PA gene. These cells are programmed to release t-PA into the culture medium, thereby facilitating the large-scale isolation and purification of the t-PA protein.

PRINCIPLES UNDERLYING THE DEVELOPMENT OF t-PA VARIANTS. A number of limitations of native t-PA were observed in early evaluations and clinical trials—resistance to reperfusion (25 per cent), reocclusion (5 to 25 per cent), delayed reperfusion, occasional significant bleeding, and short plasma half-life—which spurred interests in modifying the molecule to optimize clinical efficacy.[18,20,21] Of

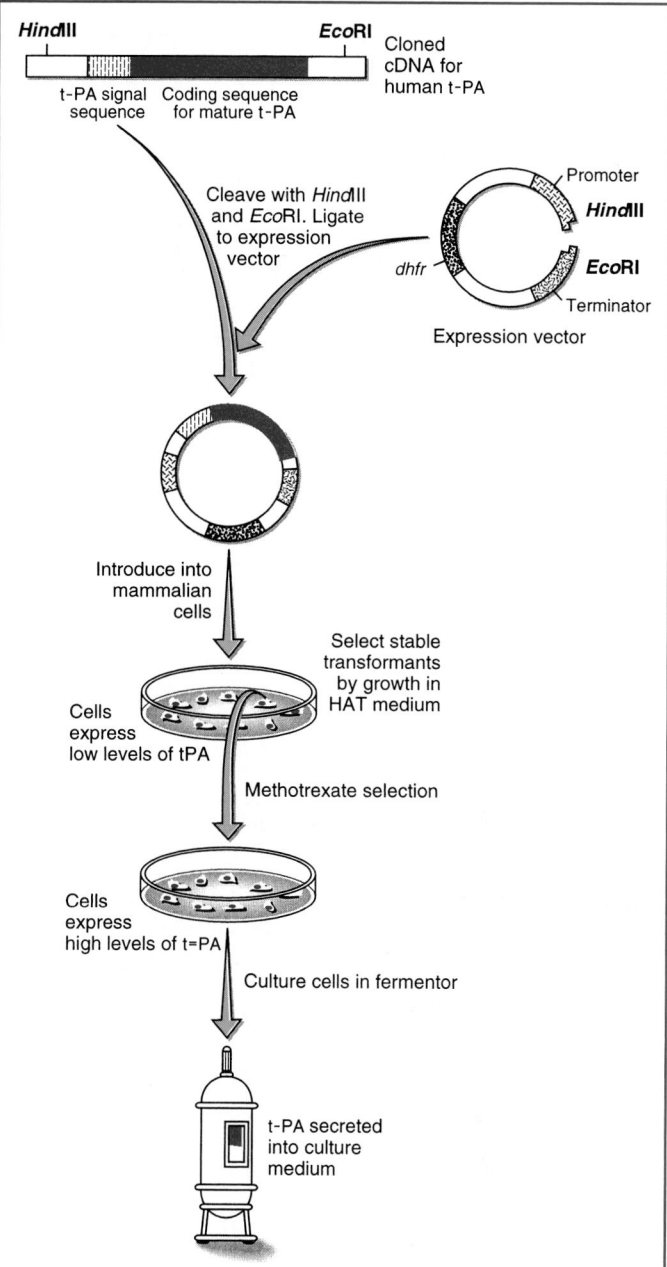

FIGURE 48–1. The production of t-PA in a mammalian cell (Chinese hamster ovary) system. The cloned cDNA for human t-PA was ligated into an expression vector under the control of a strong promoter and the vector stably transfected into the mammalian cell line (*Hind*III and *Eco*RI are endonuclease restriction sites). Initial transformants secreted low levels of t-PA into the culture medium, increased by the use of serial methotrexate selection for cells having the amplified dihydrofolate reductase *(dhfr)* gene linked to the t-PA expression cassette. High-expressing lines are grown in large-scale fermentors, with recombinant t-PA being purified from the culture medium. (Modified from Watson, J. D., Gilman, M., Witkowski, J., and Zoller, M.: Recombinant DNA. 2nd ed. © 1983, and 1992 by James D. Watson, Michael Gilman, Jan Witkowski, and Mark Zeller. New York, W. H. Freeman, 1992. Used with permission of W. H. Freeman and Co.)

course, the pressures of evolution had served to optimize t-PA only for a role in *endogenous* fibrinolysis and not for *clinical* thrombolysis. The generation of large quantities of t-PA allowed a detailed structure-function analysis of the native protein with regard to fibrin binding, catalytic action, and clearance.[10,22,23] This knowledge eventually resulted in the identification of the specific domains of the protein which account for these functional properties of the intact molecule (Fig. 48–2). Native t-PA was shown to provide a good example of a protein open to the rational application of recombinant molecular technology.[6,10,24] Par-

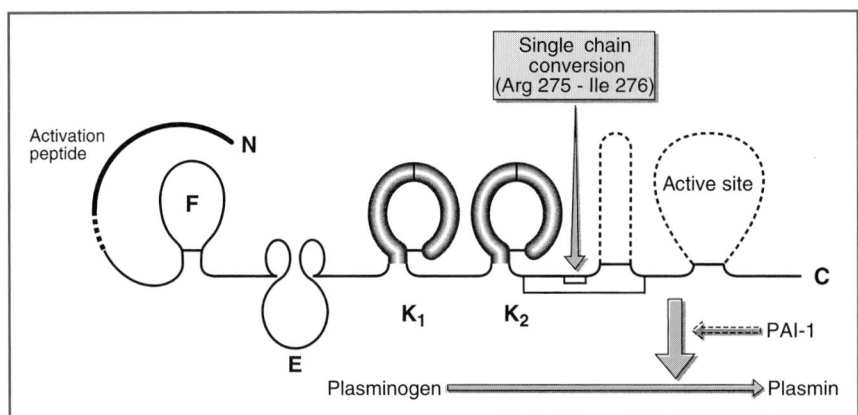

FIGURE 48–2. Structural domains of t-PA. The five distinct structural domains of the t-PA protein —finger (F) domain (residues 4 to 50 from the N-terminal region); growth factor (E) domain (residues 51 to 87); two kringle (K1/K2) domains (respectively, amino acids 87 to 176 and 176 to 262) with high-degree homology to five kringles of plasminogen; and serine protease catalytic domain (amino acids 276 to 527). These domains have structural homologies to other components of the plasminogen-plasmin system and other plasminogen activators. The finger and kringle domains confer the specificity for fibrin. Single-chain t-PA is synthesized and released from vascular endothelium; activity is further increased by conversion to the two-chain form after cleavage at Arg 275–Ile 276. The proteolytically active light chain region acts at Arg 560–Val 561 of plasminogen, resulting in the conversion to plasmin.

ticular advantages include the possession of several independent functional domains that have both independent and interdependent functions.[10,25] Improving the efficacy of the wild-type molecule was based upon the modification of the t-PA protein by site-directed mutagenesis of the structure of these domains.[25] The specific aims in re-engineering t-PA were directed at increasing efficacy by producing more rapid and persistent recanalization without rethrombosis, reducing hemorrhagic complications, and decreasing plasma clearance.[10]

Plasminogen activators all have the immediate function of cleaving plasminogen to yield fibrinolytic plasmin; the enzyme attacks fibrin to unravel a central component of the thrombotic latticework[10,22] (see p. 1815). t-PA is a serine protease catalyzing the cleavage of the common site single peptide bond (Arg560–Val561) of plasminogen.[10] The catalytic efficiency of t-PA is increased approximately 1000-fold in the presence of fibrin.[10] This is, in part, due to the high affinity of t-PA for fibrin (~ 10 nM), with selectivity being due to high-affinity fibrin-binding domains of the molecule.[10,22]

Structural analysis of human t-PA reveals a single polypeptide chain of 527 amino acids, and a complex binary and ternary structure has been predicted containing 16 disulphide bonds.[25] Five distinct structural domains are recognized: finger (F) domain (residues 4 to 50 from the N-terminal region) having homology to the fibrin affinity domain for fibronectin; growth factor (E) domain (residues 51 to 87) homologous to human epidermal growth factor; two kringle (K1/K2) domains (respectively, amino acids 87 to 176 and 176 to 262) with high-degree homology to five kringles of plasminogen; and a serine protease catalytic domain (amino acids 276 to 527). The full analysis of the three-dimensional structure of t-PA has not been achieved, although the crystal structure of the kringle-2 domain has been reported.[26] The integrated molecular structure, when solved, will facilitate understanding of how the function of the molecule is achieved in a dynamic fashion.[25]

Domain-deletion studies of t-PA have implicated the finger, growth factor, and second kringle domains in fibrin binding.[25] This fact produced attractive targets for modification using specific directed changes aimed at modifying both the structure and functional properties of t-PA and was encouraged by being ultimately therapeutically cleaner in view of preferential activation of plasminogen at the fibrin surface.[27] This contrasts with the systemic activation seen with streptokinase, anisolysated plasminogen streptokinase activated complex (APSAC), and urokinase, which could theoretically lead to a *lytic state*.[27]

t-PA MUTANTS WITH ALTERED FUNCTIONAL PROPERTIES. Despite considerable effort, the development of deletion/substitution functional domain mutants with altered properties of increased clot-specificity (targeting fibrin, uncovering either platelet epitopes or the covalent link between α_2-antiplasmin and fibrin) and decreased clearance (glycosylation, plasminogen activator inhibitor (PAI-1) resistance

and so forth) has generally been disappointing.[10,24,28] Those mutants with improved pharmacokinetics achieved by the deletion of the F, E, and K₁ domains have tended toward decreased fibrinolytic activity.[22] Recently, the successful production of mutant t-PA with theoretically improved properties has, however, been described following sequential modification of the native t-PA molecule. The addition of a glycosylation site on kringle-1, termed T-t-PA, had the most promising pharmacokinetic profile; tetra-alanine substitution at amino acids 296 to 299 improved clearance and fibrin specificity (TK-t-PA); fibrin affinity was maintained with the additional mutation N117Q yielding TNK-t-PA.[29] These variants are now undergoing clinical trials. Clues to improvement of design have also come from other sources, such as the use of the plasminogen activator from the vampire bat *(Desmodus rotundus)* which is highly fibrin-specific, homologous to human t-PA, and lacks K-2 and the plasmin cleavage site for conversion to the two-chain form.[30]

The concept behind the development of *chimeric molecules* is that they would potentially enhance targeting with fewer systemic effects.[10] These conjugate hybrid proteins have been produced by chemical cross-linking or via recombinant technology by creating fusion proteins consisting of t-PA in conjunction with elements of other peptides (e.g., single-chain urokinase) to enhance fibrin affinity or to increase catalytic activity. In addition, monoclonal antibodies directed to the Bβ chain of fibrin and $\alpha_{IIb}\beta_3$ and thrombospondin have also been used to construct chimeras to allow targets of other components that contribute to thrombus formation.[22] In general, the approach has not yet produced agents of enhanced clinical value, instead having thrombolytic properties and fibrin selectivity generally similar but not superior to those of the component parts.[10]

Further Applications of Recombinant Protein Engineering

The production of sufficient quantities of clinical-grade t-PA for widespread use in thrombolysis represented a dramatic entrance for recombinant technology into the practice of cardiology. Second-generation plasminogen activators have followed, but truly rational protein design depends on three-dimensional structural analysis,[6,10] and it is not currently possible to precisely deduce tertiary protein structure from the primary amino acid sequences.[6] However, there have been technical advances in both the practical methods of protein structure determination, using both x-ray crystallography and nuclear magnetic resonance spectroscopy (which has the advantage of allowing structure determination in solution) and parallel advances in computer modeling that now allow improved prediction of ternary structure which should enhance rational approaches to protein engineering and should prove particularly valuable in regard to multidomain proteins such as t-PA.[6] Such approaches are likely to result in improvements in mutant design of existing molecules in addition to allowing the production of other recombinant molecules.

In this regard, several other recombinant proteins have been designed for cardiovascular use and are currently being tested in the appropriate clinical settings. Hirudin was initially isolated from the medical leech, *Hirudo medicinalis,* but recognition of therapeutic potential coincided with the leech becoming endangered.[11,12,33] Hirudin is the prototypic, direct thrombin inhibitor, binding both the active catalytic site and the substrate recognition site (anion exosite) of thrombin[12,32,33] (see p. 1820). It has several putative advantages over heparin, including an ability to inactivate clot-bound thrombin, and theoretical advantages of lack of inactivation by either heparinase or platelet factor 4, and no dependence on antithrombin-III.[12] The recombinant molecule has similar in vitro and in vivo anticoagulant, antiplatelet, and antithrombotic actions to those identified in the naturally occurring molecule.[11]

In addition to agents directed to the vessel wall, the development of recombinant peptide-derived growth factors that promote angiogenesis such as the fibroblast and vascular endothelial cell growth factors (FGF, VEGF)[34] or stimulate specific hematopoietic lineages such as thrombopoietin,[8] have potential clinical utility and will be examined in clinical studies in the next several years.

One other approach to rational antagonism uses genetically engineered monoclonal antibodies produced from cell lines secreting single antibody species of desired specificity.[35,36] This technology has been advanced by the development of mutant antibodies, antibodies of dual specificity, and rodent antibodies humanized by linking rodent immunoglobulin variable regions to human constant regions (chimeric humanized antibodies), thereby reducing immunogenicity.[37] The two major categories of monoclonal antibodies applied in cardiovascular medicine—antifibrin and antiplatelet antibodies ($\alpha_{IIb}\beta_3$ and thrombospondin), have, however, not yet found widespread application (see below).

RATIONAL DESIGN AND DEVELOPMENT OF PHARMACOLOGICAL ANTAGONISTS

Pharmaceutical development has traditionally relied on large-scale screening of natural sources for the identification of candidate compounds,[38] but molecular technology now indicates a likely change of fundamental approach. Recombinant protein and therapeutic antibody technology have had a clear impact on the development of new synthetic agonists and antagonists aimed at specific molecular targets causally related to disease phenotypes.[39] The molecular cloning of target molecules has led to rapid throughput screening approaches to identify appropriate antagonists. Molecular modeling of the compound and protein targets can now be employed to maximize the efficiency of identifying structure-function relationships and designing families of related compounds.[6,38]

In this regard, although the possibility of inhibition of intracellular signal transduction molecules has been raised,[38] inhibition of the ligand-surface receptor interaction (e.g., inhibition of the $\alpha_{IIb}\beta_3$ platelet receptor) remains the common principle for the development of many drugs with cardiovascular applications and serves as a prime example of the power of this approach.[40]

$\alpha_{IIb}\beta_3$ Platelet-Specific Integrin

The search for effective inhibitors of thrombosis has been a significant challenge of modern cardiovascular therapeutics, and the platelet has become a primary therapeutic target because it is a central component of thrombotic lesions.[41] Presently available antiplatelet agents all have problems, as they target individual pathways involved in platelet aggregation, leaving other pathways open which may then compensate via biologically redundant mechanisms[42] (see p. 1818). For example, aspirin, although of proven clinical utility in certain settings, has theoretical limitations, as it inhibits only thromboxane A_2–dependent mechanisms. The ideal target would be a molecule mediating final common pathways, where inhibition totally abrogates platelet adhesion, activation, and aggregation. The molecular identification of modulatory integrin receptors on the platelet surface has therefore presented a significant therapeutic opportunity.[43]

The platelet-specific integrin, most appropriately referred to as $\alpha_{IIb}\beta_3$[40,44–47] (also termed as GPIIb/IIIa), was the first integrin to be identified, purified, expressed in recombi-

nant form, and associated with a human disease.[40] The functional importance of this molecule was first clearly shown in Glanzmann's thrombasthenia, where $\alpha_{IIb}\beta_3$ is either absent or dysfunctional and the clinical condition is characterized by mucocutaneous bleeding.[40]

The $\alpha_{IIb}\beta_3$ complex, a member of the widely distributed integrin supergene family of heterodimeric membrane proteins,[48] is an early specific marker of the megakarocyte lineage and the most abundant platelet integrin (density $\sim$ 50,000 per platelet).[40] Integrins play key roles in cell adhesion events and are important in the migration, proliferation, and differentiation of several cell types.[44,45] Integrins are divided into three families, each possessing a common β subunit, but with different α subunits; $\alpha_{IIb}\beta_3$ is a β_3-cytoadherin family member along with the vitronectin receptor.[40] The receptor complex of $\alpha_{IIb}\beta_3$ has two components: the α subunit (GPIIb) is a 136-kDa glycoprotein with light and heavy chains and a disulfide bridge (Fig. 48–3). The light chain of 22 kDa allows anchorage, and the extracellular heavy chain has homologous sequences to calmodulin and troponin C.[40] The β subunit (GPIIIa) has a molecular weight of 90 to 105 kDa and is 90 per cent extracellular, with 41 residues in the cytoplasmic domain. The structure, as established by rotary shadowing electron microscopy, has a globular head and two tails. The recognition sites and ligand binding sites have been identified, which has facilitated the development of pharmacological antagonists.[40,47]

In view of their role in cell interaction and in thrombus formation, molecular characterization of $\alpha_{IIb}\beta_3$ and the structural basis of the $\alpha_{IIb}\beta_3$-ligand interaction, have become of great interest.[40] It has been established that in unstimulated platelets, $\alpha_{IIb}\beta_3$ has a random distribution and recognizes only immobilized fibrinogen. The binding of adhesive proteins stimulates platelets and activates $\alpha_{IIb}\beta_3$ with patches of $\alpha_{IIb}\beta_3$ becoming visible on the platelet surface, with a concomitant increase in platelet binding of fibrinogen von Willebrand factor (vWF), fibronectin, and thrombo-

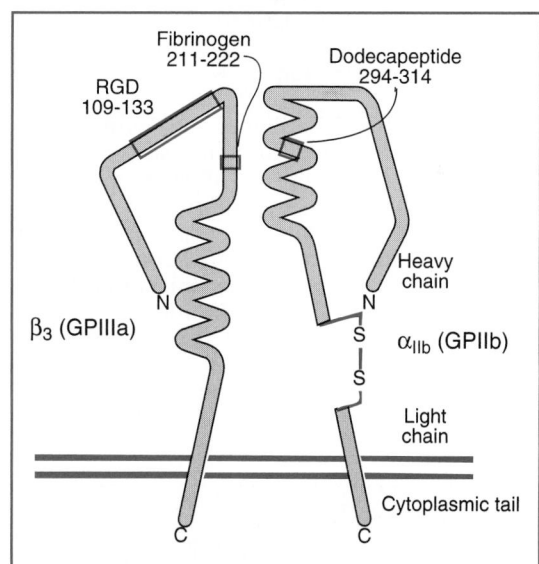

FIGURE 48–3. Schematic of structure and function of platelet membrane integrin $\alpha_{IIb}\beta_3$. Notable features of β_3 are the extracellular —NH$_2$ terminus, disulfide loop which binds —NH$_2$ to the midregion, typical transmembrane domain, and short cytoplasmic tail. α_{IIb} consists of disulfide linked heavy and light chains. The heavy chain has four Ca^{2+} binding repeats, and the light chain has a transmembrane segment and a short cytoplasmic tail. Three fibrinogen-binding sites are indicated: (1) β_3 109 to 130 has primary recognition for RGD sequences and secondary recognition for the fibrinogen gamma-chain sequence; (2) α_{IIb} 294 to 314 has the primary recognition for the gamma-chain sequence and secondary recognition for RGD; (3) β_3 211 to 222 recognition specificity has yet to be defined. The fibrinogen-binding sites provide potential targets for planned pharmacological intervention.

spondin. The dimeric structure of the molecule facilitates binding to platelets, leading to lattice formation and thrombus propagation.[40]

Two principal peptide recognition sequences on ligands interact with the platelet $\alpha_{IIb}\beta_3$ receptor complex. The arg-gly-asp (RGD) sequence was originally defined as the fibronectin sequence responsible for cell adhesion interactions[49] and has been shown to interact with a sequence localized to the amino-terminal part of the β subunit at residues 109 to 171.[47] Binding of RGD peptide recognition sequences in two molecules, vWF and fibrinogen, activates signals for the initiation of cell spreading, granular secretion, procoagulant activity, and conformational changes in the $\alpha_{IIb}\beta_3$ complex.[50] Conformational change results in exposure of the fibrinogen-binding site on the receptor complex. The second binding sequence is the lys-gln-ala-gly-asp-val sequence localized to the carboxy terminus of the γ chain of fibrinogen[47] and probably mediates the main binding mechanism for fibrinogen[40] (Fig. 48–3).

$\alpha_{IIb}\beta_3$ (II$_b$/IIIa) Inhibition

The approach to developing inhibitors of the $\alpha_{IIb}\beta_3$ system has employed a broad range of technologies, including the generation of monoclonal antibodies that can neutralize receptor function, the identification of naturally occurring antagonists,[51] and the development of synthetic antagonists based upon knowledge of the binding characteristics of the $\alpha_{IIb}\beta_3$ receptor RGD peptides, which may also function as partial agonists to generate high-affinity ligand-binding states.

Naturally occurring peptide inhibitors (disintegrins: echistatin, trigramin, apploggin, kistrin, bitan, barbourin[51–53]) isolated from puff adder and viper venoms, contain proteins, usually with the common RGD sequence that reversibly inhibits in vitro platelet aggregation. Binding is often rapid (kistrin) and has moderate affinity ($K_d \simeq 10^{-7}$ M). Barbourin displayed higher selectivity for $\alpha_{IIb}\beta_3$, which is conferred by a small change in the recognition sequence compared with other disintegrins.[54] The switch of the Lys to the Arg (KGD sequence) is responsible for this high selectivity, and the interaction of KGD with $\alpha_{IIb}\beta_3$ may be unique.[54]

Recognition of natural inhibitors and delineation of their binding characteristics and, in some cases, structural features[55] led to the development of synthetic peptides or peptidomimetics having higher affinity for the $\alpha_{IIb}\beta_3$ complex and enhanced inhibitory activity. The special properties of barbourin led to an investigation of KGD derivatives.[54] The synthetic heptapeptide, integrelin, has a modified KGD sequence and a high affinity and specificity for $\alpha_{IIb}\beta_3$.[54] The drug is potent, with a rapid onset of action and short biological half-life ($t_{1/2} \sim 10$ min), and, both in vitro and in vivo, inhibits platelet aggregation. The clinical utility of this agent is being tested clinically.[40,56] The possi-

bility of the future development of peptide-specific inhibitors based on these approaches is likely to include synthetic peptidomimetic agents (e.g., Ro43-5054),[57] which may be more potent as $\alpha_{IIb}\beta_3$ inhibitors than RGD-containing peptides. Two peptidomimetics have been tested in clinical trials (MK-383; Ro4483) but appear to be less specific.[57]

Vascular-targeted monoclonal antibodies to the $\alpha_{IIb}\beta_3$ receptor are more potent than aspirin both ex and in vivo.[40] The technology may, however, be limited by potential immunogenicity problems with repeated exposure, therefore confining use to single administrations.[40] However, clinical trials have demonstrated the value of monoclonal antibodies in the context of acute coronary angioplasty[58,59] (Table 39–2, p. 1370).

LOCALIZATION OF CARDIOVASCULAR DISEASE GENES

The ability to characterize the genetic modifiers that maintain complex cardiovascular function, as well as to identify specific cardiovascular disease genes in monogenic disorders, is a central goal in molecular cardiology. The accelerated application of molecular genetics to human cardiovascular disease is covered in Chapter 49. Here, we review general principles, indicating how genetic information is extracted and then integrated with other data sources to allow mechanistic insights into cardiovascular physiology and pathology.

Principles of Gene Localization and Gene Product Analysis

The starting point for the identification of the gene responsible for a particular phenotype is the precise definition of that phenotype. The genetic study of human disease poses several problems but has the advantage of large numbers of well-characterized wild-type and mutant phenotypes.[60,61] The identification of human disease genes can follow one of two basic strategies (Fig. 48–4). *Functional cloning* allows the identification of the disease gene on the basis of functional knowledge, and the isolation of the gene is based upon the definition of a precise, usually biochemical, defect.[60] This method is not applicable to most mutations of the cardiovascular system, which have no biochemical or cytogenetic correlate that can be readily assayed from a clinical phenotype.[62] The major cardiovascular disease phenotypes each represent a complex interaction between genetic and environmental influences.[60]

Positional cloning assumes no functional information and instead depends on defining the position of the gene on a map of the entire human genome, the identification of the primary structure of the gene, and a determination of the

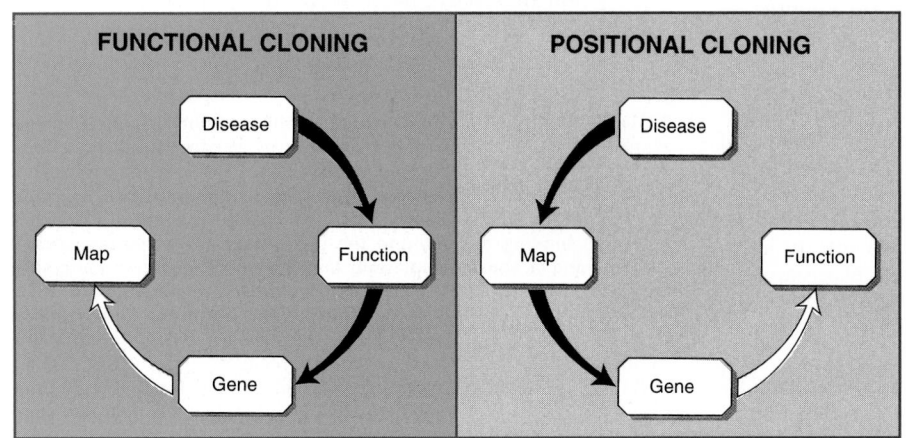

FIGURE 48–4. Paradigms for functional and positional cloning. Comparison of the functional and positional cloning of disease genes. In functional cloning, the study of the gene function precedes gene identification. In positional cloning, gene mapping precedes gene identification. The last step in each case (gene mapping and defining gene function, respectively) is not critical for the isolation of the disease gene itself. (Modified from Collins, F. S.: Positional cloning: Let's not call it reverse any more. Nature Genet. *1*:3, 1992.)

structure, tissue distribution, and expression of the gene product.[60,62] This approach had recently become dominant, but as information derived from the human genome project becomes available, the identification of candidate genes within a given region should greatly facilitate disease gene isolation (positional candidate approach).[60,62] It has been predicted that this modified approach, combining elements of both functional and positional cloning, will become the principal mode of disease gene identification.[62] This, in conjunction with appropriate biological assays for candidate gene expression, should allow further rapid advances in identifying single gene diseases that affect the cardiovascular system (Table 48–1).

THE HUMAN GENOME. The first step in the characterization of a human gene usually involves the identification of the position of that gene in the genome, the overall structure of which is best described by a map.[60] The premise upon which positional cloning is based suggests that the gene is located at a specific location on one of the chromosomes.[61] The requirement for the map is imposed by the size of the human genome.[63] The map may be physical or genetic and is constructed by observing the inheritance of markers that can be used as points of reference in offspring after well-characterized matings.[60] The quality and density of markers are the major determinants of its potential utility, but until recently markers were not ideal and the map of the human genome was characterized as being like a desert with only the occasional polymorphic oasis.[64] The first routinely used markers identified points of cleavage by restriction enzymes, known to vary within the population and termed restriction fragment length polymorphisms (RFLP).[60,65,66] These are resolved following the separation of endonuclease-generated fragments by gel electrophoresis and hybridization with appropriate probes using Southern blotting.[60]

The situation has been dramatically changed by the recognition that clusters of repeated sequences are present throughout the genome, allowing the construction of higher-resolution microsatellite-based maps.[64] These new maps, constructed around such short repeats, most notably containing cytosine and adenine (CA repeats) that occur approximately every 25 to 100 kb along the genome, are highly polymorphic.[64] In addition, they are reproducible, easily scored, and readily analyzed using amplification with the polymerase chain reaction and simple gel electrophoresis.[60,64]

POSITIONAL ASSIGNMENT. Mapping the position of a gene depends on defining the inheritance of genetic markers, along with the genes underlying the phenotype of interest. These show co-inheritance (genetic linkage) with markers in the immediate vicinity.[60,61] Conversely, genes that are far apart segregate independently, with an approximately linear relationship between the distance between genes and the probability of recombination.[60] In an individual family, the inheritance of a marker repeatedly with the disease phenotype implies a high probability that the marker is in the vicinity of the culprit gene. The concepts underlying localization are therefore simple, although in humans achieving linkage depends on prosaic considerations, particularly the size of a family pedigree and the quality of the available map.[60,61] The ideal is to develop a high-resolution map that covers the entire human genome, a goal of the Human Genome Project.[67] The delineation of such a map allows the definition of the position of any gene and thereby facilitates the analysis of the expression of that gene and, subsequently, of the gene product.[62,67] Present strategies require tracking a gene down to a chromosomal location of less than 1 to 3 million base pairs of DNA, containing only a few genes likely to be expressed in the relevant tissues. Once linkage is established, and now based on some knowledge of the disease, it is usually possible to search directly for the disease gene of interest with some likelihood of success.[60,61]

GENE CHARACTERIZATION. The identification of a specific gene location allows the nature of the genetic defect to be determined.[60] This is achieved either by identification of appropriate candidates, if known genes exist in that location, or by delivering the sequence of the gene in individuals having the disease phenotype and comparing these genotypes with normals. Sequencing can be manual but more recently has been automated with fluorescent markers and laser detection.[68] The mutation in the gene can cause the loss or change of function of a given gene via several mechanisms (deletions and duplications, base substitutions, expanding trinucleotide repeats), and these mutations provide important information, not only for the aberrant gene, but also regarding normal function and regulation.[60] Insights are then obtained into structure-function relationships of gene products and provide means to detect and analyze gene distribution in given families or in the general population.

The following sections provide two examples of the identification of important human cardiovascular disease genes and discusses recent insights gained into the relationship between the structure of the mutant protein and acquisition of the disease phenotype.

Molecular Genetics of Long Q-T Syndromes
(See also p. 1667)

The long Q-T syndromes often present clinically in the young with syncope, sudden cardiac death, abnormalities of ventricular repolarization, and torsades de pointes[69,70] (see p. 685). The condition is familial, with an autosomal dominant pattern of inheritance and high penetrance.[71] However, the incidence remains unknown, as minimal symptoms may go unrecognized, particularly in conjunction with a normal Q-T interval.[72] The gene frequency may therefore be much higher than suspected. Until recently, the electrophysiological mechanism responsible for this syndrome was unclear, and, as a result, management was empirical rather than rational.[70] This lack of a rational approach has nevertheless resulted in clinically effective approaches that have served to reduce the risks of the disease in those individuals that have been identified as being at risk.[70]

Within a single family, considerable heterogeneity in clinical presentation and electrocardiographic manifestations can be evident, thereby producing a problem in identifying affected individuals, which is the prelude to genetic dissection.[70,72] The application of a particularly stringent set of clinical criteria is usually required before successful linkage studies can be undertaken.[60] Published studies have used conservative approaches to a phenotypic assignment, characterizing patients in affected families as normal (if Q-T$_c$ interval < 410 msec); abnormal (if Q-T$_c$ interval > 450 msec with symptoms; or if asymptomatic, a Q-T$_c$ interval > 470 msec); all other patients were classified as being of uncertain phenotype.[73]

POSITIONAL ASSIGNMENT. The first gene locus for the long Q-T syndrome was located by the availability of a large, well-characterized family with the condition.[73,74] The family had been based in a small town in Utah since the arrival of two brothers from the Netherlands in the mid-nineteenth century.[73] The lineage tree was constructed and DNA from the relatives examined using restriction digestion to establish RFLP linkage. Linkage of the long Q-T locus 1 (LQ-T$_1$) to the H-ras marker on the short arm of the chromosome 11 (11p15.5) with a Lod score of +16.43 was determined (the logarithm of the odds ratio for linkage (Lod) score is a logarithmic index of the likelihood that a disease gene is not linked to a particular genetic marker; here $1/10^{16.43}$). This finding pointed strongly to the H-ras gene as a potential candidate and also provided a putative mechanistic explanation in that both the p21 ras 1 protein and GAP (GTPase-activating protein) regulate cardiac muscarinic potassium channels.[73] However, H-ras was subsequently excluded for LQ-T$_1$, both by exclusion of this candidate gene from the region containing the disease gene[75] and with the sequencing of the entire segment containing H-ras showing no mutations. Moreover, this 1 million base region contains channel (KCNA4 and KCNC1) and dopamine receptor (DRD4) genes that have also been

TABLE 48-1 GENETIC BASIS OF SOME CARDIOVASCULAR DISEASE PHENOTYPES

DISEASE	CARDIAC PHENOTYPE	DESIGNATION	GENE Location	Mutations	Product	PROBABLE MECHANISM
Myocardial Disease						
Familial hypertrophic cardiomyopathy	Cardiac hypertrophy, diastolic heart failure, arrhythmias, sudden cardiac death	CHM1 CHM2 CHM3 CHM4	14q12 1q3 15q2 11	>25 missense >6 missense >2 missense	Cardiac β-MHC Cardiac TnT α-tropomyosin	Mutations all dominant-negative; mechanisms for hypertrophy, disarray, and fibrosis unknown
Duchenne/Becker muscular dystrophy	Dilated cardiomyopathy, arrhythmias	DMD	Xp21	Deletion promoter	Dystrophin	Modified ion transport
Myotonic dystrophy	<10% clinical heart failure	MD	19	CTG repeat	Myotonin	Unknown
Long Q-T syndromes	Abnormal ECG, syncope, sudden death	LQ-T1 LQ-T2 LQ-T3	11p15.5 7q35-36 3p21-24	— Missense/ID In frame ID	— HERG SCN5A	— ⇓ Repolarizing current ⇑ Duration depolarizing current
Arrhythmogenic RV dysplasia	Monomorphic VT, sudden cardiac death	ARVD	14q23-q24	—	—	Unknown
Vascular Disease						
Marfan syndrome	Aortic root disease, valvar regurgitation	FBN1	15q21	>30 mutations	Fibrillin	⇓ Fibrillin content
Supravalvular aortic stenosis (SVAS)	SVAS, peripheral pulmonic artery stenosis	ELN	7q11.23	ID/translocation	Elastin	⇓ Elastin content with development
William's syndrome	SVAS, hypertension, systemic features	—	7q11.23	De novo deletion	Elastin	Contiguous gene disorder
Ehlers-Danlos IV	Aortic dilatation and aneurysms	COL3A1	2q24.3-q31	—	Type III collagen	Defects of type III collagen
Rendu-Weber-Osler syndrome	Telangiectasia, arteriovenous fistulae	—	9q33-34	—	—	Unknown

Data from Schwartz, K., et al.: Molecular basis of familial cardiomyopathies. Circulation *91*:532, 1995; Towbin, J., et al.: X-linked dilated cardiomyopathy: Molecular genetic evidence of linkage to the Duchenne muscular dystrophy (Dystrophin) gene at the Xp21 locus. Circulation *87*:1854, 1993; Keating, M. T.: Genetic approaches to cardiovascular disease. Circulation *92*:142, 1995; Rampazzo, A., et al.: The gene for arrhythmogenic right ventricular cardiomyopathy maps to chromosome 14q23-q24. Hum. Mol. Genet. *3*:959, 1994; Shovlin, C. L., et al.: A gene for hereditary hemorrhagic telangiectasia maps to chromosome 9q3. Nature Genet. *6*:205, 1994; Dietz, H. C., and Pyeritz, R. E.: Molecular genetic approaches to the study of human cardiovascular disease. Annu. Rev. Physiol. *56*:763, 1994. ID = intragenic deletion; MHC = myosin heavy chain; TnT = troponin T.

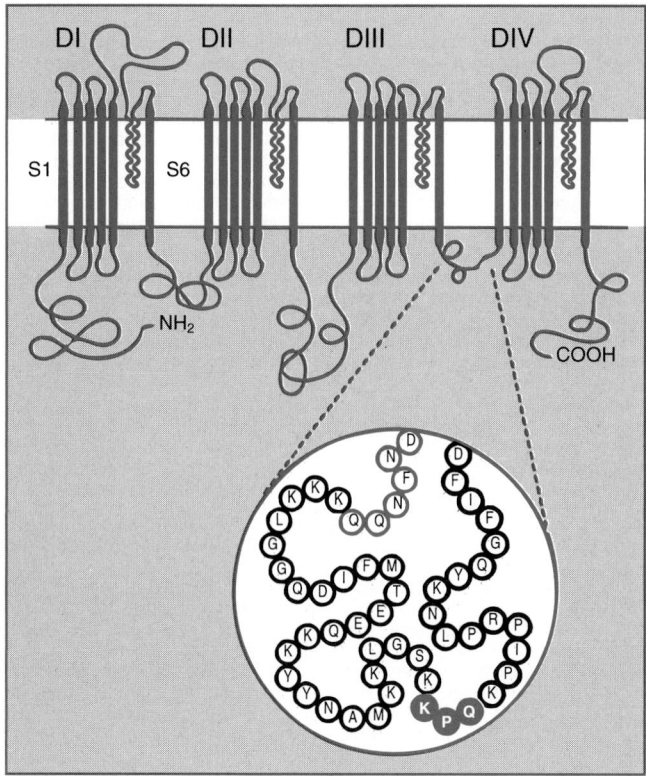

FIGURE 48–5. Mutation in the chromosome 3–linked long Q-T syndrome (LQ-T). Schematic representation of predicted topology of the protein encoded by SCN5A and the location of the LQ-T deletion. Genetic linkage was established between LQ-T3 and polymorphisms within SCN5A, the cardiac sodium channel. Single-strand conformation polymorphism and DNA sequence analyses revealed identical intragenic deletions in SCN5A in affected members of two unrelated LQ-T families. The 9-base pair deletion disrupts the coding sequence with a corresponding deletion of three conserved amino acids (Lys 1505–Pro 1506–Gln 1507; KPQ). The deleted sequences reside in the region important for channel inactivation, with the predicted phenotype being prolonged depolarizing currents accounting for the electrocardiographic phenotype of Q-T prolongation. (From Wang, Q., Shen, J., Splawski, I., et al.: SCN5A mutations associated with an inherited cardiac arrhythmia, long QT syndrome. Cell 80:805, 1995.)

excluded. Further analysis of the telomeric location of this region of chromosome 11 should reveal the defective gene.

Early reports showed linkage to 11p15.5 in all families investigated.[76] Further reports, however, identified other multigenerational families with autosomal dominant long Q-T syndrome (LQ-T) that were not linked to this locus.[77–79] To date, two additional loci have been reported with LQ-T₂ on chromosome 7q35-36 and LQ-T₃ on 3p21-24.[80] In addition, three further families not linked to any of these loci indicated the presence of additional loci, which, although initially unexpected, reflect the complexity of the process of ventricular repolarization and also imply different, albeit related, mechanisms leading to a similar phenotype.[81] The availability of the map locations opened the possibility of the identification of the disease genes, using, in this case, the candidate gene approach as the phenotype of abnormal repolarization pointed to genes encoding ion channels or modulators as likely and reasonable candidates.[80,81]

LQ-T₂. The candidates for the second locus (LQ-T₂) at chromosome location 7q35-36 included a skeletal muscle chloride channel and the cardiac muscarinic acetylcholine receptor, which were both excluded by linkage studies.[81] In *Drosophila melanogaster*, the ether-à-go-go (*eag*) gene encodes a Ca^{++}-modulated K^+ channel and, following screening of a human hippocampal cDNA library with a mouse homologue to *eag*, resulted in localization of the human equivalent gene to the short arm of chromosome 7.[82] The Human Ether-à-go-go-Related Gene (HERG) therefore became a candidate for LQ-T₂. HERG mutations were identified as a cause of LQ-T₂, as there was linkage of 7q35-36 and HERG within affected families; HERG was strongly expressed in heart and HERG mutations associated with LQ-T₂ arose de novo.[81]

Three classes of mutations were identified, including intragenic, point, and de novo. The HERG protein was later expressed in *Xenopus* oöcytes and investigated by patch-clamp analysis.[83] The biophysical properties were those of the cardiac rapidly activating delayed rectifier (I_{kr}: K^+ selective; activated with K_o^+; blocked by lanthanum).[83,84] Further evidence of this mechanism were obtained as the channel

was not blocked by the methanesulfonamilides (E-4031; MK-499), suggesting a separate, pharmacologically sensitive modulating element.[83] Pharmacological sensitivity thereby resembled that of the recently cloned cardiac K_{ATP} channel, where an additional sulfonylurea-responsive subunit is required to confer pharmacological sensitivity.[85]

LQ-T₃. The third locus at 3p21-24 (long Q-T Locus 3; LQ-T₃) initially suggested two candidates, the Ca^{++} channel gene (CACNL1A2) and the K^+ channel-modulating GTP-binding protein gene (GNA12), which were both subsequently excluded.[86] The mutation was, however, localized to another gene in this region with an intragenic deletion of the Na^+ channel gene, SCN5A, which was tightly linked to LQ-T₃ in three unrelated families.[86] This finding again provided a mechanistic basis because the deletions of the disrupted sequences, between D3 and D4, were known to be important in channel inactivation, delayed Na^+ channel inactivation, and altered voltage dependence of channel inactivation (Fig. 48–5). Thus, the deletion suggested that the LQ-T₃ phenotype may be based upon a delay in Na^+ channel inactivation. The deletion therefore is not the result of a dominant-negative electrophysiological effect and loss of function but is essentially an enhancement of normal function.[86,87]

The long Q-T syndromes are therefore apparently due to genetically heterogeneous anomalies of ion channels.[81,86,87] Phenotypic expression with delayed repolarization and predisposition to polymorphic ventricular tachycardia are, however, generally similar.[70] This molecular genetic approach therefore provides three openings in this condition: a basis for family screening; an advanced understanding of the mechanistic basis; and a point from which to devise improved management strategies. The syndrome also has become a paradigm for the molecular understanding of the genesis of arrhythmias due to ion channel dysfunction which might be present, in partial form, in some acquired arrhythmias.[88,89]

Molecular Genetics of Factor V Mutation

The Factor V mutation as seen in patients with familial thrombosis provides a contemporary example of the functional candidate approach in the identification of a gene which confers susceptibility to venous thrombosis and pulmonary thromboembolism (p. 1583).[90–92] The molecular basis of familial thrombosis was, until recently, unclear in over 90 per cent of affected kindreds, with several potential hypotheses, including resistance to activated protein C (APC), being advanced as potential thrombogenic mechanisms. Following the development of a clinically applicable assay for APC, inherited resistance to APC was identified as a significant cause of thrombophilia.[90,93,94] In the assay, the normal response to the addition of exogenous APC is increased clotting time, with APC resistance being associated with no change, following APC addition.[93,95]

The mechanism for APC resistance in affected families was initially unclear.[95] APC activity is due to specific cleavage and inactivation of the phospholipid binding factors, Va and VIIIa, resulting in the inhibition of coagulation[95,96] (Fig. 48–6). Several possible mechanisms were excluded, including mutated protease inhibitors functioning as APC inhibitors, functional protein S deficiency, mutation of the Factor VIII gene, antibodies to protein C, and antiphospholipid antibodies.[95] The exclusion of these candidate molecules led to two outstanding possibilities: deficient function of an unknown APC co-factor or a Factor V mutation. The correction of the defect following the addition of wild-type Factor V and the finding that Factor V from APC-resistant plasma transmitted the defect in vitro implicated Factor V as the molecular determinant of APC resistance.[95] This notion was subsequently supported by linkage studies in two large families which demonstrated microsatellite markers near the known location of the Factor V gene.[91,95,97,98] Sequencing of the Factor V gene then demonstrated the mutation and the replacement of Arg 506 with a glutamine residue. The site of the Factor V mutation corresponded to one of the known APC cleavage sites in Factor Va; APC cleavage of Arg 506 correlates with the loss of Factor Va activity and inhibition of coagulation.[91,95,97]

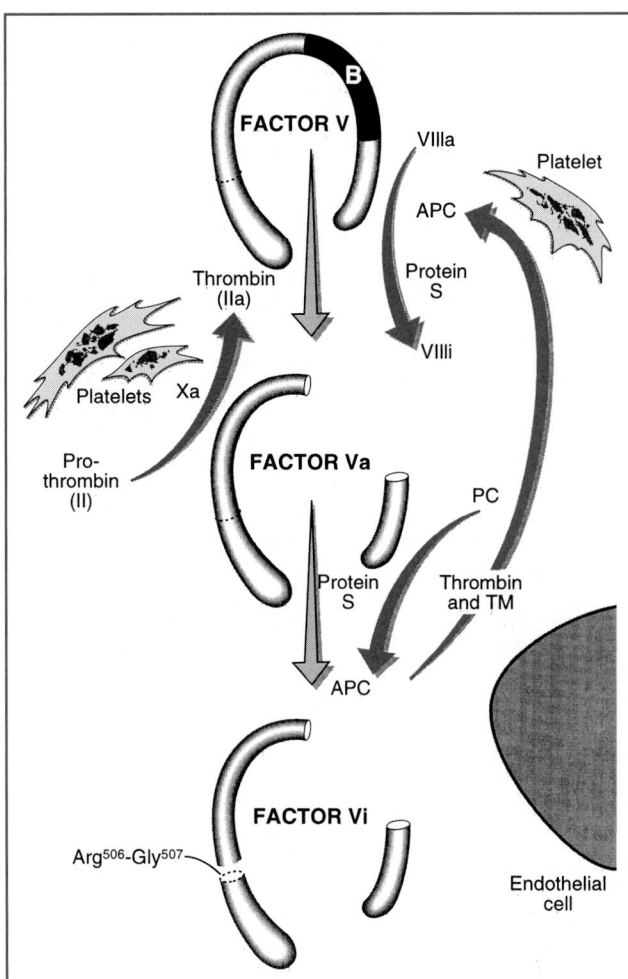

FIGURE 48-6. Activation and inactivation of Factor V and role of mutation Factor V. Factor V *(top)* is activated by excision of the B domain by thrombin, leading to the two-chain polypeptide, Factor Va *(middle)*. On the platelet surface, Factor Va markedly enhances the activation of prothrombin (Factor II) by Factor Xa. When thrombin binds to its receptor, thrombomodulin (TM), on the surface of endothelial cells, it activates protein C (PC). Factor Va augments this action. Activated protein C (APC) inactivates Factor Va, which becomes Factor Vi *(bottom)* in the presence of protein S by first cleaving the single peptide bond, Arg[506]–Gly[507] *(dotted line)* in Factor Va, leading on to the cleavage at Arg[306] responsible for inactivation (not shown). The mutation Arg[506] to Gln reduces the sensitivity to APC, thereby perpetuating the procoagulant effects of Factor Va and predisposing to thrombosis (APC resistance). (From Hajjar, K. A.: Factor V Leiden—an unselfish gene? N. Engl. J. Med. *331*:1585, 1994. Copyright Massachusetts Medical Society.)

These findings have had a major clinical impact. Most cases of APC resistance are caused by this single-point mutation of the Factor V gene, being found in more than half of all patients with inherited thrombophilia.[95] Although the thrombotic tendency is variable, estimates suggest heterozygosity in 3 to 7 per cent of the population and homozygosity in 0.02 to 0.12 per cent.[90,99,100] The mutation therefore represents the most prevalent, well-defined genetic defect associated with human disease.[95] The finding suggests that the identification of *at risk* groups is now possible prospectively, prior to high-risk situations, pointing to the need for possible directed therapy.[95,96] Despite the defect being responsible for venous thrombosis, it does not appear to confer an increased risk for arterial thrombosis.[101]

Future Impact of Molecular Genetics on Cardiovascular Disease

The long Q-T syndromes and Factor V mutation both represent single gene defects and provide useful illustrations of the dissection

of monogenic disorders. However, in general, cardiovascular disease phenotypes are complex, integrative, and polygenic.[60,102] Several genes are operative, each with a small individual contribution, and many times no single gene exerts a dominant influence. In addition, gene-environment interactions can complicate the appearance of a given disease phenotype, either positively or negatively.[61] Thus, there is no simple correspondence between genotype and phenotype, making positional cloning difficult. In addition, there are other problems with variable penetrance and phenocopy, genetic heterogeneity, polygenic inheritance, a high frequency of disease-causing alleles, and variable transmission.[60,102] However, such complex traits in humans and model organisms are now targets for genetic analysis.[102] The problem is being approached with the development of new techniques (genomic mismatch scanning, representational difference analysis), allowing rapid genome analysis, computer analysis, and the use of more sophisticated polymorphic markers.[68]

One other way forward in the analysis of complex traits is the use of parallel studies in model organisms in whom planned breeding of naturally occurring wild-type animal traits can produce models of human disease phenotypes. This approach to polygenic analysis has proven useful in hypertension, with the spontaneously hypertensive rat (SHR), the stroke-prone SHR (SHRSP), and the Dahl salt-sensitive rat being representative examples.[103] In mice, strains with phenocopies of atherosclerosis[104,105] and obesity[106] have also been generated. The major effort to generate inbred strains of mice with obesity has culminated in the isolation of a gene with a human homologue that may influence body fat stores.[107]

OBESITY-DIABETES SYNDROME. Using similar methods, at least six locations on five chromosomes producing obesity-diabetes syndromes with both recessive (diabetes [*db*], tubby [*tub*], fat [*fat*]), and dominant (agouti [*AyAvy*] adult obesity/diabetes [*db*]) mutations have been identified. The *ob* gene is the best characterized and has been cloned and sequenced.[106] *Ob* homozygous mice have morbid obesity with a three-fold increase in body weight versus controls. Positional assignment of the *ob* gene initially was to a 650-kb region on chromosome 6, containing six potential candidate genes, one of which was found to be expressed in adipose tissue of normal mice but not in the obese mice.[107] The gene *ob* encodes a 4.5-kb mRNA with a highly conserved 167 amino acid open-reading frame.

Obese mice have a premature stop codon, resulting in the truncation of the translated protein. The predicted gene product has not been identified, but sequence data predict a secreted protein.[107] In addition, there is an 84 per cent identity with the human homologous sequence.[107] The data fit well with the well-described physiological models and, based on available information, it is therefore suggested there is a signaling pathway from adipose tissue with hypothalamic action with long-term inhibition of the desire to eat regulating size of the body fat depot.[107] *Ob* mice have deficient function of the secreted protein. The function appears to be highly conserved and naturally leads on to the analysis of the function of the *ob* gene in humans.[106,108,109]

Information obtained using animal models will be interpreted in conjunction with existing information on physiology and further studies of the human genotype.[102] Ultimately, the application of information accruing from the availability of the human genetic map will make a significant difference in the isolation of disease genes. The generation of a catalog of genes will transform positional cloning to a systematic analysis of candidate genes.[60,62] Rigorous analysis and association studies could then be used to correlate functionally relevant allelic variations with disease risk. The initial intention is to obtain a high-resolution map of the human genome by the end of the decade, but the definition of the sequence map will remain some way off with less than 0.1 per cent determined to date.[62,67]

GENETIC MODELS OF HUMAN CARDIOVASCULAR DISEASE

The study of the mechanisms of disease and the design of new treatments depends, to a significant extent, on the application of animal research. Spontaneously occurring animal models of human disease[110,111] may be difficult to obtain in the numbers needed for controlled experiments, have complex phenotypes based on the actions of multiple genes, and are often expensive to raise to the point where the phenotype is tractable. Each of these characteristics make them less than ideal as experimental systems.

The development of genetic models of disease therefore represents one of the most dramatic examples of the power of molecular approaches to increase understanding of cardiovascular disease mechanisms.[112–116] Planned alterations of the murine genome allow the introduction of exogenous *human* disease genes, or their equivalents, or the deletion of endogenous genes.[117,118] The resulting models of deranged normal physiology, or of disease, allow not only the investigation of underlying mechanisms, but also the effects of specific interventions on disease processes to be defined.[119] Significant advances in coupling these techniques to the important problems of cardiovascular biology and medicine using genetically based models of developmental defects,[120] atherosclerosis,[105,121] hypertension,[122] hypertrophy, and cardiac failure,[123] in conjunction with traditional analytical techniques, can provide the details of integrated physiological mechanisms.[116,123–127]

Transgenic Technology

The development of transgenic and gene-targeting technologies has facilitated prospective genetic changes in the mouse.[112,113,114,117] Embryonic stem (ES) cells established from normal embryos can be manipulated in vitro and are derived from the inner layer of the preimplantation mouse blastocyst and remain undifferentiated under suitable tissue culture conditions.[128,129] They resume normal embryonic development following microinjection into the host embryo and subsequent incubation in a foster mother. ES cells can contribute to the germ line lineage, as well as somatic tissue in chimeric animals, allowing them to serve as vehicles for creating heritable changes.[118,128] They have several major advantages that include accessible manipulation with homologous recombination in vitro and are also amenable to several screening and selection schemes.

INSERTIONAL MUTAGENESIS. This may be achieved in two ways. The first experimental approaches required direct microinjection of DNA into fertilized oöcytes, which were then implanted into a pseudopregnant female.[117] The use of this relatively crude technique provided a tremendous amount of information but had numerous problems.[114] The exogenous gene is randomly integrated into the genome, possibly into an essential locus, with intrauterine lethality; the transgene could be variably transcribed; the copy number was unpredictable; and usually not all the founder animals passed the transgene to their progeny.[114,118] The second and more sophisticated approach, now applied, targets the gene to a specific locus, thereby avoiding the problems associated with *blind* integration.[118] Homologous recombination describes the result, which is the replacement of the native wild-type gene by the targeted homologue.[118] For the purposes of gene deletions (knockouts), the targeting construct may employ a termination codon to a critical coding exon, leading to premature translational termination or deletion of critical coding sequences.

In order to make a planned knockout of a target gene, a targeting vector is introduced into ES cells using electroporation[118] (Fig. 48–7). The cells that have integrated the DNA are then identified using standard screening methods (polymerase chain reaction, Southern blotting). The targeted ES cells are then injected into the central core of the blastocyst, which is transferred to the uterus of a foster pseudopregnant mother, where they develop to term.[118] The progeny, termed chimeras, have genetic information derived from the host blastocyst modified as a result of homologous recombination.[114,118] Crossing of these lines leads to individuals, all of whom carry the disrupted target gene. The effect on the expressed phenotype following this targeted genetic change is variable.[114,118] The deletion may, for example, be an intrauterine lethal mutation[120]; alternatively, the knockout of a clearly important gene may have no effect on the phenotype due to functional redundancy, where the function of the deleted gene is taken up by another structurally related gene.[118] The genetic background of the mice remains an important consideration in the generation and the analysis of the resulting phenotype.[121]

The alteration of the mouse genome is becoming increasingly sophisticated. Repeated targeting at a single locus may be able to convert a target to a modified form and allows secondary targeting to be carried out, e.g., "tag and exchange" and "double-replacement" strategies.[118] The gene modification may also be targeted to provide phenotypes confined to individual tissues by producing a fusion construct with a transcriptional control sequence of a gene (promoter), which drives the tissue-specific expression of a given gene. In regard to the heart, the best characterized promoters for tissue-specific expression in embryonic and adult ventricular myocardium are the myosin light chain (MLC-2)[114] and alpha-myosin heavy chain (α-MHC) genes.[130] Localization in a specific tissue location can be identified by reporter genes (*firefly luciferase, chloramphenicol acetyltransferase, β-galactosidase*), and such reporter localization serves as a prelude to the introduction of biologically active genes, facilitating the study of targeted genes and corresponding proteins in the specific cell context.[114] The development of spatial and temporal control of recombination events (conditional and tissue-specific knockouts) is being advanced by application of methods, such as the Cre-*lox* site-specific recombination method.[113,131,132]

Transgenic Phenotypes

Several cardiovascular diseases have been modeled using transgenic and gene-targeting technology.[114] Although other

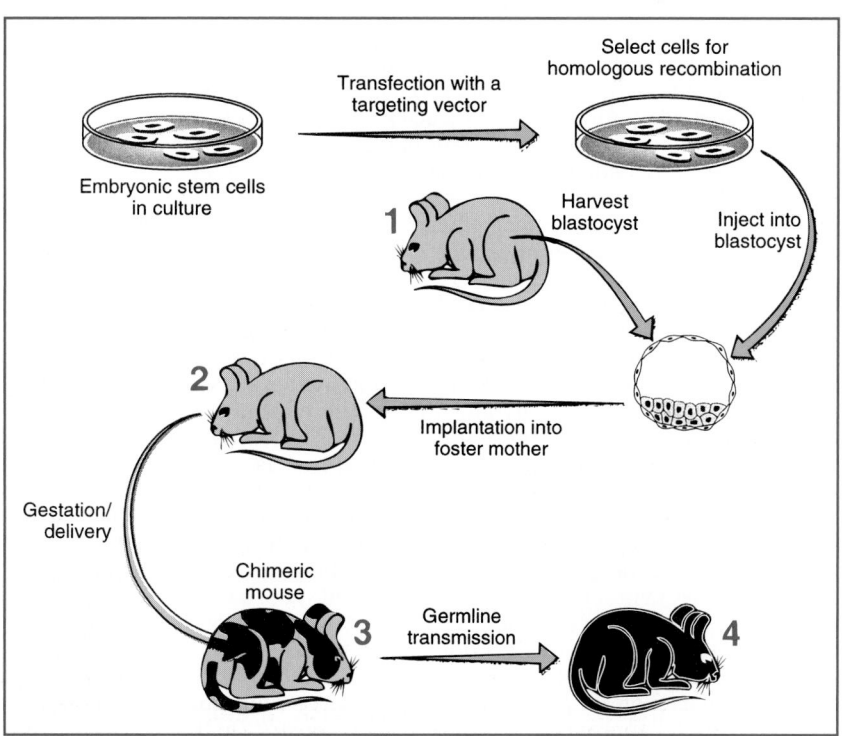

FIGURE 48–7. **Homologous recombination.** Generation of mouse germ line chimerae from embryonic stem (ES) cells containing a targeted gene disruption. The DNA sequence containing the insertion is used to replace the endogenous gene by recombination in ES cells in culture. The altered ES cells are injected into the blastocyst and implanted into a foster mother made *pseudopregnant* following coitus with a vasectomized male. The ES cell line and the blastocyst are usually derived from mouse strains with different coat colors. The resulting chimeric offspring are multicolored, indicating the presence of ES cells. The chimeric mice are bred to establish a mouse line containing the disrupted allele in the germ line.

TABLE 48–2 SOME MURINE TRANSGENIC MODELS OF ATHEROSCLEROSIS*

INTERVENTION	PHENOTYPIC FEATURES
	ATHEROSCLEROSIS-PRONE
Human apoAII overexpression	ApoAII 20% HDL protein content. Phenotype has no elevation in HDL-C. Despite normal HDL-C risk of atherosclerosis increases with fatty streak development even on low-fat diet. Indicates that qualitative features of HDL-C are also important.
Human CIII overexpression	First animal model of primary hypertryglyceridemia. Triglyceride level proportional to CIII expression. Primary abnormality decreased VLDL fractional catabolic rate.
Human AI, CIII, CETP overexpression	High triglyceride, low HDL-C phenotype. Comparable to most common lipoprotein disorder conferring susceptibility to CAD in humans.
Human apo(a) overexpression	Apo(a) mice developed 20 times greater area of lipid-rich lesions that control mice (outbred genetic background 3 months on atherogenic diet). <5% apo(a) associated with lipoprotein; suggested apo(a) produces pathology independently of LDL.
ApoE deficient	See text
LDL-receptor knockout	Homozygous mice have T_{chol} > twice normal litter mates with 7-9 times increase in LDL and IDL. Normal triglycerides. Correction with adenovirus-mediated gene transfer of LDL-R protein. Increased atherosclerosis.
	ATHEROSCLEROSIS-RESISTANT
ApoE overexpression	See text
Human LPL overexpression	LPL directed by the chick β-actin promoter produced accelerated VLDL clearance and resistance to diet-induced hypercholesterolemia.
Human LDL receptor overexpression	Radiolabeled LDL clearance increased 8-10 times compared with control mice. Resistant to high-fat high-cholesterol diet.
Human ApoAI overexpression	Major (> 70%) HDL protein. Selective doubling HDL-C. Useful model for examining effects of diet and drugs on HDL-C/apoA-I. Resistant to fatty streak development induced by atherogenic diet.

* Approximately 20 genes involved in human lipid transport have been overexpressed or knocked out in transgenic mice. Data from Breslow, J. L.: Transgenic mouse models of lipoprotein metabolism and atherosclerosis. Proc. Natl. Acad. Sci. *90*:8314, 1993; Ishibashi, S., et al.: Hypercholesterolemia in low density lipoprotein receptor knockout mice and its reversal by adenovirus-mediated gene delivery. J. Clin. Invest. *92*:883, 1993; Lawn, R. M., et al.: Atherogenesis in transgenic mice expressing human apolipoprotein (a). Nature *360*:670, 1992.

species are amenable to transgenic techniques, such as swine,[133] rabbit,[134] and rat,[122] most have been created in mice because of several intrinsic advantages, including the availability of ES cell technology, inbred strains, and the wealth of information on the mouse genome.[135] The development of apoE-deficient mice provides an example of the potential value of utilizing transgenic technology to engineer animal models of known cardiovascular disease.

Mouse Models of Atherosclerosis

The wild-type mouse, with some exceptions (e.g., strain C57BL/6), is generally resistant to atherosclerosis.[105,121,136] Nevertheless, by the creation of models with powerful analogies to human atherogenesis (Table 48–2), the mouse has become an important system for increasing our understanding of the human disease.[105,121] The generation of mouse models has been facilitated by the fact that human genes involved in lipoprotein metabolism are usually single-copy and have often been sequenced and mapped.[137,138] In addition to increasing understanding of the underlying processes,[105] these mice can also be used in the development of drugs directed against the atherosclerotic process which can be used to predict efficacy in clinical trials[119] and also for testing the applicability of other interventions directed at these processes.

The most atherogenic mouse strain is the apolipoprotein E (apoE)-deficient mouse, in which the apoE gene has been disrupted by homologous recombination.[139,140] apoE is the ligand that is responsible for LDL and chylomicron remnant uptake, playing an important role in the clearance of lipoprotein particles from the circulation.[105] The knockout of the gene for apoE results in a phenotype that is a true null mutation, with no expression of apoE, but has the considerable advantage that the homozygotes are both viable and fertile.[139,140] The pattern of disease is diet-responsive and the homozygotes fed a standard laboratory *chow diet* (0.01 per cent cholesterol, 4.5 per cent fat) have a serum cholesterol concentration of 400 to 500 mg/dl with the development of foam cell lesions at 10 weeks, whereas on a diet similar to that consumed in the United States (0.15 per cent cholesterol and 20 per cent fat) serum cholesterol rises to approximately 1800 mg/dl, mostly in the

VLDL and IDL fractions, with triglycerides being minimally raised and with foam cells as early as 8 wks.[139,140]

Animals consuming both diets develop advanced lesions of atherosclerosis, with their distribution and histology being almost indistinguishable from those of human disease[141,142] (Figs. 48–8, 48–9). These mice also provide a

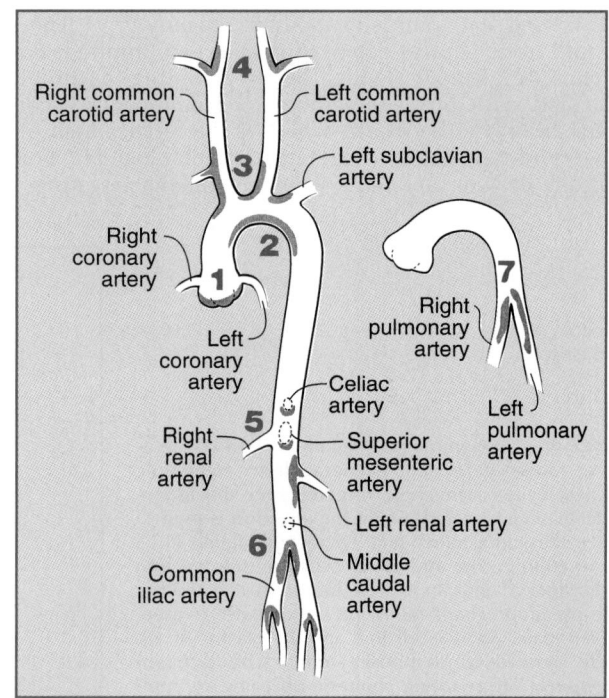

FIGURE 48–8. Extent of atheroma in the apoE-deficient mouse. Diagram of the arterial tree from apoE-deficient mice. The sites of lesion predilection are shown by shading: (1) Aortic root at the base of the valves; (2) lesser curvature of the aortic arch; (3) principal branches of the thoracic aorta; (4) carotid bifurcations; (5) principal branches of abdominal aorta; (6) aortic bifurcations and iliac arteries; (7) pulmonary arteries. The parallels to the distribution of human atheroma are clear. (From Nakashima, Y., Plump, A. S., Raines, E. W., et al.: ApoE-deficient mice develop lesions of all phases of atherosclerosis throughout the arterial tree. Arterioscler. Thromb. *14*:133, 1994. Graphics prepared by Kris Carroll.)

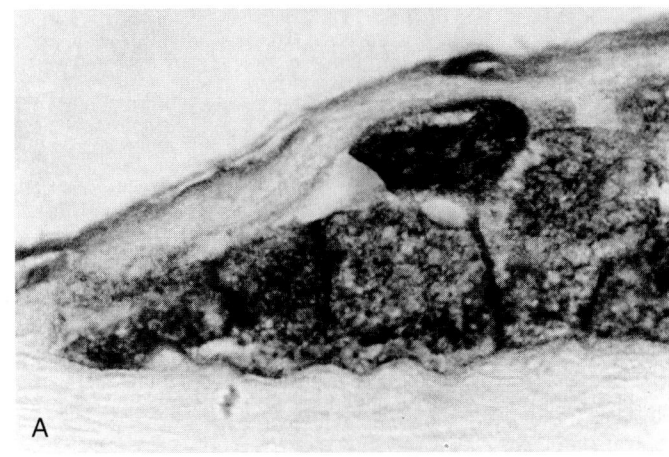

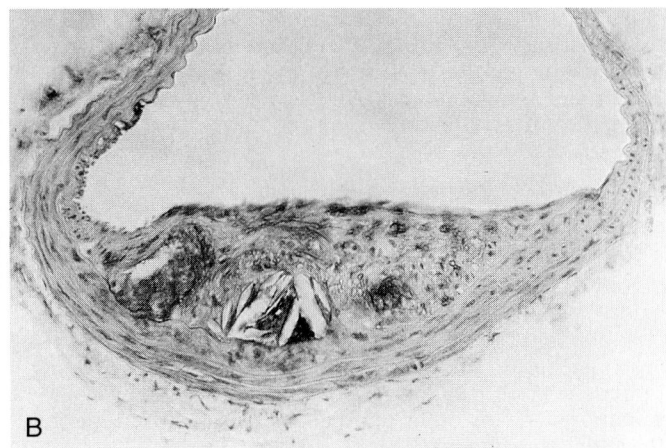

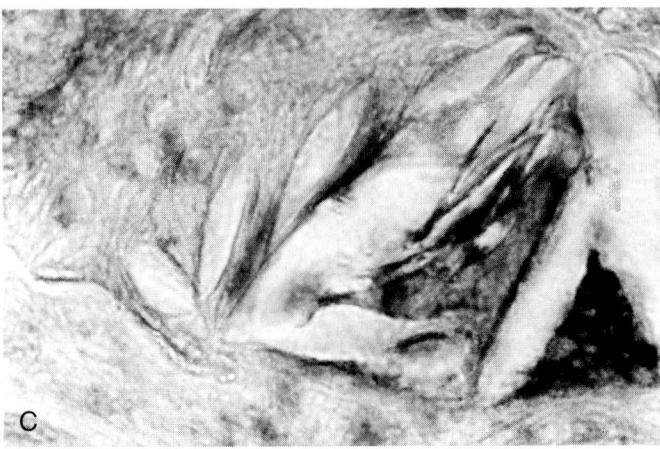

FIGURE 48–9. Photomicrographs showing histology of atherosclerosis in the apoE-deficient mouse. *A,* Transitional lesion in the aortic arch. In contrast to early lesions, consisting primarily of lipid accumulations and macrophages/macrophage-derived foam cells rich in oxidized lipoproteins, in later stages of atherosclerosis macrophages are found predominantly in the shoulder region of lesions, as shown here. *B,* Advanced lesion in the abdominal aorta immunostained for immunoglobulins G and M, showing an extensive necrotic core with cholesterol crystals. In murine models with extensive aortic lesions such as apoE- and LDL receptor-deficient mice, atherosclerotic lesions frequently involve the media, occasionally leading to aneurysms. ApoE-deficient mice have particularly high titers of circulating autoantibodies to epitopes of oxidized lipoproteins, which form immune complexes with oxidized proteins and lipoproteins within atherosclerotic lesions. *C,* Higher magnification of the necrotic core shown in *B,* showing cholesterol crystals and immunoglobulins in the vicinity of the internal elastic lamina. (Images courtesy of Wulf Palinski, M.D., adapted from Palinski, W., Ord, V. A., Plump, A. S., et al.: ApoE-deficient mice are a model of lipoprotein oxidation in atherogenesis. Arterioscler. Thromb. 14:605, 1994. Copyright American Heart Association.)

model for the study of lipoprotein oxidation, with lesion oxidation–specific epitopes and antibodies to malondialdehyde-lysine in serum.[143,144] Heterozygotes have diminished apoE with normal fasting lipids and slightly delayed postprandial lipid clearance consistent with half-normal levels of E2 being sufficient to maintain normal serum lipids.[139] Interestingly, crossing these animals with mice that display overexpression of human transgene AI leads to an elevation of apo-AI, and HDL and apparently alleviates atherogenicity, as it does also with apo(a) overexpressing mice.[145]

The physiological role of apoE is exemplified in two other models. The human apoE3 Leiden variant (tandem duplication amino acids 120 to 126) leads to type III hyperlipoproteinemia[146,147]; overexpression of this gene in so-called E3 Leiden mice leads to a phenocopy of the human disease.[146] The apoE lipoprotein has also been overexpressed in transgenic mice, leading to fourfold increase in apoE levels. These animals have a severalfold increase in radiolabeled VLDL/LDL clearance and are resistant to diet-induced hypercholesterolemia.[148]

GENE THERAPY

The concept of gene therapy encompasses a broad range of diverse technologies having as a common aim the transfer and expression of specific genes to alleviate the fundamental consequences of a disease.[149,150] These aims are inextricably linked to the development of other molecular technologies which are required for the efficient, localized, and long-term expression of the transferred gene. In addition, molecular approaches are often required to identify candidate genes that have potential therapeutic value in experimental model systems.[149] Although the potential impact of gene therapy for cardiovascular medicine is clear, to date there has been no direct demonstration of the practical use for disease targets, cardiovascular or otherwise, within the clinical context.[151,152]

Indeed, significant challenges remain if gene therapy is to become a standard form of treatment for a subset of cardiovascular diseases.[151,152] The major contemporary problem is devising technically feasible methods for gene delivery, a task that requires the coordinate development of several individual technologies with proven value in appropriate animal models that have fidelity to human disease.[151,152] Once established, the specific questions that balance efficacy and safety, in comparison to existing treatments, also need to be addressed. The denominators of the risk-benefit equation are clearly going to be different in nonterminal diseases with high morbidity, such as cardiovascular disease, versus terminal diseases, such as the acquired immunodeficiency syndrome and cancer.[151,152] In addition, the minimal requirement for gene therapy must bear comparison to those of existing treatments having appropriate risk-benefit profiles.[149,153] Herein, we consider the technical issues involved in the application of cardiovascular gene therapy and early steps toward its implementation.

Technical Aspects

Before gene therapy will be achieved in the clinical setting, it is necessary to document the feasibility of the controlled, sustained expression at the appropriate level of therapeutic gene/product for the required duration in the chosen location.[149,153] Two general approaches to somatic gene therapy have been defined: (1) gene transfer ex vivo with removal of cells, followed by gene transduction and the in vivo reimplantation of the modified cells; (2) in vivo gene transfer employing a variety of gene delivery approaches and vectors that have been applied in animal models.[149,152,153] In the context of the cardiovascular system, such an approach implies transvascular delivery for which specialized catheters have been designed.[154] This could be applied for a local effect with delivery to the vessel wall or into myocardial vasculature to facilitate improved coronary flow or might provide a source for the release of cell-derived products for systemic gene replacement therapy, e.g., Factor VIII delivery.[152]

Vector Development

The vector is the agent carrying the gene to the desired site of action, and vector choice and optimization are therefore fundamental to achieve effective gene transfer.[149,153] The ideal vector would be relatively safe, highly efficient, display tissue- or cell-type tropism, and afford high but controllable levels of expression for a long duration. Vectors fall into two general categories—viral and nonviral—with other approaches using a combination of these delivery modes.

The main viruses considered are retroviruses and adenoviruses, with most others having confounding problems with limited host range, antigenicity, pathogenicity, problems with integration, and size constraints.[149,152,153] Replication-defective retroviruses have the advantages of a high (~100 per cent) transduction rate of transported DNA into the host genome. However, they are relatively labile and inactivated in vivo in humans by complement activation. In addition, the host cell range is limited by the requirement for cell division to allow viral integration, and not all mammalian cell types are persuasive for retroviral infection.[149,152,153] There is also an additional concern about long-term expression, with the risk of oncogene activation and neoplasia.[149,152] To date, the single most important advance in improving retroviral vectors has been the development of packaging cell lines able to produce high viral titers.

Adenoviruses have become important in view of the possibility of their use in vivo.[149,152,155] The two serotypes most commonly used (Ad2, Ad5) are minimally pathogenic and have been made replication-defective by the deletion of E1A/E1B gene components.[149,152] The viruses attach to the adenoviral glycoprotein receptor and undergo receptor-mediated endocytosis, escaping lysosomal degradation, to reach the nucleus where the delivered DNA persists unintegrated.[149,152] The adenoviral vectors display several advantages, including an ability to infect nondividing cells and the capability to transfer genes in situ. In addition, recombinant adenoviruses can accommodate large amounts of DNA (36 kb-pair genome), can be produced in high titers (10^{11}/ml), and do not integrate into the genome, thereby reducing the risk of malignant transformation. The main disadvantages are transient expression due to the humoral response following in vivo use facilitated by the presence of neutralizing antibodies in greater than 20 per cent of normal individuals. Humoral immunity reduces efficacy and increases pathogenicity, with tissue inflammation being a significant problem.[149,152]

Two other viruses have been considered in cardiovascular applications. Adeno-associated viruses (AAV) are relatively small, stable, nonpathogenic, and defective viruses that cannot go into the lytic stage and have broad host-range with site-specific integration (chromosome 19) cf. retrovirus.[156] It is proposed they have applications for both in vitro packaging and ex vivo use, although producing sufficiently high titers remains a problem.[156] Haemagglutin virus of Japan (HVJ) is an inactivated paramyxovirus that has been used with a liposome-complex (viral conjugate vector) entrapping DNA and has been suggested as an efficient way of introducing DNA into vascular tissues.[157]

Physical methods exploit natural endocytosis mechanisms to deliver the DNA-ligand complexes targeted to cell-type specific receptors.[149,158] Cationic liposomes are able to form large complexes with DNA, have low toxicity, and are nonimmunogenic, allowing the possibility of repeated high-level dosing, but have problems with low efficacy and transient expression.[158] In an effort to circumvent some of these, conjugates have used the whole virus or fusogenic viral peptides to disrupt endosomes or modifications of liposomal composition.[158] Direct injection of DNA has also been shown to be capable of allowing recombinant gene expression, although this has been seen in less than 1 per cent of cells around myocardial injection sites.[152,159] The advantages suggested are that this is not ex vivo; there are no infectious vectors; plasmid DNA does not integrate; and there is, in general, muscle-specific gene expression.[159] Polymer gels applied to the adventitial aspect of blood vessels have been used for the application of antisense oligonucleotides.[160,161]

Approaches to Specific Problems

Several potential clinical targets have been identified for cardiovascular gene therapy. However, the only clinical studies with direct cardiovascular relevance have been those related to the ex vivo therapy of monogenic familial hypercholesterolemia.[162,163] Below, two additional targets are considered, on which some experimental data are available:

ANGIOGENESIS. Angiogenesis, with new vessel formation and restoration of physiological blood flow, has been identified as a potential therapeutic option in both chronic coronary artery[164] and peripheral vascular disease.[165,166] The agenda here is clearly different from that for neoplastic disease and metastasis, in which the aim is inhibition of angiogenesis.[167] Two approaches to achieving new vessel growth have been identified. First, recombinant angiogenic growth factor formulations are administered directly to the vessels related to the underperfused region, to expedite or augment collateral development.[164,168] The second approach is based on gene transfer,[165,166] which has the theoretical advantage that the secreted gene product could have significant biological effects, with only relatively few cells transfected, following site-specific arterial gene transfer.[152] The genes encoding angiogenic factors, such as FGF and VEGF, have been cloned and mechanisms of action have been established in vitro.[134] However, in vivo efficacy has yet to be definitively established. The expression of PDGF-B, FGF-1, and TGF-β_1 genes following direct transfer into porcine arteries has been shown to induce intimal hyperplasia and neointimal angiogenesis.[165] Exploring the in vivo feasibility and efficacy of this angiogenic approach will undoubtedly be one area of research in coming years.

INHIBITION OF VASCULAR SMOOTH MUSCLE CELL PROLIFERATION. Vascular smooth muscle cell proliferation following PTCA is generally perceived as a target for gene delivery, an agenda that found particular urgency in the significant absence of proven pharmacological therapy.[40,151,152,169] Inhibition of vascular smooth muscle cell proliferation has been the principal aim, with other studies being designed to define the signaling pathways that mediate in vivo proliferation of vascular smooth muscle cells.[152,170]

The feasibility of gene transfection in vivo has been suggested following studies with retroviruses[171] and liposomes, although both methods have a low (<1 per cent) efficiency of transfer.[152] Adenoviruses have been reported to display an increased efficiency of reporter-gene expression (10- to 100-fold), but transient (7 to 14 days) expression is likely to limit utility.[152,172] One of the major determinants of gene transfer with both vector systems is the state of the vessel wall, with transfection in normal vessels being restricted to vascular endothelial cells,[172] whereas in balloon-injured vessels expression in medial cells is also seen. The two approaches currently in use include direct gene transfer with balloon delivery in vivo or the implantation of grafts after ex vivo gene transfer.[152]

Two novel methods for the selective inhibition of proliferation of actively dividing cells have been reported.[173,174] The first approach employed a herpes virus–associated thymidine kinase suicide gene in an adenoviral vector which was delivered into the injured pig femoral artery. The expression of thymidine kinase gene selectively in dividing cells converts gancyclovir to an active toxic form, resulting in cell death.[174] The second approach targeted another component of the nuclear cell cycle regulatory pathway.[173] The expression of the non-phosphorylable, constitutively active form of the retinoblastoma (Rb) gene product limited vascular smooth muscle cell proliferation in both rat carotid and pig femoral arteries at greater than 3 weeks following vascular injury.[173]

ANTISENSE OLIGONUCLEOTIDES. One further potential approach to vascular proliferation is the use of antisense oligonucleotides.[175,176] These are short chain nucleic acids (10 to 39 residues) which bind to a targeted complementary region of mRNA (sense strand) and prevent translation, thereby blocking the expression of specific gene.[175,177] This approach has the theoretical advantage of the inhibition of abnormal genes, while leaving normal genes intact, but their use has been associated with several technical difficulties.[177] The oligonucleotides cross the cell membrane with low efficiency, they are degraded rapidly in the circulation, and no efficient method of drug delivery has been devised.[175] In addition, the antisense oligonucleotides often display nonspecific activity at high concentrations, which complicates interpretation of experimental results.[177]

The published studies have thus far reported biological effects but no direct relevant effects on the production of either the protein or the mRNA.[175] The use of antisense oligonucleotides to the proto-oncogenes c-myb,[160] c-myc,[161] cdc2 kinase, and proliferating cell nuclear antigen[157] have been reported. The improvement of stability facilitating administration (e.g., chemical modification, liposomal conjugates), increases in in vivo biological half-life, and improved specificity will all be required before more widespread application.[175]

Prospects for Gene Therapy

Although currently immense difficulties need to be addressed to allow routine use of in vivo gene therapy in the cardiovascular system, this approach nevertheless represents one of the areas in which the molecular sciences could impact cardiology in the next millennium. Most likely, the first application of gene therapy will be in gene replacement for patients harboring specific genetic deficiencies of circulating proteins, such as Factor VIII deficiency (hemophilia). Vascular targets may continue to be attractive with regard to the inhibition of restenosis but

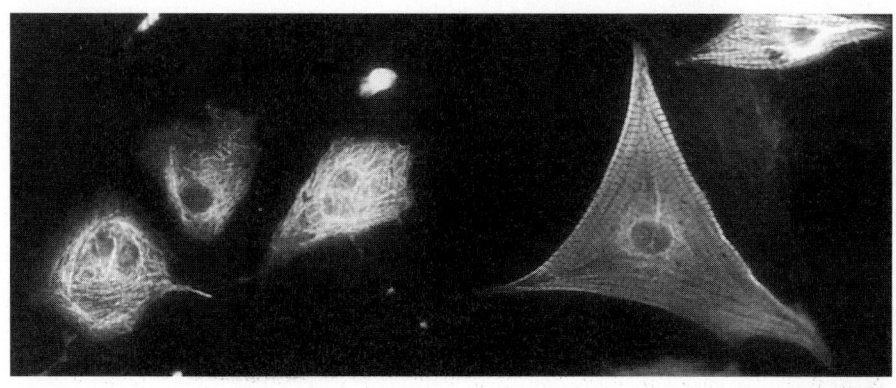

FIGURE 48–10. Hypertrophic cardiac myocyte. Alpha-adrenergic–mediated hypertrophy of cultured neonatal rat myocardial cells leads to the accumulation and assembly of individual contractile proteins into organized sarcomeric units. Myocardial cells were cultured using now standard techniques, with agonists being added to the media as required; here myocardial cells were harvested from indirect immunofluorescence analysis after 48 hours. The left panel shows control cells and the right following exposure to phenylephrine. (From Chien, K. R., Knowlton, K. U., Zhu, H., and Chien, S.: Regulation of cardiac gene expression during myocardial growth and hypertrophy: Molecular studies of an adaptive physiologic response. FASEB J. 5:3037, 1991.)

will require critical comparison with other therapeutic approaches.[152] Cardiac muscle diseases clearly will be more difficult to approach, given the requirement for the transfer and long-term expression of a given gene in sufficient numbers of muscle cells to effect a global change in chamber function, and the potentially arrhythmogenic effects of heterogeneous expression.[159]

MOLECULAR ADVANCES IN CARDIAC HYPERTROPHY

During the past decade a large body of evidence has been accumulated from both basic and clinical research which is beginning to reshape our view of the failing heart[178,179] (see also Chap. 13). The result is that the heart failure syndrome can no longer be viewed as strictly a problem of altered peripheral hemodynamics and depressed cardiac contractility.[178] Two basic elements underlie this change in perspective. The first is the realization that heart failure is heterogeneous at both the molecular and cellular levels and this heterogeneity has significant physiological and clinical

correlations. The second is that the course of both experimental and clinical heart failure is characterized by a series of physiological transitions.[178]

The activation of the cardiac hypertrophic response is characterized, and essentially defined, by increases in the size and contractile protein content of individual cardiac muscle cells[178] (see p. 399). The development of hypertrophy allows the heart to maintain cardiac work and follows as a response to several mechanical or hormonal cues.[180] It is an early milestone during the clinical course of heart failure and a significant risk factor for subsequent morbidity and mortality.[181] Agents that blunt the structural and clinical manifestations of hypertrophy may have beneficial effects on these outcomes.[181]

The pattern of hypertrophy depends on the context within which it develops. In pressure-overload hypertrophy (e.g., hypertensive heart disease, aortic stenosis), for example, additional sarcomeric proteins are assembled in parallel and the heart acquires a concentric pattern of hypertrophy with increased wall thickness, relative preservation of chamber volume, and maintained systolic function.[182] Conversely, in hypertrophy developing after chronic volume overload (e.g., aortic or mitral insufficiency), sarcomeric units become assembled in series, with increased individual myocyte length, global ventricular dilatation, and early-onset systolic dysfunction[182] (Fig. 48–10). Given such distinct morphological and physiological features, it is entirely possible that divergent signaling pathways mediate the development of these individual phenotypes[178] (Fig. 48–11).

The central importance of hypertrophy to the clinical phenotype of chronic heart failure indicates that unraveling the molecular signals that first trigger and then maintain the hypertrophic response may eventually hold the key to understanding the pathogenesis and mechanisms of progression of heart failure. Such understanding could lead to the identification of new therapeutic targets, the interruption of which may halt clinical deterioration.

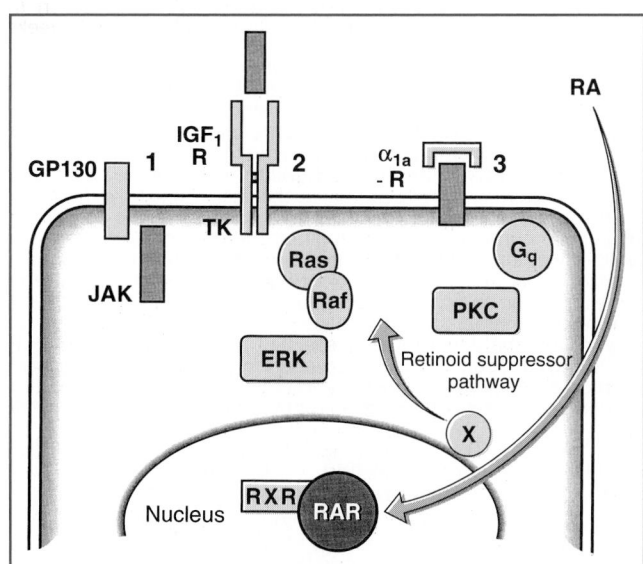

FIGURE 48–11. Signaling mechanisms of cardiac hypertrophy as identified in in vitro model. Three principal putative mechanisms (GP 130; Ras; G_q) leading to the hypertrophic phenotype are shown along with the retinoid suppressor pathway defined in vitro. Details are indicated in text. GP130 = glycoprotein cytokine signaling molecule; JAK = janus kinase; IGF_1R = insulin-like growth factor-1 receptor; TK = tyrosine kinase; α_{1a}-R = alpha-1 adrenoceptor; G_q = G protein (G_α) subunit; PKC = protein kinase C; Ras = signaling protein responsible for translocation Raf to cell membrane; Raf = principal effector of the ras pathway; ERK = mitogen activated protein kinase; RXR = retinoid X receptor; RAR = retinoid A receptor; RA = retinoids: all trans- and 9-cis retinoic acid.

Activation of Cardiac Muscle Genes During Hypertrophy

The activation of specific subsets of cardiac muscle genes is one of the first detectable phenotypic changes in the development of the hypertrophic response (Table 48–3), with the pattern of gene activation being related to the hypertrophic stimulus (pressure overload, volume overload, exercise-induced hypertrophy, hypertrophic cardiomyopathy).[178] These findings are consistent with the existence of distinct molecular phenotypes underlying clinical expressions of hypertrophy.[178] Under certain conditions, downregulation of a subset of cardiac muscle genes has also been observed, including the gene encoding the sarcoplasmic reticulum Ca^{++}-ATPase, which plays a central role in diastolic relaxation.[183]

TABLE 48–3 IN VITRO STIMULI, SIGNALING MOLECULES, AND GENE EXPRESSION THAT CHARACTERIZE THE HYPERTROPHIC RESPONSE

AGONISTS	TRANSDUCTION PATHWAYS	KINASES	NUCLEAR FACTORS	INDUCTION OF IMMEDIATE EARLY GENES	INDUCTION OF EMBRYONIC GENES	INDUCTION OF CONSTITUTIVE CONTRACTILE PROTEIN GENES
α adrenergic	ras	Protein kinase C	HF-1a/HF-1b	c-*fos*	ANF	MLC-2v
Angiotensin II	Gq	Raf-1 kinase	TEF-1	c-*jun*	Skeletal α-actin	Cardiac α-actin
Endothelin I	gp130	S6 kinase	SRF	*Egr*–1	β-MHC	
FGF		MAP kinases		*Jun*-B		
TGF-β		JAK kinases		Nur-77		
Cardiotrophin-1						
LIF						
Stretch						

Cardiac hypertrophy results in the induction of constitutively expressed sarcomeric protein genes, accounting for the increase in contractile protein content that is a necessary component of the phenotype.[178,180,182] In addition, the hypertrophic response is accompanied by ventricular reexpression of genes, which are ordinarily expressed in this location only in the fetus. In the embryonic heart, for example, atrial natriuretic factor (ANF) gene expression is observed in the atrium and ventricle.[184] Following birth there is selective downregulation of the ventricular gene, leading to restricted atrial expression.[184] However, hypertrophy invariably results in a rapid reinduction of ventricular ANF gene expression, and natriuretic peptide expression is increased in both hypertrophic[185] and dilated cardiomyopathy.[186] The constitutive activation of ANF in the hypertrophied heart is also thought to reflect the switching on of other embryonic genes.[187–189] In view of these findings, the ANF gene has become established as a well-characterized marker of the hypertrophic response in both in vitro and in vivo model systems and has been extensively used to map signaling pathways responsible for this adaptive physiological response.[124,184,190–193] These systems have also been used to identify the role of new and known growth factors in the activation of the hypertrophic response.[184,192,193]

IN VITRO ASSAY SYSTEM FOR MYOCARDIAL CELL HYPERTROPHY

Several laboratories have employed in vitro myocardial cell assays to determine which of the many phenotypic features of hypertrophy are under the control of particular signaling pathways (Table 48–4). The availability of a well-characterized cultured myocardial cell system that displays morphological and genetic features of the in vivo hypertrophic response[187,188,191,194–199] has led to the identification of a number of defined hormonal stimuli that can activate the hypertrophic phenotype in vitro, including alpha-adrenergic agonists,[195,196] angiotensin II,[197,200] and endothelin-1.[191,198,199] These systems have also been adapted to characterize specific elements of the hypertrophic response. For example, reproducible methods to stretch such cells both actively and passively have been successfully used to character-

TABLE 48–4 EXPERIMENTAL STRATEGY TO MAP SIGNALING PATHWAYS

1. Identify candidate signaling molecules and pathways in in vitro cultured myocardial cell model systems.
2. Develop and characterize a mouse-based model of hypertrophy.
3. Utilize miniaturized technology to monitor in vitro cardiac physiology in the living mouse.
4. Develop strategies for ventricular chamber–specific expression of transgenes.
5. Utilize combination of transgenic and gene-targeting approaches to assess role of individual candidate signaling molecules in in vivo hypertrophy in the mouse.

Adapted from Chien, K. R.: Cannon Award Lecture. Cardiac muscle diseases in genetically engineered mice: The evolution of molecular physiology. Am. J. Physiol. 269:H755, 1995.

ize signaling pathways activated following mechanical stimuli.[201,202] In addition, the in vitro myocardial cell assay system has been used to identify new paracrine sources of hypertrophic factors derived from cardiac fibroblasts[205]; and following transfer of the assay system to a rapid throughput, 96-well format has also allowed the isolation and cloning of a novel cytokine.[204]

Combinations of cotransfection and microinjection techniques have been used to induce or block specific component molecules[205] and led to a skeleton plan of the downstream signaling pathways capable of activating phenotypic features of hypertrophy[205,206] (Fig. 48–11). Although clearly valuable in identifying known and novel candidate genes for the hypertrophic process, such in vitro studies do not address the question of whether activation of any of these signaling pathways is sufficient to promote a hypertrophic response in vivo. For example, whether the complex in vivo physiological stimulus of pressure overload can be adequately modeled by simple mechanical stretching of myocytes in vitro must remain an open question until correlative in vivo data are available.[202] Ultimately, the detailed modeling and evaluation of the role of specific signaling molecules in clinical hypertrophy and the cardiomyopathies and in the transition from hypertrophy to dilatation and systolic failure require study in vivo.[113]

In vivo Cardiac Hypertrophy Assay System in Genetically Manipulated Mice

One difficulty faced in defining signaling pathways in in vivo models of hypertrophy has been the limited ability to manipulate or control individual elements of the in vivo physiology of myocardial hypertrophy.[190] Inhibitors of various surface receptors and enzyme systems have been used to study the development of hypertrophy, but in many cases use of inhibitors, being nonspecific, has led to secondary physiological effects that confound clear interpretation of results.[178] Thus, the ability to genetically manipulate an in vivo animal hypertrophy model represents a significant advantage.[123] The final aim has been to document how mechanical triggers orchestrate a specific set of genetic events in the adult cardiac muscle cell within a multicellular content.[190] This endpoint could be achieved by the expression of a dominantly acting gene product or the neutralization of the activity of a specific signaling molecule without, ideally, interference with other components of a highly integrated network.[113] Subsequently, assessment can be made of the effects of such genetic alteration on the acquisition of specific molecular and cellular features of hypertrophy (e.g., increase in contractile protein content, activation of embryonic genes, increase in myocyte size) in addition to other hallmarks of the integrated physiological phenotype.[124,190,207]

Advances in mouse genetics and transgenic/gene-targeting technology have resulted in the mouse becoming an important model system to study cardiac hypertrophy and failure.[124,190] The use of microsurgical approaches has led to a reproducible model of pressure-overload hypertrophy despite the diminutive size of the murine heart and great vessels (Fig. 48–12).[124,190] Creating a constriction in the ascending thoracic aorta produces a stable 35-mm Hg gradient and a 35 per cent increase in heart weight with a greater than 20-fold increase in steady-state myocardial ANF mRNA expression.[124] The pattern of immediate early gene expression during pressure-overload hypertrophy in murine myocardium is identical with that elicited in other in vivo and in vitro model systems of hypertrophy.[124] In addition, the mouse hypertrophy model recapitulates other characteristic features of ventricular hypertrophy seen both in in vitro systems and clinically.[124,190,208] The onset of hy-

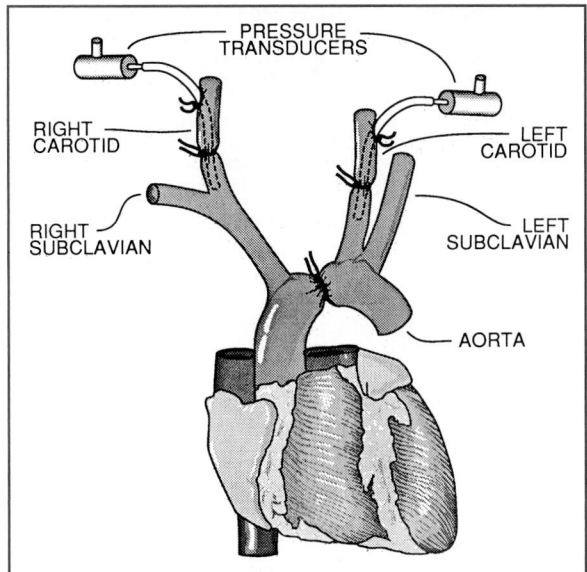

FIGURE 48–12. Microsurgical induction of transverse aortic constriction and associated cardiac hypertrophy in the mouse. Method for the production of stable transverse aortic constriction in mouse (see text for details). (From Rockman, H. A., Ross, R. S., Harris, A., et al.: Segregation of atrial specific and inducible expression of an ANF transgene in an in vitro murine model of cardiac hypertrophy. Proc. Natl. Acad. Sci. *88*:8277, 1991.)

pertrophy in the human setting, for example, is accompanied by a well-defined set of in vivo physiological phenotypes. In the initial stages of human hypertension, increased ventricular wall thickness is associated with decreased diastolic compliance and relative preservation of systolic function.[209] Subsequently, left ventricular ejection fraction decreases with ventricular dilatation and symptomatic heart failure associated with blunted beta-adrenergic responsiveness, as assessed by agonist-mediated increases in left ventricular dp/dt.[210,211] The ultimate utility of the mouse as a model system to study hypertrophic heart disease and heart failure rests upon documenting that these physiological phenotypes of impaired diastolic compliance, decreased systolic function, and basal and agonist-mediated

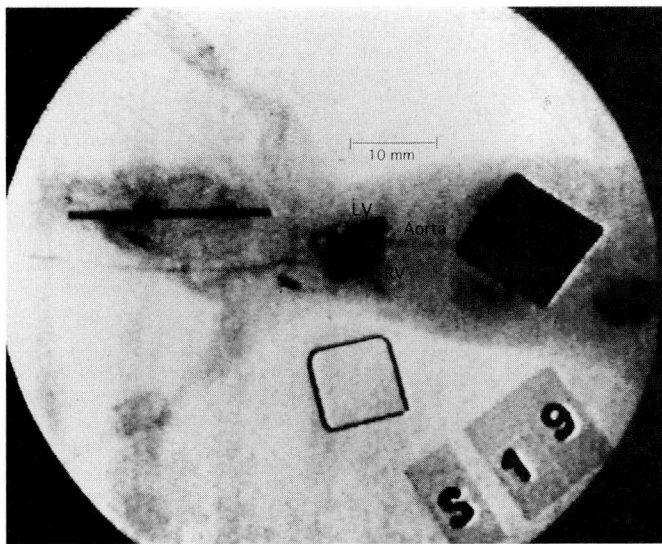

FIGURE 48–13. Digitized ventricular angiography for the in vivo assessment of hemodynamic function in the mouse. Cardiac catheter inserted from right jugular vein imaged in left anterior oblique. In addition to intracardiac opacification, renal shadow and bladder are visualized by contrast; tracheal cannula in situ. (From Chien, K. R.: Molecular advances in cardiovascular biology. Science *260*:916, 1993. Reprinted with permission, American Association for the Advancement of Science.)

increases in cardiac contractility and relaxation can be quantitatively assayed in the in vivo mouse context.[127,178] Miniaturized catheterization[207] with microangiography technology[125] to provide quantitative assays is now available and has been routinely applied to characterize such physiological phenotypes in both transgenic and gene-targeted mice (Fig. 48–13).[123,212]

Using observations from the in vitro model systems of hypertrophy, experimental strategies have been devised which should ultimately allow a definitive assessment of the roles of particular signaling molecules in the pathophysiology of cardiac hypertrophy and failure (Table 48–3). Candidate genes are identified in the in vitro model system, and their subsequent role in the in vivo context is evaluated in genetically manipulated mice produced with cardiac-specific promoters.[114,213] With the advent of tissue-specific knockout, conditional transgene expression,[131,132] and a variety of rescue strategies, future refinements in mouse genetic technology should eventually allow discrimination between primary and secondary events during the course of cardiac growth and development.[178]

Identification of Cardiac Growth Factors and Cytokines

The precise means by which hemodynamic stress is sensed by cardiac myocytes and the mechanisms of the subsequent activation of those growth-related signaling pathways that regulate the cardiac muscle gene program during myocardial hypertrophy are unknown.[178] The relative absence of hypertrophy in the right heart following aortic constriction[124] and the selective growth of the right ventricle after pulmonary artery banding[125] point against systemic circulating factors as principal mediators. The current general hypothesis is that growth factors are produced by cardiac nonmuscle cells or by myocytes themselves, in response to hemodynamic stress and, through specific signaling cascades, selectively regulate the transcription of genes leading to cardiomyocyte growth.[178,214]

The recent isolation and molecular cloning of numerous growth factors, the description of their expression in the heart, and the demonstration that cardiac myocytes are targets for peptide-derived growth factors have all supported a role for such locally produced diffusible factors initially in cardiac growth and later in myocardial failure[196,214,215] (Table 48–5). According to this perspective, the transition between compensated hypertrophy and overt cardiac dysfunction may reflect the action of different subsets of growth factors and/or cytokines. At any one time, the net structure and function of the heart might be the result of the integration of diverse paracrine stimuli that mediate distinct physiological phenotypes via control of various subsets of the cardiac gene program.[178] Under such circumstances, the pathogenesis of cardiac muscle failure could be viewed as a classical problem in growth and development, analogous to the process of cardiogenesis, in which specific molecular cues guide chamber morphogenesis with tight spatial and temporal regulation.[216,217] If such is the case, then new therapeutic approaches to heart failure could rest on the identification and manipulation of factors that promote physiological hypertrophy and inhibition of stimuli that activate phenotypic features of the failing heart.[178]

The absolute number of distinct growth factors expressed in the myocardium is not yet known, and therefore the identification of cardiac growth factors and their receptors remains an expanding area in cardiovascular research. Among those that have been identified in the heart include transforming growth factor-beta (TGF-β), insulin-like growth factor-1 (IGF-1), endothelin I, angiotensin II, and a burgeoning number of new growth factors and cytokines.[196,204,214,215] Some of the candidate growth factors that have been implicated in activating a hypertrophic response in cardiac model systems are discussed in Table 48–5.

TABLE 48–5 GROWTH FACTORS IMPLICATED IN ACTIVATING A HYPERTROPHIC RESPONSE

GROWTH FACTOR	ACTIVITY
Angiotensin II	⇑ release in in vitro stretch-induced hypertrophy ⇑ ANF, immediate early genes and skeletal α-actin expression in in vitro model ACE inhibition or AT₁ receptor antagonists block hypertrophy
Endothelin	Presence of binding sites on cardiac myocytes ⇑ mRNA pre-pro-endothelin-1 during cardiac hypertrophy ⇑ immediate early genes, ANF, and MLC$_{2v}$ in in vitro model ET$_A$ receptor antagonists block hypertrophy
TGF-β	⇑ mRNA during cardiac hypertrophy ⇑ β-MHC, α-skeletal actin, α-smooth muscle actin, ANF ⇓ α-MHC
IGF-1	⇑ IGF-1 mRNA and protein during hypertrophy ⇑ β-MHC, MLC$_{2v}$, troponin I ⇑ number of nascent myofibrils IGF-1 knockout mice show phenotype with impaired cardiac and skeletal muscle growth ⇑ Cardiac mass after in vivo administration

ANF = atrial natriuretic factor; AT = angiotensin; MLC = myosin light chain; MHC = myosin heavy chain. Adapted from Lembo, G., Hunter, J. J., and Chien, K. R.: Signaling pathways for cardiac growth and hypertrophy. Recent advances and prospects for growth factor therapy. Ann. N. Y. Acad. Sci. 752:115, 1995.

ANGIOTENSIN II

The renin-angiotensin system is one of the principal regulators of intravascular volume, natriuresis, and systemic blood pressure[218-221] (see p. 413). The activity of the circulating system is significantly determined by the proteolytic enzyme renin, which is synthesized by the kidney and secreted into the circulation, where it hydrolyzes the decapeptide, angiotensin I, from the amino-terminal end of angiotensinogen. Angiotensin I is converted to the octapeptide, angiotensin II, by the dipeptidyl carboxypeptidase, angiotensin-converting enzyme. However, renin may not be the only rate-limiting step for angiotensin II production. Enzymes that can directly cleave angiotensinogen to release angiotensin II have been described, including cathepsin G, kallikrein, and tonin, and recently a chymotrypsin-like protease has been cloned from human heart (heart chymase[222]), which has been suggested to represent an alternative pathway for the conversion of angiotensin I to angiotensin II. In the heart, angiotensin-II binding sites have been described, and the recent development of nonpeptide angiotensin II antagonists has led to the characterization of two types of angiotensin-II receptors, designated AT₁ and AT₂.[223,224] The AT₁ receptor subtype is a seven transmembrane-domain protein that transmits angiotensin II effects through G protein–coupled pathways, but the AT₂ receptor does not appear to be G protein–linked, and its biological function remains unknown.[224]

ACTIONS ON THE MYOCARDIUM. Angiotensin II has both direct and indirect actions on the myocardium, modulating both cardiac contractility and hypertrophy.[218-221,225] Clinical and experimental studies have clearly indicated that ACE inhibitors or angiotensin receptor antagonists can cause regression of cardiac hypertrophy, an effect that in some experimental models seems independent from their effect on blood pressure.[225-227] Moreover, in the past decade, mounting experimental evidence suggests that the renin-angiotensin system is not solely an endocrine system but is present in several peripheral tissues, including the heart.[219,225] Renin and angiotensinogen mRNAs have been demonstrated in the four cardiac chambers,[220,225] and AT₁ mRNA is induced more than threefold in left ventricular myocardium from hypertrophied hearts.[228] Angiotensin II can diffuse from the myocardial microvasculature through the cardiac interstitium to activate receptors on cardiac myocytes, leading to increased contractility and/or growth.

Angiotensin II increases protein synthesis in chick cardiac myocytes[226] and is able to cause hypertrophy of rat cardiac myocytes and hyperplasia of cardiac nonmyocytes, both actions mediated by the AT₁ receptor.[197,224] Furthermore, in an in vitro model of stretch-induced cardiac hypertrophy, mechanical stretch causes release of angiotensin II from cardiac myocytes and may act as an initiator of the stretch-induced hypertrophic response.[229] Electron microscopy shows that immunoreactive angiotensin II is preferentially localized in what

appear to be secretory granules in ventricular myocytes.[229] These observations are consistent with the hypothesis that locally produced angiotensin II acts as an endogenous growth factor regulating myocardial growth and, at the same time, may affect the level of expression of other growth factor genes.[218-221] However, because cardiac fibroblasts contain a high density of AT₁ receptors, whether the mechanical sensor for the stretch stimulus is within cardiac or noncardiac cells remains an open question. Gene-targeted mice with deletions of various components of the renin-angiotensin system are currently being characterized by a number of laboratories and should allow a direct evaluation of the role of this system in the hypertrophic response.[116,230]

ENDOTHELIN 1

As predicted by the primary structure of the full-length cDNA, endothelin 1 is synthesized as a pre-pro-peptide of approximately 200 residues, which is subsequently cleaved to a 38 to 39 residue big endothelin molecule.[231,232] Further proteolytic processing results in the mature, biologically active 21-amino acid peptide, which is highly conserved among species.[232] Although endothelin was initially thought to be localized exclusively in vascular endothelial cells, endothelin 1, endothelin 2, and endothelin 3 have now been found to be widely distributed in extravascular tissues.[233] Although the presence of high-affinity endothelin receptors on the surface of ventricular myocardial cells has been documented,[231] the role of endothelin 1 in the in vivo regulation of ventricular function has been the subject of some speculation, although it is clear that endothelin-1 is a potent stimulus for in vitro cardiac cell growth and hypertrophy.[191,198,199,234]

Because endothelin is released from endothelial cells that lie immediately adjacent to the myocytes within the intact myocardium, the activation of myocardial cell hypertrophy may represent another important paracrine mechanism for the regulation of cardiac growth.[178] Evidence to support such a phenomenon has been demonstrated in an animal model of coarctation of the aorta.[235] During the development of left ventricular hypertrophy, pre-pro-endothelin 1 mRNA was increased in banded compared with sham-operated control animals, peaking at 24 hours and returning to basal levels after 4 days.[235] It seems, therefore, that pressure-overload can upregulate endothelin-1 gene expression within the heart. When the animals were given a specific endothelin-1A receptor subtype antagonist (BQ123), despite the hemodynamic overload, genetic markers of cardiac hypertrophy (skeletal alpha-actin and ANF) were not induced, suggesting a specific role for endothelin-1 in the development of certain features of left ventricular hypertrophy.[235] The availability of well-characterized endothelin receptor antagonists should allow a further evaluation of the role of endothelin signaling pathways in the onset of cardiac muscle failure.[232,236]

INSULIN-LIKE GROWTH FACTOR-1 (IGF-1)

IGF-1 is a nonglycosylated, single-chain peptide of 70 amino acid residues with structural homology and biological function similar to those of proinsulin.[237] Although the pituitary secretion of growth hormone stimulates the production of IGF-1, primarily in the liver, most tissues synthesize IGF-1 locally. Recently, IGF-1 has also been shown to be a growth factor for cardiac myocytes.[238,239] In cultured cardiac myocytes, specific IGF-1 receptors are present and IGF-1 stimulation increases the mRNA for beta-MHC, MLC₂, and troponin I; protein synthesis is also enhanced by IGF-1 in adult cardiomyocytes.[240,241] More recently, it has been reported that IGF-1–treated adult cardiac myocytes showed a dramatic increase over controls in the number of nascent myofibrils.[238] An increase in both left ventricular IGF-1 mRNA and protein has been described in pressure-overload cardiac hypertrophy and in models of both high- and low-renin hypertension, suggesting that IGF-1 may be an important common mediator of an adaptive hypertrophic response.[242]

The association of IGF-1 administration in vivo with a physiological hypertrophic response in normal animals has suggested its potential value as a therapeutic agent to alter remodeling and improve global cardiac function in the setting of heart failure.[243] This supposition has been supported by the observation that IGF-1 can enhance cardiac size and improve cardiac performance during the development of experimental cardiac failure after myocardial infarction in the rat.[244] Whether these beneficial effects can be translated to improved therapy of heart failure is under investigation.[244a]

CYTOKINES INCLUDING CARDIOTROPHIN-1

The development of an in vitro assay system for myocardial cell hypertrophy has offered the possibility of isolating and characterizing both known and novel activities that might activate features of myocardial cell hypertrophy.[193,204,245] Totipotent mouse embryonic stem (ES) cells differentiate into multicellular, cystic embryoid bodies when cultured in the absence of a fibroblast feeder layer or with the removal of leukemia inhibitory factor (LIF).[246] Because these embryoid bodies spontaneously beat, display cardiac-specific markers, and are a source of ventricular myocytes, it has been suggested that they might serve as a valuable source of novel factors that can induce a hypertrophic response in vitro.[178] Embryoid bodies have now been shown to elaborate a factor that induces a hypertrophic response.[204] An expression cloning approach was used to characterize the protein responsible for this activity leading to the isolation of a cDNA clone encoding a 21.5-kDa protein, designated cardiotrophin-1 (CT-1), which can activate several features of in vitro cardiac hypertrophy.[204]

Amino acid similarity data indicate that CT-1 is a member of the leukemia inhibitory factor/ciliary neurotrophic factor/oncostatin-M/interleukin-6/interleukin-11 family of cytokines.[247] Several members of this family are known to signal through the transmembrane protein GP130 and can stimulate features of cardiac myocyte hypertrophy, in a manner similar to CT-1, suggesting the possibility that GP130-dependent signaling pathways may play a role in cardiac hypertrophy.[193] A 1.4-kb cardiotrophin-1 mRNA is expressed in the heart and several other mouse tissues.[248] Currently, a variety of experimental approaches are being taken to further evaluate the role of GP130-dependent pathways in the control of cardiac muscle cell hypertrophy in the in vivo context and define its relationship to the onset of cardiac muscle failure.[193,245,248]

Intracellular Signaling Pathways
(See also Chap. 12)

The finding that diverse growth factors and cytokines can activate distinct molecular and physiological phenotypes in cardiac myocytes has led to numerous studies examining the downstream signaling pathways, from the membrane to the nucleus, which activate specific subsets of the cardiac muscle gene program.[198,199,206,208,249,250] For the most part, these studies have focused on in vitro model systems employing cultured neonatal rat myocardial cells and well-defined downstream molecular markers, as noted previously. The cardiac muscle cell is endowed with many of the receptor-mediated signaling pathways, found in other cell types,[198,199,206,249,250] including G protein–coupled receptor pathways[251] (Fig. 12–17, p. 372), receptor tyrosine kinase pathways,[252] and GP130-dependent pathways.[193] Much of the downstream cell signaling machinery is also conserved between cardiac and other cell types, and, as such, much of this molecular machinery does not appear to be expressed in a cardiac cell–specific manner.[178] The question arises as to which of these conserved signaling pathways leads to defined phenotypic features of various forms of cardiac hypertrophy.

In this regard, recent studies in both cultured cells[206,249] and transgenic animals[123] have documented that ras-dependent pathways are sufficient to activate a hypertrophic response. p21 H-ras is a small, GTP-binding protein that functions as a critical molecular *switch* in mitogenic and differentiation signaling from a number of cell surface receptors, particularly members of the family of receptor tyrosine kinases.[253–255] Microinjection of oncogenic ras in cultured ventricular muscle cells leads to an increase in myocardial cell size, the organization of an individual contractile protein (MLC$_2$) into organized sarcomeric units, the induction of ANF gene expression, but no proliferation, all independent criteria of hypertrophy.[206,249] The questions remained as to whether ras was sufficient to activate a hypertrophic response in vivo and whether it would induce concomitant cardiac dysfunction analogous to that seen clinically.

By generating transgenic mice that harbor a MLC-ras fusion gene, direct evidence that ras is sufficient to activate in vivo cardiac hypertrophy has been obtained with appropriate structural, morphological, and genetic markers.[123] These include an increase in left ventricular mass/body weight ratio, an increase in myocardial cell size, and an increased expression of ANF and are qualitatively similar to murine pressure-overload hypertrophy[123,190] (Figs. 48–14 and 48–15). The response is massive, displaying an increase in wet heart weight (>50 per cent) comparable to that observed with a 100 mm Hg trans-stenotic gradient following thoracic aortic constriction.[190] Further, analysis of in vivo cardiac physiology in the mouse has demonstrated an effect of ras expression on diastolic dysfunction with reduced left ventricular compliance accompanied by a selective increase in left atrial size.[123] In contrast, basal and beta-adrenergic–stimulated contractile function remained intact. Moreover, as a genetically based model of cardiac

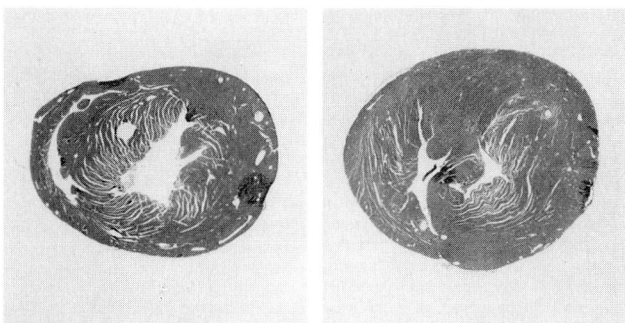

FIGURE 48–14. Hypertrophic heart in *ras* transgenic mouse. Representative histological sections from a wild-type mouse *(left)* and one harboring a MLC-2v-*ras* fusion gene *(right)*, showing increased wall thickness and ventricular chamber obliteration. (Courtesy of Dr. John Hunter, Department of Medicine, University of California, San Diego. Modified from Hunter, J. J., Tanaka, N., Rockman, H. A., et al.: Ventricular expression of an MLC-2v-*ras* fusion gene induces cardiac hypertrophy and selective diastolic dysfunction in transgenic mice. J. Biol. Chem. *270*:23173, 1995, with permission of publisher.)

muscle disease, these mice now permit dissection of the interaction of *ras* with other signaling pathways, through genetic crosses with other transgenic strains, and physiological and pharmacological manipulations that induce or impair the development of hypertrophy.[178]

The signaling pathways that lie downstream from *ras* are conserved in different eukaryotic cell types (e.g., yeast, muscle, cardiac, skeletal) and between widely divergent species (*Drosophila*, mouse, man). Since initial reports that *ras* is capable of activating a hypertrophic response,[206,249] a number of subsequent studies have suggested roles for both Raf and MAP kinase-dependent pathways using cotransfection–based approaches with well-defined reporter genes that are upregulated during the hypertrophic response.[199,256] Similarly, a role for a specific subset of the heterotrimeric G protein signaling pathways[251] via G$_q$ has been documented, which appears to be parallel and co-dominant with the *ras*-dependent pathway.[249]

The activation of protein kinase C (PKC) has long been associated with hypertrophic response in cultured cell systems and represents one potential pathway by which these signals elicited from G protein–coupled receptors could be linked with downstream signaling pathways.[178,257–259] In addition, studies have recently demonstrated that GP130-dependent pathways can activate features of hypertrophy, including the upregulation of ANF, in cultured cardiac muscle cells.[193] In other cell types, this signaling pathway works through activation of JAK/STAT signaling pathways and eventually results in the regulation of specific subsets of cellular gene responses.[247,260,261] Interestingly, angiotensin II has also been shown to

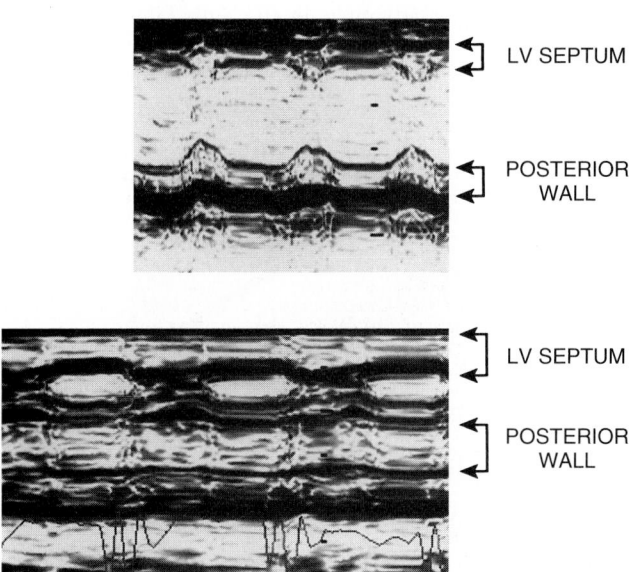

FIGURE 48–15. M-mode of ventricular hypertrophy in the *ras* overexpressing transgenic mouse. Representative M-mode echocardiograms from a wild-type mouse and one harboring a MLC-2v-*ras* fusion gene, showing increased wall thickness. (Courtesy of Dr. John Ross, Department of Medicine, University of California, San Diego.)

activate JAK/STAT pathways in cultured vascular smooth muscle cells.[262]

SPECIFICITY IN CARDIAC SIGNALING. Because much of the cell signaling machinery that lies downstream from *ras,* G$_q$, and GP130-dependent pathways appears to be in place in cardiac muscle cells, a further intriguing question is determining how specificity is conferred in cardiac signaling.[178,208] Given the conservation in the proximal signaling pathway, specificity is likely to be conferred via unique combinatorial pathways involving interaction between tissue-specific and ubiquitous transcription factors that, in turn, regulate individual cardiac muscle genes.[178] The cardiac myocyte is endowed with many quantifiable phenotypes: molecular with induction of embryonic markers[178]; physiological with changes in contractility and global function[113,190]; electrophysiological with modified conduction[89]; and biochemical with altered myofibrillar structure and function.[180] The onset of hypertrophy and the transition to overt heart failure result in changes in each of these phenotypes[178]

Future experimental challenges lie in understanding the role of specific signaling pathways in the activation of these distinct features of the hypertrophic response and how multiple signals are integrated to produce a defined phenotype. Undoubtedly, analysis of in vivo phenotypes in genetically manipulated mice will play a central role in these studies.[113,190] The development of technology for conditional, tissue-specific *knockouts* of ubiquitous signaling molecules will ultimately be required to distinguish primary versus secondary cause-effect relationships.[116,132,213] Because it will not be experimentally or economically feasible to attack all of the candidate cardiac signaling molecules, the in vitro systems should prove useful in identifying nodal points in these pathways.[178]

HYPERTROPHY SUPPRESSOR PATHWAYS

Recent studies have uncovered the presence of hypertrophy suppressor pathways that can act to suppress the onset of features of hypertrophy in the in vitro model system.[263] The first example of the existence of hypertrophy suppressor pathways has been provided by documenting that retinoids can suppress either alpha-adrenergic– or endothelin receptor–mediated hypertrophy in cultured cardiac muscle cells in vitro.[263] The suppressor pathway appears to utilize an RXR/RAR heterodimer pathway and requires the transcriptional induction of downstream cardiac muscle genes because co-transfection of the dominant-negative receptor effectively alleviates suppressor activity.[263] These studies provide evidence for cross-talk between the retinoid signaling pathways[264] and G protein–coupled receptor pathways[251] in cardiac muscle cells and could lead to the identification of a panel of retinoid-inducible hypertrophy suppressor genes. Whether these in vitro observations have any relevance to the in vivo context remains unproven but is clearly a source for future work, given the documented importance of retinoid pathways for in vivo embryonic cardiac muscle growth.[120,126] It will also become of interest to determine whether any other defined agonist or ligands can be purified on the basis of their suppressor activity in the same model system.

Familial Hypertrophic Cardiomyopathy
(See also pp. 1664–1665)

One of the major advances in the entire field of molecular cardiology has been the identification of the genetic defects responsible for familial hypertrophic cardiomyopathy (FHC).[265–269] It is now clear that FHC is a genetically heterogeneous disease, and that although several loci remain to be identified many of the disease loci fall into the class of sarcomeric proteins.[266,267] To date, most of the work has focused on the beta-myosin heavy chain mutations, most of which appear to be missense mutations localized in the head and head-rod junction[268,269] (Fig. 48–16). Because this mutation results in the expression of a myosin heavy chain with impaired function,[270] a scenario for how hypertrophy develops in this entity can now be constructed. In this manner, the expression of these mutant beta-myosin heavy chains has been proposed to serve as dominant negatives, which would act to impair cardiac function in a subtle manner by their assembly with normal sarcomeric units.[270] A secondary massive hypertrophic response in the myocardium, and markedly increased chamber pressures, would eventually lead to myocyte dropout and accompanying fibrosis.

This working model would account for much of our current clinical knowledge of this disorder, including the sporadic nature of hypertrophy, the nonuniform correlation between hypertrophy and the disease genotype, the evidence of cardiac fibrosis, and recent studies demonstrating that a phenocopy of hypertrophic cardiomyopathy can be developed by expressing a dominantly acting signaling molecule for hypertrophy in the ventricular chamber in the in vivo context in transgenic mice.[123] Although far from being proven, the possibility exists that hypertrophy in the setting of FHC may be a secondary rather than a primary phenomenon and that hypertrophy in the setting of FHC may utilize a subset of the pathways that are responsible for activating hypertrophy in other forms of the acquired disease, such as those activated during the course of chronic hypertension.[178]

Toward New Therapeutic Strategies for Heart Failure

As noted earlier, a large body of evidence suggests that cardiac muscle cells, in response to distinct hormonal, mechanical, and physiological stimuli, can activate defined subsets of the cardiac muscle gene program. In many cases, such patterns of activation may be closely linked to the distinct physiological phenotypes that are found in the hypertrophied heart.[178] Initially, these changes may be adaptive but subsequently may become maladaptive. The cardiac muscle cell is endowed with a series of complex signaling cascades that orchestrate these various elements into defined responses and may also harbor pathways to

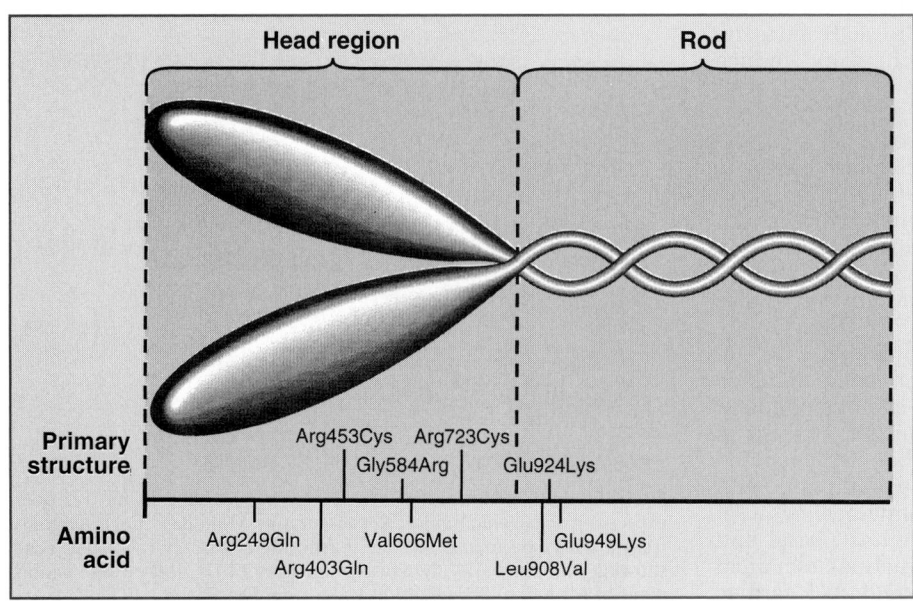

FIGURE 48–16. Location of cardiac MHC mutations in familial hypertrophic cardiomyopathy. The myosin heavy-chain dimer and the corresponding primary amino acid structure are shown in a linear format (amino acids 1 through 2002). Nine of the amino acid substitutions known to cause familial hypertrophic cardiomyopathy are shown (more than 29 beta-MHC mutations have been described). (Adapted from Kelly, D. P., and Strauss, A. W.: Inherited cardiomyopathies. N. Engl. J. Med. *330:*913, 1993. Copyright Massachusetts Medical Society.)

TABLE 48–6 ALTERED EXPRESSION OF CARDIAC GENES IN THE FAILING HUMAN HEART

GENE PRODUCT	EXPRESSION	CHARACTERISTICS
Contractile Proteins		
Myosin heavy chain	⇔	No ventricular isoform shift
		Shift α-MHC to β-MHC in atrium
Myosin light chain	⇑ ⇓	⇑ Ventricular MLC$_{2a}$ in DCM
		⇓ MLC$_{2v}$ in DCM
Actin	⇔	α-skeletal to α-cardiac actin mRNA unchanged in DCM
Troponin T	⇑ ⇓	⇑ TnT$_2$ expression
Sarcolemmal proteins		
β-adrenoceptor	⇓	⇓ β_1 radioligand binding
		⇓ mRNA in DCM
G$_{1a}$ protein	⇑	⇑ mRNA in DCM
		⇑ protein expression
G$_{sa}$ protein	⇔	Unchanged
L-type Ca^{2+} channel	⇑ ⇓	Controversial
Na$^+$, K$^+$-ATPase	⇔	Unchanged
Na$^+$/Ca^{2+} exchanger	⇑	⇑ mRNA in DCM
		⇑ protein expression
SR-Associated Proteins		
Ryanodine receptor	⇑ ⇓	Controversial
Ca^{2+}-ATPase	⇓	⇓ mRNA in DCM
		⇓ protein expression
Phospholamban	⇓	⇓ mRNA in DCM
Calsequestrin	⇔	⇔ mRNA in DCM

DCM = Dilated cardiomyopathy; MLC2a = atrial myosin light chain; MLC2v = ventricular myosin light chain; MHC = myosin heavy chains.

Adapted from Hasenfuss, G., and Just, H.: Myocardial phenotype changes in heart failure: Cellular and subcellular adaptations and their functional significance. Br. Heart J. 72:S10-17, 1994.

suppress individual signaling pathways that could lead to the appearance of distinct phenotypes. One important challenge is defining which particular subsets of factors and pathways mediate distinct phenotypes during the variable course between initiation of cardiac hypertrophy and the appearance of overt cardiac muscle failure (Table 48–6).

It is becoming increasingly apparent that the course of cardiac muscle failure with its different manifestations may largely represent a problem in cardiac growth and morphogenesis, with the morphogenic form taken being a predictor of the clinical outcome for a particular patient. Viewing this complex cardiovascular problem in this manner sets up analogies with the process of cardiogenesis itself, in which a particular signaling pathway may very well have different phenotypic outcomes depending upon the time and the place of its activation during the course of the developmental process.[216,217] In this manner, it may be appropriate to consider the problem of the heart failure syndrome after it has been broken down into stages. Individual components would then be viewed in four stages: initiation, maturation, maintenance, and finally decompensation of the hypertrophic response. The design of new molecular therapeutic approaches will depend upon elucidating the factors and the downstream signaling pathways that orchestrate transitions between stages. Given the current armamentarium of molecular, cellular, and genetic technology, there is little doubt that the definition of the characteristics of these switches will lead to molecular advances in the treatment of heart failure which should be fully apparent within the next decade.

FUTURE PERSPECTIVES

. . . the major scientific advances in medicine in the early twentieth century originated in scientific discoveries not aimed at the management of human diseases. . . . Present day cardiology

has been similarly underpinned by curiosity-driven science, the fruits of which have been taken up by physiologists and cardiologists and applied directly to clinical practice.

Sir David Weatherall[271]

The major clinical problems of interest to the cardiologist have remained largely unchanged over the course of three decades. Clearly, there has never been a greater opportunity for the generation of new, biologically targeted therapeutic strategies to attack fundamental problems in atherogenesis, hypertension, vascular disease, congenital heart disease, and cardiac hypertrophy and failure. The prospects for modern biology to impact mainstream interests of clinical cardiologists are evidenced by the discovery of the disease genes for several monogenic human cardiovascular disorders; the identification of genes that confer risk for cardiovascular disease (e.g., obesity and diabetes); the potential utility of structural biology for rational drug design; the large-scale production of low abundance recombinant proteins for gene replacement disorders (hemophilia), selected acquired diseases (erythropoietin, GM-CSF), and the promise of others (thrombopoietin); the engineering of second-generation recombinant proteins that display improved specificity, efficacy, or a lower incidence of side effects; and the generation of new, genetically manipulated animal models that offer the opportunity to intersect genetics with complex, integrative, and polygenic disorders, which account for the large majority of human cardiovascular disease.

The impending elucidation of a complete set of human cDNAs offers the prospect of mining the human genome to identify genes that cause specific cardiovascular diseases in surrogate model systems. As so aptly noted by David Weatherall,[271] these considerable advances would not be possible without the tools that have been generated through several decades of fundamental science[272] that initially was not designed for the study of human cardiovascular disease but has nevertheless laid a substantial scientific foundation for molecular cardiology.

REFERENCES

1. Chien, K. R.: Molecular advances in cardiovascular biology. Science 260:916, 1993.
2. Lewin, B.: Genes V. 5th ed. Oxford, Oxford University Press, 1994, p. 1272.
3. Watson, J. D., Gilman, M., Witkowski, J., and Zoller, M.: Recombinant DNA. 2nd ed. New York, Scientific American Books, 1992.
4. Rosenthal, N.: General principles of molecular biology. In Chien, K. (ed.): Molecular Basis of Heart Disease. Philadelphia, W. B. Saunders Company, 1997.
5. Chien, K. R. (ed.): Molecular Basis of Heart Disease. Philadelphia, W. B. Saunders Company, 1997.

RECOMBINANT PROTEIN THERAPY

6. Ward, W. H. J., Timms, D., and Fersht, A. R.: Protein engineering and the study of structure-function relationships in receptors. Trends Pharmacol. Sci. 11:280, 1990.
7. Erslev, A.: Erythropoietin. N. Engl. J. Med. 324:1339, 1991.
8. Schick, B. P.: Hope for treatment of thrombocytopenia. N. Engl. J. Med. 331:875, 1994.
9. Gerard, R. D., Chien, K. R., and Meidell, R. S.: Molecular biology of tissue plasminogen activator and endogenous inhibitors. Mol. Biol. Med. 3:449, 1986.
10. Collen, D., and Lijnen, H. R.: Basic and clinical aspects of fibrinolysis and thrombolysis. Blood 78:3114, 1991.
11. Deutsch, E., Rao, K. A., and Colman, R. W.: Selective thrombin inhibitors: The next generation of anticoagulants. J. Am. Coll. Cardiol. 22:1089, 1993.
12. Lefkovits, J., and Topol, E. J.: Direct thrombin inhibitors in cardiovascular medicine. Circulation 90:1522, 1994.
13. Astrup, T., and Permin, P. M.: Isolation of a soluble fibrinolytic activator from animal tissues. Nature 170:929, 1947.
14. Rifkin, D. B., Loe, J. N., Moore, G., and Reich, E.: Properties of plasminogen activators formed from neoplastic human cell cultures. J. Exp. Med. 139:1317, 1974.
15. Rijken, D. C., and Collen, D.: Purification and characterisation of the plasminogen activator secreted by human melanoma cells in culture. J. Biol. Chem. 256:7035, 1981.
16. Pennica, D., Holmes, W. E., Kohr, W. J., et al.: Cloning and expression

of human tissue-type plasminogen activator cDNA in *E. coli*. Nature *301*:214, 1983.

17. Sambrook, J., Hanahan, D., Rodgers, L., and Gething, M. J.: Expression of human tissue type plasminogen activator from lytic viral vectors and in established cell lines. Mol. Biol. Med. *3*:459, 1986.

18. Collen, D., and Haber, E.: Thrombolysis. *In* Chien, K. R. (ed.): Molecular Basis of Heart Disease. Philadelphia, W. B. Saunders Company, 1997.

19. Kaufman, R., Wasley, L., Spiliotes, A., et al.: Co-amplification and co-expression of human tissue type plasminogen activator and murine dihydrofolate reductase in Chinese hamster ovary cells. Mol. Cell. Biol. *5*:1750, 1985.

20. Lijnen, H. R., and Collen, D.: Strategies for the improvement of thrombolytic agents. Thromb. Hemost. *66*:88, 1991.

21. Lubin, I. M., Hayzer, D. J., and Runge, M. S.: Strategies for the design of novel thrombolytic and antithrombolytic agents. Trends Cardiovasc. Med. *2*:84, 1992.

22. Haber, E., Quertermous, T., Matsueda, G. R., and Runge, M. S.: Innovative approaches to tissue plasminogen activator therapy. Science *243*:51, 1989.

23. Baenziger, J. U.: Tissue-type plasminogen activator: A role for O-linked fucose. J. Clin. Invest. *93*:459, 1994.

24. Vaughan, D., and Loscalzo, J.: New directions in thrombolytic therapy: Molecular mutants and biochemical conjugates. Trends Cardiovasc. Med. *1*:36, 1991.

25. Bennett, W. F., Paoni, N. F., Keyt, B. A., et al.: High resolution analysis of functional determinants on human tissue-type plasminogen activator. J. Biol. Chem. *266*:5191, 1991.

26. de Vos, A., Ultsch, M. H., Kelley, R. F., et al.: Crystal structure of the kringle 2 domain of tissue plasminogen activator at 2.4-Å resolution. Biochemistry *31*:270, 1992.

27. Collen, D.: Towards improved thrombolytic therapy. Lancet *342*:34, 1993.

28. Madison, E. L., Goldsmith, E. J., Gerard, R. D., et al.: Serpin-resistant mutants of tissue-type plasminogen activator. Nature *339*:721, 1989.

29. Keyt, B. A., Paoni, N. F., Refino, C. J., et al.: A faster-acting and more potent form of tissue plasminogen activator. Proc. Natl. Acad. Sci. U.S.A. *91*:3670, 1994.

30. Gardell, S. J., Duong, L. T., Diehl, R. E., et al.: Isolation, characterisation and cDNA cloning of a vampire bat salivary plasminogen activator. J. Biol. Chem. *264*:17947, 1989.

31. Harvey, R. P., Degryse, E., Stefani, L., et al.: Cloning and expression of a cDNA coding for the anticoagulant hirudin from the bloodsucking leech, *Hirudo medicinalis*. Proc. Natl. Acad. Sci. *83*:1084, 1986.

32. Badimon, L., Merino, A., Badimon, J., et al.: Hirudin and other thrombin inhibitors: Experimental results and potential clinical applications. Trends Cardiovasc. Med. *1*:261, 1991.

33. Coughlin, S. R.: Thrombin receptor function and cardiovascular disease. Trends Cardiovasc. Med. *4*:77, 1994.

34. Ferrara, N.: Vascular endothelial growth factor. Trends Cardiovasc. Med. *3*:244, 1993.

35. Winter, G., and Milstein, C.: Man-made antibodies. Nature *349*:293, 1991.

36. Ritter, M. A., and Ladyman, H. M. (eds.): Monoclonal antibodies. Production, Engineering and Clinical Application. Cambridge, Cambridge University Press, 1995, p. 496.

37. Riechman, L., Clark, M., Waldman, H., and Winter, G.: Reshaping human antibodies for therapy. Nature *332*:323, 1988.

RATIONAL DESIGN AND DEVELOPMENT OF PHARMACOLOGICAL ANTAGONISTS

38. Brugge, J. S.: New intracellular targets for therapeutic drug design. Science *260*:918, 1993.

39. Goody, R.: Rational drug design and HIV: Hopes and limitations. Nature Med. *1*:519, 1995.

40. Lefkovits, J., Plow, E. F., and Topol, E. J.: Platelet glycoprotein IIb/IIIa receptors in cardiovascular medicine. N. Engl. J. Med. *332*:1553, 1995.

41. Shattil, S., and Ruggieri, Z.: Platelets. *In* Chien, K. R. (ed.): Molecular Basis of Heart Disease. Philadelphia, W. B. Saunders Company, 1997.

42. Jang, Y., Lincoff, A. M., Plow, E. F., and Topol, E. J.: Cell adhesion molecules in coronary artery disease. J. Am. Coll. Cardiol. *24*:1591, 1994.

43. Pyetla, R., Pierschbacher, M. D., Ginsberg, M. H., et al.: Platelet membrane glycoprotein IIb/IIIa: Member of a family of Arg-Gly-Asp-specific adhesion receptors. Science *231*:1559, 1986.

44. Hynes, R. O.: Integrins: A family of cell surface receptors. Cell *48*:549, 1987.

45. Hynes, R. O.: Integrins: Versatility, modulation, and signaling in cell adhesion. Cell *69*:11, 1992.

46. Phillips, D. R., Charo, I. F., and Scarborough, R. M.: GPIIb-IIIa: The responsive integrin. Cell *65*:359, 1991.

47. Calvete, J. J.: Clues for understanding the structure and function of a prototypic human integrin: The platelet glycoprotein IIb/IIIa complex. Thromb. Haemost. *72*:1, 1994.

48. Baldwin, H. S., and Buck, C. A.: Integrins and other cell adhesion molecules in cardiac development. Trends Cardiovasc. Med. *4*:178, 1994.

49. Pierschbacher, M. D., and Ruoslahti, E.: Cell attachment activity of fibronectin can be duplicated by small synthetic fragments of the molecule. Nature *309*:30, 1984.

50. Du, X., Plow, E. F., Frelinger, A. L., et al.: Ligands activate integrin $\alpha_{IIb}\beta_3$ (platelet GPIIb-IIIa). Cell *65*:409, 1991.

51. Dennis, M. S., Henzel, W. J., Pitti, R. M., et al.: Platelet glycoprotein IIb-IIIa protein antagonists from snake venoms: Evidence for a family of platelet aggregation inhibitors. Proc. Natl. Acad. Sci. *87*:2471, 1989.

52. Shebuski, R. J., Ramjit, D. R., Bencen, G. H., and Polokoff, M. A.: Characterisation and platelet inhibitory activity of bitistatin, a potent arginine-glycine-aspartic acid-containing peptide from the venom of the viper *Bitis arietans*. J. Biol. Chem. *264*:21550, 1989.

53. Bangs, N. U., and Clayman, M. D.: Antithrombotic agents from salivary glands of hematophagus animals. Trends Cardiovasc. Med. *2*:183, 1992.

54. Scarborough, R. M., Naughton, M. A., Teng, W., et al.: Design of potent and specific integrin antagonists. J. Biol. Chem. *268*:1066, 1993.

55. Adler, M., Lazarus, R. A., Dennis, M. S., and Wagner, G.: Solution structure of kistrin, a potent platelet aggregation inhibitor in GPIIb-IIIa antagonist. Science *253*:445, 1991.

56. Tcheng, J. E., Harrington, R. A., Kottke-Marchant, K., et al.: Multicenter, randomized, double-blind, placebo-controlled trial of platelet integrin glycoprotein IIb/IIIa blocker intergrelin in elective coronary intervention. Circulation *91*:2151, 1995.

57. Kouns, W. C., Kirchhofer, D., Hadvary, P., et al.: Reversible conformational changes induced in glycoprotein IIb-IIIa by a potent and selective peptidomimetic inhibitor. Blood *80*:2539, 1992.

58. The EPIC Investigators: Use of monoclonal antibody directed against the platelet glycoprotein IIb/IIIa receptor in high risk coronary angioplasty. N. Engl. J. Med. *330*:956, 1994.

59. Harker, L. A.: Platelets and vascular thrombosis. N. Engl. J. Med. *330*:1006, 1994.

LOCALIZATION OF CARDIOVASCULAR DISEASE GENES

60. Beaudet, A. L., Scriver, C. R., Sly, W. S., and Valle, D.: Genetics, biochemistry, and molecular basis of variant human phenotypes. *In* Scriver, C., Beaudet, A., Sly, W., and Vale, D. (eds.): The Metabolic and Molecular Bases of Inherited Disease. 7th ed. New York, McGraw-Hill, 1995, p. 53.

61. White, R., and Caskey, C. T.: The human as an experimental system in molecular genetics. Science *240*:1483, 1988.

62. Collins, F. S.: Positional cloning moves from perditional to traditional. Nature Genet. *9*:347, 1995.

63. Fields, C., Adams, M. D., White, O., and Venter, J. C.: How many genes in the human genome? Nature Genet. *7*:345, 1994.

64. Goodfellow, P. N.: Microsatellites and the new genetic maps. Curr. Biol. *3*:149, 1993.

65. Botstein, D., White, R. L., Skolnick, M., and Davis, R. W.: Construction of a genetic linkage map in man using restriction fragment length polymorphisms. Am. J. Med. Genet. *32*:314, 1980.

66. Housman, D.: Human DNA polymorphism. N. Engl. J. Med. *332*:1318, 1995.

67. Green, E. D., Cox, D. R., and Myers, R. M.: The human genome project and its impact on the study of human disease. *In* Scriver, C. R., Beaudet, A. L., Sly, W. S., and Vale, D. (eds.): The Metabolic and Molecular Bases of Inherited Disease. 7th ed. New York, McGraw-Hill, 1995, p. 401.

68. Aldhous, P.: Fast track to disease genes. Science *265*:2008, 1994.

69. Schwartz, P. J., Moss, A. J., Vincent, G. M., Crampton, R. S.: Diagnostic criteria for the long QT syndrome. Circulation *88*:782, 1993.

70. Schwartz, P. J., Locati, E. H., Napolitano, C., and Priori, S. G.: The long QT syndrome. *In* Zipes, D. P., and Jalife, J. (eds.): Cardiac Electrophysiology: From Cell to Bedside. Philadelphia, W. B. Saunders Company, 1995, p. 788.

71. Moss, A., and Robinson, J.: The long-QT syndrome: Genetic considerations. Trends Cardiovasc. Med. *2*:81, 1992.

72. Vincent, G. M., Timothy, K. W., Leppert, M., and Keating, M. T.: The spectrum of symptoms and QT intervals in carriers of the gene for the long-QT syndrome. N. Engl. J. Med. *327*:846, 1992.

73. Keating, M. T.: Linkage analysis and long QT syndrome: Using genetics to study cardiovascular disease. Circulation *85*:1973, 1992.

74. Keating, M. T., Atkinson, D., Dunn, C., et al.: Linkage of a cardiac arrhythmia, the long QT syndrome, and the Harvey ras-1 gene. Science *252*:704, 1991.

75. Roy, N., Kahlem, P., Dausse, E., et al.: Exclusion of H*ras* from long QT locus. Nature Genet. *8*:113, 1994.

76. Keating, M. T., Dunn, C., Atkinson, D., et al.: Consistent linkage of the long QT syndrome to the Harvey ras-1 locus on chromosome 11. Am. J. Hum. Genet. *49*:1335, 1991.

77. Benhorin, J., Kalman, Y. M., Medina, A., et al.: Evidence of genetic heterogeneity in the long QT syndrome. Science *260*:1960, 1993.

78. Curran, M., Atkinson, D., Timothy, K., et al.: Locus heterogeneity of autosomal dominant long QT syndrome. J. Clin. Invest. *92*:799, 1993.

79. Towbin, J. A., Li, H., Taggart, R. T., et al.: Evidence of genetic heterogeneity in Romano-Ward long QT syndrome. Circulation *90*:2635, 1994.

80. Jiang, C., Atkinson, D., Towbin, J. A., et al.: Two long QT syndrome loci map to chromosomes 3 and 7 with evidence for further heterogeneity. Nature Genet. *8*:141, 1994.

81. Curran, M. E., Splawski, I., Timothy, K. W., et al.: A molecular basis for cardiac arrhythmia: *HERG* mutations cause long QT syndrome. Cell *80*:795, 1995.

82. Warmke, J. W., and Ganetzky, B.: A family of potassium channels related to *eag* in Drosophila and mammals. Proc. Natl. Acad. Sci. U.S.A. *91*:3438, 1994.

83. Sanguinetti, M. C., Jiang, C., Curran, M. E., and Keating, M. T.: A mechanistic link between an inherited arrhythmia and an acquired cardiac arrhythmia: *HERG* encodes the I_{Kr} potassium channel. Cell 81:299, 1995.

84. Kass, R., and Freeman, L.: Potassium channels in the heart: Cellular, molecular and clinical implications. Trends Cardiovasc. Med. 3:149, 1993.

85. Ashford, M. L. J., Bond, C. T., Blair, T. A., and Adelman, J. P.: Cloning and functional expression of a rat K_{ATP} channel. Nature 370:456, 1994.

86. Wang, Q., Shen, J., Splawski, I., et al.: *SCN5A* mutations associated with an inherited cardiac arrhythmia, long QT syndrome. Cell 80:805, 1995.

87. Bennett, P. B., Yazawa, K., Makita, N., and George, A. L.: Molecular mechanism for an inherited cardiac arrhythmia. Nature 376:683, 1995.

88. Grace, A. A., and Chien, K. R.: Congenital long QT syndromes. Toward molecular dissection of arrhythmia substrates. Circulation 92:2786, 1995.

89. Marban, E.: Molecular approaches to arrhythmogenesis. *In* Chien, K. R. (ed.): Molecular Basis of Heart Disease. Philadelphia, W. B. Saunders Company, 1997.

90. Bauer, K. A.: Hypercoagulability—a new cofactor in the protein C anticoagulant pathway. N. Engl. J. Med. 330:566, 1994.

91. Majerus, P. W.: Human genetics: Bad blood by mutation. Nature 369:14, 1994.

92. Mann, K., and Rosenberg, R. D.: Thrombosis. *In* Chien, K. R. (ed.): Molecular Basis of Heart Disease. Philadelphia, W. B. Saunders Company, 1997.

93. Dahlback, B., Carlsson, M., and Svensson, P. J.: Familial thrombophilia due to a previously unrecognized mechanism characterised by poor anticoagulant response to activated protein C: Prediction of a cofactor to activated protein C. Proc. Natl. Acad. Sci. U.S.A. 90:1004, 1993.

94. Castellino, F. J.: Human protein C and activated protein C: Components of the human anticoagulation system. Trends Cardiovasc. Med. 5:55, 1995.

95. Dahlback, B.: Inherited thrombophilia: Resistance to activated protein C as a pathogenic factor of venous thromboembolism. Blood 85:607, 1995.

96. Hajjar, K.: Factor V Leiden—an unselfish gene? N. Engl. J. Med. 331:1585, 1994.

97. Bertina, R. M., Koelman, B. P. C., Koster, T., et al.: Mutation in blood coagulation factor V associated with resistance to activated protein C. Nature 369:64, 1994.

98. Zoller, B., and Dahlback, B.: Linkage between inherited resistance to activated protein C and factor V gene mutation in venous thrombosis. Lancet 343:1536, 1994.

99. Greengard, J. S., Eichinger, S., Griffin, J. H., and Bauer, K. A.: Variability of thrombosis among homozygous siblings with resistance to activated protein C due to Arg ⇒ Gln mutation in the gene for factor V. N. Engl. J. Med. 331:1559, 1994.

100. Koster, T., Rosendaal, F. R., de Ronde, H., et al.: Venous thrombosis due to poor anticoagulant response to activated protein C: Leiden thrombophilia study. Lancet 342:1503, 1993.

101. Ridker, P. M., Hennekens, C. H., Lindpainter, K., et al.: Mutation in the gene coding for coagulation factor V and the risk of myocardial infarction, stroke and venous thrombosis in apparently healthy men. N. Engl. J. Med. 332:912, 1995.

102. Lander, E. S., and Schork, N. J.: Genetic dissection of complex traits. Science 265:2037, 1994.

103. Pattengale, P. K., Steart, T. A., Leder, A., et al.: Animal models of human disease. Am. J. Pathol. 135:39, 1989.

104. Paigen, B., Morrow, A., Brandon, C., et al.: Variation in the susceptibility to atherosclerosis amongst inbred strains of mice. Atherosclerosis 57:65, 1985.

105. Breslow, J. L.: Transgenic mouse models of lipoprotein metabolism and atherosclerosis. Proc. Natl. Acad. Sci. U.S.A. 90:8314, 1993.

106. Keightley, P. D.: Chewing the fat. Nature Genet. 10:125, 1995.

107. Zhang, Y., Proenca, R., Maffei, M., et al.: Positional cloning of the mouse *obese* gene and its human homologue. Nature 372:425, 1994.

108. Rink, T. J.: In search of a satiety factor. Nature 372:406, 1994.

109. Bennett, W. I.: Beyond overeating. N. Engl. J. Med. 332:673, 1995.

GENETIC MODELS OF HUMAN CARDIOVASCULAR DISEASE

110. Yamamoto, T., Bishop, R. W., Brown, M. S., et al.: Deletion in cysteine-rich region of LDL receptor impedes transport to cell surface in WHHL rabbits. Science 232:1230, 1986.

111. Rapacz, J., Hasler-Rapascz, J., Taylor, K. M., et al.: Lipoprotein mutations in pigs are associated with elevated plasma cholesterol and atherosclerosis. Science 234:1573, 1986.

112. Chien, K. R.: Genes and physiology: Molecular medicine in genetically engineered animals. J. Clin. Invest. 97:2, 1996.

113. Chien, K. R.: Cannon Award Lecture: Cardiac muscle diseases in genetically engineered mice. Am. J. Physiol. 269:H755, 1995.

114. Doevendans, P. A., Hunter, J. J., Lembo, G., et al.: Strategies for studying cardiovascular diseases in transgenic and gene-targeted mice. *In* Monastersky, G. M., and Robl, J. M. (eds.): Strategies in Transgenic Animal Science. Washington, D. C., American Society for Microbiology, 1995, p. 107.

115. Field, L. J.: Transgenic mice in cardiovascular research. Annu. Rev. Physiol. 55:97, 1993.

116. Lin, M. C., Rockman, H. A., and Chien, K. R.: Heart and lung disease in genetically engineered mice: The evolution of molecular physiology. Nature Med. 1:749, 1995.

117. Jaenisch, R.: Transgenic animals. Science 240:1468, 1988.

118. Bronson, S. K., and Smithies, O.: Altering mice by homologous recombination using embryonic stem cells. J. Boil. Chem. 269:27155, 1994.

119. Tangirala, R. K., Casanada, F., Miller, E., et al.: Effect of antioxidant N,N′-diphenyl 1,4-phenylenediamine (DPPD) on atherosclerosis in ApoE-deficient mice. Arteriosci. Thromb. Vasc. Biol. 15:1625, 1995.

120. Sucov, H. M., Dyson, E., Gumeringer, C. L., et al.: RXRα mutant mice establish a genetic basis for vitamin A signaling in heart morphogenesis. Genes Dev. 8:1007, 1994.

121. Stoltzfus, L., and Rubin, E. M.: Atherogenesis: Insights from the study of transgenic and gene targeted mice. Trends Cardiovasc. Med. 3:130, 1993.

122. Paul, M., Wagner, J., Hoffman, S., et al.: Transgenic rats: New experimental models for the study of candidate genes in hypertension research. Annu. Rev. Physiol. 56:811, 1994.

123. Hunter, J. J., Tanaka, N., Rockman, H. A., et al.: Ventricular expression of a MLC-*2v-Ras* fusion gene induces cardiac hypertrophy and selective diastolic dysfunction in transgenic mice. J. Biol. Chem. 270:23173, 1995.

124. Rockman, H. A., Ross, R. S., Harris, A. N., et al.: Segregation of atrial-specific and inducible expression of an atrial natriuretic factor transgene in an in vivo murine model of cardiac hypertrophy. Proc. Natl. Acad. Sci. U.S.A. 88:8277, 1991.

125. Rockman, H. A., Ono, S., Ross, R. S., et al.: Molecular and physiological alterations in murine ventricular dysfunction. Proc. Natl. Acad. Sci. U.S.A. 91:2694, 1994.

126. Dyson, E., Sucov, H. M., Kubalak, S. W., et al.: Atrial-like phenotype is associated with embryonic ventricular failure in RXRα−/− mice. Proc. Natl. Acad. Sci. U.S.A. 92:7386, 1995.

127. Kubalak, S. W., Doevendans, P. A., Rockman, H. A., et al.: Molecular analysis of cardiac muscle diseases via mouse genetics. *In* Adolph, K. W. (ed.): Methods in Molecular Genetics. Orlando, FL, Academic Press, 1995.

128. Smith, A. G.: Mouse embryo stem cells: Their identification, propagation and manipulation. Semin. Cell. Biol. 3:385, 1992.

129. Evans, M. J., and Kaufman, M. H.: Establishment in culture of pluripotential cells from mouse embryos. Nature 292:154, 1981.

130. Subramaniam, A., Jones, W. K., Gulick, J., et al.: Tissue-specific regulation of the α-myosin heavy chain gene promoter in transgenic mice. J. Biol. Chem. 266:24613, 1991.

131. Sauer, B., and Henderson, N.: Site-specific DNA recombination in mammalian cells by the Cre recombinase of bacteriophage P1. Proc. Natl. Acad. Sci. U.S.A. 85:5166, 1988.

132. Gu, H., Marth, J. D., Orban, P. C., et al.: Deletion of DNA polymerase β gene segment in T cells using cell type-specific gene targeting. Science 265:103, 1994.

133. White, D., and Wallwork, J.: Xenografting: Probability, possibility, or pipe dream? Lancet 342:879, 1993.

134. Fan, J., Wang, J., Bensadoun, A., et al.: Overexpression of hepatic lipase in transgenic rabbits leads to a marked reduction of plasma high density lipoproteins and intermediate density lipoproteins. Proc. Natl. Acad. Sci. U.S.A. 91:8724, 1994.

135. Paigen, K.: A miracle enough: The power of mice. Nature Med. 1:215, 1995.

136. Luis, A.: The mouse model for atherosclerosis. Trends Cardiovasc. Med. 3:135, 1993.

137. Tall, A., and Breslow, J.: Disorders of lipoprotein metabolism. *In* Chien, K. R. (ed.): Molecular Basis of Heart Disease. Philadelphia, W. B. Saunders Company, 1997.

138. Tabas, I., and Krieger, M.: Disorders of cellular cholesterol metabolism. *In* Chien, K. R. (ed.): Molecular Basis of Heart Disease. Philadelphia, W. B. Saunders Company, 1997.

139. Plump, A. S., Smith, J. D., Hayek, T., et al.: Severe hypercholesterolemia and atherosclerosis in apolipoprotein E−deficient mice created by homologous recombination in ES cells. Cell 71:343, 1992.

140. Zhang, S. H., Reddick, R. L., Piedrahita, J. A., Maeda, N.: Spontaneous hypercholesterolemia and arterial lesions in mice lacking apolipoprotein E. Science 258:468, 1992.

141. Nakashima, Y., Plump, A. S., Raines, E. W., et al.: ApoE-deficient mice develop lesions of all phases of atherosclerosis throughout the arterial tree. Arterioscler. Thromb. 14:133, 1994.

142. Reddick, R. L., Zhang, S. H., and Maeda, N.: Atherosclerosis in mice lacking apo E: Evaluation of lesion development and progression. Arteriosci. Thromb. 14:141, 1994.

143. Palinsky, W., Ord, V. A., Plump, A. S., et al.: ApoE-deficient mice are a model of lipoprotein oxidation in atherogenesis. Arterioscler. Thromb. 14:605, 1994.

144. Steinberg, D., and Witzum, J.: The role of oxidized lipoproteins in atherogenesis. *In* Chien, K. R. (ed.): Molecular Basis of Heart Disease. Philadelphia, W. B. Saunders Company, 1997.

145. Pastzy, C., Maeda, N., Verstuyft, J., and Rubin, E. M.: Apolipoprotein AI transgene corrects apolipoprotein E deficiency-induced atherosclerosis in mice. J. Clin. Invest. 94:899, 1994.

146. Van der Maagenberg, A. M. J. M., Hofker, M. H., Krimpenfort, P. J., et al.: Transgenic mice carrying the apolipoprotein E3-Leiden gene exhibit hyperlipoproteinemia. J. Biol Chem. 268:10540, 1993.

147. Fazio, S.: Recent insights into the pathogenesis of type III hyperlipoproteinemia. Trends Cardiovasc. Med. 3:191, 1993.

148. Shimano, H., Yamada, N., Katsuki, M., et al.: Overexpression of apoli-

poprotein E in transgenic mice: Marked reduction in plasma lipoproteins except high density lipoprotein and resistance against diet-induced hypercholesterolemia. Proc. Natl. Acad. Sci. U.S.A. *89:*1750, 1992.

GENE THERAPY

149. Mulligan, R.: The basic science of gene therapy. Science *260:*926, 1993.
150. Lever, A. M. L., and Goodfellow, P. N.: Gene therapy. Br. Med. Bull. *51:*1, 1995.
151. Barr, E., and Leiden, J. M.: Somatic gene therapy for cardiovascular disease. Trends Cardiovasc. Med. *4:*57, 1994.
152. Nabel, E.: Gene therapy for cardiovascular disease. Circulation *91:*541, 1995.
153. Miller, A. D.: Human gene therapy comes of age. Nature *357:*455, 1992.
154. Riessen, R., and Isner, J. M.: Prospects for site-specific delivery of pharmacologic and molecular therapies. J. Am. Coll. Cardiol. *23:*1234, 1994.
155. Gerard, R. D., and Meidell, R. S.: Adenovirus-mediated gene transfer. Trends Cardiovasc. Med. *3:*171, 1993.
156. Muzyczka, N.: Adeno-associated virus (AAV) vectors: Will they work? J. Clin. Invest. *94:*1351, 1994.
157. Morishita, R., Gibbons, G. H., Ellison, K. E., et al.: Single intraluminal delivery of antisense cdc2 kinase and proliferating cell nuclear antigen oligonucleotides result in chronic inhibition of neointimal hyperplasia. Proc. Natl. Acad. Sci. U.S.A. *90:*8474, 1993.
158. Lasic, D., and Papahadjopoulos, D.: Liposomes revisited. Science *267:*1275, 1995.
159. Leiden, J. M., and Barr, E.: In vivo gene transfer into the heart. *In* Wolff, J. A. (ed.): Gene Therapeutics: Methods and Applications of Direct Gene Transfer. Boston, Birkhauser, 1994, p. 363.
160. Simons, M., Edelman, E. R., Dekeyser, J. L., et al.: Antisense c-*myb* oligonucleotides inhibit intimal smooth muscle cell accumulation *in vivo.* Nature *359:*67, 1992.
161. Bennett, M. R., Anglin, S., McEwan, J. R., et al.: Inhibition of vascular smooth muscle proliferation *in vitro* and *in vivo* by C-*myc* antisense oligodeoxynucleotides. J. Clin. Invest. *93:*820, 1994.
162. Grossman, M., Raper, S. E., Kozarsky, K., et al.: Successful ex vivo gene therapy directed to liver in a patient with familial hypercholesterolemia. Nature Genet. *6:*335, 1994.
163. Brown, M. S., Goldstein, J. L., Havel, R. J., and Steinberg, D.: Gene therapy for cholesterol. Nature Genet. *7:*349, 1994.
164. Yanagisawa-Miwa, A., Uchida, Y., Nakamura, F., et al.: Salvage of infarcted myocardium by angiogenic action of basic fibroblast growth factor. Science *257:*1401, 1992.
165. Nabel, E. G., Yang, Z.-Y., Plautz, G., et al.: Recombinant fibroblast growth factor-1 promotes intimal hyperplasia and angiogenesis in arteries in vivo. Nature *362:*844, 1993.
166. Isner, J. M., and Walsh, K.: Arterial gene therapy for therapeutic angiogenesis in patients with peripheral arterial disease. Circulation *91:*2687, 1995.
167. Folkmann, J.: Clinical applications of research on angiogenesis. N. Engl. J. Med. *333:*1757, 1995.
168. Takeshita, S., Zheng, L. P., Brogi, E., et al.: Therapeutic angiogenesis. J. Clin. Invest. *93:*662, 1994.
169. Cantley, L., Deuel, T., and Rosenberg, R. D.: The molecular biology of restenosis. *In* Chien, K. R. (ed.): Molecular Basis of Heart Disease. Philadelphia, W. B. Saunders Company, 1997.
170. Casscells, W., Lappi, D. A., and Baird, A.: Molecular arthrectomy for restenosis. Trends Cardiovasc. Med. *3:*235, 1993.
171. Nabel, E. G., Plautz, G., Boyce, F. M., et al.: Recombinant gene expression in vivo within endothelial cells of the arterial wall. Science *244:*1342, 1989.
172. Lemarchand, P., Jones, M., Yamada, I., and Crystal, R. G.: In vivo gene transfer and expression in normal uninjured blood vessels using replication-deficient recombinant adenovirus vectors. Circ. Res. *72:*1132, 1993.
173. Chang, M. W., Barr, E., Seltzer, J., et al.: Cytostatic gene therapy for vascular proliferative disorders with a constitutively active form of the retinoblastoma gene product. Science *267:*518, 1995.
174. Ohno, T., Gordon, D., San, H., et al.: Gene therapy for vascular smooth muscle cell proliferation after arterial injury. Science *265:*781, 1994.
175. Wagner, R.: Gene inhibition using antisense oligodeoxynucleotides. Nature *372:*333, 1994.
176. Davis, A. R.: Current potential of antisense oligonucleotides as therapeutic drugs. Trends Cardiovasc. Med. *4:*51, 1994.
177. Stein, C. A., and Cheng, Y.-C.: Antisense oligonucleotides as therapeutic agents—is the magic bullet really magical? Science *261:*1004, 1993.

MOLECULAR ADVANCES IN CARDIAC HYPERTROPHY

178. Chien, K. R., Grace, A. A., and Hunter, J. J.: Molecular basis of cardiac hypertrophy and heart failure. *In* Chien, K. R. (ed.): Molecular Basis of Heart Disease. Philadelphia, W. B. Saunders Company, 1997.
179. Chien, K. R., and Katz, A. M.: Molecular advances in cardiac hypertrophy and failure. Circulation *(in press).*
180. Morgan, H. E., and Baker, K. M.: Cardiac hypertrophy: Mechanical, neural, and endocrine dependence. Circulation *83:*13, 1991.
181. Katz, A. M.: Scientific insights from clinical studies of converting-enzyme inhibitors in the failing heart. Trends Cardiovasc. Med. *5:*37, 1995.
182. Spudich, J., and Leinwand, L.: Contractile structure and function. *In*
183. Chien, K. R. (ed.): Molecular Basis of Heart Disease. Philadelphia, W. B. Saunders Company, 1997.
183. Arai, M., Alpert, N. R., MacLennan, D. H., et al.: Alterations in sarcoplasmic reticulum gene expression in human heart failure: Possible mechanism for alterations in systolic and diastolic properties of the failing myocardium. Circ. Res. *72:*463, 1993.
184. Rosenzweig, A., and Seidman, C. E.: Atrial natriuretic factor and related peptide hormones. Annu. Rev. Biochem. *60:*229, 1991.
185. Hasegawa, K., Fujiwara, H., Doyama, K., et al.: Ventricular expression of brain natriuretic peptide in hypertrophic cardiomyopathy. Circulation *88:*372, 1993.
186. Hasegawa, K., Fujiwara, H., Doyama, K., et al.: Ventricular expression of atrial and brain natriuretic peptides in dilated cardiomyopathy: An immunohistocytochemical study of the endomyocardial biopsy specimens using specific monoclonal antibodies. Am. J. Pathol. *142:*107, 1993.
187. Iwaki, K., Sukhatme, V. P., Shubeita, H. E., and Chien, K. R.: α- and β-adrenergic stimulation induce distinct patterns of immediate early gene expression in neonatal rat myocardial cells: *fos/jun* expression is associated with sarcomere assembly; *Egr-1* induction is primarily an α-mediated response. J. Biol. Chem. *265:*13809, 1990.
188. Knowlton, K. U., Baracchini, E., Ross, R. S., et al.: Co-regulation of the atrial natriuretic factor and cardiac myosin light chain-2 genes during α-adrenergic stimulation of neonatal rat ventricular cells. J. Biol. Chem. *266:*7759, 1991.
189. Takahashi, T., Allen, P. D., and Izumo, S.: Expression of A-, B-, and C-type natriuretic peptide genes in failing and developing human ventricles. Circ. Res. *71:*9, 1992.
190. Rockman, H. A., Knowlton, K. U., Ross, J., and Chien, K. R.: In vivo murine cardiac hypertrophy: A novel model to identify genetic signaling mechanisms that activate an adaptive physiological response. Circulation *87*(Suppl. VII):VII-14, 1993.
191. Shubeita, H. E., McDonough, P. M., Harris, A. N., et al.: Endothelin induction of inositol phospholipid hydrolysis, sarcomere assembly, and cardiac gene expression in ventricular myocytes: A paracrine mechanism for myocardial cell hypertrophy. J. Biol. Chem. *265:*20555, 1990.
192. Knowlton, K. U., Rockman, H. A., Itani, M., et al.: Divergent pathways mediate the induction of ANF transgenes in neonatal and hypertrophic ventricular myocardium. J. Clin. Invest. *96:*1311, 1995.
193. Wollert, K. C., Tags, T., Kishimoto, T., et al.: Cardiotrophin-1 activates a distinct form of cardiac muscle cell hypertrophy: Assembly of sarcomeric units in series via qp130/leukemia inhibitory factor receptor dependent pathways. J. Biol. Chem. *(In press).*
194. Lee, H. R., Henderson, S. A., Reynolds, R., et al.: Alpha-1 adrenergic stimulation of cardiac gene transcription in neonatal rat myocardial cells: Effects on myosin light chain-2 gene expression. J. Biol. Chem. *263:*7352, 1988.
195. Meidell, R. S., Sen, A., Henderson, S. A., et al.: Alpha 1-adrenergic stimulation of rat myocardial cells increases protein synthesis. Am. J. Physiol. *251:*H1076, 1986.
196. Parker, T. G., and Schneider, M. D.: Growth factors, proto-oncogenes, and plasticity of the cardiac phenotype. Annu. Rev. Physiol. *53:*179, 1991.
197. Sadoshima, J., and Izumo, S.: Molecular characterization of angiotensin II-induced hypertrophy of cardiac myocytes and hyperplasia of cardiac fibroblasts. Circ. Res. *73:*413, 1993.
198. Bogoyevitch, M. A., Glennon, P. E., and Sugden, P. H.: Endothelin-1, phorbol esters and phenylephrine stimulate MAP kinase activities in ventricular cardiomyocytes. FEBS Lett. *317:*271, 1993.
199. Bogoyevitch, M. A., Glennon, P. E., Andersson, M. B., et al.: Endothelin-1 and fibroblast growth factors stimulate the mitogen-activated protein kinase signaling cascade in cardiac myocytes: The potential role of the cascade in the integration of two signaling pathways leading to myocyte hypertrophy. J. Biol. Chem. *269:*1110, 1994.
200. Sadoshima, J., and Izumo, S.: Signal transduction pathways of angiotensin II-induced c-fos gene expression in cardiac myocytes in vitro. Circ. Res. *73:*424, 1993.
201. Sadoshima, J., Takahashi, T., Jahn, L., and Izumo, S.: Roles of mechanosensitive ion channels, cytoskeleton, and contractile activity in stretch-induced immediate-early gene expression and hypertrophy of cardiac myocytes. Proc. Natl. Acad. Sci. U.S.A. *89:*9905, 1992.
202. Komuro, I., and Yazaki, Y.: Intracellular signaling pathways in cardiac myocytes induced by mechanical stress. Trends Cardiovasc. Med. *4:*117, 1994.
203. Long, S., Henrich, C. J., and Simpson, P. C.: A growth factor for cardiac myocytes is produced by cardiac nonmyocytes. Cell Regul. *2:*1081, 1991.
204. Pennica, D., King, K. L., Shaw, K. J., et al.: Expression cloning of cardiotrophin 1, a cytokine that induces cardiac myocyte hypertrophy. Proc. Natl. Acad. Sci. U.S.A. *92:*1142, 1995.
205. Shubeita, H. E., Thorburn, J., and Chien, K. R.: Microinjection of antibodies and expression vectors into living myocardial cells. Circulation *85:*2236, 1992.
206. Thorburn, A., Thorburn, J., Chen, S.-Y., et al.: HRas-dependent pathways can activate morphological and genetic markers of cardiac muscle cell hypertrophy. J. Biol. Chem. *268:*2244, 1993.
207. Milano, C. A., Allen, L. F., Rockman, H. A., et al.: Enhanced myocardial function in transgenic mice overexpressing the β$_2$-adrenergic receptor. Science *264:*582, 1994.
208. Chien, K. R., Zhu, H., Kirk, K. U., et al.: Transcriptional regulation

during cardiac growth and development. Annu. Rev. Physiol. *55*:77, 1993.

209. Little, W. C., and Downes, T. R.: Clinical evaluation of left ventricular diastolic performance. Prog. Cardiovasc. Dis. *32*:273, 1990.

210. Kiuchi, K., Shannon, R. P., Komamura, K., et al.: Myocardial beta-adrenergic receptor function during the development of pacing-induced heart failure. J. Clin. Invest. *91*:907, 1993.

211. Muntz, K. H., Zhao, M., and Miller, J. C.: Downregulation of myocardial β-adrenergic receptors. Circ. Res. *74*:369, 1994.

212. Lembo, G., Rockman, H. A., Hunter, J. J., et al.: Elevated blood pressure and enhanced myocardial contractility in mice with severe IGF-1 deficiency. J. Clin. Invest. *(in press).*

213. Hunter, J. J., Zhu, H., Lee, K. J., et al.: Targeting gene expression to specific cardiovascular cell types in transgenic mice. Hypertension *22*:608, 1993.

214. Lembo, G., Hunter, J. J., and Chien, K. R.: Signaling pathways for cardiac growth and hypertrophy: Recent advances and prospects for growth factor therapy. Ann. N.Y. Acad. Sci. *752*:115, 1995.

215. Schneider, M. D., and Parker, T. G.: Cardiac growth factors. Prog. Growth Factor Res. *3*:1, 1991.

216. Fishman, M. C., and Stainier, D. Y. R.: Cardiovascular development: Prospects for a genetic approach. Circ. Res. *74*:757, 1994.

217. Chien, K. R.: Overview: Molecular analysis of cardiac developmental phenotypes: Problems, progress and prospects. *In* Clark, E. B., Markwald, R., and Takeo, A. (eds.): Developmental Mechanisms of Heart Disease. New York, Futura, 1995, p. 3.

218. Baker, K. M., Booz, G. W., and Dostal, D. E.: Cardiac actions of angiotensin II: Role of an intracardiac renin-angiotensin system. Annu. Rev. Physiol. *54*:227, 1992.

219. Dzau, V. J., and Re, R.: Tissue angiotensin system in cardiovascular medicine: A paradigm shift? Circulation *89*:493, 1994.

220. Lindpaintner, K., and Ganten, D.: The cardiac renin-angiotensin system. Circ. Res. *68*:905, 1991.

221. Paul, M., Bachmann, J., and Ganten, D.: The tissue renin-angiotensin systems in cardiovascular disease. Trends Cardiovasc. Med. *2*:94, 1992.

222. Urata, H., Kinoshita, A., Misono, F., et al.: Identification of a highly specific chymase as the major angiotensin II-forming enzyme in the human heart. J. Biol. Chem. *265*:348, 1990.

223. Rogg, H., Scmid, A., and De Gasparo, M.: Identification and characterisation of angiotensin II receptor subtypes in rabbit ventricular myocardium. Biochem. Biophys. Res. Commun. *173*:416, 1990.

224. Timmermans, P. B. M. W. M., and Smith, R. D.: Angiotensin II receptor subtypes: Selective antagonists and functional correlates. Eur. Heart J. *15*:D79, 1994.

225. Dostal, D. E., and Baker, K. M.: Evidence for a role of an intracardiac renin-angiotensin system in normal and failing hearts. Trends Cardiovasc. Med. *3*:67, 1993.

226. Baker, K. M., and Aceto, J. F.: Angiotensin II stimulation of protein synthesis and cell growth in chick heart cells. Am. J. Physiol. *259*:H610, 1990.

227. Rockman, H. A., Wachhorst, S. P., Mao, L., and Ross, J.: ANG II receptor blockade prevents ventricular hypertrophy and ANF gene expression with pressure overload in mice. Am. J. Physiol. *266*:H2468, 1994.

228. Suzuki, J., Matsubara, H., Urakami, M., and Inada, M.: Rat angiotensin II receptor mRNA regulation and subtype expression in myocardial growth and hypertrophy. Circ. Res. *73*:439, 1993.

229. Sadoshima, J., Xu, Y., Slayter, H. S., and Izumo, S.: Autocrine release of angiotensin II mediates stretch-induced hypertrophy of cardiac myocytes in vitro. Cell *75*:977, 1993.

230. Krege, J. H., John, S. W. H., Langenbach, L. L., et al.: Male-female differences in fertility and blood pressures in ACE deficient mice. Nature *315*:146, 1995.

231. Masaki, T. S., Kimura, M., Yanagisawa, M., and Goto, K.: Molecular and cellular mechanism of endothelin regulation: Implications for vascular function. Circulation *84*:1457, 1991.

232. Rubanyi, G. M., and Polokoff, M. A.: Endothelins. Pharmacol. Rev. *46*:325, 1994.

233. Chien, K. R.: Close encounters with ET-1. J. Clin. Invest. *96*:1, 1995.

234. Ito, H., Hirata, Y., Adachi, S., et al.: Endothelin-1 is an autocrine/paracrine factor in the mechanism of angiotensin II induced hypertrophy in cultured rat cardiomyocytes. J. Clin. Invest. *92*:398, 1993.

235. Ito, H., Hiroe, Y., Hirata, H., et al.: Endothelin ET$_A$ receptor antagonist blocks cardiac hypertrophy provoked by hemodynamic load. Circulation *89*:2198, 1994.

236. Gardiner, S. M., Kemp, P. A., March, J. E., and Bennett, T.: Effects of bosentan (Ro47-0203) an ET$_A$-, ET$_B$ antagonist on regional hemodynamic responses in conscious rats. Br. J. Pharmacol. *112*:823, 1994.

237. LeRoith, D., and Roberts, C.: Insulin-like growth factors. Ann. N. Y. Acad. Sci. *692*:1, 1993.

238. Donath, M. Y., Zapf, J., Eppenberger-Eberhart, M., et al.: Insulin-like growth factor I stimulates myofibril development and decreases smooth muscle cell α-actin of adult cardiomyocytes. Proc. Natl. Acad. Sci. U.S.A. *91*:1686, 1994.

239. Sacca, L., Cittadini, A., and Fazio, S.: Growth hormone and the heart. Endocr. Rev. *15*:555, 1994.

240. Ito, H., Hiroe, M., Hirata, Y., et al.: Insulin-like growth factor-1 induces hypertrophy with enhanced expression of muscle-specific genes in cultured rat cardiomyocytes. Circulation *87*:1715, 1993.

241. Fuller, S. J., Mynett, J. R., and Sugden, P. H.: Stimulation of cardiac protein synthesis by insulin-like growth factors. Biochem. J. *282*:85, 1992.

242. Donohue, T. J., Dworkin, L. D., Lango, M. N., et al.: Induction of myocardial insulin-like growth factor-1 gene expression in left ventricular hypertrophy. Circulation *89*:799, 1994.

243. Duerr, R., Huang, S., Miraliakbar, H. R., et al.: IGF-1 enhances ventricular hypertrophy and function during the onset of experimental cardiac failure. J. Clin. Invest. *95*:619, 1995.

244. Pfeffer, J. M., Pfeffer, M. A., Fletcher, P. J., and Braunwald, E.: Progressive ventricular remodeling in rat with myocardial infarction. Am. J. Physiol. *260*:H1406, 1991.

244a. Fazio, S., Sabatini, D., Capaldo, B.: A preliminary study of growth hormone in the treatment of dilated cardiomyopathy. N. Engl. J. Med. *334*:809, 1996.

245. Pennica, D., Shaw, K. J., Swanson, T. A., et al.: Cardiotrophin 1. Biological activities and binding to the leukaemia inhibitory factor gp130 signalling complex. J. Biol. Chem. *270*:10915, 1995.

246. Robbins, J., Doetschman, T., Jones, W. K., and Sanchez, A.: Embryonic stem cells as a model for cardiogenesis. Trends Cardiovasc. Med. *2*:44, 1992.

247. Kishimoto, T., Taga, T., and Akira, S.: Cytokine signal transduction. Cell *76*:253, 1994.

248. Sheng, Z., Pennica, D., Wood, W. I., and Chien, K. R.: Cardiotrophin-1 displays early restricted expression in the murine heart tube and promotes cardiac myocyte survival. Development *122*:419, 1996.

249. LaMorte, V. J., Thorburn, J., Absher, D., et al.: G$_q$ and *ras*-dependent pathways mediate hypertrophy of neonatal rat ventricular myocytes following alpha 1-adrenergic stimulation. J. Biol. Chem. *269*:13490, 1994.

250. Lazou, A., Bogoyevitch, M. A., Clark, A., et al.: Regulation of mitogen-activated protein kinase cascade in adult rat heart preparations in vitro. Circ. Res. *75*:932, 1994.

251. Neer, E. J., and Clapham, D. E.: Signal transduction through G proteins in the cardiac myocyte. Trends Cardiovasc. Med. *2*:6, 1992.

252. Wang, J. Y. J., and McWhirter, J. R.: Tyrosine-kinase–dependent signaling pathways. Trends Cardiovasc. Med. *4*:264, 1994.

253. Hall, A.: A biochemical function for Ras—at last. Science *264*:1413, 1994.

254. Feig, L. A., and Schaffhausen, B.: The hunt for RaS targets. Nature *370*:508, 1994.

255. Boguski, M. S., and McCormick, F.: Proteins regulating RaS and its relatives. Nature *366*:643, 1993.

256. Sadoshima, J., Qiu, Z., Morgan, J. P., and Izumo, S.: Angiotensin II and other hypertrophic stimuli mediated with G protein–coupled receptors activate tyrosine kinase, MAP kinase and 90-kD S6 kinase in cardiac myocytes. Circ. Res. *76*:1, 1995.

257. Brown, J. H., and Martinson, E. A.: Phosphoinositide-generated second messengers in cardiac signal transduction. Trends Cardiovasc. Med. *2*:209, 1992.

258. Nishizuka, Y.: The molecular heterogeneity of protein kinase C and its implications for cellular regulation. Nature *334*:661, 1988.

259. Bogoyevitch, M. A., Parker, P. J., and Sugden, P. H.: Characterization of protein kinase C isotype expression in adult rat heart. Circ. Res. *72*:757, 1993.

260. Darnell, J. E., Kerr, I. M., and Stark, G. R.: Jak-STAT pathways and transcriptional activation in response to IFNs and other extracellular signaling proteins. Science *264*:1415, 1994.

261. Stahl, N., and Yancopoulos, G. D.: The alphas, betas, and kinases of cytokine receptor complexes. Cell *74*:587, 1993.

262. Marrero, M. B., Schieffer, B., Paxton, W. G., et al.: Direct stimulation of Jak/STAT pathway by angiotensin II AT$_1$ receptor. Nature *375*:247, 1995.

263. Zhou, M. D., Sucov, H. M., Evans, R. M., and Chien, K. R.: Retinoid dependent pathways suppress myocardial cell hypertrophy. Proc. Natl. Acad. Sci. U.S.A. *92*:7391, 1995.

264. Chambon, P.: The retinoid signaling pathway: Molecular and genetic analyses. Semin. Cell. Biol. *5*:115, 1994.

265. Geisterfer-Lowrance, A. A. T., Kass, S., Tanigawa, G., et al.: A molecular basis for familial hypertrophic cardiomyopathy: A beta cardiac myosin heavy chain gene missense mutation. Cell *62*:999, 1990.

266. Watkins, H., McKenna, W. J., Thierfelder, L., et al.: Mutations in the genes for cardiac troponin T and α-tropomyosin in hypertrophic cardiomyopathy. N. Engl. J. Med. *332*:1058, 1995.

267. Thierfelder, L., Watkins, H., MacRae, C. A., et al.: α-Tropomyosin and cardiac troponin T mutations cause familial hypertrophic cardiomyopathy: A disease of the sarcomere. Cell *77*:701, 1994.

268. McKenna, W. J., and Watkins, H.: Hypertrophic cardiomyopathy. *In* Scriver, C., Beaudet, A., Sly, W., and Valle, D. (eds.): The Metabolic and Molecular Basis of Inherited Disease. New York, McGraw-Hill Book Co., 1995, p. 4253.

269. Schwartz, K., Carrier, L., Guicheney, P., and Komajda, M.: Molecular basis of familial cardiomyopathies. Circulation *91*:532, 1995.

270. Sweeney, H. L., Straceski, A. J., Leinwand, L. A., et al.: Heterologous expression of a cardiomyopathic myosin that is defective in its actin interaction. J. Biol. Chem. *269*:1603, 1994.

271. Weatherall, D.: Science and the Quiet Art: The Role of Medical Research in Health Care. New York, W. W. Norton, 1995.

272. Comroe, J. H., and Dripps, R. D.: Scientific basis for the support of biomedical science. Science *192*:105, 1976.

Chapter 49
Genetics and Cardiovascular Disease

REED E. PYERITZ

GENETIC FACTORS IN DISEASE

Genes contribute to both the cause and the pathogenesis of virtually any abnormality of human physiology and behavior including, of course, disorders of the heart and vascular system. This statement carries two messages in addition to the obvious one. First, the pathology associated with even the most "environmental" of causes, such as trauma, malnutrition, and drug abuse, can be defined only in terms of the human body's response to the insult. How the stress of the initial insult is expressed (the *phenotype*) and how the patient suffers and perhaps recovers depend, to varying and as yet often poorly defined degrees, on the patient's *genotype.* This idea seems self-evident and verges on the trite, but it is frequently neglected. Some environmental insults, such as massive trauma or poisoning, are lethal to all, regardless of genotype. Nonetheless, as developments in fields such as *pharmacogenetics* and *ecogenetics* are defining genetic susceptibilities to human disease better and more simply, the physician must become increasingly attuned to the importance of the genotype.[1]

Second, the introductory statement stresses that genetic factors play roles in *both* cause and process; etiology and pathogenesis, although related, are conceptually distinct.[2] For example, the cause of sickle cell anemia is clearly a single mutant gene, whereas whether a patient homozygous for this mutation expresses all, some, or none of the manifestations of the disease depends on many other genetic and nongenetic factors. Conversely, the cause of pneumococcal pneumonia is equally evident, but the severity and resolution of the disease depend on the patient's immune competency (which in turn depends on genetic and nongenetic factors) as much as on treatment with an antibiotic.

The genotype, therefore, can be detrimental in at least two distinct ways. First, mutant genes can so upset embryology or physiology that a clinical abnormality occurs. Whereas the phenotype of any particular mutation depends on a host of factors, including which homeostatic systems are available to modulate the action of the defect, the genotype has the principal role in causing the disease. It is this class of mutations that are usually referred to as genetic diseases. Second, a mutation can facilitate the action of an extrinsic cause in producing disease. Inherited susceptibilities are part of the pathogenesis of disease and are one reason for taking the patient's family history. Until recently, the clinician could do little to pursue tantalizing facts, such as multiple relatives under age 50 suffering myocardial infarction. The long-touted prospect of detecting a patient's inherited susceptibilities and intervening before irreversible clinical sequelae occur is becoming reality.

Disorders Due to Microscopic Alterations in Chromosomes

Estimates of the total number of human genes range between 50,000 and 100,000. Two copies (termed *alleles*) of each gene are arrayed along 23 pairs of *chromosomes.* Twenty-two of the chromosomes are called *autosomes* (numbered 1 through 22), while the 23rd pair are the *sex chromosomes,* X and Y. Females have two X chromosomes and males have an X and a Y chromosome. Both autosomal alleles are potentially active in specifying RNA copies of their DNA sequences; whether a gene is active depends on the cell type, the developmental stage of the organism, and the regulatory molecules that interact with promoter and enhancer nucleotide sequences that control transcription of the gene. In cells with two X chromosomes (i.e., in all females, in the Klinefelter syndrome in which two X's and one Y occur, and in other rare conditions), only one X is active after early embryogenesis.

Human chromosomes can be examined by culturing cells capable of mitosis; T lymphocytes obtained from venous blood are the usual source, but fibroblasts, cells from chorionic villi, amniocytes, and leukocyte precursors present in bone marrow are also used clinically. Chromosomes are distinguished from one another by their size, shape (determined by the position of a constriction called the *centromere,* which functions as the attachment of the mitotic apparatus), and characteristic banding pattern as revealed by any of several staining techniques. The chromosomes are photographed, cut out, and arranged in pairs, from 1 through 22 and the sex chromosomes, in a display called the *karyotype.* This display and its interpretation are the end results of a clinical study of a patient's chromosomes. The chromosome constitution of a cell is designated by first specifying the number of chromosomes present (46 being normal in diploid cells), then specifying the sex chromosomes, and finally describing any abnormalities. For

TABLE 49–1   CONTIGUOUS GENE SYNDROMES

1651

Ch 49

	REGION	LOCUS	CARDIOVASCULAR ABNORMALITIES
Syndromes with cardiovascular involvement			
Arteriohepatic dysplasia	AHD	del 20p11.23p12.2	Peripheral pulmonic stenosis/hypoplasia
Cat-eye syndrome	CES	dup22q11	Total anomalous pulmonary venous return
DiGeorge sequence	DGS	del 22q11	Truncus arteriosus, right aortic arch, TOF, PDA
Miller-Dieker syndrome	MDS	del 17p13	Patent ductus arteriosus ± complex anomalies
Prader-Willi syndrome	PWS/AS	del 15q12	Cor pulmonale (secondary to obesity and central apnea)
WAGR syndrome		del 11p13	Hypertension (secondary to Wilms tumor)
Syndromes without frequent cardiovascular involvement			
Angelman syndrome		del 15q12*	
Smith-Magenis syndrome		del 17p11.2	

TOF = tetralogy of Fallot; PDA = patent ductus arteriosus.
WAGR = Wilms' tumor, aniridia, genitourinary, and retardation.
* The deletion is indistinguishable at the cytogenetic level from that of the Prader-Willi syndrome; genetic imprinting is thought to account in part for the phenotypic differences. In Prader-Willi, the deleted chromosome is always the chromosome 15 inherited from father, whereas in Angelman syndrome, the deletion affects the maternal chromosome 15.

example, a normal male is designated 46,XY, and a female with an extra chromosome 21 is designated 46,XX,+21.

ANEUPLOIDY. Chromosome aberrations, especially too many or too few chromosomes *(aneuploidy)*, are extremely common in human embryos; more than one-half of all conceptuses are spontaneously aborted in early pregnancy, and at least one-half of them are aneuploid. Among live-born infants, about 0.5 per cent have a chromosome aberration.

Gain or loss of chromosomes generally happens by nondisjunction, or the failure of a homologous pair of chromosomes to separate. Absence of one chromosome is termed *monosomy;* all autosomal monosomies are embryonic lethals, as is presence of only a Y sex chromosome. Presence of three chromosomes is *trisomy,* and presence of an entire extra set of chromosomes (for a total of 69) is *triploidy.* The most common autosomal aneuploidy, trisomy 21 associated with the Down syndrome, and aneuploidy for sex chromosomes are all compatible with survival into adulthood.

CHROMOSOME REARRANGEMENTS. A chromosome can break and rejoin within itself, potentially giving rise to an *inversion* of genetic material. Often no apparent phenotypic effect is seen in people with an inversion, but because inversions may disrupt chromosome pairing during meiosis, their offspring may have more profound aberrations.

DELETIONS AND DUPLICATIONS. Just as their names imply, these aberrations are losses or gains of chromosomal material. Many clinical syndromes have been associated with aberrations of specific chromosome regions.[3,4] The smallest deletion detectable by light microscopy is associated with loss of considerable DNA, on the order of one million base pairs, so more than one gene is potentially disrupted or lost.

A number of conditions, each initially thought to be due to a mutation in a single locus, are associated with small interstitial chromosome aberrations affecting a cluster of genes (Table 49–1). So rather than pleiotropic manifestations of one mutation, these conditions are likely to be due to the effects of several, and perhaps many, mutations and are therefore called *contiguous gene syndromes.*[5] Such defects are potentially heritable, and the occurrence of the disorder in a family behaves as a mendelian dominant.

Disorders Due to Changes in Single Nuclear Genes
(See also Chap. 48)

Mutations of genes located on the 22 pairs of autosomes and the two sex chromosomes produce phenotypes inherited according to the two principal tenets of Mendel: alleles segregate and nonalleles assort. The first statement refers to gametes receiving as a result of meiosis only one of the two alleles at a given locus. The second statement describes the results of recombination, the meiotic process of rearranging DNA between the two chromosomes of the pair *(homologous chromosomes);* if two loci are widely spaced along a chromosome, their chances of being separated by recombination are 50–50, and they are said to be *unlinked.*

More than 6500 individual loci have been identified on the basis of the phenotype that mutations in single genes produce. The presumption of single-gene defects is based in most instances on the pattern of inheritance in families; segregation of the phenotype according to mendelian prin-

ciples is the central piece of evidence. For an increasing number of loci, however, molecular genetic techniques have mapped the phenotype to a single gene or even revealed the actual alteration in nucleotide sequence.[6,7] The range of known mendelian variation in humans and information about gene mapping and molecular defects are routinely catalogued[8] and available on-line.[9] Based on current estimates of the size of the human genome, about 5 to 10 per cent of loci have been identified through the effects their mutations have on phenotype.

More than 2000 loci have been mapped to a restricted region of the genome. Many of these loci cause specific mendelian disorders, and the genetic map of these loci represents the "morbid anatomy of the human genome." Many of the cardiovascular and hemostatic disorders that were mapped by early 1995 are shown in Figure 49–1.

DOMINANCE AND RECESSIVENESS. These related concepts are characteristics of the phenotype, *not of the gene.* A phenotype is dominant when the patient is *heterozygous* for a mutation, i.e., when one copy of the mutant allele, and one copy of the normal allele, are present; this holds for genes on both autosomes and the X chromosome. A phenotype is recessive when the patient has two mutant alleles at the locus causing the condition. If the mutant alleles are identical, the patient is *homozygous* at that locus, a situation usually present either when the allele is identical by descent through both parents (i.e., the parents had a common ancestor and are *consanguineous*) or when the mutant allele is common in the population (e.g., the most prevalent mutation for cystic fibrosis and the mutation for sickle cell anemia). Biochemical and molecular genetic assessment of mutant alleles has shown that the majority of recessive phenotypes are due to two distinct mutant alleles, a situation termed a *genetic compound,* indicative of the widespread heterogeneity in mutations at each locus. Males have but one X chromosome, and each locus is therefore *hemizygous;* a mutant locus is always expressed in the phenotype of a male. Dominance and recessiveness for X-linked traits refer to expression in heterozygous and homozygous women, respectively.

Whether a disorder is called dominant or recessive depends on how carefully the phenotype is assessed and how it is defined. For example, familial hypercholesterolemia is a relatively common hereditary disorder due to defects in the receptor for low-density lipoprotein (LDL, p. 1134). The vast majority of patients are heterozygous for a mutant allele at the *LDLR* locus on chromosome 19,[10] and the disease is inherited as a mendelian dominant trait. However, if a man and a woman, each heterozygous for an *LDLR* mutation, mate, they have a 25 per cent risk of having a child who inherits both of the mutant alleles and thereby is either homozygous or a genetic compound for *LDLR.* Such a child has a much more severe form of familial hypercholesterolemia (see p. 1142) that is inherited as a mendelian recessive trait. Similarly, homozygosity for the sickle hemoglobin mutation at the β-globin locus on chromosome 11 produces the familiar autosomal recessive disease, sickle cell anemia. However, heterozygosity for the same mutation rarely produces disease but produces sickling of erythrocytes if they are examined under conditions of low oxygen tension; this phenotype is transmitted as a dominant trait.

AUTOSOMAL RECESSIVE INHERITANCE. Nearly all deficiencies of enzymatic activity—the classic inborn errors of metabolism first defined by Archibald Garrod in 1903—cause recessive phenotypes. Most homeostatic systems, which include all metabolic pathways, have sufficient flexibility to function well if one of the enzymatic steps

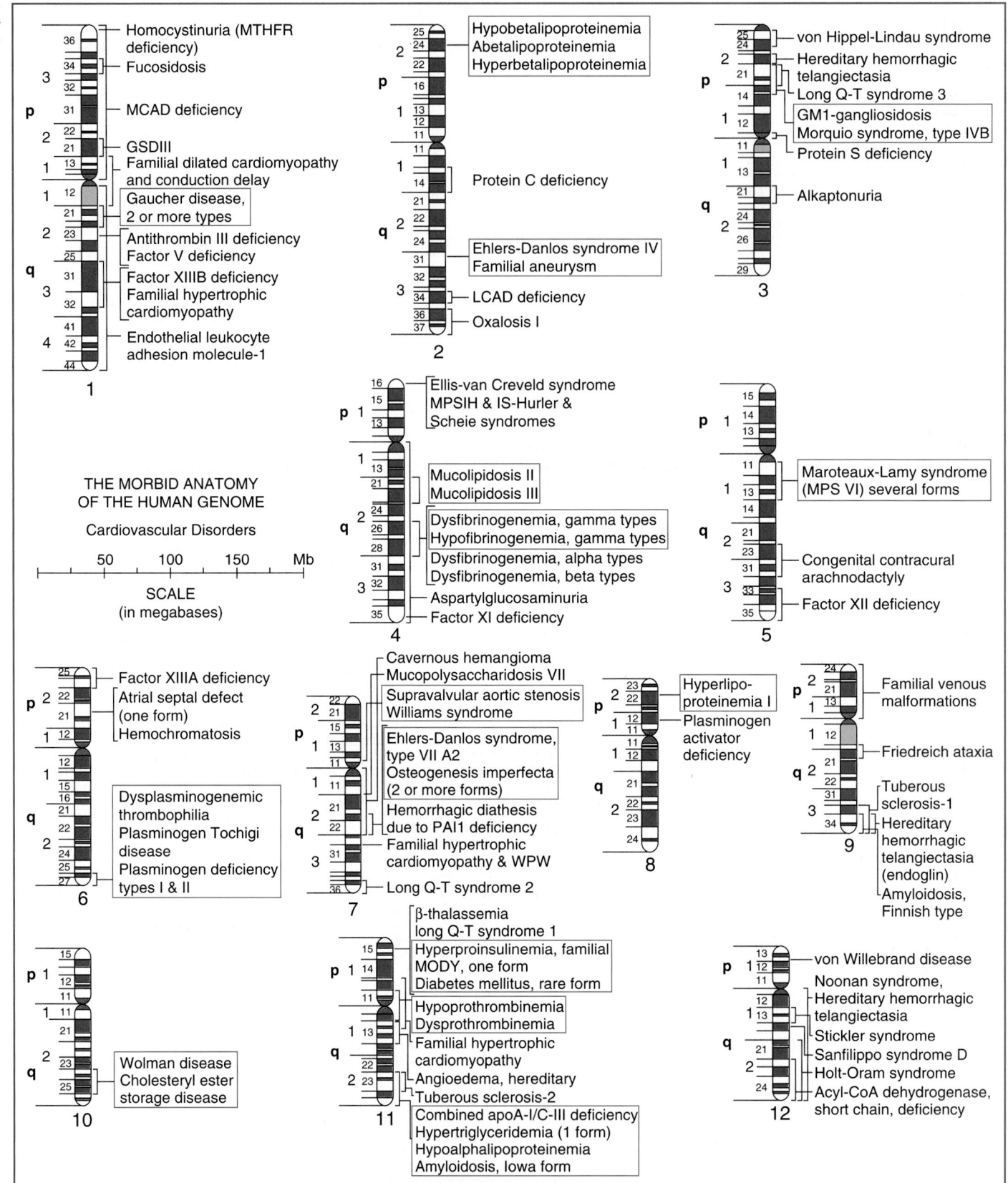

FIGURE 49–1. Chromosomal location of human genes associated with disorders of the cardiovascular system. These genes affect the structure, function, and metabolism of the heart and blood vessels and hemostasis and have been identified by the deleterious effects of mutations. Numerous additional genes that encode structural proteins important to the cardiovascular system have been identified but not yet associated with disease. In the figure, brackets next to the chromosome show the regional localization of the gene causing a particular disorder. Brackets next to two or more disorders indicate that all of the genes causing the disorders map to the same region. Disorders surrounded by boxes are caused by different mutations at the same gene.

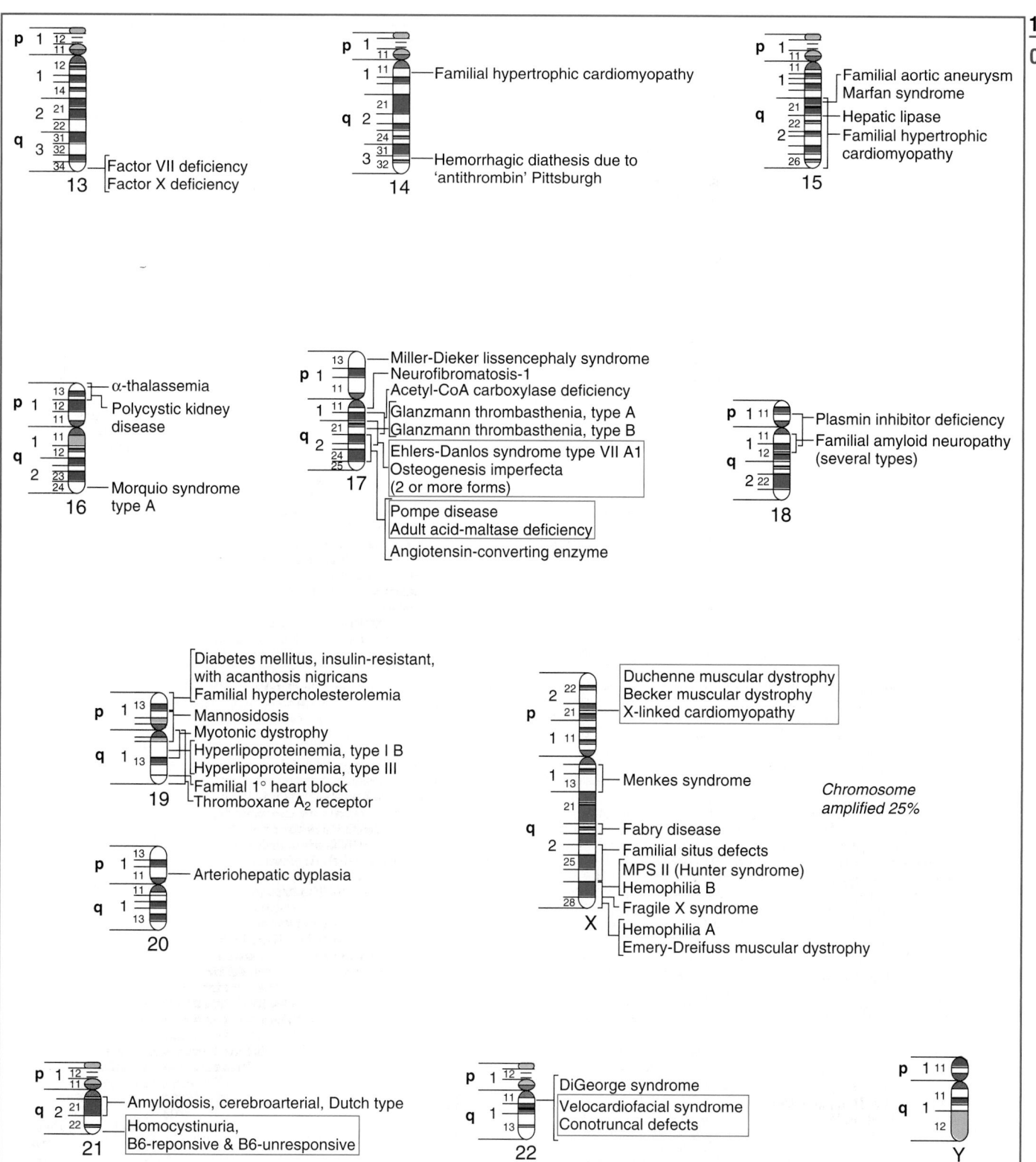

FIGURE 49–1 *See legend on opposite page*

function at half-normal efficiency, as would occur in heterozygosity for a mutant allele at a structural gene for an enzyme. However, homeostasis cannot cope if two mutant alleles cause a reduction in enzymatic activity to a few per cent or less of normal activity. The characteristics of autosomal recessive inheritance, features common to such phenotypes, and a typical pedigree are shown in Figure 49–2.

AUTOSOMAL DOMINANT INHERITANCE. Only a few enzyme deficiencies, but many disorders of development and structure, are inherited as dominant traits. The reasons for this are several. One possibility is that developmental homeostasis has a limited repertoire of responses to stress, and when a structural or regulatory macromolecule is reduced to only one-half normal amount, the system cannot cope. Another possibility, illustrated by mutations in procollagen molecules, pertains to gene products that must interact before be-

coming functional; an aberrant protein combined with a normal one would be a defective multimer, and the effect of being heterozygous for a mutation would be magnified—a *dominant-negative* effect.[7,11] The characteristics of autosomal dominant inheritance, features common to many such phenotypes, and a typical pedigree are shown in Figure 49–3.

Most human dominant traits are *incomplete*, in that the heterozygote is less severely affected than the homozygote. Defects of *LDLR* are illustrative, in which the heterozygote has classic type IIa hyperlipidemia, while the homozygote has a quantitatively worse form of the same disease.[10] It may well be that homozygosity for most alleles that cause dominant disorders is incompatible with life.

X-LINKED INHERITANCE. The characteristics of X-linked inheritance, features common to such phenotypes, and a typical pedigree are

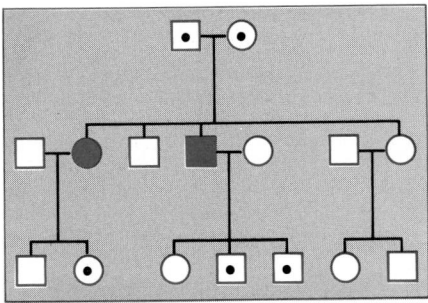

FIGURE 49–2. *Characteristics of autosomal recessive inheritance*
A single generation affected
Sexes affected equally frequently
Each parent heterozygous (a carrier)
Each offspring of two carriers has a 25% chance of being affected, a 50% chance of being a carrier, and a 25% chance of inheriting neither mutant allele
Two-thirds of clinically normal offspring are carriers
The rarer the phenotype, the greater the likelihood of consanguinity
Characteristics of autosomal recessive phenotypes
Often due to enzyme deficiencies
Often more severe than dominant disorders
Often early age of onset

shown in Figure 49–4. Whereas virtually all diseases due to mutations on the X chromosome are more severe in hemizygous males, women heterozygous for the same mutations often show some manifestations, albeit less severe and of later age of onset. For example, most women carriers of α-galactosidase A deficiency (Fabry disease) eventually develop cerebrovascular disease or renal failure due to accumulation of sphingolipid.[12]

MITOCHONDRIAL INHERITANCE. Energy generation through oxidative phosphorylation occurs in mitochondria in the cytoplasm of most cell types. Numerous mitochondria, each containing a single chromosome, exist in each cell. Some of the enzymes of oxidative phosphorylation are encoded by genes on the nuclear chromosomes and the proteins transported into the mitochondrion; the rest of the proteins are encoded by genes on the mitochondrial chromosome. Thus, genetic defects of oxidative phosphorylation can be due to mutations of genes on the autosomes or the X chromosome, and the resulting diseases behave as mendelian recessive traits, or mutations of genes on the mitochondrial chromosome, in which case the resulting diseases do not behave as mendelian traits.[13,14] The differences are explicable by the events of conception. The spermatocyte contributes virtually no mitochondria to the zygote, and the entire complement of mitochondria that will ever be present in the fetus is derived from the mitochondria already present in the cytoplasm of the oocyte. Thus, phenotypes due to mutations of the mitochondrial chromosome show *maternal inheritance,* the characteristics of which are shown in Figure 49–5.

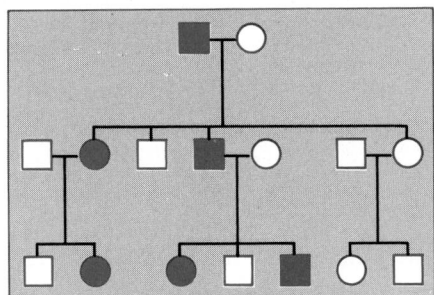

FIGURE 49–3. *Characteristics of autosomal dominant inheritance*
Multiple generations affected
Sexes affected equally frequently
In familial cases, only one parent need be affected
Male-to-male transmission occurs
Offspring of an affected parent has a 50% chance of being affected
Frequency of sporadic cases higher the more severe the condition
Paternal age effect of sporadic cases
Characteristics of autosomal dominant phenotypes
Often associated with malformations
Often pleiotropic
Usually variable
Often less severe than recessive phenotypes
Often age-dependent

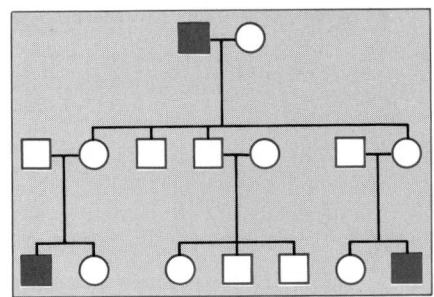

FIGURE 49–4. *Characteristics of X-linked inheritance*
No male-to-male transmission
All daughters of affected males are carriers
Sons of a carrier mother have a 50% chance of being affected; daughters have a 50% chance of being carriers
Some mothers of an affected male are not carriers, but they may have more affected sons if germinal mosaicism is present
Characteristics of X-linked phenotypes
More severe in males
Heterozygous females may be unaffected
Variable, especially in females

Principles of Clinical Genetics

PLEIOTROPY. Most mutant alleles have effects on more than one organ system, and a mendelian phenotype frequently displays multiple, often diverse, manifestations.[15] For example, the Marfan syndrome (see p. 1669) is defined by abnormalities in the eye, skeleton, skin, heart, and aorta, and until the recent recognition of a defect in extracellular microfibrils,[7] the findings could not be linked either etiologically or pathogenetically.[16]

VARIABILITY. The effects of the same mutant allele on phenotype can be different among people heterozygous (for dominant traits), homozygous (for autosomal recessive traits), or hemizygous (for X-linked traits) for the allele. Variability can be described in terms of the frequency of a particular pleiotropic manifestation among patients with the mutation; the severity of the phenotype; and the age of onset of manifestations. If a person has the mutant allele(s) but shows no phenotypic effect, the trait is called *nonpenetrant.* To an important degree, whether or not a clinical phenotype is called nonpenetrant depends on the sensitivity of the techniques employed for detection. For example, two decades ago, based on bedside examination, cardiovascular abnormalities were thought to affect about half of people with the Marfan syndrome; echocardiography now reveals aortic dilatation in more than 90 per cent. The term *incomplete penetrance* should not be used with reference to individuals but to mean a prevalence of the phenotype is less than 100 per cent of people known to carry the muta-

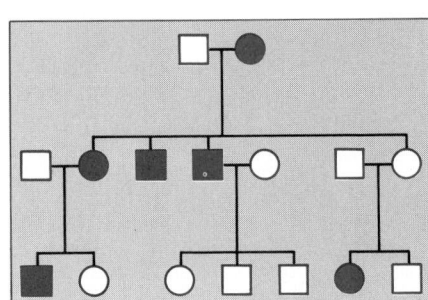

FIGURE 49–5. *Characteristics of disorders due to a mutation of the mitochondrial chromosome*
Sexes equally frequently and severely affected
Transmission only through women; offspring of affected men are unaffected
All offspring of an affected woman may be affected
Variability of expression can be extreme in a family, including apparent nonpenetrance
Phenotypes may be age-dependent

TABLE 49–2   CAUSES OF VARIABILITY OF GENE EXPRESSION

Genetic background

Age dependency

Sex influence

Sex limitation

Modifying loci: hypostasis and epistasis

Gene alteration
  Somatic mutation
  Somatic amplification
  Transpositions and rearrangements
    Mutations
    Physiological rearrangements

Variation in X-inactivation*

Endogenous complementation*

Maternal factors
  Effects of mitochondrial genome
  Intrauterine environment

Imprinting

Exogenous and ecological factors
  Ecology—temperature, diet
  Teratogens
  Medical intervention
  Chance

* Pertains to female heterozygotes for X-linked disorders.

tion(s). The Holt-Oram syndrome (see p. 1661) is an instructive example. In this autosomal dominant syndrome of reduction anomalies of the upper limb and congenital heart defect, patients in the same family can have only arm anomalies, only a heart defect, or both. Moreover, the severity of the reduction defect varies widely, from a proximally placed thumb to near total absence of the arm. The cardiac feature is incompletely penetrant because only about 50 per cent of patients have it, but in any individual with the Holt-Oram allele, the heart is either structurally normal or not.

Numerous genetic and environmental factors can affect expression of a gene (Table 49–2), and it is often impossible to determine which of these factors are most important in a specific patient or particular disease. However, the pervasiveness of variable expression emphasizes that phenotypes determined by single genes are to some extent really "multifactorial."

GENETIC HETEROGENEITY. Similar or even identical phenotypes can be due to fundamentally distinct mutations, a phenomenon termed genetic heterogeneity. For example, Marfan syndrome and homocystinuria were long thought to be the same disorder, despite what now appear in retrospect to be obvious differences in inheritance pattern and intelligence.[17] As in the case of these two disorders, the causes may lie in two different genes whose products are functionally distinct. Osteogenesis imperfecta exemplifies a disorder in which mutations in two genes, $\alpha 1(I)$ and $\alpha 2(I)$ procollagen, can each produce the same phenotype because the two proteins interact to form type I collagen.[18] Genetic heterogeneity is pervasive at the intragenic level of analysis; except for sickle cell anemia and achondroplasia, virtually all single-gene disorders are due to a variety of mutations at a given locus.[8,11]

Nonpathological Variation in the Cardiovascular System

CARDIAC STRUCTURE AND PHYSIOLOGY. All aspects of the ontogeny of the cardiovascular system are dictated by the genome. If, as seems most credible, few genes have a large effect and many have small contributions, any specific aspect of "normal" cardiovascular phenotype—size, shape, function—exhibits multifactorial inheritance. In other words, to the extent that any given phenotype can be

quantified, it shows a normal distribution within the population, and near-relatives are more similar to each other than they are to distant relatives and the rest of the population. The twin method should demonstrate a higher concordance of the trait in monozygotic than dizygotic twins. However, surprisingly few phenotypes have been examined.

Preliminary data on left ventricular dimensions measured echocardiographically showed higher correlations between parent and child than between matched controls, suggesting a genetic contribution[19]; however, as in many such studies, the effect of shared environment was not estimated. In an attempt to minimize environmental contributions, left ventricular sizes of twins who were not exercise trained were compared; the mean intrapair differences in echocardiographic dimensions were less in the monozygotic than in the dizygotic twins and nontwin sibs.[20] The caliber and branch geometry of coronary arteries show familial resemblance, and both parameters are much more similar in monozygotic twins than in other relatives.[21] Further support for the importance of genetic factors in normal development derives from studies that demonstrate ethnic differences in structure. For example, the thickness of the intima and the media of coronary arteries of children who died of noncardiovascular causes varied significantly with the ethnicity of the child.[22]

Measures of cardiac electrophysiology show familial resemblance. Studies of both nuclear families[23] and twins[24,25] suggest a genetic contribution to resting heart rate, conduction times, and repolarization time. Genetic control of normal cardiovascular function has been especially difficult to study because of the multitude of environmental (training, diet), stochastic (age), and clinical (subtle, unrecognized pathology) issues that confound comparisons of relatives and controls. Thus far, no strong genetic contribution to an individual's response to physical conditioning has emerged.[20]

VASCULAR SYSTEM. All members of certain inbred animal strains show little variation in arterial anatomy, especially branch angles, and considerable variation with other strains of the same species. Except for the studies of coronary arterial anatomy already noted[21] similar studies of humans have not been reported.

One intriguing question of clinical importance is whether certain people are predisposed to arterial spasm and whether this susceptibility has a genetic basis. An examination of hereditary pathological and polymorphic variation in factors elaborated by endothelial cells, platelets, and leukocytes to maintain patency of blood vessels, such as prostacyclin, endothelium-derived relaxing factor, and endothelin-1, may prove enlightening.[26,27] Similarly, is there genetic contribution to arterial stiffness or its variation with age and conditioning?

CARDIOVASCULAR DISORDERS ASSOCIATED WITH CHROMOSOME ABERRATIONS

Chromosome aberrations occur in 0.5 per cent of the population at birth and are common findings in tumors.[4,28] Visible alterations of the amount of chromosomal material cause primarily structural defects of the cardiovascular system that are evident in the newborn. The frequency of chromosome aberrations among live-born children with congenital heart defects has been found to range from 5 to 13 per cent.[29,30] Upward of 40 per cent of all fetuses with heart defects detected by ultrasonography at 18 to 20 weeks' gestation have chromosome aberrations; most are spontaneously aborted. Most forms of aneuploidy and most duplications and deletions of more than a chromosome band are associated with defects of the cardiovascular system[4,31] (Tables 49–1 and 49–3). Exceptions are 47,XXX, 47,XYY, and 47,XXY (Klinefelter syndrome), in which the incidence of congenital heart disease is probably not elevated over the population baseline.

ANEUPLOIDY. How the abnormal phenotypes caused by autosomal aneuploidy develop remains controversial. One view holds that disturbance of the dosage of the genes present on the specific aneuploid chromosome segments is the central issue. The other view is that any aneuploid state disturbs developmental homeostasis in a nonspecific manner. The former theory predicts some distinctiveness of phenotype among the trisomy syndromes that occur in live-born children, whereas the latter predicts shared manifestations. At a coarse level, the clinical pictures are similar, with grave problems of the craniofacies, central nervous system, genitalia, distal limbs, and heart usually present. But when a more refined examination of the phenotypes is obtained, considerable distinctiveness emerges.

The three most common autosomal trisomies—13, 18, and 21—can be distinguished readily at the bedside. In all three, membranous ventricular and atrial septal defects are common. However, the detailed accounting of cardiovascular lesions among large numbers of patients with these trisomies reveals important differences that suggest aneuploidy exerts more than a global effect on development. In

TABLE 49-3 CARDIOVASCULAR MANIFESTATIONS ASSOCIATED WITH CHROMOSOME ABERRATIONS

CHROMOSOME ABERRATION	EPONYM	CARDIOVASCULAR MANIFESTATIONS
Triploidy		
69,XXX (or XXY or XYY)		>50% have CHD: ASD and VSD
Aneuploidy		
+13	Patau	~80% have CHD; 75% of CHD is complex: PDA, VSD, ASD, PS, AS, dextro-cardia, CoA
+18	Edwards	~90% have CHD: most CHD is complex: VSD, PDA, ASD, bicuspid PV and AV, CoA
+21	Down	~40% have CHD: ECD, TOF; MVP in ~20%; AR
+8 mosaicism		~25% have CHD, most of little clinical consequence: VSD, PDA, CoA, PS
+9 mosaicism		~70% have CHD, usually complex: VSD, PDA, PLSVC
45,X	Turner	~10% have clinically important CHD: 50% of these have CoA; mild CoA is likely much more common; also AS, ARD, VSD, ASD, dextrocardia
47,XXX		CHD not increased
47,XXY	Klinefelter	CHD possibly slightly increased; ? mild conduction changes; venous thromboembolic disease
47,XYY		CHD not increased; ? mild conduction changes
Deletions		
4p-	Wolf-Hirschhorn	~50% have CHD, usually complex: VSD, ASD, PDA, PS
5p-	Cri du chat	~20% have CHD, usually single: VSD, PDA, ASD, PS
7q-		~20% have CHD, various, often complex
13q-		CHD common, often severe, but depend on region deleted
18p-		CHD uncommon
18q-		~25% have CHD, usually single, of little consequence: VSD, PDA, ASD, PS
ring 18		~20% have CHD: CoA, PA hypoplasia, HLH, PLSVC
Duplications		
4p trisomy		~10% have CHD, usually single: no defect predominates
9 p trisomy		<10% have CHD: VSD, ASD, AS, PS
10p trisomy		~30% have CHD, usually single: no defect predominates
10q24-qter trisomy		~50% have CHD, usually complex: ECD, VSD, TOF
22pter-q11 trisomy or tetrasomy	Cat eye	~50% have CHD, usually complex: TAPVR, VSD, TOF
Other Aberrations		
Marker Xq27.3	Fragile X syndrome	~55% have aortic root dilatation, MVP, or both

CHD = congenital heart defect(s); ASD = atrial septal defect; VSD = ventricular septal defect; PDA = patent ductus arteriosus; PS = valvular pulmonic stenosis; AS = aortic stenosis; CoA = coarctation of aorta; PV = pulmonic valve; AV = aortic valve; ECD = endocardial cushion defect; TOF = tetralogy of Fallot; MVP = mitral valve prolapse; AR = aortic regurgitation; PLSVC = persistence of left superior vena cava; ARD = aortic root dilatation; PA = pulmonary artery; HLH = hypoplastic left heart; TAPVR = total anomalous pulmonary venous return.

this and most other analyses of congenital heart defects, the system of classification based on the presumed pathogenetic mechanisms proves most instructive and is a useful approach to comparing different causative factors (Table 49-4).

About one-quarter of the defects in trisomies 13 and 18 are due to cell migration abnormalities, and two-thirds are flow lesions; when combined, these two mechanisms account for considerably more of these classes of defects than in the general population with congenital heart disease. By contrast, in trisomy 21 left-sided flow lesions are much less common, whereas abnormal closure of endocardial cushions is strikingly frequent; indeed, in contrast to endocardial cushion defects without a chromosome 21 anomaly, left-sided flow lesions are rarely seen in Down syndrome patients with endocardial cushion

TABLE 49-4 CLASSIFICATION OF CONGENITAL HEART DEFECTS BASED ON PATHOGENETIC MECHANISMS[35]

PATHOGENETIC MECHANISM	EXAMPLES OF DEFECTS
Embryonic blood flow defects	
Left-sided lesions	HLH; bicuspid aortic valve; IAA type A; CoA; PDA
Right-sided lesions	Secundum ASD; PS
Mesenchymal tissue migration defects	TOF; D-TGA
Extracellular matrix defects	ECD
Abnormal cellular death	Ebstein anomaly; muscular VSD
Defects of looping and situs	L-TGA
Abnormalities of targeted growth	TAPVR

HLH = hypoplastic left heart; IAA = interrupted aortic arch; CoA = coarctation of aorta; PDA = patent ductus arteriosus; ASD = atrial septal defect; PS = valvular pulmonic stenosis; TOF = tetralogy of Fallot; TGA = transposition of great arteries; ECD = endocardial cushion defect; VSD = ventricular septal defect; TAPVR = total anomalous pulmonary venous return.

defects.[29,32,38] Furthermore, the high incidence of endocardial cushion defects and low incidence of conotruncal and distal aortic anomalies have suggested a distinct pathogenetic mechanism in trisomy 21, potentially involving cell adhesiveness and the extracellular matrix.

TRISOMY 21—DOWN SYNDROME. This most common phenotype due to a human chromosome aberration occurs about once in every 600 births.[33] Most patients have trisomy 21, and the risk of this aberration is exponentially related to maternal age; the risk is lowest for young women and rises steeply after age 35, reaching 4 per cent for women over age 45. A small minority (3 per cent) of Down syndrome results from an extra copy of all or part of the long arm of chromosome 21 translocated to another chromosome. This situation is relatively more common in mothers under age 30. The phenotypes of the two forms of Down syndrome do not differ. The phenotype tends to be less severe if the trisomy is mosaic (3 per cent of Down syndrome) as a result of a mitotic nondisjunctional error in the embryo.

The most common causes of morbidity and mortality in Down syndrome patients are congenital heart defects present in 40 to 50 per cent of cases, hematological malignant disease, and duodenal atresia. If the patient either escapes or survives these problems, survival into the fifth decade and beyond is likely but is complicated by progressive dementia of the Alzheimer type. Premature aging may also affect the vasculature, although definitive studies are lacking.

The most characteristic cardiac anomaly in the Down syndrome is a defect of closure of the endocardial cushions (p. 898). Complicating the clinical problems in such patients and those with simple septal defects is a seeming predisposition to pulmonary hypertension in the face of elevated pulmonary blood flow.[36] About one-third of congenital heart defects are complex, and these patients tend not surprisingly to be the most ill patients. Mitral valve prolapse is found with a frequency exceeding that in age- and gender-matched controls.[37] The aortic and pulmonary valve cusps seem predisposed to fenestrations in adulthood.

Through the study of individuals trisomic for only a portion of the long arm of chromosome 21, the region crucial to the development of heart defects has been narrowed to 1.5 to 2.0 megabases (mb) of DNA in band 21q22.2 out of about 35 mb DNA on the entire long arm of chromosome 21 (J. R. Korenberg, personal communication).

The medical management of patients with Down syndrome has undergone evolution to more aggressive measures in recent years. Objections and hesitations on medical, societal, and ethical grounds to operative repair of heart defects in Down syndrome have been mollified substantially.[33,38] More follow-up data are becoming available, and early and late postoperative survival in Down syndrome patients appears to be no more different from that in other patients with similar defects.[36,38,39]

TRISOMY 18. *Edwards syndrome* is the second most common autosomal trisomy. Most cases are due to meiotic disjunction, and there is a strong relationship to maternal age. Routine prenatal diagnostic testing of women over age 34 would detect all aneuploid fetuses in them, but this would represent only one-third of all autosomal trisomies; less than one-half of all women of this advanced age undergo testing. Currently prenatal detection of trisomies followed by termination of pregnancy is having a small but measurable impact on decreasing the incidence of *Down, Edwards,* and *Patau* syndromes.

Although the severity of the phenotype rarely enables survival beyond a few months, 10 per cent of patients live to 1 year, and a few survive to adulthood, perhaps because of undetected mosaicism for a chromosomally normal cell line. However, central nervous system function is far less than that in the Down syndrome and leads to complex medical management and supportive care for long-term survivors.[40]
Cardiovascular defects occur in at least 90 per cent of cases and contribute to death. Complex lesions, usually involving septal defects, dysplastic valves that are rarely hemodynamically important, patent ductus arteriosus, and persistence of the left superior vena cava are common.[41,42] Right ventricular enlargement is common and may indicate not only shunting from left to right, but pulmonary hypertension due to anomalies of the pulmonary vasculature.[41] As in the Down syndrome, transposition of the great arteries is virtually unknown in trisomy 18.[42] Rarely should invasive diagnostic procedures or aggressive supportive measures be undertaken in Edwards syndrome.

TRISOMY 13. *Patau syndrome* occurs in about 0.01 per cent of live births and in progressively higher frequencies in stillbirths and spontaneous abortions. The external phenotype is usually severe, but occasionally not as characteristic as other trisomies; survival beyond a few weeks is rare, and the causes of death involve multiple organ systems, especially the heart. Cardiovascular anomalies are a bit less frequent than in trisomy 18 and have a slightly different spectrum.[31,41] Septal defects are the most common isolated lesions; dextrocardia and bicuspid semilunar valves occur in association with other anomalies.

Patients who survive beyond 1 month often are mosaic for a chromosomally normal cell line; thus, prognosis is fraught with uncertainty until detailed analysis is completed. Whether invasive cardiological studies are performed or aggressive management is undertaken can be determined by the severity of involvement of other organ systems, especially the brain, pending cytogenetic investigation.

TURNER SYNDROME. About one in every 2500 females lacks an X chromosome and has a 45,X karyotype. The frequency of a nonmosaic 45,X karyotype is much higher in spontaneous abortuses than in liveborns, and probably less than 2 per cent of such conceptuses come to term. The clinical phenotype is variable and often mild; the diagnosis is often not suspected until a child's short stature is evaluated or a woman complains of amenorrhea. Many cases are mosaic for cell lines with 46,XX or 46,XY constitutions. A variety of structural aberrations involving the X chromosome can cause partial or complete Turner syndrome.

Among patients with the 45,X karyotype, reported frequencies of congenital cardiovascular defects vary from 20 to 50 per cent, depending on how patients were ascertained. Fifty to 70 per cent of those with cardiovascular defects have clinically important aortic coarctation, usually of the postductal form.[43] As noninvasive imaging studies of asymptomatic patients became routine, the frequency of coarctation may increase. A variety of other cardiac malformations may occur, either singly or combined with coarctation. However, there is strong support for left-sided flow abnormalities as a major pathogenetic mechanism. Bicuspid aortic valve and dilatation of the

ascending aorta (with a risk of dissection and histopathology showing elastic fiber disruption) occur even in the absence of coarctation,[44,45] and hypoplastic left heart has been reported.[46] Partial anomalous pulmonary venous drainage without an atrial septal defect is fairly common and should be suspected when right ventricular overload is detected on echocardiography.[47]

Postmortem examination of mid-trimester abortuses with 45,X showed a higher incidence of left-sided flow lesions than found at birth, suggesting an association between the pathogenesis of the cardiovascular anomalies and the uniform presence of lymphatic obstruction at the base of the heart.[43]

Blood pressure elevation is common, even without coarctation or after its repair; a high frequency of renal anomalies is one likely cause, but not the sole explanation, for the prevalence of hypertension.

In about two-thirds of cases, the retained X chromosome derives from the oocyte (maternal X). Because entire chromosomes or regions of a chromosome may be differentially regulated (imprinted)[48] by passage through oogenesis versus spermatogenesis, could some of the variability in phenotype among patients with Turner syndrome be due to the origin of the retained X or the origin of the lost X? In a study of 63 patients, 10 had severe cardiovascular features, and 9 of them had retained the maternal X.[49] This is an idea worthy of further pursuit. Women with mosaic karyotypes are less likely to have cardiovascular defects.

CONGENITAL HEART DISEASE

(See Chaps. 29 and 30)

In the past few decades, the reported incidence of structural heart defects in newborns has increased from 5 to 7 per 1000 live births, probably as the result of increased diagnostic sensitivity (especially cross-sectional and Doppler echocardiography and magnetic resonance imaging).[50-54] Supporting this explanation is the lack of change over the same period in the incidence of critical defects diagnosed neonatally at 3.1 to 3.5 per 1000.[50,51] This enhanced resolving power of noninvasive methods should prove particularly useful in the study of familial structural defects, because apparently unaffected relatives can be evaluated for subclinical evidence of anomalies. Few investigations to date have capitalized on this approach.[55,56]

As is evident from the previous section, gross aberrations of chromosomes produce an extensive and varied array of structural heart disease, an observation as true for spontaneous abortuses as for liveborn children.[57] Unfortunately, the complexity and inscrutability of the human genome severely limit the insight that cytogenetic aberrations provide into etiology and pathogenesis of congenital malformations. Better understanding comes from investigating the other two mechanisms by which genes cause congenital heart defects—multifactorial processes and mutations of single genes. The latter group should prove instructive soon, as the protein products of the mutant loci are identified and their normal function and regulation are defined. In addition to the mendelian syndromes discussed below, evidence for the involvement of genes of large effect derives from studies of incidence of congenital heart disease in populations with a high rate of inbreeding. The increased occurrence of defects in offspring of consanguineous matings suggests that mutations in one or more genes, when homozygous, strongly predispose to abnormal cardiovascular development.[58]

MULTIFACTORIAL PROCESSES. The empirical risks of recurrence of congenital heart defects have increased in recent years,[59,60] in keeping with the overall higher incidence noted above. However, this conclusion has been criticized because the studies focused on the offspring of women probands, in whom the recurrence risk appears higher than in men with congenital heart defects.[61] In addition to this unexplained maternal influence, other factors may be at work. For example, improved detection of subtle lesions, more faithful reporting of patients, and the assiduousness of epidemiologists may have shown a systematic variation. It is true that some patients with cardiovascular problems now survive[60-63] to bear children because of improved medical and surgical care; their offspring might be at increased risk because of the severity of the parents' problems, but some evidence against this idea exists.[64]

The familial aggregation of congenital heart defects supports many of the predictions of the threshold liability model of multifactorial inheritance.[56,65] In most studies, whether focused on populations or families, defects were classified by their pathology; for example, all ventricular septal defects were considered as one group. There has been bias in reporting families in which one type of defect aggregates, which has led to many reports of "familial atrial septal defect," "familial cardiomyopathy," and so on, without regard to the fact that not all septal defects or cardiopathies have the same structure on careful scrutiny, let alone the same cause.

A major advance has been the movement to examine familial aggregation of defects based on presumed pathogenesis.[66-68] The scheme developed by Clark[35] and since modified and expanded[69] (Table 49-4), has become widely used. Under this approach, some anatomically distinct lesions are related by common pathogenesis; if the pathogenetic mechanism has substantial genetic control, then the occurrence of distinct defects in the same family would still be consistent with a genetic model. Alternatively, defects unrelated by pathogenesis would require a different interpretation. This model also focuses on the examination of apparently unaffected relatives and hence increases the chances of detecting subtle manifestations of defective development of cardiovascular structures.

ERRORS IN MESENCHYMAL TISSUE MIGRATION. Included in this category are a wide range of anomalies of the outflow tract, some due to failure of fusion and others due to failure of septation. Relatives of probands with interruption of the aortic arch type B or truncus arteriosus, both uncommon conotruncal malformations, had 2.5 per cent and 6.6 per cent incidences, respectively, of congenital heart defects.[70] Both recurrence rates were higher than expected. The frequency of congenital malformations was much lower in relatives of patients with other forms of interrupted aortic arch. Moreover, relatives of probands with truncus arteriosus and other defects had a recurrence rate of 13 per cent, the majority in the spectrum of conotruncal lesions. Here is an instance in which refined empirical risk data should improve the accuracy of genetic counseling.

Categorizing anatomical defects by presumed pathogenesis emphasizes that all ventricular septal defects are not alike. If there is a strong genetic component to the etiology of tetralogy of Fallot, for example, one might find in close relatives an increased risk not only of tetralogy but of truncus arteriosus and supracristal ventricular septal defects, but not of other forms of septal defects.

Conotruncal Development. Considerable progress has been made over the past few years in identifying a region of chromosome 22 which plays a major role in development of the conotruncus, the branchial arches, and the face. Interest was first stimulated by detection of small deletions involving 22q11 in patients with *DiGeorge sequence*.[71-73] This condition includes developmental anomalies of the fourth branchial arch and derivatives of the third and fourth pharyngeal pouches. Hypoplasia of the thymus and parathyroids causes immune deficiency and hypocalcemia. The cardiac defects range from tetralogy of Fallot to ventricular septal defect, truncus arteriosus, interrupted aorta type B, and right aortic arch and are often lethal.

Subsequently, patients with *velocardiofacial syndrome* (VCF, also called Shprintzen syndrome) and what has been called in Japan the *conotruncal anomaly face syndrome* were found to have deletions in the same region, albeit generally smaller ones than in DiGeorge syndrome.[74] Because the deletion is often too small to be detected by routine cytogenetics, fluorescent in situ hybridization (FISH) with a DNA probe for the region is the assay of choice. The VCF syndrome is unlike the DiGeorge syndrome and includes an abnormal but characteristic facies, cleft palate, pharyngeal insufficiency, and conotruncal cardiac defects. The acronym CATCH22 (cardiac anomaly, abnormal facies, thymic hypoplasia, cleft palate, and hypocalcemia) subsumes these related phenotypes.

This same region of chromosome 22 has been examined in patients with familial occurrence of various congenital cardiac defects and in patients with nonfamilial occurrence, nonsyndromic conotruncal defects. Although the prevalence figures are still soft, an important fraction of patients in both categories have submicroscopic deletions of 22q11.[75] Thus, a gene or genes in this region likely account for much of the recurrence risk of defects due to mesenchymal tissue migration abnormalities. Further, accurate counseling regarding recurrence risks for this broad range of defects necessitates FISH or molecular analysis for the presence of a deletion in the proband, and if present, in both parents.

Investigation of a strain of Keeshond dogs prone to conotruncal defects has shown that a single gene can be responsible for pathogenetically related defects of widely varying severity.[76]

FLOW DEFECTS. Left-sided flow lesions comprise a spectrum that includes hypoplastic left heart, congenital aortic stenosis, bicuspid aortic valve, interrupted aortic arch type A, and aortic coarctation. Various components of this spectrum can be present in the same patient.[71] Data from the Baltimore-Washington Infant Study,[51] a population-based case-control study of congenital cardiovascular malformations, were used to show that in first-degree relatives of probands with isolated hypoplastic left heart, incidence of bicuspid aortic valve was 12 per cent; most of the cases were asymptomatic and unrecognized before they were detected by echocardiography as part of this investigation.[55] In an exceptional family, four instances of aortic coarctation occurred in four generations.[77]

The association of coarctation of the aorta, bicuspid aortic valve, and dilatation of the ascending aorta, which may occur as part of the *Turner syndrome*,[44,45] is well known in the general population.[78] Several intriguing questions need to be addressed regarding the genetics and pathogenesis of this association. To what extent is the ascending aorta intrinsically abnormal, and hence predisposed to dilate, and to what extent is the dilatation simply a result of abnormal turbulence created by a bicuspid aortic valve? The fact that some patients with this association also have subtle evidence of a systemic connective tissue abnormality, reminiscent of Marfan syndrome, supports the former hypothesis. It will be of interest to extend the study of left-sided flow lesions to include probands with coarctation or congenital aortic stenosis and to evaluate close relatives with techniques capable of detecting the entire range of flow defects.

EXTRACELLULAR MATRIX ABNORMALITIES. Enough is known about the biochemistry and cell biology of cardiac embryology to state with some confidence that the extracellular matrix ("connective tissue") plays an important role. The endocardial cushions have received the most attention as an area where defects in the extracellular matrix might produce malformations.[35] The high frequency of endocardial cushion defects and atrioventricular septal defects in Down syndrome has been noted (see p. 1656). Of interest is the finding of increased adhesiveness of fibroblasts from trisomy 21 patients, a phenomenon that could reflect interaction with the extracellular matrix.[79] The distinctiveness of endocardial cushion defects in patients with normal chromosomes and in those with trisomy 21 has been suggested because of differences in associated cardiovascular malformations. However, of six families in which the proband had an endocardial cushion defect, three had recurrence of the same type of defect in a relative, including two with trisomy 21.[68]

SITUS AND LOOPING DEFECTS. This is an area fraught with difficulties of nomenclature, diagnosis, and heterogeneity of both etiology and pathogenesis. In analysis of clinical data, the most informative approach, but clearly arduous because of the large amount of data required, would be to categorize probands and their relatives by the type of situs (solitus, inversus, dextroversion, and levoversion, p. 946), and each of those by presence or absence of other cardiac and visceral defects. This has not been done on epidemiological cohorts, and in family studies relatives have rarely been subjected to evaluations sufficient to characterize their phenotypes in detail.[80] These variable phenotypes are grouped in a category, *heterotaxy*.

Several mendelian phenotypes point to single genes that have a major effect on determining laterality. In the autosomal recessive *Kartagener syndrome*, a randomization of lateralization of the heart (situs solitus and situs inversus are equally likely in homozygotes)[81] coexists with a defect in ciliary motility, which leads to sinusitis, bronchiectasis, and sperm immotility.[82]

Heterotaxy with splenic and other cardiac defects, particularly of the position of the great vessels, can be inherited as an autosomal recessive, as an autosomal dominant,[83] and as an X-linked recessive.[84] Some of the families with these apparently single-gene disorders have concordance of phenotype, but many do not, suggesting that in some cases various types of situs defects, polysplenia, and asplenia are different manifestations of the same mutation.[85,86]

In one family, complex heterotaxy involving abnormal abdominal situs, asplenia, polysplenia, simple dextrocardia, transposition, single ventricle and other cardiac anomalies, and a variety of other congenital malformations was inherited as an X-linked recessive trait.[84] The phenotype was mapped to Xq24-q27.1; still to be identified is the gene(s) responsible.

Two mouse mutants are instructive. Mice homozygous for the *iv* mutation, which maps to chromosome 12, are normal except that 50 per cent have situs inversus[87]; this is similar to the cardiac phenotype in Kartagener syndrome. Mice homozygous for a mutation at a different locus, *inv*, on chromosome 4, all have heterotaxy, with three-quarters showing situs inversus totalis.[88] Identification of the human homologues for these murine genes should further understanding of the control of human laterality.

There is a paucity of data on the recurrence risks of defects in the *cell death* (e.g., Ebstein anomaly) and *abnormal targeted growth* (e.g., anomalous pulmonary venous return) categories. Data from the Baltimore-Washington Infant Study do not show an increased risk of any cardiovascular defect in the relatives of a proband with a defect in either of these categories.[51] In one pedigree, nonsyndromic total anomalous pulmonary venous return was inherited as an autosomal

TABLE 49–5 DISORDERS OF UNCERTAIN CAUSE AND INHERITANCE THAT ARE ASSOCIATED WITH A HIGH INCIDENCE OF CARDIOVASCULAR ABNORMALITIES

DISORDER AND PHENOTYPE	MIM NO.*	CARDIOVASCULAR ABNORMALITIES†
Aase syndrome (Congenital anemia, triphalangeal thumbs)	205600	VSD
Bilateral left-sidedness sequence (Polysplenia syndrome)	208530	ASD
Bilateral right-sidedness sequence (Asplenia syndrome; Ivemark syndrome)	208530	Situs inversus, ECD, VSD
CHARGE association (Coloboma, heart anomaly, choanal atresia, retardation, genital, and ear anomalies)	214800	TOF, PDA, ECD, VSD
Cornelia de Lange syndrome (Short stature, retardation, synophrys, hypertrichosis, micromelia, genital anomalies)	122470	~20% have CHD: VSD, PDA, ASD, PLSVC, TOF
DiGeorge sequence‡ (Abnormalities of derivatives of 3rd and 4th pharyngeal pouches and 4th branchial arch: hypoplastic thymus with cellular immune deficiency, hyoplastic parathyroids with hypocalcemia)	188400	CHD in ~100%: aortic arch anomalies (especially IAA type B and right-sided aortic arch); PDA, TOF
Goldenhar syndrome (Abnormalities of derivatives of 1st and 2nd branchial arch: hemifacial microsomia, microtia, vertebral anomalies)	141400, 164210, 257700	~50% have CHD: VSD, TOF, PDA, CoA, right-sided aortic arch, PLSVC
Klippel-Feil sequence (Short neck, limited rotation of the head, cervical anomalies)	118100, 148900, 214300	Variable estimates (5–70%) of CHD: VSD, dextrocardia
"Kabuki make-up" syndrome (Dwarfism, peculiar facies, scoliosis, mental retardation)	147920	30% have CHD: ASD, VSD, TOF, CoA, PDA
Pallister-Hall syndrome (Hypothalamic hamartoblastoma, hypopituitarism, imperforate anus, postaxial polydactyly)	146510	ECD
Poland sequence (Unilateral absence of sternocostal pectoralis major, ipsilateral synbrachydactyly)	173800	~10% have dextrocardia or dextroversion
Rubinstein-Taybi syndrome (Short stature, retardation, microcephaly, characteristic facies, broad thumbs)	268600	~20% have CHD: ECD, ASD, TOF, PDA, VSD
VATER association (Vertebral defects, anal atresia, tracheo-esophageal fistula, radial dysplasia, renal anomaly)	192350	VSD

VSD = ventricular septal defect; ASD = atrial septal defect; TOF = tetralogy of Fallot; PDA = patent ductus arteriosus; ECD = endocardial cushion defect; CHD = congenital heart defect(s); PLSVC = persistence of left superior vena cava; IAA = interrupted aortic arch; CoA = coarctation of aorta; VSD = ventricular septal defect.

* None of these disorders is evidently due to a mutation in a single gene; however, most are listed in Mendelian Inheritance in Man (MIM),[8] and the MIM no. is provided as a ready source to the literature.

† Cardiovascular defects listed in approximate order of decreasing frequency.

‡ Most cases associated with del(22q11); likely a contiguous gene deletion defect.

dominant trait unassociated with other features in 14 relatives.[89] Linkage analysis localized the responsible gene to the centromere of chromosome 4 (4p13-q12).

DISORDERS OF UNCLEAR ETIOLOGY. A number of disorders include an important likelihood of malformation of the cardiovascular system but are of unclear cause (Table 49–5). Familial recurrence is so low to be *incompatible* with multifactorial inheritance. Several of these disorders deserve comment.

Certain congenital cardiac defects and other malformations occur together more frequently than expected by chance; this *association* of defects suggests a common cause, pathogenesis, or both, but the following disorders and those in Table 49–6 remain enigmatic on most of these counts. Designation as a *sequence* implies that some evidence exists for a common developmental problem to account for the features.

CHARGE Association (Table 49–5). Patients with this condition by definition have congenital heart defects.[90,91] The spectrum of cardiovascular malformations suggests not so much a common pathogenetic scheme as a common time of abnormal development. During gestational days 32 to 45, cardiac septation, fusion of the endocardial cushions and membranous ventricular septum, and formation of the outflow tracts and valves occur. An environmental insult or a breakdown in developmental homeostasis during this period could result in the malformation spectrum of this disorder. The defects in other systems could also arise during this embryological window and would be consistent with either environmental or intrinsic factors.

VATER Association (Table 49–5). This condition has expanded over the years to include *v*ertebral, *v*entricular septal, *a*nal, *t*racheo-esoph-

ageal, *r*adial, and *r*enal defects. Omitted from the mnemonic is the single umbilical artery often present.[92] Cardiac defects are present in about one-half of patients with more than two components of this association but usually are not life threatening. Although infants with this condition often fail to thrive initially, the long-term prognosis for health and mental function is good, so aggressive management of the multiple malformations is warranted. It is important to separate as soon as possible those patients who have the features of trisomy 18 or 13q- chromosome aberrations, as prognosis in these cases is distinctly unfavorable.

Mendelian Disorders

Some congenital cardiovascular defects segregate in occasional families as predicted of a mendelian phenotype. There is strong bias favoring reporting such occurrences and an equally strong temptation to conclude that, at least in some cases, the defect is caused by mutation in a single gene. However, rarely and by chance alone, a multifactorial trait recurs in a family in a pattern mimicking mendelian segregation. This potential confusion and the resultant uncertainty in counseling patients and families pertains equally well to disturbances of conduction and rhythm, to various cardiomyopathies, to vascular anomalies, and to

TABLE 49-6   CONGENITAL HEART DEFECTS OCCASIONALLY SHOWING FAMILIAL AGGREGATION CONSISTENT WITH MENDELIAN INHERITANCE

DEFECT	MIM NO.*	DEFECT	MIM NO.
Aneurysm, intracranial berry	105800	Hypoplastic left heart	140500, 241550
Aneurysm, abdominal aortic	100070	Hypoplastic right heart	277200
Angioma	106050, 106070, 206570	Lymphedema, congenital	153000, 153100, 153400, 214900, 247440
ASD, ostium primum	209400		
ASD, ostium secundum	108800, 108900, 178650	Mitral valve prolapse	157700
Bicuspid aortic valve	109730	Patent ductus arteriosus	169100
Cardiomyopathy, dilated	108770, 115200, 115250, 212110	Pulmonary venous return, anomalous	106700
Cardiomyopathy, hypertrophic	192600		
Conotruncal defect	231060	Pulmonic stenosis	126190, 178650, 193520, 265500, 265600, 270460
Dextrocardia	244400, 304750		
Ebstein anomaly	224700	Subaortic stenosis	271950, 271960
Endocardial fibroelastosis	226000, 227280, 305300	Supravalvular aortic stenosis	185500, 194050
Hemangioma	106070, 140800, 140900, 234800	Tetralogy of Fallot	187500
Hemangioma, cavernous	116860, 140850	Ventricle, single	234750

* Data from McKusick, V. A.: Mendelian Inheritance in Man. 11th ed. Baltimore, John Hopkins University Press, 1994.

hypertension, all discussed subsequently. The true cause of the cardiovascular diseases in such families may not become clarified until each is investigated in detail, in concert with efforts to map and sequence the entire human genome.

The subject of this section can therefore be parsed into three broad classes of conditions: congenital cardiac defects that occasionally seem to be inherited as mendelian traits (Table 49-6), pleiotropic mendelian syndromes that always or frequently affect the structure of the cardiovascular system (Table 49-7), and mendelian syndromes that occasionally affect the cardiovascular system (Table 49-8).

PATENT DUCTUS ARTERIOSUS (PDA). Most instances of PDA are sporadic occurrences, and there is strong association with prematurity and all of its antecedents. However, a

number of families have been reported in which PDA occurs as an autosomal dominant trait.[93] In some pedigrees, mild facial dysmorphism segregates with PDA; because the facial features differ among families, the number of syndromes remains unclear.[94,95]

FAMILIAL ATRIAL SEPTAL DEFECT. Two mendelian forms of atrial septal defect exist as autosomal dominant traits. One has no associated problems and has been described in few pedigrees.[96]

The second, and more common, condition has atrioventricular conduction delay as the only pleiotropic feature.[97,98] The defect is of the secundum type, and relatives do not seem to be at increased risk of other cardiac malformations. The severity of heart block rarely progresses to third degree. The electrocardiographic abnormality in a pa-

TABLE 49-7   MENDELIAN DISORDERS WITH CONGENITAL DEFECTS OF CARDIOVASCULAR STRUCTURE AS FREQUENT MANIFESTATIONS

DESCRIPTIVE NAME	EPONYM	MIM NO.*	CARDIOVASCULAR ABNORMALITIES
Adult polycystic kidney disease		173900	MVP, dilated aortic root, intracranial berry aneurysm
Arteriohepatic dysplasia	Alagille syndrome	118450	PPS
Cataract and cardiomyopathy		212350	HCM
Chondroectodermal dysplasia	Ellis–van Creveld syndrome	225500	ASD (ostium primum), common atrium
Deafness, mitral regurgitation, and short stature	Forney syndrome	157800	MR
Familial collagenoma syndrome		115250	DCM
Heart-hand syndrome	Holt-Oram syndrome	142900	ASD (ostium secundum), VSD, MVP, HLH
Keratosis palmoplantaris	Mal de Meleda	248300	DCM, dysrhythmia
Malignant hyperthermia and skeletal defects	King syndrome	145600	malignant hyperthermia → cardiac arrest
	Noonan syndrome	163950	PS, HCM
Pulmonic stenosis and deafness		178651	PS
	Smith-Lemli-Opitz syndrome	270400	PDA, ASD, VSD, TOF, ECD, CoA
Velocardiofacial syndrome	Shprintzen syndrome	192430	TOF, tortuous retinal vasculature

MVP = mitral valve prolapse; PPS = peripheral pulmonic stenosis; HCM = hypertrophic cardiomyopathy; ASD = atrial septal defect; MR = mitral regurgitation: DCM = dilated cardiomyopathy; VSD = ventricular septal defect; HLH = hypoplastic left heart; PS = valvular pulmonic stenosis; PDA = patent ductus arteriosus; TOF = tetralogy of Fallot; ECD = endocardial cushion defect; CoA = coarctation of aorta.

* Data from McKusick, V. A.: Mendelian Inheritance in Man. 11th ed. Baltimore, John Hopkins University Press, 1994.

TABLE 49–8 MENDELIAN DISORDERS WITH CARDIOVASCULAR ABNORMALITIES AS OCCASIONAL MANIFESTATIONS

SYNDROME	EPONYM	MIM NO.*	CARDIOVASCULAR ABNORMALITIES
Acrocephalosyndactyly type I	Apert syndrome	101200	PS, PPS, VSD, EFE
Acrocephalopolysyndactyly type II	Carpenter syndrome	201000	PDA, VSD, PS, TGA
Hereditary angioedema		106100	Coronary arteritis
Imperforate anus with hand, foot, and ear anomalies	Townes-Brocks syndrome	107480	Sporadic cases have CHD: VSD, ASD
Mandibulofacial dysostosis	Treacher Collins syndrome	154500, 248390	10% have CHD: variable
Neuronal ceroid lipofuscinosis	Batten disease	204200	HCM
Orofacial digital syndrome type II	Mohr syndrome	252100	Variable
Short rib–polydactyly syndrome	Saldino-Noonan syndrome	263530	TGA, ECD, hypoplastic right heart
Thrombocytopenia–absent radius syndrome		274000	TOF

PS = valvular pulmonic stenosis; PPS = peripheral pulmonic stenosis; VSD = ventricular septal defect; EFE = endocardial fibroelastosis; PDA = patent ductus arteriosus; TGA = transposition of great arteries; CHD = congenital heart defect(s); ASD = atrial septal defect; HCM = hypertrophic cardiomyopathy; ECD = endocardial cushion defect; TOF = tetralogy of Fallot.

* Data from McKusick, V. A.: Mendelian Inheritance in Man. 11th ed. Baltimore, John Hopkins University Press, 1994.

tient with apparently sporadic atrial septal defect should prompt a detailed family history and evaluation of close relatives. Attention should be directed to the upper limbs, particularly the thumbs, to rule out the Holt-Oram syndrome; radiographic examination of the entire limbs of the proband is helpful on this account.

When patients with atrial septal defect due to aneuploidy (a syndrome with extracardiac features), and one of the autosomal dominant forms is excluded, the recurrence risk of atrial septal defect is about 3 per cent, a value that conforms closely to the multifactorial threshold model. Several pleiotropic mendelian conditions have defects of the atrial septum as frequent manifestations.

HOLT-ORAM SYNDROME. This autosomal dominant condition, first elaborated in 1960, shows marked variability within a pedigree.[99] The cardinal manifestations are dysplasia of the upper limbs and atrial septal defect. In heterozygotes for the mutation, arm deformity ranges from undetectable through distally placed thumbs and hypoplastic thenar eminences, triphalangeal thumbs, anomalies of the carpus, and radial aplasia, to phocomelia and hypoplasia of the clavicles and shoulders. Upper extremity deformity is usually bilateral but may be asymmetrical in severity, with the left side the worse. Similarly, the atrial involvement ranges from none to a large secundum defect with early, severe hemodynamic compromise. Other cardiac malformations have been reported, with ventricular septal defects the most frequent. The skeletal and cardiac manifestations are not correlated in individuals, and how a parent is affected is not a reliable predictor of effects on offspring.[100] Prenatal diagnosis by ultrasonography was reported in a fetus with severe limb abnormalities; presumably a large septal defect could be detected as well. Other manifestations include dermatoglyphic abnormalities, pectus excavatum, hypoplastic peripheral arteries, and cardiac conduction disturbance, the last usually involving the AV node and present in patients with septal defects. Although the Holt-Oram syndrome bears some resemblance to the VATER association, the clear mendelian nature and lack of more extensive organ system involvement of the former indicate that the two conditions do not represent a pathogenetic spectrum.

The diagnosis of Holt-Oram syndrome is most likely to be missed in a patient with an unknown or unremarkable family history, a secundum septal defect, and minimal or no thumb anomaly. In any "sporadic" case of an atrial septal defect, the patient and the parents should be carefully examined for limb malformations and the family history studied in detail. Detection of a subtle limb defect alters the recurrence risk in offspring of the proband from the empirical risk of an isolated septal defect of 3 per cent to the 50 per cent of an autosomal dominant trait.

One gene for Holt-Oram syndrome has been mapped to 12q2, but the gene has not yet been identified.[100–102] In families with Holt-Oram syndrome linked to this locus, prenatal diagnosis is possible. Genetic heterogeneity exists, with some families not linked to this locus, and families with isolated atrial septal defect and conduction abnormalities without limb defects also unlinked.

ELLIS–VAN CREVELD SYNDROME (Fig. 49–6). This rare, autosomal recessive chondrodysplasia is found among the old order Amish because of a founder effect and consanguinity. Short stature, metaphyseal dysplasia, dysplastic nails and teeth, and postaxial polydactyly are the pleiotropic manifestations in addition to congenital heart disease.[103] The last is present in more than one-half of homozygotes, and most of the defects affect the atrial septum. The majority are defects of endocardial cushion closure, including ostium primum defects of widely varying size up to a single atrium. This disorder has long been thought to be due to an as yet unknown defect in the extracellular matrix, which would fit with the high frequency of endocardial cushion lesions. However, defects thought due to abnormal embryonic flow (coarctation, hypoplastic left heart, and patent ductus arteriosus) occur in about 20 per cent of cases. Ellis–van Creveld syndrome can be diagnosed prenatally by detection of polydactyly by ultrasonography.

FAMILIAL ATRIOVENTRICULAR CANAL DEFECTS. This spectrum of defects occasionally occurs in an autosomal dominant pattern in families and is unassociated with features in other systems. Because the cardiac defect is suggestive of that in the Down syndrome, linkage to chromosome 21 markers has been pursued, to no avail.[104,105]

VENTRICULAR SEPTAL DEFECT. This malformation does not seem to be inherited as an isolated mendelian malformation except when associated with CATCH22, and no syndromes include it as a common, isolated manifestation. One intriguing pedigree showed maternal transmission of a risk for atrial or ventricular septal defects to at least 11 of 13 offspring; the suggestion was made that phenotype was determined by the mitochondrial chromosome.[106] Subsequent study of the mitochondrial chromosome has not uncovered a candidate gene,[13] and the family has not been restudied.

Many other isolated defects have been described in families in patterns suggestive of mendelian inheritance, but only for supravalvular aortic stenosis and mitral valve prolapse is there convincing evidence for the action of a single mutant gene.

SUPRAVALVULAR AORTIC STENOSIS (see also p. 1662). This congenital lesion, which may be asymptomatic and detected long after birth because of an ejection murmur, occurs in at least three settings. It can be a sporadic anom-

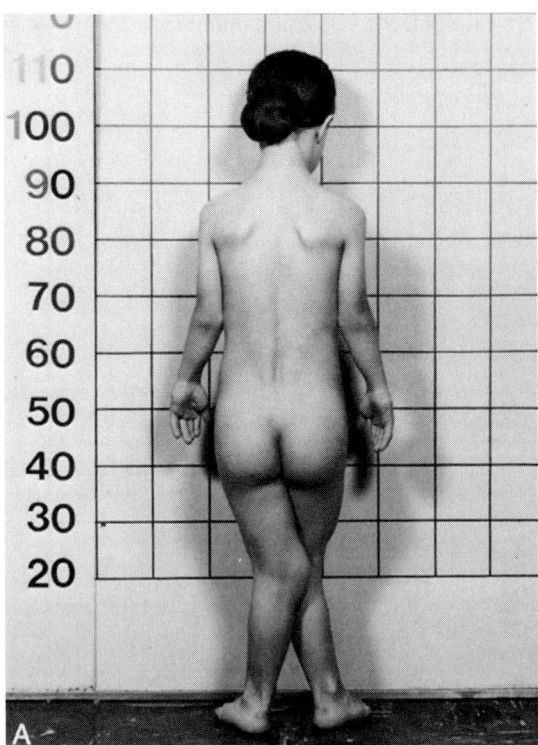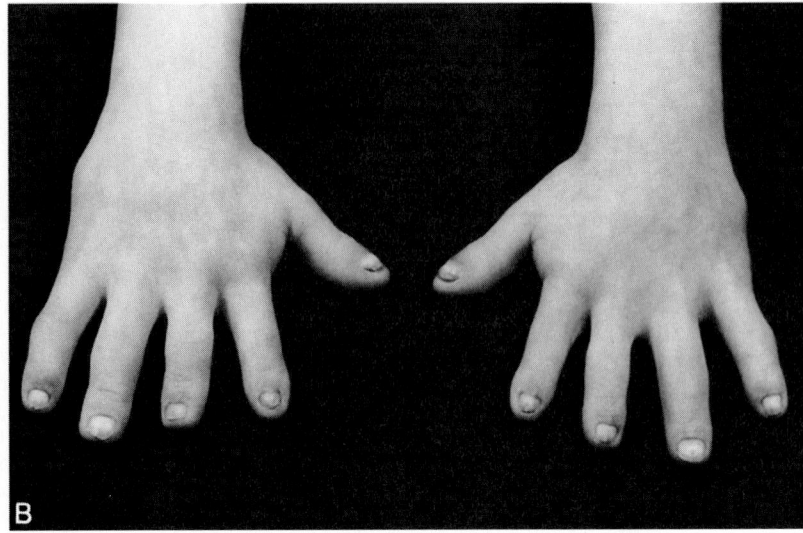

FIGURE 49–6. Ellis–van Creveld syndrome in a young woman. *A,* Note short stature, joint contractures at the elbows, and marked genu valgum. *B,* The fingers are short and the nails dysplastic. Note the protuberances along the ulnar edges of the hands where sixth digits were amputated.

aly, a component of Williams syndrome, or an autosomal dominant trait associated with peripheral pulmonic stenoses and a diffuse arteriopathy.

Williams syndrome is usually sporadic but, in more instances than previously recognized, is a highly variable autosomal dominant condition. The full spectrum includes infantile hypercalcemia, abnormal ("elfin") facies (Fig. 29–36, p. 920), mental deficiency, short stature, multiple peripheral pulmonic stenoses, and supravalvular aortic stenosis.[107] Occasional cardiovascular manifestations are mitral valve prolapse, bicuspid aortic valve, and hypertension.[108,109] Although patients usually survive the problems of infancy and show catch-up growth, progressive problems of joint contractures, genitourinary and gastrointestinal dysfunction, and psychosocial adjustment define the long-term prognosis.[110]

Supravalvular aortic stenosis (SVAS) is due to heterozygosity for a mutation in tropoelastin (see below). Because elastic fibers are intrinsic to the media of elastic and muscular arteries, a diffuse, progressive arteriopathy develops, with thickening of the wall and reduction of the lumen. The natural history of the arterial disease is just emerging as patients with Williams syndrome live longer and are followed prospectively.[111] A predisposition to cerebrovascular disease seems certain.[112,113]

Virtually all patients with Williams syndrome who have been tested have a deletion of the long arm of chromosome 7.[114] Those with SVAS have a deletion that involves the tropoelastin locus. The crucial gene(s) involved in the rest of the Williams phenotype lie telomeric to the tropoelastin locus; considerable effort is currently being directed at identifying these gene(s) that play a role in development of the face, in calcium metabolism, and in development of personality and cognitive capability.

Autosomal dominant SVAS is an entity distinct from Williams syndrome,[115–117] although some patients have subtle defects in personality and intelligence. Peripheral pulmonary artery stenoses may be present but rarely cause hemodynamic problems. The aortic lesion requires surgery in less than half of patients.

A patient with isolated SVAS was discovered to have a translocation involving chromosomes 6 and 7; although no macroscopic quantity of chromatin was apparently missing, any translocation carries the risk that the breakpoint disrupts a gene. This proved to be the case in this patient, who also had affected relatives; each person in this pedigree with SVAS also had the translocation.[118,119] Cloning of the breakpoint region showed that the tropoelastin locus at 7 was disrupted. Study of other patients, both sporadic and familial cases, none of whom had a visible chromosomal alteration, revealed that all with

SVAS had one mutation or another in the tropoelastin gene. Most of the mutations involve a deletion that results in loss of function of the allele.[120] Thus, having only one copy of a functional tropoelastin allele during embryogenesis (developmental haploinsufficiency) is sufficient to produce SVAS and peripheral pulmonic stenosis and to set the stage for a diffuse arteriopathy later in life.[120] Is this a simple dosage effect, or is the pathogenesis much more complex?

MITRAL VALVE PROLAPSE (see also p. 1029). This trait is of heterogeneous cause and pathogenesis; although it has been called the most common abnormality of human heart valves,[121] mitral valve prolapse (MVP) is equally clearly not always an "abnormality." Here only the heritable forms of MVP are discussed. These can be classified into three groups. The first is an autosomal dominant form with minimal extracardiac involvement. The second is an autosomal dominant condition that is clinically variable, and at one end of its spectrum merges with the Marfan syndrome; it could just as well be discussed as a heritable disorder of connective tissue. The third category is composed of the various mendelian syndromes that include mitral valve prolapse as a pleiotropic manifestation.

The first category, which some have called mitral valve prolapse syndrome[122] or familial mitral valve prolapse,[123] includes a condition that is centered on the mitral valve. The development of actual prolapse shows the age- and gender-dependent behavior characteristic of the "idiopathic" form so common in the general population.[123,124] Formal genetic studies confirm *autosomal dominance with variable expression.* This category has been partitioned into those patients with billowing of the mitral leaflets and those with excessive systolic mitral annular expansion; because this phenotype breeds relatively true, two distinct autosomal dominant forms may exist.[125] The cause(s) of these entities is unknown.[126] Moreover, when and how the phenotype of this condition can be distinguished from the sporadic cases of MVP and the cases with obvious evidence of a systemic disorder of connective tissue are unclear. The only consistent extracardiac manifestations are excessive arm span in women and relatively low body weight and systolic pressure.[127,128]

Many clinical geneticists and cardiologists have referred

patients with a suspicion of Marfan syndrome (see p. 1669) or Ehlers-Danlos syndrome (see p. 1672). Some of these patients do not meet minimal diagnostic criteria for a recognized connective tissue disorder[129] but clearly have extracardiac features consistent with a defect of the extracellular matrix described below. MVP is commonly but not always present; when it is, and evidence of a systemic abnormality of connective tissue is lacking, the patient should be considered to have the condition described in the preceding paragraph, what some call primary mitral valve prolapse.[130] The clinical spectrum of the patients with syndromic MVP includes abnormal striae atrophicae, excessive arm span and leg length, joint hypermobility, pectus excavatum, scoliosis, reduction in thoracic kyphosis ("straight back"), myopia, and mild aortic root dilatation.[131] Aortic dilatation beyond 3 SD above the mean for body surface area, aortic dissection, ectopia lentis, or a family history of any of these three features *removes* a patient from this category. For the remainder of patients, the acronym MASS phenotype, for *m*itral valve, *a*orta, *s*kin, and *s*keletal, describes what certainly is a heterogeneous grouping of patients and families. Aorta is mentioned specifically because of the appropriate concern that progressive dilatation and dissection will occur; in fact, neither has been the case, although prospective evaluation has been brief. Many of the associations between MVP and deformity of the thoracic cage and spontaneous pneumothorax are explained by the MASS phenotype.[132]

Finally, as described below, MVP frequently accompanies the Marfan syndrome, several of the Ehlers-Danlos syndromes, and cutis laxa and occurs more often than expected in osteogenesis imperfecta, Larsen syndrome, pseudoxanthoma elasticum, and other mendelian syndromes (see Table 49–11). In addition, occasional families with otherwise unclassified heritable disorders of connective tissue have prominent involvement of the mitral apparatus, with myxomatous deterioration or calcification, or both.[133]

NOONAN SYNDROME. Among the pleiotropic mendelian syndromes that have frequent cardiovascular involvement, the Noonan syndrome is important because of its relatively high prevalence and clinical variability. This autosomal dominant condition has been called the male Turner syndrome in the past because of the short stature, cubitus valgus, neck webbing, congenital lymphedema, and congenital heart defects that coexist in the 45,X Turner syndrome. However, the Noonan syndrome is distinct, not simply because both men and women are affected. Patients with Noonan syndrome often have an unusual deformity of the sternum, mental dullness, hypertelorism, ptosis, and cryptorchidism.[134] The cardiovascular defects, although widely varied, do not include an increased incidence of coarctation of the aorta. Because of the dysmorphism of the facies and the cardiac involvement, Noonan syndrome is often classified, along with the Williams, LEOPARD, King, and Watson syndromes, as a cardiofacial syndrome.

The entire phenotype of the Noonan syndrome is highly variable, and affected people can escape clinical problems (or accurate diagnosis), even if they have obvious manifestations.[135] Similarly, a wide range of cardiovascular involvement can occur. *Valvular pulmonic stenosis* was the first defect identified, and Noonan syndrome should always be considered in a patient with this lesion.[136] The valve cusps are thickened and dysplastic, even in the absence of hemodynamic compromise. Obstruction to right-sided flow can also occur in Noonan patients because of pulmonary artery hypoplasia or infundibular subvalvular changes. The latter finding reflects a generalized predisposition to hypertrophic cardiomyopathy, often asymmetrical, that can affect either ventricle.[137,138] *Atrial septal defect* occurs in about one-third of patients, usually in association with pulmonic stenosis. *Ventricular septal defects* and patent ductus arteriosus each occur in about 10 per cent. Congenital anomalies of coronary arteries are occasionally and unexpectedly found during evaluation of more obvious defects. The electrocardiogram often shows left anterior hemiblock and a deep precordial S wave, a pattern not common in pulmonic stenosis of other causes.

Lymphatic dysplasia, especially of the lower limbs, is common but causes clinical difficulties in less than 20 per cent.[134] While evidence of lymphedema often disappears during childhood, chylothorax and a protein-losing enteropathy represent the severe end of the spectrum.[139]

Noonan syndrome shares features with other cardiofacial syndromes, and in sporadic cases (which account for 50 per cent of Noonan syndrome) diagnosis can be difficult. All are *autosomal dominant*, so genetic counseling is somewhat easier. Affected males have

reduced reproductive capabilities because of testicular abnormalities. Susceptibility to malignant hyperthermia can be detected by family history, elevated skeletal muscle creatine kinase levels, or muscle biopsy. Despite the relatively high frequency of the Noonan syndrome, estimated up to 1 per 1000, neither its cause nor its pathogenesis is clear. One gene has been mapped to the long arm of chromosome 12, but interlocus genetic heterogeneity is likely. Intriguing issues that may shed light on these uncertainties are the overlap in phenotype with type I neurofibromatosis[140,141] (the gene for which is on chromosome 17 and has been cloned) and the frequent coexistence of Noonan syndrome and deficiency of coagulation factor XI.[142]

Teratogenic Effects

A teratogen is any agent that adversely affects embryonic or fetal development, such as infectious vectors, radiation, drugs, and other chemicals (Table 49–9). Teratogenic effects on the cardiovascular system are considered in this chapter for several reasons: (1) The phenotypes are often reminiscent of those due to chromosomal aberrations and single-gene mutations. (2) Clinical geneticists and dysmorphologists are involved in diagnosing, managing, and investigating both teratogenic and genetic syndromes. (3) How the organism responds to an encounter with a potential teratogen is largely determined by its genome. The entire field of ecogenetics and part of pharmacogenetics are concerned with these issues.

The abilities to resist disruption of normal human embryogenesis and development involve systems quite distinct from physiological homeostasis and related only in part with developmental homeostasis. Genetic susceptibilities to teratogens can be illustrated by diverse mechanisms: reduced or inaccurate repair of radiation-induced DNA damage; enhanced receptiveness to viral entry or replication; immune deficiencies that prevent inactivation of infectious vectors or maintenance of immunity; slow inactivation of a compound that exerts a direct deleterious effect; or rapid conversion of an inoffensive drug to a teratogenic metabolite. These types of hereditary variation may be determined by single genes, with susceptibility inherited as a mendelian trait, or by many genes, each of small effect. Either situation can account for the well-known fact that

TABLE 49–9   CARDIOVASCULAR DEFECTS ASSOCIATED WITH PRENATAL EXPOSURE TO TERATOGENS

TERATOGEN	CARDIOVASCULAR ABNORMALITIES*
Ethanol	~ 50% have CHD: VSD (~ 50% close spontaneously), TOF, ASD, ECD, absence of a pulmonary artery
Hydantoin	~ 10% have CHD: VSD, ASD, PS
Lithium	< 3% have Ebstein anomaly
Phenylalanine	~ 20% have CHD: TOF
Retinoic acid	> 50% have CHD: TGA, TOF, VSD, IAA
Rubella	> 50% have CHD: PDA with or without ASD, VSD, PPS, IAA
Trimethadione	~ 50% have CHD: complex combinations most frequent (involving VSD, ASD, PDA, AS, PS), VSD, TOF
Valproic acid	> 50% have CHD: left- and right-sided flow lesions: CoA, HLH, ASD, VSD, pulmonary atresia
Vitamin D	Supravalvular aortic stenosis is the cardinal manifestation; PPS
Warfarin	~ 10% have CHD: PDA, PS; rarely, intracranial hemorrhage

CHD = congenital heart defect(s); VSD = ventricular septal defect; TOF = tetralogy of Fallot; ASD = atrial septal defect; ECD = endocardial cushion defect; PS = valvular pulmonic stenosis; TGA = transposition of great arteries; IAA = interrupted aortic arch; PPS = peripheral pulmonic stenosis; PDA = patent ductus arteriosus; AS = aortic stenosis; CoA = coarctation of aorta; HLH = hypoplastic left heart.

* Among patients with the full clinical spectrum associated with each teratogen; cardiovascular defects listed in decreasing order of prevalence.

only a fraction of pregnancies exposed to a given agent are affected adversely. Variation in dose and timing of exposure also confound interpretation of epidemiological and family data. It is not surprising, then, that the actual appearance of the abnormal phenotype is not amenable to traditional pedigree analysis. Rather, examination of the biochemical susceptibilities have proved, and will continue to prove, more enlightening.

Some teratogens, such as *warfarin,* have a clear action that explains how the pleiotropic manifestations emerge. The action of other teratogens, such as alcohol, is obscure. Finally, in some teratogenic syndromes, such as that in offspring of women with diabetes mellitus, the actual offensive agent is unclear, and multiple pathogenetic mechanisms seem to pertain.[143,144] Regardless of cause and pathogenetic mechanism, the phenotypes of many teratogens often share manifestations, especially prenatal growth retardation, abnormalities of the craniofacies, and mental retardation. The following syndromes have prominent consequences on the cardiovascular system.

FETAL ALCOHOL SYNDROME. Ethanol is the most common teratogen to which the human embryo and fetus are exposed. The period of greatest vulnerability is the first trimester, and the risks are clearly related to the amount of alcohol consumed; the risk of the fetal alcohol syndrome occurring in an offspring of a chronic alcoholic woman is 30 to 50 per cent. The features are highly variable and include growth retardation, mild to moderate mental retardation, hyperactivity, short palpebral fissures, a smooth philtrum with a thin upper lip, and small distal phalanges.[145] Congenital heart defects occur in more than one-half of children with the full spectrum of the phenotype; ventricular septal defects are most common and often insignificant, but atrial septal defects, tetralogy of Fallot, and aortic coarctation can occur.

FETAL HYDANTOIN SYNDROME. Virtually all antiseizure medications can affect the fetus. Hydantoin was the first to be identified as a teratogen. The risk to the fetus depends in part on the genotype of the fetus; defects in arene oxidase predispose to the full syndrome.[146,147] The features include prenatal and postnatal growth retardation, mild mental retardation, a broad face with a short nose, short distal phalanges with small nails, and hip dislocation. Cardiovascular defects, which are an inconstant part of the syndrome, include septal defects, right- and left-sided flow defects, and a single umbilical artery.

RETINOIC ACID EMBRYOPATHY. Isotretinoin was not recognized as a teratogen until after it was licensed for the treatment of acne. The vulnerable period extends from the first week through the fourth month of gestation. The risks of miscarriage and stillbirth are elevated. The phenotype includes anomalies of the craniofacies and gross neuroanatomical disruption. Cardiovascular defects are common and emphasize a variety of conotruncal malformations.[148] Liveborn infants often succumb to the cardiac and brain anomalies. Although the mechanism of action is not certain, vitamin A derivatives such as retinoic acid function as *morphogens* during embryogenesis, serving as signals for cell migration. The fact that the cardiovascular defects are primarily those of rotation and folding suggests disruption of a normal developmental homeostatic system.

WARFARIN EMBRYOPATHY. Coumarin-related vitamin K antagonists are usually prescribed for a variety of cardiovascular problems to women of childbearing age (see p. 1859) and can cause a variety of cardiovascular and other organ damage to the fetus. Coumarin interferes with embryogenesis directly when administered during gestational weeks 6 through 9. The most pronounced effects are on cartilage because of inhibition of enzymes of extracellular matrix metabolism. Congenital cardiac defects are perhaps increased in frequency but fit no specific pathogenetic mechanism.[149] The second pattern of coumarin effects involves exposure during the second and third trimester and includes spontaneous abortion, stillbirth, and various central nervous system defects. The last are not due simply to intracranial hemorrhage as was once assumed.[149]

What predisposes to the adverse fetal effects of coumarin remains to be discovered. First, more than 75 per cent of women who take coumarin derivatives throughout pregnancy have normal offspring; reassuring most women while identifying those at risk for adverse effects has obvious advantages. Second, placing all pregnant women on a regimen of heparin is not an acceptable solution, because heparin can cause stillbirth or premature fetal loss in about 20 per cent of exposures, is not as effective as coumarin in some indications for anticoagulation, and is more trouble to administer and regulate.

MATERNAL PKU. The inborn error of metabolism phenylketonuria produces severe mental retardation unless the phenylalanine content of the diet is markedly reduced soon after birth.[150] Deficiency of phenylalanine hydroxylase in the fetus produces no harm because fetal blood levels of phenylalanine are regulated by the heterozygous mother's enzyme. Because neonatal screening for this disease is now routine in all states, virtually all patients receive treatment and grow to adulthood with average intelligence. Many patients discontinue

the rigorous dietary therapy during adolescence when the elevated phenylalanine levels have far less deleterious effects. The embryopathy occurs when a woman with homozygous deficiency for phenylalanine hydroxylase becomes pregnant and her fetus is exposed to high levels of the amino acid which overwhelm its ability to metabolize. The result is highly predictable if the mother does not restart dietary restriction of phenylalanine for the entire gestation: moderate to severe mental retardation, prenatal and postnatal growth retardation, microcephaly, and a variety of cardiovascular defects in 15 to 20 per cent.[151] This condition can largely be prevented by effective counseling of female patients with phenylketonuria.

FETAL RUBELLA EFFECTS (see p. 878). About 50 per cent of fetuses become infected with the rubella virus when the mother is infected during the first trimester. Not only does the infected fetus suffer varied and severe interference with development and organogenesis, but it acquires a chronic viral illness that can persist for years. The most common features of the embryopathy are mental deficiency, deafness, cataract, and cardiovascular defects. Patent ductus arteriosus is common, as are septal defects. Peripheral pulmonary stenosis and fibromuscular proliferation of medium and small arteries often improve postnatally.

CARDIOMYOPATHIES
(See also Chap. 41)

Each of the three clinical categories of primary cardiomyopathy—hypertrophic, dilated, and restrictive—can be caused by mutations in single genes as judged by mendelian inheritance of a consistent phenotype in multiple families. Many other mendelian and mitochondrial disorders also cause cardiomyopathies as a secondary consequence of their basic metabolic disturbance.

Hypertrophic Cardiomyopathy
(See also p. 1414)

In the more than 35 years since the recognition of hypertrophic cardiomyopathy as a clinical entity, many aspects of its natural history, pathology, and management have been substantially clarified. The phenotype is most clearly defined anatomically and histologically and consists of myocardial hypertrophy without secondary cause; cellular and myofiber disarray; myocardial fibrosis; and mediointimal proliferation of small coronary arteries. None of these features is pathognomonic; for example, myofiber disorganization is present in the normal human heart during embryogenesis and in congenital heart defects that place strain on the right-sided circulation.[152]

About half of probands with idiopathic hypertrophic cardiomyopathy of any segment of the left ventricle have affected first-degree relatives, and in those families the phenotype is inherited as an autosomal dominant, familial hypertrophic cardiomyopathy (FHC). There is wide variability of expression within a family, in part due to age-dependency of the trait.[152] Later generations of relatives in adolescence and childhood may not have developed echocardiographic evidence of hypertrophy. Hence, pedigree screening by phenotype for clinical, counseling, or investigative purposes should not be considered complete until the following criteria are satisfied: two-dimensional echocardiography is used to ensure that segmental hypertrophy is detected; a person at risk has a normal echocardiographic study and no evidence of electrocardiographic abnormality or important dysrhythmia after about age 20; and a person of any age has left ventricular hypertrophy without any other explanation, such as hypertension or aortic stenosis.

FHC is a disease of the sarcomere, with primary defects of thick and thin filaments now defined. Mutations of at least six and perhaps more loci cause FHC (Table 49–10, Fig. 41–15, p. 1417). The first locus identified was 14q1, and the cardiac β-myosin heavy chain gene was found to harbor mutations.[153] Depending on the population studied, about 50 per cent of all FHC mutations occur in this gene, *MYH7*, and more than 40 mutations have been described.[154] Patients with neither parent affected have also been shown

TABLE 49–10 FAMILIAL HYPERTROPHIC CARDIOMYOPATHY

VARIANT	MIM NO.*	GENE MAP	LOCUS	DEFECT
CMH1	192600	14q11	*MYH7*	β-Myosin HC
CMH2	115195	1 q3	*TNNT1*	Troponin T
CMH3	115196	15q2	*TPM1*	α-Tropomyosin
CMH4	115197	11p11.2	*MyBP-C*	Cardiac myosin binding protein-C
CMH5	115198	?		
CMH6		7q3	?	

* Data from McKusick, V. A.: Mendelian Inheritance in Man. 11th ed. Baltimore, Johns Hopkins University Press, 1994.

to have *MYH7* mutations, suggesting that the genetic alteration occurred in the egg or sperm of a parent.[155] Mutations that alter charge of the β-myosin heavy chain generally carry a worse prognosis in terms of age of detection, electrocardiographic abnormalities, and sudden death[156,157] (Fig. 41–16, p. 1418). Thus, defining the specific gene involved, followed by the specific mutation, has likely clinical importance. How the mutant protein interacts with other components of the sarcomere of both cardiac and skeletal muscle to produce the phenotype is another area of active research.[158]

While intergenic and intragenic heterogeneity account for much of the interfamilial variability in the FHC phenotype, there remains considerable variation among relatives who share the same mutation. Both environmental and genetic factors have impacts. A possible example of the latter is the angiotensin I-converting enzyme (ACE) genotype, with different polymorphic variants of ACE associated with more or less hypertrophy.[159]

Mutations in two genes specifying components of the thin filament, α-tropomyosin and cardiac troponin T, and in the gene encoding cardiac myosin binding protein-C, also cause FHC.[160–161b] A locus on chromosome 15q2 is associated with FHC indistinguishable from that caused by the loci with known mutations.[162] A family with Wolff-Parkinson-White syndrome and FHC shows linkage to markers at 7q3.[163] Finally, families with FHC are unlinked to any of these loci.

Dilated Cardiomyopathy
(See also p. 1407)

The prevalence of idiopathic dilated cardiomyopathy is about double that of the hypertrophic form, or about 2 to 8 per 100,000.[164–167] Although numerous occurrences of familial dilated cardiomyopathy are reported, few investigations have been conducted of an unselected series of probands for clinical and subclinical evidence of cardiac disease.[168] Thus, it is unclear what fraction of patients with idiopathic dilated cardiomyopathy have a mendelian disease, how many have a new mutation for a mendelian disease, and how many have phenocopies of nongenetic causes. Estimates of a positive family history, which could suggest a mendelian condition or a shared environmental cause, range from 7 to 30 per cent.[168–170]

Because of the risk of severe dysrhythmia in dilated cardiomyopathy, early detection of people with the disorder can be life saving.[171] Two-dimensional echocardiography is a sensitive method for detecting affected relatives with subclinical disease. Individuals who have equivocal left ventricular enlargement or dysfunction can have ambulatory electrocardiographic monitoring and, if the diagnosis is still uncertain, can have serial examinations. Certainly every patient with idiopathic dilated cardiomyopathy should have a detailed family history; about 20 per cent reveal an affected relative.[168] If any close relative has a history consistent with cardiomyopathy, dysrhythmia, or sudden death

at a relatively young age, counseling about the risk of a familial disease and the potential benefits of pedigree screening should be offered.

The majority of instances of familial occurrence fit autosomal dominant inheritance.[168,171–174] Considerable clinical variability characterizes virtually all pedigrees; variation in severity, clinical phenotype, and age of onset is typical. Recurrence of congestive cardiomyopathy of early onset in an inbred pedigree is suggestive of an autosomal recessive condition.[175]

The causes of the autosomal dominant forms of dilated cardiomyopathy are unknown. In some families with autosomal dominant disease, a mild proximal skeletal myopathy of type I fibers coexists with cardiac involvement.[172,176] Skeletal muscle changes might serve not only as an early clinical marker of heterozygosity for the mutant gene in some individuals at risk but also indicate that the search for cause should address structural components or metabolites common to both cardiac and skeletal myofibers.

In one family, cardiomyopathy developed only in association with pregnancy.[179] Although peripartum cardiomyopathy is a well-recognized, usually sporadic, disorder, its occurrence in five women in two generations suggests a hereditary predisposition. One component of muscle that is not a common cause of idiopathic dilated cardiomyopathy is dystrophin.[177]

Histological examination of myocardium generally shows nonspecific hypertrophy and fibrosis. By electron microscopy, however, mitochondria are distinctly abnormal, a finding not seen in congestive heart failure of other causes.[178] Because the inheritance pattern in these cases does not suggest a mutation of the mitochondrial genome, focus could be directed on nuclear genes that encode structural components of the mitochondrion, components of the respiratory chain found in the mitochondrion, or enzymes that regulate and facilitate free fatty acid metabolism in the mitochondrion.

A number of laboratories are conducting linkage analysis across the human genome in pedigrees showing autosomal dominant inheritance of dilated cardiomyopathy. The first success occurred in a large pedigree that is somewhat unique in that conduction disease, rather than heart failure, is usually the first manifestation of cardiovascular disease.[179] The phenotype maps to the pericentromeric region of chromosome 1 (1p1-1q1), and all of the candidate genes already mapped to this region do not appear to be at fault.[180]

Some pedigrees show convincing evidence of X-linkage of dilated cardiomyopathy. At least three loci have been identified. In *Barth syndrome,* cardiac involvement is associated with skeletal myopathy, proportionate short stature, and neutropenia; the phenotype is linked to markers at Xq28.[181,182]

Many males with *Duchenne* and some with *Becker muscular dystrophy* develop myocardial dysfunction (see p. 1867).[183] In the Becker form, right ventricular involvement may be unassociated with left ventricular dysfunction.[184] Deletion of exon 49 of the dystrophin gene predisposes to cardiomyopathy. This pleiotropic feature in a disease that presents as a skeletal myopathy prompted evaluation of the dystrophin locus in pedigrees with apparently isolated cardiomyopathy. Mutations in the 5′ end of the dystrophin gene have been found to account for some instances of X-linked dilated cardiomyopathy.[185,186] Why some dystrophin mutations are selectively expressed in cardiac muscle (and other in brain) is unclear.

Emery-Dreifuss muscular dystrophy (see p. 1872) is distinguishable clinically from the Duchenne and Becker forms by absence of pseudohypertrophy of skeletal muscle, early involvement of the arms with elbow contractures, and early onset of cardiac conduction abnormalities and atrial dysrhythmia.[181,187] Female heterozygotes are also commonly affected, albeit more mildly than males. The disease was mapped to the distal region of Xq28, and a previously unknown gene, called emerin, was found to be mutated.[188] Hearts show replacement of myocardium, especially in the atria, with fat and fibrosis. Even though the conduction system is not primarily affected histologically, sudden death is common in both hemizygous men and heterozygous women; thus, carrier detection can be life saving.[189]

Restrictive Cardiomyopathy
(See also p. 1426)

The pathogenesis of the majority of cases of restrictive cardiomyopathy involves infiltration or replacement of the myocardium or both. The causes are varied and can be nongenetic or genetic; the latter are mostly metabolic diseases with secondary effects on the heart and are summarized in Table 49–11; some are reviewed subsequently. One form of restrictive cardiomyopathy that has primary genetic forms among many other causes is endocardial fibroelastosis. Other mutations produce restriction through pericardial constriction. Isolated pedigrees of primary myocardial fibrosis without secondary cause and leading to restrictive hemodynamics are not classifiable.[190,191]

ENDOCARDIAL FIBROELASTOSIS (see also p. 991). This abnormality is characterized by thickening of the endocardium, which leads to decreased compliance and impaired diastolic function. Primary forms, discussed here, are unassociated with other cardiac anomalies (Table 49–11). When congenital, endocardial fibroelastosis accounts for somewhat under 10 per cent of childhood deaths from heart disease. In infants there is often an indolent course of failure to thrive, tachypnea, and tachycardia, until a precipitant such as an upper respiratory infection leads to rapid cardiac decompensation. Treatment of children with primary endocardial fibroelastosis is ineffective; cardiac transplantation now offers some hope. Autopsy shows enlargement of the left ventricle and perhaps other chambers, no abnormality of lung vessels, and collapse of the left lower lobe. Histopathological study reveals extensive deposition of extracellular matrix, primarily collagen and elastic fibers, in the endocardium.

X-linked recessive inheritance is the most firmly established of the single-gene causes, and even here there may be heterogeneity. Some pedigrees show mainly small, contracted cardiac chambers, whereas others have chamber dilatation; both are compatible with the functional pathophys-

iology described by the term "restrictive." Males are affected earlier and more severely by both forms, with death in infancy not unusual.[192] In other families, the ventricles are dilated, and the condition is distinguished from X-linked dilated cardiomyopathy by the presence of endocardial fibroelastosis and an immune deficiency due to defective granulocyte function, a condition termed Barth syndrome (see also p. 1665).[181,182] Morphological abnormalities of mitochondria were present on ultrastructural studies of heart and leukocytes. Insufficient longitudinal experience is recorded to know whether females heterozygous for this mutation develop a dilated restrictive cardiomyopathy later in life.

Several pedigrees suggestive of autosomal recessive inheritance of primary endocardial fibroelastosis were reported before the routine availability of laboratory methods to diagnose metabolic derangements, especially defects in fatty acid catabolism.[193] The occurrence of hydrocephalus, endocardial fibroelastosis, and neonatal cataracts may be due to a single gene mutation but could represent sequelae of a viral infection.[194] Endocardial fibroelastosis can be a prominent finding at autopsy in patients with autosomal dominant dilated cardiomyopathy[195]; whether the endocardial changes are primary, representing yet another mendelian form of this disorder, or secondary is unclear.

Restrictive cardiomyopathy often occurs with both hemodynamic evidence of impaired diastolic filling and wall thickening; any of the conditions causing pseudohypertrophy of the myocardium can eventually exhibit restrictive pathophysiology. Hemochromatosis and the amyloidoses, both hereditary and acquired forms, are especially likely to present in this manner. Connective tissue replaces myocytes or infiltrates the interstitium in a number of conditions. Fibrosis of the myocardium may cause pseudohypertrophy, but the clinical consequences are more those of restriction. Disorders in this category are those that cause coronary artery disease (*diabetes mellitus*, the *hemoglobinopathies* associated with sickling, *Fabry disease* and the *mucopolysaccharidoses*) and some of the *muscular dystrophies*, in which myocardial fibers are replaced by extracellular matrix. Finally, a number of hereditary conditions are associated with endocardial fibroelastosis (Table 49–11).

CONSTRICTIVE PERICARDITIS (see also Chap. 43). Two rare autosomal recessive disorders include fibrous thickening of the pericardium as a manifestation. In both, signs and symptoms of constrictive pericarditis develop insidiously, and treatment by pericardiotomy is life saving. One condition was first described in Finland and given the name MULIBREY nanism, a combination of a mnemonic for *muscle, liver, brain,* and *eye* and an archaic word for dwarfism (nanism). Growth failure from an early age is common, and growth does not improve once pericardial constriction is abated. Subsequently, more than a dozen patients, generally with consanguineous parents, have been reported from around the world.[196]

The *arthropathy-camptodactyly syndrome* previously had been reported because of the skeletal and rheumatological manifestations before pericardial effusion and fibrous thickening of the pericardium were recognized as manifestations.[197] Its cause is unknown.

Cardiomyopathies Secondary to Other Causes

INBORN ERRORS OF METABOLISM. These can affect the left ventricle by various mechanisms (Table 49–12) and produce diverse anatomical, histological, and functional disturbances. The most common anatomical result is an apparent hypertrophic cardiomyopathy, which is actually *pseudohypertrophic*, because the thickened walls are not due to myocardial cell hypertrophy, but to cellular or interstitial infiltration by metabolites. Abnormalities of both systolic and diastolic function result, outflow obstruction may occur, and in some cases the hemodynamic characteristics resemble a restrictive cardiomyopathy. The offending metabolite may be an incompletely degraded macromolecule such as glycogen (*glycogen storage disorder II* [Pompe's disease] and *glycogen storage disorder III*), proteoglycan and glycosaminoglycan (*mucopolysaccharidoses I, III, IV, VI, and VII*), sphingolipid (*Fabry disease, Tay-Sachs disease, Farber's disease, Refsum's disease,* and *Gaucher's disease*), glycoprotein (*fucosidosis* and *mannosidosis*), and amyloid (*familial amyloidoses I* and *III*) or a small molecule such as iron in *hemochromatosis*. Some of these disorders are discussed later. True myocardial hypertrophy occurs as a part of mendelian syndromes, such as *Noonan syndrome, von Recklinghausen neurofibromatosis*,[200] and *LEOPARD syndrome*,[201,202] and monogenic

TABLE 49–11   DISORDERS ASSOCIATED WITH RESTRICTIVE CARDIOMYOPATHY

	MIM NO.*
Primary Endocardial Fibroelastosis	
Familial endocardial fibroelastosis	226000, 305300
Faciocardiorenal syndrome	227280
Secondary Endocardial Fibroelastosis	
as a relatively common manifestation	
Maternal lupus erythematosus	
Pseudoxanthoma elasticum	177850, 264800
Systemic carnitine deficiency	212140
Trisomy 18	
as a relatively infrequent manifestation	
Cornelia de Lange syndrome	122470
Rubinstein-Taybi syndrome	268600
Secondary Infiltrative Cardiomyopathy	
Familial amyloidoses I and III	176300
Fabry disease	301500
Gaucher's disease type I	230800
Glycogen storage disorder II	232300
Glycogen storage disorder III	232400
Hemochromatosis	235200
Mucopolysaccharidosis IH	252800
Mucopolysaccharidosis II	309900

* Data from McKusick, V. A.: Mendelian Inheritance in Man. 11th ed. Baltimore, John Hopkins University Press, 1994.

errors of metabolism, notably those producing *hyperthyroidism* and *pheochromocytoma*. Any of the mendelian disorders that cause hypertension may, over time, produce true myocardial hypertrophy.

Dilated cardiomyopathy often results from inborn errors of energy production, especially fatty acid metabolism. Various disorders associated with *carnitine deficiency*, *mitochondrial* and *peroxisomal dysfunction*, and *muscle dysfunction* can present with symptoms of congestive heart failure or dysrhythmia.

PRIMARY DISORDERS OF RHYTHM AND CONDUCTION

Virtually every dysrhythmia and conduction abnormality has been reported to occur in relatives.[203] For example, *familial disturbance of conduction* occurs, without evident cause, at the sinus node,[204,205] atrioventricular node,[206,207] and bundle branches.[208,209] However, understanding the genetics of cardiac electrophysiology has been hampered by several characteristics of this extensive literature: Most families have been small, so that mode of inheritance, or even whether the inheritance is mendelian, is uncertain; many of the families show a mixture of different defects, partly because the disease is progressive[210,211]; and some specific conduction defects are associated with hereditary myocardial diseases, such as familial cardiomyopathy,[171,212] atrial cardiomyopathy,[213] and familial amyloidosis.[214] As noted earlier, there seems to be genetic control of normal electrical conduction, so it would not be surprising to find mutations in single genes that produced clinically important disturbance.

An important cause of complete heart block, although not mendelian, nonetheless involves genetic factors. The association between rheumatic diseases and heart block was clearly established when the offspring of mothers with acquired disorders of connective tissue, especially lupus erythematosus, were found to have complete heart block.[215-217] Many examples of "autosomal recessive" congenital heart block represent this familial, but nonmendelian, etiology. The risk is not related to severity of the maternal disease but is highest in children of women with antibodies to ribonucleoprotein (anti-Ro[SS-A])[218] and at least one allele for HLA-DR3.[219] Thus, it may be the maternal genotype that determines susceptibility to inflammation of the fetal heart at vulnerable periods, such as gestational weeks 3 to 4 when the atrioventricular node is forming. Genetic susceptibility to inflammation of the atrioventricular node of patients themselves is suggested by the relatively high association of HLA-B27 in adults requiring permanent pacemakers[220,221]; not all of these patients have overt evidence of HLA-B27–associated rheumatic diseases.

Familial dysrhythmia is also not uncommon. Nodal rhythm,[222] ventricular irritability,[223] and tachydysrhythmia associated with accessory atrioventricular pathways[163,224,225] have been reported in families. In one family, three generations were affected by a syndrome of ventricular extrasystoles and tachydysrhythmias with recurrent syncope, hypoplasia of the distal toes, and hypoplasia of the mandible (Robin sequence).[226] Hereditary cardiomyopathies are another cause of familial dysrhythmia, and a notable example is arrhythmogenic right ventricular dysplasia (ARVD), an autosomal dominant condition with variable expression[227,228] (see also p. 681). Although ARVD is uncommon, the familial form shows clusters of high incidence (0.4 per cent) in some regions of Italy and is an underappreciated cause of life-threatening dysrhythmia.[229] The right ventricle is involved primarily in most cases, with thinning and replacement of myocardium by fat and fibrosis (Fig. 41–2, p. 1405).[230] Dysrhythmia, usually ventricular but occasionally supraventricular, may precede signs of right ventricular dysfunction. About one-third of cases are familial, generally in an autosomal dominant pattern. Whether the primary process is homogeneous or not and whether true dysplasia, degeneration (due to a metabolic defect or muscular dystrophy), or inflammation plays the leading role are unclear. In addition to these disorders, several syndromes involving prolongation of the Q-T interval deserve comment.

WARD-ROMANO SYNDROME (see also p. 750). Familial syncope and sudden death have long been associated with ventricular dysrhythmia, but a distinct syndrome was not recognized until Ward[231] and Romano,[232] working independently three decades ago, reported the characteristic prolonged Q-T interval. Subsequent investigations of numerous families have clearly established that the defect in repolarization is inherited as an *autosomal dominant*. Although a long $Q-T_c$ is consistently present, other abnormalities of conduction also occur, although they may not be evident on the resting electrocardiogram.[233] Ward-Romano syndrome, now generally called long Q-T syndrome, is distinguished from the Jervell and Lange-Nielsen syndrome by inheritance pattern and the absence of hearing deficiency. Long Q-T syndrome is generally unassociated with systemic abnormalities, but three patients with a negative family history for long Q-T had syndactyly of multiple fingers and toes.[234]

Long Q-T syndrome is genetically heterogeneous, and mutations of at least three loci can produce similar disorders. The first locus was mapped to 11p15.5,[235] and subsequently loci at 7q35-q36 and 3p21-p24[236] were identified. Because some families show recombination of long Q-T syndrome with all of these loci, a fourth gene, at a minimum, must be involved. Use of genotype to determine unequivocally who is heterozygous for the mutation has permitted assessment of the reliability of electrocardiographic criteria for diagnosis.[237] Not unexpectedly, the criterion of a corrected Q-T interval greater than 0.44 sec is good, but less than 90 per cent sensitive and specific. Treatment with beta-adrenergic blockade or an automatic implanted defibrillator is effective. Individuals heterozygous for the mutant gene should be identified through a detailed family history, clinical assessment and, if necessary, DNA testing, and counseled appropriately.

JERVELL AND LANGE-NIELSEN SYNDROME (see also p. 750). The association of familial syncope, sudden death, and congenital deafness was codified in 1957,[238] although as with most eponymous syndromes, reports of affected individuals occurred previously. As would be expected for a rare, autosomal recessive condition, the parents of affected children are more likely than average to be consanguineous. Although heterozygotes have normal hearing and no overt primary rhythm disturbance, the $Q-T_c$ intervals may be slightly prolonged.[239] The frequency of a long $Q-T_c$ among deaf children is about 1 per 100, so routine electrocardiographic screening of anyone with congenital deafness is warranted.

Neither the cause nor the pathogenesis is known. Fright and rage clearly precipitate syncope and sudden death, leading to the proposal of autonomic dysfunction as the basic defect. However, allotransplantation of the heart, thereby causing complete denervation, failed to correct the underlying problem in one patient.[240]

DISORDERS OF CONNECTIVE TISSUE

The two broad classes of disorders of connective tissue are those due to mutations in single genes that determine or somehow affect components of the extracellular matrix and those due to extrinsic factors affecting the extracellular matrix, such as rheumatoid arthritis and systemic lupus erythematosus. The former category includes many disorders that affect the cardiovascular system. Susceptibility to so-called acquired disorders of connective tissue is, in part, determined by genes, and this specific aspect is reviewed. Disorders due to intrinsic factors acting on the extracellular matrix are discussed in Chapter 56.

TABLE 49–12   MENDELIAN ERRORS OF METABOLISM WITH MANIFESTATIONS IN THE CARDIOVASCULAR SYSTEM

DISORDER	EPONYM OR COMMON NAME	MIM NO.*	PATHOGENESIS	CARDIOVASCULAR INVOLVEMENT	BIOCHEMICAL DEFECT	GENE LOCUS†	ANIMAL MODEL‡
Aminoacidopathies							
Alkaptonuria	Ochronosis	203500	Deposition of homogentisic acid in connective tissue	AS; atherosclerosis			
Cystinosis, nephropathic type		219800	Lysosomal storage	Hypertension from renal failure, vascular wall thickening	?	?	
Homocystinuria		236200	Unknown	Early CAD; venous thrombosis; pulmonary embolism	Cystathionine-β-synthase	CBS; 21q21-q22.1	
Oxalosis I	Hyperoxaluria	259900	Vascular and tissue accumulation of oxalate	Conduction defect; vascular occlusions; Raynaud phenomenon	Peroxisomal alanine: Glyoxylate aminotransferase	AGT	
Defects in Fatty Acid Metabolism							
Carnitine transport defect	Primary carnitine deficiency	212140	Lipid myopathy; defective energy generation	DCM: ECF	?	?	Syrian hamster
MCAD deficiency		201450	Lipid myopathy; defective energy generation	DCM	Medium-chain acyl-CoA dehydrogenase	ACADM,1p	
LCAD deficiency		201460	Lipid myopathy; defective energy generation	DCM	Long-chain acyl-CoA dehydrogenase	ACADL,7	
Glycogen Storage Disorders							
GSD I	Pompe	252300	Lysosomal storage	Pseudohypertrophic CM; short P-R interval; ECF	α-1,4-glucosidase	GAA: 17q21-q25	Canine and bovine
GSD II	Adult acid maltase deficiency	232300	Lysosomal storage	Primarily skeletal muscle; respiratory insufficiency; corpulmonale	α-1,4-glucosidase		
GSD III	Forbes; debrancher deficiency	232400	Intracellular glycogen accumulation fibrosis	Pseudohypertrophic CM	Amylo-1,6-glucosidase		
Phosphorylase kinase deficiency	GSD of the heart			DCM	Phosphorylase kinase		
Glycoproteinoses							
Fucosidosis, severe		230000	Lysosomal storage	Myocardial thickening	α-fucosidase	FUCA1; 1p34	
Fucosidosis, mild		230000	Lysosomal storage	Angiokeratoma	α-fucosidase	FUCA1; 1p34	
Mannosidosis		248500	Lysosomal storage	Myocardial thickening; valvular thickening; conduction disturbance	α-Mannosidase	MANB, 19p13.2-12	
Aspartylglycosaminuria		208400	Lysosomal storage	Valvular thickening	Aspartylglycosylamine amino hydrolase	AGA, 4q21-qter	
Mucolipidoses							
ML II	I-cell	252500	Lysosomal storage	Same as MPS IH	Acetylglucosamine-1-phosphotransferase	GNPTA; 4q21-q23	
ML III	Pseudo-Hurler polydystrophy	252500	Lysosomal storage	Valvular thickening and dysfunction, esp. AS, AR	Acetylglucosamine-1-phosphotransferase	GNPTA; 4q21-q23	
Mucopolysaccharidoses							
MPS IH	Hurler	252800	Lysosomal storage	Early CAD; PH and OAD → CP; valvular dysfunction, esp. MR, AR; pseudohypertrophic CM	α-L-Iduronidase	IDUA, 22q11-pter	Canine and feline
MPS IS	Scheie	252800	Lysosomal storage	Valvular dysfunction, esp. AS	α-L-Iduronidase	IDUA, 22q11-pter	
MPS IH/S	Hurler-Scheie	252800	Lysosomal storage	Same as MPS IH	α-L-Iduronidase	IDUA, 22q11-pter	
MPS II	Hunter	209900	Lysosomal storage	Same as MPS IH; less severe in mild MPS II variant	Sulfoiduronate sulfatase	IDS, Xq28	

DISORDER	EPONYM OR COMMON NAME	MIM NO.*	PATHOGENESIS	CARDIOVASCULAR INVOLVEMENT	BIOCHEMICAL DEFECT	GENE LOCUS†	ANIMAL MODEL‡
MPS III A	Sanfilippo A	252900	Lysosomal storage	Valvular thickening and occasional dysfunction	Heparin sulfate sulfatase	?	
MPS III B	Sanfilippo B	252920	Lysosomal storage	Valvular thickening and occasional dysfunction	N-Acetyl-α-D-glucosaminidase	?	
MPS III C	Sanfilippo C	252930	Lysosomal storage	Valvular thickening and occasional dysfunction	acetyl-CoA: α-glucosaminidase N-acetyl-transferase	?	
MPS III D	Sanfilippo D		Lysosomal storage	Valvular thickening and occasional dysfunction	N-Acetylglucosamine-6-sulfatase	G6S, 12q14	
MPS IV A	Morquio A	253000	Lysosomal storage	Valvular dysfunction, esp. AR	Galactosamine-6-sulfatase		
MPS IV B	Morquio B	253010	Lysosomal storage	Milder than MPS IV A	β-Galactosidase		
MPS VI	Maroteaux-Lamy	253200	Lysosomal storage	Same as MPS IH	Arylsulfatase B	5p11-qter	Feline
MPS VII	Sly	253220	Lysosomal storage	Valvular thickening	β-Glucuronidase	GUSB;7q	Mouse and canine
Sphingolipidoses							
α-Galactosidase A deficiency	Fabry	301500	Cellular accumulation of trihexosyl ceramide, esp. endothelium	Early CAD, valvular thickening and dysfunction; pseudohypertrophic CM; short P-R interval; arteriolar occlusion; angiokeratoma	α-Galactosidase A	GLA; Xq22	
Ceramidase deficiency	Farber	228000	Histiocytic infiltration	Nodular thickening of valves	Ceramidase	?	
Glucocerebrosidase deficiency	Gaucher, adult form	230800	Cellular accumulation of glucocerebroside	PH → CP; interstitial infiltration of myocytes by Gaucher cells; constrictive pericarditis	β-Glucocerebroside	GBA; 1q21	
Miscellaneous disorders							
Acid lipase deficiency	Wolman	278000	↑ Cholesterol; foam cell infiltration	Atherosclerosis	Lysosomal acid lipase	LIPA, 10q	
Acid lipase deficiency	Cholesterol ester storage disease	278000	↑ Cholesterol, foam cell infiltration	Atherosclerosis; PH	Lysosomal acid lipase	LIPA, 10q	
Geleophysic dysplasia		231050	Lysosomal storage	Valvular dysfunction	?		
Hereditary angioedema		106100	Complement and kinin activation	Angioedema	C1 esterase inhibitor ?	CINH, 11p11.2-q13	
Multiple sulfatase deficiency	Juvenile sulfatidosis	272200	Lysosomal storage				

CAD = coronary artery disease; DCM = dilated cardiomyopathy; ECF = endocardial fibroelastosis: CM = cardiomyopathy; AS = aortic stenosis; AR = aortic regurgitation; PH = pulmonary hypertension; OAD = obstructive airway disease; CP = cor pulmonale; MR = mitral regurgitation; GSD = glycogen storage disease.

* Data from McKusick, V. A.: Mendelian Inheritance in Man. 11th ed. Baltimore, John Hopkins University Press, 1994.

† Gene symbol followed by chromosomal locus.

‡ Naturally occurring mutants; does not include transgenic and knockout rodent models.

Mendelian Disorders of the Extracellular Matrix

Close to 200 distinct phenotypes now comprise this category, which was first defined less than four decades ago with fewer than 10 disorders.[241] Several reviews and textbooks describe the phenotypes, genetics, and causes of many of the conditions (Table 49–13).[18,242–245]

Marfan Syndrome

This *autosomal dominant* disorder is relatively frequent (~ 1 per 10,000), occurs in all races and ethnic groups, and is often not diagnosed during life.[245,246] In light of the classic phenotype, failure to diagnose the Marfan syndrome may seem surprising; however, marked clinical variability,

age dependency of all of the manifestations, and a high (~ 30 per cent) rate of new mutation all conspire to make detection of mildly affected, young, sporadic patients challenging. Even with the discovery of the genetic and biochemical bases of the condition, the diagnosis of Marfan syndrome outside of families with the classic phenotype remains entirely clinical, for reasons described subsequently.[247] Current criteria (Table 49–14) depend on the manifestations in the cardinal organ systems—the eye, the skeleton, the heart, and the aorta—and other systems, and the family history[129] (Fig. 49–7). The presence of manifestations more specific for the Marfan syndrome, such as aortic dilatation, aortic dissection in a nonhypertensive young person, ectopia lentis, and dural ectasia, clearly is

TABLE 49–13 CARDIOVASCULAR MANIFESTATIONS OF HERITABLE DISORDERS OF CONNECTIVE TISSUE

DISORDER	MIM NO.*	CARDIOVASCULAR MANIFESTATIONS
Cutis laxa	219100	PS, PPS, CP
	123700	MVP
Ehlers-Danlos I	130000	MVP
II	130010	MVP
III	130020	MVP
IV	130050	Arterial rupture, MVP
VI	225400	MVP
VIII	130080	MVP
X	225310	MVP, aortic root dilatation
Osteogenesis imperfecta I	166200	MVP, mild aortic root dilatation
II	166210	CP, arterial calcification
III	259420	MVP
IV	166220	Aortic root dilatation
Marfan syndrome	154700	MVP, aortic root dilatation, aortic dissection
MASS phenotype	157700	MVP, mild aortic root dilatation
Pseudoxanthoma elasticum	177850	Arteriolar sclerosis, claudication, myocordial infarction

PS = valvular pulmonic stenosis; PPS = peripheral pulmonic stenosis; CP = cor pulmonale; MVP = mitral valve prolapse
* Data from Mendelian Inheritance in Man.[8]

TABLE 49–14 DIAGNOSTIC CRITERIA FOR THE MARFAN SYNDROME:[129] PHENOTYPIC MANIFESTATIONS*

Skeleton
  Joint hypermobility, tall stature, pectus excavatum, reduced thoracic kyphosis, scoliosis, arachnodactyly, dolichostenomelia, pectus carinatum, erosion of the lumbosacral vertebrae from dural ectasia†
Eye
  Myopia, retinal detachment, elongated globe, ectopia lentis†
Cardiovascular
  Mitral valve prolapse, endocarditis, dysrhythmia, dilated mitral annulus, mitral regurgitation, tricuspid valve prolapse, aortic regurgitation, aortic dissection†, dilatation of the aortic root†
Pulmonary
  Apical blebs, spontaneous pneumothorax
Skin and Integument
  Inguinal hernias, incisional hernias, striae atrophicae
Central Nervous System
  Attention deficit disorder, hyperactivity, verbal-performance discrepancy, dural ectasia†, anterior pelvic meningocele†

If the family history is positive for a close relative clearly affected by the Marfan syndrome, to make the diagnosis in the patient, manifestations should be present in the skeleton and one of the other organ systems, and the diagnosis confirmed by linkage analysis or mutation detection.

If the family history is negative or unknown, to make the diagnosis, the patient should have manifestations in the skeleton, the cardiovascular system, and one other system, and at least one of the manifestations indicated by †.

* Manifestations are listed within each organ system in increasing specificity for Marfan syndrome, although none is completely specific; those indicated by † are the most specific.

more important diagnostically than features common in other connective tissue disorders and in the general population, such as scoliosis, joint hypermobility, myopia, and MVP.

The most common cardiovascular features are MVP and dilatation of the sinuses of Valsalva.[246,248,249] Associated clinical problems of mitral regurgitation, aortic regurgitation, and aortic dissection account, if untreated, for most of the early mortality that results in an average age of death in the fourth and fifth decades.[250] Children tend to be more severely affected by mitral valve disease,[251–253] whereas aor-

tic problems are progressive and more likely in adolescence and beyond.

MITRAL VALVE INVOLVEMENT. MVP is age dependent and more common in women with the Marfan syndrome. The incidence reaches 60 to 80 per cent when patients are studied by two-dimensional echocardiography,[130] and generally the valve leaflets have an elongated and redundant appearance. Progression of severity, as judged by appearance or

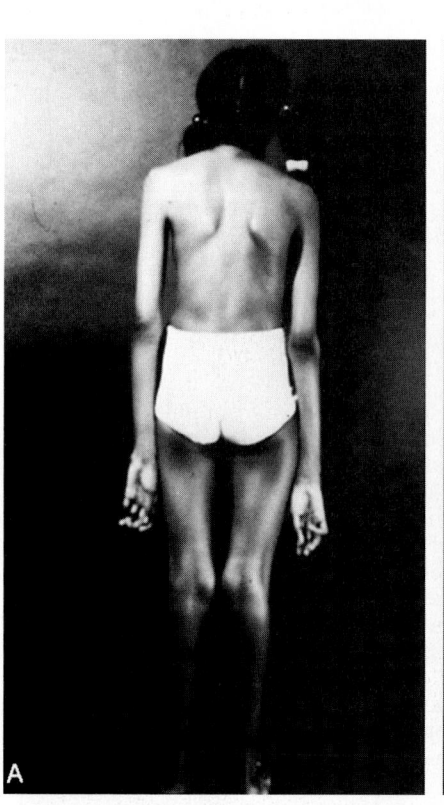
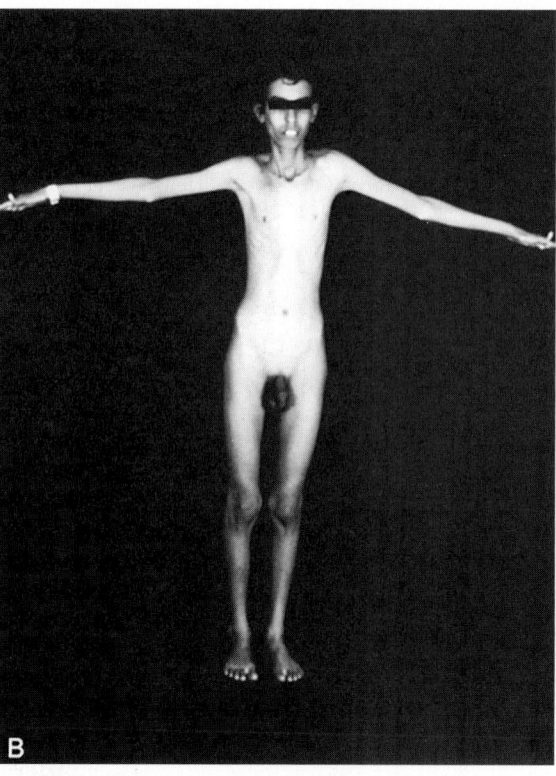

FIGURE 49–7. External phenotype of a boy with Marfan syndrome, showing long extremities and digits, tall stature, and pectus carinatum.

worsening of mitral regurgitation by clinical and echocardiographic criteria, occurs in at least one-quarter of patients,[254] a much higher rate than in MVP found in the general population.[249] The mitral annulus dilates and contributes to the regurgitation, as do stretching and occasional rupture of chordae. About 10 per cent of patients with marked prolapse have calcification of the mitral annulus. Standard treatment for chronic mitral regurgitation is indicated, but coexistent aortic root dilatation usually requires that increasing inotropy be avoided. When mitral regurgitation becomes severe enough to warrant surgical intervention, two considerations must be added to the balance: (1) Repair of the mitral apparatus is often successful and durable in the Marfan syndrome.[255,256] Repair is less easily accomplished when the cusps are extremely redundant, there is marked chordal damage, or the annulus is heavily calcified. (2) The aorta may be enlarged enough to permit concomitant replacement. We have often delayed mitral valve surgery for a time, carefully following ventricular function, until the sinuses of Valsalva dilated enough to make composite graft repair feasible. On the other hand, when operation is primarily because of aortic dilatation, a mitral annuloplasty can be performed if there is more than trivial mitral regurgitation.[257,258] In Marfan syndrome, as in virtually all of the heritable disorders of connective tissue, there is an increased susceptibility to dehiscence of prosthetic mitral valves, regardless of the care taken in placing them.

AORTIC ROOT INVOLVEMENT (see also p. 965). The sinuses of Valsalva are often dilated at birth, and the rate of progression varies widely among patients in general and also among relatives (Fig. 49–8). Thus, predicting long-term risks of developing aortic regurgitation (which is clearly positively associated with aortic root diameter[259]), suffering aortic dissection (which is less clearly associated with diameter), or requiring aortic surgery is fraught with uncertainty. Transthoracic echocardiography is sufficient for detecting and monitoring changes in diameter, because in the absence of dissection, dilatation is limited to the proximal ascending aorta, and the rate of change is slow, measured in millimeters per year. Rare exceptions of principal dilatation of the thoracic aorta can be followed with transesophageal echocardiography or magnetic resonance imaging. Patients with dilatation less than 1.5 times the mean diameter predicted for their body size[131,260] can be observed annually; as the diameter increases, more frequent evaluation is necessary. Aortic regurgitation often appears in adults at a diameter of 50 mm but may be absent at diameters of more than 60 mm.[259,261] The risk of dissection increases with the size of the aorta and fortunately occurs infrequently below

a diameter of 55 mm in the adult. Many surgeons have adopted the criterion of a 50 to 55 mm maximal aortic root dimension for performing elective composite graft repair in Marfan syndrome patients, regardless of the severity of the aortic regurgitation,[258] although patients with a family history of aortic dissection should have surgery at the lower end of this range. The perioperative results of both elective and emergency repair of the aortic root have been excellent and a marked improvement from the pre–composite graft era that ended in the mid 1970's. Long-term results of operation are limited by the problems of endocarditis and anticoagulation, common to all prosthetic valves, but in the absence of chronic aortic dissection appear favorable for patients with Marfan syndrome.[262–264]

THORACIC ABNORMALITIES. Severe *pectus excavatum* may complicate cardiovascular surgery by making exposure of the heart by median sternotomy difficult. For elective cardiovascular surgery, repair of the sternal deformity some months in advance permits sufficient healing of the costochondral junctions that a stable and functionally and cosmetically improved thoracic cage will facilitate further surgery and postoperative recovery.[265] Simultaneous repair of cardiac and sternal defects, although possible, is a long procedure, and intraoperative bleeding from bone can be considerable because of the anticoagulation associated with cardiopulmonary bypass.

AORTIC DISSECTION (see also p. 1671). This complication usually begins just above the coronary ostia (type A in the Stanford scheme) and extends the entire length of the aorta (type I in the DeBakey scheme). About 10 per cent of dissections begin distal to the left subclavian (type B or III), but rarely is dissection limited to the abdominal aorta. Angiography (Fig. 45–12, p. 1561), magnetic resonance imaging (Fig. 10–22, p. 328), and transesophageal echocardiography all have a role in the diagnosis of acute dissection in the Marfan syndrome, with the capabilities and experience of the medical center and the stability of the patient important determinants of the approach. As many acute dissections of the ascending aorta in Marfan syndrome have a stuttering course that culminates in death from rupture or hemopericardium, rapid transfer to a facility prepared to perform immediate repair is essential.

Not all acute dissections in Marfan syndrome involve severe, tearing chest pain that radiates to the back; indeed, some extensive dissections have been occult.[258] This experience reinforces the need for a high index of suspicion by physicians whenever a tall, nearsighted young person with thoracic cage deformity arrives at an emergency department with vague complaints of lightheadedness, chest or abdom-

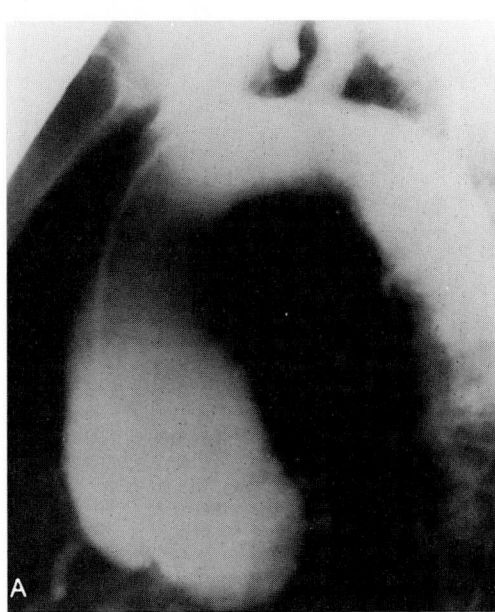 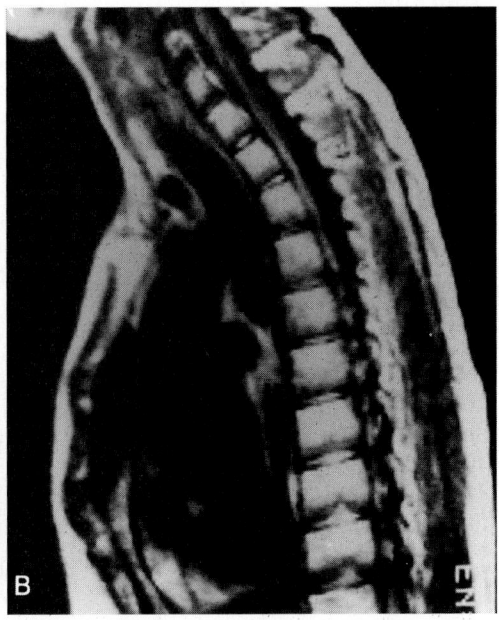

FIGURE 49–8. Dilatation of the aortic root in Marfan syndrome. *A,* Lateral angiogram of the ascending aorta showing dilatation of the sinuses of Valsalva and proximal ascending aorta and relatively normal caliber of the ascending aorta. *B,* Lateral magnetic resonance imaging of the same patient.

inal discomfort, or a murmur of aortic regurgitation. Similarly, patients known to have Marfan syndrome and their close relatives need to be educated about the signs and symptoms of aortic dissection. In general, the management of acute and chronic dissection in the Marfan syndrome follows standard practice,[266] with several departures. First, all dissections of the ascending aorta should be repaired promptly, preferably with a composite graft. Second, regular evaluation with magnetic resonance imaging is important, as the diameter of any region of dissected aorta is likely to expand over time.[267,268] Third, reduction of systolic blood pressure and administration of negative-inotropic doses of beta-adrenergic blockers should be even more strictly adhered to than in dissections without a connective tissue abnormality. In most instances, any region of the aorta should be repaired when complications of further dissection, branch vessel occlusion, or dilatation beyond about 50 mm occur. A staged approach to total replacement of the Marfan aorta is now both feasible and successful.[269]

DYSRHYTHMIAS. Some patients develop serious ventricular or supraventricular dysrhythmia. The latter often accompanies chronic mitral regurgitation, but the former may be of high grade and difficult to suppress when only MVP is present. Some patients have the syndrome of autonomic dysfunction, atypical chest pain, and palpitations seen in some patients with MVP unassociated with a flagrant connective tissue abnormality.

MANAGEMENT. The routine cardiological management of the Marfan syndrome is multifaceted: regular clinical and echocardiographic examinations; routine endocarditis prophylaxis for dental and other procedures; restriction of activity from heavy weightlifting, contact sports, and any exertion at maximal capacity; and chronic beta-adrenergic blockade form the basic approach, with individual variation often appropriate. Support for the role of beta-blockade comes from several prospective studies that show a reduction in the rate of aortic dilatation and the risk of aortic dissection in patients treated with negatively inotropic doses of propranolol or atenolol.[270,271] However, short-term administration of propranolol to patients with large sinus of Valsalva aneurysms, while reducing heart rate and peak systolic pressure, did not improve the impedance characteristics recorded in the ascending aorta.[272]

A woman with Marfan syndrome has two concerns regarding pregnancy (see also p. 1850). The first is the 50:50 risk that any child will inherit the condition; currently prenatal diagnosis can be attempted in selected situations. The second is the risk of dissection that the hemodynamic stresses of pregnancy place on the aorta. Several dozen case reports attest to the heightened incidence of dissection during the third trimester, parturition, and the first month post partum.[273,274] However, in the majority of instances, serious aortic dilatation was present. Prospective evaluation of 21 women through 45 pregnancies confirmed our earlier recommendation that the cardiovascular risks are relatively low if the aortic diameter does not exceed 40 mm and cardiac function is not compromised.[274]

ETIOLOGY. Marfan syndrome is caused by mutations in the gene that encodes fibrillin-1, the major constituent of microfibrils, components of the extracellular matrix that are widely dispersed and perform multiple function.[245,275,276]

Microfibrils form the scaffolding upon which elastin is deposited to form elastic fibers. Fragmentation and disorganization of elastic fibers in the aortic media have long been a histological marker (inappropriately called cystic medial necrosis) of Marfan syndrome,[246] although similar microscopic pathology occurs in familial aortic aneurysms and aging aortas of the normal population. A defect in microfibrils explains all of the pleiotropic manifestations of Marfan syndrome.[16,245]

After Marfan syndrome and fibrillin were mapped to the same region of chromosome 15,[277,278] it only remained to detect mutations in the *FBN1* gene to prove the cause.[279]

Subsequently, over 100 distinct mutations in this gene have been found in different families, and only a couple have occurred, by chance, in unrelated patients.[7,245,280,281] Because *FBN1* is such a large gene ($\sim 10,000$ nucleotides in the mRNA), finding a mutation is still not a simple matter. Once the mutation is identified, diagnosis in that family is straightforward. In families with multiple alive and cooperative affected people, linkage analysis can be used for presymptomatic and prenatal diagnosis.[247] The use of molecular testing is confounded, however, by the discovery that autosomal dominant ectopia lentis, familial tall stature, MASS phenotype, and familial aortic aneurysm are all phenotypes found to be due to mutations in *FBN1* and are exactly the conditions clinicians are interested in excluding in their patients of questionable diagnosis.[245,282,283]

Mutations in *FBN1* have distinct effects on microfibril formation: Some affect synthesis, others secretion, and others incorporation of fibrillin-1 monomers into the extracellular matrix.[281,284,285]

MITRAL VALVE PROLAPSE AND THE MASS PHENOTYPE. This heterogeneous group of conditions, described above (p. 1662) likely contains large numbers of patients and families who have a defect of the extracellular matrix underlying the phenotypes. Some, but not all, have mutations in *FBN1*.[245]

Ehlers-Danlos Syndrome

This group of heterogeneous conditions is linked by variable involvement of the skin and the joints, with hyperelasticity and fragility of the former occurring with hypermobility of the latter[8,18,129] (Fig. 49-9). Mitral valve prolapse is clearly increased in frequency in most of the clinical types,[243,286] but aortic root dilatation is an uncommon finding. The most serious cardiovascular problems occur in *Ehlers-Danlos type IV* in the form of spontaneous rupture of large- and medium-caliber arteries.

Various defects of type III collagen are the cause of the phenotype in virtually all patients studied.[18] In the classic syndrome, true aneurysms rarely form; rather, a rupture without dissection usually occurs

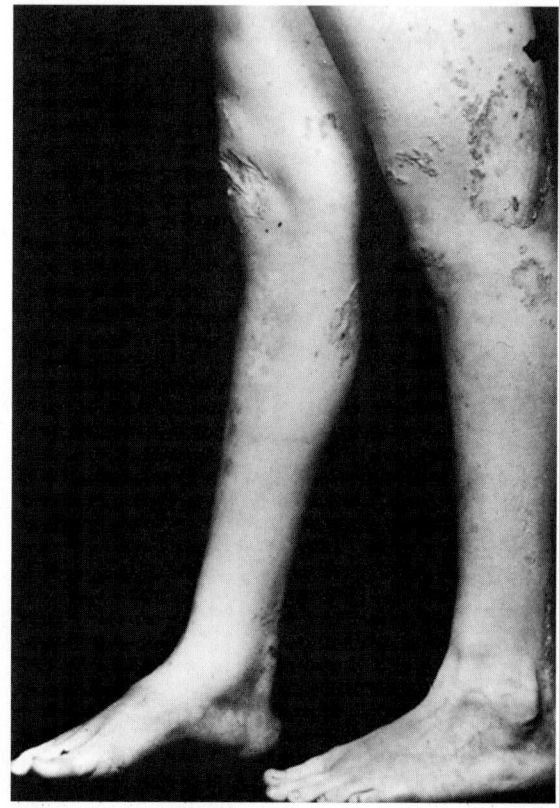

FIGURE 49–9. Legs of a patient with Ehlers-Danlos type IV who died of rupture of the subclavian artery. Note the mild joint hypermobility and the striking dermal abnormalities—elastosis perforans serpiginosa and thin, atrophic scars over areas of recurrent trauma.

as a catastrophic event. Most prone are the abdominal aorta and its branches, the great vessels of the aortic arch, and the large arteries of the limbs. False aneurysms and fistulas[18,243,287] may be one result in those patients who do not die of the initial rupture. Vascular surgery is difficult, as the normal-appearing vessels around the rent fail to hold sutures. As a consequence, elective surgery to repair vascular anomalies, such as false aneurysms, that are causing no immediate problem is contraindicated in most cases. Ehlers-Danlos type IV is often sporadic but, when familial, is usually autosomal dominant.

Prenatal diagnosis is possible by examining collagen production in amniocytes. However, pregnancy is particularly hazardous to women with Ehlers-Danlos type IV because of vascular rupture and should be avoided on medical grounds.[288]

Pseudoxanthoma Elasticum

This is a clinically variable and genetically heterogeneous disorder of unknown cause. Histopathological examination of affected tissues shows fragmentation and calcification of elastic fibers. The skin, the eye, the gastrointestinal system, and the cardiovascular system are the organs most severely affected.[129,244,289] The skin shows highly characteristic raised, yellowish papules (pseudoxanthoma) overlying areas of flexural stress, such as the neck, cubital and popliteal fossae, and groin (Fig. 49–10). Breaks in the elastic lamella, Bruch's membrane of the choroid, produce the funduscopic finding of angioid streaks. Gastrointestinal hemorrhage is common and potentially fatal; mucosal arterioles bleed, and because the calcified elastic fibers prevent effective vessel retraction, hemostasis is difficult. Selective arterial embolization was life saving in one instance.[290] The heart is affected in a number of ways. Endocardial fibroelastosis is common, but because primarily the atria are involved, a restrictive cardiomyopathy is uncommon. Mitral valve prolapse may be increased in frequency[291,292] but is rarely a clinical problem. Coronary artery disease with myocardial ischemia and infarction is the major problem and a common cause of early death.[293,294]

Elastic and muscular arteries, including the coronaries, develop a type of arteriosclerosis similar to Mönckeberg's; progressive luminal narrowing occurs and can produce complete occlusion. Initially this is most evident at the radial and ulnar arteries, where absence of pulses and a positive Allen test are noted early in the course.[293] Because narrowing progresses slowly, collaterals form, and peripheral ischemia is a late complication. Because the arterial stenoses tend to be diffuse, bypassing them often involves extensive surgery. One patient with marked endocardial fibroelastosis was helped by resection of calcified elastic bands within the left ventricle.[295] Because the basic defect is unknown (but does not involve the gene for elastin),[296] no specific treatment is available. Because of a positive association between phenotypic severity and dietary calcium intake, patients can be advised to restrict consumption of dairy products and to avoid calcium supplements.[297] Hypertension and all risk factors for atherosclerosis should be aggressively controlled.

Genetic Susceptibility to Acquired Disorders of Connective Tissue

Genetic factors are clearly implicated in the susceptibility to many of the rheumatic disorders and to specific complications of specific conditions. The cardiovascular manifestations of these disorders are particularly interesting in this regard (p. 1776). For example, study of HLA-DR antigen frequencies suggests that immune-response factors are involved in the pathogenesis of chronic rheumatic heart disease in blacks.[298]

INBORN ERRORS OF METABOLISM THAT AFFECT THE CARDIOVASCULAR SYSTEM

The hundreds of biochemical defects that affect human metabolism have direct or secondary impact on the cardiovascular system (Table 49–12). Several examples are reviewed, selected for their relevance to clinical practice or their instructive lessons about pathophysiology.

Aminoacidopathies

Inborn errors of amino acid metabolism result in the accumulation of precursors and a deficit of end products, either or both of which can be detrimental.

Alkaptonuria

An intermediate of tyrosine catabolism polymerizes to homogentisic acid, which readily accumulates in the extracellular matrix.[299] Over many years, connective tissue of cartilage, heart valves, and arteries becomes increasingly abnormal. Aortic stenosis and arteriosclerosis are the cardiological sequelae.

Homocystinuria

This condition is caused by a deficiency of cystathionine β-synthase; the pathogenesis of the pleiotropic manifestations is largely unknown.[17,300] Perhaps the amino acid sulfhydryl groups bind to collagen, fibrillin, and other macromolecules and interfere with cross-linking. The clinical features, once confused with the Marfan syndrome, include tall stature, skeletal deformity, ectopia lentis, mental retardation, psychiatric disturbances, and a predilection for venous and arterial thromboses. Those patients with mutations that render the enzyme activity able to be increased by pharmacological doses of pyridoxine are less severely affected; early treatment can prevent most aspects of the phenotype.[301] Patients unresponsive to pyridoxine can be helped by a low-protein diet to reduce intake of methionine.

Myocardial infarction, pulmonary embolism, and stroke are the most common causes of death. The pathogenesis of the vascular complications was once thought to involve abnormal platelet function, but platelet survival in untreated patients is normal.[302] Growing evidence supports a susceptibility of heterozygotes, who have none of the external phenotype of the disease, to atherosclerosis.[303–305] A variety of actions of homocysteine on endothelial receptors, stimulation of smooth muscle growth, and production of extracellular matrix components are being explored for clinical relevance.[306,307] Current therapeutic approaches are focused on maintaining physiological levels of the cofactors involved in metabolism of sulfurated amino acids—folate and vitamins B_6 and B_{12}.[308]

Disorders of Fatty Acid Metabolism

Although most organs can metabolize fatty acids when faced with hypoglycemia, only the heart depends on fatty acids as the primary source of energy generation. Thus, it is not surprising that virtually all genetic defects in fatty acid metabolism, including generalized defects in mitochondria and peroxisomes, are associated with myocardial dysfunction. Other substrates—glucose, lactate, and oxaloacetate—also generate energy in myocardial cells by entry into mitochondria and the tricarboxylic acid (Krebs) cycle. Thus, defects in conversion of pyruvate to acetyl coenzyme A and in any point along the tricarboxylic acid cycle and the respiratory chain have a major impact on myocardial energy generation. Quite likely, some sporadic and familial instances of idiopathic cardiomyopathy may represent undiagnosed or undefined metabolic disorders.

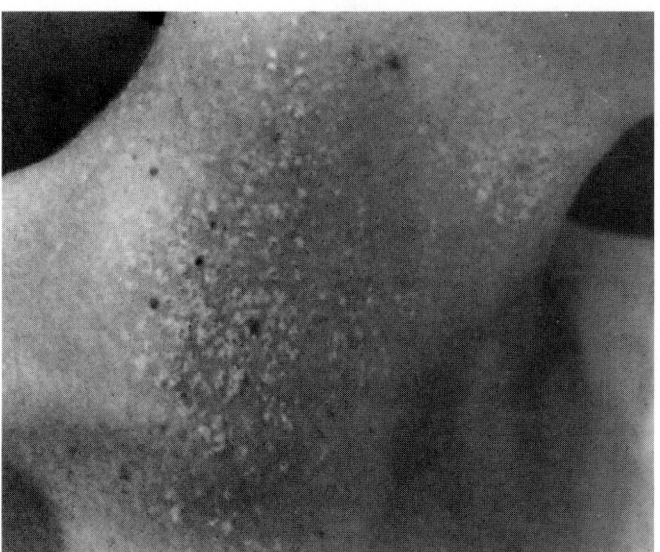

FIGURE 49–10. Skin of a young man with pseudoxanthoma elasticum. The neck is a typical location to notice the raised, yellowish papules from which the name of the condition derives.

CARNITINE DEFICIENCIES. Carnitine is a required cofactor for entry of long-chain fatty acids into mitochondria and is both synthesized endogenously and available from dietary sources.[309] Deficiency of carnitine effectively blocks metabolism of long-chain fatty acids throughout the body and hepatic metabolism of ketones. Because of their relative dependency on fatty acids, muscle cells, including myocytes, suffer out of proportion to other tissue when carnitine levels are low for any reason. Cytoplasmic inclusions of lipid are characteristic findings in myocytes and hepatocytes.

Several mendelian defects produce primary or secondary carnitine deficiency. An autosomal recessive defect in carnitine palmitoyltransferase I leads to increased plasma carnitine and a skeletal muscle myopathy with little effect on the heart.[309] So-called systemic carnitine deficiency can be due to a variety of causes: primary deficiency of intake, synthesis, or function, and secondary deficiency, the majority now known to be a result of defects in fatty acid metabolism.[309–311] The latter group of conditions usually does not respond to pharmacological doses of carnitine.[311,312]

Primary carnitine deficiency usually presents in infancy with hypoglycemia, coma, and congestive heart failure due to dilated cardiomyopathy. In the few cases reported, problems largely resolve with carnitine treatment; they can be prevented from recurring by oral supplementation with L-carnitine[312,313] (p. 1447). Primary systemic carnitine deficiency is due to a defect in carnitine transport, which leads to excessive urinary loss and which affects muscle but not liver.[311] Thus, muscle cells still may be relatively deficient in carnitine, despite supplementation, and long-term prognosis is uncertain.

DEFECTS OF BETA-OXIDATION. At least 20 steps are involved when a molecule of free fatty acid leaves the plasma, enters the beta-oxidation spiral in the mitochondrion, and generates electrons and acetyl-CoA.[309] At each turn of the oxidation spiral, two carbons are removed from the fatty acid, and the enzymes involved in this step are specific for substrates of only certain chain length: long-chain, medium-chain, and short-chain acetyl-CoA dehydrogenases, or LCAD, MCAD, and SCAD. Thus far, patients with defects in nine of the steps have been characterized.

Patients homozygous for these generally autosomal recessive disorders develop episodic hypoketotic hypoglycemia, usually associated with fasting or intercurrent illness. Deficiency of MCAD is the most common cause and occurs in about 1 of every 7000 newborns in the United States. Hypoglycemic crises can rapidly progress to coma and death, and 50 to 60 per cent of affected infants die in the first 2 years of life.[165] Because infants between episodes or before a fatal crisis appear normal, MCAD deficiency accounts for a proportion of so-called sudden infant deaths.[314] Histopathological examination shows microvesicular accumulation of fat in cardiac and skeletal muscle. One mutation in MCAD (A985G) accounts for 90 per cent of all alleles that predispose to this lethal disorder, and various approaches to newborn screening are being investigated.

MITOCHONDRIAL MYOPATHIES. All of the enzymes of fatty acid oxidation are encoded by genes located on nuclear chromosomes, but the components of the electron transport chain are encoded by both nuclear and mitochondrial genes. Several syndromes involving various types of myopathies have been shown to be due to mutations in the mitochondrial chromosome.[13] The *Kearns-Sayre* syndrome includes pigmentary degeneration of the retina, ophthalmoplegia (Fig. 60–16, p. 1876), and cardiomyopathy as its most prominent manifestation; all of the affected tissue have nearly exclusive reliance on oxidative phosphorylation for energy generation.

The *MELAS syndrome* (*myopathy, encephalopathy, lactic acidosis*, and *stroke*-like episodes) is due to mutations in mitochondrial transfer RNA genes.[315–317] In addition to the features that define the acronym, hypertrophic cardiomyopathy and diffuse coronary angiopathy are common. A variety of other mtDNA mutations are associated with hypertrophic or dilated cardiomyopathy.[318,319]

Variations in both the actual mutations and the fraction of abnormal mitochondria in the cells of the different organs (heteroplasmy) account for many of the clinical differences in phenotype, severity, and age of onset among patients with this disorder. Inheritance is maternal for patients with mitochondrial mutations; apparent autosomal recessive and dominant inheritance may indicate that mutations of nuclear genes can impair electron transport similarly to mitochondrial mutations. Some patients have been treated with moderate success over the short term with coenzyme Q[320] and with cardiac transplantation in one case.[321]

Glycogenoses

Three of the glycogen storage disorders affect cardiac muscle.

GLYCOGEN STORAGE DISEASE II (see also p. 992). This autosomal recessive condition is due to deficiency of the lysosomal enzyme α-1,4-glucosidase and results in the lysosomal accumulation of glycogen in most tissues. Several allelic variants occur.[322] The condition with infantile onset is called *Pompe disease*, and cardiac involvement is profound.[323] The infant with Pompe disease appears well initially but soon fails to thrive and develops hypotonia,

tachypnea, and tachycardia; the disease progresses during the first year to irreversible congestive heart failure and death from pneumonia or cardiopulmonary failure. Typically, auscultation reveals no murmurs until late in the course when obstruction develops, and hypoglycemia does not appear because the nonlysosomal pathway of glycogen catabolism is intact. The diagnosis is suggested by massive cardiomegaly on examination and chest radiography and by characteristic echocardiographic abnormalities of a short P-R interval and markedly increased QRS voltage.[324] Echocardiography shows tremendously thickened (pseudohypertrophic) ventricles, and Doppler interrogation or catheterization may reveal subaortic and subpulmonic pressure gradients characteristic of obstructive cardiomyopathy.

Reduced diastolic function of a restrictive cardiomyopathy develops eventually, and endocardial fibroelastosis is common.[324,325] With these findings, the diagnosis of Pompe disease is virtually certain, but it can be confirmed by analysis of α-1,4-glucosidase activity in cultured fibroblasts. Prenatal diagnosis is possible by enzymatic assay of amniocytes. Treatment is supportive, but cardiac transplantation could correct the cardiac problem; unfortunately, involvement of other organs, including the lungs, liver, and skeletal muscle, might eventually prove just as serious as the cardiomyopathy. Bone marrow transplantation might be a solution if performed early in the course. An animal model of α-1,4-glucosidase deficiency exists in cattle and develops cardiac pathology typical of human Pompe disease.[326]

Cardiomyopathy may develop in the juvenile-onset form of α-1,4-glucosidase deficiency,[327] but it is not invariable because of allelic heterogeneity. In one sibship without cardiac involvement, three brothers had extensive hepatic, skeletal muscle, and arterial smooth muscle accumulation of glycogen, and each died of rupture of a basilar artery aneurysm.[328] The adult-onset form usually presents with insidious onset of respiratory insufficiency, and clinically important cardiac disease is rare.[329]

GLYCOGEN STORAGE DISEASE III (see p. 1668). The striking clinical variability in phenotype associated with deficiency of α-1,4-glucosidase is due in large part to the extensive array of mutations that occur at the GAA locus,[330] which maps to 17q23. This autosomal recessive deficiency of amylo-1,6-glucosidase results in infantile- and juvenile-onset syndromes of muscular weakness, wasting, and hepatomegaly. Clinical cardiac disease is not common, although both cytoplasmic (nonlysosomal) and intermyofibril glycogen is routinely present in the heart and causes pseudohypertrophy and increased voltage on electrocardiography. The diagnosis has been established by enzymatic assay of an endomyocardial biopsy specimen.[331–333]

GLYCOGEN STORAGE DISEASE IV. This is caused by deficiency of α-1,4-glucan: α-1,4-glucan 6-glycosyl transferase. It usually causes a fatal disorder of early childhood characterized by hepatic failure; although extensive deposition of polysaccharide occurs in the heart, death intervenes before cardiac symptoms appear. As with all of the glycogen storage diseases, extensive allelic heterogeneity results in milder forms of the classic disorders. Patients with diagnosis later in adolescence tend to have more severe cardiomyopathy.[334,335] Liver transplant has been life saving in some cases and has, somewhat surprisingly, resulted in a reduction of glycogen deposits in the heart and skeletal muscles.[336,337]

CARDIAC PHOSPHORYLASE KINASE DEFICIENCY. Few cases of this enzyme deficiency have been reported: deposition of glycogen is confined to the heart, which may be massively thickened and enlarged, and leads to early death.[338,339]

GLYCOPROTEINOSES. As shown in Table 49–12, this group of disorders results in the lysosomal accumulation of a variety of compounds that cannot be catabolized further because of the specific enzyme deficiency. Some have prominent cardiac pathology, generally of pseudohypertrophy and valvular thickening, which present with congestive failure, valvular dysfunction, conduction defects, or dysrhythmia.

Hematological Disorders
(See Chap. 57)

HEMOCHROMATOSIS (see pp. 1430 and 1790). This is an autosomal recessive disorder of unknown cause that results in iron deposition in many tissues, including the myocardium. The manifestations include diabetes mellitus, skin hyperpigmentation, hypogonadism, hepatic failure with cirrhosis, hepatoma, and congestive heart failure; severity is considerably worse, and age of onset earlier, in women because of the autophlebotomy provided by menstruation.[340] The gene is located close to the HLA complex on chromosome 6, and presymptomatic diagnosis can be made in a family, even prenatally, by determining HLA antigen haplotypes and performing linkage analysis. Diagnosis in sporadic cases depends on finding increased serum iron, ferritin, and, especially, transferrin saturation in the absence of any obvious cause of excessive iron intake.[341] Fully 10 per cent of the population is heterozygous for the hemochromatosis mutation, suggesting that at an incidence of 2 to 3 per 1000, this disease is underdiagnosed.

Cardiac involvement often appears first as dysrhythmia or congestive heart failure. Dysrhythmia, conduction abnormalities, and low QRS voltage are typical electrocardiographic findings; cardiomegaly is seen on chest radiography, and a dilated cardiomyopathy with reduced systolic function can be documented on echocardiography.[342,343] Occasional patients have a restrictive pattern on cardiac catheterization.[344]

Treatment by repeated phlebotomy is most effective if begun before organ damage is irreversible. If a patient with congestive heart failure has not yet developed serious compromise in other organs, cardiac transplantation may be contemplated, as may combined heart-liver replacement.

HEMOGLOBINOPATHIES (see p. 1787). *Sickle cell disease* and other hemoglobinopathies associated with sickling can produce ischemia and infarction in multiple organs by occlusion of small vessels; however, the heart is relatively resistant.[345] Nonetheless, the combination of chronic hypoxemia and anemia produces a chronic high-output state that leads to congestive heart failure in many adults. The cardiovascular system can also be compromised by systemic hypertension from renal infarction, pulmonary embolism and infarction (the chest pain of which often causes concern about myocardial ischemia), pulmonary hypertension,[346] stroke, and hemosiderosis from chronic transfusions. In addition to a hyperdynamic congestive failure, iron overload is the principal risk to the myocardium in other causes of decreased erythrocyte production *(thalassemias)* and increased erythrocyte consumption *(hemolytic anemias)* requiring repeated transfusions.

Treatment with daily injections of deferoxamine can, if begun early, prevent the development of severe cardiac and hepatic disease.[347] Development of an oral iron chelator would greatly improve compliance and efficacy. Combined heart-liver transplantation has been used in a case of end-stage organ failure with homozygous β-thalassemia.[348]

Mucopolysaccharidoses and Disorders of Targeting Lysosomal Enzymes

Many of the specific disorders in these two groups share phenotypic manifestations and are caused by various defects in the ability of lysosomes to catabolize proteoglycan and glycosaminoglycan. Short stature, progressive coarsening of facial features, a skeletal dysplasia termed dysostosis multiplex, corneal clouding, and protean effects on the cardiovascular system are common[349-353] (Fig. 49-11). Only MPS IS (Scheie syndrome), the mild form of MPS IH (mild Hunter syndrome), MPS IV (Morquio syndrome), and MPS VI (Maroteaux-Lamy syndrome) have minimal or no mental impairment.

CARDIOVASCULAR MANIFESTATIONS. The cardiovascular complications (Table 49-12), which are all progressive and usually insidious, arise from engorgement of cells and tissues with macromolecular storage material.[354] First, the ventricular walls become pseudohypertrophic, and systolic function gradually deteriorates. The electrocardiogram shows reduced QRS voltages; rarely is any conduction disturbance present. Second, coronary arteries narrow because of intimal and medial thickening.[355] Myocardial infarction is common in MPS IH and the severe form of MPS II, although the patients are usually too retarded to complain of classic symptoms, and the diagnosis is made post mortem.[356] Third, valve leaflets thicken and cause progressive dysfunction that is oddly specific for individual disorders. For example, aortic stenosis is common in MPS IS, and mitral regurgitation is found frequently in MPS IH and MPS IV. Finally, narrowing of the upper and middle airways causes obstructive apnea, chronic hy-

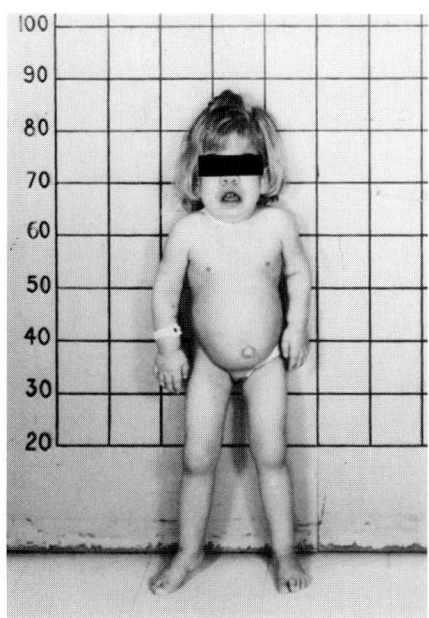

FIGURE 49-11. The Hurler syndrome in a 4-year-old girl. Note short stature and coarse facial features.

poxemia and hypercarbia, pulmonary hypertension, and eventually cor pulmonale.[357,358]

MANAGEMENT. Until recently, treatment of children with those conditions that caused mental retardation has been supportive. Increasing experience with bone marrow transplantation in many of the conditions shows that, in the relatively few survivors of the transplant, somatic accumulation of mucopolysaccharide can be reduced, with clinical improvement in cardiopulmonary function.[349,359,360] However, improvement of central nervous system function has been marginal or absent. Nonetheless, bone marrow transplantation may have a role, especially in MPS IV and MPS VI, in which cardiopulmonary compromise can greatly shorten otherwise productive lives. Attempts at cardiovascular surgery, indeed of any procedure requiring general anesthesia, are fraught with risks of difficult intubation, hyperextension of the neck with cervical cord damage (the odontoid process is often hypoplastic), and prolonged efforts to wean from mechanical ventilation.[357]

Sphingolipidoses

FABRY DISEASE (see also p. 1678). This X-linked condition deserves comment because the diagnosis is often not made until adulthood when serious end-organ damage has occurred.[12,361] As a result of deficiency of α-galactosidase A, ceramide trihexoside and other glycosphingolipids accumulate in lysosomes of many cells and organs, especially endothelial cells, glomerular and tubular cells of the kidney, and the heart. Microangiopathy causes the characteristic skin lesion, angiokeratoma, and may contribute, along with primary nerve involvement, to acroparesthesias and painful crises. Proteinuria and hypertension precede renal failure, which often has led to death in males and often leads to the fourth decade to the necessity for long-term dialysis or renal transplantation. A successful kidney allograft does not correct the systemic metabolic defect,[362] and the disease usually progresses in other organs.[349]

CARDIAC MANIFESTATIONS. Structural and functional cardiac involvement is similar qualitatively to that in the mucopolysaccharidoses. Thickening of the myocardium is pseudohypertrophy from deposition of glycosphingolipid in lysosomes; the diagnosis has been made by endocardial biopsy during the evaluation of unexplained ventricular hypertrophy or frank obstructive cardiomyopathy.[364,365] Chronic hypertension can exaggerate left ventricular dysfunction, as can ischemia and infarction from diffuse luminal narrowing of the coronary arteries. Two-dimensional echocardiography is useful for serial documentation of myocardial function.[366] Although valvular thickening and MVP are common, hemodynamically important mitral regurgitation is not.[366,367] The pulmonary vasculature becomes narrowed and right-sided pressures rise, but cor pulmonale is rarely a problem. The electrocardiogram often shows a shortened P-R interval, increased left ventricular voltages, and dysrhythmia. Medium-sized arteries throughout the body develop luminal narrowing, with cerebrovascular disease the most common cause of death after renal failure.

Heterozygous females generally show some clinical manifestations, especially in the eye, and at much later ages than hemizygous males develop renal, cerebrovascular, and cardiac disease.[12,366-368] Prenatal diagnosis is possible, and a detailed family history and genetic counseling are essential whenever the disease is found. A variety of mutations occur in the gene for α-galactosidase A and account for the clinical variability.[365,369]

Familial Amyloidoses
(See also p. 1427)

A variety of disorders, defined initially by clinical phenotype and due to progressive accumulation of amyloid in organs and tissues, are beginning to be categorized by the underlying biochemical and genetic defects.[370] The several conditions termed familial amyloidosis with polyneuropathy, and originally classified as separate autosomal dominant disorders, are now known to be due to different mutations in the same gene encoding transthyretin, a thyroxine- and retinol-binding protein also called prealbumin. Although polyneuropathy dominates the early course during young adulthood, renal failure and restrictive cardiomyopathy supervene later and cause death in most cases. The age of onset, severity, and predilection for kidney and cardiac involvement are determined by the type of mutation, with males affected earlier and more severely.[371–374]

Liver transplatation can prevent progression of the disease and potentially reverse some tissue accumulation[375]; when the myocardium is severely infiltrated, combined liver-heart transplant offers the only hope.

NEUROMUSCULAR DISORDERS
(See Chap. 60)

CARDIAC TUMORS
(See Chap. 42)

The three most common tumors that originate in the heart are myxomas, fibromas, and rhabdomyomas. All occur as part of hereditary syndromes and as sporadic events. The new occurrence of any of these tumors, especially in a child, may represent the first manifestation of a systemic condition, so a detailed general examination and family history are always indicated.[376,377] For example, 51 to 86 per cent of cardiac rhabdomyomas occur because of tuberous sclerosis.[378] Tumors due to hereditary disorders tend to be multiple and to recur after resection. An example is the NAME syndrome (see p. 1468) (for *n*evi, *a*trial myxoma, *m*yxoid neurofibromata, and *e*phelides, although the acronym ignores the multiple endocrine tumors), in which multiple myxoma can occur throughout the myocardium.[379–381]

INHERITED DISORDERS OF THE CIRCULATION

Hereditary Hemorrhagic Telangiectasia

This autosomal dominant condition, often called Osler-Rendu-Weber disease, is more common than appreciated. Because of marked intrafamilial and interfamilial variability, the condition may go undiagnosed in affected patients for years despite mild manifestations.[382,383] Mucocutaneous telangiectases, 0.5 to 3 mm in diameter, occur on the tongue, lips, and fingertips most commonly (Fig. 2–4, p. 17). Small and moderate-sized arteriovenous fistulas occur in the nose, leading to recurrent epistaxis, in the gastrointestinal system, where they cause recurrent bleeding and occult anemia, and in the lung, resulting in hypoxemia, hemoptysis, polycythemia, clubbing, paradoxical embolization through the right-to-left shunt, and a hyperdynamic circulation. Less common sites of vascular malformations are the brain,[384] liver,[385] and the kidney.[386] Diffuse ectasia of the coronary arteries was noted in one patient.[387] Bleeding is facilitated, even in the presence of normal platelet function and clotting function, because of the lack of resistance channels in the telangiectatic lesions.[388]

Patients with HHT, and their close relatives should be screened for pulmonary arteriovenous malformations through auscultation, arterial blood gas analysis, and chest radiography. A low arterial pO_2 should prompt consideration of angiography and therapeutic balloon occlusion of the feeding arteries of any sizable malformation to prevent systemic embolization, especially to the brain.[389] In a few patients, epistaxis and gastrointestinal blood loss have been reduced by antifibrinolytic therapy with danazol or aminocaproic acid.[390,392] Controlled trials of various approaches to chronic management, taking into account clinical and genetic variables, are sorely needed.

At least three genes are capable of causing HHT and two have been mapped, to 9q33-q34 and to 3p22.[393,394] The former locus encodes a transforming growth factor-β binding protein called endoglin, and a variety of mutations segregate with HHT in different families.[395] Thus, by mutation detection or linkage analysis, presymptomatic and prenatal diagnosis is available to a large number of patients with a potentially life-threatening disorder.

Von Hippel–Lindau Syndrome

The features of this autosomal dominant condition involve malformations and abnormal growth of small blood vessels. Retinal angioma, hemangioblastoma of the cerebellum, and hemangioma of the spinal cord occur in association with renal cell carcinoma, pancreatic and epididymal cystadenomas, and pheochromocytoma.[396,397] Secondary hypertension due to renal disease and pheochromocytoma, which is often bilateral, occurs and predisposes to subarachnoid hemorrhage. The cause is a tumor suppressor gene located on the short arm of chromosome 3. Patients inherit a germline mutation (and there is great diversity among families in the actual mutations) that is present in all cells. When a somatic mutation in the normal allele occurs in a susceptible cell, such as in the renal parenchyma or adrenal medulla, the cell becomes functionally homozygous for a lack of the gene product, and the cascade toward neoplasia is initiated.[398] How this gene product stimulates or permits angiomatous malformations is unclear.

Disorders Primarily Affecting Arteries

Mendelian disorders are associated with a diverse array of arterial pathology, and some have been described or catalogued earlier in this chapter. This section deals with two categories of disorders caused by a single mutant gene: pleiotropic syndromes better known for affecting organ systems other than the vasculature, and primary abnormalities of arteries.

ADULT POLYCYSTIC KIDNEY DISEASE (APKD). In the United States, this relatively common autosomal dominant disease affects 0.5 million people and accounts for 8 to 10 per cent of all long-term hemodialysis in the United States. Development of renal cysts is age dependent, and presymptomatic detection of heterozygotes, even by ultrasonography, can be uncertain into adulthood.[399,400] About one-half of patients are hypertensive, one-half have hepatic cysts, one-half eventually develop severe renal failure, and an unknown (but probably high) fraction have colonic diverticula. Elevated plasma renin levels contribute to hypertension long before renal failure occurs.[401] The cardiovascular manifestations include MVP in one-quarter, mild dilatation of the aortic root, occasional thoracic and abdominal aneurysms, and a predisposition to regurgitation of the aortic, mitral, and tricuspid valves.[402–404] The association of diverticula, organ cysts, and cardiovascular lesions reminiscent of, but milder than, the Marfan syndrome suggests some involvement of the extracellular matrix.

The most serious vascular problem is typical "berry" aneurysms of the cerebral circulation, which occur in about 10 per cent of heterozygotes but may remain asymptomatic throughout life. Hypertension predisposes to subarachnoid hemorrhage. How to screen for and treat intracranial aneurysms in patients without neurological symptoms remains controversial. Cerebral angiography carries higher risks in patients with APKD because of dissection and heightened vascular reactivity.[405] Magnetic resonance imaging detects most saccular aneurysms down to 2 to 3 mm in diameter. Whether to attempt prophylactic repair when a small aneurysm is detected has not been investigated systematically. Without question, aggressive blood pressure control is indicated in any patient with APKD.

At least three genes cause APKD. Most cases are due to mutations in a gene called *PBP* at the *PKD1* locus (16p13.3); the function of this gene is unclear.[406] In most of the rest of families, the disease maps to the *PKD2* locus in the region 4q13-q23.[407] Families affected by mutations in *PKD2* tend to develop renal failure later and have a milder course.[399] A French-Canadian family with disease typical of *PKD1* is unlinked to either locus, indicating that a *PKD3* gene exists.[408]

ARTERIOHEPATIC DYSPLASIA. An autosomal dominant disorder of marked variability, *Alagille syndrome* causes neonatal jaundice due to aplasia of intrahepatic bile ducts and congestive heart failure in the most severely affected infants but may be asymptomatic in heterozygous relatives.[409,410] The cardiovascular findings include peripheral pulmonic and systemic arterial stenoses in the majority, occasionally associated with septal defects or patent ductus arteriosus. Renal disease may produce hypertension. In some cases, a small deletion of the short arm of chromosome 20 involving the region p12.3-p11.23 occurs, suggesting that this complex phenotype is a contiguous gene deletion syndrome.[5]

ARTERIAL ANEURYSM, ECTASIA, OR DISSECTION. Pedigrees abound in which dilatation of the aortic root, aneurysm of the abdominal aorta, aortic dissection without dilatation, or a combination of these problems occurs in an autosomal dominant pattern without evidence of a recognized heritable disorder of connective tissue.[411–413] Because of the variable presentation and natural history of the aortic disease, presymptomatic detection of presumed heterozygotes is uncertain, as is reassurance of relatives at risk who are of childbearing age and would prefer not to pass this condition to offspring.

The association of dissection of the ascending aorta with bicuspid aortic valve is well known, although the cause and pathogenesis remain unclear.[414] In such cases, the aortic wall shows abnormalities of elastic fibers.[414] A person with a congenitally bicuspid aortic valve should be screened for dilatation of the aortic root, and first-degree relatives should be screened for both lesions. This recommendation is based, in part, on bicuspid aortic valve being a congenital heart defect of the left-sided flow category, with a relatively high recurrence risk (see p. 964).

Until recently, no basic defects had been identified. In two families with autosomal dominant transmission of arterial aneurysms and mild increased skin fragility and bruisability, different mutations in the gene encoding type III procollagen occurred.[415,416] Thus, depending on the mutation, deficiency of type III collagen can cause the classic syndrome of Ehlers-Danlos type IV (see p. 1672) or a form of the much subtler but just as deadly syndrome, familial arterial rupture. For these families in which the mutations have been defined, reliable presymptomatic and prenatal diagnoses are at hand. However, suggestions that mutations in type III collagen would account for the majority of aortic aneurysms, including abdominal aneurysms in the elderly, have proven unfounded.[417]

A predisposition to cervical arterial dissection in young people was found to be associated with diffuse lentiginosis in several families, with a suggestion of autosomal recessive inheritance.[418] There also is an association between cervical dissection and intracranial hemorrhage.[419]

Formal genetic analysis of 91 families ascertained through a proband with abdominal aortic aneurysm suggests that an autosomal recessive predisposition exists for late-onset aneurysms.[420] This study provides a rationale for offering ultrasound screening to sibs of patients with abdominal aortic dilatation.

FAMILIAL ARTERIAL TORTUOSITY. This is a rare, possibly autosomal recessive, condition of unknown cause. Diffuse ectasia of all systemic arteries occurs with, paradoxically, peripheral pulmonic stenoses.[421]

FAMILIAL INTRACRANIAL HEMORRHAGE. In addition to adult polycystic kidney disease, three syndromes predispose to subarachnoid or cerebral hemorrhage. *Berry aneurysms* without pleiotropic manifestations in other organs are a rare, but well documented, autosomal dominant trait.[422] A defect in type III collagen was suggested by linkage analysis, but sequence analysis of the gene in 55 unrelated patients found no mutations.[423]

The *cerebral arterial type of familial amyloidosis* (type VI) is an autosomal dominant condition due to a defect in the proteinase inhibitor cystatin C.[424] This disease is rare outside of Iceland and Holland. The walls of cerebral arteries are thickened by a material resembling amyloid, and the vessels become tortuous and fragile. Recurrent cerebral hemorrhage is common in the fifth and sixth decades.[425]

Familial hemangiomas have been reported infrequently to occur as an autosomal dominant condition.[426] The brain and retina are the principal sites of vascular malformation, although in some pedigrees, cutaneous lesions occur. The intracranial hemangioma can be large and present with varied neurological symptoms, including hemorrhage.

FAMILIAL ARTERIAL OCCLUSIVE DISEASES. *Fibromuscular dysplasia* of the renal and other arteries occurs in *von Recklinghausen neurofibromatosis*, and along with pheochromocytoma can be a cause of hypertension.[427,428] Severe deficiency of α_1-antiprotease is another cause of fibromuscular dysplasia.[429] The arterial lesion can occur by itself in families and produce stroke, myocardial infarction, intermittent claudication, and hypertension at young ages ranging down to childhood.[430] Inheritance is most consistent with autosomal dominance.[431]

Familial hypoplasia of the carotid arteries,[432] *familial arteriopathy caused by concentric thickening of systemic and pulmonic arteries*,[433]

and generalized *arterial calcification of infancy*[434] are all rare, possibly mendelian, syndromes of unknown cause.

FAMILIAL HEMIPLEGIC MIGRAINE. The migraine syndrome is commonly familial and occurs in multiple generations. A severe form, associated with recurrent hemiplegia, is inherited as an autosomal dominant trait and maps to the short arm of chromosome 9.[435] However, some families with hemiplegic migraine, and others with simple migraine, are unlinked to this locus.[436,437] In the same region of 19p is a locus causing autosomal dominant cerebral arteriopathy with subcortical infarcts.[438] Whether the two conditions are related through allelism is unclear.

FAMILIAL PULMONARY HYPERTENSION (see also p. 783). Primary pulmonary hypertension is occasionally familial.[439–441] Inheritance is most consistent with an autosomal dominant predisposition with sex influence favoring expression in females. The cause is unknown, but molecular defects favoring recurrent microemboli to the pulmonary circulation afford one area to explore.

Pulmonary hypertension can occur in *neurofibromatosis* due to pulmonary fibrosis.[442]

Disorders Primarily Affecting Veins

VARICOSE VEINS. Although a familial susceptibility to varicosities of the lower extremity clearly exists, and favors women in a ratio of 2:1, mendelian inheritance has not been confirmed. *Marfan syndrome*, various *Ehlers-Danlos syndromes*, and an autosomal recessive condition featuring distichiasis (a double row of eyelashes)[443] predispose to varicose veins.

ATRETIC VEINS. Some patients with the *Klippel-Trenaunay-Weber syndrome* of cutaneous hemangioma and hemihypertrophy have atresia of the deep venous system.[444] The concomitant superficial varicosities should not be stripped, lest the remaining venous drainage of the lower extremity be removed. This is a confusing syndrome that overlaps with several others; mendelian inheritance is uncertain. Renal arterial aneurysm and hemangioma occurred in one patient.[445]

CAVERNOUS ANGIOMAS. Cavernous angiomas represent at least 15 per cent of vascular malformations of the central nervous system, and familial occurrence is increasingly recognized.[446–450] These are not arteriovenous malformations, but primarily a tortuous collection of veins. Seizure is the most common presenting feature, followed by headache, stroke, and progressive neurologic deficit. Magnetic resonance (T_2-weighted) imaging is the procedure of choice because it is sensitive, and arteriography is not likely to detect the venous malformation. In some families, hepatic angiomas are an important feature.[451] At least one locus has been mapped.[452–453]

Disorders Primarily Affecting Lymphatics

Several forms of *hereditary lymphedema* exist, with the best studied inherited as autosomal dominants.[8] An early-onset form bears the eponym *Nonne-Milroy lymphedema* and can cause a protein-losing enteropathy and pleural effusion. *Meige lymphedema* does not appear until about the time of puberty and is most severe in the legs, although one family with late-onset edema had involvement of the arms and face.[454] The occurrence of lymphangiosarcoma in congenital[455] and late-onset lymphedema[456] suggests a predisposition to malignancy.

GENETIC FACTORS PREDISPOSING TO ATHEROSCLEROSIS

(See also Chap. 35)

A variety of genetic factors, in addition to the well-studied errors of lipid metabolism, clearly predispose to atherosclerosis. Few genes outside of those involved in lipid metabolism have such an overwhelming impact as to be identifiable from the family history. However, genes that predispose to hypertension and diabetes mellitus, control arterial diameter, reactivity, and branching angles, affect platelet adhesiveness, thrombosis, and fibrinolysis, and regulate endothelial and smooth muscle function can all be considered candidate genes for study in families predisposed to atherosclerosis.[457–459]

ESSENTIAL HYPERTENSION

(See also Chap. 26)

Blood pressure is a quantifiable trait that shows continuous variation within the population. Although many genes and environmental factors undoubtedly affect a person's blood pressure, familial transmission of some arbitrarily defined disease "hypertension" follows neither mendelian nor multifactorial inheritance.[460] A variety of cybernetic systems operate to maintain the blood pressure within tolerable limits. When this physiological homeostasis goes awry, or its limits are too lax, pathological and clinical consequences occur.[461] For example, sensitivity of the baroreflex was impaired in patients with untreated essential hypertension who had a positive family history of hypertension compared with hypertensives with no family history and to nonhypertensive controls.[462] The complexities of such systems are considerable, and two approaches have been taken in recent years to focus the analysis.[460,463-465] One involves a candidate-gene approach in humans, based on loci known to be involved in physiological pathways, and the second involves naturally occurring and experimentally created strains of animals.

STUDIES IN HUMANS. All of the classic approaches to detecting genetic influences in diseases—twin studies, familial aggregation, adoption—confirm that genes play a role. But less than 5 per cent of patients with hypertension have a defined genetic cause.[466]

Occasional families show striking mendelian segregation of hypertension without being associated with one of the identifiable syndromes listed in Table 49-13. One example, in which early, severe hypertension was inherited as an autosomal dominant trait, is *Liddle's syndrome*.[467,468] Because of hypokalemia, aldosteronism was suspected, but both aldosterone and renin levels were low. Attention then focused on sodium resorption in the distal nephron and its regulation. Mutations were discovered in the beta subunit of the epithelial sodium channel which render the channel insensitive to the usual regulators.

Another example of successful application of the candidate gene approach is investigation of *glucocorticoid-remediable aldosteronism*.[468,469] The phenotype was mapped to chromosome 8q21, a region already known to contain two candidate genes, aldosterone synthase and 11β-hydroxylase. By honing in on these loci, mutations creating a chimeric gene by unequal recombination were found to be the cause.[470] As a result of the fusion, aldosterone synthase comes under regulation of ACTH. The actual frequency of such mutational events is considerably higher than suspected in the population, and the molecular means are now available to assess the epidemiology of what will likely be a common cause of early hypertension.

Angiotensinogen, the gene for which is in the region 1q42-q43, is a logical candidate gene to investigate because of the central role of its product in blood pressure regulation. Several polymorphic variants involving single amino acid substitutions occur; at positions 174 and 235 either methionine (M) or threonine (T) can exist. The special

TABLE 49-15 MENDELIAN DISORDERS ASSOCIATED WITH ABNORMAL BLOOD PRESSURE

DISORDER	MIM NO.*	PATHOGENESIS
Primarily elevated blood pressure		
Adrenal hyperplasia IV	202010	11-β-hydroxylase deficiency → ↑ 11-deoxycorticosterone
Adrenal hyperplasia V	202110	17-α-hydroxylase deficiency → ↑ 11-deoxycorticosterone
Aldosteronism	103900	↑ Aldosterone
Alport syndrome	104200	Renal failure
	301050	
Amyloidosis, familial visceral (amyloidosis VIII)	105200	Nephropathy
Arterial calcification of infancy	208000	Arteriosclerosis
Arterial fibromuscular dysplasia	135580	Renal artery stenosis → ↑ renin
Arteriohepatic dysplasia	118450	Renal dysplasia; renal arterial stenosis
Bartter syndrome	241200	Secondary to hyperaldosteronism
Fabry disease	301500	Renal failure; renal arterial stenosis; arteriolar stenosis → ↑ peripheral resistance
Liddle syndrome	177200	Defective epithelial sodium channel → ↓ t ↓ aldosterone, ↓ renin, ↓ angiotensin
Multiple endocrine neoplasia I	131100	Adrenocortical adenoma → ↑ Cushing syndrome
Multiple endocrine neoplasia II	171400	Pheochromocytoma → ↑ catecholamines
Nail-patella syndrome	161200	Nephropathy
Neurofibromatosis type I	162200	Pheochromocytoma → ↑ catecholamines; and renal arterial fibromuscular dysplasia
Paraganglioma	168000	↑ Catecholamines Pheochromocytoma → ↑ catecholamines
Pheochromocytoma, familial	171300	↑ Catecholamines
Polycystic kidney disease, adult	173900, 173910	↑ Renin; renal failure
Porphyria, acute intermittent	176000	?, but only during acute attacks
Pseudohypoaldosteronism, type I	264350	Aldosterone receptor deficiency
Pseudohypoaldosteronism, type II	145260	Defective renal secretion of potassium
Pseudoxanthoma elasticum	177850, 264800	Arteriosclerosis
Riley-Day syndrome	223900	Dysautonomia
von Hippel–Lindau syndrome	193300	Pheochromocytoma → ↑ catecholamines
Wilms tumor	194070, 194071, 194090	?
Primarily low blood pressure†		
Dopamine β-hydroxylase deficiency	223360	↑ Synthesis of epinephrine
Fabry disease	301500	↓ Peripheral vascular tone
Hyperbradykininism	143850	↑ Bradykinin
Pelizaeus-Merzbacher, late-onset	169500	?
Peripheral motor neuropathy and dysautonomia	252320	?
Pheochromocytoma, familial	171300	↑ Catecholamines (epinephrine)
Shy-Drager syndrome	146500	Primary autonomic insufficiency

* Data from Mendelian Inheritance in Man.[8]

† Does not include hypovolemia, obstruction of blood flow, and cardiogeneic causes of hypotension, each of which subsumes numerous hereditary disorders as primary causes.

effects of these polymorphisms on activity, if any, are unclear, but persons homozygous for the 235T allele have plasma angiotensinogen levels 20 per cent higher than those with the 235M alleles. Some, but not all studies have found an association between the 174M and 235T alleles and hypertension.[471-473] Further suggestion of the relevance of this gene comes from linkage studies in families with multiple relatives with hypertension.

The *angiotensin-converting enzyme* (ACE) gene, at 17q23, contains a common insertion/deletion polymorphism, termed I and D, respectively, that permits both association and linkage studies. The three possible genotypes are DD, ID, and II, and the plasma level of ACE is highest, for unclear reasons, in people who are DD and lowest in those who are II. The DD genotype has been associated with predisposition to coronary artery disease and to myocardial infarction, which may account for a relative decrease of hypertensive patients with the DD genotype at older ages.[474,475]

STUDIES IN ANIMALS. The stroke-prone spontaneously hypertensive (SHRSP) rat is an example of an animal model for a human disease that arose in nature. The phenotype of the rat is clearly polygenic and is thus particularly relevant to much of essential hypertension in humans. Using polymorphic markers spread throughout the rat genome, it has been possible to conduct linkage analyses of hundreds of markers with hypertension when SHRSP animals were crossed with a nonhypertensive strain. Two loci have been identified, and one lies close to where ACE maps.[476] This general approach, called quantitative trait mapping or linkage (QTL), is increasingly being applied to a variety of phenotypes in animals. Determining the actual gene involved in the animal model should then suggest that the homologous locus in the human is a candidate for participation in normal and abnormal regulation of the trait.

A second approach in animals involves transgenic or knockout techniques to create and breed a new, specific genotype. In simplest terms, a given gene can be eliminated, can be mutated in a specific way, can be moved to a different strain (genetic background), or can be overexpressed. For example, eliminating function of the gene that encodes atrial natriuretic peptide in the mouse resulted in moderate elevation of blood pressure when sodium intake was low or somewhat high. Mice heterozygous for the mutation had normal blood pressure on these salt loads but became abnormally hypertensive when fed a high-salt diet.[477,478]

A number of mendelian conditions, most of which are rare, cause major deviations of blood pressure from an appropriate physiological range (Table 49-15). These disorders are likely to be underdiagnosed.

Acknowledgment

Preparation for this chapter was supported by grant HL35877 from the National Institutes of Health.

REFERENCES

GENETIC FACTORS IN DISEASE

1. Childs, B.: A logic of disease. *In* Scriver, C. R., Beaudet, A. L., Sly, W. A., and Valle, D. (eds.): The Metabolic and Molecular Bases of Inherited Disease. New York, McGraw-Hill, 1995, p. 229.
2. Murphy, E. A., and Pyeritz, R. E.: Pathogenetics. *In* Rimoin, D. L., Connor, J. M., and Pyeritz, R. E. (eds.): Principles and Practice of Medical Genetics. 3rd ed. New York, Churchill Livingstone, 1996.
3. Gardner, R. J., and Sutherland, G. R.: Chromosome Abnormalities and Genetic Counseling. New York, Oxford University Press, 1989.
4. Borgaonkar, D.: Chromosomal Variation in Man. 7th ed. New York, John Wiley & Sons, 1994.
5. Ledbetter, D. H., and Ballabio, A.: Molecular cytogenetics of continuous gene syndromes: Mechanisms and consequences of gene dosage imbalance. *In* Scriver, C. R., Beaudet, A. L., Sly, W. A., and Valle, D. (eds.): The Metabolic and Molecular Bases of Inherited Disease. New York, McGraw-Hill, 1995, p. 811.
6. Chien, K. R: Molecular advances in cardiovascular biology. Science 260:916, 1993.
7. Dietz, H. C., and Pyeritz, R. E.: Molecular genetic approaches to investigating cardiovascular disease. Ann. Rev. Physiol. 56:763, 1994.
8. McKusick, V. A.: Mendelian Inheritance in Man. 11th ed. Baltimore, Johns Hopkins University Press, 1994.
9. McKusick, V. A.: Online Mendelian Inheritance in Man [OMIM™]; contact OMIM User Support, Welch Medical Library, 1830 East Monument Street, Third Floor, Baltimore, MD 21205, Tel: 301-955-7058.
10. Goldstein, J. L., Hobbs, H. H., and Brown, M. S.: Familial hypercholesterolemia. *In* Scriver, C. R., Beaudet, A. L., Sly, W. A., and Valle, D. (eds.): The Metabolic and Molecular Bases of Inherited Disease. New York, McGraw-Hill, 1995, p. 1981.
11. Beaudet, A. L., Scriver, C. R., Sly, W. S., et al.: Genetics, biochemistry and molecular basis of variant human phenotypes. *In* Scriver, C. R., Beaudet, A. L., Sly, W. A., and Valle, D. (eds.): The Metabolic and Molecular Bases of Inherited Disease. New York, McGraw-Hill, 1995, p. 53.
12. Desnick, R. J., Ioannou, Y. A., and Eng, C. M.: α-Galactosidase a deficiency: Fabry disease. *In* Scriver, C. R., Beaudet, A. L., Sly, W. A., and Valle, D. (eds.): The Metabolic and Molecular Bases of Inherited Disease. New York, McGraw-Hill, 1995, p. 2741.
13. DiMauro, S., and Wallace, D. C.: Mitochondrial DNA in Human Pathology. New York, Raven Press, 1993.
14. Wallace, D. C.: Mitochondrial DNA sequence variation in human evolution and disease. Proc. Natl. Acad. Sci. U.S.A. 91:8739, 1994.
15. Costa, T., Scriver, C. R., and Childs, B.: The effect of mendelian disease on human health: A measurement. Am. J. Med. Genet. 21:231, 1985.
16. Pyeritz, R. E.: Pleiotropy revisited: Molecular explanations of a classic concept. Am. J. Med. Genet. 34:124, 1989.
17. Pyeritz, R. E.: Homocystinuria. *In* Beighton, P. (ed.): McKusick's Heritable Disorders of Connective Tissue. 5th ed. St. Louis, C. V. Mosby, 1993, p. 137.
18. Byers, P. H.: Disorders of collagen biosynthesis and structure. *In* Scriver, C. R., Beaudet, A. L., Sly, W. A., and Valle, D. (eds.): The Metabolic and Molecular Bases of Inherited Disease. New York, McGraw-Hill, 1995, p. 4029.
19. Diano, R., Bouchard, C., Dumesnil, J., et al.: Parent-child resemblance in left ventricular echocardiographic measurements. Can. J. Appl. Sport. Sci. 5:4, 1980.
20. Adams, T. D., Yanowitz, F. G., Fisher, A. G., et al.: Heritability of cardiac size: An echocardiographic and electrocardiographic study of monozygotic and dizygotic twins. Circulation 71:39, 1985.
21. Herrington, D. M., and Pearson, T. A.: Clinical and angiographic similarities in twins with coronary artery disease. Am. J. Cardiol. 59:366, 1987.
22. Vlodaver, Z., Kahn, H. A., and Neufeld, H. N.: The coronary arteries in early life in three different ethnic groups. Circulation 39:541, 1969.
23. Moller, P., and Heiberg, A.: Atrioventricular conduction time—a heritable trait? II. Family studies. Clin. Genet. 18:454, 1980.
24. Moller, P., Heiberg, A., and Berg, K.: The atrioventricular conduction time—a heritable trait? III. Twin studies. Clin. Genet. 21:181, 1982.
25. Hawlik, R. J., Garrison, R. J., Fabsitz, R., et al.: Variability of heart rate, P-R, QRS and QT durations in twins. J. Electrocardiol. 13:45, 1980.
26. Dinerman, J. L., and Mehta, J. L.: Endothelial, platelet and leukocyte interactions in ischemic heart disease: Insights into potential mechanisms and their clinical relevance. J. Am. Coll. Cardiol. 16:207, 1990.
27. Yang, Z., Richard, V., von Segesser, L., et al.: Threshold concentrations of endothelin-1 potentiate contractions to norepinephrine and serotonin in human arteries: A new mechanism of vasospasm? Circulation 82:188, 1990.

CARDIOVASCULAR DISORDERS ASSOCIATED WITH CHROMOSOME ABERRATIONS

28. Mitelman, F.: Catalog of Chromosome Aberrations in Cancer. 5th ed. New York, John Wiley & Sons, 1994.
29. Ferencz, C., Neill, C. A., Boughman, J. A., et al.: Congenital cardiovascular malformations associated with chromosome abnormalities: An epidemiologic study. J. Pediatr. 114:79, 1989.
30. Berg, K. A., Clark, E. B., Astemborski, J. A., et al.: Prenatal detection of cardiovascular malformations by echocardiography: An indication for cytogenetic evaluation. Am. J. Obstet. Gynecol. 159:477, 1988.
31. Schinzel, A. A.: Cardiovascular defects associated with chromosomal aberrations and malformation syndromes. Prog. Med. Genet. 5:301, 1983.
32. De Biase, L., Di Ciommo, V., Ballerini, L., et al.: Prevalence of left-sided obstructive lesions in patients with atrioventricular canal without Down syndrome. J. Thorac. Cardiovasc. Surg. 91:467, 1986.
33. Epstein, C. J.: Down syndrome (trisomy 21). *In* Scriver, C. R., Beaudet, A. L., Sly, W. A., and Valle, D. (eds.): The Metabolic and Molecular Bases of Inherited Disease. New York, McGraw-Hill, 1995, p. 749.
34. Kurnit, D. M., Aldridge, J. F., Matsuoka, R., et al.: Increased adhesiveness of trisomy 21 cells and atrioventricular canal malformations in Down syndrome: A stochastic model. Am. J. Med. Genet. 20:385, 1985.
35. Clark, E. B.: Mechanisms in the pathogenesis of congenital cardiac malformations. *In* Pierpont, M. E. M., and Moller, J. H. (eds.): Genetics of Cardiovascular Disease. Boston, Martinus Nihjoff Publishing, 1986, p. 3.
36. Clapp, S., Perry, B. L., Farooki, Z. Q., et al.: Down's syndrome, com-

plete atrioventricular canal, and pulmonary vascular obstructive disease. J. Thorac. Cardiovasc. Surg. *100*:115, 1990.

37. Goldhaber, S. Z., Rubin, I. L., Brown, W., et al.: Valvular heart disease (aortic regurgitation and mitral valve prolapse) among institutionalized adults with Down's syndrome. Am. J. Cardiol. *57*:278, 1986.

38. Schneider, D. S., Zahka, K. G., Clark, E. B., et al.: Patterns of cardiac care in infants with Down syndrome. Am. J. Dis. Child. *143*:363, 1989.

39. Greenwood, R. D., and Nadas, A. S.: The clinical course of cardiac disease in Down's syndrome. Pediatrics *58*:893, 1976.

40. Van Dyck, D. C., and Allen, M.: Clinical management considerations in long-term survivors with trisomy 18. Pediatrics *58*:893, 1976.

41. Musewe, N. N., Alexander, D. J., Teshima, I., et al.: Echocardiographic evaluation of the spectrum of cardiac anomalies associated with trisomy 13 and trisomy 18. J. Am. Coll. Cardiol. *15*:673, 1990.

42. Van Praagh, S., Truman, T., Firpo, A., et al.: Cardiac malformations in trisomy-18: A study of 41 postmortem cases. J. Am. Coll. Cardiol. *13*:1586, 1989.

43. Lacro, R. V., Lyons Jones, K., and Benirschke, K.: Coarctation of the aorta in Turner syndrome: A pathologic study of fetuses with nuchal cystic hygromas, hydrops fetalis and female genitalia. Pediatrics *81*:445, 1988.

44. Allen, D. B., Hendricks, S. A., and Levy, J. M.: Aortic dilation in Turner syndrome. J. Pediatr. *109*:302, 1986.

45. Lin, A. E., and Garver, K. L.: Genetic counseling for congenital heart defects. J. Pediatr. *113*:1105, 1988.

46. Natowicz, M., and Kelley, R. I.: Association of Turner syndrome with hypoplastic left-heart syndrome. Am. J. Dis. Child. *141*:218, 1987.

47. Moore, J. W., Kirby, W. C., Rogers, W. M., et al.: Partial anomalous pulmonary venous drainage associated with 45,X Turner's syndrome. Pediatrics *86*:273, 1990.

48. Sapienza, C., and Hall, J. G.: Genetic imprinting in human disease. *In* Scriver, C. R., Beaudet, A. L., Sly, W. A., and Valle, D. (eds.): The Metabolic and Molecular Bases of Inherited Disease. New York, McGraw-Hill, 1995, p. 437.

CONGENITAL HEART DISEASE

50. Fixler, D. E., Pastor, P., Chamberlin, M., et al.: Trends in congenital heart disease in Dallas County births: 1971–1984. Circulation *81*:137, 1990.

51. Ferencz, C., Rubin, J. D., and Loffredo, C. A. (eds.): Epidemiology of Congenital Heart Disease: The Baltimore-Washington Infant Study 1981–1989. Mt. Kisco, N.Y., Futura, 1993.

52. Helmcke, F., de Souza, A., Nanda, N. C., et al.: Two-dimensional and color Doppler assessment of ventricular septal defect of congenital origin. Am. J. Cardiol. *63*:1112, 1989.

53. Hanna, E. J., Nevin, N. C., and Nelson, J.: Genetic study of congenital heart defects in Northern Ireland (1974–1978). J. Med. Genet. *31*:858, 1994.

54. Simpson, I. A., Sahn, D. J., Valdes-Cruz, L. M., et al.: Color Doppler flow mapping in patients with coarctation of the aorta: New observations and improved evaluation with color flow diameter and proximal acceleration as predictors of severity. Circulation *77*:736, 1988.

55. Brenner, J. I., Berg, K. A., Schneider, D. S., et al.: Cardiac malformations in relatives of infants with hypoplastic left-heart syndrome. Am. J. Dis. Child. *143*:1492, 1989.

56. Pyeritz, R. E., and Murphy, E. A.: The genetics of congenital heart disease: Perspectives and prospects. J. Am. Coll. Cardiol. *13*:1458, 1989.

57. Ursell, P. C., Byrne, J. M., and Strombino, B. A.: Significance of cardiac defects in the developing fetus: A study of spontaneous abortuses. Circulation *72*:1232, 1985.

58. Sadiq, M., Stümper, O., Wright, J. G. C., et al.: Influence of ethnic origin on the pattern of congenital heart defects in the first year of life. Br. Heart J. *73*:173, 1995.

59. Whittemore, R., Hobbins, J. C., and Engle, M. A.: Pregnancy and its outcome in women with and without surgical treatment of congenital heart disease. *In* Engle, M. A., and Perloff, J. K. (eds.): Congenital Heart Disease After Surgery. New York, Yorke Medical Books, 1983, p. 362.

60. Rose, V. R., Gold, J. M., Lindsay, G., et al.: A possible increase in the incidence of congenital heart defects among the offspring of affected parents. J. Am. Coll. Cardiol. *6*:376, 1985.

61. Nora, J. J., Berg, K., and Nora, A. H.: Cardiovascular disease—genetics, epidemiology and prevention. Am. J. Hum. Genet. *50*:450, 1992.

62. Boughman, J. A.: Familial risks of congenital heart defects (letter). Am. J. Med. Genet. *29*:233, 1988.

63. Murphy, J. G., Gersh, B. J., McGoon, M. G., et al.: Long-term outcome after surgical repair of isolated atrial septal defect: Follow-up at 27 to 32 years. N. Engl. J. Med. *323*:1645, 1990.

64. Gold, R. J. M., Rose, V., and Yau, Y.: Severity and recurrence risk of congenital heart defects exemplified by atrial septal defect secundum. Clin. Genet. *32*:148, 1987.

65. Sanchez-Cascos, A.: The recurrence risk in congenital heart disease. Eur. J. Cardiol. *7*:197, 1978.

66. Corone, P., Bonaiti, C., Feingold, J., et al.: Familial congenital heart disease: How are the various types related? Am. J. Cardiol. *51*:942, 1983.

67. Boughman, J. A., Berg, K. A., Astemborski, J. A., et al.: Familial risks of congenital heart defect assessed in a population-based epidemiologic study. Am. J. Med. Genet. *26*:839, 1987.

68. Ferencz, C., Boughman, J. A., Neill, C. A., et al.: Congenital cardiovas-

cular malformations: Questions on inheritance. J. Am. Coll. Cardiol. *14*:756, 1989.

69. Maestri, N. E., Beaty, T. H., Liang, K.-Y., et al.: Assessing familial aggregation of congenital cardiovascular malformations in case-control studies: Genet. Epidemiol. *5*:343, 1988.

70. Pierpont, M. E. M., Gobel, J. W., Moller, J. H., et al.: Cardiac malformations in relatives of children with truncus arteriosus or interruption of the aortic arch. Am. J. Cardiol. *61*:423, 1988.

71. Natowicz, M., Chatten, J., Clancy, R., et al.: Genetic disorders and major extracardiac anomalies associated with the hypoplastic left heart syndrome. Pediatrics *82*:698, 1988.

72. Desmaze, C., Prieur, M., Amblard, F., et al.: Physical mapping by FISH of the DiGeorge critical region (DGCR): Involvement of the region in familial cases. Am. J. Hum. Genet. *53*:1239, 1993.

73. Wilson, D. I., Cross, I. E., and Goodship, J. A.: DiGeorge syndrome with isolated aortic coarctation and isolated ventricular septal defect in three sibs with a 22q11 deletion of maternal origin. Br. Heart J. *66*:308, 1991.

74. Matsuoka, R., Takao, A., Kimura, M., et al.: Confirmation that the conotruncal anomaly face syndrome is associated with a deletion within 22q11.2 Am. J. Med. Genet. *53*:285, 1994.

75. Wilson, D. I., Goodship, J. A., Burn, J., et al.: Deletions within chromosome 22q11 in familial congenital heart disease. Lancet *340*:573, 1992.

76. Patterson, D. F., Pexieder, T., and Schnarr, W. R., et al.: A single major-gene defect underlying cardiac conotruncal malformations interferes with myocardial growth during embryonic development: Studies in the CTD line of Keeshond dogs. Am. J. Hum. Genet. *52*:388, 1993.

77. Beekman, R. H., and Robinow, M.: Coarctation of the aorta inherited as an autosomal dominant trait. Am. J. Cardiol. *56*:818, 1985.

78. Lindsay, J., Jr.: Coarctation of the aorta, bicuspid aortic valve and abnormal ascending aortic wall. Am. J. Cardiol. *61*:182, 1988.

79. Wright, T. C., Orkin, R. W., Destrempes, M., et al.: Increased adhesiveness of Down syndrome fetal fibroblasts in vitro. Proc. Natl. Acad. Sci. U.S.A. *81*:2426, 1984.

80. Weigel, W. J., Driscoll, D. J., and Michels, V. V.: Occurrence of congenital heart defects in siblings of patients with univentricular heart and tricuspid atresia. Am. J. Cardiol. *64*:768, 1989.

81. Moreno, A., and Murphy, E. A.: Inheritance of Kartagener syndrome. Am. J. Med. Genet. *8*:305, 1981.

82. Afzelius, B. A., and Mossberg, B.: Immotile-cilia syndrome (primary ciliary dyskinesia), including Kartagener syndrome. *In* Scriver, C. R., Beaudet, A. L., Sly, W. A., and Valle, D. (eds.): The Metabolic and Molecular Bases of Inherited Disease. New York, McGraw-Hill, 1995, p. 3943.

83. Alonso, S., Pierpont, M. E., and Radtke, W.: Geterotaxia syndrome and autosomal dominant inheritance. Am. J. Med. Genet. *56*:12, 1995.

84. Casey, B., Devoto, M., Jones, K. L., et al.: Mapping a gene for familial situs abnormalities to human chromosome Xq24-q27.1 Nature Genet. *5*:403, 1993.

85. Anderson, C., Devine, W. A., Anderson, R. H., et al.: Abnormalities of the spleen in relation to congenital malformation of the heart: A survey of necropsy findings in children. Br. Heart J. *63*:122, 1990.

86. Phoon, C. K., and Neill, C. A.: Asplenia syndrome: Insight into embryology through an analysis of cardiac and extracardiac anomalies. Am. J. Cardiol. *73*:581, 1994.

87. Brueckner, M., D'Estachio, P., and Horwich, A. L.: Linkage mapping of a mouse gene, *iv*, that controls left-right asymmetry of the heart and viscera. Proc. Natl. Acad. Sci. U.S.A. *86*:5035, 1989.

88. Yokoyama, T., Copeland, N. G., Jenkins, N. A., et al.: Reversal of left-right asymmetry: A situs inversus mutation. Science *260*:679, 1993.

89. Bleyl, S., Nelson, L., Otterud, B., et al.: A gene for total anomalous pulmonary venous return (TAPVR-1) maps to the centromere of chromosome 4. Am. J. Hum. Genet. *55*(Abs.):A181, 1994.

90. Cyran, S. E., Martinez, R., Daniels, S., et al.: Spectrum of congenital heart disease in CHARGE association. J. Pediatr. *110*:576, 1987.

91. Oley, C. A., Baraitser, M., and Grant, D. B.: A reappraisal of the CHARGE association. J. Med. Genet. *25*:147, 1988.

92. Weaver, D. D., Mapstone, C. L., and Yu, P.: The VATER association: Analysis of 46 patients. Am. J. Dis. Child. *140*:225, 1986.

93. Woods, C. G., and Sheffield, L. J.: Further family with autosomal dominant patent ductus arteriosus. J. Med. Genet. *31*:659, 1994.

94. Davidson, H. R.: A large family with patent ductus arteriosus and unusual face. J. Med. Genet. *30*:503, 1992.

95. Pierpont, M. E., and Sletten, L. J.: Char syndrome: A cause of familial patent ductus arteriosus. Am. J. Hum. Genet. *55*(Abs.):A89, 1994.

96. Lynch, H. T., Bachenberg, K., Harris, R. E., et al.: Hereditary atrial septal defect: Update of a large kindred. Am. J. Dis. Child. *132*:600, 1978.

97. Kahler, R. L., Braunwald, E., Plauth, W. H., Jr., et al.: Familial congenital heart disease. Am. J. Med. *40*:384, 1966.

98. Pease, W. E., Nordenberg, A., and Ladda, R. L.: Genetic counseling in familial atrial septal defect with prolonged atrioventricular conduction. Circulation *53*:759, 1976.

99. Gall, J. C., Stern, A. M., Cohen, M. M., et al.: Holt-Oram syndrome: Clinical and genetic study of a large family. Am. J. Hum. Genet. *18*:187, 1966.

100. Basson, C. T., Cowley, G. S., Solomon, S. D., et al.: The clinical and genetic spectrum of the Holt-Oram syndrome (heart-hand syndrome). N. Engl. J. Med. *330*:885, 1994.

101. Bonnet, D., Pelet, A., Legeai-Mallet, L., et al.: A gene for Holt-Oram syndrome maps to the distal long arm of chromosome 12. Nature Genet. *6*:405, 1994.

102. Terrett, J. A., Newbury-Ecob, R., Cross, G. S., et al.: Holt-Oram syndrome is a genetically heterogeneous disease with one locus mapping to human chromosome 12q. Nature Genet. 6:401, 1994.
103. McKusick, V. A., Egeland, J. A., Eldridge, R., et al.: Dwarfism in the Amish: I. The Ellis-van Creveld syndrome. Bull. Johns Hopkins Hosp. 115:306, 1964.
104. Cousineau, A. J., Lauer, R. M., Pierpont, M. E., et al.: Linkage analysis of autosomal dominant atrioventricular canal defects: Exclusion of chromosome 21. Hum. Genet. 93:103, 1994.
105. Gennarelli, M., Novelli, G., Digilio, M. C., et al.: Exclusion of linkage with chromosome 21 in families with recurrence of non-Down's atrioventricular canal. Hum. Genet. 94:708, 1994.
106. Sherman, J., Angulo, M., Boxer, R. A., et al.: Possible mitochondrial inheritance of congenital cardiac septal defect (letter). N. Engl. J. Med. 313:186, 1985.
107. Preus, M.: The Williams syndrome: Objective definition and diagnosis. Clin. Genet. 25:422, 1984.
108. Maisuls, H., Alday, L. E., and Thuer, O.: Cardiovascular findings in the Williams-Beuren syndrome. Am. Heart J. 114:897, 1987.
109. Hallidie-Smith, K. A., and Karas, S.: Cardiac anomalies in Williams-Beuren syndrome. Arch. Dis. Child. 63:809, 1988.
110. Morris, C. A., Demsey, S. A., Leonard, C. O., et al.: Natural history of Williams syndrome: Physical characteristics. J. Pediatr. 113:318, 1988.
111. Wessel, A., Pankau, R., Kececioglu, D., et al.: Three decades of follow-up of aortic and pulmonary vascular lesions in the Williams-Beuren syndrome. Am. J. Med. Genet. 52:297, 1994.
112. Ardinger, R. H., Jr., Goertz, K. K., and Mattioli, L. F.: Cerebrovascular stenoses with cerebral infarction in a child with Williams syndrome. Am. J. Med. Genet. 51:200, 1994.
113. van Son, J. A. M., Edwards, W. D., and Danielson, G. K.: Pathology of coronary arteries, myocardium, and great arteries in supravalvular aortic stenosis: Report of five cases with implications for surgical treatment. J. Thorac. Cardiovasc. Surg. 108:21, 1994.
114. Ewart, A. K., Morris, C. A., Atkinson, D., et al.: Hemizygosity at the elastin locus in a developmental disorder, Williams syndrome. Nature Genet. 5:11, 1993.
115. Chiarella, F., Bricarelli, F. D., and Lupi, G.: Familial supravalvular aortic stenosis: A genetic study. J. Med. Genet. 26:86, 1989.
116. Ensing, G. J., Schmidt, M. A., Hagler, D. J., et al.: Spectrum of findings in a family with nonsyndromic autosomal dominant supravalvular aortic stenosis: A Doppler echocardiographic study. J. Am. Coll. Cardiol. 13:413, 1989.
117. Schmidt, M. A., Ensing, G. J., Michels, V. V., et al.: Autosomal dominant supravalvular aortic stenosis: Large three-generation family. Am. J. Med. Genet. 32:384, 1989.
118. Curran, M. W., Atkinson, D. L., Ewart, A. K., et al.: The elastin gene is disrupted by a translocation associated with supravalvular aortic stenosis. Cell 73:159, 1993.
119. Morris, C. A., Loker, J., Ensing, G., et al.: Supravalvular aortic stenosis cosegregates with a familial 6;7 translocation which disrupts the elastin gene. Am. J. Med. Genet. 46:737, 1993.
120. Ewart, A. K., Jin, W., Atkinson, D., et al.: Supravalvular aortic stenosis associated with a deletion disrupting the elastin gene. J. Clin. Invest. 93:1071, 1994.
121. Devereux, R. B., Kramer-Fox, R., Shear, M. K., et al.: Diagnosis and classification of severity of mitral valve prolapse: Methodologic, biologic, and prognostic considerations. Am. Heart J. 113:1265, 1987.
122. Wooley, C. F., and Boudoulas, H.: Mitral valve prolapse: A classification. In Boudoulas, H., and Wooley, C. F. (eds.): Mitral Valve Prolapse and the Mitral Valve Prolapse Syndrome. Mt. Kisco, N.Y., Futura, 1988, p. 3.
123. Devereux, R. B., and Kramer-Fox, R.: Inheritance and phenotypic features of mitral valve prolapse. In Boudoulas, H., and Wooley, C. F. (eds.): Mitral Valve Prolapse and the Mitral Valve Prolapse Syndrome. Mt. Kisco, N.Y., Futura, 1988, p. 109.
124. Strahan, N. V., Murphy, E. A., Fortuin, N. J., et al.: Inheritance of the mitral valve prolapse syndrome. Discussion of a three-dimensional penetrance model. Am. J. Med. 74:967, 1983.
125. Pini, R., Greppi, B., Kramer-Fox, R., et al.: Mitral valve dimensions and motion and familial transmission of mitral valve prolapse with and without mitral leaflet billowing. J. Am. Coll. Cardiol. 12:1423, 1988.
126. Henney, A. M., Schwartz, R. C., Child, A. H., et al.: Genetic evidence that mutations in the COL1A2, COL3A1 or COL5A2 collagen genes are not responsible for mitral valve prolapse. Br. Heart J. 61:292, 1989.
127. Hickey, A. J., Narunsky, L., and Wilcken, D. E. L.: Bodily habitus and mitral valve prolapse. Aust. N. Z. J. Med. 15:326, 1985.
128. Devereux, R. B., Brown, W. T., Lutas, E. M., et al.: Association of mitral valve prolapse with low body weight and low blood pressure. Lancet 2:792, 1982.
129. Beighton, P., de Paepe, A., Danks, D., et al.: International nosology of heritable disorders of connective tissue, Berlin, 1986. Am. J. Med. Genet. 29:581, 1988.
130. Roman, M. J., Devereux, R. B., Kramer-Fox, R., et al.: Comparison of cardiovascular and skeletal features of primary mitral valve prolapse and the Marfan syndrome. Am. J. Cardiol. 3:317, 1989.
131. Glesby, M. J., and Pyeritz, R. E.: Association of mitral valve prolapse and systemic abnormalities of connective tissue: A phenotypic continuum. JAMA 262:523, 1989.
132. Shamberger, R. C., Welch, K. J., and Sanders, S. P.: Mitral valve prolapse associated with pectus excavatum. J. Pediatr. 111:404, 1987.

133. Rogan, K., Sears-Rogan, P., Vermani, R., et al.: Familial myxomatous valvular disease. Am. J. Cardiol. 63:1149, 1989.
134. Mendez, H. M. M., and Opitz, J. M.: Noonan syndrome: A review. Am. J. Med. Genet. 21:493, 1985.
135. Allanson, J. E., Hall, J. G., Hughes, H. E., et al.: Noonan syndrome: The changing phenotype. Am. J. Med. Genet. 21:507, 1985.
136. Noonan, J. A., and Ehmke, D. A.: Associated noncardiac malformations in children with congenital heart disease. J. Pediatr. 63:468, 1963.
137. Phornphutkul, C., Rosenthal, A., and Nadas, A. S.: Cardiomyopathy in Noonan's syndrome. Br. Heart J. 35:99, 1973.
138. Battiste, C. E., Feldt, R. H., and Lie, J. T.: Congestive cardiomyopathy in Noonan's syndrome. Mayo Clin. Proc. 52:661, 1977.
139. Miller, M., and Motulsky, A. G.: Noonan syndrome in an adult family presenting with chronic lymphedema. Am. J. Med. 65:379, 1978.
140. Quattrin, T., McPherson, E., and Putnam, T.: Vertical transmission of the neurofibromatosis/Noonan syndrome. Am. J. Med. Genet. 26:645, 1987.
141. van der Burgt, I., Berends, E., Lommen, E., et al.: Clinical and molecular studies in a large Dutch family with Noonan syndrome. Am. J. Med. Genet. 53:187, 1994.
142. Kitchens, C. S., and Alexander, J. A.: Partial deficiency of coagulation factor XI as a newly recognized feature of Noonan syndrome. J. Pediatr. 102:224, 1983.
143. Khoury, M. J., Becerra, J. E., Cordero, J. F., et al.: Clinical-epidemiologic assessment of patterns of birth defects associated with human teratogens: Application to diabetic embryopathy. Pediatrics 83:658, 1989.
144. Beckman, D. A., and Brent, R. L.: Mechanisms of teratogenesis. Annu. Rev. Pharmacol. Toxicol. 24:483, 1984.
145. Jones, K. L.: Fetal alcohol syndrome. Pediatr. Rev. 8:122, 1986.
146. Finnell, R. H., and Chernoff, G. F.: Genetic background. The elusive component in the fetal hydantoin syndrome. Am. J. Med. Genet. 19:459, 1984.
147. Strickler, S. M., Dansky, L. V., Miller, M. A., et al.: Genetic predisposition to phenytoin-induced birth defects. Lancet 2:746, 1985.
148. Lammer, E. J.: Retinoic acid embryopathy. N. Engl. J. Med. 313:837, 1985.
149. Hall, J. G., Pauli, R. M., and Wilson, K. M.: Maternal and fetal sequelae of anticoagulation during pregnancy. Am. J. Med. 68:122, 1980.
150. Scriver, C. R., Kaufman, S., Eisensmith, R. C., et al.: The hyperphenylalaninemias. In Scriver, C. R., Beaudet, A. L., Sly, W. A., and Valle, D. (eds.): The Metabolic and Molecular Bases of Inherited Disease. New York, McGraw-Hill, 1995, p. 1015.
151. Lenke, R. R., and Levy, H. L.: Maternal phenylketonuria and hyperphenylalaninemia. N. Engl. J. Med. 303:1202, 1980.

CARDIOMYOPATHIES

152. Epstein, N. D., Lin, H. J., and Fananapazir, L.: Genetic evidence of dissociation (generational skips) of electrical from morphologic forms of hypertrophic cardiomyopathy. Am. J. Cardiol. 66:627, 1990.
153. Jarcho, J. A., McKenna, W., Pare, J. A. P., et al.: Mapping a gene for familial hypertrophic cardiomyopathy to chromosome 14q1. N. Engl. J. Med. 321:1372, 1989.
154. Watkins, H., Seidman, J. G., Seidman, C. E.: Familial hypertrophic cardiomyopathy: a genetic model of cardiac hypertrophy. Hum. Molec. Genet. 4:1721, 1995.
155. Watkins, H., Thierfelder, L., Hwang, D. S., et al.: Sporadic hypertrophic cardiomyopathy due to de novo myosin mutations. J. Clin. Invest. 90:1666, 1992.
156. Watkins, H., Rosenzweig, A., Hwang, D.-S., et al.: Characteristics and prognostic implications of myosin missense mutations in familial hypertrophic cardiomyopathy. N. Engl. J. Med. 326:1108, 1992.
157. Epstein, N. D., Cohn, G. M., Cyran, F., et al.: Differences in clinical expression of hypertrophic cardiomyopathy associated with two distinct mutations in the β-myosin heavy chain gene. Circulation 86:345, 1992.
158. Cuda, G., Fannapazir, L., Zhu, W. S., et al.: Skeletal muscle expression and abnormal function of β-myosin in hypertrophic cardiomyopathy. J. Clin. Invest. 91:2861, 1993.
159. Lechin, M., Quinones, M. A., Omran, A., et al.: Angiotensin I converting enzyme genotypes and left ventricular hypertrophy in patients with hypertrophic cardiomyopathy. Circulation 92:1808, 1995.
160. Watkins, H., MacRae, C., Thierfelder, L., et al.: A disease locus for familial hypertrophic cardiomyopathy maps to chromosome 6q3. Nature Genet. 3:333, 1993.
161. Thierfelder, L., Watkins, H., MacRae, C., et al.: α-Tropomyosin and cardiac troponin T mutations cause familial hypertrophic cardiomyopathy: A disease of the sarcomere. Cell 77:701, 1994.
161a. Watkins, H., Conner, D., Yhierfelder, L., et al.: Mutations in the cardiac myosin binding protein-C gene on chromosome 11 cause familial hypertrophic cardiomyopathy. Nature Genet. 11:434, 1995.
161b. Bonne, G., Carrier, L., Bercovici, J., et al.: Cardiac myosin binding protein-C gene splice acceptor site mutation is associated with familial hypertrophic cardiomyopathy. Nature Genet. 11:438, 1995.
162. Thierfelder, L., MacRae, C., Watkins, H., et al.: A familial hypertrophic cardiomyopathy locus maps to chromosome 15q2. Proc. Natl. Acad. Sci. U.S.A. 90:6270, 1993.
163. MacRae, C. A., Ghaisas, N., Kass, S., et al.: Familial hypertrophic cardiomyopathy with Wolff-Parkinson-White syndrome maps to a locus on chromosome 7q3. J. Clin. Invest. 96:1216, 1995.
164. Codd, M. B., Sugrue, D. D., Gersh, B. J., et al.: Epidemiology of idio-

pathic dilated and hypertrophic cardiomyopathy: A population-based study in Olmsted County, Minnesota, 1975–1984. Circulation 80:564, 1989.

165. Kelly, D. P., and Strauss, A. W.: Inherited cardiomyopathies. N. Engl. J. Med. 330:913, 1994.

166. Dec, G. W., and Fuster, V.: Idiopathic dilated cardiomyopathy. N. Engl. J. Med. 331:1564, 1994.

167. Manolio, T. A., Baughman, K. L., Rodeheffer, R., et al.: Prevalence and etiology of idiopathic dilated cardiomyopathy. Am. J. Cardiol. 69:1458, 1992.

168. Michels, V. V., Moll, P. P., Miller, F. A., et al.: The frequency of familial dilated cardiomyopathy in a series of patients with idiopathic dilated cardiomyopathy. N. Engl. J. Med. 326:77, 1992.

169. Fragola, P. V., Autore, C., Picelli, A., et al.: Familial idiopathic dilated cardiomyopathy. Am. Heart J. 115:912, 1988.

170. Valantine, H. A., Hunt, S. A., Fowler, M. B., et al.: Frequency of familial nature of dilated cardiomyopathy and usefulness of cardiac transplantation in this subset. Am. J. Cardiol. 63:959, 1989.

171. Graber, H. L., Unverferth, D. V., Baker, P. B., et al.: Evolution of a hereditary cardiac conduction and muscle disorder: A study involving a family with six generations affected. Circulation 74:21, 1986.

172. Gardner, R. J. M., Hanson, J. W., Ionasescu, V. V., et al.: Dominantly inherited dilated cardiomyopathy. Am. J. Med. Genet. 27:61, 1987.

173. Maclennan, B. A., Tsoi, E. Y., Maguire, C., et al.: Familial idiopathic congestive cardiomyopathy in three generations: A family study with eight affected members. Q. J. Med. 63:335, 1987.

174. Schmidt, M. A., Michels, V. V., Edwards, W. D., et al.: Familial dilated cardiomyopathy. Am. J. Med. Genet. 31:135, 1988.

175. Goldblatt, J., Melmed, J., and Rose, A. G.: Autosomal recessive inheritance of idiopathic dilated cardiomyopathy in a Madeira Portuguese kindred. Clin. Genet. 31:249, 1987.

176. Caforio, A. L. P., Rossi, B., and Risaliti, R.: Type 1 fiber abnormalities in skeletal muscle of patients with hypertrophic and dilated cardiomyopathy: Evidence of subclinical myogenic myopathy. J. Am. Coll. Cardiol. 14:1464, 1989.

177. Michels, V. M., Pastores, G. M., Moll, P. P., et al.: Dystrophin analysis in idiopathic dilated cardiomyopathy. J. Med. Genet. 30:955, 1993.

178. Urie, P. M., and Billingham, M. E.: Ultrastructural features of familial cardiomyopathy. Am. J. Cardiol. 62:325, 1988.

179. Voss, E. G., Reddy, C. V. R., Detrano, R., et al.: Familial dilated cardiomyopathy. Am. J. Cardiol. 54:456, 1984.

180. Kass, S., McRae, C., Graber, H. L., et al.: A gene defect that causes conduction system disease and dilated cardiomyopathy maps to chromosome 1p1-q1. Nature Genet. 7:546, 1994.

181. Barth, P. G., Scholte, J. A., Berden, J. A., et al.: An X-linked mitochondrial disease affecting cardiac muscle, skeletal muscle and neutrophil leukocytes. J. Neurol. Sci. 62:327, 1983.

182. Christodoulou, J., McInnes, R. R., Jay, V., et al.: Barth syndrome: Clinical observations and genetic linkage studies. Am. J. Med. Genet. 50:255, 1994.

183. Worton, R. G., and Brooke, M. H.: The X-linked muscular dystrophies. In Scriver, C. R., Beaudet, A. L., Sly, W. A., and Valle, D. (eds.): The Metabolic and Molecular Bases of Inherited Disease. New York, McGraw-Hill, 1995, p. 4195.

184. Melacini, P., Fanin, M., Danieli, G. A., et al.: Cardiac involvement in Becker muscular dystrophy. J. Am. Coll. Cardiol. 22:1927, 1993.

185. Muntoni, F., Cau, M., Ganau, A., et al.: Deletion of the dystrophin muscle-promoter region associated with X-linked dilated cardiomyopathy. N. Engl. J. Med. 329:921, 1993.

186. Towbin, J. A., Hejtmancik, J. F., Brink, P., et al.: X-linked dilated cardiomyopathy: Molecular genetic evidence of linkage to the Duchenne muscular dystrophy (dystrophin) gene at the Xp21 locus. Circulation 87:1854, 1993.

187. Fishbein, M. C., Siegel, R. J., Thompson, C. E., et al.: Sudden death of a carrier of X-linked Emery-Dreifuss muscular dystrophy. Ann. Intern. Med. 119:900, 1993.

188. Bione, S., Maestrini, E., Rivella, S., et al.: Identification of a novel X-linked gene responsible for Emery-Dreifuss muscular dystrophy. Nature Genet. 8:323, 1994.

189. Östavik, K. H., Skjörten, F., Hellebostad, M., et al.: Possible X-linked congenital mitochondrial cardiomyopathy in three families. J. Med. Genet. 30:269, 1993.

190. Aroney, C., Bett, N., and Radford, D.: Familial restrictive cardiomyopathy. Aust. N. Z. J. Med. 18:877, 1988.

191. Fitzpatrick, A. P., Shapiro, L. M., Richards, A. F., et al.: Familial restrictive cardiomyopathy with atrioventricular block and skeletal myopathy. Br. Heart J. 63:114, 1990.

192. Hodgson, S., Child, A., and Dyson, M.: Endocardial fibroelastosis: Possible X-linked inheritance. J. Med. Genet. 24:210, 1987.

193. Opitz, J. M.: Genetic aspects of endocardial fibroelastosis. Am. J. Med. Genet. 11:92, 1982.

194. Devi, A. S., Eisenfeld, L., Uphoff, D., et al.: New syndrome of hydrocephalus, endocardial fibroelastosis, and cataracts (HEC) syndrome. Am. J. Med. Genet. 56:62, 1995.

195. Ross, R. S., Bulkley, B. H., Hutchins, G. M., et al.: Idiopathic familial myocardiopathy in three generations: A clinical and pathologic study. Am. Heart J. 96:170, 1978.

196. Voorhees, M. L., Hussan, G. S., and Blackman, M. S.: Growth failure with pericardial constriction: The syndrome of mulibrey nanism. Am. J. Dis. Child. 130:1146, 1976.

197. Martinez-Lavin, M., Buendia, A., Delgado, E., et al.: A familial syndrome of pericarditis, arthritis and camptodactyly. N. Engl. J. Med. 309:224, 1983.

198. Laxer, R. M., Cameron, B. J., Chaisson, D., et al.: The camptodactyly-arthropathy-pericarditis syndrome: Case report and literature review. Arthritis Rheum. 29:439, 1986.

199. Bulutlar, G., Yazici, H., Ozdogan, H., et al.: A familial syndrome of pericarditis, arthritis, camptodactyly, and coxa vara. Arthritis Rheum. 29:436, 1986.

200. Fitzpatrick, A. P., and Emanuel, R. W.: Familial neurofibromatosis and hypertrophic cardiomyopathy. Br. Heart J. 60:247, 1988.

201. Sommer, A., Contras, S. B., Craenen, J. M., et al.: A family study of the LEOPARD syndrome. Am. J. Dis. Child. 121:520, 1971.

202. St. John Sutton, M. G., Tajik, A. J., Giuliani, E. R., et al.: Hypertrophic obstructive cardiomyopathy and lentiginosis: A little known neural ectodermal syndrome. Am. J. Cardiol. 47:214, 1981.

203. Marks, M. L., and Keating, M. T.: Familial dysrhythmias. In Rimoin, D. L., Connor, J. M., and Pyeritz, R. E. (eds.): Principles and Practice of Medical Genetics. 3rd ed. New York, Churchill Livingstone, 1995.

DISORDERS OF RHYTHM AND CONDUCTION

204. Gambetta, M., Weese, J., Ginsburg, M., et al.: Sick sinus syndrome in a patient with familial PR prolongation. Chest 64:520, 1973.

205. Surawicz, B., and Hariman, R. J.: Follow-up of the family with congenital absence of sinus rhythm. Am. J. Cardiol. 61:467, 1988.

206. Balderston, S. M., Shaffer, E. M., Sondheimer, H. M., et al.: Hereditary atrioventricular conduction defect in a child. Pediatr. Cardiol. 10:37, 1989.

207. Wolkowicz, J., and Burgess, J. H.: Complete heart block in an Inuit family. Can. J. Cardiol. 4:352, 1988.

208. Stephan, E.: Hereditary bundle branch system defect: Survey of a family with four affected generations. Am. Heart J. 95:89, 1978.

209. Lorber, A., Maisuls, E., and Naschitz, J.: Hereditary right axis deviation: Electrocardiographic pattern of pseudo left posterior hemiblock and incomplete right bundle branch block. Int. J. Cardiol. 20:399, 1988.

210. Van Der Merwe, P.-L., Weymar, H. W., Torrington, M., et al.: Progressive familial heart block (type I): A follow up study after 10 years. S. Afr. Med. J. 73:275, 1988.

211. Torrington, M., Weymar, H. W., van der Merwe, P.-L., et al.: Progressive familial heart block: Pt I. Extent of the disease. S. Afr. Med. J. 70:354, 1986.

212. Kothari, S. S., Agrawal, S. M., and Kirshnaswami, S.: Familial complete heart block in hypertrophic cardiomyopathy. Int. J. Cardiol. 20:294, 1988.

213. Stables, R. H., Bailey, C., and Ormerod, O. J. M.: Idiopathic familial atrial cardiomyopathy with diffuse conduction block. Q. J. Med. 264:325, 1989.

214. Olofsson, B.-V., Eriksson, P., and Eriksson, A.: The sick sinus syndrome in familial amyloidosis with polyneuropathy. Int. J. Cardiol. 4:71, 1983.

215. Winkler, R. B., Nora, A. H., and Nora, J. J.: Familial congenital complete heart block and maternal systemic lupus erythematosus. Circulation 56:1103, 1977.

216. McCue, C. M., Mantakas, M. E., Tingelstad, J. B., et al.: Congenital heart block in newborns of mothers with connective tissue disease. Circulation 56:82, 1977.

217. Chameides, L., Truex, R. C., Vetter, V., et al.: Association of maternal systemic lupus erythematosus with congenital complete heart block. N. Engl. J. Med. 297:1204, 1977.

218. Scott, J. S., Maddison, P. J., Taylor, P. V., et al.: Connective-tissue disease, antibodies to ribonucleoprotein, and congenital heart block. N. Engl. J. Med. 309:209, 1983.

219. Lockshin, M. D., Gibofsky, A., Peebles, C. L., et al.: Neonatal lupus erythematosus with heart block: Familial study of a patient with anti-SS-A and SS-B antibodies. Arthritis Rheum. 26:210, 1983.

220. Bergfeldt, L., and Möller, E.: Complete heart block—another HLA B27 associated disease manifestation. Tissue Antigens 21:385, 1983.

221. Bergfeldt, L., Vallin, H., and Edhag, O.: Complete heart block in HLA B27 associated disease. Electrophysiological and clinical characteristics. Br. Heart J. 51:184, 1984.

222. Bacos, J. M., Eagan, J. T., and Orgain, E. S.: Congenital familial nodal rhythm. Circulation 22:887, 1960.

223. Gault, J. H., Cantwell, J., Lev, M., et al.: Fetal familial cardiac arrhythmias. Am. J. Cardiol. 29:548, 1972.

224. Chia, B. L., Yew, F. C., Chay, S. O., et al.: Familial Wolff-Parkinson-White syndrome. J. Electrocardiol. 15:195, 1982.

225. Vidaillet, H. J., Pressley, J. C., Henke, E., et al.: Familial occurrence of accessory atrioventricular pathways: Preexcitation syndrome. N. Engl. J. Med. 317:65, 1987.

226. Stoll, C., Kieny, J.-R., Dott, B., et al.: Ventricular extrasystoles with syncopal episodes, perodactyly, and Robin sequence in three generations: A new inherited MCA syndrome? Am. J. Med. Genet. 42:480, 1992.

227. Laurent, M., Descases, C., Biron, Y., et al.: Familial form of arrhythmogenic right ventricular dysplasia. Am. Heart J. 113:827, 1987.

228. Ruder, M. A., Winston, S. A., Davis, J. C., et al.: Arrhythmogenic right ventricular dysplasia in a family. Am. J. Cardiol. 56:799, 1985.

229. Wiesfeld, A. C. P., Crijns, J. G. M., Van Dijk, R., et al.: Potential role for endomyocardial biopsy in the clinical characterization of patients with idiopathic ventricular fibrillation. Am. Heart J. 127:1421, 1993.

230. McKenna, W. J., Thiene, G., Nava, A., et al.: Diagnosis of arrhythmo-

genic right ventricular dysplasia/cardiomyopathy. Br. Heart J. 72:215, 1994.

231. Ward, O. C.: A new familial cardiac syndrome in children. J. Ir. Med. Assoc. 54:103, 1964.

232. Romano, C.: Congenital cardiac arrhythmia. Lancet 1:658, 1965.

233. Greenspon, A. J., Kidwell, G. A., Barrasse, L. D., et al.: Hereditary long QT syndrome associated with cardiac conduction system disease. PACE 12:479, 1989.

234. Marks, M. L., Whisler, S. L., Clericuzio, C., et al.: A new form of long QT syndrome associated with syndactyly. J. Am. Coll. Cardiol. 25:59, 1995.

235. Keating, M., Atkinson, D., Dunn, C., et al.: Linkage of a cardiac arrhythmia, the long QT syndrome and Harvey ras-1 gene. Science 252:704, 1991.

236. Jiang, C., Atkinson, D., Towbin, J. A., et al.: Two long QT syndrome loci map to chromosome 3 and 7 with evidence for future heterogeneity. Nature Genet. 8:141, 1994.

237. Vincent, G. M., Timothy, K. W., Leppert, M., et al.: The spectrum of symptoms and QT intervals in carriers of the gene for the long-QT syndrome. N. Engl. J. Med. 327:846, 1992.

238. Jervell, A., and Lange-Nielsen, F.: Congenital deaf-mutism, functional heart disease with prolongation of Q-T interval and sudden death. Am. Heart J. 54:59, 1957.

239. Fraser, G. R., Froggatt, P., and Murphy, T.: Genetical aspects of the cardioauditory syndrome of Jervell and Lange-Nielsen (congenital deafness and electrocardiographic abnormalities). Ann. Hum. Genet. 28:133, 1964.

240. Till, J. A., Shinebourne, E. A., Pepper, J., et al.: Complete denervation of the heart in a child with congenital long QT and deafness. Am. J. Cardiol. 62:1319, 1988.

DISORDERS OF CONNECTIVE TISSUE

241. McKusick, V. A.: Heritable Disorders of Connective Tissue. St. Louis, C. V. Mosby Co., 1956.

242. Royce, P. M., and Steinmann, B. (eds.): Connective Tissue and Its Heritable Disorders: Molecular, Genetic and Medical Aspects. New York, Wiley-Liss, 1993.

243. Pyeritz, R. E.: Heritable disorders of connective tissue. In Pierpont, M. E., and Moller, J. H. (eds.): The Genetics of Cardiovascular Disease. Boston, Martinus Nijhoff Publishing, 1987, p. 265.

244. Beighton, P. (ed.): McKusick's Heritable Disorders of Connective Tissue. 5th ed. St. Louis, C. V. Mosby Co., 1993.

245. Pyeritz, R. E.: Disorders of fibrillins and microfibrilogenesis: Marfan syndrome, MASS phenotype, contractural arachnodactyly and related conditions. In Rimoin, D. L., Connor, J. M., and Pyeritz, R. E. (eds.): Principles and Practice of Medical Genetics. 3rd ed. New York, Churchill Livingstone, 1996.

246. McKusick, V. A.: The cardiovascular aspects of Marfan's syndrome: A heritable disorder of connective tissue. Circulation 11:321, 1955.

247. Pereira, L., Levran, O., Ramirez, F., et al.: A molecular approach to the stratification of cardiovascular risk in families with Marfan's syndrome. N. Engl. J. Med. 331:148, 1994.

248. Marsalese, D. L., Moodie, D. S., Vacante, M., et al.: Marfan's syndrome: Natural history and long-term follow-up of cardiovascular involvement. J. Am. Coll. Cardiol. 14:422, 1989.

249. Child, J. S., Perloff, J. K., and Kaplan, S.: The heart of the matter: Cardiovascular involvement in Marfan's syndrome. J. Am. Coll. Cardiol. 14:429, 1989.

250. Murdoch, J. L., Walker, B. A., Halpern, B. L., et al.: Life expectancy and causes of death in the Marfan syndrome. N. Engl. J. Med. 286:804, 1972.

251. Sisk, H. E., Zahka, K. G., and Pyeritz, R. E.: The Marfan syndrome in early childhood: Analysis of 15 patients diagnosed less than 4 years of age. Am. J. Cardiol. 52:353, 1983.

252. Gross, D. M., Robinson, L. K., Smith, L. T., et al.: Severe perinatal Marfan syndrome. Pediatrics 84:83, 1989.

253. Morse, R. P., Rockenmacher, S., Pyeritz, R. E., et al.: Diagnosis and management of Marfan syndrome in infants. Pediatrics 86:888, 1990.

254. Pyeritz, R. E., and Wappel, M. A.: Mitral valve dysfunction in the Marfan syndrome. Am. J. Med. 74:797, 1983.

255. Crawford, E. S., and Coselli, J. S.: Marfan's syndrome: Combined composite valve graft replacement of the aortic root and transaortic mitral valve replacement. Ann. Thorac. Surg. 45:296, 1988.

256. Cohn, L. H., DiSesa, V. J., Couper, G. S., et al.: Mitral valve repair for myxomatous degeneration and prolapse of the mitral valve. J. Thorac. Cardiovasc. Surg. 98:987, 1989.

257. Gillinov, A. M., Hulyalkar, A., Cameron, D. E., et al.: Mitral valve operation in patients with the Marfan syndrome. J. Thorac. Cardiovasc. Surg. 107:724, 1994.

258. Gott, V. L., Cameron, D. E., Pyeritz, R. E., et al.: Composite graft repair of Marfan aneurysm of the ascending aorta: Results in 150 patients. J. Card. Surg. 9:482, 1994.

259. Lima, S. D., Lima, J. A. C., Pyeritz, R. E., et al.: Relationship of mitral valve prolapse to left ventricular size in Marfan's syndrome. Am. J. Cardiol. 55:739, 1985.

260. Henry, W. L., Gardin, J. M., and Ware, J. H.: Echocardiographic measurements in normal subjects from infancy to old age. Circulation 62:1054, 1980.

261. Roman, M. J., Rosen, S. E., Kramer-Fox, R., et al.: Prognostic signifi-

cance of the pattern of aortic root dilation in the Marfan syndrome. J. Am. Coll. Cardiol. 22:1470, 1993.

262. Crawford, E. S.: Marfan's syndrome: Broad spectral surgical treatment: cardiovascular manifestations. Ann. Surg. 198:487, 1983.

263. Svensson, L. G., Crawford, E. S., Coselli, J. S., et al.: Impact of cardiovascular operation on survival in the Marfan patient. Circulation 80:233, 1988.

264. Silverman, D. I., Burton, K. J., Gray, J., et al.: Life expectancy in the Marfan syndrome. Am. J. Cardiol. 75:157, 1995.

265. Arn, P. H., Scherer, L. R., Haller, J. A., Jr., et al.: Outcome of pectus excavatum in patients with Marfan syndrome and in the general population. J. Pediatr. 115:954, 1989.

266. deSanctis, R., Doroghazi, R. M., Austen, W. G., et al.: Aortic dissection. N. Engl. J. Med. 317:1060, 1987.

267. Schaefer, S., Peshock, R. M., Malloy, C. R., et al.: Nuclear magnetic resonance imaging in Marfan's syndrome. J. Am. Coll. Cardiol. 9:70, 1987.

268. Soulen, R. L., Fishman, E., Pyeritz, R. E., et al.: Evaluation of the Marfan syndrome: MR imaging versus CT. Radiology 165:697, 1987.

269. Crawford, E. S., Crawford, J. L., Stowe, C. L., et al.: Total aortic replacement for chronic aortic dissection occurring in patients with and without Marfan's syndrome. Ann. Surg. 199:358, 1984.

270. Shores, J., Berger, K. R., Murphy, E. A., et al.: Chronic β-adrenergic blockade protects the aorta in the Marfan syndrome: A prospective, randomized trial of propranolol. N. Engl. J. Med. 330:1335, 1994.

271. Salim, M. A., Alpert, B. S., Ward, J. C., et al.: Effect of beta-adrenergic blockade on aortic root rate of dilation in the Marfan syndrome. Am. J. Cardiol. 74:629, 1994.

272. Yin, F. C. P., Brin, K. P., Ting, C.-T., et al.: Arterial hemodynamics in the Marfan syndrome. Circulation 79:854, 1989.

273. Pyeritz, R. E.: Maternal and fetal complications of pregnancy in the Marfan syndrome. Am. J. Med. 71:784, 1981.

274. Rossiter, J. P., Morales, A. J., Repke, J. T., et al.: A prospective longitudinal evaluation of pregnancy in the Marfan syndrome. Am. J. Obstet. Gynecol. 173:1599, 1995.

275. Hollister, D. W., Godfrey, M., Sakai, L. Y., et al.: Marfan syndrome: Immunohistologic abnormalities of the elastin-associated microfibrillar fiber system. N. Engl. J. Med. 323:152, 1990.

276. Sakai, L. Y., Keene, D. R., and Engvall, E.: Fibrillin, a new 350-kD glycoprotein, is a component of extracellular microfibrils. J. Cell. Biol. 103:2499, 1986.

277. Kainulainen, K., Pulkkinen, L., Savolainen, A., et al.: The gene defect causing Marfan syndrome is located on chromosome 15. N. Engl. J. Med. 323:935, 1990.

278. Dietz, H. C., Pyeritz, R. E., Hall, B. D., et al.: The Marfan syndrome locus: Confirmations of assignment to chromosome 15 and identification of tightly linked markers at 15q15-q21.3. Genomics 9:355, 1991.

279. Dietz, H. C., Cutting, G. R., Pyeritz, R. E., et al.: Marfan syndrome caused by a recurrent de novo missense mutation in the fibrillin gene. Nature 352:337, 1991.

280. Dietz, H. C., McIntosh, I., Sakai, L. Y., et al.: Four novel FBN1 mutations: Significance for mutant transcript level and EGF-like domain calcium binding in the pathogenesis of Marfan syndrome. Genomics 17:468, 1993.

281. Kielty, C. M., Rantamaki, T., Child, A. H., et al.: Cystein-to-arginine mutation in a 'hybrid' eight-cysteine domain of FBN1: Consequences for fibrillin aggregation and microfibril assembly. J. Med. Genet. (in press).

282. Milewicz, D. M., Grossfield, J., Cao, S.-N., et al.: A mutation in FBN1 disrupts profibrillin processing and results in isolated skeletal features of the Marfan syndrome. J. Clin. Invest. 95:2373, 1995.

283. Francke, U., Berg, M. A., Tynan, K., et al.: A Gly1127Ser mutation in an EGF-like domain of the fibrillin-1 gene is a risk factor for ascending aortic aneurysm and dissection in the absence of the Marfan syndrome. Am. J. Hum. Genet. 56:1287, 1995.

284. Milewicz, D. Mc. G., Pyeritz, R. E., Crawford, E. S., et al.: Marfan syndrome: Defective synthesis, secretion and extracellular matrix formation of fibrillin by cultured dermal fibroblasts. J. Clin. Invest. 89:79, 1992.

285. Aoyama, T., Francke, U., Dietz, H., et al.: Quantitative differences in biosynthesis and extracellular deposition of fibrillin in cultured fibroblasts distinguish five groups of Marfan syndrome patients and suggest distinct pathogenetic mechanisms. J. Clin. Invest. 94:130, 1994.

286. Leier, C. V., Call, T. D., Fulkerson, P. K., et al.: The spectrum of cardiac defects in the Ehlers-Danlos syndrome, types I and III. Ann. Intern. Med. 92:171, 1980.

287. Fox, R., Pope, F. M., Narcisi, P., et al.: Spontaneous carotid cavernous fistula in Ehlers-Danlos syndrome. J. Neurol. Neurosurg. Psychiatry 51:984, 1988.

288. Rudd, N. L., Nimrod, C., Holbrook, K. A., et al.: Pregnancy complications in type IV Ehlers-Danlos syndrome. Lancet 1:50, 1983.

289. Viljoen, D. L., Pope, F. M., and Beighton, P.: Heterogeneity of pseudoxanthoma elasticum: Delineation of a new form? Clin. Genet. 32:100, 1987.

290. Cunningham, J. R., Lippman, S. M., Renie, W. A., et al.: Pseudoxanthoma elasticum: Treatment of gastrointestinal hemorrhage by arterial embolization and observations of autosomal dominant inheritance. Johns Hopkins Med. J. 147:168, 1980.

291. Lebwohl, M. G., Distefano, D., Prioleau, P. G., et al.: Pseudoxanthoma elasticum and mitral-valve prolapse. N. Engl. J. Med. 307:228, 1982.

292. Pyeritz, R. E., Weiss, J. L., Renie, W. A., et al.: Pseudoxanthoma elasticum and mitral-valve prolapse. N. Engl. J. Med. *307*:1451, 1982.

293. Goodman, R. M., Smith, E. W., Paton, D., et al.: Pseudoxanthoma elasticum: A clinical and histopathological study. Medicine *42*:297, 1963.

294. Lebwohl, M., Halperin, J., and Phelps, R. G.: Occult pseudoxanthoma elasticum in patients with premature cardiovascular disease. N. Engl. J. Med. *329*:1237, 1993.

295. Challenor, V. F., Conway, N., and Monro, J. L.: The surgical treatment of restrictive cardiomyopathy in pseudoxanthoma elasticum. Br. Heart J. *59*:266, 1988.

296. Raybould, M. C., Birley, A. J., Moss, C., et al.: Exclusion of an elastin gene (ELN) mutation as the cause of pseudoxanthoma elasticum (PXE) in one family. Clin. Genet. *45*:48, 1994.

297. Renie, W. A., Pyeritz, R. E., Combs, J., et al.: Pseudoxanthoma elasticum: High calcium intake in early life correlates with severity. Am. J. Med. Genet. *19*:235, 1984.

298. Maharaj, B., Hammond, M. G., Appadoo, B., et al.: HLA-A, B, DR, and DQ antigens in black patients with severe chronic rheumatic heart disease. Circulation *76*:259, 1987.

INBORN ERRORS OF METABOLISM THAT AFFECT THE CARDIOVASCULAR SYSTEM

299. La Du, B. N.: Alkaptonuria: *In* Scriver, C. R., Beaudet, A. L., Sly, W. A., and Valle, D. (eds.): The Metabolic and Molecular Bases of Inherited Disease. New York, McGraw-Hill, 1995, p. 1371.

300. Mudd, S. H., Levy, H. L., and Skovby, F.: Disorders of transsulfuration. *In* Scriver, C. R., Beaudet, A. L., Sly, W. A., and Valle, D. (eds.): The Metabolic and Molecular Bases of Inherited Disease. New York, McGraw-Hill, 1995, p. 1279.

301. Mudd, S. H., Skovby, F., Levy, H. L., et al.: The natural history of homocystinuria due to cystathionine beta-synthase deficiency. Am. J. Hum. Genet. *37*:1, 1985.

302. Hill-Zobel, R. L., Pyeritz, R. E., Scheffel, U., et al.: Kinetics and biodistribution of ^{111}In-labeled platelets in homocystinuria. N. Engl. J. Med. *307*:781, 1982.

303. Selhub, J., Jacques, P. F., Bostom, A. G., et al.: Association between plasma homocysteine concentrations and extracranial carotid-artery stenosis. N. Engl. J. Med. *332*:286, 1995.

304. Kang, S.-S., Passen, E. L., Ruggie, N., et al.: Thermolabile defect of methylenetetrahydrofolate reductase in coronary artery disease. Circulation *88*:1463, 1993.

305. Rolland, P. H., Friggi, A., Barlatier, A., et al.: Hyperhomocysteinemia-induced vascular damage in the minipig captopril-hydrochlorothiazide combination prevents elastic alterations. Circulation *91*:1161, 1995.

306. Hajjar, K. A.: Homocysteine-induced modulation of tissue plasminogen activator binding to its endothelial cell membrane receptor. J. Clin. Invest. *91*:2873, 1993.

307. Majors, A., Ehrhart, L. A., Pezacka, E. H.: Homocysteine as a risk factor for vascular disease: Enhanced collagen production and accumulation by smooth muscle cells. Proc. Natl. Acad. Sci. USA *(in press)*.

308. Stampfer, M. J., and Manilow, M. R.: Can lowering homocysteine levels reduce cardiovascular risk? N. Engl. J. Med. *332*:328, 1995.

309. Roe, C. R., and Coates, P. M.: Mitochondrial fatty acid oxidation disorders. *In* Scriver, C. R., Beaudet, A. L., Sly, W. A., and Valle, D. (eds.): The Metabolic and Molecular Bases of Inherited Disease. New York, McGraw-Hill, 1995, p. 1501.

310. Rebouche, C. J., and Engel, A. G.: Carnitine metabolism and deficiency syndrome. Mayo Clin. Proc. *58*:533, 1983.

311. Treem, W. R., Stanley, C. A., Finegold, D. N., et al.: Primary carnitine deficiency due to a failure of carnitine transport in kidney, muscle, and fibroblasts. N. Engl. J. Med. *319*:1331, 1988.

312. Waber, L. J., Valle, D., Neill, C., et al.: Carnitine deficiency presenting as familial cardiomyopathy: A treatable defect in carnitine transport. J. Pediatr. *101*:700, 1982.

313. Tripp, M. E., Katcher, M. L., Peters, H. A., et al.: Systemic carnitine deficiency presenting as familial endocardial fibroelastosis. N. Engl. J. Med. *305*:385, 1981.

314. Sato, W., Tanaka, M., Sugiyama, S., et al.: Cardiomyopathy and angiopathy in patients with mitochondrial myopathy, encephalopathy, lactic acidosis, and strokelike episodes. Am. Heart J. *128*:733, 1994.

315. Brackett, J. C., Sims, H. F., Steiner, R. D., et al.: A novel mutation in medium chain Acyl-CoA dehydrogenase causes sudden neonatal death. J. Clin. Invest. *94*:1477, 1994.

316. Anan, R., Nakagawa, M., Miyata, M., et al.: Cardiac involvement in mitochondrial diseases. A study of 17 patients with documented mitochondrial DNA defects. Circulation *91*:955, 1995.

317. Merante, F., Tein, I., Benson, L., et al.: Maternally inherited hypertrophic cardiomyopathy due to a novel T-to-C transition at nucleotide 9997 in the mitochondrial tRNA[glycine] gene. Am. J. Hum. Genet. *55*:437, 1994.

318. Van Hove, J. L. K., Shanske, S., Ciacci, F., et al.: Mitochondrial myopathy with anemia, cardiomyopathy and lactic acidosis: A distinct late onset mitochondrial disorder. Am. J. Med. Genet. *51*:115, 1994.

319. Wallace, D. C.: Mitochondrial genetics: A paradigm for aging and degenerative diseases? Science *256*:628, 1992.

320. Ogashara, S., Engel, A. G., Frens, D., et al.: Muscle coenzyme Q deficiency in familial mitochondrial encephalomyopathy. Proc. Natl. Acad. Sci. U.S.A. *86*:2379, 1989.

321. Channer, K. S., Channer, J. L., Campbell, M. J., et al.: Cardiomyopathy in the Kearns-Sayre syndrome. Br. Heart J. *59*:486, 1988.

322. Chen, Y.-T., and Burchell, A.: Glycogen storage diseases. *In* Scriver, C. R., Beaudet, A. L., Sly, W. A., and Valle, D. (eds.): The Metabolic and Molecular Bases of Inherited Disease. New York, McGraw-Hill, 1995, p. 935.

323. Ehlers, K. H., Hagstrom, J. W. C., Lukas, D. S., et al.: Glycogen-storage disease of the myocardium with obstruction to left ventricular outflow. Circulation *25*:96, 1962.

324. Bharati, S., Serratto, M., Du Brow, I., et al.: The conduction system in Pompe's disease. Pediatr. Cardiol. *2*:25, 1982.

325. Bonnici, F., Shapiro, R., Joffe, H. S., et al.: Angiocardiographic and enzyme studies in a patient with type II glycogenosis. S. Afr. Med. J. *58*:860, 1980.

326. Robinson, W. F., Howell, J. M., and Dorling, P. R.: Cardiomyopathy is generalised glycogenosis type II in cattle. Cardiovasc. Res. *17*:238, 1982.

327. Suzuki, Y., Tsuji, A., Omura, K., et al.: Km mutant of acid alpha-glucosidase in a case of cardiomyopathy without signs of skeletal muscle involvement. Clin. Genet. *33*:376, 1988.

328. Makos, M. M., McComb, R. D., Hart, M. N., et al.: Alpha-glucosidase deficiency and basilar artery aneurysm: Report of a sibship. Ann. Neurol. *22*:629, 1987.

329. Kretzschmar, H. A., Wagner, H., Hubner, G., et al.: Aneurysm and vacuolar degeneration of cerebral arteries in late-onset acid maltase deficiency. J. Neurol. Sci. *98*:169, 1990.

330. Martiniuk, F., Mehler, M., Tzall, S., et al.: Extensive genetic heterogeneity in patients with acid alpha glucosidase deficiency as detected by abnormalities of DNA and mRNA. Am. J. Hum. Genet. *47*:73, 1990.

331. Olson, L. J., Reeder, G. S., Noller, K. L., et al.: Cardiac involvement in glycogen storage disease III. Morphologic and biochemical characterization with endomyocardial biopsy. Am. J. Cardiol. *53*:980, 1984.

332. Coleman, R. A., Winter, H. S., Wolf, B., et al.: Glycogen debranching enzyme deficiency: Long-term study of serum enzyme activities and clinical features. J. Inherit. Metab. Dis. *15*:869, 1992.

333. Talente, G. M., Coleman, R. A., Alter, C., et al.: Glycogen storage diseases in adults. Ann. Intern. Med. *120*:218, 1994.

334. Servidei, S., Metlay, L. A., Chodosh, J., et al.: Fatal infantile cardiopathy caused by phosphorylase b kinase deficiency. J. Pediatr. *113*:82, 1988.

335. Schroder, J. M., May, R., Shin, Y. S., et al.: Juvenile hereditary polyglucosan body disease with complete branching enzyme deficiency (type IV glycogenosis). Acta Neuropathol. *85*:419, 1993.

336. Howell, R. R.: Continuing lessons from glycogen storage diseases. N. Engl. J. Med. *324*(Edit.):55, 1991.

337. Selby, R., Starzl, T. E., Yunis, E., et al.: Liver transplantation for type IV glycogen storage disease. N. Engl. J. Med. *324*:39, 1991.

338. Eishi, Y., Takemura, T., Sone, R., et al.: Glycogen storage disease confined to the heart with deficient activity of cardiac phosphorylase kinase: A new type of glycogen storage disease. Hum. Pathol. *16*:193, 1987.

339. Elleder, M., Shin, Y. S., Zuntova, A., et al.: Fatal infantile hypertrophic cardiomyopathy secondary to deficiency of heart specific phosphorylase b kinase. Virchows Arch. A *423*:303, 1993.

340. Bothwell, T. H., Charlton, R. W., and Motulsky, A. G.: Hemochromatosis. *In* Scriver, C. R., Beaudet, A. L., Sly, W. A., and Valle, D. (eds.): The Metabolic and Molecular Bases of Inherited Disease. New York, McGraw-Hill, 1995, p. 2237.

341. Edwards, C. Q.: Early detection of hereditary hemochromatosis. Ann. Intern. Med. *101*:707, 1984.

342. Olson, L. J., Baldus, W. P., and Tajik, A. J.: Echocardiographic features of idiopathic hemochromatosis. Am. J. Cardiol. *60*:885, 1987.

343. Porter, J., Cary, N., and Schofield, P.: Haemochromatosis presenting as congestive cardiac failure. Br. Heart J. *73*:73, 1995.

344. Cutler, D. J., Isner, J. M., Bracey, A. W., et al.: Hemochromatosis heart disease: An unemphasized cause of potentially reversible restrictive cardiomyopathy. Am. J. Med. *69*:923, 1980.

345. Weatherall, D. J., Clegg, J. B., Higgs, D. R., et al.: The hemoglobinopathies. *In* Scriver, C. R., Beaudet, A. L., Sly, W. A., and Valle, D. (eds.): The Metabolic and Molecular Bases of Inherited Disease. New York, McGraw-Hill, 1995, p. 3417.

346. Sutton, L. L., Castro, O., Cross, D. J., et al.: Pulmonary hypertension in sickle cell disease. Am. J. Cardiol. *74*:626, 1994.

347. Brittenham, G. M., Griffith, P. M., Nienhuis, A. W., et al.: Efficacy of deferoxamine in preventing complications of iron overload in patients with thalassemia major. N. Engl. J. Med. *331*:567, 1994.

348. Olivieri, N. F., Liu, P. P., Sher, G. D., et al.: Combination liver and heart transplantation for end-stage iron-induced organ failure in an adult with homozygous beta-thalassemia. N. Engl. J. Med. *330*:1125, 1994.

349. Neufeld, E. F., and Muenzer, J.: The mucopolysaccharidoses. *In* Scriver, C. R., Beaudet, A. L., Sly, W. A., and Valle, D. (eds.): The Metabolic and Molecular Bases of Inherited Disease. New York, McGraw-Hill, 1995, p. 2465.

350. Johnson, G. L., Vine, D. L., Cottrill, C. M., et al.: Echocardiographic mitral valve deformity in the mucopolysaccharidoses. Pediatrics *67*:401, 1981.

351. Gross, D. M., Williams, J. C., Caprioli, C., et al.: Echocardiographic abnormalities in the mucopolysaccharide storage diseases. Am. J. Cardiol. *61*:170, 1988.

352. John, R. M., Hunter, D., and Swanton, R. H.: Echocardiographic abnormalities in type IV mucopolysaccharidosis. Arch. Dis. Child. *65*:746, 1990.

353. Pyeritz, R. E.: Storage disorders. *In* Pierpont, M. E., and Moller, J. H.

(eds.): The Genetics of Cardiovascular Disease. Boston, Martinus Nijhoff Publishing, 1987, p. 215.

354. Nelson, J., Shields, M. D., and Mulholland, H. C.: Cardiovascular studies in the mucopolysaccharidoses. J. Med. Genet. 27:94, 1990.

355. Brosius, F. C., III, and Roberts, W. C.: Coronary artery disease in the Hurler syndrome: Qualitative and quantitative analysis of the extent of coronary narrowing at necropsy in six children. Am. J. Cardiol. 47:649, 1981.

356. Renteria, V. G., Ferrans, V. J., and Roberts, W. C.: The heart in the Hurler syndrome: Gross, histologic and ultrastructural observations in five necropsy cases. Am. J. Cardiol. 38:487, 1976.

357. Semenza, G. L., and Pyeritz, R. E.: Respiratory complications of the mucopolysaccharide storage disorders. Medicine 67:209, 1988.

358. Young, I. D., and Harper, P. S.: Long-term complications in Hunter's syndrome. Clin. Genet. 16:125, 1979.

359. Armitage, J. O.: Bone marrow transplantation. N. Engl. J. Med. 330:827, 1994.

360. Whitley, C. B., Belani, K. G., Chang, P.-N., et al.: Long-term outcome of Hurler syndrome following bone marrow transplantation. Am. J. Med. Genet. 46:209, 1993.

361. Morgan, S. H., and Crawfurd, M. d'A.: Anderson-Fabry disease. A commonly missed diagnosis. BMJ 297:872, 1988.

362. Spence, M. W., MacKinnon, K. E., Burgess, J. K., et al.: Failure to correct the metabolic defect by renal allotransplantation in Fabry's disease. Ann. Intern. Med. 84:13, 1976.

363. Kramer, W., Thormann, J., Mueller, K., et al.: Progressive cardiac involvement by Fabry's disease despite successful renal allotransplantation. Int. J. Cardiol. 7:72, 1985.

364. Colucci, W. S., Lorell, B. H., Schoen, F. J., et al.: Hypertrophic obstructive cardiomyopathy due to Fabry's disease. N. Engl. J. Med. 307:926, 1982.

365. von Scheidt, W., Eng, C. M., Fitzmaurice, T. F., et al.: An atypical variant of Fabry's disease with manifestations confined to the myocardium. N. Engl. J. Med. 324:395, 1991.

366. Goldman, M. E., Cantor, R., Schwartz, M. F., et al.: Echocardiographic abnormalities and disease severity in Fabry's disease. J. Am. Coll. Cardiol. 7:1157, 1986.

367. Sakuraba, H., Yanagawa, Y., Igarashi, T., et al.: Cardiovascular manifestations in Fabry's disease: A high incidence of mitral valve prolapse in hemizygotes and heterozygotes. Clin. Genet. 29:276, 1986.

368. Mutoh, T., Senda, Y., Sugimura, K., et al.: Severe orthostatic hypotension in a female carrier of Fabry's disease. Arch. Neurol. 34:468, 1988.

369. Bernstein, H. S., Bishop, D. F., Astrin, K. H., et al.: Fabry disease: Six gene rearrangements and an exonic point mutation in the alpha-galactosidase gene. J. Clin. Invest. 83:1390, 1989.

370. Benson, M. D., and Wallace, M. R.: Amyloidosis. In Scriver, C. R., Beaudet, A. L., Sly, W. S., and Valle, D. (eds.): The Metabolic Basis of Inherited Disease. 6th ed. New York, McGraw-Hill Book Co., 1989, p. 2439.

371. Benson, M. D.: Amyloidosis. In Scriver, C. R., Beaudet, A. L., Sly, W. A., and Valle, D. (eds.): The Metabolic and Molecular Bases of Inherited Disease. New York, McGraw-Hill, 1995, p. 4157.

372. Backman, C., and Olofsson, B. O.: Echocardiographic features in familial amyloidosis with polyneuropathy. Acta Med. Scand. 214:273, 1983.

373. Eriksson, A., Eriksson, P., Olofsson, B.-O., et al.: The cardiac atrioventricular conduction system in familial amyloidosis with polyneuropathy: A clinico-pathologic study of six cases from Northern Sweden. Acta Pathol. Microbiol. Immunol. Scand. 91:343, 1983.

374. Booth, D. R., Tan, S. Y., Hawkins, P. N., et al.: A novel variant of transthyretin, 59$^{Thr→Lys}$, associated with autosomal dominant cardiac amyloidosis in an Italian family. Circulation 91:962, 1995.

375. Skinner, M., Lewis, W. D., Jones, L. A., et al.: Liver transplantation as a treatment for familial amyloidotic polyneuropathy. Ann. Intern. Med. 120:133, 1994.

376. Vidaillet, H. J., Jr.: Cardiac tumors associated with hereditary syndromes. Am. J. Cardiol. 61:1355, 1988.

377. Burke, A. P., Rosado-de-Christenson, M., Templeton, P. A., et al.: Cardiac fibroma: Clinicopathologic correlates and surgical treatment. J. Thorac. Cardiovasc. Surg. 108:862, 1994.

378. Harding, C. O., and Pagon, R. A.: Incidence of tuberous sclerosis in patients with cardiac rhabdomyoma. Am. J. Med. Genet. 37:443, 1990.

379. Liebler, G. A., Magovern, G. J., Park, S. B., et al.: Familial myxomas in four siblings. J. Thorac. Cardiovasc. Surg. 71:605, 1976.

380. Carney, J. A., Gordon, H., Carpenter, P. C., et al.: The complex of myxomas, spotty pigmentation, and endocrine overactivity. Medicine 64:270, 1985.

381. Handley, J., Carson, D., Sloan, J., et al.: Multiple lentigines, myxoid tumours and endocrine overactivity: Four cases of Carney's complex. Br. J. Dermatol. 126:367, 1992.

INHERITED DISORDERS OF THE CIRCULATION

382. Peery, W. H.: Clinical spectrum of hereditary hemorrhagic telangiectasia (Osler-Weber-Rendu disease). Am. J. Med. 82:989, 1987.

383. Guttmacher, A. E., McKinnon, W. C., and Upton, M. D.: Hereditary hemorrhagic telangiectasia: A disorder in search of the genetics community. Am. J. Med. Genet. 52:252, 1994.

384. Guillén, B., Guizar, J., de la Cruz, J., et al.: Hereditary hemorrhagic telangiectasia: Report of 15 affected cases in a Mexican family. Clin. Genet. 39:214, 1991.

385. Nikolopoulos, N., Xynos, E., and Vassilakis, J. S.: Familial occurrence

386. Cooke, D. A. P.: Renal arteriovenous malformation demonstrated angiographically in hereditary haemorrhagic telangiectasia (Rendu-Osler-Weber disease). J. R. Soc. Med. 79:744, 1986.

387. Kurnik, P. B., and Heymann, W. R.: Coronary artery ectasia associated with hereditary hemorrhagic telangiectasia. Arch. Intern. Med. 149:2357, 1989.

388. Braverman, I. M., Keh, A., and Jacobson, B. S.: Ultrastructure and three-dimensional organization of the telangiectases of hereditary hemorrhagic telangiectasia. J. Invest. Dermatol. 95:422, 1990.

389. Terry, P. B., White, J. I., Jr., Barth, K. H., et al.: Pulmonary arteriovenous malformations: Physiologic observations and results of therapeutic balloon embolization. N. Engl. J. Med. 308:1197, 1983.

390. Haq, A. U., Glass, J., Netchvolodoff, C. V., et al.: Hereditary hemorrhagic telangiectasia and danazol. Ann. Intern. Med. 109:171, 1988.

391. Saba, H. I., Morelli, G. A., and Logrono, L. A.: Treatment of bleeding in hereditary hemorrhagic telangiectasia with aminocaproic acid. N. Engl. J. Med. 330:1789, 1994.

392. Phillips, M. D.: Stopping bleeding in hereditary telangiectasia. N. Engl. J. Med. 330:1822, 1994.

393. McDonald, M. T., Papenberg, K. A., Ghosh, S., et al.: A disease locus for hereditary haemorrhagic telangiectasia maps to chromosome 9q33-34. Nature Genet 6:197, 1994.

394. Shovlin, C. L., Hughes, J. M. B., Tuddenham, E. G. D., et al.: A gene for hereditary haemorrhagic telangiectasia maps to chromosome 9q3. Nature Genet. 6:205, 1994.

395. McAllister, K. A., Grogg, K. M. M., Johnson, D. W., et al.: Endoglin, a TGF-β binding protein of endothelial cells, is the gene for hereditary haemorrhagic telangiectasia type 1. Nature Genet. 8:345, 1994.

396. Jennings, A. M., Smith, C., Cole, D. R., et al.: Von Hippel-Lindau disease in a large British family: Clinicopathological features and recommendations for screening and follow-up. Q. J. Med. 66:233, 1988.

397. Lamiell, J. M., Salazar, F. G., and Hsia, Y. E.: Von Hippel-Lindau disease affecting 43 members of a single kindred. Medicine 68:1, 1989.

398. Latif, F., Troy, K., Gnarra, J., et al.: Identification of the von Hippel-Landau disease tumor suppressor gene. Science 260:1317, 1993.

399. Parfrey, P. S., Bear, J. C., Morgan, J., et al.: The diagnosis and prognosis of autosomal dominant polycystic kidney disease. N. Engl. J. Med. 323:1085, 1990.

400. Gabow, P. A.: Autosomal dominant polycystic kidney disease. N. Engl. J. Med. 329:332, 1993.

401. Chapman, A. B., Johnson, A., Gabow, P. A., et al.: The renin-angiotensin aldosterone system and autosomal dominant polycystic kidney disease. N. Engl. J. Med. 323:1091, 1990.

402. Leier, C. V., Baker, P. B., Kilman, J. W., et al.: Cardiovascular abnormalities associated with adult polycystic kidney disease. Ann. Intern. Med. 100:683, 1984.

403. Hossack, K. F., Leddy, C. L., Johnson, A. M., et al.: Echocardiographic findings in autosomal dominant polycystic kidney disease. N. Engl. J. Med. 319:907, 1988.

404. Chapman, J. R., and Hilson, A. J. W.: Polycystic kidneys and abdominal aortic aneurysms. Lancet 1:646, 1980.

405. Chapman, A. B., Rubinstein, D., Hughes, R., et al.: Intracranial aneurysms in autosomal dominant polycystic kidney disease. N. Engl. J. Med. 327:916, 1992.

406. European Polycystic Kidney Disease Consortium: The polycystic kidney disease 1 gene encodes a 14 kb transcript and lies within a duplicated region on chromosome 16. Cell 77:881, 1994.

407. Peters, D. J. M., Spruit, L., Saris, J. J., et al.: Chromosome 4 localization of a second gene for autosomal dominant polycystic kidney disease. Nature Genet. 5:359, 1993.

408. Daoust, M. C., Reynold, D. M., Bichet, D. G., et al.: Evidence for a third genetic locus for autosomal dominant polycystic kidney disease. Genomics 25:733, 1995.

409. Shulman, S. A., Hyams, J. S., Gunta, R., et al.: Arteriohepatic dysplasia (Alagille syndrome): Extreme variability among affected family members. Am. J. Med. Genet. 19:325, 1984.

410. Dhorne-Pollet, S., Deleuze, J.-F., Hadchouel, M., et al.: Segregation analysis of Alagille syndrome. J. Med. Genet. 31:453, 1994.

411. Nicod, P., Bloor, C., Godfrey, M., et al.: Familial aortic dissecting aneurysms. J. Am. Coll. Cardiol. 13:811, 1989.

412. Toyama, M., Amano, A., and Kameda, T.: Familial aortic dissection: A report of rare family cluster. Br. Heart J. 61:204, 1989.

413. Bixler, D., and Antley, R. M.: Familial aortic dissection with iris anomalies—a new connective tissue disease syndrome? Birth Defects 12(5):229, 1976.

414. Roberts, C. S., and Roberts, W. C.: Dissection of the aorta associated with congenital malformation of the aortic valve. J. Am. Coll. Cardiol. 17:712, 1994.

415. Kontusaari, S., Tromp, G., Kuivaniemi, H., et al.: Inheritance of RNA splicing mutation (G^{+1} IVS$_{20}$) in the type III procollagen gene (COL3AI) in a family having aortic aneurysms and easy bruisability: Phenotypic overlap between familial arterial aneurysms and Ehlers-Danlos syndrome type IV. Am. J. Hum. Genet. 47:112, 1990.

416. Kontusaari, S., Tromp, G., Kuivaniemi, H., et al.: A mutation in the gene for type III procollagen (COL3AI) in a family with aortic aneurysms. J. Clin. Invest 86:1465, 1990.

417. Tromp, G., Wu, Y., Prockop, D. J., et al.: Sequencing of cDNA from 50 unrelated patients reveals that mutations in the triple-helical domain of

type III procollagen are an infrequent cause of aortic aneurysms. J. Clin. Invest. *91*:2539, 1993.

418. Schievink, W. I., Michaels, V. V., Mokri, B., et al.: A familial syndrome of arterial dissections with lentiginosis. N. Engl. J. Med. *332*:576, 1995.

419. Majamaa, K., Portimojarvi, H., Sotaniemi, K. A., et al.: Familial aggregation of cervical artery dissection and cerebral aneurysm. Stroke *25*:1704, 1994.

420. Majumder, P. P., St. Jean, P. L., Ferrell, R. E., et al.: On the inheritance of abdominal aortic aneurysm. Am. J. Hum. Genet. *48*:164, 1991.

421. Pletcher, B. A., Fox, J. E., Boxer, R. A., et al.: Three siblings with arterial tortuosity syndrome: Description and review of the literature. Am. J. Med. Genet. *(in press)*.

422. Halal, F., Mohr, G., Toussi, T., et al.: Intracranial aneurysms: A report of a large pedigree. Am. J. Med. Genet. *15*:89, 1983.

423. Kuivaniemi, H., Prockop, D. J., Wu, Y., et al.: Exclusion of mutations in the gene for type III collagen (COL3A1) as a common cause of intracranial aneurysms or cervical artery dissections: Results from sequence analysis of the coding sequences of type III collagen from 55 unrelated patients. Neurology *43*:2652, 1993.

424. Abrahamson, M.: Human cysteine proteinase inhibitors: Isolation, physiological importance, inhibitory mechanism, gene structure and relation to hereditary cerebral hemorrhage. Scand. J. Clin. Lab. Invest. *48*:21, 1988.

425. Wattendorf, A. R., Bots, G. T. A. M., Went, L. N., et al.: Familial cerebral amyloid angiopathy presenting as recurrent cerebral haemorrhage. J. Neurol. Sci. *55*:121, 1982.

426. Pasyk, K. A., Argenta, L. C., and Erickson, R. P.: Familial vascular malformations: Report of 25 members of one family. Clin. Genet. *26*:221, 1984.

427. Stanley, J. C.: Arterial fibrodysplasia. Arch. Surg. *110*:561, 1975.

428. Kousseff, B. G., and Gilbert-Barness, E. F.: Vascular neurofibromatosis and infantile gangrene. Am. J. Med. Genet. *34*:221, 1989.

429. Schievink, W. I., Björnsson, J., Parisi, J. E., et al.: Arterial fibromuscular dysplasia associated with severe α_1-antitrypsin deficiency. Mayo Clin. Proc. *69*:1040, 1994.

430. Petit, H., Bouchez, B., Destee, A., et al.: Familial form of fibromuscular dysplasia of the internal carotid artery. J. Neuroradiol. *10*:15, 1983.

431. Rushton, A. R.: The genetics of fibromuscular dysplasia. Arch. Intern. Med. *140*:233, 1980.

432. Austin, J. G., and Stears, J. C.: Familial hypoplasia of both internal carotid arteries. Arch. Neurol. *24*:1, 1971.

433. McDonald, A. H., Gerlis, L. M., and Somerville, J.: Familial arteriopathy with associated pulmonary and systemic arterial stenoses. Br. Heart J. *31*:375, 1969.

434. Van Dyck, M., Proesmans, W., VanHollebeke, E., et al.: Idiopathic infantile arterial calcification with cardiac, renal and central nervous system involvement. Eur. J. Pediatr. *148*:374, 1989.

435. Joutel, A., Bousser, M-G., Biuosse, V., et al.: A gene for familial hemiplegic migraine maps to chromosome 19. Nature Genet. *5*:40, 1993.

436. Joutel, A., Ducros, A., Vahedi, K., et al.: Genetic heterogeneity of familial hemiplegic migraine. Am. J. Hum. Genet. *55*:1166, 1994.

437. Hovatta, I., Kallela, M., Färkkilä, M., et al.: Familial migraine: Exclusion of the susceptibility gene from the reported locus of familial hemiplegic migraine on 19p. Genomics *23*:707, 1994.

438. Tournier-Lasserve, E., Joutel, A., Melki, J., et al.: Cerebral autosomal dominant arteriopathy with subcortical infarcts and leukoencephalopathy maps to chromosone 19q12. Nature Genet. *3*:256, 1993.

439. Melmon, K. L., and Braunwald, E.: Familial pulmonary hypertension. N. Engl. J. Med. *269*:770, 1963.

440. Kingdon, H. S., Cohen, L. S., Roberts, W. C., et al.: Familial occurrence of primary pulmonary hypertension. Arch. Intern. Med. *118*:422, 1966.

441. Loyd, J. E., Primm, R. K., and Newman, J. H.: Familial primary pulmonary hypertension: Clinical patterns. Am. Rev. Respir. Dis. *129*:194, 1984.

442. Porterfield, J. K., Pyeritz, R. E., and Traill, T. A.: Pulmonary hypertension and interstitial fibrosis in von Recklinghausen neurofibromatosis. Am. J. Med. Genet. *25*:531, 1986.

443. Goldstein, S., Qazi, Q. H., Fitzgerald, J., et al.: Distichiasis, congenital heart defects and mixed peripheral vascular anomalies. Am. J. Med. Genet. *20*:283, 1985.

444. Lindenauer, S. M.: The Klippel-Trenaunay-Weber syndrome: Varicosity, hypertrophy and hemangioma with no arteriovenous fistula. Ann. Surg. *162*:303, 1965.

445. Campistol, J. M., Agusti, C., Torras, A., et al.: Renal hemangioma and renal artery aneurysm in the Klippel-Trenaunay syndrome. J. Urol. *140*:134, 1988.

446. Bicknell, J. M.: Familial cavernous angioma of the brain stem dominantly inherited in Hispanics. Neurosurgery *24*:102, 1989.

447. Dellemijn, P. L. I., and Vanneste, J. A. L.: Cavernous angiomatosis of the central nervous system: Usefulness of screening the family. Acta Neurol. Scand. *88*:259, 1993.

448. Dobyns, W. B., Michels, V. V., Groover, R. V., et al.: Familial cavernous malformations of the central nervous system and retina. Ann. Neurol. *21*:578, 1987.

449. Rigamonti, D., Hadley, M. N., Drayer, B. P., et al.: Cerebral cavernous malformations: Incidence and familial occurrence. N. Engl. J. Med. *319*:343, 1988.

450. Steichen-Gersdorf, E., Felber, S., Fuchs, W., et al.: Familial cavernous angiomas of the brain: Observations in a four generation family. Eur. J. Pediatr. *151*:861, 1992.

451. Drigo, P., Mammi, I., Battistella, P. A., et al.: Familial cerebral, hepatic, and retinal cavernous angiomas: A new syndrome. Child's Nerv. Sys. *10*:205, 1994.

452. Dubovsky, J., Zabramski, J. M., Kurth, J., et al.: A gene responsible for cavernous malformations of the brain maps to chromosome 7q. Hum. Molec. Genet. *4*:453, 1995.

452a. Gunel, M., Awad, I. A., Anson, J., et al.: Mapping a gene causing cerebral cavernous malformation to 7q11.2-q21. Proc. Nat. Acad. Sci. U.S.A. *92*:6620, 1995.

453. Marchuk, D. A., Gallione, C. J., Morrison, L. A., et al.: A locus for cerebral cavernous malformations maps to chromosome 7q in two families. Genomics *28*:311, 1995.

454. Herbert, F. A., and Bowen, P. A.: Hereditary late-onset lymphedema with pleural effusion and laryngeal edema. Arch. Intern. Med. *143*:913, 1983.

455. Offori, T. W., Platt, C. C., Stephens, M., et al.: Angiosarcoma in congenital hereditary lymphoedema (Milroy's disease). Clin. Exp. Dermatol. *18*:174, 1993.

456. Anderson, H. C., Parry, D. M., and Mulvihill, J. J.: Lymphangiosarcoma in late-onset hereditary lymphedema: Case report and nosological implications. Am. J. Med. Genet. *56*:72, 1995.

457. Cambien, F., Poirier, O., Lecerf, L., et al.: Deletion polymorphism in the gene for angiotensin-converting enzyme is a potent risk factor for myocardial infarction. Nature *359*:641, 1992.

458. Fowkes, F. G. R., Connor, J. M., Smith, F. B., et al.: Fibrinogen genotype and risk for peripheral atherosclerosis. Lancet *339*:693, 1992.

459. Ishigami, T., Umemura, S., Iwamoto, T., et al.: Molecular variant of angiotensinogen gene is associated with coronary atherosclerosis. Circulation *91*:951, 1995.

460. Burke, W., and Motulsky, A. G.: Hypertension. *In* King, R. A., Rotter, J. I., and Motulsky, A. G. (eds.): The Genetic Basis of Common Diseases. New York, Oxford University Press, 1992, p. 170.

461. Murphy, E. A., and Pyeritz, R. D.: Homeostasis: VII. A conspectus. Am. J. Med. Genet. *24*:735, 1986.

462. Parmer, R. J., Cervenka, J. H., and Stone, R. A.: Baroflex sensitivity and heredity in essential hypertension. Circulation *85*:497, 1992.

463. Lifton, R. P.: Genetic factors in hypertension. Curr. Opin. Nephrol. Hyperten. *2*:258, 1993.

464. Jeunemaitre, X., and Corvol, P.: Hypertension. *In* Rimoin, D. L., Connor, J. M., and Pyeritz, R. E. (eds.): Principles and Practice of Medical Genetics. 3rd ed. New York, Churchill Livingstone, 1996.

465. Lindpainter, K.: Genes, hypertension and cardiac hypertrophy. N. Engl. J. Med. *330*:1678, 1994.

466. McKusick, V. A.: Genetics and the nature of essential hypertension. Circulation *22*:857, 1960.

467. Shimkets, R. A., Warnock, D. G., Bositis, C. M., et al.: Liddle's syndrome: Heritable human hypertension caused by mutations in the β subunit of the epithelial sodium channel. Cell *79*:407, 1994.

468. Gordon, R. G., Klemm, S. A., Tunny, T. J., et al.: Primary aldosteronism: Hypertension with a genetic basis. Lancet *340*:159, 1992.

469. Gordon, R. D.: Heterogeneous hypertension. Nature Genet. *11*:6, 1995.

470. Lifton, R. P., Dluhy, R. G., Powers, M., et al.: A chimeric 11β-hydroxylase/aldosterone synthase gene causes glucocorticoid-remediable aldosteronism and human hypertension. Nature *355*:262, 1992.

471. Hata, A., Namikawa, C., Sasaki, M., et al.: Angiotensinogen as a risk factor for essential hypertension in Japan. J. Clin. Invest. *93*:1285, 1994.

472. Jeunemaitre, X., Soubrier, F., Kotelevtsev, Y. V., et al.: Molecular basis of human hypertension: Role of angiotensinogen. Cell *71*:169, 1992.

473. Caulfield, M., Lavendar, P., Farral, M., et al.: Linkage of the angiotensinogen gene to essential hypertension. N. Engl. J. Med. *33*:1629, 1994.

474. Barley, J., Carter, N., Crews, D., et al.: Angiotensin 1 converting enzyme (ACE) polymorphism in different groups and its association with hypertension, plasma renin activity and aldosterone. J. Med. Genet. *31*:172, 1994.

475. Morris, B. J., Zee, R. Y. L., and Schrader, A. P.: Different frequencies of angiotensin-converting enzyme genotypes in older hypertensive individuals. J. Clin. Invest. *94*:1085, 1994.

476. Jacob, H. J., Lindpainter, K., Lincoln, S. E., et al.: Genetic mapping of a gene causing hypertension in the stroke-prone spontaneously hypertensive rat. Cell *67*:213, 1991.

477. John, S. W. M., Krege, J. H., Oliver, P. M., et al.: Genetic decreases in atrial natriuretic peptide and salt-sensitive hypertension. Science *267*:679, 1995.

478. Cohen, L. S., Friedman, J. M., Jefferson, J. W., et al.: A reevaluation of risk of in utero exposure to lithium. JAMA *271*:146, 1994.

Chapter 50
The Aging Heart: Structure, Function, and Disease

EDWARD G. LAKATTA, GARY GERSTENBLITH, MYRON L. WEISFELDT

STRUCTURE AND FUNCTION OF THE AGING HEART

AGING IN ANIMAL MODELS

Cellular and molecular mechanisms that account for age-associated changes in myocardial performance have been studied largely in rodents (see reference 34 for review). In the normotensive rat, cardiac fibrosis increases with aging,[1,2] the number of myocytes decreases (Fig. 50–1D),[2,3] and myocyte size increases.[4] Variable degrees of left ventricular hypertrophy occur,[5,6] depending on the rodent strain, and this is due to ventricular dilatation with apparent preservation of normal ventricular wall thickness.[1] Functional, biophysical/biochemical, pharmacological, and molecular changes occur in the aging rat heart (Table 50–1).

There are coordinated changes in several key steps of excitation-contraction coupling that result in a prolonged Ca_i transient and a prolonged contraction. The transmembrane action potential (Fig. 50–1A) is prolonged approximately twofold in cardiac muscle isolated from senescent 24-month rats, compared with younger adult 6- to 8-month rats.[8–10] The L type sarcolemmal Ca^{++} current is not substantially increased in magnitude but inactivates more slowly[10] and could possibly account, in part, for the prolonged transmembrane action potential. However, it is likely that changes in outwardly directed K^+ currents[10] substantially contribute to the transmembrane AP prolongation. The cytosolic Ca^{++} transient following excitation (Fig. 50–1C) is prolonged in senescent rats.[16] The rate of Ca^{++} sequestration by the sarcoplasmic reticulum decreases in the senescent myocardium (Fig. 50–2A), and this may in part explain the prolonged Ca_i transient (Fig. 12–12, p. 368).[17,18] A reduction in the mRNA coding for the sarcoplasmic reticular Ca^{++}-ATPase[29,30] suggests that the diminished Ca^{++} accumulation rate could, in part, be secondary to a decrease in the sarcoplasmic reticular pump site density.[18] The myofilament force response to Ca^{++} is not altered by age.[34] However, marked shifts occur in the myosin heavy chain in rodents, i.e., the β or V_3 isozyme becomes predominant in senescent rat (85 per cent β versus 15 per cent α). Steady-state messenger RNA levels for α- and β-MHC parallel the age-associated changes in the myosin heavy chain proteins V_1 and V_3, and thus the isoenzyme shift appears to be transcriptionally regulated. The myosin Ca^{++}-ATPase activity declines (Fig. 50–3A) with the decline in V_i content. The altered cellular profile, which results in a contraction that exhibits a reduced velocity (Fig. 50–3B) and a prolonged time course (Fig. 50–1B), can be considered to be adaptive rather than degenerative in nature because the reduced velocity is energy efficient and

prolonged contraction permits continued ejection for a longer period.[8,9,11,33]

Aggregate age-associated alterations in cytosolic Ca^{++} concentration, the Na-Ca exchanger, Na-K pump, and the sarcoplasmic reticular Ca^{++} pump, possibly in conjunction with nonspecific changes in sarcolemmal membrane ionic permeabilities, may predispose senescent myocardium to altered cell Ca^{++} homeostasis. Intriguingly, aged myocardium (and that chronically exposed to pressure overload) is more susceptible to Ca^{++} overload and spontaneous sarcoplasmic reticulum Ca^{++} release than is young adult myocardium.[17,33,35] Aged myocardium demonstrates a reduced Ca^{++} threshold for diastolic afterdepolarizations and for ventricular fibrillation.[35] The former is caused by and the latter is preceded by an increase in spontaneous sarcoplasmic reticular oscillatory Ca^{++} release.[35]

Studies in isolated left ventricular muscle (Fig. 50–4A) and in individual rat ventricular cardiocytes, similar to recent studies in humans,[36,37] (Fig. 50–4B) indicate that a reduced contractile response to β_1-AR stimulation occurs with aging. This is due to failure of the intracellular Ca^{++} transient to increase in cells of senescent hearts to the same extent to which it increases in cells from younger adult hearts.[26] The blunted increase in the Ca^{++} transient in cells from the aged heart is attributed to a decrease in the ability of β_1-AR stimulation to increase L type sarcolemmal Ca^{++} channel availability in cells from senescent versus younger adult hearts[26] (Fig. 50–4B). The richly documented age-associated reduction in the postsynaptic response of myocardial cells to β_1-AR stimulation appears to be due to multiple changes in molecular and biochemical receptor coupling and postreceptor mechanisms rather than to a major modification of a single rate-limiting step, as might occur, for example, in a genetic defect (see reference 33 for review).

The multiple changes in cardiac excitation, myofilament activation, contraction mechanisms, and gene expression that occur with aging (Figs. 50–1 through 50–4 and Table 50–1) are interrelated. Many of these can be interpreted as adaptive in nature because they also occur in the hypertrophied myocardium of younger animals adapted to experimentally induced chronic hypertension[11,25,38–44] (Table 50–2). There is some evidence to suggest that the adaptive response to chronic passive loading declines with aging,[45–51] possibly in part because some of the adaptive capacity of the heart is used as a response to the aging process per se. Chronic exercise in older animals reverses some of the alterations in the cardiac function (prolonged contraction, reduced sarcoplasmic reticular function) that occur with aging.[12,18,23,43,52–55] Other aspects of cardiac func-

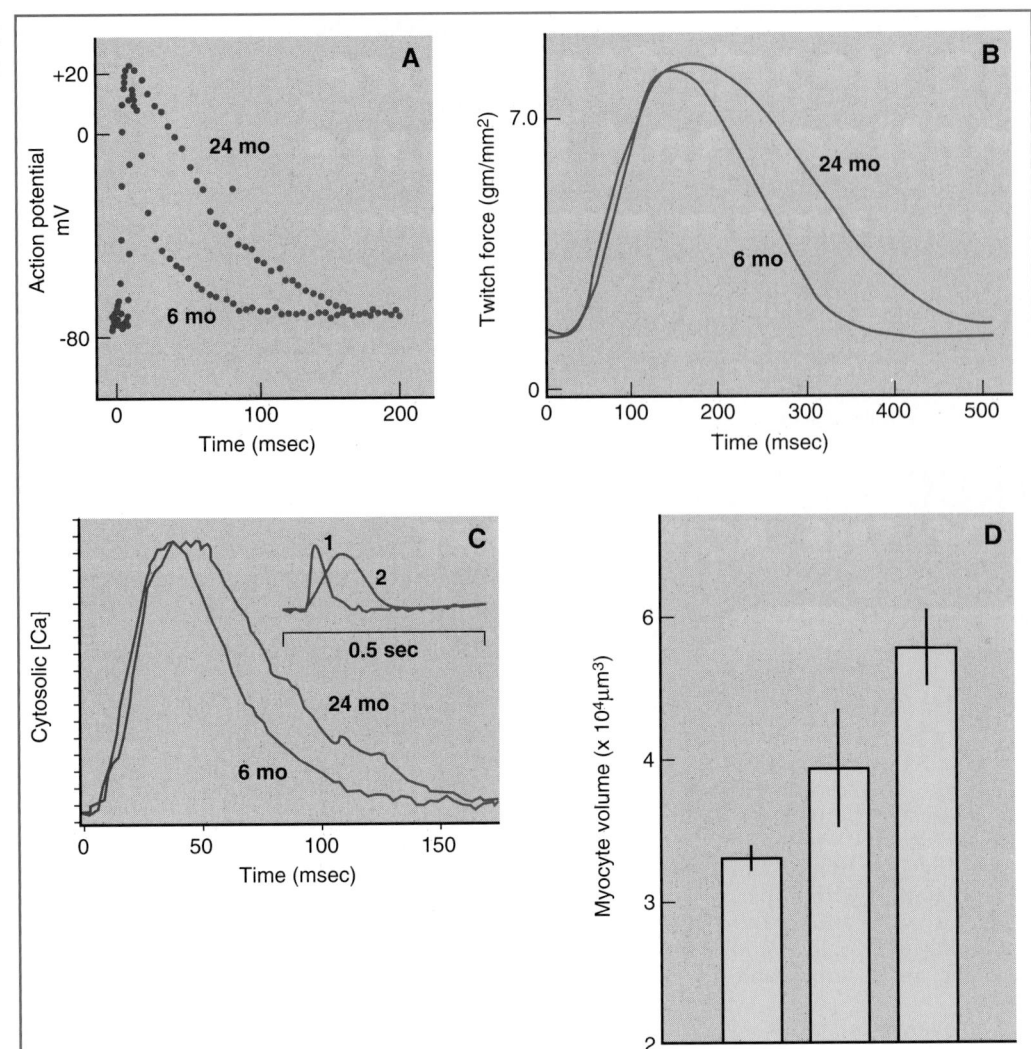

FIGURE 50–1. Action potential (Panel A), isometric twitch (Panel B), and Ca$_i$ transient (Panel C), measured via aequorin luminescence, in isometric right ventricular papillary muscles isolated from the hearts of young adult and senescent Wistar rats. Inset in Panel C indicates the time course of the Ca$_i$ transient[1] relative to that of the contraction.[2] (Panels A and B from Wei, J. Y., Spurgeon, H. A., and Lakatta, E. G.: Excitation-contraction in rat myocardium: Alterations with adult aging. Am. J. Physiol. *246*:H784, 1984. Panel C from Orchard, C. H., and Lakatta, E. G.: Intracellular calcium transients and developed tensions in rat heart muscle. A mechanism for the negative interval-strength relationship. J. Gen. Physiol. *86*:637, 1985.) Panel D, Left ventricular cell volume (single cells, isolated via collagenase dissection of hearts) measured via Coulter Counter technique increases with age. (Panel D from Fraticelli, A., Josephson, R., Danziger, R., et al.: Morphological and contractile characteristics of rat cardiac myocytes from maturation to senescence. Am. J. Physiol. *257*:H259, 1989.)

TABLE 50–1   MYOCARDIAL CHANGES WITH ADULT AGING

STRUCTURAL Δ	FUNCTIONAL Δ	IONIC, BIOPHYSICAL/BIOCHEMICAL MECHANISM(S)	MOLECULAR MECHANISMS
↑ Myocyte size[4]	Prolonged contraction[7–9]	Prolonged cystosolic Ca^{++} transient[16]	
↓ Myocyte number[2,3]		↓ SR Ca^{++} pumping rate[17,18]	↓ SR Ca^{++} pump mRNA[29,30]
		↓ Pump site density[18]	No Δ calsequestrin mRNA[29]
	Prolonged action[8–10] potential	↓ I$_{Ca}$ inactivation[10]	
		↓ I$_{To}$ density[10]	
	Diminished contraction[11] velocity	↓ α MHC protein[19,20]	↓ α MHC mRNA[17,19,31,32]
		↑ β MHC protein[19,20]	↑ β MHC mRNA[19,31,32]
		↓ Myosin ATPase activity[8,18,20,21]	No Δ actin mRNA[33]
	Diminished β-adrenergic contractile response	↓ Coupling BAR-acyclase[22,23]	
		↓ TNI phosphorylation[24]	
		↓ Phospholamban phosphorylation[25]	
		↓ I$_{Ca}$ augmentation[26]	
		↓ Ca$_i$ transient augmentation[26]	
		↑ Enkephalin peptides[27]	↑ Proenkephalin mRNA[27]
↑ Matrix connective tissue[1,2]	↑ Myocardial stiffness[12–15]	↑ Atrial natriuretic peptide[28]	↑ Atrial natriuretic peptide mRNA[28]

Δ = change; ↑ = increased; ↓ = decreased.

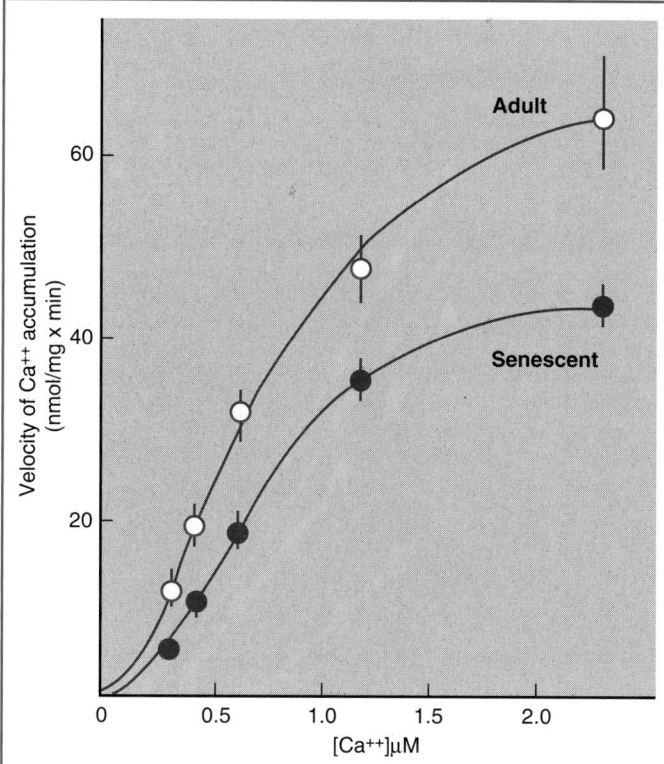

FIGURE 50–2. The effect of age on Ca⁺⁺ accumulation velocity by sarcoplasmic reticulum isolated from senescent and adult Wistar rat hearts. (From Froehlich, J. P., Lakatta, E. G., Beard, E., et al.: Studies of sarcoplasmic reticulum function and contraction duration in young adult and aged rat myocardium. J. Mol. Cell. Cardiol. *10:*427, 1978.)

tion that change with aging (e.g., prolonged action potential, altered myosin isoform expression[18]) are not affected by chronic exercise.

NORMAL AGING HUMANS

Age changes in cardiac function in humans can be understood only by strictly segregating normal aging from the interplay of aging and disease. This is of importance be-

TABLE 50–2 ALTERED MYOCARDIAL GENE EXPRESSION IN ADVANCED AGE, HYPERTENSION, HEART FAILURE, OR AFTER GROWTH FACTORS*

| | RODENT | | GROWTH FACTORS† | | |
| | | | | FGF | |
	Aging	Hypertension	TGFβ	Acidic	Basic
SR Ca⁺⁺-ATPase	↓	↓	↓	↓	↓
Calsequestrin	↔		↔		
Phospholamban		↑ (rabbit)			
α-Major histocompatibility complex	↓	↓	↓	↓	↓
β-Major histocompatibility complex	↑	↑	↑	↑	↑
β Tropomyosin	↓	↑ ‡			
α Skeletal actin	↓	↑ §	↑	↓	↑
Atrial natriuretic factor	↑	↑	↑	↑	↑
Proenkephalin	↑				

* See references 33 and 34 for review.
† In neonatal cultured cardiocytes.
‡ In atrial tissue.
§ Only transient changes occur in situ following cardiac pressure loading.
SR = Sarcoplasmic reticulum.

cause most forms of acquired heart disease increase in frequency and severity with age.

Observed age changes in cardiovascular function in human subjects selected for the absence of demonstrable cardiovascular disease are direct extensions of the principal physiological changes that are documented in the experimental laboratory.[33] The major features of cardiac physiology in experimental animals that are well maintained with age are intrinsic cardiac muscle function under conditions of moderate stress and coronary perfusion. In males, studies using echocardiography and gated blood pool scans consistently show, in well-selected populations, only a small age-associated increase in left ventricular end-diastolic volume and end-systolic volume at rest, and therefore little change in ejection fraction.[56] Women show no increase in end-diastolic or end-systolic volume with age. During beta-adrenergic blockade there are no major age differences at rest.[57] Recent studies in several catheterization laboratories[58] measuring coronary sinus blood flow in subjects without coronary artery disease or other forms of heart disease show that maximal coronary vasodilating capacity or flow is unchanged with age. At rest, probably due to mild hypertrophy, coronary blood flow may increase slightly with age under physiological noncoronary vasodilated states.[58] Endothelial-dependent vasodilation is reduced with age, but the response to direct smooth muscle vasodilators is unchanged.[59]

In humans, as in experimental animals, there is evidence of modest left ventricular hypertrophy with age[60] (Fig. 50–5). In animal models, pressure load or impedance-induced hypertrophy results in prolonged cardiac muscle relaxation and the expected decrease in early left ventricular diastolic filling and maximal diastolic filling rates. The age-associated increase in impedance to left ventricular ejection is associated with left ventricular hypertrophy and prolonged relaxation. This age change in relaxation has important implications when the issue of aging and disease is addressed. With regard to normal cardiac physiology and response to exercise, there is no evidence that this prolonged relaxation has any detrimental effects on overall left ventricular function and capacity to augment cardiac performance during exercise. This is in part related to the slower heart rate during exercise, which allows a longer diastolic filling time and some sympathetic-induced increased relaxation rate during exercise. As a result, there is less potential for incomplete left ventricular relaxation between contractions.

As discussed in detail below, there are major and obvious age-associated changes in the hemodynamic response to exercise in humans without cardiovascular disease. These are entirely consistent with the two underlying mechanisms described in animals with age. The first is an age-associated increase in left ventricular load or impedance that results from stiffening of the central arterial system and the second is a decrease in general beta-sympathetic response leading to reduced augmentation of heart rate and contractility, or inotropic state, of ventricular myocardium and to diminished arterial vasodilation.

Increased Impedance to Left Ventricular Ejection

One of the most universally documented age changes in humans is the increase in pulse wave velocity within the arterial system (Fig. 50–6). The pulse wave is the rise in arterial pressure in the central aorta during left ventricular ejection of blood. This pressure wave travels in the central arterial system toward the brain, arms, and feet much faster in older than in younger individuals. This increase is quite linear with age, beginning essentially at birth and extending beyond 80 years of age.[61,62] Such changes in pulse wave velocity have been measured in many civilizations and cultures, both in populations in which hypertension and

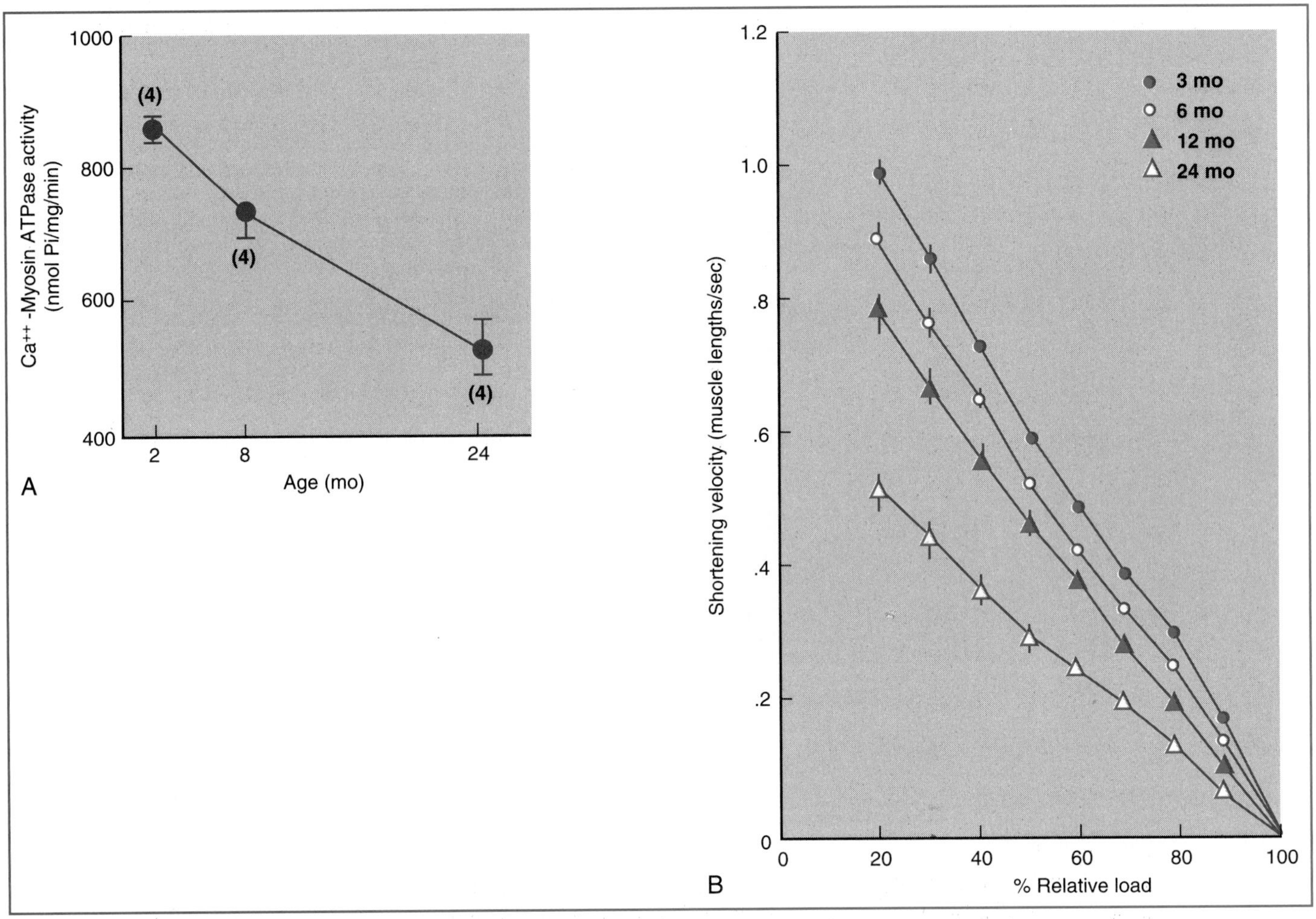

FIGURE 50–3. Panel A, Ca⁺⁺-activated myosin ATPase activity of Wistar rat hearts decreases with age. (From Effron, M. B., Bhatnagar, G. M., Spurgeon, H. A., et al.: Changes in myosin isoenzymes, ATPase activity, and contraction duration in rat cardiac muscle with aging can be modulated by thyroxine. Circ. Res. *60:*238, 1987.) Panel B, The velocity of shortening during lightly loaded isotonic contractions in isolated cardiac muscle from younger and older rats decreases with aging. (From Capasso, J. M., Malhotra, A., Remily, R. M., et al.: Effects of age on mechanical and electrical performance of rat myocardium. Am. J. Physiol. *245:*H72, 1983.)

atherosclerotic disease are prevalent and populations in which these disorders of the arterial vasculature are unusual.

This increase in pulse wave velocity is a reflection of changes in the compliance properties of the central arteries[63] due to age-associated alterations in the precise structure and composition of the collagen and ground substance in and around the blood vessels themselves. Some age-associated dilation of these arteries also occurs.[60] Thus, the artery functions on a stiffer portion of its pressure-volume relationship. Although one might speculate that these changes in aortic stiffness are due to alterations in the smooth muscle structure or function or to properties of the central arterial system, this evidence against this idea exists in experimental animals. Aortic and arterial rings have equal vasodilating properties when the arteries are stimulated with nitrates or other stimulants of the effects of endothelial-derived relaxing factor on vascular tone. There is some evidence of decreased endothelial-mediated vasodilation,[59] thus implying decreased endothelial vasodilator production, not response, with age.

Because the left ventricle is ejecting blood into a stiffer central aorta, the systolic blood pressure tends to be higher in older individuals, even the absence of disease. The higher systolic pressure in older individuals is even greater in the central aorta than it is in the periphery. This is because of the central superimposition of the direct pressure wave from ejection of blood from the left ventricle and

the reflected wave returning to the central aorta from the periphery. O'Rourke demonstrated quite clearly in humans that the forward pulse wave in the arterial system reflects off the iliac bifurcation much like an ocean wave reflects off a dock.[64] In the case of the iliac bifurcation, the reflected wave moves backwards toward the central aorta. The actual movement of the direct pulse wave, as well as the reflected wave, is so much faster than in the central aorta there is superimposition of the direct and reflected waves *during* left ventricular ejection. In younger individuals, the reflected wave does not return to the central aorta until after aortic valve closure.

EFFECTS OF EXERCISE. The increase in left ventricular load is greater with age during exercise because of diminished arterial vasodilation mediated by beta-adrenergic receptor. Studies in chronically instrumented animals demonstrate that in the younger animal arterial vasodilation prevents an increase in impedance to left ventricular ejection during exercise, whereas in the older animal there is a further increase in impedance to ejection as exercise progresses (Fig. 50–7). This reflects a failure of beta-sympathetic–induced arterial vasodilatation.[65] After pharmacological beta blockade, young animals as well show an increase in impedance to left ventricular ejection of blood during exercise (Fig. 50–7). In a number of important respects exercise response is quite similar in adult and aged animals following beta-adrenergic blockade. This also appears to be the case in humans.

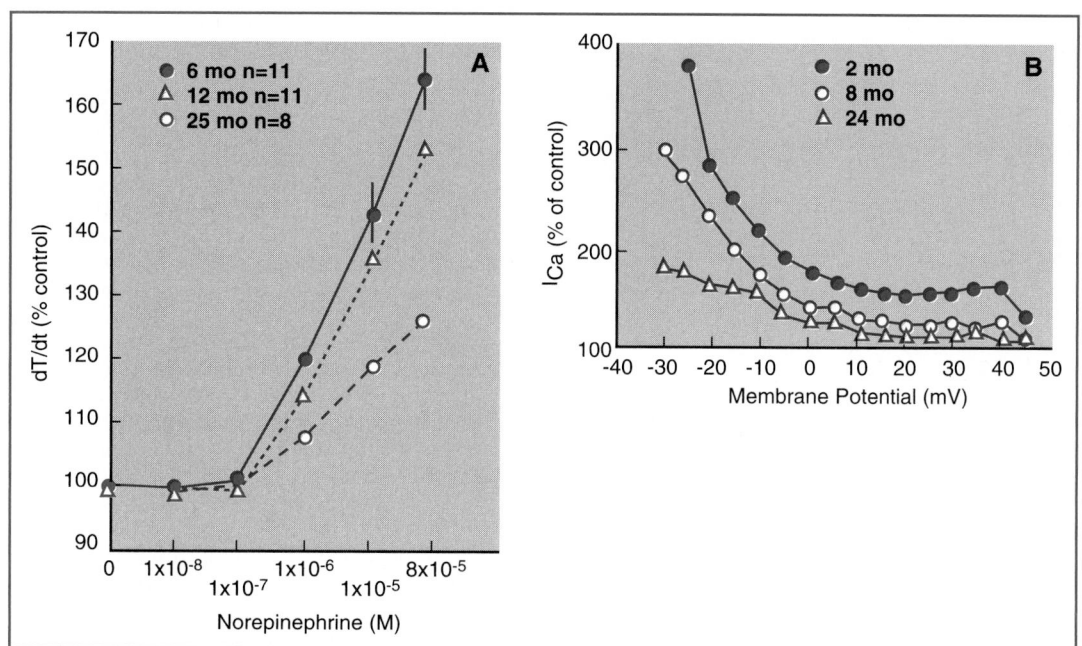

FIGURE 50–4. *A,* The effect of norepinephrine on the maximum rate of isometric tension development in isolated trabeculae from hearts of varying age. (Reproduced with permission from Lakatta, E. G., Gerstenblith, G., Angell, C. S., et al.: Diminished inotropic response of aged myocardium to catecholamines. Circ. Res. *36:*262, 1975. Copyright 1975 American Heart Association.) *B,* The effect of norepinephrine to increase the L type sarcolemmal channel current (I_{Ca}) across a range of activating steps to different membrane potentials in single vascular cells potential decline with aging, the norepinephrine concentration was 1×10^{-7} M. (From Xiao, R.-P., Spurgeon, H. A., O'Connor, F., and Lakatta, E. G.: Age-associated changes in β-adrenergic modulation on rat cardiac excitation-contraction coupling. J. Clin. Invest. *94:*2051, 1994, by permission of the American Society for Clinical Investigation.)

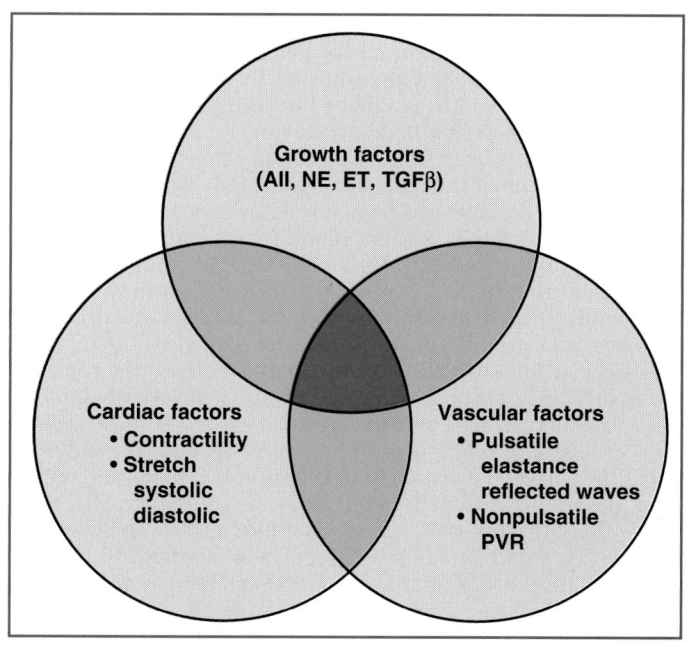

FIGURE 50–5. Acute and chronic regulation of myocardial function and structure. Cardiac factors (Ca^{++} activation of myofilaments, in part, regulated by fiber stretch prior to excitation) and vascular factors (peripheral vascular resistance [PVR], arterial elastance, and reflexed pulse waves) interact to determine the acute workload placed upon the heart and thus acutely modulate cardiac performance. Chronic increases in cardiac workload, due to any of the specific entities depicted within the cardiac and vascular factors, and growth factors interact to determine cardiac mass and long-term changes in cardiac function that accompany changes in cardiac structure. (AII = angiotensin II, NE = norepinephrine; ET = endothelin; TGFβ = transforming growth factor beta.)

STUDY OF AGE CHANGES IN CARDIAC FUNCTION IN THE ABSENCE OF DISEASE

Studies of "normal aging" are handicapped by an understandable reluctance to use invasive methodology in people who are thought to be free of cardiovascular disease. This resulted in two major limitations in some earlier work. First, it was difficult to exclude patients with occult coronary disease. This is an important consideration because the prevalence of autopsy-documented disease is much higher than the presence of clinically obvious disease.[66] Many individuals thought to be free of coronary disease on screening using routine history, physical examination, and resting electrocardiogram undoubtedly were not, and many older study participants with asymptomatic coronary disease were probably included as normal in the

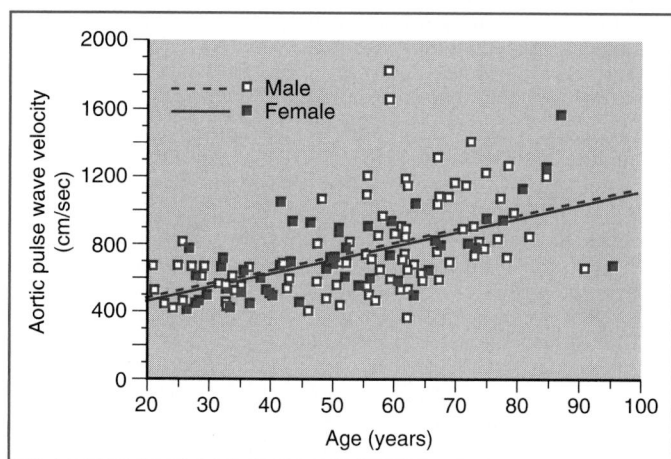

FIGURE 50–6. Aortic pulse wave velocity, an index of aortic stiffness, increases with age in healthy participants. (Reproduced with permission from Vaitkevicius, P. V., Fleg, J. L., Engel, J. H., et al.: Effects of age and aerobic capacity on arterial stiffness in healthy adults. Circulation *88:*1456, 1993. Copyright 1993 American Heart Association.)

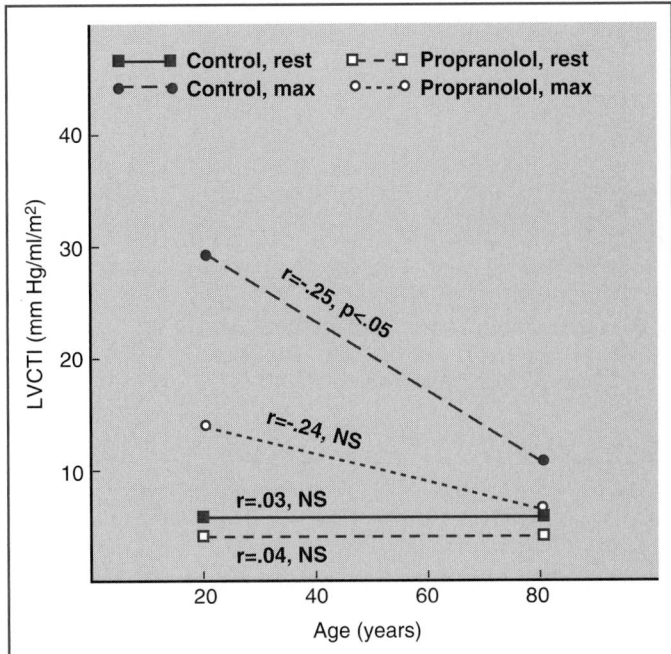

FIGURE 50–7. Left ventricular contractility index (LVCTI) measured as the ratio of end-systolic arterial pressure and end-systolic volume index. Lines are the best fit, linear regressions at rest and during exercise in the presence and absence of β-adrenergic blockade with propranolol. (From Fleg, J. L., O'Connor, F., Gerstenblith, G., et al.: Impact of age on the cardiovascular response to dynamic upright exercise in healthy men and women. J. Appl. Physiol. *78:*890, 1995.)

study protocols. This problem was overcome in a series of studies on well-selected and tested members of the Baltimore Longitudinal Study of Aging at the National Institute of Aging.[67,68]

The second limitation resulting from the hesitancy to use invasive methodology was an inability to measure central circulatory function (stroke volume or its determinants, left ventricular end-diastolic and end-systolic volumes) in relatively large numbers and volunteers. Previous studies used mainly Fick principle determination of cardiac output and derived only stroke volume. The introduction of nuclear cardiology and echocardiographic techniques, and the use of thallium scintigraphy to diagnose the presence of coronary disease, led to remarkable progress. Echocardiography and gated blood pool scans are able to estimate cardiac volume throughout the cardiac cycle at rest and during exercise, and thus have provided significant information concerning the effect of normal aging on cardiac function at rest and during stress.[56,69-72]

Hemodynamics at Rest

Although studies performed 30 years ago indicated that aging is associated with a decline in cardiac output at rest in men,[73] these results may have been due to selection of subjects not free of disease. Several of the studies involved hospitalized or disabled subjects not known to have alterations in resting cardiac function that are not age-related but rather condition-related. Studies using both echocardiography and gated blood pool scans at rest with and without beta-adrenergic blockade show that seated men at rest show a modest increase in the end-diastolic, end-systolic, and stroke volumes with age, but these volumes are not changed by aging in females (Fig. 50–8A). Once more, it should be emphasized that the most significant age-associated change in resting cardiovascular parameters is the increase in systolic blood pressure (Fig. 50–8F) with aortic dilation. As discussed above, this change is secondary to the age-associated increase in arterial stiffness and is likely responsible, at least in part, for the mild left ventricular hypertrophy associated with aging. Thus, the near-normal left ventricular volumes and preserved ejection fraction in seated persons at rest reflect the balance between the mild hypertrophy and the increase in vascular load and left ventricular size. At least in theory, normalized left ventricular

wall stress may be preserved through this mild left ventricular hypertrophy.

Prolonged relaxation of cardiac muscle at rest with aging is reflected in these same studies using gated cardiac blood pool scanning techniques.[74] There is a decrease in the maximum rate of early diastolic filling, and, similarly, Doppler-recorded velocity of blood flow through the mitral valve during early diastole is also reduced.[75] Slowed early diastolic filling with age leads to greater contribution of atrial contraction to diastolic filling and the appearance of the "normal" S_4 sound and atrial enlargement.

Exercise Performance in the Elderly

One of the most universally accepted changes with aging is a decline in maximum work performance, which has as a consequence a decline in maximum oxygen consumption.[76] Many have interpreted this age-associated decrease in maximum work capacity and oxygen consumption to be a reflection of diminished cardiovascular performance and the ability of the heart to augment cardiac output during exercise. The reduction in maximum heart rate during exercise in older individuals, even following endurance training, support this.[77] However, noncardiac factors also contribute to the age-associated decline in maximum work capacity. These include a decline in maximum skeletal muscle performance parameters, a greater sense of muscle fatigue and discomfort, and/or a marked increase in the sensation of the work of breathing or dyspnea. Cardiovascular function is thought to limit oxygen consumption when oxygen consumption does not consistently increase at the highest levels of exercise. With aging, oxygen consumption often increases progressively with increasing workload performance. Data of this type raise the possibility that maximum work capacity in the elderly is limited by either skeletal muscle fatigue (or sense of fatigue) or the increased work of breathing. It is possible that differences in muscle mass, less diversion of blood flow to the exercising muscle, and/or reduced oxygen extraction may also be limiting factors. Age differences in maximum oxygen consumption are minimized when the values are adjusted for lean body mass.[78]

The mechanism for achieving the augmentation of cardiac output differs markedly with age. First, younger individuals augment heart rate considerably more than do older individuals, reflecting the age-associated decrease in the chronotropic response to beta-sympathetic stimulation (Fig. 50–8D). With gated cardiac blood pool scans, it is clear that the stroke volume in both male and female older individuals is maintained by end-diastolic dilatation. In contrast, end-diastolic volume in younger individuals does not increase measurably during vigorous exercise. Also, end-diastolic volume becomes exceedingly small in the younger individual, almost at the limits of the measurement techniques, whereas end-systolic volume in older individuals fails to decrease markedly (Fig. 50–8B). In younger individuals the marked sympathetic response at maximum workload maintains a small heart size and a high heart rate. Even though systemic blood pressure rises, end-systolic volume is small because of increased contractility. This response in the young is also aided by beta-sympathetic–central arterial vasodilatation, decreasing the impedance to left ventricular ejection of blood during exercise. The marked augmentation of heart rate (Fig. 50–8D) and relaxation velocity by beta-sympathetic stimulation allows the heart rate of the younger individual to increase from approximately one beat per second to three beats per second without compromising filling, and with each beat essentially ejecting the entire contents of the left ventricle into the aorta.

Age-Related Changes in Sympathetic Modulation

The impact of beta-adrenergic modulation of heart rate and cardiac volume during exercise can be determined

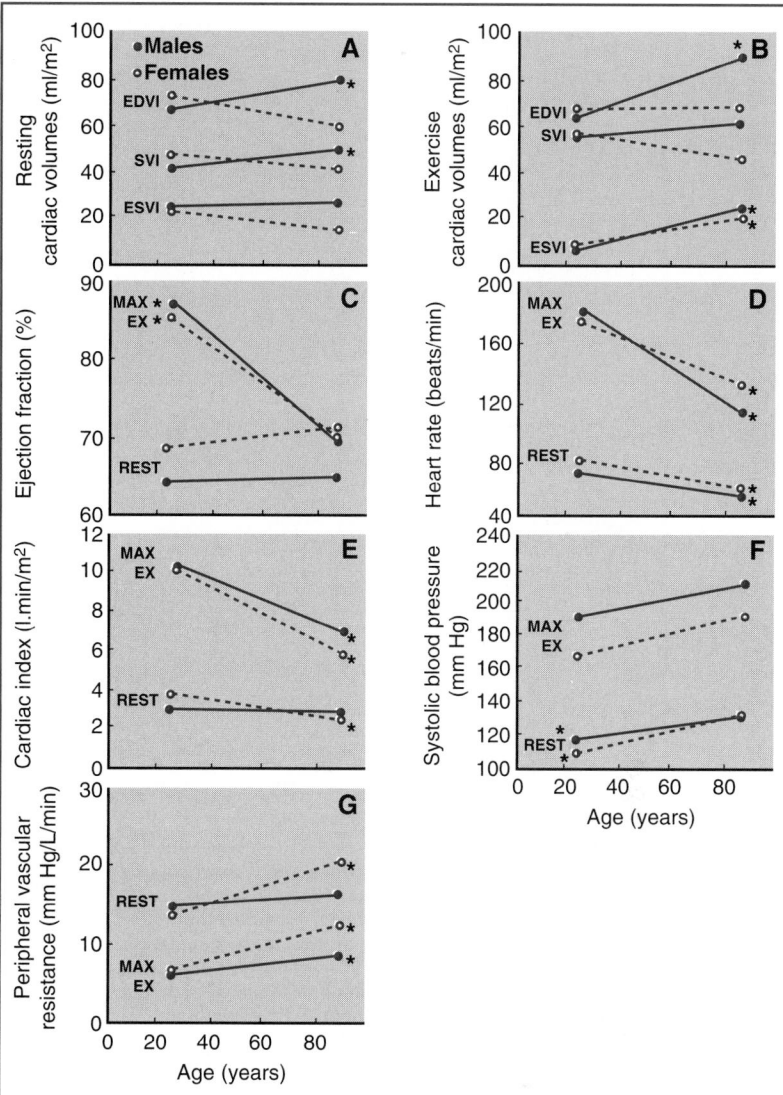

FIGURE 50–8. Linear regression on age of cardiac volume indices (A, at rest; B, during exercise) and ejection fraction (C), heart rate (D), cardiac index (E), systolic arterial pressure (F), and peripheral vascular resistance (G) at rest and during maximum cycle ergometry in the upright position. Study participants were healthy, sedentary male (n = 95, closed symbols) and female (n = 50, open symbols), community-dwelling volunteers who had been rigorously screened to exclude clinical hypertension and occult coronary artery disease. Cardiac volumes were measured via gated blood-pool scans. *Linear regression on age within sex is statistically significant. EDVI = end-diastolic volume index, ESVI = end-systolic volume index, SVI = stroke volume index, MAX EX = maximum exercise. (Age-gender interactions are described in Fleg, J. L., O'Connor, F., Gerstenblith, G., et al.: Impact of age on the cardiovascular response to dynamic upright exercise in healthy men and women. J. Appl. Physiol. *78*:890, 1995.)

when exercise is performed in the presence of beta adrenergic blockade. In young individuals, the same cardiac output is achieved during upright cycle exercise in the presence and absence of acute beta blockade with propranolol, but the hemodynamic profile differs: The increment in heart rate and the reduction in end-systolic volume are markedly less in the presence of beta blockade. However, the end-diastolic volume increases substantially during beta blockade, permitting a larger stroke volume.[57] The rate of early left ventricular filling and myocardial contractility are reduced. This altered hemodynamic pattern during acute beta blockade indicates the interaction among parameters that maintain cardiac output when a deficit in adrenergic modulation is present. Cardiac dilatation at end diastole augments stroke volume, which compensates for a reduction in heart rate.

An age-associated diminution in the effectiveness of sympathetic modulation of the cardiovascular response to exercise could contribute to many of the changes identified in the cardiovascular response to exercise in healthy older humans (Figs. 50–7, 50–8, and 50–9), including the decline in maximum heart rate, the increases in left ventricular end-diastolic and end-systolic volume indices, and decreased ejection fraction and left ventricular contractility. A recent study, in fact, demonstrated that the age-associated changes in left ventricular end-diastolic volume and stroke volume indices during upright cycle exercise do not occur in the presence of blockade and that the age-associated reduction in heart rate is markedly attenuated because of a

greater effect of beta-adrenergic blockade to decrease heart rate and increase heart size in younger, rather than in older, subjects.[57] Age differences in the early diastolic filling rate and left ventricular contractility (Fig. 50–7) during exercise are also reduced or abolished when exercise is performed during beta-adrenergic blockade.[74] Thus, during stress the older heart is confronted with an increased impedance to ejection and greater venous return. The response is increased work performance, despite decreased contractility and heart rate, by left ventricular dilation during diastole. The Frank-Starling mechanism operates to augment stroke work and volume and meet the peripheral demands for increased blood flow (Fig. 50–9).

INTEGRATED RESPONSE TO EXERCISE

Thus, the overall picture of the cardiovascular response to exercise is entirely consistent with animal and human studies approaching aging as a selective process. Coronary perfusion and left ventricular function are well maintained with age, predicting that older individuals should be able to employ the Frank-Starling mechanism to augment cardiac function when other mechanisms fail. Cellular hypertrophy with age is clearly a helpful factor in maintaining left ventricular function. Although prolonged relaxation and delayed filling are present, in association with pressure overload hypertrophy, there is no evidence that left ventricular filling during exercise is compromised. Because end-diastolic volume is greater, end-diastolic pressure may be higher, and contribute to dyspnea and the increased work of breathing in older individuals. Finally, stiffening of central arteries with age and greater pulse wave velocity and earlier reflected waves increase the left ventricular workload during exercise more in the elderly than in the younger individual. This increase in load also reflects the diminished beta-sympathetic arterial vasodilat-

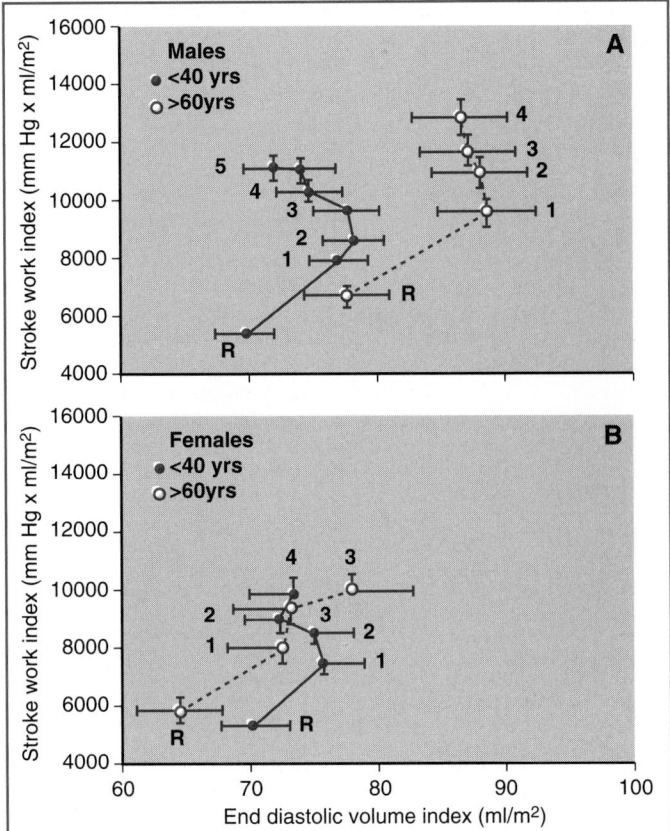

FIGURE 50–9. Left ventricular stroke work index (SWI) measured as the product of stroke volume index (SVI) and brachial systolic pressure at rest and during graded exercise in younger (< 40 yr) and older (>60 yr) men *(top),* and women *(bottom)* of the study population depicted in Figure 17.7. R = seated rest. 1–5 = progressive increases in submaximal workload affected by increasing resistance to peddling on a cycle ergometer. (From Fleg, J. L., O'Connor, F., Gerstenblith, G., et al.: Impact of age on the cardiovascular response to dynamic upright exercise in healthy men and women. J. Appl. Physiol. *78*:890, 1995.)

ing response. In summary, the lower heart rate response and inotropic response and the increase in left ventricular workload due to arterial stiffness is compensated for by the intrinsic Frank-Starling mechanism in a remarkable and predictable manner in the elderly. During the transition from normal aging to aging and disease, it can easily be conceptualized that the older heart, using the Frank-Starling mechanism during exercise, has no further reserve. All of the compensatory mechanisms available to augment cardiac output are used during normal exercise. Thus, it would not be surprising if older individuals with a given severity of cardiovascular disease did worse during exercise than younger individuals who can utilize the Starling reserve mechanism after sympathetic reserve is exhausted.

EJECTION FRACTION AT REST AND DURING EXERCISE. It is of clinical interest that left ventricular ejection fraction increases during exercise in both young and old individuals who are free of disease. The exercise ejection fraction is greater in younger individuals, 80 to 90 per cent, than in older individuals, 60 to 80 per cent, respectively. This difference is due to a greater decrease in end-systolic volume in younger individuals than in older individuals during exercise. Recent studies in men and women during exercise at various ages indicate that the changes described above are more pronounced in older men than in older women.[51] It is not clear whether hormonal factors have an influence in the specific populations under study. In both young and old, a decline in ejection fraction during exercise is an abnormal response and is suggestive of the presence of disease.

Finally, the age-associated alterations in exercise response are not attributable to decreased catecholamine elaboration during exercise, because plasma levels of catecholamines are higher, not lower, in older humans during exercise.[79]

EFFECTS OF CHRONIC PHYSICAL CONDITIONING ON AEROBIC RESERVE

There is mounting evidence that some of the cardiovascular structural and functional changes that occur with aging in healthy humans can be modified by chronic exercise. The age-associated increases in pulse wave velocity and carotid pulse pressure augmentation are blunted in exercise-trained older individuals.[61,80] Additionally, it has recently been shown that arterial stiffness varies inversely with aerobic capacity in a healthy sedentary study population across a broad age range. This inverse relationship occurred over and above the effects of age to increase arterial stiffness and to decrease aerobic capacity.[61]

ENDURANCE TRAINING. In younger men, endurance training blunts the baroreceptor response, measured as the change in heart rate relative to arterial pressure during phenylephrine infusion or during lower body negative pressure.[81] In contrast, in healthy, rigorously screened sedentary middle-aged and older men, strenuous prolonged endurance training, sufficient to elicit large increases in maximal exercise capacity and small reductions in resting heart rate, appears to increase cardiac vagal tone at rest and not to alter arterial baroreflex control of heart rate, but it does result in a diminished forearm vasoconstrictor response to reductions in baroreflex sympatho-inhibition.[82] In endurance-trained older (60 to 80 years) individuals during lower body negative pressure, end-diastolic volume, stroke volume, and arterial pressure are better preserved than in age-matched controls.[83] This contrasts with a reduction in stroke volume during lower body negative pressure in young endurance-trained versus young sedentary individuals.[84]

In most[74,85–88] but not all studies, early diastolic left ventricular filling in chronically endurance-trained older men is slowed and similar to their sedentary age peers. Thus, slowed early diastolic filling appears to be intrinsic to normative aging and not secondary to the reduction in aerobic capacity accompanying the aging process.

Changes in both central and peripheral reflex mechanisms utilized during acute dynamic exercise occur with chronic endurance training in older individuals.[70,89,90] After high-intensity training of older (60 to 69 years of age) individuals for 10 months to 1 year, $\dot{V}O_{2max}$ increased by about 20 per cent (25.4 to 32.9 ml/kg/min). This was achieved primarily by an increase in peripheral oxygen utilization during treadmill exercise, manifested by an increase in estimated arteriovenous oxygen difference, with little increase in estimated maximum cardiac output.[77] In contrast, a study using the acetylene rebreathing method reported that stroke volume at peak *treadmill* exercise increased by 15 per cent in older (64 years) men following 12 months of endurance training.[53] This was accompanied by a 7 per cent increase in arteriovenous O_2 difference. In women, in contrast to men, increased $\dot{V}O_{2max}$ accompanying the training effect was achieved exclusively by an increase in exercise arteriovenous O_2 difference, as neither peak stroke volume nor maximum heart rate increased.[89]

In another study, similarly aged individuals (60 to 70 years), whose $\dot{V}O_{2max}$ increased by about 25 per cent (29.6 to 37.2 ml/kg/min) following training, had an 18 per cent increase in maximum cardiac output during *supine* cycle exercise. This increase in cardiac output following chronic endurance training was achieved by an increase in stroke volume, due to an increase in end-diastolic volume and to a greater reduction in end-systolic volume, resulting in augmentation of the ejection fraction achieved during exercise. As arterial pressure during the supine exercise testing was not affected by conditioning, the enhanced ejection fraction and reduced end-systolic volume after conditioning have been interpreted to reflect an increase in myocardial contractility induced by conditioning. A peculiarity of this study is that the estimated arteriovenous oxygen did not increase following exercise, in contrast to observations in similar training paradigms.[77] This may relate to the supine body position during this more recent study.[89] In contrast to the above study, less intense exercise paradigms in older individuals may not enhance cardiac performance (increased ejection fraction or reduced end-systolic volume) during cycle ergometry.[90]

In summary, it is quite clear that the aerobic capacity of both middle-aged and older individuals can increase following endurance training and that this is mediated by adaptations in both peripheral and cardiac mechanisms.

Conclusions

The mechanisms involved in the cardiovascular response to exercise are directly related to the age-associated alterations in central arterial stiffness and diminished sympathetic response. This is also true for the response to disease states such as congestive heart failure in which there is an increased emphasis on the importance of vasodilation in the elderly. Impedance to left ventricular ejection is markedly increased with age and dominates the clinical picture and potentially the therapeutic options available. The aging heart with its modest hypertrophy and consequent prolonged relaxation is, as most pressure-hypertrophied hearts, perhaps more sensitive to ischemic injury with more profound consequences.

The fact that cardiac function of younger individuals in the presence of beta blockade appears similar to that of older individuals supports the conclusion that the major factor contributing to age change in the cardiovascular system is a decreased beta-sympathetic response. During beta-adrenergic blockade, the cardiovascular response to exercise in young and old is very similar, with the Frank-Starling mechanism available to augment stroke volume.

Finally, the aged heart may be slower, or may have decreased capacity to hypertrophy and modify structure in response to long-term changes in load. This decreased hypertrophy response to hemodynamic stress may result in the decreased ability of the older heart to tolerate obstructive aortic valvular disease and/or alterations in left ventricular function such as acute myocardial infarction. Many other factors may change with age to a modest degree that does not interfere with physiological function. The fundamental mechanisms for the age-associated decrease in beta-sympathetic response and the decrease in hypertrophy response to stress remain to be entirely elucidated, although with regard to the sympathetic response, there appear to be mechanisms operating on a number of different levels, both at the receptor and within the myocardial or smooth muscle cell.

HEART DISEASE IN THE ELDERLY

Cardiovascular diseases, e.g., atherosclerosis, hypertension, heart failure, and stroke, reach epidemic proportions among older persons and, in this regard, are indicative of a failure of modern cardiology and medicine. One way to conceptualize why the clinical manifestations and the prognosis of these diseases worsen with age is that in older individuals the specific pathophysiological mechanisms that cause clinical disorders are superimposed on heart and vascular substrates that are modified by aging per se (Fig. 50–10). Imagine that age increases as one moves from the lower to the upper part of the figure, and that the line bisecting the top and bottom parts represents the clinical practice "threshold" for disease recognition. Thus, entities above the line are presently classified as "diseases" and lead to heart and brain failure. The vascular and cardiac changes presently thought to occur as a result of the "normal aging process" (i.e., those addressed in the previous sections) are depicted below the line. These age-associated changes in cardiac and vascular properties alter the substrate upon which cardiovascular disease is superimposed in several ways. First, they lower the extent of disease severity required to cross the threshold that results in clinically significant signs and symptoms. For example, a mild degree of ischemia-induced relaxation abnormalities that may be asymptomatic in a younger individual may cause dyspnea in an older individual, who, by virtue of age alone, has preexisting slowed and delayed early diastolic relaxation.

Age-associated changes may also alter the manifestations and presentation of common cardiac diseases. This usually occurs in patients with acute infarction in whom the diagnosis is delayed because of atypical symptoms resulting in increased time to onset of therapy. Age-associated changes, including those in beta-adrenergic responsiveness and in vascular stiffness, also influence the response to and therefore the selection of different therapeutic inventions in older individuals with cardiovascular disease. In one sense those processes below the line in Figure 50–10 ought not

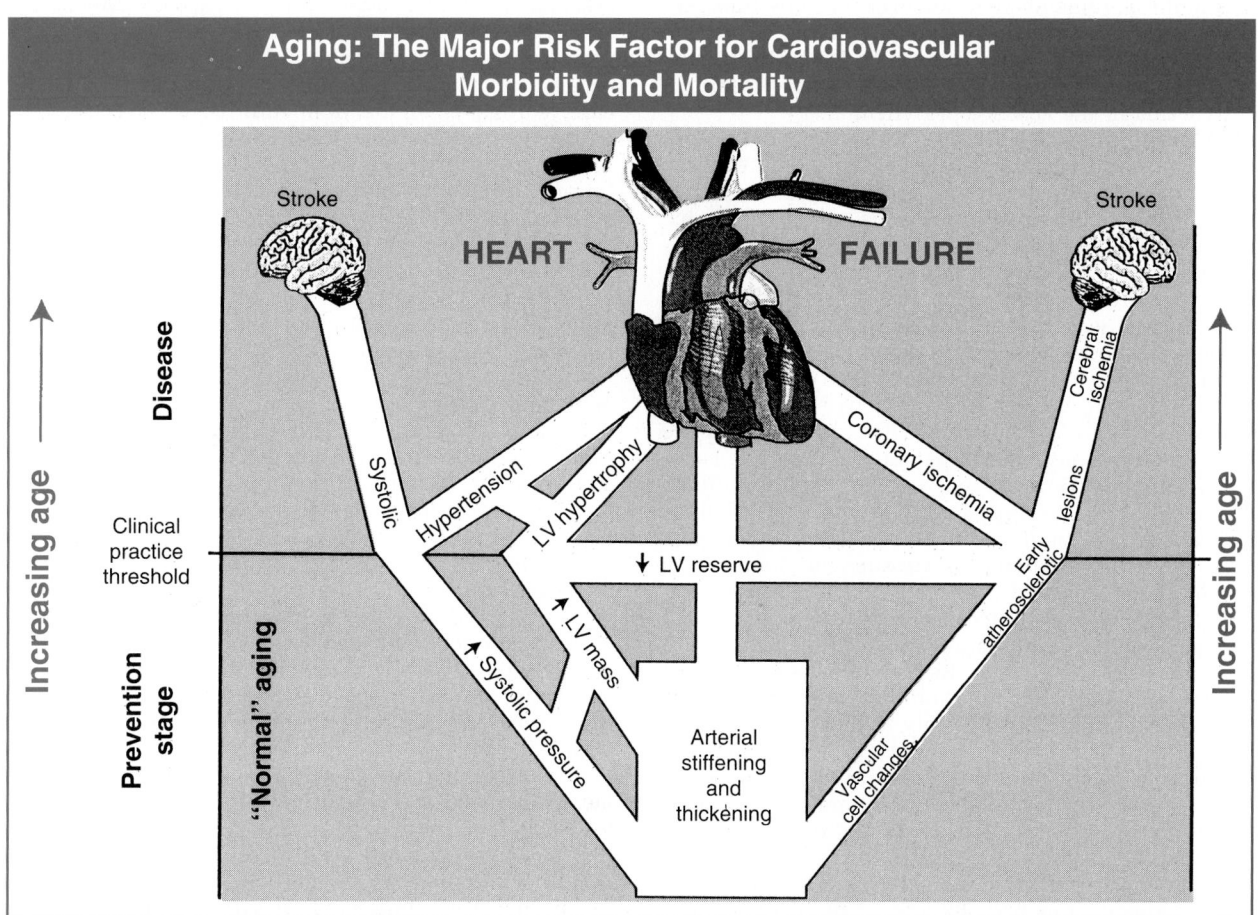

FIGURE 50–10. Changes in the vasculature and heart with aging in health may also be construed as risk factors for cardiovascular disease, leading to heart and brain disorders in older age (see text for details). (From Lakatta, E. G.: Aging effects on the vasculature in health. Risk factors for cardiovascular disease. Am. J. Geriatr. Cardiol. 3:11–17, 1994.)

to be considered to reflect "normal" aging. Rather, they might be construed as specific risk factors for the diseases that they relate to, and thus might be targets of interventions designed to decrease the occurrence and/or manifestations of cardiovascular disease at later ages. Such a strategy would thus advocate treating "normal" aging. Additional studies of the specific risks of each "normal" age-associated change are required. In the following section the question of how aging influences the presentation and approach to the treatment of common cardiovascular diseases is reviewed, focusing on the influence and impact of the age-associated changes described above.

Chronic Ischemic Heart Disease
(See also Chap. 38)

DIAGNOSIS. Clinical Findings. The prevalence and severity of coronary atherosclerosis increase so dramatically with age that more than one-half of all deaths in persons aged 65 years or older are due to coronary disease and about three-fourths of all deaths from ischemic heart disease occur in older individuals.[91] The diagnosis of ischemic heart disease may be more difficult in the older individual since the prevalence of diagnosed disease is only one-third to one-half the prevalence of autopsy-documented significant atherosclerosis. The lack of classic symptomatology may be related to an age-associated decline in physical activity to the point at which ischemic symptoms are not present. In addition, dyspnea, rather than pain, may be the most prominent feature of the clinical picture in angina, as well as infarction, possibly because of the age-related changes in myocardial compliance and diastolic relaxation discussed above. The physical examination is of limited usefulness in the diagnosis of ischemic heart disease (see p. 1292). It should be remembered, however, that the transient features associated with acute ischemia (i.e., an S_4 gallop, reversed splitting of the second sound, and a systolic murmur secondary to mitral regurgitation) are often present in older individuals in the absence of ischemia.

Stress Testing (see also p. 1296). Stress tests are useful in the diagnosis of older patients with suspected coronary disease, although with certain caveats. The presence of resting ST-segment abnormalities or the use of digitalis, both of which are more common in the elderly, may invalidate the interpretation of the stress electrocardiogram and, in this setting, stress testing using thallium scintigraphy[92] or echocardiography is helpful. These techniques are also useful when the stress electrocardiogram is unexpectedly negative in an older individual whose history suggests the presence of ischemia, because the predictive accuracy of a negative test is low in a population with a high prevalence of disease. Finally, many elderly patients may not be capable of exercising to 85 to 90 per cent of their predicted maximum heart rate. In this setting a thallium scan or echocardiogram in conjunction with a pharmacological stress test using dipyridamole, adenosine, or dobutamine may provide diagnostic and prognostic information similar to that of an exercise examination. Echocardiography can also be used in the initial assessment of patients with known or suspected coronary disease to evaluate global and regional left ventricular function, left ventricular mass, and valve abnormalities, and possibly to distinguish nonviable from stunned or hibernating regions of left ventricular dysfunction. In a recent report, the sensitivity and specificity of exercise echocardiography were 88 and 82 per cent, respectively, and are comparable to values obtained using exercise thallium imaging. The sensitivities of dobutamine and dipyridamole echocardiography were 82 and 74 per cent, and the specificities were 82 and 77 per cent, respectively.[93]

MANAGEMENT. The treatment of angina in older and younger patients is similar (see p. 1299). After diagnosis, reversible factors should be identified and treated. Of these, anemia, hyperthyroidism, hypertension, congestive heart failure, and noncompliance with medication may all be more common and more difficult to diagnose in the elderly. It should also be remembered that atherosclerosis is a progressive disease, and although it has sometimes been stated that risk factor reduction is less important in the older patient, more recent evidence suggests that both successful treatment of hypertension[94-96] and cessation of smoking[97] decrease cardiovascular mortality in the elderly.

The goals of antiischemic medical therapy and the use of specific antiischemic agents are generally similar to those in the younger population. Older individuals may be more susceptible to symptoms related to any hypotensive effects of some antiischemics because of decreased sympathetic responsiveness. The degree to which ischemia may be mediated via a heart rate or contractility response to beta-adrenergic stimulation, and therefore the extent to which benefit may be achieved with beta blockers, may be decreased by the same age-associated change in sympathetic responsiveness. Although there are no controlled secondary prevention trials of aspirin in older populations, its effectiveness in the middle-aged group[98] and the low side effect profile support the use of low-dose therapy in the elderly with known coronary disease.

If medical therapy fails to control symptoms adequately, percutaneous transluminal coronary angioplasty (PTCA) should be considered in patients with appropriate anatomy (see Chap. 39). In the more elderly individuals, whose life span is limited regardless of therapy, and whose activity is restricted by other disease, treatment goals should be directed toward symptom alleviation and continuation of an independent life style. Although immediate success and complication rates in those 65 to 80 years of age are often similar to those in the younger age groups when angioplasty is performed by experienced individuals,[99,99a,99b] it is associated with a lower clinical success rate and higher vascular and cardiac complication rates in those over 80 years of age. This probably relates to more difficult access because of increased likelihood of peripheral vascular disease, coronary calcification, multivessel disease, renal impairment, and cerebrovascular complications. Angioplasty in one group of 26 patients over 90 years from seven institutions indicated a clinical success rate of only 65 per cent and six in-hospital deaths, four of which were related to the procedure.[100] A higher complication rate is also reported for rotational coronary atherectomy in those over 80 years of age.[101] There is also a distinction between success of coronary bypass surgery in those younger and older than 80 years.[102] This may relate again to the increased likelihood and severity of coexisting illnesses, including diabetes and pulmonary and renal disease as well as peripheral vascular and cerebrovascular disease. As is true of randomized trials in the general population, retrospective studies in those over 70 years undergoing PTCA and bypass surgery indicate that bypass surgery is associated with fewer recurrent symptoms and repeat procedures than is angioplasty.[103]

PREVENTION (see also Chap. 35). The importance of cholesterol screening and cholesterol-lowering therapy in the elderly is uncertain. The biphasic increase in cholesterol levels with advanced age, the high rate of coronary disease and outcomes in the elderly, and the most recent guidelines from the National Cholesterol Education Program,[104] which include age as a risk factor for coronary disease and which recommend screening and treatment of elevated levels in the older population all suggest that cholesterol-lowering therapy may be useful. It is also important to note that since the absolute risk of coronary events is so high in the older populations, a small decrease in *relative* risk may result in large numbers of avoided events. Several recent analyses, however, found no statistically significant relationship between elevated cholesterol levels and coronary outcomes in older individuals without known coronary disease. The analyses by Manolio,[105] Framingham data,[106] and Krumholz[107] suggest that the relationship declines over age 65 and that there may be no relationship between coronary outcomes and cholesterol levels in those over 80 years of age. In older individuals with known disease, however, the recent Scandinavian Simvastatin Survival Study results indicate that treatment of elevated cholesterol significantly reduces cardiovascular mortality and morbidity.[108] It seems reasonable, therefore, to screen and treat those older individuals with known coronary disease but not those without coronary artery disease, except for possibly men in their 70's with other known risk factors.[109]

Other prevalent risk factors in the older population are obesity and in women estrogen deficiency. A recent analysis of over 40,000 older women reported that the relationship between the waist to hip ratio and cardiovascular outcomes, as well as other causes of death, is strong and monotonic[110] (see p. 1706). The waist to hip ratio, but not the body mass index, was also the best marker for the metabolic hazards of obesity, including lipid levels and insulin resistance. There are several studies indicating that estrogen replacement therapy is associated with a decrease in the development of cardiovascular disease and cardiovascular mortality in postmenopausal women[111] (see p. 1708). Although the benefits of estrogen are often attributed to a favorable influence on the lipid profile, the Nurses' Health Study demonstrated a significant decrease in the development of cardiovascular disease, even after risk factor adjustment.[112] Other benefits of estrogen may include inhibition of endothelial hyperplasia[113] and, as demonstrated by Reis et al.,[114] attenuation of inappropriate coronary vasoconstriction in the setting of endothelial dysfunction. The latter may be particularly important because aging itself, i.e., in the absence of coronary disease and risk factors, is associated with decreased endothelium-dependent coronary vasodilation.[115]

Acute Myocardial Infarction
(See also Chap. 37)

MANAGEMENT. The treatment of acute infarction should be undertaken with the realization that in-hospital and subsequent mortality, reinfarction, and complications are all increased in the elderly. Although the large randomized thrombolytic trials show a survival benefit with thrombolysis in this age group, fewer older individuals are eligible for and actually receive thrombolytic therapy. Furthermore, in those who do not receive thrombolytic therapy, the age-related increase in mortality (of about 1.6 per cent per year), congestive heart failure, and recurrent infarctions is still present.[116–119] This may be related in part to atypical and delayed presentation, a higher incidence of non–Q-wave infarcts, and increased perceived and real rates of bleeding.[116–118,120] A recent analysis of GISSI-2 data, in which all participants received thrombolytic therapy, indicates that although the size of the first infarction is not increased with age, the degree of left ventricular dysfunction is.[119] Electromechanical dissociation was a more common mechanism for death in the older-age group and ventricular fibrillation was less common. Autopsy data indicated no relation between age and the extent of fixed coronary atherosclerotic disease in this population of patients with a first infarction, but there was a marked increase in cardiac rupture, which was found in 86 per cent of those over age 70 at autopsy.

Analysis of the Thrombolysis in Myocardial Infarction-II (TIMI-II) data indicates an age-related increase in complications, mortality, and recurrent infarction in this population as well.[121] This may be explained, in part, by delay of administration of thrombolytics in the older-age groups and by the fact that fewer are eligible to receive beta blockers, probably because of coexisting illnesses. This analysis also indicated no difference in outcomes between the older individuals who were randomized to an early "invasive" strategy with routine catheterization and prophylactic re-

vascularization following thrombolytic therapy, and those randomized to a "conservative" strategy, in which patients underwent these procedures only if there was subjective or objective evidence of recurrent ischemia during the early postinfarction period.

There are many limitations of thrombolytic therapy in the older population. More older individuals have relative or absolute contraindications to these agents, particularly hypertension, history of stroke, and gastrointestinal bleeding. In a subset analysis from the Global Utilization of Streptokinase and Tissue Plasminogen Activator for Occluded Coronary Arteries I (GUSTO I) trial, outcomes in 3600 patients 75 years of age or older showed that there was significantly increased risk of intracranial bleeding in the tissue plasminogen activatory (t-PA) group.[122] Thrombolysis is unsuccessful in about 20 per cent of patients, and less than 60 per cent achieve brisk flow in the infarct-related artery. These considerations prompted randomized trials of primary angioplasty versus thrombolysis for acute infarction.[123] A meta-analysis of some of these studies, performed by O'Neill, indicated a survival advantage in those over age 70 with primary angioplasty.[124] Of particular interest to those caring for older individuals is that a cerebrovascular accident occurred in 3.5 per cent of those in the thrombolytic groups and in none of those in the primary angioplasty groups.

Aging may also be associated with architectural or remodeling changes occurring subsequent to an infarction, including regional thinning at the site of the infarction and hypertrophy in regions remote from the infarction. These may result from preexisting changes in left ventricular wall thickness, increased peripheral impedance, increased collagen content of the infarct and remote areas, decreased capability of the remote region to undergo hypertrophy, and changes in the inflammatory and healing response of the infarct itself. It should also be noted that the elderly benefit as much as younger patients from the secondary prevention effects of beta blockade[125] and that reduction in fatal and nonfatal events following infarction in patients with ejection fractions of 40 per cent or less treated with angiotensin-converting enzyme inhibitors was the same in those over and under 65 years of age.[126]

Arrhythmias
(See also Chap. 22)

Because of the increasing prevalence of hypertension and coronary disease, arrhythmias occur more frequently and are more often associated with hemodynamic compromise in the older age groups. However, in one study, the incidences of supraventricular and ventricular ectopic activity (>100 beats/24 hr of ambulatory monitoring) were 26 and 17 per cent, respectively, in 98 healthy subjects 60 to 85 years of age.[127] Ventricular couplets occurred in 11 per cent but ventricular tachycardia in only 4 per cent of the population. In a larger population from the Cardiovascular Health Study, 15 per cent of women and 25 per cent of men over age 65 had ventricular arrhythmias, while 57 per cent of women and 58 per cent of men had supraventricular arrhythmias during 24 hours of ambulatory monitoring.[128] Although these are often asymptomatic in healthy individuals, they may be more ominous in the presence of disease. Any compromise of cardiac output and blood pressure may, in turn, be associated with more critical decreases in cerebral flow in older patients because of impaired beta-adrenergic cardiovascular responsiveness, an increased likelihood of preexisting cerebrovascular disease, and increased vascular stiffness. Older patients may also experience significant symptoms at a slower rate of ventricular tachycardia than do younger individuals because of prolonged relaxation time and because they are more dependent on atrial contribution to diastolic filling, which is lost in ventricular tachycardia.

ATRIAL FIBRILLATION (see p. 654). This is the most common supraventricular tachyarrhythmia in persons over 65 years of age, occurring in one study in 4.8 per cent of women and 6.2 per cent of men.[129] It is associated with chronic cardiovascular disease including hypertension, ischemia, and failure, and also acute illnesses such as pneumonia and other infections, surgery, and acute infarction. Atrial fibrillation may precipitate or worsen failure or ischemic symptoms in older patients and is associated with an increased risk of adverse long-term cardiovascular outcomes, particularly stroke.[130] The goals of therapy include decreasing the likelihood of systemic embolization (see p. 1582) and correction of hemodynamic compromise, which may require slowing the ventricular rate and restoring sinus rhythm. Echocardiographic predictors of stroke in atrial fibrillation include mitral annular calcification, left atrial size, and left ventricular dysfunction.[131,132]

A pooled analysis of five randomized controlled trials of antithrombotic therapy in atrial fibrillation indicates that age, a history of hypertension, diabetes, and a prior transient ischemic attack or stroke are associated with increased risk of stroke in the control groups[133] (see p. 1830). Warfarin decreased the annual stroke rate from 4.5 per cent in the control groups to 1.4 per cent.[133] The annual rate for major hemorrhage was 1.0 per cent in the control groups and 1.3 per cent in the warfarin groups. Hemorrhage was associated with age, excessive anticoagulation, and poorly controlled hypertension.[134] Although the risk of hemorrhage is age related, the benefit of warfarin outweighs the risk and it should be generally used in the older population. However, the target INR (International Normalized Ratio) should be kept below 3.0, and those with contraindications to anticoagulation and those who cannot reliably take medication should be treated with aspirin.

Although several agents may help in maintaining sinus rhythm, for reasons that are unclear a meta-analysis indicated increased mortality associated with quinidine.[135] *Flecainide* is useful for patients with supraventricular arrhythmias, but side effects preclude its use in patients with other forms of organic heart disease, which are usually present in the older age groups. *Sotalol* may also be considered but may be associated with undesirable side effects in patients with systolic dysfunction.[136] Low-dose *amiodarone* therapy, however, has been shown to preserve sinus rhythm with relatively few side effects over both short- and long-term follow-up periods.[137] It also has the advantage of slowing the ventricular response if atrial fibrillation does recur. If medical therapy is unsuccessful and/or not tolerated, atrioventricular functional ablation with radiofrequency energy or direct current (see p. 619) was reported to be 100 per cent successful in 37 patients 70 years of age or older with a complication rate of only 3 per cent.[138]

The diagnosis of an arrhythmia in an older patient differs only in that the index of suspicion should perhaps be higher for any complaints relating to transient cerebral ischemia, angina, heart failure, or mental status changes. Long-term ambulatory monitoring, particularly with loop recorders, is often useful. The urgency of therapy depends on the associated hemodynamic changes, and emergency treatment is the same in all age groups.

The routine work-up should include a search for associated and/or precipitating factors. Some of these, including electrolyte imbalance, digitalis excess, clinical or subclinical hyperthyroidism,[139] anemia, pulmonary embolism, and congestive heart failure, are more common in the older population. Specific therapy for the arrhythmia is guided by the severity of associated symptoms, the presence and type of underlying heart disease, and recognition of the age-associated changes in the pharmacokinetics of the antiarrhythmic drugs, as discussed below.

BRADYARRHYTHMIAS (see also p. 645). Sinus bradycardia is often present in older individuals in the presence or absence of cardiac disease. It may be related to age-associated histological changes in the sinus node, a hypersensitive carotid sinus reflex, or medications. Evaluation should be undertaken if the patient is symptomatic and, since other causes for neurological symptoms are often present in the elderly, to determine whether, in fact, the transient symptoms are related to the bradycardia. Long-term ambulatory monitoring, often with loop recorders, is most useful in this regard. There is also a group of older individuals with postprandial hypotension significant enough to result in syncope,[140] possibly from impaired postprandial autonomic modulation of systemic vascular resistance and heart rate.[141]

If the patient is symptomatic from the bradycardia, immediate therapy is dependent on the degree of hemodynamic compromise. Temporary emergency measures, including administration of atropine and isoproterenol and insertion of a temporary pacemaker, can be used. If no reversible factors are present, the only effective long-term therapy is permanent pacing. Pacemakers that allow for proper sequencing of atrial and ventricular events are particularly useful in the elderly because of increased reliance on late diastolic filling and hence atrial systole. This pacing mode is also associated with a decreased likelihood of stroke and development of atrial fibrillation in some patient subsets.[142] Idiopathic heart block without evidence of structural heart disease is also more common in older persons, probably because of age-associated fibrosis within the conducting system.

Valvular Disease
(See also Chap. 32)

The diagnosis of valvular disease in the elderly is often obscured by age-related but benign systolic murmurs, changes in S_2, and increased stiffness of the central arteries. The latter may prevent the appearance of the slow anacrotic shoulder and small pulse pressure that would otherwise be seen in significant aortic stenosis. The other findings, however, particularly the presence of a late peaking systolic murmur, electrocardiographic evidence of left ventricular hypertrophy, and echocardiographic demonstration of valve narrowing and calcification all retain their significance. Doppler examination may be particularly useful in assessing the severity of obstruction. The usual causes are calcification of a congenital bicuspid valve, and in those over 75 years of age, degenerative calcification.

Aortic valve replacement should be recommended for the usual indications, i.e., syncope, angina, and heart failure, and is often associated with low mortality and excellent quality of life. Older individuals with calcific aortic stenosis should be observed closely because hemodynamic compromise may develop rapidly with little hypertrophy. In patients over 70 years of age, operative mortality for aortic valve replacement is about 4 per cent[143] and 5-year actuarial survival in a group of patients over 80 years undergoing aortic valve replacement was 76 per cent.[54] Risk factors for operative mortality include left ventricular dysfunction, lack of sinus rhythm, associated cardiac procedures, and emergency status.[143–145] Aortic valvuloplasty provides only palliative relief in patients with aortic stenosis,[146] but should be considered in those with definite contraindications to surgery. The diagnosis of aortic regurgitation is not more difficult in the older age groups but the timing of aortic valve replacement may be, because of the often benign course of the disease. Surgery is usually recommended for those patients who continue to be symptomatic with medical therapy.

Mitral stenosis in the elderly is usually due to rheumatic disease, while regurgitation can be due to rheumatic disease as well as calcification of the mitral annulus, mitral valve prolapse, and ischemic papillary muscle dysfunction. Survival time is considerably shortened in the presence of atrial fibrillation and heart failure, and the results of mitral valve surgery are satisfactory in the elderly. Mitral valve repair is also associated with low operative mortality (3.8 per cent), successful elimination of mitral regurgitation (>90 per cent), and good long-term survival at 5 years without embolism, hemorrhage, or need for reoperation.[147] Balloon mitral valvuloplasty is associated with higher morbidity and mortality in elderly patients with heavily calcified valves than it is in younger patients with pliable valves and no subvalvular stenosis.[148]

Hypertension
(See also Chap. 26)

The importance of the diagnosis and effective treatment of hypertension in the elderly cannot be overemphasized.[149] The incidence of hypertension in the Third National Health and Nutrition Examination Survey was 54 per cent in those 65 to 74 years of age.[94] A recent meta-analysis of nine major trials that included more than 15,000 individuals 60 years of age or older demonstrated that antihypertensive therapy significantly improves survival and decreases stroke and cardiac mortality and morbidity in this population.[95] Isolated systolic hypertension, i.e., systolic elevations in the presence of normal pressure, accounts for 65 per cent of hypertension in the elderly.[94] The Systolic Hypertension in the Elderly Program (SHEP) trial demonstrated that treating those over age 60 with a systolic pressure of over 160 mm Hg but a normal diastolic pressure reduced nonfatal infarctions by 33 per cent, left ventricular failure by 54 per cent, and stroke by 36 per cent over a 4.5-year follow-up period.[96]

In considering the diagnosis of hypertension, it is important to note that pseudohypertension, due to increased stiffening of the brachial artery, and pseudohypotension, due to atherosclerotic disease in the subclavian artery, may be more common in the elderly. In older patients who suddenly develop severe pressure elevations despite their disease having been previously well controlled with a modest regimen, the possibility of a renovascular cause on the basis of atherosclerotic renal artery disease should be investigated.[150] It is also important to measure the pressure in the upright position before deciding to intensify any antihypertensive regimen since older individuals are more likely to experience orthostatic falls in pressure and because of age-related changes in cerebrovascular autoregulation that render them less able to compensate for any abrupt decline in perfusion pressure.

The target pressures for older patients are not clearly defined. Borderline isolated systolic hypertension, defined as systolic pressure between 140 and 159 mm Hg with diastolic pressure below 90 mm Hg is also common in those over 60 years of age and is associated with an increased risk of cardiovascular disease. The fifth report of the Joint National Committee on Detection, Evaluation, and Treatment of High Blood Pressure[94] (see p. 809) recommends considering treatment for those with systolic pressure greater than 150 mm Hg, although prospective trials have not yet demonstrated that antihypertensive therapy decreases risk for systolic levels between 150 and 160 mm Hg. The SHEP trial, which, as noted above, did demonstrate significant decreases in cardiovascular outcomes, targeted a pressure of less than 160 mm Hg for those with systolic pressure greater than 180 mm Hg and a reduction of 20 mm Hg for those with a pressure of 160 to 180 mm Hg. Although it is generally agreed that the target diastolic pressure should be less than 90 mm Hg, there are reports of a "J-shaped" relationship between treated diastolic pressure and clinical outcomes,[151] although this was not true of the SHEP results. Any J-shaped relationship may be due, in part, to the fact that most of coronary flow occurs in diastole and that such flow may be compromised by a lower diastolic pressure in individuals with obstructive coronary disease.

Antihypertensive therapy should consider not only the appropriate blood pressure goals but also the fact that hypertension is associated with other risk factors that independently predict cardiovascular outcomes. These include left ventricular hypertrophy, hyperlipidemia, and insulin resistance. Regarding specific therapy, it should be noted that thiazides were used as the step one antihypertensive agent in all of the major trials that documented a decline in cardiovascular morbidity and mortality. An increased incidence of cardiovascular deaths in hypertensive patients taking thiazides was not present in those also using potassium-sparing agents.[152] This benefit could not be mimicked by the addition of potassium supplements. It is not clear whether this is related to noncompliance with potassium supplements, the inability of supplements to adequately replete and/or maintain intracellular stores, or to other effects of thiazides.

Although beta blockers are effective antihypertensive agents in some populations, elderly patients respond less often than young hypertensives when beta blockers are used as single agents. In addition, beta blockers should be used cautiously in patients with systolic dysfunction, obstructive pulmonary disease, and peripheral vascular disease. Calcium channel blockers may be used in older hypertensives with associated ischemic disease, hypertrophy, and diastolic dysfunction; angiotensin-converting enzyme inhibitors in those with systolic dysfunction and diabetes; and alpha blockers in those with prostatic hypertrophy.

Congestive Heart Failure
(See also Chap. 17)

The evaluation and treatment of left ventricular dysfunction is an important consideration in the older population for several reasons. The incidence of congestive heart failure (9 per cent for those 80 to 89 years of age)[153] is the final common pathway of ischemic, hypertensive, and valvular disease and accounts for a large number of hospital admissions and office visits in this population. Congestive heart failure has a significant impact on survival as well as work status and quality of life. The mortality associated with congestive heart failure is approximately 50 per cent within 5 years of the diagnosis.[154] Although age-adjusted mortality due to coronary disease and that due to stroke have decreased in the older age groups over the past 20 years, the mortality due to congestive heart failure has increased significantly—by 29 per cent in those 65 to 74 years of age and by 45 per cent in those 75 to 84 years.[155]

The evaluation of symptoms suggestive of heart failure in older persons should include a determination of whether there is a predominant systolic or diastolic component (p. 447). This is particularly important in the older-age groups because up to 40 per cent of those over 60 years with these symptoms have normal systolic function. The distinction cannot be made easily by the history, the examination, or the chest film since both pathophysiological states often present with dyspnea, rales, and congestion on roentgenography. The distinction is best made with the echocardiogram or the gated blood pool examination. In the patient with predominant systolic dysfunction the cavity is dilated, the walls often thin, and the ejection fraction low. In the patient with predominant diastolic dysfunction, cavity size is normal, the walls often thick, and the ejection fraction normal or above normal, but indices of diastolic filling are reduced.

The evaluation should also consider whether there is an easily reversible precipitating factor, which is likely to be a superimposed illness in older persons. Pneumonia, anemia, renal failure, and supraventricular arrhythmia, for example, may all be present in the elderly with cardiac decompensation. Treating any superimposed illness may reverse the decompensation. An evaluation of underlying cardiac disorders should also be considered, and in the older individual, this is most likely to be hypertension and/or ischemic disease.

DIASTOLIC DYSFUNCTION. Predominant diastolic dysfunction often occurs in the presence of hypertension and is marked primarily by decreased early diastolic filling rates, elevated diastolic pressures, and increased dependence on atrial contribution. It is important to avoid antihypertensives that increase heart rate and thus compromise diastolic filling time. Although these patients often show evidence of a steep pressure/volume chamber and vascular relationship, and dramatic improvement with short-term diuretic and vasodilator administration, it is also necessary, as part of any long-term strategy, to maintain the preload that is needed to fill the stiff diastolic ventricle (see p. 378). Regression of left ventricular mass and improved diastolic function are often best achieved using long-term therapy with a calcium channel blocker or angiotensin-converting enzyme inhibitor. A report by Schulman et al. indicated that in hypertensive patients over 60 years of age a calcium channel blocker was better able to induce regression of left ventricular mass than was the beta blocker atenolol.[156] In this study, regression was associated with improved diastolic filling and did not impair either cardiac output or ejection fraction at rest or during mild upright bicycle exercise.

SYSTOLIC DYSFUNCTION. This occurs often in the setting of ischemic disease. In these patients, it is useful to keep in mind the entity of the "hibernating" myocardium (see p. 388) and that antiischemic interventions in this setting, including revascularization, may improve not only angina, but left ventricular function and failure symptoms as well. There are several goals of medical therapy. One is to decrease neurohormonal activation. Studies with angiotensin-converting enzyme inhibitors indicate improved survival and decreased morbidity in older, as well as younger, patients with systolic dysfunction.[156] Another goal is to favorably influence hemodynamics, primarily by decreasing preload and afterload. Diuretics are very useful, although it is usually necessary to use a higher dose to achieve a given efficacy in older patients because of age-associated decreases in glomerular filtration and tubular secretion.

Digitalis improves clinical outcomes in patients with systolic dysfunction, including those with sinus rhythm. Studies in experimental models indicate that the therapeutic/toxic window for digitalis is narrower in the older-age groups because of a decreased inotropic effect without a change in arrhythmogenic potential. Because of age-associated changes in renal function and pharmacokinetics, the maintenance dose of digitalis should be decreased in those over 70 years of age.

One particular problem in patients with congestive heart failure is frequent and early readmission. Close follow-up of weights and compliance with the medical and dietary regimens, as well as insuring that appropriate doses of the indicated agents are used, may be particularly useful.

Drug Use in the Elderly

As a consequence of the increased prevalence of cardiovascular and other diseases in the elderly, cardiovascular agents make up a higher fraction of total drug expenditure for older persons than they do in the general population. In considering the effects of age on the pharmacokinetics and pharmacodynamics of cardiovascular agents[157] it is important to note the heterogeneity of response in the older population. There are no strict age-related rules that apply to the entire geriatric population, and it is clear that the commitment of the physician to carefully assess the therapeutic results and side effects of medical therapy must be greater in older- than in younger-age groups.

Although age-related changes in gastric pH and absorptive surface are described, these have relatively unimportant effects for most cardiovascular drugs. The distribution of cardiovascular agents, however, is affected by age-associated decreases in serum albumin[158] and lean body mass[159] and increases in alpha-1-acid glycoproteins[160] and body fat.[159] A decrease in albumin results in increased free drug for those agents that are highly protein bound, which will, in turn, increase plasma concentrations for those agents whose metabolism is independent of the available free drug (e.g., lidocaine and propranolol). An increase in alpha-1-acid glycoprotein results in a decrease in the free fractions of acidic drugs. A change in body mass results in an increased distribution volume for fat-soluble drugs and a decreased distribution volume for water-soluble agents.

The effect of age on metabolism and excretion relates to age effects on renal and hepatic function. The influence of age on renal function has been extensively studied and a diminished glomerular filtration rate over a broad age range has been shown.[161] Decreased renal tubular secretion and concentration ability have also been demonstrated. Because lean body mass decreases with age, renal function cannot be indexed using serum creatinine alone in older persons. These age-related changes in renal function result in decreased clearance of quinidine, procainamide, digoxin, and the water-soluble beta blocker atenolol. Diminished tubular secretion of furosemide results in a diminished diuretic response to this drug and presumably other agents that act on the luminal side of the kidney tubule. The effect of age on hepatic metabolism has been evaluated less extensively, but it is undoubtedly affected by the decrease in hepatic mass, blood flow, and activity of the microsomal oxidizing system. These changes result in increased half-lives of lidocaine and the lipid-soluble beta blockers, including propranolol.

In addition to its effects on pharmacokinetics, aging may also influence the cardiac response to any given level of drug. Thus, a diminished response to beta agonists, beta blockers, and digitalis preparations is observed in human and/or animal models. The increased prevalence of other diseases associated with aging may render the older individual more sensitive to the side effect profile of cardiovascular agents as well. Preexisting decreased plasma volume and decreased baroreflex activity may render older patients more susceptible to the hypotensive effects of nitrates and diuretics. Preexisting conduction system disease or left ventricular dysfunction may also increase the likelihood of side effects of beta blockers and of some calcium antagonists.

In summary, the characterization of those cardiovascular changes in humans that are due to aging alone is difficult because of the age-related increasing prevalence of overt and latent cardiovascular disease and sedentary life style. It appears, however, that age does not significantly alter left ventricular performance except in the presence of superimposed stress, which can take the form of severe exercise or disease, particularly ischemia, a tachycardic arrhythmia, and hypertension. In these instances, impaired diastolic relaxation and systolic emptying, probably related to diminished responsiveness to beta-adrenoceptor stimulation, may occur. The diagnostic and therapeutic principles used in the management of cardiac disease do not differ in older and younger patients. The presence of other associated diseases, changed life style habits, and altered pharmacokinetics and pharmacodynamics, however, require more careful, skilled, conscientious, and often time-consuming application of these principles in the treatment of older patients.

REFERENCES

AGING IN ANIMAL MODELS

1. Weisfeldt, M. L., Loeven, W. A., and Shock, N. W.: Resting and active mechanical properties of trabeculae carneae from aged male rats. Am. J. Physiol. *220*:1921, 1971.

2. Anversa, P., Palackal, T., Sonnenblick, E. H., et al.: Myocyte cell loss and myocyte cellular hyperplasia in the hypertrophied aging rat heart. Circ. Res. 67:871, 1990.

3. Anversa, P., Hiler, B., Ricci, R., et al.: Myocyte cell loss and myocyte hypertrophy in the aging rat heart. J. Am. Coll. Cardiol. 8:1441, 1986.

4. Fraticelli, A., Josephson, R., Danziger, R., et al.: Morphological and contractile characteristics of rat cardiac myocytes from maturation to senescence. Am. J. Physiol. 257:H259, 1989.

5. Yin, F. C. P., Spurgeon, H. A., Rakusan, K., et al.: Use of tibial length to quantify cardiac hypertrophy: Application in the aging rat. Am. J. Physiol. 243:H941, 1982.

6. Yin, F. C., Spurgeon, H. A., Weisfeldt, M. L., and Lakatta, E. G.: Mechanical properties of myocardium from hypertrophied rat hearts. A comparison between hypertrophy induced by senescence and by aortic banding. Circ. Res. 46:292, 1980.

7. Lakatta, E. G., Gerstenblith, G., Angell, C. S., et al.: Prolonged contraction duration in aged myocardium. J. Clin. Invest. 55:61, 1975.

8. Capasso, J. M., Malhotra, A., Scheuer, J., and Sonnenblick, E. H.: Myocardial biochemical, contractile and electrical performance after imposition of hypertension in young and old rats. Circ. Res. 58:445, 1986.

9. Wei, J. Y., Spurgeon, H. A., and Lakatta, E. G.: Excitation-contraction in rat myocardium: Alterations with adult aging. Am. J. Physiol. 246:H784, 1984.

10. Walker, K. E., Lakatta, E. G., and Houser, S. R.: Age associated changes in membrane currents in rat ventricular myocytes. Cardiovasc. Res. 27:1968, 1993.

11. Capasso, J. M., Malhotra, A., Remily, R. M., et al.: Effects of age on mechanical and electrical performance of rat myocardium. Am. J. Physiol. 245:H72, 1983.

12. Spurgeon, H. A., Steinbach, M. F., and Lakatta, E. G.: Chronic exercise prevents characteristic age-related changes in rat cardiac contraction. Am. J. Physiol. 244:H513, 1983.

13. Spurgeon, H. A., Thorne, P. R., Yin, F. C. P., et al.: Increased dynamic stiffness of trabeculae carneae from senescent rats. Am. J. Physiol. 232:H373, 1977.

14. Starnes, J. W., and Rumsey, W. L.: Cardiac energetics and performance of exercised and food-restricted rats during aging. Am. J. Physiol. 254:H599, 1988.

15. Templeton, G. H., Platt, G. H., Willerson, J. T., and Weisfeldt, M. L.: Influence of aging on left ventricular hemodynamics and stiffness in beagles. Circ. Res. 44:189, 1979.

16. Orchard, C. H., and Lakatta, E. G.: Intracellular calcium transients and developed tensions in rat heart muscle. A mechanism for the negative interval-strength relationship. J. Gen. Physiol. 86:637, 1985.

17. Froehlich, J. P., Lakatta, E. G., Beard, E., et al.: Studies of sarcoplasmic reticulum function and contraction duration in young adult and aged rat myocardium. J. Mol. Cell. Cardiol. 10:427, 1978.

18. Tate, C. A., Taffet, G. E., Hudson, E. K., et al.: Enhanced calcium uptake of cardiac sarcoplasmic reticulum in exercise-trained old rats. Am. J. Physiol. 258:H431, 1990.

19. Buttrick, P. A., Malhotra, A., Factor, S., et al.: Effect of aging and hypertension on myosin biochemistry and gene expression in the rat heart. Circ. Res. 68:645, 1991.

20. Effron, M. B., Bhatnagar, G. M., Spurgeon, H. A., et al.: Changes in myosin isoenzymes, ATPase activity, and contraction duration in rat cardiac muscle with aging can be modulated by thyroxine. Circ. Res. 60:238, 1987.

21. Bhatnagar, G. M., Effron, M. B., Ruano-Arroyo, G., et al.: Dissociation of myosin Ca²⁺-ATPase activity from myosin isoenzymes and contractile function in rat myocardium. Fed. Proc. 44(Abs.):826, 1985.

22. Scarpace, P. J., and Abrass, I. B.: Decreased beta-adrenergic agonist affinity and adenylate cyclase activity in senescent rat lung. J. Gerontol. 38:143, 1983.

23. Scarpace, P. J.: Forskolin activation of adenylate cyclase in rat myocardium with age: Effects of guanine nucleotide analogs. Mech. Ageing Dev. 52:169, 1990.

24. Sakai, M., Danziger, R. S., Staddon, J. M., et al.: Decrease with senescence in the norepinephrine-induced phosphorylation of myofilament proteins in isolated rat cardiac myocytes. J. Mol. Cell. Cardiol. 21:1327, 1989.

25. Jiang, M. T., Moffat, M. P., and Narayanan, N.: Age-related alterations in the phosphorylation of sarcoplasmic reticulum and myofibrillar proteins and diminished contractile response to isoproterenol in intact rat ventricle. Circ. Res. 72:102, 1993.

26. Xiao, R.-P., Spurgeon, H. A., O'Connor, F., and Lakatta, E. G.: Age-associated changes in β-adrenergic modulation on rat cardiac excitation-contraction coupling. J. Clin. Invest. 94:2051, 1994.

27. Boluyt, M. O., Younes, A., Caffrey, J. L., et al.: Age-associated increase in rat cardiac opioid production. Am. J. Physiol. 265:H212, 1993.

28. Younes, A., Boluyt, M. O., O'Neill, L., et al.: Age-associated alterations in atrial natiuretic factor gene expression in rat. Am. J. Physiol. 269:H1003, 1995.

29. Lompre, A. M., Lambert, F., Lakatta, E. G., and Schwartz, K.: Expression of sarcoplasmic reticulum Ca²⁺-ATPase and calsequestrin genes in rat heart during ontogenic development and aging. Circ. Res. 69:1380, 1991.

30. Maciel, L. M. Z., Polikar, R., Rohrer, D., et al.: Age-induced decreases in the messenger RNA coding for the sarcoplasmic reticulum Ca²⁺-ATPase of the rat heart. Circ. Res. 67:230, 1990.

31. O'Neill, L., Holbrook, N. J., Fargnoli, J., and Lakatta, E. G.: Progressive

changes from young adult age to senescence in mRNA for rat cardiac myosin heavy chain genes. Cardioscience 2:1, 1991.

32. Schuyler, G. T., and Yarbrough, L. R.: Comparison of myosin and creatine kinase isoforms in left ventricles of young and senescent Fischer 344 rats after treatment with triiodothyronine. Mech. Ageing Dev. 56:39, 1990.

33. Lakatta, E. G.: Cardiovascular regulatory mechanisms in advanced age. Physiol. Rev. 73:413, 1993.

34. Bhatnagar, G. M., Walford, G. D., Beard, E. S., et al.: ATPase activity and force production in myofibrils and twitch characteristics in intact muscle from neonatal, adult, and senescent rat myocardium. J. Mol. Cell. Cardiol. 16:203, 1984.

35. Hano, O., Bogdanov, K. Y., Sakai, M., et al.: Reduced threshold for myocardial cell calcium intolerance in the rat heart with aging. Am. J. Physiol. 269:H1607, 1995.

36. White, M., Roden, R., Minobe, W., et al.: Age-related changes in β-adrenergic neuroeffector systems in the human heart. Circulation 90:1225, 1994.

37. Harding, S. E., Jones, S. M., O'Gara, P., et al.: Isolated ventricular myocytes from failing and non-failing human heart: The relation of age and clinical status of patients to isoproterenol response. J. Mol. Cell. Cardiol. 24:549, 1992.

38. Jacob, R., Kissling, G., Ebrecht, G., et al.: Adaptive and pathological alterations in experimental cardiac hypertrophy. In Chazov, E., Saks, V., and Rona, G. (eds.): Advances in Myocardiology. New York, Plenum, 1983, p. 55.

39. Lakatta, E. G.: Regulation of cardiac muscle function in the hypertensive heart. In Cox, R. H. (ed.): Cellular and Molecular Mechanisms of Hypertension. New York, Plenum, 1991, p. 149.

40. Lecarpentier, Y., Bugaisky, L. B., Chemla, D., et al.: Coordinated changes in contractility, energetics, and isomyosins after aortic stenosis. Am. J. Physiol. 252:H275, 1987.

41. Michel, J. B., Heudes, D., Michel, O., et al.: Effect of chronic ANG I-converting enzyme inhibition on aging processes: II. large arteries. Am. J. Physiol. 267:R-124, 1994.

42. Nagai, R., Zarain-Herzberg, A., Brandl, C. J., et al.: Regulation of myocardial Ca²⁺-ATPase and phospholamban mRNA expression in response to pressure overload and thyroid hormone. Proc. Natl. Acad. Sci. USA 86:2966, 1989.

43. Swynghedauw, B.: Remodelling of the heart in response to chronic mechanical overload. Eur. Heart J. 10:935, 1989.

44. Yazaki, Y., and Komuro, I.: Molecular analysis of cardiac hypertrophy due to overload. J. Mol. Cell. Cardiol. (Suppl. III) 21(Abs.):S.29, 1989.

45. Bing, O. H. L., Brooks, W. W., Conrad, C. H., et al.: Intracellular calcium transient in myocardium from spontaneously hypertensive rats during the transition to heart failure. Circ. Res. 68:1390, 1991.

46. Boluyt, M. O., Opiteck, J. A., Esser, K. A., and White, T. P.: Cardiac adaptations to aortic-constriction in adult and aged rats. Am. J. Physiol. 257:H643, 1989.

47. Isoyama, S., Grossman, W., and Wei, J. Y.: Effect of age on myocardial adaptation to volume overload in the rat. J. Clin. Invest. 81:1850, 1988.

48. Kuroha, M., Isoyama, S., Ito, N., and Takishima T.: Effects of age on right ventricular hypertrophic response to pressure-overload in rats. J. Mol. Cell. Cardiol. 23:1177, 1991.

49. Takahashi, T., Schunkert, H., Isoyama, S., et al.: Age-related differences in the expression of proto-oncogene and contractile protein genes in response to pressure overload in the rat myocardium. J. Clin. Invest. 89:939, 1992.

50. Walford, G. D., Spurgeon, H. A., and Lakatta, E. G.: Diminished cardiac hypertrophy and muscle performance in older compared to younger adult rats with chronic atrioventricular block. Circ. Res. 63:502, 1988.

51. Pfeffer, J. M., Pfeffer, M. A., Fishbein, M. C., and Frohlich, E. D.: Cardiac function and morphology with aging in the spontaneously hypertensive rat. Am. J. Physiol. 237:H461, 1979.

52. Gwathmey, J. K., Slawsky, M. T., Perreault, C. L., et al.: The effect of exercise conditioning on excitation-contraction coupling in aged rats. J. Appl. Physiol. 69:1366, 1990.

53. Farrar, R. P., Starnes, J. W., Cartee, G. D., et al.: Effects of exercise on cardiac myosin isozyme composition during the aging process. J. Appl. Physiol. 64:880, 1988.

54. Oscai, L. B., Mole, P. A., and Holloszy, J. O.: Effects of exercise on cardiac weight and mitochondria in male and female rats. Am. J. Physiol. 220:1944, 1971.

55. Starnes, J. W., Beyer, R. E., and Edington, D. W.: Myocardial adaptations to endurance exercise in aged rats. Am. J. Physiol. 245:H560, 1983.

NORMAL AGING HUMANS

56. Fleg, J. L., O'Connor, F., Gerstenblith, G., et al.: Impact of age on the cardiovascular response to dynamic upright exercise in healthy men and women. J. Appl. Physiol. 78:890, 1995.

57. Fleg, J. L., Schulman, S., O'Connor, F., et al.: Effects of acute β-adrenergic receptor blockage on age-associated changes in cardiovascular performance during dynamic exercise. Circulation 90:2333, 1994.

58. Czernin, J., Muller, P., Chan, S., et al.: Influence of age and hemodynamics on myocardial blood flow and flow reserve. Circulation 88:62, 1993.

59. Celermajer, D. S., Sorensen, K. E., Spiegelhalter, D. J., et al.: Aging is

associated with endothelial dysfunction in healthy men years before the age-related decline in women. J. Am. Coll. Cardiol. *24*:471, 1994.

60. Gerstenblith, G., Frederiksen, J., Yin, F. C. P., et al.: Echocardiographic assessment of a normal adult aging population. Circulation *56*:273, 1977.
61. Vaitkevicius, P. V., Fleg, J. L., Engel, J. H., et al.: Effects of age and aerobic capacity on arterial stiffness in healthy adults. Circulation *88*:1456, 1993.
62. Avolio, A. P., Chen, S. G., Wang, R. P., et al.: Effects of aging on changing arterial compliance and left ventricular load in a northern Chinese urban community. Circulation *68*:50, 1983.
63. Nichols, W. W., O'Rourke, M. F., Avolio, A. P., et al.: Effects of age-ventricular-vascular coupling. Am. J. Cardiol. *55*:1179, 1985.
64. O'Rourke, M. F.: Arterial Function in Health and Disease. New York, Churchill Livingstone, 1982, p. 275.
65. Yin, F. C. P., Weisfeldt, M. L., and Milnor, W. R.: Role of aortic input impedance in the decreased cardiovascular response to exercise with aging in dogs. J. Clin. Invest. *68*:28, 1981.
66. Elveback, L., and Lie, J. T.: Continued high incidence of coronary artery disease at autopsy in Olmsted County, Minnesota, 1950 to 1979. Circulation *70*:345, 1984.
67. Fleg, J. L., Gerstenblith, G., Zonderman, A. B., et al.: Prevalence and prognostic significance of exercise-induced silent myocardial ischemia detected by thallium scintigraphy and electrocardiography in asymptomatic volunteers. Circulation *81*:423, 1990c.
68. Fleg, J., Schulman, S. P., Gerstenblith, G., et al.: Additive effects of age and silent myocardial ischemia on the left ventricular response to upright cycle exercise. J. Appl. Physiol. *75*:499, 1993.
69. Ehsani, A. A., Ogawa, T., Miller, T. R., et al.: Exercise training improves left ventricular systolic function in older men. Circulation *83*:96, 1991.
70. Ogawa, T., Spina, R. J., Martin, W. H., III, et al.: Effects of aging, sex and physical training on cardiovascular responses to exercise. Circulation *86*:494, 1992.
71. Stratton, J. R., Cerqueira, M. D., Schwartz, R. S., et al.: Differences in cardiovascular responses to isoproterenol in relation to age and exercise training in healthy men. Circulation *86*:504, 1992.
72. Spina, R. J., Ogawa, R., Kohrt, W. M., et al.: Differences in cardiovascular adaptations to endurance exercise training between older men and women. J. Appl. Physiol. *75*:849, 1993.
73. Brandfonbrener, M., Landowne, M., and Shock, N. W.: Changes in cardiac output with age. Circulation *12*:557, 1955.
74. Schulman, S., Lakatta, E. G., Fleg, J. L., et al.: Age-related decline in left ventricular filling at rest and exercise. Am. J. Physiol. *263* (Heart Circ. Physiol. *34*):H1932, 1992.
75. Swinne, C. J., Shapiro, E. P., Lima, S. D., and Fleg, J. L.: Age-associated changes in left ventricular diastolic performance during isometric exercise in normal subjects. Am. J. Cardiol. *69*:823, 1992.
76. Bruce, R. A., and Hornsten, T. R.: Exercise stress testing in evaluation of patients with ischemic heart disease. Prog. Cardiovasc. Dis. *11*:371, 1969.
77. Seals, D. R., Hagberg, J. M., Hurley, B. F., et al.: Endurance training in older men and women. I. Cardiovascular responses to exercise. J. Appl. Physiol. *57*:1024, 1984.
78. Fleg, J. L., and Lakatta, E. G.: Role of muscle loss in the age-associated reduction in VO_{2max}. J. Appl. Physiol. *65*:1147, 1988.
79. Fleg, J. L., Tzankoff, S. P., and Lakatta, E. G.: Age-related augmentation of plasma catecholamines during dynamic exercise in healthy males. J. Appl. Physiol. *59*:1033, 1985.
80. Haber, P., Honiger, B., Klicpera, M., and Niederberger, M.: Effects in elderly people 67–76 years of age of three-month endurance training on a bicycle ergometer. Eur. Heart J. *5*(Suppl. E):37, 1984.
81. Smith, M. L., Graitzer, H. M., Hudson, D. L., and Raven, P. B.: Baroreflex function in endurance- and static exercise-trained men. J. Appl. Physiol. *64*:585, 1988.
82. Seals, D. R., and Chase, P. B.: Influence of physical training on heart rate variability and baroreflex circulatory control. J. Appl. Physiol. *66*:1886, 1989.
83. Fortney, S., Tankersley, C., Lightfoot, J. T., et al.: Cardiovascular response to lower body negative pressure in trained and untrained older men. J. Appl. Physiol. *73*:2693, 1992.
84. Smith, M. L., and Raven, P. B.: Cardiovascular responses to lower body negative pressure in endurance and static exercise-trained men. Med. Sci. Sports Exer. *18*:545, 1986.
85. Fleg, J. L., Shapiro, E. P., O'Connor, F., et al.: Failure of intensive long-term aerobic conditioning to prevent the age-associated decline in left-ventricular diastolic filling performance (*in press*).
86. Forman, D. E., Manning, W. J., Hauser, R., et al.: Enhanced left ventricular diastolic filling associated with long-term endurance training. J. Gerontol. Med. Sci. *47*:M56, 1992.
87. Levy, W. C., Cerqueira, M. D., Abrass, I. B., et al.: Endurance training augments diastolic filling at rest and during exercise in healthy young and older men. Circulation *88*:116, 1993.
88. Takemoto, K. A., Bernstein, L., Lopez, J. F., et al.: Abnormalities of diastolic filling of the left ventricle associated with aging are less pronounced in exercise trained individuals. Am. Heart J. *124*:143, 1992.
89. Ehsani, A. A., Ogawa, T., Miller, T. R., et al.: Exercise training improves left ventricular systolic function in older men. Circulation *83*:96, 1991.

90. Schocken, D. D., Blumenthal, J. A., Port, S., et al.: Physical conditioning and left ventricular performance in the elderly: Assessment by radionuclide angiocardiography. Am. J. Cardiol. *52*:359, 1983.
91. National Center for Health Statistics. Vital statistics of the United States, 1988, vol 2, mortality, part A. Washington, DC, Public Health Service, 1991.
92. Lam, J. Y. T., Chaitman, B. R., Glaenzer, M., et al.: Safety and diagnostic accuracy of dipyridamole-thallium imaging in the elderly. J. Am. Coll. Cardiol. *11*:585, 1988.
93. Beleslin, B. D., Ostojic, M., Stepanovic, J., et al.: Stress echocardiography in the detection of myocardial ischemia. Head-to-head comparison of exercise, dobutamine, and dipyridamole tests. Circulation *90*:1168, 1994.
94. Joint National Committee on Detection, Evaluation, and Treatment of High Blood Pressure: The fifth report of the Joint National Committee on Detection, Evaluation and Treatment of High Blood Pressure (JNC V). Arch. Intern. Med. *153*:154, 1993.
95. Insua, J. T., Sacks, H. S., Lau, T. S., et al.: Drug treatment of hypertension in the elderly: A meta-analysis. Ann. Intern. Med. *121*:355, 1994.
96. SHEP Cooperative Research Group: Prevention of stroke by antihypertensive drug treatment in older persons with isolated systolic hypertension. Final results of the Systolic Hypertension in the Elderly Program (SHEP). JAMA *265*:3255, 1991.
97. LaCroix, A. Z., Lang, J., Scherr, P., et al.: Smoking and mortality among older men and women in three communities. N. Engl. J. Med. *324*:1619, 1991.
98. Antiplatelet Trialists' Collaboration: Secondary prevention of vascular disease by prolonged antiplatelet treatment. Br. Med. J. *296*:320, 1988.
99. Thompson, R. C., Holmes, D. R., Gersh, B. J., and Bailey, K. R.: Predicting early and intermediate-term outcome of coronary angioplasty in the elderly. Circulation *88*:1579, 1993.
99a. Laster, S. B., Rutherford, B. D., Giorgi, L. V., et al.: Results of direct percutaneous transluminal coronary angioplasty in octogenarians. Am. J. Cardiol. *77*:10, 1996.
99b. Thompson, R. C., Holmes, D. R. Jr., Grill, D. E., et al.: Changing outcomes of angioplasty in the elderly. J. Am. Coll. Cardiol. *27*:8, 1996.
100. Weyrens, F. J., Goldenberg, I., Mooney, J. F., et al.: Percutaneous transluminal coronary angioplasty in patients aged ≥ 90 years. Am. J. Cardiol. *74*:397, 1994.
101. Henson, K. D., Popma, J. J., Leon, M. B., et al.: Efficacy and safety of rotational coronary atherectomy in elderly patients. J. Am. Coll. Cardiol. *21*:214A, 1993.
102. Edmunds, L. H., Jr., Stephenson, L. W., Edie, R. N., et al.: Open-heart surgery in octogenarians. N. Engl. J. Med. *319*:131, 1988.
103. O'Keefe, J. H., Sutton, M. B., McCallister, B. D., et al.: Coronary angioplasty versus bypass surgery in patients >70 years old matched for ventricular function. J. Am. Coll. Cardiol. *24*:425, 1994.
104. Expert Panel on the Detection, Evaluation, and Treatment of High Blood Cholesterol in Adults: Summary of the second report of the National Cholesterol Education Program (NCEP) Expert Panel on Detection, Evaluation, and Treatment of High Blood Cholesterol in Adults (Adult Treatment Panel II). JAMA *269*:3015, 1993.
105. Manolio, T. A., Pearson, T. A., Wenger, N. K., et al.: Cholesterol and heart disease in older persons and women: Review of an NHLBI workshop. Ann. Epidemiol. *2*:161, 1992.
106. Krommal, R. A., Cain, K. C., Ye, Z., et al.: Total serum cholesterol levels and mortality risk as a function of age. A report based on the Framingham data. Arch. Intern. Med. *153*:1065, 1993.
107. Krumholz, H. M., Seeman, T. E., Merrill, S. S., et al.: Lack of association between cholesterol and coronary heart disease mortality and morbidity and all-cause mortality in persons older than 70 years. JAMA *272*:1335, 1994.
108. Scandinavian Simvastatin Survival Study Group: Randomised trial of cholesterol lowering in 4444 patients with coronary heart disease: The Scandinavian Simvastatin Survival Study (4S). Lancet *344*:1383, 1994.
109. Hulley, S. B., and Newman, T. B.: Cholesterol in the elderly. Is it important? JAMA *272*:1372, 1994.
110. Folsom, A. R., Kaye, S. A., Sellers, T. A., et al.: Body fat distribution and 5-year risk of death in older women. JAMA *269*:483, 1993.
111. Stampfer, M. J., and Colditz, G. A.: Estrogen replacement therapy and coronary heart disease: A quantitative assessment of the epidemiologic evidence. Prev. Med. *20*:47, 1991.
112. Stampfer, M. J., Colditz, G. A., Willett, W. C., et al.: Postmenopausal estrogen therapy and cardiovascular disease. Ten year follow-up from the Nurses' Health Study. N. Engl. J. Med. *325*:756, 1991.
113. Fischer, G. M., Cherian, K., and Swain, M. L.: Increased synthesis of aortic collagen and elastin in experimental atherosclerosis: Inhibition by contraceptive steroids. Atherosclerosis *39*:463, 1981.
114. Reis, S. E., Gloth, S. T., Blumenthal, R. S., et al.: Ethinyl estradiol acutely attenuates abnormal coronary vasomotor responses to acetylcholine in postmenopausal women. Circulation *89*:52, 1994.
115. Egashira, K., Inou, T., Hirooka, Y., et al.: Effect of age on endothelium-dependent vasodilation of resistance coronary artery by acetylcholine in humans. Circulation *88*:77, 1993.
116. Weaver, W. D., Litwin, P. E., Martin, J. S., et al.: Effect of age on use of thrombolytic therapy and mortality in acute myocardial infarction. J. Am. Coll. Cardiol. *18*:657, 1991.
117. Goldberg, R. J., Gurwitz, J., Yarzebski, J., et al.: Patient delay and re-

ceipt of thrombolytic therapy among patients with acute myocardial infarction from a community-wide perspective. Am. J. Cardiol. *70*:421, 1992.

118. Gore, J., Becker, R., Tiefenbrunn, A., et al.: The National Registry of Myocardial Infarction (NRMI) Investigators: Current trends in the treatment of elderly patients with acute myocardial infarction. J. Am. Coll. Cardiol. *21*:481A, 1993.

119. Maggioni, A. P., Maseri, A., Fresco, C., et al.: Age-related increase in mortality among patients with first myocardial infarction treated with thrombolysis. N. Engl. J. Med. *329*:1442, 1993.

120. Simoons, M. L., Maggioni, A. P., Knatterud, G., et al.: Individual risk assessment for intracranial haemorrhage during thrombolytic therapy. Lancet *342*:1523, 1993.

121. Aguirre, F. V., McMahon, R. P., Mueller, H., et al.: Impact of age on clinical outcome and postlytic management strategies in patients treated with intravenous thrombolytic therapy. Results from the TIMI II Study. Circulation *90*:78, 1994.

122. The GUSTO Investigators: An international randomized trial comparing four thrombolytic strategies for acute myocardial infarction. N. Engl. J. Med. *329*:673, 1993.

123. Grines, C. L., Browne, K. F., Marco, J., et al.: A comparison of immediate angioplasty with thrombolytic therapy for acute myocardial infarction. N. Engl. J. Med. *328*:673, 1993.

124. Grines, C. L., Griffin, J. J., Brodie, B. R., et al.: The second primary angioplasty for myocardial infarction study (PAMI-II): Preliminary Report. Circulation *90*(Suppl. I):433, 1994.

125. Gundersen, T., Abrahamsen, A. M., Kjekshus, J., et al.: Timolol-related reduction in mortality and reinfarction in patients ages 65–75 years surviving acute myocardial infarction. Circulation *66*:1179, 1982.

126. Pfeffer, M. A., Braunwald, E., Moye, L. A., et al.: Effect of captopril on mortality and morbidity in patients with left ventricular dysfunction after myocardial infarction. N. Engl. J. Med. *327*:669, 1992.

127. Fleg, J. L., and Kennedy, H. L.: Cardiac arrhythmias in a healthy elderly population: Detection by 24 hour ambulatory electrocardiography. Chest *81*:302, 1982.

128. Manolio, T. A., Furberg, C. D., Rautaharju, P. M., et al.: Cardiac arrhythmias on 24-hr ambulatory electrocardiography in older women and men: The Cardiovascular Health Study. J. Am. Coll. Cardiol. *23*:916, 1994.

129. Furberg, C. D., Psaty, B. M., Manolio, T. A., et al.: Prevalence of atrial fibrillation in elderly subjects (the Cardiovascular Health Study). Am. J. Cardiol. *74*:236, 1994.

130. Onundarson, P. T., Thorgeirsson, G., Jonmundsson, E., et al.: Chronic atrial fibrillation: Epidemiologic features and 14 year follow-up: A case-control study. Eur. Heart J. *8*:521, 1987.

131. Benjamin, E. F., Plehn, J. F., D'Agostino, R. B., et al.: Mitral annular calcification and the risk of stroke in an elderly cohort. N. Engl. J. Med. *327*:374, 1992.

132. The Stroke Prevention in Atrial Fibrillation Investigators: Predictors of thromboembolism in atrial fibrillation: II. Echocardiographic features of patients at risk. Ann. Intern. Med. *116*:6, 1992.

133. Atrial Fibrillation Investigators: Risk factors for stroke and efficacy of antithrombotic therapy in atrial fibrillation. Analysis of pooled data from five randomized controlled trials. Arch. Intern. Med. *154*:1449, 1994.

134. Albers, G. W.: Atrial fibrillation and stroke. Arch. Intern. Med. *154*:1443, 1994.

135. Coplen, S. E., Antman, E. M., Berlin, J. A., et al.: Efficacy and safety of quinidine therapy for maintenance of sinus rhythm after cardioversion. A meta-analysis of randomized control trials. Circulation *82*:1106, 1990.

136. Hohnloser, S. H., and Woosley, R. L.: Sotalol. N. Engl. J. Med. *331*:31, 1994.

137. Gosselink, A. T. M., Crijns, H. J. G. M., Van Gelder, I. C., et al.: Low-dose amiodarone for maintenance of sinus rhythm after cardioversion of atrial fibrillation or flutter. JAMA *267*:3289, 1992.

138. Epstein, L. M., Chiesa, N., Wong, M. N., et al.: Radiofrequency catheter ablation in the treatment of supraventricular tachycardia in the elderly. J. Am. Coll. Cardiol. *23*:1356, 1994.

139. Sawin, C. T., Geller, A., Wolf, P. A., et al.: Low serum thyrotropin concentrations as a risk factor for atrial fibrillation in older persons. N. Engl. J. Med. *331*:1249, 1994.

140. Vaitkevicius, P. V., Esserwein, D. M., Maynard, A. K., et al.: Frequency and importance of postprandial blood pressure reduction in elderly nursing-home patients. Ann. Intern. Med. *115*:865, 1991.

141. Lipsitz, L. A., Ryan, S. M., Parker, J. A., et al.: Hemodynamic and autonomic nervous system responses to mixed meal ingestion in healthy young and old subjects and dysautonomic patients with postprandial hypotension. Circulation *87*:391, 1993.

142. Sgarbossa, E. B., Pinski, S. L., Maloney, J. D., et al.: Chronic atrial fibrillation and stroke in paced patients with sick sinus syndrome. Relevance of clinical characteristics and pacing modalities. Circulation *88*:1045, 1993.

143. Aranki, S. F., Rizzo, R. J., Couper, G. S., et al.: Aortic valve replacement in the elderly. Effect of gender and coronary artery disease on operative mortality. Circulation *88*(Suppl. II):II-17, 1993.

144. Elayda, M. A., Hall, R. J., Reul, R. M., et al.: Aortic valve replacement in patients 80 years and older. Operative risks and long-term results. Circulation *88*(Suppl. II):II-11, 1993.

145. Logeais, Y., Langanay, T., Roussin, R., et al.: Surgery for aortic stenosis in elderly patients. A study of surgical risk and predictive factors. Circulation *90*:2891, 1994.

146. Litvack, F., Jakubowski, A. T., Buchbinder, N. A., and Eigler, N.: Lack of sustained clinical improvement in an elderly population after percutaneous aortic valvuloplasty. Am. J. Cardiol. *62*:270, 1088.

147. Jebara, V. A., Dervanian, P., Acar, C., et al.: Mitral valve repair using Carpentier techniques in patients more than 70 years old: Early and late results. Circulation *86*(Suppl. II):II-53, 1992.

148. Le Feuvre, C., Bonan, R., Lachurie, M. L., et al.: Balloon mitral commissurotomy in patients aged ≥ 70 years. Am. J. Cardiol. *71*:233, 1993.

149. Bennet, N. E.: Hypertension in the elderly. Lancet *344*:447, 1994.

150. Derkx, F. H. M.: Renal artery stenosis and hypertension. Lancet *344*:237, 1994.

151. Farnett, L., Mulrow, C. D., Linn, W. D., et al.: The J-curve phenomenon and the treatment of hypertension: Is there a point beyond which pressure reduction is dangerous? JAMA *265*:489, 1992.

152. Siscovick, D. S., Raghunathan, T. E., Psaty, B. M., et al.: Diuretic therapy for hypertension and the risk of primary cardiac arrest. N. Engl. J. Med. *330*:1852, 1994.

153. Kannel, W. B., and Belanger, A. J.: Epidemiology of heart failure. Am. Heart J. *121*:951, 1991.

154. Massie, B. M., and Conway, M.: Survival of patients with congestive heart failure: Past, present, and future prospects. Circulation *75*(Suppl. IV):IV-11, 1987.

155. Yusuf, S., Thom, T., and Abbott, R. D.: Changes in hypertension treatment and in congestive heart failure mortality in the United States. Hypertension *13*(Suppl. I):I-74, 1989.

156. Schulman, S. P., Weiss, J. L., Becker, L. C., et al.: The effects of antihypertensive therapy on left ventricular mass in elderly hypertensive patients. N. Engl. J. Med. *322*:1350, 1990.

157. Montamat, S. C., Cusack, B. J., and Vestal, R. E.: Management of drug therapy in the elderly. N. Engl. J. Med. *321*:303, 1989.

158. Dybkaer, R., Lauritzen, M., Krakauer, R., et al.: Relative reference values for clinical chemical and haematological quantities in "healthy" elderly people. Acta Med. Scand. *209*:1, 1981.

159. Bruce, A., Andersson, M., Arvidsson, B., and Isaksson, B.: Body composition. Prediction of normal body potassium, body water and body fat in adults on the basis of body height, body weight and age. Scand. J. Clin. Lab. Invest. *40*:461, 1980.

160. Abernathy, E. R., and Kerzner, L.: Age effects on alpha-1-acid glycoprotein concentration and imipramine plasma protein binding. J. Am. Geriatr. Soc. *32*:705, 1984.

161. Rowe, J. W., Andres, R., Tobin, J. D., et al.: Age-adjusted standards for creatinine clearance. Ann. Intern. Med. *84*:567, 1976.

Chapter 51
Coronary Artery Disease in Women

PAMELA S. DOUGLAS

For most of this century, cardiovascular disease has been the most common cause of death and disability in women of all ethnic and racial groups in the United States (Fig. 51–1).[1–3] The prevalence of cardiovascular disease in women increases dramatically with age (Fig. 51–2); as the population ages and women's life expectancy increases, the importance of these diseases will also increase.

While similar in many respects, men and women with coronary artery disease (CAD) demonstrate striking and clinically important differences in epidemiology, diagnosis, prognosis, treatment, and prevention. Clinical care is rapidly changing as evidence accumulates to suggest that estrogen has the potential to be among the most powerful cardiovascular drugs available. Proving this, understanding the underlying mechanisms of hormones' interaction with the cardiovascular system, and learning to use them optimally will take many years. An equally important challenge, however, involves recognition by both patients and their physicians of the enormous health risk that cardiovascular diseases pose for women.

EVALUATION OF CHEST PAIN

CLINICAL SYNDROMES. It has long been assumed that the clinical expression of CAD is similar in men and women, yet available information suggests that gender differences in presentation and disease manifestations exist and should be considered in the evaluation of the patient with chest pain. Several studies document that women are more likely than men to present with angina and less likely to present with a myocardial infarction as either the first or subsequent manifestations of CAD.[4,5] Further, women are on average 10 years older at the time of presentation. These results are closely linked to the finding that chest pain is a poor predictor of epicardial coronary disease in women. Perhaps even more than in men, the prevalence of angiographic coronary disease varies dramatically according to the nature of the chest pain, the patient's age, and the presence of coronary risk factors[6–8] (Fig. 51–2). This underlines the importance of good history taking and careful cardiovascular risk factor assessment in the evaluation of women with chest pain.

A variety of factors influence the evaluation of chest pain in women.[9] Although women seek medical care more often than men do, they also drastically underestimate their own risk of CAD. In addition, a woman's presentation style alters physicians' estimates of the likelihood of CAD, so that a woman whose demeanor was more business-like was judged to have a much higher probability of disease than one who behaved histrionically.[11] Compared with men, women with chronic stable angina are older and more likely to have hypertension, diabetes, and congestive heart failure but less likely to have had a myocardial infarction or revascularization.[10] While equally likely to have effort angina, such women are more likely to experience pain at rest, during sleep, or with mental stress. This patient pro-

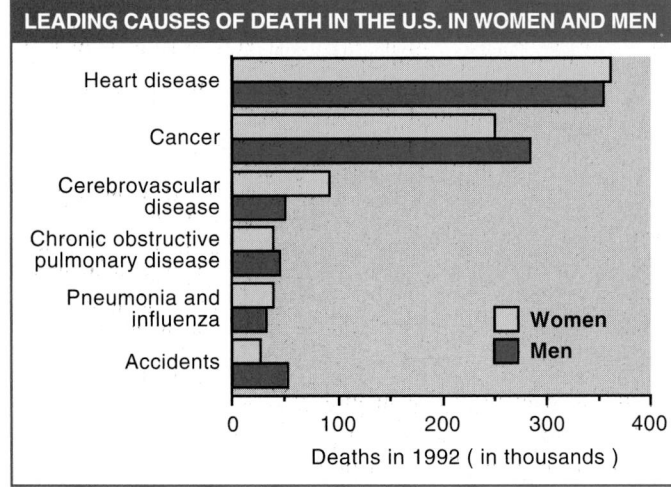

FIGURE 51–1. Number of deaths due to the six leading causes of death in women and men in the U.S. in 1992, ranked in order for women. (Data from Advance Report of Final Mortality Statistics for 1992, National Center for Health Statistics, 1995.)

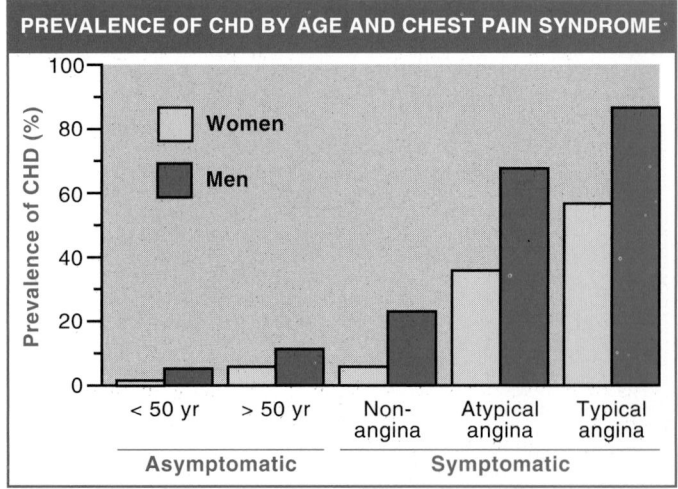

FIGURE 51–2. Prevalence of angiographically documented coronary heart disease in men and women according to age and chest pain syndrome. (Modified from DeSanctis, R.W.: Clinical manifestations of coronary artery disease: Chest pain in women. *In* Wenger, N.K., Speroff, L. and Packard, B. [eds.]: Cardiovascular Health and Disease in Women. Greenwich, CT, Le Jacq Communications, 1993, p. 68.)

file makes the evaluation of a new symptom or disability more complex.

The mechanisms by which ischemia is produced may help explain differences in anginal patterns. Women have higher prevalences than men do of vasospastic angina and of microvascular angina,[7,8,12] both of which are associated with atypical chest pain patterns, are often treated differently, and have a more favorable prognosis than epicardial coronary disease (Chap. 38). Even in the presence of angiographically documented disease, gender differences in plaque components, (more cellular and fibrous tissue in women) endothelial function (estrogen-induced coronary vasodilation) and hemostasis (higher fibrinogen and Factor VII levels in women) may influence the pathophysiology and therefore the clinical manifestations of coronary disease.[13,14] Finally, women more commonly have noncoronary chest pain syndromes, further complicating their clinical assessment.

NATURAL HISTORY AND PROGNOSIS. Women with angina are less likely to experience a subsequent myocardial infarction or coronary death than men.[5,15,16] Although overall age-adjusted rates of death or myocardial infarction in women with angina are less than those in men,[15] of subjects over age 65, women and men with exertional chest pain have the same relative risks of CAD death (2.7 vs 2.4).[17] Other data suggesting that the prognosis of coronary disease is not more benign in women include the similar (if not worse) early mortality after myocardial infarction in women.[18]

Thus, determination of the etiology of chest pain in women can be difficult, hampered by the onset of CAD later in life, the more common appearance of symptoms such as rest angina in patients with otherwise stable patterns, the poor predictive value of angina for angiographic coronary disease, and the higher likelihood of alternative mechanisms of chest pain and ischemia.

Noninvasive and Invasive Diagnostic Testing

While noninvasive diagnostic testing for CAD does not fully resolve the difficulties inherent in evaluating chest pain in women, careful test selection and interpretation can provide valuable information regarding the presence and severity of CAD in women. The general principles underlying noninvasive diagnostic testing do not differ in men and women (see Chap. 5). The simplest diagnostic test, the resting electrocardiogram, reveals a higher prevalence of repolarization (ST-T wave) abnormalities in women with suspected coronary disease than in men (32 vs 23 per cent).[6,19]

Treadmill exercise testing carries a higher false-positive rate in women, ranging from 38 to 67 per cent, than in men, 7 to 44 per cent in the same studies,[19] in part because of a lower pretest likelihood of disease.[7] However, women have a low false-negative rate (12 to 22 per cent) that compares favorably to that in men (12 to 40 per cent), and suggests that routine testing reliably *excludes* the presence of CAD in women with negative tests. The exercise electrocardiogram also provides useful prognostic information in women.[20] Variables contributing to test accuracy are resting ST-T wave abnormalities, peak exercise heart rate, number of diseased vessels, typical angina, age, gender, drug use (digitalis, diazepam, methyldopa), hyperventilation, conduction abnormalities, left ventricular hypertrophy, mitral valve prolapse, vasospasm, and hormonal influences. Although less common in women, false-negative studies may be contributed to by gender-specific characteristics including reduced exercise tolerance and the higher prevalence of single vessel disease in women.

The failure of many normal women to increase their ejection fraction during exercise directly affects the interpretation of the exercise radionuclide angiogram,[21] since disease detection is based on ejection fraction augmentation during exercise (see p. 434).

The addition of imaging to electrocardiographic stress testing markedly improves its accuracy in women. Planar thallium scans during treadmill exercise testing suggest moderate increases in sensitivity and specificity in women[22-31] (Table 51–1). The use of single-photon emission computed tomography (SPECT) may not improve accuracy in women as it does in men.[26] Much of the inaccuracy of thallium scanning in women has been attributed to breast attenuation, but the benefit of higher energy isotopes such as technetium-^{99m}-sestamibi has not yet been proved. Coupling exercise testing with echocardiographic visualization of wall motion (i.e., exercise echocardiography) also improves diagnostic accuracy in women[28,29,29a] (Table 51–1). This is particularly true when the resting electrocardiogram is abnormal or uninterpretable. The use of pharmacological stress agents (adenosine, dipyridamole dobutamine) in women coupled with either echocardiographic or nuclear imaging shows substantial improvements in test performance over electrocardiographic results alone.

Since few direct comparisons between exercise echocardiography and exercise-thallium or sestamibi testing have been reported, and none with adequate numbers of women, there is little objective basis for selecting one modality over another, and both appear more accurate than routine exercise electrocardiography testing. One approach,[23] which reduced both the number of thallium scans and angiographic procedures necessary without a loss of diagnostic accuracy, was the performance of treadmill exercise testing first in all women referred for noninvasive testing, with subsequent

TABLE 51–1 INCREMENTAL VALUE OF IMAGING TO EXERCISE STRESS TESTING FOR THE DIAGNOSIS OF CORONARY HEART DISEASE IN WOMEN

STUDY, YEAR, REFERENCE	STRESS MODALITY	STRESS ECG ALONE		IMAGING MODALITY	WITH IMAGING	
		Sensitivity (%)	Specificity (%)		Sensitivity (%)	Specificity (%)
Hung 1984[22]	Treadmill	73	59	Planar thallium	75	91
Melin 1985[23]	Bicycle	61	78	Planar thallium	70	93
Friedman 1982[24]	Treadmill	32	41	Planar thallium	75	88
Goodgold 1987[25]	Treadmill	N/A	N/A	Planar thallium	93	85
Fintel 1989[26]	N/A	N/A	N/A	Planar thallium	84	90*
				SPECT thallium	86	90*
Chae 1993[27]	Treadmill	66	60	SPECT thallium	71	65
Sawada 1989[28]	Treadmill/bicycle	29	83	Echo	86	86
Williams 1994[29]	Bicycle	67	51	Echo	88	84
Masini 1988[30]	Bicycle	72	52	Dipyridamole echo	79	93
Kong 1992[31]	N/A	N/A	N/A	Dipyridamole thallium	87	58

* Preset from receiver operator curves.

exercise thallium examination only in the 30 per cent with post test probabilities between 10 and 90 per cent (i.e., those in whom a reasonably certain diagnosis of CAD could not be reached or excluded on the basis of history, risk factors, and exercise electrocardiography. A recent theoretical analysis of accuracy and cost-effectiveness[32] considered seven different diagnostic testing strategies and suggested that one employing exercise *echocardiography* as the first test might be superior.

Coronary Angiography

Few studies have examined gender differences in invasive diagnostic testing. While it is reasonable to assume that the assessment of the extent and severity of angiographic coronary narrowing is similar in men and women, it has been suggested that coronary vasoconstriction is a more important mechanism of ischemia in women.[7,8,12] Women are more likely than men to experience vascular and renal complications from diagnostic angiography, possibly due to more advanced age and smaller body size[33]; the incidence of myocardial infarction, stroke, and death are similar.

GENDER BIAS. A 1987 study reporting that men with positive nuclear exercise tests were 6.3 times more likely to be referred to cardiac catheterization than women[34] gave rise to concerns that female patients were receiving inadequate or inappropriate care, a conclusion that has been supported by several subsequent studies. Coronary angiography is performed 28 to 45 per cent more often and revascularization 15 to 27 per cent more often in men than in women with a diagnosis of CAD.[35] In the Systolic Hypertension in the Elderly Program (SHEP), men with incident coronary disease were more likely to undergo revascularization by angioplasty or surgery than were women (26 vs 9 per cent in patients between 60 and 75; 6 vs. 2 per cent in those age 75 or older).[36] Other studies have suggested that gender differences in care may be due to overtreatment of low-risk men.[37,38]

It has been proposed that different treatment strategies in women might represent optimal care,[39] given the known differences in disease prevalence and the difficulties in noninvasively diagnosing coronary disease in women. This question has been addressed recently by examining the outcomes of patients undergoing diagnostic stress testing.[40] Although women were equally likely to have a positive stress electrocardiogram (29 per cent in women vs 30 per cent in men) or stress thallium examination (23 vs 27 per cent), they were less commonly referred for additional noninvasive testing (4 vs 20 per cent) or catheterization (34 vs 45 per cent). However, subsequent event rates were higher in women, whether they had a normal initial test (1.6 per cent/year death or myocardial infarction vs 0.8 per cent in men) or an abnormal one (14.3 per cent/year vs 6.0 per cent/year). Both male and female patients who did undergo revascularization had no events, while women who were not revascularized had a worse prognosis than similarly untreated men. These data demonstrate not only a gender-based difference in clinical practice but a worse patient outcome in women treated less aggressively.

CARDIAC RISK FACTORS AND THEIR MODIFICATION

(See also Chap. 35)

In the broadest sense, those factors associated with higher cardiac risk in men are also associated with increased cardiac risk in women, including age, family history, smoking, hypertension, lipoproteins, and diabetes mellitus.[41,42] However, they may have a different relative importance, and additional factors, such as hormonal status, are equally powerful predictors of CAD.

LIPIDS. In contrast to men, elevated total cholesterol and low-density lipoprotein (LDL) levels are only weakly associated with CAD in women, and only in women 65 years old or younger.[42-44] Instead, high-density lipoprotein (HDL) cholesterol is closely and inversely associated with CAD risk.[45] Triglycerides are an independent predictor of CAD in older women[46-48] but not in men. Lp(a), a composite of LDL, apo B-100, and apo(a), is also associated with higher cardiac risk in women.

Modification of lipoproteins is generally accomplished by the same life style changes and medications in men and women, although such interventions may be less effective in women.[50] While clinical trials have generally not included women in sufficient numbers for independent analysis, several recent studies employing aggressive, multifactorial treatment for lipid lowering have documented an equal or greater effect in women,[51-53] including angiographic regression of coronary atherosclerosis and reduction in coronary events, but not death.

In general, recommended dietary and pharmacological lipid-lowering strategies are similar in men and women. However, hormone replacement therapy may be a preferred primary therapy for postmenopausal women with low HDL and high LDL.[54] Effects of estrogen may be additive to or event supplant those of conventional lipid-lowering medications.[52] However, estrogen increases triglycerides in 20 to 25 per cent of women, particularly those with elevated baseline levels,[55] who may therefore be less likely to benefit from hormone replacement therapy. An elevated baseline level therefore mandates careful monitoring of lipid levels following institution of hormonal therapy.

Current recommendations for initiation of treatment and therapeutic goals (NCEP-II) are similar in men and women and are based on LDL levels[54] (see Table 35–6, p. 1138). Despite the fact that HDL is a more powerful determinant of CAD risk in women, the NCEP-II guidelines do not include HDL or triglyceride levels except as modifying factors. It is not clear how well these recommendations address the needs of women or the very elderly, who are predominantly female.[56]

DIABETES AND OBESITY (see also Chap. 60). Diabetes is a risk factor for the presence and severity of coronary heart disease in both men and women but carries a greater incremental risk in women, completely eliminating the "female advantage."[47,57] Even more than in men, diabetes dramatically increases the mortality of myocardial infarction in women.[58a]

Non–insulin-dependent diabetes is associated with obesity, abdominal and upper body fat distribution, hypertension, and insulin resistance, all of which have been associated with higher coronary heart disease risk.[57] It has been hypothesized that this complex of abnormalities may be causally related to high circulating insulin levels, but this remains unproved. More so than in men, obesity and body fat distribution appear to be independent coronary heart disease risk factors in women.[58a] Diabetes is also linked with the presence of hyperlipidemia (elevated triglycerides, reduced HDL), especially in women,[57] and the lipoprotein response to adequate diabetic treatment is variable.[59] Overall, it is unclear what effect diabetic treatment or weight loss have (if any) in modifying cardiovascular risk in women.

HYPERTENSION (see also Chap. 26). The prevalence of hypertension in women greatly increases with age so that nearly 80 per cent of women over age 75 are hypertensive.[60] Hypertension carries an independent coronary heart disease risk for both men and women and substantially enhances the risks associated with hyperlipidemia, smoking, obesity, and diabetes. While the benefits of antihypertensive treatment have not been well studied in women, it appears that therapy may reduce both overall mortality and cardiac morbidity as well as the incidence of stroke; these effects are most striking in the elderly.[61]

SMOKING. Smoking is a strong independent risk factor for coronary heart disease in both men and women; although smoking rates in the United States are falling overall, they are currently increasing among women.[62] This risk is present even with minimal exposure (1 to 4 cigarettes/day) and is not improved by use of low-yield cigarettes.[63] Smoking risk is strikingly synergistic with that of oral contraceptive use, especially in women over age 35, and often leads to an earlier menopause, another coronary heart disease risk unique to women.[64] Cessation of smoking appears to gradually eliminate the excess risk in women,[65] although women more often smoke to lose or maintain body weight and find it harder to quit than do men.

HEMOSTASIS. Elevated fibrinogen levels appear to be an independent cardiac risk factor in men and women, although women have not been as well studied.[66] The mechanism(s) by which fibrinogen enhances risk are poorly understood, although high fibrinogen levels have been associated with other CAD risk factors, including hypertension, diabetes, smoking, obesity, hyperlipidemia, and menopause, and lower levels have been associated with exercise, hormone replacement therapy, and high HDL.[67] Gender differences in platelet function and hemostasis are virtually unexplored.[68]

EXERCISE. A sedentary life style is associated with CAD in both men and women, although the data for women are sparse.[69] The reported beneficial effects of exercise on coronary heart disease risk profile are less marked in women compared with men,[69,70] with lesser increases in HDL and less weight loss resulting from similar exercise training. In prospective observational studies, a lower fitness level has been associated with a 4.7 fold-increased risk for all-cause mortality in women,[71] and higher activity levels have been associated with decreased relative risks for CAD (0.44) and stroke (0.51) compared with lower activity levels.[72] These results were independent of other vascular risk factors.[72]

PSYCHOSOCIAL. The interaction of psychosocial and biobehavorial factors and heart disease are complex, but perhaps have been more extensively studied in women than in men.[73–75] Several of the cardiovascular risk factors discussed above are related to behavior (obesity, smoking, exercise) and are treated with its modification. Perceived stress and its balance with situational control has been found to affect CAD risk in women as well as in men. Social networks and support influence CAD outcome both independently and through the likelihood of compliance with therapeutic strategies (e.g., cardiac rehabilitation). The lack of social support has been associated with a worse outcome in both men and women, but its impact may be greater in women.

HORMONES AND HORMONAL THERAPY

The ovary produces both estrogenic and androgenic hormones until the menopause, when production decreases gradually over several years but does not fully cease. The risk of CAD in women rises thereafter, equaling that in men by age 75. Women who have an early menopause and/or bilateral oophorectomy experience an accelerated risk of CAD. Menopause, or estrogen deprivation, is associated with detrimental changes in cardiovascular risk factors that help explain the increased risk. Chief among these is an increase in LDL cholesterol, a small decrease in HDL, and an increased total ratio of cholesterol to HDL.[76,77] Natural menopause seems to have little immediate effect on blood pressure, glucose tolerance, insulin levels, body weight, or physical activity other than that of advancing age.[77]

Oral contraceptives are perhaps the most commonly prescribed hormones today and generally contain a synthetic estrogen, such as ethinyl estradiol, and a synthetic progestin. Currently used low-dose oral contraceptives pose only a very neglible cardiovascular risk for most patients.[76] The risk of arterial and venous thrombosis is low in current low-dose formulations but is magnified by advancing age and especially by smoking. The risk of myocardial infarction is not increased by oral contraceptives unless the patient is over age 35 and/or smokes cigarettes,[78,79] and appears to be entirely caused by thromboembolism rather than by coronary atherosclerosis, since the angiographic coronary plaque burden is actually lower in oral contraceptive users.[80]

Because most regimens employ a combination of hormones, the effect of any given oral contraceptive on circulating lipoproteins represents the sum of estrogenic effects (higher HDL and triglycerides, lower LDL) and progestogenic effects (higher LDL, lower HDL). Newer agents such as norethindrone gestodine, desogestrel, and norgestinate have beneficial effects on lipoprotein levels as well as enhancing plasminogen levels, fibrinolytic activity, and platelet aggregation reduction.[81]

Estrogen and Cardiac Risk Factor Modification

Postmenopausal estrogen replacement has been proposed for the primary and secondary prevention of CAD in both men and women. Clinical trials of estrogen therapy in men in the 1950's and 1960's used high-dose conjugated estrogens (up to 10 mg/day) and generally uncovered poor drug tolerance, little in the way of favorable risk factor modification, and an excess of thrombophlebitis, cholecystitis, and embolic events without evidence of cardioprotection. Randomized trials in women are only now being undertaken; results will not be available for several years. Currently, the use of hormonal replacement therapy in women is based on its prospectively demonstrated beneficial effects on cardiac risk factors and observational evidence of primary protection.

In postmenopausal women, exogenous estrogen results in higher HDL (especially HDL_2, and apo AI, and lower LDL and apo B-100 and perhaps Lp (a)[76,82–85] (Table 51–2). Importantly, the PEPI trial showed that the addition of a progestin to estrogen did not interfere with the LDL cholesterol-lowering effect of the latter. The use of micronized progestin was associated with an increase in HDL cholesterol.[82] Triglycerides and LDL are often increased in a dose-dependent manner, and although the magnitude of these increases are highly variable, they may limit the use of estrogen in some patients. Transdermal estrogens appear to have lesser effects on all lipoproteins, suggesting that first-pass liver metabolism is important in mediating these effects, and that this mode of drug delivery may be preferred in women with marked triglyceride elevations in response to the oral route.[86]

Other effects of estrogen replacement include a relative decrease in thrombotic potential.[82,87] Reports of an idiosyncratic elevation of blood pressure and improved insulin sensitivity have not been confirmed by more recent studies.[82,85,88] Unopposed estrogen markedly increases the risk of endometrial hyperplasia, although the concomitant use of a progestin largely prevents this.[82]

Recently, important physiological effects of estrogen have been demonstrated in vascular smooth muscle and endothelium. Estrogen receptors are present in vascular smooth muscle cells in both men and women and are capable of altering gene transcription, suggesting a possible role of estrogen in the regulation of vascular smooth muscle cell proliferation.[89] Estrogen also acutely decreases the paradox-

TABLE 51–2 ALTERATIONS IN LIPOPROTEIN LEVELS WITH HORMONE REPLACEMENT THERAPY (%)

	PLACEBO	E ALONE	E + PA (CYCLIC)	E + PA (CONTINUOUS)	E + PA (CYCLIC)
TC	−11	−20	−36	−36	−20
LDL	−11	−37	−46	−43	−38
HDL	−3	+14	+4	+3	+11
Triglycerides	−4	+15	+14	+13	+15

E = conjugated equine estrogen 0.625 mg daily; E + PA (cyclic) = conjugated equine estrogen 0.625 mg daily plus medroxy progesterone acetate 10 mg/day for 12 days each month; E + PA (continuous) = E + PA 2.5 mg/day; E + P (cyclic) = E + micronized progesterone, 200 mg/d for 12 days each month.

Adapted from The Postmenopausal Estrogen/Progestin Interventions (PEPI) Trial: Effects of estrogen or estrogen/progestin regimens on heart disease risk factors in postmenopausal women. JAMA *273*:199, 1995. Copyright 1995 American Medical Association.

ical coronary vasoconstriction response to acetylcholine[90,91] and potentiates the endothelium-dependent vasodilation of conductance and resistance coronary beds and forearm vessels in women.[92,93] Estrogen decreases the atherogenic oxidation of LDL both in vivo and in vitro and decreases the incorporation of lipids into the vessel wall, suggesting additional protective mechanisms for estrogen replacement.[94,95] At present, which of the many beneficial effects of estrogen are most important for the prevention of coronary heart disease has not been determined.

PREVENTION OF CAD WITH ESTROGEN. To date, over 30 epidemiological studies have examined the utility of estrogen in the primary prevention of CAD, and the vast majority report a significant benefit.[76,96–98] The largest of these studies, the Nurses' Health Study, reported a relative risk of 0.56 for myocardial infarction or death in women currently using estrogen and 0.83 in ever-users, after adjustment for age and risk factors.[99] Recent meta-analyses[96,98] have determined composite relative risks of 0.50 to 0.65 for both the development of and death from CAD in estrogen users.

Other documented benefits of estrogen therapy include the alleviation of menopausal symptoms and prevention of osteoporosis and fatal hip fracture (relative risk for death from this common disease is 0.75 for users of estrogen).[76,96,97] A possible protective effect against stroke has been noted in several studies[100] but is not significant in others, including the large Nurses' Health Study (relative risk 0.97 for current users) and another recent meta-analysis.[96] It is possible that the relatively young cohorts examined may have influenced these findings (median age for stroke in women is 83 years).

The beneficial effect of reproductive hormones also extends to tamoxifen, an estrogen agonist/antagonist, which has been shown to have salutory effects on circulating lipoproteins[101] and to reduce the number of hospital admissions resulting from CAD, and death due to myocardial infarction and vascular causes.[102,103]

Only a very small number of studies have evaluated the utility of estrogen in the secondary prevention of coronary heart disease. Women who were current or ever-users of estrogen had less severe angiographic coronary artery disease than never-users, even after correction for age, cholesterol, smoking, diabetes, and hypertension.[104,105] Long-term survival in women with a similar extent of angiographically documented coronary disease or after coronary artery bypass grafting is greater in women taking estrogen (Table 51–3).[106,107]

While the benefits may seem large, there are methodological limitations in all available studies as well as significant risks associated with estrogen use and logistic problems with its prescription. Chief among the risks of estrogen use is *endometrial cancer*, for which unopposed estrogen therapy carries a five- to eightfold increased risk, associated with an estimated threefold increased risk of death.[96,97,97a] While the risk of this complication is obviously zero in women without a uterus, it has been proposed that the addition of a progestin also nullifies it. A potential detrimental effect on the cardioprotective action of estrogen of adding progestins is anticipated because of their androgenic effect on circulating lipids; however, recent studies suggest that this factor may have negligible effects or may even be beneficial.[82,97,98]

BREAST CANCER. Estrogen may increase breast cancer risk, with meta-analyses showing little increased risk for short-term therapy, whereas a higher relative risk, up to 1.5, has been associated with long-term use (over 10 years) in the Nurses' Health Study.[96,109,109a] If confirmed, this

TABLE 51–3 NET CHANGE IN LIFE EXPECTANCY FOR A 50-YEAR-OLD WHITE WOMAN TREATED WITH LONG-TERM HORMONE REPLACEMENT

CLINICAL CHARACTERISTICS	UNTREATED LIFE EXPECTANCY (YEARS)	NET CHANGE IN LIFE EXPECTANCY WITH RX		
		Estrogen**	E + P††	E + P‡‡
No cardiac risk factors, intact	82.8	+0.9	+1.0	+0.1
No risk factors and hysterectomy	82.8	+1.1	N/A	N/A
With history of CAD*	76.0	+2.1	+2.2	+0.9
With 1 or more CAD risk factors†	79.6	+1.5	+1.6	+0.6
At risk for breast cancer‡	82.3	+0.7	+0.8	−0.5
At risk for hip fracture§	82.4	+1.0	+1.1	+0.2

* Relative risk of dying of recurrent CAD estimated at 5.0.
† Relative risk of CAD death estimated as 2.5, as with smoking, hypertension, diabetes, or a sedentary life style.
‡ Breast cancer risk estimated as 2.0, as for a woman with a family history of breast cancer.
§ Hip fracture risk estimated as 3.0, as for a woman with low bone mineral density.
** Net change in life expectancy assumes that estrogen therapy carries the following relative risks; endometrial cancer death 3.0, breast cancer death 1.25, coronary heart disease death 0.65, hip fracture death 0.75, and death due to stroke 0.96.
†† E + P = Estrogen plus progesterone. These figures assume that the addition of progesterone to estrogen does not alter any relative risks, except to fully prevent the increased risk for endometrial cancer death (relative risk = 1.0).
‡‡ These figures assume that the addition of progesterone to estrogen reduces by one-third the benefit for CAD risk reduction (relative risk for CAD becomes 0.8) and that the relative risk for breast cancer increases to 2.0.

From Grady, D., Rubin, S. M., Pettiti, D. B., et al.: Hormone therapy to prevent disease and prolong life in postmenopausal women. Ann. Intern. Med. *117*:1016, 1992.

would represent a deterrent to estrogen replacement, especially in women with a personal or family history of breast cancer and a low likelihood of (i.e., no risk factors for) CAD. On the other hand, women with established CAD or with risk factors and no family history of breast cancer are the best candidates for estrogen replacement. The effects of the addition of progestins to estrogen in the incidence of breast cancer are unknown, but they appear to be minimal.[109a]

A recent meta-analysis of estrogen replacement reviewed all available data on its effects on endometrial and breast cancers, hip fracture, stroke, and coronary heart disease.[96] Combining these data with other information regarding the incidence and mortality of these diseases, detailed estimates of the gain/loss in life expectancy with hormone therapy for a hypothetical 50-year-old white woman with a variety of health risks were derived (Table 51-3). In most cases, estrogen replacement enhanced longevity.

BALANCING RISKS AND BENEFITS. Other considerations in the decision to use estrogen replacement include the drug's side effects, such as vaginal bleeding, the need for careful monitoring for breast and uterine cancers and endometrial hyperplasia, and the costs of therapy and of monitoring.[96,97,110,111] Thrombophlebitis is not a problem at the doses currently employed.[112] Compliance with estrogen replacement therapy taken to relieve menopause symptoms is poor; there is no reason to think that this will improve in asymptomatic women taking estrogen for the prevention of future disease.[113]

A full evaluation of the risks and benefits of estrogen replacement cannot be made without considering the methodological flaws inherent in all available data, and those crucial areas in which information is lacking. The lack of available results from any large observational studies raises issues of selection bias, especially because women using estrogen are more likely to see their physicians frequently, to adopt healthy behaviors such as exercise, prudent diet, and smoking cessation, and to be of higher socioeconomic status.[114]

The most commonly used estrogen is conjugated equine estrogens at a daily dose of 0.625 mg. There is no evidence that cardioprotection is enhanced or even preserved at a higher dose and side effects are often worse. In contrast, the optimal formulation, dosage, and regimen for progestins are unclear. The optimal timing of estrogen replacement is also unknown. Some workers suggest starting drug at menopause and continuing indefinitely for women at high risk. The usefulness of beginning therapy at a more advanced age (for example, with the first manifestation of CAD) is unknown, but this practice is likely to be of some benefit to those who have not been treated earlier.[115]

GUIDELINES FOR ESTROGEN REPLACEMENT THERAPY. The American College of Physicians recently published guidelines for counseling postmenopausal women about preventive hormone therapy that are well grounded in available knowledge.[116] These guidelines suggest that, based on available data, it is reasonable to state that estrogen replacement is likely of value in women with a high risk of developing osteoporosis or CAD and for secondary prevention in any woman currently with cardiovascular disease who is not at high risk for breast cancer. Because this includes all women with documented ischemia or infarction or those undergoing revascularization, this proposal represents an enormous potential change in cardiovascular therapeutics and practice. It is important to recognize that while salutary effects of estrogen replacement on lipids have been demonstrated in prospective randomized trials, clinical benefits thus far are limited to observational studies. Ongoing randomized trials of primary and secondary prevention will prove whether the wide use of estrogen replacement in postmenopausal women is a viable strategy.

Chronic Coronary Artery Disease
(See also Chap. 38)

Medical Therapy

Because few studies have examined the medical treatment of chronic CAD in women, there is little evidence as to whether women and men respond similarly to conventional therapy. Cross-sectional studies reveal that women with CAD are more likely than men to be receiving nitrates, calcium channel blockers, sedatives, diuretics, and other antihypertensive agents but are equally or less likely to have been prescribed aspirin and beta blockers.[10,40] The impact, if any, of these differences on the prognosis of coronary disease is unknown, although the Coronary Artery Surgery Study (CASS), shows that women treated medically had better 12-year survival with angiographically documented zero-, one-, or two-vessel disease than did men with similar anatomy.[117]

The use of aspirin is not as well proved in women as it is in men, and results cannot simply be extrapolated to women because gender may affect the antithrombotic and endothelial effects of aspirin.[14,18] The few observational studies in women have reported conflicting results regarding the effectiveness of aspirin for primary prevention. The most favorable, the Nurse's Health Study, showed a reduction in myocardial infarction risk of borderline statistical significance for women over 50 years taking one to six aspirin per week[119] but not in younger women or those taking higher doses. Other large studies have shown an increase in CAD risk in women with aspirin use.[120,121,121a] No study has yet demonstrated effective secondary prevention with aspirin in women.

Revascularization

In contrast to the paucity of data regarding medical therapy for CAD in women, many studies have addressed the relative effectiveness of revascularization procedures (angioplasty and coronary artery bypass grafting [CABG]) in men and women. Unfortunately, comparisons of the results of medical and invasive and operative management are few. Instead, these studies have focused on gender differences in the population under study, making difficult the application of these data to the optimal care of individual patients. Virtually all data for both angioplasty and CABG have been derived from post hoc subgroup analysis of studies designed to address other issues.

ANGIOPLASTY (see also p. 1371). Virtually all angioplasty studies note a greater prevalence of comorbidities in women, including advanced age, hypertension, congestive heart failure, diabetes, severe concomitant noncardiac disease, and hypercholesterolemia.[118,122–127] The severity of angina is also greater in women, the condition being more likely to be unstable or to be of Canadian Class III or IV severity.[122,124–126]

The likelihood of *angiographic success* of the application of balloon angioplasty or of new devices is similar in men and women in current series,[124–126] with lower success rates in women reported only in the older studies. In contrast, women experience higher complication and mortality rates, including groin complications, acute closure and death, but not myocardial infarction or emergency coronary artery bypass grafting[123] (Table 51-4). The difference in outcome has been variously attributed to women's older age, smaller body size, greater severity of angina, more fragile vessels, and perhaps greater comorbidity.[126]

The late outcome of angioplasty appears to be similar in men and women, with women more likely to experience angina and men more likely to experience cardiac events (myocardial infarction, revascularization, or death).[123–125,]

TABLE 51-4   GENDER DIFFERENCES IN EARLY OUTCOME OF ANGIOPLASTY

STUDY, YEAR, REFERENCE	SERIES	ANGIOGRAPHIC SUCCESS (%)		COMPLICATIONS (%)		MORTALITY (%)	
		W	M	W	M	W	M
Cowley 1985[122]	NHLBI 1978–82	56.6	56.6	27.2	19.4	1.7	0.3
Kelsey 1993[123]	NHLBI 1985–86	89	89	29	20	2.6	0.3
Arnold 1994[124]	Cleveland Clinic 1980–88	93.6	93.3	9	7	1.1	0.3
Weintraub 1994[125]	Emory 1980–91	90.8	89.7	—	—	0.7	0.1
Bell 1993[126]	Mayo 1979–87	83	82	—	—	1.0	1.2
	Mayo Clinic 1988–90	87	90	—	—	2.9	1.4
Welty 1994[127]	Deaconess 1981–89	89.6	91.2	—	—	0.6	0.9

[127,128] Gender differences in angiographic restenosis rates have not been carefully examined.

CORONARY ARTERY BYPASS GRAFTING. Gender differences in outcome following CABG are well established.[118,129–135] As with angioplasty, virtually every study has shown women to have more comorbidities and less favorable patient characteristics preoperatively. Women are also more likely than men to undergo urgent or emergent surgery.[129,131,133] Women and men undergoing CABG are equally symptomatic but women are more likely to have preserved ventricular function and less likely to have multivessel or three-vessel disease.[129,130,132]

The mortality of women is higher than of men, with a risk ratio of 1.4 to 4.4.[118,129–135] In addition, women are less likely to receive internal mammary grafts or undergo complete revascularization and are more likely to experience the complications of heart failure, perioperative infarction, and hemorrhage.[129,131]

The causes of this higher mortality appear to be multiple, including technical factors such as smaller body size and coronary diameter, advanced age, comorbidities such as diabetes and hypertension, and clinical factors such as the urgency of the procedure.[129,130,132–134] Disease-related factors such as the extent and severity of angiographic stenoses and left ventricular dysfunction are also important in determining outcome, yet these factors tend to be more favorable in women. As with angioplasty, patient-related factors and comorbidities seem increasingly important to outcome, with more recent studies reporting widening gender differences in outcome.[130,134]

Women have a lower likelihood of being free of angina than do men[130] and experience greater physical disability and less return to work. Rates of long-term survival, infarction, and reoperation are similar.[130,132,135]

Acute Myocardial Infarction
(See also Chap. 37)

Although little is known of the pathophysiology underlying gender differences in acute myocardial infarction, it is clear that women have a different clinical presentation and respond differently to both medical and procedural therapies.

CLINICAL SYNDROMES. Women suffering from an acute myocardial infarction are likely to be older and more likely to have a history of hypertension, diabetes, unstable angina, hyperlipidemia, and congestive heart failure and are less likely to be smokers than their male counterparts.[136,139,141–150] Women are also more likely to experience neck and shoulder pain, abdominal pain, nausea, vomiting, fatigue, and dyspnea in addition to chest pain,[151] and are more likely to have silent infarctions.[5] Perhaps due in part to these more atypical symptoms, women seek medical attention more slowly[152] and even after hospital arrival may experience greater delays in receiving care.[145,147,153] Women are more likely to have experienced a nontransmural infarction.[141,150] Women with infarction have more serious

presentations, with greater prevalences of tachycardia, rales, heart block, and a higher Killip class on initial presentation.[145,147,149,150,152] Nevertheless, women are less likely to receive thrombolysis (even after controlling for eligibility)[136,152,154,155,155a] and receive it later than do men.[147] Women are also less likely to be admitted to a coronary care unit[152,156] or to be hospitalized in an institution in which catheterization is available.[150] Most[150,151,153,154,156] but not all[137,157] women with acute infarction are less likely to undergo diagnostic catheterization during their hospital stay, even after controlling for age and a variety of clinical characteristics. Most studies have reported equal or near equal rates of angioplasty and bypass surgery among catheterized patients,[137,147,148,151,153] so that differences in treatment disappear once disease is documented angiographically.[158]

Women have higher rates of in-hospital complications from infarction, including bleeding, stroke, shock, myocardial rupture, and recurrent chest pain, than do men, although most of these differences disappear on correction for controlling for age and comorbidities.[138,141,147,148] Women with acute infarction are more likely to be treated with nitrates, digoxin, and diuretics than are men and are less likely to receive thrombolytics, antiarrhythmics, antiplatelet agents, and beta blockers.[141,146,152] Even after discharge,

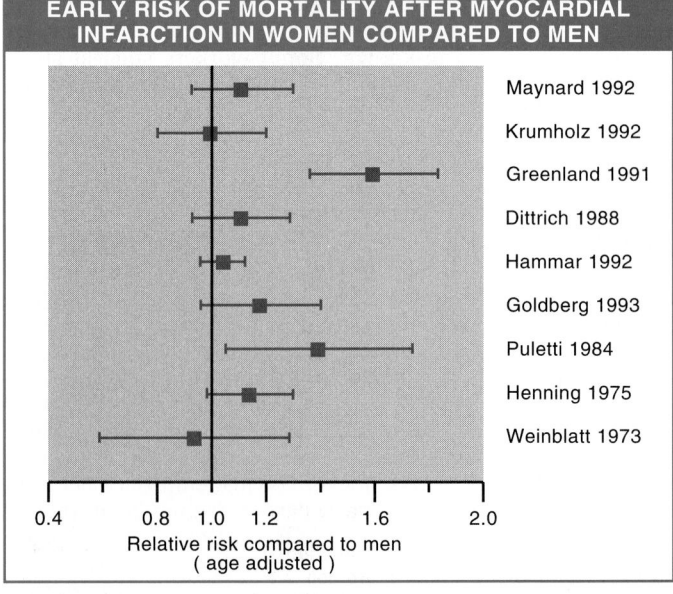

FIGURE 51–3. Relative risk of early mortality (in-hospital or first month) after myocardial infarction in women as compared to men. Data are shown as relative risk with 95% confidence interval. Three additional studies did not report 95% confidence intervals but were not significant. (Modified from Vaccarino, V., Krumholz, H.M., Berkman, L.F., Horvitz, R.I.: Sex differences in mortality after myocardial infarction. Circulation *91:*1861, 1995. Copyright 1995 American Heart Association.)

women are less likely to be scheduled for exercise tests or referred for cardiac rehabilitation, and recovery from infarction appears delayed with slower return to work and full resumption of all activities, with more sleep disturbance and psychiatric and psychosomatic complaints experienced.[159]

MORTALITY. Although early or in-hospital mortality in women appears to be greater than in men, most studies have shown that adjustment for age and/or clinical characteristics serves to reduce this difference but not to eliminate it fully (Fig. 51–3).[18,136–144,160] Mortality 1 to 3 years after hospital discharge is similar in men and women, and when adjustments are made for age and other baseline characteristics, women may actually do better.[18,139]

TREATMENT. Comparison of benefits from thrombolysis in men and women with acute myocardial infarction are difficult, but it appears that the reductions in mortality are similar (Fig. 51–4).[161–165] The efficacy of thrombolysis also appears similar in men and women with similar rates of infarct-related artery patency[145,148] and left ventricular function.[145,148,166] However, complication rates, particularly hemorrhagic stroke and recurrent myocardial infarction, appear to be higher in women.[147,148,167,168] Information on primary angioplasty is limited, but in the PAMI trial the improvement in women was impressive (Fig. 51–4).[170]

Medical treatment after hospital discharge appears to carry somewhat different benefits for men and women. Aspirin (see above) has not yet been proved to prevent reinfarction in women and calcium channel blockers have not been evaluated. Two studies suggest that men may experience more benefit than women when treated with angiotensin-converting enzyme inhibitors postinfarction.[171,172] In contrast, beta blockade clearly provides a substantial

improvement in postinfarction survival in women that is equal to, if not greater than, that seen in men.[173–175] Unfortunately, women are less likely to be discharged on beta-blockers.[146,149,152]

CONCLUSIONS

The time-honored observation of demographic differences in heart disease in men and women is now well supported by newer findings of gender-based differences in the clinical presentation, evaluation, and treatment of heart disease. While principles of diagnostic and therapeutic management of women are similar to those in men, the differences in diagnostic test characteristics and outcomes of interventions mandate careful consideration of risks and benefits for each individual.

Hormones and hormone replacement status are unique and important considerations of heart disease in women. The available epidemiological evidence suggests that such treatment should be a consideration in women at risk for cardiac disease or its recurrence. These clinical observations and elucidation of the underlying pathophysiology suggest new ways to improve upon all aspects of cardiovascular care for women.

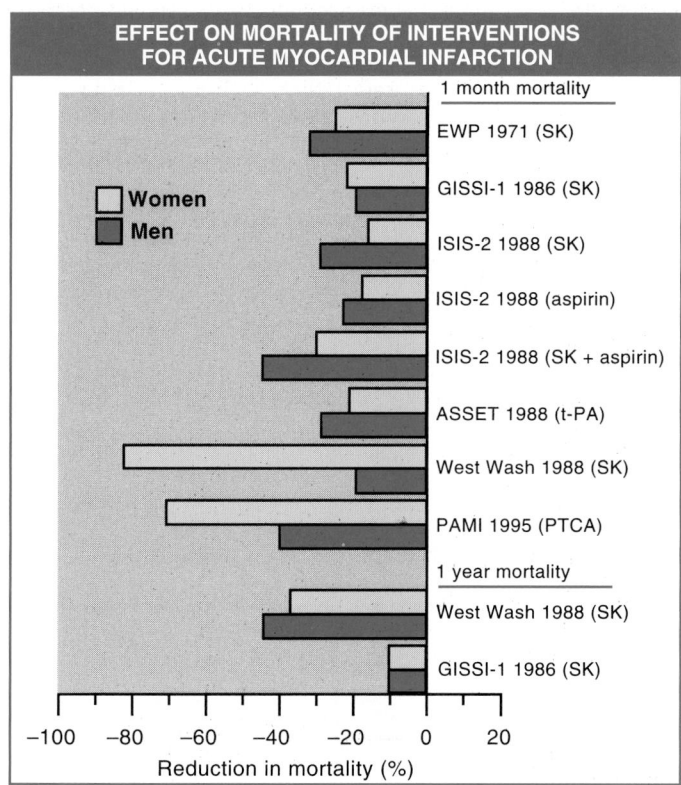

FIGURE 51–4. Comparison of reductions in early and late mortality after myocardial infarction in women and men with thrombolysis, aspirin and primary angioplasty. (EWP = European Working Party; GISSI-1 = Gruppo Italiano per lo Studio della Streptochinasi Nell' infarto Miocardico; ISIS-2 = Second International Study of Infarct Survival; ASSET = Anglo-Scandanavian Study of Early Thrombolysis; West Wash = Western Washington Intravenous Streptokinase in Acute Myocardial Infarction Trial; PAMI = Primary Angioplasty in Myocardial Infarction; SK = Streptokinase; t-PA = Tissue Plasminogen Activator.)

REFERENCES

1. Eaker, E. D., Chesebro, J. H., Sacks, F. M., et al.: Cardiovascular disease in women. Circulation 88:1999, 1993.
2. Higgins, M., and Thom, T.: Cardiovascular disease in women as a public health problem. In Wenger, N. K., Speroff, L., Packard, B. (eds.): Cardiovascular Health and Disease in Women. Greenwich, CT, Le Jacq Communications, Inc., 1993, p. 15.
3. Advance Report of Final Mortality Statistics for 1992 National Center for Health Statistics, 1995.
4. Reunanen, A., Suhonen, O., Aromaa, A., et al.: Incidence of different manifestations of coronary heart disease in middle-aged Finnish men and women. Acta Med. Scand. 218:19, 1985.
5. Lerner, D. J., and Kannel, W. B.: Patterns of coronary heart disease morbidity and mortality in the sexes: 26-year follow-up of the Framingham population. Am. Heart J. 111:383, 1986.
6. Weiner, D. A., Ryan, T. J., McCabe, C. H., et al.: Correlations among history of angina, ST-segment response and prevalence of coronary artery disease in the coronary artery surgery study (CASS). N. Engl. J. Med. 301:230, 1979.
7. DeSanctis, R. W.: Clinical manifestations of coronary artery disease: Chest pain in women. In Wenger, N. K., Speroff, L., Packard, B. (eds.): Cardiovascular Health and Disease in Women. Greenwich, CT, Le Jacq Communications, Inc., 1993, p. 67.
8. Sullivan, A. K., Holdright, D. R., Wright, C. A., et al.: Chest pain in women: Clinical, investigative, and prognostic features. Br. Med. J. 308:883, 1994.
9. Fields, S. K., Savard, M. A., and Epstein, K. R.: The female patient. In Douglas, P. S. (ed.): Cardiovascular Health and Disease in Women. Philadelphia, W. B. Saunders Company, 1993, p. 3.
10. Pepine, C. J., Abrams, J., Marks, R. G., et al.: Characteristics of a contemporary population with angina pectoris. Am. J. Cardiol. 74:226, 1994.
11. Birdwell, B. G., Herbers, J. E., and Kroenke, K.: Evaluating chest pain. Arch. Intern. Med. 153:1991, 1993.
12. Cannon, R. O., Camici, P. G., and Epstein, S. E.: Pathophysiological dilemma of syndrome X. Circulation 85:883, 1992.
13. Mautner, S. L., Lin, F., Mautner, G. C., and Roberts, W. C.: Comparison in women versus men of composition of atherosclerotic plaques in native coronary arteries and in saphenous veins used as aortocoronary conduits. J. Am. Coll. Cardiol. 21:1312, 1992.
14. Weksler, B. B.: Hemostasis and thrombosis. In Douglas, P. S. (ed.): Cardiovascular Health and Disease in Women. Philadelphia, W. B. Saunders Company, 1993, p. 231.
15. Murabito, J. M., Evans, J. C., Larson, M. G., and Levy, D.: Prognosis after the onset of coronary heart disease. An investigation of differences in outcome between the sexes according to initial coronary disease presentation. Circulation 88:2548, 1993.
16. Orencia, A., Bailey, K., Yawn, B. P., and Kottke, T. E.: Effect of gender on long-term outcome of angina pectoris and myocardial infarction/sudden unexpected death. JAMA 269:2392, 1993.
17. LaCroix, A. Z., Guralnik, J. M., Curb, J. D., et al.: Chest pain and coronary heart disease mortality among older men and women in three communities. Circulation 81:437, 1990.
18. Vaccarino, V., Krumholz, H. M., Berkman, L. F., and Horwitz, R. I.: Sex differences in mortality after myocardial infarction. Circulation 91:1861, 1995.
19. Gibbons, R. F.: Exercise ECG testing with and without radionuclide

studies. *In* Wenger, N. K., Speroff, L., Packard, B. (eds.): Cardiovascular Health and Disease in Women. Greenwich, CT, Le Jacq Communications, Inc., 1993, p. 73.

20. Weiner, D. A., Ryan, T. J., Parsons, L., et al.: Long-term prognostic value of exercise testing in men and women from the coronary artery surgery study (CASS) registry. Am. J. Cardiol. *75*:865, 1995.

21. Higgenbotham, M. B., Morris, K. G., Coleman, E., et al.: Sex-related differences in normal cardiac response to supine exercise assessed by radionuclide angiography. J. Am. Coll. Cardiol. *13*:624, 1989.

22. Hung, J., Chaitman, B. R., Lam, J., et al.: Noninvasive diagnostic test choices for the evaluation of coronary artery disease in women: A multivariate comparison of cardiac fluoroscopy, exercise electrocardiography and exercise thallium myocardial perfusion scintigraphy. J. Am. Coll. Cardiol. *4*:8, 1984.

23. Melin, J. A., Wijns, W., Vanbutsele, R. J., et al.: Alternative diagnostic strategies for coronary artery disease in women: Demonstration of the usefulness and efficiency of probability analysis. Circulation *71*:535, 1985.

24. Friedman, T. D., Greene, A. C., Iskandrian, A. S., et al.: Exercise thallium-201 myocardial scintigraphy in women: Correlation with coronary arteriography. Am. J. Cardiol. *49*:1632, 1982.

25. Goodgold, H. M., Rehder, J. G., Samuels, L. D., and Chaitman, B. R.: Improved interpretation of exercise T1-201 myocardial perfusion scintigraphy in women: Characterization of breast attenuation artifacts. Radiology *165*:361, 1987.

26. Fintel, D. J., Links, J. M., Brinker, J. A., et al.: Improved diagnostic performance of exercise thallium-201 single photon emission computed tomography over planar imaging in the diagnosis of coronary artery disease: A receiver operating characteristic analysis. J. Am. Coll. Cardiol. *13*:600, 1989.

27. Chae, S. C., Heo, J., Iskandrian, A. S., et al.: Identification of extensive coronary artery disease in women by exercise single-photon emission computer tomographic (SPECT) thallium imaging. J. Am. Coll. Cardiol. *21*:1305, 1993.

28. Sawada, S. G., Ryan, T., Fineberg, N. S., et al.: Exercise echocardiographic detection of coronary artery disease in women. J. Am. Coll. Cardiol. *14*:1440, 1989.

29. Williams, M. J., Marwick, T. H., O'Gorman, D., and Foale, R. A.: Comparison of exercise echocardiography with an exercise score to diagnose coronary artery disease in women. Am. J. Cardiol. *74*:435, 1994.

29a. Marwick, T. H., Anderson, T., Williams, M. J., et al.: Exercise echocardiography is an accurate and cost-efficient technique for detection of coronary artery disease in women. J. Am. Coll. Cardiol. *26*:335, 1995.

30. Masini, M., Picano, E., Lattanzi, F., et al.: High-dose dipyridamole-echocardiography test in women: Correlation with exercise-electrocardiography test and coronary arteriography. J. Am. Coll. Cardiol. *12*:682, 1988.

31. Kong, B. A., Shaw, L., Miller, D. D., and Chaitman, B. R.: Comparison of accuracy for detecting coronary artery disease and side effect profile of dipyridamole thallium-201 myocardial perfusion imaging in women versus men. Am. J. Cardiol. *70*:168, 1992.

32. Anderson, T., Marwick, T., Williams, M. J., et al.: Exercise echocardiography is more cost efficient than exercise ECG as an initial test for evaluation of cardiac symptoms in women. J. Am. Coll. Cardiol. *25*:17A, 1995.

33. Steen, M. K., Jacobs, A. K., Freney, D., et al.: Gender related differences in complications during coronary angiography. Circulation 86 (Suppl I):254, 1992.

34. Tobin, J. N., Wassertheil-Smoller, S., Wexler, J. P., et al.: Sex bias in considering coronary bypass surgery. Ann. Intern. Med. *107*:19, 1987.

35. Ayanian, J. Z., and Epstein, A. M.: Differences in the use of procedures between women and men hospitalized for coronary heart disease. N. Engl. J. Med. *325*:221, 1991.

36. Bearden, D., Allman, R., McDonald, R., et al.: Age, race, and gender variation in the utilization of coronary artery bypass surgery and angioplasty in SHEP. SHEP cooperative research group. Systemic hypertension in the elderly program. J. Am. Geriatr. Soc. *42*:1143, 1994.

37. Bickell, N. A., Pieper, K. S., Lee, K. L., et al.: Referral patterns for coronary artery disease treatment: Gender bias or good clinical judgment? Ann. Intern. Med. *116*:791, 1992.

38. Green, L. A., and Ruffin, M. T.: A closer examination of sex bias in the treatment of ischemic cardiac disease. J. Fam. Pract. *39*:331, 1994.

39. Laskey, W. K.: Editorial. Gender differences in the management of coronary artery disease: Bias or good clinical judgment? Ann. Intern. Med. *116*:869, 1992.

40. Shaw, L. J., Miller, D. D., Romeis, J. C., et al.: Gender differences in the noninvasive evaluation and management of patients with suspected coronary artery disease. Ann. Intern. Med. *120*:559, 1994.

41. Kannel, W. B., and Vokonas, P. S.: Demographics of the prevalence, incidence, and management of coronary heart disease in the elderly and in women. Ann. Epidemiol. *2*:5, 1992.

42. Detection, Evaluation, and Treatment of High Blood Cholesterol in Adults (Adult Treatment Panel II). Circulation *89*:1329, 1994.

42a. Rich-Edwards, J. W., Manson, J. E., Hennekens, C. H., et al.: The primary prevention of coronary heart disease in women. N. Engl. J. Med. *332*:1758, 1995.

43. LaRosa, J. C.: Lipoproteins and lipid disorders. *In* Douglas, P. S. (ed.): Cardiovascular Health and Disease in Women. Philadelphia, W. B. Saunders Company, 1993, p. 175.

44. Eaker, E. D., and Castelli, W. P.: Coronary heart disease and its risk factors among women in the Framingham Study. *In* Eaker, E. D.,

Packer, B., Wenger, N., et al. (eds.): Coronary Heart Disease in Women. New York, Haymarket Doyma, 1987, p. 122.

45. Miller, V. T.: Lipids, lipoproteins, women and cardiovascular disease. Atherosclerosis *108*:S73, 1994.

46. Criqui, M. H., Heiss, G., Cohn, R., et al.: Plasma triglyceride level and mortality from coronary heart disease. N. Engl. J. Med. *328*:1220, 1993.

47. Wang, X. L., Tam, C., McCredie, R. M., and Wilcken, D. E. L.: Determinants of severity of coronary artery disease in Australian men and women. Circulation *89*:1974, 1994.

48. Bengtsson, C., Bjorkelund, C., Lapidus, L., and Lissner, L.: Associations of serum lipid concentrations and obesity with mortality in women: 20 year follow up of participants in prospective population study in Gothenburg, Sweden. Br. Med. J. *307*:1385, 1993.

49. Boston, A. G., Gagnon, D. R., Cupples, A., et al.: A prospective investigation of elevated lipoprotein (a) detected by electrophoresis and cardiovascular disease in women: The Framingham Heart Study. Circulation *90*:1688, 1994.

50. Bush, T. L., Fried, L. P., and Barrett-Connor, E.: Cholesterol, lipoproteins, and coronary heart disease in women. Clin. Chem. *34*:B60, 1988.

51. Kane, J. P., Malloy, M. J., Ports, T. A., et al.: Regression of coronary atherosclerosis during treatment of familial hypercholesterolemia with combined drug regimens. JAMA *264*:3007, 1990.

52. Blankenhorn, D. H., Azen, S. P., Kramsch, D. M., et al. and the MARS research group: The monitored atherosclerosis regression study (MARS): Coronary angiographic changes with lovastatin therapy. Ann. Intern. Med. *119*:969, 1993.

53. Scandinavian Simvastatin Survival Study Group (4S): Randomized trial of cholesterol lowering in 4444 patients with coronary heart disease: The Scandinavian Simvastatin survival study. Lancet *344*:1383, 1389, 1994.

54. Summary of the Second Report of the National Cholesterol Education Program (NCEP) Expert Panel on Detection, Evaluation, and Treatment of High Blood Cholesterol in Adults (Adult Treatment Panel II): Expert Panel on Detection, Evaluation and Treatment of High Blood Cholesterol in Adults. JAMA *269*:3015, 1993.

55. Walsh, B. W., Schiff, I., Rosner, B., et al.: Effects of postmenopausal estrogen replacement on the concentrations and metabolism of plasma lipoproteins. N. Engl. J. Med. *325*:1196, 1991.

56. Krumholz, H. M., Seeman, T. E., Merrill, S. S., et al.: Lack of association between cholesterol and coronary heart disease mortality and morbidity and all-cause mortality in persons older than 70 years. JAMA *272*:1335, 1994.

57. Spelsberg, A., Ridker, P. M., and Manson, J. E.: Carbohydrate metabolism, obesity, and diabetes. *In* Douglas, P. S. (ed.): Cardiovascular Health and Disease in Women. Philadelphia, W. B. Saunders Company, 1993, p. 191.

58. Zuanetti, G., Latini, R., Maggioni, A. P., et al.: Influence of diabetes on mortality in acute myocardial infarction: Data from the GISSI-2 study. J. Am. Coll. Cardiol. *22*:1788, 1993.

58a. Manson, J. E., Colditz, G. A., Stampfer, M. J., et al.: A prospective study of obesity and risk of coronary heart disease in women. N. Engl. J. Med. *322*:882, 1990.

59. Diabetes Control and Complications Trial Research Group: The effect of intensive treatment of diabetes on the development and progression of long-term complications in insulin-dependent diabetes mellitus. N. Engl. J. Med. *329*:977, 1993.

60. Bittner, V., and Oparil, S.: Hypertension. *In* Douglas, P. S. (ed.): Cardiovascular Health and Disease in Women. Philadelphia, W. B. Saunders Company, 1993, p. 63.

61. Dahloef, B., Lindholm, L., Hansson, L., et al.: Morbidity and mortality in the swedish trial in old patients with hypertension (STOP-hypertension). Lancet *338*:1281, 1991.

62. Fried, L. P., and Becker, D. M.: Smoking and cardiovascular disease. *In* Douglas, P. S. (ed.): Cardiovascular Health and Disease in Women. Philadelphia, W. B. Saunders Company, 1993, p. 217.

63. Colditz, G. A., Bonita, R., Stampfer, M. J., et al.: Cigarette smoking and risk of stroke in middle-aged women. N. Engl. J. Med. *318*:937, 1988.

64. Shapiro, S., Sloane, D., Rosenberg, L., et al.: Oral contraceptive use in relation to myocardial infarction. Lancet *1*:743, 1979.

65. Hermanson, B., Omenn, G. S., Kronmal, R. A., et al.: Beneficial six-year outcome of smoking cessation in older men and women with coronary artery disease. Results from the CASS registry. N. Engl. J. Med. *319*:1365, 1988.

66. Ernst, E., and Resch, K. L.: Fibrinogen as a cardiovascular risk factor: A meta-analysis and review of the literature. Ann. Intern. Med. *118*:956, 1993.

67. Kannel, W. B., Wolf, P. A., Castelli, W. P., and D'Agostino, R. B.: Fibrinogen and risk of cardiovascular disease. JAMA *258*:1183, 1987.

68. Weksler, B. B.: Hemostasis and Thrombosis. *In* Douglas, P. S. (ed.): Cardiovascular Health and Disease in Women. Philadelphia, W. B. Saunders Company, 1993, p. 231.

69. O'Toole, M. L.: Exercise and physical activity. *In* Douglas, P. S. (ed.): Cardiovascular Health and Disease in Women. Philadelphia, W. B. Saunders Company, 1993, p. 253.

70. Krummel, D., Etherton, T. D., Peterson, S., and Kris-Etherton, P. M.: Effects of exercise on plasma lipids and lipoproteins of women. Soc. Exp. Biology Med. *204*:123, 1993.

71. Blair, S. N., Kohl, H. W., Paffenbarger, R. S., et al.: Physical fitness and all-cause mortality. A prospective study of healthy men and women. JAMA *262*:2395, 1989.

72. Manson, J. E., Stampfer, M. J., Willet, W. C., et al.: Physical activity and

incidence of coronary heart disease and stroke in women. Circulation 91:927, 1995.

73. Haynes, S. G., and Czajkowski, S. M.: Psychosocial and environmental correlates of heart disease. In Douglas, P. S. (ed.): Cardiovascular Health and Disease in Women. Philadelphia, W. B. Saunders Company, 1993, p. 269.

74. Frank, E., and Taylor, C. B.: Psychosocial influences on diagnosis and treatment plans of women with coronary heart disease. In Wenger, N. K., Speroff, L., Packard, B. (eds.): Cardiovascular Health and Disease in Women. Greenwich, CT, Le Jacq Communications, Inc., 1993, p. 231.

75. Berkman, L. F., Vaccarino, V., and Seeman, T.: Gender differences in cardiovascular morbidity and mortality: The contribution of social networks and support. In Wenger, N. K., Speroff, L., Packard, B. (eds.): Cardiovascular Health and Disease in Women. Greenwich, CT, Le Jacq Communications, Inc., 1993, p. 217.

76. Lobo, R. A.: Hormones, hormone replacement therapy, and heart disease. In Douglas, P. S. (ed.): Cardiovascular Health and Disease in Women. Philadelphia, W. B. Saunders Company, 1993, p. 153.

77. Matthews, K. A., Meilahn, E., Kuller, L. H., et al.: Menopause and risk factors for coronary heart disease. N. Engl. J. Med. 321:641, 1989.

78. Croft, P., and Hannaford, P. C.: Risk factors for acute myocardial infarction in women: Evidence from the Royal College of General Practitioners' oral contraception study. Br. Med. J. 298:165, 1989.

79. Stampfer, M. J., Willett, W. C., Colditz, G. A., et al.: A prospective study of past use of oral contraceptive agents and risk of cardiovascular diseases. N. Engl. J. Med. 319:1313, 1988.

80. Engel, H. J., Engel, E., and Lichtlen, P. R.: Coronary atherosclerosis and myocardial infarction in young women—role of oral contraceptives. Eur. Heart J. 4:1, 1983.

81. Daly, L., and Bonnar, J.: Comparative studies of 30 μg ethinyl estradiol combined with gestodene and desogestrel on blood coagulation, fibrinolysis, and platelets. Am. J. Obstet. Gynecol. 163:430, 1990.

82. The Writing Group for the PEPI Trial: Effects of estrogen or estrogen/progestin regimens on heart disease risk factors in postmenopausal women. The Postmenopausal Estrogen/Progestin Interventions (PEPI) Trial. JAMA 273:199, 1995.

83. Manolio, T. A., Furberg, C. D., Shemanski, L., et al.: Associations of postmenopausal estrogen use with cardiovascular disease and its risk factors in older women. The CHS Collaborative Research Group. Circulation 88:2163, 1993.

84. Hong, M. K., Romm, P. A., Reagan, K., et al.: Effects of estrogen replacement therapy on serum lipid values and angiographically defined coronary artery disease in postmenopausal women. Am. J. Cardiol. 69:176, 1992.

85. Nabulsi, A. A., Folsom, A. R., White, A., et al.: Association of hormone-replacement therapy with various cardiovascular risk factors in postmenopausal women. The Atherosclerosis Risk in Communities Study Investigators. N. Engl. J. Med. 328:1069, 1993.

86. Crook, D., Cust, M. P., Gangar, K. F., et al.: Comparison of transdermal and oral estrogen-progestin replacement therapy: Effects on serum lipids and lipoproteins. Am. J. Obstet. Gynecol. 166:950, 1992.

87. Gebara, O. C., Mittleman, M. A., Sutherland, P., et al.: Association between increased estrogen status and increased fibrinolytic potential in the Framingham Offspring Study. Circulation 91:1952, 1995.

88. Barrett-Connor, E., and Laakso, M.: Ischemic heart disease risk in postmenopausal women. Effects of estrogen use on glucose and insulin levels. Arteriosclerosis 10:531, 1990.

88a. Gerhard, M., and Ganz, M.: How do we explain the clinical benefits of estrogen? Circulation 92:5, 1995.

89. Karas, R. H., Patterson, B. L., and Mendelsohn, M. E.: Human vascular smooth muscle cells contain functional estrogen receptor. Circulation 89:1943, 1994.

90. Herrington, D. M., Braden, G. A., Williams, J. K., and Morgan, T. M.: Endothelial-dependent coronary vasomotor responsiveness in postmenopausal women with and without estrogen replacement therapy. Am. J. Cardiol. 73:951, 1994.

91. Reis, S. E., Gloth, S. T., Blumenthal, R. S., et al.: Ethinyl estradiol acutely attenuates abnormal coronary vasomotor responses to acetylcholine in postmenopausal women. Circulation 89:52, 1994.

92. Gilligan, D. M., Quyyumi, A. A., and Cannon, R. O. III: Effects of physiological levels of estrogen on coronary vasomotor function in postmenopausal women. Circulation 89:2545, 1994.

93. Lieberman, E. H., Gerhard, M. D., Uehata, A., et al.: Estrogen improves endothelium-dependent, flow-mediated vasodilation in postmenopausal women. Ann. Intern. Med. 121:936, 1994.

94. Sack, M. N., Rader, D. J., and Cannon, R. O. III: Oestrogen and inhibition of oxidation of low-density lipoproteins in postmenopausal women. Lancet 343:269, 1994.

95. Keaney, J. F., Jr., Shwaery, G. T., Xu, A., et al.: 17-beta-estradiol preserves endothelial vasodilator function and limits low-density lipoprotein oxidation in hypercholesterolemic swine. Circulation 89:2251, 1994.

96. Grady, D., Rubin, S. M., Petitti, D. B., et al.: Hormone therapy to prevent disease and prolong life in postmenopausal women. Ann. Intern. Med. 117:1016, 1992.

97. Ravnikar, V. A.: Hormone replacement therapy in the primary prevention of cardiovascular disease: Benefits, risks, and compliance issues. In Wenger, N. K., Speroff, P., and Packard, B. (eds.): Cardiovascular Health and Disease in Women. Greenwich, CT, Le Jacq Communications, Inc., 1993, p. 181.

97a. Grady, D., Gebretsadik, T., Kerlikowske, K., et al.: Hormone replacement therapy and endometrial cancer risk: A meta-analysis. Obstet. Gynecol. 85:304, 1995.

98. Stampfer, M. J., and Colditz, G. A.: Estrogen replacement therapy and coronary heart disease: A quantitative assessment of the epidemiologic evidence. Prev. Med. 20:47, 1991.

99. Stampfer, M. J., Colditz, G. A., Willett, W. C., et al.: Postmenopausal estrogen therapy and cardiovascular disease. Ten-year follow-up from the Nurses' Health Study. N. Engl. J. Med. 325:756, 1991.

100. Finucane, F. F., Madans, J. H., Bush, T. L., et al.: Decreased risk of stroke among postmenopausal hormone users. Results from a national cohort. Arch. Intern. Med. 153:73, 1993.

101. Love, R. R., Newcomb, P. A., Wiebe, D. A., et al.: Effects of tamoxifen therapy on lipid and lipoprotein levels in postmenopausal patients with node-negative breast cancer. J. Natl. Cancer Inst. 82:1327, 1990.

102. Rutqvist, L. E., and Mattsson, A.: Cardiac and thromboembolic morbidity among postmenopausal women with early-stage breast cancer in a randomized trial of adjuvant tamoxifen. The Stockholm Breast Cancer Study Group. J. Natl. Cancer Inst. 85:1398, 1993.

103. Early Breast Cancer Trialists' Collaborative Group: Systemic treatment of early breast cancer by hormonal, cytotoxic, or immune therapy. 133 randomized trials involving 31,000 recurrences and 24,000 deaths among 75,000 women. Lancet 339:1, 71, 1992.

104. Sullivan, J. M., Vander Zwaag, R., Lemp, G. F., et al.: Postmenopausal estrogen use and coronary atherosclerosis. Ann. Intern. Med. 108:358, 1988.

105. Gruchow, H. W., Anderson, A. J., Barboriak, J. J., and Sobocinski, K. A.: Postmenopausal use of estrogen and occlusion of coronary arteries. Am. Heart J. 115:954, 1988.

106. Sullivan, J. M., Vander Zwaag, R., Hughes, J. P., et al.: Estrogen replacement and coronary artery disease. Effect on survival in postmenopausal women. Arch. Intern. Med. 150:2557, 1990.

107. Sullivan, J. M., El-Zeky, F., Vander Zwaag, R., and Ramanathan, K. K.: Estrogen replacement therapy after coronary artery bypass surgery: Effect on survival. Circulation 345:669, 1995.

108. Bilezikian, J. P.: Major issues regarding estrogen replacement therapy in postmenopausal women. J. Women's Health 3:273, 1994.

109. Henrich, J. B.: The postmenopausal estrogen/breast cancer controversy. JAMA 268:1900, 1992.

109a. Colditz, G. A., Hankinson, S. E., Hunter, D. J., et al.: The use of estrogens and progestins and the risk of breast cancer in postmenopausal women. N. Engl. J. Med. 332:1589, 1995.

110. Belchetz, P. E.: Hormonal treatment of postmenopausal women. N. Engl. J. Med. 330:1062, 1994.

111. Martin, K. A., and Freeman, M. W.: Postmenopausal hormone-replacement therapy. N. Engl. J. Med. 328:1115, 1993.

112. Devor, M., Barrett-Connor, E., Renvall, M., et al.: Estrogen replacement therapy and the risk of venous thrombosis. Am. J. Med. 92:275, 1992.

113. Barrett-Connor, E.: Prevalence, initiation, and continuation of hormone replacement therapy. J. Women's Health 4:143, 1995.

114. Posthuma, W. F. M., Westendorp, R. G. J., and Vandenbroucke, J. P.: Cardioprotective effect of hormone replacement therapy in postmenopausal women: Is the evidence biased? Br. Med. J. 308:1268, 1994.

115. Henderson, B. E., Paganini-Hill, A., and Ross, R. K.: Estrogen replacement therapy and protection from acute myocardial infarction. Am. J. Obstet. Gynecol. 159:312, 1988.

116. American College of Physicians: Guidelines for counseling postmenopausal women about preventive hormone therapy. Ann. Intern. Med. 117:1038, 1992.

117. Edmond, M., Mock, M. B., Davis, K. B., et al.: Long-term survival of medically treated patients in the coronary artery surgery study (CASS) registry. Circulation 90:2645, 1994.

118. Eysmann, S. B., and Douglas, P. S.: Coronary heart disease: Therapeutic principles. In Douglas, P. S. (ed.): Cardiovascular Health and Disease in Women. Philadelphia, W. B. Saunders Company, 1993, p. 43.

119. Manson, J. E., Stampfer, M. J., Colditz, G. A., et al.: A prospective study of aspirin use and primary prevention of cardiovascular disease in women. J. Am. Med. Assoc. 266:521, 1991.

120. Paganini-Hill, A., Chao, A., Ross, R. K., and Henderson, B. E.: Aspirin use and chronic diseases: A cohort study of the elderly. Br. Med. J. 299:1247, 1989.

121. Hammond, E. C., and Garfinkel, L.: Aspirin and coronary heart disease: Findings of a prospective study. Br. Med. J. 2:269, 1975.

122. Cowley, M. J., Mullin, S. M., Kelsey, S. F., et al.: Sex differences in early and long-term results of coronary angioplasty in the NHLBI PTCA registry. Circulation 71:90, 1985.

123. Kelsey, S. F., James, M., Holubkov, A. L., et al.: Results of percutaneous transluminal coronary angioplasty in women: 1985-1986 NHLBI coronary angioplasty registry. Circulation 87:720, 1993.

124. Arnold, A. M., Mick, M. J., Piedmonte, M. R., and Simpfendorfer, C.: Gender differences for coronary angioplasty. Am. J. Cardiol. 74:18, 1994.

125. Weintraub, W. S., Wenger, N. K., Kosinski, A. S., et al.: Percutaneous transluminal coronary angioplasty in women compared with men. J. Am. Coll. Cardiol. 24:81, 1994.

126. Bell, M. R., Holmes, D. R., Berger, P. B., et al.: The changing in-hospital mortality of women undergoing percutaneous transluminal coronary angioplasty. JAMA 269:2091, 1993.

127. Welty, F. K., Mittleman, M. A., Healy, R. W., et al.: Similar results of percutaneous transluminal coronary angioplasty for women and men with postmyocardial infarction ischemia. J. Am. Coll. Cardiol. 23:35, 1994.

128. Greenberg, M. A., and Mueller, H. S.: Why the excess mortality in women after PTCA? Circulation 87:1030, 1993.

129. King, K. B., Clark, P. C., and Hicks, G. L.: Patterns of referral and recovery in women and men undergoing coronary artery bypass grafting. Am. J. Cardiol. 69:179, 1992.

130. Rahimtoola, S. H., Bennett, A. J., Grunkemeier, G. L., et al.: Survival at 15 to 18 years after coronary bypass surgery for angina in women. Circulation 88:II-71, II-78, 1993.

131. O'Connor, G. T., Morton, J. R., Diehl, M. J., et al. for the Northern New England Cardiovascular Disease Study Group: Differences between men and women in hospital mortality associated with coronary artery bypass graft surgery. Circulation 88:2104, 1993.

132. Eaker, E. D., Kronmal, R., Kennedy, J. W., and Davis, K.: Comparison of the long-term, postsurgical survival of women and men in the Coronary Artery Surgery Study (CASS). Am. Heart J. 117:71, 1989.

133. Hannan, E. L., Bernard, H. R., Kilburn, H. C., and O'Donnell, J. F.: Gender differences in mortality rates for coronary artery bypass surgery. Am. Heart J. 123:866, 1992.

134. Weintraub, W. S., Wenger, N. K., Jones, E. L., et al.: Changing clinical characteristics of coronary surgery patients: Differences between men and women. Circulation 88:II-79, II-86, 1993.

135. Caracciolo, E. A., Davis, K. B., Sopko, G., et al.: Comparison of surgical and medical group survival in patients with left main coronary artery disease: Long-term CASS experience. Circulation 91:2325, 1995.

136. Maynard, C., Litwin, P. E., Martin, J. S., and Weaver, W. D.: Gender differences in the treatment and outcome of acute myocardial infarction: Results from the myocardial infarction triage and intervention registry. Arch. Intern. Med. 152:972, 1992.

137. Krumholz, H. M., Douglas, P. S., Lauer, M. S., and Pasternak, R. C.: Selection of patients for coronary angiography and coronary revascularization early after myocardial infarction: Is there evidence for a gender bias? Ann. Intern. Med. 116:785, 1992.

138. Greenland, P., Reicher-Reiss, H., Goldbourt, U., and Behar, S.: In-hospital and 1-year mortality in 1,524 women after myocardial infarction: Comparison with 4,315 men. Circulation 83:484, 1991.

139. Dittrrich, D., Gilpin, E., Nicod, P., et al.: Acute myocardial infarction in women: Influence of gender on mortality and prognostic variables. Am. J. Cardiol. 62:1, 1988.

140. Hammar, N., Larsen, F. F., Sandberg, E., et al.: Time trends in survival from myocardial infarction in Stockholm County 1976-1984. Int. J. Epidemiol. 21:1090, 1992.

141. Goldberg, R. J., Gorak, E. J., Yarzebski, J., et al.: A communitywide perspective of sex differences and temporal trends in the incidence and survival rates after acute myocardial infarction and out-of-hospital deaths caused by coronary heart disease. Circulation 87:1947, 1993.

142. Puletti, M., Sunseri, L., Curione, M., et al.: Acute myocardial infarction: Sex-related differences in prognosis. Am. Heart J. 108:63, 1984.

143. Henning, R., and Lundman, T.: The Swedish Cooperative Study, Part I: A description of the early stage. Acta Med. Scand. 586:27, 1975.

144. Weinblatt, E., Shapiro, S., and Frank, C. W.: Prognosis of women with newly diagnosed coronary heart disease: A comparison with causes of disease among men. Am. J. Public Health 63:577, 1973.

145. Jenkins, J. S., Flaker, G. C., Nolte, B., et al.: Causes of higher in-hospital mortality in women than in men after acute myocardial infarction. Am. J. Cardiol. 73:319, 1994.

146. Wilkinson, P., Laji, K., Ranjadayalan, K., et al.: Acute myocardial infarction in women: Survival analysis in first six months. Br. Med. J. 309:566, 1994.

147. White, H. D., Barbash, G. I., Modan, M., et al.: After correcting for worse baseline characteristics, women treated with thrombolytic therapy for acute myocardial infarction have the same mortality and morbidity as men except for a higher incidence of hemorrhagic stroke. The Investigators of the International Tissue Plasminogen Activator/Streptokinase Mortality Study. Circulation 88:2097, 1993.

148. Lincoff, A. M., Califf, R. M., Ellis, S. G., et al.: Thrombolytic therapy for women with myocardial infarction: Is there a gender gap? Thrombolysis and angioplasty in myocardial infarction study group. J. Am. Coll. Cardiol. 22:1780, 1993.

149. Fiebach, N. H., Viscoli, C. M., and Horwitz, R. I.: Differences between women and men in survival after myocardial infarction: Biology or methodology? JAMA 263:1092, 1990.

150. Kostis, J. B., Wilson, A. C., O'Dowd, K. O., et al.: Sex differences in the management and long-term outcome of acute myocardial infarction: A statewide study. Circulation 90:1715, 1994.

151. Maynard, C., and Weaver, W. D.: Treatment of women with acute MI: New findings from the MITI registry. J. Myocardial Ischemia 4:27, 1992.

152. Clarke, K. W., Gray, D., Keating, N. A., and Hampton, J. R.: Do women with acute myocardial infarction receive the same treatment as men? Br. Med. J. 309:563, 1994.

153. Behar, S., Gottlieb, S., Hod, H., et al.: Influence of gender in the therapeutic management of patients with acute myocardial infarction in Israel. Am. J. Cardiol. 73:438, 1994.

154. Dellborg, M., and Swedberg, K.: Acute myocardial infarction: Difference in the treatment between men and women. Qual. Assur. Health Care 5:261, 1993.

155. Pashos, C. L., Normand, S-L. T., Garfinkle, J. B., et al.: Trends in the use of drug therapies in patients with acute myocardial infarction: 1988 to 1992. J. Am. Coll. Cardiol. 23:1023, 1994.

155a. Yarzebski, J., Col, N., Pagley, P., et al.: Gender differences and factors associated with the receipt of thrombolytic therapy in patients with acute myocardial infarction. A community-wide perspective. Am. Heart J. 131:43, 1996.

156. Adams, J. N., Jamieson, M., Rawles, J. M., et al.: Women and myocardial infarction: Agism rather than sexism? Br. Heart J. 73:87, 1995.

157. Funk, M., and Griffey, K. A.: Relation of gender to the use of cardiac procedures in acute myocardial infarction. Am. J. Cardiol. 74:1170, 1994.

158. Healy, B.: The Yentl syndrome. N. Engl. J. Med. 325:274, 1991.

159. Hamilton, G. A.: Recovery from acute myocardial infarction in women. Cardiology 77(Suppl 2):58, 1990.

160. Lee, K. L., Woodlief, L. H., Topol, E. J., et al.: Predictors of 30-day mortality in the era of reperfusion for acute myocardial infarction: Results from an international trial of 41,021 patients. Circulation 91:1659, 1995.

161. European Working Party: Streptokinase in recent myocardial infarction: A controlled multicentre trial. Br. Med. J. 3:325, 1971.

162. Gruppo Italiano per lo studio della Streptochinasi nell'infarto miocardico (GISSI): Effectiveness of intravenous thrombolytic treatment in acute myocardial infarction. Lancet 1:397, 1986.

163. ISIS-2 (Second International Study of Infarct Survival) Collaborative Group: Randomised trial of intravenous Streptokinase, oral aspirin, both, or neither among 17,187 cases of suspected acute myocardial infarction: ISIS-2. Lancet 1:349, 1988.

164. Wilcox, R. G., Olsson, C. G., Skene, A. M., et al.: Trial of tissue plasminogen activator for mortality reduction in acute myocardial infarction: Anglo-Scandinavian Study of Early Thrombolysis (ASSET). Lancet 2:525, 1988.

165. Kennedy, J. W., Martin, G. V., Davis, K. B., et al.: The Western Washington intravenous streptokinase in acute myocardial infarction randomized trial. Circulation 77:345, 1988.

166a. The GUSTO Angiographic Investigators: The effects of tissue plasminogen activator, streptokinase, or both on coronary-artery patency, ventricular function, and survival after acute myocardial infarction. N. Engl. J. Med. 329:1615, 1993.

167. Maggioni, A. P., Franzosi, M. G., Santoro, E., et al., and the Gruppo Italiano per lo studio della sopravvivenza nell'infarto miocardico II (GISSI-2), and the International Study Group: The risk of stroke in patients with acute myocardial infarction after thrombolytic and antithrombotic treatment. N. Engl. J. Med. 327:1, 1992.

168. Becker, R. C., Terrin, M., Ross, R., et al., and the Thrombolysis in Myocardial Infarction Investigators: Comparison of clinical outcomes for women and men after acute myocardial infarction. Ann. Intern. Med. 120:638, 1994.

169. Grines, C. L., Browne, K. F., Marco, J., et al., for the Primary Angioplasty in Myocardial Infarction Study Group: A comparison of immediate angioplasty with thrombolytic therapy for acute myocardial infarction. N. Engl. J. Med. 328:673, 1993.

170. Stone, G. W., Grines, C. L., Browne, K. F., et al.: A comparison of in-hospital outcome in men versus women treated by either thrombolytic therapy or primary coronary angioplasty for acute myocardial infarction. Am. J. Cardiol. 75:987, 1995.

171. Pfeffer, M. A., Braunwald, E., Moyé, L. A., et al., on behalf of the SAVE investigators: Effect of Captopril on mortality and morbidity in patients with left ventricular dysfunction after myocardial infarction: Results of the survival and ventricular enlargement trial. N. Engl. J. Med. 327:669, 1992.

172. ISIS-4 (Fourth International Study of Infarct Survival) Collaborative Group: ISIS-4: A randomised factorial trial assessing early oral captopril, oral mononitrate, and intravenous magnesium sulphate in 58,050 patients with suspected acute myocardial infarction. Lancet 345:669, 1995.

173. Rodda, B. E.: The Timolol myocardial infarction study: An evaluation of selected variables. Circulation 67:I-101, I-106, 1983.

174. ISIS-1 Collaborative Group: Randomised trial of intravenous atenolol among 16,027 cases of suspected acute myocardial infarction. Lancet ii:57, 1986.

175. Yusuf, S., Peto, R., Lewis, J., et al.: Beta-blockade during and after myocardial infarction: An overview of the randomized trials. Progr. Cardiovasc. Dis. 27:335, 1985.

Chapter 52
Medical Management of the Patient Undergoing Cardiac Surgery

ELLIOTT M. ANTMAN

Several advances have occurred in cardiac surgery that make the operative repair of a variety of cardiac lesions a viable therapeutic alternative for an increasing number of patients with cardiovascular diseases. These include improvements in surgical and anesthesia techniques for myocardial revascularization, valve repair and replacement, and repair of complex congenital cardiac defects, as well as new approaches to management of patients with left ventricular dysfunction and cardiac arrhythmias.[1–8] In addition, perioperative medical and surgical supportive measures have progressed, including the proliferation of transesophageal echocardiography, ventricular assist devices, new inotropic agents, and new hemostatic drugs. Evidence suggests that translation of these improvements into routine surgical practice and institution of regular quality control surveillance measures have led to a reduction of risk-adjusted operative mortality for coronary artery bypass grafting (CABG) to less than 3 per cent for the general population and 5 to 6 per cent for the Medicare population.[9–13] However, the profile of patients referred for surgery has also changed, characterized by greater proportions of patients with advanced age, depressed left ventricular function, multiple comorbidities, prior revascularization operations, and failed acute interventional procedures leading to higher mortality rates in tertiary care referral centers that are called upon to operate on such cases with greater frequency.[14–22]

This chapter summarizes the information required by the cardiologist, whose important responsibilities include collaboration with the surgical team for both preoperative and postoperative care, especially of the medical complications that may develop. The indications for the operation, surgical options (e.g., valve repair versus replacement), and the relative advantages, costs, and limitations of surgery versus an interventional catheterization option (see Chap. 39) all must be considered.[23–28] The details of the decision process for referral for surgery are discussed in the chapters on the individual forms of heart disease.

PREOPERATIVE EVALUATION

The preoperative interview should be used to provide a sensitive and thoughtful review of the indications for the operation and an explanation of the postoperative procedures as well as to assess the patient's potential ability to comply with postoperative medical issues such as anticoagulation and follow-up procedures for permanent pacemakers and implanted defibrillators (see Chap. 23). Serious language barriers and lack of a family support system, especially in the elderly patient, can turn a surgical success into a postoperative failure.[29,30]

GENERAL MEDICAL CONDITION. Except for life-threatening conditions (e.g., proximal aortic dissection,[31] cardiogenic shock caused by ruptured papillary muscle in acute myocardial infarction, penetrating wound of the heart), it behooves the consulting cardiologist to assess the overall medical condition of the patient and advise the surgical team if postponement of the operation seems warranted (Tables 52–1 and 52–2).[32–43] Particular attention should be paid to the patient's potential for developing one or more of the following complications; (1) bleeding on cardiopulmonary bypass while heparinized or while anticoagulated after insertion of a mechanical heart valve prosthesis[44,45]; (2) deterioration of renal function; (3) development of arrhythmias because of electrolyte imbalance; (4) sepsis because of incompletely treated pulmonary, urinary tract, or dental infections, or dermatologic infections over the sternum or saphenous vein harvest site; (5) the need for prolonged ventilatory support postoperatively because of underlying pulmonary disease and preoperative malnutrition; and (6) development of exacerbation of a neurological deficit because of carotid artery disease or prior stroke.[35] Where perioperative intra-aortic balloon pump support may be needed, the status of the iliofemoral circulation should be assessed bilaterally. Of note, the risk of limb ischemia may be reduced by the use of sheathless, small-caliber balloon pump catheters.[46] Despite the increased risk of perioperative morbidity and mortality, recent data indicate that patients with combined coronary artery disease and peripheral vascular disease have greater likelihood of long-term survival and freedom from myocardial infarction with CABG surgery versus medical therapy, particularly in the presence of two- and three-vessel coronary artery disease.[47]

The *protein-calorie malnutrition* associated with cardiac cachexia has been shown to compromise cardiac function and is associated with a greater risk of respiratory failure, sepsis, and prolonged hospitalization.[30] If the clinical situation allows, patients diagnosed as having cardiac cachexia should receive 1 to 2 weeks of preoperative nutritional support before undergoing elective cardiac surgery. The general principles of nutritional support in cardiac surgical patients are outlined in Table 52–3.

The risk factors for morbidity and mortality after coronary revascularization surgery have been analyzed extensively.[48–53] A commonly employed, simple clinical severity scoring system is shown in Table 52–4.[48] Although patients with low risk scores (< 3) may be considered candidates for "fast-track" cost saving measures such as admission on the day of surgery or early extubation postoperatively, those with higher risk scores (>6) are likely to require a longer intensive care unit stay and more consultations by specialists and consume a greater proportion of **1715**

TABLE 52–1 IMPORTANT ASPECTS OF PHYSICAL EXAMINATION IN PATIENTS SCHEDULED FOR CARDIAC SURGERY

PORTION OF PHYSICAL EXAMINATION	ABNORMAL FINDING	COMMENT
Head, eyes, ears, nose, throat	Dental caries, ENT infection	Risk of endocarditis in valvular surgery
Chest	Prior radical mastectomy	Previous mastectomy (especially left) may compromise thoracic blood supply[32] and therefore contraindicates use of internal mammary artery as conduit because of lack of patency or possible inadequate sternal wound healing.
Cardiovascular	Murmur of aortic regurgitation	Aortic regurgitation may worsen during cardiopulmonary bypass because of a jet from aortic cannulation; left ventricular distention may ensue. Intra-aortic balloon pump contraindicated.
Abdomen	Abdominal aortic aneurysm	Presence of abdominal aortic aneurysm or significant atherosclerosis may contraindicate use of intra-aortic balloon pump.
Extremities	1. Peripheral arterial insufficiency	1. May complicate use of intra-aortic balloon pump
	2. Extensive venous varicosities in lower extremities	2. Insufficient venous conduits may be available in lower extremities, necessitating use of arm veins. If this is the case, intravenous lines should not be inserted in the arm veins that will be harvested. For reoperation cases, cardiac catheterization should include imaging of the left internal mammary artery; noninvasive venous mapping of the lower extremities is advisable.
	3. Tinea pedis	3. Increased risk of lower-extremity cellulitis
Neurological	1. Carotid bruits	1. Cerebrovascular accident may occur perioperatively. Perform noninvasive studies of carotids preoperatively and consider combined carotid endarterectomy/CABG in symptomatic patients and those with history of prior stroke, severe bilateral carotid stenoses, or contralateral carotid occlusion.[33,34] Role of a combined or staged procedure in asymptomatic patients is unclear, but many surgeons opt for a combined procedure if high-grade carotid stenoses are present (> 75%).[35,36]
	2. Preoperative neurological deficit(s)	2. Neurological status may deteriorate postoperatively because of compromised cerebral perfusion.

medical resources. By assembling and reviewing the data necessary for an accurate assessment of a patient's operative risk, cardiologists can help with the appropriate triage of patients to contain hospital costs and to facilitate consultations with other medical specialists (e.g., dialysis team) as needed. Patients at increased risk of mediastinal infection include the elderly and those suffering from diabetes mellitus, malnutrition, severe pulmonary disease that is likely to lead to prolonged postoperative ventilatory support, and macromastia in women.[54–56]

HEMODYNAMIC COMPENSATION. An especially important aspect of the preoperative evaluation of the cardiac surgical patient involves estimating the extent of underlying ventricular dysfunction. Evidence exists that unrevascularized viable myocardium after myocardial infarction serves as a substrate for recurrent ischemic events.[57–63] Also, patients with severe multivessel disease and akinetic myocardial zones who suffer from chronic congestive heart failure due to hibernating myocardium (see p. 1215) experience improved ventricular function after CABG.[57,60,61] Contemporary techniques that should be used for assessing myocardial viability in dysfunctional regions include imaging procedures that correlate perfusion with cell membrane integrity, metabolic activity, or contractile reserve.[57–58a] Because no large-scale randomized studies comparing PET scanning with stress-echocardiography are available for the preoperative evaluation of patients, clinicians should rely on those imaging modalities with which they are most familiar and which are available at their institution (see p. 1946).

Careful consideration should be given to the possibility of *right ventricular dysfunction* (Table 52–2), which should be suspected in patients with preoperative elevation of pulmonary artery systolic pressure (> 60 mm Hg), a history of inferoposterior left ventricular infarction (which may be associated with right ventricular infarction), and longstanding tricuspid regurgitation. Patients with right ventricular dysfunction should be placed on maintenance digitalis and receive supplemental oxygen perioperatively in an attempt to lower pulmonary vascular resistance and improve right

ventricular systolic performance. Intravenous nitrate infusions in the perioperative period also have been shown to reduce pulmonary hypertension and ameliorate right ventricular failure.

Patients with mitral regurgitation and severe heart failure should undergo preoperative afterload reduction with such agents as oral angiotensin-converting enzyme (ACE) inhibitors and intravenous sodium nitroprusside to a systolic pressure of about 90 to 100 mm Hg. Potential contraindications to such preoperative afterload reduction include concomitant severe aortic stenosis and hemodynamically significant cerebral or renal vascular disease.

RISK OF MYOCARDIAL ISCHEMIA. Acute thrombolytic and interventional catheterization treatment regimens for acute myocardial infarction may not successfully restore coronary perfusion because of inadequate thrombolysis, reocclusion of the infarct-related artery following initially successful thrombolysis, or dissection/acute thrombosis of the target vessel during angioplasty.[64–66] Identification of patients for referral for emergency bypass surgery and decisions regarding the timing of such surgery remain a challenging clinical problem, particularly in view of the high perioperative mortality rate for patients who require surgery within 24 to 48 hours of thrombolysis.[66–66a]

Potential indications for emergency bypass surgery following failed attempts at reperfusion in acute myocardial infarction include significant left main stenosis and inability to maintain patency of the infarct-related artery, severe multivessel coronary artery disease with anatomy unsuitable for angioplasty and ischemic dysfunction of noninfarct zones, and inability to maintain patency of an infarct-related artery that places a large amount of myocardium in jeopardy (proximal left anterior descending) in patients presenting with an infarct of less than 6 hours duration.[64–66] Although some clinical reports suggest that patients with cardiogenic shock who undergo urgent revascularization have an improved survival compared with those who are not revascularized, these series suffer from potential selection bias, and definitive recommendations regarding the management of cardiogenic shock and acute myo-

PREOPERATIVE LABORATORY TEST	ABNORMAL FINDING	COMMENT
Complete blood count	1. Anemia, especially Hct < 35%	1. Anticipate that hemodilution will occur on cardiopulmonary bypass and blood loss will occur intraoperatively. Preoperative RBC transfusions may be needed. In addition, patients with unstable angina, congestive heart failure, aortic stenosis, and left main coronary artery disease should be advised against autologous donation of blood in the preoperative period.
	2. WBC > 10,000	2. Search for possible infection.
Coagulation screen	1. Prolonged bleeding time 2. Elevated PT and/or PTT 3. Thrombocytopenia	All of these laboratory abnormalities suggest that the patient is at risk for bleeding postoperatively and may have excessive chest tube drainage. Corrective measures (e.g., vitamin K, fresh frozen plasma, platelet transfusions) should be considered preoperatively, and surgery may need to be postponed. Hematological consultation may be required if an inherited defect in coagulation (e.g., von Willebrand's factor deficiency) is suspected.
Chemistry profile	1. Elevated BUN/creatinine	1. Abnormal renal function that may worsen in perioperative period (caused by nonpulsatile flow on cardiopulmonary bypass and potential low flow postoperatively); this may necessitate temporary or even permanent hemodialysis.
	2. Potassium < 4.0 mEq/liter and/or magnesium < 2.0 mEq/liter	2. Electrolyte deficits may place the patient at risk of arrhythmias perioperatively and should be corrected before induction of anesthesia.
	3. Abnormal liver function tests	3. Patient may clear anesthetic agents as well as other cardioactive drugs more slowly. Low albumin level may indicate a state of relative malnutrition that may need to be corrected with nutritional support perioperatively.
Stool hematest	Positive for occult blood	Because heparinization will take place while on cardiopulmonary bypass apparatus, the patient may be at risk for gastrointestinal (GI) bleeding perioperatively. The source of GI heme loss should be investigated preoperatively, if clinical circumstances permit. The potential for bleeding in the future may influence the choice of prosthetic valve inserted.
Pulmonary function	Reduced VC or prolonged FEV₁	Anticipate longer than usual process of weaning from ventilator postoperatively if FEV$_1$ < 65% VC or FEV$_1$ < 1.5–2.0 liters. Obtain baseline arterial blood gas analysis on room air to help guide respiratory management postoperatively.
Thyroid function	These tests are not ordered routinely but should be drawn in cases of suspected hypothyroidism or hyperthyroidism, known thyroid dysfunction on replacement therapy, and in patients with atrial fibrillation who have not undergone evaluation of thyroid function.	1. Hypothyroid patients require prolonged period of ventilatory support postoperatively because of slower clearance of anesthetic agents. 2. Hyperthyroid patients have a hypermetabolic state that places them at increased risk of myocardial ischemia, vasomotor instability, and poorly controlled ventricular rate in atrial fibrillation.
Cardiac catheterization	1. Elevated left ventricular end-diastolic pressure and pulmonary capillary wedge pressure	1. These may remain elevated in the early postoperative period and indicate a need for careful attention to maintenance of adequate preload postoperatively.
	2. Elevated right atrial pressure	2. This may reflect tricuspid regurgitation or right ventricular dysfunction from prior infarction. Such patients require vigorous volume expansion postoperatively to maintain an adequate cardiac output.
	3. Elevated pulmonary artery pressure (and pulmonary vascular resistance)	3. Fixed pulmonary vascular resistance should be suspected when the pulmonary artery diastolic pressure exceeds the mean pulmonary capillary wedge pressure. Vigorous oxygenation and pharmacological support with a pulmonary vasodilator (isoproterenol, prostaglandin E$_1$) are important in such cases. Patients with a pulmonary artery diastolic pressure equal to the pulmonary capillary wedge pressure usually have a more rapid resolution of pulmonary hypertension postoperatively.
	4. Left ventricular mural thrombus	4. Increased risk of stroke perioperatively.
	5. Status of internal mammary arteries	5. Highly desirable arterial conduits for planned revascularization surgery.[38–42] Particular care required during reoperation if patent internal mammary artery bypass is in place from previous surgery.
	6. Status of saphenous vein grafts	6. "Pseudoextravasation" of dye outside lumen in patent graft with slow flow probably represents thrombus-filled atherosclerotic aneurysm of graft.[43]

Hct, hematocrit; RBC, red blood cell; PT, prothrombin time; PTT, partial thromboplastin time; BUN, blood urea nitrogen; VC, vital capacity; FEV₁, volume of air expired at 1 second.

cardial infarction patients must await the results of ongoing randomized trials.[64,65]

Patients who are referred for emergency revascularization surgery should be supported by an intra-aortic balloon pump and, if technically feasible, an intracoronary perfusion catheter. Other methods for mechanical assistance of the failing circulation are described in Chapter 19. Because

patients who undergo emergency bypass surgery within 6 to 12 hours of administration of a thrombolytic agent are at greater risk for intraoperative and postoperative hemorrhage, they should receive a hemostatic agent such as aprotinin (2 million KIU over 20 minutes followed by a continuous infusion of 500,000 KIU per hour).[67]

Patients with other presentations of an acute coronary

TABLE 52–3 PRINCIPLES OF NUTRITIONAL SUPPORT IN CARDIAC SURGICAL PATIENTS

I. RECOGNIZE NUTRITIONALLY DEFICIENT PATIENT
Current weight < 10% of ideal body weight or unintentional, significant weight loss (≥ 10%) over past 6 months; inadequate daily caloric intake (< 1000 calories) for ≥ 1 week, serum albumin < 3.0 related to malnutrtion.

II. CALCULATE DAILY CALORIE REQUIREMENTS
  A. Determine basal energy expenditure (BEE) in kcal/24 hr from the following Harris-Benedict formulae* (where W is body weight in kg, H is height in cm, and A is age in years):
$$BEE_{men} = 66.5 + (13.8 \times W) + (5 \times H) - (6.8 \times A)$$
$$BEE_{women} = 655.1 + (9.6 \times W) + (1.8 \times H) - (4.7 \times A)$$
  B. Adjust for level of activity
    1. Add (1.2 × BEE) for normal postoperative state.
    2. Do not apply activity "factor" for patients who are at a reduced level of physical activity such as those who are on ventilators or comatose.
  C. Adjust for stress (e.g., fever)
    1. Add (0.13 × BEE) for each 1°C rise in temperature above normal (use [0.07 × BEE]/1°F).
    2. Septic patients may need as much as (1.2–1.8 × BEE) added to their daily caloric intake.
  D. Add additional calories if weight gain is desired (e.g., to treat cardiac cachexia); 500 kcal/day will result in a weight gain of 1 lb/wk.

III. CALCULATE PROTEIN REQUIREMENTS
  A. For general cardiac surgical patient: 1.0 gm protein/kg body weight.
  B. For nutritionally deficient or malnourished patient: 1.2–1.5 gm protein/kg body weight.
  C. With renal or hepatic failure patient: may need to adjust protein.

IV. DETERMINE ROUTE FOR NUTRITIONAL SUPPORT
  A. Functioning gastrointestinal tract
    1. Adequate oral intake: Provide calculated calories in a diet that is 15–20% protein, 50–60% carbohydrate, and the remainder as fat.
    2. Inadequate oral intake: Use enteral feeding to deliver daily caloric requirement (e.g., Osmolite = 1 cal/ml; Ensure Plus = 1.5 cal/ml). If renal or hepatic failure is present, use modified enteral feeding.
  B. Nonfunctioning gastrointestinal tract or intolerance of enteral feedings
    1. Insert sterile central line for parenteral nutrition and prescribe central parenteral nutrition in consultation with nutritional support service. Prescription may need to be modified daily.
    2. For short-term feeding, peripheral parenteral nutrition (PPN) may be indicated. Should have normal renal function and be able to tolerate 2500 ml/day.

* The Harris-Benedict equation has recently been shown to overestimate BEE by 10–15%.

Adapted from data in Jeejeebhoy, K. N.: Nutrition in critical illness. In Shoemaker, W. C., Ayres, S., Grenovik, A., et al. (eds.): Textbook of Critical Care. Philadelphia, W. B. Saunders Co., 1989, pp. 1093–1118; Mifflin, M. D., St. Jeor, S. T., et al.: A new predictive equation for resting energy expenditure in healthy individuals. Am. J. Clin. Nutr. 51:241, 1990.

TABLE 52–4 PREOPERATIVE RISK FACTORS FOR ADVERSE OUTCOMES IN PATIENTS UNDERGOING CARDIAC SURGERY: A CLINICAL SEVERITY SCORING SYSTEM

PREOPERATIVE FACTORS	SCORE
Emergency case	6
Serum creatinine	
≥ 1.6 and ≤ 1.8 mg/dl	1
≥ 1.9 mg/dl	4
Severe left ventricular dysfunction	3
Reoperation	3
Operative mitral valve insufficiency	3
Age ≥ 65 and ≤ 74 years	1
Age ≥ 75 years	2
Prior vascular surgery	2
Chronic obstructive pulmonary disease	2
Anemia (hematocrit ≤ 0.34)	2
Operative aortic valve stenosis	1
Weight ≤ 65 kg	1
Diabetes, on oral or insulin therapy	1
Cerebrovascular disease	1

From Higgins, T., Estafanous, F., Lloyd, F., et al.: Stratification of morbidity and mortality outcome by preoperative risk factors in coronary artery bypass patients. A clinical severity score. JAMA 267:2344, 1992. Copyright 1992, the American Medical Association.

chapter and are available in other sources.[70,71] High-dose synthetic narcotics, such as fentanyl and sufentanil, that do not cause vasodilatation have replaced morphine in many centers. Recently, early extubation has been proposed for patients with preserved ventricular function. Advocates of early extubation argue that the advantages include a decrease in respiratory complications, a decrease in ventilatory support, and a decrease in the length of stay in the Intensive Care Unit. In order to achieve early extubation within 6 hours of surgery, anesthetic techniques have included combinations of inhalational anesthetics—enflurane and isoflurane—together with low to moderate amounts of intravenous opioids—fentanyl and sufentanil—along with the intravenous anesthetic propofol. The newer, inhaled anesthetics that have replaced nitrous oxide still have the potential to cause vasodilatation. Patients with critical aortic stenosis, critical mitral stenosis, and large right-to-left shunts may experience a dramatic reduction in cardiac output as ventricular stroke volume falls with a reduction in preload. Preoperative volume expansion and even administration of vasopressor agents may be necessary to avoid this problem.

Cardiac Rhythm[72-89]

Although supraventricular arrhythmias after cardiac surgery are seldom life-threatening, they frequently provoke disturbing symptoms, may jeopardize hemodynamic stability, and are associated with an increased incidence of postoperative stroke, increased length of stay in the intensive care unit, and increased hospital costs.[72-74]

In the past it was a common preoperative practice in many institutions to administer digitalis prophylactically to all patients undergoing cardiac surgery, not only for inotropic support but also for "control" of the ventricular rate if atrial fibrillation occurred postoperatively.[74] There is little reason to believe that digoxin prevents the development of atrial fibrillation; indeed, clinical trials do not clearly substantiate either a lower incidence of atrial fibrillation or a slower ventricular rate in atrial fibrillation in patients

syndrome such as active unstable angina may also be in a tenuous hemodynamic balance as they proceed to the operating room, particularly if significant left main coronary artery stenosis or severe three-vessel coronary artery disease associated with left ventricular dysfunction and/or mitral regurgitation is present. Delays while awaiting surgery and the time between the induction of anesthesia and the institution of cardiopulmonary bypass are high-risk periods during which a vicious spiral of myocardial ischemia and low-output syndrome can rapidly develop. Such patients should also be protected by an intra-aortic balloon pump inserted preoperatively and infusion of nitroglycerin intraoperatively.

ANESTHESIA FOR CARDIAC SURGERY. The details of the practice of cardiac anesthesia are beyond the scope of this

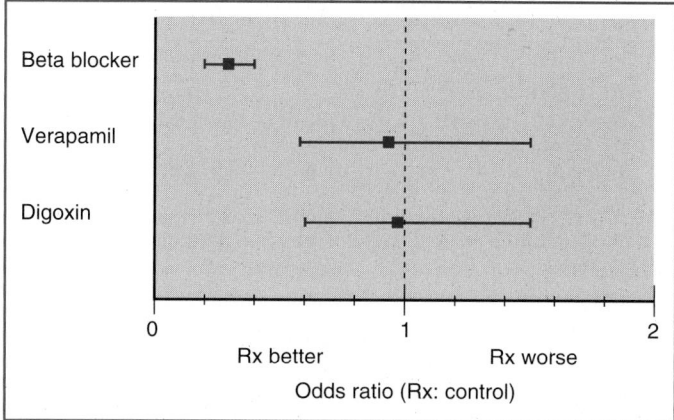

FIGURE 52–1. Meta-analysis of randomized control trials of therapies for prophylaxis against supraventricular arrhythmias in patients undergoing coronary artery bypass surgery. The pooled odds ratio for the development of supraventricular arrhythmias for treatment (Rx) with digoxin, verapamil, or beta blockers is shown. The width of the horizontal lines indicates the 95 per cent confidence intervals for the estimates of the odds ratios. (Reproduced with permission from Andrews, T. C., Reimold, S. C., Berlin, J. A., and Antman, E. M.: Prevention of supraventricular arrhythmias after coronary artery bypass surgery. A meta-analysis of randomized control trials. Circulation 84:[Suppl. III]:236, 1991. Copyright 1991 American Heart Association.)

treated prophylactically with digoxin[75] (Fig. 52–1). Furthermore, hypoxia, hypokalemia, elevated catecholamine levels, and reduced clearance of digoxin are common postoperatively, and these may predispose the patient to digoxin toxicity.

ATRIAL FIBRILLATION

Because of the hazards of postoperative atrial fibrillation, considerable effort has been devoted to identifying preoperative factors associated with an increased risk of postoperative arrhythmia.[74] The preoperative factors most consistently found to be associated with an increased risk of this arrhythmia include advanced age and male gender. Recently it has been proposed that a prolonged P-wave duration recorded on a signal-averaged electrocardiogram and a greater than 70 per cent narrowing of the lumen of the right coronary artery are associated with an increased risk of postoperative atrial fibrillation.[76,77] However, for a substantial number of patients with postoperative atrial fibrillation, no apparent preoperative risk factor can be identified. Cox has presented clinical data suggesting that about one-third of patients undergoing cardiac operations are vulnerable to postoperative atrial fibrillation because of a mild nonuniformity in the distribution of their atrial refractory periods.[78] Intraoperative atrial ischemia associated with rapid rewarming of the atria during prolonged periods of cold cardioplegic arrest may increase the dispersion of refractoriness in the atria of such patients, increasing the risk of postoperative atrial fibrillation.

Because of difficulties in reliably identifying patients at risk of atrial fibrillation preoperatively, it is common clinical practice to provide prophylactic therapy to the majority of patients undergoing coronary artery bypass graft surgery. Beta-adrenoceptor blocking agents are most suitable for prophylaxis against atrial fibrillation.[74,75] This stems from a number of considerations: (1) A rebound phenomenon after withdrawal of such agents at the time of surgery may contribute to the appearance of arrhythmias in the postoperative period; (2) there is a heightened level of sympathetic nervous system tone in the postoperative period that may provoke supraventricular arrhythmias; and (3) the therapeutic index for digitalis glycosides is narrow.

Clinical trials with several beta blockers have shown statistically significant reductions not only in the frequency of supraventricular arrhythmias but also in the severity (duration, speed of ventricular response) of the arrhythmia when it does occur. In the *absence* of an ejection fraction less than 30 per cent, severe bronchospastic lung disease, or bradyarrhythmias, we advocate the use of prophylactic beta blockers in patients undergoing coronary artery bypass grafting.[75]

BRADYARRHYTHMIAS AND ATRIOVENTRICULAR AND INTRAVENTRICULAR BLOCK. Patients with high-grade (third-degree

or type II second-degree) atrioventricular block and hemodynamic compromise (systolic pressure < 90 mm Hg) are at high risk for general anesthesia unless a temporary transvenous pacemaker wire is inserted preoperatively.

In patients in whom a permanent pacemaker has been implanted, its specifications (model, mode, and settings) and, if possible, a statement as to the pacemaker dependency of the patient should be noted in the medical record. The possibility of postoperative malfunction in the permanent pacing system should be anticipated because of the effects of anesthesia, electrocautery, and surgical manipulation of the leads (e.g., during caval cannulation).[88,89] Clinicians should have the appropriate pacemaker programming equipment available postoperatively because many problems (e.g., reversion to the VOO mode [see p. 728] because of electromagnetic interference from the electrocautery apparatus) can be quickly resolved by interrogation of the generator and reprogramming in the recovery area. It is currently recommended that all patients with a Telectronics AccuFIX atrial J lead have the lead removed at the time of atriotomy, regardless of fracture, because of the risk of retention wire fracture and protrusion.

The risk of permanent, complete heart block postoperatively is increased with multiple valve replacements, particularly in patients who have had previous valve surgery. However, there is rarely a need for implantation of a permanent epicardial pacing lead at the time of surgery because of the ease of implantation of a transvenous endocardial system postoperatively. An exception to this would be patients who are undergoing tricuspid valve replacement with a mechanical prosthesis, especially if they are simultaneously undergoing an aortic or mitral valve operation. Because of the contraindication to passing a transvenous lead through the mechanical tricuspid prosthesis, the surgical team should be alerted to the need for placement of permanent epicardial leads intraoperatively.

Patients with previously implanted cardioverter-defibrillator devices should have their unit disabled prior to surgery to minimize the risk of inappropriate shocks from sensing of electrocautery signals intraoperatively. Until the device is reactivated in the postoperative period, equipment for rapid external defibrillation should be available.

Perioperative Drug Therapy

With the exception of oral anticoagulation with warfarin, most medications can and should be continued up to the time of surgery. Clinical trials of patients receiving saphenous vein bypass grafts have demonstrated the importance of initiating antiplatelet therapy in the perioperative period.[90] Because of the increased risk of postoperative bleeding, some surgical groups discontinue aspirin for several days preoperatively in elective cases.[29,30] Many cardiologists are concerned about the risk of "breakthrough" episodes of ischemia if aspirin is discontinued preoperatively and prefer to continue it up to the time of operation, relying on preoperative donations of autologous red cells, cell-saver techniques, autotransfusion of shed blood intraoperatively and postoperatively, and drugs such as aprotinin to minimize the need for and potential hazards of homologous blood transfusion.[91] If asprin is witheld preoperatively, it should be restarted within 48 hours of surgery to reduce the risk of vein graft occlusion.[90] Warfarin therapy should be stopped 2 days preoperatively and, if necessary, treatment with heparin or low molecular weight dextran initiated.

Calcium antagonists previously prescribed for control of ischemic heart disease should be continued up to the time of operation to reduce the chance of myocardial ischemia from withdrawal of the drug. In the case of diltiazem and verapamil, the dose may need to be reduced because these agents may provoke bradycardia and a low-output syndrome postoperatively, especially if a beta blocker or amiodarone is given concurrently or the patient is elderly. Profound atropine- and isoproterenol-resistant bradyarrhythmias may occur postoperatively in patients on these calcium antagonists, particularly when the patient has not yet recovered from the hypothermia that is imposed intraoperatively; temporary dual-chamber pacing support should be available to manage such patients.

PROPHYLAXIS. Insufficient data are available to provide definitive recommendations for prophylaxis against atrial fibrillation in patients undergoing valve surgery. We individualize our recommendations for prophylaxis in such cases and usually do not start beta blockers in patients who have not received them chronically preoperatively. Patients under the age of 40 years undergoing isolated repair of an atrial septal defect or patent ductus arteriosus also need not receive prophylactic beta blockers preoperatively because they are likely to tolerate a postoperative supraventricular arrhythmia during the time it takes to initiate measures to slow the ventricular rate or terminate the arrhythmia.

Suggested doses of beta-adrenoceptor blockers for prophylaxis against atrial fibrillation are as follows: propranolol, 10 to 40 mg every 6 hours; metoprolol, 50 mg every 6 to 12 hours. For patients with depressed left ventricular function who cannot tolerate the negative inotropic effects of beta blockers, digoxin (0.25 to 0.375 mg/day) is frequently prescribed, although convincing data on its prophylactic benefit are limited.

Although oral verapamil (40 to 120 mg every 8 hours) or diltiazem (30 to 90 mg every 8 hours) also may be considered for prophylaxis against supraventricular arrhythmias, their use for that purpose is less well studied.[74,75] More commonly, intravenous verapamil or diltiazem is used for the acute postoperative management of supraventricular arrhythmias that may occur despite prophylaxis with other drugs.

HYPOMAGNESEMIA AND POSTOPERATIVE ARRHYTHMIAS. It has been shown that cardiopulmonary bypass produces hypomagnesemia postoperatively and that this is associated with an increased incidence of atrial dysrhythmias.[79] This observation has led to several small studies, the results of which suggest that maintenance of normomagnesemia (≥ 2.0 mEq/liter) by supplemental administration of magnesium perioperatively reduces the risk of postoperative atrial and ventricular arrhythmias.[80-83] These intriguing findings require confirmation in large-scale randomized trials to ascertain whether inclusion of magnesium in the cardiopulmonary bypass pump-priming solution or the routine administration of supplemental magnesium postoperatively is indicated for all patients undergoing coronary artery bypass surgery to prevent atrial fibrillation or only for specific subgroups of patients. At present, it seems prudent to correct any magnesium (and potassium) deficits preoperatively, monitor the patient's electrolytes carefully postoperatively, and promptly replete any electrolyte deficits that are determined.

CONTINUATION OF ANTIARRHYTHMICS. With the exception of amiodarone, antiarrhythmic drugs that have been prescribed for hemodynamically compromising or life-threatening ventricular tachyarrhythmias should be continued up to the time of operation because of the risk of "breakthrough" of a potentially lethal ventricular arrhythmia in the preoperative period.

Patients with a documented history of resuscitation from sudden cardiac death receiving amiodarone (see p. 613) should continue to receive this drug up to the time of operation. However, in cases where amiodarone was prescribed for a less overtly life-threatening arrhythmia (e.g., atrial fibrillation), the maintenance dosage has been >200 mg/day, and the patient has a history of lung disease, we recommend at least a 3-month period off the drug before subjecting the patient to elective cardiopulmonary bypass.

INTRAOPERATIVE MANAGEMENT

Important intraoperative surgical advances that have improved patient outcome, especially in cases of repeat CABG, include aortic root surface scanning with echo probes, transesophageal echocardiography, femoral cannulation for bypass, minimal dissection before bypass, antegrade and retrograde blood cardioplegia, and performance of all vascular anastomoses with a single aortic cross-clamp under cardioplegic arrest.[1,16,92-97a]

To achieve hemostasis more effectively, surgeons frequently use antifibrinolytic agents (tranexamic acid and aminocaproic acid), serine protease inhibitors (aprotinin), and bioactive surface-coated devices to which heparin is covalently bonded (Carmeda).[91,98-102] Table 52-5 pro-

TABLE 52-5   GENERAL SEQUENCE OF ELECTIVE CARDIAC OPERATIONS

1. Preoperative medications (anxiolytic and narcotic) administered on call to operating room

2. Insertion/positioning of the following devices:
   a. Arterial line (usually radial artery)
   b. Central venous pressure or pulmonary artery catheter
   c. Urinary catheter
   d. ECG electrodes for oscilloscopic monitoring
   e. Grounding plate for electrocautery apparatus (over buttock)

3. Induction of anesthesia and endotracheal intubation

4. Skin preparation and draping of patient

5. Transesophageal echocardiogram may be performed for assessment of LV function and mitral valve insufficiency

6. Median sternotomy (with simultaneous harvesting of greater saphenous vein if coronary revascularization is to be performed)

7. Mobilization of internal mammary artery (usually left) if coronary revascularization is to be performed

8. Heparinization

9. Cannulation for cardiopulmonary bypass usually by one of the following routes:
   Venous: Right atrium, superior/inferior vena cava, femoral
   Arterial: ascending aorta; femoral artery

10. Initiation of cardiopulmonary bypass

11. Systemic cooling of patient to desired temperature

12. Cross-clamping of aorta

13. Myocardial protection: topical cooling, cold potassium cardioplegia solution injected by cannulae in root of aorta (antegrade cardioplegia) and coronary sinus (retrograde cardioplegia)

14. Operative procedure*

15. Initiate ventilation and begin weaning from extracorporeal circulation: rewarming by means of cardiopulmonary bypass apparatus, evacuation of air from left ventricle and aorta if heart has been entered. Discontinuation of bypass occurs by means of a gradual reduction of venous return and incremental volume loading of the heart. Reversal of anticoagulation by protamine with guidance by activated clotting time results intraoperatively. Removal of bypass cannulae

16. Placement of the following devices:
    a. Atrial, ventricular, and ground (subcutaneous) pacing electrodes
    b. Additional monitoring lines: right atrial, left atrial catheters (variable)
    c. Anterior and posterior mediastinal chest tubes; pleural tube if needed

17. Wire closure of sternum and skin closure

18. Transportation of recovery facility by team consisting of surgeon, anesthesiologist, and nurse. Temporary pacing box and defibrillator available during transportation

* The precise sequence of operative procedures such as valve replacement, aneurysm resection, and coronary revascularization is variable. Coronary revascularization usually is accomplished according to the following scheme: Distal venous anastomoses are performed (frequently followed by supplemental injection of cardioplegia solution down graft). Distal end of internal mammary artery is directly anastomosed to target coronary vessel. Aortic cross-clamp is removed. Proximal venous anastomoses to ascending aorta are performed. (The precise sequence is variable, with some surgeons preferring to perform the proximal and distal venous anastomoses first followed by internal mammary anastomosis.)

vides a summary of the general sequence of cardiac surgical procedures, and Figures 52-2 and 52-3 provide examples of pump oxygenators and the usual monitoring devices in place when the patient returns from the operating room.

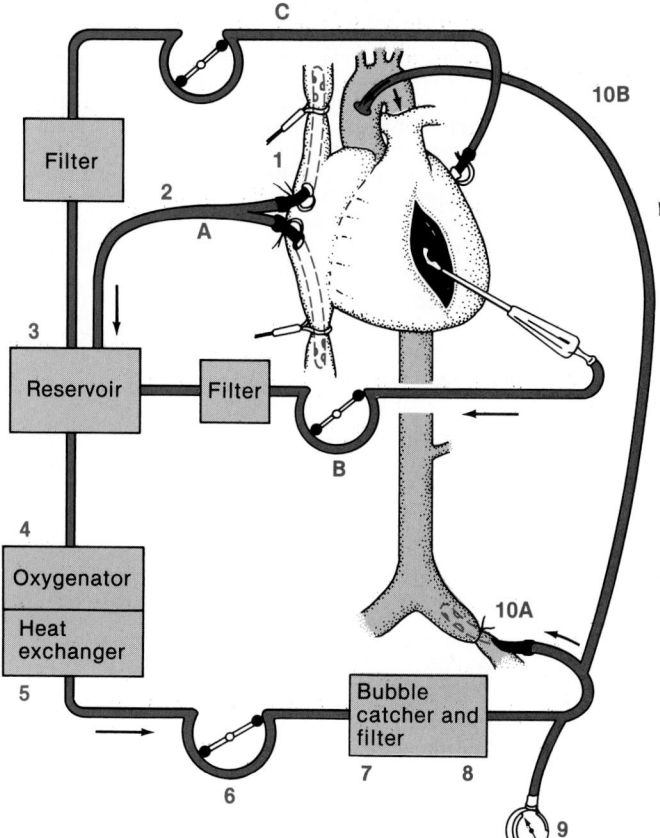

FIGURE 52–2. Schematic diagram of a typical cardiopulmonary bypass circuit. Blood is drained by gravity from the venae cavae (1) through venous cannula (2) into a venous reservoir (3). Blood from surgical field suction and from a ventricular vent (if used during operation) is pumped (*B, C*) into a cardiotomy reservoir (3). Venous blood is oxygenated (4), temperature adjusted (5), raised to arterial pressure (6), filtered (7–8), and returned to the patient by way of a cannula either in the aorta (10*B*) or femoral artery (10*A*). Arterial line pressure is monitored (9). (Modified from Nose, Y.: The Oxygenator. Vol. II. St. Louis, C. V. Mosby, 1973.)

POSTOPERATIVE MANAGEMENT

Fluid, Electrolyte, and Acid-Base Balance

After extracorporeal circulation there is an increase in extracellular fluid and total exchangeable sodium, along with a decrease in exchangeable potassium.[30] The cumulative experience in many centers has led to the following basic principles of management:

1. For the first 48 hours after operation, free water is limited to about 1000 ml/day and intravenous fluids are in the form of 5 per cent glucose in water. Sodium replacement varies with volume needs.

2. Serum potassium levels can fluctuate dramatically, and therefore frequent measurement of serum potassium is indicated, especially in diabetics. We attempt to maintain the serum potassium in the range of 4.5 ± 0.5 mEq/liter and magnesium at 2.0 mEq/liter or greater to minimize the chance of cardiac arrhythmias.

3. Serum glucose levels are frequently elevated (250–400 mg/dl), resulting from glucose-containing intravenous solutions and surgically induced increases in cortisol and catecholamine levels. In nondiabetic patients insulin therapy usually is not required, whereas it is routinely used in insulin-requiring diabetic patients to avoid uncontrolled hyperglycemia.

4. Mild metabolic acidosis or metabolic alkalosis may be present for the first 24 hours postoperatively, particularly during rewarming. These acid-base abnormalities usu-

ally do not require correction in the absence of preoperative renal dysfunction or acute renal failure developing postoperatively.[103]

5. Serum total calcium, phosphorus, and magnesium levels are frequently depressed for about 24 to 48 hours in the normally convalescing patient, owing in part to the effects of hemodilution. These electrolyte abnormalities usually are self-correcting, and replacement therapy usually is not required. A possible exception is hypomagnesemia, which may predispose to the development of cardiac arrhythmias.[74]

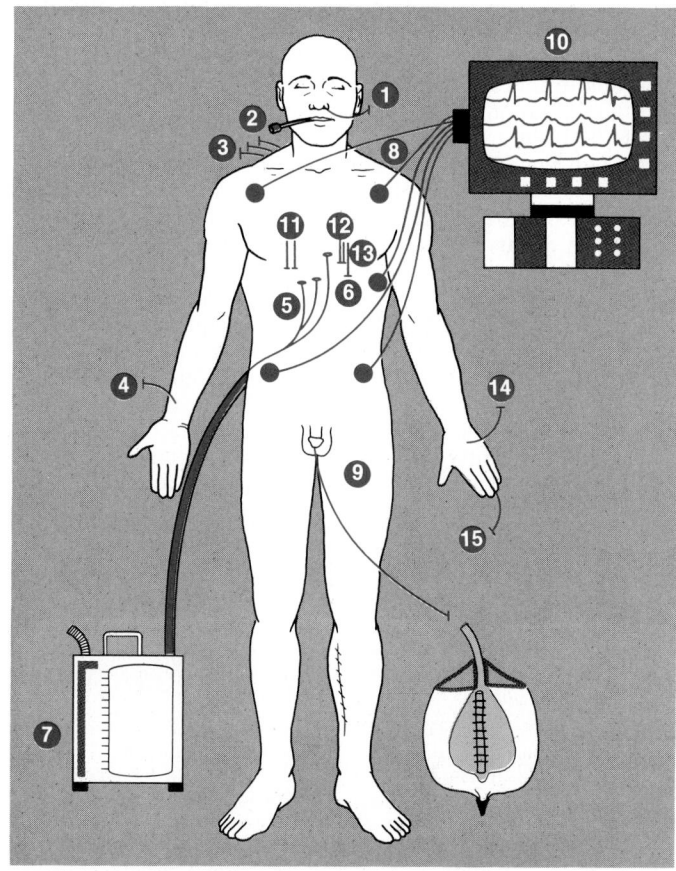

FIGURE 52–3. Schematic diagram of the various devices commonly used after cardiac surgery. (1) Nasogastric tube. (2) Endotracheal tube. (3) Central venous access catheter. This may have multiple ports for the simultaneous measurement of central venous pressure, pulmonary arterial pressure, and pulmonary capillary wedge pressure. Through a sheath introducer a triple-lumen catheter for drug administration and hyperalimentation also may be inserted. (4) Radial arterial pressure monitoring line. (5) Mediastinal chest tubes. One tube is positioned in the anterior mediastinum and the other in the posterior mediastinum. (6) Left pleural chest tube (the left pleural space having been entered during mobilization of the left internal mammary artery for bypass surgery). (7) Chest tube drainage apparatus. (8) Multiple-lead electrocardiograph cable. (9) Urinary drainage catheter. (10) Oscilloscopic monitor capable of the simultaneous recording of multiple electrocardiographic leads and pressures (systemic arterial, pulmonary arterial, central venous). Many contemporary monitoring systems provide modules for calculation of cardiac output by the thermodilution method, automated temperature, end-tidal CO_2 pressure measurements, and on-line help screens for calculations of the infusion rate of various medications and important hemodynamic variables, such as systemic and pulmonary vascular resistance. (11) Right atrial pacing wires. (12) Right ventricular pacing wires. (13) Subcutaneous "ground" (indifferent) pacing wire. The median sternotomy has been secured with stainless steel wires (not shown). The skin wounds from the median sternotomy and saphenous vein harvest site (left leg in this diagram) are typically covered with dry sterile dressings for the first several days postoperatively. (14) Peripheral intravenous line. (15) Pulse oximeter monitoring line. (Diagram courtesy of Cheryl Warrick-Brooks, R. N., Brigham and Women's Hospital, Boston.)

EFFECTS OF ANESTHESIA, STERNOTOMY, AND CARDIOPULMO-NARY BYPASS ON PULMONARY FUNCTION. Four broad areas should be considered, as outlined in Table 52–6.[104,105] Almost all patients experience alveolar dysfunction after open-heart surgery because of right-to-left intrapulmonary shunting of blood from various intrinsic alveolar abnormalities (e.g., atelectasis, edema, infection) and pulmonary vascular events (e.g., extravasation of fluid, inhibition of hypoxia-induced vasoconstriction). Central respiratory drive and respiratory muscle function are depressed postoperatively because of a combination of pharmacological effects and mechanical derangements of thoracic function. Patients with preexisting pulmonary disease may experience a more profound depression of respiratory function, necessitating vigorous pulmonary toilette and an extended period of ventilatory support.

VENTILATORS. Principles. Although most patients receive between 6 and 18 hours of ventilatory support, as already stated, early extubation (< 6 hours) is possible if low-dose synthetic narcotics (e.g., fentanyl) and inhaled anesthetic agents are used, muscle relaxants are reversed, the total cardiopulmonary bypass time is less than 100 minutes, and the patient is hemodynamically stable and mentally alert and has a vital capacity equal to or greater than 10 cc/kg.[106] While intubated, the patient should be ventilated in the intermittent mandatory ventilation (IMV) mode, and arterial blood gases should be checked every hour for the first 8 hours to ensure adequate oxygenation and less frequently thereafter.[30] Positive end-expiratory pressure (PEEP), which is used to minimize the number of collapsed alveolar segments, should be applied cautiously

TABLE 52–6 ABNORMALITIES OF RESPIRATORY FUNCTION AFTER CARDIAC SURGERY

EFFECTS OF ANESTHESIA, THORACIC SURGERY, AND CARDIOPULMONARY BYPASS ON PULMONARY FUNCTION	POTENTIAL CAUSES
Alveolar dysfunction (e.g., widened alveolar-arterial oxygen gradient because of right-to-left intrapulmonary shunting)	a. Scattered regions of atelectasis with preserved perfusion b. Pulmonary edema (e.g., cardiogenic, noncardiogenic "post pump" alveolar capillary leak) c. Infection d. Inhibition of hypoxic pulmonary vasoconstriction by anesthetic agents e. Exacerbation of ventilation/perfusion mismatch by vasodilating agents used postoperatively (e.g., nitroprusside)
Decreased central respiratory drive	a. General anesthetics b. Narcotic analgesics c. Cerebral insult in perioperative period
Decreased respiratory muscle function	a. Thoracic pain (incision, chest tubes) b. Persistent effects of muscle relaxants c. Age d. Obesity e. Depressed cardiac function f. Primary diaphragmatic dysfunction (e.g., phrenic nerve injury)
Exacerbation of underlying chronic pulmonary disease	a. Increase in airway resistance b. Increased secretions and worsening bronchitis c. Pneumonia

TABLE 52–7 CRITERIA FOR SUCCESSFUL WEANING FROM VENTILATORY SUPPORT*

Tests of Mechanical Capability

A. Vital capacity > 10–15 cc/kg body weight
B. Forced expiratory volume in 1 sec > 10 cc/kg body weight
C. Peak inspiratory pressure > − 20 to − 30 cm H_2O
D. Resting minute ventilation < 10 liters/min (can be doubled with maximal voluntary ventilation)
E. Spontaneous respiratory rate under 25 on intermittent mandatory ventilation (IMV) of 6 while resting comfortably, and no apparent increase in work of breathing

Tests of Oxygenation Capability

A. Alveolar-arterial gradient on 100% O_2 < 300–500 torr
B. Arterial Po_2 > 80 torr in the absence of intracardiac right-to-left shunting when the FIO_2 is ≤ 0.5
C. Arterial Pco_2 < 45 and pH > 7.37
D. Shunt fraction (Q_s/Q_t) < 10–20%
E. Dead space/tidal volume (V_d/V_t) < 0.55–0.60

* Modified from Snow, J. C.: Respiration and respiratory care. *In* Snow, J. C. (ed.): Manual of Anesthesia. Boston, Little, Brown and Co., 1977, pp. 317–331; Kirklin, J. K., Daggett, W. M., and Lappas, D. G.: Postoperative care following cardiac surgery. *In* Johnson, R. A., Haber, E., and Austen, W. G.: The Practice of Cardiology. The Medical and Surgical Cardiac Units at the Massachusetts General Hospital. Boston, Little, Brown and Co., 1980, pp. 110–113; and Yang, K., and Tobin, M.: A prospective study of indexes predicting the outcome of trials of weaning from mechanical ventilation. N. Engl. J. Med. *324*:1445, 1991.

in patients with obstructive pulmonary disease (risk of pneumothorax from air trapping and barotrauma), and is contraindicated in patients who have undergone operative procedures in which elevation of the right atrial pressure would be undesirable (e.g., total transposition of venous return, Fontan procedure, superior vena caval–right atrial anastomosis). PEEP may not be tolerated in patients with relative hypovolemia and inadequate preload (see p. 428).[107]

Guidelines for Weaning. Suggested guidelines for identifying the patient who is ready to be weaned from the ventilator are shown in Table 52–7. Additional factors that may influence the decision to not extubate a patient, even if the pulmonary criteria are satisfied, include hemodynamic instability, recurrent malignant ventricular arrhythmias, postoperative bleeding that may require reoperation, ineffective cough, inadequate oxygen-carrying capacity of the blood (hemoglobin ≤ 10 gm/dl) and significant atelectasis, lobar consolidation, or pleural effusion on chest radiograph.[104–106]

During weaning, the IMV setting is progressively reduced to about two to four breaths per minute, and then the patient may be given a brief trial of T-tube ventilation (with or without continuous positive airway pressure or pressure support) before extubation occurs.

SPECIAL PROBLEMS

An increased alveolar-arterial (A-a) gradient postoperatively is a serious problem that demands a thorough evaluation. The ventilator settings should be checked and a chest radiograph obtained to ascertain the position of the tip of the endotracheal tube (to exclude, for example, intubation of the right mainstem bronchus) and to rule out pneumothorax, lobar atelectasis or pneumonia, or a large pleural effusion. Hemodynamic monitoring by means of a pulmonary artery catheter can cause pulmonary hemorrhage because of overinflation of the balloon, and bronchoscopy may need to be performed to diagnose and manage the problem (e.g., occlusion of the bronchus draining the bleeding segment of the lung).

PULMONARY EDEMA (see also Chap. 15). The most common cause of pulmonary edema postoperatively is elevated pulmonary venous pressure arising from left ventricular dysfunction and/or a valvular lesion (e.g., mitral regurgitation). Such patients require aggressive diuresis and vasodilator and inotropic support. Mechanical ventilation with PEEP is used until the patient's ventricular function improves. Repeat operation may be needed if pulmonary edema persists despite attempts to control severe mitral regurgitation medically.

In a minority of patients postcardiac surgery pulmonary edema is due to the adult respiratory distress syndrome (ARDS). In its most extreme form, this disorder is associated with a generalized whole-body *postpump syndrome,* characterized by increased capillary permeability, interstitial edema, fever, leukocytosis, renal dysfunction, and hemodynamic collapse. Although the inciting cause of ARDS in some patients may be sepsis, transfusion reactions, or anaphylaxis, in most cases it is the adverse consequences of exposure of the blood to foreign surfaces during prolonged cardiopulmonary bypass. Included among these are platelet clumping and capillary blockage by embolization, protein denaturation, liberation of free fat by lipoproteins, and activation of the coagulation cascade, fibrinolytic system, complement system (by way of C3a and C5a), and the kallikrein-bradykinin system. Generation of the anaphylatoxins C3a and C5a mediates leukocyte chemotaxis, aggregation, and enzyme release.[108-110] Pulmonary sequestration of activated leukocytes and platelets occurs with attendant damage to the pulmonary endothelium.[60]

There is a direct relation between the duration of cardiopulmonary bypass and administration of blood products and the development of the derangements of pulmonary and vascular integrity noted above.[104,105] Important early clues to the presence of ARDS are a diminished pulmonary compliance as determined by ventilator, elevated alveolar-arterial gradient with a clear chest radiograph, and increasing difficulty maintaining oxygenation utilizing conventional mechanical ventilatory modes.[104] Management of ARDS includes mechanical ventilation with PEEP (often for extended periods), minimization of the pulmonary capillary wedge pressure without compromising cardiac output, and nutritional support as needed (Table 52-3). Extreme cases may require extracorporeal membrane oxygenator support (ECMO).[111]

UNDERLYING CHRONIC LUNG DISEASE. General surgical preparation of patients with obstructive lung disease, including antibiotics, bronchodilators, and cessation of cigarette smoking, may help minimize the risk of respiratory failure from postoperative atelectasis and pneumonia.[104,105] Inhaled bronchodilators should be continued postoperatively. Refractory patients may require a short course of corticosteroids (e.g., methylprednisolone, 0.5 mg/kg every 6 hours for 3 days) to be weaned from the ventilator.[104] Previous enthusiasm for intravenous methylxanthines has waned because of evidence of limited efficacy and the risk of agitation, arrhythmias, and grand mal seizures.[112] Intravenous theophylline should therefore be reserved for extremely refractory cases and should be administered in a dose of 0.4 mg/kg/hr with careful monitoring of plasma levels to maintain them in the range of 10 to 15 μg/ml.

Patients with chronic obstructive pulmonary disease should be weaned from the ventilator slowly. It is helpful to maintain the arterial carbon dioxide tension close to the patient's baseline level to ensure an adequate respiratory drive.

DIAPHRAGMATIC FAILURE. Diaphragmatic dysfunction after cardiac surgical procedures usually occurs as a result of injury to the phrenic nerve(s). An elevated hemidiaphragm may be seen on postoperative roentgenograms in 25 per cent of patients who undergo myocardial preservation, including a topical ice slush and harvesting of an internal mammary artery.[113] A simple bedside test of diaphragmatic function is to ask the patient to protrude his or her umbilicus, a movement that requires diaphragmatic functional integrity. Of note, an elevated hemidiaphragm usually is not associated with increased postoperative morbidity or mortality; recovery of the hemidiaphragm to normal position occurs in 80 per cent of patients at 1 year and nearly all patients by 2 years postoperatively. Less than 1 per cent of patients develop clinically important diaphragmatic dysfunction after cardiac surgery because of unilateral or bilateral phrenic nerve injury.

Evidence of diaphragmatic failure includes the inability to wean the patient from the ventilator, a vital capacity less than 500 cc, and paradoxical movement of the diaphragm on fluoroscopy (abnormal "sniff" test[104]) or ultrasonography. Because it may take up to 6 weeks for an injured phrenic nerve to recover function, management includes a more prolonged period of mechanical ventilation and, for some patients, transition to a rocking bed.[114] In cases of permanent unilateral phrenic nerve damage, plication of the diaphragm may help to improve respiratory function.[115]

PROLONGED VENTILATORY INSUFFICIENCY. Patients who fail to wean from the ventilator within 48 hours require special attention. Such patients should be sedated and consideration given to neuromuscular blockade if the patient is not breathing synchronously with the respirator. Because of the risk of stress-induced gastritis, an H_2-receptor blocker (e.g., ranitidine, 50 mg intravenously every 8 to 12 hours) is administered. To maintain hemodynamic stability, such patients frequently receive large volumes of intravenous fluids; packed red blood cells should be used to maintain an adequate oxygen-carrying capacity. Nutritional support in the form of tube feedings (preferably as a continuous infusion with the patient positioned in the right lateral decubitous position) or parenteral feedings is critical to provide adequate metabolic needs and prevent catabolism of skeletal muscles (e.g., respiratory muscles) (Table 52-3).

If the patient remains intubated beyond 10 to 14 days, the risks of tracheal stenosis, vocal cord damage, retropharyngeal abscess formation, and tracheoesophageal fistula

increase. High-compliance, low-pressure cuffs on endotracheal tubes have reduced the risk of such complications and permit patients to remain intubated continuously for up to 20 or even 30 days, provided that the cuff pressures are maintained below 20 mm Hg and meticulous respiratory care technique is used. Placement of a tracheostomy tube is not a trivial decision because it can be associated with a number of complications that may offset the advantages of improved endotracheal suctioning and reduced risk of upper airway damage, but tracheostomy usually is desirable if it is clear that the patient will remain intubated beyond 3 weeks.

Hypertension
(See also p. 830)

Postoperative hypertension has been defined variably in the literature,[116] but we consider it to be present if the systolic pressure exceeds 140 mm Hg.[117] The incidence of postoperative hypertension ranges from 40 to 60 per cent of patients.[118] It occurs more commonly in patients with a preoperative history of hypertension, prior maintenance therapy with a beta blocker, and well-preserved left ventricular function.[119] Postoperative hypertension is especially frequent after coronary artery bypass grafting and surgical relief of left ventricular outflow tract obstruction (e.g., aortic valve replacement, correction of coarctation of the aorta).[120]

The mechanism of postoperative hypertension probably varies from patient to patient, but usually includes: (1) a "rebound" effect from withdrawal of beta blockade administered preoperatively; (2) excessive sympathetic nervous system activity with elevations of circulating catecholamine levels (especially norepinephrine)[121]; (3) pressor reflexes originating in the heart, great vessels, or coronary arteries[122]; and (4) following correction of aortic coarctation, a drop in the aortic pressure proximal to the site of the prior coarctation with resultant stimulation of aortic and carotid baroreceptors by apparent "hypotension." The renin-angiotensin system is stimulated and peripheral resistance is increased. The sudden exposure of vascular beds downstream to the coarctation to "undamped" aortic pressure also has been reported to cause mesenteric arteritis.

The adverse consequences of elevated systemic pressure include an increased risk of postoperative bleeding, suture line disruption, and aortic dissection[103]; elevated left ventricular afterload and consequent reduction of left ventricular output; injury to aortocoronary bypass grafts and postoperative stroke.

MANAGEMENT. Although a variety of agents may be used for treating acute postoperative hypertension, we prefer those that are rapidly acting and titratable and have a short half-life. Such drugs include sodium nitroprusside (0.5 to 2.0 μg/kg/min), esmolol (50 to 250 μg/kg/min), labetalol (1 to 2 mg/min), and nitroglycerin (25 to 300 μg/min).[103,123] Initial reports suggest that an infusion of the dihyrdopyridine calcium antagonist isradipine (8–50 μg/min) is also a safe and effective means of treating postoperative hypertension.[124] Many centers are starting to use closed-loop systems designed to titrate the intravenous infusion rate of a drug to a preset pressure level that is constantly being monitored invasively.[125] The need for transition to oral antihypertensive therapy is assessed on an individual basis; chronic treatment usually is required only in the patient with a preoperative history of hypertension.

Perioperative Myocardial Infarction

Despite modern intraoperative myocardial protection and improvements in surgical techniques, some degree of ischemia occurs nearly uniformly during coronary artery bypass surgery. Only a minority of patients (5 to 15 per cent of patients undergoing coronary artery bypass graft surgery),

TABLE 52-8 DIAGNOSIS OF MYOCARDIAL INFARCTION AFTER CARDIAC SURGERY

DIAGNOSTIC FINDING	COMMENT
Symptoms	
Early (< 48 hr postop)	Not reliable because of residual effects of anesthesia and postoperative analgesics
Late (> 48 hr postop)	Potentially reliable but may be confused with incisional pain and pleuritic pain from chest tubes, pericarditis
Electrocardiogram	
New, persistent Q waves	This is the most reliable diagnostic finding but only if the Q waves persist on serial ECGs over several days.
Evolutionary ST-T changes	Supportive data favoring the diagnosis of MI only if a typical evolutionary pattern is observed. Because of the effects of cardiopulmonary bypass, hypothermia, postoperative pericarditis, mediastinal chest tubes, and medications (e.g., digitalis), a variety of nonspecific ST-T wave abnormalities may be seen and should not be relied on for diagnosing a perioperative MI.
Myocardial Specific Enzymes	
Total CK	Elevated total CK levels postoperatively may arise from multiple sources, including skeletal muscle in the thorax and calf as well as myocardium.
CK-MB	Myocardial-specific CK may be released from ischemia occurring during cardiopulmonary bypass as well as myocardial and aortic incisions made intraoperatively (e.g., right atrium for cannulation of cavae). Because of the nearly universal release of CK-MB, a diagnosis of MI should not be made unless the CK-MB is significantly elevated (e.g., > 30 units/liter).
Echocardiogram	A regional wall motion abnormality is a helpful finding, particularly if it can be shown to be a new finding by comparison with a peroperative study. Paradoxical motion of the high anterior portion of the interventricular septum is a common finding postoperatively in the absence of MI and should not be taken as the sole evidence of new perioperative myocardial necrosis.

MI, myocardial infarction; CK, creatine kinase.

however, actually experience a *perioperative myocardial infarction*, even in tertiary care centers currently operating on higher risk patients, including those with failed interventional procedures.[126–129] The potential causes of myocardial ischemia and infarction in the perioperative period include incomplete revascularization; diffuse atherosclerotic disease of the distal coronary arteries; spasm, embolism, or thrombosis of the native coronary vessels or bypass grafts[130,131]; technical problems with graft anastomoses; inadequate myocardial preservation intraoperatively; increased myocardial oxygen needs, as in left ventricular hypertrophy; and hemodynamic derangements in the postoperative period (e.g., hypotension, hypertension, tachycardia). Although initially one might suspect that perioperative myocardial infarction results from occlusion of bypass grafts placed to diseased coronary arteries, autopsy studies have shown that bypass grafts usually are patent in patients dying of a perioperative myocardial infarction.[132] This observation lends support to the concept that a mismatch between myocardial oxygen supply and demand in the operating room accounts for much of the infarction noted postoperatively.

DIAGNOSIS. The diagnosis of a myocardial infarction after cardiac surgery is more difficult than at other times because of the nonspe-

cific ST-T wave abnormalities on the electrocardiogram and nearly universal elevation of creatine-kinase (CK) levels postoperatively.[126] A number of diagnostic findings (Table 52-8) must be carefully interpreted and then integrated along the lines of the algorithm shown in Table 52-9.

A 12-lead electrocardiogram should be obtained immediately on the patient's arrival in the intensive care unit after operation and no less frequently than once every 24 hours for the first 3 postoperative days. Measurements of total CK and CK-MB should be made every 8 hours for the first 24 hours and every 24 hours thereafter for the first 3 postoperative days. If there is clinical suspicion of a perioperative myocardial infarction, the CK measurements are made more frequently (every 8 hours) during the second and third postoperative days.

TROPONIN (see also p. 1203). Experience with newer, more sensitive serum markers of cardiac injury, such as troponin I and troponin T, is limited.[133–134] However, initial reports suggest that cardiac-specific troponin I and troponin T are elevated postoperatively in virtually all patients who undergo coronary artery bypass graft surgery. Those patients who experience a perioperative myocardial infarction release greater quanitities of troponin such that serum measurements may remain 10- to 20-fold higher than the upper limit of the reference interval for at least 4 to 5 days postoperatively. Even in patients not experiencing perioperative myocardial infarctions by conventional diagnostic criteria, the relative increase in proteins such as cardiac troponin I over preoperative baseline values is greater than that of CK-MB, suggesting that troponin measurements can detect small amounts of myocardial tissue damage that are not detected by CK-MB. The clinical significance of detection of such episodes of minor myocardial damage postoperatively requires further investigation,

TABLE 52-9 ALGORITHM FOR DIAGNOSIS OF PERIOPERATIVE MI AFTER CARDIAC SURGERY

NEW Qs ON ECG	CK-MB > 30 IU/LITER	NEW RWMA ON ECHO*	DIAGNOSIS	COMMENT
Yes	Yes	Yes	Definite MI	
Yes	Yes	No	Probable MI	New zone of necrosis not evident on echo. The persistence of new Q waves and abnormally elevated CK-MB suggests that Q waves are not a "benign" postoperative finding.
Yes	No	Yes	Definite MI	CK-MB peak probably missed because of infrequent sampling.
Yes	No	No	Possible MI	New Q waves may be false-positive finding.
No	Yes	Yes	Probable MI	Non–Q wave MI.
No	Yes	No	MI unlikely	Small non–Q wave MI cannot be entirely excluded.
No	No	Yes	MI unlikely	Removal of "restraining" effect of pericardium may result in new RWMAs, especially in high anterior septal area.
No	No	No	No MI	Although small patchy areas of necrosis may be seen histologically, these are probably not of clinical significance.

* Perioperative echocardiography is not *required* for the diagnosis of a perioperative MI but can provide useful supportive data or aid in the diagnosis in unclear cases, especially if obtained acutely. RWMA, regional wall motion abnormality; MI, myocardial infarction.

and formal criteria for the diagnosis of a perioperative myocardial infarction using troponin I and troponin T have not been firmly established.

ECHOCARDIOGRAPHY. Beside echocardiograms (transthoracic and if necessary transesophageal) play an important role in establishing the diagnosis of a perioperative myocardial infarction by detecting new regional wall motion abnormalities in cases in which the electrocardiogram or serum marker measurements are unclear. It is especially helpful to compare new echocardiograms with the preoperative studies that are almost always available.

ELECTROCARDIOGRAPHY. The electrocardiogram is the most reliable tool for diagnosing a perioperative myocardial infarction. New and persistent Q waves accompanied by new, persistent, and evolutionary ST-T wave abnormalities are the most helpful criteria. Pathological Q waves owing to perioperative myocardial infarction may appear with an earlier time course (i.e., immediately on arrival from the operating room) than in the nonrevascularized patient; they should be considered diagnostic, however, only if they are seen on serial electrocardiograms once the early postoperative hypothermia, axis shifts, and any potentially reversible myocardial ischemia have resolved.[126]

RISKS AND CONSEQUENCES OF PERIOPERATIVE INFARCTION. Variables that have been found to correlate with the development of a perioperative myocardial infarction in patients undergoing coronary artery bypass grafting include emergency surgery, aortic cross-clamp time greater than 100 minutes, a recent myocardial infarction (within the prior week), and a history of previous revascularization (either PTCA or CABG surgery).[129] Earlier reports suggesting that an increased number of grafts are also correlated with myocardial infarction have not been substantiated in more recent series.

Although the unique circumstances of perioperative myocardial infarction (early reperfusion, revascularization of adjacent ischemic zones, potential for early intervention if complications should arise) may lessen the potential adverse impact of myocardial infarction on ventricular function, most patients with a perioperative myocardial infarction have an increased hospital mortality (about 10 to 15 per cent) compared with patients undergoing coronary bypass grafting who have not sustained a perioperative myocardial infarction (about 1 per cent).[129,135]

Characteristics of patients who are especially at risk of increased short-term mortality after a perioperative myocardial infarction include age over 65 years, unstable angina preoperatively, a myocardial infarction within 1 week before operation, left ventricular aneurysm, intraventricular conduction disturbance (e.g., left bundle branch block), and the need for reoperation for bleeding. About two-thirds of the postoperative mortality is due to pump failure and one-third is due to malignant ventricular tachyarrhythmias.[135] Perioperative myocardial infarction also adversely affects long-term prognosis, particularly if associated with inadequate revascularization and depressed left ventricular function.[136]

Low-Output Syndrome and Shock States

RECOGNITION. Sometimes diagnosis of the low-output syndrome and a shock state after cardiac surgery is difficult. Because cold extremities and mottled skin may result from hypothermia postoperatively, these observations lack sufficient specificity. Although reduced systolic pressure is the most striking manifestation of this disorder, a low-output syndrome may be present even if the arterial systolic pressure exceeds 100 mm Hg because an increased systemic vascular resistance (>1500 dynes-sec-cm^{-5}) may be supporting the peripheral perfusion pressure. It is important to recognize this syndrome because of the strong relation between the cardiac index in the early postoperative period and the probability of cardiac death after surgery. Common clinical features of the low-output syndrome and shock states after cardiac surgery include cold extremities, mottled skin, reduced systolic pressure (<90 mm Hg), decreased urine output (<30 ml/hr), low cardiac index (<2.0 liter/min/m^2), low mixed venous oxygen saturation (<50 per cent), and acidosis.

One should make careful hemodynamic measurements and integrate them with bedside echocardiographic recordings to confirm the diagnosis of a low-output syndrome and attempt to segregate the findings into one of the patterns (*reduced preload, cardiogenic,* or *septic*) in Table 52–10. Although there is overlap of the hemodynamic findings among these patterns, and coexistence of multiple disorders (e.g., bradycardia and hypovolemia) may blur the distinctions between patterns, they offer a clinically useful approach to the evaluation of the patient with a low-output syndrome. In addition to the specific treatment measures discussed below, a number of general measures are applicable to all patients who are in a shocklike condition after cardiac surgery, including prompt correction of any electrolyte and acid-base disturbances, transfusion to a hematocrit over 30 per cent for improved oxygen-carrying capacity of the blood, and a "low threshold" for mechanical ventilatory support to minimize the work of breathing and thereby reduce total body oxygen needs.

REDUCED PRELOAD. Hypovolemia. Low ventricular filling pressures, a normal systemic vascular resistance, and a reduced cardiac index, coupled with echocardiographic demonstration of small ventricular volumes with preserved systolic function, are indicative of *hypovolemia*. Possible causes include bleeding, excessive diuresis, the "leaky capillary state" associated with the postpump syndrome, and, less frequently, inadequate vascular volume because of insufficient return of fluids at the conclusion of cardiopulmonary bypass. Rarely, adrenal cortical insufficiency owing to perioperative hemorrhage into the adrenals has been reported as a cause of hypovolemic hypotension after cardiac surgery.

Therapeutic maneuvers include administration of intravenous fluids (normal saline solution, lactated Ringer's solution) transfusion with packed red blood cells if the hemoglobin is less than 10 gm/dl, and administration of colloid-type volume expanders. It also is important to discontinue any vasodilators or antihypertensives that may have been prescribed during a period when the patient was hypertensive. While waiting for the above measures to take effect, the patient may require a transient infusion of an inotropic pressor agent, usually dopamine (see p. 502).

Vasodilatation. Inhibition of sympathetic tone by the effects of anesthetic agents may cause peripheral vasodilatation. In combination with increased venous capacitance that may occur during rewarming, a low-output syndrome may develop owing to a markedly reduced systemic vascular resistance (<1000 dynes-sec-cm^{-5}). This situation is best treated by an infusion of a vasoconstrictor such as norepinephrine in a dose of 1 to 10 μg/min until the systemic vascular resistance returns to a normal level.

CARDIOGENIC SHOCK. When the right ventricular and left ventricular filling pressures are in the normal range and systemic vascular resistance is not reduced, a frequent cause of a cardiac index less than 2 liters/min/m^2 is *bradycardia*. Because cardiac index is the product of stroke volume and heart rate, this abnormality is easily corrected by atrial or atrioventricular pacing at 85 to 100 beats/min.

Left Ventricular Failure. The pattern of predominant *left ventricular failure* in the early postoperative state is characterized by a disproportionately elevated pulmonary capillary wedge pressure compared with right atrial pressure, low cardiac index, and normal or elevated systemic vascular resistance. Echocardiography usually reveals a dilated, poorly contractile left ventricle, often exhibiting multiple regional wall motion abnormalities. The differential diagnosis of left ventricular failure after cardiac surgery includes the following conditions (which may coexist in the same patient): preoperative left ventricular dysfunction, inadequate surgical correction of the cardiac lesion (e.g., persistent aortic valve gradient owing to mismatch between the patient's aortic ring and prosthesis, residual left ventricular outflow tract obstruction after repair of idiopathic

TABLE 52–10 LOW-OUTPUT SYNDROME AND SHOCK STATES AFTER CARDIAC SURGERY

	REDUCED PRELOAD			CARDIOGENIC SHOCK			SEPTIC
Causes	Hypovolemia	Vasodilatation	Bradycardia (Inappropriately slow HR postoperatively)	LV failure	RV failure	Cardiac tamponade	Sepsis
Hemodynamics							
RA	<8	<8	≤10	≥10	>10	>15	<10
PCW	<15	<15	<15	≥20	≤15*	>15	<15
CI	<2.0	<2.0	<2.0	<2.0	<2.0	<2.0	≥2.0
SVR	>1200	<1000	>1200	>1000	>1000	>1000	<1000
Other			HR < 60		PCW > 15 if LV failure is present	RA = PCW = PAd (within 5 mm Hg) unless "asymmetric" tamponade occurs due to pericardial clots	Narrow AVO$_2$ difference
Echocardiogram	Small ventricular chambers with vigorous systolic contraction unless LV dysfunction was present preoperatively	Small ventricular chambers with normal systolic contraction unless LV dysfunction was present preoperatively	Normal-sized ventricular chambers with vigorous systolic contraction, albeit at a slow rate	Dilated LV with reduced systolic performance; regional wall motion abnormalities may reflect old or new myocardial ischemia and/or infarction.	Dilated RA and RV with reduced RV systolic contraction. TR often present on Doppler study. The contractile performance of LV is variable.	Small cardiac chambers with diastolic collapse of RA and RV. Systolic contraction of RV and LV usually normal unless dysfunction was present preoperatively or coexistent LV or RV failure has occurred postoperatively.	Small ventricular chambers with normal or slightly depressed contractile function (myocardial depressant factor)
Management	IV fluids Transfusion if Hgb < 10 inotropes	Vasopressors	Cardiac pacing	Search for correctible lesion, offending agent, or laboratory abnormality inotropes Vasopressors and vasodilators Mechanical assistance	Supplemental O$_2$ Pulmonary vasodilators inotropes Mechanical assistance	Reexploration Supportive measures: IV fluids, inotropes	IV fluids Antibiotics Vasopressors inotropes

LV, left ventricular; RV, right ventricular; RA, right atrial; PCW, pulmonary capillary wedge; CI, cardiac index; SVR, systemic vascular resistance; TR, tricuspid regurgitation.

hypertrophic subaortic stenosis, residual atrial or ventricular septal defect), complication of surgical procedure (e.g., prosthetic valve leak or thrombosis, depression of stroke volume after correction of mitral regurgitation caused by the elevation of afterload), dysrhythmia, depressant effect of pharmacological agent (e.g., antiarrhythmic drug), acid-base or electrolyte disturbance, or myocardial ischemia and/or infarction. Bedside echocardiography usually can help to identify mechanical disorders such as prosthetic valve dysfunction and dysrhythmias, and metabolic abnormalities and toxic drug levels can be readily recognized by electrocardiogram and laboratory measurements.[96a]

MANAGEMENT. The objectives of hemodynamic management of patients with *left ventricular failure* postoperatively are to correct hypotension if present, increase forward left ventricular output, and return left and right ventricular filling pressures to the normal range. These parameters are intimately related, and treatment may require careful titration of several intravenous agents for pharmacological support of the failing circulation. Boluses of calcium chloride (0.5 to 1.0 gm) increase myocardial contractility, but the effect is modest and short-lived. A continuous infusion of dopamine (5 to 10 µg/kg/min) is preferable if the primary goal is to increase systemic arterial pressure and cardiac output. Dobutamine (2 to 5 µg/kg/min), amrinone (bolus of 0.75 mg/kg and infusion of 5 to 10 µg/kg/min), or milrinone (bolus of 50 µg/kg/min and infusion of 0.375 to 0.75 µg/kg/min) also both augment cardiac output and should be selected if reduction of ventricular filling pressure is desired; systemic arterial pressure is usually unchanged or may even drop slightly because of the peripheral vasodilatory effects of these drugs.[103,123,137] A commonly used combination is dopamine (2 µg/kg/min) to achieve greater renal perfusion in conjunction with dobutamine (2 to 5 µg/kg/min) for augmentation of cardiac output. If the arterial pressure is equal to or greater than 90 mm Hg, vasodilator therapy with sodium nitroprusside or nitroglycerin increases forward cardiac output and lowers the pulmonary capillary wedge pressure further. When hypotension is profound (e.g., systolic pressure < 70 mm Hg), norepinephrine, 1 to 10 µg/min, may be necessary to prevent coronary hypoperfusion.[103,123]

We prefer to use an intra-aortic balloon pump (Chap. 19) for mechanical support of the circulation along with pharmacotherapy early in the course of management of postoperative left ventricular failure that does not respond to the initial pharmacological maneuvers already discussed. This has the advantages of avoiding a continuous upward titration of the dose of sympathomimetic inotropic agents and vasoconstrictors associated with downregulation of beta adrenoceptors and diminished perfusion of the renal, mesenteric, and coronary vascular beds. Also, intra-aortic balloon counterpulsation does not increase myocardial oxygen demand. The intra-aortic balloon pump is particularly helpful if significant mitral regurgitation is present but is contraindicated in the presence of aortic regurgitation and if an abdominal aortic aneurysm is present. If the patient fails to improve despite a combination of intra-aortic balloon pumping and pharmacotherapy, a left ventricular assist device may be inserted for temporary support or as a "bridge" to cardiac transplantation until a donor is located.[138,139] Serial evaluations of left ventricular function over time and under different loading conditions and supportive measures are best obtained with transesophageal echocardiograms.[140]

RIGHT VENTRICULAR FAILURE. The pattern of predominant *right ventricular failure* is characterized by a disproportionate elevation of the right atrial pressure in comparison with the pulmonary capillary wedge pressure. In severe cases of postoperative right ventricular failure, the right atrial pressure may exceed 20 mm Hg while the pulmonary capillary wedge pressure remains equal to or less than 15 mm Hg. When left ventricular failure is present simultaneously, the difference between the right atrial and pulmonary capillary wedge pressures lessens and differentiation from cardiac tamponade becomes difficult. Bedside echocardiography is useful for making a proper diagnosis (Table 52–10).

Postoperatively, predominant right ventricular failure may be seen as a result of one or more of the following conditions: elevated pulmonary vascular resistance (persistently elevated from preoperative elevations of pulmonary artery pressure; postoperative hypoxia, pulmonary embolus, or pneumothorax), primary right ventricular ischemia/infarction[141] or a mechanical lesion (tricuspid regurgitation, residual shunt flow, right ventriculotomy).

Massive pulmonary embolism is a rare occurrence after cardiac surgery (Chap. 46). The diagnosis should be suspected when sudden deterioration in oxygenation occurs in association with systemic hypotension, tachycardia, electrocardiographic abnormalities (unexplained right axis deviation, right bundle branch block, and right ventricular strain pattern), and elevation of right atrial pressure. Angiographic confirmation of the diagnosis is usually not necessary. Expeditious noninvasive confirmation by echocardiography is advisable in those patients in whom the diagnosis remains uncertain. Management consists of immediate intravenous heparin and emergency pulmonary embolectomy. Pulmonary emboli that cause limited hemodynamic compromise (right atrial pressure < 15 mm Hg, arterial pressure > 90 mm Hg, cardiac index ≥ 2 liters/min/m²) can be treated with anticoagulation alone. An inferior vena caval filter should be inserted if venography reveals lower-extremity venous thrombosis and recurrences are detected, or if, after the index event, it is felt that the patient could not survive a recurrent embolus. Because a caval filter does not prevent embolization from right atrial or right ventricular thrombi, an echocardiogram should be performed with consideration of surgical removal of any large mobile, nonsessile right heart thrombi.

Management. Hemodynamic management of predominant right ventricular failure should focus on improvement of right ventricular output to allow adequate filling of the left ventricle. Supplemental oxygen is provided to lower the pulmonary artery pressure. Bradycardia (<60 beats/min) is corrected by atrial or atrioventricular pacing. Isoproterenol (1 to 2 μg/min in the average adult) increases right ventricular contractility and also causes pulmonary vasodilatation. Pulmonary hypertension also may be reduced by prostaglandin E₁[142] and intravenous nitroglycerin.[68] Further reduction in right ventricular afterload can be achieved by an infusion of dobutamine to decrease the pulmonary capillary wedge pressure and lower the driving force across the pulmonary vascular circuit.

Profound hypotension caused by right ventricular failure that does not respond to the above measures can be treated with an infusion of a pulmonary vasodilator (isoproterenol, phentolamine) directly into the pulmonary artery by way of a Swan-Ganz catheter or inhalation of nitric oxide.[143] Insertion of a counterpulsation balloon catheter directly into the pulmonary artery has been reported, but the survival rate in such cases has been poor. Mechanical support of the failing right ventricle is now being used more frequently. Rarely, pulmonary embolectomy may be considered in the presence of refractory failure or shock (see p. 1597).

Cardiac Tamponade (see p. 1486). Postoperative echocardiography has shown that virtually all patients have a pericardial effusion after cardiac surgery and that many such effusions are asymmetrical and loculated.[144,145] Even with mediastinal drains in place, it is possible for a patient to develop cardiac tamponade postoperatively; recognition of this condition requires a high index of suspicion and assessment of hemodynamics at the bedside.[146]

RECOGNITION. Important clinical features of tamponade, such as diminished heart sounds and pulsus paradoxus, may be obscured by mechanical ventilation. Asymmetrical, loculated accumulation of blood and clots in the mediastinum and pericardial space may cause isolated tamponade of one or two cardiac chambers, producing unusual elevations of diastolic pressures (e.g., right atrial tamponade with elevation of central venous pressure without an increase in right ventricular end-diastolic pressure or pulmonary capillary wedge pressure).[147] Bedside two-dimensional transthoracic and transesophageal echocardiography is extremely helpful for diagnosing pericardial effusions and assessing the hemodynamic significance of fluid collections.[148] Diastolic collapse of the right atrium and right ventricle is an indication of a hemodynamically significant external compressive force and should prompt urgent treatment.

TREATMENT. Although pericardiocentesis may be helpful in nonsurgical tamponade, it is unlikely to be successful in evacuating the organized pericardial and mediastinal material that develops after cardiac surgery; subxiphoid drainage and/or emergency sternotomy is preferred. Supportive measures that can be attempted in the interim include volume expansion with intravenous fluids (Plasmanate, whole blood), and inotropic agents (dobutamine).

SEPTIC SHOCK. Low ventricular filling pressures, a markedly reduced systemic vascular resistance, and a normal or unexpectedly high cardiac index in the setting of hypotension and a shocklike state should raise the suspicion of the early stages of *sepsis*. With progression of septic shock, a capillary leak syndrome develops (hypovolemia) and myocardial depression may occur, resulting in a somewhat reduced contractile pattern of the ventricles on echocardiography. Combined therapy with intravenous fluids, antibiotics, and inotropic agents is required to interrupt the vicious cycle of hypotension, acidosis, and diminished coronary perfusion. Most patients who are septic during the first 48 hours after cardiac surgery are infected with a skin organism (incision, monitoring lines) or from seeding the bloodstream from a pulmonary or urinary source. Broad antibiotic coverage with one of the following combinations should be instituted: vancomycin plus an aminoglycoside, or ampicillin plus oxacillin and an aminoglycoside. Because the offending organism is likely to be resistant to the prophylactic antibiotic given preoperatively, it is wise not to include it as one of the empiric antibiotics selected to treat sepsis.

Arrhythmias

EVALUATION AND TREATMENT. There appear to be two peaks in the incidence of arrhythmias perioperatively: the first occurs in the operating room (most commonly during induction of anesthesia, weaning from cardiopulmonary bypass, rewarming) and the second occurs in the intensive care unit between the second and fifth postoperative days. The electrophysiological mechanisms underlying perioperative arrhythmias are incompletely understood, but they can probably be ascribed to a combination of the effects of circulating catecholamines, alterations in autonomic nervous system tone, transient electrolyte imbalances, myocardial ischemia or infarction, and mechanical irritation of the heart.

The physician caring for the postoperative cardiac surgical patient is frustrated by the lack of clinical data on which to base treatment decisions. Most of the emphasis in the literature is placed on prophylaxis against supraventricular tachyarrhythmias with digoxin and extrapolation of the early (and now outdated) coronary care unit guidelines for treating "warning" ventricular arrhythmias to the postoperative cardiac surgical patient. The availability of newer antiarrhythmic agents (verapamil, diltiazem, esmolol, adenosine) with efficacy against supraventricular arrhythmias coupled with published reports of the successful use of atrial pacing techniques provide a more rational approach to *supraventricular arrhythmias*. The management of *ventricular arrhythmias* remains controversial, especially in light of data from the nonsurgical ischemic heart disease population that prophylactic and suppressive antiarrhythmic therapy for the asymptomatic or minimally symptomatic patient may be associated with an increased mortality (see Chap. 37). Studies of the prognostic significance of ventricular arrhythmias after cardiac surgery and the impact of antiarrhythmic therapy on postoperative mortality are limited.[74,149,150]

APPROACH TO THE PATIENT. In the absence of more definitive data, clinicians can only cautiously apply the information gleaned from arrhythmia-intervention trials in nonsurgical patients and individualize treatment decisions based on the specifics of the patient's medical history and the circumstances present in the intensive care unit. For example, a patient with depressed left ventricular function and a preoperative history of resuscitation from sudden cardiac death who has just undergone coronary revascularization requires an aggressive approach to prevent recurrent ventricular tachycardia or ventricular fibrillation. Alternatively, a young patient with normal left ventricular function who has undergone closure of an atrial septal defect or mitral valve repair for ruptured chordae tendineae probably does not require suppression of ventricular arrhythmias in the absence of sustained ventricular tachycardia causing hemodynamic compromise.

Several factors may predispose to the development of arrhythmias, including ventilatory dysfunction, fever, electrolyte imbalance (hypokalemia, hypomagnesemia, hypocalcemia), anemia, myocardial ischemia or infarction, low cardiac output and reflex increase in sympathetic tone, hypertension, pericardial inflammation, and toxic effects of cardioactive medications (e.g., digitalis toxicity, bradycardia induced by diltiazem).[74,149] *Every effort should be made to look for and eliminate any of the factors that may be provoking the arrhythmia.*

Although antiarrhythmic drug therapy and direct-current cardioversion are traditional methods for treating postoperative arrhythmias, cardiac pacing techniques have a number of advantages. These include a more rapid onset and offset of action, avoidance of potential drug toxicity—especially proarrhythmia, elimination of the need for anesthesia (required for cardioversion), reduced anxiety for the patient, greater safety in patients receiving digitalis, and, perhaps most important, the ability to repeat the pacing protocol if the arrhythmia should recur, a not infrequent event. In addition to terminating arrhythmias, cardiac pacing can be used to suppress arrhythmias in many patients by atrial, atrioventricular sequential, or ventricular stimulation at a critical rate (e.g., 85 to 100 beats/min).

Surface Electrocardiogram. The value of a 12-lead electrocardiogram and simultaneously recorded multiple standard electrocardiograph lead rhythm strips cannot be overemphasized if one is attempting to analyze a wide-complex tachycardia. Unfortunately, a number of the criteria for differentiating supraventricular tachycardia with aberrant conduction from ventricular tachycardia (see p. 678) may not be applicable to postoperative patients because of previous or newly acquired infarction patterns, transient conduction defects (seen in 5 to 15 per cent of patients in the early recovery period), and nonspecific repolarization patterns. Although carotid sinus massage and specialized electrocardiograph lead recordings to detect atrial activation may be helpful, it is important to take advantage of the additional recording capabilities provided by the atrial and ventricular epicardial electrodes placed at the conclusion of cardiopulmonary bypass (Fig. 52–4).

Epicardial Electrodes. It is desirable to place two wires high on the free wall of the right atrium to allow for bipolar atrial recording and pacing. The advantages of bipolar pacing include a smaller stimulus artifact, the ability to record a bipolar atrial electrogram during ventricular pacing, and a reduced likelihood of precipitating undesired atrial arrhythmias if an atrial wire is used as the indifferent electrode during unipolar ventricular pacing.[151] Schematic diagrams showing the suggested intrathoracic positioning of the right atrial wires and recordings of unipolar and bipolar atrial electrocardiograms are shown in Figures 52–5 and 52–6.

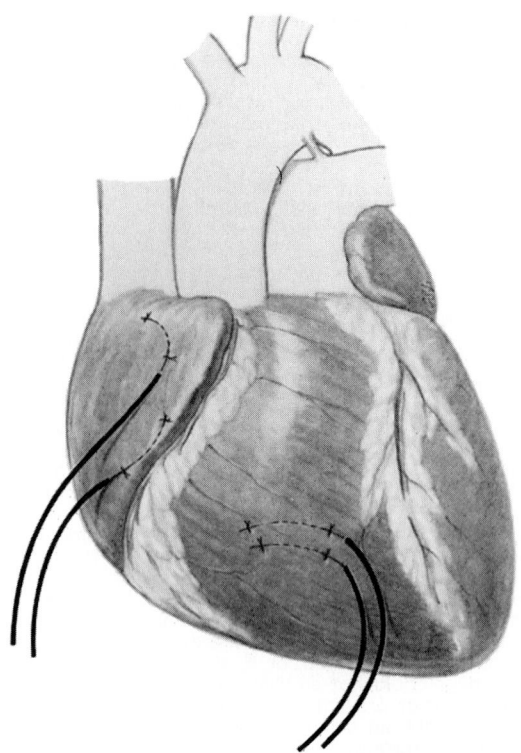

FIGURE 52–5. Placement of atrial and ventricular pacing wires during cardiac surgery. Although two atrial and ventricular electrodes are shown in this diagram (allowing bipolar recording and pacing), some surgeons place only one electrode in each of the sites (restricting recording and pacing to a unipolar configuration). Not shown in this diagram is an indifferent (ground) electrode that is placed in a subcutaneous position. The distal ends of the pacing wires are brought out to the skin through small stab wounds and positioned as shown in Figure 52–3. (From Behrendt, D. M., and Austen, W. G.: Patient Care in Cardiac Surgery. 4th ed. Boston, Little, Brown and Co., 1985.)

Atrial Electrograms

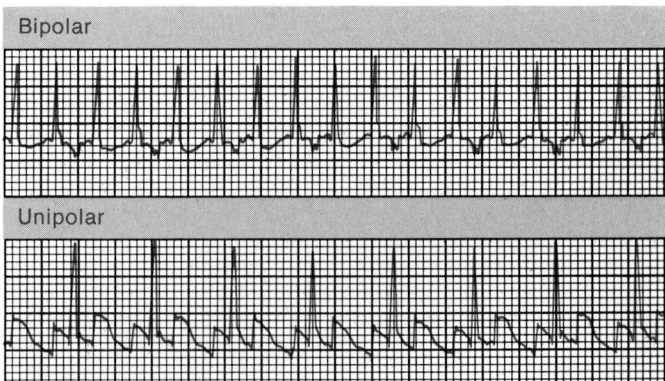

FIGURE 52–6. Simultaneous recording of bipolar and unipolar atrial electrograms utilizing a two-channel electrocardiograph machine with the standard right and left arm leads of the electrocardiograph patient cable attached to the two atrial wires and the recording selector set to the standard lead I (bipolar atrial electrogram) and standard lead II (unipolar atrial electrogram) positions. The rhythm disorder is type I (classical) atrial flutter with an atrial rate of 280 beats/min and 2:1 AV conduction. This type of atrial flutter is easily treated with rapid atrial pacing techniques. More rapid forms of atrial flutter (atrial rate 340 to 430 beats/min) are less responsive to atrial pacing and have been designated type II flutter. (From Waldo, A. L., and MacLean, W. A. H.: Diagnosis and Treatment of Cardiac Arrhythmias Following Cardiac Surgery. Mt. Kisco, N.Y., Futura Publishing Co., 1980.)

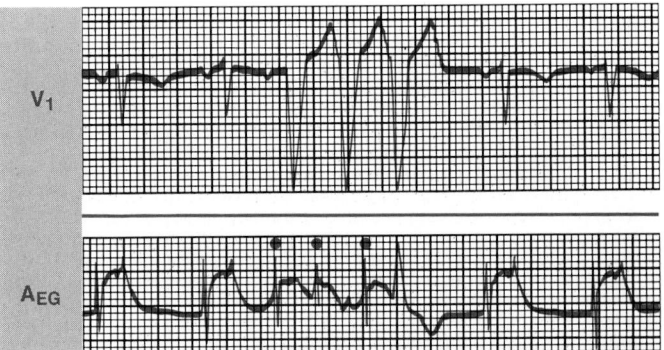

FIGURE 52–4. Simultaneous recordings of electrocardiographic lead V_1 and a bipolar atrial electrogram (A_{EG}). The three consecutive beats with wide QRS complexes recorded in the electrocardiogram do not represent ventricular tachycardia, but are due to aberrant ventricular conduction of three premature atrial beats (dots), as documented in the bipolar atrial electrogram. The appearance of a small ventricular complex after each atrial complex in the bipolar atrial electrogram recording helps to confirm the diagnosis. (From Waldo, A. L., and MacLean, W. A. H.: Diagnosis and Treatment of Cardiac Arrhythmias Following Cardiac Surgery. Mt. Kisco, N.Y., Futura Publishing Co., 1980.)

Supraventricular Arrhythmias

ATRIAL PREMATURE DEPOLARIZATIONS (see also p. 658). The hemodynamic consequences of atrial premature depolarizations are almost always minor, and one should resist the urge to suppress them with antiarrhythmic drugs. Instead, they should be considered a signal that the patient is possibly hypoxic or that an electrolyte imbalance is present, and a warning that the patient is at risk of developing a more serious arrhythmia, such as atrial fibrillation or atrial flutter. In the absence of such correctable abnormalities, one may want to administer a beta blocker to inhibit the effects of circulating catecholamines and also to slow the ventricular rate if atrial fibrillation should develop.

ATRIAL FLUTTER (see also p. 652). Control of the ventricular rate in atrial flutter is more difficult than atrial fibrillation because of the limited number of ventricular responses to atrial activation (usually 2:1, 4:1, but rarely an odd-numbered multiple). Atrial flutter may be difficult to terminate with antiarrhythmic agents. Cardioversion with an energy of 25 to 50 watt-seconds delivered as a single discharge can be expected to terminate atrial flutter in more than 90 per cent of patients.

Atrial flutter can also be terminated by rapid atrial pacing using the temporary epicardial atrial wires placed at the time of operation. The likelihood of success is increased if one uses sufficiently rapid rates of pacing (up to 140 per cent of the spontaneous atrial rate), a sufficient duration of pacing (10 to 30 seconds) with adequate strength (5 to 20 mA), and pretreats the patient with procainamide.[151,152] To achieve the high drive rates required, a special stimulator is utilized.[151] A bipolar pacing mode is preferred, although unipolar pacing can be attempted but with a lower chance of success. Difficulty also may be encountered if the spontaneous atrial rate is particularly rapid (i.e., >350 beats/min) and when pacing stimuli are delivered at a distance from the focus initiating the arrhythmia. In the latter instance the pacing protocol may be unable to penetrate and depolarize a portion of the reentrant circuit, allowing the flutter mechanism to persist. Examples of the diagnostic usefulness of atrial electrograms and the successful use of rapid atrial pacing for the termination of atrial flutter are shown in Figures 52–6 and 52–7.

ATRIAL FIBRILLATION (see also p. 654). Despite the fact that atrial fibrillation is an extremely common arrhythmia following cardiac surgery, the optimal management strategy has not been established. Despite prophylactic therapy with beta-adrenoceptor blockers, transient symptomatic atrial fibrillation occurs in at least 25 to 30 per cent of patients following coronary artery bypass grafting and 50 per cent of patients following valvular surgery, appearing with greatest incidence on the second or third postoperative day.[74]

Management. Unless hemodynamic collapse is present, in which case direct current cardioversion should be performed, the initial treatment of choice in the postoperative patient is to slow the ventricular rate. Although some textbooks and manuals of patient care continue to list digitalis glycosides as the drugs of choice, the therapeutic index is especially narrow in the postoperative patient and the likelihood of achieving a desired level of control of the ventricular rate is reduced in the presence of high circulating catecholamine levels. Provided that the patient's ventricular function is adequate, acute intravenous administration of beta blockers (e.g., metoprolol, 5 mg every 5 minutes for up to three doses), verapamil (e.g., 5-mg bolus every 5 to 10 minutes for three or four doses), or diltiazem (e.g., 0.25 to 0.35 mg/kg bolus over 2 minutes) are more desirable options. Esmolol, an ultrashort-acting cardioselective beta blocker, when administered intravenously in a dose of 50 to 250 μg/kg/min, provides the option of rapid onset; in the event of hemodynamic deterioration the effects of the drug are usually dissipated within 15 to 30 minutes after discontinuation of the infusion. In addition, the probability of conversion to sinus rhythm with esmolol appears to be better than with other agents such as verapamil.[153]

ANTICOAGULANTS. Epidemiological observations suggest that the development of postoperative atrial fibrillation is associated with a marked increase in the risk of stroke (odds ratio 3.0) and a prolonged hospitalization.[72–74,154] There is no consensus regarding the anticoagulation recommendations in patients with postoperative atrial fibrillation. The risks of hemorrhage in the early postoperative period must be weighed against the risk of systemic thromboembolism.[155] The level of risk for systemic embolization varies with the underlying cardiovascular pathology (valvular heart disease, dilated or hypertrophic cardiomyopathy, and CHF > nonvalvular heart disease > lone atrial fibrillator).[156] When atrial fibrillation develops beyond the second postoperative day, we generally advocate adherence to the guidelines established for nonsurgical patients and initiate anticoagulation (intravenous heparin followed by oral warfarin) in patients who have been in the arrhythmia for more than 48 hours, especially if the patient has a history of systemic embolism, or mitral valve disease or cardiomyopathy is present.[156]

Beyond the control of the ventricular rate acutely, the two treatment strategies for management of postoperative atrial fibrillation are similar to those for the nonsurgical patient: chronic anticoagulation while administering rate-controlling agents versus restoration of sinus rhythm and attempts at suppression of recurrences of atrial fibrillation. Because large-scale clinical trial data are not available to guide decision making in this area, therapeutic approaches must be individualized.[155] Although procainamide is frequently used for the treatment of atrial fibrillation after open heart surgery, evidence exists that it has limited effectiveness at suppressing recurrences of atrial fibrillation.[155a] Furthermore, any treatment decision formulated during hospitalization should be readdressed at the first postoperative visit (typically 4 to 6 weeks) to determine if it is still a desirable course of action once the inflammation and metabolic alterations of the postoperative state have dissipated.

Patients with depressed left ventricular function or striking ventricular hypertrophy who experience troublesome dyspnea and/or hypotension when in atrial fibrillation postoperatively are suitable candidates for a trial of restoration of sinus rhythm. It has been our experience that patients undergoing isolated coronary artery bypass surgery who have normal left ventricular function and no preoperative history of atrial fibrillation are likely to undergo spontaneous reversion to sinus rhythm by the time of the first postoperative visit and may therefore be adequately treated with a regimen of an oral beta-adrenoceptor blocker and a short term (1 to 2 months) of oral anticoagulation with warfarin (INR 1.5 to 2.0).

For those patients for whom a decision is made to attempt to restore sinus rhythm, we prefer to postpone the cardioversion procedure until 5 to 7 days postoperatively, when the risk of recurrent atrial fibrillation is decreased because pericardial and mediastinal inflammation have resolved somewhat and the level of sympathetic tone has decreased. Approximately 48 hours prior to cardioversion, antiarrhythmic treatment to possibly restore sinus rhythm pharmacologically (albeit successfully in only 5 to 15 per cent of patients) and suppress recurrences of atrial fibrillation is started. Because patients are most likely to relapse back into atrial fibrillation during the

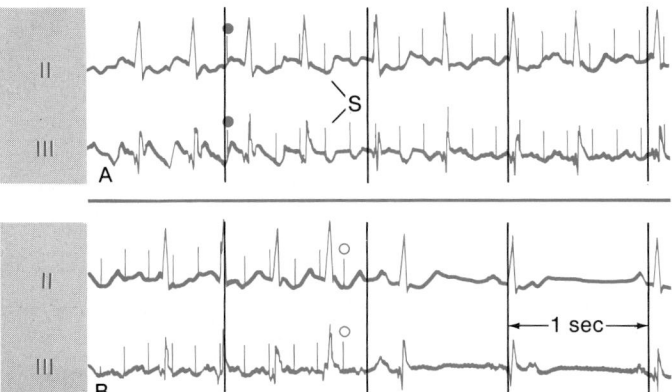

FIGURE 52–7. Recording of electrocardiographic leads II and III in a patient with atrial flutter. Panels A and B are not continuous tracings. The dots in Panel A mark the onset of rapid atrial pacing at 350 beats/min using a pacing stimulator capable of high drive rates. The morphology of the atrial complexes changes dramatically, such that by the end of the trace in Panel A, the atrial complexes are positive in leads II and III. Panel B shows the termination of 30 seconds of atrial pacing at 350 beats/min. The circles represent the last paced atrial beat. With abrupt termination of the rapid atrial pacing, sinus rhythm appears. S = stimulus artifact. Time lines are at 1-second intervals. (From Waldo, A. L., and MacLean, W. A. H.: Diagnosis and Treatment of Cardiac Arrhythmias Following Cardiac Surgery. Mt. Kisco, N.Y., Futura Publishing Co., 1980.)

first 1 to 2 months following cardioversion, it is important to administer suppressive antiarrhythmic therapy and oral anticoagulation during that period and then consider addressing the long-term need for further treatment.[156,157]

PERMANENT SUPPRESSIVE ANTIARRHYTHMIC THERAPY. This is often still necessary in patients with rheumatic heart disease and a preoperative history of atrial fibrillation despite successful aortic or mitral valve surgery even if sinus rhythm is present during the early postoperative period. Such patients typically have scarring of enlarged atria which places them at continued risk for intra-atrial reentry and atrial fibrillation. Patients with nonrheumatic mitral regurgitation (e.g., ruptured chordae tendineae) who have undergone mitral valve repair or replacement may not have a long-term need for suppressive antiarrhythmic therapy despite a preoperative history of atrial fibrillation because relief of the hemodynamic burden may decrease their propensity to atrial premature depolarizations and atrial fibrillation.

PAROXYSMAL SUPRAVENTRICULAR TACHYCARDIA (see p. 1763). The reentrant forms of paroxysmal supraventricular tachycardia (PSVT)—atrioventricular nodal reentry tachycardia and atrioventricular reentry tachycardia—occur less frequently in the postoperative patient than atrial fibrillation or atrial flutter, but fortunately retain their responsiveness to vagal maneuvers and pharmacotherapy to inhibit atrioventricular nodal conduction. The antiarrhythmic agent adenosine (see p. 619), an endogenous nucleoside, has a number of features that make it the drug of choice for treating PSVT in the postoperative patient.[158] A rapid (2 seconds) intravenous bolus of 6 mg terminates about 60 per cent of episodes of PSVT within 20 seconds; a subsequent bolus of 12 mg administered 1 to 2 minutes later terminates PSVT in virtually all those cases that failed to respond to the lower dose. Because adenosine is rapidly transported into the cell or degraded enzymatically to inosine, the physiological effects of adenosine are dissipated in less than 5 minutes. Untoward reactions such as flushing, chest pain, or dyspnea, although common, are mild and short-lived.

PSVT also may be diagnosed by atrial recordings, and terminated by burst atrial pacing or randomly delivered atrial or ventricular premature depolarizations that invade the reentrant circuit and interrupt the arrhythmia. The automatic form of PSVT (i.e., ectopic automatic atrial tachycardia) is sufficiently unusual postoperatively that its presence should strongly raise the suspicion of digitalis toxicity.

Ventricular Arrhythmias

VENTRICULAR PREMATURE DEPOLARIZATIONS (see p. 675). Isolated ventricular premature depolarizations (VPDs) commonly occur after cardiac surgery. There may be an increase in the density of VPDs in patients with a preoperative history of VPDs, or they may appear de novo in patients with no history of ventricular arrhythmias. Although there may be a fall in arterial pressure associated with isolated VPDs, this usually is extremely brief and of no significant hemodynamic consequence to the patient unless prolonged periods of bigeminy occur.

The emergence of frequent VPDs should trigger a search for any potentially correctable factors. Such a search would include measurement of serum electrolyte levels (potassium, calcium, magnesium), hematocrit, and blood pressure; assessment of the level of oxygenation; estimation of volume status (central venous pressure, pulmonary capillary wedge pressure, urine output); and screening for possible toxic levels of cardioactive agents (digitalis, theophylline).

As is the case with VPDs in acute myocardial infarction, there is no conclusive evidence that complex VPDs are harbingers of ventricular tachycardia (VT)/ventricular fibrillation (VF) or a poor outcome in the postoperative patient.[159,160] Nor is there evidence that prophylactic suppression of VPDs improves postoperative outcome.[161]

Sustained VT and VF in the early postoperative period are infrequent events and probably most often the result of transitory electrolyte disturbances or myocardial ischemia/infarction. Therefore, aggressive correction of electrolyte deficits and anti-ischemic therapy with intravenous nitroglycerin and beta blockers alone may be effective for preventing VF without exposing the patient to the potential hazards of antiarrhythmic therapy (myocardial depression, torsades de pointes).[74]

Management. We advocate a conservative approach focusing on prompt detection and correction of provocative factors, liberal use of beta blockers in patients with an ejection fraction greater than 30 per cent, overdrive atrial or atrioventricular sequential pacing between 85 and 100 beats/min, and restriction of suppressive antiarrhythmic therapy to patients with a preoperative history of serious ventricular

tachyarrhythmias.[74] If the decision is made to suppress VPDs in a patient without a history of symptomatic ventricular arrhythmias, the treatment period should be brief (6 to 24 hours) and the patient should not be automatically converted to an oral antiarrhythmic drug regimen without careful reconsideration of the indications for treatment.

VENTRICULAR TACHYCARDIA (see p. 677). Many of the same arguments cited above for isolated VPDs can be applied for paroxysms of nonsustained VT. No definitive guidelines are available, but we believe that episodes of VT lasting for 15 to 30 seconds or more in the absence of correctable factors and attempts at overdrive atrial or atrioventricular sequential pacing are indications for antiarrhythmic therapy, especially if the episodes are associated with hemodynamic compromise. *Sustained VT* is a serious emergency that should be handled with an orderly approach. If the clinical situation permits, a 12-lead electrocardiogram should be obtained for future reference and confirmation of the diagnosis; simultaneous recording of surface electrocardiographic leads with electrograms from the epicardial wires may be helpful in establishing the mechanism of a wide complex tachycardia (Fig. 52–8).

Acute attempts at conversion of the tachycardia include the following maneuvers in the sequence listed: thumpversion, burst ventricular pacing (see p. 680), and boluses of antiarrhythmic agents (lidocaine, 100 mg; procainamide, up to 500 to 1000 mg over 20 minutes; bretylium, 500 to 1000 mg over 5 to 10 minutes; or amiodarone, 75 to 150 mg; infused over 10 minutes). In urgent circumstances synchronized direct-current cardioversion with a low-energy shock (25 to 50 watt-seconds) may be used. Unsynchronized shocks of 100 to 200 watt-seconds should be used if the tachycardia rate is greater than 160 beats/min and/or has a sinusoidal waveform on the electrocardiogram. After conversion a search for correctable disorders should be undertaken, and if none is found a continuous infusion of lidocaine (2 mg/min), procainamide (2 mg/min), bretylium (1 to 2 mg/min), or amiodarone (1.0 mg/min for 6 hours followed by maintenance infusion of 0.5 mg/min) is started.

VENTRICULAR FIBRILLATION (see p. 686). As in the nonsurgical patient, VF must be promptly treated with an unsynchronized direct-current shock. Extrapolating from experience in the electrophysiology laboratory, where VF frequently is provoked iatrogenically, it often can be reverted with shocks of 200 watt-seconds, provided the intervention is performed promptly. It should be possible to defibrillate postoperative patients in the intensive care unit expeditiously; therefore, the higher energies (360 to 400 watt-seconds) used in the "field" probably are unnecessary—at least initially. Emergency cardiopulmonary bypass in

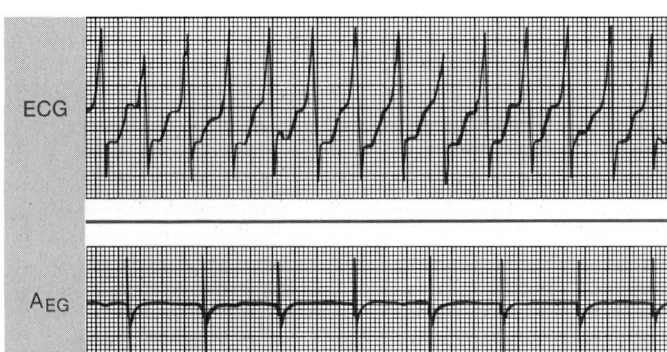

FIGURE 52–8. Monitor electrocardiographic lead recorded simultaneously with bipolar atrial electrogram (A_{EG}) during a wide QRS complex tachycardia at 155 beats/min. The A_{EG} demonstrates the presence of sinus rhythm at 90 beats/min. This observation in conjunction with AV dissociation and fusion beats (second and ninth QRS complexes) establishes that the wide QRS complex tachycardia is ventricular in origin. (From Waldo, A. L., and MacLean, W. A. H.: Diagnosis and Treatment of Cardiac Arrhythmias Following Cardiac Surgery. Mt. Kisco, N.Y., Futura Publishing Co., 1980.)

the cardiac surgical intensive care unit should be considered a potential life-saving measure in patients suffering postoperative cardiac arrest due to intractable VF.[162] Owing to the small number of patients experiencing unexpected sustained hemodynamically compromising VT or VF, epidemiological data on provocative factors and the prognosis of these arrhythmias are difficult to evaluate.[74,150,163] Evidence suggests that unexplained VT or VF occurring within 24 hours of coronary artery bypass graft surgery is associated with a very high in-hospital mortality, probably resulting from perioperative ischemia, infarction, and/or pump failure.[150] Episodes of VT or VF occurring more than 24 hours following bypass surgery have a slightly less ominous prognosis and may be due to reperfusion of previously ischemic zones or transmembrane shifts of electrolytes during the process of recovery.[164]

Risk stratification of patients experiencing VT or VF postoperatively should include assessment of left ventricular function, coronary arteriography if ischemia/infarction is suspected, and consideration of an electrophysiologic study to establish the most appropriate course of therapy.[164a] Because of the numerous metabolic fluxes taking place in the early postoperative period, electrophysiologic study should, if possible, be postponed until at least 5 to 7 days following surgery.[74]

ATRIOVENTRICULAR JUNCTIONAL RHYTHMS. Nonparoxysmal atrioventricular junctional rhythms (rate >45 beats/min) can be seen after mitral or aortic valve surgery. Trauma and tissue swelling from surgical debridement and suture placement are believed to be the provocative mechanisms. Such rhythms typically are transient (≤48 hours) and easily treated with atrial or atrioventricular sequential pacing at a rate above that of the intrinsic junctional mechanism.[165]

Bradyarrhythmias (See p. 1349)

Sinus bradycardia or sinus arrest with emergence of a slow atrioventricular junction escape rhythm may be seen postoperatively when one or more of the following factors are present: advanced age, hypothermia, drug effects (diltiazem, beta blocker, digitalis, procainamide), preoperative sinus node dysfunction, intraoperative trauma to the sinus node, and postoperative elevation of vagal tone.[166] In addition to modifying the dose or discontinuing offending drugs (such as those noted above), atrial pacing at 85 to 100 beats/min should be initiated to maintain an adequate cardiac output and urine flow. Checks of the intrinsic heart rate every 6 hours during the first 24 to 48 hours indicate when pacing may be discontinued.

Although up to 45 per cent of patients may develop a new conduction defect following cardiac surgery, the majority are usually transient and are related to the extensive use of cold cardioplegia, hypothermia, perioperative electrolyte shifts, or surgical trauma during valve repair/replacement or closure of septal defects.[167–169] Complete heart block occurs infrequently following CABG surgery.[169]

In the absence of a low cardiac output syndrome related to bradycardia, the development of a new fascicular block or bundle branch alone is not necessarily an indication for initiation of temporary pacing (although it is a common practice in many centers to attach the epicardial wires to an external generator that is either turned off or programmed in the VVI mode with a low escape rate, in the unlikely event that complete heart block occurs). As with nonsurgically related conduction defects, the prognosis of patients with postoperative conduction defects is closely related to the underlying ventricular function.

MANAGEMENT. The decision to insert a permanent pacemaker after cardiac surgery should be based on the hemodynamic consequences of bradycardia in the individual patient rather than on a specific heart rate. Most new conduction defects resolve in the early postoperative period, but some persist for as long as 2 weeks. Few data are available to guide the decision about timing of implantation of a permanent pacemaker. Although we are willing to observe a younger patient (<65 years) following CABG surgery with a temporary pacing system postoperatively to see if a conduction defect resolves, we have a low threshold for implanting a permanent pacemaker following aortic or mitral valve surgery or if antiarrhythmic therapy or beta blocker treatment is contemplated because these pharmacological measures might "stress" a diseased conduction system. We advocate early insertion of a permanent pacemaker in elderly patients with symptomatic bradycardia because the recuperative process is facilitated, the period of relative immobilization and electrocardiographic monitoring is minimized, and hospital stay is shortened.[170] Finally, we are more aggressive about implantation of permanent pacemakers in patients with persistent advanced atrioventricular block as compared to patients with isolated sinus bradycardia.

Cardioversion (See p. 619)

Direct-current cardioversion should be used in the postsurgical patient with the following additional considerations. The recent cardiotomy with resultant pericardial and mediastinal inflammation, presence of chest tubes and/or pleural effusions, and elevated catecholamine levels after surgery may all contribute to higher energy requirements for reversion of arrhythmias such as atrial fibrillation than are commonly required in patients who have not recently undergone cardiac surgery. To achieve the maximum trans-cardiac spread of current after a median sternotomy, the anterior paddle should be placed to the *right* of the sternum between the third and sixth intercostal spaces, and the other paddle should be positioned in the fourth to sixth intercostal space as far in the left axilla as possible or in a posterior location under the tip of the left scapula. Firm pressure is applied to the paddles to maintain contact with the chest wall as the discharge buttons are depressed.

Hemostatic Disturbances
(See Chap. 58)

All patients who undergo cardiopulmonary bypass develop a multifactorial derangement of the hemostatic system. These abnormalities are caused by exposure of the blood to artificial surfaces, hemodilution, and the effects of heparin (Table 52–11).[110,171–178] Platelet dysfunction is the most significant hemostatic abnormality that occurs after cardiopulmonary bypass, although diminution of coagulation factor levels may assume greater significance in patients with preoperative deficiencies of hemostasis. Administration of the following drugs before surgery may predispose the patient to excessive bleeding: aspirin, nonsteroidal anti-inflammatory agents, thrombolytic agents,[174] certain antibiotics (carbenicillin, ticarcillin, moxalactam, cefamandole, third-generation cephalosporins), dextran, amrinone, quinidine, cytotoxic agents, gold, phenylbutazone, and fish oils.[174] In some institutions, for patients who are undergoing a reoperation or are polycythemic (p. 1792), when the risk of early postoperative bleeding is increased, two units of fresh frozen plasma are administered prophylactically after cardiopulmonary bypass.

The most obvious evidence of bleeding in the postoperative cardiac surgical patient is by means of chest tube drainage. "Acceptable" rates of bleeding are usually less than 100 ml/hr. In our institution, guidelines for returning to the operating room because of excessive bleeding include more than 500 ml/hr for 1 hour, more than 300 ml/hr for 3 hours, and 200 to 300 ml/hr for 5 hours. These guidelines may be tempered by correctable extenuating circumstances, such as uncontrolled hypertension postoperatively, failure to achieve normothermia, or an abnormal coagulation status that is being corrected. Emergency medi-

TABLE 52–11 HEMOSTATIC DISTURBANCES FOLLOWING CARDIOPULMONARY BYPASS

ABNORMALITY	CAUSE
Exposure of blood to artificial surfaces	
1. Platelet dysfunction A. Prolonged bleeding time B. Decreased adhesiveness	1. Depletion of platelet alpha granules, reduced response to wound, and increased plasma levels of platelet factor 4 and beta-thromboglobulin.[171]
2. Inflammatory response	2. Activation of the complement, coagulation, fibrinolytic, and kallikrein cascades; activation of neutrophils with degranulation and protease enzyme release; oxygen free radical production; and synthesis of cytokines (tumor necrosis factor, interleukin-1, interleukin-6, interleukin-8).[110,172]
Hemodilution	
1. Thrombocytopenia	1. Priming of extracorporeal bypass circuit with crystalloid solutions. Heparin-mediated immune thrombocytopenia may occur in about 5% of patients.[173]
2. Coagulation factor depletion	2. Most coagulation factor levels are reduced by hemodilution by about 50%; Factor V is reduced to 20–30% of normal and Factor VIII is relatively unaffected. Factor levels usually return to normal within 12 hours after completion of cardiopulmonary bypass. Although plasminogen and fibrinogen levels are decreased by about 50%, fibrin degradation products usually do not appear in the plasma during bypass.[174]
Heparinization	Thrombus formation is inhibited and excessive bleeding is avoided intraoperatively by maintaining the activated clotting time (ACT) between 400–480 seconds.

* Note: reversal of heparin effects is accomplished with protamine sulfate. Vascular collapse has been reported in some patients during protamine treatment.[175] To avoid the problem of heparin induced thrombocytopenia and because heparin may not effectively inhibit all the thrombin generated during cardiopulmonary bypass ("heparin rebound"), novel antithrombins are being evaluated as alternatives to heparin during surgery.[176-178]

cal maneuvers that can be attempted after sending coagulation studies to the laboratory include the use of PEEP up to 10 cm H$_2$O for mediastinal tamponade; empirical "correction" of putative platelet dysfunction with desmopressin acetate (DDAVP, a synthetic analog of arginine vasopressin that increases plasma levels of von Willebrand factor), 0.3 μg/kg, infused over 15 to 30 minutes; and empirical administration of a small dose of protamine sulfate, 25 to 50 mg, because heparin may be liberated from the patient's fat stores as rewarming occurs.[179]

Once the coagulation profile returns, additional therapy in the form of platelet transfusions for a platelet count less than 100,000/mm^3 and fresh frozen plasma to correct an elevated prothrombin time can be prescribed. Recent reports suggest that aprotinin (2 × 10^6 KIU loading bolus followed by infusion of 0.5 × 10^6 KIU/hr for 4 hours) is helpful in cases of excessive postoperative bleeding by virtue of its ability to inhibit fibrinolysis and replenish platelet GPIb receptors and von Willebrand factor activity.[180,180a] When monitoring bleeding from a chest tube, it is important to be alert to a sudden cessation of hemorrhage. This may indicate that the chest tubes have clotted and the fluid is now draining into the mediastinum or the pleural spaces. Serial chest radiographs may be helpful while observing a patient during a bleeding episode. With correct medical management, only about 5 per cent of patients need to return to the operating room for control of bleeding; this should be accomplished within 3 to 4 hours of the original surgery, before hemodynamic destabilization occurs and large volumes of blood products are administered.

ANTITHROMBOTIC THERAPY IN PATIENTS WITH PROSTHETIC HEART VALVES (see pp. 1061 and 1834). Patients who have undergone implantation of a prosthetic heart valve are exposed to a lifelong risk of thromboembolism. The degree of risk varies with the type of valve implanted (mechanical > bioprosthetic), valve location (mitral > aortic), the presence of atrial fibrillation, the size of the left atrium, a history of thromboembolism or the presence of left atrial thrombi at the time of operation, and the adequacy of anticoagulation. For mechanical prosthetic heart valves it is strongly recommended that all patients undergoing implantation of a second-generation bileaflet or disc valve receive lifelong warfarin therapy to a target INR of 2.5 to 3.5.[181] (Patients with first-generation mechanical valves such as Starr-Edwards, standard Bjork-Shiley, and Omniscience should be anticoagulated to a target INR of 3.5 to 4.5.)[181]

Patients with bioprosthetic valves appear to be at greatest risk of thromboembolism in the first 3 months after valve implantation. For patients in sinus rhythm who have a bioprosthetic valve placed in the mitral position, we prescribe warfarin for 3 months, designed to prolong the prothrombin time to 1.3 to 1.5 times control; if atrial fibrillation persists, warfarin is continued permanently. We usually do not anticoagulate patients with bioprosthetic valves inserted in the aortic position, provided that the patient is in sinus rhythm.

Infection

FEVER. Despite its nonspecific nature, fever is the most common initial clinical sign of a postoperative infection.[182] It should be emphasized, however, that patients who experience a normal course of convalescence continue to show an elevated temperature for up to 6 days postoperatively.[183] In the absence of infection such early fevers are believed to be caused by alterations in blood components after cardiopulmonary bypass. In addition to infectious causes, fevers that occur beyond 6 days may be due to drug reactions, phlebitis at the site of intravenous lines, atelectasis, pulmonary emboli, or the postpericardiotomy syndrome.

WOUND AND INCISION. Leg. Infections of the leg wound typically present with fever, induration, pain, erythema, local warmth, and drainage from the suture line. The usual infectious agents include *Staphylococcus*, *Streptococcus*, and aerobic gram-negative bacilli. Wound aspiration and Gram's stain should be used to guide antibiotic treatment. More advanced cases require wound debridement and open drainage. Recurrent bacterial cellulitis in the leg used for saphenous vein harvest may be a recalcitrant problem that appears months to years after operation.[184] Antibiotic courses directed against staphylococcus and streptococcus species for each individual occurrence may be insufficient, and a long-term course of antibiotic therapy may be needed. It is important to search for evidence of superficial fungal infections in the affected leg because persistent tinea pedis infection has been reported to cause recurrent lower-extremity cellulitis.[185] If a fungal infection is identified, treatment with topical miconazole or clotrimazole should be given in addition to antibacterial therapy. Persistent fungal infections (owing to breaks in integrity of the dermal barrier) should be treated with either oral ketoconazole or griseofulvin.

Mediastinitis. Mediastinitis and sternal osteomyelitis are among the most serious complications of a median sternotomy.[54,186,187] If one excludes operations that occur after thoracic trauma, it is estimated that mediastinitis occurs in about 2 per cent of patients who undergo median sternotomy.

Most cases present within 2 weeks after sternotomy. Important diagnostic features of patients who develop mediastinitis early after cardiac surgery include persistent fever in excess of 101°F beyond the fourth postoperative day, a systemic toxic condition, leukocytosis, bacteremia, and a purulent discharge from the sternal wound. Wound erythema, abnormal sternal tenderness or instability, and mediastinal widening may all be absent or clinically unapparent early in the development of mediastinitis. Recognition of mediastinitis requires a high index of suspicion and a vigorous, repetitive search for evidence of sternal wound drainage in patients who are persistently febrile late into the first week after surgery and in whom there is no other obvious focus of infection, such as pneumonia or urinary tract infection.[188] The diagnosis can be confirmed by needle aspiration from the subxiphoid approach followed by Gram's stain and culture.

RISK FACTORS AND DIAGNOSIS. There are a number of intraoperative and postoperative risk factors for the development of mediastinitis. These include prolonged cardiopulmonary bypass time, excessive postoperative bleeding with reexploration for control of hemorrhage, and diminished cardiac output in the postoperative period. There is an increase in the development of mediastinitis when both internal mammary arteries are mobilized bilaterally for use as bypass conduits.[189] For that reason many surgeons prefer to use only the left internal mammary artery, particularly in elderly diabetic patients who may already be predisposed to delayed sternal wound healing.

The spectrum of microorganisms that cause mediastinitis includes *Staphylococcus* (*aureus* and *epidermidis*) in about 50 per cent of patients and a variety of gram-negative bacilli in about 40 per cent of cases.[188–191] Mixed infections and fungal infections are rare. The organism isolated frequently is resistant to the prophylactic antibiotic used preoperatively, especially if the isolate includes a gram-negative bacillus or a β-lactamase–producing *S. aureus*.

Definitive diagnosis of a sternal wound infection requires exploration of the wound and culture of suspicious areas. Specialized radiological techniques such as CT and MRI scanning also have been reported to be helpful in localizing the sites of infection. Although both closed and open methods of treatment of mediastinitis have been reported, most authorities comment on the need for experienced surgical judgment if the closed approach (debridement, reclosure, and antibiotic irrigation) is utilized. The open approach is more frequently used for chronic or extensive infections and often entails removal of involved bony or cartilaginous structures. Although previously the wound was allowed to heal by secondary intention, current strategy involves formation of a myocutaneous flap over the sternal area.[192] The patient is treated with nutritional (Table 52–3) and respiratory support as needed. With both the closed and open method, intravenous antibiotics and sternal antibiotic irrigation are continued for at least 10 to 14 days; 4 to 6 weeks of treatment may be needed in cases of documented sternal osteomyelitis.

The reported mortality associated with mediastinitis varies greatly and appears to be related to the delay in initiation of treatment; patients diagnosed and treated aggressively within 1 month of surgery have a mortality of about 10 per cent, whereas those treated later have a mortality of about 25 per cent.[188,190] Surprisingly, the presence of a mediastinal infection does not appear to reduce the likelihood of patency of coronary artery bypass grafts.[193]

INFECTIVE ENDOCARDITIS
(See Chap. 33)

It has been convincingly shown that perioperative antibiotic prophylaxis is of benefit in patients undergoing cardiac surgery.[194] Although the antibiotic regimen varies, in part related to local differences in microbiological flora and personal preference, it is directed against gram-positive cocci (the most frequent causative pathogen in infections after cardiac surgery) and usually contains a cephalosporin. The regimen utilized in our institution consists of 1 gm of cefazolin intravenously 30 minutes before the skin incision and then repeated at 8-hour intervals for 48 hours after operation.

Cardiac surgery does not appear to increase the risk of endocarditis in patients with abnormal native valves that are not repaired or replaced during the operative procedure, in patients with intracardiac shunts, or in patients with intravascular devices (e.g., permanent pacemaker wires or renal dialysis shunts).[195] Assuming no infection is present preoperatively, such patients need only receive the standard antibiotic prophylaxis regimen in force at the institution in which the surgery is being performed.

PROSTHETIC VALVE ENDOCARDITIS (see p. 1079). Prosthetic valve endocarditis is a rare but extremely serious complication of cardiac surgery, frequently arising from nosocomial bacteremias.[196–198] It is estimated to occur in only 2 to 4 per cent of patients; about half of the cases are classified as "early" (<60 days from the date of operation) and half as "late" (>60 days from the date of operation).[196–199] The pooled data from several series indicate that the organism responsible for early prosthetic valve endocarditis includes a *Staphylococcus* species in about 50 per cent of cases.[199] The remainder of early cases of prosthetic valve endocarditis are caused by gram-negative bacilli, diphtheroids, and fungi.

The microbiological spectrum of late prosthetic valve endocarditis is more characteristic of that seen with native valve endocarditis. Only 30 per cent of cases are due to either *S. epidermidis* or *S. aureus*, and slightly more than one-third are caused by *Streptococcus* species (group D streptococci and *Streptococcus pneumoniae*).

The nature of the pathology in prosthetic valve endocarditis varies, depending on the type of prosthesis.[199] Mechanical valves typically show a ring abscess or myocardial abscess, whereas porcine heterografts more commonly develop valvar stenosis or regurgitation as a result of the endocarditis.

Management. Features of prosthetic valve endocarditis that have been associated with increased mortality include invasive infection (i.e., extension into the myocardium), congestive heart failure resulting from dysfunction of the prosthesis, and the presence of antibiotic-resistant, virulent microorganisms or a fungal organism.[199] Appropriate antibiotic therapy for prosthetic valve endocarditis is discussed in Chapter 33.

Advances in the treatment of congestive heart failure and the current generation of antibiotics may allow postponement of surgery to achieve a healed status in the absence of any compelling indication for urgent operation.[200] Transthoracic and if needed transesophageal echocardiography should be employed to clarify the severity of the hemodynamic lesion and search for any endocarditis-associated complications such as vegetations and paravalvular abscesses that may influence the timing of operation and the choice of prosthesis at surgery (e.g., unstented aortic homograft if extensive aortic root reconstruction is required).[5] The following clinical characteristics indicate the need for early operative intervention: (1) moderate to severe congestive heart failure caused by prosthetic valve dysfunction (incompetence or stenosis); (2) signs of extension of the infection into the perivalvular tissue or formation of a myocardial abscess (new electrocardiographic conduction abnormalities, pericarditis, valve dehiscence, persistent unexplained fever beyond 10 days of antibiotic treatment); (3) infection caused by aggressive, invasive organisms or those that are difficult to eradicate (fungi, *S. aureus*, some cases of *S. epidermidis*); (4) persistently positive blood cultures despite appropriate antibiotic therapy; (5) relapse of the clinical syndrome of endocarditis after appropriate antibiotic therapy; and (6) recurrent systemic emboli.

VIRAL. Viral infections that occur after cardiac surgery are almost exclusively the result of infectious complications of transfusion therapy, and with the exception of human immunodeficiency virus, primarily result in hepatitis. The incidence of viral infections after cardiac operations is decreasing as a result of a reduction in the number of transfusions of blood bank products (e.g., cell-saver techniques and preoperative autologous blood donations) and improved screening techniques in contemporary blood bank practice. CMV infection is a febrile syndrome that typically presents 1 month postoperatively. It is characterized by high-spiking fevers, abnormalities of liver function tests, and arthralgias. A self-limited illness, it is best treated with antipyretics and supportive fluid therapy.

Hepatitis C is caused by an RNA virus and is characterized by a protracted course with fluctuating transaminase levels.[201] About 50 per cent of patients respond to a course of interferon therapy with a reduction in transaminase levels; half of the responders relapse over the long term.[202,203]

FUNGAL. Fungal infections that involve the heart are rare. They typically are seen in cases of fungemia and usually are fatal. Although the problem of fungemia is well described in the immunocompromised host (e.g., heart transplant recipient), in an autopsy study of 60 patients with fungal infections of the heart 25 per cent of cases occurred in association with conventional valvular surgery.[204] About half of fungal infections of the heart are confined to the endocardium, and half involve both the endocardium and the myocardium. Extracardiac involvement is common, with spread of the infection to the lungs, cerebrospinal fluid, urine, and skin. The most commonly encountered organisms, in descending order of frequency, are *Candida, Aspergillus,* and *Cryptococcus* species. Patients who appear at particular risk of fungal involvement of the heart are those who have received corticosteroids and long courses of antibiotic treatment postoperatively.

Peripheral Vascular Complications

Most adults who undergo cardiac surgery—especially coronary revascularization—have atherosclerosis of the peripheral vasculature (e.g., ileofemoral system) and may experience lower-extremity ischemia after surgery because of low flow in the perioperative period with in situ thrombosis, embolism from the heart or aorta, or vascular compromise from an intra-aortic balloon pump catheter. Management consists of anticoagulation and removal of indwelling catheters, if clinically feasible. Thrombectomy and even revascularization surgery of the lower extremities (e.g., femorofemoral, femoropopliteal, or axillofemoral bypass) may be required to salvage threatened limbs.

Asymptomatic deep venous thrombosis of the calf can develop before hospital discharge in about one-third to one-half of patients who receive saphenous vein bypass grafts. Occasionally, these thrombi propagate to the proximal leg veins; only rarely do they cause massive pulmonary embolism.[45,205] The best strategy is rigorous perioperative prophylaxis against venous thromboembolism in all such patients. "Minidose unfractionated heparin" (5000 units subcutaneously initiated 2 hours preoperatively and continued every 8 to 12 hours postoperatively) appears to be efficacious.

Other Complications

PERICARDITIS (see Chap. 43). Postoperative tamponade is discussed on p. 152. Pericardial friction rubs frequently are audible in the early postoperative period and probably are the result of mechanical irritation from the mediastinal chest tubes. They usually disappear by the second or third postoperative day and are asymptomatic because of the narcotic analgesics prescribed at that stage of recovery. Although some patients develop pericardial rubs toward the end of the first postoperative week, these usually are benign, do not indicate a need for prolongation of hospitalization, and do not require treatment. A separate clinical syndrome that appears late in the first postoperative month is the *postpericardiotomy syndrome* (p. 230).[206] The relation between the postpericardiotomy syndrome and chronic constrictive pericarditis is not firmly established, but a number of patients with *postoperative constrictive pericarditis*[144] have a history of postpericardiotomy syndrome.

RENAL FAILURE (see Chap. 62). All patients who undergo cardiac surgery experience a reduction in renal blood flow and glomerular filtration rate (GFR) as a consequence of both anesthesia and cardiopulmonary bypass. Risk factors for the development of persistent renal failure after cardiac surgery include a preoperative history of renal dysfunction or left ventricular dysfunction, prolonged bypass time (>180 minutes), prolonged aortic cross-clamping (>40 minutes), perioperative hypotension, advanced age (>70 years), and the development postoperatively of medical complications.[207]

Most cases of acute renal failure after cardiac surgery result from renal ischemia that lowers the GFR directly (prerenal disease) or, if severe or prolonged, can induce acute tubular necrosis. Possible additional contributory factors include sepsis, nephrotoxic drugs, radiocontrast material injections, cholesterol plaque embolization to the renal circulation, increased urine free hemoglobin levels from hemolysis while on cardiopulmonary bypass, and the effects of ACE inhibitors on glomerular capillary pressure.[208] The detrimental effects of ACE inhibitors are most likely to occur when renal perfusion pressure is low because of renal artery stenosis or systemic hypotension caused by cardiac failure.

Urine output is variable in patients with postoperative acute renal failure. Anuria is uncommon and, if present, should raise the suspicion of urinary tract obstruction (e.g., occluded Foley catheter). More commonly patients are either oliguric (<400 mg/day) or nonoliguric. Oliguric acute renal failure occurs less frequently than nonoliguric renal failure, usually reflects more severe renal injury, and is associated with a greater probability of requiring dialysis during the acute phase.[208]

Differentiation Between Prerenal Azotemia and Acute Tubular Necrosis. Important diagnostic studies in all patients with acute renal failure include a urinalysis and estimation of pulmonary capillary wedge pressure and cardiac output by means of pulmonary artery catheterization. Prerenal azotemia should be suspected if the urine sodium level is less than 20 mEq/liter, the fractional excretion of sodium is less than 1 per cent, and the urine osmolality level is greater than 500 mOsm/liter. Acute tubular necrosis should be suspected if the urine sodium level is greater than 40 mEq/liter, the fractional excretion of sodium is greater than 2 per cent, and the urine osmolality level is less than 350 mOsm/liter.[208]

Treatment. Essential elements of treatment for both prerenal azotemia and acute tubular necrosis include optimization of intravascular fluid volume and cardiac output. The latter is best accomplished with vasodilators and inotropic agents (see p. 1935) rather than with vasopressors, to avoid further reductions in renal blood flow. Experimental studies suggest that several modalities may protect against the development of progressive renal failure in models of acute renal ischemic injury (e.g., renal artery clamping that simulates the effects of suprarenal aortic cross-clamping while on cardiopulmonary bypass). Mannitol (which washes out obstructing casts), a loop diuretic (which decreases energy requirements in the thick ascending limb of the loop of Henle, thereby decreasing ischemic injury), and the combination of dopamine and atrial natriuretic peptide (but neither alone) have all been effective.[209] There are, however, no good clinical trials to confirm the efficacy of these interventions. Several uncontrolled observations suggest that those patients who appear to be protected by a loop diuretic, mannitol, or dopamine were all treated within 12 to 24 hours of the onset of renal dysfunction.[208]

It is prudent to undertake a trial of furosemide and mannitol (only if the patient can tolerate the volume load of the latter) within the first 12 to 24 hours after the development of oliguria. The aim of such therapy is to increase urine output. Because of the renal vasodilating effects of dopamine (3 μg/kg/min), patients with both oliguric and nonoliguric renal failure may experience an increase in urine output.[210] There is, however, no evidence that dopamine alone given in this setting is helpful for recruiting salvageable but nonfunctioning nephrons.

If oliguria persists beyond 12 hours, a number of supportive measures must be activated, including careful attention to electrolyte balance, specifically avoiding hyperkalemia; excessive free water administration that might lead to hyponatremia; correction of acidosis (adding bicarbonate to daily fluids); and adjustment of medication dosages for delayed excretion if the drug is cleared by renal mechanisms. There seems little benefit to instituting dialysis prophylactically for a given level of blood urea nitrogen or creatinine. Rather, dialysis should be carried out for pericarditis, refractory hyperkalemia, uremic encephalopathy, or colitis. Continuous arteriovenous hemofiltration is a simpler modality that can be used to remove excess fluid.

Cardiac Surgery in the Patient with Chronic Renal Failure. Finally, the patient with chronic renal failure who undergoes surgery is at increased risk of exacerbation of renal dysfunction perioperatively. This may require temporary or even permanent hemodialysis, and these eventualities should be addressed with the patient and the cardiac surgical team preoperatively. Surgery can be safely performed in patients who are already on hemodialysis, but careful coordination of the surgical and dialysis schedules is essential to minimize postoperative problems with fluid and electrolyte management. Ultrafiltration can be performed while on cardiopulmonary bypass, to help minimize the intraoperative fluid load received by the patient.

GASTROINTESTINAL COMPLICATIONS (Table 52–12).[211–213] Serious gastrointestinal complications after cardiac surgery are rare (occurring in about 1 per cent of patients) and usually can be handled by a conservative approach. Only about 0.5 per cent of patients who undergo cardiac surgery require a general surgical operation for a gastrointestinal complication.[212–214] Patients with circulatory compromise and those who require intra-aortic balloon pump support are more likely to develop gastrointestinal complications. Despite their relative rarity, gastrointestinal complications are associated with a significant mortality (approaching 40 per cent in some series), highlighting the need for careful monitoring and repeated physical examination in high-risk patients.[212–213] Most complications occur within 7 days of surgery.

NEUROLOGICAL. Neurological complications after cardiac surgery are quite common, particularly in the elderly, if one is attentive to the subtle cognitive (short-term memory loss, lack of concentration) and psychological (depression, increased sense of dependency) changes seen early after operation.[35,215] A positive and supportive attitude on the part of the staff and enlistment of the aid of family members help to minimize these problems. Although many patients return to their postoperative state by 4 to 6 weeks after surgery, about 10 per cent continue to show deterioration of their neuropsy-

TABLE 52–12 GASTROINTESTINAL COMPLICATIONS AFTER CARDIAC SURGERY

COMPLICATIONS	COMMON CAUSES	EVALUATION	TREATMENT	COMMENT
Hyperbilirubinemia				
Early (1–10 days)	"Shock liver" syndrome	Check full chemistry profile	Maximize cardiac output, BP, and oxygenation	Markedly elevated enzyme levels are seen early after onset of shock state
	Hemolysis on cardiopulmonary bypass	↑ Plasma free hemoglobin	Observe	Isolated elevation of direct and indirect bilirubin without enzyme elevation
	Right heart failure	Chest x-ray, hemodynamic monitoring	Digitalis, diuretics, oxygen, consider isoproterenol infusion	Elevated direct bilirubin and alkaline phosphatase but without enzyme elevation
Late (10–90 days)	Infection (cytomegalovirus, hepatitis C)	Viral serology	Observe	Consider interferon for hepatitis C
	Cholecystitis	Ultrasound, biliary isotopic scan (e.g., HIDA, PIPIDA)	General surgical consultation	May require ERCP, cholecystectomy, cholesystotomy
Gastroduodenal disease				
Hemorrhage	Stress gastritis	Nasogastric aspirate (pH and Hematest), CBC	Nasogastric tube, antacids, H$_2$-receptor antagonists, transfusions	Because of the increased risk of developing this complication, it is important to provide prophylactic treatment (antacids, H$_2$-receptor antagonists) to patients with COPD and postoperative hypotension, bleeding, or reoperation. Early endoscopy and consideration of surgical intervention are strongly advised if supportive medical care is unsuccessful.
	Peptic ulcer disease	Nasogastric aspirate (pH and Hematest), CBC	Nasogastric tube, antacids, H$_2$-receptor antagonists, transfusions	Early endoscopy and consideration of surgical intervention are strongly advised if supportive medical care is unsuccessful.
Mesenteric ischemia	Combination of low cardiac output, embolization of atherosclerotic debris or thrombi, and vascular dissection by intra-aortic balloon pump	High index of suspicion and early surgical consultation	Early laparotomy with resection of affected bowel and embolectomy when possible	Mortality rate remains high.
Pancreatitis	Hypotension, thromboembolism of vascular supply, splanchnic vasoconstriction	Serum amylase measurements serially, abdominal ultrasonogram	Nasogastric suction and fluid support	Hyperamylasemia is common after cardiac surgery, but clinical pancreatitis is rare. Severe fulminating acute pancreatitis in postcardiac surgical patients has a poor prognosis despite aggressive surgical treatment.
Miscellaneous				
Intra-abdominal bleeding	Trauma (intraop, chest tubes) Preexisting lesion (e.g., hamartoma)	Abdominal lavage	General surgical consultation	
Lower gastrointestinal tract bleed	Colonic pathology (e.g., polyp)	Plain film of abdomen, colonoscopy		
Ileus	Narcotics Adhesions	Plain film of abdomen	Nasogastric suction	

CBC, complete blood count; COPD, chronic obstructive pulmonary disease; ERCP, endoscopic retrograde cholangiopancreatography.

chrological function over the next 6 months, especially if they are over age 65.[35,215] More serious neurological complications, such as stroke (Table 52–13), occur in 1 to 5 per cent of patients, but may be seen in as many as 10 per cent of patients over age 65.[35]

Symptomatic visual defects may be seen after cardiac surgery and result from retinal emboli, occipital lobe infarction, or anterior ischemic optic neuropathy. Risk factors for cerebrovascular accident (CVA) or transient ischemic attack (TIA) after cardiac surgery include preoperative carotid bruit, previous CVA or TIA, postoperative atrial fibrillation, prolonged cardiopulmonary bypass (>2 hours), and preoperative left ventricular mural thrombus.[35,216,217]

Neuropathies in the upper extremities have been reported after cardiac operations. The pattern of injury involving predominantly the ulnar nerve and medial antebrachial cutaneous nerve suggests that the lesion involves a brachial plexus compression or traction injury.[218] The average duration of symptoms after such an injury is 2 months, but some patients show a slower time course of improvement extending over 6 to 12 months.

CHYLOTHORAX, CHYLOPERICARDIUM. These are rare postcardiac surgical complications in adults, occurring in less than 0.5 per cent of cases. Treatment of chylothorax consists of prolonged chest tube drainage and dietary support with medium-chain triglycerides. Refractory cases of chylothorax have been successfully treated by the creation of a pleuroperitoneal shunt.[219] Chylopericardium may cause cardiac tamponade (see p. 1522) and is treated by creation of a pericardial window into the pleural space and management as above for chylothorax.[220] Persistent chyle leaks may necessitate thoracic duct ligation.

REHABILITATION AND PREPARATION FOR DISCHARGE

(See Chap. 40)

A coordinated, multidisciplinary cardiac exercise program is essential to overcome the physical deconditioning

TABLE 52–13 POSSIBLE CAUSES OF STROKE AFTER CARDIAC SURGERY[35,212,216]

Embolism
Debridement or replacement of calcified aortic valve
Dislodgment of atherosclerotic plaque during cannulation of aorta
Introduction of air into the arterial circulation intraoperatively
Dislodgment of atherosclerotic plaque from carotid artery stenosis by means of "jet effect" from aortic inflow cannula
Arrhythmia (e.g., atrial fibrillation)
Thrombosis of mechanical prosthetic valve
Dissection of aorta during cannulation
Left ventricular thrombus
Dislodgment of fragment of left atrial myxoma
Endocarditis
Microaggregate formation on cardiopulmonary bypass
Hemorrhage
Anticoagulation perioperatively
Hypertension
Hypotension
Hypoperfusion of cerebral circulation while on cardiopulmonary bypass
Hypoperfusion of cerebral circulation during period of postoperative shock

and psychosocial upheaval associated with cardiac surgery.[220a] Emphasis should be placed on early mobilization and progressively more patient self-care, including in the intensive care unit during the first 48 hours postoperatively. After transfer out of the intensive care unit, the patient should be encouraged to engage in low-density (2 to 3 METS) isotonic activities such as walking and range-of-motion exercises.[221] The nursing staff should monitor the patient's progress, being alert to any undue acceleration of the heart rate (>120 beats/min) or hemodynamically compromising arrhythmias.

Patients should also participate in an education program focusing on instructions regarding postoperative medications and initiation of secondary measures targeted at preventing graft occlusion and progression of atherosclerosis (Table 52–14).[90,222,223] Because of the overwhelming evidence indicating that platelet inhibition is critical to prevention of graft occlusion, all patients undergoing bypass surgery should receive long-term therapy with aspirin unless contraindicated. Ticlopidine may be useful in aspirin-intolerant patients, but there is no evidence of significant benefit from the routine use of either dipyridamole or sulfinpyrazone. Finally, innovative strategies are needed to encourage patients to return to work and society to accept postcardiac surgical patients back into the work force.

TABLE 52–14 ASSESSMENT OF RISK FACTORS AND THERAPEUTIC GOALS IN THE PATIENT WHO HAS UNDERGONE CORONARY REVASCULARIZATION

RISK FACTOR	ASSESSMENT	THERAPEUTIC GOAL
Elevated LDL cholesterol	Fasting lipid profile	<100 mg/dl (<2.6 mmol/L)
Decreased HDL cholesterol	Fasting lipid profile	>35 mg/dl (>0.9 mmol/L)
Hypertension	Blood pressures confirmed on two visits	<140/90 mm Hg
Physical inactivity	Interview	>20 min of physical activity or level walking, 1.5–2 miles/day, three times per week as a minimum
Smoking	Interview	Complete cessation
Obesity	Body weight for height	<130% of ideal body weight
Diabetes	Fasting blood glucose	<140 mg/dl
Stress	Interview	Improved coping skills

LDL, low density lipoprotein; HDL, high density lipoprotein.
Adapted from Pearson, T., Rapaport, E., Criqui, M., et al.: Optimal risk factor management in the patient after coronary revascularization. A statement for healthcare professionals from an American Heart Association Writing Group. Circulation 90:3125, 1994. Copyright 1994 American Heart Association.

REFERENCES

1. Savage, E. B., and Cohn, L. H.: 'No Touch' dissection, antegrade-retrograde blood cardioplegia, and single aortic cross-clamp significantly reduce operative mortality of reoperative CABG. Circulation 90:II-140, 1994.
1a. Cameron, A., Davis, K. B., Green, G., et al.: Coronary bypass surgery with internal thoracic artery grafts—effects on survival over a 15 year period. N. Engl. J. Med. 334:216, 1996.
2. Manapat, A., McCarthy, P., Lytle, B., et al.: Gastroepiploic and inferior epigastric arteries for coronary artery bypass: Early results and evolving applications. Circulation 90:II-144, 1994.
3. Horvath, K., Mannting, F., and Cohn, L.: Improved myocardial perfusion and relief of angina after transmyocardial laser revascularization. Circulation 90:I-640, 1994.
3a. Frazier, O. H., Cooley, D. A., Kadipasaoglu, K. A., et al.: Myocardial revascularization with laser: Preliminary findings. Circulation 92:58, 1995.
3b. Robinson, C. L., Gross, D. R., Zeman, W., et al.: Minimally invasive coronary artery bypass grafting: A new method using an anterior mediastinotomy. J. Card. Surg. 10:529, 1995.
4. Jamieson, W. R.: Modern cardiac valve devices—bioprostheses and mechanical prostheses: State of the art. J. Cardiac Surg. 8:89, 1993.
5. Petrou, M., Wong, K., Albertucci, M., et al.: Evaluation of unstented aortic homografts for the treatment of prosthetic aortic valve endocarditis. Circulation 90:II-198, 1994.
5a. Cohn, L. C., Kowalker, W., Bhatia, S., et al.: Comparative morbidity of mitral valve repair versus replacement for mitral regurgitation with and without coronary artery disease. Ann. Thorac. Surg. 60:1452, 1995.
5b. Cohn, L. H., Rizzo, R. J., Adams, D. H., et al.: The effect of pathophysiology on the surgical treatment of ischemic mitral regurgitation: operative and late risks of repair versus replacement. Eur. J. Cardiothorac. Surg. 9:568, 1995.
6. Carpentier, A., and Chachques, J.: Clinical dynamic cardiomyoplasty: Method and outcome. Semin. Thorac. Cardiovasc. Surg. 3:136, 1991.
7. Bellotti, G., Moraes, A., Bocchi, E., et al.: Late effects of cardiomyoplasty on left ventricular mechanics and diastolic filling. Circulation 88:II-304, 1993.
8. Glick, D. B., and Ferguson, T. B.: Surgery for cardiac arrhythmias. Curr. Opin. Cardiol. 9:222, 1994.
9. Hannan, E., Kilburn, H., Racz, M., et al.: Improving the outcomes of coronary artery bypass surgery in New York state. JAMA 271:761, 1994.
10. Rahimtoola, S., Bennett, A., Grunkemeier, G., et al.: Survival at 15-18 years after coronary bypass surgery for angina in women. Circulation 88:II-71, 1993.
11. Peterson, E., Jollis, J., Bebchuk, J., et al.: Changes in the mortality after myocardial revascularization in the elderly: The national Medicare experience. Ann. Intern. Med. 121:919, 1994.
12. Nugent, W., Schults, W., Plume, S., et al.: Designing an instrument panel to monitor and improve coronary artery bypass grafting. J. Clin. Outcomes Management 1:57, 1994.
13. Hannan, E., Siu, A., Kumar, D., et al.: The decline in coronary artery bypass graft surgery mortality in New York state: The role of surgeon volume. JAMA 273:209, 1995.
14. Aranki, S. F., and Cohn, L. H.: Coronary artery bypass grafting in the elderly. J. Myocard. Ischemia 6:1, 1994.
15. Aranki, S., Rizzo, R., Couper, G., et al.: Aortic valve replacement in the elderly: Effect of gender and coronary artery disease on operative mortality. Circulation 88:II-17, 1993.
16. Frank, R. A., and Mills, N. L.: Reoperative coronary artery bypass grafting. Curr. Opin. Cardiol. 9:680, 1994.
17. Lieberman, E., Wilson, J., Harrison, J., et al.: Aortic valve replacement in adults after balloon aortic valvuloplasty. Circulation 90:II-205, 1994.
18. Jones, E., Weintraub, W., Craver, J., et al.: Coronary bypass surgery: Is the operation different today? J. Thorac. Cardiovasc. Surg. 101:108, 1991.
19. Zehr, K., Lee, P., Poston, R., et al.: Two decades of coronary artery bypass graft surgery in young adults. Circulation 90:II-133, 1994.
20. Beyersdorf, F., Mitrev, Z., Sarai, K., et al.: Changing patterns of patients undergoing emergency surgical revascularization for acute coronary occlusion: Importance of myocardial protection techniques. J. Thorac. Cardiovasc. Surg. 106:137, 1993.
21. Disch, D., O'Connor, G., Birkmeyer, J., et al.: Changes in patients undergoing coronary artery bypass grafting. Ann. Thorac. Surg. 57:416, 1994.
22. Edwards, F., Clark, R., and Schwartz, M.: Coronary artery bypass grafting: The Society of Thoracic Surgeons National Database experience. Ann. Thorac. Surg. 57:12, 1994.

23. Komeda, M., David, T., Rao, V., et al.: Late hemodynamic effects of the preserved papillary muscles during mitral valve replacement. Circulation 90:II-190, 1994.
24. Mauldin, P., Weintraub, W., and Becker, E.: Predicting hospital costs for first-time coronary artery bypass grafting from preoperative and postoperative variables. Am. J. Cardiol. 74:772, 1994.
25. Marwick, C.: Coronary bypass grafting economics, including rehabilitation. Curr. Opin. Cardiol. 9:635, 1994.
26. Taylor, G., Mikell, F., Moses, H., et al.: Determinants of hospital charges for coronary artery bypass surgery: The economic consequences of postoperative complications. Am. J. Cardiol. 65:309, 1990.
27. Smith, L., Milano, C., Molter, B., et al.: Preoperative determinants of postoperative costs associated with coronary artery bypass graft surgery. Circulation 90:II-124, 1994.
28. Sculpher, M., Seed, P., Henderson, R., et al.: Health service costs of coronary artery angioplasty and coronary artery bypass surgery: The Randomised Intervention Treatment of Angina (RITA) trial. Lancet 334:927, 1994.

PREOPERATIVE EVALUATION

29. Wagner, E., and Trexler, S.: Preoperative evaluation. In Baumgartner, W., Owens, S., Cameron, D., and Reitz, B. (eds.): The Johns Hopkins Manual of Cardiac Surgical Care. St. Louis, C. V. Mosby, 1994, p. 27.
30. Vlahakes, G. J., Lemmer, J. H., Behrendt, D. M., and Austen, W. G.: Handbook of Patient Care in Cardiac Surgery. Boston, Little, Brown and Co., 1994.
31. Rizzo, R., Aranki, S., Aklog, L., et al.: Rapid noninvasive diagnosis and surgical repair of acute ascending aortic dissection. J. Thorac. Cardiovasc. Surg. 108:567, 1994.
32. Hanet, C., Marchand, E., and Keyeux, A.: Left internal mammary artery occlusion after mastectomy and radiotherapy. Am. J. Cardiol. 65:1044, 1990.
33. Rizzo, R., Whittemore, A., Couper, G., et al.: Combined carotid and coronary revascularization; The preferred approach to the severe vasculopath. Ann. Thorac. Surg. 54:1099, 1992.
34. Vassilidze, T., Cernaianu, A., Gaprindashvili, T., et al.: Simultaneous coronary artery bypass and carotid endarterectomy. Texas Heart Inst. J. 21:119, 1994.
35. Hornick, P., Smith, P., and Taylor, K.: Cerebral complications after coronary bypass surgery. Curr. Opin. Cardiol. 9:670, 1994.
36. Barnett, H. J. M., Eliasziw, M., and Meldrum, H. E.: Drugs and surgery in the prevention of ischemic stroke. N. Engl. J. Med. 332:238, 1995.
37. Moore, W., Barnett, H., Beebe, H., et al.: Guidelines for carotid endarterectomy: A multidisciplinary consensus statement from the ad hoc committee, American Heart Association. Circulation 91:566, 1995.
38. Acinapura, A., Jacobowitz, I., Kramer, M., et al.: Internal mammary artery bypass: Thirteen years of experience: Influence of angina and survival in 5125 patients. J. Cardiovasc. Surg. 33:554, 1992.
39. Velebit, V., Christenson, J., Maurice, J., et al.: A patent internal mammary artery graft decreases the risk of reoperative coronary artery bypass surgery. Texas Heart Inst. J. 21:125, 1994.
40. Lytle, B. W., McElroy, D., McCarthy, P., et al.: Influence of arterial coronary bypass grafts on the mortality in coronary reoperations. J. Thorac. Cardiovasc. Surg. 107:675, 1994.
41. Cameron, A., Green, G., Brogno, D., and Thornton, J.: Internal thoracic artery grafts: 20-year clinical follow-up. J. Am. Coll. Cardiol. 25:188, 1995.
42. Edwards, F., Clark, R., and Schwartz, M.: Impact of internal mammary artery conduits on operative mortality in coronary revascularization. Ann. Thorac. Surg. 57:27, 1994.
43. Liang, B., Antman, E., Taus, R., et al.: Atherosclerotic aneurysms of aortocoronary vein grafts. Am. J. Cardiol. 61:185, 1988.
44. Cannegieter, S., Rosendaal, F., and Briet, E.: Thromboembolic and bleeding complications in patients with mechanical heart valve prostheses. Circulation 90:635, 1994.
45. Kondo, N. I., Maddi, R., Ewenstein, B. M., and Goldhaber, S. Z.: Anticoagulation and hemostasis in cardiac surgical patients. J. Cardiac Surg. 9:443, 1994.
46. Tatar, H., Cicek, S., Demirkilic, U., et al.: Vascular complications of intraaortic balloon pumping: Unsheathed versus sheathed insertion. Ann. Thorac. Surg. 55:1518, 1993.
47. Rihal, C., Eagle, K., Mickel, M., et al.: Surgical therapy for coronary artery disease among patients with combined coronary artery and peripheral vascular disease. Circulation 91:46, 1995.
48. Higgins, T., Estafanous, F., Lloyd, F., et al.: Stratification of morbidity and mortality outcome by preoperative risk factors in coronary artery bypass patients: A clinical severity score. JAMA 267:2344, 1992.
49. Craddock, D., Iyer, V. S., and Russell, W. J.: Factors influencing mortality and myocardial infarction after coronary artery bypass grafting. Curr. Opin. Cardiol. 9:664, 1994.
50. Findlay, I. N.: Coronary bypass surgery in women. Curr. Opin. Cardiol. 9:650, 1994.
51. Latimer, R., and Mahmood, N.: Predicting the outcome from cardiac surgery: Trial or tribulation. Curr. Opin. Anaesthesiol. 7:39, 1994.
52. Iyer, V., Russell, W., Leppard, P., and Craddock, D.: Mortality and myocardial infarction after coronary artery surgery: A review of 12003 patients. Med. J. Aust. 159:166, 1993.
53. Tu, J. V., Jaglal, S. B., Naylor, C. D., and the Steering Committee of the Provincial Adult Cardiac Care Network of Ontario: Multicenter valida-

54. Loop, F. D., Lytle, B. W., Cosgrove, D. M., et al.: Sternal wound complications after isolated coronary artery bypass grafting: Early and late mortality, morbidity, and cost of care. Ann. Thorac. Surg. 49:179, 1990.
55. Copeland, M., Senkowski, C., Ulcickas, M., et al.: Breast size as a factor for sternal wound complications following cardiac surgery. Arch. Surg. 129:757, 1994.
56. He, G. W., Ryan, W. H., Acuff, T. E., et al.: Risk factors for operative mortality and sternal wound infection in bilateral internal mammary artery grafting. J. Thorac. Cardiovasc. Surg. 107:196, 1994.
57. Palazzo, R., and Barner, H. B.: Surgery for ischemic heart disease. Curr. Opin. Cardiol. 9:216, 1994.
58. Ritchie, J. L., Bateman, T. M., Bonow, R. O., et al.: Guidelines for clinical use of cardiac radionuclide imaging. J. Am. Coll. Cardiol. 25:521, 1995.
58a. Vanoverschelde, J.-L. J., Gerber, B. L., D'Hondt, A.-M., et al.: Preoperative selection of patients with severely impaired left ventricular function for coronary revascularization: Role of low-dose dobutamine echocardiography and exercise-redistribution-reinjection thallium SPECT. Circulation 92:37, 1995.
59. Lee, K., Marwick, T., Cook, S., et al.: Prognosis of patients with left ventricular dysfunction, with and without viable myocardium after myocardial infarction: Relative efficacy of medical therapy and revascularization. Circulation 90:2687, 1994.
60. vom Dahl, J., Eitzman, D., Al-Aouar, Z., et al.: Relation of regional function, perfusion, and metabolism in patients with advanced coronary artery disease undergoing surgical revascularization. Circulation 90:2356, 1994.
61. Edmond, M., Mock, M., Davis, K., et al.: Long-term survival of medically treated patients in the coronary artery surgery study (CASS) registry. Circulation 90:2645, 1994.
62. Lomboy, C., Schulman, D., Grill, H., et al.: Rest-redistribution thallium-201 scintigraphy to determine myocardial viability early after myocardial infarction. J. Am. Coll. Cardiol. 25:210, 1995.
63. Foster, E., O'Kelly, B., LaPidus, A., et al.: Segmental analysis of resting echocardiographic function and stress scintigraphic perfusion: Implications for myocardial viability. Am. Heart J. 129:7, 1995.
64. Kereiakes, D., Topol, E., George, B., et al.: Emergency coronary artery bypass surgery preserves global and regional left ventricular function after intravenous tissue plasminogen activator therapy for acute myocardial infarction. J. Am. Coll. Cardiol. 11:899, 1988.
65. Moosvi, A. R., Khaja, F., Villanueva, L., et al.: Early revascularization improves survival in cardiogenic shock complicating acute myocardial infarction. J. Am. Coll. Cardiol. 19:7, 1992.
66. Tardiff, B., Califf, R., Morris, D., et al.: Coronary revascularization surgery following myocardial infarction: Effect of bypass surgery on survival following thrombolysis (in press).
66a. Braxton, J. H., Hammond, G. L., Letsou, G. V., et al.: Optimal timing of coronary artery bypass graft surgery after acute myocardial infarction. Circulation 92:66, 1995.
67. Mannucci, P.: Nontransfusional modalities. In Loscalzo, J., and Schafer, A. (eds.): Thrombosis and Hemorrhage. Boston, Blackwell Scientific Publications, 1994, p. 1117.
68. Parsons, R. S., Mohandas, K., and Riaz, N.: The effects of an intravenous infusion of isosorbide dinitrate during open heart surgery. Eur. Heart J. 9(Suppl. A):195, 1988.
69. Gersh, B. J., Chesebro, J. H., Braunwald, E., et al.: Coronary artery bypass graft surgery after thrombolytic therapy in the Thrombolysis in Myocardial Infarction Trial, Phase II (TIMI II). J. Am. Coll. Cardiol. 23:395, 1995.
70. Lappas, D.: Anesthesia in cardiac and noncardiac surgery: Overview. Coronary Artery Dis. 4:399, 1993.
71. Kirklin, J., and Barratt-Boyes, B.: Anesthesia for cardiovascular surgery. In Kirklin, J., and Barratt-Boyes, B. (eds.): Cardiac Surgery. New York, Churchill Livingstone, 1993, p. 167.
72. Creswell, L., Schuessler, R., Rosenbloom, M., and Cox, J.: Hazards of postoperative atrial arrhythmias. Ann. Thorac. Surg. 56:539, 1993.
73. Aranki, S., Shaw, D., Adams, D., et al.: Predictors of atrial fibrillation following coronary artery surgery: Current trends and impact on hospital resources. Circulation (in press).
74. Lauer, M., and Eagle, K.: Arrhythmias following cardiac surgery. In Podrid, P., and Kowey, P. (eds.): Cardiac Arrhythmia. Mechanisms, Diagnosis, and Management. Baltimore, Williams and Wilkins, 1995, p. 1206.
75. Andrews, T. C., Reimold, S. C., Berlin, J. A., and Antman, E. M.: Prevention of supraventricular arrhythmias after coronary artery bypass surgery: A meta-analysis of randomized control trials. Circulation 84(Suppl. III):236, 1991.
76. Steinberg, J., Zelenkofske, S., Wong, S., et al.: Value of the P wave signal-averaged ECG for predicting atrial fibrillation after cardiac surgery. Circulation 88:2618, 1993.
77. Mendes, L., Connelly, G., McKenney, P., et al.: Right coronary artery stenosis: An independent predictor of atrial fibrillation after coronary artery bypass surgery. J. Am. Coll. Cardiol. 25:198, 1995.
78. Cox, J.: A perspective on postoperative atrial fibrillation in cardiac operations. Ann. Thorac. Surg. 56:405, 1993.
79. Aglio, L. S., Stanford, G. G., Maddi, R., et al.: Hypomagnesemia is common following cardiac surgery. J. Cardiothorac. Vasc. Anesth. 5:201, 1991.
80. Katholi, R., Woods, W., Womack, K., et al.: MgCl$_2$ replacement after

tion of a risk index for mortality, intensive care unit stay, and overall hospital length of stay after cardiac surgery. Circulation 91:677, 1995.

bypass surgery to prevent atrial fibrillation: A double blind, randomized trial. Circulation 82:III-58, 1990.

81. England, M. R., Gordon, G., Salem, M., and Chernow, B.: Magnesium administration and dysrhythmias after cardiac surgery: A placebo-controlled double-blind, randomized trial. JAMA 268:2395, 1992.

82. Fanning, W. J., Thomas, C., Jr., Roach, A., et al.: Prophylaxis of atrial fibrillation with magnesium sulfate after coronary artery bypass grafting. Ann. Thorac. Surg. 52:529, 1991.

83. Casthely, P. A., Yoganathan, T., Komer, C., and Kelly, M.: Magnesium and arrhythmias after coronary artery bypass surgery. J. Cardiothorac. Vasc. Anesth. 8:188, 1994.

84. Chassard, D., George, M., Giuraud, M., et al.: Relationship between preoperative amiodarone treatment and complications observed during anaesthesia for valvular cardiac surgery. Can. J. Anaesth. 37:251, 1990.

85. Nalos, P. C., Kass, R. M., Gang, E. S., et al.: Life-threatening postoperative pulmonary complications in patients with previous amiodarone pulmonary toxicity undergoing cardiothoracic operations. J. Thorac. Cardiovasc. Surg. 93:904, 1987.

86. Kupferschmid, J. P., Rosengart, T. K., McIntosh, C. L., et al.: Amiodarone-induced complications after cardiac operation for obstructive hypertrophic cardiomyopathy. Ann. Thorac. Surg. 48:359, 1989.

87. Barbieri, E., Conti, F., Zampieri, P., et al.: Amiodarone and desethyl-amiodarone distribution in the atrium and adipose tissue of patients undergoing short- and long-term treatment with amiodarone. J. Am. Coll. Cardiol. 8:210, 1986.

88. Lamas, G., Rebecca, G., Braunwald, N., and Antman, E.: Pacemaker malfunction after nitrous oxide anesthesia. Am. J. Cardiol. 56:995, 1985.

89. Lamas, G., Antman, E., Gold, J., et al.: Pacemaker back-up mode reversion and injury during cardiac surgery. Ann. Throac. Surg. 41:155, 1986.

90. Pearson, T., Rapaport, E., Criqui, M., et al.: Optimal risk factor management in the patient after coronary revascularization: A statement for healthcare professionals from an American Heart Association writing group. Circulation 90:3125, 1994.

91. Murkin, J. M., Lux, J., Shannon, N. A., et al.: Aprotinin significantly decreases bleeding and transfusion requirements in patients receiving aspirin and undergoing cardiac operations. J. Thorac. Cardiovasc. Surg. 107:554, 1994.

INTRAOPERATIVE MANAGEMENT

92. Kirklin, J. W., and Barratt-Boyes, B. G.: Cardiac Surgery. Morphology, Diagnostic Criteria, Natural History, Techniques, Results, and Indications. 2nd ed. New York, Churchill Livingstone, 1993.

93. D'Ambra, M.: Is intraoperative echocardiography a useful monitor in the operating room? Ann. Thorac. Surg. 56:S83, 1993.

94. Aranki, S., Rizzo, R., Adams, D., et al.: Single-clamp technique: An important adjunct to myocardial and cerebral protection in coronary operations. Ann. Thorac. Surg. 58:296, 1994.

95. Krukenkamp, I., Burns, P., Calderone, C., and Levitsky, S.: Perfusion and cardioplegia. Curr. Opin. Cardiol. 9:247, 1994.

96. Hines, R. L.: Transesophageal echocardiography: Is it for everyone? J. Cardiac Surg. 5:240, 1990.

96a. Joffe, I. I., Jacobs, L. E., Lampert, C., et al.: Role of echocardiography in perioperative management of patients undergoing open heart surgery. Am. Heart J. 131:162, 1995.

97. Horvath, K., Smith, W., Laurence, R., et al.: Recovery and viability of an acute myocardial infarct after transmyocardial laser revascularization. J. Am. Coll. Cardiol. 25:258, 1995.

97a. Flameng, W.: New strategies for intraoperative myocardial protection. Curr. Opin. Cardiol. 10:577, 1995.

98. Aranki, S.: Cardiovascular surgery in the elderly. In Homburger, F. (ed.): The Rational Use of Advanced Medical Technology with the Elderly. New York, Springer-Verlag, 1994, p. 132.

99. Aprotinin to decrease bleeding in cardiac surgery. Med. Lett. 36:50, 1994.

100. Videm, V., Svennevig, J., Fosse, E., et al.: Reduced complement activation with heparin-coated oxygenator and tubings in coronary bypass operations. J. Thorac. Cardiovasc. Surg. 103:806, 1992.

101. Jones, D., Hill, R., Hollingsed, M., et al.: Use of heparin-coated cardiopulmonary bypass. Ann. Thorac. Surg. 56:556, 1993.

102. Leung, J. M., Stanley, T. R., Mathew, J., et al.: An initial multicenter, randomized controlled trial on the safety and efficacy of acadesine in patients undergoing coronary artery bypass graft surgery: SPI Research Group. Anesth. Analg. 78:420, 1994.

POSTOPERATIVE MANAGEMENT

103. Kirklin, J., and Barratt-Boyes, B.: Postoperative care. In Kirklin, J., and Barratt-Boyes, B. (eds.): Cardiac Surgery. New York, Churchill Livingstone, 1993, p. 195.

104. Lippmann, M., Goldberg, S., and Walkenstein, M.: Pulmonary complications of open heart surgery. In Kotler, M., and Alfieri, A. (eds.): Cardiac and Noncardiac Complications of Open Heart Surgery: Prevention, Diagnosis, and Treatment. Mt. Kisco, N.Y., Futura, 1992, p. 239.

105. Walden, S., and Meyer, P.: Pulmonary management. In Baumgartner, W., Owens, S., Cameron, D., and Reitz, B. (eds.): The Johns Hopkins Manual of Cardiac Surgical Care. St. Louis, C. V. Mosby, 1994, p. 161.

106. Quasha, A. C., Loeber, N., Feeley, T. W., et al.: Postoperative respiratory care: A controlled trial of early and late extubation following coronary artery bypass grafting. Anesthesiology 52:135, 1980.

107. Cambier, B., Missault, L., Kockx, M., et al.: Influence of the breathing mode on the time course and amplitude of the cyclic inter-atrial pressure reversal in postoperative coronary bypass surgery patients. Eur. Heart J. 14:920, 1993.

108. Svennevig, J., Geiran, O., Karlsen, J., et al.: Complement activation during extracorporeal circulation: In vitro comparison of duraflo-II heparin-coated and uncoated oxygenator circuits. J. Thorac. Cardiovasc. Surg. 106:466, 1993.

109. Shafique, T., Johnson, R., Dai, H., et al.: Altered pulmonary microvascular reactivity after total cardiopulmonary bypass. J. Thorac. Cardiovasc. Surg. 106:479, 1993.

110. Butler, J., Rocker, G. M., and Westaby, S.: Inflammatory response to cardiopulmonary bypass. Ann. Thorac. Surg. 55:552, 1993.

111. Aranki, S., Adams, D., Rizzo, R., et al.: Femoral veno-arterial extracorporeal life support with minimal or no heparin. Ann. Thorac. Surg. 56:149, 1993.

112. Lam, A., and Newhouse, M.: Management of asthma and chronic airflow limitation. Chest 98:44, 1990.

113. Curtis, J. J., Weerachai, N., Walls, J. T., et al.: Elevated hemidiaphragm after cardiac operations: Incidence, prognosis, and relationship to the use of topical ice slush. Ann. Thorac. Surg. 48:764, 1989.

114. Abd, G., Braun, N., Baskin, M., et al.: Diaphragmatic dysfunction after open heart surgery: Treatment with a rocking bed. Ann. Intern. Med. 111:881, 1989.

115. Graham, D. R., Kaplan, D., Evans, C. C., et al.: Diaphragmatic plication for unilateral diaphragmatic paralysis: A 10-year experience. Ann. Thorac. Surg. 49:248, 1990.

116. Weiss, S. J., and Longnecker, D. E.: Perioperative hypertension: An overview. Coronary Artery Dis. 4:401, 1993.

117. Gray, R. J., Bateman, T. M., Czer, L. S., et al.: Use of esmolol in hypertension after cardiac surgery. Am. J. Cardiol. 56:56, 1985.

118. Estafanous, F., and Tarazi, R.: Systemic arterial hypertension associated with cardiac surgery. Am. J. Cardiol. 46:685, 1980.

119. Cooper, T. J., Clutton, B. T. H., Jones, S. N., et al.: Factors relating to the development of hypertension after cardiopulmonary bypass. Br. Heart J. 54:91, 1985.

120. Rocchini, A., Rosenthal, A., Barger, A., et al.: Pathogenesis of paradoxical hypertension after coarctation resection. Circulation 54:382, 1976.

121. O'Dwyer, J. P., Yorukoglu, D., and Harris, M. N.: The use of esmolol to attenuate the haemodynamic response when extubating patients following cardiac surgery—a double-blind controlled study. Eur. Heart J. 14:701, 1993.

122. James, T., Hageman, G., and Urthaler, F.: Anatomic and physiologic considerations of a cardiogenic hypertensive reflex. Am. J. Cardiol. 44:852, 1979.

123. Baumgartner, W., Owens, S., Cameron, D., and Reitz, B.: The Johns Hopkins Manual of Cardiac Surgical Care. St. Louis, C. V. Mosby, 1994, p. 546.

124. Leslie, J., Brister, N., Levy, J., et al.: Treatment of postoperative hypertension after coronary artery bypass surgery: Double-blind comparison of intravenous isradipine and sodium nitroprusside. Circulation 90:II-256, 1994.

125. Ruiz, R., Borches, D., Gonzalez, A., and Corral, J.: A new sodium-nitroprusside-infusion controller for the regulation of arterial blood pressure. Biomed. Instrum. Technol. 27:244, 1993.

126. Bruss, J., Meyerowitz, C., Greenspan, A., and Spielman, S.: The significance of the electrocardiogram after open heart surgery. In Kotler, M., and Alfieri, A. (eds.): Cardiac and Noncardiac Complications of Open Heart Surgery: Prevention, Diagnosis, and Treatment. Mt. Kisco, N.Y., Futura, 1992, p. 39.

127. Hamm, C. W., Reimers, J., Ischinger, T., et al.: A randomized study of coronary angioplasty compared with bypass surgery in patients with symptomatic multivessel coronary disease: German Angioplasty Bypass Surgery Investigation (GABI). N. Engl. J. Med. 331:1037, 1994.

128. King, S. E., Lembo, N. J., Weintraub, W. S., et al.: A randomized trial comparing coronary angioplasty with coronary bypass surgery: Emory Angioplasty versus Surgery Trial (EAST). N. Engl. J. Med. 331:1044, 1994.

129. Greaves, S., Rutherford, J., Aranki, S., et al.: Current incidence and determinants of perioperative myocardial infarction in coronary artery surgery. Am. Heart J. (in press).

130. Lemmer, J. H., Jr., and Kirsh, M. M.: Coronary artery spasm following coronary artery surgery. Ann. Thorac. Surg. 46:108, 1988.

131. Obarski, T. P., Loop, F. D., Cosgrove, D. M., et al.: Frequency of acute myocardial infarction in valve repairs versus valve replacement for pure mitral regurgitation. Am. J. Cardiol. 65:887, 1990.

132. Bulkley, B. H., and Hutchins, G. M.: Myocardial consequences of coronary artery bypass graft surgery: The paradox of necrosis in areas of revascularization. Circulation 56:906, 1977.

133. Katus, H., Schoeppenthau, M., Tanzeem, A., et al.: Non-invasive assessment of perioperative myocardial cell damage by circulating cardiac troponin T. Br. Heart J. 65:259, 1991.

134. Mair, J., Larue, C., Mair, P., et al.: Use of cardiac troponin I to diagnose perioperative myocardial infarction in coronary artery bypass grafting. Clin. Chem. 40:2066, 1994.

135. Bateman, T., Matloff, J., and Gray, R.: Myocardial infarction during coronary artery bypass surgery-benign event or prognostic omen? Int. J. Cardiol. 6:259, 1984.

136. Force, T., Hibberd, P., Weeks, G., et al.: Perioperative myocardial infarction after coronary artery bypass surgery. Circulation 82:903, 1990.

137. Feneck, R. O.: Intravenous milrinone following cardiac surgery: I. Ef-

fects of bolus infusion followed by variable dose maintenance infusion: The European Milrinone Multicentre Trial Group. J. Cardiothorac. Vasc. Anesth. 6:554, 1992.

138. Lee, W. A., Gillinov, A. M., Cameron, D. E., et al.: Centrifugal ventricular assist device for support of the failing heart after cardiac surgery. Crit. Care Med. 21:1186, 1993.

139. Oz, M., Rose, E., and Levin, H.: Selection criteria for placement of left ventricular assist devices. Am. Heart J. 129:173, 1995.

140. Reichert, C. L., Koolen, J. J., and Visser, C. A.: Transesophageal echocardiographic evaluation of left ventricular function during intraaortic balloon pump counterpulsation. J. Am. Soc. Echocardiogr. 6:490, 1993.

141. Reichert, C. L., Visser, C. A., Van den Brink, R. B., et al.: Prognostic value of biventricular function in hypotensive patients after cardiac surgery as assessed by transesophageal echocardiography. J. Cardiothorac. Vasc. Anesth. 6:429, 1992.

142. Mikawa, K., Maekawa, N., Goto, R., et al.: Use of prostaglandin E1 to treat perianaesthetic pulmonary hypertension associated with mitral valve disease. J. Int. Med. Res. 21:161, 1993.

143. Rich, G. F., Murphy, G. D., Jr., Roos, C. M., and Johns, R. A.: Inhaled nitric oxide: Selective pulmonary vasodilation in cardiac surgical patients. Anesthesiology 78:1028, 1993.

144. D'Cruz, I. A., Overton, D. H., and Pai, G. M.: Pericardial complications of cardiac surgery: Emphasis on the diagnostic role of echocardiography. J. Cardiac Surg. 7:257, 1992.

145. Pepi, M., Muratori, M., Barbier, P., et al.: Pericardial effusion after cardiac surgery: Incidence, site, size, and haemodynamic consequences. Br. Heart J. 72:327, 1994.

146. Chuttani, K., Tischler, M. D., Pandian, N. G., et al.: Diagnosis of cardiac tamponade after cardiac surgery: Relative value of clinical, echocardiographic, and hemodynamic signs. Am. Heart J. 127:913, 1994.

147. Russo, A. M., O'Connor, W. H., and Waxman, H. L.: Atypical presentations and echocardiographic findings in patients with cardiac tamponade occurring early and late after cardiac surgery. Chest 104:71, 1993.

148. Schoebrechts, B., Herregods, M. C., Van, D. W. F., and De, G. H.: Usefulness of transesophageal echocardiography in patients with hemodynamic deterioration late after cardiac surgery. Chest 104:1631, 1993.

149. Moore, S. L., and Wilkoff, B. L.: Rhythm disturbances after cardiac surgery. Semin. Thorac. Cardiovasc. Surg. 3:24, 1991.

150. Gottipaty, V., Kocovic, D., Kinchla, N., et al.: Timing and impact on survival of in-hospital cardiac arrest after coronary artery bypass graft surgery. Circulation 88:I-166, 1993.

151. Waldo, A. L., and MacLean, W. A.: Treatment of cardiac arrhythmias with emphasis on cardiac pacing. In Diagnosis and Treatment of Cardiac Arrhythmias Following Open Heart Surgery: Emphasis on the Use of Atrial and Ventricular Epicardial Wire Electrodes. Mt. Kisco, N.Y., Futura, 1980, p. 115.

152. Olshansky, B., Okumura, K., Hess, P. G., et al.: Use of procainamide with rapid atrial pacing for successful conversion of atrial flutter to sinus rhythm. J. Am. Coll. Cardiol. 11:359, 1988.

153. Platia, E. V., Fitzpatrick, P., Wallis, D., et al.: Esmolol vs verapamil for the treatment of recent-onset atrial fibrillation/flutter. J. Am. Coll. Cardiol. 11:170, 1988.

154. Reed, G. L., Singer, D. E., and Pilard, E. H.: Stroke following coronary artery bypass surgery: A case control estimate of the risk of carotid bruits. N. Engl. J. Med. 319:1246, 1988.

155. Eckman, M. H., Levine, H. J., and Pauker, S. G.: Making decisions about antithrombotic therapy in heart disease: Decision analytic and cost-effectiveness issues. Chest 108:457S, 1995.

155a. Raitt, M. H., Dolack, G. L., Kino, K., et al.: Procainamide has limited effectiveness for the treatment of atrial fibrillation after open heart surgery. Circulation 90(Supp. 1):376, 1994.

156. Laupacis, A., Albers, G. W., Dalen, J. E., et al.: Antithrombotic therapy in atrial fibrillation. Chest 108:352S, 1995.

157. Raitt, M., Dolack, G., Kino, K., et al.: Procainamide has limited effectiveness for the treatment of atrial fibrillation after open heart surgery. Circulation 90:I-376, 1994.

158. Ganz, L., and Friedman, P.: Medical progress: Supraventricular tachycardia. N. Engl. J. Med. 332:162, 1995.

159. Rubin, D., Nieminski, K., Monteferrante, J., et al.: Ventricular arrhythmias after coronary artery bypass graft surgery: Incidence, risk factors and long-term prognosis. J. Am. Coll. Cardiol. 6:307, 1985.

160. Smith, R., Leung, J., Keith, F., et al.: Ventricular dysrhythmias in patients undergoing coronary artery bypass graft surgery: Incidence, characteristics, and prognostic significance. Am. Heart J. 123:73, 1992.

161. Johnson, R., Goldberger, A., Thurer, R., et al.: Lidocaine prophylaxis in coronary revascularization patients: A randomized prospective trial. Ann. Thorac. Surg. 55:1180, 1993.

162. Rousou, J., Engelman, R., Flack, J., III., et al.: Emergency cardiopulmonary bypass in the cardiac surgical unit can be a lifesaving measure in postoperative cardiac arrest. Circulation 90(Suppl. II):280, 1994.

163. Carlson, M., Biblo, L., and Waldo, A.: Post open heart surgery ventricular arrhythmias. Cardiovasc. Clin. 22:241, 1992.

164. Holman, W., Spruell, R., Vicente, W., and Pacifico, A.: Electrophysiological mechanisms for postcardioplegia reperfusion ventricular fibrillation. Circulation 90:II-293, 1994.

164a. Costeas, X. F., and Schoenfeld, M. H.: Usefulness of electrophysiologic studies for new-onset sustained ventricular tachyarrhythmias shortly after coronary artery bypass grafting. Am. J. Cardiol. 72:1291, 1993.

165. Scott, W. A.: Temporary DDD pacing after surgically induced heart block. Am. J. Cardiol. 71:1123, 1993.

166. Hippeläinen, M., Mustonen, P., Manninen, H., and Rehnberg, S.: Pre-

dictors of conduction disturbances after coronary bypass grafting. Ann. Thorac. Surg. 57:1284, 1994.

167. Baerman, J., Kirsh, M., de Buitleir, M., et al.: Natural history and determinants of conduction defects following coronary artery bypass surgery. Ann. Thorac. Surg. 44:150, 1987.

168. Tuzcu, E. M., Emre, A., Goormastic, M., et al.: Incidence and prognostic significance of intraventricular conduction abnormalities after coronary bypass surgery. J. Am. Coll. Cardiol. 16:607, 1990.

169. Emlein, G., Huang, S., Pires, L., et al.: Prolonged bradyarrhythmias after isolated coronary artery bypass graft surgery. Am. Heart J. 126:1084, 1993.

170. Tsai, T., and Matloff, J.: Cardiac surgery in the elderly. In Matloff, R. G. A. J. (ed.): Medical Management of the Cardiac Surgical Patient. Baltimore, Williams and Wilkins, 1990, p. 27.

171. Kestin, A. S., Valeri, C. R., Khuri, S. F., et al.: The platelet function defect of cardiopulmonary bypass. Blood 82:107, 1993.

172. Kalfin, R., Engelman, R., Rousou, J., et al.: Induction of interleukin-8 expression during cardiopulmonary bypass. Circulation 88:II-401, 1993.

173. Cines, D. B., Tomaski, A., and Tannenbaum, S.: Immune endothelial-cell injury in heparin-associated thrombocytopenia. N. Engl. J. Med. 316:581, 1987.

174. Kajani, M., and Waxman, H.: Hematologic problems after open heart surgery. In Kotler, M., and Alfieri, A. (eds.): Cardiac and Noncardiac Complications of Open Heart Surgery: Prevention, Diagnosis, and Treatment. Mt. Kisco, N.Y., Futura, 1992, p. 219.

175. Cormack, J. G., and Levy, J. H.: Adverse reactions to protamine. Coronary Artery Dis. 4:420, 1993.

176. Brister, S. J., Ofosu, F. A., and Buchanan, M. R.: Thrombin generation during cardiac surgery: Is heparin the ideal anticoagulant? Thromb. Haemost. 70:259, 1993.

177. Walenga, J., Bakhos, M., Messmore, H., et al.: Potential use of recombinant hirudin as an anticoagulant in a cardiopulmonary bypass model. Ann. Thorac. Surg. 51:271, 1991.

178. Mossad, E., and Estafanous, F.: Blood use in cardiac surgery and the limitations of hemodilution. Curr. Opin. Cardiol. 10:584, 1995.

179. Baumgartner, W., and Owens, S.: Hemorrhage and tamponade. In Baumgartner, W., Owens, S., Cameron, D., and Reitz, B. (eds.).: The Johns Hopkins Manual of Cardiac Surgical Care. St. Louis, C. V. Mosby, 1994, p. 183.

180. Kallis, P., Tooze, J. A., Talbot, S., et al.: Aprotinin inhibits fibrinolysis, improves platelet adhesion and reduces blood loss: Results of a double-blind randomized clinical trial. Eur. J. Cardiothorac. Surg. 8:315, 1994.

180a. Royston, D.: Aprotinin in patients having coronary artery bypass graft surgery. Curr. Opin. Cardiol. 10:591, 1995.

181. Stein, P. D., Alpert, J. S., Copeland III, J. G., et al.: Antithrombotic therapy in patients with mechanical and biological prosthetic heart valves. Chest 108:371S, 1995.

182. Verkkala, V., Valtonen, V., Jarvinen, A., and Tolppanen, E.: Fever, leukocytosis and C-reactive protein after open-heart surgery and their value in the diagnosis of postoperative infections. Thorac. Cardiovasc. Surg. 35:78, 1987.

183. Livelli, F., Johnson, R., McEnany, M., et al.: Unexplained in-hospital fever following cardiac surgery: Natural history, relationship to postpericardiotomy syndrome, and a prospective study of therapy with indomethacin versus placebo. Circulation 57:968, 1978.

184. Baddour, L., and Bisno, A.: Recurrent cellulitis after saphenous venectomy for coronary bypass surgery. Ann. Intern. Med. 97:493, 1982.

185. Greenberg, J., DeSanctis, R. W., and Mills, R. M. J.: Vein-donor-leg cellulitis after coronary bypass surgery. Ann. Intern. Med. 97:565, 1982.

186. Spencer, F. C., and Grossi, E. A.: Mediastinitis after cardiac operations. Ann. Thorac. Surg. 49:506, 1990.

187. Demmy, T. L., Park, S. B., Liebler, G. A., et al.: Recent experience with major sternal wound complications. Ann. Thorac. Surg. 49:458, 1990.

188. Greenblatt, J., and Fischer, R.: Complications of cardiac surgery: Infections. In Kotler, M., and Alfieri, A. (eds.): Cardiac and Noncardiac Complications of Open Heart Surgery: Prevention, Diagnosis, and Treatment. Mt. Kisco, N.Y., Futura, 1992, p. 145.

189. Kouchoukos, N. T., Wareing, T. H., Murphy, S. F., et al.: Risks of bilateral internal mammary artery bypass grafting. Ann. Thorac. Surg. 49:210, 1990.

190. Bor, D. H., Rose, R. M., Modlin, J. F., et al.: Mediastinitis after cardiovascular surgery. Rev. Infect. Dis. 5:885, 1983.

191. Kernodle, D. S., Classen, D. C., Burke, J. P., and Kaiser, A. B.: Failure of cephalosporins to prevent Staphylococcus aureus surgical wound infections. JAMA 263:961, 1990.

192. Omura, K., Misaki, T., Takahashi, H., et al.: Omental transfer for the treatment of sternal infarction after cardiac surgery: Report of three cases. Surg. Today 24:67, 1994.

193. Macmanus, Q., and Okies, J. E.: Mediastinal wound infection and aortocoronary graft patency. Am. J. Surg. 132:558, 1976.

194. Hall, J., Christiansen, K., Carter, M., et al.: Antibiotic prophylaxis in cardiac operations. Ann. Thorac. Surg. 56:916, 1993.

195. Keys, T. F.: Antimicrobial prophylaxis for patients with congenital or valvular heart disease. Mayo Clin. Proc. 57:171, 1982.

196. Threlkeld, M., and Cobbs, C.: Infectious disorders of prosthetic valves and intravascular devices. In Mandell, G., Douglas, R., and Bennett, J. (eds.): Principles and Practice of Infectious Diseases. New York, Churchill-Livingstone, 1990, p. 706.

197. Hall, T., and Reitz, B.: Valve replacement and repair. In Baumgartner,

1739

Ch 52

W., Owens, S., Cameron, D., and Reitz, B. (eds.): The Johns Hopkins Manual of Cardiac Surgical Care. St. Louis, C. V. Mosby, 1994, p. 365.

198. Fang, G., Keys, T., Gentry, L., et al.: Prosthetic valve endocarditis resulting from nosocomial bacteremia: A prospective multicenter study. Ann. Intern. Med. *119:*560, 1993.

199. Cowgill, L. D., Addonizio, V. P., Hopeman, A. G., and Harken, A. H.: A practical approach to prosthetic valve endocarditis. Ann. Thorac. Surg. *43:*450, 1987.

200. Aranki, S., Santini, F., Adams, D., et al.: Aortic valve endocarditis: Determinants of early survival and late morbidity. Circulation *90:*II-175, 1994.

201. Tremolada, F., Casarin, C., Alberti, A., et al.: Long-term follow-up of non-A, non-B (type C) post-transfusion hepatitis. J. Hepatol. *16:*273, 1992.

202. Davis, G., Balart, L., Schiff, E., et al.: Treatment of chronic hepatitis C with recombinant interferon alfa: A multicenter randomized, controlled trial. N. Engl. J. Med. *321:*1501, 1989.

203. DiBisceglie, A. M., Martin, P., Kassiandes, C., et al.: Recombinant interferon ALFA therapy for chronic hepatitis C. N. Engl. J. Med. *321:*1506, 1989.

204. Atkinson, J. B., Connor, D. H., Robinowitz, M., et al.: Cardiac fungal infections: Review of autopsy findings in 60 patients. Hum. Pathol. *15:*935, 1984.

205. Gillinov, A. M., Davis, E. A., Alberg, A. J., et al.: Pulmonary embolism in the cardiac surgical patient. Ann. Thorac. Surg. *53:*988, 1992.

206. Khan, A. H.: The postcardiac injury syndromes. Clin. Cardiol. *15:*67, 1992.

207. Kellerman, P. S.: Perioperative care of the renal patient. Arch. Intern. Med. *154:*1674, 1994.

208. Kobrin, S., and Tobias, S.: Renal complications of open heart surgery. *In* Kotler, M., and Alfieri, A. (eds.): Cardiac and Noncardiac Complications of Open Heart Surgery: Prevention, Diagnosis, and Treatment. Mt. Kisco, N.Y., Futura, 1992, p. 311.

209. Rose, B.: Acute renal failure-prerenal disease versus acute tubular necrosis. *In* Rose, B. (ed.): Pathophysiology of Renal Disease. New York, McGraw-Hill Book Co., 1987, p. 63.

210. Casale, A., and Ulrich, S.: Complications in other organ systems. *In* Baumgartner, W., Owens, S., Cameron, D., and Reitz, B. (eds.): The Johns Hopkins Manual of Cardiac Surgical Care. St. Louis, C. V. Mosby, 1994, p. 271.

211. Kelberman, I., and Levine, G.: Gastroenterologic complications of open heart surgery. *In* Motler, M., and Alfieri, A. (eds.): Cardiac and Noncardiac Complications of Open Heart Surgery: Prevention, Diagnosis, and Treatment. Mt. Kisco, N.Y., Futura, 1992, p. 177.

212. Egleston, C. V., Wood, A. E., Gorey, T. F., and McGovern, E. M.: Gastrointestinal complications after cardiac surgery. Ann. R. Coll. Surg. Engl. *75:*52, 1993.

213. Tsiotos, G. G., Mullany, C. J., Zietlow, S., and Van, H. J. A.: Abdominal complications following cardiac surgery. Am. J. Surg. *167:*553, 1994.

214. Zeithofer, J., Asenbaum, S., Spiss, C., et al.: Central nervous system function after cardiopulmonary bypass. Eur. Heart J. *14:*885, 1993.

215. Kallis, P., Unsworth-White, J., Munsch, C., et al.: Disability and distress following cardiac surgery in patients over 70 years of age. Eur. J. Cardiothorac. Surg. *7:*306, 1993.

216. Taylor, G. J., Malik, S. A., Colliver, J. A., et al.: Usefulness of atrial fibrillation as a predictor of stroke after isolated coronary artery bypass grafting. Am. J. Cardiol. *60:*905, 1987.

217. Kuroda, Y., Uchimoto, R., Kaieda, R., et al.: Central nervous system complications after cardiac surgery: A comparison between coronary artery bypass grafting and valve surgery. Anesth. Analg. *76:*222, 1993.

218. Seyfer, A. E., Grammer, N. Y., Bogumill, G. P., et al.: Upper extremity neuropathies after cardiac surgery. J. Hand. Surg. [Am.] *10:*16, 1985.

219. Murphy, M. C., Newman, B. M., and Rodgers, B. M.: Pleuroperitoneal shunts in the management of persistent chylothorax. Ann. Thorac. Surg. *48:*195, 1989.

220. Chan, B. B., Murphy, M. C., and Rodgers, B. M.: Management of chylopericardium. J. Pediatr. Surg. *25:*1185, 1990.

220a. Pearson, S. D., Goulart-Fisher, D., and Lee, T. H.: Critical pathways as a strategy for improving care: Problems and potential. Ann. Intern. Med. *123:*941, 1995.

REHABILITATION AND PREPARATION FOR DISCHARGE

221. Fletcher, G., Balady, G., Froelicher, V., et al.: Exercise standards: A statement for healthcare professionals from the American Heart Association. Circulation *91:*580, 1995.

222. van der Meer, J., Hillege, H., Koostra, G., et al.: Prevention of one-year vein-graft occlusion after aortocoronary-bypass surgery: A comparison of low-dose aspirin, low-dose aspirin plus dipyridamole, and oral anticoagulants. Lancet *342:*257, 1993.

223. Daida, H., Yokoi, H., Miyano, H., et al.: Relation of saphenous vein graft obstruction to serum cholesterol levels. J. Am. Coll. Cardiol. *25:*193, 1995.

Chapter 53
Cost-Effective Strategies in Cardiology

LEE GOLDMAN

The availability of an increasing number of diagnostic and therapeutic technologies, coupled with concerns over the rising costs of health care, has generated growing interest in determining the cost and effectiveness of cardiological care. Cost-effectiveness analysis, which initially had been used principally by economists and policymakers, is a potentially useful technique for evaluating how best to diagnose, prevent, and treat medical illnesses. Such analyses highlight the important issues that should guide the physician-decision maker. They can help in identifying gaps in knowledge and establishing priorities for research to be carried out by clinical investigators. To appreciate the implications of the emerging literature on cost-effectiveness in cardiology, it is important to understand the basic concepts that underlie formal cost-effectiveness analysis.

QUANTITATIVE ANALYSES OF COSTS AND EFFECTIVENESS

Analysts commonly distinguish between *cost-benefit analysis,* in which both costs and benefits are expressed in the same units (such as dollars), and *cost-effectiveness analysis,* in which the costs are commonly expressed in monetary terms while the effectiveness is expressed in terms of the health benefit.[1] The health benefit commonly is measured in units such as the number of lives that are saved, the years of life gained, the quality-adjusted years of life saved,[1-7] the days of disability avoided, or other suitable measurements.

SENSITIVITY ANALYSIS. Cost-effectiveness analyses are critically dependent on the accuracy of the assumptions on which they are based. Therefore, the analysis should include a "sensitivity analysis," in which the calculations are repeated with varying assumptions to determine whether the conclusions are altered.[1-4] It is vital to determine whether the final conclusions are critically dependent on a tenuous estimate by determining whether reasonable variations in important assumptions make major differences in the results of the analysis.

For example, in an analysis of the cost-effectiveness of admitting patients with chest pain and possible uncomplicated acute myocardial infarction in the absence of ST-segment elevation to a full-fledged coronary care unit as opposed to a nonintensive care unit bed with telemetry monitoring, it would be critical to estimate the relative difference, if any, in the rate of successful resuscitation from primary ventricular fibrillation in the two settings. The larger the estimated difference, the more cost-effective the coronary care unit would appear. If the two settings were assumed to be equally effective, the additional cost of the coronary care unit would not yield additional effectiveness for this purpose. Because no randomized controlled data address this issue, any analysis of the relative cost-effectiveness of care of patients with possible myocardial infarction in these two settings depends on the estimates that are made. When a sensitivity analysis was performed, the nonintensive care bed with telemetry monitoring remained the more cost-effective option for patients whose probability of acute myocardial infarction was about 20 per cent or less. Only patients with ST-segment elevation or with ischemic ST-T changes had probabilities sufficiently high to warrant a coronary care unit to rule out a myocardial infarction, unless other complications requiring intensive care were already evident.[8]

THE CLINICAL DECISION TREE. Some cost-effectiveness analyses address difficult clinical problems for which no clear agreement exists, often because available data are not adequate even for the experienced clinician. In such situations, cost-effectiveness analysis may not yield clear answers, usually because the relative differences between competing strategies are small. For example, it may be difficult to decide whether or not to implant a permanent pacemaker in an elderly patient who has symptoms that are suggestive of a pacemaker-responsive arrhythmia but in whom the relation between arrhythmia and symptoms has not been proved. The therapeutic options can be displayed using a decision tree (Fig. 53–1) that explicitly outlines the various possibilities.[9] In this decision analysis, estimates about the relative cost-effectiveness of various therapeutic strategies would depend on the patient's subjective assessment of the quality of life under different scenarios, including persistent symptoms and no pacemaker, persistent symptoms despite a pacemaker, and the pacemaker without symptoms. Because small changes in the assessment of quality of life[10] under these different circumstances would alter the preferred strategy, this particular analysis could not provide a definitive solution for all cases involving this therapeutic dilemma. Nevertheless, this analysis demonstrated that empirical pacing was an attractive option in an elderly patient with unexplained syncope even when there was only about a 25 per cent chance that the syncope was caused by a pacemaker-responsive arrhythmia.

The goal of cost-effectiveness analysis is not to find the greatest possible benefit for the lowest possible cost, because it is not possible to achieve both simultaneously.[2,11] Instead, it is necessary either to determine the resources that are available and then find the greatest possible effectiveness that can be purchased for those resources or to determine the desired effectiveness and then find the lowest cost to achieve it. In either case, it is important to have a preconceived idea of the desirable or acceptable relative ratio of cost to effectiveness. Although cost-effectiveness analyses determine the ratio of cost to effectiveness, two strategies with the same ratio may have quite different absolute costs and absolute effectiveness. For example, a pro-

1741

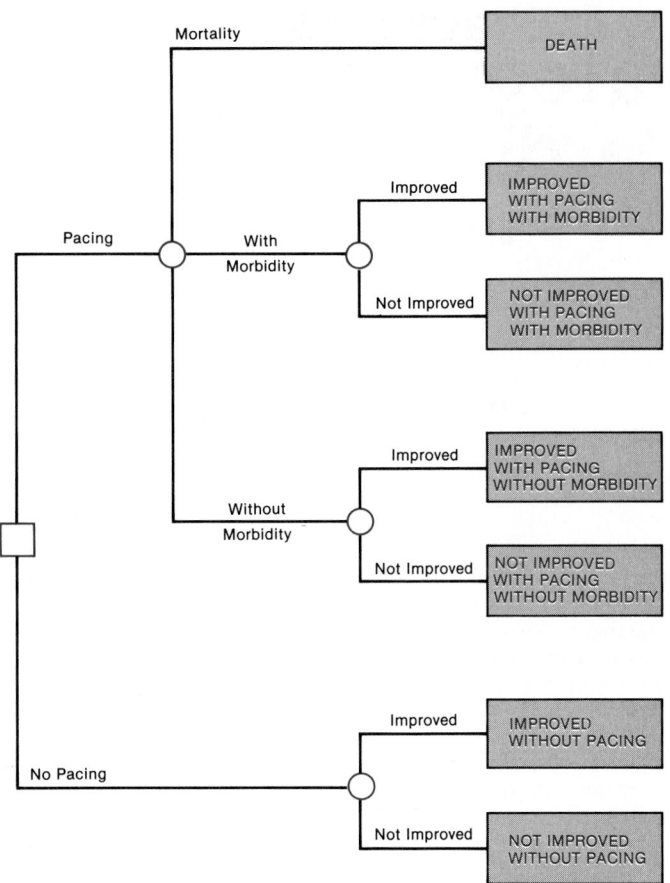

FIGURE 53–1. Decision tree for whether or not to perform empirical pacing in the elderly patient with syncope that may or may not be caused by a pacemaker-responsive arrhythmia. Branches of this decision tree explicitly detail the potential outcomes from the various options. The square denotes the outcome of decisions that the physician must make, whereas the circles denote events over which the physician has no control, i.e., occur "by chance." In constructing the decision tree, physicians would use either their own judgment or probabilities derived from the literature to estimate the likelihood of each of the events that can occur at a "chance" node. The sum of the probabilities of these chance events is always 100 per cent. In a cost-effectiveness analysis, each of the potential outcomes, as displayed in the rectangles in the right column, would be assigned a cost and a "utility." The utility would denote how highly the outcome is valued compared with perfect health, which traditionally has a value of 1.0, versus death, which traditionally has a value of 0. Cost-effectiveness calculations would compute the average expected costs and utilities for each of the various options that might be chosen by the physician, in this case the "pacing" and "no pacing" options that emanate from the initial square node. (From Kwoh, C. K., Beck, J. R., and Pauker, S. G.: Repeated syncope with negative diagnostic evaluation. Med. Decis. Making 4:351, 1984.)

gram that saves 100 lives for $10,000 has the same cost-effectiveness ratio as one that saves 10,000 lives for $1,000,000, but the two programs' absolute costs and absolute effectiveness vary 100-fold. In cost-effectiveness analyses, any potentially new strategy usually is compared with the current, or baseline, strategy by calculating the *incremental cost/incremental effectiveness* ratio.[1–3]

Calculation of Costs

In determining costs, several types must be considered.[1–3] *Operating costs* may include both direct costs such as salaries and indirect costs such as overhead, including utilities and maintenance. Costs also can be categorized as *fixed* versus *variable* costs. For example, the first 100 cardiac scans carried out in an imaging center may cost $100,000 for an average cost of $1000 per scan because of the high capital costs of the equipment. If the laboratory were to

"increase its output," the incremental cost for the next 100 scans would be much less than the cost for the first 100 scans because the capital costs of the equipment would be nearly the same regardless of whether 100 scans or 200 scans were performed. Thus one could distinguish between the *incremental* cost of performing the second 100 scans versus the *average* cost of all 200 scans. In many medical analyses, true costs are not available, and charges are used in the calculation of "cost" effectiveness. Because charges often are the same regardless of volume, they usually do not consider fully the important differences between average and incremental costs.

In calculating net health care costs, a useful approach is shown in Table 53–1. Unfortunately many cost-effectiveness analyses have concentrated only on direct medical costs, without fully taking into account the other terms in the equation.

DISCOUNTING. In virtually all cost analyses, it is important to consider the time frame during which costs and effects will be achieved. Because current dollars or benefits are more highly valued than a promise of future dollars or health benefits, a cost or benefit achieved immediately is more highly valued than one that is achieved later.[1] For example, one would be more willing to spend $10,000 today to prevent a death that otherwise would occur tomorrow than to spend $10,000 today to prevent a death that otherwise would occur in 10 years, even if there were no inflation and if there were no interest to be earned on the dollars. There is a preference to achieve an immediate benefit for several reasons. First, other events may intercede so that the projected future death may not occur or might be avoided as a consequence of newly available options that cost less than $10,000. Second, another illness could terminate life during the intervening period. Also, the $10,000 might be spent during the intervening 10 years in ways that are deemed more valuable. Furthermore, there is always a lingering doubt that the money spent now will not actually achieve the desired effect 10 years hence. This principle, by which the promise of future events is less valued than known immediate events, is termed "discounting," and is independent of monetary inflation. It is common practice to "discount" both future costs and future benefits by about 5 per cent per year.

In discussions of costs and effectiveness, several common misconceptions occur.[11] Cost-effective should not be equated with cost-saving because one often must spend to achieve a real benefit. Although a strategy that saves money *and* achieves an equal or better outcome is obviously cost-effective, a program is also cost-effective if it yields an additional benefit that is worth the additional cost. The definition of "worth the cost" may be somewhat arbitrary because it is difficult to place a monetary value on years of life and productivity. In many analyses, the approximately $35,000 to $40,000 per year cost in 1995 dollars of renal dialysis,[12] a program that the United States has decided to support with tax dollars, has been used as the benchmark for the amount of cost that the public appears willing to bear to prolong useful life by 1 year.

Although physicians must be aware of the relative cost-

TABLE 53–1   CALCULATION OF NET HEALTH CARE COSTS FOR A PROGRAM

Net costs = direct medical costs*
+ health care costs associated with the adverse effects of treatment
− savings of health care, rehabilitation, and custodial costs owing to prevention or alleviation of disease
+ costs of treating disease that would not have occurred if the patient had not lived longer as a result of the original treatment

* Costs of hospitalization, physician time, medications, laboratory services, and other ancillary services.

effectiveness of various diagnostic and therapeutic options if they are to make optimal choices for their patients, decisions about the number of dollars that *should* be spent to achieve specific health care benefits will ultimately be determined by society. Physicians have a critical role to play in developing appropriate data on cost-effectiveness issues, but the individual physician's primary responsibility is to the patient, within the confines of the economic limitations that may be imposed on both the physician and the patient by society.

One example of societal constraints on medical care expenditures is the diagnosis-related groups (DRG) system of prospective reimbursement. By defining in advance the number of dollars that a hospital will be reimbursed for the care of certain types of patients, the physician, the hospital, and the patient may all become more concerned with issues of cost-effectiveness. In an analogous manner, capitation systems, in which physicians are prepaid a fixed sum to assume the care of a patient, place an increased emphasis on the determination of cost-effective strategies.

DIAGNOSTIC TESTING

Modern cardiology includes an impressive armamentarium of diagnostic tests. Good clinical judgment requires that the physician choose tests in a cost-effective manner, in which the tests individually or sequentially may lead to improved diagnosis and management. The cost-effective use of diagnostic tests requires the physician to proceed logically through evaluation of the patient, selection of diagnostic tests, integration of the test with clinical data, and formulation of management strategies.[13,14] Each of these steps must be carefully considered for the proper utilization of diagnostic testing.

THE ESTIMATION OF CLINICAL PROBABILITIES. Regardless of the condition in question, the physician must utilize data from the medical history and physical examination to estimate the likelihood of its presence. For example, in evaluating the patient with chest pain, the physician may consider the patient's age and gender, as well as the typicality of the discomfort for angina pectoris.[13,14] The symptom may be categorized as typical angina pectoris, atypical angina pectoris, or nonanginal chest discomfort on the basis of its character, location, provocation, and response to rest or nitroglycerine (see p. 1290). Similarly, in estimating the probability of the presence of hemodynamically significant aortic stenosis in an adult with a systolic murmur, one would consider factors such as the intensity, location, and radiation of the murmur, the volume and rate of upstroke of the carotid arterial pulse, and the second heart sound (see p. 1039). Although these estimates of clinical probabilities can be based on the judgment of an experienced physician, in some circumstances, the physician can be aided by accumulated data from large series of patients in whom the clinical probability of conditions such as significant coronary artery disease[15] or acute myocardial infarction[16,17] has been determined.

ORDERING A DIAGNOSTIC TEST. When considering ordering a test, the physician must determine whether the test is effective and sufficiently accurate for indications for which it is being considered, that no other test with acceptable efficacy is less hazardous or less expensive, and that this is the most appropriate time for ordering the test.[13,18] In one such study carried out in 1977, soon after cardiac nuclear medicine scans became clinically available, 35 per cent were found *not* to have been ordered appropriately.[18] By comparison, the utility of two-dimensional echocardiograms was substantially better when studied in the 1990's, well after the test had been widely used and appreciated by clinicians.[19]

Tests may be ordered for such indications as to plan or monitor therapy, to establish a diagnosis, to define the ex-

tent of a known disease, to estimate prognosis, or to reassure the physician or the patient.[18,20] Although each of these indications can be a legitimate reason for ordering a diagnostic test, test results that may influence therapeutic action usually are the most valued and are certainly the most cost-effective.

When assessing the accuracy of a test, one must understand terms such as sensitivity, specificity, and positive predictive value (see Table 5–2, p. 161).[13] For some tests, such as a thallium scintiscan, the result is often dichotomized into "normal" versus "abnormal," even though it is understood that the precise distinction between normal and abnormal may be difficult and somewhat arbitrary. Other tests, such as the ejection fraction, commonly are reported on a continuous scale. In some circumstances, such as with the exercise electrocardiogram, a continuous result (e.g., the extent of ST-segment depression) often is dichotomized into normal or abnormal to facilitate the test's interpretation. When a continuous result is dichotomized, an increase in its sensitivity, or the likelihood of a positive test result among patients with the condition, can be obtained only at the expense of decreasing specificity, or the likelihood of a normal test result in patients without the condition.[13] For example, the sensitivity of the exercise electrocardiogram for detecting patients with coronary artery disease can be increased by reducing the depth of ST-segment depression required for a "positive" test result. However, as the definition of a "positive" test result is changed from 2 mm of ST-segment depression to 1 mm of ST-segment depression, the resulting increase in apparent sensitivity will be at the expense of a decreased specificity because patients who have between 1 and 2 mm of ST-segment depression and who do not have coronary artery disease now will be misclassified.

In an era of cost consciousness, the physician often must be asked to decide between two tests that may offer similar types of information. For example, a radionuclide ventriculogram may provide a more accurate assessment of the left ventricular ejection fraction than a two-dimensional echocardiogram, but the latter frequently provides a sufficiently accurate estimate of left ventricular function to obviate the need for the more expensive radionuclide study.

INTEGRATING THE TEST RESULT WITH CLINICAL DATA. To use diagnostic tests efficiently, the physician should decide the threshold probability above or below which the future diagnostic or management strategy would be altered.[14,21] For example, consider that a patient has recurrent chest pain, and on the basis of history and physical examination, the physician estimates that there is a 50 per cent probability that it is caused by coronary artery disease. The physician also knows that coronary arteriography would be required to decide whether coronary artery bypass grafting or percutaneous transluminal coronary angioplasty should be carried out if coronary artery disease were present. For cost-effective test ordering, the physician then must estimate how unlikely coronary artery disease would have to be for this strategy to be altered. If the physician would proceed with catheterization provided that the probability of coronary artery disease were as low as 10 per cent (or higher), then a test such as an exercise radionuclide ventriculogram, whose negative result might reduce the probability of coronary artery disease to 30 per cent, would not be helpful in decision-making.

Threshold Approach. This concept has been called the "threshold approach" to test utilization and decision-making.[13,21] In essence, it emphasizes that a test is potentially helpful only if its result would change the pretest probability of disease to a degree that could be sufficient to alter the approach to the patient. If it is highly unlikely that the available diagnostic test could move the probability of disease across such a threshold, the test would not be cost-effective and ordinarily would not be ordered. In some situations, the diagnostic threshold may be redefined because of

Header: 1743 Ch 53

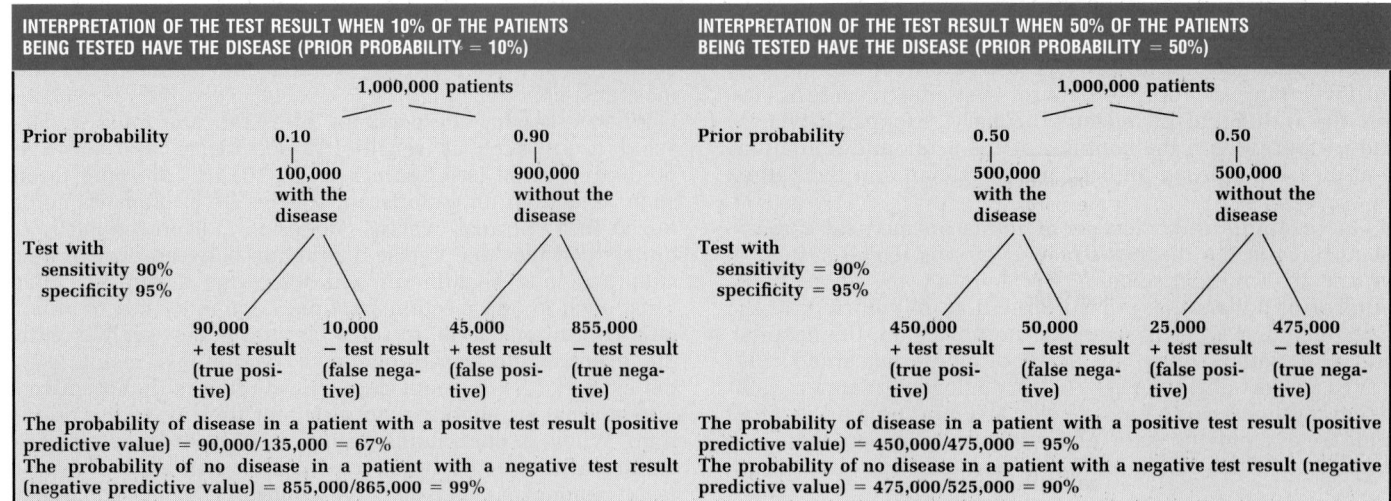

TABLE 53–2   HOW THE POSITIVE AND NEGATIVE PREDICTIVE VALUES OF THE SAME TEST VARY DEPENDING ON THE PRIOR PROBABILITY OF DISEASE

INTERPRETATION OF THE TEST RESULT WHEN 10% OF THE PATIENTS BEING TESTED HAVE THE DISEASE (PRIOR PROBABILITY = 10%)	INTERPRETATION OF THE TEST RESULT WHEN 50% OF THE PATIENTS BEING TESTED HAVE THE DISEASE (PRIOR PROBABILITY = 50%)
1,000,000 patients	1,000,000 patients

Prior probability — 0.10 / 0.90
100,000 with the disease / 900,000 without the disease

Test with sensitivity 90% specificity 95%

90,000 + test result (true positive) / 10,000 − test result (false negative) / 45,000 + test result (false positive) / 855,000 − test result (true negative)

The probability of disease in a patient with a positve test result (positive predictive value) = 90,000/135,000 = 67%
The probability of no disease in a patient with a negative test result (negative predictive value) = 855,000/865,000 = 99%

Prior probability — 0.50 / 0.50
500,000 with the disease / 500,000 without the disease

Test with sensitivity = 90% specificity = 95%

450,000 + test result (true positive) / 50,000 − test result (false negative) / 25,000 + test result (false positive) / 475,000 − test result (true negative)

The probability of disease in a patient with a positive test result (positive predictive value) = 450,000/475,000 = 95%
The probability of no disease in a patient with a negative test result (negative predictive value) = 475,000/525,000 = 90%

From Goldman, L.: Quantitative aspects of clinical reasoning. *In* Wilson, J. D., et al. (eds.): Harrison's Principles of Internal Medicine. 13th ed. New York, McGraw-Hill Book Co., 1994. © 1994 The McGraw-Hill Companies, Inc.

the special characteristics of the patient at hand. For example, it would be considered important to rule out significant coronary artery disease in an otherwise healthy airline pilot who has atypical chest pain. In this situation, the combination of a normal exercise electrocardiogram and a normal exercise thallium scintiscan would make the presence of coronary disease unlikely. If it were argued that the airline pilot's occupational responsibilities would require even a greater degree of certainty, it would be preferable to proceed directly to the test that usually is considered the benchmark, in this case, coronary arteriography, if it were necessary to be as certain as possible that coronary disease was not present.

BAYES' THEOREM (see p. 162). One way to understand the concepts of prior probability, thresholds, and the impact of diagnostic tests is through Bayes' theorem.[1,13] When the prior probability (prevalence) of the disease is known in patients who are similar to the patient under consideration, and when the sensitivity and specificity of the test to be ordered are known, the post-test probability that the disease is present can be calculated. Table 53–2 emphasizes how the physician must consider both the prior (pretest) probability that the patient has a disease and the test result in estimating the post-test probability. For example, if a test has a sensitivity of 90 per cent and a specificity of 95 per cent, a patient whose prior probability of disease was 10 per cent and who has a positive test result would have a 67 per cent probability of disease after the test. By

comparison, the same test result in a patient whose prior probability was 50 per cent would yield a post-test probability of 95 per cent.

A test is potentially useful if it changes the probability of disease sufficiently to cross the threshold for decision-making. Unfortunately, available data do not always provide precise guidelines for establishing such appropriate thresholds for diagnostic decision-making. Nevertheless, common clinical judgment is often a sufficient guide. For example, using pooled data from the literature, the effects of exercise electrocardiography and exercise thallium testing can be estimated for a patient with typical angina pectoris (Fig. 53–2), a patient with atypical angina (Fig. 53–3), and a patient with presumably nonanginal chest pain (Fig. 53–4). These estimated probabilities correspond well to the actual probability of disease in patients who have been evaluated.[22]

NONINVASIVE TESTING IN PATIENTS WITH POSSIBLE ANGINA PECTORIS (see p. 1295). The patient with symptoms typical for angina pectoris already has a high probability of coronary artery disease on the basis of the history alone (80 to 85 per cent); the probability becomes even higher (95 per cent) if the exercise electrocardiogram is positive and becomes overwhelming (99 per cent) after a confirmatory exercise thallium scan. For diagnosing the presence or absence of coronary disease, however, the exercise thallium scan adds little to the results of the exercise test. Although the exercise thallium test appears to have additional prog-

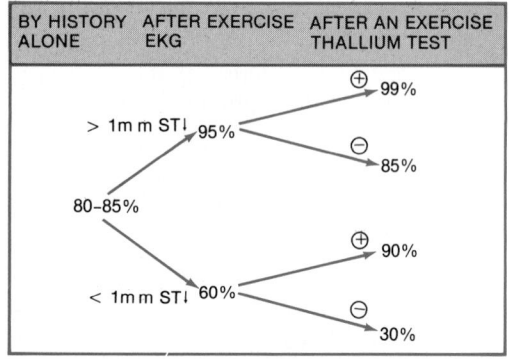

FIGURE 53–2. Approximate probabilities of coronary artery disease in a patient with typical angina pectoris before and after the sequential use of an exercise electrocardiogram and an exercise thallium test. (From Lee, T. H., and Goldman, L.: Non-invasive tests in cardiology. *In* Branch, W., Jr. [ed.]: Office Practice of Medicine. 3rd ed. Philadelphia, W. B. Saunders Company, 1994.)

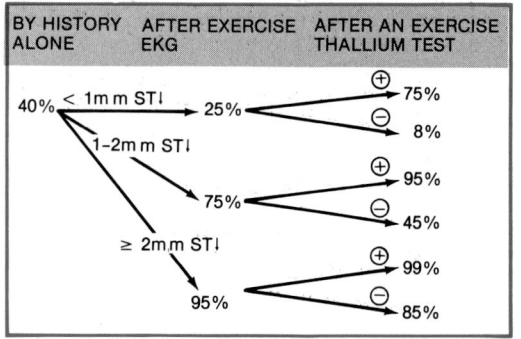

FIGURE 53–3. Approximate probabilities of coronary artery disease in a patient with atypical anginal symptoms before and after the sequential use of an exercise electrocardiogram and an exercise thallium test. (From Lee, T. H., and Goldman, L.: Non-invasive tests in cardiology. *In* Branch, W., Jr. [ed.]: Office Practice of Medicine. 3rd ed. Philadelphia, W. B. Saunders Company, 1994.)

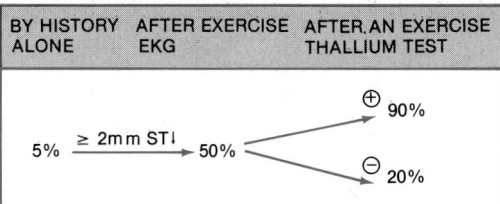

BY HISTORY ALONE	AFTER EXERCISE EKG	AFTER AN EXERCISE THALLIUM TEST

5% $\xrightarrow{\geq 2\,mm\,ST\downarrow}$ 50% $\nearrow$ ⊕ 90%
$\searrow$ ⊖ 20%

FIGURE 53–4. Approximate probabilities of coronary artery disease in an asymptomatic subject in the coronary artery disease age range before and after the sequential use of an exercise electrocardiogram and an exercise thallium test. (From Lee, T. H., and Goldman, L.: Non-invasive tests in cardiology. *In* Branch, W., Jr. [ed.]: Office Practice of Medicine. 3rd ed. Philadelphia, W. B. Saunders Company, 1994.)

nostic value,[23,24] in most situations, the results of the exercise thallium test would be unlikely to add substantial independent information regarding the diagnosis of the presence of coronary artery disease. If the exercise electrocardiogram and exercise thallium test give conflicting information, the probability of coronary artery disease in the patient with typical angina pectoris remains similar to what it was before either test was obtained (80 to 90 per cent). If both tests are negative, the patient with typical angina pectoris still has a reasonable probability of having significant coronary artery disease (30 per cent). Thus even two negative tests have not "ruled out" coronary artery disease in a patient with typical angina to an extent to which one could simply reassure the patient, even though they imply a favorable prognosis if coronary artery disease should be present.[23–25] Thus, if one were trying to rule out coronary artery disease in a patient with typical angina pectoris, coronary arteriography still would be required.[14,26]

In the patient with atypical angina (Fig. 53–3), positive results on both exercise electrocardiography and exercise thallium testing would raise the probability of coronary artery disease from 40 to 95 to 99 per cent. Conversely, negative results on both tests would lower the probability of coronary artery disease substantially (to 8 per cent), perhaps to a low enough level that one would not feel compelled to obtain coronary arteriography except in unusual circumstances. If the two tests give conflicting results, the probability of the disease has not been altered appreciably by the two tests.

In asymptomatic healthy people, a resting electrocardiogram appears to have little value as a screening test.[27] Similarly, screening exercise tests have too small a yield to justify their use in healthy people.[28] If, however, an asymptomatic subject who is in the age range in which coronary disease usually occurs has a strongly positive exercise electrocardiogram, the probability of coronary disease is increased substantially (from about 5 to about 50 per cent), and a subsequent negative exercise thallium test is not sufficiently reassuring to eliminate the possibility of coronary disease. Thus one cannot simply use the negative exercise thallium scan to "prove" that the exercise electrocardiogram was a false-positive result. Coronary arteriography is required to determine whether the exercise electrocardiogram was a true- or false-positive result, and this frequent need to proceed to invasive testing greatly increases the cost of any program that uses screening exercise electrocardiography.

It is beyond scope of this chapter to discuss the precise guidelines for the most cost-effective use of each of the various types of cardiac diagnostic tests for each possible indication. Nevertheless, test ordering becomes more cost-effective if the physician estimates the pretest probability of disease, orders the appropriate test, and properly integrates the test results with the available clinical information. A test is helpful only to the extent that it provides nonredundant information (i.e., information above and beyond what was previously available).[13] It must be em-

phasized, however, that a test can add incremental information regardless of whether its result is "positive" or "negative."[13,29]

Cost-effective medicine requires that tests be ordered only if their incremental information will have a positive impact on patient care. The finding that major variations in resource utilization often do not correlate with discernible differences in health outcome suggests that many tests and treatments do not meet such criteria.[30,31] Substantial financial savings can be realized by reducing the utilization of low- or moderate-cost tests as well as by reducing the utilization of expensive procedures.[32]

PREVENTION AND TREATMENT

The current and projected future costs of heart disease are substantial. The rate of death from coronary heart disease has been declining in the United States since the late 1960's,[33–35] but the increase in the total population and especially its age portends a rise in the total absolute number of cases of coronary heart disease unless there are major declines in risk factors.[36] Furthermore, the high cost of medical care for prevalent cases of coronary heart disease indicates that coronary disease will remain a major cost for the American public.[36,37]

Among the various preventive and therapeutic modalities in cardiology, some have been studied by means of formal cost-effectiveness analysis, whereas others have been studied in a more qualitative manner. In evaluating the cost-effectiveness of any program, it must be compared with a baseline or standard current approach. In the following sections, selected data on the costs and effectiveness of several modalities for the diagnosis, prevention, and treatment of heart disease are considered.

Detection and Treatment of Hyperlipidemia
(See also Chap. 35)

Substantial data indicate that the serum cholesterol level is significantly correlated with the risk of coronary artery disease (see p. 1127), and after controlling for the cholesterol level, the triglyceride level probably is not an important independent predictor.[38–40] The ratio of the high-density lipoprotein cholesterol fraction to the low-density lipoprotein fraction is more important than either level alone[41] for prediction. For primary care settings, a prudent screening technique is to obtain a total serum cholesterol level. If it is elevated, fasting levels of total cholesterol, low-density and high-density lipoprotein cholesterol, and triglycerides can be obtained to define risk more precisely and to determine the hyperlipidemia pattern to guide future dietary and perhaps drug therapy.[38,39]

The increased risk of hypercholesterolemia begins by early adulthood,[42] leading some to suggest screening by this age.[39] Others, however, argue against early screening because the risk of coronary events remains low until men reach their 40's and women reach their 50's and because intervention to lower cholesterol is efficacious within about 2 years.[38,43] Most agree that children and adolescents should not be screened except when the family history is compelling.[43–45]

Cholesterol is clearly a risk factor for coronary disease in women under age 65.[46] However, because coronary disease is not a dominant cause of death in younger women, cholesterol is not as strong a correlate of total mortality in middle-aged women as in middle-aged men.[47]

Despite some data and opinions to the contrary,[48,49] cholesterol appears to be a risk factor in the elderly. Even though the relative risk associated with hypercholesterolemia appears to be somewhat lower in the elderly,[46] their higher absolute risk of coronary disease implies that the incremental risk attributable to cholesterol is at least as high in the elderly.

The potential noncoronary hazards of low cholesterol and of reducing an individual's cholesterol level are unclear[47,50-52] but are proportionately of more potential relevance in persons with lower risks for coronary disease such as women and younger men, individuals without other coronary risk factors, and those with moderate hypercholesterolemia.[53-55] Furthermore, even small decrements in quality of life from being labeled as having hypercholesterolemia, from dietary changes, or from side effects of medications could outweigh the benefits of cholesterol screening and treatment in people with only mildly elevated risk.[56]

Despite these caveats, much is to be gained by addressing cholesterol abnormalities because each 1 per cent reduction in serum cholesterol is associated with at least a 2 per cent reduction in coronary risk,[57-60] and each 1 per cent increase in HDL cholesterol is associated with a 2 to 3 per cent decrease in risk.[61] Coronary risk reductions of similar magnitude have been observed in randomized intervention trials for both primary and secondary prevention.[62-71] Because up to 52 million Americans may be candidates for dietary interventions to reduce cholesterol and 13 million might be candidates for drug therapy,[39,72] cost-effectiveness assessments are of substantial relevance.[40]

A number of analyses have assessed the cost-effectiveness of interventions to lower serum cholesterol.[40,73-78] The most cost-effective use of medications for cholesterol-lowering is for secondary prevention in patients with existing coronary disease. In this setting, cholesterol reduction clearly reduces the risks of coronary disease and lowers all-cause mortality.[63-68] Because patients with existing coronary disease are at high risk for recurrent events and death, aggressive cholesterol-lowering therapy can sometimes save costs as well as lives and tends to be well worth the cost across a wide range of secondary prevention settings (Table 53-3). Of note is that the predicted benefits and favorable cost-effectiveness ratios for secondary prevention are relatively unaffected by varying assumptions regarding possible noncoronary hazards of lowering cholesterol, because about 80 per cent of deaths in patients with existing coronary disease are caused by coronary events.[63]

By comparison, aggressive cholesterol-lowering therapy has relatively less favorable cost-effectiveness ratios when used for primary prevention in individuals without coro-

TABLE 53-4   COST-EFFECTIVENESS RATIO (DOLLARS PER YEAR OF LIFE SAVED) OF 20 mg/d OF LOVASTATIN FOR PRIMARY PREVENTION OF CORONARY HEART DISEASE

	AGE (YEARS)				
	35-44	45-54	55-64	65-74	75-84
Men, pretreatment cholesterol level > 300 mg/dl					
High risk*	24,000	13,000	15,000	23,000	66,000
Moderate risk*	130,000	49,000	29,000	32,000	92,000
Low risk*	330,000	110,000	58,000	58,000	150,000
Women, pretreatment cholesterol level > 300 mg/dl					
High risk*	195,000	62,000	34,000	39,000	67,000
Moderate risk*	480,000	140,000	62,000	46,000	87,000
Low risk*	1,500,000	320,000	130,000	68,000	110,000

* High risk = diastolic blood pressure > 105 mm Hg, smoker, weight > 130% of ideal; moderate risk = diastolic blood pressure 95-104 mm Hg, nonsmoker, weight 110-129% of ideal; low risk = diastolic blood pressure < 95 mm Hg, nonsmoker, weight < 110% of ideal.

From Goldman, L., et al.: The cost-effectiveness of programs to lower serum cholesterol. *In* Rifkind, B. M. (ed.): Lowering Cholesterol in High-Risk Individuals and Populations. New York, Marcel Dekker, 1995, p. 311.

nary disease. The risks of coronary disease and hence the expected benefits from cholesterol reduction depend not only on the cholesterol level but also on the presence of other risk factors, such as age, gender, cigarette smoking, hypertension, and glucose intolerance. When cholesterol reduction for primary prevention is specifically targeted at individuals with multiple coronary risk factors or with marked elevation of serum cholesterol,[71,74,76-79] the effectiveness of treatment increases and cost-effectiveness ratios are more reasonable (Table 53-4). Cost-effectiveness ratios tend to be more favorable with more efficacious medications, such as HMG-CoA reductase inhibitors, than with less efficacious and equally expensive drugs, such as cholestyramine. Cost-effectiveness ratios are more favorable when medications become less expensive, such as substituting bulk cholestyramine for the drug in packets,[77] or if the costs of medications fall because of competition or when generic formulations become available.[79] In general, nicotinic acid and HMG-CoA reductase inhibitors have been estimated to be more cost-effective than other medications.

Because aggressive medications are not cost-effective in the primary prevention setting except in very high risk individuals, an alternative approach is population-based interventions. Such programs are especially attractive because half or more of the cases of new coronary disease occur in individuals with serum cholesterol levels below 250 mg/dl.[80] Population-wide education programs in northern California and in Finland were able to reduce serum cholesterol levels by up to 4 per cent, combined with other favorable changes in other risk factors, and at an estimated annual cost of less than $10 per person.[81,82] Unless it is assumed that there are major negative effects on noncardiac mortality in reducing cholesterol levels, population-wide cholesterol reduction programs emphasizing dietary interventions appear to have very favorable cost-effectiveness ratios.[40,78]

Although existing analyses are limited by the fact that they have not considered how medications or the avoidance of coronary events affects quality of life, they nevertheless provide reasonable economic guidelines to hypercholesterolemia: aggressive medications for secondary prevention and targeted medications for primary prevention in very high risk individuals superimposed on population-wide programs for everyone. These recommendations based on cost-effectiveness results suggest strategies that are somewhere between those recommended by Canadian and American consensus groups[38,39] and support the screening strategies discussed previously.[38,39,83]

TABLE 53-3   ESTIMATED COST (IN DOLLARS) PER YEAR OF LIFE SAVED FOR LOVASTATIN AS SECONDARY PREVENTION

	AGE (YEARS)				
	35-44	45-54	55-64	65-74	75-84
Pretreatment cholesterol level ≥ 250 mg/dl					
Men					
Lovastatin 20 mg/d	*	*	1,600	10,000	19,000
Lovastatin 40 mg/d	14,000	86,000	17,000	27,000	38,000
Women					
Lovastatin 20 mg/d	4,500	3,500	8,100	12,000	15,000
Lovastatin 40 mg/d	49,000	30,000	29,000	30,000	29,000
Pretreatment cholesterol level < 250 mg/dl					
Men					
Lovastatin 20 mg/d	38,000	16,000	17,000	25,000	30,000
Lovastatin 40 mg/d	120,000	57,000	48,000	53,000	58,000
Women					
Lovastatin 20 mg/d	210,000	73,000	36,000	30,000	23,000
Lovastatin 40 mg/d	310,000	150,000	81,000	62,000	45,000

* Therapy estimated to save both lives and money.

From Goldman, L., et al.: The cost-effectiveness of programs to lower serum cholesterol. *In* Rifkind, B. M. (ed.): Lowering Cholesterol in High-Risk Individuals and Populations. New York, Marcel Dekker, 1995, p. 311.

Detection and Treatment of Hypertension

(See also Chaps. 26 and 27)

Most epidemiological data emphasize that the systolic blood pressure is an independent significant predictor of coronary heart disease but that the diastolic blood pressure is not (after controlling for the systolic blood pressure). Nevertheless, it has been common practice to define the threshold for treating hypertension on the basis of the diastolic blood pressure, and, until recently, virtually all treatment trials used definitions that were based on the diastolic blood pressure level.

An estimated 50 million Americans have hypertension, defined as a systolic blood pressure of 140 mm Hg or above, or a diastolic blood pressure of 90 mm Hg or above, or the use of antihypertensive medication.[84] Current recommendations of the US Joint National Committee are that all people with moderate hypertension (systolic blood pressure 160 to 169 mm Hg or diastolic blood pressure of 100 to 109 mm Hg) and mild hypertension (systolic blood pressure 140 to 159 mm Hg or diastolic blood pressure 90 to 99 mm Hg) be treated.[84]

Recent research has emphasized the importance of even mild systolic hypertension. Individuals with systolic blood pressures of 140 to 159 mm Hg and diastolic blood pressures below 90 mm Hg have elevated relative risks of about 1.5 for cardiovascular disease, 1.4 for coronary heart disease, 1.4 for stroke or transient ischemic attacks, 1.6 for congestive heart failure, and 1.6 for cardiovascular death (all $P < 0.05$) compared with age-matched normotensive controls.[85] The striking results of the Systolic Hypertension in the Elderly Program (SHEP) Trial emphasized the benefits of treating isolated systolic hypertension.[86]

Although physicians have historically been hesitant to treat hypertension aggressively in the elderly, three randomized trials[86-88] of about 10,000 patients have shown that treatment with diuretics or beta-adrenoceptor blockers, with added medications when needed, can reduce all-cause mortality by 12 per cent, stroke mortality by 36 per cent, and coronary mortality by 25 per cent.[89] Of note is that only about 20 elderly patients had to be treated for 5 years to avoid one cardiac or cerebrovascular event.[90]

Early studies that first demonstrated the benefit of antihypertensive medications for reducing cerebrovascular events tended not to show any benefit in terms of coronary events. However, cumulative meta-analysis of these large trials for the treatment of mild to moderate hypertension demonstrates that treated patients have a relative risk of 0.84 for coronary heart disease events, 0.84 for coronary heart disease death, 0.62 for cerebrovascular attacks, and 0.79 for all-vascular mortality (all $P < 0.01$).[91] The inability of the individual studies to find such differences in coronary mortality was probably based on their small sample size and relatively short duration of follow-up.

Although nonpharmacological therapy for hypertension is inherently attractive, medications are truly preferable to placebo.[92] Monotherapy is often successful in patients with mild to moderate hypertension.[92] Diltiazem may be somewhat more efficacious in African-Americans, captopril in young whites, and beta-blockers in elderly whites, but these differences are modest and cannot predict responses in individuals. Of note is that angiotensin-converting enzyme inhibitors at low doses are generally no more effective, and sometimes less effective, than low doses of diuretics.[93]

Screening to detect and treat hypertension appears to be relatively cost-effective for men and women of all ages.[94] The marginal cost per quality-adjusted year of life gained ranged from about $8000 for men aged 60 to about $29,000 for men aged 20. For women, the cost ranged from about $12,000 at age 60 to about $44,000 at age 20. The results of the analysis were affected relatively little when the authors varied many of the assumptions inherent in their analysis,

except that the results were dependent on the cost of medication.

Weinstein and Stason used data from the Framingham Heart Study to calculate the cost-effectiveness of the treatment of mild hypertension.[95] They concluded that the reduction in direct medical care costs for stroke and coronary heart disease would offset about 22 per cent of the cost of treating moderate to severe diastolic hypertension (105 mm Hg and above) and about 15 per cent of the cost for treating mild hypertension (95 to 104 mm Hg), an estimate similar to those made by Stokes and Carmichael.[96] These cost-effectiveness estimates also are similar to those of Littenberg et al.,[94] who found that a program that would screen for hypertension and treat if the diastolic blood pressure was 95 mm Hg or greater would cost about $41,000 per quality-adjusted year of life gained. Treatment programs aimed at people with diastolic blood pressures of 105 mm Hg or greater would be more cost-effective: The cost would be only about $20,000 per year of life gained.

Edelson et al. reported that the cost of primary prevention to treat people 35 to 60 years of age with diastolic blood pressures of 95 mm Hg or greater and no known coronary heart disease was about $11,000 per year of life saved for propranolol and about $16,000 for hydrochlorothiazide.[97] Once again, however, cost-effectiveness was highly dependent on the cost of the medication, and the costs per year of life saved were not estimated to be nearly as favorable for the newer, more expensive medications.

Thus several analyses indicate that screening and treating people with hypertension is reasonably cost-effective and is in the range of the annual cost of hemodialysis for chronic renal failure.[12] Although hypertension detection and treatment are most cost-effective when performed by the patients' own physicians as part of routine medical care,[94,98] worksite programs for the detection and treatment of hypertension can more than pay for themselves by reducing direct medical costs and absenteeism.[99]

Cigarette Smoking

(See also Chap. 35)

Cigarette smoking is an independently significant correlate of the risk of developing coronary heart disease (p. 1147) and also is a major risk factor for several types of cancer. Many of these risks appear to be reversed after smokers stop smoking. Tsevat used data from a variety of sources to estimate that smoking cessation could increase life expectancy by 2 to 5 years.[100]

Although it is not possible to design a trial in which patients are randomized to continue smoking or to guarantee smoking cessation, substantial data confirm that discontinuing smoking improves prognosis.[101-105]

There are a variety of interventions to reduce smoking. On average, about 5 per cent of smokers discontinue the habit for 1 year after receiving a physician's advice, although the rate of quitting is higher in more highly motivated cohorts.[106,107] Nicotine gum or transdermal patches may increase the 1-year likelihood of smoking cessation by 30 to 100 per cent,[108,109] suggesting that the cost of a physician's advice plus the availability of nicotine gum per year of life saved will range from about $5700 to $9200 in men aged 35 to 69 and from about $9800 to $13,000 in women aged 35 to 69 in 1990 dollars.[110-113]

Group counseling can increase rates of quitting.[113,114] Public programs also are effective, with television advertisements against smoking among the most cost-effective.[115,116] Physicians should not be discouraged by the relatively low rate of quitting that occurs immediately after their advice because this advice is among the most cost-effective of all the interventions and may be a necessary psychological prelude to the patient's response to subsequent interventions. Nurse-managed smoking cessation programs may be especially effective and may cost as little as $220 per year of life saved when utilized in survivors of a myocardial infarction.[117]

Obesity

In long-term follow-up of the Framingham cohort,[118] obesity emerged as an independently significant risk factor for the development of coronary artery disease (see p. 0000). Unfortunately, it is extremely difficult for most adults to lose weight and to maintain the weight loss over the long term. Programs in schools or at the worksite commonly can help to achieve weight losses of 2 to 5 kg at costs that are about $10 to $30 per kilogram lost, which would be highly cost-effective.[119,120] Lay organizations such as Weight Watchers also can aid in producing similar losses at similar costs and are clearly cost-effective despite the high attrition rate. More intensive weight-loss programs for motivated people may still be very cost-effective for those people for whom simpler measures are ineffective.[121] Although physicians may become discouraged over the inability of their patients to lose weight, the usual effects of these other programs are not substantially greater than what may be achieved simply by a physician's advice. Furthermore, it often is a physician's advice that influences patients to try other interventions that might not be considered if the physician had not identified overweight as a medical problem.

Physical Activity
(See Chap. 40)

Substantial data indicate that physical activity reduces coronary heart disease and all-cause mortality, partly because of its beneficial effects on other risk factors but apparently partly independently.[122–128] Unfortunately, physicians often do not recommend exercise for their patients. Many patients, however, both want and expect their physicians to make recommendations regarding physical activity, and a substantial proportion of active people ascribed their activity in large part to the advice of a physician.

Worksite exercise programs also are potentially cost-effective independent of their possible effect on the development of clinical coronary artery disease. In one study, employees in the experimental exercise program group missed fewer days of work, were more likely to remain employed, and had fewer hospital days and fewer medical claims, thus resulting in substantial health care savings.[129,130] In fact, some employers have decided to pay their employees directly for participating in exercise programs, such as jogging, and some managed health care plans include membership in health clubs as one of their covered services. Unlike antismoking campaigns, media campaigns advocating exercise seem to encourage people to seek out other programs in the community but not to lead to direct changes in behavior by themselves.[131] Thus it appears that a physician's encouragement of increased physical activity, especially if combined with direct guidance on how to implement the suggestion, can lead to major changes in health behavior. Although it is difficult to determine the exact degree of effectiveness to be gained for the cost, there are substantial data linking physical activity to other cardiovascular risk factors and apparently independently to cardiovascular and all-cause mortality.[122–128] These data suggest that efforts to increase physical activity have the potential for being highly cost-effective.[132]

Cardiac rehabilitation in patients who have suffered a myocardial infarction (see Chap. 40) appears to lower by about 25 per cent the subsequent rates of reinfarction, cardiovascular mortality, and total mortality.[133] These programs improve the functional and symptomatic status of patients, and the exercise programs themselves are associated with a very small risk of major adverse events.[133]

Such programs also can help patients return to work earlier after uncomplicated myocardial infarction,[134] and, as a result, can both reduce costs of medical care and increase productivity.[135] Thus the combination of cardiac rehabilitation services and occupational work evaluations appears to be very cost-effective for the post-myocardial infarction patient.

Prevention of Infective Endocarditis in Valvular Heart Disease
(See also Chaps. 32 and 33)

By extrapolation from cost-effectiveness analyses, penicillin prophylaxis to prevent bacterial endocarditis in patients with rheumatic valvular heart disease appears to have a cost-effectiveness of about $13,000 per year of life gained.[136,137] In patients with prosthetic heart valves, in whom the risk of endocarditis is higher, the cost-effectiveness is likely to be even more favorable. By comparison, two detailed cost-effectiveness analyses indicate that penicillin prophylaxis before dental work to prevent bacterial endocarditis is *not* cost-effective for patients with mitral valve prolapse[136,137] (see p. 1035). Using the most likely assumptions, people are as likely to die of penicillin reactions as they are to die of endocarditis, and even given the most optimistic assumptions, it is estimated that routine penicillin prophylaxis for dental procedures in patients with mitral valve prolapse would cost more than $1 million to save a year of life. In most studies of mitral valve prolapse, the risk of endocarditis is substantially higher in patients with murmurs of mitral regurgitation. Although the cost-effectiveness in this subpopulation of patients with mitral valve prolapse is unclear, the use of prophylactic antibiotics in the presence of a murmur of mitral valve prolapse is often recommended.[138]

Prehospital Emergency Services
(See also Chaps. 24 and 37)

Prehospital emergency services range from basic life support to advanced life support services. Advanced life support programs, which include interventions such as defibrillation, endotracheal intubation, and intravenous or intramuscular medications, have been instituted throughout much of the United States. Because about 60 per cent of patients whose death certificates list the cause of death as myocardial infarction die outside of the hospital, advances in prehospital emergency services, such as better training in the community or dispatcher-assisted instruction, could have a substantial impact on survival.[139]

Prehospital emergency care appears to be extremely successful in patients who have ventricular fibrillation and who are seen very soon after cardiac arrest (see p. 761). For example, in pooled data, about two-thirds of patients who are seen within 5 minutes of a ventricular fibrillation arrest survive to leave the hospital.[140–142] Unfortunately, many arrests are not caused by ventricular fibrillation, and even the most successful prehospital emergency services often cannot deliver care within 5 minutes. Thus, results in many urban and rural areas have been disappointing.[143–146] Only about 15 to 20 per cent of prehospital cardiac arrest patients commonly survive to leave the hospital in even the best programs,[141,142] and the rates are 1 to 5 per cent in many parts of the country.[143–146] Higher success rates are achieved principally through advanced life support programs utilizing paramedics, which appear to increase the likelihood of reaching the hospital alive from about 19 to 34 per cent and the likelihood of being discharged alive from the hospital from 7 to 17 per cent,[147] and through very rapid response times. However, the prognosis after hospital discharge of patients who were resuscitated from prehospital arrest is only about 75 per cent as high as age-

and sex-matched comparison groups who have survived myocardial infarction without prehospital arrest, and it is only about 60 per cent as high as for age- and gender-adjusted members of the general population.[141]

The cost-effectiveness of prehospital emergency programs is difficult to estimate. One analysis estimated that a mobile coronary care unit has an incremental cost of about $25,000 (in 1991 dollars) per life saved above and beyond the cost of the ambulance system itself.[142] Another analysis estimated that the incremental cost-effectiveness of a mobile coronary care unit was about $100,000 (in 1991 dollars) per life saved and $50,000 (in 1991 dollars) per year of life saved, but this analysis included only the incremental costs of the mobile coronary care unit program and not the costs of the existing emergency medical technician and community training program to which it was added.[148]

Analyses of the cost-effectiveness of prehospital emergency services depend on assumptions about the mean response time and the patients' prognoses, both in terms of life expectancy and in terms of quality of life and neurological impairment.[149] For example, the longer the response time, the more likely it is that survivors of prehospital cardiac arrest will have neurological impairment. If the years of life expectancy that are gained are compromised by such neurological impairment, then the *quality* of those years of life will not be the same as the quality of the years of life that might be gained from preventive measures that delay the onset of disease. Thus, when the calculation of cost-effectiveness is adjusted for the years of life that are gained without major neurological impairment, the apparent benefit of prehospital resuscitation is reduced. Furthermore, patients whose lives are saved by prehospital emergency services are likely to require careful medical follow-up, sometimes including expensive interventions such as coronary bypass grafting. Most studies[150–152] have not clearly considered the fact that the survivors of out-of-hospital cardiac arrest will have costs other than those included in the first term of the equation in Table 53–1, such as the costs for rehabilitative and custodial care and the costs for additional diagnosis and therapy of the substantial coronary disease that may have precipitated the arrest. When these costs are taken into account, the relative cost-effectiveness of prehospital emergency services programs becomes less appealing, although upgrading to paramedic services, either as the first responder or as the second part of a two-tier system, appears to be worthwhile from a cost-effectiveness standpoint.[153]

Acute Myocardial Infarction
(See also Chap. 37)

CORONARY CARE UNITS (see also p. 1226). These were originally designed to provide the ready availability of resuscitative services to patients with obvious acute myocardial infarction, for which there were no other therapies known to be effective at the time. The mission of coronary care units subsequently broadened in several ways. First, large numbers of patients were admitted with a suspicion of myocardial infarction so that they might have access to resuscitative facilities should they develop definitive evidence of infarction. Second, coronary care units became cardiac intensive care units, where patients could receive acute interventions to treat ischemia, pump failure, or other complications. The advent of thrombolysis and the availability of emergency percutaneous transluminal coronary angioplasty (PTCA) have further redefined the modern coronary care unit. At the same time, financial considerations have led to the development of alternative management strategies for low-risk patients who need diagnostic or monitoring facilities rather than intensive interventions.

REPERFUSION THERAPY (see also p. 1213). Reperfusion therapy with thrombolytic agents is most successful when it is given as soon as possible after the onset of symptoms in patients with acute myocardial infarction. Prehospital thrombolysis, which provides treatment about 55 minutes earlier, on average, than treatment that begins in the hospital, can significantly reduce both the cardiac death rate and overall mortality from the acute myocardial infarction by about 17 per cent compared with treatment begun in the hospital.[154] Although precise cost data are not currently available, intravenous thrombolysis provided either at home in systems such as are available in Great Britain[155] or in an ambulance[154,156,157] appears to afford benefits that are likely to be well worth the cost.

Meta-analysis[158] indicates a benefit from thrombolysis when it is administered as late as 7 to 12 hours after the onset of symptoms. Among patients treated more than 12 hours after the onset of symptoms, results remain inconclusive.[158–160] Although the costs of thrombolysis are higher and the relative benefits somewhat lower in the elderly, the higher absolute mortality rates from acute myocardial infarction in the elderly translate into overall benefits that are easily equivalent to those found in younger patients.[161]

Accelerated tissue plasminogen activator (t-PA) appears to be somewhat more efficacious than streptokinase for opening the infarct-related artery[162] at 90 minutes and hence has been associated with a lower mortality rate than streptokinase.[163] Despite substantial ongoing debate,[164,165] these incremental benefits would translate into a cost of about $25,000 to $30,000 per year of life saved.[166]

Although the methods have varied among different cost-effectiveness analyses for acute thrombolytic therapy, all have shown intravenous thrombolysis with streptokinase to be well worth the cost under a variety of assumptions in patients of all age ranges[161] and even in high-risk patients in whom an acute myocardial infarction could not be definitively diagnosed at the time the treatment was begun.[161,167–171] The incremental cost-effectiveness of t-PA compared with streptokinase is also more appealing in higher risk patients, in whom its relative advantages would translate into larger absolute benefits.[166]

PRIMARY PERCUTANEOUS TRANSLUMINAL CORONARY ANGIOPLASTY (see also p. 1221). Emergent primary PTCA appears to result in an even higher rate of effective reperfusion than intravenous thrombolysis.[172] As a result, it is not surprising that primary PTCA has been associated with a significant reduction in mortality in several randomized trials.[173–175] Most notably, primary PTCA was not more costly because patients tended to be discharged from the hospital more quickly.[174] Although feasibility of extending primary PTCA to an increased proportion of the population remains uncertain at the present time, this treatment appears to be the most effective and cost-effective option when it can be provided immediately by a highly skilled physician.[172]

An analysis of these various recent studies indicates that the benefits of prehospital versus in-hospital thrombolysis result in about a 17 per cent reduction in mortality, each hour earlier that the thrombolysis is administered results in about a 10 to 15 per cent relative mortality reduction, and accelerated t-PA versus streptokinase results in about a 12 per cent relative mortality reduction. Emergent PTCA on demand by highly skilled operators, on average at about 1 hour after hospital arrival and thus no more than 1 hour later than thrombolysis would have been given, results in about a 63 per cent relative reduction in mortality. Each of these mortality reductions appears to be worth the cost, based on currently available data. The choices among them and decisions regarding the development of the most appropriate system depend on local factors and the results of future research.

SUBSEQUENT TREATMENT AND RISK STRATIFICATION AFTER ACUTE MYOCARDIAL INFARCTION (see also p. 1258). After thrombolysis, conservative treatment, in which invasive procedures are used only for patients with symptoms such as recurrent ischemia, is just as good as routine cardiac catheterization followed by revascularization of significant stenoses.[176] Although post-myocardial infarction risk stratification is widely recommended,[177] formal testing with rest and exercise electrocardiograms, stress thallium scintigraphy, radionuclide ventriculograms, and 24-hour electrocardiographic recordings is limited by the abilities of any of these tests to predict which patients will subsequently have a clinical event.[178,179] Substantially less aggressive strategies, such as practiced in Canada, result in rates of survival and reinfarction equivalent to those with more aggressive United States practices, although patients treated in Canada tend to have a higher frequency of angina that limits their activities.[180] The relative cost-effectiveness of various strategies to stratify risk and base therapies upon these risks in the post-myocardial infarction patient is not well defined.

LONG-TERM TREATMENT. In addition to the known beneficial effects of cholesterol reduction therapy for secondary prevention in patients after myocardial infarction,[63,68] other therapies appear to be effective and cost-effective. Oral anticoagulation with warfarin or coumarin derivatives reduces recurrent cardiac deaths,[181] but there is no evidence that such therapy is more effective than aspirin, which is less expensive and probably safer.[182,183] Treatment with angiotensin-converting enzyme inhibitors, beginning acutely soon after a myocardial infarction or up to 6 weeks later, results in a 19 to 27 per cent benefit in reducing mortality at 30 to 48 months after the infarction,[184–186] and this treatment saves a year of life for less than $25,000 in most patients.[187] Long-term therapy with beta-adrenoceptor inhibitors confers a 25 per cent or so reduction in the relative risk of reinfarction and cardiac death and is associated with a cost-effectiveness ratio of well less than $10,000 per year of life saved for high- and medium-risk patients and no more than $30,000 per year of life saved in even the lowest risk patients.[188]

POTENTIAL COST-EFFECTIVE ALTERNATIVES TO CORONARY CARE UNIT ADMISSION. Patients who are evaluated for symptoms that may potentially represent acute myocardial infarction present a difficult diagnostic and therapeutic dilemma: Should they be admitted to intensive facilities for diagnosis and monitoring even though the risks of complications are low, or can they be managed in lower cost ways that do not appreciably increase their risk? In general, admission to a coronary intensive care unit is not a cost-effective alternative unless the probability of myocardial infarction is close to 20 per cent. This suggests that such an option be limited to patients who have electrocardiographic evidence of acute myocardial infarction or acute cardiac ischemia, unless the patient has an otherwise uninterpretable electrocardiogram (for example, left bundle branch block or a paced rhythm) and has very high risk clinical characteristics.[8] Clinical algorithms that are based on routine information from the history, physical examination, and electrocardiogram can stratify patients into various risk groups.[16,17,189,190] Decisions based on these predictive probabilities can improve coronary care unit admission practices[17,189–191] and help guide which patients should be admitted to less intensive units, where they will receive more cost-effective care.[192,193] Although echocardiography[194,195] and technetium-99m sestamibi myocardial imaging can also be used to identify higher versus lower risk patients,[196,197] the logistics and cost-effectiveness of these approaches remain uncertain at this time.

Newer enzymatic assays show great promise in improving the rapid diagnosis of acute myocardial infarction.[198,199] Measurements of CK isoforms,[200] troponin I,[201] or troponin T[202] can result in more sensitive and specific diagnoses of

acute myocardial infarction or complicated unstable angina more quickly than conventional CK-MB isoenzyme assays. Although the true costs of these new enzyme assays are not yet clearly known, the potential to use these assays to shorten the diagnostic evaluation period for patients with suspected myocardial ischemia suggests that they are likely to have favorable cost-effectiveness ratios and ultimately to replace currently used enzyme assays.

In patients who are at low risk for acute myocardial infarction but are admitted to the hospital, the absence of major complications or a definitive diagnosis of acute myocardial infarction within 12 to 24 hours implies a low-risk status and the safety of discharge from the coronary care unit. In patients whose initial risk for an acute myocardial infarction is below about 10 per cent, a 12-hour or perhaps even a 6-hour period of sequential electrocardiograms and cardiac enzymes to rule out acute myocardial infarction is adequate.[16,17,203–204] After thrombolysis, low-risk patients can be discharged from the hospital as early as 4 days after admission.[205] Use of practice guidelines and reminders is an effective way to increase the early transfer of patients from more intensive to less intensive settings and to facilitate early hospital discharge.[206–208]

Coronary Artery Revascularization
(See also Chap. 39)

Directional atherectomy can result in a greater increase in coronary lumen than traditional PTCA (see p. 1376) but with early complication rates that are about twofold higher.[209,210] Rates of clinical restenosis may be slightly lower for directional atherectomy, but death rates and costs do not appear to be significantly different between the two procedures.[209,210]

Coronary stenting with balloon-expandable stents also can increase the postprocedure coronary diameter and reduce the rate of clinical restenosis.[211,212] However, the initial larger coronary diameter is achieved at the cost of a higher rate of acute complications and of longer hospital admissions.[211,212] The cost-effectiveness of stenting may be worthwhile[213] when compared with routine PTCA, but longer-term clinical and economic follow-up is required to derive precise cost-effectiveness ratios.

Although coronary artery bypass grafting (CABG) has probably accounted for only about 3 per cent of the decline in coronary heart disease mortality,[214] the benefits of CABG compared with medical treatment in many subgroups of patients is clear.[215] However, many CABG procedures are performed for indications in which the benefits are uncertain, even though few are used in truly inappropriate situations.[216,217] Centers that perform a large volume of procedures generally have better outcomes,[217,218] and feedback of information regarding coronary artery bypass mortality can result in marked improvements in outcome.[219]

For single-vessel disease, PTCA results in better symptomatic status than medical treatment (see p. 1373).[220] When PTCA is compared with coronary bypass grafting for patients with single-vessel or multivessel disease, the PTCA

TABLE 53–5 ESTIMATED APPROXIMATE COST PER GAIN IN ONE QUALITY-ADJUSTED YEAR OF LIFE FOR CORONARY ARTERY BYPASS GRAFTING

	ONE-VESSEL	TWO-VESSEL	THREE-VESSEL	LEFT MAIN DISEASE
Very mild angina	*	$86,000	$14,000	$6,300
Mild angina	$850,000	$55,000	$13,500	$6,600
Severe angina	$55,000	$32,000	$13,000	$7,000

* Quality-adjusted life expectancy is reduced.
From Weinstein, M. C., and Stason, W. B.: Cost-effectiveness of coronary artery bypass surgery. Circulation 66(Suppl. III):56, 1982.

patients generally have higher rates of repeat revascularization and angina but similar rates of death, myocardial infarction, employment, and overall costs.[221-224] Nonrandomized data from a large data bank suggest that CABG may be better than PTCA for improving the survival of patients with three-vessel disease or severe two-vessel disease, whereas the choice is between PTCA and medical treatment in patients with less severe disease.[225] The estimated cost-effectiveness of CABG depends on the patient's symptomatic status and extent of disease (Table 53-5).[226]

SUMMARY

The gratifying reduction in mortality from ischemic heart disease usually is regarded as testimony to the effectiveness of a variety of primary and secondary preventive and therapeutic measures. It will be necessary, however, for current and future interventions to be carefully analyzed, so that the benefit of medical care to reduce cardiovascular morbidity and mortality can be maximized within the constraints of the resources that will be available.

Physicians should not view the current emphasis on cost-effective care as contradictory to excellent care. Patients should not be treated as numbers, and optimal medical care cannot be routinely derived from equations. The physician's principal responsibility is to render the best possible medical care to the patient as an individual. An understanding of the principles of cost-effectiveness should allow the physician to improve the choice of diagnostic and therapeutic strategies, and it should assist the physician's ability to determine strategies that are optimal in the aggregate and to adopt or adapt them for the person at hand. In such a context, more cost-effective care implies better care for the individual patient as well as the conservation of resources to improve care for the population as a whole.

REFERENCES

QUANTITATIVE ANALYSES OF COSTS AND EFFECTIVENESS

1. Weinstein, M. C., and Fineberg, H. V.: Clinical Decision Analysis. Philadelphia, W. B. Saunders Co., 1980.
2. Weinstein, M. C., and Stason, W. B.: Foundations of cost-effectiveness analysis for health and medical practices. N. Engl. J. Med. 296:716, 1977.
3. Detsky, A. S., and Naglie, J. G.: A clinician's guide to cost-effectiveness analysis. Ann. Intern. Med. 113:147, 1990.
4. Kupersmith, J., Holmes-Rovner, M., Hogan, A., et al.: Cost-effectiveness analysis in heart disease, Part I: General principles. Prog. Cardiovasc. Dis. 37:161, 1994.
5. Udvarhelyi, I. S., Colditz, G. A., Rai, A., and Epstein, A. M.: Cost-effectiveness and cost-benefit analyses in the medical literature. Ann. Intern. Med. 116:238, 1992.
6. Russell, L. B.: Some of the tough decisions required by a national health plan. Science 246:892, 1989.
7. Goldman, L. G.: Cost awareness in medicine. In Isselbacher, K. J., et al. (eds.): Harrison's Principles of Internal Medicine. 13th ed. New York, McGraw-Hill Book Co., 1994, p. 38.
8. Tosteson, A. N. A., Goldman, L., Udvarhelyli, I. S., and Lee, T. H.: Cost-effectiveness of a coronary care unit versus a stepdown unit for emergency department patients with acute chest pain. Circulation (In press).
9. Kwoh, C. K., Beck, J. R., and Pauker, S. G.: Repeated syncope with negative diagnostic evaluation. To pace or not to pace? Med. Decis. Making 4:351, 1984.
10. Fryback, D. G., Dasbach, E. J., Klein, R., et al.: The Beaver Dam Health Outcomes Study: Initial catalog of health-state quality factors. Med. Decis. Making 13:89, 1993.
11. Doubilet, P., Weinstein, M. D., and McNeil, B. J.: Use and misuse of the term "cost-effective" in medicine. N. Engl. J. Med. 314(Edit):253, 1986.
12. Iglehart, J. K.: The American health care system. The end-stage renal disease program. N. Engl. J. Med. 328:366, 1993.

DIAGNOSTIC TESTING

13. Goldman, L.: Quantitative aspects of clinical reasoning. In Isselbacher, K. J., et al. (eds.): Harrison's Principles of Internal Medicine. 13th ed. New York, McGraw-Hill Book Co., 1994, p. 43.
14. Goldman, L.: Noninvasive tests in cardiology. In Branch, W. T., Jr. (ed.): Office Practice of Medicine. 3rd ed., Philadelphia, W. B. Saunders Company, 1994, p. 40.
15. Diamond, G. A., Staniloff, H. M., Forrester, J. S., et al.: Computer-assisted diagnosis in the noninvasive evaluation of patients with suspected coronary artery disease. J. Am. Coll. Cardiol. 1:444, 1983.
16. Lee, T. H., Juarez, G., Cook, E. F., et al.: Ruling out acute myocardial infarction: Prospective multicenter validation of a 12 hour strategy for low risk patients. N. Engl. J. Med. 324:1239, 1991.
17. Goldman, L., Cook, E. F., Brand, D.A., et al.: A computer protocol to predict myocardial infarction in emergency department patients with chest pain. N. Engl. J. Med. 318:797, 1988.
18. Goldman, L., Feinstein, A. R., Batsford, W. P., et al.: Ordering patterns and clinical impact of cardiovascular nuclear medicine procedures. Circulation 62:680, 1980.
19. Krumholz, H., Douglas, P. S., Goldman, L., and Waksmonski, C.: Clinical utility of transthoracic two-dimensional and Doppler echocardiography. J. Am. Coll. Cardiol. 24:125, 1994.
20. Sox, H. C., Margulies, I., and Sox, C. H.: Psychologically mediated effects of diagnostic tests. Ann. Intern. Med. 95:680, 1981.
21. Pauker, S. G., and Kassirer, J. P.: The threshold approach to clinical decision-making. N. Engl. J. Med. 302:1109, 1980.
22. Weintraub, W. S., Madeira, S. W., Bodenheimer, M. M., et al.: Critical analysis of the application of Bayes' theorem to sequential testing in the noninvasive diagnosis of coronary artery disease. Am. J. Cardiol. 54:43, 1984.
23. Pamelia, F. X., Gibson, R. S., Watson, D. D., et al.: Prognosis with chest pain and normal thallium-201 exercise scintigrams. Am. J. Cardiol. 55:920, 1985.
24. Zaret, B. L., and Wachers, F. J.: Nuclear cardiology. N. Engl. J. Med. 329:775, 1993.
25. Gordon, D. J., Ekelund, L., Karon, J. M., et al.: Predictive value of the exercise tolerance test for mortality in North American men: The Lipid Research Clinics Mortality Follow-up Study. Circulation 74:252, 1986.
26. Patterson, R. E., Eng, C., Horowitz, S. F., et al.: Bayesian comparison of cost-effectiveness of different clinical approaches to diagnose coronary artery disease. J. Am Coll. Cardiol. 4:278, 1984.
27. Sox, H. C., Garber, A. M., and Littenberg, B.: The resting electrocardiogram as a screening test: A clinical analysis. Ann. Intern. Med. 111:489, 1989.
28. Sox, H. C., Littenberg, B., and Garber, A. M.: The role of exercise testing in screening for coronary artery disease. Ann. Intern. Med. 110:456, 1989.
29. Gorry, G. A., Pauker, S. G., and Schwartz, W. B.: The diagnostic importance of the normal finding. N. Engl. J. Med. 298:486, 1978.
30. Wennberg, J. E., Freeman, J. L., and Culp, W. J.: Are hospital services rationed in New Haven or over-utilised in Boston? Lancet 1:1185, 1987.
31. Fineberg, H. V., and Hiatt H. H.: Evaluation of medical practices. The case for technology assessment. N. Engl. J. Med. 301:1086, 1979.
32. Eagle, K. S., Mulley, A. G., Field, T. S., et al.: Variation in intensive care unit practices in two community hospitals. Med. Care 29:1237, 1991.
33. Gillum, R. F.: Trends in acute myocardial infarction and coronary heart disease death in the United States. J. Am. Coll. Cardiol. 23:1273, 1993.
34. DeStefano, F., Merritt, R. K., Anda, R. F., et al.: Trends in nonfatal coronary heart disease in the United States, 1980 through 1989. Arch. Intern. Med. 153:2489, 1993.

PREVENTION AND TREATMENT

35. Sytkowski, P. A., Kannel, W. B., and D'Agostino, R. B.: Changes in risk factors and the decline in mortality from cardiovascular disease. The Framingham Heart Study. N. Engl. J. Med. 322:1635, 1990.
36. Weinstein, M. C., Coxson, P. G., Williams, L. W., et al.: Forecasting coronary heart disease incidence, mortality, and cost: The coronary heart disease policy model. Am. J. Public Health 77:1417, 1987.
37. Wittels, E. H., Hay, J. W., and Gotto, A. M.: Medical costs of coronary artery disease in the United States. Am. J. Cardiol. 65:432, 1990.
38. Canadian Task Force on the Periodic Health Examination: Periodic health examination, 1993 update: 2. Lowering the blood total cholesterol level to prevent coronary heart disease. Can. Med. Assoc. J. 148:521, 1993.
39. Expert Panel on Detection, Evaluation, and Treatment of High Blood Cholesterol in Adults: Summary of the Second Report of the National Cholesterol Education Program (NCEP) Expert Panel on Detection, Evaluation, and Treatment of High Blood Cholesterol in Adults (Adult Treatment Panel II). JAMA 269:3015, 1993.
40. Goldman, L., Gordon, D.J., Rifkind, B. M., et al.: Cost and health implications of cholesterol lowering. Circulation 85:1960, 1992.
41. Stampfer, M. J., Sacks, F. M., Salvini, S., et al.: A prospective study of cholesterol, apolipoproteins, and the risk of myocardial infarction. N. Engl. J. Med. 325:373, 1991.
42. Klag, M. J., Ford, D. E., Mead, L. A., et al.: Serum cholesterol in young men and subsequent cardiovascular disease. N. Engl. J. Med. 328:313, 1993.
43. Hulley, S. B., Newman, T. B., Grady, D., et al.: Should we be measuring blood cholesterol levels in young adults? JAMA 269:1416, 1993.
44. Newman, T. B., Browner, W. S., and Hulley, S. B.: Childhood cholesterol screening: Contraindications. JAMA 267:100, 1992.

45. Newman, T., Browner, W., and Hulley, S.: The case against childhood cholesterol screening. JAMA 264:3039, 1990.

46. Manolio, T. A., Pearson, T. A., Wenger, N. K., et al.: Cholesterol and heart disease in older persons and women. Review of an NHLBI Workshop. Ann. Epidemiol. 2:161, 1992.

47. Jacobs, D., Blackburn, H., Higgins, M., et al.: Report of the Conference on Low Blood Cholesterol: Mortality Associations. Circulation 86:1046, 1992.

48. Krumholz, H. M., Seeman, T. E., Merrill, S. S., et al.: Lack of association between cholesterol and coronary heart disease mortality and morbidity and all-cause mortality in persons older than 70 years. JAMA 272:1335, 1994.

49. Hulley, S. B., and Newman, T. B.: Cholesterol in the elderly. Is it important? JAMA 272:1372, 1994.

50. Stamler, J., Stamler, R., Brown, W. V., et al.: Serum cholesterol. Doing the right thing. Circulation 88:1954, 1993.

51. Jacobs, D. R., and Blackburn, H.: Models of effects of low blood cholesterol on the public health. Implications for practice and policy. Circulation 87:1033, 1993.

52. LaRosa, J. C.: Cholesterol lowering, low cholesterol, and mortality. Am. J. Cardiol. 72:776, 1993.

53. Smith, G. D., Song, F., and Sheldon, T. A.: Cholesterol lowering and mortality: The importance of considering initial level of risk. Br. Med. J. 306:1367, 1993.

54. Frank, J. W., Reed, D. M., Grove, J. S., and Benfante, R.: Will lowering population levels of serum cholesterol affect total mortality? Expectations from the Honolulu heart program. J. Clin Epidemiol. 45:333, 1992.

55. McIsaac, W. J., Naylor, C. D., and Basinski, A.: Mismatch of coronary risk and treatment intensity under the National Cholesterol Education Program Guidelines. J. Gen. Intern. Med. 6:518, 1991.

56. Krahn, M., Naylor, C. D., Basinski, A. S., and Detsky, A. S.: Comparison of an aggressive (U.S.) and a less aggressive (Canadian) policy for cholesterol screening and treatment. J. Gen. Intern. Med. 115:248, 1991.

57. Stamler, J., Wentworth, D., and Neaton, J. D.: Is relationship between serum cholesterol and risk of premature death from coronary heart disease continuous and graded? Findings in 356,222 primary screenees of the Multiple-Risk Factor Intervention Trial (MRFIT). JAMA 256:2823, 1986.

58. MacMahon, S., Peto, R., Cutler, J., et al.: Blood pressure, stroke, and coronary heart disease: Part I. Prolonged differences in blood pressure: Prospective observational studies corrected for the regression dilution bias. Lancet 335:765, 1990.

59. Lipid Research Clinics Program: The Lipid Research Clinics Coronary Primary Prevention Trial results. II. The relationship of reduction in incidence of CHD to cholesterol lowering. JAMA 251:365, 1984.

60. Davis, C. E., Rifkind, B. M., Brenner, H., and Gordon, D. J.: A single cholesterol measurement underestimates the risk of coronary heart disease. JAMA 264:3044, 1990.

61. Gordon, D. J., Probstfield, J. L., Garrisons, R. J., et al.: High-density lipoprotein cholesterol and cardiovascular disease. Four prospective American studies. Circulation 79:8, 1989.

62. Lipid Research Clinics Program: The Lipid Research Clinics Coronary Primary Prevention Trial results: I. Reduction in incidence of coronary heart disease. JAMA 251:351, 1984.

63. Roussouw, F. E., Lewis, B., and Rifkind, B. M.: The value of lowering cholesterol after myocardial infarction. N. Engl. J. Med. 323:1112, 1990.

64. Brown, G., Albers, J. J., Fisher, L. D., et al.: Regression of coronary artery disease as a result of intensive lipid-lowering therapy in men with high levels of apolipoprotein B. N. Engl. J. Med. 323:1289, 1990.

65. Buchwald, H., Varco, R. L., Matts, J. P., et al.: Effect of partial ileal bypass surgery on mortality and morbidity from coronary heart disease in patients with hypercholesterolemia. N. Engl. J. Med. 323:946, 1990.

66. Cashin-Hemphill, L., Mack, W. J., Pagoda, J. M., et al.: Beneficial effects of colestipol-niacin on coronary atherosclerosis. JAMA 264:3013, 1990.

67. Kane, J. P., Malloy M. J., Ports, T., et al.: Regression of coronary atherosclerosis during treatment of familial hypercholesterolemia with combined drug regimens. JAMA 264:3007, 1990.

68. Scandinavian Simvastatin Survival Study Group: Randomised trial of cholesterol lowering in 4444 patients with coronary heart disease: The Scandinavian Simvastatin Survival Study (4S). Lancet 344:1383, 1994.

69. Canner, P. L., Berge, K. G., Wenger, N. K., et al.: Fifteen year mortality in coronary drug project patients; long-term benefits with niacin. J. Am. Coll. Cardiol. 8:1245, 1986.

70. Frick, M. H., Elo, O., Haapa, K., et al.: Helsinki Heart Study: Primary-prevention trial with gemfibrozil in middle-aged men with dyslipidemia. N. Engl. J. Med. 317:1237, 1987.

71. Shepherd, J., Cobbe, S. M., Ford, I., et al.: Prevention of coronary heart disease with pravastatin in men with hypercholesterolemia. N. Engl. J. Med. 333:1301, 1995.

72. Sempos, C. T., Cleeman, J. I., Carroll, M. D., et al.: Prevalence of high blood cholesterol among US adults. An update based on guidelines from the Second Report of the National Cholesterol Education Program Adult Treatment Panel. JAMA 269:3009, 1993.

73. Schulman, K. A., Kinosian, B., Jacobson, T. A., et al.: Reducing high blood cholesterol level with drugs: Cost-effectiveness of pharmacologic management. JAMA 264:3025, 1990.

74. Oster, G., and Epstein, A. M.: Cost-effectiveness of antihyperlipemic therapy in the prevention of coronary heart disease: The case of cholestyramine. JAMA 258:2381, 1987.

75. Goldman, L., Weinstein, M. C., Goldman, P. A., and Williams, L. W.: Cost-effectiveness of HMG-CoA reductase inhibition for primary and secondary prevention of coronary heart disease. JAMA 265:1145, 1991.

76. Hay, J. W., Wittels, E. H., and Gotto, A. M.: An economic evaluation of lovastatin for cholesterol lowering and coronary artery disease reduction. Am. J. Cardiol. 67:780, 1991.

77. Kinosian, B. P., and Eisenberg, J. M.: Cutting into cholesterol: Cost-effective alternatives for treating hypercholesterolemia. JAMA 259:2249, 1988.

78. Kristiansen, I. S., Eggen, A. E., and Thelle, D. S.: Cost-effectiveness of incremental programmes for lowering serum cholesterol concentration: Is individual intervention worthwhile? Br. Med. J. 302:1119, 1991.

79. Goldman, L., Goldman, P., Williams, L., and Weinstein, M. C.: Cost-effectiveness considerations in the treatment of heterozygous familial hypercholesterolemia with medications. In Proceedings of the National Heart, Lung, and Blood Institute Workshop on Identification and Management of Heterozygous Familial Hypercholesterolemia. Am. J. Cardiol. 72:75D, 1993.

80. Goldman, L., Weinstein, M. C., and Williams, L. W.: Relative impact of targeted versus populationwide cholesterol interventions on the incidence of coronary heart disease. Circulation 80:254, 1989.

81. Farquhar, J. W., Fortmann, S. P., Flora, J. A., et al.: Effects of community-wide education on cardiovascular disease risk factors. The Stanford Five-City Project. JAMA 264:359, 1990.

82. Puska, P., Salonen, J. T., Nissinen, A., et al.: Change in risk factors for coronary heart disease during 10 years of a community intervention programme (North Karelia project). Br. Med. J. 287:1840, 1983.

83. Garber, A. M., Sox, H. C., and Littenberg, B.: Screening asymptomatic adults for cardiac risk factors: The serum cholesterol level. Ann. Intern. Med. 110:622, 1989.

HYPERTENSION

84. The Fifth Report of the Joint National Committee on Detection, Evaluation, and Treatment of High Blood Pressure (JNC V). Arch. Intern. Med. 153:154, 1993.

85. Sagie, A., Larson, M. G., and Levy, D.: The natural history of borderline isolated systolic hypertension. N. Engl. J. Med. 329:1912, 1993.

86. SHEP Cooperative Research Group: Prevention of stroke by antihypertensive drug treatment in older persons with isolated systolic hypertension: Final results of the Systolic Hypertension in the Elderly Program (SHEP). JAMA 265:3255, 1991.

87. Dahlof, B., Lindholm, L. H., Hansson, L., et al.: Morbidity and mortality in the Swedish Trial in Old Patients with Hypertension (STOP-Hypertension). Lancet 338:1281, 1991.

88. Medical Research Council Working Party: MRC trial of treatment of mild hypertension: Principal results. Br. Med. J. 291:97, 1985.

89. Insua, J. T., Sacks, H. S., Lau, T., et al.: Drug treatment of hypertension in the elderly: A meta-analysis. Ann. Intern. Med. 121:355, 1994.

90. Mulrow, C. D., Cornell, J. A., Herrera, C. R., et al.: Hypertension in the elderly. Implications and generalizability of randomized trials. JAMA 272:1932, 1994.

91. Hebert, P. R., Joser, M., Mayer, J., et al.: Recent evidence on drug therapy of mild to moderate hypertension and decreased risk of coronary heart disease. Arch. Intern. Med. 153:578, 1993.

92. Materson, B. J., Reda, D. J., Cushman, W. C., et al.: Single-drug therapy for hypertension in men: A comparison of six antihypertensive agents with placebo. N. Engl. J. Med. 328:914, 1993.

93. Neaton, J. D., Grimm, R. H., Prineas, R. J., et al.: Treatment of mild hypertension study: Final results. JAMA 270:713, 1993.

94. Littenberg, B., Garber, A. M., and Sox, H. C.: Screening for hypertension. Ann. Intern. Med. 112:192, 1990.

95. Weinstein, M. C., and Stason, W. B.: Hypertension: A Policy Perspective. Cambridge, Mass., Harvard University Press, 1976.

96. Stokes, J., III, and Carmichael, D. C.: A Cost-Benefit Analysis of Model Hypertension Control. Bethesda, National Heart, Lung and Blood Institute, 1975.

97. Edelson, J. T., Weinstein, M. C., Tosteson, A. N. A., et al.: Long-term cost-effectiveness of various initial monotherapies for mild to moderate hypertension. JAMA 263:408, 1990.

98. Three-Community Hypertension Control Program. V. Cost-effectiveness of intervention. Mayo Clin. Proc. 56:11, 1981.

99. Hannan, E. L., and Graham, J. K.: A cost-benefit study of hypertension screening and treatment program at the work setting. Inquiry 15:345, 1978.

100. Tsevat, J.: Impact and cost-effectiveness of smoking interventions. Am. J. Med. 93(Suppl. 1A):43, 1992.

101. Hermanson, B., Omenn, G. S., Kronmal, R. A., and Gersh, B. J.: Beneficial six-year outcome of smoking cessation in older men and women with coronary artery disease. N. Engl. J. Med. 319:1365, 1988.

102. Rosenberg, L., Palmer, J. R., and Shapiro, S.: Decline in the risk of myocardial infarctions among women who stop smoking. N. Engl. J. Med. 322:213, 1990.

103. Bartecchi, C. E., MacKenzie, T. D., and Schrier, R. W.: The human costs of tobacco use (first of 2 parts). N. Engl. J. Med. 330:907, 1994.

104. MacKenzie, T. D., Bartecchi, C. E., and Schrier, R. W.: The human costs of tobacco use (second of 2 parts). N. Engl. J. Med. 330:975, 1994.

105. Grover, S. A., Gray-Donald, K., Joseph, L., et al.: Life expectancy fol-

lowing dietary modification or smoking cessation. Estimating the benefits of a prudent lifestyle. Arch. Intern. Med. 154:1697, 1994.

106. Cohen, S. J., Stookey, G. K., Katz, B. P., et al.: Encouraging primary care physicians to help smokers quit. Ann. Intern. Med. 110:648, 1989.

107. Cummings, S. T., Coates, T. J., Richard, R. J., et al.: Training physicians in counseling and smoking cessation: A randomized trial of the "Quit for Life" program. Ann. Intern. Med. 110:640, 1989.

108. Silagy, C., Mant, D., Fowler, G., and Lodge, M.: Meta-analysis on efficacy of nicotine replacement therapies in smoking cessation. Lancet 343:139, 1994.

109. Kenford, S. L., Fiore, M. C., Jorenby, D. E., et al.: Predicting smoking cessation. Who will quit with and without the nicotine patch? JAMA 271:589, 1994.

110. Oster, G., Huse, D. M., Delea, T. E., and Colditz, G. A.: Cost effectiveness of nicotine gum as an adjunct to physician's advice against cigarette smoking. JAMA 256:1315, 1986.

111. Hughes, J. R., Gust, S. W., Keenan, R. M., et al.: Nicotine vs placebo gum in general medical practice. JAMA 261:1300. 1989.

112. Abelin, T., Muller, P., Buehler, A., et al.: Controlled trial of transdermal nicotine patch in tobacco withdrawal. Lancet 1:7, 1989.

113. Tonnesen, P., Fryd, V., Hansen, M., et al.: Effect of nicotine chewing gum in combination with group counseling on the cessation of smoking. N. Engl. J. Med. 318:15, 1988.

114. Lando, H. A., McGovern, P. G., Barrios, F. X., and Etringer, B. D.: Comparative evaluation of American Cancer Society and American Lung Association smoking cessation clinics. Am. J. Public Health 80:554, 1990.

115. Danaher, B. G., Berkanovic, E., and Gerger, B.: Mass media-based health behavior change: Televised smoking cessation program. Addict. Behav. 9:245, 1984.

116. Pierce, J. P., Macaskill, P., and Hill, D.: Long-term effectiveness of mass media led antismoking campaigns in Australia. Am. J. Public Health 80:565, 1990.

117. Krumholz, H. M., Cohen, B. J., Tsevat, J., et al.: Cost-effectiveness of a smoking cessation program after myocardial infarction. J. Am. Coll. Cardiol. 22:1697, 1993.

118. Hubert, H. B., Feinleib, M., McNamara, P. M., and Castelli, W. P.: Obesity as an independent risk factor for cardiovascular disease: A 26-year follow-up of participants in the Framingham Heart Study. Circulation 67:968, 1983.

119. Brownell, K. D., and Kaye, F. S.: A school-based behavior modification, nutrition, education, and physical activity program for obese children. Am. J. Clin. Nutr. 35:277, 1982.

120. Brownell, K. D., Stunkard, A. J., and McKeon, P. E.: Weight reduction at the worksite: A promise partially fulfilled. Am. J. Psychiatry 142:47, 1985.

121. Stunkard, A. J.: The current status of treatment for obesity in adults. In Stunkard, A. J., and Stellar, E. (eds.): Eating and Its Disorders. New York, Raven Press, 1984.

122. Blair, S. N., Kohl, H. W., Paffenbarger, R. S., et al.: Physical fitness and all-cause mortality: A prospective study of healthy men and women. JAMA 262:2395, 1989.

123. Slattery, M. L., Jacobs, D. R., and Nichaman, M. Z.: Leisure time physical activity and coronary heart disease death. The US Railroad Study. Circulation 79:304, 1989.

124. Ekelund, L. G., Haskell, W. L., Johnson, J. L., et al.: Physical fitness as a predictor of cardiovascular mortality in asymptomatic North American men. N. Engl. J. Med. 310:1379, 1988.

125. Paffenbarger, R. S., Jr., Hyde, R. T., Wing, A. L., et al.: The association of changes in physical-activity level and other lifestyle characteristics with mortality among men. N. Engl. J. Med. 328:538, 1993.

126. Sandvik, L., Erikssen, J., Thaulow, E., et al.: Physical fitness as a predictor of mortality among healthy, middle-aged Norwegian men. N. Engl. J. Med. 328:533, 1993.

127. Lakka, T. A., Venalainen, J. M., Rauramaa, R., et al.: Relation of leisure-time physical activity and cardiorespiratory fitness to the risk of acute myocardial infarction in men. N. Engl. J. Med. 330:1549, 1994.

128. Rodriguez, L., Curb, J. D., Burchfiel, C. M., et al.: Physical activity and 23-year incidence of coronary heart disease morbidity and mortality among middle-aged men. The Honolulu Heart Program. Circulation 89:2540, 1994.

129. Cox, M., Shepard, R. J., and Corey, P.: Influence of an employee fitness programme upon fitness, productivity, and absenteeism. Ergonomics 24:795, 1981.

130. Shepard, R. J., Corey, P., Renzland, P., and Cox, M.: The influence of an employee fitness and lifestyle modification upon medical care costs. Can. J. Public Health 73:259, 1982.

131. Oldridge, N. B.: Adherence to adult exercise fitness programs. In Matarazzo, J. D., Miller, N. E., Herd, J. A., and Weiss, S. M. (eds.): Behavioral Health: A Handbook of Health Enhancement and Disease Prevention. New York, John Wiley and Sons, 1984, pp. 467–487.

132. Hatziandreu, E. I., Koplan, J. P., Weinstein, M. C., et al.: A cost-effectiveness analysis of exercise as a health promotion activity. Am. J. Public Health 78:1417, 1988.

133. Oldridge, N. B., Guyatt, G. H., Fischer, M. E., and Rimm, A. A.: Cardiac rehabilitation after myocardial infarction. Combined experience of randomized clinical trials. JAMA 260:945, 1988.

134. Dennis, C. A., Houston-Miller, N., Schwartz, R. G., et al.: Early return to work after uncomplicated myocardial infarction: Results of a randomized trial. JAMA 260:214, 1988.

135. Picard, M. H., Dennis, C., Schwartz, R. G., et al.: Cost-benefit analysis of early return to work after uncomplicated acute myocardial infarction. Am. J. Cardiol. 63:1308, 1989.

136. Bor, D. H., and Himmelstein, D. U.: Endocarditis prophylaxis for patients with mitral valve prolapse. A quantitative analysis. Am. J. Med. 76:711, 1984.

137. Clemens, J. D., and Ransohoff, D. F.: A quantitative assessment of predental antibiotic prophylaxis for patients with mitral valve prolapse. J. Chron. Dis. 37:531, 1984.

138. Durack, D. T.: Prevention of infective endocarditis. N. Engl. J. Med. 332:38, 1995.

139. Kellerman, A. L., Hackman, H. B., and Somes, G.: Dispatcher-assisted cardiopulmonary resuscitation—validation of efficacy. Circulation 80:1231, 1989.

140. Crampton, R. S., Aldrich, R. F., Gascho, J. A., et al.: Reduction of prehospital, ambulance, and community coronary death rates by the community-wide emergency cardiac care system. Am. J. Med. 58:151, 1975.

141. Eisenberg, M. S., Hallstrom, A., and Bergner, L.: Long-term survival after out-of-hospital arrest. N. Engl. J. Med. 306:1340, 1982.

142. Cummins, R. O., and Eisenberg, M. S.: Prehospital cardiopulmonary resuscitation: Is it effective? JAMA 253:2408, 1985.

143. Bachman, J. W., McDonald, G. S., and O'Brien, P. C.: A study of out-of-hospital cardiac arrests in Northeastern Minnesota. JAMA 256:477, 1986.

144. Lombardi, G., Gallagher, J., and Gennis, P.: Outcome of out-of-hospital cardiac arrest in New York City. The Pre-Hospital Arrest Survival Evaluation (PHASE) study. JAMA 271:678, 1994.

145. Becker, L. B., Ostrander, M. P., Barrett, J., and Kondos, G. T.: Outcome of CPR in a large metropolitan area. Where are the survivors? Ann. Emerg. Med. 20:48, 1991.

146. Solomon, N. A.: What are representative survival rates for out-of-hospital cardiac arrest? Insights from the New Haven (Conn) Experience. Arch. Intern. Med. 153:1218, 1993.

147. Eisenberg, M. S., Bergner, L., and Hallstrom, A.: Out-of-hospital cardiac arrest: Improved survival with paramedic services. Lancet 1:812, 1980.

148. Urban, N., Bergner, L., and Eisenberg, M. S.: The costs of a suburban paramedic program in reducing deaths due to cardiac arrest. Med. Care 19:379, 1981.

149. Roine, R. O., Kajaste, S., and Kaste, M.: Neuropsychological sequelae of cardiac arrest. JAMA 269:237, 1993.

150. Ornato, J. P., Craren, E. J., Gonzalez, E. R., et al.: Cost-effectiveness of defibrillation by emergency medical technicians. Am. J. Emerg. Med. 6:108, 1988.

151. Valenzuela, T. D., Criss, E. A., Spaite, D., et al.: Cost-effectiveness analysis of paramedic emergency medical services in the treatment of prehospital cardiopulmonary arrest. Ann. Emerg. Med. 19:1407, 1990.

152. Jakobsson, J., Nyquist, O., Rehnqvist, N., and Norberg, K. A.: Cost of a saved life following out-of-hospital cardiac arrest resuscitated by specially trained ambulance personnel. Acta Anaesthesiol. Scand. 31:426, 1987.

153. Weisfeldt, M. L., Kerber, R. E., McGoldrick, P., et al.: American Heart Association report on the Public Access Defibrillation Conference, December 8–10, 1994. Circulation 92:2740, 1995.

ACUTE MYOCARDIAL INFARCTION

154. The European Myocardial Infarction Project Group: Prehospital thrombolytic therapy in patients with suspected acute myocardial infarction. N. Engl. J. Med. 329:383, 1993.

155. GREAT Group: Feasibility, safety, and efficacy of domiciliary thrombolysis by general practitioners: Gramian region early anistreplase trial. Br. Med. J. 305:548, 1992.

156. Arntz, H.-R., Stern, R., Linderer, T., and Schroder, R.: Efficiency of a physician-operated mobile intensive care unit for prehospital thrombolysis in acute myocardial infarction. Am. J. Cardiol. 70:4170, 1992.

157. Weaver W. D., Cerqueira, M., Halstrom, A. P., et al.: Prehospital-initiated vs hospital-initiated thrombolytic therapy. The Myocardial Infarction Triage and Intervention Trial. JAMA 270:1211, 1993.

158. Fibrinolytic Therapy Trialists' Collaborative Group: Indications for fibrinolytic therapy in suspected acute myocardial infarction: Collaborative overview of early mortality and major morbidity results from all randomised trials of more than 1000 patients. Lancet 343:311, 1994.

159. EMERAS (Estudio Multicentrico Estreptoquinasa Republicas de America del Sur) Collaborative Group: Randomised trial of late thrombolysis in patients with suspected acute myocardial infarction. Lancet 342:767, 1993.

160. LATE Study Group: Late Assessment of Thrombolytic Efficacy (LATE) study with Alteplase 6-24 hours after onset of acute myocardial infarction. Lancet 342:759, 1993.

161. Krumholz, H. M., Pasternak, R. C., Weinstein, M. C., et al.: Cost-effectiveness of thrombolytic therapy with streptokinase in elderly patients with suspected acute myocardial infarction. N. Engl. J. Med. 327:7, 1992.

162. The GUSTO Angiographic Investigators: The effects of tissue plasminogen activator, streptokinase, or both on coronary-artery patency, ventricular function and survival after acute myocardial infarction. N. Engl. J. Med. 329:1615, 1993.

163. The GUSTO Investigators: An international randomized trial comparing four thrombolytic strategies for acute myocardial infarction. N. Engl. J. Med. 329:673, 1993.

164. Lee, K. L., Califf, R. M., Simes, J., et al. for the GUSTO Investigators: Holding GUSTO up to the light. Ann. Intern. Med. 120:876, 1994.

165. Ridker, P. M., O'Donnell, C. J., Marder, V. J., and Hennekens, C. H.: A response to "Holding GUSTO up to the light." Ann. Intern. Med. 120:882, 1994.

166. Mark, D. B., Hlatky, M. A., Califf, R. M., et al.: Cost-effectiveness of thrombolytic therapy with tissue plasminogen activator as compared with streptokinase for acute myocardial infarction. N. Engl. J. Med. 332:1418, 1995.

167. Goel, V., and Naylor, C. D.: Potential cost-effectiveness of intravenous tissue plasminogen activator versus streptokinase for acute myocardial infarction. Can. J. Cardiol. 8:31, 1992.

168. Simoons, M. L., Vos, J., and Martens, L. L.: Cost-utility analysis of thrombolytic therapy. Eur. Heart J. 12:694, 1991.

169. Brody, B., Wray, N., Bame, S., et al.: The impact of economic considerations on clinical decisionmaking: The case of thrombolytic therapy. Med. Care 29:899, 1991.

170. Midgett, A. S., Wong, J. B., Beshansky, J. R., et al.: Cost-effectiveness of streptokinase for acute myocardial infarction: A combined meta-analysis and decision analysis of the effects of infarct location and of likelihood of infarction. Med. Decis. Making 14:108, 1994.

171. Laffel, G. L., Fineberg, H. V., and Braunwald, E.: A cost-effectiveness model for coronary thrombolysis/reperfusion therapy. J. Am. Coll. Cardiol. 10:79, 1987.

172. Goldman, L.: Cost and quality of life: Thrombolysis and primary angioplasty. J. Am. Coll. Cardiol. 25:38s–41s, 1995.

173. Grines, C. L., Browne, K. F., Marco, J., et al.: A comparison of immediate angioplasty with thrombolytic therapy for acute myocardial infarction. N. Engl. J. Med. 328:673, 1993.

174. Zijlstra, F., de Boer, M. J., Hoorntje, J. C. A., et al.: A comparison of immediate coronary angioplasty with intravenous streptokinase in acute myocardial infarction. N. Engl. J. Med. 328:680, 1993.

175. Gibbons, R. J., Holmes, D. R., Reeder, G. S., et al. for the Mayo Coronary Care Unit and Catheterization Laboratory Groups: Immediate angioplasty compared with the administration of a thrombolytic agent followed by conservative treatment for myocardial infarction. N. Engl. J. Med. 328:685, 1993.

176. Williams, D. O., Braunwald, E., Knatterud, G., et al.: One-year results of the Thrombolysis in Myocardial Infarction Investigation (TIMI) Phase II Trial. Circulation 85:533, 1992.

177. Pitt, B.: Evaluation of the postinfarct patient. Circulation 91:1855, 1995.

178. Myers, M. G., Baigrie, R. S., Charlat, M. L., and Morgan, C. D.: Are routine noninvasive tests useful in prediction of outcome after myocardial infarction in elderly people? Lancet 342:1069, 1993.

179. Moss, A. J., Goldstein, R. E., Hall, W. J., et al.: Detection and significance of myocardial ischemia in stable patients after recovery from an acute coronary event. JAMA 69:2379, 1993.

180. Rouleau, J. L., Moye, L. A., Pfeffer, M. A., et al.: A comparison of management patterns after acute myocardial infarction in Canada and the United States. N. Engl. J. Med. 328:779, 1993.

181. Anticoagulants in the Secondary Prevention of Events in Coronary Thrombosis (ASPET) Research Group: Effect of long-term oral anticoagulant treatment on mortality and cardiovascular morbidity after myocardial infarction. Lancet 343:499, 1994.

182. van Bergen, P. F. M. M., Jonker, J. J. C., van Hout, B. A., et al.: Costs and effects of long-term oral anticoagulant treatment after myocardial infarction. JAMA 273:925, 1995.

183. Cairns, J. A., and Markham, B. A.: Economics and efficacy in choosing oral anticoagulants or aspirin after myocardial infarction. JAMA 273(Edit.):965, 1995.

184. Pfeffer, M. A., Braunwald, E., Moye, L. A., et al.: Effect of captopril on mortality and morbidity in patients with left ventricular dysfunction after myocardial infarction: Results of the Survival and Ventricular Enlargement Trial. N. Engl. J. Med. 327:669, 1992.

185. The Acute Infarction Ramipril Efficacy (AIRE) Study Investigators: Effect of ramipril on mortality and morbidity of survivors of acute myocardial infarction with clinical evidence of heart failure. Lancet 342:821, 1993.

186. Gruppo Italiano per lo Studio della Sopravvivenza nell'Infarto Miocardico (GISSI):GISSI-3: Effects of lisinopril and transdermal glyceryl trinitrate singly and together on 6-week mortality and ventricular function after acute myocardial infarction. Lancet 343:1115, 1994.

187. Tsevat, J., Duke, D., Goldman, L., et al.: Cost-effectiveness of captopril therapy after myocardial infarction. J. Am. Coll. Cardiol. 26:914, 1995.

188. Goldman, L., Sia, S. T. B., Cook, E. F., et al.: Cost-effectiveness of routine long-term beta-adrenergic antagonist therapy following acute myocardial infarction. N. Engl. J. Med. 319:152, 1988.

189. Pozen, M. W., D'Agostino, R. B., Mitchell, J. B., et al.: The usefulness of a predictive instrument to reduce inappropriate admissions to the coronary care unit. Ann. Intern. Med. 92:238, 1980.

190. Pozen, M. W., D'Agostino, R. B., Selker, H. P., et al.: A predictive instrument to improve coronary-care-unit admission practices in acute ischemic heart disease: A prospective multicenter clinical trial. N. Engl. J. Med. 310:1273, 1984.

191. Sarasin, F. P., Reymond, J.-M., Griffith, J. L., et al.: Impact of the Acute Cardiac Ischemia Time-Insensitive Predictive Instrument (ACI-TIPI) on the speed of triage decision making for emergency department patients presenting with chest pain. A controlled clinical trial. J. Gen. Intern. Med. 9:187, 1994.

192. Gaspoz, J. M., Lee, T. H., Cook, E. F., et al.: Outcomes of rule-out myocardial infarction patients admitted to a new short-stay unit. Am. J. Cardiol. 68:1459, 1991.

193. Gaspoz, J. M., Lee, T. H., Weinstein, M. C., et al.: Cost-effectiveness of a new short-stay unit to "rule-out" acute myocardial infarction in low risk patients. J. Am. Coll. Cardiol. 24:1249, 1994.

194. Berning, J., Launbjerg, J., and Appleyard, M.: Echocardiographic algorithms for admission and predischarge prediction of mortality in acute myocardial infarction. Am. J. Cardiol. 69:1538, 1992.

195. Fleischmann, K. E., Goldman, L., Robiolio, P., et al.: Echocardiographic correlates of survival in chest pain patients. J. Am. Coll. Cardiol. 23:1390, 1994.

196. Hilton, T. C., Thompson, R. C., Williams, H. J., et al.: Technetium-99m sestamibi myocardial perfusion imaging in the emergency room evaluation of chest pain. J. Am. Coll. Cardiol. 23:1016, 1994.

197. Varetto, T., Cantalupi, D., Altieri, A., and Orlandi, C.: Emergency room technetium-99m sestamibi imaging to rule out acute myocardial ischemic events in patients with nondiagnostic electrocardiograms. J. Am. Coll. Cardiol. 22:1804, 1993.

198. Adams, J. E., III, Abendschein, D. R., and Jaffe, A. S.: Biochemical markers of myocardial injury. Is MB creatine kinase the choice for the 1990s? Circulation 88:750, 1993.

199. Roberts, R., and Kleiman, N. S.: Earlier diagnosis and treatment of acute myocardial infarction necessitates the need for a "new diagnostic mind-set." Circulation 89:872, 1994.

200. Puleo, P. R., Meyer, D., Wathen, C., et al.: Use of a rapid assay of subforms of creatine kinase MB to diagnose or rule out acute myocardial infarction. N. Engl. J. Med. 331:561, 1994.

201. Adams, J. E., III, Bodor, G. S., Davila-Roman, V. G., et al.: Cardiac troponin I. A marker with high specificity for cardic injury. Circulation 88:101, 1993.

202. Hamm, C. W., Ravkilde, J., Gerhardt, W., et al.: The prognostic value of serum troponin T in unstable angina. N. Engl. J. Med. 327:146, 1992.

203. Lee, T. H., Rouan, G. W., Weisberg, M. C., et al.: Sensitivity of routine clinical criteria for diagnosing myocardial infarction within 24 hours of hospitalization. Ann. Intern. Med. 106:181, 1987.

204. Mulley, A. G., Thibault, G. E., Hughes, R. A., et al.: The course of patients with suspected myocardial infarction: The identification of low-risk patients for early transfer from intensive care. N. Engl. J. Med. 302:943, 1980.

205. Mark, D. B., Sigmon, K., Topol, E. J., et al.: Identification of acute myocardial infarction patients suitable for early hospital discharge after aggressive interventional therapy. Results from the Thrombolysis and Angioplasty in Acute Myocardial Infarction Registry. Circulation 83:1186, 1991.

206. Weingarten, S., Ermann, B., Bolus, R., et al.: Early "step-down" transfer of low-risk patients with chest pain. Ann. Intern. Med. 113:283, 1990.

207. Weingarten, S. R., Riedinger, M. S., Conner, L., et al.: Practice guidelines and reminders to reduce duration of hospital stay for patients with chest pain. Ann. Intern. Med. 120:257, 1994.

208. Ellrodt, A. G., Conner, L., Riedinger, M., and Weingarten, S.: Measuring and improving physician compliance with clinical practice guidelines. Ann. Intern. Med. 122:277, 1995.

209. Topol, E. J., Leya, F., Pinkerton, C. A., et al.: A comparison of directional atherectomy with coronary angioplasty in patients with coronary artery disease. N. Engl. J. Med. 329:221, 1993.

210. Adelman, A. G., Cohen, E. A., Kimball, B. P., et al.: A comparison of directional atherectomy with balloon angioplasty for lesions of the left anterior descending coronary artery. N. Engl. J. Med. 329:228, 1993.

211. Serruys, P. W., de Jaegere, P., Kiemeneij, F., et al.: A comparison of balloon-expandable-stent implantation with balloon angioplasty in patients with coronary artery disease. N. Engl. J. Med. 331:489, 1994.

212. Fischman, D. L., Leon, M. B., Baim, D. S., et al. for the Stent Restenosis Study Investigators: A randomized comparison of coronary-stent placement and balloon angioplasty in the treatment of coronary artery disease. N. Engl. J. Med. 331:496, 1994.

213. Cohen, D. J., Breall, J. A., Ho, K. K., et al.: Evaluating the potential cost-effectiveness of stenting as a treatment for symptomatic single-vessel coronary disease: Use of a decision-analytic model. Circulation 89:1859, 1994.

214. Doliszny, K. M., Luepker, R. V., Burke, G. L., et al.: Estimated contribution of coronary artery bypass graft surgery to the decline in coronary heart disease mortality: The Minnesota Heart Survey. J. Am. Coll. Cardiol. 24:95, 1994.

215. Yusuf, S., Zucker, D., Peduzzi, P., et al.: Effect of coronary artery bypass graft surgery on survival: Overview of 10-year results from randomised trials by the Coronary Artery Bypass Graft Surgery Trialists Collaboration. Lancet 344:565, 1994.

216. Bernstein, S. J., Hilborne, L. H., Leape, L. L., et al.: The appropriateness of use of coronary angiography in New York State. JAMA 269:766, 1993.

217. Leape, L. L., Hilborne, L. H., Park, R. E., et al.: The appropriateness of use of coronary artery bypass graft surgery in New York State. JAMA 269:753, 1993.

218. Cromwell, J., Mitchell, J. B., and Stason, W. B.: Learning by doing in CABG surgery. Med. Care 28:6, 1990.

219. Hannan, E. L., Kilburn, H., Racz, M., et al.: Improving the outcomes of coronary artery bypass surgery in New York State. JAMA 271:761, 1994.

220. Parisi, A. F., Folland, E. D., and Hartigan, P. on behalf of the Veterans

Affairs ACME Investigators: A comparison of angioplasty with medical therapy in the treatment of single-vessel coronary artery disease. N. Engl. J. Med. *326:*10, 1992.

221. RITA Trial Participants: Coronary angioplasty versus coronary artery bypass surgery: The Randomised Intervention Treatment of Angina (RITA) trial. Lancet *341:*573, 1993.

222. Goy, J. J., Eeckhout, E., Burnand, B., et al.: Coronary angioplasty versus left internal mammary artery grafting for isolated proximal left anterior descending artery stenosis. Lancet *343:*1449, 1994.

223. Hamm, C. W., Reimers, J., Ischinger, T., et al. for the German Angioplasty Bypass Surgery Investigation: A randomized study of coro-

nary angioplasty compared with bypass surgery in patients with symptomatic multivessel coronary disease. N. Engl. J. Med. *331:*1037, 1994.

224. King, S. B., III, Lembo, N. J., Weintraub, W. S., et al.: A randomized trial comparing coronary angioplasty with coronary bypass surgery. N. Engl. J. Med. *331:*1044, 1994.

225. Mark, D. B., Nelson, C. L., Califf, R. M., et al.: Continuing evolution of therapy for coronary artery disease. Initial results from the era of coronary angioplasty. Circulation *89:*2015, 1994.

226. Weinstein, M. C., and Stason, W. B.: Cost-effectiveness of coronary artery bypass surgery. Circulation *66*(Suppl. III):56, 1982.

Part V

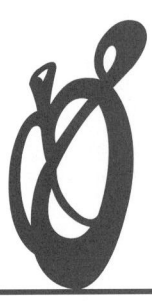

Heart Disease and Disorders of Other Organ Systems

Chapter 54

General Anesthesia and Noncardiac Surgery in Patients with Heart Disease

LEE GOLDMAN

The cardiovascular system of patients undergoing general anesthesia and noncardiac surgical procedures is subject to multiple stresses owing to depression of myocardial contractility and respiration as well as fluctuations in temperature, arterial pressure, ventricular filling pressures, blood volume, and activity of the autonomic nervous system. Complications of anesthesia and operation, such as hemorrhage, infection, fever, pulmonary embolism, and myocardial infarction, impose additional burdens on the cardiovascular system. The patient with cardiac disease who is compensated preoperatively may be unable to meet these increased demands during the perioperative period, in which case arrhythmias, myocardial ischemia, and/or heart failure may develop.[1-3] As a consequence, a substantial proportion of all deaths in most series of noncardiac operations results from cardiovascular complications.

Because both the frequency and the seriousness of cardiovascular complications of general anesthesia and operation are considerably increased in the patient with known cardiovascular disease, the magnitude of these risks must be appreciated to decide on the advisability of noncardiac surgery in the cardiac patient. In addition, both the life expectancy and the quality of life of the patient must be taken into account. For instance, a noncardiac surgical procedure with a high risk, directed to correct a disorder that is not life threatening, may be difficult to justify if the patient's cardiac condition precludes a survival period sufficient to allow the patient to reap the benefits of the operation. Obviously the dangers and disability of the disease for which an operation is being proposed must also be balanced against the risk of the operation itself.

ANESTHESIA

Changes in cardiovascular function during general anesthesia are due to many factors, including direct effects of the anesthetic agent(s) and indirect effects mediated primarily through the autonomic nervous system. In addition, if respiration is inadequately maintained, the resulting hypoxemia, hypercarbia, and acidosis may further depress myocardial contractility and increase cardiac irritability. The interplay of these several variables may produce changes in arterial and central venous pressures, cardiac output, and rate and rhythm. To minimize the risk of operation in the patient with a compromised cardiovascular system, it is essential to minimize these changes.[3]

The choice of the anesthetic approach and the specific anesthetic agents to be used should be made by a qualified anesthesiologist, commonly after careful evaluation of the patient's medical and cardiac condition and often after consultation with the surgeon and the internist or cardiologist. Different anesthesiologists may prefer different anesthetic techniques, and the anesthesiological literature clearly indicates that there is little, if any, correlation between the anesthetic route or agents and the likelihood of major clinical complications. Thus, the skill and experience of the anesthesiologist, including the ability to monitor hemodynamics and respond quickly, are far more important than the specific agent that is used. Although the cardiological consultant should not expect to dictate the anesthetic approach, the quality of the consultation will be improved if the consultant appreciates the clinical pharmacology of the anesthetic agent and the effects of intubation and extubation.

General Anesthesia

The induction of anesthesia is usually accomplished with intravenous anesthetics. With the exception of ketamine, the agents used for the induction of anesthesia commonly lower systemic arterial pressure by about 20 to 30 per cent in healthy patients, but sometimes by a greater amount in hypertensive patients.[4] During laryngoscopy and tracheal intubation, blood pressure can increase by 20 to 30 mm Hg,[4] but such increases can be avoided by adequate topical anesthesia or by nasal intubation because the hypertension appears to be caused by the laryngoscopy rather than by the passage of a tube into the trachea.

INHALATION AGENTS. These agents enter the bloodstream by way of the alveoli and are excreted across the alveoli essentially unchanged. In most major operations a combination of inhalation agents and/or intravenous anesthetics is used.[5]

Nitrous oxide usually is used to supplement other intravenous or inhalation agents. It causes a modest decrease of about 15 per cent in cardiac output but usually does not cause substantial hypotension because of reflex vasoconstriction.

Halothane and related agents also cause a reduction in myocardial contractility,[6] but unlike nitrous oxide, they are not associated with substantial reflex vasoconstriction. Thus, when halothane is added to nitrous oxide, there are often further reductions in arterial pressure because of reductions in cardiac output without concomitant vasoconstriction. Halothane also appears to sensitize the myocardium to catecholamines, sometimes resulting in arrhythmias. *Enflurane* has properties similar to halothane; it appears to result in less sensitization to catecholamines but potentially more risks of hypotension than with halothane. *Isoflurane* appears to have less of a negative inotropic effect than halothane or enflurane, but it can be associated with marked decreases in systemic vascular resistance, and hence a fall in systemic blood pressure.

INTRAVENOUS ANESTHETICS. Among the narcotic analgesics, *morphine* is generally well tolerated, although it does cause venodilation, thereby decreasing preload and cardiac output. *Fentanyl* is less likely to cause as much hypotension or vasodilation as morphine, and it has a shorter duration of action.[7] Like morphine, it tends not to have major effects on myocardial contractility, but it is more likely than morphine to cause bradycardia. *Sufentanil* and *alfentanil* have cardiovascular effects that are generally similar to those of fentanyl.

Short-acting barbiturates, especially *thiopental,* often cause a fall in blood pressure because of depressive actions on myocardial contractility and sympathetic tone.[8] In patients who have severe hypovolemia or severe cardiac dysfunction, serious reductions in cardiac output can occasionally occur after a small dose of thiopental.

Benzodiazepines, including midazolam, can achieve adequate sedation with only mild cardiovascular depression. However, occasionally patients may become apneic or hypotensive after small doses. *Droperidol* causes vasodilation because of its alpha-adrenergic blocking action and its effect on the central nervous system.

Ketamine is unlike other commonly used intravenous anesthetics in that it does not cause cardiovascular depression. Although it does cause some direct myocardial depression, this is commonly counterbalanced by direct stimulation of the central nervous system and by an increase in circulating catecholamines.

MUSCLE RELAXANTS. Drugs used for muscle relaxation also may have cardiovascular effects. *Succinylcholine* can cause bradycardia, which can be reversed or prevented by the administration of atropine. In patients anesthetized with halothane, *pancuronium* and *gallamine* cause an increase in heart rate, arterial pressure, and cardiac output, while *tubocurarine* and *metocurine* result in a fall in mean arterial pressure with mild elevations in heart rate and little, if any, change in cardiac output. *Vecuronium* has essentially no cardiovascular side effects.

Spinal and Epidural Anesthesia

Spinal and epidural anesthesia cause sympathetic denervation, which produces peripheral arteriodilation and venodilation. Systemic vascular resistance may be reduced by 10 to 15 per cent. Venodilation may cause a marked reduction in right ventricular preload as a consequence of sympathetic denervation. Under these circumstances, right ventricular preload depends critically on the effects of gravity on the patient's position, and on the total blood volume.

REGIONAL AND LOCAL ANESTHESIA. Regional and local anesthesia cause cardiovascular effects only to the extent that the agents are absorbed into the bloodstream or where there is sympathetic blockade accompanying the local sensory block. A major concern with local or regional anesthesia is whether the technique is adequate for the planned procedure; the cardiological consultant should not underestimate the cardiovascular consequences of inadequate anesthesia.

Complications of General Anesthetics

In a prospective randomized trial comparing enflurane, fentanyl, halothane, and isoflurane carried out in over 17,000 patients, severe ventricular arrhythmias were more common with halothane, severe hypertension was more common with fentanyl, and severe tachycardia was more common with isoflurane. However, these four agents were not associated with significantly different overall rates of death, myocardial infarction, or stroke, perhaps because the rates of these events were so low.

As of this writing, the potential benefit of regional anesthesia compared with general anesthesia is uncertain,[10–12] in part because the decline in systemic blood pressure from regional anesthesia can cause transient myocardial ischemia.[13] Combined epidural and general anesthesia and analgesia can attenuate sympathetic nervous system hyperactivity, reduce the need for parenteral analgesia, reduce coagulation abnormalities, improve postoperative ventilatory function, and reduce the duration of intensive care unit stay in patients undergoing major vascular surgery.[14,15] In a randomized trial of 173 patients, however, there were no differences in cardiac complications among patients who underwent abdominal aortic surgery with combined epidural and light general anesthesia compared with general anesthesia alone.[16]

Intraoperative Hemodynamics and Arrhythmias

During the operative procedure, it is not uncommon for systolic blood pressure to fall into the range of 95 to 105 mm Hg. Such blood pressure reductions are often brief and may respond to a lightening of the anesthesia or, in 20 to 30 per cent of patients, either to a brisk fluid challenge or the use of intravenous sympathomimetic agents. Any severe reduction in arterial pressure in patients with ischemic heart disease can reduce coronary flow and precipitate myocardial ischemia. In general, such reductions in blood pressure are not associated with major cardiac complications, such as myocardial infarction, unless they are marked and sustained. For example, increased complication rates have been reported for reductions in systolic arterial pressures that exceed approximately 33 per cent of the preoperative blood pressure and that persist for 10 or more minutes, or are more than 50 per cent below the preoperative blood pressure, or for mean arterial pressure reductions of 20 mm Hg or greater for 60 or more minutes, or for 20-mm Hg increases in mean arterial pressure sustained for 15 or more minutes.[17–19] Fluids that are administered to maintain intraoperative blood pressure can potentially cause postoperative fluid overload.

The risk of unplanned intraoperative hypotension is at least as great with spinal or epidural anesthesia as with general anesthesia.[20] However, because spinal and epidural anesthesia are not direct myocardial depressants, they may be advantageous in patients with very severe myocardial dysfunction; but even in those circumstances, well-balanced general anesthesia, sometimes including ketamine, has been used successfully.

Transient bradycardias, such as sinus bradycardia and junctional rhythm, may occur during periods of vagal stimulation. These bradyarrhythmias commonly respond to a lightening of the anesthesia or to the administration of atropine or beta$_1$-adrenoceptor agonists such as isoproterenol or epinephrine. Tachyarrhythmias may result from hypovolemia or vasodilation as well as from sensitization of the myocardium to catecholamines that are circulating and/or released by sympathetic nerve endings in the heart. Tachycardia is poorly tolerated by patients with mitral stenosis (see p. 1007) and may cause myocardial ischemia in patients with coronary artery disease. Therapy with specific antiarrhythmic medications is usually indicated only when the arrhythmia causes circulatory compromise and does not respond to changes in the depth of anesthesia or to attention to problems such as hypoxemia, hypovolemia, hypotension, or the potentially precipitating surgical manipulation.

Positive-pressure ventilation during general anesthesia reduces the return of blood to the right side of the heart and tends to reduce ventricular preload. Fluid that is administered during positive-pressure ventilation does not increase preload to the extent that it would in the patient who is ventilating spontaneously. When the positive-pressure ventilation of general anesthesia ceases, ventricular preload increases, often abruptly, and hypertension or pulmonary congestion may result. Analogous physiological changes can occur with the cessation of spinal or epidural anesthesia because the venodilation caused by these agents also reduces right ventricular preload.

MONITORING. In patients with severe underlying heart disease undergoing noncardiac surgery, it is mandatory to monitor cardiac function during anesthesia,[21] including cardiac rate and rhythm and directly recorded arterial blood pressure. A radial artery line permits not only monitoring of intra-arterial pressure but also frequent sampling for determination of blood gases. In the presence of peripheral vasoconstriction, indirect (cuff) blood pressure measurements may greatly underestimate true arterial pressure. Monitoring of the pulmonary artery (or, preferably, pulmonary artery wedge) pressure and cardiac output is often desirable in patients who are critically ill, who have marginal cardiovascular reserve, who are to undergo prolonged operative procedures in which major blood losses might occur, and in whom hypotensive anesthesia is to be used. Both pulmonary artery wedge pressure and cardiac output can be measured with the aid of a multiple-lumen balloon flotation catheter (Swan-Ganz) and the thermodilution method (see Chap. 6). For detection of intraoperative myocardial ischemia, multiple-lead electrocardiography is preferable and data suggest that transesophageal echocardiography can be reserved for patients with a recent myocardial infarction, unstable angina, advanced heart failure, tight aortic stenosis, or a thoracic aortic aneurysm. Pulmonary capillary wedge pressure is a poor marker of ischemia, but the pulmonary capillary wedge pressure remains the best index of fluid balance.[22] In one randomized, unblinded study, aggressive preoperative optimization of cardiac hemodynamics was associated with a reduced risk of postoperative cardiac morbidity and graft occlusion after peripheral vascular surgery, but the regimen provoked a preoperative myocardial infarction in 2 of 68 patients.[23] In

seriously ill patients, urine output should be monitored with a Foley catheter.

The Operation

Just as consultant cardiologists must understand the pharmacological effects of anesthesia, they must also recognize the physiological effects of the operation and the expected responses to postoperative recuperation.

NATURE OF THE OPERATION. Although ophthalmological surgery[24] and transurethral prostatic resection[25] long have been known almost always to be safe, even in patients with a history of serious cardiac disease, general surgical mortality is often 25 to 50 per cent higher in patients with underlying cardiovascular conditions than in patients with normal cardiac function.[17,20,26–29] Among noncardiac surgical procedures, the highest cardiovascular complication rates are commonly associated with abdominal aortic aneurysm surgery,[26,30] which causes substantial myocardial stress because of aortic cross-clamping and major shifts in fluid and electrolytes. The risk of cardiac complications is also higher in other major abdominal and thoracic procedures than in procedures on the extremities, in large part because of the more difficult postoperative course. Patients who undergo operation for aortic aneurysm, carotid arterial disease, or peripheral vascular disease often have substantial coronary artery disease as well, and the extent of the latter may be underestimated because of the limitations caused by the peripheral arterial disease.

DURATION. The risk of cardiovascular mortality and morbidity is generally correlated with the duration of anesthesia, but this is principally because the longest operations are more often on the aorta or in the abdomen or chest than on the extremities. The risk of major cardiovascular complications does not appear to correlate with the duration of surgery after controlling for the type of surgery, unless the operation is prolonged because of intraoperative complications.

EMERGENCY OPERATION. When an operation is carried out under emergency conditions, it is associated with greatly increased mortality in patients with cardiovascular disease. The risk of postoperative cardiac complications, including postoperative myocardial infarction or cardiac death, is increased anywhere from 2.5- to 4-fold in emergency compared with elective surgery.[20,26,28,31] Part of this increased risk is because patients undergoing emergency operations may often have poorly controlled or unappreciated general medical problems, such as fluid and electrolyte imbalance or hepatic dysfunction.[26,28] However, emergency surgery appears to be an important correlate of postoperative complications, even after controlling for the underlying medical disease.[26,28,31]

The application of careful selection criteria and aggressive hemodynamic monitoring to noncardiac surgical procedures in patients with severe underlying heart disease may reduce the risk of intraoperative and postoperative cardiovascular complications. Thus the risk of a new infarction was reduced by about 40 per cent or more when patients with a history of infarction were aggressively monitored compared with when minimal invasive monitoring was used in the period from 1973 to 1976.[32,33] Although these nonrandomized studies did not control for other secular changes in medical care, it should not be surprising that the application of cardiovascular anesthesiological techniques to noncardiac surgery would have a beneficial effect. Thus, in patients who have suffered a myocardial infarction within the past 3 months, who have angina that is more severe than Canadian Class II (see pp. 12, 13), who have severe heart failure, or who are at very high risk based on indices such as the multifactorial index of cardiac risk in noncardiac surgery[26,28,34–36] (see p. 1765), available data support the use of intra-arterial and pulmonary artery catheters for careful hemodynamic monitoring. In other patients, even those undergoing abdominal aortic surgery, the value of pulmonary artery catheters is unproven.[37–39]

INFLUENCE OF UNDERLYING CARDIOVASCULAR DISEASE

Ischemic Heart Disease

Assessment of Risk

CLINICAL. Ischemic heart disease is a major determinant of perioperative morbidity and mortality. The incidence of perioperative myocardial infarction is increased 10- to 50-fold in patients who have previously suffered infarcts compared with patients who do not have a clinical history of coronary disease.

During the 1970's, several studies reported about a 30 per cent risk of reinfarction or cardiac death when patients were operated on within 3 months of the previous myocardial infarction, about a 15 per cent risk when the operation was performed 3 to 6 months after a prior infarction, and about a 5 per cent risk when the operation was performed more than 6 months after the infarction.[17,20] However, more recent data indicate that the application of invasive hemodynamic monitoring and careful regulation of oxygenation, electrolytes, volume status, and the hematocrit have markedly reduced the complication rate. For example, Rao et al.[32] reported only a 6 per cent reinfarction rate within 3 months after preoperative myocardial infarction and only a 2 per cent reinfarction rate between 3 and 6 months after a myocardial infarction, and then confirmed these low risks in a subsequent report.[33]

Obviously, truly life-saving procedures must be performed almost regardless of the cardiac risk, and purely elective surgery should commonly be delayed for 6 months after infarction, when the cardiovascular risks will have returned to a stable, long-term baseline risk. The more difficult issue is in patients in whom the operation is not truly emergent but is also not purely elective, for example, a patient with severe symptomatic peripheral vascular disease or a patient with a potentially resectable malignant tumor. In such situations one would like to delay operation sufficiently long for cardiac risk to be reduced but not wait a full 6 months. Because full healing of a myocardial infarction usually takes about 4 to 6 weeks, one rational approach is to evaluate the patient with post-myocardial infarction prognostic studies, such as a submaximal exercise tolerance test (Chap. 5)[37] and to use the patient's clinical and cardiological conditions as the guide for surgery sometime between 4 weeks and 3 months after the infarction.

A recent preoperative myocardial infarction increases a patient's relative risk of reinfarction with operation, but the absolute risk depends on a variety of factors in addition to the timing of the infarction. In general, one should be influenced less by whether or not a preoperative myocardial infarction was associated with the development of new Q waves than by the state of left ventricular function and the severity of preoperative angina. Thus, patients who have good exercise tolerance and left ventricular function after infarction and who can resume normal activity levels within 4 to 6 weeks after infarction should be able to undergo operation with relatively small absolute risks, even if their relative risk might be slightly lower if one could wait the full 6 months. By comparison, risks are likely to be substantially higher in patients who have postinfarction angina, large reversible defects on thallium scintigraphy, reduced left ventricular function, marked ST-segment depression with exercise, or other evidence of easily induced ischemia (see p. 1260).

When the patient with angina pectoris is evaluated, the patient's current (preoperative) exercise tolerance should be ascertained and an assessment made as to whether the anginal pattern is stable or unstable (see p. 1290). In patients who can carry objects such as two grocery bags or a young child up a flight of stairs without stopping and without appreciable symptoms, most surgical procedures are generally well tolerated.[40] Physicians should avoid relying on the *frequency* of angina because patients who voluntarily reduce their activity level may also greatly reduce their symptoms. This phenomenon is especially true in patients whose surgical conditions, such as orthopedic disorders or peripheral vascular disease, limit ambulation.

LABORATORY. *Exercise treadmill testing* is an objective means for assessing exercise tolerance and is especially beneficial if the history is unreliable. Unfortunately, the limited sensitivity and specificity of standard electrocardiographic exercise tolerance testing limit the use of this test for diagnosing coronary artery disease (see Chap. 5). In two studies of vascular surgery patients,[41,42] postoperative cardiac complications were significantly less in patients who exercised to higher heart rates and cardiac workloads. The prognostic value of limited exercise tolerance has also been reported in persons over age 65[43,44] in whom the inability to perform 2 minutes of bicycle exercise in a supine position and to raise the heart rate above 99 beats per minute

was an independent important predictor of cardiac complications in noncardiac surgery. Of note was that poor exercise capacity was an independent predictor of cardiac complications, but electrocardiographic changes with exercise were not. Although some investigators have used radionuclide ventriculography to predict risk,[45] in other studies data from resting and/or exercise radionuclide ventriculography did not add important independent information for predicting overall perioperative cardiac risk.[43,46–48]

In patients who are unable to exercise because of noncardiac disability (e.g., intermittent claudication or orthopedic abnormalities), dipyridamole thallium imaging, ambulatory ischemia monitoring, or stress echocardiography can be used to assess perioperative risk. Dipyridamole thallium imaging (see Chap. 10) has been successful in identifying high-risk patients among selected subgroups of patients who are referred for the test prior to undergoing vascular surgery, and it is especially appealing for patients who have abnormal resting electrocardiograms or are taking medications such as digoxin that make electrocardiographic monitoring unreliable for the detection of ischemia.

Among 1410 patients in the five largest series of such patients,[49–53] a reversible defect on thallium scintigraphy had a sensitivity of 85 per cent for predicting postoperative cardiac complications and a specificity of 60 per cent; the relative risk of cardiac complications in a patient with a reversible defect was 9.0. However, when dipyridamole thallium scintigraphy was used in *unselected,* consecutive patients having abdominal aneurysm or major vascular surgery, it was *not* proven useful for predicting perioperative myocardial infarction, myocardial ischemia, or cardiac death.[48,54] In the largest single series of 451 *consecutive,* unselected patients, the presence of a reversible thallium defect had a sensitivity of just 36 per cent, a specificity of 65 per cent, and a relative risk of 1.0 (i.e., it was of no value whatsoever) for predicting major perioperative cardiac events.

Ambulatory electrocardiographic (Holter) monitoring can identify up to 90 per cent of patients who will develop major postoperative ischemic complications.[55] Patients with asymptomatic preoperative ischemia or asymptomatic postoperative ischemia have as high as a 30 per cent risk of developing a clinical event, including myocardial infarction, unstable angina, ischemic pulmonary edema, or cardiac death.[55–57] In contrast, asymptomatic intraoperative ischemia is less predictive.[57,58] Asymptomatic postoperative ischemia, which is found in a substantial minority of patients with or at risk for atherosclerotic disease,[59,60] commonly precedes a clinical event by an hour or more[58,61]; longer episodes of postoperative ischemia are associated with a higher risk of a major clinical event.[61] Patients with perioperative ischemia also have more late cardiac events well after surgery.[58,62]

Although routine transthoracic echocardiography adds little for the prediction of postoperative complications,[63] stress echocardiography after exercise or agents such as dipyridamole or dobutamine can be used to identify patients at markedly increased risk based on the provocation of left ventricular wall motion abnormalities with stress.[64–68] Stress echocardiography appears to be at least as good as dipyridamole thallium scintigraphy or ambulatory ischemia monitoring for predicting complications.

The utility of dipyridamole thallium imaging, ambulatory ischemia monitoring, and stress echocardiography can be improved when these techniques are used in appropriate patient subsets, such as patients with known coronary disease or patients who are undergoing major vascular surgery *and* are over age 70, have ventricular ectopic activity requiring treatment, or have diabetes mellitus requiring treatment.[49] In other types of patients, the lower risk of complications and the lower predictive values of the tests lead to unattractive cost-effectiveness ratios, especially because good results have been reported in series in which preoperative testing has been limited to patients with unstable angina pectoris, uncontrolled arrhythmias, or severe congestive heart failure.[69]

PRIOR CORONARY REVASCULARIZATION. Patients who have undergone successful coronary revascularization can undergo major noncardiac surgical procedures with a low mortality rate,[70] except perhaps in the first 30 days postoperatively. An alternative is percutaneous transluminal coronary angioplasty (PTCA),[71] which can more easily be performed during the course of the same admission.[72] It must be remembered, however, that the operative mortality rate for major noncardiac surgery in patients with stable angina and good exercise tolerance is relatively low, usually in the range of 2 per cent. No randomized controlled trials are available to assess the value of coronary artery bypass grafting or PTCA preoperatively in patients with stable angina pectoris who are about to undergo noncardiac surgery. An analysis of patients in the Coronary Artery Surgery Study registry[70] showed that total operative mortality was 2.4 per cent in 458 patients who had significant coronary artery disease and underwent noncardiac operations without prior coronary artery bypass grafting. By comparison,

operative mortality was 0.9 per cent among 399 patients who had had a coronary artery bypass grafting procedure performed before noncardiac surgery. The mortality was higher in patients who had more severe left ventricular dysfunction or dyspnea on exertion and in patients who used nitrates, were older, and had diabetes. The risk of myocardial infarction, however, was not significantly different between the patients with and without preoperative coronary artery bypass grafting, and the cardiac death rates were only 1.3 per cent and 0.4 per cent, respectively, in the two groups. Furthermore, if one considers the mortality associated with coronary artery bypass grafting, which was 1.4 per cent in the Coronary Artery Surgery Study, the overall mortality from combined coronary artery bypass grafting and noncardiac surgery (2.3 per cent) would be as high as for the noncardiac surgery done in the non-bypassed group (2.4 per cent). Thus the data do not argue in favor of prophylactic coronary artery bypass grafting for patients whose symptoms would not otherwise warrant revascularization, who have stable angina with good exercise tolerance, and who do not have other factors that define a high-risk status (Table 54–1).

TABLE 54–1 RECOMMENDATIONS FOR SPECIAL PERIOPERATIVE CARDIAC EVALUATION AND MANAGEMENT*

	PREOPERATIVE DIAGNOSTIC RECOMMENDATIONS	SPECIAL PERIOPERATIVE CARDIAC TREATMENT RECOMMENDATIONS
1. No known CAD Good cardiac functional status† Class I-II on the cardiac risk index[28] or its equivalent (regardless of CAD risk factors or type of surgery)	None	None
2. Known stable CAD with good (Class I or early Class II) functional status†	None	**Conservative treatment** Continue cardiac medications Postoperative electrocardiogram day 1 and again prior to hospital discharge and to rule out myocardial infarction after any suspicious perioperative events
3. Known CAD, functional status unclear	**Noninvasive testing** Exercise thallium testing if patient can exercise Other tests (dipyridamole thallium, stress echocardiography, or ambulatory ischemia monitor) if patient cannot exercise	If test is negative: Conservative treatment (see above) If test is positive: Aggressive medical treatment or angiography 1. Intensify preoperative CAD medications, identify and address non-CAD risk factors, and consider repeating noninvasive test if major changes have been made (if now negative, use conservative treatment; if still positive, proceed to 2 or 3). 2. More intensive perioperative monitoring and perioperative medications to control blood pressure and pulse or 3. Coronary angiography and revascularization as indicated
4. Known CAD, poor cardiac functional status	None	Aggressive medical treatment or angiography (see above)
5. Poor noncardiac functional status, no CAD or CAD status unclear 　No or few risk factors‡ 　Multiple risk factors	 None Noninvasive testing (see above)	 None If test is negative: Conservative treatment (see above) If test is positive: Aggressive medical treatment or angiography (see above)
6. CAD and Class III or IV on the cardiac risk index or its equivalent	None	Aggressive medical treatment or angiography (see above)

* Does not include procedure-specific decisions regarding routine use of intraoperative electrocardiographic monitoring, arterial catheters, and so on.

† Cardiac functional Class I or early Class II—can walk up a flight of stairs carrying objects weighing 10 to 20 pounds without cardiac symptoms.

‡ Risk factors include age over 70, diabetes mellitus, congestive heart failure, important atrial or ventricular arrhythmias, known vascular disease, or aortic, abdominal, or thoracic surgery.

CAD = coronary artery disease defined as a clinical diagnosis of angina, a prior myocardial infarction, or a positive coronary angiogram.

From Mangano, D. T., and Goldman, L.: Preoperative assessment of the patient with known or suspected coronary disease. N. Engl. J. Med. *333*:1750, 1995. Copyright 1995 Massachusetts Medical Society.

APPROACH TO RISK ASSESSMENT. A practical approach to the patient with known ischemic heart disease or with specified high-risk characteristics[49] should utilize information from the history as well as diagnostic tests.[73-77] If the patient's history indicates reliably that Class I or Class II activities can be performed (see p. 1741), the patient will commonly be raising the double product (the heart rate multiplied by the systolic blood pressure) above the range to be expected with general anesthesia and surgery, and hence should be able to withstand the stress of the procedure.[40,70] If the history is unreliable, exercise testing to assess physical function[41-44] will aid in risk assessment. If the patient is unable to exercise because of noncardiac conditions, ambulatory ischemia monitoring (in a patient with a normal resting electrocardiogram who is not receiving medication such as digoxin), dipyridamole thallium imaging, or stress echocardiography should be used.

Patients who can exercise to Class I or II levels, or who have normal ambulatory ischemia monitoring, dipyridamole thallium imaging, or stress echocardiography can undergo most operations with acceptable risk. Patients who cannot perform Class I or II activities or who have positive ambulatory ischemia monitoring or dipyridamole thallium images should have their medical regimens intensified, if possible, and then have repeat testing. If tests remain positive or physical functioning remains limited after optimization of medical management, coronary arteriography will usually be indicated prior to elective surgery to determine whether coronary revascularization, with either PTCA or coronary bypass surgery, would be feasible.[74] The decision to proceed with revascularization depends more on the functional limitations that result from the coronary lesions than on their anatomical severity. Although the latter is important for long-term prognosis, the former is probably the more relevant correlate of perioperative risk.

USE OF BETA BLOCKERS, CALCIUM ANTAGONISTS, AND NITRATES. Although some concern has been expressed about the use of general anesthesia in patients receiving beta-adrenocepter blocking agents and calcium antagonists, no clinical data indicate that such medications should routinely be discontinued preoperatively. Intravenous esmolol is clearly effective for reducing perioperative tachycardia and hypertension,[78,79] although it is less effective in preventing perioperative ischemia.[78] Aggressive perioperative medication regimens, with special emphasis on beta-adrenoceptor blockers and nitrates, may reduce clinical ischemic events in patients with asymptomatic perioperative ischemia.[80] Intravenous beta-adrenoceptor blockers should be used in patients with a prior history of severe angina that required beta-adrenoceptor blocking agents for its control or in patients who have evidence of postoperative myocardial ischemia or otherwise unexplained hypertension or tachycardia.

Nifedipine can be given sublingually, and nitrates can be given sublingually, topically, or intravenously, to aid in the management of the early postoperative patient with angina. However, these agents cannot substitute for beta-adrenoceptor blockers in patients who have relied on the latter for the control of their ischemic heart disease.

Hypertension

Several studies have documented that patients with hypertension have higher risks of suffering major cardiac complications during or shortly after noncardiac operation than do patients who have always been normotensive. However, most, if not all, of this increased risk is because of the ischemic heart disease, left ventricular dysfunction, renal failure, or other abnormalities that often occur in patients with hypertension. Thus, in patients with mild to moderate hypertension, diastolic pressures below 100 mm Hg, and no evidence of serious end-organ damage, general anesthesia and major noncardiac surgery are generally well

tolerated.[18] Halothane anesthesia may be more likely than other anesthetic agents to induce intraoperative hypotension in patients with a history of hypertension,[18] and hypertensive patients are at higher risk for labile blood pressures and for hypertensive episodes during surgery and especially just after extubation.

Although uncontrolled early studies suggested that the continuation of any hypertensive agents might increase the risk of perioperative hypotension, substantial subsequent data from more careful studies indicate that patients whose hypertension is well controlled do at least as well, if not better, if their medications are, in fact, continued up to the time of operation.[18,81] Thus, although it is neither mandatory nor desirable to delay noncardiac operation for the weeks or months that may be required to achieve ideal blood pressure control in the stable patient with mild to moderate hypertension who has no complications of the hypertension, there is also no apparent benefit, and some potential harm, from discontinuing successful antihypertensive therapy before surgery.

Thiazide and other diuretics cause some degree of chronic volume depletion, and patients receiving these drugs may require more fluid administration early during the operative procedure. If severe perioperative hypertension develops in a patient who has previously been receiving clonidine, and if the clonidine cannot be given orally, it can be administered intramuscularly in doses about one-half as large as the patient's usually daily dose or it can be administered topically,[82] or the patient can be treated with sublingual captopril, with methyldopa, or with a beta blocker. Although it may be desirable to use propranolol, metoprolol, or esmolol intravenously in patients who rely on beta-adrenoceptor blockers for the control of ischemic heart disease, these agents usually need not be given intravenously for prophylaxis in patients who take them for their antihypertensive effects. Intravenous esmolol,[83] labetalol,[84] or nitroprusside can be used for acute episodes of hypertension and methyldopa for nonacute situations.

Valvular Heart Disease and Cardiomyopathy

Patients with valvular heart disease undergoing anesthesia and noncardiac operation are subject to many potential hazards: heart failure, infection, tachycardia, and embolization. As might be expected, patients with no or only mild limitation of activity (i.e., those in Class I or II) tolerate operation well[85] and probably require little more than careful perioperative care and prophylaxis for infective endocarditis (see p. 1099). Those with more serious impairment of cardiac reserve (i.e., those in Class III or IV) tolerate major noncardiac operations poorly, and their prognosis for surviving major surgery is distinctly worse,[20,29] although as is the case for patients with rheumatic heart disease who face the stress of pregnancy (see p. 1848), the risk of operation depends on the functional state of the heart. Patients with symptomatic critical aortic[28] or mitral stenosis are especially prone to sudden death or acute pulmonary edema during the perioperative period; this may occur if demands on cardiac output are suddenly increased or if atrial fibrillation and a rapid ventricular rate are precipitated by anesthesia or operation. Every effort should be made to treat heart failure preoperatively. Patients with severe stenotic or regurgitant valve disease should undergo corrective valvular surgery before an elective operation, whereas those who require an emergency noncardiac operation may benefit from intraoperative hemodynamic monitoring, afterload reduction, and preload augmentation.[86] In some patients with mitral or aortic stenosis, balloon valvuloplasty (see p. 1385) may offer relief of severe obstruction at a low risk when it might not be desirable to carry out valve replacement.[87,88]

HYPERTROPHIC CARDIOMYOPATHY. Patients with hypertrophic cardiomyopathy are intolerant of hypovolemia, which may lead to both a reduction in the elevated preload necessary to maintain cardiac output and an increase in the obstruction to left ventricular outflow (see p. 1414). With careful perioperative, intraoperative, and postoperative care, however, the risk of major cardiac complications in such patients is small. In one series of 56 operations in patients with hypertrophic cardiomyopathy, there were no deaths and the only major complication was a myocardial infarction with congestive heart failure in a patient who also had underlying coronary artery disease. Intraoperative or postoperative hypotension requiring vasoconstrictors occurred in less than 10 per cent of patients.[81,89] It has been suggested that spinal anesthesia may be relatively contraindicated in patients with hypertrophic obstructive cardiomyopathy because of its tendency to reduce systemic vascular resistance and increase venous pooling and thereby increase the severity of obstruction to outflow.[89] Hemodynamic monitoring is not routinely required but may be helpful when these patients undergo major aortic, abdominal, or thoracic procedures.

PROSTHETIC HEART VALVES. Most patients with mechanical prosthetic heart valves receive anticoagulants on a long-term basis to prevent thromboembolic complications (see p. 1066). If these medications are continued through the period of noncardiac operation, hemostasis, hematoma formation, and persistent postoperative bleeding may ensue. Anticoagulants can be temporarily discontinued during the perioperative period with minimal risk of thrombosis. In one study,[90] no thromboembolic complications occurred in 159 patients with prosthetic valves undergoing 180 noncardiac operations when warfarin was discontinued an average of 2.9 days preoperatively and resumed 2.7 days postoperatively.[90] Using a similar approach, Katholi et al. did not observe thromboembolic complications in 25 noncardiac operations on patients with prosthetic aortic valves[91]; however, two such complications occurred in the 10 patients with mitral valve prostheses when anticoagulants were discontinued for noncardiac operations, although these patients had Kay-Shiley caged-disc valves, which are associated with a somewhat higher risk of thromboembolic complications. Because there is a distinct risk of hemorrhagic complications in patients whose anticoagulants have been discontinued for only 2 or 3 days,[90] prothrombin time should be restored to within 20 per cent of normal before one proceeds with the noncardiac surgery.[92] Low molecular weight dextran can be used in the postoperative period to minimize thrombotic complications during the 2 to 3 days when the risk of hemorrhagic complications from resuming anticoagulation is relatively higher. In patients with prostheses that are at high risk for thrombosis, such as caged-disc valves, we recommend discontinuing warfarin, allowing the prothrombin time to come to within about 2 to 3 seconds of normal, using intravenous heparin until about 6 hours before the operation, restarting the heparin about 36 to 48 hours after surgery, and switching to warfarin about 2 to 5 days later. Recent analyses indicate that these various anticoagulation regimens are cost-effective provided that they do not result in lengthening the hospitalization.[93] Even one day of additional hospitalization is relatively costly, and the daily risk of thromboembolic complications is low. Thus, perioperative anticoagulation management should focus on regimens that provide reasonable protection from thromboembolic disease but that permit the patient to be discharged when the surgical condition itself permits.[93]

ENDOCARDITIS PROPHYLAXIS. Patients with valvular heart disease and those with prosthetic heart valves should receive prophylactic antibiotics for surgical procedures likely to be complicated by bacteremias.[94] These include incision and drainage of an infected site; oral, lower gastrointestinal, and gallbladder surgery; and genitourinary procedures. Penicillin can be used before operation involving the upper respiratory tract, with erythromycin or vancomycin an acceptable alternative for patients with a penicillin allergy. For gastrointestinal and genitourinary surgery, which can be complicated by either enterococci or gram-negative bacteremia, gentamicin or streptomycin is required in addition to penicillin. (Suggested doses are given on p. 1099.)

The value of antibiotic prophylaxis before noncardiac operation in patients with *mitral valve prolapse* is controversial (see p. 1035). Most studies indicate that patients with this condition who have murmurs of mitral regurgitation are at substantially higher risk than patients who do not have murmurs,[95] and cost-effectiveness analyses argue *against* routine antibiotic prophylaxis in patients without a murmur.[96,97] At the present time a reasonable compromise is to use antibiotic prophylaxis before surgery in patients with mitral valve prolapse who have clinical evidence of mitral regurgitation.

Congenital Heart Disease

Depending on the nature of the malformation, the patient with congenital heart disease may be subject to one or more potentially serious complications, such as infection, bleeding, hypoxemia, and paradoxical embolization during general anesthesia and operation. As is the case for patients with valvular heart disease, patients with congenital heart disease who are to undergo a surgical procedure require prophylaxis to prevent infective endocarditis (see p. 1098). Patients with cyanotic congenital heart disease and secondary polycythemia are at increased risk of intraoperative and postoperative hemorrhage as a consequence of coagulation defects and thrombocytopenia (see p. 884); this risk can be reduced with careful preoperative phlebotomy, usually to a hematocrit of 50 to 55 per cent.[93]

Patients with cyanotic congenital heart disease tolerate systemic hypotension poorly because this increases the right-to-left shunt and the severity of hypoxemia. In one large series, induction was commonly accomplished using ketamine or fentanyl to avoid hypotension, and anesthesia was maintained with morphine and nitrous oxide or with large doses of fentanyl with or without nitrous oxide. Halothane in very low concentrations can be used in patients with less severe degrees of cyanosis.[99] With use of careful anesthetic techniques, the risk of major anesthetic complications is extremely low even in very ill and cyanotic patients. However, spinal anesthesia, which causes peripheral arterial vasodilation and reduces venous return, can have deleterious hemodynamic effects in patients with cyanotic congenital heart disease. Occasionally, infusion of a vasoconstrictor such as phenylephrine may be required to raise systemic vascular resistance and thereby decrease the magnitude of the right-to-left shunt. Because patients with right-to-left shunts are subject to the risk of paradoxical emboli, including air emboli, meticulous techniques with regard to intravenous solutions and injections are mandatory to prevent such complications.

Congestive Heart Failure

Congestive heart failure is a major determinant of perioperative risk, irrespective of the nature of the underlying cardiac disorder. Mortality with noncardiac surgery increases with worsening cardiac class[20,40] and with the presence of pulmonary congestion,[20,26] especially when a third heart sound is noted.[28] Because the perioperative mortality rate appears to depend more on the patient's condition at the time of operation than on the most severe depression of cardiovascular status the patient has ever experienced, it is clearly advisable to treat the congestive heart failure before the contemplated major elective noncardiac surgery. However, because such a therapeutic regimen almost always includes a diuretic, both hypovolemia and hypokalemia are potential problems for patients treated just before operation. It is therefore desirable, if possible, to stabilize the patient's condition by treating heart failure for approximately 1 week rather than for only 1 or 2 days before the contemplated operation. Also, great care should be taken to avoid dehydration because hypovolemic patients may be especially likely to experience marked hypotension during the early phases of anesthesia. Perioperative cardiogenic pulmonary edema develops in about 2 per cent of patients over age 40 undergoing major noncardiac surgery without prior congestive heart failure, in about 6 per cent of patients whose heart failure is well controlled, and in about 16 per cent of patients whose heart failure persists on physical examination or chest radiograph before surgery.[20]

Although digitalis can counteract the myocardial depressant actions of many general anesthetic agents,[93] the value of digitalis in patients with congestive heart failure appears to be limited to certain subsets of patients, especially those who have a third heart sound.[94] Digitalis is one of the most common causes of iatrogenic complications in hospitalized patients, and it may be associated with a higher risk of intraoperative bradyarrhythmias.[20] Therefore, preoperative digitalization is *not* recommended except in patients whose congestive heart failure is sufficiently severe that they would normally meet the criteria for long-term digitalization (see p. 499).

Arrhythmias

Arrhythmias may be a manifestation of the severity of underlying left ventricular dysfunction and of coronary artery disease and hence are frequently markers for the likelihood of perioperative cardiac complications. Because patients who have ventricular premature contractions but no evidence of underlying heart disease on detailed examination have an apparently normal cardiac prognosis,[102] ventricular premature contractions in the *absence* of underlying heart disease should not be considered a risk factor for cardiac complications with noncardiac surgery. Atrial arrhythmias are often a manifestation of atrial enlargement, and a supraventricular rhythm other than sinus appears to be a risk factor for the development of perioperative complications.[28]

Although it would be ideal for arrhythmias to be well controlled preoperatively, the risks associated with arrhythmias appear to be related more to the underlying cardiac disease than to the arrhythmias per se. Therefore, there currently is no evidence that asymptomatic ventricular premature contractions require aggressive preoperative control or prophylactic intraoperative suppression. Similarly, in the patient with well-controlled atrial fibrillation, cardioversion need not be carried out specifically because of planned noncardiac surgery if such a management option would not otherwise be appropriate.

Patients who are most at risk for the development of postoperative supraventricular tachyarrhythmias include elderly patients undergoing pulmonary surgery, patients with subcritical valvular stenoses, and patients with prior histories of supraventricular tachyarrhythmias. Although data are less than decisive, digitalis may reduce the risk of the development of postoperative supraventricular tachycardia in such patients,[103] and the rate of the supraventricular tachycardia may be slower in the digitalized patient.[20] Thus, prophylactic preoperative digitalization is reasonable in elderly patients undergoing major pulmonary surgery, patients with subcritical valvular stenoses, and patients with a prior history of symptomatic supraventricular tachycardias, except if the latter are already taking other medications for the control of such arrhythmias. Another alternative is to use verapamil or adenosine to treat arrhythmias acutely when they occur.

CONDUCTION DEFECTS. The patient with *complete heart block* (see p. 687) must respond to the demands for an increased cardiac output by augmenting stroke volume, but this compensatory response is prevented in many patients by a concurrent impairment of cardiac contractility. In addition, most anesthetic agents depress myocardial contractility and/or produce peripheral vasodilatation. Furthermore, anesthesia may cause further depression of the automaticity, and therefore the ventricular rate, of the patient with heart block. Thus patients with untreated complete heart block may be unable to meet the increased demands placed on the cardiovascular system by anesthesia and operation, and a permanent or temporary pacemaker should be inserted before general anesthesia, even in asymptomatic patients (Chap. 24).

Another problem is presented by the patient with *chronic bifascicular block* (see p. 121).[20,104] A significant fraction of patients developing this abnormality in the course of an acute myocardial infarction progress to complete heart block, often accompanied by sudden severe hemodynamic compromise (see p. 1233). In several series, progression from bifascicular to complete heart block has not been documented during the perioperative period in patients without a previous history of third-degree heart block. Therefore, we do *not* recommend prophylactic pacemaker placement for such patients or for patients with first-degree atrioventricular (AV) block or type I second-degree AV block (Wenckebach), although a pacemaker should always be available in the operating room for emergency placement. However, in patients who have bifascicular block, and either type II second-degree AV block or a history of unexplained syncope or transient third-degree AV block, the risk of development of complete heart block is much higher, and a temporary pacemaker should be inserted preoperatively.

THE PATIENT WITH A PERMANENT PACEMAKER. When a patient with a permanent pacemaker in situ is about to undergo operation, the device should be carefully evaluated to ensure that it is functioning properly preoperatively (Chap. 24). Demand pacemakers are sensitive to electromagnetic interference, such as that produced by the electrocautery, which may result in failure to pace. The danger of this potentially hazardous interaction can be reduced by placing the indifferent plate of the cautery unit as far as possible from the lead and pulse generator, and the electrocautery should be used in brief bursts rather than continuously. Also, a magnet should be available in the operating room to convert the pacemaker from the demand to the fixed-rate mode. Because the cautery may also interfere with the electrocardiographic monitor and render it temporarily uninterpretable, arterial pressure should be monitored directly when the cautery is being used on patients with permanent pacemakers.

In general, a prophylactic *temporary pacemaker* should be inserted before noncardiac operations only if the patient meets the indications for permanent pacemaker insertion (see p. 707) and the operation should not be delayed for the time required for a permanent pacemaker insertion, or if the operative course is likely to be complicated by transient bacteremia. In such situations a temporary pacemaker should be placed initially, and the permanent pacemaker can be inserted after the operation. The occasional exception is the patient who has a severe bradycardic response to vagal stimuli and who might be difficult to manage during a major operation without a pacemaker.

General Medical Problems

Patients with heart disease whose general medical status is complicated by diabetes, renal insufficiency, hepatic abnormalities, hypoxemia, or electrolyte abnormalities have a higher risk of cardiac complications, presumably because these nonmedical conditions exacerbate the stress placed on the heart by the operation.[20,26,28] Morbidity is also higher in markedly obese patients[105] because obesity is often associated with abnormal cardiorespiratory function, metabolic function, and hemostasis. Every effort should be made to correct any of these noncardiac problems before operation, and the potential long-term benefits of surgery must also be interpreted in light of the patient's general prognosis.

POSTOPERATIVE COMPLICATIONS

MYOCARDIAL INFARCTION. Transient intraoperative ischemia does not appear to be a major correlate of postoperative ischemic events in patients undergoing noncardiac surgery,[57,58] but most clinical postoperative ischemic events are preceded by asymptomatic episodes of postoperative ischemia that can be detected by ambulatory ischemic monitoring.[56–59,61] Although series from before 1980 showed a peak in the risk of myocardial infarction on about the third postoperative day,[106] more recent series show that a combination of frequent electrocardiograms and cardiac enzymes detects many non–Q-wave infarctions in the first 24 hours postoperatively.[55,107–110] Although care must be taken in interpreting cardiac enzymes in the perioperative period,[109] it may be that supply-demand imbalances cause an early peak in non–Q-wave postoperative infarctions, whereas the hypercoagulable postoperative state leads to a later (3 to 5 days postoperatively) peak in Q-wave infarctions. For both types of infarction, postoperative stresses include general surgical complications, hypoxia and other pulmonary complications, fluid and electrolyte abnormalities, and the stresses of modern postoperative ambulation protocols. Substantial data indicate that prophylactic anticoagulation with low-dose heparin reduces the risk of postoperative thromboembolic complications,[111] and such therapy is routinely indicated in most cardiac patients who undergo noncardiac operations. In fact, such anticoagulation regimens may permit a more gradual postoperative ambulation protocol in cardiac patients, and hence possibly lower the incidence of postoperative myocardial infarction.

Myocardial infarction occurring in the perioperative period is often painless. Obviously, then, the incidence of perioperative infarction is underestimated if electrocardiograms and serial estimations of serum creatine kinase isoenzyme (MB fraction) are not obtained routinely during the postoperative period in high-risk patients.[106]

HYPERTENSION. Postoperative hypertension is most likely to occur soon after the cessation of positive-pressure ventilation or in the recovery room, and it is more common after carotid endarterectomy and major abdominal vascular procedures.[18]

Common precipitants include fluid overload after cessation of positive-pressure ventilation, hypoxemia, anxiety, and pain. The principal therapeutic approaches should therefore concentrate on assuring adequate oxygenation, pain control, and fluid control. In general, supplemental oxygen, morphine, and diuretics are the mainstays of the treatment of postoperative hypertension. Nitroprusside (see p. 858) and labetalol[84] (see p. 854) are the preferred medications for more severe hypertension. Intravenous hydralazine in small doses is effective for treating postoperative hypertension, but it has the potential of precipitating supraventricular tachyarrhythmias.

CONGESTIVE HEART FAILURE. Although postoperative heart failure may be precipitated by myocardial infarction or ischemia, a substantial proportion of the cases are directly caused by excess fluid administration. Heart failure tends to occur soon after cessation of positive-pressure ventilation and again at about 24 to 48 hours after operation, when the fluid that was given in the perioperative period is mobilized from the extravascular sites. Diuretics, often given intravenously, and rarely supplemented by digitalis glycosides, are usually sufficient therapy for postoperative congestive heart failure.

POSTOPERATIVE ARRHYTHMIAS. Arrhythmias are common after operation and are often a manifestation of a noncardiac complication, such as bleeding, infection, or an acid-base or electrolyte imbalance occurring in a patient with heart disease. Management of such arrhythmias often requires recognition and correction of extracardiac factors.

In one study of 916 patients with sinus rhythm throughout the course of major noncardiac surgery, 35 patients (4 per cent) developed new supraventricular tachyarrhythmias postoperatively.[112] Of these 35 patients, 46 per cent had acute cardiac conditions, 31 per cent had major infections, 29 had preexisting hypotension, 26 per cent had anemia, 23 per cent had metabolic derangements, 23 per cent had received new parenteral drugs that could be implicated, and 20 per cent were hypoxic. Forty per cent of the patients required no new therapy with cardiac medications, and only two patients required electrical cardioversion; the arrhythmias of all treated patients reverted to sinus rhythm. No deaths were related to the supraventricular tachyarrhythmias per se, but a substantial proportion of the patients in whom these arrhythmias occurred died as a result of the concurrent medical problems. Thus, a new postoperative supraventricular tachyarrhythmia should prompt a search for remediable medical problems. Direct antiarrhythmic therapy is often unnecessary and is usually secondary in importance to correction of the underlying cause of the arrhythmia.

Sinus tachycardia is the most common rhythm disturbance in the postoperative patient. Multiple noncardiac etiological factors have been identified, including pain, hypovolemia, hypervolemia, fever, anemia, hypoxemia, pulmonary emboli, anxiety, infection, hypotension, and electrolyte abnormalities (especially hypokalemia). These noncardiac factors are much more common causes of sinus tachycardia in the postoperative cardiac patient than is either myocardial infarction or heart failure. Sinus tachycardia not caused by congestive heart failure does not slow with cardiac glycosides. The therapeutic/toxic ratio of these drugs is actually reduced by most of the above-mentioned noncardiac causes of sinus tachycardia, and therefore digitalis glycosides are not considered appropriate for postoperative patients unless the sinus tachycardia is caused by impaired cardiac function.

Atrial fibrillation is also a common postoperative arrhythmia. Atrial dilatation, which lowers the threshold for development of this arrhythmia, may result from heart failure, mitral valve disease, and/or hypervolemia. Noncardiac precipitants include pneumonia, atelectasis, and pulmonary emboli. Initially, the postoperative patient with atrial fibrillation should be treated with a digitalis glycoside or verapamil; in addition, a beta-adrenoceptor blocker can be used to help gain rapid control of the ventricular rate. Cardioversion is usually delayed until the precipitating factors have been eliminated, because in the patient who has cardioversion before clearing of the atelectasis or pneumonia there is frequently reversion to atrial fibrillation, whereas in the patient whose pulmonary problem or congestive heart failure is adequately treated there is often spontaneous reversion to sinus rhythm.

Atrial flutter is often poorly tolerated because of the rapid ventricular rate and the difficult pharmacological management. Cardioversion is the treatment of choice.

IMPLICATIONS OF POSTOPERATIVE COMPLICATIONS FOR LONG-TERM MANAGEMENT. When a patient develops a perioperative myocardial infarction, the evaluation and the recuperative process generally should be analogous to when a myocardial infarction occurs in other patients (see Chap. 37). Because postoperative congestive heart failure is commonly precipitated by iatrogenic fluid overload, the patient commonly does not need long-term therapy for congestive heart failure. Similarly, perioperative arrhythmias are often precipitated by specific stimuli, and the patient with a postoperative arrhythmia should not automatically be consigned to long-term antiarrhythmic therapy. In patients who develop either postoperative congestive heart failure or arrhythmias, it is often appropriate to discontinue new cardiac therapies several days before discharge and observe the patient to see whether long-term therapy is indicated.

THE ROLE OF THE MEDICAL CONSULTANT

The physician called on to evaluate the status of a patient with suspected or overt cardiac disease before elective or emergency noncardiac surgery must first determine whether cardiovascular disease is present and, if it is, must identify those factors that may increase the risk of operation. It may be necessary to invest considerable time and effort to prepare the patient for operation. In addition, the patient must be followed carefully after operation to detect and manage the cardiac problems that frequently complicate the postoperative period.

ESTIMATION OF RISK. A few patients have such compelling reasons for operation (e.g., rupturing aortic aneurysm, perforated or necrotic bowel, life-threatening hemorrhage, or some forms of intestinal obstruction) that estimation of operative risk is an academic exercise, because failure to operate almost certainly will result in the patient's death. Often, however, the timing or even the performance of an operation is elective, and under these circumstances estimation of risk is an important aspect of the medical consultant's role. Certain cardiovascular problems, such as recent myocardial infarction (less than 1 month), inadequately treated congestive heart failure, and severe mitral or aortic stenosis, are *absolute contraindications* to *elective* surgery. *Relative contraindications,* which commonly require further clinical or laboratory evaluation or treatment before elective surgery, include more remote myocardial infarction (1 month to 6 months previously), angina pectoris, mild heart failure, cyanotic congenital heart disease with severe polycythemia, and a coagulation abnormality. Several other problems should be recognized and treated before operation: anemia, hypovolemia, polycythemia, pulmonary disease causing hypoxemia, adrenal hyporesponsiveness secondary to long-term administration of adrenal steroids, hypertension, electrolyte abnormalities, as well as the entire gamut of cardiac arrhythmias. Considerable judgment must be exercised when one or more of the above-mentioned problems are present and when a patient requires prompt surgical treatment but the situation is not a true emergency, as for neoplastic disease.

To identify those preoperative factors associated with the development of cardiac complications after major noncardiac operation in patients over 40 years of age, one analysis[20] identified nine independently significant correlates of life-threatening and fatal cardiac complications. When these factors were weighted based on their relative significance as predictors of cardiac outcome, a multifactorial index was developed for predicting perioperative risk. Other investigations of relatively unselected patients have noted similar risk factors[26,35] (Table 54–2).

The value of the information in this index has been confirmed in large prospective series of general surgical patients,[26,34,35] in a large series of patients who had prior coronary or valvular heart surgery,[113] and in several other studies.[43,107,114,115] In one series,[35] risk stratification was equally good when several minor modifications were made in point assignment and when a prior history of Class III or IV angina, unstable angina, and pulmonary edema was included in the index.

However, because the index was derived from unselected general surgical patients above age 40, it appears to underestimate risk by about 40 per cent in patients who undergo

TABLE 54–2 THREE COMMONLY USED CARDIAC RISK INDICES

FACTOR	ORIGINAL INDEX (Goldman et al.)[28]		DETSKY et al†[35]		LARSEN et al‡[26]	
	Definition	Points	Definition	Points	Definition	Points
1. Ischemic heart disease	MI within 6 months	10	MI within 6 months	10	MI within 3 months	11
			MI more than 6 months ago	5	No, but older infarction and/or angina pectoris	3
			Canadian Cardiovascular Society angina			
			Class III	10		
			Class IV	20		
			Unstable angina within 6 months	10		
2. Congestive heart failure	S₃ gallop or jugular venous distention	11	Pulmonary edema		Persistent pulmonary congestion	12
			Within 1 week	10	No, but previous pulmonary edema	8
			Ever	5	Neither, but previous heart failure	4
3. Cardiac rhythm	Rhythm other than sinus or PACs on last preoperative ECG	7	Rhythm other than sinus or sinus plus PACs on last preoperative ECG	5		
	>5 PVCs/min documented at any time before operation	7	>5 PVCs/min at any time prior to surgery	5		
4. Valvular heart disease	Important aortic stenosis	3	Suspected critical aortic stenosis	20		
5. General medical status	pO₂ < 60 or pCO₂ > 50 mm Hg, K < 3.0 or HCO₃ < 20 mEq/L, BUN > 50 or Cr > 3.0 mg/dl, abnormal AST, signs of chronic liver disease or bedridden from noncardiac causes	3	Same as for original	5	Serum creatinine above 0.13 mmol/L⁻¹	2
					Diabetes mellitus	3
6. Age	Age > 70 yr	5	Age over 70	5		
7. Type of surgery	Intraperitoneal, intrathoracic, or aortic operation	3	Emergency operation	10	Emergency operation	3
					Aortic operation	5
	Emergency operation	4			Other intraperitoneal/pleural operation	3

MI = myocardial infarction; PAC = premature atrial contraction; PVC = premature ventricular contraction.
* Derived from 1001 consecutive unselected patients over age 40 undergoing major noncardiac surgery using multivariable analysis.
† Modification of original index based on the clinical judgments of the authors.
‡ Derived from 2609 patients over age 40 undergoing non-minor noncardiac surgery using multivariable analysis.
Complications were defined as myocardial infarction, cardiogenic pulmonary edema, sustained ventricular tachycardia or ventricular fibrillation, or cardiac death.
Grouping and outcomes for the various indices—original index: Class I = 0 to 35 points, Class II = 6 to 12 points, Class III = 13 to 25 points, Class IV = >25 points (see Fig. 54–1); Detsky et al.: points integrated with prior probability to compute a continuous score; Larsen et al.: 0 to 5 points = 11 (0.5%) complications in 2022 patients; 6 to 7 points = 12 (3.8%) complications in 317 patients; 8 to 14 points = 27 (11%) complications in 239 patients; > 15 points = 18 (58%) complications in 31 patients. For the original index, the area under the receiver operating characteristic curve (ROC) (a summary measure of both sensitivity and specificity where 1.0 indicates perfect discrimination of complicated versus uncomplicated patients, while a value of 0.5 indicates discrimination that is not better than chance) was 0.81 in the original derivation set of patients, 0.80 (34) and 0.77 (26) (estimated) in other studies of unselected consecutive patients, 0.81 in patients with prior coronary or valvular surgery (113), 0.69 in patients having medical consultations (35,116), and 0.63 in patients undergoing abdominal aortic aneurysm surgery (30). All of these ROC values were significantly better than chance. From Mangano, D. T., and Goldman, L.: Preoperative assessment of the patient with known or suspected coronary disease. N. Engl. J. Med. *333*:1750, 1995.

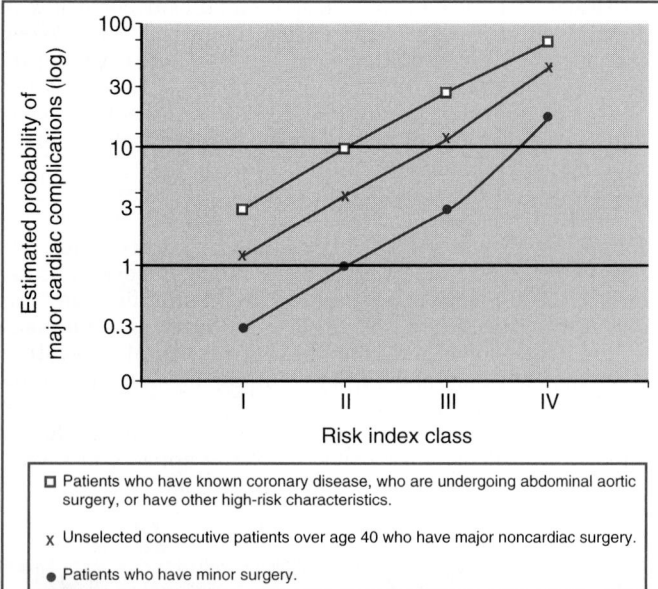

FIGURE 54–1. Approximate risk of major cardiac complications in different types of patients as adjusted using the original multifactorial index.[28] The risks of major complications, which are defined as pulmonary edema and arrhythmic cardiac arrest, as well as myocardial infarction and cardiac death, were calculated by multiplying the prior odds of complications times the likelihood ratio for each class. Classes are defined as follows: Class I = 0 to 5 points; Class II = 6 to 12 points; Class III = 13 to 25 points; and Class IV = 26 or more points. Points are calculated as follows: myocardial infarction within 6 months = 10; age over 70 = 5; S_3 gallop or jugular venous distention = 11; important aortic stenosis = 3; rhythm other than sinus or sinus plus APBs on last preoperative ECG = 7; more than 5 premature ventricular beats per minute at any time preoperatively = 7; poor general medical status [pO_2 < 60 mm Hg; pCO_2 > 50 mm Hg; K^+ < 3.0 mEq/L; HCO_3 < 20 mEq/L; BUN > 50 mg/dl (18 mmol/L); creatinine > 3 mg/dl (260 mmol/L); abnormal SGOT or signs of liver disease; bedridden from noncardiac causes] = 3; intraperitoneal, intrathoracic, or aortic surgery = 3; emergency operation = 4. (From Mangano, D. T., and Goldman, L.: Preoperative assessment of the patient with known or suspected coronary disease. N. Engl. J. Med. *333*:1750, 1995. Copyright Massachusetts Medical Society.)

resection of an abdominal aortic aneurysm,[30] and it also underestimates risk in patients who are selected on the basis of any high-risk status such as patients with stable coronary artery disease, in whom the risk of a major event is 2 to 4 per cent, even in the absence of other risk factors. One way to take into account the fact that some patients have higher baseline risks is to know the baseline probability of cardiac complications for specific types of patients or types of surgery and then to modify these "pre-test" probabilities on the basis of the patient's cardiac condition.[35,73,74,116,117] As shown in Figure 54–1, this can be a useful approach to estimating the risk of major cardiac complications. Even at its best, however, any index for predicting cardiac complications should be viewed as an aid and not as a crutch; it should supplement, not substitute for, clinical judgment.

PREPARATION OF THE PATIENT FOR ANESTHESIA AND OPERATION. Careful preparation of the cardiac patient for operation may diminish the frequency and seriousness of intraoperative and postoperative complications. The medical consultant should, after appropriate discussion with the surgeon, be prepared to urge postponement or cancellation of an elective operation or to insist on sufficient time to institute any measures that are necessary to minimize risk. The consultant should attempt to be brief and to the point, and to provide a limited number of explicit, relevant sug-

gestions.[118] The cardiological consultant should work closely with the anesthesiologist and the surgeon so that their talents may be combined to maximize the likelihood of a favorable outcome.

REFERENCES

ANESTHESIA

1. Breslow, M. J., Miller, C. F., and Rogers, M. (eds.): Perioperative Management. St. Louis, C. V. Mosby Co., 1990.
2. Mangano, D. T. (ed.): Perioperative Cardiac Assessment. Philadelphia, J. B. Lippincott Co., 1990.
3. Rogers, M. C., Tinker, J. H., Covino, B. G., and Longnecker, D. E. (eds.): Principles and Practice of of Anesthesiology. St. Louis, Mosby-Year Book, 1993.
4. Derbyshire, D. R., Chmielewski, A., Fell, D., et al.: Plasma catecholamine responses to endotracheal intubation. Br. J. Anaesth. *55*:855, 1983.
5. Longnecker, D. E., and Miller, F. L.: Pharmacology of inhalational anesthetics. *In* Rogers, M. C., Tinker, J. H., Covino, B. G., and Longnecker, D. E. (eds.): Prinicples and Practice of Anesthesiology. St. Louis, Mosby-Year Book, 1993, p. 1053.
6. Rusy, B. F., and Komai, H.: Anesthetic depression of myocardial contractility: A review of possible mechanisms. Anesthesiology *67*:745, 1987.
7. Philbin, D. M., Rosow, C. E., Schneider, R. C., et al.: Fentanyl and sufentanil anesthesia revisited: How much is enough? Anesthesiology *73*:5, 1990.
8. White, P. F.: Clinical uses of intravenous anesthetic and analgesic infusions. Anesth. Analg. *68*:161, 1989.
9. Forrest, J. B., Cahalan, M. K., Redher, K., et al.: Multicenter study of general anesthesia. II. Results. Anesthesiology *72*:262, 1990.
10. Scott, N. B., and Kehlet, H.: Regional anaesthesia and surgical morbidity. Br. J. Surg. *75*:299, 1988.
11. Yeager, M. P.: Regional anesthesia for the patient with heart disease. Pro: Regional anesthesia is preferable to general anesthesia for the patient with heart disease. J. Cardiothorac. Anesth. *3*:793, 1989.
12. Beattie, C.: Regional anesthesia for the patient with heart disease. Con: Regional anesthesia is not preferable to general anesthesia for the patient with heart disease. J. Cardiothorac. Anesth. *3*:797, 1989.
13. Saada, M., Duval, A. M., Bonnet, F., et al.: Abnormalities in myocardial segmental wall motion during lumbar epidural anesthesia. Anesthesiology *71*:26, 1989.
14. Her, C., Kizelshteyn, G., Walker, V., et al.: Combined epidural and general anesthesia for abdominal aortic surgery. J. Cardiovasc. Anesth. *4*:552, 1990.
15. Tuman, K. J., McCarthy, R. J., March, R. J., et al.: Effects of epidural anesthesia and analgesia on coagulation and outcome after major vascular surgery. Anesth. Analg. *73*:696, 1991.
16. Baron, J. F., Bertrand, M., Barre, E., et al.: Combined epidural and general anesthesia versus general anesthesia for abdominal aortic surgery. Anesthesiology *75*:611, 1991.
17. Steen, P. A., Tinker, J. H., and Tarhan, S.: Myocardial reinfarction after anesthesia and surgery. JAMA *239*:2566, 1978.
18. Goldman, L., and Caldera, D. L.: Risks of general anesthesia and elective surgery in the hypertensive patient. Anesthesiology *50*:285, 1979.
19. Charlson, M. E., MacKenzie, C. R., Gold, J. P., et al.: The preoperative and intraoperative hemodynamic predictors of postoperative myocardial infarction or ischemia in patients undergoing noncardiac surgery. Ann. Surg. *210*:637, 1989.
20. Goldman, L., Caldera, D. L., Southwick, F. S., et al.: Cardiac risk factors and complications in non-cardiac surgery. Medicine *57*:357, 1978.
21. Eisenberg, M. J., London, M. J., Leung, J. M., et al.: Monitoring for myocardial ischemia during noncardiac surgery. A technology assessment of transesophageal echocardiography and 12-lead electrocardiography. JAMA *268*:210, 1992.
22. Van Daele, M. E. R. M., Sutherland, G. R., Mitchell, M. M., et al.: Do changes in pulmonary capillary wedge pressure adequately reflect myocardial ischemia during anesthesia? Circulation *81*:865, 1990.
23. Berlauk, J. F., Abrams, J. H., Gilmour, I. J., et al.: Preoperative optimization of cardiovascular hemodynamics improves outcome in peripheral vascular surgery. A prospective, randomized clinical trial. Ann. Surg. *214*:289, 1991.
24. Backer, C. L., Tinker, J. H., Robertson, D. M., and Vliestra, R. E.: Myocardial reinfarction following local anesthesia for ophthalmic surgery. Anest. Analg. *59*:257, 1980.
25. Erlik, D., Valero, A., Birkhan, J., and Gersh, I.: Prostatic surgery and the cardiovascular patient. Br. J. Urol. *40*:53, 1968.
26. Larsen, S. F., Olesen, K. H., Jacobsen, E., et al.: Prediction of cardiac risk in non-cardiac surgery. Eur. Heart J. *8*:179, 1987.
27. Ashton, C. M., Petersen, N. J., Wray, N. P., et al.: The incidence of perioperative myocardial infarction in men undergoing noncardiac surgery. Ann. Intern. Med. *118*:504, 1993.
28. Goldman, L., Caldera, D. L., Nussbaum, R. R., et al.: Multifactorial index of cardiac risk in noncardiac surgical procedures. N. Engl. J. Med. *297*:845, 1977.
29. Forrest, J. B., Rehder, K., Cahalan, M. K., and Goldsmith, C. H.: Multi-

center study of general anesthesia. III. Predictors of severe perioperative adverse outcomes. Anesthesiology 76:3, 1992.

30. Jeffrey, C. C., Kunsman, J., Cullen, D. J., and Brewster, D. C.: A prospective evaluation of cardiac risk index. Anesthesiology 58:462, 1983.

31. Shah, K. B., Kleinman, B. S., Rao, T. L. K., et al.: Angina and other risk factors in patients with cardiac diseases undergoing noncardiac operations. Anesth. Analg. 70:240, 1990.

32. Rao, T. L. K., Jacobs, K. H., and El-Etr, A. A.: Reinfarction following anesthesia in patients with myocardial infarction. Anesthesiology 59:499, 1983.

33. Shah, K. B., Kleinman, B. S., Sami, H., et al.: Reevaluation of perioperative myocardial infarction in patients undergoing noncardiac operations. Anesth. Analg. 71:231, 1990.

INFLUENCE OF UNDERLYING CARDIOVASCULAR DISEASE

34. Zeldin, R. A.: Assessing cardiac risk in patients who undergo noncardiac surgical procedures. Can. J. Surg. 27:402, 1984.

35. Detsky, A. S., Abrams, H. B., McLaughlin, J. R., et al.: Predicting cardiac complications in patients undergoing non-cardiac surgery. J. Gen. Intern. Med. 1:211, 1986.

36. Shah, K., Kleinman, B., Rao, T., et al.: Reduction in mortality from cardiac causes in Goldman class IV patients. J. Cardiothorac. Anesth. 2:789, 1988.

37. Isaacson, I. J., Lowdon, J. D., Berry, A. J., et al.: The value of pulmonary artery and central venous monitoring in patients undergoing abdominal aortic reconstructive surgery: A comparative study of two selected, randomized groups. J. Vasc. Surg. 12:754, 1990.

38. Garnett, R. L.: Pro: A pulmonary artery catheter should be used in all patients undergoing abdominal aortic surgery. J. Cardiothorac. Vasc. Anesth. 7:750, 1993.

39. Ellis, J. E.: Con: Pulmonary artery catheters are not routinely indicated in patients undergoing elective abdominal aortic reconstruction. J. Cardiothorac. Vasc. Anesth. 7:753, 1993.

40. McPhail, N., Menkis, A., Shariatmadar, A., et al.: Statistical prediction of cardiac risk in patients who undergo vascular surgery. Can. J. Surg. 28:404, 1985.

41. McPhail, N., Calvin, J. E., Shariatmadar, A., et al.: The use of preoperative exercise testing to predict cardiac complications after arterial reconstruction. J. Vasc. Surg. 7:60, 1988.

42. Cutler, B. S., Wheeler, H. B., Paraskos, J. A., and Cardullo, P. A.: Applicability and interpretation of electrocardiographic stress testing in patients with peripheral vascular disease. Am. J. Surg. 141:501, 1981.

43. Gerson, M. C., Hurst, J. M., Hertzberg, V. S., et al.: Cardiac prognosis in noncardiac geriatric surgery. Ann. Intern. Med. 103:832, 1985.

44. Gerson, M. C., Hurst, J. M., Hertzberg, V. S., et al.: Prediction of cardiac and pulmonary complications related to elective abdominal and noncardiac thoracic surgery in geriatric patients. Am. J. Med. 88:101, 1990.

45. Pasternack, P. F., Imparato, A. M., Riles, T. S., et al.: The value of the radionuclide angiogram in the prediction of perioperative myocardial infarction in patients undergoing lower extremity revascularization procedures. Circulation 72(Suppl. 2):13, 1985.

46. Franco, C. D., Goldsmith, J., Veith, F. J., et al.: Resting gated pool ejection fraction: A poor predictor of perioperative myocardial infarction in patients undergoing vascular surgery for infrainguinal bypass grafting. J. Vasc. Surg. 10:656, 1989.

47. McCann, R. L., and Wolfe, W. G.: Resection of abdominal aortic aneurysm in patients with low ejection fractions. J. Vasc. Surg. 10:240, 1989.

48. Baron, J. F., Mundler, O., Bertrand, M., et al.: Dipyridamole-thallium scintigraphy and gated radionuclide angiography to assess cardiac risk before abdominal aortic surgery. N. Engl. J. Med. 330:663, 1994.

49. Eagle, K. A., Coley, C. M., Newell, J. B., et al.: Combining clinical and thallium data optimizes preoperative assessment of cardiac risk before major vascular surgery. Ann. Intern. Med. 110:859, 1989.

50. Brown, K. A., and Rowen, M.: Extent of jeopardized viable myocardium determined by myocardial perfusion imaging best predicts perioperative cardiac events in patients undergoing noncardiac surgery. J. Am. Coll. Cardiol. 21:325, 1993.

51. Hendel, R. C., Whitfield, S. S., Villegas, B. J., et al.: Prediction of late cardiac events by dipyridamole thallium imaging in patients undergoing elective vascular surgery. Am. J. Cardiol. 70:1243, 1992.

52. Lette, J., Waters, D., Cerino, M., et al.: Preoperative coronary artery disease risk stratification based on dipyridamole imaging and a simple three-step, three-segment model for patients undergoing noncardiac vascular surgery or major general surgery. Am. J. Cardio. 69:1553, 1992.

53. Bry, J. D. L., Belkin, M., O'Donnell, T. F., Jr., et al.: An assessment of the positive predictive value and cost-effectiveness of dipyridamole myocardial scintigraphy in patients undergoing vascular surgery. J. Vasc. Surg. 19:112, 1994.

54. Mangano, D. T., London, M. J., Tubau, J. F., et al.: Dipyridamole thallium-201 scintigraphy as a preoperative screening test. A re-examination of its predictive potential. Circulation 84:493, 1991.

55. Raby, K. E., Goldman, L., Creager, M. A., et al.: Correlation between preoperative ischemia and major cardiac events after peripheral vascular surgery. N. Engl. J. Med. 321:1296, 1989.

56. Pasternack, P. F., Grossi, E. A., Baumann, F. G., et al.: Silent myocardial ischemia monitoring predicts late as well as perioperative cardiac events in patients undergoing vascular surgery. J. Vasc. Surg. 16:171, 1992.

57. Mangano, D. T., Browner, W. S., Hollenberg, M., et al.: Association of perioperative myocardial ischemia with cardiac morbidity and mortality in men undergoing noncardiac surgery. N. Engl. J. Med. 323:1781, 1990.

58. Raby, K. E., Barry, J., Creager, M. A., et al.: Detection and significance of intraoperative and postoperative myocardial ischemia in peripheral vascular surgery. JAMA 268:222, 1992.

59. Mangano, D. T., Hollenberg, M., Fegert, G., et al.: Perioperative myocardial ischemia in patients undergoing noncardiac surgery—I. Incidence and severity during the 4 day perioperative period. J. Am. Coll. Cardiol. 17:843, 1991.

60. Mangano, D. T., Wong, M. G., London, M. J., et al.: Perioperative myocardial ischemia in patients undergoing noncadiac surgery—II. Incidence and severity during the first week after surgery. J. Am. Coll. Cardiol. 17:851, 1991.

61. Landesberg, G., Luria, M. H., Cotev, S., et al.: Importance of long-duration postoperative ST-segment depression in cardiac morbidity after vascular surgery. Lancet 341:715, 1993.

62. Mangano, D. T., Browner, W. S., Hollenberg, M., et al., for the McSPI Research Group: Long-term cardiac prognosis following noncardiac surgery. JAMA 268:233, 1992.

63. Halm, E. A., Browner, W. S., Tubau, J. F., et al., for the McSPI Research Group: Echocardiography for preoperative assessment of cardiac risk in noncardiac surgery. J. Gen. Intern. Med. 9:31, 1994.

64. Tischler, M. D., Lee, T. H., Hirsch, A. T., et al.: Prediction of major cardiac events after peripheral vascular surgery using dipyridamole echocardiography. Am. J. Cardiol. 68:593, 1991.

65. Langan, A. M., Youkey, J. R., Franklin, D. P., et al.: Dobutamine stress echocardiography for cardiac risk assessment before aortic surgery. J. Vasc. Surg. 18:905, 1993.

66. Poldermans, D., Fioretti, P. M., Forster, T., et al.: Dobutamine stress echocardiography for assessment of perioperative cardiac risk in patients undergoing major vascular surgery. Circulation 87:1506, 1993.

67. Poldermans, D., Arnese, M., Fioretti, P. M., et al.: Improved cardiac risk stratification in major vascular surgery with dobutamine-atropine stress echocardiography. J. Am. Coll. Cardiol. 26:648, 1995.

68. Davila-Roman, V. G., Waggoner, A. D., Sicard, G. A., et al.: Dobutamine stress echocardiography predicts surgical outcome in patients with an aortic aneurysm and peripheral vascular disease. J. Am. Coll. Cardiol. 21:957, 1993.

69. Taylor, L. M., Yeager, R. A., Moneta, G. L., et al.: The incidence of perioperative myocardial infarction in general vascular surgery. J. Vasc. Surg. 15:52, 1991.

70. Foster, E. D., Davis, K. B., Carpenter, J. A., et al.: Risk of noncardiac operation in patients with defined coronary disease. The Coronary Artery Surgery Study (CASS) registry experience. Ann. Thorac Surg. 41:42,1986.

71. Elmore, J. R., Hallett, J. W., Jr., Gibbons, R. J., et al.: Myocardial revascularization before abdominal aortic aneurysmorrhaphy: Effect of coronary angioplasty. Mayo Clin. Proc. 68:637, 1993.

72. Huber, K. C., Ebans, M. A., Bresnahan, J. F., et al.: Outcome of noncardiac operations in patients with severe coronary artery disease successfully treated preoperatively with coronary angioplasty. Mayo Clin. Proc. 67:15, 1992.

73. Goldman, L.: Cardiac risk in noncardiac surgery: An update. Anesth. Anal. 80:810, 1995.

74. Mangano, D. T., and Goldman, L.: Preoperative assessment of the patient with known or suspected coronary disease. N. Engl. J. Med. 333:1750, 1995.

75. Fleisher, L. A., and Barash, P. G.: Preoperative cardiac evaluation for noncardiac surgery: A functional approach. Anesth. Analg. 74:586, 1992.

76. Granieri, R., and Macpherson, D. S.: Perioperative care of the vascular surgery patient. The perspective of the internist. J. Gen. Intern. Med. 7:102, 1992.

77. Wong, T., and Detsky, A. S.: Preoperative cardiac risk assessment for patients having peripheral vascular surgery. Ann. Intern. Med. 116:743, 1992.

78. Neustein, S. M., Bronheim, D. S., Lasker, S., et al.: Esmolol and intraoperative myocardial ischemia: A double-blind study. J. Cardiothorac. Vasc. Anesth. 8:273, 1994.

79. Kataja, J. H. K., Kukinen, S., Vinamaki, O. V. K., et al.: Esmolol for treatment of hypertension and tachycardia in patients during and after abdominal aortic surgery. J. Cardiothorac. Anesth. 4:37, 1990.

80. Andrews, T. C., Goldman, L., Creager, M. A., et al.: Identification and treatment for myocardial ischemia in patients undergoing peripheral vascular surgery. J. Vasc. Med. Biol. 5:8, 1994.

81. Prys-Roberts, C.: Hypertension and anesthesia—fifty years on. Anesthesiology 50:281, 1979.

82. Bruce, D. L., Croley, T. F., and Lee, J. S.: Preoperative clonidine withdrawal syndrome. Anesthesiology 51:90, 1979.

83. Kataria, B., Dubois, M., Lea, D., et al.: Evaluation of intravenous esmolol for treatment of postoperative hypertension. J. Cardiothorac. Anesth. 4:13, 1990.

84. Orlowski, J. P., Vidt, D. G., Walker, S., and Haluska, J. F.: The hemodynamic effects of intravenous labetalol for postoperative hypertension. Cleve. Clin. J. Med. 56:29, 1989.

85. O'Keefe, J. H., Shub, C., and Rettke, S. R.: Risk of noncardiac surgical procedures in patients with aortic stenosis. Mayo Clin. Proc. 64:400, 1989.

86. Stone, J. G., Hoar, P. F., Calabro, J. R., et al.: Afterload reduction and preload augmentation improve the anesthetic management of patients with cardiac failure and valvular regurgitation. Anesth. Analg. 59:737, 1980.

87. Hayes, S. N., Holmes, D. R., Jr., Nishimura, R. A., and Reeder, G.S.: Palliative percutaneous aortic balloon valvuloplasty before noncardiac operations and invasive diagnostic procedures. Mayo Clin. Proc. 64:753, 1989.

88. Roth, R. B., Palacios, I. F., and Block, P. C.: Percutaneous aortic balloon valvuloplasty: Its role in the management of patients with aortic stenosis requiring major noncardiac surgery. J. Am Coll. Cardiol. 13:1039, 1989.

89. Thompson, R. C., Liberthson, R. R., and Lowenstein, E.: Perioperative anesthetic risk of noncardiac surgery in hypertrophic obstructive cardiomyopathy. J.A.M.A. 254:2419, 1985.

90. Tinker, J. H., and Tarhan, S.: Discontinuing anticoagulant therapy in surgical patients with cardiac valve prostheses. J.A.M.A. 239:738, 1978.

91. Katholi, R. E., Nolan, S. P., and McGuire, L. B.: Living with prosthetic heart valve. Subsequent noncardiac operations and the risk of thromboembolism or hemorrhage. Am. Heart J. 92:162, 1976.

92. Tinker, J. H., Noback, C. R., Vliestra, R. E., and Frye, R. L.: Management of patients with heart disease for noncardiac surgery. J.A.M.A. 246:1348, 1981.

93. Eckman, M. H., Beshansky, J. R., Durand-Zaleski, I., et al.: Anticoagulation for noncardiac procedures in patients with prosthetic heart valves. J.A.M.A. 263:1513, 1990.

94. Durack, D. T.: Prevention of infective endocarditis. N. Engl. J. Med. 332:38, 1995.

95. Clemens, J. D., Horwitz, R. I., Jaffe, C. C., et al.: A controlled evaluation of the risk of bacterial endocarditis in persons with mitral-valve prolapse. N. Engl. J. Med 307:776, 1982.

96. Bor, D. H., and Himmelstein, D. U.: Endocarditis prophylaxis for patients with mitral valve prolapse. Am. J. Med. 76:711, 1984.

97. Clemens, J. D., and Ransohoff, D. F.: A quantitative assessment of predental antibiotic prophylaxis for patients with mitral valve prolapse. J. Chronic Dis. 37:531, 1984.

98. Sommerville, J., McDonald, L., and Edgill, M.: Postoperative haemorrhage and related abnormalities of blood coagulation in cyanotic congenital heart disease. Br. Heart J. 27:440, 1965.

99. Hickey, P. R., Hansen, D. D., Norwood, W. I., and Castaneda, A. R.: Anesthetic complications in surgery for congenital heart disease. Anesth. Analg. 63:657, 1984.

100. Goldberg, A. H., Maling, H. M., and Gaffney, T. E.: The value of prophylactic digitalization in halothane anesthesia. Anesthesiology 23:207, 1962.

101. Lee, D. C., Johnson, R. A., Bingham, J. B., et al.: Heart failure in outpatients. A randomized trial of digoxin versus placebo. N. Engl. J. Med. 306:699, 1982.

102. Kennedy, H. L., Whitlock, J. A., Sprague, M. K., et al.: Long-term follow-up of asymptomatic healthy subjects with frequent and complex ventricular ectopy. N. Engl. J. Med. 312:193, 1985.

103. Bergh, N. P., Dottori, O., and Malmberg, R.: Prophylactic digitalis in thoracic surgery. Scand. J. Resp. Dis. 48:197, 1967.

104. Pastore, J. O., Yurchak, P. M., Janis, K. M., et al.: The risk of advanced heart block in surgical patients with right bundle branch block and left axis deviation. Circulation 57:677, 1978.

105. Pasulka, P. S., Bistrian, B. R., Benotti, P. N., and Blackburn, G. L.: The risks of surgery in obese patients. Ann. Intern. Med. 104:540, 1986.

POSTOPERATIVE COMPLICATIONS

106. Salem, D. N., Homans, D. C., and Isner, J. M.: Management of cardiac disease in the general surgical patient. In Harvey, W. P. (ed.): Current Problems in Cardiology. Vol. 5. Chicago, Year Book Medical Publishers, 1980.

107. Charlson, M. E., MacKenzie, C. R., Ales, K. L., et al.: Surveillance for postoperative myocardial infarction after noncardiac operations. Surg. Gynecol. Obstet. 167:407, 1988.

108. Charlson, M. E., MacKenzie, C. R., Ales, K. L., et al.: The post-operative electrocardiogram and creatine kinase: Implications for diagnosis of myocardial infarction after non-cardiac surgery. J. Clin. Epidemiol. 42:25, 1989.

109. Rettke, S. R., Shub, C., Naessens, J. M., et al.: Significance of mildly elevated creatine kinase (myocardial band) activity after elective abdominal aortic aneurysmectomy. J. Cardiothorac. Vasc. Anesth. 5:425, 1991.

110. Adams, J. E., III, Scicard, G. A., Allen, B. T., et al.: Diagnosis of perioperative myocardial infarction with measurement of cardiac troponin I. N. Engl. J. Med. 330:670, 1994.

111. Oster, G., Tuden, R. L., and Colditz, G. A.: Prevention of venous thromboembolism after general surgery. Cost-effectiveness analysis of alternative approaches to prophylaxis. Am. J. Med. 82:889, 1987.

112. Goldman, L.: Supraventricular tachyarrhythmias in hospitalized adults after surgery. Chest 73:450, 1978.

THE ROLE OF THE MEDICAL CONSULTANT

113. Michel, L. A., Jamart, J., Bradpiece, H. A., and Malt, R. A.: Prediction of risk in noncardiac operations after cardiac operations. J. Thorac. Cardiovasc. Surg. 100:595, 1990.

114. Perry, M. O., and Calcagno, D.: Abdominal aortic aneurysm surgery: The basic evaluation of cardiac risk. Ann. Surg. 208:738, 1988.

115. Rivers, S. P., Scher, L. A., Gupta, S. K., and Veith, F. J: Safety of peripheral vascular surgery after recent acute myocardial infarction. J. Vasc. Surg. 11:70, 1990.

116. Detsky, A. S., Abrams, H. B., Forbath, N., et al.: Cardiac assessment for patients undergoing noncardiac surgery. A multifactorial clinical risk index. Arch. Intern. Med. 146:2131, 1986.

117. Goldman, L.: Multifactorial index of cardiac risk in noncardiac surgery: Ten-year status report. J. Cardiothorac. Anesth. 1:237, 1987.

118. Lee, T. H., and Goldman, L.: Role of consultant. In Breslow, M. J., Mullen, C. F., and Rogers, M. (eds.): Perioperative Management. St. Louis, C. V. Mosby Co., 1990.

Rheumatic fever (RF) is generally classified as a connective tissue or collagen-vascular disease. Its anatomical hallmark is damage to collagen fibrils and to the ground substance of connective tissue. The rheumatic process is expressed as an inflammatory reaction that involves multiple organs: primarily the heart, the joints, and the central nervous system. The clinical manifestations of acute RF follow a group A streptococcal (GAS) infection of the tonsillopharynx after a latent period of approximately 3 weeks. The major importance of acute RF is its ability to cause fibrosis of heart valves, leading to crippling hemodynamics of chronic heart disease.

RF is the most common cause of acquired heart disease in children and young adults worldwide. Although the incidence of RF declined sharply in many developed countries, the disease remains a major problem in many developing countries. The precise reasons for the fluctuations in the incidence of the disease remain only partly understood. Although RF has been studied extensively, the pathogenesis of the disease is not well defined.

Epidemiology

The incidence of RF and prevalence of rheumatic heart disease are markedly variable in different countries.[1,2] At the turn of the century, the incidence of RF in the United States was over 100 per 100,000 population, ranged between 40 and 65 per 100,000 between 1935 and 1960, and is currently estimated at less than 2 per 100,000. Beginning in 1984, several outbreaks of acute RF were reported from a number of geographically distinct areas in the United States.[3-14] These focal outbreaks were not associated with a national increase in the incidence of RF.[15] The decline in the incidence of RF in the industrialized countries is in sharp contrast to the persistent high incidence of the disease in nonindustrialized countries.

In many developing countries, the incidence of acute RF approaches or exceeds 100 per 100,000.[1] In keeping with the falling incidence of RF in industrialized countries, the prevalence of rheumatic heart disease has declined. Table 55-1 compares the prevalence of rheumatic heart in school-age children in different regions of the world.

The decline in incidence of RF and prevalence of rheumatic heart disease has been attributed to several factors. Although the decline preceded the introduction of antimicrobial agents for the treatment of streptococcal pharyngitis, some reports suggest that the use of these agents may have enhanced the rate of this decline.[16] Improved economic standards, better housing conditions, decreased crowding in homes and schools, and access to medical care are often credited, at least in part, for the marked decline in RF.[1] Epidemiological observations in the United States[17] and the United Kingdom[18] show periodic shifts in the appearance and disappearance of specific M types in a particular geographical location. Such shifts may be another explanation for the decline and resurgence of RF in some parts of the world.

Because of the causal relationship between RF and GAS pharyngitis, the epidemiologies of the two illnesses are very similar. Initial attacks of RF occur most commonly between the ages of 6 and 15 years, and RF is rarely seen before the age of 5 years.[19] The risk of RF is increased in populations at high risk for streptococcal pharyngitis such as military recruits, persons living in crowded conditions, and those in close contact with school-age children.[20] The incidence of RF is equal in male and female patients. The seasonal incidence of RF also parallels that of streptococcal pharyngitis. The peak incidence of RF in Europe and the United States is in spring. Although RF used to be considered a disease of temperate climates, it is now more common in warm tropical climates, particularly in developing countries.

Pathogenesis

The evidence that GAS is the agent causing initial and recurrent attacks of RF is strong but indirect. It is based on clinical, epidemiological, and immunological observations. Factors that contribute to the pathogenesis of RF are related to both the putative causative agent and the host (Table 55-2).

THE ETIOLOGICAL AGENT. An untreated GAS tonsillopharyngitis is the antecedent event that precipitates RF.[21,22] RF does not follow streptococcal skin infection (impetigo). Proper antimicrobial treatment of the streptococcal pharyngitis with eradication of the organism virtually eliminates the risk of RF.[21] In situations conducive to epidemic streptococcal pharyngitis (such as the military population, crowding), as many as 3 per cent of untreated acute streptococcal sore throats may be followed by rheumatic fever.[23] Endemic infections result in much lower attack rates. It has been well documented that about one-third of all cases of acute RF follow mild, almost asymptomatic, pharyngitis. The lack of symptomatic pharyngitis was particularly striking in most of the recent outbreaks of acute RF in which

TABLE 55-1 RHEUMATIC HEART DISEASE IN SCHOOL-AGE CHILDREN

LOCATION	PREVALENCE PER 1000
United States	0.6
Japan	0.7
Asia (other)	0.4–21.0
Africa	0.3–15.0
South America	1.0–17.0

TABLE 55-2 PATHOGENESIS OF RHEUMATIC FEVER

GROUP A STREPTOCOCCUS
Tonsillopharyngeal infection, not other sites
Intensity of the infection
Brisk antibody response
Persistence of the organism
Rheumatogenic strains
M types 1, 3, 5, 6, 14, 18, 19, 27, and 29
Distinct structural characteristics of M proteins
Long terminal antigenic domain
Epitopes that are shared with human heart tissue
Heavily encapsulated, forming mucoid colonies
Resist phagocytosis
Do not produce opacity factor

SUSCEPTIBLE HOST
Genetic predisposition
Presence of specific B cell alloantigen
High incidence of class II HLA antigens

the majority of patients (58 per cent) had no history of pharyngitis.[2] This is an alarming observation, because the primary prevention of acute RF relies on the identification and proper treatment of streptococcal pharyngitis.

The major factors that are related to the risk of RF are the magnitude of the immune response to the antecedent streptococcal pharyngitis and persistence of the organism during convalescence.[23] Variations in the rheumatogenicity of GAS strains are a factor influencing the attack rate of RF.[24] The concept that RF is associated with infections due to virulent encapsulated (mucoid) strains capable of inducing strong type-specific immune responses to M protein and other streptococcal antigens[25] has been strengthened by observations made during the outbreaks of acute RF in the mid 1980's. The streptococci isolated from patients with RF and their sibling contacts during these outbreaks were primarily strains belonging to M types 1, 3, 5, 6, and 18.[26] M proteins of rheumatogenic streptococci show distinct structural characteristics: they share a long terminal antigenic domain[27] and contain epitopes that are shared with human heart tissue, particularly sarcolemmal membrane proteins and cardiac myosin.[28,29]

THE HOST. Although only a small proportion of individuals with untreated streptococcal pharyngitis may develop RF (3 per cent), the incidence of the disease following streptococcal pharyngitis in patients who have had a previous episode of RF is substantially more (about 50 per cent). Numerous epidemiological studies also indicate familial predisposition to the disease. These observations and more recent studies strongly suggest a genetic basis for susceptibility to RF. A specific B-cell alloantigen, identified by monoclonal antibodies, has been described in almost all patients (99 per cent) with RF but only in a small number (14 per cent) of controls.[30] Furthermore, susceptibility to RF has been linked with HLA-DR 1, 2, 3, and 4 haplotypes in various ethnic groups.[31]

Pathology

The acute phase of RF is characterized by exudative and proliferative inflammatory reactions involving connective or collagen tissue. Although the disease process is diffuse, it affects primarily the heart, joints, brain, and cutaneous and subcutaneous tissues. A generalized vasculitis affecting small blood vessels is commonly noted, but unlike the vasculitis of some other connective tissue disorders, thrombotic lesions are not seen in RF.

The basic structural change in collagen is fibrinoid degeneration. The interstitial connective tissue becomes edematous and eosinophilic, with fraying, fragmentation, and disintegration of collagen fibers. This is associated with infiltration of mononuclear cells including large modified fibrohistiocytic cells (Aschoff cells). Some of the histiocytes are multinucleated and form Aschoff giant cells.

The Aschoff nodule in the proliferative stage is considered pathognomonic of rheumatic carditis. These nodules have been described almost invariably in the autopsies of patients who died of rheumatic carditis; however, more recent observations indicate that the Aschoff nodules are observed in only 30 per cent to 40 per cent of biopsies from patients with primary or recurrent episodes of RF.[32] Aschoff bodies may be seen in any area of the myocardium but not in other affected organs such as joints or brain. They are most often noted in the interventricular septum, the wall of the left ventricle, or the left atrial appendage. Aschoff nodules persist for many years after a rheumatic attack, even in patients with no evidence of recent or active inflammation.

Inflammation of valvular tissue accounts for the more commonly recognized clinical manifestations of rheumatic carditis. Initial inflammation leads to valvular insufficiency. The histological findings in endocarditis consist of edema and cellular infiltration of the valvular tissue and the chordae tendineae. Hyaline degeneration of the affected valve leads to the formation of verrucae at its edge, preventing total approximation of the leaflets. Fibrosis and calcification of the valve occur if inflammation persists. Eventually, this process may lead to valvular stenosis.

DIAGNOSIS

There is no specific clinical, laboratory, or other test that establishes the diagnosis of RF. In 1944, T. Duckett Jones formulated his criteria for the diagnosis of RF[33]; these criteria are still valuable. The criteria have been modified, revised, edited, and updated by the Committee on Rheumatic Fever, Endocarditis, and Kawasaki Disease of the Council on Cardiovascular Disease in the Young (American Heart Association).[34] The most recent guidelines (Table 55–3) emphasize the diagnosis of *initial attacks* of RF. Dividing clinical and laboratory findings into major and minor manifestations is based on the diagnostic importance of a particular finding. If supported by evidence of preceding GAS infection, the presence of two major manifestations or of one major and two minor manifestations indicates a high probability of acute RF.

Major Clinical Manifestations

CARDITIS. Rheumatic carditis is a pancarditis affecting the endocardium, myocardium, and pericardium to varying degrees. Clinically, rheumatic carditis is almost always associated with a murmur of valvulitis. The severity of carditis is variable. In its most severe form, death from cardiac failure may occur. More commonly, carditis is less intense, and the predominant effect is subsequent scarring of the heart valves. Evidence of carditis may be very subtle; signs of valvular involvement may be mild and transient and may be easily missed on auscultation. Baseline studies, including electrocardiographs and echocardiographs, should be obtained in patients in whom RF is suspected. Patients who show no clear evidence of carditis on initial examination should be monitored closely over a few weeks to assess cardiac involvement.

Carditis is often regarded as the most specific manifestation of RF. It is noted in at least 50 per cent of patients with acute RF (Fig. 55–1). Recent outbreaks in the United States suggested that the frequency of carditis was somewhat higher than traditionally reported and may be in part due to more sophisticated diagnostic methods.[2] In one report,[3] carditis was diagnosed in 72 per cent of cases by auscultation and in 91 per cent of cases by Doppler ultrasonography. The risk of overdiagnosing valvular incompetence by echocardiography should be emphasized, and over-reliance on this tool in diagnosing rheumatic carditis should be avoided.

Valvulitis (endocarditis) involving mitral and aortic valves and the chordae of the mitral valve is the most characteristic component of rheumatic carditis. Mitral in-

TABLE 55–3   GUIDELINES FOR THE DIAGNOSIS
OF INITIAL ATTACKS OF RHEUMATIC FEVER
(JONES CRITERIA, UPDATED 1992)

MAJOR MANIFESTATIONS	MINOR MANIFESTATIONS
Carditis	Clinical findings
Polyarthritis	Arthralgia
Chorea	Fever
Erythema marginatum	Laboratory findings
Subcutaneous nodules	Elevated acute phase reactants
	Erythrocyte sedimentation rate
	C-reactive protein
	Prolonged P–R interval
SUPPORTING EVIDENCE OF ANTECEDENT GROUP A STREPTOCOCCAL INFECTION	
Positive throat culture or rapid streptococcal antigen test Elevated or rising streptococcal antibody titer	

From Dajani, A. S., Ayoub, E. M., Bierman, F. Z., et al.: Guidelines for the diagnosis of rheumatic fever: Jones Criteria, updated 1992. JAMA *268:*2069, 1992. Copyright 1992 American Medical Association.

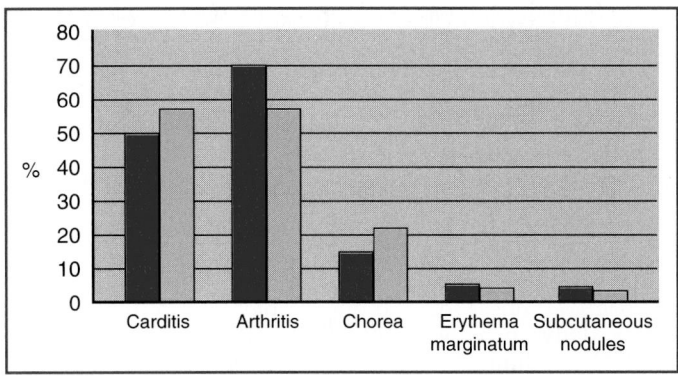

FIGURE 55–1. Relative frequency of major manifestations of rheumatic fever in earlier *(dark bars)* and more recent reports in the 1980s *(light bars)*.

sufficiency is the hallmark of rheumatic carditis. Aortic insufficiency is less common and usually associated with mitral insufficiency. The pulmonic and tricuspid valves are rarely involved. Residual valvular damage is a major concern in patients with RF and may lead to intractable cardiac failure requiring surgical intervention.

Myocarditis or pericarditis in the *absence* of valvulitis is *not* likely to be due to RF. Tachycardia is an early sign of myocarditis but may also be due to fever or cardiac failure. Transient arrhythmias may occur in patients with myocarditis. Severe myocarditis or valvular insufficiency may lead to cardiac failure. Cardiac enlargement occurs when severe hemodynamic changes result from valvular, myocardial, or pericardial disease. Inflammation of the visceral and parietal surfaces of the pericardium occurs, resulting in pericarditis and the accumulation of pericardial fluid.

ARTHRITIS. Polyarthritis is the most common major manifestation of RF (Fig. 55–1), but the least specific. It is almost always asymmetric, migratory, and involves larger joints (knees, ankles, elbows, and wrists). Characteristically there is swelling, redness, heat, severe pain, limitation of motion, and tenderness to touch. The arthritis of RF is benign and does not result in permanent joint deformity. Joint fluid shows findings characteristic of inflammation (not infection). In untreated cases, arthritis usually lasts 2 to 3 weeks. A striking feature of rheumatic arthritis is its dramatic response to salicylates. Indeed, if a patient does not improve substantially after 48 hours of adequate salicylate treatment, the diagnosis of RF should be in doubt.

Some patients may develop arthritis and other multisystem manifestations following acute streptococcal pharyngitis that do not fulfill the Jones criteria for the diagnosis of acute RF. This "syndrome" has been referred to as post-streptococcal reactive arthritis (PSRA). The arthritis of PSRA does not respond dramatically to anti-inflammatory agents. Some patients with PSRA may have silent or delayed-onset carditis[35]; therefore, these patients should be observed carefully for several months for the subsequent development of carditis.

CHOREA. Sydenham's chorea, St. Vitus' dance, or chorea minor occurs in about 20 per cent of patients with RF (see Fig. 55–1). The rheumatic inflammatory process in the central nervous system specifically involves the basal ganglia and caudate nuclei. Chorea is a *delayed* manifestation of RF, usually appearing in 3 months or longer after the onset of the precipitating streptococcal infection. This is in sharp contrast to the latent period of carditis or arthritis, which is usually 3 weeks. As such, chorea is frequently the only manifestation of RF. Furthermore, evidence of a recent GAS infection may be difficult to document and other supporting historical, clinical, or laboratory findings to fulfill the Jones criteria may be lacking. The diagnosis of RF can be made in a patient with chorea without strictly adhering to the Jones criteria.

Sydenham's chorea is characterized clinically by purposeless and involuntary movements, muscular incoordination and weakness, and emotional lability. The manifestations are more evident when the patient is awake and under stress and may disappear during sleep. All muscles may be involved, but primarily muscles of the face and extremities. Speech may be affected, being explosive and halting. Handwriting deteriorates, and the patient becomes uncoordinated and easily frustrated. The symptoms of Sydenham's chorea must be distinguished from tics, athetosis, conversion reactions, hyperkinesis, and behavior problems. Symptoms usually resolve in 1 to 2 weeks, even without treatment.

ERYTHEMA MARGINATUM. This distinctive rash is a rare manifestation of RF occurring in less than 5 per cent of patients. It is an evanescent, erythematous, macular, nonpruritic rash with pale centers and rounded or serpiginous margins. Lesions vary greatly in size and occur mainly on the trunk and proximal extremities, not on the face. The rash may be induced by application of heat.

SUBCUTANEOUS NODULES. These are firm, painless, freely movable nodules that measure 0.5 to 2 cm. They are rarely seen in patients with RF (about 3 per cent); when present, they are most seen in patients with carditis. They are usually located over extensor surfaces of the joints (particularly elbows, knees, and wrists), in the occipital scalp, or over spinous processes. The overlying skin is freely movable, shows no discoloration, and is not inflamed.

Minor Manifestations

CLINICAL FINDINGS. Fever and arthralgia are nonspecific, common findings in patients with acute RF. Their diagnostic value is limited because they are encountered commonly in a variety of other diseases. They are used to support the diagnosis of RF when only a single major manifestation is present. Fever is noted during the acute stages of the disease and has no characteristic pattern. Arthralgia is pain in one or more large joints without objective findings on examination and must not be considered a minor manifestation if arthritis is present. Epistaxis and abdominal pain may also occur but are not included as minor diagnostic criteria for RF.

LABORATORY FINDINGS. Elevated acute phase reactants offer objective but nonspecific indications of tissue inflammation. The erythrocyte sedimentation rate (ESR) and C-reactive protein (CRP) level are almost always elevated during the acute stages of the disease in patients with carditis or polyarthritis, but are usually normal in patients with chorea. The ESR is very useful in following the course of the disease; it usually returns to normal as the rheumatic activity subsides. The ESR may be elevated in patients with anemia and may be suppressed to normal levels in patients with congestive cardiac failure. Unlike the ESR, the CRP is unaffected by anemia or cardiac failure.

A common finding in patients with acute RF is a prolonged P-R interval for age and rate on electrocardiography. This finding alone is not diagnostic of carditis and does not correlate with the ultimate development of chronic rheumatic cardiac disease. Other findings on electrocardiography include tachycardia, atrioventricular block, and QRS–T changes suggestive of myocarditis; these changes are not considered minor manifestations.

Leukocytosis may be observed in the acute stages of RF, but the leukocyte count is variable and not dependable. Anemia is usually mild or moderate and normocytic normochromatic in morphology (anemia of chronic inflammation). Chest roentgenograms are useful in assessing cardiac size; however, a normal chest roentgenogram does not exclude the presence of carditis. Pericarditis, pulmonary edema, and increased pulmonary vascularity are also detected by this examination. Echocardiography may be helpful in detecting endocardial, myocardial, and pericardial involvement.

Antecedent Group A Streptococcal (GAS) Infection

A number of illnesses mimic acute RF, and there is no laboratory test or tests that allow the specific diagnosis of RF. It is therefore important to establish an antecedent streptococcal infection in the form of demonstrating a GAS in the tonsillopharynx or an elevated or rising streptococcal antibody titer. *Evidence of an antecedent streptococcal infection is required for the confirmation of the initial diagnosis of acute RF.*

At the time of diagnosis of acute RF, only about 11 per cent of patients have throat cultures positive for group A streptococci.[2] The paucity of positive cultures is due, in part, to elimination of the organism by host defense mechanisms during the latent period between the onset of the infection and the subsequent development of RF. Several rapid GAS antigen detection tests are commercially available. These tests vary in methodology. Most of these tests have a high degree of specificity but a low sensitivity in a clinical setting. A negative test does not exclude the presence of group A streptococci in the pharynx. A positive throat culture or rapid antigen test does not distinguish between a recent infection that can be associated with acute RF and chronic pharyngeal carriage of the organism.

Because the presence of GAS in the pharynx may not represent active infection, elevated or rising antistreptococcal antibody titers provide more reliable evidence of a recent streptococcal infection than a positive culture or a positive rapid antigen test. The most commonly used antibody tests are the antistreptolysin O (ASO) and antideoxyribonuclease B (anti-DNase B). The ASO test is usually obtained first, and if not elevated, the anti-DNase B test is done. Elevated titers for both tests may persist for several weeks or months. ASO titers rise and fall more rapidly than anti-DNase B. A slide agglutination test is commercially available and measures antibodies to several streptococcal antigens. It is simple to perform, rapid, and widely available; however, the test is not well standardized and not very reproducible and is not recommended as a definitive test for evidence of a preceding GAS infection.

TREATMENT

GENERAL. Whenever possible, the patient should be admitted to a hospital for close observation and appropriate work-up. Bed rest is generally considered important because it lessens joint pain. The duration of bed rest may be variable and individually determined. Ambulation may be attempted once fever abates and acute phase reactants return to normal. The patient should be allowed to return to a reasonably active life with normal physical activity. Strenuous physical exercise should be avoided, however, particularly if carditis was present. Although throat cultures are rarely positive for GAS at the time of onset of rheumatic fever, the patient should receive a 10-day course of penicillin therapy. Patients allergic to penicillin should be treated with erythromycin.

If heart failure is present, the patient should receive diuretics, oxygen, and digitalis and be on a restricted sodium diet. Digitalis preparations should be used cautiously because cardiac toxicity may occur with conventional dosages.

ANTIRHEUMATIC THERAPY. There is no specific treatment for the inflammatory reactions initiated by rheumatic fever. Supportive therapy is aimed at reducing constitutional symptoms, controlling toxic manifestations, and improving cardiac function.

Patients with mild or no carditis usually respond well to salicylates. Salicylates are particularly effective in relieving joint pain; such pain usually abates within 24 hours of starting salicylates. Indeed, if joint pain persists after salicylate treatment, the diagnosis of rheumatic fever may be questionable, and the patient should be reevaluated. Because no specific diagnostic tests for rheumatic fever exist, anti-inflammatory therapy should be withheld until the clinical picture has become sufficiently clear to allow for a diagnosis. Early administration of anti-inflammatory agents may suppress clinical manifestations and prevent appropriate diagnosis. For optimal anti-inflammatory effect, serum salicylate levels around 20 mg per cent are required. Aspirin, at doses of 100 mg/kg/day, given four to five times daily, usually results in adequate serum levels to achieve a clinical response. Optimal salicylate therapy must be individualized, however, to assure adequate response and avoid toxicity. Tinnitus, nausea, vomiting, and anorexia are common dose-related toxicities associated with salicylism. Side effects may subside after a few days of treatment despite continuation of the medication.

Patients with significant cardiac involvement—particularly those with pericarditis or congestive heart failure—respond more promptly to corticosteroids than to salicylates.[36] Indeed, steroids may be life-saving in very ill patients. Occasionally, patients who do not respond to adequate doses of salicylates may benefit from a trial course of corticosteroids. Prednisone, 1 to 2 mg/kg/day, is the usual dose.

There is no evidence that salicylate or corticosteroid therapy affects the course of carditis or diminishes the incidence of residual heart disease. Therefore, the duration of therapy with anti-inflammatory agents is arbitrarily based on an estimate of the severity of the episode and the promptness of the clinical response.

Mild attacks with little or no cardiac involvement may be treated with salicylates for about 1 month or until there is sufficient clinical and laboratory evidence of inflammatory inactivity. In more severe cases, therapy with corticosteroids may be continued for 2 to 3 months. The medication is then gradually reduced over the next 2 weeks. Even with prolonged therapy, some patients (approximately 5 per cent) will continue to demonstrate evidence of rheumatic activity for 6 or more months. A "rebound," manifested by the reappearance of mild symptoms or of acute phase reactants, may occur in some patients after anti-inflammatory medications have been discontinued, usually within 2 weeks. Modest symptoms usually subside without treatment; more severe symptoms may require treatment with salicylates. Some physicians recommend the use of salicylates (aspirin, 75 mg/kg/day) during the period when corticosteroids are being tapered and believe that such an approach may reduce the likelihood of a rebound.

Information about the use of salicylates other than aspirin is very limited. There is no evidence that the nonsteroidal anti-inflammatory agents are more effective than aspirin. In patients who cannot tolerate aspirin or who are allergic to it, a trial of the nonsteroidal agents may be warranted. Aspirin preparations that are coated, or that contain alkali or buffers, may also be tried; however, there is little evidence that such preparations are better tolerated and some may have undesirable side effects.

PREVENTION

Primary Prevention

Prevention of primary attacks of rheumatic fever depends on the prompt recognition and proper treatment of GAS tonsillopharyngitis. Eradication of GAS from the throat is essential. Although appropriate antimicrobial therapy started up to 9 days after the onset of acute streptococcal pharyngitis is effective in preventing primary attacks of rheumatic fever,[21] early therapy is advisable because it reduces both morbidity and the period of infectivity. In selecting a regimen for the treatment of GAS pharyngitis, various factors should be considered, including bacteriological and clinical efficacy; ease of adherence to the recommended regimen (frequency of daily administration, duration of therapy, palatability); cost; spectrum of activity of the selected agent; and potential side effects.[37]

Penicillin is the antimicrobial agent of choice for the treatment of GAS, except in patients with history of allergy to penicillin.[38-40] Penicillin has a narrow spectrum of activity, a longstanding proven efficacy, and is the least expensive regimen. GAS resistant to penicillin has not been documented.[41] Penicillin may be administered intramuscularly or orally (Table 55-4) depending on the patient's likely adherence to an oral regimen.

Intramuscular benzathine penicillin G is preferred, particularly for patients who are unlikely to complete a 10-day course of oral therapy and patients with a personal or family history of RF or rheumatic heart disease. Benzathine penicillin G injections should be given as a single dose in a large muscle mass. This formulation is painful; injections that contain procaine penicillin in addition to benzathine penicillin G are less painful. Less discomfort is associated with intramuscular benzathine penicillin G if the medication is warmed to room temperature before administration.

The oral antibiotic of choice is penicillin V (phenoxymethyl penicillin). Patients should take oral penicillin regularly for an entire 10-day period, although they are likely to be asymptomatic after the first few days. Although the broader-spectrum amoxicillin is often used for treatment of GAS pharyngitis, it offers no microbiological advantage over penicillin.

Oral erythromycin is acceptable for patients allergic to penicillin. Treatment should also be prescribed for 10 days. Erythromycin estolate (20 to 40 mg/kg/day in two to four divided doses), or erythromycin ethyl succinate (40 mg/kg/day in two to four divided doses) is effective in treating streptococcal pharyngitis; however, efficacy of a twice-daily

regimen in adults requires further study. The maximal dose of erythromycin is 1 g/day. Although strains of GAS resistant to erythromycin are prevalent in some areas of the world and have resulted in treatment failures,[42] they are uncommon in most parts of the United States.[41]

The new macrolide azithromycin has similar susceptibility pattern to that of erythromycin against GAS but may cause fewer gastrointestinal side effects. Azithromycin can be administered once daily and produces high tonsillar tissue concentrations. A 5-day course of azithromycin is approved by the Food and Drug Administration as a second-line therapy for the treatment of patients 16 years of age or older with GAS pharyngitis. The recommended dosage is 500 mg as a single dose on the first day followed by 250 mg once daily for 4 days.[43]

A 10-day course of an oral cephalosporin is an acceptable alternative, particularly for penicillin-allergic patients. Narrower-spectrum cephalosporins, such as cefadroxil or cephalexin, are probably preferable to the broader-spectrum cephalosporins such as cefaclor, cefuroxime, cefixime, and cefpodoxime. Some penicillin-allergic persons (< 15 per cent) are also allergic to cephalosporins, and these agents should not be used in patients with immediate (anaphylactic-type) hypersensitivity to penicillin.

Several reports indicate that a 10-day course with an oral cephalosporin is superior to 10 days of oral penicillin in eradicating GAS from the pharynx.[44-47] Recent reports suggest that a 5-day course with selected oral cephalosporins is comparable to a 10-day course of oral penicillin in eradicating GAS from the pharynx.[48-51] Such regimens are not currently approved by the Food and Drug Administration, and further studies are warranted to expand and confirm these observations.

Certain antimicrobials are not recommended for treatment of streptococcal upper respiratory tract infections.[40] Tetracyclines should not be used because of the high prevalence of resistant strains. Sulfonamides and trimethoprim-sulfamethoxazole will not eradicate GAS in patients with pharyngitis and should not be used to treat active infections. Chloramphenicol is not recommended because of unpredictable efficacy and potential serious toxicity.

Secondary Prevention

A patient with a previous attack of RF who develops streptococcal pharyngitis is at high risk for a recurrent attack of rheumatic fever. A GAS infection need not be symptomatic to trigger a recurrence. Furthermore, RF recurrence can occur even when a symptomatic infection is optimally treated. For these reasons, prevention of recurrent RF requires continuous antimicrobial prophylaxis rather than recognition and treatment of acute episodes of streptococcal pharyngitis. Continuous prophylaxis is recommended for patients with a well-documented history of rheumatic fever (including cases manifested solely by Sydenham's chorea) and those with definite evidence of rheumatic heart disease. Such prophylaxis should be initiated as soon as acute RF or rheumatic heart disease is diagnosed. A full therapeutic course of penicillin (as outlined in Table 4) should first be given to patients with acute rheumatic fever to eradicate residual GAS even if a throat culture is negative at that time. Streptococcal infections occurring in family members of rheumatic patients should be treated promptly.

CONTINUOUS ANTIMICROBIAL PROPHYLAXIS. This provides the most effective protection from rheumatic fever recurrences. Risk of recurrence depends on several factors. Risk increases with multiple previous attacks, whereas the risk decreases as the interval since the most recent attack lengthens. The likelihood of acquiring a streptococcal upper respiratory tract infection is an important consideration. Patients with increased exposure to streptococcal infections include children and adolescents, parents of young children, teachers, physicians, nurses, and allied health

TABLE 55-4   PREVENTION OF RHEUMATIC FEVER

AGENT	DOSE	MODE	DURATION
Primary Prevention			
Benzathine penicillin G	600,000 units for patients ≤ 27 kg 1,200,000 units for patients > 27 kg	IM	Once
OR			
Penicillin V	Children: 250 mg 2–3 times daily Adolescents and adults: 500 mg 2–3 times daily	PO	10 days
For patients allergic to penicillin:			
Erythromycin	40 mg/kg/day 2–4 times daily (maximum 1 g/day)	PO	10 days
Secondary Prevention			
Benzathine penicillin G	1,200,000 units every 3–4 weeks	IM	See Table 5
OR			
Penicillin V	250 mg twice daily	PO	See Table 5
OR			
Sulfadiazine	0.5 g once daily for patients ≤ 27 kg (60 lb) 1.0 g once daily for patients > 27 kg (60 lb)	PO	See Table 5
For patients allergic to penicillin and sulfadiazine:			
Erythromycin	250 mg twice daily	PO	See Table 5

IM = intramuscularly; PO = orally
Modified from Dajani, A. S., Taubert, K., Ferrieri, P., et al.: Treatment of streptococcal pharyngitis and prevention of rheumatic fever. Pediatrics 96:758, 1995; with permission.

personnel in contact with children, military recruits, and others in crowded housing. A higher risk of of recurrences in economically disadvantaged populations has been demonstrated.

Physicians must consider each individual situation when determining appropriate duration of prophylaxis. Patients who have had rheumatic carditis are at a relatively high risk for recurrences of carditis and are likely to sustain increasingly severe cardiac involvement with each recurrence. Therefore, patients who have had rheumatic carditis should receive long-term antibiotic prophylaxis, perhaps for life. Duration of prophylaxis depends on whether residual valvular disease is present or absent (Table 55–5). Prophylaxis should continue even after valve surgery, including prosthetic valve replacement. Patients who have had rheumatic fever without carditis are at considerably less risk of cardiac involvement with a recurrence. Therefore, prophylaxis may be discontinued in these individuals after several years.[52] In general, prophylaxis should continue until 5 years have elapsed since the last rheumatic fever attack or age 21 years, whichever is longer. The decision to discontinue prophylaxis or reinstate it should be made after discussion with the patient of potential risks and benefits and careful consideration of the epidemiological risk factors enumerated above.

An injection of 1,200,000 units of this long-acting penicillin preparation every 4 weeks is the recommended regimen for secondary prevention in most circumstances in the United States (see Table 55–4). In countries where the incidence of RF is particularly high, in special circumstances, or in certain high-risk individuals, such as patients with residual rheumatic carditis, the administration of benzathine penicillin G every 3 weeks is recommended.[53,54] Long-acting penicillin is of particular value in patients with a high risk of recurrence of RF. The advantages of benzathine penicillin G must be weighed against inconvenience to the patient and pain of injection, which causes some patients to discontinue prophylaxis.

Successful oral prophylaxis depends primarily on patient adherence to prescribed regimens. Patients need careful and repeated instructions about the importance of continuing prophylaxis. Most failures of prophylaxis occur in nonadherent patients. Even with optimal patient adherence, risk of recurrence is higher in individuals receiving oral prophylaxis compared to those receiving intramuscular benzathine penicillin G.[37] Oral agents are more appropriate for patients at lower risk for rheumatic recurrence. Accordingly, some physicians switch patients to oral prophylaxis when they have reached late adolescence or young adulthood and have remained free of rheumatic attacks for at least 5 years.

Penicillin V is the preferred oral agent (see Table 55–4). There are no published data about the use of other penicillins, macrolides, or cephalosporins for the secondary prevention of rheumatic fever. Although sulfonamides are not effective in eradication of GAS, they do prevent infection. Sulfadiazine and sulfisoxazole appear to be equivalent; the

TABLE 55–5 DURATION OF SECONDARY PROPHYLAXIS IN PATIENTS WITH RHEUMATIC FEVER

CATEGORY	DURATION
Rheumatic fever with carditis and residual valvular disease	At least 10 years after last episode and at least until age 40. Sometimes lifelong prophylaxis
Rheumatic fever with carditis but no residual valvular disease	10 years or well into adulthood, whichever is longer
Rheumatic fever without carditis	5 years or until age 21, whichever is longer

From Dajani, A. S., Taubert, K., Ferrieri, P., et al.: Treatment of streptococcal pharyngitis and prevention of rheumatic fever. Pediatrics, 96:758, 1995; with permission.

use of sulfisoxazole is acceptable based on extrapolation from data demonstrating that sulfadiazine has proven effectiveness in secondary prophylaxis. The recommended dose of sulfisoxazole is the same as that for sulfadiazine. Sulfonamide prophylaxis is contraindicated in late pregnancy because of transplacental passage of the drugs and potential competition with bilirubin for albumin-binding sites. Erythromycin is recommended for the patient who is allergic to penicillin and sulfisoxazole.

Bacterial Endocarditis Prophylaxis
(See also Chap. 33)

Patients with rheumatic valvular heart disease also require additional short-term antibiotic prophylaxis before certain surgical and dental procedures to prevent possible development of bacterial endocarditis. Patients with prosthetic valves or previous endocarditis are at particularly high risk. *Antibiotic regimens used to prevent recurrences of acute rheumatic fever are inadequate for prevention of bacterial endocarditis.* The current recommendations of the American Heart Association concerning prevention of bacterial endocarditis should be followed.[55] Because alpha-hemolytic streptococci in the oropharynx may have developed resistance to oral penicillin being used for secondary prevention of rheumatic fever, the agent selected to prevent endocarditis should not be a penicillin. Patients who have had rheumatic fever but do not have evidence of rheumatic heart disease do not need endocarditis prophylaxis.

REFERENCES

1. World Health Organization: Rheumatic fever and rheumatic heart disease. W. H. O. Technical Report Series 764. Geneva, World Health Organization, 1988.
2. Dajani, A. S.: Current status of nonsuppurative complications of group A streptococci. Pediatr. Infect. Dis. J. 10:S25, 1991.
3. Veasy, L. G., Wiedmeier, S. E., Orsmond, G. S., et al.: Resurgence of acute rheumatic fever in the intermountain area of the United States. N. Engl. J. Med. 316:421, 1987.
4. Congeni, B., Rizzo, C., Congeni, J., et al.: Outbreak of acute rheumatic fever in northeast Ohio. J. Pediatr. 111:176, 1987.
5. Wald, E. R., Dashefsky, B., Feidt, C., et al.: Acute rheumatic fever in western Pennsylvania and the tristate area. Pediatrics 80:371, 1987.
6. Hosier, D. M., Craenen, J. M., Teske, D. W., et al.: Resurgence of acute rheumatic fever. Am. J. Dis. Child. 141:730, 1987.
7. Centers for Disease Control: Acute rheumatic fever at a Navy training center-San Diego, California. M. M. W. R. 37:101, 1988.
8. Centers for Disease Control: Acute rheumatic fever among army trainees-Fort Leonard Wood, Missouri, 1987–1988. M.M.W.R. 37:519, 1988.
9. Wallace, M. R., Garst, P. D., Papadimos, T. J., et al.: The return of acute rheumatic fever in young adults. JAMA 262:2557, 1989.
10. Westlake, R. M., Graham, T. P., and Edwards, K. M.: An outbreak of acute rheumatic fever in Tennessee. Pediatr. Infect. Dis. J. 9:97, 1990.
11. Griffiths, S. P., and Gersony, W. M.: Acute rheumatic fever in New York City (1969–1988): A comparative study of two decades. J. Pediatr. 116:882, 1990.
12. Leggiadoro, R. J., Birnbaum, S. T., Chase, N. A., et al.: A resurgence of acute rheumatic fever in a mid-south children's hospital. South. Med. J. 83:1418, 1990.
13. Zangwill, K. M., Wald, E. R., and Londino, A. V.: Acute rheumatic fever in western Pennsylvania: A persistent problem into the 1990s. J. Pediatr. 118:561, 1991.
14. Veasy, L. G., Tani, L. Y., and Hill, H. R.: Persistence of acute rheumatic fever in the intermountain area of the United States. J. Pediatr. 124:9, 1994.
15. Taubert, K. A., Rowley, A. H., and Shulman, S. T.: Seven-year national survey of Kawasaki disease and acute rheumatic fever. Pediatr. Infect. Dis. J. 13:704, 1994.
16. Massell, B. F., Chute, C. G., Walker, A. M., et al.: Penicillin and the marked decrease in morbidity and mortality from rheumatic fever in the United States. N. Engl. J. Med. 318:280, 1988.
17. Schwartz, B., Facklam, R. R., and Breiman, R. F.: Changing epidemiology of group A streptococcal infection in the USA. Lancet 336:1167, 1990.
18. Colman, G., Tanna, A., Efstatiou, A., et al.: The serotypes of *Streptococcus pyogenes* present in Britain during 1980–1990 and their association with disease. J. Med. Microbiol. 39:165, 1993.
19. Bland, E. F., and Jones, T. D.: Rheumatic fever and rheumatic heart disease: A twenty-year report on 1000 patients followed since childhood. Circulation 4:836, 1951.
20. Gordis, L., Lilienfeld, A., and Rodriguez, R.: Studies in the epidemiology and preventability of rheumatic fever. I. demographic factors and the incidence of acute attacks. J. Chron. Dis. 21:645, 1969.
21. Denny, F. W., Wannamaker, L. W., Brink, W. R., et al.: Prevention of

rheumatic fever: Treatment of the preceding streptococcal infection. JAMA *143*:151, 1950.

22. Catanzaro, F. J., Stetson, C. A., Morris, A. J., et al.: Symposium on rheumatic fever and rheumatic heart disease. Am. J. Med. *17*:749, 1954.

23. Siegel, A. C., Johnson, E. E., and Stollerman, G. H.: Controlled studies of streptococcal pharyngitis in a pediatric population. I. Factors related to the attack rate of rheumatic fever. N. Engl. J. Med. *265*:559, 1961.

24. Stollerman, G. H.: Rheumatogenic group A streptococci and the return of rheumatic fever. Adv. Intern. Med. *35*:1, 1990.

25. Stollerman, G. H.: Rheumatogenic streptococci and autoimmunity. Clin. Immunol. Immunopathol. *61*:131, 1991.

26. Kaplan, E. L., Johnson, D. R., and Cleary, P. P.: Group A streptococcal serotypes isolated from patients and sibling contacts during the resurgence of rheumatic fever in the United States in the mid-1980s. J. Infect. Dis. *159*:101, 1989.

27. Bessen, D., Jones, K. F., and Fischetti, V. A.: Evidence for two distinct classes of streptococcal M protein and their relationship to rheumatic fever. J. Exp. Med. *169*:269, 1989.

28. Krisher, K., and Cunningham, M. W.: Myosin: A link between streptococci and heart. Science *227*:413, 1985.

29. Dale, J. B., and Beachey, E. H.: Sequence of myosin cross-reactive epitopes of streptococcal M protein. J. Exp. Med. *164*:1785, 1986.

30. Khanna, A. K., Buskirk, D. R., Williams, R. C., et al.: Presence of non-HLA B cell antigen in rheumatic fever patients and their families as defined by a monoclonal antibody. J. Clin. Invest. *83*:1710, 1989.

31. Ayoub, E. M., Barrett, D. J., Maclaren, N. K., et al.: Association of class II human histocompatibility leukocyte antigens with rheumatic fever. J. Clin. Invest. *77*:2019, 1986.

32. Narula, J., Chopra, P., Talwar, K. K., et al.: Does endomyocardial biopsy aid in the diagnosis of active rheumatic carditis? Circulation *88*:2198, 1993.

DIAGNOSIS AND TREATMENT

33. Jones, T. D.: Diagnosis of rheumatic fever. JAMA *126*:481, 1944.

34. Dajani, A. S., Ayoub, E. M., Bierman, F. Z., et al.: Guidelines for the diagnosis of rheumatic fever: Jones criteria, updated 1992. JAMA *268*:2069, 1992.

35. Schaffer, F. M., Agarwal, R., Helm, J., et al.: Poststreptococcal reactive arthritis and silent carditis: A case report and review of the literature. Pediatrics *93*:837, 1994.

36. Czoniczer, G., Amezcua, F., Pelargonio, S., et al.: Therapy of severe rheumatic carditis: Comparison of adrenocortical steroids and aspirin. Circulation *29*:813, 1964.

PREVENTION

37. Dajani, A. S.: Adherence to physicians' instructions as a factor in managing streptococcal pharyngitis. Pediatrics, (*In press*).

38. Bass, J. W.: Antibiotic management of group A streptococcal pharyngotonsillitis. Pediatr. Infect. Dis. J. *10*:S43, 1991.

39. Markowitz, M., Gerber, M. A., and Kaplan, E. L.: Treatment of streptococcal pharyngotonsillitis: Reports of penicillin's demise are premature. J. Pediatr. *123*:679, 1993.

40. Dajani, A. S., Taubert, K., Ferrieri, P., et al.: Treatment of streptococcal pharyngitis and prevention of rheumatic fever. Pediatrics, *96*:758, 1995.

41. Coonan, K. M., and Kaplan, E. L.: In vitro susceptibility of recent North American group A streptococcal isolates to eleven oral antibiotics. Pediatr. Infect. Dis. J. *13*:630, 1994.

42. Seppala, H., Nissinen, A., Jarvinen, H., et al.: Resistance to erythromycin in group A streptococci. N. Engl. J. Med. *326*:292, 1992.

43. Hooton, T. M.: A comparison of azithromycin and penicillin V for the treatment of streptococcal pharyngitis. Am. J. Med. *91*:23S, 1991.

44. Pichichero, M. E., and Margolis, P. A.: A comparison of cephalosporins and penicillin in the treatment of group A streptococcal pharyngitis: A meta-analysis supporting the concept of microbial copathogenicity. Pediatr. Infect. Dis. J. *10*:275, 1991.

45. Block, S. L., Hedrick, J. A., and Tyler, R. D.: Comparative study of the effectiveness of cefixime and penicillin V for the treatment of streptococcal pharyngitis in children and adolescents. Pediatr. Infect. Dis. J. *11*:919, 1992.

46. Gooch, W. M., McLinn, S. E., Aronovitz, G. H., et al.: Efficacy of cefuroxime axetil suspension compared with that of penicillin V suspension in children with group A streptococcal pharyngitis. Antimicrob. Agents Chemother. *37*:159, 1993.

47. Dajani, A. S., Kessler, S. L., Mendelson, R., et al.: Cefpodoxime proxetil vs penicillin V in pediatric streptococcal pharyngitis/tonsillitis. Pediatr. Infect. Dis. J. *12*:275, 1993.

48. Pichichero, M. E., Gooch, W. M., Rodriguez, W., et al.: Effective short-course treatment of acute group A beta-hemolytic streptococcal tonsillo-pharyngitis: Ten days of penicillin V vs 5 days or 10 days of cefpodoxime therapy in children. Arch. Pediatr. Adolesc. Med. *148*:1053, 1994.

49. Aujard, Y., Boucut, I., Brahimi, N., et al.: Comparative efficacy and safety of four-day cefuroxime axetil and 10-day penicillin treatment of group A beta-hemolytic streptococcal pharyngitis in children. Pediatr. Infect. Dis. J. *14*:295, 1995.

50. Dajani, A. S.: Pharyngitis/tonsillitis: European and United States experience with cefpodoxime proxetil. Pediatr. Infect. Dis. J. *14*:S7, 1995.

51. Still, J. G.: Management of pediatric patients with group A beta-hemolytic *Streptococcus* pharyngitis: Treatment options. Pediatr. Infect. Dis. J. *14*:S57, 1995.

52. Berrios, X., del Campo, E., Guzman, B., et al.: Discontinuing rheumatic fever prophylaxis in selected adolescents and young adults. Ann. Intern. Med. *118*:401, 1993.

53. Lue, H. C., Wu, M. H., Hsieh, K. H., et al.: Rheumatic fever recurrences: Controlled study of a 3-week versus 4-week benzathine penicillin prevention program. J. Pediatr. *108*:299, 1986.

54. Lue, H. C., Wu, M. H., Wang, J. K., et al.: Long-term outcome of patients with rheumatic fever receiving benzathine penicillin G prophylaxis every three weeks versus every four weeks. J. Pediatr. *125*:812, 1994.

55. Dajani, A. S., Bisno, A. L., Chung, K. J., et al.: Prevention of bacterial endocarditis: Recommendations by the American Heart Association. JAMA *264*:2919, 1990.

Chapter 56
Rheumatic Diseases and the Heart

JONATHAN S. COBLYN, MICHAEL E. WEINBLATT

The rheumatic diseases are a protean group of illnesses whose manifestations primarily occur in bones, joints, and connective tissues. Many of these illnesses have striking systemic features that may dominate the clinical course. This chapter will outline the cardiac manifestations of the systemic rheumatic diseases. As there is no unifying pathogenesis for this group of illnesses, there is no pathobiological mechanism to explain the cardiac manifestations of each disease. The immune mechanisms of cardiac disease are reviewed in Chapter 41, and further elucidation of the cardiac myocyte's response to immune injury may help clarify the differing cardiac manifestations of the rheumatic diseases.[1]

RHEUMATOID ARTHRITIS

Rheumatoid arthritis is the most common systemic rheumatic disease, affecting approximately 1 per cent of the population. The various cardiac manifestations of rheumatoid arthritis include pericarditis, valvular disease, coronary arteritis, myocarditis, conduction pathway disease, aortic arch disease, and pulmonary hypertension (Table 56–1).

PERICARDITIS (See also p. 1518). The most common lesion seen in the hearts of patients with rheumatoid arthritis is pericarditis, which occurs in 11 to 50 per cent of

TABLE 56–1 CARDIAC MANIFESTATIONS OF RHEUMATOID ARTHRITIS

PERICARDITIS
  Constrictive pericarditis
  Cardiac tamponade
  Septic pericarditis

VALVULAR DISEASE
  Mitral and aortic regurgitation predominate
  Stenotic lesions rare

CORONARY ARTERITIS
  Small and large vessels

MYOCARDIAL DYSFUNCTION
  Myocarditis/fibrosis
  Amyloidosis
  Drug-induced-Chloroquine/Hydroxychloroquine

CONDUCTION SYSTEM ABNORMALITIES
  Varying degrees including complete heart block
  Fibrosis/rheumatoid nodule

AORTITIS
  Thoracic and abdominal

PULMONARY HYPERTENSION
  "Primary" pulmonary hypertension
  Pulmonary fibrosis/vasculitis

patients. In patients with known pericarditis, chest pain is often the chief complaint as well as peripheral edema and orthopnea.[2]

The *electrocardiogram* is often nondiagnostic with no abnormality or first-degree heart block being the most common manifestation, reflecting underlying involvement of the conduction system. *Chest radiographs* usually reveal cardiomegaly and/or pleural effusions.[2] Diagnosis is most often confirmed by *echocardiography*, which shows pericardial effusion in up to 30 per cent of patients.[3]

PERICARDIAL FLUID AND PATHOLOGY. A low pericardial fluid glucose, leukocyte counts ranging from 156 to 33,650/MM³, and often low complement values may be seen.[2] The pathology of pericarditis in rheumatoid arthritis includes fibrinous pericarditis, fibrous adhesions, fibrocellular changes similar to rheumatoid synovitis and rheumatoid nodule/granuloma formation, or combinations of these.

TREATMENT. Pericarditis generally resolves with aggressive treatment of the underlying arthritis. Such treatment may include nonsteroidal antiinflammatory drugs (NSAIDs), corticosteroids, or disease-modifying drugs such as gold salts or methotrexate. The daily steroid dosage needed to treat serositis (pleuritis, pericarditis) usually is less than 0.5 mg/kg of prednisone, but in life-threatening situations, high-dose corticosteroids (1 to 2 mg/kg prednisone) may be initiated.

CARDIAC COMPRESSION AND CONSTRICTIVE PERICARDITIS. The distinction between constrictive pericarditis and cardiac tamponade is often blurred in patients with rheumatoid pericarditis. The term *cardiac compression* refers to both patients with tamponade and pericardial constriction.[4] Presenting features include edema, dyspnea, chest pain, pulsus paradoxus, and a pericardial rub. Diagnosis is made generally by echocardiography, but cardiac catheterization is often required. Once the diagnosis of cardiac compression is made, treatment is almost uniformly surgical. Pericardiocentesis may be life saving in the setting of tamponade physiology, but surgical decompression is the treatment of choice.

Constrictive pericarditis in rheumatoid arthritis occurs more commonly than cardiac tamponade. The prevalence of constrictive pericarditis in rheumatoid arthritis is less than 1 per cent.[5] The treatment of constrictive pericarditis is surgical.[4] Therapy with steroids or disease-modifying drugs is not indicated.

VALVULAR DISEASE. In autopsy studies, the prevalence of rheumatoid granulomata involving the heart valves ranges from 3 per cent to 5 per cent.[6] Heart valve lesions in rheumatoid arthritis involve the valve leaflets and valve rings and may be pathologically identical to rheumatoid nodules. There may also be nongranulomatous valve inflammation (Fig. 56–1) with subsequent fibrosis and thickening of valve leaflets. The order of frequency of valvular involvement is similar to rheumatic fever: mitral, aortic, tricuspid, and pulmonary.[7] The process appears to begin within the core of the valve leaflet preserving the peripheral portions; this differs from rheumatic valvular disease in which the entire leaflet is involved. In an echocardiographic study of 101 patients with rheumatoid arthritis, 13 per cent of patients had abnormalities of the mitral valve including mitral valve prolapse and mitral annular calcification.[8]

Despite the relative rarity of hemodynamic valve incompetence, numerous cases of progressive aortic insufficiency have been reported. Rarely, patients may require mitral and/or aortic valve replacement.

CORONARY ARTERY DISEASE. Coronary arteritis has been detected in up to 20 per cent of autopsies of patients with

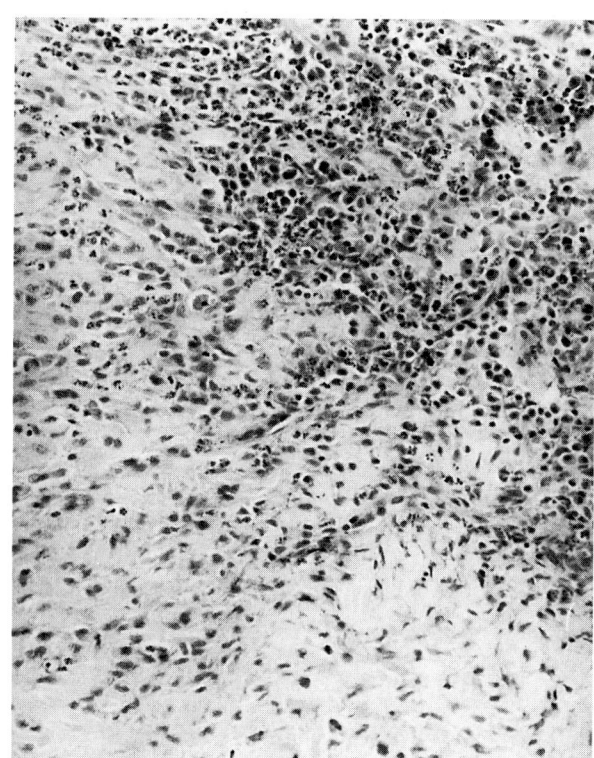

FIGURE 56-1. Aortic valve in a patient with rheumatoid arthritis with florid chronic active inflammation including numerous plasma cells, lymphocytes and polymorphonuclear leukocytes. (H&E, × 175). (Courtesy of Frederick J. Schoen, M.D., Ph.D.)

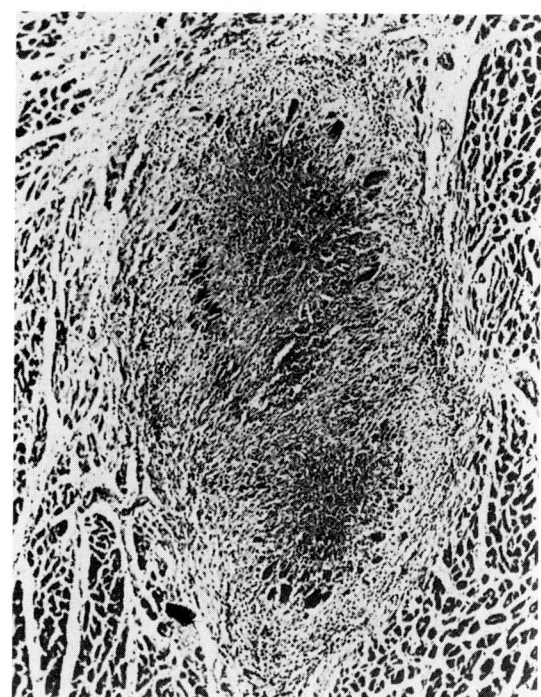

FIGURE 56-2. Rheumatoid granuloma in a section of myocardium. A central zone of fibrinoid necrosis is surrounded by histiocytes and fibroblasts as well as interspersed multinucleated giant cells. The outer zone of fibrosis contains chronic inflammatory cells (H&E, × 35). (From McAllister, H.A.: Collagen vascular diseases and the cardiovascular system. *In* Silver, M.D. [ed.]: Cardiovascular Pathology. New York, Churchill Livingstone, 1983.)

rheumatoid arthritis, but involvement tends to be restricted to smaller intramyocardial arteries.[6] Intense mononuclear cell infiltration of the left anterior descending artery has been described in a patient with pancarditis, and, in another patient, a percutaneous endomyocardial biopsy revealed immunoglobulin M (IgM) deposits in small blood vessels resulting in small vessel arteritis.[9,10] If coronary vasculitis is confirmed, aggressive treatment with corticosteroids and/or immunosuppressive agents is suggested, although this manifestation is a rare clinical problem.

MYOCARDITIS. The myocarditis of rheumatoid arthritis is usually nonspecific, and although it occurs in up to 20 per cent of patients, it rarely causes significant myocardial dysfunction.[6] The pathology reveals granulomatous involvement or nonspecific interstitial inflammatory cells (Fig. 56-2). Rarely, amyloid deposition contributes to myocardial dysfunction. In patients with large- and small-vessel vasculitis, myocarditis and congestive heart failure have been observed.

CONDUCTION SYSTEM DISEASE. Varying degrees of heart block occur in 10 per cent of patients.[6] First-degree atrioventricular block is the most common conduction system abnormality in rheumatoid arthritis, but fascicular blocks and atrial arrhythmias have been described. Complete heart block rarely occurs. The conduction system abnormalities are usually due to rheumatoid nodules involving the conduction system but, rarely, may be from extension of inflammation from the aortic or mitral valves, hemorrhage into a rheumatoid nodule, or amyloidosis.[10] A permanent pacemaker may be required.

AORTITIS (see also p. 1575). The incidence of aortitis in rheumatoid arthritis may be higher than previously thought, occurring in 10 of 188 (5 per cent) consecutive cases examined by autopsy.[11] Three of these 10 cases showed definite involvement of the intima by aortitis, and the remaining seven had a lymphoplasmacytic infiltrate confined to the media and adventitia (Fig. 56-3). The thoracic aorta was most commonly involved, although in-

volvement of both the thoracic and abdominal aorta was present in four cases. Aneurysm formation was present in three cases, and one patient died of a ruptured aortic aneurysm.

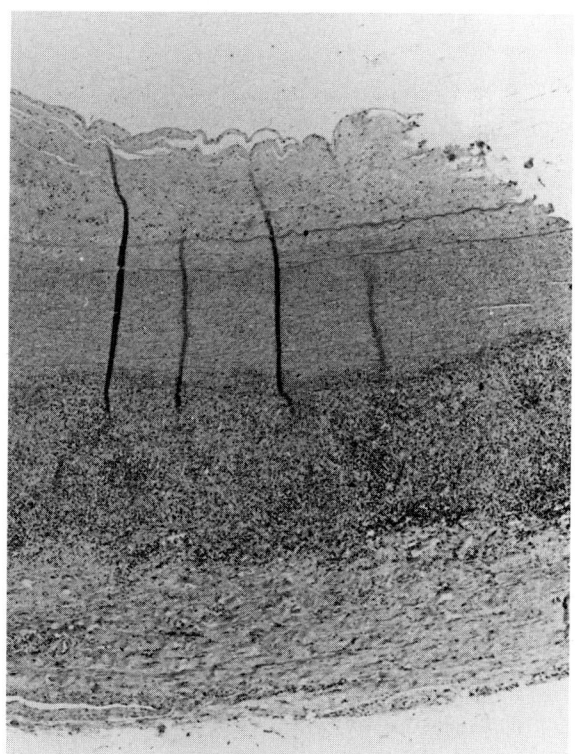

FIGURE 56-3. Panmural aortitis in a patient with rheumatoid arthritis, demonstrating fibrosis and inflammation of the intima (top) and adventitia (bottom) and a dense lymphoplasmacytic infiltrate in the media with disruption of elastic fibers. Hematoxylin and eosin. (Courtesy of Ellen Gravallese, M.D.)

UNUSUAL CARDIAC MANIFESTATIONS. *Pulmonary hypertension* due to pulmonary vasculitis is an uncommon complication of rheumatoid arthritis. Chloroquine or hydroxychloroquine therapy, disease-modifying drugs used in rheumatoid arthritis, may occasionally result in the development of *cardiomyopathy.* Endomyocardial biopsy is diagnostic with characteristic curvilinear bodies, myelin bodies, and large secondary lysosomes demonstrated upon electron microscopy.[12]

STILL'S DISEASE. Still's disease (systemic onset juvenile arthritis) is an uncommon inflammatory disorder occurring in children and rarely in adults. As in adult rheumatoid arthritis, the most common cardiac manifestation is pericarditis, which may lead to tamponade. Other rare manifestations include myocarditis, dilated cardiomyopathy, and symptomatic aortic and mitral valve disease. Aggressive treatment of the underlying illness with corticosteroids and disease-modifying drugs, with appropriate surgical intervention for tamponade or valve replacement, may be necessary.[13]

SYSTEMIC LUPUS ERYTHEMATOSUS

The cardiac manifestations of systemic lupus erythematosus (SLE) are varied (Table 56–2) and are found more commonly at autopsy than clinically. William Osler first noted cardiac involvement as part of the group of diseases called *exudative erythema,* which clinically describes patients with SLE.[14] The incidence of cardiac involvement varies with the mode of detection. With two-dimensional and Doppler echocardiography, 57 per cent of patients had echocardiographic abnormalities including valvular abnormalities, pericardial disease, and myocardial abnormalities.[15] The incidence of coronary artery involvement differs between the pre- or post-steroid era, with a marked acceleration of coronary atherosclerosis in the post-steroid era.[16] Although the cardiac lesions in SLE are presumably due to immune deposits in the walls of blood vessels, the myocardium, or the pericardium,[17] newer studies have sought to define an association between SLE and antiphospholipid antibodies.[18]

PERICARDITIS. The most common cardiac manifestation of SLE is pericarditis, presenting in up to 30 per cent of patients with active disease.[16,19] Pericarditis may be asymptomatic or may present with typical chest pain, pericardial rub, fever, and tachycardia. Electrocardiograms may demonstrate diffuse ST-segment elevation, but sinus tachycardia and atrial arrhythmias are often seen. Symptomatic pa-

TABLE 56–2 CARDIAC MANIFESTATIONS OF SYSTEMIC LUPUS ERYTHEMATOSUS

PERICARDITIS
Cardiac tamponade
Constrictive pericarditis
Drug-induced pericarditis

MYOCARDITIS
Rare manifestation
? Association with myositis, anti-RNP

ENDOCARDIAL/VALVULAR LESIONS
Libman-Sacks endocarditis
Regurgitant and stenotic lesions (aortic and mitral)
Secondary bacterial endocarditis, embolization
Inflammatory valvulitis (vasculitis)

CORONARY ARTERY DISEASE
Coronary arteritis uncommon
Increased artherogenesis
Coronary artery spasm

CONDUCTION SYSTEM ABNORMALITIES
Varying degrees of atrioventricular block
Complete heart block
Anti-Ro/La-associated fetal heart block

PULMONARY HYPERTENSION

ANTIPHOSPHOLIPID ANTIBODY SYNDROME
Valvular (regurgitant) lesions
Cerebrovascular events
Coronary artery disease
Pulmonary hypertension
Dilated cardiomyopathy
Endocardial thrombi

tients usually have pericardial effusions. Pericardial tamponade may occur in SLE, but the incidence of this complication is less than 1 per cent. Serum hypocomplementemia and/or high-titer antinuclear antibody/anti-DNA antibodies uniformly accompany this complication.[20] Pericardial fluid is often exudative and may be hypocomplementemic. The pathology of the pericardium may show fibrosis and acute inflammation, but frank vasculitis also may be seen.[16,19]

Drug-induced SLE causes pericarditis, presumably due to pathogenic mechanisms similar to those in native SLE. Constrictive pericarditis is very rare in SLE and has been reported in both native SLE and drug-induced SLE.[20]

Management. The treatment of pericarditis in SLE depends on the degree of hemodynamic compromise. NSAIDs are quite effective. For symptomatic serositis 10 to 20 mg per day of prednisone is usually sufficient. In the setting of tamponade, aggressive treatment, including daily systemic corticosteroids at doses of 1 to 2 mg per kg of prednisone and pericardiocentesis to normalize hemodynamics, is recommended. Most patients will require pericardiotomy or a pericardial window for long-term relief.

MYOCARDITIS. Myocarditis is clinically diagnosed in up to 10 per cent of patients with SLE.[21] The incidence of myocarditis in autopsy studies, however, approaches 40 per cent.[20,22] Immunofluorescent findings in cardiac tissue are more diffuse and more frequent than histological findings. Immune deposits are found in myocardial vessels, suggesting a role for immune complex deposition as a factor in myocardial injury.[17] Echocardiographic studies in SLE confirm the relative lack of clinically active myocarditis.

In a retrospective review of 140 consecutive patients with SLE, five had myocarditis, and each also had skeletal myositis. The most striking finding was the presence of antibodies to nuclear ribonucleoprotein (RNP) in all five patients.[21] Endomyocardial biopsies in patients with SLE myocarditis show moderate-to-marked lymphocytic infiltrate in the interstitium and fibrous tissue around blood vessels.[23] The treatment of myocarditis is similar to treatment of other cardiomyopathies. However, aggressive therapies with prednisone, and possibly immunosuppressive drugs, should also be administered.

ENDOCARDITIS. In 1924, Libman and Sacks first described endocardial involvement in SLE.[24] Libman-Sacks endocarditis is present in up to 50 per cent of hearts at autopsy, but clinical manifestations are rare.[22] Verrucous vegetations 3 to 4 mm in size may appear on the valvular or mural endocardial surface; any valve may be involved, but the posterior leaflet of the mitral valve is the most common site (Fig. 56–4). Mitral and aortic regurgitation are the most common clinically important lesions, although mitral stenosis, aortic stenosis and tricuspid stenosis, and regurgitation have all been described. Despite the appearance of fragility, these vegetations rarely embolize to the brain or the coronary arteries.[22]

The pattern and outcome of patients with endocardial damage secondary to SLE appears to be changing with the advent of steroid therapy, valve replacement, and the increased longevity of these patients. In a classic autopsy series, Bulkley and Roberts report that in the post-steroid era, the Libman-Sacks type of endocardial lesions were smaller, fewer in number, mainly left sided, and pathologically were either partly or completely healed.[16] Other causes of valve dysfunction in SLE include valvulitis, vasculitis in valve tissue, thrombus formation upon the valve, and nodular calcification within the valve.[25]

The frequency of valvular involvement in SLE ranges from 18 per cent using standard echocardiography (Fig. 56–5) to as high as 74 per cent using transesophageal echocardiography.[26,27] Patients with valve thickening and dysfunction, rather than classic verrucous lesions, may have more hemodynamic compromise and a higher incidence of associated antiphospholipid antibodies.[26,27] The presence of endocardial lesions in patients with SLE may increase the likelihood of bacterial endocarditis and possible embolic disease.[27] Steroids have no role in the treatment of valve disease per se and may, in fact, exacerbate outcomes.[25]

Management of the valve disease is dependent on the

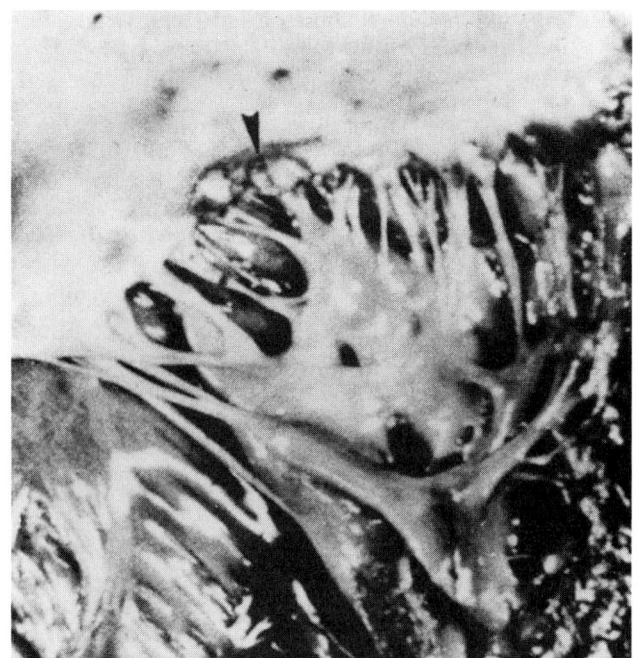

FIGURE 56–4. Verrucous endocarditis of Libman and Sacks involving the chordal attachments of an atrioventricular valve in a patient with systemic lupus erythematosus. The vegetations are usually 1 to 4 mm in diameter, may occur in clusters, and involve mural endocardium as well as valvular tissue. (From McAllister, H.A.: Collagen vascular diseases and the cardiovascular system. *In* Silver, M.D. [ed.]: Cardiovascular Pathology. New York, Churchill Livingstone, 1983.)

extent of hemodynamic compromise. Some series report that the mortality and morbidity from valve replacement in patients with SLE is quite high, but others report an improving outcome.[25,28]

CORONARY ARTERY DISEASE. In the pre-steroid era, myocardial infarction and coronary artery disease (CAD) were quite rare. In a major pathological comparison of SLE patients pre- and post-steroid use, there were no atherosclerotic plaques in patients treated less than 1 year with steroids, but plaques were found in over 40 per cent of

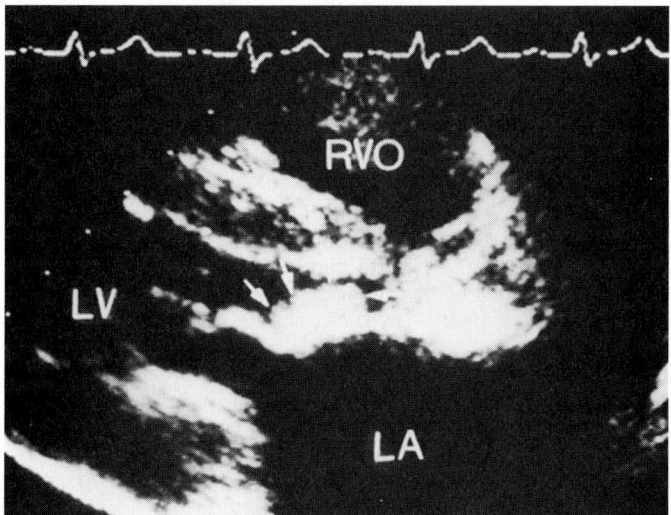

FIGURE 56–5. Parasternal long-axis view of the heart from a patient with systemic lupus erythematosus and high levels of anticardiolipin antibodies. A massive vegetation on ventricular surface of the anterior mitral leaflet *(arrows)* not interfering with the valve mobility, is clearly visualized. LA = left atrium, LV = left ventricle, RVO = right ventricular outflow. (Reproduced with permission from Nihoyannopoulos, N., et al.: Cardiac abnormalities in systemic lupus erythematosus: Association with raised anticardiolipin antibodies. Circulation *82:*369, 1990. Copyright 1990 American Heart Association.)

those patients treated more than 1 year with steroids.[16] Whether corticosteroids have an independent role in atherogenesis is unclear. Increased atherogenesis may be due to hypertension, hyperlipidemia, and prolonged survival, all possibly related to the use of corticosteroids.[29,30]

Coronary artery involvement in SLE may also be due to active arteritis, which, in one small series, occurred in 50 per cent of patients.[31] Other causes of CAD in patients with SLE include coronary artery spasm and the hypercoagulable state secondary to antiphospholipid antibodies.[32] Management of patients with CAD and SLE requires attempts to decrease the dosage of prednisone and control hypercholesterolemia, hypertension, obesity, and other coronary risk factors.[30]

CONDUCTION SYSTEM ABNORMALITIES/CONGENITAL HEART BLOCK. Heart block of all degrees is a relatively rare manifestation of SLE. Atrial arrhythmias and, occasionally, ventricular arrhythmias, may be associated with accompanying myocarditis, coronary artery disease, or pericarditis.

Neonatal lupus may present as complete heart block; women who carry anti-Ro and anti-La antibodies have increased risk of giving birth to children with complete heart block.[33] Myocardial inflammation and fibrosis of the conduction system occur in infants with this syndrome.[34] The treatment of a fetus with congenital heart block secondary to maternal anti-Ro/La antibodies may include treatment of the mother with steroids and/or intravenous gamma globulin or a temporary or permanent pacemaker in the neonate.[35] Although the risk for developing complete heart block in the offspring of an anti-Ro–positive mother is quite low, mothers at risk for such an occurrence should be closely monitored with the use of fetal ultrasounds to detect complete heart block or myocarditis before delivery.

MISCELLANEOUS. Cardiac manifestations of SLE also include pulmonary hypertension, which has been estimated to occur in up to 5 per cent of patients. This may be related to vasospasm and/or vasculitis, and cor pulmonale may result.

ANTIPHOSPHOLIPID ANTIBODY SYNDROME. Clinical manifestations of this syndrome (which may occur independent of SLE) include thrombotic disorders including venous and arterial thrombosis, fetal loss in the late first trimester and second trimester, thrombocytopenia, premature stroke, and other neurological and cardiac manifestations. Patients with SLE who possess antiphospholipid antibodies or the lupus anticoagulant have an apparent increased risk of cardiac abnormalities. Valvular involvement is more common in patients with the antiphospholipid antibody and SLE. SLE valvular lesions tend to be both regurgitant and stenotic. Valve lesions in antiphospholipid antibody syndrome (APS) are more often regurgitant.[27,36–38] In patients with APS, there is an increased risk of embolic cerebrovascular complications.[36,39]

Approximately 5 per cent of patients with APS may develop myocardial infarction, especially patients under age 45.[39] Other cardiac manifestations of APS with SLE include pulmonary hypertension and cardiomyopathy, with bland thrombotic occlusions of the microcirculation without vasculitis. Anticoagulation in the setting of regurgitant disease, myocardial infarction, and pulmonary hypertension is indicated, and it is suggested that the international normalized ratio should be greater than 3.0.[40]

Polymyositis/Dermatomyositis

The cardiac manifestations of polymyositis and dermatomyositis include electrocardiographic changes with varying degrees of atrioventricular and interventricular block, atrial and ventricular tachyarrhythmias, sick sinus syndrome, congestive heart failure secondary to acute myocarditis, and/or end-stage myocardial fibrosis. Rare manifestations of polymyositis include coronary vasculitis, acute pericarditis and tamponade, and constrictive pericarditis.[41,42]

Numerous studies in the past two decades have revealed that cardiac involvement is common in polymyositis and may be associated with a poor prognosis.[41] In a series of 20 autopsy cases, myocarditis was detected in six patients; four had congestive heart failure.[43] In another autopsy series of 16 patients with polymyositis/dermatomyositis syndromes, 43 per cent had congestive heart failure, 25 per cent with histological evidence of myocarditis and 25 per cent with focal myocardial fibrosis.[44]

CONDUCTION SYSTEM INVOLVEMENT. In an electrocardiographic study of 77 patients with polymyositis, 32 per cent had an abnormal electrocardiogram; 13 per cent had left anterior hemiblock, and 9 per cent had right-bundle branch block.[45] Other electrocardiographic abnormalities, including atrioventricular conduction disturbances, atrial and ventricular arrhythmias, sick sinus syndrome, progressive fascicular block requiring pacemaker therapy, atrial fibrillation, and ventricular tachycardia, have been observed, but these are only rarely the cause of death.[46]

MYOCARDITIS. Myocardial involvement similar to that in skeletal muscle can result in congestive heart failure but is only rarely a cause of serious morbidity. Heart failure may be due to atherosclerotic disease and/or corticosteroid- and hypertension-related disorders or myocarditis. Pathology of heart failure includes myocardial fibrosis, inflammatory myocarditis, or, rarely, vasculitis with small vessel involvement.[43,44] The onset of heart failure secondary to myocarditis usually occurs in patients with active peripheral muscle involvement. However, it may rarely be the presenting symptom of polymyositis or may develop in the setting of improving peripheral myositis.[47]

If myocarditis is confirmed, treatment with prednisone or its equivalent at 1 to 1.5 mg/kg/day for at least 6 to 8 weeks is recommended. If there is no response, methotrexate should be added, although other drugs such as azathioprine, cyclophosphamide, and cyclosporin have been used.[46] Endomyocardial biopsy should be performed if myocarditis is the initial presenting manifestation or to clarify the degree of myocardial inflammation or fibrosis. If fibrosis predominates, steroids and immunosuppressive agents may be withheld.

OTHER CARDIAC MANIFESTATIONS. Pericarditis and/or pericardial effusions diagnosed by echocardiography may be found in up to 25 per cent of patients.[41] However, the incidence of pericarditis is greater in patients who have overlap syndromes and significantly higher in children with dermatomyositis.[48] Rarely, dermatomyositis has been associated with constrictive pericarditis and pericardial tamponade.[42,48] Clinical pericardial involvement is rare; treatment with nonsteroidal agents and/or corticosteroids (less than 0.5 mg/kg/day) may be beneficial.

Other manifestations of polymyositis heart disease include mitral valve prolapse, unexplained high-output cardiac failure, pulmonary hypertension, and systemic vasculitis. Complete heart block secondary to polymyositis induced by D-penicillamine has been described.[49] Cardiac involvement is one of the most significant clinical factors associated with impaired prognosis in polymyositis.

SPONDYLOARTHROPATHIES

The inflammatory aspect of cardiac disease in this group of diseases differs from rheumatoid arthritis by the higher frequency of aortic valve involvement, the relative lack of pericardial involvement, and relatively characteristic echocardiographic findings in a small subset of patients with aortic insufficiency.

Ankylosing Spondylitis

It was not until 1958 that ankylosing spondylitis and rheumatoid arthritis were recognized as distinct clinical entities. Therefore, pathological data regarding cardiac involvement before this time was based upon mixed data from patients with various inflammatory polyarthropathies.

AORTIC FINDINGS (see also p. 1575). The seminal pathological description of the cardiac manifestations of ankylosing spondylitis was published in 1973.[50] In this study, the pathological findings were described in eight patients with combined ankylosing spondylitis and aortic regurgitation. The aorta in ankylosing spondylitis is histologically similar to that in syphilitic aortitis. There is adventitial scarring, intimal proliferation with scarring of the media, and the vasa vasora are narrowed and surrounded by lymphocytes and plasma cells. The adventitial scarring extends below the base of the aortic valve. This thickening is particularly prominent behind the commissures of the aortic valve cusp and form a fibrous commissural bump.[50] Aortic regurgitation therefore results from shortening and thickening of the aortic valve cusps, displacement of the cusps by the "fibrous tissue bump," and dilatation of the aortic root. Similarly, one can rarely observe mitral regurgitation secondary

to dilatation of the left ventricle from aortic regurgitation and from thickening of the basal portion of the anterior mitral valve leaflet.[50] In an echocardiographic study of patients who had ankylosing spondylitis greater than 10 years, 29 per cent had cardiac abnormalities.[51] This included aortic insufficiency (8 per cent), conduction system abnormalities (12 per cent), and pericardial effusions (4 per cent).

VALVULAR INVOLVEMENT. Aortic valve disease has been reported in up to 10 per cent in patients with ankylosing spondylitis[52] (Fig. 56–6). Rarely, aortic insufficiency may be the presenting manifestation. Subacute infective endocarditis is an uncommon complication. Aortic regurgitation may be progressive and require aortic valve replacement. Mitral regurgitation is relatively uncommon in ankylosing spondylitis; it may be secondary to mitral valve prolapse[53] as well as the extension of the "subaortic ridge or bump" affecting the basal portion of the anterior leaflet of the mitral valve.[54] Mitral valve replacement may be required if there is no improvement with standard medical therapy.

CONDUCTION SYSTEM DISORDER. Cardiac conduction disturbances are quite frequent in ankylosing spondylitis, occurring in up to 33 per cent of patients, and are more frequently observed in patients with aortic valve disease.[52] Conduction system abnormalities may be associated with the HLA-B27 antigen; the frequency of HLA-B27–positive men without spondylitis with permanent pacemakers is higher than in controls, suggesting an increased prevalence of heart block associated with this antigen alone.[55] Pathological changes in the aorta of patients with HLA-B27 heart disease without spondylitis are identical to the changes seen in patients with ankylosing spondylitis. The atrioventricular node and the bundle are distorted by fibrous tissue, consistent with extension of the same fibrotic process.[50,56] There is a wide spectrum of cardiac conduction disturbances, including Wolff-Parkinson-White syndrome, to all degrees of atrioventricular block.[57,58] These conduction system abnormalities may be intermittent, asymptomatic, and may spontaneously resolve.

It is speculated that although fibrosis contributes to the conduction system lesions, inflammatory infiltrates also contribute.[58] A trial of aggressive antiinflammatory medication may therefore be advisable to see if the inflammatory component resolves before permanent pacemaker implantation in those patients with complete heart block.

OTHER CARDIAC MANIFESTATIONS. Myocardial disease has been recognized as part of the spectrum of ankylosing

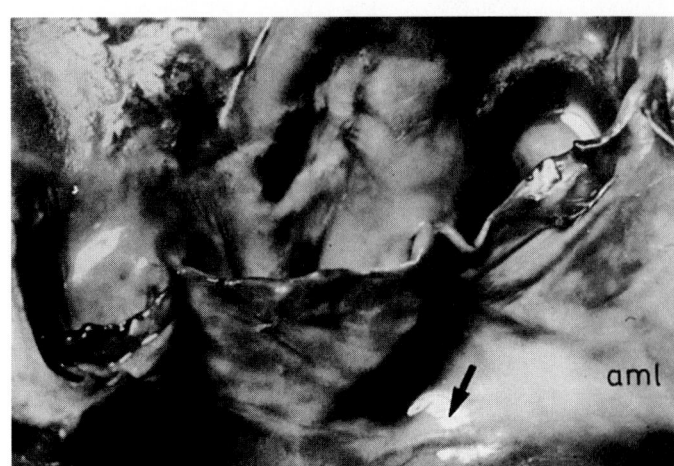

FIGURE 56–6. The aortic valve and sinus of Valsalva cut open in a patient with ankylosing spondylitis who was HLA-B27–positive. The base of the cusps is thickened. The orifice of the right coronary artery is distorted. Aortic regurgitation had been present during life. aml = anterior mitral leaflet. (From Bergfeldt, L.: HLA-B-27–associated heart disease. Am. J. Med. 77:961, 1984.)

spondylitis. In one echocardiographic study, 53 per cent of patients, although asymptomatic, had left ventricular abnormalities. The left ventricular dysfunction is presumably related to excess connective tissue in the myocardium.[59] Significant left ventricular dysfunction has been reported in less than 1 per cent of patients. Pericarditis, cor pulmonale, and aortic arch syndromes may occur rarely.

REITER'S SYNDROME. The cardiac manifestations of Reiter's syndrome are similar to those of ankylosing spondylitis. Although unusual, aortitis and aortic regurgitation have been described in Reiter's syndrome. Fulminant aortic regurgitation requiring aortic valve replacement has been observed.[60] The pathology of the aorta is similar to that in ankylosing spondylitis, with aortic dilatation leading to aortic regurgitation. Reiter's syndrome rarely will present with angina, with aortitis leading to narrowing of the coronary ostia.[61]

Varying degrees of heart block, including complete heart block, are common in Reiter's syndrome and may be an early manifestation. Indeed, 25 per cent of patients with Reiter's syndrome develop conduction system abnormalities.[62] Pericarditis may occur at a somewhat higher frequency than in ankylosing spondylitis. As with ankylosing spondylitis, treatment depends upon the severity of the manifestations. Corticosteroids and/or NSAIDs may forestall the need for permanent pacemaker therapy in the setting of acute Reiter's syndrome and complete heart block.

PSORIATIC ARTHRITIS. Isolated aortitis causing aortic regurgitation potentially requiring aortic valve replacement has been described in psoriatic arthritis, although this complication is exceedingly rare.[63] Mitral valve prolapse has also been reported to occur at an increased frequency in psoriatic arthritis.[64]

PROGRESSIVE SYSTEMIC SCLEROSIS AND ITS VARIANTS

In 1943 it was recognized that cardiac dysfunction occurred in scleroderma and characteristic myocardial lesions were seen in a classic autopsy study.[65] Scleroderma may also cause pulmonary hypertension and/or systemic hypertension; cardiac manifestations may be difficult to interpret because one may not be able to differentiate primary myocardial disease from changes secondary to systemic and/or pulmonary hypertension. Pathological observations in scleroderma do show significant primary myocardial lesions, with a clear increase in myocardial fibrosis compared to controls, especially in patients who died in their fourth decade.[66]

PATHOGENESIS. The pathogenesis of the cardiac lesion in scleroderma is controversial. An intriguing concept is one of repetitive vascular insults secondary to cold induced perfusion changes. Classic pathological changes of contraction band necrosis seen in scleroderma are similar to the findings in hearts subjected to prolonged ischemia and subsequent reperfusion.[67] There appears to be a reversible component to myocardial perfusion deficits, and calcium channel blockers can, to some extent, blunt these responses.[68]

PERICARDIAL INVOLVEMENT. Autopsy series report pericardial involvement in up to 50 per cent of patients with systemic sclerosis. Pericardial involvement includes fibrinous pericarditis, pericardial adhesions, and pericardial effusions. Symptomatic pericarditis, however, was present in only 16 per cent of patients with diffuse scleroderma but was present in over 30 per cent of patients with CREST syndrome (*c*alcinosis, *R*aynaud's, *e*sophageal dysfunction, *s*clerodactylia, *t*elangiectasia) or limited scleroderma. Clinical presentation varies from chest pain, fever, and dyspnea to, rarely, tamponade and/or constrictive pericarditis.[69,70] Pericardial fluid may be exudative, but there is no evidence for autoantibodies or complement depletion in the fluid implying a different pathogenesis than that in rheumatoid arthritis or SLE.[71]

The treatment of acute pericarditis is therapy with NSAIDs with careful observation of renal function. Corticosteroids may be used, but their use is of concern in patients with scleroderma. Patients rarely need pericardiocentesis or surgical intervention.

MYOCARDIAL INVOLVEMENT. Myocardial lesions and fibrosis, which are found in up to 80 per cent of patients upon autopsy, may be patchy, may present in both ventricles, and may bear no relationship to myocardial perfusion.[66,69] In an autopsy study of nine patients with progressive systemic sclerosis and sudden cardiac death, extensive myocardial necrosis was found in seven and scarring in nine although the coronary arteries were otherwise normal; seven patients had contraction-band necrosis.[72]

Myocardial dysfunction occurs often, although clinical congestive heart failure occurs in less than 5 per cent of patients with progressive systemic sclerosis. Using extensive noninvasive techniques, left ventricular dysfunction and myocardial perfusion defects can be detected in up to 75 per cent of patients[73] (Fig. 56-7). Restrictive and dilated cardiomyopathies rarely occur in adults and children with diffuse scleroderma. Inflammatory myocarditis may occur but is rare.[74]

MANAGEMENT. The treatment of patients with scleroderma heart disease is not unlike the treatment of cardiomyopathy or congestive heart failure of other causes. Steroids are usually withheld in severe scleroderma for the fear of potentiating renal crisis, but in the setting of proven myocarditis, they may be life saving. Additionally, the use of D-penicillamine and immunosuppressive agents, such as methotrexate or azathioprine, has been suggested, but there is no convincing evidence that these agents will prevent further myocardial damage. The main therapeutic advance in the treatment of scleroderma myocardial dysfunction has been the aggressive control of hypertension, particularly with an angiotensin-converting enzyme (ACE) inhibitor. Calcium antagonists have been shown to improve perfusion defects (Fig. 56-8).

CONDUCTION SYSTEM DISEASE. The electrocardiogram may be abnormal in 50 per cent of patients with scleroderma.[75] A wide variety of electrocardiographic abnormalities have been described and include all degrees of heart block, septal infarction pattern, ventricular tachycardia, and supraventricular tachycardias.[72] The extent of the electrocardiographic abnormality correlates with the degree of presumed myocardial fibrosis.

OTHER CARDIAC MANIFESTATIONS. Valvular abnormalities in progressive systemic sclerosis include nonspecific thickening of the mitral and aortic valves.[66,67] Pulmonary hypertension is a leading cause of morbidity and mortality in patients with scleroderma (diffuse and localized).

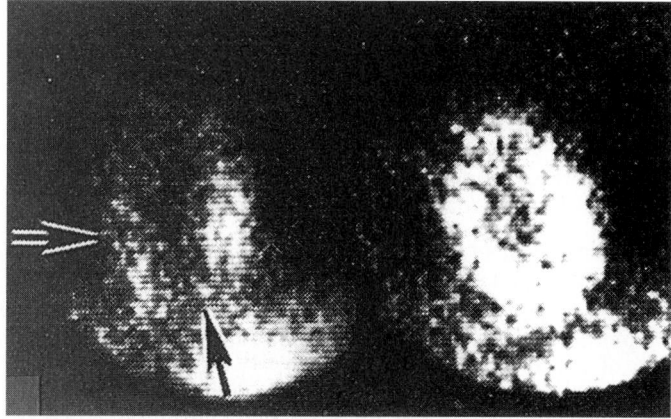

FIGURE 56-7. Thallium scintigrams obtained from a patient with scleroderma obtained immediately after immersion of the patient's hand in ice water for 2 minutes (*left*) and after 3 hours of redistribution (*right*). Images were obtained in the 40° left anterior oblique view and demonstrate a septal and inferoapical perfusion defect (*arrows*) that completely resolved with redistribution. (Modified from Alexander, E.L., et al.: Reversible cold-induced abnormalities in myocardial perfusion and function in systemic sclerosis. Ann. Intern. Med. 105:661–668, 1986.)

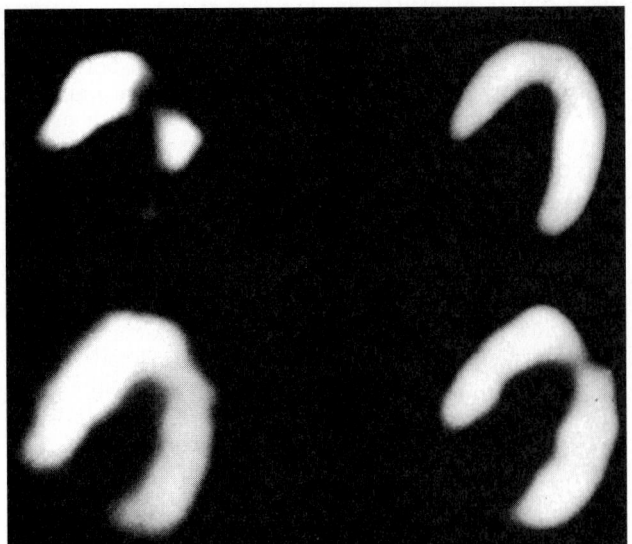

FIGURE 56–8. Positron emission tomographic images of a mid-left ventricular slice in a representative patient with systemic sclerosis showing ³⁸K myocardial uptake at baseline *(upper left)*. ³⁸K myocardial uptake after treatment with nifedipine *(lower left)*. These reflect increased perfusion and erduced ischemia, respectively. ¹⁸F-Fluorodeoxyglucose (¹⁸FDG) myocardial uptake at baseline *(upper right)* and ¹⁸FDG myocardial uptake after treatment with nifedipine *(lower right)*. An increase in ³⁸K myocardial uptake and a decrease in ¹⁸FDG myocardial uptake are seen after treatment with nifedipine. (From Duboc, D., et al.: The effect of nifedipine on myocardial perfusion and metabolism in systemic sclerosis. Arthritis Rheum. *34*:198, 1991; with permission.)

MIXED CONNECTIVE TISSUE DISEASE

The cardiac pathology of mixed connective tissue disease (MCTD) is similar to scleroderma. These patients often develop significant pulmonary hypertension as a result of an underlying pulmonary vasculopathy with marked intimal proliferation and luminal narrowing of the small pulmonary arterioles.[76] Pericarditis, pleuritis, massive pericardial effusions, myocarditis, and arrhythmias, have also been described.[77]

SJÖGREN'S SYNDROME

The incidence of primary myocardial and pericardial involvement in Sjögren's syndrome is low. Primary Sjögren's syndrome can result in verrucous endocarditis, similar to that seen in SLE. Conduction defects may also develop and fetal heart block may occur in the offspring of mothers' with primary Sjögren's syndrome who are anti-Ro positive.[78]

SYSTEMIC VASCULITIS

The clinical manifestations of vasculitis depend primarily on the size of the blood vessel involved and its location. A high index of suspicion for cardiac disease in any patient with pathologically defined vasculitis must be considered.

Large Vessel Involvement/Giant Cell Arteritis
(See also p. 1573)

Cardiac involvement in giant cell arteritis includes inflammation of the aorta with dilatation and/or inflammation of the aortic valve and its cusps, coronary arteritis, as well as pericarditis and myocarditis. The incidence of involvement of the aorta or its major branches approaches 13 per cent in some studies.[79] Inflammation of the vessel wall may become extensive enough to weaken the wall and produce a thoracic aortic aneurysm, and subsequent dilation may lead to aortic insufficiency. Prolonged inflammation of the vessel wall may lead to aortic rupture and death.[79,80] Occlusion of the aorta or its branches can occur along the course of the ascending, thoracic, or descending aorta, producing an aortic arch syndrome. Initial symptoms of tho-

racic aortic aneurysms secondary to giant cell arteritis (GCA) include exertional dyspnea and other symptoms of congestive heart failure, chest pain secondary to aortic dissection, angina, limb claudication and arterial bruits. In one study of patients with thoracic aortic aneurysms, 34 per cent were asymptomatic when the aneurysm was discovered.[81] The vast majority had GCA for an average of 2 years. Mortality from aortic dissection was 50 per cent. Patients with GCA or polymyalgia rheumatica should be examined carefully to ascertain that there are no pulse deficits, thoracic symptoms, or any symptoms or signs of limb ischemia.

Aortic regurgitation can rarely occur in giant cell arteritis, as an initial or a late complication.[82] The aortic regurgitation is usually due to aortitis resulting in destruction of elastic fibers within the arterial wall with marked inflammation and/or giant cells (Fig. 56–9). This inflammation leads to dilatation and distortion of the valve ring and the aortic root causing aortic regurgitation. When the aortic regurgitation is severe, aortic valve replacement is necessary and may be life saving.

Treatment of giant cell arteritis consists of high-dose corticosteroids (1 to 1.5 mg/kg/day of prednisone) and if there is no sign of improvement within 6 to 8 weeks, and if large vessel symptoms are suspected, cytotoxic therapies should be used.

Coronary vasculitis may rarely occur in giant cell arteritis. The pathology reveals granulomatous arteritis of epicardial coronary arteries and of intramural branches of the coronary arteries and arterioles.[83] Pericarditis and myocarditis are rare manifestations of giant cell arteritis. The treatment of these cardiac manifestations are similar to the treatment of GCA alone.

Behçet's Disease

Cardiac manifestations of Behçet's disease have classically included occlusion of the subclavian artery, aneu-

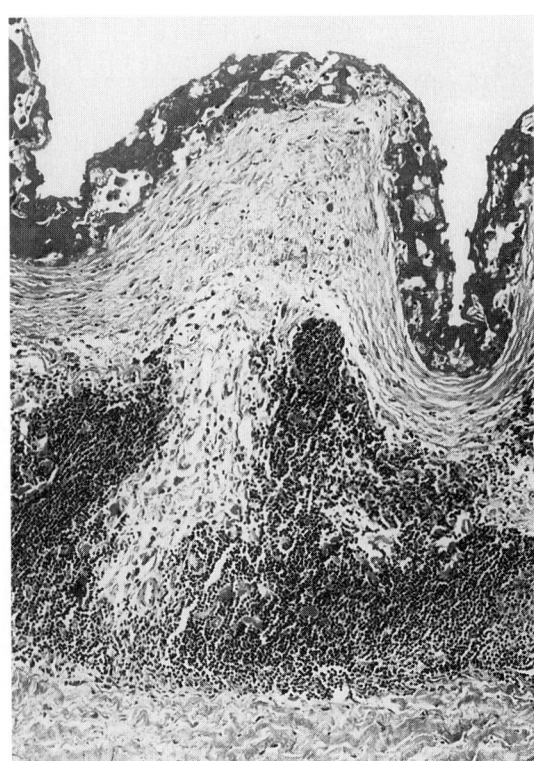

FIGURE 56–9. Active aortitis with perivascular lymphoplasmacytic infiltrate in the adventitia, unorganized periadventitial fibrin and secondary infarcts and patchy scarring involving approximately 50 per cent of the media in giant cell arteritis. (Courtesy of Frederick J. Schoen, M.D., Ph.D.)

rysms of the common carotid artery, aortic arch syndromes, and abdominal aortic aneurysms.[84] Diffuse aortitis with resultant proximal aortic dilatation may lead to severe aortic regurgitation requiring valve replacement.[85] The aortic wall pathology reveals endarteritis obliterans, with a normal aortic valve cusp. Other manifestations of Behçet's include pericarditis, myocarditis, conduction-system abnormality, and, rarely, formation of spontaneous arterial aneurysm, resulting in myocardial infarction or rupture.[86,87] The incidence of cardiac abnormalities in Behçet's disease is unclear. Recent studies using echocardiography in 65 patients revealed no significant difference in the prevalence of cardiac findings between a group of patients with Behçet's disease and controls, putting the true incidence of cardiac involvement in Behçet's disease in doubt.[88]

Medium Size Vessel Involvement

Polyarteritis Nodosa

The incidence of cardiac involvement in polyarteritis nodosa (PAN) has been misunderstood because it is confused with other medium-size vasculitides. In a clinicopathologic study of PAN, 50 per cent of patients had either active or healed coronary arteritis.[89] Of this group, only 19 per cent had evidence of active coronary arteritis of multiple vessels. The vessels involved usually included small subepicardial vessels rather than deep intramyocardial arteries. Formation of aneurysm was also seen; arteritis observed in the heart was milder than observed in other organs. Interstitial myocarditis was occasionally observed. Gross infarcts were identified in only 11 per cent. Pericarditis appeared in 19 per cent of these patients, but all had renal involvement.

In the past, cardiac involvement was commonly cited as a leading cause of death in patients with PAN; more recent studies discount this involvement.[89] It is possible that the combined use of corticosteroids and immunosuppressive drug therapies, as well as improved treatment of resultant hypertension, congestive heart failure, and renal insufficiency, have contributed to increased longevity.

CHURG-STRAUSS SYNDROME. Cardiac manifestations of the Churg-Strauss syndrome include acute pericarditis, chronic constrictive pericarditis, tamponade, cardiac failure, arrhythmias, and myocardial infarction.[90] The frequency of cardiac involvement in the steroid era is probably greater than 50 per cent, with cardiac disease accounting for one-half of deaths caused by Churg-Strauss syndrome.

Myocardial involvement includes either an obliterative or restrictive type of cardiomyopathy that later may develop into endomyocardial fibrosis. The myocardium may also show eosinophilic myocarditis, vasculitis, or fibrosis. Endomyocardial biopsy may help guide treatment by determining the degree of inflammation or fibrosis present. Appropriate steroids and immunosuppressive therapy (cyclophosphamide) has resulted in reversal of myocardial impairment.[91] Coronary artery involvement may occur in Churg-Strauss syndrome in the setting of systemic vasculitis or as an isolated eosinophilic coronary arteritis.

WEGENER'S GRANULOMATOSIS. Cardiac involvement is rare in Wegener's granulomatosis. Pericarditis may occur in 6 per cent of patients.[92] This only rarely requires pericardiocentesis and pericardiectomy.[92] Retrospective reviews, prior to the advent of C-antineutrophil cytoplasmic antibody (C-ANCA) reveal more frequent cardiac involvement including coronary arteritis, myocarditis, valvulitis of the mitral or aortic valve, varying degrees of heart block, and myocardial infarction.[93] With the advent of earlier diagnosis and aggressive treatment with cyclophosphamide, cardiac manifestations are quite rare.

SMALL VESSEL VASCULITIDES. Cardiac involvement in the small vessel vasculitides is rare and includes pericarditis, tamponade, and aortic and mitral regurgitation.[94,95]

MISCELLANEOUS VASCULITIDES

COGAN'S SYNDROME. This is a rare disease manifested by interstitial keratitis and hearing loss, tinnitus, and vertigo. Aortic regurgitation is the most severe cardiac lesion. Valvulitis or aortitis may occur in up to 10 per cent of cases.[96] Rare cases of aortitis have been associated with myocardial infarction due to either vasculitis or embolization.

RELAPSING POLYCHONDRITIS. This condition may involve noncartilage-containing tissues, such as the aorta and sclera, which have a

high content of mucopolysaccharide. Loss of the supporting structures and elastic tissue from the aortic root lead to aneurysmal dilatation at the aorta, with dilatation of the valve ring and secondary aortic regurgitation. However, relapsing polychondritis may also be associated with significant arterial inflammation with inflammatory aortic aneurysms and systemic vasculitis.

The most significant cardiac manifestations of relapsing polychondritis include aortic aneurysms and aortic regurgitation, which may include significant necrotizing inflammation of the cardiac valves and coronary arterial vasculitis.[97] Aortic regurgitation may occur in up to 6 per cent of patients with relapsing polychondritis and may be progressive, requiring aortic valve replacement. This may occur when the disease itself seems to be inactive.[98] Myxomatous degeneration of the mitral valve, pericarditis, myocarditis, myocardial ischemia, and complete heart block may occur rarely.[97,98]

The treatment of relapsing polychondritis must be aggressive if cardiac disease and vasculitis is suspected. There is a significant morbidity rate with aortic valve replacement due to involvement of supporting structures. Treatment with corticosteroids and/or immunosuppressive therapies should be considered for patients with life-threatening organ involvement.

REFERENCES

1. Lange, L. G., and Schreiner, G. F.: Immune mechanisms of cardiac disease. N. Engl. J. Med. 330:1129, 1994.

RHEUMATOID ARTHRITIS

2. Hora, K. S., Ballard, D. J., Ilstrup, D. M., et al.: Rheumatoid pericarditis: Clinical features and survival. Medicine 69:81, 1990.
3. Maione, S., Valentin, G., Giunta, A., et al.: Cardiac involvement in rheumatoid arthritis. Cardiology 83:234, 1993.
4. Escalonte, A., Kaufman, R. L., Quismorio, F. P., and Beardmore, T. D.: Cardiac compression in rheumatoid pericarditis. Semin. Arthritis Rheum. 20:148, 1990.
5. Thould, A. K.: Constrictive pericarditis in rheumatoid arthritis. Ann. Rheum. Dis. 45:89, 1986.
6. Leibowitz, W. B.: The heart in rheumatoid arthritis. Ann. Intern. Med. 58:102, 1963.
7. Roberts, W. C., Kehoe, J. A., Carpenter, D. F., and Golden, A.: Cardiac valvular lesions in rheumatoid arthritis. Arch. Intern. Med. 122:141, 1968.
8. Mody, G., Stevens, J. E., and Meyers, O. L.: The heart in rheumatoid arthritis: A clinical and echocardiographic study. Q. J. Med. 247:921, 1987.
9. Slack, J. D., and Waller, B.: Acute congestive heart failure due to the arteritis of rheumatoid arthritis. Early diagnosis by endocardial biopsy: A case report. Angiology 37(6):477, 1986.
10. Ahern, M., Lever, J. V., and Cosh, J.: Complete heart block in rheumatoid arthritis. Ann. Rheum. Dis. 42:389, 1983.
11. Gravallese, E., Corson, J., Coblyn, J. S., et al.: Rheumatoid aortitis: A rarely recognized but clinically significant entity. Medicine 68:95, 1989.
12. Ratliff, N. B., Estes, M. L., Myles, J. L., et al.: Diagnosis of chloroquine cardiomyopathy by endomyocardial biopsy. N. Engl. J. Med. 316:191, 1987.
13. Goldenberg, J., Ferraz, M. B., Fonseca, A. S., et al.: Symptomatic cardiac involvement in juvenile rheumatoid arthritis. Int. J. Cardiol. 34:57, 1992.

SYSTEMIC LUPUS ERYTHEMATOSUS

14. Osler, W.: On the visceral manifestations of the erythema group of skin diseases. Am. J. Med. Sci. 127:629, 1895.
15. Cervera, R., Font, J., Paré, C., et al.: Cardiac disease in systemic lupus erythematosus: Prospective study of 70 patients. Ann. Rheum. Dis. 51:156, 1992.
16. Roberts, W. C., and Bulkley, B. H.: The heart in systemic lupus erythematosus and the changes induced in it by corticosteroid therapy: A study of 36 necropsy patients. Am. J. Med. 58:243, 1975.
17. Bidani, A. K., Roberts, J. L., Schwartz, M. M., and Lewis, E. J.: Immunopathology of cardiac lesions in fatal systemic lupus erythematosus. Am. J. Med. 69:849, 1980.
18. Nihoyannopoulos, P., Gomez, P. M., Joshi, J., et al.: Cardiac abnormalities in systemic lupus erythemotosus: Association with raised anticardiolipin antibodies. Circulation 82:369, 1990.
19. Kahl, L.: The spectrum of pericardial tamponade in systemic lupus erythematosus. Arthritis Rheum. 35:1343, 1992.
20. Doherty, N. E., and Siegel, R. J.: Cardiovascular manifestations of systemic lupus erythematosus. Am. Heart J. 110:1257, 1985.
21. Bornstein, D. G., Fye, W. B., Arnett, F. C., and Stevens, M. B.: The myocarditis of systemic lupus erythematosus: Association with myositis. Ann. Intern. Med. 89(Part I):619, 1978.
22. Ansari, A., Larson, P. H., and Bates, B. D.: Cardiovascular manifestations of systemic lupus erythematosus. Prog. Cardiovasc. Dis. 27:421, 1985.
23. Fairfax, M. J., Osborn, J. G., Williams, G. A., et al.: Endomyocardial biopsy in patients with systemic lupus erythematosus. J. Rheumatol. 15:593, 1988.

24. Libman, E., and Sacks, B.: A hitherto undescribed form of valvular and mural endocarditis. Arch. Intern. Med. *33*:701, 1924.

25. Straaton, K. V., Chatham, W. W., Reveille, J. D., et al.: Clinically significant valvular heart disease in systemic lupus erythematosus. Am. J. Med. *85*:645, 1988.

26. Galve, E., Condill-Riera, J., Pigrau, C., et al.: Prevalence, morphologic types, and evolution of cardiac valvular disease in systemic lupus erythematosus. N. Engl. J. Med. *319*:817, 1988.

27. Roldan, C., Shirley, B., Lau, C. C., et al.: Systemic lupus erythematosus valve disease by transesophageal echocardiography and the role of antiphospholipid antibodies. J. Am. Coll. Cardiol. *20*:1127, 1992.

28. Alameddine, A. K., Schoen, F. J., Yaragi, H., et al.: Aortic or mitral valve replacement in systemic lupus erythematosus. Am. J. Cardiol. *70*:955, 1992.

29. Haidir, Y. S., and Roberts, W. C.: Coronary arterial disease in systemic lupus erythematosus: Quantification of degrees of narrowing in 22 necropsy patients (21 women) aged 16 to 37 years. Am. J. Med. *70*:775, 1981.

30. Petri, M., Spence, D., Bone, L., and Hochberg, M. C.: Coronary artery disease risk factors in the Johns Hopkins Lupus Cohort: Prevalence, recognition by patients and preventive practices. Medicine *71*:291, 1992.

31. Homcy, C. J., Liberthson, R. P., Fallon, J. J., et al.: Ischemic heart disease in systemic lupus erythematosus in the young patient: Report of six cases. Am. J. Med. *49*:478, 1982.

32. Wilson, V. E., Eck, S. L., and Bates, E. R.: Evaluation and treatment of acute myocardial infarction complicating systemic lupus erythematosus. Chest *101*:420, 1992.

33. Scott, J. S., Maddison, P. J., Taylor, P. V., et al.: Connective tissue-disease, antibodies to ribonucleoprotein, and congenital heart block. N. Engl. J. Med. *309*:209, 1983.

34. Silverman, E., Mamula, M., Hardin, J. A., and Laxer, R.: Importance of the immune response to the Ro/La particle in the development of congenital heart block and neonatal lupus erythematosus. J. Rheumatol. *18*:120, 1991.

35. Kaaja, R., Julkuren, H., Ammala, P., et al.: Congenital heart block: Successful prophylactic treatment with intravenous gamma globulin and corticosteroid therapy. Am. J. Obstet. Gynecol. *165*:1333, 1991.

36. Kaplan, S. D., Chartash, E. K., Pizzarello, R. A., and Furie, R. A.: Cardiac manifestations of the antiphospholipid syndrome. Am. Heart. J. *124*:1331, 1992.

37. Galve, E., Ord, J., Barquinero, J., et al.: Valvular heart disease in primary antiphospholipid syndrome. Ann. Intern. Med. *116*:293, 1992.

38. Vianna, J. L., Khamashta, M. A., Ordi-Ros, J., et al.: Comparison of the primary and secondary antiphospholipid syndrome: A European multicenter study of 114 patients. Am. J. Med. *96*:3, 1994.

39. Asherson, R. A., and Cervera, R.: Antiphospholipid antibodies and the heart: Lessons and pitfalls for the cardiologist. Circulation *84*:920, 1991.

40. Khamashta, M. A., Cuadrado, M. J., Mujic, F., et al.: The management of thrombosis in the anti-phospholipid-antibody syndrome. N. Engl. J. Med. *332*:993, 1995.

POLYMYOSITIS/DERMATOMYOSITIS

41. Askari, A. D.: Inflammatory disorders of muscle: Cardiac abnormalities. Clin. Rheum. Dis. *10*:131, 1984.

42. Yale, S. H., Adlakha, A., and Stanton, M. S.: Dermatomyositis with pericardial tamponade and polymyositis with pericardial effusion. Am. Heart J. *126*:997, 1993.

43. Denbow, C. E., Lie, J. J., Tancredi, R. G., and Burch, J. W.: Cardiac involvement in polymyositis: A clinicopathologic study of 20 autopsied patients. Arthritis Rheum. *27*:1088, 1979.

44. Haupt, H. M., and Hutchins, G. M.: The heart and cardiac conduction system in polymyositis-dermatomyositis: A clinicopathologic study of 16 autopsied patients. Am. J. Cardiol. *50*:998, 1982.

45. Stern, R., Godbold, J. H., Chess, Q., and Kagen, L.: ECG abnormalities in polymyositis. Arch. Intern. Med. *144*:2185, 1984.

46. Plotz, P. H., Dalakas, M., Leff, R. L., et al.: Current concepts in the idiopathic inflammatory myopathies: Polymyositis, dermatomyositis and related disorders. Ann. Intern. Med. *111*:143, 1989.

47. Rechavia, E., Rotenberg, Z., Fuch, J., and Strasberg, B.: Polymyositis heart disease. Chest *88*:309, 1985.

48. Tami, L. F., and Bhasin, S.: Polymorphism of the cardiac manifestations in dermatomyositis. Clin. Cardiol. *16*:260, 1992.

49. Wright, C. D., Wilson, C., and Bell, A.: D-Penicillamine-induced polymyositis causing complete heart block. Clin. Rheum. Dis. *13*:80, 1994.

SPONDYLOARTHROPATHIES

50. Bulkley, B. H., and Roberts, W. C.: Ankylosing spondylitis and aortic regurgitation: Description of the characteristic cardiovascular lesion from study of eight necropsy patients. Circulation *48*:1014, 1973.

51. O'Neill, T. W., King, G., Graham, J. M., et al.: Echocardiographic abnormalities in ankylosing spondylitis. Ann. Rheum. Dis. *5*:652, 1992.

52. O'Neill, T. W.: The heart in ankylosing spondylitis. Ann. Rheum. Dis. *51*(6):705, 1992.

53. Alves, M. G., Espirito-Santo, J., Queiroz, M. V., et al.: Cardiac alterations in ankylosing spondylitis. Angiology *39*:567, 1988.

54. Shah, A.: Echocardiographic features of mitral regurgitation due to ankylosing spondylitis. Am. J. Med. *82*:353, 1987.

55. Bergfeldt, L., and Moller, E.: Complete heart block: Another HLA-B27 associated disease manifestation. Tissue Antigens *21*:385, 1983.

56. Bergfeldt, L., Edhay, O., and Rajs, J.: HLA-B27 associated heart disease: Clinicopathologic study of three cases. Am. J. Med. *77*:961, 1984.

57. Bergfeldt, L., Vallin, H., Edhay, O.: Complete heart block in HLA-B27 associated disease: Electrophysiological and clinical characteristics. Br. Heart. J. *51*:184, 1984.

58. Bergfeldt, L., Edhay, O., and Vallin, H.: Cardiac conduction disturbances: An underestimated manifestation in ankylosing spondylitis. Acta Med. Scand. *212*:217, 1982.

59. Brewerton, D. A., Goddard, D. H., Moore, R. B., et al.: The myocardium in ankylosing spondylitis: A clinical echocardiographic and histopathologic study. Lancet *1*(8540):995, 1987.

60. Misukiewicz, P., Carlson, R. W., Rowan, L., et al.: Acute aortic insufficiency in a patient with presumed Reiter's syndrome. Ann. Rheum. Dis. *51*(5):686, 1992.

61. Hoagland, Y. T., Alexander, E. P., Patterson, R. H., et al.: Coronary artery stenosis in Reiter's syndrome: A complication of aortitis. J. Rheumatol. *21*(4):757, 1994.

62. Havermain, J. F., Albada-Kuipers, G. A. V., Dohmen, H. J. M., and Dijkmons, B. A. C.: Atrioventricular conduction disturbance as an early feature of Reiter's syndrome. Ann. Rheum. Dis. *47*:1017, 1988.

63. Muna, W. F., Roller, D. H., Craft, J., et al.: Psoriatic arthritis and aortic regurgitation. JAMA *244*:363, 1980.

64. Pines, A., Ehrenfeld, M., Fishman, E. Z., et al.: Mitral valve prolapse in psoriatic arthritis. Arch. Intern. Med. *146*:1371, 1986.

PROGRESSIVE SYSTEMIC SCLEROSIS AND ITS VARIANTS

65. Weiss, S., Stead, E. A., Warren, J. V., and Bailey, O. T.: Scleroderma heart disease, with a consideration of certain other visceral manifestations of scleroderma. Arch. Intern. Med. *71*:749, 1943.

66. D'Angelo, W. A., Fries, J. F., Masi, A. T., and Shulman, L. E.: Pathologic observations in systemic sclerosis: A study of 58 autopsy cases and 58 matched controls. Am. J. Med. *46*:428, 1969.

67. Bulkley, B. H., Rudolfi, R. L., Salyer, W. R., and Hutchins, G. M.: Myocardial lesions of progressive systemic sclerosis: A cause of cardiac dysfunction. Circulation *53*:483, 1976.

68. Ellis, W. W., Baer, A. N., Robertson, R. M., et al.: Left ventricular dysfunction induced by cold exposure in patients with systemic sclerosis. Am. J. Med. *80*:385, 1986.

69. Botstein, G. R., and LeRoy, E. C.: Primary heart disease in systemic sclerosis (scleroderma): Advances in clinical and pathologic features, pathogenesis, and new therapeutic approaches. Am. Heart J. *102*:913, 1981.

70. Satter, M. A., Guindi, R. T., and Vajcik, J.: Pericardial tamponade and limited cutaneous systemic sclerosis (CREST syndrome). Br. J. Rheumatol. *29*:306, 1990.

71. Gladman, P. D., Gordon, D. A., Urowitz, M. B., and Levy, H. L.: Pericardial fluid analysis in scleroderma (systemic sclerosis). Am. J. Med. *60*:1064, 1976.

72. Bulkley, B. H., Klacsmann, P. G., and Hutchins, G. M.: Angina pectoris, myocardial infarction and sudden cardiac death with normal coronary arteries: A clinicopathologic study of nine patients with progressive systemic sclerosis. Am. Heart J. *95*:563, 1978.

73. Anuari, A., Graninger, W., Schneider, B., et al.: Cardiac involvement in systemic sclerosis. Arthritis Rheum. *35*:1356, 1992.

74. Kerr, L. D., and Spiera, H.: Myocarditis as a complication in scleroderma patients with myositis. Clin. Cardiol. *16*:895, 1993.

75. Follansbee, W. P., Curtiss, E. I., Rahko, P. S., et al.: The electrocardiogram in systemic sclerosis: Study of 102 consecutive cases with functional correlations and review of the literature. Am. J. Med. *79*:183, 1985.

76. Suzuki, M., Homada, M., Semkiya, M., et al.: Fatal pulmonary hypertension in a patient with mixed connective tissue disease: Report of an autopsy case. Intern. Med. *31*:74, 1992.

77. Beier, J. M., Neilsen, H. L., and Nielsen, D.: Pleuritis-pericarditis-an unusual manifestation of mixed connective tissue disease. Eur. Heart J. *13*:859, 1992.

78. Veille, J. C., Sunderland, C., and Bennett, R. M.: Complete heart block in fetus associated in the maternal Sjogren's Syndrome. Am. J. Obstet. Gynecol. *151*:660, 1985.

SYSTEMIC VASCULITIS

79. Klem, R. G., Hunder, G. G., Stenson, A. W., and Sheps, S. G.: Large artery involvement in giant cell (temporal) arteritis. Ann. Intern. Med. *83*:806, 1975.

80. Hunder, G. G.: Giant cell (temporal) arteritis. Clin. Rheumatol. *16*:399, 1990.

81. Evans, J. M., Bowles, C. A., Bjornsson, J., et al.: Thoracic aortic aneurysms and rupture in giant cell arteritis. Arthritis Rheum. *37*:1539, 1994.

82. Costello, J. M., and Nicholson, W. J.: Severe aortic regurgitation as a late complication of temporal arteritis. Chest *98*:875, 1990.

83. Lie, J. T., Failoni, D. D., and Davis, D. C.: Temporal arteritis with giant cell aortitis, coronary arteritis, and myocardial infarction. Arch. Pathol. Lab. Med. *110*:857, 1986.

84. Shimizu, T., Ehrlich, G. E., Inaba, G., and Hayash, K.: Behçet's disease (Behçet's syndrome). Semin. Arthritis Rheum. 8:223, 1979.

85. Tai, Y.-T., Fong, P. C., Ng, W. F., et al.: Diffuse aortitis complicating Behçet's disease leading to severe aortic regurgitation. Cardiology 79:156, 1991.

86. Jones, D. G., and Thomson, A.: Recognition of the diverse cardiovascular manifestations in Behçet's disease. Am. Heart J. 82:457, 1982.

87. Bowles, C. A., Nelson, A. M., Hammill, S. C., and O'Duffy, J. D.: Cardiac involvement in Behçet's disease. Arthritis Rheum. 28:345, 1985.

88. Ozkon, M. D., Emil, O., Ozdemir, M., et al.: M-mode, 2-D and Doppler echocardiographic study in 65 patients with Behçet's syndrome. Eur. Heart J. 13:638, 1992.

89. Schrader, M. L., Hochman, J. S., and Bulkley, B. H.: The heart in polyarteritis nodosa: A clinicopathologic study. Am. Heart J. 109:1313, 1985.

90. Hasley, P. G., Follansbee, W. P., and Coulehan, J. L.: Cardiac manifestation of Churg-Strauss syndrome: Report of a case and review of the literature. Am. Heart J. 120:996, 1990.

91. Renaldini, E., Spandrio, S., Cerudilli, B., et al.: Cardiac involvement in Churg-Strauss syndrome: A follow-up of three cases. Eur. Heart J. 14:1717, 1993.

92. Hoffman, G. S., Kerr, G. S., Leavitt, R. Y., et al.: Wegener's granulomatosis: An analysis of 158 patients. Ann. Intern. Med. 116:488, 1992.

93. Grant, S. C. D., Levy, R. D., Venning, M. C., et al.: Wegener's granulomatosis and the heart. Br. Heart J. 71:82, 1994.

94. Babajanianis, A., Chung-Park, M., and Visnieski, J.: Recurrent pericarditis and cardiac tamponade in a patient with hypocomplementemic urticarial vasculitis syndrome. J. Rheumatol. 18:752, 1991.

95. Palazzo, E., Bourgeois, P., Meyer, O., et al.: Hypocomplementemic urticarial vasculitis syndrome, Jaccoud's syndrome, valvulopathy: A new syndrome combination. J. Rheumatol. 20:7:1236, 1993.

96. Vollerstein, R. S.: Vasculitis and Cogen's syndrome. Rheum. Dis. Clin. North Am. 16:433, 1990.

97. Bowness, P., Hawley, I. C., Morris, T., et al.: Complete heart block and severe aortic incompetence in relapsing polychondritis: Clinicopathologic findings. Arthritis Rheum. 34:97, 1991.

98. Buckley, L. M., and Ades, P.: Progressive aortic inflammation occurring despite apparent remission of relapsing polychondritis. Arthritis Rheum. 35:812, 1992.

Chapter 57
Hematological-Oncological Disorders and Heart Disease

LAWRENCE N. SHULMAN, EUGENE BRAUNWALD, DAVID S. ROSENTHAL

The higher frequency of cardiovascular abnormalities in patients with hematological and neoplastic disorders and, conversely, of blood disorders in patients being treated for a variety of cardiovascular diseases has led to increasing interaction between cardiologists and hematologist-oncologists. Blood dyscrasias often complicate the use of cardiac medications and prosthetic heart valves and cardiovascular surgery. Hematologist-oncologists must often consult cardiologists regarding clinical problems that range from interpreting abnormal physical findings and electrocardiographic and echocardiographic changes in their patients to obtaining advice about how to treat heart failure, pericardial effusion, or other cardiac complications common among patients with anemia and hematological malignant diseases.

ANEMIA AND CARDIOVASCULAR DISORDERS

(See also p. 460)

Anemia is one of the most common causes of increased cardiac output and when extremely severe sometimes results in heart failure due to a high-output state in the absence of heart disease. As discussed in Chapter 15, tissue hypoxia combined with reduced blood viscosity leads to a reduction in systemic vascular resistance, which is associated with an increase in cardiac output.[1] Acutely induced anemia lowers coronary vascular resistance, whereas chronic anemia enhances formation of intercoronary collaterals and causes increases in preload and reduction of afterload.[2] When the normal hemoglobin concentration is restored, all signs and symptoms of cardiovascular disease usually disappear. The gradual development of severe anemia may lead to cardiac hypertrophy, by causing vasodilation, which increases venous return (and thereby preload) and causes volume overload. It reduces peripheral resistance (and thereby afterload). Left ventricular end-diastolic volume is increased in patients with chronic anemia, and afterload reduction, as reflected in left ventricular end-systolic stress, has been demonstrated. Such changes may favor maintaining a sufficiently high stroke volume (Chap. 14). Another mechanism of enhanced left ventricular function in chronic anemia has been attributed to increased levels of catecholamine and noncatecholamine inotropic factors in plasma.[3]

CARDIAC SYMPTOMS OF ANEMIA. The severity of reduction of cardiac reserve, of fatigue, exertional dyspnea, and edema depend on the severity of the anemia and the presence of an underlying cardiovascular disorder such as myocardial, coronary arterial, or valvular heart disease. Severely anemic patients without heart disease have few if any cardiac symptoms. When hemoglobin values decline below 9 gm/dl, resting cardiac output increases.[4,5] Symptoms also depend on the rapidity with which the anemia develops, as well as the physical activity of the patient. For example, if the anemia develops gradually in a normal person, patients with hemoglobin levels as low as 7 gm/dl may be able to carry out all but the most strenuous activities, whereas in the presence of coronary artery disease, anemia lowers the threshold for development of angina pectoris, so that patients with mild anemia may develop intensified angina.

Although uncommon, congestive heart failure with pulmonary edema can occur *solely* on the basis of very severe anemia (Hb < 4 gm/dl) even in the absence of underlying heart disease. It may be difficult to distinguish congestive heart failure secondary to chronic anemia from that related to myocardial iron infiltration secondary to transfusion-related hemosiderosis (see p. 1790). However, the symptoms of reduced cardiac reserve secondary to anemia alone are usually relieved when the anemia is corrected and a normal red cell mass has been restored.

Electrocardiographic findings are not uncommon as the anemia progresses. With hemoglobin levels below 7 gm/dl, T-wave depression and inversion may be found, simulating myocardial disease. With transfusions, these findings usually return to normal.

Studies in anesthetized dogs have shown that maximal myocardial oxygen delivery far exceeds the supply at all levels of hematocrit. When one is plotting maximum oxygen transport against hematocrit, an "inverted U-shaped" relationship results (Fig. 57–1).[6] In otherwise normal subjects, the gradual occurrence of severe anemia rarely if ever results in myocardial hypoxia, because of several compensatory mechanisms, including the development of coronary collaterals and increased concentration of 2,3-diphosphoglycerate (2,3-DPG) in red cells, and its effect on the hemoglobin-oxygen dissociation curve,[7] as described below.

OXYGEN DISSOCIATION AND LEVELS OF 2,3-DIPHOSPHOGLYCERATE IN RED CELLS

Normally, 1 gm of hemoglobin binds 1.34 ml of O_2. With a hemoglobin concentration of 15 gm/dl, 100 ml of arterial blood contains 20 ml of O_2. As can be calculated from the Hb-O_2 dissociation curve (Fig. 57–2), 100 ml of mixed venous blood having a PO_2 of 40 mm Hg will contain 15.5 ml of O_2. The difference (i.e., 4.5 ml of O_2 per 100 ml of arterial blood) would be available for delivery to tissues.

SHIFTS OF THE HEMOGLOBIN-OXYGEN DISSOCIATION CURVE. In most patients with anemia, the Hb-O_2 dissociation curve shifts to the right, and more oxygen is released from hemoglobin as the PO_2 declines. The red cell concentrations of 2,3-diphosphoglycerate (2,3-DPG) profoundly affect the binding and release of O_2 by hemoglobin.[7] Deoxygenated hemoglobin, which is more alkaline than oxyhemoglobin, stimulates the production of 2,3-DPG, a byproduct of glycolysis. As a consequence, the intraerythrocytic ratio of deoxyhemoglobin to oxyhemoglobin serves as a critical regulator of 2,3-DPG concentration. For example, the decreased oxygen affinity present in chronic anemia can be accounted for by this increase in red cell 2,3-DPG. At a normal

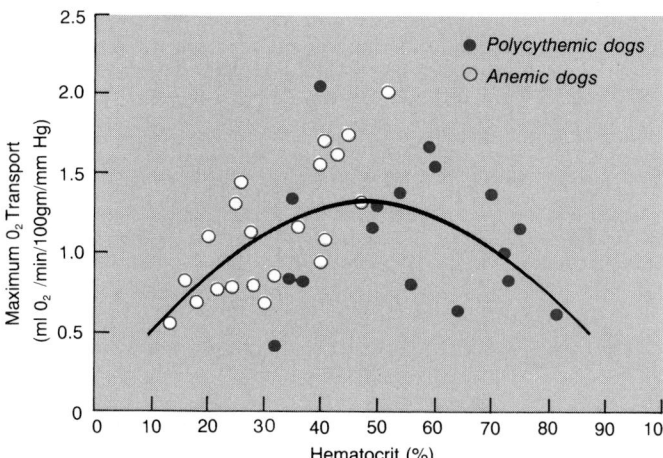

FIGURE 57–1. Maximum oxygen transport adjusted per unit perfusion pressure is shown as a function of hematocrit in anemic and polycythemic dogs. (From Baer, R. W., et al.: Maximum myocardial oxygen transport during anemia and polycythemia in dogs. Am. J. Physiol. *252*:H1086, 1987.)

arterial PO_2, arterial oxygen saturation remains high despite the reduction in oxygen affinity. However, at the lower PO_2 in the venous blood, elevated 2,3-DPG displaces the Hb-O_2 dissociation curve to the right, enabling greater release of oxygen from the cells at any level of PO_2. Oski et al. have calculated that decreased oxygen affinity mediated by increased red cell 2,3-DPG may compensate for up to half the oxygen deficit in anemia.[8] High levels of 2,3-DPG have also been found in subjects exposed to altitude[9] and in patients with pulmonary disease.[10]

The position of the Hb-O_2 dissociation curve can be expressed by the value of P_{50}, i.e., the partial pressure of O_2 at which hemoglobin is 50 per cent saturated. A reduction of the oxygen affinity of hemoglobin, i.e., a shift of the dissociation curve to the right, is reflected in an elevation of P_{50}. With a P_{50} of 34 mm Hg (instead of the normal P_{50} of 26.5 mm Hg), 3.3 ml of O_2 is unloaded per 100 ml of blood. As a consequence, an anemic individual with a 50 per cent reduction in red cell mass would suffer only a 27 per cent reduction in oxygen unloading.

RESPONSE TO HYPOXIA. Figure 57–2 summarizes the factors responsible for oxygenation in response to hypoxia. O_2 delivery to the metabolizing tissues depends directly on three principal factors: (1) blood flow; (2) hemoglobin concentration (i.e., the O_2-carrying capacity of the blood), and (3) the O_2 unloaded per unit of blood, as represented by the difference between arterial and venous blood oxygen saturations. Each of these three factors varies independently. Blood flow to any tissue is a function of total cardiac output and its fractional distribution. The red cell mass is regulated by erythropoietin in response to tissue oxygenation. The position of the Hb-O_2 dissociation curve is determined primarily by red cell 2,3-DPG levels and blood pH. Chronic anemia is usually well tolerated when these compensatory mechanisms operate effectively, i.e., with an increased cardiac output, redistribution of blood flow, and decreased O_2 affinity.

CARDIAC EXAMINATION. The cardiac enlargement that develops with severe, chronic anemia usually results from dilatation and eccentric hypertrophy with a normal ratio of

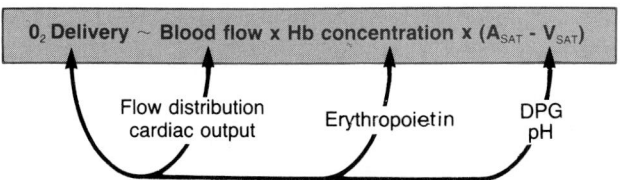

FIGURE 57–2. Oxygen delivered to an organ or tissue is directly proportional to blood flow, hemoglobin concentration, and the difference in oxygen saturation between arterial and venous blood. Patients with various types of hypoxia may compensate in the following ways: (1) Blood flow distribution may be altered to maintain oxygenation of vital organs, with an increase in total cardiac output when hypoxia is severe. (2) Increased erythropoietin production may stimulate erythropoiesis. (3) Oxygen unloading may be enhanced by a shift to the right in the oxygen dissociation curve, mediated by an increase in red cell 2,3-DPG. (From Bunn, H. F.: Pathophysiology of the anemias. *In* Isselbacher, K. J., et al. [eds.]: Harrison's Principles of Internal Medicine. 13th ed. New York, McGraw-Hill, 1994, p. 1720. © 1994 The McGraw-Hill Companies, Inc.)

wall thickness to cavity diameter, as occurs in other forms of volume overload (see Fig. 13–10, p. 401). The precordium is usually hyperactive, not unlike that in mitral regurgitation. Third and fourth heart sounds are frequently present, and a midsystolic murmur, maximal at the left sternal border, is usually audible.[11] The murmur is probably secondary to the combined effects of increased velocity of blood flow across the pulmonic and aortic valve orifices and reduced blood viscosity. Less frequently, an early, midsystolic rumbling murmur may be heard at the apex or along the left sternal border. This diastolic murmur is probably related to the increase in blood flow across the mitral or tricuspid valves and may be difficult to distinguish from the murmurs of mitral or tricuspid stenosis, although the murmur follows a third heart sound rather than an opening snap. Accurate diagnosis may require echocardiography as well as reexamination after correction of the anemia.

In patients with chronic anemia whose hearts are compensated at a reduced concentration of hemoglobin, blood volume expansion achieved by the transfusion of whole blood may be poorly tolerated. Expanding the blood volume and augmenting left ventricular filling pressure will risk precipitating or aggravating heart failure. Therefore, the slow infusion of packed red blood cells accompanied by the administration of a diuretic is desirable.

Cardiac Disorders Associated With Hemolytic Anemia

Cardiomegaly, congestive heart failure, and sudden death have been reported frequently in patients with chronic hemolytic anemias such as sickle cell disease and thalassemia. In addition, hemolysis secondary to cardiac disease (see below) may cause cardiac failure.

Hemoglobinopathies

SICKLE CELL DISEASE. Sickle hemoglobin results from a mutation in the codon for the sixth amino acid of the beta globin chain from glutamic acid to valine. This single mutation causes sickle hemoglobin to polymerize when it becomes deoxygenated, leading to all the manifestations of the disease as described.[12,13] It is likely that the sickle gene was selected during evolution in central Africa because persons with sickle trait (one affected beta globin gene) appear to be more resistant to the effects of falciparum malaria. In central Africa the sickle gene frequency may be as high as 20 per cent. Eight to 10 per cent of black Americans are heterozygous for this trait.

PATHOPHYSIOLOGY OF SICKLE CELL DISEASE. When sickle hemoglobin becomes deoxygenated it polymerizes, giving sickle cells their characteristic shape. The degree of sickling is related to both the intracellular concentration of sickle hemoglobin and the intracellular oxygen tension. Polymerization is initially reversible, and if the cell is quickly and sufficiently reoxygenated, hemoglobin will return to its normal configuration and sickling will resolve. With prolonged deoxygenation polymerization and sickling become irreversible.

The propensity of a cell to sickle is affected by the concentration of sickle hemoglobin. When one beta gene is mutated to produce sickle hemoglobin (sickle trait) there is insufficient sickle hemoglobin to polymerize, except in the most hypoxic of conditions. Therefore, patients with sickle trait (AS) are generally not anemic and do not suffer the complications of sickle cell anemia. On the other hand, if both genes are affected, as in sickle cell disease (SS), red cells will sickle in minimally hypoxic circumstances, often in the venous capillary bed leading to microvascular occlusion.

Classical sickle cell anemia (SS disease) is a severe disease manifested by significant anemia and sickle crises from an early age. Generally patients have hematocrits of 20 to 22 per cent, with reticulocyte counts of 5 to 20 per cent. Variations of sickle cell disease occur when one beta chain has the sickle mutation and the other beta chain has another abnormal gene such as hemoglobin C or a thalassemic variant. SC disease is not as severe as SS disease, and the sickle-thalassemia syndromes vary depending on the amount of beta globin produced by the thalassemic gene. Particularly in the case of the sickle–beta thalassemia syndromes, because of the reduction in beta chain production from the thalassemic gene, intracellular hemoglobin concentrations are reduced. In turn, the propensity for these cells to sickle under hypoxic conditions is decreased.

In addition, many blacks are heterozygous for alpha-thalassemia and the concurrence of alpha-thalassemia trait and sickle cell disease makes the sickle cell disease less severe because of more balanced globin chain production, and because the red cell hemoglobin concentration is lower, resulting in less sickling.

The clinical manifestations of sickle cell disease relate to the effects of sickled cells and their propensity to become sequestered in the microvasculature, and to their short life span resulting in a chronic hemolytic anemia.

When sickling occurs in the capillary bed, the sickled cells become trapped in the microvasculature, leading to vascular occlusion. This is the result of both the rigid nature of sickle cells making transport through the microcirculation difficult, and the fact that sickled cells have a membrane that is particularly sticky, leading the cells to adhere to vessel walls. When additional cells become trapped they become progressively deoxygenated. If not quickly released from the microcirculation to become re-oxygenated in the pulmonary bed, they become irreversibly sickled. When they become permanently entrapped in the microcirculation a sickle cell crisis may result due to vascular insufficiency in the area of vascular occlusion. This is associated with severe pain and can be associated with local tissue damage such as bone infarcts, strokes, and pulmonary infarcts.

Red cells from patients with homozygous sickle disease (SS) that are not entrapped in the microcirculation nevertheless become damaged because of polymerized hemoglobin and membrane alterations. These cells have a very short half-life and are rapidly destroyed in the spleen or other reticuloendothelial organs. Therefore, patients with homozygous sickle cell disease are chronically anemic, in spite of vigorous red cell production as demonstrated by high reticulocyte counts. Otherwise well patients with sickle cell anemia (SS disease) maintain hematocrits between 19 and 22 per cent with a high compensatory reticulocyte count, but in cases of bone marrow suppression due to bacterial or viral infections, a suppression of the reticulocyte count can lead to an acute worsening of the anemia.

Cardiopulmonary Manifestations. The cardiopulmonary system is frequently involved in sickle cell anemia.[14-17] As in other chronic anemias, both cardiac output and oxygen extraction by tissues are increased, and the reduced oxygen content of these red cells leads to further sickling. A normal left ventricle is able to tolerate the volume overload of chronic, moderately severe anemia for indefinite periods with no deterioration in functional capacity.[16] The increased preload and decreased afterload characteristic of chronic anemia (Fig. 57–3) compensate for any left ventricular dysfunction and maintain a normal ejection fraction and high cardiac output in sickle cell anemia.[17] When cardiac decompensation occurs in patients with sickle cell anemia, it is usually the result of other coexisting complications of the SS disease or the presence of underlying cardiovascular abnormalities. Deaths secondary to congestive heart failure occurring in children and young adults with sickle cell anemia are usually precipitated by chronic renal failure, pulmonary thrombosis, or infections.[18]

Acute myocardial infarction is a rare complication of sickle cell disease and has been confirmed at postmortem examination in a few patients without significant coronary atherosclerosis.[14,19] More O_2 is extracted by the myocardium than by any other tissue, and transmural infarction due to in situ thrombosis by sickled cells is rare. However, infarction of the papillary muscles of the heart does occur.

This should not be surprising, since the papillary muscles are at the terminal portion of the coronary circulation, where collateral vessels are scant and hypoxia is marked.

Pulmonary infarction, a common complication of sickle cell anemia, is probably due to thrombosis in situ rather than to embolization.[20,21] Although infrequent, fat and bone marrow emboli to the lungs have been reported, the latter resulting from necrosis caused by sickling within the marrow sinusoids. Patients with sickle cell anemia are unusually susceptible to infection. In addition, damage to the lung caused by repeated vascular insults creates a suitable milieu for bacterial growth; as a consequence, pneumonia is a frequent and serious complication. Mortality and morbidity are high in the setting of pneumonia and hypoxia, so that treatment of these complications must be immediate and vigorous. However, it may be difficult to differentiate pulmonary infection from infarction in patients with sickle cell anemia. Although impaired pulmonary function in sickle cell anemia is common, pulmonary hypertension and cor pulmonale are rarely encountered.

In almost all patients with sickle cell anemia the heart ultimately becomes enlarged, and at autopsy strikingly high heart weights are noted in a majority of patients despite the absence of other causes of cardiomegaly such as hypertension, atherosclerosis, or coronary artery disease.[1] In patients who have received multiple blood transfusions, myocardial iron deposition (hemosiderosis) may contribute both to the cardiac enlargement and to the associated impairment of cardiac function. However, this complication occurs much less frequently in sickle cell anemia than in homozygous thalassemia (see below). Histological studies have suggested that the increase in heart weight is secondary to fibrosis, presumably caused by the combination of anemia and papillary muscle infarction. With time, children with sickle cell disease exhibit progressive cardiac chamber enlargement with a progressive increase in left ventricular mass.[21]

There are no specific electrocardiographic changes in sickle cell anemia. However, almost 80 per cent of patients with sickle cell anemia have an abnormal electrocardiogram. These abnormalities include left ventricular hypertrophy and first-degree atrioventricular (AV) block as well as nonspecific ST-segment and T-wave changes and abnormal septal Q waves; this last finding is believed to be secondary to excessive septal thickness.[22] Arrhythmias rarely occur with sickle cell anemia, although continuous electrocardiographic monitoring during painful crises has revealed both atrial and ventricular arrhythmias in the majority of patients.[23] Echocardiographic measurements in patients with cardiac symptoms are useful in documenting both cardiac hyperactivity and depressed left ventricular performance.[24] Radiological studies may be entirely normal. With exercise, cardiac dysfunction may be manifested by an abnormal ejection fraction response, abnormalities of wall motion, and slowed left ventricular filling.[24-26] M-mode echocardiographic studies demonstrated an incidence of mitral valve prolapse in 25 per cent of SS patients,[15,27] far in excess of that expected. More recent two-dimensional echo and Doppler ultrasonography performed in adult patients with SS disease demonstrated a 22 per cent incidence of diastolic murmurs but no instances of myxomatous valvular degeneration or mitral valve prolapse.[15]

THALASSEMIC SYNDROMES. The thalassemic syndromes are a group of inherited disorders caused by mutations of either the alpha or beta globin genes resulting in a decrease in the production of the respective globin chain.[28] Hemoglobin is composed of two alpha and two beta chains. This tetramer binds iron and carries oxygen. There are four alpha genes and a mutation of one or more of them will cause a decrease in alpha chain production, resulting in alpha-thalassemia. There are two beta genes, and abnormalities in one or both will result in a beta thalassemia syndrome. Alpha thalassemia is primarily a disease of the Far East, though alpha-thalassemia trait can occur in Africans. Beta-thalassemia is a disease concentrated in those ethnic groups from the Mediterranean area.

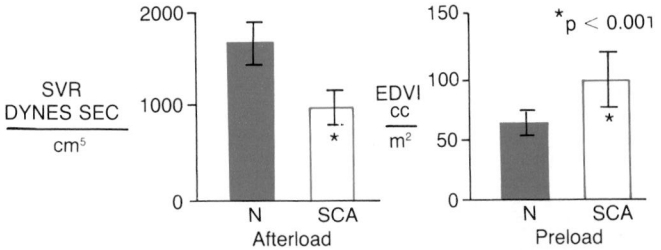

FIGURE 57–3. Loading conditions in 11 patients with sickle cell anemia (SCA) and 11 normal subjects (N). *Left,* Afterload, as indicated by systemic vascular resistance (SVR), was significantly decreased in patients with SCA. *Right,* Preload, as indicated by end-diastolic volume index (EDVI), was significantly increased in patients with SCA. (From Dennenberg, B. S., et al.: Cardiac function in sickle cell anemia. Am. J. Cardiol. *51:*1675, 1983.)

In each case, when production of one of the globin chains is reduced, there are reduced levels of hemoglobin and an imbalance in beta and alpha chain production. The red cells are hypochromic reflecting the reduced concentration of hemoglobin, and are often misshapen due to precipitated globin chains, which are removed with excess red cell membrane by the reticuloendothelial system.

The severity of the thalassemic syndromes depends on the degree of reduction of either alpha or beta chain production. In the case of alpha-thalassemia, the deletion of one or two of the four genes results in microcytosis, but not in substantial anemia. Mutations in three of the four alpha genes leads to severe anemia. Total absence of the four alpha globin genes usually results in fetal or neonatal death.

The mutations that occur in the beta genes are variable, some leading to no beta chain production (β^0) or a reduced beta chain production (β^+). Beta-thalassemia can range from mild, when only one beta chain is affected, resulting in microcytosis but no significant anemia, to very severe, when both beta genes are affected and produce little beta globin (thalassemia major, or Cooley's anemia).

The clinical manifestations of the severe thalassemias relate to the significant degree of anemia. Thalassemic red cells can have a very short life span due to their low hemoglobin concentration, excess membrane, and globin chain precipitates caused by imbalanced alpha and beta chain production. Extreme erythroid hyperplasia is present in the bone marrow, causing bone marrow expansion, often pronounced in the facial bones. Transfusions are often required to correct the anemia, resulting in iron overload, and because of the severe anemia, iron is also hyperabsorbed by the small intestine. Iron overload is one of the important complications of the disease, particularly in relation to the heart, as described below. The combination of hemosiderosis of the heart, and severe anemia requiring increased cardiac output, leads to cardiac morbidity and mortality as a prime cause of illness and death in these patients.

CARDIAC ABNORMALITIES IN THALASSEMIA.

Cardiac complications are the major cause of death in patients with thalassemia.[29-31] As with sickle cell disease, these events may be due in part to chronic anemia. In addition, cardiac siderosis is a frequent problem in thalassemia, unlike the situation in sickle cell anemia or many other chronic anemias.[32,33] Iron overload results from a combination of extravascular hemolysis, frequent transfusions, and an inappropriate increase in intestinal iron absorption. Consequently, heart failure and arrhythmias are the common causes of death in children with this condition.[28] Although anemia per se undoubtedly contributes to cardiomegaly, iron overload of the heart, with its attendant impairment of systolic and diastolic function, is the most likely cause of myocardial damage.[33-35]

Prior to the era of hypertransfusion and chelation therapy,[1] patients with transfusion-dependent, chronic, severe refractory thalassemia regularly manifested serious cardiac involvement, usually by the second decade of life. Although most died within months of the development of congestive heart failure, occasionally patients died suddenly, presumably secondary to an arrhythmia. Intensive treatment of heart failure and antiarrhythmic therapy do not appear to change the natural history. At postmortem examination, widespread iron deposition characteristic of hemochromatosis is found in all viscera, including the heart, which is hypertrophied and sometimes twice its normal weight; it is often a deep brown, with large quantities of iron in myocardial cells, demonstrated by staining with Prussian blue dye. The sinoatrial node is usually spared, but the AV node is frequently involved. Apparently cardiac dysfunction depends on the quantity of iron deposited in the ventricles, and it has been suggested that myocardial damage results from iron-induced release of acid hydrolases from lysosomes.[10]

Pericarditis occurs in about half of all patients with thalassemia and is often recurrent and associated with fever, precordial pain, and electrocardiographic changes characteristic of acute pericarditis (see p. 1481). Pericardial effusion is common; in rare cases, creation of a pericardial window is necessary to relieve tamponade or a recurrent effusion.

The *electrocardiogram* often shows left ventricular hypertrophy, nonspecific ST-segment and T-wave abnormalities, supraventricular or ventricular premature contractions, and first- or second-degree AV block. The His bundle elec-

trogram may show prolongation of the P-R interval, signifying abnormal conduction through the AV node. The chest roentgenogram may show slight to moderate cardiac enlargement, and *echocardiographic* assessment may disclose increased left ventricular end-diastolic, left atrial, and aortic root dimensions as well as a thickened left ventricular wall[44] and diastolic abnormalities. At cardiac catheterization, the usual findings comprise a normal or elevated cardiac index with moderate elevations in left ventricular end-diastolic pressure and volume and end-systolic volume with a reduced ejection fraction.

There has been considerable interest in defining abnormalities of cardiac performance noninvasively in asymptomatic patients. Valdes-Cruz et al. have reported that in asymptomatic children with thalassemia major[36] the left ventricular posterior wall thinned more slowly than normal during diastole. Utilizing the relationship between ventricular fractional shortening and end-systolic pressure (see p. 430), Borow et al. identified preclinical left ventricular dysfunction (Fig. 57-4),[37,38] an approach that may be useful in the serial assessment of left ventricular contractility in response to chelation therapy.

Management. Supportive therapy consisting primarily of an adequate transfusion program (and even hypertrans-

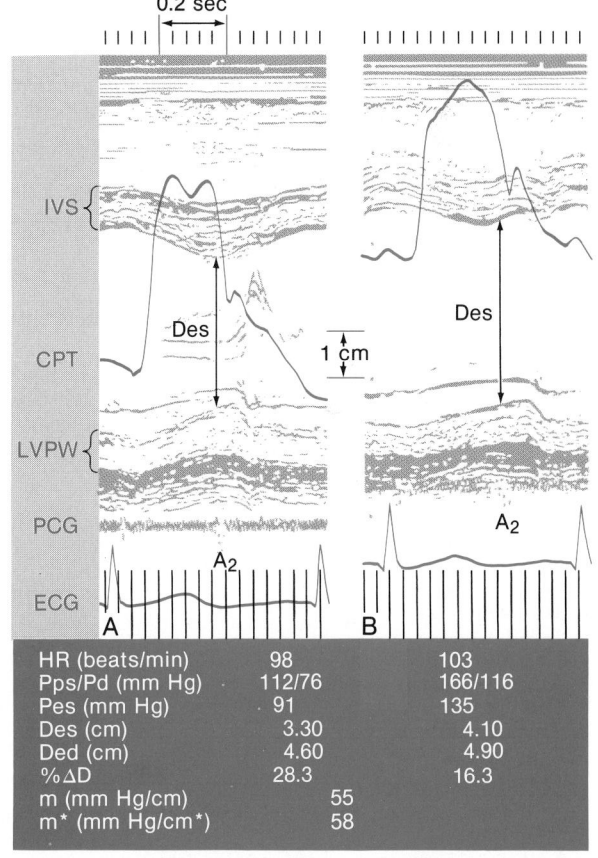

FIGURE 57-4. Recordings from a 16-year-old patient with thalassemia major during baseline conditions (A) and at peak methoxamine effect (B). Both the actual and corrected slope values (m and m*) were abnormal despite normal resting fractional shortening (%ΔD). The 44-mm Hg increase in end-systolic pressure (Pes) resulted in a 0.80-cm increase in end-systolic dimension (Des). For the control population, a comparable change in Pes resulted in a 0.40 ± 0.05-cm increase in Des. IVS = interventricular septum; LVPW = left ventricular posterior wall; A$_2$ = aortic component of the second heart sound; HR = heart rate; Pps = peak systolic pressure; Pd = aortic diastolic pressure; %ΔD = per cent fractional shortening; m = slope; m* = corrected slope. (Reproduced with permission from Borow, K. M., et al.: The left ventricular end-systolic pressure-dimensions relation in patients with thalassemia major. A new noninvasive method for assessing contractile state. Circulation 66:980, 1982. Copyright 1982 American Heart Association.)

fusions), splenectomy, and early treatment of infections has prolonged the life of many patients with thalassemia.[1,28] Roentgenographic evidence of cardiomegaly in children often regresses when hemoglobin is maintained above 10 gm/dl. Indeed, in one study, in four of seven patients with significant cardiomegaly, heart size returned to normal 1 week after multiple transfusions restored hemoglobin to near-normal levels. The use of chelating agents for both treatment and prevention of iron overload and left ventricular systolic function is necessary and is discussed on page 1792).

HEMOLYTIC ANEMIA IN PATIENTS WITH VALVULAR HEART DISEASE. In 1964, Dameshek described an interesting patient with aortic, mitral, and tricuspid stenosis and mitral regurgitation who had hemolytic anemia with distorted and fragmented red cells, including helmet cells, burr cells, and schistocytes.[39] At autopsy, numerous calcified excrescences were present on the mitral valve and the free margins of the aortic valve. The presence of excess iron deposits in the kidney suggested intravascular hemolysis, but it could not be established whether the cardiac abnormalities were the cause. Subsequently, shortened red cell survival was demonstrated in other patients with aortic valve disease, some of whom had anemia.[40] In patients with rheumatic aortic valve disease with mild hemolytic anemia, red cell survival may be significantly reduced during periods of exercise.[44] Although this form of hemolytic anemia is probably uncommon, it should be considered in patients with valvular heart disease and unexplained anemia.

HEMOLYTIC ANEMIA AFTER CARDIAC SURGERY. The potentially serious nature of the hemolytic anemia associated with an intracardiac prosthesis was not really appreciated until chronic and severe hemolytic anemia characterized by microangiopathic red cell changes (consisting of fragmented red cells, burr cells, and schistocytes) was noted after a Teflon patch repair of an ostium primum atrial septal defect.[41] Chromium-51 red cell survival studies confirmed that the half-life of not only autologous red cells but also of donor cells was shortened, indicating a defect extrinsic to the red cell. In keeping with intravascular hemolysis, high concentrations of hemoglobin in the plasma and urine were noted along with hemosiderinuria. At reoperation a jet of blood was found regurgitating through a cleft in the mitral valve that had been impinging on the prosthetic interatrial Teflon patch. Part of the septum had become denuded of endothelium and had formed a small cul-de-sac in contact with the jet of blood. With repair of the cul-de-sac and reendothelialization of the area, hemolysis ceased. Torn cusps of porcine mitral valve or dehiscence of an implanted mitral ring can also cause the sudden onset of a hemolytic anemia.[42,43]

MICROANGIOPATHIC HEMOLYTIC ANEMIA. This condition has now been reported in association with many cardiac defects (Table 57–1). Its incidence after valve surgery depends on many variables, including the specific operation,

the surgical technique, and the tests used to determine hemolysis, and varies widely. In many instances, diurnal variations occur, with greater intravascular hemolysis during physical activity.[44]

Clinical Presentation. With newer surgical techniques and prosthetic valves, the incidence of microangiopathic hemolytic anemia appears to be declining.[45] Symptoms and signs may develop suddenly or gradually, usually with no associated splenomegaly. Rarely, a vicious circle develops in a patient with a perivalvular leak: the resultant shear stress produces hemolytic anemia, increasing stroke volume and shear stress, and in turn intensifying the anemia. While it is agreed that direct mechanical trauma to the red cells is the cause of hemolysis, the relative contributions of valve closure, denuded endothelium, turbulence, and the development of antierythrocyte autoantibodies are still not clear and probably vary among patients. In some instances, the hemolytic anemia observed in the early postoperative period is probably due simply to multiple intraoperative transfusions or to the lymphocyte-splenomegaly syndrome (post–pump-oxygenator syndrome) associated with cytomegaloviral infection.

Excessive blood turbulence is the most common feature of all hemolytic anemias associated with valvular disease and cardiac surgery. For example, after insertion of a prosthetic valve, perivalvular regurgitation will increase the stroke volume and therefore the turbulence of flow through the narrowed orifice.

Definitive treatment of the hemolytic syndrome secondary to turbulence consists of surgical repair of the cardiac abnormality, i.e., either replacement or correction of the prosthesis or correction of the perivalvular leak. If a patient is not readily operable, rest should alleviate the condition, and iron and folate replacement may be helpful.

HEMOCHROMATOSIS AND HEMOSIDEROSIS

(See also p. 1430)

Normal iron homeostasis is carefully protected by the body, in both its absorption and its storage. Iron deficiency can cause anemia, and a number of important enzymes utilize iron as a cofactor. Excess iron is stored in tissues in ferritin. The liver, heart, pancreas, brain, skin, and other tissues become iron overloaded when body iron stores are very high, and excess iron in these tissues is a highly toxic state that can lead to local cellular damage.

Iron overload occurs either as a result of an inappropriate excess iron absorption, as in the case of primary hemochromatosis, or due to multiple transfusions. In some cases of chronic anemia, such as thalassemia, there is intestinal hyperabsorption of iron related to the chronic anemia. Some of the more common conditions leading to hemochromatosis are shown in Table 57–2.

NONCARDIAC MANIFESTATIONS OF IRON OVERLOAD. In the iron overload state iron is stored as ferritin in many body organs including the skin, liver, pancreas, brain, and heart (Fig. 57–5). Cellular damage results from release of lysoso-

TABLE 57–1 CAUSES OF MACROVASCULAR HEMOLYTIC ANEMIA

A. Without Surgery
1. Aortic stenosis
2. Ruptured sinus of Valsalva
3. Ruptured chordae tendineae
4. Coarctation of aorta
5. Aortic aneurysm

B. Following Surgery
1. "Patching" operations
   a. Ostium primum repair, especially if mitral regurgitation present
   b. Aortic aneurysm repair (aortofemoral bypass)
   c. Hemodialysis shunt
2. Valvular replacement
   a. Uncomplicated
      (1) Outflow too small
      (2) Large area of exposed plastic
      (3) Cloth-covered struts
      (4) Two or more valves replaced
      (5) Xenograft
   b. Complicated
      (1) Ball variance
      (2) Regurgitation around seating of valve
      (3) Rupture of cloth-covered strut

From Erslev, A. J.: Traumatic cardiac hemolytic anemia. *In* Williams, W. J., et al. (eds.): Hematology. 4th ed. New York, McGraw-Hill Book Co., 1990, p. 656.

TABLE 57–2 CAUSES OF IRON OVERLOAD

PRIMARY
A. Primary hemochromatosis–genetically transmitted
   1. Men affected more severely than women
   2. Alcohol increases iron absorption and worsens disease

SECONDARY
A. Transfusion-related with intestinal hyperabsorption
   1. Thalassemias, alpha and beta
B. Transfusion related without intestinal hyperabsorption
   1. Aplastic anemia
   2. Pure red cell aplasia
   3. Refractory anemia (myelodysplastic syndrome)

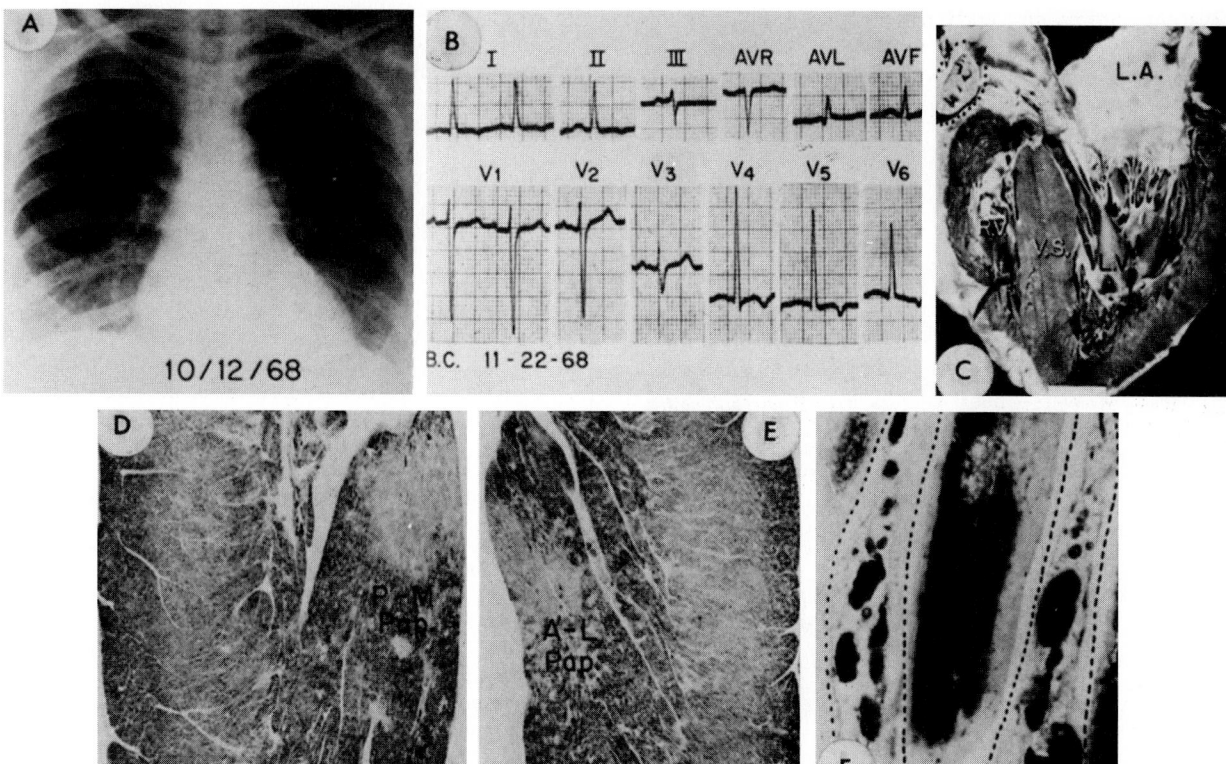

FIGURE 57–5. Observations in a 42-year-old woman with sickle cell anemia who developed congestive heart failure after cumulative transfusions of 260 units of blood. By the time of death, she had received a total of 359 units of blood (90 gm iron). A, Chest roentgenogram 2 weeks prior to death, showing cardiomegaly. B, Ischemic ST-segment and T-wave changes can be seen on the electrocardiogram. C, At autopsy the walls of the right (R.V.) and left (L.V.) ventricles and left atrium (L.A.) and the atrial and ventricular (V.S.) septa were rusty brown, owing to extensive iron deposits. The right atrial wall (partially enclosed by dotted line), in contrast, was tan; only minute particles of iron were present on microscopic examination. D and E, Large areas of replacement fibrosis (pale areas) were present in both left ventricular papillary muscles. F, Severely degenerated myocardial fibers (enclosed by dotted lines) that also contained iron deposits were often found adjacent to viable myocardial fibers. (Prussian blue stains.) (From Buja, L. M., and Roberts, W. C.: Iron in the heart. Am. J. Med. 51:209, 1971.)

mal acid hydrolases.[46] Patients develop a "bronzed" appearance from the accumulation of iron in the skin. Liver failure due to cirrhosis ensues, and patients with hemochromatosis involving the liver are at risk for the development of malignant hepatomas. Pancreatic involvement may lead to diabetes, and pituitary involvement can lead to loss of libido and other endocrine abnormalities.

CARDIAC MANIFESTATIONS. Cardiac abnormalities develop when there is sufficiently high myocardial iron concentrations over prolonged periods of time. Cardiac manifestations are significant in about one-third of patients with hemochromatosis,[31] and about that percentage of patients with hemochromatosis die of cardiac complications. Both atrial and ventricular arrhythmias and heart block are common in these patients, presumably due to both myocardial dysfunction and iron deposition in the AV node and conduction system.[47,48] Biventricular enlargement and heart failure eventually ensue with characteristics of a restrictive cardiomyopathy.[49,50]

Cardiac manifestations of early stages of hemochromatosis can be reversed by reduction in myocardial iron content. Because body stores of iron are in equilibrium with serum iron, this is accomplished by the removal of serum iron either by phlebotomy, as in the case of primary hemochromatosis or chelation therapy, as in the case of transfusional related hemochromatosis, as discussed below. In either case, reduction in total body iron stores may result in improvement in the cardiac manifestations of hemochromatosis, making early recognition and treatment of this entity essential.[30,50–57]

DIAGNOSIS. The diagnosis of hemochromatosis is suggested by an elevated serum ferritin and increased ratio of iron to total iron binding capacity (TIBC). There are no definitive values for either of these tests that confirm the diagnosis, and the most definitive test is measurement of iron concentration in the liver by liver biopsy. Magnetic resonance imaging (MRI) scans can also be suggestive because of the "blackness" of iron laden organs as seen on these scans, but the specificity of this test is still uncertain. Some studies have shown good correlations between MRI scans of the liver, serum ferritin values, and liver biopsy iron concentrations.[58,59] MRI is also used as a diagnostic tool for cardiac involvement[60] (Fig. 57–6).

Cardiac iron deposition can be assessed by endomyocardial biopsy.[61] Although cardiac dysfunction can be evaluated on echocardiography, findings are nonspecific and similar to those of other cardiomyopathies.[62]

PRIMARY HEMOCHROMATOSIS. This is a genetic disorder of increased intestinal absorption of iron (see also p. 1674). The gene has been localized to chromosome 6, close to the HLA locus, and exhibits variable expression.[63] The disease is almost never evident before the age of 20, because children are chronically iron deficient as they grow and expand their red cell mass. Environmental factors, such as alcohol intake and dietary iron intake, affect iron absorption and therefore the severity of disease. Alcohol, which increases iron absorption, is a particularly significant risk factor for the development of hemochromatosis in persons bearing an affected gene. Women are relatively protected until menopause because of blood (and iron) loss from menses, and therefore men tend to be more severely affected and affected at younger ages.

Treatment. The iron overload state of primary hemochromatosis as well as its complications can be easily

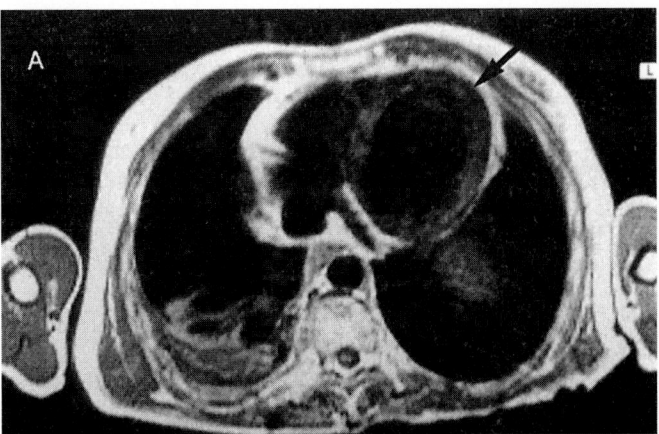

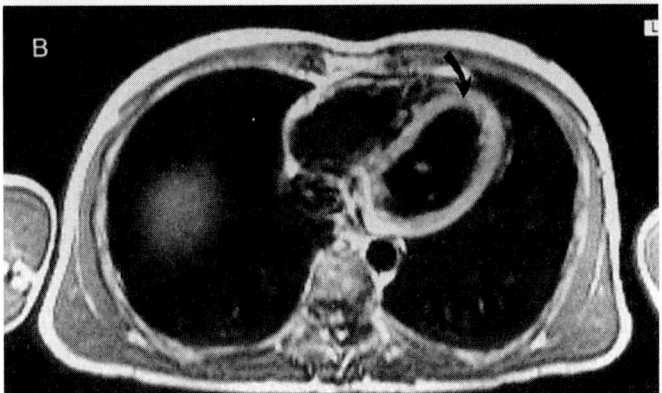

FIGURE 57-6. *A,* MRI shows signal hypointensity of left ventricular myocardium resulting from susceptibility effect (arrow) in hemochromatosis. Signal value = 280; myocardial/skeletal ratio = 0.59. Incidental right pleural effusion is visualized. *B,* MRI of healthy control shows normal signal intensity of left ventricular myocardium (arrow). (From Waxman, S., et al.: Myocardial involvement in primary hemochromatosis demonstrated by magnetic resonance imaging. Am. Heart J. *128:*1047, 1994.)

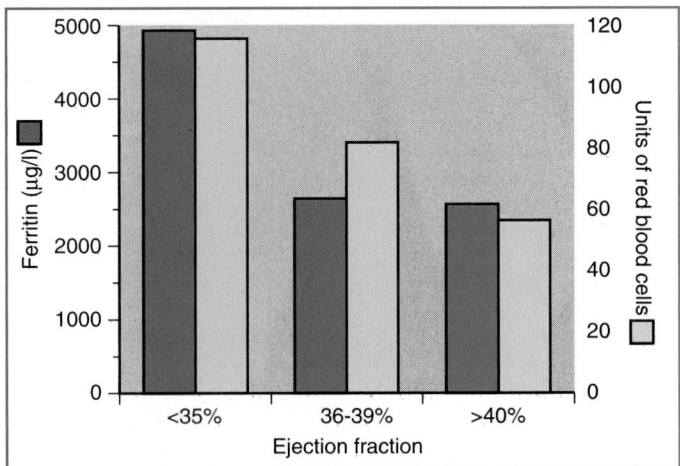

FIGURE 57-7. Correlation of cardiac ejection fraction with serum ferritin and number of transfusions in patients with iron overload. (From Bridges, K. R., and Seligman, P. A.: Disorders of iron metabolism. *In* Handin, R. I., et al. [eds.]: Blood: Principles and Practice of Hematology. Philadelphia, Lippincott-Raven, 1995, pp. 1433–1472.)

moval is inefficient, it is difficult to remove sufficient amounts of iron if it is begun when iron overload is extreme. Ascorbic acid may enhance the removal of iron by desferrioxamine; the latter must be administered parenterally and over extended periods of time (8- to 15-hour infusions) on a regular basis (3 to 7 times/week) to chelate sufficient iron, which makes this therapy a burden for the patient. On the other hand, it provides life-saving relief from the effects of iron overload, as shown in Figure 57–8. Oral chelators are currently under trial in Europe but are not available in the United States.[59]

DISORDERS ASSOCIATED WITH INCREASED BLOOD VISCOSITY

As discussed on p. 1786, delivery of oxygen to an organ or tissue is directly proportional to blood flow, hemoglobin concentration, and the difference in oxygen saturation between arterial and venous blood (Fig. 57–2). In anemic patients, an increase in blood flow, due in part to reduced blood viscosity, and enhanced oxygen delivery through elevated levels of red cell 2,3-DPG compensate for the reduced hemoglobin levels. In contrast, conditions associated with increased viscosity cause an increase in resistance to flow and a reduction in blood flow. Disorders with increased viscosity and abnormal blood rheology include the erythrocytoses, such as polycythemia vera, and disease states associated with hypergammaglobulinemia, such as multiple myeloma and cryoglobulinemia.

Polycythemia

Polycythemia is characterized by an increase in red cells, as determined by hematocrit, hemoglobin, and/or red blood cell count.[64] However, the terms *polycythemia* and its synonym *erythrocytosis* do not refer to a specific disease entity but to a variety of conditions. *Absolute* polycythemias refer to conditions in which there is an absolute increase in red cell mass (as measured by ^{51}Cr labeling or other dilution techniques). The absolute erythrocytoses are subclassified as primary or secondary, depending whether the elevation in red cell mass is autonomous (primary) or under hormonal (erythropoietin) control. *Primary* polycythemia, i.e., polycythemia vera, is part of the spectrum of myeloproliferative disorders. *Secondary* polycythemia is further classified into those disorders which cause an appropriate increase in erythropoietin secretion (e.g., disorders associated with hypoxemia, such as cyanotic forms of congenital heart

prevented by repeated phlebotomy. This is particularly true if the disease is identified early, before there is accumulation of high levels of iron in tissues. Even if early organ damage is present, iron unloading by phlebotomy can result in improved organ function. Because red blood cell production is intact, the patient replaces those red cells removed by phlebotomy. Each unit removed results in the loss of approximately 200 to 250 mg of iron. Phlebotomy is performed as frequently as required to maintain the body stores of iron in a normal range, which can be assessed by serum ferritin levels.

SECONDARY OR TRANSFUSION-RELATED HEMOCHROMATOSIS. Patients with severe anemia that is caused by poor red cell production and increased destruction, such as in the thalassemias or in bone marrow failure states such as aplastic anemia or refractory anemia, require frequent red cell transfusions to maintain the hematocrit in a reasonable range. Even with transfusion they tend to remain significantly anemic, and this, in combination with iron overload and its resultant cardiomyopathy, can cause life-threatening cardiac failure.

Each unit of transfused red blood cells contains 200 to 250 mg of iron, and between 50 and 100 units of red cells lead to a severe iron overload state and progressive impairment of left ventricular function (Fig. 57–7). Because these patients have defective red cell production and require red cell transfusions to remain compensated from the hemodynamic point of view, phlebotomy is not an option for treatment. Chronic iron chelation with the parenteral drug desferrioxamine can remove modest amounts of iron; this treatment must be initiated early in the disease to prevent organ damage.[30,31,54,56–58] Because this method of iron re-

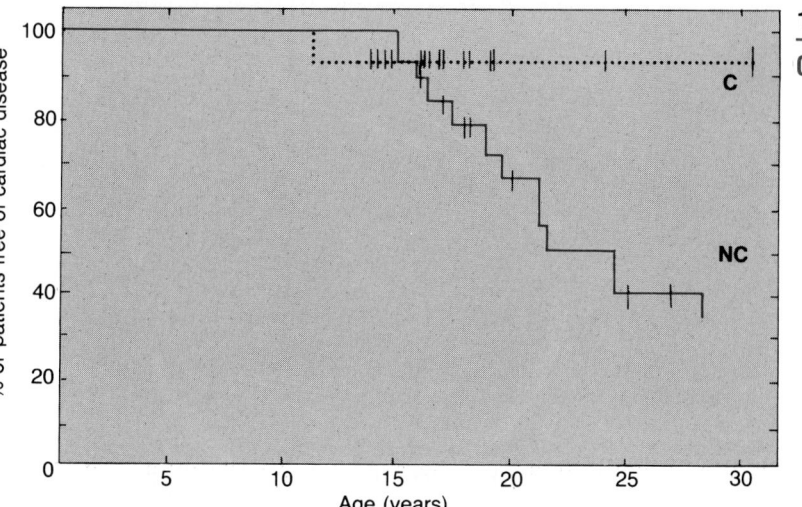

FIGURE 57–8. Life-table depiction of survival free of cardiac disease in patients with thalassemia major treated with desferrioxamine. Dotted line represents the compliant group (C) and solid line represents the current ages of patients still free of cardiac disease. (Reprinted by permission from Wolfe, L., et al.: Prevention of cardiac disease by subcutaneous desferrioxamine in patients with thalassemia major. N. Engl. J. Med. *312*:1600, 1985. Copyright Massachusetts Medical Society.)

disease and pulmonary disease) and those which cause an inappropriate increase in erythropoietin production, as occurs with tumors and a variety of renal diseases. In the *relative* polycythemias, red cell mass is normal but plasma volume is decreased, causing hematocrit, hemoglobin, and red cell values to be elevated.

Although the symptoms of polycythemia depend on the underlying disease state, they are also usually a consequence of increased blood volume and viscosity; the latter increases exponentially with increased hematocrit.[1] When flow rate through a capillary tube is determined at various levels of hematocrit, flow decreases as an essentially linear function of hematocrit (Fig. 57–9). The product of flow rate and arterial oxygen content provides a relative measure of the rate of oxygen transport through a single blood vessel; optimal hematocrit is just below 40 per cent. Delivery of oxygen to the body depends on the product of total blood flow and the oxygen content of arterial blood, which tends to be high in polycythemia vera, in which blood volume, cardiac output, and arterial blood oxygen content are all increased, despite the increase in viscosity. Although the increases in oxygen content, blood volume, and cardiac output in polycythemia vera are not required for adequate tissue oxygenation, in the polycythemias secondary to hypoxemia the increases in blood oxygen content and cardiac output represent an attempt to improve oxygen delivery.

POLYCYTHEMIA VERA

Polycythemia vera is a clonal, malignant proliferation of an early hemopoietic stem cell, and is classified as a myeloproliferative disorder because increased numbers of mature cells are produced.[65] In polycythemia vera there is disregulated clonal growth not only of red cells but also of neutrophils and platelets. Splenomegaly is usually present owing to the presence of extramedullary hematopoiesis. In addition to an elevated red cell mass, leukocytosis, thrombocytosis, and elevations of the leukocyte alkaline phosphatase, LDH, and serum B_{12} are common findings in this disease.

CLINICAL MANIFESTATIONS. Patients often complain of sweats, fevers, and weight loss, hypermetabolic symptoms due to an increased bone marrow mass. In addition, pruritus—often exacerbated by hot showers—can be severe. The major symptoms and morbidity and mortality of the disease result from polycythemia and abnormal platelet function. With increased hematocrit, there is increased blood viscosity and decreased oxygen transport. Blood viscosity rises quickly as hematocrits rise above 50 per cent, and it has been shown that reduction of the hematocrit below 45 per cent results in improved blood flow, particularly in the brain.[66] Severe polycythemia can cause headache and/or confusion, plethora and dyspnea, as well as stroke.

Thrombotic and hemorrhagic events can occur as well.[66a] Thrombosis occurs due to increased viscosity and blood stasis, and hemorrhage can occur from local ischemia due to reduced or absent blood flow and vascular break down. Thrombosis and hemorrhage can still occur when the hematocrit has been reduced to normal levels because platelets in polycythemia vera are derived from the malignant clone and aggregate abnormally. They can behave unpredictably, particularly when the platelet count is high, and in some circumstances thrombosis and hemorrhage will occur simultaneously.

TREATMENT. Patients with significant polycythemia should undergo urgent phlebotomy to hematocrits of 45 per cent or less, particularly if symptoms or signs of polycythemia are present. In addition, treatment with antiproliferative agents such as hydroxyurea reduces the platelet count and red blood cell production, decreasing the need for phlebotomy. More importantly, it has been shown that treatment with agents such as hydroxyurea also significantly reduce the risk of thrombosis and hemorrhage.[67] However, some of these agents, such as chlorambucil and radioactive phosphorus, can also cause polycythemia vera to undergo a leukemic transformation. It is not certain whether hydroxyurea increases the likelihood of conversion to acute leukemia. Nonetheless, in cases of advanced polycythemia vera patients should rapidly undergo phlebotomy to an hematocrit level of under 45 per cent, and many physicians would recommend simultaneous treatment with hydroxyurea.

SECONDARY POLYCYTHEMIAS

The secondary polycythemias may be divided into two subgroups: (1) those in which the increased red cell mass compensates for a reduction in oxygen transport with appropriate stimulation by erythropoietin and (2) those in which erythrocytosis is associated with an inappropriate increase in erythropoietin production. It has been suggested that any hypoxic stimulus will cause production of the enzyme erythrogenin in the kidney, which generates erythropoietin by acting enzymatically on a proposed plasma protein substrate, possibly of hepatic origin (Fig. 57–10). If an individual living at sea level is transported to a high altitude, hemoglobin concentrations will rise[68]

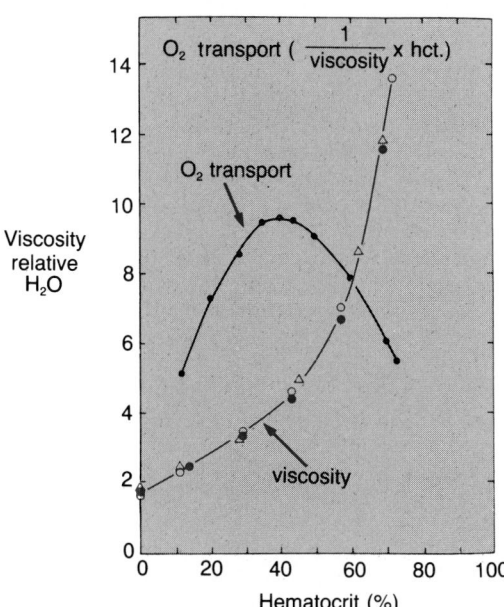

FIGURE 57–9. Viscosity of heparinized normal blood related to hematocrit. Viscosity was measured with an Ostwald viscosimeter at 37°C and expressed in relation to viscosity of water. Oxygen transport was calculated from the product of hematocrit and 1/viscosity and is recorded in arbitrary units. (From Williams, W. J. [ed.]: Hematology. 4th ed. New York, McGraw-Hill, 1990, p. 351.)

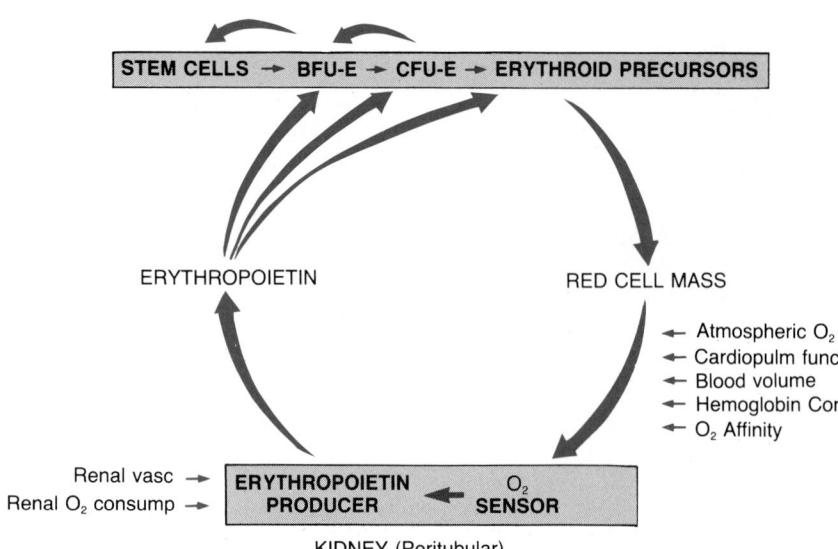

STEM CELLS → BFU-E → CFU-E → ERYTHROID PRECURSORS

ERYTHROPOIETIN

RED CELL MASS

← Atmospheric O₂
← Cardiopulm func
← Blood volume
← Hemoglobin Conc
← O₂ Affinity

Renal vasc →
Renal O₂ consump →

ERYTHROPOIETIN
PRODUCER

O₂
SENSOR

KIDNEY (Peritubular)
Liver (Kupffer cells?)
Macrophages?

FIGURE 57–10. Feedback circuit linking an oxygen sensor in the kidney with erythroid progenitor cells in the bone marrow. The circuit is moved in one direction by red cells containing oxygen and in the opposite direction by erythropoietin. Oxygen sensing and erythropoietin production may also take place in the liver and in some macrophages. The target for erythropoietin is primarily the erythropoietin-dependent progenitor cells (CFU-E), with milder actions on the burst-forming progenitor cells (BFU-E) and the precursor cells. (From Erslev, A. J.: Production of erythrocytes. *In* Williams, W. J., et al. [eds.]: Hematology. 4th ed. New York, McGraw-Hill, 1990, p. 395. © 1990 The McGraw-Hill Companies, Inc.)

accompanied by an increase in erythropoietin. Similarly, with severe degrees of chronic hypoxemia in chronic obstructive pulmonary disease, an arterial PO₂ less than 60 mm Hg usually leads to an increase in red cell mass. In cyanotic congenital heart disease, red cell mass increases as resting arterial oxygen saturation falls (see p. 891). Hematocrits as high as 86 per cent may be seen with red blood cell masses almost three times normal.[69] Although plasma volume may be diminished, total blood volume remains significantly elevated because of the striking increase in red cell mass.

CLINICAL MANIFESTATIONS. Signs and symptoms of hyperviscosity generally occur as hematocrit exceeds 60 per cent; cardiac function may be compromised because of the combination of hypervolemia and the constant volume load and augmented vascular resistance secondary to the increased viscosity of the blood. Ruddy cyanosis, headache, dizziness, roaring in the ears, thrombotic episodes, and bleeding are the major clinical findings and may be treated with phlebotomy.[65] Careful monitoring of arterial pressure, heart rate, and general condition is necessary during phlebotomy, and the acute reduction in blood volume may have to be avoided by the simultaneous administration of plasma expanders.[70] After isovolemic phlebotomy to reduce the hematocrit from the 70's to the 60's, cardiac output rises, and despite the fall in arterial oxygen content, systemic oxygen transport usually increases. These favorable changes are attributed to the reduced blood viscosity and vascular resistance. Although the erythrocytosis is a homeostatic mechanism compensating for the chronic arterial hypoxemia, greatly increased hematocrits are generally undesirable. Studies by Erslev and Caro suggest that secondary polycythemia is not necessarily a boon but could be a burden, and that secondary erythrocytosis cannot always be considered optimal for overall oxygen transport.[71] Secondary polycythemia due to cyanotic congenital heart disease has been reported to cause myocardial infarction without manifestations of coronary atherosclerosis.[72]

MANAGEMENT (see also p. 972). Phlebotomy, or preferably erythropheresis, in secondary polycythemia reduces blood viscosity, increases systemic oxygen transport without lowering peripheral oxygen consumption, and simultaneously increases effective renal plasma flow.[73] The optimal hematocrit for patients with cyanotic congenital heart disease and other chronically hypoxemic states is poorly defined and presents an interesting and perplexing dilemma. The clinical presentation of the patient must be carefully considered. Cerebral blood flow is reduced in secondary erythrocytosis as well as in polycythemia vera and improves with phlebotomy.[74] As might be expected from the decreased oxygen transport associated with right-to-left shunts, P₅₀ and red cell 2,3-DPG are increased, but the relationship between decreased arterial PO₂ and the rise in P₅₀ and red cell 2,3-DPG varies greatly.[75] Successful surgical correction of the cardiac defect will result in normal saturation and obviate the adaptive mechanism, and hematocrit and blood volume will return to normal.

HEMOGLOBIN VARIANTS WITH INCREASED AFFINITY FOR OXYGEN. In 1966, it was first recognized that a hemoglobin variant with *increased* oxygen affinity could be associated with erythrocytosis.[76] These variants, which generally have amino acid substitutions at structural sites crucial to hemoglobin function and individually are quite rare, now number over 40. They are transmitted in an autosomal dominant fashion and cause a shift in the oxygen dissociation curve to the left with reduced levels of P₅₀.

RELATIVE POLYCYTHEMIA. This is a distinct and commonly encountered entity that is also referred to as spurious polycythemia, *Gaisböck syndrome*, and *stress erythrocytosis*. It is not a primary disease process and may be merely a physiological state in which the plasma

volume is slightly reduced and the red cell mass is slightly increased. Hematocrit rarely exceeds 60 per cent, and other blood constituents are normal. Patients are often hypertensive, prone to thromboembolic complications,[77,78] and obese; however, these complications appear to be unrelated to the hematological changes, so that reducing the red cell mass by phlebotomy, radiation therapy, or chemotherapy is not appropriate. When present, hypertension and thromboembolic complications should be treated in the usual manner.

THROMBOCYTOSIS

Occasionally thrombocytosis value may be seen alone as a manifestation of a myeloproliferative disorder without an increased hematocrit. Essential thrombocytosis has been associated in several instances of sudden catastrophic events such as massive arterial thrombosis in the cerebral and coronary arteries, occurring even in young adults without underlying atherosclerosis.[79–82] Such complications rarely occur in the thrombocytosis secondary to nonmyeloproliferative states such as iron deficiency or postsplenectomy states unless coexistent with severe anemia.

CARDIAC MANIFESTATIONS OF NEOPLASTIC DISEASE

INCIDENCE. Primary tumors of the heart, which are discussed in Chap. 42, are rare, occurring in less than 0.1 per cent of autopsies. Here we deal with tumors metastatic to the pericardium or heart, which are far more common, ranging from 1.5 to 20.6 per cent (average 6 per cent) of autopsies on patients with malignant diseases.[83–87] The frequency with which various tumors metastasize to the heart is shown in Figure 57–11 and the frequency at which various tumors are represented among cardiac metastases are shown in Figure 57–12. Prolonged survival of cancer patients may be the reason for this higher incidence. Usually the metastases involve the pericardium and myocardium, with the valves or endocardium rarely affected, and the right side of the heart appears to be affected more frequently than the left.[88,89] Solitary metastases to the heart are rare. Although metastatic nodules in the heart are generally multiple (Fig. 57–13), they may become diffuse and lead to the manifestations of restrictive cardiomyopathy (see p. 1426). The mode of spread to the heart may be by direct extension, as occurs in lung cancer; via the hematogenous route,[90] as in malignant melanoma; or through lymphatic channels, as in lymphoma.

The most common primary tumor producing cardiac metastases is carcinoma of the lung (Fig. 57–13), with carcinoma of the breast, malignant melanoma, lymphomas, and leukemias next in order of frequency (Table 57–3). At autopsy, 15 to 35 per cent of patients dying with primary

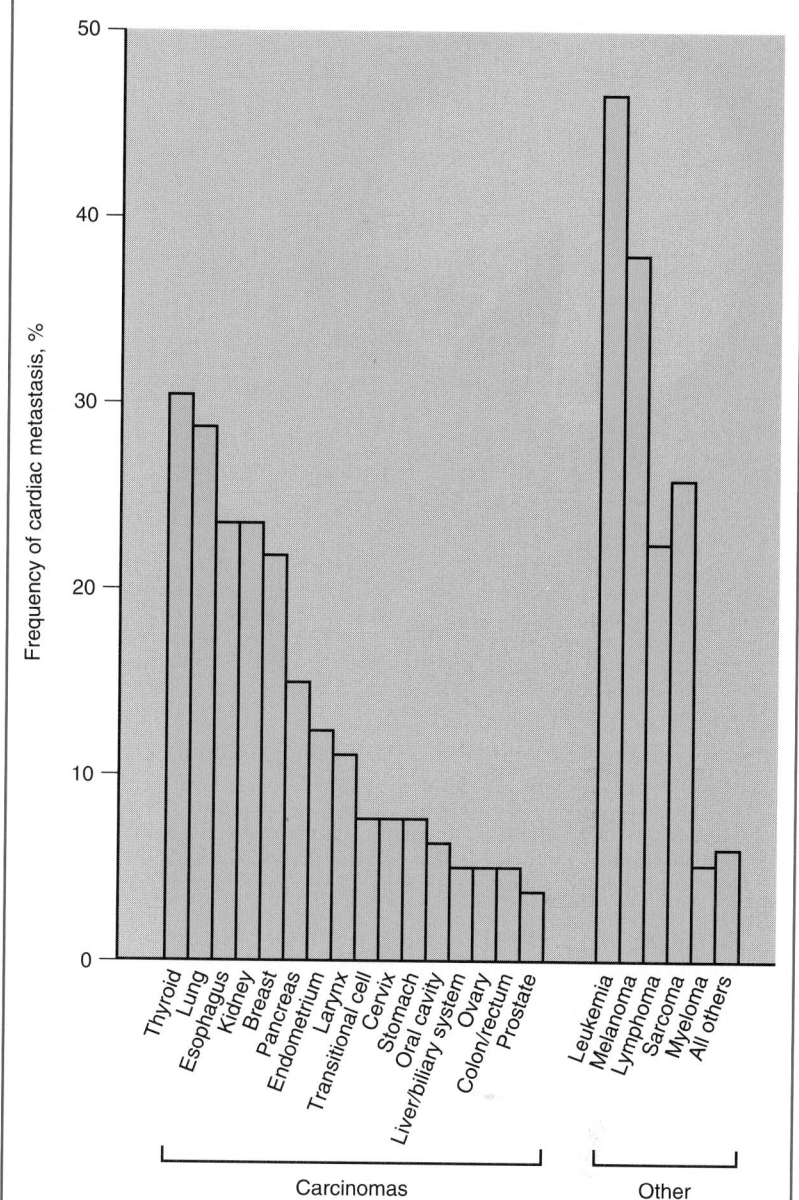

FIGURE 57–11. Frequency of metastatic tumors of the heart and pericardium found in one large autopsy series between 1950 and 1970 in one metropolitan area of the United States. (From English, J. C., et al.: Metastatic tumors of the heart. *In* Goldhaber, S. Z. [ed.]: Cardiopulmonary Diseases and Cardiac Tumors. *In* Braunwald, E. (series ed.): Atlas of Heart Diseases. Vol. 3. Philadelphia, Current Medicine, 1995, pp. 116.1–116.16. Adapted from McAllister, H. A., and Fenoglio, J. J.: Tumors of the cardiovascular system. *In* Atlas of Tumor Pathology. 2nd ed. Washington, D.C., Armed Forces Institute of Pathology, 1978, pp. 111–119.)

lung cancer show cardiac involvement, while over 60 per cent of patients with melanoma have cardiac metastases.[90] Hematological malignant tumors, especially lymphomas, have been reported to account for 15 per cent of all cardiac and pericardial metastases,[91] and about 15 per cent of patients dying of malignant lymphomas show metastases to the heart. Metastatic cardiac lesions secondary to mesothe-lioma and sarcoma, as well as melanoma and breast cancer, are all increasing in number.

Clinical Manifestations

Many metastatic cardiac lesions are clinically silent and are found only at necropsy. For example, despite massive heart involvement with melanoma ("charcoal heart"), sometimes there is surprisingly little evidence of cardiac dysfunction.[92] Specific clinical manifestations of cardiac involvement by cancer may be divided into those due to pericardial, myocardial, or endocardial involvement; cardiac compression by extracardiac tumors; indirect consequences of tumor complications of circulating mediators; embolization in patients in a hypercoagulable state; or the effects of specific tumor therapy, such as chemotherapy and radiation therapy (Table 57–4).[89] The most common clinical manifestations result from pericardial effusion with tamponade, tachyarrhythmias, AV block,[93] or congestive heart failure.[94] Metastatic cardiac disease is rarely the presenting symptom of a tumor. The mode of spread may be by direct extension, the hematogenous route, or through

TABLE 57–3 TUMORS ASSOCIATED WITH PERICARDIAL INVOLVEMENT

TUMORS OF THE THORAX, OFTEN WITH DIRECT EXTENSION TO PERICARDIUM
1. Lung cancer, non-small-cell and small-cell carcinoma
2. Large-cell lymphoma of the mediastinum
3. Hodgkin's disease with mediastinal involvement
4. Malignant mesothelioma

EXTRATHORACIC TUMORS MANIFESTING PERICARDIAL INVOLVEMENT—HEMATOGENOUS SPREAD OF TUMOR TO PERICARDIUM
1. Breast cancer
2. Metastatic malignant melanoma
3. Pancreatic cancer
4. Gastric cancer

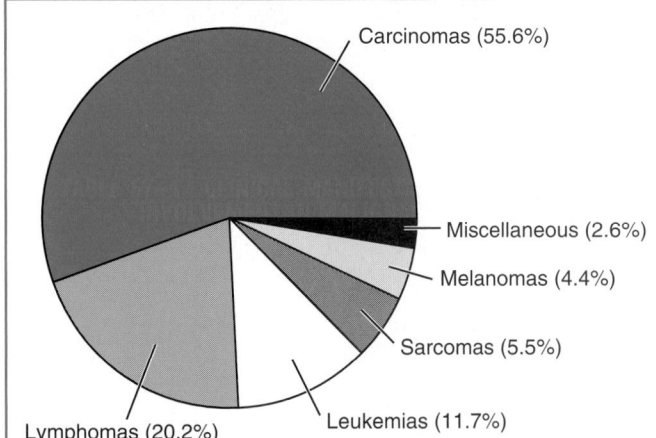

FIGURE 57–12. When the frequency of tumors that have metastasized to the heart is evaluated according to the type of tumor, carcinomas—themselves common—were clearly the most common metastases to the heart (56 per cent). Lymphomas (about 20 per cent) and leukemias (about 12 per cent) were the second and third most common types of neoplasia found during evaluation for metastasis. (From English, J. C., et al.: Metastatic tumors of the heart. *In* Goldhaber, S. Z. [ed.]: Cardiopulmonary Diseases and Cardiac Tumors. *In* Braunwald, E. (series ed.): Atlas of Heart Diseases. Vol. 3. Philadelphia, Current Medicine, 1995, pp. 116.1–116.16.)

lymphatic channels. Routine chest radiographs, computed chest tomography, magnetic resonance imaging, echocardiography, and/or radionuclide imaging with gallium or thallium are often helpful in diagnosis (Chap. 10). Osteogenic sarcoma, which may metastasize to the heart, is unique because the metastases contain bone and may be radiographically visible.[94]

PERICARDIAL INVOLVEMENT (see also p. 1514). Pericardial involvement can occur from direct extension of tumor from the lung or mediastinum, or from hematogenous spread. Involvement from direct extension is often seen in lung cancer and lymphoma (Hodgkin's disease or non-Hodgkin's lymphoma) involving the mediastinum. Hematogenous spread is frequently a complication of malignant metastatic melanoma and metastatic breast cancer. Recently, subclinical pericardial involvement may be more frequently recognized early in the course of malignancy since CT scans have become an integral part of staging evaluations for patients with systemic cancer such as lung cancer and lymphoma.

Malignant pericardial involvement can take several forms. The pericardium can be minimally involved with tumor, retaining its relative elasticity, but a large primarily reactive effusion can be present. The pericardium can be extensively involved with tumor and thickened but not adherent to the myocardium, causing both an effusion and a restrictive picture even without a large volume of pericar-

TABLE 57–4 CLINICAL MANIFESTATIONS OF CARDIAC
INVOLVEMENT IN MALIGNANT DISEASE

Pericardial involvement
Pericarditis
Cardiac tamponade
Superior vena caval syndrome
Arrhythmias
Supraventricular tachycardia
Carotid sinus syncope
Atrioventricular block
Cardiomegaly and congestive heart failure
Unexplained heart murmur
Unexplained hypotension
Noninfective (marantic) endocarditis

dial fluid. The pericardium can be thickened and adherent to the myocardium, sometimes with direct infiltration of the myocardium leading to constrictive pericardial tamponade as well as myocardial dysfunction, often with little or no pericardial fluid present.

Etiology. Lung cancer and breast cancer are the most frequent causes of malignant pericardial disease.[95] Lymphomas of the mediastinum also frequently involve the pericardium, with 50 per cent of patients with large cell lymphoma of the mediastinum demonstrating pericardial involvement in one series.[96] Tumors which most frequently involve the pericardium are shown in Table 57–3.

Symptoms and Signs. Dyspnea is by far the most common symptom of patients with malignant pericardial involvement. Dyspneic symptoms may worsen dramatically with exertion because the heart cannot increase its cardiac output to meet the increased oxygen demand of exercise. Unexplained tachycardia is also a frequent sign of tamponade, and minimal exertion can substantially increase the heart rate. In the patient with dyspnea and tachycardia who has a relatively normal resting oxygen saturation, pericardial tamponade should be suspected. Cough and chest pain can also be signs of pericardial involvement with tumor. Pulsus paradoxus and paradoxical movement of the jugular venous pulse are important clinical signs of

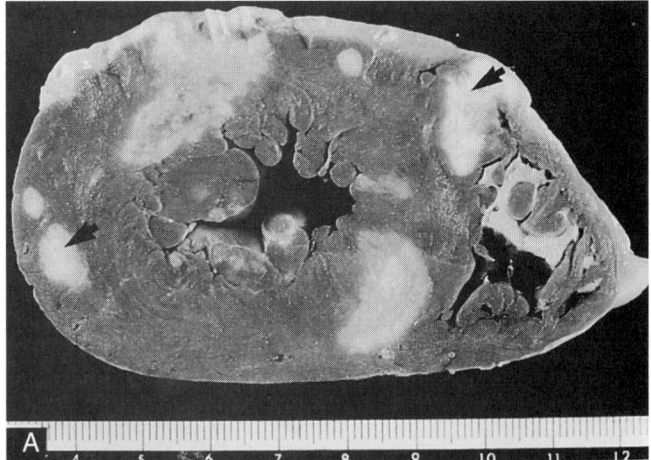

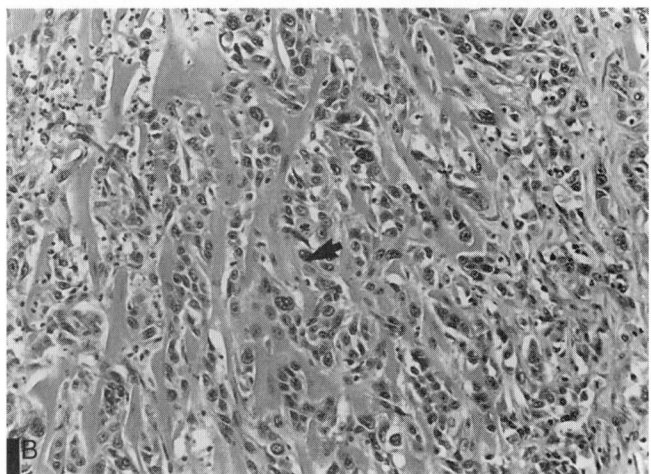

FIGURE 57–13. *A,* Transverse section of the left and right ventricular myocardium shows extensive involvement of the myocardium by several well-circumscribed tumor nodules in a patient with carcinoma of the thyroid (arrows). *B,* Photomicrograph of a representative tumor nodule in the myocardium showing a poorly differentiated carcinoma with marked cellular pleomorphism and evident mitotic activity (arrow; hematoxylin and eosin × 100). (From English, J. C., et al.: Metastatic tumors of the heart. *In* Goldhaber, S. Z. [ed.]: Cardiopulmonary Diseases and Cardiac Tumors. *In* Braunwald, E. (series ed.): Atlas of Heart Diseases. Vol. 3. Philadelphia, Current Medicine, 1995, pp. 116.1–116.16.)

tamponade but are not invariably present, even when tamponade is significant. The cardiac impulse is usually imperceptible. Frequently only some symptoms or signs of tamponade are present, and the clinician must have a high suspicion of tamponade in the patient with a known malignancy.[97] It is possible for the patient to be asymptomatic, without any clinical signs of tamponade until cardiac decompensation occurs.

Diagnosis. The diagnosis is almost always confirmed by echocardiography, which can demonstrate an effusion or pericardial thickening. Physiological signs of tamponade can be evaluated on echocardiography. As intrapericardial pressure rises, right atrial collapse will occur. With further increase in pressure, right ventricular collapse occurs, and this correlates well with clinically significant tamponade.[97]

Rarely, CT scans will demonstrate pericardial involvement not seen by echocardiography, although echocardiography can better delineate the functional compromise of pericardial involvement whereas CT scan cannot.[98] CT scans are particularly helpful in cases of pericardial thickening and constriction without effusion. Because CT scans are frequently used as staging procedures for many malignancies, they are often the first test to suggest pericardial involvement (Fig. 10–41, p. 341).

In the patient with a pericardial effusion who has previously received chest radiation therapy, malignant pericardial involvement must be distinguished from radiation induced pericardial effusion. Malignant effusions tend to be larger and are more likely to cause tamponade physiology than radiation induced effusions.[99,100] Radiation induced effusions can occur any time after radiation therapy but most frequently occur within the first year, as discussed later.

Treatment. Management of malignant pericardial disease depends on the severity of the effusion, the type of tumor, and previous treatment.[101–102a] In a patient with untreated mediastinal large cell lymphoma and minimal signs of tamponade, chemotherapy usually results in rapid resolution of the effusion and signs of tamponade. Malignant pericardial disease caused by lung cancer, on the other hand, almost always requires surgical drainage. Percutaneous catheter drainage can be a temporizing procedure but rarely results in lasting relief of tamponade in patients with malignant effusions.[103,104] Thoracotomy, subxiphoid pericardiectomy, and video-assisted thoracoscopic surgical (VATS) approaches have all been successfully utilized. Subxiphoid pericardiectomy appears to be more effective and safer than anterior thoracotomy. In one nonrandomized series comparing the subxiphoid approach with anterior thoracotomy, no patients undergoing the subxiphoid approach had recurrent effusions or major complications.[105] Fifty per cent of patients undergoing anterior thoracotomy had major complications including pulmonary embolism, disseminated intravascular coagulation, acute renal failure, pneumonia, and recurrent pericardial and pleural effusions. Although this was not a randomized study, the patient groups undergoing these two procedures appeared comparable.

VATS, a more recent procedure, has been highly effective as reported in one series in which all 22 patients treated had relief of their effusions without morbidity or mortality.[106] The ability to open both the anterior and posterior pericardium may be an advantage to this procedure as well.

MYOCARDIAL METASTASES. Direct myocardial or endocardial involvement by tumor such as lung cancer, lymphoma, or melanoma may result in arrhythmias, congestive heart failure, ventricular outflow tract obstruction, and peripheral emboli.[91,107] Cardiac metastases can be detected on two-dimensional echocardiography (Figs. 57–14 and 57–15),[136] computed tomography, and magnetic resonance imaging (Fig. 10–17, p. 326).[108]

VENA CAVAL OBSTRUCTION. Tumors of the mediastinum, including lung cancer, and Hodgkin's and non-Hodgkin's lymphoma, can compress the superior vena cava resulting in obstruction, frequently leading to thrombosis of the vena

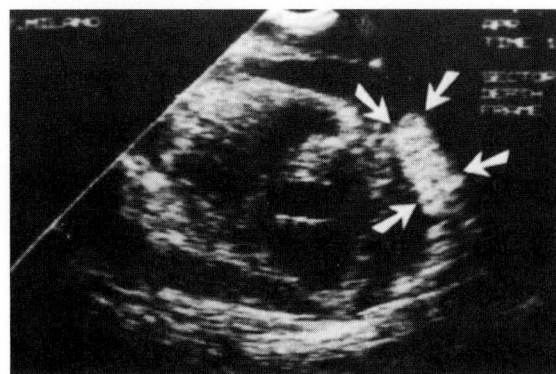

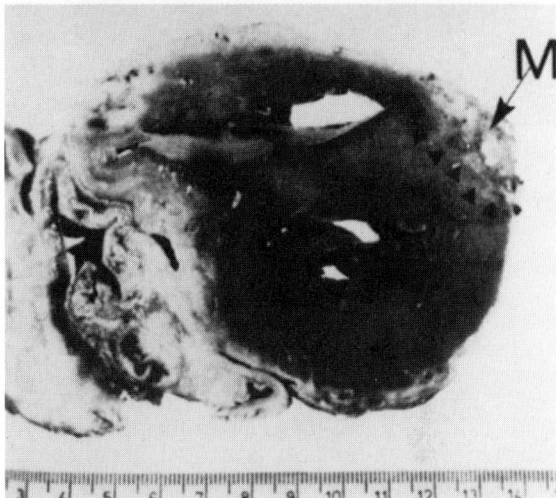

FIGURE 57–14. *Top,* Echocardiogram in parasternal short-axis view. A large echogenic mass *(arrows)* infiltrates the left lateral ventricular wall and the septum. *Bottom,* Postmortem specimen (cross section). The neoplastic mass (M) infiltrates the epicardium and the subepicardial myocardium. (From Lestuzzi, C., et al.: Secondary neoplastic infiltration of the myocardium diagnosed by two-dimensional echocardiography in seven cases with anatomic confirmation. J. Am. Coll. Cardiol. 9:439, 1987.)

cava.[109,110] Facial plethora and headache are frequent signs. Facial and arm edema occur, and collateral vessels become more prominent and numerous, as can be ascertained on examination of the anterior chest wall. Rarely is superior vena caval obstruction life-threatening, although it can result in impeded filling of the right atrium and ventricle when severe, and particularly if accompanied by inferior vena caval obstruction, which can occur from retroperitoneal, hepatic, and renal tumors. Treatment of the obstruction by radiation therapy and/or chemotherapy may or may not relieve the symptoms and signs of vena caval obstruction, depending on whether thrombosis is also present.

CARDIAC AMYLOIDOSIS (see also p. 1427). The heart is involved in the majority of cases of primary amyloidosis and also in many instances of amyloidosis secondary to multiple myeloma. Symptoms often include congestive heart failure, hypotension, arrhythmias, and conduction disturbances.[111,112] Echocardiographic examination, contrast tomography, and endomyocardial biopsy have made it easier to confirm this diagnosis. A low myocardial density on contrast-aided tomography, diffuse myocardial thickening, and diffuse hypokinetic wall motion may be the result of cardiac amyloidosis and may simulate hypertrophic cardiomyopathy. Endomyocardial biopsy may be necessary to confirm the diagnosis.[113]

ELECTROCARDIOGRAPHIC AND ROENTGENOGRAPHIC FINDINGS. Arrhythmias and a wide variety of electrocardiographic changes are common in patients with metastatic disease. Although they may certainly be caused by tumor involvement of the heart, they are more often due to concomitant factors, such as altered electrolyte concentrations, anemia,

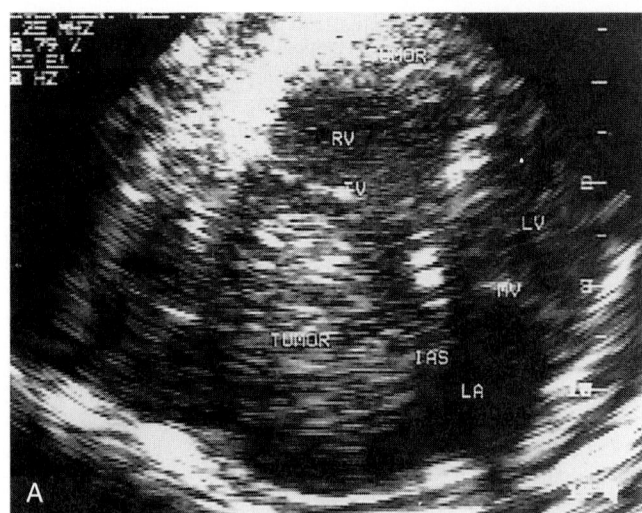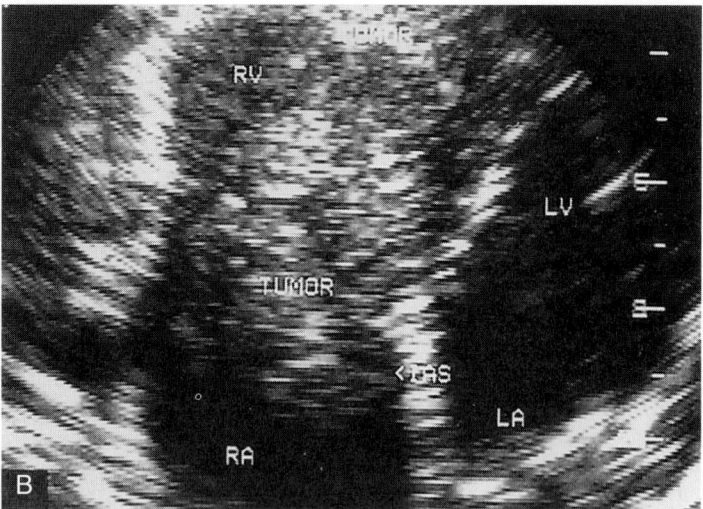

FIGURE 57–15. Echocardiograms of carcinoma that has metastasized from the cervix. *A,* The four-chamber view demonstrates that the tumor virtually fills the right atrium (RA); an attachment point on the interatrial septum (IAS) can be seen. Additional tumor mass can also be visualized in the right ventricular (RV) apex. *B,* In diastole, the atrial tumor mass prolapses through the tricuspid valve (TV) to contact the RV apical tumor mass. (From English, J. C., et al.: Metastatic tumors of the heart. *In* Goldhaber, S. Z. [ed.]: Cardiopulmonary Diseases and Cardiac Tumors. *In* Braunwald, E. (series ed.): Atlas of Heart Diseases. Vol. 3. Philadelphia, Current Medicine, 1995, pp. 116.1–116.16.)

and hypoxia. Nonspecific ST-segment and T-wave changes, low voltage, and sinus tachycardia are frequent electrocardiographic abnormalities and cannot be considered diagnostic.[114] Clinically it may be difficult to determine whether any such abnormality is attributable to cardiac metastases or is due to an associated cardiac problem, irradiation, or the cardiotoxic effects of drugs. Atrial arrhythmias, such as fibrillation and flutter, may occur secondary to either neoplastic involvement of autonomic fibers supplying the atria or tumor invasion of the coronary arteries perfusing the atria, with resulting atrial infarction, or to neoplastic infiltration of the atrial myocardium or sinus node. Similarly, electrocardiographic changes of acute myocardial infarction can be produced by tumor infiltration or hemorrhage into the ventricle or occlusion of one of the coronary arteries. Occasionally, the exact area of tumor involvement may be pinpointed based on the acute electrocardiographic changes.[115] Involvement of the AV node is a rare cause of complete heart block but may be the presenting symptom of the tumor.[116] In addition, tumor involvement of cervical lymph nodes without mediastinal involvement has been associated with carotid sinus syncope.[117]

Roentgenographic evidence of cardiac enlargement and the development of congestive heart failure may be the only clinical signs of malignant involvement of the heart. New systolic murmurs may occur with intraluminal invasion or external compression of the carotid or pulmonary arteries by the tumor. In addition to coincidental atherosclerosis, coronary artery disease in cancer patients can be caused by tumor emboli, extrinsic compression of the coronary arteries or ostia, or thromboemboli brought about by tumor-associated coagulation disorders.

If myocardial metastases are suspected from clinical or electrocardiographic data, a two-dimensional echocardiogram is often helpful diagnostically.

MYOCARDIAL INFARCTION. In a necropsy study of 816 patients with solid tumors, 33 (4 per cent) died of myocardial infarction.[118] Patients with carcinoma of the lung, malignant lymphoma, and leukemia are most commonly afflicted; less frequently affected were patients with cancer of the breast and gastrointestinal tract and malignant melanoma.[119] The etiology of coronary artery disease in patients with cancer is most frequently coincidental spontaneous atherosclerosis.[120] The most common cause of tumor-related myocardial infarction is extrinsic compression of a coronary artery, occurring in 60 per cent of cases, whereas

tumor emboli are responsible for about 35 per cent.[119,121] Widespread thromboses, including coronary artery thromboses due to disseminated intravascular coagulation, occasionally occur in patients with metastatic tumors, most commonly mucin-secreting adenocarcinomas. Rarely, cardiac metastases present as acute myocardial infarction.[122] Approximately half of all patients with acute myocardial infarction secondary to malignant disease had a history of typical chest pain prior to death. An acute myocardial infarction in a patient with advanced malignant disease is a particularly poor prognostic sign, since more than two-thirds of such patients die within 3 weeks of the event.

VALVULAR EFFECTS: NONBACTERIAL THROMBOTIC ENDOCARDITIS (NBTE). Metastatic tumors may affect cardiac valves in a variety of ways, including direct invasion of valves, interference with valvular function by compression, valvular dysfunction secondary to malignant carcinoid (see p. 1434), but most commonly by NBTE.[123–125] Although the pathogenesis is unclear, this condition is associated with adenocarcinomas—especially of the pancreas and lung—as well as hematological malignant disease and lymphomas.[125] It has been suggested that immune complexes elicited by the underlying malignant process play a role in the formation of thrombi.[126] Other causes of NBTE include disseminated intravascular coagulation and non-neoplastic causes of debilitation and cachexia.[126] The fibrin matrix is attached to, but does not destroy, valve leaflets that may be normal or show degenerative changes.[123] NBTE involves principally the aortic and mitral valves equally. (The pulmonic valve may be involved in patients with catheters in place for long periods in the right heart and pulmonary artery.[127])

Patients may have clinical evidence of arterial embolization and microembolic events resembling those of infective endocarditis (see p. 1083), and changing murmurs, often without fever or leukocytosis (unless an unrelated infection is present). The most serious complications are cerebral emboli with neurological sequelae. Rarely coronary embolization may occur, causing myocardial infarction.

The diagnosis is aided immensely by two-dimensional echocardiography. Antiplatelet therapy with aspirin or anticoagulants has been employed to prevent recurrent embolization, but its effectiveness has yet to be demonstrated.

THE HYPEREOSINOPHILIC SYNDROMES WITH ENDOCARDIAL INVOLVEMENT (see also p. 1432). The hypereosinophilic syndromes are a group of diseases characterized by hypereosinophila in the peripheral blood, as well as tissue infiltration with eosinophils. The etiology of these diseases is not understood, and the course and prognosis is very variable. When severe, the bone marrow as well as other organs including the heart are infiltrated. In a series of 50 patients from the National Institutes of Health, 54 per cent had cardiac involvement, 64 per cent neurologic involvement, 56 per cent skin involvement, 40 per cent pulmonary involvement and 32 per cent hepatic involvement.[128] The NIH also prospectively followed 26 patients with hypereosinophilic syndrome and related cardiac disease and found that 42 per cent of patients complained of dyspnea and 27 per cent of chest pain.[129] Thirty-five per cent of patients developed cardiomegaly and 38 per cent developed signs of congestive heart failure. Echocardiography demonstrated cardiomegaly with increased left ventricular wall thickness and signs of restrictive cardiomyopathy. Pathologically there was endomyocardial infiltration with eosinophils and myocardial fibrosis. Left ventricular mural thrombi were also common.

CARDIAC EFFECTS OF RADIATION THERAPY AND CHEMOTHERAPY

With the advent of intensive radiation therapy and aggressive chemotherapy, cardiac toxicity of antitumor treatment has increased greatly. Formerly, the heart was considered one of the most radioresistant organs and seemed to be spared most of the side effects of chemotherapy. However, radiation can cause myocardial damage. The incidence of cardiovascular complications has risen sharply with the use of curative forms of radiation therapy for Hodgkin's disease and non-Hodgkin's lymphoma involving the mediastinum and the addition of one of the most potent classes of chemotherapeutic agents, the anthracyclines. The addition of growth factors and cytokines such as interferon and interleukin-2 to the armamentarium of the therapist has also brought on unexpected cardiac complications.

Radiation Therapy

Therapeutic radiation can cause acute and chronic cardiac damage. The pericardium, myocardium, endocardium, valves and coronary arteries can be affected by radiation (Table 57-5).[130-134] The successful treatment of Hodgkin's disease frequently using chest (mantle) radiation, and other childhood cancers successfully treated with radiation has left a large number of adults who are long-term survivors and are at risk for the development of cardiac abnormalities from radiation. It has been estimated that 15 per cent of all patients with cardiomyopathy had received treatment for cancer during childhood, and that as many of 40% of those

TABLE 57-5 CLASSIFICATION OF RADIATION-RELATED CARDIAC DISEASE

1. Acute pericarditis (caused by necrosis of tumor adjacent to the heart)
2. Delayed pericarditis
   a. Acute radiation-induced pericarditis, without effusion
   b. Acute radiation-induced pericarditis, without effusion, with/without cardiac tamponade
   c. Chronic effusive pericarditis
   d. Effusive constrictive pericarditis
   e. Chronic pericardial constriction
   f. Occult constrictive pericarditis
3. Myocardial fibrosis
4. Occlusive coronary artery disease
5. Conduction abnormalities
6. Valvular regurgitation or stenosis

patients treated with mediastinal radiation have some demonstrable cardiac abnormality.[135]

Radiation can cause cardiac damage by two mechanisms: (1) It can produce direct cellular damage, resulting in a loss of myocardial tissue; (2) it can also cause endothelial damage, which can lead to microvascular changes resulting in ischemia, secondary cellular loss and progressive fibrosis.

PERICARDIAL EFFECTS (see also p. 1516). Acute and delayed pericarditis can occur in association with radiation therapy. Of 635 patients below the age of 21 years treated at Stanford University, 19 per cent had cardiac events, including 12 patients with fatal events and 106 with non-fatal cardiac events.[136] Eight patients developed acute pericarditis during radiation therapy and 30 patients developed pericardial disease 3 months to 18 years (mean 6 years) after treatment for an incidence of pericardial disease of 6 per cent. Twelve patients required pericardiectomy for symptomatic tamponade. The finding that pericardial effusion can occur very late after radiation therapy has been confirmed by others.

In a group of 49 patients treated for Hodgkin's disease studied with pulsed Doppler echocardiography, 39 per cent had pericardial thickening, although none had demonstrable effusions.[137] This suggests that pericardial damage is common after mediastinal radiation, but in only a minority of patients does it become clinically significant.

MYOCARDIAL, VASCULAR AND VALVULAR EFFECTS OF RADIATION. Radiation therapy can have profound effects on the heart leading to microvascular cardiomyopathy, coronary artery disease and valvular disease. Accelerated coronary artery narrowing unassociated with atherosclerotic plaque and composed of intima fibrous thickening and adventitial scarring suggests that radiation damage causes vascular lesions sufficient to result in myocardial infarction and sudden death.[130-134,138-142] In young patients examined at autopsy, proximal portions of the coronary arteries are more severely narrowed than distal portions.[139] It is possible that this is due to the design of mediastinal radiation ports that often extend over the base of the heart and the origins of the coronary arteries, but not lower.

Children appear to be particularly sensitive to the effects of irradiation. Stanford reported follow-up of 635 children below the age of 21 years treated for Hodgkin's disease and found the relative risk of death from acute myocardial infarction to be 41.5 (95 per cent) CI 18.1–82.1).[136] For males it was 35.6 (95 per cent CI 13.0–79.1) and for females 70.4 (95 per cent CI 11.7–23.3). The absolute risk was 10.4 excess cases per 10,000 patient-years.

Cardiac effects can also be seen in children irradiated for diseases other than Hodgkin's disease. In a group of children between the ages of 2 and 12 years receiving spinal radiation that included the heart, 75 per cent had maximal cardiac indices below the fifth percentile.[143]

Adults appear less sensitive to the effects of cardiac irradiation, but those who receive mediastinal irradiation do have a significantly increased risk of both acute myocardial infarction and sudden death. In a series of 4665 patients from several centers the relative risk of acute myocardial infarction was 4.09 (95 per cent CI 1.54–10.89).[144] Age at time of radiation, sex, interval between radiation and cardiac event, and standard cardiac risk factors such as smoking and hypertension did not significantly alter the relative risk in these patients.

Using pulsed Doppler echocardiography on patients treated for Hodgkin's disease, reduced ejection fraction can be demonstrated in 14 per cent of patients in one series, as well as valvular thickening in 42 per cent.[137]

Chemotherapy

Since the late 1960's there have been major advances in the management of a variety of neoplastic disorders using combination chemotherapy. Therapies have become more intensive and new agents have been introduced, resulting in significant responses and longer survival. Unfortunately, concomitant with this increased response rate has been an increase in toxicity. Although most complications due to drugs are limited to rapidly proliferating tissues such as the bone marrow and gastrointestinal tract, cardiotoxicity, both early and late, has been recognized with increasing frequency (Table 57–6).[145–149,149a]

For many years, the only notable cardiopulmonary complications of chemotherapy for neoplastic disease were orthostatic hypotension and the rare myocardial infarctions that occurred in the course of therapy with vincristine, a periwinkle alkaloid, and the interstitial lung disease and mild pulmonary hypertension secondary to pulmonary fibrosis created by bleomycin or busulfan. However, with the use of higher doses of conventional therapy for curative intent and the addition of the anthracycline group of drugs (doxorubicin, daunorubicin), the incidence of cardiac toxicity as a consequence of chemotherapy for neoplastic disease has increased greatly.

Anthracycline Cardiotoxicity

The anthracyclines (doxorubicin, daunorubicin, and idarubicin) and the anthracenedione mitoxantrone have become important and widely used agents in the treatment of cancer. These drugs are crucial in the treatment of the acute leukemias, Hodgkin's and non-Hodgkin's lymphoma, and breast cancer, all of which can occur in young people and can be cured. The importance of these agents in cancer therapy cannot be overstated, and not only are they being used with increasing frequency but they are being given in higher dosages in an attempt to improve treatment results.

These agents intercalate into DNA, therefore interfering with both DNA and RNA polymerase activity. They must be administered intravenously and are metabolized in the liver.

MECHANISM OF TOXICITY. The exact mechanism of anthracycline-induced myocardial cell injury is not known, but it may relate to the production of free radicals, reactive oxygen species leading to speculation that free-radical scavengers such as vitamin E and the bispiperazine ICRF-187 might be protective of this toxicity, although this remains controversial.[150] Anthracyclines may also interfere with the sarcolemmal sodium-potassium pump and may hinder the mitochondrial electron-transport chain. This may explain the propensity for myocardial toxicity from the anthracyclines because the heart is a mitochondrial-rich

organ and also may be poorly suited to combat oxidative damage by free radicals because its peroxide-reducing potential resides solely in the glutathione-glutathione peroxidase cycle.[150,151]

On pathological analysis of the myocardium after exposure to anthracyclines myocytes are partially or totally devoid of myofibrillar content.[152] Swelling of the sarcoplasmic reticulum can lead to their coalescence into vacuoles. These findings are shown in Figure 57–16. With more severe injury there is mitochondrial and nuclear degeneration. Several grading systems have been devised to classify the severity of injury, and one is shown in Table 57–7.

Acute injury can be demonstrated on endomyocardial biopsy after a single injection of doxorubicin.[153] Increased nuclear chromatin clumping and abnormal nucleoli with fewer fibrillar centers and less evident nucleolonema were most evident four hours after drug administration, and many of these abnormalities resolved by 24 hours suggesting cellular repair. With additional exposure to doxorubicin these changes may become irreversible.

CLINICAL ASPECTS OF TOXICITY. With very high single

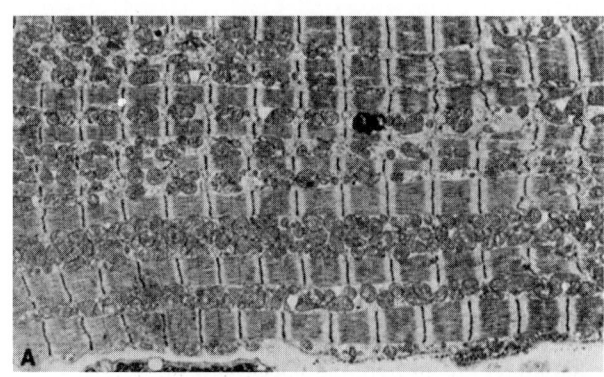
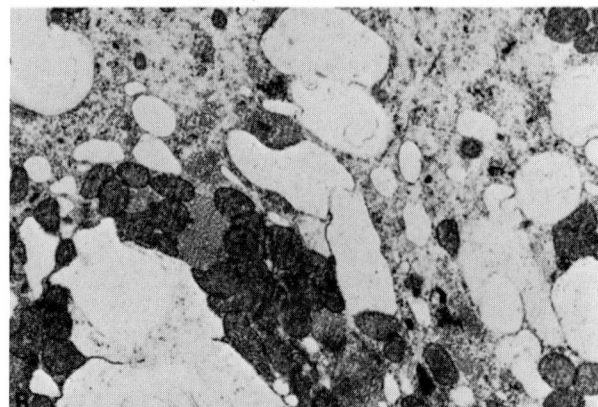
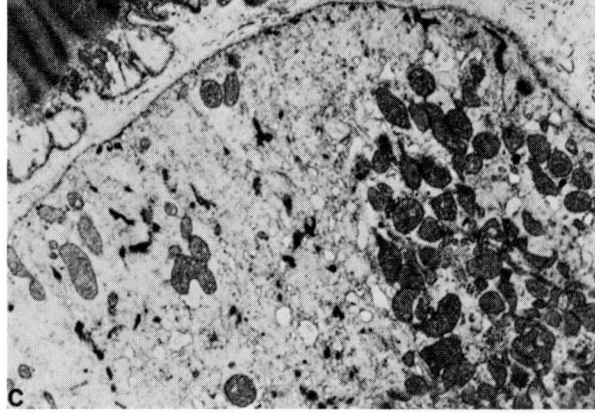

FIGURE 57–16. Electron microscopic images of cardiac biopsy specimens. *A,* Normal cardiac muscle fiber (grade O). *B,* Vacuolation. *C,* Myofibrillar dropout (× 3,575). *B* and *C* follow doxorubicin treatment. (From Ali, M. D., and Ewer, M. S.: Cancer and the Cardiopulmonary System. New York, Raven Press, 1984, pp. 62 and 63.)

TABLE 57–6 MAJOR CARDIOVASCULAR COMPLICATIONS OF CHEMOTHERAPEUTIC AGENTS

AGENT	CARDIAC TOXICITY
Amsacrine	Arrhythmia, cardiomyopathy
Busulfan	Pulmonary fibrosis
	Pulmonary hypertension
	Endocardial fibrosis
Cisplatin	ECG changes, vaso-occlusion
Cyclophosphamide	Cardiac necrosis, cardiomyopathy
Cytosine arabinoside	Congestive heart failure
	Pericarditis
Diethylstilbestrol	Cardiovascular deaths
Doxorubicin	ECG changes, cardiomyopathy
Etoposide	Myocardial infarction
5-Fluorouracil	Vaso-occlusion, myocarditis
Methotrexate	ECG changes
Mitomycin	Myocardial damage
Mitoxantrone	Cardiomyopathy
Vincristine	Hypotension

TABLE 57–7 SEMIQUANTITATIVE SCALE OF BIOPSY-DETERMINED ANTHRACYCLINE MYOCARDIAL DAMAGE

BIOPSY GRADE	HISTOPATHOLOGICAL FEATURES
0	No detectable change from normal
1	Scant number of cells ($\leq 5\%$) showing distended sarcoplasmic reticulum and/or early myofibrillar loss
1.5	Small numbers of cells (5 to 15%), some showing definite cytoplasmic vacuolization and/or myofibrillar loss
2	Groups of cells (16 to 25%), some showing definite cytoplasmic vacuolization and/or myofibrillar loss
	Biopsy grades up to 2 carry < 10% risk of heart failure with 100 mg/m² incremental dose of doxorubicin
2.5	Groups of cells (26 to 35%), some showing definite cytoplasmic vacuolization and/or marked myofibrillar loss
	Biopsy grade of 2.5 carries a 10 to 25% risk of heart failure with 100 mg/m² incremental dose of doxorubicin
3	Diffuse cell injury (>35%) showing advanced loss of organelles, total loss of myofibrils, and mitochondrial and nuclear degeneration
	Biopsy grade 3 is associated with >25% risk of heart failure if more doxorubicin is given

From Fowles, R. E.: Cardiac catheterization and endomyocardial biopsy. In Kapoor, A. S. (ed.): Cancer and the Heart. New York, Springer-Verlag, 1986, p. 48.

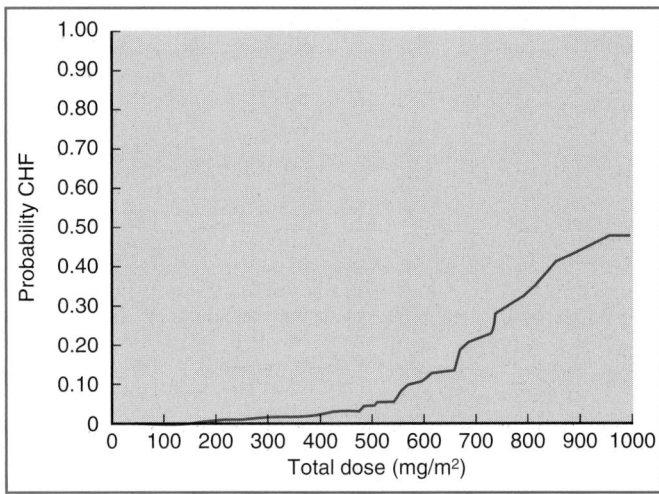

FIGURE 57–17. Cumulative probability of developing doxorubicin-induced congestive heart failure versus total cumulative dose of doxorubicin in 3941 patients of whom 88 developed congestive heart failure. (From Von Hoff, D. D., et al.: Risk factors for doxorubicin-induced congestive heart failure. Ann. Intern. Med. *91:*710, 1979.)

doses, there can be acute cardiac toxicity usually manifested by atrial and ventricular arrhythmias. More commonly, a cardiomyopathy results from myocyte damage as described above, leading to congestive heart failure.

Anthracycline cardiomyopathy is clearly related to total cumulative exposure to these agents, as well as acute peak levels, age at exposure, and the concurrent administration of other cardiotoxic antineoplastic agents. Factors known to be associated with the development of cardiac toxicity from these agents are shown in Table 57–8.

The most powerful predictor of anthracycline cardiotoxicity is the total cumulative dosage administered (Fig. 57–17). Clinically apparent cardiotoxicity due to doxorubicin is rare below cumulative doses of 400 mg/m², then becomes increasingly frequent with higher dosages. However, subclinical cardiac toxicity can be demonstrated by more sensitive testing, with high frequency, at much lower cumulative doses. Bristow et al. studied 33 patients receiving doxorubicin using echocardiography, cardiac catheterization, and endomyocardial biopsy.[152] Twenty-seven of 29 patients receiving greater than 272 mg/m² had endomyocardial biopsies showing myocyte damage, although one patient had biopsy-proved evidence of doxorubicin-induced damage after only 45 mg/m². Another patient had no evidence of myocyte damage on biopsy after receiving 400 mg/m². On the other hand, preejection period to left ventricular ejection time ratio (PEP/LVET) was increased only in patients who had received greater than 400 mg/m² of doxorubicin.

Gottdiener et al. studied 32 patients with radionuclide cineangiography who had been treated with between 480 and 550 mg/m² of doxorubicin for sarcomas.[154] All patients were asymptomatic, without signs of cardiomyopathy. The mean ejection fraction at rest for all patients was 49 per cent as compared with 57 per cent for normal controls. With maximal exercise, patients treated with doxorubicin had a mean ejection fraction of 52 per cent compared with 71 per cent for normal subjects, suggesting that these patients had a moderate decrease in ejection fraction after treatment with doxorubicin. The relative reduction in ejection fraction during maximal exercise suggests that the doxorubicin-treated heart is less able to keep up with increased demand than is the normal heart. In another study 18 patients were examined by radionucleotide angiography before and after treatment with 500 mg/m² of doxorubicin.[155] Pretreatment ejection fractions averaged 60.4 per cent and post-treatment ejection fractions averaged 49.8 per cent, a difference that was highly significant. Myocardial damage was assessed using monoclonal antibodies to myosin labeled with indium 111. Abnormal uptake was present in all patients, but only those with high uptake were likely to have a decreased ejection fraction and/or clinically apparent congestive heart failure. This supports the hypothesis that all patients receiving doxorubicin have some evidence of myocardial damage, but in only a subset is this clinically significant.

MONITORING OF PATIENTS RECEIVING ANTHRACYCLINES. Because anthracyclines have become such an integral part of cancer chemotherapy and are often best used in high cumulative doses, considerable effort has been expended in determining criteria to evaluate those patients suitable for anthracycline therapy, particularly among patients with known heart disease and to evaluate patients during therapy to reduce the risk of developing congestive heart failure. This is important because the total cumulative dose of an anthracycline that can lead to heart failure in an individual patient is highly variable. Grading systems for severity of heart failure have been proposed, though most studies do not report their results using these recommendations. One such system is shown in Table 57–9.

Investigators at Yale reviewed records of 1487 patients undergoing chemotherapy who had serial radionuclide angiocardiograms and identified 282 patients who were thought to be at high risk for developing anthracycline-in-

TABLE 57–8 RISK FACTORS FOR THE DEVELOPMENT OF ANTHRACYCLINE CARDIOTOXICITY

1. High total cumulative dose of drug administered
2. High peak serum levels of drug
3. Previous or concurrent mediastinal or heart irradiation
4. Concurrent administration of other cardiotoxic antineoplastic drugs such as high-dose cyclophosphamide
5. Age at time of exposure—very young and very old are most susceptible
6. History of cardiac disease, particularly coronary artery disease

TABLE 57–9 HEMODYNAMIC GRADING OF PATIENTS UNDERGOING DOXORUBICIN CHEMOTHERAPY

GRADE	HEMODYNAMIC FINDINGS
0 Normal	Mean RA < 7 mm Hg RVEDP < 8 mm Hg LVEDP/Mean PAW < 12 mm Hg Cardiac index > 2.5 L/min/m² Exercise factor > 5.0

1 Mildly abnormal	Any of the following:
	  Mean RA = 7 to 10 mm Hg
	  RVEDP = 8 to 12 mm Hg at rest
	    with increase on exercise = 5 to 9
	    mm Hg
	  LVEDP/Mean PAW = 12 to 15
	    mm Hg at rest with increase on
	    exercise = 5 to 11 mm Hg
	  Cardiac index = 2.2 to 2.5 L/min/m²
	  Exercise factor = 4.0 to 5.0

2 Moderately abnormal	Any of the following:
	  Two or more grade 1 features
	  Mean RA = 10 to 15 mm Hg
	  RVEDP = 12 to 17 mm Hg at rest
	    with increase on exercise ≥ 9
	    mm Hg
	  Cardiac index = 1.8 to 2.2 L/min/m²
	  Exercise factor < 4.0

3 Severely abnormal	Any of the following:
	  Two or more grade 2 features
	  Mean RA ≥ 16 mm Hg
	  RVEDP ≥19 mm Hg
	  LVEDP/Mean PAW ≥ 20 mm Hg
	  Cardiac index < 1.8 L/min/m²

RA = right atrium; RVEDP and LVEDP = right and left end-diastolic pressure, respectively; PAW = pulmonary artery wedge pressure. Abnormal cardiac index is accompanied by elevated AV oxygen content difference (>5 vol%). Exercise factor = increase in cardiac output (ml/min)/increase in total body oxygen consumption.

From Bristow, M. R., et al.: Efficacy and the cost of cardiac monitoring in patients receiving doxorubicin. Cancer 50:32, 1982. Copyright © 1982 American Cancer Society.

TABLE 57–10 GUIDELINES FOR ADMINISTRATION AND MONITORING OF PATIENTS RECEIVING DOXORUBICIN

1. **Patients with pre-treatment LVEF ≥ 50%**
   A. Repeat LVEF after 350–300 mg/m².
   B. Repeat LVEF after 400 mg/m² in patients with known heart disease, heart irradiation or cyclophosphamide therapy, or after 450 mg/m² in patients without these risk factors.
   C. Repeat LVEF measurements after each subsequent dose of doxorubicin.
   D. Discontinue doxorubicin therapy if LVEF declines by ≥ 10% to a value of less than 50%.

2. **Patients with pre-treatment LVEF < 50%**
   A. Do not administer doxorubicin at all to patients with baseline LVEF of ≤ 30%.
   B. In patients with LVEF of between 30 and 50%, repeat LVEF prior to each dose.
   C. Discontinue doxorubicin therapy if LVEF declines by ≥ 10% and/or to a value of less than 30%.

LVEF = Left ventricular ejection fraction, measured by radionuclide cardioangiography

Adapted from Schwartz, R. G., et al.: Congestive heart failure and left ventricular dysfunction complicating doxorubicin therapy: Seven-year experience using serial radionucleotide angiocardiography. Am. J. Med. 82:1112, 1987.

duced cardiomyopathy.[156] High-risk patients were defined as those with either a decline of ≥ 10 per cent in absolute left ventricular ejection fraction (LVEF) from a normal baseline to an LVEF of 50 per cent or less, a total cumulative dose of doxorubicin of 450 mg/m² or more, or a pretreatment LVEF of < 50 per cent. Clinically apparent heart failure occurred in 49 patients (17 per cent). The 49 patients who developed heart failure received total cumulative doses of doxorubicin of between 75 to 1,095 mg/m² as compared with those who did not develop heart failure who received doses between 30 and 880 mg/m², demonstrating that total doxorubicin dose alone is insufficient to predict the development of this complication. Pretreatment LVEF was similar in patients who developed CHF as compared with those who did not—57 and 58 per cent, respectively. Decline in LVEF during therapy was greater in those patients developing CHF than in those who did not; 23 and 12 per cent.

Guidelines for administration and monitoring of doxorubicin therapy are shown in Table 57–10. When these guidelines were applied to the cohort of 282 patients at high risk for the development of doxorubicin cardiomyopathy there was fourfold reduced risk of developing heart failure in the group treated according to these guidelines as compared with those whose management was discordant with the guidelines as shown in Figure 57–18.

OUTCOME OF PATIENTS WITH ANTHRACYCLINE CARDIOMYOPATHY. It was once thought that anthracycline cardiomyopathy was uniformly rapidly progressive and fatal for most patients.[157] Others have suggested some patients will do well with conventional heart failure management. Of 46 patients studied by Schwartz et al., 87 per cent improved with standard therapy for heart failure, whereas 11 per cent

remained stable and only one patient worsened.[156] In another series, 19 patients with anthracycline-induced heart failure were evaluated and followed.[158] The mean onset from the last dose of anthracycline to the development of heart failure was 4 weeks with a range of 1 to 17 weeks. For the 7 patients who died of heart failure, the median time to death was 6 weeks with a range of 1 to 15 weeks. Sixty-three per cent of patients survived with improved symptomatology with a median follow-up of 3 years. The authors could not identify any predisposing factors which would predict fatal outcome from anthracycline-induced heart failure, although none of the patients who died had cumulative anthracycline doses of < 300 mg/m², whereas 5 of 12 of the survivors were given doses below this value.

A number of case reports exist suggesting that viral illnesses or other stresses can have severe and sometimes fatal outcomes in patients with seemingly well-compensated anthracycline-induced heart failure indicate that these patients have little cardiac reserve to compensate for these stresses or that minimal additional cardiac toxicity can cause a patient with well-compensated heart failure to decompensate and die.

ANTHRACYCLINE CARDIOTOXICITY IN CHILDREN. It is now known that children are at particular risk for the late de-

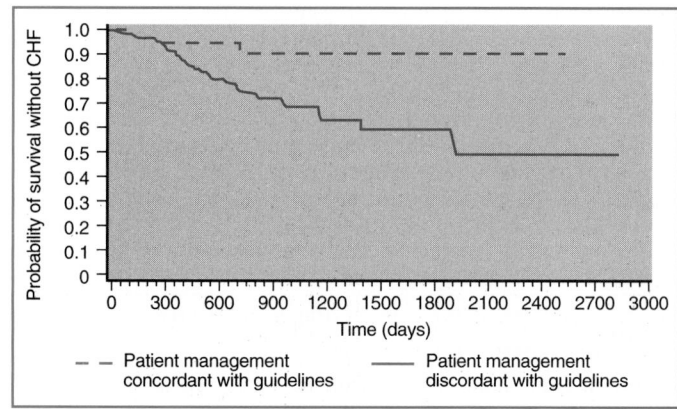

FIGURE 57–18. Kaplan-Meier plot demonstrating the probability of survival without congestive heart failure in patients whose management was either concordant or discordant with guideline criteria shown in Table 57–10. (From Schwartz, R. G., et al.: Congestive heart failure and left ventricular dysfunction complicating doxorubicin therapy: Seven-year experience using serial radionuclide angiocardiography. Am. J. Med. 82:1109, 1987.)

velopment of cardiotoxicity from anthracyclines, and those who receive anthracyclines before the age of 4 years may be at specially high risk.[159] Eleven (10 per cent) of 115 children between the ages of 7 months and 19 years treated with doxorubicin for acute lymphoblastic leukemia developed heart failure. All patients improved with standard heart failure therapy and eventually all were able to discontinue cardiac medications. Five of the 11 patients had recurrent heart failure 3 to 10 years after the initial episode and two patients required cardiac transplantation. Similar results have been observed in another series of 30 children between the ages of 4 and 16 years treated with a mean of 317 mg/m^2 of doxorubicin.[160] Fractional shortening declined from pretreatment levels of 34.9 to 32.0 (p < .0001) at the conclusion of chemotherapy, although all of these children were clinically well at this time. However, seven of these patients developed late cardiac decompensation, five during an acute viral illness, raising concern about the role of viral illnesses in causing cardiac decompensation in these patients.

Among children treated with anthracyclines, females are much more sensitive to the cardiotoxic effects of this agent than males, although the reason for this is unknown. In a study of 120 patients who had received doxorubicin during childhood for either acute lymphoblastic leukemia or osteogenic sarcoma, for any given cumulative dose of doxorubicin females had a higher probability of depressed left ventricular contractility.[160a] This difference was most marked at higher cumulative doses of doxorubicin.

REDUCED ANTHRACYCLINE-INDUCED CARDIAC TOXICITY FROM LOW-DOSE OR INFUSIONAL REGIMENS. It has been suggested that either more frequent lower-dose doxorubicin schedules or continuous infusion schedules would produce less cardiotoxicity for any given cumulative dose without compromising antitumor activity.[161-166] The mechanism of reduction of cardiotoxicity for these regimens is not known, although it has been hypothesized that toxicity is related in part to peak serum levels.

Doxorubicin toxicity was compared by endomyocardial biopsy in 98 patients receiving standard doses every 3 weeks, and 27 patients receiving lower doses weekly.[164] In both groups total cumulative dose was predictive of myocardial damage on biopsy specimens, but for any given total cumulative dose, patients receiving low dose weekly doxorubicin had less damage. Another study compared doxorubicin given by standard bolus injection every 3 weeks to patients receiving infusional doxorubicin over 48 or 96 hours.[165] Patients receiving continuous infusion received higher total cumulative doses of doxorubicin than those receiving bolus administration, and for any given total cumulative dose of doxorubicin, less severe myocardial changes were seen on biopsy in the patients receiving infusional therapy. Shorter infusions, over 6 hours for instance, have not shown cardiac sparing effects.[166]

5-Fluorouracil

Vaso-occlusive complications, including acute myocardial infarction, often occur in patients with malignant tumors. There is increasing suspicion that chemotherapeutic agents such as 5-fluorouracil (5-FU)[149,167,168] may be the sole precipitating factor of this complication in a small but significant percentage of cases.

The incidence and severity of these complications, and the link to 5-FU itself has been difficult to discern because this agent is often administered in conjunction with other antineoplastic agents, and often to patients who are very ill from manifestations of their malignancy. In a recent review of 135 cases of suspected 5-FU cardiotoxicity angina and electrocardiographic changes occurred in the majority of patients and congestive heart failure occurred transiently in 33 patients.[168] The patients who developed heart failure responded well to therapy. The overall incidence of these events, and their effect on quality and duration of survival

of cancer patients remains unclear since the denominator from which these 135 cases were drawn is not known.

Cyclophosphamide

As noted in Table 57–7, cardiomyopathies have been reported secondary to high doses of intravenous cyclophosphamide.[146,168-170] In contrast to doxorubicin, the cardiotoxicity of cyclophosphamide is acute and not due to cumulative doses. It causes reductions in ECG voltage and systolic function and an increase in myocardial mass, presumably secondary to edema. Cyclophosphamide may also cause acute pericarditis. A prior history of heart failure and a pretreatment ejection fraction less than 50 per cent correlate with clinical cardiotoxicity. Although mortality is appreciable, survivors exhibit no residual cardiac abnormalities.[171]

Ifosfamide, an active compound related to cyclophosphamide, may also cause cardiac side effects in the form of supraventricular arrhythmias and ST-T wave changes.[172] When administered in high doses, between 10 and 18 mg/m^2, arrhythmias and congestive heart failure are common. Of 52 consecutive patients treated at the NIH with this agent at these doses, 9 developed heart failure between 6 and 23 days after drug administration.[173] Eight required admission to an intensive care unit. One patient died of cardiogenic shock, and one had pulseless ventricular tachycardia requiring emergent cardioversion and survived. Of the eight patients who survived their heart failure, all recovered cardiac function in 1 to 2 weeks, and three patients who are long-term survivors had return of normal cardiac function.

Other Antineoplastic Agents

Ischemic coronary complications have also been reported after treatment with cisplatinum,[146,173] bleomycin,[174] and vinca alkaloids,[175] such as vincristine, vinblastine, and VP-16-213 (etoposide). Acute endothelial injury, vasospasm and/or autonomic dysfunction, hypomagnesemia, autoimmune response, increases in platelet aggregability, and a synergistic effect of irradiation to the heart are all possible mechanisms. *Amsacrine* (AMSA) has been associated with acute cardiac arrhythmias and cardiomyopathy. Although AMSA-related cardiac events are frequent, they are less common than those due to doxorubicin. Manifestations of toxicity include ECG abnormalities, sudden death, and congestive heart failure. Hypokalemia appears to be a risk factor for the development of severe arrhythmias with this agent.[176-178]

Bone marrow transplantation, either allogeneic or autologous, involves the combination of large doses of whole-body irradiation therapy with high-dose chemotherapy. Cardiac complications are frequent during these transplant procedures and may be an important factor in limiting the success rate.[179] Fatal cardiomyopathies, pericarditis, and significant arrhythmias are not infrequent. High-dose cyclophosphamide and cytosine arabinoside are commonly associated with cardiotoxicity. In addition, the effect of whole-heart irradiation in conjunction with anthracycline drugs and cyclophosphamide appears to be additive.

The glycoproteins of the interferon and interleukin family are used with increasing frequency in treating many refractory cancers. Interferon alpha is effective against hairy cell leukemia, chronic myelogenous leukemia, and condyloma acuminatum and also is approved for use in treating Kaposi's sarcoma. In high doses, interferon can cause a severe congestive cardiomyopathy with severe myocardial dysfunction, usually reversible with discontinuation of the agents.[179-182]

BIOLOGIC RESPONSE MODIFIERS. Biologic response modifiers such as interleukin-2, now FDA approved for the treatment of renal cancer, and the investigational agent interleukin-1 have become part of the oncologist's armamentarium. These agents have potent effects on the immune system, but also have significant toxicity. Both cause fever and myalgias. More importantly, both cause capillary leak syndromes that can result in tissue edema, vascular hypovolemia and hypotension, noncardiogenic pulmonary edema, myocardial infarction, and renal failure.[183-185] These effects are largely dose dependent but can, even at low doses, result in death. Aggressive fluid and pressor support is often required during periods of administration of these agents.

HEMATOLOGICAL ABNORMALITIES RELATED TO CARDIAC DRUGS

Blood dyscrasias are frequent complications of drugs used to treat cardiac disorders. The development of unexplained anemia, leukopenia, or thrombocytopenia in a patient receiving a diuretic, antihypertensive, or antiarrhythmic agent should immediately raise the suspicion that a drug used in the treatment of cardiac disease might be responsible.

Many different types of blood dyscrasias occur secondary to drug ingestion. The anemias may be of the aplastic, hemolytic, megaloblastic, or sideroblastic type; other disorders may include granulocytopenia and agranulocytosis, thrombocytopenia, thrombocytosis, defects of platelet function, and a variety of miscellaneous disorders (Table 57–11). Underlying mechanisms include suppression of one or more of the three cellular elements in the bone marrow as well as a variety of immune phenomena with increased peripheral destruction of the formal elements. The drug effect may be dose related or idiosyncratic.

APLASTIC ANEMIA. Many chemical agents are capable of suppressing marrow function and producing hypoplasia or aplasia. Chloramphenicol, benzene, cytostatic agents used in the treatment of malignant disease, and phenylbutazone are the drugs most commonly implicated. Less frequently involved, and perhaps less well documented, are antibiotics such as sulfonamides, hypoglycemic agents, and insecticides. Among drugs used to treat cardiovascular disease, the antiarrhythmic agent phenytoin (see p. 608), the diuretic agent acetazolamide, and the angiotensin-converting enzyme inhibitor captopril[186] (see p. 855) have been reported, on rare occasion, to lead to such reactions. The onset of aplastic anemia is usually insidious, and the symptoms are directly related to the degree of pancytopenia. If the causative agent is immediately discontinued upon detection of the blood dyscrasia, the latter can often be reversed.

MEGALOBLASTIC ANEMIA. A pancytopenia characterized by macrocytic red cells due to impairment of DNA synthesis may be caused by vitamin B_{12} or folate deficiency or by purine and pyrimidine inhibitors. Most commonly, drugs cause megaloblastic anemia by impairing the absorption of folic acid or acting as folate antagonists. Phenytoin, oral contraceptives, and a variety of other drugs can impair folate absorption by interfering with the liver conjugases needed to break down the polyglutamate structure of naturally occurring folates to the monoglutamate form appropriate for absorption by the gastrointestinal tract. Triamterene, a potassium-sparing diuretic (see p. 477), is a pteridine analog that exhibits antifolate activity, similar to aminopterin, in vitro. Its propensity to produce a megaloblastic anemia appears to be dose related.

IMMUNOHEMOLYTIC ANEMIAS. There are four different causes for the development of a positive direct Coombs' or antiglobulin test, two of which involve cardiac medications: the first mechanism, which is uncommon, involves some drugs that bind to plasma protein and thereby become antigenic, including quinidine and the sulfonamides. The resultant antigen-antibody complex may deposit on the red cell surface and cause agglutinability by anticomplement sera. Hemolysis may be severe, but rapid improvement follows withdrawal of the drug.

The second type of reaction that results in a positive Coombs' test involves the antihypertensive drug alpha-methyldopa[187] (see p. 852). The mechanism of antibody formation is unknown, but presumably antibody induced by alpha-methyldopa has an affinity for the Rh locus of the red cell, similar to that of IgG antibodies in idiopathic

TABLE 57–11 BLOOD DYSCRASIAS ASSOCIATED WITH CARDIAC MEDICATIONS

	ANEMIA			NEUTROPENIA	THROMBOCYTOPENIA	OTHER
	Aplastic	Megaloblastic	Hemolytic			
Antiarrhythmics						
Digitoxin	–	–	–	–	+	L
Phenytoin	+	+	–	+	+	L, P
Procainamide	–	–	–	+(A)	–	–
Propranolol	–	–	–	+	–	–
Quinidine	–	–	+	+	+	–
Tocainide	+	–	–	+(A)	–	–
Moricizine	–	–	–	–	+	–
Propafenone	–	–	–	+(A)	–	–
Anticoagulants						
Heparin	+*	–	–	–	+	–
Phenindione	–	–	–	+	–	–
Antihypertensives						
Captopril	+	–	–	+	+	–
Glutethimide	+*	–	–	–	–	P
Hydralazine	–	–	–	–	+	L
Methyldopa	–	–	+	+	+	P
Reserpine	–	–	–	–	+	–
Diuretics						
Acetazolamide	+	–	–	+	+	–
Chlorothiazide	–	–	–	–	+	–
Chlorthalidone	–	–	–	+	+	–
Diazoxide	–	–	–	–	+	–
Ethacrynic acid	–	–	–	+	–	–
Hydrochlorothiazide	–	–	–	+	–	–
Mercurials	–	–	–	+	+	–
Spironolactone	–	–	–	+	+	–
Triamterene	–	+	–	–	–	–
Coronary Dilators						
Amyl nitrite	–	–	–	–	–	M
Nitroglycerin	–	–	–	–	–	M
Other						
Amrinone	–	–	–	–	+	–

* Pure red cell aplasia.
L = lupus-like syndrome; P = porphyria; A = agranulocytosis; M = methemoglobinemia.

immunohemolytic anemia. The frequency of positive results on Coombs' test varies from 11 per cent for patients who are receiving 0.75 gm per day for over 3 months to 40 per cent for those receiving 2 gm per day for the same time. Fortunately, the affinity of the alpha-methyldopa antibody for red cells is low, and fewer than 1 per cent of patients whose antiglobulin test is positive will manifest significant hemolytic anemia. Nonetheless, alpha-methyldopa surpasses all other drugs in causing immunohemolytic anemia. On withdrawal of the drug, hemolysis improves within 1 or 2 weeks, with full recovery in 1 month, although the positive Coombs' test may persist for 6 to 24 months. A positive Coombs' test without hemolysis is not an indication to discontinue alpha-methyldopa if its administration is otherwise indicated in the treatment of hypertension.

The other two mechanisms of drug-related positive antiglobulin reactions do not involve cardiovascular drugs. The third is represented by penicillin, in which the drug binds to the red cell membranes, creating a cell-drug complex and antigenic stimulation of an IgG antibody. The fourth mechanism involves cephalothin, which is bound to the red cell membrane; normal serum proteins adhere nonspecifically to red cell membranes.

GRANULOCYTOPENIA AND AGRANULOCYTOSIS. A reduction in circulating neutrophils is the most toxic hematological effect of drugs. It may be secondary to depression of the marrow, or it may be an immune mechanism causing peripheral destruction. When there is immune suppression, examination of the marrow reveals active myeloid precursors, whereas the absence of myeloid elements suggests suppression of synthesis. The marrow-depressive effect is dose related. Anticoagulants such as phenindione, antiarrhythmics such as procainamide and tocainide,[188,189] antihypertensives such as captopril, and diuretics such as the thiazides have all been reported to produce granulocytopenia. Procainamide and its relative tocainide are the most dangerous and most frequently implicated cardiac drugs in granulocytopenia.[190] Presenting symptoms may include a sore throat, ulcerations of mucous membranes, fever, malaise, fatigue, and weakness. Discontinuation of the drug may be followed by a rebound in the white blood cell count and occasionally a leukemoid picture. Because laboratory tests are not conclusive for white cell antibodies, an accurate definition of the immune mechanism responsible for white cell destruction remains unclear.

DRUG-INDUCED THROMBOCYTOPENIA. Many of the drugs used to treat cardiovascular disorders may cause thrombocytopenia, either by a direct effect on the bone marrow or by inducing formation of drug-specific antibody.[191] For example, the thiazide diuretics (p. 849) directly suppress megakaryocyte production. Thiazide-induced thrombocytopenia is usually mild, with the platelet count rarely falling below 50,000/μl. This condition is unique, since it persists for 6 to 8 weeks after drug withdrawal. Thrombocytopenia caused by amrinone, a positive inotropic agent with vasodilator properties (see p. 484), is less well studied but is clearly related to the total dose of drug administered and to peripheral destruction of platelets.[192] Other common agents like alcohol and some estrogen preparations may cause thrombocytopenia by a direct depressant effect on the bone marrow.

Shortened platelet survival secondary to antibody or complement binding to platelets can cause severe thrombocytopenia and life-threatening hemorrhage. The onset is abrupt and is not related to the dose of medication or the duration of its use. In most cases of immunological thrombocytopenia, the offending agent induces a specific antibody. The resulting drug-antibody complex then binds to the platelet, thereby shortening its survival. Quinidine, one of the first cardiac drugs to produce this response, has been well studied as a cause of thrombocytopenia. The defect can be transferred to a normal individual by administering serum from a patient with quinidine-induced thrombocytopenia, followed by a quinidine challenge to the normal subject. A similar defect can be caused by antibodies to quinine, including the small quantities present in tonic drinks. Acetaminophen (a common analgesic given to cardiac patients), acetazolamide, digitoxin, phenytoin, ethacrynic acid, alpha-methyldopa, and spironolactone have all been implicated in various cases of suspected drug-induced thrombocytopenia, although the mechanism has not always been well defined.

Although in vitro laboratory tests for drug-dependent platelet antibody are available, the results do not always correlate with clinical events. The best proof of drug-induced thrombocytopenia is prompt recovery of the platelet count after drug withdrawal followed by a second episode of thrombocytopenia upon readministration of the suspected drug. (Because of this potential hazard, the drug challenge is not advised.) If serious hemorrhage persists after the drug is withdrawn, treatment with 1 mg/kg prednisone or its equivalent may be necessary. Corticosteroids may hasten the return of a normal platelet count and may also protect capillaries and small vessels even without altering the platelet count. Platelet transfusions are not usually helpful but can be tried in desperate situations in which hemorrhage is life threatening. They are most useful if thrombocytopenia persists well after the drug-antibody complex has been cleared. In this situation, a gratifying elevation in platelet count sometimes occurs.

HEPARIN-INDUCED THROMBOCYTOPENIA (see also p. 1594). Treatment with this drug is one of the most important causes of thrombocytopenia in cardiac patients. The incidence of thrombocytopenia in patients receiving heparin has been reported from 0 to 30 per cent.[193] A review of pooled data from the literature estimates the incidence of heparin-induced thrombocytopenia at 1.1 per cent for porcine heparin and 2.9 per cent for beef heparin.[194]

The heparin-induced thrombocytopenia (HIT) syndromes have been divided into two types, Type I HIT, and Type II HIT on the basis of both severity of disease, and pathophysiology.[195-197] Type I HIT is a mild disease, with platelet counts often between 100,000 and 150,000/mm³. This syndrome is likely due to direct heparin-induced platelet aggregation. Thromboembolic phenomena are usually not seen.[198] No treatment is required and the thrombocytopenia will usually resolve even if heparin is continued. Heparin is usually stopped, however, because of the inability to distinguish, early on, this from type II HIT.

Type II HIT is more severe than type I HIT, with greater degrees of thrombocytopenia, and frequent thromboembolic complications from platelet thrombi. This has clearly been shown to be an autoimmune disease, with production of IgG that binds to platelets and causes both clearance of platelets by the reticuloendothelial system, and platelet activation leading to platelet aggregation and microthrombotic complications.[199] In cases of type II HIT, heparin must be stopped, and oral anticoagulants or thrombolytic agents must be substituted depending on the clinical needs.

OTHER HEMATOLOGICAL ABNORMALITIES CAUSED BY CARDIAC DRUGS. Amyl nitrite, sodium nitrite, and nitroglycerin can oxidize hemoglobin to methemoglobin, which cannot effectively carry oxygen. The patient with methemoglobinemia appears cyanotic but has a normal arterial PO_2, and oxygen therapy will not improve the pallor. Although symptomatic methemoglobinemia may occur in adults, most cases are seen in children who accidentally ingest medications prescribed for adults. Occasionally, adults with mild congenital methemoglobinemia will become markedly symptomatic when exposed to small doses of these same medications. With the increasing use of intravenous nitroglycerin, this complication may become more frequent.[194] If venous blood is chocolate brown and this color persists after the blood is shaken in air, the diagnosis of methemoglobinemia is almost certain. The diagnosis is confirmed by the addition of a few drops of 10 per cent potassium cyanide, which results in the rapid production of the bright red cyanmethemoglobin. Symptoms are nonspecific and consist of dyspnea, headache, fatigue, and dizziness. They are usually self-limited if the responsible drugs are discontinued, since normal red cells can enzymatically reduce the methemoglobin. In severe cases or in patients with enzyme defects, methylene blue may be administered to stimulate reduction of the methemoglobin.

Other medications may interfere with oxygen delivery to tissues. For example, sodium nitroprusside used to treat hypertensive emergencies and to reduce afterload in the management of heart failure may cause fatigue, nausea, abnormal behavior, and muscle spasm as the agent reacts with oxyhemoglobin, producing cyanmethemoglobin and free cyanide ions.[195]

Hydralazine (p. 1052), procainamide (p. 594), and rarely phenytoin (p. 1051) can cause a lupus erythematosus-like syndrome, with urticaria, erythema multiforme, photosensitivity, delirium, and immune-mediated blood cell destruction.[196] Although patients with drug-induced lupus have positive antinuclear antibody tests and many of the clinical manifestations of the systemic form, renal function is not usually impaired, and all these manifestations usually remit within several months if the drugs are discontinued. The syndrome is of particular importance in cardiac patients, since the onset of chest pain, pleurisy, or pericardial effusion in the patient with heart disease could lead to an erroneous diagnosis unless drug-induced lupus is suspected.

REFERENCES

ANEMIA AND CARDIOVASCULAR DISORDERS

1. Handin, R. I., Lux, S. E., and Stossel, T. P.: Blood: Principles and Practice of Hematology. Philadelphia, J. B. Lippincott, 1995.
2. Eckstein, R. W.: Development of interarterial coronary anastomoses by chronic anemia. Disappearance following correction of anemia. Circ. Res. 3:306, 1955.
3. Florenzano, F., Diaz, G., Regonesi, C., and Escobar, E.: Left ventricular function in chronic anemia: Evidence of noncatecholamine positive inotropic factor in the serum. Am. J. Cardiol. 54:638, 1984.
4. Varat, M. A., Adolph, R. J., and Fowler, N. O.: Cardiovascular effects of anemia. Am. Heart J. 83:415, 1972.
5. Asimacopoulos, P. J., Groves, M. D., Fischer, D. K., et al.: Pernicious anemia manifesting as angina pectoris. South. Med. J. 87:671, 1994.
6. Baer, R. W., Vlahakes, G. J., Uhlig, P. N., and Hoffman, I. E.: Maximum myocardial oxygen transport during anemia and polycythemia in dogs. Am. J. Physiol. 252:H1086, 1987.
7. Torrance, J. D., Jacobs, P., Restrepo, A., et al.: Intraerythrocyte adaptation to anemia. N. Engl. J. Med. 283:165, 1970.
8. Oski, F. A., Marshall, B. D., Cohen, P. J., et al.: Exercise with anemia. The role of the left or right shifted oxygen-hemoglobin equilibrium curve. Ann. Intern. Med. 74:44, 1971.
9. Lenfant, C., Torrance, J., English, E., et al.: Effect of altitude on the oxygen binding by hemoglobin and on organic phosphate levels. J. Clin. Invest. 47:2652, 1968.

10. Oski, F. A., Gottlieb, A. J., Delivoria-Papadopoulos, M., and Miller, W. W.: Red-cell 2,3-diphosphoglycerate levels in subjects with chronic hypoxemia. N. Engl. J. Med. 280:1165, 1969.
11. Harris, T. N., Friedman, S., Tuncali, M. T., and Hallidie-Smith, K. A.: Comparison of innocent murmur of childhood with cardiac murmurs in high output states. Pediatrics 33:341, 1964.
12. Bunn, H. F.: Disorders of hemoglobin. In Wilson, J., and Braunwald, E., et al. (eds.): Harrison's Principles of Internal Medicine, 12th ed. New York, McGraw-Hill, 1991, pp. 1543–1552.
13. Buchanan, G. R.: Sickle cell disease: Recent advances. Curr. Probl. Pediatr. 23:219, 1993.
14. Powars, D. R.: Sickle cell anemia and major organ failure. Hemoglobin 14:573, 1990.
15. Simmons, B. E., Santhanam, V., Castaner, A., et al.: Sickle cell heart disease. Two dimensional echo and doppler ultrasonographic findings in the hearts of adult patients with sickle cell anemia. Arch. Intern. Med. 148:1526, 1988.
16. Gaffney, J. W., Bierman, F. Z., Donnelly, C. M., et al.: Cardiovascular adaptation to transfusion/chelation therapy of homozygote sickle cell anemia. Am. J. Cardiol. 62:121, 1988.
17. Estrade, G., Pointrineau, D., Bernasconi, F., et al.: Left ventricular function and sickle-cell anemia. Echocardiographic Study. Arch. Mal. Coeur 82:1975, 1989.
18. Gerry, J. L., Bulkley, B. H., and Hutchins, G. M.: Clinicopathologic analysis of cardiac dysfunction in 52 patients with sickle cell anemia. Am. J. Cardiol. 42:211, 1978.
19. McCormick, W. F.: Massive nonatherosclerotic myocardial infarction in sickle cell anemia. Am. J. Forensic Med. Pathol. 9:151, 1988.
20. Francis, R. B., Jr.: Platelets, coagulation and fibrinolysis in sickle cell disease: Their possible role in vascular occlusion. Blood Coagul. Fibrinolysis 2:341, 1991.
21. Balfour, I. C., Covitz, W., Davis, H., et al.: Cardiac size and function in children with sickle cell anemia. Am. Heart J. 108:345, 1984.
22. Lippman, S. M., Niemann, J. T., Thigpen, T., et al.: Abnormal septal Q waves in sickle cell disease. Prevalence and causative factors. Chest 88:543, 1985.
23. Maisel, A., Friedman, H., Flint, J., et al.: Continuous electrocardiographic monitoring in patients with sickle cell anemia during pain crisis. Clin. Cardiol. 6:339, 1983.
24. Covitz, W., Eubig, C., Balfour, I. C., et al.: Exercise-induced cardiac dysfunction in sickle cell anemia. Radionuclide study. Am. J. Cardiol. 51:570, 1983.
25. Manno, B. V., Burka, E. R., Hakki, A., et al.: Biventricular function in sickle cell anemia: Radionuclide angiographic and thallium-201 scintigraphic evaluation. Am. J. Cardiol. 52:584, 1983.
26. Willens, H. J., Lawrence, C., Frishman, W. H., and Strom, J. A.: A noninvasive comparison of left ventricular performance in sickle cell anemia and chronic aortic regurgitation. Clin. Cardiol. 6:542, 1983.
27. Lippman, S. M., Ginzton, L. E., Thigpen, T., et al.: Mitral valve prolapse in sickle cell disease: Presumptive evidence for a linked connective tissue disorder. Arch. Intern. Med. 145:435, 1985.
28. Forget, B. G., and Pearson, H. A.: Hemoglobin synthesis and the thalassemias. In Handin, R. I., Lux, S. E., and Stossel, T. P. (eds.): Blood: Principles and Practice of Hematology. Philadelphia, J. B. Lippincott, 1995.
29. Sanakul, D., Thakerngpol, K., and Pacharee, P.: Cardiac pathology in 76 thalessemic patients. Birth Defects 23:177, 1988.
30. Wacker, P., Halperin, D. S., Balmer-Ruedin, D., et al.: Regression of cardiac insufficiency after ambulatory intravenous deferoxamine in thalassemia major. Chest 103:1276, 1993.
31. Aldouri, M. A., Wonke, B., Hoffbrand, A. V., et al.: High incidence of cardiomyopathy in betathalassaemia patients receiving regular transfusion and iron chelation: Reversal by intensified chelation. Acta Haematol. 84:113, 1990.
32. Ehlers, L. H., Levin, A. R. Klein, A. A., et al.: The cardiac manifestations of thalassemia major: Natural history, noninvasive cardiac diagnostic studies, and results of cardiac catheterization. In Engle, M. A. (ed.): Pediatric Cardiovascular Disease. Cardiovascular Clinics II. Philadelphia, F. A. Davis Co., 1981, pp. 171–186.
33. Spirito, P., Lupi, G., Melevendi, C., and Vecchio, C.: Restrictive diastolic abnormalities identified by Doppler echocardiography in patients with thalassemia major. Circulation 82:88, 1990.
34. Sapoznikov, D., Lewis, N., Rachmilewitz, E. A., et al.: Left ventricular filling and emptying patterns in anemia due to beta-thalassemia. A computer-assisted echocardiographic study. Cardiology 69:276, 1982.
35. Lau, K. C., Li, A.M.C., Hui, P. W., and Yeung, C. Y.: Left ventricular function in β thalassemia major. Arch. Dis. Child 64:1046, 1989.
36. Valdes-Cruz, L. M., Reinecke, C., Rutkowski, M., et al.: Preclinical abnormal segmental cardiac manifestations of thalassemia major in children on transfusion-chelation therapy: Echographic alterations of left ventricular posterior wall contractions and relaxation patterns. Am. Heart J. 103:505, 1982.
37. Borow, K. M., Propper, R., Bierman, F. Z., et al.: The left ventricular end-systolic pressure-dimensions relation in patients with thalassemia major. A new noninvasive method for assessing contractile state. Circulation 66:980, 1982.
38. Canale, C., Terrachini, V., Vallebena, A., et al.: Thalassemic cardiomyopathy: Echocardiographic difference between major and intermediate thalassemia at rest and during isometric effort: Yearly follow-up. Clin. Cardiol. 11:563, 1988.
39. Dameshek, W., and Roth, S. I.: Case Records of the Massachusetts General Hospital—Weekly Clinicopathological exercises. Case 52. N. Engl. J. Med. 271:148, 1964.
40. Westring, D. W.: Aortic valve disease and hemolytic anemia. Ann. Intern. Med. 65:203, 1966.
41. Sonaer, D. H., Cheng, T. O., and Aaron, B. L.: Hemolytic anemia and acute mitral regurgitation caused by a torn cusp of a porcine mitral prosthetic valve 7 years after its implantation. Am. Heart J. 113:404, 1987.
42. Enzenauer, R. J., Berenberg, J. L., and Cassell, P. F., Jr.: Microangiopathic hemolytic anemia as the initial manifestation of porcine valve failure. South. Med. J. 83:912, 1990.
43. Mok, P., Lieberman, E. H., Lilly, L. S., et al.: Severe hemolytic anemia following mitral valve repair. Am. Heart J. 117:1171, 1989.
44. Sears, A. D., and Crosby, W. H.: Intravascular hemolysis due to intracardiac prosthetic devices. Diurnal variations related to activity. Am. J. Med. 39:341, 1965.
45. DiSosa, V. J., Collins, J. J., Jr., and Cohn, C. H.: Hematological complications with the St. Jude valve and reduced-dose coumadin. Ann. Thorac. Surg. 48:280, 1989.

HEMOCHROMATOSIS AND HEMOSIDEROSIS

46. Schafer, A. I.: Iron overload. In Fairbanks, V. F. (ed.): Current Hematology. New York, John Wiley and Sons, 1981, pp. 191–218.
47. Rosenqvist, M., and Hultcrantz, R.: Prevalence of haemochromatosis among men with clinically significant bradyarrhythmias. Eur. Heart J. 10:473, 1989.
48. James, T. N.: Pathology of the cardiac conduction system in hemochromatosis. N. Engl. J. Med. 271:92, 1964.
49. Wasserman, A. J., Richardson, D. W., Baird, C. L., and Wyso, E. M.: Cardiac hemochromatosis simulating constrictive pericarditis. Am. J. Med. 32:316, 1962.
50. Westra, W. H., Hruban, R. H., Baughman, K. L., et al.: Progressive hemochromatotic cardiomyopathy despite reversal of iron deposition after liver transplantation. Am. J. Clin. Pathol. 99:39, 1993.
51. Rivers, J., Garrahy, P., Robinson, W., and Murphy, A.: Reversible cardiac dysfunction in hemochromatosis. Am. Heart J. 113:216, 1987.
52. Wolfe, L., Olivieri, N., Sallan, D., et al.: Prevention of cardiac disease by subcutaneous deferoxamine in patients with thalassemia major. N. Engl. J. Med 312:1600, 1985.
53. Maurer, H. S., Lloyd-Still, J. D., Ingrisano, C., et al.: A prospective evaluation of iron chelation therapy in children with severe beta-thalassemia. A six year study. Am. J. Dis. Child. 142:287, 1988.
54. Freeman, A. P., Giles, R. W., Berdoukas, V. A., et al.: Sustained normalization of cardiac function by chelation therapy in thalassemia major. Clin. Lab. Haematol. 11:299, 1989.
55. Strack, M. F., and Hannah, E. E.: Venesection responsive cardiomyopathy in a patient with idiopathic haemochromatosis. N. Z. Med. J. 105:360, 1992.
56. Lerner, N., Blei, F., Bierman, F., et al.: Chelation therapy and cardiac status in older patients with thalassemia major. Am. J. Pediatr. Hematol. Oncol. 12:56, 1990.
57. Russo, G.: Iron chelating therapy in thalassemia: Current problems. Haematologica 75(Suppl. 5):84, 1990.
58. Jensen, P. D., Jensen, F. T., Christensen, T., and Ellegaard, J.: Non-invasive assessment of tissue iron overload in the liver by magnetic resonance imaging. Br. J. Haematol. 87:171, 1994.
59. Kaltwasser, J. P., Gottschalk, R., Schalk, K. P., and Hartl, W.: Non-invasive quantitation of liver iron-overload by magnetic resonance imaging. Br. J. Haematol. 74:360, 1990.
60. Wasman, S., Eustace, S., and Hartnell, G. G.: Myocardial involvement in primary hemochromatosis demonstrated by magnetic resonance imaging. Am. Heart J. 128:1047, 1994.
61. Olson, L. J., Edwards, W. D., Holmes, D. R., et al.: Endomyocardial biopsy in hemochromatosis: Clinicopathologic correlates in six cases. J. Am. Coll. Cardiol. 13:116, 1989.
62. Candell-Riera, J., Permanger-Miralda, G., and Soler-Soler, J.: Cardiac hemochromatosis. Primary Cardiol. 12(October):123, 1986.
63. Edwards, C. Q., Griffen, L. M., Goldgar, D., et al.: Prevalence of hemochromatosis among 11,065 presumably healthy blood donors. N. Engl. J. Med. 318:1355, 1988.
64. Venegoni, P., and Cyprus, G.: Polycythemia and the heart. Tex. Heart Inst. J. 21:198, 1994.
65. Fruchtman, S. M., and Berk, P. D.: Polycythemia vera and agnogenic myeloid metaplasia. In Handin, R. I., Lux, S. E., and Stossel, T. P.: Blood: Principles and Practice of Hematology. Philadelphia, J. B. Lippincott, 1995.

DISORDERS ASSOCIATED WITH ABNORMAL BLOOD FLOW DISTRIBUTION OR INCREASED VISCOSITY

66. Thomas, D. J., Marshall, J., Russell, R. W., et al.: Effect of hematocrit on cerebral blood flow in man. Lancet 2:941, 1977.
66a. Al-Saif, S., Bhat, R. P., Hijazi, A.: Left ventricular and aortic valve thrombosis caused by polycythemia rubra vera successfully treated with streptokinase. Am. Heart J. 131:397, 1996.
67. Kaplan, M. E., Mack, K., Goldberg, J. D., et al.: Long-term management of polycythemia vera with hydroxyurea: A progress report. Semin. Hematol. 23:167, 1986.
68. Messinezy, M., Aubry, S., O'Connell, G., et al.: Oxygen desaturation in apparent and relative polycythaemia. BMJ 302:216, 1991.

69. Rosenthal, A., Button, L. N., and Nathan, D. G.: Blood volume changes in cyanotic congenital heart disease. Am. J. Cardiol. *29:*162, 1971.

70. Rosenthal, A., Nathan, D. G., Marty, A. T., et al.: Acute hemodynamic effects of red cell production in polycythemia of cyanotic congenital heart disease. Circulation *42:*197, 1970.

71. Erslev, A. J., and Caro, J.: Secondary polycythemia: A boon or a burden? Blood Cells *10:*177, 1984.

72. Grant, P., Patel, P., and Singh, S.: Acute myocardial infarction secondary to polycythemia in a case of cyanotic congenital heart disease. Int. J. Cardiol. *9:*108, 1985.

73. Wallis, P. J., Skehan, J. D., Newland, A. C., et al.: Effects of erythropheresis on pulmomary hemodynamics and oxygen transport in patients with secondary polycythemia and cor pulmonale. Clin. Sci. *70:*91, 1986.

74. York, E. L., Junes, R. L., Menon, D., and Sproule, B. J.: Effects of secondary polycythemia on cerebral flood flow in chronic obstructive pulmonary disease. Am. Rev. Respir. Dis. *121:*813, 1980.

75. Rosenthal, A., Mentzer, W. C., and Eisenstein, E. B.: The role of red blood cell organic phosphates in adaptation to congenital heart disease. Pediatrics *47:*537, 1971.

76. Charache, S., Weatherall, D. J., and Clegg, J. B.: Polycythemia associated with hemoglobinopathy. J. Clin. Invest. *45:*813, 1966.

77. Weinreb, N. J., and Shih, C. F.: Spurious polycythemia. Semin. Hematol. *12:*397, 1975.

78. Schwarcz, T. H., Hogan, L. A., Endean, E. D., et al.: Thromboembolic complications of polycythemia: polycythemia vera versus smokers' polycythemia. J. Vasc. Surg. *17:*518, 1993.

79. Saffitz, J. E., Phillips, E. R., Temesy-Armos, P. N., and Roberts, W. C.: Thrombocytosis and fatal coronary heart disease. Am. J. Cardiol. *52:*651, 1983.

80. Koh, K. K., Cho, S. K., Kim, S. S., et al.: Coronary vasospasm, multiple coronary thrombosis, unstable angina, and essential thrombocytosis. Int. J. Cardiol. *41:*168, 1993.

81. Mitus, A. J., Barbui, R., Shulman, L. N., et al.: Hemostatic complications in young patients with essential thrombocythemia. Am. J. Med. *88:*371, 1990.

82. Rosenthal, D. S., and Murphy, S.: Thrombocytosis. *In* Handin, R. I., Lux, S. E., Stossel, T. P. (eds.): Blood: Principles and Practice of Hematology. Philadelphia, J. B. Lippincott, 1995.

83. McAllister, H. A., and Fenoglio, J. J.: Tumors of the cardiovascular system. *In* Atlas of Tumor Pathology. 2nd ed. Washington, D.C.: Armed Forces Institute of Pathology; 1978.

84. MacGee, W.: Metastatic and invasive tumors involving the heart in a geriatric population: A necropsy study. Virchows Arch. A. Pathol. Anat. Histopathol. *419:*183, 1991.

85. Abraham, J. M.: Neoplasms metastatic to the heart: Review of 3314 consecutive autopsies. Am. J. Cardiovasc. Pathol. *3:*195, 1990.

86. Lam, K. Y., Dickens, P., and Chan, A.C.L.: Tumors of the heart: A 20-year experience with a review of 12,485 consecutive autopsies. Arch. Pathol. Lab. Med. *117:*1027, 1993.

87. English, J. C., Allard, M. F., Babul, S., and McManus, B. M.: Metastatic tumors of the heart, *In* Goldhaber, S. Z.: Cardiopulmonary Diseases and Cardiac Tumors, Atlas of Heart Diseases. Vol. 3. Philadelphia, Current Medicine, 1995.

CARDIAC MANIFESTATIONS OF NEOPLASTIC DISEASE

88. Israeli, A., Rein, A.J.J.T., Kriski, M., et al.: Right ventricular outflow tract obstruction due to extracardiac tumors: A report of three cases diagnosed and followed up by echocardiographic studies. *149:*2105, 1989.

89. Kapoor, A. S.: Clinical manifestations of neoplasia of the heart. *In* Kapoor, A. S. (ed.): Cancer and the Heart. New York, Springer-Verlag, 1986, pp. 21–25.

90. Roberts, W. C., Glancy, D. L., and DeVita, V. T.: Heart in malignant lymphoma. A study of 196 autopsy cases. Am. J. Cardiol. *22:*85, 1968.

91. Petersen, C. D., Robinson, Q. A., and Kurnich, J. E.: Involvement of the heart and pericardium in the malignant lymphomas. Am. J. Med. Sci. *272:*161, 1976.

92. Waller, B. F., Gottdiener, J. S., Virmni, R., and Roberts, W. C.: Structure-function correlations in cardiovascular and pulmonary diseases. The charcoal heart. Chest *77:*671, 1980.

93. Almange, C., Lebrestec, T., Louvet, M., et al.: Bloc auriculo-ventriculaire complet par metastase cardiaque: A propos dune observation. Sem. Hop. Paris *54:*1419, 1978.

94. Seibert, K. A., Rettenmier, C. W., Waller, B. F., et al.: Osteogenic sarcoma metastatic to the heart. Am. J. Med. *73:*136, 1982.

95. Kralstein, J., and Frishman, W.: Malignant pericardial disease: Diagnosis and treatment. Am. Heart J. *113:*785, 1987.

96. Kirn, D., Mauch, P., and Shaffer, K., et al.: Large-cell and immunoblastic lymphoma of the mediastinum: Prognostic features and treatment outcome in 57 patients. J. Clin. Oncol. *11:*1336, 1993.

97. Singh, S., Wann, S., Schuchard, G. H., et al.: Right ventricular and right atrial collapse in patients with cardiac tamponade: A combined echocardiographic and hemodynamic study. Circulation *70:*966, 1984.

98. Isner, J. M., Carter, B. L., Bankoff, M. S., et al.: Computed tomography in the diagnosis of pericardial heart disease. Ann. Intern. Med. *97:*473, 1982.

99. Buck, M., Ingle, J. N., Giuliani, E. R., et al.: Pericardial effusion in women with breast cancer. Cancer *60:*263, 1987.

100. Posner, M. R., Cohen, G. I., and Skarin, A. T.: Pericardial disease in patients with cancer. The differentiation of malignant from idiopathic and radiation-induced pericarditis. Am. J. Med. *71:*407, 1981.

101. Hancock, E. W.: Neoplastic pericardial disease. Cardiol. Clin. *8:*673, 1990.

102. Press, O. W., and Livingston, R.: Management of malignant pericardial effusion and tamponade. JAMA *256:*2301, 1987.

102a. Laham, R. J., Cohen, D. J., Kuntz, R. E.: Pericardial effusion in patients with cancer: Outcome with contemporary management strategies. Heart *75:*67, 1996.

103. Snow, N., and Lucas, A.: Subxiphoid pericardiotomy: A safe, accurate, diagnostic and therapeutic approach to pericardial and intrapericardial disease. Am. Surg. *49:*249, 1983.

104. Osuch, J. R., Khandekar, J. D., and Fry, W. A.: Emergency subxiphoid pericardial decompression for malignant pericardial effusion. Am. Surg. *51:*298, 1985.

105. Park, J. S., Tentschler, R., and Wilbur, D.: Surgical management of pericardial effusion in patients with malignancies. Cancer *67:*76, 1991.

106. Mack, M. J., Landreneau, R. J., Hazelrigg, S. R., and Acuff, T. E.: Video thoracoscopic management of benign and malignant pericardial effusions. Chest *103:*390s, 1993.

107. Gouldesbrough, D. R., and Carder, P. J.: Rapidly progressive cardiac failure due to lymphomatous infiltration of the myocardium. Postgrad. Med. J. *65:*668, 1989.

108. Lestuzzi, C., Biasi, S., Nicolosi, G. L., et al.: Secondary neoplastic infiltration of the myocardium diagnosed by two-dimensional echocardiography in seven cases with anatomic confirmation. J. Am. Coll. Cardiol. *9:*439, 1987.

109. Perez, C. A., Presant, C. A., and Amburg, A. L.: Management of superior vena caval syndrome. Semin. Oncol. *5:*123, 1978.

110. Lopez, M. I., and Vincent, R. J.: Malignant superior vena cava syndrome. *In* Kapoor, A. S. (ed.): Cancer and the Heart. New York, Springer-Verlag, 1986, p. 206.

111. Wahlin, A., Olofsson, B., Eriksson, A., and Backman, C.: Myeloma-associated cardiac amyloidosis. Acta Med. Scand. *215:*189, 1984.

112. Alpert, M. A.: Cardiac amyloidosis. *In* Kapoor, A. S. (ed.): Cancer and the Heart. New York, Springer-Verlag, 1986, p. 162.

113. Ursell, P. C., and Fenogolio, J. J.: Spectrum of cardiac disease diagnosed by endomyocardial biopsy. Pathol. Annu. *19:*197, 1984.

114. Koiwaya, Y., Nakamura, M., and Yamamoto, K.: Progressive ECG alterations in metastatic cardiac mural tumor. Am. Heart J. *105:*339, 1983.

115. Hartman, R. B., Clark, P. I., and Schulman, P.: Pronounced and prolonged ST segment elevation. A pathognomonic sign of tumor invasion of the heart. Arch. Intern. Med. *142:*1917, 1982.

116. Cole, T. O., Attah, E. B., and Onyemelukwe, G. C.: Burkitt's lymphoma presenting with heart block. Br. Heart J. *37:*94, 1975.

117. Ballentyne, F., VanderArk, C. R., and Holick, M.: Carotid sinus syncope and cervical lymphoma. Wis. Med. J. *74:*91, 1975.

118. Inagaki, R., Rodriguez, V., and Brody, G. P.: Causes of death in cancer patients. Cancer *33:*568, 1974.

119. Kopelson, G., and Herwig, K. J.: The etiologies of coronary artery disease in cancer patients. Int. J. Radiat. Oncol. Biol. Phys. *4:*895, 1978.

120. Stewart, J. R., and Fajardo, L. F.: Cancer and coronary artery disease. Int. J. Radiat. Oncol. Biol. Phys. *4:*915, 1978.

121. Ackerman, D. M., Hyma, B. A., and Edwards, W. D.: Malignant neoplastic emboli to the coronary arteries. Report of two cases and review of the literature. Hum. Pathol. *18:*955, 1987.

122. Kountz, D. S.: Isolated cardiac metastasis from cervical carcinoma: Presentation as acute anteroseptal myocardial infarction. South. Med. J. *86:*228, 1993.

123. Parker, B. M.: Valvular involvement in cancer. *In* Kapoor, A. S. (ed.): Cancer and the Heart. New York, Springer-Verlag, 1986, p. 64.

124. Blanchard, D. G., Ross, R. S., and Dittrich, H. C.: Nonbacterial thrombotic endocarditis. Assessment by transesophageal echocardiography. Chest *102:*954, 1992.

125. Chino, F., Kodama, A., Otake, M., and Dock, D. S.: Nonbacterial thrombotic endocarditis in a Japanese autopsy sample. A review of eighty cases. Am. Heart J. *90:*190, 1975.

126. Gonzalez Quintela, A., Candela, M. J., Vidal, C., et al.: Nonbacterial thrombotic endocarditis in cancer patients. Acta Cardiologica *XLVI:*1, 1991.

127. Lehto, V. P., Stenman, S., and Somer, T.: Immunohistological studies on valvular vegetations in nonbacterial thrombotic endocarditis. Arch. Pathol. Microbiol. Scand. *90:*207, 1982.

128. Fauci, A. S., Harley, J. B., Roberts, W. C., et al.: The idiopathic hypereosinophilic syndrome: Clinical, pathophysiologic, and therapeutic considerations. Ann. Intern. Med. *97:*78, 1982.

129. Parrillo, J. E., Borer, J. S., Henry, W. L., et al.: The cardiovascular manifestations of the hypereosinophilic syndrome: Prospective study of 26 patients, with review of the literature. Am. J. Med. *67:*572, 1979.

CARDIAC EFFECTS OF RADIATION THERAPY AND CHEMOTHERAPY

130. Geist, B. J., Lauk, S., Bornhausen, M., and Trott, K.-R.: Physiologic consequences of local heart irradiation in rats. Int. J. Radiat. Oncol. Biol. Phys. *18:*1107, 1990.

131. Om, A., Ellahham, S., and Vetrovec, G. W.: Radiation-induced coronary artery disease. Am. Heart J. *124:*1598, 1992.

132. Carlson, R. G., Mayfield, W. R., Normann, S., and Alexander, J. A.: Radiation-associated valvular disease. Chest *99:*538, 1991.

133. Arsenian, M. A.: Cardiovascular sequelae of therapeutic thoracic radiation. Prog. Cardiovasc. Dis. *33:*299, 1991.

134. Schultz-Hector, S.: Radiation-induced heart disease: Review of experi-

mental data on dose response and pathogenesis. Int. J. Radiat. Biol. 61:149, 1992.

135. Lipshultz, S. E., and Sallan, S. E.: Cardiovascular abnormalities in long-term survivors of childhood malignancy. J. Clin. Oncol. 11:1199, 1993.

136. Hancock, S. L., Donaldson, S. S., and Hoppe, R. T.: Cardiac disease following treatment of Hodgkin's disease in children and adolescents. J. Clin. Oncol. 11:1208, 1993.

137. Kreuser, E.-D., Voller, H., Behles, C., et al.: Evaluation of late cardiotoxicity with pulsed Doppler echocardiography in patients treated for Hodgkin's disease. Br. J. Haematol. 84:614, 1993.

138. McReynolds, R. A., Gold, G. L., and Roberts, W. C.: Coronary heart disease after mediastinal irradiation for Hodgkin's disease. Am. J. Med. 60:39, 1976.

139. Brosius, F. C., Waller, B. F., and Roberts, W. C.: Radiation heart disease: Analysis of 16 young (aged 15 to 33 years) necropsy patients who received over 3500 rads to the heart. Am. J. Med. 7:519, 1981.

140. Joesuu, H.: Acute myocardial infarction after heart irradiation in young patients with Hodgkin's disease. Chest 95:388, 1989.

141. Green, D., Gingell, R. L., Pearce, J., et al.: The effect of mediastinal irradiation on cardiac function of patients treated during childhood and adolescence for heart disease. J. Clin. Oncol. 5:239, 1987.

142. O'Donnell, L. O., O'Neill, T., Toner, M., et al.: Myocardial hypertrophy, fibrosis and infarction following exposure of the heart to radiation for Hodgkin's disease. Postgrad. Med. J. 62:1055, 1986.

143. Boivin, J.-F., Hutchison, G. B., Lubin, J. H., and Mauch, P.: Coronary artery disease mortality in patients treated for Hodgkin's disease. Cancer 69:1241, 1992.

144. Jakacki, R. I., Goldwein, J. W., Larsen, R. L., et al.: Cardiac dysfunction following spinal irradiation during childhood. J. Clin. Oncol. 11:1033, 1993.

145. Perry, M. C.: Effects of chemotherapy on the heart. In Kapoor, A. S. (ed.): Cancer and the Heart. New York, Springer-Verlag, 1986, p. 223.

146. Icli, F., Karaoguz, H., Dincol, D., et al.: Severe vascular toxicity associated with cisplatin-based chemotherapy. Cancer 72:587, 1993.

147. Ayash, L. J., Wright, J. E., Tretyakov, O., et al.: Cyclophosphamide pharmacokinetics: Correlation with cardiac toxicity and tumor response. J. Clin. Oncol. 10:995, 1992.

148. Watts, R. G.: Severe and fatal anthracycline cardiotoxicity at cumulative doses below 400 mg/m²: Evidence for enhanced toxicity with multi-agent chemotherapy. Am. J. Hematol. 36:217, 1991.

149. de Forni, M., and Armand, J. P.: Cardiotoxicity of chemotherapy. Curr. Opin. Oncol. 6:340, 1994.

149a. Frishman, W. H., Sung, H. M., Yee, H. C. M., et al.: Cardiovascular toxicity with cancer chemotherapy. Curr. Prob. Cardiol. 21:225, 1996.

150. Doroshow, J. H.: Doxorubicin-induced cardiac toxicity. N. Engl. J. Med. 324:843, 1991.

151. Doroshow, J. H., Locker, G. Y., and Myers, C. E.: Enzymatic defenses of the mouse heart against reactive oxygen metabolites: Alterations produced by doxorubicin. J. Clin. Invest. 65:128, 1980.

152. Bristow, M. R., Mason, J. W., Billingham, M. E., and Daniels, J. R.: Doxorubicin cardiomyopathy. Evaluation by phonocardiography, endomyocardial biopsy, and cardiac catheterization. Ann. Intern. Med. 88:168, 1978.

153. Unverferth, B. J., Magorien, R. D., Balcerzak, S. P., et al.: Early changes in human myocardial nuclei after doxorubicin. Cancer 52:215, 1983.

154. Gottdiener, J. S., Mathisen, D. J., Barer, J. S., et al.: Doxorubicin cardiotoxicity: Assessment of late left ventricular dysfunction by radionuclide cineangiography. Ann. Intern. Med. 94:430, 1981.

155. Estorch, M., Carrio, I., Martinez-Duncker, D., et al.: Myocyte cell damage after administration of doxorubicin or mitoxantrone in breast cancer patients assessed by indium 111 antimyosin monoclonal antibody studies. J. Clin. Oncol. 7:1264, 1993.

156. Schwartz, R. G., McKenzie, W. B., Alexander, J., et al.: Congestive heart failure and left ventricular dysfunction complicating doxorubicin therapy. Seven-year experience using serial radionuclide angiocardiography. Am. J. Med. 82:1109, 1987.

157. Von Hoff, D. D., Layard, M. W., Basa, P., et al.: Risk factors for doxorubicin-induced congestive heart failure. Ann. Intern. Med. 91:710, 1979.

158. Moreb, J. S., and Oblon, D. J.: Outcome of clinical congestive heart failure induced by anthracycline chemotherapy. Cancer 70:22637, 1992.

159. Lipshultz, S. E., Colan, S. D., Gelber, R. D., et al.: Late cardiac effects of doxorubicin therapy for acute lymphoblastic leukemia in childhood. N. Engl. J. Med. 324:808, 1991.

160. Ali, M. K., Ewer, M. S., Gibbs, H. R., et al.: Late doxorubicin-associated cardiotoxicity in children: The possible role of intercurrent viral infection. Cancer 74:182, 1994.

160a. Lipshultz, S. E, Lipsitz, S. R., Mone, S. M., et al.: Female sex and higher drug dose as risk factors for late cardiotoxic effects of doxorubicin therapy for childhood cancer. N. Engl. J. Med. 332:1738, 1995.

161. Anders, R. J., Shanes, J. G., and Zeller, F. P.: Lower incidence of doxorubicin cardiomyopathy by one-a-week low-dose administration. Am. Heart J. 111:755, 1986.

162. Shapira, J., Gotfried, M., Lishner, M., et al.: Reduced cardiotoxicity of doxorubicin by a 6-hour infusion regimen. A prospective randomized evaluation. Cancer 65:870, 1990.

163. Valdirieso, M., Burgess, M. A., Awer, M. S., et al.: Increased therapeutic index of weekly doxorubicin in the therapy of non small cell lung cancer: A prospective randomized study. J. Clin. Oncol. 2:207, 1984.

164. Torti, F. M., Bristow, M. R., Howes, A. E., et al.: Reduced cardiotoxicity of doxorubicin delivered on a weekly schedule: Assessment by endomyocardial biopsy. Ann. Intern. Med. 99:745, 1983.

165. Legla, S. S., Benjamin, R. S., MacKay, B., et al.: Reduction of doxorubi-

cin cardiotoxicity by prolonged continuous intravenous infusion. Ann. Intern. Med. 96:133, 1982.

166. Speyer, J. L., Green, M. D., Dubin, N., et al.: Prospective evaluation of cardiotoxicity during a six-hour doxorubicin infusion regimen in women with adenocarcinoma of the breast. Am. J. Med. 78:555, 1985.

167. Ensley, J. F., Patel, B., Kloner, R., et al.: The clinical syndrome of 5-fluorouracil cardiotoxicity. Invest. New Drugs 7:101, 1989.

168. Robben, N. C., Pippas, A. W., and Moore, J. O.: The syndrome of 5-fluorouracil cardiotoxicity: An elusive cardiopathy. Cancer 71:493, 1993.

169. Goldberg, M. A., Antin, J. H., Guinan, E. C., and Rappeport, J. M.: Cyclophosphamide cardiotoxicity. An analysis of dosing as a risk factor. Blood 68:1114, 1986.

170. Braverman, A. C., Antin, J. H., Plappert, M. T., et al.: Cyclophosphamide cardiotoxicity: A prospective evaluation of new dosing regimens. (Submitted for publication.)

171. Gottdiener, J. S., Applebaum, F. R., Ferrans, V. J., et al.: Cardiotoxicity associated with high dose cyclophosphamide therapy. Arch. Intern. Med. 141:758, 1981.

172. Kandylis, K., Vassilomanolakis, M., Tsoussis, S., and Efremidis, A. P.: *Ifosfamide* cardiotoxicity in humans. Cancer Chemother. Pharmacol. 24:395, 1989.

173. Quezado, Z. M. N., Wilson, W. H., Cunnion, R. E., et al.: High-dose ifosfamide is associated with severe, reversible cardiac dysfunction. Ann. Intern. Med. 118:31, 1993.

174. Burkhardt, A., Haltje, W. J., and Gebbens, J. O.: Vascular lesions following perfusion with bleumycin: Electron-microscopic observations. Virchows Arch. Pathol. Anat. 372:227, 1976.

175. Aisner, J., VanEcho, D. A., Whitacre, M., and Wiernik, P. H.: A phase-I trial of continuous infusion VP-16-213 (etoposide). Cancer Chemother. Pharmacol. 7:157, 1982.

176. Steinherz, L. J., Steinherz, P. G., Mangiacasale, D., et al.: Cardiac abnormalities after AMSA administration. Cancer Treat. Rep. 66:483, 1982.

177. Lindpainter, K., Lindpainter, L. S., Wentworth, M., and Burns, C. P.: Acute myocardial necrosis during administration of amsacrine. Cancer 57:1284, 1986.

178. Weiss, R. B., Grillo-Lopez, A. J., Marsoni, S., et al.: Amsacrine-associated cardiotoxicity: An analysis of 82 cases. J. Clin. Oncol. 4:919, 928, 1986.

179. Cazin, V., Gorin, C., Laport, J. P., et al.: Cardiac complications after bone marrow transplantation. A report on a series of 63 consecutive transplantations. Cancer 57:2061, 1986.

180. Cohen, M. C., Huberman, M. S., and Nesto, R. W.: Recombinant alpha-2 interferon-related cardiomyopathy. Am. J. Med. 85:549, 1988.

181. Deyton, L. R., Walker, R. E., Kovacs, J. A., et al.: Reversible cardiac dysfunction associated with interferon alpha therapy in AIDS patients with Kaposi's sarcoma. N. Engl. J. Med. 321:1246, 1989.

182. Schechter, D., and Nagler, A.: Recombinant interleukin-2 and recombinant interferon-alpha immunotherapy cardiovascular toxocity (editorial). Am. Heart J. 123:1736, 1992.

183. Rosenberg, S. A., Lotze, M. T., Muul, L. M., et al.: A progress report on the treatment of 157 patients with advanced cancer using lympho-kineactivated hilar cells and interleukin-2 or high dose interleukin-2 alone. N. Engl. J. Med. 316:889, 1987.

184. Osanto, S., Cluitman, F. H. M., Franks, C. R., et al.: Myocardial injury after interleukin-2 therapy. Lancet 2:48, 1988.

185. Nora, R., Abrams, J. S., Tait, N. S., et al.: Myocardial toxic effects during recombinant interleukin-2 therapy. J. Natl. Cancer Inst. 81:59, 1989.

HEMATOLOGICAL ABNORMALITIES RELATED TO CARDIAC DRUGS

186. Gavras, F., Graff, L. G., Rose, B. D., et al.: Fatal pancytopenia associated with the use of captopril. Ann. Intern. Med. 94:58, 1981.

187. Lundh, B., and Hasselgren, K. H.: Hematological side effects from antihypertensive drugs. Acta Med. Scand. (Suppl.)628:73, 1979.

188. Soff, G. A., and Kadin, M. E.: Tocainide-induced reversible agranulocytosis and anemia. Arch. Intern. Med. 147:598, 1987.

189. Morrill, G. B., and Gibson, S. M.: Tocainide-induced aplastic anemia (letter). Drug Intell. Clin. Pharm. 23:90, 1989.

190. Volosin, K., Greenberg, R. M., and Grenspon, A. J.: Tocainide-associated agranulocytosis. Am. Heart J. 109:1392, 1985.

191. Hackett, T., Kelton, J. G., and Powers, P.: Drug-induced platelet destruction. Semin. Thromb. Hemostas. 8:116, 1982.

192. Ansell, J., McCue, J., Tiarks, C., et al.: Amrinone-induced thrombocytopenia. Blood 58(Suppl. 1):187a, 1981.

193. Bell, W. R., and Royall, R. M.: Heparin-associated thrombocytopenia: A comparison of three heparin preparations. N. Engl. J. Med. 303:902, 1980.

194. Schmitt, P. B., and Adelman, B.: Heparin-associated thrombocytopenia: A critical review and a pooled analysis. Am. J. Med. Sci. 305:208, 1993.

195. Green, D.: Heparin-induced thrombocytopenia. Med. J. Aust. 144:37, 1986.

196. Chong, B. H.: Heparin-induced thrombocytopenia. Aust. N. Zeal. J. Med. 22:145, 1992.

197. Chong, B. H.: Heparin-induced thrombocytopenia. Br. J. Haematol. 89:431, 1995.

198. Salzman, E. W., Rosenberg, R. D., Smith, M. H., et al.: Effect of heparin and heparin fractions on platelet aggregation. J. Clin. Invest. 65:64, 1980.

199. Warkentin, T. E., and Kelton, J. G.: Heparin-induced thrombocytopenia. Ann. Rev. Med. 40:31, 1989.

Chapter 58
Hemostasis, Thrombosis, Fibrinolysis, and Cardiovascular Disease

VALENTIN FUSTER, MARC VERSTRAETE

Over the last 2 decades, much evidence has indicated that thrombosis plays a crucial role in many cardiovascular events. It also is becoming apparent that variations in plasma levels of coagulation and fibrinolytic components may determine the individual's response to vascular changes, including fissuring of atherosclerotic plaques. Such cardiovascular patients could benefit from antithrombotic drugs, while thrombolytic agents are indicated in others with acute vascular occlusions. In the first section of this chapter, relevant aspects of the normal coagulation and fibrinolytic systems and their main defects associated with cardiovascular disorders are discussed; this section includes a discussion of registered antithrombotic and thrombolytic drugs. In the second section, the recent antithrombotic and thrombolytic clinical trials are reviewed and the specific approaches to antithrombotic and thrombolytic therapy are discussed.

HEMOSTASIS, FIBRINOLYSIS, ANTITHROMBOTICS, AND THROMBOLYTICS

HEMOSTASIS

The Vessel Wall With Focus on the Endothelium

The vast majority of blood vessels are capillaries that have no smooth muscle cells, and hemostasis depends on direct sealing. The first event in hemostasis (Fig. 58–1) in response to vascular injury of arterioles and venules is contraction of smooth muscle cells, soon followed by local perivascular and intravascular activation of platelets and coagulation components.

One of the unsolved mysteries of hemostasis and thrombosis is why platelets do not, or hardly ever, adhere to normal (unstimulated) endothelial cells in vivo. One possible answer is that both platelets and endothelium have a negative charge and thus would be mutually repulsive. The negative electric charge of endothelial cells is due to a pronounced glycocalyx, consisting of proteoglycans, of which heparan sulfate (a heparin-like substance that binds

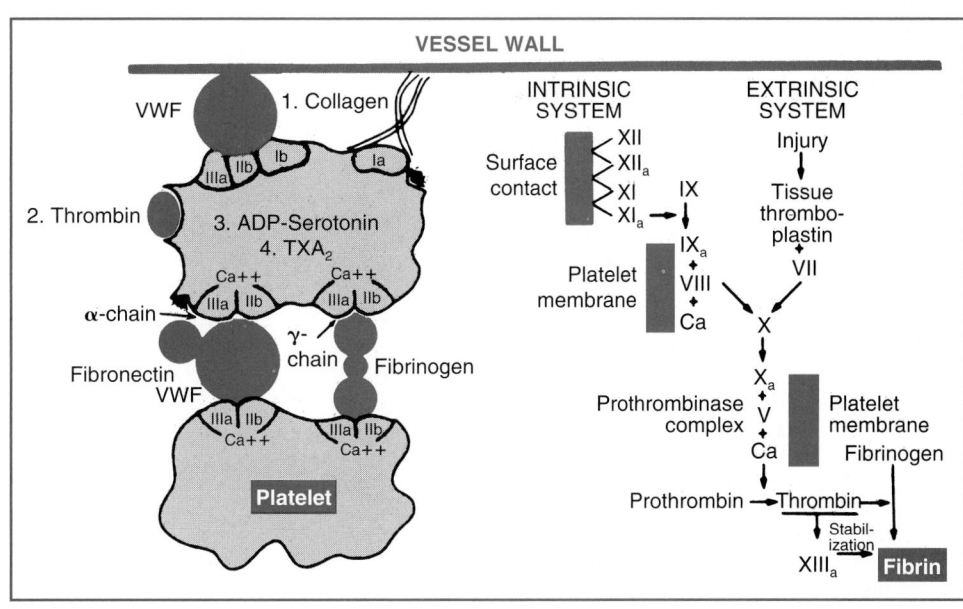

FIGURE 58–1. Interactions among platelet membrane receptors (glycoproteins Ia, Ib, and IIb/IIIa), adhesive macromolecules, and the disrupted vessel wall *(left)* and a flow chart of the intrinsic and extrinsic systems of the coagulation cascade *(right)*. On the left, Arabic numerals indicate the pathways of platelet activation that are dependent on collagen (1), thrombin (2), ADP and serotonin (3), and thromboxane A$_2$ (TXA$_2$) (4); there are also some reports that suggest the binding of von Willebrand factor (VWF) (polymeric protein) to collagen or heparin. Note the interaction at the right between clotting factors (XII, XIIa, XI, XIa, IX, IXa, VII, VIII, X, Xa, V, and XIIIa) and the platelet membrane. (From Fuster, V., et al.: N. Engl. J. Med. *326:*315, 1992. Copyright Massachusetts Medical Society.)

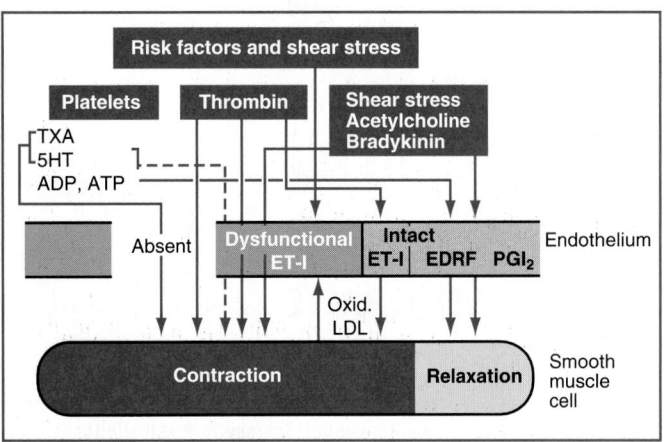

FIGURE 58–2. The effects of shear stress, acetylcholine, and brady-kinin lead intact endothelium to generate and release endothelium-derived relaxing factor (EDRF) and prostacyclin (PGI$_2$), which in turn causes relaxation of the smooth muscle. The effect of thrombin leads the intact endothelium to generate endothelin-1 (ET-1), which causes vasoconstriction of the smooth muscle. After minor endothelial injury or damage (i.e., induced by risk factors), dysfunctional endothelium may not generate relaxing substances; in these circumstances, all of the above-mentioned stimulants exert a vasoconstrictive effect, either through the enhancement of endothelium-derived contracting factors or directly. As a result of severe endothelial injury or damage in areas of deendothelialization (Absent), thrombin and the platelet products thromboxane A$_2$ and serotonin (5-HT) induce direct vasoconstriction of the smooth muscle. (Modified from Fuster, V., et al.: The pathogenesis of coronary artery disease and the acute coronary syndrome. N. Engl. J. Med. *326*:313, 1992. Copyright Massachusetts Medical Society.)

antithrombin III) is the most important. Stimulated or injured endothelial cells lose their negative surface charge or anionic property.

Normal endothelial cells are much more than a semipermeable barrier between the blood and the vascular smooth muscle. They can be regarded as a highly active metabolic and endocrine organ that plays a major role in maintaining a proper balance between the formation of hemostatic plugs and the avoidance of intraluminal thrombi (see p. 1121). Endothelial cells inactivate vasoactive substances and have an important function on vasomotor tone.[1,2] For instance, carrier mechanisms in their cell membrane specifically transport serotonin, adenosine, and adenine nucleotides into the cell where they are metabolized. Angiotensin-converting enzyme on the outer surface of the cell inactivates bradykinin, a potent vasodilator. Perhaps a more crucial function is the synthesis of active substances that intervene in important physiological and pathological processes (Fig. 58–2).[3] Larger substances than those depicted in Figure 58–2 include fibronectin, heparan sulfate, tissue plasminogen activator, interleukin-1, and various growth factors. Smaller molecules synthesized by endothelial cells include prostacyclin (PGI$_2$), endothelium-derived relaxing factor (EDRF or nitric oxide, NO), endothelium-derived constricting factor(s) (endothelin-1), and platelet activating factor (PAF).

The production of prostacyclin by endothelium is stimulated by contact with activated platelets or leukocytes, by stretching of the arterial wall (pulsatile pressure), and by some drugs. Prostacyclin has strong antiplatelet and vasodilator properties and thus acts as the biological antagonist of thromboxane A$_2$. A direct link between impaired biosynthesis of prostacyclin in the vessel wall and thrombosis or atherosclerosis is suggested by the decreased capacity of endothelium to generate prostacyclin with age, atherosclerosis, and risk factors such as high cholesterol, heavy smoking, and diabetes. EDRF is formed from L-arginine by an oxidation pathway that requires several co-factors. EDRF relaxes smooth muscle cells through stimulation of guanylate cyclase, which in turn generates cyclic guanosine mon-

ophosphate (cyclic GMP).[3] By the same mechanism it is also a potent inhibitor of adhesion and aggregation of platelets. There is a clear synergism between prostacyclin and EDRF in preventing platelet activation. EDRF is effective only in the immediate vicinity of its site of release because hemoglobin almost immediately inactivates any EDRF that enters the bloodstream. It has been suggested that a deficiency in EDRF production contributes to the pathogenesis of atherosclerosis and to the development of complications of diabetes. Endothelin-1 is a 21-residue peptide that is slowly released from endothelial cells by various stimuli and acts as a local hormone to induce vasodilation at low concentrations and vasoconstriction at high concentrations. Cleavage of a larger propeptide (big endothelin) by a putative endopeptidase (endothelin-converting enzyme) produces the active peptide. Its possible role in the pathophysiology of cardiovascular diseases is currently under intense scrutiny. Synthesis of platelet-activating factor (PAF), a strong stimulator of platelet aggregation, may be activated by thrombin that is locally generated if a break occurs in the endothelial lining. Thrombomodulin is a transmembranous protein that serves as an endothelial receptor for free thrombin.[4] In the complex that is formed and that does not require calcium, thrombin loses its procoagulant activity and expresses its anticoagulant role by activating protein C.

Thus, apart from a metabolic function with respect to the synthesis of vasoactive substances, the primary role of endothelium is in maintaining the patency of the blood vessels and the fluidity of blood. However, endothelium also has the potential to enhance and amplify the formation of a hemostatic plug initiated by a local endothelial lesion.

Platelets

In normal conditions, platelets are quiescent and circulate freely in the blood, because they do not attach to normally functioning endothelium. Vessel injury, however, exposes subendothelial connective tissue with various elements to which platelets can adhere.[5,6] Collagen and fibronectin interact readily with platelets, particularly with their membrane glycoproteins Ia/IIa and Ic/IIa (Fig. 58–3). von Willebrand factor, which has two collagen-binding sites, is an absolute requirement for platelets in flowing blood to adhere to the vascular wall. Adhered platelets lose their discoid shape, form pseudopods, and spread out over the injured surface. Through the action of activators such as collagen and eventually thrombin and norepinephrine, the adhered platelets soon become activated, which in turn expresses other platelet receptors and releases several mediators.[7] Phospholipase C hydrolyzes platelet membrane

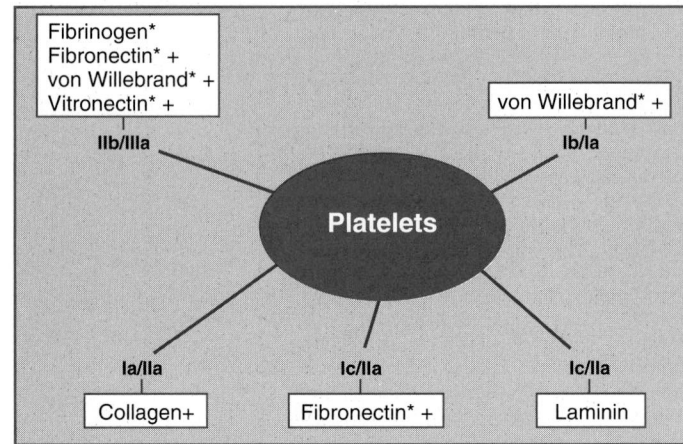

FIGURE 58–3. Stimulated platelets express on their membrane different glycoprotein receptors (integrins) that bind to ligands present in plasma (*) or in endothelial basement membranes (+). GPIa-IIa = VLA-2 or $\alpha_2\beta$ii; Ic/IIa = VLA-5 or $\alpha_5\beta$ii; IIB/IIIA = $\alpha_{11}\beta\beta_3$.

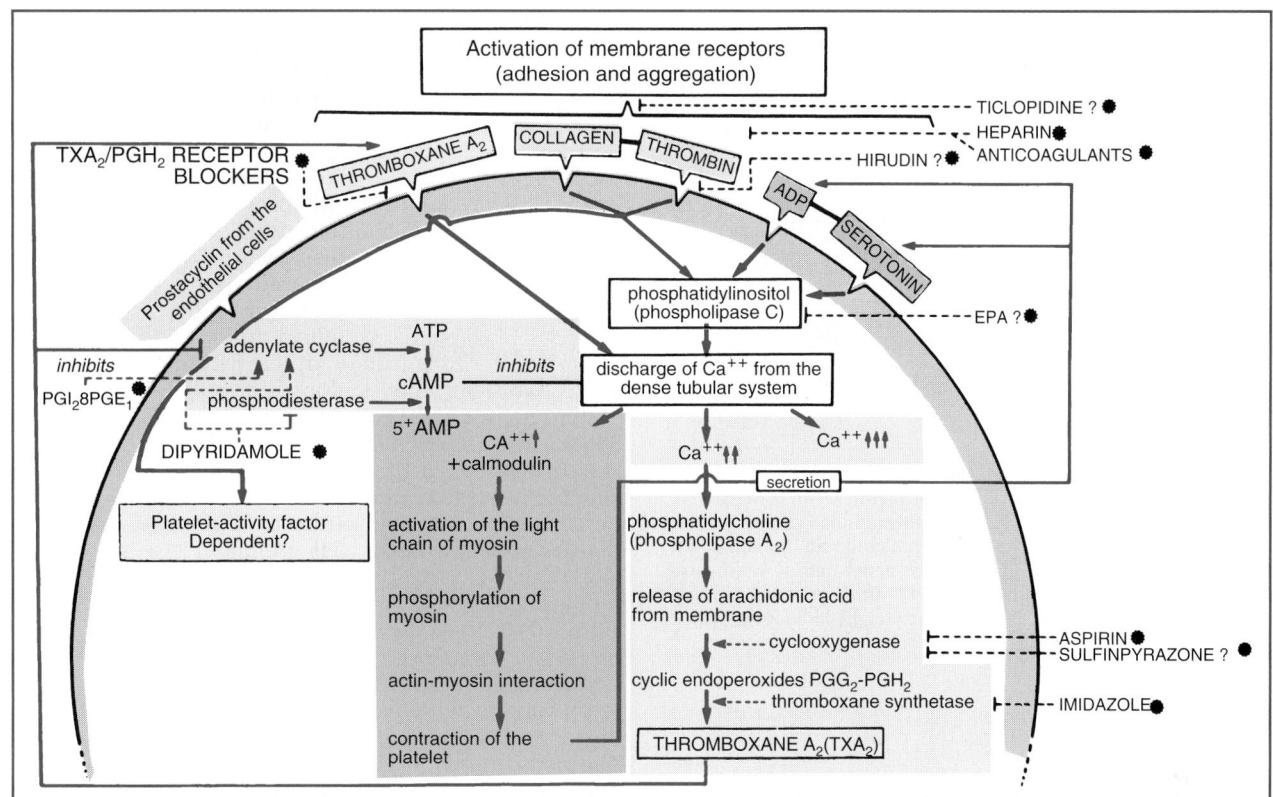

FIGURE 58–4. Mechanisms of platelet activation and presumed sites of action of various platelet inhibitor agents. Platelet agonists lead to the mobilization of calcium (Ca++), which functions as a mediator of platelet activation through metabolic pathways dependent on adenosine diphosphate (ADP), thromboxane A_2 (TXA$_2$), thrombin, and collagen. Cyclic adenosine monophosphate (cAMP) inhibits calcium mobilization from the dense tubular system. Note that thrombin and collagen may independently activate platelets by means of platelet activating factor. • = a platelet inhibitor. Dashed line = a presumed site of drug action. ATP = adenosine triphosphate; EPA = eicosapentaenoic acid; PGE$_1$ = prostaglandin E$_1$; PGH$_2$ = prostaglandin H$_2$; PGI$_2$ = prostaglandin I$_2$ or prostacyclin. (From M. Verstraete and J. Vermylen: Thrombosis. Pergamon Press, 1984, p. 11. Modified by Stein, B., et al.: Platelet inhibitor agents in cardiovascular disease: An update. Reprinted by permission from the American College of Cardiology. J. Am. Coll. Cardiol. *14*:813, 1989.)

phosphatidylinositol, which leads to release of calcium from the dense tubular system (Fig. 58–4). Calcium in turn activates a protein kinase that phosphorylates intra-platelet regulatory proteins; activation of the actin-myosin system results in platelet contraction with release of adenosine diphosphate (ADP) and serotonin from the platelet dense granules and of thromboxane A$_2$.[8,9]

These potent inducers of platelet aggregation are capable of recruiting circulating platelets, which in turn adhere and transform the initial monolayer of platelets into an aggregate. The platelet glycoproteins IIb-IIIa on the platelet membrane undergo a conformational change in the activation process, so that they can interact with plasma fibrinogen and other adhesive proteins as fibronectin and endothelial thrombospondin, which serve to link platelets together into a tighter aggregate.[10,11] In addition, phospholipase A$_2$ acts on phosphatidylcholine to release arachidonic acid from the platelet membrane (Fig. 58–4). Arachidonic acid is converted to proaggregating prostaglandin endoperoxide intermediates (prostaglandins G$_2$ and H$_2$) by cyclooxygenase. Thromboxane A$_2$ is formed by the action of thromboxane synthase on prostaglandin H$_2$; it further promotes platelet activation, thrombus growth and local vasoconstriction. On the other hand, the vascular endothelial cells synthesize prostacyclin (PGI$_2$) starting from arachidonic acid or from platelet derived prostaglandin G$_2$. Prostacyclin stimulates adenylate cyclase and leads to an increased level of cyclic adenosine monophosphate (cyclic AMP) in the platelet. Cyclic AMP, in turn, inhibits the discharge of calcium from the dense tubular system and thus prevents platelet aggregation and secretion. Phosphodiesterase enhances the breakdown of cyclic AMP.

Coagulation

Activated platelets rearrange their surface lipoproteins so that phospholipids, on which coagulation factors can concentrate, are now exposed to the bloodstream. Thus, activated platelets, which lose their electronegativity in the process, markedly accelerate the formation of thrombin. Thrombin occupies a central position in the coagulation process. It is formed as the end result of a chain of reactions that transform, in sequence, a number of coagulation factors present as precursors (zymogens) in plasma into activated factors. The reactions occur mainly on the membrane of activated platelets and other stimulated cells and on tissue factor (a membrane protein that is exposed to the blood, e.g., after trauma) on which coagulation factors bind. Because of the low concentration of these factors in plasma and because of the abundant presence of circulating inhibitors, the interaction of procoagulants and their subsequent activation would proceed only slowly in the fluid phase of blood.

The traditional coagulation scheme distinguishes an "intrinsic" from an "extrinsic" activation pathway.

THE "INTRINSIC" PATHWAY OF THE COAGULATION SYSTEM. All factors participating in the intrinsic pathway are present in the circulating blood, and the reaction sequence is initiated by contact of platelets and/or coagulation components with a subendothelial tissue. Antigen-antibody complexes and activated platelets may serve this purpose, as can fissured atherosclerotic plaques and foreign surfaces such as those in an extracorporeal circulation or renal dialysis. This initial contact phase involves the interaction of factor XII (Hageman factor), prekallikrein, and high molec-

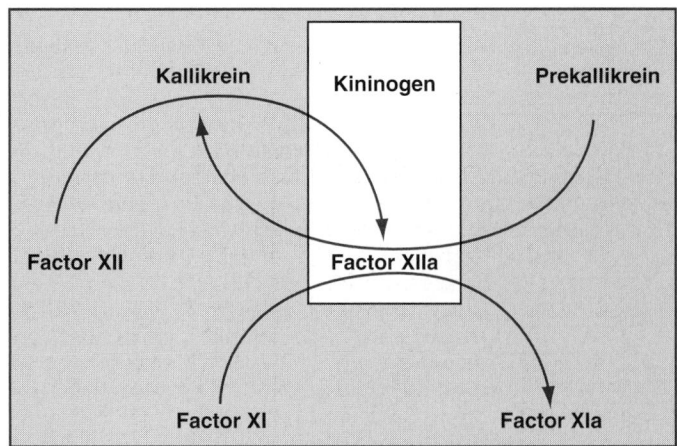

FIGURE 58–5. The contact phase of the intrinsic activation pathway. The initial event in vitro is the adsorption of factor XII to a negatively charged surface where it undergoes a conformational change to expose its active site. Factor XIIa converts prekallikrein to kallikrein. Additional factor XIIa and kallikrein are then generated by reciprocal activation. Factor XIIa also activates factor IX. Both prekallikrein and factor XI bind to a co-factor, high molecular weight kininogen, which serves to anchor them to the charged surface.

ular weight kininogen. However, the precise mechanism of the initial firing spark triggering the contact activation remains elusive.

Factor XII circulates in plasma; its heavy chain has great affinity for negatively charged surfaces such as glass and kaolin. Upon adsorption, bound factor XII now exerts traces of biological activity (Figs. 58–5 and 58–6). The actual activation of factor XII is facilitated by kallikrein. Factor XIIa converts the next factor of the coagulation cascade, factor XI, from its zymogen form to its enzymatic constellation (factor XIa).

Factor XIa bound to the surfaces by high molecular weight kininogen interacts upon activation with factor IX in a calcium-dependent two-step reaction. Activated factor IX, thrombin-modified factor VIII, negatively charged phospholipid (i.e., phospholipids of activated platelets), and calcium ions form a complex called tenase because it activates factor X (Fig. 58–6).

THE "EXTRINSIC" PATHWAY OF THE COAGULATION SYSTEM. In the "extrinsic" system, membrane-bound tissue factor starts off the chain of events by forming a complex with factor VII in the presence of calcium ions (Fig. 58–6). The tissue factor–factor VIIa complex then combines with the substrate (factor X), producing a further conformational change in factor VIIa, so that it binds still more tightly to tissue factor, precluding dissociation of factor VIIa from tissue factor.[12] The tissue factor–factor VIIa complex activates primarily factor X but also factors IX and XI, which interconnects the intrinsic and extrinsic activation pathways and plays a "prima ballerina" role in the activation of coagulation.[13] It should be noted that phospholipids of the platelet membrane, in conjunction with factor Xa, can also activate factor VII—another bridge between the intrinsic and extrinsic pathways. Thus, the earlier concepts of clearly separate intrinsic and extrinsic activation systems are becoming obsolete.

THE PATHWAY IN COMMON: THE FORMATION OF PROTHROMBINASE, THE ENZYME CONVERTING PROTHROMBIN TO THROMBIN. Factor X stands at the intersection of the so-called extrinsic and intrinsic activation pathways.[14,15] This means that factor X can be activated either by the tenase complex or by the tissue factor–factor VIIa complex. The presence of proteolytically modified factor VIII (whether by thrombin, factor Xa, or factor IXa) enhances 10,000-fold the rate of activation of factor X by factor IXa. Factor VIII is thus a helper protein (a co-factor).[16]

To be fully active, factor Xa has to form a stoichiometric 1:1 complex with factor Va; the latter molecule enhances the activation of prothrombin by factor Xa 300,000-fold. The association of factor Va with factor Xa on an anionic phospholipid is termed prothrombinase and has been reported to position the active site at a proper distance above the membrane for optimal enzymatic activity.

THE ACTION OF PROTHROMBINASE ON PROTHROMBIN. Prothrombinase initially cleaves the Arg-IIe bond in the prothrombin molecule, producing thrombin. This intermediate molecule remains membrane bound through the retained glutamic acid (Gla)-domain linkage and activates protein C but lacks procoagulant properties either on platelets or on fibrinogen. To obtain the latter property, another arginine bond (Arg-Thr) has to be cleaved, yielding alpha-thrombin.

THE PIVOTAL ROLE OF THROMBIN. Thrombin represents the culmination of the coagulation cascade; its action on fibrinogen is most dramatic because thrombus formation is a visible process. Thrombin itself is responsible for its own nonlinear generation caused by positive feedback activation, whereby thrombin enhances new formation of throm-

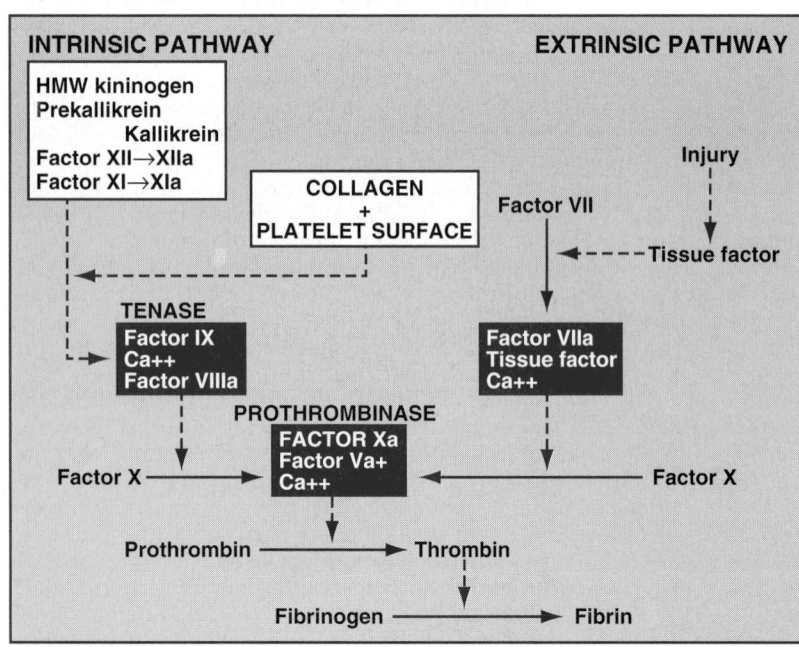

FIGURE 58–6. Clotting factor interactions. Coagulation is initiated by either an intrinsic or extrinsic pathway. In the intrinsic pathway, negatively charged surfaces initiate the contract activation and the phospholipid is furnished by platelets. In the extrinsic system, the phospholipid portion of tissue thromboplastin functions in conjunction with factor VIIa on the activation of factor X. From factor Xa on, both pathways converge upon a common path. Omitted from the diagram are inhibitors of the various steps, the augmentation of action of each pathway by activated factors, and the interaction between the intrinsic and extrinsic systems.

bin. In addition, thrombin is a pivotal molecule for numerous other functions (Fig. 58–7). The action of thrombin on platelets results in the release of platelet factor V exteriorization and in the transbilayer movement of its inner membrane surface (flip-flop reaction). Thrombin activates three of the four co-factor or helper proteins (factors V and VIII, thrombomodulin, but not tissue factor). Thrombin furthermore activates factor XIII, which increases the strength and renders the fibrin more resistant to thrombolysis; thrombin also releases prostacyclin, nitric oxide (NO, endothelial-derived relaxing factor), von Willebrand factor, and ADP from the normal endothelium, protecting the microcirculation against thrombosis. Thrombin inhibits its own production by a negative feedback mechanism via the thrombomodulin proteins C and S system.

THE CONVERSION OF FIBRINOGEN TO FIBRIN. Fibrinogen is a large paired molecule held together by disulfide bridges. Each symmetrical half-molecule consists of one set of three different polypeptide chains termed Aα, Bβ, and Gγ. Thrombin splits an arginine-glycine bond, first at the amino end of the two Aα chains and later at the amino end of each of the two Bβ chains so that each molecule releases two small aminopeptides A (FPA) and two small fibrinopeptides B (FPB) from fibrinogen and thus converts this molecule to fibrin monomers that are still soluble. The fibrinopeptide A release exposes a polymerization site in the central region of the fibrinogen molecule (E domain) that subsequently aligns with a complementary site in the outer region (D domain) of another fibrin monomer to form staggered overlapping two-stranded fibrils. Coupled monomers of fibrin, called polymers, are still soluble unless they become too large and precipitate; the resulting gel of fibrin forms the skeleton of a thrombus and traps red and white cells.

The structural stability of the fibrin network is achieved through covalent crosslinking.[17] Thrombin activates factor XIII, a transglutaminase that in the presence of calcium forms peptide bonds between side chains of suitable lysine (donors) and glutamic acid (acceptors) residues. The result of such a lysine crosslink is that the thrombus becomes firmer and more resistant to thrombolysis. It should be noted that fibrin-bound thrombin (approximately 40 per cent of the thrombin generated) retains its coagulant and platelet activating properties and is protected from inactivation by heparin-antithrombin III).[18] During thrombolysis, fibrin-bound thrombin is released and can cause rethrombosis. Hirudin, hirulog, and similar synthetic compounds that are smaller than heparin can inhibit fibrin-bound thrombin.

CONNECTIONS BETWEEN THE INTRINSIC AND EXTRINSIC PATHWAYS. The strict separation of the coagulation system into the intrinsic and extrinsic pathways of activation that merge in a common pathway from the activation of factor X is a didactic schematization that is rendered obsolete by more recent findings.[13] It is obvious that both systems are interconnected. For example, the factor VIIa–tissue factor complex can activate factors IX and XI directly; factor IXa and Xa can activate factor VII.

COAGULATION—SURFACE-CATALYZED EVENTS. The coagulation factors are present in the fluid phase of blood at very low concentrations, with the exception of fibrinogen, prothrombin, and plasminogen. Their encounter in solution is possible and their interaction slow, though this can be accelerated up to 100,000-fold after adsorption and concentration on surfaces. Modified endothelium, stimulated platelets, denuded subendothelial structures (e.g., collagen), and fissured atherosclerotic plaques and foreign surfaces (extracorporeal circulation conduits) allow attachment of passing platelets (adhesion) and adsorption of coagulation proteins. Assembly on surfaces increases the local concentration of clotting factors considerably and creates an optimal steric relationship (better alignment) for their interaction. Inhibitors of activated coagulation factors are much less effective in binding to phospholipid surfaces, and thus binding of activated coagulation factors to such a surface protects them from being inhibited.[19]

REGULATION OF THE COAGULATION PROCESS. A number of proteins circulate in the blood to inhibit the coagulation process at various stages of the cascade. Two of them appear particularly important in preventing thrombosis: antithrombin III and protein C.

Antithrombin III is an inhibitor of thrombin and of factor Xa.[20] Thrombin forms a tightly bound complex with antithrombin III; this occurs at a relatively slow rate that is enormously enhanced by heparin (see below) and also appreciably by heparan sulfate, a substance very similar to heparin that is found on the intraluminal surface of vascular endothelial cells. The inhibition of factor Xa is the result of the formation of a binary complex between antithrombin III and factor Xa.

Protein C is a proenzyme formed in the liver; vitamin K is required in its synthesis. Protein C is activated by thrombin to become a serine protease that inhibits factor Va and VIIIa (Fig. 58–8). Complex formation between thrombin and thrombomodulin, a potent co-factor present on the endothelial surface, catalyzes the activation of protein C. Protein S is another vitamin K-dependent protein that functions as a co-factor for activated protein C by facilitating its binding to membrane phospholipids.[21] In addition to being a powerful anticoagulant, activated protein C initiates fibrinolysis by releasing tissue plasminogen activator (t-PA) from the endothelium and neutralizing plasminogen activator inhibitor.

FIGURE 58–7. Thrombin is the pivotal enzyme in coagulation, responsible for positive feedback activation, rapid activation of platelets and endothelial cells, and indirectly via thrombomodulin for its own activation.

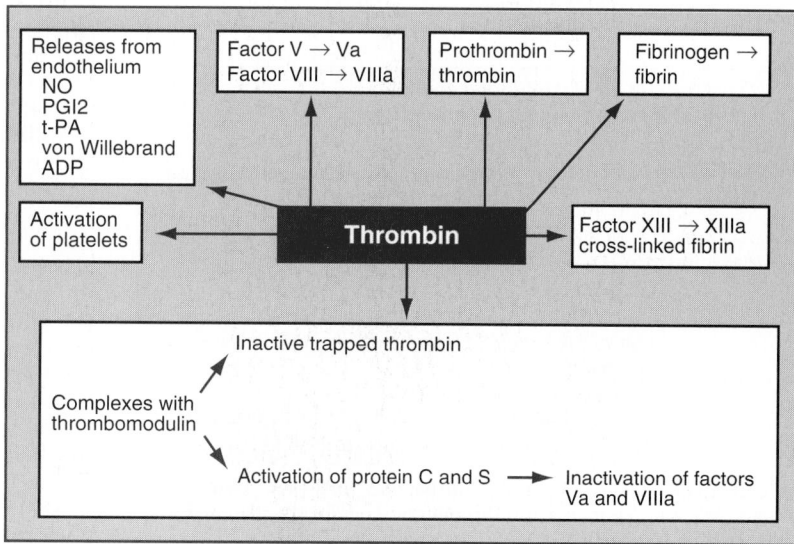

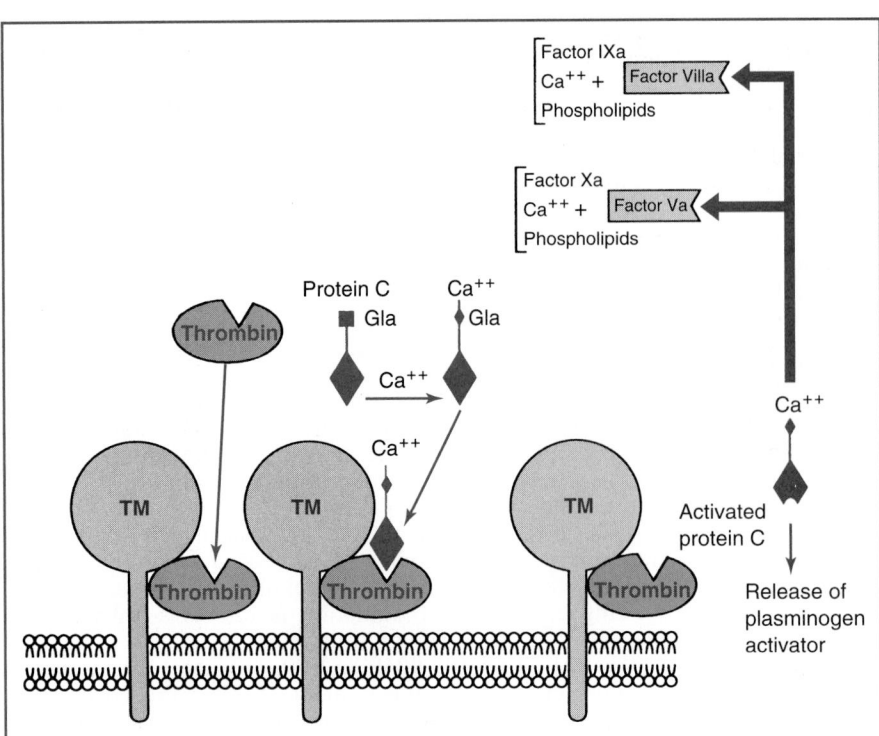

FIGURE 58–8. Thrombin forms a complex with the endothelium-bound protein thrombomodulin (TM). This complex activates circulating protein C, which inhibits factor Va and VIIIa and releases tissue-plasminogen activator from the endothelial cells. Binding of activated protein C to phospholipids is facilitated by protein S. Gla = γ-carboxyglutamic acid.

Tissue factor–factor VII complex is inactivated by the tissue factor pathway inhibitor (TFPI).[13,14,19,22] Factor VIIa cannot be neutralized effectively unless it is bound to tissue factor.[13] This is in contrast to other coagulation components, which are neutralized more effectively as free reactants than after they interact in complexes.[22]

THE FIBRINOLYTIC SYSTEM AND ITS CONTROL

Components of the Fibrinolytic System
(Fig. 58–9)

PLASMINOGEN. Plasminogen is present in human plasma at a concentration of about 2 μM, which is about twice the concentration of α_2-antiplasmin. The native molecule is a single-chain glycoprotein, organized in seven structural domains (Fig. 58–10).[23] From the NH2-terminal end, there is a "preactivation peptide" (amino acid residues 1–77), five sequential homologous kringle domains (about 90 residues each), and the proteinase domain (residues 562–791) with the catalytic site composed of His603, Asp646, and Ser741.[24–26] Plasminogen is converted to the two-chain serine proteinase plasmin by cleavage of a single Arg561-Val562 peptide bond between kringle 5 and the proteinase domain.

PLASMINOGEN ACTIVATORS. Tissue-type plasminogen activator (t-PA) is a 70 kDa serine proteinase, which consists of a single polypeptide chain in its native form. t-PA is converted by plasmin to a two-chain form by hydrolysis of the Arg275-Ile276 peptide bond. In contrast to most single-chain forms of serine proteinases, single-chain t-PA possesses significant catalytic activity. The aminoterminal region is composed of several domains with homologies to other proteins: a finger domain (residues 4-50), a growth factor domain (residues 50-87), and two kringles (residues 87–176 and 176–262) (Fig. 58–11).[27,28] The region constituted by residues 276-527 represents the serine proteinase part with the catalytic site.

Single-chain urokinase-type plasminogen activator (scu-PA) is a 54 kDa glycoprotein containing 411 amino acids. The plasma concentration of scu-PA is about 2 ng/ml. Upon proteolytic cleavage of the Lys158-Ile519 peptide bond, the molecule is converted to a two-chain derivative (tcu-PA, urokinase). The u-PA receptor is essential for localization of u-PA–mediated plasmin formation to the pericellular environment.[29,30] A low molecular weight scu-PA (32 kDa) can be generated by proteolytic cleavage of the Glu143–Leu144 peptide bond.[28]

INHIBITORS. Alpha$_2$-antiplasmin (α-plasmin inhibitor) and plasminogen activator inhibitors belong to the serine proteinase inhibitor superfamily (serpins).[31] Alpha$_2$-antiplasmin is present in plasma at a concentration of about 1 μM. It is a 67 kDa glycoprotein containing 464 amino acids and about 13 per cent carbohydrate.[32] The reactive site of the inhibitor is the Arg364-Met365 peptide bond. Alpha$_2$-antiplasmin (plasminogen-binding form) becomes partly converted in the circulating blood to a non-plasminogen-binding, less reactive form (about 30 per cent of the total), that lacks the 26 carboxyterminal residues. Two forms of alpha$_2$-antiplasmin are present in about equal amounts in purified preparations of the inhibitor.

The two most important plasminogen activator inhibitors (PAI's) are PAI-1 and PAI-2. PAI-1 is a 52 kDa single-chain glycoprotein consisting of 379 amino acids.[33,34] The reactive

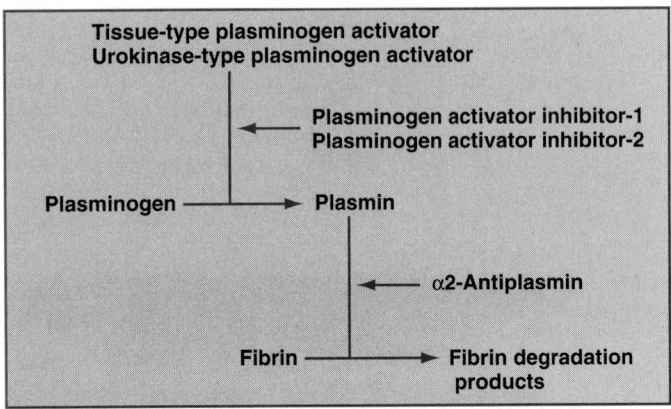

FIGURE 58–9. Overview of the fibrinolytic pathways. (From Verstraete, M., and Vermylen, J.: Thrombosis. London, Pergamon Press, 1984, p. 41.)

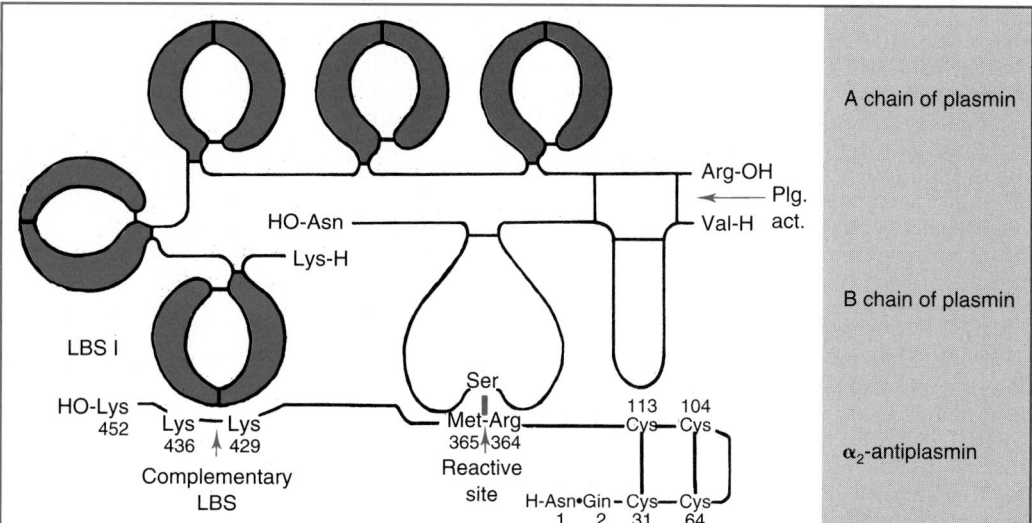

FIGURE 58-10. Structure of the plasminogen molecule and the interaction between plasmin and α_2-antiplasmin. LBS indicates lysine-binding sites. Plg.act. is where the plasminogen molecule is cleaved by activators. The heavy or A chain originates from the amino-terminal part of the molecule; the light or B chain constitutes the COOII-terminal part; the latter contains the active serine site.

site of the inhibitor is the Arg346-Met347 peptide bond. PAI-1 is stabilized by a tight binding to the cell adhesive protein vitronectin. PAI-2 exists in two different forms with comparable kinetic properties and is detected only in pregnant women.[35]

UROKINASE RECEPTOR. The specific cell surface receptor for urokinase plasminogen activator (u-PAR) is a heterogeneously glycosylated protein of 50–60 kDa synthesized as a 313 amino acid polypeptide.[36–38]

Regulation of the Fibrinolytic System

The physiologic fibrinolytic system is regulated by controlled activation and inhibition (Fig. 58–9). Activation of plasminogen by t-PA is enhanced in the presence of fibrin or at the endothelial cell surface. Inhibition of fibrinolysis may occur at the level of plasminogen activation or at the level of plasmin. Fibrinolysis is also regulated as a result of increased or decreased synthesis and/or secretion of t-PA

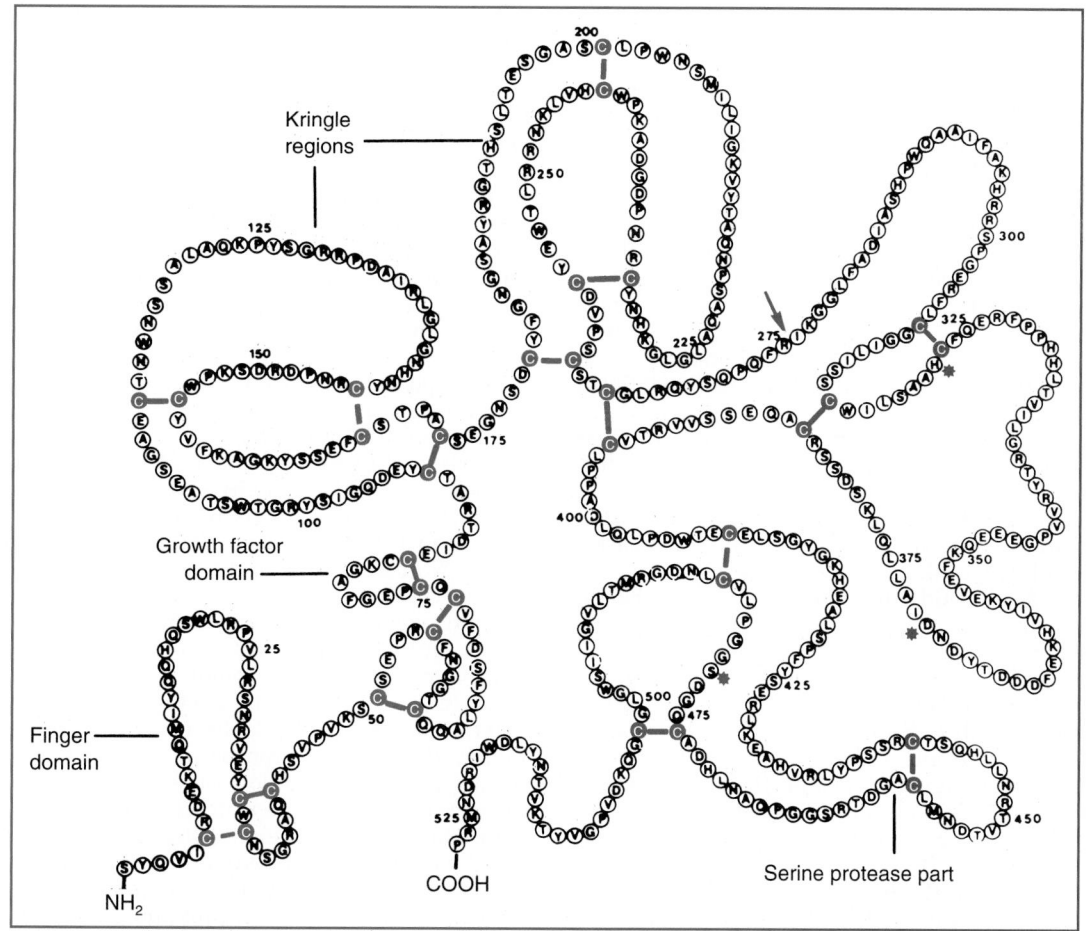

FIGURE 58-11. Primary structure of t-PA. The amino acids are represented by their single-letter symbols, and the black bars indicate disulfide bonds. * = active site residues His[322], Asp[371], and Ser[478]; arrow = plasmin cleavage site for conversion of single-chain t-PA to two-chain t-PA.

and of PAI-1 from the vessel wall,[39] or by changes in their rates of elimination by the liver.[40]

SYNTHESIS AND SECRETION OF t-PA. Vascular endothelial cells synthesize and secrete t-PA into the circulating blood.[39] The plasma concentration of free t-PA is less than 1 ng/ml. The half-life of t-PA in the circulation is only about 5 minutes because of rapid hepatic clearance; some t-PA is inactivated by PAI-1. Various stimuli, such as venous occlusion, physical exercise, catecholamines, brady-kinin, or desmopressin, produce a rapid increase (within minutes) in the level of t-PA in the blood. This response is too rapid to represent increased synthesis, but may reflect release of t-PA from cellular storage pools as well as decrease in hepatic clearance due to reduced hepatic blood flow.[41-43] A storage pool of t-PA in endothelial cells has not been conclusively identified.[42]

SYNTHESIS AND SECRETION OF PAI-1. PAI-1 is found in plasma, platelets, placenta, and in the extracellular matrix.[44] The concentration in plasma is in the picomolar range, but may increase to about 2 nM during pregnancy, most likely as a result of release of the inhibitor from placenta. Both active and latent PAI-1 are cleared rapidly, with half-lives in rabbits of approximately 15 and 5 minutes, respectively.[45,46] For unknown reasons, PAI-1 exhibits a circadian variation; the plasma concentration peaks in the morning and reaches a trough in the late afternoon and evening[47]; t-PA exhibits a diurnal variation, which is opposite to that observed for PAI-1.

INHIBITION OF PLASMIN BY ALPHA$_2$-ANTIPLASMIN. Alpha$_2$-antiplasmin forms an inactive 1:1 stoichiometric complex with plasmin. The half-life of plasmin molecules on the fibrin surface, which have both their lysine-binding sites and active site occupied, is estimated to be 2 to 3 orders of magnitude longer than that of free plasmin.

INHIBITION OF PLASMINOGEN ACTIVATORS BY PAI-1. PAI-1 reacts very rapidly with single-chain and two-chain t-PA and with two-chain u-PA (tcu-PA).[48,49] PAI-2 primarily inhibits tcu-PA.[48]

Like other serpins, PAI-1 inhibits its target proteinases by formation of a 1:1 stoichiometric reversible complex, followed by covalent binding between the hydroxyl group of the active site serine residue of the proteinase and the carboxyl group of the P1 residue at the reactive center ("bait region") of the serpin. The rapid inhibition of both t-PA and u-PA by PAI-1 involves a reversible high-affinity second-site interaction that does not depend on a functional active site. In the presence of fibrin, single-chain t-PA is protected from rapid inhibition by PAI-1. It has, however, also been reported that PAI-1 binds to fibrin and that fibrin-bound PAI-1 may inhibit t-PA–mediated fibrin clot lysis.[50]

The active form of PAI-1 converts to a latent form that can be partially reactivated by denaturing agents. In addition, inhibitory PAI-1 may not only convert to latent PAI-1, which can be reactivated, but also to substrate PAI-1, which may be irreversibly degraded by target proteinases, including t-PA, u-PA, and thrombin.[51]

PLASMINOGEN ACTIVATION BY t-PA AT THE FIBRIN SURFACE. The main role of t-PA most likely is in the dissolution of fibrin.[52] t-PA is a poor enzyme in the absence of fibrin, but the presence of fibrin strikingly enhances the activation rate of plasminogen.[53] Plasmin formed on the fibrin surface has both its lysine-binding sites and active site occupied and is thus only slowly inactivated by alpha$_2$-antiplasmin (half-life of about 10–100 s); in contrast, free plasmin, when formed, is rapidly inhibited by alpha$_2$-antiplasmin (half-life of about 0.1 s).

During fibrin clot lysis, single-chain t-PA is converted to two-chain t-PA at the fibrin surface. This conversion is probably of little physiological relevance, since the activity of single-chain t-PA and two-chain t-PA is enhanced to the

same extent in the presence of fibrin or fragment X-polymer.[54]

Binding studies,[55,56] as well as kinetic studies, have revealed that Lp(a) competes with plasminogen for binding to fibrin, as a result of binding of Lp(a) to fibrin via its lysine-binding domains. As for plasminogen, binding of Lp(a) to fibrin is enhanced by partial proteolytic degradation of the fibrin surface.[55] As a functional consequence of the competition between Lp(a) and plasminogen for binding to fibrin, the fibrin-dependent enhancement of plasminogen by t-PA is inhibited.[56,57]

Pathophysiology of Fibrinolysis

Increased levels of PAI-1 activity resulting in decreased fibrinolytic capacity have been reported in several thrombotic disease states, including venous thromboembolism, obesity, sepsis, coronary artery disease, and acute myocardial infarction.[47,56] Increased levels of PAI-1 have also been found in association with the insulin resistance syndrome (see p. 1340), in which significant correlation was found between plasma PAI-1 levels and body mass index, triglyceride levels, insulin levels, and systolic blood pressure.[57] Obese people—particularly those with android obesity—also have high PAI-1 levels.[57]

Increased plasma levels of PAI-1 are one of the major disturbances of the hemostatic system in patients with coronary heart disease, and multiple interrelations with established metabolic risk factors have been observed. Increased PAI-1 levels have also been demonstrated in atherosclerotic lesions within the vessel wall. Therefore, both systemically and locally increased PAI-1 concentrations could have a pathogenic role in the development of atherosclerotic disease.[41,58-60]

Many case-control or cross-sectional studies have demonstrated high plasma PAI-1 levels in patients who have had a myocardial infarction or have had unstable angina. A relationship between deficient fibrinolysis due to high PAI activity levels and recurrent (within 3 years) myocardial infarction was demonstrated in young men who had survived a first myocardial infarction.[61] On the other hand, PAI activity was not predictive of recurrent infarction (nor was t-PA antigen) in a group of older patients followed over 5 years. In a cohort of patients with angina pectoris, high basal t-PA antigen levels were found to be associated with an increased risk of myocardial infarction, while no correlation was observed with PAI activity.[62]

Attempts to demonstrate a relationship between plasma PAI-1 levels and the severity of vessel wall damage have led to conflicting results in cross-sectional studies.[59] Recent analysis of the data of the ECAT angina pectoris study[63] demonstrated that there was a weak distinction between patients with and patients without significant coronary stenosis; the former had significantly higher plasma levels of PAI-1. No association could be observed with the extent of coronary atherosclerosis.

There are multiple interrelations between plasma PAI-1 levels and other risk factors of atherothrombosis such as those involved in the metabolic syndrome of insulin resistance. In the ECAT angina pectoris study, in which insulin determination was available for almost 1500 patients, two-fold to threefold differences in PAI-1 levels were observed when comparing the lowest and the highest quintile of insulin, body mass index, or triglyceride.[64]

In addition, lipoprotein(a) (Lp[a]) was shown to enhance PAI-1 synthesis by endothelial cells in culture, and it was suggested that Lp(a) binding to endothelium and subsequent increased PAI-1 expression may contribute to the generation of a specific prothrombotic endothelial phenotype.[65]

ANTITHROMBOTIC DRUGS

Unfractionated Heparin, Low Molecular Weight Heparins, and Heparinoids

UNFRACTIONATED HEPARIN (Table 58–1). The term *heparin* refers not to a single structure but rather to a family of mucopolysaccharide chains of varying length and composition.[65a] Heparin by itself has no anticoagulant property. It accelerates the action of two naturally occurring plasma inhibitors, forming a 1:1 stoichiometric complex with antithrombin III (an inhibitor of thrombin and activated factors X, IX, and XI) and, at very high doses, with heparin co-factor II, which acts only on thrombin decay. Heparin contains a unique pentasaccharide that has a high-affinity binding sequence for antithrombin III. This sequence is present in only one-third of heparin molecules and is not required for binding to heparin co-factor II.

Factor Xa bound to platelets and thrombin bound to the endothelium or to fibrin (thrombus) are protected from inactivation by heparin-antithrombin III complex.[66,67] In plasma, approximately 20 times more heparin is needed to inactivate fibrin-bound thrombin than to inactivate free thrombin.[66] This explains why more heparin is needed to prevent the extension of venous thrombosis than to prevent formation of the initial thrombus.

Heparin is not absorbed by the gastrointestinal mucosa. When in the bloodstream after parenteral administration, heparin binds to endothelial cells, mononuclear macrophages, and numerous plasma proteins. Some of these neutralize anticoagulant activity (e.g., platelet factor 4, vitronectin), while others such as von Willebrand factor lose their function. Elevated levels of these heparin-binding proteins explain the different individual heparin dose requirements to obtain the same antithrombotic effect and the so-called heparin resistance in patients with inflammatory and malignant diseases.[67] Binding of heparin to the endothelium and various plasma proteins reduces bioavailability at low concentrations and causes variability of response to fixed doses of anticoagulant.[67]

The pharmacokinetics of heparin are complicated; suffice it to say that the anticoagulant response increases disproportionately in intensity and duration as the dose increases. This explains why the anticoagulant effect of heparin has to be closely monitored. At present, no completely satisfactory test measuring the generation of thrombin and the levels of antithrombin is available. The most commonly used test is the activated partial thromboplastin time (APTT), which is sensitive to the inhibitory effect of heparin on thrombin, factor X, and factor IX. Unfortunately, the different commercial APTT reagents vary in their response to heparin, and there are technical variables. The therapeutic level of the APTT should therefore be established in each clinical laboratory to correspond to 0.2 to 0.4 units of heparin per milliliter plasma by protamine titration[67] or to 0.2 to 0.7 units of factor Xa per milliliter plasma by the chromogenic substrate assay for the determination of anti-factor Xa activity.[68] A nomogram may help, but should be adapted to the responsiveness of the reagent and APTT test system in use in the local laboratory.[68]

The most common and major side effect of heparin is bleeding. The risk is higher when unfractionated heparin is given by intermittent (14.2 per cent) rather than continuous infusion (6.8 per cent) or subcutaneous route (4.1 per cent). Also, the dose of heparin, the patient's anticoagulant response, serious concurrent illness, and chronic consumption of alcohol may predispose to bleeding. Heparin-induced thrombocytopenia (HIT) occurs in 2.4 per cent of patients receiving therapeutic heparin and 0.3 per cent receiving prophylactic heparin. In addition, vascular occlusion occurs in 0.4 per cent.[67] Rare complications are osteoporosis, alopecia, skin necrosis, urticaria, and transient increase of hepatic transaminases.

LOW MOLECULAR WEIGHT HEPARINS. Some of the limitations of unfractionated heparin can be overcome with low molecular weight (LMW) heparins (mean MW 4000 to 5000; range 1000 to 10,000) (Table 58–1). These LMW heparins produce their major anticoagulant effect by binding to antithrombin III through the same high-affinity pentasaccharide sequence of unfractionated heparin, which, however, is present in only one-third of the LMW molecules. A minimum additional chain length of 15 saccharides (MW > 5400) is required for the inactivation of thrombin, but the inactivation of factor X requires only the pentasaccharide. Unfractionated heparin has by definition an antifactor Xa to antithrombin-III ratio of 1:1, which is between 4:1 and 2:1 for the various LMW heparins. Drugs with high antifactor Xa activity were indeed designed based on the hypothesis that inhibition of earlier steps in the blood coagulation system would be associated with a more potent antithrombotic effect than inhibiting subsequent steps. This is because of the amplification process inherent in the coagulation cascade; that is, a single factor Xa molecule can lead to the generation of multiple thrombin molecules.

The advantages of LMW heparins over unfractionated heparin are numerous (Table 58–1). Factor Xa bound to the platelet membrane in the prothrombinase complex is resistant to inactivation by unfractionated heparin, but is not resistant to inactivation by LMW heparins. Also, LMW heparins have lesser binding characteristics to platelet factor 4, other plasma proteins, and endothelial cells, resulting in higher bioavailability (after subcutaneous injection > 90

TABLE 58–1 COMPARISON OF SOME PROPERTIES OF UNFRACTIONATED HEPARIN, LMW HEPARIN AND HIRUDIN

UNFRACTIONATED HEPARIN	LMW HEPARIN	HIRUDIN
Inhibits to the same extent thrombin and factor VII, much less IXa and XIa	Inhibits mainly factor Xa, thrombin to some extent	Specific and potent inhibitor of thrombin
Antithrombin III-dependent	Antithrombin III-dependent	Antithrombin III-independent
Neutralized by heparinase, several plasma proteins, platelet factor 4, and endothelium	Neutralized by heparinase, weak endothelium, binding	Not neutralized by heparinase, endothelium, macrophages, fibrin monomer, and plasma proteins
Does not inactivate clot-bound thrombin and factor VII	Does not inactivate clot-bound thrombin and factor VII	Inactivates clot-bound thrombin
Inhibits platelet function	Inhibits platelet function	Prevents thrombin-induced aggregation but not other platelet agonists
Induced thrombocytopenia not rare	Can induce thrombocytopenia	Does not induce thrombocytopenia
Bioavailability after sc injection 30%	Bioavailability after sc injection > 90%	Good bioavailability after sc injection, about 85%
Poor dose-effect response	Fair dose-effect response	Fair dose-effect response
Not immunogenic	Not immunogenic	Not or barely immunogenic
Transient increase of liver enzymes common	Transient increase of liver enzymes possible	No liver toxicity
Increases vascular permeability	No increase of vascular permeability	No increase of vascular permeability

LMW = low molecular weight; SC = subcutaneous.

versus 30 per cent for unfractionated heparin); reduced plasma clearance, which is independent of dose and plasma concentration; a longer half-life (anti-Xa activity between 3 and 4 hours for LMW heparins versus 30 to 150 minutes for unfractionated heparin); and less interindividual variability of the anticoagulant response.[70] LMW heparins have lower affinity for von Willebrand factor,[71] increase vascular permeability less than unfractionated heparin, and have a weak effect on platelet function. These differences could explain why LMW heparins produce less bleeding than unfractionated heparin with equivalent or higher antithrombotic effect in experimental animals[70] and in some clinical studies.[72–75]

The long half-life of LMW heparins and their predictable anticoagulant response to weight-adjusted doses allow once-daily subcutaneous administration without laboratory monitoring.[70]

It has been observed that thrombocytopenia is more common with unfractionated heparin than with low molecular weight heparin.[76,77]

HEPARINOIDS: MIXTURE OF LOW MOLECULAR WEIGHT SULFATE GLYCOSAMINOGLYCANS. Danaparoid sodium (Org 10172) is a low molecular weight heparinoid (6 kDa) and consists of a polydisperse mixture comprising sulfated glycosaminoglycuronans derived from animal mucosa, heparan sulfate (83 per cent w/w), of which 4 to 5 per cent has high affinity for antithrombin III dermatan sulfate (12 per cent w/w) and a minor amount of chondroitin sulfate (5 per cent w/w).[78–81] Its anticoagulant profile is characterized by a high ratio of anti-factor Xa/antithrombin activity (14 over < 0.5), resulting in effective inhibition of thrombin generation. The anti-Xa activity is mediated by antithrombin III and is not inactivated by endogenous heparin-neutralizing factors. The low antithrombin activity is mediated by heparin co-factor II and antithrombin III. In contrast to heparin, danaparoid sodium shows hardly any or no effect on blood platelet function in vitro or in vivo. Danaparoid sodium is essentially free of contaminating heparin, has minimal cross reactivity in in vitro assays for HIT, and has been used successfully in patients with this complication.

After intravenous and subcutaneous administration of danaparoid sodium the antithrombin activity half-life of danaparoid sodium is shorter (1.8 hours) than its anti-factor Xa half-life (17.6 hours). Danaparoid sodium has absolute bioavailability of 100 per cent after subcutaneous administration.

Danaparoid sodium is effective in the prevention of deep vein thrombosis in patients with thrombotic stroke and after elective hip surgery or hip fracture.[82] The long half-life of danaparoid sodium, which is not effectively neutralized by protamine, has been rather difficult to manage clinically.

Coumarin-Type Oral Anticoagulants

Warfarin sodium and related coumarin congeners are effective antithrombotic compounds that differ in speed in their inhibition of vitamin K-2,3 epoxide within hepatic chromosomes.[65a] These compounds depress the synthesis of four vitamin K–dependent procoagulants (factors II, VII, IX, and X) and of two natural inhibitor proteins, C and S. The plasma concentration of these proteins will decrease in accord with their half-life. The coagulation components with the shortest half-life are the procoagulant factor VII and the endogenous anticoagulant protein C. This may cause frank imbalance at the start of treatment and lead to thrombosis of skin capillaries and venules with cutaneous necrosis.[83]

MONITORING OF COUMARIN THERAPY. The intensity of the effect of warfarin on the synthesis of coagulation factors differs among patients; moreover, in the same individual it may, over time, vary considerably. This explains the need for close monitoring by having daily blood tests in the first week of treatment with warfarin. The test used is the *prothrombin time,* a term that leads to confusion because the assay depends in fact on the global activity of five coagulation factors (prothrombin, factors V, VII, IX and X). Among the six factors whose synthesis is inhibited by coumarin derivatives, three (prothrombin and factors VII and X) are effectively measured by this test, but not factor IX and the anticoagulant proteins C and S. On the other hand, the prothrombin time is also sensitive to factor V, a coagulation protein independent of vitamin K.

To determine the prothrombin time a tissue extract (thromboplastin) and calcium are added to citrated plasma, and the time to fibrin formation is measured. Commercial thromboplastin reagents extracted by different methods from various organs and species vary extensively in their sensitivity to reductions in levels of vitamin K–dependent factors. To standardize prothrombin time determinations, and thus allow direct comparison of results obtained with different thromboplastins, the International Normalized Ratio (INR) is recommended but not yet universally applied.[84]

At the start of warfarin treatment the prothrombin time is first prolonged by factor VII depletion because factor VII has a half-life much shorter than the other vitamin K–dependent coagulation factors (II, IX, and X). Thus, in the beginning of warfarin treatment, the prothrombin time is prolonged while the intrinsic and common coagulation pathways are still uninfluenced. This explains why in switching from heparin to warfarin, heparin should be continued unabated for at least 1 day after the prothrombin time (INR) has reached therapeutic values. Also, during long-term warfarin therapy, prothrombin times should be checked regularly, as many drugs and foods can enhance or decrease the warfarin effect. Certain intercurrent diseases (hepatic failure, heart failure, hyperthyroidism) may also modify warfarin dose requirements. Bleeding is the most important side effect, and the risk may vary from patient to patient, depending upon the presence of co-morbid conditions (hypertension, malignant disease, older age, recent surgery) and the intensity of anticoagulation. Patients with intensive anticoagulation (INR 2.5 to 4) have during the first 3 months a risk of clinically important bleeding over 2 times greater (14 versus 6 per cent) than those with less intensive anticoagulation (INR 2.0 to 2.5).[85] On average, the overall annual risk of bleeding is 6 per cent, with major and fatal bleeding incidence estimated to be 2 and 0.8 per cent, respectively.

A rare, nonhemorrhagic side effect of warfarin is coumarin-induced skin necrosis, an unexplained complication that occurs between the third and eighth day of therapy. The rapid decline in protein C level is postulated to play a role in the obscure pathogenesis of thrombosis of skin venules and capillaries within the subcutaneous fat, usually in the lower part of the body.[83] Coumarin drugs readily cross the placenta and may be teratogenic, particularly during the first trimester of pregnancy.[86]

In conclusion, vitamin K antagonists are effective antithrombotic drugs with a narrow risk/benefit ratio that require regular monitoring and a disciplined patient. Their main virtues are oral administration and low cost.

Inhibitors of Platelet Function

Several strategies are currently being used to reduce platelet function[65a] (Fig. 58–4). These include inhibition of platelet enzyme prostaglandin synthase (aspirin, sulfinpyrazone, flurbiprofen, indobufen), inhibition of thromboxane synthase, blockade of endoperoxide-thromboxane receptors or inhibition of the activation pathway of GPIIb/IIIa (ticlopidine, clopidogrel). Inhibition of platelet function was also obtained by modulation of platelet adenylate or guanylate cyclase (stable prostacyclin analogs), interference with the function of the platelet glycoprotein Ib-IX receptor (monoclonal antibodies to GP1b-IX, synthetic peptides to the A1 von Willebrand factor domain, recombinant von Willebrand fragments covering the A1 domain, aurin tricarboxylic acid), specific blockers of the IIb/IIIa receptor (monoclonal antibodies, natural antagonists, synthetic peptides containing the Arg-Gly-Asp [RGD] sequence or nonpeptide inhibitors), and peptides that bind to but do not activate the platelet-receptor domain that interacts with thrombin. In this chapter, only platelet inhibitors that have been investigated in therapeutic trials are discussed. Several reviews on inhibitors of platelet function have recently been published.[87-91]

ASPIRIN. Several pathways lead to platelet aggregation (Fig. 58-12). Aspirin very selectively inhibits thromboxane (TXA2) formation but only partially impedes platelet aggregation induced by ADP, collagen, and low concentrations of thrombin. Aspirin does not inhibit adherence of the initial layer of platelets to the subendothelium or atherosclerotic plaques, and the release of granule contents is not opposed. Thus the effects of platelet-derived growth factors and other mitogens on smooth muscle cells are not inhibited (Table 58-2).[92]

The ideal dose of aspirin for primary or secondary prevention of cardiovascular disease is not determined. Doses between 324 and 1300 mg daily seem to induce a similar reduction of cardiovascular complications, while doses between 1 and 2 mg/kg daily produce virtually complete inhibition of cyclo-oxygenase–dependent platelet aggregation.[93] Slow-release aspirins are associated with few gastrointestinal side effects, particularly when an enteric coated preparation is used. There is increasing evidence that the antithrombotic effect of aspirin is due not only to its inhibition of platelet oxygenase. Aspirin also impairs thrombinogenesis by a mechanism that seems to be unrelated to platelet cyclo-oxygenase; for instance, the acetylation of GTP-binding proteins, thrombin receptors, and prothrombin.[94,95] The salicylate moiety of aspirin also antagonizes the lipoxygenase pathway of arachidonate metabolism in platelets, and the demonstration of two cyclo-oxygenase enzymes (COX-1, COX-2)[96] may further elucidate the antithrombotic mechanism of aspirin.[97]

TICLOPIDIN, CLOPIDOGREL. These two thienopyridine derivatives can be considered bioprecursors, since they are inactive in vitro but potent antiaggregating agents in vivo, indicating the importance of at least one active transient metabolite. Ticlopidine and its chemical analog clopidogrel are noncompetitive but selective antagonists of ADP-induced platelet aggregation and act by specifically blocking glycoprotein IIb/IIIa (GPIIb/IIIa) activation specific for the ADP pathway (Fig. 58-4). Since the two compounds are chemically related, their mechanism of action is considered similar.[98,99] The binding of fibrinogen to GPIIb/IIIa complex, triggered by ADP, is dramatically inhibited; this inhibition is not due to direct modification of the glycoprotein complex.[100]

TABLE 58–2 ASPIRIN AS PLATELET INHIBITOR
Inhibits only TXA₂ pathway; much less inhibition of platelet activation by thrombin, ADP, and collagen and not by PAF
Provides no inhibition of platelet adhesion
Has no effect on smooth muscle cell proliferation
Prolongs bleeding time
Can induce gastrointestinal problems
Can induce allergy (rare)

ADP = adenosine diphosphate; PAF = platelet activating factor.

Clopidogrel is approximately 40 to 100 times as active as ticlopidine in inhibiting ADP-induced platelet aggregation in animal models, but about 6 times as potent as ticlopidine in inhibition of ADP-induced aggregation of human platelets.

The effectiveness of ticlopidine has been convincingly demonstrated in patients at high risk of arterial thromboembolic events, i.e., those with transient ischemic cerebral attacks and stroke, peripheral arterial or ischemic heart disease.[101-103] A trial in more than 3000 patients has shown that ticlopidine has a more pronounced effect on death from all causes or nonfatal stroke than aspirin.[104,105]

The most potentially serious problem of ticlopidine is bone marrow depression (leukopenia, thrombocytopenia, pancytopenia); close monitoring is therefore essential for at least the first 12 weeks of ticlopidine therapy.[101] Ticlopidine has also been associated with an increase in total cholesterol levels by 9 per cent.[104] Clopidogrel was developed because this compound was not toxic to bone marrow pluripotent stem cells in the mouse (Till and McCullogh test).

THROMBOXANE SYNTHASE INHIBITORS. Thromboxane synthase inhibitors have been developed with the expectation of not only suppressing TXA₂ biosynthesis but also sparing or even enhancing the formation of prostacyclin (PGI₂) by the vascular endothelium (Fig. 58-4). Most thromboxane synthase inhibitors have moderate potency and short duration of action and do not result in sufficiently sustained inhibition of TXA₂ production to be clinically effective.[106] Although thromboxane synthase inhibitors have shown some benefit in experimental models, their effects in clinical trials in patients with coronary artery disease have been disappointing.

THROMBOXANE RECEPTOR BLOCKERS. The more recently developed thromboxane receptor blockers specifically impede the action of both TXA₂ and endoperoxides on their presumed common receptors on platelets and prevent vasoconstriction induced by TXA₂ (Fig. 58-4). These agents leave the normal pattern of thromboxane and PGI₂ for-

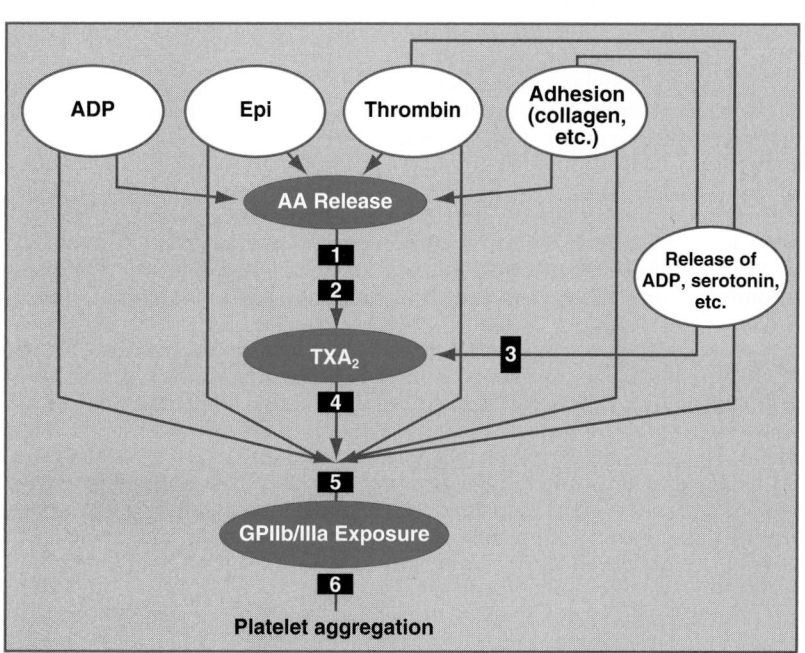

FIGURE 58–12. Pathways of platelet activation. Exposure of GPIIb/IIIa receptors at the platelet surface is the final common endpoint of all pathways. AA = arachidonic acid; ADP = adenosine diphosphate; Epi = epinephrine; TXA₂ = thromboxane A₂.

mation unaltered. Thromboxane receptor antagonists prolong bleeding time more than thromboxane synthase inhibitors. As expected, TXA$_2$ synthesis is not inhibited, and PGI$_2$ generation is not augmented by specific thromboxane/endoperoxide receptor antagonists.[106]

Several of the thromboxane/endoperoxide receptor blockers are relatively short acting, and the magnitude of their blockade is modest.[106]

COMBINED THROMBOXANE SYNTHASE INHIBITORS AND RECEPTOR BLOCKERS. Some compounds have a dual activity. Ridogrel is a potent TXA$_2$ synthase inhibitor with modest additional TXA$_2$/prostaglandin endoperoxide receptor antagonist properties (at least 100-fold less).[107] Although the animal pharmacology was very promising, the preclinical evaluation has been disappointing.[106] Picotamide is a rather weak thromboxane synthase inhibitor and receptor blocker.[108]

BLOCKERS OF THE PLATELET GLYCOPROTEIN IIb/IIIa RECEPTOR

(Figs. 58–1 and 58–12). Exposure of GPIIb/IIa receptors at the platelet surface is the final common endpoint of all pathways leading to platelet aggregation (Fig. 58–1).

Monoclonal Antibodies (7E3). The first platelet GPIIb/IIIa antagonists to be developed were murine monoclonal antibodies.[109] In vitro, these antibodies completely inhibit platelet aggregation and, in animal models of angioplasty injury and thrombolysis, prevent thrombosis and augment the activity of thrombolytic agents. Because of concerns about their immunogenicity, the derivative product chimeric monoclonal 7E3Fab (c7E3Fab, abciximab) was created via genetic recombination. This new molecule consists of the mouse-derived variable regions from the original molecule linked to the constant region derived from human immunoglobulin IgG. Data from a dose-escalation study[110] and a pilot therapeutic trial[111] suggested an abciximab dosing regimen that was evaluated in patients with high-risk percutaneous transluminal coronary angioplasty (PTCA)[112,113] (Table 39–2, p. 1370). As compared with placebo, an abciximab bolus of 0.25 mg/kg followed by an infusion of 10 μg/kg/hour for 12 hours in 2099 patients resulted in a 35 per cent reduction in the rate of the primary endpoints (death, nonfatal myocardial infarction, unplanned surgical revascularization, unplanned repeat PTCA, stent or balloon pump for refractory ischemia.) However, bleeding episodes and transfusions were more frequent in patients treated with abciximab. At 6 months, the absolute difference in patients with a major ischemic event or elective revascularization was 8.1 per cent between the placebo group and abciximab bolus-plus-infusion group.

To be effective, more than 90 per cent of the GPIIb/IIIa receptors have to be blocked. This is associated with a very prolonged bleeding time and risk of bleeding without an antidote being available. Moreover, even chimeric monoclonal antibodies contain some murine proteins and can still be immunogenic.

The same drawbacks prevail for cysteine-rich single-chain snake venom peptides binding to GPIIb/IIIa, which, moreover, have a lower potency than chimeric monoclonal abciximab. Their shorter half-life may be an advantage in case of bleeding.

Synthetic IIb/IIIa Inhibitors. The synthetic antiplatelet peptides, particularly those in cyclic configuration, are potent antithrombotic agents when tested in platelet-mediated thrombosis in various experimental animals. While short cyclic synthetic peptides have a higher potency, they also lack specificity for the GPIIb/IIIa receptors and recognize receptors on several integrins. The most potent compounds, at doses required for effective inhibition of in vivo thrombus formation, also induce a hemorrhagic tendency as witnessed by marked prolongation of the bleeding time.[114] Structure-activity studies have resulted in partial dissociation between the inhibition of ex vivo platelet aggregation and bleeding time prolongation and suggest that it might be possible to obtain GPIIb/IIIa antagonists with an optimized antithrombotic versus hemorrhagic ratio.[114]

The nonpeptide inhibitors are reversible antagonists and have obvious advantages compared to monoclonal antibodies as their effects are much shorter (3 hours for tirofiban

[MK-383] versus 3 days for abciximab), they have no immunogenicity and have the potential to be active orally. Lamifiban (RO43-5054) is a nonpeptide, low molecular weight GPIIb/IIIa antagonist almost 1000 times more active than RGDS (Arg-Gly-Asp-Ser) in inhibiting platelet aggregation in human platelet-rich plasma.[115]

SC-5468A is a prodrug of a nonpeptide mimetic of the tetrapeptide RGDS. The active metabolite SC-54701A, is a potent inhibitor of GPIIb/IIIa receptors and exhibits specificity for this receptor with respect to other integrins.[116] Fradafibran (BIBU 104XX) is the orally available prodrug of the GPIIb/IIIa receptor antagonist BIBU 52 and has a mean residence time of approximately 12 hours.[117] At these oral doses GPIIb/IIIa receptors were blocked by more than 80 per cent in a reversible and dose-proportional manner.

Specific Thrombin Inhibitors

HIRUDIN (Table 58–1). Natural hirudin is a single-chain, carbohydrate-free polypeptide containing three intramolecular disulfide bridges and a sulfated tyrosine residue. The polypeptide chain contains 65 amino acids with a molecular weight of approximately 7000 daltons. Recombinant hirudin has been obtained using *Escherichia coli* and yeast. With both methods, hirudin is expressed as desulfatohirudin lacking the sulfate residue on tyrosine 63. The nonsulfated molecules result in about a 10-fold reduction in thrombin affinity.[118] Unlike heparin, which requires endogenous co-factors for activity (mainly antithrombin III, heparin co-factor II), hirudin does not need a co-factor for its anticoagulant activity and therefore is still active in states of deficiency of these proteins.

Hirudin is a specific potent inhibitor of thrombin to which it binds with extraordinary tightness (KD 2 $\times$ 10 $-$ 14 M) near the active center at the substrate recognition site. In addition, there are multiple other contacts between hirudin and thrombin over an extended area of the molecule forming a highly stable noncovalent complex. All known functions of thrombin are inhibited.

The terminal half-life of r-hirudin in healthy young volunteers is 50 to 65 minutes, with a half-life of its effect on the APTT of about 2 hours.[119-122] Recombinant hirudin appears to be a weak allergen. Hirudin-specific IgE antibodies were rarely seen in 163 immunocompetent healthy volunteers receiving recombinant hirudin twice at an interval of 1 month.[123]

In contrast to unfractionated and LMW heparins, hirudin penetrates the thrombus and neutralizes thrombin bound to fibrin. Hirudin, but not heparin, reduces platelet deposition and thrombus growth on deep wall injury at both low- and high-shear rate conditions. As hirudin is not inhibited by plasma proteins and endothelium, while unfractionated heparin is, the anticoagulant effect of hirudin is more predictable. Hirudin, a specific inhibitor of thrombin, prevents platelet aggregation induced by thrombin but does not oppose platelet aggregation by other agonists. Unfractionated and LMW heparins can induce thrombocytopenia; this untoward effect has not been observed with hirudin.

On the negative side, there is no antidote for hirudin. Furthermore, hirudin inhibits also the interaction between thrombin and thrombomodulin, a prerequisite for activation of the endogenous coagulation inhibitory proteins C and S.

HIRULOG. Hirulog is a bifunctional 20-amino acid peptide designed on the structure of hirudin. It combines a fragment of the C-terminus of hirudin (interacting with the anion-binding exosite of thrombin) with an N-terminus fragment [D-Phe-Pro-Arg-Pro(Gly)], which interacts with the catalytic site of thrombin.[124,125] There is no antidote for hirulog.

ARGATROBAN. This arginine derivative that binds to thrombin with intermediate affinity (KD 3.9 $\times$ 10 $-$ 8 M) is a competitive antagonist inhibiting fibrinogen cleavage and platelet activation by thrombin. Compared to heparin, argatroban is significantly more effective in the prevention of platelet-rich thrombi after vascular injury and was effective at APTTs of only 2 to 3 × baseline control.[126,127]

THROMBOLYTIC DRUGS

STREPTOKINASE. This is a nonenzyme protein produced by several strains of hemolytic streptococci; it consists of a single polypeptide chain of 414 amino acids with a molecular weight of 47,000 to 50,000. Streptokinase cannot directly cleave peptide bonds, but it activates plasminogen to plasmin indirectly, following a three-step mechanism.[128] In the first step, streptokinase forms an equimolar complex with plasminogen. This complex undergoes a conformational change resulting in the exposure of an active site in the plasminogen moiety. In the second step, this active site catalyzes the activation of plasminogen to plasmin. In a third step, plasminogen-streptokinase molecules are converted to plasmin-streptokinase complexes.[129] The active site residues in the plasmin-streptokinase complex are the same as those in the plasmin molecule. However, plasmin is unable to activate plasminogen, whereas the plasmin(ogen)-streptokinase complex is not inhibited by alpha$_2$-antiplasmin.

Most individuals have measurable circulating streptokinase-neutralizing antibodies, which may result from previous infections with beta-hemolytic streptococci. Therefore, during thrombolytic therapy, sufficient streptokinase must be infused to neutralize these antibodies. A few days after streptokinase administration, the antistreptokinase titer rises rapidly to 50 to 100 times the preinfusion value and remains high for 4 to 6 months, during which period renewed treatment with streptokinase is impracticable.[130]

ANISOYLATED PLASMINOGEN-STREPTOKINASE COMPLEX. Anisoylated plasminogen-streptokinase activator complex (APSAC, anistreplase) was constructed with the aim of controlling the enzymatic activity of the plasmin(ogen)-streptokinase complex by a specific reversible chemical protection of its catalytic center (i.e., by titration with a p-anisoyl group).[131] Deacylation of anistreplase uncovers the catalytic center, which converts plasminogen to plasmin. A plasma half-life of 70 minutes was found for anistreplase compared with 25 minutes for the plasminogen-streptokinase complex formed in vivo after administration of streptokinase.[132] Patients with a high titer of streptokinase antibodies do not respond to anistreplase, and anistreplase causes a marked increase in the streptokinase antibody titer within 2 to 3 weeks, which persists for months.

UROKINASE. Two-chain urokinase-type plasminogen activator (tcu-PA), a trypsin-like serine proteinase composed of two polypeptide chains (Mr 20,000 and 34,000) has been isolated from human urine[133] and from cultured human embryonic kidney cells.[134] Extensive plasminogen activation and depletion of α_2-antiplasmin may occur following treatment of thromboembolic diseases with tcu-PA, leading to degradation of several plasma proteins, including fibrinogen, factor V, and factor VIII.

PROUROKINASE. Single-chain urokinase-type plasminogen activator (scu-PA, pro-urokinase) is a naturally occurring human protein first isolated from natural sources and then produced through recombinant DNA technology.[135,136] scu-PA is the native zymogenic precursor of urokinase. Limited hydrolysis by plasmin or kallikrein of the Lys158-Ile159 peptide bond converts the molecule to two-chain urokinase-type plasminogen activator (tcu-PA, urokinase), which is held together by one disulfide bond that is essential for the thrombolytic activity. A fully active tcu-PA derivative is obtained after additional proteolysis at position Lys135-Lys136.

TISSUE-TYPE PLASMINOGEN ACTIVATOR (see also p. 1816). Native tissue-type plasminogen activator (t-PA) is a serine proteinase with a molecular weight of about 70,000, composed of one polypeptide chain containing 527 amino acids with serine as aminoterminal amino acid[137] (Fig. 58-11). t-PA is converted by plasmin to a two-chain form by hydrolysis of the Arg275-Ile276 peptide bond. The two-chain form is held together by one interchain disulfide bond. t-PA for clinical use is presently produced by recombinant DNA technology (Activase, Genentech Inc., or Actilyse, Boehringer Ingelheim GmbH, Germany) and consists mainly of the single-chain form.

The activation of plasminogen by t-PA, both in the presence and in the absence of fibrin, follows Michaelis-Menten kinetics.[53] Although different kinetic constants were obtained by several investigators, there is a consensus that the presence of fibrin enhances the efficiency of plasminogen activation by t-PA by 2 to 3 orders of magnitude.[53] The kinetic data support a mechanism in which fibrin provides a surface to which t-PA and plasminogen adsorb in a sequential and ordered way, yielding a cyclic ternary complex. Fibrin essentially increases the local plasminogen concentration by creating an additional interaction between t-PA and its substrate. The high affinity of t-PA for plasminogen in the presence of fibrin thus allows efficient activation on the fibrin clot, while no efficient plasminogen activation by t-PA occurs in plasma.

Plasmin formed on the fibrin surface has both its lysine-binding sites and active sites occupied and is thus only slowly inactivated by α_2-antiplasmin (half-life about 10 to 100 s); free plasmin, when formed, is rapidly inhibited by α_2-antiplasmin (half-life about 0.1 s). The fibrinolytic process thus seems to be triggered by and confined to fibrin.

MUTANTS AND VARIANTS OF t-PA

Several mutants of recombinant tissue-type plasminogen activator (rt-PA) have been constructed with interesting properties, including slower clearance from the circulation, more selective binding to fibrin, stronger stimulation by fibrin, and resistance to plasma protease inhibitors.[138,139]

RETEPLASE. This is a single-chain nonglycosylated deletion variant of r-PA consisting only of the kringle 2 and the protease domain of human t-PA. Production of reteplase in *Escherichia coli* leads to formation of inactive protein aggregates (inclusion bodies). The isolation of the inclusion bodies, the refolding, and the chromatographic purification of reteplase have been described.[140,141] The active site of the protease domain of reteplase and of t-PA, and their plasminogenolytic activity in the absence of a stimulator, do not differ, but the plasminogenolytic activity of reteplase in the presence of CNBr fragments of fibrinogen as a stimulator was fourfold lower compared to t-PA, whereas the binding of reteplase to fibrin was five times lower. These differences in plasminogenolytic activity and fibrin binding between the two molecules might possibly be due to the missing finger domain in reteplase. It is known that fibrin binding is mediated through both the finger domain and the lysine-binding site in the kringle 2 domain of t-PA.

Reteplase and t-PA are inhibited by PAI-1 to a similar degree, but the affinity of reteplase for binding to endothelial cells and monocytes is reduced, probably as a consequence of deletion of the finger and epidermal growth factor domains in reteplase, which seem to be involved in the interaction with endothelial cell receptors. The thrombolytic properties of reteplase and alteplase (recombinant t-PA) were compared in the rabbit jugular vein thrombosis model. The effective dose for 50 per cent thrombolysis (ED50) was 163 kU/kg (0.28 mg/kg) for reteplase, and 871 kU/kg (1.09 mg/kg) for alteplase, indicating 5.3 (3.9)-fold higher potency of reteplase. At equipotent doses (50 per cent thrombolysis), the residual concentration of fibrinogen was 74.2 per cent with reteplase and 76.5 per cent with alteplase. Pharmacokinetic analysis of plasma activity at a dose of 400 kU/kg in the rabbit revealed a half-life of 18.9 ± 1.5 minutes for reteplase and 2.1 ± 0.1 minutes for alteplase. Plasma clearance for reteplase was 4.3-fold slower than for alteplase (4.7 versus 1.2 ml/min/kg). One may therefore conclude that the higher potency of reteplase is due to its slower clearance.[141] An initial half-life of 14 to 18 minutes was also observed with reteplase in healthy human volunteers[142,143] and in patients with acute myocardial infarction.[144]

Dose-ranging studies of bolus reteplase were performed in a multicenter trial.[145] With a dose of 10 million units (MU) of reteplase, a patent infarct-related coronary artery (TIMI-3) was obtained at 30 minutes in 46 per cent, at 60 minutes in 48 per cent, at 90 minutes in 52 per cent, and at 24 to 48 hours in 88 per cent of patients with acute myocardial infarction. With 15 MU a higher angiographic patency rate at the same time intervals was obtained (38, 58, 69, and 85 per cent). Because there was a 20 per cent (10 MU) and 12.5 per cent (15 MU) reocclusion rate between the 30-minute and 90-minute angiogram, the administration of a second smaller bolus of reteplase (5 MU) 30 minutes after the initial bolus (10 MU) was investigated in an open uncontrolled study.[146] Patency rates (TIMI-3) reached 50 per cent at 60 minutes, 58 per cent at 90 minutes, and 84 per cent at 24 to 48 hours. Only 1 of the 50 patients studied had reocclusion in the first 24 to 48 hours. In a controlled study in 605 patients with acute myocardial infarction, different bolus doses of reteplase (single dose of 15 MU, 10 MU and 5 MU 30 minutes later, 10 MU and 10 MU 30 minutes later) were compared with the conventional-dose regimen of alteplase (100 mg over 3 hours). TIMI-3 patency rates at 90 minutes were obtained with the given reteplase regimen in 42.7, 45.4, 62.9 per cent, respectively, and in 47.6 per cent of patients treated with alteplase.[147] The difference between the 10 MU + 10 MU reteplase and alteplase arms is significant (p = 0.01). Recently, a direct comparison of reteplase versus frontloading t-PA (100 mg over 90 minutes) was completed. A large-scale, double-blind trial in 6010 patients with acute myocardial infarction demonstrates that there is a nonsignificant difference between 35-day mortality in patients treated with streptokinase (1.5 MU over 60 minutes) and reteplase (two boluses of 10 MU given 30 minutes apart [9.53 and 9.02 per cent, respectively]).[148]

rt-PA-TNK. An rt-PA mutant in which Thr103 is substituted by Asn (code rt-PA-T) and the sequence Lys296-His-Arg-Arg is mutagenized to Ala-Ala-Ala-Ala (code rt-PA-K) was found to have both a prolonged half-life and resistance to PAI-1.[149] This mutant has increased potency on platelet-rich arterial thrombi (rich in PAI-1) in a canine model of coronary thrombosis. Additional substitution in this mutant of Asn117 by Gln (code rt-PA-N) resulted in a t-PA variant with 8-fold slower clearance and 200-fold enhanced resistance to PAI-1. These three combinations in a single molecule are referred to as rt-PA-TNK. In in vivo models of thrombolysis in rabbits, rt-PA-TNK was shown to have increased thrombolytic potency on platelet-rich clots, to conserve fibrinogen, and to be effective upon bolus administration at half the dose of rt-PA.[149] Similar results were obtained in a combined arterial and venous thrombosis model in the dog.[150] A pilot dose-finding clinical trial was recently completed (TIMI 10) and large scale clinical trials in patients with acute myocardial infarction are planned.

RECOMBINANT CHIMERIC PLASMINOGEN ACTIVATORS. Recombinant chimeric plasminogen activators have been constructed primarily using different regions of t-PA and scu-PA, although several alternative combinations have been evaluated to some extent.[138,139] Only a small feasibility study of coronary thrombolysis with K1K2Pu has been performed in patients with acute myocardial infarction.[151]

DESMODUS SALIVARY PLASMINOGEN ACTIVATOR. The subsistence of vampire bats on a diet of fresh blood is apparently contingent on their ability to interfere with the hemostatic system of the blood donor. The saliva of vampire bats contains a variety of factors that presumably satisfy two essential requirements: to maintain prolonged bleeding from the wound and to preserve blood fluidity following ingestion of a meal.[152] Different molecular forms of the *Desmodus* salivary plasminogen activator (DSPA) have been purified, characterized, cloned, and expressed.[153]

STAPHYLOKINASE. Mature staphylokinase consists of 136 amino acids in a single polypeptide chain without disulfide bridges. Staphylokinase, like streptokinase, is not an enzyme, but it forms a 1:1 stoichiometric complex with plasmin(ogen) that activates other plasminogen molecules.[154] Streptokinase and plasminogen produce a complex that exposes the active site in the plasminogen molecule without proteolytic cleavage, whereas generation of plasmin is required for exposure of the active site in the complex with staphylokinase.[154] Pilot trials with recombinant staphylokinase are presently being conducted in patients with acute myocardial infarction and recent occlusion of leg arteries.[154a,b]

ANTITHROMBOTIC AND THROMBOLYTIC THERAPY IN CARDIAC DISEASE

Risk Stratification—The Concept of Relative Versus Absolute Reduction of Events

Preexisting cardiovascular disease is considered a most powerful risk factor for coronary events.[155] For example, as shown in the Lipid Research Clinics Program Prevalence Study, high LDL or low HDL in preexisting cardiovascular disease predicts subsequent mortality in men 40 to 69 years of age to a much greater extent than high LDL or low HDL in an otherwise healthy population.[156] Accordingly, the impact of lipid-modifying strategies is much more evident in secondary prevention or in patients with known cardiovascular disease than in primary prevention or in the general apparently healthy population.[156–158] Similar rationale should apply to antithrombotic therapy for the prevention of coronary events.[159]

Conceptually, and assuming no use of antithrombotic agents (aspirin or anticoagulants), in 1989 we defined patients with coronary artery disease at high risk for coronary events as those with an acute coronary syndrome, in whom the incidence of a recurrent event of coronary occlusion is higher than 6 per cent per year (Table 58–3). We defined patients at medium risk as those with stable angina, when the incidence of a coronary event is about 2 to 6 per cent per year. And finally, we defined patients at low risk as those without previous evidence of cardiovascular disease, in whom the incidence of a coronary event is less than 2 per cent per year.[160] If these three groups of patients are treated with aspirin, we assume that there will be about a 25 to 30 per cent relative reduction of coronary events (i.e., 10 per cent becomes about 7 per cent in high-risk patients, 4 per cent becomes about 3 per cent in medium-risk patients, and 1 per cent becomes about 0.7 per cent in the

TABLE 58–3 RISK STRATIFICATION IN CARDIOVASCULAR DISEASE: ROLE OF ASPIRIN AND ANTICOAGULANTS

PATHOGENESIS	THROMBOEMBOLIC RISK		
	High (> 6%/yr)	Medium (2–6%/yr)	Low (< 2%/yr)
Arterial Platelets and fibrin (PI and/or A/C)	ACS, PTCA ASA + A/C	Stable CAD ASA or A/C	Primary prevention PI?
Chambers	A-fib-emboli A-fib-M. stenosis	A-fib-valv, nonvalv Anterior MI-early Dilated cardiomyopathy	A-fib—lone Chronic LV aneurysm
Fibrin (A/C)	INR 2.5–3.5	INR 2.0–3.0	No therapy
Prostheses Fibrin more than platelets	Old mechanical Previous emboli Extensive atherosclerosis	Recent mechanical Bioprosthesis.-A-fib	Biopr.-NSR
(A/C > PI)	INR 3.0–4.5 or INR 2.5–3.5 + ASA	Mech-INR 2.5–3.5 Bio-INR 2.0–3.0	No therapy

Modified from Stein, B., Fuster, V., Halperin, J. L., Chesebro, J. H.: Antithrombotic therapy in cardiac disease: An emerging approach based on pathogenesis and risk. Circulation *80*:1501, 1989.

PI = platelet inhibitor (i.e., aspirin); A/C = anticoagulants; ACS = acute coronary syndrome; PTCA = percutaneous transluminal coronary angioplasty; ASA = aspirin; CAD = coronary artery disease; A-fib = atrial fibrillation; MI = myocardial infarction; LV = left ventricle; INR = international normalized ratio.

low-risk subset). In other words, with aspirin use, the *relative* decrease of coronary events is about the same regardless of risk.[93,160] However, the *absolute* reduction or clinical impact is very different; thus, a decrease in events from 10 to 7 per cent—or for each 1000 patients treated, 30 are benefited—in the high-risk population with an acute coronary syndrome is much more striking than a decrease from 1 to 0.7 per cent—or for each 1000 treated patients only 3 benefited—in the lowest-risk patients without previous evidence of cardiovascular disease. Thus, what matters most is *not* the proportional reduction in risk, but the absolute reduction in risk. Furthermore, conceptually, because of the high incidence of events, the clinical impact in the high-risk population could even be improved by combining aspirin and anticoagulants, while in the low-risk population even the use of aspirin alone might be debatable in terms of risk/benefits.

We further defined the pathogenesis of thrombosis and thromboembolic risk in various cardiovascular entities (Table 58–3).[160] Thrombosis within the coronary arteries involves activation of both platelets and the coagulation system. With fibrin deposition, thromboembolism in patients with diseases of the cardiac chambers (i.e., atrial fibrillation or ventricular dysfunction) or valves (i.e., prosthetic devices) is related primarily to hemodynamic abnormalities, in which activation of the coagulation system with fibrin deposition predominates over that of platelets. Finally, thrombosis within the venous system is mostly related to blood stasis and endothelial damage, leading to activation of the clotting system. A systemic approach to the patient at risk for a thromboembolic event has been proposed,[160] allowing the selection of the most appropriate antithrombotic therapy based on pathogenetic principles and the risk of thromboembolism. In general, the higher the risk, the more intensive the recommended antithrombotic approach.

ANTITHROMBOTIC THERAPY IN CORONARY ARTERY DISEASE

Unstable Angina
(See also p. 1331)

EFFICACY OF ANTIPLATELET AGENTS ALONE (Table 58–4). Antiplatelet agents have been found to reduce acute myocardial infarction and short- and long-term death in four large trials of unstable angina. In the Veterans Administration Cooperative Study, men with unstable angina were randomized to receive aspirin or placebo for 12 weeks. During the treatment period the aspirin group demonstrated a risk reduction of 51 per cent, and the overall benefits of aspirin were maintained during the 1-year follow-up period.[161] In the Canadian Multicenter Trial, patients with unstable angina were randomized to receive aspirin, sulfinpyrazone, the combination of both, or placebo. The incidence of death and myocardial infarction was reduced in the aspirin groups from 17 to 8.6 per cent or a 51 per cent reduction; sulfinpyrazone demonstrated no benefit.[162]

TABLE 58–4   MAJOR ASPIRIN TRIALS IN UNSTABLE ANGINA

STUDY	NO. PATIENTS	DOSE (mg/day)	DURATION OF FOLLOW-UP	RELATIVE RISK REDUCTION (%)
Lewis et al.[161]	1338	324	3 months	51
Cairns et al.[162]	555	1300	24 months	51
Theroux et al.[163]	479	650	6 days	72
RISC[164]	796	75	5 days	57
			3 months	68

In the Montreal Heart Institute Study, aspirin reduced the rate of myocardial infarction by 72 per cent compared to placebo.[163] In the European RISC study group,[164] patients with unstable angina or non-Q-wave infarction were randomized to receive 75 mg/day of aspirin for 3 months, intravenous heparin for 5 days, both, or neither. At the end of 3 months, the incidence of death or myocardial infarction was significantly reduced by aspirin and, to a greater extent, by the combination of aspirin and heparin.

EFFICACY OF ANTICOAGULANTS (HEPARIN) ALONE AND WITH ASPIRIN (Table 58–5). The use of heparin for the treatment of unstable angina was suggested by Teleford and Wilson.[165] They demonstrated an 80 per cent reduction in myocardial infarction in patients with unstable angina treated with heparin for 7 days. The most convincing evidence comes from the Montreal Heart Institute Study[163] in which heparin reduced the total cardiac event rate by 57 per cent (P = 0.001) and fatal and nonfatal myocardial infarction by 85 per cent. (Aspirin also reduced the incidence of fatal and nonfatal myocardial infarction by 72 per cent, as mentioned previously.) The combination of aspirin and heparin was superior to aspirin alone, but had no increased benefit compared to heparin alone (Fig. 38–24, p. 1337). There was a trend toward less frequent myocardial infarction in the heparin group compared to the aspirin group. An extension of this study was subsequently performed that randomized patients to either aspirin or heparin. The combined results of these studies demonstrated the greater reduction in the rate of myocardial infarction with heparin over aspirin.[166]

It is important to be aware of a rebound phenomenon that may occur when heparin is discontinued. This effect may be blunted when aspirin is given as concomitant therapy.[164] The RISC[167] study examined patients with unstable angina or non-Q-wave myocardial infarction. Patients were randomized to receive aspirin and/or intermittent intravenous heparin. Aspirin therapy compared to no aspirin therapy significantly reduced the risk ratios of fatal or nonfatal myocardial infarction. Heparin did not show such benefit. However, the group treated with combination heparin and aspirin showed the lowest event rate at 5 days. The more recent ATACS trial[168] randomized patients, with either unstable angina or non-Q-wave myocardial infarction, to receive aspirin alone or aspirin plus anticoagulation (Fig. 58–13). There was significant reduction in total ischemic events in the combination group versus aspirin (3.8 versus 8.3 per cent, P = 0.004) at the end of 14 days. At the end of 12 weeks, there was a trend toward reduction in total ischemic events (13 versus 25 per cent, P = 0.06). In a more recent British trial, the combination of aspirin and heparin did not reveal further benefit than aspirin alone.[169]

Ticlopidine was examined in patients with unstable angina.[170] The administration of ticlopidine in a dose of 250 mg twice a day for 6 months was found to reduce the incidence of death and myocardial infarction by 46 per cent.

In *summary,* there is ample evidence to suggest that the use of aspirin or heparin in the early phase of unstable angina reduces the incidence of death and myocardial infarction. The combination of aspirin and heparin in unstable angina and non-Q-wave myocardial infarction may be more effective than either drug alone in reducing total ischemic events in the early phase of such unstable syndromes.[171]

DIRECT THROMBIN INHIBITORS AND IIb/IIIa PLATELET RECEPTOR BLOCKERS. Given the central role of thrombin in the coagulation process, there is much enthusiasm for the development of direct thrombin inhibitors for use in acute coronary syndromes. Several small studies have examined the efficacy of these agents in unstable angina.[172–174] Results of these studies were encouraging. However, the larger studies of hirudin, GUSTO II[175] in unstable angina and other acute coronary syndromes, and TIMI-9[176] in acute

TABLE 58–5   MAJOR ANTICOAGULANT (HEPARIN) TRIALS IN UNSTABLE ANGINA

TRIAL	NO. PATIENTS	FOLLOW-UP	DRUG	REDUCTION IN DEATH OR MI (%)	P
Teleford and Wilson[165]	214	7 days	Heparin	80	< .05
Theroux et al.[163–167]	479	6 days	Heparin	85	< .001
			Heparin + aspirin	88	.001
RISC[164]	796	3 months	Heparin	5	NS
			Heparin + aspirin	68	< .0005
ATACS[168]	214	5 days	Aspirin	—	—
			Heparin + aspirin	46	.06
Holdright et al.[169]	285	6 days	Aspirin	—	—
			Heparin + aspirin	—	NS

MI = myocardial infarction.

myocardial infarction required reduction of the planned dose because of an observed increase in hemorrhagic stroke. In addition, HIT III[177] in acute myocardial infarction was terminated because of excessive bleeding with hirudin. With a change in dosage, the large trials GUSTO IIb and TIMI 9B have been completed and the results are being tabulated.

Most importantly, following the promising pilot studies in variable angina,[177a–c] platelet receptor blockade (c7E3) has just been preliminarily reported to be of most benefit in patients with refractory unstable angina (the CAPTURE study).

THROMBOLYTICS. At the present time there is little experimental evidence to support the use of thrombolytic therapy in unstable angina. There are many small and inconclusive studies conducted during the 1980–1990 period evaluating the use of thrombolytic therapy in unstable angina.[178] Many of these studies are difficult to evaluate because of different patient populations, timing of angiography, dose, and route of administration of the thrombolytic agent.

Two large recent trials evaluating thrombolytics give important insight into the issue of thrombolytic agents in unstable angina. The Unstable Angina Study using Eminase (UNASEM) trial was a large, randomized, placebo-controlled trial designed to evaluate both the angiographic and clinical outcome of the use of APSAC in unstable angina.[179] The improvement with APSAC of the occluded arteries (26 per cent of the APSAC group and 18 per cent of the placebo group had total occlusion of the artery) accounted for a favorable statistical difference in degree of stenosis before and after therapy. Despite a possible difference in angiographic appearance between the two groups, there was no significant difference in clinical outcome in the two groups. The TIMI-IIIB[180] study was designed to evaluate the use of t-PA and early angiography and revascularization for patients with unstable angina. At 42 days and 1 year, there were no differences in death and infarction between the two groups.

Possible reasons for the failure of thrombolytic therapy to improve outcome in unstable angina as opposed to acute infarction relate to pathophysiological observations in unstable angina. In unstable angina, the incidence of total occlusion of the culprit vessel is significantly lower than in acute myocardial infarction. In addition, Falk[181] found partial organization and layering of the thrombus in patients with unstable angina. Thus much of the thrombus formation in unstable angina may be beneath the fibrous cap, rather than within the lumen of the artery. This may allow only small amounts of thrombus to be accessible to the thrombolytic agent.

RECOMMENDATIONS. All patients with unstable angina should immediately receive at least 75 mg of chewable aspirin and intravenous heparin (bolus followed by continuous infusion in doses sufficient to raise the PTT to approximately 85 seconds). The combination of aspirin and heparin is probably more efficacious than either agent alone.[182] This is particularly true when one takes into account aspirin's ability to blunt the rebound phenomenon at the time of discontinuation of heparin. Ticlopidine can be used as an alternative treatment in patients intolerant or allergic to aspirin. At the present time there is little clinical evidence to recommend the administration of thrombolytic therapy to patients with unstable angina.

Acute Myocardial Infarction

Thrombolytic Therapy
(See also p. 1215)

INTRAVENOUS THROMBOLYTIC VERSUS CONVENTIONAL THERAPY[183] (Fig. 58–14). A definitive overview[184] of 24 trials of intravenous thrombolytic therapy conducted between 1959 and 1979 found that the pooled odds reduction of mortality was 22 ± 5 per cent (P < 0.001). However, generalizations to clinical practice were of uncertain relevance, and subsequent trials were designed to be of sufficient size individually to allow the evaluation of mortality.

Three published, well-designed prospective trials have demonstrated mortality reduction by intravenous streptoki-

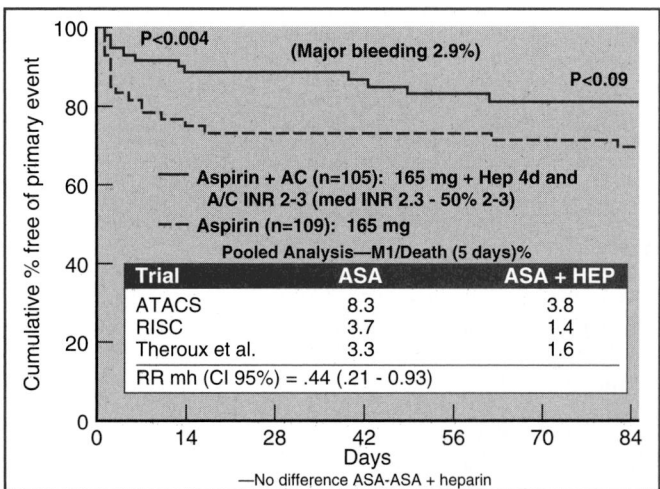

FIGURE 58–13. Data from the ATACS trial examining the use of aspirin versus aspirin plus anticoagulation in unstable angina and non-Q-wave myocardial infarction demonstrates improvement in event-free survival in the combination therapy group. Pooled analysis from ATACS, RISC, and the Theroux study groups demonstrates relative risk reduction (RR) of 0.44 in the combination group. ASA = aspirin; Hep = heparin. (From Holdright, D., Patel, D., Cunningham, D., et al.: Comparison of the effect of heparin and aspirin versus aspirin alone on transient myocardial ischemia and in-hospital prognosis in patients with unstable angina. J. Am. Coll. Cardiol. *24:*39, 1994. Reprinted by permission from the American College of Cardiology.)

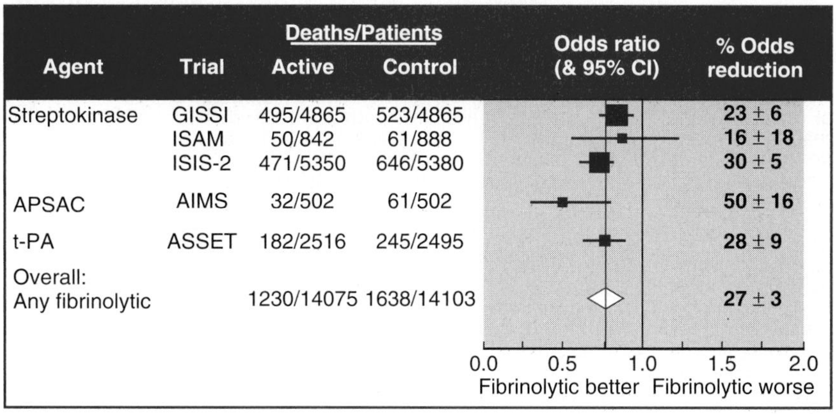

FIGURE 58–14. Reduction in mortality (3–5 weeks) among patients with myocardial infarction treated within 6 hours of symptom onset in the five major placebo-controlled trials of thrombolytic therapy. ci = confidence interval. (From Granger, et al.: Thrombolytic therapy for acute myocardial infarction: A review. Drugs 44(3):293, 1992. With permission.)

nase (SK).[185–187] The GISSI-I study[185] randomized patients to SK or conventional therapy (i.e., no placebo control). Hospital mortality was significantly reduced from 13.0 to 10.7 per cent, an 18 per cent risk reduction. The ISIS-II study,[186] using placebo controls, randomized patients to SK, aspirin (160 mg enteric coated daily for 1 month, the first tablet chewed at the time of study entry), both, or neither, according to factorial design. The 5-week vascular mortality was significantly reduced from 12.0 to 9.2 per cent, a 23 per cent risk reduction by SK when compared with no SK, and from 13.2 to 8 per cent, a 39 per cent risk reduction by the combination of SK and ASA when compared to no SK or aspirin. The ISAM Study with SK showed 16 per cent risk reduction.[187]

The AIMS[188,189] randomized patients to APSAC or placebo, and 30-day mortality was significantly reduced from 12.1 to 6.4 per cent, a 50.5 per cent odds reduction of mortality. However, the trial was stopped early by the Data Monitoring Committee, so the magnitude of the true benefit may have been overestimated.

The ASSET trial[190,191] randomized patients to intravenous rt-PA or placebo. All patients received intravenous heparin for 24 hours. The 1-month all-cause mortality was significantly reduced by rt-PA from 9.8 to 7.2 per cent, a 28 per cent odds reduction. The European Cooperative Trial[192] randomized patients to rt-PA (100 mg single chain) or placebo infusion over 3 hours, all patients receiving heparin and low-dose aspirin. At 21 days, there was a nonsignificant difference in mortality (3.7 per cent with rt-PA versus 6.8 per cent with placebo).

The Fibrinolytic Therapy Trialists' (FTT) Collaborative Group reported on an overview of the results of all trials of fibrinolytic therapy versus control that randomized more than 1000 patients with suspected acute myocardial infarction.[193] Among the 58,600 patients included in these trials, mortality at 35 days was reduced from 11.5 to 9.6 per cent, and 18 per cent odd reduction (Fig. 37–26, p. 1217).

STUDIES COMPARING INTRAVENOUS THROMBOLYTIC AGENTS[182] (Table 58–6). The clot specificity of rt-PA compared to SK offered the promise of greater efficacy and fewer complications from bleeding, hypotension, and allergic reaction. APSAC also offered promise because of its relative clot specificity compared to SK. However, no distinct advantages of any available thrombolytic agent emerged from the individual placebo-controlled trials, and it became clear that direct comparisons in large trials were necessary to determine relative efficacies and side effect profiles.

GISSI-2 TRIAL. This was a multi-center, randomized open-label trial designed to compare SK to alteplase (single-chain rt-PA).[194] In this 2 × 2 factorial design, patients were also randomly allocated to heparin (12,500 units subcutaneously, beginning at 12 hours, and repeated every 12 hours to hospital discharge) or usual therapy. Oral acetylsalicylic acid (ASA) (300 to 325 mg/day) was recommended for all patients. Hospital mortality was not significantly different at 8.6 per cent with SK and 9 per cent with rt-PA. Use of heparin did not alter the results. The International TPA/SK Mortality Trial[195] was a collaboration of the Italian GISSI-2 centers and those in several additional countries following the GISSI-2 protocol. Again there was no differ-

ence in hospital mortality between patients treated with SK and rt-PA.

ISIS-3. This was a multi-center, randomized trial, designed to address the following questions[196]: (1) Which of the three commonly used thrombolytic agents (SK, APSAC, and rt-PA), if any, is the most effective? (2) What are the effects of adding heparin to thrombolytic/aspirin regimens? Patients were further randomized in a factorial design to calcium heparin (12,500 units subcutaneously, the first dose about 4 hours postrandomization, and then every 12 hours for 7 days), or no heparin. All patients were expected to receive ASA (162 mg/day). Among the patients randomized, the vascular mortality rates at 35 days postrandomization were not as significant among the three groups: rt-PA, 10.3 per cent; SK, 10.6 per cent; APSAC, 10.5 per cent. Mortality was similar among the heparin-treated patients at 10.3 per cent, and the non-heparin-treated patients at 10.6 per cent. An overview[196] of the GISSI-2 and ISIS-3 data, based upon an analysis of 48,293 patients, found that 35 day mortality was 10.5 per cent with both rt-PA and SK.

GUSTO-I. The Global Utilization of Streptokinase and Tissue plasminogen activator for Occluded coronary arteries (GUSTO) trial[197] sought to determine whether a regimen designed to produce rapid and sustained infarct vessel recanalization was associated with improved survival. All patients received chewable aspirin, two 80 mg tablets, as soon as possible. They were randomized to one of four regimens: (1) rt-PA (alteplase) intravenous 15-mg bolus, then 0.75 mg/kg over 30 minutes, not to exceed 50 mg, then 0.5 mg/kg over 60 minutes, not to exceed 35 mg, the total dose not to exceed 100 mg. Simultaneously, heparin was begun with a 5000-unit intravenous bolus, followed by a continuous infusion of 1000 to 1200 units/hour for at least 48 hours, maintaining APTT at 60 to 85 seconds; (2) streptokinase 1.5 million units (MU) intravenously over 1 hour plus heparin intravenously in an identical regimen to that for the rt-PA group; (3) SK 1.5 MU intravenously over 1 hour plus heparin 12,500 units subcutaneously beginning 4 hours after initiation of SK and repeated every 12 hours for 7 days (or until prior discharge); (4) rt-PA 1.0 mg/kg intravenously over 60 minutes, maximum total dose 90 mg, including an initial bolus of 10 per cent of the total amount, plus simultaneously SK 1.0 intravenously over 60 minutes, plus heparin in an identical regimen to that for the rt-PA group. Mortality at 24 hours and 30 days was, respectively, for rt-PA 2.3 and 6.3 per cent; for rt-PA/SK 2.8 and 7.0 per cent; for SK (subcutaneous heparin) 2.8 and 7.2 per cent; and for SK (intravenous heparin) 2.9 and 7.4 per cent. The relative mortality reduction with accelerated rt-PA versus the SK alone group

TABLE 58–6 DEATH, TOTAL STROKE, AND CEREBRAL HEMORRHAGE IN THREE LARGE-SCALE MORTALITY TRIALS

	DEATH (%)	TOTAL STROKE (%)	HEMORRHAGE CEREBRAL (%)
GISSI-2 (n = 20,891)			
SK	9.2	0.94	0.29
t-PA	9.6	1.33	0.42
ISIS-3 (n = 41,299)			
SK	10.6	1.04	0.24
t-PA	10.3	1.39	0.66
APSAC	10.5	1.26	0.55
GUSTO-1 (n = 41,021)			
SK + SC heparin	7.2	1.22	0.49
t-PA + IV heparin	6.3	1.55	0.72
SK + IV heparin	7.4	1.40	0.54
t-PA + SK + IV heparin	7.0	1.64	0.94

From Hennekens, C. H., et al.: Current issues concerning thrombolytic therapy for acute myocardial infarction. Reprinted with permission from the American College of Cardiology. J. Am. Coll. Cardiol. 25(Suppl. 1):18S, 1995.

was 14 per cent, and the absolute mortality reduction was 1 per cent, which was significant. As shown in Table 8–6, hemorrhagic and total stroke were significantly more common with the accelerated rt-PA than the SK alone groups (0.72 per cent versus 0.52 per cent, P = 0.03), and 1.55 per cent versus 1.31 per cent). The composite outcome of death or nonfatal disabling stroke was less with accelerated rt-PA than SK (6.9 per cent versus 7.8 per cent). Major bleeding was not different among the four regimens.

The findings of the GUSTO trial suggest that for 1000 patients with evidence of acute myocardial infarction, treated within 6 hours of onset using accelerated rt-PA rather an SK, there would be ten fewer deaths, or nine fewer occurrences of a composite of death or nonfatal disabling stroke. However, the relative benefit is less evident in patients older than 75 years with inferior myocardial infarction, when therapy is initiated after 6 hours of infarct onset.[197]

TIMI-4. This trial[198] randomized patients to front-loaded rt-PA (GUSTO regimen), APSAC 30 units intravenously over 2 to 5 minutes, or a combination of a lower-dose rt-PA plus APSAC 20-unit bolus. All patients received aspirin and heparin. In-hospital mortality was 2.2 per cent with rt-PA, 8.8 per cent with APSAC, and 7.2 per cent with the combination (rt-PA versus APSAC, significant; rt-PA versus combination, nonsignificant).

RECOMMENDATIONS. As of this writing, according to the above information and taking into account the higher cost of rt-PA, accelerated rt-PA would appear to offer reasonably cost-effective therapy and be preferable to SK for patients under age 75 years with large infarctions, when therapy can be initiated within 6 hours of onset of acute myocardial infarction.[183,199]

TIME DELAY TO THROMBOLYTIC THERAPY.[183] There is considerable clinical evidence to indicate that thrombolytic therapy begun within the first few hours after the onset of acute myocardial infarction results in greater benefit than when it is begun many hours after the onset (Fig. 37–28, p. 1219). Indeed, the highest priority in the thrombolytic treatment of myocardial infarction is to minimize the delays in the initiation of therapy, regardless of the agent used. In regard to late initiation of thrombolytic treatment, patients seen between 6 and 12 hours may still be good candidates for therapy, particularly those with anterior or large infarctions.[199]

Adjuvant Antithrombotic Therapy

ASPIRIN. The rationale for the use of aspirin along with thrombolytic therapy lies in the relatively high risk of reocclusion of 5 to 30 per cent, and a rate of reinfarction of about 4 per cent when aspirin is not used.[199] The ISIS-2 trial,[186] reviewed above, demonstrated a 5-week significant reduction in the odds of death of 23 per cent with aspirin, 25 per cent with SK, and 42 per cent with the combination. Among patients receiving SK, the reinfarction rate was reduced from 4 to 2 per cent. The addition of aspirin to SK caused less than a 1 per cent absolute increase of minor bleeding and no increase in major bleeding, while stroke incidence fell significantly. Although there has been no evaluation of the contribution of aspirin to the treatment with APSAC or rt-PA, the combined use has become standard. The Antiplatelet Trialists' overview[93] indicated that aspirin may be expected to reduce the odds of vascular mortality by about 15 per cent, and of fatal and nonfatal vascular events by about 25 per cent over an approximate 2-year period following the in-hospital phase of acute myo-

cardial infarction. These observations indicate that additional benefits of aspirin may be anticipated if it is continued beyond the 1 month protocol of the ISIS-2 study.

HEPARIN (Table 58–7). Low-dose, subcutaneous heparin (i.e., 7500 units), given until full ambulation, reduces calf vein thrombosis among patients with acute myocardial infarction, particularly those at risk (i.e., cardiac failure, late ambulation).[182]

The International Study Group,[195] and ISIS-3,[196] reviewed above, revealed minimal evidence for a benefit of subcutaneous heparin over placebo in patients treated with SK, rt-PA, or APSAC. Concerns that the heparin regimens employed in GISSI-2 and ISIS-3 may have been suboptimal prompted the use of aggressive intravenous regimens along with three of the four thrombolytic regimens evaluated in the GUSTO trial.[197] Heparin as a bolus of 5000 units intravenously was given immediately and followed by an infusion of 1000 to 1200 units/hour to maintain APTT at 60 to 85 seconds, in the accelerated rt-PA, the rt-PA/SK combination, and in one SK group. The other SK group received heparin subcutaneously according to the ISIS-3 protocol. Among the SK-treated patients, there was no difference in mortality, reinfarction, major hemorrhage, cerebral hemorrhage, patency, or reocclusion in relation to the heparin regimen. Hence, there was no evidence to indicate that intravenous heparin is superior to subcutaneous heparin among patients receiving SK.

RECOMMENDATIONS. According to the above information, there is no reason to routinely administer heparin along with SK, and it appears rational to reserve its use for those patients at high risk of systemic embolization because of congestive heart failure, large infarction, or atrial fibrillation. There has been no study among patients receiving rt-PA that has assessed the value of adjunctive heparin in relation to important patient outcomes. However, the results from the angiographic trials,[200–202] together with the short half-life and lesser systemic fibrinolytic effect of rt-PA, provide a rationale for adjunctive heparin for about 48 hours following administration of rt-PA.

Coronary Revascularization Procedures[203]
(See also Chaps. 38 and 39)

Atherothrombosis is not only the basis of coronary disease leading to the need for coronary artery bypass grafting and percutaneous coronary angioplasty, but it is also an important factor in the early complication rate of such interventions.

SAPHENEOUS VEIN BYPASS GRAFT DISEASE (see p. 1317) Vein graft disease can be divided into three phases: an early postoperative phase, within 1 month of thrombotic occlusion; an intermediate phase, within the first postoperative year, characterized by intimal hyperplasia resulting in a form of accelerated atherosclerosis that may have a superimposed thrombotic tendency; and a late phase, after the first postoperative year, composed of graft atherosclerosis similar to that affecting the native coronary arteries.[204] Accordingly, in the original Mayo Clinic trial on saphenous

TABLE 58–7   DATA FROM DIRECT COMPARISON OF ANTITHROMBOTIC REGIMENS: GISSI-2, ISIS-3, AND GUSTO-1

| Outcome | GISSI-2 AND ISIS-3 (ASA PLUS ANY THROMBOLYTIC AGENT) | | GUSTO-1 (ASA PLUS SK) | |
	No Heparin (n = 31,050)	SC Heparin (n = 31,017)	SC Heparin (n = 9971)	IV Heparin (n = 10,377)
Death	10.2	10.0	7.2	7.4
Reinfarction	3.3	3.0	3.4	4.0
Total stroke	1.2	1.2	1.3	1.4
Hemorrhagic stroke	0.4	0.5	0.5	0.5
Major bleeding	0.7	1.0	0.3	0.5

From O'Donnell, C. J., et al.: Antithrombotic therapy for acute myocardial infarction. J. Am. Coll. Cardiol. *25*(Suppl. I):23S, 1995.
ASA = aspirin; SK = streptokinase; SC = subcutaneous; IV = intravenous.

vein bypass grafting, patients received dipyridamole (100 mg four times daily) for 2 days before surgery, followed by aspirin (325 mg) and dipyridamole (75 mg) three times daily, starting 7 hours after surgery and continuing for 1 year. There was no increased incidence of bleeding complications in the treatment group. At vein graft angiography 1 month after surgery, there was significant reduction in graft occlusion in the treated group, from 10 per cent to 2 per cent distal graft anastomosis, and from 22 to 6 per cent per patient.[205,206] Reviews of all reported studies to date have convincingly demonstrated the importance of initiating platelet inhibitor therapy in the perioperative period, preferably before but not later than 48 hours after surgery. Indeed, when therapy was not started 48 hours after surgery, no reduction in the vein graft occlusion rate was observed.[207]

In the Veterans Administration Cooperative Study, patients receiving saphenous vein grafts were randomly assigned into five groups, taking 325 mg aspirin per day, 325 mg aspirin three times daily, 325 mg aspirin plus 75 mg dipyridamole three times daily, 267 mg sulfinpyrazone three times daily, or placebo. Early graft patency at a median of 9 days was significantly higher in the aspirin-treated group (92 per cent) than in those given placebo (85 per cent).[208] At 1 year, benefit was seen only in patients at high risk of graft occlusion (those with vein grafts placed to vessels ≤1.5 mm in diameter) taking aspirin.[209] It is important to note that one daily dose of aspirin was as effective as three daily doses. Dipyridamole conferred no additional benefit over aspirin alone.

In another Veterans Affairs Cooperative Study, preoperative aspirin use was associated with increased bleeding complications and no additional benefit in early vein graft patency compared with aspirin started 6 hours after surgery.[210] Other trials of antithrombotic therapy within the first year of saphenous vein bypass grafting have provided information of some interest: (1) Aspirin also, at the low dose of 100 mg/day, was found by Lorenz and colleagues[211] to be effective in reducing vein graft closure. (2) In one study, ticlopidine (250 mg twice daily), started on the second postoperative day, significantly reduced the incidence of vein graft occlusion by approximately 40 per cent, as assessed angiographically at 10, 180, and 360 days after surgery.[212] (3) Indobufen, a reversible inhibitor of platelet cyclooxygenase, in two recent 1-year studies appeared to be as effective as the combination of aspirin and dipyridamole in maintaining graft patency and was associated with a lower incidence of gastrointestinal side effects.[213,214] (4) Heparin and oral anticoagulants have been shown to be of some benefit for the prevention of graft occlusion in various trials[215,216]; however, the perioperative use of anticoagulants may be undesirable because of the risk of surgical bleeding.[216]

RECOMMENDATIONS. Platelet inhibitor therapy appears mandatory for prevention of early thrombotic occlusion of saphenous vein bypass grafts.[216] Aspirin should be started immediately after surgery and continued for at least 1 year and probably indefinitely. Ticlopidine can be used as an alternative treatment in patients intolerant or allergic to aspirin. No currently available agent prevents graft atherosclerosis, although control of risk factors such as hyperlipidemia and cigarette smoking may be beneficial.[217,218] In a new trial sponsored by the National Institutes of Health for

prevention of vein graft atherosclerosis, the use of aspirin and lipid-lowering therapy, either alone or in combination, is being tested.

OCCLUSION FOLLOWING CORONARY ANGIOPLASTY. As discussed in more detail in Chapter 39, thrombosis plays a major role among the several multifactorial pathophysiological processes responsible for early occlusion after percutaneous transluminal coronary angioplasty (which without technical and pharmacological precautions occurs in about 7 to 20 per cent of patients).[219]

RECOMMENDATIONS. Based on six reported studies, pretreatment with aspirin, combined with adequate heparinization throughout the procedure, is strongly recommended.[220] Ticlopidine can be used as alternative treatment in patients intolerant or allergic to aspirin. The results of clinical trials of use of different antiplatelet drugs and anticoagulant agents aimed at reducing the re-stenosis rate have been disappointing. However, interest in using the class of agents that act by inhibiting fibrinogen binding to the platelet GP IIb/IIIa receptor has been stimulated by a recent report (the EPIC study) that showed a reduced incidence of acute complications and delayed complications, including restenosis, following PTCA in the group of patients receiving the 7E3 antibody directed against the GPIIb/IIIa receptor complex.[112,113] This approach should be considered in patients at "high risk" for ischemic complications following angioplasty.[220] However, preliminary data on an interventional study (the EPILOG study) also suggest significant benefit in "lower-risk" patients.

In patients undergoing stent implantation, the use of aspirin and heparin, followed by short-term coumadin, is presently recommended. Less aggressive anticoagulation regimens, including only antiplatelet therapy (i.e., aspirin alone or in combination with ticlopidine), are not recommended in patients at high risk for subacute thrombosis after stent replacement.[220]

Postmyocardial Infarction and Stable Coronary Disease

Survivors of acute myocardial infarction are at moderate risk of recurrent infarction or cardiac death. Because morbidity and mortality following a mycoardial infarction may be related to arrhythmias, left ventricular dysfunction, and recurrent myocardial infarction, proving that antithrombotic therapy is beneficial in these patients has been difficult.

ASPIRIN AND OTHER PLATELET INHIBITORS (Table 58–8). Multiple trials examining the use of aspirin for the secondary prevention of myocardial infarction have been

TABLE 58–8 ASPIRIN IN CARDIOVASCULAR DISEASE

CATEGORY OF TRIAL	NO. TRIALS	MI, STROKE, OR VASCULAR DEATH Antiplatelet (%)	Controls (%)	Odds Ratio and Confidence Interval	% Odds Reduction (SD)
Prior MI	11	13.5	17.1		25 (4)
Acute MI	9	10.6	14.4		29 (4)
Prior stroke/TIA	18	18.4	22.2		22 (4)
Other high risk	104	6.9	9.2		32 (4)
All high risk (4 main categories)	142	11.4	14.7		27 (2)
All low risk (primary prevention)	3	4.46	4.85		10 (6)
All trials (high or low risk)	145	9.5	11.9		25 (2)

0   0.5   1.0   1.5   2.0
better | worse
Treatment effect 2P < 0.00001

Data from Antiplatelet Trialists' Collaboration: Collaborative overview of randomised trials of antiplatelet therapy: I. Prevention of death, myocardial infarction, and stroke by prolonged antiplatelet therapy in various categories of patients. Br. Med. J. *306*:81, 1994. With permission.
SD = standard deviation; MI = myocardial infarction; TIA = transient ischemic attack.

conducted. However, no single study has provided definitive results. The results of a meta-analysis that included more than 18,000 patients revealed that platelet inhibitor therapy reduced cardiovascular mortality by 13 per cent, nonfatal reinfarction by 31 per cent, and nonfatal stroke by 42 per cent,[93] with overall risk reduction of 25 per cent. Aspirin alone was at least as effective as the combination of aspirin and dypyridamole and more effective than sulfinpyrazone. Available data do not justify the additional cost and frequency of administration of drugs other than aspirin in this group of patients. Medium-dose aspirin (75 to 325 mg) was as efficacious as higher-dose aspirin. No studies on the use of ticlopidine for secondary prevention are available.

Evidence from a 5-year trial of aspirin (975 mg/day) plus dipyridamole (225 mg/day) for prevention of progression of coronary disease in patients with stable angina revealed that these platelet inhibitors reduced new lesion formation as detected angiographically (with no effect on the progression of existing lesions) and reduced the incidence of myocardial infarction from 12 to 4 per cent (a 67 per cent reduction).[221] In a study of 333 men with chronic stable angina, aspirin alone (125 mg every other day) reduced the incidence of myocardial infarction by 87 per cent compared with placebo; there was only a slight trend toward decreased mortality, but the risk of stroke, presumed to be hemorrhagic, increased.[222] Similar favorable effects of aspirin in patients with stable coronary disease were reported in another study.[223]

ANTICOAGULANTS. Numerous studies have assessed the usefulness of anticoagulants in the secondary prevention of cardiovascular disease after myocardial infarction. The Warfarin and Reinfarction Study (WARIS) is the second largest study to date of anticoagulants in the secondary prevention of myocardial infarction (Fig. 58–15).[224] In this placebo-controlled, double-blind trial, patients were randomized after initial acute myocardial infarction to warfarin (target INR 2.8–4.8) or placebo. Patients were advised not to take aspirin during the trial. At mean follow-up of 37 months, warfarin resulted in significant reductions of mortality, total reinfarctions, nonfatal infarctions, and total strokes. Although four fatal intracranial hemorrhages occurred in the warfarin group compared to none in the placebo group, ten nonhemorrhagic fatal strokes occurred in the placebo group compared to none in the warfarin group.

The ASPECT trial,[225] the largest study of anticoagulants in secondary prevention following myocardial infarction,

was conducted concurrently with the WARIS trial, but was completed at a later date. Patients were randomized to phenprocoumon or acenocoumarol or placebo. The anticoagulant therapy was titrated to achieve an INR of 2.8 to 4.8, and the mean follow-up was 37 months. There was a significant reduction in recurrent myocardial infarction in the anticoagulant-treated group compared to the placebo-treated group (114 versus 242 patients; risk reduction, 53 per cent). There was, however, no significant difference in mortality between the placebo and anticoagulant groups. The anticoagulant-treated group experienced a larger number of hemorrhagic events than the placebo-treated group, and gastrointestinal-related bleeding accounted for half of the major bleeding episodes.

To study anticoagulation for patients with stable coronary disease, the Sixty Plus Reinfarction Study involved patients over 60 years of age who had been taking anticoagulants for a median time of 6 years after infarction. Patients were randomly assigned to continue anticoagulant therapy or placebo substitute for 2 more years. By intention-to-treat analysis, patients receiving anticoagulant therapy had a 26 per cent lower death rate (11.6 per cent compared with 15.7 per cent) and an impressive 51 per cent lower rate of reinfarction (4.1 per cent compared with 8.4 per cent) than patients taking placebo. A trend toward reduced frequency of cerebrovascular events was observed in the group receiving anticoagulant therapy.[226]

Two clinical trials compared warfarin with aspirin in secondary prevention of myocardial infarction. In the German-Austrian Myocardial Infarction Study (GAMIS), patients were randomized after acute myocardial infarction to open label phenprocoumon (target INR 2.5 to 5.0), aspirin 1.5 mg/day, or placebo.[227] No difference in mortality or reinfarction was observed between groups. The French Enquete de Prevention Secondaire de l'Infarctus de Myocarde (EPSIM)[228] revealed no difference in death or reinfarction in patients receiving either oral anticoagulants or aspirin. However, there was 54 per cent more patients with gastrointestinal events with aspirin and four times more severe hemorrhagic events with warfarin.

In the Aspirin Versus Coumadin in the Prevention of Reocclusion and Recurrent Ischemia After Successful Thrombolysis (APRICOT) trial, patients were randomized to either 325 mg/day of aspirin or to heparin followed by warfarin (target INR 2.8 to 4.0) after an initial angiogram < 48 hours after acute myocardial infarction revealed a patent infarct-related artery.[229] At 3 months there was no significant difference in reocclusion rates among the aspirin, warfarin, and placebo arms (25, 30, and 32 per cent, respectively). Aspirin significantly reduced reinfarction in comparison to placebo, but not to warfarin (3, 11, and 8 per cent respectively). Mortality did not differ between the groups.

Currently there are two randomized studies examining the unsolved issue of the combination of anticoagulants and antiplatelet regimens after acute myocardial infarction.[230] The CARS trial is studying patients randomized to three treatment regimens: (1) 160 mg/day of aspirin; (2) 80 mg/day of aspirin plus 3 mg of warfarin; (3) a combination pill of 80 mg of aspirin plus 1 mg of warfarin per day. The CHAMP study is randomizing patients to receive either 160 mg/day of aspirin or 80 mg of aspirin plus Coumadin to achieve an INR of 1.5 to 2.5.

RECOMMENDATIONS. When the results of trials of aspirin and anticoagulant therapy for secondary prevention in survivors of myocardial infarction and in patients with stable coronary disease are analyzed together, both treatments appear to confer protection against death and reinfarction. Thus, for most patients the advantage of aspirin over anticoagulant agents is not higher effectiveness but lower costs, ease of administration, and less need for monitoring. For patients intolerant of aspirin, at risk of embolism from the left ventricle (i.e., those with mural thrombi or severe myo-

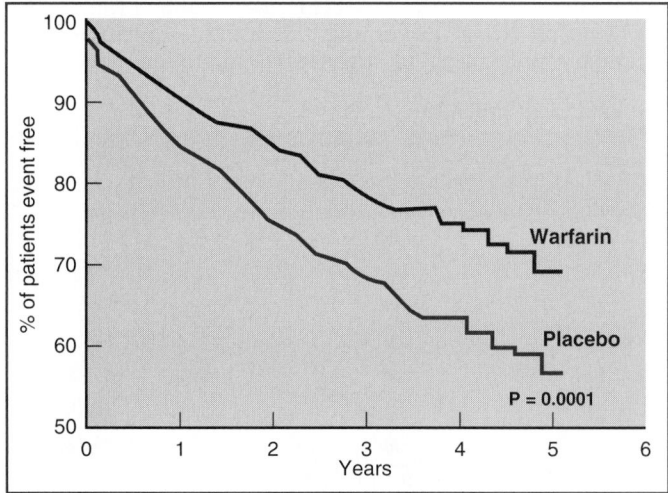

FIGURE 58–15. The WARIS Trial Study of anticoagulants in the secondary prevention of myocardial infarction. Cumulative rates (Kaplan-Meier) of total mortality, recurrent myocardial infarction, and stroke. (From Smith, P., Arnesen, H., and Holme, I.: The effect of warfarin on mortality and reinfarction after myocardial infarction. N. Engl. J. Med. *323:*147, 1990. Copyright Massachusetts Medical Society.)

ENDPOINT	REDUCTION (% ± SD)			P VALUE
	U.S. Physicians' Health Study	British Doctors' Trials	Overview of Both Trials	
Nonfatal myocardial infarction	39 ± 9	3 ± 19	32 ± 8	< 0.0001
Nonfatal stroke	↑ 19 ± 15	↑ 13 ± 24	↑ 18 ± 13	NS
Total cardiovascular deaths	2 ± 15	7 ± 14	5 ± 10	NS
Any vascular event	18 ± 7	4 ± 12	13 ± 6	P < .05

Hennekens, C. H., Buring, J. E., Sandercock, P., et al.: Aspirin and other antiplatelet agents in the secondary and primary prevention of cardiovascular disease. Circulation 80:749, 1989.

cardial dysfunction) or left atrium (i.e., those with atrial fibrillation), or with prior embolism, oral anticoagulant treatment is preferred.

Primary Prevention

ASPIRIN. Because aspirin has a significant protective effect in secondary prevention of vascular disease, the possible benefit of aspirin in primary prevention has also been tested. Two randomized trials, the United States Physicians' Health Study[231,232] and the British Doctors' Trial,[233] have been conducted (Table 58–9).

Results from the United States trial of more than 22,000 male physicians, aged 40 to 84 years, assigned to receive aspirin (325 mg every other day) or placebo for 5 years, revealed a 44 per cent reduction in the incidence of myocardial infarction, from approximately 0.4 per cent to 0.2 per cent per year. This effect was limited to those older than 50 years. Over the 5-year period, the incidence of cardiovascular death was similar in the aspirin and placebo groups; in the aspirin-treated group there was a slight increase in hemorrhagic stroke that was not statistically significant (0.2 per cent in the aspirin group compared with 0.1 per cent in the placebo group), but there was a significant increase in gastrointestinal hemorrhage requiring transfusion (0.5 per cent in the aspirin group compared with 0.3 per cent in the placebo group).

In the British primary prevention trial of more than 5000 male physicians, ages 50 to 78 years, two-thirds were randomly assigned to take aspirin (500 mg/day) and one-third were instructed to avoid it (no placebo used). After 6 years, no difference in the rate of myocardial infarction or cardiovascular death was detected; however, as in the American study, there was a slight increase in disabling strokes among those assigned to aspirin.

Overall, the prevalence of cardiovascular events was quite low among the relatively healthy physicians who participated in these primary prevention trials. Even analyzing the most striking data, such as the rate of nonfatal myocardial infarction in the American study being reduced by 44 per cent, the absolute risk reduction was less than two events per 1000 per year. Thus, as previously discussed, there are clear problems in reporting risk reduction as a percentage when the absolute prevalence of events is low. Furthermore, in the more favorable American study, for the combined endpoints of all important cardiovascular events (myocardial infarction, stroke, and death), the risk reduction favoring aspirin was only 18 per cent. Therefore, based on these studies the use of aspirin in an overall healthy population for primary prevention of coronary events is not justified.

Although in these relatively low-risk apparently healthy populations the per cent reduction in the rate of myocardial infarction was similar whether or not risk factors for coronary disease were present, it seems important to consider the absolute prevalence of events. The rate of myocardial infarction was consistently higher among patients with these risk factors than among those without—ranging from 1.4-fold in those with a parental history of coronary disease to 5-fold in those with diabetes, with intermediate incre-

ments associated with smoking, hypercholesterolemia, and hypertension. Thus, in primary prevention the absolute impact is greater in groups with a high-risk factor profile.[234]

RECOMMENDATIONS. Given the available data, it now seems reasonable to advocate the use of aspirin in a dose of 75 to 325 mg/day (body weight may be a guide) or every other day in patients with clinical manifestations of coronary disease, if no specific contraindications are present.[182] For primary prevention, aspirin should be considered only in men over the age of 50 with uncontrolled risk factors for the development of coronary events.[182] However, aspirin should be used cautiously, if at all, in patients with poorly controlled hypertension. Furthermore, aspirin should be viewed as a possible adjunct, rather than as an alternative to the management of coronary risk factors. Most important, although the short-term benefit of aspirin in these populations appears to outweigh its risk, the long-term advantages and toxicity of the drug remain uncertain.

Observational epidemiological studies in primary prevention have suggested a possible benefit of aspirin in women[235]; however, definitive recommendations for women, particularly in those with uncontrolled risk factors, will have to await the results of the Women's Health Study, a large randomized trial of low-dose aspirin use among more than 40,000 female nurses 45 years old and older. In an ongoing thrombosis prevention trial among men at high risk of coronary heart disease,[236,237] the effects of low-dose aspirin (75 mg/day), low-dose warfarin, and the combination of both agents in being evaluated. The results of this trial will define further the role of antithrombotic agents in primary prevention.

ANTITHROMBOTIC THERAPY FOR CARDIAC CHAMBER THROMBOEMBOLISM

(Table 58–3)

Atrial Thrombosis

Atrial thrombosis occurs in patients with valvular heart disease and with nonvalvular atrial fibrillation. The pathogenesis is probably dominated by stasis and the generation of fibrin, but endocardial abnormalities and activation of platelets may contribute under some circumstances. Standard techniques are much less reliable for detecting thrombi in the atrium than in the ventricle. Two-dimensional echocardiography detected 30 to 60 per cent of thrombi in the body of the left atrium[238,239] but did not detect thrombosis in the left atrial appendage and most small thrombi in the body of the atrium. Transesophageal echocardiography has permitted excellent imaging of both atria and atrial appendages and appears to be sensitive for the detection of thrombi.[240] However, this technique has not been used to determine the frequency of atrial thrombi in large-scale clinical studies. Consequently the prevalence of left atrial thrombosis in various cardiovascular disease is uncertain. On the basis of autopsy studies in patients with rheumatic heart disease, about half of patients with atrial fibrillation have atrial thrombi (range 24.5 to 55.2 per cent) compared with 15 per cent of patients with sinus rhythm (range 6.5 to 22 per cent).[241] With the use of transesophageal echocardiography, new insights may be gained into the prevalence of atrial thrombosis and risk of thromboembolism in valvular heart disease and nonvalvular atrial fibrillation.

Valvular Heart Disease

MITRAL STENOSIS (see p. 1009). The incidence of thromboembolism complicating mitral stenosis is reported to be 1.5 to 4.7 per cent per year.[242] Up to 75 per cent of clinically significant embolic episodes involve the cerebral circulation, and this may be the initial manifestation of disease in more than 10 per cent of cases. The risk of emboli increases with age and correlates inversely with cardiac output, but it is unrelated to left atrial size, valve area, or functional class.[242,243] The most significant risk factors are atrial fibrillation and previous embolism. The risk of embolism in mitral stenosis increases by 7-fold to 18-fold with the onset of atrial fibrillation, and nearly 75 per cent of the patients who have emboli have chronic atrial fibrillation.[242,243] Up to 30 per cent of emboli occur in the first month of onset of atrial fibrillation, and 66 per cent occur within the first year.[242,243] Thus, it is important to anticipate atrial fibrillation, or detect it early, so that prophylactic anticoagulant therapy can be administered. There is recurrence of emboli in up to 65 per cent of cases, mostly in the first 6 to 12 months, resulting in a substantial mortality.[242,243]

No prospective randomized studies have evaluated the effectiveness of anticoagulants in preventing systemic thromboemboli in mitral stenosis. However, several descriptive studies report that warfarin appears to be effective in preventing recurrent emboli.[242]

MITRAL REGURGITATION (see p. 1020). This valvular lesion is associated with a somewhat lower risk of systemic emboli than is mitral stenosis.[242,243] Systemic embolism occurred at the rate of one to 2 events per 100 patient years when the lesion is relatively mild and isolated, but it occurred at the rate of up to 4 events per 100 patient years when regurgitation was severe, or when mixed stenosis and regurgitation were present.[242,243] Up to 14 to 18 per cent of such patients may ultimately suffer thromboembolic complications. In the Mayo Clinic study of patients with severe isolated mitral regurgitation, a moderately high incidence of 2.9 thromboembolic events per 100 patient years was found.[244] The risk of embolism with mitral regurgitation is much higher in the presence of atrial fibrillation. In the series of Coulshed and associates of over 800 patients with rheumatic mitral disease, 7.7 per cent of those with predominant regurgitation with sinus rhythm had emboli, compared with 22 per cent of patients with atrial fibrillation. In contrast, when mitral stenosis was the dominant lesion, 8 per cent of patients with sinus rhythm had emboli, compared with 32 per cent with atrial fibrillation.[243]

MITRAL VALVE PROLAPSE (see p. 1031). This condition is very prevalent in the general population; it is usually well tolerated and asymptomatic. In a small percentage of patients, however, serious symptoms may occur, including transient or permanent cerebral ischemic events, which may be recurrent.[242,245] The pathogenesis of these adverse events has been linked to abnormalities of the valvular endocardium detected at autopsy, including thickening, endocardial denudation, and inflammatory changes.[242] Deposits of fibrin and platelet aggregates have been detected on the surface of valves in patients dying of embolic complications.[242] Echocardiographically these changes are manifested as valvular leaflet redundancy, which in one study was suggested to predict embolic risk.[246] Nevertheless, in this study, of 10 patients with embolism, only 2 experienced embolic complications in the absence of other risk factors, including atrial fibrillation, left ventricular thrombus, or infective endocarditis. This latter observation supports the common view that there is a low risk of thromboembolism with mitral valve prolapse in the absence of other predisposing conditions. Accordingly, routine prophylaxis is unwarranted in patients with mitral valve prolapse in the absence of other conditions that predispose to thromboembolism, such as atrial fibrillation or left ventricular dysfunction.

AORTIC VALVE DISEASE (see p. 1037). Very few long-term studies are available to define what appears to be a very low incidence of thromboembolism in aortic valve disease. In one study, 68 patients with moderate to severe aortic regurgitation were observed for 10 years; embolic complications occurred in 4.4 per cent for a low overall event rate of 0.083 per cent per 100 patient years.[247] In aortic stenosis, accurate diagnosis of embolic events may be confounded by the frequent occurrence of neurological symptoms due to abnormal hemodynamics or arrhythmias. Additionally, many of the emboli that are detected are probably calcific. Calcareous emboli have been found in up to 19 per cent of cases at autopsy[248]; although clinically significant embolic events have been reported involving the retinal circulation,[249] most calcific emboli are probably small and subclinical.

RECOMMENDATIONS.[242,250] 1. Patients with mitral regurgitation or mixed lesions (stenosis and regurgitation) with atrial fibrillation are at moderate risk for systemic embolism and should receive long-term oral anticoagulation to maintain the INR at 2.0 to 3.0. Patients with mitral stenosis and atrial fibrillation, and those with valvular heart disease and a prior thromboembolic event, are at higher risk and should receive anticoagulants with an INR of about 2.5 to 3.5.

2. In patients with mitral valve prolapse, if a transient ischemic attack (TIA) occurs, aspirin may be advised at a dose of 325 mg daily. However, in such cases, other causes of the cerebral symptoms should first be excluded. Few data are available upon which to base antithrombotic recommendations in the setting of clinically convincing recurrent TIAs or a definitive cerebral embolus in the patient with mitral valve prolapse; long-term anticoagulation with warfarin is justified in such cases at the lower intensity of an INR 2.0 to 3.0.

3. Routine anticoagulant therapy is not warranted in patients with aortic valve disease in the absence of other risk factors, such as atrial fibrillation.

4. Anticoagulant therapy is not warranted in infective endocarditis of a native valve. On the other other hand, anticoagulant therapy is recommended in nonbacterial thrombotic endocarditis.

Nonvalvular Atrial Fibrillation

Atrial fibrillation is a common cardiac arrhythmia of the elderly (p. 654), and stroke is its most devastating complication. The high risks of thromboembolism in atrial fibrillation associated with mitral stenosis and prosthetic mitral valves have long been appreciated (Table 58–3). However, atrial fibrillation carries a substantially increased risk of ischemic stroke even in the absence of these valvular disorders.[251] The rate of ischemic stroke among elderly people with atrial fibrillation averages 5 per cent a year, about six times that of people without atrial fibrillation.[252,253] Considering transient ischemic attacks (often causing radiographic evidence of brain infarction) and clinically occult stroke detected radiographically, the rate of brain ischemia accompanying nonvalvular atrial fibrillation exceeds 7 per cent a year—an impressive threat to the brain.[254,255] However, the absolute rate of stroke varies importantly with patient age and coexistent cardiovascular disease.[256-258] Stratification of atrial fibrillation patients into those at high and low risk of thromboembolism is a crucial determinant of optimal antithrombotic prophylaxis, as discussed in detail below.

Most ischemic strokes associated with atrial fibrillation

are probably due to embolism of stasis-induced thrombi forming in the left atrium, and particularly its appendage. Transesophageal echocardiography shows left atrial thrombi to be more frequent in atrial fibrillation patients who have suffered an ischemic stroke compared with atrial fibrillation patients without a stroke. However, perhaps 25 per cent of atrial fibrillation–associated stroke is due to associated intrinsic cerebrovascular diseases, other cardiac sources of embolism, or aortic arch atheroma.[259,260] Thus, about half of elderly atrial fibrillation patients have chronic hypertension, a major risk factor for primary cerebrovascular disease.[253] About 12 per cent of elderly atrial fibrillation patients harbor cervical carotid artery stenosis, but the frequency of carotid artery stenosis is not substantially greater in atrial fibrillation patients with stroke, suggesting that carotid artery stenosis is a minor contributor to atrial fibrillation–associated stroke.[251]

ATRIAL FIBRILLATION PATIENTS WITH HIGH AND LOW RATES OF THROMBOEMBOLISM (Table 58–10). The absolute rate of ischemic stroke in atrial fibrillation patients is crucially influenced by coexistent cardiovascular disease.[252] Identification of subpopulations of atrial fibrillation patients who have relatively high or low absolute rates of stroke determine which patients gain the greatest benefit from anticoagulant therapy. Two prospective studies included sufficient numbers of patients and stroke, analyzed by multivariable techniques, and provide the most reliable stratification schemes available.[253,254] The differences in the two schemes (presence of age versus heart failure) are not contradictory or even substantially conflicting, as clinical variables overlap (age is related to heart failure, hypertension, and diabetes). Interestingly, intermittent (i.e., paroxysmal) atrial fibrillation was *not* an independent predictor of thromboembolic risk in either study. In summary, the five clinical variables listed in Table 58–10 are independently predictive of thromboembolic risk and are clinically useful in characterizing atrial fibrillation patients with high and low risks for stroke.

Echocardiographic predictors of increased thromboembolic risk in atrial fibrillation are enlarged left atrial size (mitigated by mitral regurgitation) and impaired left ventricular function.[258,259] Impaired left ventricular function may contribute further to stasis within the left atrium in patients with atrial fibrillation.[260] Indeed, transthoracic echocardiographic findings can be combined with clinical risk stratifiers to identify atrial fibrillation patients with very low inherent rates of thromboembolism.[258] Transesophageal echocardiography offers better visualization of the left atrium and its appendage than conventional transthoracic echocardiography. With use of transesophageal echocardiography, left atrial appendage thrombi and spontaneous echogenic densities ("smoke"), possibly indicative of stasis, are more often found in atrial fibrillation patients with thromboembolism.[240] However, the predictive value of transesophageal echocardiographic findings for subsequent stroke has yet to be validated by adequate clinical studies.

ANTITHROMBOTIC THERAPEUTIC METHODS TO PREVENT STROKE. Anticoagulation with oral vitamin K antagonists such as warfarin is highly effective for reducing ischemic stroke in atrial fibrillation patients.[252,252a] Five recent randomized clinical trials using INR ranges of approximately 1.8 to 4.2 showed a mean reduction in ischemic stroke of nearly 70 per cent of patients assigned anticoagulation (Fig. 58–16); on-therapy analysis indicated an even greater benefit.[253] Furthermore, warfarin is particularly effective in subgroups of atrial fibrillation patients with a high inherent risk of thromboembolism (see Table 58–10).[253,261] The incremental risk of serious bleeding was < 1 per cent/year among anticoagulated patients selected for participation in these clinical trials and who were followed carefully on protocols. Low-intensity anticoagulation (INR 2.0 to 3.0) clearly confers benefit.[253,262]

The safety and tolerability of long-term anticoagulation titrated to conventional levels has not been well defined in the very elderly (age > 75 years), the age group encompassing perhaps half of atrial fibrillation–associated stroke. All but one of the placebo-controlled trials testing anticoagulation enrolled atrial fibrillation patients with a mean age in the late 60s.[253] The single placebo-controlled trial involving atrial fibrillation patients with a mean age of 75 years reported a 38 per cent withdrawal rate from anticoagulation after 1 year.[253,263] A relatively recent clinical trial comparing anticoagulation in atrial fibrillation patients under and over age 75 years found that the risk of major hemorrhage during anticoagulation (INR range 2.0 to 4.5, mean INR = 2.7) was substantially increased in patients over 75 years compared with younger ones anticoagulated to similar intensities.[253] While the very elderly have a

TABLE 58–10 RISK STRATIFICATION IN ATRIAL FIBRILLATION*: INDEPENDENT PREDICTORS OF THROMBOEMBOLIC RISK

	SPAF-I PLACEBO PATIENTS[118]	AFI POOLED ANALYSIS[114]
Number of patients	568	1236
Number of events	46	81
High-risk variables	History of hypertension Prior stroke/TIA Diabetes Recent heart failure	History of hypertension Prior stroke/TIA Diabetes Age > 65 years
Thromboembolic rate (95% CI)		
Low risk	1.4%/yr (0.05–3.7)	1.0%/yr (0.3–3.1)
High risk	> 7%/yr	> 5%/yr
Percentage of cohort "low risk"	38%	15%

* Large, prospectively acquired data sets analyzed by multivariable techniques. The SPAF-I placebo data set[118] was included in the pooled analysis of clinical trials by the Atrial Fibrillation Investigators.[114]

SPAF = Stroke Prevention in Atrial Fibrillation study, AFI = Atrial Fibrillation Investigators, CI = confidence interval.

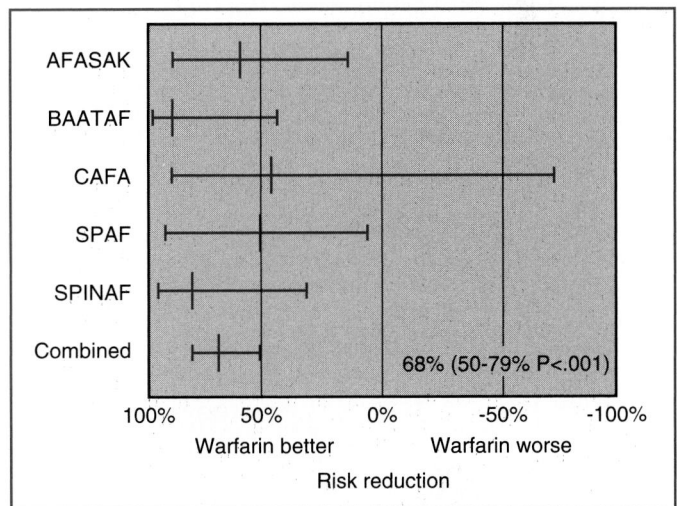

FIGURE 58–16. Risk-reduction plot of the results of five randomized clinical trials comparing warfarin with control for prevention of ischemic stroke in atrial fibrillation patients. Horizontal lines indicate the 95% confidence intervals around the point estimates (vertical lines) for each trial. The combined risk reduction was 68% (95% confidence interval, 50% to 79%; P < 0.991). See Atrial Fibrillation Investigators' pooled analysis for specific data. AFASAK = Atrial Fibrillation, Aspirin and Anticoagulant Therapy study; BAATAF = Boston Area Anticoagulation Trial for Atrial Fibrillation; CAFA = Canadian Atrial Fibrillation Anticoagulation study; SPAF = Stroke Prevention in Atrial Fibrillation study; and SPINAF = Stroke Prevention in Nonrheumatic Atrial Fibrillation study.

greater risk of atrial fibrillation–associated stroke, the benefit of anticoagulation was offset somewhat by the greater risk of bleeding in this age group. However, lower-intensity anticoagulation may be as effective and is certainly safer[262]; pending results of ongoing clinical trials, a target INR of 2.0 seems sensible in atrial fibrillation patients over age 75.

The efficacy of aspirin, an antiplatelet agent, for stroke prevention in atrial fibrillation patients is less clear and remains controversial.[252,253] The effects of aspirin in doses between 75 and 325 mg/day has been assessed in three randomized, placebo-controlled clinical trials with statistically significant risk reduction of about 25 per cent (range 14 to 44 per cent) in aspirin-treated patients, based upon pooled data.[254,264,265] However, aspirin was significantly less effective than anticoagulation in two of these clinical trials,[264,265] and also by secondary on-therapy analysis of the third trial (Fig. 58–17).[261] There is no compelling evidence that the specific dose of aspirin between 75 and 325 mg/day confers more or less benefit. In short, aspirin has some degree of efficacy for preventing atrial fibrillation–associated stroke, but it is clearly less than that of anticoagulation. Indeed, aspirin has a greater effect of noncardioembolic stroke than on those presumed to be cardioembolic.[266,267] Thus, it may be particularly effective in atrial fibrillation patients < 75 years old with a history of diastolic hypertension, who are at special risk for noncardioembolic stroke.[267] Most atrial fibrillation–related strokes, particularly in women, are due to cardiogenic embolism, and these strokes are more effectively prevented by anticoagulation.[266,268]

RECOMMENDATIONS.[252,269] Pending further clinical studies now ongoing, "low-risk" atrial fibrillation patients (Tables 58–3 and 58–10) may be given aspirin 325 mg/day to prevent stroke and carefully observed; this can be more specifically recommended for low-risk atrial fibrillation patients ≤ 75 years with a history of diastolic hypertension or coronary disease.[261,267] "Higher-risk" patients who can safely receive anticoagulation should be treated with warfarin. For higher risk atrial fibrillation patients ≤ 75 years, an INR range of 2.0 to 3.0 is safe and effective; for those over age 75, a lower target INR of 2.0 is recommended. Patients with atrial fibrillation who cannot safely receive anticoagulation

should be given aspirin. The value of other antiplatelet agents has not been assessed in patients with fibrillation.

SECONDARY PREVENTION OF STROKE IN ATRIAL FIBRILLATION PATIENTS. The risk of early recurrent stroke (within 2 weeks) is relatively low in atrial fibrillation patients.[270] Initiating oral anticoagulation within a few days in submassive cerebral infarcts seems reasonable; a delay in starting warfarin of 1 week or more in atrial fibrillation patients with large infarcts may be prudent to avoid accentuating secondary brain hemorrhage. The long-term rate of recurrent stroke is high, exceeding 10 per cent a year.[264] A large randomized trial demonstrated chronic anticoagulation (INR 2.5 to 4.0) to be highly effective (significantly more effective than aspirin) and relatively safe.[264] Because of the substantial rate of recurrent stroke, the absolute risk reduction by anticoagulation for secondary prevention clearly favors its use in most patients, with a recommended INR of 2.5 to 3.5 (Table 58–3).[264] Aspirin offers a lesser benefit for those who cannot receive anticoagulants for secondary prevention.[264]

ANTICOAGULATION FOR CARDIOVERSION. Systematic embolism is a complication of electric and pharmacological cardioversion of atrial fibrillation to sinus rhythm. Unfortunately there have been no randomized, prospective clinical trials to evaluate the usefulness of anticoagulant therapy to prevent emboli. The recommendations that follow are based on observations regarding intraatrial thrombus formation and noncontrolled published observations.[271,272]

A newly formed thrombus may take at least 2 weeks to become firmly attached to the atrial myocardium.[271] Further, after cardioversion, forceful atrial contractions may not resume for 2 weeks or longer.[271,273,274] Thus, in patients who have atrial fibrillation of unknown duration or for more than 48 hours, anticoagulation therapy should be given for 3 weeks prior to cardioversion (electric or pharmacological) and continued for at least 3 to 4 weeks after cardioversion[271,273,274]; that is, if not indicated permanently by the above-mentioned guidelines. Minimal data are available regarding embolic risk in patients with atrial fibrillation of short duration (< 48 hours). In most instances, anticoagulation prior to cardioversion may not be required, although it appears safer first to rule out left atrial thrombus by transesophageal echocardiography.[275] Indeed, the role of transesophageal echocardiography and the meaning of spontaneous echogenic diversities ("smoke") to guide anticoagulant therapy are now evolving.[277]

Ventricular Thrombosis

ACUTE MYOCARDIAL INFARCTION (see also p. 1256). The use of heparin in acute myocardial infarction may prevent the occurrence of left ventricular thrombus formation. Left ventricular thrombus develops in approximately 30 per cent of patients with anterior myocardial infarction and is associated with increased risk of subsequent arterial embolization.[278] Indeed, thrombus formation almost always occurs in the anterior wall, particularly the anteroapical areas of akinesis or dyskinesis.[279] Less than 5 per cent of patients with infarctions in other areas develop thrombus.[242] Other factors that predict left ventricular thrombus formation are ejection fraction, size of the infarct, and atrial fibrillation.[242] When thrombi occur, they usually do so by the end of the first week, with peak incidence at 4 to 5 days of the infarct.[242] Echocardiography has 90 per cent specificity and 75 to 90 per cent sensitivity for detection of thrombus.[242]

Stroke. Combining the data from several large series, the incidence of stroke from any cause following myocardial infarction averages 2.9 per cent[242,280]; however, with the use of antithrombotic and thrombolytic therapy, the incidence of stroke within the first year after myocardial infarction has been estimated to be 1 per cent by the

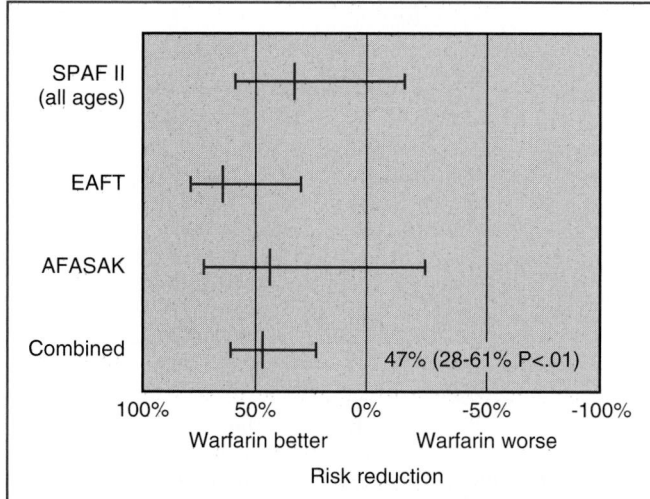

FIGURE 58–17. Risk-reduction plot of the results of three randomized clinical trials comparing warfarin with aspirin for prevention of ischemic stroke in atrial fibrillation patients. Horizontal lines indicate the 95% confidence intervals around the point estimates (vertical lines) for each trial. The combined estimated risk reduction from published results (intent to treat) was 47% (95% confidence interval, 28% to 61%) by warfarin relative to aspirin. SPAFII = Stroke Prevention in Atrial Fibrillation Trial II; and AFASAK = Atrial Fibrillation, Aspirin and Anticoagulant Therapy study.

SPRINT (Secondary Prevention Reinfarction Israeli Nifedipine Trial) Study Group.[281] In most, but not all, studies, the frequency of stroke has been reported to be higher in patients with larger infarcts. The risk of cerebral infarction in patients with known left ventricular thrombus not treated with anticoagulants ranges from 5 to 27 per cent (average 16 per cent), which is much higher than in those without left ventricular thrombosis, about 1.2 per cent. Within the group of patients with left ventricular thrombosis, high embolic risk is predicted by mobility of the thrombus on real-time echocardiography, or when the thrombus appears pedunculated and protrudes into the left ventricular cavity.[242] The risk of embolism in patients with left ventricular thrombosis is greatest in the first week to 3 months following myocardial infarction. Embolic risk may persist beyond this period, however, particularly in patients with severe left ventricular dysfunction (ejection fraction (EF) < 35 per cent), in those with persistence of mobile or protruding thrombi, and in those with a positive indium-111-labeled platelet scan.[242,280]

Vaitkus and Barnathan performed a meta-analysis of 19 studies with a total of more than 1000 patients, addressing efficacy of anticoagulants, platelet inhibitors, and thrombolytics on left ventricular thrombi and systemic emboli[282] (Fig. 58–18). There was no randomization to therapy, and the investigators were not blinded. This meta-analysis demonstrated significant reduction in the risk of embolism in patients recovering from a myocardial infarction who were treated with anticoagulants (Fig. 58–18). The effect of subcutaneous heparin on the incidence of intracardiac thrombosis was evaluated in two of these studies in which patients receiving 12,500 units every 12 hours were compared with either an untreated group or patients receiving 5000 units subcutaneously every 12 hours. In these two trials the incidence of mural thrombosis detected by 2-dimensional echocardiography was 72 and 58 per cent lower, respectively, in patients taking moderate doses (12,500 units) of heparin.[283,284]

RECOMMENDATIONS.[182] (1) During hospitalization, the use of moderate doses of subcutaneous heparin (12,500 units twice daily) is recommended in all patients with anterior myocardial infarction. (2) At the time of hospital discharge, medium-term (3 months) anticoagulants with Coumadin to an INR of 2.0 to 3.0 is recommended in patients with remaining large anterior myocardial infarction and in those patients who have visible left ventricular thrombus at echocardiography. (3) Indications of long-term anticoagulation in patients with left ventricular aneurysm and mural thrombi, and in postinfarction or ischemic cardiomyopathy, are discussed below.

LEFT VENTRICULAR ANEURYSM (see also p. 1347). Layers of thrombus are commonly found in left ventricular aneurysms.[242] Intraaneurysmal thrombi have been reported in 46 to 99 per cent of patients undergoing surgery and in 49 per cent of patients at autopsy.[242] The presence of a left ventricular aneurysm is a risk factor for persistence of a thrombus formed during the acute phase of myocardial infarction and for its recurrence after discontinuation of anticoagulants.[285] About 10 per cent of patients with intraaneurysmal thrombi will experience systemic embolization, the majority in the early weeks to 3 months following myocardial infarction. In a study of patients with chronic left ventricular aneurysm (more than 3 months following infarction), the incidence of emboli was reported to be very low, occurring in only 1 of 69 patients followed for 288 patient years (0.3 per cent per year).[286] Presumably this incidence is low because the organized thrombus is sequestered within the aneurysm and isolated from the dynamic forces of the circulation. The situation is different for patients with left ventricular aneurysm and a poor ejection fraction, or protruding thrombi,[287] in whom the risk of thromboemboli may continue long term.

Recommendations. (1) Because of the low risk of embolization in patients with chronic left ventricular aneurysm, it is likely that the risk of hemorrhage with oral anticoagulants would outweigh the benefits. Therefore, no anticoagulant therapy is advised beyond the first 3 months after infarction. (2) Patients with chronic left ventricular aneurysm and global severe left ventricular dysfunction, protruding thrombi, or prior embolism should be considered for long-term anticoagulant therapy at an INR of 2.0 to 3.0.

DILATED CARDIOMYOPATHY (see also p. 1407). Autopsy studies indicate that there is a high incidence of mural thrombi in patients with nonischemic dilated cardiomyopathy.[242] In one series, thrombus was found in 53 per cent of patients who died from dilated cardiomyopathy[288]; 45 per cent of thrombi were in the left ventricle, 25 per cent in the right ventricle, 20 per cent in the right atrium, and 8 per cent in the left atrium. Nearly 30 per cent of cases showed evidence of thrombosis in more than one cardiac chamber. In one study, a 36 per cent incidence of left ventricular thrombus was demonstrated echcoardiographically, with an 11 per cent incidence of systemic embolism in 192 patient years of follow-up.[289] In the Mayo Clinic study,[290] patients not receiving anticoagulants had an overall 18 per cent incidence of ischemic embolism—

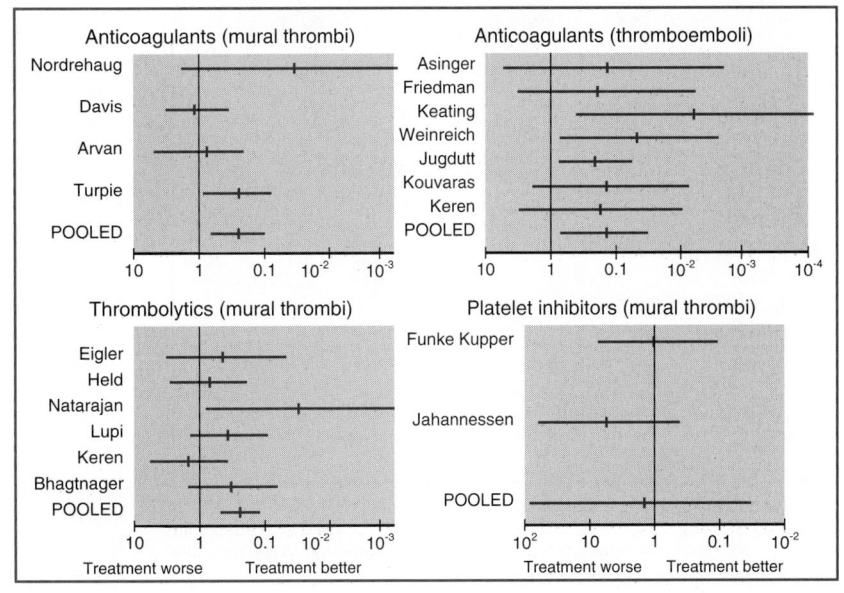

FIGURE 58–18. Meta-analysis of 19 studies of antithrombotic and thrombolytic therapy for the prevention of mural thrombus and systemic emboli after a myocardial infarction. (Modified from Vaitkus, P. T., and Barnathan, E. S.: Embolic potential, prevention and management of mural thrombus complicating anterior myocardial infarction. A meta-analysis. J. Am. Coll. Cardiol. *22*:1004, 1993. Reprinted with permission from the American College of Cardiology.)

thromboembolic rate at 3.5 events per 100 patient years—occurring in 14 per cent of patients with sinus rhythm and 33 per cent of patients with atrial fibrillation. Overall, in retrospective uncontrolled studies, great variation has been reported in the annual incidence of clinically apparent embolization, which ranged from less than 1 per cent to 12 per cent.[290-294] The risk is greatest in patients with severe left ventricular dysfunction (ejection faction ≤ 35 per cent), established or paroxysmal atrial fibrillation, a history of thromboembolism, or echocardiographic evidence of thrombus.[291,294]

Pulmonary embolism is reported to occur with a frequency of 5 to 11 per cent[295,296] and is associated with significant mortality.[296,297] No prospective randomized trials of anticoagulation in dilated cardiomyopathy have been conducted. However, in the Mayo Clinic study, patients receiving anticoagulants had no thromboembolic events in 101 patient years of follow-up[290]; other observational studies suggest similar protective effects of anticoagulants (Table 58–11).

In ischemic cardiomyopathy, the incidence of systemic emboli appears to be significantly lower than in nonischemic cardiomyopathy,[298] perhaps because in ischemic cardiomyopathy akinetic regions predispose to thrombosis and not to emboli, while in nonischemic cardiomyopathy myocardial dysfunction and stasis predispose to thrombosis,[298] and also to emboli because of some degree of global contractility.[291,293,299] This different pathophysiology may explain in part the controversy in left ventricular failure whether anticoagulants are of benefit (nonischemic cardiomyopathy?)[290,291,294] or whether they are not (ischemic cardiomyopathy?).[300-302]

Recommendations. (1) In nonischemic dilated cardiomyopathy, in view of the moderate risk of embolism in these patients and the apparent efficacy of anticoagulants in its prevention, medium-intensity anticoagulant therapy (INR 2.0 to 3.0) is recommended pending further studies; this indication is stronger in the presence of atrial fibrillation, significant left ventricular dysfunction and/or failure, or history of thromboembolism and/or left ventricular thrombus at echocardiography. (2) In patients with ischemic dilated cardiomyopathy, cardiac failure alone may not be an indication for anticoagulation, unless there is atrial fibrillation or history of thromboembolism and/or left thrombus at echocardiography.[242,280]

TABLE 58–11 THROMBOEMBOLISM IN NONISCHEMIC CARDIOMYOPATHY

AUTHOR	SYSTEMIC EMBOLI INCIDENCE	
	% NO A/C	% A/C
Fuster, V., et al.[290] (n = 104)	18	0
Gottdiener, J. S., et al.[289] (n = 123)	11	
Kyrle, P. A., et al.[290a] (1985) (n = 38)	44	0
Roberts, W. C. et al.[290b] (1987) (n = 152 autopsy)	39 (clinical)	
Ciaccheri, M., et al.[290c] (1989) (n = 126)	8	0
Yokota, Y., et al.[290d] (1989) (n = 40) (n = 17 autopsy)	20	0

A/C = anticoagulants.

Modified from Falk, R. H., Foster, E., and Coats, M. H.: Ventricular thrombi and thromboembolism in dilated cardiomyopathy: A prospective follow-up study. Am. Heart J. *123*:136, 1992.

ANTITHROMBOTIC THERAPY IN PROSTHETIC HEART VALVE REPLACEMENT

Incidence of Thromboembolism With and Without Appropriate Anticoagulation
(See also pp. 1835 to 1836)

The overall incidence of ischemic thromboembolism in patients taking anticoagulants, as expressed per 100 patients times years of exposure, is about 2.5 per cent for the Starr-Edwards and Omniscience prostheses, 2 per cent for the Medtronic Hall prosthesis, 1.5 per cent for the St. Jude Medical prosthesis, and 1 per cent for the pericardial and porcine bioprostheses.[303,304] Without anticoagulation, the incidence tends to double. The incidence of thromboembolism is cumulative, and the risk is persistent throughout the years of follow-up. However, recent observations have revealed that the highest incidence of thromboembolism is within the first 30 postoperative days (being particularly high within the first 10 days) for both bioprosthetic and mechanical prosthetic valves.[305,306] Patients with a prior embolus are also at great risk for recurrence. In the Mayo Clinic series, 20 per cent of patients with mitral prostheses and 27 per cent with aortic prostheses had recurrent embolism.[304] A history of an embolus preceding surgery was also predictive of an increased risk of postoperative embolus.[304] This has also been found in patients with nonvalvular trial fibrillation and suggests that some persons may be predisposed in some way to thromboembolic complications. Overall there has been a decreasing risk of thromboembolism after valve replacement in recent years, probably as a result of factors involving both patients and valves.[304] Patients now are usually operated on when their disease is less advanced than in the past. This means that the incidence of atrial fibrillation is generally lower, left atrial size is smaller, and left ventricular function is better at operation. Also, the mechanical prosthetic valves themselves have been improved, with design modifications that result in less turbulent flow and better hemodynamics.

Maintenance of adequate anticoagulation is also critical in the prevention of valvular thrombosis. In patients who were not treated or were inadequately treated with anticoagulants, valvular thrombosis has been reported in approximately 5 to 6 per cent of Bjork-Shiley valves in the mitral position and 2 to 3 per cent of such valves in the aortic position.[304] Even the St. Jude Medical valve, which is widely held to be less thrombogenic than other mechanical prostheses, was associated with a 5 per cent rate of valve thrombosis in patients who did not receive anticoagulants.[304] In contrast, adequately treated patients have a risk of valve thrombosis of 0.2 to 1.8 per cent per year, regardless of valve model or position.[304,307]

OPTIMIZATION OF ORAL ANTICOAGULANTS. The optimal anticoagulant regimen may be defined as that intensity of anticoagulation that leads to the lowest incidence of valve thrombosis, or systemic embolism, with the minimum number of bleeding episodes. It appears from retrospective studies of late postoperative thromboembolic and bleeding complications that the generally recommended INR of 3.0 to 4.5 may not be necessary after aortic and/or mitral valve replacement with mechanical prostheses.[308,309] Thus, for mechanical prostheses, an INR of 2.5 to 3.5 may be adequate (Table 58–3) (Fig. 58–19); a lower level of anticoagulation with an INR of 2.0 to 3.0 may suffice in bioprosthetic valves in atrial fibrillation or no anticoagulation at all (sinus rhythm) in bioprosthetic valves in sinus rhythm. A large-scale, prospective, randomized trial (GELIA) has been started, therefore, to provide conclusive evidence regarding the optimum level of anticoagulation after valve replacement with the St. Jude Medical prosthesis.

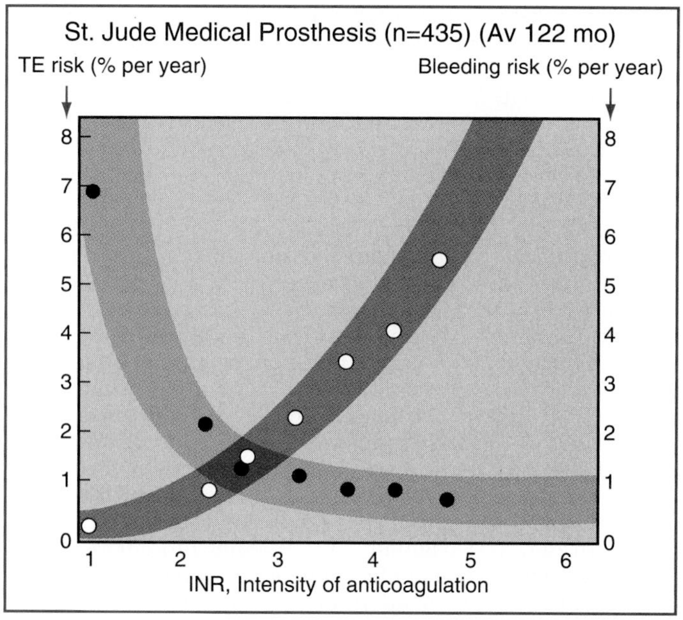

St. Jude Medical Prosthesis (n=435) (Av 122 mo)

TE risk (% per year)   Bleeding risk (% per year)

INR, Intensity of anticoagulation

FIGURE 58–19. Thromboembolic and bleeding risks with different anticoagulation regimens in 435 consecutive patients with St. Jude valve replacement. (Modified from Piper, C., Schulte, H. D., and Horstkotte, D.: Optimization of oral anticoagulation for patients with mechanical heart valve prostheses. J. Heart Valve Dis. 4:127, 1995. With permission.)

PLATELET INHIBITOR THERAPY ALONE AND COMBINED WITH ANTICOAGULANTS. No randomized placebo-controlled clinical trials have tested the use of platelet inhibitors alone as an antithrombotic regimen in mechanical heart valve replacement. However, the use of combination antiplatelet therapy with dipyridamole and aspirin, or pentoxifylline and aspirin, was associated with a significantly higher incidence of thromboembolism when compared with warfarin in an open prospective randomized trial of patients with mitral or aortic Starr-Edwards valves.[310] In addition, in other nonrandomized series, aspirin alone, dipyridamole alone, or the combination of both did not show a significant protective effect.[242] Results in several small nonrandomized trial suggest that platelet inhibitors may provide adequate protection for children with normal sinus rhythm and mechanical prostheses in the aortic position, but such findings must be considered preliminary pending further investigation.[304] Once again, data are very limited concerning the use of platelet inhibitors in patients with bioprosthetic heart valve replacements, and no randomized or placebo-controlled study has been conducted.

Although consistent and optimal anticoagulant therapy is critical for patients with mechanical heart valve prostheses, there is still a relatively high residual risk of systemic thromboembolism. As a result, five randomized controlled trials have been conducted comparing the antithrombotic efficacy of warfarin plus dipyridamole versus warfarin alone in recipients of mechanical ball or tilting disc valves. In three trials, combination therapy was significantly better than warfarin alone, resulting in a 70 to 92 per cent reduction in embolic events. In two other trials the addition of dipyridamole to the warfarin regimen resulted in a 40 to 50 per cent decrease in embolic episodes compared with warfin therapy alone. However, with relatively low event rates in both groups, as is characteristic of more recently operated-on patients, these differences did not achieve statistical significance.[304] Aspirin did lead to a decrease in systemic embolism in three trials when combined with warfarin in doses of 500 to 1000 mg/day.[304]

In each of these trials, this combination led to a significant increase in serious hemorrhage requiring blood transfusion, and the combination of warfarin with high-dose

aspirin (500 to 1000 mg) is, therefore, not recommended. However, a very interesting recent study by Turpie et al.[311] tested the combination of anticoagulation with warfarin (INR 3.0 to 4.5) with aspirin in doses of 100 mg/daily. This trial studied 370 patients with prosthetic heart valves implanted between 1987 and 1991, 75 per cent of whom had mechanical heart valve prostheses. A comparison of the combination of warfarin and aspirin with warfarin alone showed a statistically significant reduction in annualized event rates for the endpoints of major systemic embolism and vascular death (1.9 versus 8.5 per cent, P < 0.01) and death alone (2.8 versus 7.4 per cent, P = 0.01). Although the risk of hemorrhagic events was higher in the combination therapy group compared to warfarin alone (35 per cent per year versus 22 per cent per year, P = 0.02), this difference was largely the result of minor bleeding, and the rates of major hemorrhagic events were not significantly different.

Several interesting points emerged from this study: The addition of aspirin to warfarin led to a highly significant reduction in embolism and vascular death, even in patients operated on with late-model prosthetic heart valves, usually a lower-risk cohort. Critical review of the data suggests that a main effect of aspirin might have been a decrease in myocardial infarction in a population at risk for coronary events. In fact, the annual rate of major systemic embolism or death in the warfarin group appears relatively high. Although the intended INR was 3.0 to 4.5, the actual mean INR was only 3.1 in the warfarin group and 3.0 in the combination group, perhaps an attempt to lower hemorrhagic complications; whether this contributed to a higher thrombotic risk in patients without adjunctive platelet inhibition is unclear. Similar conclusions can be drawn from a recent Japanese study in which warfarin was combined with dipyridamole, aspirin, or ticlopidine.[312]

Special Situations Concerning the Use of Antithrombotic Therapy

(Prosthetic valve endocarditis and anticoagulation during pregnancy are described in Chapters 33 and 59, respectively.)

REQUIREMENTS FOR NONCARDIAC SURGERY. In patients with prosthetic heart valves, temporary discontinuation of oral anticoagulants for 7 to 10 days appears to be associated with low overall risk when a patient requires noncardiac therapy.[313] However, as noted previously, in many series most thromboembolic events have occurred when anticoagulants were temporarily discontinued or the level of anticoagulation had fallen to a suboptimal range. Thus, in the high-risk patient, it is advisable either to lower anticoagulation to an INR of about 2.0[314] or to stop oral anticoagulants 3 to 4 days before surgery and start intravenous heparin to maintain the activated partial thromboplastin time at twice the control level; the heparin may be infused up to 4 to 5 hours before surgery and resumed as soon as possible after surgery until oral anticoagulant therapy can be reestablished at optimal levels.

ANTICOAGULATION AFTER AN EMBOLIC EVENT. A difficult clinical decision is the appropriate time to begin anticoagulation when a patient with a prosthetic heart valve experiences an aseptic cardiogenic cerebral embolus. Aggregate data suggest that up to 12 per cent of patients will have a recurrent embolus within the first 2 weeks, the risk being equally distributed over this period at approximately 1 per cent per day.[304,315] Aggregate data from nonrandomized and retrospective series suggest that immediate anticoagulation may decrease this risk, but immediate anticoagulation is associated with an increased risk of hemorrhagic transformation of cerebral infarction.[304,315] However, patients with large cerebral infarcts seem to be at greatest risk of hemorrhagic transformation, which occurs most commonly in the first 48 hours, although it may occur later.[315]

In view of the above data, continuation of anticoagulant therapy in patients with prosthetic heart valves appears advisable after a small-to-moderate size stroke, if CT of the brain at 24 and 48 hours does not detect hemorrhage and if acute hypertension (blood pressure 180/100 mm Hg or more) is not present.[316] Patients with larger infarctions may be at especially high risk for delayed hemorrhagic transformation, and anticoagulants should be withheld for 5 to 7 days after the event and until a second scan of the head can be obtained.[315]

PROSTHETIC VALVE THROMBOSIS. The incidence of valve thrombosis and total thromboembolism with coumarin therapy in general is 0.2 and 1.8 per 100 patient years, respectively,[317] and as much as 20 per cent in patients with valve prostheses in the tricuspid position.[318] Surgery has been the traditional treatment for prosthetic valve thrombosis; however, reported operative mortality ranges between 8 and 60 per cent, depending on clinical functional class.[318,319] Fibrinolytic therapy appears to be an attractive alternative to surgical treatment.[318,319] It is the treatment of choice in patients with valve prostheses in the tricuspid position.[318-320] However, because of the risk of cerebral embolism, its use is still controversial in left-sided prosthetic valve thrombosis. Based on a literature search, 200 cases of left-sided prosthetic valve thrombolysis have been reported with 82 per cent initial success rate, an overall embolic rate of 17 per cent, stroke rate of 5 per cent, with 6 per cent fatalities, 5 per cent major bleeding episodes, and 11 per cent recurrences.[318] Therefore, thrombolysis may be a useful therapeutic alternative for left-sided prosthetic valve thrombosis in patients with a perceived contradiction to surgery (i.e., Class III–Class IV).[318,319,321] Transesophageal echocardiography has recently been reported to be the diagnostic technique of choice in selected candidates for safe and efficacious thrombolytic treatment of mitral prosthetic valve thrombosis.[318]

RECOMMENDATIONS (Tables 58–3 and 58–12). **Mechanical Prostheses.** All patients with mechanical heart valve prostheses should be treated with anticoagulants. Intravenous or high-dose subcutaneous heparin may be given once the chest tubes are removed and continued until oral anticoagulation of adequate intensity has been achieved.[242] Warfarin therapy may be initiated in most situations within 24 to 48 hours after the operation. Although the optimal intensity of anticoagulation may vary in some situations, a target INR of 2.5 to 3.5 is advised.[242,322] The consistency with which anticoagulation is maintained at the target intensity is very important, and the prothrombin time should be carefully monitored, every 3 to 4 weeks and at additional times if drugs are added or dietary changes are made that may interact with warfarin. Routine-risk patients may be treated with anticoagulants alone. High-risk patients include those with mechanical heart valves implanted before

the mid-1970s and those with prior embolic complications. Such patients could receive either higher-intensity oral anticoagulants (INR 3.0 to 4.5) or medium-intensity oral anticoagulants (INR 2.5 to 3.5) with a platelet inhibitor, either aspirin at 100 mg/day (ideally, in patients with coronary or cerebrovascular disease) or dipyridamole at 100 mg four times daily.[242,322] Patients with hemorrhagic complications during therapeutic anticoagulation with warfarin should receive lower-intensity anticoagulation (INR of about 2.0) in combination with dipyridamole or aspirin, and medical evaluation of the source of bleeding should be completed.

Platelet inhibitor agents alone are not advisable as the sole antithrombotic therapy in the patient with a mechanical heart valve prosthesis. However, in the event that an absolute contraindication to oral anticoagulant therapy develops after implantation of a mechanical prosthesis, the combination of dipyridamole, 100 mg four times daily, and aspirin 325 mg daily, or ticlopidine 250 mg twice a day may be tried empirically. In patients with recurrent cerebrovascular emboli, despite maximal antithrombotic therapy with oral anticoagulants and platelet inhibitors, causes other than embolic and/or hypercoagulable states should be investigated before consideration of reoperation for implantation of a bioprosthetic valve.[242]

Biological Heart Valve Prostheses. All patients with bioprosthetic heart valve replacement should ideally receive postoperative, low-intensity, oral anticoagulant therapy to an INR of 2.0 to 3.0 beginning as soon as possible after surgery and continuing for more than 3 months postoperatively.[242,322] Patients with bioprostheses who are at higher risk for systemic embolism, including those with atrial fibrillation, previous embolism, or severe left ventricular dysfunction, should receive oral anticoagulant therapy indefinitely.[242,322]

TABLE 58–12 ANTITHROMBOTIC THERAPY FOR PROSTHETIC HEART VALVES

GRADE-SITUATION	THERAPY
Mechanical Valve	
Routine	MD Warfarin
Old prosthesis, TE, other	HD Warfarin
	MD Warfarin + LD ASA or + Dip
ACRx problems (bleeding)	LD Warfarin + Dip
	LD Warfarin + LD ASA
Recurrent embolism	Consider other causes
Bioprosthetic Valve	
Routine—NSR	LD Warfarin for 3 mo (then ASA?)
AF, LA thrombus, TE	MD Warfarin for 3 mo, then LD warfarin

TE = thromboembolism; Dip = dipyridamole; LD = low dose; MD = medium dose; HD = high dose; Warfarin: HD = INR 3.0–4.5; MD = INR 2.5–3.5; LD = INR 2.0–3.0; ASA MD = 325 mg/d; LD = 100 mg/d. ACRx = Anticoagulant treatment; NSR = normal sinus rhythm; AF = atrial fibrillation.

REFERENCES

HEMOSTASIS

1. Vane, J. R., Anggard, E. E., and Botting, R. M.: Regulatory functions of the vascular endothelium. N. Engl. J. Med. 323:27, 1990.
2. Jaffe, E. A.: Endothelial cell structure and function. In Hoffmann, R., Benz, E. J., Shattil, S. J., et al. (eds.): Hematology: Basic Principles and Practice. New York, Churchill Livingstone, 1991, pp. 1198–1212.
3. Furchgott, R. F., and Vanhoutte, P. M.: Endothelium-deriving relaxing and contracting factors. F.A.S.E.B. J. 3:2007, 1989.
4. Esmon, C. T.: The roles of protein C and thrombomodulin in the regulation of blood coagulation. J. Biol. Chem. 264:4743, 1989.
5. Harker, L. A.: Pathogenesis of thrombosis. In Williams, W. J. (ed.): Hematology. 4th ed. New York, McGraw-Hill, 1990, pp. 1559–1569.
6. Ruoslahti, E.: Integrins. J. Clin. Invest. 87:1, 1991.
7. Kieffer, N., and Philips, D. R.: Platelet membrane glycoproteins: Functions in cellular interactions. Ann. Rev. Cell. Biol. 6:329, 1990.
8. Lapetina, E. G.: The signal transduction induced by thrombin in human platelets. F.E.B.S. Lett. 268:400, 1990.
9. Rhee, S. G.: Inositol phospholipid-specific phospholipase C: Interaction of γ1 isoform with tyrosine kinase. Trends Biochem. Sci. 16:297, 1991.
10. Kieffer, N., and Philips, D. R.: Platelet membrane glycoproteins: Functions in cellular interactions. Ann. Rev. Cell. Biol. 6:329, 1990.
11. Turitto, V. T., and Baumgartner, H. R.: Platelet-surface interactions. In Colman, R. W., Hirsh, J., Marder, V. J., Salzman, E. W. (eds.): Hemostasis and Thrombosis: Basic Principles and Clinical Practice. 2nd ed. Philadelphia, J. B. Lippincott Co., 1987, pp. 555–571.
12. Edgington, T. S.: The structural biology of expression and function of tissue factor. Thromb. Haemost. 66:67, 1991.
13. Rapaport, S. I., and Rao, L. V. M.: The tissue factor pathway: How it has become a "prima ballerina?" Thromb. Haemost. 74:7, 1995.
14. Davie, E. W.: Biochemical and molecular aspects of the coagulation cascade. Thromb. Haemost. 74:1, 1995.
15. Mann, K. G., Jenny, R. J., and Krishnaswamy, S.: Cofactor proteins in the assembly and expression of blood clotting enzyme complexes. Annu. Rev. Biochem. 57:915, 1988.
16. Gilbert, G. E., Furie, B. C., and Furie, B.: Binding of human factor VIII to phospholipid vesicles. J. Biol. Chem. 265:815, 1990.
17. Mosesson, M. W.: Fibrin polymerization and its regulatory role in hemostasis. J. Lab. Clin. Med. 116:8, 1990.
18. Hogg, P. J., and Jackson, C. M.: Fibrin monomer protects thrombin from inactivation by heparin-antithrombin III: Implications for heparin efficacy. Proc. Natl. Acad. Sci. U.S.A. 86:3619, 1989.
19. Harker, L. A., and Mann, K. G.: Thrombosis and fibrinolysis. In Fuster, V., and Verstraete, M. (eds.): Thrombosis in Cardiovascular Disorders. Philadelphia, W. B. Saunders Company, 1992, pp. 1–16.

20. Rosenberg, R. D. and Baurka: The heparin-antithrombin system: A natural anticoagulant mechanism. *In* Colman, R. W., Hirsh, J., Marder, V. J., and Salzman, E. W. (eds.): Hemostasis and Thrombosis: Basic Principles and Clinical Practice. Philadelphia, J. B. Lippincott, 1994, pp. 837–860.

21. Dahlbäck, B.: Protein S and C4b-binding protein: Components involved in the regulation of the protein C anticoagulant system. Thromb. Haemost. *66*:49, 1991.

22. Rapaport, S. R.: The extrinsic pathway inhibitor: A regulator of tissue-factor-dependent blood coagulation. Thromb. Haemost. *66*:6, 1991.

THE FIBRINOLYTIC SYSTEM AND ITS CONTROL

23. Petersen, T. E., Martzen, M. R., Ichinose, A., and Davie, E. W.: Characterization of the gene for human plasminogen, a key proenzyme in the fibrinolytic system. J. Biol. Chem. *265*:6104, 1990.

24. Collen, D.: On the regulation and control of fibrinolysis. Thromb. Haemost. *43*:77, 1980.

25. Plow, E. F., Felez, J., and Miles, L. A.: Cellular regulation of fibrinolysis. Thromb. Haemost. *66*:32, 1991.

26. Thorsen, S.: The mechanism of plasminogen activation and the variability of the fibrin effector during tissue-type plasminogen activator-mediated fibrinolysis. Ann. N.Y. Acad. Sci. *667*:52, 1992.

27. Pennica, D., Holmes, W. E., Kohr, W. J., et al.: Cloning and expression of human tissue-type plasminogen activator cDNA in E. coli. Nature *301*:214, 1983.

28. Lijnen, H. R., and Collen, D.: Strategies for the improvement of thrombolytic agents. Thromb. Haemost. *66*:88, 1991.

29. Blasi, F.: Urokinase and urokinase receptor: A paracrine/autocrine system regulating cell migration and invasiveness. BioEssays *15*:105, 1993.

30. Bachmann, F.: The plasminogen-plasmin enzyme system. *In* Colman, R. W., Hirsch, J., Marder, V. J., and Salzman, E. W. (eds.): Hemostasis and Thrombosis: Basic Principles and Clinical Practice. 3rd ed. Philadelphia, J. B. Lippincott Co., 1994, pp. 1592–1622.

31. Huber, R., and Carrell, R. W.: Implications of the three-dimensional structure of α1-antitrypsin for structure and function of serpins. Biochemistry *28*:8951, 1989.

32. Sumi, Y., Ichikawa, Y., Nakamura, Y., et al.: Expression and characterization of α_2-plasmin inhibitor. J. Biochem. (Tokyo) *106*:703, 1989.

33. Pannekoek, H., Veerman, H., Lambers, H., et al.: Endothelial plasminogen activator inhibitor (PAI): A new member of the serpin gene family. E.M.B.O. J. *5*:2539, 1986.

34. Kruithof, E. K. O., Vassalli, J. D., Schleuning, W. D., et al.: Purification and characterization of plasminogen activator inhibitor from the histiocytic lymphoma cell line U-937. J. Biol. Chem. *261*:11207, 1986.

35. Bachmann, F.: The enigma PAI-2 gene expression, evolutionary and functional aspects. Thromb. Haemost. *74*:172, 1995.

36. Ploug, M., Ronne, E., Behrendt, N., et al.: Cellular receptor for urokinase plasminogen activator. Carboxyl-terminal processing and membrane anchoring by glycosyl-phosphatidylinositol. J. Biol. Chem. *266*:1926, 1991.

37. Behrendt, N., Ploug, M., Patthy, L., et al.: The ligand-binding domain of the cell surface receptor for urokinase-type plasminogen activator. J. Biol. Chem. *266*:7842, 1991.

38. Hajjar, K. A.: Cellular receptors in the regulation of plasmin generation. Thromb. Haemost. *74*:294, 1995.

39. Van Hinsbergh, V. W. M., Kooistra, T., Emeis, J. J., and Koolwijk, P.: Regulation of plasminogen activator production by endothelial cells: role in fibrinolysis and local proteolysis. Int. J. Radiat. Biol. *60*:261, 1991.

40. Chandler, W. L., Levy, W. C., Veith, R. C., Stratton, J. R.: A kinetic model of the circulatory regulation of tissue plasminogen activator during exercise, epinephrine infusion, and endurance training. Blood *81*:3293, 1993.

41. Collen, D., and Lijnen, H. R.: Molecular basis of fibrinolysis, as relevant for thrombolytic therapy. Thromb. Haemost. *74*:167, 1995.

42. Lijnen, H. R., and Collen, D.: Regulation of the fibrinolytic system. Year Book on Thrombolytic Therapy, Amsterdam: Excerpta Medica, 1995, pp. 1–30.

43. Jaklitsch, M. T., Biro, S., Casscells, W., and Dichek, D. A.: Transduced endothelial cells expressing high levels of tissue plasminogen activator have an unaltered phenotype in vitro. J. Cell. Physiol. *154*:207, 1993.

44. Loskutoff, D. J.: Regulation of PAI-1 gene expression. Fibrinolysis *5*:197, 1991.

45. Mayer, E. J., Fujita, T., Gardell, S. J., et al.: The pharmacokinetics of plasminogen activator inhibitor-1 in the rabbit. Blood *76*:1514, 1990.

46. Racanelli, A. L., Diemer, M. J., Dobies, A. C., et al.: Distribution and pharmacokinetics of active recombinant plasminogen activator inhibitor-1 in the rat and rabbit. Fibrinolysis *6*:187, 1992.

47. Wiman, B.: Plasminogen activator inhibitor 1 (PAI-1) in plasma: its role in thrombotic disease. Thromb. Haemost. *74*:71, 1995.

48. Kruithof, E. K. O.: Plasminogen activator inhibitors—a review. Enzyme *40*:113, 1988.

49. Thorsen, S., Philips, M., Selmer, J., et al.: Kinetics of inhibition of tissue-type and urokinase-type plasminogen activator by plasminogen-activator inhibitor type 1 and type 2. Eur. J. Biochem. *175*:33, 1988.

50. Reilly, C. F., and Hutzelmann, J. E.: Plasminogen activator inhibitor-1 binds to fibrin and inhibits tissue-type plasminogen activator-mediated fibrin dissolution. J. Biol. Chem. *267*:17128, 1992.

51. Declerck, P. J., De Mol, M., Vaughan, D. E., and Collen, D.: Identification of a conformationally distinct form of plasminogen activator inhibitor-1, acting as a non-inhibitory substrate for tissue-type plasminogen activator. J. Biol. Chem. *267*:11693, 1992.

52. Collen, D.: On the regulation and control of fibrinolysis. Thromb. Haemost. *43*:77, 1980.

53. Hoylaerts, M., Rijken, D. C., Lijnen, H. R., and Collen, D.: Kinetics of the activation of plasminogen by human tissue plasminogen activator. Role of fibrin. J. Biol. Chem. *257*:2912, 1982.

54. Andreasen, P. A., Petersen, L. C., and Danø, K.: Diversity in catalytic properties of single chain and two chain tissue-type plasminogen activator. Fibrinolysis *5*:207, 1991.

55. Harpel, P. C., Gordon, B. R., and Parker, T. S.: Plasmin catalyzes binding of lipoprotein (a) to immobilized fibrinogen and fibrin. Proc. Natl. Acad. Sci. U.S.A. *86*:3847, 1989.

56. Juhan-Vague, I., Valadier, J., Alessi, M. C., et al.: Deficient t-PA release and elevated PA inhibitor levels in patients with spontaneous or recurrent deep venous thrombosis. Thromb. Haemost. *57*:67, 1987.

57. Juhan-Vague, I., Alessi, M. C., and Vague, P.: Increased plasma plasminogen activator inhibitor 1 levels. A possible link between insulin resistance and atherothrombosis. Diabetologia *34*:457, 1991.

58. Juhan-Vague, I., and Alessi, M. C.: Plasminogen activator inhibitor 1 and atherothrombosis. Thromb. Haemost. *70*:138, 1993.

59. Wiman, B., and Hamsten, A.: The fibrinolytic enzyme system and its role in the etiology of thromboembolic disease. Semin. Thromb. Hemost. *16*:207, 1990.

60. Prins, M. H., and Hirsh, J.: A critical review of the relationship between impaired fibrinolysis and myocardial infarction. Am. Heart J. *122*:545, 1991.

61. Hamsten, A., De Faire, U., Walldius, G., et al.: Plasminogen activator inhibitor in plasma: Risk factor for recurrent myocardial infarction. Lancet *2*:3, 1987.

62. Jansson, J. J., Nilsson, T. K., and Johnson, O.: Von Willebrand factor in plasma: A novel risk factor for recurrent myocardial infarction and death. Br. Med. J. *66*:351, 1991.

63. Thompson, S. G., and van de Loo, J. C. W.: ECAT angina pectoris study. Baseline associations of haemostatic factors with extent of coronary arteriosclerosis and other coronary risk factors in 3,000 patients with angina pectoris undergoing coronary angiography. Eur. Heart J. *14*:8, 1993.

64. Juhan-Vague, I., Thompson, S., and Jespersen, J.: Involvement of the hemostatic system in insulin resistance. A study of 1,500 patients with angina pectoris. Arterioscl. Thromb. *13*:1865, 1993.

65. Etingin, O. R., Hajjar, D. P., Hajjar, K. A., et al.: Lipoprotein (a) regulates plasminogen activator inhibitor-1 expression in endothelial cells. A potential mechanism in thrombogenesis. J. Biol. Chem. *266*:2459, 1991.

65a. Majerus, P. W., Broze, G. J. Jr., Miletich, J. P., and Tollefsen, D. M.: Anticoagulant, thrombolytic, and antiplatelet drugs. *In* Hardman, J. G., et al. (eds.): Goodman & Gilman's The Pharmacological Basis of Therapeutics, 9th ed. New York: McGraw-Hill, 1996, pp. 1341–1360.

ANTITHROMBOTIC DRUGS

66. Weitz, J. L., Hudoba, M., Massel, D., et al.: Clot-bound thrombin is protected from inhibition by heparin-antithrombin III but is susceptible to inactivation by antithrombin III-independent inhibitors. J. Clin. Invest. *86*:3619, 1990.

67. Hirsh, J., and Fuster, V.: Guide to anticoagulant therapy. Part 1: Heparin. Circulation *89*:1449, 1994.

68. Kandrotas, R. J.: Heparin pharmacokinetics and pharmacodynamics. Clin. Pharmacokinet. *22*:359, 1992.

69. Glimelius, B., Busch, C., and Hook, M.: Binding of heparin on the surface of cultured human endothelial cells. Thromb. Res. *12*:773, 1978.

70. Hirsh, J., and Levine, M. N.: Low molecular weight heparin. Blood *79*:1, 1992.

71. Sobel, M., McNeill, P. M., Carlson, P. L., et al.: Heparin inhibition of von Willebrand factor-dependent platelet function in vitro and in vivo. J. Clin. Invest. *87*:1787, 1991.

72. Hartle, P., Brucke, P., Dienstl, E., and Vinazzer, H.: Prophylaxis of thromboembolism in general surgery: Comparison between standard heparin and Fragmin. Thromb. Res. *57*:577, 1991.

73. Eriksson, B. I., Kalebo, P., Anthmyr, B. A., et al.: Comparison of low-molecular weight heparin and unfractionated heparin in the prevention of deep vein thrombosis and pulmonary embolism after total hip replacement. J. Bone Joint Surg. *73*:484, 1991.

74. Albada, J., Nieuwenhuis, H. K., and Sixma, J. J.: Treatment of acute venous thromboembolism with low molecular weight heparin (Fragmin): results of a double-blind randomized study. Circulation *80*:935, 1989.

75. Simonneau, G., Charbonnier, D., Decousus, H., et al.: Subcutaneous low-molecular-weight heparin compared with continuous intravenous unfractionated heparin in the treatment of proximal deep vein thrombosis. Arch. Intern. Med. *153*:1541, 1993.

76. Hull, R. D., Raskob, G. E., Pineo, G. F., et al.: Subcutaneous low-molecular-weight heparins compared with continuous intravenous heparin in the treatment of proximal vein thrombosis. N. Engl. J. Med. *326*:975, 1992.

77. Warkentin, T. E., Levine, M. N., Roberts, R. S., et al.: Heparin induced thrombocytopenia is more common with unfractionated heparin than

with low molecular weight heparin. Thromb. Haemost. *69*(Abs.):911, 1993.

78. Van Dedem, G., and de Leeuw den Bouter, H.: The nature of the glucosaminoglycan in Orgaran (Org 10172). Thromb. Haemost. *69*(Abs.):652, 1993.

79. Meuleman, D. G.: Orgaran (Org 10172): its pharmacological profile in experimental models. Haemost. *22*:58, 1992.

80. Zammit, A., and Dawes, J.: Low-affinity material does not contribute to the antithrombotic activity of Orgaran (Org 10172) in human plasma. Thromb. Haemost. *71*:759, 1994.

81. Stiekema, J. C., Wynand, H. P., Van Danther, T. G., et al.: Safety and pharmacokinetics of the low molecular weight heparinoid ORG 10172 administered to healthy elderly volunteers. Br. J. Clin. Pharmacol. *27*:39, 1989.

82. Nurmohamed, M. T., Fareed, J., Hoppensteadt, T. J. M., et al.: Pharmacological and clinical studies with Lomoparan, a low molecular weight glycosaminoglycan. Sem. Thromb. Hemost. *7*:205, 1991.

83. Comp, P. C.: Coumarin-induced skin necrosis. Incidence, mechanisms, management and avoidance. Drug Safety *8*:128, 1993.

84. Hirsh, J., and Fuster, V.: Guide to anticoagulant therapy. Part 2: Oral anticoagulants. Circulation *89*:1469, 1994.

85. Turpie, A. G. G., Gunstenen, J., Hirsh, J., et al.: Randomized comparison of two intensities of oral anticoagulant therapy after tissue heart valve replacement. Lancet *1*:1242, 1988.

86. Ginsberg, J. S., and Hirsh, J.: Anticoagulants during pregnancy. *In* Fuster, V., and Verstraete, M. (eds.): Thrombosis in Cardiovascular Disorders. Philadelphia, W. B. Saunders Company, 1992, pp. 485–490.

87. Patrono, C.: Aspirin as an antiplatelet drug. N. Engl. J. Med. *3*:1287, 1994.

88. Lekkovits, J., Plow, E. F., and Topol, E. J.: Platelet glycoprotein IIb/IIIa receptors in cardiovascular medicine. N. Engl. J. Med. *332*:1553, 1995.

89. Verstraete, M., and Zoldhelyi, P.: Novel antithrombotic drugs in development. Drugs *49*:856, 1995.

90. Harker, L. A., Hanson, S. R., and Kelly, A. B.: Antithrombotic benefits and hemorrhagic risks of direct thrombin antagonists. Thromb. Haemost. *74*:464, 1995.

91. Verstraete, M.: The long search towards ideal antithrombotic drugs in hypercoagulable state: Biological aspects and clinical management. *In* Seghatchian, J., Samama, M., and Hecker, S. (eds.): Hypercoagulable State: Biological Aspects and Clinical Management. CRC Press, Boca Raton, *(in press)*.

92. Clowes, A. W.: Prevention and management of recurrent disease after arterial reconstruction: A new prospect for pharmacological control. Thromb. Haemost. *66*:62, 1991.

93. Antiplatelet Trialist Collaboration: Collaborative overview of randomised trials of antiplatelet therapy: I. Prevention of death, myocardial infarction, and stroke by prolonged antiplatelet therapy in various categories of patients. Br. Med. J. *308*:81, 1994.

94. Szczeklik, A., Krzanowski, M., Gora, P., and Randwan, J.: Antiplatelet drugs and generation of thrombin in clotting blood. Blood *80*:2006, 1992.

95. Szczeklik, A.: Thrombin generation in myocardial infarction and hypercholesterolemia: Effects of aspirin. Thromb. Haemost. *74*:77, 1995.

96. Meade, E. A., Smith, W. L., and DeWitt, D. L.: Differential inhibition of prostaglandin endoperoxide anti-inflammatory drugs. J. Biol. Chem. *268*:610, 1993.

97. Marcus, A. J., Safier, L. B., Broekman, J., et al.: Thrombosis and inflammation as multicellular processes: Significance of cell-cell interactions. Thromb. Haemost. *74*:213, 1995.

98. Mills, D. C. B., Puri, R., Hu, C. J., et al.: Clopidogrel inhibits the binding of ADP analogues to the receptor mediating inhibition of platelet adenylate cyclase. Arterioscler. Thromb. *12*:430, 1992.

99. Schrör, K.: The basic pharmacology of ticlopidine and clopidogrel. Platelets *4*:252, 1993.

100. Gachet, C., Stierlé, A., Cazenave, J. P., et al.: The thienopyridine PCR 4099 selectively inhibits ADP-induced platelet aggregation and fibrinogen binding without modifying the membrane glycoprotein IIb-IIIa complex in rat and in man. Biochem. Pharmacol. *40*:229, 1990.

101. McTavish, D., Faulds, D., and Goa, K. L.: Ticlopidine. An updated review of its pharmacology and therapeutic use in platelet-dependent disorders. Drugs *40*:238, 1990.

102. Verstraete, M.: Risk factors, interventions and therapeutic agents in the prevention of atherosclerotic related ischaemic diseases. Drugs *42*:22, 1991.

103. Verhaeghe, R.: Prophylactic antiplatelet therapy in peripheral arterial disease. Drugs *42*:51, 1991.

104. Hass, W. K., Eaton, J. D., Harold, P., et al. for the Ticlopidine Aspirin Stroke Study: A randomized trial comparing ticlopidine hydrochloride with aspirin for the prevention of stroke in high-risk patients. N. Engl. J. Med. *21*:501, 1989.

105. Easton, J. D.: Antiplatelet therapy in the prevention of stroke. Drugs *42*:39, 1991.

106. Verstraete, M.: Thromboxane synthase inhibition, thromboxane/endoperoxide receptor blockade and molecules with the dual property. Drugs Today *29*:221, 1993.

107. De Clerck, F., Beertens, J., De Chaffoy de Courcelles, D., et al.: R68070: Thromboxane A2 synthetase inhibition and thromboxane A2/prostaglandin endoperoxide receptor blockade combined in one molecule. I. Biochemical profile in vitro. Thromb. Haemost. *61*:35, 1989.

108. Berrettini, M., De Cunto, M., Parisi, F., et al.: In vitro and ex vivo effects of picotamide, a combined thromboxane A2-synthase inhibitor

and -receptor antagonist, on human platelets. Eur. J. Clin. Pharmacol. *39*:495, 1990.

109. Coller, B. S.: A new murine monoclonal antibody reports an activation-dependent change in the conformation and/or microenvironment of the platelet glycoprotein IIb/IIIa complex. J. Clin. Invest. *6*:101, 1985.

110. Tcheng, J. E., Ellis, S. G., George, B. S., et al.: Pharmacodynamics of chimeric glycoprotein IIb/IIIa integrin antiplatelet antibody Fab 7E3 in high-risk coronary angioplasty. Circulation *90*:1757, 1994.

111. Kleiman, N. S., Ohman, E., Califf, R. M., et al.: Profound inhibition of platelet aggregation with monoclonal antibody 73E Fab after thrombolytic therapy. Results of the Thrombolysis and Angioplasty in Myocardial Infarction (TAMI) 8 Pilot Study. J. Am. Coll. Cardiol. *22*:381, 1993.

112. The EPIC Investigators: Use of a monoclonal antibody directed against the platelet glycoprotein IIb/IIIa receptor in high-risk coronary angioplasty. N. Engl. J. Med. *330*:956, 1994.

113. Topol, E. J., Califf, R. M., Weisman, H. F., et al. on behalf of the EPIC Investigators: Randomised trial of coronary intervention with antibody against platelet GPIIb/IIIa integrin for reduction of clinical restenosis: results at 6 months. Lancet *343*:881, 1994.

114. Collen, D., Lu, H. R., Stassen, J.-M., Vreys, I., et al.: Antithrombotic effects and bleeding time prolongation with synthetic platelet GPIIb/IIIa inhibitors in animal models of platelet-mediated thrombosis. Thromb. Haemost. *71*:95, 1994.

115. Carteaux, J. P., Steiner, B., and Roux, S.: R044-9883, a new non-peptide GPIIb-GPIIIa antagonist prevents platelet loss in a guinea pig model of extracorporeal circulation. Thromb. Haemost. *70*:817, 1993.

116. Hartman, G. D., Egbertson, M. S., Halczenko, W., et al.: Non-peptide fibrinogen receptor antagonists: Discovery and design of exosite inhibitors. J. Med. Chem. *36*:4640, 1992.

117. Müller, T. H., Weisenberger, H., Brickl, R., et al.: Pharmacodynamics and kinetics of BIBU52, a platelet glycoprotein (GP) IIb/IIIa antagonist, and its orally active prodrug BIBU104 in man. Thromb. Haemost. *73*:1445, 1995.

118. Hofsteenge, J., Stone, S. R., Donella-Deane, A., and Pinna, L. A.: The effect of substituting phosphotyrosine for sulphotyrosine on the activity of hirudin. Eur. J. Biochem. *188*:55, 1990.

119. Dahlbäck, B., and Stenflo, J.: A natural anticoagulant pathway. Biochemistry and physiology of proteins C, S, C4b-binding protein and thrombomodulin. *In* Bloom, A. L., Forbes, C. D., Thomas, D. P., and Tuddenham, E. S. D. (eds.): Haemostasis and Thrombosis. 3rd ed. New York, Churchill Livingstone, 1994, pp. 671–698.

120. Talbot, M. D., Ambler, J., Butler, K. D., et al.: Recombinant desulfatohirudin (CGP 39393) anticoagulant and antithrombotic properties in vivo. Thromb. Haemost. *61*:77, 1991.

121. Marbet, G. A., Verstraete, M., Kienast, J., et al.: Clinical pharmacology of intravenously administered recombinant desulfatohirudin (CGP 39393) in healthy volunteers. J. Cardiovasc. Pharmacol. *22*:364, 1993.

122. Verstraete, M., Nurmohamed, M., Kienast, J., et al. on behalf of the European Hirudin in Thrombosis Group: Biologic effects of recombinant hirudin (CGP 39393) in human volunteers. J. Am. Coll. Cardiol. *22*:1080, 1993.

123. Close, P., Bichler, J., Kerry, R., et al. on behalf of the European Hirudin in Thrombosis Group (HIT Group): Weak allergenicity of recombinant hirudin CGP 39393 (TMRevasc) in immunocompetent volunteers. Coron. Art. Dis. *5*:943, 1994.

124. Fox, I., Dawson, A., Loynds, P., et al.: Anticoagulant activity of hirulog, a direct inhibitor of thrombin. Thromb. Haemost. *69*:157, 1993.

125. Cannon, C. P., Maraganore, J. M., Loscalzo, J., et al.: Anticoagulant effect of hirulog, a novel thrombin inhibitor, in patients with coronary artery disease. Am. J. Cardiol. *71*:778, 1993.

126. Imura, Y., Stassen, J.-M., and Collen, D.: Comparative antithrombotic effects of heparin, recombinant hirudin, and argatroban in a hamster femoral vein platelet-rich mural thrombus model. J. Pharmacol. Exper. Ther. *261*:895, 1992.

127. Jang, I., Gold, H. K., Ziskind, A. A., et al.: Prevention of platelet-rich arterial thrombosis by selective thrombin inhibition. Circulation *18*:219, 1990.

THROMBOLYTIC DRUGS

128. Jackson, K. W., and Tang, J.: Complete amino acid sequence of streptokinase and its homology with serine protease. Biochemistry *21*:6620, 1982.

129. Reddy, K. N. N.: Streptokinase—biochemistry and clinical application. Enzyme *40*:78, 1988.

130. Battershill, P. E., Benfield, P., and Goa, K. L.: Streptokinase. A review of its pharmacology and therapeutic efficacy in acute myocardial infarction in older patients. Drugs Aging *4*:36, 1994.

131. Smith, R. A. G., Dupe, R. J., English, P. D., and Green, J.: Fibrinolysis with acyl-enzymes: A new approach to thrombolytic therapy. Nature *290*:505, 1981.

132. Monk, J. P., and Heel, R. C.: Anisoylated plasminogen streptokinase activator complex (APSAC). A review of its mechanism of action, clinical pharmacology and therapeutic use in acute myocardial infarction. Drugs *34*:25, 1987.

133. White, W. F., Barlow, G. H., and Mozen, M. M.: The isolation and characterization of plasminogen activators (urokinase) from human urine. Biochemistry *5*:2160, 1966.

134. Barlow, G. H.: Urinary and kidney cell plasminogen activator (urokin-

ase). *In* Lorand, L. (ed.): Methods in Enzymology. Vol. 45. San Diego Academic Press, 1976, pp. 239–247.

135. Nolli, M. L., Sarubbi, E., Corti, A., et al.: Production and characterization of human recombinant single chain urokinase-type plasminogen activator from mouse cells. Fibrinolysis 3:101, 1989.

136. Holmes, W. E., Pennica, D., Blaber, M., et al.: Cloning and expression of the gene for pro-urokinase in Escherichia coli. Biotechnology 3:923, 1985.

137. Pennica, D., Holmes, W. E., Kohr, W. J., et al.: Cloning and expression of human tissue-type plasminogen activator cDNA in E. coli. Nature 301:214, 1983.

138. Lijnen, H. R., and Collen, D.: Strategies for the improvement of thrombolytic agents. Thromb. Haemost. 66:88, 1991.

139. Madison, E. L.: Probing structure-function relationships of tissue-type plasminogen activator by site-specific mutagenesis. Fibrinolysis 8:221, 1994.

140. Kohnert, U., Rudolph, R., Verheijen, J. H., et al.: Biochemical properties of the kringle 2 and protease domains are maintained in the refolded t-PA deletion variant BM 06.022. Prot. Engineer. 5:93, 1992.

141. Stern, A., Kohnert, U., Rudolph, R., et al.: Gewebs-Plasminogenaktivator-Derivat. Eur. Patent. Appl. 38217, 1989.

142. Martin, U., Fischer, S., Kohnert, U., et al.: Thrombolysis with an Escherichia coli-produced recombinant plasminogen activator (BM 06.022) in the rabbit model of jugular vein thrombosis. Thromb. Haemost. 65:560, 1991.

143. Martin, U., van Möllendorf, E., Akpan, W., et al.: Dose-ranging study of the novel recombinant plasminogen activator BM 06.022 in healthy volunteers. Clin. Pharmacol. Ther. 50:429, 1991.

144. Martin, U., Köhler, J., Sponer, G., et al.: Pharmacokinetics of the novel recombinant plasminogen activator BM 06.022 in rats, dogs, and non-human primates. Fibrinolysis 6:39, 1992.

145. Neuhaus, K. L., von Essen, R., Vogt, A., et al.: Dose finding with a novel recombinant plasminogen activator (BM 06.022) in patients with acute myocardial infarction: results of the German recombinant plasminogen activator study. J. Am. Coll. Cardiol. 24:55, 1994.

146. Tebbe, U., von Essen, R., Smolarz, A., et al.: Open, noncontrolled dose-finding study with a novel recombinant plasminogen activator (BM 06.022) given as a double bolus in patients with acute myocardial infarction. Am. J. Cardiol. 72:518, 1993.

147. Smalling, R. W., Bode, C., Kalbfleisch, J., et al.: For the RAPID Investigators. Improvement of global and regional LV function by the bolus administration of recombinant plasminogen activator (r-PA) in acute myocardial infarction: A comparison with standard dose alteplase. Circulation 90(Abs.):562, 1994.

148. International Joint Efficacy Comparison of Thrombolytics: Randomised, double-blind comparison of reteplase double-bolus administration with streptokinase in acute myocardial infarction (INJECT): Trial to investigate equivalence. Lancet 346:329, 1995.

149. Keyt, B., Paoni, N. F., Refino, C. J., et al.: A faster-acting and more potent form of tissue plasminogen activator. Proc. Natl. Acad. Sci. U.S.A. 91:3670, 1994.

150. Collen, D., Stassen, J. M., Yasuda, T., et al.: Comparative thrombolytic properties of tissue-type plasminogen activator and of a plasminogen activator inhibitor-1-resistant glycosylation variant, in a combined arterial and venous thrombosis model in the dog. Thromb. Haemost. 72:98, 1994.

151. Van de Werf, F., Lijnen, H. R., and Collen, D.: Coronary thrombolysis with K1K2Pu, a chimeric tissue-type and urokinase-type plasminogen activator. A feasibility study in six patients with acute myocardial infarction. Coron. Art. Dis. 4:929, 1993.

152. Gardell, S. J., Duong, L. T., Diehl, R. E., et al: Isolation, characterization, and cDNA cloning of a vampire bat salivary plasminogen activator. J. Biol. Chem. 264:17947, 1989.

153. Bergum, P. W., and Gardell, S. J.: Vampire bat salivary plasminogen activator exhibits a strict and fastidious requirement for polymeric fibrin as its cofactor, unlike human tissue-type plasminogen activator. J. Biol. Chem. 267:17726, 1992.

154. Collen, D., and Lijnen, H. R.: Staphylokinase, a fibrin-specific plasminogen activator with therapeutic potential? Blood 84:680, 1994.

154a. Vanderschueren, S., Stockx, L., Wilms, G., et al.: Thrombolytic therapy of peripheral arterial occlusion with recombinant staphylokinase. Circulation 92:2040, 1995.

154b. Vanderschueren, S., Barrios, L., Kerdsinchai, P., et al.: A randomized trial of recombinant staphylokinase versus alteplase for coronary artery patency in acute myocardial infarction. Circulation 92:2044, 1995.

ANTITHROMBOTIC AND THROMBOLYTIC THERAPY IN CARDIAC DISEASE

155. Summary of the second report of the National Cholesterol Education Program (NCEP) Expert Panel on Detection: Evaluation and treatment of high blood cholesterol in adults (Adult Treatment Panel II). JAMA 269:3015, 1993.

156. Pekkanen, J., Lin, S., Heiss, G., et al.: Ten-year mortality from cardiovascular disease in relation to cholesterol level among men with and without preexisting cardiovascular disease. N. Engl. J. Med. 322:1700, 1990.

157. Rader, D. J., Hoeg, J. M., and Brewer, H. B., Jr.: Quantitation of plasma apolipoproteins in the primary and secondary prevention of coronary artery disease. Ann. Intern. Med. 120:1012, 1994.

158. Scandinavian Simvastatin Survival Study Group: Randomised trial of cholesterol lowering in 4,444 patients with coronary heart disease: the Scandinavian Simvastatin Survival Study (4S). Lancet 344:1383, 1994.

159. Fuster, V., and Chesebro, J. H.: Aspirin for primary prevention of coronary disease. Eur. Heart J. *(in press).*

160. Stein, B., Fuster, V., Halperin, J. L., and Chesebro, J. H.: Antithrombotic therapy in cardiac disease: An emerging approach based on pathogenesis and risk. Circulation 80:1501, 1989.

ANTITHROMBOTIC THERAPY IN CORONARY ARTERY DISEASE

161. Lewis, H., Davis, J., Archibald, D., Steinke, W., et al.: Protective effects of aspirin against acute myocardial infarction and death in men with unstable angina: Results of a Veterans Administration Cooperative Study. N. Engl. J. Med. 309:396, 1983.

162. Cairns, J., Gent, M., Singer, J., et al.: Aspirin, sulfinpyrazone or both in unstable angina. N. Engl. J. Med. 313:1349, 1985.

163. Theroux, P., Ouimet, H., and McCanu, T.: Aspirin, heparin or both to treat acute unstable angina. N. Engl. J. Med. 319:1105, 1988.

164. RISC Investigators: Risk of myocardial infarction and death during treatment with low-dose aspirin and intravenous heparin in men with unstable coronary artery disease. Lancet 336:827, 1990.

165. Teleford, A., and Wilson, C.: Trial of heparin versus atenolol in prevention of myocardial infarction in intermediate coronary syndromes. Lancet 1:1225, 1981.

166. Hirsh, J., and Fuster, V.: AHA Medical/Scientific Statement Guide to Anticoagulant Therapy. Part I: Heparin. Circulation 89:1449, 1994.

167. Theroux, P., Walters, D., Lam, J., et al.: Reactivation of unstable angina after discontinuation of heparin. N. Engl. J. Med. 327:141, 1992.

168. Cohen, M., Adams, P., Parry, G., et al.: Combination of antithrombotic therapy in unstable rest angina and non-Q wave infarction in nonprior aspirin users. Primary endpoint analysis from the ATACS trial. Circulation 89:81, 1994.

169. Holdright, D., Patel, D., Cunningham, D., et al.: Comparison of the effect of heparin and aspirin versus aspirin alone on transient myocardial ischemia and in-hospital prognosis in patients with unstable angina. J. Am. Coll. Cardiol. 24:39, 1994.

170. Balsano, F., Rizzon, P., Violoi, F., et al.: Antiplatelet treatment with ticlopidine in unstable angina: A controlled, multicenter clinical trial. The Studio della Ticlopidina nell'Angina Instabile Group. Circulation 82:17, 1990.

171. Braunwald, E., Jones, R. H., Mark, D. B., et al.: Diagnosing and managing unstable angina. Circulation 90:613, 1994.

172. Sharma, G., Lapsely, D., Vita, J., et al.: Safety and efficacy of hirulog in patients with unstable angina. Circulation 86:1, 1992.

173. Fuchs, J., McCabe, C., Antman, E., et al.: Hirulog in the treatment of unstable angina: Results of the Thrombin Inhibition in Myocardial Ischemia (TIMI) 7 Trial. Circulation 92:727, 1995.

174. Topol, E., Fuster, V., Harrington, R., Califf, R., et al.: Recombinant hirudin for unstable angina pectoris: A multicenter, randomized angiographic trial. Circulation 89:1557, 1994.

175. The Global Use of Strategies to Open Occluded Coronary Arteries (GUSTO) IIa Investigators: Randomized trial of intravenous heparin versus recombinant hirudin for acute coronary syndromes. Circulation 90:1631, 1994.

176. Antman, E. M. for the TIMI 9A Investigators: Safety Report from the Thrombolysis and Thrombin Inhibition in Myocardial Infarction (TIMI) 9A Trial. Circulation 90:1624, 1994.

177. Neuhaus, K.-L., Van Essen, R., Tebbe, U., et al.: Safety observations from the pilot phase of the randomized r-hirudin for improvement of thrombolysis (HIT III) study. A study of the arbeitsgemeinschaft leitender kardiologischer krankenhausarzte (ALKK). Circulation 90:1638, 1994.

177a. Théroux, P., White, H., David, D., et al.: A heparin-controlled study of MK-383 in unstable angina (abstract). Circulation 90:I-231, 1994.

177b. Théroux, P., Kouz, S., Knudtson, M., et al.: A randomized double-blind controlled trial with the non-peptidic platelet GPIIb/IIIa antagonist RO 44-9883 in unstable angina (abstract). Circulation 90:I-231, 1994.

177c. Simoons, M., Jan de Boer, M., van den Brand, M. J. B. M., et al.: Randomized trial of a GPIIb/IIIa platelet receptor blocker in refractory unstable angina. Circulation 89:596, 1994.

178. Fuster, V., Ip, J., Jang, I., et al.: Antithrombotic therapy in cardiac disease. *In* Parmley, W., and Chatterjee, K. (eds.): Cardiology-Physiology, Pharmacology, Diagnosis. Philadelphia, J. B. Lippincott Co., 1990, pp. 1–40.

179. Bar, F., Verheugt, F., Col, J., et al.: Thrombolysis in patients with unstable angina improves the angiographic but not the clinical outcome. Results of UNASEM. Circulation 86:131, 1992.

180. TIMI-IIIB Investigators: Effects of tissue plasminogen activator and a comparison of early invasive and conservative strategies in unstable angina and non-Q wave myocardial infarction. Results of the TIMI-IIIB trial. Circulation 89:1545, 1994.

181. Falk, E.: Unstable angina with fatal outcome: Dynamic coronary thrombosis leading to infarction and/or sudden death: Autopsy evidence of recurrent mural thrombosis and peripheral embolization culminating in total vascular occlusion. Circulation 71:699, 1985.

182. Cairns, J. A., Lewis, H. D., Meade, T. W., Sutton, G. C., and Theroux, P.: Antithrombotic agents in coronary artery disease. Chest 108(4 Suppl.): 3805, 1995.

183. Cairns, J. A., Fuster, V., Gore, J., and Kennedy, J. W.: Coronary thrombolysis. Chest 108(4 Suppl.):4015, 1995.

184. Yusuf, S., Collins, R., Peto, R., et al.: Intravenous and intracoronary fibrinolytic therapy in acute myocardial infarction: Overview of results on mortality, reinfarction and side effects from 33 randomized controlled trials. Eur. Heart J. 6:556, 1985.

185. Gruppo Italiano per lo Studio della Streptokinase nell'Infarcto Miocardico: (GISSI-I) Effectiveness of intravenous thrombolytic treatment in acute myocardial infarction. Lancet 1:397, 1986.

186. ISIS-II (Second International Study of Infarct Survival) Collaborative Group: Randomised trial of intravenous streptokinase, oral aspirin, both or neither among 17,187 cases of suspected acute myocardial infarction. Lancet 2:349, 1988.

187. ISAM Study Group: A prospective trial of intravenous streptokinase in acute myocardial infarction (ISAM). N. Engl. J. Med. 314:1465, 1986.

188. AIMS Trial Study Group: Effect of intravenous APSAC on mortality after acute myocardial infarction: Preliminary report of a placebo-controlled clinical trial. Lancet 1:545, 1988.

189. AIMS Trial Study Group: Long-term effects of intravenous antistreplase in acute myocardial infarction: Final report of the AIMS Study. Lancet 335:427, 1990.

190. Wilcox, R. G., Van der Lippe, G., Olsson, C. G., et al.: Trial of tissue plasminogen activator for mortality reduction in acute myocardial infarction. Anglo-Scandinavian Study of early thrombolysis (ASSET). Lancet 2:525, 1988.

191. Wilcox, R. G., Van der Lippe, G., Olsson, C. G., et al.: Effects of alteplase in acute myocardial infarction: Six-month results from the ASSET Study. Lancet 335:1175, 1990.

192. Van de Werf, F., and Arnold, A. E. R.: Intravenous tissue plasminogen activator and size of infarct, left ventricular function, and survival in acute myocardial infarction. Br. Med. J. 287:1374, 1988.

193. Fibrinolytic Therapy Trialists' (FTT) Collaborative Group: Indications for fibrinolytic therapy in suspected acute myocardial infarction: Collaborative overview of early mortality and major morbidity results from all randomised trials of more than 1,000 patients. Lancet 343:311, 1994.

194. Gruppo Italiano per lo Studio della Sopravvivenza nell'infarcto Miocardico: GISSI-2: A factorial randomized trial of alteplase and heparin versus no heparin among 12,490 patients with acute myocardial infarction. Lancet 336:65, 1990.

195. The International Study Group: In-hospital mortality and clinical course of 20,891 patients with suspected acute myocardial infarction randomized between alteplase and streptokinase with or without heparin. Lancet 336:71, 1990.

196. ISIS-3 Collaborative Group: ISIS-3: A randomized comparison of streptokinase vs tissue plasminogen activator vs antistreplase and os aspirin plus heparin vs aspirin alone among 41,299 cases of suspected acute myocardial infarction. Lancet 339:753, 1992.

197. The GUSTO Investigators: An international randomized trial comparing four thrombolytic strategies for acute myocardial infarction. N. Engl. J. Med. 329:673, 1993.

198. Cannon, C. P., McCabe, C. H., Diver, D. J., et al.: Comparison of front-loaded recombinant tissue-type plasminogen activator, antistreplase and combination thrombolytic therapy for acute myocardial infarction: Results of the Thrombolysis in Myocardial Infarction (TIMI) 4 trial. J. Am. Coll. Cardiol. 24:1602, 1994.

199. Fuster, V.: Coronary thrombolysis: A perspective for the practicing physician (editorial). N. Engl. J. Med. 329:723, 1993.

200. The Heparin-Aspirin Reperfusion Trial (HART) Investigators: A comparison between heparin and low-dose aspirin as adjunctive therapy with tissue-type plasminogen activator for acute myocardial infarction. N. Engl. J. Med. 323:1434, 1990.

201. Bleich, S. D., Nichols, T. C., Schumacher, R. R., et al.: Effect of heparin on coronary arterial patency after thrombolysis with tissue plasminogen activator in acute myocardial infarction. Am. J. Cardiol. 66:1412, 1990.

202. De Bono, D. P., Simoons, M. L., Tijssen, J., and the European Cooperative Study Group (ECSG): The effect of early intravenous heparin on coronary patency, infarct size and bleeding complications after alteplase thrombolysis: Results of randomized, double-blind European Cooperative Study Group trial. Br. Heart J. 67:122, 1992.

203. Fuster, V., Dyken, M. L., Vokonas, P. S., and Hennekens, C.: Aspirin as a therapeutic agent in cardiovascular disease. Circulation 87:659, 1993.

204. Fuster, V., and Chesebro, J. H.: Role of platelets and platelet inhibitors in aortocoronary artery vein-graft disease. Circulation 73:227, 1986.

205. Chesebro, J. H., Fuster, V., Elveback, L. R., et al.: Effects of dipyridamole and aspirin on late vein-graft patency after coronary bypass operations. N. Engl. J. Med. 310:209, 1984.

206. Chesebro, J. H., Clements, I. P., Fuster, V., et al.: A platelet-inhibitor-drug trial in coronary-artery bypass operation: Benefit of perioperative dipyridamole and aspirin therapy on early vein-graft patency. N. Engl. J. Med. 307:73, 1982.

207. Chesebro, J. H., and Goldman, S.: Coronary artery bypass surgery. In Fuster, V., and Verstraete, M. (eds.): Thrombosis in Cardiovascular Disorders. Philadelphia, W. B. Saunders Company, 1992, pp. 375–388.

208. Goldman, S., Copeland, J., Mortiz, T., et al.: Improvement in early saphenous vein graft patency after coronary artery bypass surgery with antiplatelet therapy: Results of a Veterans Administration Cooperative Study. Circulation 77:1324, 1988.

209. Goldman, S., Copeland, J., Mortiz, T., et al.: Saphenous vein graft patency one year after coronary artery bypass surgery and effects of antiplatelet therapy: Results of a Veterans Administration Cooperative Study. Circulation 80:1190, 1989.

210. Goldman, S., Copeland, J., Mortiz, T., et al., and the Department of Veterans Affairs Cooperative Study Group: Starting aspirin therapy after operation: Effects on early graft patency. Circulation 84:520, 1991.

211. Lorenz, R. L., Schacky, C. V., Weber, M., et al.: Improved aortocoronary bypass patency by low-dose aspirin (100 mg daily): Effects on platelet aggregation and thromboxane formation. Lancet 1:1261, 1984.

212. Limet, R., David, J. L., Magotteaux, P., et al.: Prevention of aortocoronary bypass graft occlusion: Beneficial effect of ticlopidine on early and late patency rates of venous coronary bypass grafts. A double blind-study. J. Thorac. Cardiovasc. Surg. 94:773, 1987.

213. Rajah, S. M., Rees, M., Walker, D., et al.: Effects of antiplatelet therapy with indobufen or aspirin-dipyridamole on graft patency one year after coronary artery bypass grafting. J. Thorac. Cardiovasc. Surg. 107:1146, 1994.

214. The SINBA Group: Indobufen versus aspirin plus dipyridamole after coronary artery bypass surgery. Cor. Art. Dis. 2:897, 1991.

215. Israel, D. H., Adams, P. C., Stein, B., et al.: Antithrombotic therapy in the coronary vein graft patient. Clin. Cardiol. 14:283, 1991.

216. Stein, P. D., Dalen, J. E., Goldman, S., et al.: Antithrombotic therapy in patients with spontaneous vein and internal mammary artery bypass grafts. Chest 108(Suppl. Oct):424S, 1995.

217. Solymoss, B. C., Nadeau, P., Millette, D., and Campeau, L.: Late thrombosis of saphenous vein coronary bypass grafts related to risk factors. Circulation 78:140, 1988.

218. Blankenhorn, D. H., Nessim, S. A., Johnson, R. L., et al.: Beneficial effects of combined colestipolniacin therapy on coronary atherosclerosis and coronary venous bypass grafts. JAMA 257:3233, 1987.

219. Califf, R. M., and Willerson, J. T.: Percutaneous transluminal coronary angioplasty: Prevention of occlusion and restenosis. In Fuster, V., and Verstraete, M. (eds.): Thrombosis in Cardiovascular Disorders. Philadelphia, W. B. Saunders Company, 1992, pp. 389–408.

220. Popma, J. J., Coller, B. S., Ohman, E. M., et al.: Antithrombotic therapy in patients undergoing coronary angioplasty. Chest 108(Suppl. Oct):486S, 1995.

221. Chesebro, J. H., Webster, M. W. I., Zolhelyi, P., et al.: Antithrombotic therapy and progression of coronary artery disease. Circulation 86(Suppl. III):III-100, 1992.

222. Ridker, P. M., Manson, J. E., Gaziano, J. M., et al.: Low-dose aspirin therapy for chronic stable angina: A randomized, placebo-controlled clinical trial. Ann. Intern. Med. 114:835, 1991.

223. Juul-Moller, S., Edvardsson, N., Jahnmatz, B., et al., for the Swedish Angina Pectoris Aspirin Trial (SAPAT): Double-blind trial of aspirin in primary prevention of myocardial infarction in patients with stable chronic angina pectoris. Lancet 340:1421, 1992.

224. Smith, P., Arnesen, H., and Holme, I.: The effect of warfarin on mortality and reinfarction after myocardial infarction. N. Engl. J. Med. 323:147, 1990.

225. The ASPECT Research Group: The effect of long term oral anticoagulant treatment on mortality and cardiovascular morbidity after myocardial infarction. Lancet 343:499, 1994.

226. Report of the Sixty Plus Reinfarction Study Research Group: A double-blind trial to assess long-term oral anticoagulant therapy in elderly patients after myocardial infarction. Lancet 2:989, 1980.

227. Breddin, D., Loew, D., Lechner, K., et al.: The German-Austrian Aspirin Trial: A comparison of aspirin, placebo and phenprocoumon in secondary prevention of myocardial infarction. Circulation 62:63, 1980.

228. The EPSIM Research Group: A controlled comparison of aspirin and oral anticoagulants in prevention of death after myocardial infarction. N. Engl. J. Med. 307:701, 1982.

229. Meijer, A., Verheug, F., and Werter, C.: Aspirin versus coumadin in the prevention of reocclusion and recurrent ischemia after successful thrombolysis: A prospective placebo-controlled angiographic study. Results of the APRICOT study. Circulation 87:1524, 1993.

230. Cairns, J. A., and Markham, B. A.: Economics and efficacy in choosing oral anticoagulants or aspirin after myocardial infarction. JAMA 273:965, 1995.

231. Steering Committee of the Physicians' Health Study Research Group: Preliminary report: Findings from the aspirin components of the ongoing Physicians' Health Study. N. Engl. J. Med. 318:262, 1988.

232. Steering Committee of the Physicians' Health Study Research Group: Final report on the aspirin component of the ongoing Physicians' Health Study. N. Engl. J. Med. 321:129, 1989.

233. Peto, R., Gray, R., Collins, R., et al.: Randomized trial of prophylactic daily aspirin in British male doctors. Br. Med. J. 296:313, 1988.

234. Fuster, V., Cohen, M., and Halperin, J.: Aspirin in the prevention of coronary disease. N. Engl. J. Med. 321:183, 1989.

235. Manson, J. E., Stampler, M. J., Colditz, G. A., et al.: A prospective study of aspirin use and primary prevention of cardiovascular disease in women. JAMA 266:521, 1991.

236. Made, T., Wilkes, H. C., Stirling, Y., et al.: Randomised controlled trial of low-dose warfarin in the primary prevention of ischaemic heart disease in men at high-risk: Design and pilot study. Eur. Heart J. 9:836, 1988.

237. Meade, T. W.: Low-dose warfarin and low-dose aspirin in the primary prevention of ischemic heart disease. Am. J. Cardiol. 65:76, 1990.

238. Schweizer, P., Bardos, P., Erbel, R., et al.: Detection of left atrial thrombi by echocardiography. Br. Heart J. 45:148, 1981.

ANTITHROMBOTIC THERAPY FOR CARDIAC THROMBOEMBOLISM

239. Shrestha, N. K., Moreno, F. L., Narciso, F. V., et al.: Two-dimensional echocardiographic diagnosis of left atrial thrombus in rheumatic heart disease: A clinicopathologic study. Circulation 67:341, 1983.

240. Chimowitz, M. I., DeGeorgia, M. A., Poole, R. M., et al.: Left atrial spontaneous echo contrast is highly associated with previous stroke in patients with atrial fibrillation. Stroke 24:1015, 1993.

241. Askey, J. M., and Cherry, C. B.: Thromboembolism associated with auricular fibrillation. Continuous anticoagulant therapy. JAMA 144:97, 1950.

242. Israel, D. H., Fuster, V., Ip, J. H., et al.: Intracardiac thrombosis and systemic embolization. In Colman, R. W., Hirsh, J., Marder, V. J., Salzman, E. W. (eds.): Hemostasis and Thrombosis: Basic Principles and Clinical Practice. 3rd ed. Philadelphia, J. B. Lippincott Co., 1994, pp. 1452–1468.

243. Coulshed, N., Epstein, E. J., McKendrick, C. S., et al.: Systemic embolism in mitral valve disease. Br. Heart J. 32:26, 1970.

244. Pumphrey, C. W., Fuster, V., and Chesebro, J. H.: Systemic thromboembolism in valvular heart disease and prosthetic heart valves. Mod. Con. Cardiovasc. Dis. 51:131, 1982.

245. Barrett, H. J. M., Boughner, D. R., and Taylor, D. W.: Further evidence relating mitral valve prolapse to cerebral ischemic events. N. Engl. J. Med. 302:139, 1980.

246. Nishimura, R. A., McGoon, M. D., Shub, C., et al.: Echocardiographically documented mitral valve prolapse. Long-term follow-up of 237 patients. N. Engl. J. Med. 313:1305, 1985.

247. Wood, J. C., and Conn, H. L.: Prevention of systemic arterial embolism in chronic rheumatic heart disease by means of protracted anticoagulant therapy. Circulation 10:517, 1954.

248. Holley, K. E., Bahn, R. C., McGoon, D. C., and Mankin, H. T.: Spontaneous calcific embolization associated with calcific aortic stenosis. Circulation 27:197, 1963.

249. Brockmeier, L. B., Adolph, R. J., Gustin, B. W., et al.: Calcium emboli to the retinal artery in calcific aortic stenosis. Am. Heart J. 101:32, 1981.

250. Levine, H. J., Pauker, S. G., and Eckman, M. H.: Antithrombotic therapy in valvular heart disease. Chest 108(Suppl. Oct):360S, 1995.

251. Wolf, P. A., Abbot, R. D., and Kannel, W. B.: Atrial fibrillation as an independent risk factor for stroke. The Framingham Study. Stroke 22:983, 1991.

252. Prystowsky, E. N., Benson, Jr., D. W., Fuster, V., et al.: AHA Medical/Scientific Statement. Special report: Management of patients with atrial fibrillation. A report for health professionals from the Subcommittee on Electrocardiography and Electrophysiology, American Heart Association. Circulation 93:1262, 1996.

252a. Shivkumar, K., Jafri, S. M., and Gheorghide, M.: Antithrombotic therapy in atrial fibrillation: A review of randomized trials with special reference to the Stroke Prevention in Atrial Fibrillation II (SPAF II) Trial. Progr. Cardiovasc. Dis. 38:337, 1996.

253. Atrial Fibrillation Investigators: Risk factors for stroke and efficacy of antithrombotic therapy in atrial fibrillation. Analysis of pooled data from five randomized trials. Ann. Intern. Med. 154:1449, 1994.

254. Stroke Prevention in Atrial Fibrillation Investigators: The Stroke Prevention in Atrial Fibrillation Study: Final results. Circulation 84:527, 1991.

255. Feinberg, W. M., Seeger, I. F., Carmody, R. F., et al.: Epidemiologic features of asymptomatic cerebral infarction in patients with nonvalvular atrial fibrillation. Arch Intern. Med. 150:2340, 1990.

256. Kopecky, S. L., Gersh, B. J., McGoon, M. D., et al.: The natural history of lone atrial fibrillation. A population-based study over three decades. N. Engl. J. Med. 317:669, 1987.

257. Stroke Prevention in Atrial Fibrillation Investigators: Predictors of thromboembolism in atrial fibrillation: I. Clinical features of patients at risk. Ann. Intern. Med. 116:1, 1992.

258. Stroke Prevention in Atrial Fibrillation Investigators: Predictors of thromboembolism in atrial fibrillation: II. Echocardiographic features of patients at risk. Ann. Intern. Med. 116:6, 1992.

259. Blackshear, J. L., Peace, L. A., Asinger, R., et al.: Mitral regurgitation associated with reduced thromboembolic events in high-risk patients with atrial fibrillation. J. Am. Coll. Cardiol. 72:840, 1993.

260. Rosenthal, M. S., and Halperin, J. L.: Thromboembolism in nonvalvular atrial fibrillation: The answer may be in the ventricle. Int. J. Cardiol. 37:277, 1992.

261. Stroke Prevention in Atrial Fibrillation Investigators: Warfarin versus aspirin for prevention of thromboembolism in atrial fibrillation: Stroke prevention in atrial fibrillation II study. Lancet 343:687, 1994.

262. Veterans Affairs Stroke Prevention in Nonrheumatic Atrial Fibrillation Investigators: Warfarin in the prevention of stroke associated with nonrheumatic atrial fibrillation. N. Engl. J. Med. 327:1406, 1992.

263. Petersen, P., Boysen, G., Godtfredsen, J., et al.: Placebo-controlled, randomized trial of warfarin and aspirin prevention of thromboembolic complications in chronic atrial fibrillation. Lancet 1:175, 1989.

264. EAFT Study Group: European Atrial Fibrillation Trial: Secondary prevention of vascular events in patients with nonrheumatic atrial fibrillation and recent transient ischemic attack or minor stroke. Lancet 342:1255, 1993.

265. Petersen, P., and Boysen, G.: Prevention of stroke in atrial fibrillation. N. Engl. J. Med. 323:482, 1990.

266. Miller, V. T., Feinberg, W. M., Pearce, L. A., et al.: Differential effect of aspirin versus warfarin on clinical stroke types in patients with atrial fibrillation. Neurology 46:238, 1996.

267. Stroke Prevention in Atrial Fibrillation Investigators: A differential effect of aspirin for prevention of stroke in atrial fibrillation. J. Stroke Cerebrovasc. Dis. 3:181, 1993.

268. D'Olhaberriague, L., Hernandez-Vidal, A., Molina, L., et al.: A progressive study of atrial fibrillation and stroke. Stroke 20:1648, 1989.

269. Laupacis, A., Albers, G., Dalen, J., et al.: Antithrombotic therapy in atrial fibrillation. Chest 108(Suppl. Oct):352S, 1995.

270. Vangerhoets, F., Bogousslavsky, J., Regli, F., and VanMelle, G.: Atrial fibrillation after acute stroke. Stroke 24:26, 1993.

271. Stein, B., Halperin, J. L., and Fuster, V.: Should patients with atrial fibrillation be anticoagulated prior to cardioversion? Cardiovasc. Clinics 21:231, 1990.

272. Moreyra, E., Finkelhor, R. S., and Cebul, R. D.: Limitations of transesophageal echocardiography in the risk assessment of patients before nonanticoagulated cardioversion from atrial fibrillation and flutter: An analysis of pooled trials. Am. Heart J. 129:71, 1995.

273. Black, I. W., Fatkin, D., Sagar, K. B., et al.: Exclusion of atrial thrombus by transesophageal echocardiography does not preclude embolism after cardioversion of atrial fibrillation. A multicenter study. Circulation 89:2509, 1994.

274. Manning, W. J., Silverman, D. I., Katz, S. E., et al.: Impaired left atrial function after cardioversion: Relation to the duration of atrial fibrillation. J. Am. Coll. Cardiol. 23:1535, 1994.

275. Toddard, M. F., Dawkins, P. R., Prince, C. R., and Ammash, N. M.: Left atrial appendage thrombus is not uncommon in patients with acute atrial fibrillation and a recent embolic event: A transesophageal echocardiographic study. J. Am. Coll. Cardiol. 25:452, 1995.

276. Merino, A., Hauptman, P., Badimon, L., et al.: Echocardiographic "smoke" is produced by an interaction of erythrocytes and plasma proteins modulated by shear forces. J. Am. Coll. Cardiol. 20:1661, 1992.

277. Mugge, A., Kuhn, H., Nikutta, P., et al.: Assessment of left atrial appendage function by biplane transesophageal echocardiography in patients with nonrheumatic atrial fibrillation: Identification of a subgroup of patients at increased embolic risk. J. Am. Coll. Cardiol. 23:599, 1994.

278. Kontny, F., Dale, J., Hegren, L., et al.: Left ventricular thrombosis and arterial embolism after thrombolysis in acute anterior myocardial infarction: Predictors and effects of adjunctive antithrombotic therapy. Eur. Heart J. 14:1489, 1993.

279. Visser, C., Kan, G., David, K., et al.: Two-dimensional echocardiography in the diagnosis of left ventricular thrombus. Chest 83:228, 1993.

280. Huggins, G., and Fuster, V.: Left ventricular thromboembolism after myocardial infarction. Heart Disease and Stroke 3:355, 1994.

281. Tanne, D., Goldbourt, U., Zion, M., et al. of the SPRINT Study Group: Frequency and prognosis of stroke/TIA among 4,808 survivors of acute myocardial infarction. Stroke 24:1490, 1993.

282. Vaitkus, P. T., and Barnathan, E. S.: Embolic potential, prevention and management of mural thrombus complicating anterior myocardial infarction: A meta-analysis. J. Am. Coll. Cardiol. 22:1004, 1993.

283. The SCATI Group: A randomized controlled trial of subcutaneous calcium heparin in acute myocardial infarction. Lancet 2:182, 1989.

284. Turpie, A., Robinson, J., and Doyle, D.: A comparison of high-dose with low-dose subcutaneous heparin to prevent left ventricular mural thrombosis in patients with acute transmural anterior myocardial infarction. N. Engl. J. Med. 320:352, 1989.

285. Keren, A., Goldberg, S., Gottlieb, S., et al.: Natural history of left ventricular thrombi: Their appearance and resolution in the post-hospitalization period of acute myocardial infarction. J. Am. Coll. Cardiol. 15:790, 1990.

286. Lapeyre, III, A. C., Steele, P. M., Kazmier, F. J., et al.: Systemic embolism in chronic left ventricular aneurysm: Incidence and the role of anticoagulation. J. Am. Coll. Cardiol. 6:534, 1985.

287. Stratto, J. R., and Resnick, A. D.: Increased embolic risk in patients with left ventricular thrombi. Circulation 75:1004, 1987.

288. Roberts, W. C., and Ferran, V. J.: Pathologic aspects of certain cardiomyopathies. Circ. Res. 34:128, 1974.

289. Gottdiener, J. S., Gay, J. A., VanVoorhees, L., et al.: Frequency and embolic potential of left ventricular thrombus in dilated cardiomyopathy: Assessment by two-dimensional echocardiography. Am. J. Cardiol. 52:1281, 1983.

290. Fuster, V., Gersh, B. J., Giuliani, E. R., et al.: The natural history of idiopathic dilated cardiomyopathy. Am. J. Cardiol. 47:525, 1981.

290a. Kyrle, P. A., Korninger, C., Gossinger, H., et al.: Prevention of arterial and pulmonary embolism by oral anticoagulants in patients with dilated cardiomyopathy. Thromb. Haemost. 54:521, 1985.

290b. Roberts, W. C., Siegel, R. J., McManus, B. M.: Idiopathic dilated cardiomyopathy: analysis of 152 necropsy patients. Am. J. Cardiol. 60:1340, 1987.

290c. Ciaccheri, M., Castelli, G., Cecchi, F., et al.: Lack of correlation between intracavitary thrombosis detected by cross-sectional echocardiography and systemic emboli in patients with dilated cardiomyopathy. Br. Heart J. 62:26, 1989.

290d. Yokota, Y., Kawanishi, H., Hayakawa, M., et al.: Cardiac thrombus in dilated cardiomyopathy: relationship between left ventricular pathophysiology and left ventricular thrombus. Jpn. Heart J. 30:1, 1989.

291. Dec, G. W., and Fuster, F.: Idiopathic dilated cardiomyopathy. N. Engl. J. Med. 331:1564, 1994.

292. Diaz, R. A., Obasohan, A., and Oakley, C. M.: Prediction of outcome in dilated cardiomyopathy. Br. Heart J. 58:393, 1987.

293. Dunkman, W. B., Johnson, G. R., Carson, P. E., et al.: Incidence of thromboembolic events in congestive heart failure. Circulation 87(Suppl. VI):VI-94, 1993.

294. Falk, R. H., Foster, E., and Coats, M. H.: Ventricular thrombi and thromboembolism in dilated cardiomyopathy: A prospective follow-up study. Am. Heart J. 123:136, 1992.

295. Hatle, L., Orjavik, O., and Storstein, O.: Chronic myocardial disease: I.

Clinical picture related to long-term prognosis. Acta. Med. Scand. *199:*399, 1976.

296. Hamby, R. J.: Primary myocardial disease. Medicine *49:*55, 1970.
297. The European Working Group on Echocardiography: The European Co-operative Study on clinical significance of right heart thrombi. Eur. Heart J. *10:*1046, 1989.
298. Yamamoto, K., Ikeda, U., Furuhashi, K., et al.: The coagulation system is activated in idiopathic cardiomyopathy. J. Am. Coll. Cardiol. *25:*1634, 1995.
299. Sawada, S. G., Ryan, T., Segar, D., et al.: Distinguishing ischemic cardiomyopathy from nonischemic dilated cardiomyopathy with coronary echocardiography. J. Am. Coll. Cardiol. *19:*1223, 1992.
300. Tsevat, J., Eckman, M. H., McNutt, R. A., and Pauker, S. G.: Warfarin for dilated cardiomyopathy: A bloody tough pill to swallow? Med. Decis. Making *9:*162, 1989.
301. Baker, D. W., and Wright, R. F.: Management of heart failure: IV. Anticoagulation for patients with heart failure due to left ventricular systolic dysfunction. JAMA *272:*1614, 1994.
302. Richardson, W. S., and Detsky, A. S., for the Evidence-Based Medicine Working Group: Users' guides to the medical literature. VII. How to use a clinical decision analysis. A. Are the results of the study valid? JAMA *273:*1292, 1995.

ANTITHROMBOTIC THERAPY IN PROSTHETIC HEART VALVE REPLACEMENT

303. Fuster, V., Badimon, L., Badimon, J. J., and Chesebro, J. H.: Prevention of thromboembolism induced by prosthetic heart valves. Semin. Thromb. Hemost. *14:*50, 1988.
304. Israel, D. H., Sharma, S. K., and Fuster, V.: Antithrombotic therapy in prosthetic heart valve replacement. Am. Heart J. *127:*400, 1994.
305. Heras, M., Chesebro, J. H., Fuster, V., et al.: High risk of thromboembolic early after bioprosthetic cardiac valve replacement. J. Am. Coll. Cardiol. *25:*1111, 1995.
306. Butchart, E. G.: Thrombogenicity, thrombosis and embolism. *In* Butchart, E. G., Bodnar, E. (eds.): Current Issues in Heart Valve Disease: Thrombosis, Embolism and Bleeding. London, ICR Publishers, 1992, p. 293.
307. Horstkotte, D., and Burckhardt, D.: Prosthetic valve thrombosis. J. Heart Valve Dis. *4:*141, 1995.
308. Piper, C., Schulte, H. D., and Horstkotte, D.: Optimization of oral anti-coagulation for patients with mechanical heart valve prostheses. J. Heart Valve Dis. *4:*127, 1995.
309. Butchart, E. G.: Rationalizing antithrombotic management for patients with prosthetic heart valves. J. Heart Valve Dis. *4:*106, 1995.
310. Mok, D. C., Boey, J., Wang, R., et al.: Warfarin versus dipyridamole-aspirin and pentoxifylline-aspirin for the prevention of prosthetic heart valve thromboembolism: A prospective randomized clinical trial. Circulation *72:*1059, 1985.
311. Turpie, A. G. G., Gent, M., Laupacis, A., et al.: A comparison of aspirin with placebo in patients treated with warfarin after heart valve replacement. N. Engl. J. Med. *329:*524, 1993.
312. Hayashi, J. I., Nakazawa, S., Oguma, F., et al. Combined warfarin and antiplatelet therapy after St. Jude Medical valve replacement for mitral valve disease. J. Am. Coll. Cardiol. *23:*672, 1994.
313. Tinker, J. H., and Tarhan, S.: Discontinuing anticoagulation therapy in surgical patients with cardiac valve prostheses: Observation in 180 operations. JAMA *239:*738, 1978.
314. Butchart, E. G.: Anticoagulation management during non-cardiac surgery—time for common sense. J. Heart Valve Dis. *3:*313, 1994.
315. Sherman, D. G., Dyken, M. L., Gent, M., et al.: Antithrombotic therapy in cerebrovascular disorders. Chest *108*(Suppl. Oct):371S, 1995.
316. Hoylaerts, M., Kijken, D. C., Lijnen, H. R., and Collen, D.: Kinetics of the activation of plasminogen by human tissue plasminogen activator. Role of fibrin. J. Biol. Chem. *257:*2912, 1982.
317. Canneigieter, S. C., and Rosendaal, F. R.: Thromboembolic and bleeding complications in patients with mechanical heart valve prostheses. Circulation *89:*635, 1994.
318. Lengyel, M., Fuster, V., Keltai, M., et al.: Guidelines for the management of left-sided prosthetic valve thrombosis. Am. J. Cardiol. *(submitted for publication.)*
319. Roudaut, R., Labbe, T., Lorient-Roudaut, M. F., et al.: Mechanical cardiac valve thrombosis. Is fibrinolysis justified? Circulation *86:*8, 1992.
320. Vilanyi, J., Wladika, Z. S., Bartek, I., and Lengyel, M.: Diagnosis and treatment of tricuspid mechanical prosthetic valve dysfunction. Eur. Heart J. *13:*2190, 1992.
321. Birdi, I., Angelini, G. D., and Bryan, A. J.: Thrombolytic therapy for left-sided prosthetic heart valve thrombosis. J. Heart Valve Dis. *4:*154, 1995.
322. Stein, P. D., Albert, J. S., Copeland, J., et al.: Antithrombotic therapy in patients with mechanical and biological prosthetic heart valves. Chest *108*(Suppl. Oct):371S, 1995.

Chapter 59
Pregnancy and Cardiovascular Disease

URI ELKAYAM

CARDIOVASCULAR PHYSIOLOGY DURING PREGNANCY AND THE PUERPERIUM

Pregnancy and the peripartum period are associated with substantial cardiocirculatory changes. In the woman with heart disease, these changes can lead to rapid clinical deterioration. The approach to the cardiac patient during pregnancy therefore requires an understanding of the alteration in cardiovascular physiology during gestation, labor, delivery, and the puerperium. Hemodynamic changes occurring during pregnancy are summarized in Table 59–1.

BLOOD VOLUME. Blood volume increases substantially during pregnancy, starting as early as the sixth week, rising rapidly until midpregnancy, when the rise continues, but at a much slower rate.[1] The degree of volume expansion varies considerably in the individual patient (20 to 100 per cent) and averages 50 per cent. This increase is reported to correlate with fetal weight, placental mass, weight of the products of conception, neonatal weight, and maternal weight. A higher increment in blood volume is reported in multigravidas and in women with multiple pregnancies.[1]

Because increase in blood volume is more rapid than increase in red blood cell mass (Fig. 59–1), hemoglobin concentration falls during pregnancy, causing the "physiological anemia of pregnancy."[2] Hematocrit and hemoglobin levels are frequently as low as 33 to 38 per cent and 11 to 12 gm/100 ml, respectively, and can be partially corrected with iron therapy.[1] Changes in blood volume during pregnancy are attributable to estrogen-mediated stimulation of the renin-aldosterone system,[3] which results in sodium and water retention.[2] Chorionic somatomammotropin, a hormone-like substance in the placenta, may also be a factor.

CARDIAC OUTPUT, STROKE VOLUME, AND HEART RATE. Augmentation of blood volume alters stroke volume and cardiac output (Table 59–1). Cardiac output during pregnancy is estimated to exceed the output during the nonpregnant state by 30 to 50 per cent.[1,2,4] It begins to rise around the fifth week and peaks between the middle of the second and the third trimesters, when it plateaus. Body position can substantially influence cardiac output, with levels rising in the lateral position and declining in the supine position, owing to caval compression by the gravid uterus and decrease in venous return to the heart. The increase in cardiac output early in pregnancy is predominantly due to augmentation in stroke volume, whereas in the third trimester it is largely due to an accelerated heart rate, while stroke volume declines toward prepregnancy values as a result of caval compression.

Rise in heart rate peaks during the third trimester with an average increase of 10 to 20 beats/min,[4,5] although on occasion it may be markedly faster. Pregnancy of multiple fetuses is associated with an even higher heart rate. The heart rate may decrease slightly in the lateral position in comparison with the supine position.[1]

BLOOD PRESSURE AND SYSTEMIC VASCULAR RESISTANCE. Systemic arterial pressure begins to fall during the first trimester, reaches a nadir in midpregnancy, and returns

TABLE 59–1 HEMODYNAMIC CHANGES DURING NORMAL PREGNANCY

PARAMETER	1st TRIMESTER	2nd TRIMESTER	3rd TRIMESTER
Blood volume	↑	↑↑	↑↑↑
Cardiac output	↑	↑↑ to ↑↑↑	↑↑↑ to ↑↑
Stroke volume	↑	↑↑↑	↑, ↔, or ↓
Heart rate	↑	↑↑	↑↑ or ↑↑↑
Systolic blood pressure	↔	↓	↔
Diastolic blood pressure	↓	↓↓	↓
Pulse pressure	↑	↑↑	↔
Systemic vascular resistance	↓	↓↓↓	↓↓

Modified from Elkayam, U., and Gleicher, N.: Hemodynamics and cardiac function during normal pregnancy and the puerperium. *In* Elkayam, U., and Gleicher, N. (eds.): Cardiac Problems in Pregnancy: Diagnosis and Management of Maternal and Fetal Disease. 2nd ed. New York, Alan R. Liss, Inc., 1990, p. 5. Copyright © 1990. Reprinted by permission of John Wiley & Sons, Inc.

↔ = no change compared with nonpregnant level; ↑ = small increase; ↑↑ = moderate increase; ↑↑↑ = large increase; ↓ = small decrease; ↓↓ = moderate decrease; ↓↓↓ = large decrease.

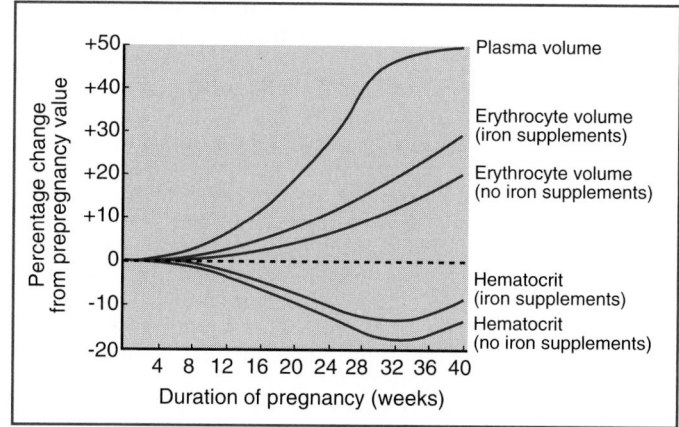

FIGURE 59–1. Changes in plasma volume, erythrocyte volume, and hematocrit during pregnancy. Increase in plasma volume is more rapid than increase in erythrocyte volume, causing the "physiological anemia of pregnancy," which can be partially corrected with iron supplements. (From Pitkin, R. M.: Nutritional support in obstetrics and gynecology. Clin. Obstet. Gynecol. 19:489, 1976, with permission.)

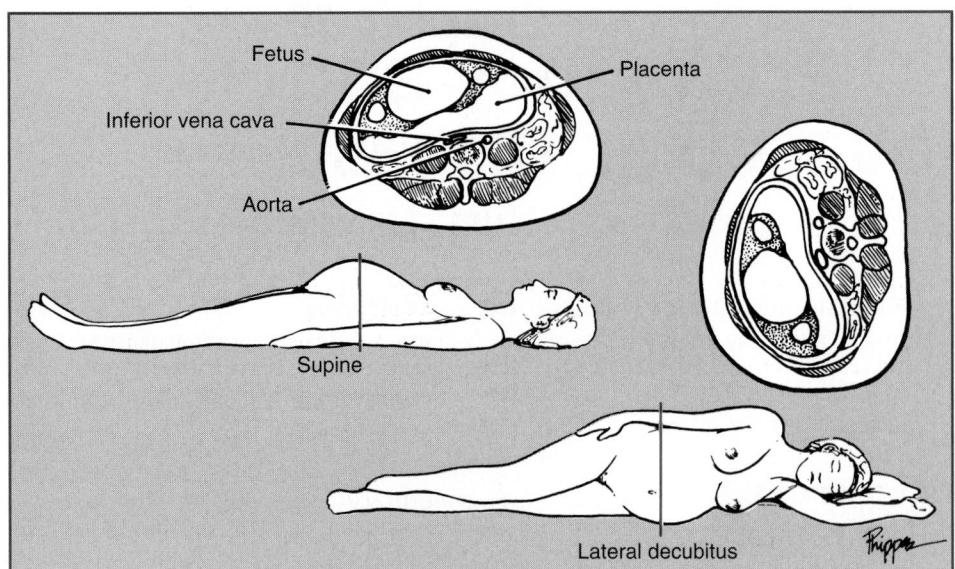

FIGURE 59–2. Venocaval compression of the inferior vena cava and abdominal aorta by the gravid uterus can lead to decreased cardiac output due to reduced venous return and to supine hypotensive syndrome. (From Lee, W., Shah, P. K., Amin, D. K., et al.: Hemodynamic monitoring of cardiac patients during pregnancy. *In* Elkayam, U., Gleicher, N. [eds.]: Cardiac Problems in Pregnancy, 2nd ed., New York, Alan R. Liss, Inc., 1990, p. 61.)

toward pregestational levels before term.[1] Because diastolic blood pressure decreases substantially more than systolic pressure, the pulse pressure widens.[1,6] Reduction in blood pressure is caused by a decline in systemic vascular resistance due to vasodilation,[1] probably mediated by (1) gestational hormonal activity, increased levels of circulating prostaglandins,[7] and atrial natriuretic factor[8]; (2) increased heart production by the developing fetus; and (3) the creation of low-resistance circulation in the pregnant uterus. A phenomenon unique to pregnancy and described as the supine hypotensive or the uterocaval syndrome of pregnancy occurs with significant decreases in heart rate and blood pressure in up to 11 per cent of pregnant women.[1] These hemodynamic changes are associated with weakness, lightheadedness, nausea, dizziness, and even syncope and are explained by acute occlusion of the inferior vena cava by the enlarged uterus (Fig. 59–2). When the supine position is abandoned, these hemodynamic effects and symptoms usually are promptly relieved.

HEMODYNAMIC CHANGES DURING LABOR AND DELIVERY. Anxiety, pain, and uterine contractions all alter hemodynamics substantially during labor and delivery. Oxygen consumption increases threefold. Cardiac output rises by up to 50 per cent during contractions, mainly owing to changes in stroke volume,[9] and it is higher in the lateral position than in the supine position. The effect of uterine contractions on the heart rate varies[13] and may be influenced by body position during labor and the form of sedation used. Both systolic and diastolic blood pressures increase markedly during contractions, with greater augmentation during the second stage.[1,9] Hemodynamic changes during labor and delivery are greatly influenced by the form of anesthesia and analgesia.[10] Reduction of pain and apprehension by local and caudal anesthesia may limit the rise in oxygen consumption, hemodynamic changes, and cardiac output, but does not prevent the increase in cardiac output related to uterine contractions.

HEMODYNAMIC EFFECTS OF CESAREAN SECTION. To avoid the hemodynamic changes associated with vaginal delivery, cesarean section is frequently recommended for women with cardiovascular disease. However, this form of delivery can also be associated with considerable hemodynamic fluctuation related largely to intubation, the technique, and drugs used for anesthesia and analgesia[10]; extent of blood loss; abdominal surgery; the relief of caval compression; extubation; and postoperative awakening.[1,10]

HEMODYNAMIC CHANGES POST PARTUM. Clinical status often deteriorates in the immediate postpartum period when venous return increases after the fetus is removed and caval compression is relieved.[1] In addition, blood

shifting from the contracting, emptied uterus into the systemic circulation (autotransfusion) increases the preload. This change in effective blood volume occurs despite blood loss during delivery and leads to a substantial rise in ventricular filling pressure, stroke volume, and cardiac output immediately after delivery. Within the first hour, however, the reduction in heart rate decreases cardiac output, which falls to prepregnancy levels 24 hours post partum as stroke volume normalizes.[9]

HEMODYNAMIC RESPONSE TO EXERCISE. Exercise-mediated increase in cardiac output is limited during gestation and in the third trimester may be more than 20 per cent lower than it is in nonpregnant women.[11] This attenuated rise in cardiac output is due to the lower responses of heart rate and stroke volume; the latter is probably the result of reduction in venous return during pregnancy. Uterine blood flow is also reduced (25 per cent) in the third trimester during mild exercise. Such reductions may be associated with fetal hypoxia, manifested by brief episodes of fetal bradycardia.[12] Strenuous physical activity may therefore be associated with fetal compromise and is not recommended during pregnancy.

CARDIAC EVALUATION DURING PREGNANCY

The evaluation of cardiac disease in pregnancy may be complicated by the normal anatomical and functional changes of the cardiovascular system. Such changes may result in signs and symptoms that can either simulate or obscure heart disease.[13] It is therefore imperative in many cases to use additional diagnostic tools to obtain objective and reliable information about cardiac status. The selection of such diagnostic tools should be influenced by the potential risk to the fetus posed by certain methods.

History and Physical Examination
(Table 59–2).

Normal pregnancy is often accompanied by symptoms of fatigue, decreased exercise capacity, hyperventilation, dyspnea, lightheadedness, and even syncope.[14,15] In addition, distention of the jugular veins due to increased blood volume and leg edema, often observed in late pregnancy, could lead to an erroneous diagnosis of heart failure or overestimation of its severity. Systemic arterial pulses are full and collapsing and are similar to those palpated in patients with aortic regurgitation or hyperthyroidism. A left ventricular impulse is easily detected in most women in late pregnancy; usually it is hyperactive and brisk. The

TABLE 59–2 CARDIAC SYMPTOMS AND PHYSICAL FINDINGS DURING NORMAL PREGNANCY

SYMPTOMS
  Decreased exercise capacity
  Tiredness
  Dyspnea
  Orthopnea
  Lightheadedness
  Syncope

PHYSICAL FINDINGS
  Inspection
    Hyperventilation
    Peripheral edema
    Distended neck veins with prominent A and V waves and brisk x and y descents
    Capillary pulsation
  Precordial palpation
    Brisk, diffuse, and displaced left ventricular impulse
    Palpable right ventricular impulse
    Palpable pulmonary trunk impulse
  Auscultation
    Increased S_1 with exaggerated splitting
    Persistent splitting of S_2
    Midsystolic ejection-type murmurs at lower left sternal edge and/or over pulmonary area radiating to left side of neck
    Continuous murmurs (cervical venous hum, mammary souffle)
    Diastolic murmurs (rare)

Modified from Elkayam, U., and Gleicher, N.: Changes in cardiac findings during normal pregnancy. *In* Elkayam, U., and Gleicher, N. (eds.): Cardiac Problems in Pregnancy: Diagnosis and Management of Maternal and Fetal Disease. 2nd ed. New York, Alan R. Liss, Inc., 1990, p. 31. Copyright © 1990. Reprinted by permission of John Wiley & Sons, Inc.

quality of the impulse may simulate a volume overload state such as that seen in aortic or mitral valve regurgitation. The pulmonary trunk, right ventricle, and pulmonic valve closure are often palpable, and this group of findings may result in difficulty in assessing the presence and/or severity of pulmonary hypertension.

CARDIAC AUSCULTATION. Especially after the first trimester, auscultation often reveals an increased first heart sound (S_1) with exaggerated splitting that may be misinterpreted as S_4 or as a systolic click.[13] The physiological increase in the amplitude of the second component of S_1 with inspiration should help differentiate it from an abnormal auscultatory event. S_2 is often increased in late pregnancy and may exhibit persistent splitting when the patient is examined in the lateral position. These changes in S_2 may be interpreted as signs of pulmonary hypertension (loud S_2) or atrial septal defect (fixed splitting of S_2). Auscultation of S_3 and S_4 sounds is uncommon in normal pregnancy, and their presence warrants further investigation to detect possible underlying disease.[13]

Innocent Systolic Murmurs. These can be heard in most pregnant women and are the result of the hyperkinetic circulation of pregnancy.[13] Murmurs are usually midsystolic and soft, heard best at the lower left sternal edge and over the pulmonic area, radiating to the suprasternal notch and to the left and, at times, also to the right side of the neck.[13,16] Not uncommonly the benign murmur of pregnancy may be louder or longer and may sound like those associated with atrial septal defect or stenosis of one of the semilunar valves.[16] In such cases an echocardiographic and Doppler evaluation is warranted to rule out an abnormal cardiac condition. Two benign continuous murmurs that may be heard during gestation are the cervical venous hum and the mammary souffle. The venous hum is usually heard maximally over the right supraclavicular fossa but can radiate to the contralateral area and sometimes to the area below the clavicle. The mammary souffle may be either systolic or continuous, is heard over the breast late in gestation or in the lactating woman, and is caused by increased flow in the mammary vessels. Characteristically the murmur decreases or vanishes when pressure is applied to

the stethoscope or when the patient moves into the upright position.[13] Diastolic murmurs may be heard in normal pregnant women due to increased blood flow through the atrioventricular valve.[13] Such a finding, however, is infrequent in the healthy pregnant woman and therefore requires careful diagnostic work-up to rule out organic disease.

Increases in blood volume and flow across the various cardiac valves may augment systolic murmurs of aortic or pulmonic stenosis and the diastolic murmur of mitral stenosis. In contrast, the murmurs associated with mitral or aortic regurgitation may decrease in intensity because of a reduction in systemic vascular resistance during pregnancy. In addition, the change in volume may abolish the systolic click and murmur commonly heard in patients with mitral valve prolapse[17] and may decrease the systolic murmur typical of obstructive hypertrophic cardiomyopathy.[18]

Laboratory Examinations

ELECTROCARDIOGRAPHY (Table 59–3). In normal pregnancy, QRS axis may shift to either the left or the right, but it usually stays within normal limits.[13] Slight ST-segment depressions and T-wave changes may be seen. A small Q wave and an inverted P wave in lead III that vary with respiration as well as a greater R-wave amplitude in lead V_2 are often present. A high incidence of ST-segment depression mimicking myocardial ischemia but not associated with wall motion abnormalities has been described relatively recently in patients undergoing cesarean section.[19] Increased susceptibility to arrhythmias during pregnancy can be manifested by the frequent finding of sinus tachycardia and atrial and/or ventricular premature beats.[20]

CHEST RADIOGRAPHY (Table 59–3). Although the radiation dose associated with a routine chest X-ray examination is minimal (the average dose to the skin in the primary beam is 70 to 150 mrad, while the estimated dose to the uterus is 0.2 to 43.0 mrad),[21] this diagnostic test is best avoided during pregnancy because of the potential for adverse biological effects from any amount of radiation. When chest radiography is performed, the pelvic area should be shielded by protective lead material.

Changes seen on chest films in normal pregnancy may simulate cardiac disease and should be interpreted with caution.[13,14] Straightening of the left upper cardiac border because of prominence of the pulmonary conus is often seen. The heart may seem enlarged because of its horizontal positioning secondary to the elevated diaphragm. In addition, an increase in lung markings may simulate a pattern of flow redistribution seen with increased pulmonary venous pressure due to left ventricular failure or mitral valve disease. Pleural effusion is often found early post partum[22]; it is usually small and resorbs 1 to 2 weeks after delivery.

DOPPLER ECHOCARDIOGRAPHY (Table 59–3). Gestational use of both

TABLE 59–3 FINDINGS ON ELECTROCARDIOGRAM, CHEST X-RAY, AND ECHO-DOPPLER DURING NORMAL PREGNANCY

ELECTROCARDIOGRAM
  QRS-axis deviation
  ST-segment and T-wave changes
  Small Q wave and inverted P wave in lead III (abolished by inspiration)
  Increased R-wave amplitude in lead V_2
  Frequent sinus tachycardia
  Increased incidence of arrhythmias

CHEST X-RAY
  Straightening of left upper cardiac border
  Horizontal position of heart
  Increased lung marking
  Small pleural effusion early post partum

ECHO-DOPPLER
  Increased left and right ventricular dimensions
  Unchanged or slightly increased size and systolic function of left ventricle
  Mild increase in left and right atrial size
  Small pericardial effusion
  Increased diameter of tricuspid annulus
  Functional tricuspid, pulmonary, and mitral insufficiency

Modified from Elkayam, U., and Gleicher, N.: Changes in cardiac findings during normal pregnancy. *In* Elkayam, U., and Gleicher, N. (eds.): Cardiac Problems in Pregnancy: Diagnosis and Management of Maternal and Fetal Disease. 2nd ed. New York, Alan R. Liss, Inc., 1990, p. 31. Copyright © 1990. Reprinted by permission of John Wiley & Sons, Inc.

maternal and fetal cardiac ultrasound is considered safe.[23] Transesophageal echocardiography has been increasingly used in pregnancy and seems to be well tolerated by both mother and fetus.[24] Normal gestational changes in the cardiovascular system are reflected echocardiographically and should be taken into consideration. Examination in the left lateral position often shows enlarged dimensions of cardiac chambers, especially the right atrium and ventricle.[5,25,26] These changes progress with the pregnancy but return to baseline dimensions post partum. Left ventricular systolic dimensions and function are either unchanged or slightly increased during pregnancy.

Pericardial effusion, usually small or minimal, has been noted in 40 per cent of normal pregnant women late in pregnancy.[27] Studies have demonstrated mild regurgitation of the tricuspid and pulmonary valves in the majority of normal pregnant women at term and of the mitral valve in approximately one-third.[25,26] These findings seem to be related to chamber enlargement and dilatation of the valve annulus. Repeat examination 3 to 6 weeks post partum still demonstrated tricuspid and pulmonary regurgitation in 70 to 80 per cent of women.[26] These findings, although not clinically important, need to be considered in the interpretation of Doppler echocardiograms obtained during pregnancy.

STRESS TESTING. An exercise test using bicycle ergometry or a treadmill may be carried out during pregnancy to help establish the diagnosis of ischemic heart disease and to assess functional capacity and cardiac reserve. The safety of such testing in pregnancy has not been fully established. Because fetal bradycardia has been reported with maximal but not with submaximal exercise,[12] a low-level exercise protocol allowing heart rate increase to 75 per cent of maximal predicted heart rate with fetal monitoring is recommended when stress testing is indicated.[13]

RADIONUCLIDE IMAGING. A potential limitation of these techniques during pregnancy is radiation exposure to the fetus. The dose estimated to reach the fetus with the radiopharmaceuticals generally used for cardiac imaging is equal to or less than 800 mrad.[28] However, calculations of the dose to the fetus are only approximations and can vary from person to person owing to differences in the uptake of radionuclides by maternal organs and in placental uptake and transfer. Because of these uncertainties and the potential risk, use of radionuclide imaging during gestation and in particular during the first trimester should be limited to cases in which the information desired cannot be obtained by other noninvasive techniques.

MAGNETIC RESONANCE IMAGING. Magnetic resonance imaging has been used in pregnancy for the assessment of congenital heart disease and aortic dissection.[29,30] Experience with this technique is limited, however, and its safety has not been fully established. This technique should therefore be used only when evaluation cannot be delayed until after pregnancy, and if possible after the first trimester.[31]

PULMONARY ARTERY CATHETERIZATION. Hemodynamic monitoring with the aid of a pulmonary artery catheter can be of great help in managing patients at high risk during pregnancy, labor, delivery, and the postpartum period. The ability to insert and position the flotation catheter under pressure monitoring without the need for fluoroscopy makes it particularly attractive for use during pregnancy.[32] Hemodynamic monitoring can provide useful diagnostic and prognostic information and therapeutic guidance and should be used without hesitation at any time during pregnancy if a noninvasive cardiac work-up does not provide conclusive information.

Hemodynamic monitoring is recommended throughout labor and delivery for any patient with symptomatic cardiac disease during pregnancy or with the potential for deterioration due to valvular, vascular, myocardial, or ischemic heart disease. Since significant circulatory changes that may lead to hemodynamic deterioration occur in the early postpartum period,[1] hemodynamic monitoring should be continued for at least several hours after delivery to assure stability.

CARDIAC CATHETERIZATION. When cardiac decompensation occurs during pregnancy, particularly if cardiac surgery, coronary angioplasty, or balloon valvuloplasty is being considered, cardiac catheterization may be required. Although this technique provides high-quality images, it is associated with a relatively high dose of radiation. The median dose to the skin is 47 rads per examination with 10 to 15 per cent exposure to an unshielded abdomen and approximately 500 mrad estimated dose to the conceptus, even with an appropriate pelvic shield.[21]

The potentially deleterious effect of ionizing radiation is linearly proportional to the absorbed dose and is present at all times after fertilization. The type and likelihood of this effect vary with the stage of fetal development and the dose of radiation. Increased incidence of fetal malformation appears to be highly unlikely with doses below 5 rads, even when these are delivered at a time when the induction of any specific type of maldevelopment is critical.[33] In general, radiation exposure during the first week of pregnancy may result in absorption or resorption of the preimplanted blastocyst, whereas the risk of teratogenic effects predominates during the second to sixth weeks of gestation. Developing brain cells can be affected by radiation during the seventh to fifteenth weeks, which may lead to alterations in neurological function or behavior. In addition, irradiation at any time during the entire pregnancy may increase the risk for child-

hood cancer[34]; this risk seems to be higher with exposure during the first trimester.

Cardiac catheterization during gestation should be performed only if information cannot be obtained by alternative noninvasive methods. To minimize radiation to the pelvic and abdominal areas, the brachial rather than the femoral approach is preferred. Appropriate shielding should be used, and roentgen exposure should be kept to a minimum. To minimize the use of ionizing radiation, as much information as possible should be obtained by noninvasive techniques such as contrast[35] and Doppler echocardiography.

CONGENITAL HEART DISEASE (CHD)

(See also Chaps. 29 and 30)

PRECONCEPTION COUNSELING. This should include an accurate diagnostic and functional evaluation and counseling of both the patient and her family regarding contraceptive alternatives, potential maternal and fetal risks of pregnancy, and, when appropriate, expected long-term maternal morbidity and survival as well as the risk of transmitting CHD to the offspring. In addition, guidance concerning anticoagulation and prophylactic antibiotics, if needed, should be provided.[36,37]

MATERNAL AND FETAL OUTCOME. In general, a good maternal outcome can be expected in most cases with noncyanotic congenital heart disease. Maternal outcome is determined by the nature of the disease, surgical repair, presence and severity of cyanosis, level of hemoglobin, increased pulmonary vascular resistance, and functional capacity.[36-38] Unfavorable outcome, including development of congestive heart failure, arrhythmias, and hypertension, is commonly seen in patients with impaired functional status and with cyanosis.[38] Other reported complications include angina, infective endocarditis, and thromboembolic phenomena. Factors that may increase likelihood of cardiovascular deterioration include exercise, heat, humidity, anemia, infections, and cardiac arrhythmias.[39]

Maternal functional capacity and cyanosis also determine fetal outcome. Fetal wastage was reported in 45 per cent of cyanotic mothers compared with 20 per cent in acyanotic mothers with CHD.[38] Low birth weight for gestational age and prematurity are common in cyanotic mothers and correlate with maternal hemoglobin and hematocrit values.[40] Risk of CHD is increased for the offspring of mothers with CHD with a reported incidence of about 10 per cent (3.4 to 16.1 per cent).[38-42] In addition, there are a greater number of noncardiac abnormalities as well as mental and physical impairments in children born to mothers with CHD.[38]

LABOR AND DELIVERY. Elective induction of labor when fetal maturity is confirmed may be used in high-risk patients for better planning of hemodynamic monitoring and availability of expert personnel.[39] Cesarean section is not indicated in most patients with CHD[36,38,39] and should be performed primarily for obstetrical reasons or in response to deteriorating maternal status. Oxygen should be given to hypoxemic mothers, and hemodynamic as well as blood gas monitoring is recommended in patients with impaired functional capacity, cardiac dysfunction, pulmonary hypertension, and cyanotic malformations.[32]

ANTIBIOTIC PROPHYLAXIS. Official recommendations by the American Heart Association do *not* include patients with CHD undergoing uncomplicated vaginal delivery unless they have a prosthetic heart valve or a surgically constructed systemic-to-pulmonary shunt.[43] Because of the difficulties in predicting complicated deliveries and the potential devastating consequences of endocarditis, we recommend antibiotic prophylaxis for vaginal delivery for patients with CHD, with the exception of those with an isolated secundum type of atrial septal defect and those ≥6 months after ligation and division of a patent ductus arteriosus. There is no need for antibiotic prophylaxis for cesarean section delivery.

Specific Malformations
(See also p. 976)

ATRIAL SEPTAL DEFECT (ASD) (see also pp. 966 and 970). This condition is usually well tolerated in pregnancy, even among patients with large left-to-right shunts. The development of pulmonary hypertension and atrial arrhythmias rarely occurs in the childbearing age. Because endocarditis is rare, antibiotic prophylaxis is not indicated in patients with secundum-type ASD. Recommendations concerning pregnancy in patients with ASD should be made on an individual basis, considering accompanying lesions, functional status, and the level of pulmonary vascular resistance.[42]

VENTRICULAR SEPTAL DEFECT (VSD) (see also p. 967). Women with isolated VSD usually tolerate pregnancy well, although congestive heart failure and arrhythmias have been reported.[42] The risk posed by pregnancy after closure of an uncomplicated VSD should not differ from that in patients without heart disease. The incidence of CHD in offspring of women with VSD was found to be as high as 22 per cent among live-born offspring in one report; 50 per cent of them had VSD.[38] Marked reduction in blood pressure during or after delivery as a result of blood loss or anesthesia may lead to shunt reversal in patients with pulmonary hypertension. The use of vasopressors and volume replacement to stabilize blood pressure promptly should prevent further complications.

PATENT DUCTUS ARTERIOSUS (PDA) (see p. 966). Maternal outcome in patients with PDA with left-to-right shunt is usually favorable[36,42]; however, clinical deterioration and congestive heart failure may occur in some patients.[42] There were no maternal deaths among a large number of patients with PDA.[36,42,44] The occasional patient with heart failure should be treated with bed rest, diuretics, digitalis, and vasodilators. The need for surgical intervention during pregnancy is rare. A fall in systemic vascular resistance during gestation and hypotension early post partum may lead to shunt reversal in women with pulmonary hypertension. Peripartum decrease in systemic blood pressure should be corrected by means of vasopressor agents.

CONGENITAL AORTIC VALVE DISEASE (see p. 969). These abnormalities may lead to significant aortic stenosis and regurgitation in women of childbearing age. Obstruction of left ventricular outflow can also result from unicuspid or tricuspid valve stenosis or supravalvular and subvalvular obstruction. Aortic stenosis, especially if mild, can easily be missed on physical examination, because murmur may be attributed to the flow-related systolic murmur commonly heard in the normal pregnant woman. The presence of a sustained left ventricular impulse, aortic ejection sound, maximum murmur intensity heard in the second right intercostal space, S_4, and radiation of the murmur to both sides of the neck should raise the level of suspicion.

Most patients with aortic stenosis should have favorable outcome of pregnancy provided that they receive early diagnosis and appropriate care, including hemodynamic monitoring during labor and delivery, and appropriate anesthesia.[42] At the same time, however, worsening of symptoms during pregnancy, especially in women with severe aortic stenosis, is not uncommon.[45–48] Symptoms usually develop in the second or third trimester and may include exertional dyspnea, chest pain, lightheadedness, syncope, and pulmonary edema. A high incidence (20 per cent) of cardiac defects has been reported in live-born infants of mothers with left ventricular outflow obstruction.[38] Because of the risk involved, patients with severe aortic stenosis (aortic valve area < 1.0 cm²) should undergo valve replacement prior to pregnancy. Optional management of a pregnant patient with severe aortic stenosis includes (1) early abortion followed by valve replacement and repeat pregnancy and (2) continuation of pregnancy and plan for percutaneous balloon valvuloplasty or surgical intervention in

patients who show clinical deterioration not controlled by medical therapy.

Both replacement of aortic valve and percutaneous balloon valvuloplasty have been performed successfully in pregnant women with aortic stenosis.[46–49] These procedures, however, are not free of complications. While valvuloplasty obviates the general anesthesia and cardiopulmonary bypass required for surgery, it can be associated with prolonged radiation exposure and hemodynamic fluctuations that may lead to immediate and late fetal complications. Surgical replacement of the aortic valve during pregnancy may be associated with increased incidence of fetal loss.[49] For these reasons, these procedures should be considered only in patients with severe disease and symptoms not manageable with medical therapy, and they should be avoided when possible during the first trimester.

COARCTATION OF THE AORTA (see p. 971). Available information[38] as well as our experience indicates a favorable outcome of pregnancy in most women with uncomplicated coarctation. At the same time, however, complications such as hypertension, congestive heart failure, and angina have been reported. In addition, aortic dissection and rupture, as well as rupture of an aneurysm of the circle of Willis,[36] have also been associated with coarctation of the aorta during pregnancy. Also, a higher incidence of infective endocarditis in the mother and of CHD in the fetus has been shown in cases with surgically uncorrected compared with corrected coarctation.[36,38] For all of these reasons, it seems advisable to correct aortic coarctation prior to pregnancy.

Treatment to reduce the incidence of aortic rupture and cerebral aneurysms during pregnancy consists of limiting physical activity and controlling blood pressure. Excessive blood pressure reduction, however, may compromise uteroplacental blood flow and should be avoided. Surgical correction of coarctation has been performed successfully during pregnancy[50] and may be indicated in patients with severe uncontrollable systolic hypertension or heart failure.

PULMONIC STENOSIS (see also p. 965). Although complications such as congestive heart failure and syncope have been described, women with pulmonic valve stenosis, even if severe, usually tolerate pregnancy well.[36,51,52] When possible, however, severe stenosis should be corrected prior to conception. In the rare instance of progressive right ventricular failure or symptoms clearly related to the stenotic valve despite appropriate drug therapy, surgical or percutaneous balloon valvotomy should be considered.

TETRALOGY OF FALLOT (see p. 968). Hemodynamic changes associated with pregnancy may become severe and cause clinical deterioration in women with surgically uncorrected or only partially corrected tetralogy of Fallot. Increases in blood volume and venous return to the right atrium raise right ventricular pressure, which combined with a fall in systemic vascular resistance can produce or exacerbate a right-to-left shunt and cyanosis.

Maternal hematocrit above 60 per cent, arterial oxygen saturation below 80 per cent, right ventricular hypertension, and syncopal episodes are poor prognostic signs. Close monitoring of systemic blood pressure and blood gases during labor and delivery is recommended for cyanotic or symptomatic patients. Although reports of pregnancies in 37 women with corrected tetralogy of Fallot described no maternal deaths,[38] worsening of the clinical condition necessitating interruption of the pregnancy is not uncommon. Incidence of cardiac defects reported in born infants ranges between 3 and 17 per cent.

Because maternal and fetal outcomes seem to be markedly improved after surgical repair, this procedure should be performed prior to conception.[36] Patients who have undergone only palliative procedures or who have significant residual defects after repair are still at higher risk during pregnancy. Although mortality associated with complete repair is slightly increased in older patients who have previously undergone a palliative procedure,[38] surgical repair is recommended prior to pregnancy. Since revision of an incompletely repaired defect is recommended in patients with residual VSD when the pulmonary/systemic flow ratio is greater than 1.5:1, in those with right ventricular outflow obstruction (right ventricular systolic pressure > 60 mm Hg), and in those with right ventricular failure due to pulmonic regurgitation, such revision should be performed prior to conception in a woman who plans to conceive.[42]

Inhalation analgesia and paracervical or pudendal block have been recommended for labor and vaginal delivery.[53] Epidural block could result in systemic hypotension and shunt reversal and should therefore be used with great care. To minimize potential hemodynamic problems, a segmental epidural block for the first stage of labor with pudendal or caudal block for the second stage has been recommended along with opiates to decrease the concentration of anesthetics injected epidurally.

EISENMENGER'S SYNDROME (see p. 799). This condition continues to be associated with high risk for maternal morbidity and mortality. A relatively recent review of 24 women with this syndrome revealed a mortality rate of 38 per cent.[42] Several cases published since 1990 confirm the risk associated with pregnancy in patients with this syndrome.[41,54–58] Maternal mortality often occurs in the first few days after delivery and is preceded by desaturation and hemodynamic deterioration. Eisenmenger's syndrome is also associated with a poor fetal outcome and a high incidence of fetal loss, prematurity, intrauterine growth retardation, and perinatal death.[42,54,57,59]

Because of the high risk of maternal mortality, patients with Eisenmenger's syndrome should be advised against pregnancy. Abortion should be recommended for patients who are already pregnant. Management of a patient who decides to proceed to term must include close follow-up for early detection of clinical deterioration and restriction of physical activity to minimize the hemodynamic burden. Because of the increased incidence of peripartum thromboembolic events—which are often fatal in such patients[42,59]—anticoagulent therapy seems indicated for at least the third trimester of gestation and for 4 weeks post partum. Since premature delivery is common, women with Eisenmenger's syndrome should be hospitalized for any sign of premature uterine activity. For this reason and to assure restriction of activity and close follow-up, early elective hospitalization is recommended. Spontaneous labor is preferred to induction and should lower the chance of prematurity or the need for cesarean section. Blood pressure, electrocardiographic, and blood gas monitoring are essential during labor and delivery to ensure early detection and correction of problems; high concentrations of oxygen may be helpful. Most patients in stable condition will tolerate vaginal delivery; however, an attempt should be made to shorten the second stage of labor by the use of forceps or vacuum extraction.

Because epidural anesthesia may lead to peripheral vasodilation and increased shunting from right to left, epidural block should be titrated carefully with local anesthetics.[53] Delivery has been successful with lumbar epidural block for the first stage of labor and caudal block for delivery; other authors have preferred the use of systemic medications, inhalation analgesia, and paracervical or pudendal block. For cesarean section, general anesthesia with drugs having a minimal negative inotropic effect is recommended. In addition, segmental epidural anesthesia has been used successfully for cesarean section in patients with Eisenmenger's syndrome.[53]

EBSTEIN'S ANOMALY. Most patients with Ebstein's anomaly survive to childbearing age. Long-term prognosis depends on the severity of tricuspid regurgitation, the presence of right ventricular failure, and the presence and degree of cyanosis due to shunting from right to left. Successful pregnancies have been reported in the majority of patients with Ebstein's anomaly.[60] However, complications such as right ventricular failure, infective endocarditis, and paradoxical em-

bolism can occur.[42] The incidence of maternal and fetal complications is increased among cyanotic patients.[38] The approach to labor and delivery in symptomatic or cyanotic patients with Ebstein's anomaly includes antibiotic prophylaxis, oxygen administration, hemodynamic and blood gas monitoring, and efforts to prevent a drop in systemic blood pressure in response to peripheral vasodilation or blood loss.

COMPLEX CYANOTIC CHD. The more widespread use of palliative and corrective surgical procedures for complex cyanotic congenital cardiac anomalies has allowed more women who are so affected to reach childbearing age.[42] Although successful pregnancies have been reported in patients with partially corrected and uncorrected cyanotic heart disease including pulmonary and tricuspid atresia,[41,54] transposition of the great vessels,[41,61] truncus arteriosus,[54,62] single ventricle,[41,63] double-outlet right ventricle,[64] and double-inlet left ventricle,[65] pregnancy is associated with increased risk in these patients. A recent report[41] of 96 pregnancies in 44 patients with cyanotic heart disease but without Eisenmenger's reaction demonstrated cardiovascular complications in 32 per cent of the patients. These complications included heart failure, thromboembolic events, supraventricular tachycardia, and peripartum bacterial endocarditis resulting in postpartum maternal death in one patient. In addition, a high incidence of fetal wastage (57 per cent), premature deliveries, small-for-gestational-age newborns, and both cardiac and noncardiac congenital malformations has been reported.[38,41]

Hemoglobin and arterial oxygen saturation prior to pregnancy were found to be best predictors for fetal outcome.[41] When serious risk to the mother is predicted, pregnancy should be discouraged prior to conception or should be interrupted early if it has already begun. If the patient wishes to continue the pregnancy, restriction of physical activity and early detection and management of heart failure and/or arrhythmias are essential. Because of potential for severe thromboembolic events,[41,55] anticoagulation is recommended at least during the third trimester and 1 month post partum. Diuretics, if indicated, should be used carefully because of rise of hemoconcentration in the cyanotic patients. Antibiotic prophylaxis and oxygen therapy are strongly recommended for delivery,[41] as well as hemodynamic and blood gas monitoring. Although vaginal delivery appears to be tolerated by most women,[41,42,65] attempts should be made to shorten the second stage by the use of forceps or vacuum extraction.

During labor and delivery, systemic hypotension due to vasodilation or blood loss should be expeditiously corrected to avoid increasing right-to-left shunt.[42,63] Regional anesthetic techniques should be used cautiously. Systemic medications, inhalation analgesia, nerve blocks, and intrathecal morphine have been recommended.[53,56]

RHEUMATIC HEART DISEASE

Although the incidence of rheumatic heart disease is declining in the United States, the disease continues to be prevalent in many parts of the world and may be associated with significant morbidity and even mortality during pregnancy.[66–68]

ACUTE RHEUMATIC FEVER (see Chap. 55). This disease occurs most commonly in children, before puberty, and may recur during pregnancy. Acute rheumatic fever associated with carditis and congestive heart failure may be fatal in the pregnant woman.[66] The incidence of Sydenham's chorea, like acute rheumatic fever itself, has been reported to be increased in pregnancy (chorea gravidarum) and can cause preterm labor and fetal and maternal death. Because of the problems faced by women with recurrent rheumatic fever during pregnancy, it is prudent to continue antibiotic prophylaxis against streptococcal infection in the pregnant patient with a history of this condition. The recommended antibiotic regimen is discussed in detail on page 1773.

Chronic Rheumatic Valvular Disease
(See also Chap. 32)

Patients with chronic rheumatic valvular disease should be managed individually according to the site and severity of the lesion. However, certain general guidelines apply to the care of all patients. These include restriction of physical activity in symptomatic patients, to reduce cardiovascular load and prevent hemodynamic and symptomatic worsening, and prophylactic antibiotic treatment to prevent streptococcal infection and recurrence. Although antibiotic prophylaxis during labor and delivery has not been uniformly recommended,[43] it is commonly used for vaginal and abdominal deliveries.[66] Hemodynamic monitoring is strongly recommended from the onset of labor to approxi-

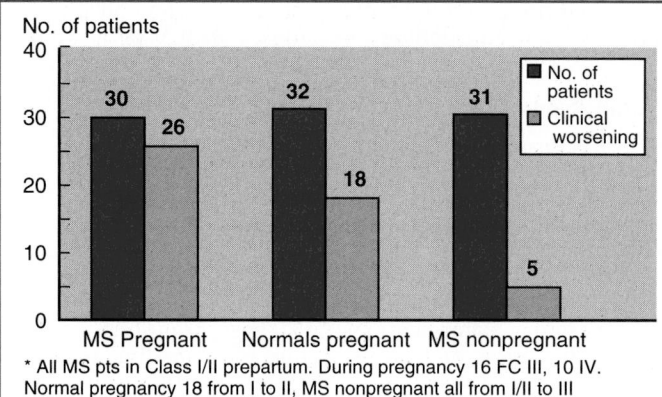

FIGURE 59–3. Worsening in functional classification in patients with mitral stenosis (MS). Twenty-six of 30 patients with MS reported worsening of symptoms during pregnancy. However, more than 50 per cent of women without heart disease also described similar symptoms and impairment of functional capacity during normal pregnancy. Only 5 of 31 nonpregnant patients with MS reported clinical worsening over a similar period. (Modified from Avila, W. S., Grinberg, M., Cardoso, L. F., et al.: Course of pregnancy and puerperium in women with mitral valve stenosis. Rev. Assoc. Med. Bras. *38:*195, 1992.)

mately 24 hours post partum in any patient who experiences symptoms of heart failure during pregnancy and for those with severe valvular disease, left ventricular dysfunction, or pulmonary hypertension.[32]

MITRAL STENOSIS. This condition is the most common rheumatic valvular lesion in pregnancy.[44,68] The majority of patients with moderate to severe mitral stenosis demonstrate worsening of clinical status during gestation (Fig. 59–3).[69] Although mitral stenosis is often accompanied by some degree of mitral regurgitation, hemodynamic problems are related predominantly to flow obstruction. The pressure gradient across the narrowed mitral valve may increase greatly secondary to the physiological increase in heart rate and blood volume of pregnancy.[1] Increased left atrial pressure may result in atrial flutter or fibrillation, substantially accelerating ventricular rate and further elevating left atrial pressure. In addition, decreased serum colloid osmotic pressure during pregnancy and excessive peripartum intravenous fluid administration can both predispose to pulmonary edema.

The therapeutic approach to patients with significant mitral stenosis should aim to reduce the heart rate and decrease blood volume. Both heart rate and symptoms can be controlled effectively by restricting physical activity and administering beta-adrenergic receptor blockers.[69,70] In patients with atrial fibrillation, digoxin may also be useful for control of ventricular rate. Blood volume can be decreased through restriction of salt intake and the use of oral diuretics; aggressive use of diuretic agents should, however, be avoided to prevent hypovolemia and reduction of uteroplacental perfusion.

Vaginal delivery can be permitted in most patients with mitral stenosis. In symptomatic patients or those with moderate or severe stenosis (mitral valve area < 1.5 cm²), hemodynamic monitoring is recommended during labor and delivery. Initiation of monitoring at onset of labor allows hemodynamic optimization by means of intravenous diuretics, digoxin (in case of atrial fibrillation), beta blockers, or nitroglycerin and prevention of a rise in left atrial pressure during labor and delivery.[71] With delivery and thus relief of venocaval obstruction due to the gravid uterus, there is an immediate increase in venous return, which may lead to a substantial increase in pulmonary artery wedge pressure.[32] For this reason, hemodynamic monitoring should be continued for at least several hours post partum.

Epidural anesthesia is the most appropriate form of analgesia in patients with mitral stenosis[53,71,72] for both vaginal and abdominal delivery. This form of anesthesia is often associated with a significant fall in pulmonary arterial and left atrial pressures due to systemic vasodilation. With this approach, the great majority of patients with mitral stenosis, even if it is severe, can be delivered with few complications.

Mitral Valve Repair or Replacement. My experience with a large number of patients with moderate and severe mitral stenosis as well as experience of other investigators indicates that careful medical therapy, with particular emphasis on lowering the heart rate,[70] allows successful completion of pregnancy in the great majority of women without the need for valve correction or replacement during pregnancy (Fig. 59–4). Repair or replacement of the valve during pregnancy, however, may be indicated in some patients with severe symptomatic mitral stenosis in spite of adequate medical therapy.[67,70,72] In both mitral valve commissurotomy (open or closed) and replacement, the risk in pregnant patients is comparable to that in nonpregnant patients. In contrast, however, open commissurotomy and valve replacement are likely to result in increased fetal loss.[68] Closed mitral commissurotomy is associated with only minimal risk to the fetus; it is therefore preferable to the open technique.[73] However, it should be recommended only in centers where it is performed routinely.

Percutaneous Mitral Balloon Valvuloplasty (see also p. 1386). The use of this procedure during pregnancy has recently been reported in an increasing number of pregnant patients with mitral stenosis.[74–79] In the majority of cases, hemodynamic and symptomatic improvement has been achieved without apparent untoward maternal and fetal effects. At the same time, however, serious complications have occasionally been reported, including initiation of uterine contraction,[76] maternal arrhythmia leading to fetal distress,[78] cardiac tamponade requiring surgical intervention, and systemic embolization.[79] In addition, this procedure is associated with some risk to the fetus secondary to unavoidable ionizing radiation. This information suggests that percutaneous mitral balloon valvuloplasty is an attractive alternative to surgery during pregnancy, but is limited by the exposure to radiation and possible complications that may result in fetal distress or require surgical intervention during pregnancy.

For all of the aforementioned reasons, mitral valve repair or replacement during pregnancy should be considered only in cases with severe mitral stenosis (mitral valve area < 1.0 cm²) refractory to optimal medical therapy and should be avoided if possible during the first trimester.[80]

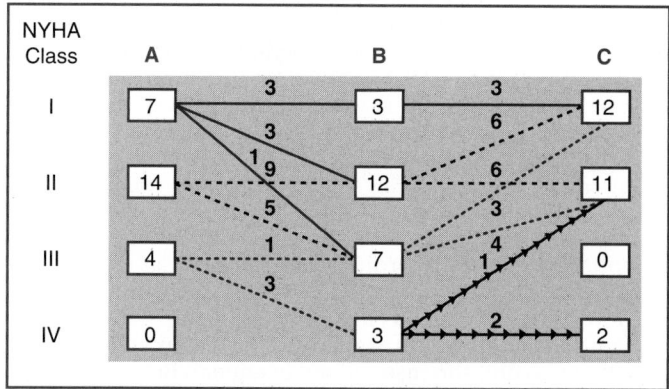

FIGURE 59–4. Effect of beta-blockade therapy on New York Heart Association functional class in 25 pregnant patients with symptomatic mitral stenosis (mean valve area 1.1 ± 0.25 cm²). *A,* before pregnancy; *B,* during pregnancy before initiation or increase of beta-blockade therapy; *C,* during pregnancy with adequate beta blockade. (From Al Kasab, S. M., Sabag, T., Al Zaibag, et al.: B-adrenergic receptor blockade in the management of pregnant women with mitral stenosis. Am. J. Obstet. Gynecol. *169:*37, 1990.)

Balloon valvuloplasty should be done under echocardiographic guidance if possible and with abdominal and pelvic shielding if fluoroscopy is used. When valve replacement is indicated, selection of the type of prosthesis should be based on its hemodynamic profile and durability and the need for anticoagulation.

MITRAL REGURGITATION. This condition is usually well tolerated in pregnancy, presumably because of left ventricular unloading secondary to the physiological fall in systemic vascular resistance. In symptomatic patients, drug therapy with diuretics is indicated, and digoxin may be useful in those with impaired left ventricular systolic function. Because hydralazine has been shown to be safe for use during pregnancy,[81] it may be used for further reduction of left ventricular afterload and prevention of hemodynamic worsening associated with isometric exercise during labor.[82]

Bicuspid aortic valve is the most common cause for aortic valve disease during gestation.[68] Rheumatic aortic valve involvement occurs in conjunction with mitral valve disease in approximately 5 per cent of pregnant patients with rheumatic valvular disease.[68]

AORTIC STENOSIS. Although most patients with aortic stenosis and valve area greater than 1.0 cm² tolerate pregnancy well, patients with more severe stenosis may demonstrate clinical deterioration with exertional dyspnea, near-syncope, or syncope and pulmonary edema.[83–85] Development of serious symptoms during pregnancy, especially if resistant to medical therapy, may require termination of pregnancy or repair of valve either surgically (valve replacement) or by percutaneous balloon valvuloplasty.[83–86]

AORTIC REGURGITATION. Similar to mitral regurgitation, aortic regurgitation is also well tolerated during pregnancy, probably because of reduced systemic vascular resistance and increased heart rate, which results in shortening of diastole. In symptomatic patients, diuretics, digoxin, and hydralazine for afterload reduction can be safely used. Since hydralazine has been shown to prevent an increase in pulmonary artery wedge pressure during isometric exercise in patients with aortic regurgitation,[87] it may be used for this purpose during labor and delivery.

OTHER CONDITIONS AFFECTING THE VALVES, AORTA, AND MYOCARDIUM

Mitral Valve Prolapse (MVP)
(See also p. 1029)

Diagnosed by M-mode echocardiography, MVP was reported in approximately 15 per cent of women of childbearing age. However, when the diagnosis was based on two-dimensional (2-D) echocardiographic criteria, the incidence was reported to be only about 2 per cent.[17] In a review of heart disease in pregnancy, MVP was found in only two of 145 pregnant women and suspected in 1.2 per cent of women examined in prenatal clinics.[17] A combined experience involving 158 pregnant women showed that MVP has no effect on maternal or fetal outcome.[17,88,89]

Pregnancy may reduce the incidence of prolapse-related auscultatory and echocardiographic changes as a result of an increase in left ventricular end-diastolic volume.[17] For the few patients with MVP with chest pain or cardiac arrhythmias, the emphasis should be on reassurance and attempts to avoid the use of medications. Beta-adrenergic blocking agents are recommended when therapy is indicated,[89] with periodic reassessment of the need to continue drug therapy. Patients with MVP, especially those with a thickened mitral valve and mitral regurgitation, are at increased risk for infective endocarditis. Although antibiotic prophylaxis for uncomplicated vaginal delivery has not been uniformly recommended, the development of bacteremia during vaginal delivery and cesarean section cannot

always be predicted. For this reason, I recommend prophylaxis for labor and delivery in patients with MVP accompanied by valve thickening and/or regurgitation.

Marfan Syndrome
(See also p. 1672)

Pregnancy in women with Marfan syndrome poses a twofold problem: a potential catastrophic and often lethal acute aortic dissection and a risk of having a child who will inherit the condition.[90] Review of available literature published since 1980 reveals the description of 15 cases of pregnancy in Marfan patients, the majority of whom had cardiovascular complications.[90,91] These complications included dilatation of the ascending aorta leading to aortic regurgitation and heart failure and proximal and distal aortic dissections (Fig. 59–5). The majority of patients developed their complications in the later phase of pregnancy. Aortic dissection resulted in maternal death in three cases; in three other cases live babies were delivered by cesarean section before successful surgery; and in two cases surgery was performed during pregnancy. In contrast to these selected reports of complications, a retrospective analysis of 105 unselected pregnancies among 26 women with this syndrome revealed only one death from endocarditis in a patient with severe mitral regurgitation.[92]

The management of pregnancy in women with Marfan syndrome should include preconception counseling to discuss potential maternal and fetal risks.[90] Women with significant cardiac involvement—in particular, dilatation of the aorta—are at high risk for complications during gestation and should be advised against conception or, if they are already pregnant, to have an early abortion. In contrast, the risk is significantly lower in patients without cardiac complications and a normal aortic diameter. Still, a favorable outcome is not guaranteed, and aortic dissection can

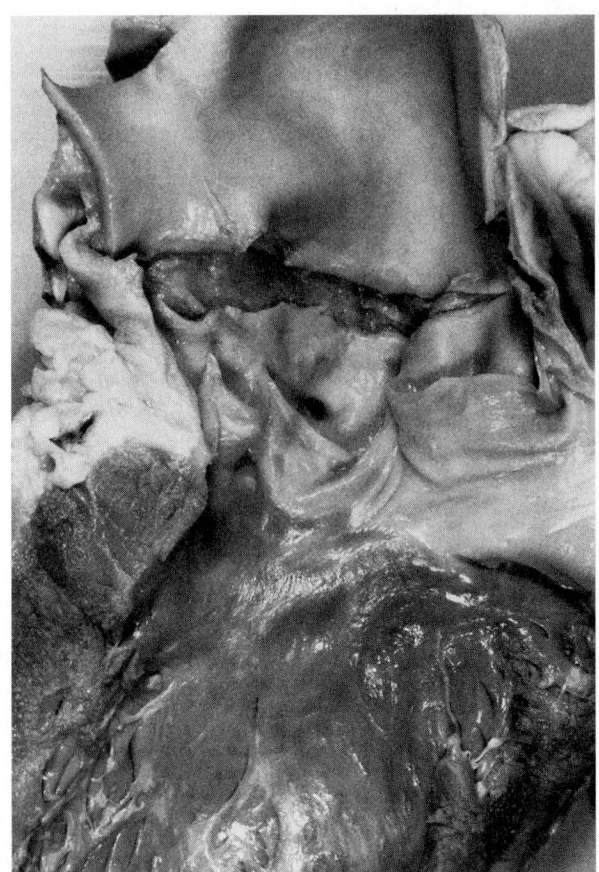

FIGURE 59–5. Just above the cusps of the aortic valve is a transverse tear across nearly the entire diameter of the ascending aorta in a 34-year-old woman with the Marfan syndrome who died suddenly 2 days post partum.

occur, albeit infrequently, in patients with a normal sized aorta.[90] Preconceptual echocardiographic assessment of the aorta and periodic follow-up during pregnancy are highly recommended. Since aneurysm and dissection of the aorta can occasionally involve the descending aorta, the use of transesophageal seems preferred to transthoracic echocardiography.[93] During pregnancy, physical activity should be limited. Beta blockers, which have been shown to reduce the rate of aortic dilatation and the risk of complications in patients with the Marfan syndrome, should be administered.[94] In case of substantial dilatation of the aorta during pregnancy, therapeutic abortion or surgical intervention should be considered.[90,95] In women with aortic dilatation, aortic dissection, or other cardiac complications, abdominal delivery by cesarean section should be the preferred mode of delivery to minimize hemodynamic changes associated with vaginal delivery.

Cardiomyopathies

HYPERTROPHIC CARDIOMYOPATHY (HC) (see also p. 1414). Reported experience in 89 pregnancies among 42 patients with hypertrophic cardiomyopathy (HC) reveals a favorable outcome in most cases but at the same time a potential for increased morbidity and even mortality.[96–100] New onset or worsening of congestive heart failure has been reported in 25 per cent of cases, and a few patients experienced chest pain, palpitations, dizzy spells, and syncope. Three patients had ventricular arrhythmias, which proved fatal in one,[96] and in one patient sudden death occurred at 28 weeks while she was running upstairs.[99] Fetal outcome in most cases does not seem to be affected by maternal HC; however, premature labor and delivery have been reported.[97,100] In addition, the risk of inheriting the disease may be as high as 50 per cent in familial cases and less in sporadic cases.[96]

The therapeutic approach to the pregnant patient with HC depends on the presence of symptoms and left ventricular outflow obstruction. In the symptomatic patient with obstructive HC, blood loss during delivery, vasodilation, and sympathetic stimulation during anesthesia must be avoided. Indications for drug therapy include symptoms and the presence of arrhythmias. Symptoms associated with elevated left ventricular filling pressure should be treated with beta-adrenergic blocking agents, with diuretics and calcium antagonists added if beta blockers alone are not sufficient.[99] Dual-chamber pacemaker may be considered in the patients who develop symptoms in the early phase of pregnancy.[100] Because of the arrhythmogenic effect of pregnancy, implantation of an automatic defibrillator should be considered in patients with HC with a history of sudden death, syncope, or life-threatening arrhythmias.

Vaginal delivery has been shown to be safe in women with HC.[96] In those with symptoms or outflow obstruction, the second stage of labor may be shortened by the use of forceps. The use of prostaglandins to induce uterine contractions may be unfavorable in a patient with obstructive HC owing to their vasodilatory effect, whereas oxytocin should be well tolerated. Since tocolytic agents with beta-adrenergic receptor activity may aggravate left ventricular outflow tract obstruction, magnesium sulfate is preferred. Similarly, spinal and epidural anesthetics should be used with great caution in obstructive HC because of their vasodilatory effect, and excessive blood loss should be avoided or replaced promptly with intravenous fluid or blood.[96]

Because the risk for infective endocarditis is increased in HC, especially the obstructive form, and in patients with mitral valve abnormality, antibiotic prophylaxis should be considered for labor and delivery.

PERIPARTUM CARDIOMYOPATHY. Peripartum cardiomyopathy (PPCM) is a form of dilated cardiomyopathy (see p. 1407) with left ventricular systolic dysfunction that results

in signs and symptoms of heart failure. Symptoms usually occur during the last trimester of gestation, and diagnosis is usually made in the peripartum period (Fig. 59–6).[101] Since there is no specific test available for the diagnosis of PPCM, it is established by exclusion of other causes of left ventricular dilatation and systolic dysfunction. The reported incidence of the disease in the United States is approximately 1 in 10,000, with a higher incidence—up to 1 in 100—in certain parts of Africa.[102]

Common symptoms and signs are shortness of breath, fatigue, chest pain, palpitations, weight gain, peripheral edema, and occasionally peripheral or pulmonary embolization.[101–108] Physical examination often reveals an enlarged heart, S_3, and murmurs of mitral and tricuspid regurgitation.[102] The electrocardiogram may show left ventricular hypertrophy, ST-T changes, conduction abnormalities, and arrhythmias. Chest x-ray examination may reveal cardiomegaly, pulmonary venous congestion with interstitial or alveolar edema, and occasionally pleural effusion. Doppler echocardiography shows that all four chambers are enlarged, with marked reduction in left ventricular systolic function. Small-to-moderate pericardial effusion and mitral, tricuspid, and pulmonic regurgitation may be evident. The clinical presentation and hemodynamic changes are indistinguishable from those found in other forms of dilated cardiomyopathy.[101,107] A few patients with high-output heart failure have been reported.[109]

The incidence of PPCM is greater in women with twin pregnancies, in multiparas, in women over 30 years of age, and in African-American women.[102] Although the etiology of PPCM is still unknown, the unique nature of this syndrome is suggested by its occurrence at a relatively young age when compared with other forms of dilated cardiomyopathy, the recovery of cardiac size and function in a large number of patients, and its relation to pregnancy.[107] It has been postulated that PPCM may be due to nutritional deficiency, small-vessel coronary artery abnormalities, hormonal effects, toxemia, maternal immunological response to fetal antigen, or myocarditis. The association between myocarditis and PPCM was suggested by some investigators who reported a high incidence of myocarditis documented by endomyocardial biopsy.[110] Later reports, however, have indicated a low incidence of myocarditis in patients with PPCM that was comparable to that found in an age- and sex-matched nonpregnant, control population with idiopathic dilated cardiomyopathy.[104,107,108,111]

The clinical course of PPCM varies with approximately 50 to 60 per cent of patients showing complete or near-complete recovery of clinical status and cardiac function,

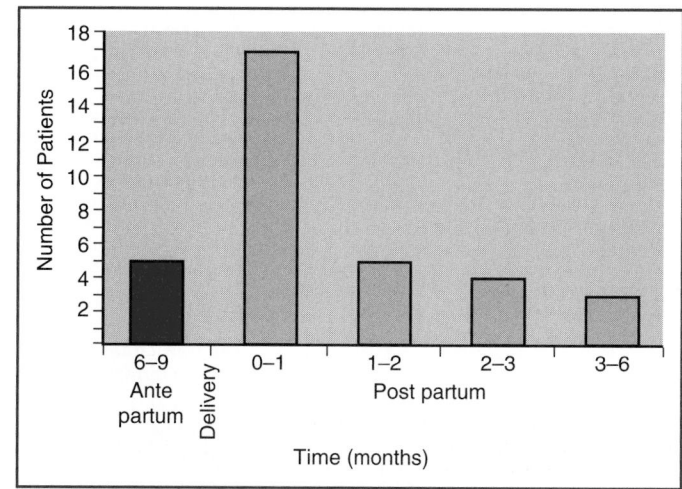

FIGURE 59–6. Time of onset of symptoms in relation to time of delivery in 34 patients with peripartum cardiomyopathy. (From Rizeq, M. N., Rickenbacher, P. R., Fowler, M. B., et al.: Incidence of myocarditis in peripartum cardiomyopathy. Am. J. Cardiol. 74:474, 1994.)

usually within the first 6 months post partum[106]; the rest of the patients demonstrate either continuous clinical deterioration, leading to cardiac transplantation or early death, or persistent left ventricular dysfunction and chronic heart failure.[102,104–106]

Management. Acute heart failure should be treated vigorously with oxygen, diuretics, digitalis, and vasodilator agents. The use of hydralazine as an afterload-reducing agent is safe during pregnancy.[81] The use of organic nitrates, dopamine, dobutamine, or milrinone has been reported in pregnancy in a limited number of cases. Nitroprusside has been used successfully during pregnancy, but experiments in animals have shown the potential for fetal toxicity.[112] Angiotensin-converting enzyme inhibitors have a teratogenic effect on the fetus, may cause fetal renal dysfunction, and should therefore not be used during pregnancy (see p. 1859).[113] Because of the increased incidence of thromboembolic events in PPCM, anticoagulant therapy is recommended. Since the disease may be reversible, the temporary use of an intraaortic balloon pump or left ventricular assist device may help stabilize the patient's condition pending improvement.[114]

Although a beneficial effect of immunosuppressive therapy has been suggested in patients with PPCM, reported failure of such treatment even in patients with histological evidence of myocarditis[107] and clinical as well as cardiac improvement in patients given supportive therapy alone raise doubt regarding the efficacy of immunosuppression in patients with this disease. Predictors for clinical deterioration post partum are older age, higher parity, severe left ventricular dilatation, later onset of symptoms after delivery, high pulmonary arterial and pulmonary artery wedge pressures, and conduction defects on the surface ECG.[106] Because of the high risk of mortality and morbidity among patients who do not recover early, such patients should be considered for cardiac transplantation.[114,115]

Subsequent pregnancies in women with PPCM are often associated with relapses and a high risk for maternal morbidity and mortality. Although the likelihood of such relapse is greater in patients with persistently abnormal heart size and/or function,[101,116] it has also been reported in women in whom left ventricular function is restored after the first episode.[105,117] For these reasons, subsequent pregnancies should be discouraged in patients with PPCM who have persistent cardiac dysfunction; women with recovered cardiac function after an episode of PPCM should be informed that subsequent pregnancy may not be risk free.

Hypertension in Pregnancy

(See also p. 830)

Hypertension in pregnancy is defined as increments in systolic and diastolic blood pressure of ≥ 30 and ≥ 15 mm Hg respectively or a diastolic pressure of ≥ 90 mm Hg as measured on more than one occasion.[118,119] Hypertension complicates 8 to 10 per cent of all pregnancies and is an important cause of maternal mortality and morbidity, including abruptio placentae, disseminated intravascular coagulation, cerebral hemorrhage, hepatic failure, and acute renal failure. The recommended classification by the working group on high blood pressure in pregnancy[119] identified the following categories: (1) chronic hypertension; (2) preeclampsia-eclampsia; (3) preeclampsia-eclampsia superimposed on chronic hypertension; and (4) transient hypertension.

CHRONIC HYPERTENSION. Defined as blood pressure $\geq 140/90$ mm Hg diagnosed (1) prior to pregnancy; (2) before the 20th gestational week; and (3) during pregnancy and persisting beyond the 42nd postpartum day. Chronic hypertension is associated with increased complications (15 per cent) such as fetal growth retardation, premature delivery, abruption, acute renal failure, and hypertensive crisis; most of these complications occur in patients older than 30 years with a longer duration of hypertension or those who develop superimposed preeclampsia. Drug therapy is recommended for diastolic pressure ≥ 100 mm Hg or ≥ 90 mm Hg in patients with renal disease or evidence of end-organ involvement. Guidelines for antihypertension drug therapy for chronic hypertension in pregnancy are shown in Table 59–4.

PREECLAMPSIA-ECLAMPSIA. Preeclampsia usually occurs after 20 weeks' gestation in the first pregnancy and near term in multiparous women. It is characterized by hypertension accompanied by proteinuria (≥ 0.3 gm/24 hours), edema, or both. Hypertension in this condition is defined as (1) increased systolic blood pressure ≥ 30 mm Hg; or (2) increased diastolic blood pressure ≥ 15 mm Hg from values before 20 weeks' gestation. If prior blood pressure is not known, values $\geq 140/90$ mm Hg after 20 weeks' gestation are diagnostic. Preeclampsia is always associated with increased risk to both mother and fetus; certain signs and symptoms are predictors for complications and are listed in Table 59–5.[118,120] Preeclampsia may progress to eclampsia, a life-threatening convulsive phase. Preeclampsia usually regresses within 24 to 48 hours post partum. In the minor-

TABLE 59–4 ANTIHYPERTENSIVE DRUGS USED TO TREAT CHRONIC HYPERTENSION IN PREGNANCY

DRUG	COMMENT
α_2-Adrenergic receptor agonists	Methyldopa is the most extensively used drug in this group, its safety and efficacy supported in randomized trials, and there is a 7.5-yr follow-up study of children born to treated mothers. Methyldopa is the drug of choice recommended by the Working Group.
β-Adrenergic receptor antagonists	These drugs, especially atenolol and metoprolol, appear safe and efficacious in late pregnancy, but fetal growth retardation has been noted when treatment was started in early or midgestation. Fetal bradycardia can occur, and animal studies suggest the fetus' ability to tolerate hypoxic stress may be compromised.
α- and β-Adrenergic receptor antagonists	Labetalol appears as effective as methyldopa, but there is little or no follow-up information on children born to mothers treated with labetalol, and there is concern for maternal hepatotoxicity.
Arteriolar vasodilators	Hydralazine is used frequently as adjunctive therapy with methyldopa and β-adrenergic receptor antagonists. Rarely, neonatal thrombocytopenia has been reported. Trials with calcium channel blockers look promising. Experience with minoxidil is limited; this drug is not recommended.
Converting enzyme inhibitors	Captopril causes fetal death in diverse animal species, and several converting enzyme inhibitors have been associated with renal failure in the newborn when administered to humans. Do not use in pregnancy.
Diuretics	Many authorities discourage their use, but others continue these medications if they were prescribed before gestation or if a chronic hypertensive patient appears quite salt sensitive. The latter views have been endorsed by the Working Group.

From Lindheimer, M. D.: Hypertension in pregnancy. Hypertension *22*:127, 1993.

TABLE 59-5 PREDICTORS FOR HIGH RISK IN WOMEN WITH PREECLAMPSIA

1. Systolic blood pressure ≥160 mm Hg or diastolic blood pressure ≥110 mm Hg

2. New proteinuria ≥2.0 gm/24 hr (2+ or 3+ on qualitative examination)

3. New increased serum creatinine levels (>2.0 mg/dl)

4. Platelet count <100,000/liter or evidence of microangiographic hemolytic anemia (e.g., schistocytes and/or increased lactic acid dehydrogenase and direct bilirubin levels)

5. Elevated hepatic enzymes (alanine aminotransferase or aspirate aminotransferase)

6. Upper abdominal pain (especially epigastric and right upper quadrant)

7. Headache and other cerebral or visual disturbances

8. Cardiac decompensation (e.g., pulmonary edema)

9. Retinal hemorrhage, exudates, or papilledema*

10. Intrauterine growth retardation and decreased urine volumes

Modified from Lindheimer, M. D.: Hypertension in pregnancy. Hypertension 22:127, 1993.
* Unlikely to occur without other major signs of severity.

ity of cases, postpartum eclampsia with hypertension, proteinuria, and convulsions occurs within 10 days post partum.

Hospitalization is recommended in preeclamptic patients. If the patient is near term (34 to 36 weeks), labor should be induced after control of hypertension and preventive antieclamptic treatment; if the fetus is immature, delay of delivery should be considered. Patients with severe hypertension in spite of 24 to 48 hours of therapy and any high-risk manifestations (Table 59–5) should be delivered regardless of gestational age. Drug therapy is recommended if diastolic blood pressure is 105 to 110 mm Hg,[118] which should be reduced to 90 to 104 mm Hg. Guidelines for drug treatment of severe hypertension near term or during labor are shown in Table 59–6.

TRANSIENT HYPERTENSION. Defined as the development of elevated blood pressure during pregnancy or in the first 24 hours post partum without preexisting hypertension and without other signs of preeclampsia. This condition is predictive for future development of hypertension.

PREGNANCY AFTER CARDIAC TRANSPLANTATION

A recent study conducted to determine the outcome of pregnancy in cardiac allograft recipients identifed 30 such cases.[121] Maternal hemodynamic changes during gestation were well tolerated by all pa-

tients, and rejection episodes were rare. At the same time, however, a high incidence of maternal complications was reported, including chronic hypertension, preeclampsia, and infections.[121-123] Although fetal death did not occur, fetal growth retardation was found in 20 per cent, and 40 per cent of births were preterm. None of the newborns was found to have congenital malformations, supporting a lack of teratogenic effect of immunosuppressive agents.[123] There were no maternal deaths during pregnancy, but three patients died within 30 months after delivery. This limited information suggests, therefore, that pregnancy in women after cardiac transplantation is not associated with increased maternal mortality; however, it results in increased maternal morbidity, preterm deliveries, and fetal growth retardation. In addition, the patients and their families should be informed regarding potential limited life span after delivery in patients after heart transplantation.

CORONARY ARTERY DISEASE

PATHOGENESIS. Coronary artery disease (CAD) is rare among women of childbearing age, and the occurrence of peripartum acute myocardial infarction (AMI) is anecdotal.[124]

Risk factors for CAD in women under the age of 50 years include high levels of total plasma cholesterol, low levels of high-density lipoproteins, cigarette smoking, diabetes mellitus, hypertension, a family history of CAD, toxemia of pregnancy, and the use of oral contraceptives.[125] The combination of heavy smoking and concurrent use of oral contraceptives has been shown to be a powerful predictor of AMI.[126] In addition, increased risk has been related to the patient's age at the time of her first delivery (below the age of 20 years)[127] and to a lifelong irregular pattern of menstruation.[128]

Several mechanisms have been proposed to explain the relationship between oral contraceptives and AMI. These drugs may trigger clot formation and embolization, as suggested by the increased incidence of venous thrombosis, pulmonary embolism, and cerebral thromboembolism.[124] In addition, oral contraceptives may raise serum levels of triglycerides, total cholesterol, and low-density lipoprotein; lower the level of high-density lipoprotein; increase the incidence of hypertension; and precipitate the ulceration of atherosclerotic plaques.[124] To reduce the risk for AMI, oral contraceptives should be avoided or formulations with lower effective doses of estrogen should be used in women over the age of 35, cigarette smokers, and those who develop hypertension while using this form of birth control.

Peripartum AMI is often associated with normal coronary angiographic findings[129-133] and may be due to a decrease in coronary perfusion caused by spasm or in situ thrombosis. Although the cause of spasm is not clear, it has often been associated with pregnancy-induced hypertension and in some instances with the use of ergot derivatives—oxytocin,[132] and prostaglandin[134]—to suppress lactation or uterine bleeding.[134,135] Coronary arterial dissection during pregnancy or immediately post partum is another relatively common cause of peripartum AMI[136-139] (Fig. 59–7). The dissection involves the left anterior descending artery in approximately 80 per cent of cases and the right coronary artery in most other cases.[138] Multiple coronary artery dissections have been recently reported in two cases (Fig. 59–8).[137,139] Other potential causes of AMI during pregnancy have been collagen vascular disease,[140,141] Kawasaki's disease,[142] sickle cell anemia,[143] and pheochromocytoma.[144]

DIAGNOSIS. The diagnostic approach to ischemic myocardial disease in pregnancy is influenced to some extent

TABLE 59-6 GUIDELINES FOR TREATING SEVERE HYPERTENSION NEAR TERM OR DURING LABOR

REGULATION OF BLOOD PRESSURE

The degree to which blood pressure should be decreased is disputed. The Working Group's Consensus Report recommends maintaining diastolic levels between 90 and 105 mm Hg.[119]

DRUG THERAPY

1. Hydralazine administered intravenously is the drug of choice. Start with low doses (5 mg IV bolus), then administer 5 to 10 mg every 20 to 30 min to avoid precipitous decreases. Side effects include tachycardia and headache. Neonatal thrombocytopenia has been reported.
2. Diazoxide is recommended for the occasional patient whose hypertension is refractory to hydralazine. Use 30 mg miniboluses because precipitous hypotension may result with higher doses. Side effects include arrest of labor and neonatal hypoglycemia.
3. Experience with labetalol is growing, and some use this agent instead of diazoxide as a second-line drug.
4. Favorable results have been reported with calcium channel blockers. However, if magnesium sulfate is being infused, the magnesium ion may potentiate the effect of the calcium channel blockers, resulting in precipitous and severe hypotension.
5. Refrain from using nitroprusside, because fetal cyanide poisoning has been reported in animal models. However, in the final analysis, maternal well-being will dictate therapy choice.

The Working Group retained parenteral magnesium sulfate as the drug of choice for preventing impending eclamptic convulsions. Therapy should continue for 12 to 24 hr into the puerperium, because one-third of patients with eclampsia have their convulsion after childbirth.

From Lindheimer, M. D.: Hypertension in pregnancy. Hypertension 22:127, 1993.

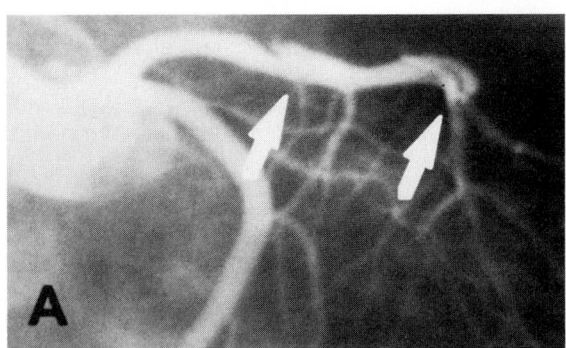

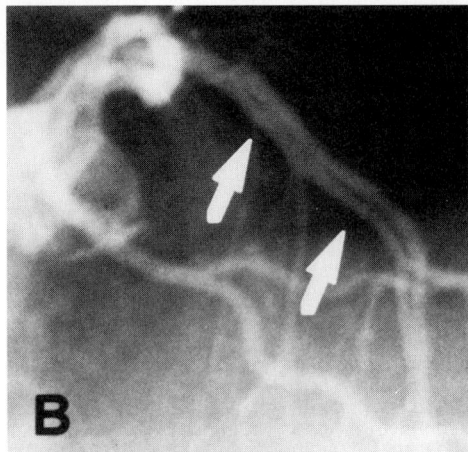

FIGURE 59–7. *A* and *B*, A long dissection in the left anterior descending artery (arrows) in a 44-year-old woman with acute anterior myocardial infarction in the early postpartum period. (Courtesy of Y. Almagor, M. D., and S. Goldberg, M. D.)

by whether a diagnostic procedure could harm the fetus and by normal changes seen during pregnancy that may mimic pathological changes. T-wave inversion, Q wave in lead III, and increased R/S ratio in lead V_2 are commonly seen in normal pregnancy.[13] ST-segment depression not associated with chest pain or echocardiographic wall motion abnormalities has been described during elective cesarean section and can mimic myocardial ischemia (Fig. 59–8).[19] Since fetal bradycardia has been reported during maximal exercise in normal women, a submaximal exercise protocol with fetal monitoring is recommended for the evaluation of ischemic myocardial disease during pregnancy.[13] Radionuclide myocardial perfusion scans and radionuclide ventriculography expose the fetus to radiation and should be used only when the potential benefits seem to outweigh fetal risk.[13] For similar reasons, cardiac catheterization involving fluoroscopy and cineangiography should be used only when relevant information cannot be obtained by other, noninvasive methods. It should be noted that the diagnosis of myocardial ischemia and infarction has been reported to be delayed during pregnancy because of the low level of suspicion.[132]

MANAGEMENT. Both maternal and fetal considerations should influence the therapeutic approach to ischemic heart disease during pregnancy. Because of their safety in pregnancy, beta blockers appear to be the most appropriate drugs of choice. The use of organic nitrates and calcium antagonists in patients with acute myocardial ischemia or infarction has been described in a limited number of patients.[131,135,137,145–147] These drugs should be given cautiously to prevent maternal hypotension and potential fetal distress.[145,148,149] Use of high-dose aspirin during pregnancy is debatable, since it has been reported to cause bleeding in the neonate and in the mother,[150] as well as growth retardation in the fetus.[151] Use of low-dose aspirin, however, is safe during pregnancy.[148,150] Although only lim-

ited experience is available regarding thrombolytic therapy during pregnancy, it has been safely used in several cases[151,152] and should be considered in high-risk patients with AMI. Coronary reperfusion by means of percutaneous transluminal coronary angioplasty or coronary artery bypass graft surgery has been reported to be successful during pregnancy,[154] although experience is still limited. Such procedures should be avoided during the first trimester, if possible, owing to the potential deleterious fetal effects due to ionizing radiation as well as cardiopulmonary bypass.

Risk stratification after AMI during pregnancy should be determined by noninvasive methods. Coronary angiography should be done only in cases in which coronary angioplasty or bypass surgery seems indicated during pregnancy.[149,155] Management should focus on reducing cardiovascular stress during pregnancy and the peripartum period. Termination of pregnancy may be required in patients with intractable ischemia or heart failure in the early phase of gestation.[147] Pulmonary artery catheterization with hemodynamic monitoring can help in the early detection and correction of hemodynamic abnormalities during labor and delivery.[146,147,155] During labor, adequate analgesia and supplemental oxygen should be given, and if desired, cardiac output can be increased by placing the patient in the left lateral decubitus position (Fig. 59–2). Labor in the supine position, however, may decrease venous return and thus reduce right atrial and left ventricular filling pressures. Low forceps can be used to shorten the second stage of labor.

Although elective cesarean section is not indicated in every case, it should be used in patients with active ischemia or hemodynamic instability despite adequate medical therapy.[146] Epidural anesthesia can reduce hemodynamic fluctuations during labor and is associated with left ventricular unloading due to vasodilation. If general anesthesia is indicated, halothane should be avoided in patients with depressed left ventricular systolic function. In addition, atropine and ketamine should be used with caution to prevent tachycardia. Continued hemodynamic monitoring is advisable for several hours post partum to detect hemodynamic worsening associated with the postpartum hemodynamic changes described earlier.

ARRHYTHMIAS

Pregnancy is associated with an increased incidence of arrhythmias in women both with and without organic heart disease.[155–157] In healthy women, multiple and even frequent atrial and ventricular premature beats may occur, usually without effect on either the mother or the fetus. Although palpitations, dizziness, and even syncope are relatively common in pregnancy, a relation to arrhythmias can be found in only the minority of cases.[156] At the same time, however, symptomatic and hemodynamically significant ventricular and supraventricular tachycardia have been reported in patients with a normal heart during gestation.[157] Reduction in blood pressure occasionally associated with such arrhythmias may result in fetal bradycardia[160] and necessitate immediate treatment with antiarrhythmic drugs, electric cardioversion, or immediate cesarean section. New onset or exacerbation of an arrhythmia has been demonstrated during pregnancy in patients with an antepartum history of arrhythmias,[158] preexcitation,[159] and other forms of acquired congenital heart disease.[161]

ATRIAL FLUTTER AND FIBRILLATION. These arrhythmias are rare during normal pregnancy and are usually associated with rheumatic mitral valve disease. Recent reports have described atrial fibrillation during gestation accompanied by treatment with magnesium sulfate[162] and in a patient with preexcitation.[163] Ventricular tachycardia or fibrillation is also rare in pregnancy and is usually associated with structural heart disease, drugs,[164,165] electrolyte abnormalities,[166] or

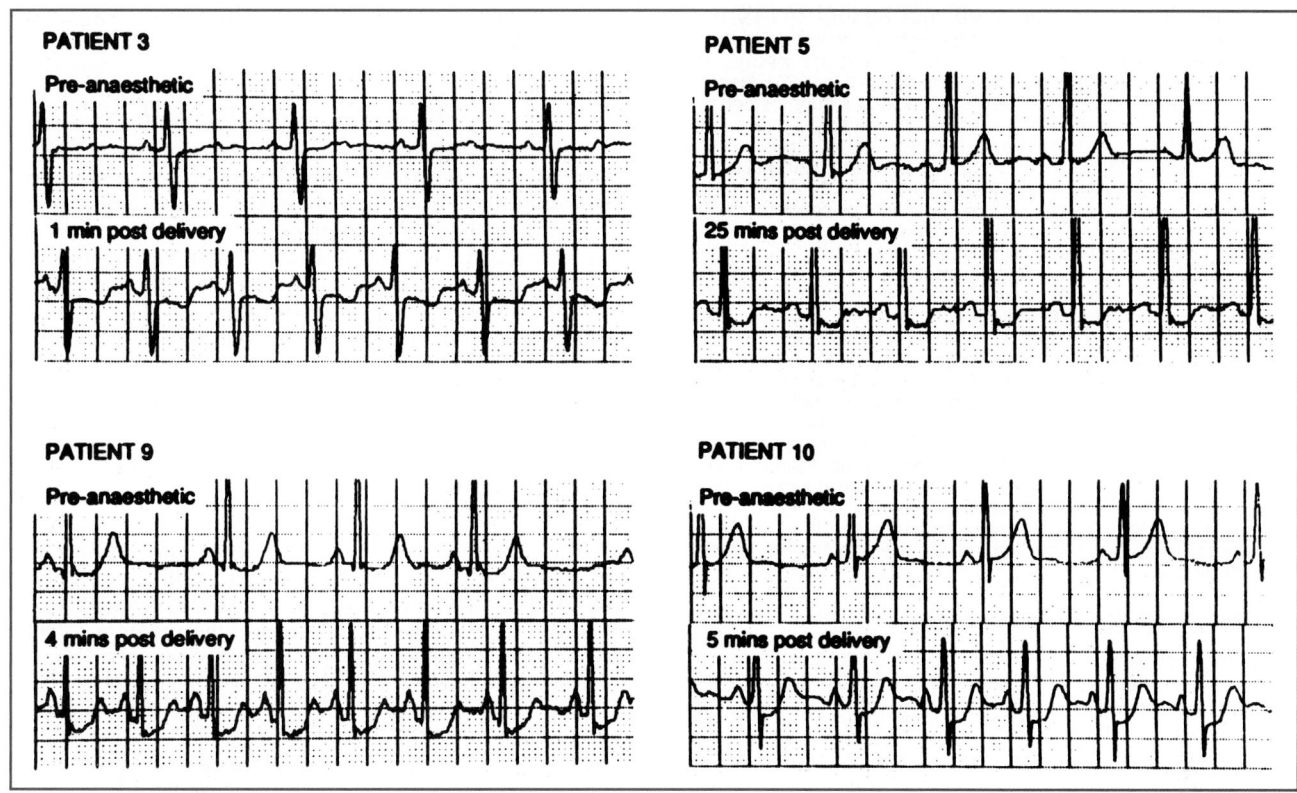

FIGURE 59–8. ST-segment depression recorded in healthy women during cesarean section. These changes were not associated with ventricular wall motion abnormalities. (From McLintic, A. J., Pringle, S. D., Lilley, S., et al.: Electrocardiographic changes during cesarean section under regional anesthesia. Anesth. Analg. *74*:51, 1992.)

eclampsia.[167] Uneventful pregnancy has been reported in women with long QT syndrome.[168,169]

COMPLETE HEART BLOCK. This condition has been described during pregnancy; although usually congenital,[170–172] it can be acquired as a result of myocarditis, congenital heart disease, acute myocardial infarction, or infective endocarditis.[173,174] Patients with complete heart block may remain asymptomatic during pregnancy and have an uncomplicated labor and delivery without treatment.[170] Improvement of atrioventricular nodal conduction during two successive uncomplicated pregnancies in a patient with congenital heart block has been reported.[175] Symptomatic patients with conduction abnormalities, including bifascicular block,[176] second-degree atrioventricular block,[177] and complete heart block,[170,173] have been treated during pregnancy with either temporary or permanent pacemakers, and numerous pregnancies have been reported in patients after pacemaker implantation.[174,178] A rate-adaptive pacemaker seems to be indicated in women of childbearing age.[166] In an attempt to reduce exposure to ionizing radiation, placement of a pacemaker during pregnancy has been done with electrocardiographic and echocardiographic guidance.[171,177] Reports of skin irritation and ulceration at the implant site due to enlargement of the breast and abdomen during pregnancy have led to placement of the battery under the breast in such women.

A complete evaluation is indicated in a case of arrhythmias during pregnancy to rule out either a cardiac or a noncardiac cause such as electrolyte imbalance, thyroid disease, and arrhythmogenic effects of drugs, alcohol, caffeine, and cigarette smoking. An identified cause should be treated and antiarrhythmic drug therapy initiated only if arrhythmia is symptomatic, hemodynamically important, or life threatening. When drug therapy seems necessary, the smallest therapeutic dose of drugs known to be safe for the fetus should be used. Therapeutic blood levels and the indication for continuous drug therapy should be reevaluated periodically. In cases of persistent arrhythmias resulting in symptoms and/or hemodynamic effect that do not respond to short-term drug intervention, electric cardioversion can be performed.[161,165,179–181] Electrophysiological evaluation is usually postponed till the postpartum period but can be performed under echocardiographic guidance if indicated during pregnancy.[182] Because of the unpredicta-

ble exposure to ionizing radiation, catheter ablation procedures should be performed after delivery.[161]

OTHER CARDIOVASCULAR DISORDERS

Aortic Dissection
(See also p. 1556)

A predisposition to aortic dissection during gestation has been suggested.[30] Over the last 50 years, approximately 200 cases of aortic dissection in association with pregnancy have been reported. The incidence is increased among multiparous women older than 30 years with coarctation of the aorta and the Marfan syndrome. Pregnancy-related aortic dissection seems to occur most often during the third trimester and peripartum period.

Transesophageal echocardiography provides a powerful and safe tool for establishing the diagnosis of aortic dissection during pregnancy. This method is preferable to computed tomography, which involves radiation exposure, and to magnetic resonance imaging, the safety of which during gestation has not been fully established.

The combination of nitroprusside and propranolol is currently recommended for the control of hypertension in nonpregnant patients with aortic dissection. Since nitroprusside may result in fetal toxicity it should be used only post partum or in patients refractory to other drugs during pregnancy. Hydralazine should be substituted for nitroprusside for blood pressure reduction in pregnant women with aortic dissection. To avoid blood pressure elevation associated with labor and vaginal delivery in women with aortic dissection, cesarean section using epidural anesthesia is recommended.[30]

TAKAYASU'S ARTERITIS (see p. 1572). Our review of the literature revealed 118 pregnancies in 91 women with Takayasu's disease.[183–185] Cerebral hemorrhage, heart failure, and even death have been reported in some pregnant patients with this disorder.[183] Low birth weights were noted in cases with complications, including retinopathy, hypertension, aortic regurgitation, or arterial aneurysms. The management of pregnant patients with Takayasu's arteritis includes treatment of hypertension to prevent complications such as congestive heart failure and cerebral hemorrhage. However, to avoid compromising uteroplacental blood flow, blood pressure should not be reduced excessively in patients with aortic narrowing. Adrenal glucocorticoids have been used in some cases of Takayasu's arteritis during pregnancy[184]; however, since pregnancy does not seem to change the inflammatory activity of this disorder, glucocorticoids should be reserved for patients who become pregnant during the acute phase of the disease. Prophylactic antibiotics may be given for labor and delivery in patients with aortic regurgitation and vascular stenoses.

Vaginal delivery is likely to be tolerated in the majority of patients with Takayasu's arteritis. However, a marked increase in systolic blood pressure during uterine contractions may occur and should be anticipated and treated.[183,184] Abdominal delivery may be considered for those with severe systemic hypertension and heart failure not responding to medical therapy. Vacuum extraction or forceps should be used to shorten the second stage of labor in patients with hypertension. In patients with substantial aortic narrowing, epidural anesthesia should be used with caution to prevent blood pressure reduction and compromise of placental perfusion.

The use of oral contraceptives may accelerate the progression of Takayasu's arteritis[183] and should therefore be avoided in patients with this condition.

Primary Pulmonary Hypertension (PPH)

PPH (see p. 783) is one of the few cardiovascular conditions in which pregnancy may be associated with a high maternal mortality rate. A review of the literature as well as of our own experience has revealed peripartum maternal mortality of approximately 40 per cent.[186–189] Clinical deterioration or death during pregnancy cannot always be predicted on the basis of the patient's preconceptual clinical status. Symptomatic deterioration usually occurs in the second trimester and is manifested by fatigue, dyspnea, syncope, chest pain, and right ventricular failure. Death occurs most often during late gestation or in the early postpartum period. Because hemodynamic or electrocardiographic information has not been available, the exact cause of death in patients with PPH is not clear. However, right ventricular ischemia and failure, cardiac arrhythmias, and pulmonary embolism are likely mechanisms. In addition to high maternal risk, PPH is associated with poor fetal outcome with high incidence of fetal loss, prematurity, and fetal growth retardation.

Because of the potentially deleterious effect of pregnancy both on mothers with PPH and their fetuses, pregnancy should be avoided in these patients. Since an etiological link between pulmonary hypertension and estrogen-containing oral contraceptives has been suggested, this form of birth control is not recommended for women with PPH.[190] Tubal ligation should provide maximum protection against the undesired risks of pregnancy. Early abortion is indicated in PPH patients who become pregnant. If the patient elects to continue the pregnancy, physical exertion should be restricted to reduce the circulatory load. The incidence of premature deliveries is increased in patients with PPH and should be anticipated.

Because of the beneficial effect of anticoagulation in patients with PPH[191] and the increased incidence of thromboembolism during pregnancy, such therapy is recommended throughout gestation or at least during the third trimester and early postpartum phase. Hemodynamic monitoring and blood gas measurements should be performed continuously during labor and delivery. Oxygen should be provided to prevent hypoxemia, and every effort should be made to prevent or immediately replace blood lost during delivery.[186]

Segmental epidural anesthesia and intrathecal morphine have been successful in relieving pain in these patients.[186,192] Because right ventricular dysfunction is likely, anesthetics having a negative inotropic effect should be avoided in patients with PPH. Most patients can tolerate vaginal delivery, and spontaneous labor is preferable to induction. Because of the high rate of early postpartum

maternal death,[186,187] close monitoring is recommended for several days post partum.

Cardiac Surgery during Pregnancy

Since heart disease that requires surgery is usually diagnosed and treated prior to pregnancy, cardiac surgery during gestation is uncommon, and the experience continues to be anecdotal.[193–197] In general, cardiac surgery in the pregnant woman is not associated with increased maternal risk, but may lead to fetal wastage.[193] The effects of anesthesia and the surgical procedure, especially cardiopulmonary bypass, on the uteroplacental circulation and fetal outcome are not well understood. Therefore, surgery should be recommended only for patients who do not respond to medical therapy, and procedures not requiring cardiopulmonary bypass are preferred. To minimize the risk of teratogenicity, surgery should be avoided during the first trimester. Because heart surgery is indicated when medical therapy has not led to satisfactory improvement, many of these patients will be hemodynamically unstable and will require hemodynamic monitoring for stabilization and careful anesthetic technique. Anesthetic agents should be selected on the basis of their hemodynamic effects and fetal safety. When the patient is at or near term, abdominal delivery by cesarean section can be performed at the same time as cardiac surgery, once fetal maturity has been confirmed. Fetal monitoring is essential for early detection of fetal bradycardia commonly seen in surgery involving cardiopulmonary bypass. This finding most likely indicates fetal distress due to a decrease in placental blood flow and can frequently be managed by increasing the flow rate.[198]

Pregnancy in Patients with Valve Prostheses

The risk of pregnancy in women with a valve prosthesis is multifactorial and should be assessed and discussed with the patient and her family prior to conception. Potential problems may be related to an increased hemodynamic load, the hypercoagulable state of pregnancy with increased likelihood of thromboembolic events, accelerated deterioration of bioprostheses, and risk to the fetus due to anticoagulants and other cardiovascular drugs. Most patients with NYHA functional classes I and II with an adequately functioning valve prosthesis, including those with two and three prosthetic valves, can tolerate the hemodynamic load of pregnancy.[152,199,200] Pregnancy with a higher functional class or severe cardiac dysfunction is risky and should be avoided. In questionable cases, evaluation of exercise capacity before conception may be used to predict whether a patient with a prosthetic heart valve can tolerate the increased hemodynamic load of pregnancy.

VALVE SELECTION (see also p. 1065). The selection of a prosthetic valve for pregnant patients or women of childbearing age involves a number of difficult issues. Because it is desirable to avoid anticoagulation during pregnancy, the use of tissue valves is often recommended.[199] However, the long-term durability of these valves is limited, resulting in the need for reoperation within several years. In addition, there is strong and increasing evidence for pregnancy-related accelerated deterioration of tissue valves, leading to the need for valve replacement either during pregnancy or shortly after.[152,201] A mechanical valve is recommended for patients who are willing to follow a strict regimen of anticoagulation and for those who require anticoagulation therapy for other conditions such as thrombophlebitis, atrial fibrillation, rheumatic mitral valve disease with enlargement of the left atrial diameter, intracardiac thrombus, or a history of pulmonary embolism. It should be noted, however, that significant changes in the levels of coagulation factors increase the risk for thrombosis during gestation.[202] Thrombosis of prosthetic valves during pregnancy has been reported in several cases despite anticoagulation.[152,199,200] Salazar et al.[199] and Iturbe-Alessio et al.[200] reported thromboembolic events in 6 of 165 pregnant patients with mechanical mitral prostheses (3.6 per cent) and in none of 37 patients with aortic prostheses.[203] A recent retrospective survey reported thromboembolic events in 19 of 141 pregnancies (13.5 per cent) in women with a mechanical prosthesis in spite of anticoagulation; 12 women had mitral valve thrombosis, 4 cases were fatal, 5 required emergency surgery, and 4 were managed medically with thrombolytic therapy.[152] Ten of the patients were treated with heparin; the level of anticoagulation was not reported. The majority of these patients had first-generation mechanical valves (Starr-Edwards, Björk-Shiley).

Based on the available information, it seems therefore that there is no safe method of anticoagulation during pregnancy in women with a mechanical heart valve. The use of oral anticoagulation may be associated with an increased incidence of spontaneous abortion, prematurity, and still birth and a 4 to 10 per cent risk of fetal deformity (coumadin embryopathy),[199,200,204,205] while the subcutaneous use of adjusted-dose heparin may result in a higher incidence of valve thrombosis.[152] The potential limitations of the various approaches to anticoagulation in pregnancy should be discussed with the patient prior to conception. Because of the disturbing increased risk of valve thrombosis and death with use of heparin, the use of oral anticoagulation throughout pregnancy, aiming at an INR between 2.0 and 3.0, with in-hospital intravenous administration of heparin for the last 3 to 4 weeks of gestation may be considered in high-risk patients, including women with first-generation mechanical valves in the mitral position and patients with a history of thromboembolism.[206] Patients with an aortic mechanical prosthesis and newer generation mechanical valves in the mitral position may be treated with adjusted subcutaneous doses of heparin to maintain a partial thromboplastin time (PTT) at 2.0 to 2.5 times the control from conception to week 13 and during the last 3 to 4 weeks of gestation. The patient should be admitted to the hospital for initiation and adjustment of heparin therapy, and the dose of heparin should be adjusted to achieve prolongation of activated PTT

to twice the control value at midinterval 6 hours after the morning dose. PTT should be carefully and frequently checked, and the dose of heparin adjusted accordingly.

Because of the potential limitations and risk involved in the selection of anticoagulation regimen, the choice of treatment should involve the patient and her family.

Heparin should be withdrawn at the onset of labor. If onset of labor occurs when the patient is treated with oral anticoagulation, performance of a cesarean section to avoid fetal bleeding associated with vaginal delivery is recommended. If there are no hemorrhages, heparin administration can be resumed a few hours post delivery. Breast feeding is permitted in the mother treated with anticoagulation, since coumadin does not affect the newborn.

CARDIOVASCULAR DRUGS IN PREGNANCY

Because of their potentially unfavorable effects on the developing fetus, all drugs should be avoided, if possible, during pregnancy. When drugs are needed, however, risk/benefit ratio must be evaluated carefully, and the smallest effective dose should be used (Table 59–7). Another source of concern is the transfer of drugs into breast milk and subsequently to the neonate during lactation. Generally, 1 to 2 per cent of the maternal dose appears in breast milk.[207] Most data regarding drug excretion in human milk are anecdotal, and except for some drugs that are clearly contraindicated, there is not enough information to permit or prohibit breast feeding in mothers receiving medications. Because the mechanisms involved in drug excretion into breast milk are complex, the various models and formulas used to estimate plasma:milk ratios are of limited clinical value. Close monitoring of the infant's ingested dose and plasma levels, as well as close observation for adverse effects or toxicity, is necessary to ensure safety.

CARDIAC GLYCOSIDES
Digoxin alone or combined with other drugs has been employed to treat maternal as well as fetal supraventricular arrhythmias and con-

TABLE 59–7 SAFETY AND ADVERSE EFFECTS OF CARDIOVASCULAR DRUGS DURING PREGNANCY

DRUG	POTENTIAL FETAL ADVERSE EFFECTS	SAFETY
Digoxin	Low birth weight	Safe
Quinidine	Toxic dose may induce premature labor and damage to fetal eighth cranial nerve	Safe
Procainamide	None reported	*
Disopyramide	May initiate uterine contractions	*
Lidocaine	In high blood levels and fetal acidosis may cause central nervous system depression	Safe
Mexiletine	Fetal bradycardia, IUGR, low Apgar score, neonatal hypoglycemia, neonatal bradycardia, and neonatal hypothyroidism	*
Flecainide	One reported fetal death	*
Propafenone	None reported	*
Adenosine	None reported. Use during first trimester limited to a few patients.	Safe
Amiodarone	IUGR, prematurity, hypothyroidism	Unsafe
Calcium antagonists	Fetal distress due to maternal hypotension	*
Beta-adrenergic blocking agents	IUGR, apnea at birth, bradycardia, hypoglycemia, hyperbilirubinemia; beta$_2$ blockade may initiate uterine contractions	Safe
Sodium nitroprusside	Potential thiocyanate toxicity with high dose, fetal mortality in animal studies	Potentially unsafe
Organic nitrates	Fetal heart rate deceleration and bradycardia	*
ACE inhibitors	Skull ossification defect, IUGR, premature deliveries, low birth weight, oligohydramnios, neonatal renal failure, anemia and death, limb contractures, patent ductus arteriosus	Unsafe
Diuretic agents	Impairment of uterine blood flow, thrombocytopenia, jaundice, hyponatremia, bradycardia	Potentially unsafe

* To date, only limited information is available, and safety during pregnancy cannot be established.
IUGR = intrauterine growth retardation.

gestive heart failure.[208,209] The fetomaternal serum digoxin concentration ratio has been shown to range from 0.5 to 1.0.[208] Pregnancy, especially when complicated by hypertension, is associated with increased levels of digoxin-like substances,[208,209] which can cause errors of up to 2 μg/ml in measurements of digoxin serum concentration.

Gestational use of digoxin is considered safe and without teratogenic effect. Caution is advised in digitalis administration, however, since overdose can be detrimental to the mother and may be lethal to the fetus. Potential side effects of cardiac glycosides in pregnancy include low birth weight, which has been postulated to be secondary to digoxin effect on amino acid transport through the placenta, with consequent growth retardation.[209] However, since the duration of pregnancy has been noted to be shorter in mothers with long-term digoxin therapy, it is possible that low birth weight has been due to prematurity rather than intrauterine growth retardation.

Digoxin is excreted in breast milk with a reported milk/plasma ratio ranging from 0.59 to 0.90.[206] The total amount of digoxin ingested daily by the infant has been estimated to be approximately 1/100 of the pediatric recommended dose. No apparent clinical effects have been demonstrated in newborns, so digoxin therapy of the mother should not affect breast feeding decisions.

ANTI-ARRHYTHMICS

QUINIDINE. Substantial clinical experience with quinidine for the treatment of maternal as well as fetal supraventricular arrhythmias[210,211] has established both its efficacy and safety. Potential side effects include fetal thrombocytopenia and minimal oxytocic activity reported mostly during development of spontaneous uterine contractions. Toxic doses of quinidine, however, may cause premature labor, abortion, or damage to the fetal eighth cranial nerve. Quinidine is secreted in breast milk, with a milk/plasma ratio of 0.71.[207] The calculated total dose of quinidine likely to be ingested by the infant is far below the recommended therapeutic daily pediatric dose.

PROCAINAMIDE. The drug has been successfully used to treat maternal and fetal supraventricular tachycardia.[210-212] Fetomaternal drug level ratios have been found to be 0.28 and 1.32 in two different patients. No teratogenic effects have been reported; however, because of limited experience with procainamide, quinidine should be used as the IA antiarrhythmic drug of choice during pregnancy.

A milk/plasma ratio of 4.3 ± 2.4 was reported for procainamide and 3.8 ± 1.8 for *N*-acetylprocainamide (NAPA). Although the high ratio may indicate accumulation in the milk, the amount of both procainamide and NAPA ingested daily by the infant is considered to be clinically insignificant.[210]

DISOPYRAMIDE. Reports regarding disopyramide treatment in pregnancy are limited to only several patients treated for ventricular and supraventricular arrhythmias.[210,213] The drug crosses the placenta, and the fetal/maternal ratio is 0.39.[214] No teratogenic effects have been described; however, disopyramide was reported to trigger uterine contractions[215] in one patient.

Disopyramide is secreted in breast milk in concentrations similar to those in plasma.[213] The estimated dose likely to be ingested by the infant is less than 2 mg/kg/day.[209] The drug is probably safe for use during pregnancy[210]; however, because of limited available information, disopyramide should be used in patients not tolerating or not responding to treatment with quinidine.

LIDOCAINE. This drug has been used during pregnancy mainly for epidural or local anesthesia; occasional reports have described its use as an antiarrhythmic agent[210,211,215] or in acute myocardial infarction.[216] The fetomaternal plasma concentration ratio of lidocaine is 0.5 to 0.7. The available data indicate that lidocaine is safe for use during pregnancy as long as blood levels are closely monitored. Elevated lidocaine levels may cause infant central nervous system depression and apnea, hypotonia, dilation of pupils, seizures and bradycardia. As a weak base, lidocaine may be trapped by an acidic environment. Caution should be exercised, therefore, in cases with fetal distress when fetal acidosis is likely and may be associated with increased blood levels of the drug and likelihood of toxicity. Lidocaine use during pregnancy has not been associated with teratogenic effects.

MEXILETINE. A limited number of pregnant women have been treated with mexiletine in doses between 600 and 800 mg/day.[217,218] The reported fetomaternal ratio ranged from 0.7 to 1.0. Fetal bradycardia, infants small for gestational age, low Apgar score, and neonatal hypoglycemia have all been reported in cases of maternal treatment with mexiletine. Despite these concerns, no teratogenic or long-term adverse effects have been reported. Mexiletine was found in breast milk in concentrations equal to or higher than that in maternal plasma (milk/plasma ratio varied between 0.8 and 1.9)[207]; however, the calculated daily quantity ingested by the infant appears to be below the therapeutic range, and drug levels were undetectable in infants' blood. Owing to very limited information and its reported untoward effects, mexiletine cannot be recommended for use during gestation; its safety must be investigated further.

FLECAINIDE. This drug has been used during pregnancy for both maternal and fetal tachyarrhythmias.[219-221] The drug seems to be effective for conversion of fetal supraventricular tachycardia and devoid of teratogenic effects. One reported fetal death[221]; however, raises some questions regarding its safety, although the death could

not be attributed with certainty to flecainide. More information is needed before the safety of flecainide can be established.

PROPAFENONE. Teratogenicity studies in animals have been negative.[210] In humans this drug has been used in a few cases during the second and third trimester of pregnancy for the treatment of maternal arrhythmias.[210,211,222] There is a clear evidence that propafenone and its metabolite, 5-hydroxypropafenone, cross the placenta, reaching approximately 30 to 40 per cent of maternal blood levels. Because of the limited available data, the safety of propafenone during pregnancy is unknown.

AMIODARONE. The use of amiodarone during pregnancy for the treatment of maternal and fetal arrhythmias has been reported by several investigators.[207,223-225] Transplacental transfer of amiodarone and its metabolite desethylamiodarone has been reported to be 10 to 25 per cent.

In a review of 34 pregnancies associated with amiodarone therapy,[223] 53 per cent of the neonates had an uncomplicated course and 15 per cent had minor side effects, including bradycardia and prolonged Q-T interval. However, a substantial number of neonates showed more serious complications such as hypothyroidism (9 per cent), prematurity (12 per cent), and small for gestational age (21 per cent), casting doubts on amiodarone's safety during pregnancy. Pending further studies, amiodarone should be used only in refractory cases of maternal or fetal tachyarrhythmias. Close monitoring of maternal and neonatal thyroid size and function is important for early detection of abnormalities.

Amiodarone is secreted in breast milk in quantities significant enough to be detected in the infant's blood.[207] The effect of long-term amiodarone exposure in infants is unknown; however, because of the well-known potential side effects of this drug, breast feeding is not recommended in women being treated with amiodarone.

CALCIUM ANTAGONISTS

VERAPAMIL. This drug has been used in pregnancy for maternal and fetal supraventricular arrhythmias, premature labor, preeclampsia, and severe gestational proteinuric hypertension.[226-228]

Rapid intravenous injection of verapamil may cause maternal hypotension and fetal distress and should be avoided.[210] More data are required to establish the safety of long-term therapy during pregnancy. Verapamil is excreted in breast milk[210]; its concentration ranges from 23 to 94 per cent of maternal blood level. The estimated total amount of verapamil secreted in milk is less than 0.01 to 0.04 per cent of the administered dose, and no pharmacological effects have been observed in neonates.

NIFEDIPINE. There is increasing experience with the use of nifedipine during pregnancy, mainly in long-term treatment of hypertension but also in preeclampsia, hypertensive emergencies, myocardial ischemia, and tocolysis.[155,229-231] Multiple studies have suggested the efficacy and safety of this drug. Sublingual administration of nifedipine in one case, however, resulted in maternal hypotension and fetal distress.[150]

DILTIAZEM. Use of this drug during pregnancy has been reported in a limited number of patients, primarily for relief of myocardial ischemia and treatment of supraventricular arrhythmias and hypertension.[211,232,233] No adverse effects on the fetus have been described. Diltiazem is secreted in breast milk. In a single reported case, maternal blood and milk concentrations closely correlated, and peak milk concentration exceeded 200 μg/liter.[235]

BETA-ADRENOCEPTOR BLOCKING AGENTS

PROPRANOLOL. This drug has been extensively used in pregnancy for treatment of cardiac arrhythmias, hypertrophic cardiomyopathy, mitral stenosis, and hyperthyroidism.[69,210,235] Propranolol readily crosses the placenta; at delivery, fetal serum concentrations are equal to or lower than maternal concentrations. Because of decreased hepatic metabolism and altered protein binding, serum concentration and half-life may be increased in the neonate during the first 10 days of life. Several adverse effects on the fetus and neonate have been reported, including intrauterine growth retardation, delayed onset of respiration in the newborn, bradycardia, hypoglycemia, and hyperbilirubinemia. Although increasing experience with the use of propranolol in pregnancy has demonstrated the rarity of these side effects, they should be anticipated by the clinician. Since blockade of myometrial beta$_2$-adrenergic receptors with propranolol may stimulate uterine contractions, selective beta$_1$-receptor blockers may be preferable for use during gestation.

Propranolol is excreted in breast milk, with a milk/plasma ratio of approximately 0.5 to 1.0.[209] No adverse effects were observed in infants breast-fed by mothers treated with propranolol. However, careful observation of such infants is recommended, since propranolol may accumulate as a result of the immature hepatic microsomal enzyme system of the neonate.

METOPROLOL. The use of metoprolol in pregnancy is primarily to control hypertension or tachyarrhythmias without causing teratogenic or major side effects.[235] Since metoprolol's metabolism is increased during pregnancy, its half-life serum concentration and bioavailability are decreased. The drug crosses the placenta, and the fetomaternal serum concentration ratio is approximately 1.0. Use of metoprolol in the treatment of hypertension was not associated with fetal growth retardation. Metoprolol is secreted in breast milk[209]; however, the daily quantity ingested by the neonate is very small. Unless hepatic function in the newborn is markedly impaired, breast feeding is probably safe.

ATENOLOL. Several studies have reported the use of atenolol in the treatment of hypertension during gestation.[235] Transplacental transfer of atenolol has been well documented with a fetomaternal ratio of 1.0.[209] Although available data indicate that the safety of atenolol during pregnancy is similar to that of other beta blockers, some of the published studies have reported low birth weight in association with its use during pregnancy.[112] Atenolol is secreted in breast milk. No adverse effects have been noted, however, in babies exposed to breast milk of women treated with atenolol, so that breast feeding need not be discontinued.

SOTALOL. This drug has been used during pregnancy in several cases for treatment of maternal hypertension and maternal and fetal arrhythmias.[236] The drug has been shown to cross the placenta, and levels in the fetal circulation have been found to be approximately 85 per cent of the maternal circulation.[237] Sotalol is secreted in breast milk, and the milk–serum concentration has been found to be 1.57 to 5.64. Breast feeding was not associated with fetal bradycardia.[237]

VASODILATORS

SODIUM NITROPRUSSIDE. During pregnancy, nitroprusside (NP) has been used to control blood pressure and heart failure in patients with intracranial aneurysm or in those undergoing surgery.[112] Data concerning the effect of NP on uterine blood flow are conflicting. The drug has been demonstrated to cross the placenta, both in animals and in humans. In pregnant ewes, maternal and fetal levels achieved equilibrium within 20 minutes. In the limited number of patients treated with NP during pregnancy, no unfavorable drug-related effect on the fetus was noticed. A large dose of NP in animals, however, resulted in significant accumulation of maternal and fetal cyanide and in fetal death. NP has been employed in pregnancy mostly in severely ill patients, and the data available are minimal. Until further studies clarify its safety during pregnancy, caution is recommended.

ORGANIC NITRATES. Intravenous as well as oral nitrates have been used in pregnancy for the treatment of hypertension, myocardial ischemia, and heart failure and for uterine relaxation in the postpartum patient with retained placenta.[133,155,215,216,233,238,239] In two patients in whom blood pressure was suddenly lowered with nitroglycerin, fetal heart rate deceleration, bradycardia, and attenuation of spontaneous beat-to-beat variability were reported. It appears, therefore, that as with the use of other vasodilators, careful monitoring of systemic blood pressure is required when nitrates are used during pregnancy.

ANGIOTENSIN-CONVERTING ENZYME (ACE) INHIBITORS

Numerous reports both in animals and in humans have been published in the last decade describing use of ACE inhibitors in pregnancy.[113,240] There is evidence in humans that captopril, enalapril, and lisinopril cross the placenta. Available experience indicates a high degree of morbidity and even mortality in fetuses or newborns exposed to ACE inhibitors during pregnancy. Reported complications include oligohydramnios, intrauterine growth retardation, premature labor, fetal and neonatal renal failure, bony malformations, limb contractures, persistent patent ductus arteriosus, pulmonary hypoplasia, respiratory distress syndrome, prolonged hypotension, and neonatal death. The FDA recently has warned against the use of ACE inhibitors during the second and third trimester of pregnancy.[241] Even more recently, Shotan et al. extended this warning to all trimesters of pregnancy and recommended discontinuation of the drugs prior to anticipated conception.[113]

DIURETIC AGENTS

Diuretics have been used in pregnancy for the management of hypertension, heart failure, and fluid retention and to prevent preeclampsia.[81,112] Because of the benign nature of dependent edema in pregnancy and the potential impairment of uterine blood flow and placental perfusion due to decreased blood volume, diuretics are not recommended for dependent edema. The prophylactic use of diuretics has not been proved effective in patients with preeclampsia; moreover, further volume restriction with these drugs may be deleterious. Because of the potential for a decrease in placental perfusion, initiation of treatment with diuretics during pregnancy is not recommended. However, continuation of diuretic therapy initiated prior to conception does not seem unfavorable. Although no teratogenic effects have been described, case reports of neonatal thrombocytopenia, jaundice, hyponatremia, and bradycardia have been reported with the use of thiazides. Recent data have shown, however, that thiazide diuretics are safe and effective when used in combination with methyldopa. Placental transfer of both hydrochlorothiazide and furosemide has been documented, with similar maternal and fetal serum levels.

ANTITHROMBOTIC AGENTS

Antithrombotic therapy may be necessary to prevent or control the following cardiovascular conditions during pregnancy; venous thrombophlebitis, hypertension, pulmonary embolism, rheumatic mitral valve disease, prosthetic heart valves, peripartum cardiomyopathy, primary pulmonary hypertension, ischemic heart disease, complex congenital heart disease, and Eisenmenger's syndrome.[242] However, the use of both antithrombotic agents, i.e., coumadin and heparin, may not be without complications, both for the mother and the fetus.[152,242]

COUMADIN. Because of its large molecular size, heparin does not cross the placenta, is relatively safe for the fetus[243] and is therefore the drug of choice during pregnancy. The use of Coumadin during pregnancy is associated with substantial risk, including fetal wastage due to spontaneous abortion and stillbirths; central nervous system disease such as optic nerve atrophy and blindness, mental retardation, microcephaly, and spasticity; and even death secondary to intracranial hemorrhage.[242] Use of this drug during the first trimester has been associated with "coumarin embryopathy" in 4 to 10 per cent of newborns.[180,200,201,204] This syndrome includes nasal bone hypoplasia and epiphyseal stippling (chondrodysplasia punctata).[242] Labor and delivery while the patient is taking Coumadin places both the mother and fetus at risk of hemorrhage and is an indication for cesarean section. Because the half-life is longer in the fetus, the effect of Coumadin may persist for 7 to 10 days after its discontinuation.

HEPARIN. Patients of childbearing age who are taking anticoagulants on a long-term basis should be advised prior to conception regarding the maternal and fetal risks of these agents. If pregnancy is planned, close monitoring and early diagnosis of pregnancy are essential. As soon as pregnancy is diagnosed, oral anticoagulants should be discontinued and subcutaneous heparin started. A brief period of hospitalization is advisable to establish the required heparin dose and ensure continuity of effective anticoagulation. Self-injection of an adjusted dose of heparin subcutaneously for the duration of pregnancy is the preferred approach in all cases, except in patients with mechanical heart valve. Heparin is administered into the lower abdominal subcutaneous tissue at 12-hour intervals, with dose adjustment to prolong the activated partial thromboplastin time to 1.5 to 2.0 times normal. To reduce pain, concentrated heparin (20,000 units/ml) should be used.

Complications related to long-term heparin therapy may occur and include sterile abscesses and hematomas in the abdominal wall, thrombocytopenia, and osteoporosis.[242,243] To reduce the risk of bleeding at delivery, subcutaneous heparin should be replaced in the hospital with intravenous heparin at 36 weeks' gestation. If needed, heparin can be substituted with oral Coumadin, adjusted to increase INR 2.0 to 3.0 times normal value, at the end of the first trimester. Heparin and Coumadin should be given concomitantly until a therapeutic level of Coumadin is achieved.

Heparin should be discontinued at the onset of labor to prevent bleeding during and after delivery and to allow safe prudential and epidural anesthesia. Hemostatic stitches should be used to avoid bleeding in patients undergoing episiotomy, and uterine contraction

TABLE 59–8 ANTIBIOTIC PROPHYLAXIS FOR LABOR AND DELIVERY

DRUG	DOSAGE REGIMEN
	STANDARD REGIMEN
Ampicillin, gentamicin, and amoxicillin	Intravenous or intramuscular administration of ampicillin, 2.0 gm, plus gentamicin, 1.5 mg/kg (not to exceed 80 mg), 30 min before procedure; followed by amoxicillin, 1.5 gm orally 6 hr after initial dose; alternatively, parenteral regimen may be repeated once 8 hr after initial dose
	AMPICILLIN/AMOXICILLIN/PENICILLIN–ALLERGIC PATIENT REGIMEN
Vancomycin and gentamicin	Intravenous administration of vancomycin, 1.0 gm, over 1 hr plus intravenous or intramuscular administration of gentamicin, 1.5 mg/kg (not to exceed 80 mg), 1 hr before procedure; may be repeated once 8 hr after initial dose
	ALTERNATE LOW-RISK PATIENT REGIMEN
Amoxicillin	3.0 gm orally 1 hr before procedure; then 1.5 gm 6 hr after initial dose

From Dajani, A. S., Bisno, A. L., Chung, K. J.: Prevention of endocarditis recommendations by the American Heart Association. JAMA *264*:2919, 1990.

should be stimulated after delivery by massage and Pitocin or ergot derivatives. It should be noted that heparin therapy may cause persistent anticoagulation for up to 28 hours after administration.[244] For this reason, discontinuation of heparin therapy 24 hours before elective induction of labor or judicious use of protamine sulfate to reduce the risk of bleeding and allow the use of epidural analgesia has been recommended.[150] Intravenous administration of heparin can be resumed after delivery once hemostasis is deemed adequate, and oral anticoagulation therapy can be started 24 hours post partum after bleeding and hemorrhage have been ruled out.[242] Low molecular weight heparin has been used during pregnancy mostly for the treatment of deep vein thrombosis.[245-247] The safety and efficacy of this drug need to be further established before it can be recommended for use in pregnancy and the lactating period. Both regular heparin and oral anticoagulation can be safely used after delivery, even in lactating women.[150] For recommendations of anticoagulation in the patient with prosthetic valves during pregnancy, see page 1066.

PROPHYLACTIC ANTIBIOTICS

Antibiotics are indicated to prevent recurrent acute rheumatic fever in patients with a history of this disease and to prevent bacterial endocarditis in patients with certain types of underlying heart disease.

The recommended regimen for the prevention of rheumatic fever is the same as in the nongravid state and includes 1.2 million units of benzathine penicillin G intramuscularly every 4 weeks, 250,000 units of oral penicillin V twice a day, or 1 gm/day of sulfadiazide.[248] Because of predisposition to kernicterus with the use of sulfadiazine, these drugs are not recommended during the third trimester of pregnancy and in women with a previous history of children with neonatal jaundice or blood-group incompatibility.

As in the nongravid state, antibiotic prophylaxis for infective endocarditis is indicated during gestation in patients with prosthetic heart valves, previous bacterial endocarditis, most congenital cardiac malformations, rheumatic valvular disease, obstructive hypertrophic cardiomyopathy, and mitral valve prolapse with thickened mitral valve and mitral insufficiency who are undergoing procedures likely to result in bacteremia.[43] Since the incidence of bacteremia associated with uncomplicated vaginal delivery has been reported to be low (0 to 5 per cent), the Committee on Bacterial Endocarditis, formed by the American Heart Association, has recommended routine prophylaxis for vaginal delivery in the presence of infection but not for uncomplicated vaginal delivery and for cesarean section. Despite these recommendations, and since complications and bacteremia are not always predictable, we routinely administer prophylactic antibiotics for vaginal delivery to all patients susceptible to bacterial endocarditis. The antibiotic regimens recommended for labor and delivery are shown in Table 59-8.

REFERENCES

CARDIOVASCULAR PHYSIOLOGY DURING PREGNANCY AND THE PUERPERIUM

1. Elkayam, U., and Gleicher, N.: Hemodynamics and cardiac function during normal pregnancy and the puerperium. In Elkayam, U., and Gleicher, N. (eds.): Cardiac Problems in Pregnancy: Diagnosis and Management of Maternal and Fetal Disease. 2nd ed. New York, Alan R. Liss, Inc., 1990, p. 5.
2. Longo, L. D.: Maternal blood volume and cardiac output during pregnancy: A hypothesis of endocrinologic control. Am. J. Physiol. 245:R720, 1983.
3. Plouin, P. F., Cudek, P., Arnal, J. F., et al.: Immunoradiometric assay of active renin versus determination of plasma renin activity in the clinical investigation of hypertension, congestive heart failure, and liver cirrhosis. Horm. Res. 34:138, 1990.
3a. Cheek, D. B., Petrucco, O. M., Gillespie, A., et al.: Muscle cell growth and the distribution of water and electrolyte in human pregnancy. Early Hum. Dev. 11:293, 1985.
4. Robson, S. C., Hunter, S., Boys, R. J., et al.: Serial study of factors influencing changes in cardiac output during human pregnancy. Am. J. Physiol. 256:H1060, 1989.
5. Metcalfe, J., and Ueland, K.: Maternal cardiovascular adjustments to pregnancy. Prog. Cardiovasc. Dis. 16:363, 1974.
6. Creasy, P. K., and Resnik, R.: Maternal-fetal medicine: Principles and Practice. 2nd ed. Philadelphia, W. B. Saunders Co., 1989.
7. Gerber, J. G., Payne, N. A., Murphy, R. R., et al.: Prostacyclin produced by the pregnant uterus in the dog may act as a circulating vasodepressor substance. J. Clin. Invest. 67:632, 1981.
8. Itoh, H., Sagawa, N., Mori, T., et al.: Plasma brain natriuretic peptide level in pregnant women with pregnancy-induced hypertension. Obstet. Gynecol. 82:71, 1993.
9. Robson, S. C., Dunlop, W., Boys, R. J., et al.: Cardiac output during labour. Br. Med. J. 295:1169, 1987.
10. Morgan, M.: Anesthetic choice for the cardiac obstetric patient. N. Engl. J. Anesth. 10:621, 1990.
11. Artal, R.: Cardiopulmonary responses to exercise in pregnancy. In Elkayam, U., and Gleicher, N. (eds.): Cardiac Problems in Pregnancy: Diagnosis and Management of Maternal and Fetal Disease. 2nd ed. New York, Alan R. Liss, Inc., 1990, p. 25.

12. Carpenter, M. W., Sady, S. P., Hoegsberg, B., et al.: Fetal heart rate response to maternal exertion. JAMA 259:3006, 1988.

CARDIAC EVALUATION DURING PREGNANCY

13. Elkayam, U., and Gleicher, N.: The evaluation of the cardiac patient. In Gleicher, N. (ed.): Principles and Practice of Medical Therapy in Pregnancy. 2nd ed. Norwalk, Conn., Appleton and Lange, 1992, p. 759.
14. Avila, W. S., Grinberg, M., Cardoso, L. F., et al.: Course of pregnancy and puerperium in women with mitral valve stenosis. Rev. Assoc. Med. Bras. 38:195, 1992.
15. Zeldis, S. M.: Dyspnea during pregnancy: Distinguishing cardiac from pulmonary causes. Clin. Chest Med. 13:567, 1992.
16. Mishra, M., Chambers, J. B., and Jackson, G.: Murmurs in pregnancy: An audit of echocardiography. Br. Med. J. 304:1413, 1992.
17. Rayburn, W. F.: Mitral valve prolapse and pregnancy. In Elkayam, U., and Gleicher, N. (eds.): Cardiac Problems in Pregnancy: Diagnosis and Management of Maternal and Fetal Disease. 2nd ed. New York, Alan R. Liss, Inc., 1990, p. 181.
18. Kumar, A., and Elkayam, U.: Hypertrophic cardiomyopathy in pregnancy: In Elkayam, U., and Gleicher, N. (eds.): Cardiac Problems in Pregnancy: Diagnosis and Management of Maternal and Fetal Disease. 2nd ed. New York, Alan R. Liss, Inc., 1990, p. 129.
19. McLintic, A. J., Pringle, S. D., Lilley, S., et al.: Electrocardiographic changes during cesarean section under regional anesthesia. Anesth. Analg. 74:51, 1992.
20. Widerhorn, J., Rahimtoola, S. H., and Elkayam, U.: Cardiac rhythm disorders. In Gleicher, N. (ed.): Principles and Practice of Medical Therapy in Pregnancy. 2nd ed. Norwalk, Conn., Appleton and Lange, 1992, p. 135.
21. Wagner, C. K., Leser, R. G., and Saldana, L. R.: Exposure of the pregnant patient to diagnostic radiation. A Guide to Medical Management. Philadelphia, J. B. Lippincott Co., 1985, p. 52.
22. Austin, J. H. M.: Postpartum pleura effusions. Ann. Intern. Med. 98:555, 1983.
23. Bioeffects Committee of the American Institute of Ultrasound in Medicine. J. Ultrasound Med. Biol. 2:R14, 1983.
24. Stoddard, M. F., Longaker, R. A., Vuocolo, L. M., and Dawkins, P. R.: Transesophageal echocardiography in the pregnant patient. Am. Heart. J. 124:785, 1992.
25. Limacher, M. C., Ware, J. A., O'Meara, M. E., et al.: Tricuspid regurgitation during pregnancy. Am. J. Cardiol. 55:1059, 1985.
26. Campos, O., Andrade, J. L., Bocanegra, J., et al.: Physiological multivalvular regurgitation during pregnancy: A longitudinal Doppler echocardiographic study. Intern. J. Cardiol. 40:265, 1993.
27. Enein, M., Aziz, A., Zima, A., et al.: Echocardiography of the pericardium in pregnancy. Obstet. Gynecol. 69:851, 1987.
28. Kereiakes, J. J., and Rosenstein, M.: Handbook of radiation doses in nuclear medicine and diagnostic x-ray. Boca Raton, Fla., CRC Press, 1980, p. 70.
29. Kupferminc, M. J., Lessing, J. B., Vidne, B. A., and Peyser, M. R.: Feto-maternal blood flow measurements and management of combined coarctation and aneurysm of the thoracic aorta in pregnancy. Acta Obstet. Gynecol. Scand. 72:398, 1993.
30. Elkayam, U., and Shotan, A.: Aortic dissection. In Gleicher, N., Elkayam, U., Galbraith, R. M., et al. (eds.): Principles of Medical Therapy in Pregnancy. 2nd ed. Norwalk, Conn., Appleton and Lange, 1992, p. 823.
31. Colletti, P. M., and Platt, L. D.: Obstetric MRI acceptable under specific criteria. Diagn. Radiol. 11:84, 1989.
32. Lee, W., Shah, P. K., Amin, D. K., and Elkayam, U.: Hemodynamic monitoring of cardiac patients during pregnancy. In Elkayam, U., and Gleicher, N. (eds.): Cardiac Problems in Pregnancy: Diagnosis and Management of Maternal and Fetal Disease. 2nd ed. New York, Alan R. Liss, Inc., 1990, p. 47.
33. Medical Radiation Exposure of Pregnant and Potentially Pregnant Women: Recommendations of the National Council on Radiation Protection and Measurements. Washington, National Council on Radiation Protection and Measurements, 1977, p. 13.
34. Bithell, J. F., and Steward, A. M.: Prenatal irradiation and childhood malignancy: A review of British data from the Oxford survey. Br. J. Cancer 31:271, 1975.
35. Elkayam, U., Kawanishi, D., Reid, C. L., et al.: Contrast echocardiography to reduce ionizing radiation associated with cardiac catheterization during pregnancy. Am. J. Cardiol. 52:213, 1983.

CONGENITAL HEART DISEASE

36. Perloff, J. K.: Congenital heart disease. In Gleicher, N. (ed.): Principles and Practice of Medical Therapy in Pregnancy, 2nd ed., Norwalk, Conn., Appleton and Lange, 1992, p. 788.
37. Uzark, K.: Counseling adolescents with congenital heart disease. J. Cardiovasc. Nurs. 6:65, 1992.
38. Whittemore, R., Hobbins, J. C., and Engle, M. A.: Pregnancy and its outcome in women with and without surgical treatment of congenital heart disease. Am. J. Cardiol. 50:641, 1982.
39. Pitkin, R. M., Perloff, J. K., Koos, B. J., and Beall, M. H.: Pregnancy and congenital heart disease. Ann. Intern. Med. 112:445, 1990.
40. Presbeterio, P., Somerville, J., Stone, S., et al.: Pregnancy in cyanotic congenital heart disease: Outcome of mother and fetus. Circulation 89:2673, 1994.

41. Weiss, B. M., and Atanassoff, P. G.: Cyanotic congenital heart disease and pregnancy: Natural selection, pulmonary hypertension and anesthesia. J. Can. Anesth. 5:332, 1993.

42. Elkayam, U., Cobb, T., and Gleicher, N.: Congenital heart disease and pregnancy. In Elkayam, U., and Gleicher, N. (eds.): Cardiac Problems in Pregnancy: Diagnosis and Management of Maternal and Fetal Disease. 2nd ed. New York, Alan R. Liss, Inc., 1990, p. 73.

43. Dajani, A. S., Bisno, A. L., Chung, K. J., et al.: Prevention of bacterial endocarditis. Recommendations by the American Heart Association. JAMA 264:2191, 1990.

44. McFaul, P. B., Dorman, J. C., Lamki, H., et al.: Pregnancy complicated by maternal heart disease. A review of 519 women. Br. J. Obstet. Gynecol. 95:861, 1988.

45. Easterling, T., Chadwick, H. S., Otto, C., and Benedetti, T.: Aortic stenosis in pregnancy. Obstet. Gynecol. 72:1131, 1988.

46. Banning, A. P., Pearson, J. F., and Hall, R. J. C.: Role of balloon dilatation of the aortic valve in pregnant patients with severe aortic stenosis. Br. Heart. J. 70:544, 1993.

47. Lao, T. T., Sermer, M., MaGee, L., et al.: Congenital aortic stenosis and pregnancy—a reappraisal. Am. J. Obstet. Gynecol. 169:540, 1993.

48. Lao, T. T., Adelman, A. G., Sermer, M., and Colman, J. M.: Balloon valvuloplasty for congenital aortic stenosis in pregnancy. Br. J. Obstet. Gynaecol. 100:1141, 1993.

49. Ben-Ami, M., Battino, S., Rosenfeld, T., et al.: Aortic valve replacement during pregnancy: A case report and review of the literature. Acta Obstet. Gynecol. Scand. 69:651, 1990.

50. Kupferminc, M. J., Lessing, J. B., Jaffa, A., et al.: Fetomaternal blood flow measurements and management of combined coarctation and aneurysm of the thoracic aorta in pregnancy. Acta Obstet. Gynecol. Scand. 72:398, 1993.

51. Togo, T., Sugishita, Y., Tamura, T., et al.: Uneventful pregnancy and delivery in a case of multiple peripheral pulmonary stenosis. Acta Cardiol. 18:143, 1983.

52. Larsen-Disney, P., Price, D., Meredith, I.: Undiagnosed maternal Fallot tetralogy presenting in pregnancy. Aust. N. Z. J. Obstet. Gynaecol. 32:169, 1992.

53. Geller, E., Rudick, V., and Niv, D.: Analgesia and anesthesia during pregnancy. In Elkayam, U., and Gleicher, N. (eds.): Cardiac Problems in Pregnancy: Diagnosis and Management of Maternal and Fetal Disease. 2nd ed. New York, Alan R. Liss, Inc., 1990, p. 283.

54. Patton, D. E., Lee, W., Cotton, D. B., et al.: Cyanotic maternal heart disease in pregnancy. Obstet. Gynecol. Surv. 45:594, 1990.

55. Fong, J., Druzin, M., Gimbel, A. A., and Fisher, J.: Epidural anaesthesia for labour and caesarean section in a parturient with a single ventricle and a transposition of the great arteries. Can. J. Anaesth. 37:680, 1990.

56. Gilman, D. H.: Caesarean section in undiagnosed Eisenmenger's syndrome. Anaesthesia 46:371, 1991.

57. Jackson, G. M., Dildy, G. A., Varner, M. W., and Clark, S. L.: Severe pulmonary hypertension in pregnancy following successful repair of ventricular septal defect in childhood. Obstet. Gynecol. 82:680, 1993.

58. Jeyamalar, R., Sivanesaratnam, V., and Kuppuvelumani, P.: Eisenmenger syndrome in pregnancy. Aust. N. Z. J. Obstet. Gynaecol. 32:275, 1992.

59. Pollack, K. L., Chestnut, D. H., and Wenstrom, K. D.: Anesthetic management of a parturient with Eisenmenger's syndrome. Anesth. Analg. 70:212, 1990.

60. Connolly, H. M., and Warnes, C. A.: Ebstein's anomaly: Outcome of pregnancy. J. Am. Coll. Cardiol. 23:1194, 1994.

61. Megerian, G., Bell, J. G., Huhta, J. C., et al.: Pregnancy outcome following mustard procedure for transposition of the great arteries: A report of five cases and review of the literature. Obstet. Gynecol. 83:512, 1994.

62. Perry, C. P.: Childbirth after surgical repair of truncus arteriosus. J. Reprod. Med. 5:65, 1990.

63. Sumner, D., Melville, C., Smith, C. D. R., et al.: Successful pregnancy in a patient with a single ventricle. Eur. J. Obstet. Gynecol. Reprod. Biol. 44:239, 1992.

64. Rowbottom, S. J., Gin, T., and Cheung, L. P.: General anesthesia for caesarean section in a patient with uncorrected complex cyanotic heart disease. Anaesth. Intensive Care 22:74, 1994.

65. Walsh, T., Savage, R., and Hess, D. B.: Successful pregnancy in a patient with a double inlet left ventricle treated with a septation procedure. South. Med. J. 83:358, 1990.

RHEUMATIC HEART DISEASE

66. Ueland, K.: Rheumatic heart disease and pregnancy. In Elkayam, U., and Gleicher, N. (eds.): Cardiac Problems in Pregnancy: Diagnosis and Management of Maternal and Fetal Disease. 2nd ed. New York, Alan R. Liss, Inc., 1990, p. 99.

67. Stephen, S. J.: Changing patterns of mitral stenosis in childhood and pregnancy in Sri Lanka. J. Am. Coll. Cardiol. 19:1276, 1992.

68. Guleria, R., Vasisht, K., Dhall, G. I., et al.: Pregnancy with heart disease: Experience at Postgraduate Institute of Medical Education and Research, Chandigarh. J. Assoc. Physicians India, 38:902, 1990.

69. Avila, W. S., Grinberg, M., D'ecourt, L. V., et al.: Clinical course of women with mitral valve stenosis during pregnancy and puerperium. Arq. Bras. Cardiol. 58:359, 1992.

70. Al Kasab, S. M., Sabag, T., Al Zaibag, M., et al.: B-adrenergic receptor blockade in the management of pregnant women with mitral stenosis. Am. J. Obstet. Gynecol. 163:37, 1990.

71. Jacobi, P., Adler, Z., Zimmer, E. Z., et al.: Effect of uterine contractions on left atrial pressure in pregnant women with mitral stenosis. Br. J. Med. 298:27, 1989.

72. Ziskind, Z., Etchin, A., Frenkel, Y., et al.: Epidural anesthesia with the Trendelenburg position for cesarean section with or without a cardiac surgical procedure in patients with severe mitral stenosis: A hemodynamic study. J. Cardiothorac. Anesth. 4:354, 1990.

73. De Swiet, M., and Deverall, P.: Editorial note: Pregnancy—Still an indication for closed mitral valvotomy. Int. J. Cardiol. 26:323, 1990.

74. Esteves, C. A., Ramos, A. I. O., Braga, S. L. N., et al.: Effectiveness of percutaneous balloon mitral valvotomy during pregnancy. Am. J. Cardiol. 68:930, 1991.

75. Farhat, M. B., Maatouk, F., Betbout, F., et al.: Percutaneous balloon mitral valvuloplasty in eight pregnant women with severe mitral stenosis. Eur. Heart. J. 13:1658, 1992.

76. Lung, B., Cormier, B., Elias, J., et al.: Usefulness of percutaneous balloon commissurotomy for mitral stenosis during pregnancy. Am. J. Cardiol. 73:398, 1994.

77. Ribeiro, P. A., Fawzy, M. E., Awad, M., et al.: Balloon valvotomy for pregnant patients with severe pliable mitral stenosis using the Inoue technique with total abdominal and pelvic shielding. Am. Heart. J. 124:1558, 1992.

78. Glantz, J. C., Pomerantz, R. M., Cunningham, M. J., and Woods, J. R.: Percutaneous balloon valvuloplasty for severe mitral stenosis during pregnancy: A review of therapeutic options. Obstet. Gynecol. Surv. 48:503, 1993.

79. Sharma, S., Loya, Y. S., Desai, D. M., and Pinto, R. J.: Percutaneous mitral valvotomy in 200 patients using Inoue balloon—immediate and early haemodynamic results. Indian Heart J. 45:169, 1993.

80. Ribiero, P. A., and Al Zaibag, M.: Mitral balloon valvotomy in pregnancy (editorial). J. Heart Valve Dis. 1:206, 1992.

81. Myers, S. A.: Antihypertensive drug use during pregnancy. In Elkayam, U., and Gleicher, N. (eds.): Cardiac Problems in Pregnancy: Diagnosis and Management of Maternal and Fetal Disease. 2nd ed. New York, Alan R. Liss, Inc., 1990, p. 381.

82. Roth, A., Shotan, A., and Elkayam, U.: A randomized comparison between the hemodynamic effects of hydralazine and nitroglycerin alone and in combination at rest and during isometric exercise in patients with chronic mitral regurgitation. Am. Heart J. 125:155, 1993.

83. Banning, A. P., Pearson, J. F., and Hall, R. J. C.: Role of balloon dilatation of the aortic valve in pregnant patients with severe aortic stenosis. Br. Heart J. 70:544, 1993.

84. McIvor, R. A.: Percutaneous balloon aortic valvuloplasty during pregnancy. Int. J. Cardiol. 32:1, 1991.

85. Peterson, J. J., Owen, J., and Aldrich, M.: The antepartum patient in the CCU: Educational preparation for nursing staff. Crit. Care Nurse 11:82, 1991.

86. Lao, T. T., Sermer, M., MaGee, L., et al.: Congenital aortic stenosis and pregnancy—A reappraisal. Am. J. Obstet. Gynecol. 169:540, 1993.

87. Elkayam, U., McKay, C. R., Weber, L., et al.: Favorable effects of hydralazine on the hemodynamic response to isometric exercise in chronic severe aortic regurgitation. Am. J. Cardiol. 53:1603, 1984.

OTHER CONDITIONS AFFECTING THE VALVES, AORTA, AND MYOCARDIUM

88. Tank, L. C. H., Chan, S. Y. W., Wong, V. C. W., et al.: Pregnancy in patients with mitral valve prolapse. Int. J. Gynaecol. Obstet. 23:217, 1985.

89. Kral, J., Spacil, J., Hradec, J., and Cech, E.: Pregnancy and labor in women with mitral valve prolapse. Cas. Lek. Cesk. 129:1029, 1990.

90. Elkayam, U., Ostrzega, E., Shotan, A., and Mehra, A.: Cardiovascular problems in pregnant women with the Marfan syndrome. Ann. Int. Med. (in press).

91. Kotter-Thomsen, I., Weisner, D., Lehmann-Willenbrock, E., et al.: Marfan-syndrom und Schwangerschaft, kompliziert durch das aneurysma dissecans. Geburtshilfe Frauenheilkd. 51:653, 1991.

92. Pyeritz, R. E.: The Marfan syndrome. Am. Fam. Physician 34:83, 1986.

93. Simpson, I. A., deBelder, M. A., Treasure, T., et al.: Cardiovascular manifestations of Marfan's syndrome: Improved evaluation by transesophageal echocardiography. Br. Heart J. 69:104, 1993.

94. Shores, J., Berger, K. R., Murphy, E. A., and Pyeritz, R. E.: Progression of aortic dilatation and the benefit of long-term beta adrenergic blockade in Marfan's syndrome. N. Engl. J. Med. 330:1335, 1994.

95. Treasure, T.: Elective replacement of the aortic root in Marfan's syndrome. Br. Heart J. 69:101, 1993.

96. Kumar, A., and Elkayam, U.: Hypertrophic cardiomyopathy in pregnancy. In Elkayam, U., and Gleicher, N. (eds.): Cardiac Problems in Pregnancy: Diagnosis and Management of Maternal and Fetal Disease. 2nd ed. New York, Alan R. Liss, Inc., 1990, p. 129.

97. van Kasteren, Y. M., Kleinhout, J., Smit, M. A., et al.: Hypertrophic cardiomyopathy and pregnancy: A report of three cases. Eur. J. Obstet. Gynecol. Reprod. Biol. 38:63, 1990.

98. Tessler, M. J., Hudson, R., Naugler-Colville, M. A., and Biehl, D. R.: Pulmonary edema in two parturients with hypertrophic obstructive cardiomyopathy (HOCM). Can. J. Anaesth. 37:469, 1990.

99. Pelliccia, F., Cianfrocca, C., Gaudig, C., and Reale, A.: Sudden death during pregnancy in hypertrophic cardiomyopathy. Eur. Heart. J. 13:421, 1992.

100. Rowe, T.: Hypertrophic cardiomyopathy in pregnancy: A case study. J. Cardiovasc. Nurs. 8:69, 1994.

101. Elkayam, U., Ostrzega, E., and Shotan, A.: Peripartum cardiomyopathy. In Gleicher, N. (ed.): Principles and Practice of Medical Therapy in Pregnancy. 2nd ed. Norwalk, CT, Appleton and Lange, 1992, p. 131.

102. Ribner, H. S., and Silverman, R. I.: Peripartal cardiomyopathy. In Elkayam, U., and Gleicher, N. (eds.): Cardiac Problems in Pregnancy: Diagnosis and Management of Maternal and Fetal Disease. 2nd ed. New York, Alan R. Liss, Inc., 1990, p. 115.

103. Rolfe, M., Tang, C. M., Walker, R. W., et al.: Peripartum cardiac failure in the Gambia. J. Trop. Med. Hyg. 95:192, 1992.

104. Leonard, R. B., Schwartz, E., Allen, D. A., and Alson, R. L.: Peripartum cardiomyopathy: A case report. J. Emerg. Med. 10:157, 1992.

105. Nwosu, E. C., and Burke, M. F.: Cardiomyopathy of pregnancy. Br. J. Obstet. Gynecol. 100:1145, 1992.

106. Ravikishore, A. G., Kaul, U. A., Sethi, K. K., and Khalilullah, M.: Peripartum cardiomyopathy: Prognostic variables at initial evaluation. Int. J. Cardiol. 32:377, 1991.

107. van Hoevan, K. H., Kitsis, R. N., Katz, S. D., and Factor, S. M.: Peripartum versus idiopathic dilated cardiomyopathy in young women—A comparison of clinical, pathological and prognostic features. Int. J. Cardiol. 40:57, 1993.

108. Oakley, C. M., and Nihoyannopoulos, P.: Peripartum cardiomyopathy with recovery in a patient with coincidental Eisenmenger ventricular septal defect. Br. Heart J. 67:190, 1992.

109. Marin-Neto, J. A., Maciel, B. C., Teran Urbanetz, L. L., et al.: High output failure in patients with peripartum cardiomyopathy: A comparative study with dilated cardiomyopathy. Am. Heart J. 121:134, 1990.

110. Midei, M. C., DeMent, S. H., Feldman, A. M., et al.: Peripartum myocarditis and cardiomyopathy. Circulation 81:922, 1990.

111. Rizeg, M. N., Rickenbacher, P. R., Fowler, M. B., and Billingham, M. E.: Incidence of myocarditis in peripartum cardiomyopathy. Am. J. Cardiol. 74:474, 1994.

112. Widerhorn, J., Widerhorn, A. L. M., and Elkayam, U.: Cardiovascular pharmacotherapy in pregnancy and lactation. In Gleicher, N. (ed.): Principles and Practice of Medical Therapy in Pregnancy. 2nd ed. Norwalk, CT, Appleton and Lange, 1992, p. 767.

113. Shotan, A., Widerhorn, J., Hurst, A., and Elkayam, U.: Risks of angiotensin-converting enzyme inhibition during pregnancy: Experimental and clinical evidence, potential mechanisms, and recommendations for use. Am. J. Med. 96:451, 1994.

114. Hovsepian, P. G., Ganzel, B., Sohi, G. S., et al.: Peripartum cardiomyopathy treated with a left ventricular assist device as a bridge to cardiac transplantation. South Med. J. 82:527, 1989.

115. Liljestrand, J., Lindstrom, B.: Chidlbirth after post partum cardiac insufficiency treated with cardiac transplant. Acta Obstet. Gynecol. Scand. 72:406, 1993.

116. St. John Sutton, M. S. J., Cole, P., Plappert, M., et al.: Effects of subsequent pregnancy on left ventricular function in peripartum cardiomyopathy. Am. Heart J. 121:1776, 1991.

117. Garla, P. G. N.: Epidural fentanyl for cesarean section in postpartal cardiomyopathy. W. Va. Med. J. 86:11, 1990.

118. Lindheimer, M. D.: Hypertension in pregnancy. Hypertension 22:127, 1993.

119. National High Blood Pressure Education Program Working Group Report on High Blood Pressure in Pregnancy. Am. J. Obstet. Gynecol. 163:1689, 1990.

120. Svenson, A.: Hypertension in pregnancy. Clin. Exp. Hypertens. 15:1353, 1993.

121. Scott, J. R., Wagoner, L. E., Olsen, S. E., et al.: Pregnancy in heart transplant recipients: Management and outcome. Obstet. Gynecol. 82:324, 1993.

122. Liljestrand, J., and Lindstrom, B.: Childbirth after post partum cardiac insufficiency treated with cardiac transplant. Acta Obstet. Gynecol. Scand. 72:406, 1993.

123. Laifer, S. A.: Pregnancy after transplantation. In Lee, R. V., Barron, W. M., Cotton, D. B., et al. (eds.): Current Obstetric Medicine, Vol. 2. St. Louis, C. V. Mosby, 1993, p. 1.

CORONARY ARTERY DISEASE

124. Goldman, M. E., and Meller, J.: Coronary artery disease in pregnancy. In Elkayam, U., and Gleicher, N. (eds.): Cardiac Problems in Pregnancy: Diagnosis and Management of Maternal and Fetal Disease. 2nd ed. New York, Alan R. Liss, Inc., 1990, p. 153.

125. La Vecchia, C., Franceschi, S., Decarli, A., et al.: Risk factors for myocardial infarction in young women. Am. J. Epidemiol. 125:832, 1987.

126. Croft, P., and Hannaford, P. C.: Risk factors for acute myocardial infarction in women: Evidence from the Royal College of General Practitioners' Oral Contraception Study. Br. Med. J. 298:165, 1989.

127. La Vecchia, C., Decarli, A., Franceschi, S., et al.: Menstrual and reproductive factors and the risk of myocardial infarction in women under fifty-five years of age. Am. J. Obstet. Gynecol. 157:1108, 1987.

128. Raymond, R., Lynch, J., Underwood, E., et al.: Myocardial infarction and normal coronary arteriography: A 10-year clinical and risk analysis of 74 infants. J. Am. Coll. Cardiol. 11:471, 1988.

129. Donnelly, S., McKenna, P., McGing, P., and Sugrue, D.: Myocardial infarction during pregnancy. Br. J. Obstet. Gynaecol. 100:781, 1993.

130. Etienne, Y., Jobic, Y., Houel, J. F., et al.: Papillary fibroelastoma of the aortic valve with myocardial infarction: Echocardiographic diagnosis and surgical excision. Am. Heart J. 127:443, 1994.

131. Maekawa, K., Ohnishi, H., Hirase, T., et al.: Acute myocardial infarction during pregnancy caused by coronary artery spasm. J. Intern. Med. 235:489, 1994.

132. Menegakis, N. E., and Amstey, M. S.: Case report of myocardial infarction in labor. Am. J. Obstet. Gynecol. 165:1383, 1991.

133. Skeikh, A. U., and Harper, M. A.: Myocardial infarction during pregnancy: Management and outcome of two pregnancies. Am. J. Obstet. Gynecol. 169:279, 1993.

134. Delay, M., Genestal, M., Carrie, D., et al.: Arrêt cardiocirculatoire après administration de l'association mifepristone (Mifegyne) sulprostone (Nalador) pour interruption de grossesse. Arch. Mal. Coeur. 85:105, 1992.

135. Liao, J. K., Cockrill, B. A., and Yurchak, P. M.: Acute myocardial infarction after ergonovine administration for uterine bleeding. Am. J. Cardiol. 68:823, 1991.

136. Efstratiou, A., and Singh, B.: Combined spontaneous postpartum coronary artery dissection and pulmonary embolism with survival. Cathet. Cardiovasc. Diagn. 31:29, 1994.

137. Emori, T., Goto, Y., Maeda, T., et al.: Multiple coronary artery dissections diagnosed in vivo in a pregnant woman. Chest 104:289, 1993.

138. Kearney, P., Singh, H., Hutter, J., et al.: Spontaneous coronary artery dissection: A report of three cases and review of the literature. Postgrad Med. J. 69:940, 1993.

139. Verkaaik, A. P. K., Visser, W., Deckers, J. W., Lotgering, F. K.: Multiple coronary artery dissections in a woman at term. Br. J. Anaesth. 71:301, 1993.

140. Rallings, P., Exner, I., and Abraham, R.: Coronary artery vasculitis and myocardial infarction associated with antiphospholipid antibodies in a pregnant woman. Aust. N. Z. J. Med. 19:347, 1989.

141. Parry, G., Goudevenos, J., and Williams, D. O.: Coronary thrombosis postpartum in a young woman with Still's disease. Clin. Cardiol. 15:305, 1992.

142. Nolan, T. E., and Savage, R. W.: Peripartum myocardial infarction from presumed Kawasaki's disease. South. Med. J. 83:1360, 1990.

143. Van Enk, A., Visschers, G., Jansen, W., and Van Eps, L. W. S.: Maternal death due to sickle cell chronic lung disease. Br. J. Obstet. Gynaecol. 99:162, 1992.

144. Jessurun, C. R., Adam, K., Moise, K. J., and Wilansky, S.: Pheochromocytoma-induced myocardial infarction in pregnancy. A case report and literature review. Tex. Heart Inst. J. 20:120, 1993.

145. Hands, M. E., Johnson, M. D., Saltzman, D. H., and Rutherford, J. D.: The cardiac, obstetric and anesthetic management of pregnancy complicated by acute myocardial infarction. J. Clin. Anesth. 2:258, 1990.

146. Kannan, P., Raman, S., Ramani, V. S., and Jeyamalar, R.: Myocardial infarction in a young Indian grandmultipara. Aust. N. Z. J. Obstet. Gynaecol. 33:424, 1993.

147. Sheikh, A. U., and Harper, M. A.: Myocardial infarction during pregnancy: Management and outcome of two pregnancies. Am. J. Obstet. Gynecol. 169:279, 1993.

148. Viinikka, L., Hartikainen-Sorri, A. L., Lumme, R., et al.: Low dose aspirin in hypertensive pregnant women: Effect on pregnancy outcome and prostacyclin-thromboxane balance in mother and newborn. Br. J. Obstet. Gynaecol. 100:809, 1993.

149. Impey, L.: Severe hypotension and fetal distress following sublingual administration of nifedipine to a patient with severe pregnancy induced hypertension at 33 weeks. Br. J. Obstet. Gynaecol. 100:959, 1993.

150. Ginsberg, J. S., and Hirsch, J.: Use of antithrombotic agents during pregnancy. Chest 108:305S, 1995.

151. Corby, D. G.: Aspirin in pregnancy and fetal effects. Pediatrics 62:930, 1978.

151a. Shores, J., Berger, K. R., Murphy, E. A., and Pyeritz, R. E.: Progression of aortic dilatation and the benefit of long-term beta adrenergic blockade in Marfan's syndrome. N. Engl. J. Med. 330:1335, 1994.

152. Sbarouni, E., and Oakley, C. M.: Outcome of pregnancy in women with valve prostheses. Br. Heart J. 71:196, 1994.

153. Tissot, H., Vergnes, C., Rougier, P., et al.: Fibrinolytic treatment with urokinase and streptokinase for recurrent thrombosis in two valve prostheses for the aortic and mitral valves during pregnancy. J. Gynecol. Obstet. Biol. Reprod. 20:1093, 1991.

154. Cowan, N. C., de Belder, M. A., and Rothman, M. T.: Coronary angioplasty in pregnancy. Br. Heart J. 59:588, 1988.

155. Shalev, Y., Ben-Hur, H., Hagay, Z., et al.: Successful delivery following myocardial ischemia during the second trimester of pregnancy. Clin. Cardiol. 16:754, 1993.

ARRHYTHMIAS

156. Mehra, A., Ostrzega, E., Widerhorn, J., et al.: Arrhythmias in pregnancy: Prevalence and effect on fetal and maternal outcome in a large group of asymptomatic women. Clin. Res. (Abs)39:79a, 1991.

157. Brodsky, M., Doria, R., Allen, B., et al.: New-onset ventricular tachycardia during pregnancy. Am. Heart J. 123:933, 1992.

158. Tawam, M., Levine, J., Mendelson, M., et al.: Effect of pregnancy on paroxysmal supraventricular tachycardia. Am. J. Cardiol. 72:838, 1993.

159. Widerhorn, J., Widerhorn, A. L. M., Rahimtoola, S. H., and Elkayam, U.: WPW syndrome during pregnancy: Increased incidence of supraventricular arrhythmias. Am. Heart J. 124:796, 1992.

160. Field, L. M., Barton, F. L.: The management of anaesthesia for caesarean section in a patient with paroxysmal ventricular tachycardia. Anaesthesia 48:593, 1993.

161. Gras, D., Mabo, P., Kermarrec, A., et al.: Radiofrequency ablation of

162. Oettinger, M., and Pelitz, Y.: Asymptomatic paroxysmal atrial fibrillation during intravenous magnesium sulfate treatment in preeclampsia. Gynecol. Obstet. Invest. *36*:244, 1993.

163. Penkala, M., and Hancock, E. W.: Wide-complex tachycardia in pregnancy. Hos. Pract. Jul. 63, 1993.

164. Feldman, J. M.: Cardiac arrest after succinylcholine administration in a pregnant patient recovered from Guillain-Barré syndrome. Anesthesiology *72*:942, 1990.

165. Swartjes, J. M., Schutte, M. F., and Bleker, O. P.: Management of eclampsia: Cardiopulmonary arrest resulting from magnesium sulfate overdose. Eur. J. Obstet. Gynaecol. Reprod. Biol. *47*:73, 1992.

166. Varon, M. E., Sherer, D. M., Abramowicz, J. S., and Akiyama, T.: Maternal ventricular tachycardia associated with hypomagnesemia. Am. J. Obstet. Gynecol. *167*:1352, 1992.

167. Naidoo, D. P., Bhorat, I., Moodley, J., et al.: Continuous electrocardiographic monitoring in hypertensive crises in pregnancy. Am. J. Obstet. Gynecol. *164*:530, 1991.

168. Plotz, J., Heidegger, H., von Hugo, R., et al.: Hereditary prolonged QT interval (Romano-Ward syndrome) in a female patient with nonelective cesarean section. Anaesthetist *41*:88, 1992.

169. Wilkinson, C., Gyaneschwar, R., and McCusker, C.: Twin pregnancy in a patient with idiopathic long QT syndrome. Case report. Br. J. Obstet. Gynecol. *98*:1300, 1991.

170. Dalvi, B. V., Chaudhuri, A., Kulkarni, H. L., and Kale, P. A.: Therapeutic guidelines for congenital complete heart block presenting in pregnancy. Obstet. Gynecol. *79*:802, 1992.

171. Lau, C. P., Lee, C. P., Wong, C. K., et al.: Rate responsive pacing with a minute ventilation sensing pacemaker during pregnancy and delivery. PACE *13*:158, 1990.

172. Ramsewak, S., Persad, P., Perkins, S., and Narayansingh, G.: Twin pregnancy in a patient with complete heart block. Clin. Exp. Obstet. Gynecol. *19*:166, 1992.

173. Rosen, A., Klein, M., Ambros, O., and Pfemeter, G.: Implantation eines herzschrittmachers in der 25.SSW bei erworbenem AV block III. Grades. Gerburtshilfe Frauenheilkd. *51*:239, 1991.

174. Walsh, T., Savage, R., and Hess, D. B.: Successful pregnancy in a patient with a double inlet left ventricle treated with a septation procedure. South. Med. J. *83*:358, 1990.

175. Holdright, D. R., and Sutton, G. C.: Restoration of sinus rhythm during two consecutive pregnancies in a woman with congenital complete heart block. Br. Heart J. *64*:338, 1990.

176. Emori, T., Goto, Y., Maeda, T., et al.: Multiple coronary artery dissections diagnosed in vivo in a pregnant woman. Chest *104*:289, 1993.

177. Jordaens, L. J., Vandenbogaerde, J. F., Van De Bruaene, P., and De Buyzere, M.: Transesophageal echocardiography for insertion of a physiological pacemaker in early pregnancy. PACE *13*:955, 1990.

178. Terhaar, M., and Schakenbach, L.: Care of the pregnant patient with a pacemaker. J. Perinat. Neonat. Nurs. *5*:1, 1991.

179. Elkayam, U., Goodwin, T. M.: Adenosine therapy for supraventricular tachycardia during pregnancy. Am. J. Cardiol. *75*:521, 1995.

179a. Gilson, G. J., Knieriem, K. J., Smith, J. F., et al.: Short-acting beta-adrenergic blockade and the fetus. A case report. J. Reprod. Med. *37*:277, 1992.

180. Doig, J. C., McComb, J. M., and Reid, D. C.: Incessant atrial tachycardia accelerated by pregnancy. Br. Heart J. *67*:266, 1992.

181. Treakle, K., Kostic, B., and Hulkower, S.: Supraventricular tachycardia resistant to treatment in a pregnant woman. J. Fam. Pract. *35*:581, 1992.

182. Lee, M. S., Evans, S. J. L., Blumberg, S., et al.: Echocardiographically guided electrophysiologic testing in pregnancy. J. Am. Soc. Echocardiogr. *7*:182, 1994.

OTHER CARDIOVASCULAR DISORDERS

183. Elkayam, U., Rose, J., Jamison, M.: Vascular aneurysms and dissections during pregnancy. *In* Elkayam, U., and Gleicher, N. (eds.): Cardiac Problems in Pregnancy: Diagnosis and Management of Maternal and Fetal Disease. 2nd ed. New York, Alan R. Liss, Inc., 1990, p. 215.

184. Del Corso, L., De Marco, S., Vannini, A., and Pentimone, F.: Takayasu's arteritis: Low corticosteroid dosage and pregnancy—A case report. Angiology *44*:827, 1993.

185. Hampl, K. F., Schneider, M. C., Skarvan, K., et al.: Spinal anesthesia in a patient with Takayasu's disease. Br. J. Anaesth. *72*:129, 1994.

186. Elkayam, U., and Gleicher, N.: Primary pulmonary hypertension and pregnancy. *In* Elkayam, U., and Gleicher, N. (eds.): Cardiac Problems in Pregnancy: Diagnosis and Management of Maternal and Fetal Disease. 2nd ed. New York, Alan R. Liss, Inc., 1990, p. 189.

187. Pfisterer, J., Runge, H. M., Kommoss, F., et al.: Primare pulmonale hypertronie und Schwangerschaft. Gerburtshilfe Frauenheilkd. *51*:236, 1991.

188. Torres, P. J., Gratacos, E., Magrina, J., et al.: Primary pulmonary hypertension and pre-eclampsia: A successful pregnancy. Br. J. Obstet. Gynaecol. *101*:163, 1994.

189. Kiss, H., Egarter, C., Asseryanis, E., et al.: Primary pulmonary hypertension in pregnancy: A case report. Am. J. Obstet. Gynecol. *172*:1052, 1995.

190. Wilson, N. J., and Neutze, J. M.: Adult congenital heart disease: Principles and management guidelines. Part I. Aust. N. Z. J. Med. *23*:498, 1993.

191. Fuster, V., Steele, P. M., Edwards, W. D., et al.: Primary pulmonary hypertension: Natural history and the importance of thrombosis. Circulation *70*:580, 1984.

192. Abboud, T. K., Raya, J., Noueihed, R., et al.: Intrathecal morphine for relief of labor pain in a parturient with severe pulmonary hypertension. Anesthesiology *59*:477, 1983.

193. Gazzaniga, A.: Cardiac surgery during pregnancy. *In* Elkayam, U., and Gleicher, N. (eds.): Cardiac Problems in Pregnancy: Diagnosis and Management of Maternal and Fetal Disease. 2nd ed. New York, Alan R. Liss, Inc., 1990, p. 259.

194. Kupferminc, M. J., Lessing, J. B., Vidne, B. A., and Peyser, M. R.: Fetomaternal blood flow measurements and management of combined coarctation and aneurysm of the thoracic aorta in pregnancy. Acta Obstet. Gynecol. Scand. *72*:398, 1993.

195. Pamulapati, M., Treague, S., Stelzer, P., and Thadani, U.: Successful surgical repair of a ruptured aneurysm of the sinus of Valsalva in early pregnancy. Ann. Intern. Med. *115*:880, 1991.

196. Said, S. A. M., Veerbeek, A., van der Wieken, L. R.: Dextrocardia, situs inversus and severe mitral stenosis in a pregnant woman: Successful closed commissurotomy. Eur. Heart J. *12*:825, 1991.

197. Westaby, S., Parry, A. J., Forfar, J. C.: Reoperation for prosthetic valve endocarditis in the third trimester of pregnancy. Ann. Thorac. Surg. *53*:263, 1992.

198. Levy, D. L., Warriner, R. A., and Burgess, G. E.: Fetal response to cardiopulmonary bypass. Obstet. Gynecol. *56*:112, 1980.

199. Salazar, E., Zajarias, A., Guiterrez, N., et al.: The problem of cardiac valve prosthesis, anticoagulants and pregnancy. Circulation *70*(Suppl. 1):169, 1984.

200. Iturbe-Alessio, I., Del Carmen Fonseca, M., Mutchinik, O., et al.: Risks of anticoagulant therapy in pregnant women with artificial heart valve. N. Engl. J. Med. *315*:1390, 1986.

201. Lee, C. N., Wu, C. C., Lin, P. Y., et al.: Pregnancy following cardiac prosthesis valve replacement. Obstet. Gynecol. *83*:353, 1994.

202. Bick, R. L., and Pegram, M.: Syndrome of hypercoagulability and thrombosis: A review. Semin. Thromb. Hemost. *20*:109, 1994.

203. Elkayam, U., and Gleicher, N.: Anticoagulation in pregnant women with artificial heart valves. N. Engl. J. Med. *316*:1663, 1987.

204. Sareli, P., England, M. J., Berk, M. R., et al.: Maternal and fetal sequelae of anticoagulation during pregnancy in patients with mechanical heart valve prostheses. Am. J. Cardiol. *63*:1462, 1989.

205. Born, D., Martinez, E. E., Almeida, P. A. M., et al.: Pregnancy in patients with prosthetic heart valves: The effects of anticoagulation on mother, fetus, and neonate. Am. Heart J. *124*:413, 1992.

206. Ad Hoc Committee of the Working Group on Valvular Heart Disease, European Society of Cardiology: Guidelines for prevention of thromboembolic events in valvular heart disease. J. Heart Valve Dis. *2*:298, 1993.

CARDIOVASCULAR DRUGS IN PREGNANCY

207. Mitani, G. M., Steinberg, I., Lien, E., et al.: The pharmacokinetics of antiarrhythmic agents in pregnancy and lactation. Clin. Pharmacokinet. *12*:253, 1987.

208. Gleicher, N., and Elkayam, U.: Intrauterine therapy of rhythm and rate disorders and heart failure. *In* Elkayam, U., and Gleicher, N. (eds.): Cardiac Problems in Pregnancy: Diagnosis and Management of Maternal and Fetal Disease. 2nd ed. New York, Alan R. Liss, Inc., 1990, p. 749.

209. Mitani, G. M., Harrison, E. C., Steinberg, I., et al.: Digitalis glycosides in pregnancy. *In* Elkayam, U., and Gleicher, N. (eds.): Cardiac Problems in Pregnancy: Diagnosis and Management of Maternal and Fetal Disease. 2nd ed. New York, Alan R. Liss, Inc., 1990, p. 417.

210. Cox, J. L., and Gardner, M. J.: Treatment of cardiac arrhythmias during pregnancy. Prog. Cardiovasc. Dis. *36*:137, 1993.

211. Widerhorn, J., Shotan, A., Widerhorn, A. L. M., et al.: Antiarrhythmias. *In* Lee, R. V., Garner, P. R., Barron, W. M., et al. (eds.): Curr. Obstet. Med. *3*:95, 1995.

212. Treakle, K., Kostic, B., and Hulkower, S.: Supraventricular tachycardia resistant to treatment in a pregnant woman. J. Fam. Pract. *35*:581, 1992.

213. Ellsworth, A. J., Horn, J. R., Raisys, V. A., et al.: Disopyramide and N-monodesalkyl disopyramide in serum and breast milk. Drug Intell. Clin. Pharm. *23*:56, 1989.

214. Tadmor, O. P., Keren, A., Rosenak, D., et al.: The effect of disopyramide on uterine contractions during pregnancy. Am. J. Obstet. Gynecol. *162*:482, 1990.

215. Juneja, M. M., Ackerman, W. E., Kaczorowski, D. M., et al.: Continuous epidural lidocaine infusion in the parturient with paroxysmal ventricular tachycardia. Anesthesiology *71*:305, 1989.

216. Hands, M. E., Johnson, M. D., Saltzmann, D. H., and Rutherford, J. D.: The cardiac, obstetric and anesthetic management of pregnancy complicated by acute myocardial infarction. J. Clin. Anesth. *2*:258, 1990.

217. Lownes, H. E., and Ives, T. J.: Mexiletine use in pregnancy and lactation. Am. J. Obstet. Gynecol. *157*:446, 1987.

218. Gregg, A. R., and Tomich, P. G.: Mexiletine use in pregnancy. J. Perinat. *8*:33, 1988.

219. Wagner, X., Jouglard, J., Moulin, M., et al.: Coadministration of flecainide acetate and sotalol during pregnancy: Lack of teratogenic effects, passage across the placenta, and excretion in human breast milk. Am. Heart J. *119*:700, 1990.

220. Perry, J. C., Ayres, N. A., Carpenter, R. J.: Fetal supraventricular tachycardia treated with flecainide acetate. J. Pediatr. *118*:303, 1991.

221. Allan, L. D., Chita, S. K., Sharland, G. K., et al.: Flecainide in the treatment of fetal tachycardia. Br. Heart J. *65*:46, 1991.

222. Libardoni, M., Piovan, D., Busato, E., and Padrini, R.: Transfer of propafenone and 5-OH-propafenone to foetal plasma and maternal milk. Br. J. Clin. Pharmacol. *32*:527, 1991.

223. Widerhorn, J., Bhandari, A. K., Bughi, S., et al.: Fetal and neonatal adverse effects profile of amiodarone treatment during pregnancy. Am. Heart J. *122*:1162, 1991.

224. Plomp, T. A., Vulsma, T., and Vijlder, J. J. M.: Use of amiodarone during pregnancy. Eur. J. Obstet. Gynaecol. Reprod. Biol. *43*:2017, 1992.

225. Valensise, H., Civitella, V., and Garzetti, G. G.: Amiodarone treatment in pregnancy for dilatative cardiomyopathy with ventricular malignant extrasystole and normal maternal and neonatal outcome. Prenat. Diagn. *12*:705, 1992.

226. Mariani, P.: Pharmacotherapy of pregnancy-related SVT. Ann. Emerg. Med. *21*:229, 1992.

227. Schwingshandl, J., Stein, J. I., and Hausler, M.: Successful intrauterine treatment of a supraventricular tachycardia-induced hydrops fetalis with digoxin and verapamil. Wien. Klin. Wochensch. *103*:73, 1991.

228. Belfort, M. A., and Moore, J.: Verapamil in the treatment of severe postpartum hypertension. S. Afr. Med. J. *74*:265, 1988.

229. Childress, C. H., and Katz, V. L.: Nifedipine and its indications in obstetrics and gynecology. Obstet. Gynecol. *83*:616, 1994.

230. Ismail, A. A., Medhat, I., Tawfic, T. A., and Kholeif, A.: Evaluation of calcium antagonist (nifedipine) in the treatment of pre-eclampsia. Int. J. Gynecol. Obstet. *40*:39, 1993.

231. Lindow, S. W., Davies, N., Davey, D. A., and Smith, J. A.: The effect of sublingual nifedipine on uteroplacental blood flow in hypertensive pregnancy. Br. J. Obstet. Gynecol. *95*:1276, 1988.

232. Lubbe, W. F.: Use of diltiazem during pregnancy. N. Z. Med. J. *100*:121, 1987.

233. Maekawa, K., Ohnishi, H., Hirase, T., et al.: Acute myocardial infarction during pregnancy caused by coronary artery spasm. J. Intern. Med. *235*:489, 1994.

234. Okada, M., Inoue, H., Nakamura, Y., and Kishimoto, M. L.: Excretion of diltiazem in human milk. N. Engl. J. Med. *312*:992, 1985.

235. Frishman, W. H., and Chesner, M.: Use of beta-adrenergic blocking agents in pregnancy. *In* Elkayam, U., and Gleicher, N. (eds.): Cardiac Problems in Pregnancy: Diagnosis and Management of Maternal and Fetal Disease. 2nd ed. New York, Alan R. Liss, Inc., 1990, p. 351.

236. Blake, S., and MacDonald, D.: The prevention of the maternal manifestation of preeclampsia by intensive antihypertensive treatment. Br. J. Obstet. Gynecol. *98*:244, 1993.

237. Hackett, L. P., Wojnar-Horton, R. E., Dusci, L. J., et al.: Excretion of sotalol in breast milk. Br. J. Clin. Pharmacol. *29*:277, 1990.

238. Kannan, P., Raman, S., Ramani, V. S., and Jeyamalar, R.: Myocardial infarction in a young Indian grandmultipara. Aust. N. Z. J. Obstet. Gynaecol. *33*:424, 1993.

239. Peng, A. T. C., Gorman, R. S., Shulman, S. M., et al.: Intravenous nitroglycerin for uterine relaxation in the post partum patient with retained placenta. Anesthesiology *71*:172, 1989.

240. Bhatt-Mehta, V., and Deluga, K. S.: Fetal exposure to lisinopril: Neonatal manifestations and management. Pharmacotherapy *13*:515, 1993.

241. Nightingale, S. L.: Warning on the use of ACE inhibitors in second and third trimester of pregnancy. JAMA *267*:2445, 1992.

242. McGehee, W.: Anticoagulation in pregnancy. *In* Elkayam, U., and Gleicher, N. (eds.): Cardiac Problems in Pregnancy: Diagnosis and Management of Maternal and Fetal Disease. 2nd ed. New York, Alan R. Liss, Inc., 1990, p. 397.

243. Ginsberg, J. S., Kowalchuk, G., Hirsh, J., et al.: Heparin therapy during pregnancy: Risks to the fetus and mother. Arch. Intern. Med. *149*:2233, 1989.

244. Anderson, D. R., Ginsberg, J. S., Burrows, R., et al.: Subcutaneous heparin therapy during pregnancy: A need for concern at the time of delivery. Thromb. Haemost. *65*:248, 1991.

245. Manoharan, A.: Use of low molecular weight heparin during pregnancy. J. Clin. Pathol. *47*:94, 1994.

246. Nelson-Piercy, C.: Low molecular weight heparin for obstetric thromboprophylaxis. Br. J. Obstet. Gynaecol. *101*:6, 1994.

247. Sturridge, F., De Swiet, M., and Letsky, E.: The use of low molecular weight heparin for thromboprophylaxis in pregnancy. Br. J. Obstet. Gynaecol. *101*:69, 1994.

248. Cesario, T. C.: Antibiotic therapy in pregnancy. *In* Elkayam, U., and Gleicher, N. (eds.): Cardiac Problems in Pregnancy: Diagnosis and Management of Maternal and Fetal Disease. 2nd ed. New York, Alan R. Liss, Inc., 1990, p. 437.

Chapter 60

Neurological Disorders and Heart Disease

JOSEPH K. PERLOFF

Cardiovascular disorders occur as consequences of diseases of the nervous system, and disorders of the nervous system occur secondary to diseases of the heart and circulation. This chapter deals with the complex and varied interplay between the circulatory and nervous systems and focuses upon six general topics: (1) major heredofamilial neuromyopathical disorders of which cardiac disease is an inherent part, (2) less common neuromyopathic disorders that are sometimes associated with diseases of the heart, (3) acute cerebral disorders accompanied by cardiovascular abnormalities, (4) cardiac complications of drugs used for the treatment of neuromuscular diseases, (5) neuromuscular complications of drugs used for the treatment of cardiovascular diseases; and (6) the autonomic nervous system and cardiac denervation. Neurological complications associated with congenital and acquired heart disease are discussed in the chapters dealing with those disorders. Cardiac syncope is discussed in Chapter 28.

HEREDOFAMILIAL NEUROMYOPATHIC DISORDERS

Cardiac involvement is inherent in three major categories of heredofamilial neuromyopathic disorders: the progressive muscular dystrophies, myotonic muscular dystrophy, and Friedreich's ataxia.[1-5] The majority of nonmyotonic progressive muscular dystrophies are classified as follows:

1. X-linked
   a. Early-onset, rapidly progressive (classic Duchenne dystrophy)
   b. Late-onset, slowly progressive (Becker muscular dystrophy)
2. Limb–girdle dystrophy of Erb
3. Facioscapulohumeral dystrophy of Landouzy-Dejerine

Duchenne Muscular Dystrophy

GENETICS. Classic Duchenne muscular dystrophy (Fig. 60–1) is an X-linked recessive disorder, transmitted by the mother to one half of her sons as overt disease and to one-half of her daughters as a carrier state.[6,7] Incidence in the general population is approximately 1 in 3500 male births, making Duchenne dystrophy the most common lethal X-linked disease in humans.[8,9] The prevalence of the disease reflects the relatively high sporadic mutation rate that accounts for approximately one-third of new cases of affected boys in families with no other examples of neuromuscular disease.[8] Duchenne dystrophy is a myopathic disorder that involves striated muscle fibers (skeletal, cardiac), smooth muscle fibers (vasculature), and nervous system (neurons of central nervous system and cortex).[10]

The Duchenne muscular dystrophy gene has been identified on the Xp21 locus of the short arm of the X chromosome[8,11-14] (see p. 1632). The gene is the largest known, and the high mutation rate has been ascribed to its great size.[8,15] Cloning of the Duchenne muscular dystrophy gene and identification of its protein product, *dystrophin*, set the stage for understanding the genetic and biochemical basis of the neuromuscular disorder, but the function of dystrophin and the pathogenesis of the disease remain to be established.[12,15-17] The protein product is believed to form a network on the cytoplasmic face of the plasma membrane and may serve to stabilize the membrane or anchor or modulate the membrane proteins to which dystrophin binds.[10,14,16-18] More precisely, dystrophin is localized to the cytoplasmic surface of the sarcolemma and T tubules.[19] These observations fit Roland's "membrane hypothesis" of Duchenne dystrophy.[20] The molecule is composed of four domains, three of which share many features with the membrane's cytoskeletal proteins spectrin and actinin.[21] Skeletal muscle dystrophin is associated with a complex of six glycoproteins, including a 156-kd glycoprotein that is localized to the extracellular surface of the cell membrane.[22,23] The 156-kd dystrophin-associated glycoprotein is markedly reduced in mdx (muscular dystrophy, X-linked) mice and in patients with Duchenne dystrophy, suggesting that the absence of dystrophin may be accompanied by reductions in other proteins, the functions of which have not been established.

PATHOGENESIS. Dystrophin is present on the sarcolemma of normal muscle fibers, but is virtually absent from the cell surface of Duchenne muscular dystrophy fibers.[10,14-16,24] Antidystrophin antibodies have been successfully employed to determine the cell types normally containing dystrophin and, conversely, the cell types in Duchenne dystrophy that are dystrophin deficient.[10,16] Dystrophin expression appears to be limited to myogenic cells in every tissue tested with the exception of the central nervous system.[10] Similar levels of dystrophin have been identified in all physiological muscle types including "fast" skeletal, "slow" skeletal, cardiac, smooth, and embryonic muscle.[10] The very low dystrophin levels in nonmuscle tissues correspond to the smooth muscle content (vasculature) of each tissue except the central nervous system.[10] Assays of dystrophin content in cell cultures of neurons or astrocytes indicate that central nervous system dystrophin probably results from expression in neurons.[10] Importantly, dystrophin deficiency does not lead to myofiber necrosis until myofibers become vulnerable (sensitized) relatively late in their development.[10] Fetal and adult myofibers, which con-

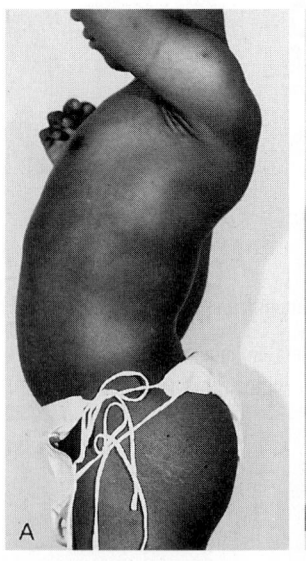
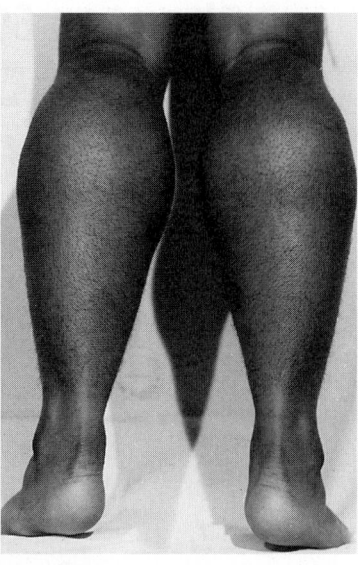

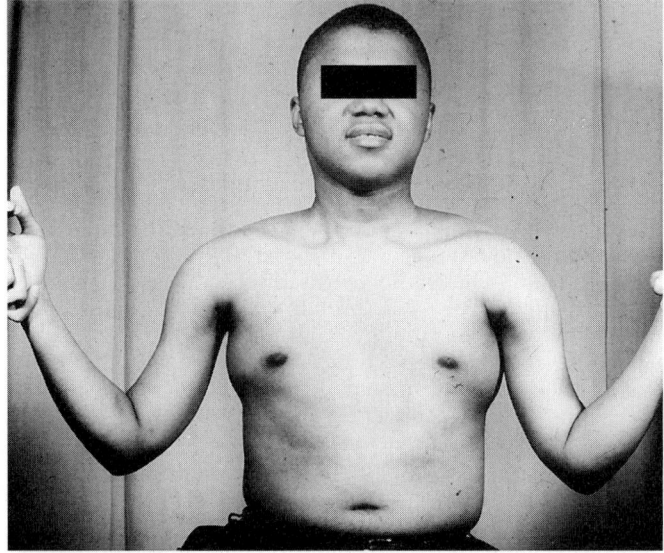

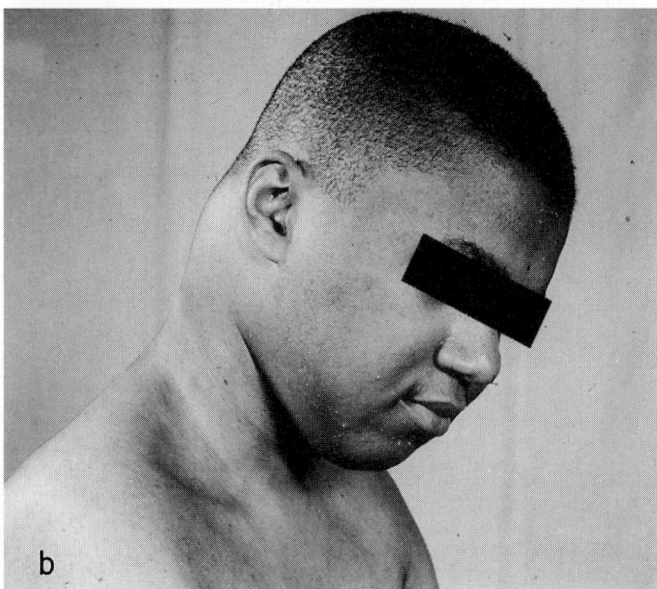

FIGURE 60–1. *A,* Classic X-linked muscular dystrophy. *Left,* exaggerated lumbar lardosis. *Right,* calf pseudohypertrophy and shortening of the Achilles tendons. *B,* Seventeen-year-old male with Duchenne muscular dystrophy. *Upper,* there is striking enlargement (hypertrophy/pseudohypertrophy) of the deltoid and pectoralis major muscles and *(lower)* of the trapezius. There was also striking enlargement of both calves, not shown.

tain similar amounts of dystrophin, should be equally vulnerable to necrosis based upon dystrophin content per se, but that clearly is not the case.[10]

Polyclonal antibodies used to assess the quantity and quality of dystrophin not only provide a laboratory method for the diagnosis of Duchenne dystrophy, but represent a major step forward in identification of female carriers.[9,22] Highly accurate prenatal diagnosis is now possible with Southern analysis using Duchenne muscular dystrophy cDNA and genomic clones.[9]

Rare cases of clinical Duchenne muscular dystrophy in female patients have been attributed to X translocation of a single mutant gene.[25,26] The normal X is inactivated, so the mutant X-linked recessive gene expresses itself.

CLINICAL MANIFESTATIONS. Overt clinical manifestations of Duchenne muscular dystrophy typically begin in the second year of life, although there is histological and enzymatic evidence that the disease is present at birth.[6] Skeletal muscle enzymes are copiously released into the plasma. Creatinine kinase (CK) elevations are present at birth, peak in 1 to 2 years, and precede the onset of overt clinical disease. Because the disorder exists at birth, it is present in utero.[27] Distinctive profiles of an isozyme such as MB-CK cannot be used to identify myocardial dystrophy because the isozyme originates in dystrophic skeletal muscle, compromising the specificity of the determination.[28,29]

In a child just learning to walk, the clumsy, waddling gait and frequent falls may go unnoticed, and the boy's difficulty in rising from the floor using the device of "climbing up" himself (Gowers' sign) tends to be ignored initially by parents and physicians. Because of what is interpreted as good muscle development (early enlargement of the calves) (Fig. 60–1A), reduced strength is not ascribed to an abnormality of skeletal muscle. Rarely, regional muscle enlargement (hypertrophy/pseudohypertrophy) in Duchenne dystrophy is striking in muscle groups other than the calves (Fig. 60–1B). Lumbar lordosis, hyperextension of the knees, and shortening of the Achilles tendons contribute to a precarious balance on the toes (Fig. 60–1A). Kyphoscoliosis becomes progressively more marked, and in the terminal stages of the disease, the patient sits in a wheelchair, twisted like a pretzel, with the head lolling unsupported because of inadequate neck-muscle strength.

Dystrophy of thoracic muscles and diaphragm together with kyphoscoliosis compromise coughing and breathing. Diaphragmatic dysfunction together with respiratory muscle weakness may result in hypercapnia that profoundly worsens with the use of supplemental oxygen therapy.[30] Patients are likely to succumb to pulmonary infection in the second decade, although cardiac involvement is an important and sometimes dramatic cause of death. Rapidly progressive preterminal heart failure may follow years of circulatory stability during which the chief, if not only, suspicion of cardiac involvement is the typical electrocardiogram (Fig. 60–2). Pulmonary emboli have been reported in patients with end-stage Duchenne dystrophy, and systemic emboli sometimes originate in a dilated, hypokinetic left ventricle.[31,32]

Physical examination. There are thoracic deformities and a high diaphragm of diaphragmatic dystrophy, features confirmed in the chest roentgenogram. A reduction in anteroposterior chest dimension is often striking and is commonly responsible for a systolic impulse at the left sternal border, a grade 1-3/6 short impure midsystolic murmur in the second left interspace, and a relatively loud pulmonary component of the second heart sound. These signs should not be mistaken for evidence of pulmonary hypertension, which if present at all, occurs in the terminal stage of the disease in conjunction with respiratory failure.[33] An increase in transverse heart size in the chest roentgenogram is more often than not caused by the high diaphragm and decreased anteroposterior chest dimen-

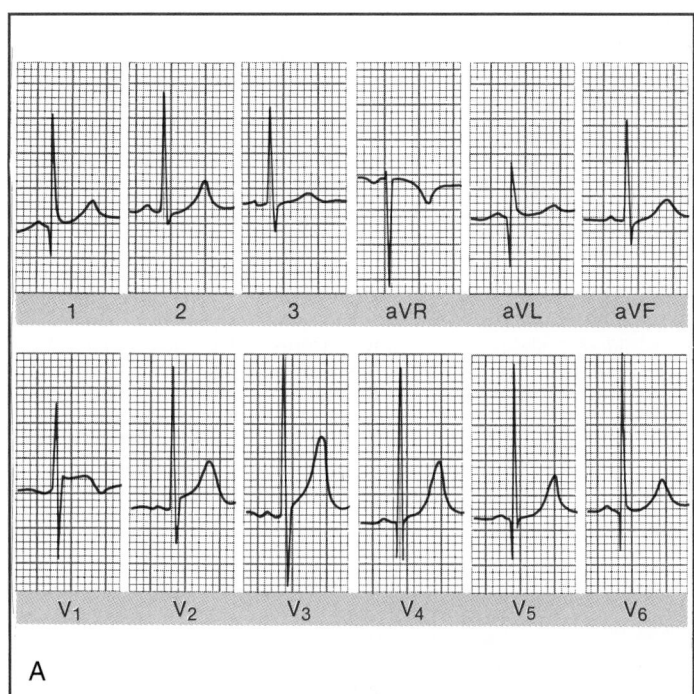

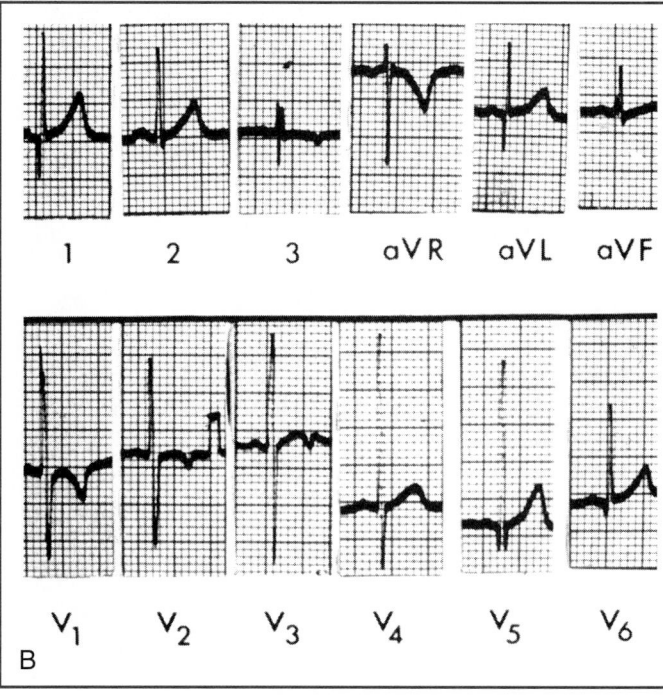

FIGURE 60–2. Electrocardiogram from a 10-year-old boy with classic Duchenne muscular dystrophy. The P–R interval is short (100 msec in lead 2). The QRS complex is typical of Duchenne dystrophy, showing an anterior shift in the right precordial leads and deep but narrow Q waves in leads I, aVL, and V_{4-6}. (From Perloff, J. K.: Cardiac rhythm and conduction in Duchenne's muscular dystrophy. Reprinted by permission of the American College of Cardiology. J. Am. Coll. Cardiol. 3:1263, 1984.) B, Twelve-lead scalar electrocardiogram in an obligate female carrier of the Duchenne muscular dystrophy gene. The tracing is similar, if not identical, to the typical scalar electrocardiogram in boys who overtly express Duchenne muscular dystrophy. The tall right precordial R waves and deep but narrow Q waves in leads I, aVL, and V_5 reflect posterolateral left ventricular extension of myocardial dystrophy in the female carrier. (From Perloff, J. K.: Cardiac manifestations of neuromuscular disease. In Abelmann, W. H. [ed.]: Cardiomyopathies, Myocarditis, and Pericardial Disease. In Braunwald, E. (series ed.): Atlas of Heart Diseases. Vol. 2. Philadelphia, Current Medicine, 1995, pp. 6.1–6.19.)

sion rather than by ventricular dilatation.[1] The murmur of mitral regurgitation has a relatively firm anatomical basis related to dystrophic involvement of the posterior papillary muscle and contiguous posterobasal left ventricular wall.[34,35]

CK quantification is a useful but limited means of identifying female carriers and families with Duchenne dystrophy.[36,37] Female carriers sometimes manifest occult or overt muscle weakness and mild calf pseudohypertrophy[37] in addition to electrocardiographic evidence of cardiac involvement.[36-40] Electrocardiograms in female carriers differ significantly from those of normal adult women, with larger R/S ratios in leads V_{1-2} in the carrier group.[37,41] Cardiac involvement in female carriers is occasionally expressed overtly as dilated cardiomyopathy.[38,40,41]

The standard scalar *electrocardiogram* is the simplest and most reliable tool for detecting cardiac involvement in Duchenne dystrophy.[1,34,42,43] Abnormal electrocardiograms are present in early childhood.[43,44] Tall right precordial R waves and increased R/S amplitude ratios together with deep Q waves in leads 1, aVL, and $V_{5,6}$ are characteristic of the classic, rapidly progressive pseudohypertrophic X-linked dystrophy of Duchenne (Fig. 60–2).[34,45-47] A reduction or loss of electromotive force caused by myocardial dystrophy in the posterobasal left ventricular wall (anterior shift of the QRS) and contiguous lateral wall (deep Q waves in leads 1, aVL and $V_{5,6}$) is believed to be responsible for the characteristic electrocardiogram.[1,34,45] At necropsy, these regions are the initial and most extensive sites of myocardial dystrophy (Fig. 60–3),[34,45,46] which is preceded by ultrastructural (subcellular) abnormalities.[40]

Electron microscopic examination of right ventricular endomyocardial biopsy specimens has identified abnormalities of mitochondria, C bands, sarcoplasmic reticulum, and nuclei.[48] The initial posterobasal involvement spreads to the epicardial third of the contiguous lateral left ventricular free wall, with transmural progression and fibrous replacement.[45,49] There is relative sparing of the ventricular septum and comparatively little involvement of right ventricular and atrial myocardium.[34,45,49] Duchenne dystrophy is an unusual form of heart disease characterized by a predilection for specific regions of the myocardium: the posterobasal and posterolateral left ventricular walls.[1,34,45,47,50] Relevant to this discussion are the scalar electrocardiographic abnormalities in the dystrophic hamster[51] and particularly in the canine model of Duchenne dystrophy.[52] Dystrophic dogs have deep Q waves and tall right precordial R waves that develop in animals older than 6 months, corresponding to hyperechoic regions in the posterobasal left ventricular wall in two-dimensional echocardiograms.[52]

ANATOMICAL CHANGES. The following hypothesis has been proposed to explain the posterobasal localization of myocardial involvement in Duchenne muscular dystrophy.[50] Cardiac myocytes are mononuclear and branched, whereas skeletal myocytes are multinuclear and linear. Skeletal muscle generates force exclusively along its major axis because of its linear configuration. Cardiac muscle generates force radially because of its branched configuration, although the vector of force is principally along its major axis. The force generated by cardiac myocytes is also distributed around the cell, owing to its rich sarcolemmal connections to fibroblasts and collagen. Because the forces acting upon skeletal myocytes are directed almost entirely axially, whereas the forces acting upon cardiac myocytes are more broadly distributed, strain upon the sarcolemma is more uniformly directed in skeletal muscle than in cardiac muscle.

In the anterior wall of the left ventricle, the muscle bundles are "mesh-like," whereas in the posterior wall, the bundles run in a parallel manner, especially in the epicardial half of the posterior wall, which is the site of orgin of myocardial involvement in Duchenne muscular dystrophy. Longitudinal shortening in the posterior wall is far greater during ventricular systole than in the anterior wall. If the role of dystrophin is to reinforce the sarcolemma against axial force, then absence of dystrophin (as in Duchenne muscular dystrophy), would cause a loss in structural integrity of those myocytes with the highest degree of axial forces. It is therefore postulated that the

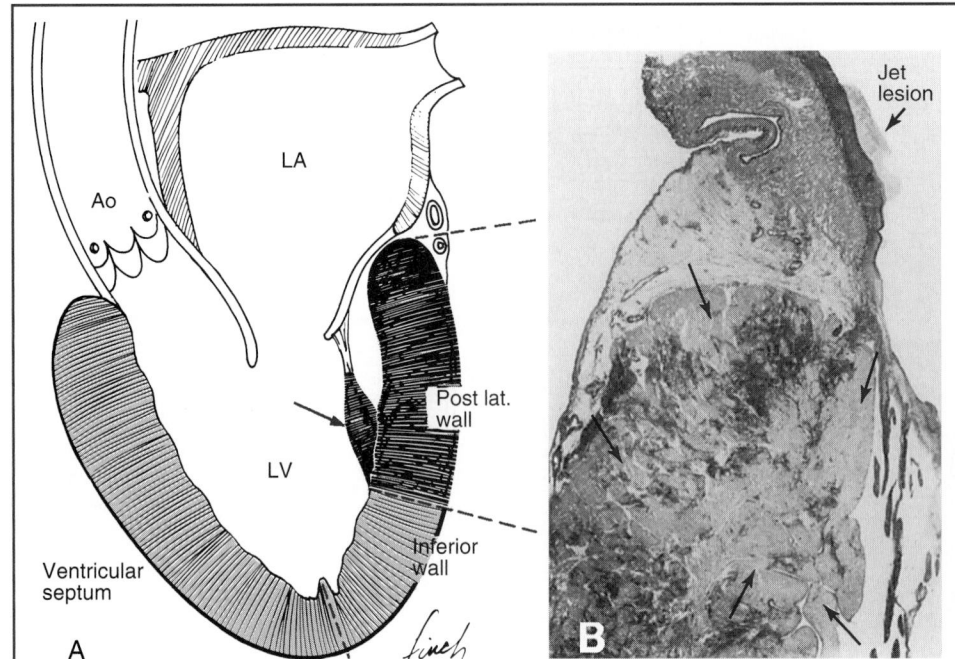

FIGURE 60–3. *A,* Schematic illustration showing the typical posterobasal myocardial involvement with lateral extension in classic Duchenne muscular dystrophy. The posterolateral papillary muscle is involved (arrow). LA = left atrium; LV = left ventricle; Ao = aorta. *B,* Necropsy section showing posterobasal involvement (arrows) of the left ventricle (LV) in a boy with classic Duchenne muscular dystrophy. The posterolateral papillary muscle was involved resulting in mitral regurgitation and the jet lesion shown in the upper right.

posterior left ventricular wall is the initial site of cardiac involvement in Duchenne muscular dystrophy.[50]

POSITRON EMISSION TOMOGRAPHY. Accelerated use of exogenous glucose ([18]Fluorodeoxyglucose) in the posterobasal and contiguous lateral left ventricular walls (Fig. 60–4) provide evidence of a regional myocardial metabolic abnormality in Duchenne dystrophy.[2,53] [13]NH$_3$ activity is reduced in wall segments in which uptake of exogenous glucose is accelerated (Fig. 60–4). These wall segments correspond to the sites of primary initial dystrophic involvement found at necropsy as described above.[34,45,46]

THALLIUM SCINTIGRAPHY. Regional perfusion defects demonstrated by thallium scintigraphy and thallium-201 myocardial SPECT are sometimes detected in older patients with Duchenne dystrophy.[2,54,55] Necropsy studies (light microscopy) have not identified luminal narrowing of extramural or intramural coronary arteries in these involved segments, despite the existence of a small vessel coronary arteriopathy.[34] Although reduction or loss of posterobasal/posterolateral left ventricular electrical forces is believed to be the cause of the distinctive electrocardiogram in Duchenne dystrophy,[1,34,45] this loss of forces does not require transmural replacement of myocardium by connective tissue. Increased [18]Fluorodeoxyglucose concentrations in these regions together with normal regional wall motion imply the presence of abnormal but viable (metabolically active) contracting myofibers or the preservation of a sufficient population of normal myofibers.[2]

Investigations of cardiac involvement in classic progressive X-linked Duchenne muscular dystrophy have focused chiefly upon gross morphological, histological, ultrastructural, and regional metabolic abnormalities of ventricular myocardium. Disorders of impulse formation and conduction arising or potentially arising from specialized cardiac tissue have received less attention, and there is only scant morphological information on the cardiac impulse and conduction system.[45,56–58] The following remarks focus upon the electrophysiological expressions related to impulse formation and conduction in Duchenne dystrophy.

ELECTROPHYSIOLOGICAL FINDINGS. At least two fundamental variables are relevant to cardiac electrophysiological involvement in Duchenne dystrophy, namely, the small vessel coronary arteriopathy, and abnormalities believed to originate in specialized cardiac tissues. There is a small vessel coronary arteriopathy characterized principally by striking hypertrophy of media with luminal narrowing (Fig. 60–5), less commonly by coexisting cystic degeneration and mucopolysaccharide material in the vessel wall, including small arteries that supply the sinus node and atrioventricular nodes.[34] Dystrophin content of vascular smooth muscle cells has been found to be similar to that of striated myofibers.[10]

An unanswered question is why the dystrophin deficiency in vascular smooth muscle expresses itself chiefly as hypertrophy rather than necrosis. It may be relevant that the earliest clinical expression (phenotype) of human Duchenne muscular dystrophy in skeletal muscle is enlargement of the calves, generally termed "pseudohypertrophy," because the enlargement results from extensive infiltration if not replacement with connective tissues and fat. However, before 2 years of age, connective tissue and fat are often minimal in enlarged calves that almost certainly exhibit true hypertrophy rather than pseudohypertrophy.[11] Rarely, regional muscle enlargement (hypertrophy/pseudohypertrophy) in Duchenne dystrophy can be striking in muscle groups other than the calves. Interestingly, in the cat model of Du-

chenne dystrophy, hypertrophy is especially striking in skeletal muscle in animals that exhibit dramatic elevations of serum CK but little evidence of overt muscle necrosis.[59] Whether vascular smooth muscle shares in the hypertrophy of the cat model is not clear. Relevant to our concerns is whether a relationship exists between the coronary arteriopathy (medial smooth muscle hypertrophy) and certain electrophysiologic disorders.

A second concern fundamental to an understanding of cardiac electrophysiological involvement in Duchenne muscular dystrophy centers upon the *specialized cardiac tissues.*[56] Specialized cardiac tissues and cardiac muscle have close embryologic origins, although the specialized tissues are believed to be so designated ab origine in the embryonic heart.[60] If there is an embryologic kinship between cardiac muscle and specialized cardiac tissue, does the plasma membrane of the latter normally contain dystrophin as does the cell membrane of cardiac muscle? Immunocytochemical staining has identified dystrophin localized to the membrane surface of normal human cardiac Purkinje fibers.[61,62] Little or no light has been shed upon this question, but if cell membranes of normal cardiac specialized tissues contain dystrophin, it is reasonable to hypothesize that in Duchenne dystrophy, cell membranes of specialized tissues may be dystrophin deficient.[56,61] Should that be the case, how might dystrophin deficiency affect specialized tissue viability, and how might that interplay manifest itself as overt electrophysiological disturbances? The presence of well-defined plasma cell membranes in neurogenic and myogenic specialized cardiac tissues provide a morphological basis that lends credence to a dystrophin-deficiency hypothesis for certain electrophysiological disorders in Duchenne dystrophy.

CARDIAC ARRHYTHMIAS

The electrophysiological abnormalities that have been documented in human Duchenne dystrophy are expressed as disturbances in rhythm and conduction.[56–58,63] The most common rhythm disturbance is inappropriate sinus tachycardia (rate acceleration without discernible cause).[64] Two types of sinus tachycardia occur: (1) persistent sinus acceleration (minimal heart rate during a 24-hour period of not less than 100 beats/min in patients older than 12 years of age or not less than 110 beats/min in younger patients) and (2) labile sinus tachycardia during waking hours or sleep, so designated because a labile rate acceleration without change in P-wave morphology is unprovoked by a definable circumstantial cause. Episodes of labile sinus tachycardia are either gradual in onset (brief warm-up) or abrupt (within one beat). The mechanism(s) of sinus tachycardia, persistent or labile, gradual or abrupt, have not been established, but may reflect an increase in sympathetic activity and/or a decrease in parasympathetic activity.[56] Studies of the autonomic nervous system, although less than ideal, thus far have not provided convincing evidence of autonomic dysfunction, and observations of sleep hypoxemia have shed little or no light on the sinus tachycardia.[56]

Heart rate variability in the time and frequency domain[64] may yield further information. Mild-to-marked sinus arrhythmia (not necessarily sleep related) is common in Duchenne dystrophy.[63] Morphological observations also leave the above disturbances in sinus rhythm unresolved. The nutrient artery to the sinus node has been described in a limited number of patients as thick-walled (medial hypertrophy with small lumen), less commonly as having cystic medial degeneration and endothelial proliferation.[34] Histological observations on the sinus

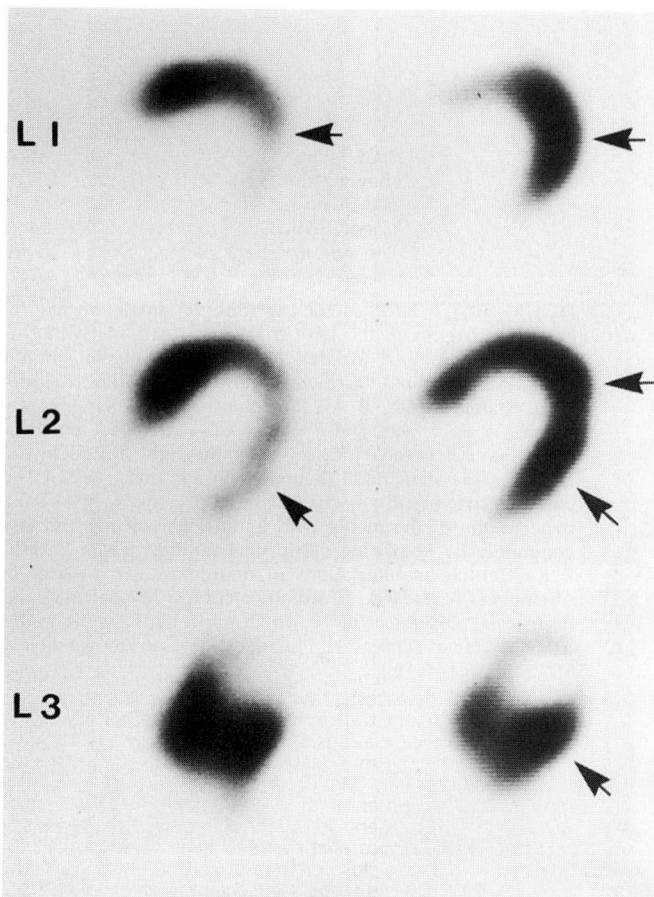

A   **B**

L 1

L 2

L 3

FIGURE 60–4. Regional myocardial uptake of $^{13}NH_3$ (A) and ^{18}F fluorodeoxyglucose (B) visualized in three contiguous positron CT images (L1, L2, L3) of left ventricular myocardium in a 24-year-old man with classic Duchenne dystrophy. There is a segmental decrease in $^{13}NH_3$ activity in the posterolateral wall (arrows) with a discordant increase in ^{18}F fluorodeoxyglucose concentration in the same region (arrows). This patient had a moderate posterolateral thallium-201 defect, posterolateral akinesis on technetium-99m radionuclide imaging, and a left ventricular ejection fraction of 46 per cent. (Reproduced by permission from Perloff, J. K., et al.: Alterations in regional myocardial metabolism, perfusion, and wall motion in Duchenne muscular dystrophy studied by radionuclide imaging. Circulation *69:*33, 1984. Copyright 1984 The American Heart Association.)

node have disclosed occasional mild fibrosis.[58] In a limited study, sinus node myofibers varied in size and showed vacuolization, fatty encroachment, and nuclear pyknosis, with focal areas of fibrosis in the presence of a normal sinus node artery.[57] It is unclear whether the morphological changes in the sinus node cause an increase in intercellular resistance, reduce electrotonic effects, and accelerate pacemaker activity, producing sinus tachycardia.

The most important disturbance in atrial rhythm is flutter, a rare tachyarrhythmia in children, but a relatively common preterminal tachyarrhythmia in Duchenne muscular dystrophy.[34,63,65] In addition, atrial premature beats, intermittent atrial ectopic rhythms, intermittent junctional rhythm, and sustained supraventricular tachycardia have been observed.[51,56] Recall the focal areas of fibrosis at the cellular level and a loss of thick and thin myofilaments at the subcellular level together with P terminal force evidence of prolonged intra-atrial conduction.[57,63] Focal areas of fibrosis are associated with increased intracellular resistance and slowed conduction, which facilitate reentrant arrhythmias.[66–68] Slowed intra-atrial conduction is the electrophysiologic substrate associated with atrial fibrillation and atrial flutter.[68,69]

The incidence of ventricular electrical instability appears to be increased in Duchenne dystrophy, especially in older

patients with depressed left ventricular function.[63,70–72] Ventricular ectopic rhythms include premature ventricular complexes (uniform or multiform), couplets, and nonsustained ventricular tachycardia. The clinical substrate for an increased incidence of ventricular ectopic rhythms appears to be duration of disease and depressed left ventricular function.[70–72] But what are the morphological and electrophysiological substrates of ventricular ectopic rhythms? There is little evidence that the metabolically abnormal but viable posterobasal left ventricular myocardium in young patients (Fig. 60–3) is electrically unstable even though the zone generates decreased electromotive force. In the late stages of the disease, these regional zones of abnormal but viable myocardium are replaced with connective tissue containing islands of muscle cells. The left ventricle and ventricular septum then have focal areas with variability of myofibrillar size, some atrophic fibers surrounded by fibrosis and islands of fat, some adjacent fibers that are normal and others hypertrophic. In addition, degenerative changes have been reported in the peripheral conduction tissue fibers (Purkinje).[58] Do areas of regional or focal myocardial scarring result in slow conduction that provides the electrophysiological substrate for reentrant ventricular tachycardia as has been shown to be the case with ventricular tachycardia originating from myocardial infarction scars? Late potentials recorded on signal-averaged electrocardiograms in older patients with Duchenne muscular dystrophy have been found to be associated with left ventricular wall-motion abnormalities and left ventricular dysfunction. The significance of these late potentials in Duchenne dystrophy is not clear; a correlation with ventricular tachcyardia or sudden death has not been established.[71]

Procainamide and phenytoin may reinforce muscle weakness, and intravenous verapamil has resulted in fatal respiratory arrest.[65,73] Malignant hyperthermia and cardiac arrest have occurred during anesthesia in a number of children with Duchenne muscular dystrophy after the use of halothane, suxamethonium, isoflurane, and succinylcholine.[74,75]

Now let us turn to *abnormalities of conduction.* The terminal force of the P wave, especially in lead V_1, may be abnormal or less commonly, the P wave in lead 2 may be broad and notched, implying prolongation of interatrial or left-atrial conduction. Focal areas of fibrosis at the cellular level, and minimal loss of thick and thin myofilaments at the subcellular level occur in the left atrium and have been proposed as explanations for prolonged left-atrial conduction and abnormal P waves.[57,63]

Early reports of atrioventricular conduction in Duchenne dystrophy commented upon an increase in the P-R interval,[1] an observation that has been confirmed in the relatively late stage of the disease.[2] More systematic observations have disclosed a prevalence of short P-R intervals indicating accelerated AV conduction.[2,45,57] As in the case of the sinus node, the short P-R interval in Duchenne dystrophy may reflect accelerated conduction from intrinsic properties within the AV node.

Intranodal conduction defects take the form of minor right ventricular conduction delay, left posterior fascicular block, left anterior fascicular block, right bundle branch block, and exceptionally bifascicular block.[2,57] Histopathological studies of the atrioventricular bundle have disclosed abnormalities that varied from mild fibrosis and fatty infiltration to focal areas of fibrosis and vascular degeneration involving the penetrating portion and branching portion of AV node.[57,58]

Becker Muscular Dystrophy

Becker muscular dystrophy is considered a milder allelic variant of Duchenne muscular dystrophy, but the clinical expression—both the phenotype and the presence and degree of cardiac involvement—are much more variable.[76–79] Becker dystrophy and Duchenne muscular dystrophy are

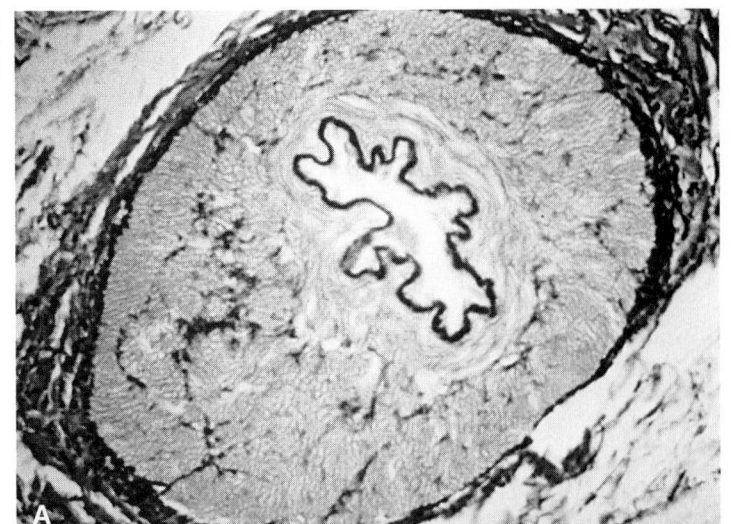

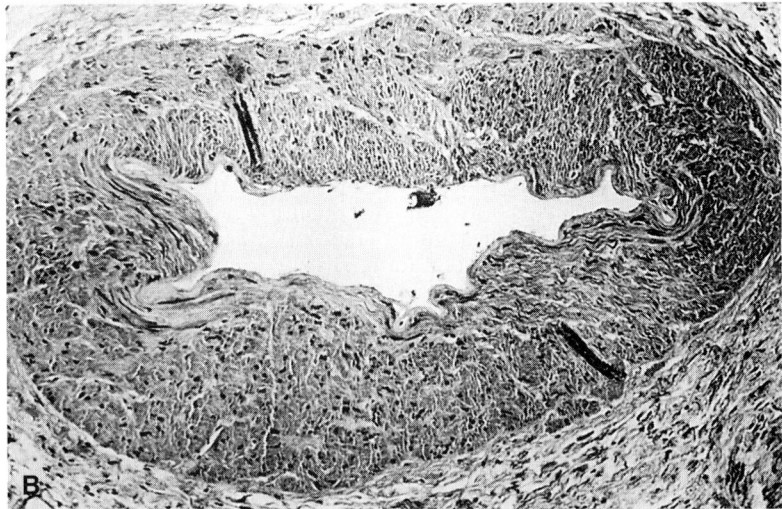

FIGURE 60–5. Histological sections of small intramural coronary arteries in the left atria of two patients with Duchenne dystrophy. *A,* Striking hypertrophy of medial smooth muscle with luminal narrowing (Verhoeff-von-Gieson elastic tissue stains, ×260). *B,* Medial smooth muscle hypertrophy causing a thick wall and a moderately narrowed lumen in an intramural coronary artery from the right atrium in the region of the sinus node (hematoxylin and eosin, ×25). The coronary arteriopathy is characterized principally by striking hypertrophy of the media with luminal narrowing, and less commonly by coexisting cystic degeneration (From Perloff, J. K.: Cardiac manifestations of neuromuscular disease. *In* Abelmann, W. H. [ed.]: Cardiomyopathies, Myocarditis, and Pericardial Disease. Vol. 2. *In* Braunwald, E. (series ed.): Atlas of Heart Diseases. Philadelphia, Current Medicine, 1995, pp. 6.1–6.19.)

both believed to be caused by mutations of the Duchenne muscular dystrophy gene.[24,80] Mutations have different effects on dystrophin expression and clinical severity, reflecting a number of functional roles for the dystrophin domains.[79] The Becker dystrophy gene is expressed in both skeletal muscle and cardiac muscle.[24,76,78,81] Becker dystrophy can be distinguished from Duchenne dystrophy by immunohistochemical dystrophin assays of skeletal muscle biopsies.[79,80] In Becker dystrophy, dystrophin is present in skeletal muscle but is abnormal in molecular weight, whereas in Duchenne dystrophy, the protein product is absent or scanty but is of normal molecular weight.[10,22] The dystrophin abnormality has been identified with immunostaining of endomyocardial biopsies in patients with Becker muscular dystrophy.[82]

Becker dystrophy is later in onset and slower in progression than Duchenne dystrophy. Most patients remain ambulant into adulthood[6,83] (Fig. 60–6), but Becker dystrophy exhibits a considerable variation in clinical expression, both in skeletal and cardiac muscle.[76–78] Cardiac involvement may occur at an early age and is unrelated to the extent of the musculoskeletal disorder.[78,84,85] Appreciable cardiac involvement can occur in patients without significant muscular disability,[79,86–88] while other patients with progressive muscular atrophy and weakness have comparatively little cardiac involvement, at least overtly.[77,79] X-linked dilated cardiomyopathy without clinical signs of skeletal myopathy is believed to be due, at least in part, to the Becker gene on the short arm of the X chromosome.[89,90] Severe familial dilated cardiomyopathy occurs in the context of Becker progressive muscular dystrophy.[91]

Because the diagnosis of Becker dystrophy was not se-

cure before the advent of current molecular diagnostic techniques, reports on the incidence and type of associated heart disease have been open to question. The severity of cardiac involvement is not related to age,[84] but patients who reach adulthood generally have cardiomyopathy and may succumb to it.[86,88,91] Involvement of both ventricles culminates in dilatation and failure (Fig. 60–7*A,B*).[86–88] Abnormalities of the His bundle and of infranodal conduction express themselves as fascicular block, right bundle branch block, left bundle branch block, and complete heart block[86–88] (Fig. 60–5*C*). Defective dystrophin expression in specialized cardiac tissues may be responsible for these conduction defects in Becker dystrophy, as hypothesized for Duchenne dystrophy.[56,61] Serious ventricular arrhythmias have been documented in patients with Becker dystrophy and are believed to play a role in sudden death.

LIMB-GIRDLE DYSTROPHY OF ERB

Neuromuscular disorders designated "limb-girdle dystrophy" represent a poorly defined group within the major muscular dystrophies. The term *limb-girdle syndromes* has sometimes been applied.[6,92] There is variation in mode of inheritance, age of onset, progression of illness, and distribution of muscle weakness. Two forms of autosomal dominant limb-girdle muscular dystrophy have been proposed. One variety, Bethlem myopathy,[93] is well documented but rare and thus far has been devoid of cardiac involvement.[78] The other variety is relatively heterogeneous with late onset and slow progression.[94] The pelvic girdle is chiefly affected, the upper limbs and shoulder girdle less so, and the face is spared. Because of disproportionate pelvic involvement, patients are often confined to a wheelchair.[6] Limb-girdle dystrophy with calf pseudohypertrophy can now be distinguished from Becker dystrophy by dystrophin and molecular genetic analysis.[95,96]

The type and prevalence of heart disease are uncertain because the diagnosis of limb-girdle dystrophy has been poorly defined. If cardiac

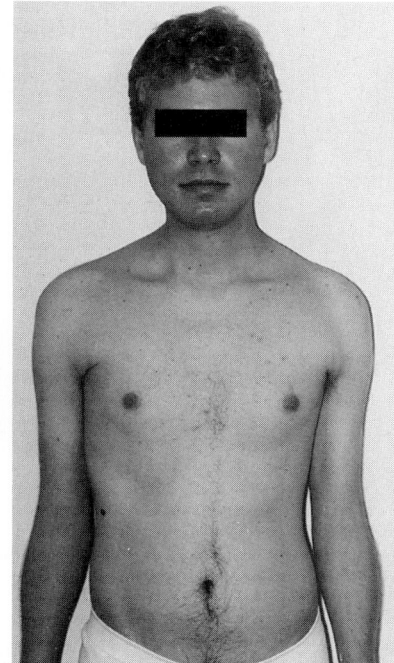
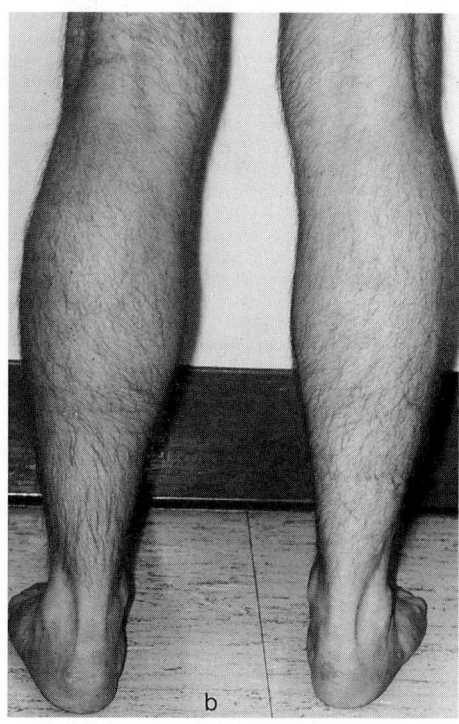

FIGURE 60–6. A 22-year-old man with late onset, slowly progressive Becker muscular dystrophy. *A,* There is dystrophy of the shoulder girdle, arms, and pelvic girdle (latter not shown). *B,* Asymmetric calf pseudohypertrophy, greater on the left than on the right. Dystrophy of proximal leg muscles is not shown.

involvement occurs, it is generally occult (asymptomatic).[96] Disorders of cardiac conduction have been reported, especially intraventricular conduction defects and fascicular block.[96,97] A unique case of limb-girdle dystrophy with dilated cardiomyopathy has been described.[98]

FACIOSCAPULOHUMERAL DYSTROPHY OF LANDOUZY-DEJERINE

Facioscapulohumeral dystrophy is inherited as an autosomal dominant with strong penetrance and an incidence estimated at one in 20,000.[99] The genetic locus has been mapped to the long arm of chromosome 4 in the region of 4q35.[100,101] The disease typically becomes overt at the end of the first decade or the beginning of the second decade. Facial weakness may be signaled by no more than an

inability to whistle or drink through a straw. More distinctive and troublesome is the inability to close the eyes, even during sleep. The face ultimately becomes smooth and the forehead unlined; loss of the normal upward curvature of the lower lip creates a pouting appearance, and the only marks on an otherwise expressionless face are the dimples on either side of the angles of the mouth, creating an enigmatic smile (Fig. 60–8A). Concurrently, the muscles of the arms and shoulders (scapulohumeral) are involved, and winging of the scapulae become apparent (Fig. 60–8B). Infrequently, the disease expresses itself in infancy and runs a rapid course with death in adolescence.[102] Asymptomatic or minimally affected parents may have severely affected offspring with the infantile form of the disease.[102]

Cardiac Findings. The type of cardiac abnormality previously ascribed to the adult form of facioscapulohumeral dystrophy was a unique variety of heart disease: permanent atrial paralysis. However,

FIGURE 60–7. Gross and microscopic cardiac pathological specimens and the electrocardiogram from a 45-year-old man with late-onset, slowly progressive Becker muscular dystrophy. *A,* Dilated, flabby left ventricle with focal endocardial thickening. *B,* Microscopic section from the left ventricle shows marked confluent scarring with variations in fiber size; there was no significant coronary artery disease. *C,* Electrocardiogram recorded at age 40 years. The 12-lead tracing shows left-axis deviation, a QRS of 0.14 sec, small Q waves in leads I and aVL and loss of R waves in leads V₂ and V₃. The lower tracings, taken 4 years later (a year before death), show complete heart block with a variable QRS configuration. (Reproduced by permission from Perloff, J. K., et al.: The cardiomyopathy of progressive muscular dystrophy. *Circulation 33:*625, 1966. Copyright 1966 The American Heart Association.)

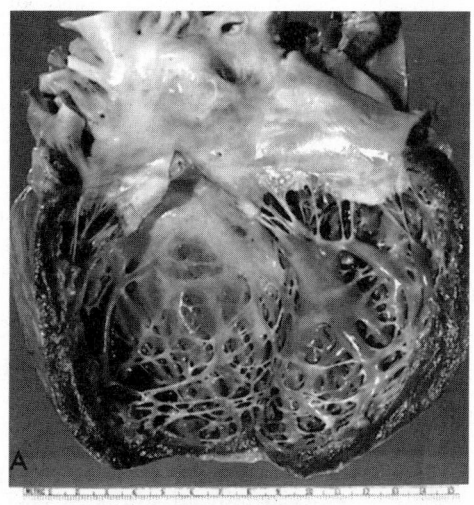
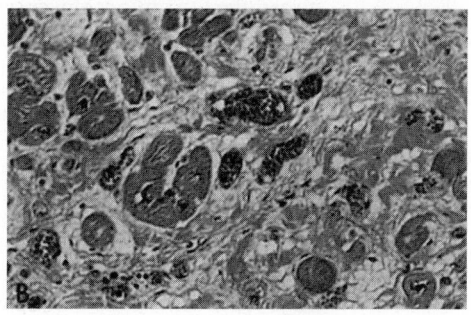
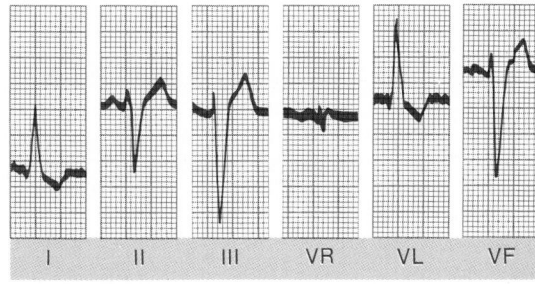
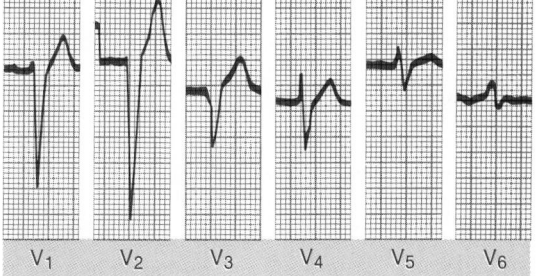
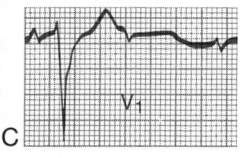
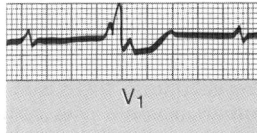

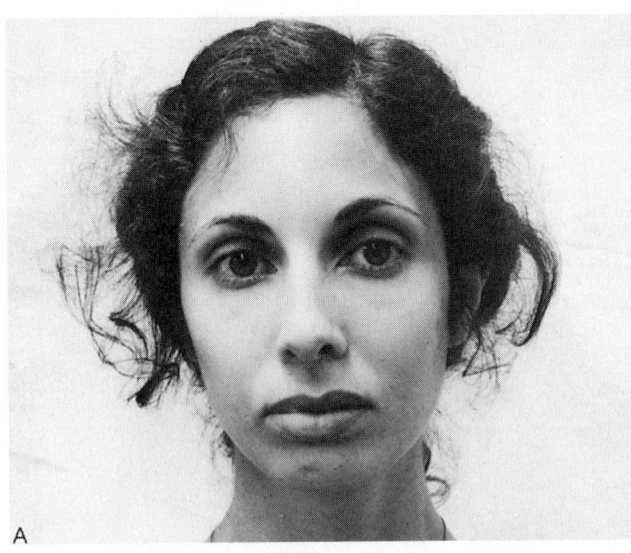
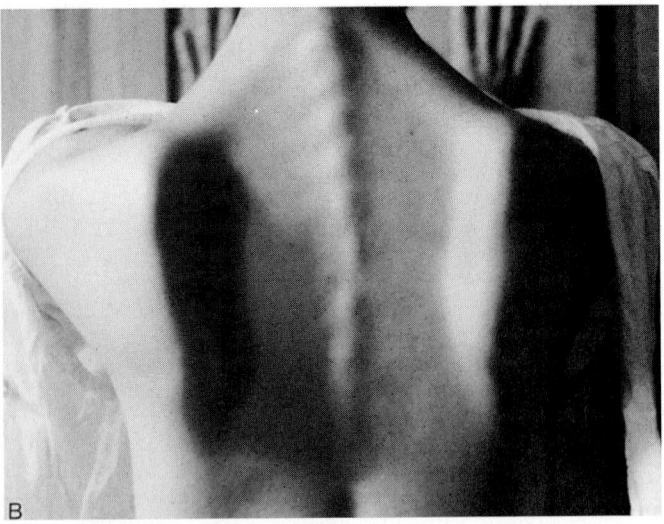

FIGURE 60–8. Facioscapulohumeral muscular dystrophy in a 32-year-old woman. *A,* The face is in repose (myopathic) with dimpling of the corners of the mouth. *B,* Typical winging of the scapulae.

the cases that were reported as facioscapulohumeral dystrophy[103-105] are now believed to have been Emery-Dreifuss dystrophy.[106] Cardiac involvement in facioscapulohumeral dystrophy takes the form of electrophysiological abnormalities of the atria and AV node, and of infranodal conduction.[106] There is a relatively high susceptibility to induced atrial flutter or fibrillation during electrophysiological study, together with less frequent evidence of abnormal sinus-node function and abnormal AV nodal or infranodal conduction.[106] It has been hypothesized that the genetic marker for facioscapulohumeral dystrophy results in a form of cardiac involvement analogous to but much more benign than that in phenotypically similar but genetically different Emery-Dreifuss dystrophy and its variants.[106]

EMERY-DREIFUSS MUSCULAR DYSTROPHY

Emery-Dreifuss dystrophy has been distinguished from facioscapulohumeral dystrophy, which it superficially resembles.[107-109] Scapulohumeral and scapuloperoneal muscular dystrophy are believed to be genetic variants of the Emery-Dreifuss form, which is an X-linked disorder—Xq28[110]—characterized by slowly progressive muscle wast-

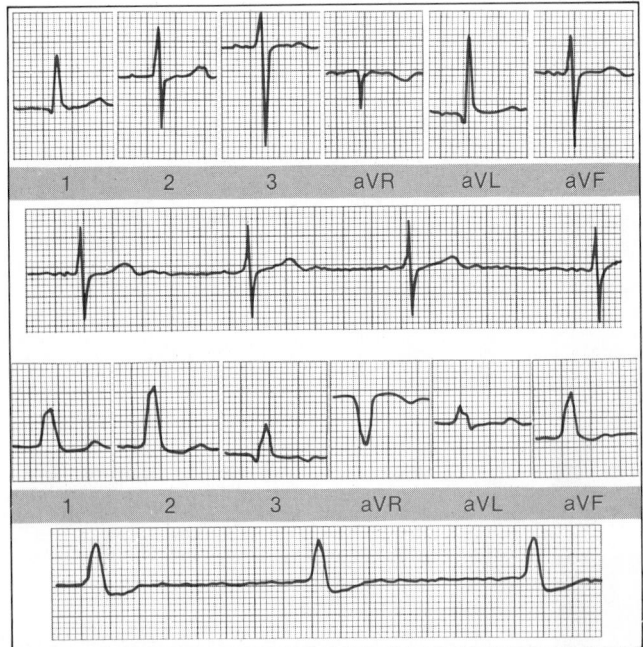

FIGURE 60–9. Limb leads and rhythm strips from two patients, a 16-year-old male *(upper)* and his 38-year-old father *(lower)* with Emery-Dreifuss muscular dystrophy. The son's tracing shows left anterior fascicular block. The P waves are low voltage and bifid, and the rate is bradycardiac. The father's tracing shows complete left bundle branch block. There is fine atrial fibrillation (not to be confused with atrial standstill) with a slow ventricular response. A pacemaker was inserted a month later.

ing and weakness with humeral peroneal distribution and early contractures of the elbows, Achilles tendons, and postcervical muscles.[111-114]

CARDIAC ARRHYTHMIAS. Permanent paralysis of the atria (atrial standstill) is the unusual if not unique form of electrophysiological heart disease that sometimes occurs in Emery-Dreifuss dystrophy. As an isolated disorder, partial or permanent atrial standstill has been reported in adults, rarely in children, and occasionally in families.[115-120] Criteria for the diagnosis of atrial paralysis include absence of P waves on scalar, esophageal, and intracardiac electrocardiograms; lack of response to direct (intracardiac) electrical or mechanical stimulation of the atria; absence of an *a* wave in the jugular venous pulse and in the right atrial pressure pulse; a supraventricular QRS; and immobility of the atria on fluoroscopy or on two-dimensional echocardiography.[117] The entire atrial myocardium ultimately becomes inexcitable, but before that stage is reached, atrial standstill appears to be regional, with certain focal areas that are inert, whereas others are subject to enhanced atrial electrical activity (atrial tachycardia or flutter).[116,118-120]

While permanent atrial paralysis, atrial fibrillation and atrial flutter are features of Emery-Dreifuss dystrophy, the greatest threats are abnormalities of infranodal conduction with slow junctional rhythms or complete atrioventricular block (Fig. 60–9).[108,112,121-126] A permanent pacemaker is often required. Emery-Dreifuss dystrophy puts patients at risk because of the cardiac involvement, not because of the systemic neuromuscular disease. In addition to defects in rhythm and conduction in Emery-Dreifuss dystrophy and its genetic variants, myocardial fibrosis has been described at necropsy[127] and on myocardial biopsy.[112]

Female carriers may exhibit age-related disturbances in cardiac rhythm and conduction similar to those in male patients with overt Emery-Dreifuss dystrophy.[128] Sinus bradycardia, first-degree heart block, or complete heart block may require pacemaker support, which should be ventricular because of concern regarding nonresponsive atrial myocardium.[128]

Myotonic Muscular Dystrophy

GENETICS AND PATHOGENESIS. Myotonic muscular dystrophy (Steinert's disease) is a multisystem disorder inherited as an autosomal dominant with an estimated incidence of three to five per 100,000, making it a relatively common neuromuscular disease and the most common muscular dystrophy in adults.[129-132] The diagnosis is made by neuromuscular examination, electromyography, muscle biopsy and DNA analysis.[129,133] Myotonic dystrophy is caused by an increased number of cytosine-thymine-guanine (CTG) trinucleotide repeats in the untranslated region of a protein kinase gene located on the q13.3 band of chromosome 19.[133,134] There is believed to be a significant correlation between clinical severity and the number of trinucleotide repeats.[135]

An early feature is weakness of the flexor muscles of the neck. Atrophy of the sternocleidomastoid muscles often progresses to virtual disappearance. The phenotype of the adult with myotonic dystrophy is characteristic.[6,130] Myotonia (delayed relaxation after contraction) is provoked by voluntary, mechanical, or electrical stimulation of muscles of the hands, forearms, tongue, and jaw.[132] Myotonic responses are best elicited by tapping the thenar eminence (percussion myotonia), especially after having the patient rapidly open and close the fist. Myotonic dystrophy is a systemic disease with important nonmyotonic/nonmyopathic features, including cataracts, testicular atrophy, premature baldness, mental deterioration and involvement of smooth muscle (esophagus, colon, uterus).[130,132,136]

Because specialized cardiac tissues and myocardium have close embryological origins, it is not surprising that both are affected. Cardiac involvement is therefore an integral part of myotonic dystrophy, especially targeting the infranodal conduction system, to a lesser extent the sinus node, and still less specifically the myocardium.[3,133-143]

CARDIAC MANIFESTATIONS. Clinically important cardiac manifestations generally reside in specialized tissues rather than in myocardium.[3,137-141] Involvement is relatively specific, primarily assigned to the His-Purkinje system. The most frequent histopathological lesions of the cardiac conduction system are fibrosis, fatty infiltration, and atrophy involving the sinus node, AV node, His bundle, and bundle branches.[142] Involvement of cardiac muscle, generally occult, takes the form of dystrophy and is not selective, appearing with approximately equal distribution in all four chambers.[3]

Myocardial dystrophy may be responsible for atrial and ventricular arrhythmias including sinus bradycardia, premature atrial beats, atrial flutter (Fig. 60-10), atrial fibrillation, premature ventricular beats, and ventricular tachycardia.[144-147] Preferential selection of the His-Purkinje system (80 per cent of patients) is reflected in intraventricular conduction defects, prolongation of the H-V interval and of the effective refractory period of the right bundle branch, right bundle branch block, and abnormal responses to atrial pacing or extrastimuli.[3,139-141] The most common electrocardiographic abnormalities—prolongation of the P-R interval, left anterior fascicular block, increased QRS duration—reflect His-Purkinje disease that can progress

rapidly, although neither the scalar electrocardiogram nor a single H-V interval determination predicts the rate of progression.[148,149] His-Purkinje disease can culminate in fatal Stokes-Adams episodes unless anticipated by insertion of pacemaker (Fig. 60-8).[145,149-151] Although sudden death caused by AV block is relatively rare, it is the most grave cardiac threat in myotonic dystrophy.[149] Ventricular tachycardia has also been responsible for sudden death.[146,147] Signal-averaging electrocardiography identified abnormal ventricular late potentials that correlated directly with cytosine-thymine-guanine expansion, an important observation because abnormal late potentials are caused by slowed, fragmented myocardial conduction that represents a substrate for malignant reentrant ventricular arrhythmias.[152]

The myocardium is seldom involved extensively enough to cause clinical signs or symptoms.[3] Less than 10 per cent of patients have overt evidence of heart failure.[142] On one occasion, pregnancy in a patient with myotonic dystrophy was associated with severe congestive heart failure.[153] Occult involvement of the myocardium can sometimes be identified by radionuclide ventriculography during exercise.[3,154] The electrocardiogram is a sensitive determinant of involvement of specialized cardiac tissues but not of myocardium. Nevertheless, abnormal Q waves with normal coronary arteries indicate regional myocardial dystrophy (Fig. 60-11). Light microscopic examination of the myocardium varies from few or no changes to focal or diffuse fatty infiltration and fibrosis in all four cardiac chambers.[145,155-157]

Myotonia in skeletal muscle indicates inability of the muscle cell membrane to reestablish its resting membrane potential quickly after contraction.[132] Interestingly, there is evidence of myocardial myotonia, albeit subtle, based upon ultrasound analysis of the rate of early diastolic relaxation defined as diastolic endocardial velocity maximum of the left ventricular posterior wall.[158]

An important variation from the adult pattern occurs in the offspring of mothers with myotonic dystrophy.[130,159] The disorder expresses itself in infants as hypotonia and facial paralysis without myotonia, at least initially. Respiratory distress is largely responsible for neonatal death from congenital myotonic dystrophy.[130,159] Af-

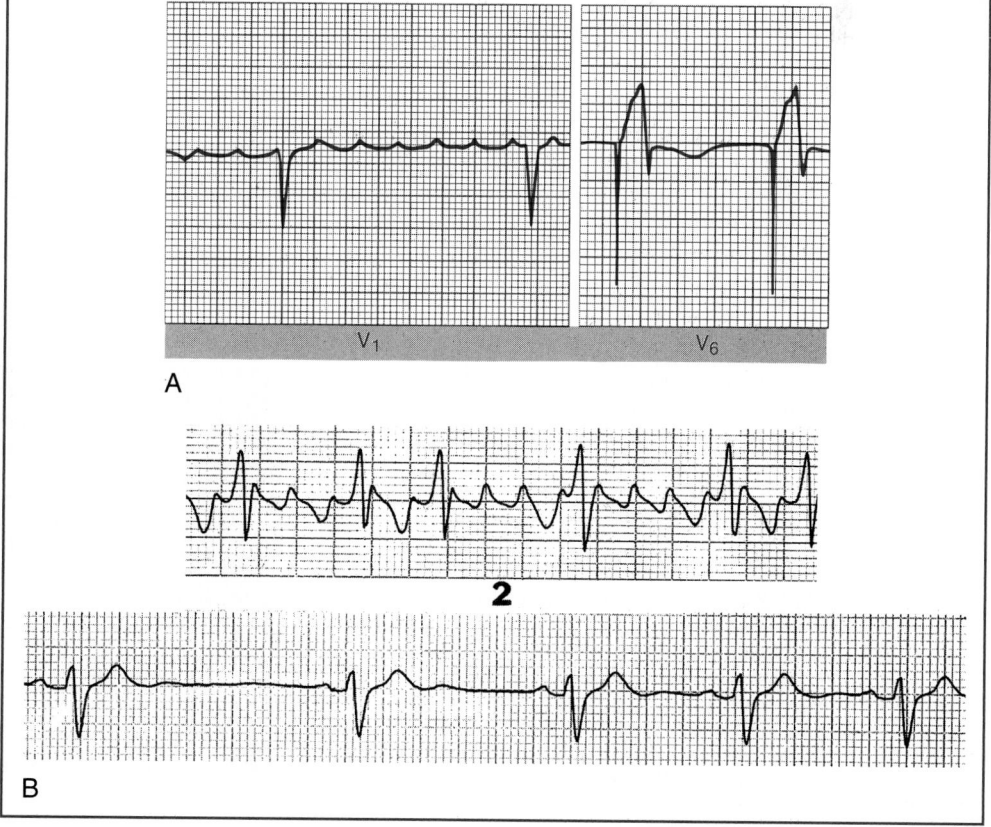

FIGURE 60-10. *A,* Rhythm strip from a 34-year-old man with myotonic muscular dystrophy. Lead V₁ shows atrial flutter with high-degree heart block. A syncopal episode prompted insertion of a right ventricular pacemaker (lead V₆). *B,* Rhythm strips (lead 2) from a 54-year-old man with myotonic muscular dystrophy. *Upper,* atrial flutter with 2:1 and 4:1 atrioventricular conduction. *Lower,* reversion to sinus rhythm was accompanied by bradycardia with marked sinus arrhythmia.

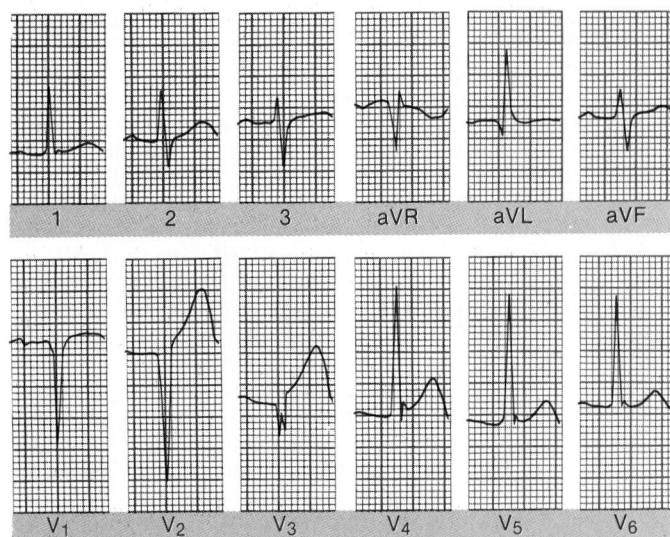

FIGURE 60–11. Electrocardiogram from a 38-year-old man with myotonic muscular dystrophy. Prominent QS deformities are present in leads V1-3. The P–R interval is 0.21 sec, and the frontal plane QRS axis is horizontal. (From Perloff, J. K., et al.: Cardiac involvement in myotonic muscular dystrophy [Steinert's disease]: A prospective study of 25 patients. Am. J. Cardiol. *54*:1074, 1984.)

fected children have characteristic facies with the upper lip forming a cupid's bow. Studies on cardiac involvement in these children are limited, but have reportedly disclosed atrioventricular and intraventricular conduction defects, less commonly reduced left ventricular systolic function.[159,160] Apart from genetic transmission from the mother (cytoplasmic inheritance), pregnancy is hazardous to the gravida with myotonic dystrophy.[130,153]

MYOTONIA CONGENITA (THOMSEN'S DISEASE) AND PARAMYOTONIA CONGENITA. This must be distinguished from myotonic muscular dystrophy.[130,132] Thomsen's disease is characterized by myotonia without dystrophy and by skeletal muscles that are well developed, even hypertrophied.[6,130] Because the natural history of Thomsen's disease is benign, longevity permits conclusions regarding cardiac involvement, which is conspicuously absent, although in a single case, cardiac conduction abnormalities similar to those found in myotonic dystrophy were reported.[161] Paramyotonia congenita is an uncommon to rare autosomal dominant disorder characterized by a prolonged myotonic reaction to cold.[6,132,162,163] Dystrophy of skeletal muscle is absent, and cardiac involvement is unknown.

Friedreich's Ataxia

The hereditary ataxias are divided into (1) the spinocerebellar ataxia of Friedreich, (2) ataxia with muscular atrophy (Roussy-Lévy syndrome), (3) spinocerebellar ataxia, and (4) olivopontocerebellar atrophy.[164] Despite a century of lively interest, Friedreich's ataxia has resisted precise clinical and biochemical definition, and there is still disagreement on where this spinocerebellar degenerative disease fits into the complex framework of the hereditary ataxias.[164–166] It is important to underscore that the disorder is essentially neurological rather than myopathic.[164–166] Friedreich's ataxia is inherited as an autosomal recessive trait and is characterized by ataxia of the limbs and trunk, absence of tendon reflexes, extensor plantar responses, and loss of proprioceptive sensations in the limbs.[166] There are no remissions; instead, ataxia of gait and weakness of muscle progress relentlessly, affecting first the lower limbs and then all four extremities. Pes cavus (Friedreich's foot) (Fig. 60–12) and kyphoscoliosis develop within a few years of onset.

CARDIAC MANIFESTATIONS. When strict neurological and genetic criteria were used to identify a clinically homogeneous group of patients with Friedreich's ataxia, the incidence of cardiac involvement exceeded 90 per cent.[4,167–173] Severe ataxia occurs long before overt heart disease, and there is no relationship between the degrees of neurological and cardiac involvement.[4] Nevertheless, cardiac disease is often the cause of death.[4,174] There is reason to believe that phenotypically identical Friedreich patients are not genetically homogeneous, so the cardiac expressions might be expected to vary. This proved to be the case in a prospective study of 75 patients.[4] Cardiac involvement, usually occult and asymptomatic, is the rule.[174,175] Scalar electrocardiography and echocardiography detected one or more abnormalities in 95 per cent of study patients.[4]

HYPERTROPHIC CARDIOMYOPATHY. The most common echocardiographic finding is concentric (symmetrical) left ventricular hypertrophy (Fig. 60–13). Asymmetric septal thickening occurs, but less frequently.[169,171,176–178] Left ventricular outflow gradients are present in some cases with disproportionate septal thickness[171] but not in others.[169] Importantly, septal cellular disarray—the histological hallmark of genetic hypertrophic cardiomyopathy (see p. 1664)—has been absent or only focal in necropsy studies of Friedreich's ataxia.[167,170,179,180] The potentially malignant ventricular arrhythmias common in genetic hypertrophic cardiomyopathy are essentially unknown in Friedreich's ataxia.[181] In the hypertrophic cardiomyopathy of Friedreich's ataxia, systolic ventricular function is normal, not supernormal, and diastolic function is not depressed as in genetic hypertrophic cardiomyopathy.[182,183]

DILATED CARDIOMYOPATHY. A second and much less common form of cardiac involvement in Friedreich's ataxia is dilated cardiomyopathy, which may initially express itself as global hypokinesis with normal left ventricular internal dimensions (Fig. 60–14).[4,178] There is one report of dilated cardiomyopathy, chiefly involving the right ventricle, with ventricular tachyarrhythmias.[184] In contrast to the favorable prognosis of Friedreich's ataxia with hypertrophic cardiomyopathy, the outlook is poor in dilated cardiomyopathy patients who experience relentless, progressive cardiac deterioration.[4,178] There is convincing evidence that the dilated form of cardiomyopathy in Friedreich's ataxia is distinct from the hypertrophic form: i.e., not a transition from one to the other, and that it represents a fundamentally different type of cardiac involvement designated dystrophic.[4] This view is supported by the flabby myocardium with normal wall thickness in necropsy cases that exhibited premortem progression on echocardiography from normal to dilated globally hypofunctional left ventricles with normal wall thickness (Fig. 60–14).[4] The initial force deformities on electrocardiograms and vectorcardiograms (Fig. 60–15)[4,172] are believed to represent areas of regional ventricular myocardial dystrophy which, if sufficiently widespread, might result in depressed systolic function.[4] Atrial arrhythmias (flutter, fibrillation) and ventricular arrhythmias are features of the dilated cardiomyopathy of Friedreich's ataxia.[4,184] Disease of the coronary arteries, especially small intramural coronary arteries, has been reported,[180] but a relationship between the coronary arteriopathy and regional wall abnormalities has not been established.

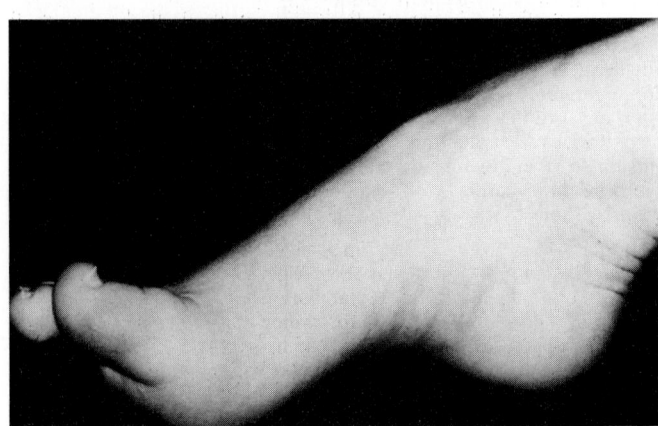

FIGURE 60–12. Pes cavus with hammer toe: Friedreich's foot.

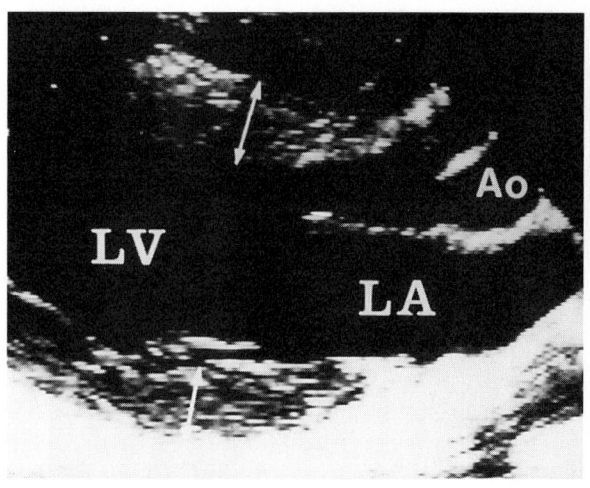 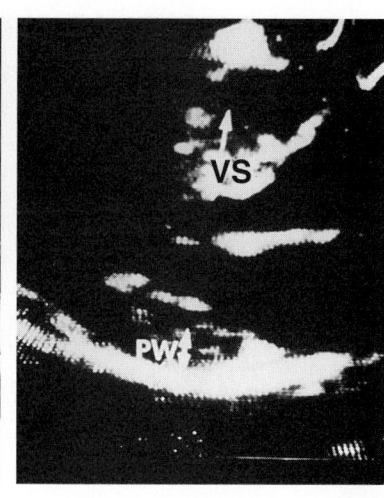

FIGURE 60–13. *A,* Two-dimensional echocardiogram (parasternal long axis diastolic frames) from a 14-year-old girl with Friedreich's ataxia and concentric hypertrophy (arrows) of the left ventricle (LV). *B,* Two-dimensional echocardiogram (parasternal long axis) from a 17-year-old boy with Friedreich's ataxia and hypertrophic cardiomyopathy characterized by disproportionate thickness (arrows) of the ventricular septum (VS) compared with the posterior wall (PW). Ao = aorta; LA = left atrium. (From Perloff, J. K.: Cardiac manifestations of neuromuscular disease. *In* Abelmann, W. H. [ed.]: Cardiomyopathies, Myocarditis, and Pericardial Disease. Vol. 2. *In* Braunwald, E. (series ed.): Atlas of Heart Diseases. Philadelphia, Current Medicine, 1995, pp. 6.1–6.19.)

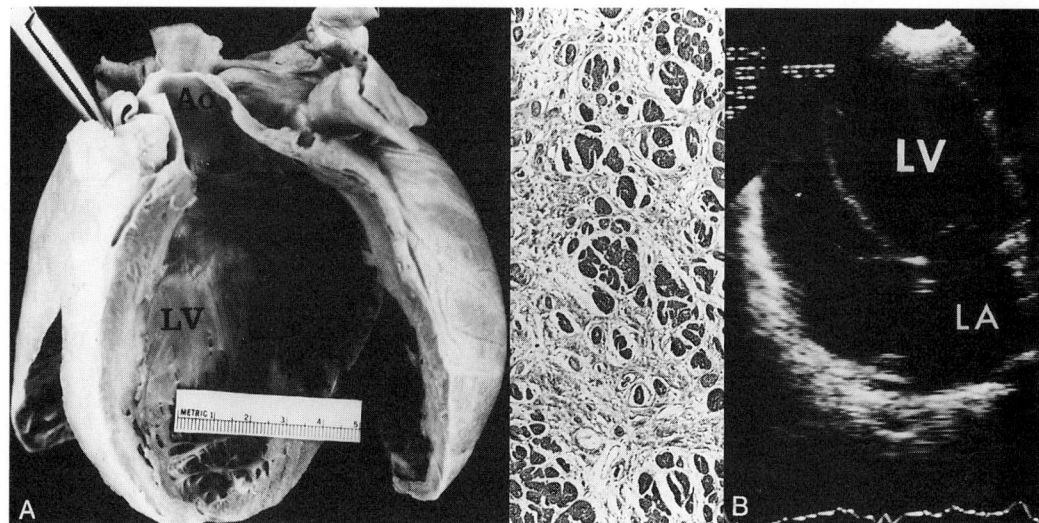

FIGURE 60–14. *A,* Gross and histological specimens from a 17-year-old boy with Friedreich's ataxia whose echocardiogram progressed from normal at age 13 years to a minimally dilated, hypocontractile left ventricle 3 to 4 years later. The gross specimen shows a mildly dilated left ventricle (LV) with normal wall thickness; the walls were flabby. The microscopic section from the left ventricular free wall shows marked connective tissue replacement. Although specifically sought, small-vessel coronary artery disease was not identified. *B,* Two-dimensional echocardiogram (apical window) showing the mildly dilated, thin-walled left ventricle (LV). LA = left atrium. (From Child, J. S., et al.: Cardiac involvement in Friedreich's ataxia. Reprinted by permission of the American College of Cardiology. J. Am. Coll. Cardiol. *7:*1370, 1986.)

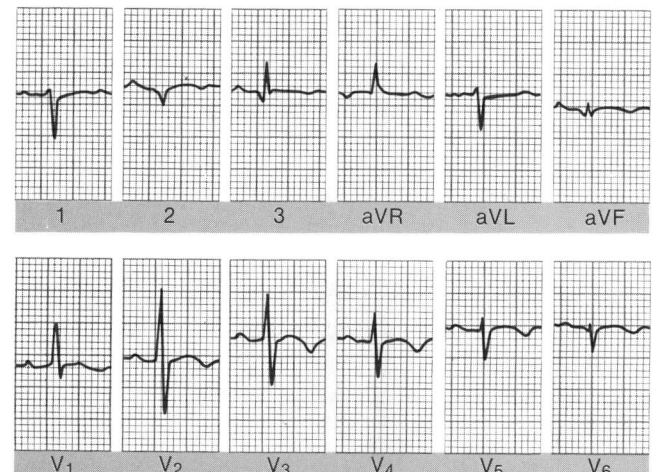

FIGURE 60–15. Electrocardiogram in a 28-year-old man with Friedreich's ataxia. The QRS shows marked right-axis deviation. There are 40-msec Q waves in leads 2, 3, and aVL. A prominent 60-msec R wave appears in lead V1. A vectorcardiogram and echocardiogram showed no evidence of right ventricular hypertrophy. The electrocardiograph pattern reflects loss of inferior and posterior electrical forces without a corresponding regional wall motion abnormality on echocardiography. (From Child, J. S., et al.: Cardiac involvement in Friedreich's ataxia. Reprinted by permission of the American College of Cardiology. J. Am. Coll. Cardiol. *7:*1370, 1986.)

Other Neuromyopathic Diseases Associated with Heart Disease

PERONEAL MUSCULAR ATROPHY (CHARCOT-MARIE-TOOTH SYNDROME). Peroneal muscular atrophy includes several genetic disorders (the hereditary motor and sensory neuromyopathies) characterized by distal weakness of the legs with predilection for muscles innervated by the peroneal nerves, particularly the everters of the foot and occasionally intrinsic muscles of the hands.[185] Peroneal muscular atrophy is autosomal dominant. One type begins during the first 20 years of life, whereas the other type begins later, sometimes not until middle age. Arrhythmias, conduction abnormalities and dilated heart failure have been sporadically reported in patients with peroneal muscular atrophy,[186–190] but are believed to be chance associations.[191]

MYOTUBULAR MYOPATHY (CENTRONUCLEAR MYOPATHY). Centronuclear myopathy typically exhibits internal nuclei that structurally resemble fetal myotubes (rows of nuclei separated by spaces).[192,193] The disorder is characterized clinically by slow but progressive wasting and weakness of skeletal muscle beginning at birth. Ptosis is the rule. Patients are hyporeflexic or areflexic. Few examples are available for study, but presumptive evidence indicates that myotubular myopathy can be associated with extensive myocardial fibrosis, cardiac dilatation, and early death.[192] In an illustration in one report on skeletal muscle in "idiopathic cardiomyopathy," numerous internal nuclei could be seen.[194] Centronuclear myopathy had apparently presented as cardiomyopathy before the neuromuscular disease was identified.

CARDIAC INVOLVEMENT IN MITOCHONDRIAL DISEASES. Mitochondrial diseases are important from a genetic point of view because mitochondria contain their own DNA and are capable of synthesizing a small but vital set of proteins.[195] The vast majority of mitochondrial proteins are encoded by nuclear DNA and have to be imported from the cytoplasm into mitochondria through a complex translocation

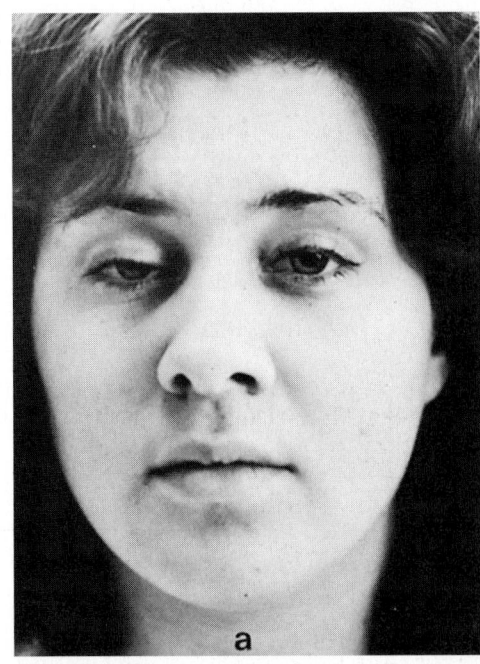 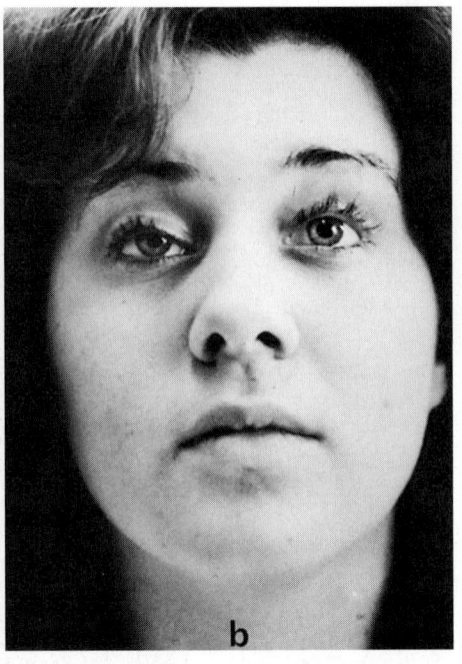

FIGURE 60–16. An 18-year-old girl with Kearns-Sayre syndrome and bilateral asymmetrical ptosis. Within 24 months, her electrocardiogram changed from normal to bifascicular block (complete right bundle branch block, and left anterior fascicular block). *A,* The asymmetrical ptosis when the patient looks straight ahead. *B,* Ptosis of the right lid persists when the patient looks up. She also had typical pigmentary retinopathy.

machinery which is under the control of the nuclear genome.[195] The human mitochondrial genome is a circular double-stranded DNA.[196] Mitochondrial myopathy, defined as a disease caused by mitochondrial DNA mutations, has been proposed, and is believed to represent a state of premature cardiac aging wherein the somatic mutations of mitochondrial DNA are abnormally accelerated because of a patient's germ-aligned mutations.[197] Mutations of mitochondrial DNA are responsible for human mitochondrial diseases that involve many but not all organ systems.[196] Examples include Kearns-Sayre syndrome, ocular myopathy, myoclonic epilepsy with ragged red fibers, and mitochondrial myopathy, encephalopathy, lactic acidosis, and stroke-like episodes.[196]

KEARNS-SAYRE SYNDROME. The most important of these mitochondrial diseases, certainly from the point of view of cardiac involvement, is Kearns-Sayre syndrome, characterized by progressive external ophthalmoplegia (Fig. 60–16), pigmentary retinopathy, and heart block.[198–200] Morphological alterations in skeletal muscle can be identified in the trichrome stain as ragged-red fibers.[198] Cardiac involvement primarily afflicts the specialized conduction pathways.[201,202] Clinically overt myocardial disease is the exception, despite well-documented myocardial ultrastructural abnormalities, especially of mitochondria.[203–205] Occasionally patients exhibit dilated cardiomyopathy with progressive heart failure,[203–205] but the chief risk resides in abnormalities of the specialized conduction pathways.

Two derangements in cardiac conduction coexist: (1) gradually progressive impairment of infranodal conduction (left anterior hemiblock, right bundle branch block, complete heart block) (Fig. 60–17), and (2) concomitant enhancement of AV nodal conduction.[201,206] The morphological basis for impaired infranodal conduction lies in extensive distal His bundle abnormalities that extend to the origins of the bundle branches.[206] Evidence of enhanced AV nodal conduction has been identified by His bundle electrocardiograms (Fig. 60–15).[201] A short or relatively short P-R interval cannot be used as evidence against risk inherent in the trifascicular disease of patients with Kearns-Sayre syndrome, right bundle branch block and left anterior hemiblock.[201] Pacemaker implantation is often necessary.

GUILLAIN-BARRÉ SYNDROME. This disorder is the most common of the acquired demyelinative neuropathies.[207] The incidence gradually increases with age, but the disease may occur at any age, and both sexes are equally affected. The syndrome often appears days to weeks after a viral respiratory or gastrointestinal infection, with neurological symptoms consisting of symmetrical weakness of the limbs often accompanied by paresthesias. The incidence af the acute polyneuropathy is higher in patients with Hodgkin's disease, and the disorder may be precipitated by pregnancy, general surgery, or vaccinations. Myocardial infarction was believed to be the precipitating cause in two cases.[208] Important and characteristic features of the syndrome are flaccid motor paralysis with a distinctive tendency to ascend (Landry's ascending paralysis), together with elevation of cerebrospinal fluid protein without an increase in the number of white blood cells. Involvement of thoracic muscles often requires assisted ventilation. Despite respiratory support, the Guillain-Barré syndrome is fatal in approximately 20 per cent of children when there is significant involvement of trunk muscles and associated pulmonary insufficiency.[209]

Cardiac Findings. Postmortem studies have shed little or no light on the cause of sudden death in Guillain-Barré syndrome. There is substantial evidence, however, that deaths are often not invariably related to cardiac arrhythmias.[209–211] Bradyarrhythmias (sinus arrest,

complete heart block) and tachyarrhythmias (supraventricular and ventricular) as well as premature atrial and ventricular beats are common and are increased by the use of a respirator.[210] Autonomic dysfunction, especially sympathetic hyperactivity, is manifested by orthostatic hypotension, transient hypertension, wide fluctuations in blood pressure and heart rate, and variations in the R-R interval.[212–214] Pacemaker support may be required because of recurrent syncope.[210] Tracheal aspiration has produced an idioventricular rhythm of 40 beats/min that reverted to sinus rhythm when aspiration ceased.[209] Cardiac monitoring is advisable, especially when the Guillain-Barré syndrome is sufficiently severe to warrant assisted ven-

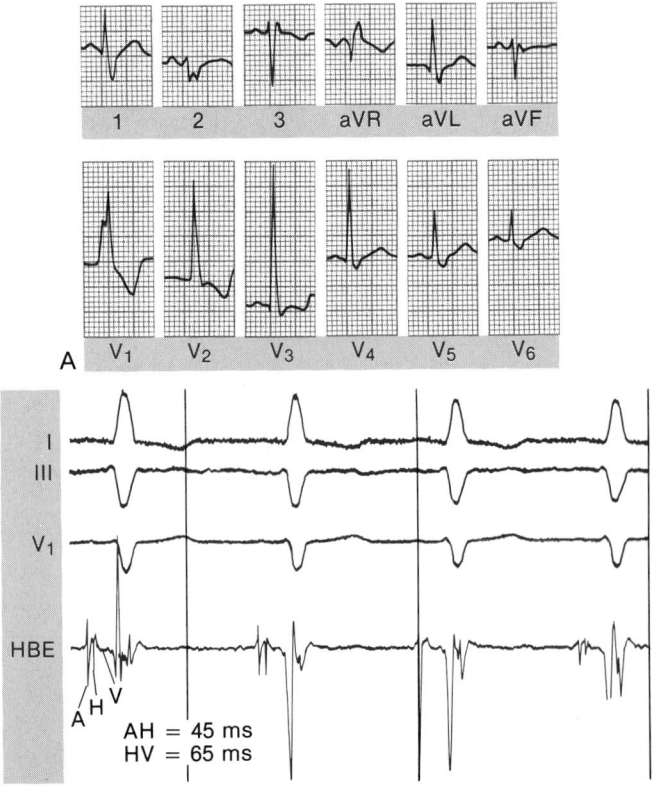

FIGURE 60–17. *A,* Electrocardiogram from a 13-year-old boy with Kearns-Sayre syndrome. There is a short P–R interval (110 msec), left anterior hemiblock, and complete right bundle branch block. *B,* Leads I, III, and V₁ with His bundle electrogram (HBE) in a 21-year-old woman with Kearns-Sayre syndrome. Time lines are at 1-sec intervals. The A-H interval is 45 msec (short) and the H–V interval is 65 msec (prolonged). (From Roberts, J. K., et al.: Cardiac conduction in Kearns-Sayre syndrome. Am. J. Cardiol. *44*:1396, 1979).

tilation.[209] The electrocardiogram occasionally shows widespread, deep T-wave inversions.[214]

NEMALINE MYOPATHY. This disorder is characterized by myriad small, rodlike particles in striated muscle.[215-217] Inheritance is either autosomal dominant or recessive, with occasional sporadic cases. The most common clinical manifestation is hypotonia with diffuse weakness of limbs and trunk beginning at an early age. Children are often dysmorphic with an elongated, narrow face, high arched palate, and slender musculature.[6] Alternatively, symptoms may begin in adolescence or adult life and are characterized by scapuloperoneal weakness and footdrop.[218] Nemaline myopathy is only rarely associated with cardiac involvement, but nemaline rods have been found in the myocardium and in cardiac conduction tissues, and held responsible for ventricular dilatation and conduction defects.[219,220]

MYASTHENIA GRAVIS. This is a "neuroimmunological" disease caused by an abnormality of neuromuscular transmission due to antibodies to acetylcholine receptors.[221,222] The abnormality may become manifest at any age, but is most common in the second to fourth decades. Overt pathological evidence of myasthenia gravis resides primarily in the thymus, which shows lymphoid hyperplasia and numerous lymphoid follicles with germinal centers in the medulla. Ocular muscles are affected first. Weakness characteristically fluctuates during the course of a single day, sometimes within minutes. The association of myocardial disease with thymoma, especially malignant thymoma, is generally accepted, whereas the association of myasthenia gravis with heart disease is less clear despite a considerable body of suggestive evidence.[223] Specific cardiac involvement is unproved even though clinical, electrocardiographic, and vectorcardiographic data implicate the myocardium.[223]

Early in this century, quinine was used as a provocative diagnostic test for myasthenia gravis. Quinidine and procainamide, like quinine, have anticholinergic properties that depress neuromuscular conduction.[224] These antiarrhythmic agents can unmask previously unsuspected myasthenia gravis and can exacerbate symptoms in well-controlled patients.[224,225] Accordingly, quinidine and procainamide should be avoided.

McARDLE SYNDROME. This is a disorder of myophosphorylase deficiency.[6,226] A defect in the enzyme prevents use of glycogen as an energy source during heavy or intensive short-term exercise when glycogen is normally the chief substrate.[6,226] McArdle's disease was the first enzyme defect suspected on clinical grounds. It is inherited as an autosomal recessive, or rarely as an autosomal dominant, and is more common in male children. Mild aching in the legs usually begins before age 10 years, ultimately becomes severe, and is provoked by the mildest exercise. Pain may last for hours, and is accompanied by Burgundy-colored urine because of myoglobinuria. The typical cardiac manifestation is rapid inappropriate acceleration of heart rate (sinus tachycardia) and hyperventilation immediately after the onset of exercise[5,189] (Fig. 60–18). Less commonly, the scalar electrocardiogram reveals sinus bradycardia, increased QRS voltage, and PR interval prolongation. The precise diagnosis depends upon biochemical and histochemical documentation that phosphorylase is absent in skeletal muscle.

KUGELBERG-WELANDER SYNDROME. The proximal spinal muscular atrophies are autosomal recessive.[227] The childhood form is subdivided into the acute Werdnig-Hoffmann, the intermediate Werdnig-Hoffmann, and the Kugelberg-Welander.[227] The latter variety is characterized by onset in childhood or adolescence, atrophy and weakness principally of proximal limb muscles, a slowly progressive course, development of fasciculations, and evidence of neurogenic changes in the electromyogram and on muscle biopsy. There are a few reports of cardiac involvement in the Kugelberg-Welander syndrome including atrial fibrillation, atrial standstill, conduction defects (H-V prolongation, complete AV block), and dilated heart failure.[228]

POLIOMYELITIS. Cardiac involvement is believed to occur only rarely in childhood poliomyelitis, but may be clinically occult.[229,230] In adults, the infrequency of symptomatic involvement of the heart contrasts with a relatively high incidence of electrocardiographic abnormalities, especially of rhythm and conduction.[229,230] Disturbances of rhythm take the form of premature beats (atrial and ventricular), atrial fibrillation or atrial flutter. Disturbances in conduction are manifested by impaired AV conduction (first-, second-, and third-degree heart block) and abnormalities of infranodal conduction (left-axis deviation and bundle branch block).[229,230] Respiratory failure can provoke hypoxemia-induced pulmonary hypertension[231] and multifocal atrial tachycardia.

At necropsy, the sinoatrial node, distal His bundle, and left and right bundle branches show infiltration, degeneration, and fibrous replacement that wholly or in part account for the conduction defects.[229,230] Pathological changes in the myocardium tend to be similar to those in skeletal muscle, including diffuse mononuclear cell infiltration and myofibril degeneration, regeneration, and fibrosis.

PERIODIC PARALYSIS. The disorder is characterized by recurrences of flaccid weakness and by either abnormally high or abnormally low levels of serum potassium.[232,233] *Hypokalemic attacks* typically begin in late childhood or adolescence, usually occur at night, tend to be severe, and last a day or longer.[233] *Hyperkalemic attacks* have their onset at a younger age. Episodes occur more frequently than with hypokalemia, but tend to be milder and shorter (minutes or hours). Many features are common to both varieties of periodic paralysis, including familial recurrence (autosomal dominant inheritance),

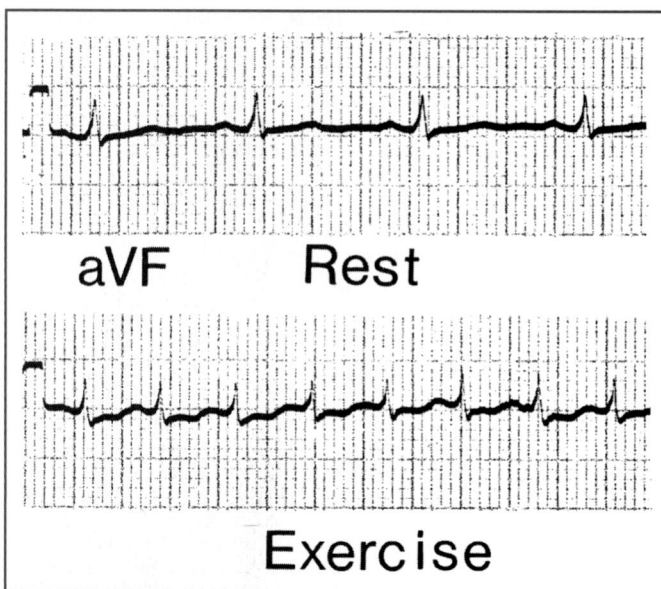

FIGURE 60–18. Rhythm strip (aVF) from a 37-year-old woman with McArdle disease. At the very onset of exercise, there was a sudden sustained acceleration of cardiac rate represented by sinus tachycardia *(lower strip)* accompanied by hyperventilation and aching in the leg muscles.

heightened susceptibility immediately after ceasing strenuous exercise, termination of incipient attacks by *mild* exercise, onset of weakness in the lower extremities with progression to arm muscles but not to respiratory muscles, intensification by cold, and persistent weakness between attacks even though potassium levels may be normal.[232,234] During hyperkalemia, the electrocardiogram exhibits peaked T waves. During hypokalemia, the T waves are low voltage, and there is digitalis sensitivity.

More important are the cardiac arrhythmias that accompany periodic paralysis including ventricular ectopic beats, ventricular bigeminy, and fusion beats producing multiform complexes.[233-235] Of particular interest is bidirectional tachycardia that is believed to originate in the left ventricle, is refractory to antiarrhythmic therapy, occurs independent of attacks of muscle weakness, exhibits no correlation with serum electrolytes, and is consistently converted to sinus rhythm with mild exercise.[236,237] Hypokalemic episodes are best treated with oral potassium and hyperkalemic episodes with glucose and insulin, but it should be underscored that administration of potassium does not necessarily suppress ventricular electrical instability during hypokalemic attacks.[235]

ALCOHOLIC CARDIOMYOPATHY (see also p. 1412). Dilated cardiomyopathy associated with chronic ingestion of large amounts of ethyl alcohol may be accompanied by clinically occult skeletal myopathy.[238,239] Alcohol withdrawal is occasionally accompanied by "rum fits."[240] The teratogenic potential of alcohol, exemplified by the fetal alcohol syndrome, afflicts the fetal central nervous system but not the myocardium, although congenital malformations of the heart are not uncommon in the offspring of alcoholic mothers.[241]

ACUTE CEREBRAL DISORDERS CAUSED BY CARDIOVASCULAR ABNORMALITIES

Acute cerebral injury can provoke cardiovascular abnormalities, and abnormalities of the heart can set the stage for acute cerebral injury. A connection between certain acute cerebral events—subarachnoid hemorrhage, intracranial hemorrhage—and overt cardiovascular abnormalities has been recognized for nearly a century, and a relationship between head trauma and cardiac abnormalities was proposed more than 60 years ago.[242] In 1938, Aschenbrenner and Bodechtel reported that neurological lesions could be associated with electrocardiographic abnormalities in young patients without heart disease,[243] and in 1947 Byer, Ashman, and Toth described large upright T waves and long Q-T intervals following subarachnoid hemorrhage.[244] A more systematic study was published in 1954 by Burch,[245] who concluded that the principal offending cerebral lesions were intracerebral or subarachnoid hemorrhage, and that the principal electrocardiographic abnormalities were prolongation of the Q-T interval, increased amplitude and duration of T waves and abnormal U waves.

Neurogenic pulmonary edema occurs with a variety of disorders of the central nervous system[246,247] and with brain-stem hemorrhage. A rise in systemic blood pressure in response to cerebral injury[248] was known to Harvey Cushing at the turn of the century (the Cushing pressor response),[249] and experimentally induced intense cerebral compression in rats evokes a marked increase in systemic vascular resistance, a profound decrease in cardiac output, and hemorrhagic pulmonary edema.[246] In human subjects, interest has also focussed upon myocardial injury, especially severe brain damage caused by craniocerebral trauma.[250-255]

Arrhythmias, Conduction Defects, and Repolarization Abnormalities

Approximately 90 per cent of patients with acute cerebral accidents—especially intracerebral or subarachnoid hemorrhage or acute cerebral trauma—exhibit electrocardiographic abnormalities that consist chiefly of disturbances of cardiac rhythm and repolarization.[253,254,256-267] Abnormalities in rhythm include sinus bradycardia (sometimes profound), sinus tachycardia, atrial arrhythmias (ectopic beats, fibrillation, flutter, or supraventricular tachycardia), junctional rhythms, and ventricular arrhythmias (ectopic beats, ventricular tachycardia, or fibrillation).[259,268,269] Repolarization abnormalities closely resemble those of ischemic heart disease and consist chiefly of abnormalities of ST segments and T waves in addition to prominent U waves, and prolonged Q-T interval.[256,257,262,269] ST segments may be dramatically elevated and T waves dramatically inverted (Fig. 60–19). Conduction disturbances include first-, second-, or third-degree AV block.[254]

There is little information in human subjects regarding a relationship between specific stroke location and disturbances in cardiac rhythm, conduction and repolarization,[257] but some experimental evidence is available.[270,271] The left insular cortex of the rat contains a site of cardiac chronotropic representation.[270] Prolonged phasic stimulation within the insular cortex of the rat results in atrioventricular block, prolongation of the Q-T interval, and ST-segment depression.[271]

Because the left insular cortex of the rat contains a site of cardiac representation, Oppenheimer postulated that there might be a difference in cardiac expression between right- and left-sided lesions.[257] There is evidence that asymmetries in brain function influence the heart through ipsilateral pathways, and there is a reported association between right-hemisphere strokes and tachyarrhythmias of supraventricular origin and left hemisphere strokes and arrhythmias of ventricular origin.[272] More recent reports call attention to the cardiovascular effects of human insular cortex stimulation,[273] and there is a reported association between

a neurosurgical intervention in the region of the left insular cortex, premature ventricular complexes, and prolonged Q-T interval.[274] (The insular cortex in humans lies beneath the frontoparietal and superior temporal opercula.)

Migraine-related stroke—migrainous cerebral infarction—has been firmly established.[275] Less well known and perhaps less firmly established are atrial arrhythmias—atrial fibrillation, sinoatrial block—that are believed to be provoked by the autonomic discharge accompanying migraine headache.[276]

MYOCARDIAL INJURY. There is substantial evidence that the "catecholamine storm"—characterized by copious release of norepinephrine from cardiac beta-1 receptor sites—during acute cerebral accidents is responsible for myocardial damage, reflected in a rise of cardiac enzymes (CK-MB), left-ventricular wall motion abnormalities,[255] evidence of myofibrillar degeneration on light microscopy, and subendocardial injury.[248,252,265] Steroids combined with catecholamines have been implicated in the genesis of myocardial stress injury.[259] The myocardial damage associated with acute cerebral injury puts patients at additional risk. Subarachnoid hemorrhage can be associated with abnormal myocardial perfusion[277] and reversible left-ventricular wall motion abnormalities.[278] It is important to emphasize that the major sources of donor organs for heart and heart and lung transplantation are victims of motor vehicle accidents or gunshot wounds that cause acute cerebral damage. Those patients have necessarily suffered massive cerebral injury and, in all probability, have varying degrees of catecholamine- and stress-induced myocardial and lung injury.[253,275]

NEUROGENIC PULMONARY EDEMA AND CARDIOPULMONARY ARREST. Cerebrogenic hemorrhagic pulmonary edema has been experimentally induced by cranial compression in rats,[246] and neurogenic pulmonary edema sometimes accompanies acute cerebral injury in patients[246,247,256] (see p. 466). Myocardial damage may aggravate the pulmonary edema but is not necessary for its genesis. Respiratory arrest without circulatory collapse is more common than cardiac arrest in response to acute cerebral injury.[279] Cardiac arrest is likely to be triggered by disturbances in ventricular rhythm. Cerebrogenic arrhythmias and neurogenic pulmonary edema occasionally follow generalized tonic-clonic epileptic seizures without acute cerebral injury.[280,281] Acute injury to the cervical spinal cord without cerebral damage is frequently accompanied by disturbances in cardiac rhythm and conduction and occasionally by sudden death.[282] Bradyarrhythmias are most common, but supraventricular and ventricular tachyarrhythmias and AV block also occur in addition to marked hypotension. The cardiac abnormalities are believed to arise from acute autonomic imbalance imposed on the heart by the cervical cord injury.[282]

COEXISTING CEREBROVASCULAR AND CORONARY HEART DISEASE

The preceding section emphasized that acute cerebrovascular accidents in patients with normal hearts—i.e., without coronary artery disease—were often accompanied by electrocardiographic abnormalities resembling those of myocardial ischemia or infarction, by release of MB-creatinine phosphokinase (CPK) and by abnormal myocardial perfusion. In older patients experiencing an acute cerebrovascular accident, however, the same abnormalities may in fact represent an acute myocardial ischemic event caused by coexisting atherosclerotic coronary artery disease.[283] Because ST-segment elevations, deep T-wave inversions, and a rise in MB-CPK occur with cerebrovascular accidents in patients *without* ischemic heart disease, these criteria cannot be relied upon to diagnose ischemic injury due to coexisting coronary artery obstruction.

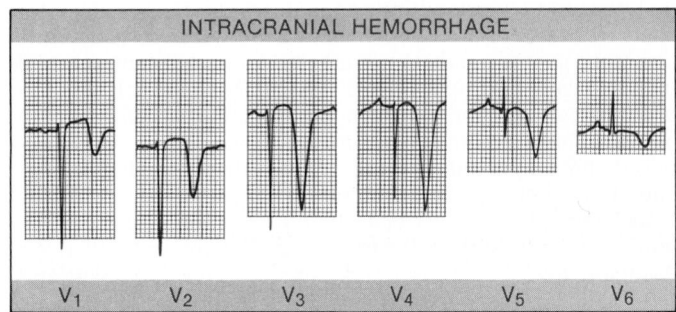

FIGURE 60–19. Deep, symmetrical T-wave inversions in precordial leads of a patient with a cerebral hemorrhage. (Courtesy of John H. Phillips, M. D., Tulane Medical Center, New Orleans, Louisiana.)

Although earlier estimates of the incidence of acute myocardial infarction in patients with acute cerebrovascular accidents were less than reliable,[285] it is now clear that cerebrovascular disease and coronary artery disease have similar risk factors and often coexist.[286] Differential diagnosis is important, because mortality is high in patients who simultaneously experience an acute cerebrovascular accident and acute myocardial infarction. After presentation with threatened stroke, patients may be at higher risk for a subsequent myocardial infarction than for stroke. However, the presence of coronary artery disease adversely affects survival in stroke patients.[286] Another important relationship is the prevalence of significant coronary artery disease and coronary events among patients with transient ischemic attacks, small strokes, asymptomatic carotid arterial murmurs, or carotid stenosis.[286]

One of the mechanisms believed to be responsible for transient ischemic attacks is embolization from carotid plaques.[287] Recent attention has focused upon ulcerated plaques in the ascending aorta and aortic arch as a source of cerebral embolic events.[288] Nearly one-half of patients with either symptomatic or asymptomatic cerebrovascular disease as just defined were found to have abnormal thallium-201 scans induced by exercise or pharmacological stress.[286] The primary cause of death following the onset of transient ischemic attacks is coronary artery disease.[287]

CAROTID ARTERIAL DISEASE AND CORONARY ARTERY DISEASE. Patients with symptomatic atherosclerotic coronary artery disease may have occult carotid artery disease, and patients with symptomatic carotid artery disease may have occult atherosclerotic coronary artery disease.[286] Cervical arterial murmurs have been found in 4.4 to 12.6 per cent of subjects 45 years of age and older with no history of stroke, transient cerebral ischemia, or overt ischemic heart disease.[289-291] The incidence of asymptomatic cervical murmurs (asymptomatic atherosclerotic carotid artery disease) increases with age. Thirty per cent of persons over age 50 years have some evidence of carotid artery disease.[292] The prevalence of carotid disease relates to the same risk factors as coronary artery disease, especially hypertension, cigarette smoking, hyperlipidemia, and diabetes mellitus.[293] Nevertheless, it is important to distinguish between mild carotid stenosis with an exceedingly low risk of stroke and severe carotid stenosis in which the risk of even nonfatal cerebral infarction is appreciable.[291,294,295] An early Framingham study called attention to the relative frequency of cerebral infarction in vascular territories different from those predicted by an asymptomatic carotid arterial murmur.[293] Embolization from ulcerated carotid or proximal aortic plaques may in part account for this observation.[287,288,293]

Symptoms ascribed to carotid artery lesions represented by stenosis or plaque ulceration include transient or persistent monocular visual loss, hemispheric transient ischemic attacks, and frank ischemic stroke.[293] Patients with transient ischemic attacks related to severe carotid stenosis confront stroke risk at a rate of 12 per cent within the first year after onset of symptoms, and a cumulative stroke risk of 30 to 35 per cent at 5 years.[293] After an initial stroke, the risk of subsequent cerebral events is approximately 7 per cent per year, with approximately 35 per cent of patients experiencing another stroke within 5 years after the original event.[293]

Auscultation should be routinely used for the detection of carotid arterial murmurs, but the presence of a murmur does not identify a critical carotid lesion, and a critical carotid lesion is not always associated with a murmur.[293] Ultrasound technology using color-coded Doppler and B-mode ultrasonography should be used as a screening test. However, carotid arteriography is required for precise definition because ultrasonographic measurements are currently less than precise.[292]

MANAGEMENT. Expert opinion regarding the indications for carotid endarterectomy to prevent stroke has varied widely[295] and has resulted in many retrospective reviews, natural history studies, position papers, and, more recently, in prospective randomized trials.[292,293] Relevant to this chapter is the problem of the coexistence of carotid artery stenosis and coronary artery disease. A number of relatively current and well conceived publications address this problem,[296-298] but optimal strategy for the management of patients with *combined* coronary artery stenosis and carotid disease awaits a well-designed prospective randomized trial.[293] In patients with combined carotid and coronary disease, surgical options include operating upon the carotid lesion first with an increased risk of morbidity and mortality from myocardial infarction; coronary artery bypass grafting first with an increased risk of perioperative stroke; or operating upon both lesions at the same time.[293] Meta-analysis findings indicate that perioperative stroke rate was similar if carotid and coronary surgery were combined or if carotid surgery preceded coronary bypass grafting.[293] The frequency of stroke was significantly greater if coronary bypass grafting preceded carotid surgery, and the frequency of myocardial infarction and death was greater when carotid surgery preceded coronary bypass grafting.[293] Simultaneous performance of coronary artery bypass grafting and carotid endarterectomy carries an increased risk that is warranted when patients present with recent symptoms of severe carotid artery stenosis and a compelling reason for coronary artery bypass grafting.[292,293,296,297,299] If a patient presents with symptomatic severe carotid artery stenosis, carotid endarterectomy should be done initially, and a month later, if necessary, the coronary artery disease can be addressed by bypass grafting or balloon dilatation.[292] If a patient with asymptomatic cerebrovascular disease that requires carotid endarterectomy needs urgent coronary revascularization, a staged procedure commencing with the latter can be carried out. Often, coronary angioplasty can be performed first, followed in 2 to 4 weeks by carotid endarterectomy. Patients who have simultaneous unstable coronary and carotid arterial disease can be considered for a combined procedure.

NEUROLOGICAL COMPLICATIONS OF CORONARY BYPASS SURGERY. An important corollary is the incidence of neurological complications unassociated with obstruction of the carotid artery in patients undergoing coronary artery bypass grafting.[297,299-302] These complications are in addition to and apart from those accompanying open-heart surgery.[303,304] Major central nervous system events are associated with coronary bypass operations in 1 to 2 per cent of cases.[299,301,302] The majority of these cerebral events are related to embolization of atheromatous material from the ascending aorta or to embolization from a postinfarction left ventricular mural thrombus.[299,302]

Cardiogenic Brain Embolism

Aggregate clinical data regarding cardiac sources of embolic stroke include "nonvalvular" atrial fibrillation, ischemic heart disease (acute myocardial infarction, healed myocardial infarction with ventricular aneurysm), mechanical prosthetic valves, and rheumatic heart disease (mitral stenosis)[305,306] (see p. 1009). Important but less common sources of cardiogenic embolism to the brain include nonischemic dilated cardiomyopathy, infective endocarditis, nonbacterial thrombotic vegetations, myxomatous mitral valve, paradoxical embolism, atrial septal aneurysm, left atrial myxoma, mitral annular calcification, and calcific aortic stenosis.[305,306] Nonvalvular atrial fibrillation encompasses a wide spectrum from "lone atrial fibrillation" that occurs without other clinical evidence of heart disease to atrial dilatation with congestive heart failure. Nonvalvular atrial fibrillation is the most common cardiac substrate for cardiogenic embolism, accounting for almost one-half of cardiogenic embolic strokes.[305-309] Both warfarin anticoagulation and aspirin are effective in reducing the risk of systemic embolism in patients with nonvalvular atrial fibrillation.[306,308,309] The approximate reduction achieved with warfarin anticoagulation is 70 per cent; the approximate reduction achieved with aspirin is 42 per cent.[306,309] Aspirin is safer, cheaper, and easier to administer than warfarin and has been recommended in patients 75 years or younger[308] (see Fig. 58-17, p. 1832).

Embolic stroke from left ventricular mural thrombi accompanies acute myocardial infarction generally within the first weeks (see p. 1256). In 90 per cent of cases, the infarct is anterior.[305] Persistent left ventricular dyskinesis or ventricular aneurysm in healed myocardial infarction are also important sources of ventricular mural thrombi and cardiogenic cerebral embolism.[305]

In patients with mechanical prosthetic heart valves, the risk of embolism is 2 to 4 per cent per year, with higher rates for mitral prostheses, especially in the presence of atrial fibrillation[305,306] (see p. 655). Focal neurological signs occasionally occur in patients with myxomatous mitral valves (mitral valve prolapse) (see p. 1032) and are believed to be embolic (platelet aggregates, sterile thrombi).[306,310,311] Aspirin is recommended as the initial antithrombotic therapy.[306]

Left atrial myxoma results in peripheral emboli in about 45 per cent of cases, and the brain is involved in one-half (see p. 867). Patients with left atrial myxoma are sometimes seen first by a neurologist because of presenting neurological manifestations.[312]

Nonischemic dilated cardiomyopathy with mural thrombi is more likely to cause cerebral emboli than are mural thrombi associated with myocardial infarction.[238] Infants with endocardial fibroelastosis of the dilated type suffer strokes caused by emboli from left ventricular endocardial thrombi.[313]

Atheromatous plaques or platelet-fibrin aggregates originating in the ascending aorta[288] or in the carotid arteries[287] are important and often unrecognized sources of cardiogenic brain embolism. Transient ischemic attacks associated with carotid disease often originate from plaques rather than impaired perfusion.[287]

INFECTIVE ENDOCARDITIS. This condition gives rise to a host of neurological complications including cerebral embolic events (transient ischemic attacks/stroke), intraparenchymal hemorrhage, subarachnoid hemorrhage, meningitis/meningoencephalitis, cerebral abscess, mycotic aneurysm, seizures and encephalopathy[314-318] (see p. 1085). *Prosthetic valve infective endocarditis* (see p. 1079) typically involves mechanical prostheses, especially in the mitral location, and is associated with high mortality.[315,317] The incidence of focal neurological events ranges from 11 to 44 per cent in patients with prosthetic valve infective endocarditis, much higher than the thromboembolic rate of 1 to 4 per cent per year for anticoagulated patients with prosthetic valves but without infective endocarditis.[315] Neurological complications are of special concern because of the risk of intracranial hemorrhage associated with anticoagulation. Septic cerebral emboli may result in intracranial hemorrhage or cerebral abscess after a misleading quiescent interval. A septic cerebral aneurysm is potentially catastrophic because of rupture.[318]

In patients with nonbacterial thrombotic vegetations, bland cerebral emboli are not uncommon.[319] The aortic valve is the usual site of the noninfectious thrombotic vegetations.

Drug abuse not only causes infective endocarditis but, depending on the drug and vehicle (embolization from foreign matter), may be associated with intracranial or subarachnoid hemorrhage, cerebral emboli, and ischemic stroke.[320]

PARADOXICAL EMBOLI. These reach the brain when peripheral venous blood enters the systemic arterial circulation via right-to-left shunts of cyanotic congenital heart disease.[313,321] An important variation on this theme are paradoxical emboli in acyanotic patients with interatrial communications: patent foramen ovale or ostium secundum atrial septal defect.[322–324,324a] Inferior vena caval streaming directs blood toward the midportion of the atrial septum and —in the presence of a defect—into the left atrium and systemic circulation. Especially vulnerable are pregnant women with an ostium secundum atrial septal defect and an increased incidence of emboli from peripheral and pel-

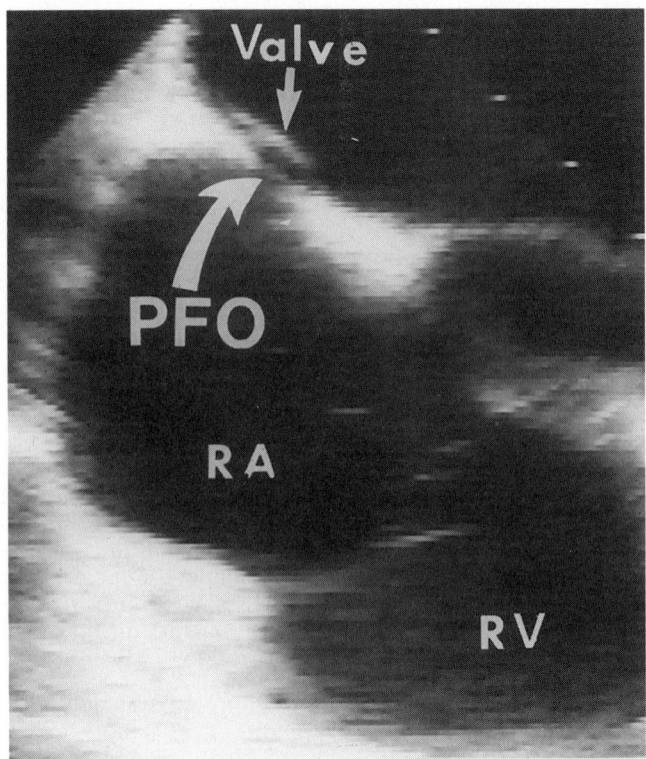

FIGURE 60–20. Transesophageal echocardiogram from a 22-year-old woman who came to attention because of a transient cerebral event. A patent foramen ovale (PFO) guarded by its valve were identified. Following a Valsalva maneuver, transient right-to-left shunting was identified with color flow imaging. RA = right atrium; RV = right ventricle.

vic veins.[325] Recent interest has focused upon younger adults with embolic stroke caused by paradoxical emboli through a patent foramen ovale[322,326] (Fig. 60–20). The incidence of patent foramen ovale in a necropsy study of 965 autopsy specimens of human hearts was 27.3 per cent ranging from 34.3 per cent during the first three decades of life to 22.2 per cent during the ninth and tenth decades.[327] Another source of cerebral embolization is from an atrial septal aneurysm, a highly mobile malformation of the interatrial septum that briskly oscillates from right atrium to left atrium.[324,328]

Focal neurological deficits are well known sequelae of cerebral emboli. Less well known are diffuse cerebral symptoms believed to result from recurrent multiple small cortical emboli that cause agitated confusion, dulled sensorium, and seizures.[329]

NEUROLOGICAL DISORDERS IN PATIENTS WITH CONGENITAL HEART DISEASE

(See Chap. 29)

NEUROLOGICAL COMPLICATIONS AFTER CARDIAC ARREST

Neurological outcomes vary considerably, ranging from complete recovery to a vegetative state.[330-333] A reversible "metabolic encephalopathy" occurs in patients with brief episodes of circulatory arrest and mild degrees of cerebral hypoxia. Recovery is rapid and complete. In contrast, patients with severe cerebral hypoxia suffer structural damage to specific areas of the brain as if they had a stroke and, on awakening, manifest permanent focal or multifocal motor, sensory, and intellectual deficits.[330,331,333] Patients with more widespread brain injury remain hospitalized in a state of wakefulness without awareness (vegetative) or die a neurological (brain) death. Serious neurologic deficits occur in only about 10 per cent of patients who are discharged because severe postarrest neurological complications so often culminate in in-hospital or preadmission death.[332] Preexisting neurological deficits are ominous for survivors of cardiopulmonary resuscitation. Early return of consciousness and return of cranial nerve function and electroencephalographic function imply a better cerebral prognosis but do not guarantee a good outcome.[332] Delayed electroencephalographic return signifies a poor neurologic prognosis.

CARDIAC COMPLICATIONS OF DRUGS USED IN TREATING NEUROMUSCULAR DISEASE

Methysergide prescribed for migraine headache is occasionally accompanied by inflammatory retroperitoneal fibrosis and by a similar fibrotic disease of pleura, systemic arteries, cardiac valves, endocardium, and pericardium.[334-336] Methysergide-induced lesions cause little or no damage to underlying cardiac structures but result in a layer of fresh collagen upon the surfaces of otherwise unharmed cardiac tissue.[335] The aortic valve disorder induced by methysergide is stenosis or regurgitation, whereas the mitral lesion generally causes regurgitation. If the drug is continued, the valvular abnormalities generally progress. Regression or complete disappearance (at least of the cardiac murmurs) may follow discontinuation of methysergide.[335]

In *Parkinson's disease*, neurons are selectively destroyed and cannot release the neurotransmitter dopamine.[337] Accordingly, levodopa (L-dopa), the precursor of dopamine, is used in treatment. A relatively large dose is required for a therapeutic response because only a small percentage of oral L-dopa crosses the blood-brain barrier. Large doses are seldom tolerated without side effects. Cardiovascular effects are mediated by the action of L-dopa on the central and peripheral nervous systems. L-Dopa provokes hypotension (supine and postural) as well as ventricular ectopic beats.[337] The drug must therefore be used cautiously in patients with cerebral ischemia, angina pectoris, recent myocardial infarction, or cardiac arrhythmias, although after weeks (sometimes months) of use, tolerance improves and side effects diminish.

Bromocriptine, an ergot derivative, stimulates dopamine-sensitive receptors and is also useful in parkinsonism.[337] In high doses, the drug may cause a significant postural fall in blood pressure. The hypotensive effect may persist for as long as 6 weeks. Rarely, severe hypotension, both supine and erect, occurs after the initial dose of bromocriptine.

NEUROLOGICAL COMPLICATIONS OF THERAPY FOR CARDIOVASCULAR DISEASE

Certain therapies for cardiovascular disease can result in serious neurological impairment such as the sequelae of cardiac arrest and resuscitation. Systemic emboli related to cardioversion for chronic atrial fibrillation can occur either at the time of reversion to sinus rhythm or upon recurrence of atrial fibrillation. If an anticoagulant is used, it must precede cardioversion and be maintained until stable sinus rhythm seems assured.[338]

Cyclosporine neurotoxicity is only one of the neuropathological concerns in the management of cardiac transplantation.[339,340] Cyclosporine may produce a wide range of neurological disorders including coma, encephalopathy, cortical blindness, tremor, ataxia, peripheral neuropathy, and paraparesis.[339,340] There is no necessary correlation between blood levels and neurotoxic effects of the drug. However, withdrawal of cyclosporine or dose reduction generally results in resolution of the signs and symptoms, but cases of fatal convulsions and coma have been reported.[339] Perioperative neurological complications of cardiac transplantation (first 2 weeks) include cerebrovascular disorders, encephalopathy, acute psychosis, and mononeuropathy.[341,342] Late neurological complications are related primarily to the use of chronic immunosuppression, with cerebrovascular disorders becoming less frequent.[341,342]

Several commonly used cardiac drugs have important, although relatively rare, central or peripheral nervous system effects. The adverse responses to quinidine and procainamide in patients with myasthenia gravis were mentioned earlier. *Lidocaine neurotoxicity* (see p. 607) includes drowsiness, dizziness, dysarthria, blurred vision, muscular fasciculations, and occasionally convulsions.[343] Beta-adrenoceptor blockers (see p. 1306), in addition to causing drowsiness and lightheadedness, sometimes result in mental depression. Even digitalis glycosides are not exempt from neurotoxic effects[344] (see p. 484). William Withering reported that, "The Foxglove when given in very large and quickly repeated doses occasions giddiness, confused vision, objects appearing green or yellow . . . cold sweats, convulsions, syncope, death."[345]

CARDIAC DENERVATION

The most common cause of cardiac denervation is transplantation of the heart (see Chap. 18). Less well known is the remarkable denervation of the heart's intrinsic nervous system that occurs with Chagas' disease (see p. 1442).[346,347] Chagasic dysautonomia is associated with pathological changes in the cardiovascular, digestive, and autonomic nervous systems.[347] The cardioneuropathy is characterized by bradycardia, absent postural reflexes, hypotension, and an abnormal hyperventilatory response.[347] The increased capacity of the coronary arteries (judged at necropsy by the volume of barium sulfate-gelatin mass occupied by the coronary arterial bed relative to heart weight) has been attributed to relative sympathetic overdrive.[346]

REFERENCES

HEREDOFAMILIAL NEUROMYOPATHIC DISORDERS

1. Perloff, J. K., deLeon, A. C., and O'Doherty, D.: The cardiomyopathy of progressive muscular dystrophy. Circulation 33:625, 1966.

2. Perloff, J. K., Henze, E., and Schelbert, H. R.: Alterations in regional myocardial metabolism, perfusion and wall motion in Duchenne muscular dystrophy studied by radionuclide imaging. Circulation 69:33, 1984.

3. Perloff, J. K., Stevenson, W. G., Roberts, N. K., et al.: Cardiac involvement in myotonic muscular dystrophy (Steinert's disease): A prospective study of 25 patients. Am. J. Cardiol. 54:1074, 1984.

4. Child, J. S., Perloff, J. K., Bach, P. M., et al.: Cardiac involvement in Friedreich's ataxia. J. Am. Coll. Cardiol. 7:1370, 1986.

5. Melacini, T., Fanin, M., Danieli, G. A., et al.: Cardiac involvement in Becker muscular dystrophy. Am. J. Cardiol. 22:1927, 1993.

6. Brooke, M. H.: A Clinician's View of Neuromuscular Disease. 2nd ed. Baltimore, Williams and Wilkins Co., 1986.

7. Kunkel, L. M.: Analysis of deletions in DNA from patients with Becker and Duchenne muscular dystrophy. Nature 322:73, 1986.

8. Koenig, M., Hoffman, E. P., Bertelson, C. J., et al.: Complete cloning of the Duchenne muscular dystrophy (DMD) cDNA and preliminary genomic organization of the DMD gene in normal and affected individuals. Cell 50:509, 1987.

9. Chamberlain, J. S., Gidbs, R. A., Rainier, J. E., et al.: Deletion screening of the Duchenne muscular dystrophy locus via multiplex DNA amplification. Nucleic Acids Res. 16:11, 141, 1988.

10. Worton, R.: Muscular dystrophies: Diseases of the dystrophin-glycoprotein complex. Science 270:755, 1995.

11. Hoffman, E. P., and Gorospe, M.: The animal models of Duchenne muscular dystrophy: Windows on the pathophysiological consequences of dystrophin deficiency. Curr. Top. Membr. 38:113, 1991.

12. Lansman, J. B., and Franco, A.: What does dystrophin do in normal muscle. Muscle Res. Cell Motil. 12:409, 1991.

13. Hoffman, E. P., and Kunkel, L. M.: Dystrophin abnormalities in Duchenne/Becker muscular dystrophy. Neuron 2:1019, 1989.

14. Towbin, J. A., Hejtmanck, F., Brink, P., et al.: X-linked dilated cardiomyopathy: Molecular genetic evidence of linkage to the Duchenne muscular dystrophy (dystrophin gene at the Xp21 locus). Circulation 87:1154, 1993.

15. Rojas, C. V., and Hoffman, E. P.: Recent advances in dystrophin research. Curr. Opin. Neurobiol. 1:420, 1992.

16. Hoffman, E. P., Brown, R. H., and Kunkel, L. M.: Dystrophin: The protein product of the Duchenne muscular dystrophy locus. Cell 51:919, 1987.

17. Koenig, M., Monaco, A. P., and Kunkel, L. M.: The complete sequence of dystrophin predicts a rod-shaped cytoskeletal protein. Cell 53:219, 1988.

18. Love, D. R., Morris, G. E., Ellie, J. M., et al.: Tissue distribution of the dystrophin-related gene product and expression in the mdx and dy mouse. Proc. Natl. Acad. Sci. USA 88:3243, 1991.

19. Bonilla, E., Samitt, C. E., Mirande, A. F., et al.: Duchenne muscular dystrophy: Deficiency of dystrophin at the muscle cell surface. Cell 54:447, 1988.

20. Roland, L. P.: Biochemistry of muscle membranes in Duchenne muscular dystrophy. Muscle Nerve 3:3, 1980.

21. Pons, F., Augier, N., Heilig, R., et al.: Isolated dystrophin molecules as seen by electron microscopy. Proc. Natl. Acad. Sci. USA 87:7851, 1990.

22. Ervasti, J. M., Ohlendieck, K., Kahl, S. D., Gaver, M. G., and Campbell, K. P.: Deficiency of a glycoprotein component of the dystrophin complex in dystrophic muscle. Nature 345:315, 1990.

23. Ervasti, J. M., and Campbell, K. P.: Membrane organization of the dystrophin-glycoprotein complex. Cell 66:1121, 1991.

24. Hoffman, E. P., Fishbeck, K. H., Brown, R. H., et al.: Characterization of dystrophin in muscle-biopsy specimens from patients with Duchenne's or Becker's muscular dystrophy. N. Engl. J. Med. 318:1363, 1988.

25. Boyd, Y., Buckle, V., Holt, S., Munro, E., Hunter, D., and Craig, I.: Muscular dystrophy in girls with X; autosome translocations. J. Med. Genet. 23:484, 1986.

26. Boyd, Y. and Buckle, V. J.: Cytogenetic heterogeneity of translocations associated with Duchenne muscular dystrophy. Clin. Genet. 29:108, 1986.

27. Valentine, B. A., Cooper, B. J., deLahunta, A., et al.: Canine X-linked muscular dystrophy. Neurol. Sci. 88:69, 1988.

28. Pennington, R. J. T.: Serum enzymes. In Rowland, L. P. (ed.): Pathogenesis of Human Muscular Dystrophies. Amsterdam-Oxford, Excerpta Medica, 1977, p. 341.

29. Sutton, T. M., O'Brien, J. F., Kleinberg, F., et al.: Serum levels of creatine phosphokinase and its isoenzymes in normal and stressed neonates. Mayo Clin. Proc. 56:150, 1981.

30. Gay, P. C., and Edmonds, L. C.: Severe hypercapnia after low-flow oxygen therapy in patients with neuromuscular disease and diaphragmatic dysfunction. Mayo Clin. Proc. 70:327, 1995.

31. Riggs, T.: Cardiomyopathy and pulmonary emboli in terminal Duchenne's muscular dystrophy. Am. Heart J. 119:690, 1990.

32. Gaffney, J. F., Kingston, W. J., Metlay, L. A., and Gramiak, R.: Left ventricular thrombus and systemic emboli complicating the cardiomyopathy of Duchenne's muscular dystrophy. Arch. Neurol. 46:1249, 1989.

33. Yotsukura, M., Miyagawa, M., Tsuya, T., Ishihara, T., and Ishikawa, K.: Pulmonary hypertension in progressive muscular dystrophy of the Duchenne type. Jpn. Circ. J. 52:321, 1988.

34. Perloff, J. K., Roberts, W. C., deLeon, A. C., and O'Doherty, D.: The distinctive electrocardiogram of Duchenne's progressive muscular dystrophy. Am. J. Med. 42:179, 1967.

35. Sanyal, S. K., Johnson, W. W., Dische, M. R., et al.: Dystrophic degeneration of papillary muscle and ventricular myocardium: A basis for

mitral valve prolapse in Duchenne's muscular dystrophy. Circulation 62:430, 1980.

36. Yoshioka, M.: Clinically manifesting carriers in Duchenne muscular dystrophy. Clin. Genet. 20:6, 1981.

37. Lane, R. J. M., Gardner-Medwin, D., and Roses, A. D.: Electrocardiographic abnormalities in carriers of Duchenne muscular dystrophy. Neurology 30:497, 1980.

38. Mann, O., deLeon, A. C., Perloff, J. K., et al.: Duchenne's muscular dystrophy: The electrocardiogram in female relatives. Am. J. Med. Sci. 255:376, 1968.

39. Paillonry, M., Citron, B., Hersch, B., et al.: Electrocardiograms of women carriers of Duchenne-type muscular dystrophy. Ann. Cardiol. Angiol. 31:47, 1982.

40. Wiegand, V., Rahlf, G., Meinck, M., and Kreuzer, H.: Cardiomyopathy in female carriers of the Duchenne gene. Z. Kardiol. 73:188, 1984.

41. Mirabella, M., Serbidei, S., Manfredi, G., et al.: Cardiomyopathy may be the only clinical manifestation in female carriers of Duchenne muscular dystrophy. Neurology 43:342, 1993.

42. Skyring, A., and McKusick, V. A.: Clinical, genetic and electrocardiographic studies in childhood muscular dystrophy. Am. J. Med. Sci. 242:54, 1961.

43. Slucka, C.: The electrocardiogram in Duchenne's progressive muscular dystrophy. Circulation 38:933, 1968.

44. Fitch, C. W., and Ainger, L. E.: The Frank vectorcardiogram and the electrocardiogram in Duchenne muscular dystrophy. Circulation 35:1124, 1967.

45. Sanyal, S. K., Johnson, W. W., Thapar, M. K., and Pitner, S. E.: An ultrastructural basis for the electrocardiographic alterations associated with Duchenne's progressive muscular dystrophy. Circulation 57:1122, 1978.

46. Rubler, S., Perloff, J. K., and Roberts, W. C.: Clinical Pathological Conference—Duchenne's muscular dystrophy. Am. Heart J. 94:776, 1977.

47. Ronan, J. A., Perloff, J. K., Bowen, P. J., and Mann, O.: The vectorcardiogram in Duchenne's progressive muscular dystrophy. Am. Heart J. 84:588, 1972.

48. Wakai, S., Minami, R., Kameda, K., et al.: Electron microscopic study of the biopsied cardiac muscle in Duchenne muscular dystrophy. J. Neurol. Sci. 84:167, 1988.

49. Frankel, K. A., and Rosser, R. J.: The pathology of the heart in progressive muscular dystrophy. Hum. Pathol. 7:375, 1976.

50. Cziner, D. G., and Levin, R. I.: The cardiomyopathy of Duchenne's muscular dystrophy and the function of dystrophin. Med. Hypotheses 40:169, 1993.

51. Bhattacharya, S. K., Crawford, A. J., and Pate, J. W.: Electrocardiographic, biochemical, and morphologic abnormalities in dystrophic hamsters with cardiomyopathy. Muscle Nerve 10:168, 1987.

52. Moise, N. S., Valentine, B. A., Brown, C. A., et al.: Duchenne's cardiomyopathy in a canine model: Electrocardiographic and echocardiographic studies. Am. Coll. Cardiol. 17:812, 1991.

53. Schelbert, H. R., Benson, L., Schwaiger, M., and Perloff, J. K.: Positron emission tomography. Cardiol. Clin. 1:501, 1983.

54. Nagamachi, S., Jinnouchi, S., Ono, S., et al.: Tl-201 myocardial SPECT in patients with Duchenne's muscular dystrophy: A long-term follow-up. Clin. Nucl. Med. 14:827, 1989.

55. Tamura, T., Shivuya, N., Hashiba, K., et al.: Evaluation of myocardial damage in Duchenne's muscular dystrophy with thallium-201 myocardial SPECT. Jpn. Heart J. 34:51, 1993.

56. Perloff, J. K., Moise, N. S., Stevenson, W. G., and Gilmour, R. F.: Cardiac electrophysiology in Duchenne muscular dystrophy: From basic science to clinical expression. J. Cardiovasc. Electrophysiol. 3:394, 1992.

57. Sanyal, S. K., Johnson, W. W.: Cardiac conduction abnormalities in children with Duchenne progressive muscular dystrophy: Electrocardiographic features and morphologic correlates. Circulation 66:853, 1982.

58. Nomura, H., Hizawa, K.: Histopathological study of the conduction system of the heart in Duchenne progressive muscular dystrophy. Acta Pathol. Jpn. 32:1027, 1982.

59. Gaschen, F. P., Hoffman, E. P., Goroscope, M. Jr., et al.: Dystrophin deficiency causes lethal muscle hypertrophy in cats. J. Neurosci. 110:149, 1992.

60. James, T. N.: Cardiac conduction system: Fetal and postnatal development. Am. J. Cardiol. 25:213, 1970.

61. Bies, R. D., Friedman, D., Roberts, R., et al.: Expression and localization of dystrophin in human cardiac Purkinje fibers. Circulation 86:147, 1992.

62. Pons, F., Robert, A., Fabbricio, E., et al.: Utrophin localization in normal and dystrophin-deficient heart. Circulation 90:369, 1994.

63. Perloff, J. K.: Cardiac rhythm and conduction in Duchenne's muscular dystrophy. J. Am. Coll. Cardiol. 3:1263, 1984.

64. Bigger, J. T. Jr., Fleiss, J. L., Steinman, R. C., et al.: Frequency domain measures of heart rate period variability and mortality after myocardial infarction. Circulation 85:164, 1992.

65. Zalman, F., Perloff, J. K., Durant, N. N., and Campion, D. S.: Acute respiratory failure following intravenous verapamil in Duchenne's muscular dystrophy. Am. Heart J. 105:510, 1983.

66. Spach, M. S., and Dolber, P. C.: Relating intracellular potentials and their derivatives to anisotropic propagation at a microscopic level in human cardiac muscle. Circ. Res. 58:356, 1986.

67. Ursell, P. C., Gardner, P. I., Alvala, A., et al.: Structural and electro-physiological changes in the epicardial border zone of canine myocardial infarcts during infarct healing. Circ. Res. 56:436, 1985.

68. Shimizu, A., Nobaki, A., Rudy, Y., et al.: Onset of induced atrial flutter in the canine pericarditis model. J. Am. Coll. Cardiol. 17:1223, 1991.

69. Cosio, F. G., Aribas, F., Placios, J., et al.: Fragmented electrocardiograms and continuous electrical activity in atrial flutter. Am. J. Cardiol. 57:1309, 1986.

70. D'Orsogna, L., O'Shea, L. P., and Miller, G.: Cardiomyopathy of Duchenne muscular dystrophy. Pediatr. Cardiol. 9:205, 1988.

71. Yotsukura, M., Ishizuka, T., Shimada, T., et al.: Late potentials in progressive muscular dystrophy of the Duchenne type. Am. Heart J. 121:1137, 1991.

72. Mori, H., Utsunomiya, T., Ishijima, M., et al.: The relationship between 24-hour total heart beats or ventricular arrhythmias and cardiopulmonary function in patients with Duchenne's muscular dystrophy. Can. Anaesth. Soc. J. 33:492, 1986.

73. Ilan, Y., Hillman, M., Oren, R.: Intravenous verapamil for tachyarrhythmia in Duchenne's muscular dystrophy. Pediatr. Cardiol. 11:177, 1990.

74. Chalkiadis, G. A., and Branch, K. G.: Cardiac arrest after isoflurane anaesthesia in a patient with Duchenne's muscular dystrophy. Anaesthesia 45:22, 1990.

75. Sethna, N. F., and Rockoff, M. A.: Cardiac arrest following inhalation induction of anaesthesia in a child with Duchenne's muscular dystrophy. Can. Anaesth. Soc. J. 33:799, 1986.

76. Beggs, A. H., Hoffman, E. P., Snyder, J. R., et al.: Exploring the molecular basis for variability among patients with Becker muscular dystrophy: Dystrophin gene and protein studies. Am. J. Hum. Genet. 49:54, 1991.

77. Yoshiba, K., Ikeda, S., Nakamura, A., et al.: Molecular analysis of the Duchenne muscular dystrophy gene in patients with Becker muscular dystrophy presenting with dilated cardiomyopathy. Muscle Nerve 16:1161, 1993.

78. de Visser, M., de Voogt, W. G., la Riviere, G. V.: The heart in Becker muscular dystrophy, facioscapulohumeral dystrophy, and Bethlem myopathy. Muscle Nerve 15:591, 1992.

79. Comi, G. T., Prelle, A., Bresolin, N., et al.: Clinical variability in Becker muscular dystrophy: Genetic, biochemical and immunohistochemical correlates. Brain 117:1, 1994.

80. Hoffman, E. P., and Kunkel, L. M.: Dystrophin abnormalities in Duchenne/Becker muscular dystrophy. Neuron 2:1019, 1989.

81. Anan, R., Higuchi, I., Ichinari, K., et al.: Myocardial patchy staining of dystrophin in Becker's muscular dystrophy associated with cardiomyopathy. Am. Heart J. 123:1088, 1992.

82. Maeda, M., Nakao, S., Miyacato, H., et al.: Cardiac dystrophin abnormalities in Becker muscular dystrophy assessed by endomyocardial biopsy. Am. Heart J. 129:702, 1995.

83. Markand, O. N., North, R. R., D'Agostino, A. N., and Daly, D. D.: Benign sex-linked muscular dystrophy. Neurology 19:617, 1969.

84. Steare, S. E., Dubowitz, V., and Banater, A.: Subclinical cardiomyopathy in Becker muscular dystrophy. Br. Heart J. 68:304, 1992.

85. Nigro, G., Comi, L. I., Politano, L., et al.: Evaluation of the cardiomyopathy in Becker muscular dystrophy. Muscle Nerve 18:283, 1995.

86. Yazawa, M., Ikeda, S., Owa, M., et al.: A family of Becker's progressive muscular dystrophy with severe cardiomyopathy. Eur. Neurol. 27:13, 1987.

87. Levin, R. N., and Narahara, K. A.: Right axis deviation and anterior wall thallium-201 defect in Becker's muscular dystrophy. Am. J. Cardiol. 56:203, 1985.

88. Melacini, P., Fanin, M., Danieli, D. A., et al.: Cardiac involvement in Becker muscular dystrophy. J Am. Coll. Cardiol. 22:1927, 1993.

89. Towbin, J. A., Hejtmancik, F., Drink, P., et al.: X-linked dilated cardiomyopathy: Molecular genetic evidence of linkage to the Duchenne muscular dystrophy (dystrophin) gene at the Xp21 locus. Circulation 87:1854, 1993.

90. Muntoni, F., Cau, M., Ganau, A., et al.: Deletion of the dystrophin muscle-promoter region associated with X-linked dilated cardiomyopathy. N. Engl. J. Med. 329:921, 1993.

91. Nigro, G., Comi, L. I., Limonselli, F. M., et al.: Prospective study of X-linked progressive muscular dystrophy in Campania. Muscle Nerve 6:253, 1983.

92. Panegyres, P. K., Mastaglia, F. L., and Kakulas, B. A.: Limb-girdle syndromes: Clinical, morphological and electrophysiological studies. J. Neurol. Sci. 95:201, 1990.

93. Bethlem, J., and Wijngaarden, G. K.: Benign myopathy with autosomal dominant inheritance. Brain 99:91, 1976.

94. Manconi, G., Pizzi, A., Arimondi, C. G., et al.: Limb-girdle muscular dystrophy with autosomal dominant inheritance. Acta Neurol. Scand. 83:234, 1991.

95. Miller, G., Beggs, A. H., and Towfighi, J.: Early onset autosomal dominant progressive muscular dystrophy presenting in childhood as a Becker phenotype: The importance of dystrophin and molecular genetic analysis. Neuromuscl. Disord. 2:121, 1992.

96. Stubegen, J.: Limb-girdle muscular dystrophy: A non-invasive cardiac evaluation. Cardiology 83:324, 1993.

97. Hoshio, A., Kotake, H., Saitoh, M., et al.: Cardiac involvement in a patient with limb-girdle muscular dystrophy. Heart Lung 16:439, 1987.

98. Kawashima, S., Ulno, M., Kondo, T., et al.: Marked cardiac involvement in limb girdle muscular dystrophy. Am. J. Med. Sci. 299:411, 1990.

99. Lunt, P. W., and Harper, P. S.: Genetic counseling in facioscapulohumeral muscular dystrophy. J. Med. Genet. 28:655, 1991.

100. Wijmenga, C., Sandkuijl, L. A., Moerer, P., et al.: Genetic linkage map of facioscapulohumeral muscular dystrophy and five polymorphic loci on chromosome 4q35-qter. Am. J. Hum. Genet. *51*:411, 1992.

101. Haraguchi, Y., Chung, A. B., Torroni, A., et al.: Genetic mapping of human heart-skeletal muscle adenine nucleotide translocator and its relationship to the facioscapulohumeral muscular dystrophy locus. Genomics *61*:479, 1993.

102. Bailey, R. O., Marzulo, D. C., and Hans, M. B.: Infantile facioscapulohumeral muscular dystrophy: New observations. Acta Neurol. Scand. *74*:51, 1986.

103. Bloomfield, D. A., and Sinclair-Smith, B. C.: Persistent atrial standstill. Am. J. Med. *39*:335, 1965.

104. Caponnetto, S., Patorini, C., and Tirelli, G.: Persistent atrial standstill in a patient affected with facioscapulohumeral dystrophy. Cardiologia *53*:341, 1968.

105. Baldwin, A. J., Talley, R. C., Johnson, C., and Nutter, O.: Permanent paralysis of the atrium in a patient with facioscapulohumeral muscular dystrophy. Am. J. Cardiol. *31*:649, 1973.

106. Stevenson, W. G., Perloff, J. K., Weiss, J. N., and Anderson, T. L.: Facioscapulohumeral muscular dystrophy: Evidence for selective, genetic electrophysiologic cardiac involvement. J. Am. Coll. Cardiol. *15*:292, 1990.

107. Emery, A. E. H., and Dreifuss, F. E.: Unusual type of benign X-linked muscular dystrophy. J. Neurol. Neurosurg. Psychiatr. *29*:338, 1966.

108. Emery, A. E. H.: X-linked muscular dystrophy with early contractures and cardiomyopathy (Emery-Dreifuss type). Clin. Genet. *32*:360, 1987.

109. Hopkins, L. C., Jackson, J. A., and Elsas, L. J.: Emery-Dreifuss humeroperoneal muscular dystrophy: An X-linked myopathy with unusual contractures and bradycardia. Ann. Neurol. *10*:230, 1981.

110. Bialer, M. G., and Kelly, T. E.: Localization of the gene for Emery-Dreifuss muscular dystrophy to X-q28. Am. J. Hum. Genet. *45*:(Suppl A)130, 1989.

111. Fenichel, G. M., Sul, Y. C., Kilroy, A. W., and Blouin, R.: An autosomal-dominant dystrophy with humeropelvic distribution and cardiomyopathy. Neurology *32*:1399, 1982.

112. Takamoto, K., Hirose, K., and Nonaka, I.: A genetic variant of Emery-Dreifuss disease. Arch. Neurol. *41*:1292, 1984.

113. Tanaka, K., Yoshimura, T., Muratani, H., et al.: Familial myopathy with scapulohumeral distribution, rigid spine, cardiomyopathy and mitochondrial abnormality. J. Neurol. *236*:52, 1989.

114. Bergia, B., Sybers, H. D., and Butler, I. J.: Familial lethal cardiomyopathy with mental retardation and scapuloperoneal muscular dystrophy. J. Neurol. *49*:1423, 1986.

115. Wooliscroft, J., and Tuna, N.: Permanent atrial standstill: The clinical spectrum. Am. J. Med. *49*:2037, 1982.

116. Ward, D. E., Ho, S. Y., and Shinebourne, E. A.: Familial atrial standstill and inexcitability in childhood. Am. J. Cardiol. *53*:965, 1984.

117. Disertori, M., Guarnerio, M., Vergara, G., et al.: Familial endemic persistent atrial standstill in a small mountain community. Eur. Heart J. *4*:354, 1983.

118. Levy, S., Pouget, B., Bemurat, M., et al.: Partial atrial electrical standstill: Report of three cases and review of clinical and electrophysiological features. Eur. Heart J. *1*:107, 1980.

119. Effendy, F. N., Bolognesi, R., Bianchi, G., and Visioli, O.: Alternation of partial and total atrial standstill. J. Electrocardiol. *12*:121, 1979.

120. Shah, M. K., Subramanyan, R., Tharakan, J., et al.: Familial total atrial standstill. Am. Heart J. *123*:1379, 1992.

121. Miller, R. G., Layzer, R. B., Mellenthin, M. A., et al.: Emery-Dreifuss muscular dystrophy with autosomal dominant transmission. Neurology *35*:1230, 1985.

122. Rowland, L. P., Fetell, M., Alarte, M., et al.: Emery-Dreifuss muscular dystrophy. Ann. Neurol. *5*:111, 1979.

123. Dickey, P. P., Ziter, F. A., and Smith, R. A.: Emery-Dreifuss muscular dystrophy. J. Pediatr. *104*:555, 1984.

124. Oswald, A. H., Goldblatt, J., Horak, A. R., and Beighton, P.: Lethal cardiac conduction defects in Emery-Dreifuss muscular dystrophy. S. Afr. Med. J. *72*:567, 1987.

125. Wyse, D. G., Nath, F. C., and Brownell, A. K. W.: Benign X-linked (Emery-Dreifuss) muscular dystrophy is not benign. PACE *10*:533, 1987.

126. Yoshioka, M., Saida, K., Itagaki, Y., and Kamiya, T.: Follow up study of cardiac involvement in Emery-Dreifuss muscular dystrophy. Arch. Dis. Child. *64*:713, 1989.

127. Hopkins, L. C., Jackson, J. H., and Elsas, L. J.: Emery-Dreifuss humeroperoneal muscular dystrophy: An X-linked myopathy with unusual contractures and bradycardia. Ann. Neurol. *10*:230, 1981.

128. Bialer, M. G., McDaniel, N. L., and Kelly, T. E.: Progression of cardiac disease in Emery-Dreifuss muscular dystrophy. Clin. Cardiol. *14*:411, 1991.

129. Bartlett, R. J., Pericak-Vance, M. A., Yamaoka, L., et al.: A new probe for the diagnosis of myotonic muscular dystrophy. Science *235*:1648, 1987.

130. Harper, P. S.: Myotonic Dystrophy. 2nd ed. Philadelphia, W. B. Saunders Co., 1989.

131. Wieringa, B., Brunner, H., Hulsebos, T., et al.: Genetic and physical demarcation of the locus for dystrophia myotonica. Adv. Neurol. *48*:47, 1988.

132. Rudel, R., and Lehmann-Horn, F.: Membrane changes in cells from myotonic patients. Physiol. Rev. *65*:310, 1985.

133. Mahadevan, M., Tsilfidis, C., Sabourin, L., et al.: Myotonic muscular dystrophy mutation: An unstable CTG repeat in the 3′ untranslated region of the gene. Science *255*:1253, 1992.

134. Annane, D., Duboc, D., Mazoyer, B., et al.: Correlation between decreased myocardial glucose phosphorylation and the DNA mutation size in myotonic dystrophy. Circulation *90*:2629, 1994.

135. Tokgozoglu, L. S., Ashizaina, T., Pacifico, A., et al.: Cardiac involvement in a large kindred with myotonic dystrophy. Quantitative assessment and relation to size of CTG repeat expansion. JAMA *274*:813, 1995.

136. Ono, S., Inoue, K., Mannen, T., et al.: Neuropathological changes of the brain in myotonic dystrophy: Some new observations. Neurol. Sci. *81*:301, 1987.

137. Bharati, S., Bump, F. T., Bauernfeind, R., and Lev, M.: Dystrophica myotonia: Correlative electrocardiographic, electrophysiologic and conduction system study. Chest *86*:444, 1984.

138. Moorman, J. R., Coleman, R. E., Packer, D. L., et al.: Cardiac involvement in myotonic muscular dystrophy. Medicine *64*:371, 1985.

139. Fragola, P. V., Luzi, M., Calo, L., et al.: Cardiac involvement in myotonic dystrophy. Am. J. Cardiol. *74*:1070, 1994.

140. Fragola, P. V., Autore, C., Magni, G., et al.: The natural course of cardiac conduction disturbances in myotonic dystrophy. Cardiology *79*:93, 1991.

141. Hawley, R. J., Milner, M. R., Gottdiener, J. S., and Cohen, A.: Myotonic heart disease: A clinical follow-up. Neurology *41*:259, 1991.

142. Nguyen, H. H., Wolfe, J. T. III, Holmes, D. R. Jr., and Edwards, W. D.: Pathology of the cardiac conduction system in myotonic dystrophy: A study of 12 cases. J. Am. Coll. Cardiol. *11*:662, 1988.

143. Hiromasa, S., Ikeda, T., Kubota, K., et al.: Myotonic dystrophy: Ambulatory electrocardiogram, electrophysiologic study, and echocardiographic evaluation. Am. Heart J. *113*:1482, 1987.

144. Hiromasa, S., Ikeda, T., Kubota, K., et al.: A family with myotonic dystrophy associated with diffuse cardiac conduction disturbances as demonstrated by His bundle electrocardiography. Am. Heart J. *111*:85, 1986.

145. Olofsson, B., Forsberg, H., Andersson, S., et al.: Electrocardiographic findings in myotonic dystrophy. Br. Heart J. *59*:47, 1988.

146. Grigg, L. E., Chan, W., Mond, H. G., et al.: Ventricular tachycardia and sudden death in myotonic dystrophy: Clinical, electrophysiologic and pathologic features. Am. J. Cardiol. *6*:254, 1985.

147. Hiromasa, S., Ikeda, T., Kubota, K., et al.: Ventricular tachycardia and sudden death in myotonic dystrophy. Am. Heart J. *115*:914, 1988.

148. Prystowsky, E. N., Pritchett, E. L. C., Roses, A. D., and Gallagher, J. J.: The natural history of conduction system disease in myotonic muscular dystrophy as determined by serial electrophysiologic studies. Circulation *60*:1360, 1979.

149. Melacini, T., Buja, G., Fasoli, G., et al.: The natural history of cardiac involvement in myotonic dystrophy: An eight-year follow-up in 17 patients. Clin. Cardiol. *11*:231, 1988.

150. Uemura, N., Tanaka, H., Niimura, T., et al.: Electrophysiological and histological abnormalities of the heart in myotonic dystrophy. Am. Heart J. *86*:616, 1973.

151. Petkovitch, N. J., Dunn, M., and Reed, W.: Myotonia dystrophica with AV dissociation and Stokes-Adams attacks. Am. Heart J. *68*:391, 1964.

152. Melacini, P., Villanova, C., Menegazzo, E., et al.: Correlation between cardiac involvement and CTG trinucleotide repeat length in myotonic dystrophy. J. Am. Coll. Cardiol. *25*:239, 1995.

153. Fall, L. H., Young, W. W., Power, J. A., et al.: Severe congestive heart failure and cardiomyopathy as a complication of myotonic dystrophy in pregnancy. Obstet. Gynecol. *76*:481, 1990.

154. Hartwig, G. R., Ran, K. R., Radoff, F. M., et al.: Radionuclide angiocardiographic analysis of myocardial function in myotonic muscular dystrophy. Neurology *33*:657, 1983.

155. Motta, J., Guilleminault, C., Billingham, M., et al.: Cardiac abnormalities in myotonic dystrophy: Electrophysiologic and histopathologic studies. Am. J. Med. *67*:467, 1979.

156. Ludatscher, R. M., Kerner, H., Amikam, S., and Gellei, B.: Myotonia dystrophica with heart involvement: An electron microscopic study of skeletal, cardiac, and smooth muscle. J. Clin. Pathol. *31*:1057, 1978.

157. Tanaka, N., Tanaka, H., Takeda, M., et al.: Cardiomyopathy in myotonic dystrophy: A light and electron microscopic study of the myocardium. Jpn. Heart J. *14*:202, 1973.

158. Child, J. S., and Perloff, J. K.: Diastolic properties of the left ventricle in myotonic muscular dystrophy (Steinert's disease). Am. Heart J. *129*:982, 1995.

159. Forsberg, H., Olofsson, B., Eriksson, A., and Andersson, S.: Cardiac involvement in congenital myotonic dystrophy. Br. Heart J. *63*:119, 1990.

160. Forsberg, H., Olofsson, B., Eriksson, A., and Andersson, S.: Cardiac involvement in congenital myotonic dystrophy. Br. Heart J. *63*:119, 1990.

161. Anderson, M.: Probable Thomsen's disease with cardiac involvement. J. Neurol. *214*:301, 1977.

162. Subramony, S. H., Malhotra, C. P., and Mishra, S. K.: Distinguishing paramyotonia congenital and myotonia congenita by electromyography. Muscle Nerve *6*:374, 1983.

163. Streib, F. W., Sun, S. F., and Hanson, M.: Paramyotonia congenita: Clinical and electrophysiologic studies. Electromyogr. Clin. Neurophysiol. *23*:315, 1983.

164. Rosenberg, R. N.: Hereditary ataxias. *In* Rowland, L. P. (ed.): Merritt's Textbook of Neurology. Philadelphia, Lea and Febiger, 1984, p. 499.

165. Barbeau, A.: Friedreich's ataxia 1980. Our overview of the pathophysiology. J. Can. Sci. Neurol. 7:455, 1980.

166. Harding, A. E.: Friedreich's ataxia: A clinical and genetic study of 90 families with an analysis of early diagnostic criteria and intrafamilial clustering of clinical features. Brain 104:589, 1981.

167. Brumback, R. A., Panner, B. J., and Kingston, W. J.: The heart in Friedreich's ataxia. Arch. Neurol. 43:189, 1986.

168. Grenadier, E., Goldberg, S. J., Stern, L. Z., and Feldman, J.: M-mode and two-dimensional echocardiographic examination of patients with Friedreich's ataxia. J. Cardiovasc. Ultrasonogr. 3:5, 1984.

169. Gottdiener, J. S., Hawley, R. J., Maron, B. J., et al.: Characteristics of the cardiac hypertrophy in Friedreich's ataxia. Am. Heart J. 103:525, 1982.

170. Barbeau, A.: Pathophysiology of Friedreich's ataxia. In Matthews, W. B., and Glaser, G. H. (eds.): Recent Advances in Clinical Neurology, No. 3. Edinburgh, Churchill Livingstone, 1982, p. 129.

171. Pastertac, A., Drol, R., Petitclerc, R., et al.: Hypertrophic cardiomyopathy in Friedreich's ataxia: Symmetric or asymmetric? J. Can. Sci. Neurol. 7:379, 1980.

172. Harding, A. E., and Hewer, R. L.: The heart disease of Friedreich's ataxia: A clinical and electrocardiographic study of 115 patients, with an analysis of serial electrocardiographic changes in 30 cases. Q. J. Med. 28:489, 1983.

173. Zimmermann, M., Gabathuler, J., Adamec, R., and Pinget, L.: Unusual manifestations of heart involvement in Friedreich's ataxia. Am. Heart J. 111:184, 1986.

174. Barbeau, A.: Quebec cooperative study of Friedreich's ataxia. J. Can. Sci. Neurol. 3:2779, 1976.

175. Unverferth, D. V., Schmidt, W. R., Baker, P. B., and Wooley, C. F.: Morphologic and functional characteristics of the heart in Friedreich's ataxia. Am. J. Med. 82:5, 1987.

176. Smith, E. R., Sangalang, V. E., Heffernan, L. P., et al.: Hypertrophic cardiomyopathy: The heart disease of Friedreich's ataxia. Am. Heart J. 94:428, 1977.

177. Hawley, R. J., and Gottdiener, J. S.: Five-year follow-up of Friedreich's ataxia cardiomyopathy. Arch. Intern. Med. 146:483, 1986.

178. Alboliras, E. T., Shub, C., Gomez, M. R., et al.: Spectrum of cardiac involvement in Friedreich's ataxia: Clinical, electrocardiographic and echocardiographic observations. Am. J. Cardiol. 58:518, 1986.

179. Pentland, B., and Fox, K. A. A.: The heart in Friedreich's ataxia. J. Neurol. Neurosurg. Psychiatr. 46:1138, 1983.

180. James, T. N., Cobbs, B. W., Coghlan, H. C., et al.: Coronary disease, cardioneuropathy, and conduction system abnormalities in the cardiomyopathy of Friedreich's ataxia. Br. Heart J. 57:446, 1987.

181. Spach, N. S., and Kootsey, J. M.: The nature of electrical propagation in cardiac muscle. Am. J. Physiol. 244:H3, 1983.

182. Palagi, B., Picozzi, R., Casazza, F., et al.: Biventricular function in Friedreich's ataxia: A radionuclide angiographic study. Br. Heart J. 59:692, 1988.

183. Giunta, A., Maione, S., Biagini, R., et al.: Noninvasive assessment of systolic and diastolic function in 50 patients with Friedreich's ataxia. Cardiology 75:321, 1988.

184. Zimmermann, M., Gabathuler, J., Adamec, R., and Pinget, L.: Unusual manifestations of heart involvement in Friedreich's ataxia. Am. Heart J. 111:184, 1986.

185. Pleasure, D. E., and Schotland, D. L.: Hereditary neuropathies. In Rowland, L. P. (ed.): Merritt's Textbook of Neurology. Philadelphia, Lea and Febiger, 1984.

186. Leak, D.: Paroxysmal atrial flutter in peroneal muscular atrophy. Br. Heart J. 23:326, 1961.

187. Littler, W. A.: Heart block and peroneal muscular atrophy. Q. J. Med. 39:431, 1970.

188. Kaj, J. M., Littler, W. A., and Meade, J. B.: Ultrastructure of the myocardium in familial heart block and peroneal muscular atrophy. Br. Heart J. 34:1081, 1972.

189. Lowry, P. I., and Littler, W. A.: Peroneal muscular atrophy associated with cardiac conduction tissue disease. Postgrad. Med. J. 59:530, 1983.

190. Martin-Du Pan, R. C., Juse, C., and Perrenoud, J. J.: Congestive cardiomyopathy and pyruvate elevation in a case of Charcot-Marie-Tooth disease. Schweiz. Med. Wochenschr. 5:114, 1984.

191. Isner, J. M., Hawley, R. J., Weintraub, A. B., and Engel, W. K.: Cardiac findings in Charcot-Marie-Tooth disease. Arch. Intern. Med. 139:1161, 1979.

192. Spiro, A. J., Shy, G. M., and Gonatas, N. K.: Myotubular myopathy. Arch Neurol. 14:1, 1966.

193. Verhiest, W., Brucher, J. M., Goddeeris, P., et al.: Familial centronuclear myopathy associated with cardiomyopathy. Br. Heart J. 38:504, 1976.

194. Shafiq, S. A., Sande, M. A., Carruthers, R. R., et al.: Skeletal muscle in idiopathic cardiomyopathy. J. Neurol. Sci. 15:303, 1972.

195. di Mauro, S., and Moraes, C. T.: Mitochondrial encephalomyopathies. Arch. Neurol. 50:1197, 1993.

196. Anan, R., Nakagawa, M., Miyata, M., et al.: Cardiac involvement in mitochondrial diseases: A study on 17 patients with documented mitochondrial DNA defects. Circulation 91:955, 1995.

197. Ozawa, T., Katsumata, K., Hayakawa, M., et al.: Genotype and phenotype of severe mitochondrial cardiomyopathy: A recipient of heart transplantation and the genetic control. Biochem. Biophys. Res. Commun. 207:613, 1995.

198. Berenberg, R. A., Pellock, J. M., DiMauro, S., et al.: Lumping or split-

199. Lowes, M.: Chronic progressive external ophthalmoplegia, pigmentary retinopathy and heart block (Kearns-Sayre syndrome). Acta Ophthalmol. 53:610, 1975.

200. Charles, R., Holt, S., Kay, J. M., et al.: Myocardial ultrastructure and the development of atrioventricular block in Kearns-Sayre syndrome. Circulation 63:214, 1981.

201. Roberts, N. K., Perloff, J. K., and Kark, P.: Cardiac conduction in Kearns-Sayre syndrome. Am. J. Cardiol. 44:1396, 1979.

202. Schwartzkopff, B., Frenzel, H., Losse, B., et al.: Heart involvement in progressive external ophthalmoplegia (Kearns-Sayre syndrome): Electrophysiologic, hemodynamic and morphologic findings. Z. Kardiol. 75:161, 1986.

203. Schwartzkopff, B., Frenzel, H., Breithardt, G., et al.: Ultrastructural findings in endomyocardial biopsy of patients with Kearns-Sayre syndrome. J. Am. Coll. Cardiol. 12:1522, 1988.

204. Channer, K. S., Channer, J. L., Campbell, M. J., and Rees, J. R.: Cardiomyopathy in the Kearns-Sayre syndrome. Br. Heart J. 59:486, 1988.

205. Kenny, D., and Wetherbee, J.: Kearns-Sayre syndrome in the elderly: Mitochondrial myopathy with advanced heart block. Am. Heart J. 120:440, 1990.

206. Clark, D. S., Myerburg, R. J., Morales, R. R., et al.: Heart block and Kearns-Sayre: Electrophysiologic-pathologic correlation. Chest 68:727, 1975.

207. Pleasure, D. E., and Schotland, D. L.: Acquired neuropathies. In Rowland, L. P. (ed.): Merritt's Textbook of Neurology. 7th ed. Philadelphia, Lea and Febiger, 1984.

208. McDonagh, A. J. G., and Dawson, J.: Guillain-Barré syndrome after myocardial infarction. Br. Med. J. 294:613, 1987.

209. Emmons, P. R., Blume, W. T., and DuShane, J. W.: Cardiac monitoring and demand pacemaker in Guillain-Barré syndrome. Arch. Neurol. 32:59, 1975.

210. Greenland, P., and Griggs, R. C.: Arrhythmic complications in the Guillain-Barré syndrome. Arch. Intern. Med. 140:1053, 1980.

211. Narayam, D., Huang, M. T., and Matthew, P. K.: Bradycardia and asystole requiring pacemaker in Guillain-Barré syndrome. Am. Heart J. 108:426, 1984.

212. Fagius, J., and Wallin, B. G.: Microneurographic evidence of excessive sympathetic outflow in the Guillain-Barré syndrome. Brain 106:589, 1983.

213. Persson, A., and Solders, G.: R–R variations in Guillain-Barré syndrome: A test of autonomic dysfunction. Acta Neurol. Scand. 67:294, 1983.

214. Palferman, T. G., Wright, I., Doyle, D. V., and Amiel, S.: Electrocardiographic abnormalities and autonomic dysfunction in Guillain-Barré syndrome. Br. Med. J. 284:1231, 1982.

215. Shy, G. M., Engel, W. K., Somers, J. E., and Wanko, T.: Nemaline myopathy; A new congenital myopathy. Brain 86:793, 1963.

216. Conen, P. E., Murphy, G. E., and Donohue, W. L.: Light and electron microscopic studies of "myogranules" in a child with hypotonia and muscle weakness. Can. Med. Assoc. J. 89:983, 1963.

217. Ishibashi-Veda, H., Imakita, M., Yutani, C., et al.: Congenital nemaline myopathy with dilated cardiomyopathy: An autopsy study. Hum. Pathol. 21:77, 1990.

218. Kinoshita, M., and Satoyoshi, E.: Type I fiber atrophy and nemaline bodies. Arch. Neurol. 31:423, 1974.

219. Meier, C., Gertsch, M., Zimmerman, A., et al.: Nemaline myopathy presenting as cardiomyopathy. N. Engl. J. Med. 308:1536, 1983.

220. Meier, C., Voellmy, W., Gertsch, M., et al.: Nemaline myopathy appearing in adults as cardiomyopathy: A clinicopathologic study. Arch. Neurol. 41:443, 1984.

221. Penn, A. S., and Rowland, L. P.: Neuromuscular junction. In Rowland, L. P. (ed.): Merritt's Textbook of Neurology. 7th ed. Philadelphia, Lea and Febiger, 1984, p. 561.

222. Barnes, D. M.: Nervous and immune system disorders linked in a variety of diseases. Science 232:160, 1985.

223. Gibson, T. C.: The heart in myasthenia gravis. Am. Heart J. 90:389, 1975.

224. Kornfeld, P., Horowitz, S. H., Genkins, G., and Papatestas, A.: Myasthenia gravis unmasked by antiarrhythmic agents. Mt. Sinai J. Med. 43:10, 1976.

225. Niakan, E., Bertorini, T. E., Acchiardo, S. R., and Werner, M. F.: Procainamide-induced myasthenia-like weakness in a patient with peripheral neuropathy. Arch. Neurol. 38:378, 1981.

226. Ratinov, G., Baker, W. P., and Swaiman, K. F.: McArdle's syndrome with previously unreported electrocardiographic and serum enzyme abnormalities. Ann. Intern. Med. 62:328, 1965.

227. Melki, J., Abdelhak, S., Sheth, P., et al.: Gene for chronic proximal spinal muscular atrophies maps to chromosome 5q. Nature 344:767, 1990.

228. Kimura, S., Yokota, H., Tateda, K., et al.: A case of the Kugelberg-Welander syndrome complicated with cardiac lesions. Jpn. Heart J. 21:417, 1980.

229. Gottdiener, J. S., Sherber, H. S., Hawley, R. J., and Engel, W. K.: Cardiac manifestations in polymyositis. Am. J. Cardiol. 41:1141, 1978.

230. Singsen, B., Goldreyer, B., Stanton, R., and Hanson, V.: Childhood polymyositis with cardiac conduction defects. Am. J. Dis. Child. 131:72, 1976.

231. Farber, H. W., and Make, B.: Physiologic closure of a symptomatic

patent foramen ovale with oxygen therapy. Am. Rev. Respir. Dis. *131*:181, 1985.

232. Lisak, R. P., Lebeau, J., Tucker, S. H., and Rowland, L. P.: Hyperkalemic periodic paralysis and cardiac arrhythmias. Neurology *22*:810, 1972.

233. Buruma, O. J., Schipperheyn, J. J., and Bots, G. T.: Heart muscle disease in familial hypokalemic periodic paralysis. Circulation *64*:12, 1981.

234. Klein, R., Ganelin, R., Marks, J. F., et al.: Periodic paralysis with cardiac arrhythmia. J. Pediatr. *62*:371, 1963.

235. Kastor, J. A., and Goldreyer, B. N.: Ventricular origin of bidirectional tachycardia. Circulation *48*:897, 1973.

236. Karpawich, P. P., Hart, Z. H., Perry, B. L., et al.: Childhood periodic paralysis with dysrhythmias: Electrophysiologic and histopathologic evaluation. Am. Heart J. *114*:186, 1987.

237. Fukuda, K., Ogawa, S., Yokozuka, H., et al.: Long-standing bidirectional tachycardia in a patient with hypokalemic periodic paralysis. J. Electrocardiol. *21*:71, 1988.

238. Perloff, J. K. (ed.): The Cardiomyopathies. Philadelphia, W. B. Saunders Co., 1988.

239. Rubin, E.: Alcoholic myopathy in heart and skeletal muscle. N. Engl. J. Med. *301*:28, 1979.

240. Meyer, J. G., and Urban, K.: Electrolyte changes and acid-base balance after alcohol withdrawal. With special reference to rum fits and magnesium depletion. J. Neurol. *215*:135, 1977.

241. Clarren, S. K., and Smith, D. W.: The fetal alcohol syndrome. N. Engl. J. Med. *298*:1063, 1978.

ACUTE CEREBRAL DISORDERS

242. Bramwell, C.: Can head injury cause auricular fibrillation? Lancet *1*:8, 1934.

243. Aschenbrenner, R., and Bodechtel, G.: Ueber EKG veranderungen veihirntumorkranken. Klin. Wochenschr. *17*:298, 1938.

244. Byer, E., Ashman, R., Toth, L. A.: Electrocardiogram with large upright T waves and long QT intervals. Am. Heart J. *33*:796, 1947.

245. Burch, G. E., Meyers, R., Abildskov, J. A.: A new electrocardiographic pattern observed in cerebrovascular accidents. Circulation *9*:719, 1954.

246. Chen, H. I., Liao, J. F., and Ho, S. T.: Centrogenic pulmonary hemorrhagic edema induced by cerebral compression in rats. Circ. Res. *47*:366, 1980.

247. Schell, A. R., Shenoy, M. M., Friedman, S. A., and Patel, A. R.: Pulmonary edema associated with subarachnoid hemorrhage. Arch. Intern. Med. *147*:591, 1987.

248. Robertson, C. S., Clifton, G. L., Taylor, A. A., and Grossman, R. G.: Treatment of hypertension associated with head injury. J. Neurosurg. *59*:455, 1983.

249. Cushing, H.: Concerning a definite regulatory mechanism of the vasomotor center which controls blood pressure during cerebral compression. Bull. Johns Hopkins Hosp. *12*:390, 1901.

250. Sciarra, D.: Head injury. *In* Rowland, L. P. (ed.): Merritt's Textbook of Neurology. 7th ed. Philadelphia, Lea and Febiger, 1984, p. 277.

251. Hackenberry, L. E., Miner, M. E., Rea, G. L., et al.: Biochemical evidence of myocardial injury after severe head trauma. Crit. Care Med. *10*:641, 1982.

252. Clifton, G. L., Robertson, C. S., Kyper, K., et al.: Cerebrovascular response to severe head injury. J. Neurosurg. *59*:447, 1983.

253. McLeod, A. A., Neil-Dwyer, G., Meyer, C. H. A., et al.: Cardiac sequelae of acute head injury. Br. Heart J. *47*:221, 1982.

254. Tobias, S. L., Bookatz, B. J., and Diamond, T. H.: Myocardial damage and electrocardiographic changes in acute cerebrovascular hemorrhage: A report of three cases and review. Heart Lung *16*:521, 1987.

255. Pollick, C., Cujec, B., Parker, S., and Tator, C.: Left ventricular wall motion abnormalities in subarachnoid hemorrhage: An echocardiographic study. J. Am. Coll. Cardiol. *12*:600, 1988.

256. Yamour, B. J., Sridharan, M. R., Rice, J. F., and Flowers, N. C.: Electrocardiographic changes in cerebrovascular hemorrhage. Am. Heart J. *99*:294, 1980.

257. Oppenheimer, S. M., and Hachinski, V. C.: The cardiac consequences of stroke. Neurol. Clin. *10*:167, 1992.

258. Baur, H. R., Gobel, F. L., and Pierach, C. A.: Electrocardiographic changes after cervical laminectomy. Int. J. Cardiol. *1*:37, 1981.

259. Samuels, M. A.: Electrocardiographic manifestations of neurologic disease. Semin. Neurol. *4*:453, 1984.

260. Carruth, J. E., and Silverman, M. E.: *Torsades de pointes* atypical ventricular tachycardia complicating subarachnoid hemorrhage. Chest *78*:886, 1980.

261. Mikolich, J. R., Jacobs, W. C., and Fletcher, G. F.: Cardiac arrhythmias in patients with acute cerebrovascular accidents. JAMA *246*:1314, 1981.

262. Goldberger, A. L.: Recognition of ECG pseudoinfarct patterns. Mod. Concepts Cardiovasc. Dis. *49*:13, 1980.

263. Taylor, A. L., and Fozzard, H. A.: Ventricular arrhythmias associated with CNS disease. Arch. Intern. Med. *142*:232, 1982.

264. Gould, L., Reddy, R. C., Kollali, M., et al.: Electrocardiographic normalization after cerebral vascular accident. J. Electrocardiol. *14*:191, 1981.

265. Myers, M. G., Norris, J. W., Hachinski, V. C., et al.: Cardiac sequelae of acute stroke. Stroke *13*:838, 1982.

266. Stober, T., Anstätt, T., Sen, S., et al.: Cardiac arrhythmias in subarachnoid haemorrhage. Acta Neurochir. *93*:37, 1988.

267. Rudehill, A., Olsson, G. L., Sundqvist, K., and Gordon, E.: ECG abnormalities in patients with subarachnoid haemorrhage and intracranial tumours. J. Neurol. Neurosurg. Psychiatr. *50*:1375, 1987.

268. Melin, J., and Fogelholm, R.: Electrocardiographic findings in subarachnoid hemorrhage. Acta Med. Scand. *213*:5, 1983.

269. Gascon, P., Ley, T. J., Toltzis, R. J., and Bonow, R. O.: Spontaneous subarachnoid hemorrhage simulating acute transmural myocardial infarction. Am. Heart J. *105*:511, 1983.

270. Oppenheimer, S. M., and Cechetto, D. F.: Cardiac chronotropic organization of the rat insular cortex. Brain Res. *533*:66, 1990.

271. Oppenheimer, S. M., Wilson, J. X., Guiraudon, C., et al.: Insular cortex stimulation produces lethal cardiac arrhythmias: A mechanism of sudden death? Brain Res. *550*:115, 1991.

272. Lane, R. D., Wallace, J. D., Petrosky, P. P., et al.: Supraventricular tachycardia in patients with right hemisphere strokes. Stroke *23*:362, 1992.

273. Oppenheimer, S. M., Gelvagirvin, J. P., et al.: Cardiovascular effects of human insular cortex stimulation. Neurology *42*:1727, 1992.

274. Svigelj, V., Grad, A., and Tekavcic, I.: Cardiac arrhythmia associated with reversible damage to insula in a patient with subarachnoid hemorrhage. Stroke *25*:1053, 1994.

275. Welch, K. M. A., and Levine, S. R.: Migraine-related stroke in the context of the International Headache Society classification of head pain. Arch. Neurol. *47*:458, 1990.

276. Oppenheimer, S. M., Cechetto, D. F., and Hachinski, V. C.: Cerebrogenic cardiac arrhythmias: Cerebral electrocardiographic influences and their role in sudden death. Arch. Neurol. *47*:513, 1990.

277. Szabo, M. D., Crosby, G., Hurford, W. E., and Strauss, H. W.: Myocardial perfusion following acute subarachnoid hemorrhage in patients with an abnormal electrocardiogram. Anesth. Analg. *76*:253, 1993.

278. Handlin, L. R., Kindred, L. H., Beauchamp, G. D., et al.: Reversible left ventricular dysfunction after subarachnoid hemorrhage. Am. Heart J. *126*:235, 1993.

279. Tabbaa, M. A., Ramirez-Lassepas, M., and Snyder, B. D.: Aneurysmal subarachnoid hemorrhage presenting as cardiorespiratory arrest. Arch. Intern. Med. *147*:1661, 1987.

280. Fredberg, U., Bøtker, H. E., and Rømer, F. K.: Acute neurogenic pulmonary oedema following generalized tonic clonic seizure: A case report and a review of the literature. Eur. Heart J. *9*:933, 1988.

281. Oppenheimer, S. M., Cechetto, D. F., and Hachinski, V. C.: Cerebrogenic cardiac arrhythmias. Arch. Neurol. *47*:513, 1990.

282. Lehmann, K. G., Lane, J. G., Piepmeier, J. M., and Batsford, W. P.: Cardiovascular abnormalities accompanying acute spinal cord injury in humans: Incidence, time course and severity. J. Am. Coll. Cardiol. *10*:46, 1987.

283. Komrad, M. S., Coffey, C. E., Coffey, K. S., et al.: Myocardial infarction and stroke. Neurology *34*:1403, 1984.

284. Chin, P. L., Kaminski, J., and Rout, N.: Myocardial infarction coincident with cerebrovascular accidents in the elderly. Age Ageing *6*:29, 1977.

285. Gillum, R. F., Fortmann, S. P., Prineas, R. J., and Kottke, T. E.: International diagnostic criteria for acute myocardial infarction and acute stroke. Am. Heart J. *108*:150, 1984.

286. Love, B. S., Grover-McKay, M., Biller, J., et al.: Coronary artery disease and cardiac events with asymptomatic and symptomatic cerebrovascular disease. Stroke *23*:939, 1992.

287. Scheinberg, P.: Transient ischemic attacks: An update. J. Neurol. Sci. *101*:133, 1991.

288. Davila-Roman, V. G., Barzilai, B., Waring, T. H., et al.: Atherosclerosis of the ascending aorta: Prevalence and role as an independent predictor of cerebrovascular events in cardiac patients. Stroke *25*:2010, 1994.

289. Sandok, B. A., Whisnant, J. P., Furlan, A. J., and Mickell, J. L.: Carotid arterial bruits. Mayo Clin. Proc. *57*:224, 1982.

290. Heyman, A., Wilkinson, W. E., Heyden, S., et al.: Risk of stroke in asymptomatic persons with cervical arterial bruits. N. Engl. J. Med. *302*:838, 1980.

291. Sundt, T. M. Jr., Whisnant, J. P., Houser, O. W., and Fode, N. C.: Prospective study of the effectiveness and durability of carotid endarterectomy. Mayo Clin. Proc. *65*:625, 1990.

292. Barnett, H. J. M., Eliasziw, M., and Meldrum, H. E.: Drugs and surgery in the prevention of ischemic stroke. N. Engl. J. Med. *332*:238, 1995.

293. Moore, W. S., Barnett, H. J. M., Beebe, H. G., et al.: Guidelines for carotid endarterectomy: A multidisciplinary consensus statement from the ad hoc committee, American Heart Association. Circulation *91*:566, 1995.

294. Busuttil, R. W., Baker, J. D., Davidson, R. K., and Machleder, H. I.: Carotid arterial stenosis: Hemodynamic significance and clinical course. JAMA *245*:1438, 1981.

295. Matchar, D. B.: Decision making in the face of uncertainty: The case of carotid endarterectomy. Mayo Clin. Proc. *65*:756, 1990.

296. Chang, B. B., Darling, C., Shah, D. M., et al.: Carotid endarterectomy can be safely performed with an acceptable mortality and morbidity in patients requiring coronary artery bypass grafts. Am. J. Surg. *168*:94, 1994.

297. Kaul, T. K., Fields, B. L., Wyatt, D. A., et al.: Surgical management in patients with coexisting coronary and cerebrovascular disease. Chest *106*:1349, 1994.

298. Kouchoukos, N. T., Daily, B. B., Wareing, T. H., and Murphy, S. F.:

Hypothermic circulatory arrest for cerebral protection during combined carotid and cardiac surgery in patients with bilateral carotid artery disease. Ann. Surg. *219*:699, 1994.

299. Vermeulen, F. E. E., Hamerlijnck, R. P. H. M., Defau, H. A. M., and Ernest, S. M. G. P.: Synchronous operation for ischemic cardiac and cerebrovascular disease: Early results and long-term follow-up. Ann. Thorac. Surg. *53*:381, 1992.

300. Breuer, A. C., Hanson, M. R., Furlan, A. J., et al.: Central nervous system complications of myocardial revascularization: A prospective analysis of 400 patients. Stroke *11*:136, 1980.

301. Gonzalez-Scarano, F., and Hurtig, H. I.: Neurologic complications of coronary artery bypass grafting: Case-control study. Neurology *31*:1032, 1981.

302. Bojar, R. M., Najafi, H., De Laria, G. A., et al.: Neurological complications of coronary revascularization. Ann. Thorac. Surg. *36*:427, 1983.

303. Sotaniemi, K. A.: Brain damage and neurological outcome after open heart surgery. J. Neurol. Neurosurg. Psychiatr. *43*:127, 1980.

304. Ferry, P. C.: Neurologic sequelae of cardiac surgery in children. Am. J. Dis. Child. *141*:309, 1987.

305. Cardiogenic brain embolism: Cerebral embolism task force. Arch. Neurol. *43*:71, 1986.

306. Hart, R. G.: Cardiogenic embolism to the brain. Lancet *339*:589, 1992.

307. Kopecky, S. L., Gersh, B. J., McGoon, M. D., et al.: The natural history of lone atrial fibrillation. N. Engl. J. Med. *317*:669, 1987.

308. Stroke Prevention in Atrial Fibrillation Study Group Investigators: Preliminary report of the stroke prevention in atrial fibrillation study. N. Engl. J. Med. *322*:863, 1990.

309. Maladies attributed to myxomatous mitral valve. Circulation *83*:328, 1991.

310. Perloff, J. K., and Child, J. S.: Clinical and epidemiological issues in mitral valve prolapse. Am. Heart J. *113*:1324, 1987.

311. Wolf, P. A., and Sila, C. A.: Cerebral ischemia with mitral valve prolapse. Am. Heart J. *113*:1308, 1987.

312. Yufe, R., Karpati, G., and Carpenter, S.: Cardiac myxoma: A diagnostic challenge for the neurologist. Neurology *26*:1060, 1976.

313. Perloff, J. K.: The Clinical Recognition of Congenital Heart Disease. 4th ed. Philadelphia, W. B. Saunders Co., 1994, p. 302.

314. Selky, A. K., and Roos, K. L.: Neurologic complications of infective endocarditis. Semin. Neurol. *12*:225, 1992.

315. Tunkel, A. R., and Kaye, D.: Neurologic complications of infective endocarditis. Neurol. Clin. *11*:419, 1993.

316. Kanter, M. C., and Hart, R. G.: Neurologic complications of infective endocarditis. Neurology *41*:1015, 1991.

317. Kaeyser, D. L., Biller, J., Coffman, T. T., and Adams, H. P.: Neurologic complications of late prosthetic valve endocarditis. Stroke *21*:472, 1990.

318. Meyer, F. B., Morita, A., Puumala, M. R., and Nichols, D. A.: Medical and surgical management of intracranial aneurysms. Mayo Clin. Proc. *70*:153, 1995.

319. Fujishima, S., Okada, Y., Irie, K., et al.: Multiple brain infarction and hemorrhage by nonbacterial thrombotic endocarditis in occult lung cancer. Angiology *45*:161, 1994.

320. Caplan, L. R., Hier, D. B., and Banks, G.: Stroke and drug abuse. Curr. Concepts Cerebrovasc. Dis. *17*:9, 1982.

COEXISTING CEREBROVASCULAR AND CORONARY HEART DISEASE

321. Biller, J., Johnson, M. R., Adams, H. P. Jr., et al.: Further observations on cerebral or retinal ischemia in patients with right-left intracardiac shunts. Arch. Neurol. *44*:740, 1987.

322. Lechat, P., Mas, J. L., Lascault, G., et al.: Prevalence of patent foramen ovale in patients with stroke. N. Engl. J. Med. *318*:1148, 1988.

323. Harvey, J. R., Teague, S. M., Anderson, J. L., et al.: Clinically silent atrial septal defects with evidence for cerebral embolization. Ann. Intern. Med. *105*:695, 1986.

324. Cabanes, L., Mas, J. L., Cohen, A., et al.: Atrial septal aneurysm and patent foramen ovale as risk factors for cryptogenic stroke in patients less than 55 years of age. Stroke *24*:1865, 1993.

324a. Stone, D. A., Godard, J., Corretti, M. C., et al.: Patent foramen ovale: Association between the degree of shunt by contrast transesophageal echocardiography and the risk of future ischemic neurologic events. Am. Heart J. *131*:158, 1996.

325. Perloff, J. K.: Congenital heart disease and pregnancy. Clin. Cardiol. *17*:579, 1994.

326. Karnik, R., Stollberger, C., Valentin, A., et al.: Detection of patent foramen ovale by transcranial contrast Doppler ultrasound. Am. J. Cardiol. *69*:560, 1992.

327. Hagen, P. T., Scholz, D. G., and Edwards, W. D.: Incidence and size of patent foramen ovale during the first ten decades of life: An autopsy study of 965 normal hearts. Mayo Clin. Proc. *59*:17, 1984.

328. Schneider, B., Hanrath, P., Vogel, P., and Meinertz, T.: Improved morphologic characterization of atrial septal aneurysm by transesophageal echocardiography: Relation to cerebrovascular events. J. Am. Coll. Cardiol. *16*:1000, 1990.

329. Dodge, R. P., Richardson, E. P., and Victor, M.: Recurrent convulsive seizures as a sequel to cerebral infarction. Brain *77*:610, 1959.

330. Rosenberg, M., Wang, C., Hoffman-Wilde, S., and Hickman, D.: Results of cardiopulmonary resuscitation. Arch. Intern. Med. *153*:1370, 1993.

331. McIntyre, K. M.: Failure of "predictors" of cardiopulmonary resuscitation outcomes to predict cardiopulmonary resuscitation outcomes. Arch. Intern. Med. *153*:1293, 1993.

332. Bircher, N. G.: Neurologic management following cardiac arrest. Neurol. Crit. Care *5*:773, 1989.

333. Bircher, N. G.: Brain resuscitation. Resuscitation *18*:S1, 1989.

334. Orlando, R. C., Moyer, P., and Barnett, T. B.: Methysergide therapy and constrictive pericarditis. Ann. Intern. Med. *88*:213, 1978.

335. Bana, D. S., MacNeal, P. S., LeCompte P. M., et al.: Cardiac murmurs and endocardial fibrosis associated with methysergide therapy. Am. Heart J. *88*:640, 1974.

336. Dorne, H. L., and Satin, R.: Methysergide-induced lower extremity arterial insufficiency. J. Can. Assoc. Radiol. *37*:210, 1986.

337. Yahr, M. D.: Parkinsonism. *In* Rowland, L. P. (ed.): Merritt's Textbook of Neurology, 7th ed. Philadelphia, Lea and Febiger, 1984, p. 526.

338. Francis, D. A., Heron, J. R., and Clarke, M.: Ambulatory electrocardiographic monitoring in patients with transient focal cerebral ischaemia. J. Neurol. Neurosurg. Psychiatr. *47*:256, 1984.

339. de Prada, J. A. V., Nartin-Duran, R., Garcia-Monco, C., et al.: Cyclosporine neurotoxicity in heart transplantation. J. Heart Lung Transplant *9*:581, 1990.

340. McManus, R. P., O'Hair, D. P., Schweiger, S., et al.: Cyclosporine-associated central neurotoxicity after heart transplantation. Ann. Thorac. Surg. *53*:326, 1992.

341. Hotson, J. R., and Enzmann, D. R.: Neurologic complications of cardiac transplantation. Neurol. Clin. *6*:349, 1988.

342. Ang, L. C., Gillett, J. M., and Kaufmann, J. C. E.: Neuropathology of heart transplantation. Can. J. Neurol. Sci. *16*:291, 1989.

343. Benorvitz, N. L.: Clinical applications of the pharmacokinetics of lidocaine. Cardiovasc. Clin. *6*:77, 1974.

344. Weidler, D. J., Jallad, N. S., Keener, D. B., et al.: The effects of acute focal cerebral ischemia on digoxin toxicity and pharmacokinetics. Pharmacology *20*:188, 1980.

345. Withering, W.: An Account of the Foxglove. *In* Willius, F. A., and Keys, T. E.: Classics of Cardiology. Vol. 1. Malabar, Fla., Robert E. Krieger Publishing Co., 1983, p. 244.

346. Oliveira, J. S. M., dos Santos, J. C. M., Muccillo, G., and Ferreira, A. L.: Increased capacity of the coronary arteries in chronic Chagas' heart disease: Further support for the neurogenic pathogenetic concept. Am. Heart J. *109*:304, 1985.

347. Iosa, D., DeQuattro, V., Lee, D. D., et al.: Plasma norepinephrine in Chagas' cardioneuromyopathy: A marker of progressive dysautonomia. Am. Heart J. *117*:882, 1989.

Chapter 61
The Heart in Endocrine and Nutritional Disorders

GORDON H. WILLIAMS, LEONARD S. LILLY, ELLEN W. SEELY

In 1835, Robert Graves described "three cases of violent and long-continued palpitation in females" with thyrotoxicosis.[1] Twenty years later, Thomas Addison reported that patients with disease of the "suprarenal capsules" had a "pulse, small and feeble . . . excessively soft and compressible." As the disease progressed, "the body wastes . . . the pulse becomes smaller and weaker, and . . . the patient at length gradually sinks and expires."[2] Thus, since the mid-19th century, it has been known that deranged hormonal secretion can significantly alter cardiovascular function. The purpose of this chapter is to summarize the more important cardiovascular manifestations of endocrine and nutritional diseases.

ACROMEGALY

The anterior pituitary gland secretes at least seven polypeptide hormones. Four (ACTH and related peptides, FSH, LH, and TSH) primarily produce their biological effect indirectly by altering hormonal secretion from a specific target gland (adrenal cortex, gonad, or thyroid). Thus, the pathophysiological manifestations of a derangement in their secretion are the same as those of their target organs and will be discussed later. There are no cardiovascular manifestations of altered prolactin secretion, but acromegaly (growth hormone excess) is associated with a number of clinical signs and symptoms related to the cardiovascular system.

ACTIONS OF GROWTH HORMONE. Growth hormone is only one of a family of peptides whose overall function is to regulate growth of the organism.[3,4] Two hormones secreted by the hypothalamus (somatotropin-releasing hormone and somatostatin) regulate the release of growth hormone from the anterior pituitary.[5,6] After growth hormone is released into the circulation, it stimulates the production of insulin-like growth factors (IGF-I and IGF-II).[7] Thus, growth hormone can exert its effect on tissues both directly and via the production of IGF-I and IGF-II.

In humans, the gene for IGF-I is located on chromosome 12 and that for IGF-II on chromosome 11 near the insulin gene. Expression of mRNAs from these genes occurs in many tissues, particularly in the fetus. They are homologues of the pro-insulin molecule and therefore have biological effects that are qualitatively similar to those of insulin.[8] Post-partum, mRNA levels are highest in the liver but also are found in a number of other tissues. IGF is synthesized in the liver in response to growth hormone and, for the most part, is bound to one of four specific binding proteins. Because the production of these binding proteins can be regulated by growth factors, they may play a functional role by producing a readily available circulating reservoir of growth factors. It is uncertain whether either or both IGFs can be produced in the absence of growth hormone, although currently available data suggest that at least IGF-II, the weaker growth-promoting hormone, may not require growth hormone for

synthesis. Thus, it is likely that IGF-I (somatomedin C) may be the major final mediator of growth hormone's biological effects.[3] It feeds back on the pituitary, modifying mRNA levels in the pituitary and growth hormone secretion.[9] In this chapter, by convention the term *growth hormone effects* is used, although most of these effects are probably mediated by the insulin-like growth factors, particularly somatomedin C.

Growth hormone effects influence many metabolic processes, but the net effect is anabolic. Thus, when growth hormone is administered to a growth hormone–deficient individual, positive nitrogen balance, with retention of calcium, sodium, potassium, magnesium, and chloride, is manifest within days.[3,4]

Growth hormone also induces changes in both fat and carbohydrate metabolism.[3,4] When administered for a short time, it increases the uptake and utilization of glucose by fat cells, thus increasing lipogenesis. However, when administered over a long period, it promotes lipolysis, thus increasing plasma free fatty acid levels and their oxidation and promoting ketogenesis, particularly in diabetic patients or animals. Growth hormone reduces glucose uptake by fat and muscle cells, increases gluconeogenesis, and increases peripheral resistance to insulin; as a consequence, plasma glucose levels rise. Because of this reduced tissue uptake of glucose and the increased blood levels of free fatty acids and ketones, those tissues, like the myocardium, that are able to use these latter compounds as energy substrates do so. Interestingly, if IGF-I is administered to patients with non–insulin-dependent diabetes mellitus, glycemic control improves and insulin sensitivity increases, in contrast to the effects of growth hormone administration.[11] Thus, it is unclear what mediates the reduced insulin sensitivity associated with excess growth hormone production. Growth hormone also increases the synthesis and/or accumulation of sulfated mucopolysaccharides in connective tissue.

EFFECT OF GROWTH HORMONE AND SOMATOSTATIN ON THE HEART. Animal studies have clarified both the acute and chronic effects of growth hormone administration. Growth hormone or IGF-I induces the expression of genes for specific contractile proteins and also those responsible for myocyte hypertrophy. Growth hormone also increases the force of contraction and shifts the myosin form to the low ATPase activity V_3 isoform[10] (see p. 406). Short-term administration of growth hormone to normal subjects, which produces changes in growth hormone levels similar to those observed in patients with mild acromegaly, increases heart rate and myocardial contractility, the latter reflected in fractional shortening of the left ventricle and mean circumferential shortening of velocity, determined by echocardiography.[12] There is no effect on mean arterial blood pressure. In adults with growth hormone deficiency, replacement therapy also modifies cardiac function, but the changes differ from those observed in normal subjects given growth hormone. Left ventricular mass, stroke volume, and cardiac output increase significantly, whereas total peripheral resistance and arterial pressure decrease. However, systolic blood pressure does not change either at rest or during exercise.[13]

Somatostatin has an effect on the heart beyond that induced by its effect on growth hormone secretion. Infusion of somatostatin causes bradycardia and a fall in cardiac output. Furthermore, in some cases of supraventricular arrhythmias somatostatin administration restores sinus rhythm.[14] Finally, cardiac nerves have been shown to contain somatostatin, suggesting that this hormone may be an important physiological regulator of cardiac conduction.[15]

CLINICAL AND BIOCHEMICAL MANIFESTATIONS. Acromegaly is almost invariably the result of a growth hormone–producing chromophobic or eosinophilic pituitary adenoma, although rarely it may be secondary to ectopic production of growth hormone or somatotropin-releasing hormone.[16,17]

A derangement in carbohydrate metabolism is the most common metabolic consequence of chronic overproduction of growth hormone. Impaired glucose tolerance is found in half the patients, and hyperinsulinism is present in nearly all; thus a state of insulin resistance exists. However, clinical diabetes mellitus is present in only 20 to 30 per cent of patients, which suggests that only those who are predisposed and have limited insulin reserve actually develop overt disease.[16] The insulin-resistant state also may contribute to other features of the disease, e.g., the hypertension. Nearly three-quarters of the subjects are overweight. Thus, it might be anticipated that hyperlipidemia would be common in acromegaly. Yet, it is in fact infrequently observed except in patients with clinical diabetes mellitus.[3,4,17] Even in these patients, it is probably secondary to the decreased secretion of insulin rather than to the increased secretion of growth hormone.

Cardiovascular Manifestations

The cardiac manifestations of acromegaly include cardiac enlargement that is greater than would be anticipated for the generalized organomegaly. In addition, the frequency of a number of other cardiovascular disorders is increased in acromegaly: hypertension, premature coronary artery disease, congestive heart failure, and cardiac arrhythmias, particularly frequent ventricular premature beats and intraventricular conduction defects.[10,18] Indeed, because of the frequent occurrence of congestive heart failure and cardiac arrhythmias in patients who otherwise have no predisposing factors (e.g., no hypertension or arteriosclerosis), it has been suggested that a specific acromegalic cardiomyopathy exists[19] (see below).

CARDIOMEGALY. Nearly all patients with acromegaly have cardiomegaly (Fig. 61–1), particularly after the fifth decade.[10,18,20] Echocardiographic assessment suggests that frequently there is an increase in cardiac mass, particularly asymmetrical septal hypertrophy, and in a sizable minority left ventricular dilatation and a reduced ejection fraction.[18,20,21] Although the cardiomegaly may be related to the generalized effect of growth hormone on protein synthesis, some data suggest that other factors may also be important. For example, enlargement of the heart is often greater than that of other organs. Furthermore, there is no direct relationship between the degree of cardiomegaly and the level of circulating growth hormone.[18,20] Although there is a correlation between the duration of acromegaly and the severity of cardiac hypertrophy,[19] other factors that may be important in the genesis of cardiomegaly include hypertension and atherosclerosis, both of which occur with increased frequency in acromegaly. Focal cardiac interstitial fibrosis and a myocarditis with lymphocytic infiltrate also

have been reported in the majority of cases.[10,19] The former is probably due to the effect of growth hormone on collagen synthesis. Additionally, small-vessel disease of the myocardium occasionally may be present.[19] The resultant dysfunction in cardiac contraction secondary to any of these pathological changes could also contribute to the cardiac enlargement. Finally, the cardiomyopathy characteristic of acromegaly may also contribute to the cardiomegaly.

HYPERTENSION. This is the most common cardiovascular manifestation of acromegaly, occurring in 25 to 50 per cent of patients if individuals with hypopituitarism are excluded. Hypertensive acromegalic patients tend to be older and to have had their acromegaly longer than nonhypertensive acromegalic patients. The underlying pathophysiology is uncertain. However, the hypertension usually is mild, uncomplicated, and readily responsive to drugs.[17] Most investigators either have searched for factors other than growth hormone that could cause hypertension or have attempted to determine how growth hormone itself may produce hypertension. In many respects, in patients with acromegaly there appears to be volume expansion; the presence of an increase in glomerular filtration rate, renal plasma flow, extracellular fluid volume and sodium space, and reduction in plasma renin activity all support this hypothesis.[4,22–24] Indeed, there is a striking increase in plasma volume in active acromegaly that is reduced following treatment.

A number of studies have suggested that growth hormone itself may be responsible for the hypertension. Thus, pituitary irradiation or hypophysectomy significantly reduces arterial pressure in hypertensive acromegalic patients, even when full glucocorticoid replacement is carried out, unless growth hormone levels are not normalized.[20] Indeed, the apparent volume expansion may be directly related to the elevated growth hormone levels because administration of growth hormone can produce retention of sodium, expansion of extracellular fluid volume, and abnormalities in white blood cell sodium transport.[25] It has been proposed that the pathophysiology of the hypertension in acromegaly may be similar to that in essential hypertension. In both conditions, there may be initial elevation of cardiac output secondary to expansion of extracellular fluid volume (see Chap. 26). This could elevate arterial pressure and lead ultimately to changes in the peripheral vasculature producing fixed hypertension.

ATHEROSCLEROSIS. In view of the alterations in carbohydrate and lipid metabolism caused by growth hormone (see above) as well as the high incidence of hypertension, it is not surprising that premature atherosclerosis occurs in pa-

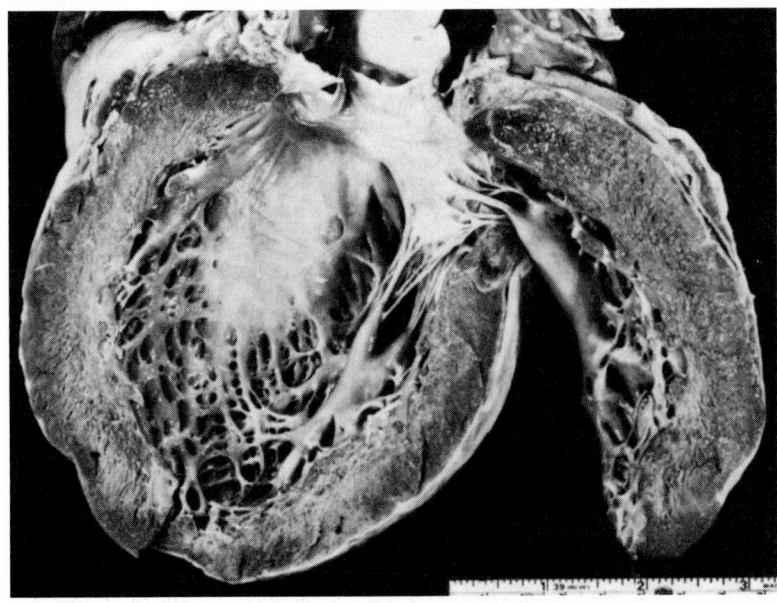

FIGURE 61–1. Opened left ventricle of the heart of an acromegalic patient showing the marked dilatation and hypertrophy, with fibrosis in the left septal endocardium. (From Rossi, L., et al.: Dysrhythmias and sudden death in acromegalic heart disease. A clinicopathologic study. Chest 72:496, 1977.)

tients with acromegaly. What is uncertain is its frequency.[19] Coronary atherosclerosis could also contribute to the cardiomegaly observed in these patients.

Acromegalic Cardiomyopathy

Some patients with acromegaly without evidence of hypertension or atherosclerosis have significant cardiac dysfunction.[19] They primarily have cardiomegaly, congestive heart failure, and/or cardiac dysrhythmias[10,26]; the congestive heart failure is particularly resistant to conventional therapy. It has been suggested that these are manifestations of an acromegalic cardiomyopathy which is related to the higher collagen content per gram of heart than in normal myocardium.[19] Histological observations show cellular hypertrophy, patchy fibrosis, and myofibrillar degeneration (Fig. 61–2). Sudden death has been associated with inflammatory and degenerative damage to the sinoatrial perinodal nerve plexus and degeneration of the AV node.

It is not clear whether acromegalic cardiomyopathy is a specific entity. The evidence favoring this view, although indirect, comes from five types of observations: (1) Nearly 50 per cent of acromegalic patients have electrocardiographic abnormalities.[26,27] The most common findings are ST-segment depression with or without T-wave abnormalities, patterns consistent with left ventricular hypertrophy, intraventricular conduction disturbances—specifically, bundle branch block—and, supraventricular or ventricular ectopic rhythms. Indeed, in one controlled study, 48 per cent of acromegalic patients had Lown grade III or IV complex ventricular arrhythmias, compared with 12 per cent of normal subjects. Although no correlation has been found between the severity of ventricular arrhythmias and growth hormone levels, the frequency of premature ventricular contractions increases with the duration of acromegaly.[26] Although hypertension or signs of atherosclerosis are present in many, 10 to 20 per cent of patients with acromegaly and electrocardiographic changes have no evidence of these conditions. (2) Ten to 20 per cent of acromegalics have overt congestive heart failure. In perhaps a fourth of these there is no known predisposing cause. (3) The major-

ity of patients with acromegaly but without hypertension or atherosclerosis have subclinical evidence for cardiac, particularly diastolic, dysfunction.[18] (4) Approximately half of all patients with acromegaly, including patients without hypertension, have echocardiographic evidence of left and right ventricular hypertrophy.[18,29,30] These patients have growth hormone levels that are significantly higher than those of patients without left ventricular hypertrophy. Half of the patients with left ventricular hypertrophy exhibit asymmetrical septal hypertrophy, and these patients have a significantly greater percentage of internal dimensional shortening during systole than either the patients with concentric hypertrophy or those without left ventricular hypertrophy.

(5) The most compelling evidence for a specific effect of growth hormone hypersecretion inducing cardiac abnormalities comes from the impact of administration of a somatostatin analog, octreotide, which inhibits secretion of growth hormone on cardiac function. In one study, seven patients with acromegaly, three of whom had refractory congestive heart failure, were given octreotide subcutaneously three times daily. Right heart catheterization performed before and after 3 months of therapy showed an 18 per cent increase in stroke volume and a return of the cardiac index to normal. Within 40 days of treatment, the three patients with congestive heart failure had a dramatic clinical improvement, which was sustained for up to 3 years.[31] In a second study, within 1 week of initiating octreotide therapy, left ventricular mass was reduced, as assessed by echocardiography.[32] In a third study in 11 normotensive patients with active acromegaly, 6 months of octreotide therapy produced a significant reduction in left ventricular mass index, mean wall thickness, and isovolumic relaxation time, as well as a significant increase in the ratio of early to late peak velocity of right ventricular filling. This improvement in diastolic function was not accompanied by significant differences in systolic function indices.[33] However, improvement in left ventricular function does not universally occur following correction of the excess growth hormone production. In some patients who have had longstanding active acromegaly, left ventricular

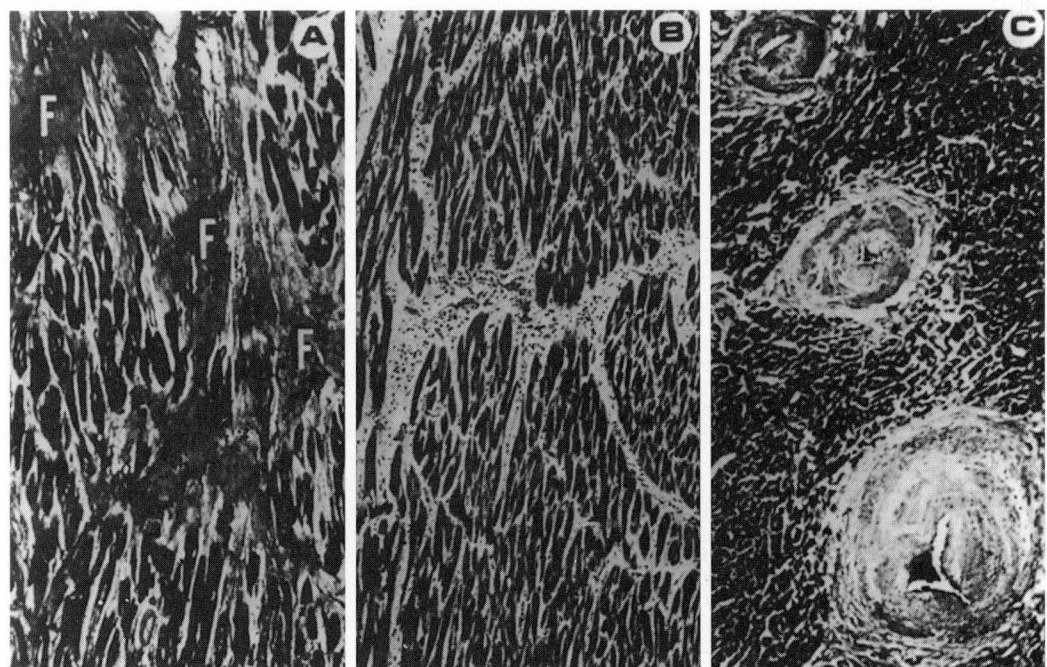

FIGURE 61–2. Histopathological features of acromegalic heart disease. *A,* Nonspecific myocardial hypertrophy and interstitial fibrosis (F). *B,* Myocarditis with predominantly lymphomononuclear cell infiltrate. *C,* Small-vessel disease (proliferative fibrous wall thickening) or intramural coronary artery branches. (Reproduced with permission from Lie, J. T.: Acromegaly and heart disease. Primary Cardiol. 7:53, 1981. Copyright PW Communications, Inc.)

filling abnormalities may be only partly reversible. In these patients, presumably nonreversible interstitial fibrosis prevents the correction of the growth hormone–induced cardiomyopathy.[34]

DIAGNOSIS AND TREATMENT

The *diagnosis* of acromegaly is established by documenting the nonsuppressibility of serum growth hormone levels following glucose loading.[3,4] In most laboratories, growth hormone concentrations in normal subjects are less than 2 ng/ml 120 minutes after the oral administration of 100 gm of glucose. It is also important to evaluate the integrity of the other pituitary hormones, and, in hypertensive patients, to rule out an associated pheochromocytoma or aldosteronoma. The presence of sinus tachycardia or atrial fibrillation in a patient with acromegaly warrants a careful search for coexisting hyperthyroidism.

Surgery and irradiation remain the mainstays of treatment. The surgical approach is more often transsphenoidal rather than transfrontal; heavy particle (proton beam) instead of conventional irradiation is often used.[3] Because of the delayed reduction in growth hormone levels with the latter method, progression of cardiovascular disease in acromegalics continues even though growth hormone levels are falling if they are not normal.[20] The secretion of growth hormone can be suppressed in some acromegalics with the dopamine agonist bromocriptine and somatostatin, the latter with considerable success.[31–33] Whether these agents have any effect on tumor growth, however, is unclear.

Acromegalic patients with cardiovascular abnormalities usually respond to conventional therapeutic measures for hypertension, heart failure, and arrhythmias. Two caveats: (1) those with hypertension appear to be particularly responsive to volume-depleting maneuvers, i.e., diuretics and sodium restriction, perhaps even more so than patients with essential hypertension; (2) on the other hand, some patients with congestive heart failure, primarily those *without* underlying hypertensive heart disease (i.e., those who are considered to have acromegalic cardiomyopathy), appear to be particularly resistant to therapy.

THYROID DISEASE

Thyroid hormone has a profound effect on a number of metabolic processes in virtually all tissues, with the heart being particularly sensitive to its effects. Therefore, it is not surprising that thyroid dysfunction can produce dramatic cardiovascular effects, often mimicking primary cardiac disease.

ACTION OF THYROID HORMONE. Two biologically active hormones are secreted by the thyroid: thyroxine (T$_4$) and tri-iodothyronine (T$_3$). Most studies support the hypothesis that T$_3$ is the final mediator and that T$_4$ is a prohormone, primarily because of the universal presence of T$_3$ but not T$_4$ nuclear receptors in tissues responsive to thyroid hormone, specifically the heart.[35–38]

Nuclear-Mediated Effects of Thyroid Hormone. Investigations over the past decade have established that the majority of thyroid hormone's effects are mediated via a change in expression of responsive genes. This process begins with the diffusion of T$_4$ and T$_3$ across the plasma membrane because of their lipid solubility. In the cytosol, T$_4$ is converted into T$_3$ by the action of 5' monodelodinase, the concentration of which varies from tissue to tissue in direct relationship to the tissue's responsiveness to thyroid hormone. Then the circulating and newly synthesized T$_3$ passes through the nuclear membrane to bind to specific thyroid hormone receptors (THRs), which are attached to chromatin tissue. The THR is part of the nuclear receptor superfamily of proteins, which also include proteins that act as receptors for steroids, vitamin D, and retinoic acid.

There are at least two thyroid hormone receptor genes—one located on chromosome 17 and the other on chromosome 3. The predominant THR form in the heart is the alpha-1, whereas the predominant receptor form in the pituitary and liver is the beta isoform. Several other isoforms also have been reported, the functions of which are unclear.[39] The thyroid hormone receptor is located almost exclusively within the nucleus. After interacting with T$_3$ and other protein transcription factors, the entire complex binds to thyroid response elements (TREs) located on the promoter region on specific genes (for additional details, the reader is referred to the review by Tsai and O'Malley[40]).

Thyroid hormone's effect on the synthesis of specific proteins can be either direct or indirect. Indirect effects include a change in production of an intermediate factor necessary for the function or activity of a more distant targeted protein. Thyroid hormone can have a positive or negative effect on regulating gene transcription. Positive effects have been documented for the following genes: myosin heavy-chain alpha[41]; Ca^{2+} ATPase[42]; Na$^+$, K$^+$-ATPase[43]; beta$_1$-adrenergic receptor[44]; glucose transporter (Glut-4)[45]; cardiac troponin I[46,47]; and atrial natriuretic protein.[48] Thyroid hormone also can negatively regulate genes, e.g., myosin heavy-chain beta and the glucose transporter Glut-1, at least neonatally.[45]

Thyroid Extranuclear Actions. Whereas the predominant effects of thyroid hormone are via its effect in regulating gene expression as noted above, there has been clear documentation that thyroid hormone also has extranuclear effects. For example, T$_3$ increases both glucose and calcium uptake by the heart. Although some of these effects could be nuclear-mediated events, some studies suggest that thyroid hormone must also have a membrane effect. Evidence supporting this includes the rapid onset (for calcium uptake, maximum effect is achieved within 30 seconds); independence from new protein synthesis; and thyroid hormone specificity in that analogs of thyroid hormone which have no biological effect do not produce similar changes.[37,49,50]

In summary, thyroid hormone's nuclear and extranuclear effects on the heart lead to changes in the proportion of myosin heavy chain protein from beta to alpha, thereby increasing myosin V$_1$ and decreasing myosin V$_3$ isoenzyme levels (see p. 363), leading to an increased velocity of contraction and diastolic relaxation. It also increases transcription of the calcium ATPase gene. Extranuclear effects include thyroid hormone's direct effect on calcium current and cytosolic calcium changes induced by inotropic factors, including isoproterenol and external calcium concentration.[51,52]

As a secondary event, thyroid hormone also increases ATP consumption. However, less of the chemical energy is used in the contractile process and more is dissipated as heat, resulting in less efficient myocardial metabolism.[35,51,52]

RELATION BETWEEN THE THYROID AND THE SYMPATHETIC NERVOUS SYSTEM

While the effects of thyroid hormone on the heart are varied and complex, it has been proposed that some of them are indirect, being secondary to changes in the activity of the sympathetic nervous system (Table 61–1). For example, many of the cardiovascular effects of hyperthyroidism, i.e., tachycardia, systolic hypertension, increased cardiac output, and myocardial contractility, can be abolished or re-

TABLE 61–1 CLINICAL FEATURES OF HYPERTHYROIDISM

DIRECT THYROID HORMONE EFFECT†	BETA-ADRENERGIC-LIKE EFFECT†
Resting heart rate > 90/min (90%)	Resting heart rate > 90/min (90%)
Palpitations (85%)	Palpitations (85%)
Atrial fibrillation (10%)	Exertional dyspnea (80%)
Pedal edema (30%)	Increased pulse pressure (systolic hypertension)
Increased oxygen consumption (basal metabolism)	Active apical impulse
Weight loss	Loud first heart sound and pulmonic component of second heart sound
Skeletal muscle myopathy	
Increased bone turnover (occasional osteoporosis or hypercalcemia)	Midsystolic murmur, usually basal
Fair skin	Third heart sound (occasional)
Fine brittle hair	Means-Lerman scratch (rare)‡
Brittle nails	Tremor
Oligomenorrhea or amenorrhea	Brisk reflexes
Increased bowel frequency	Increased perspiration
	Heat intolerance
	Insomnia
	Anxiety
	Stare, lid lag§

The numbers in parentheses are approximate prevalences of the findings, compiled from several large series. Goiter is almost always present, although in elderly patients the thyroid enlargement may be minimal or absent.

† Both types of effects contribute to the tachycardia and palpitations.

‡ A systolic scratch or click in the second left intercostal space that is probably generated by the pleura and pericardium rubbing together.

§ These reflect upper-lid retraction. Infiltrative ophthalmyopathy with exophthalmos is found only when Graves' disease is the cause of the hyperthyroidism and is not related to the hyperthyroid state per se.

Reproduced with permission from Kaplan, M. M.: The thyroid and the heart: How do they interact? J. Cardiovasc. Med. 7:893, 1982.

duced by blocking the activity of the sympathetic nervous system.[53] It has been proposed that thyroid hormone may alter the relationship between the sympathetic nervous and cardiovascular systems, either by increasing the activity of the sympathoadrenal system or by enhancing the response of cardiac tissue to normal sympathetic stimulation.[54] Also, it has been suggested that sympathetic stimuli merely exert a direct additive effect on cardiovascular function above that produced by thyroid hormone. On the other hand, there is also evidence that hyperthyroidism reduces the sensitivity of cardiac tissue to sympathetic stimuli.[55]

Thus the results of experiments on the relationship between the sympathoadrenal system and hyperthyroidism have evoked considerable controversy. Three areas have been explored in an attempt to unravel the conflicting data: thyroid hormone's effect on adrenergic output; thyroid hormone's effect on adrenergic receptors; and thyroid hormone's action on adrenergic transduction mechanisms. The plasma and urine levels of norepinephrine, epinephrine, dopamine, and beta-hydroxylase are either low or normal in hyperthyroidism and either normal or elevated in hypothyroidism.[56] These data suggest that the sympathomimetic features of hyperthyroidism cannot be due simply to an overall increase in adrenergic activity but rather are due to a change in the affinity of catecholamines for their receptors or to a modification of a postreceptor mechanism. Previously such changes were difficult to document, primarily because thyroid hormone appears to have different effects on adrenoceptors in different tissues. For example, the effect of thyroid hormone in the rat liver is different from that in the rat heart. Thyroid hormones reduce beta-adrenoceptor number in the rat liver, and hypothyroid animals show an increase in these receptors.[57] In contrast, in the rat heart, which has been the organ most extensively studied, administration of thyroid hormone causes both an increase in the number of receptors and their affinity for their ligand, while hypothyroidism induces the opposite effect.[54,58] Finally is the documentation that thyroid hormone increases the mRNA level for the beta$_1$-adrenergic receptor.[44]

These changes in receptor number and affinity lead to appropriate changes in sensitivity of the myocardium to beta-adrenoceptor agonists. For example, stimulation of adenylate cyclase activity by isoproterenol is increased in hyperthyroidism and reduced in hypothyroidism. Finally, there are also changes in the force of contraction with increased sensitivity of the ventricular muscle to isoproterenol-induced contraction in hyperthyroidism and reduction in hypothyroidism.[54] That this effect is specific is shown by an unaltered change in calcium-stimulated contractility in hypothyroid animals. These effects were also observed in vivo in dogs in which propranolol-induced reductions of heart rate and myocardial contractility were greater in hyperthyroid than in euthyroid animals.[59]

Further support comes from the study by Guarnieri et al., who showed that hyperthyroid rats have enhanced activation of protein kinase and contractile response following administration of a threshold dose of the beta-adrenoceptor agonist isoproterenol.[60] In the aforementioned study in conscious hyperthyroid dogs,[59] however, no alteration in the sensitivity of the inotropic response to isoproterenol and norepinephrine was found.

Circulating blood elements have also provided additional evidence in support of the concept that thyroid hormone "up-regulates" beta-adrenoceptors. When patients are used as their own control, both the number of beta-adrenoceptors and the sensitivity of adenylate cyclase to isoproterenol stimulation in mononuclear cells are increased by thyroid hormone.[61] Additionally, in circulating reticulocytes of hypothyroid animals, the number of receptors is decreased.[62]

The evidence supporting an additional effect of thyroid hormone in modifying the transduction mechanisms mediating adrenergic effects is less clear. In cultured developing rat myocardial cells, the addition of T$_3$ increased the level of G$_{s\alpha}$ protein while reducing G$_{i\alpha}$ and the β subunits of G proteins. These results suggest that thyroid hormone elevates G protein subunits that activate adenylate cyclase and suppresses those that inhibit it. However, Levine et al. could not document an effect of thyroid hormone on G$_{s}\alpha$ subunits using adult rat ventricles, although an apparent inhibitory effect of thyroid hormone on G$_{i\alpha}$ 2 and 3, and Gβ 1 and 2 protein, polypeptide, and mRNA levels was confirmed.[64] Similar effects have been reported for adipose tissue,[65] probably explaining the reduced lipolytic response to catecholamines in hypothyroidism.[66] Thus, thyroid hormone has a complex interaction with the adrenergic nervous system. Hyperthyroidism increases the number, and potentially the affinity, of beta-adrenergic receptors and also modifies the intracellular G protein milieu so as to enhance the transduction potential of agonists binding to the adrenergic receptor.

Effect of Thyroid Hormone on the Heart

There is abundant evidence that thyroid hormone may alter cardiac function directly, as noted above. Additionally, the increased heart rate and myocardial contractility observed in experimental hyperthyroidism are not completely reversed by either sympathetic or parasympathetic blockade.[55,59] Finally, T$_4$ enhances the rate of contraction of cardiac muscle even in the presence of adrenergic block-

ade.[67] Right ventricular papillary muscles isolated from cats rendered hyperthyroid exhibited augmented myocardial contractility, as reflected in an upward shift of the myocardial force-velocity curve,[55] with a greatly increased velocity of myocardial fiber shortening, a reduced time to peak tension during isometric contraction, and an augmented peak tension development. Single ventricular myocytes isolated from hyperthyroid rats exhibited a marked augmentation of twitch velocity and abbreviated both the time required for contraction and relaxation.[68] Prior catecholamine depletion by pretreatment of the hyperthyroid cats with reserpine did not alter this inotropic effect of hyperthyroidism, providing further evidence for a direct cardiac effect.[55] This hypothesis has been assessed in intact conscious animals. The results suggest that the major actions of T$_4$ on the left ventricle are (1) a direct positive inotropic effect and (2) an increase in the size of the ventricular cavity without a change in the end-diastolic pressure or length of the sarcomere in diastole, although hypothyroidism does not necessarily impair pump function.[69]

The available data suggest that the direct effect of thyroid hormone on the heart is primarily mediated via a change in protein synthesis, as described above. Specifically, there is a change in synthesis of the myosin heavy chains from the β to the α form, thereby increasing the level of the more mobile myosin isoenzyme (V$_1$). With the reduction in mRNA level for the beta myosin heavy chain, the slower V$_3$ myosin isoform is substantially reduced. Goto et al. demonstrated in the hyperthyroid rabbit heart that the increase in myosin isoform V$_1$/V$_3$ ratio is associated with decreased contractile efficiency and increased energy cost of excitation-contraction coupling.[70] This change produces a less efficient system, thereby leading to more heat production per contractile response.

Thyroid hormone's effect on cardiac contractility also appears to be mediated in part by changes in intracellular calcium handling. Thyroid hormone increases the expression of the sodium-calcium-ATPase, which augments trans-sarcolemmal calcium influx in cultured ventricular cells.[71]

In ferret ventricular muscle, hypothyroidism reduces peak tension and prolongs the duration of contraction in association with changes in cytosolic calcium that are decreased and prolonged in relation to ventricular muscle obtained from euthyroid animals (Fig. 61–3). Hyperthyroidism produces the opposite changes. Thus, alteration in intracellular calcium handling, specifically related to recycling of calcium by the sarcoplasmic reticulum, may account for the thyroid-induced changes in myocardial contractile function.[72,73] Finally, the effect of thyroxine on myosin isoenzyme appears to be localized primarily to the ventricles, with atrial isoenzymes relatively unaltered by changes in thyroid hormone.[74] Thus, while thyroid hormone itself has a major direct effect on modifying protein synthesis, the changes in cardiac workload may also contribute. Studies using heterotrophic cardiac isografts suggest that the changes in myosin enzyme levels may in part be secondary to changes in workload.[75]

The tachycardia observed in hyperthyroidism appears to be due to a combination of an increased rate of diastolic depolarization and a decreased duration of the action potential in the sinoatrial node cells.[76] The propensity for the development of atrial fibrillation may be due to the shortened refractory period of atrial cells.[77]

Hyperthyroidism

Hyperthyroidism is the clinical state resulting from the excess production of T$_3$, T$_4$, or both. The most common cause is a diffuse toxic goiter (Graves' disease). Although the etiology of this condition is still unknown, the hyperproduction of T$_4$ and T$_3$ is thought to result from circulating IgG autoantibodies that bind to the thyrotropin receptor on the thyroid gland. The second most common form of hyperthyroidism is nodular toxic goiter, a condition in which localized areas of the gland function excessively and autonomously.[78]

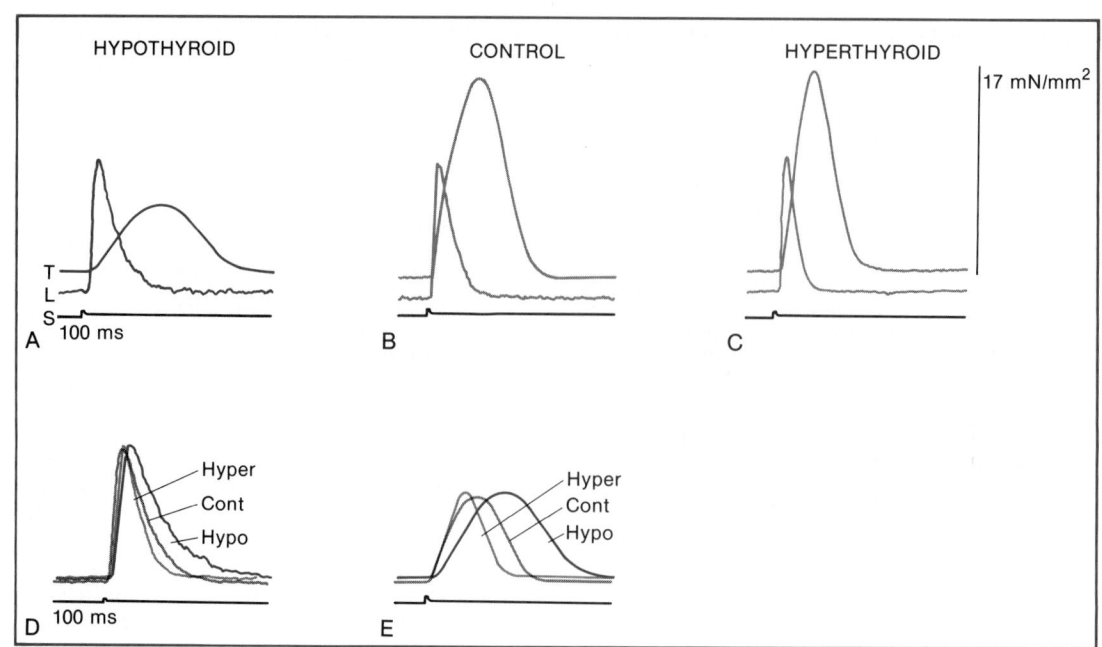

FIGURE 61–3. The thyroid state influences the time course of the isometric contraction and the Ca⁺⁺ transient. The isometric tension (T) and the aequorin light signal, reflecting intracytoplasmic [Ca]⁺⁺ (L), were recorded from myocardium obtained from a hypothyroid (A), euthyroid (B), and hyperthyroid (C) ferret at 30°C; 0.33 Hz stimulation. I is expressed in milliNewtons/m² muscle cross-sectional area. The Ca⁺⁺ transients (aequorin signals) are scaled to equal amplitudes and superimposed in D. In E, the tensions have been scaled to equal amplitudes and superimposed. The time from the beginning of the stimulus sweep (S) to the stimulus represents 100 msec. (Reproduced with permission from MacKinnon, R., et al.: Modulation by the thyroid state of intracellular calcium and contractility in ferret ventricular muscle. Circ. Res. *63:*1084, 1988. Copyright 1988 American Heart Association.)

Hyperthyroidism is a relatively common disease, occurring four to eight times more commonly in women than in men, with a peak incidence in the third and fourth decades. The commonly associated signs and symptoms (Table 61–1) include fatigue, hyperactivity, insomnia, heat intolerance, palpitations, dyspnea, increased appetite with weight loss, nocturia, diarrhea, oligomenorrhea, muscle weakness, tremor, emotional lability, increased heart rate, systolic hypertension, hyperthermia, warm moist skin, lid lag, stare, and brisk reflexes. T_3 levels are invariably elevated, and serum T_4 levels are usually increased as well.

CARDIOVASCULAR MANIFESTATIONS. The heart is among the most responsive organs in thyroid disease, and cardiovascular signs and symptoms are therefore important clinical features of hyperthyroidism.[78,79] Palpitations, dyspnea, tachycardia, and systolic hypertension are common findings. Diastolic hypertension can also occur. Typically, there is a hyperactive precordium with a loud first heart sound, an accentuated pulmonic component of the second heart sound, and a third heart sound; occasionally, a systolic ejection click is heard. Midsystolic murmurs along the left sternal border are common, and a systolic scratch, the so-called Means-Lerman scratch, is occasionally heard in the second left intercostal space during expiration. It is presumed to be secondary to the rubbing together of normal pleural and pericardial surfaces by the hyperdynamic heart.

As would be anticipated, and as described on page 447, cardiac and stroke volume index, mean systolic ejection rate, velocity and extent of wall shortening (Fig. 61–4), and coronary blood flow[80] are all increased, the systolic ejection period and preejection period are abbreviated, the pulse pressure is widened, and systemic vascular resistance is reduced in hyperthyroidism.[81] The changes in left ventricular performance induced by thyroid hormone appear to be secondary to augmented contractility rather than to alterations in loading conditions or change in heart rate.[82] If the hyperthyroidism is relatively mild, many of the indices of left ventricular function are normal, with exercise needed to bring out abnormalities.[79,83] It has been suggested that many of the changes in cardiac function are secondary to

the increased metabolic demands of peripheral tissue. However, the increase in cardiac output is greater than would be predicted on the basis of the increased total body oxygen consumption, supporting the view that thyroid hormone exerts a direct cardiac stimulant action independent of its effect on general tissue metabolism, as noted above. Furthermore, normalization of myocardial contractile response to exercise may not occur until several months after normalization of thyroid function.[84] However, it is likely that the overall pathological consequences associated with

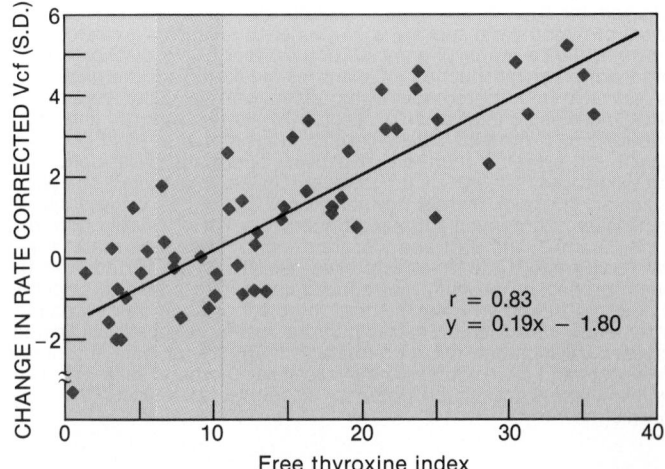

FIGURE 61–4. Rate-corrected velocity of shortening (V_{cf}) in SD units from the normal mean regression line obtained from 11 patients at varying levels of the free thyroxine index. There is a strong positive correlation between the level of thyroid hormone and the change in contractile state. The shaded area represents the normal range for serum free thyroxine index. (From Feldman, T., et al.: Myocardial mechanics in hyperthyroidism: Importance of left ventricular loading conditions, heart rate and contractile state. By permission of the American College of Cardiology. J. Am. Coll. Cardiol. *7:*972, 1986.)

thyrotoxicosis result from an interaction between the effect of thyroid hormone on the heart and its effect on the circulation (Fig. 61–5).

Roentgenographic and electrographic changes are common but are nonspecific in hyperthyroidism.[79] Thus the left ventricle, the aorta, and the pulmonary artery are prominent, and, in some cases, there is generalized cardiac enlargement, which may be accompanied by signs and symptoms of heart failure. In patients with sinus rhythm, the magnitude of the tachycardia, in general, parallels the severity of the disease. Sinus tachycardia, i.e., a rate exceeding 100 beats/min, is present in 40 per cent of patients with hyperthyroidism, occurring most frequently in the younger age groups, and often at night.[85] Fifteen to 25 per cent of patients with hyperthyroidism have persistent atrial fibrillation, which is often heralded by one or more transient episodes of this arrhythmia.[86] There is shortening of the A-V conduction time and functional refractory period, resulting in an increased frequency at which the A-V conduction system transmits rapid atrial impulses.[86] Intra-atrial conduction disturbances, manifested by prolongation or notching of the P wave and prolongation of the P-R interval in the absence of treatment with digitalis, occur in 15 per cent and 5 per cent of patients with hyperthyroidism, respectively. Occasionally, second- or third-degree heart block may result. The cause of the A-V conduction disturbance is not clear because animal experiments have shown that the functional refractory period of the A-V conduction system and the conduction time were shortened in dogs with hyperthyroidism and prolonged in dogs with hypothyroidism.[87] Intraventricular conduction disturbances, most commonly right bundle branch block, occur in about 15 per cent of patients with hyperthyroidism without associated heart disease of other etiology. Paroxysmal supraventricular tachycardia and flutter are rare in hyperthyroidism. Finally, occult thyrotoxicosis may underlie either chronic or paroxysmal isolated atrial fibrillation.[86,88]

Both angina pectoris and heart failure occur in patients with hyperthyroidism, and for many years it was assumed that these were seen only in the presence of underlying cardiovascular disease. Support for this position came primarily from the absence of these symptoms in young persons with significant hyperthyroidism. More recently, however, five lines of evidence have suggested otherwise: (1) Congestive heart failure has been produced in experimental animals by simply administering T_4. (2) Children with thy-

rotoxicosis without underlying cardiac disease may develop congestive heart failure.[89] (3) Angina has been reported in a hyperthyroid patient with normal coronary arteries, presumably secondary to thyroid-induced coronary artery spasm.[90] (4) Abnormal left ventricular function observed during exercise in hyperthyroid subjects is not reversed by beta blockade but is reversed by treating the hyperthyroidism.[91] (5) Finally, Ebisawa et al. reported that the cardiomyopathy in patients with thyrotoxicosis may be irreversible. Four patients with this condition had increased left ventricular end-diastolic volumes and reduced ejection fractions, even 13 to 15 years following treatment of their hyperthyroidism. Myocardial biopsies, performed in two patients, showed no specific light microscopic abnormalities.[92]

Thus, when it is severe and persistent, thyrotoxicosis can overtax even the normal heart, although, in most instances, the development of clinical manifestations of heart failure and myocardial ischemia in patients with hyperthyroidism signifies the presence of underlying cardiac or coronary vascular disease. There is also increased frequency of hyperthyroidism in patients with familial hypertrophic cardiomyopathy. In one kindred, 3 of 17 members with hypertrophic cardiomyopathy also had hyperthyroidism.[93] Finally, in one study hyperthyroidism was associated with mitral value prolapse in more than a third of cases.[94]

TREATMENT OF CARDIOVASCULAR DISEASE IN HYPERTHYROIDISM. Hyperthyroid patients with cardiovascular disease are particularly resistant to therapy. For example, it has been well documented that both heart failure and arrhythmias are resistant to conventional doses of the cardiac glycosides. Although the specific mechanisms underlying these altered responses remain obscure, they may be related to both systemic and local effects.[95] First, serum levels of cardiac glycosides are diminished in hyperthyroidism, not because there is an augmentation of its metabolism but because there is an increase in its volume of distribution. Second, experimental hyperthyroidism reduces the enhancement of the myocardial contractile force and the prolongation of the atrioventricular nodal refractory period produced by these agents.[95] Because of this decreased sensitivity to cardiac glycosides, toxicity may develop at a dose that has relatively little therapeutic effect.

DIAGNOSIS AND THERAPY OF HYPERTHYROIDISM

The diagnosis is made on the basis of a suppressed TSH level (reflecting elevated levels of thyroid hormone in the blood). Because only serum T_3 is increased in some individuals, it is important to obtain serum levels of *both* T_3 and T_4 and an index of the thyroid-binding capacity of the patient's serum (resin thyroxine uptake).

The definitive treatment of hyperthyroidism is surgical removal of the gland or irradiation using radioactive iodide. In severely ill patients, particularly those with thyroid storm or significant cardiovascular symptoms or both, neither of these therapies is appropriate. Thus, medical therapy is directed at reducing both the production and biological effect of thyroid hormone.[96] Because many of the cardiovascular symptoms of thyrotoxicosis are related to increased beta-adrenoceptor activity, treatment with beta-adrenoceptor blocking agents has been useful.[97] Tachycardia, palpitations, tremor, restlessness, muscle weakness, and heat intolerance are reversed by these agents, which offer the additional benefit of inhibiting the conversion of T_4 to the biologically active T_3 in peripheral tissues.

TREATMENT OF CARDIOVASCULAR MANIFESTATIONS OF HYPERTHYROIDISM. Prompt treatment of the hyperthyroid state can significantly reduce, if not eliminate, the associated cardiovascular symptoms. About half of patients with concurrent onset of hyperthyroidism and angina pectoris experience complete remission of this symptom after treatment of hyperthyroidism.[98,99] Furthermore, in 62 per cent of 163 thyrotoxic patients with atrial fibrillation sustained for 1 week or longer, spontaneous reversion to sinus rhythm was found when they became euthyroid.[100,101] In elderly patients with apathetic hyperthyroidism, cardiovascular manifestations, specifically atrial fibrillation and/or congestive heart failure, predominate, and therefore evaluation of thyroid function in such patients is particularly

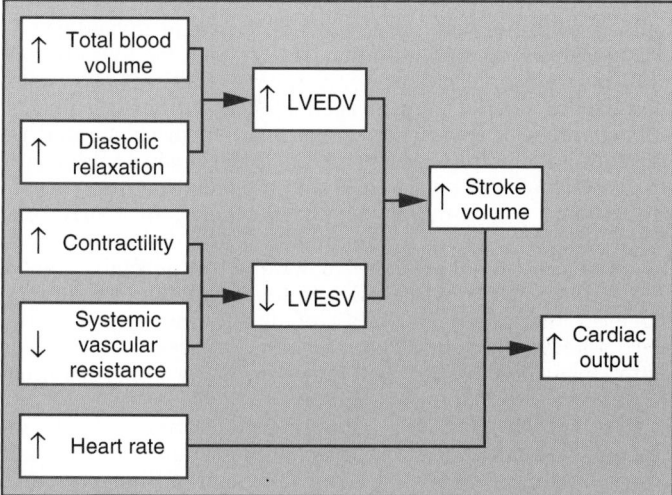

FIGURE 61–5. Cardiovascular effects of hyperthyroidism. Cardiac output is increased as a result of thyroid hormone augmentation of the hemodynamic parameters indicated in the figure. LVEDV = Left ventricular end-diastolic volume; LVESV = left ventricular end-systolic volume. (Modified from Woeber, K. A.: Thyrotoxicosis and the heart. N. Engl. J. Med. 327:94, 1992. Copyright Massachusetts Medical Society.)

important. However, it should be noted that these individuals are particularly resistant to cardiac glycosides.

Beta blockers (see p. 502) can be administered orally or intravenously, but because these drugs interfere with the effects of sympathetic stimulation on the heart, they must be used with caution in patients with congestive heart failure. However, if the heart failure is in part related to the tachycardia, beta blockade may be beneficial.[97] Beta-blocking drugs and cardiac glycosides act synergistically to slow ventricular rate in atrial fibrillation. Correction of the basic metabolic defect requires specific therapy directed at reducing the production of thyroid hormone.[97,99] The most useful agents are the thionamides, such as propylthiouracil,[96] which inhibit thyroid hormone synthesis. Iodine inhibits the release of thyroid hormones from the thyrotoxic gland, and its beneficial effects occur more rapidly than the thionamides. It is therefore useful in the rapid amelioration of the hyperthyroid state in patients with thyroid heart disease. Ipodate may be particularly useful for this purpose.[102] Iodine may also be utilized along with antithyroid agents to control thyrotoxicosis following ^{131}I treatment until the radioactive iodide has had time to take effect. Most hyperthyroid patients, however, escape from the effects of iodide after 10 to 14 days.

Hypothyroidism

Hypothyroidism results from reduced secretion of both T_4 and T_3, occurring in most cases as a consequence of destruction of the thyroid gland itself, usually by an inflammatory process. In some cases, it is secondary to decreased secretion of TSH, due to either pituitary or hypothalamic disease. In secondary hypothyroidism, the signs and symptoms associated with deficiency of other pituitary hormones are also usually present. The incidence of hypothyroidism peaks between the ages of 30 and 60 years, and it is twice as common in women as in men. The following signs and symptoms are common: cold intolerance, dryness of the skin, weakness, impairment of memory, personality changes, shortness of breath, constipation, hoarseness, menorrhagia and other forms of menstrual dysfunction, and, occasionally, heart failure.

EFFECTS OF AMIODARONE ON THYROID FUNCTION. The antiarrhythmic agent amiodarone (see p. 613) has three effects on thyroid function. Its first effect is to antagonize thyroid hormone action on pituitary cells by binding to the intranuclear thyroid hormone receptor, and it thereby inhibits T_3-induced changes in mRNA levels and TSH response to TRH.[103,104] Its second effect is to inhibit peripheral conversion of T_4 to T_3. Thus, in nearly all patients who receive long-term treatment with this drug, there is reduction in serum T_3 levels and a transient rise in TSH. Within a few days to weeks this causes an increase in serum T_4 levels and a return of serum TSH to normal. Clinically and metabolically, these patients are euthyroid even though their T_4 levels are elevated.[105] Amiodarone's third effect is due to its high iodide content (35 per cent by weight). Thus, when it is metabolized there is a massive increase in the available inorganic iodide, resulting in acute inhibition of thyroid organification. Depending upon the state of iodine intake before its administration, patients may develop either hypothyroidism (common in the United States) or thyrotoxicosis (more common in Europe).[105-107]

In susceptible individuals this agent can also induce a marked increase in Ia-positive T cells (an abnormality found in patients with spontaneous Graves' disease). These T-cell abnormalities disappear after discontinuation of the amiodarone. Thus, amiodarone may induce T-cell abnormalities leading to an autoimmune state.[108] Because of amiodarone's long half-life, the biochemical and clinical abnormalities can persist for months after it is stopped.

CARDIOVASCULAR MANIFESTATIONS (Fig. 61–6). The heart in overt myxedema is often pale, flabby, and grossly dilated. Histological examination discloses myofibrillar swelling, loss of striations, and interstitial fibrosis. With the early detection and treatment of hypothyroidism, the classic findings of cardiac enlargement, cardiac dilatation, significant bradycardia, weak arterial pulses, hypotension, distant heart sounds, low electrocardiographic voltages, nonpitting facial and peripheral edema, and evidence of congestive heart failure, such as ascites, orthopnea, and paroxysmal dyspnea, are now seen only infrequently. However, exertional dyspnea and easy fatigability continue to be common complaints.

Myxedema is associated with increased capillary permeability and subsequent leakage of protein into the intersti-

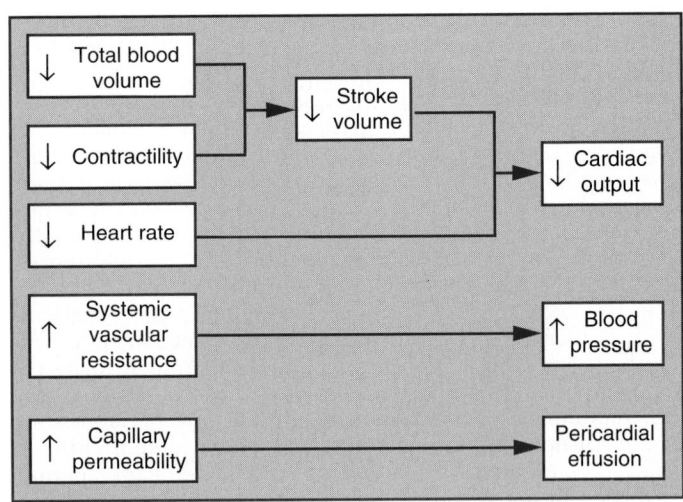

FIGURE 61–6. Cardiovascular effects of hypothyroidism. Cardiac output is decreased because of diminished total blood volume, impaired left ventricular contractility, and bradycardia. Hypertension results from increased systemic vascular resistance. Pericardial effusion results from increased capillary permeability and interstitial protein leak.

tial space, resulting in pericardial effusion, a common clinical finding in overt myxedema, occurring in about one-third of all patients (see p. 1521). Rarely, it is complicated by cardiac tamponade.[109] Echocardiography is the most useful method of establishing the diagnosis (see p. 93). The effusions disappear with thyroid replacement therapy.[110] Myxedema-associated cardiogenic shock has also rarely been reported. It, too, responds to thyroid replacement therapy.[111]

The electrocardiographic changes include sinus bradycardia and prolongation of the Q-T interval. The P-wave amplitude is usually very low. It is possible that hypothermia may contribute to reentrant ventricular arrhythmias.[112] The incidence of atrioventricular and intraventricular conduction disturbances is about three times greater in patients with myxedema than in the general population. Incomplete or complete right bundle branch block has been observed, and a primary myocardial abnormality suggestive of a cardiomyopathy has been reported.[113] Other electrocardiographic changes are those associated with pericardial effusion[110] (see p. 1485).

There is increased frequency of hypertension in patients with hypothyroidism, although not in severe myxedema.[114] In one study of 477 patients, 15 per cent of hypothyroid subjects had a blood pressure greater than 160/95, compared with 5.5 per cent in age-matched euthyroid subjects. Replacement of thyroid hormone resulted in substantial reduction in blood pressure in the hypertensive patients.[115] In a study of 688 consecutive hypertensive patients, hypothyroidism was found in 25 (3.5 per cent). In nearly one-third of this subgroup, treatment of the hypothyroidism lowered the blood pressure to within the normal range.[114] Thus, individuals with mild to moderate hypothyroidism have an increased possibility of developing hypertension, particularly diastolic hypertension, whereas individuals with severe hypothyroidism are more likely to have normal or slightly low blood pressures.[114-116]

MYOCARDIAL EFFECTS. Hypothyroid patients have reduced cardiac output, stroke volume, and blood and plasma volumes.[117,118] Right and left heart filling pressures are usually within normal limits unless they are elevated by a pericardial effusion. There is a redistribution of blood flow with mild reductions in cerebral and renal flow and significant reductions in cutaneous flow. Ventricular isovolumetric relaxation time is prolonged and is normalized during T_4 replacement.[119,120] The impact of hypothyroidism on cardiac function can occur quickly in patients rendered hypothyroid for assessment of thyroid status in the treatment of thyroid cancer. Two weeks after discontinuing thyroid medication the left ventricular end-diastolic diameter and peak velocity of early diastolic filling, as well as heart rate, were reduced. There were no changes in systolic or diastolic blood pressure.[121]

Cardiac muscle isolated from cats with experimentally produced hypothyroidism exhibited reduced contractility, characterized by a depression of the myocardial force-velocity curve, a reduction of the rate of tension development, and a prolongation of the contractile response.

There is little evidence that congestive heart failure is common in myxedema or that it occurs in the absence of other cardiac disease.[122] Presumably the depressed myocardial contractility is sufficient to sustain the reduced workload placed on the heart in hypothyroidism. However, it may be difficult to distinguish between symptoms of myxedema and heart failure. Dyspnea, edema, effusions, cardiomegaly, and T-wave changes occur in both conditions. In left heart failure, pulmonary arterial pressure is usually elevated during exercise, cardiac output fails to rise normally, and the Valsalva response is normal, whereas the opposite occurs in myxedema.[122] Also, the hemodynamic changes in myxedema respond to thyroid hormone administration.

Cardiac catecholamine levels are not reduced in hypothyroidism. Neither the sensitivity of the mechanical performance of the heart to sympathetic nerve stimulation nor the response of the cardiac adenylate cyclase to norepinephrine is altered in hypothyroidism. However, there is a reduction in the total number of myocardial beta receptors.[62,63] Both isoproterenol-stimulated contractility and the accumulation of cyclic AMP are reduced in hearts obtained from hypothyroid rats.[123] In experimental hypothyroidism, calcium in isolated myocardial sarcoplasmic reticulum particles is reduced, which may explain the altered contractile state.[70]

ATHEROSCLEROSIS. It has been suggested that patients with hypothyroidism are at increased risk of developing atherosclerosis, because this disease is accompanied by significant changes in lipid metabolism. Thus, hypercholesterolemia and hypertriglyceridemia, which are associated with the development of premature coronary artery disease, are found in patients with hypothyroidism.[124] Furthermore, treatment of patients with hypothyroidism corrects the abnormal lipid pattern. For example, Arem and Patsch noted a 22 per cent reduction in mean LDL cholesterol concentration after 4 months of thyroid replacement therapy.[125] HDL cholesterol levels did not change appreciably. Support for a connection between hypothyroidism and atherosclerosis has come from several sources, including the documentation that the latter occurs with twice the frequency in patients with myxedema than in age- and sex-matched controls and that the development of atherosclerosis in cholesterol-fed animals is enhanced by the presence of hypothyroidism and reduced when thyroid hormone is administered.[126,127] Yet myocardial infarction and angina pectoris are relatively uncommon in hypothyroidism. The latter was present in only 7 per cent of a group of such patients.[128] This low frequency of cardiac complications from atherosclerosis may simply reflect the decreased metabolic demand on the myocardium in hypothyroidism. However, the known effects of hypothyroidism on serum enzyme concentrations do complicate the assessment of chest pain in patients with myxedema.[129]

DIAGNOSIS AND TREATMENT OF HYPOTHYROIDISM

Caution must be exercised in treating hypothyroid patients who are elderly and who may have underlying heart disease, to avoid precipitating myocardial infarction or severe congestive heart failure; a slow replacement program is indicated in these individuals.

The treatment of congestive heart failure is particularly difficult in patients with myxedema, both because of the effect of thyroid hormone on the heart and because the heart's response to cardiac gly-

cosides is altered.[95] Patients with severe angina pectoris and untreated myxedema pose a difficult clinical dilemma because angina may be exacerbated by thyroid hormone replacement, and the usual medical management of angina with beta blockers may induce severe bradycardia. Coronary arteriography often shows severe coronary artery disease in these patients, and an excellent surgical team can perform successful coronary revascularization with minimal thyroid replacement. Full thyroid replacement can then be safely achieved during the postoperative period, without the recurrence of angina.[130-132]

DISEASES OF THE ADRENAL CORTEX

Since Addison's description in 1849 of adrenal insufficiency,[2] it has been appreciated that steroids secreted by the adrenal cortex exert a significant effect on the cardiovascular system, primarily by altering blood pressure. Adrenal insufficiency is characterized by significant hypotension, whereas excessive production of adrenal steroids is often accompanied by hypertension.

Three classes of steroids are secreted by the adrenal cortex: glucocorticoids, e.g., cortisol; mineralocorticoids, e.g., aldosterone; and androgens, e.g., dehydroepiandrosterone. In this section, the physiology and pathophysiology of glucocorticoid and mineralocorticoid secretion are addressed.

HORMONE ACTIONS

CORTISOL. The primary glucocorticoid, cortisol, is synthesized from cholesterol in the inner layers of the adrenal cortex. Its average plasma concentration is 15 μg/dl in the morning, falling to 5 μg/dl by early evening.[133] The fundamental mechanism of action of the glucocorticoids is similar to that of other steroid hormones. They enter a target tissue by diffusion and combine with a specific high-affinity cytoplasmic receptor protein. The receptor-cortisol complex is then transferred to specific acceptor sites on nuclear chromatin tissue (promoter region) where it produces an increase in RNA and later protein synthesis. The major action of glucocorticoids is to promote gluconeogenesis, and, in that respect, they are both catabolic and anti-insulin.

Glucocorticoids also have anti-inflammatory properties related to their effects on both the microvasculature and the lymphatic system. They maintain normal vascular responsiveness to circulating vasoconstrictors, such as norepinephrine, and have a major effect on both the distribution and excretion of body water.

ALDOSTERONE. The major mineralocorticoid produced by the human adrenal gland is aldosterone. It is also synthesized from cholesterol but almost exclusively in the outer layer (glomerulosa) of the adrenal cortex. Aldosterone has two important functions: (1) it is a major regulator of extracellular fluid volume by its effect on sodium retention, and (2) it is a major determinant of potassium metabolism. Aldosterone acts predominantly on the distal convoluted tubule and/or collecting duct of the kidney, where it promotes the reabsorption of sodium. Potassium then diffuses into the lumen of the tubules because of the change in electrochemical gradient produced by the active reabsorption of the positively charged sodium ion. Hydrogen ion may also be more freely excreted because of this change in the electrochemical gradient. Although aldosterone also acts on salivary and sweat glands and on the endothelial cells of the gastrointestinal tract, these have little impact on total body sodium and potassium homeostasis.

There are three well-defined control mechanisms for aldosterone release.[133,134]

1. The renin-angiotensin system is the major system for the control of extracellular fluid volume by regulating aldosterone secretion. Aldosterone is linked in a negative feedback loop with the renin-angiotensin system. Thus, during periods registered as volume deficiency there is increased release of the enzyme renin from the juxtaglomerular cells of the kidney. Renin then increases the production of angiotensin I from its substrate. Angiotensin I is rapidly converted into the biologically active angiotensin II, which increases aldosterone secretion. Angiotensin II also produces vasoconstriction, thereby raising blood pressure and reducing blood flow to a variety of tissues, especially the kidney.

2. Potassium ion also regulates aldosterone secretion independent of the renin-angiotensin system; elevation of potassium concentration increases aldosterone secretion and vice versa. The adrenal cortex is very sensitive to changes in potassium concentration with as little as 0.1 mEq/liter increment producing significant changes in the plasma aldosterone levels.

3. ACTH also has been documented to affect aldosterone secretion profoundly. However, because the control of aldosterone release is not appreciably altered in patients who have been on a long-term regimen of steroid therapy, ACTH probably has a smaller role than the other two factors in maintaining normal aldosterone secretion.

In addition to these major stimuli controlling aldosterone secretion, salt-losing hormones such as atrial natriuretic peptide (see p. 1917) and dopamine inhibit aldosterone secretion, particularly in response to angiotensin II.[134] Finally, the poor dietary intake of both sodium and potassium alters the magnitude of the aldosterone response to acute stimulation, sodium restriction, and potassium loading, both enhancing the response of the adrenal, perhaps by modifying the local (adrenal) renin-angiotensin system.[133,134]

Diseases of the adrenal cortex, therefore, primarily affect the cardiovascular system via changes in blood pressure or volume homeostasis. However, aldosterone, and perhaps angiotensin II itself, also can have a direct effect on collagen metabolism in cardiac fibroblasts. In both primary aldosteronism and renal vascular hypertension, there is a reactive perivascular and interstitial fibrosis that does not seem to be due to pressure overload alone. Documentation of this effect has been provided by in vitro studies using cardiac fibroblasts. Both angiotensin II and aldosterone increase the collagen synthesis and collagenase activity. These effects could be completely abolished by either type I or type II angiotensin II receptor antagonists or the competitive aldosterone antagonist, spironolactone.[135]

Cushing's Syndrome
(See also p. 829)

In 1932 Harvey Cushing reported a syndrome characterized by truncal obesity, hypertension, fatigue, weakness, amenorrhea, hirsutism, purple abdominal striae, glucosuria, edema, and osteoporosis.[136] The majority of cases are secondary to bilateral adrenal hyperplasia, with the predominant feature being excess production of glucocorticoids and androgens.[133] Some cases are due to ACTH-producing tumors of either the pituitary gland (Cushing's disease) or nonendocrine tissue (ectopic ACTH production). Fifteen to 20 per cent of the cases are due to primary adrenal neoplasia, either adenoma or carcinoma. Most patients have the typical body habitus: central obesity and slender extremities with proximal muscle weakness. Hypertension is present in 80 to 90 per cent of patients, and diabetes occurs in 20 per cent, probably in those individuals with a predisposition.[133] Evidence of androgen excess may also be present, including hirsutism, amenorrhea, and clitoromegaly.

Laboratory tests disclose evidence of excess production of both glucocorticoids and androgens in the majority of cases. Thus, urinary metabolites of these steroids, 17-ketosteroids and 17-hydroxysteroids, are characteristically increased. Most patients show some evidence of glycosuria or hyperglycemia.

CARDIOVASCULAR MANIFESTATIONS. Prior to the development of effective treatment for Cushing's syndrome, accelerated atherosclerosis was a common finding. Early death usually occurred from myocardial infarction, congestive heart failure, or stroke. Even with more effective treatment, the mortality of patients with Cushing's syndrome is still significantly higher than in the general population, primarily owing to an increased risk of cardiovascular disease.[137] Although the pathophysiology of the accelerated atherosclerosis is not clear, the hypertensive process probably contributes. Chronic excess production of cortisol leads to hyperlipidemia and hypercholesterolemia, both of which may promote the development of atherosclerosis.[133]

The pathophysiology of the hypertension in Cushing's syndrome has been much debated. Early studies suggested that it was secondary to volume expansion due to cortisol's mineralocorticoid properties. Support for this comes from the demonstration of increased levels of atrial natriuretic hormone in patients with Cushing's syndrome, suggesting a volume-expanded state.[138] However, recent studies have not supported this hypothesis. Alternative hypotheses include glucocorticoid potentiation of response of vascular smooth muscle to vasoconstrictive agents and ACTH- or cortisol-induced increases in renin substrate.[133] The latter thesis suggests that the increased blood pressure is secondary to increased generation of angiotensin II. Support for the potentiation hypothesis comes from a documented increased vascular response to both angiotensin II and catecholamines in patients with Cushing's syndrome compared with normal subjects.[139,140] Thus, the pathophysiology of the hypertension may be multifactorial, being related to volume expansion, increased production of vasoactive agents, e.g., angiotensin II, and increased sensitivity of vascular smooth muscle to vasoactive agents.

The hemodynamic, electrocardiographic, and roentgenographic studies of patients with Cushing's syndrome have revealed no specific abnormalities except those that are, in general, associated with either hypertension or hypokalemia. The P-R intervals tend to be shorter than normal.

Echocardiograms have shown ventricular hypertrophy with asymmetrical septal thickening. The frequency of these abnormalities is greater than that of those seen in patients with essential hypertension with equivalent levels of blood pressure.[141]

Over the past several years, a new familial syndrome has been described: Cushing's syndrome and cardiac myxoma occurring in the same individual (see p. 1467). In addition to having these two conditions, 80 per cent of the patients have a cutaneous abnormality. In most it is a pigmented lesion; in some it is a subcutaneous myxoma. Histologically the adrenal glands show nodular hyperplasia.[142]

DIAGNOSIS AND TREATMENT. The diagnosis of Cushing's syndrome is established by the lack of appropriate suppression of cortisol secretion by dexamethasone. The best screening test is the administration of 1 mg of dexamethasone at bedtime with measurement of plasma cortisol between 7 and 10 the next morning.[133] In normal subjects cortisol levels are less than 5 μg/dl. Some patients, particularly the obese, may have false-positive responses, but false-negative responses occur only rarely. The definitive diagnosis of Cushing's syndrome is made by administration of 0.5 mg of dexamethasone every 6 hours for 2 days, with measurement either of plasma cortisol levels at the end of the second day (normal < 5 μg/dl) or of the 24-hour cortisol excretory rate on the second day of dexamethasone suppression (normal < 30 μg/24 hours).[133]

Therapy of Cushing's syndrome is usually directed at the specific cause. Thus, patients with adrenal carcinoma or adenoma or an ACTH-producing pituitary tumor are treated surgically. In some cases, patients with adrenal carcinoma have nonresectable lesions, and therefore surgery is combined with chemotherapy. The treatment of patients with bilateral hyperplasia without an evident ACTH-producing tumor is controversial, because the cause is often unknown. In some centers, bilateral adrenalectomy is the treatment of choice, while more commonly, therapy directed at the pituitary (either surgery or irradiation) is used.[133]

The treatment of the *cardiovascular abnormalities* associated with Cushing's syndrome is directed at lowering blood pressure and correcting the hypokalemia if present. Caution should be exercised in treating the hypertension with potassium-losing diuretics because of the tendency for these patients to develop hypokalemia. Thus, potassium-sparing diuretics or potassium supplements are often required. As in all clinical conditions in which hypokalemia may be present, cardiac glycosides should be used with caution in patients with Cushing's syndrome.

The hypertension is often resistant to conventional antihypertensive programs. Fallo et al. reported that only 15 per cent of their hypertensive patients with Cushing's syndrome had control of blood pressure using conventional medications: diuretics, calcium antagonists, angiotensin-converting enzyme inhibitors either as single agents or in combination. In 12 patients who failed conventional therapy, treatment with ketoconazole, an adrenal enzyme inhibitor, normalized blood pressure in all but one subject. In that one subject cortisol levels were not decreased. Thus, specific therapy directed at lowering cortisol production appears to be more effective than conventional antihypertensive therapy in controlling the hypertension in patients with Cushing's syndrome.[143]

Hyperaldosteronism
(See also p. 827)

CLINICAL AND BIOCHEMICAL MANIFESTATIONS. Aldosteronism is a syndrome associated with hypersecretion of aldosterone. Primary aldosteronism signifies that the stimulus for the excess aldosterone production resides within the adrenal. In secondary aldosteronism, the stimulus is of extra-adrenal origin.

In patients with primary aldosteronism, which most commonly is due to an aldosterone-producing adrenal adenoma, hypertension, hypokalemia, and metabolic alkalosis are common.[133,144] Polyuria may exist because of the hypokalemia, and glucose intolerance is increased in frequency. Muscle cramps due to the hypokalemia may be present, but little else distinguishes this from other forms of hypertension. Laboratory studies confirm the presence of hypokalemic alkalosis with a low specific gravity of urine and normal levels of adrenal glucocorticoids. The incidence of primary aldosteronism is between 0.5 and 2 per cent of the hypertensive population and it occurs twice as frequently in females as in males, with an initial presentation usually between the ages of 30 and 50 years.[133]

CARDIOVASCULAR MANIFESTATIONS. Many of the cardiovascular effects of aldosteronism are nonspecific, being related to aldosterone's effect on atrial pressure and potassium balance. Thus, T-wave flattening or U-wave prominence on the electrocardiogram and the presence of premature ventricular contractions and other arrhythmias due to hypokalemia are observed.[27] Evidence of left ventricular hypertrophy, either on the electrocardiogram or by echocardiography, may also be present in patients with longstanding hypertension and hyperaldosteronism. Malignant hypertension and changes in renal function secondary to severe hypertensive angiopathy are infrequent.

DIAGNOSIS AND TREATMENT. The diagnosis of primary aldosteronism is made by the presence of diastolic hypertension without edema, hypersecretion of aldosterone that fails to suppress appropriately during volume expansion, hyposecretion of renin, and hypokalemia with inappropriate urinary potassium loss during salt loading. The state of the renin-angiotensin system is often used to distinguish primary aldosteronism from other conditions that produce hypertension and hypokalemia. For example, hypertension and hypokalemia may be part of the clinical picture of secondary aldosteronism that accompanies malignant or accelerated hypertension or is associated with renal artery stenosis. Secondary aldosteronism can be readily distinguished from primary aldosteronism by the plasma renin activity, which is increased in the former and reduced in the latter. However, the combination of hypertension and a low plasma renin activity does not necessarily mean primary aldosteronism. Between 15 and 30 per cent of patients with essential hypertension have low renin levels, so-called low-renin essential hypertension.[144] The possibility of excess mineralocorticoid secretion has been extensively evaluated in these patients; however, no definitive evidence for such exists (Chap. 26).

Another entity that mimics primary aldosteronism is glucocorticoid-remediable aldosteronism (GRA) (see p. 827). This condition is an inherited hypertensive disorder with dysregulation of aldosterone secretion secondary to a gene mutation. The mutation is a fusion gene product between two genes coding for the enzymes responsible for the last step in biosynthesis of aldosterone and cortisol, i.e., 11β-hydroxylase/aldosterone synthase. This chimeric enzyme is expressed in the fasciculata cells, thereby leading to ACTH control of aldosterone synthase—a condition that normally does not occur. These patients can be distinguished by either genetic assessment or measurement of unique 18-hydroxycortisol steroids in the urine.[145]

The principal treatment for primary aldosteronism is surgical removal of the aldosterone-producing adenoma. In some cases, this is not possible because of the excessive risk imposed by the general physical status of the patient; then, spironolactone, which pharmacologically blocks the effects of aldosterone, is used long term. This form of therapy may be of limited benefit in men because compliance is reduced by the undesirable side effects of gynecomastia and impotence, particularly when doses greater than 200 mg per day are required.[133]

In some patients, primary aldosteronism is due not to a solitary adenoma but to bilateral hyperplasia.[144] Although the clinical characteristics of these two conditions are similar, their responses to surgery are different. In both cases hypokalemia is corrected, but patients with bilateral hyperplasia often do not exhibit reduction in arterial pressure.

Patients with bilateral hyperplasia are best treated with spironolactone and other antihypertensive agents. Thus, preoperative distinction between bilateral hyperplasia and an adrenal adenoma, using adrenal venography or adrenal scanning, is important.

Adrenal Insufficiency

Clinically, patients with adrenal insufficiency can be divided into four types:[133] (1) the most common, primary insufficiency (Addison's disease); (2) secondary insufficiency due to a lack of ACTH; (3) selective hypoaldosteronism; and (4) enzyme deficiency (congenital adrenal hyperplasia).

Addison's disease may occur at any age and affects both genders equally. It is commonly due to a destructive process involving both adrenal glands; this process is sometimes infectious, but most often it is autoimmune.[146] Nearly all patients with primary adrenal insufficiency have weakness, increased skin pigmentation, significant weight loss, anorexia, nausea, vomiting, and hypotension, particularly postural. As the disease progresses, there is a gradual reduction in serum levels of sodium, chloride, and bicarbonate and an increase in potassium levels.

CARDIOVASCULAR MANIFESTATIONS. The most common cardiovascular finding in adrenal insufficiency is arterial hypotension. In severe cases the pressure may be in the range of 80/50 mm Hg, with postural accentuation. Indeed, syncope occurs in a significant percentage of patients. In severe cases, heart size and peripheral pulses decrease. The most common electrocardiographic abnormalities are low or inverted T waves, sinus bradycardia, prolonged Q-T_c interval, and low voltage. Conduction defects also occur, with first-degree block present in 20 per cent of patients. Changes secondary to the hyperkalemia are not common, and cardiac failure is unusual.[147,148]

DIAGNOSIS AND TREATMENT. Decreased response of the adrenal cortex to ACTH establishes the diagnosis of Addison's disease. The best screening test is the administration of synthetic ACTH (cosyntropin), 0.25 mg intramuscularly or intravenously, with measurement of plasma cortisol levels 30 to 60 minutes later. Cortisol levels double or increase by 10 μg/dl in normal subjects. Definitive evaluation is by prolonged (usually 24-hour) infusion of ACTH with assessment of either plasma cortisol or excretion of cortisol or both.[133]

It is possible to differentiate primary adrenal insufficiency from secondary adrenal insufficiency, isolated hypoaldosteronism, or congenital adrenal hyperplasia because one of the adrenal hormonal functions is normal in each of the latter three conditions.

An increasingly common form of hypoaldosteronism is that associated with *hyporeninism*. Most commonly this syndrome is observed in older diabetic patients with a mild degree of renal impairment and hypertension; acidosis is also common. Usually these patients present with unexplained hyperkalemia. The cause is unknown but may be secondary to damage to the juxtaglomerular apparatus and/or reduced conversion of a renin precursor into the active enzyme.[149] This clinical syndrome is particularly important in the presence of cardiovascular diseases. Furthermore, commonly used drugs (beta blockers and calcium antagonists) can exacerbate this condition by further compromising aldosterone release.[150]

The treatment of adrenal insufficiency is accomplished by replacement of the deficient steroid. In adults with primary or secondary insufficiency, hydrocortisone, 20 to 30 mg daily, is administered in divided doses, usually two-thirds in the morning and one-third in midafternoon. In those patients with associated aldosterone deficiency, 9α-fluorohydrocortisone, 0.05 to 0.10 mg daily, is given. During periods of significant stress (surgery, infection, or trauma), the dose of glucocorticoids should be increased.[151,152]

PHEOCHROMOCYTOMA
(See also p. 829)

Effects of Catecholamines on the Cardiovascular System

The adrenal medulla and sympathetic nervous system are linked morphologically, biochemically, and physiologically and are often referred to as the sympathoadrenal system.[153,154] In addition to their important effects on the cardiovascular system, catecholamines also have significant metabolic effects, stimulating glycogenolysis and gluconeogenesis, that is, increasing the production of glucose from glycogen and amino acid precursors and stimulating lipolysis.

CLINICAL AND BIOCHEMICAL MANIFESTATIONS. A pheochromocytoma is a catecholamine-producing tumor derived from chromaffin cells. Those arising from extra-adrenal chromaffin cells are called nonadrenal pheochromocytomas or paragangliomas. Probably less than 0.1 per cent of patients with hypertension have a pheochromocytoma. Despite the fact that it is an uncommon disease, pheochromocytomas generate a great deal of interest, largely because the morbidity and mortality associated with these tumors are significant, with detection often resulting in cure. Pheochromocytomas are highly vascular tumors; less than 10 per cent are malignant as indicated by local invasion or metastasis, but, as with other endocrine tumors, malignancy cannot always be determined by microscopic appearance alone.

Although the vast majority of tumors occur sporadically, approximately 5 per cent are inherited as an autosomal trait, by which they are often part of a pluriglandular neoplastic syndrome,[153] which, in addition to pheochromocytoma, may consist of medullary carcinoma of the thyroid, parathyroidadenoma, and retinal or cerebellar hemangioblastomas. Most pheochromocytomas are solitary adrenal tumors, with 10 per cent being bilateral and 10 per cent nonadrenal. However, in the familial form of pheochromocytoma nearly half the patients have bilateral adrenal tumors.

CARDIOVASCULAR MANIFESTATIONS. Hypertension is the major cardiovascular manifestation of pheochromocytoma. The features that suggest pheochromocytoma in hypertensive patients are (1) paroxysmal attacks of any kind, (2) headaches, (3) excessive sweating, (4) signs of hypermetabolism, (5) orthostatic hypotension, and (6) unusual blood pressure elevations due to trauma or operation.[154] Many of the features are similar to those of hyperthyroidism. Although paroxysmal attacks are the hallmark of pheochromocytoma, more than half the patients have fixed hypertension and nearly 10 per cent are normotensive.

The lability of blood pressure in patients with pheochromocytoma has been suggested to be due not only to episodic discharge of catecholamines but also to a reduction in plasma volume, as well as to impaired sympathetic reflexes. A number of observations suggest that chronic volume depletion is present.[155] For example, alpha-adrenoceptor blockade or removal of the tumor produces severe hypotension, which is correctable by volume expansion.[153] Cardiac output has been reported to be normal, whereas heart rate is increased, and orthostatic hypotension is accompanied by decreased stroke volume and inadequate adjustments in peripheral vascular resistance indicative of impaired peripheral vascular reflexes.[155] An occasional patient has markedly elevated central aortic pressure and severe systemic hypotension due to severe arterial vasoconstriction. Patients with pheochromocytoma may also have acute pulmonary edema.[156] In some patients with pheochromocytoma, hemodynamic features are indistinguishable from those with essential hypertension. These results suggest that long-term exposure to high circulating levels of catecholamines may produce a different clinical picture than that observed with acute administration. These differences may be due to desensitization induced by chronic exposure to catecholamines.[157]

The electrocardiogram is abnormal in as many as 75 per cent of patients with pheochromocytoma.[27] The changes consist of T-wave inversion, left ventricular hypertrophy, sinus tachycardia, and, in some cases, other alterations in rhythm, such as frequent supraventricular ectopic beats or paroxysmal supraventricular tachycardia.[158] An occasional patient has a short P-R interval and a narrow QRS complex, suggesting that catecholamines are modifying the A-V conduction system. When arterial pressure increases markedly, changes suggestive of myocardial damage, including transient ST-segment elevations, marked diffuse T-wave inversions, and depression of ST segments, are present. These changes are usually transient, and the electrocardiographic pattern reverts to normal after removal of the tumor or pharmacological blockade.[153,159] Some of the electrocardiographic abnormalities are presumably due to hypertensive heart disease or myocardial ischemia. However, a specific catecholamine-induced myocarditis and/or cardiomyopathy has also been suggested.[160,161] Interestingly, a patient with catecholamine-induced cardiomyopathy was treated with captopril, with resolution of the cardiomyopathy within 2

weeks.[162] In rats with pheochromocytomas, treatment with captopril also markedly attenuated the cardiomyopathy but did not modify contraction of isolated rings of the thoracic aorta in response to either epinephrine or angiotensin II.[163] The mechanism by which captopril produced these beneficial effects is unclear but could be related to inhibiting angiotensin II–induced cardiac fibrosis.[135]

The echocardiogram often shows left ventricular hypertrophy with normal left ventricular systolic function.[164] During a hypertensive crisis it may show systolic anterior involvement of the anterior mitral leaflet, paradoxical septal motion, and proximal excursion of the posterior wall.[165]

Myocarditis. Pathologically, the myocarditis consists of focal necrosis with infiltration of inflammatory cells, perivascular inflammation, and contraction band necrosis[166] (Fig. 61–7), finally resulting in fibrosis. In some studies, 50 per cent of patients who died of pheochromocytoma had myocarditis, usually accompanied by left ventricular failure and pulmonary edema. Although coronary atherosclerosis is usually present, medial thickening is the most characteristic lesion of the coronary arteries. When norepinephrine is infused into the rabbit, there is sustained coronary vasoconstriction that within 48 hours leads to histologically documented myocardial damage.[167] Occasionally, patients with pheochromocytoma have manifestations of cardiomyopathy which may be reversed when the tumor is removed[160,161] (Fig. 61–8). The myositis is not necessarily limited to the myocardium, as it also may occur in skeletal muscle.[168]

DIAGNOSIS AND TREATMENT. The diagnosis of pheochromocytoma is established by documenting increased urinary or plasma levels of catecholamines or one of their metabolites.[153] Three tests are commonly employed: (1) total catecholamines, (2) vanillylmandelic acid (VMA), and (3) metanephrine. The last two are metabolites of catecholamine and were first used to screen for pheochromocytoma because they are present in greater quantities. When reliably performed, these tests are probably equivalent in accuracy. The probability of pheochromocytoma being present in a hypertensive patient with a single normal urine level is less than 5 per cent. It is most desirable to measure both the catecholamines and one of the two metabolites, preferably metanephrine, in screening for pheochromocytoma. If the blood pressure fluctuates, it is particularly important to collect the urine at a time when the pressure is elevated. Specific pharmacological tests to screen for pheochromocytoma are of limited benefit, usually hazardous, and therefore warranted only in unusual circumstances. Clonidine has been proposed as a useful definitive test for pheochromocytoma, although it is necessary only in unusual cases. Catecholamine levels are suppressed in normal subjects via stimulation of central alpha-adrenoceptors; following clonidine administration in patients with pheochromocytoma they are not.[153] Unfortunately, profound and prolonged hypotension has been reported in some patients during the course of this test.

Once the diagnosis of pheochromocytoma is established, specific pharmacological blockade should be initiated.[153] Administration of phenoxybenzamine hydrochloride should be begun, with the initial dosage 10 mg every 12 hours; the dose is then gradually increased every 2 to 3 days until the arterial pressure is restored to normal. Alternatively, prazosin may be used. However, it should be noted that alpha-adrenoceptor blockade may induce a decline in arterial pressure accompanied by serious postural hypotension, presumably because of the vasodilatation occurring in the presence of hypovolemia. This hypotensive response can be prevented by adequate sodium intake; if the response is very striking, infusion of saline may be required. Adequate control of arterial pressure is essential prior to any arteriographic procedure before initiating beta-adrenoceptor blockade, and before operation. Calcium an-

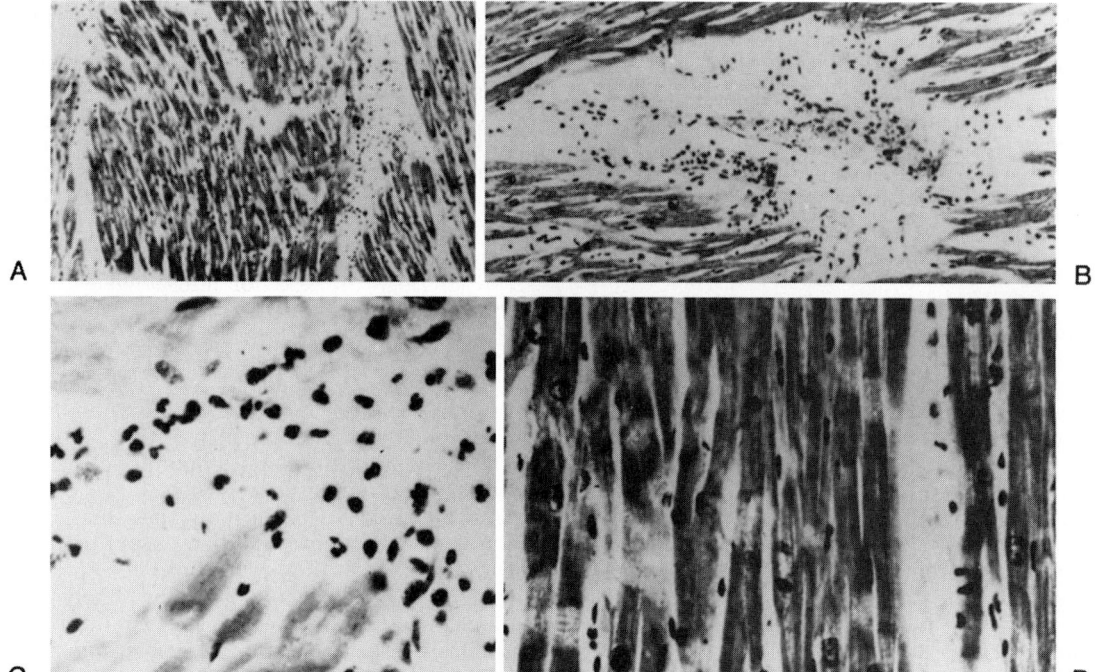

FIGURE 61–7. Left ventricular myocardium with acute myocarditis and contraction band necrosis in a patient with pheochromocytoma dying of catecholamine crisis. *A*, Diffuse infiltration by inflammatory cells through myocardium. *B*, Perivascular inflammation. *C*, Close-up of the inflammatory infiltrate. *D*, Contraction-band necrosis of myocytes. H&E; original magnification × 20 *(A)*, × 45 *(B)*, × 540 *(C)*, × 330 *(D)*. (From McManus, B. M., et al.: Fatal catecholamine crisis in pheochromocytoma: Curable cause of cardiac arrest. *Am. Heart J. 102:*930, 1981.)

tagonists may be useful both in treating the hypertension associated with pheochromocytoma and in reducing catecholamine production.[169]

Beta-adrenoceptor blockade is useful in patients with pheochromocytoma who have significant tachycardia, palpitations, and catecholamine-induced arrhythmias. However, beta blockade with a drug affecting beta$_2$ receptors must not be initiated prior to inadequate alpha blockade, since severe *hypertension* may occur as a result of unopposed alpha-stimulating activity of the circulating catecholamines.

Definitive treatment is surgical removal of the tumor, usually after localization with computed tomography, arteriography, or scanning using a radioactive iodide derivative of guanethidine as the scanning agent.[153] Scanning may be particularly important in localizing extra-adrenal, e.g., thoracic, pheochromocytomas. Precise definition of the anatomical boundaries of this tumor is important preoperatively if surgery is to be successful.[170] In those patients with inoperable lesions, long-term use of the combination of alpha- and beta-adrenoceptor blockers has been helpful.

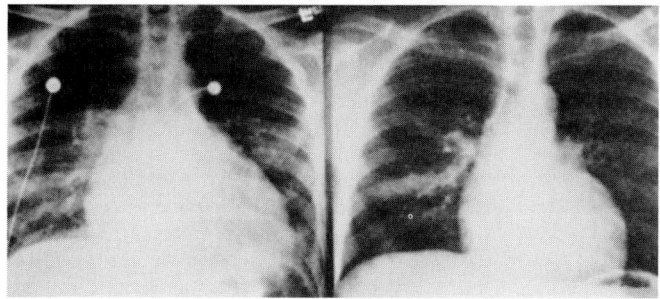

FIGURE 61–8. Pheochromocytoma-induced cardiomyopathy. *Left,* Chest x-ray on admission. Cardiomegaly, right pleural effusion, and signs of congestive heart failure. *Right,* One month after removal of the tumor. No signs of congestion and significant decrease of the heart size. (From Velasquez, G., et al.: Phaeochromocytoma and cardiomyopathy. *Br. J. Radiol. 57:*89, 1984.)

Drugs that inhibit the biosynthesis of catecholamines, such as alpha-methyltyrosine, and generalized chemotherapeutic agents have also been used in patients with malignant pheochromocytoma.[153] Although rare, of particular importance to the cardiologist is the presence of a cardiac pheochromocytoma (see p. 1897).

PARATHYROID DISEASE

Disordered parathyroid secretion is associated with two cardiovascular disturbances, cardiac arrhythmias and hypertension. Changes in calcium metabolism as well as a direct effect of parathyroid hormone on the cardiovascular system appear to be responsible.

CLINICAL AND BIOCHEMICAL MANIFESTATIONS. Parathyroid hormone (PTH) is a single-chain polypeptide of 84 amino acids. Its major biological effect is to increase mobilization of calcium into the extracellular fluid from a variety of tissues; this action is linked in a negative feedback loop with serum unbound calcium concentration. Thus, an increase in serum calcium concentration reduces PTH release and vice versa.[171] PTH also increases urinary excretion of phosphate, augments bone resorption, and reduces the urinary excretion of calcium.

Primary hyperparathyroidism, the excess production of PTH, is usually secondary to a solitary parathyroid adenoma. Occasionally, generalized parathyroid hyperplasia exists, and infrequently, carcinoma of the parathyroid gland is found. The signs and symptoms of primary hyperparathyroidism are related to direct effects of PTH on kidney or bone or those associated with the hypercalcemia. Nearly half the patients have signs and symptoms of renal dysfunction, such as polyuria, nocturia, renal stones, and, in severe cases, nephrocalcinosis and renal failure.

Cardiac hypertrophy is found with increased frequency in patients with hyperparathyroidism, even in the absence of hypertension. In one study, 5 of 18 patients with hypertrophic cardiomyopathy had raised serum PTH levels but normal serum calcium levels. In contrast, left ventricular hypertrophy did not occur in six patients with hypercalcemia alone.[171]

Cardiovascular Manifestations of Parathyroid Diseases

(See also p. 830)

CARDIAC EFFECTS. Although most of the effects of PTH on the heart are probably secondary to a change in extracellular calcium, PTH also has a direct effect on the heart, resulting in an increased beating rate of isolated heart cells and a positive inotropic action.[172–175] These effects are probably mediated by PTH binding to specific receptors, leading to increased entry of calcium into cardiac cells, and by the PTH increasing the release of endogenous myocardial norepinephrine. The direct effect of PTH may be deleterious, because it causes necrosis of rat myocytes and may be directly responsible for the increased accumulation of calcium in dystrophic muscles and for the heart damage found in uremia.[172,174] However, Gafter et al. did not find an improvement in cardiac performance in patients with end-stage renal disease following parathyroidectomy for hyperparathyroidism.[175] On the other hand, hypoparathyroidism may cause a dilated cardiomyopathy, presumably secondary to the hypocalcemia. However, because longstanding hypocalcemia does not necessarily produce left ventricular dysfunction,[176] hypomagnesemia and reduced circulating PTH may also be involved.[177] PTH also has a direct effect on vascular smooth muscle, causing vasodilatation.

Chronic hypercalcemia from a variety of causes is associated with increased deposition of calcium in the fibrous skeleton of the heart and valvular cusps as well as in coronary arteries and in myocardial fibers[179] (Fig. 61–9). Chronic hypercalcemia also may be a risk factor for accelerated coronary atherosclerosis.[180,181]

The plateau of the action potential of cardiac fibers is prolonged by low and shortened by high extracellular calcium concentrations (Chap. 20). The changes in duration of action potential are accompanied by corresponding changes in the duration of the refractory period, of the ST segment, and of the Q-T interval.[27] Thus the major electrocardiographic change in hypercalcemia is shortening of the Q-T interval. Less frequently, disorders of intraventricular conduction have been reported with shortening of the P-R interval.[27] Complete heart block occurs only rarely.

Hypocalcemia produces the opposite effect on the electrocardiogram with prolongation of the Q-T interval and nonspecific ST- and T-wave changes. Normal contractile function of cardiac muscle requires calcium, and heart failure has been reported in patients with chronic hypocalcemia secondary to hypoparathyroidism.[182]

HYPERTENSION. Hypercalcemic patients detected by routine serum calcium screening techniques have higher arterial pressure than do matched normocalcemic subjects.[183] Yet in patients with hyperparathyroidism, the level of serum calcium is similar in those who are normotensive and those who have hypertension, suggesting that hypercalcemia per se is not the dominant cause for the hypertension. Thus, the pathophysiology of the hypertension is uncertain[184] and it may be multifactorial. Hypercalcemia produces nephrocalcinosis, which may lead to renal failure and hypertension. Thus, reversal of hypertension after successful parathyroid surgery is more likely to occur when renal function is normal. Increased serum calcium also increases myocardial contractility, peripheral resistance, and release of or vascular sensitivity to vasoconstrictor agents, such as angiotensin II and norepinephrine. Although hypercalcemia can increase cardiac contractility and arterial pressure acutely, it is unlikely that this action produces a significant alteration in cardiac output or performance on a long-term basis in the absence of PTH.[184] Thus an elevation of peripheral resistance is the most likely cause of the hypertension associated with hyperparathyroidism. Although PTH itself is a vasodilator, characteristic changes in other hormones that occur in hyperparathyroidism may contribute to the hypertension. For example, PTH increases 1 α-hydroxylation of 25(OH) vitamin D, leading to higher levels of 1,25(OH)$_2$ vitamin D. 1,25(OH)$_2$ Vitamin D enhances vascular reactivity,[185] and the higher levels in hyperparathyroidism could contribute to hypertension. Finally, a circulating hypertensive factor produced in the parathyroid gland has been identified. It is termed "parathyroid hypertensive factor (PHF)."[186] This factor appears to be at least partially peptidic in composition.[187] PHF is distinct from PTH and has the ability to increase intracellular calcium concentration in vascular smooth muscle cells primarily via opening L-type calcium channels.[188] PHF was first found in the parathyroid glands of spontaneously hypertensive rats[187] but has since been found in the circulation of essential hypertensives, especially those who are salt-sensitive and have low renin levels.[189] Elevated levels have been reported to predict a beneficial response to calcium channel blockers.[190] However, further support for the existence and physiological role of PHF is required.

DIAGNOSIS AND TREATMENT

An elevated or even a normal concentration of PTH in the presence of hypercalcemia establishes the diagnosis of hyperparathyroidism; many patients with this condition manifest hypercalcemia for the first time after starting thiazide therapy for the associated hypertension. Treatment consists of surgical removal of the parathyroid tumor or hyperplastic glands.

Patients with hypertension should have a determination of serum calcium levels before therapy is begun. If thiazide diuretics are used in treatment, serum calcium levels should be determined every 6 months. If thiazide-induced hypercalcemia occurs, the serum calcium should be determined for 2 to 3 months after discontinuation of the thiazides. Persistence of the hypercalcemia suggests that the patient has primary hyperparathyroidism.[182]

Patients with hypoparathyroidism and hypocalcemia usually are treated with calcium supplementation and vitamin D or one of its metabolites, calcitriol (1,25 dihydroxyvitamin D).

DIABETES MELLITUS

Diabetes mellitus is one of the leading public health problems in the industrialized world, and it has a profound effect on the cardiovascular system. Nearly 10 million people are afflicted with this disease in the United States; it is the eighth health-related cause of death. Nearly all the increased morbidity from diabetes is related to cardiovascular dysfunction secondary to coronary artery disease, congestive heart failure, and hypertension or renal failure secondary to microvascular disease.

ACTIONS OF INSULIN. Insulin is a double-chain polypeptide derived from proinsulin, which is synthesized in the islet cells of the pancreas. Many stimuli, such as glucose, glucagon, amino acids, catechol-

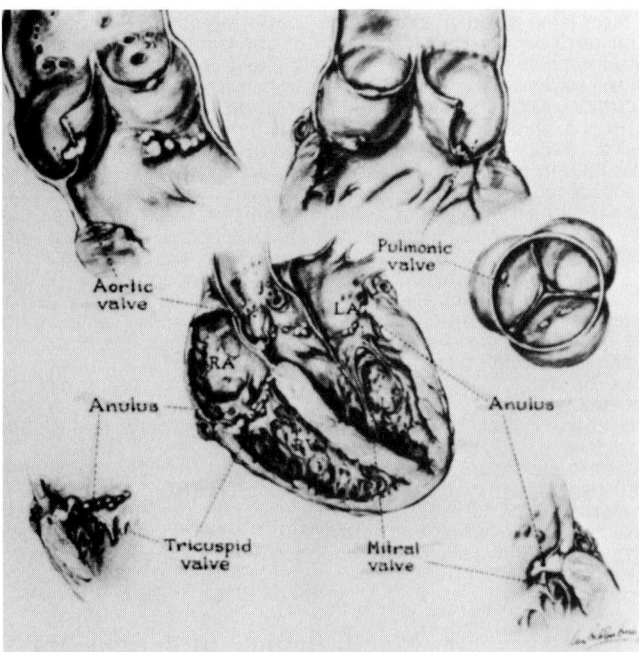

FIGURE 61–9. Heart showing distribution of calcific deposits in the tricuspid and mitral valve annuli and at the bases of both pulmonic and aortic valve cusps in a 43-year-old woman with hypercalcemia secondary to primary hyperparathyroidism. (From Roberts, W. C., and Waller, B. F.: Effect of chronic hypercalcemia on the heart: An analysis of 18 necropsy patients. Am. J. Med. 71:371, 1981.)

amines, and gastrointestinal hormones, can promote insulin secretion, which occurs in two phases. The rapid early phase releases preformed insulin stored in granules in the beta cells while the late phase results from increased biosynthesis of insulin.[191]

Insulin is an anabolic hormone affecting all metabolic substrates, i.e., carbohydrates, fats, and proteins, as well as nucleic acids. All target tissues for insulin have specific membrane-bound receptors; thus, binding to the receptor is the first step in initiating its metabolic effect. The ingestion of fuel substrates provokes a rapid rise in the concentration of circulating insulin, which then facilitates the transfer of these substances into their respective depots.

In the patient with diabetes, because insulin release is decreased in response to the ingested fuel, there is a delay in the uptake and the disposal of these fuels into their respective depots, which leads to abnormal circulating levels of the substrates. The increased concentrations of lipids in the circulation may be the underlying pathophysiological effect producing a number of the clinical complications of diabetes mellitus.

ETIOLOGY AND BIOCHEMICAL MANIFESTATIONS. Several lines of evidence suggest that in many instances the insulin-dependent (IDDM) form may be infectious or autoimmune in origin, whereas in most cases the non-insulin dependent form (NIDDM) is probably the result of a genetic predisposition.[192]

Most of the signs and symptoms of this disease either are related to the increased levels of blood glucose or are secondary to changes in the cardiovascular system. Thus, the classic presenting symptoms (observed in about 25 per cent of IDDM patients) are polyuria, polydipsia, and polyphagia, all due to the glucosuria. The major pathophysiological consequence of diabetes mellitus is related to changes in the vascular system. The specific target organs include the heart, the eye, the kidney, the autonomic nervous system, and the peripheral vasculature.

Cardiovascular Changes in Diabetes

PATHOLOGY. The vascular disease associated with diabetes mellitus can be nonspecific (atherosclerosis and arteriosclerosis) or specific (microangiopathic or endothelial proliferative changes of arterioles). The former primarily involves large vessels (especially in the lower extremities), heart, and brain of older patients, whereas the latter is localized to small vessels and may be seen in patients of all ages. The microangiopathy produces a characteristic thickening of the basement membrane of the capillaries in the retina, conjunctiva, glomerulus, brain, pancreas, and myocardium.[192] In some cases there is also proliferation of the epithelial cells, leading to occlusion of small arterioles similar to that observed in immune arteritis.

CORONARY ARTERY DISEASE. Coronary heart disease is the leading cause of death among adult diabetics and accounts for about three times as many deaths among diabetics as among nondiabetics.[192a] The incidence of coronary artery disease correlates more closely with the duration of diabetes than with its severity. Certainly, diabetes should be considered to be a separate risk factor for coronary heart disease[193] (see p. 1150). Of note, however, is that diabetes has a greater impact on the incidence of congestive heart failure than coronary artery disease. More diffuse coronary artery disease and greater involvement of smaller caliber vessels and microaneurysms are characteristic of diabetes.[194] Because each risk for vascular disease is thought to add independently (although not equally) to the likelihood for the development of ischemic disease, the diabetic should be considered a high-risk patient in whom all correctable factors should be managed.[195,196] Hypertension occurs more frequently in diabetics than nondiabetics and is a major contributor to cardiovascular disease in this population. Cigarette smoking and even moderate elevation of blood pressure and plasma lipids should be approached more intensively in diabetic than in nondiabetic patients. The use of contraceptive hormonal drugs must be carefully considered because they may contribute to the metabolic abnormalities that underlie increased risk for vascular disease. The obese diabetic patient should lose weight; this is often accompanied by gratifying improvement of hypertension, hyperglycemia, hyperinsulinemia, and hypertriglyceridemia.

MYOCARDIAL INFARCTION. Not only is the frequency of acute myocardial infarction increased in diabetic pa-

tients,[193,195] but also the treatment of the infarct is more complicated than in the nondiabetic patient. For many years it was thought that diabetics had a greater frequency of "silent" myocardial infarctions than the general population.[196] More recently this belief has been challenged. The 30-year follow-up of the Framingham Study showed no increased incidence of unrecognized myocardial infarction in diabetics.[197] Patients with acute myocardial infarction, regardless of the control of their diabetes before hospital admission, exhibit significantly higher mortality and morbidity than do nondiabetics.[194,195] Several factors contribute to the increased mortality of diabetic patients with acute myocardial infarction. The size of the infarct tends to be greater in diabetics, who have a greater frequency of both congestive heart failure and shock than do nondiabetics; and the patient is often in a precarious metabolic status compounded by the difficulty of adjusting insulin therapy to prevent ketoacidosis while not precipitating hypoglycemia.[194,198] Also, survival after infarction is more limited than in the nondiabetics, with fatality rates being as high as 25 per cent during the first year after infarction.[194,195] Recurrent infarction, heart failure, and dysrhythmias all contribute to the higher death rate.[193-195,198] Administration of beta blockers to diabetics appears to reduce the overall mortality, at least in the immediate post–myocardial infarction period, similar to what has been reported in nondiabetics.

The occurrence of myocardial infarction may have an adverse effect on carbohydrate and fat metabolism and often leads to stimulation of the sympathetic nervous system and increased catecholamine concentration[200] (p. 1197). Subsequent increases in circulating free fatty acid levels and reductions in glucose tolerance appear to be related to a number of physiological functions—adipose tissue lipolysis, hepatic and muscle glycogenolysis, catecholamine-induced suppression of insulin release, and increased circulating concentrations of growth hormone and cortisol. The net result is that carbohydrate intolerance is common after myocardial infarction, even in nondiabetics.

AUTONOMIC DYSFUNCTION. Peripheral somatic neuropathy is a commonly recognized complication of diabetes mellitus. Autonomic neuropathy also occurs in the diabetic, leading to diarrhea, vomiting, and other gastrointestinal disturbances. A form of autonomic dysfunction involves the heart and is termed *cardiac autonomic dysfunction*.[201] Cardiac autonomic dysfunction may be diagnosed by abnormalities in two or more of the following: (1) resting heart rate (after 15 minutes rest) of 100 beats/min or more; (2) lack of beat-to-beat variability on electrocardiographic recording ≤ 10 beats/min; (3) a ratio of the longest R-R interval to the shortest of 1.10 or less during Valsalva maneuver; and/or (4) a ratio of the R-R interval of the 30th beat to 15th beat after standing of 1 or less; (5) a fall in systolic blood pressure of 30 mm Hg or more after 1 minute of standing.[202] The anginal threshold may be increased, presumably as a consequence of autonomic and sensory neuropathies.[203] In two large series cardiac autonomic neuropathy was present in more than a third of the patients and accompanied by depression of left ventricular function. The severity of cardiac dysfunction was directly related to the severity of the cardiac autonomic neuropathy.[204] Occasionally it may be present before clinical symptoms of generalized autonomic neuropathy are demonstrable. Furthermore, the neuropathy may involve the sympathetic nervous system and/or the parasympathetic nervous system. Indeed, it may become so severe as to lead to total cardiac denervation. These changes in adrenergic nervous system function result in a fixed, rapid heart rate that barely responds to physiological stimuli, such as the Valsalva maneuver, carotid sinus pressure, or tilting,[205] or to drugs, such as phenylephrine, atropine, or propranolol. Rarely, these denervated hearts develop arrhythmias. There is a markedly decreased survival with an increased risk of

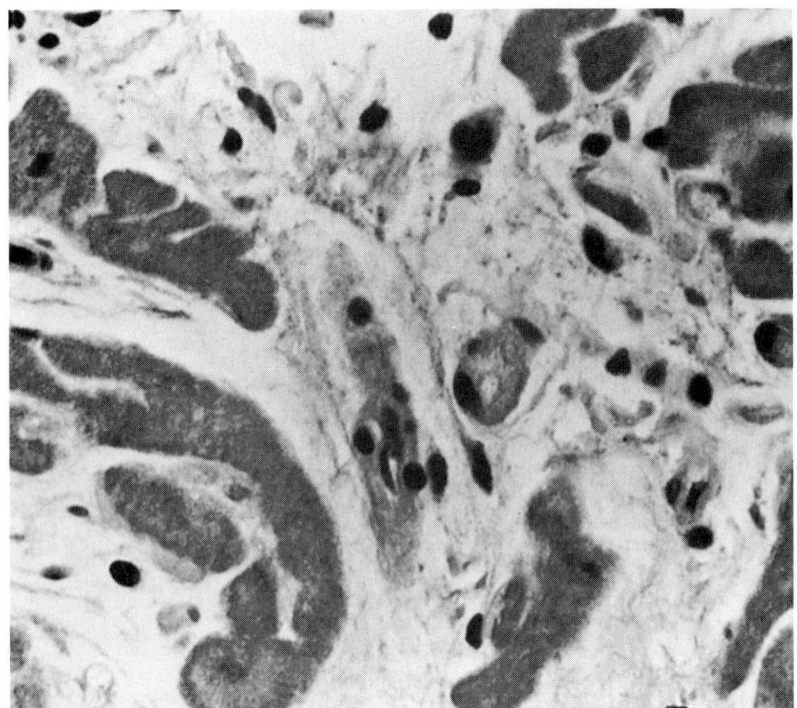

FIGURE 61–10. Myocardium of diabetic patient showing atrophied myocytes on right side (compare with more normal fibers on left), increased interstitial fibrous tissue, and thickening of small arteriolar walls. H & E × 300. (From Sutherland, C. G. G., et al.: Endomyocardial biopsy pathology in insulin-dependent diabetic patients with abnormal ventricular function. Histopathology 14:596, 1989.)

sudden death in diabetics with abnormal autonomic function tests.[206]

CONGESTIVE HEART FAILURE. Diabetes mellitus appears to increase the likelihood of the development of congestive heart failure from all causes. The role of diabetes in congestive heart failure was analyzed in the Framingham Study,[196] and the risk of developing heart failure was found to be increased substantially. Even when patients with prior coronary or rheumatic heart disease were excluded, diabetic subjects had a four- to fivefold increased risk of congestive heart failure. Furthermore, this increased risk persisted after age, blood pressure, weight, and cholesterol values, as well as coronary heart disease, were taken into account. On the basis of these findings it appeared that the excessive risk of heart failure in diabetic patients is caused by factors other than accelerated atherogenesis and coro-

nary heart disease. One suggested possibility is a diabetes-induced cardiomyopathy.

Diabetic Cardiomyopathy. There is a substantial increase in the coincidence of diabetes mellitus and cardiomyopathy. The cardiomyopathy may occur in patients who have no evidence of large-vessel disease or abnormalities in myocardial capillary basal lamina documented by endomyocardial biopsies.[206,207] The most common histological abnormalities are interstitial fibrosis (Fig. 61-10) and arteriolar hyalinization (Fig. 61–11). Evidence supporting the presence of cardiomyopathy even in children with diabetes mellitus has been reported. Both systolic and diastolic dysfunctions have been observed. The severity of dysfunction is related to the degree of metabolic control, even when there is no clinical evidence of cardiovascular or microvascular disease.[208] Taken together, these studies strongly sug-

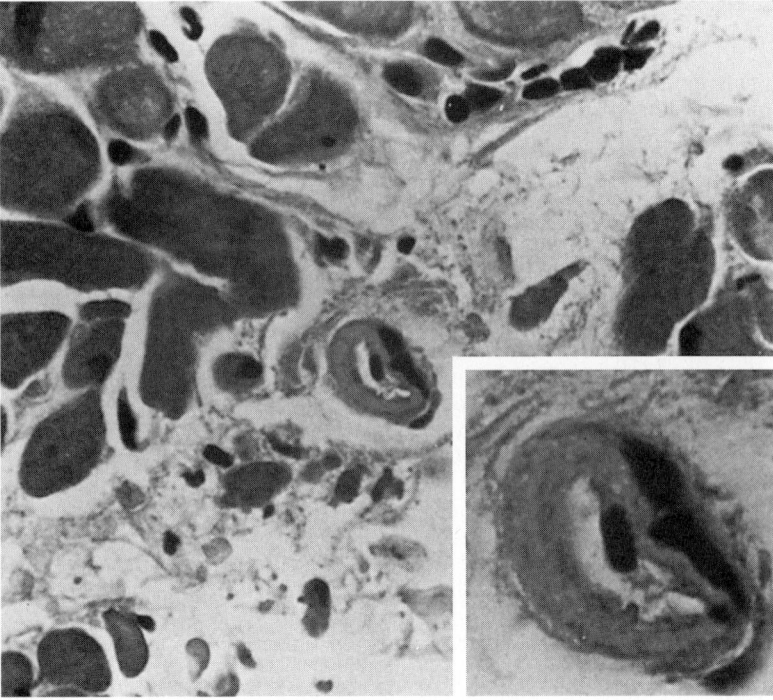

FIGURE 61–11. Hyalinization without luminal narrowing of small arteriole in myocardium of diabetic patient. H&E, × 300. Inset, Same arteriole. (H&E, × 750). (From Sutherland, C. G. G., et al.: Endomyocardial biopsy pathology in insulin-dependent diabetic patients with abnormal ventricular function. Histopathology 14:597, 1989.)

gest that in some diabetic patients there is a nonischemic cardiomyopathic process.

ABNORMALITIES OF VENTRICULAR FUNCTION. Several abnormalities of ventricular function, using echocardiographic techniques, have been reported in diabetics.

In young asymptomatic patients, the ratio of early to peak filling velocity is significantly decreased while atrial filling velocity is significantly increased (Fig. 61-12). There is no relationship between the left ventricular diastolic filling abnormalities and evidence of severity of the diabetes, i.e., retinopathy, nephropathy, or peripheral neuropathy.[209] Other reported abnormalities in diabetic subjects include left ventricular asynergy on two-dimensional echocardiograms,[209,210] reduction in the peak diastolic filling rate[211]; an abnormal left ventricular ejection fraction in response to exercise[212,213]; and evidence of diastolic dysfunction, even in normotensive diabetic patients.[214,215]

Several factors have been reported to contribute to the abnormalities in left ventricular function in diabetics: (1) The role of hypertension with a concomitant increase in left ventricular mass.[216] (2) The potential role of growth hormone. Patients with difficult-to-control diabetes often have increased growth hormone levels. Several investigators have reported that this metabolic abnormality could account for the increased collagen levels present in the left ventricular wall of diabetic humans and animals[217] (Fig. 61-12). Regan et al., however, have reported that in experimental diabetes induced in dogs the

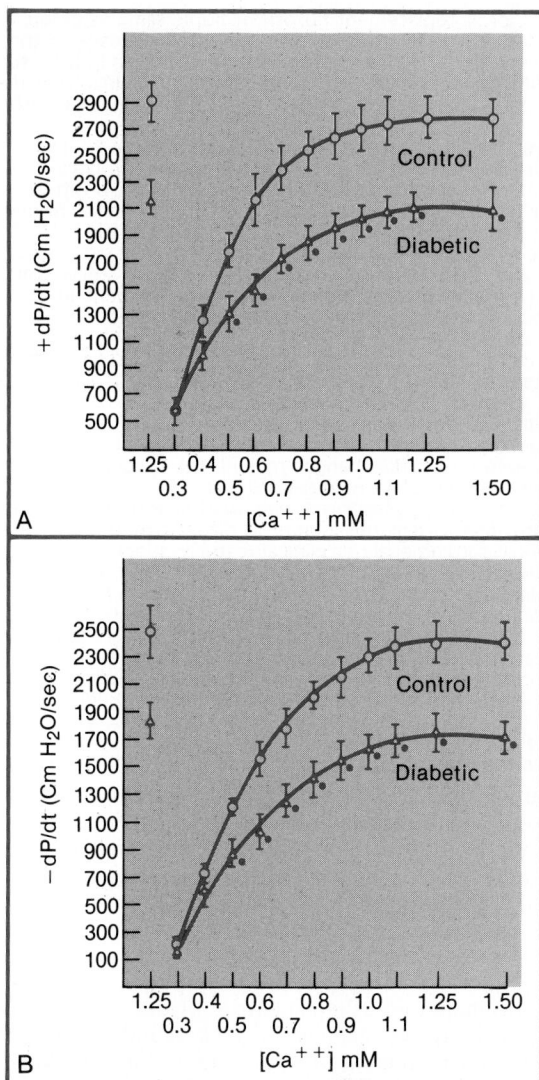

FIGURE 61–13. Effect of non–insulin-dependent diabetes mellitus on myocardial contractility (+ dp/dt). Hearts from 12-month-old diabetic rats (triangles) and the age-matched controls (circles) were perfused during the initial 20-minute stabilization period with Krebs-Henseleit buffer. Each data point represents mean ± SE of five to seven hearts. Similar reductions in − dp/dt (an index of relaxation) were noted in diabetic hearts. Significant difference from control ($P < .05$). (From Schaffer, S. W., et al.: Basis for myocardial mechanical defects associated with non–insulin-dependent diabetes. Am. J. Physiol. *256*:E27, 1989. Reproduced by permission of the American Physiological Society.)

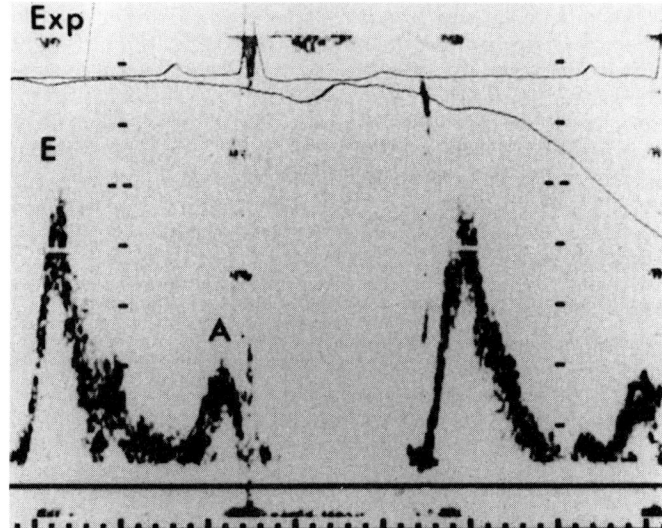

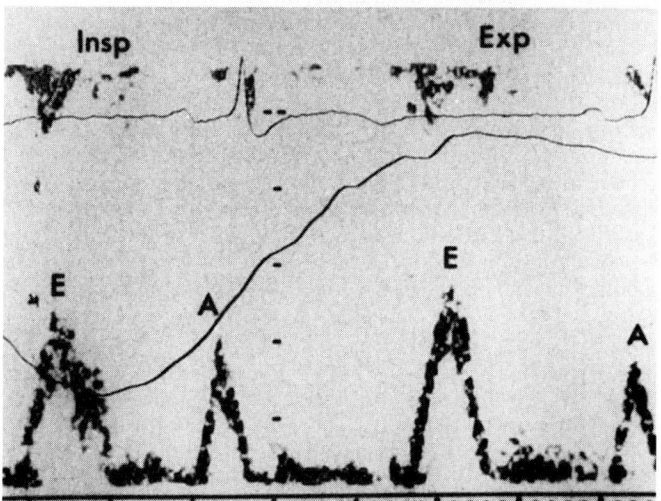

FIGURE 61–12. *A*, Transmitral Doppler echocardiogram obtained from a normal adolescent patient. The early phase of ventricular filling (E wave) is greater than the late diastolic A wave. *B*, In this diabetic adolescent, the early phase of atrial filling (E wave) is less prominent and the late diastolic A wave is taller, with a lower E/A ratio than in the normal patient. These findings are consistent with impaired diastolic filling in the diabetic patient. Exp = End-expiration; Insp = end-inspiration. (From Riggs, T. W., and Transue, D.: Doppler echocardiographic evaluation of left ventricular diastolic function in adolescents with diabetes mellitus. Am. J. Cardiol. *65*:899, 1990. Copyright 1990 by Excerpta Medica Inc.)

collagen accumulation in the myocardium is not related to or dependent on an increase in plasma growth hormone levels.[218] (3) The increased cardiac sorbitol level.[219] (4) The impairment in Ca^{2+} handling with hypersensitivity of the myocardium to Ca^{2+} secondary to increased sarcolemmal Ca^{2+} ATPase activity[220,221] (Fig. 61-13). In a rat model of non–insulin-dependent diabetes mellitus, the abnormalities in myocardial Ca^{2+} ATPase activity have also been demonstrated.[222] Further support for this hypothesis comes from the beneficial effect of a calcium antagonist (verapamil), which prevented diabetes-induced myocardial changes in experimental diabetes.[223] (5) Finally, Okumura et al. have suggested that increased 1,2-diacylglycerol levels with resultant activation of protein kinase C may underlie the cardiomyopathy, at least in experimentally induced diabetes.[224] Despite these observations in experimental models, it should be noted that when insulin is administered, the cardiac abnormality is not necessarily corrected. Thus, the relationship between the hyperglycemic state and the abnormalities in myocardial function and metabolism present in experimental diabetes is still unclear.

PATHOLOGICAL CHANGES. In postmortem studies of 11 diabetic patients, 9 of whom were without significant obstructive disease of the proximal coronary arteries and had died of cardiac failure, all exhibited positive periodic acid-Schiff (PAS) staining material in the interstitium, but none had luminal narrowing of the intramural vessels. Collagen accumulation was present in perivascular loci, between the myofibers, or as replacement fibrosis. Multiple samples of left ventricle and septum revealed abnormally increased deposits of triglyceride and cholesterol.[225] Thus these observations, taken in toto, suggest that a diffuse abnormality, either extravascular or involving the microvasculature, may be the basis for the cardiomyopathic features of diabetes.

However, a recent morphological study casts some doubt on small-vessel disease as the producer of cardiac myopathy, because similar findings have been reported in NIDDM subjects. Unsitupa et al., studying 133 patients with NIDDM (type 2), found a high incidence of impaired left ventricular function already present at the time of initial diagnosis.[226] Hypertension appears to accelerate this process, both in humans and animals, as severe interstitial fibrosis, focal scars, and myocytolytic activity were significantly more frequent in hypertensive diabetics with chronic heart failure examined post mortem than in normotensive diabetics.[227]

Other (nondiabetic) cardiomyopathies may exhibit similar hemodynamic abnormalities; an abnormal rise of ventricular filling pressure without a stroke volume increase in response to afterload increments has also been observed in the preclinical phase of alcoholic cardiomyopathy, in which the interstitium is also altered.[227] More severely altered interstitial changes may be the predominant lesion in the incipient stages of amyloid heart disease.[228]

Diabetes mellitus is associated with another form of cardiomyopathy. Approximately half the infants of diabetic mothers have either radiographic cardiomegaly or clinical features suggesting congestive heart failure[229] (see p. 992). The cardiomyopathy in these infants may be transient and secondary to hematological, respiratory, and metabolic problems or a more protracted form of nonobstructive or obstructive hypertrophic cardiomyopathy, which appears to be secondary to maternal hormonal influences and to be reversible.

Electrocardiographic changes are commonly observed in patients with diabetes.[27] Although many of the changes are predictable on the basis of the associated hypertension or coronary artery disease, in some there is an unexplained diffuse T-wave abnormality that may be related to the cardiomyopathy.

VASCULAR DISEASE. Peripheral vascular disease is a frequent and significant manifestation of diabetes mellitus, sometimes leading to gangrene and requiring amputation. The smaller arteries below the knee are more likely to be involved in patients with diabetes, in contrast to iliac or femoral artery disease in nondiabetic patients. Cerebral vascular disease is also more frequent, with a greater incidence of cerebral infarction although not cerebral hemorrhage. The increased atherosclerosis of the cerebral vessels and the proliferative changes in the cerebral arterioles both contribute to this increased rate of infarction. In addition to the direct effect of diabetes on cardiac function, insulin itself can cause salt and water retention by mechanisms still obscure. In most cases this fluid retention is self-limiting. However, in individuals who have underlying cardiovascular disease it may lead to overt cardiac failure.[230]

The renal vasculature is affected in a number of ways: Atherosclerosis is common in the larger vessels, with proliferative endothelial changes occurring in small vessels. Capillary basement membrane thickening is common, particularly in the glomerular tuft where a pathognomonic change—nodular glomerulosclerosis—is often found. These vascular changes, in concert with parenchymal changes secondary to pyelonephritis and altered renal hemodynamics (increased glomerular pressure),[231,232] lead to a variety of renal disorders, including the nephrotic syndrome, hypertension, and renal failure.

The mechanism underlying the accelerated development of atherosclerosis in diabetes is multifactorial (see p. 1150). Hyperinsulinemia itself has been shown to enhance lipid synthesis in arterial walls and may be a major factor contributing to the macroangiopathy.[233] Most studies have reported an increased incidence of hypertension in diabetes. Indeed, more than one-third of diabetic patients have hypertension, an incidence that is higher than that of the general population.[234] The hypertension is in part related to the increased frequency of renal disease. Volume overload may be an additional factor.

The association of hypertension with both diabetes and obesity has led some investigators to propose that insulin resistance is the causal link between these conditions. Resistance to the metabolic actions of insulin is a prominent feature of NIDDM. It has been suggested that the increased frequency of hypertension in this condition is secondary to selective insulin resistance—the autonomic nervous system and/or the kidney is not insulin-resistant. Elevated levels of insulin acting on the kidney induces volume retention, whereas an increased insulin effect on the adrenergic nervous system increases sympathetic outflow. Either of these can then lead to elevation of blood pressure.[235,236] Treatment of hypertension in diabetics involves weight loss, exercise, and antihypertensive agents. Converting-enzyme inhibitors have theoretical advantages both in terms of glucose control and in retarding the deterioration of renal function. Thus, they are the treatment of choice for hypertension in diabetics.[231,237,238]

Treatment of Diabetes

It is generally agreed that therapy directed at the control of excessive fatty acid mobilization and oxidation and protein catabolism is essential in diabetes mellitus. Whether "tight" control of glucose levels is essential has been controversial until recently. The Diabetes Control and Complications trial (DCCT) studied more than 1440 patients with IDDM for a mean of 6.5 years. Patients were randomized to either conventional treatment or intensive treatment ("tight control"). Those patients who received tight control experienced a reduction in incidence and progression of retinopathy and in the incidence of microalbuminuria and clinical neuropathy compared with those receiving conventional therapy. This study is a landmark in resolving the debate over the benefit of tight control. In terms of cardiovascular disease there was a reduction in the frequency of elevated LDL cholesterol levels (>160 mg/dl) with tight control. The overall reduction in cardiovascular and peripheral vascular disease induced by tight control was 41 per cent but was not statistically significant. However, the average age of the patients was 26 to 27 years, which may explain the lack of statistical significance. Therefore, tight control is the goal of treatment to reduce long-term complications of diabetes.[239]

Diet, insulin, and oral hypoglycemic agents have been the mainstays of treatment. However, a controversy has arisen concerning the efficacy and safety of oral hypoglycemic agents, such as the sulfonylureas.[240] Although hyperglycemia is better controlled with these agents than it is with diet alone, an increased frequency of myocardial infarction has been reported with the first-generation agents. Although the interpretation and implications of these findings are controversial, some experimental evidence suggests that some sulfonylureas may have an adverse effect on the myocardium. Wu and colleagues have reported increased "stiffness" of the myocardium secondary to interstitial accumulation of PAS-staining material that reduced left ventricular function in dogs treated with tolbutamide.[241] This association has not been seen with second-generation agents.

On the basis of available information, patients with diabetes who should use oral hypoglycemic agents, preferably one of the second-generation agents (glyburide or glipizide),[242] are those who are not ketosis prone and whose hyperglycemia cannot be controlled with diet alone.[243] The recent approval of metformin by the FDA provides another oral agent to treat diabetes. Metformin lowers glucose but lowers lipids as well, which may provide an additional cardiovascular benefit. Metformin may be added to the regimen of a diabetic whose glucose is not optimally controlled on a second-generation agent. It should not be used in patients with renal insufficiency. If this combination fails, the patient should be switched to insulin. It should also be recognized that beta-adrenoceptor blockers reduce the hyperglycemic reaction to stress, and it is possible that beta-adrenoceptor blocker therapy may require a downward adjustment of insulin dosage because patients receiving beta blockers may be more susceptible to hypoglycemia, particularly in the elderly.[242] Because many of the symptoms of which the hypoglycemic patient is aware are due to the effects of the epinephrine that is released, both physician and patient must be alert to the possibility that hypoglycemia occurring in the beta blocker-treated diabetic may be relatively asymptomatic. Because certain diuretics, such as the thiazides and furosemide, may result in hypokalemia, and because hypokalemia can inhibit insulin release, these drugs may intensify the glucose intolerance of diabetic patients.

In patients with diabetes mellitus and impairment of left ventricular function, a sudden change in the glucose concentration of extracellular fluid, as occurs with the development of insulin deficiency, may result in the movement of fluid from the intracellular to the extracellular space and the intensification of heart failure. The hyperosmolar state has been shown experimentally to reduce cardiac contractility.[244]

OBESITY

(See also p. 1634)

There are two types of obesity: adult onset and lifelong. Adult-onset obesity is extremely common, probably occurring to a varying extent in nearly all individuals in developed countries. Its clinical course consists of normal weight patterns during childhood and adolescence, with a gradual increase in weight beginning between 20 and 40 years of age; it reflects an imbalance between caloric intake and utilization.[245] Much less common is lifelong obesity, characterized by the development of obesity early in childhood, with significant increase in weight during adolescence and, in women, during and after pregnancy. These individuals are usually grossly obese, weighing more than 150 per cent of their ideal weight as adults. The underlying cause of obesity in either condition is unclear.

Hirsch has documented an increase in both the size and the number of adipose cells in individuals with lifelong obesity, whereas in adult-onset obesity only an increase in cell size occurs.[246] With weight reduction the size of the adipose cells decreases in both conditions; however, the number does not change in either. Whether the increased number of adipose cells in lifelong obesity is determined by genetic or environmental factors is uncertain. However, it has been documented that there is no significant change in the number of adipose cells when obesity develops after late childhood in both experimental animals and humans. On the other hand, some evidence suggests that early infant feeding habits may significantly alter their number.[246] The metabolic consequences of obesity include decreased sensitivity to insulin, with resultant hyperinsulinemia, glucose intolerance, hypercholesterolemia, hypertriglyceridemia, and hyperaminoacidemia.

Cardiovascular Consequences of Severe Obesity

During the past decade the health risk of obesity has been intensively studied. A conference analyzing data from two national health and nutrition surveys and the Framingham 30-year follow-up study concluded that a significant excess in mortality is evident in individuals with a body mass index (weight in kilograms/height in meters²) greater than 27. A value greater than this is present in 34 million adult United States citizens. There is a direct correlation between the levels of blood pressure and cholesterol and the degree of obesity.[247]

OBESITY AND CARDIOVASCULAR HEMODYNAMICS. Evidence of circulatory dysfunction in the massively obese, associated with cardiac enlargement during life and at autopsy, was first described by Smith and Willius in 1933.[248] It is now widely appreciated that massive obesity is accompanied by a marked increase in blood volume and cardiac output, which are proportional to the excess of body weight and the duration of obesity.[192a,249–251]; the hematocrit is often slightly elevated as well. The increased cardiac output is secondary to increased end-diastolic left ventricular volume[249–251] and stroke volume, because heart rate is normal; the cardiac output rises normally during exercise.

Left ventricular filling pressures are at or close to the upper limits of normal in the supine position in the basal state, but increase with passive leg raising and reach strikingly elevated levels during exercise. These increases in ventricular filling pressure are associated with a high resting central blood volume, which also increases significantly with exertion. A tendency to leftward deviation of the electrical axis correlates significantly with increasing obesity independent of age and blood pressure. However, this association is usually confined to the normal QRS-axis range. Thus, left-axis deviation is not necessarily a reflection of obesity.[252] The maximum velocity of myocardial fiber shortening and the ratio of stroke work index to left ventricular end-diastolic pressure were reduced, even in relatively young obese persons, without any other evidence of heart disease[249] (Fig. 61-14). Massive edema may occur as a consequence of the elevated ventricular filling pressure, despite elevation of the cardiac output.

PATHOLOGY. Examination of the gross and microscopic anatomy of the heart in patients with marked chronic obesity showed heart weight to be considerably greater than predicted for ideal body weight, with left ventricular dilatation and eccentric hypertrophy and, in a few instances, right ventricular hypertrophy as well[253,254] (Fig. 61-15). Left atrial abnormalities (increased size and reduced emptying index) also have been reported.[255] This increase in cardiac weight is not due to excess epicardial fat and fatty infiltration of the myocardium, which were previously considered to be the principal features of the obese heart. Obesity-induced cardiac hypertrophy is different from that induced by hypertension. Instead of the concentric left ventricular hypertrophy associated with hypertension, the hypertrophy is eccentric, with chamber dilatation and some wall thickening, as seen in other conditions in which cardiac output is chronically increased (Fig. 61-16). Also, in contrast to the increased afterload associated with systemic hypertension, obesity produces an elevated preload. When hypertension accompanies severe obesity, a combination of concentric and eccentric hypertrophy is present. Obese patients with clinically evident ventricular hypertrophy have an increased propensity to ectopy, in comparison with obese persons without left ventricular hypertrophy or with lean persons.[255] In part, this increased ectopy may be secondary to cardiac autonomic dysfunction.[256] Thus, when these clinical, hemodynamic, and pathological observations are taken together, it appears that manifestations of myocardial dysfunction occur in very obese subjects without

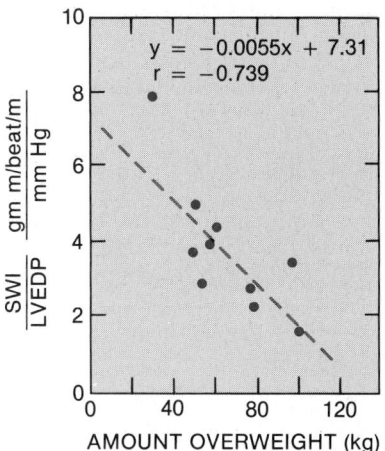

FIGURE 61–14. The significant negative correlation between the ratio of the stroke work index (SWI) to the left ventricular end-diastolic pressure (LVEDP) and the amounts of overweight shows that the higher the degree of obesity, the greater the impairment of left ventricular function. (Reproduced by permission from Divitiis, O., et al.: Obesity and cardiac function. Circulation 64:477, 1981. Copyright 1981 American Heart Association.)

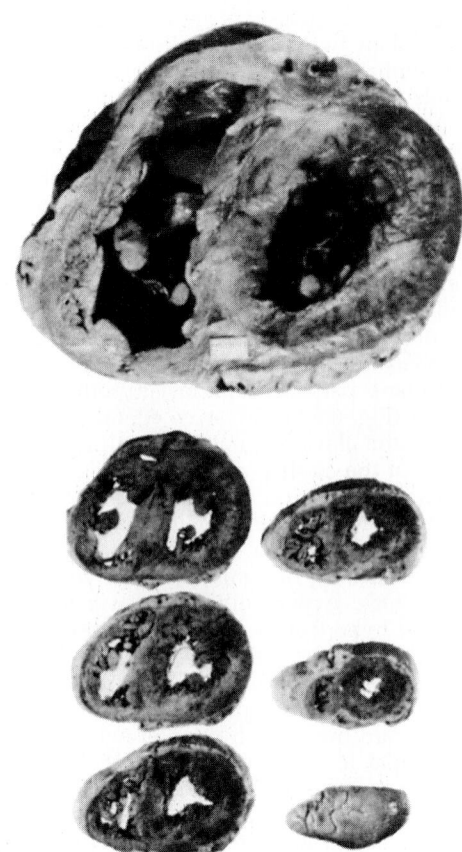

FIGURE 61–15. Cross section of the heart of a 34-year-old man who weighed more than 500 lbs. Both ventricular walls are hypertrophied and both cavities are dilated. The heart weight (825 gm) was greatly increased. (From Warnes, C. A., and Roberts, W. C.: The heart in massive [more than 300 pounds or 136 kilograms] obesity: Analysis of 12 patients studied at necropsy. Am. J. Cardiol. *54:*1090, 1984. Copyright 1984 by Excerpta Medica Inc.)

evidence of other heart disease and that, in the absence of the obesity hypoventilation syndrome, which may also complicate obesity (see p. 801), cor pulmonale is not a presenting feature.

HYPERTENSION. Hypertension is common in the obese,[247] although it must be recognized that indirect measurement of blood pressure frequently leads to overestimation of the arterial pressure by the standard cut-off method. Nonetheless, direct measurement of arterial pressure frequently shows moderate elevations. The Second National Health and Examination Survey (NHANES II) demonstrated an increased risk of hypertension of 2.9 times in overweight compared with normal weight individuals.[257] This increased risk may be secondary to the accompanying hyperinsulinemia, resulting in increased tubular reabsorption of sodium, increased catecholamine activity, and altered cellular ion transport.[258] *Syndrome X* has been defined as insulin resistance, hyperlipidemia, and obesity and is frequently associated with hypertension. This syndrome appears to play an important role in coronary artery disease.[259]

CORONARY ARTERY DISEASE. Obesity is associated with coronary artery disease by increasing several of its risk factors. These include hypertension, hyperinsulinemia, hyperlipidemia, and diabetes mellitus. Obesity may also have an independent effect that differs depending on the location of the body fat (see p. 1152). A study of more than 7600 individuals in the Honolulu Heart Program demonstrated that central obesity was a risk factor for coronary heart disease independent of body mass index.[260] In addition, analysis of data from the Nurses' Health Study demonstrated an increased risk of coronary heart disease (myocardial infarction and angina) in mildly to moderately overweight women.[261]

CONGESTIVE HEART FAILURE. Heart failure in the markedly obese is usually chronic. The pulmonary and systemic congestion with symptoms of dyspnea and edema are, at first, simply related to the reductions in ventricular compliance and elevations of filling pressures. Later, these symptoms are related also to increases in ventricular end-diastolic volume and the reduction of myocardial contractility. Thus, the marked chronic increase in cardiac work, i.e., in cardiac output and arterial pressure, ultimately leads to heart failure.

CARDIAC BENEFITS OF WEIGHT LOSS. Fortunately, weight reduction is beneficial in the majority of patients.[261a] It usually improves the exercise capacity of patients with chronic exogenous obesity and decreases total body oxygen uptake, the cardiothoracic ratio on chest roentgenogram, systemic arterial pressure, blood volume, cardiac output, arteriovenous oxygen difference, and left ventricular filling pressure at rest.[262] MacMahon et al. have documented that weight loss of as little as 8 kg is associated with a significant decrease in left ventricular mass, particularly the thickness of the posterior and central walls.[263] Alpert and colleagues, studying cardiac function in grossly obese individuals, noted a substantial reduction in left ventricular chamber enlargement and an improvement in systolic function with an average weight loss of 55 kg.[264] However, they were unable to show a change in septal or posterior wall thickness, suggesting that some of the beneficial effects of weight loss on cardiac function may occur only if the obesity is mild or of short duration. Supporting this conclusion is the persistence of elevated left ventricular filling pressure with exercise in obese patients following weight reduction.[265]

BLOOD PRESSURE BENEFITS OF WEIGHT LOSS. The Framingham Study has shown a decrease in systolic blood pressure by 10 per cent with a 15 per cent decrease in body weight in men. In the Evans County longitudinal study, an 8-kg weight loss was associated with a 13 mm Hg decrease in diastolic blood pressure. A fall in blood pressure can occur even if ideal body weight is not achieved.[266]

Treatment

Most cases of adult-onset obesity are the result of imbalance between intake and output. Thus, reduction of intake

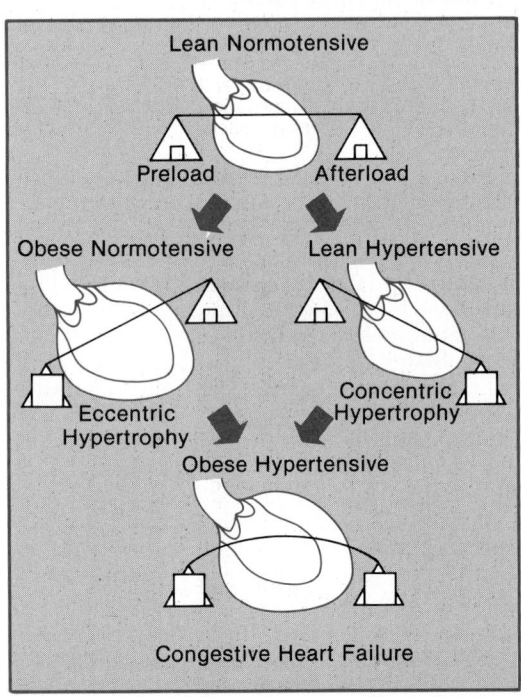

FIGURE 61–16. Adaptation of the heart to obesity and hypertension. (From Messerli, F. H.: Cardiovascular effects of obesity and hypertension. Lancet *1:*1165, 1982. © by The Lancet Ltd.)

is the most significant factor in treating this disease. Although abnormalities in endocrine function, particularly of the thyroid or adrenal, have often been implicated in the pathophysiology of obesity, this thesis is rarely substantiated by detailed evaluation. The quantity and rate of weight loss with a given level of caloric restrictions depend on the degree of energy expenditure. Energy expenditure depends on both the physical activity and mass of the individual. Thus, with a fixed level of intake and activity, the rate of weight loss decreases as the total weight decreases. There is no evidence that a specific type of diet has any intrinsic benefit except as it is related to its caloric regimen.

CARDIAC COMPLICATIONS OF WEIGHT LOSS. Rapid weight loss has been associated with cardiac arrhythmias and sudden death.[267] In some cases, this is probably secondary to inadequate electrolyte supplementation. In others, it may be related to a reduction in myocardial protein and cardiac atrophy, similar to what has been reported in severe malnutrition[268] (see below). Although initially associated with a liquid protein diet, sudden death may occur under any circumstance in which there is rapid weight loss.[269] In nearly all cases, prolongation in the Q-T interval as well as ventricular arrhytmias has been reported, providing strong support for the need for an electrocardiogram in any patient undergoing significant rapid weight loss.

MALNUTRITION

Malnutrition, particularly protein-calorie deficiency, is prevalent in many underdeveloped areas of the world. However, in recent years, it has also become a concern in developed countries in those individuals who have chronic diseases, in whom it exists as a result of both anorexia and hypermetabolism and in otherwise healthy individuals with anorexia nervosa. The clinical picture is similar to that of adult kwashiorkor reported from underdeveloped countries, described below.

Protein-calorie malnutrition of childhood refers to syndromes of nutritional deficiency, which range from marasmus to kwashiorkor and which result from a stress like a serious infection superimposed upon an inadequate diet.[270] *Marasmus* is a state of malnutrition in an infant who has been weaned early and fed a diet grossly deficient in calories, protein, and other essential nutrients. *Kwashiorkor* usually occurs in children 1 to 4 years of age and is due to deficiency of protein relative to calories.

CARDIAC CHANGES IN MALNUTRITION. The circulatory status of patients with severe nutritional depletion and electrolyte imbalance is precarious; the cardiac output, systolic pressure, and pulse pressure are abnormally low, and there may be massive, generalized edema; the P-R interval may be shortened (Table 61-2). There is loss of subcutaneous fat and general wasting and atrophy of most organs, including the heart, which is thin-walled, pale, and flabby on gross

TABLE 61–2 SPECTRUM OF CARDIAC EFFECTS DUE TO STARVATION AND ANOREXIA NERVOSA

| **Cellular** |
| Diminished protein synthesis |
| Activation of calcium-dependent proteinase |
| Mitochondrial swelling |
| Decreased glycogen content |
| Interstitial edema |
| Myofibrillar atrophy and destruction |
| **Physiological** |
| Decreased contractile force |
| Decreased cardiac output |
| Diminished diastolic compliance |
| **Clinical** |
| Bradycardia |
| Relative hypertension |
| Nonspecified electrocardiographic changes |
| Ectopic rhythms |
| Mitral valve prolapse |
| Diminished exercise capacity |
| Heart failure, worsened or precipitated by refeeding |

Adapted from Schocken, D. D., Holloway, J. D., and Powers, P. S.: Weight loss and the heart. Effects of anorexia nervosa and starvation. Arch. Intern. Med. *149*:878, 1989.

examination. Histological study reveals atrophy of the muscle fibers, sometimes with interstitial edema. In experimental chronic protein-calorie undernutrition, not only is the heart atrophic, but also left ventricular function may be normal. In the dog there are reductions in left ventricular compliance and contractility, the latter secondary to loss of cardiac tissue, not altered function,[271] whereas in the rat this apparently does not occur, although there is striking atrophy of the heart.[272] The treatment of the dehydrated or severely anemic patient with protein-calorie malnutrition involves correction of hematological, fluid, and electrolyte imbalance and the treatment of infection. Congestive failure can be avoided if care is taken to avoid overloading with sodium, water, or blood. Digitalis must be given cautiously when these patients are in heart failure because of their sensitivity to glycosides.

In parts of the world where pediatric kwashiorkor is common, there are also cases of adults with similar clinical features. These include loss of subcutaneous fat and muscle with edema, weakness, depression, anorexia, diarrhea, abdominal distention, hair loss, and thinning of the skin. Classically, plasma albumin and amino acid levels are low, as are serum concentrations of sodium, magnesium, and phosphorus. Urinary excretion of nitrogen is reduced, as is total body potassium. On the other hand, total body and extracellular water and plasma volume are usually increased. The primary pathophysiological event is protein malnutrition. All the clinical signs and symptoms are related to this basic defect.

Anorexia Nervosa. This condition is more frequently observed in developed countries but produces symptoms similar to those observed in kwashiorkor. Hypomagnesemia with hypocalcemia and hypokalemia frequently occurs in this condition, resulting in arrythmias, heart failure, and sometimes sudden death.[273] Compared with normal weight or constitutionally thin women, in women with anorexia nervosa, cardiac index is decreased secondary to low stroke index and heart rate. There also are reduced left ventricular mass, systolic dysfunction, and mitral valve motion abnormalities.[274] Sinus bradycardia is common and appears to be secondary to increased vagal tone.[275] Anorexia nervosa also has been associated with a prolonged Q-T interval compared with age- and gender-matched controls. The prolonged Q-T interval may predispose to arrhythmias.[276] Congestive heart failure may occur, particularly in the early refeeding phases, probably secondary to an exacerbation of the hypophosphatemia when hyperalimentation and/or oral intake is rich in glucose.

MALNUTRITION IN CARDIAC DISEASE. The protein-calorie nutritional status in cardiac patients has not been extensively evaluated. However, there has been increasing awareness that some patients with cardiovascular disease have clinical features similar to those with primary malnutrition described above. In these cases, instead of involuntary protein deprivation, anorexia plays a significant role. For example, chronic heart failure leads to cellular hypoxia as well as hypermetabolism. Gastrointestinal hypoxia produces anorexia, which then initiates a vicious circle. Decreased protein intake produces cardiac atrophy, increased right atrial pressure, tricuspid regurgitation, and increasing heart failure, which produces more cellular hypoxia, greater anorexia, and finally death.[277]

A similar condition has been described in some patients undergoing open-heart surgery for correction of rheumatic valvular disease. In some malnourished patients the mortality reaches 20 per cent, significantly greater than the 1 to 2 per cent in normally nourished patients undergoing the same procedure. The underlying pathophysiology is uncertain but probably includes (1) decreased cardiac mass, (2) impairment of this biosynthetic activity of liver, (3) poor healing due to reduced levels of substrate, and (4) impairment of cell-mediated immunity.[278] As a result, wound healing is retarded, skin ulcers occur, and requirements for artificial ventilation are prolonged. Abel and colleagues have suggested that hyperalimentation in the immediate postoperative period does not significantly alter the increased morbidity.[279] This has led Blackburn et al. to suggest that both preoperative and concurrent nutritional support are necessary.[278]

Cardiovascular Manifestations of Vitamin Deficiency

THIAMINE DEFICIENCY

(See p. 461)

OTHER VITAMIN DEFICIENCIES. Deficiencies of other vitamins have not led to specifically definable cardiovascular abnormalities, except for the hypocalcemia-accompanied vitamin D deficiency. However, vitamin deficiencies, particularly of the B group and folic acid, have been diagnosed with increasing frequency in patients with cardiovascular disease. For example, nearly a third of infants and children with congenital heart disease have been reported to be deficient in a number of the B vitamins.[280] Folic acid deficiency has been documented in a significant number of patients with congestive heart failure. Although the deficient state may simply be related to decreased intake, abnormal intestinal absorption or increased rates of excretion may also contribute.

THE HEART AND GONADAL HORMONES

There are no specific cardiovascular abnormalities associated with altered gonadal function except for occasional cardiac structural abnormalities in Kallman's syndrome, a genetic form of hypogonadotropic hypogonadism, and a rare form of cardiomyopathy associated with primary hypogonadism. Men have an increased risk of coronary heart disease of approximately twice that of women, as demonstrated in the 26-year follow-up of the Framingham population. With increasing age, the coronary heart disease mortality rate in women approaches that of men, becoming almost equal by age 75[281] (see p. 1707). Of note, however, is the dramatic increase in coronary heart disease in women that occurs at age 45 to 55. Because these years encompass the average time of menopause in the United States, it is postulated that hormones of the premenopausal woman are protective against coronary heart disease. Several risk factors for coronary heart disease increase following menopause, including hypertension and a more atherogenic lipid profile, which may be secondary to the loss of estrogen. Estrogens increase HDL cholesterol, which represented much of its cardiovascular benefit in the Lipid Research Clinics Trial.[282] Natural estrogen may also lower blood pressure.[283] Much of the belief to the contrary is based on outdated oral contraceptive literature, which used higher doses of estrogens and various progestins. In addition, estrogen may have direct effects that impact on coronary heart disease. For example, estrogens may act as direct vasodilators in the coronary vessels and thereby improve ischemia in women with coronary heart disease.[284] Finally, estrogen appears to lower levels of plasminogen activator inhibitor (PAI-1), which could lead to greater fibrinolytic activity.[285]

In 1985, two major conflicting studies were published addressing the issue of hormone replacement therapy's effect on cardiovascular disease. Whereas analysis of the Framingham population demonstrated an increased risk of coronary heart disease without a concomitant increased mortality associated with estrogen use,[286] analysis of the Nurses' Health Study[287] showed a benefit for the use of estrogen. The majority of prospective studies, however, have found a *reduction* in risk of coronary heart disease with estrogen use (reviewed in ref. 288). The more recent analysis of 10 years of follow-up in the Nurses' Health Study supported the earlier finding of a benefit of estrogen on cardiovascular disease.[289] Of the 48,470 women followed prospectively, those who were current users of estrogen for hormone replacement therapy had an approximately 50 per cent lower risk of fatal cardiovascular disease with no increase in stroke, compared with those who had never used estrogen. The reason for the discrepancy between the Framingham Study and the majority of other studies is unclear. The Framingham population did report higher estrogen doses than those of other studies. This conflict illustrates the potential limitations of epidemiological *versus* clinical trial approaches to answer critical therapeutic questions.

In summary, most studies demonstrate a benefit for estrogen use against coronary heart disease. In practice, however, estrogen is given with a progestin to protect against endometrial hyperplasia in women who have not undergone hysterectomy. The effect of the use of both an estrogen and progestin on coronary heart disease has been less well studied. A recent cross-sectional study of 4958 postmenopausal women taking estrogen alone, and women taking estrogen and progestin, demonstrated persistent or even greater benefit in terms of lipid profiles with the addition of progestin.[290]

A prospective 3-year study of 875 postmenopausal women who received estrogen alone or in combination with a progestin confirmed the results of the cross-sectional study. Women who received estrogen alone and those who received both estrogen and a progestin showed an improvement in lipoprotein profiles and a lowering in fibrinogen levels, whereas the former group alone had a high rate of endometrial hyperplasia not seen in the latter.[291] Treatment with estrogen alone also led to a greater increase in HDL cholesterol. Future studies of the impact of the combined use of estrogen and progestin on actual coronary heart disease are necessary.

TAMOXIFEN. This drug, an estrogen receptor partial agonist with antiestrogenic activity on the breast, is frequently used for the treatment of breast cancer, particularly in postmenopausal women. Several studies have suggested a cardiovascular benefit to tamoxifen. A retrospective review of women in the Scottish adjuvant tamoxifen trial, compared 1070 women who were randomized to tamoxifen given as adjuvant prophylactically versus only on recurrence. The incidence of fatal myocardial infarction was significantly lower in the women given adjuvant tamoxifen for at least 5 years. The Stockholm Breast Cancer Study group found that in over 1000 women receiving tamoxifen, there was a significant decrease in hospital admissions for cardiac disease compared with 1000 who were not. There was greater benefit seen with 5 than with 2 years of use.[293] One mechanism whereby tamoxifen may provide cardiovascular benefit is through a fall in total cholesterol and LDL, as demonstrated in the Wisconsin Tamoxifen Study.[294]

ORAL CONTRACEPTIVES. The literature on the association between oral contraceptive use and coronary heart disease is controversial. The controversy is due in large part to the decreasing estrogen content in oral contraceptives over the past 40 years as well as the incorporation of varying progestins with different androgenic potencies. The changing spectrum of oral contraceptive composition also makes it difficult to extend data based on earlier agents to today's preparations. Several studies have shown an increased risk of myocardial infarction in oral contraceptive users.[295-297] However, prior oral contraceptive use does not confer an increased risk for cardiovascular disease.[298] Studies of the effect of newer contraceptive agents are not available.

BLOOD PRESSURE EFFECTS OF ORAL CONTRACEPTIVES AND HORMONAL REPLACEMENT THERAPY

Oral contraceptive use has been associated with a rise in blood pressure since their widespread use in the 1960's. When blood pressure rises, it usually remains within the normotensive range; rarely, it increases into the hypertensive (> 140/90 mm Hg) range. Even with the earlier generation oral contraceptives, which used higher estrogen dose and varied progestins, there were conflicting data as to whether blood pressure rises or not.[299-301] Differences in responses to oral contraceptives may depend on quantity of estrogen, type of progestin, and race and genetic background of the user. Studies of the new generation of oral contraceptives, which contain no greater than 35 μg ethinyl estradiol and less androgenic progestins, are more limited. Available data on desogestrel-containing oral contraceptives include a multicenter trial of more than 1600 women followed over 23,000 cycles. No significant change in mean blood pressure over 2 years of use was observed and only a 0.3 per cent incidence of hypertension was noted.[302] Other studies of this agent have revealed similar results.[303,304] Although activation of the renin-angiotensin-aldosterone axis occurs in oral contraceptive users, the degree of activation may be greater in those who remain normotensive than those who became hypertensive.[305] Thus, the etiology of oral contraceptive–induced hypertension remains unclear.

The belief that estrogens used for hormone replacement therapy induce hypertension is largely based on the older oral contraceptive literature. In fact, the use of estrogen in many trials is associated with no change in blood pressure. It is likely that estrogens differ in their effect on blood pressure. Estrone, a natural estrogen, may actually lead to a fall in blood pressure.[306]

REFERENCES

1. Graves, R. J.: Clinical lectures. London Med. Surg. J. (Part II) 7:516, 1835.
2. Addison, T.: On the constitutional and local effects of diseases of the suprarenal capsules. London, Highley, 1855.

3. Daughaday, W. H.: Growth hormone, insulin-like growth factors, and acromegaly. In DeGroot, L. J., et al. (eds.): Endocrinology, Vol. 1. 3rd ed. Philadelphia, W.B. Saunders Company, 1995, p. 303.

4. Strobl, J. S., and Thomas, M. J.: Human growth hormone. Pharmacol. Rev. 46:1, 1994.

5. Hartman, M. L., Veldhuis, J. D., and Thorner, M. O.: Normal control of growth hormone secretion. Horm. Res. 40:37, 1993.

6. Wass, J. A. H.: Somatostatin. In DeGroot, L. J., et al. (eds.): Endocrinology, Vol. 1. 3rd ed. Philadelphia, W.B. Saunders Company, 1995, p. 266.

7. Rotwein, P.: Structure, evolution, expression and regulation of insulin-like growth factors I and II. Growth Factors 5:3, 1991.

8. Clemmons, D. R.: Insulin-like growth factor binding proteins. Trends Endocrin. Metab. 1:412, 1990.

9. Yamashita, S., Weiss, M., and Melmed, S.: Insulin-like growth factor I regulates growth hormone secretion and messenger ribonucleic acid levels in human pituitary cells. J. Clin. Endocrinol. Metab. 62:730, 1986.

10. Sacca, L., Cittadini, A., and Fazio, S.: Growth hormone and the heart. Endocr. Rev. 15:55, 1994.

11. Froesch, E. R., Zenobi, P. D., and Hussain, M.: Metabolic and therapeutic effects of insulin-like growth factor I. Horm. Res. 42:66, 1994.

12. Thuesen, L., Christiansen, J. S., Sorensen, J. O. L., et al.: Increased myocardial contractility following growth hormone administration in normal man. Danish Med. Bull. 35:183, 1988.

13. Caidahl, K., Eden, S., and Bengtsson, B. A.: Cardiovascular and renal effects of growth hormone. Clin. Endocrinol. 40:393, 1994.

14. Greco, A. V., Ghirlanda, G., Barone, C., et al.: Somatostatin in the paroxysmal supraventricular and junctional tachycardia. Br. Med. J. 288:28, 1984.

15. Day, S. M., Gu, J., Polak, J. M., and Bloom, S. R.: Somatostatin in the human heart and comparison with guinea pig and rat heart. Br. Heart J. 53:153, 1985.

16. Thorner, M. O., Perryman, R. L., Cronin, M. J., et al.: Somatotroph hyperplasia: Successful treatment of acromegaly by removal of a pancreatic islet tumor secreting a growth hormone–releasing factor. J. Clin. Invest. 70:965, 1982.

17. Ezzat, S., Forster, M. J., Berchtold, P., et al.: Acromegaly. Clinical and biochemical features in 500 patients. Medicine 73:233, 1994.

18. Fazio, S., Cittadini, A., Cuocolo, A., et al.: Impaired cardiac performance is a distinct feature of uncomplicated acromegaly. J. Clin. Endocrinol. Metab. 79:441, 1994.

19. Lie, J. T., and Grossman, S. J.: Pathology of the heart in acromegaly: Anatomic findings in 27 autopsied patients. Am. Heart J. 100:41, 1980.

20. Hradec, J., Marek, J., Kral, J., et al.: Long-term echocardiography follow-up of acromegalic heart disease. Am. J. Cardiol. 72:204, 1993.

21. Cuocolo, A., Nicolai, E., Fazio, S., et al.: Impaired left ventricular diastolic filling in patients with acromegaly: Assessment with radionuclide angiography. J. Nucl. Med. 36:196, 1995.

22. Deray, G., Chanson, P., Maistre, G., et al.: Atrial natriuretic factor in patients with acromegaly. Eur. J. Clin. Pharmacol. 38:409, 1990.

23. Kraatz, C., Benker, G., Weber, F., et al.: Acromegaly and hypertension: Prevalence and relationship to the renin-angiotensin-aldosterone system. Klin. Wochenschr. 68:583, 1990.

24. Moore, T. J., Thein-Wai, W., Dluhy, R. G., et al.: Abnormal adrenal and vascular responses to angiotensin II and an angiotensin antagonist in acromegaly. J. Clin. Endocrinol. Metab. 51:215, 1980.

25. Ng, L. L., and Evans, D. L.: Leukocyte sodium transport in acromegaly. Clin. Endocrinol. 26:471, 1987.

26. Kahaly, G. Olshausen, K. V., Mohr-Kahaly, S., et al.: Arrhythmia profile in acromegaly. Eur. Heart J. 13:51, 1992.

27. Surawicz, B., and Mangiardi, M. L.: Electrocardiogram in endocrine and metabolic disorders. In Rios, J. G. (eds.): Clinical Electrocardiographic Correlations. Philadelphia, F. A. Davis Co., 1977, p. 243.

28. Hayward, R. P., Emanuel, R. W., and Navarro, J. D. N.: Acromegalic heart disease: Influence of treatment of the acromegaly on the heart. Q. J. Med. 62:41, 1987.

29. Rodrigues, E. A., Caruana, M., Lahiri, A., et al.: Subclinical cardiac dysfunction in acromegaly: Evidence for a specific disease of heart muscle. Br. Heart J. 62:185, 1989.

30. Fazio, S., Cittadini, A., Sabatini, D., et al.: Evidence for biventricular involvement in acromegaly: A Doppler echocardiographic study. Eur. Heart J. 14:26, 1993.

31. Chanson, P., Timsit, J., Masquet, C., et al.: Cardiovascular effects of the somatostatin analog octreotide in acromegaly. Ann. Intern. Med. 113:921, 1990.

32. Lim, M. J., Barkan, A. L., and Buda, A. J.: Rapid reduction of left ventricular hypertrophy in acromegaly after suppression of growth hormone hypersecretion. Ann. Intern. Med. 117:719, 1992.

33. Merola, B., Cittadini, A., Colao, A., et al.: Chronic treatment with the somatostatin analog octreotide improves cardiac abnormalities in acromegaly. J. Clin. Endocrinol. Metab. 77:790, 1993.

34. Rossi, E., Zuppi, P., Pennestri, F., et al.: Acromegalic cardiomyopathy. Left ventricular filling and hypertrophy in active and surgically treated disease. Chest 102:1204, 1992.

35. Dillmann, W. H.: Biochemical basis of thyroid hormone action in the heart. Am. J. Med. 88:626, 1990.

36. Polikar, R., Burger, A. G., Scherrer, U., and Nicod, P.: The thyroid and the heart. Circulation 87:1435, 1993.

37. Davis, P. J., and Davis, F. B.: Acute cellular actions of thyroid hormone and myocardial function. Ann. Thorac. Surg. 56:S16, 1993.

38. Dillmann, W. H.: Cardiac function in thyroid disease: Clinical features and management considerations. Ann. Thorac. Surg. 56:S9, 1993.

39. Lazar, M. A.: Thyroid hormone receptors: Multiple forms, multiple possibilities. Endocrinol. Rev. 14:184, 1993.

40. Tsai, M. J., and O'Malley, B. W.: Molecular mechanisms of action of steroid/thyroid receptor superfamily members. Ann Rev. Biochem. 63:451, 1994.

41. Tsika, R. W., Bahl, J. J., Leinwand, L. A., and Morkin, E.: Thyroid hormone regulates expression of a transfected human α-myosin heavy chain fusion gene in fetal rat heart cells. Proc. Natl. Acad. Sci. U.S.A. 87:379, 1990.

42. Zarain-Herzberg, A., Marques, J., Sukovich, D., and Periasamy, M.: Thyroid hormone receptor modulates the expression of the rabbit cardiac sarco (endo) plasmic reticulum Ca(2+)-ATPase gene. J. Biol. Chem. 269:1460, 1994.

43. Orlowski, J., and Lingrell, J. B.: Thyroid and glucocorticoid hormones regulate the expression of multiple Na, K-ATPase genes in cultured neonatal rat cardiac myocyte. J. Biol. Chem. 265:3462, 1990.

44. Bahouth, S. W.: Thyroid hormones transcriptionally regulate the β-1 adrenergic receptor gene in cultured ventricular myocyte. J. Biol. Chem. 266:15863, 1991.

45. Castello, A., Rodriguez-Manazaneque, J. C., Camps, M., et al.: Perinatal hypothyroidism impairs the normal transition of GLUT4 and GLUT1 glucose transporters from fetal to neonatal levels in heart and brown adipose tissue. Evidence for tissue-specific regulation of GLUT4 expression by thyroid hormone. J. Biol. Chem. 269:5905, 1994.

46. Averyhart-Fullard, V., Fraker, L. D., Murphy, A. M., and Solaro, R. J.: Differential regulation of slow-skeletal and cardiac troponin I mRNA during development and by thyroid hormone in rat heart. J. Mol. Cell Cardiol. 26:609, 1994.

47. Dieckman, L. J., and Solaro, R. J.: Effect of thyroid status on thin-filament Ca^{2+} regulation and expression of troponin I in perinatal and adult rat hearts. Circ. Res. 67:344, 1990.

48. Fullerton, M. J., Stuchbury, S., Krozowski, Z. S., and Funder, J. W.: Altered thyroidal status and the in vivo synthesis of atrial natriuretic peptide in the rat heart. Mol. Cell Endocrinol. 69:227, 1990.

49. Segal, J.: Acute effect of thyroid hormone on the heart: An extranuclear increase in sugar uptake. J. Mol. Cell Cardiol. 21:323, 1989.

50. Segal, J.: Calcium is the first messenger for the action of thyroid hormone at the level of the plasma membrane: First evidence for an acute effect of thyroid hormone on calcium uptake in the heart. Endocrinology 126:2693, 1990.

51. Morgan, J. P.: Thyroid hormone effects on intracellular calcium and inotropic responses of rat ventricular myocardium. Am. J. Physiol. 267:H1112, 1994.

52. Han, J., Leem, C., So, I., et al.: Effects of thyroid hormone on the calcium current and isoprenaline-induced background current in rabbit ventricular myocytes. J. Mol. Cell. Cardiol. 26:925, 1994.

53. Levey, G. S., and Klein, I.: Catecholamine-thyroid interactions and the cardiovascular manifestation of hyperthyroidism. Am. J. Med. 88:642, 1990.

54. Hammond, H. K., White, F. C., Buxton, I. L. O., et al.: Increased myocardial beta-receptors and adrenergic responses in hyperthyroid pigs. Am. J. Physiol. 252:H283, 1987.

55. Buccino, R. A., Spann, J. F., Pool, P. E., and Braunwald, E.: Influence of the thyroid state on the intrinsic contractile properties and the energy stores of the myocardium. J. Clin. Invest. 46:1669, 1967.

56. Nishizawa, Y., Hamada, N., Fujii, S., et al.: Serum dopamine beta-hydroxylase activity in thyroid disorders. J. Clin. Endocrinol. Metab. 39:599, 1974.

57. Malbon, C. C., and Greenberg, M. L.: 3, 3',5'-Triiodothyronine administration in vivo modulates the hormone sensitive adenylate cyclase system of rat hepatocytes. J. Clin. Invest. 69:414, 1982.

58. Whitsett, J. A., Pollinger, J., and Matz, S.: β-Adrenergic receptors and catecholamine-sensitive adenylate cyclase in developing rat ventricular myocardium: Effect of thyroid status. Pediatr. Res. 16:463, 1982.

59. Rutherford, J. P., Vatner, S. F., and Braunwald, E.: Adrenergic control of myocardial contractility in conscious hyperthyroid dogs. Am. J. Physiol. 237:590, 1980.

60. Guarnieri, T., Filburn, C. R., Beard, E. S., and Lakatta, E. G.: Enhanced contractile response and protein kinase activation to threshold levels of β-adrenergic stimulation in hyperthyroid rat heart. J. Clin. Invest. 65:861, 1980.

61. Andersson, R. G. G., Nilsson, O. R., and Kuo, J. F.: β-Adrenoreceptor adenosine 3'-5'-monophosphate system in human leukocytes before and after treatment for hyperthyroidism. J. Clin. Endocrinol. Metab. 56:42, 1993.

62. Stiles, G. L., Stadel, J. M., DeLean, A., and Lefkowitz, R. J.: Hypothyroidism modulates beta-adrenergic receptor adenylate cyclase interactions in rat reticulocytes. J. Clin. Invest. 68:1450, 1981.

63. Bahouth, S. W.: Regulation of steady-state levels of beta-adrenergic re-

ceptors and G-proteins by thyroid hormones in cultured rat myocardial cells. FASEB J. *4:*A1779, 1990.

64. Levine, M. A., Feldman, A. M., Robishaw, J. D., et al.: Influence of thyroid hormone status on expression of genes encoding G protein subunits in the rat heart. J. Biol. Chem. *265:*3553, 3560, 1990.

65. Rapiejko, P. J., Watkins, D. C., Ros, M., and Malbon, C. C.: Thyroid hormones regulate G-protein beta-subunit mRNA expression in vivo. J. Biol. Chem. *264:*16183, 1989.

66. Ling, E., O'Brien, P. J., Salerno, T., et al.: Effects of different thyroid treatments on the biochemical characteristics of rabbit myocardium. Can. J. Cardiol. *4:*301, 1988.

67. Murayama, M., and Goodkind, M. J.: Effect of thyroid hormone on the frequency-force relationship of atrial myocardium from the guinea pig. Circ. Res. *23:*743, 1968.

68. Josephson, R. A., Spurgeon, H. A., and Lakatta, E. G.: The hyperthyroid heart: An analysis of systolic and diastolic properties in single rat ventricular myocytes. Circ. Res. *66:*773, 1990.

69. Goldman, S., Olajos, M., Friedman, H., et al.: Left ventricular performance in conscious thyrotoxic calves. Am. J. Physiol. *242:*H113, 1982.

70. Goto, Y., Slinker, B. K., and LeWinter, M. M.: Decreased contractile efficiency and increased nonmechanical energy cost in hyperthyroid rabbit heart: Relation between O₂ consumption and systolic pressure-volume area or force-time interval. Circ. Res. *66:*999, 1990.

71. Kim, D., Smith, T. W., and Marsh, J. D.: Effect of thyroid hormone on slow calcium channel function in cultured chick ventricular cells. J. Clin. Invest. *80:*88, 1987.

72. MacKinnon, R., Gwathmey, J. K., Allen, P. D., et al.: Modulation by the state of intracellular calcium and contractility in ferret ventricular muscle. Circ. Res. *63:*1080, 1988.

73. Poggesi, C., Everets, M., Polla, B., et al.: Influence of thyroid state on mechanical restitution of rat myocardium. Circ. Res. *60:*142, 1987.

74. Samuel, J. L., Rappaport, L., Syrovy, L., et al.: Differential effect of thyroxine on atrial and ventricular isomyosins in rats. Am. J. Physiol. *250:*H333, 1986.

75. Korecky, B., Zak, R., Schwartz, K., et al.: Role of thyroid hormone in regulation of isomyosin composition, contractility, and size of heterotypically isotransplanted rat heart. Circ. Res. *60:*824, 1987.

76. Johnson, P. N., Freedberg, A. S., and Marshall, J. M.: Action of thyroid hormone on the transmembrane potentials from sinoatrial cells and atrial muscle cells in isolated atria of rabbits. Cardiology *58:*273, 1973.

77. Arnsdorf, M. D., and Childers, R. W.: Atrial electrophysiology in experimental hyperthyroidism in rabbits. Circ. Res. *26:*575, 1970.

78. McKenzie, J. M., and Zakarija, M.: Hyperthyroidism. *In* DeGroot, J. L., et al. (eds.): Endocrinology, Vol. 1. 3rd ed. Philadelphia, W.B. Saunders Company, 1995, p. 676.

79. Woeber, K. A.: Thyrotoxicosis and the heart. N. Engl. J. Med. *327:*94, 1992.

80. Talafih, K., Briden, K. L., and Weiss, H. R.: Thyroxine-induced hypertrophy of the rabbit heart. Effect on regional oxygen extraction, flow and oxygen consumption. Circ. Res. *52:*272, 1983.

81. Friedman, M. J., Okada, R. D., Ewy, G. A., and Hellman, D. J.: Left ventricular systolic and diastolic function in hyperthyroidism. Am. Heart J. *104:*1303, 1982.

82. Feldman, T., Borow, K. M., Sarne, D. H., et al.: Myocardial mechanics in hyperthyroidism: Importance of left ventricular loading conditions, heart rate and contractile state. J. Am. Coll. Cardiol. *7:*967, 1986.

83. Maciel, B. C., Gallo, L., Marin-Neto, J. A., et al.: Autonomic control of heart rate during dynamic exercise in human hyperthyroidism. Clin. Sci. *75:*209, 1988.

84. Forfar, J. C., Matthews, D. M., and Toft, D. A.: Delayed recovery of left ventricular function after antithyroid treatment: Further evidence for reversible abnormalities on contractility in hyperthyroidism. Br. Heart J. *52:*215, 1984.

85. Olshausen, K., Bischoll, S., Kahaly, G., et al.: Cardiac arrhythmias and heart rate in hyperthyroidism. Am. J. Cardiol. *63:*930, 1989.

86. Ciaccheri, M., Cecchi, F., Arcangeli, C., et al.: Occult thyrotoxicosis in patients with chronic and paroxysmal isolated atrial fibrillation. Clin. Cardiol. *7:*413, 1984.

87. Goel, B. G., Hanson, C. S., and Han, J.: A-V conduction in hyper- and hypothyroid dogs. Am. Heart J. *83:*504, 1972.

88. Seibers, M. J., Drinka, P. J., and Vergauwen, C.: Hyperthyroidism as a cause of atrial fibrillation in long-term care. Arch. Intern. Med. *152:*2063, 1992.

89. Cavallo, A., Joseph, C. J., and Casta, A.: Cardiac complications in juvenile hyperthyroidism. Am. J. Dis. Child. *138:*479, 1984.

90. Featherstone, H. J., and Stewart, D. K.: Angina in thyrotoxicosis: Thyroid-related coronary artery spasm. Arch. Intern. Med. *143:*554, 1983.

91. Forfar, J. C., Muir, A. L., Sawers, S. A., and Toft, A. D.: Abnormal left ventricular function in hyperthyroidism: Evidence for a possible reversible cardiomyopathy. N Engl. J. Med. *307:*1165, 1982.

92. Ebisawa, K., Ikeda, U., Maruta, M., et al.: Irreversible cardiomyopathy due to thyrotoxicosis. Cardiology *84:*274, 1994.

93. Wilson, R., Gibson, T. C., Terrien, C. M., and Levy, A. M.: Hyperthyroidism and familial hypertrophic cardiomyopathy. Arch. Intern. Med. *143:*378, 1983.

94. Noah, M. S., Sulimani, R. A., Famuyiwa, F. O., et al.: Prolapse of the mitral valve in hyperthyroid patients in Saudi Arabia. Int. J. Cardiol. *19:*217, 1988.

95. Morrow, D. H., Gaffney, T. E., and Braunwald, E.: Studies on digitalis: VIII. Effect of autonomic innervation and of myocardial catecholamine

stores upon the cardiac action of ouabain. J. Pharmacol. Exp. Ther. *140:*236, 1963.

96. Klein, I., Becker, D. V., and Levey, G. S.: Treatment of hyperthyroid disease. Ann. Intern. Med. *121:*281, 1994.

97. Geffner, D. L., and Hershman, J. M.: β-Adrenergic blockade for the treatment of hyperthyroidism. Am. J. Med. *93:*61, 1992.

98. Sandler, G., and Wilson, G. M.: The nature and prognosis of heart disease in thyrotoxicosis. A review of 150 patients treated with ¹³¹I. Q.J. Med. *28:*347, 1959.

99. Ladenson, P. W.: Recognition and management of cardiovascular disease related to thyroid dysfunction. Am. J. Med. *88:*638, 1990.

100. Nakazawa, H. K., Sakurai, K., Hamada, N., et al.: Management of atrial fibrillation in the post-thyrotoxic state. Am. J. Med. *72:*903, 1982.

101. Staffurth, J. S., Gibberd, M. C., and Fui, S. T.: Arterial embolism in thyrotoxicosis with atrial fibrillation. Br. Med. J. *2:*688, 1977.

102. Chopra, I. J., Huang, T.-S., Hurd, R. E., and Solomon, D. H.: A study of cardiac effects of thyroid hormones: Evidence for amelioration of the effects of thyroxine by sodium ipodate. Endocrinology *114:*2039, 1984.

103. Norman, M. F., and Lavin, T. N.: Antagonism of thyroid hormone action by amiodarone in rat pituitary tumor cells. J. Clin. Invest. *83:*306, 1989.

104. Lambert, M., Burger, A. G., DeNayer, P., et al.: Decreased TSH response to TRH induced by amiodarone. Acta Endocrinol. *118:*449, 1988.

105. Gammage, M. D., and Franklyn, J. A.: Amioradone and the thyroid. Q.J. Med. *62:*83, 1987.

106. Martino, E., Bartalena, L., Mariotti, S., et al.: Radioactive iodine thyroid uptake in patients with amioradone iodine-induced thyroid dysfunction. Acta Endocrinol. *119:*167, 1988.

107. Kasim, S. E., Bagchi, N., Brown, T. R., et al.: Effect of amiodarone on serum lipids, lipoprotein lipase, and hepatic triglyceride lipase. Endocrinology *120:*1991, 1987.

108. Rabinowe, S. L., Larsen, P. R., Antman, E. M., et al.: Amioradone therapy and autoimmune thyroid disease. Am. J. Med. *81:*53, 1986.

109. Zimmerman, J., Yahalom, J., Bar-On, H.: Clinical spectrum of pericardial effusion as the presenting feature of hypothyroidism. Am. Heart J. *106:*770, 1983.

110. Khaleeli, A. A., and Memon, N.: Factors affecting resolution of pericardial effusions in primary hypothyroidism: A clinical, biochemical and echocardiographic study. Postgrad. Med. J. *58:*1073, 1982.

111. Mackerrow, S. D., Osborn, L. A., Levey, H., et al.: Myxedema-associated cardiogenic shock treated with intravenous thyronine. Ann. Intern. Med. *117:*1014, 1992.

112. Kumar, A., Bhandari, A. K., and Rahimtoola, S. H.: Torsade de pointes and marked QT prolongation in association with hypothyroidism. Ann. Intern. Med. *106:*712, 1987.

113. Shenoy, M. M., and Goldman, J. M.: Hypothyroid cardiomyopathy: Echocardiographic documentation of reversibility. Am. J. Med. Sci. *294:*1, 1987.

114. Streeten, D. H. P., Andersen, G. H., Howland, T., et al.: Effects of thyroid function on blood pressure: Recognition of hypothyroid hypertension. Hypertension *11:*78, 1988.

115. Saito, I., Kunihiko, I., and Saruta, T.: Hypothyroidism as a cause of hypertension. Hypertension *5:*112, 1983.

116. Fouron, J. C., Bourgin, J. H., Letarte, J., et al.: Cardiac dimensions and myocardial function of infants with congenital hypothyroidism: An echocardiographic study. Br. Heart J. *47:*584, 1982.

117. Graettinger, J. S., Muenster, J. J., and Checchia, C.: A correlation of clinical and hemodynamic studies in patients with hypothyroidism. J. Clin. Invest. *37:*502, 1958.

118. Wieshammer, S., Keck, F. S., Waitzinger, J., et al.: Left ventricular function at rest and during exercise in acute hypothyroidism. Br. Heart J. *60:*204, 1988.

119. Vora, J., O'Malley, B. P., Petersen, S., et al.: Reversible abnormalities of myocardial relaxation in hypothyroidism. J. Clin. Endocrinol. Metab. *61:*269, 1985.

120. Hillis, W. S., Bremmer, W. F., Lawrie, T. D. V., and Thomson, J. A.: Systolic time intervals in thyroid disease. Clin. Endocrinol. *4:*617, 1975.

121. Grossman, N. G., Wieshammer, S., Keck, F. S., et al.: Doppler echocardiographic evaluation of left ventricular diastolic function in acute hypothyroidism. Clin. Endocrinol. *40:*227, 1994.

122. McBrion, D. J., and Hindle, W.: Myxedema and heart failure. Lancet *1:*1065, 1994.

123. Levey, G. S., Skelton, C. L., and Epstein, S. E.: Decreased myocardial adenyl cyclase activity in hypothyroidism. J. Clin. Invest. *48:*2244, 1969.

124. Elder, J., McLelland, A., O'Reilly, D. S., et al.: The relationship between serum cholesterol and serum thyrotropin, thyroxine and tri-iodothyronine concentrations in suspected hypothyroidism. Ann. Clin. Biochem. *36:*110, 1990.

125. Arem, N., and Patsch, W.: Lipoprotein and apolipoprotein levels in subclinical hypothyroidism. Arch. Intern. Med. *150:*2097, 1990.

126. Steinberg, A. D.: Myxedema and coronary artery disease—a comparative autopsy study. Ann. Intern. Med. *68:*338, 1968.

127. Karlsberg, R. P., Friscia, D. A., Aronow, W. S., and Sekhon, S. S. Deleterious influence of hypothyroidism on evolving myocardial infarction in conscious dogs. J. Clin. Invest. *67:*1024, 1981.

128. Keating, F. R., Parkin, T. W., Selby, J. B., and Dickinson, L. S.: Treatment of heart disease associated with myxedema. Prog. Cardiovasc. Dis. *3:*364, 1960.

129. Griffiths, P. D.: Serum enzymes in diseases of the thyroid gland. J. Clin. Pathol. 18:660, 1965.
130. Drucker, D. J., and Burrow, G. N.: Cardiovascular surgery in the hypothyroid patient. Arch. Intern. Med. 145:1585, 1985.
131. Hamblin, P. S., Dyer, S. A., Mohr, V. S., et al.: Relationship between thyrotropin and thyroxine changes during recovery from severe hypothyroxinemia of critical illness. J. Clin. Endocrinol. Metab. 62:717, 1986.
132. Brent, G. A., and Hershman, J. M.: Thyroxine therapy in patients with severe nonthyroidal illnesses and low serum thyroxine concentration. J. Clin. Endocrinol. Metab. 63:1, 1986.

DISEASES OF THE ADRENAL CORTEX

133. Williams, G. H., and Dluhy, R. G.: Diseases of the adrenal cortex. *In* Isselbacher, K., et al. (eds.): Harrison's Principles of Internal Medicine. 13th ed. New York, McGraw-Hill Book Co., 1994, p. 1953.
134. Mortensen, R. M., and Williams G. H.: Aldosterone action: Physiology. *In* DeGroot, L. J., et al. (eds.): Endocrinology, Vol. 1. 3rd ed. Philadelphia, W.B. Saunders Company, 1995, p. 1668.
135. Brilla, C. G., Zhou, G., Matsubara, L., and Weber, K. T.: Collagen metabolism in cultured rat cardiac fibroblasts: Response to angiotensin II and aldosterone. J. Mol. Cell Cardiol. 26:809, 1994.
136. Cushing, H.: The basophil adenomas of the pituitary body and their clinical manifestations (pituitary basophilism). Bull. Johns Hopkins Hosp. 50:137, 1932.
137. Etxabe, J., and Vazquez, J. A.: Morbidity and mortality in Cushing's disease: An epidemiological approach. Clin. Endocrinol. 40:479, 1994.
138. Soszynski, P., Slowinska-Srzednicka, J., Kasperlik-Zaluska, A., and Zglicaynski, S.: Endogenous natriuretic factors: Atrial natriuretic hormone and digitalis-like substance in Cushing's syndrome. J. Endocrinol. 129:453, 1991.
139. Mantero, F., and Boscaro, M.: Glucocorticoid-dependent hypertension. J. Steroid Biochem. Mol. Biol. 43:409, 1992.
140. Yasuda, G., Shionoiri, H., Umeura, S., et al.: Exaggerated blood pressure response to angiotensin II in patients with Cushing's syndrome due to adrenocortical adenomas. Eur. J. Endocrinol. 131:582, 1994.
141. Sugihara, N., Shimizu, M., Kita, Y., et al.: Cardiac characteristics and post-operative courses in Cushing's syndrome. Am. J. Cardiol. 69:1475, 1992.
142. Carney, J. A., Gordon, H., Carpenter, P. C., et al.: The complex of myxomas, spotty pigmentation, and endocrine overactivity. Medicine 64:270, 1985.
143. Fallo, F., Paoletta, A., Tona, F., et al.: Response of hypertension to conventional antihypertensive treatment and/or steroidogenesis inhibitors in Cushing's syndrome. J. Intern. Med. 234:595, 1993.
144. Conlin, P. R., Dluhy, R. G., and Williams, G. H.: Disorders of the renin-angiotensin-aldosterone system. *In* Schrier, R. W. (ed.): Renal and Electrolyte Disorders. 4th ed. Boston, Little, Brown & Co., 1992, p. 405.
145. Lifton, R. P., Dluhy, R. G., Powers, M., et al.: A chimeric 11 β-hydroxylase/aldosterone synthase gene causes glucocorticoid-remediable aldosteronism in human hypertension. Nature 355:262, 1992.
146. Rabinowe, S. L., Jackson, R. A., Dluhy, R. G., and Williams, G. H.: Ia-positive T lymphocytes in recently-diagnosed idiopathic Addison's disease. Am. J. Med. 77:597, 1984.
147. Knowlton, A. L., and Baer, L.: Cardiac failure in Addison's disease. Am. J. Med. 74:829, 1983.
148. Dorin, R. I., and Kearns, P. J.: High output circulatory failure in acute adrenal insufficiency. Crit. Care Med. 16:296, 1988.
149. Schambelan, M., Sebastian, A., and Biglieri, E. G.: Prevalence, pathogenesis and functional significance of aldosterone deficiency in hyperkalemic patients with chronic renal insufficiency. Kidney Int. 17:89, 1980.
150. Lee, T. H., Salomon, D. R., Rayment, C. M., and Antman, E.: Hypotension and sinus arrest with exercise-induced hyperkalemia and combined verapamil/propranolol therapy. Am. J. Med. 80:1203, 1986.
151. Mannisi, J. A., Weisman, H. F., Bush, D. E., et al.: Steroid administration after myocardial infarction promotes early infarct expansion. J. Clin. Invest. 79:1431, 1987.
152. Alford, W. C., Meador, C. K., Mihalevich, J., et al.: Acute adrenal insufficiency following cardiac surgical procedures. J. Thorac. Cardiovasc. Surg. 78:489, 1979.

PHEOCHROMOCYTOMA

153. Gifford, R. W., Manger, W. M., and Bravo, E. L.: Pheochromocytoma. Endocrinol. Metab. Clin. North. Am. 23:387, 1994.
154. Wurtman, R. J., and Axelrod, J.: Control of enzymatic synthesis of adrenaline in the adrenal medulla by adrenal cortical steroids. J. Biol. Chem. 241:2301, 1966.
155. Levenson, J. A., Safar, M. E., London, G. M., and Simon, A. C.: Haemodynamics in patients with phaeochromocytoma. Clin. Sci. 58:349, 1980.
156. Sardesai, S. H., Marinde, A. J., Sivathandon, Y., et al.: Phaeochromocytoma and catecholamine-induced cardiomyopathy presenting as heart failure. Br. Heart J. 63:234, 1990.
157. Bravo, E., Fouad-Tarazi, F., Rossi, G., et al.: A reevaluation of the hemodynamics of pheochromocytoma. Hypertension 15:I128, 1990.
158. Strenson, G., and Swedberg, K.: QRS amplitudes, QT intervals, and ECG abnormalities in pheochromocytoma patients before, during and after treatment. Acta Med. Scand. 224:231, 1988.
159. Haas, G. J., Tzagournis, M., and Boudoulas, H.: Pheochromocytoma: Catecholamine-mediated electrocardiographic changes mimicking ischemia. Am. Heart J. 116:1363, 1988.
160. Scott, I., Parkes, R., and Cameron, D. P.: Pheochromocytoma and cardiomyopathy. Med. J. Aust. 148:94, 1988.
161. Behrana, A. J., Haselton, P., Leen, C. I. S., et al.: Multiple extra-adrenal paragangliomas associated with catecholamine cardiomyopathy. Eur. Heart J. 10:182, 1989.
162. Slathe, M., Weiss, P., and Ritz, R.: Rapid reversal of heart failure in a patient with phaeochromocytoma and catecholamine-induced cardiomyopathy who was treated with captopril. Br. Heart J. 68:527, 1992.
163. Hu, Z. W., Billingham, M., Tuck, M., and Hoffman, B. B.: Captopril improves hypertension and cardiomyopathy in rats with pheochromocytoma. Hypertension 15:210, 1990.
164. Schub, C., Gueto-Garcia, L., Sheps, S. G., et al.: Echocardiographic findings in pheochromocytoma. Am. J. Cardiol. 57:971, 1986.
165. Cueto, L., Arriaga, J., and Zinser, J.: Echocardiographic changes in pheochromocytoma. Chest 76:600, 1979.
166. McManus, B. M., Fleury, T. A., Roberts, W. C.: Fatal catecholamine crisis in pheochromocytoma. Curable form of cardiac arrest. Am. Heart J. 102:930, 1981.
167. Simons, M., and Downing, S. E.: Coronary vasoconstriction and catecholamine cardiomyopathy. Am. Heart J. 109:297, 1985.
168. Bhatnagar, D., Carey, P., and Pollard, A.: Focal myositis and elevated creatinine kinase levels in a patient with phaeochromocytoma. Postgrad. Med. J. 62:197, 1986.
169. Serfas, D., Shoback, D. M., and Lorrell, B. H.: Phaeochromocytoma and hypertrophic cardiomyopathy: Apparent suppression of symptoms and noradrenaline secretion by calcium-channel blockade. Lancet 2:711, 1983.
170. Jebara, V. A., Uva, M. S., Farge, A., et al.: Cardiac pheochromocytomas. Ann. Thorac. Surg. 53:356, 1992.
171. Brown, E. M.: Physiology of calcium metabolism. *In* Becker, K. L. (ed.): Principles and Practice of Endocrinology and Metabolism. Philadelphia, J. B. Lippincott, Co., 1990, p. 423.
172. Bogin, E., Massry, S. G., and Harary, I.: Effect of parathyroid hormone on rat heart cells. J. Clin. Invest. 67:1215, 1981.
173. Katoh, Y., Klein, K. L., Kaplan, R. A., et al.: Parathyroid hormone has a positive inotropic action in the rat. Endocrinology 109:2252, 1981.
174. Palmieri, G. M., Nutting, D. F., Bhattacharya, S. K., et al.: Parathyroid ablation in dystrophic hamsters: Effects of Ca content and histology of heart, diaphragm, and rectus femoris. J. Clin. Invest. 68:646, 1981.
175. Gafter, U., Battler, A., Eldar, M., et al.: Effect of hyperparathyroidism on cardiac function in patients with end-stage renal disease. Nephron 41:30, 1985.
176. Vered, I., Vered, Z., Perez, J. E., et al.: Normal left ventricular performance documented by Doppler echocardiography in patients with long-standing hypocalcemia. Am. J. Med. 86:413, 1989.
177. Giles, T. D., Iteld, B. J., and Rires, K. L.: The cardiomyopathy of hypoparathyroidism. Chest 79:225, 1981.
178. Ellison, D. H., and McCarron, D. A.: Structural prerequisites for the hypotensive action of parathyroid hormone. Am. J. Physiol. 246:F551, 1984.
179. Roberts, W. C., and Waller, B. F.: Effect of chronic hypercalcemia on the heart: An analysis of 18 necropsy patients. Am. J. Med. 71:371, 1981.
180. Roberts, W. C., and Waller, B. F.: Chronic hypercalcemia as a risk factor for coronary atherosclerosis. Cardiovasc. Rev. Rep. 4:1275, 1983.
181. Slavich, G. A., Antonucci, F., and Sponza, E.: Primary hyperparathyroidism and angina pectoris. Int. J. Cardiol. 19:266, 1988.
182. Csanady, M., Forster, T., and Julesz, J.: Reversible impairment of myocardial function in hypoparathyroidism causing hypocalcaemia. Br. Heart J. 63:58, 1990.
183. Kleerekoper, M., Rao, D. S., and Frame, B.: Hypercalcemia, hyperparathyroidism and hypertension. Cardiovasc. Med. 3:1283, 1978.
184. Daniels, J., and Goodman, A. D.: Hypertension and hyperparathyroidism: Inverse relation of sodium phosphate level and blood pressure. Am. J. Med. 75:17, 1983.

PARATHYROID DISEASE

185. Hatton, D. C., Xue, H., DeMerritt, J. A., and McCarron, D. A.: 1,25(OH)$_2$ vitamin D$_3$-induced alterations in vascular reactivity in the spontaneously hypertensive rat. Am. J. Med. Sci. 307:S154, 1994.
186. Benishin, C. G., Lewanczuk, R. Z., and Pang, P. K.: Purification of parathyroid hypertensive factor from plasma of spontaneously hypertensive rats. Proc. Natl. Acad. Sci. U.S.A. 88:6372, 1991.
187. Benishin, C. G., Labeda, T., Guo, D. D., et al.: Identification and purification of parathyroid hypertensive factor from organ culture of parathyroid glands from spontaneously hypertensive rats. Am. J. Hypertens. 6:134, 1993.
188. Pang, P. K., Benishin, C. G., Shan, J., and Lewanczuk, R. Z.: PHF: The new parathyroid hypertensive factor. Blood Press. 3:148, 1994.
189. Lewanczuk, R. Z., Benishin, C. G., Shan, J., and Pang, P. K.: Clinical aspects of parathyroid hypertensive factor. J. Cardiovasc. Pharmacol. 23:S23, 1994.
190. Lewanczuk, R. Z., Resnick, L. M., Ho, M. S., et al.: Clinical aspects of parathyroid hypertensive factor. J. Hypertens. (Suppl). 12:S11, 1994.

191. Halban, P. A., and Weir, G. C.: Islet cell hormones: Production and degradation. *In* Becker, K. L. (ed.): Principles and Practice of Endocrinology and Metabolism. Philadelphia. J. B. Lippincott Co., 1990, p. 1068.

192. Eisenbarth, G. S., and Kahn, C. R.: Etiology and pathogenesis of diabetes mellitus. *In* Becker, K. L. (ed.): Principles and Practice of Endocrinology and Metabolism. Philadelphia, J. B. Lippincott Co., 1990, p. 1074.

192a. Aronson, D., and Rayfield, E. J.: Diabetes and obesity. *In* Fuster, V., Ross, R., and Topol, E. J. (eds.): Atherosclerosis and Coronary Artery Disease. Philadelphia, Lippincott-Raven, 1996, pp. 327–362.

193. Woods, K. L., Samanta, A., and Burden, A. C.: Diabetes mellitus as a risk factor for acute myocardial infarction in Asians and Europeans. Br. Heart J. *62*:118, 1989.

194. Stone, P. H., Muller, J. E., Hartwell, T., et al.: The effect of diabetes mellitus on prognosis and serial left ventricular function after acute myocardial infarction: Contribution of both coronary disease and diastolic left ventricular dysfunction to the adverse prognosis. J. Am. Coll. Cardiol. *14*:49, 1989.

195. Herlitz, J., Malmberg, K., Karlson, B. W., et al.: Mortality and morbidity during a five-year follow-up of diabetics with myocardial infarction. Acta Med. Scand. *224*:31, 1988.

196. Bradley, R. F., and Schanfield, H.: Diminished pain in diabetic patients with acute myocardial infarction. Geriatrics *17*:322, 1962.

197. Kannel, W. B.: Silent myocardial ischemia and infarction: Insights from the Framingham study. Cardiol. Clin. *4*:583, 1986.

198. Savage, M. P., Krolewski, A. S., Kenien, G. G., et al.: Acute myocardial infarction in diabetes mellitus and significance of congestive heart failure as a prognostic factor. Am. J. Cardiol. *62*:665, 1988.

199. Gunderson, T., and Kjekshus, J.: Timolol treatment after myocardial infarction in diabetic patients. Diabetes Care *6*:285, 1983.

200. Ceremuzynski, L.: Hormonal and metabolic reactions evoked by acute myocardial infarction. Circ. Res. *48*:767, 1981.

201. Roy, T. M., Peterson, H. R., Snider, H. L., et al.: Autonomic influence on cardiovascular performance in diabetic subjects. Am. J. Med. *87*:382, 1989.

202. Ewing, D. J., and Clarke, B. F.: Diagnosis and management of diabetic autonomic neuropathy. Br. Med. J. *285*:916, 1982.

203. Ambepitiya, G., Kopelman, P. G., Ingram, D.: Exertional myocardial ischemia in diabetes: A quantitative analysis of anginal perceptual threshold and the influence of autonomic function. J. Am. Coll. Cardiol. *15*:72, 1990.

204. Zola, B., Kahn, J. K., Juni, J. E., and Vinik, A. I.: Abnormal cardiac function in diabetic patients with autonomic neuropathy in the absence of ischemic heart disease. J. Clin. Endocrinol. Metab. *63*:208, 1986.

205. Weise, F., Heydenreich, F., Gehrig, W., and Runge, U.: Heart rate variability in diabetic patients during orthostatic load—a spectral analytic approach. Klin. Wochenschr. *68*:26, 1990.

206. Zoneraich, S.: Diabetes and the Heart. Springfield, Ill., Charles C Thomas, Publisher, 1978, p. 303.

207. Sutherland, C. G. G., Fisher, B. M., Frier, B. M., et al.: Endomyocardial biopsy pathology in insulin-dependent diabetic patients with abnormal ventricular function. Histopathology *14*:593, 1989.

208. Hausdorf, G., Rieger, U., and Koepp, P.: Cardiomyopathy in childhood diabetes mellitus: Incidence, time of onset, and relation to metabolic control. Int. J. Cardiol. *19*:225, 1988.

209. Zarich, S. W., Arbuckle, B. E., Cohen, L. R., et al.: Diastolic abnormalities in young asymptomatic diabetic patients assessed by pulsed Doppler echocardiography. J. Am. Coll. Cardiol. *12*:114, 1988.

210. Takenakam, K., Sakamoto, T., Amano, K., et al.: Left ventricular filling determined by Doppler echocardiography in diabetes mellitus. Am. J. Cardiol. *61*:1139, 1988.

211. Ruddy, T. D., Shumak, S. L., Liu, P. P., et al.: The relationship of cardiac diastolic dysfunction to concurrent hormonal and metabolic status in Type I diabetes mellitus. J. Clin. Endocrinol. Metab. *66*:113, 1988.

212. Mustonen, J. N., Usitupa, M. I. J., Tahvanainen, K., et al.: Impaired left ventricular systolic function during exercise in middle-aged insulin-dependent and noninsulin-dependent diabetic subjects without clinically evident cardiovascular disease. Am. J. Cardiol. *62*:1273, 1988.

213. Danielsen, R., Nordrehaug, J. E., and Vik-Mo, H.: Left ventricular function in young long-term Type I (insulin-dependent) diabetic men during exercise assessed by digitized echocardiography. Eur. Heart J. *9*:395, 1988.

214. Bouchard, A., Sanz, N., Botvinick, E. H., et al.: Noninvasive assessment of cardiomyopathy in normotensive diabetic patients between 20 and 50 years old. Am. J. Med. *87*:160, 1989.

215. Paillole, C., Dahan, M., Paycha, F., et al.: Prevalence and significance of left ventricular filling abnormalities determined by Doppler echocardiography in young Type I (insulin-dependent) diabetic patients. Am. J. Cardiol. *64*:1010, 1989.

216. Danielsen, R.: Factors contributing to left ventricular diastolic dysfunction in long-term Type I diabetic subjects. Acta Med. Scand. *224*:249, 1988.

217. Ramandaham, S., Rodrigues, B., and McNeill, J. H.: Growth hormone and diabetes-induced cardiomyopathy. J. Lab. Clin. Med. *110*:257, 1987.

218. Regan, T. J., Altszuler, N., Eaddy, C., et al.: Relation of growth hormone and myocardial collagen accumulation in experimental diabetes. J. Lab. Clin. Med. *110*:274, 1987.

219. Nakada, T., and Kwee, I. L.: Sorbitol accumulation in heart: Implication for diabetic cardiomyopathy. Life Sci. *45*:2491, 1989.

220. Schaffer, S. W., Mozaffari, M. S., Artman, M., et al.: Basis for myocardial mechanical defects associated with noninsulin-dependent diabetes. Am. J. Physiol. *256*:E25, 1989.

221. Borda, E., Pascual, J., Wald, M., et al.: Hypersensitivity to calcium associated with an increased sarcolemmal Ca^{++}-ATPase activity in diabetic rat heart. Can. J. Cardiol. *4*:97, 1988.

222. Pierce, G. N., Lockwood, K., and Eckhert, C. D.: Cardiac contractile protein ATPase activity in a diet induced model of noninsulin dependent diabetes mellitus. Can. J. Cardiol. *5*:117, 1989.

223. Afzal, N., Ganguly, P. K., Dhalla, K. S., et al.: Beneficial effects of verapamil in diabetic cardiomyopathy. Diabetes *37*:936, 1988.

224. Okumura, K., Akiyama, N., Hashimoto, H., et al.: Alteration of 1,2 diacyglycerol content in myocardium from diabetic rats. Diabetes *37*:1168, 1988.

225. Sunni, S., Bishop, S. P., Kent, S. P., and Geer, J. C.: Diabetic cardiomyopathy. Arch. Pathol. Lab. Med. *110*:375, 1986.

226. Unsitupa, M., Siitonen, O., Pyorala, K., and Lansimies, E.: Left ventricular function in newly diagnosed noninsulin-dependent (type 2) diabetes evaluated by systolic time intervals and echocardiography. Acta Med. Scand. *217*:379, 1985.

227. Fein, F. S., Capasso, J. M., Aronson, R. S., et al.: Combined renovascular hypertension and diabetes in rats: A new preparation of congestive cardiomyopathy. Circulation *70*:318, 1984.

228. Regan, T. J., Wu, C. F., Weisse, A. B.: Acute myocardial infarction in toxic cardiomyopathy without coronary obstruction. Circulation *51*:453, 1975.

229. Deorari, A. K., Saxena, A., Singh, M., et al.: Echocardiographic assessment of infants born to diabetic mothers. Arch. Dis. Child. *64*:721, 1989.

230. Sheehan, J. P., Sisam, D. A., and Schumacher, O. P.: Insulin-induced cardiac failure. Am. J. Med. *79*:147, 1985.

231. Zatz, R., Dunn, B. R., Meyer, T. W., et al.: Prevention of diabetic glomerulopathy by pharmacological amelioration of glomerular capillary hypertension. J. Clin. Invest. *77*:1925, 1986.

232. Marre, M., Leblanc, H., Suarez, L., et al.: Converting enzyme inhibition and kidney function in normotensive diabetic patients with persistent microalbuminuria. Br. Med. J. *294*:1448, 1987.

233. Sowers, J. R., Sowers, P. S., and Peuler, J. D.: Role of insulin resistance and hyperinsulinemia in development of hypertension and atherosclerosis. J. Lab. Clin. Med. *123*:647, 1994.

234. The Working Group on Hypertension in Diabetes: Statement on hypertension in diabetes mellitus. Final report. Arch. Intern. Med. *147*:830, 1987.

235. Ferrannini, E., and DeFronzo, R. A.: The association of hypertension, diabetes, and obesity: A review. J. Nephrol. *1*:3, 1989.

236. Reaven, G. M., and Hoffman, B. B.: Hypertension as a disease of carbohydrate and lipoprotein metabolism. Am. J. Med. *87*:2S, 1989.

237. Williams, G. H.: Converting enzyme inhibitors in the treatment of hypertension. N. Engl. J. Med. *319*:1517, 1988.

238. Houston, M. C.: Treatment of hypertension in diabetes mellitus. Am. Heart. J. *118*:819, 1989.

239. The Diabetes Control and Complications Trial Research Group: The effect of intensive treatment of diabetes on the development and progression of long-term complications in insulin-dependent diabetes mellitus. N. Engl. J. Med. *329*:977, 1993.

240. University Group Diabetes Program: A study of the effects of hypoglycemic agents on vascular complications in patients with adult onset diabetes. V. Evaluation of phenoformin therapy. Diabetes *24*(Suppl. I):65, 1975.

241. Wu, C. F., Haider, B., Ahmed, S. S., et al.: The effects of tolbutamide on the myocardium in experimental diabetes. Circulation *55*:200, 1977.

242. Regan, T. J.: Cardiac disease in the older diabetic: Management considerations. Geriatrics *44*:91, 1989.

243. United Kingdom Prospective Diabetes Study Group: United Kingdom prospective diabetes study (UKPDS) 13: Relative efficacy of randomly allocated diet, sulphonylurea, insulin, or metformin in patients with newly diagnosed non-insulin dependent diabetes followed for three years. Br. Med. J. *310*:83, 1995.

244. Bielefeld, D. R., Pace, C. S., and Boshell, B. R.: Hyperosmolarity and cardiac function in chronic diabetic rat heart. Am J. Physiol. *245*:E568, 1983.

OBESITY

245. Salan, S.: The obesities. *In* Felig, P., et al. (eds.): Endocrinology and Metabolism. 2nd ed. New York, McGraw-Hill Book Co., 1987, p. 1203.

246. Hirsch, J.: The adipose cell hypothesis. N. Engl. J. Med. *294*:389, 1976.

247. Foster, W. R., and Burton, B. T. (eds.): Health implications of obesity: NIH consensus development conference. Ann. Intern. Med. *103*:979, 1985.

248. Smith, H. L., and Willius, R. A.: Adiposity of the heart. A clinical and pathological study of one hundred and thirty-six obese patients. Ann. Intern. Med. *52*:911, 1933.

249. De Divitis, O., Fazio, S., Petitto, M., et al.: Obesity and cardiac function. Circulation *64*:477, 1981.

250. Egan, B., Fitzpatrick, M. A., Juni, J., et al.: Importance of overweight in studies of left ventricular hypertrophy and diastolic function in mild systemic hypertension. Am. J. Cardiol. *64*:752, 1989.

251. Nakajima, T., Fujioka, S., Tokunaga, K., et al.: Correlation of intraab-

dominal fat accumulation and left ventricular performance in obesity. Am. J. Cardiol. *64:*369, 1989.

252. Zack, P. M., Wiens, R. D., and Kennedy, H. L.: Left-axis deviation and adiposity: The United States health and nutrition examination survey. Am. J. Cardiol. *53:*1129, 1984.

253. Ventura, H. O., Messerli, F.H., Dunn, F. G., and Frohlich, E. D.: Left ventricular hypertrophy in obesity: Discrepancy between echo and electrocardiogram. J. Am. Coll. Cardiol. *1:*682, 1983.

254. Warnes, C. A., and Roberts, W. C.: The heart in massive (more than 300 pounds or 136 kilograms) obesity: Analysis of 12 patients studied at necropsy. Am. J. Cardiol. *54:*1087, 1984.

255. Lavie, C. J., Amodeo, C., Ventura, H. O., et al: Left atrial abnormalities indicating diastolic ventricular dysfunction in cardiopathy of obesity. Chest *92:*1042, 1987.

256. Rossi, M., Marti, G., Ricordi, L., et al.: Cardiac autonomic dysfunction in obese subjects. Clin. Sci. *76:*567, 1989.

257. National High Blood Pressure Education Program: The Fifth Report of the Joint National Committee on detection, evaluation and treatment of high blood pressure. Bethesda, MD, NIH Publication No. 93-1088.

258. Reaven, G. M.: Role of insulin resistance in human disease. Diabetes *37:*1495, 1988.

259. Reaven, G. M.: Insulin resistance and compensatory hyperinsulinemia: Role in hypertension, dyslipidemia, and coronary heart disease. Am. Heart J. *121:*1283, 1991.

260. Donahue, R. P., Abbott, R. D., Bloom, E., et al.: Central obesity and coronary heart disease in men. Lancet *1:*821, 1987.

261. Manson, J. E., Colditz, G. A., Stampher, M. J., et al.: A prospective study of obesity and risk of coronary heart disease in women. N. Engl. J. Med. *322:*882, 1990.

261a. Himeno, E., Nishino, K., Nakashima, Y., et al.: Weight reduction regresses left ventricular mass regardless of blood pressure level in obese subjects. Am. Heart J. *131:*313, 1996.

262. Reisin, E., Frohlich, E. D., Messerli, F. H., et al.: Cardiovascular changes after weight reduction in obesity hypertension. Ann. Intern. Med. *98:*315, 1983.

263. MacMahon, S. W., Wilcken, D. E. L., and Macdonald, G. J.: The effect of weight reduction on left ventricular mass: A randomized controlled trial in young, overweight hypertensive patients. N. Engl. J. Med. *314:*334, 1986.

264. Alpert, M. A., Terry, B. E., and Kelley, D. L.: Effect of weight loss on cardiac chamber size, wall thickness and left ventricular function in morbid obesity. Am. J. Cardiol. *55:*783, 1985.

265. Backman, L., Freyschuss, U., Hallberg, D., and Melcher, A.: Reversibility of cardiovascular changes in extreme obesity: Effects of weight reduction through jejunoileostomy. Acta Med. Scand. *205:*367, 1979.

266. Pi-Sunyer, F. X.: Short-term medical benefits and adverse effects of weight loss. Ann. Intern. Med. *119:*722, 1993.

267. Frank, A., Graham, C., and Frank, S.: Fatalities on the liquid protein diet: An analysis of possible causes. Int. J. Obes. *5:*243, 1981.

MALNUTRITION

268. Webb, J. G., Kiess, M. C., and Chan-Yan, C. C.: Malnutrition and the heart. Can. Med. Assoc. J. *135:*753, 1986.

269. Pringle, T. H., Scobie, I. N., Murray, R. G., et al.: Prolongation of the QT interval during therapeutic starvation: A substrate for malignant arrhythmias. Int. J. Obes. *7:*253, 1983.

270. Bergman, J. W., Human, D. G., DeMoor, M. M. A., et al.: Effect of kwashiorkor on the cardiovascular system. Arch. Dis. Child. *63:*1359, 1988.

271. Alden, P. B., Madoff, R. D., Stahl, T. J., et al.: Left ventricular function in malnutrition. Am. J. Physiol. *253:*H380, 1987.

272. Nutter, D. O., Murray, T. G., Heymsfield, S. T., and Fuller, E. O.: The effect of chronic protein-calorie undernutrition in the rat on myocardial function and cardiac function. Circ. Res. *45:*144, 1979.

273. Isner, J. M., Roberts, W. C., Heymsfield, S. B., and Yager, J.: Anorexia nervosa and sudden death. Ann. Intern. Med. *102:*49, 1985.

274. de Simone, G., Scalfi, L., Galderisi, M., et al.: Cardiac abnormalities in young women with anorexia nervosa. Br. Heart J. *71:*287, 1994.

275. Kollai, M., Bonyhay, I., Jokkel, G., and Szanyi, L.: Cardiac vagal hyperactivity in adolescent anorexia nervosa. Eur. Hypertens. J. *15:*113, 1994.

276. Cooke, R. A., Chambers, T. B., Singh, R., et al.: Q T interval in anorexia nervosa. Br. Heart J. *72:*69, 1994.

THE HEART AND GONADAL HORMONES

277. Carr, J. G., Stevenson, L. W., Walden, J. A., et al.: Prevalence and hemodynamic correlates of malnutrition in severe congestive heart failure secondary to ischemic or idiopathic dilated cardiomyopathy. Am. J. Cardiol. *63:*709, 1989.

278. Blackburn, G. L., Gibbons, G. W., Bothe, A., et al.: Nutritional support in cardiac cachexia. J. Thorac. Cardiovasc. Surg. *73:*489, 1977.

279. Abel, R. M., Fischer, J. E., Buckley, M. J., et al.: Malnutrition in cardiac surgical patients. Arch. Surg. *111:*45, 1976.

280. Steier, M., Lopez, R., and Cooperman, J. M.: Riboflavin deficiency in infants and children with hearth disease. Am. Heart J. *92:*139, 1976.

281. Lerner, D. J., and Kannel, W. B.: Patterns of coronary heart disease, morbidity and mortality in the sexes: A 26 year follow-up of the Framingham population. Am. Heart J. *111:*383, 1986.

282. Bush, T. L., Barrett-Connor, E., Cowan, L. D., et al.: Cardiovascular mortality and non-contraceptive use of estrogen in women. Results from the Lipid Research Clinics Program follow-up. Circulation *75:*1102, 1987.

283. Wren, B. G.: The effect of estrogen on the female cardiovascular system. Med. J. Aust. *157:*204, 1992.

284. Rosano, G. M. C., Sarrel, P. M., Poole-Wilson, P. A., and Collins, P.: Beneficial effect of oestrogen on exercise-induced myocardial ischemia in women with coronary artery disease. Lancet *342:*133, 1993.

285. Gebara, O. C. E.: Association between increased estrogen status and increased fibrinolytic potential in the Framingham Offspring Study. Circulation *91:*1952, 1995.

286. Gordon, T., Kannel, W. B., Hjortland, M. C., and McNamara, P. M.: Menopause and coronary heart disease. The Framingham Study. Ann. Intern. Med. *89:*157, 1978.

287. Stampfer, M. J., Willett, W. C., Colditz, C. A., et al.: A prospective study of post-menopausal estrogen therapy and coronary heart disease. N. Engl. J. Med. *313:*1044, 1985.

288. Stampfer, M. J., and Colditz, C. A.: Estrogen replacement therapy and coronary heart disease: A quantitative assessment of the epidemiologic evidence. Prev. Med. *20:*47, 1991.

289. Stampfer, M. J., Colditz, G. A., Willett, W. C., et al.: Postmenopausal estrogen therapy and cardiovascular disease. Ten-year follow-up from the Nurses' Health Study. N. Engl. J. Med. *325:*756, 1991.

290. Nabulsi, A. A., Folsom, A. R., White, A., et al.: Association of hormone-replacement therapy with various cardiovascular risk factors in post-menopausal women. N. Engl. J. Med. *328:*1069, 1993.

291. The Writing Group for the PEPI Trial: Effects of estrogen or estrogen/progestin regimens on hearty disease risk factors in post-menopausal women. The post-menopausal estrogen/progestin interventions (PEPI) trial. JAMA *273:*199, 1995.

292. McDonald, C. C., and Stewart, H. J.: Fatal myocardial infarction in the Scottish adjuvant tamoxifen trial. The Scottish Breast Cancer Committee. BMJ *303:*435, 1991.

293. Rutqvist, L. E., and Mattsson, A.: Cardiac and thromboembolic morbidity among postmenopausal women with early-stage breast cancer in a randomized trial of adjuvant tamoxifen. The Stockholm Breast Cancer Study Group. J. Natl. Cancer Inst. *85:*1298, 1993.

294. Love, R. R., Wiebe, D. A., Newcomb, P. A., et al.: Effects of tamoxifen on cardiovascular risk factors in post-menopausal women. Ann. Intern. Med. *115:*860, 1991.

295. Webber, L. S., Hunter, S. M., Baugh, J. G., et al.: The interaction of cigarette smoking, oral contraceptive use, and cardiovascular risk factor variables in children: The Bogalusa Heart Study. Am. J. Publ. Health *72:*266, 1982.

296. Jaffe, M. D.: Effect of oestrogens on postexercise electrocardiogram. Br. Heart J. *38:*1299, 1976.

297. Merians, D. R., Haskell, W. L., Vranizan, K. M., et al.: Relationship of exercise, oral contraceptive use, and body fat to concentrations of plasma lipids and lipoprotein cholesterol in young women. Am. J. Med. *78:*913, 1985.

298. Stampfer, M. J., Willett, W. C., Colditz, G. A., et al.: A prospective study of past use of oral contraceptive agents and risk of cardiovascular diseases. N. Engl. J. Med. *319:*1313, 1988.

299. Ramcharan, S., Pellegrin, F. A., and Hoag, E. J.: The occurrence and course of hypertensive disease in users and nonusers of oral contraceptive drugs. In The Walnut Creek Contraceptive Drug Study: A prospective study of the side effects of oral contraceptives, Vol. 2. Edited by Ramcharan, S. U.S. Department of Health, Education, and Welfare Publications No. (NIH) 76-563. Washington, DC, Government Printing Office, 1976, p. 1.

300. Prentice, R. L.: On the ability of blood pressure effects to explain the relation between oral contraceptives and cardiovascular disease. Am. J. Epidemiol. *127:*213, 1988.

301. Blumenstein, B. A., Douglas, M. B., and Hall, W. D.: Blood pressure changes and oral contraceptive use: A study of 2676 black women in the southeastern United States. Am. J. Epidemiol. *112:*539, 1980.

302. Rekers, H.: Multicenter trial of a monophasic oral contraceptive containing ethinyl estradiol and desogestrel. Acta Obstet. Gynecol. Scand. *67:*171, 1988.

303. Walling, M.: A multicenter efficacy and safety study of an oral contraceptive containing 150 μg desogestrel and 30 μg ethinyl estradiol. Contraceptive *46:*313, 1992.

304. Shoupe, D.: Multicenter randomized comparison of two low-dose triphasic combined oral contraceptive containing desogestrel or norethindrone. Obstet. Gynecol. *83:*679, 1994.

305. Laragh, J. H., Sealey, J. E., Ledingham, J. G. G., and Newton, M. A.: Oral contraceptives: Renin, aldosterone, and high blood pressure. JAMA *201:*918, 1967.

306. Wren, B. G., and Routledge, D. A.: Blood pressure changes: Oestrogens in climacteric women. Med. J. Aust. *2:*528, 1981.

Chapter 62
Renal Disorders and Heart Disease

CARL V. LEIER, HARISIOS BOUDOULAS

The kidney can be viewed as a component of the circulatory system. Within this integrated system, the function, regulation, and adjustments of the heart and vasculature are closely linked to those of the kidneys. Renal dysfunction and failure adversely affect cardiovascular function, frequently leading to a cardiovascular disorder or failure and, consequently, further impairment of renal performance. Cardiovascular disease, dysfunction, and failure, in turn, can disturb renal function, occasionally to the point of evoking acute or chronic renal failure, which then causes further deterioration of the cardiovascular condition. Clinicians have for years appreciated the fact that failure of one component of the cardiorenal system (e.g., renal failure) greatly amplifies the difficulty in clinical management of the failure of another component (e.g., heart failure).

This chapter presents the principal cardiovascular disorders that commonly affect renal performance and the primary renal conditions responsible for altering cardiovascular structure and function.

CARDIOVASCULAR CONDITIONS THAT AFFECT RENAL FUNCTION

HEART FAILURE

The development of cardiac dysfunction and failure evokes a series of pathophysiological events affecting renal function. The renal responses to these events in turn contribute heavily to the overall pathophysiology and clinical manifestations of congestive heart failure. The nature and degree of renal involvement is largely related to the acuity and severity of cardiac decompensation.

Chronic Low-Output Congestive Heart Failure

The principal pathophysiological forces that bring the kidney into the syndrome of chronic congestive heart failure (CHF) are a reduction in renal blood flow (Fig. 62–1) and progressive activation of a number of hormonal and other regulatory systems (e.g., sympathetic nervous system, renin-angiotensin-aldosterone axis, atrial natriuretic peptide [ANP], arginine vasopressin) (Table 62–1). The mechanisms controlling and activating these events, systems, and factors in CHF are presented in more detail in Chapter 15.

Cardiovascular and Systemic Events Influencing Renal Function in Chronic Heart Failure

DISTRIBUTION OF CARDIAC OUTPUT TO THE KIDNEYS (RENAL BLOOD FLOW). For most CHF patients, the fall in effective renal blood flow is proportional to the reduction in cardiac output. Renal blood flow in normal subjects (age range of 20 to 80 years) averages 600 to 660 ml/min/m², comprising 14 to 20 per cent of simultaneously measured cardiac output.[1,2] Within a wide spectrum of CHF severity (and without intrinsic renal disease), renal blood flow is depressed to an average range of 250 to 450 ml/min/m², but still representing 12 to 18 per cent of the cardiac output.[1,3–5] These data indicate that for human chronic CHF, renal vascular resistance increases to a similar extent as overall systemic vascular resistance, and that for most patients with this condition, the renal share of cardiac output is not substantially redistributed to other "more vital" organs or regions.

Although not precisely delineated in human heart failure, renal blood flow in this condition appears to be strongly influenced by systemic and intrarenal renin-angiotensin and by autonomic nervous system tone. Major modulation of renal blood flow by angiotensin II is supported by the finding that angiotensin-converting enzyme inhibition substantially augments renal blood flow in chronic heart failure.[4,6] Renal flow, in striking contrast to hepatosplanchnic and limb blood flow, is influenced only modestly by alpha-adrenergic blockade.[7] This indicates that the mechanisms (or the relative contribution of each mechanism) adjusting renal vascular resistance and blood flow in human chronic heart failure are not the same as those influencing the vascular resistance and blood flow in other regions of the body. The findings that renal blood flow on an average does not fall below its usual share of cardiac output and that it may plateau as cardiac output drops below 2.0 liters/m²/min[1] support the view that renal blood flow in chronic heart failure is also influenced by a number of local mechanisms and substances, including endothelial modulators of vascular tone (e.g., nitric oxide [EDRF], endothelin], prostaglandin (PGE₂, PGI₂) production and release, tubuloglomerular feedback, myogenic tone, and other "autoregulatory" responses.

Renal blood flow should not be equated with renal function. The functional reserve of the kidneys is such that renal blood flow can be chronically reduced by at least 30 to 40 per cent without substantially affecting overall renal performance. For most patients with chronic heart failure, the disparity between renal blood flow and renal function is related to the relative dissociation of renal blood flow and glomerular filtration rate[4,5,8] (Fig. 62–1). As heart failure evolves and renal blood flow falls, glomerular filtration rate is maintained by enhanced constriction of the efferent arteriole (postglomerulus) relative to the afferent arteriole (preglomerulus). Thus, filtration fraction (ratio of glomerular filtration rate to renal plasma flow) tends to rise as patients advance from mild to moderately severe stages of chronic CHF.

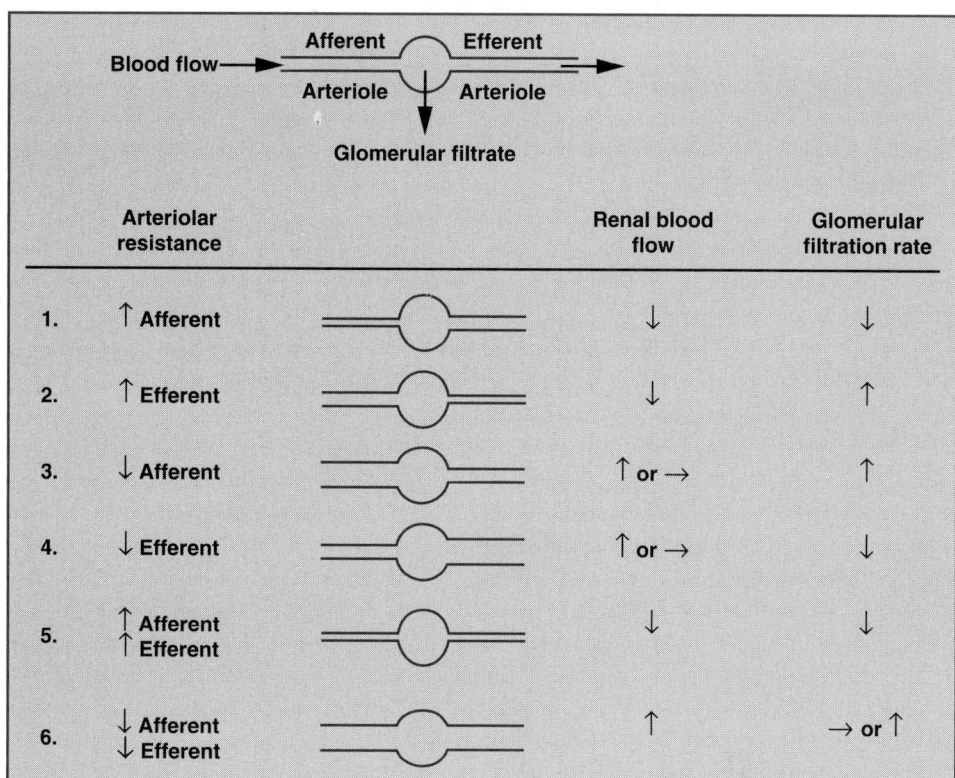

FIGURE 62–1. The renal vascular determinants of renal blood flow are not necessarily the same as those adjusting glomerular filtration rate. Situation 2 applies to most patients with heart failure, a condition accompanied by activation of systemic and intrarenal renin-angiotensin, elevated plasma atrial natriuretic peptide levels, and increased intrarenal prostaglandin activity. Situations 1 and 5 apply to patients with severe reduction in renal perfusion and marked increase of sympathetic nervous system activity and endothelin release, as seen in terminal, end-stage heart failure and/or circulatory shock. Converting enzyme inhibitors can evoke responses 4 and 6 in congestive heart failure. (Adapted from Leier, C. V., and Boudoulas, H.: Cardiorenal Disorders and Diseases. Armonk, N.Y., Futura Publishing Co., 1992.)

Preferential constriction of the efferent arteriole by angiotensin II and dilation of the afferent arteriole by ANP and prostaglandins appear to be the major mechanisms for maintaining glomerular filtration rate (GFR) as renal blood flow declines[4,9-11]; this also explains why GFR and overall renal function can decrease despite a rise in renal blood flow in some CHF patients receiving angiotensin-converting enzyme inhibitors (resultant ↓ angiotensin II).[12,13]

ADVANCED HEART FAILURE. The extremely advanced, terminal stage of chronic CHF is usually accompanied by marked reduction in cardiac output and renal blood flow. At this stage, substantial vasoconstriction of the afferent arteriole occurs to depress glomerular filtration rate (Fig. 62–1). Renal dysfunction in this setting is exacerbated by a concomitant fall in mean systemic blood pressure below 70 to 75 mm Hg and consequent drop in renal perfusion pressure.[14] Low urine output, fluid volume retention, and edema refractory to standard orally administered medication and azotemia now complicate the clinical setting.

Management. Higher doses of diuretics and combined use of loop and tubule diuretics (e.g., furosemide and thiazide) are frequently required (see Chap. 17). Strategies to enhance renal function by increasing renal blood flow and glomerular filtration rate are still generally limited to drugs requiring intravenous administration. Dopamine at doses ≤ 5.0 μg/kg/min can augment renal blood flow and function via stimulation of renal dopaminergic receptors (renal arteriolar dilatation) and some increase in cardiac output.[15,16] In certain instances, vasopressor doses of dopamine (≥ 6.0 μg/kg/min) may be required to bring renal perfusion pressure into an acceptable range (mean systemic arterial pressure ≥ 70 mm Hg). Dobutamine and nitroprusside can improve renal blood flow and function, principally by increasing cardiac output and perhaps, by evoking some renal vasodilation in severely vasoconstricted states.[15,17-19] It is reasonable to employ dobutamine-dopamine or nitroprusside-dopamine combinations in these desperate clinical situations in an attempt to optimally improve cardiac output, renal hemodynamics and function, and renal responsiveness to diuretic therapy. For the patient on a heart transplant waiting list, the failure to respond adequately to these interventions often necessitates the placement of a mechanical assist device. Unless complicated by considerable renal dysfunction and failure, he-

modialysis and related methods have not yet earned a role in the long-term management of chronic CHF.

HORMONAL AND OTHER ENDOGENOUS SUBSTANCES MODULATING RENAL FUNCTION. Heart failure activates a number of hormonal and regulatory systems, which greatly influence renal function. The major hormones and systems so affected and their regulation and renal effects in heart failure are presented in Table 62–1. Basically, as patients move from mild heart failure to moderate to severe stages, the protective vasodilatory and natriuretic properties of increased ANP (and perhaps renal prostaglandins and bradykinin) are overwhelmed by the vasoconstricting and salt and water–retaining effects of the progressively activated sympathetic nervous system, renin-angiotensin-aldosterone axis, arginine vasopressin, and adrenocorticotropin-corticosteroid axis.[20-36] This imbalance is exacerbated in heart failure by gradual attenuation of the vascular and renal responses to atrial natriuretic peptide and by development of a disordered vascular endothelium (increased endothelin production and release with loss of endothelium-derived vasodilation).[37,38]

Renal Responses in Chronic Congestive Heart Failure

The renal responses to the aforementioned cardiovascular-systemic consequences of chronic low-output CHF are reduced excretion of salt, water, and metabolic products (e.g., BUN, creatinine) and enhanced urinary loss of potassium and magnesium. These renal responses account for many of the clinical manifestations and for the "congestive" component of CHF. In untreated chronic CHF, whole-body sodium increases 5 to 40 per cent and water 5 to 45 per cent above normal and whole-body potassium decreases by 5 to 20 per cent.[24,39]

SODIUM RETENTION. The avid retention of sodium by the kidney in CHF is multifactorial in mechanism and basically a result of the antinatriuretic forces in this clinical condition overwhelming the natriuretic properties of circulating ANP and renal prostaglandins (Table 62–1 and Fig. 62–2).

Intrarenal physical factors and fluid dynamics contribute to sodium retention in CHF. A fall in cardiac output, effective blood volume, and renal blood flow is accompanied by activation of specific substances (e.g., angiotensin II, ANP,

TABLE 62–1 MAJOR HORMONAL AND OTHER ENDOGENOUS SUBSTANCES AFFECTING RENAL FUNCTION IN HUMAN HEART FAILURE

SUBSTANCE	INCREASED PRODUCTION RELEASE	DECREASED PRODUCTION RELEASE	RENAL EFFECTS	OTHER PROPERTIES RELEVANT TO RENAL FUNCTION
RENIN-ANGIOTENSIN-ALDOSTERONE SYSTEM				
Renin	Reduced renal perfusion pressure Reduced "effective" blood volume Low sodium diet Beta-adrenergic stimulation Reduced NaCl delivery to macula densa Prostaglandins (PGE$_2$, PGI$_2$) ACTH Endothelin Diuretic therapy Certain vasodilators ACE inhibitors	Normal or increased renal perfusion pressure Alpha-adrenergic stimulation Increased NaCl delivery to macula densa Increased serum [K+] Angiotensin II ANP Vasopressin Dopamine Digitalis Beta-adrenergic blockade	Mediated via increases in intrarenal and vascular angiotensin II production and elevated circulating angiotensin II and aldosterone levels	Converts angiotensinogen to angiotensin I, which is converted to angiotensin II by circulating and local tissue (e.g., vascular, renal)-converting enzyme
Angiotensin II	Renin	ACE inhibitors	Maintains glomerular filtration rate as renal blood flow falls by preferentially vasoconstricting efferent arteriole (> afferent arteriole) Promotes sodium reabsorption by proximal tubule Counters many renal actions of atrial natriuretic peptide Promotes renal vascular remodeling Possibly increases renal interstitial fibrosis	Increases production and release of aldosterone from adrenal gland May evoke release of arginine vasopressin from CNS May stimulate thirst center Augments sympathetic nervous system effects Proximal tubule produces angiotensinogen, and brush border contains converting enzyme
Aldosterone	Angiotensin II ACTH Vasopressin Increased serum [K+] Endothelin Beta-endorphin	ANP Dopamine ACE inhibitors Angiotensin II inhibitors	Increases sodium reabsorption by distal tubule and collecting duct Evokes potassium and magnesium loss from distal tubule	Increases whole body NaCl-H$_2$O content, and lowers whole body potassium
SYMPATHETIC NERVOUS SYSTEM TONE				
Norepinephrine Release	Activation of high- and low-pressure baroreceptors by reduced blood pressure, volume, or flow "Ineffective" blood volume Angiotensin II Certain vasodilators	Central alpha-adrenergic agonists and other sympatholytic agents ACE inhibitors Digitalis	Increases renin production and release Increases sodium reabsorption by proximal tubule Evokes modest kaliuresis Intense SNS activation: a. Reduces renal blood flow and GFR by vasoconstricting afferent (> efferent) arteriole b. May shift cortical blood flow to medullary region	Evokes production and release of: Arginine vasopressin ANP ACTH Corticosteroids Intrarenal prostaglandins Endothelin
Arginine Vasopressin	Various nonosmotic stimuli in heart failure, including: a. Sympathetic nervous system activation and catecholamines b. Reduction in blood pressure, flow or volume or "ineffective" blood volume c. Angiotensin II	Hypo-osmolar state	Acts on V$_2$ receptor of distal tubule and collecting duct to allow water reabsorption from tubular filtrate	Antagonistic to tubular effects of renal prostaglandins

SUBSTANCE	INCREASED PRODUCTION RELEASE	DECREASED PRODUCTION RELEASE	RENAL EFFECTS	OTHER PROPERTIES RELEVANT TO RENAL FUNCTION
	d. Parasympathetic withdrawal(?) Reduced hypo-osmolar negative feedback Reduced clearance Elevation of serum osmotic pressure Endothelin(?)			
Atrial Natriuretic Peptide	Elevation of intraatrial pressure and atrial dilatation Vasopressin, endothelin, and increased sympathetic nervous system activity(?)	Interventions that improve central hemodynamics and lower atrial pressures and volume	Renal vasodilation with afferent > efferent arteriolar dilatation: ↑ Renal blood flow ↑ GFR Relaxation of mesangium Suppression of: Renin release Angiotensin II production and renal effects Inhibition of tubular sodium channels and sodium transport to reduce NaCl reabsorption Inhibition of tubuloglomerular feedback	Some afterload-preload reduction via vasodilatory and renal effects Cardiovascular and renal effects of ANP become attenuated in moderate to severe chronic CHF
Renal prostaglandins (PGE₂, PGI₂)	Renal vasoconstriction Reduced renal blood flow and perfusion pressure Reduced or "ineffective" blood volume Renin-angiotensin Norepinephrine Vasopressin Bradykinin	Cyclo-oxygenase inhibitors (e.g., acetylsalicylic acid, nonsteroidal antiinflammatory drugs)	Renal vasodilation with afferent > efferent arteriolar dilatation: ↑ Renal blood flow ↑ GFR Inhibition of tubular NaCl reabsorption Inhibition of vasopressin-mediated water uptake by tubule and collecting duct	Possible augmentation of renin production and release
Endothelin	Increased experimentally by a rise in local concentrations of: Norepinephrine Angiotensin II Arginine vasopressin Bradykinin Various cytokines Thrombin Platelet-activating factor Changes in blood flow over endothelial cells Local ischemia		Increases renal vascular resistance with preferential afferent (> efferent) arteriolar constriction: ↓ Renal blood flow ↓ GFR ↓ Sodium excretion ↓ Urine volume Mesangial contraction	Acts on local endothelial cells to increase production of prostacyclin and nitric oxide(?) Contributes heavily to development of acute renal failure in cardiogenic-shock states(?) Elevates: Renin Aldosterone Arginine vasopressin Atrial natriuretic peptide

ACE = angiotensin-converting enzyme; ANP = atrial natriuretic peptides; (?) = possible but unproven; CHD = congestive heart disease; GFR = glomerular filtration rate; SNS = sympathetic nervous system.

and renal prostaglandins) that augment the vascular tone of the glomerular efferent arteriole relative to that of the afferent arteriole (Fig. 62–1). The perfusion pressure in the glomerular capillaries is thereby maintained, thus preserving glomerular-tubular filtrate (as measured by the glomerular filtration rate [GFR]); filtration fraction, defined as glomerular filtration rate/renal blood flow, increases.[20,23,26,40] The increase in filtration fraction leads to a substantial rise in the oncotic pressure and a fall in the hydrostatic pressure of blood leaving the glomerulus to enter the peritubular capillaries. These physical factors (elevated oncotic and reduced hydrostatic pressures) lead to enhanced NaCl-H₂O uptake into the postglomerular peritubular capillary network from the proximal renal tubules and adjacent interstitial space.

Several other local events contribute to sodium retention. If the balance of afferent to efferent arteriolar tone fails to maintain GFR at an adequate level, a fall in GFR delivers less NaCl-H₂O into the tubule, allowing greater proximal tubular reabsorption of sodium via aforementioned physical and hormonal (e.g., angiotensin II, catecholamines) mechanisms. At this point, tubuloglomerular feedback likely serves as a countermeasure[20,23,40,41]; reduced tubular filtrate and flow evoke feedback augmentation of efferent > afferent arteriolar tone to try to increase and maintain GFR. Second, as filtrate and sodium delivery to the distal tubule falls, it is believed that the macula densa cells of the distal tubule send a signal to adjacent juxtaglomerular cells to secrete more renin (with consequent increase of angiotensin II and aldosterone), further intensifying the vascular (glomerular), physical, and hormonal forces promoting sodium reabsorption.[41] Third, although not proven in human chronic CHF, it is possible that in severe stages some of the cortical blood flow is shifted to medullary nephrons, which have an even greater capacity to reabsorb NaCl-H₂O.[14,42]

ROLE OF HORMONES (Table 62–1). Elevated concentrations of certain hormones in CHF constitute powerful mechanisms for sodium retention.[11,20,21,43] Increased aldosterone concentrations cause NaCl reabsorption by the distal tubule and collecting duct, while angiotensin II and norepinephrine augment sodium reabsorption by the proxi-

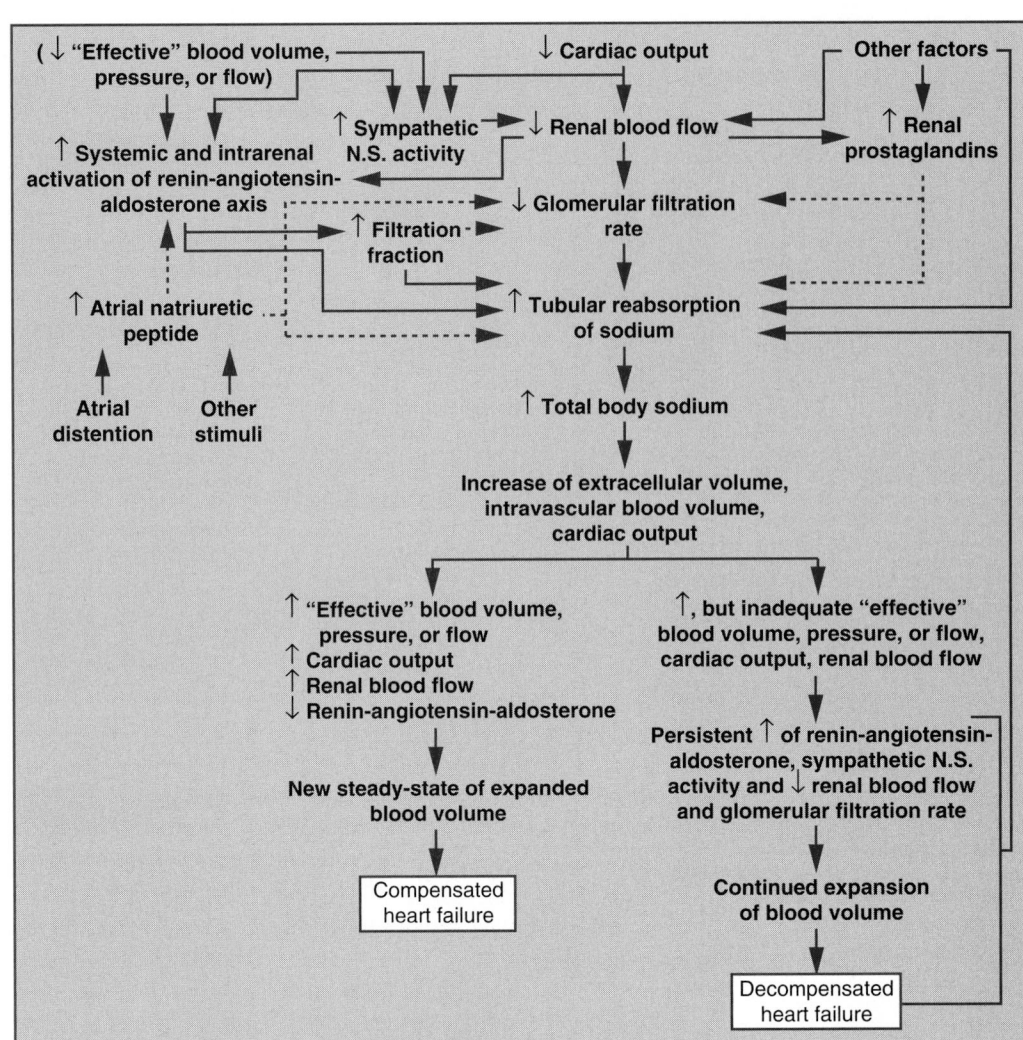

FIGURE 62–2. Schema of the known major mechanisms for enhanced sodium retention in congestive heart failure. Solid connecting lines indicate positive influence or stimulus, and dashed lines indicate negative input or feedback. N.S. = nervous system (Adapted from Leier, C. V., and Boudoulas, H.: Cardiorenal Disorders and Diseases. Armonk, N.Y., Futura Publishing Co., 1992.)

mal tubule. When elevated, circulating corticosteroids retain sodium at the distal tubule. In severe CHF, increased circulating concentrations and enhanced local release of endothelin probably contribute to the fall in glomerular filtration rate and sodium clearance.[34,35]

Elevated circulating ANP levels and intrarenal production of PGE_2 and PGI_2 represent the primary endogenous natriuretic forces in CHF.[28–30,32,36] Experimentally, ANP inhibits renin, aldosterone, arginine vasopressin, and norepinephrine release; inhibits the renal effects of angiotensin II, aldosterone, and arginine vasopressin, and tubular sodium reabsorption; and favorably affects glomerular arteriolar tone (preferential relaxation of afferent arteriole) and GFR (Table 62–1). PGE_2 and PGI_2 augment renal blood flow, preferentially dilate afferent glomerular arterioles to increase GFR, and inhibit tubular $NaCl$-H_2O reabsorption and the renal effects of arginine vasopressin. In mild CHF, ANP, PGE_2, and PGI_2 probably contribute substantially to proper NaCl balance and overall cardiovascular compensation. As CHF advances, the favorable effects of ANP wane and the antinatriuretic forces intensify, resulting in a progressive rise in whole-body $NaCl$-H_2O content and an expanded extracellular volume.

WATER RETENTION. The major mechanisms responsible for water retention in CHF[20,26,27,44–46] are presented in Figure 62–3. In health and disease, water is an obligatory component of NaCl reabsorption. In CHF, local renal factors enhance water uptake; these include a reduction in the delivery of filtrate to the distal tubule and, as filtration fraction increases, a fall in the hydrostatic pressure and rise in oncotic pressure of postglomerular blood as it enters peritubular capillaries. Water retention in moderate to severe heart failure is also mediated by an absolute or relative increase in circulating arginine vasopressin[20,45,46]; this represents the predominant mechanism for excessive water retention (often greater than sodium retention) by the kidneys, even in the presence of reduced serum sodium concentrations and serum osmolality. In other words, the various nonosmotic stimuli for vasopressin release (Table 62–1) become quite prominent and overwhelm osmotic-os-

moreceptor mechanisms. Suppression of arginine vasopressin with a water load and the kidney's capacity to eliminate a water load are also significantly reduced in CHF patients.[46] Thirst, provoked in large part by elevated angiotensin II levels, exacerbates the water imbalance with continued water intake in the face of hypo-osmolality, dilutional hyponatremia, and whole body fluid volume overload.

These mechanisms and derangements intensify as CHF increases in severity and account for the rather common occurrence of hyponatremia in advanced stages of the condition.[44–47] Therefore, hyponatremia in CHF usually indicates more severe stages of CHF, marked activation of sympathetic nervous, renin-angiotensin-aldosterone, and arginine vasopressin systems, and if one includes the entire spectrum of CHF patients, probably a higher mortality rate as well.[44,45,47] The hyponatremic CHF patient depends heavily on the renin-angiotensin-aldosterone and vasopressin systems for support of central and peripheral hemodynamics, blood pressure, renal perfusion, and GFR and thus is quite susceptible to the hypotensive and potentially adverse renal effects (fall in GFR, azotemia) of angiotensin-converting enzyme inhibitors.[48]

LOSS OF POTASSIUM AND MAGNESIUM. Excessive urinary loss of potassium is a consistent feature of CHF[24,39] (Fig. 62–4). Aldosterone-induced sodium reabsorption by the distal tubule is accompanied by a 1:1 exchange for potassium or hydrogen ion and consequent urinary loss. Respiratory and metabolic alkalosis, not uncommon in CHF, further augments potassium loss by causing the distal tubule to preferentially retain hydrogen ions. Interventions that increase delivery of sodium to the distal tubule (e.g., diuretics) invariably enhance exchange for potassium and thereby promote kaliuresis.

Thus a number of factors predispose the CHF patient to potassium depletion and its threatening consequences (e.g., dysrhythmias). Potassium supplementation (KCl), potas-

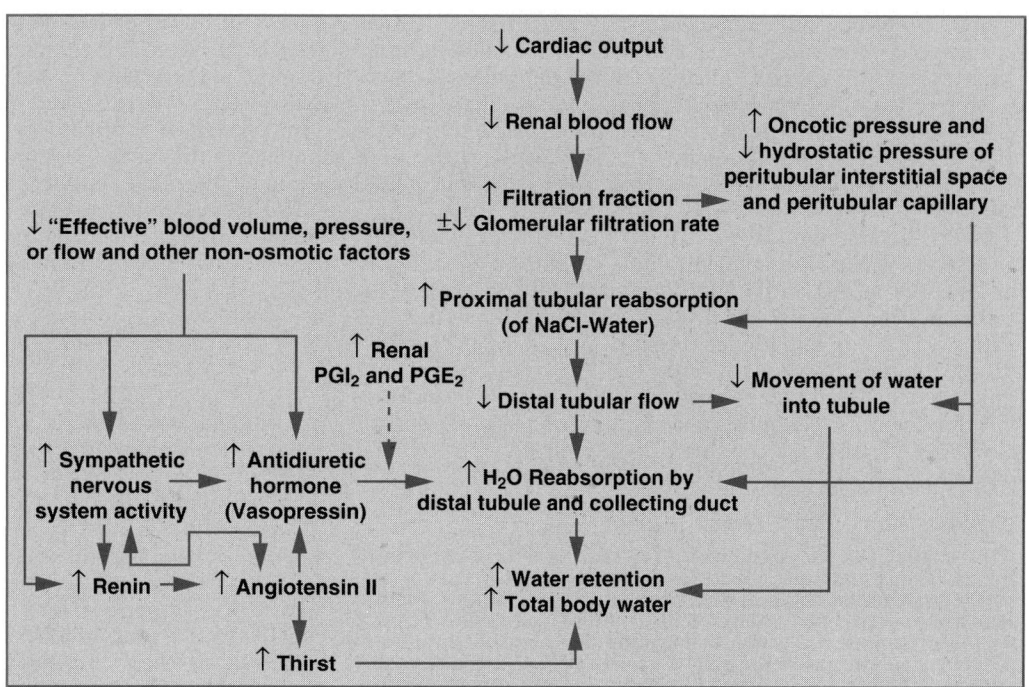

FIGURE 62–3. Major mechanisms for enhanced water retention in heart failure. In advanced stages of heart failure, the degree of water retention can exceed that of sodium retention to cause hyponatremia. Dashed connecting line indicates inhibition or negative feedback. (Adapted from Leier, C. V., and Boudoulas, H.: Cardiorenal Disorders and Diseases. Armonk, N.Y., Futura Publishing Co., 1992.)

sium-sparing diuretics, and angiotensin-converting enzyme inhibitors (by reducing aldosterone) are strategies used to treat this complication of CHF and CHF management.

Generally, the renal loss of magnesium is not quite as problematic for most CHF patients.[49] However, excessive loss and hypomagnesemia do occur in patients with advanced CHF, particularly when treated with high-dose diuretics for an extended period.

AZOTEMIA. Azotemia (increased blood urea nitrogen [BUN]) can occur in moderate to severe CHF or as a consequence of CHF therapy.[24,39,50] A common clinical situation in chronic CHF is in the patient in a state of decompensation who enters the hospital with an elevated BUN (generally > 30 mg/dl), which steadily falls toward normal values with supportive therapy and hemodynamic improvement, but progressively rises again as a phase of inadvertent overdiuresis (relative volume depletion) is entered or a state of decompensation returns.

Tubular urea movement generally follows that of water. Therefore, as renal uptake of NaCl-H$_2$O increases in CHF, more urea is retained by the kidneys. BUN levels will still generally remain in the normal range or increase only slightly as long as GFR, tubular flow, and urine output are maintained within a near-normal range. A fall in GFR and

urine output, as may occur in severe CHF or as a consequence of certain therapeutic measures, will be accompanied by a rise in BUN. Excretion of creatinine occurs via filtrate plus active tubular secretion. Because renal elimination of creatinine is less dependent on tubular flow, serum creatinine will generally not increase until GFR falls below 30 ml/min. Therefore, unless a patient has intrinsic renal disease or marked depression of GFR, the azotemia of CHF is invariably "prerenal" in character, that is, greater retention of BUN than of creatinine with a serum BUN to creatinine ratio of >10:1.

Because of the physiological adjustments required of the kidneys to maintain adequate renal function in heart failure, this organ system in CHF is quite vulnerable to any type of pharmacological, hemodynamic, or structural disturbance. As noted, for patients with moderate to severe heart failure, maintenance of GFR in the face of reduced renal blood flow depends on the proper balance of afferent to efferent arteriolar tone.

ROLE OF THERAPEUTIC AGENTS IN EXACERBATING AZOTEMIA. Angiotensin II plays a major role in this compensatory mechanism by preferentially vasoconstricting the efferent arteriole. By lowering angiotensin II, converting enzyme inhibitors can lower GFR in spite of a concomitant increase in renal blood flow. For most CHF patients, this response will not significantly reduce overall renal performance, or it may increase BUN modestly. However, in the face of severe CHF or low-output hypotension (when GFR and renal function are greatly dependent on angiotensin II), hyponatremia (indicative of high renin-angiotensin and vasopressin activity), relative volume depletion (diuretics), or intrinsic renal disease (e.g., concomitant diabetes mellitus, longstanding systemic hypertension), a reduction of angiotensin II following angiotensin-converting enzyme inhibition, particularly if accompanied by a significant fall in systemic blood pressure and renal perfusion, will often evoke a substantial rise in BUN.[10,12,13,48,51,52] However, converting enzyme inhibitors are still indicated in these situations, but dosing must be initiated at a lower level with appropriate adjustment of diuretic therapy (usually lowered until the dosage of the converting enzyme inhibitor is optimized).

Renal function in CHF is vulnerable to diuretic therapy (see p. 480). Even closely monitored diuretic therapy is associated with additional activation of neurohormonal systems (probably via reduced "effective" blood volume, flow, or pressure, and if overdiuresis occurs, significant reduction in renal blood flow and GFR results and is manifested as a rising BUN.[50,53] In moderate to severe heart failure, renal performance also depends on activation of its prostaglandin system (to dilate the afferent arteriole and reduce tubular NaCl-H$_2$O reabsorption). It is not uncommon in a CHF patient for clinical decompensation to result from fluid retention, and for azotemia to develop and occasionally advance to renal failure after the administration of cyclo-oxygenase inhibitors (e.g., nonsteroidal antiinflammatory drugs).[54]

Management of Azotemia in Heart Failure. The general approach to azotemia in CHF is optimization of therapy to provide the best central and renal hemodynamic status possible and elimination of precipitating factors (e.g., overdiuresis, cyclo-oxygenase inhibitors). If the azotemia (and often accompanying refractory edema) is substantial, is secondary to hemodynamic decompensation, and does not re-

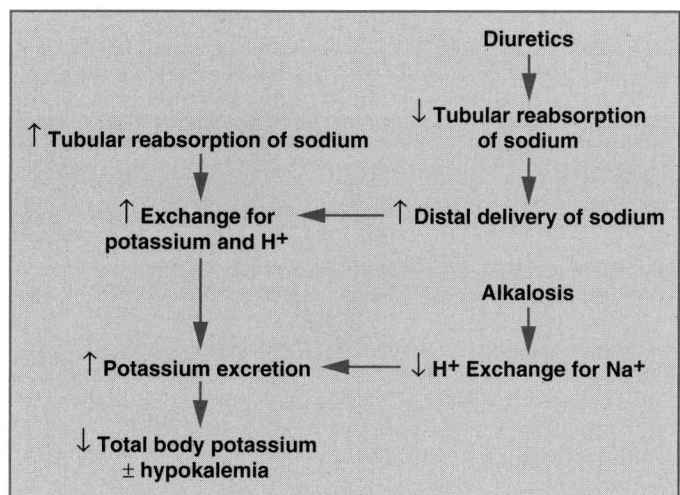

FIGURE 62–4. Major events promoting kaliuresis in congestive heart failure. (Adapted from Leier, C. V., and Boudoulas, H.: Cardiorenal Disorders and Diseases. Armonk, N.Y., Futura Publishing Co., 1992.)

spond to optimal adjustment of orally administered drugs, intravenous drug support (e.g., dopamine, dobutamine) may be required[15,16,18]; this clinical situation generally portends a poor prognosis. Dosage of drugs primarily cleared by the kidney (e.g., digoxin, potassium, certain antiarrhythmic and antibiotic agents) must be adjusted downward as the CHF kidney becomes more dysfunctional, GFR falls, and azotemia develops.

Unless accompanied by intrinsic renal disease, the BUN and serum creatinine concentrations in chronic CHF rarely exceed 100 mg/dl and 4 mg/dl, respectively. It is also uncommon for patients who have azotemia secondary to chronic CHF to experience uremic symptoms. Therefore, dialysis is rarely necessary in the patient with chronic CHF unless excessive fluid retention or threatening hyperkalemia refractory to therapy, renal failure, or perhaps marked elevation of BUN (≥ 100 mg/dl) complicates the clinical course.

CHRONIC HIGH-OUTPUT HEART FAILURE

This condition is discussed on pages 460 to 462. A number of mechanisms gradually convert the initial asymptomatic condition of persistent high cardiac output (e.g., vascular fistulas, chronic anemia) into high-output heart failure.[19,20,55,56] A major contributor is renal NaCl-H_2O retention. Detection by low- and high-pressure baroreceptors of a state of "ineffective" blood volume, pressure, and flow, and in some instances, the diversion of blood flow away from the kidneys provoke chronic activation of the sympathetic nervous system, the renin-angiotensin-aldosterone axis, and arginine vasopressin. Chronic volume overload secondary to renal NaCl-H_2O retention, continuous neurohormonal activation, and persistent increase of myocardial work and energy expenditure gradually cause ventricular enlargement, remodeling, and failure.

Many of the high-output conditions, if untreated, eventually evolve into chronic low-output heart failure with the accompanying renal pathophysiology described above for chronic CHF. Needless to say, the optimal therapeutic approach is to eradicate the underlying cause for the persistently increased cardiac output as soon as it is identified and before it leads to irreversible cardiac dysfunction and failure.

The kidney itself can serve as a primary cause of high-output heart failure.[19,55,56] The kidney is one of the more common sites for arteriovenous fistula formation; this lesion can occur as a complication of renal biopsy and surgery, arterial aneurysmal penetration, and renal neoplasia. Because of concomitant anemia, a sizable arteriovenous access shunt, and chronic tachycardia, the clinical course of chronic renal failure can be further complicated by the development of high-output heart failure.

Acute Heart Failure

The systemic and hormonal responses just described for chronic CHF are also activated in acute heart failure,[57–60] but at a far faster rate of recruitment. Although not well studied in acute human heart failure, the full pathophysiological expression of acute renin-angiotensin-aldosterone activation—particularly that of aldosterone—is not likely to develop within the first 1 to 2 hours of the acute precipitating event. Whole body fluid volume overload is thus not a major component of the very early course but does become important thereafter if the precipitating lesion and acute heart failure are not corrected and as the full impact of acute renin release takes hold. Therefore, the very early, often dramatic, clinical presentation is predominantly related to the extent of myocardial damage or disruption, the intensity of consequent sympathetic nervous system activation, and the circulating and tissue levels of angiotensin II, endothelin, and other vasoactive substances at that point. However, many of these patients do have markedly elevated ventricular filling pressures, acute "congestive" heart failure, and pulmonary edema within minutes of the cardiac event, suggesting that central blood volume (albeit not whole body fluid volume) is indeed excessive at this stage; the mechanisms include peripheral-to-central redistribution of blood volume and an acute rise in ventricular afterload, superimposed on significant cardiac disruption (e.g., large infarct, valvular regurgitation).

The kidney via renal artery stenosis (and consequent re-lease of renin) can serve as the precipitating cause of acute heart failure. This diagnosis should be suspected in the aging patient with a recent history of poorly controlled severe hypertension and new onset or episodic acute pulmonary edema. In this setting, renal insufficiency or asymmetry, a dramatic reduction in blood pressure or the occurrence of renal failure following angiotensin-converting enzyme inhibitor therapy, evidence of atherosclerotic vascular disease elsewhere, or an upper abdominal bruit should also arouse clinical suspicion of renal artery stenosis.

Cardiogenic Shock
(See also p. 1725)

Prerenal azotemia is a common feature of cardiogenic shock and near-shock. The mechanisms causing prerenal azotemia in this setting are generally similar to those discussed above for severe chronic CHF. Unfortunately, acute renal failure is also an occasional complication of cardiogenic shock. For the oliguric or azotemic shock patient, distinguishing between prerenal causation and acute renal failure is important for the optimal management of these critically ill individuals. Prerenal azotemia is approached by treating the reversible conditions that elevate BUN and by agents and methods that improve renal perfusion. Acute renal failure in this setting is managed by avoiding fluid volume, potassium, and protein overload and with dialysis for problematic fluid volume overload, hyperkalemia, uremic symptoms, or plasma creatinine levels ≥ 7.0 mg/dl.

Table 62–2 presents the laboratory studies useful in distinguishing the azotemia and oliguria of prerenal causes from those of acute renal failure. The principal structural defect of acute renal failure in cardiogenic shock is tubular injury and necrosis. As such, the characteristics of the urine in acute renal failure generally approach those of glomerular filtrate, because the filtrate is modified little by the defective tubules. Thus, urinary sodium content will be high (>40 mEq/liter) and osmolality low (<350 mOsm) despite the oliguric state, and the urinary concentrations of BUN and creatinine will be low despite elevated serum values, because of the inability of the tubules to reabsorb, secrete, and/or concentrate (reduced water uptake) these metabolites. The plasma BUN:creatinine ratio will usually remain at $\leq 10:1$, with an average daily increase of 15 to 20 mg/dl and 1.5 to 2.0 mg/dl respectively. In contrast, prerenal azotemia and oliguria are characterized by laboratory findings indicative of intense NaCl-H_2O retention by normally functioning tubules, which are under considerable stimulation from an activated renin-angiotensin-aldo-

TABLE 62–2 LABORATORY FINDINGS USED TO DISTINGUISH AZOTEMIA AND OLIGURIA OF PRERENAL CAUSES (E.G., HEART FAILURE) FROM AZOTEMIA AND OLIGURIA OF ACUTE RENAL FAILURE

LABORATORY PARAMETER	PRERENAL*	RENAL FAILURE
Urine		
Osmolality	>400 mOsm	<350 mOsm
Na$^+$ content	<15 mEq/liter	>40 mEq/liter
Sediment	Normal or a small number of non-pigmented granular or hyaline casts	Substantial number of renal tubular cell casts and/or pigmented casts
Urine/plasma ratios of		
BUN	>8	<3
Creatinine	>40	<20
Serum		
BUN:Creatinine	$>10:1$	$10:1$

* These laboratory results can be substantially altered by diuretic therapy and/or underlying renal disease.

sterone axis and increased vasopressin. The urine will therefore have a low sodium concentration (<15 to 20 mEq/liter), high osmolality, and high urea and creatinine concentrations. Plasma creatinine levels stay normal unless renal perfusion and GFR fall considerably or the patient has intrinsic renal disease. With the reduction in urine flow, BUN rises to increase the serum BUN:creatinine ratio to >10:1. A not unusual urinary sediment or a small number of granular, proteinaceous, or hyaline casts is typical for prerenal azotemia, whereas the sediment of acute renal failure often shows pigmented or tubular cell casts.

Two situations commonly distort the aforementioned laboratory findings. First, diuretics or concomitant renal disease can increase the urinary sodium and water content of patients with prerenal azotemia such that the urinary sodium and osmolality data can be difficult to interpret. Second, oliguria (urine flow <600 ml/24 hr) is not a mandatory feature of acute renal failure. Nonoliguric renal failure is a variant of acute renal failure; these patients have a urine output of 1000 to 6000 ml/24 hr, accompanied by a steady rise in serum BUN and creatinine indicative of ongoing renal failure. Although high urine output can occasionally occur in the early phase of acute renal failure, it usually follows a period of oliguric renal failure. Urinary sodium concentration is still elevated and urinary osmolality depressed in nonoliguric acute renal failure, rendering the pathophysiological impression that the nephrons have reestablished flow, but the tubular cells remain dysfunctional.

Following reversal of cardiogenic shock, the usual clinical course of shock-induced acute renal failure consists of a 1- to 8-week period of intermittent dialysis and eventual recovery. The status of an occasional patient, particularly one with previous renal disease or one who experienced a prolonged period of renal hypoperfusion-ischemia, may proceed into permanent renal failure requiring long-term dialysis or renal transplantation. Although acute renal failure still carries a mortality rate of 10 to 15 per cent, the long-term clinical course and prognosis in patients who experience acute renal failure secondary to cardiogenic shock are usually related to the nature, extent, and reversibility of the cardiac injury and the residual cardiovascular function.

MECHANISM OF RENAL FAILURE. The precise mechanisms leading to the development of acute renal failure during cardiogenic shock in humans have not yet been definitively established.[34,61-63] The potential pivotal role of endothelin in the pathogenesis of acute renal failure in shock conditions is suggested by the results of preliminary studies in animal models, which indicate that inhibition of this substance significantly reduces the prevalence and severity of ischemia-induced renal failure.[34,63] The drop in cardiac output and renal blood flow, intense activation of the sympathetic nervous system, increased circulating and intrarenal renin-angiotensin, and the endothelial release of endothelin can reduce renal blood flow in cardiogenic shock to ≤15 per cent of normal with possible diversion of flow from the renal cortex to medulla as well. Low tissue oxygen tension and depleted energy substrate depress tubular function and membrane transport. Renal tubular cells undergo ischemic injury and death and aggregate with tubular filtrate and proteinaceous exudation (across glomeruli or from the interstitium) to obstruct the tubules and collecting ducts. An increase in interstitial edema and pressure leads to compression of nephrons with additional impairment of tubular flow.

INFECTIVE ENDOCARDITIS

(See also Chap. 33)

In the preantibiotic era, 10 to 15 per cent of deaths from infective endocarditis were attributable to renal failure. Early recognition, precise identification of the infecting organism, and prompt, aggressive antibiotic therapy specifically directed at the offending organism have greatly reduced the renal complications of infective endocarditis, particularly renal failure. Nevertheless, more than 60 per cent of patients with documented infective endocarditis have clinical, laboratory, or biopsy evidence of renal involvement.[64-66] The manifestations of endocarditic renal disease range from none to hematuria, pyuria, proteinuria, and occasional renal failure; the prevalence and severity of these manifestations are generally related to the duration of endocarditis prior to cure.

The deposition of immune complex material in glomeruli represents the most common mechanistic link between infective endocarditis and its renal consequences. Circulating immune complexes and their subsequent deposition in kidneys (and elsewhere) account for the common laboratory finding of reduced serum levels of certain complements (e.g., C3, C4, C1q) in affected individuals. The resultant glomerular lesions are generally proliferative in histological type with demonstrable immune deposits of IgG, IgM, and C3 along the basement membrane and in the mesangium. The distribution of the glomerular lesions ranges from focal/segmental to diffuse and their clinical behavior from subclinical to rapidly progressive.

FOCAL/SEGMENTAL PROLIFERATIVE GLOMERULONEPHRITIS. This is the most commonly encountered glomerulopathy in bacterial endocarditis and represents a wide spectrum of involvement, including focal inflammation of single tufts of glomeruli, sporadic glomerular inflammation and fibrosis, and inflammation and fibrosis of most glomeruli within a renal segment(s) in the midst of normal appearing kidney.[64,65] In addition to neutrophil and round cell infiltration and varying degrees of fibrosis, glomerular pathology often includes focal necrosis, fibrin deposition, enlargement and proliferation of endothelial, epithelial, and mesangial cells, and occasional crescent formation. The demonstration of immune complex components in the involved glomeruli and the observation that similar glomerular lesions can occur in isolated right-heart endocarditis, nonendocarditic infections, and noninfectious inflammatory conditions implicate immunological mechanisms as the cause for the focal/segmental glomerulonephritis of infective endocarditis. The focal/segmental glomerulonephritis can be rather widespread, such that occasionally it is indistinguishable using clinical, laboratory, and biopsy criteria from diffuse proliferative glomerulonephritis. Although the urine of focal/segmental glomerulonephritis may not be unusual, it customarily shows microscopic hematuria, sterile pyuria, or mild proteinuria. Moderate to marked proteinuria (over 2 gm/24 hr), systemic hypertension, or renal failure can develop in extensive or recurrent focal/segmental glomerulonephritis, but these manifestations are more commonly associated with diffuse proliferative glomerulonephritis.

DIFFUSE PROLIFERATIVE GLOMERULONEPHRITIS. This lesion, viewed by many to simply represent a more severe and extensive form of focal/segmental glomerulonephritis, attacks most glomeruli with a very proliferative cellular process, usually involving the entire glomerulus. The clinical consequences of systemic hypertension, nephritic proteinuria, and chronic renal failure are considerably more prevalent with the diffuse forms of proliferative glomerulonephritis. Hematuria, sterile pyuria, proteinuria, and heme or red blood cell casts are common features on urinalysis.

Renal biopsy reveals considerable proliferation and swelling of endothelial, epithelial, and mesangial cells, giving the typically involved glomerulus a packed cellular, even avascular, appearance. Neutrophils and round cells can be scattered throughout the glomerulus and interstitium. Fibrous replacement of the glomerulus and tubular atrophy and loss are common histological findings in more advanced stages. Immunofluorescent staining shows deposition of IgG, IgM, and C3 in subendothelial, subepithelial, and mesangial regions. Rapidly progressive glomerulonephritis with widespread glomerular crescent formation can occasionally occur in infective endocarditis and is often the explanation for rapid loss of renal function.

MANAGEMENT. Prompt identification and aggressive antibiotic treatment of the infecting organism are the principal means of preventing endocarditic renal disease. Antibiotic therapy has lowered the incidence of diffuse proliferative glomerulonephritis during infective endocarditis from 55 to 80 per cent to less than 15 per cent.[64,65] Pharmacological control of systemic hypertension and dialysis for renal failure occasionally are necessary supportive measures.

RENAL EMBOLIZATION. While evidence of renal embolization is found at necropsy in 60 to 70 per cent of patients who die of infective endocarditis, less than 25 per cent have clinically recognizable renal emboli.[64,65] Hematuria is the most common sign of renal emboli. Back or flank pain and renal hemorrhage, rarely fatal, can occur with a large embolus and sizable renal infarction. Larger emboli most often originate from prosthetic valves or from valvular infections caused by *Staphylococcus aureus, Neisseria gonococcus, Streptococcus pneumoniae,* or fungi. On rare occasions, an infected embolus can evolve into a renal abscess.

Cortical necrosis may occur when infective endocarditis is complicated by a coagulopathy, and acute tubular necrosis can be precipitated by concomitant cardiogenic shock or the use of nephrotoxic agents. Interstitial nephritis can occur in infective endocarditis, but generally in combination with glomerulonephritis. If interstitial nephritis develops as the predominant renal lesion in this clinical setting, a reaction to drug therapy must be considered.

CAUSES. Table 62–3 presents the major cardiovascular conditions responsible for renal embolization. Because 14 to 20 per cent of cardiac output passes through the kidneys and because of their direct proximity to the commonly diseased aorta, the kidneys represent favorite targets for arterial embolization.[67–73] The atherosclerotic aorta is a common source of fibrin, plaque, and cholesterol emboli. Suprarenal aneurysms, aortic surgery, intraaortic balloon counterpulsation, cardiac or aortic catheterization, anticoagulation, and thrombolytic therapy increase the risk of renal embolization from the atherosclerotic aorta (see p. 1570). Massive embolization to skeletal muscle can exacerbate or cause renal dysfunction and failure via myoglobinemia-myoglobinuria. The more common cardiac conditions serving as embolic sources are atrial fibrillation, mural thrombi of the left ventricle, mitral stenosis, and prosthetic heart valves (Table 62–3).

Renal pathology ranges from isolated occlusion of an arteriole with minimal histological change, to segmental infarction ("white infarcts" and scarring), to complete occlusion of a renal artery with unilateral loss of renal function and mass. Cholesterol clefts and calcified debris are histological features of atherosclerotic emboli. Capsular rupture and retroperitoneal hemorrhage can complicate a large infarction.

Similar to embolization elsewhere, the majority are not likely to be detected clinically. Clinical manifestations include varying degrees of hematuria, proteinuria, back or flank pain, systemic hypertension (secondary to elevated plasma renin), and renal dysfunction. Extensive embolization to both kidneys or a large embolus of a sole functioning kidney can result in anuria. Eosinophilia, depressed serum levels of C3 and C4, and rarely, lipid droplets floating in a urine sample can occur with cholesterol emboli.

TABLE 62–3 MAJOR CARDIOVASCULAR SOURCES, CAUSES, AND PREDISPOSING FACTORS FOR EMBOLIZATION TO KIDNEYS

AORTA
Atherosclerotic disease
Extensive atherosclerotic plaque formation; rupture, thrombus and cholesterol embolization
Suprarenal aortic aneurysm
Cardiac and aortic catheterization
Intraaortic balloon counterpulsation therapy
Anticoagulation
Thrombolytic therapy
Aortic surgery

ATRIA
Atrial fibrillation
Atrial enlargement
Cardiomyopathy
Atrial septal aneurysms
Paradoxical embolization
Myxoma (less commonly located in ventricles and on valves)
States of hypercoagulation (e.g., neoplastic diseases; protein C, protein S, or antithrombin III deficiency)

VENTRICLES
Mural thrombus
    Myocardial infarction
    Cardiomyopathy
Cardiac tumors
States of hypercoagulation (see Atria above)

VALVES
Mitral stenosis (via atrial or valvular thrombus)
Prosthetic valves
Endocarditis
    Infective
    Marantic (noninfective thrombotic)
Mitral annular calcification

The renal manifestations of atherosclerotic or cholesterol emboli are commonly part of an embolic multisystem "polyarteritis" presentation. Clinical suspicion of renal emboli is raised in patients with an obvious predisposition (e.g., prosthetic heart valve, atherosclerotic aorta, aortic surgery, recent cardiovascular catheterization). Perfusion defects secondary to large emboli are detectable with renal radionuclide scanning. Renal arteriography generally shows a cutoff sign at the point of occlusion with few vascular markings distal to the occlusion. The "rim sign" (subcapsular contrast overlying regions of noncontrast) may be seen with extensive or large embolization.

MANAGEMENT. This is generally directed at correcting the source of embolization with supportive therapy for accompanying systemic hypertension or renal failure. For large renal emboli, local thrombolytic therapy, angioplasty, retrieval via catheter, or surgical embolectomy are the principal interventional options.[72,73] The approach to atherosclerotic-cholesterol emboli is somewhat limited; an obvious source (e.g., suprarenal atherosclerotic aortic disease or aneurysm) should be considered for resection with the understanding that the aorta is usually diffusely involved with atherosclerosis and that further embolization may occur during and after surgery. Whether long-term anticoagulation for atheroembolic renal disease offers effective therapy or exacerbation of the problem remains unresolved; prolonged aspirin therapy is a reasonable option and skirts this controversy.

OTHER CARDIOVASCULAR CONDITIONS

Aortic Aneurysm and Dissection
(See also Chap. 45)

The atherosclerotic aneurysm can threaten renal function in a number of ways including thromboembolism from a suprarenal location (see Thromboembolic disease, above), reduction of renal blood flow by local involvement or encroachment, rupture with hypovolemic shock, aortorenal vein fistula, ureteral obstruction, and the consequences of its surgical repair.[67,74–76] Ten to 20 per cent of atherosclerotic aortic aneurysms are complicated by renal artery stenosis. Clinical suspicion of renal involvement by an atherosclerotic aneurysm is prompted by recent onset or acceleration of systemic hypertension, location near the renal arteries, hematuria, proteinuria, occasional eosinophilia (in cases of atheroemboli), and renal dysfunction and failure. Aneurysmectomy with renal revascularization (when renal arteries are involved) is generally the treatment of choice.

Renal involvement by aortic dissection takes the form of renal artery occlusion or renal dysfunction secondary to compromised hemodynamics from hemorrhagic-hypovolemic shock, cardiac tamponade, or acute heart failure caused by acute aortic valvular insufficiency or acute myocardial infarction.[77] Partial or total renal artery occlusion can occur via an ostial flap or displacement of the intima-media into the lumen as the dissecting hematoma moves into the renal artery. Renal manifestations can include proteinuria, hematuria, systemic hypertension (high plasma renin), renal infarction, azotemia, and renal failure. Anuria should bring bilateral renal artery occlusion (unilateral for a sole functioning kidney) into consideration. Operative correction of the dissection with renal revascularization remains the intervention of choice in most instances.

Congenital Heart Disease

CYANOTIC CONGENITAL DISEASE. The clinical course of cyanotic congenital heart disease is often accompanied by the development of renal dysfunction.[78–80] Although the mechanism for the renal dysfunction is not known, its severity appears to be related to the level and duration of arterial desaturation, the degree of polycythemia, age, severity of right-heart failure, and elevation of systemic venous pressure. Histologically, the glomeruli enlarge ("glomerulomegaly") with mesangial hypercellularity, capillary congestion, focal glomerulosclerosis, and localized thickening of the basement membrane. Functionally, the disorder behaves as a glomerulopathy with proteinuria occurring in 30 per cent and microscopic hematuria in 15 to 20 per cent of patients.[79] Five to 10 per cent develop considerable proteinuria and occasionally the nephrotic syndrome, usually after the age of 21 years.[79,80] Tubular dysfunction can occur. Because of increased uric acid production during polycythemia and the tubular dysfunction, hyperuricemia is a common metabolic complication of cyanotic heart disease. A reduction in renal blood flow, GFR, and urea clearance also occurs over time. Most of the glomerular lesions, renal dysfunction, and urinary findings are reversible and usually return toward normal after successful surgical correction of the cardiac defect and subsequent improvement in hemodynamics, oxygen delivery, and hematocrit.

COARCTATION OF THE AORTA. This malformation has a significant impact on renal physiology and function.[81-83] The lower renal perfusion pressure (distal to the coarctation) evokes sustained release of renin, which contributes to the characteristic hypertension present in the vascular system located above the coarctation. Depending somewhat on the age of the patient and duration of the condition, surgical or angioplasty correction usually does not immediately lower systemic blood pressure (in fact, it may initially increase) and systemic hypertension can persist long-term after correction in up to one-third of the patients.[81,82] Congestive heart failure, infective endocarditis, and aortic dissection are other complications of coarctation, which in addition to post-repair systemic hypertension, can adversely affect renal function. Fibromuscular dysplasia and developmental hypoplasia of the renal arteries have been reported in association with coarctation or hypoplasia of the abdominal aorta.[83]

EFFECTS OF RENAL FAILURE ON THE CARDIOVASCULAR SYSTEM

CARDIAC FAILURE CAUSED BY RENAL FAILURE

Left ventricular dysfunction and CHF are common complications of chronic renal failure.[19,84-92] Factors that contribute to myocardial damage and dysfunction in patients with this condition are depicted in Figure 62–5. Because it is usually difficult to attribute a predominant causative role to any one of these factors or events, the term *uremic cardiomyopathy* is often used to identify the cardiac disorder resulting from the integration of the various disruptive factors of chronic renal failure.

Factors Contributing to the Development of Congestive Heart Failure

The conditions contributing to the development of CHF in patients with chronic renal failure are presented in Figure 62-6.

VOLUME OVERLOAD. Loss of renal function allows salt and fluid retention and the development of volume overload. Other factors that contribute to volume overload are chronic anemia and the arteriovenous (AV) access fistula. Normochromic, normocytic anemia is common in chronic renal failure, with nontreated hematocrits ranging from 20 to 30 per cent and hemoglobin from 7 to 9 gm/dl; the introduction of erythropoietin therapy in chronic renal failure has reduced the degree and consequences of anemia. In general, the overall hemodynamic effect of the typical upper extremity AV access fistula is small; however, the fistula may contribute to the development of CHF in patients with left ventricular (LV) dysfunction.

The contribution of volume overload to the development of CHF in chronic renal failure is related to the magnitude and time course of volume expansion and to the concomitant status of cardiac function. A sudden rise in plasma volume can increase LV end-diastolic pressure to levels that produce pulmonary edema, even in the presence of normal resting LV systolic function. In contrast, a gradual increase in plasma volume can allow compensatory ventricular dilatation and hypertrophy with less immediate elevations in LV diastolic pressure.

PRESSURE OVERLOAD. Systemic hypertension, a common finding in patients with chronic renal failure, contributes considerably to the generation of acute and chronic CHF by placing an excessive afterload burden on the dysfunctional heart. Increased afterload in chronic renal failure is also a result of reduced compliance of the aorta and large arteries.[93] Renal artery stenosis with secondary or concomitant chronic renal failure can cause episodic, marked systemic hypertension and consequently evoke intermittent acute heart failure and pulmonary edema.[94]

NEGATIVE INOTROPIC EFFECTS. Several factors in chronic renal failure may decrease myocardial contractility. These include hypoxemia (often present during hemodialysis), subendocardial ischemia, certain buffers (e.g., acetate) added to the hemodialysis fluid, elevated parathormone levels, various metabolic and electrolyte abnormalities, and "uremic toxins."

EFFECTS OF DIALYSIS AND RENAL TRANSPLANTATION ON THE HEART

DIALYSIS. During dialysis, changes in preload, afterload, arterial pO_2, adrenergic activity, concentrations of electrolytes, ionized calcium, "uremic toxins," and other metabolites and the composition of the dialysis solution affect cardiac-ventricular performance (Fig. 62-7).[19,84] The baseline status of LV function prior to the initiation of dialysis therapy is a major determinant of LV performance during dialysis. In general, patients with normal LV function experience little change or a modest decrease in LV performance during dialysis, whereas LV performance in those with baseline systolic dysfunction often improves during the procedure. These observations are due in part to the fact that the preload reduction of dialysis has less effect on LV systolic performance in the dysfunctional (systolic) LV com-

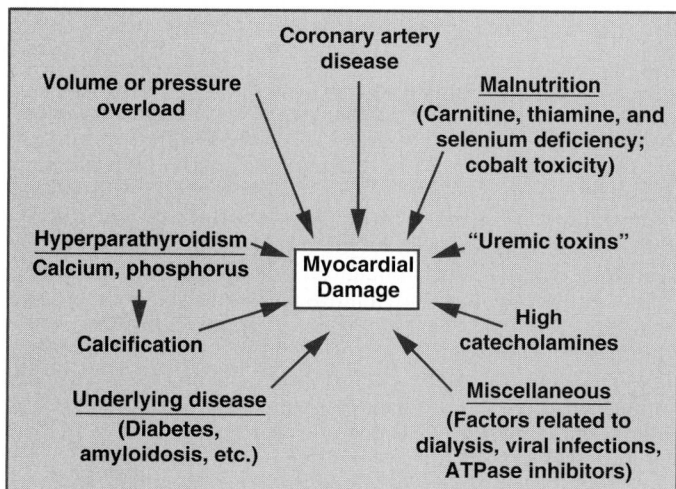

FIGURE 62–5. Factors contributing to myocardial damage in patients with chronic renal failure. (Modified from Leier, C. V., and Boudoulas, H.: Cardiorenal Disorders and Diseases. Armonk, N.Y., Futura Publishing Co., 1992.)

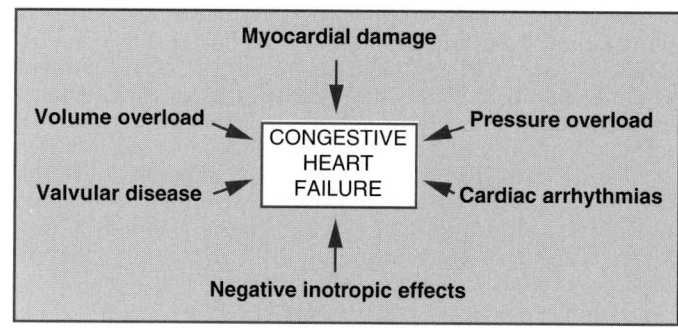

FIGURE 62–6. Factors contributing to the development of congestive heart failure in patients with chronic renal failure. (Modified from Leier, C. V., and Boudoulas, H.: Cardiorenal Disorders and Diseases. Armonk, N.Y., Futura Publishing Co., 1992.)

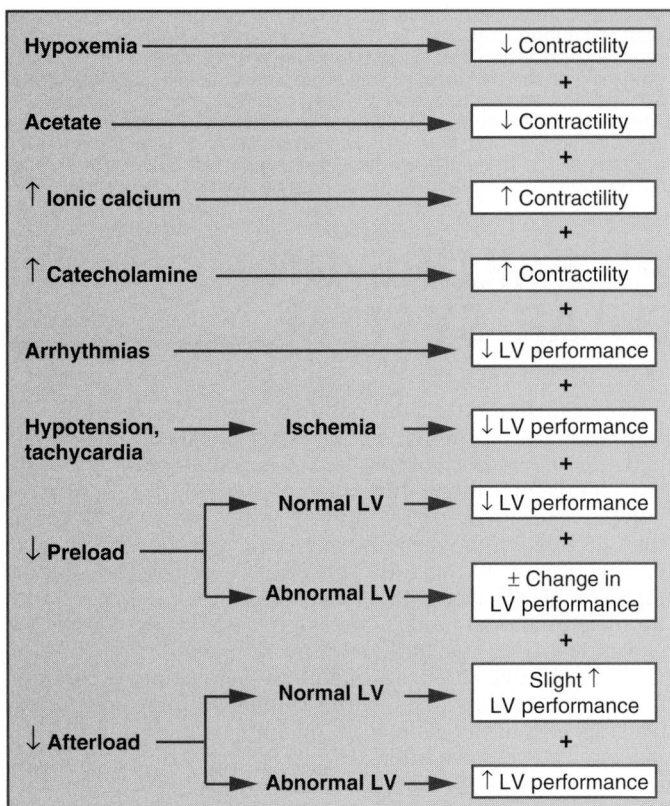

FIGURE 62–7. Effects of multiple factors and events during dialysis on left ventricular (LV) performance. (Modified from Leier, C. V., and Boudoulas, H.: Cardiorenal Disorders and Diseases. Armonk, N.Y., Futura Publishing Co., 1992.)

pared to the normal LV, while the opposite responses occur during shifts in afterload. Preload reduction during dialysis can adversely affect LV systolic performance and overall hemodynamics in patients with predominant LV diastolic dysfunction.

Changes in preload and afterload during peritoneal dialysis are more gradual and less in magnitude, and thus its effects on LV performance are not as marked as those of hemodialysis. However, large amounts of intraperitoneal fluid can impair LV systolic performance by reducing venous return and raising afterload.

RENAL TRANSPLANTATION. LV systolic and diastolic volumes and ventricular mass decrease and ejection fraction generally increases over 3 to 4 months after renal transplantation. These changes are likely related to favorable alterations of LV preload and afterload, an increase in hematocrit value, and correction of the various metabolic/endocrinological abnormalities already discussed.[19,88,89] Because commonly used immunosuppressive agents (e.g., cyclosporine) can evoke systemic hypertension, blood pressure should be checked regularly and treated appropriately in the post-transplant patient.

Management of Heart Failure in Patients with Renal Failure

The clinical presentation and evaluation of CHF in chronic renal failure patients are similar to those of patients without this condition (see Chap. 15). As in patients without chronic renal failure, the principles of CHF management in CRF include correcting remediably reversible lesions (e.g., operable occlusive coronary disease), improving contributory conditions (e.g., severe anemia), and optimizing preload, afterload, and cardiac rhythm. Restriction of dietary sodium to ≤2 gm/day is recommended. Angiotensin-converting enzyme inhibitors, digitalis, and vasodilators are often useful in this setting.[19] The duration of dialysis may be lengthened to increase fluid removal or to remove the usual amount of fluid volume more gradually and thus avoid hypotension. Peritoneal dialysis should be considered if problematic hypotension occurs during hemodialysis in the CRF patient with CHF. Erythropoietin is an effective and safe means of increasing the hematocrit of

CRF anemia, and an oversized AV access shunt may have to be modified. Long-term administration of 1α-hydrocholecalciferol may improve LV performance by reducing circulating parathormone and improving cellular calcium, phosphorous, and magnesium metabolism. Renal transplantation usually improves LV performance, hemodynamics, and CHF symptoms. In select patients with end-stage myocardial and kidney disease, combined cardiac and renal transplantation, preferably from the same donor, should be considered.[88,95]

HYPERTROPHIC CARDIOMYOPATHY

For yet undetermined reasons, hypertrophic cardiomyopathy and asymmetrical septal hypertrophy are not uncommon complications of CRF.[19] Patients with CRF with hypertrophic cardiomyopathy also invariably have LV diastolic dysfunction, which, when combined with a LV outflow tract gradient, makes them particularly vulnerable to the occurrence of systemic hypotension during hemodialysis. Special care must be taken to avoid volume depletion during hemodialysis in these patients, with consideration for peritoneal dialysis in those who experience problematic hypotension. If symptoms or complications during dialysis appear to be exacerbated by high adrenergic tone, beta-adrenergic blockade is a reasonable option.

ACCELERATED CORONARY ATHEROSCLEROSIS

Atherogenic Factors in Chronic Renal Failure

CHRONIC RENAL FAILURE AND DIALYSIS. Cardiovascular mortality remains high in these patients. This is in large part related to aging of the affected population and to the increased number of diabetic patients undergoing long-term dialysis. Thirty to 35 per cent of patients on long-term dialysis management have overt diabetes mellitus. Women with chronic renal failure develop coronary artery disease (CAD) as frequently and severely as age-matched men with chronic renal failure, perhaps because of earlier menopause and alterations in the pituitary-gonadal axis in these women.[19,89–92] For yet unknown reasons, patients with chronic pyelonephritis or interstitial renal disease develop CAD more frequently than patients with other forms of chronic renal failure.

Carbohydrate and lipid abnormalities occur early in chronic renal insufficiency (serum creatine levels >3 mg/dl) and persist as the patient's condition advances into end-stage renal failure and necessitates long-term dialysis. Glucose intolerance and insulin resistance have been demonstrated in a large proportion of chronic renal failure patients who are not overtly diabetic, and patients undergoing long-term dialysis develop carbohydrate and lipid disturbances similar to those of diabetes mellitus (insulin resistance, glucose intolerance, increased triglycerides). While the total cholesterol concentration in serum of chronic renal failure patients on maintenance dialysis can be normal, the level of the high-density lipoproteins is usually depressed. Caucasian men with chronic renal failure have lower levels of high-density lipoproteins than African-American men so affected, which may account for the higher incidence of CAD in the former group.[19,96–102] Other abnormalities that likely augment the atherosclerotic process include carnitine deficiency (adversely affects lipoprotein metabolism), secondary hyperparathyroidism, vascular calcification, increased homocystine, various states of hypercoagulation, and enhanced fibrin and platelet deposition (Fig. 62–8). Depressed endothelium-derived vasodilation and elevated local and circulating levels of endothelin in

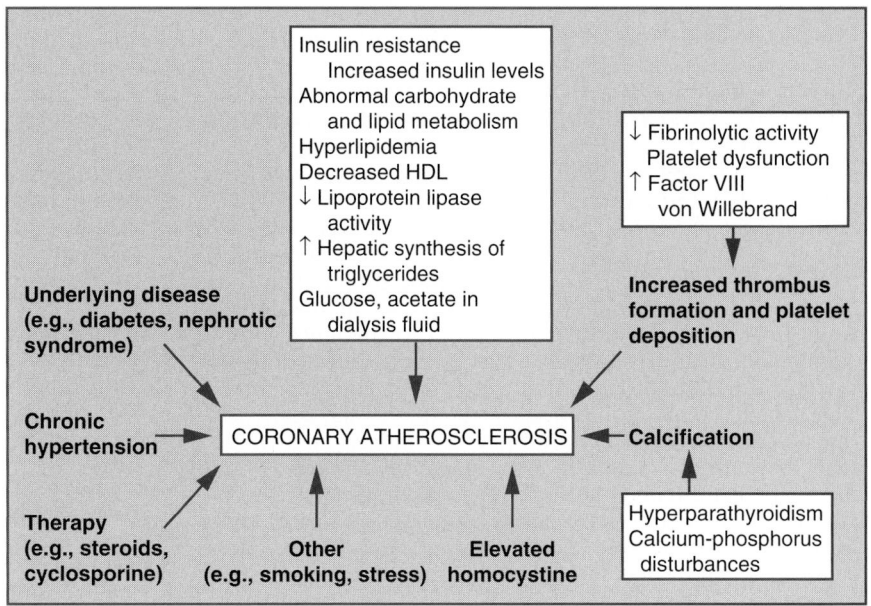

FIGURE 62–8. Factors contributing to the development and acceleration of coronary atherosclerosis in patients with chronic renal failure. HDL = high-density lipoproteins. (Modified from Leier, C. V., and Boudoulas, H.: Cardiorenal Disorders and Diseases. Armonk, N.Y., Futura Publishing Co., 1992.)

patients with chronic renal failure may also play a role.[103,104]

NEPHROTIC SYNDROME. Elevation of serum lipid values is a major feature of the nephrotic syndrome. Total cholesterol and low-density lipoprotein cholesterol concentrations are generally elevated, and high-density lipoprotein cholesterol is normal or low.[105] These lipid derangements can persist for some time after remission of the nephrotic syndrome, particularly in children. Chronic hypertension and corticosteroid therapy further accelerate atherosclerosis in this subgroup of patients.

RENAL TRANSPLANTATION. Cardiovascular disease contributes heavily to mortality following kidney transplantation. Many chronic renal failure patients have generalized arteriosclerosis-atherosclerosis at the time of transplantation and thus their pre-transplant and post-transplant cardiovascular disease represents a continuum, perpetuated by the persistence, worsening, and accumulation of risk factors (e.g., age, hypertension, diabetes, hyperlipidemia, immunosuppressive drugs)[19,106,107] (Fig. 62–8). The number of acute rejection episodes is also linked as an independent risk factor to the development of cardiovascular disease.[19] Significant proteinuria occurs in 10 to 15 per cent of transplantation patients and usually indicates varying degrees of graft rejection or failure; urinary protein excretion > 0.5 gm daily in the post-transplant patient is associated with a significant rise in low-density and very low-density lipoprotein cholesterol and in total triglycerides. Immunosuppressive therapy with corticosteroids evokes insulin resistance and hyperlipoproteinemia. Cyclosporine increases

total cholesterol by elevating the level of low-density lipoprotein cholesterol.[106,107] Therefore the cumulative atherogenic risk factors—long-term dialysis, renal transplantation, and periodic graft rejection—account for the high prevalence of morbid cardiovascular disease in renal transplant patients.

FACTORS AFFECTING MYOCARDIAL OXYGEN SUPPLY AND DEMAND IN CHRONIC RENAL FAILURE

Although the general determinants of myocardial oxygen supply and demand in these patients are similar to those of patients without renal failure (see p. 381), chronic renal failure adds several conditions that can evoke myocardial ischemia, even without occlusive CAD. Chronic renal failure adversely affects coronary perfusion pressure, diastolic perfusion time, and oxygen-carrying capacity of blood (Fig. 62–9). Volume and pressure overload increase ventricular diastolic pressure and thus can decrease coronary perfusion pressure (coronary perfusion pressure during diastole equals coronary artery pressure minus LV diastolic pressure). In the presence of occlusive coronary artery disease, coronary artery pressure distal to a high-grade obstruction is not only low but is also not affected significantly by the usual changes in aortic diastolic pressure. Therefore, distal to an obstruction, only changes in LV diastolic pressure can significantly alter coronary perfusion pressure in that region of the heart. An increase in heart rate (as occurs with dialysis, AV shunt, or anemia) reduces myocardial blood flow simply by decreasing diastolic perfusion time.

Since the majority of coronary blood flow occurs in diastole and the duration of diastole (diastolic perfusion time) has a nonlinear inverse relationship with heart rate, even small increases in heart rate can substantially reduce diastolic perfusion time.[108] Anemia, a common feature of chronic renal failure, reduces the oxygen-carrying capacity of blood. Hemodialysis with accompanying hypotension, tachycardia, and leftward shift in the arterial hemoglobin-oxygen dissociation curve can be especially threatening to myocardial oxygena-

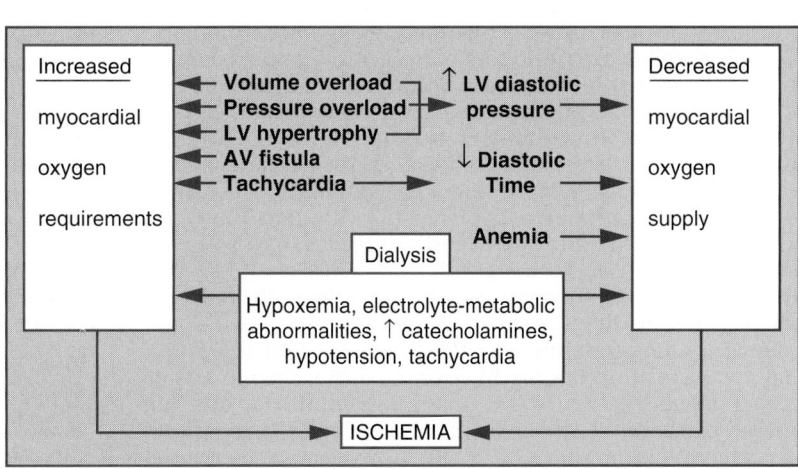

FIGURE 62–9. Factors affecting myocardial oxygen supply and oxygen requirements in patients with chronic renal failure. AV = arteriovenous, LV = left ventricle. (Modified from Leier, C. V., and Boudoulas, H.: Cardiorenal Disorders and Diseases. Armonk, N.Y., Futura Publishing Co., 1992.)

tion. Coronary blood flow has been shown to decrease in some patients during hemodialysis.[109]

Chronic Coronary Artery Disease

CLINICAL PRESENTATION AND DIAGNOSTIC EVALUATION.
CRF modifies the clinical presentation of chronic CAD with a greater prevalence of painless ischemia, partially attributable to a large proportion of chronic renal failure patients with diabetes mellitus, and with chest pain secondary to a variety of nonischemic causes (e.g., uremic pericarditis, neuritis).[19,110] Electrocardiographic findings similar to those of myocardial ischemia (e.g., ST-segment depression, T-wave inversion) are present in many CRF patients without significant CAD (especially during and after dialysis), thereby limiting the specificity of this diagnostic method. The sensitivity of radionuclide exercise testing for detecting obstructive CAD in chronic renal failure is low, perhaps because of generally poor exercise capacity,[111] and there are insufficient data in this condition regarding the sensitivity and specificity of radionuclide-perfusion imaging after dipyridamole administration. Dobutamine-stress echocardiography has recently been shown to be a promising means of detecting significant CAD in chronic renal failure.[112] Coronary arteriography is often required in these patients with suspected or problematic CAD to define their coronary artery anatomy and pathology and to develop the most appropriate management plan.

USE OF CONTRAST RADIOGRAPHY.
To minimize the renal complications of radiocontrast angiography in patients with serum creatinine concentrations greater than 2 mg/dl who are not yet undergoing long-term dialysis, preprocedural hydration and postprocedural volume replacement (saline solution for urine volume) are the most effective interventions.[113] The routine administration of 20 per cent mannitol solution is no longer advocated in this clinical setting. The smallest possible amount of radiocontrast agent should be used, because the degree of nephrotoxicity is closely related to the quantity injected. Patients with renal artery stenosis are especially susceptible to contrast-induced nephropathy. The osmotic and volume load of radiocontrast material can also provoke acute pulmonary edema in chronic renal failure patients with underlying volume overload or LV dysfunction. Nonionic contrast material evokes less intravascular volume expansion and should generally be employed in chronic renal failure. To further reduce the amount and risk of administered radiocontrast agent, information regarding ventricular size and function should be obtained via two-dimensional echocardiography or radionuclide angiography.

MANAGEMENT.
The general management approach to CAD in chronic renal failure is similar to that of patients without this condition (Ch. 38); management aspects unique to chronic renal failure patients are presented below.[19,114–117] A diet weighted with polyunsaturated fats and a carbohydrate content of approximately 20 per cent of total caloric intake is generally recommended. Lipid-lowering agents are usually effective in this clinical setting, and HMG-CoA reductase inhibitors are generally better tolerated in CRF than most other agents. Because of an increased risk of developing skeletal myopathy and rhabdomyolysis, the HMG-CoA reductase inhibitors must be used with caution in patients receiving cyclosporine. Disturbed calcium-phosphorus metabolism and resultant peripheral and coronary vascular calcification are approached with long-time oral administration of phosphate-binding agents (e.g., calcium carbonate, calcium acetate). For problematic CAD, it is often necessary to administer erythropoietin to keep hemoglobin ≥ 10 gm/dl.

Oxygen administration at a flow rate of 2 to 3 liters/min may be useful in reducing hypoxemia and ischemic events during hemodialysis. When possible, sodium bicarbonate instead of sodium acetate should be employed as the dialysis buffer. This produces resultant improvement in arterial oxygenation, less provocation of hypotension, and reduction in the tendency of this procedure to precipitate myocardial ischemia. Certain patients with severe CAD and ventricular dysfunction cannot tolerate hemodialysis because of problematic dialysis-induced reduction in cardiac output or blood pressure; some of these patients require cardioactive drug support (e.g., dopamine, dobutamine) during hemodialysis, and others are best managed with peritoneal dialysis.

Percutaneous transluminal coronary angioplasty (PTCA) can be performed in these patients; however, the restenosis rate is rather high.[115] Chronic renal failure patients, whether or not they are undergoing long-term dialysis and prerenal or postrenal transplantation, can undergo coronary artery bypass surgery with acceptable risk and with an expectation for significant improvement of ischemic symptoms, exercise tolerance, and, perhaps for some, survival.[114,117]

PERIOPERATIVE MANAGEMENT

Table 62–4 lists the major recommendations for the perioperative management of the chronic renal failure patient undergoing cardiac surgery. Intravascular volume, serum potassium, hematocrit, and drug administration must be carefully monitored during the perioperative period.[19,114,117] Preoperatively, daily dialysis (usually of shorter duration) against a low potassium bath should be considered to control serum and whole body potassium content. Hemoglobin and hematocrit should be raised to ≥ 10 gm/dl and ≥ 30 per cent, respectively, with erythropoietin administration or via red cell transfusion during dialysis in more urgent situations. The patient should go to surgery at near "dry weight." Intravenously administered fluids are kept to a minimum with little or no potassium administration. To prevent excessive hemodilution during cardiopulmonary bypass, both blood and Ringer's lactated solution are used to prime the extracorporeal pump. Beta-adrenergic blockade should be continued throughout the perioperative period to avert the myocardial and dysrhythmic complications of the hyperadrenergic state of cardiac surgery. Intraoperative hemofiltration can be used to treat any excessive intravascular volume accumulated during cardiopulmonary bypass.

Postoperatively, dialysis is employed to reverse hyperkalemia, significant azotemia, or volume overload. Regional heparinization or citration should be considered during the first 5 to 10 postoperative days as a means of controlling bleeding complications during hemodialysis. The perioperative management used for CRF patients undergoing lengthy dialysis also applies to nondialyzed CRF patients undergoing cardiac surgery; renal function in the latter patients may have to be supported with dialysis over several postoperative days, but function usually returns to its preoperative status by 10 to 15 days after surgery. Patients with a functioning transplanted kidney can be managed in a near-routine (nonchronic renal failure) manner with special attention directed at providing adequate corticosteroid support, avoiding nephrotoxic drugs, and maintaining adequate urine output.

Pericarditis is a common complication; total pericardiectomy

TABLE 62–4 PERIOPERATIVE MANAGEMENT OF CHRONIC RENAL FAILURE IN PATIENTS UNDERGOING CARDIAC SURGERY

PREOPERATIVE
Dental evaluation and correction
Decrease intake of sodium, potassium, and fluid volume
Short dialysis daily (low potassium bath)
Beta-blockade therapy throughout perioperative period
Antibiotic prophylaxis (start immediately before surgery and continue for 2 days after surgery)
Raise hemoglobin/hematocrit above 10 gm per dl/30 per cent

INTRAOPERATIVE
Keep fluid administration to minimum
Do not administer potassium
Special effort to preserve arm vessels and AV access fistula
Hemodynamic monitoring (during and after surgery) as needed

POSTOPERATIVE
Determine serum potassium levels and arterial blood gases every 4 hr during first 24 hr
Perform dialysis as indicated
Use regional anticoagulation during dialysis over first 5 to 10 postoperative days

AV = arteriovenous.

should be considered as a reasonable elective addition to the cardiac surgical procedure in patients with chronic renal failure.

Acute Myocardial Ischemic Syndromes

The clinical presentation, diagnostic steps, and therapeutic measures for these patients with acute ischemic syndromes are generally similar to those directed at patients without chronic renal failure (Ch. 37). Unfortunately, chronic renal failure patients also frequently exhibit abnormal electrocardiographic ST-segment and T-wave abnormalities and elevated serum cardiac enzyme values in the absence of myocardial ischemia-necrosis. Because of impaired renal clearance, total creatine phosphokinase (CPK) and lactic dehydrogenase levels are often elevated. However, the total CPK is usually composed of brain band CPK (CPK-BB, increased in about 30 per cent of patients with CRF) or skeletal muscle band (CPK-MM). Therefore, when myocardial ischemia and infarction is suspected, careful monitoring of the myocardial band (CPK-MB) over the ensuing 24 to 48 hours becomes important; new or transient elevation of the CPK-MB fraction can usually be regarded as an indication of acute myocardial necrosis.[118]

In the chronic renal failure patient with acute myocardial infarction who has end-stage renal disease or is nonresponsive to intravenous administration of loop diuretics in moderate to high doses, fluid overload is approached with dialysis. Hemodynamic monitoring with a flow-directed indwelling pulmonary artery catheter is appropriate when a low perfusion state or heart failure develops. Electrolyte and metabolic abnormalities are controlled with dietary measures and dialysis as needed.

CARDIOVASCULAR CALCIFICATION

Dystrophic (metastatic) calcification commonly occurs in CRF patients receiving maintenance dialysis and can involve all tissues, including heart, vasculature, and kidneys. Hyperphosphatemia with elevation of the calcium X phosphorus product, shifts in plasma and tissue pH during and following dialysis, and secondary hyperparathyroidism are regarded as the most important factors responsible for tissue calcification in CRF (Table 62–5).[19,119] The calcification is exacerbated by excessive intake of milk, use of certain antacids, and calcium extraction from calcium polystyrene materials and surfaces (e.g., certain dialysis units).

The mitral annulus and valve and aortic valve are the preferential cardiac sites for dystrophic calcification in chronic renal failure (Table 62–5). Consequently, hemody-

TABLE 62–5 METASTATIC CALCIFICATION OF CHRONIC RENAL FAILURE: CONTRIBUTING FACTORS AND COMMON CARDIOVASCULAR SITES OF INVOLVEMENT

POSSIBLE CONTRIBUTING FACTORS	CARDIOVASCULAR SITES
Hyperphosphatemia	Mitral annulus and valve
Increased ionized calcium	Aortic valve
Increased calcium-phosphorus product	Atrioventricular node/conduction system
Increased parathormone levels	Myocardium
Acute changes in blood pH	Interventricular septum
Increased calcium ingestion	Coronary arteries
Certain antacids	Pericardium
Extraction from calcium-containing polymers and materials	
Vitamin D preparations	

Modified from Leier, C. V., and Boudoulas, H.: Cardiorenal Disorders and Diseases. Armonk, N. Y., Futura Publishing Co., 1992.

namically significant valvular stenosis and/or regurgitation, usually manifested clinically as murmurs and occasionally as symptoms and signs of heart failure, are common complications of cardiac calcification in chronic renal failure. Myocardial calcification can evoke conduction abnormalities (most commonly atrioventricular or bundle branch block), various arrhythmias, ventricular dysfunction, and CHF. Significant annular, valvular, and coronary artery calcification and regions of dense calcification elsewhere in the heart are usually detectable by image-amplified fluoroscopy, echocardiography, or magnetic resonance imaging. Technetium pyrophosphate scintigraphy may demonstrate uptake in areas of myocardial calcification. Diffuse myocardial calcification can occasionally be detected with special histological processing of myocardial biopsy specimens. Pericardial calcification, usually microscopic in degree, contributes to the pathological process of uremic pericarditis. Dense pericardial calcification is not a feature of chronic renal failure and implicates another disease process.

Prevention of cardiovascular calcification is an important component of chronic renal failure management. Phosphate-binding agents and dietary measures (restriction of phosphate and avoidance of excessive calcium intake) are employed for this purpose. Regression of nonvisceral calcification has been achieved by lowering serum phosphorus with oral phosphate-binding agents, parathyroidectomy, and renal transplantation; visceral calcification (including cardiovascular) does not appear to be as readily reversible. Management of the congestive heart failure, atrioventricular block, and cardiac arrhythmias caused by cardiac calcification is directed at controlling symptoms.

HEART MURMURS AND VALVULAR HEART DISEASE

Heart murmurs and acquired valvular abnormalities are common in these patients. Dystrophic calcification, infectious and noninfectious endocarditis, and certain renal diseases (e.g., polycystic kidney disease) are associated with structural abnormalities of heart valves.[19,120-122] However, heart murmurs are frequently noted in chronic renal failure without obvious underlying valvular abnormalities and are probably evoked by anemia, the AV access fistula, hyperadrenergic tone, and volume and pressure overload. Early diastolic murmurs of functional aortic or pulmonic regurgitation, generally related to pressure and volume overload, can appear during advanced stages of renal failure and often disappear following hemodialysis. An occasional murmur audible over the anterior chest may be transmitted from an AV access fistula located in the upper limb. In patients with forearm shunt access, bruits can be heard in the ipsilateral axillary, clavicular, and cervical regions. Cervical venous hums are also common in these patients. Thus, murmurs in chronic renal failure can represent valvular disease, functional pulmonic or aortic valvular flow or regurgitation, transmission from an AV fistula, or a venous hum.

As in other conditions, each murmur requires clinical assessment to define the underlying cause, and if associated with valvular or congenital heart disease, evaluation of the severity of the lesion. A precordial systolic murmur secondary to high flow or transmission from the AV fistula can be easily distinguished from other murmurs by observing the response of the murmur to transient obstruction of the fistula. Functional murmurs secondary to pressure or volume overload decrease considerably with control of hypertension, reduction of fluid overload, correction of anemia, and so forth. Venous hums are usually audible throughout the cardiac cycle; are loudest at the base of the neck, in the upright position and during inspiration; and are abolished by compression of the neck veins or by the Valsalva maneuver.

Laboratory evaluation and overall management of valvular heart disease in affected patients is similar to that recommended for patients without chronic renal failure (see Ch. 32). Cardiac valve replacement can be done with acceptable operative mortality and reasonably good cardiac rehabilitation in patients undergoing prolonged hemodialysis. Long-term survival for most of these patients is still limited by the clinical course and complications of chronic renal failure, but quality of life is generally improved after valve replacement.

Preoperative dental evaluation is mandatory, and dental treatment should be completed several weeks before cardiac surgery. The patient should arrive at operation at near "dry weight," and with a hematocrit of ≥30 per cent and a serum potassium level of 3.5 to 4.5 mEq/liter (Table 62–4). Serum potassium and arterial blood gases should be measured every 4 to 6 hours during the first postoperative day. Hemodialysis may be required to manage fluid overload, azotemia, or hyperkalemia. Chronic renal failure patients undergoing open-heart surgery—especially placement of prosthetic heart valves—are at high risk for infective endocarditis. In the perioperative period, *Staphylococcus aureus*, coagulase-negative staphylococci, and diphtheroids are the most common infecting organisms. No single antibiotic agent is effective against all of these organisms, and prolonged use of broad-spectrum antibiotics predisposes patients to superinfection with unusual or resistant organisms. Thus, antibiotic prophylaxis at the time of valvular surgery is primarily directed against staphylococci and should be started immediately before the operative procedure and continued postoperatively for approximately 2 days. The choice of mechanical versus bioprosthetic valve for replacement in chronic renal failure remains controversial.[19,121,122] When technically feasible, reconstructive valvular repair should be considered for problematic mitral regurgitation.[120,121]

PERICARDIAL DISEASE

Pericardial disease remains a relatively common complication in these patients. The contributory factors are depicted in Figure 62–10, and the evaluation and management of pericardial disorders are presented in Chapter 43.

SYSTEMIC HYPERTENSION

HYPERTENSION ASSOCIATED WITH CHRONIC RENAL FAILURE (see also p. 824). Systemic hypertension occurs in more than 80 per cent of these patients prior to initiation of dialysis. Chronic renal failure patients who remain normotensive most often have tubular and interstitial disease or obstructive uropathy as the underlying pathological process. In contrast, arterionephrosclerosis and glomerulonephritis are usually associated with hypertension, often marked. The various factors that likely contribute to the development of systemic hypertension in chronic renal failure are presented in Figure 62–11.

HYPERTENSION ASSOCIATED WITH RENAL TRANSPLANTATION. The incidence of systemic hypertension after renal transplantation varies widely (25 to 80 per cent) and is highest during the early months after transplantation. The incidence 5 years after transplantation is about 40 to 50 per cent. Renal graft failure is increased considerably in the

setting of poorly controlled systemic hypertension.[123] Renal artery stenosis (of the transplanted kidney or native kidneys), chronic rejection, native kidney disease, therapy with corticosteroids or cyclosporine, and essential hypertension prior to transplantation are the leading causes for systemic hypertension in the post-transplant patient. Recipients of cadaveric kidneys from donors with a family history of essential hypertension are also more likely to experience post-transplant hypertension. On the other hand, essential hypertension can undergo remission for up to 8 to 10 years after successful transplantation of a kidney from a normotensive donor.

MANAGEMENT. Diagnostic studies should be undertaken in patients with renal failure and hypertension to exclude a reversible renovascular cause (see Chap. 26) and determine the nature of the underlying renal disease. Distinguishing hypertension secondary to renal parenchymal disease from essential hypertension with resultant hypertensive renal disease is often quite difficult at this stage. The medical history may identify patients who have had longstanding essential hypertension and a familial tendency for such, diabetes mellitus, or an episode of glomerulonephritis prior to developing renal failure.

The treatment of systemic hypertension in patients with active glomerulonephritis and/or chronic renal failure is similar to that of essential hypertension (Chap. 27). However, for chronic renal failure patients, the dosage schedule of drugs cleared by the kidney has to be modified to match renal function to avoid the deleterious effects of accumulated drug or metabolite. Dialysis should be considered in patients with a substantial reduction of renal function and hypertension refractory to medical management (Fig. 62–12). Early initiation of dialysis decreases the consequences of uremia, allows easier control of hypertension, and reduces the complications of chronic hypertension.

Bilateral nephrectomy is reserved for the severely hypertensive chronic renal failure patient whose hypertension is refractory to aggressive hemodialysis and optimal drug therapy. The results of nephrectomy are best in patients with markedly elevated plasma renin activity. The major, but correctable, disadvantages of nephrectomy are a further drop in the hemoglobin and hematocrit (reduced erythropoietin) and exacerbation of renal osteodystrophy (depressed generation of certain forms of vitamin D). The availability of potent oral antihypertensive agents, such as central sympatholytic drugs (e.g., clonidine), high-dose angiotensin-converting enzyme inhibitors, and minoxidil, has now made bilateral nephrectomy an uncommon procedure in chronic renal failure.

The management of systemic hypertension is often complicated by concomitant drug therapy; this is particularly relevant to the post-transplant patient.[19,124] Corticosteroids adversely affect hypertension control by increasing blood volume and insulin resistance and blunting responsiveness to antihypertensive drugs. Cyclosporine commonly provokes or exacerbates systemic hypertension, occasionally to extremely high levels of blood pressure; calcium channel blocking drugs are usually effective in controlling cyclosporine-induced hypertension. A marked and often refractory increase in systemic blood pressure and occasionally renal interstitial disease can follow the administration of nonsteroidal antiinflammatory agents.

Because spontaneous improvement of systemic hypertension in post-transplant patients with obstructing renal artery lesions (usually at the site of vascular anastomosis) is not uncommon, conservative management is generally recommended of the transplantation patient with stable, adequate renal function whose hypertension is amenable to medications. When stenosis-induced hypertension becomes difficult to control or renal function falls, percutaneous transluminal angioplasty of the arterial lesion becomes a therapeutic option. Surgical intervention may become necessary if angioplasty is not feasible or is unsuccessful. Effective treatment of post-transplant hypertension is very important for the long-term health and survival of both graft and patient.[123]

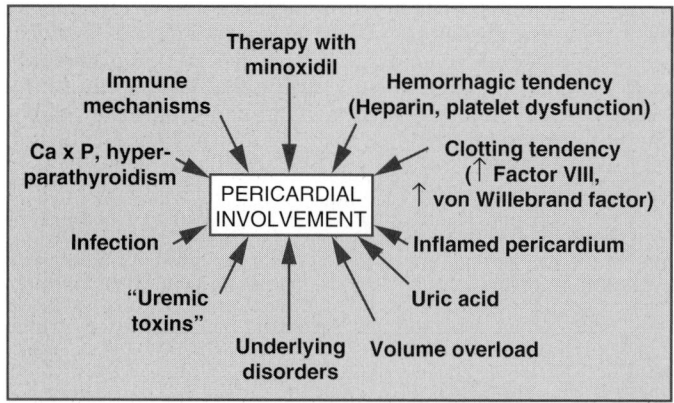

FIGURE 62–10. Factors contributing to the development of pericardial disease in patients with chronic renal failure. Ca = calcium, P = phosphorus. (Modified from Leier, C. V., and Boudoulas, H.: Cardiorenal Disorders and Diseases. Armonk, N.Y., Futura Publishing Co., 1992.)

CARDIAC ARRHYTHMIAS

Cardiac arrhythmias constitute a major clinical problem in chronic renal failure because of their increased prevalence and potentially serious complications; their episodic nature also makes identification and characterization difficult. A multicenter study of longstanding hemodialyzed pa-

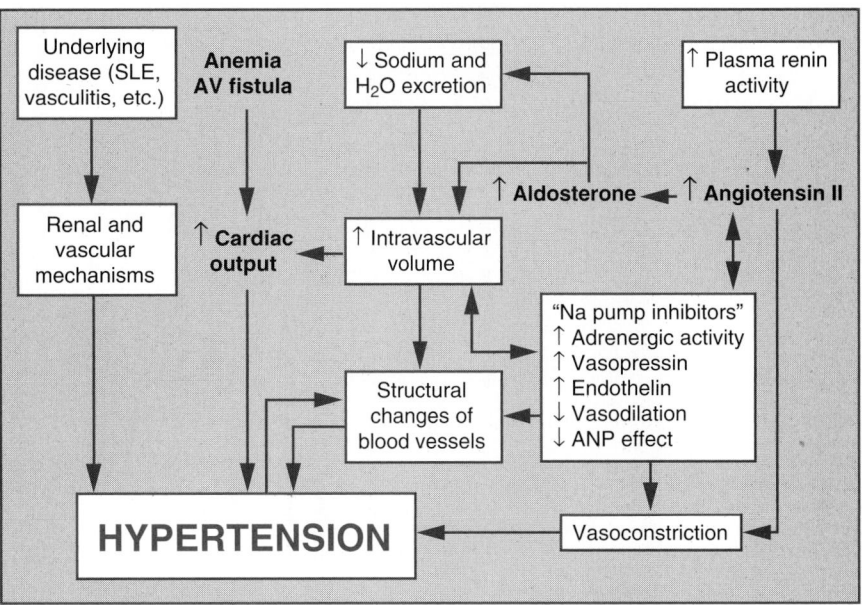

FIGURE 62-11. Pathophysiological mechanisms contributing to the development of systemic hypertension in patients with parenchymal renal disease and failure. ANF = atrial natriuretic peptide, SLE = systemic lupus erythematosus. (Modified from Leier, C. V., and Boudoulas, H.: Cardiorenal Disorders and Diseases. Armonk, N.Y., Futura Publishing Co., 1992.)

tients showed that ventricular arrhythmias, as assessed by 48-hour ambulatory monitoring, were present in 76 per cent of patients[125]; 39 per cent had two or more events of two or more sequential ventricular ectopic beats (i.e., couplets or nonsustained ventricular tachycardia) per hour. The frequency of ventricular arrhythmias rose significantly after the second hour of hemodialysis and lasted up to 5 hours following dialysis. The independent risk factors for the presence of ventricular arrhythmias were age over 55 years and LV dysfunction. The frequency of ventricular ectopic beats also appeared to vary directly with resting heart rate. 69 per cent of the CRF patients undergoing long-term dialysis had supraventricular arrhythmias, mostly nonsustained. Table 62-6 lists the major factors in chronic renal failure likely to contribute to the development of cardiac arrhythmias.

MANAGEMENT. While a detailed discussion of arrhythmia management is not within the scope of this chapter, a few general principles are important in managing these patients. As in other patients, the initial approach is directed at treating remedial cardiac disease and at reversing contributory factors (Table 62-6). Caffeine and other cardiac stimulants should be avoided by CRF patients with tachyarrhythmias. If arrhythmias are related to hemodialysis, attention should be directed to the potassium concentration of the dialysis bath. A low

potassium concentration of the dialysate can lead to hypokalemia and serious rhythm disturbances, particularly in patients who are receiving digitalis or are afflicted with CAD, LV hypertrophy, or LV dysfunction. A dialysate potassium concentration of 3.5 mEq/liter usually abolishes dialysis-related ventricular arrhythmias. If the dialysate potassium concentration exceeds 3.5 mEq/liter, dietary potassium restriction is usually necessary between hemodialysis runs to prevent life-threatening hyperkalemia. Arrhythmias secondary to pericarditis tend to respond to treatment of the inflammatory component, when present.

PREDISPOSITION FOR CARDIOVASCULAR INFECTIONS

Infections are common in patients with end-stage renal disease. Because these patients undergo dialysis 100 to 180 times a year, it is not surprising that infections often involve the AV access site or the abdominal catheter in patients receiving peritoneal dialysis. It is estimated that up to 6 per cent of hemodialysis patients will develop infective endocarditis sometime during the course of their disease; the most common culprit organism is *Staphylococcus aureus*, followed by *Streptococcus viridans* and enterococci; the aortic valve is the usual target followed by the mitral valve.[19]

Proper sterile technique during the entire dialysis procedure is mandatory to prevent infectious disease in this very susceptible patient population. Patients should maintain good oral health and personal hygiene to reduce other potential sources for bacteremia and infective endocarditis. Skin flora of the dialysis patient and the dialysis staff should be controlled with bactericidal soap. The staff (via nasal discharge, skin, and other sites) is not an uncommon source for culprit organisms.[126] Patients undergoing long-term hemodialysis who have prosthetic valves and those who have had renal transplantation should receive antibiotics prophylactically.

Recurrent or prolonged bacteremia and septicemia in chronic renal failure patients receiving dialysis implicates persistent infection of the access shunt or catheter or infective endocarditis. Appropriate antibiotic therapy, based on blood culture and antibiotic-sensitivity data, should be initiated as soon as possible in these patients. Surgi-

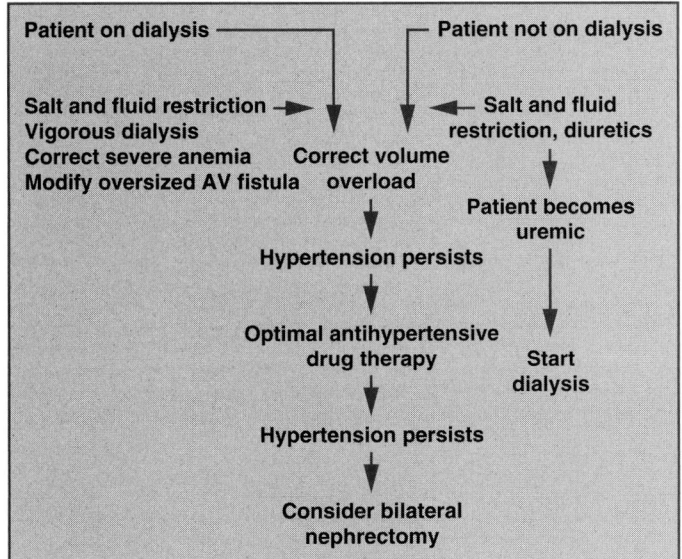

FIGURE 62-12. General management of arterial hypertension caused by renal parenchymal disease. AV = arteriovenous. (Modified from Leier, C. V., and Boudoulas, H.: Cardiorenal Disorders and Diseases. Armonk, N.Y., Futura Publishing Co., 1992.)

TABLE 62-6 FACTORS CONTRIBUTING TO DEVELOPMENT OF CARDIAC ARRHYTHMIAS IN PATIENTS WITH CHRONIC RENAL FAILURE

UNDERLYING CARDIAC DISEASE
Myocardial disease (left ventricular hypertrophy, left ventricular dysfunction)
Coronary artery disease—myocardial ischemia
Pericardial disease—myocardial inflammation
Cardiac calcification

HEMODIALYSIS
Rapid changes in serum electrolytes
Rapid changes in blood pH
Hypoxemia

HYPERADRENERGIC STATE

HIGH CALCIUM X PHOSPHORUS PRODUCT

HIGH PARATHORMONE LEVELS(?)

From Leier, C. V., and Boudoulas, H.: Cardiovascular Disorders and Diseases. Armonk, N. Y., Futura Publishing Co., 1992, with permission.

Text continues on page 1935

TABLE 62–7 CARDIOVASCULAR DRUG THERAPY IN RENAL FAILURE

DRUG	THERAPEUTIC RANGE/ml (PLASMA LEVELS)	ELIMINATION AND METABOLISM	HALF-LIFE — hr Normal	HALF-LIFE — hr Renal Failure	PROTEIN BINDING % Normal	PROTEIN BINDING % Renal Failure	ADJUSTMENT FOR RENAL FAILURE	REMOVAL BY DIALYSIS	COMMENTS
CARDIAC GLYCOSIDES									
Digoxin	0.8–2.0 ng	75% Renal	45	72–96	25	18	Yes	No	Radioimmunoassay may overestimate serum levels in renal failure
Digitoxin	20–35 ng	95% Hepatic	145	Unchanged	90–97	86–97	Decrease dose when creatinine clearance < 10 ml/min	No	8% converted to digoxin; protein binding decreases slightly by dialysis
ANTIARRHYTHMIC AGENTS									
Procainamide	4.0–10.0 µg	50% Renal 50% Hepatic	3–4	11–20	15–20	Unchanged	Yes	Yes, hemodialysis	Some patients require higher plasma concentrations (10–25 µg/ml)
N-Acetylprocainamide	10–20 µg	Renal	6–8	35–70	10	Unchanged	Yes	Yes, hemodialysis	Active metabolite of procainamide
Quinidine	2.0–5.0 µg	85% Hepatic 15% Renal	6	5–14	80–85	↑	No	Yes, hemodialysis	May increase serum digoxin levels
Disopyramide	0.5–2.0 µg	60% Renal 40% Hepatic	5–7	10–18	40–90	—	Yes	Yes, hemodialysis	Protein binding concentration dependent
Lidocaine	1.5–5.0 µg	90% Hepatic	1.2–2.2	1.3–3	60–66	Unchanged	No	No	Protein binding may be concentration dependent
Tocainide	4–10 µg	40% Renal	15	—	10	—	Yes	—	—
Mexiletine	2–7 µg	Hepatic Renal	7–11	↑	57–69	—	Yes	—	—
Phenytoin	10.0–18.0 µg	Hepatic	24	May be shorter	90–95	70–85	No	No	Protein binding in renal failure decreased
Encainide	250 µg	Hepatic (93% population) Hepatic-Renal (7% population)	2.3 / 11.3	—	60–80 / 70–80	—	No / Yes	—	—
a. O-desmethylencainide	30 µg	Hepatic (90%) Renal	3.5	—	—	—	Yes	—	—
b. 3-Methoxy-O-desmethylencainide	100 ng	Hepatic Renal	6.4	—	—	—	Yes	—	—
Flecainide	0.4–0.8 µg	Hepatic Renal (40%)	8–14	↑	50–70	—	Yes	—	—
Propafenone	—	Hepatic	2–10	—	85–87	—	—	—	—
Moricizine	—	Hepatic	—	—	85	—	Yes	—	—
Amiodarone	0.5–3.0 µg	Hepatic	53 days	—	>95	—	—	—	—
Bretylium	—	80% Renal 20% Nonrenal	6.0	13.6	—	—	Yes	—	Avoid when creatinine clearance < 10 ml/min

TABLE 62-7 CARDIOVASCULAR DRUG THERAPY IN RENAL FAILURE (continued)

DRUG	THERAPEUTIC RANGE/ml (PLASMA LEVELS)	ELIMINATION AND METABOLISM	HALF-LIFE—hr Normal	HALF-LIFE—hr Renal Failure	PROTEIN BINDING % Normal	PROTEIN BINDING % Renal Failure	ADJUSTMENT FOR RENAL FAILURE	REMOVAL BY DIALYSIS	COMMENTS
BETA-ADRENERGIC BLOCKERS									
Acebutolol	—	Hepatic	8	22	15–20	—	No	Yes, hemodialysis	Accumulation of active metabolite diacetolol
Alprenolol	—	Hepatic	1–3	2–3	85	—	No	—	—
Atenolol	—	Renal	6–9	15–35	< 5	—	Yes	Yes, hemodialysis	Significant accumulation in renal failure
Metoprolol	—	Hepatic	2.5	4.5	12	—	No	Yes, hemodialysis	—
Nadolol	—	Renal	14–24	45	25–30	—	Yes	Yes, hemodialysis	Significant accumulation in renal failure
Oxprenolol	—	Hepatic	2–3	2–3	80	—	No	—	—
Pindolol	—	Hepatic Renal	3–4	3–4	40–55	—	No	—	—
Propranolol	—	Hepatic	2–4	2–4	90–95	—	No	Yes, hemodialysis	Active metabolites may accumulate
Sotalol	—	Renal (60%) Hepatic	8	15–50	50	—	Yes	Yes, hemodialysis	—
Timolol	—	Hepatic	4–6	4–6	10	—	No	Yes, hemodialysis	—
Esmolol	—	Hepatic	.06–2	—	55	—	No	No	For IV use only
Labetolol	—	Mostly hepatic	6–8	—	50	—	—	—	—
Carteolol	—	60–70% Renal	6	—	23–30	—	Yes	—	—
Penbutolol	—	Hepatic	5	5	80–98	—	—	—	—
Betaxolol	—	Primarily hepatic, renal	14–22	30–40	50	—	Yes	Small amount	—
CALCIUM CHANNEL BLOCKERS									
Verapamil	—	Hepatic	3	?7	90	≈ 90	No	Yes	—
Diltiazem	—	Hepatic	2	?8	83	—	No	—	—
Nifedipine	—	Hepatic	4	?5.5	95	—	No	—	—
Nicardipine	—	Hepatic	1–1.6	—	89–99	—	No	—	—
Nimodipine	—	Hepatic	8–9	—	95; binding concentration dependent	—	No	—	—
Bepridil hydrochloride	—	Liver 70%; urine excretion of metabolites	Early 2 Terminal 26–64	—	99	—	—	—	Type 1A antiarrhythmic properties
Isradipine	—	Hepatic	Early 1.5–2 Terminal 8	—	95	—	—	—	—
Felodipine	—	Hepatic	11–16	—	> 99	—	No	—	—

TABLE 62-7 CARDIOVASCULAR DRUG THERAPY IN RENAL FAILURE *(continued)*

DRUG	THERAPEUTIC RANGE/ml (PLASMA LEVELS)	ELIMINATION AND METABOLISM	HALF-LIFE—hr		PROTEIN BINDING %		ADJUSTMENT FOR RENAL FAILURE	REMOVAL BY DIALYSIS	COMMENTS
			Normal	Renal Failure	Normal	Renal Failure			
ANTIHYPERTENSIVES									
Methyldopa	—	Mostly renal	5–8	7–16	<15	—	May be necessary when creatinine clearance <50 ml/min	Yes, peritoneal and hemodialysis	Retention of active metabolites in renal failure
Clonidine	—	Renal	6–23	39–42	20–40	—	Yes, when creatinine clearance <10 ml/min	No	Rebound hypertension can occur if drug stopped abruptly
Guanfacine	—	Hepatic Renal	12–24	—	—	—	—	—	Withdrawal syndrome may appear
Guanabenz	—	Hepatic	4–6	—	—	—	—	—	—
Trimethaphan	—	—	—	—	—	—	—	—	Ganglionic blocking drug for IV use with short duration of action
Mecamylamine	—	Renal	—	—	—	—	Contraindicated in uremic patients	—	—
Guanethidine	—	Mostly renal, less nonrenal	48–72	96–196	0	—	Yes	—	Orthostatic hypotension common side effect
Reserpine	—	Hepatic, nonrenal	50–170	87–320	40	—	Avoid when creatinine clearance <10 ml/min	No	Long biologic half-life
Minoxidil	—	Hepatic	2.8–4.2	—	0	—	No	Yes, hemodialysis	May induce pericardial effusion and pericarditis
Hydralazine	—	Hepatic, nonrenal	2.5–5	7–16	87	—	May be necessary when creatinine clearance <50 ml/min	No	—
Diazoxide	—	Mostly renal	17–31	>30	>90	Decreased	No	Yes, peritoneal dialysis, hemodialysis	May produce sodium and water retention and hyperglycemia; protein binding decreased in renal failure
Prazosin	—	Mostly hepatic, some renal	2–3	—	97	—	No	No	—
Doxazosin	—	Liver	22	—	98	—	—	Yes	—
Terazosin	—	10% Urine	12	—	90–94	—	—	—	—
Nitroglycerin (sublingual)	—	Hepatic	2–4 (min)	2–4 (min)	—	—	No	—	—
Isosorbide-2-mononitrate	—	Hepatic	1.5–2.4	—	—	—	Yes	—	—
Isosorbide-5-mononitrate	—	Hepatic	4.0–5.0	—	—	—	—	—	—
Nitroprusside	—	Nonrenal	<10 min.	<10 min.	—	—	No	Hemodialysis	Thiocyanate and cyanide may accumulate

TABLE 62-7 CARDIOVASCULAR DRUG THERAPY IN RENAL FAILURE (continued)

DRUG	THERAPEUTIC RANGE /ml (PLASMA LEVELS)	ELIMINATION AND METABOLISM	HALF-LIFE—hr Normal	HALF-LIFE—hr Renal Failure	PROTEIN BINDING % Normal	PROTEIN BINDING % Renal Failure	ADJUSTMENT FOR RENAL FAILURE	REMOVAL BY DIALYSIS	COMMENTS
CONVERTING ENZYME INHIBITORS									
Captopril	—	Mostly renal, some hepatic	1.9	Prolonged	25–30	—	May be necessary when creatinine clearance <10 ml/min	Yes, hemodialysis	Deterioration of renal function in patients with bilateral renal artery stenosis
Enalapril	—	Mostly renal	11	—	—	—	When creatinine clearance <30 ml/min	—	Deterioration of renal function in patients with bilateral renal artery stenosis
Lisinopril	—	Renal	12	—	—	—	When creatinine clearance <30 ml/min	—	—
Enalaprilat	—	Renal	11	—	—	—	When creatinine clearance <30 ml/min	Yes	For IV injection
Benazepril	—	—	10–11	96.7	—	—	When plasma creatinine >3 mg/dl	—	—
Fosinopril sodium	—	50% Urine	12	≥95	—	—	No	—	—
Ramipril	—	60% Urine	13–17	—	—	—	When plasma creatinine >2.5 mg/dl	—	—
DIURETICS									
Thiazides	—	Renal	1–2	4–6	70	—	Yes	—	May be ineffective when creatinine clearance <30 ml/min
Metolazone	—	—	—	—	—	—	—	—	Can produce marked diuresis
Furosemide	—	Mostly renal	1	3	95	—	—	Yes, hemodialysis	Large doses necessary in renal failure
Ethacrynic acid	—	Renal, hepatic	3	—	90	—	Yes	Yes, hemodialysis	Large doses necessary in renal failure
Bumetanide	—	Renal, hepatic	1	—	90	—	No	—	Can be effective in patients with renal failure
Acetazolamide	—	Renal	8	Prolonged	80	—	Yes	—	Ineffective when GFR <10 ml/min
Amiloride	—	Renal	7.5	Prolonged	Low	—	Yes	—	May cause hyperkalemia
Triamterene	—	Hepatic, renal	2–12	10	60	Decreased	Yes, avoid when creatinine clearance <30 ml/min	—	Active metabolites have long half-life; may cause hyperkalemia
Spironolactone	—	Hepatic	10–35	10–35	98	—	Yes, avoid when creatinine clearance <30 ml/min	—	May cause hyperkalemia
Indapamide	—	Mostly renal, some hepatic	14	—	71–79	—	—	—	Oral antihypertensive-diuretic; has little or no diuretic effect in renal failure
ANTICOAGULANTS									
Heparin	—	Nonrenal	0.3–2.0	0.5–3.0	>90	—	No	Yes, hemodialysis and peritoneal dialysis	May potentiate uremic bleeding
Warfarin	—	Hepatic	40	40	99	Decreased	No	—	May decrease protein binding of other drugs; may potentiate uremic bleeding

TABLE 62–7   CARDIOVASCULAR DRUG THERAPY IN RENAL FAILURE (continued)

DRUG	THERAPEUTIC RANGE/ml (PLASMA LEVELS)	ELIMINATION AND METABOLISM	HALF-LIFE—hr		PROTEIN BINDING %		ADJUSTMENT FOR RENAL FAILURE	REMOVAL BY DIALYSIS	COMMENTS
			Normal	Renal Failure	Normal	Renal Failure			
THROMBOLYTICS									
Streptokinase	—	—	0.38	—	—	—	No	—	May potentiate uremic bleeding
Anistreplase	—	—	1–2	—	—	—	—	—	May potentiate uremic bleeding
Urokinase	—	Hepatic	0.33	—	—	—	—	—	May potentiate uremic bleeding
Tissue plasminogen activators (t-PA)	—	Hepatic	0.05	—	—	—	—	—	May potentiate uremic bleeding
LIPID-LOWERING AGENTS									
Cholestyramine	—	Not absorbed	—	—	—	—	No	—	May cause hyperchloremic acidosis
Colestipol	—	Not absorbed	—	—	—	—	No	—	May cause hyperchloremic acidosis
Clofibrate	—	Renal (40–60%), hepatic	17	46–110	96	—	Yes	Hemodialysis	Restricted use because of high profile of adverse effects
Gemfibrozil	—	Renal, fecal	1.5	—	Low	—	Yes	—	—
Nicotinic acid	—	Hepatic, renal	0.5–1.0	—	—	—	Yes	—	Frequent adverse effects in patients with renal failure; aspirin may reduce flushing
Lovastatin	—	Hepatic Renal	—	—	95	—	—	—	—
Probucol	—	Hepatic	—	—	—	—	—	—	—

Modified from Leier, C. V., and Boudoulas, H.: Cardiovascular Disorders and Diseases. Armonk, N. Y., Futura Publishing Co., 1992, with permission.

cal consultation is indicated when access shunts show abscess or aneurysm formation, thrombosis, or bleeding. Clinical recognition of infective endocarditis in the setting of chronic renal failure is often difficult, because many features (e.g., recurrent bacteremia, anemia, and encephalopathy) can occur in patients with end-stage renal failure without infective endocarditis. It is prudent to suspect infective endocarditis in any such patient with fever, leukocytosis, or bacteremia, particularly if associated with an infected access site. The appearance of new murmurs or changes in murmurs increases the likelihood of infective endocarditis. Demonstration of valvular vegetations by echocardiography is most informative and can be diagnostic in the presence of other clinical manifestations of infective endocarditis.

AUTONOMIC DYSFUNCTION

Derangements of the autonomic nervous system in chronic renal failure, most commonly manifested as postural or dialysis-induced hypotension, abnormal hemodynamic responses to Valsalva and other maneuvers, impairment of perspiration, and alterations in gastric motility, can evoke major symptoms and disability. The cause of autonomic dysfunction in these patients is multifactorial and attributable in some cases to the underlying cause of chronic renal failure (e.g., diabetic mellitus, amyloidosis), antihypertensive drugs (e.g., sympatholytic agents), aluminum intoxication from certain antacids, and the uremic syndrome itself.[127–129] Determination of the specific type of autonomic dysfunction can be difficult and may require additional diagnostic testing (e.g., nerve conduction, bladder and sphincter function, tilt studies). Informative yet simple and inexpensive clinical maneuvers include blood pressure and heart rate responses to upright posture or the Valsalva maneuver and heart rate response to normal and deep inspiration.[127] In general, specific therapy for the autonomic dysfunction of renal disease is rather limited, and symptomatic therapy is employed in most instances.

CARDIOVASCULAR DRUG THERAPY IN PATIENTS WITH RENAL DISEASE

Patients with renal failure are often treated with drugs primarily cleared or metabolized by the kidneys. In comparison to patients with normal renal function, any dose or dosage schedule of such agents in patients with renal failure usually produces higher plasma concentrations for longer duration. In addition, patients with renal failure can react unpredictably and atypically to pharmacological agents; thus, the adverse effects of a drug in this clinical setting are often related to factors other than plasma drug concentration. For example, nausea and vomiting after ingestion of certain agents (e.g., analgesics, potassium elixirs) occur more frequently in chronic renal failure patients because of preexisting chronic inflammation of the gastrointestinal mucosa, and the adverse effects of digitalis and antiarrhythmic agents are exacerbated by abnormalities in serum potassium, magnesium, and calcium; hypoxemia; and the hyperadrenergic state of renal disease and dialysis. Side effects of a drug must always be considered when a chronic renal failure patient experiences unexpected or unusual symptoms.

Renal failure often modifies the pharmacokinetics and pharmacodynamics of a drug[19,130–133]; many of these variations, however, are not directly linked to the simple reduction in renal function and GFR. The pharmacokinetic-pharmacodynamic modifications of chronic renal failure are also related to greater variability in drug absorption, protein binding, metabolism, and receptor affinity, sensitivity, and responsiveness. Lower protein binding for many agents is related to hypoproteinemia or hypoalbuminemia, an alteration of the protein molecule, or competition for protein-binding sites by endogenous substances and other types of CRF therapy. Nonesterified fatty acids, increased in chronic renal failure and with heparin administration, can displace certain drugs from their binding sites. Anemia with reduced red cell binding increases the plasma concentration of certain drugs. Patients with renal failure are commonly treated with several agents; drug-drug interactions can affect gastrointestinal absorption, protein binding, tissue distribution, drug metabolism and clearance, and pharmacodynamic properties.

For drugs cleared by the kidney, dosing is adjusted for renal function. Three dosing modifications can be employed: the dosing interval can be lengthened without altering the dose amount, the dose amount can be lowered without changing the dosing schedule, or a combination of both. The second approach is preferable in most patients because it averts wide swings in plasma drug concentration. Precise adjustment of dosing is usually not necessary for drugs with few adverse effects and a large therapeutic index (safety margin). Pharmacokinetic and dose-adjustment information for the use of the more commonly employed cardiovascular drugs in renal disease is presented in Table 62–7. In most instances, the application and monitoring of drug therapy in chronic renal failure is based on pharmacodynamic and clinical responses, occasionally supplemented by determination of the drug's plasma concentration (e.g., digitalis) or another laboratory endpoint (e.g., prothrombin time for warfarin).

The therapeutic objectives are fairly well defined for most cardiovascular drugs. For example, for drugs used to control systemic hypertension or edema, the therapeutic endpoints are clear (decrease arterial pressure, reduce edema) and are best followed by clinical observations (blood pressure, physical examination, body weight) for proper drug and dose selection. Angiotensin-converting enzyme inhibitors, most vasodilators, and calcium channel blockers have reasonably well defined clinical endpoints (e.g., decrease arterial pressure, reduce pulmonary congestion, improve symptoms of heart failure, control angina pectoris). The therapeutic objectives of beta-adrenergic blocking drugs can be followed clinically in most patients (e.g., reduce arterial pressure, myocardial ischemia, and angina; control cardiac rhythms). For digitalis and antiarrhythmic drugs the clinical endpoints are more elusive and are threatened by potentially serious adverse effects; determination of plasma drug concentrations for such agents often becomes an important component of optimally effective, safe dosing.

CARDIOVASCULAR COMPLICATIONS DURING DIALYSIS

SYSTEMIC HYPOTENSION. Removal of fluid volume, redistribution of plasma volume, baroreceptor disturbances, dysfunction of the autonomic nervous system, depressed responsiveness to alpha-adrenergic receptor stimulation, concomitant drug therapy (e.g., antihypertensive agents), and LV diastolic dysfunction contribute to the propensity of the chronic renal failure patient to develop hypotension during hemodialysis. Interestingly, some renal disease patients with dialysis-induced hypotension have higher plasma concentrations of atrial natriuretic peptide and lower norepinephrine levels compared to chronic renal failure patients without hypotension.[134]

Symptomatic depletion of fluid volume during dialysis can be averted by allowing a modest amount of weight gain between dialysis treatments. When feasible, antihypertensive therapy and other potential hypotension-inducing drugs (e.g., nitrates) can be withheld 4 to 6 hours before dialysis to minimize their contribution to the problem. Of the antihypertensive agents, minoxidil is least likely to cause unpredictable changes in blood pressure during hemodialysis; however, drug-induced hirsutism and occasional pericarditis make this drug unacceptable to some patients, particularly females. Small doses of noncardioselective beta-adrenergic blocking drugs can be effective in maintaining acceptable arterial pressure; the beta$_1$- and beta$_2$-receptor blockade allows circulating norepinephrine to evoke unopposed alpha-adrenergic receptor stimulation and vasoconstriction. Either peritoneal dialysis or renal transplantation is the best option for chronic renal failure patients who poorly tolerate hemodialysis because of hypotension.

HYPOXEMIA. The mechanisms for hemodialysis-induced hypoxemia have not been definitively established; leading explanations include nonbicarbonate buffers (e.g., acetate) used in the dialysis bath, Cupraphane membranes, and pulmonic ventilation and perfusion mismatch elicited by systemic hypotension. Acetate buffer evokes a significant leftward shift in the hemoglobin-oxygen dissociation curve and can disturb ventilation/perfusion of the lungs through its vasodilatory properties. Activation of complement along Cupraphane exchange membranes can result in sequestration of leukocytes within pulmonary vessels, ventilation and perfusion abnormalities, and hypoxemia; this complication has been reduced considerably with the use of biocompatible dialyzers.

ELECTROLYTE AND OTHER METABOLIC ABNORMALITIES. Electrolyte disturbances, metabolic acidosis, and other metabolic abnormalities likely contribute to the development of various cardiovascular derangements in chronic renal failure (e.g., cardiac arrhythmias, depression of myocardial contractility). The rate of change in pH, electrolyte concentrations, and other metabolic factors during dialysis is probably as important as the actual degree of change with respect to the clinical consequences of these disturbances. The most common and crucial electrolyte disturbances in patients undergoing hemodialysis involve potassium. Hyperkalemia is a common problem in these patients, and plasma and whole body potassium levels can be dramatically altered by hemodialysis. The dialysis buffer, acetate, transiently decreases serum bicarbonate, and with repeated dialysis the chronic renal failure patient can become depleted of bicarbonate; bicarbonate has now largely replaced acetate as the dialysis buffer at most modern facilities.

COMPLICATIONS OF THE ARTERIOVENOUS ACCESS FISTULA DURING HEMODIALYSIS. The external access vascular shunt is employed when a patient is expected to require only short-term dialysis (days to a few weeks). Because of fewer complications (e.g., lower infection rate and less thrombogenic) over time, the surgically constructed subcutaneous AV fistula is used for long-term dialysis management. In certain patients, particularly the elderly and those with peripheral vascular disease or diabetes mellitus, reduction of blood flow distal to the fistula can lead to local ischemia and infarction, occasionally requiring amputation of a digit or distal extremity.[19] An infrequent complication during hemodialysis involves a "steal syndrome," which may occur when the radial artery distal to a forearm fistula has not been ligated; this vascular arrangement can allow blood to flow from the ulnar artery through the palmar arch (as non-nutritive flow), retrograde into the radial artery and access fistula.

OTHER DIALYSIS-INDUCED COMPLICATIONS. Air embolization and hemolysis, although rare, are serious complications. Hemolysis can occur from improper composition or chemical contamination of the dialysate. Severe illness and death have resulted from dialysate contaminated with excessive aluminum, calcium, or fluoride.[19,135] Other substances, such as polyvinylchloride, have been leached from membranes, dialyzer shells, and tubing to cause systemic and cardiovascular toxicity.[136] With the use of high-flux polyacrylonitrile AN 69 exchange membranes, CRF patients receiving angiotensin-converting enzyme inhibitors appear to be somewhat more susceptible to anaphylactoid reactions during hemodialysis.[137]

REFERENCES

CARDIOVASCULAR CONDITIONS THAT AFFECT RENAL FUNCTION

1. Leithe, M. E., Magorien, R. D., Hermiller, J. B., et al.: Relationship between central hemodynamics and regional blood flow in normal subjects and in patients with congestive heart failure. Circulation 69:57, 1984.
2. Wade, O. L., and Bishop, J. M.: The distribution of the cardiac output in normal subjects at rest. In Wade, O. L., and Bishop, J. M. (eds.): Cardiac Output and Regional Blood Flow. Oxford, Blackwell Scientific Publications, 1962, p. 86.
3. Merrill, A. J.: Edema and decreased renal blood flow in patients with chronic congestive heart failure: Evidence for "forward failure" as the primary cause of edema. J. Clin. Invest. 25:389, 1946.
4. Creager, M. A., Halperin, J. L., Bernard, D. B., et al.: Acute regional circulatory and renal hemodynamic effects of converting-enzyme inhibition in patients with congestive heart failure. Circulation 64:483, 1981.
5. Elkayam, U., Weber, L., Campese, V. M., et al.: Renal hemodynamic effects of vasodilation with nifedipine and hydralazine in patients with heart failure. J. Am. Coll. Cardiol. 4:1261, 1984.
6. Levine, T. B., Oliveri, M. T., Garberg, U., et al.: Hemodynamic and clinical response to enalapril, a long-acting converting enzyme inhibitor in patients with congestive heart failure. Circulation 69:548, 1984.
7. Magorien, R. D., Triffon, D. W., Desch, C. E., et al.: Prazosin and hydralazine in congestive heart failure: Regional hemodynamic effects in relation to dose. Ann. Intern. Med. 95:5, 1981.
8. Lameiere, N. H., Lifshitz, M. D., and Stein, J. H.: Heterogenicity of renal function. Anu. Rev. Physiol. 39:159, 1977.
9. Frega, N. S., Davalos, M., and Leaf, A.: Effect of endogenous angiotensin on the efferent glomerular arteriole of rat kidney. Kidney Int. 18:323, 1980.
10. Packer, M., Lee, W. H., and Kessler, P. D.: Preservation of glomerular filtration rate in human heart failure by activation of the renin-angiotensin system. Circulation 74:766, 1986.
11. Hall, J. E., Guyton, A. C., Jackson, T. E., et al.: Control of glomerular filtration rate by renin-angiotensin system. Am. J. Physiol. 233:F366, 1977.
12. Mujias, S. K., Fouad, F. M., Textor, S. C., et al.: Transient renal dysfunction during initial inhibition of converting enzyme in congestive heart failure. Br. Heart J. 52:63, 1984.
13. Parker, M., Lee, W. H., and Kessler, P.: Functional renal insufficiency during long-term therapy with captopril and enalapril in severe chronic heart failure. Ann. Intern. Med. 106:346, 1987.

14. Pomeranz, B. H., Birtch, A. G., and Barger, A. C.: Neural control of intrarenal blood flow. Am. J. Physiol. 215:1067, 1968.
15. Leier, C. V., Heban, P. T., Huss, P., et al.: Comparative systemic and regional hemodynamic effects of dopamine and dobutamine in patients with cardiomyopathic heart failure. Circulation 58:466, 1978.
16. McDonald, R. H., Jr., Goldberg, L. I., McNay, et al.: Effect of dopamine in man: Augmentation of sodium excretion, glomerular filtration rate, and renal plasma flow. J. Clin. Invest. 43:116, 1964.
17. Cogan, J. J., Humphreys, M. H., Carlson, J., and Rapaport, E.: Renal effects of nitroprusside and hydralazine in patients with congestive heart failure. Circulation 61:316, 1980.
18. Leier, C. V., Bambach, D., Thompson, M. J., et al.: Central and regional hemodynamic effects of intravenous isosorbide dinitrate, nitroglycerin, and nitroprusside in patients with congestive heart failure. Am. J. Cardiol. 48:1115, 1981.
19. Leier, C. V., and Boudoulas, H.: Cardiorenal Disorders and Diseases. Mount Kisco, N.Y., Futura Publishing Co., 1992.
20. Schrier, R. W.: Pathogenesis of sodium and water retention in high output and low output cardiac failure, nephrotic syndrome, cirrhosis, and pregnancy. N. Engl. J. Med. 319:1065, 1988.
21. Dzau, V. J., Colucci, W. S., Hollenberg, N. K., and Williams, G. H.: Relation of the renin-angiotensin-aldosterone system to clinical state in congestive heart failure. Circulation 63:645, 1981.
22. Levine, T. B., Francis, G., Goldsmith, S. R., et al.: Activity of the sympathetic nervous system and renin-angiotensin system assessed by plasma hormone levels and their relation to hemodynamic abnormalities in congestive heart failure. Am. J. Cardiol. 49:1659, 1982.
23. Ichikawa, I., Pfeffer, J. M., Pfeffer, M. A., et al.: Role of angiotensin II in the altered renal function of congestive heart failure. Circ. Res. 55:669, 1984.
24. Anand, I. S., Ferrari, R., Kalra, G. S., et al.: Edema of cardiac origin: Studies of body water and sodium, renal function, hemodynamic indices and plasma hormones in untreated congestive heart failure. Circulation 80:299, 1989.
25. Pederson, E. B., Danielsen, H., Jensen, T., et al.: Angiotensin II, aldosterone, and arginine vasopressin in plasma in congestive heart failure. Eur J. Clin. Invest. 16:56, 1986.
26. Yamane, Y.: Plasma ADH levels in patients with chronic congestive heart failure. Jpn. Circ. J. 32:745, 1968.
27. Rouleau, J. L., Kortas, C., Bichet, D., and DeChamplain, J.: Neurohumoral and hemodynamic changes in congestive heart failure: Lack of correlation and evidence of compensatory mechanisms. Am. Heart J. 116:746, 1988.
28. Nakaoka, H., Imataka, K., Amano, M., et al.: Plasma levels of atrial natriuretic factor in patients with congestive heart failure. N. Engl. J. Med. 313:892, 1985.
29. Francis, G. S., Benedict, C., Johnson, D. E., et al.: Comparison of neuroendocrine activation in patients with left ventricular dysfunction with and without congestive heart failure. Circulation 82:1724, 1990.
30. Wei, C. M., Heublein, D. M., Perrella, M. A., et al.: Natriuretic peptide system in human heart failure. Circulation 88:1004, 1993.
31. Rodeheffer, R. J., Naruse, M., Atkinson, J. B., et al.: Molecular forms of atrial natriuretic factor in normal and failing human myocardium. Circulation 88:364, 1993.
32. Logan, M. G.: Renal effects of atrial natriuretic factor. Annu. Rev. Physiol. 52:699, 1990.
33. Schunkert, H., Ingelfinger, J.R., Hirsch, A. T., et al.: Evidence for tissue-specific activation of renal angiotensinogen mRNA expression in chronic stable experimental heart failure. J. Clin. Invest. 90:1523, 1992.
34. Simonson, M. S., and Dunn, M. J.: Endothelin peptides and the kidney. Annu. Rev. Physiol. 55:249, 1993.
35. We, C. M., Lerman, A., Rodeheffer, R. J., et al.: Endothelin in human congestive heart failure. Circulation 89:1580, 1994.
36. Packer, M.: Interaction of prostaglandins and angiotensin II in the modulation of renal function in congestive heart failure. Circulation 77:I, 1988.
37. Kubo, S. H., Rector, T. S., Bank, A. J., Williams, R. E., and Heifetz, S. M.: Endothelium-dependent vasodilation is attenuated in patients with heart failure. Circulation 84:1589, 1991.
38. Katz, S. D., Schwarz, M., Yuen, J., and LeJemtel, T. H.: Impaired acetylcholine-mediated vasodilation in patients with congestive heart failure. Circulation 88:55, 1993.
39. Cleland, J. G. F., Dargie, H. J., Robertson, I., et al.: Total body electrolyte composition in patients with heart failure: A comparison with normal subjects and patients with untreated hypertension. Br. Heart J. 58:230, 1987.
40. Ichikawa, I., and Brenner, B. M.: Importance of efferent arteriolar vascular tone in regulation of proximal tubular reabsorption and glomerulotubular balance in the rat. J. Clin. Invest. 65:1192, 1980.
41. Wright, F. S., and Briggs, J. P.: Feedback control of glomerular blood flow, pressure, and filtration rate. Physiol. Rev. 59:958, 1979.
42. Kilcoyne, M. M., Schmidt, D. H., and Cannon, P. J.: Intrarenal blood flow in congestive heart failure. Circulation 47:786, 1973.
43. Schunkert, H., Tang, S. S., Litwin, S. E., et al.: Regulation of intrarenal and circulating renin-angiotensin systems in severe heart failure in the rat. Cardiovasc. Res. 27:731, 1993.
44. Levine, T. B., Franciosa, J. A., Vrobel, T., and Cohn, J. N.: Hyponatremia as a marker for high renin heart failure. Br. Heart J. 47:161, 1982.
45. Anderson, R. J., Chung, H. M., Kluge, R., and Schrier, R. W.: Hyponatremia: A prospective analysis of its epidemiology and the pathogenic role of vasopressin. Ann. Intern. Med. 102:164, 1985.

46. Goldsmith, S. R., Francis, G. S., and Cowley, A. W., Jr.: Arginine vasopressin and the renal response to water loading in congestive heart failure. Am. J. Cardiol. *58*:295, 1986.

47. Lee, W. H., and Parker, M.: Prognostic importance of serum sodium and its modification by converting enzyme inhibition in patients with severe heart failure. Circulation *73*:257, 1986.

48. Parker, M., Lee, W. H., Kessler, P. D., et al.: Identification of hyponatremia as a risk factor for the development of functional renal insufficiency in severe chronic heart failure. J. Am. Coll. Cardiol. *10*:837, 1987.

49. Ralston, M. A., Murnane, M. R., Kelley, R. E., et al.: Magnesium content of serum, circulating mononuclear cells, skeletal muscle and myocardium in congestive heart failure. Circulation *80*:573, 1989.

50. Badr, K. F., and Ichikawa, I. I.: Pre-renal failure: A deleterious shift from renal compensation to decompensation. N. Engl. J. Med. *319*:623, 1988.

51. Pierpont, G. L., Francis, G. S., and Cohn, J. N.: Effect of captopril on renal function in patients with congestive heart failure. Br. Heart J. *46*:522, 1981.

52. Packer, M., Lee, W. H., Medina, N., et al.: Influence of diabetes mellitus on changes in ventricular performance and renal function produced by converting enzyme inhibition in patients with severe chronic heart failure. Am. J. Med. *82*:1119, 1987.

53. Bayliss, J., Norell, M., Canepo-Anson, R., et al.: Untreated heart failure: Clinical and neuroendocrine effects of diuretics. Br. Heart J. *57*:17, 1987.

54. Gottlieb, S. S., Robinson, S., Krichten, C. M., and Fisher, M. L.: Renal response to indomethacin in congestive heart failure. Am. J. Cardiol. *70*:890, 1992.

55. Epstein, F. H., Post, R. S., and McDowell, M.: The effect of an arteriovenous fistula on renal hemodynamics and electrolyte excretion. J. Clin. Invest. *32*:233, 1953.

56. Ahearn, D. J., and Maher, J. F.: Heart failure as a complication of hemodialysis arteriovenous fistula. Ann. Intern. Med. *77*:201, 1972.

57. Tomoda, H.: Atrial natriuretic peptide in acute myocardial infarction. Am. J. Cardiol. *62*:1122, 1988.

58. Rouleau, J. L., DeChamplain, J., Klein, M., et al.: Activation of neurohumoral systems in postinfarction left ventricular dysfunction. J. Am. Coll. Cardiol. *22*:390, 1993.

59. Karlsberg, R. P., Cryer, P. E., and Roberts, R.: Serial plasma catecholamine response early in the course of clinical acute myocardial infarction: Relation to infarct extent and mortality. Am. Heart J. *102*:24, 1981.

60. Tomoda, H.: Plasma endothelin-1 in acute myocardial infarction with heart failure. Am. Heart J. *125*:667, 1993.

61. Myers, B. D., and Moran, S. M.: Hemodynamically mediated acute renal failure. N. Engl. J. Med. *314*:97, 1986.

62. Matsumoto, H., Terashita, Z. I., Kondo, K., and Nishikawa, K.: Pathophysiological role of endothelin in acute renal failure. Life Sci. *46*:1611, 1990.

63. Gellai, M., Jugus, M., Fletcher, T., et al.: Reversal of postischemic acute renal failure with selective endothelin-A receptor antagonist in the rat. J. Clin. Invest. *93*:900, 1994.

64. Neugarten, J., and Baldwin, D. S.: Glomerulonephritis in bacterial endocarditis. Am. J. Med. *77*:297, 1984.

65. Feinstein, E. I., Eknoyan, G., Lister, B. J., et al.: Renal complications of bacterial endocarditis. Am. J. Nephrol. *5*:457, 1985.

66. Morel-Maroger, L., Sraer, J. D., Herreman, G., and Godeau, P.: Kidney in subacute endocarditis: Pathological and immunofluorescent findings. Arch. Pathol. *94*:205, 1972.

67. Kassirer, J. P.: Atheroembolic renal disease. N. Engl. J. Med. *280*:812, 1969.

68. Iliopoulis, J. I., Zdon, M. J., Crawford, B. G., et al.: Renal microembolization syndrome: A cause for renal dysfunction after abdominal aortic reconstruction. Am. J. Surg. *146*:779, 1983.

69. Gupta, B. K., Spinowitz, B. S., Charytan, C., and Wahl, S. J.: Cholesterol crystal embolization-associated renal failure after therapy with recombinant tissue-type plasminogen activator. Am. J. Kidney Dis. *21*:659, 1993.

70. Hyman, B. T., Landas, S. K., Ashman, R. F., et al.: Warfarin-related purple toes syndrome and cholesterol microembolization. Am J. Med. *82*:1233, 1987.

71. Meltzer, R. S., Visser, C. A., and Fuster, V.: Intracardiac thrombi and systemic embolization. Ann. Intern. Med. *104*:689, 1986.

72. Salam, T. A., Lumsden, A. B., and Martin, L. G.: Local infusion of fibrinolytic agents for renal artery thromboembolism. Ann. Vasc. Surg. *7*:21, 1993.

73. Bonttier, S., Valverde, J. P., Lacombe, M., et al.: Renal artery emboli: The role of surgical treatment. Ann. Vasc. Surg. *2*:161, 1988.

74. Spittel, J. A., Jr., and Hunt, J. C.: Abdominal aortic aneurysm and the kidney. Med. Clin. North Am. *50*:1021, 1966.

75. Moore, H. D.: Abdominal aortic aneurysm. J. Cardiovasc. Surg. *17*:47, 1976.

76. Celoria, G. M., Friedmann, P., Rhee, S. W., and Berman, J.: Fistulas between the aorta and the left renal vein. J. Vasc. Surg. *6*:191, 1987.

77. DeSanctis, R. W., Doroghazi, R. M., Austen, W. G., and Buckley, M. J.: Aortic dissection. N. Engl. J. Med. *317*:1060, 1987.

78. Burke, J. R., Glasgow, E. F., McCredie, D. A., and Powell, H. R.: Nephropathy in cyanotic congenital heart disease. Clin. Nephrol. *7*:38, 1977.

79. Flanagan, M. F., Hourihanm, M., and Keane, J. F.: Incidence of renal dysfunction in adults with cyanotic congenital heart disease. Am. J. Cardiol. *68*:403, 1991.

80. Krull, F., Ehrich, J. H., Wurster, U., et al.: Renal involvement in patients with congenital cyanotic heart disease. Acta Pediatr. Scand. *80*:1214, 1991.

81. Liberthson, R. R., Pennington, D. G., Jacobs, M. L., and Dagger, W. M.: Coarctation of the aorta: Review of 234 patients and clarification of management problems. Am. J. Cardiol. *43*:835, 1979.

82. Cohen, M., Fuster, V., Steele, P. M., et al.: Coarctation of the aorta: Long-term follow-up and prediction of outcome after surgical correction. Circulation *80*:840, 1989.

83. Hallett, J. W., Brewster, D. C., Darling, R. C., and O'Hara, P. J.: Coarctation of the abdominal aorta. Ann. Surg. *191*:430, 1980.

EFFECTS OF RENAL FAILURE ON THE CARDIOVASCULAR SYSTEM

84. Gupta, S., Vishva, D., Kumar, M. V., and Dash, S. C.: Left ventricular diastolic function in end-stage renal disease and the impact of hemodialysis. Am. J. Cardiol. *71*:1427, 1993.

85. Ma, K. W., Greene, E. L., and Raij, L.: Cardiovascular risk factors in chronic renal failure and hemodialysis populations. Am. J. Kidney Dis. *19*:505, 1992.

86. Hörl, W. H., and Riegel, W.: Cardiac depressant factors in renal disease. Circulation *87*(suppl IV):77, 1993.

87. Sohn, H. J., Stokes, G. S., and Johnston, H.: An Na, K ATPase inhibitor from ultrafiltrate obtained by hemodialysis of patients with uremia. J. Lab. Clin. Med. *120*:264, 1992.

88. Burt, R. K., Gupta-Burt, S., Suki, W. N., et al.: Reversal of left ventricular dysfunction after renal transplantation. Ann. Int. Med. *111*:635, 1989.

89. Rostand, S. G., Brunzell, J. D., Cannon, R. O., and Victor, R. G.: Cardiovascular complications in renal failure. J. Am. Soc. Nephrol. *2*:1053, 1991.

90. Brancati, F. L., Whittle, J. C., Whelton, P. K., et al.: The excess incidence of diabetic end-stage renal disease among blacks. JAMA *268*:3079, 1992.

91. Consensus Development Conference Panel: Morbidity and mortality of renal dialysis: An NIH Consensus Conference. Ann. Int. Med. *121*:62, 1994.

92. Khan, I. H., Catto, G. R. D., Edward, N., et al.: Influence of coexisting disease on survival on renal-replacement therapy. Lancet *1*:415, 1993.

93. London, G. M., Pannier, B., Guerin, A. P., et al.: Cardiac hypertrophy, aortic compliance, peripheral resistance, and wave reflection in end-stage renal disease: Comparative effects of ACE inhibitors and calcium channel blockade. Circulation *90*:2786, 1994.

94. Pickering, T. G., Devereux, R. B., James, G. D., et al.: Recurrent pulmonary oedema in hypertension due to bilateral renal artery stenosis: Treatment by angioplasty or surgical revascularization. Lancet *2*:551, 1988.

95. Hüting, J.: Course of left ventricular hypertrophy and function in end-stage renal disease after renal transplantation. Am. J. Cardiol. *70*:1481, 1992.

96. Cressman, M. D., Hoogwerf, B. J., Schreiber, M. J., and Cosentino, F. A.: Lipid abnormalities and end-stage renal disease: Implications for atherosclerotic cardiovascular disease. Miner. Electrolyte Metab. *19*:180, 1993.

97. Joven, J., Vilella, E., Ahmad, S., et al.: Lipoprotein heterogeneity in end-stage renal disease. Kidney Int. *43*:410, 1993.

98. Heimann, P., Josephson, M. A., Fellner, S. K., et al.: Elevated lipoprotein (a) levels in renal transplantation and hemodialysis patients. Am. J. Nephrol. *11*:470, 1991.

99. Sakurai, T., Oka, T., Hasegawa, H., et al.: Comparison of lipids, apoproteins and associated enzyme activities between diabetic and nondiabetic end-stage renal disease. Nephron *61*:409, 1992.

100. Senti, M., Romero, R., Pedro-Botet, J., Pelegri, A., Nogues, X., and Rubies-Prat, J.: Lipoprotein abnormalities in hyperlipidemic and normolipidemic men on hemodialysis with chronic renal failure. Kidney Int. *41*:1394, 1992.

101. Burrell, D. E., Antignani, A., Goldwasser, P., Mittman, N., Fein, P. A., Slater, P. A., Gan, A., and Avram, M. M.: Lipid abnormalities in black renal patients. N. Y. State J. Med. *91*:192, 1991.

102. Attman, P. O., and Alaupovic, P.: Lipid and apolipoprotein profiles of uremic dyslipoproteinemia—relation to renal function and dialysis. Nephron *57*:401, 1991.

103. Tolins, J. P.: Mechanisms of glucagon-induced renal vasodilation: Role of prostaglandins and endothelium-derived relaxing factor. J. Lab. Clin. Med. *120*:941, 1992.

104. Moore, K., Wendon, J., Frazer, M., et al.: Plasma endothelin immunoreactivity in liver disease and the hepatorenal syndrome. N. Engl. J. Med. *327*:1774, 1992.

105. Wanner, C., Rader, D., Bartens, W., et al.: Elevated plasma lipoprotein(a) in patients with the nephrotic syndrome. Ann. Intern. Med. *119*:263, 1993.

106. Webb, A. T., Reaveley, D. A., O'Donnell, M., et al.: Does cyclosporin increase lipoprotein(a) concentrations in renal transplant recipients? Lancet *1*:268, 1993.

107. Burke, J. F., Jr., Pirsh, J. D., Ramos, E. L., et al.: Long-term efficacy and safety of cyclosporine in renal-transplant recipients. N. Engl. J. Med. *331*:358, 1994.

108. Boudoulas, H., Rittgers, S. E., Lewis, R. P., et al.: Changes in diastolic

time with various pharmacologic agents. Implications for myocardial perfusion. Circulation *60:*164, 1979.

109. Kenny, A., Sutters, M., Evans, D. B., and Shapiro, L. M.: Effects of hemodialysis on coronary blood flow. Am. J. Cardiol. *74:*291, 1994.

110. Kremastinos, D., Paraskevaidis, I., Voudiklari, S., et al.: Painless myocardial ischemia in chronic hemodialysed patients: A real event? Nephron *60:*164, 1992.

111. Holley, J. L., Fenton, R. A., and Arthur, R. S.: Thallium stress testing does not predict cardiovascular risk in diabetic patients with end-stage renal disease undergoing cadaveric renal transplantation. Am. J. Med. *90:*563, 1991.

112. Reis, G., Marcovitz, P. A., Leichtman, A. B., et al.: Usefulness of dobutamine stress echocardiography in detecting coronary artery disease in end-stage renal disease. Am. J. Cardiol. *75:*707, 1995.

113. Soleman, R., Werner, C., Mann, D., et al.: Effects of saline, mannitol, and furosemide on acute decreases in renal function induced by radiocontrast agents. N. Engl. J. Med. *331:*1416, 1994.

114. Manske, C. L., Wang, Y., Rector, T., et al.: Coronary revascularization in insulin-dependent diabetic patients with chronic renal failure. Lancet *340:*998, 1992.

115. Reusser, L. M., Orebon, L. A., White, H. J., et al.: Increased morbidity after coronary angioplasty in patients on chronic hemodialysis. Am. J. Cardiol. *73:*965, 1994.

116. Thomas, M. E., Harris, K. P., Ramaswamy, C., Hattersley, J. M., Wheeler, D. C., Varghese, Z., Williams, J. D., Walls, J., and Moorhead, J. F.: Simvastatin therapy for hypercholesterolemic patients with nephrotic syndrome or significant proteinuria. Kidney Int. *44:*1124, 1993.

117. Ilson, B. E., Bland, P. S., Jorkasky, D. K., et al.: Intraoperative versus routine hemodialysis in end-stage renal disease patients undergoing open-heart surgery. Nephron *61:*170, 1992.

118. Adams, J. E., Abendschein, D. R., and Jaffe, A. S.: Biochemical markers of myocardial injury: Is MB creatinine kinase the choice for the 1990s? Circulation *88:*750, 1993.

119. Wade, M. R., Chen, Y. J., Soliman, M., et al.: Myocardial texture and cardiac calcification in uremia. Miner. Electrolyte Metab. *19:*21, 1993.

120. Sim, E. K., Mestres, C. A., Lee, C. N., and Adebo, O.: Mitral valve repair in patients on chronic hemodialysis. Ann. Thorac. Surg. *52:*341, 1992.

121. Straumann, E., Meyer, B., Misteli, M., et al.: Aortic and mitral valve disease in patients with end-stage renal failure on long-term haemodialysis. Br. Heart J. *67:*236, 1992.

122. Lucke, J. C., Samy, R. N., Atkins, Z., et al.: Results of valve replacement with mechanical versus biological prosthesis in patients on chronic renal dialysis. J. Am. Coll. Cardiol. *25*(Abs.):429, 1995.

123. Cosio, F. G., Dillon, J. J., Falkenhain, M. E., et al.: Racial differences in renal allograft survival: The role of systemic hypertension. Kidney Int. *47:*1136, 1995.

124. Carter, P. L.: Dosing of antihypertensive medications in patients with renal failure. J. Clin. Pharmacol. *35:*81, 1995.

125. Gruppo Hemodialisi E Pathologie Cardiovascolari: Multicenter, cross-sectional study of ventricular arrhythmias in chronically hemodialyzed patients. Lancet *2:*305, 1988.

126. Luzar, M. R., Coles, G. A., Faller, B., et al.: Staphylococcus aureus nasal carriage and infection in patients on continuous ambulatory peritoneal dialysis. N. Engl. J. Med. *322:*505, 1990.

127. Robertson, D., Hollister, A. S., Biaggioni, I., et al.: The diagnosis and treatment of baroreflex failure. N. Engl. J. Med. *329:*1449, 1993.

128. Converse, R. L., Jr., Jacobsen, T. N., Toto, R. D., et al.: Sympathetic overactivity in patients with chronic renal failure. N. Engl. J. Med. *327:*1912, 1992.

129. Crum, R., Fairchild, R., Bronsther, O., et al.: Neuroendocrinology of chronic renal failure and renal transplantation. Transplantation *52:*818, 1991.

CARDIOVASCULAR DRUG THERAPY IN RENAL FAILURE

130. Hoyer, J., Schulte, K. L., and Lentz, T.: Clinical pharmacokinetics of angiotensin converting enzyme (ACE) inhibitors in renal failure. Clin. Pharmacokinet. *24:*230, 1993.

131. Ujhelyi, M. R., Robert, S., Cummings, D. M., et al.: Influence of digoxin immune fab therapy and renal dysfunction on the disposition of total and free digoxin. Ann. Intern. Med. *119:*273, 1993.

132. Kovarik, J. M., Mueller, E. A., Gaber, M., et al.: Pharmacokinetics of cyclosporine and steady-state aspirin during coadministration. J. Clin. Pharmacol. *33:*513, 1993.

133. Talbert, R. L.: Drug dosing in renal insufficiency. J. Clin. Pharmacol. *34:*99, 1994.

134. Morrissey, E. C., Wilner, K. D., Barager, R. R., et al.: Atrial natriuretic factor in renal failure and posthemodialytic postural hypotension. Am. J. Kidney Dis. *12:*510, 1988.

135. Arnow, P., Bland, L. A., Garcia-Houchings, S., et al.: An outbreak of fatal fluoride intoxication in a long-term hemodialysis unit. Ann. Intern. Med. *121:*339, 1994.

136. Burhop, K. E., Johnson, R. J., Simpson, J., et al.: Biocompatibility of hemodialysis membranes: Evaluation in an ovine model. J. Lab. Clin. Med. *121:*276, 1993.

137. Verresen, L., Waer, M., Vanrenterghen, Y., and Michaelson, P.: Angiotensin converting enzyme inhibitors and anaphylactoid reaction to high-flux membrane dialysis. Lancet *2:*136, 1990.

Chapter 63
Practice Guidelines in Cardiovascular Medicine

THOMAS H. LEE

In recent years, practice guidelines in cardiovascular medicine have become ubiquitous for a number of reasons, the most prominent of which is intense pressure for cost-containment. Health services research has demonstrated marked variability in the rate of performance of cardiovascular procedures among patient subsets, types of facilities, and regions.[1–10] Practice guidelines seek to standardize management around strategies likely to lead to high-quality, cost-effective care.[11]

Although this basic theme underlies most practice guidelines, there is considerable variability in their sources, specific goals, and methods of application. Agencies of the federal government such as the United States Agency for Health Care Policy and Research have convened multidisciplinary expert panels to develop practice guidelines for unstable angina[12] and congestive heart failure.[13] An extensive series of guidelines in cardiovascular medicine has been formulated by expert panels convened by the American College of Cardiology, the American Heart Association, and other professional societies. Insurance companies and for-profit companies have also developed guidelines aimed at assessing the appropriateness of hospital admissions and procedures as well as targeting lengths of stay. Additionally, as financial risk for health care is progressively transferred to the actual providers of health care, an increasing number of physicians and their organizations have developed their own guidelines and algorithms for the care of specific clinical syndromes.

These different types of guidelines often bear little resemblance to each other, in part because the organizations behind them have different goals. The guidelines that are the focus of this chapter seek to define *optimal care*—that is, management strategies that yield the best possible patient outcomes while reducing inappropriate and possibly harmful use of tests and therapies. These guidelines are evidence-based, that is, derived from analysis of published studies and emphasizing, when available, randomized trials. When data are not available, expert opinion is invoked.

Guidelines developed by task forces sponsored jointly by the American College of Cardiology and American Heart Association generally divide indications into three classes according to their appropriateness: Class I conditions are those for which there is general agreement that a test or procedure is useful. Class II conditions are those for which the test or procedure is often used, but for which there is disagreement as to its appropriateness. Class III indications are those for which there is general agreement that the test or procedure is inappropriate.

In many instances, the expert panels that developed and approved such guidelines have been exclusively or pre-

dominantly cardiovascular specialists. The guidelines are often highly detailed because of the perceived need to define most or all circumstances in which use of cardiovascular resources would be reasonable; as a result, such guidelines tend to err on the side of minimizing the percentage of cases for which care would be called "inappropriate."

In contrast, guidelines that have been developed or applied by payers do not seek to define the optimal management of patients with a syndrome. Instead, these guidelines are intended to serve as a *screening test* to detect patients for whom further evaluation should occur before planned procedures or other resources are used. When applied retrospectively to the medical records of patients who have already received cardiovascular services, these guidelines can be used to identify physicians whose practice patterns differ from those of their colleagues. For example, an appropriateness protocol for cardiac catheterization[14–16] could be used to identify physicians or hospitals with unusually low thresholds for performing this procedure.

Like any medical test, these "appropriateness protocols" have a sensitivity and a specificity and false-positive and -negative rates.[17] For example, when an appropriateness protocol for the use of a cardiac procedure is applied to a patient population, there will inevitably be some percentage of patients for whom a cardiac procedure is potentially beneficial but for whom the procedure will be categorized by the protocol as inappropriate. Similarly, there will be some patients for whom the procedure is actually inappropriate, yet it will be classified as appropriate by the protocol.

Just as physicians should weigh the sensitivity and specificity of a diagnostic test in interpreting its results, organizations that use appropriateness protocols as screening tests should consider their "performance characteristics" before adopting them. Extremely "tight" criteria for appropriateness—that is, guidelines that are highly sensitive for the detection of unnecessary resource use—reduce the chances that inappropriate procedures will be performed but have a high "false-positive" rate and therefore increase the percentage of cases that must be reviewed and discussed. On the other hand, "loose" criteria that identify only the most inappropriate use of resources are likely to allow approval of many referrals and procedures that are equivocal at best.

Yet another form of practice guideline is a *critical pathway,* also known by other names such as *clinical pathways* and *care maps.* These pathways attempt to define an optimal management strategy in detail, including time frames for specific outcomes and actions.[18] By achieving consensus around these plans, and collecting data on the frequency and causes of deviations from the pathways, critical pathways can help decrease length of stay and overall costs while improving quality of care by standardizing management.

Although practice guidelines are now extremely common in cardiovascular medicine, their impact has been highly variable.[19-22] In some cases, physicians disagree with the content of the guidelines,[23] suspect that they could be used against them in malpractice litigation,[24] or believe that these guidelines might compromise professional autonomy and satisfaction with medical practice.[25] Nevertheless, practice guidelines are likely to continue to proliferate, and a literature about the methods of their development is emerging.[26-28] They are used increasingly by payers and assessors of the quality of care.

This chapter summarizes the principal features of the guidelines for the use of important cardiovascular tests and procedures, as well as the management of major clinical syndromes. The series of practice guidelines jointly developed by the American College of Cardiology and American Heart Association are emphasized. For the complete guidelines, readers are referred to the original references, which are given in the text.*

---

* An up-to-date listing and copies of the American College of Cardiology/American Heart Association and other American College of Cardiology guidelines can be obtained by calling 800-247-4740 or by Internet (http://acc.org).

NONINVASIVE TESTS AND PROCEDURES

ELECTROCARDIOGRAPHY

(See Chap. 4)

Electrocardiograms are among the most commonly performed tests in medicine and are "the procedure of first choice" in the evaluation of chest pain, syncope, or dizziness.[29] Beyond diagnosis of cardiovascular conditions, electrocardiograms can be used to detect metabolic abnormalities, including side effects of some medications. Electrocardiograms also are frequently obtained to establish a "baseline" against which future tracings can be compared.

Guidelines published in 1992 by a task force of the American College of Cardiology and American Heart Association described conditions for which there is general agreement that electrocardiograms are useful (Class I), conditions for which opinion diverges with respect to their usefulness (Class II); and conditions for which general agreement exists that electrocardiograms are of little or no use (Class III). These guidelines addressed categories of patients defined by whether they had (1) known, (2) suspected, or (3) no evidence of cardiovascular disease. For each category of patients, the guidelines evaluated the use of the electrocardiogram as a baseline test, as a measure of response to therapy for follow-up, and before surgery.

PATIENTS WITH KNOWN CARDIOVASCULAR DISEASE OR DYSFUNCTION. The electrocardiogram is so crucial to the evaluation of all cardiovascular conditions that this test was considered appropriate (Class I) for all patients during the initial evaluation and to evaluate the short- and long-term responses to therapy known to produce electrocardiographic changes. The guidelines offer no specific recommendations about the frequency of follow-up electrocardiograms, but note that, for several acute cardiovascular problems, serial electrocardiograms are warranted until the patient has returned to a stable condition. Even in the absence of new symptoms or signs, ECGs are considered appropriate for follow-up of patients with several conditions, including syncope or near-syncope, chest pain, and unexplained fatigue. The electrocardiogram was not considered appropriate for patients with mild chronic cardiovascular conditions that were not considered likely to progress (e.g., mild mitral valve prolapse). Obtaining electrocardiograms at *each* visit was considered inappropriate for patients with stable heart disease who were seen frequently (e.g., within 4 months) and had no evidence of clinical change.

The ACC/AHA guidelines considered electrocardiograms appropriate before cardiac or noncardiac surgery, for all patients with known cardiovascular disease or dysfunction except those with significant or mild conditions such as mild systemic arterial hypertension.

PATIENTS WITH SUSPECTED OR AT HIGH RISK FOR DEVELOPING CARDIOVASCULAR DISEASE. The electrocardiogram was considered an appropriate baseline test for all patients with suspected cardiovascular conditions and those at high risk for developing such conditions. It was also considered an appropriate test after administration of any drug known to influence cardiac structure of function. Follow-up electrocardiograms more often than once per year were not recommended for patients who remained clinically stable, as long as they had not been previously demonstrated to have cardiac disease. However, for patients known to be at increased risk for the development of heart disease, electrocardiograms every 1 to 5 years were considered appropriate (Class I). Electrocardiograms were considered appropriate before cardiac or noncardiac surgery for all patients in this population.

PATIENTS WITHOUT KNOWN OR SUSPECTED HEART DISEASE. For patients without evidence suggesting cardiovascular disease, electrocardiograms were considered appropriate during the baseline evaluation in the ACC/AHA guidelines for those aged 40 or more years. The ACC/AHA guidelines also recommended electrocardiograms for patients for whom drugs with a high incidence of cardiovascular effects (e.g., chemotherapy) or exercise testing are planned, and for people of any age in occupations with high cardiovascular demands or whose cardiovascular status might affect the well-being of many other people (e.g., airline pilots).

These guidelines are similar to those of the U.S. Preventive Services Task Force,[30] which suggested electrocardiographic screening for persons at increased risk for coronary disease and for those with occupations in which their cardiovascular health might jeopardize the lives of others. The U.S. Preventive Services Task Force guidelines specifically state that electrocardiograms are not necessary for young adults who have no evidence of heart disease and are about to embark on an athletic program.

Different guidelines for the use of the baseline ECG have been offered by other organizations. A different expert panel commissioned by the American Heart Association recommended in 1987 that ECGs be obtained at ages 20, 40, and 60 years in persons with normal blood pressure,[31] while a task force assembled by the Canadian government has discouraged the use of *any* screening electrocardiograms.[32] The frequency of follow-up electrocardiograms in asymptomatic people without evidence of cardiovascular disease is not explicitly addressed in any guidelines.

The practice of obtaining electrocardiograms before any surgical procedure in patients of all ages does not draw support from any of the major guidelines. Before cardiac or noncardiac surgery, the ACC/AHA guidelines recommend electrocardiograms for all people aged 40 years or more,[29] and electrocardiograms are considered equivocal in appropriateness (Class II) for surgical patients aged 30 to 40 years. Guidelines issued from the American College of Physicians[33] recommend electrocardiograms preoperatively and upon hospital admission for men age 40 years or more and women age 50 years or more, as well as for all patients having elective intrathoracic, intraperitoneal, or aortic surgery; elective major neurosurgery; or emergency operations under general or regional anesthesia.

EXERCISE TESTING

(See Chap. 5)

Exercise testing is performed for several reasons, including to diagnose coronary artery disease, to assess prognosis, to determine functional capacity, and to evaluate the effects of therapy. Exercise electrocardiography is safe and inexpensive compared with invasive technology for diagnosis of coronary disease. However, the interpretation of exercise electrocardiography results and subsequent management is often variable, and "false-positive" exercise tests can lead to coronary angiography and even revascularization procedures in patients who have a low risk for complications of ischemic heart disease. Therefore, managed care organizations have sought to ensure the appropriateness of use of exercise tests. At least some health maintenance organizations have experimented with a strategy in which only cardiologists are allowed to order exercise tests and other noninvasive cardiology tests. A more common trend is the use of guidelines for the appropriateness of exercise tests.

One of the first sets of guidelines developed by ACC/AHA task forces focused on exercise testing and was published in 1986.[34] These guidelines rate the appropriateness of this test in various patient subsets according to three levels of appropriateness (Table 63–1), including condi-

TABLE 63–1 ACC/AHA GUIDELINES FOR EXERCISE TESTING

	CLASS I (APPROPRIATE)	CLASS II (POSSIBLY APPROPRIATE)	CLASS III (INAPPROPRIATE)
Patients with symptoms or signs suggestive of coronary artery disease or with known coronary artery disease	**1.** To assist in the diagnosis of coronary disease in male patients with symptoms that are atypical for myocardial ischemia. **2.** To assess functional capacity and to aid in assessing the prognosis of patients with known coronary disease. **3.** To evaluate patients with symptoms consistent with recurrent, exercise-induced cardiac arrhythmias.	**1.** To assist in the diagnosis of coronary disease in women with a history of typical or atypical angina pectoris. **2.** To assist in the diagnosis of coronary disease in patients taking digitalis. **3.** To assist in the diagnosis of coronary disease in patients with complete right bundle branch block. **4.** To evaluate the functional capacity and response to therapy with cardiovascular drugs in patients with coronary disease or heart failure. **5.** To evaluate patients with variant angina. **6.** To follow serially (at 1 year or longer intervals) patients with known coronary disease.	**1.** To evaluate patients with simpler premature ventricular depolarizations on the resting ECG but no other evidence of coronary disease. **2.** To evaluate functional capacity serially in the course of an exercise cardiac rehabilitation program. **3.** To assist in the diagnosis of coronary artery disease in patients who demonstrate preexcitation (Wolff-Parkinson-White) syndrome or complete left bundle branch block on the resting ECG.
Screening apparently healthy individuals	None	**1.** To evaluate asymptomatic male patients over age 40 in special occupations (pilots, firemen, police officers, bus or truck drivers, railroad engineers). **2.** To evaluate asymptomatic male patients over age 40 with two or more of the following increased risk factors for coronary artery disease: • serum cholesterol > 240 mg/dl • blood pressure ≥ 160/ ≥ 90 • cigarette smoking • diabetes mellitus • family history of coronary disease with onset under the age of 55 years **3.** To evaluate male patients over age 40 who are sedentary and plan to enter a vigorous exercise program.	**1.** To evaluate asymptomatic, apparently healthy men or women with no risk factors for coronary artery disease. **2.** To evaluate men or women with a history of chest discomfort not thought to be of cardiac origin.
Patients with hypertension or cardiac pacemakers	None	To evaluate the blood pressure response of patients being treated for systemic arterial hypertension who wish to engage in vigorous dynamic or static exercise.	**1.** To evaluate patients with severe, uncontrolled systemic hypertension. **2.** To evaluate the blood pressure response to exercise in patients treated for hypertension who are not engaging in vigorous exercise. **3.** To evaluate pacemaker function in patients with cardiac pacemakers.

Class I: Conditions for which or patients for whom there is general agreement that exercise testing is useful.
Class II: Conditions for which or patients for whom exercise testing is frequently used but there is divergence of opinion with respect to its usefulness (possibly appropriate).
Class III: Conditions for which or patients for whom there is general agreement that exercise testing is of little or no usefulness.
From Schlant, R. C., Blomqvist, C. G., Brandenburg, R. O., et al.: Guidelines for exercise testing. A report of the American College of Cardiology/American Heart Association Task Force on Assessment of Cardiovascular Procedures (Subcommittee on Exercise Testing). Reprinted with permission from the American College of Cardiology. J. Am. Coll. Cardiol. 8:725, 1986.

tions for which or patients for whom there is general agreement that exercise testing is useful (Class I), conditions for which or patients for whom exercise testing is frequently used but there is divergence of opinion with respect to its usefulness (Class II), and conditions for which or patients for whom there is general agreement that exercise testing is of little or no usefulness (Class III).

PATIENTS WITH KNOWN OR SUSPECTED CORONARY ARTERY DISEASE. The ACC/AHA guidelines for exercise testing reflect the lower positive predictive value for this test in women compared with men (see p. 169). According to the guidelines, exercise testing is appropriate (Class I) for assessment of male patients with symptoms atypical for myocardial ischemia, but of equivocal appropriateness (Class II) in women with a history of typical or atypical angina pectoris. Use of the exercise test is also of uncertain value (Class II) in other settings in which its diagnostic performance is less than ideal, such as in patients who take digitalis or who have right bundle branch block on their baseline electrocardiogram. It is considered an *inappropriate* test for the diagnosis of coronary disease in patients with preexcitation syndrome or complete left bundle branch block because of the difficulties of interpreting electrocardiographic changes.

The exercise test is considered valuable for assessment of prognosis for patients with coronary disease, and the guidelines indicate that repetition at approximately 1-year intervals is a reasonable if unproven (Class II) strategy. The use of exercise tests to evaluate the response to therapy with cardiovascular drugs is also considered a Class II indication. However, the ACC/AHA task force *discouraged* the use of serial exercise tests to assess functional capacity in the course of an exercise rehabilitation program.

APPARENTLY HEALTHY INDIVIDUALS. Because the specificity of the exercise test is about 90 per cent in apparently healthy individuals, the positive predictive value of an abnormal exercise test result is poor when it is applied to patients at low risk for coronary artery disease. Therefore, the ACC/AHA guidelines do not support the use of exercise testing in any setting to screen apparently healthy individuals or those with chest discomfort not thought to be of cardiac origin. However, the guidelines acknowledge that the test may have a role (Class II) in evaluation of asymptomatic patients with special occupations or of those over the age of 40 with two or more major risk factors for coronary artery disease. The exercise test is also considered to be of equivocal appropriateness for patients over age 40 who are sedentary and about to embark on a vigorous exercise program.

AFTER MYOCARDIAL INFARCTION (see p. 165). Exercise testing before hospital discharge for patients with acute myocardial infarction was still a relatively recent innovation when the ACC/AHA guidelines were published in 1986, and the guidelines refer to predischarge testing as occurring 10 to 14 days after uncomplicated infarction. Over a decade later, the average hospital length of stay for patients with uncomplicated myocardial infarctions is half that time at many hospitals, and predischarge exercise tests must therefore be performed on the fourth hospital day or even earlier. The ACC/AHA guidelines caution against performance of this test in patients who are unstable because of ischemia, left ventricular dysfunction, or arrhythmias. In these patients, whose clinical data indicate a high risk for complications, exercise testing frequently will not alter management. The task force indicated that the greatest contribution of postinfarction exercise testing was in patients with a low clinical risk for complications.

Performance of a limited exercise test before discharge from the hospital does not preclude the use of exercise testing several weeks later. The guidelines do not directly support the use of both predischarge and postdischarge exercise testing but note that predischarge exercise tests are often halted when a patient reaches a specified level of exertion (e.g., 5 METS). In contrast, a full, symptom-limited test performed a few weeks later presumably has greater sensitivity for detecting ischemic myocardium. The guidelines supported performance of symptom-limited tests 21 days or more after infarction. Patients whose exercise tests did not indicate ischemia at a workload of at least 7 METS after an uncomplicated acute myocardial infarction were considered generally capable of resuming their usual occupational tasks within the next 2 to 3 weeks. For patients whose occupations demand heavy physical effort, exercise testing 6 to 8 weeks after infarction was supported by the guidelines.

AFTER ANGIOPLASTY OR CARDIAC SURGERY. The ACC/AHA task force considered exercise testing appropriate for evaluation of coronary artery revascularization either by surgery or coronary angioplasty. These tests can be used to document that improvement has occurred and to serve as a baseline against which later tests can be compared. Full, symptom-limited exercise testing should usually be delayed for at least 3 months after surgery, so that chest and leg wounds do not cause pain during testing. Exercise testing can be performed with safety 2 to 5 days after angioplasty, according to these guidelines. Exercise testing at 3 and 6 months can be used to identify patients who have had restenosis.

PATIENTS WITH OTHER CONDITIONS. Exercise testing is not supported for routine use in patients with valvular heart disease, hypertension, or cardiac pacemakers. The ACC/AHA guidelines caution against use of exercise tests for patients with symptomatic critical aortic valve stenosis, hypertrophic obstructive cardiomyopathy, and uncontrolled hypertension, all of which are considered Class III indications because of the danger of complications during testing. An equivocal (Class II) indication for exercise testing is evaluation of functional capacity in patients with valvular heart disease, because serial exercise tests at 1- to 3-year intervals might demonstrate a decline in exertional capacity that is not detected through the patient history. Another Class II indication for exercise testing is assessment of blood pressure response with exertion in patients with hypertension who wish to engage in an exercise program.

ECHOCARDIOGRAPHY

(See also Chap. 3)

Echocardiography has evolved in many ways into an ideal testing technology: it is portable, provides information on cardiovascular structure and function, and, particularly when performed via the transthoracic approach, causes minimal discomfort and no risk to the patient. This test is regarded as so useful that guidelines published by an ACC/AHA task force in 1991[35] did not identify any disease states in which use of echocardiography was regarded as inappropriate except borderline hypertension without evidence of heart disease (Table 63–2). According to the guidelines, echocardiography is an appropriate test for patients with any valvular heart disease or other structural abnormalities, such as cardiac masses and possible primary myocardial diseases.

Echocardiography is not a test that should be performed for every patient, however, in part because of its personnel and equipment costs. Echocardiography and other noninvasive tests also prolong hospitalization when performed on patients with low risk for complications, therefore incurring additional costs beyond those of the test itself.[36] Furthermore, there are now various forms of echocardiography, including transesophageal and exercise echocardiography. These variations provide different types of information, although at higher costs and with additional risks and discomfort for the patient. There are few data on selection of cases in which these newer echocardiographic-based tests should be used instead of more traditional tests such as transthoracic echocardiography.

Another cause of difficulty in defining appropriate use of echocardiography is the lack of standardization in what strategies physicians pursue in response to echocardiographic data. There have been no randomized trials in which outcomes were compared in patients who did and did not undergo echocardiography. Nevertheless, guidelines for performance of this test are based on the assumption that echocardiography is likely to be used more appropriately under two conditions: (1) when physicians have a specific question to be answered by the test, and (2) if results from the test might alter management.

The ACC/AHA guidelines consider echocardiography to be the noninvasive technique of choice for several issues, including evaluation of valvular heart disease, detection of intracardiac thrombi, and detection of the cardiac effects of hypertension. For many questions, such as detection of ischemic heart disease, echocardiography must compete with other techniques, and the superiority of echocardiography has not been demonstrated.

EVALUATION OF SYMPTOMS. The appropriateness of echocardiography for diagnosis of the etiology of various symptom complexes is less clear than when echocardiography is used for evaluation of specific disease states. The ACC/AHA guidelines stress the importance of a careful history and physical examination and do not recommend echocardiography if, on the basis of that evaluation, the physician considers the probability of cardiac abnormalities to be low.

For example, echocardiographic abnormalities are often present in patients with *dyspnea* due to pulmonary disease, and the echocardiogram can provide important information in patients with dyspnea due to congestive heart failure, such as chamber sizes and myocardial and valvular function. However, dyspnea is a common symptom in patients without heart disease, and the ACC/AHA task force therefore concludes that this test is *not* recommended as an initial diagnostic study in patients with normal blood pressure and physical examinations.

For patients with *chest pain,* echocardiography can sometimes contribute to diagnosis and prediction of risk of future complications. The task force noted, however, that most patients with coronary artery disease have essentially normal findings on rest echocardiography; hence, echocardiography does little to exclude this diagnosis. At some medical centers, echocardiography is used for patients with acute chest pain as part of the emergency department or chest pain observation protocols.[37,38] However, because of the costs of this test, the logistic difficulties of providing echocardiography in the emergency department, and the high frequency of acute chest pain, this test is not part of routine care for patients with acute chest pain at most institutions.

Stress echocardiography is now in use at an increasing number of institutions; the stress used to induce ischemia can be exercise or pharmacological (see p. 86). The ACC/AHA guidelines note, however, that the addition of echocardiography substantially increases the cost of a routine stress test.

For patients with *heart murmurs,* routine clinical data are usually sufficient to determine its cause and significance. The ACC/AHA guidelines emphasize that patients with murmurs and a low probability of heart disease do not routinely require echocardiography. However, echocardiography can be an appropriate test when used in patients with probable organic heart disease and can provide information on coexisting abnormalities such as left ventricular dysfunction. In patients with a low probability of coronary artery disease, cardiac valve surgery can often be safely performed on the basis of data from the echocardiogram without prior cardiac catheterization (see section on cardiac catheterization).

Emboli originating in the heart are believed to account for 15 per cent of *cerebrovascular ischemic strokes*[39] (see p. 1878), and echocardiography is therefore an appropriate test for patients with cerebral embolism and clinical evidence of heart disease. Because of a lower likelihood of cerebrovascular atherosclerosis as a cause of ischemic stroke in younger patients, echocardiography is also considered an appropriate test in patients with a cerebrovascular event who are younger than age 45. In such patients, potential embolic sources include mitral valve prolapse or an intraatrial communication.

A major unresolved question is whether transesophageal echocardiography should be used instead of transthoracic echocardiography, because the transesophageal approach provides better images of the left atrium, left atrial appendage, and mitral valve. The optimal use of these testing techniques is uncertain and not addressed by the ACC/AHA guidelines. One algorithm has been proposed by DeRook et al., although it has not been formally tested.[40]

The ACC/AHA guidelines do not support routine use of echocardiography for all patients with *syncope* (Chap. 28). This test is considered appropriate (Class I) for patients with murmurs consistent with significant valvular heart disease or hypertrophic obstructive cardiomyopathy, but these are rare causes compared with vasodepressor reflexes or cardiac arrhythmias. Even rarer cardiac causes of syncope such as atrial myxoma may be detected with echocardiography (see p. 94), but these guidelines recommend that echocardiography should not be a "first-line" test for patients with syncope.

CARDIAC RADIONUCLIDE IMAGING

(See also Chap. 9)

Guidelines for the use of cardiac radionuclide imaging have been difficult to develop and apply for several reasons. As is true for most diagnostic tests, there have been no randomized trials comparing outcomes for patients who did and those who did not undergo nuclear cardiology tests, nor have there been large trials comparing these tests with competing techniques. Furthermore, there has been rapid evolution in radionuclide imaging techniques, which has increased both the number and the complexity of choices for clinicians.

These tests are considerably more expensive than treadmill exercise electrocardiography or echocardiography, however, and therefore interest in increasing the appropriateness of their use has intensified in recent years. An ACC/AHA task force initially published guidelines for cardiac radionuclide imaging in 1986[41]; because of developments, including pharmacological stress testing, new isotopes (technetium- and rubidium-based perfusion agents), and progress in single-photon emission computed tomography (SPECT) and positron emission tomography (PET), the ACC/AHA task force issued revised guidelines in 1995.[42] These guidelines are scheduled to be reviewed in 1997 and yearly thereafter—a reflection of the rate of change in this discipline.

As is true of most ACC/AHA guidelines, this task force designated some indications for cardiac radionuclide imaging as generally appropriate (Class I) and generally inappropriate (Class III). However, these guidelines subdivided the equivocal indications for nuclear cardiology tests into two groups: Class IIa (weight of evidence in favor of usefulness); and Class IIb (can be helpful but not well established by evidence).

TABLE 63-2 ACC/AHA GUIDELINES FOR ECHOCARDIOGRAPHY

SETTING	CLASS I (APPROPRIATE)	CLASS II (EQUIVOCAL)	CLASS III (INAPPROPRIATE)
Valvular heart disease	1. Native cardiac valve disease. 2. Prosthetic cardiac valve disease. 3. Suspected or proven infective endocarditis.	None	None
Ischemic heart disease	1. *Rest echocardiography:* Myocardial infarction when there is a specific question that can be resolved by echocardiography. 2. *Stress echocardiography:* None	1. *Rest echocardiography:* Clinical evidence of coronary artery disease. 2. *Stress echocardiography:* Whenever there is a high pretest probability that an indicated standard exercise stress test would be inadequate, nondiagnostic, or false-positive.	1. *Rest echocardiography:* Screening test for coronary disease in the general population. 2. *Stress echocardiography:* Routine screening of the general population without significant coronary risk factors.
Disease of the heart muscle	1. Establishment of the morphological diagnosis and assessment of hemodynamic status of patients with cardiomyopathies. 2. Systemic illness associated with cardiac involvement, with clinical symptoms. 3. Exposure to cardiotoxic agents.	1. Systemic illness with high incidence of cardiac involvement but no clinical evidence of cardiac involvement. 2. Clinical evidence suggesting cardiomyopathy. 3. Family history of genetically transmitted cardiac disease.	Systemic illness with low incidence of cardiac involvement and no clinical evidence of cardiac involvement.
Pericardial disease	Patients with clinical manifestations of or suspected pericardial disease.	Follow-up studies	None
Cardiac masses	Evaluation of patients with suspected cardiac masses.	None	None
Diseases of the great vessels	1. Acute aortic root dilation or clinical suspicion of aortic dissection. 2. First-degree relatives of patients with genetically transmitted connective tissue disorders.	1. Chronic aortic root dilation. 2. Suspected connective tissue disorder in athletes. 3. All other suspected disease of the great vessels.	None
Pulmonary disease	1. Unexplained pulmonary hypertension. 2. Pulmonary emboli and suspected clots in the right atrium or ventricle.	1. Lung disease with clinical suspicion of cardiac involvement. 2. Pulmonary emboli	None
Hypertension	Hypertension with clinical evidence of heart disease	Hypertension without signs or symptoms of heart disease.	Borderline hypertension without signs or symptoms of heart disease.

ACUTE MYOCARDIAL INFARCTION (see Chap. 37). The ACC/AHA guidelines indicate that nuclear cardiology tests have a limited role in the diagnosis of acute myocardial infarction, and should be used only when the history, electrocardiogram, and chemistry tests are less reliable. Technetium-99m pyrophosphate scanning is considered potentially useful (Class IIa) for patients who present more than 24 hours and less than 7 days after the onset of symptoms, and radionuclide angiography can be used to support the diagnosis of right ventricular infarction by demonstrating a reduced right ventricular ejection fraction and right ventricular asynergy. However, nuclear tests are considered inappropriate for routine use for diagnosis.

For evaluation of prognosis after acute myocardial infarction, stress myocardial perfusion imaging is considered appropriate (Class I) to assess whether more myocardium is in jeopardy (Table 63-3). The stress used to provoke ischemia can be physical exercise or pharmacological, although these guidelines noted that the safety of dipyridamole and adenosine testing that is performed 2 to 3 days after admission remains to be established. The guidelines do not address settings in which radionuclide imaging would be preferred over standard exercise electrocardiography.

Radionuclide angiography is considered useful for assessment of ventricular function after acute myocardial infarction and also can help detect aneurysms and mechanical complications such as an infarct-related ventricular septal defect. However, the ACC/AHA guidelines imply that, for assessment of mechanical complications, nuclear cardiology tests are second-choice techniques that should be used when echocardiography is not available or definitive.

UNSTABLE ANGINA (see Chap. 38). The ACC/AHA task force identified two principal issues for which radionuclide imaging techniques are potentially useful in patients with unstable angina: assessment of myocardial viability and prediction of future cardiac events in patients whose angina is successfully stabilized with medical therapy. Therefore, the two indications considered clearly appropriate (Class I) are use of stress myocardial perfusion imaging to detect ischemia and use of radionuclide angiography to assess baseline left ventricular function. Myocardial perfusion imaging is also considered potentially useful (Class IIa) for patients with ongoing ischemia who undergo imaging at rest. The use of rest myocardial perfusion imaging is considered less proven (Class IIb) in patients in whom the diagnosis of myocardial ischemia was uncertain after consideration of routinely available clinical data.

CHRONIC ISCHEMIC HEART DISEASE (see Chap. 38). The ACC/AHA guidelines considered exercise or pharmacological myocardial perfusion imaging to be appropriate (Class I) for identification of the extent and severity of ischemia and localization of ischemia in patients with chronic ischemic heart disease. The guidelines consider thallium-201 and technetium-99m to be sufficiently similar to be used interchangeably in this patient population.[43]

SETTING	CLASS I (APPROPRIATE)	CLASS II (EQUIVOCAL)	CLASS III (INAPPROPRIATE)
Dyspnea	None	**1.** Dyspnea with clinical evidence or suspicion of heart disease. **2.** Unexplained dyspnea.	**1.** Dyspnea without clinical evidence of heart disease, pulmonary hypertension or significant lung disease. **2.** Hyperventilation syndrome.
Chest pain	Chest pain with clinical evidence of valvular, pericardial or primary myocardial disease.	Known or suspected coronary artery disease.	Noncardiac chest pain
Murmurs	**1.** An organic murmur in a patient with cardiorespiratory symptoms. **2.** A murmur in an asymptomatic patient if the clinical features indicate at least a moderate probability that the murmur is organic.	A murmur in an asymptomatic patient in whom there is low probability of heart disease but in whom the diagnosis of heart disease cannot be reasonably excluded by standard cardiovascular clinical evaluation.	A typically innocent murmur in an asymptomatic patient without any other reason to suspect heart disease.
Neurological ischemic syndromes	**1.** Patients with cerebral embolism and clinical evidence of heart disease. **2.** Patients <45 with a cerebrovascular event.	Patients >45 with suspicion of cardiogenic brain embolism but without clinical evidence of heart disease.	Patients with known noncardiac causes of the neurological disorder.
Syncope	Patients with a murmur suggestive of significant valvular heart disease or obstructive cardiomyopathy.	Patients without clinical evidence of heart disease and normal findings on evaluation for noncardiac causes of syncope.	Patients with known noncardiac causes of syncope.
Evaluation of ventricular function	**1.** To evaluate global left ventricular function. **2.** To evaluate regional left ventricular function. **3.** Qualitative right ventricular function.	Diastolic left ventricular function	Quantitative right ventricular function (except in children).
Screening	Patients with a family history of cardiovascular disease that is clearly inheritable.	Competitive athletes	General population

Class I: Conditions for which or patients for whom there is general agreement that echocardiography is appropriate.
Class II: Conditions for which or patients for whom echocardiography is frequently used but there is a divergence of opinion with respect to its appropriateness.
Class III: Conditions for which or patients for whom there is general agreement that echocardiography is not appropriate.
From Ewy, G. A., Appleton, C. P., Demaria, A. N., et al.: ACC/AHA guidelines for the clinical application of echocardiography. A report of the American College of Cardiology/American Heart Association Task Force on Assessment of Diagnostic and Therapeutic Cardiovascular Procedures (Subcommittee to Develop Guidelines for the Clinical Application of Echocardiography). Reprinted with permission from the American College of Cardiology. J. Am. Coll. Cardiol. *16*:1505, 1990.

TABLE 63–3 INDICATIONS FOR USE OF EXERCISE OR PHARMACOLOGICAL MYOCARDIAL PERFUSION IMAGING

CLASS I (APPROPRIATE)

1. Prognostic stratification after acute myocardial infarction.

2. Identification of ischemia in patients with unstable angina.

3. Identification of extent and severity of ischemia in symptomatic patients and selected patients with asymptomatic myocardial ischemia.

4. Planning PTCA—identifying lesions causing myocardial ischemia if not otherwise known.

5. Risk stratification for selected patients before noncardiac surgery.

6. Assessment for restenosis after PTCA for symptomatic patients.

7. Assessment of ischemia in symptomatic patients after CABG.

8. Assessment of selected asymptomatic patients after PTCA or CABG, such as patients with an abnormal electrocardiographic response to exercise or those with rest electrocardiographic changes precluding identification of ischemia during exercise.

CLASS IIA

1. Identification of severity/extent of disease in patients whose angina is satisfactorily stabilized with medical therapy.

2. Diagnosis of anomalies of coronary circulation in adults with congenital heart disease.

3. Detection and assessment of functional significance of concomitant coronary artery disease in valvular heart disease patients.

CLASS IIB

1. Assessment of drug therapy upon myocardial perfusion.

2. Assessment of coronary arteriopathy after cardiac transplantation.

CLASS III (INAPPROPRIATE)

1. Screening of asymptomatic patients with low likelihood of ischemic heart disease.

From Guidelines for Clinical Use of Cardiac Radionuclide Imaging. A Report of the American College of Cardiology/American Heart Association Task Force on Assessment of Cardiovascular Procedures (Committee on Nuclear Imaging). Reprinted with permission from the American College of Cardiology. J. Am. Coll. Cardiol. *25*:521, 1995.

The difficult question of when radionuclide tests should be used instead of exercise electrocardiography was addressed in a separate set of guidelines issued in 1990 by a subcommittee of the American College of Physicians.[44] This group concluded that thallium scintigraphy is most clearly preferable to exercise electrocardiography alone when the resting electrocardiogram shows abnormalities impairing interpretation of changes or when information on the reversibility of ischemia in specific myocardial segments is needed to evaluate the potential impact of revascularization therapy.

Because of marked differences in complexity and costs, choices among scanning techniques are reviewed in the ACC/AHA guidelines. SPECT is considered preferable to planar imaging, although the task force noted that SPECT gamma cameras are not always available, and many patients cannot tolerate lying on the SPECT table. Positron emission tomography scanning using dipyridamole and either rubidium-92 or N-13 ammonia has been found in some studies to offer better diagnostic accuracy than thallium SPECT[45,46]; however, a review of available data by an American Heart Association committee in 1991 concluded that PET had *not* been demonstrated to be clearly superior to SPECT.[47] Noting the high costs of PET technology, the ACC/AHA task force concluded that PET should be considered for routine diagnostic purposes only if its costs are equivalent to or less than the costs of SPECT imaging in the same community.

Review of data on the three most commonly used agents in pharmacological perfusion imaging (dipyridamole, adenosine, and dobutamine) led the ACC/AHA task force to conclude that their diagnostic performances are in the same range as exercise testing.

ASYMPTOMATIC PATIENTS. The ACC/AHA guidelines do *not* consider cardiac radionuclide imaging an appropriate routine test for diagnosis of coronary artery disease in patients who are not symptomatic. However, a stress radionuclide test (either perfusion imaging or radionuclide angiography) can be useful for determining the need for coronary angiography in asymptomatic patients with positive exercise electrocardiography tests. The use of a stress radionuclide test can also be valuable in asymptomatic patients with known coronary artery disease to determine the presence and severity of inducible ischemia.

BEFORE NONCARDIAC SURGERY. Several studies have demonstrated that abnormal dipyridamole or adenosine thallium-201 scintigraphy identifies patients at increased risk for cardiovascular complications associated with noncardiac surgery (see Chap. 54). Most of these investigations have focused on vascular surgery procedures, but some data indicate that these tests can also be expected to help stratify patients according to the risk associated with other types of major operations.[48] However, because the overall risk of elective noncardiac surgery is low, the positive predictive value of abnormal tests is only between 15 and 30 per cent.[42] Therefore the ACC/AHA guidelines conclude that noninvasive testing is not needed in most patients undergoing nonvascular surgery if their cardiac risk is low.

BEFORE AND AFTER REVASCULARIZATION INTERVENTIONS. Myocardial perfusion imaging can be useful in planning percutaneous transluminal coronary angioplasty (PTCA) procedures by providing insight into the functional impact of single or multiple coronary artery stenoses. These tests can also be used after PTCA to assess whether restenosis has occurred and for patients who are symptomatic after coronary artery bypass graft (CABG) surgery to determine whether grafts may have occluded. However, the ACC/AHA guidelines do *not* endorse routine testing for patients who are asymptomatic after PTCA or CABG because of the lack of data that outcomes are improved with this approach.

MYOCARDITIS AND CARDIOMYOPATHIES (see Chap. 41).

With the exception of assessment of ventricular function with radionuclide angiography, there are *no* indications for the use of nuclear cardiology tests in patients with myocarditis and cardiomyopathies that are considered clearly appropriate (Class I) by the ACC/AHA task force. Thallium-201 scintigraphy is believed to be potentially useful (Class IIa) for the purpose of differentiating ischemic and dilated cardiomyopathy and assessment of myocardial ischemia in patients with hypertrophic cardiomyopathy. Other indications for testing in patients with myocarditis or cardiomyopathies, such as gallium-67 imaging to demonstrate myocardial inflammation, are considered possibly useful but are unproven.

OTHER CONDITIONS. Echocardiography is the imaging technique of choice for patients with congenital heart disease; first-pass radionuclide angiography and lung perfusion scanning can be used to detect, localize, and quantify shunts. For patients who have undergone cardiac transplantation, the use of radionuclide tests to detect rejection or coronary arteriopathy is not well established (Class IIb). Similarly, cardiac nuclear tests are not considered to be directly useful for assessment of valvular heart disease, except for left ventricular function.

AMBULATORY ELECTROCARDIOGRAPHY
(See also p. 1345)

Ambulatory electrocardiography is often used for confirmation of arrhythmias as the cause of patients' symptoms; it is also used for the evaluation of the efficacy of therapy, assessment of prognosis, and detection of myocardial ischemia. For many of the "endpoints" for which ambulatory electrocardiography is ordered, there are no "gold standards." Hence, data on the sensitivity, specificity, and cost-effectiveness of this test in various settings are sparse. The lack of certainty about the impact of ambulatory electrocardiography and the heterogeneity of the outcomes of patients who undergo this test leads to considerable variability in its application. Therefore, an ACC/AHA task force published guidelines in 1989[49] that described conditions for which there was general agreement that ambulatory electrocardiography is useful and reliable (Class I); for which there was divergence of opinions about its usefulness (Class II); and for which there was agreement that the test is not useful (Class III) (Table 63–4). Similar recommendations were issued by a subcommittee of the American College of Physicians in 1990.[50]

Among patients who undergo ambulatory electrocardiography for assessment of symptoms that may be related to arrhythmias, the positive predictive value of abnormal findings depends on the nature of the symptoms. Therefore the ACC/AHA and the American College of Physicians guidelines consider ambulatory electrocardiography an appropriate test for symptoms such as palpitation, syncope, or dizziness, which have a high likelihood of being due to arrhythmia. However, the indications for this test are considered by the ACC/AHA task force to be less certain (Class II) for symptoms that are less frequently caused by arrhythmia, such as shortness of breath, chest pain, and fatigue.

Regardless of whether symptoms of arrhythmia are present, the ACC/AHA task force considers ambulatory electrocardiography useful for patients who have medical conditions associated with life-threatening arrhythmias. Therefore, this test is considered appropriate (Class I) for patients with idiopathic hypertrophy and patients with left ventricular dysfunction after acute myocardial infarction. The American College of Physicians guidelines, however, noted that antiarrhythmic therapy in asymptomatic patients is of unproven value; hence, these guidelines discourage use of ambulatory monitoring after acute myocardial infarction in asymptomatic patients.

SETTING	CLASS I (APPROPRIATE)	CLASS II (EQUIVOCAL)	CLASS III (INAPPROPRIATE)
Symptoms	1. Palpitation 2. Syncope 3. Dizziness	1. Shortness of breath 2. Chest pain or fatigue not otherwise explained, episodic and strongly suggestive of arrhythmia as the cause because of a relation of the symptom with palpitation.	Symptoms not reasonably expected to be due to arrhythmia.
Assessment of R-R interval characteristics	1. Sleep apnea. 2. Visceral diabetic neuropathy.	For prognostic assessment of R-R interval in coronary artery disease.	None
Prognostic stratification in patients with and without symptoms of arrhythmia	1. Patients with idiopathic hypertrophic cardiomyopathy, with or without symptoms. 2. Postmyocardial infarction patients with left ventricular dysfunction.	1. Patients with known stable coronary artery disease or who have undergone coronary bypass surgery or angioplasty and have evidence for myocardial dysfunction or arrhythmia. 2. Wolff-Parkinson-White syndrome 3. Long Q-T intervals 4. Documented significant aortic valve disease and symptoms suggestive of arrhythmia. 5. Patients with dilated cardiomyopathy and symptoms suggestive of arrhythmia.	1. Patients with known coronary artery disease without evidence for myocardial dysfunction or arrhythmia. 2. Asymptomatic mitral valve prolapse. 3. Asymptomatic persons without known heart disease about to embark on an exercise program. 4. Asymptomatic persons who require assessment of risk for potentially disabling arrhythmias because their occupation might place others in jeopardy if an arrhythmia were to occur.
Assessment of efficacy of antiarrhythmic therapy	Patients with baseline high-frequency, reproducible sustained symptomatic premature ventricular complexes, supraventricular arrhythmias, or ventricular tachycardia.	1. Patients with known episodic or reverted atrial fibrillation to determine efficacy of arrhythmia control. 2. Patients with premature ventricular complexes of variable frequency and complexity or relatively infrequent brief salvos of ventricular or supraventricular arrhythmias. 3. Patients with Wolff-Parkinson-White syndrome. 4. Assessment of proarrhythmia effects. 5. Assessment of tachycardias, bradycardias and conduction defects related to drug administration.	None
Detection of myocardial ischemia in patients with chest pain	Patients with chest pain suggestive of Prinzmetal's angina.	Symptomatic patients who are unable to be tested by treadmill or bicycle.	1. Patients whose description of chest pain is classic for angina pectoris and who have one or more risk factors for coronary artery disease. 2. Patients with atypical chest pain and one or more risk factors. 3. Patients with chest pain atypical for myocardial ischemia in the absence of coronary artery disease risk factors.
Detection of ischemia in the asymptomatic individual	None	None	1. Primary detection of ischemia in the asymptomatic individual with known risk factors for coronary artery disease. 2. Detection of ischemia in the asymptomatic individual without identifiable coronary artery disease risk factors.
Primary detection of asymptomatic ischemia in the patient with known coronary artery disease	None	1. Postmyocardial infarction patients who have been known to have premature ventricular complexes. 2. Patients with chronic stable angina to assess efficacy of antiischemic therapy.	1. For routine use after acute myocardial infarction. 2. For routine use in the postrevascularization patient. 3. For patients entering a cardiovascular rehabilitation program.

Class I: Conditions for which or patients for whom there is general agreement that an ambulatory electrocardiogram is a useful and reliable test.
Class II: Conditions for which or patients for whom ambulatory electrocardiography is frequently used but there is a divergence of opinion with respect to its usefulness.
Class III: Conditions for which or patients for whom there is general agreement that ambulatory electrocardiography is not a useful test.

From Knoebel, S. B., Crawford, M. H., Dunn, M. I., et al.: Guidelines for ambulatory electrocardiography. A report of the American College of Cardiology/American Heart Association Task Force on Assessment of Diagnostic and Therapeutic Cardiovascular Procedures (Subcommittee on Ambulatory Electrocardiography). Reprinted with permission from the American College of Cardiology. J. Am. Coll. Cardiol. 13:249, 1989.

Both task forces discourage the test in persons with low risks for arrhythmic complications, e.g., those with known coronary disease without complicating left ventricular dysfunction or arrhythmia, or asymptomatic mitral valve prolapse. In the ACC/AHA guidelines, equivocal (Class II) indications include conditions that carry an intermediate risk for major arrhythmic complications, such as Wolff-Parkinson-White syndrome.

The ACC/AHA guidelines do *not* support the use of ambulatory electrocardiography for asymptomatic persons in occupations in which others might be endangered if an arrhythmia occurs. Major arrhythmic events are so uncommon in this population that the capability of ambulatory electrocardiography to identify high-risk patients is very limited.

Ambulatory electrocardiography is also used to assess prognosis in several ways. Several studies have shown that beat-to-beat changes in heart rate or cycle length (R-R intervals) provide information on prognosis for patients with myocardial infarction and other cardiovascular conditions.[51,52] R-R interval variability can also contribute to evaluation of sleep apnea and visceral diabetic neuropathy, in which abrupt marked changes in heart rate may occur.

This test is considered an appropriate strategy by both the ACC/AHA and the American College of Physicians task forces for assessing the impact of pharmacological therapy for ventricular arrhythmias that cause symptoms or appear life threatening. The underlying assumption for this recommendation is that a decrease in the frequency of arrhythmias detected with ambulatory electrocardiography is associated with either a decrease in symptomatic events or improved survival. However, subsequent data from the Electrophysiologic Study Versus Electrocardiographic Monitoring (ESVEM) Trial have raised questions about this assumption. In this trial,[53] suppression of spontaneous ventricular ectopy did *not* identify patients with a better outcome. Furthermore, there is no agreement as to which magnitude of reduction in arrhythmia constitutes a reasonable target. Therefore, evaluation of the efficacy of antiarrhythmic therapy remains a difficult challenge, with ambulatory electrocardiography the most easily performed of imperfect alternative tests.

Pacemaker function is also often assessed with ambulatory electrocardiography, which has the advantage over other technologies of providing data on pacemaker function as the patient performs activities of daily living. The appropriateness of ambulatory electrocardiography is considered uncertain (Class II) for routine evaluation of pacemaker function immediately after implantation and other routine follow-up of patients with pacemakers.

DETECTION OF ISCHEMIA. Modifications of ambulatory electrocardiography that allow accurate measurement of ST-segment deviation have introduced new functions for this technique—diagnosis and prognostic stratification of ischemic heart disease. The ACC/AHA guidelines consider ambulatory electrocardiography an appropriate test for patients with suspected Prinzmetal's angina, since exercise stress tests or even coronary angiography might miss this diagnosis. Ambulatory electrocardiography is also considered a potential test for the diagnosis of ischemia in patients who are unable to perform exercise tests (Class II).

The dominant theme of the ACC/AHA comments on the use of ambulatory electrocardiography for detection of ischemia is that there are too few data to recommend routine use of this test in many settings, especially for patients with atypical chest pain or for asymptomatic patients. The American College of Physicians guidelines also do not support routine use of this technique for either diagnosis or management of coronary disease. These assessments of the role of ambulatory electrocardiography for detection of ischemia may be subject to revision as a result of subsequent research demonstrating the usefulness of ambulatory electrocardiography in settings such as before major vascular surgery.[54] The use of this test would also likely increase markedly if research supports benefit from treatment of asymptomatic ischemia[55-57] (see p. 1345).

IN-HOSPITAL CARDIAC MONITORING
(See also p. 1226)

Few data are available on the value and limitations of in-hospital cardiac monitoring,[58-63] and most published studies have been rendered outdated by technological advances and the transition of coronary care to settings outside the coronary care unit, such as intermediate care units and chest pain emergency units. The availability of electrocardiographic monitoring in a variety of settings has been accompanied by a trend toward the use of monitors in many patients with a low risk for arrhythmic complications. Although the per-diem costs of monitors are low, the costs of personnel who are appropriately trained to observe monitors are high. Therefore, an ACC committee recommended guidelines for the use of this method that were published in 1991.[63] These guidelines assume that there is adequate surveillance of the monitors 24 hours a day by personnel trained and qualified in electrocardiographic recognition of cardiac rhythm disturbances.

Cardiac monitoring is considered to be appropriate (Class I indication) for most if not all patients because of a high risk of immediate, life-threatening arrhythmias. Although in general these guidelines do not specify the duration for which monitoring should be continued, the guidelines endorse monitoring for the first 3 days of hospitalization for patients with acute myocardial infarction or who undergo cardiac surgery. For patients who suffer clinically important complications after myocardial infarction, monitoring for 2 or more days is considered appropriate.

Monitoring is also considered to be appropriate for patients with a variety of other conditions associated with arrhythmias, including suspected myocardial infarction, until that diagnosis had been excluded; ingestion of agents with cardiac toxicity; myocarditis; and, for patients with potentially life-threatening arrhythmias, during initiation of therapy with Type I or Type III antiarrhythmic drugs. Electrocardiographic monitoring is recommended for patients with unstable angina and those with high-risk coronary artery lesions who are scheduled for urgent revascularization.

The use of monitoring was less clear-cut in populations with a lower risk of complications, such as patients with acute myocardial infarction who were without complications during their first 3 hospital days; patients with a non-life-threatening arrhythmia undergoing initiation of Type I or Type III antiarrhythmic agents; and patients with pericarditis without myocarditis. Syncope and other neurological events that might have a cardiac cause are also considered equivocal (Class II) indications for electrocardiographic monitoring, implying that some but not all such patients should receive this care.

The guidelines specify only a few situations in which monitoring is not indicated, as in patients who have undergone routine uncomplicated coronary angiography, patients with chronic stable atrial fibrillation, and patients with stable asymptomatic ventricular premature contractions. After uncomplicated surgery, young patients and obstetrical patients often do not need monitoring, according to these guidelines. The guidelines indicate that monitoring can be stopped for patients whose cardiac syndrome has been stabilized and who have been free of arrhythmia for 3 days.

CARDIAC CATHETERIZATION AND CORONARY ANGIOGRAPHY

(See also Chaps. 6 and 8)

Because of high costs and rising rates of utilization, cardiac catheterization and coronary angiography have been the focus of numerous guidelines. The developers of these guidelines include national organizations[64,65] as well as individual provider and payer organizations. One goal of these guidelines is to ensure appropriate use of these procedures, because investigations have demonstrated considerable variability in their use. Therefore, some guidelines seek to standardize which patients are considered appropriate for cardiac catheterization.[14–16]

In addition to *who* undergoes cardiac catheterization, guidelines also seek to decrease variability in *how* the procedure is performed. In many regions of the United States, cardiac catheterization laboratories have been almost totally unregulated, and these facilities are used for a widening range of diagnostic and interventional procedures. Ambulatory cardiac catheterizations are now frequently performed in many laboratories, including facilities that do not have surgical back-up on site. Mobile cardiac catheterization laboratories are also used for performance of cardiac catheterization in regions without hospital-based facilities. Finally, guidelines from professional organizations have addressed specific issues related to cardiac catheterization, including the volume of procedures that operators must perform to maintain clinical skills and use of non-ionic contrast agents.

Appropriateness of Coronary Angiography

Detailed guidelines for the use of coronary angiography were published in 1987 by a task force of the American College of Cardiology and American Heart Association.[64] (The process of revising these guidelines began in 1995.)

The two principles underlying these guidelines are:

1. Coronary angiography should be performed for patients in whom the presence or absence of coronary disease should be determined with reasonable probability in order to improve management.

2. Patients who are at high risk for complications of ischemic heart disease should be identified.

Although accurate diagnosis of coronary disease is believed to contribute to improved management, the guidelines note that performance of coronary angiography in all patients with suspected coronary disease would be very costly, and that noninvasive tests can be used to establish diagnoses and assess prognosis in many patients. The noninvasive criteria for "high risk" were adopted from a joint ACC/AHA Task Force report.[66] These high-risk criteria were chosen for their correlation with poor overall prognosis, left main or multivessel coronary artery disease, and with impaired left ventricular function (Table 63–5).

ASYMPTOMATIC PATIENTS. Asymptomatic patients are considered to have "known" coronary disease if they have had a previous myocardial infarction or have undergone coronary bypass surgery or angioplasty. Asymptomatic patients have "suspected" coronary disease if they have rest- or exercise-induced electrocardiographic abnormalities suggesting "silent" ischemia.

Among these, coronary angiography is considered an appropriate procedure in those with markedly abnormal noninvasive tests for ischemic heart disease (Table 63–6).

For patients in whom noninvasive tests indicate a high probability of coronary disease but in whom these "high-risk" criteria are not present, there were varying opinions about the appropriateness of coronary angiography among

---

TABLE 63–5   EXERCISE TEST PARAMETERS ASSOCIATED WITH POOR PROGNOSIS AND/OR INCREASED SEVERITY OF CORONARY ARTERY DISEASE

EXERCISE ELECTROCARDIOGRAM

Duration of symptom-limited exercise
- Failure to complete Stage II of Bruce protocol or equivalent work load ($\leq$ 6.5 METS) with other protocols

Exercise heart rate at onset of limiting symptoms
- Failure to attain heart rate $\geq$ 120/min (off beta blockers)

Time of onset, magnitude, morphology and postexercise duration of abnormal horizontal or downsloping ST-segment depression
- Onset at heart rate < 120/min or $\leq$ 6.5 METS
- Magnitude $\geq$ 2.0 mm
- Postexercise duration $\geq$ 6 min
- Depression in multiple leads

Systolic blood pressure response during or following progressive exercise
- Sustained decrease of > 10 mm Hg or flat blood pressure response ($\leq$ 130 mm Hg) during progressive exercise

Other potentially important determinants
- Exercise-induced ST-segment elevation in leads other than AVR
- Angina pectoris during exercise
- Exercise-induced U wave inversion
- Exercise-induced ventricular tachycardia

THALLIUM SCINTIGRAPH

Abnormal thallium distribution in more than one vascular region at rest or with exercise that redistributes at another time
- Abnormal distribution associated with increased lung uptake produced by exercise in the absence of severely depressed left ventricular function at rest.
- Enlargement of the cardiac pool of thallium with exercise.

RADIONUCLIDE VENTRICULOGRAM
- A fall in left ventricular ejection fraction of $\geq$ 0.10 during exercise
- A rest or exercise left ventricular ejection fraction of < 0.50, when suspected to be due to coronary artery disease.

Data from Schlant, R. C., Blomqvist, C. G., Brandenburg, R. O., et al.: Guidelines for exercise testing. A report of the American College of Cardiology/American Heart Association Task Force on Assessment of Cardiovascular Procedures (Subcommittee on Exercise Testing). J. Am. Coll. Cardiol. 8:725, 1986.

From Pepine, C. J., Allen, H. D., Bashore, T. M., et al.: ACC/AHA Guidelines for cardiac catheterization and cardiac catheterization laboratories. American College of Cardiology/American Heart Association Ad Hoc Task Force on Cardiac Catheterization. Reprinted with permission from the American College of Cardiology. J. Am. Coll. Cardiol. 18:1149, 1991.

TABLE 63–6 ACC/AHA GUIDELINES FOR CORONARY ANGIOGRAPHY

SETTING	CLASS I (APPROPRIATE)	CLASS II (EQUIVOCAL)	CLASS III (INAPPROPRIATE)
Asymptomatic patients with known or suspected coronary disease	**1.** Evidence of high risk on noninvasive testing (see Table 63–5). **2.** Individuals whose occupation involves the safety of others. **3.** Individuals in certain occupations that frequently require sudden vigorous activity. **4.** After successful resuscitation from cardiac arrest that occurred without obvious precipitating cause when a reasonable suspicion of coronary artery disease exists.	**1.** Presence of ≥ 1 but < 2 mm of ischemic ST depression during exercise, confirmed as ischemia by an independent noninvasive stress test. **2.** Presence of two or more major risk factors and a positive exercise test in male patients without known coronary heart disease. **3.** Presence of prior myocardial infarction with normal left ventricular function at rest and evidence of ischemia by noninvasive testing, but without high-risk criteria. **4.** Before high-risk noncardiac surgery in patients with evidence of ischemia by noninvasive testing.	**1.** As a screening test for coronary artery disease in patients who have not had appropriate noninvasive testing. **2.** After coronary bypass surgery or percutaneous transluminal angioplasty when there is no evidence of ischemia, unless with informed consent for research purposes. **3.** Presence of an abnormal ECG exercise test alone, excluding categories listed in Classes I and II.

Symptomatic patients with known or suspected coronary artery disease	**1.** Angina pectoris that is *inadequately responsive* to medical treatment, percutaneous transluminal angioplasty, thrombolytic therapy, or coronary bypass surgery.
	2. Unstable angina pectoris
	3. Prinzmetal's or variant angina pectoris
	4. Angina pectoris in association with any of the following:
	  • Evidence of high risk on noninvasive testing
	  • Intolerance to medical therapy because of uncontrollable side effects
	  • Occupation or lifestyle that involves unusual risk or "need to know" for insurance or job-related purposes
	5. Before major vascular surgery if angina pectoris or objective evidence of myocardial ischemia is present.
	6. After resuscitation from cardiac arrest or sustained ventricular tachycardia in absence of acute myocardial infarction.
		1. Angina pectoris in the following groups:
		  • Female patients < 40 years of age with objective evidence of myocardial ischemia by noninvasive testing.
		  • Male patients < 40
		  • Patients < 40 with previous myocardial infarction.
		  • Patients requiring major nonvascular surgery if there is objective evidence of myocardial ischemia.
		  • Patients showing a progressively abnormal exercise ECG or other noninvasive stress test on serial testing.
		2. Patients who cannot be risk stratified by other means; e.g., those unable to exercise because of amputation, arthritis, limb deformity, or peripheral vascular disease.
			1. The presence of mild, clinically stable (Canadian Class I or II) angina pectoris in patients who do not have impaired ventricular function, or exercise studies suggesting high-risk or other criteria listed under Classes I and II.
			2. The presence of well-controlled angina pectoris (Canadian Class I or II) in patients who are clearly not candidates for bypass surgery or angioplasty because of age or life expectancy limited by other illnesses.

Atypical chest pain of uncertain origin	**1.** Atypical chest pain when ECG or radionuclide stress tests indicate that high-risk coronary disease may be present. **2.** When the presence of atypical chest pain due to coronary artery spasm is suspected. **3.** When there are associated symptoms or signs of abnormal left ventricular function or failure.	**1.** Atypical chest pain when noninvasive studies are equivocal or cannot be adequately performed. **2.** When noninvasive tests are negative but symptoms are severe and management requires that significant coronary artery disease be excluded.	Atypical chest pain in patients without objective signs of ischemia who have had an earlier technically satisfactory normal coronary angiogram for the same chest pain.
Completed myocardial infarction (after the initial 6 hours up to but not including pre-discharge evaluation)	**1.** Recurrent episodes of ischemic chest pain, particularly if accompanied by ECG changes. **2.** Suspected mitral regurgitation or ruptured interventricular septum causing heart failure or shock. **3.** Suspected subacute cardiac rupture (pseudoaneurysm)	**1.** Thrombolytic therapy during the evolving phase, particularly with evidence of reperfusion.* **2.** Congestive heart failure or hypotension or both, during intensive medical therapy. **3.** Recurrent ventricular tachycardia or ventricular fibrillation, or both, during intensive antiarrhythmic therapy. **4.** Cardiogenic shock	Myocardial infarction in which no acute mechanical or surgical intervention is contemplated.

SETTING	CLASS I (APPROPRIATE)	CLASS II (EQUIVOCAL)	CLASS III (INAPPROPRIATE)
Valvular heart disease	**1.** When valve surgery is being considered in the adult patient with chest discomfort or ECG changes, or both, suggesting coronary artery disease. **2.** When valve surgery is being considered in male patients ≥35 years of age. **3.** When valve surgery is being considered in postmenopausal female patients.	**1.** During left heart catheterization when aortic or mitral valve surgery is being considered in male patients <35 years of age. **2.** During left heart catheterization when aortic or mitral valve surgery is being considered in female patients ≥40. **3.** When one or more major risk factors for coronary artery disease are present in adult patients of any age being considered for valve surgery.	**1.** When cardiac surgical treatment is planned for infective endocarditis in patients who are <35 and have no evidence of coronary embolization. **2.** When aortic or mitral valve surgery is being considered in female patients <40 who have no evidence suggesting coronary artery disease.
Known or suspected congenital heart disease	**1.** Evaluation of patients with congenital heart disease who have signs or symptoms suggesting associated atherosclerotic coronary artery disease. **2.** Suspected congenital coronary anomalies such as congenital coronary artery stenosis, coronary arteriovenous fistula, supravalvular aortic stenosis, an anomalous origin of left coronary artery, provided that aortography is not diagnostic. **3.** When corrective open heart surgery for congenital heart disease is being planned in male patients >40 or postmenopausal female patients.	The presence of forms of congenital heart disease frequently associated with coronary artery anomalies that may complicate surgical management (e.g., tetralogy of Fallot, truncus arteriosus, transposition complexes, and corrected [levo] transposition), provided that aortography is not diagnostic.	Coronary angiography is not routinely indicated in the evaluation of congenital heart disease.

* Subsequent trials suggest revision of these recommendations may be appropriate. See text.
Class I: Conditions for which or patients for whom there is general agreement that coronary angiography is justified.
Class II: Conditions for which or patients for whom coronary angiography is frequently used but there is a divergence of opinion with respect to its justification in terms of value and appropriateness.
Class III: Conditions for which or patients for whom there is general agreement that coronary angiography is not ordinarily justified.
From Ross, J., Jr., Brandenburg, R. O., Dinsmore, R. E., et al.: Guidelines for coronary angiography. A report of the American College of Cardiology/American Heart Association Task Force on Assessment of Diagnostic and Therapeutic Cardiovascular Procedures (Subcommittee on Coronary Angiography). Reprinted with permission from the American College of Cardiology. J. Am. Coll. Cardiol. *10*:935, 1987.

the developers of these guidelines. Hence, test results such as ST depression more than 1 mm but less than 2 mm are considered Class II indications for coronary angiography. In these patients, occupation and life style are important determinants of the appropriateness of angiography. Coronary angiography is considered appropriate (Class I) among individuals whose occupation involves the safety of others (such as airline pilots, bus drivers, truck drivers, air traffic controllers) and individuals in occupations that frequently require sudden vigorous activity (such as firefighters, police officers, and athletes).

Coronary angiography is also considered appropriate for survivors of cardiac arrest, because such patients frequently have extensive coronary disease. Particularly if the cardiac arrest has occurred outside the setting of an acute myocardial infarction, these patients are at high risk for recurrent sudden death[67]; hence, an invasive evaluation is considered appropriate for planning therapy for such patients.

The use of coronary angiography varies markedly for patients undergoing major noncardiac surgery (e.g., abdominal or thoracic aneurysmectomy, ileofemoral bypass surgery). There continues to be progress in noninvasive techniques for the identification of high-risk patients, and patients with normal results with preoperative noninvasive tests such as dipyridamole thallium scintigraphy and ambulatory ischemia monitoring have a low risk for major cardiac complications (see Chap. 54). Strategies for preoperative use of these invasive and noninvasive tests remain uncertain; therefore the appropriateness of coronary angiography in this setting is considered Class II.

Coronary angiography is considered *inappropriate* (Class III) as a screening test in patients who had not undergone appropriate noninvasive testing, or did not have evidence of ischemia on such tests sufficiently severe to place them in Classes I or II.

SYMPTOMATIC PATIENTS. ACC/AHA guidelines for the use of coronary angiography among symptomatic patients reflect the high probability of relief of severe symptoms with coronary artery bypass graft surgery or percutaneous transluminal coronary angioplasty. Coronary angiography is therefore considered appropriate in patients for whom medical or invasive therapy has proved inadequate—that is, when "patient and physician agree that angina significantly interferes with a patient's occupation or ability to perform his or her usual activities."[64] *All* of the "high-risk" noninvasive criteria in Table 63–5 are considered Class I indications for coronary angiography in patients with symptoms of coronary disease, including failure to complete Stage II of the Bruce protocol or equivalent workload (≤6.5 METS). Coronary angiography is also considered appropriate for patients with unstable or variant angina, and for patients with even mild angina who have high-risk occupations or are to undergo major vascular surgery. Another Class I indication is evaluation after resuscitation from cardiac arrest or sustained ventricular tachycardia that occurred outside the setting of acute myocardial infarction.

The appropriateness of coronary angiography is considered more equivocal (Class II) in patients with angina pectoris if they are under age 40 or have responded well to medical therapy. The guidelines also acknowledge that coronary angiography is frequently performed before major nonvascular surgery in patients with evidence of myocardial ischemia, in patients with progressively more abnormal noninvasive tests for ischemia, and in patients who cannot undergo risk stratification using noninvasive tests. However, these patients are considered to be at lower risk for poor outcomes than those in Class I patient subsets; hence these settings are considered Class II indications for coronary angiography.

Coronary angiography is considered *inappropriate* in patients with mild angina who do not have adverse prognostic factors such as high-risk exercise test results. The guidelines also do *not* support use of coronary angiography in patients with well-controlled angina who are not candidates for revascularization because of diseases limiting life expectancy, such as malignant disease, or because of advanced "biological" age.

ATYPICAL CHEST PAIN. Coronary angiography is considered appropriate (Class I) for patients with atypical chest pain, i.e., "single or recurrent episodes of chest pain suggestive, but not typical, of the pain of myocardial ischemia," with high-risk noninvasive tests using the same criteria as for asymptomatic patients with known or suspected coronary disease. Coronary angiography is also considered appropriate for patients in whom coronary spasm is suspected or patients with left ventricular dysfunction associated with atypical chest pain. In such cases, coronary angiography might prove useful in defining the pathophysiology.

Coronary angiography is considered to be equivocally appropriate (Class II) in patients in whom the diagnosis of coronary disease could not be adequately excluded with noninvasive tests or in patients with intractable symptoms in whom definitive demonstration of normal coronary arteries might be useful.

ACUTE MYOCARDIAL INFARCTION. The 1987 ACC/AHA guidelines considered coronary angiography to be of uncertain appropriateness (Class II) during the initial hours of acute myocardial infarction, whether or not thrombolytic therapy had been carried out. However, since the publication of these guidelines, randomized trials have demonstrated excellent and possibly superior outcomes for patients treated with primary angioplasty for acute myocardial infarction.[68-70] Therefore, revisions of these guidelines can be expected to consider coronary angiography to be appropriate in the early hours after the onset of infarction, assuming that the goal of the procedure is to identify patients for whom angioplasty can be performed.

After the initial 6 hours, when the myocardial infarction can be considered "complete," coronary angiography has the goal not of reducing infarct size but of identifying patients at high risk for poor outcomes, and whose outcomes can be improved with revascularization. Therefore, coronary angiography is considered appropriate for patients with evidence of recurrent ischemia, hemodynamic dysfunction due to acute mitral regurgitation or rupture of the interventricular septum, or suspected subacute cardiac rupture.

The guidelines also acknowledge that coronary angiography is frequently used in other settings after acute myocardial infarction, including routinely after thrombolytic therapy or in patients with hemodynamic dysfunction or life-threatening arrhythmia. However, because the role of coronary angiography is not clearly established in such patients, these indications are considered equivocal (Class II). Since the publication of the ACC/AHA guidelines, studies[71-73] have shown that routine early PTCA does *not* improve outcome and actually increases the need for urgent coronary artery bypass surgery. Furthermore, the TIMI II study showed that the strategy of elective catheterization and PTCA did not improve outcomes compared with "watchful waiting"[74] (see Chap. 37). Therefore, future revisions of these guidelines are *unlikely* to recommend *routine* coronary angiography in patients without clinical indications of increased risk for poor outcomes during the hospitalization. However, some data indicate that "rescue" PTCA may improve outcome for patients with persistent

occlusion of the infarct-related artery after thrombolytic therapy,[75,76] so that the use of coronary angiography in this patient population is likely to be considered possibly appropriate.

In the convalescent period after myocardial infarction (i.e., from hospital discharge up to 8 weeks), coronary angiography is again considered most appropriate for patients who demonstrate clinical evidence of increased risk, including those with angina pectoris at rest or with minimal activities, evidence indicative of myocardial ischemia on noninvasive tests, heart failure, or non-Q-wave infarction. The appropriateness of the procedure is considered equivocal (Class II) in patients with mild angina. Coronary angiography is considered inappropriate for patients for whom revascularization is unlikely to improve survival, such as patients with a poor prognosis due to noncardiac disease.

VALVULAR HEART DISEASE. The ACC/AHA guidelines for the use of coronary angiography for patients with valvular heart disease reflect two key facts: (1) Patients with significant coronary disease that is not treated with coronary artery bypass graft surgery at the time of cardiac valvular procedures have higher rates of adverse outcomes[77] and (2) many patients with valvular heart disease who have concomitant coronary artery disease do not have angina pectoris. Therefore, coronary angiography is considered appropriate (Class I) in any adult in whom valve surgery is being considered who has clinical evidence suggestive of ischemic heart disease, who is a male over the age of 35 years or a postmenopausal woman. Coronary angiography is often performed before major valvular surgery in younger patients without evidence of ischemic coronary disease, but the guidelines considered the appropriateness of such procedures equivocal (Class II). Coronary angiography is considered *inappropriate* (Class III) in women patients younger than age 40 without clinical evidence of coronary artery disease and in patients younger than age 35 who require operation for infective endocarditis without signs of coronary artery embolization.

KNOWN OR SUSPECTED CONGENITAL HEART DISEASE. Patients with congenital heart disease are at increased risk for congenital coronary anomalies that can cause symptoms and complications, including sudden death after exertion without warning (see Chaps. 29 and 30). Coronary angiography is therefore considered appropriate (Class I) in patients with congenital disease with symptoms suggestive of atherosclerotic coronary artery disease or any other evidence of coronary anomalies.

The use of coronary angiography in patients with congenital heart disease is also directed at ensuring the safe performance of corrective cardiac surgery; hence, coronary angiography is considered appropriate before surgery in male patients over age 40 years and in postmenopausal female patients. Anomalous coronary artery positions may also lead to injury of the vessels at the time of corrective surgery; therefore, preoperative coronary angiography is often performed when aortography does not allow definitive localization of the site of the coronary arteries.

OTHER CONDITIONS. The ACC/AHA guidelines consider coronary angiography an appropriate procedure when surgery is planned for other cardiac and major vascular conditions in which patients have a high risk of coronary artery disease, such as patients with aortic aneurysms. The guidelines do not consider coronary angiography necessary for all patients with aortic dissection, whereas they note that definition of coronary anatomy may be important for patients with dissections of the ascending aorta because of the risk of involvement of the origins of the coronary arteries.

Coronary angiography is also considered potentially appropriate for patients with other vascular diseases that may involve the coronary arteries (e.g., Takayasu's arteritis, Kawasaki disease). Whether coronary angiography should be performed in patients with Kawasaki disease who have coronary artery aneurysms detected by echocardiography is uncertain (Class II).

Coronary angiography is considered potentially appropriate for other patients in whom the etiology of anginal symptoms or congestive heart failure is uncertain. Thus, Class I indications for coronary angiography include normal left ventricular systolic function but clinical evidence of left ventricular failure. Coronary angiography is also considered appropriate for patients with hypertrophic cardiomyopathy if they are men over age 35 years or postmenopausal women in two settings: (1) if they have symptoms of angina pectoris uncontrolled by medical therapy and (2) if surgery is planned to relieve outflow obstruction. On the other hand, coronary angiography is *not* considered to be clearly appropriate for routine evaluation of dilated cardiomyopathy. Coronary angiography is frequently performed in this patient population to determine whether the left ventricular dysfunction results from coronary disease and therefore might improve with revascularization. However, the ACC/AHA guidelines note that the distinction between ischemic and idiopathic cardiomyopathy can usually be made on the basis of available clinical data. The most appropriate role for coronary angiography in this population is in patients with dilated cardiomyopathy who also have symptoms of angina pectoris or left ventricular aneurysm or evidence of reversible ischemia.

Site of Cardiac Catheterization

ACC/AHA guidelines for cardiac catheterization and cardiac catheterization laboratories that were published in 1991 cover a broad range of topics related to the provision of these procedures, with particular emphasis on the site of cardiac catheterization.[65] This focus was stimulated by the increasing performance of ambulatory cardiac catheterization and the use of mobile laboratories. These "nontraditional" strategies and settings for cardiac catheterization have the potential to reduce costs for procedures and make cardiac catheterization more accessible to patients who live or are hospitalized in rural areas. However, these advantages must be weighed against the possible increase in risk for complications and the potential for overuse of catheterization for patients who have low probability of benefiting from this procedure.

These guidelines therefore attempt to define which patients can safely undergo coronary angiography in which settings. "Ambulatory" patients are those who do not stay in the hospital overnight either before or after the proce-

dure. In general, these patients should be those who are at low risk for complications from the procedure and also have low probability of instability due to the underlying disease process. These guidelines dictate that ambulatory catheterization can be considered for diagnostic coronary angiography or evaluation of valvular, congenital, or myocardial disease. However, the guidelines indicate that PTCA should not be performed on an outpatient basis and, as a general rule, endorse ambulatory catheterization only for patients with stable cardiovascular symptomatic status.

Previous studies of ambulatory cardiac catheterization have reported that postprocedure hospitalizations occur frequently even among "low-risk" patients.[78,79] Therefore, no guidelines can identify a patient population for whom outpatient catheterization can be expected to be completely free of complications. As a result, the ACC/AHA guidelines stress that formal protocols for urgent hospitalization and special care are essential to the performance of ambulatory catheterization.

Several clinical conditions were identified that render the patient *inappropriate* (Class III) or of *uncertain appropriateness* (Class II) for ambulatory cardiac catheterization (Table 63–7). These conditions reflect predictors of complications during cardiac catheterization. Some of these factors (e.g., morbid obesity and severe peripheral vascular disease) increase a patient's risk for vascular complications. Others reflect increased risk for systemic complications (e.g., severe insulin-dependent diabetes mellitus and renal insufficiency).

Ambulatory cardiac catheterization should also be used with caution in patients whose underlying cardiovascular disease places them at increased risk for hemodynamic and other cardiovascular complications after coronary angiography. Therefore, the guidelines consider patients with noninvasive tests suggestive of high risk (see Table 63–6), recent cerebrovascular events, or severe pulmonary hypertension to be *inappropriate* for ambulatory cardiac catheterization.

The guidelines for use of outpatient catheterizations that were published in 1991 by the ACC/AHA are similar in content to those reported in 1992 by the Society for Cardiac Angiography and Interventions.[80] These latter guidelines describe in detail standards for the preprocedural preparation and the performance of the procedure itself. In addition to the conditions that were cited by the ACC/AHA task force as rendering patients inappropriate for outpatient cardiac catheterization, the Society for Cardiac Angiogra-

TABLE 63–7 ACC/AHA CRITERIA FOR EXCLUSION FROM AMBULATORY CARDIAC CATHETERIZATION

CLASS II (EQUIVOCAL)
1. History of contrast material allergy
2. Older than age 75
3. Severe obesity
4. Generalized debility or dementia
5. Frequent ventricular arrhythmia
6. Renal insufficiency (serum creatinine more than 2 mg/dl)

CLASS III (INAPPROPRIATE)
1. Geographic remoteness (> 1-hour drive) from laboratory with inadequate or unreliable follow-up likely over next 24 hours.
2. Interventional therapeutic procedure (e.g., PTCA, valvuloplasty)
3. Infancy
4. Noncandidacy for cardiac catheterization because of other circumstances (e.g., fever, active infection, severe anemia or electrolyte imbalance, bleeding diathesis, uncontrolled systemic hypertension, or digitalis toxicity).
5. Transient cerebral ischemic episodes or recent stroke (less than one month before).
6. Suspected severe pulmonary hypertension
7. Severe peripheral vascular disease
8. Severe insulin dependent diabetes
9. Noninvasive testing data suggesting that detected ischemia may be associated with a high risk for adverse outcome (see Table 63–5).

From Pepine, C. J., Allen, H. D., Bashore, T. M., et al.: ACC/AHA Guidelines for cardiac catheterization and cardiac catheterization laboratories. American College of Cardiology/American Heart Association Ad Hoc Task Force on Cardiac Catheterization. Reprinted with permission from the American College of Cardiology. J. Am. Coll. Cardiol. *18*:1149, 1991.

phy and Interventions added (1) ventricular ectopy requiring antiarrhythmic prophylaxis, (2) severe aortic stenosis, (3) known bleeding disorders, and (4) emotional lability.

CATHETERIZATION IN DIFFERENT TYPES OF FACILITIES. The ACC/AHA guidelines indicate that stricter criteria should be used to identify candidates for ambulatory catheterization in settings with less capability to treat complications. In this respect, hospital-based facilities without surgical support are intermediate in capability between full-service hospitals and mobile catheterization laboratories. Hospital-based facilities permit prolonged monitoring of patients after the procedure and ready access to at least noncardiac surgical management of vascular complications.

For *suspected coronary artery disease,* patients with severe symptoms of ischemia or congestive heart failure are considered *inappropriate* for ambulatory catheterization, as are those with acute myocardial infarction within the last 7 days or a history of pulmonary edema thought due to transient ischemia. These guidelines consider the indications for ambulatory catheterization to be equivocal (Class II) for patients with noninvasive test data suggestive of high-risk coronary disease, if the procedure is performed in a full-service institution. However, catheterization of such patients in a hospital-based facility without immediate cardiac surgical capability is considered *inappropriate* (Class III).

For patients with suspected *valvular heart disease,* the ACC/AHA guidelines consider ambulatory catheterization *inappropriate* in *any* facility for patients with conditions including poor functional class, severe right ventricular failure or pulmonary hypertension, suspected severe aortic valve disease, active endocarditis, and need for continuous anticoagulation. Left ventricular puncture should be performed only at full-service hospitals. Transseptal procedures (Class II), as well as catheterizations in patients with an ejection fraction less than or equal to 35 per cent, are considered inappropriate for facilities without immediate access to cardiac surgical services.

OTHER ISSUES RELATED TO CARDIAC CATHETERIZATION. The ACC/AHA and other organizations have also recommended that physicians who perform cardiac catheterization in adults maintain a caseload of approximately 150 cases per year.[65,81] The guidelines note that, in some cases, the laboratory director may decide that a physician's skills are such that this minimum number of cases is not mandatory. The guidelines also recommend that physicians who begin performing cardiac catheterization after a prolonged hiatus first undergo a period of preceptorship involving at least 25 cases with a variety of diagnoses.

PERCUTANEOUS TRANSLUMINAL CORONARY ANGIOPLASTY

(See also Chaps. 38 and 39)

The development of guidelines for percutaneous transluminal coronary angioplasty (PTCA) is complicated by several trends, including technological innovations (e.g., stents, rotational and directional atherectomy), broadening of the patient population to which this procedure is applied, and the lack of data identifying populations in which PTCA confers a survival advantage. As physicians have become more expert in performing this procedure, they have also become more aggressive, and PTCA is now frequently used for patients with acute myocardial infarction and patients with multivessel coronary artery disease. An additional reason for uncertainty over the optimal role for PTCA is that it is an alternative to more than one major strategy—medical therapy or coronary artery bypass graft surgery. Hence, trials in which PTCA is directly compared with one other strategy[82-86] do not address the full range of choices for the clinicians.

Available guidelines do not address the issue whether patients with coronary disease requiring revascularization should undergo PTCA or CABG (see Chap. 38). Therefore, available guidelines do not present the optimal management for various subsets of patients with coronary disease. Instead, guidelines provide expert opinion on the yes-no question whether PTCA is likely to be regarded as appropriate (Class I), equivocal (Class II), or inappropriate (Class III).

An ACC/AHA task force published guidelines for PTCA in 1993[87] (Table 63–8) that defined contraindications to *elective* angioplasty, which include the relative contraindications to coronary angiography. These guidelines stress that PTCA may be appropriate even in patients with these contraindications who are severely symptomatic and not candidates for coronary bypass surgery.

Absolute contraindications include:

1. Absence of a lesion that causes a 50 per cent or greater reduction in coronary diameter;
2. Presence of significant left main coronary disease unless this coronary distribution is protected by at least one nonobstructed bypass graft;
3. Absence of a formal cardiac surgical program in the institution.

Relative contraindications include:

1. Conditions associated with unacceptable risks of serious bleeding or thrombotic occlusion or a recently dilated vessel;
2. Diffusely diseased saphenous vein grafts without a focal dilatable lesion;
3. Diffusely diseased native coronary arteries with distal vessels suitable for bypass grafting;
4. The vessel under consideration is the sole remaining source of myocardial perfusion;
5. Chronic total occlusions with clinical features suggesting a very low anticipated success rate;
6. Borderline stenotic lesion (usually less than 50 per cent stenosis);
7. Procedure proposed for a non-infarct-related artery in patients with multivessel disease who are undergoing direct angioplasty for acute myocardial infarction.
8. ACC/AHA guidelines also consider anatomical features that increase the risk for abrupt closure (see Chap. 39) to be relative contraindications to PTCA.

Many of these absolute and relative contraindications to PTCA will require reevaluation before new guidelines for this procedure are issued because of changes in interventional techniques. Coronary stents can prevent abrupt closure after attempted dilations of complex lesions, and new devices such as rotational atherectomy catheters have the potential to address lesions that previously would have been considered unlikely to yield to a balloon catheter. The guidelines that are described in this section were developed for balloon angioplasty, and it seems unlikely that they can or should be extended without change to these new techniques.

Because of the risk for complications with angioplasty, the ACC/AHA guidelines consider mandatory for all *elective* PTCA procedures the presence of an experienced cardiovascular surgical team within the hospital to perform emergency coronary bypass surgery should the need arise. However, the task force considers PTCA reasonable under some circumstances even if surgical back-up is not available. For patients at high risk for acute myocardial infarction in whom thrombolytic therapy is contraindicated, emergency PTCA is deemed "acceptable treatment" even if the patient cannot be transferred expeditiously to a center with surgical back-up. However, the guidelines note that patients with unstable angina should usually be transferred to an institution with a cardiac surgical program before consideration of PTCA.

SETTING	CLASS I (APPROPRIATE)	CLASS II (EQUIVOCAL)	CLASS III (INAPPROPRIATE)
Single-vessel coronary artery disease — Asymptomatic or mildly symptomatic patients with or without medical therapy	Patients who have a significant ($\geq 50\%$) lesion in a major epicardial artery that subtends a *large* area of viable myocardium, and who: 1. Show evidence of severe myocardial ischemia during laboratory testing, i.e., ischemia induced by low-level exercise (Bruce Stage I or < 4.0 METS, or heart rate < 100 beats/min) 2. Have been resuscitated from cardiac arrest or from sustained ventricular tachycardia in the absence of acute myocardial infarction, or 3. Must undergo high-risk noncardiac surgery, if angina is present or there is objective evidence of ischemia as described above.	Patients with mild or no symptoms, single-vessel coronary disease in a major epicardial artery that subtends at least a *moderate-sized* area of viable myocardium, and show objective evidence of myocardial ischemia during laboratory testing[†] and • Have at least a moderate likelihood of successful dilation, and • Have a low risk of abrupt vessel closure, and • Are at low risk for morbidity and mortality.	Patients with mild or no symptoms and single-vessel coronary disease who do not meet Class I or Class II criteria; e.g., those who: 1. Have only a small area of viable myocardium at risk, or 2. Do not manifest evidence of myocardial ischemia during laboratory testing,[†] 3. Have borderline lesions (50 to 60% diameter reduction) and have no inducible ischemia, or 4. Are at moderate or high risk for morbidity and mortality.
Single-vessel coronary artery disease — Symptomatic patients with angina pectoris (functional Classes II to IV, unstable angina) with medical therapy	Patients who have a significant lesion in a major epicardial artery that subtends at least a moderate-sized area of viable myocardium and who: 1. Show evidence of myocardial ischemia while on medical therapy (including ECG monitoring at rest), or 2. Have angina pectoris inadequately responsive to medical treatment, or 3. Are intolerant of medical therapy because of uncontrollable side effects.	Patients who have a significant lesion in a major epicardial artery that subtends at least a moderate-sized area of viable myocardium and who: 1. Show evidence of myocardial ischemia during laboratory testing[†] and have one or more complex (type B or C morphology) lesions in the same vessel or its branches or 2. Have disabling symptoms and a small area of viable myocardium at risk.	All other symptomatic patients with single-vessel disease who do not fulfill criteria for Class I or Class II. Examples include patients who: 1. Have no or only a small area of viable myocardium at risk in the absence of disabling symptoms, or 2. Have clinical symptoms not likely to be indicative of ischemia, or 3. Have a very low likelihood of successful dilation, or 4. Are at high risk for morbidity and mortality, or 5. Have no symptoms or objective evidence of myocardial ischemia during high-level stress testing (≥ 12 METS)
Multivessel coronary artery disease — Asymptomatic or mildly symptomatic patients with or without medical therapy	Patients who have one significant lesion in a major epicardial artery that could result in nearly complete revascularization because the additional lesion subtends a small viable or nonviable area of myocardium. Also, patients in this category must: 1. Have a *large* area of viable myocardium at risk, and 2. Show evidence of severe myocardial ischemia while on medical therapy during laboratory testing, or 3. Have been resuscitated from cardiac arrest or from sustained ventricular tachycardia in the absence of acute myocardial infarction.	1. Patients who are similar to those in Class I but who: • Have a *moderate-sized* area of viable myocardium at risk, or • Have objective evidence of myocardial ischemia during laboratory testing, or 2. Who have significant lesions in two or more major epicardial arteries, each of which subtends at least a *moderate-sized* area of viable myocardium.	All other patients with multivessel disease and mild or no symptoms who do not fulfill the above criteria for Class I or Class II. Examples include patients who: 1. Have only a small area of viable myocardium at risk, or 2. Have chronic total occlusions in major epicardial vessels subtending moderate or large areas of viable myocardium, or 3. Are at high risk for morbidity or mortality.
Multivessel coronary artery disease — Symptomatic patients with angina pectoris (functional Classes II to IV, unstable angina) with medical therapy	Patients who have significant lesions in two or more major epicardial arteries both subtending at least *moderate-sized* areas of viable myocardium and who: 1. Show evidence of myocardial ischemia while on medical therapy during laboratory testing[†] 2. Have unstable angina or angina pectoris that has proved inadequately responsive to medical therapy, or 3. Are intolerant of medical therapy because of uncontrollable side effects.	Patients who have significant lesions in two or more major epicardial arteries that subtend at least *moderate-sized* areas of viable myocardium and who: 1. Are similar to patients in Class I but who are at moderate risk for morbidity and mortality, or have angina pectoris but do not necessarily have objective evidence of myocardial ischemia during laboratory testing. 2. Have disabling angina proved inadequately responsive to medical therapy, and are considered poor candidates for surgery because of advanced physiologic age or coexisting medical disorders	All other symptomatic patients with multivessel disease who do not fulfill the preceding criteria in Class I or Class II. Examples include patients who: 1. Have only a small area of myocardium at risk in the absence of disabling symptoms, or 2. Have lesion morphology with a low likelihood of successful dilation and subtending moderate or large areas of viable myocardium, or 3. Are at high risk for morbidity or mortality, or both.

Table continues on the following page

TABLE 63–8 ACC/AHA GUIDELINES FOR PERCUTANEOUS TRANSLUMINAL CORONARY ANGIOPLASTY—*Continued*

SETTING	CLASS I (APPROPRIATE)	CLASS II (EQUIVOCAL)	CLASS III (INAPPROPRIATE)
Direct immediate coronary angioplasty for evolving acute myocardial infarction	Patients who can be managed in the *appropriate laboratory setting* and who: **1.** Are within 0 to 6 hours of onset of a myocardial infarction **2.** Are within 6–12 hours of onset of a myocardial infarction but who have continued symptoms of ongoing myocardial ischemia, or **3.** Are in cardiogenic shock with or without previous thrombolytic therapy and within 12 hours after onset of symptoms.	Patients who: **1.** Are within 6–12 hours of onset of an acute myocardial infarction and have no symptoms of myocardial ischemia but have a large area of myocardium at jeopardy and/or are in a higher-risk clinical category **2.** Are within 12–24 hours of onset of an acute myocardial infarction but who have continued symptoms of ongoing myocardial ischemia.	**1.** Angioplasty of a non-infarct-related artery at the time of acute myocardial infarction. **2.** Patients who are at more than 12 hours after onset of acute myocardial infarction at the time of admission and who have no symptoms of myocardial ischemia, or **3.** Patients who have had successful thrombolytic therapy within the past 24 hours and have no symptoms of myocardial ischemia.
After acute myocardial infarction (Angioplasty during initial hospitalization)	Patients who have one or more lesions that predict a high (>90) success rate and are at low risk for morbidity and mortality, and: **1.** Have recurrent episodes of ischemic chest pain, particularly if accompanied by ECG changes (postinfarction angina), or **2.** Show objective evidence of myocardial ischemia during laboratory testing performed before discharge from the hospital, or **3.** Have recurrent sustained ventricular tachycardia or ventricular fibrillation, or both, while receiving intensive medical therapy.	Patients who: **1.** Are similar to patients in Class I but: • Have more complex lesions with at least a moderate likelihood of successful dilation, or • undergo multivessel angioplasty. **2.** Have survived cardiogenic shock in the period before discharge or **3.** Are asymptomatic but have a significant residual lesion in the infarct-related artery supplying a large or moderate area of angiographically functioning myocardium, or **4.** Have had a non-Q-wave myocardial infarction, and have a large area at risk or objective evidence of myocardial ischemia.	All other patients in the immediate postinfarction period who do not fulfill the criteria for Class I and Class II. Examples include: **1.** Dilation of borderline residual lesions (50 to 60% diameter reduction) in the absence of spontaneous or stress-induced ischemia, or **2.** Dilation of chronic total occlusions subtending nonviable myocardium, or **3.** Angioplasty in patients at high risk for morbidity and mortality.

† Evidence for myocardial ischemia during laboratory testing includes the following, with or without exercise-induced angina pectoris:
a. Ischemic ST segment depression ≥ 1 mm, or
b. One or more stress-induced reversible nuclear perfusion defects and/or exercise-induced reduction in the ejection fraction and/or wall motion abnormalities on radionuclide ventriculographic or stress echocardiographic studies.

Class I: Conditions for which there is general agreement that coronary angioplasty is justified. A Class I indication does not mean that coronary angioplasty is the only acceptable therapy.
Class II: Conditions for which there is a divergence of opinion with respect to the justification for coronary angioplasty in terms of value and appropriateness.
Class III: Conditions for which there is general agreement that coronary angioplasty is not ordinarily indicated.

From Ryan, T. J., Bauman, W. B., Kennedy, J. W., et al.: Guidelines for percutaneous transluminal coronary angioplasty. A report of the American College of Cardiology/American Heart Association Task Force on Assessment of Diagnostic and Therapeutic Cardiovascular Procedures (Subcommittee on Percutaneous Transluminal Coronary Angioplasty). Reprinted with permission from the American College of Cardiology. J. Am. Coll. Cardiol. *22*:2033, 1993.

The experience of the operator is also a crucial factor in determining the outcome for PTCA. Therefore, several task forces have provided similar recommendations for the minimum number of cases during PTCA training and for the minimum annual volume required to maintain competency.[87–90] All recommend that a structured fellowship program in PTCA involve a minimum of 125 coronary angioplasty procedures, including at least 75 in which the trainee was the primary operator. Estimates of the number of PTCA cases per year required to maintain competency range from 50 to 75. The ACC/AHA task force recommends that PTCA operators who did not meet these requirements be required to discontinue performance of the procedure. The task force also recommends that institutions offering PTCA perform at least 200 such procedures annually and indicates that an initial success rate of 90 per cent or more for single-lesion dilations is a reasonable expectation.

Indications for PTCA

The ACC/AHA task force developed assessments of the appropriateness of PTCA in various clinical settings according to the same three classes used in other ACC/AHA guidelines.[87]

SINGLE-VESSEL CORONARY DISEASE. For patients who are *asymptomatic* or only mildly symptomatic, regardless whether they have received medical therapy, PTCA is considered appropriate (Class I) in those who have a lesion resulting in a 30 per cent or greater reduction in the diameter of a coronary artery that supplies a large area of viable myocardium *and* myocardial ischemia induced by low levels of exercise during noninvasive testing (Bruce Stage 1 or less or less than 4.0 METS, *or* heart rate less than 100 beats/min). Other Class I indications for PTCA include prior cardiac arrest or sustained ventricular tachycardia in the absence of acute myocardial infarction; and the need to undergo major vascular surgery (such as aortic aneurysm repair, iliofemoral bypass, or carotid artery surgery) in patients with clinical evidence of ischemic heart disease.

The appropriateness of single-vessel angioplasty is less clear-cut in asymptomatic patients with less myocardium in jeopardy. PTCA is considered inappropriate (Class III) for patients with only a small area of viable myocardium at risk, or no evidence of ischemia, or a moderate-to-high risk for complications.

For patients who are *symptomatic* from single-vessel coronary disease despite medical therapy, the ACC/AHA guidelines consider PTCA appropriate (Class I) even if only a moderate amount of myocardium is supplied by the stenosed vessel—if they exhibit ischemia despite medical therapy, have angina pectoris that is inadequately responsive to medical treatment, or are intolerant of medical therapy. "Inadequately responsive" indicates that angina significantly interferes with the patient's occupation or ability to perform usual activities. These patients should have at least a moderate likelihood of successful dilation and be at low or moderate risk for morbidity and mortality for PTCA to be considered clearly appropriate.

PTCA is considered to be of equivocal appropriateness (Class II) in patients with increased risk for complications or failure of the procedure. The ACC/AHA guidelines do not deem PTCA to be appropriate in patients with no or only a small area of myocardium at risk in the absence of disabling symptoms or in patients with a high risk of procedural failure or complications.

MULTIVESSEL CORONARY DISEASE. For *asymptomatic* patients with multivessel disease, the guidelines indicate that PTCA is appropriate (Class I) if dilation of a single major coronary artery could lead to nearly complete revascularization, and the patients have a moderate or high chance of success. PTCA is considered inappropriate (Class IV) if patients had only a small amount of viable myocardium at risk, had chronic total occlusions, or had a high risk for complications.

For *symptomatic* patients with multivessel coronary disease, appropriate (Class I) indications for PTCA are similar to those for symptomatic patients with single-vessel disease except that these indications include lesions in two or more major arteries affecting at least moderate-sized areas of viable myocardium.

DIRECT CORONARY ANGIOPLASTY FOR EVOLVING ACUTE MYOCARDIAL INFARCTION. This topic is also addressed in guidelines for management of acute myocardial infarction (see p. 1221), and current recommendations reflect findings from recent randomized trials comparing direct angioplasty with intravenous thrombolytic therapy in patients with acute myocardial infarction.[68-70]

The 1993 guidelines for PTCA by the ACC/AHA task force reflect the promise as well as the uncertainty of this procedure for patients with evolving myocardial infarction. Percutaneous transluminal coronary angioplasty is considered appropriate for patients with continuing symptoms of ischemia within the first 6 hours after the onset of myocardial infarction, and from 6 to 12 hours after onset. It is also regarded as an effective therapy for patients within 12 hours of the onset of infarction who are in cardiogenic shock, even if they have had thrombolytic therapy.

The appropriateness of PTCA according to the ACC/AHA guidelines diminishes as time elapses; hence the use of this procedure 6 to 12 hours after the onset of infarction is considered an equivocal (Class II) indication, and its use more than 12 hours after the onset of infarction is considered inappropriate unless the patients have symptoms of ongoing ischemia. To minimize PTCA-related complications, the ACC/AHA guidelines recommend against the dilatation of non-infarct related arteries at the time of PTCA for acute infarction.

AFTER ACUTE MYOCARDIAL INFARCTION. Data from several trials do not support a strategy of routine performance of coronary angiography and PTCA after successful thrombolytic therapy for acute myocardial infarction.[71-74] Other studies, however, have shown that PTCA can be performed successfully in most patients in whom thrombolytic therapy has failed[75,76] and that patients with evidence of recurrent ischemia or other complications after myocardial infarction have a poorer prognosis. Therefore, the ACC/AHA guidelines for use of PTCA consider it appropriate for patients with evidence of ischemia or life-threatening arrhythmias if they have lesions that suggest a high success rate for the procedure.

For patients with coronary lesions associated with a worse success rate or greater complication rate, the indications for PTCA after myocardial infarction are considered uncertain (Class II). The guidelines also consider the use of PTCA equivocal for patients who are asymptomatic but have a large or moderate area of myocardium threatened by a residual lesion in the infarct-related artery, and for pa-

tients with a non-Q-wave myocardial infarction and further myocardium at risk.

CORONARY ARTERY BYPASS GRAFT SURGERY

(See also Chap. 38)

Coronary artery bypass graft surgery (CABG) is indicated for relief of symptoms that are unresponsive to medical treatment (or to coronary angioplasty), and for some patient subsets, to increase life expectancy. Guidelines published by an ACC/AHA task force on performance of CABG in 1991[91] are based on the comparative benefits of surgery versus medical therapy. These benefits are assumed to be dependent on (1) the number and type of coronary arteries whose stenoses can be "neutralized" by bypass surgery and (2) the expected survival of the patient with medical therapy. An implication of this approach is that CABG may be most beneficial in patient subsets with high surgical mortality if outcomes with medical therapy are even worse. Conversely, patient subsets with low surgical mortality often have excellent outcomes with medical therapy—implying that the comparative benefit from CABG may be low. For example, patients with left ventricular dysfunction have higher surgical mortality but a greater potential benefit from CABG than patients without left ventricular dysfunction.

These guidelines preceded trials published in 1993–1994 comparing outcomes for patients with multivessel disease who were randomized to CABG or PTCA[82-85]; they do not provide direct guidance on which form of revascularization should be used for specific patient subsets. However, subsequent data have not demonstrated clear differences in outcomes, such as ability to return to work, for CABG or PTCA for most patient subsets that could reasonably be considered for either approach[92]; hence the choice between these two alternatives must continue to be determined on a case-by-case basis.

The ACC/AHA guidelines are summarized in Table 63–9. These tables were developed to apply to patients with an ejection fraction greater than 20 per cent, because the benefits of surgery versus medical therapy in patients with lower ejection fractions have not been well defined in prospective trials. Class I indications are those for which surgery has a demonstrated advantage over medical treatment either in terms of longevity or relief of symptoms or both. Class II indications are those for which surgery is acceptable treatment, but for which its advantages over medical therapy have not been defined. Class III indications are those for which the operation is usually considered not indicated. Exceptions to the overall appropriateness classification system are made for patients with severe proximal stenoses of the left anterior descending coronary artery, which have a more serious prognostic implication than lesions more distal in this artery or in the left circumflex or right coronary artery.[93-95] Therefore, in the ACC/AHA guidelines, surgery is generally considered more appropriate for patients with severe proximal left anterior descending coronary artery obstructions than for patients with stenoses in other locations.

INDICATIONS FOR PATIENT SUBSETS. Certain subsets of coronary anatomy have been found to have better prognoses with surgical than medical therapy and therefore are considered indications for CABG regardless of the patient's symptomatic status and severity of ischemia on noninvasive testing (Table 63–9). In the ACC/AHA guidelines, CABG surgery is considered appropriate (Class I) for all patients with any of these criteria: (1) significant stenosis (greater than 50 per cent) of the left main coronary artery, (2) three-vessel disease and moderate to severe left ventric-

TABLE 63-9 ACC/AHA GUIDELINES FOR CORONARY ARTERY BYPASS GRAFT SURGERY: INDICATION CLASSES

CORONARY DISEASE	LEFT VENTRICULAR DYSFUNCTION			
	None	Mild	Moderate	Severe (but Ejection Fraction > 0.20)
I. Asymptomatic Patients				
1. No or Mild Myocardial Ischemia With Noninvasive Stress Testing				
Left main	I	I	I	I
3 vessel	II[a]	II[a]	I	I
2 vessel	III[b]	III[b]	II	II
1 vessel	III[b]	III[b]	III[b]	III[b]
2. Moderate or Severe Myocardial Ischemia With Noninvasive Stress Testing				
Left main	I	I	I	I
3 vessel	II[c]	II[c]	I	I
2 vessel	II[c]	II[c]	II[c]	II[c]
1 vessel	III[b]	III[b]	II[c]	II[c]
II. Patients With Chronic Stable Class I or II Angina				
1. No or Mild Myocardial Ischemia With Noninvasive Stress Testing				
Left main	I	I	I	I
3 vessel	II[c]	II[c]	I	I
2 vessel	II[c]	II[c]	II[c]	II[c]
1 vessel	III[b]	III[b]	II[c]	II[c]
2. Moderate or Severe Myocardial Ischemia With Noninvasive Stress Testing				
Left main	I	I	I	I
3 vessel	I	I	I	I
2 vessel	II[c]	II[c]	II[c]	II[c]
1 vessel	III[b]	III[b]	II[c]	II[c]
III. Patients With Chronic Stable Class III or IV Angina (regardless of severity of ischemia on exercise testing)				
Left main	I	I	I	I
3 vessel	I	I	I	I
2 vessel	II[c]	II[c]	II[c]	II[c]
1 vessel	II[c]	II[c]	II[c]	II[c]

[a] Class I if there is severe proximal large left anterior descending and left circumflex coronary artery stenoses.
[b] Class II if there is severe proximal stenosis in a large left anterior descending coronary artery.
[c] Class I if there is severe proximal stenosis in a large left anterior descending coronary artery.
Class I: Conditions for which the operation is indicated on the basis of a demonstrated advantage over medical treatment in terms of longevity or relief of symptoms, or both.
Class II: Conditions for which the operation is acceptable treatment but for which its advantages over medical therapy have not yet been fully defined.
Class III: Conditions for which the operation is not generally considered to be indicated.
From Kirklin, J. W., Akins, C. W., Blackstone, E. H., et al.: Guidelines and indications for coronary artery bypass graft surgery. A report of the American College of Cardiology/American Heart Association Task Force on Assessment of Diagnostic and Therapeutic Cardiovascular Procedures (Subcommittee on Coronary Artery Bypass Graft Surgery). Reprinted with permission from the American College of Cardiology. J. Am. Coll. Cardiol. 17:543, 1991.

ular dysfunction, and (3) three-vessel disease that includes a severe proximal left anterior descending stenosis, regardless of the severity of left ventricular dysfunction. For patients with asymptomatic coronary disease and no or only mild evidence of ischemia on exercise testing, this last criterion is modified so that three-vessel disease must include involvement of both the proximal left anterior *and* the left circumflex coronary arteries.

Asymptomatic Patients. The ACC/AHA task force considers CABG *inappropriate* for most asymptomatic patients with one- or two-vessel disease with no or only mild myocardial ischemia on noninvasive stress testing. Exceptions are patients with severe proximal left anterior descending coronary artery stenoses or a combination of two-vessel disease and moderate to severe left ventricular dysfunction.

For these patients, CABG was considered acceptable but unproven (Class II).

A lower threshold for performing CABG is described for asymptomatic patients who have moderate or severe myocardial ischemia with exercise testing. In this population the ACC/AHA task force considers surgery appropriate (Class I) if there is two-vessel disease involving the proximal left anterior descending coronary artery. Surgery is considered *inappropriate* (Class III) for patients with one-vessel disease and good left ventricular function, as long as there is no involvement of the proximal left anterior descending coronary artery. Otherwise, CABG is considered acceptable if unproven (Class II) for such patients with one- or two-vessel disease.

Patients with Chronic Stable Class I or II Angina.

Relief of symptoms is not usually justification for operation in patients with stable mild angina. Therefore the ACC/AHA task force concludes that the indications for CABG in this population should be dictated by the same factors as in asymptomatic patients.

For patients with moderate or severe myocardial ischemia with noninvasive stress testing, however, surgery is considered appropriate (Class I) for patients in several major categories, including all patients with (1) left main disease, (2) three-vessel disease, (3) two-vessel disease with proximal left anterior descending coronary artery involvement, (4) isolated left anterior descending coronary artery involvement associated with moderate to severe left ventricular dysfunction.

Surgery is considered *inappropriate* only for patients with good left ventricular function and one-vessel disease that does not involve the proximal left anterior descending coronary artery.

Patients with Chronic Stable Class III or IV Angina. Patients with Class III or IV angina usually represent failures of medical therapy and often cannot undergo noninvasive stress testing because of concern of risk for complications. In this population, CABG can often improve symptomatic status, and therefore surgery is *not* considered inappropriate for any patient subset. The ACC/AHA guidelines deem surgery to be clearly appropriate (Class I) for all patients except those with one- or two-vessel disease that does not include involvement of the left anterior descending coronary artery.

Unstable Angina. The ACC/AHA guidelines recommend CABG on an emergency basis only when intensive medical management fails to relieve the unstable angina. (See p. 1336 for unstable angina guidelines.) Once medical therapy has led to control of anginal symptoms, recent unstable angina predisposes a patient to further cardiovascular complications.[96] Therefore the ACC/AHA task force concludes that a recent history of unstable angina should lower the threshold for performing CABG.

Acute Myocardial Infarction. The ACC/AHA guidelines discourage use of CABG for patients with uncomplicated Q wave acute myocardial infarction, and recommend that patients with non-Q-wave infarctions be considered for bypass surgery according to the same criteria as patients with unstable angina. For patients with hemodynamic deterioration after acute myocardial infarction, the ACC/AHA guidelines recognize that an aggressive approach including CABG surgery probably improves outcomes in comparison with noninterventional strategies.

CARE OF PATIENTS AFTER CABG. The ACC/AHA task force makes several explicit recommendations aimed at optimization of the patient's recovery after surgery, promotion of graft patency, and control of risk factors. These include (1) cessation of cigarette smoking, (2) a program of daily exercise, (3) antiplatelet therapy, and (4) counseling about risk factor reduction. Although formal cardiac rehabilitation is described as often useful, it is not endorsed for routine care. Electrocardiographic stress testing is considered *possibly useful* 6 weeks to 6 months after surgery, particularly for patients who had silent ischemia.

ORGANIZATIONAL CONSIDERATIONS. The ACC/AHA guidelines offer specific recommendations about the responsibilities and qualifications of key personnel. The cardiac surgeon usually should be certified by the American Board of Thoracic Surgery or an equivalent certifying body, and a CABG surgery program should include at least two qualified cardiac surgeons. A minimum case load of 200 to 300 cases per year was recommended by the Inter-Society Commission for Heart Disease Resources in 1972,[97] the American College of Surgeons in 1984,[98] and the ACC/AHA task force in 1991.[91] Individual surgeons should perform a minimum of 100 to 150 open-heart operations, the majority of which are CABG operations. The ACC/AHA guidelines rec-

ognize that surgeons in densely and in sparsely populated areas may require different guidelines.

ELECTROPHYSIOLOGICAL PROCEDURES

(See also Chap. 21)

ACC/AHA guidelines for the use of intracardiac electrophysiological procedures were first published in 1989.[99] Because of rapid evolution in this field, these guidelines were revised in 1995.[100] This version of these guidelines reflects the emerging importance of catheter ablation as a primary treatment option for most forms of paroxysmal supraventricular tachycardias and preexcitation syndromes, and in patients with monomorphic ventricular tachycardia and structurally normal hearts. The new guidelines also demonstrate progress in understanding the role of electrophysiological studies for risk stratification of patients with tachyarrhythmias, while emphasizing consideration of whether or not the test is likely to influence management decisions.

The ACC/AHA task force identifies a narrow list of indications for which electrophysiological testing is clearly appropriate for guiding drug therapy (Table 63–10): sustained ventricular tachycardia or cardiac arrest, especially among patients with prior myocardial infarction, and supraventricular tachyarrhythmias associated with reentry loops and/or accessory pathways. However, the ACC/AHA guidelines reflect the increasing importance of electrophysiological testing as a prelude to interventions such as the insertion of implantable electric devices and catheter ablation.

EVALUATION OF SINUS NODE FUNCTION. Clinical evaluation of sinus node function is often difficult because of the episodic nature of symptomatic abnormalities and the finding that asymptomatic patients frequently have wide variability in sinus node rates. Invasive tests of sinus node function can assess the ability of the sinus node to recover from overdrive suppression (sinus node recovery time) and assess sinoatrial conduction by introducing atrial extrastimuli or by atrial pacing. These tests can be used to complement data from noninvasive testing, including ambulatory electrocardiography, exercise testing, and tilt-table testing to assess chronotropic incompetence.

The ACC/AHA guidelines consider electrophysiological studies of sinus node function most appropriate for patients in whom dysfunction is suspected but not proven despite noninvasive evaluation; conversely, such studies would be inappropriate (Class III) when bradyarrhythmias had been proven the cause of symptoms, and electrophysiological studies would not alter treatment. When bradyarrhythmias are recognized as the cause of the patient's symptoms, electrophysiological studies are considered to have possible but uncertain appropriateness (Class II) when data might refine treatment choices. These procedures are deemed inappropriate for asymptomatic patients who have bradyarrhythmias observed only during sleep.

ACQUIRED ATRIOVENTRICULAR BLOCK. Electrophysiological studies permit evaluation of conduction above, within, and below the His bundle. This information can be useful to clinicians because patients with atrioventricular (AV) block that is lower in the conduction system tend to have a worse prognosis. Both prognosis and the level at which AV block is occurring often can be predicted from the surface electrocardiogram, however. Therefore the ACC/AHA guidelines emphasize that electrophysiological studies are inappropriate (Class III) when electrocardiographic findings correlate with symptoms, and the findings from electrophysiological studies are unlikely to alter therapy. For example, if a patient warrants implantation of a pacemaker because of documented symptomatic advanced AV block (see p. 687), documentation of His bundle conduction will rarely contribute to management. Similarly, electrophysio-

TABLE 63–10   ACC/AHA GUIDELINES FOR CLINICAL INTRACARDIAC ELECTROPHYSIOLOGICAL STUDIES

SETTING	CLASS I (APPROPRIATE)	CLASS II (EQUIVOCAL)	CLASS III (INAPPROPRIATE)
Evaluation of sinus node function	Symptomatic patients in whom sinus node dysfunction is suspected to be the cause of symptoms but a causal relation between an arrhythmia and the symptoms has not been established after appropriate evaluation.	1. Patients who have documented sinus node dysfunction in whom evaluation of AV or VA conduction or susceptibility to arrhythmias may aid in selection of the most appropriate pacing modality. 2. Patients with electrocardiographically documented sinus bradyarrhythmias to determine if abnormalities are due to intrinsic disease, autonomic nervous system dysfunction, or the effects of drugs to help select therapeutic options.	1. Symptomatic patients in whom an association between symptoms and a documented bradyarrhythmia has been established and the choice of therapy would not be affected by EP study results. 2. Asymptomatic patients with sinus bradyarrhythmias or sinus pauses observed only during sleep, including sleep apnea.
Patients with acquired atrioventricular block	1. Symptomatic patients in whom His-Purkinje block, suspected as a cause of symptoms, has not been established. 2. Patients with 2nd- or 3rd-degree AV block treated with a pacemaker who remain symptomatic, and in whom another arrhythmia is suspected as a cause of symptoms.	1. Patients with 2nd or 3rd degree AV block, in whom knowledge of the site of block or its mechanism, or response to pharmacological or other temporary intervention, may help to direct therapy or assess prognosis. 2. Patients with premature concealed junctional depolarizations suspected as a cause of 2nd or 3rd degree AV block pattern (i.e., pseudo AV block).	1. Symptomatic patients in whom the symptoms and the presence of AV block are correlated by ECG findings. 2. Asymptomatic patients with transient AV block associated with sinus slowing (e.g., nocturnal type I 2nd degree AV block).
Patients with chronic intraventricular conduction delay	Symptomatic patients in whom the cause of the symptoms is not known.	Asymptomatic patients with bundle branch block in whom pharmacological therapy is contemplated with a drug that could increase the conduction delay or produce heart block.	1. Asymptomatic patients with intraventricular conduction delay. 2. Symptomatic patients in whom the symptoms can be correlated with, or excluded by, ECG events.
Patients with a narrow QRS tachycardia (QRS complex < 0.12 sec)	1. Patients with frequent or poorly tolerated episodes of tachycardia not adequately responding to drug therapy in whom information about site of origin, mechanism, and electrophysiological properties of the tachycardia pathways is essential for choosing appropriate therapy (drugs, catheter ablation, pacing, or surgery). 2. Patients who prefer ablative therapy to pharmacological management.	Patients with frequent episodes of tachycardia requiring drug treatment in whom there is concern about proarrhythmia or the effects of the antiarrhythmic drug on the sinus node or on AV conduction.	Patients whose tachycardias are easily controlled by vagal maneuvers and/or well-tolerated drug therapy and who are not candidates for nonpharmacological forms of therapy.
Patients with wide complex tachycardias	Patients with wide QRS tachycardias when the correct diagnosis is unclear after analysis of available ECG tracings and knowledge of the correct diagnosis is necessary for appropriate patient care.	None	Patients with ventricular tachycardia or SVT with aberrant conduction or preexcitation syndromes diagnosed with certainty by ECG criteria and in whom invasive electrophysiological data would not influence therapy. Data obtained at baseline electrophysiological study in these patients might be appropriate to guide subsequent therapy (see sections on therapy).
Patients with ventricular premature complexes, couplets, and nonsustained ventricular tachycardia	None	1. Patients with other risk factors for future arrhythmic events, e.g., a low ejection fraction, positive signal-averaged ECG, and nonsustained ventricular tachycardia on ambulatory ECG recordings. 2. Patients with highly symptomatic, uniform morphology ventricular premature complexes, couplets, and nonsustained ventricular tachycardia.	Asymptomatic or mildly symptomatic patients with premature ventricular complexes, couplets, and nonsustained ventricular tachycardia without other risk factors for sustained arrhythmias.
Patients with unexplained syncope	Patients with syncope that remains unexplained after appropriate evaluation, and who have suspected structural heart disease.	Patients with recurrent unexplained syncope without structural heart disease and a negative head-up tilt test.	Patients with known cause of syncope in whom treatment will not be guided by electrophysiological testing.
Survivors of cardiac arrest	1. Patients surviving an episode of cardiac arrest without evidence of an acute Q-wave myocardial infarction. 2. Patients surviving an episode of cardiac arrest occurring ≥ 48 hours after acute myocardial infarction.	1. Patients surviving cardiac arrest due to bradyarrhythmia. 2. Patients surviving cardiac arrest thought to be associated with a congenital repolarization abnormality (long Q-T syndrome) in whom the results of noninvasive diagnostic testing are equivocal.	1. Patients surviving a cardiac arrest that occurred during the acute phase (< 48 hours) of myocardial infarction. 2. Patients with cardiac arrest resulting from clearly definable specific causes such as reversible ischemia, severe valvular aortic stenosis, or noninvasively defined congenital or acquired long Q-T syndrome.

SETTING	CLASS I (APPROPRIATE)	CLASS II (EQUIVOCAL)	CLASS III (INAPPROPRIATE)
Guidance of drug therapy	**1.** Patients with sustained ventricular tachycardia or cardiac arrest, especially those with prior myocardial infarction. **2.** Patients with atrioventricular nodal reentrant tachycardia, AV reentrant tachycardia using an accessory pathway or atrial fibrillation associated with an accessory pathway in whom chronic drug therapy is involved.	**1.** Patients with sinus node reentrant tachycardia, atrial tachycardia, atrial fibrillation or atrial flutter without ventricular preexcitation syndrome in whom chronic drug therapy is planned. **2.** Patients with arrhythmias not inducible during control electrophysiologic study in whom drug therapy is planned.	**1.** Patients with isolated atrial or ventricular premature complexes. **2.** Patients with ventricular fibrillation with a clearly identified reversible cause.
Patients who are candidates for, or who have, implantable electrical devices	**1.** Patients with tachyarrhythmias, prior to and during implantation, and final (predischarge) programming of an electrical device, to confirm ability of the system to perform as anticipated. **2.** Patients in whom an electrical antitachyarrhythmia device has been implanted in whom changes in status or therapy may have influenced continued safety and efficacy of the device.	Patients with previously documented indications for pacemaker implantation to test for the most appropriate chronic pacing mode and sites to optimize symptomatic improvement and hemodynamics.	Patients who are not candidates for device therapy.
Indications for catheter ablation procedures	**1.** Patients with symptomatic atrial tachyarrhythmias who have inadequately controlled ventricular rates *unless* primary ablation of the atrial tachyarrhythmia is possible. **2.** Patients with symptomatic atrial tachyarrhythmias such as those in No. 1 above but when drugs are not tolerated, or the patient does not wish to take them, even though the ventricular rate can be controlled. **3.** Patients with symptomatic nonparoxysmal junctional tachycardia that is drug resistant, drugs are not tolerated, or the patient does not wish to take them. **4.** Patients resuscitated from sudden cardiac death due to atrial flutter or atrial fibrillation with a rapid ventricular response in the absence of an accessory pathway.	Patients with a dual chamber pacemaker and pacemaker-mediated tachycardia that cannot be treated effectively by drugs or by reprogramming the pacemaker.	Patients with atrial tachyarrythmias responsive to drug therapy that is acceptable to the patient.
Radiofrequency catheter ablation for AV nodal reentrant tachycardia, (AVNRT)	Patients with symptomatic sustained AVNRT that is drug resistant or when the patient is drug intolerant or does not desire long-term drug therapy.	**1.** Patients with sustained AVNRT identified during electrophysiological study or catheter ablation of another arrhythmia. **2.** The finding of dual AV nodal pathway physiology and atrial echos but without AV nodal reentrant tachycardia during electrophysiological study in a patient suspected to have AV nodal reentrant tachycardia clinically.	**1.** Patients with AVNRT that is responsive to drug therapy, that is well tolerated and preferred by the patient to ablation. **2.** The finding of dual AV nodal pathway physiology (with or without echo complexes) during electrophysiological study in a patient in whom AV nodal reentrant tachycardia is not suspected clinically.
Ablation of atrial tachycardia, flutter, and fibrillation: atrium/atrial sites	**1.** Patients with atrial tachycardia that is drug resistant or when the patient is drug intolerant or does not desire long-term drug therapy. **2.** Patients with atrial flutter that is drug resistant or when the patient is drug intolerant or does not desire long-term drug therapy.	**1.** Atrial flutter/atrial tachycardia associated with paroxysmal atrial fibrillation when the tachycardia is drug resistant or when the patient is drug intolerant or does not desire long-term drug therapy. **2.** Patients with atrial fibrillation in whom there is evidence of (a) localized site(s) of origin when the tachycardia is drug resistant or when the patient is drug intolerant or does not desire long-term drug therapy.	**1.** Patients with atrial arrhythmia that is responsive to well-tolerated drug therapy that the patient prefers to ablation. **2.** Patients with multiform atrial tachycardia.

Table continues on the following page

SETTING	CLASS I (APPROPRIATE)	CLASS II (EQUIVOCAL)	CLASS III (INAPPROPRIATE)
Ablation of atrial tachycardia, flutter, and fibrillation: accessory pathways	1. Patients with symptomatic AV reentrant tachycardia that is drug resistant or when the patient is drug intolerant or does not desire long-term drug therapy. 2. Patients with atrial fibrillation (or other atrial tachyarrhythmia) and a rapid ventricular response via the accessory pathway when the tachycardia is drug resistant or when the patient is drug intolerant or does not desire long-term drug therapy.	1. Patients with AV reentrant tachycardia or atrial fibrillation with rapid ventricular rates identified during electrophysiological study of another arrhythmia. 2. Asymptomatic patients with ventricular preexcitation whose livelihood, profession, important activities, insurability, mental well-being, or the public safety would be affected by spontaneous tachyarrhythmias or by ECG abnormality. 3. Patients with atrial fibrillation and a controlled ventricular response via the accessory pathway. 4. Patients with a family history of sudden cardiac death.	Patients who have accessory pathway-related arrhythmias responsive to drug therapy that is well tolerated and preferable to ablation by the patient.
Ablation of ventricular tachycardia	1. Patients with symptomatic sustained monomorphic ventricular tachycardia when the tachycardia is drug resistant or when the patient is drug intolerant or does not desire long-term drug therapy. 2. Patient with bundle branch ventricular reentrant tachycardia. 3. Patients with sustained monomorphic ventricular tachycardia and an implantable cardioverter-defibrillator who are receiving multiple shocks not manageable by reprogramming or concomitant drug therapy.	Nonsustained ventricular tachycardia that is symptomatic when the tachycardia is drug resistant or when the patient is drug intolerant or does not desire long-term drug therapy.	1. Patients with ventricular tachycardia that is responsive to drug, ICD, or surgical therapy and that therapy is well tolerated and preferable to ablation by the patient. 2. Unstable, or rapid, or multiple, or polymorphic ventricular tachycardia that cannot be adequately localized by present mapping techniques. 3. Asymptomatic and clinically benign nonsustained ventricular tachycardia.

Class I: Conditions for which there is general agreement that the electrophysiological study provides information that is useful and important for patient management. Experts agree that patients with these conditions are likely to benefit from electrophysiological studies.

Class II: Conditions for which electrophysiological studies are frequently performed but there is less certainty regarding the usefulness of the information that is obtained. Experts are divided in their opinion as to whether these conditions are likely to benefit from electrophysiological study.

Class III: Conditions for which there is general agreement that electrophysiological studies do not provide useful information. Experts agree that electrophysiological studies are not warranted in patients with these conditions.

From Zipes, D. P., DiMarco, J. P., Gillette, P. C., et al.: Guidelines for Clinical Intracardiac Electrophysiological Studies and Catheter Ablation Procedures. A report of the American College of Cardiology/American Heart Association Task Force on Practice Guidelines (Subcommittee to Assess Clinical Intracardiac Electrophysiological and Catheter Ablation Procedures). Reprinted with permission from the American College of Cardiology. J. Am. Coll. Cardiol. *26:*555, 1995.

logical studies are not appropriate for asymptomatic patients with mild degrees of AV block who are not likely to warrant pacemaker implantation. According to these guidelines, electrophysiological studies of AV conduction *should* be performed when the relationship between symptoms and AV block has not been proven; in such patients, another arrhythmia could be the cause of symptoms.

CHRONIC INTRAVENTRICULAR CONDUCTION DELAY. Patients with prolonged H-V intervals have an increased risk for developing complete trifascicular block, but the specificity of the H-V interval for predicting the development of complete block among patients with bifascicular block is only about 63 per cent.[101] The use of rapid atrial pacing can improve the specificity of this test, but the annual incidence of progression to complete trifascicular block is low. Therefore, the main role for electrophysiological testing in this population, according to the ACC/AHA guidelines, is not to predict future complications but to determine whether symptoms of arrhythmia are due to conduction delays or some other arrhythmia.

The only Class I (clearly appropriate) indication for electrophysiological testing in patients with intraventricular conduction delays according to the guidelines is in the determination of the cause of symptoms. The guidelines *discourage* the use of electrophysiological testing in asymptomatic patients with conduction system delays.

NARROW AND WIDE COMPLEX QRS TACHYCARDIAS. In narrow QRS tachycardia, the site of abnormal impulse formation or the reentry circuit can be located in the sinus node, the atria, or in the AV node–His bundle axis. The correct diagnosis can often be made using information from the 12-lead surface electrocardiogram, particularly when the electrocardiogram is combined with vagal maneuvers. In contrast, wide QRS tachycardias can be caused by ventricular or supraventricular arrhythmias, and identifying the site of origin of the tachycardia is frequently impossible using electrocardiographic tracings alone. As a result, electrophysiological testing plays different roles in these two types of tachycardias. In patients with *wide complex tachycardias,* electrophysiological testing permits accurate diagnosis in virtually all patients. Because knowledge of the mechanism of the arrhythmia is essential for the selection of the best therapeutic strategy, use of electrophysiological testing is considered appropriate (Class I) by the ACC/AHA task force for diagnosis of wide complex tachycardias. However, when the diagnosis is already clear from other data, electrophysiological testing is unlikely to influence therapy, and these procedures are not generally useful.

In patients with narrow QRS tachycardias, electrophysiological testing is considered more appropriate as a guide to therapy than as a tool for diagnosis. Therefore, the Class I indications for such testing include poorly controlled tachycardia in which data from electrophysiological testing may help clinicians choose among drug therapy, catheter ablation, pacing, and surgery. The ACC/AHA task force, however, does not believe that electrophysiological testing is useful for patients who have narrow complex tachycardias that are well controlled with medications and who are not candidates for nonpharmacological therapy.

OTHER CONDITIONS. Prolonged Q-T Intervals.

The ACC/AHA task force concludes that electrophysiological testing has a limited role in the evaluation of congenital or acquired forms of prolonged Q-T syndrome. The results of such testing have only modest predictive value.[102] Whether catecholamine infusion during testing can unmask patients who are at high risk for complications[103] or whether electrophysiological testing can be used to evaluate proarrhythmic effects[104] in this population is unclear. Therefore, no indication for electrophysiological testing for this problem is clearly appropriate.

Wolff-Parkinson-White Syndrome. Electrophysiological studies can be used in patients with this syndrome to determine the mechanism of arrhythmia, to assess the electrophysiological properties of the accessory pathway, and to evaluate the location and response to drugs of accessory pathways. Therefore, electrophysiological studies are considered appropriate by the ACC/AHA task force for patients who were candidates for catheter or surgical ablation, who have had cardiac arrest or unexplained syncope, or whose management might be altered by knowledge of the electrophysiological properties of the accessory pathway and normal conduction system. For asymptomatic patients, however, electrophysiological testing was deemed inappropriate except in special situations, such as patients with high-risk occupations and those with a family history of sudden cardiac death.

Nonsustained Ventricular Tachycardia. The usefulness of electrophysiological testing is compromised by the lack of therapeutic strategies that have been shown to improve outcome in patients with ventricular premature beats, couplets, and nonsustained ventricular tachycardia. There are no indications in this patient population for which the ACC/AHA task force agreed that electrophysiological testing is clearly useful. Therefore, these tests are considered inappropriate for patients with no symptoms or only mild ones.

Unexplained Syncope. Arrhythmia is an important cause of syncope—and a worrisome prognostic sign in patients with structural heart disease. Therefore, electrophysiological testing is highly useful for evaluation of syncope in this patient population. In contrast, among patients without structural heart disease, an arrhythmic cause of syncope is uncommon, and the yield of electrophysiological testing is low.[105] Consequently the ACC/AHA guidelines recommend a higher threshold for use of electrophysiological testing in patients without known heart disease and suggest that head-up tilt-testing may provide more useful data in this population.

Survivors of Cardiac Arrest. In patients who have survived cardiac arrest, electrophysiological testing is frequently used to assess prognosis and identify drugs that suppress inducible arrhythmia. The assumption that these data can be used to improve patient outcome has been called into question by data from the ESVEM trial.[53] Nevertheless, electrophysiological testing is considered appropriate by the ACC/AHA task force for patients who have survived cardiac arrest without evidence that the event was directly provoked by ischemia or myocardial infarction. These tests are deemed *inappropriate* when the cardiac arrest was closely associated with acute ischemic syndromes or other specific causes.

Unexplained Palpitations. The procedure of choice to determine the cause of palpitations, according to the ACC/AHA guidelines, is ambulatory electrocardiography. Electrophysiological testing should be reserved for patients with associated syncope or those in whom ambulatory electrocardiography has failed to capture a cause of palpitations but who have been noted by medical personnel to have a rapid pulse rate. Electrophysiological testing is of equivocal value in patients whose symptoms are so sporadic that they cannot be documented while ambulatory electrocardiography is being performed.

Appropriateness of Catheter Ablation Procedures

Catheter ablation of the AV junction or accessory pathways is a rapidly advancing technique that has been reviewed in guidelines and position papers from several organizations, including the American Medical Association,[106] the American College of Cardiology,[107] the North American Society of Pacing and Electrophysiology,[108] and an ACC/AHA task force.[100] The ACC/AHA task force identified several conditions for which they consider catheter ablation an appropriate strategy (Table 63–10). The characteristics that are common among appropriate indications include supraventricular arrhythmias that are symptomatic; that cannot be controlled with medications either because of limited effectiveness, side effects, or inconvenience; or that have caused sudden cardiac death. Catheter ablation is also useful for some patients with ventricular tachycardia, although patients with extensive structural heart disease tend to have multiple sites of origin of their arrhythmia and therefore are poor candidates for this procedure.

PACEMAKERS, ANTIARRHYTHMIA DEVICES, AND IMPLANTED AUTOMATIC DEFIBRILLATORS

(See also Chaps. 21 and 23)

INDICATIONS FOR PERMANENT CARDIAC PACING. Cardiac pacemakers are implanted to relieve symptoms and prevent sudden death. These goals are reflected in ACC/AHA guidelines published in 1991,[109] which evaluate potential indications for pacemaker implantation (Table 63–11). For patients with acquired AV block, bifascicular or trifascicular block, or sinus node dysfunction, permanent pacing is considered appropriate when the abnormality causes complications and is not precipitated by a drug that could be discontinued. Examples of complications include symptomatic bradycardia, congestive heart failure, and confusional states. Permanent pacing is also deemed appropriate for asymptomatic patients at high risk for the subsequent development of complications, such as patients with complete heart block and periods of asystole of 3 seconds or more or a slow escape rate or patients with bifascicular or trifascicular block with intermittent second-degree AV block.

Indications for permanent pacing for patients who do not have symptoms or complications are less certain. In asymptomatic patients, complete heart block with a ventricular escape rate of 40 or more beats/min or type II second-degree AV block are considered equivocal (Class II) indications for permanent pacing. Bifascicular or trifascicular block in patients with syncope is also not a clear indication for permanent pacing but is regarded as acceptable if unproven if other possible causes for syncope cannot be identified. Pacemakers are explicitly discouraged for patients with mild asymptomatic conduction abnormalities, such as type I second-degree AV block at the supra-His level; fascicular block with no or only first-degree AV block, and sinus node dysfunction.

Symptoms do not play as important a role in determination of the appropriateness of permanent pacing after acute myocardial infarction because of poor prognosis and the high incidence of sudden death in postinfarction patients with conduction system disturbances. The ACC/AHA task force has emphasized that the requirement for temporary pacing after acute myocardial infarction (see p. 1252) is not in itself an indication for permanent pacing, but it considers pacemakers to be appropriate for patients with persistent advanced-degree AV block or complete heart block with block in the His-Purkinje system. Although the usefulness of permanent pacemakers for patients with advanced block at the AV node is less clear (Class II), permanent

TABLE 63–11   ACC/AHA GUIDELINES FOR IMPLANTATION OF CARDIAC PACEMAKERS AND ANTIARRHYTHMIA DEVICES

SETTING	CLASS I (APPROPRIATE)	CLASS II (EQUIVOCAL)	CLASS III (INAPPROPRIATE)
Permanent pacing in acquired AV block in adults	**A.** Complete heart block, permanent or intermittent, at any anatomical level, associated with any one of the following complications: **1.** Symptomatic bradycardia **2.** Congestive heart failure **3.** Ectopic rhythms and other medical conditions that require drugs that suppress the automaticity of escape pacemakers and result in symptomatic bradycardia. **4.** Documented periods of asystole ≥3.0 sec or any escape rate <40 beats/min in symptom-free patients. **5.** Confusional states that clear with temporary pacing. **6.** Post AV junction ablation, myotonic dystrophy. **B.** 2nd degree AV block, permanent or intermittent, regardless of the type or the site of block, with symptomatic bradycardia. **C.** Atrial fibrillation, atrial flutter or rare cases of supraventricular tachycardia with complete heart block or advanced AV block, bradycardia, and any of the conditions described under A. The bradycardia must be unrelated to digitalis or drugs known to impair AV conduction.	**A.** Asymptomatic complete heart block, permanent or intermittent, at any anatomical site, with ventricular rates of 40 beats/min or faster. **B.** Symptomatic type II second degree AV block, permanent or intermittent. **C.** Asymptomatic type I second degree AV block at intra-His or infra-His levels.	**A.** 1st degree AV block **B.** Asymptomatic type I 2nd degree AV block at the supra-His (AV node) level.
Permanent pacing after myocardial infarction	**A.** Persistent advanced 2nd degree AV block or complete heart block after acute myocardial infarction with block in the His-Purkinje system (bilateral bundle branch block). **B.** Patients with transient advanced AV block and associated bundle branch block.	Patients with persistent advanced AV block at the AV node.	**A.** Transient AV conduction disturbances in absence of intraventricular conduction defects. **B.** Transient AV block in the presence of isolated left anterior hemiblock. **C.** Acquired left anterior hemiblock in absence of AV block. **D.** Patients with persistent 1st degree AV block in the presence of bundle branch block not demonstrated previously.
Permanent pacing in bifascicular and trifascicular block	**A.** Bifascicular block with intermittent complete heart block associated with symptomatic bradycardia. **B.** Bifascicular or trifascicular block with intermittent type II second degree AV block without symptoms attributable to the heart block.	**A.** Bifascicular or trifascicular block with syncope not proved to be due to complete heart block, but other possible causes for syncope are not identifiable. **B.** Markedly prolonged HV (>100 msec). **C.** Pacing-induced infra-His block.	**A.** Fascicular block without AV block or symptoms. **B.** Fascicular block with 1st degree AV block without symptoms.
Permanent pacing in sinus node dysfunction	Sinus node dysfunction with documented symptomatic bradycardia.	Sinus node dysfunction, occurring spontaneously as a result of necessary drug therapy, with heart rates <40 beats/min when a clear association between significant symptoms consistent with bradycardia and the actual presence of bradycardia has not been documented.	**A.** Sinus node dysfunction in asymptomatic patients, including those in whom substantial sinus bradycardia (heart rate <40 beats/min) is a consequence of long-term drug treatment. **B.** Sinus node dysfunction in patients in whom symptoms suggestive of bradycardia are clearly documented not to be associated with a slow heart rate.

SETTING	CLASS I (APPROPRIATE)	CLASS II (EQUIVOCAL)	CLASS III (INAPPROPRIATE)
Permanent pacing in hypersensitive carotid sinus and neurovascular syndromes	Recurrent syncope associated with clear, spontaneous events provoked by carotid sinus stimulation; minimal carotid sinus pressure induces asystole of >3 sec duration in the absence of any medication that depresses the sinus node or AV conduction.	A. Recurrent syncope without clear provocative events and with a hypersensitive cardioinhibitory response. B. Syncope with associated bradycardia reproduced by a head-up tilt with or without isoproterenol or other forms of provocative maneuvers and in which a temporary pacemaker and a second provocative test can establish the likely benefits of a permanent pacemaker.	A. A hyperactive cardioinhibitory response to carotid sinus stimulation in the absence of symptoms. B. Vague symptoms (e.g., dizziness or lightheadedness or both) with a hyperactive cardioinhibitory response to carotid sinus stimulation. C. Recurrent syncope, lightheadedness, or dizziness in the absence of a cardioinhibitory response.
Pacing for tachyarrhythmia Permanent pacemakers that automatically detect and pace to terminate tachycardias	A. Symptomatic recurrent supraventricular tachycardia when drugs fail to control arrhythmia or produce intolerable side effects. B. Symptomatic recurrent ventricular tachycardia after an automatic defibrillator has been implanted or incorporated in the device and recurrence of ventricular tachycardia is not prevented by drug therapy or when no other therapy is applicable.	Recurrent supraventricular tachycardia as an alternative to drug therapy.	A. Tachycardias accelerated or converted to fibrillation by pacing. B. The presence of accessory pathways having the capacity for rapid anterograde conduction whether or not the pathways participate in the mechanism of the tachycardia.
Pacing for tachyarrhythmia Externally manually activated antitachyarrhythmia devices that act to terminate tachycardia	Recurrent, symptomatic ventricular tachycardia uncontrolled by drugs when surgery, catheter ablation, or the implantation of an automatic pacemaker or cardioverter-defibrillator is not indicated.	None	Recurrent tachycardia that produces syncope.
Pacing for tachyarrhythmia Overdrive or atrial synchronous ventricular pacemakers intended to prevent tachycardia occurrence	Atrioventricular reentrant or AV node reentrant supraventricular tachycardia unresponsive to medical therapy.	A. Sustained ventricular tachycardia in other conditions when all other therapies are ineffective or inapplicable and efficacy of pacing is thoroughly documented. B. Long Q-T syndrome	A. Frequent or complex ventricular ectopic activity without sustained ventricular tachycardia associated with coronary artery disease, cardiomyopathy, mitral valve prolapse; or a normal heart and in the absence of long Q-T syndrome. B. Long Q-T syndrome due to remediable causes.
Implantation of automatic defibrillator devices	A. One or more documented episodes of hemodynamically significant ventricular tachycardia or ventricular fibrillation in a patient in whom electrophysiological testing and ambulatory monitoring cannot be used to accurately predict efficacy of therapy. B. One or more documented episodes of hemodynamically significant ventricular tachycardia or ventricular fibrillation in a patient in whom no drug was found to be effective or no drug currently available and appropriate was tolerated. C. Continued inducibility at electrophysiological study of hemodynamically significant ventricular tachycardia or ventricular fibrillation despite the best available drug therapy or despite surgery or catheter ablation if drug therapy has failed.	A. One or more documented episodes of hemodynamically significant ventricular tachycardia or ventricular fibrillation in a patient in whom drug efficacy testing is possible. B. Recurrent syncope of undetermined origin in a patient with hemodynamically significant ventricular tachycardia or ventricular fibrillation induced at electrophysiological study in whom no effective or no tolerated drug is available or appropriate.	A. Recurrent syncope of undetermined cause in a patient without inducible tachyarrhythmias. B. Arrhythmias not due to hemodynamically significant ventricular tachycardia or ventricular fibrillation. C. Incessant ventricular tachycardia or fibrillation.
Single-chamber pacemakers Atrial-AAI	Symptomatic sinus node dysfunction (sick sinus syndrome), provided AV conduction is shown to be adequate by appropriate studies.	Hemodynamic enhancement through rate adjustment in patients with bradycardia and symptoms of impaired cardiac output, provided AV conduction is shown to be adequate by appropriate tests.	A. Preexisting AV conduction delay or block or if decremental AV conduction is demonstrated by appropriate tests. B. Inadequate intracavitary atrial complexes.

Table continues on the following page

TABLE 63–11 ACC/AHA GUIDELINES FOR IMPLANTATION OF CARDIAC PACEMAKERS AND ANTIARRHYTHMIA DEVICES—*Continued*

SETTING	CLASS I (APPROPRIATE)	CLASS II (EQUIVOCAL)	CLASS III (INAPPROPRIATE)
Single-chamber pacemakers Ventricular-VVI	Any symptomatic bradyarrhythmia but particularly when there is: 1. No significant atrial hemodynamic contribution (persistent or paroxysmal atrial flutter/fibrillation, giant atria). 2. No evidence of pacemaker syndrome due to loss of atrial contribution or negative atrial kick.	Symptomatic bradycardia where pacing simplicity is a prime concern in cases of: 1. Senility (for life-sustaining purposes only) 2. Terminal disease 3. Domicile remote from a follow-up center 4. Absent retrograde ventriculoatrial (VA) conduction	A. Known pacemaker syndrome or symptoms produced by temporary ventricular pacing at the time of initial pacemaker implantation. B. The need for maximum atrial contribution because of 1. Congestive heart failure 2. Special need for rate response
Dual-chamber pacemakers VDD	Requirements for ventricular pacing when adequate atrial rates and adequate intracavitary atrial complexes are present. This includes the presence of complete AV block when: A. Atrial contribution is needed for hemodynamic benefit. B. Pacemaker syndrome had existed or is anticipated.	Normal sinus rhythm and normal AV conduction in patients needing ventricular pacing intermittently.	A. Frequent or persistent supraventricular tachyarrhythmias, including atrial fibrillation or flutter. B. Inadequate intracavitary atrial complexes. C. Intact VA conduction.
Dual-chamber pacemakers DVI	A. The need for synchronous atrial-ventricular contraction in symptomatic bradycardia and a slow atrial rate. B. Previously documented pacemaker syndromes.	A. Frequent supraventricular arrhythmias in which combined pacing and drugs have been shown to be therapeutically effective. B. Bradycardia-tachycardia syndrome, provided adjustment of atrial rate and AV interval terminates or prevents the emergence of supraventricular arrhythmias with or without concomitant drug administration.	Frequent or persistent supraventricular tachyarrhythmias, including atrial fibrillation or flutter.
Dual-chamber pacemakers DDD	Requirement for AV synchrony over a wide range of rates such as A. The active or young patient with atrial rates responsive to clinical need. B. Significant hemodynamic need. C. Pacemaker syndrome during previous pacemaker experience or a reduction in systolic blood pressure >20 mm Hg during ventricular pacing at the time of pacemaker implantation (with or without evidence of VA conduction).	A. Complete heart block or sick syndrome and stable atrial rates. B. When simultaneous control of atrial and ventricular rates can be shown to inhibit tachyarrhythmias or when the pacemaker can be adjusted to a mode designed to interrupt the arrhythmia.	A. Frequent or persistent supraventricular tachyarrhythmias, including atrial fibrillation or flutter. B. Inadequate intracavitary atrial complexes. C. Angina pectoris aggravated by rapid heart rates.

Class I: Conditions for which there is general agreement that permanent pacemakers or antitachycardia devices should be implanted, or that a mode of pacing is appropriate.

Class II: Conditions for which permanent pacemakers or antitachycardia devices are frequently used but there is divergence of opinion with respect to the necessity of their insertion, or for which a given mode of pacing may be used but there is divergence of opinion with respect to the necessity of that mode of pacing.

Class III: Conditions for which there is general agreement that pacemakers or antitachycardia devices are unnecessary or that such a mode of pacing is inappropriate.

From Dreifus, L. S., Fisch, C., Griffin, J. C., et al.: Guidelines for implantation of cardiac pacemakers and antiarrhythmia devices. A report of the American College of Cardiology/American Heart Association Task Force on Assessment of Diagnostic and Therapeutic Cardiovascular Procedures (Committee on Pacemaker Implantation). Reprinted with permission from the American College of Cardiology. J. Am. Coll. Cardiol. *18*:1, 1991.

Addenda

Atrial-AAI: Atrial pacing inhibited by sensed atrial activity

Ventricular-VVI: The classic prototypical pacing mode; ventricular pacing inhibited by sensed spontaneous ventricular activity.

VDD: Ventricular pacing in synchrony with sensed atrial activity inhibited by sensed ventricular activity.

DVI: Pacing of both chambers at a preselected rate with both outputs inhibited by ventricular but not atrial complexes.

DDD: Pacing of both chambers, sensing of both chambers, inhibition of atrial or ventricular output by sensed atrial or ventricular activity; triggering of ventricular output by sensed atrial activity.

pacing is discouraged if the sole indication is transient AV conduction disturbances or left anterior hemiblock.

The ACC/AHA guidelines also define explicit criteria for appropriateness of permanent pacing in patients with hypersensitive carotid sinus and neurovascular syndromes. The only Class I indication is recurrent syncope associated with clear, spontaneous events provoked by carotid sinus stimulation. In such patients, minimal carotid sinus pressure should induce asystole of 3 seconds or more in the absence of medications that depress the sinus node.

ANTITACHYCARDIA DEVICES. Antitachycardia devices include permanent pacemakers that can be programed to interrupt reentrant arrhythmias or prevent their occurrence, and automatic defibrillator devices. The ACC/AHA guidelines stress that these devices should be implanted only after careful evaluation by experienced electrophysiologists.

Permanent pacemakers are recommended for use for recurrent supraventricular tachycardias in symptomatic patients whose arrhythmias cannot be controlled with drug therapy. For patients with symptomatic ventricular tachycardia, permanent pacemakers are considered appropriate only after an automatic defibrillator has been implanted, and symptoms cannot be controlled by drug therapy. If such patients remain symptomatic even after a permanent pacemaker has been implanted, use of an externally manually activated antitachycardia device is considered appropriate. These devices are considered inappropriate in settings in which pacing might lead to complications such as conversion of a tachyarrhythmia to fibrillation.

The threshold for implanting automatic defibrillator devices has been decreasing because of three major developments: disappointing data on the lack of beneficial impact on survival of antiarrhythmic medications; inability of ambulatory electrocardiographic monitoring or electrophysiological testing data to predict subsequent efficacy of therapy[53]; and the availability of new defibrillator systems that do not require a thoracotomy for implantation. Because of rapid evolution and the promise of this technique, the ACC/AHA task force defined indications that it termed fairly liberal, implying an expectation that the range of appropriate indications for these devices will continue to expand. However, the task force stressed that patients should not be considered for an automatic defibrillator unless they have experienced an arrhythmia that has been demonstrated to be life threatening by producing sudden death, syncope, or severe hemodynamic compromise. Furthermore, remedial causes of the arrhythmia such as drugs, electrolyte imbalances, or ischemia must be excluded.

A special case directly addressed by the ACC/AHA task force is that of the patient who has been resuscitated from a documented sudden death episode who does not have an inducible arrhythmia during subsequent electrophysiological testing. The guidelines consider an automatic defibrillator appropriate (Class I) in such patients even if electrophysiological testing and ambulatory monitoring cannot be used to predict the efficacy of the therapy. Because the ability of such tests to predict drug efficacy is in question,[53] future guidelines might consider automatic defibrillators appropriate for most patients who have documented hemodynamically significant sustained ventricular tachycardia or ventricular fibrillation. However, these devices are not considered appropriate for patients who have these arrhythmias incessantly, because of the intolerable effects of repeated discharges of the defibrillators.

CHOICE OF PACING MODE AND DEVICE. Clinicians can choose among several types of pacemakers and modes of pacing to seek the best functional outcome for patients. However, the costs for different types of pacemakers vary markedly, and pacemakers that adapt their rate in response to physical, chemical, or other stimuli are particularly expensive. Therefore, ACC/AHA guidelines seek to identify patients most likely to benefit from the more advanced techniques. A key unresolved issue in this effort is whether dual-chamber pacing can increase life expectancy by decreasing the incidence of atrial fibrillation and stroke. Research to address this issue is currently under way, and, if dual-chamber pacing is found to improve survival, the indications for its use can be expected to broaden considerably.

The ACC/AHA guidelines recommend that the decision between pacemakers with and without adaptive rate functions be based on factors including the nature of the conduction abnormality, comorbid medical conditions, presence of coronary heart disease and angina, degree of left ventricular dysfunction, impact of drug therapy, level of anticipated activity, availability of support services, expertise of implant teams, and costs. The primary goal of adaptive-rate pacemakers is to permit the heart rate to increase in the absence of an appropriate spontaneous rise in heart rate; the definition of chronotropic incompetence used by this group is failure of the heart rate to reach 100 beats/min in response to an exercise test. In general, adaptive-rate pacemakers are recommended for patients with an anticipated moderate to high level of physical activity but are contraindicated in settings in which they might precipitate tachyarrhythmias via retrograde VA conduction or aggravate angina pectoris or congestive heart failure.

Single-chamber pacing is recommended by the ACC/AHA task force as a "default" for patients with symptomatic bradyarrhythmias that are not due to medications or other reversible causes. Ventricular single-chamber pacing is considered particularly appropriate when there is no significant atrial hemodynamic contribution, as is the case in patients with atrial flutter or fibrillation. Ventricular pacing is also recommended for patients without evidence of "pacemaker syndrome," which includes lightheadedness, syncope, episodic weakness, inadequate cardiac output, or patient awareness of beat-to-beat variation in cardiac contractile sequence related to absence of AV asynchrony.

When patients have a high likelihood of benefiting from AV synchrony and single-chamber atrial pacing cannot achieve that goal, dual-chamber pacing is appropriate. The choice among various dual-chamber pacing modes should be made by an experienced pacemaker specialist, but the ACC/AHA guidelines emphasize that patients with frequent or persistent supraventricular tachyarrhythmias, including atrial fibrillation, are generally inappropriate choices for these devices.

CLINICAL SYNDROMES

ACUTE CHEST PAIN

(See also Chap. 37)

In patients with acute myocardial infarction who are discharged from the emergency department the short-term mortality is about 25 per cent—about double what might be expected with inpatient care.[110] As a result, missed myocardial infarctions are the greatest source of dollar losses in emergency department malpractice cases,[111] and admission of patients with myocardial infarction to a coronary care unit or intermediate care unit where they undergo electrocardiographic monitoring is generally considered an accepted standard of care.[112] Researchers have studied a wide range of issues related to increasing the efficiency of management of this patient population, including the development of decision aids,[112-116] the use of intermediate care units and special chest pain evaluation units for patients who are at low risk of needing the facilities and personnel of a coronary care unit,[117-121] shorter "rule-out" protocols for low-risk patients,[122] and the early use of diagnostic techniques for risk stratification.[123-126]

The major emphasis from this recent research is rapid identification of which patients are *safe* for discharge; however, a risk that is inherent in any strategy that seeks to accomplish earlier discharges and shorter lengths of hospital stay is that patients with unstable ischemic syndromes might suffer preventable complications. Many standards for the initial evaluation and subsequent management aimed at reducing that risk for patients with chest pain are addressed in guidelines developed by a multidisciplinary panel sponsored by the Agency for Health Care Policy and Research (AHCPR).[12] The recommendations regarding the entry of the patient with chest pain into medical care include:

1. The initial evaluation of symptoms that suggest a possible acute ischemic syndrome should not be carried out over the telephone but in a facility equipped to perform electrocardiography.

2. Patients with duration of symptoms longer than 20 minutes, hemodynamic instability, or recent loss of consciousness should generally be referred to an emergency department (as opposed to an outpatient office).

Emergency Department Evaluation

Standards of care of the initial evaluation in the patient with acute chest pain are provided in a "policy statement" issued by the American College of Emergency Physicians (ACEP) in 1990 and revised in 1995[127] (Table 63–12). The statement stresses that the decision to admit the patient must be based primarily on clinical judgment. This policy statement does not make recommendations about levels of care (coronary care unit versus intermediate care or chest pain unit) for different patient subsets.

The ACEP statement provide "rules" and "guidelines" about the data that should be obtained and recorded as part of the evaluation and the actions that should follow from certain findings. *Rules* are considered actions that reflect principles of good practice in most situations. When circumstances dictate that these rules cannot be followed, the ACEP statement asserts, the deviation from the rule should be justified in writing. *Guidelines* in the ACEP document are actions that should be considered but are not always followed; there is no implication that failure to follow a guideline is improper care.

The ACEP policy indicates that routine evaluation of nontraumatic chest pain should include a history that obtains data on character of pain, age, associated symptoms, and past history. The physical examination should include vital signs, a cardiovascular examination, and a pulmonary examination. Recommendations and rules for what tests should be performed—and initial responses to some data—are summarized in Table 63–12. An electrocardiogram is recommended for men over 33 years of age, women over age 40, and patients with risk factors for coronary disease,

but the electrocardiogram is considered standard care (i.e., a rule) for patients with a prior history of coronary disease.

The National Heart Attack Alert Program (NHAAP) report also includes guidelines for specific functions related to evaluation and treatment in patients with chest pain; they are aimed at improving the speed with which patients with acute myocardial infarction are identified and treated,[95] including recommendations for which patient subsets should be placed on the acute myocardial infarction protocol. For registration staff, the NHAAP guidelines recommend that patients over age 30 with the following chief complaints receive immediate assessment by the triage nurse and be referred for further evaluation:

- Chest pain, pressure, tightness, or heaviness. Radiating pain in neck, jaw, shoulders, back, or one or both arms
- Indigestion or "heartburn"/nausea and/or vomiting
- Persistent shortness of breath
- Weakness, dizziness, lightheadedness, loss of consciousness

The triage nurse should immediately assess patients for initiation of the myocardial infarction protocol and obtain an electrocardiogram if they have any of the following:

- Chest pain
- Associated dyspnea
- Associated nausea/vomiting
- Associated diaphoresis

For physicians, the NHAAP guidelines offer several clinical recommendations and explicitly note that use of a "GI cocktail" (usually including an antacid) as a diagnostic test to differentiate between gastrointestinal and cardiac causes of the patient's symptoms is "inappropriate," because it frequently leads to erroneous conclusions.

Initial Triage and Management

The actions in response to the data that are collected during this evaluation are intended to lead to timely care for patients with acute myocardial infarction, unstable an-

TABLE 63–12 EVALUATION OF ACUTE CHEST PAIN; EXCERPTS FROM THE CLINICAL POLICY OF THE AMERICAN COLLEGE OF EMERGENCY PHYSICIANS (ACEP)

VARIABLE	FINDING	RULE (STANDARD)	GUIDELINE (RECOMMENDED)
Pain	Ongoing and severe and crushing and substernal or same as previous pain diagnosed as myocardial infarction.	IV access Supplemental oxygen ECG Aspirin Nitrates Management of ongoing pain Admit	Serum cardiac markers Chest X-ray Anticoagulation
	Severe or pressure or substernal or exertional or radiating to jaw, neck, shoulder, or arm.	ECG	IV access Supplemental oxygen Cardiac monitor Serum cardiac markers Chest X-ray Nitrates Management of ongoing pain Admit
	Tearing, severe, radiating to back	Large-bore IV access Supplemental oxygen Cardiac monitor Chest X-ray ECG	Differential upper extremity blood pressures Aortic imaging Management of ongoing pain Admit
	Similar to that of previous pulmonary embolus	IV access Supplemental oxygen Cardiac monitor ABG and oximetry Anticoagulation Pulmonary vascular imaging ECG	Chest X-ray Admit

TABLE 63–12 EVALUATION OF ACUTE CHEST PAIN; EXCERPTS FROM THE CLINICAL POLICY OF THE AMERICAN COLLEGE OF EMERGENCY PHYSICIANS (ACEP)—*Continued*

1969

Ch 63

VARIABLE	FINDING	RULE (STANDARD)	GUIDELINE (RECOMMENDED)
	Indigestion or burning epigastric	None	ECG
	Pleuritic	None	Chest X-ray ECG
Age	Male > 33 years Female > 40 years	None	ECG
Associated symptoms	Syncope or near-syncope	ECG	Cardiac monitor Hct.
	Shortness of breath, dyspnea on exertion, paroxysmal nocturnal dyspnea, or orthopnea	ECG	ABG/oximetry Chest X-ray
Past medical history	Previous myocardial infarction, coronary artery bypass surgery, angioplasty, cocaine use within last 96 hours, previous positive cardiac diagnostic studies	ECG	
	Major risk factors for coronary artery disease		ECG
Assessment	Unstable angina—new-onset, exertional	ECG, aspirin	IV access Supplemental oxygen Cardiac monitor Nitrates Consult/Admit
	Unstable angina—Ongoing or recurrent ischemia ECG showing new ST-segment depressions or T-wave inversions consistent with ischemia	IV access Supplemental oxygen Cardiac monitor Anticoagulation Aspirin Nitrates Management of ongoing pain Admit	Serial serum cardiac markers Chest X-ray Cardiac imaging Serial ECGs Beta blockers
	High clinical suspicion of myocardial infarction with nondiagnostic ECG	IV access Supplemental oxygen Cardiac monitor Anticoagulation Aspirin Nitrates Management of ongoing pain Admit	Serial serum cardiac markers Chest X-ray Cardiac imaging Serial ECGs Magnesium therapy Beta blockers
	High clinical suspicion of myocardial infarction with diagnostic ECG or bundle branch block	IV access Supplemental oxygen Cardiac monitor Anticoagulation Assessment for thrombolytic therapy or other reperfusion techniques Anticoagulation Aspirin Nitrates Management of ongoing pain Admit	Serial serum cardiac markers Chest X-ray Cardiac imaging Serial ECGs Magnesium therapy if not given thrombolytics Beta blockers
	Aortic dissection	Large-bore IV access Supplemental oxygen Cardiac monitor Blood type and crossmatch ECG Management of blood pressure/cardiac contractility Management of ongoing pain Immediate surgical consultation Admit	Aortic imaging
	Pericarditis/myocarditis	ECG	Serum cardiac markers Chest X-ray/echocardiography Consult/admit

From American College of Emergency Physicians. Clinical policy for the initial approach to adults presenting with a chief complaint of chest pain, with no history of trauma. Ann. Emerg. Med. *25*:274, 1995.

gina, aortic dissection, and pulmonary embolus. Patients with possible or probable acute myocardial infarction as suggested by the description of their pain or electrocardiographic findings are expected to be admitted and receive interventions, including aspirin, nitrates, and—in the presence of ST-segment elevation on the electrocardiogram—anticoagulation, thrombolysis, and/or other therapy aimed at achieving reperfusion.

Performance of electrocardiography and initiation of aspirin therapy are strongly recommended for patients with new-onset angina that is exertional, but admission is not considered mandatory in the ACEP policy statement. The AHCPR guidelines also indicate that not all patients with unstable angina require admission but recommend that patients with unstable angina be monitored electrocardiographically during their evaluation and that those with ongoing rest pain should be placed at bed rest during the initial phase of stabilization[12] (see p. 1336).

Admission should be considered but is also not a rule for pericarditis and myocarditis. The ACEP policy statement indicates that patients who are discharged should be provided a referral for follow-up care and instructions regarding treatment and circumstances that require a return to the emergency department.

The ACEP policy statement includes in its appendix forms that can be used to assess compliance with their rules and to remind clinicians of their content.

ACUTE MYOCARDIAL INFARCTION

(See also Chap. 37)

Advances in the treatment of acute myocardial infarction have accelerated in recent years, with a particularly intense focus on the beneficial impact of thrombolytic therapy and percutaneous transluminal angioplasty in the early hours after the onset of infarction. Recent research, however, has also provided important insights into the limitations of interventions such as routine performance of angioplasty after myocardial infarction. To define practice patterns likely to achieve the optimal patient outcomes without subjecting patients to unnecessary procedures, guidelines for the management of acute myocardial infarction have been developed by the National Heart Attack Alert Program (NHAAP)[128] and an ACC/AHA task force.[129] These guidelines have complementary focuses: The NHAAP guidelines define a goal for time-to-treatment with thrombolytic therapy and provide practical strategies for reaching that goal. These recommendations from the NHAAP are essentially a "critical path" for treatment of acute myocardial infarction that defines time frames for the performance of specific tasks. The ACC/AHA task force examines a range of interventions that might be considered for patients with acute myocardial infarction and classifies them according to their appropriateness.

DIAGNOSIS OF MYOCARDIAL INFARCTION. Several alternative markers for myocardial injury are now available, but the ACC/AHA guidelines recommend basing the diagnosis of myocardial infarction upon creatine kinase (CK) -MB determinations in combination with serial electrocardiograms and a chest X-ray study. According to these guidelines, electrocardiograms should be obtained daily until the nature of evolution of the infarction is clear, and longer if patients have complications. Sampling of total CK and CK-MB is recommended at 6-hour intervals for the first 24 hours, and then daily until the diagnosis is established. Routine use of other enzyme assays, such as lactate dehydrogenase, is not recommended. The AHCPR guidelines for unstable angina[12] (see Tables 63–15, 63–16 and 63–17) offer slightly different, but qualitatively similar, recommendations:

> Total CK and CK-MB measured every 6 to 8 hours for the first 24 hours

Serial lactate dehydrogenase (LDH) isoenzymes should be considered for patients presenting 24 to 72 hours after symptom onset if CK and CK-MB levels are normal.

More conservative recommendations for the use of cardiac enzyme assays are endorsed by the American College of Physicians.[130] These guidelines recommend a sampling interval of 12 hours, and do not support measurement of cardiac enzymes each day or until abnormal levels return to baseline. However, patients with unstable angina or electrocardiographic changes suggestive of active ischemic syndromes have a higher probability of acute myocardial infarction than the general population of patients with acute chest pain, and a strategy with increased frequency of enzyme sampling that is more sensitive for detecting CK-MB elevations is reasonable for a higher-risk population.

Initial Triage and Use of Thrombolytic Therapy

The NHAAP was initiated by the National Heart, Lung, and Blood Institute to promote rapid identification and treatment of acute myocardial infarction. The multidisciplinary expert panel examined the factors responsible for delay in administration of thrombolytic therapy and focused its main recommendations on decreasing the time between the patient's presentation at the hospital and the administration of thrombolytic therapy to 30 minutes or less. This target is similar to the 30- to 60-minute goal recommended by the American Heart Association.[131] The long-range goal of the NHAAP is to decrease the time from onset of symptoms to treatment to 60 minutes, but that effort will require community interventions that lead to earlier presentation to the hospital of patients with myocardial infarction.

Although these time targets have been described as guidelines, they more appropriately might be called recommended goals. Administration of thrombolytic therapy *more* than 30 minutes after presentation of a patient with acute myocardial infarction would not represent a deviation from a guideline or a variation from the standard of care. These time goals are instead intended to be used by institutions to understand whether they need to improve their system of care. To achieve this goal, the NHAAP recommends measuring the time at which four specific events occur for patients with acute myocardial infarction:

1. Presentation to the emergency department
2. Recording of the electrocardiogram
3. Decision whether to administer thrombolytic therapy
4. Actual infusion of the thrombolytic agent

These four time points can be used to define three intervals. In one multicenter thrombolytic trial, the median time from emergency department arrival to recording the electrocardiogram was 6 minutes; from recording the electrocardiogram to decision to use thrombolytic therapy, 20 minutes; from decision to drug administration, 20 minutes.[132]

Another crucial issue is who gives the order to administer thrombolytic therapy. ACEP guidelines recommend that emergency department physicians be given the authority to administer thrombolytic therapy.[127]

ELIGIBILITY FOR THROMBOLYTIC THERAPY. Eligibility criteria for administration of thrombolytic therapy according to the NHAAP guidelines are presented in Table 63–13. Similar criteria are endorsed by the AHCPR guidelines for unstable angina.[12] The eligibility criteria supported by the ACC/AHA task force[129] (see Table 63–14) recommend a lower threshold for administration of thrombolytic therapy for patients less than age 70 years and for those presenting in less than 6 hours after the onset of pain. There was little support for the use of thrombolytic therapy more than 6 hours after the onset of symptoms in these 1990 guidelines. Since then, a meta-analysis of studies of thrombolytic therapy concluded that mortality rates were significantly re-

1. ELIGIBILITY CRITERIA

Clinical:
Chest pain or chest-pain-equivalent syndrome consistent with acute myocardial infarction ≤ 12 hours from symptom onset with:

ECG
- ≥ 1 mm ST elevation in ≥ 2 contiguous limb leads
- ≥ 2 mm ST elevation in ≥ 2 contiguous precordial leads
- New bundle branch block

Cardiogenic shock: emergency catheterization and revascularization if possible; consider thrombolysis if catheterization not immediately available.

2. CONTRAINDICATIONS

Absolute contraindications
- Altered consciousness
- Active internal bleeding
- Known spinal cord or cerebral arteriovenous malformation or tumor
- Recent head trauma
- Known previous hemorrhagic cerebrovascular accident
- Intracranial or intraspinal surgery within 2 months
- Trauma or surgery within 2 weeks, which could result in bleeding in a closed space
- Persistent blood pressure > 200/120 mm Hg
- Known bleeding disorder
- Pregnancy
- Suspected aortic dissection
- Previous allergy to streptokinase (but not a contraindication to use of other thrombolytic agents)

Relative contraindications
- Active peptic ulcer disease
- History of ischemic or embolic cerebrovascular accident
- Current use of oral anticoagulants
- Major trauma or surgery > 2 weeks, < 2 months
- History of chronic, uncontrolled hypertension (diastolic > 100 mm Hg), treated or untreated
- Subclavian or internal jugular venous cannulation

From National Heart Attack Alert Program Coordinating Committee 60 Minutes to Treatment Working Group. Emergency Department: Rapid Identification and Treatment of Patients with Acute Myocardial Infarction. NIH Publication No. 93-3278. Washington, D.C., National Heart, Lung and Blood Institute, Public Health Service, U.S. Department of Health and Human Services, Sept. 1993.

duced by this therapy for patients treated 7 to 12 hours after the onset of symptoms (11.1 versus 12.7 per cent), while the difference was not significant for patients treated 13 to 24 hours after onset of symptoms.[133]

The NHAAP contraindications to thrombolytic therapy[128] (Table 63–13) are similar to those noted by the ACC/AHA task force,[129] which also include as absolute contraindications prolonged or traumatic cardiopulmonary resuscitation and diabetic hemorrhagic retinopathy or other hemorrhagic ophthalmic condition. Significant liver dysfunction is included as a relative contraindication to thrombolytic therapy by the ACC/AHA guidelines.

Both NHAAP and ACC/AHA guidelines were written before the publication of the Global Utilization of Streptokinase and Tissue Plasminogen Activator for Occluded Coronary Arteries (GUSTO) study, which demonstrated a 1 per cent reduction in mortality for patients treated with accelerated tissue plasminogen activator (t-PA) versus streptokinase.[134] Two 1995 cost-effectiveness analyses based on data from GUSTO concluded that the cost-effectiveness of t-PA compares favorably with that of other accepted medical interventions.[135,136] Therefore, future guidelines may directly comment on the choice between these two agents.

Other Specific Interventions

ACC/AHA guidelines addressing several specific interventions often used for treatment of acute myocardial infarction were first published in 1990 and were undergoing revision in 1996. Like most ACC/AHA guidelines, the 1990 recommendations identify class I (appropriate) and class III (inappropriate) indications, but divide the class II interventions, which are considered acceptable but of uncertain efficacy, into two subclasses. Class IIa interventions are those for which the weight of evidence is in favor of their usefulness; Class IIb interventions are those that are not well established by evidence, may be useful, and probably are not harmful. Recommendations for interventions are summarized in Table 63–14.

ELECTROCARDIOGRAPHIC MONITORING. The duration of electrocardiographic monitoring in patients with uncomplicated myocardial infarction is a major determinant of cost, since the need for monitoring often dictates the level of care (and intensity of nursing) for the patient. The ACC/AHA guidelines recommend 48 to 72 hours of electrocardiographic monitoring, with longer periods for patients who have hemodynamic, ischemic, or arrhythmic complications. These guidelines consider 12 to 36 hours of monitoring appropriate for patients who are admitted with suspected myocardial infarction. Recent research indicates that shorter periods are safe for selected low-risk patients[120,125]; hence this guideline should not be interpreted as indicating that monitoring periods of 12 hours or more to "rule out" myocardial infarction are mandatory for all patients who are admitted.

HEMODYNAMIC MONITORING. Although hemodynamic monitoring with a balloon flotation right-heart catheter and/or arterial pressure line can provide useful data for management of patients with hypotension and other hemodynamic complications, both of these interventions are associated with a risk of vascular complications. Therefore, the ACC/AHA guidelines do not support use of hemodynamic monitoring in patients who are hemodynamically stable. Balloon flotation right-heart catheters are considered possibly useful (Class IIb) for patients with evidence of mild pulmonary congestion and probably useful (Class IIa) for patients with hypotension not responding to fluid administration, even in the absence of evidence of pulmonary congestion. Use of an arterial line is considered appropriate (Class I) or usually indicated (Class IIa) in patients receiving vasopressor, vasodilator, or inotropic agents.

LIDOCAINE. Lidocaine is the drug of choice for management of ventricular arrhythmias after acute myocardial infarction, but trials have failed to demonstrate that this therapy reduces overall mortality.[137] Furthermore, lidocaine can cause side effects, including sinus arrest and central nervous system depression. Therefore, the ACC/AHA guide-

Text continues on page 1978

TABLE 63–14 ACC/AHA GUIDELINES FOR THE EARLY MANAGEMENT OF ACUTE MYOCARDIAL INFARCTION

ISSUE	CLASS I—USUALLY INDICATED	CLASS II—ACCEPTABLE, OF UNCERTAIN EFFICACY		CLASS III—NOT INDICATED
		A. Evidence Favors Efficacy	B. Not Well Established By Evidence	
Atropine use in first 6 to 8 hours after onset of myocardial infarction	**1.** Sinus bradycardia with evidence of low cardiac output and peripheral hypoperfusion or frequent premature ventricular contractions at onset of symptoms of acute myocardial infarction. **2.** Acute inferior infarction with symptomatic type I 2nd degree AV block. **3.** Bradycardia and hypotension after nitroglycerin administration. **4.** For nausea and vomiting associated with morphine administration. **5.** Asystole	**1.** Administration concomitantly with (before or after) morphine in the presence of sinus bradycardia, even without evidence of low cardiac output or peripheral hypoperfusion. **2.** Asymptomatic patients with inferior infarction and type I 2nd degree heart block or 3rd degree heart block at the level of the AV node (see Class III-2.)	None	**1.** Sinus bradycardia >40 beats/min without signs or symptoms of hypoperfusion or frequent premature ventricular contractions. **2.** AV block at the His-Purkinje level (i.e., type II AV block and 3rd degree AV block with new wide QRS complex).
Electrocardiographic monitoring	**1.** Patients with acute myocardial infarction during the initial 48 to 72 hours. **2.** Patients >72 hours after acute myocardial infarction who have hemodynamic instability, persistent ischemia, or arrhythmia. **3.** Patients with suspected myocardial infarction ("rule out" myocardial infarction) during the initial 12 to 36 hours. **4.** Patients who have a temporary transvenous pacemaker.	**1.** Patients >72 hours after acute myocardial infarction with a high likelihood of intermittent ischemia or complex ventricular arrhythmias. **2.** Patients with chest pain in whom there is a low likelihood of myocardial infarction.	Monitoring >72 hours after myocardial infarction, particularly if the patient has undergone thrombolysis or angioplasty.	Patients with or without known heart disease in whom there is no evidence of myocardial ischemia, recent infarction, or arrhythmia.
Right heart catheterization	**1.** Severe or progressive congestive heart failure. **2.** Cardiogenic shock or progressive hypotension. **3.** Mechanical complications of acute infarction, such as a ventricular septal defect or papillary muscle rupture.	**1.** Hypotension not responding rapidly to fluid administration in a patient without evidence of pulmonary congestion. **2.** Before giving a fluid challenge in a patient with circulatory insufficiency and suspected pulmonary congestion. **3.** As a diagnostic tool when there is suspicion of an intracardiac shunt, acute mitral insufficiency, or pericardial tamponade.	Patients with acute myocardial infarction who are hemodynamically stable but have evidence of mild pulmonary congestion.	Patients with acute myocardial infarction who are hemodynamically stable and without evidence of cardiac or pulmonary congestion.
Intraarterial pressure monitoring	**1.** Patients with severe hypotension (systolic <80 mm Hg) or cardiogenic shock. **2.** Patients receiving vasopressor agents.	**1.** Patients receiving intravenous nitroprusside or other powerful arterial dilating agents. **2.** Hemodynamically stable patients receiving intravenous vasodilators for myocardial ischemia. **3.** Patients receiving intravenous inotropic agents. **4.** Patients with life-threatening arrhythmias.	None	Patients with acute myocardial infarction who are hemodynamically stable.

Lidocaine use	**1.** In patients with acute myocardial ischemia or infarction, or both, with ventricular premature beats that are:
	  a. frequent (>6/min)
	  b. closely coupled (R on T),
	  c. multiform in configuration, or
	  d. occurring in short bursts of three or more in succession.
		In patients with suspected acute myocardial infarction or ischemia or both, with indications as in Class I.	Prophylactic administration in the presence of uncomplicated acute myocardial ischemia or infarction or both, without ventricular premature beats in patients <70 and within the first 6 hours of onset of symptoms.	Patients with proved allergic or hypersensitivity reactions to lidocaine.

ISSUE	CLASS I—USUALLY INDICATED	CLASS II—ACCEPTABLE, OF UNCERTAIN EFFICACY		CLASS III—NOT INDICATED
		A. Evidence Favors Efficacy	B. Not Well Established By Evidence	
Lidocaine use— *Continued*	2. In patients with ventricular tachycardia or ventricular fibrillation or both, in association with defibrillation and cardiopulmonary resuscitation as indicated.			
Temporary pacemaker implantation	1. Asystole 2. Complete heart block 3. Right bundle branch block with left anterior or left posterior hemiblock developing in acute myocardial infarction. 4. Left bundle branch block developing in acute myocardial infarction. 5. Type II 2nd degree AV block. 6. Symptomatic bradycardia not responsive to atropine.	1. Type I 2nd degree AV block with hypotension not responsive to atropine. 2. Sinus bradycardia with hypotension not responsive to atropine. 3. Recurrent sinus pauses not responsive to atropine. 4. Atrial or ventricular overdrive pacing for incessant ventricular tachycardia.	1. Left bundle branch block with 1st degree heart block of unknown duration. 2. Bifascicular block of unknown duration.	1. First degree heart block. 2. Type I 2nd degree AV block with normal hemodynamics. 3. Accelerated idioventricular rhythm causing AV dissociation. 4. Bundle branch block known to exist before the myocardial infarction.
Transfer to a tertiary care facility equipped for angioplasty and cardiovascular surgery	1. Patients with recurrent pain. 2. Patients with hemodynamic instability as manifested by persistent congestive heart failure, arterial hypotension or cardiogenic shock. 3. Patients with resistant, recurrent ventricular arrhythmias (ventricular tachycardia or fibrillation).	1. Patients with high-risk myocardial infarction and contraindications to thrombolytic therapy but in whom it is reasonable to expect that reperfusion can be accomplished by percutaneous transluminal coronary angioplasty or coronary artery bypass grafting within 6 hours. 2. Patients who are stable late in initial hospitalization but who are to be evaluated for angioplasty or bypass grafting before discharge. 3. Patients in the early hours of acute myocardial infarction who have had prior bypass grafting and who may be candidates for angioplasty or regrafting.	1. Patients in stable condition in the early hours of acute myocardial infarction after thrombolysis but are in a facility in which coronary angioplasty or surgery cannot be performed. 2. Stable patients with early acute transmural infraction and extensive ST-T changes.	
Echocardiography in the early phase of acute myocardial infarction	1. Myocardial infarction associated with shock or profound pump failure consistent with extensive myocardial dysfunction or a potentially surgically remediable lesion. 2. Myocardial infarction associated with extensive infarction (ECG localization and peak MB CK > 150 IU/liter [or total CK > 1.000 IU/liter]). 3. Myocardial infarction accompanied by clinical complications suggestive of pump failure, refractory angina or pericardial tamponade, associated valvular or congenital heart disease, or suspected pericarditis or pericardial effusion, or in patients being or to be treated with calcium antagonists or beta blockers in whom left ventricular function may be compromised.	1. Myocardial infarction superimposed on previous infarction or associated with ECG phenomena such as left bundle branch block or posterior locus that may obscure diagnosis, in which case delineation of regional wall motion abnormalities may help confirm the diagnosis and provide prognostically important information. 2. Myocardial infarction with suspected concomitant right ventricular infarction (such as true posterior infarction) to define the severity of right ventricular involvement as a guide to management and to exclude pericardial tamponade.	Myocardial infarction of modest extent without clinical complications for evaluation of prognosis.	None

Table continues on the following page

TABLE 63–14   ACC/AHA GUIDELINES FOR THE EARLY MANAGEMENT OF ACUTE MYOCARDIAL INFARCTION—*Continued*

ISSUE	CLASS I—USUALLY INDICATED	CLASS II—ACCEPTABLE, OF UNCERTAIN EFFICACY		CLASS III—NOT INDICATED
		A. Evidence Favors Efficacy	B. Not Well Established By Evidence	
Early IV beta blockade	**1.** Patients, including those receiving thrombolytic therapy, with reflex tachycardia or systolic hypertension or both, without signs of congestive heart failure or contraindication to beta blockade. **2.** Patients with continuing or recurrent ischemic pain, tachyarrhythmias such as atrial fibrillation with a rapid ventricular response, or an enzyme elevation thought to represent recurrent injury with no contraindication to beta blockade. **3.** Postinfarction angina while awaiting study in patients without contraindications.	**1.** Other patients without contraindication to beta blockade who can be treated within the first 12 hours from the onset of chest pain. **2.** Non-Q-wave myocardial infarction	None	Patients with moderate to severe left ventricular failure and other contraindications to beta blockade.
Long-term beta blockade in secondary prevention	All but low-risk patients who do not have a clear contraindication to beta blockade. Treatment should ordinarily begin within the first few days of infarction and should be continued for at least 2 years.	Low-risk patients who do not have a clear contraindication to beta blockade.	None	Patients with contraindications to beta blockade.
Calcium channel blockers	Symptomatic treatment of postinfarction angina while awaiting cardiac catheterization and therapy based on angiographic findings.	**1.** Diltiazem in patients with non-Q-wave infarction in whom no contraindication exists. **2.** After angioplasty, a calcium channel blocker to prevent coronary vasospasm.	A calcium channel blocker may be used in transmural (Q-wave) infarction for treatment of postinfarction angina, especially if contraindications to proceeding with coronary arteriography and more definitive treatment exist.	Calcium channel blockers that suppress ventricular function in patients with myocardial infarction complicated by pulmonary congestion or left ventricular dysfunction.
Anticoagulation and platelet inhibitory agents Prevention of deep vein thrombosis and pulmonary embolism	**1.** Immediate subcutaneous heparin (5,000 U every 12 hours) for the first 24 to 48 hours unless full-dose anticoagulant therapy has been initiated in association with thrombolytic therapy or for the prevention of systemic emboli. **2.** Continued low-dose subcutaneous heparin in high-risk patients (age >70, large acute myocardial infarction, previous myocardial infarction, heart failure or shock, necessity for immobilization for >3 days, prior deep venous thrombosis or pulmonary emboli, obesity, or evidence of chronic venous insufficiency) until fully ambulatory.	None	None	None
Anticoagulation and platelet inhibitory agents Prevention of arterial embolism	**1.** Immediate high-dose SC or IV heparin in a dosage sufficient to prolong the activated partial thromboplastin time to 1.5 to 2.0 times control in patients with a large anterior transmural myocardial infarction. Heparin should be continued until discharge. **2.** Oral anticoagulants administered at a dose sufficient to prolong the prothrombin time to 1.3 to 1.5 times the control value (INR = 2.0 to 3.0) after heparin in patients who have a	Long-term (indefinite) oral anticoagulant therapy in patients with a diffusely dilated and poorly contracting left ventricle. (Prolong prothrombin time to 1.3 to 1.5 times the control value, or INR = 2.0 to 3.0.)	In patients with anterior myocardial infarction requiring anticoagulation up to 3 months for the prevention of systemic emboli, low-dose aspirin (80 to 160 mg/day) to prevent coronary events may be added to the anticoagulants and then continued alone indefinitely.	None

ISSUE	CLASS I—USUALLY INDICATED	CLASS II—ACCEPTABLE, OF UNCERTAIN EFFICACY		CLASS III—NOT INDICATED
		A. Evidence Favors Efficacy	B. Not Well Established By Evidence	
	ventricular mural thrombus or a large akinetic region of the apex of the left ventricle. Anticoagulant therapy should be continued for at least 3 months.			
Anticoagulation and platelet inhibitory agents The reduction of early recurrence or extension of myocardial infarction and mortality in patients not receiving thrombolytic therapy	Short-term aspirin begun immediately and continued for at least 1 month at a dose of 160 mg/day. After 1 month, aspirin should be continued at a dose of 160 to 325 mg/day.	Heparin followed by oral anticoagulant therapy for at least 1 month after infarction (prolong prothrombin time to 1.3 to 1.5 times control value).	None	None
Anticoagulation and platelet inhibitory agents Reduction in early reocclusion and in mortality after successful reperfusion with thrombolytic therapy	**1.** Aspirin (160 mg/day) started as soon as the patient is admitted and given daily until hospital discharge, at which time it can be continued at 160 to 325 mg daily. **2.** Heparin should be administered together with or immediately after thrombolysis to maintain the activated partial thromboplastin time approximately 1.5 to 2.0 times the control value for 24 to 72 hours.	None	None	None
Anticoagulation and platelet inhibitory agents Secondary prevention of late recurrence of myocardial infarction and death	Aspirin (160 to 325 mg daily) if not associated with significant side effects.	Oral anticoagulant therapy with warfarin (prothrombin time 1.3 to 1.5 times the control value, or INR = 2.0 to 3.0) rather than aspirin for long-term prevention of myocardial infarction recurrence.	None	None
Percutaneous transluminal coronary angioplasty Angioplasty after IV thrombolysis	Dilation of a significant lesion suitable for coronary angioplasty in the infarct-related artery in patients who are in the low-risk group for angiographic-related morbidity and mortality who have a type A lesion and: **1.** Have recurrent episodes of ischemic chest pain particularly if accompanied by ECG changes (postinfarction angina). **2.** Show evidence of myocardial ischemia while on optimal medical therapy during submaximal stress testing performed before hospital discharge or on maximal stress testing in the early posthospital period. **3.** Have recurrent ventricular tachycardia or ventricular fibrillation or both, convincingly related to ischemia while on antiarrhythmic therapy.	Dilation of significant lesions in patients who: **1.** Are similar to those in class I but who have type B lesions (anticipated success rate 60 to 85%). **2.** Are within 18 hours of onset of acute infarction and have cardiogenic shock or pump failure. **3.** Before hospital discharge in those who have survived cardiogenic shock or pump failure.	Dilation of a lesion in patients who: **1.** Have an occluded coronary artery after attempted thrombolytic therapy. **2.** Require multivessel angioplasty. **3.** Have >90% diameter proximal narrowing of an infarct-related artery with a large area of viable myocardium still at risk.	All patients in the immediate postinfarct period who do not fulfill Class I or II criteria such as: **1.** Patients within the early hours of an evolving myocardial infarction and have <50% residual stenosis of the infarct-related artery after receiving a thrombolytic agent. **2.** Lesions in vessels other than the infarct-related artery within early hours of infarction. **3.** Residual lesions that are borderline in severity (50 to 70% diameter narrowing) of the infarct-related artery without demonstration of ischemia on functional testing.

Table continued on the following page

TABLE 63–14 ACC/AHA GUIDELINES FOR THE EARLY MANAGEMENT OF ACUTE MYOCARDIAL INFARCTION—*Continued*

ISSUE	CLASS I—USUALLY INDICATED	CLASS II—ACCEPTABLE, OF UNCERTAIN EFFICACY		CLASS III—NOT INDICATED
		A. Evidence Favors Efficacy	B. Not Well Established By Evidence	
Intraaortic balloon counterpulsation or other circulatory assist devices	**1.** Cardiogenic shock or pump failure not responding promptly to pharmacological therapy. **2.** Right ventricular infarction with pump failure or shock not responding to volume infusion and appropriate pharmacological therapy. **3.** Refractory postinfarction angina for stabilization before and during angiography. **4.** Intractable recurrent tachycardia in patients with hemodynamic instability during the arrhythmia.	**1.** Ventricular septal rupture **2.** Acute mitral insufficiency **3.** Persistent ischemic pain **4.** Progressive congestive heart failure despite pharmacological therapy, particularly as a bridge to more definitive therapy.	None	**1.** A patient who is reasonably stable and in whom balloon insertion may delay more definitive therapy. **2.** Severe peripheral vascular disease and fewer indications than in Class I.
Emergency or urgent coronary bypass surgery in early management of myocardial infarction	**1.** Failed angioplasty with persistent pain or hemodynamic instability. **2.** Postinfarct angina with left main or 3-vessel disease or where coronary angioplasty is not indicated, with 2-vessel disease involving the proximal left anterior descending coronary artery or 2-vessel disease and poor left ventricular function.	**1.** At the time of surgical repair of ventricular septal defect or acute mitral insufficiency. **2.** Cardiogenic shock not suitable for angioplasty.	None	Where the available surgical mortality rate exceeds the mortality rate associated with appropriate medical therapy.
Emergency or urgent cardiac repair	**1.** Papillary muscle rupture (emergency). **2.** Ventricular septal defect or free wall rupture (urgent). **3.** Aneurysmal infarction with intractable ventricular arrhythmias or pump failure (urgent), or both. **4.** Acute mitral insufficiency with intractable failure (urgent). **5.** Intractable ventricular tachycardia (urgent).	**1.** Ventricular septal defect or free wall rupture (emergency). **2.** Severe mitral insufficiency with controlled failure (urgent).	None	**1.** Acute infarctectomy in hemodynamically stable patients. **2.** Surgery when the operative mortality rate exceeds the expected mortality rate associated with conservative therapy.
Implantable ventricular assist devices	None	None	As a bridge in a patient with intractable pump failure who would be a reasonable candidate for cardiac transplantation.	None
Noninvasive evaluation of patients at low risk by clinical indicators†	**1.** Stress ECG **a.** Before discharge for prognostic assessment (submaximal at 6 to 10 days or symptom-limited at 10 to 14 days). **b.** Early after discharge for prognostic assessment and functional capacity (3 weeks). **c.** Late after discharge (3 to 8 weeks) for functional capacity and prognosis if early stress was submaximal. **2.** Exercise thallium-201 scintigraphy (whenever baseline abnormalities of the ECG compromise its interpretation).	**1.** Exercise thallium-201 scintigraphy; before discharge for prognostic assessment with symptom-limited exercise at 10 to 14 days. **2.** Dipyridamole thallium-201 scintigraphy (before discharge for prognostic assessment in patients judged to be unable to perform exercise). **3.** Exercise radionuclide ventriculography predischarge at 10 to 14 days or early after discharge for prognostic assessment. **4.** Exercise two-dimensional echocardiography (before discharge or early after discharge for prognostic assessment).	**1.** Stress ECG **a.** In patients with baseline ECG abnormalities or coexisting medical problems that limit ability to achieve maximal exertion. **b.** Before discharge or early after discharge to evaluate patients who have sustained complicated myocardial infarction but who have subsequently "stabilized" and for whom a decision for invasive evaluation has not been made. **2.** Exercise thallium-201 myocardial scintigraphy (late after discharge at 6 to 8 weeks for prognostic assessment).	**1.** Stress ECG **a.** Within 72 hours of acute myocardial infarction. **b.** At any time to evaluate patients having unstable postinfarction angina pectoris. **c.** At any time to evaluate patients with acute myocardial infarction who have uncompensated congestive heart failure, cardiac arrhythmia, or noncardiac conditions that severely limit their ability to exercise. **d.** Before discharge to evaluate patients who have already been selected for cardiac catheterization.

ISSUE	CLASS I—USUALLY INDICATED	CLASS II—ACCEPTABLE, OF UNCERTAIN EFFICACY		CLASS III—NOT INDICATED
		A. Evidence Favors Efficacy	B. Not Well Established By Evidence	
Noninvasive evaluation of patients at low risk by clinical indicators†— *Continued*			3. Dipyridamole thallium or dobutamine thallium before discharge in patients judged unable to exercise.	
Rest radionuclide ventriculography	Predischarge rest radionuclide ventriculography to determine the high-risk subset unless determination of ventricular function has been made by other means.	For shunt detection in patients with suspected ventricular septal defect (pulmonary artery injection).	None	1. Predischarge radionuclide ventriculography to detect left ventricular thrombus. 2. Where similar information can be derived from other tests already performed or scheduled.
Two-dimensional echocardiography at rest	Detection or confirmation of suspected complications of infarction; tissue rupture, aneurysm or pseudoaneurysm formation, infarct extension or expansion, mural thrombus, and right ventricular infarction.	For evaluation of left ventricular function in predicting a low-risk subgroup for ambulation and early discharge from CCU.	Prediction of patients with multivessel coronary artery disease by the detection of remote asynergy.	Where similar information has been obtained from other tests already performed or scheduled.
Ambulatory electrocardiographic monitoring	None	After myocardial infarction, in patients with moderate to severe left ventricular dysfunction, or with significant ventricular ectopic activity in the CCU or stepdown telemetry unit for prognostic assessment.	1. After myocardial infarction, in patients to determine heart rate variability for prognostic assessment. 2. In high-risk postmyocardial infarction as screened for silent ischemia.	Uncomplicated ambulatory patients after discharge as a routine screen.
Coronary angiography Late evolving MI (after the initial 6 hours)	1. Patients with recurrent episodes of ischemic chest pain, particularly if accompanied by ECG changes. 2. Patients suspected of acute mitral regurgitation or a ruptured interventricular septum causing heart failure or shock. 3. Patients suspected of developing subacute cardiac rupture (pseudoaneurysm). 4. Patients with cardiogenic shock or severe pump failure.	1. Patients with congestive heart failure during intensive medical therapy. 2. Patients with recurrent ventricular tachycardia or ventricular fibrillation or both during intensive antiarrhythmic therapy.	Asymptomatic patients who were given thrombolytic therapy during the evolving phase.	Patients with uncomplicated completed myocardial infarction in whom no acute mechanical or surgical intervention is contemplated.
Coronary angiography Convalescent myocardial infarction (immediate predischarge up to 8 weeks after discharge)	1. Postinfarction angina pectoris. 2. Patients with evidence of myocardial ischemia on laboratory testing.	1. Patients with the need to return to unusually active and vigorous physical employment. 2. Patients with a left ventricular ejection fraction < 40%.	1. As a routine in patients receiving thrombolytic therapy during the evolving phase of infarction. 2. Otherwise uncomplicated and asymptomatic patients who are < 45. 3. Patients with uncomplicated non-Q-wave infarction without evidence of myocardial ischemia on noninvasive laboratory testing.	1. Patients judged to have a debilitating disease or conditions that preclude invasive intervention. 2. Patients with very advanced left ventricular dysfunction (ejection fraction < 20%) in the absence of angina pectoris or evidence of ischemia. 3. Patients with ventricular arrhythmias who have no evidence of ischemia symptomatically or during exercise testing, well-preserved exercise tolerance, and no suggestion of aneurysm formation.

* Likely to be affected by subsequent randomized trials.   † Timing likely to be modified by trend toward shorter hospital stay.
Class I: Usually indicated, always acceptable, and considered useful/effective.
Class II: Acceptable, of uncertain efficacy and may be controversial. a: Weight of evidence usefulness/efficacy. b: Not well established by evidence; can be helpful, probably not harmful.
Class III: Not indicated and may be harmful.
From Gunnar, R. M., Bourdillon, P. D. V., Dixon, D. W., et al.: Guidelines for the early management of patients with acute myocardial infarction. A report of the ACC/AHA Task Force on Assessment of Diagnostic and Therapeutic Cardiovascular Procedures. Reprinted with permission from the American College of Cardiology. J. Am. Coll. Cardiol. *16*:249, 1990.
Addenda: Long-term beta blockers: Treatment to begin within the first few days of infarction and continued for at least 2 years. Decisions concerning beta blockade withdrawal (or dose reduction) because of drug side effects should take into account the risk status of the individual patient (that is, the decision to reduce or discontinue should be controlled by weighing side effects more heavily as one moves from high- to low-risk patients).

lines consider lidocaine therapy appropriate (Class I) for patients with acute myocardial ischemia or infarction who have ventricular premature beats with characteristics that suggest a high risk for cardiac arrest. Use of lidocaine is discouraged (Class IIb) in uncomplicated acute myocardial ischemia or infarction without ventricular premature beats in patients less than 70 years of age and within the first 6 hours of the onset of symptoms.

USE OF TEMPORARY PACEMAKERS. The ACC/AHA guidelines recommend temporary pacemakers for patients with asystole and complete heart block or with conduction disturbances with a high risk of progressing to these catastrophic arrhythmias. Pacemakers are also supported for bradycardia that causes symptoms or hypotension and is not responsive to atropine. The ACC/AHA task force also considers use of pacemakers to overdrive incessant ventricular tachycardia an acceptable if unproven strategy (Class IIa). However, these guidelines do not support the use of pacemakers for conduction abnormalities that do not cause symptoms or hemodynamic compromise. Guidelines for the use of permanent pacemakers are reviewed on page 1963.

TRANSPORTATION. The decision to transfer a patient to a facility that can perform interventions such as angioplasty and coronary artery bypass graft surgery requires weighing potential benefits against the risk of complications during the transfer. The ACC/AHA guidelines support transfer to a tertiary care facility of patients with major ischemic, hemodynamic, or arrhythmic complications, all of which are deemed Class I indications for transfer. This task force considers transfer acceptable and probably beneficial (Class IIa) for patients who might benefit from reperfusion therapy with either angioplasty or coronary artery bypass graft surgery either early or late in the hospitalization. However, routine transfer of stable patients to tertiary facility is not recommended.

BETA-ADRENERGIC BLOCKING DRUGS. Randomized trials have now demonstrated that beta-adrenergic blocking agents can both limit myocardial damage when administered during the first few hours of infarction and reduce the risk of reinfarction or death when administered after infarction. The ACC/AHA guidelines therefore are generally supportive of the early and late use of beta blockers after myocardial infarction in patients without contraindications. Specific *contraindications* to beta blockers include:

- Heart rate less than 60 beats/min
- Systolic blood pressure less than 100 mm Hg
- Moderate to severe left ventricular failure
- Signs of peripheral hypoperfusion
- P-R interval more than 0.22 second
- Type I and II AV block or complete heart block
- Severe chronic obstructive pulmonary disease

Relative contraindications include history of asthma, severe peripheral vascular disease, and difficult to control insulin-dependent diabetes.

The guidelines do not express a preference between cardioselective and nonselective beta blockers, but recommend avoiding agents with intrinsic sympathomimetic activity. Daily dosages of the beta blockers, such as 180 mg to 240 mg/day of propranolol, have been high in randomized trials,[138] but studies have not defined the lowest possible dose that is efficacious. A period of treatment of at least 2 years is supported by the guidelines.

CALCIUM CHANNEL BLOCKERS. Randomized trials have not demonstrated that calcium channel blocking agents are beneficial after acute myocardial infarction[139] except in the subset of patients with non-Q-wave infarction in which early reinfarction and recurrent angina were reduced in patients given diltiazem 90 mg every 6 hours.[140] Therefore, the ACC/AHA guidelines do not support use of this class of drugs after myocardial infarction except for patients with postinfarction angina. Acceptable other indications (Class IIa) include use of diltiazem after angioplasty to prevent coronary spasm and in patients with non-Q-wave infarction. In the latter setting, diltiazem should be started during the first 48 hours and continued through the hospital phase and the first postinfarction year.

ANTICOAGULATION AND PLATELET INHIBITORY AGENTS. The ACC/AHA guidelines support administration of intravenous heparin and aspirin for several indications in patients with acute myocardial infarction:

- To prevent reocclusion of the infarct artery: Intravenous heparin and aspirin are both considered appropriate (Class I) for patients who receive thrombolytic therapy.
- To prevent deep venous thrombosis: Immediate subcutaneous heparin is recommended for the first 24 to 48 hours, with continued treatment for patients at increased risk for venous thrombosis.
- To prevent arterial embolism: "Therapeutic" anticoagulation for periods up to 3 months is considered appropriate for patients with large anterior transmural myocardial infarctions, ventricular mural thrombus, or a large akinetic region of the apex of the left ventricle (Table 63–14). For patients at high risk for arterial embolism, continued anticoagulation is recommended for at least 3 months.
- Reduction of early and late recurrence or extension of myocardial infarction: For patients who do not receive thrombolytic therapy, immediate initiation of aspirin is considered appropriate. Continued use of aspirin is endorsed for patients who do not have side effects from this medication. Anticoagulation with heparin followed by warfarin therapy is considered acceptable and probably useful (Class IIa).

PERCUTANEOUS TRANSLUMINAL CORONARY ANGIOPLASTY. The ACC/AHA guidelines for acute myocardial infarction and for PTCA were both developed before publication of randomized trials indicating that primary PTCA was effective and potentially superior therapy for acute myocardial infarction compared with thrombolysis.[68-70] The 1990 ACC/AHA guidelines considered primary PTCA clearly appropriate only for patients in whom thrombolytic therapy is clearly contraindicated, and only when a large amount of myocardium is at risk. Revisions of the myocardial infarction guidelines can be expected to provide more support for primary PTCA. The choice between thrombolytic therapy and PTCA when both therapies are available should be influenced by the time frame in which PTCA can be performed. The 1990 ACC/AHA guidelines for acute myocardial infarction considered performance of PTCA within 1 hour "acceptable" (Class IIb), but subsequent and future research may provide better insight into what can be considered an appropriate time goal for invasive revascularization. See previous section of guidelines for PTCA for further discussion of more recent (1993) ACC/AHA guidelines for the role of PTCA after acute myocardial infarction (see p. 1954).

INTRAAORTIC BALLOON COUNTERPULSATION OR OTHER CIRCULATORY ASSIST DEVICES. Pump failure and cardiogenic shock indicate a poor prognosis for patients with acute myocardial infarction, and ACC/AHA guidelines for acute myocardial infarction recommend that all patients with pump failure be transferred to facilities equipped to perform angioplasty and cardiovascular surgery, particularly if the patient is seen during the first 12 to 24 hours after onset of infarction. These guidelines emphasize that these patients need early angiographic evaluations so that interventions can be undertaken before hemodynamic deterioration becomes irreversible.

Intraaortic balloon counterpulsation or other circulatory assist devices can be used to stabilize the condition of patients until such evaluations can be completed. The ACC/AHA guidelines consider use of these devices appropriate in patients with cardiogenic shock that does not respond promptly to pharmacological therapy, and for patients with refractory postinfarction angina or recurrent ventricular tachycardia leading to hemodynamic instability. The use of these devices is considered acceptable and probably useful (Class IIb) for mechanical complications such as ventricular septal rupture and acute mitral insufficiency and for patients with persistent ischemic pain or progressive congestive heart failure. The guidelines do not support use of these devices in patients whose condition was stable after myocardial infarction.

CORONARY ARTERY BYPASS SURGERY. The use of emergency coronary artery bypass graft surgery as primary therapy for acute myocardial infarction is discouraged by both the 1990 ACC/AHA guidelines for acute myocardial infarction and the 1991 ACC/AHA guidelines for coronary artery bypass graft surgery. Thrombolysis and angioplasty are instead regarded as first choice strategies, with CABG reserved for patients with failed PTCA or postinfarction angina that is found to be due to coronary anatomy configurations that do not lend themselves to angioplasty. CABG is also considered appropriate for patient subsets in which this procedure has been found to increase survival, compared with medical therapy.

Coronary bypass surgery is endorsed, however, as an emergent or urgent treatment for severe mechanical or arrhythmic complications. The use of ventricular assist devices as bridge therapy for patients who might be candidates for cardiac transplantation is considered acceptable but unproven (Class IIb).

Postinfarction Evaluation

The ACC/AHA guidelines for acute myocardial infarction describe three strategies for risk stratification of patients after infarction, all of which are based on identifying patients whose clinical characteristics place them at high risk for subsequent complications, directing them toward early invasive evaluations. For risk stratification of other patients, the next step in the evaluation is a submaximal exercise test performed before discharge or a full symptom-limited test after discharge from the hospital. These 1990 guidelines were based on the assumption that patients without major complications remain in the hospital for 7 to 14 days, whereas shorter stays have become more common in recent years. Therefore, revisions of these guidelines can be expected to modify the time frame in which exercise tests are performed.

Choices among the techniques used to detect ischemia (electrocardiography, radionuclide imaging, echocardiography) and the methods used to provoke ischemia (exercise, pharmacological agent) are not the subject of explicit recommendations in the ACC/AHA guidelines. These guidelines also do not address directly which patients *should* undergo which tests (if any) to assess left ventricular function or the presence of asymptomatic arrhythmia. Instead, the guidelines endorse as appropriate or acceptable the use of these techniques in various clinical settings in which the probability of detecting abnormalities is greater.

The appropriateness of coronary angiography in the early or late periods after acute myocardial infarction is directly related to the appropriateness of revascularization procedures such as PTCA. The ACC/AHA guidelines discourage coronary angiography for patients having uncomplicated courses or as routine after intravenous thrombolytic therapy. Coronary angiography is also not supported for patients with cardiac or noncardiac conditions that render them unlikely to benefit from invasive revascularization therapy.

(See also Chap. 38)

Practice guidelines for the treatment of unstable angina were issued in 1994 by a multidisciplinary panel sponsored by the Agency for Health Care Policy and Research (AHCPR). These guidelines differ qualitatively from the series of guidelines developed by the ACC/AHA task forces, which tend to rate the appropriateness of use of an intervention in various settings. In contrast, the AHCPR guidelines seek to describe optimal overall management strategies and to rate the strength of the evidence supporting specific recommendations. Hence the AHCPR guidelines include flow sheets that schematically summarize management plans, and use the following grading scale to describe the data addressing a specific issue:

- A = at least one randomized controlled trial as part of a body of literature of overall good quality and consistency
- B = well-conducted clinical studies but no randomized clinical trials
- C = absence of directly applicable clinical studies of good quality

These guidelines include a broad spectrum of illness under the topic of unstable angina. Three basic presentations include symptoms of angina at rest, usually prolonged for more than 20 minutes, new-onset (less than 2 months) exertional angina that is Canadian Cardiovascular Society Class (CCSC) III or IV in severity, and recent (less than 2 months) acceleration of angina, with an increase in severity of at least one CCSC class to CCSC class III or IV. Variant angina, non-Q-wave myocardial infarction, and angina occurring more than 24 hours after acute myocardial infarction are also considered unstable angina.

The overall management strategy of the AHCPR guidelines is summarized in Figure 63–1. Principal conclusions of the guidelines include:

1. Many patients suspected of having unstable angina can be discharged home after adequate initial evaluation. Further outpatient evaluation should be concluded within 72 hours after initial evaluation.

2. Patients with unstable angina who are judged to be at intermediate or high risk of complications should be hospitalized and receive aspirin, heparin, nitroglycerin, and beta blocker therapy.

3. Intravenous thrombolytic therapy should not be administered to patients without evidence of acute myocardial infarction.

4. Noninvasive testing can often guide therapy selection.

Initial Evaluation and Treatment

The AHCPR guidelines rely on early assessment of the probability that a patient has coronary disease and the patient's risk of death or myocardial infarction. Combinations of features that place patients in groups with high, intermediate, and low probabilities of these outcomes are summarized in Tables 63–15 and 63–16. As noted in the section on Acute Chest Pain (see p. 1967), the guidelines emphasize that ECG data are crucial for this assessment; hence this evaluation cannot be made over the telephone. In patients with prolonged pain (more than 20 minutes), hemodynamic instability, or symptoms of arrhythmia, evaluation should take place in an emergency department. The guidelines recommend that evaluation in such patients, including the electrocardiogram, be completed within 20 minutes of arrival at the medical facility. In the absence of these adverse prognostic signs, the evaluation can sometimes be performed in an outpatient office.

During the initial evaluation, the guidelines recommend the use of continuous electrocardiographic monitoring, and

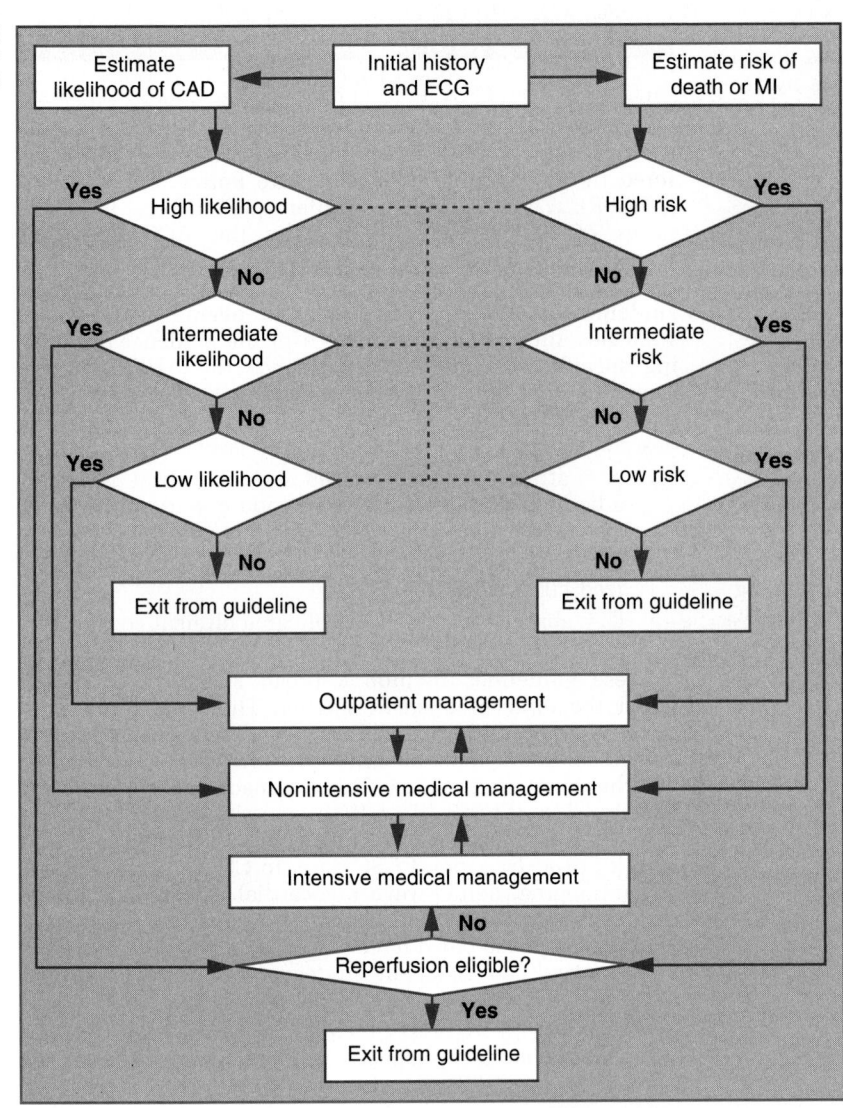

FIGURE 63–1. Overall strategy for diagnosis and risk stratification for patients with unstable angina according to AHCPR guidelines.

TABLE 63–15   LIKELIHOOD OF SIGNIFICANT CORONARY ARTERY DISEASE IN PATIENTS WITH SYMPTOMS SUGGESTING UNSTABLE ANGINA

HIGH LIKELIHOOD (e.g., 0.85–0.99)	INTERMEDIATE LIKELIHOOD (e.g., 0.15–0.84)	LOW LIKELIHOOD (e.g., 0.01–0.14)
Any of the following features:	**Absence of high likelihood features and any of the following:**	**Absence of high or intermediate likelihood features but may have:**
History of prior MI or sudden death or other known history of CAD	Definite angina: males <60 or females <70	Chest pain classified as probably not angina
Definite angina: males ≥60 or females ≥70	Probable angina: males ≥60 or females ≥70	One risk factor other than diabetes
Transient hemodynamic or ECG changes during pain	Chest pain probably not angina in patients with diabetes	T-wave flattening or inversion <1 mm in leads with dominant R waves
Variant angina (pain with reversible ST-segment elevation)	Chest pain probably not angina and two or three risk factors other than diabetes	Normal ECG
ST-segment elevation or depression ≥1 mm	Extracardiac vascular disease	
Marked symmetrical T-wave inversion in multiple precordial leads.	ST depression 0.05 to 1 mm or T-wave inversion ≥1 mm in leads with dominant R waves	

From Braunwald, E., Mark, D. B., Jones, R. H., et al.: Unstable Angina: Diagnosis and Management. Clinical Practice Guideline Number 10 (amended). AHCPR Publication No. 94-0602. Rockville, Md., Agency for Health Care Policy and Research and the National Heart, Lung, and Blood Institute, Public Health Service, US Department of Health and Human Services, May 1994.

TABLE 63–16 SHORT-TERM RISK OF DEATH OR NONFATAL MYOCARDIAL INFARCTION IN PATIENTS WITH UNSTABLE ANGINA

HIGH RISK	INTERMEDIATE RISK	LOW RISK
At least one of the following features must be present:	No high-risk feature but must have any of the following:	Absence of high or intermediate likelihood features but may have any of the following features:
Prolonged ongoing (≥20 min) rest pain	Prolonged (>20 min) rest angina, now resolved, with moderate or high likelihood of coronary artery disease	Increased angina frequency, severity, or duration
Pulmonary edema, most likely related to ischemia	Rest angina (>20 min or relieved with rest or sublingual nitroglycerin)	Angina provoked at a lower threshold
Angina at rest with dynamic ST changes ≥1 mm	Nocturnal angina	New-onset angina with onset 2 weeks to 2 months before presentation
Angina with new or worsening mitral regurgitation murmur	Angina with dynamic T-wave changes	Normal or unchanged ECG
Angina with S3 or new/worsening rales	New-onset Canadian Cardiovascular Society Class III or IV angina in the past 2 weeks with moderate or high likelihood of CAD	
Angina with hypotension	Pathological Q waves or resting ST depression ≤1 mm in multiple lead groups (anterior, inferior, lateral)	
	Age >65 years	

From Braunwald, E., Mark, D. B., Jones, R. H., et al.: Unstable Angina: Diagnosis and Management. Clinical Practice Guideline Number 10 (amended). AHCPR Publication No. 94-0602. Rockville, Md., Agency for Health Care Policy and Research and the National Heart, Lung, and Blood Institute, Public Health Service, US Department of Health and Human Services, May 1994.

for patients with ongoing rest pain, placement at bed rest. If it is concluded that a patient has unstable angina, aspirin should be given unless there is contraindication, such as evidence of ongoing major hemorrhage, a significant risk for bleeding complications, or a clear history of severe hypersensitivity to aspirin.

The guidelines recommend that antiischemia medications should be initiated in the emergency department for patients with unstable angina and titrated to dosages that are adequate to relieve symptomatic ischemia without causing excessive bradycardia or hypotension. For patients at high or intermediate risk of complications (Table 63–16), intravenous heparin is recommended. The guidelines suggest an initial dose of 80 units/kg by intravenous bolus followed by an infusion of 18 units/kg/hour, maintaining the activated partial thromboplastin time (aPTT) at 1.5 to 2.5 times control. The use of thrombolytic therapy is not supported in the absence of acute ST-segment elevation or left bundle branch block.

A major theme of the AHCPR guidelines is involvement of patients in their care, and the initial treatment recommendations urge that patients be encouraged to participate in monitoring the relief of symptoms. Throughout the course of treatment, the guidelines specifically recommend that the health care team should keep the patient and the patient's family informed of the probable diagnosis, most reasonable treatment strategies, and most likely outcomes.

After initial treatment and stabilization, the AHCPR guidelines recommend triage of patients with a high risk for complications (Table 63–16) if possible to an ICU bed, while intermediate-risk patients can be managed in an ICU or other monitored bed. The guidelines support management of patients who fall into low-risk subsets as outpatients, however. These low-risk patients should undergo follow-up outpatient evaluations within 72 hours.

Outpatient Care of Low-Risk Patients

Patients with unstable angina who are at low risk for complications tend to be those with new-onset angina or with worsening of symptoms due to ischemia, but without severe, prolonged, or rest pain. At the follow-up evaluation, the guidelines recommend that the physician determine whether a patient's symptoms have worsened, in which

case the patient should be admitted. A search for noncardiac causes of pain should be undertaken, but if the leading diagnosis is still ischemic heart disease, the evaluation should be directed at further risk stratification.

Exercise or pharmacological stress testing usually should be part of this evaluation but need not be performed for patients with a very low probability of coronary disease or complications from ischemic disease. Conversely, stress testing would be excessively risky for patients who have a high clinical risk for complications, such as those with significant left ventricular dysfunction or worsening of symptoms despite medical therapy. In such cases, referral of the patient for coronary angiography may be the most appropriate course. The guidelines recognize that coronary angiography may be useful for some low-risk patients who believe their symptoms are due to ischemia despite reassurance and noninvasive test results to the contrary.

The treatment guidelines for low-risk patients recommend beginning with instruction in the proper use of sublingual nitroglycerin tablets, followed by oral beta blockers. The guidelines suggest starting with one major antianginal medication, preferably a long-acting preparation, and adding a second only if the symptoms are not adequately controlled. For most low-risk outpatients, therapy with aspirin and one antianginal medication is sufficient initial treatment. Patients with contraindications to aspirin can be treated with ticlopidine 250 mg twice a day as an alternative.

Intensive Medical Treatment

Patients with unstable angina and either intermediate or high risk for complications should receive intensive medical therapy aimed at relieving their symptoms. According to the AHCPR guidelines, this therapy should include beta blockers and nitrate preparations, including intravenous nitroglycerin for nonhypotensive patients with high-risk unstable angina (Table 63–17). A patient whose pain cannot be controlled should be referred for catheterization and revascularization.

Patients whose angina is controlled for 24 hours by intravenous nitroglycerin can be switched to other nitrate preparations. Whereas prolonged exposure to nitrates can cause tolerance to their effects, responsiveness to nitrates can be

TABLE 63–17 SELECTED RECOMMENDATIONS AND STRENGTH OF EVIDENCE FOR MANAGEMENT OF UNSTABLE ANGINA (AHCPR)

TOPIC	RECOMMENDATION	STRENGTH OF EVIDENCE
Initial treatment	• All patients with unstable angina should receive regular ASA 160 to 324 mg as soon as possible after presentation unless a definite contraindication is present.	A
	• IV heparin should be started as soon as a diagnosis of intermediate- or high-risk unstable angina is made.	A
Triage	• High-risk unstable angina patients should be admitted initially to an ICU bed whenever possible.	B
	• Intermediate-risk unstable angina patients should be admitted to an ICU or monitored cardiac bed.	C
	• Low-risk unstable angina patients may be managed as outpatients with planned early follow-up evaluations.	C
Intensive medical treatment: Nitrates	• Patients whose symptoms are not fully relieved with three sublingual nitroglycerin (NTG) tablets and initiation of beta blocker therapy (when possible), as well as all nonhypotensive high-risk unstable angina patients, may benefit from IV NTG. IV NTG should be started at a dose of 5 to 10 μg/min by continuous infusion and titrated up by 10 μg/min every 5 to 10 min until relief of symptoms or limiting side effects occur.	B
	• Patients on IV NTG should be switched to oral or topical nitrate therapy once they have been symptom-free for 24 hours.	C
Morphine sulfate	Morphine sulfate at a dose of 2 to 5 mg IV is recommended for any patient whose symptoms are not relieved after three serial sublingual NTG tablets or whose symptoms recur with adequate antiischemic therapy unless contraindicated by hypotension or intolerance. Morphine may be repeated every 5 to 10 min as needed to relieve symptoms and maintain patient comfort.	C
Beta blockers	IV (for high-risk patients) or oral (for intermediate- and low-risk patients) beta blockers should be started in the absence of contraindications.	B
Calcium channel blockers	• Calcium channel blockers may be used to control ongoing or recurring ischemic symptoms in patients already on adequate doses of nitrates and beta blockers or in patients unable to tolerate adequate doses of one or both of these agents or in patients with variant angina. Calcium channel blockers should be avoided in patients with pulmonary edema or evidence of LV dysfunction.	B
	• Nifedipine should not be used in the absence of concurrent beta blockage.	A
Aspirin	ASA to be taken once/day at a dose of 80 to 324 mg, should be continued indefinitely following presentation with unstable angina.	A
Ticlopidine and other antiplatelet agents	• Patients unable to take ASA may be started on ticlopidine 250 mg twice per day as a substitute.	B
	• Heparin infusion should be continued for 2 to 5 days or until revascularization is performed.	C
Laboratory testing	• Total CK and CK-MB should be measured every 6 to 8 hours for the first 24 hours after admission.	C
	• Lactate dehydrogenase isoenzymes may be useful in patients presenting 24 to 72 hours after symptom onset if serial CK and CK-MB levels are normal.	
	• Serum lipid levels within 24 hours of admission unless patients have had a recent determination or are on chronic therapy for hyperlipidemia.	
	• Follow-up ECG 24 hours after admission and whenever the patient has recurrent symptoms or a change in clinical status.	
	• Chest film.	
	• Assessment of left ventricular function within 72 hours.	
Emergency/urgent cardiac catheterization	If chest discomfort with objective evidence of ischemia persists for $\geq$ 1 hour after aggressive medical therapy, triage to emergency cardiac catheterization should be strongly considered.	B
	Urgent cardiac catheterization should be considered in patients with unstable angina who have recurrent ischemic episodes despite appropriate medical therapy or who have high-risk unstable angina.	B
Acute revascularization	Acute revascularization is indicated for patients with refractory pain ($\geq$ 1 hour on aggressive medical therapy) who are found at catheterization to have an acutely occluded major coronary vessel, or severe subtotal occlusion of a culprit vessel, or severe multivessel disease with impaired LV function.	B
Use and timing of noninvasive tests	Exercise or pharmacological stress testing should generally be an integral part of the outpatient evaluation of low-risk patients with unstable angina.	B
	Unless cardiac catheterization is indicated, noninvasive exercise or pharmacological stress testing should be performed in low- or intermediate-risk patients (see Table 63–16) hospitalized with unstable angina who have been free of angina and congestive heart failure for a minimum of 48 hours.	B

TOPIC	RECOMMENDATION	STRENGTH OF EVIDENCE
Selection of stress testing modality	The exercise treadmill test should be the standard mode of stress testing employed in patients with a normal ECG who are not taking digoxin. Patients with widespread resting ST depression (≥ 1 mm), ST changes secondary to digoxin, left ventricular hypertrophy, LBBB/significant intraventricular conduction deficit (IVCD), or preexcitation usually should be tested using an imaging modality. Patients unable to exercise due to physical limitations should undergo pharmacological stress testing in combination with an imaging modality.	B
Use of noninvasive test results in patient management	• Patients with a low-risk exercise test result (predicted average annual cardiac mortality $< 1\%$/year) can be managed medically without need for referral to cardiac catheterization.	B
	• Patients with a high-risk exercise test result (predicted average annual cardiac mortality $\geq 4\%$/year) should be referred for prompt cardiac catheterization.	B
	• Patients with intermediate-risk exercise test result (predicted average annual cardiac mortality 2–3%/year) should be referred for additional testing, either cardiac catheterization or an (alternative) exercise imaging study	C
	• A stress test result of intermediate risk combined with evidence of left ventricular dysfunction should prompt referral to cardiac catheterization.	C
Cardiac catheterization	• *Early invasive strategy:* cardiac catheterization is performed routinely in all hospitalized patients without contraindications, usually within 48 hours of presentation.	A
	• *Early conservative strategy:* cardiac catheterization is performed routinely in patients admitted to the hospital with unstable angina who are candidates for a revascularization procedure and have one or more of the following high-risk indicators: prior revascularization (PTCA or CABG); associated congestive heart failure or depressed left ventricular function (EF < 0.50) by noninvasive study; malignant ventricular arrhythmia; persistent or recurrent pain/ischemia; and/or a functional study indicating high risk.	A
Myocardial revascularization	• Patients found at catheterization to have significant left main disease ($\geq 50\%$) or significant ($\geq 70\%$) 3-vessel disease with depressed left ventricular function (EF < 0.50) should be referred promptly for CABG surgery.	A
	• Patients with 2-vessel disease with proximal severe subtotal stenosis ($\geq 95\%$) of the left anterior descending artery and depressed left ventricular function should be referred promptly for CABG or PTCA.	B C
	• Patients with significant coronary artery disease should be considered for prompt revascularization (PTCA or CABG) if they have any of the following: failure to stabilize with medical treatment; recurrent angina/ischemia at rest or with low-level activities; and/or ischemia accompanied by congestive heart failure symptoms, and S3 gallop, new or worsening mitral regurgitation, or definite ECG changes.	B
	• For patients with significant coronary artery disease not included in the above recommendations, two strategies are possible: early invasive and early conservative. In early invasive strategy, revascularization is performed only on those patients meeting criteria for failure of initial therapy necessitating cardiac catheterization. Medical therapy without revascularization is continued for patients without criteria for failure of therapy.	S
Discharge from hospital and postdischarge care	Patients should continue on ASA, 80 mg to 324 mg per day, indefinitely after discharge.	B

From Braunwald, E., Mark, D. B., Jones, R. H., et al.: Unstable Angina: Diagnosis and Management. Clinical Practice Guideline Number 10 (amended). AHCPR Publication No. 94-0602. Rockville, Md., Agency for Health Care Policy and Research and the National Heart, Lung, and Blood Institute, Public Health Service, US Department of Health and Human Services, May 1994. (For definition of A, B, C and S see p. 1979.)

restored by increasing the dose or giving the patient topical, oral, or buccal nitrates with a 6- to 8-hour nitrate-free interval. Morphine sulfate can be used to relieve symptoms in patients whose pain is not controlled with three sublingual nitroglycerin tablets or whose symptoms recur.

Beta blockers can be given orally for most patients with unstable angina, but intravenous administration should be considered for patients who are at high risk for complications. A patient at risk for adverse effects from beta blockers because of pulmonary disease, left ventricular dysfunction, or severe bradycardia should be treated initially with a short-acting beta blocker. The value of beta blockers is sufficiently impressive that the guidelines recommend a trial of a short-acting agent at a reduced dose (e.g., 2.5 mg metoprolol intravenously, 12.5 mg metoprolol orally, or 25 ug/kg/min esmolol as initial doses), rather than complete avoidance of beta blocker therapy, in patients with mild wheezing or a history of chronic obstructive pulmonary disease.

Calcium channel blockers are the next class of drugs used to control symptoms after nitrates and beta blockers. This class of drugs can relieve ischemic symptoms[141] but does not appear to change mortality or rates of nonfatal myocardial infarction.[142,143] Because of the negative inotropic effects of these agents, the AHCPR guidelines discourage their use in patients with pulmonary edema or left ventricular dysfunction. The guidelines also recommend that nifedipine not be used in patients who are not also receiving a beta blocker because of randomized trial data demonstrating an increased risk of myocardial infarction or recurrent angina in such settings.[144]

As noted above, the AHCPR guidelines also recommend that all patients with unstable angina receive aspirin or other antiplatelet agents unless they have contraindications to such drugs. Intravenous heparin therapy should be continued for at least 2 days.

Laboratory Testing

Guidelines from the AHCPR, ACC/AHA, and American College of Physicians for the use of cardiac enzyme assays are reviewed on page 1970. None of these guidelines provides recommendations regarding the use of newer markers such as cardiac troponin I and T,[123,124] which may be useful markers for myocardial injury. For example, troponin T appears to improve risk stratification of patients with unstable angina,[124] and troponin I has demonstrated high specificity for cardiac damage.[123] These new markers are just beginning to enter the market, however, and strategies for their use have not yet been addressed by guidelines.

The AHCPR guidelines recommend serial CK and CK-MB sampling for 24 hours, and an electrocardiogram 24 hours after admission. This 24-hour period exceeds the duration of hospitalizations currently used for many patients admitted for acute chest pain,[122] but these shorter observation periods were developed and evaluated for patients with a low risk for acute myocardial infarction and cardiovascular complications. Data support the use of a 24-hour observation period for patients with electrocardiographic changes or worsening of ischemic syndromes, and even longer enzyme sampling periods for patients who have recurrent ischemic pain in the hospital.[122]

The AHCPR guidelines support obtaining a chest film upon admission, particularly in patients with hemodynamic instability, and suggest assessment of left ventricular function with either echocardiography or radionuclide ventriculography within 72 hours of admission unless the patient undergoes early cardiac catheterization. These data can provide insight into the patient's left ventricular function, which is an important predictor of prognosis and therefore a factor in the consideration of who should undergo coronary angiography.

Initiation of secondary prevention strategies during the hospitalization is a major priority of the AHCPR guidelines, but these interventions can get overlooked when the focus of management is on questions such as whether or not the patient needs coronary revascularization. The AHCPR guidelines therefore recommend measurement of serum lipid levels within 24 hours of admission unless there has been a recent determination or the patient is receiving long-term therapy for hyperlipidemia. Levels obtained later in the hospitalization may not reflect the patient's usual lipid profile.

Early Assessment and Management

The goal of initial therapy for patients with unstable angina is to institute a regimen that includes aspirin, intravenous heparin adjusted to maintain an aPTT value of 1.5 to 2.5 times control, plus nitrates and a beta blocker. Calcium blockers should be considered for patients with refractory ischemia, significant hypertension, or variant angina, according to the AHCPR. Failure of these measures to control ischemia should prompt consideration of urgent cardiac catheterization.

For patients who have ischemia refractory to medical management, *intraaortic balloon pumping* may be useful if coronary angiography is not possible or for stabilization until the patient can reach the catheterization laboratory or operating room. *Urgent or emergency cardiac catheterization* is recommended if patients have evidence of ischemia persisting for more than 1 hour after institution of aggressive medical therapy, and in patients who have recurrent ischemic episodes despite appropriate treatment or who have high-risk unstable angina. Acute revascularization with either PTCA or CABG should be used for patients with refractory pain and acute vessel occlusions, severe subtotal occlusion of a culprit vessel, or severe multivessel disease with impaired left ventricular function.

For patients whose course is uncomplicated for at least 24 hours, the AHCPR guidelines recommend that intravenous medications can be switched to nonparenteral regimens. As the patient is mobilized, counseling should include assessment of the patient's life situation, anxiety level, and coping skills. The guidelines recommend that the health care team observe the patient as activity is increased to a level that allows performance of activities of daily living. During this period, the patient and family should receive education about and begin working toward risk-factor modification goals.

Use of Noninvasive Testing

The AHCPR guidelines support use of exercise or pharmacological stress testing to improve risk stratification of patients with unstable angina once they are sufficiently stable to undergo such testing. For low-risk patients who may not have been admitted to the hospital or who were discharged early, the guidelines recommend that these tests be performed within 72 hours. For hospitalized patients with a low or intermediate risk for complications, the guidelines recommend testing when the patient has been free of angina and congestive heart failure for 48 hours. The guidelines recommend exercise electrocardiography as the first-choice method for noninvasive assessment of ischemic heart disease. When electrocardiographic abnormalities such as left bundle branch block render the electrocardiogram an unreliable test for ischemia, an imaging method should be used; when patients are unable to exercise, a pharmacological stressor should be employed.

Data from the noninvasive tests help determine the subsequent management strategy for patients whose condition remains clinically stable. The AHCPR guidelines include a nomogram for prediction of annual mortality on the basis of exercise-induced ST-segment deviation, the degree of angina observed during exercise, and the duration of exercise[145] (Fig. 5–12, p. 166). Medical therapy without cardiac catheterization is recommended for patients with a predicted annual cardiac mortality of less than 1 per cent per year, while prompt catheterization is recommended for those with an estimated average annual mortality of 4 per cent or more. For patients with an intermediate risk after exercise testing, the AHCPR guidelines suggest cardiac catheterization if those patients have left ventricular dysfunction; in the absence of left ventricular dysfunction, the guidelines recommend further risk stratification either with cardiac catheterization or alternative noninvasive tests.

Early Invasive and Conservative Strategies

The AHCPR guidelines proposed two alternative treatment strategies, which were termed early invasive and early conservative strategies. Published research has not demonstrated an advantage of one approach over the other, so the guidelines recommend basing the decision of which strategy to use on factors including the patient's estimated risk of complications, available facilities, and patient preferences. In the early invasive strategy, patients admitted to the hospital for unstable angina routinely undergo coronary angiography, usually within 48 hours of presentation. In the conservative strategy, catheterization is performed in admitted patients who have at least one of several high-risk indicators (Table 63–17). Cardiac catheterization is *not* performed in patients who are not candidates for revascularization or who have extensive comorbidity that would render them unlikely to benefit from the procedure.

Figure 63–2 shows a schematic integration of early invasive and conservative strategies and the recommended management according to the results of the coronary angiograms. Coronary artery bypass graft surgery is recommended for patients with left main coronary disease or significant three-vessel disease with depressed left ventricular function. Revascularization with PTCA or CABG should be performed for patients with two-vessel disease

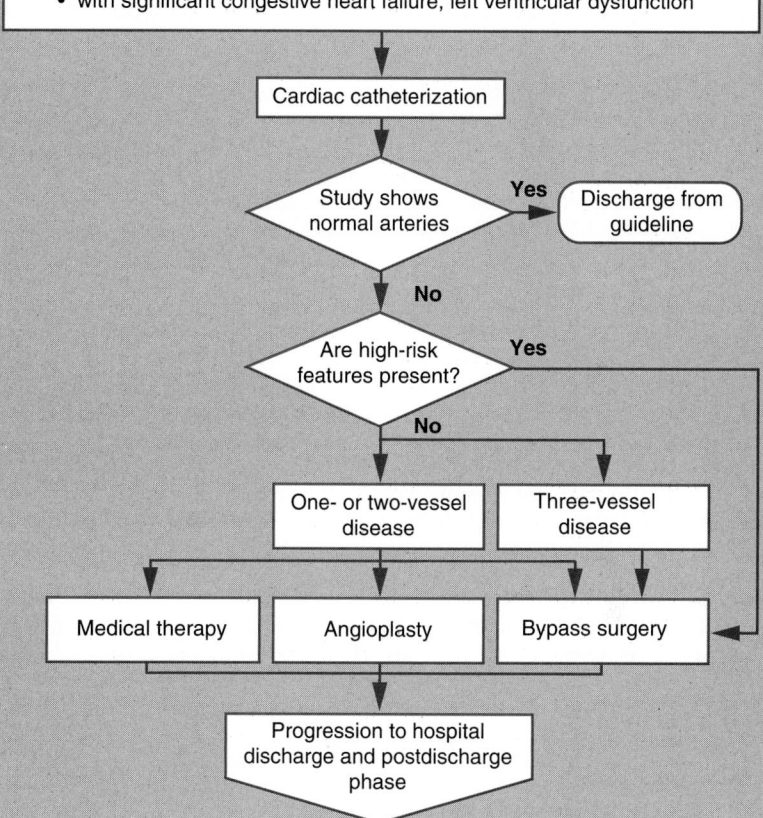

Patients who are candidates for cardiac catheterization and revascularization include those:
- opting for early invasive strategy
- failing to stabilize with medical therapy
- with prior angioplasty, bypass surgery, or myocardial infarction
- with high-risk clinical findings or noninvasive test results
- with significant congestive heart failure, left ventricular dysfunction

FIGURE 63–2. Cardiac catheterization and myocardial revascularization in unstable angina according to AHCPR guidelines. (From Braunwald, E., Mark, D. B., Jones, R. H., et al.: Unstable Angina: Diagnosis and Management. Clinical Practice Guideline Number 10 [amended]. AHCPR Publication No. 94-0602. Rockville, Md., Agency for Health Care Policy and Research and the National Heart, Lung, and Blood Institute, Public Health Service, US Department of Health and Human Services, May 1994.)

with proximal severe subtotal stenosis of the left anterior descending coronary artery and depressed left ventricular function. These procedures should also be performed for other patients with coronary disease if they have high-risk factors (Table 63–17). For patients without these high-risk factors, the patient and physician should choose between an early invasive strategy, in which revascularization is performed, and an early conservative strategy, in which revascularization is performed only if the patient's symptoms are not controlled with medical therapy.

Hospital Discharge and Postdischarge Care

Throughout the hospitalization—and after discharge—patients and their families should be kept fully informed of the patient's status, crucial issues, options, and probable outcomes. In the absence of contraindications, the AHCPR guidelines recommend use of aspirin indefinitely, as well as continuation of medications needed to achieve adequate symptom control. Those patients with signs or symptoms of ischemia should receive instruction in the use of sublingual nitroglycerin. Patients with successful revascularization without recurrent ischemia do not require postdischarge antianginal therapy.

The AHCPR guidelines recommend that low-risk patients and patients with successful CABG or PTCA be seen in an outpatient facility at 2 to 6 weeks, and higher-risk patients should return in 1 to 2 weeks. Follow-up care should emphasize secondary prevention, with appropriate continued management of risk factors including hypertension, hyperlipidemia, smoking, and physical inactivity. Patients should be given advice on specific physical activities, including resumption of work, driving, and sexual activity.

The guidelines recommend consideration of an outpatient cardiac rehabilitation program but gave a low grade (C) to the strength of evidence supporting this intervention for patients with unstable angina.

HEART FAILURE

(See also Chap. 17)

Heart failure was one of the first three topics chosen by the AHCPR for the development of practice guidelines; these guidelines were released in 1994. Among the reasons for choosing heart failure were its high prevalence, poor prognosis, and high costs. More than two million Americans suffer from heart failure, and 5-year mortality rates are in the range of 50 per cent. The estimated cost to society exceeds $10 billion per year.[13] Research has demonstrated that improved management can decrease mortality and improve functional status for patients with heart failure, and there is considerable variation in the strategies used by physicians in the care of heart failure.[146] Among the common errors in management and testing cited by the AHCPR panel are:

- Overuse of testing techniques
- Inadequate treatment of coexistent hypertension
- Inadequate education for patient, family, and caregivers
- Inappropriate treatment of heart failure not due to systolic dysfunction
- Suboptimal patient involvement in care and compliance

- Delayed referral for transplantation
- Underutilization of exercise prescriptions
- Underutilization of ACE inhibitors
- Inadequate dosing of diuretics in patients with persistent volume overload
- Failure of clinicians to appreciate adverse effects of medications

To reduce the frequency of these errors, the AHCPR panel formulated recommendations for a wide range of topics[13] (excerpted in Table 63–18). The multidisciplinary group that developed these guidelines used an A-B-C system to grade the strength of evidence to support their recommendations similar to that used for the AHCPR unstable angina guidelines (p. 1979).[12] The focus of the AHCPR guidelines was on patients with left ventricular systolic dysfunction leading to volume overload or inadequate tissue perfusion, but one of their most specific recommendations was aimed at preventing this syndrome—the guidelines recommend use of ACE inhibitors in patients with moderately or severely reduced left ventricular systolic function even if they are asymptomatic.

Guidelines for care of patients with heart failure associated with left ventricular dysfunction were also developed by the American College of Cardiology/American Heart Association Task Force on Practice Guidelines.[147] These guidelines address management of chronic and acute heart failure, whereas the AHCPR guidelines focus more on the management and prevention of chronic heart failure.

Initial Evaluation

As summarized in the ACC/AHA guidelines, the initial evaluation in patients with heart failure should seek to distinguish diastolic from systolic function and to determine the cause. Of particular importance is excluding ischemic heart disease as the cause of heart failure, since patients with coronary disease might benefit from revascularization.

The AHCPR guidelines identify symptoms that should trigger consideration of an evaluation for heart failure, the most crucial of which are paroxysmal nocturnal dyspnea, orthopnea, or new-onset dyspnea on exertion. Unless the patient has clear evidence of a noncardiac cause for these symptoms, the AHCPR guidelines indicate that echocardiography or radionuclide ventriculography should be used to evaluate left ventricular function—even if physical signs of heart failure are not present. Other symptoms that suggest this diagnosis are lower extremity edema, decreased exercise tolerance, unexplained confusion or fatigue, and abdominal symptoms associated with ascites and/or hepatic engorgement.

Several tests are recommended by both AHCPR and ACC/AHA guidelines for the initial evaluation of patients with heart failure, and the goals of this testing include assessment of severity and identification of causes of the myocardial dysfunction (Table 63–18). If the patients would be candidates for revascularization, the ACC/AHA guidelines recommend performance of a noninvasive stress test to detect ischemia in two groups of patients: (1) patients without angina but with a high probability of coronary artery disease and (2) patients with a previous infarction but with no angina. Performance of noninvasive stress testing to detect ischemia in all patients with unexplained heart failure who are potentially candidates for revascularization was considered to be of uncertain appropriateness (Class II). These guidelines also consider exercise testing, usually with respiratory gas analysis, to determine whether patients are candidates for heart transplantation, to be an appropriate test for patients with severe heart failure.

The ACC/AHA guidelines were equivocal (Class II) about the appropriateness of coronary arteriography for *all* patients with unexplained heart failure who might be candidates for revascularization but considered catheterization appropriate (Class I) for patients with heart failure and with angina or large areas of ischemic or hibernating myocardium, as well as patients at risk for coronary artery disease who are to undergo surgical correction of noncoronary cardiac lesions. These guidelines deemed cardiac catheterization and stress testing to be inappropriate (Class III) if patients have previously had coronary disease excluded as a cause of left ventricular dysfunction and no objective evidence of ischemia has developed.

Both sets of guidelines emphasize that screening evaluations for arrhythmias such as ambulatory electrocardiography should not be performed routinely for all patients with heart failure; instead, this test should be reserved for patients with a history of syncope, near-syncope, or other symptoms suggestive of arrhythmia. This recommendation is supported by data from the Cardiac Arrhythmia Suppression Trial,[148,149] which found increased mortality in patients with ejection fractions of 40 per cent or less who were treated with moricizine, encainide, and flecainide. These findings have led to reservations about treating any but the most serious ventricular arrhythmias in this patient population.

One arrhythmia that may be *undertreated* in patients with heart failure is atrial fibrillation. The AHCPR guidelines recommend attempting cardioversion for patients with left atrial diameter less than 50 mm and less than a 1-year history of atrial fibrillation. No recommendations are offered on the drug of choice, although the guidelines comment that amiodarone may emerge as the preferred agent.

Routine use of myocardial biopsy was not supported by *both* guidelines because of lack of evidence that this information leads to improved management or outcomes. The ACC/AHA guidelines were uncertain (Class II) about the appropriateness of endomyocardial biopsy for patients (1) with recent onset of rapidly deteriorating cardiac function or other clinical indications of myocarditis; (2) receiving chemotherapy with Adriamycin or other myocardial toxic agents; and (3) with a systemic disease and possible cardiac involvement.

The ACC/AHA guidelines also considered measurement of circulating neurohormone levels to be of little value in routine management and evaluation.

Inpatient and Outpatient Management

The AHCPR guidelines provide specific criteria for admission to the hospital and also offer standards for outcomes to be achieved before patients with heart failure are discharged from the hospital (Table 63–18). These recommendations reflect the importance of discharge planning and an adequate system of outpatient care. Readmission rates as high as 57 per cent within 90 days have been reported in elderly patients with heart failure.[150] In that study, factors associated with readmission were failed social support systems, inadequate follow-up, failure to seek medical attention promptly when symptoms recurred, and noncompliance with diet and medications. Such findings led to a series of recommendations regarding patient and family education and counseling. Many of these interventions, such as support groups, have not been part of the traditional focus of physicians; hence, these guidelines imply close collaboration of a team of providers for patients with heart failure. Among the topics for patient education specifically cited were:

- Nature of heart failure
- Drug regimens
- Dietary restrictions
- What to do if symptoms occur
- Prognosis
- Completion of advanced directives
- Smoking and chewing of tobacco

TABLE 63-18 SELECTED RECOMMENDATIONS FROM GUIDELINES FOR HEART FAILURE (AHCPR)

TOPIC	RECOMMENDATION	STRENGTH OF EVIDENCE
Prevention in asymptomatic patients	Asymptomatic patients with moderately or severely reduced left-ventricular systolic function (ejection fraction <35–40%) should be treated with an angiotensin-converting enzyme (ACE) inhibitor to reduce the chance of developing clinical heart failure.	A
Initial evaluation	Patients with symptoms highly suggestive of heart failure should undergo echocardiography or radionuclide ventriculography to measure left ventricular function even if physical signs of heart failure are absent.	C
Diagnostic testing	Practitioners should perform a chest x-ray; ECG; complete blood count (CBC); serum electrolytes, serum creatinine, serum albumin, liver function tests; and urinalysis for all patients with suspected or clinically evident heart failure. A T_4 and thyroid-stimulating hormone (TSH) level should also be checked in all patients over age 65 with heart failure and no obvious etiology, and in patients who have atrial fibrillation or other signs or symptoms of thyroid disease. Routine use of myocardial biopsy is not recommended.	C
Screening for arrhythmias	Screening evaluation for arrhythmias such as ambulatory electrocardiography is not routinely warranted.	A
Hospital admission criteria	Presence or suspicion of heart failure and any of the following findings usually indicates a need for hospitalization: • Clinically or ECG evidence of acute myocardial ischemia. • Pulmonary edema or severe respiratory distress. • Oxygen saturation below 90% (not due to pulmonary disease). • Severe complicating medical illness (e.g., pneumonia). • Anasarca. • Symptomatic hypotension or syncope. • Heart failure refractory to outpatient therapy. • Inadequate social support for safe outpatient management.	C
Hospital discharge criteria	Patients with heart failure should be discharged from the hospital only when: • Symptoms of heart failure have been adequately controlled. • All reversible causes of morbidity have been treated or stabilized. • Patients and caregivers have been educated about medications, diet, activity and exercise recommendations, and symptoms of worsening heart failure. • Adequate outpatient support and follow-up care have been arranged.	C
Activity recommendations	Regular exercise should be encouraged for all patients with stable NYHA Class I-III heart failure.	B
Cardiac rehabilitation	There is insufficient evidence at this time to recommend the routine use of supervised rehabilitation programs for patients with heart failure.	C
Diet	Dietary sodium should be restricted to as close to 2 grams per day as possible.	C
	People who drink alcohol should be advised to consume no more than one drink per day.	C
Discussion of prognosis	All patients should be encouraged to complete a durable power of attorney for health care or another form of advanced directive.	N/A
The initial pharmacological management	Patients with heart failure and signs of significant volume overload should be started immediately on a diuretic. Patients with mild volume overload can be managed adequately on thiazide diuretics, whereas those with more severe volume overload should be started on a loop diuretic.	C
ACE inhibitors	Patients with heart failure due to left ventricular systolic dysfunction should be given a trial of ACE inhibitors unless specific contraindications exist: (1) history of intolerance or adverse reactions to these agents, (2) serum potassium greater than 5.5 mEq/liter that cannot be reduced, or (3) symptomatic hypotension. Patients with systolic blood pressure less than 90 mm Hg have a higher risk of complications and should be managed by a physician experienced in utilizing ACE inhibitors in such patients. Caution and close monitoring are also required for patients who have a serum creatinine greater than 3.0 mg/dl or an estimated creatinine clearance of less than 30 ml/min; half the usual dose should be used in this setting.	B
Digoxin	Digoxin should be used routinely in patients with severe heart failure and should be added to the medical regimen of patients with mild or moderate heart failure who remain symptomatic after optimal management with ACE inhibitors and diuretics.	C
Hydralazine/isosorbide dinitrate	Isosorbide dinitrate and hydralazine is an appropriate alternative in patients with contraindications or intolerance to ACE inhibitors.	B
Anticoagulation	Routine anticoagulation is not recommended.	C
Beta blockers	This form of treatment should be considered experimental at this time.	B
Patient follow-up	Patients should be instructed to call if they experience an unexplained weight gain greater than 3–5 pounds since their last clinical evaluation.	C

From Konstam, M., Dracup, K., Baker, D., et al.: Heart Failure: Evaluation and care of patients with left-ventricular systolic dysfunction. Clinical Practice Guideline No. 11. AHCPR Publication No. 94-0612. Rockville, Md.; Agency for Health Care Policy and Research, Public Health Service, U.S. Department of Health and Human Services, June 1994. (For definition of A, B, & C see p. 1979.)

- Importance of influenza and pneumococcal vaccination
- Sexual activity
- Alcohol use

Regular physical activity programs are recommended for all patients except those with NYHA Class IV heart failure, but the guidelines do not explicitly endorse the use of cardiac rehabilitation programs for all patients with heart failure.

Management

Both the ACC/AHA and AHCPR guidelines provide a strong endorsement of the use of angiotensin-converting enzyme (ACE) inhibitors for patients with left ventricular systolic dysfunction in the absence of specific contraindications (Table 63–18), and make similar recommendations regarding several other medications. Diuretic use for patients with signs of volume overload should be immediate according to both sets of guidelines, and the AHCPR guidelines also suggest that patients with mild volume overload can be managed adequately with thiazide diuretics, which cause a less acute diuresis than does furosemide.[150,151] For patients without volume overload, ACE inhibitors may be considered as the sole initial therapy. The prominent roles of ACE inhibitors and diuretics in the AHCPR guidelines are reflected in its flow sheet summarizing pharmacological management (Fig. 63–3).

The guidelines also support use of digoxin, despite the uncertainty regarding its impact on mortality. The ACC/AHA guidelines considered routine use of digoxin for all patients with left ventricular systolic function to be of uncertain appropriateness (Class II). Because of data demonstrating that digoxin can improve physical function and decrease symptoms in at least some patients with heart failure,[152] both sets of guidelines recommend that it be used routinely for patients with heart failure who remain symptomatic despite diuretics and ACE inhibitors. The ACC/AHA guidelines also note that digoxin is appropriate (Class I) for patients with heart failure and atrial fibrillation.

The AHCPR task force concludes that anticoagulation is not justifiable as part of routine therapy for heart failure, but that it should be reserved for patients with thromboembolic disease, atrial fibrillation, or mobile left ventricular thrombi. The guidelines also do not support use of beta-

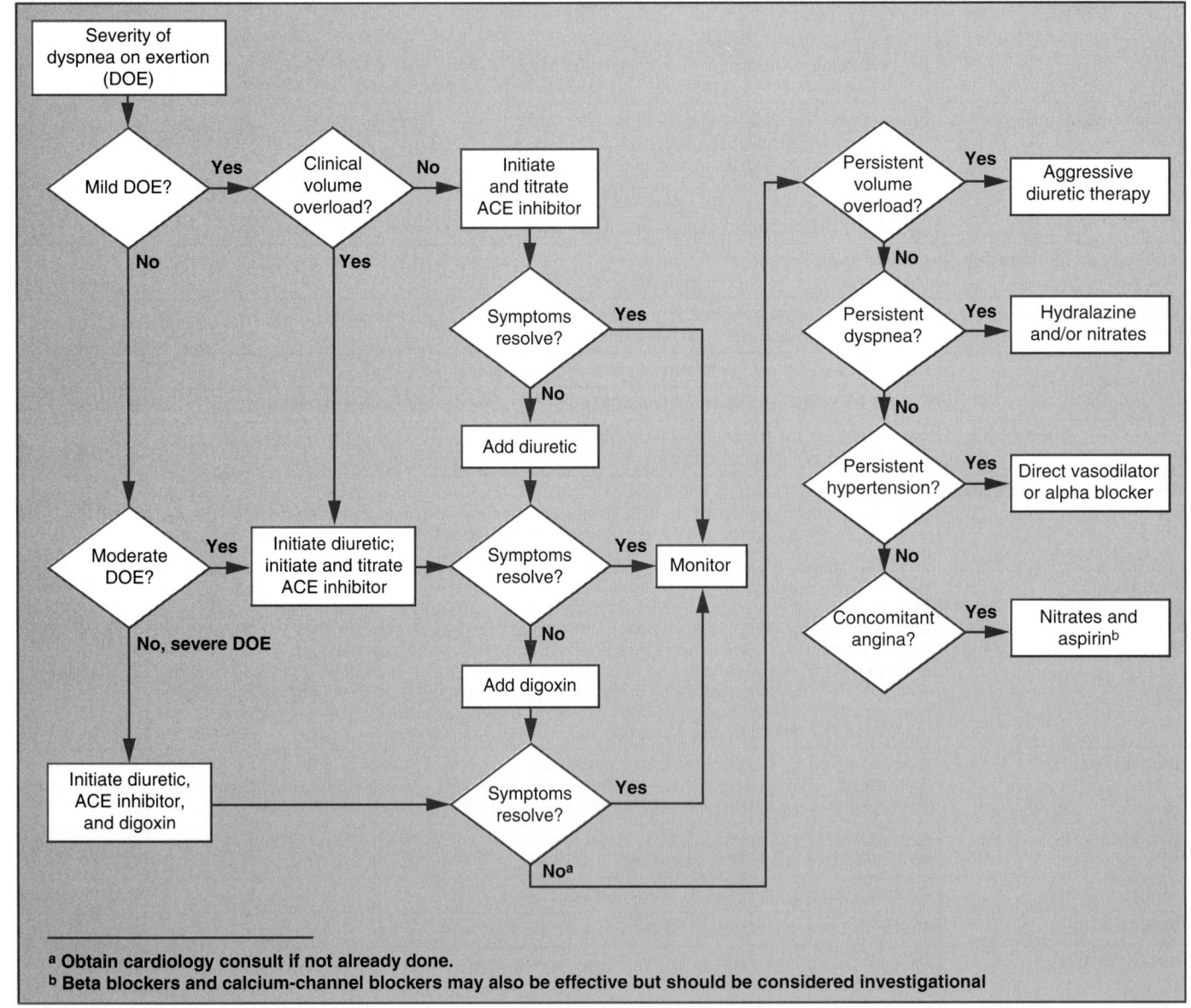

a Obtain cardiology consult if not already done.
b Beta blockers and calcium-channel blockers may also be effective but should be considered investigational

FIGURE 63–3. Flow sheet from AHCPR guidelines for heart failure describing strategy for using pharmacological measures. (From Konstam, M., Dracup, K., Baker, D., et al.: Heart Failure: Evaluation and Care of Patients with Left-Ventricular Systolic Dysfunction. Clinical Practice Guideline Number 11. AHCPR Publication No. 94-0612. Rockville, Md., Agency for Health Care Policy and Research and the National Heart, Lung, and Blood Institute, Public Health Service, US Department of Health and Human Services, June 1994.)

adrenergic blockers, despite the promising findings from some studies. Which patients are appropriate for trials of beta blockers remains uncertain; hence, the guidelines conclude that beta blockers are "an experimental, albeit promising, therapy." Similar conclusions were reached by the ACC/AHA expert panel, which also commented that use of calcium channel blockers in the absence of coexisting angina or hypertension was inappropriate.

Although revascularization of ischemic myocardium either by PTCA or CABG does not directly improve heart failure in most patients, this strategy can improve survival because patients with severe coronary disease and left ventricular dysfunction have a poor prognosis with medical therapy alone. Therefore, the guidelines support performance of coronary angiography in heart failure patients with exercise-limiting angina, rest angina, or recurrent episodes of acute pulmonary edema.

Should left ventricular function be irreversibly and severely damaged, patients may be considered for cardiac transplantation. The AHCPR guidelines do not provide recommendations for the evaluation of this patient population.

Even though the ACC/AHA guidelines also focus on systolic dysfunction, these guidelines make specific recommendations for the treatment of diastolic dysfunction. These guidelines considered appropriate (Class I) the use of diuretic drugs, nitrates, drugs suppressing AV conduction to control ventricular rate in patients with atrial fibrillation, and anticoagulation in patients with atrial fibrillation or prior embolization. Class II therapy included calcium channel blockers, beta blockers, ACE inhibitors, and anticoagulation in patients with intracardiac thrombus. Class III (inappropriate) interventions included drugs with positive inotropic effects in the absence of systolic dysfunction and treatment of asymptomatic arrhythmia.

Interventions for Acutely III Patients

The ACC/AHA guidelines offer recommendations regarding the management of patients with acute syndromes including pulmonary edema and cardiogenic shock. In addition to the tests already described, these guidelines comment that cardiac catheterization is appropriate for patients with acute pulmonary edema and suspected coronary artery disease (1) if acute intervention for myocardial injury or infarction is anticipated, or (2) to determine the cause for refractory pulmonary edema.

Pulmonary artery balloon catheters are recommended for consideration in patients with pulmonary edema: (1) if the patient's condition is deteriorating; (2) recovery from the acute presentation is not occurring as anticipated; (3) high-dose nitroglycerin or nitroprusside is required; (4) dobutamine or dopamine is needed to augment systemic blood pressure and peripheral perfusion; or (5) there is uncertainty regarding the diagnosis. Indwelling arterial cannula and transesophageal echocardiography are of uncertain (Class II) appropriateness.

For patients with cardiogenic shock, the ACC/AHA guidelines recommend a rapid infusion of intravenous fluids unless there is evidence of volume overload. If there is not a satisfactory response to this infusion, hemodynamic monitoring should include a pulmonary artery balloon flotation catheter and an indwelling arterial cannula. Intraaortic balloon counterpulsation is also considered appropriate (Class I) for patients with cardiogenic shock or pulmonary edema who do not respond to fluid volume or pharmacological therapy and in patients with acute heart failure accompanied by refractory ischemia.

Outcome Assessment and Follow-up

The most important judge of whether therapeutic interventions have led to improvement is the patient, not a noninvasive test. Therefore, the AHCPR guidelines emphasize the importance of follow-up of patient data such as physical functioning, mental health, sexual function, and the ability to perform usual work and social activities. Between visits to their physicians, patients should keep track of their own weight, and contact their provider if their weight goes up more than 3 to 5 pounds.

PERIOPERATIVE CARDIOVASCULAR EVALUATION FOR NONCARDIAC SURGERY

An ACC/AHA task force issued guidelines in 1996 for the evaluation and management of patients undergoing noncardiac surgery.[153] Few issues related to this topic have been subjected to randomized or controlled trials; thus, these guidelines do not classify many interventions as clearly appropriate or inappropriate. Instead, these guidelines synthesize the literature and offer recommendations for some common clinical issues. A theme that characterizes these recommendations is that interventions are rarely necessary simply to reduce the risk for complications during noncardiac surgery unless the intervention is indicated as part of the routine care of the patient.

These guidelines also emphasize that the goal of the evaluation is not to "clear" the patient but to perform an evaluation of the patient's medical status and to make recommendations regarding the risk of cardiac problems over the entire perioperative period. A specific recommendation is that coronary bypass surgery and coronary angioplasty are almost never appropriate unless they would otherwise be indicated to improve survival and quality of life.

Tests are discouraged unless they are likely to influence patient management. Preoperative noninvasive evaluation of left ventricular function, for example, is considered appropriate (Class I) in these guidelines for patients with current or poorly controlled congestive heart failure, but of equivocal (Class II) appropriateness in other patients with heart failure and patients with dyspnea of unknown etiology.

For most patients who are candidates for noninvasive tests for ischemia, the guidelines conclude that the "test of choice" is exercise electrocardiography, which can provide data on functional status as well as detection of ischemia. For patients who cannot undergo this test because of abnormal electrocardiograms, no specific recommendation is issued regarding the choice of stress echocardiography versus myocardial perfusion imaging. The guidelines do not support the use of ambulatory electrocardiography as the only diagnostic test to identify candidates for coronary angiography.

Indications for coronary angiography before noncardiac surgery are summarized in Table 63–19. These are adapted from 1987 ACC/AHA guidelines for the use of coronary angiography[64] and incorporate the nature of the procedure to be undertaken. "High-risk" procedures are those with a reported cardiac risk that is usually over 5 per cent, including emergency major operations, particularly in the elderly, aortic and other major vascular procedures, and operations with an anticipated large fluid shift and/or blood loss. "Intermediate-risk" procedures include carotid endarterectomy, head and neck surgery, intraperitoneal and intrathoracic procedures, orthopedic procedures, and prostate operations. The guidelines for coronary angiography also rely on stratification of patients according to their risk for complications, with major predictors of risk including unstable coronary syndromes, decompensated heart failure, significant arrhythmias, and severe valvular disease.

Recommendations for the use of revascularization procedures before noncardiac surgery are tempered by the lack of data demonstrating beneficial impact from revascularization. Therefore, the ACC/AHA guidelines conclude that the timing of revascularization procedures in patients for whom they are otherwise indicated must be determined by the urgency of the noncardiac procedure. Revascularization

TABLE 63–19   INDICATIONS FOR CORONARY ANGIOGRAPHY IN THE PERIOPERATIVE EVALUATION OF PATIENTS WITH SUSPECT OR PROVEN CORONARY ARTERY DISEASE*

I. APPROPRIATE

1. High-risk results on noninvasive testing.
2. Angina pectoris unresponsive to adequate medical therapy.
3. Most patients with unstable angina pectoris.
4. Nondiagnostic or equivocal noninvasive test in a high-risk patient undergoing a high-risk noncardiac surgical procedure.

II. EQUIVOCAL

1. Intermediate risk results on noninvasive testing.
2. Nondiagnostic or equivocal noninvasive test in a lower-risk patient undergoing a high-risk noncardiac surgical procedure.
3. Urgent noncardiac surgery in a patient convalescing from acute myocardial infarction.
4. Perioperative myocardial infarction.

III. INAPPROPRIATE

1. Low-risk noncardiac surgery in a patient with known coronary artery disease and low-risk results on noninvasive testing.
2. Screening for coronary artery disease without appropriate noninvasive testing.
3. Asymptomatic after coronary revascularization, with excellent exercise capacity ($\geq$ 7 METS).
4. Mild stable angina in patients with good left ventricular function, low-risk noninvasive test results.
5. Patient not candidate for coronary revascularization because of concomitant medical illness.
6. Prior technically adequate normal coronary angiogram within 5 years.
7. Severe left ventricular dysfunction and patient not considered candidate for revascularization procedure.
8. Patient unwilling to consider coronary revascularization procedure.

* If results will affect management.
Modified from Eagle, K. A., Brundage, B. H., Chaitman, B. R., et al.: Guidelines for perioperative cardiovascular evaluation for noncardiac surgery. Report of the American College of Cardiology/American Heart Association Task Force on Practice Guidelines (Committee on Perioperative Cardiovascular Evaluation for Noncardiac Surgery). Reprinted with permission from the American College of Cardiology. J. Am. Coll. Cardiol. *27*:910, 1996.

before noncardiac elective surgical procedures of high or intermediate risk was supported for patients who are found to have high-risk coronary anatomy in whom long-term outcome would likely be improved by PTCA or CABG.

Specific recommendations were not made for the use of intraoperative pulmonary artery catheters, computerized ST-segment monitoring, or intraaortic balloon counterpulsation. Routine testing to detect evidence of myocardial injury after surgery was discouraged. In patients with known or suspected coronary disease who undergo surgical procedures with a high risk for complications, the ACC/AHA guidelines recommend electrocardiograms at baseline, immediately after the procedure, and daily on the first 2 postoperative days. Measurement of cardiac enzymes is recommended for high-risk patients or those who demonstrate clinical evidence of cardiovascular dysfunction.

PREVENTION OF CORONARY ARTERY DISEASE

SECONDARY PREVENTION OF CORONARY ARTERY DISEASE

(See also Chap. 35)

Although many guidelines described in this chapter have the goal of decreasing the use of tests and procedures by defining appropriate indications, some guidelines seek to decrease *underutilization* of interventions that may improve patient outcome through prevention. Clinical trial data are now available to support several measures aimed at preventing or slowing the progression of coronary artery disease, and these interventions are generally most cost-effective when used for secondary prevention, that is, for patients with known coronary disease.[154] Secondary prevention tends to be more cost-effective than primary prevention—that is, intervention for patients without known coronary disease—because patients with known disease are at higher risk of subsequent complications and therefore have a higher probability of benefiting from an effective preventive measure.

Specific recommendations for the use of preventive interventions were provided in a 1995 consensus panel statement from the American Heart Association,[155] which was also endorsed by the American College of Cardiology. These recommendations provide explicit goals for a wide range of topics including smoking cessation, lipid management, physical activity, weight management, blood pressure control, and the use of several key medications. Particularly noteworthy are recommendations that:

• Patients with coronary disease start the American Heart Association Step II Diet ($\leq$ 30 per cent fat, < 7 per cent saturated fat, < 200 mg/dl cholesterol), as recommended by the National Cholesterol Education Program (NCEP) Adult Treatment Panel II[156]

• For cholesterol management, drug therapy should be added to diet for coronary disease patients with LDL cholesterol levels greater than 130 mg/dl and considered for those with LDL cholesterol levels between 100 and 130 mg/dl (Fig. 35–4, p. 1138). This recommendation is also consistent with the NCEP definitions of desirable levels of serum lipids in patients with known coronary disease as an LDL cholesterol level less than 100 mg/dl, HDL cholesterol level greater than 35 mg/dl, and triglycerides less than 200 mg/dl.[156]

• Patients perform a minimum of 30 to 60 minutes of moderate-intensity activity three or four times weekly, supplemented by an increase in daily life style activities

• Aspirin 80 mg to 325 mg per day should be started in the absence of contraindications.

- The goal of blood pressure management is to reduce systolic pressure below 140 mm Hg and diastolic pressure below 90 mm Hg.

A similar but separate set of preventive guidelines directed specifically at patients who had undergone coronary revascularization were issued by an AHA panel in 1994.[157]

HIGH BLOOD CHOLESTEROL

(See also Chap. 35)

The most influential guidelines for detection and treatment of serum lipid abnormalities were revised and published by the National Cholesterol Education Program (NCEP) in 1993.[156] As was true in previous guidelines from this NHLBI-sponsored group, LDL cholesterol is the most important determinant of cholesterol-lowering strategy. However, these revisions emphasize the emerging recognition of age and low HDL cholesterol as important risk factors for coronary heart disease and describe different strategies for groups at various risks of ischemic complications.

In the revised guidelines, screening evaluations of HDL cholesterol level are recommended, and HDL cholesterol levels below 35 mg/dl are considered a major risk factor for coronary heart disease. High HDL cholesterol levels (>60 mg/dl) are considered a "negative" risk factor that reduces the count of total risk factors.

Age also influences risk assessment in the new guidelines. Men below age 35 years and premenopausal women are considered to be at low risk for coronary heart complications, and delays in initiation of drug therapy for LDL cholesterol levels in the range of 160 to 220 mg/dl are recommended. (Pharmacotherapy is supported for patients in these age groups who have higher LDL cholesterol levels.) In contrast, age over 45 years for men and over 55 years for women is considered a major risk factor for coronary heart disease. Other major risk factors include family history of premature coronary heart disease, cigarette smoking, hypertension, and diabetes mellitus.

These risk factors and the patient's history are used to divide patients into one of three risk categories:

1. Patients with high blood cholesterol who are otherwise at low risk
2. Patients without evidence of coronary heart disease who are at increased risk because of high blood cholesterol together with multiple other risk factors
3. Patients with known coronary heart disease or other atherosclerotic disease

Different thresholds and goals for initiation of diet and drug therapy for these three groups are recommended in the NCEP guidelines.

The guidelines also encourage more stringent dietary measures for higher-risk patients. The NCEP's eating pattern recommendation for the general public is similar to an American Heart Association Step I diet. This diet includes an intake of saturated fat of 8 to 10 per cent of total calories, 30 per cent or less of calories from total fat, and cholesterol intake less than 300 mg/day.

For patients with known coronary heart disease or other atherosclerotic disease, the guidelines recommend a Step II diet. This diet calls for saturated fat intake of less than 7 per cent of total calories, and total cholesterol intake of less than 200 mg/day. The Step II Diet generally requires intervention by a trained nutritionist. Patients who are unable to meet lipid goals with the Step I Diet and other nonpharmacological goals should also attempt the Step II Diet.

With these diets, total cholesterol levels should be measured and adherence assessed after 4 to 6 weeks and at 3 months of therapy. The guidelines recommend a minimum of 6 months of intensive dietary therapy and counseling before initiation of drug therapy, unless patients have severe elevations of LDL cholesterol ($\geq$ 220 mg/dl).

Although the NCEP guidelines do not make explicit recommendations about the sequence in which drugs are tried, they note that there are fewer long-term data available on the safety and efficacy of the statins compared with older agents such as the bile acid sequestrants and nicotinic acid. However, recent data demonstrating decreased mortality with this class of drugs may lead to more support for statins as an initial choice in future versions of these guidelines.

HYPERTENSION

(See also Chap. 26)

Guidelines for the treatment of high blood pressure in adults have been issued periodically for more than 20 years by the Joint National Committee on Detection, Evaluation, and Treatment of High Blood Pressure, which published its fifth report (also known as JNC-V) in 1994.[158] These guidelines include a new classification system (Table 63–20) for blood pressure that replaced the traditional terms of "mild" and "moderate" hypertension with stages. "Optimal" blood pressure is systolic blood pressure less than 120 mm Hg and diastolic blood pressure less than 80 mm Hg. Classifications should be based on two or more readings taken at each of two or more visits following initial screening.

The response to an initial elevated blood pressure reading—and the timing of that response—should be dictated by factors including the magnitude of the blood pressure elevation, presence of cardiovascular disease, and risk factors. The JNC-V guidelines for follow-up that are summarized in Table 63–21 provide recommendations for when patients should get immediate treatment (systolic pressure $\geq$ 210 mm Hg and/or diastolic pressure $\geq$ 120 mm Hg), and how quickly other patients should be asked to return for further evaluation. During these evaluations, recommended tests include urinalysis; complete blood count; blood glucose, potassium, calcium, creatinine, uric acid, total and high-density lipoprotein cholesterol and triglyceride levels; and electrocardiography.

TABLE 63–20   CLASSIFICATION OF BLOOD PRESSURE FOR ADULTS (JNC-5)

CATEGORY	SYSTOLIC (mm Hg)	DIASTOLIC (mm Hg)
Normal	<130	<85
High normal	130–139	85–89
Stage 1 (mild) hypertension	140–159	90–99
Stage 2 (moderate) hypertension	160–179	100–109
Stage 3 (severe) hypertension	180–209	110–119
Stage 4 (very severe) hypertension	$\geq$210	$\geq$120

When systolic and diastolic pressures fall into different categories, the higher category should be selected to classify the individual's blood pressure status.
From National High Blood Pressure Education Program: The Fifth Report of the Joint National Committee on Detection, Evaluation, and Treatment of High Blood Pressure. Bethesda, Md., National Heart, Lung, and Blood Institute, 1993. U.S. Department of Health, Education, and Welfare publication NIH 93-1088.

TABLE 63–21   RECOMMENDATIONS FOR FOLLOW-UP BASED ON INITIAL SET OF BLOOD PRESSURE MEASUREMENTS (JNC-5)

INITIAL SCREENING BLOOD PRESSURE (mm Hg*)		
Systolic	Diastolic	Follow-up Recommended
< 130	< 85	Recheck in 2 years
130–139	85–89	Recheck in 1 year
140–159	90–99	Confirm within 2 months
160–179	100–109	Evaluate or refer to source of care within 1 month
180–209	110–119	Evaluate or refer to source of care within 1 week
≥ 210	≥ 120	Evaluate or refer to source of care immediately

* If the systolic and diastolic categories are different, follow recommendation for the shorter time follow-up.
From National High Blood Pressure Education Program: The Fifth Report of the Joint National Committee on Detection, Evaluation, and Treatment of High Blood Pressure. Bethesda, Md., National Heart, Lung, and Blood Institute, 1993. U.S. Department of Health, Education, and Welfare publication NIH 93-1088.

A more explicit set of recommendations for the definition and management of mild hypertension (systolic pressure 140 to 180 mm Hg and/or diastolic pressure 90 to 105) was revised and published in 1993 by the World Health Organization/International Society of Hypertension Liaison Committee[159] (Fig. 63–4). These guidelines suggest repeat measurement to confirm the diagnosis on at least two occasions over a 4-week period, with regular follow-up for patients whose blood pressure was below 140/90 on remeasurement. Drug treatment is recommended for those whose repeat measurements show diastolic blood pressures greater than 100 mm Hg or systolic pressures greater than 160 to 180 mm Hg with diastolic pressures of 95 or more. For patients with blood pressure between these two levels, observation periods with non-drug antihypertensive measures were recommended. The threshold for initiation of drug therapy varies according to blood pressure levels and presence of other coronary risk factors.

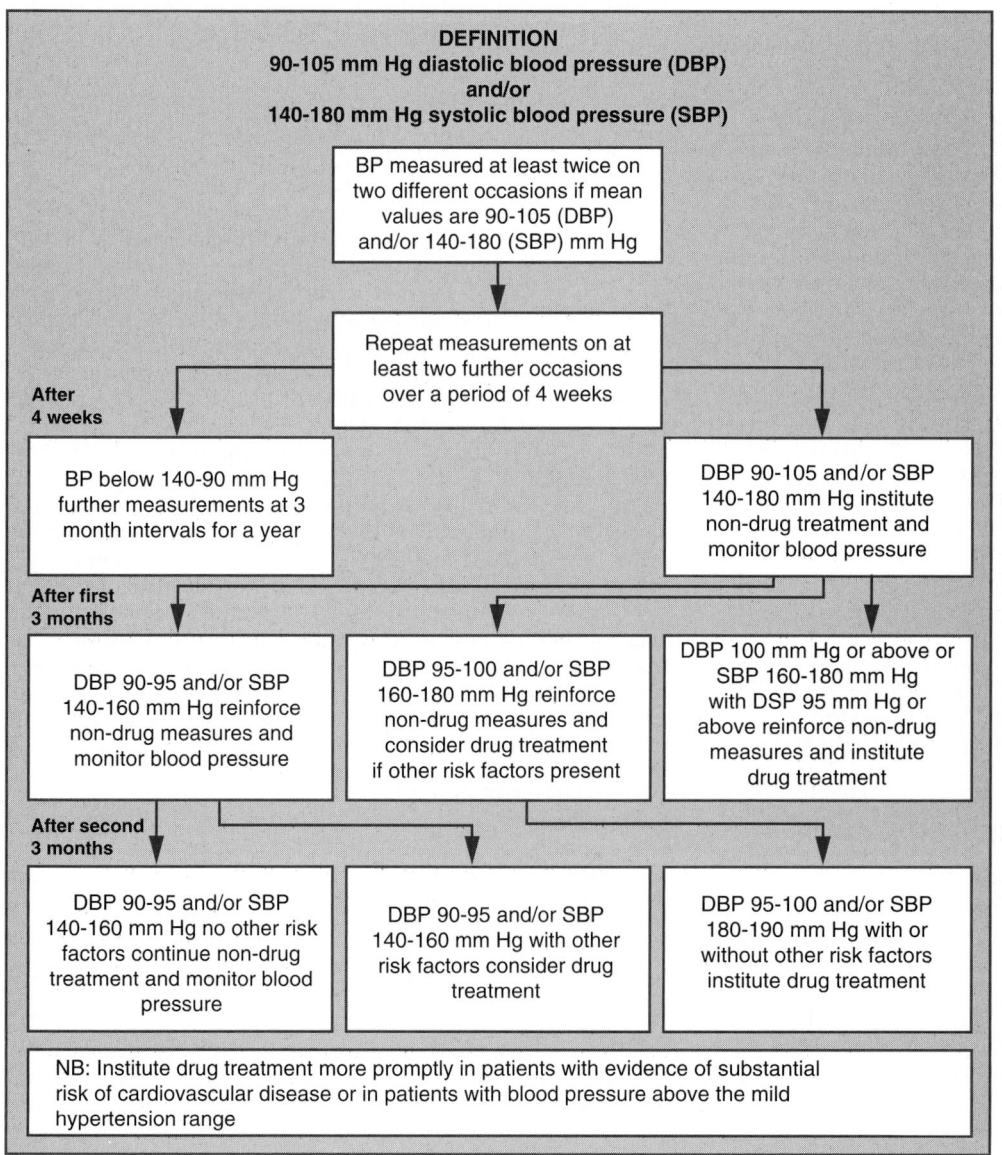

FIGURE 63–4. Recommendations or the definition and management of mild hypertension (systolic pressure 140 to 180 mm Hg and/or diastolic pressure 90 to 105). (Reproduced by permission from The Guidelines Subcommittee of the WHO/ISH Mild Hypertension Liaison Committee: 1993 guidelines for the management of mild hypertension. Memorandum from a World Health Organization/International Society of Hypertension meeting. Hypertension 22:392, 1993. Copyright 1993 American Heart Association.)

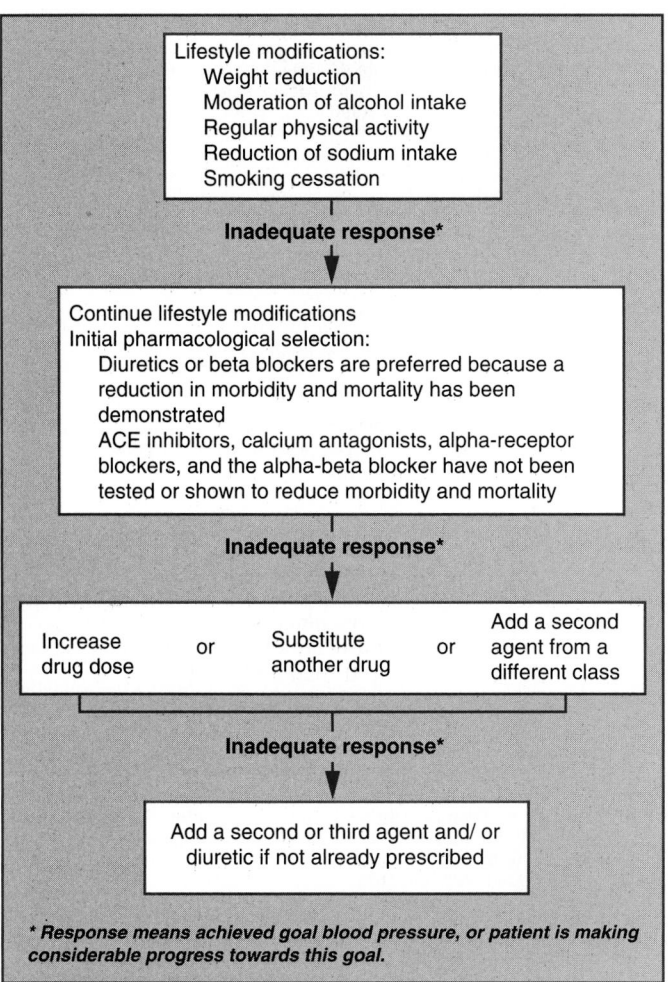

FIGURE 63–5. JNC-5 guidelines for initiation of antihypertensive therapy. (From National High Blood Pressure Education Program: The Fifth Report of the Joint National Committee on Detection, Evaluation, and Treatment of High Blood Pressure. Bethesda, Md.: National Heart, Lung, and Blood Institute, 1993. US Department of Health, Education, and Welfare publication NIH 93-1088.)

The JNC-V guidelines for initiation of therapy (Fig. 63–5) also emphasize a trial of nonpharmacological measures and, if these measures do not lead to satisfactory reduction in blood pressure, initiation of drug therapy. These guidelines recommend diuretics or beta blockers as first-choice agents, because trials have demonstrated reduction in morbidity and mortality with these agents.[160] Alternative drugs include calcium antagonists, ACE inhibitors, alpha₁-receptor blockers, and an alpha-beta blocker. Should the chosen agents not reduce blood pressure to the target level during the next 1 to 3 months, the clinician has three options, including increasing the drug dose, substituting another drug, and adding a second agent from a different class.

REFERENCES

1. Chassin, M. R., Brook, R. H., Park, R. E., et al.: Variations in the use of medical and surgical services by the Medicare population. N. Engl. J. Med. *314:*285, 1986.
2. Wenneker, M. B., and Epstein, A. M.: Racial inequalities in the use of procedures for patients with ischemic heart disease in Massachusetts. JAMA *261:*253, 1989.
3. Ayanian, J. Z., Udvarhelyi, I. S., Gastonis, C. A., Pashos, C. L., and Epstein, A. M.: Racial differences in the use of revascularization procedures after coronary angiography. JAMA *269:*2642, 1993.
4. Whittle, J., Conigliaro, J., Good, C. B., and Lofgren, R. P.: Racial differences in the use of invasive cardiovascular procedures in the Department of Veterans Affairs medical system. N. Engl. J. Med. *329:*600, 1993.
5. Johnson, P. A., Lee, T. H., Cook, E. F., et al.: Effect of race on the presentation and management of patients with chest pain. Ann. Intern. Med. *118:*593, 1993.
6. Ayanian, J. Z., and Epstein, A. M.: Differences in the use of procedures between women and men hospitalized for coronary heart disease. N. Engl. J. Med. *325:*1221, 1991.
7. Tobin, J. N., Wassertheil-Smoller, S., Wexler, J. P., et al.: Sex bias in considering coronary bypass surgery. Ann. Intern. Med. *107:*19, 1987.
8. Wenneker, M. B., Weissman, J. S., and Epstein, A. M.: The association of payer with utilization of cardiac procedures in Massachusetts. JAMA *264:*1255, 1990.
9. Rouleau, J. L., Moye, L. A., Pfeffer, M. A., et al.: A comparison of management patterns after acute myocardial infarction in Canada and the United States. N. Engl. J. Med. *328:*779, 1993.
10. Every, N. R., Larson, E. B., Litwin, P. E., et al.: The association between on-site cardiac catheterization facilities and the use of coronary angiography after acute myocardial infarction. N. Engl. J. Med. *329:*546, 1993.
11. Institute of Medicine Committee to Advise the Public Health Service on Practice Guidelines: Clinical Practice Guidelines: Directions for a New Agency. Washington, D.C., National Academy Press, 1990.
12. Braunwald, E., Mark, D. B., Jones, R. H., et al.: Unstable Angina: Diagnosis and Management. Clinical Practice Guideline Number 10 (amended). AHCPR Publication No. 94-0602. Rockville, Md., Agency for Health Care Policy and Research and the National Heart, Lung, and Blood Institute, Public Health Service, US Department of Health and Human Services, May 1994.
13. Konstam, M., Dracup, K., Baker, D., et al.: Heart Failure: Evaluation and Care of Patients with Left-Ventricular Systolic Dysfunction. Clinical Practice Guidelines No. 11. AHCPR Publication No. 94-0612. Rockville, Md., Agency for Health Care Policy and Research and the National Heart, Lung, and Blood Institute, Public Health Service, US Department of Health and Human Services, June 1994.
14. Bernstein, S. J., Hilborne, L. H., Leape, L. L., et al.: The appropriateness of use of coronary angiography in New York State. JAMA *269:*766, 1993.
15. Brook, R. H., Park, R. E., Chassin, M. R., et al.: Predicting the appropriate use of carotid endarterectomy, upper gastrointestinal endoscopy, and coronary angiography. N. Engl. J. Med. *323:*1173, 1990.
16. Bernstein, S. J., Laouri, M., Hilborne, L. H., et al.: Coronary Angiography. A literature review and ratings of appropriateness and necessity. Santa Monica, Calif., RAND, 1992.
17. Phelps, C. E.: The methodological foundations of studies of the appropriateness of medical care. N. Engl. J. Med. *329:*1241, 1993.
18. Pearson, S. D., Goulart-Fisher, D., and Lee, T. H.: Critical pathways: potential and pitfalls. Ann. Intern. Med. *123:*941, 1995.
19. Lomas, J., Anderson, G. M., Domnick-Pierre, K., et al.: Do practice guidelines guide practice? The effect of a consensus statement on the practice of physicians. N. Engl. J. Med. *321:*1306, 1989.
20. Kosecoff, J., Kanouse, D. E., Rogers, W. H., et al.: Effects of the National Institutes of Health Consensus Development Program on physician practice. JAMA *258:*2708, 1987.
21. Hill, M. N., Levine, D. M., and Whelton, P. K.: Awareness, use and impact of the 1984 Joint National Committee Consensus Report on High Blood Pressure. Am. J. Public Health. *78:*1190, 1988.
22. Ellrodt, A. G., Conner, L., Riedinger, M., and Weingarten, S.: Measuring and improving physician compliance with clinical practice guidelines. A controlled interventional trial. Ann. Intern. Med. *122:*277, 1995.
23. Zyzanski, S. J., Stange, K. C., Kelly, R., et al.: Family physicians' disagreements with the US Preventive Services Task Force recommendations. J. Fam. Pract. *39:*140, 1994.
24. Hyams, A. L., Brandenburg, J. A., Lipsitz, S. R., et al.: Practice guidelines and malpractice litigation: a two-way street. Ann. Intern. Med. *122:*450, 1995.
25. Tunis, S. R., Hayward, R. S., Wilson, M. C., et al.: Internists' attitudes about clinical practice guidelines. Ann. Intern. Med. *120:*956, 1994.
26. Woolf, S. H.: Practice guidelines: A new reality in medicine: I. Recent developments. Arch. Intern. Med. *150:*1811, 1990.
27. Woolf, S. H.: Practice guidelines: A new reality in medicine: II. Methods of developing guidelines. Arch. Intern. Med. *152:*946, 1992.
28. Audet, A. M., Greenfield, S., and Field, M.: Medical practice guidelines: Current activities and future directions. Ann. Intern. Med. *113:*709, 1990.

NONINVASIVE TESTS AND PROCEDURES

29. Schlant, R. C., Adolph, R. J. DiMarco, J. P., et al.: Guidelines for electrocardiography. A report of the American College of Cardiology/American Heart Association Task Force on Assessment of Diagnostic and Therapeutic Cardiovascular Procedures (Committee on Electrocardiography. J. Am. Coll. Cardiol. *19:*473, 1992.
30. U.S. Preventive Task Force Guide to Clinical Preventive Services. Baltimore, Williams and Wilkins, 1989.
31. Grundy, S. M., Greenland, P., Herd, A., et al.: Cardiovascular and risk factor evaluation of healthy American adults: A statement for physicians by an ad hoc committee appointed by the Steering Committee, American Heart Association. Circulation *75:*1340A, 1987.
32. Hayward, R. S. A., Steinberg, E. P., Ford, D. E., et al.: Preventive care guidelines: 1991. Ann. Intern. Med. *114:*758, 1991.
33. Goldberger, A. L., and O'Konski, M. S.: Utility of the routine electrocardiogram before surgery and on general hospital admission. Critical re-

view and new guidelines. *In* Sox, H. C., Jr. (ed.): Common Diagnostic Tests. Use and Interpretation. 2nd ed. Philadelphia, American College of Physicians, 1990, pp. 67–78.

34. Schlant, R. C., Blomqvist, C. G., and Brandenburg, R. O., et al.: Guidelines for exercise testing. A report of the American College of Cardiology/American Heart Association Task Force on Assessment of Cardiovascular Procedures (Subcommittee on Exercise Testing). J. Am. Coll. Cardiol. *8*:725, 1986.

35. Ewy, G. A., Appleton, C. P., Demaria, A. N., et al.: ACC/AHA guidelines for the clinical application of echocardiography. A report of the American College of Cardiology/American Heart Association Task Force on Assessment of Diagnostic and Therapeutic Cardiovascular Procedures (Subcommittee to Develop Guidelines for the Clinical Application of Echocardiography). J. Am. Coll. Cardiol. *16*:1505, 1990.

36. Udvarhelyi, I. S., Goldman, L., Komaroff, A. L., and Lee, T. H.: Determinants of resource utilization for patients admitted for evaluation of acute chest pain. J. Gen. Intern. Med. *7*:1, 1992.

37. Gibler, W. B., Runyon, J. P., Levy, R. C., et al.: Evaluation of patients with chest pain in an emergency department rapid diagnosis and treatment unit. Ann. Emerg. Med. *25*:1, 1995.

38. Sabia, P., Abott, R. D., Afrookteh, A., et al.: Importance of two-dimensional echocardiographic assessment of left ventricular systolic function in patients presenting to the emergency room with cardiac-related symptoms. Circulation *84*:1615, 1991.

39. Cardiogenic brain embolism. Cerebral Embolism Task Force. Arch. Neurol. *43*:71, 1986.

40. DeRook, F. A., Komess, K. A., Albers, G. W., and Popp, R. L.: Transesophageal echocardiography in the evaluation of stroke. Ann. Intern. Med. *117*:922, 1992.

41. Guidelines for Clinical Use of Cardiac Radionuclide Imaging, December 1986.: A Report of the American College of Cardiology/American Heart Association Task Force on Assessment of Cardiovascular Procedures. J. Am. Coll. Cardiol. *8*:1471, 1986.

42. Ritchie, J. L., Bateman, T. M., Bonow, R. O., et al.: Guidelines for clinical use of cardiac radionuclide imaging. Report of the American College of Cardiology/American Heart Association Task Force on Assessment of Diagnostic and Therapeutic Cardiovascular Procedures (Committee on Radionuclide Imaging), developed in collaboration with the American Society of Nuclear Cardiology. J. Am. Coll. Cardiol. *25*:521, 1995.

43. Maddahi, J., Kiat, H., Friedman, J. D., et al.: Technetium-99m-sestamibi myocardial perfusion imaging for evaluation of coronary artery disease. *In* Zaret, B. L. and Beller, G. A., (eds.): Nuclear Cardiology: State of the Art and Future Directions. St. Louis, C. V. Mosby, 1993, pp. 191–200.

44. American College of Physicians.: Efficacy of exercise thallium-201 scintigraphy in the diagnosis and prognosis of coronary artery disease. Ann. Intern. Med. *113*:703, 1990.

45. Go, R. T., Marwick, T. H., MacIntyre, W. J., et al.: A prospective comparison of rubidium-82 PET and thallium-201 SPECT myocardial perfusion imaging utilizing a single dipyridamole stress in the diagnosis of coronary artery disease. J. Nucl. Med. *31*:1899, 1990.

46. Stewart, R. E., Schwaiger, M., Molina, E., et al.: Comparison of rubidium-82 positron emission tomography and thallium-201 SPECT imaging for detection of coronary artery disease. Am. J. Cardiol. *67*:1303, 1991.

47. Bonow, R. O., Berman, D. S., Gibbons, R. J., et al.: Cardiac positron emission tomography: A report for health professionals from the Committee on Advanced Cardiac Imaging and Technology of the Council on Clinical Cardiology, American Heart Association. Circulation *84*:447, 1991.

48. Shaw, L., Miller, D. D., Kong, B. A., et al.: Determination of perioperative cardiac risk by adenosine thallium-201 myocardial imaging. Am. Heart J. *124*:861, 1992.

49. Knoebel, S. B., Crawford, M. H., Dunn, M. I., et al.: Guidelines for ambulatory electrocardiography. A report of the American College of Cardiology/American Heart Association Task Force on Assessment of Diagnostic and Therapeutic Cardiovascular Procedures (Subcommittee on Ambulatory Electrocardiography). J. Am. Coll. Cardiol. *13*:249, 1989.

50. American College of Physicians.: Ambulatory electrocardiographic (Holter) monitoring. Ann. Intern. Med. *113*:77, 1990.

51. Kleiger, R. E., Miller, J. P., Bigger, J. T., Moss, A. J., and The Multicenter Post-Infarction Research Group.: Decreased heart rate variability and its association with increased mortality after acute myocardial infarction. Am. J. Cardiol. *59*:256, 1987.

52. Martin, G. J., Magid, N. M., Myers, G., et al.: Heart rate variability and sudden death. Am. J. Cardiol. *59*:256, 1987.

53. Reiter, M. J., Mann, D. E., Reiffel, J. E., et al.: Significance and incidence of concordance of drug efficacy predictions by Holter monitoring and electrophysiological study in the ESVEM Trial. Electrophysiologic Study versus Electrocardiographic Monitoring. Circulation *91*:1988, 1995.

54. Raby, K. E., Goldman, L., Creager, M. A., et al.: Correlation between preoperative ischemia and major cardiac events after peripheral vascular surgery. N. Engl. J. Med. *321*:1296, 1989.

55. Pepine, C. J., Cohn, P. F., Deedwania, P. C., et al.: Effects of treatment on outcome in mildly symptomatic patients with ischemia during daily life. The Atenolol Silent Ischemia Study. Circulation *90*:762, 1994.

56. Knatterud, G. L., Bourassa, M. G., Pepine, C. J., et al.: Effects of treatment strategies to suppress ischemia in patients with coronary artery disease; 12-week results of the Asymptomatic Cardiac Ischemia Pilot (ACIP) Study. J. Am. Coll. Cardiol. *24*:11, 1994.

57. Stone, P. H., Gibson, R. S., Glasser, S. P., et al.: Comparison of propranolol, diltiazem, and nifedipine in the treatment of ambulatory ischemia in patients with stable angina. Differential effects on ambulatory ischemia, exercise performance, and angina symptoms. The ASIS Study Group. Circulation *82*:1962, 1990.

58. Hubner, P. J. B., Goldberg, M. J., and Lawson, C. W.: Value of routine cardiac monitoring in the management of acute myocardial infarction outside a coronary care unit. Br. Med. J. *1*:815, 1969.

59. Macy, J., and James, T. N.: The value and limitations of computer monitoring in myocardial infarction. Prog. Cardiovasc. Dis. *13*:495, 1971.

60. Lindsay, J., and Bruckner, N. V.: Conventional coronary care unit monitoring—nondetection of transient rhythm disturbances. JAMA *232*:51, 1975.

61. Lipskis, D. J., Dannehl, K. N., and Silverman, M. E.: Value of radiotelemetry in a community hospital. Am. J. Cardiol. *53*:1284, 1984.

62. Vismara, L. A., DeMaria, A. N., Hughes, J. L., et al.: Evaluation of arrhythmias in the late hospital phase of acute myocardial infarction compared to coronary care unit ectopy. Br. Heart J. *37*:598, 1975.

63. Jaffe, A. S., Atkins, J. M., Field, J. M., et al.: Recommended guidelines for in-hospital cardiac monitoring of adults for detection of arrhythmia. J. Am. Coll. Cardiol. *18*:1431, 1991.

INVASIVE TESTS AND PROCEDURES

64. Ross, J., Jr., Brandenburg, R. O., Dinsmore, R. E., et al.: Guidelines for coronary angiography. A report of the American College of Cardiology/American Heart Association Task Force on Assessment of Diagnostic and Therapeutic Cardiovascular Procedures (Subcommittee on Coronary Angiography). J. Am. Coll. Cardiol. *10*:935, 1987.

65. Pepine, C. J., Allen, H. D., Bashore, T. M., et al.: ACC/AHA Guidelines for cardiac catheterization and cardiac catheterization laboratories. American College of Cardiology/American Heart Association Ad Hoc Task Force on Cardiac Catheterization. J. Am. Coll. Cardiol. *18*:1149, 1991.

66. ACC/AHA Task Force on Assessment of Cardiovascular Procedures.: Guidelines for Exercise Testing. J. Am. Coll. Cardiol. *8*:725, 1986.

67. Schaffer, W. A., and Cobb, L. A.: Recurrent ventricular fibrillation and modes of death in survivors of out-of-hospital ventricular fibrillation. N. Engl. J. Med. *293*:259, 1975.

68. Grines, C. L., Browne, K. F., Marco, J., et al. for the Primary Angioplasty in Myocardial Infarction Study Group.: A comparison of immediate angioplasty with thrombolytic therapy for acute myocardial infarction. N. Engl. J. Med. *328*:673, 1993.

69. Zijlstra, F., de Boear, M. J., Hoornthje, J. C. A., et al.: A comparison of immediate coronary angioplasty with intravenous streptokinase in acute myocardial infarction. N. Engl. J. Med. *328*:680, 1993.

70. Gibbons, R. J., Holmes, D. R., Reeder, G. S., et al., for the Mayo Coronary Care Unit and Catheterization Laboratory Groups.: Immediate angioplasty compared with the administration of a thrombolytic agent followed by conservative treatment for myocardial infarction. N. Engl. J. Med. *328*:685, 1993.

71. Topol, E. J., Califf, R. M., George, B. S., et al.: A randomized trial of immediate versus delayed elective angioplasty after intravenous tissue plasminogen activator in acute myocardial infarction. N. Engl. J. Med. *317*:581, 1987.

72. Simoons, M. L., Arnold, A. E. R., Betriu, A., et al.: Thrombolysis with tissue plasminogen activator in acute myocardial infarction: No additional benefit from immediate percutaneous coronary angioplasty. Lancet *1*:197, 1988.

73. Rogers, W. J., Baim, D. S., Gore, J. M., et al.: Comparison of immediate invasive, delayed invasive, and conservative strategies after tissue-type plasminogen activator. Results of the Thrombolysis in Myocardial Infarction (TIMI). Phase II—A trial. Circulation *81*:1457, 1990.

74. The TIMI Study Group.: Comparison of invasive and conservative strategies after treatment with intravenous tissue plasminogen activator in acute myocardial infarction. Results of the Thrombolysis in Myocardial Infarction (TIMI) Phase II Trial. N. Engl. J. Med. *320*:618, 1989.

75. Ellis, S. G., Ribeiro da Silva, E., Heyndrickx, G. R., et al.: Final results of the randomized RESCUE study evaluating PTCA after failed thrombolysis for patients with anterior infarction. Circulation *88*:I-106, 1993.

76. Belenkie, I., Traboulsi, M., Gall, C. A., et al.: Rescue angioplasty during myocardial infarction has a beneficial effect on mortality: A tenable hypothesis. Can. J. Cardiol. *8*:357, 1992.

77. Czer, L. S., Gray, R. J., DeRoberts, M. A., et al.: Mitral valve replacement: Impact of coronary artery disease and determinants of prognosis after revascularization. Circulation *70* (suppl. I):I-198, 1984.

78. Block, P. C., Ockene, I., Goldberg, R. J., et al.: A prospective randomized trial of outpatient versus inpatient cardiac catheterization. N. Engl. J. Med. *319*:1251, 1988.

79. Klinke, W. P., Kubac, G., Talibi, T., and Lee, S. J. K.: Safety of outpatient cardiac catheterizations. Am. J. Cardiol. *56*:639, 1985.

80. Clark, D. A., Moscovich, M. D., Vetrovec, G. W., and Wexler, L.: Guidelines for the performance of outpatient catheterization and angiographic procedures. Cathet. Cardiovasc. Diagn. *27*:5, 1992.

81. Society for Cardiac Angiography, Laboratory Performance Standards Committee.: Guidelines for approval of professional staff for privileges in the cardiac catheterization laboratory. Cathet. Cardiovasc. Diagn. *10*:199, 1984.

82. Rodriguez, A., Boullon, F., Perez-Balino, N., et al.: Argentine randomized trial of percutaneous transluminal coronary angioplasty versus coronary artery bypass surgery in multivessel disease (ERACI): In-hospital results and 1-year follow-up. J. Am. Coll. Cardiol. 22:1060, 1993.

83. Hamm, C. W., Reimers, J., Ischinger, T., et al., for the German Angioplasty Bypass Surgery Investigation.: A randomized study of coronary angioplasty compared with bypass surgery in patients with symptomatic multivessel coronary disease. N. Engl. J. Med. 331:1037, 1994.

84. Hamptom, J. R., Henderson, R. A., Julian, D. G., and the RITA trial participants.: Coronary angioplasty versus coronary artery bypass surgery: The Randomised Intervention Treatment of Angina (RITA) trial. Lancet 341:573, 1993.

85. King, S. B., III, Lembo, N. J., Weintraub, W. S., et al.: A randomized trial comparing coronary angioplasty with coronary bypass surgery: The Emory Angioplasty versus Surgery Trail. N. Engl. J. Med. 331:1044, 1994.

86. Parisi, A. F., Folland, E. D., and Hartigan, P., for the Veterans Affairs ACME Investigators.: A comparison of early invasive and conservative strategies in unstable angina and non-Q-wave myocardial infarction. Circulation 89:1545, 1994.

87. Ryan, T. J., Bauman, W. B., Kennedy, J. W., et al.: Guidelines for percutaneous transluminal coronary angioplasty. A report of the American College of Cardiology/American Heart Association Task Force on Assessment of Diagnostic and Therapeutic Cardiovascular Procedures (Subcommittee on Percutaneous Transluminal Coronary Angioplasty). J. Am. Coll. Cardiol. 22:2033, 1993.

88. Society for Cardiac Angiography.: Guidelines for credentialing and facilities for performance of coronary angioplasty. Cathet. Cardiovasc. Diagn. 15:136, 1988.

89. Ryan, T. J., Klocke, F. J., and Reynolds, W. A.: Clinical competence in percutaneous transluminal coronary angioplasty: A statement for physicians from the ACP/ACC/AHA Task Force on Clinical Privileges in Cardiology. J. Am. Coll. Cardiol. 15:1469, 1990.

90. 17th Bethesda Conference: Adult Cardiology Training. November 1–2, 1985. J. Am. Coll. Cardiol. 7:1191, 1986.

91. Kirklin, J. W., Akins, C. W., Blackstone, E. H., et al.: Guidelines and indications for coronary artery bypass graft surgery. A report of the American College of Cardiology/American Heart Association Task Force on Assessment of Diagnostic and Therapeutic Cardiovascular Procedures (Subcommittee on Coronary Artery Bypass Graft Surgery) J. Am. Coll. Cardiol. 17:543, 1991.

92. Mark, D. B., Lam, L. C., Lee, K. L., et al.: Effects of coronary angioplasty, coronary bypass surgery, and medical therapy on employment in patients with coronary artery disease. A prospective comparison study. Ann. Intern. Med. 120:111, 1994.

93. Varnauskas, E., and the European Coronary Surgery Study Group: Twelve-year follow-up of survival in the randomized European Coronary Surgery Study. N. Engl. J. Med. 319:332, 1988.

94. Chaitman, B. R., Davis, K. B., Kaiser, G. C., et al.: The role of coronary bypass surgery for 'left main equivalent' coronary disease: The Coronary Artery Surgery Study Registry. Circulation 74 (suppl. III):III-17, 1986.

95. Chaitman, B. R., Davis, K., Fisher, L. D., et al.: A life table and Cox regression analysis of patients with combined proximal left anterior descending and proximal left circumflex coronary artery disease: Non-left main equivalent lesions (CASS). Circulation 68:1163, 1983.

96. Parisi, A. F., Khuri, S., Deupree, R. H., et al.: Medical compared with surgical management of unstable angina; five-year mortality and morbidity in the Veterans Administration study. Circulation 80:1176, 1989.

97. Wright, I. S., and Fredrickson, D. T. (eds.): Cardiovascular Disease. Guidelines for Prevention and Care. Reports of the Inter-Society Commission for Heart Disease Resources. Washington, D. C., U. S. Government Printing Office, 1972.

98. Subcommittee on Cardiac Surgery Standards of the Cardiovascular Committee and the Advisory Council for Cardiothoracic Surgery of the American College of Surgeons.: Guidelines for minimal standards in cardiac surgery. ACS Bulletin, 1984, pp. 67–69.

99. Zipes, D. P., Akhtar, M., Denes, P., et al.: Guidelines for clinical intracardiac electrophysiologic studies. A report of the American College of Cardiology/American Heart Association Task Force on Assessment of Diagnostic and Therapeutic Cardiovascular Procedures (Subcommittee to Assess Clinical Intracardiac Electrophysiologic Studies). J. Am. Coll. Cardiol. 14:1827, 1989.

100. Zipes, D. P., DiMarco, J. P., Gillette, P. C., et al.: Guidelines for clinical intracardiac electrophysiologic and catheter ablation procedures. A report of the American College of Cardiology/American Heart Association Task Force on Practice Guidelines (Subcommittee on Clinical Intracardiac Electrophysiologic and Catheter Ablation Procedures). J. Am. Coll. Cardiol. 26:555, 1995.

101. Dhingra, R. C., Palileo, E., Strasberg, B., et al.: Significance of the HV interval in 517 patients with chronic bifascicular block. Circulation 64:1265, 1981.

102. Bhandari, A. K., Shapiro, W. A., Morady, F., et al.: Electrophysiologic testing in patients with the long QT syndrome. Circulation 71:63, 1985.

103. Jackman, W. M., Friday, K. J., Anderson, J. L., et al.: The long QT syndromes: A critical review, new clinical observations, and a unifying hypothesis. Prog. Cardiovasc. Dis. 31:115, 1988.

104. Myerburg, R. J., Kessler, K. M., Kimura, S., and Castellanos, A.: Sudden cardiac death: Future approaches based upon identification and control of transient risk factors. J. Cardiovasc. Electrophysiol. 3:626, 1992.

105. Gulamhusein, S., Naccarelli, G. V., and Ko, P. T.: Value and limitations of clinical electrophysiologic study in assessment of patients with unexplained syncope. Am. J. Med. 73:700, 1982.

106. Diagnostic and therapeutic technology assessment (DATTA).: Radiofrequency catheter ablation of aberrant conducting pathways of the heart. JAMA 268:2091, 1992.

107. Fisher, J. D.: American College of Cardiology Cardiovascular Technology Assessment Committee. Catheter ablation for cardiac arrhythmias: Clinical applications, personnel and facilities. J. Am. Coll. Cardiol. 24:828, 1994.

108. Scheinman, M. M.: Catheter ablation for cardiac arrhythmias, personnel and facilities. North American Society of Pacing and Electrophysiology Ad Hoc Committee on Catheter Ablation. PACE Pacing Clin. Electrophysiol. 15:715, 1992.

109. Dreifus, L. S., Fisch, C., Griffin, J. C., et al.: Guidelines for implantation of cardiac pacemakers and antiarrhythmia devices. A report of the American College of Cardiology/American Heart Association Task Force on Assessment of Diagnostic and Therapeutic Cardiovascular Procedures (Committee on Pacemaker Implantation) J. Am. Coll. Cardiol. 18:1, 1991.

CLINICAL SYNDROMES

110. Lee, T. H., Rouan, G. W., Weisberg, M. C., et al.: Clinical characteristics and natural history of patients with acute myocardial infarction sent home from the emergency room. Am. J. Cardiol. 60:219, 1987.

111. Rusnak, R. A., Stair, T. O., Hansen, K., and Fastow, J. S.: Litigation against the emergency physician: Common features in cases of missed myocardial infarction. Ann. Emerg. Med. 14:1029, 1989.

112. Lee, T. H., and Goldman, L.: The coronary care unit turns 25: Historical trends and future directions. Ann. Intern. Med. 108:887, 1988.

113. Goldman, L., Cook, E. F., Brand, D. A., et al.: A computer protocol to predict myocardial infarction in emergency department patients with chest pain. N. Engl. J. Med. 318:797, 1988.

114. Pozen, M. W., D'Agostino, R. B., Selker, H. P., et al.: A predictive instrument to improve coronary-care-unit admission practices in acute ischemic heart disease. A prospective multicenter clinical trial. N. Engl. J. Med. 310:1273, 1984.

115. Selker, H. P., Griffith, J. L., and D'Agostino, R. B.: A tool for judging coronary care unit admission appropriateness, valid for both real-time and retrospective use. A time-insensitive predictive instrument (TIPI) for acute cardiac ischemia: a multicenter study. Med. Care. 29:610, 1991.

116. Baxt, W. G.: Use of an artificial neural network for the diagnosis of myocardial infarction. Ann. Intern. Med. 115:843, 1991.

117. Fiebach, N. H., Cook, E. F., Lee, T. H., et al.: Outcomes of patients with myocardial infarction who are initially admitted to stepdown units: data from the Multicenter Chest Pain Study. Am. J. Med. 89:15, 1990.

118. Gaspoz, J. M., Lee, T. H., Cook, E. F., et al.: Outcome of patients who were admitted to a new short-stay unit to "rule-out" myocardial infarction. J. Am. Coll. Cardiol. 68:145, 1991.

119. Gaspoz, J. M., Lee, T. H., Weinstein, M. C., et al.: Cost-effectiveness of a new short-stay unit to rule out acute myocardial infarction in low risk patients. J. Am. Coll. Cardiol. 24:1249, 1994.

120. Gibler, W. B., Runyon, J. P., Levy, R. C., et al.: A rapid diagnostic and treatment center for patients with chest pain in the emergency department. Ann. Emerg. Med. 25:1, 1995.

121. Graff, L., Zun, L. S., Leikin, J., et al.: Emergency department observation beds improve patient care: Society for Academic Emergency Medicine debate. Ann. Emerg. Med. 21:967, 1992.

122. Lee, T. H., Juarez, G., Cook, E. F., et al.: Ruling out acute myocardial infarction. A prospective multicenter validation of a 12-hour strategy for patients at low risk. N. Engl. J. Med. 324:1239, 1991.

123. Adams, J. E., III, Bodor, G. S., Davila-Roman, V. G., et al.: Cardiac troponin I: A marker with high specificity for cardiac injury. Circulation 88:101, 1993.

124. Hamm, C. W., Ravkilde, J., Gerhardt, W., et al.: The prognostic value of serum troponin T in unstable angina. N. Engl. J. Med. 327:146, 1992.

125. Lewis, W. R., et al.: Utility and safety of immediate exercise testing of low risk patients admitted to the hospital for suspected acute myocardial infarction. Am. J. Cardiol. 74:987, 1994.

126. Sabia, P., Afrookteh, A., Touchstone, D. A., et al.: Value of regional wall motion abnormality in the emergency room diagnosis of acute myocardial infarction. A prospective study using two-dimensional echocardiography. Circulation 84 (suppl. I):I-85, 1991.

127. American College of Emergency Physicians.: Clinical policy for the initial approach to adults presenting with a chief complaint of chest pain, with no history of trauma. Ann. Emerg. Med. 25:274, 1995.

128. National Heart Attack Alert Program Coordinating Committee 60 Minutes to Treatment Working Group.: Emergency Department: Rapid Identification and Treatment of Patients with Acute Myocardial Infarction. NIH Publication No. 93-3278. National Heart, Lung and Blood Institute, Public Health Service, U.S. Department of Health and Human Services. September 1993.

129. Gunnar, R. M., Bourdillon, P. D. V., Dixon, D. W., et al.: Guidelines for the early management of patients with acute myocardial infarction. A report of the American College of Cardiology/American Heart Association Task Force on Assessment of Diagnostic and Therapeutic Cardiovascular Procedures (Subcommittee to Develop Guidelines for the Early Management of Patients with Acute Myocardial Infarction). J. Am. Coll. Cardiol. 16:249, 1990.

130. Lee, T. H., and Goldman, L.: Serum enzyme assays in the diagnosis of acute myocardial infarction. Recommendations based on a quantitative analysis. *In* Sox, H. C., Jr., (ed.): Common Diagnostic Tests. Use and Interpretation. 2nd ed. Philadelphia, American College of Physicians, 1990, pp. 36–66.

131. American Heart Association/Emergency Cardiac Care Committee and Subcommittees: Guidelines for cardiopulmonary resuscitation and emergency cardiac care, III: Adult advanced cardiac life support. JAMA *268*:2199, 1992.

132. Gonzalez, E. R., Jones, L. A., Ornato, J. P., et al. (Virginia Thrombolytic Study Group): Hospital delays and problems with thrombolytic administration in patients receiving thrombolytic therapy: A multicenter prospective assessment. Ann. Emerg. Med. *21*:1215, 1992.

133. Fibrinolytic Therapy Trialists' Collaborative Group.: Indications for fibrinolytic therapy in suspected acute myocardial infarction: Collaborative overview of early mortality and major morbidity results from all randomized trials of more than 1000 patients.Lancet *343*:311, 1994.

134. The GUSTO Investigators: An international randomized trial comparing four thrombolytic strategies for acute myocardial infarction. N. Engl. J. Med. *329*:673, 1993.

135. Mark, D. B., Hlatky, M. A., Califf, R. M., et al.: Cost-effectiveness of thrombolytic therapy with tissue plasminogen activator as compared with streptokinase for acute myocardial infarction. N. Engl. J. Med. *332*:1418, 1995.

136. Kalish, S. C., Gurwitz, J. H., Krumholz, H. M., and Avorn, J.: A cost-effectiveness model of thrombolytic therapy for acute myocardial infarction. J. Gen. Intern. Med. *10*:321, 1995.

137. MacMahon, S., Collins, R., Peto, R., et al.: Effects of prophylactic lidocaine in suspected acute myocardial infarction: An overview of results from the randomized controlled trials. JAMA *260*:1910, 1988.

138. Beta-Blocker Heart Attack Trial Research Group.: A randomized trial of propranolol in patients with acute myocardial infarction: I. Mortality results. JAMA *247*:1707, 1982.

139. Moss, A. J.: Secondary prevention with calcium channel-blocking drugs in patients after myocardial infarction: A critical review. Circulation *75*(Suppl. V):V-148, 1987.

140. The Multicenter Diltiazem Postinfarction Trial Research Group.: The effect of diltiazem on mortality and reinfarction after myocardial infarction. N. Engl. J. Med. *319*:385, 1988.

141. Theroux, P., Taeymans, Y., Morissette, D., et al.: A randomized study comparing propranolol and diltiazem in the treatment of unstable angina. J. Am. Coll. Cardiol. *5*:717, 1985.

142. Held, P. H., Yusuf, S., and Furberg, C. D.: Calcium channel blockers in acute myocardial infarction and unstable angina: An overview. Br. Med. J. *299*:1187, 1989.

143. Yusuf, S., Wittes, J., and Friedman, L.: Overview of results of randomized clinical trials in heart disease: II. Unstable angina, heart failure, primary prevention with aspirin, and risk factor modification. JAMA *260*:2259, 1988.

144. Lubsen, J., and Tijssen, J. G.: Efficacy of nifedipine and metoprolol in the early treatment of unstable angina in the coronary care unit: Findings from the Holland Interuniversity Nifedipine/metoprolol Trial (HINT). Am. J. Cardiol. *60*:18A, 1987.

145. Mark, D. B., Shaw, L., Harrell, F. E., et al.: Prognostic value of a treadmill exercise score in outpatients with suspected coronary disease. N. Engl. J. Med. *325*:849, 1991.

146. Fleg, J. L., Hinton, P. C., Lakatta, E. G., et al.: Physician utilization of laboratory procedures to monitor outpatients with congestive heart failure. Arch. Intern. Med. *149*:393, 1989.

147. Williams, J. F., Bristow, M. R., Fowler, M. B., et al.: Guidelines for the evaluation and management of heart failure. Report of the American College of Cardiology/American Heart Association Task Force on Practice Guidelines (Committee on Evaluation and Management of Heart Failure). J. Am. Coll. Cardiol. *26*:1376, 1995.

148. The Cardiac Arrhythmia Suppression Trial II Investigators.: Effect of the antiarrhythmic agent moricizine on survival after myocardial infarction. N. Engl. J. Med. *327*:227, 1992.

149. The Cardiac Arrhythmia Suppression Trial (CAST) Investigators.: Preliminary report: Effect of encainide and flecainide on mortality in a randomized trial of arrhythmia suppression after myocardial infarction. N. Engl. J. Med. *321*:406, 1989.

150. Vinson, J. M., Rich, M. W., Sperry, J. C., et al.: Early readmission of elderly patients with congestive heart failure. J. Am. Geriatr. Soc. *38*:1290, 1990.

151. Kupper, A. J., Fintelman, H., Huige, M. C., et al.: Cross-over comparison of the fixed combination of hydrochlorothiazide and triamterene and the free combination of furosemide and triamterene in the maintenance treatment of congestive heart failure. Eur. J. Clin. Pharmacol. *30*:341, 1986.

152. Packer, M., Gheorghiade, M., Young, D., et al.: Withdrawal of digoxin from patients with chronic heart failure treated with angiotensin-converting-enzyme inhibitors. N. Engl. J. Med. *329*:1, 1993.

153. Eagle, K. A., Brundage, B. H., Chaitman, B. R., et al.: Guidelines for perioperative cardiovascular evaluation for noncardiac surgery. Report of the American College of Cardiology/American Heart Association Task Force on Practice Guidelines (Committee on Perioperative Cardiovascular Evaluation for Noncardiac Surgery). J. Am. Coll. Cardiol. *27*:910, 1996.

PREVENTION OF CORONARY ARTERY DISEASE

154. Tengs, T. O., Adams, M. E., Pliskin, J. S., et al.: Five-hundred life-saving interventions and their cost-effectiveness. Risk Analysis *15*:369, 1995.

155. Smith, S. C., Blair, S. N., Criqui, M. H., et al.: Preventing heart attack and death in patients with coronary disease. J. Am. Coll. Cardiol. *26*:292, 1995.

156. Summary of the Second Report of the National Cholesterol Education Program (NCEP) Expert Panel on Detection, Evaluation, and Treatment of High Blood Cholesterol in Adults (Adult Treatment Panel II). JAMA *269*:3015, 1993.

157. Pearson, T. D., Rapaport, E., Criqui, M., et al.: Optimal risk factor management in the patient after coronary revascularization: A statement for healthcare professionals from an American Heart Association writing group. Circulation *90*:3215, 1994.

158. National High Blood Pressure Education Program.: The Fifth Report of the Joint National Committee on Detection, Evaluation, and Treatment of High Blood Pressure. Bethesda, Md.: National Heart, Lung, and Blood Institute, 1993. U. S., Department of Health, Education, and Welfare publication NIH 93-1088.

159. The Guidelines Subcommittee of the WHO/ISH Mild Hypertension Liaison Committee. 1993 guidelines for the management of mild hypertension. Memorandum from a World Health Organization/International Society of Hypertension meeting. Hypertension *22*:392, 1993.

160. Alderman, M. H.: Which antihypertensive drugs first—and why! JAMA *267*:2786, 1992.

Index

Note: Page numbers in *italics* indicate illustrations; those followed by t indicate tables. **Boldface page numbers** indicate main discussion. **Plate numbers** indicate color plates.

Sinus tachycardia (Continued)
 postoperative, 1764
 radiofrequency catheter ablation in, 624–627, 625
Situational syncope, 864–865. See also Syncope.
Situs ambiguus, 946
Situs inversus, 946
 dextrocardia with, in adult, 966
  noncardiac surgery and, 981
Situs solitus, 946
 dextrocardia with, in adult, 966
Six-minute walk test, for exercise stress testing, 156
 in heart failure, 452, 452
Size, cardiac, on radiograph, 215, 217
Sjögren's syndrome, 1782
Skin, coumarin-induced necrosis of, 1818
 examination of, 16, 17
 in cholesterol embolization syndrome, 1571
 warfarin-associated necrosis of, 1595
Sleep apnea syndrome, etiology of, 1615
 in cor pulmonale, 1614–1615
 in hypertension, 821
 management of, 1615
Sly syndrome, 1669t
Small vessel vasculitides, 1783
Smith-Lemli-Opitz syndrome, genetic factors in, 1660t
Smith-Magenis syndrome, 1651t
Smooth muscle cells, 1108–1110, 1109
 collagen formation by, 1109, 1109
 contractile phenotype of, 1109, 1109
 embryogenesis of, 1109
 gene therapy–induced inhibition of, 1638
 injury to, 1109–1110
 lipid accumulation in, 1109
 phenotypes of, 1109, 1109
 receptors of, 1109
Snake bite, myocardial effects of, 1448
Sneeze syncope, 864–865. See also Syncope.
Sodium, dietary, in hypertension, 844–845, 845
 myocardial concentration of, 554t
 renal retention of, in heart failure, 1915, 1917–1918, 1918
 in hypertension, 817–818, 817t
 serum, in heart failure, 548
Sodium (Na⁺), chloride (Cl⁻) symporter, in heart failure, 477–478, 477t
Sodium (Na⁺), potassium (K⁺)-ATPase pump, cardiac glycoside effect on, 480–481
Sodium azide, myocardial effects of, 1448
Sodium channel, in action potential phase 0, 557–559, 557, 559
 inactivation of, 558, 559
 lidocaine effects on, 559, 560
Sodium polystyrene sulfonate (Kayexalate), in pediatric cardiology, 1002t
Sodium (Na⁺), potassium (K⁺), chloride (2Cl) symport, inhibitors of, in heart failure, 476–477, 477t
Sodium pump, in contraction-relaxation cycle, 371–372
Sodium-bicarbonate cotransporter, in contraction-relaxation cycle, 371
Sodium-calcium exchanger, in contraction-relaxation cycle, 370–371, 370, 371
 in heart failure, 406
Sodium-proton exchanger, in contraction-relaxation cycle, 371, 371
Solu-Medrol (methylprednisolone), in pediatric cardiology, 1001t
Somatostatin, in acromegaly, 1887
Sones technique, for coronary artery catheterization, 185
Sotalol, adverse effects of, 616
 dosage of, 616
 electrophysiological actions of, 615–616
 hemodynamics of, 616
 in arrhythmias, 610–613, 611t, 615–616
 in elderly, 1698
 in hypertrophic cardiomyopathy, 1426
 in pregnancy, 1859
 in renal failure, 1931t
 indications of, 616
 pharmacodynamic properties of, 487t
 pharmacokinetics of, 616
Space constant, of cable, 564
Sphingolipidoses, 1669t, 1675–1676
Sphygmomanometry, for arterial pressure measurement, 20

Sphygmomanometry (Continued)
 for intracardiac pressure measurement, 422–423
Spider cell, of rhabdomyoma, 1470
Spider sting, myocardial effects of, 1448
Spiral wave model of reentry, 571, 572
Spirochetes, in pericarditis, 1511
Spironolactone (Aldactone), hematological abnormalities with, 1804t
 in congenital heart disease–related heart failure, 890t
 in heart failure, 477t, 890t
 in pediatric cardiology, 1002t
 in renal failure, 1933t
Splanchnic circulation, in heart failure, 410
Spleen, abscess of, in infective endocarditis, 1095–1096
 congenital disorders of, cardiac anomalies with, 946
 enlargement of, 18
  in infective endocarditis, 1085
 examination of, 18
Splinter hemorrhages, 17
 in infective endocarditis, 1085, 1085
Spondyloarthropathy, 1780–1781, 1780
Springwater cysts, 1522
Sputum, in differential diagnosis, 10
Square root sign, in restrictive cardiomyopathy, 1427
Squatting posture, auscultatory effects of, 48, 48
 in congenital heart disease, 885
ST alternans, 140
 in ischemic heart disease, 131–132
ST segment, 113, 139, 139t
 after percutaneous transluminal coronary angioplasty, 171
 digitalis effect on, 142
 during cesarean section, 854, 1855
 in coronary artery disease, 1296
 in early repolarization, 136, 138
 in exercise stress testing, 157–160, 157–160, 163
 in hyperkalemia, 137
 in ischemia, 127, 127
 in left bundle branch block, 148
 in left ventricular hypertrophy, 139
 in myocardial infarction, 129–131, 130, 131, 134, 134–135, 149, 166, 714, 1205–1206, 1206, 1208–1210, 1256
 in pericarditis, 1483–1484, 1483, 1483t
 in posterior left ventricular infarction, 134–135
 in Prinzmetal's variant angina, 137, 1341
 in right bundle branch block, 121
 in right ventricular hypertrophy, 118
 in right ventricular infarction, 134, 134, 149
 in silent myocardial ischemia, 1345, 1345
 in unstable angina, 1334, 1334
ST segment/heart rate slope, in exercise stress testing, 163
Standing, sudden, in hypertrophic cardiomyopathy evaluation, 1423
Staphylococcus aureus, in infective endocarditis, 1078, 1081, 1086, 1088, 1091–1092, 1092t, 1095
Staphylococcus epidermidis, in infective endocarditis, 1081
Staphylococcus lugdunensis, in infective endocarditis, 1081
Staphylococcus pneumoniae, in infective endocarditis, 1078, 1086
Staphylokinase, 1822
Stare, 15
Starr-Edwards valve, 1061, 1062, 1065
Stenosis, coronary artery, arteriography of, 255–257, 256, 257
 compensation for, 1172–1173, 1173
 congenital, 260
 coronary blood flow effects of, 1171–1174, 1171–1173
 diameter of, 1172–1173, 1172
 eccentric, arteriography of, 256–257, 257
 length of, 1172
 magnetic resonance imaging of, 321, 322
 myocardial blood flow in, positron emission tomography of, 307
 pressure drop across, 1171
 radiation-induced, 1349
 severity of, 1172
 valvular. See Aortic stenosis; Mitral stenosis; Pulmonic stenosis; Tricuspid stenosis.

Stenosis flow reserve, 200
Stenosis resistance, 1171–1172
Stents, intracoronary, 1378–1382, 1379, 1380, 1380t
 cost-effectiveness analysis of, 1750
 implantation of, 1381–1382, 1381
Sternum, postoperative infection of, 1732–1733
Steroids, in rheumatic fever, 1772
 in uremic pericarditis, 1513
Still's disease, 1778
Still's murmur, 37–38, 37
Stool hematest, preoperative, 1717t
Straight back syndrome, 24
Streinert's disease, 1872–1874, 1873, 1874
Strength-duration curve, of pacemaker, 710–711, 711
Streptococci, in infective endocarditis, 1080–1082, 1089–1090, 1090t
 in myocarditis, 1440
Streptococcus adjacens, 1081
Streptococcus agalactiae, 1081
Streptococcus anginosus, 1081
Streptococcus bovis, 1080, 1081, 1089–1090, 1090t
Streptococcus constellatus, 1081
Streptococcus defectivus, 1080, 1081
Streptococcus intermedius, 1081
Streptococcus milleri, 1080, 1081
Streptococcus mitior, 1080
Streptococcus pneumoniae, 1081, 1090, 1090t
Streptococcus pyogenes, 1090, 1090t
Streptococcus salivarius, 1080
Streptococcus sanguis, 1080
Streptokinase, 1218–1219, 1219, 1821. See also Thrombolytic therapy.
 in myocardial infarction, 1824–1826, 1825, 1825t, 1970–1971, 1971t
 in renal failure, 1934t
 vs. tissue-type plasminogen activator, 1220–1221
Streptomycin, myocardial effects of, 1449
Stress, in coronary artery disease, 1154, 1166
 in heart failure, 449
 in hypertension, 818–819, 818, 819
 in myocardial infarction, 1198
 in stable angina pectoris, 1293
 reduction of, in cardiac rehabilitation, 1398
 silent ventricular dysfunction with, 302
Stress erythrocytosis, 1794
Stretch receptors, in contraction-relaxation cycle in, 376
 in heart failure, 410
Stroke, after coronary artery bypass surgery, 1319–1320
 diastolic blood pressure and, 812–813, 812
 hypertension in, 815
 in atrial fibrillation, 655–656
 in myocardial infarction, 1198
Stroke volume, 425, 425t
 computed tomography of, 336
 in myocardial infarction, 1195, 1200
 in pregnancy, 1843, 1843t
 magnetic resonance imaging of, 331
 myocardial oxygen consumption and, 1162, 1162
Stroke work–end-diastolic volume relation, 432, 433
Stroke-prone spontaneously hypertensive rat, 1679
ST-T segment, 139, 139t
 in coronary artery disease, 1295
Stunned myocardium, 388–389, 388t, 389, 1176, 1176
 after coronary artery bypass surgery, 1327
 echocardiography of, 89
Subaortic obstruction, echocardiography in, 80, 80, 81
Subaortic stenosis, congenital, 918–919, 919
Subclavian artery, left, on plain chest radiography, 204, 206
Subclavian flap arthroplasty, in juxtaductal coarctation, 913, 913
Subcutaneous nodules, in rheumatic fever, 1771
Submaximal exercise, in exercise stress testing, 164
Submitral obstruction, echocardiography in, 81, 81
Subpulmonic infundibular stenosis, 928
 in intraventricular right ventricular obstruction, 928

ISBN 0-7216-5666-8

90071

9 780721 656663